The Pediatric Risk of Mortality (PRISM III)

Cardiovascular, Neurologic, Vital Signs

Systolic Blood Pressure (mm Hg)	Score = 3	Score = 7
Neonate	40-55	<40
Infant	45-65	<45
Child	55-75	<55
Adolescent	65-85	<6̲5̲

Temperature	Score = 3	
	<33°C (91.4°F) or >40°C (1̲…	

Mental Status	Score = 5	
	Stupor/coma or GCS<8	

Heart Rate (beats per minute)	Score = 3	Sco̲
Neonate	215-225	>225
Infant	215-225	>225
Child	185-205	>205
Adolescent	145-155	>155

Pupillary Reflexes	Score = 7	Score = 11
	One fixed	Both fixed

Acid-Base, Blood Gases

Acidosis (pH or Total CO_2)	Score = 2	Score = 6
pH or	7.0-7.28	<7.0
Total CO_2	5-16.9	<5

pH	Score = 2	Score = 3
	7.48-7.55	>7.55

PCO_2 (mm Hg)	Score = 1	Score = 3
	50-75	>75

Total CO_2 (mmol/L)	Score = 4	
	>34	

PaO_2 (mm Hg)	Score = 3	Score = 6
	42-49	<42

Chemistry Tests

Glucose	Score = 2
	>200 mg/dL or >11 mmol/L

Potassium (mmol/L)	Score = 3
	>6.9

Blood Urea Nitrogen (BUN)	Score = 3
Neonate	>11.9 mg/dL or >4.3 mmol/L
All other ages	>14.9 mg/dL or >5.4 mmol/L

Creatinine	Score = 2
Neonate	>0.85 mg/dL or >75 µmol/L
Infant	>0.90 mg/dL or >80 µmol/L
Child	>0.90 mg/dL or >80 µmol/L
Adolescent	>1.30 mg/dL or >115 µmol/L

Hematology Tests

White Blood Cell Count (cells/mm³)	Score = 4		
	<3,000		

Platelet Count (× 10³ cells/mm³)	Score = 2	Score = 4	Score = 5
	100-200	50-99	<50

Prothrombin Time (PT) or Partial Thromboplastin Time (PTT)	Score = 3
Neonate	PT>22.0 or PTT>85.0
All other ages	PT>22.0 or PTT>57.0

Other Factors: Nonoperative cardiovascular disease, chromosomal anomaly, cancer, previous PICU admission, pre-ICU CPR, postoperative, acute diabetes (e.g., DKA), admit from inpatient unit.

From Pollack MM, Patel KM, Ruttimann EU: PRISM III: An updated pediatric risk of mortality score. Crit Care Med 1996;24:743-752.

Metric Unit Conversions

1 cm = 0.3937 in	1 kg = 2.2 lb
1 in = 2.54 cm	1 lb = 0.4545 kg
°C = [(°F − 32) × 5]/9	1 gm = 0.03527 oz
°F = [(°C × 9)/5] + 32	1 oz = 28.35 g

The Pediatric Risk of Mortality (PRISM III)

Cardiovascular, Neurologic, Vital Signs

Systolic Blood Pressure (mm Hg)	Score = 3	Score = 7
Neonate	40-55	<40
Infant	45-65	<45
Child	55-75	<55
Adolescent	65-85	<65

Temperature	Score = 3
	<33°C (91.4°F) or >40°C (…)

Mental Status	Score = 5
	Stupor/coma or GCS<8

Heart Rate (beats per minute)	Score = 3	Score = …
Neonate	215-225	>225
Infant	215-225	>225
Child	185-205	>205
Adolescent	145-155	>155

Pupillary Reflexes	Score = 7	Score = 11
	One fixed	Both fixed

Acid-Base, Blood Gases

Acidosis (pH or Total CO_2)	Score = 2	Score = 6
pH or	7.0-7.28	<7.0
Total CO_2	5-16.9	<5

pH	Score = 2	Score = 3
	7.48-7.55	>7.55

PCO_2 (mm Hg)	Score = 1	Score = 3
	50-75	>75

Total CO_2 (mmol/L)	Score = 4
	>34

PaO_2 (mm Hg)	Score = 3	Score = 6
	42-49	<42

Chemistry Tests

Glucose	Score = 2
	>200 mg/dL or >11 mmol/L

Potassium (mmol/L)	Score = 3
	>6.9

Blood Urea Nitrogen (BUN)	Score = 3
Neonate	>11.9 mg/dL or >4.3 mmol/L
All other ages	>14.9 mg/dL or >5.4 mmol/L

Creatinine	Score = 2
Neonate	>0.85 mg/dL or >75 µmol/L
Infant	>0.90 mg/dL or >80 µmol/L
Child	>0.90 mg/dL or >80 µmol/L
Adolescent	>1.30 mg/dL or >115 µmol/L

Hematology Tests

White Blood Cell Count (cells/mm³)	Score = 4
	<3,000

Platelet Count ($\times 10^3$ cells/mm³)	Score = 2	Score = 4	Score = 5
	100-200	50-99	<50

Prothrombin Time (PT) or Partial Thromboplastin Time (PTT)	Score = 3
Neonate	PT>22.0 or PTT>85.0
All other ages	PT>22.0 or PTT>57.0

Other Factors: Nonoperative cardiovascular disease, chromosomal anomaly, cancer, previous PICU admission, pre-ICU CPR, postoperative, acute diabetes (e.g., DKA), admit from inpatient unit.

From Pollack MM, Patel KM, Ruttimann EU: PRISM III: An updated pediatric risk of mortality score. Crit Care Med 1996;24:743-752.

Metric Unit Conversions

1 cm = 0.3937 in	1 kg = 2.2 lb
1 in = 2.54 cm	1 lb = 0.4545 kg
°C = [(°F – 32) × 5]/9	1 gm = 0.03527 oz
°F = [(°C × 9)/5] + 32	1 oz = 28.35 g

Textbook of
CRITICAL
CARE
FIFTH
EDITION

Textbook of CRITICAL CARE

FIFTH EDITION

Mitchell P. Fink, MD

Professor and Chair
Department of Critical Care Medicine
Watson Professor of Surgery
University of Pittsburgh School of Medicine
Pittsburgh, Pennsylvania

Edward Abraham, MD

Roger Sherman Mitchell Professor of Pulmonary and Critical Care Medicine
Vice Chair, Department of Medicine
Head, Division of Pulmonary Sciences and Critical Care Medicine
University of Colorado Health Sciences Center
Denver, Colorado

Jean-Louis Vincent, MD, PhD

Professor of Intensive Care
Faculty of Medicine
Free University of Brussels
Head, Department of Intensive Care
Erasme University Hospital
Brussels, Belgium

Patrick M. Kochanek, MD

Director, Safar Center for Resuscitation Research
Professor and Vice Chairman, Department of Critical Care Medicine
Professor of Pediatrics and Anesthesiology
University of Pittsburgh School of Medicine and
Children's Hospital of Pittsburgh
Pittsburgh, Pennsylvania

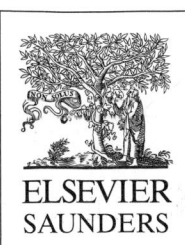

ELSEVIER
SAUNDERS

ELSEVIER
SAUNDERS

The Curtis Center
170 S Independence Mall W 300E
Philadelphia, Pennsylvania 19106

TEXTBOOK OF CRITICAL CARE · ISBN 0-7216-0335-1

NOTICE

Critical care is an ever-changing field. Standard safety precautions must be followed, but as new research and clinical experience broaden our knowledge, changes in treatment and drug therapy may become necessary or appropriate. Readers are advised to check the most current product information provided by the manufacturer of each drug to be administered to verify the recommended dose, the method and duration of administration, and contraindications. It is the responsibility of the treating physician, relying on experience and knowledge of the patient, to determine dosages and the best treatment for each individual patient. Neither the publisher nor the editor assumes any liability for any injury and/or damage to persons or property arising from this publication.

The Publisher

Library of Congress Cataloging-in-Publication Data

Textbook of critical care.--5th ed. / [edited by] Mitchell P. Fink ... [et al.].
   p. ; cm.
  Includes bibliographical references and index.
  ISBN 0-7216-0335-1
   1. Critical care medicine. I. Fink, M. P. (Mitchell P.)
  [DNLM: 1. Critical Care. 2. Intensive Care Units. WX 218 T355 2005]
  RC86.7.T453 2005
  616.02'8--dc22   2004061426

Publisher: Natasha Andjelkovic

Senior Developmental Editor: Joanne Husovski

Publishing Services Manager: Tina Rebane

Designer: Elsevier Staff

Marketing Manager: Emily McGrath-Christie

Multimedia Producer: David Wisner

Printed in the United States of America

Last digit is the print number: 9   8   7   6   5   4   3   2   1

DEDICATION

To my beloved wife, Ian, and my two wonderful children, Emily and Matt, for tolerating my long hours away from home; and to my wonderful parents, Walter and Betty Fink, for providing me with a stable and supportive environment during my formative years.

–Mitchell P. Fink

To Norma-May, the love of my life, and to Claire and Erin, who bring me the greatest joy each day.

–Edward Abraham

To Hac and Amélie, hoping for better care of the critically ill throughout the world.

–Jean-Louis Vincent

To my parents, Stella and Julius Kochanek, for leading by example on the value of hard work; to my wife, Denise, and my children, Ashley, Stanton, and Jillian, for their many sacrifices; and to the late Dr. Peter Safar, for encouraging each of us to bring promising new therapies to the bedside of the critically ill.

–Patrick M. Kochanek

Edward Abraham, MD

Roger Sherman Mitchell Professor of Pulmonary and Critical Care Medicine; Vice Chair, Department of Medicine; Head, Division of Pulmonary Sciences and Critical Care Medicine, University of Colorado Health Sciences Center, Denver, Colorado

Regulation of Gene Expression

Kareem Abu-Elmagd, MD

University of Pittsburgh Health System, Pittsburgh, Pennsylvania

Intestinal and Multiple Organ Transplantation

Yasir Abu-Omar, MB, ChB

Department of Cardiothoracic Surgery, MRI of the Brain, John Radcliffe Hospital, Oxford, United Kingdom

Atheromatous Embolization

Carlos Agustí, MD, PhD

Consultor, Servei Pneumologia, Hospital Clinic, Barcelona, Spain

Pulmonary Infections in the Acute Immunocompromised Patient

William C. Aird, MD

Department of Medicine, Beth Israel Deaconess Medical Center and Harvard Medical School, Boston, Massachusetts

Thrombocytopenia; Coagulopathy

Louis H. Alarcon, MD

Assistant Professor, Departments of Critical Care Medicine and Surgery, University of Pittsburgh School of Medicine, Pittsburgh, Pennsylvania

Paracentesis and Diagnostic Peritoneal Lavage

Jorge E. Albina, MD

Professor, Brown University School of Medicine; Director, Division of Surgical Research, Department of Surgery, Rhode Island Hospital, Providence, Rhode Island

Apoptosis in the Critically Ill

Rakesh Alva, MD

Fellow in Critical Care Medicine, Department of Critical Care Medicine, Montefiore Medical Center, Albert Einstein College of Medicine, Bronx, New York

Disaster Medicine for the ICU Physician

Derek C. Angus, MD, MPH

Professor of Critical Care Medicine and Health Services Administration, and Vice-Chair of Research, Department of Critical Care Medicine, University of Pittsburgh, Pittsburgh, Pennsylvania

Evidence-Based Critical Care

Nicole T. Ansani, PharmD

Clinical Education Consultant, Pfizer, Inc., Pittsburgh, Pennsylvania

Principles of NSAID Therapy in Critical Care Medicine

Massimo Antonelli, MD

Associate Professor of Intensive Care and Anesthesiology and Director, General Intensive Care Unit, Policlinico Universitario A. Gemelli, Universita Cattolica del Sacro Cuore; Associate Editor of *Intensive Care Medicine*, Rome, Italy

Fiberoptic Bronchoscopy

Anastasia Antoniadou, MD, PhD

Lecturer of Internal Medicine, Athens University Medical School; Infectious Diseases Specialist and Attending Physician, 4th Department of Internal Medicine, Attikon University General Hospital, Athens, Greece

Infectious Endocarditis

Anupam Anupam, MBBS

Attending Physician, Department of Medicine, Advocate Illinois Masonic Medical Center, Chicago, Illinois

Sudden Deterioration in Neurologic Status

Andrew Charles Argent, MD

Associate Professor, Division of Paediatric Critical Care and Children's Heart Disease, School of Child and Adolescent Health, University of Cape Town; Medical Director, Paediatric Intensive Care, Red Cross War Memorial Children's Hospital, Cape Town, South Africa

Metabolic and Endocrine Crises in the Pediatric Intensive Care Unit

John H. Arnold, MD

Associate Professor, Department of Anesthesia (Pediatrics), Harvard Medical School; Associate Director, Medical Surgical ICU, Children's Hospital; Medical Director, Department of Respiratory Care, Children's Hospital, Boston, Massachusetts

Acute Parenchymal Disease in Infants and Children

Vicente Arroyo, MD
Professor, Department of Medicine, University of Barcelona; Chief of Liver Unit, Hospital Clinic; Research Member, IDIBAPS, Barcelona, Spain
Hepatorenal Syndrome

Karen Ashworth, MD
Senior Registrar in Anesthesia and Intensive Care, Chelsea and Westminster Hospital, London, United Kingdom
Bedside Pulmonary Artery Catheterization

Mark E. Astiz, MD
Professor of Medicine, New York Medical College; Chief, Section of Critical Care Medicine, Saint Vincent's Hospital, New York, New York
Pathophysiology and Classification of Shock States

Todd L. Astor, MD
Assistant Professor of Pediatrics; Medical Director, Lung Transplant Program; Assistant Professor, Section of Pulmonary Medicine, Columbus Children's Hospital, The Ohio State University, Columbus, Ohio
Oxidative Lung Injury

Alfred Ayala, PhD
Professor, Brown University School of Medicine, Division of Surgical Research, Rhode Island Hospital, Providence, Rhode Island
Apoptosis in the Critically Ill

Iyad M. Ayoub, MD
Research Instructor, Department of Medicine, Rosalind Franklin University of Medicine and Science, North Chicago Veterans Affairs Medical Center, North Chicago, Illinois
Transvenous and Transcutaneous Cardiac Pacing

Élie Azoulay, MD, PhD
Service de Réanimation Médicale, Hôpital St. Louis, Paris, France
Specific Facets of Managing Neutropenic Cancer Patients in the Intensive Care Unit; Hematologic Malignancies in the Intensive Care Unit; Organ Toxicity of Cancer Chemotherapy

David B. Badesch, MD
Professor of Medicine, Clinical Director, Pulmonary Hypertension Center, Division of Pulmonary Sciences and Critical Care Medicine, University of Colorado Health Sciences Center, Denver, Colorado
Pulmonary Hypertension

Anna Kathryn Baer, MD
Fellow in Cardiovascular Medicine, Department of Internal Medicine, Division of Cardiology, University of Virginia Health System, Charlottesville, Virginia
Acute Coronary Syndromes: Pathophysiology and Diagnosis

Omer A. Bajwa, MD
Senior Fellow, Department of Critical Care Medicine, University of Pittsburgh; Pulmonary Fellow, Department of Pulmonary Medicine, Allegheny General Hospital, Pittsburgh, Pennsylvania
The Management of Gastrointestinal Bleeding

Marie R. Baldisseri, MD
Associate Professor of Critical Care Medicine, University of Pittsburgh School of Medicine; Medical Director, Intensive Care Unit, Magee-Women's Hospital, Pittsburgh, Pennsylvania
Cardiovascular and Endocrinologic Changes Associated with Pregnancy; Hypertensive Disorders in Pregnancy; Postpartum Hemorrhage

Zsolt Balogh, MD
Assistant Professor, Department of Traumatology, University of Szeged, Hungary
Abdominal Compartment Syndrome

Rasheed A. Balogun, MD
Assistant Professor of Medicine, Division of Nephrology, University of Virginia; Medical Director, Renal Unit and Extracorporeal Therapies, University of Virginia Health Systems, Charlottesville, Virginia
Lithium

Vishal Bansal, MD
Chief Resident, University of Pittsburgh Medical Center, Pittsburgh, Pennsylvania
Ileus; Diarrhea; Ileus and Mechanical Small Bowel Obstruction

Joel Edward Barbato, MD
General Surgical Resident, University of Pittsburgh Medical Center, Pittsburgh, Pennsylvania
Thrombolytics

Carol A. Barch, MN, CRNP, CNRN
Program Coordinator, Stroke Institute, University of Pittsburgh Medical Center, Pittsburgh, Pennsylvania
Management of Acute Ischemic Stroke

Philip Steven Barie, MD
Professor of Surgery and Public Health, Departments of Surgery and Public Health, Weill Medical College of Cornell University, New York, New York
Peritonitis and Intra-abdominal Abscess

Brendan J. Barrett, MB, MSc, MRCPI, FRCPC
Professor of Medicine, Division of Nephrology and Clinical Epidemiology Unit, Memorial University of Newfoundland; Active Staff, Internal Medicine and Nephrology, Health Care Corporation of St. John's, St. John's, Newfoundland, Canada
Contrast Dye-Induced Nephropathy

John G. Bartlett, MD

Professor of Medicine, Department of Medicine, Johns Hopkins University School of Medicine; Chief, Infectious Diseases, Johns Hopkins Hospital, Baltimore, Maryland

Clostridium difficile Colitis

Robert H. Bartlett, MD

Professor, Department of Surgery; Director, Surgical Intensive Care Unit; Division Chief, Critical Care, University of Michigan Health Systems, Ann Arbor, Michigan

Extracorporeal Life Support

Sarice L. Bassin, MD

Clinical Assistant Professor, The Queens Medical Center, Neuroscience Center, Honolulu, Hawaii

Seizures in the Critically Ill; Lumbar Puncture; Intracranial Pressure Monitoring

Daniel G. Bausch, MD, MPH

Associate Professor, Department of Tropical Medicine, Tulane School of Public Health and Tropical Medicine, Department of Medicine, Section of Infectious Diseases, Tulane University School of Medicine, New Orleans, Louisiana

Malaria and Other Tropical Infections in the Intensive Care Unit

Hülya Bayır, MD

Assistant Professor, Department of Critical Care Medicine, University of Pittsburgh School of Medicine, Pittsburgh, Pennsylvania

Key Issues in Pediatric Neurointensive Care

David T. Bearden, PharmD

Clinical Assistant Professor, Department of Pharmacy Practice, College of Pharmacy, Oregon State University, Portland, Oregon

Macrolides

Yanick Beaulieu, MD

Fellow, Department of Critical Care Medicine, University of Pittsburgh School of Medicine, Pittsburgh, Pennsylvania

Bedside Ultrasonography

Gregory J. Beilman, MD

Associate Professor, Department of Surgery and Anesthesia, University of Minnesota; Director of Surgical Critical Care, Fairview University Medical Center, Minneapolis; Director of Trauma Research, North Memorial Health Center, Robbinsdale, Minnesota

Management of Patients with Kidney, Pancreas, or Kidney-Pancreas Transplantation

Giuseppe Bello, MD

Research Fellow, Istituto di Anestesiologia e Rianimazione, Policlinico Universitario A. Gemelli, Universita Cattolica del Sacro Cuore, Rome, Italy

Fiberoptic Bronchoscopy

Rinaldo Bellomo, MBBS, MD, FAACP, FRACP

Associate Professor, Department of Intensive Care, Austin and Repatriation Medical Centre, University of Melbourne, Heidelberg, Melbourne, Australia

Renal Replacement Therapy in the ICU

E. David Bennett, MD

Professor of Intensive Care Medicine, Department of Intensive Care, St. George's Hospital, London, United Kingdom

Hemodynamic Monitoring

Tomas Berl, MD

Professor of Medicine, Department of Medicine, and Head, Division of Renal Disease, University of Colorado, Denver, Colorado

Disorders of Water Balance

Gordon R. Bernard, MD

Professor of Medicine, Allergy, Pulmonary and Critical Care Medicine, Vanderbilt University Medical Center, Nashville, Tennessee

Acute Lung Injury and Acute Respiratory Distress Syndrome

Anatole Besman, MD

Assistant Professor of Surgery, University of Connecticut School of Medicine, Hartford Hospital, Hartford, Connecticut

Pelvic and Major Long Bone Fractures

Joost Bierens, MD

Department of Anesthesiology, VU University Medical Center; Professor of Emergency Medicine, Medical Commission International Life-Saving Federation; Advisory Board Member Maatschappij tot Reding van Drenkelingen, Amsterdam, The Netherlands

Drowning

Walter L. Biffl, MD

Chief, Division of Trauma and Surgical Critical Care, Rhode Island Hospital; Associate Professor of Surgery, Brown University School of Medicine, Providence, Rhode Island

Apoptosis in the Critically Ill; Thoracic Trauma

Thomas P. Bleck, MD, FCCM

Louise Nerancy Eminent Scholar in Neurology and Professor of Neurology, Neurological Surgery, and Internal Medicine, and Director, Neuroscience Intensive Care Unit, University of Virginia, Charlottesville, Virginia

Seizures in the Critically Ill; Neuromuscular Disorders in the ICU; Botulism; Lumbar Puncture; Intracranial Pressure Monitoring; Determination of Death by Neurologic Criteria

Thomas A. Bledsoe, MD

Clinical Assistant Professor, Brown University School of Medicine, Providence, Rhode Island

Ethical Issues in the Intensive Care Unit

Karen C. Bloch, MD, MPH

Assistant Professor of Medicine and Preventive Medicine, Vanderbilt University School of Medicine, Nashville, Tennessee

Central Nervous System Infections

Frank Bloos, PhD, UWO

Senior Physician, Department of Anesthesiology and Critical Care Medicine, University Hospital Jena; Member of the Medical Study Coordination for the German Compedence Network Sepsis (SEPNET)

Pathophysiology of Sepsis and Multiple Organ Dysfunction

Desmond J. Bohn, MB, BCh, MRCP, FRCPC, FRA

Professor of Pediatrics and Anesthesia, University of Toronto; Chief, Department of Critical Care Medicine, The Hospital for Sick Children, Toronto, Ontario, Canada

Fluids and Electrolytes in Pediatrics

Nicole C. Bouchard, MD

New York City Poison Control Center, New York, New York

Opioids

Arthur Boujoukos, MD

Associate Professor of Critical Care Medicine; Director, Cardiovascular Intensive Care Unit; Vice Chair, Clinical Operations, Department of Critical Care Medicine, University of Pittsburgh School of Medicine, Pittsburgh, Pennsylvania

Tachycardia and Bradycardia; Management of Patients after Heart and Lung Transplants

Alessandro Bozzano, MD

Tutor (Cardiology Specialization), Department of Clinical Medicine, Prevention, and Applied Biotechnologies, University of Milan-Bicocca, Milan; Cardiologist, Cardiology and Coronary Care Department, San Gerardo Hospital, Monza (Mi), Italy

Pericardiocentesis

William J. Brady, MD

Associate Professor of Emergency Medicine and Clinical Internal Medicine, and Vice Chair, Department of Emergency Medicine, University of Virginia School of Medicine; Medical Director, Life Support Learning Center, University of Virginia Health System, Charlottesville, Virginia

Acute Coronary Syndromes: Pathophysiology and Diagnosis

Serge Brimioulle, MD, PhD

Associate Professor of Medicine, School of Medicine, Free University of Brussels; Staff Physician, Department of Intensive Care, Erasme University Hospital, Brussels, Belgium

Diabetes Insipidus

Daniel E. Brooks, MD

Assistant Professor, University of Pittsburgh Medical Center; Medical Toxicologist, Pittsburgh, Pennsylvania

Calcium Channel Blocker Toxicity

Richard C. Brundage, PharmD, PhD

Associate Professor and Director, Center for Drug Forecasting, College of Pharmacy, Graduate Program in Experimental and Clinical Pharmacology, University of Minnesota, Minneapolis, Minnesota

General Principles of Pharmacokinetics and Pharmacodynamics

Frank Martin Brunkhorst, MD

Oberarzt, Friedrich Schiller University, University Hospital Jena, Jena, Germany

Pathophysiology of Sepsis and Multiple Organ Dysfunction

D. Patrick Bryant, MD

Assistant Professor of Surgery, Penn State University, College of Medicine, Penn State M.S. Hershey Medical Center, Hershey, Pennsylvania

Hypomagnesemia

Timothy G. Buchman, MD, PhD

Professor, Department of Surgery, Washington University School of Medicine, St. Louis, Missouri

Indications for and Management of Tracheostomy

Jeffrey P. Burns, MD, MPH

Clinical Director, Medical-Surgical ICU; Program Director, Fellowship in Pediatric Critical Care Medicine, Children's Hospital; Associate Professor of Anesthesia and Pediatrics, Harvard Medical School, Boston, Massachusetts

Ethical Controversies in Pediatric Critical Care

Belén Cabello, MD

Resident, Critical Care, Medica Intensiva, Hospital San Pau, Barcelona, Spain

Acute Weaning from Mechanical Ventilation

Karen Calhoun, MD

Professor and Chair, Department of Otolaryngology, Head and Neck Surgery, University of Missouri, Columbia, Missouri

Epistaxis

Clifton W. Callaway, MD

Center for Emergency Medicine, Department of Emergency Medicine, Safar Center for Resuscitation Research, University of Pittsburgh, Pittsburgh, Pennsylvania

Cardiopulmonary-Cerebral Resuscitation

Peter M. A. Calverley, MD, MBChB, FRCP

Professor of Pulmonary Medicine, Department of Medicine, University of Liverpool; Honorary Consultant Physician, University Hospital Aintree, Liverpool, United Kingdom

Chronic Obstructive Pulmonary Disease

A. John Camm, MD, FRCP, QHP, FESC, FACC, FAHA

Professor of Clinical Cardiology, and Division Head, Division of Cardiac and Vascular Sciences, St. George's Hospital Medical School, London, United Kingdom

Supraventricular Arrhythmias

Sean M. Caples, DO

Division of Pulmonary and Critical Care Medicine, Mayo Clinic College of Medicine, Rochester, Minnesota

Respiratory System Mechanics and Respiratory Muscle Function

Diane M. Cappelletty, PharmD

Associate Professor of Pharmacy Practice, University of Toledo, College of Pharmacy, Toledo, Ohio

Agents with Primary Activity Against Gram-Positive Bacteria

Joseph A. Carcillo, MD

Associate Professor, Department of Critical Care Medicine, University of Pittsburgh School of Medicine, Associate Director, PICU, Children's Hospital of Pittsburgh, Pittsburgh, Pennsylvania

Sepsis and Multiple Organ System Failure in Children

Franco N. Carnevale, RN, PhD

Associate Professor, Faculty of Medicine (Pediatrics); Associate Professor, School of Nursing; Adjunct Professor, Counselling Psychology; and Affiliate Member, Biomedical Ethics Unit, McGill University, Montreal, Quebec, Canada

Key Issues in Critical Care Nursing

Emily E. Castelli, PharmD

Assistant Professor of Pharmacy and Therapeutics, University of Pittsburgh; Clinical Pharmacist, University of Pittsburgh Medical Center, Pittsburgh, Pennsylvania

Digitalis

Edward D. Chan, MD

Associate Professor of Medicine, University of Colorado Health Sciences Center; Staff Physician, National Jewish Medical and Research Center, Denver, Colorado

Tuberculosis

Jean Chastre, MD

Professor of Medicine, University Paris; Medical ICU, Groupe Hospitalier Pitie Salpetriere, Paris, France

Nosocomial Pneumonia; Bronchoalveolar Lavage and Protected Specimen Bronchial Brushing

Robert Chavko, MD

Fellow, Department of Critical Care Medicine, University of Pittsburgh School of Medicine, Pittsburgh, Pennsylvania

Management of the Brain-Dead Organ Donor

Lakshmipathi Chelluri, MD

Associate Professor, Departments of Critical Care Medicine and Medicine, University of Pittsburgh Medical Center, Pittsburgh, Pennsylvania

Acute Respiratory Failure

Augustine M.K. Choi, MD

Professor of Medicine, and Chief, Pulmonary, Allergy, and Critical Care Medicine, University of Pittsburgh School of Medicine, Pittsburgh, Pennsylvania

Carbon Monoxide and Heme Oxygenase-1

Chun-Shiang Chung, MD

Division of Surgical Research, Assistant Professor of Surgery, Department of Surgery, Brown University School of Medicine and Rhode Island Hospital, Providence, Rhode Island

Apoptosis in the Critically Ill

T. Philip Chung, MD

Department of Surgery, Division of General Surgery, Washington University School of Medicine, St. Louis, Missouri

Molecular and Biochemical Monitoring

Robert S.B. Clark, MD

Associate Professor, Department of Critical Care Medicine, University of Pittsburgh School of Medicine, Pittsburgh, Pennsylvania

Biochemical, Cellular, and Molecular Mechanisms of Neuronal Death and Secondary Brain Injury in Critical Care; Key Issues in Pediatric Neurointensive Care

J. Perren Cobb, MD

Associate Professor of Surgery, Washington University; Injury Genomics Group, Cellular Injury and Adaptation Laboratory, St. Louis, Missouri

Molecular and Biochemical Monitoring

Jonathan D. Cohen, MD

General Intensive Care Department, Rabin Medical Center, Beilinson Campus, Petah Tiqwa, Israel

Indirect Calorimetry and Metabolic Monitoring

Steven M. Cohen, MD

Dr. Witten B. Russ Professor and Chairman, Department of Surgery, University of Texas Health Science Center, San Antonio, Texas

Traumatic Brain Injury

Stephen M. Cohn, MD, FACS

The Robert Zeppa Professor of Surgery, and Chief, Divisions of Trauma and Surgical Critical Care; Medical Director, Ryder Trauma Center, University of Miami School of Medicine, Miami, Florida

Anemia of Critical Illness

John Cole, MD

Assistant Professor, Emergency Medicine, University of Pittsburgh School of Medicine; Medical Director, STATMed EVAC, Center for Emergency Medicine, University of Pittsburgh Medical Center, Pittsburgh, Pennsylvania

Transport Medicine

Deborah J. Cook, MD

Professor of Medicine and Clinical Epidemiology and Biostatistics, McMaster University, Hamilton, Ontario, Canada

Venous Thromboembolism in Medical-Surgical Critically Ill Patients

James A. Cook, PhD

Professor, Departments of Physiology and Neuroscience, Medical University of South Carolina, Charleston, South Carolina

Prostaglandins, Thromboxanes, Leukotrienes, and Other Products of Arachidonic Acid

Robert N. Cooney, MD

Professor of Surgery, Chief of General Surgery, Milton S. Hershey Medical Center, Hershey, Pennsylvania

Hypomagnesemia; Hypocalcemia and Hypercalcemia

Susan J. Corbridge, RN, MS, CNP

Clinical Instructor, College of Nursing, University of Illinois at Chicago; Nurse Practitioner, Pulmonary Medicine, University of Illinois Chicago Medical Center, Chicago, Illinois

Severe Asthma Exacerbation

Thomas C. Corbridge, MD, FCCP

Associate Professor of Medicine, Northwestern University Feinberg School of Medicine; Director, Medical Intensive Care, Northwestern Memorial Hospital, Chicago, Illinois

Severe Asthma Exacerbation

Howard L. Corwin, MD

Section of Critical Care Medicine, Department of Anesthesiology, Dartmouth-Hitchcock Medical Center, Lebanon, New Hampshire

Hypernatremia and Hyponatremia

Gad Cotter, MD

Assistant Professor of Medicine, Duke University Medical Center, Durham, North Carolina

Pulmonary Edema

Barry G. Crowe, MD

Instructor in Surgery, Saint Louis University, St. Louis, Missouri

Mediastinitis

Mark A. Crowther, MD

Associate Professor, Department of Medicine, McMaster University; St. Joseph's Hospital, Hamilton, Ontario, Canada

Venous Thromboembolism in Medical-Surgical Critically Ill Patients

Burke A. Cunha, MD

Chief, Infectious Disease Division, Winthrop-University Hospital, Mineola; Professor of Medicine, State University of New York School of Medicine, Stony Brook, New York

Rashes

Joseph M. Darby, MD

Professor of Critical Care Medicine and Surgery, University of Pittsburgh School of Medicine; Medical Director, Trauma ICU, UPMC-Presbyterian Hospital, Pittsburgh, Pennsylvania

Sudden Deterioration in Neurologic Status; Management of the Brain-Dead Organ Donor

Michaël Darmon, MD

Fellow, Faculty of Medicine, University of Paris VII; Service de Réanimation Médicale, Hôpital St. Louis, Paris, France

Specific Facets of Managing Neutropenic Cancer Patients in the Intensive Care Unit

Joseph F. Dasta, MSc

Professor of Pharmacy, The Ohio State University College of Pharmacy, Columbus, Ohio

Pharmacoeconomics in Critical Care

R. Phillip Dellinger, MD

Professor of Medicine, Robert Wood Johnson Medical School; Director, Section of Critical Care Medicine, Department of Medicine, Cooper University Hospital, Camden, New Jersey

Hyperkalemia and Hypokalemia; Hypophosphatemia and Hyperphosphatemia; Arterial Blood Gas Interpretation

Mark Dershwitz, MD, PhD

Professor and Vice Chair of Anesthesiology, and Professor of Biochemistry and Molecular Pharmacology, University of Massachusetts Medical School, Worcester, Massachusetts

Antipsychotics

Michael A. DeVita, MD

Associate Professor, Departments of Critical Care Medicine and Internal Medicine, University of Pittsburgh School of Medicine, Associate Medical Director, UPMC-Presbyterian Hospital, Pittsburgh, Pennsylvania

Non-Heartbeating Organ Donation

Vincenzo D'Intini, MBBS, FRNCP, FRACP

Research Fellow, Department of Nephrology, Dialysis and Transplantation, San Bortolo Hospital, Vicenza, Italy

Renal Replacement Therapy in the ICU

Michael N. Diringer, MD, FCCM

Professor, Departments of Neurology, Neurological Surgery, and Occupational Therapy, Washington University; Director, Neurology/Neurosurgical ICU, Barnes-Jewish Hospital, St. Louis, Missouri

Nontraumatic Intracerebral and Subarachnoid Hemorrhage

Peter Doelken, MD

Assistant Professor, Division of Pulmonology, Allergy and Clinical Immunology, Medical University of South Carolina, Charleston, South Carolina

Thoracentesis

Michael Donahoe, MD

Associate Professor of Medicine, and Associate Chief, Division of Pulmonary, Allergy, and Critical Care Medicine, University of Pittsburgh School of Medicine; Director, Medical ICU, UPMC, Pittsburgh, Pennsylvania

Very High Systemic Arterial Blood Pressure

Richard Donnelly, MD, PhD, FRCP, FRACP

Professor and Associate Dean (Graduate-Entry Medicine), University of Nottingham; Director of Research and Development, Southern Derbyshire Acute Hospitals Trust, The Medical School, Derby City General Hospital, Derby, United Kingdom

Peripheral Arteriopathies Including Embolism

Gregory P. Downey, MD

Division of Respiratory Medicine, Department of Pediatrics, The Hospital for Sick Children; Department of Medicine, Division of Respirology, The University of Toronto, The Toronto General Hospital Research Institute of University Health Network, Toronto, Ontario, Canada

The Neutrophil: Balancing Antimicrobial Effectiveness and the Potential for Damage to the Host

Howard R. Doyle, MD

Attending Physician, Critical Care Medicine, Montefiore Medical Center, Bronx, New York

Balloon Tamponade

Thomas D. DuBose, Jr., MD

Professor and Chair, Department of Internal Medicine, and Professor of Physiology and Pharmacology, Wake Forest University Health Sciences; Chief of Internal Medicine Service, North Carolina Baptist Hospital, Winston-Salem, North Carolina

Metabolic Acidosis and Alkalosis

Amy Durtschi, PhD

College of Pharmacy, The Ohio State University; Assistant Director, Abbott Laboratories, GPRD Center for Pharmaceutical Appraisals and Customer Research, Columbus, Ohio

Pharmacoeconomics in Critical Care

Susan Duthie, MD

Assistant Director, Pediatric Critical Care, Children's Hospital, San Diego, California

Pediatric Trauma

Brian K. Eble, MD

Instructor, Baylor College of Medicine, Texas Children's Hospital, Houston, Texas

Pediatric Intensive Care Procedures

Philippe Eggimann, MD

Department of Internal Medicine, Medical ICU, and Infection Control Program, University of Geneva Hospitals, Geneva, Switzerland

Acute Bacteremia

Frederick J. Ehlert, PhD

Department of Pharmacology, College of Medicine, University of California, Irvine, Irvine, California

Receptor Physiology

E. Wesley Ely, MD

Associate Professor, Division of Allergy, Pulmonary, and Critical Care Medicine, Department of Medicine, Vanderbilt University School of Medicine; Veterans Affairs Tennessee Valley, Geriatric Research, Education, and Clinical Care, Nashville, Tennessee

Agitation and Delirium; Management of Pain, Anxiety, and Delirium

Guillaume Emeriaud, MD

Chef de Clinique (Clinical Assistant), Faculte de Medicine, Universite Joseph Fourier; Assistant (Hospital Assistant), Service de Reanimation Pediatrique, Departement de Pediatrie, CHU Grenoble, Grenoble, France

Hematology and Oncology in Children

Angels Escorsell, MD

Staff Member, Liver Unit, Digestive Diseases Institute, Institut D'Investigacions Biomediques August R. Sunyer (IDIBAPS), Hospital Clinic, Barcelona, Spain

Hepatorenal Syndrome

Charles T. Esmon, PhD

Cardiovascular Biology Research Program, Oklahoma Medical Research Foundation, Departments of Pathology and Biochemistry and Molecular Biology, University of Oklahoma Health Sciences Center, Howard Hughes Medical Institute, Oklahoma City, Oklahoma

Coagulation

Joel Ettinger, BA, MHA

Principal, Pugh, Ettinger, and McCarthy Associates, LLC, Pittsburgh, Pennsylvania

The Pursuit of Performance Excellence

Josh Ettinger, BS

Center for Innovation in Quality Patient Care, Johns Hopkins University School of Medicine, Johns Hopkins Outpatient Center, Baltimore, Maryland; Principal, Pugh, Ettinger, and McCarthy Associates, LLC, Pittsburgh, Pennsylvania

The Pursuit of Performance Excellence

Gregory T. Everson, MD

Professor of Medicine, Director of Hepatology, University of Colorado School of Medicine, Denver, Colorado

Hepatic Encephalopathy

Derek V. Exner, MD

Associate Professor, University of Calgary, Calgary, Alberta, Canada

Sudden Cardiac Death: Implantable Cardioverter-Defibrillators

M. Charlene Fabrizio, MD

Director, Perfusion Services, University of Pittsburgh Medical Center, Pittsburgh, Pennsylvania

Cannulation for Extracorporeal Membrane Oxygenation

Jean-Yves Fagon, MD

Professor of Medicine, University of Paris V; Head, Medical ICU, Hôpital Europeen Georges Pompidou, Paris, France

Nosocomial Pneumonia; Bronchoalveolar Lavage and Protected Specimen Bronchial Brushing

Ronald J. Falk, MD

Professor, Department of Medicine, Doc J. Thurston Professor of Medicine, and Professor of Pathology and Laboratory Medicine, University of North Carolina at Chapel Hill and University of North Carolina Hospitals, Chapel Hill, North Carolina

Glomerulonephritis and Interstitial Nephritis in the ICU

Hongkuan Fan, PhD

Departments of Physiology and Neuroscience, Medical University of South Carolina, Charleston, South Carolina

Prostaglandins, Thromboxanes, Leukotrienes, and Other Products of Arachidonic Acid

Jeremy Farrar, BSc, MBBS, FRCP, DPhil

Clinical Reader, Oxford University, Oxford, United Kingdom; Director, The Oxford University Clinical Research Unit, The Hospital for Tropical Diseases, Ho Chi Minh City, Vietnam

Dengue Hemorrhagic Fever

Alan P. Farwell, MD

Associate Professor of Medicine, Division of Endocrinology, Department of Medicine, University of Massachusetts Medical School; Staff Physician, University of Massachusetts Memorial Health Care, Worcester, Massachusetts

Thyroid Gland Disorders

Florence Fenollar, MD

Unite des Rickettsies, Faculte de Medecine, Universite de le Mediterranee, Marseille, France

Rickettsial Diseases

Michael B. Fessler, MD

Assistant Professor, University of Colorado School of Medicine, National Jewish Medical and Research Center, Denver, Colorado

Cellular Signaling

Ericka L. Fink, MD

Fellow, Department of Critical Care Medicine, University of Pittsburgh School of Medicine, Pittsburgh, Pennsylvania

Key Issues in Pediatric Neurointensive Care

Mitchell P. Fink, MD

Professor and Chair, Department of Critical Care Medicine, and Watson Professor of Surgery, University of Pittsburgh School of Medicine, Pittsburgh, Pennsylvania

Fever and Hypothermia; Hyperbilirubinemia; Cytopathic Hypoxia: Mitochondrial Dysfunction in Sepsis

Douglas N. Fish, PharmD

Associate Professor of Pharmacy, University of Colorado Health Sciences Center; Clinical Specialist in Critical Care/Infectious Diseases, University of Colorado Hospital, Denver, Colorado

Antimicrobials in Chemotherapy Strategy; Fluoroquinolones

Bradley D. Freeman, MD

Assistant Professor of Surgery, Washington University School of Medicine, St. Louis, Missouri

Indications for and Management of Tracheostomy

John J. Fung, MD, PhD

Chairman, Department of General Surgery, and Director, Transplant Center, The Cleveland Clinic Foundation, Cleveland, Ohio

Clinical Use of Immunosuppressants

Richard L. Gamelli, MD, FACS

The Robert J. Freeark Professor and Chairman, Department of Surgery; Director, The Burn Shock Trauma Institute; Chief, The Burn Center, Loyola University Medical Center, Maywood, Illinois

Burns and Inhalation Injury

Raúl J. Gazmuri, MD, PhD, FCCM

Professor, Department of Medicine; Associate Professor, Physiology and Biophysics, Rosalind Franklin University of Medicine and Science; Section Chief, Critical Care Medicine; ICU Director, North Chicago Veterans Affairs Medical Center, North Chicago, Illinois

Ventricular Arrhythmias; Cardioversion and Defibrillation; Transvenous and Transcutaneous Cardiac Pacing

Robert Geelkerken, MD

Vascular Surgeon, Medisch Spectrum Twente, Department of Surgery, Enschede, The Netherlands

Splanchnic Ischemia

Todd W.B. Gehr, MD

Professor of Medicine, Division of Nephrology, Virginia Commonwealth University Health System, Richmond, Virginia

Clinical Assessment of Renal Function

Herwig Gerlach, MD

Professor of Anesthesiology, Critical Care Medicine, and Physiology, Humboldt University; Director and Chairman, Department of Anesthesiology, Critical Care, and Pain Management, Vivante-Klinikum Neukoelln, Berlin, Germany

Adrenal Insufficiency

Chris A. Ghaemmaghami, MD
Associate Professor of Emergency Medicine and Clinical Internal Medicine, University of Virginia School of Medicine, Charlottesville, Virginia
Acute Coronary Syndromes: Pathophysiology and Diagnosis

Helen Giamarellou, MD, PhD
Professor of Internal Medicine, Infectious Diseases Specialist, and Head, 4th Department of Internal Medicine, Athens University Medical School, Athens, Greece
Infectious Endocarditis

Fredric Ginsberg, MD
Assistant Professor of Medicine, Robert Wood Johnson Medical School at Camden, University of Medicine and Dentistry of New Jersey (UMDNJ), Camden, New Jersey
Myocarditis in the Intensive Care Unit

Debbie S. Gipson, MD, MS
Assistant Professor, Division of Nephrology and Hypertension, Departments of Medicine and Pediatrics; Adjunct Assistant Professor, Department of Epidemiology, School of Public Health, University of North Carolina at Chapel Hill, Chapel Hill, North Carolina
Glomerulonephritis and Interstitial Nephritis in the ICU

Andrew Githaiga, MD
Department of Medicine, University of Pittsburgh Medical Center, Pittsburgh, Pennsylvania
Infections in the Immunocompromised Patient

Thomas Gleason, MD
Division of Cardiothoracic Surgery, Department of Surgery, University of Pennsylvania School of Medicine, Philadelphia, Pennsylvania
Mechanical Support in Cardiogenic Shock

Jacques P. Goldstein, MD, PhD
Professor, Department of Cardiac Surgery, AZ Vrije Universiteit Brussels, Brussels, Belgium
Cardiac Surgery: Indications and Complications

Rene M. Gonzales, MD
Staff Anesthesiologist, St. Luke's Coordinated Health Network, Bethlehem, Pennsylvania
Difficult Airway Management for Intensivists

Prabhakaran P. Gopalakrishnan, MD
Hospitalist, John Peter Smith Hospital, Fort Worth, Texas
Ventricular Arrhythmias

John Gorcsan III, MD
Associate Professor of Medicine, Director of Echocardiography, University of Pittsburgh School of Medicine, Pittsburgh, Pennsylvania
Bedside Ultrasonography

Yaacov Gozal, MD
Senior Lecturer in Anesthesiology, Anesthesiology and Critical Care Medicine, Hebrew University–Hadassah Medical School; Director, Operating Room and PACU, Anesthesiology and Critical Care Medicine, Hadassah University Hospital, Ein Karem, Jerusalem, Israel
Arterial Cannulation and Invasive Blood Pressure Measurement

Jeremy D. Gradon, MD, FACP, FIDSA
Associate Professor of Medicine, Johns Hopkins University School of Medicine; Attending Physician, Department of Medicine, Division of Infectious Diseases, Sinai Hospital, Baltimore, Maryland
Head and Neck Infections

Cornelia R. Graves, MD
Associate Professor, Director, Critical Care Obstetrics, and Chief, Maternal Medicine, Division of Maternal-Fetal Medicine, Department of Obstetrics and Gynecology, Vanderbilt University, Nashville, Tennessee
Acute Pulmonary Complications in Pregnancy

Cesare Gregoretti, MD
Servizio di Anestesiologia e Rianimazione, Dipartimento di Discipline Medico-Chirurgiche, Universita di Torino, Ospedale S. Giovanni Battista, Torino, Italy
Patient-Ventilator Interaction

Robin L. Gross, MD
Assistant Professor of Medicine, Robert Wood Johnson Medical School; Division of Pulmonary and Critical Care Medicine, Cooper University Hospital, Camden, New Jersey
Arterial Blood Gas Interpretation

Michael R. Grounds, MD
Reader in Intensive Care Medicine, St. George's Hospital, London, United Kingdom
Hemodynamic Monitoring

Patricia S. Grutkoski, PhD
Instructor, Brown University School of Medicine; Division of Surgical Research, Rhode Island Hospital, Providence, Rhode Island
Apoptosis in the Critically Ill

Paul O. Gubbins, PharmD
Associate Professor, Department of Pharmacy Practice, College of Pharmacy, University of Arkansas for Medical Sciences, Little Rock, Arkansas
Fungal Infections

Kyle J. Gunnerson, MD
Assistant Professor, Department of Anesthesiology and Critical Care and Department of Emergency Medicine, VCURES Laboratory (VCU Reanimation Engineering Shock Center), Virginia Commonwealth University Health System, Richmond, Virginia
Low Systemic Arterial Blood Pressure

Weidun Alan Guo, MD, PhD

Surgical Critical Care Resident, Department of Surgery, Ohio State University, Columbus, Ohio

Infections of Skin, Muscle, and Soft Tissue

Ali Hallal, MD

Surgical Critical Care and Trauma Surgery Fellow, University of Miami, Ryder Trauma Center, Miami, Florida

Anemia of Critical Illness

Mitchell L. Halperin, MD

Division of Nephrology, St. Michael's Hospital, University of Toronto, Toronto, Ontario, Canada

Disorders of Plasma Potassium Concentration

Perry V. Halushka, MD, PhD

Dean, College of Graduate Studies, and Professor, Departments of Pharmacology and Medicine, Medical University of South Carolina, Charleston, South Carolina

Prostaglandins, Thromboxanes, Leukotrienes, and Other Products of Arachidonic Acid

Brian G. Harbrecht, MD

Associate Professor of Surgery, and Medical Director, Trauma Services, University of Pittsburgh School of Medicine, Pittsburgh, Pennsylvania

Chest Tube Placement, Care, and Removal

Mary E. Hartman, MD

Fellow, Department of Critical Care Medicine, University of Pittsburgh School of Medicine, Pittsburgh, Pennsylvania

Evidence-Based Critical Care

Maurene A. Harvey, RN, MPH, CCRN, FCCM

President, Educator, Consultant, Consultants in Critical Care Inc., Glenbrook, Nevada

Building Bedside Collaborative Practice

Michelle Hayes, MD

Consultant in Anaesthesia and Intensive Care, Chelsea and Westminster Hospital, London, United Kingdom

Bedside Pulmonary Artery Catheterization

Jan A. Hazelzet, MD, PhD

Sophia Children's Hospital, Erasmus University Medical Center, Rotterdam, The Netherlands

Sepsis and Multiple Organ System Failure in Children

Stephen O. Heard, MD

Chair, Department of Anesthesiology, University of Massachusetts Medical School, and Chairman, Department of Anesthesiology, University of Massachusetts Memorial Medical Center, Worcester, Massachusetts

Management of Acute Pain in the Intensive Care Unit

Paul C. Hébert, MD

University of Ottawa Center for Transfusion Research and the Clinical Epidemiology Program of the Ottawa Health Research Institute, Ottawa, Ontario, Canada

Anemia and Red Blood Cell Transfusion in Critically Ill Patients

John A. Henry, MD, FRCP, FFAEM

Professor, Academic Department of Accident and Emergency Medicine, Imperial College School of Medicine at St. Mary's, and Honorary Consultant, Department of Accident and Emergency, St. Mary's Hospital, London, United Kingdom

Hydrocarbons

Elizabeth D. Hermsen, PharmD, MBA

Adjunct Assistant Professor, University of Nebraska Medical Center College of Pharmacy, and Antimicrobial Pharmacist and Research Associate, The Nebraska Medical Center, Omaha, Nebraska

Metronidazole and Other Antibiotics for Anaerobic Infections

Daniel Herzig, MD

Chief Resident, Department of Surgery, Brown University Medical School, Providence, Rhode Island

Thoracic Trauma

Daren K. Heyland, MD, FRCPC, MSc

Department of Medicine, Queen's Hospital, Kingston, Ontario, Canada

Critical Care Nutrition

Robert W. Hickey, MD

Associate Professor of Pediatrics, Division of Emergency Medicine, Children's Hospital of Pittsburgh, Pittsburgh, Pennsylvania

Key Issues in Pediatric Neurointensive Care

Thomas L. Higgins, MD, MBA

Associate Professor of Medicine and Anesthesiology, Tufts University School of Medicine, Boston; Chief, Critical Care Division, Departments of Medicine, Surgery, and Anesthesia, Baystate Medical Center, Springfield, Massachusetts

Severity of Illness Indices and Outcome Prediction: Development and Evaluation

Nicholas S. Hill, MD

Chief, Pulmonary Critical Care, and Sleep Division, Tufts-New England Medical Center; Professor of Medicine, Tufts University School of Medicine, Boston, Massachusetts

Noninvasive Positive-Pressure Ventilation

Roman Hlatky, MD

Assistant Professor, University of Texas Health Science Center, San Antonio, Texas

Advanced Bedside Neuromonitoring; Jugular Venous and Brain Tissue Oxygen Tension Monitoring

Steven M. Hollenberg, MD

Professor of Medicine, Robert Wood Johnson Medical School/UMDNJ; Director, Coronary Care Unit, Cooper Hospital/University Medical Center, Camden, New Jersey

Acute Coronary Syndromes: Management and Complications

Nathaniel L. Holzman, MD

Department of Surgery, Tufts-New England Medical Center, Tufts University School of Medicine, Boston, Massachusetts

Gastrointestinal Hemorrhage

David T. Huang, MD, MPH

Assistant Professor, Departments of Critical Care Medicine and Emergency Medicine, University of Pittsburgh; Attending Physician, University of Pittsburgh Medical Center, Pittsburgh, Pennsylvania

Chest Pain

Rolf D. Hubmayr, MD

Professor of Medicine, Division of Pulmonary and Critical Care Medicine, Mayo Clinic College of Medicine, Rochester, Minnesota

Respiratory System Mechanics and Respiratory Muscle Function

John T. Huggins, MD

Assistant Professor of Medicine, Medical University of South Carolina; Senior Fellow, Division of Pulmonary and Critical Care Medicine, Allergy and Clinical Immunology, Medical University of South Carolina, Charleston, South Carolina

Pleural Disease in the Intensive Care Unit

Russell D. Hull, MBBS, MSc

Professor of Medicine, and Director, Thrombosis Research Unit, University of Calgary, Foothills Hospital, Calgary, Alberta, Canada

Pulmonary Embolism

Sabah N.A. Hussain, MD, PhD

Professor of Medicine, Critical Care and Respiratory Divisions, Department of Medicine, McGill University Hospital Centre, Montreal, Quebec, Canada

Nitric Oxide

James P. Isbister, MD

Consultant in Haematology and Transfusion Medicine, Royal North Shore Hospital of Sydney; Clinical Professor of Medicine, University of Sydney; Adjunct Professor, University of Technology, Sydney, St. Leonards, NSW, Australia

Blood Component Therapy

Rao R. Ivatury, MD

Professor, Department of Surgery, Virginia Commonwealth University, Medical College of Virginia, Richmond, Virginia

Peritonitis and Intra-abdominal Abscess

Connie A. Jastremski, RN, MS, MBA, ANP

Chief Nursing Officer and Vice President, Patient Care Services, Bassett Healthcare, Cooperstown, New York

Building Bedside Collaborative Practice

Larry Jenkins, PhD

Associate Professor, Department of Neurosurgery, University of Pittsburgh School of Medicine, Pittsburgh, Pennsylvania

Biochemical, Cellular, and Molecular Mechanisms of Neuronal Death and Secondary Brain Injury in Critical Care

Mariell Jesup, MD

Division of Cardiothoracic Surgery, Departments of Surgery and Medicine, University of Pennsylvania School of Medicine, Philadelphia, Pennsylvania

Mechanical Support in Cardiogenic Shock

Paul Jodka, MD, BS

Assistant Professor of Anesthesiology and Medicine, Tufts University School of Medicine, Boston; Attending Physician, Adult Critical Care Division, Baystate Medical Center, Springfield, Massachusetts

Management of Acute Pain in the Intensive Care Unit

Robert G. Johnson, MD

C. Rollins Hanlon Professor and Chair, St. Louis University; Chief of Surgery, Saint Louis University Hospital/Tenet, St. Louis, Missouri

Mediastinitis

Vern C. Juel, MD

Associate Professor of Medicine, Division of Neurology, Duke University Medical Center, Durham, North Carolina

Neuromuscular Disorders in the ICU; Botulism

Rose Jung, PharmD

Assistant Professor, Department of Clinical Pharmacy, School of Pharmacy, University of Colorado Health Sciences Center, Denver, Colorado

Aminoglycosides

Allen B. Kaiser, MD

Professor and Vice-Chairman, Department of Medicine, Vanderbilt University School of Medicine, Nashville, Tennessee

Central Nervous System Infections

Richard Kallet, MS, RRT, FAARC

Clinical Research Coordinator, Critical Care and Respiratory Care Division, Department of Anesthesia and Perioperative Care, University of California at San Francisco General Hospital; Clinical Resident Coordinator, Cardiovascular Resident Institute, University of California, San Francisco, San Francisco, California

Bedside Monitoring of Pulmonary Function

Edo Kaluski, MD, FACC
Cardiology Department, Assaf-Harofeh Medical Center, Zerifin; Sackler Faculty of Medicine, Tel-Aviv University, Tel Aviv, Israel
Pulmonary Edema

Kamel S. Kamel, MD
Associate Professor of Medicine, University of Toronto; Attending Staff, Chief, Division of Nephrology, Department of Medicine, Toronto, Ontario, Canada
Disorders of Plasma Potassium Concentration

Sandra Kane-Gill, PharmD, MSc
Assistant Professor, Center for Pharmacoinformatics and Outcomes Research, University of Pittsburgh, Pittsburgh, Pennsylvania
Pharmacoeconomics in Critical Care

Jeffrey P. Kanne, MD
Department of Radiology, Harborview Medical Center, University of Washington, Seattle, Washington
Imaging of the Chest in the ICU

Lionel Karlin, MD
Medical Intensive Care Unit, Hôpital Saint Louis and Paris University VII, Paris, France
Organ Toxicity of Cancer Chemotherapy

Manoj Karwa, MD
Assistant Professor of Medicine, Department of Critical Care Medicine, Montefiore Medical Center, Albert Einstein College of Medicine, Bronx, New York
Disaster Medicine for the ICU Physician

Kenneth D. Katz, MD
Assistant Professor, University of Pittsburgh Medical Center, Pittsburgh, Pennsylvania
Calcium Channel Blocker Toxicity

David Charles Kaufman, MD, FCCM
Associate Professor of Surgery, Medicine, Anesthesia and Medical Humanities, University of Rochester; Medical Director, Surgical Intensive Care Unit, Strong Memorial Hospital, Rochester, New York
Hepatopulmonary Syndrome

Catherine Kelleher, MD
Assistant Professor of Medicine, Denver Health Medical Center, Denver, Colorado
Hypertensive Crisis and Urgency

John A. Kellum, MD
Associate Professor of Critical Care Medicine, University of Pittsburgh; Staff Intensivist, University of Pittsburgh School of Medicine, Pittsburgh, Pennsylvania
Polyuria; Oliguria; Acid-Base Disorders; Evidence-Based Critical Care

Aktar S. Khan, MD
Assistant Professor of Surgery, Thomas E. Starzl Transplantation Institute, University of Pittsburgh School of Medicine, Pittsburgh, Pennsylvania
Management of the Brain-Dead Organ Donor

Richard J. King, MD
Fellow, Surgical Critical Care, Penn State/M.S. Hershey Medical Center, Hershey, Pennsylvania
Hypocalcemia and Hypercalcemia

Rick Kingston, PharmD
Vice President/Senior Clinical Toxicologist with the PROSAR International Poison Center; Associate Professor of Pharmacy at the University of Minnesota, College of Pharmacy, Department of Clinical and Experimental Pharmacology, Minneapolis, Minnesota
Pesticides and Herbicides

Orlando Kirton, MD, FACS, FCCM, FCCP
Ludwig J. Pyrtek Chair in Surgery, and Director of Surgery and Chief, Division of General Surgery, Hartford Hospital; Professor of Surgery and Associate Program Director, Integrated General Surgery Residency, and Vice Chair, Department of Surgery, University of Connecticut School of Medicine, Hartford, Connecticut
Pelvic and Major Long Bone Fractures

Jason Knight, MD
Physician, Department of Emergency Medicine, Maricopa Medical Center, Phoenix, Arizona
Conduction Disturbances and Cardiac Pacemakers

Patrick M. Kochanek, MD
Director, Safar Center for Resuscitation Research; Professor and Vice Chairman, Department of Critical Care Medicine, Professor of Pediatrics and Anesthesiology, University of Pittsburgh School of Medicine and Children's Hospital of Pittsburgh, Pittsburgh, Pennsylvania
Key Issues in Pediatric Intensive Care; Biochemical, Cellular, and Molecular Mechanisms of Neuronal Death and Secondary Brain Injury in Critical Care

W. Andrew Kofke, MD, MBA, FCCM
Professor, Anesthesia and Neurosurgery, and Director of Neuroanesthesia, Department of Anesthesia, University of Pennsylvania, Philadelphia, Pennsylvania
Critical Neuropathophysiology

Jeroen J. Kolkman, MD
Gastroenterologist, Medisch Spectrum Twente, Enschede, The Netherlands
Splanchnic Ischemia

Robert L. Kormos, MD

Director, Thoracic Transplantation and Artificial Heart Program, Medical Director, McGowan Institute for Regenerative Medicine, University of Pittsburgh, Pittsburgh, Pennsylvania

Ventricular Assist Devices

Larry W. Kraiss, MD

Associate Professor of Surgery, and Chief, Division of Vascular Surgery, University of Utah School of Medicine, Salt Lake City, Utah

Endothelial Function

David J. Kramer, MD

Professor of Medicine, Mayo Clinic College of Medicine; Director, Transplant Critical Care, Mayo Clinic, Jacksonville, Florida

Liver Transplantation

John W. Kreit, MD

Associate Professor of Medicine, Division of Pulmonary, Allergy, and Critical Care Medicine, University of Pittsburgh School of Medicine, Pittsburgh, Pennsylvania

Antidepressant Drug Overdose

James A. Kruse, MD

Chief, Critical Care Services, Mary Imogene Bassett Hospital, Cooperstown, New York

Ethanol, Methanol, and Ethylene Glycol

Vladimir Kvetan, MD

Professor of Anesthesiology and Clinical Medicine, Associate Professor of Surgery, and Director of Critical Care Medicine Service and Fellowship, Department of Critical Care Medicine, Montefiore Medical Center, Bronx, New York

Disaster Medicine for the ICU Physician

Jacques R. Lacroix, MD

Professor of Pediatrics, Universite de Montreal; Pediatrician, Hospital Sainte-Justine, Montreal, Quebec, Canada

Hematology and Oncology in Children

Yi-Chen Lai, MD

Research Scholar, Physical Care Medicine, NRSA Fellow, NICHD/NIH, University of Pittsburgh Medical Center, Pittsburgh, Pennsylvania

Biochemical, Cellular, and Molecular Mechanisms of Neuronal Death and Secondary Brain Injury in Critical Care

Fred J. Laine, MD

Radiology Associates of Richmond, Richmond, Virginia

Neuroimaging

David Laithwaite, MD

Clinical Research Fellow, Division of Vascular Medicine, University of Nottingham, Southern Derbyshire Acute Hospitals Trust, Derby, United Kingdom

Peripheral Arteriopathies Including Embolism

Gilles Lebuffe, MD, PhD

Anesthesiologist and Intensivist, Clinique d'Anesthésie et de Réanimation, Hôpital Claude Huriez, Centre Hospitalier Universitaire de Lille, Lille, France

Resuscitation from Circulatory Shock

James A. Lederer, MD

Associate Professor, Harvard Medical School; Associate Professor of Surgery, and Brook Investigator, Brigham and Women's Hospital, Boston, Massachusetts

Lymphocyte Function after Injury

Moshe Levi, MD

Division of Renal Diseases and Hypertension, Department of Medicine, University of Colorado Health Sciences Center, and Denver Veterans Affairs Medical Center, Denver, Colorado

Disorders of Calcium and Magnesium Metabolism

Allan D.O. Levi, MD, PhD

Chief of Neurosurgical Services, University of Miami School of Medicine, Miami, Florida

Spinal Cord Injury

Phillip D. Levin, MA, MB, BChir

Research Fellow, Department of Critical Care, Sunnybrook and Women's College Health Sciences Centre, Toronto, Ontario, Canada; Staff Anesthetist, Department of Anesthesiology and Critical Care Medicine, Hadassah Hebrew University Hospital, Jerusalem, Israel

Arterial Cannulation and Invasive Blood Pressure Measurement; Beyond Technology: Caring for the Critically Ill

Mitchell M. Levy, MD

Brown University School of Medicine; and Rhode Island Hospital, Department of Pulmonary and Critical Care Medicine, Providence, Rhode Island

Ethical Issues in the Intensive Care Unit; End-of-Life Issues in the Intensive Care Unit

Scott Liebman, MD

Assistant Professor of Medicine, University of Rochester School of Medicine and Dentistry; Assistant Professor of Medicine, Strong Memorial Hospital, Rochester, New York

Urinary Tract Obstruction

Stuart L. Linas, MD

Director, Renal Fellowship Program, Rocky Mountain Kidney Research Center, University of Colorado Health Sciences Center; Chief of Nephrology, Denver Health Medical Center, Denver, Colorado

Hypertensive Crisis and Urgency

Peter K. Linden, MD

Professor, Department of Critical Care Medicine, University of Pittsburgh School of Medicine; Director, Abdominal Organ Transplant ICU, University of Pittsburgh Medical Center, Pittsburgh, Pennsylvania,

Fulminant Hepatic Failure Including Acetaminophen Toxicity

Krishna Lingam, MD

Consultant Vascular Surgeon, Derby Hospitals NHS Foundation Trust, Derby, United Kingdom

Peripheral Arteriopathies Including Embolism

Gregory Y.H. Lip, MD, FRCP

Professor of Cardiovascular Medicine, University of Birmingham, and University Department of Medicine, City Hospital, Birmingham, United Kingdom

Severe Heart Failure

Pamela A. Lipsett, MD, FACS

Professor of Surgery, Anesthesia, Critical Care Medicine, and Nursing, Johns Hopkins University Schools of Medicine and Nursing; Fellowship Director, Surgical Critical Care, and Co-Director, Surgical Intensive Care Units, Johns Hopkins Hospital, Baltimore, Maryland

Acute Pancreatitis

Alan Lisbon, MD

Assistant Professor of Anesthesia, Harvard Medical School; Department of Anesthesia and Critical Care, Beth Israel Deaconess Medical Center, Boston, Massachusetts

Management of the Postoperative Cardiac Surgical Patient

Raghu S. Loganathan, MD

Fellow in Critical Care Medicine, Department of Critical Care Medicine, Montefiore Medical Center, Albert Einstein College of Medicine, Bronx, New York,

Disaster Medicine for the ICU Physician

Adriana M. Lopez, MD

Pediatric Critical Care Fellow, University of Arkansas for Medical Sciences, Arkansas Children's Hospital, Little Rock, Arkansas

Pediatric Intensive Care Procedures

John M. Luce, MD

Professor of Medicine, Division of Pulmonary and Critical Care Medicine, Department of Medicine, University of California, San Francisco, School of Medicine; Associate Director, Medical and Surgical Intensive Care Units, San Francisco General Hospital, San Francisco, California

Human Immunodeficiency Virus Infection

Courtney H. Lyder, ND, GNP, FAAN, RN

Professor of Nursing, Professor of Internal Medicine and Geriatrics, Acting Chair of the Department of Acute and Specialty Care, and Gerontology Consultant, University of Virginia Medical Center, Charlottesville, Virginia

Pressure Ulceration

Andrew I.R. Maas, MD

Department of Neurosurgery, Erasmus Medical Center, Rotterdam, The Netherlands

Intensive Care after Neurosurgery

Neil R. MacIntyre, MD

Professor of Medicine, Duke University Medical Center, Durham, North Carolina

Assist-Control Mechanical Ventilation

Duncan J. Macrae, MBChB, BMSc, FRCA, FRCPCH

Director of Paediatric Intensive Care, Royal Brompton Hospital; Honorary Senior Lecturer, Imperial College, University of London, London, United Kingdom

Acquired and Congenital Heart Disease in Children

Stefano Maggiolini, MD

Tutor (Cardiology Specialization), University Department of Clinical Medicine, Prevention, and Applied Biotechnologies, University of Milan-Bicocca, Milan; Cardiologist, Cardiology and Coronary Care Unit Department, San Gerardo Hospital, Monza (Mi), Italy

Pericardiocentesis

Vinay Maheshwari, MD

Clinical Associate, Pulmonary, Critical Care and Sleep Medicine, Tufts-New England Medical Center; Clinical Instructor, Tufts University School of Medicine, Boston, Massachusetts

The Hematopoietic Stem Cell Transplantation Patient

Bernhard Maisch, MD, FESC, FACC

Professor and Chairman, Department of Internal Medicine and Cardiology, and Dean of Medical Faculty, Phillips University; Director of the University Hospital Departments of Internal Medicine and Cardiology, Marburg, Germany

Pericardial Diseases

Ajai K. Malhotra, MD

Assistant Professor, Trauma, Virginia Commonwealth University's Medical College of Virginia Hospitals, Richmond, Virginia; Clinical Instructor in Surgery, University of Tennessee, Memphis, Tennessee

Peritonitis and Intra-abdominal Abscess

Jordi Mancebo, MD

Associate Professor, Department of Medicine, Universitat Autonoma de Barcelona; Unit Chief, Medicina Intensiva, Hospital San Pau, Barcelona, Spain

Acute Weaning from Mechanical Ventilation

Henry J. Mann, MD

Professor, College of Pharmacy, and Director, Center for Excellence in Critical Care, University of Minnesota, Minneapolis, Minnesota

General Principles of Pharmacokinetics and Pharmacodynamics

John A. Mannick, MD
Moseley Distinguished Professor of Surgery, Harvard Medical School; attending, Brigham and Women's Hospital, Boston, Massachusetts
Lymphocyte Function after Injury

Sanjay Manocha, MD
Post-Doctoral Fellow of the CIHR IMPACT Program and Michael Smith Foundation for Health Research, Critical Care Research Laboratories, Centre for Cardiovascular and Pulmonary Research, St. Paul's Hospital, Vancouver, British Columbia, Canada
Adjunctive Respiratory Therapy

Eric L. Marderstein, MD
Department of Surgery and Critical Care Medicine, University of Pittsburgh Health System, Pittsburgh, Pennsylvania
Placement of Feeding Tubes

Daniel R. Margulies, MD
Director of Trauma, Department of Surgery, Cedars-Sinai Medical Center; Assistant Clinical Professor of Surgery, David Geffen School of Medicine, University of California, Los Angeles, Los Angeles, California
Percutaneous Dilatational Tracheostomy

Paul E. Marik, MD, FCCM, FCCP
Professor, Pulmonary and Critical Care Medicine, Thomas Jefferson University; Chief, Pulmonary and Critical Care Medicine, Jefferson Medical College, Philadelphia, Pennsylvania
The Management of Gastrointestinal Bleeding; Aspiration Pneumonitis and Pneumonia

John J. Marini, MD
Professor of Medicine, University of Minnesota, Minneapolis; Director of Translational Research, Regions Hospital, St. Paul, Minnesota
Principles of Gas Exchange

Donald W. Marion, MD, FACS
Senior Research Fellow, The Brain Trauma Foundation, New York, New York
Traumatic Brain Injury

Steven J. Martin, PharmD, BCPS, FCCM
Associate Professor of Pharmacy, and Co-Director, The Infectious Disease Research Laboratory, Department of Pharmacy Practice, College of Pharmacy, University of Toledo, Toledo, Ohio
Beta-Lactam Drugs Used in Critical Care

Mark L. Martinez, MD
Fellow, Department of Internal Medicine, Division of Pulmonary and Critical Care, University of Utah School of Medicine, Salt Lake City, Utah
Endothelial Function

Michael A. Matthay, MD
Professor of Medicine and Anesthesia; Senior Associate, Cardiovascular Research Institute; Associate Director, Intensive Care; and Director, Critical Care Medicine Training Program, Department of Medicine, University of California, San Francisco, San Francisco, California
Lung Epithelial Function

Gary R. Matzke, BS Pharm, PharmD
Vice-Chairman and Professor, Department of Pharmacy and Therapeutics, School of Pharmacy; Professor, Renal and Electrolyte Division, Department of Medicine, School of Medicine, University of Pittsburgh, Pittsburgh, Pennsylvania
Drug Dosing in the Patient with Renal Failure

Addison K. May, MD
Associate Professor of Surgery, Department of Surgery, Vanderbilt University, Nashville, Tennessee
Peritonitis and Intra-abdominal Abscess

George V. Mazariegos, MD
University of Pittsburgh Health System, Division of Transplant Surgery, Pittsburgh, Pennsylvania
Intestinal and Multiple Organ Transplantation

Clyde E. McAuley, MD, FACS
Associate Professor, Department of Surgery, Northeastern Ohio Universities College of Medicine, Rootstown; Trauma Surgeon, St. Elizabeth Health Center, Youngstown, Ohio
Vascular Catheter-Related Infections

Stephen A. McClave, MD
Professor of Medicine, Division of Gastroenterology/Hepatology, Department of Medicine, Louisville School of Medicine, Louisville, Kentucky
Critical Care Nutrition

Michael McCready, MD
Chief Cardiology Fellow, Department of Cardiovascular Sciences, University of Calgary, Calgary, Alberta, Canada
Sudden Cardiac Death: Implantable Cardioverter-Defibrillators

Kenneth R. McCurry, MD
Assistant Professor of Surgery, University of Pittsburgh; Director, Adult Lung and Heart-Lung Transplantation; Surgical Director, Pediatric Lung and Heart-Lung Transplantation, University of Pittsburgh Medical Center, Pittsburgh, Pennsylvania
Cannulation for Extracorporeal Membrane Oxygenation

John K. McIlwaine, MD
Section of Critical Care Medicine, Department of Anesthesiology, Dartmouth-Hitchcock Medical Center, Lebanon, New Hampshire
Hypernatremia and Hyponatremia

Dieter Mesotten, MD, PhD

Resident, Department of Intensive Care Medicine, University Hospital Gasthuisberg, Catholic University of Leuven, Leuven, Belgium

Hyperglycemia and Blood Glucose Control in the Intensive Care Unit

Isabelle Michaud, MD

Senior Instructor, Department of Medicine, Pulmonary and Critical Care, University of Rochester Medical Center, Rochester, New York

Hepatopulmonary Syndrome

Eric B. Milbrandt, MD, MPH

Assistant Professor, Department of Critical Care Medicine, University of Pittsburgh School of Medicine, Pittsburgh, Pennsylvania

Agitation and Delirium; Management of Pain, Anxiety, and Delirium

Marek Mirski, MD, PhD

Director, Neuroscience Critical Care Unit; Chief, Division of Neuroanesthesiology; Associate Professor of Anesthesiology and Critical Care, Johns Hopkins Medical Institutions, Baltimore, Maryland

Anticonvulsants in the Intensive Care Unit

Xavier Monnet, MD

Assistant Professor, Paris XI University; Medical Intensive Care Unit, Bicêtre University Hospital, Paris, France

Inotropic Therapy in the Critically Ill

Frederick A. Moore, MD

Chief, General Surgery and Trauma/Critical Care Medicine, and Professor and Vice-Chairman, University of Texas at Houston Medical School, Houston, Texas

Abdominal Compartment Syndrome

Theo J. Morales, MD

Division of Respiratory Medicine, Department of Pediatrics, The Hospital for Sick Children, and Department of Medicine, Division of Respirology, The University of Toronto, The Toronto General Hospital Research Institute of University Health Network, Toronto, Ontario, Canada

The Neutrophil: Balancing Antimicrobial Effectiveness and the Potential for Damage to the Host

Delphine Moreau, MD

Assistant Professor, University of Paris VII; Medical Intensive Care Unit, Saint Louis Hospital, Paris, France

Hematologic Malignancies in the Intensive Care Unit

Alison Morris, MD, MS

Assistant Professor of Medicine, Division of Pulmonary and Critical Care Medicine, Department of Medicine, Keck School of Medicine, University of Southern California, Los Angeles, California; Adjunct Assistant Professor of Medicine, Division of Pulmonary, Allergy, and Critical Care Medicine, University of Pittsburgh, Pittsburgh, Pennsylvania

Human Immunodeficiency Virus Infection

Michele Moss, MD

Professor and Vice Chair of Pediatrics, University of Arkansas for Medical Sciences, Arkansas Children's Hospital, Little Rock, Arkansas

Pediatric Intensive Care Procedures

Claus-Martin Muth, MD

Assistant Professor of Anesthesiology and Staff Anesthesiologist, Sektion Anesthesiologische, Pathophysiologie und Verfahrensentwicklung, Universitaet Ulm; Assistant Professor of Anesthesiology, Universitaetsklinik für Anesthesiologie, Universitaetsklinikum, Ulm, Germany

Other Embolic Syndromes

Kurt G. Naber, MD

Professor and Head of Urology, Hospital St. Elisabeth, Teaching Hospital of the Technical University Munich, Straubing, Germany

Infections of the Urogenital Tract

Lena M. Napolitano, MD

Professor of Surgery, University of Maryland School of Medicine; Division Chief, Surgical Critical Care and General Surgery, and Deputy Chief, Surgical Care Clinical Center, Virginia-Maryland Healthcare System, Baltimore, Maryland

Ascites

Stanley A. Nasraway, Jr., MD

Associate Professor, Departments of Surgery, Medicine and Anesthesia, Tufts University School of Medicine; Director, Surgical Critical Care, Tufts-New England Medical Center, Boston, Massachusetts

Gastrointestinal Hemorrhage

Magdaline Ndirangu, MD

Department of Medicine, University of Pittsburgh Medical Center, Pittsburgh, Pennsylvania

Infections in the Immunocompromised Patient

Lewis S. Nelson, MD

Department of Emergency Medicine, New York University, and New York City Poison Control Center, New York, New York

Opioids

Jerry A. Nick, MD
Associate Professor, National Jewish Medical and Research Center, University of Colorado Health Sciences Center, Denver, Colorado
Cellular Signaling

Michael S. Niederman, MD
Chairman, Department of Medicine, Winthrop University Hospital, Mineola; Professor of Medicine and Vice-Chairman, Department of Medicine, SUNY at Stony Brook, Stony Brook, New York
Community-Acquired Pneumonia

Scott Norwood, MD, FACS, FCCP
Clinical Associate Professor of Surgery, Department of Surgery, University of Texas School of Medicine, Houston; Director, Trauma Services, Department of Surgery, East Texas Medical Center, Tyler, Texas
Vascular Catheter-Related Infections

Beatrice Nyakonu-Schwake, PharmD
Critical Care Resident, Regions Hospital, St. Paul, Minnesota
Toxic Inhalations

Juan B. Ochoa, MD
Associate Professor, Departments of Surgery and Critical Care Medicine, University of Pittsburgh School of Medicine, Pittsburgh, Pennsylvania
Ileus; Diarrhea; Ileus and Mechanical Small Bowel Obstruction; Placement of Feeding Tubes

Mark D. Okusa, MD
Professor of Internal Medicine and Attending Physician, University of Virginia Health System, Charlottesville, Virginia
Lithium

Keith M. Olsen, PharmD, FCCP, FCCM
Professor of Pharmacy, Department of Pharmacy Practice, University of Nebraska Medical Center, Omaha, Nebraska
Theophylline and Other Methylxanthines

James P. Orlowski, MD
Division of Pediatrics, Department of Pediatric Critical Care Medicine, University Community Hospital, and Department of Pediatrics, Critical Care Medicine and Medical Ethics, University of South Florida, Tampa, Florida
Drowning

Richard Orr, MD
Associate Professor, Departments of Critical Care Medicine and Pediatrics, University of Pittsburgh School of Medicine; Associate Director, Pediatric Intensive Care, and Medical Director, Pediatric Critical Care Transplant, Children's Hospital of Pittsburgh, Pittsburgh, Pennsylvania
Transport Medicine

Catherine M. Otto, MD
Professor of Medicine and Director, Cardiology Fellowship Training Programs, University of Washington School of Medicine; Co-Director, Adult Congenital Heart Disease Program, and Associate Director, Echocardiography Laboratory, University of Washington Medical Center, Seattle, Washington
Emergent Valvular Disorders

Heleen M. Oudemans-van Straaten, MD, PhD
Internist-Intensivist, Department of Intensive Care, Onze Lieve Vrouwe Gasthuis, Amsterdam, The Netherlands
Toxic Megacolon in Critically Ill Patients

Joseph E. Parrillo, MD, FCCM
Professor of Medicine, Robert Wood Johnson Medical School at Camden, UMDNJ; Head, Division of Cardiovascular Disease and Critical Care Medicine, and Director, Cooper Heart Institute and Cardiovascular and Critical Care Services, Cooper University Hospital, Camden, New Jersey
Myocarditis in the Intensive Care Unit

Amit Patel, MD
Department of Cardiac Surgery, University of Pittsburgh Medical Center, Pittsburgh, Pennsylvania
Ventricular Assist Devices

David L. Paterson, MD
Department of Medicine, University of Pittsburgh School of Medicine, Pittsburgh, Pennsylvania
Infections in the Immunocompromised Patient; Acute Viral Syndromes

Donna M. Paulnock, PhD
Professor, Department of Medical Microbiology and Immunology, University of Wisconsin Medical School, Madison, Wisconsin
Macrophage Function

Andrew B. Peitzman, MD
Professor, Department of Surgery, University of Pittsburgh School of Medicine, Pittsburgh, Pennsylvania
Abdominal Trauma

Judith Pepe, MD
Associate Professor of Surgery, University of Connecticut School of Medicine, Farmington; Associate Director, Surgical Critical Care, Hartford Hospital, Hartford, Connecticut
Central Venous Catheterization

Andrew D. Perron, MD
Attending Physician and Program Director, Department of Emergency Medicine, Maine Medical Center, Portland, Maine
Acute Coronary Syndromes: Pathophysiology and Diagnosis

Bradley Peterson, MD, FCCM

Director, Pediatric Intensive Care Unit, Children's Hospital of San Diego, San Diego, California

Pediatric Trauma

Graham F. Pineo, MD

Professor of Medicine and Director, Thrombosis Research Unit, University of Calgary; Acting Head, Division of Hematology, Foothills Hospital, Calgary, Alberta, Canada

Pulmonary Embolism

Michael R. Pinsky, MD

Professor, Departments of Critical Care Medicine, Bioengineering and Anesthesiology, University of Pittsburgh School of Medicine; Attending Physician, University of Pittsburgh Medical Center and Magee Women's Hospital, Pittsburgh, Pennsylvania

Heart-Lung Interactions

Didier Pittet, MD, MS

Professor, Faculty of Medicine, University of Geneva; Director, Infection Control Program, and Professor, Division of Infectious Diseases, Department of Internal Medicine, University of Geneva Hospitals, Geneva, Switzerland

Acute Bacteremia

Fred Plum, MD

Professor Emeritus, Department of Neurology and Neuroscience, Weill Medical College of Cornell University, New York, New York

Coma

Murray M. Pollack, MD, MBA

Executive Director, Center for Hospital Based Specialties; Division Chief, Critical Care Medicine, Children's National Medical Center; and Professor of Pediatrics, The George Washington University School of Medicine, Washington, DC

Evaluating Pediatric Critical Care

Brian D. Poole, MD

Division of Renal Diseases and Hypertension, University of Colorado School of Medicine, Denver, Colorado

Acute Renal Failure

Mordecai M. Popovtzer, MD, FACP

Professor of Clinical Medicine, Department of Medicine, Section of Renal Disease, University of Arizona Health Sciences Center; Professor of Clinical Medicine, Southern Arizona Veterans Affairs Health Care System, Tucson, Arizona

Disorders of Calcium and Magnesium Metabolism

Stephen M. Prescott, MD

Department of Internal Medicine, University of Utah; Executive Director, Huntsman Cancer Center Institute, Salt Lake City, Utah

Endothelial Function

Peter J. Pronovost, MD

Associate Professor, Departments of Anesthesiology and Critical Care, Surgery, and Health Policy and Management, and Medical Director, Center for Innovations in Quality Patient Care, The Johns Hopkins University School of Medicine, Baltimore, Maryland

The Pursuit of Performance Excellence

Juan Carlos Puyana, MD

Associate Professor, Departments of Critical Care Medicine and Surgery, University of Pittsburgh School of Medicine; Director, Surgical/Trauma Intensive Care Unit, University of Pittsburgh Medical Center, Pittsburgh, Pennsylvania

Resuscitation of Hypovolemic Shock

Murugan Raghavan, MD, MRCP(UK)

Fellow, Critical Care Medicine, Department of Critical Care Medicine, University of Pittsburgh Medical Center, Pittsburgh, Pennsylvania

Fulminant Hepatic Failure Including Acetaminophen Toxicity

Thomas G. Rainey, MD

Director, Critical Care, Suburban Hospital; Chairman, Idealized Design of the Intensive Care Unit, Institute for Healthcare Improvement/Voluntary Hospitals of America; and President, Critical Medical Inc., Bethesda, Maryland

The Pursuit of Performance Excellence

Thomas Rajan, MD

Fellow, Pulmonary Critical Care and Sleep Division, Tufts-New England Medical Center, Tufts University School of Medicine, Boston, Massachusetts

Noninvasive Positive-Pressure Ventilation

V. Marco Ranieri, MD

Universita di Torina, Dipartimento di Discipline Medico-Chirurgiche, Sezione di Anestesiologia e Rianimazione, Ospedale S. Giovanni Battista, Torino, Italy

Patient-Ventilator Interaction

Ana Rañó, MD, PhD

Intensive Care Unit, Fundacio Althaia, Hospital General de Mannresa, Barcelona, Spain

Pulmonary Infections in the Acute Immunocompromised Patient

Didier Raoult, MD

Unite des Rickettsies, Faculte de Medecine, Universite de le Mediterranee, Marseille, France

Rickettsial Diseases

Jill A. Rebuck, PharmD, BCPS

Clinical Assistant Professor, Department of Surgery, University of Vermont, Fletcher Allen Health Care, Burlington, Vermont

Digitalis

Christina G. Rehm, MD, FACS, FCCM, FCCP
Clinical Associate Professor of Surgery, Oregon Health
Sciences University; Medical Director, Surgery Intensive
Care Unit, Veterans Affairs Medical Center,
Portland, Oregon
Bedside Laparoscopy in the ICU

Konrad Reinhart, MD
Professor and Director of Anesthesiology, Klinik für
Anesthesiologie und Intensivtherapie,
Klinikum der Friedrich-Schiller-Universität Jena,
Jena, Germany
Pathophysiology of Sepsis and Multiple Organ Dysfunction

Jorge D. Reyes, MD
Professor, Surgery, Division of Transplant Surgery, and
Chief, Division of Transplant Surgery, University of
Washington, Seattle, Washington
Intestinal and Multiple Organ Transplantation

Andrew Rhodes, MD
Consultant in Intensive Care Medicine, St. George's
Hospital, London, United Kingdom
Hemodynamic Monitoring

Christian Richard, MD
Professor of Critical Care Medicine, Paris XI University;
Chief of Department, Medical Intensive Care Unit,
Bicêtre University Hospital, Paris, France
Inotropic Therapy in the Critically Ill

Niels C. Riedemann, MD
Research Fellow, Medizinische Hochschule Hannover,
Unfallchirurgische Klinik, Hannover, Germany
Complement

Sophie Rigaudeau, MD
Medical Intensive Care Unit, Saint Louis Teaching
Hospital and Paris VII University, Paris, France
Organ Toxicity of Cancer Chemotherapy

Arsen D. Ristić, MD
Assistant Professor of Internal Medicine-Cardiology,
University of Belgrade Medical School, and Institute for
Cardiovascular Diseases of the Clinical Center of Serbia,
Belgrade, Serbia and Montenegro
Pericardial Diseases

Claudia Robertson, MD
Professor, Department of Neurosurgery, Baylor College
of Medicine; Director, Neurosurgical Intensive Care
Unit, Department of Neurosurgery, Ben Taub General
Hospital, Houston, Texas
*Advanced Bedside Neuromonitoring; Jugular Venous and
Brain Tissue Oxygen Tension Monitoring*

Paul Rogers, MD
Professor, Department of Critical Care Medicine; Vice
Chair, Education for Critical Care; Director,
Multidisciplinary Critical Care Program; Director,
Medical Student Education Program, University of
Pittsburgh School of Medicine,
Pittsburgh, Pennsylvania
*Respiratory Distress with Arterial Hypoxemia; Teaching
Critical Care*

Claudio Ronco, MD
Professor and Director of Nephrology, Dialysis and
Transplantation, San Bortolo Hospital, Vicenza, Italy
Renal Replacement Therapy in the ICU

Kimberly Roth, MD
Chief Fellow, Pediatric Emergency Medicine,
Department of Pediatrics, Division of Pediatric
Emergency Medicine, Children's Hospital of Pittsburgh
and University of Pittsburgh Medical Center,
Pittsburgh, Pennsylvania
Transport Medicine

John C. Rotschafer, PharmD, FCCP
Professor and Head, Department of Experimental and
Clinical Pharmacology, University of Minnesota; Section
of Clinical Pharmacology, Regions Hospital,
St. Paul, Minnesota
*Metronidazole and Other Antibiotics for
Anaerobic Infections*

Stephen A. Rowe, MD
Assistant Professor, Trauma, Burn, and Critical Care,
University of Michigan, Ann Arbor, Michigan
Extracorporeal Life Support

Gordon D. Rubenfeld, MD
Division of Pulmonary and Critical Care Medicine,
University of Washington, and Harborview Medical
Center, Seattle, Washington
Resource Allocation in the Intensive Care Unit

Lewis J. Rubin, MD
Professor of Medicine and Director, Pulmonary
Hypertension Clinic/Program, University of California,
San Diego; Perlman Ambulatory Care Center,
La Jolla, California
Pulmonary Hypertension

Olga Rubio, MD
Resident, Critical Care, Medica Intensiva, Hospital
San Pau, Barcelona, Spain
Acute Weaning from Mechanical Ventilation

Randall A. Ruppel, MD
Assistant Professor, Department of Critical Care
Medicine, Saint Vincent Hospital, Indianapolis, Indiana
Key Issues in Pediatric Neurointensive Care

Laura T. Russo, RD, CSP, LD

Critical Care Clinical Dietician, Children's Memorial Hospital, Chicago, Illinois

Nutrition Issues in Critically Ill Children

Steven A. Sahn, MD

Professor of Medicine and Director, Division of Pulmonary and Critical Care Medicine, Allergy and Clinical Immunology, Medical College of South Carolina, Charleston, South Carolina

Pleural Disease in the Intensive Care Unit; Thoracentesis

John A. Sarko, MD, PhD

Attending Physician, Department of Emergency Medicine, Maricopa Medical Center, Phoenix, Arizona

Conduction Disturbances and Cardiac Pacemakers

Irina Savelieva, MD

Senior Fellow in Cardiology, Division of Cardiac and Vascular Sciences, St. George's Hospital Medical School, London, United Kingdom

Supraventricular Arrhythmias

John J. Schaefer, MD

Department of Anesthesiology, Montefiore Hospital, Pittsburgh, Pennsylvania

Difficult Airway Management for Intensivists

Dennis E. Schellhase, MD

Associate Professor of Pediatrics, University of Arkansas for Medical Sciences, Arkansas Children's Hospital, Little Rock, Arkansas

Pediatric Intensive Care Procedures

Clemens M. Schirmer, MD

Resident in Surgery, Tufts University School of Medicine, Tufts-New England Medical Center, Boston, Massachusetts

Gastrointestinal Hemorrhage

Benoit Schlemmer, MD

Service de Réanimation Médicale, Hôpital St. Louis, Paris, France

Hematologic Malignancies in the Intensive Care Unit

Kristine S. Schonder, PharmD

Assistant Professor, University of Pittsburgh School of Pharmacy; Clinical Pharmacist, Thomas E. Starzl Transplantation Institute, Pittsburgh, Pennsylvania

Clinical Use of Immunosuppressants

Anton C. Schoolwerth, MD, MSHA

Visiting Professor, Department of Nephrology and Medicine, Dartmouth-Hitchcock Medical Center, Lebanon, New Hampshire

Clinical Assessment of Renal Function

Robert W. Schrier, MD

Division of Renal Diseases and Hypertension, University of Colorado School of Medicine, Denver, Colorado

Acute Renal Failure

Vaishali Dixit Schuchert, MD

Assistant Professor of Surgery and Critical Care Medicine, University of Pittsburgh Medical Center, Pittsburgh, Pennsylvania

Abdominal Trauma

Carl Schulman, MD

Assistant Professor of Surgery, University of Miami School of Medicine, Miami, Florida

Anemia of Critical Illness

Donna Seger, MD, FAACT, FACEP, ABMT

Assistant Professor of Medicine and Emergency Medicine, Vanderbilt University Medical Center; Medical Director, Tennessee Poison Center, Nashville, Tennessee

Poisoning: Overview of Approaches for Evaluation and Treatment

Frank W. Sellke, MD

Johnson & Johnson Professor of Surgery, Harvard Medical School; Chief of Cardiothoracic Surgery, Beth Israel Deaconess Medical Center, Boston, Massachusetts,

Aortic Dissection

Soman Sen, MD

General Surgery Resident, Department of Surgery, Loyola University Medical Center, Maywood, Illinois

Burns and Inhalation Injury

Jigme Sethi, MD

Assistant Professor of Medicine, Division of Pulmonary, Allergy, and Critical Care, University of Pittsburgh School of Medicine, Pittsburgh, Pennsylvania

Carbon Monoxide and Heme Oxygenase-1

F. Kay Seymour, MD, MA, MB, BCUC, MRCS, DOHNS

Honorary Research Registrar, Academic Department of Accident and Emergency Medicine, Imperial College School of Medicine at St. Mary's, London, United Kingdom

Hydrocarbons

M. Michael Shabot, MD, FACS, FCCM, FACMI

Professor of Surgery, University of California, Los Angeles; Chief of Staff, Office of Medical Affairs; Director, Surgical Intensive Care Unit; and Medical Director, Enterprise Information Services, Cedars-Sinai Medical Center, Los Angeles, California

Percutaneous Dilational Tracheostomy

Erik S. Shank, MD

Assistant Professor, Department of Anesthesia, Harvard Medical School; Associate Chief, Pediatric Anesthesia, Department of Anesthesiology and Critical Care, Massachusetts General Hospital, Boston, Massachusetts

Other Embolic Syndromes

Robert L. Sheridan, MD

Associate Professor of Surgery, Harvard Medical School; Chief of Burn Surgery, Shriners Hospital for Children; Co-Director, Burn Unit, Massachusetts General Hospital, Boston, Massachusetts

Burns

Fernanda Silveira, MD

Infectious Diseases Fellow, Department of Medicine, University of Pittsburgh School of Medicine, Pittsburgh, Pennsylvania

Acute Viral Syndromes

Pierre Singer, MD

The Sakler School of Medicine, Tel Aviv University, Tel Aviv; General Intensive Care Department, Rabin Medical Center, Beilinson Campus, Petah Tikva, Israel

Indirect Calorimetry and Metabolic Monitoring

Jeffrey M. Singh, MD, FRCPC

Fellow, Adult Critical Care Medicine, University of Toronto, Toronto, Ontario, Canada

High-Frequency Ventilation

Leo J. Sioris, PharmD

Professor, Department of Experimental and Clinical Pharmacology, College of Pharmacy, University of Minnesota, Minneapolis; Senior Toxicologist, SafetyCall International, Minnetonka, Minnesota

Heavy Metals

Elizabeth Sizer, MD

Liver Intensive Therapy Unit, King's College Hospital, London, United Kingdom

Portal Hypertension

Debra J. Skaar, PharmD

Assistant Professor, Department of Experimental and Clinical Pharmacology, University of Minnesota College of Pharmacy, Minneapolis, Minnesota

Sedatives and Hypnotics

Anthony D. Slonim, MD, MPH

Assistant Professor of Pediatrics and Internal Medicine, The George Washington University School of Medicine; Medical Director, Performance Improvement, Patient Safety, and Clinical Resource Management, and Attending Physician, Children's National Medical Center, Washington, DC

Evaluating Pediatric Critical Care

Teresa L. Smith, MD

Clinical Assistant Professor, Western Michigan University College of Human Medicine; Neurointensivist, Bronson Memorial Hospital, Kalamazoo, Michigan

Determination of Death by Neurologic Criteria

Michael D. Sosin, MRCP

Research Fellow, University Department of Medicine, City Hospital, Birmingham, United Kingdom

Severe Heart Failure

Christian Spaulding, MD

Professor of Cardiology, Rene Descartes University, and Director, Cardiology Catheterization Laboratory, Cochin Hospital, Paris, France

Invasive Cardiac Procedures: Percutaneous Transluminal Coronary Angioplasty, Mitral and Aortic Valvuloplasty

Kathryn Lee Springer, MD

Division of Infectious Diseases, University of Colorado Health Sciences Center, Denver, Colorado

Tuberculosis

Charles L. Sprung, MD

Department of Anesthesia and Critical Care Medicine, Hadassah Hebrew University Hospital, Jerusalem, Israel

Beyond Technology: Caring for the Critically Ill

Vincenzo Squadrone, MD

Universita di Torino, Dipartimento di Discipline Medico-Chirurgiche, Sczione di Anestesiologia e Rianimazione, Ospedale S. Giovanni Battista, Torino, Italy

Patient-Ventilator Interaction

Terence Starz, MD

University of Pittsburgh Medical Center and Arthritis and Internal Medicine Associates, Pittsburgh, Pennsylvania

Principles of NSAID Therapy in Critical Care Medicine

Thomas E. Starzl, MD, PhD

University of Pittsburgh School of Pharmacy, Thomas E. Starzl Transplantation Institute, University of Pittsburgh School of Medicine, Pittsburgh, Pennsylvania

Clinical Use of Immunosuppressants; Intestinal and Multiple Organ Transplantation

Steven Steinberg, MD

Professor of Surgery, The Ohio State University, Columbus, Ohio

Infections of Skin, Muscle, and Soft Tissue

David M. Steinhorn, MD

Associate Professor of Pediatrics, Northwestern University Feinberg School of Medicine; Attending Physician, Division of Pulmonary and Critical Care, Children's Memorial Hospital, Chicago, Illinois

Nutrition Issues in Critically Ill Children

Eric J. Stern, MD

Department of Radiology, Harborview Medical Center, University of Washington, Seattle, Washington

Imaging of the Chest in the ICU

Thomas E. Stewart, MD, FRCPC

Associate Professor of Medicine and Anesthesia, University of Toronto; Director of Critical Care, University Health Network and Mount Sinai Hospital, Toronto, Ontario, Canada

High-Frequency Ventilation

Nino Stocchetti, MD

Physician, Terapia Intensiva Neuroscienze, Universita di Milano, Ospedale Maggiore Policlinico, Milano, Italy

Intensive Care after Neurosurgery

Joerg-Patrick Stübgen, MD, FRCPC

Associate Professor, Clinical Neurology, Department of Neurology and Neuroscience, Weill Medical College of Cornell University; Associate Attending Neurologist, Department of Neurology, New York-Presbyterian Hospital and Hospital for Special Surgery, New York, New York

Coma

Sanjay Subramanian, MD

Hospitalist and Intensivist, The Everett Clinic, Everett, Washington

Oliguria

Tomoko Suzuki, MD, PhD

Division of Respiratory Medicine, Department of Pediatrics, The Hospital for Sick Children; Department of Medicine, Division of Respirology, University of Toronto, Toronto General Hospital Research Institute of University Health Network, Toronto, Ontario, Canada

The Neutrophil: Balancing Antimicrobial Effectiveness and the Potential for Damage to the Host

David Szpilman, MD

Head, Adult Intensive Care Unit, Hospital Municipal Migvel Couto; Physician, Drowning Resuscitation Center-GMAR; Founder, Brazilian Life Saving Society, Medical Commission of International Life-Saving Federation, Brazilian Resuscitation Council, Rio de Janeiro, Brazil

Drowning

David P. Taggart, MD (Hon), PhD

Professor of Cardiovascular Surgery, Oxford University; Consultant Cardiothoracic Surgeon, John Radcliffe Hospital, Oxford, United Kingdom

Atheromatous Embolization

Daniel Talmor, MD, MPH

Associate Professor of Anesthesia, Harvard Medical School; Department of Anesthesia and Critical Care, Beth Israel Deaconess Medical Center, Boston, Massachusetts

Management of the Postoperative Cardiac Surgical Patient

Julin F. Tang, MD, MS

Associate Professor of Anesthesia, Department of Anesthesia and Perioperative Care, and Medical Director of Respiratory Care Services, University of California, San Francisco, at San Francisco General Hospital, San Francisco, California

Bedside Monitoring of Pulmonary Function

Jeremy Taylor, MD

Assistant Professor, University of Rochester, Strong Memorial Hospital, Rochester, New York

Disorders of Water Balance

Jean-Louis Teboul, MD

Professor of Therapeutic and Critical Care Medicine, Paris XI University; Medical Intensive Care Unit, Bicêtre University Hospital, Paris XI University, Paris, France

Inotropic Therapy in the Critically Ill

Isaac Teitelbaum, MD

Professor of Medicine, University of Colorado School of Medicine; Director, Acute and Home Dialysis Programs, University of Colorado Hospital, Denver, Colorado

Urinary Tract Obstruction

Stephen R. Thom, MD, PhD

Professor of Emergency Medicine and Chief, Hyperbaric Medicine, University of Pennsylvania, Philadelphia, Pennsylvania

Hyperbaric Oxygen in Critical Care

David B. Thomas, MD

Assistant Professor, Department of Pathology and Laboratory Medicine, University of North Carolina School of Medicine at Chapel Hill, and University of North Carolina Hospitals, Chapel Hill, North Carolina

Glomerulonephritis and Interstitial Nephritis in the ICU

Nisa Thoongsuwan, MD

Department of Radiology, University of Washington, Harborview Medical Center, Seattle, Washington

Imaging of the Chest in the ICU

C. Louise Thwaites, BSc, MBBS, MRCP(UK)

Wellcome Trust Training Fellow, Oxford University Clinical Research Unit, Hospital for Tropical Diseases, Ho Chi Minh City, Viet Nam; Clinical Research Fellow, Centre for Tropical Medicine, Centre for Clinical Vaccinology and Tropical Medicine, Churchill Hospital, Oxford, United Kingdom

Tetanus

Jean-François Timsit, MD

Assistant Professor, Service de Réanimation Médicale et des Maladies Infectieuses, Hôpital Bichat-Claude-Bernard, Faculté de Medecine de Grenoble, Paris, France

Infectious Endocarditis

Alan Tinmouth, MD, MSc, FRCPC

University of Ottawa Centre for Transfusion Research and the Clinical Epidemiology Program of the Ottawa Health Research Institute, Ottawa, Ontario, Canada

Anemia and Red Blood Cell Transfusions in Critically Ill Patients

Samuel A. Tisherman, MD

Associate Professor, Departments of Surgery and Critical Care Medicine, University of Pittsburgh; Attending Physician, University of Pittsburgh Medical Center-Presbyterian University Hospital, Pittsburgh, Pennsylvania

Calculous and Acalculous Cholecystitis; Trauma in the Gravid Patient

Antoni Torres, MD, PhD

Director, Institut Clinic de Pneumologia ICPCT, Hospital Clinic, Barcelona, Spain

Pulmonary Infections in the Acute Immunocompromised Patient

Robert D. Truog, MD

Professor of Anesthesia and Pediatrics, Harvard Medical School; Chief, Division of Critical Care Medicine, Children's Hospital, Boston, Massachusetts

Ethical Controversies in Pediatric Critical Care

Stephen Trzeciak, MD

Assistant Professor of Medicine and Emergency Medicine, Robert Wood Johnson Medical School; Section of Critical Care Medicine and the Department of Emergency Medicine, Cooper University Hospital, Camden, New Jersey

Hypophosphatemia and Hyperphosphatemia

Suzanne J. Tschida, PharmD, BCPS

Director, Clinical Services, Chronimed Statscript Pharmacy, Minnetonka, Minnesota

Toxic Inhalations

Edith Tzeng, MD

Assistant Professor, Department of Surgery, University of Pittsburgh School of Medicine, Pittsburgh, Pennsylvania

Thrombolytics

Benoit Vallet, MD

Professor of Anesthesiology and Intensive Care Medicine, Clinique d'Anesthésie et de Réanimation, Hôpital Claude Huriez, Centre Hospitalier Universitaire de Lille, Lille, France

Resuscitation from Circulatory Shock

Greet Van den Berghe, MD, PhD

Professor of Medicine and Chair, Department of Intensive Care Medicine, Catholic University of Leuven, Leuven, Belgium

Hypoglycemia; Hyperglycemia and Blood Glucose Control in the Intensive Care Unit

P. Vernon van Heerden, MD

Clinical Associate Professor, University of Western Australia; Senior Intensive Care Specialist, Sir Charles Gairdner Hospital, Perth, Western Australia

Hyperglycemic Comas

Olivier Varenne, MD, PhD

Associate Director, Cardiac Catheterization Laboratory, Cardiology Department, Cochin Hospital, Rene Descartes University, Paris, France

Invasive Cardiac Procedures: Percutaneous Transluminal Coronary Angioplasty, Mitral and Aortic Valvuloplasty

Ramesh Venkataraman, MD

Assistant Professor, Critical Care Medicine, University of Pittsburgh School of Medicine, Pittsburgh, Pennsylvania

Polyuria; Oliguria

Kathleen M. Ventre, MD

Fellow, Anesthesia/Critical Care Medicine, Children's Hospital Boston, Harvard Medical School, Boston, Massachusetts

Acute Parenchymal Disease in Infants and Children

Zvi Vered, MD, FACC, FESC

Director, Cardiology Department, Assaf-Harofeh Medical Center, Zerifin; Sackler Faculty of Medicine, Tel-Aviv University, Tel Aviv, Israel

Pulmonary Edema

Vasundhara Vidyarthi, MD

Cardiology Fellow, Department of Medicine, Finch University of Health Sciences, The Chicago Medical School, North Chicago, Illinois

Cardioversion and Defibrillation

Jean-Louis Vincent, MD, PhD

Professor of Intensive Care, Faculty of Medicine, Free University of Brussels; Head, Department of Intensive Care, Erasme University Hospital, Brussels, Belgium

Septic Shock

Giovanni Vitale, MD

Anesthesiologist, Anesthesia and Intensive Care Department, San Gerardo Hospital, Monza (Mi), Italy

Pericardiocentesis

Elizabeth A. Vitarbo, MD

Chief Resident, Department of Neurological Surgery, University of Miami, Miami, Florida

Spinal Cord Injury

Stefanie N. Vogel, PhD

Professor, Department of Microbiology and Immunology and Department of Medicine, University of Maryland School of Medicine, Baltimore, Maryland

Macrophage Function

Florian M.E. Wagenlehner, MD

Urologic Clinic, Hospital St. Elisabeth, Teaching Hospital of the Technical University Munich, Straubing, Germany

Infections of the Urogenital Tract

Keith R. Walley, BSc, MD, FRCPC
Professor of Medicine, University of British Columbia;
Associate Director, Intensive Care Unit,
St. Paul's Hospital, Vancouver, British Columbia, Canada
Adjunctive Respiratory Therapy

Peter A. Ward, MD
Chairman and Professor, Department of Pathology,
University of Michigan Medical School, University of
Michigan Hospitals, Ann Arbor, Michigan
Complement

Nicholas S. Ward, MD
Assistant Professor, Department of Medicine,
Brown University School of Medicine;
Department of Pulmonary and Critical Care Medicine,
Rhode Island Hospital, Providence, Rhode Island
End-of-Life Issues in the Intensive Care Unit

Lorraine B. Ware, MD
Assistant Professor of Medicine, Department of Allergy,
Pulmonary and Critical Care Medicine, Vanderbilt
University Medical Center, Nashville, Tennessee
Acute Lung Injury and Acute Respiratory Distress Syndrome

Gregory A. Watson, MD
University of Pittsburgh Medical Center-Presbyterian
University Hospital, Pittsburgh, Pennsylvania
Chest Tube Placement, Care, and Removal

Pierre Wauthy, MD
Resident, Department of Cardiac Surgery,
CHU Brugmann, Brussels, Belgium
Cardiac Surgery: Indications and Complications

Robert J. Weber, MS, FASHP
University of Pittsburgh School of Pharmacy,
Thomas E. Starzl Transplantation Institute,
University of Pittsburgh School of Medicine,
Pittsburgh, Pennsylvania
Clinical Use of Immunosuppressants

Lawrence R. Wechsler, MD
Director, Stroke Institute, and Professor of Neurology
and Vice Chair, Department of Neurology,
University of Pittsburgh Medical School,
Pittsburgh, Pennsylvania
Management of Acute Ischemic Stroke

David Weill, MD
Associate Professor of Medicine, Division of Pulmonary
and Critical Care Sciences, Lung Transplant Program,
University of Colorado Health Sciences Center, Denver,
Colorado
Oxidative Lung Injury; Lung Transplantation

Craig R. Weinert, MD, PhD
Assistant Professor of Medicine, Division of Pulmonary,
Allergy, and Critical Care Medicine, University of
Minnesota, Minneapolis, Minnesota
Sedatives and Hypnotics

Dov Weissberg, MD
Associate Clinical Professor Emeritus of Surgery,
Department of Surgery, Tel Aviv University Sackler
School of Medicine, Tel Aviv; Emeritus Chief,
Department of Surgery (Thoracic and General),
E. Wolfson Medical Center, Holon, Israel
Pleural Disease in the Intensive Care Unit

Julia Wendon, MD
Liver Intensive Therapy Unit, King's College Hospital,
London, United Kingdom
Portal Hypertension

Alexander C. White, MD
Associate Professor of Medicine, Tufts University School
of Medicine; Attending Physician, Pulmonary, Critical
Care and Sleep Division, Tufts-New England Medical
Center, Boston, Massachusetts
The Hematopoietic Stem Cell Transplantation Patient

Eric Wiel, MD
Anesthesiologist and Intensivist, Clinique d'Anesthésie
et de Réanimation, Hôpital Claude Huriez, Centre
Hospitalier Universitaire de Lille, Lille, France
Resuscitation from Circulatory Shock

Lawrence Scott Wilner, MD
Clinical Assistant Professor, Department of Medicine,
Section of Palliative Care and Medical Ethics,
University of Pittsburgh School of Medicine,
Pittsburgh, Pennsylvania
*Non-Heartbeating Organ Donation
(Donation after Cardiac Death)*

Michel Wolff, MD
Assistant Professor, Service de Réanimation Médicale et
des Maladies Infectieuses, Hôpital Bichat-
Claude-Bernard, Faculté Xavier-Bichat, Paris, France
Infectious Endocarditis

Richard G. Wunderink, MD
Professor of Medicine, Pulmonary and Critical Care
Division, Northwestern University Feinberg School of
Medicine, Chicago, Illinois
*Genetics of Critical Illness; Prevention and Control of
Nosocomial Infection*

Lam M. Yen, MD, MSc
Director, Tetanus Unit, Hospital for Tropical Diseases,
Ho Chi Minh City, Viet Nam
Tetanus

Mesut Yilmaz, MD
Cerrahpasa Medical Faculty, Infectious Diseases and
Clinical Microbiology, University of Istanbul,
Istanbul, Turkey
Acute Viral Syndromes

Sergio Zanotti-Cavazzoni, MD
Assistant Professor of Medicine,
Cooper University Hospital, Robert Wood Johnson
Medical School, University of Medicine and
Dentistry of New Jersey,
Cooper Health System, Camden, New Jersey
Hyperkalemia and Hypokalemia

Allyson R. Zazulia, MD
Assistant Professor, Departments of Neurology and
Radiology, Washington University; Attending Physician,
Barnes-Jewish Hospital,
St. Louis, Missouri
Nontraumatic Intracerebral and Subarachnoid Hemorrhage

Xiaopeng Zhang, MD
Visiting Research Associate,
Safar Center for Resuscitation Research, University of
Pittsburgh Medical Center, Pittsburgh, Pennsylvania
*Biochemical, Cellular, and Molecular Mechanisms of
Neuronal Death and Secondary Brain Injury in
Critical Care*

Guy A. Zimmerman, MD
Professor, Department of Internal Medicine, and
Director, The Program in Human Molecular Biology
and Genetics, University of Utah Medical Center,
Salt Lake City, Utah
Endothelial Function

PREFACE

The fifth edition of the *Textbook of Critical Care* continues the tradition of excellence established by the earlier editions but embodies a number of new features that should make it easier to use by both trainees and experienced clinicians and more likely to remain up-to-date. Several features of the fifth edition warrant special comment.

- Because critical care medicine is now a mature specialty that is practiced all over the world, the experts selected to write chapters for the fifth edition are an international group.
- The opening section of the book consists of short chapters that provide a brief overview of clinical problems, such as acute respiratory failure or diarrhea, that are commonly encountered in the management of patients with critical illness.
- Although the book contains extensive citations to the medical literature, both the bulk and the cost of the resulting volume have been decreased by providing most of the references on a CD-ROM rather than in the text per se. The most important citations are provided in the text with some annotation to help readers understand why the selected references are particularly noteworthy.
- Most chapters include a list of key points. A quick glance at this list will help readers remember the "take home" messages for the chapter.
- New pediatric content of the textbook is also international in scope and addresses key topics within each area of pediatric critical care that are germane to the broader readership of the book.
- Because the basic science that underlies the practice of critical care medicine is advancing rapidly, the editors have included an entire section devoted to key topics in areas of fundamental biology that are relevant to the field.

A new feature of the fifth edition is a dedicated website, www.criticalcaretext.com, which has been launched at the same time the book published. This website will be updated every week throughout the life of this edition. The website features the full text and illustrations of the fifth edition of the *Textbook of Critical Care* and is fully searchable. You can even download the illustrations to PowerPoint to enhance your presentations or lectures. Another added-value feature on the website is the inclusion of critical care calculators. References are linked to Medline or directly to full-text articles where available, which will expand your search capabilities. However, the absolute key feature of the website is the regular weekly updates from experts in the field, so that the text is consistent with the best information available in the scientific literature. The latest issues of the major medical journals might contain an article that will fundamentally change the standard of care for the management of a disease or syndrome encountered in the care of critically ill patients. If this happens, the relevant chapter(s) will be updated immediately, so that this work can stay current year after year. The book and the website can be purchased either separately or together as an **e dition** package, giving you unprecedented reference power.

The fifth edition of this textbook would not have been possible without the enormous contributions made by the prior editors. We express our gratitude to Will Shoemaker, Steve Ayers, Ake Grenvik, and Peter Holbrook for the opportunity and great honor to follow in their footsteps.

We want to thank the many people who were instrumental in helping us assemble the text you are now holding in your hands. Specifically, we wish to thank Ms. Janice Knapp, editorial assistant to Dr. Fink; Marci Provins, editorial assistant to Dr. Kochanek; Dr. Karen Pickett and Ms. Marie-Rose Andre, who assisted Dr. Vincent; and Kelly Kast and Katie Overdier, who assisted Dr. Abraham.

Mitchell P. Fink, MD
Edward Abraham, MD
Jean-Louis Vincent, MD
Patrick M. Kochanek, MD

CONTENTS

Pediatric chapters within each section edited by
Patrick M. Kochanek

SECTION III
CENTRAL NERVOUS SYSTEM
Section Editor: Patrick M. Kochanek

SECTION IV
RESPIRATORY DISORDERS
Section Editor: Edward Abraham

SECTION V
CARDIOVASCULAR DISORDERS
Section Editor: Jean-Louis Vincent

SECTION VI
HEPATIC DISORDERS, GASTROINTESTINAL DISORDERS, AND NUTRITIONAL SUPPORT
Section Editor: Mitchell P. Fink

SECTION XV
ETHICAL AND END-OF-LIFE ISSUES
Section Editor: Edward Abraham

SECTION XVI
ORGANIZATION, MANAGEMENT, AND EDUCATION
Section Editor: Patrick M. Kochanek

Section I

COMMON PROBLEMS

Chapter 1

SUDDEN DETERIORATION IN NEUROLOGIC STATUS

Joseph M. Darby • Anupam Anupam

Patients admitted to the intensive care unit (ICU) with critical illness or injury are at risk for neurologic complications.[1-5] A sudden or unexpected change in the neurologic condition of a critically ill patient often heralds a complication that may cause direct injury to the central nervous system (CNS). Alternatively, such changes may simply be neurologic manifestations of the underlying critical illness or treatment that necessitated ICU admission (e.g., sepsis). These complications can occur in patients admitted to the ICU without neurologic disease and in those admitted for the management of primary CNS problems (e.g., stroke). Neurologic complications also can occur as a result of invasive procedures and therapeutic interventions performed. Commonly, the recognition of neurologic complications is delayed or missed entirely because ICU treatments (e.g., intubation, drugs) interfere with the physical examination or confound the clinical picture. In other cases, neurologic complications are not recognized because of a lack of sensitive methods to detect the problem (e.g., delirium). Morbidity and mortality are increased among patients who develop neurologic complications; therefore, the intensivist must be vigilant in the evaluation of all critically ill patients for changes in neurologic status.

Despite the importance of neurologic complications of critical illness, few studies have specifically assessed their incidence and impact on outcome among ICU patients. Available data are limited to medical ICU patients; data regarding neurologic complications in general surgical and other specialty ICU populations must be extracted from other sources. In studies of medical ICU patients, the incidence of neurologic complications is 12.3% to 33%.[1,2] Patients who develop neurologic complications have increased morbidity, mortality, and ICU length of stay. Sepsis is the most common problem associated with the development of neurologic complications (sepsis-associated encephalopathy). In addition to encephalopathy, other common neurologic complications associated with critical illness include seizures and stroke. As the complexity of ICU care has increased, so has the risk of neurologic complications. Neuromuscular disorders are now recognized as a major source of morbidity in severely ill patients.[6] Recognized neurologic complications occurring in selected medical, surgical, and neurologic ICU populations are shown in Table 1–1.[7-41]

IMPAIRMENT IN CONSCIOUSNESS

Global changes in CNS function, best described in terms of impairment in consciousness, are generally referred to as encephalopathy or altered mental status. An acute change in

TABLE 1–1. NEUROLOGIC COMPLICATIONS IN SELECTED SPECIALTY POPULATIONS

Medical

Bone marrow transplantation[7,8]	CNS infection, stroke, subdural hematoma, brainstem ischemia, hyperammonemia, Wernicke's encephalopathy
Cancer[9]	Stroke, intracranial hemorrhage, CNS infection
Fulminant hepatic failure[10]	Encephalopathy, coma, brain edema, increased ICP
HIV/AIDS[11,12]	Opportunistic CNS infection, stroke, vasculitis, delirium, seizures, progressive multifocal leukoencephalopathy
Pregnancy[13,14]	Seizures, ischemic stroke, cerebral vasospasm, intracranial hemorrhage, cerebral venous thrombosis, hypertensive encephalopathy, pituitary apoplexy

Surgical

Cardiac surgery[15-19]	Stroke, delirium, brachial plexus injury, phrenic nerve injury
Vascular surgery[20,21]	
Carotid	Stroke, cranial nerve injuries (recurrent laryngeal, glossopharyngeal, hypoglossal, facial), seizures
Aortic	Stroke, paraplegia
Peripheral	Delirium
Transplantation[10,22-25]	
Heart	Stroke
Liver	Encephalopathy, seizures, opportunistic CNS infection, intracranial hemorrhage, Guillain-Barré syndrome, central pontine myelinolysis
Renal	Stroke, opportunistic CNS infection, femoral neuropathy
Urologic surgery (TURP)[26]	Seizures and coma (hyponatremia)
Otolaryngologic surgery[27,28]	Recurrent laryngeal nerve injury, stroke, delirium
Orthopedic surgery[29]	
Spine	Myelopathy, radiculopathy, epidural abscess, meningitis
Knee and hip replacement	Delirium (fat embolism)
Long bone fracture/nailing	Delirium (fat embolism)

Neurologic

Stroke[30-34]	Stroke progression or extension, reocclusion after thrombolysis, bleeding, seizures, delirium, brain edema, herniation
Intracranial surgery[35]	Bleeding, edema, seizures, CNS infection
Subarachnoid hemorrhage[32,36-38]	Rebleeding, vasospasm, hydrocephalus, seizures
Traumatic brain injury[32,39,40]	Intracranial hypertension, bleeding, seizures, stroke (cerebrovascular injury), CNS infection

Continued

TABLE 1–1. NEUROLOGIC COMPLICATIONS IN SELECTED SPECIALTY POPULATIONS—CONT'D

| Cervical spinal cord injury[41] | Ascension of injury, stroke (vertebral artery injury) |

CNS, central nervous system; HIV/AIDS, human immunodeficiency virus/acquired immunodeficiency syndrome; ICP, intracranial pressure; TURP, transurethral prostatic resection.

the level of consciousness undoubtedly is the most common neurologic complication that occurs after ICU admission. Consciousness is defined as a state of awareness (arousal or wakefulness) and the ability to respond appropriately to changes in environment.[42] For consciousness to be impaired, global hemispheric dysfunction or dysfunction of the brainstem reticular activating system must be present.[43] Altered consciousness may result in a sleeplike state (coma) or a state characterized by confusion and agitation (delirium) (Table 1–2).

When an acute change in consciousness is noted, the patient should be evaluated, keeping in mind the patient's age, the presence or absence of coexisting organ system dysfunction, the patient's metabolic status and medication list, and the presence or absence of infection (Table 1–3). In patients with a primary CNS disorder, deterioration in the level of consciousness (e.g., from stupor to coma) frequently represents the development of brain edema, increasing intracranial pressure, new or worsening intracranial hemorrhage, hydrocephalus, CNS infection, or cerebral vasospasm. In patients without a primary CNS diagnosis, an acute change in consciousness is often due to the development of infectious complications (i.e., sepsis-associated encephalopathy), drug toxicities, or the development or exacerbation of organ system failure. Nonconvulsive status epilepticus is increasingly being recognized as a cause of impaired consciousness in critically ill patients.[44-53]

States of altered consciousness manifesting as impairment in wakefulness or arousal (i.e., coma and stupor) and their causes are well defined.[42,43,54,55] Much confusion remains, however, regarding the diagnosis and management of delirium, perhaps the most common state of impaired CNS functioning in critically ill patients at large. When dedicated instruments are used, delirium can be diagnosed in more than 80% of critically ill patients, making this condition the most common neurologic complication of critical illness.[56-58] Much of the difficulty in establishing the diagnosis of delirium stems from the belief that delirium is a state characterized mainly by confusion and agitation and that such states are expected consequences of the unique environmental factors and sleep deprivation that characterize the ICU experience. Terms previously used to describe delirium in critically ill patients include ICU

TABLE 1–2. STATES OF ACUTELY ALTERED CONSCIOUSNESS

State	Description
Coma	Closed eyes, sleeplike state with no response to external stimuli (pain)
Stupor	Responsive only to vigorous or painful stimuli
Lethargy	Drowsy, arouses easily and appropriately to stimuli
Delirium	Acute state of confusion with or without behavioral disturbance
Catatonia	Eyes open, unblinking, unresponsive

TABLE 1–3. GENERAL CAUSES OF ACUTELY IMPAIRED CONSCIOUSNESS IN THE CRITICALLY ILL

Infection

Sepsis encephalopathy
CNS infection

Drugs

Narcotics
Benzodiazepines
Anticholinergics
Anticonvulsants
Tricyclic antidepressants
Selective serotonin uptake inhibitors
Phenothiazines
Steroids
Immunosuppressants (cyclosporine, FK506, OKT3)
Anesthetics

Electrolyte and Acid-Base Disturbances

Hyponatremia
Hypernatremia
Hypercalcemia
Hypermagnesemia
Severe acidemia and alkalemia

Organ System Failure

Shock
Renal failure
Hepatic failure
Pancreatitis
Respiratory failure (hypoxia, hypercapnea)

Endocrine Disorders

Hypoglycemia
Hyperglycemia
Hypothyroidism
Hyperthyroidism
Pituitary apoplexy

Drug Withdrawal

Alcohol
Opiates
Barbiturates
Benzodiazepines

Vascular Causes

Shock
Hypotension
Hypertensive encephalopathy
CNS vasculitis
Cerebral venous sinus thrombosis

CNS Disorders

Hemorrhage
Stroke
Brain edema
Hydrocephalus
Increased intracranial pressure
Meningitis
Ventriculitis
Brain abscess
Subdural empyema
Seizures
Vasculitis

Seizures

Convulsive and nonconvulsive status epilepticus

Continued

TABLE 1–3. GENERAL CAUSES OF ACUTELY IMPAIRED CONSCIOUSNESS IN THE CRITICALLY ILL—CONT'D

Miscellaneous

Fat embolism syndrome
Neuroleptic malignant syndrome
Thiamine deficiency (Wernicke's encephalopathy)
Psychogenic unresponsiveness

CNS, central nervous system.

psychosis, acute confusional state, encephalopathy, and post-operative psychosis. It is now recognized that ICU psychosis is a misnomer; delirium is a more accurate term.[59]

The currently accepted criteria for the diagnosis of delirium include an abrupt onset of impaired consciousness, disturbed cognitive function, fluctuating course, and the presence of a medical condition that could impair brain function.[60] Subtypes of delirium include hyperactive (agitated) delirium and the more common hypoactive or quiet delirium.[58] Impaired consciousness may be apparent as a reduction in awareness, psychomotor retardation, agitation, or impairment in attention (increased distractability or vigilance). Cognitive impairment can include disorientation, impaired memory, and perceptual aberrations (hallucinations or illusions).[61] Autonomic hyperactivity and sleep disturbances may be features of delirium in some patients (e.g., those with drug withdrawal syndromes, delirium tremens). Delirium in critically ill patients is associated with increased morbidity, mortality, and ICU length of stay.[62-64] In general, sepsis and drugs should be the primary etiologic considerations in critically ill patients who develop delirium.

As has been noted, nonconvulsive status epilepticus is increasingly recognized as an important cause of impaired consciousness in critically ill patients. Although the general term can encompasses other entities, such as absence and partial complex seizures, in critically ill patients, nonconvulsive status epilepticus is often referred to as "status epilepticus of epileptic encephalopathy."[53] It is characterized by an alteration in consciousness or behavior associated with electroencephalographic evidence of continuous or periodic epileptiform activity without overt motor manifestations of seizures. In one study of comatose patients without overt seizure activity, nonconvulsive status epilepticus was evident in 8%.[51] Nonconvulsive status epilepticus can precede or follow an episode of generalized convulsive status epilepticus; it can also occur in patients with traumatic brain injury, subarachnoid hemorrhage, global brain ischemia or anoxia, sepsis, and multiple organ failure. Despite the general consensus that nonconvulsive status epilepticus is a unique entity responsible for impaired consciousness in some critically ill patients, there is no general consensus on the electroencephalographic criteria for its diagnosis or the optimal approach to treatment.[65]

STROKE AND OTHER FOCAL NEUROLOGIC DEFICITS

The new onset of a major neurologic deficit that manifests as a focal impairment in motor or sensory function (e.g., hemiparesis) or results in seizures usually indicates a primary problem referable to the cerebrovascular circulation. In a study evaluating the value of computed tomography (CT) in medical ICU patients, ischemic stroke and intracranial bleeding were the most common abnormalities associated with the new onset of a neurologic deficit or seizures.[66] Overall, the frequency of new-onset stroke is between 1% and 4% in medical ICU patients.[1,2] Among general surgical patients, the frequency of perioperative stroke ranges from 0.3% to 3.5%.[67] Patients undergoing cardiac or vascular surgery and surgical patients with underlying cerebrovascular disease can be expected to have an increased risk of perioperative stroke.[19]

The frequency of new or worsening focal neurologic deficits in patients admitted with a primary neurologic or neurosurgical disorder varies. For example, as many as 30% of patients with aneurysmal subarachnoid hemorrhage develop delayed ischemic neurologic deficits.[36] Patients admitted with stroke often develop worsening or new symptoms as a result of stroke progression, bleeding, or reocclusion of vessels previously opened with interventional therapy. In patients who have undergone elective intracranial surgery, postsurgical bleeding or infectious complications are the main causes of new focal deficits. In trauma patients, unrecognized injuries to the cerebrovascular circulation can cause new deficits. Patients who have sustained spinal cord injuries, and those who have undergone surgery of the spine or of the thoracic or abdominal aorta, can develop worsening or new symptoms of spinal cord injury. Early deterioration of CNS function after spinal cord injury usually occurs as a consequence of medical interventions to stabilize the spine, whereas late deterioration is usually due to hypotension and impaired cord perfusion. Occasionally, focal weakness or sensory symptoms in the extremities occur as a result of occult brachial plexus injury or compression neuropathy. New cranial nerve deficits in patients without primary neurologic problems can occur after neck surgery or carotid endarterectomy.

SEIZURES

The new onset of motor seizures occurs in 0.8% to 4% of critically ill medical ICU patients.[1,2,68] The new onset of seizures in general medical-surgical ICU patients is typically caused by narcotic withdrawal, hyponatremia, drug toxicities, or previously unrecognized structural abnormalities.[3,68] New stroke, intracranial bleeding, and CNS infection are other potential causes of seizures after ICU admission. The frequency of seizures is higher in patients admitted to the ICU with a primary neurologic problem, such as traumatic brain injury, aneurysmal subarachnoid hemorrhage, stroke, or CNS infection.[69] Because nonconvulsive status epilepticus may be more common than was previously appreciated, this problem should also be considered in the differential diagnosis of patients developing new, unexplained, or prolonged alterations in consciousness.

GENERALIZED WEAKNESS AND NEUROMUSCULAR DISORDERS

Generalized muscle weakness often becomes apparent in ICU patients as previous impairments in arousal are resolving or sedative and neuromuscular blocking agents are being discontinued or tapered. Polyneuropathy and myopathy associated

Eric B. Milbrandt • E. Wes Ely

Agitation and delirium are commonly encountered in the intensive care unit (ICU). They are more than an inconvenience; these conditions can have deleterious effects on patient and staff safety and contribute to poor outcomes. It is important for clinicians to have an organized approach for the evaluation and management of agitation and delirium.

AGITATION

Agitation is a state of extreme arousal, irritability, and motor restlessness that results from an internal sense of discomfort or tension. It is the behavioral response to physical or emotional distress, including pain, dyspnea, and anxiety, although the most common cause of agitation in the ICU is probably delirium.[1] Agitation is characterized by repetitive, nonproductive movements that may appear purposeless, although careful observation of the patient sometimes reveals an underlying intent. Agitation may be mild, characterized by increased movements and an apparent inability to get comfortable. Severe agitation can be life-threatening, leading to removal of life-saving devices as well as hypoxia, barotrauma, and hypotension due to patient-ventilator asynchrony. Indeed, recent studies have shown that agitation contributes to ventilator asynchrony, increased oxygen consumption, and inadvertent removal of devices and catheters.[2-5]

DELIRIUM

Delirium is an acute, fluctuating change in mental status, with inattention and altered level of consciousness. Delirium is an objective sign of cerebral insufficiency or acute cognitive dysfunction. It should be thought of as a form of organ dysfunction, much like shock and hypoxemia are considered evidence of dysfunction of the cardiovascular and pulmonary systems, respectively. Delirium has myriad causes, including pain and anxiety, medications, toxins, and metabolic derangements. Also known as acute encephalopathy[6] or ICU psychosis,[7] delirium occurs in as many as 80% of mechanically ventilated ICU patients and has recently been shown to be associated with increased length of stay, medical complications, and poor outcomes, including an increased 6-month mortality.[8-12] Furthermore, delirium can adversely affect the quality of life in survivors of critical illnesses, because a significant percentage of individuals who develop delirium in the hospital continue to demonstrate symptoms of delirium after discharge.[13-16] These patients manifest decreased cerebral activity and increased cognitive deterioration, and they are more likely to develop dementia than are patients without delirium. Finally, patients who develop delirium have a greater rate of decline on cognitive tests than do nondelirious patients.[13-16]

Delirium can be hypoactive or hyperactive. Patients with hypoactive delirium are calm but inattentive, and they manifest decreased mobility. Patients with hyperactive delirium are agitated and combative. Inattention is the hallmark feature of both types of delirium. Patients with hyperactive delirium are at risk for self-extubation, loss of catheters, and patient-ventilator asynchrony. Because of these risks, patients are often given high doses of sedatives that commit them to continued mechanical ventilation. Despite the dangers of hyperactive delirium, hypoactive delirium may actually be associated with a worse prognosis.[17-20]

Because the majority of patients manifest hypoactive delirium instead of the more obvious hyperactive type,[18,21-25] delirium frequently goes unrecognized in the ICU. Furthermore, up to 40% of alert or easily arousable patients who are usually assumed to be "cognitively intact" by ICU personnel may actually be delirious.[10] Even when ICU delirium is recognized, most clinicians consider it an expected event that is often iatrogenic and without consequence.[26]

CAUSES AND RISK FACTORS

The list of causes and risk factors for agitation and delirium is long, and the causes of the two conditions overlap to a large extent (Table 2–1). Fortunately, there are several mnemonics that can aid clinicians in recalling the list; two common ones are IWATCHDEATH and DELIRIUM (Table 2–2). In practical terms, the risk factors can be divided into three categories: the acute illness itself, patient factors, and iatrogenic or environmental factors. Importantly, a number of medications that are commonly used in the ICU are associated with the development of agitation and delirium (Table 2–3). A thorough approach to the treatment and support of the acute illness (e.g., controlling sources of sepsis and giving appropriate antibiotics), as well as minimizing the iatrogenic component (e.g., avoiding excessive sedation), can help reduce the incidence and magnitude of delirium and its attendant complications.

ASSESSMENT

There are many scales available for the assessment of agitation and sedation, including the Ramsay Scale,[27] the Riker Sedation-Agitation Scale (SAS),[28] the Motor Activity Assessment Scale (MAAS),[29] and the Richmond Agitation-Sedation Scale (RASS).[30] Each has good reliability and validity

TABLE 2–1. CAUSES OF AND RISK FACTORS FOR AGITATION AND DELIRIUM

Age >70 years	BUN/creatinine ratio ≥18
Transfer from a nursing home	Renal failure, creatinine >2.0 mg/dL
History of depression	Liver disease
History of dementia, stroke, or epilepsy	Congestive heart failure
Alcohol abuse within past month	Cardiogenic or septic shock
Tobacco use	Myocardial infarction
Drug overdose or illicit drugs	Infection
HIV infection	Central nervous system pathology
Medications	Urinary retention or fecal impaction
Hypo- or hypernatremia	Tube feeding
Hypo- or hyperglycemia	Rectal or bladder catheters
Hypo- or hyperthyroidism	Physical restraints
Hypothermia or fever	Central line catheters
Hypertension	Malnutrition or vitamin deficiencies
Hypoxia	Procedural complications
Acidosis or alkalosis	Visual or hearing impairment
Pain	Sleep disruption
Fear and anxiety	

BUN, blood urea nitrogen; HIV, human immunodeficiency virus.

among adult ICU patients and can be used to set targets for goal-directed sedative administration. The SAS, which scores agitation and sedation using a 7-point system, has excellent interrater reliability (kappa = 0.92), and it is highly correlated (r^2 = 0.83 to 0.86) with other scales. The RASS (Table 2–4), however, is the only method that has been shown to detect variations in the level of consciousness over time or in response to changes in sedative and analgesic drug use.[31,32] The 10-point Richmond scale has discrete criteria to distinguish levels of agitation and sedation. Patient evaluation consists of a three-step process. First, a patient is observed to determine whether he or she is alert, restless, or agitated (0 to +4). If the patient is not spontaneously alert, the patient's name is called and the duration of eye contact is measured (−1 to −3). If there is no eye contact with verbal stimulation,

TABLE 2–2. MNEMONICS FOR REMEMBERING CAUSES OF DELIRIUM AND AGITATION: IWATCHDEATH AND DELIRIUM

IWATCHDEATH	DELIRIUM
Infection	Drugs
Withdrawal	Electrolyte and physiologic abnormalities
Acute metabolic	Lack of drugs (withdrawal)
Trauma/pain	Infection
Central nervous system pathology	Reduced sensory input (blindness, deafness)
Hypoxia	Intracranial problems (CVA, meningitis, seizure)
Deficiencies (vitamin B$_{12}$, thiamine)	Urinary retention and fecal impaction
Endocrinopathies (thyroid, adrenal)	Myocardial problems (MI, arrhythmia, CHF)
Acute vascular (hypertension, shock)	
Toxins/drugs	
Heavy metals	

CHF, congestive heart failure; CVA, cerebrovascular accident; MI, myocardial infarction.

TABLE 2–3. COMMONLY USED DRUGS ASSOCIATED WITH DELIRIUM AND AGITATION

Benzodiazepines	Antibiotics
Opiates (especially meperidine)	Corticosteroids
Anticholinergics	Metoclopramide
Antihistamines	Muscle relaxants
H$_2$ blockers	Lidocaine

the shoulder is shaken or the sternum is rubbed, and the response is noted (−4 or −5). This assessment takes less than 20 seconds and correlates well with other measures of sedation (e.g., Glasgow Coma Scale, bispectral electroencephalography, neuropsychiatric ratings).

Until recently, there was no valid and reliable way to assess delirium in critically ill patients, many of whom are nonverbal owing to sedation or mechanical ventilation. The Confusion Assessment Method for the ICU (CAM-ICU) (Table 2–5) is a delirium measurement tool that was developed by a team of specialists in critical care, psychiatry, neurology, and geriatrics.[8-12] Administered by a nurse, the evaluation takes only 1 to 2 minutes to conduct and is 98% accurate for detecting

TABLE 2–4. RICHMOND AGITATION-SEDATION SCALE

+4	Combative	Combative, violent, immediate danger to staff
+3	Very agitated	Pulls or removes tube(s) or catheter(s); aggressive
+2	Agitated	Frequent nonpurposeful movement; fights ventilator
+1	Restless	Anxious, apprehensive, but movements not aggressive or vigorous
0	Alert and calm	
−1	Drowsy	Not fully alert but has sustained (>10 sec) awakening (eye opening/contact) to voice
−2	Light sedation	Drowsy; briefly (<10 sec) awakens to voice or physical stimulation
−3	Moderate sedation	Movement or eye opening (but no eye contact) to voice
−4	Deep sedation	No response to voice, but movement or eye opening to physical stimulation
−5	Unarousable	No response to voice or physical stimulation

Procedure for Assessment

1. Observe patient
   Is patient alert, restless, or agitated? **(Score 0 to +4)**
2. If not alert, state patient's name and tell him or her to open eyes and look at speaker.
   Patient awakens, with sustained eye opening and eye contact. **(Score −1)**
   Patient awakens, with eye opening and eye contact, but not sustained. **(Score −2)**
   Patient does not awaken (no eye contact) but has eye opening or movement in response to voice. **(Score −3)**
3. Physically stimulate patient by shaking shoulder and/or rubbing sternum.
   No response to voice, but response (movement) to physical stimulation. **(Score −4)**
   No response to voice or physical stimulation **(Score −5)**

From Sessler CN, Gosnell MS, Grap MJ, et al: The Richmond Agitation-Sedation Scale: Validity and reliability in adult intensive care unit patients. Am J Respir Crit Care Med 2002;166:1338-1344; Ely EW, Truman B, Shintani A, et al: Monitoring sedation status over time in ICU patients: Reliability and validity of the Richmond agitation-sedation scale (RASS). JAMA 2003;289:2983-2991.

TABLE 2–5. CONFUSION ASSESSMENT METHOD FOR THE INTENSIVE CARE UNIT

	Absent	Present
1. Acute Onset or Fluctuating Course		

A. Is there evidence of an acute change in mental status from baseline?

OR

B. Did the (abnormal) behavior fluctuate during the past 24 hours, that is, tend to come and go or increase and decrease in severity, as evidenced by fluctuation on a sedation scale (e.g., Richmond Agitation-Sedation Scale), Glasgow Coma Scale, or previous delirium assessment?

	Absent	Present
2. Inattention		

Did the patient have difficulty focusing attention, as evidenced by a score of less than 8 on either the auditory or visual component of the Attention Screening Examination?

	Absent	Present
3. Disorganized Thinking		

Is there evidence of disorganized or incoherent thinking, as evidenced by incorrect answers to 2 or more of the 4 questions or the inability to follow commands?

Questions (use either set A or set B):

Set A
1. Will a stone float on water?
2. Are there fish in the sea?
3. Does 1 pound weigh more than 2 pounds?
4. Can you use a hammer to pound a nail?

Set B
1. Will a leaf float on water?
2. Are there elephants in the sea?
3. Do 2 pounds weigh more than 1 pound?
4. Can you use a hammer to cut wood?

Other:
1. Are you having any unclear thinking?
2. Hold up this many fingers. (Examiner holds two fingers in front of patient.)
3. Now do the same thing with the other hand. (Do not repeat the number of fingers.)

	Absent	Present
4. Altered Level of Consciousness		

Is the patient's level of consciousness anything other than alert, such as vigilant, lethargic, or stuporous (i.e., Richmond agitation-sedation score other than 0 at time of assessment)?

Alert: spontaneously fully aware of environment and interacts appropriately
Vigilant: hyperalert
Lethargic: drowsy but easily aroused; unaware of some elements in the environment or not spontaneously interacting appropriately with the interviewer; becomes fully aware and appropriately interactive when prodded minimally
Stuporous: becomes incompletely aware when prodded strongly; can be aroused only by vigorous and repeated stimuli, and as soon as the stimulus ceases, lapses back into the unresponsive state

	Yes	No
Overall Assessment: Presence of Features 1 and 2 and Either Feature 3 or Feature 4?		

delirium as compared with a full *Diagnostic and Statistical Manual of Mental Disorders* IV assessment by a geriatric psychiatrist.[8,10] Delirium is diagnosed when a patient demonstrates an acute change or fluctuating changes in mental status, inattention, and either disorganized thinking or altered level of consciousness. National guidelines recommend the routine use of this method for delirium assessment in all critically ill patients.[32]

MANAGEMENT

Agitation is expected in a newly intubated patient. However, when agitation or delirium develops in a previously comfortable patient, a search for the underlying cause should be undertaken before attempting pharmacologic intervention. A rapid assessment should be performed, including vital signs and physical examination, to rule out life-threatening problems (e.g., hypoxia, self-extubation, pneumothorax, hypotension) or other acutely reversible physiologic causes (e.g., hypoglycemia, metabolic acidosis, stroke, seizure, pain). The previously mentioned IWATCHDEATH and DELIRIUM mnemonics can be particularly helpful in guiding this initial evaluation.

After correcting any identifiable contributing factors, pharmacologic treatment is often required. If pain is present, an analgesic should be the initial drug of choice. Although benzodiazepines are the most commonly used drugs for the treatment of agitation, they are not recommended for the management of delirium because they can paradoxically exacerbate confusion. Patients who manifest delirium should be treated with a traditional antipsychotic medication (e.g., haloperidol). When given intravenously, these medications exert a calming effect, flattening the affect and diminishing psychomotor agitation without suppressing respiratory drive or affecting hemodynamics. Haloperidol and related drugs achieve this effect by blocking dopamine receptors in the central nervous system. With acute delirium, haloperidol should be given in doses of 2 to 10 mg i.v. every 20 to 30 minutes until delirium is controlled. Subsequently, 25% of the total loading dose should be administered every 6 hours.[32] The dose should then be tapered over several days. Despite their favorable safety profile, antipsychotic medications can cause extrapyramidal reactions, neuroleptic malignant syndrome, and QT interval prolongation leading to torsades de pointes. These adverse effects are thought to be dose related, leading some experts to question the safety of the rapid-loading approach. According to this view, patients should receive no more than 20 mg/day of haloperidol.[33] Anecdotally, the use of atypical antipsychotics, such as risperidone, olanzapine, or ziprasidone,[34] is in vogue. However, their effectiveness in treating ICU delirium has not been evaluated systematically and, like haloperidol, these agents have the potential for QT interval prolongation.

For nondelirious agitated patients, benzodiazepines and propofol are the drugs of choice in the ICU. These agents are most effectively administered using standardized nurse-driven protocols with a clearly stated target level for sedation. Benzodiazepines bind to gamma-aminobutyric acid receptors in the central nervous system, leading to sedation, anxiolysis, hypnosis, muscle relaxation, anticonvulsant activity, and amnesia.[35] Benzodiazepines do not relieve pain, but their anxiolytic and amnestic properties may improve pain tolerance by moderating the anticipatory pain response.[36] Benzodiazepines can cause hypotension when given as a bolus dose, particularly in hypovolemic patients who may not tolerate the reduction in sympathetic vascular tone associated with benzodiazepine-induced anxiolysis. Further, by reducing inhibitions, these agents can sometimes cause paradoxical increases in agitation and aggressiveness. Of the benzodiazepines that are currently available, diazepam, midazolam, and lorazepam are the preferred agents in the ICU. The onset of action of diazepam is 2 to 5 minutes, making it useful for rapidly sedating acutely agitated patients. However, its long half-life makes prolonged sedation a risk with repeated use, particularly in patients with renal or hepatic dysfunction. To control acute agitation, it is given in doses of 2 to 6 mg every 5 to 15 minutes until the event is controlled. Continuous infusions are not recommended. Midazolam is also useful for acute agitation because it has a rapid onset (2 to 5 minutes) and short duration of action. It is given as bolus injections of 2 to 5 mg every 5 to 15 minutes. When used for long-term sedation (>48 to 72 hours), it tends to produce unpredictable awakening times, especially in patients who are obese or who have low serum albumin concentrations or renal failure.[32] Lorazepam has a slower onset of action (5 to 20 minutes), making it less helpful for acute agitation; however, it is less lipid-soluble and has no active metabolite, making it the preferred agent for long-term administration in most critically ill patients. Intermittent doses of 1 to 4 mg are given every 2 to 6 hours, or continuous infusions may be used.

Propofol is an intravenous anesthetic whose mechanism of action is not known. It is quite popular in the ICU owing to its rapid onset of action (1 to 2 minutes) and short duration of action (2 to 8 minutes). It is the preferred sedative when rapid awakening is important, such as for neurologic assessment or pending extubation.[32] When used for long-term (>48 to 72 hours) sedation, the short duration of action does not translate into a reduced duration of mechanical ventilation or a shorter ICU stay.[37] Propofol can cause hypotension due to vasodilatation-related loss of preload and myocardial depression.[38] High-dose continuous infusions have been associated with lactic acidosis in children and with metabolic acidosis, arrhythmias, and cardiac arrest in adults.[39-41] Consequently, providers should consider alternative sedative agents for any patient receiving high-dose propofol infusions who develops unexplained metabolic acidosis, arrhythmias, or cardiac failure.

At times, mechanical restraints may be needed to ensure patient and staff safety while waiting for medications to take effect. It is important to keep in mind, however, that restraints can actually increase agitation and delirium, and their use may have adverse consequences, including strangulation, nerve injury, skin breakdown, and other complications of immobilization.

SUMMARY

Agitation and delirium are very common in the ICU, where their occurrence puts patients at risk for self-injury and poor clinical outcomes. Through a systematic approach, life-threatening problems and other acutely reversible physiologic causes can be rapidly identified and remedied. Recognizing and treating agitated delirium with antipsychotic medications may reduce the use of sedative medications and decrease the risk of prolonging the ICU stay due to oversedation.

Chapter 3

MANAGEMENT OF ACUTE PAIN IN THE INTENSIVE CARE UNIT

Paul Jodka • Stephen O. Heard

Acute pain often occurs in patients who are cared for in the intensive care unit (ICU). Acute pain and discomfort can have multiple causes in this setting, including surgical and post-traumatic wounds and injuries, the use of invasive monitoring devices and mechanical ventilators, prolonged immobilization, and routine nursing care (e.g., dressing changes, airway suctioning).[1-4] Pain is defined as "an unpleasant sensory and emotional experience associated with actual or potential tissue damage."[5] The experience of pain and any related suffering differs among patients,[6,7] but the physiologic sequelae of inadequately treated pain are relatively predictable and potentially deleterious. Such physiologic responses to acute pain and stress are mediated by neuroendocrine activation and increased sympathetic tone. As a consequence, the patient develops tachycardia, increased myocardial oxygen consumption, immunosuppression, hypercoagulability, persistent catabolism, and numerous other metabolic alterations.[8,9] Additional morbidity may be incurred by pain-related functional limitations affecting, for example, pulmonary mechanics[10] and the timing of ambulation.

ACUTE PAIN ASSESSMENT

A variety of scales, such as the visual analog scale and the numeric rating scale, have been used as pain assessment tools in the ICU, although they have not been formally validated for such use (Fig. 3–1). Unfortunately, many ICU patients cannot provide full (or even partial) information regarding their pain. As a consequence, caregivers must sometimes use signs of heightened sympathetic activity (e.g., hypertension, tachycardia, lacrimation, diaphoresis, restlessness) as surrogate markers for the presence of pain; trends in such signs provide a measure of the success of a given intervention. Behavioral-physiologic scales have been described and compared with the visual analog and numeric rating scales.[11,12] These scales, however, are not specific enough to eliminate the subjective component of pain assessment in ICU patients. Thus, pain assessment in critically ill patients remains an inexact science requiring an individualized approach. Assessments must be made consistently and repeatedly and documented in the medical record.

OPTIONS FOR ACUTE PAIN THERAPY

Acute pain is triggered by stimulation of peripheral nociceptors in the skin or deeper structures and is a complex process, involving multiple mediators at various levels of the neuraxis (Fig. 3–2).[5] Different parts of the pain pathway can be targeted either individually or as part of a comprehensive strategy aimed at multiple sites for additive or synergistic effects. Thus, nociception can be influenced peripherally by the use of nonsteroidal anti-inflammatory drugs (NSAIDs) and nerve blocks, at the spinal cord level by the use of epidural or intrathecal medications, and centrally by the use of systemic medications.

NONSTEROIDAL ANTI-INFLAMMATORY DRUGS

Drugs in this class inhibit cyclooxygenase (COX) enzymes, which are involved in prostaglandin synthesis and related inflammation in response to injury. COX-1 is a constitutive enzyme that is present in most tissues and, through the production of prostaglandins E_2 and I_2, serves homeostatic and protective functions.[13] COX-2 is an inducible enzyme that is expressed in response to inflammation. Nonsteroidal anti-inflammatory drugs (NSAIDs) are commonly used in conjunction with other agents, such as opioids, to take advantage of different side effect profiles and possible synergistic efficacy. As a class, NSAIDs may cause adverse effects that include nausea, gastrointestinal bleeding, inhibition of platelet function, operative site bleeding, renal insufficiency, and bronchospasm in aspirin-sensitive patients (triad of asthma, nasal polyposis, and aspirin allergy).[1,5,14,15]

Currently, ketorolac tromethamine (Toradol) is the only parenteral NSAID available in the United States. It has been

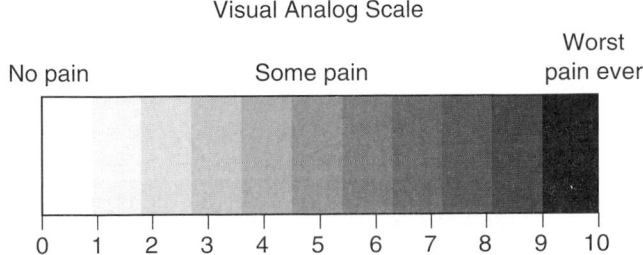

FIGURE 3–1. Visual analog scale. Pain can be rated between 0 (no pain) and 10 (extreme pain). Use of a graphic such as this allows an intubated patient to indicate his or her level of discomfort by pointing. Other scales use cartoon faces that are either smiling or frowning. (From Higgins TL, Jodka PG, Farid A: Pharmacologic approaches to sedation, pain relief and neuromuscular blockade in the intensive care unit. Part II. Clin Intensive Care 2003;14[3-4]:91-98.)

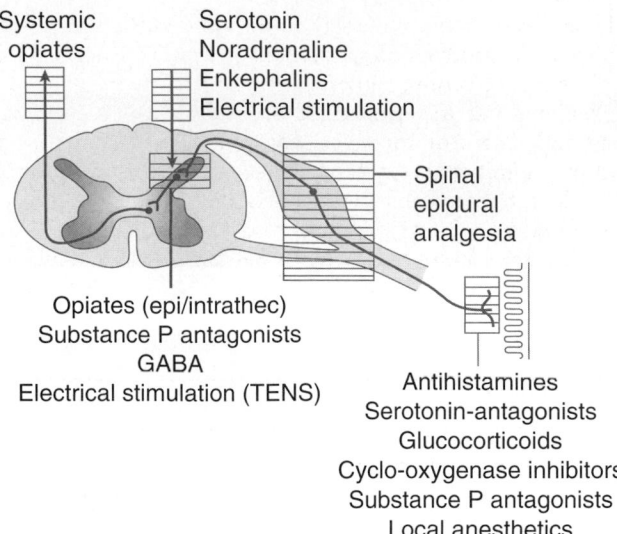

Systemic
opiates

Serotonin
Noradrenaline
Enkephalins
Electrical stimulation

Spinal
epidural
analgesia

Opiates (epi/intrathec)
Substance P antagonists
GABA
Electrical stimulation (TENS)

Antihistamines
Serotonin-antagonists
Glucocorticoids
Cyclo-oxygenase inhibitors
Substance P antagonists
Local anesthetics

FIGURE 3–2. A "map" of the path of nociceptive information from the periphery to the central nervous system. Modification of that information can occur at any point of information transfer. GABA, gamma-aminobutyric acid; stim, stimulation; TENS, transcutaneous electric nerve stimulation. (From Kehlet H: Modification of responses to surgery by neural blockade: Clinical implications. In Cousins MJ, Bridenbaugh PO [eds]: Neural Blockade in Clinical Anesthesia and Pain Management, 2nd ed. Philadelphia, Lippincott, 1988, p 145.)

shown to reduce postoperative opioid requirements and does not cause respiratory depression.[16,17] However, prolonged use has been associated with a significant incidence of the aforementioned side effects (primarily bleeding and renal failure)[18,19]; consequently, ketorolac therapy should be limited to a maximum of 5 days.[1] In addition, ketorolac should be used at decreased dosages, or avoided altogether, in patients at higher risk of such complications owing to advanced age, hypovolemia, and preexisting renal insufficiency. This caution also applies to enterally administered NSAIDs.

Selective COX-2 inhibitors such as celecoxib (Celebrex) and rofecoxib (Vioxx) are available for enteral administration, and injectable COX-2 agents are being studied primarily for the management of acute postoperative pain.[13] The main advantage of these agents over their nonselective relatives lies in the promise of decreased gastrointestinal side effects. However, because COX-2 inhibitors reduce the formation of prostaglandin I_2 (a vasodilating prostaglandin) without affecting the production of thromboxane A_2 (a vasoconstricting prostaglandin), the potential for cardiovascular toxicity exists.[13] Clinical trials are under way to determine the efficacy, cost-effectiveness, and safety of these drugs in the perioperative arena. As with NSAIDs overall, this class of drugs has yet to be formally evaluated in the ICU setting.

OPIOID ANALGESICS

A number of opioids are available(Table 3–1), and this drug class remains the mainstay of ICU analgesia. Morphine, hydromorphone (Dilaudid), and fentanyl are commonly used in ICUs in the United States and have been recommended as first-line narcotic analgesic agents.[1] Opioids bind to a variable degree with various opioid receptor subtypes (μ, δ, κ) located in the brain, spinal cord, and peripheral sites and modulate the transmission and processing of nociceptive signals.[5] The clinical and pharmacologic properties of opioids depend on several variables, such as chemical and solubility properties, dosing regimen (dose, route, and duration of administration), patient characteristics (Table 3–2), and presence of active metabolites. Drugs that are often thought of as short-acting (e.g., fentanyl) actually have a markedly prolonged duration of action if given repeatedly or as an infusion (Fig. 3–3).

Opioids are excellent analgesics, but they are not amnestic agents. As a class, opioids can suppress respiratory drive and promote sedation, gastrointestinal symptoms (ileus, nausea and vomiting, constipation), urinary retention, pruritus, or hypotension. Morphine can cause hypotension by triggering the release of histamine. High doses of meperidine can cause myocardial depression and lead to hypotension on this basis. Hypotension can also be caused by the ablation of pain-mediated sympathetic stimulation, or it may be multifactorial.[20] In actual practice, however, opioids are relatively neutral regarding their hemodynamic effects, if they are used judiciously in euvolemic patients. Of note, coadministration of other central nervous system–active agents (such as benzodiazepines) tends to accentuate opioid-induced side effects, specifically those of sedation, respiratory depression, and hypotension.

Opioids are most commonly administered intravenously in critically ill patients and titrated to effect, either on a scheduled, intermittent basis or as a continuous infusion following a loading dose to achieve analgesia.[1] This strategy avoids concerns regarding unpredictable bioavailability associated with intramuscular, enteral, or transdermal administration and favors more stable analgesic drug concentrations. The benefits of administering analgesics (and sedatives) in such a fashion are several, but they must be balanced against the possibility of inadvertent excess dosing, which may result in prolonged mechanical ventilation and longer hospital stays.[21] It has been reported, however, that scheduled daily interruption of sedative-analgesic drug infusions can help minimize this problem and may actually lead to a shorter duration of mechanical ventilation and a shorter ICU stay.[22]

Morphine is a naturally occurring narcotic analgesic.[1,20] It is metabolized mainly by the liver to an active compound (morphine-6-glucuronide) that can cause a prolonged drug

TABLE 3–1. COMMONLY USED OPIOIDS

Agent	Intermittent Dose	Continuous Dose	Metabolism	Precautions
Fentanyl	0.35–1.5 µg/kg i.v. q 0.5–1 h	0.7–10 µg/kg/h	Oxidation	Rigidity with high doses
Hydromorphone	10–30 µg/kg i.v. q 1–2 h	7–15 µg/kg/h	Glucuronidation	
Morphine	0.01–0.15 mg/kg i.v. q 1–2 h	0.07–0.5 mg/kg/h	Glucuronidation	Histamine release
Meperidine	Not recommended	Not recommended	Demethylation and hydroxylation	Avoid with MAOIs and SSRIs

MAOI, monoamine oxidase inhibitor; SSRI, selective serotonin reuptake inhibitor.

TABLE 3–2. FACTORS INFLUENCING NARCOTIC PHARMOCOKINETICS

Age (increased sensitivity in elderly)
Acid-base status (increased arterial pH increases brain penetration)
Cardiopulmonary bypass (prolongs elimination half-life)
Liver disease
Renal disease (active metabolites may accumulate)
Other central nervous system depressants
Acute and chronic tolerance

effect in patients with renal insufficiency. Onset of action after intravenous administration is relatively slow (5 to 10 minutes) owing to low lipid solubility, and the duration of clinical effect is long enough to permit its use as either an intermittent injection or an infusion. Morphine can cause histamine release and vasodilatation, resulting in hypotension, so it should be used with caution in hypovolemic and hemodynamically unstable patients. Dosing requirements vary significantly from patient to patient and must be individualized (see Table 3–1).

Hydromorphone is a semisynthetic narcotic that, compared with morphine, has a similar duration of action, is a more potent analgesic, does not release histamine, and lacks an active metabolite. These properties make it an attractive alternative to morphine in patients with hemodynamic instability or significant renal impairment.[1] Hydromorphone is also best administered by either infusion or intermittent injection.

Fentanyl is a synthetic narcotic with a potency about 100 times that of morphine. Fentanyl does not cause histamine

release, has no active metabolites, and generally has minimal effects on hemodynamics. It is very lipophilic, leading to a rapid onset of action. Fentanyl can accumulate in fat, however, giving rise to a prolonged drug effect if it is given in very high doses or for a lengthy period, even in patients without significant renal or hepatic dysfunction.[1] Rapid high-dose fentanyl injection can cause chest rigidity that may interfere with ventilation, even in intubated patients, necessitating temporary use of a paralytic agent. On balance, however, fentanyl is a good choice for the analgesic needs of unstable ICU patients, provided the aforementioned pharmacokinetic properties are kept in mind.[1]

Meperidine (Demerol) is a synthetic opioid that is about one tenth as potent as morphine. Meperidine is metabolized by the liver into several compounds that are cleared by the kidneys; these compounds tend to accumulate in the setting of renal insufficiency or after repeated administration in patients with normal renal function. Normeperidine is a primary and neuroexcitatory metabolite of meperidine that has been reported to cause seizures.[23] Additionally, meperidine can cause tachycardia[24] due to anticholinergic effects and also may cause myocardial depression at higher doses. Given these concerns and the ready availability of alternative agents, it is difficult to justify the use of meperidine in the ICU.

OTHER NARCOTIC ANALGESICS

Many other opioids are available for clinical use, such as alfentanil, sufentanil, and remifentanil. Comparative data on the use of these drugs in critically ill patients are lacking, and the use of a given agent is determined largely by a given practitioner's experience and practice patterns.

NEURAXIAL ANALGESIC TECHNIQUES

The administration of narcotics, local anesthetics, and other agents via intrathecal or epidural catheters targets the processing of pain signals at the level of the spinal cord or nerve root.[5,25] Intrathecal analgesic techniques are most appropriate for the acute perioperative setting, with limited applicability to the general ICU population. The use of epidural catheters for regional analgesia in ICU patients may be quite useful, assuming that the pain pattern is regionalized and that there are no contraindications to catheter placement (e.g., coagulopathy, uncontrolled infection, unstable spinal skeletal structures). In some patients, epidural analgesia may be preferable to intravenously administered medications, because this approach affords dense regional pain control[5] while largely avoiding the sedative and respiratory side effects of systemic medications. Because there are multiple factors related to the feasibility and utility of neuraxial techniques in ICU patients, consultation with a pain management specialist is advised when such an approach is being considered.

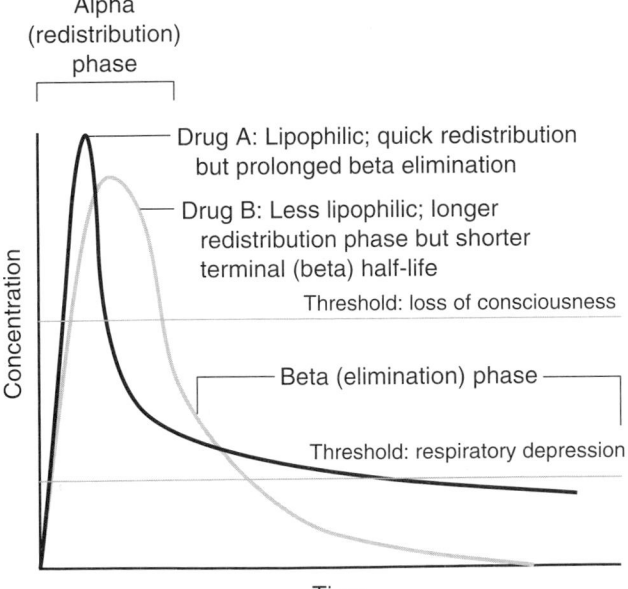

FIGURE 3–3. Pharmacokinetics. A lipophilic drug (drug A) may have a rapid onset and an initially quick distribution but a prolonged beta-elimination (metabolism) phase, resulting in respiratory depression with repeated doses or constant infusion. A less lipophilic drug (drug B) may take longer to redistribute, giving the impression of a prolonged initial duration of action, but does not accumulate, owing to a shorter elimination half-life. Fentanyl is like drug A, whereas morphine is more similar to drug B. (From Higgins TL, Jodka PG, Farid A: Pharmacologic approaches to sedation, pain relief and neuromuscular blockade in the intensive care unit. Part II. Clin Intensive Care 2003;14[3-4]:91-98.)

Labels in figure:
Alpha (redistribution) phase
Concentration
Time
Drug A: Lipophilic; quick redistribution but prolonged beta elimination
Drug B: Less lipophilic; longer redistribution phase but shorter terminal (beta) half-life
Threshold: loss of consciousness
Beta (elimination) phase
Threshold: respiratory depression

ANNOTATED REFERENCES

Carroll KC, Atkins PJ, Herold GR, et al: Pain assessment and management in critically ill postoperative and trauma patients: A multisite study. Am J Crit Care 1999;8:105-117.

A descriptive, correlational study of pain management in 213 patients in 13 ICUs. The authors found that patients were generally satisfied with their pain management, despite being in pain. They concluded that patient satisfaction alone is not a reliable means of gauging the effectiveness of pain management.

Desbiens NA, Wu AW, Broste SK, et al: Pain and satisfaction with pain control in seriously ill hospitalized adults: Findings from the SUPPORT research investigations. Study to Understand Prognoses and Preferences for Outcomes and Risks of Treatment. Crit Care Med 1996;24:1953-1961.

In the Study to Understand Prognoses and Preferences for Outcomes and Risks of Treatment (SUPPORT), approximately 50% of patients experienced pain, 15% reported extreme or moderate amounts of pain, and 15% were dissatisfied with their pain management. Patients were more likely to be dissatisfied if they had severe pain, greater anxiety, depression, and alteration of mental status.

Gilron I, Milne B, Hong M: Cyclooxygenase-2 inhibitors in postoperative pain management: Current evidence and future directions. Anesthesiology 2003; 99:1198-1208.

An up-to-date review of COX-2 inhibitors for analgesia in the postoperative period.

Jacobi J, Fraser GL, Coursin DB, et al: Clinical practice guidelines for the sustained use of sedatives and analgesics in the critically ill adult. Crit Care Med 2002;30:119-141.

A review of pain assessment and analgesic therapy in the critically ill patient promulgated by a task force of the American College of Critical Care Medicine of the Society of Critical Care Medicine. Recommendations are made (and graded), based on a critical evaluation of the literature.

Kress JP, Pohlman AS, O'Connor MF, Hall JB: Daily interruption of sedative infusions in critically ill patients undergoing mechanical ventilation. N Engl J Med 2000;342:1471-1477.

A classic study showing that the daily interruption of sedatives and analgesics can decrease the duration of mechanical ventilation.

Novaes MA, Knobel E, Bork AM, et al: Stressors in ICU: Perception of the patient, relatives and health care team. Intensive Care Med 1999;25: 1421-1426.

The ICU environmental stressor scale was administered to patients, families, and ICU professionals during a patient's first week of care. Pain, inability to sleep, and having tubes in the mouth were the most important stressors identified by the three groups.

Chapter 4

FEVER AND HYPOTHERMIA

Mitchell P. Fink

Fever is defined as an increase in body temperature. Normal body temperature is $36.8 \pm 0.4°$ C. Normally, body temperature varies in a circadian fashion by about $0.6°$ C, being lowest in the morning and highest in the late afternoon or early evening. Fever is triggered by the release of various cytokines—notably, interleukin-1 beta, tumor necrosis factor, and interleukin-6—that are capable of causing secretion of prostaglandin E_2 in the hypothalamus. Prostaglandin E_2 binds to prostaglandin receptors on neurons in the ventromedial preoptic area and the median preoptic nucleus.[1,2] Activation of these receptors triggers a number of neurohumoral and physiologic changes that lead to increased body temperature.

Body temperature can be measured using an oral, axillary, or rectal mercury-filled glass thermometer. These traditional approaches, however, have been largely replaced by a variety of safer and more environmentally friendly methods. These approaches use thermistors located on catheters or probes situated in the pulmonary artery, distal esophagus, urinary bladder, or external ear canal.[3] Infrared detectors can also be used to measure tympanic membrane temperature. Forehead skin temperature can be measured using a temperature-sensitive patch. A core (i.e., rectal, pulmonary artery, esophageal, bladder, or tympanic membrane) temperature greater than $38.3°$ C should be regarded as evidence of fever.

Fever is a cardinal sign of infection. Accordingly, the new onset of fever should trigger a careful diagnostic evaluation, looking for a source of infection. The diagnostic evaluation should be thorough and tailored to the recent history of the patient. For example, the possibility of a central nervous system infection should receive greater attention in a patient with recent or ongoing central nervous system instrumentation. By the same token, if a patient recently underwent a gastrointestinal surgical procedure, the clinician should have a high index of suspicion for an intra-abdominal source of infection. Key elements in the assessment of new-onset fever in the intensive care unit (ICU) are listed in Table 4–1. Common sources of infection in ICU patients are listed in Table 4–2.

Although fever in the ICU is most commonly due to infection, myriad noninfectious causes of systemic inflammation can also result in hyperthermia. Important noninfectious causes of fever in ICU patients are listed in Table 4–3. Some authors claim that noninfectious causes of fever rarely result in a core temperature greater than $38.9°$ C,[4,5] although rigorous data in support of this view are lacking. By the same token, infections are rarely, if ever, associated with core temperatures greater than $41.1°$ C. When the core temperature is this high, the clinician should suspect malignant hyperthermia, neuroleptic malignant syndrome, or heat stroke.

In general, fever should not be treated using antipyretics. This view is based on data that suggest that hyperthermia is an adaptive response that enhances the host's ability to fight infection.[6,7] In addition, body temperature is an unreliable clinical parameter when patients are receiving antipyretic therapy. These considerations notwithstanding, antipyretic therapy should be administered to selected patients with fever. Among such patients are those with acute coronary syndromes (i.e., myocardial infarction or unstable angina), because the tachycardia that usually accompanies the febrile response can exacerbate imbalances between myocardial oxygen delivery and demand. Febrile patients with head trauma, subarachnoid hemorrhage, or stroke should receive antipyretics to prevent temperature-related increases in cerebral oxygen utilization. Children with temperatures greater than $40°$ C or a history of seizures should also be treated.

Hypothermia blankets are often used to lower the core temperature in febrile ICU patients; however, hypothermia

TABLE 4–1. KEY ELEMENTS IN THE EVALUATION OF NEW-ONSET FEVER IN ICU PATIENTS

Be familiar with the patient's history. Pay particular attention to possible predisposing causes of fever.

Perform a careful physical examination. Pay particular attention to surgical wounds and vascular access sites. Look for evidence of pressure-induced skin ulceration. In patients with recent median sternotomy, evaluate the stability of the chest closure. Perform a careful abdominal examination.

Obtain or review a recent chest x-ray, looking for evidence of new infiltrates or effusions.

Obtain appropriate laboratory studies. At a minimum, these studies should include a peripheral white blood cell count and cultures of blood and urine. If the patient is endotracheally intubated or has a tracheotomy, obtain a sample of sputum for Gram stain. In some centers, sputum is routinely cultured. In other centers, bronchoalveolar lavage or bronchial brushing for quantitative microbiology is performed using blind or bronchoscopic methods.

Central venous catheters that have been in place for longer than 96 h should be removed. The tip should be submitted for semiquantitative microbiology.

In patients receiving antibiotics for more than 3 days, a stool sample should be analyzed for the presence of *Clostridium difficile* toxin.

More extensive diagnostic evaluation should be considered in a graded fashion based on history, physical examination findings, laboratory results, persistence of fever despite presumably appropriate antimicrobial chemotherapy, or clinical instability. These additional tests and procedures include diagnostic thoracentesis, paracentesis, and lumbar puncture. Imaging studies should be considered, including abdominal or cardiac ultrasonography and head, chest, or abdominal computed tomography.

TABLE 4–2. COMMON INFECTIOUS CAUSES OF FEVER

Central nervous system
  Meningitis
  Encephalitis
  Brain abscess
  Epidural abscess
Head and neck
  Acute suppurative parotitis
  Acute sinusitis
  Parapharyngeal and retropharyngeal space infections
  Acute suppurative otitis media
Cardiovascular
  Catheter-related infection
  Endocarditis
Pulmonary and mediastinal
  Pneumonia
  Empyema
  Mediastinitis
Hepatobiliary and gastrointestinal
  Diverticulitis
  Appendicitis
  Peritonitis (spontaneous or secondary)
  Intraperitoneal abscess
  Perirectal abscess
  Infected pancreatitis
  Acute cholecystitis
  Cholangitis
  Hepatic abscess
  Acute viral hepatitis
Genitourinary
  Bacterial or fungal cystitis
  Pyelonephritis
  Perinephric abscess
  Tubo-ovarian abscess
  Endometritis
  Prostatitis
Breast
  Mastitis
  Breast abscess
Cutaneous and muscular
  Cellulitis
  Suppurative wound infection
  Necrotizing fasciitis
  Bacterial myositis or myonecrosis
  Herpes zoster
Osseous
  Osteomyelitis

TABLE 4–3. NONINFECTIOUS CAUSES OF FEVER

Central nervous system
  Subarachnoid hemorrhage
  Intracerebral hemorrhage
  Infarction
Cardiac
  Myocardial infarction
  Pericarditis
Pulmonary
  Atelectasis
  Pulmonary embolism
  Fibroproliferative phase of acute respiratory distress syndrome
Hepatobiliary and gastrointestinal
  Acalculous cholecystitis
  Acute pancreatitis
  Active Crohn's disease
  Toxic megacolon
  Alcoholic hepatitis
Rheumatologic syndromes
  Vasculitides (e.g., polyarteritis nodosa, temporal arteritis, Wegener's syndrome)
  Systemic lupus erythematosus
  Rheumatoid arthritis
  Goodpasture's syndrome
Endocrine
  Hyperthyroidism
  Adrenal insufficiency
  Pheochromocytoma
Other
  Drug reactions ("drug fever")
  Transfusion reactions
  Neoplasms (especially lymphoma, hepatoma, renal cell carcinoma)
  Malignant hyperthermia
  Neuroleptic malignant syndrome
  Serotonin syndrome
  Opioid withdrawal syndrome
  Ethanol withdrawal syndrome
  Transient endotoxemia or bacteremia associated with procedures
  Devitalized tissue secondary to trauma
  Hematoma

blankets are no more effective in cooling patients than are antipyretic agents.[8] Hypothermia blankets can cause large temperature fluctuations and are associated with rebound hyperthermia when removed.[8] Additionally, external cooling can augment hypermetabolism and actually promote persistent fever. Lenhardt and colleagues demonstrated that active external cooling in volunteers with induced fever increased oxygen consumption by 35% to 40% and was associated with a significant increase in circulating epinephrine and norepinephrine concentrations.[9]

In view of the preceding, when treatment of fever is warranted, administration of an antipyretic agent is the recommended approach. Commonly used antipyretics include isoform nonselective cyclooxygenase inhibitors, such as ibuprofen or aspirin, or acetaminophen. Although acetaminophen is not a cyclooxygenase inhibitor, it is converted in the central nervous system to a metabolite with activity against this enzyme. Cyclooxygenase inhibitors treat fever by inhibiting the formation of prostaglandin E_2. Because corticosteroids, such as hydrocortisone or methylprednisolone, are potent anti-inflammatory agents, these drugs can suppress the febrile response to infection. Other anti-inflammatory agents have a similar effect. Therefore, absence of fever should not be used to rule out infection, especially in patients receiving corticosteroids or other potent anti-inflammatory drugs.

A reasonable approach for evaluating fever in ICU patients was described by Marik.[4] As depicted in Figure 4–1, blood cultures should be obtained whenever an ICU patient develops a new fever. A comprehensive physical examination should be carried out, and a chest x-ray obtained and reviewed. Noninfectious causes of fever should be excluded. In patients with an obvious focus of infection, a directed diagnostic evaluation is necessary. However, if there is no obvious source of infection and the patient is not deteriorating clinically, it is reasonable to obtain blood cultures and observe the patient for 48 hours before ordering additional diagnostic studies or starting empirical antibiotics. This approach is not reasonable, however, if new fever is accompanied by other signs of worsening clinical status such as arterial hypotension, oliguria, increasing confusion, rising serum lactate concentration, falling platelet count, or worsening coagulopathy. Nor is this approach reasonable if the core temperature is greater than 39° C but less than 41.1° C. Patients in this category should receive empirical antimicrobial chemotherapy while aggressive attempts are made to diagnose the source of infection. All febrile neutropenic patients should receive broad-spectrum empirical antimicrobial chemotherapy after appropriate cultures are obtained.

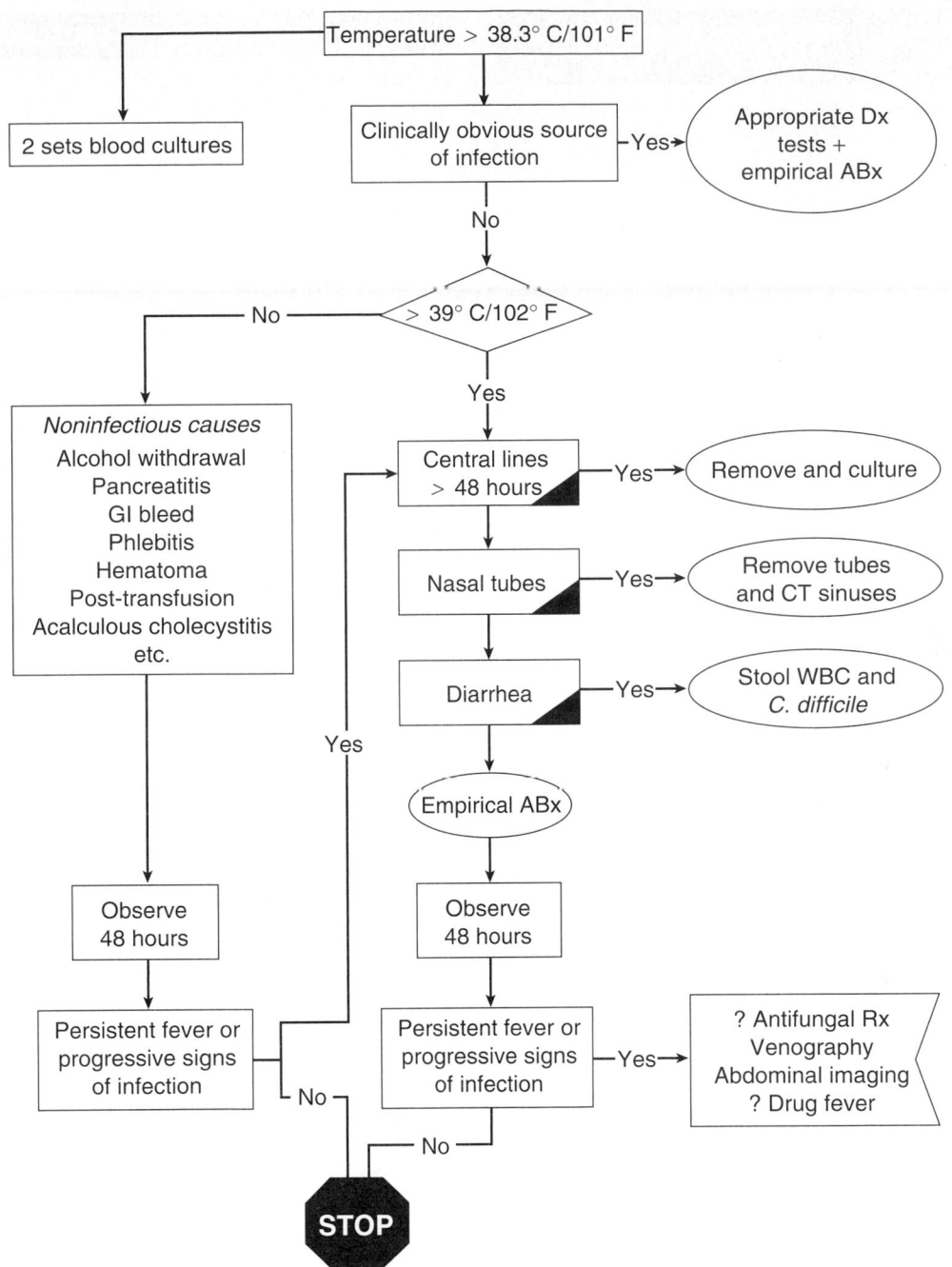

FIGURE 4–1. Approach to evaluating patients with fever in the intensive care unit. ABx, antibiotics; CT, computed tomography; Dx, diagnostic; GI, gastrointestinal; Rx, prescription; WBC, white blood cell. (From Marik PE: Fever in the ICU. Chest 2000;117:855-869.)

Chapter 5

VERY HIGH SYSTEMIC ARTERIAL BLOOD PRESSURE

Michael Donahoe

Very high systemic arterial blood pressure is a common problem in the ICU. The intensivist must distinguish conditions requiring prompt intervention from clinical situations in which aggressive blood pressure control could lead to an adverse outcome. This distinction cannot be based solely on the level of arterial blood pressure elevation.

The Joint National Committee on Prevention, Detection, Evaluation, and Treatment of High Blood Pressure described two acute conditions of elevated systemic arterial pressure.[1] A *hypertensive emergency* is a rare clinical situation that requires immediate blood pressure reduction (not necessarily to normal ranges) within minutes to hours. Hypertensive emergencies are defined by the presence of new or progressive end-organ damage of the neurologic, cardiovascular, or renal systems (Table 5-1).

In contrast, *hypertensive urgencies* are characterized by elevated systemic arterial pressure without evidence of end-organ damage. In these cases, a gradual reduction of blood pressure over several hours to days is the goal because there is no proven benefit to more rapid reduction of blood pressure in asymptomatic patients. Cerebral or myocardial ischemia or infarction can be induced by aggressive antihypertensive therapy if the blood pressure decreases to less than a level that supports adequate tissue perfusion.[2] Hypertensive urgencies are not to be ignored, however, because they can progress to end-organ damage if blood pressure remains uncontrolled over a sustained interval.

Another term, *accelerated hypertension*, also implies end-organ damage. In this case, the clinical markers of damage are pathophysiologic changes involving the retina of the eye, including exudates, hemorrhages, arteriolar narrowing, and spasm. The term *malignant hypertension* is characterized by the additional retinal finding of papilledema. Both of these conditions are often associated with vascular injury to the kidney, termed *malignant nephrosclerosis*, and to other target organs. Two large series confirmed that specific retinal findings do not predict the outcome in patients with elevated systemic arterial pressure.[3,4] This chapter uses the term *hypertensive emergency* to identify acute increases in systemic blood pressure that mandate prompt intervention by the intensivist.

PATHOPHYSIOLOGY

An acute elevation in systemic arterial blood pressure most frequently results from increased systemic vascular resistance. Increased vascular resistance can be precipitated by increased circulating concentrations of catecholamines, increased activity of the sympathetic nervous system, or activation of the renin-angiotensin system. Less commonly, hypertension occurs in the setting of significant volume expansion or augmented contractility of the left ventricle or both.

Two crucial components in the pathophysiology of organ dysfunction associated with accelerated hypertension include the development of obliterative vascular lesions and disordered vasoregulation. The vascular changes of the retina, in accelerated and malignant hypertension, are mirrored by similar changes in the kidney and other organs, leading to a proliferative arteritis and, in advanced stages of the process, fibrinoid necrosis. Presumably, vasoactive mediators play a key role in this process, but the mechanisms underlying these pathologic changes due to severe hypertension remain to be elucidated. A state of relative ischemia is produced in affected organs, resulting in end-organ dysfunction. Early recognition and control of elevated blood pressure are crucial to prevent progression to this more advanced stage of disease.

Aggressive control of elevated systemic arterial blood pressure must be undertaken with caution. There is a rightward shift of the pressure-flow relationship in the central nervous system in patients with long-standing hypertension.[5] Normally, cerebrovascular arteriolar tone is adjusted over a range of perfusion pressures to maintain a constant blood flow. In normal individuals, normal flow is maintained over a range of mean arterial pressure from approximately 60 to 150 mm Hg. A rightward shift in this relationship results in the loss of autoregulation at higher mean arterial pressure values. Aggressive lowering of the blood pressure in patients with an altered autoregulation curve can lead to compromised organ perfusion and ischemia. These pathophysiologic observations are supported by numerous clinical observations. The lower limit of autoregulation is about 20% to 25% below the resting mean arterial pressure. A safe level of blood pressure reduction in the acute setting has been proposed as a 25% reduction of mean arterial pressure or a diastolic blood pressure in the 100 to 110 mm Hg range. This regulated level of blood pressure reduction should maintain critical organ perfusion even in patients with long-standing hypertension.

CEREBROVASCULAR DISEASE

HYPERTENSIVE ENCEPHALOPATHY

Acute elevations in systemic arterial blood pressure can lead to hypertensive encephalopathy. The most common presenting

TABLE 5–1. HYPERTENSIVE EMERGENCIES

Cerebrovascular

Hypertensive encephalopathy
Acute stroke
Subarachnoid hemorrhage

Cardiovascular

Acute coronary syndrome
Acute left ventricular dysfunction
Acute aortic dissection
Accelerated/malignant hypertension

Renovascular

Acute glomerulonephritis
Scleroderma renal crisis
Post–kidney transplantation

Excess Catecholamine States

Pheochromocytosis
Pharmacologically mediated
  Monoamine oxidase inhibitor–tyramine interaction
  Antihypertensive withdrawal
  Alpha-stimulant intoxication
Autonomic hyperreflexia post–spinal cord injury

Miscellaneous Conditions

Eclampsia/preeclampsia
Postoperative hypertension

clinical manifestations include headache, nausea and vomiting, visual disturbances, focal neurologic findings, and seizures. If left untreated, the condition can progress to coma and death. Most patients with hypertensive encephalopathy have a mean arterial pressure significantly greater than the patient's baseline blood pressure, although not in the range typically associated with hypertensive emergency. Retinal findings, including arteriolar spasm, exudates or hemorrhages, and papilledema, are often present. Absence of these findings does not exclude the diagnosis of hypertensive encephalopathy, however. Neuroimaging studies suggest that edema involving the subcortical white matter of the parieto-occipital regions is a characteristic feature of hypertensive encephalopathy; this finding is termed *posterior leukoencephalopathy.*[6] Although the exact mechanism is debated, disordered regulation of vascular flow is believed to contribute to the clinical and radiographic findings. Hypertensive encephalopathy must be distinguished from other acute neurologic conditions associated with hypertension by a thorough evaluation. In general, the neurologic symptoms of stroke or intracranial hemorrhage have a more acute onset than the symptoms associated with hypertensive encephalopathy. The diagnosis of hypertensive encephalopathy is confirmed by the absence of other conditions and the prompt resolution of symptoms with effective blood pressure control. The failure of a patient to improve within 6 to 12 hours of blood pressure reduction should prompt an investigation for an alternative cause of the mental status changes. In most cases, the condition is entirely reversible with no observable adverse outcomes.

ACUTE STROKE

Hypertension is reportedly present in 80% of patients with an acute stroke.[7] The incidence of hypertension is higher in patients with primary intracerebral hemorrhage compared with ischemic disorders.[8,9] Current data suggest that hypertension in the setting of acute stroke is associated with a poor functional outcome.[8,10] Despite this knowledge, the treatment of elevated systemic arterial pressure in acute stroke is poorly investigated and complex.

Two important clinical features complicate the management of hypertension in acute stroke. First, during acute stroke, cerebral autoregulation may be compromised, and lowering of blood pressure may compromise cerebral blood flow further and extend ischemic injury.[11] Second, medications used to treat hypertension may lead to cerebral vasodilation, resulting in increased cerebral blood flow and progression of cerebral edema.[12] Ideally a "correct" level of mean arterial pressure should be maintained in each patient to maintain cerebral perfusion pressure without risking worsening cerebral edema or progression of the lesion, but the clinical determination of this "ideal" value is difficult.

Data are lacking from randomized clinical trials to guide antihypertensive therapeutic decisions in acute stroke. Only a few drug classes have been investigated in this condition, and the total number of patients studied is small. Published guidelines are not based on solid evidence. Using available information, only modest reductions in mean arterial pressure (10% to 15%) are advised in the acute setting of an ischemic stroke. The natural history is for the blood pressure to begin declining shortly after the onset of the acute event and to stabilize within the first 24 hours. Agents that allow titration of therapy (i.e., intravenous medications) may be preferred over oral agents when treatment is necessary, provided that the patient can be monitored carefully in a stroke unit. Also, many patients are unable to tolerate oral medications because of stroke-induced swallowing dysfunction.

For patients with hemorrhagic strokes, the general recommendation is that blood pressure should be reduced to prevent hematoma progression and rebleeding. Even this recommendation is not based on carefully controlled clinical trials, however. Similar cautions to limit the extent of blood pressure reduction (i.e., 15% to 20%) are advised.

SUBARACHNOID HEMORRHAGE

A patient with aneurysmal subarachnoid hemorrhage provides the challenge of an acute neurologic syndrome secondary to an initial insult, followed by the ongoing risk of additional insults over time. These additional insults can include hydrocephalus, rebleeding, and vasospasm. Hemodynamic management is complicated by the competing goals of lowering blood pressure to minimize the rebleeding risk and elevating blood pressure to minimize the risk of cerebral vasospasm and infarction.[13] In general, hypertension is not treated aggressively in this population for fear of precipitating cerebral ischemia. Treatment can be guided by the neurologic condition. For a patient with a normal neurologic picture, small reductions in blood pressure can be accomplished to minimize the risk of rebleeding. For a neurologically impaired patient, aggressive control of blood pressure is avoided to maintain cerebral perfusion pressure.

CARDIOVASCULAR DISEASE

ACUTE CORONARY SYNDROME

Patients presenting with acute myocardial ischemia or infarction frequently have elevated systemic arterial pressure.

The increased afterload increases myocardial oxygen demand. A reduction in myocardial work, achieved by decreasing heart rate and blood pressure, favorably reduces myocardial oxygen demand and infarct size in these patients. A reduction of high systemic arterial pressure in this setting should be done cautiously, however. Potent systemic vasodilation, without coronary vasodilation, can lead to a reduced coronary artery perfusion pressure and infarct extension. For this reason, nitroglycerin, a potent coronary and arterial vasodilator, is often the antihypertensive agent of choice in acute coronary syndromes. In combination with beta blocker therapy, this approach to reduction in arterial pressure can reduce cardiac workload significantly in the setting of ischemia. Careful monitoring of hemodynamic indices during treatment is paramount.

ACUTE LEFT VENTRICULAR DYSFUNCTION

High systemic arterial blood pressure in a patient with acute pulmonary edema contributes to an increased myocardial workload and diastolic dysfunction. The hypertension may be a primary event with secondary myocardial dysfunction or secondary to the sympathoadrenal response to hypoxemia, increased work of breathing, and anxiety in the setting of acute left ventricular dysfunction. Regardless of the cause, efforts to control elevated systemic arterial pressure are essential. For a critically ill patient, infusion of sodium nitroprusside permits rapid titration of blood pressure. Angiotensin-converting enzyme (ACE) inhibitors, which are available in oral and intravenous forms, are associated with acute and long-term beneficial effects in patients with left ventricular failure.[14,15] Aggressive diuresis before blood pressure control may not be advised. Patients with hypertensive emergencies in particular may have had a natriuresis resulting in elevated levels of renin production by the kidney and increased circulating levels of the potent endogenous vasoconstrictor angiotensin II. Further reduction in renal perfusion can lead to increased production of angiotensin II. Medications that increase cardiac work (e.g., hydralazine) or impair cardiac contractility (e.g., labetalol) also may be contraindicated in this setting.

In contrast, nicardipine, a calcium antagonist, has been associated with reduced systemic arterial pressure with preservation of coronary blood flow, favoring the use of this medication in acute left ventricular dysfunction.[16] Likewise, fenoldopam, a dopamine-1 receptor antagonist, has been associated with preservation of coronary blood flow during treatment to reduce systemic arterial pressure.[17]

ACUTE AORTIC DISSECTION

Aortic dissection is believed to result from an intimal tear in the aortic wall. The primary morbidity and mortality result from extension of that tear. This extension is promoted by factors that increase the rate of change of aortic pressure (dP/dt), including elevation in blood pressure, heart rate, and myocardial stroke volume. Blood pressure should be reduced promptly to near-normal levels. Aggressive control of blood pressure with a vasodilator could precipitate a reflex tachycardia, increasing dP/dt. Combined-modality therapy to promote vasodilation (sodium nitroprusside) and control cardiac contractility (beta blocker) is advocated for this disorder. Alternatively, drugs that do not increase dP/dt,

such as trimethaphan, can be used effectively to control blood pressure.

RENOVASCULAR DISEASE

The kidney is a source of the mediators that promote hypertension (i.e., angiotensin II) and a target of high systemic arterial pressure. Chronic hypertension is secondary only to diabetes mellitus as a cause of renal insufficiency. In younger patients, the presence of severe hypertension suggests the possibility of intrinsic renal disease, such as poststreptococcal glomerulonephritis and IgA nephropathy. Renovascular disease is noted in 30% of white patients with severe hypertension and retinopathy.[18]

Elevated systemic arterial pressure should be regulated in patients with underlying renal insufficiency, and a comprehensive workup should be initiated to determine the cause-and-effect relationship. Traditional vasodilator medications, such as labetalol and sodium nitroprusside, are preferred to ACE inhibitors in the acute setting because ACE inhibitors can compromise renal function.[19] The risk of ACE inhibitor–induced renal dysfunction is particularly great in patients with hyperkalemia and acute uremia.[19]

SCLERODERMA RENAL CRISIS

Scleroderma renal crisis is characterized by the development of acute renal failure associated with moderate-to-severe hypertension and a normal to minimally abnormal urine sediment. The most significant risk factor for scleroderma renal crisis is the presence of the diffuse skin involvement characteristic of the disease. The disorder results in marked activation of the renin-angiotensin system. Aggressive control of blood pressure using ACE inhibitors, particularly early in the disease process, can control blood pressure in 90% of patients and promote a greater rate of recovery in renal function.[20] Captopril has been the most extensively studied agent used for treatment of this hypertensive emergency.

POST–KIDNEY TRANSPLANTATION

Hypertension after renal transplantation occurs in a high percentage of patients. In the immediate post-transplantation period, hypertension usually is a manifestation of graft rejection, ischemia, or medication toxicity. Corticosteroids and calcineurin inhibitors promote the development of hypertension. In addition, renal artery stenosis can complicate allograft function and should be evaluated in any patient with resistant hypertension. In the immediate post-transplant period, blood pressure should be regulated at the upper limits of normal to preserve graft function. In the later post-operative period, even more strict control of blood pressure is preferred.[21] The therapy of choice for post–kidney transplantation hypertension is controversial. Calcium channel blockers may reverse cyclosporine-induced renal vasoconstriction; however, outcome trials in this area showed conflicting results.[22,23] ACE inhibitors have the potential to exacerbate renal dysfunction and augment the hyperkalemia induced by calcineurin inhibitors. Either category of medication for blood pressure control could be used with careful monitoring for toxicity.

EXCESS CATECHOLAMINE STATES

PHEOCHROMOCYTOMA

Pheochromocytoma can result in the production of circulating mediators leading to catecholamine excess. These mediators result in hypertension, diaphoresis, tachycardia, and paresthesias of the hands and feet. These attacks can last minutes to days and occur several times a day or once per month. Operative manipulation of the tumor can result in perioperative hypertension. The treatment of hypertension in this disorder must avoid the use of isolated therapy with a beta blocker, a strategy that can lead to unopposed alpha-adrenergic stimulation with the risk of further vasoconstriction and blood pressure elevation. The preferred agent for treatment of hypertension due to pheochromocytoma is phentolamine, a potent alpha-adrenergic antagonist. If necessary, this medication can be combined with a beta blocker, or a combined alpha/beta blocker, such as labetalol, can be used safely.

PHARMACOLOGICALLY MEDIATED

Clonidine withdrawal can mimic the crisis of pheochromocytoma. Clonidine is a centrally acting stimulant of alpha-adrenergic receptors that reduces peripheral adrenergic system activation. Rapid withdrawal or tapering of therapy with this agent has been associated with a hyperadrenergic state, characterized by hypertension, diaphoresis, headache, and anxiety.[24] The syndrome can best be treated by restarting treatment with clonidine. If the symptoms are extreme, treatment can be initiated as outlined for patients with pheochromocytoma. Hypertension also can occur during the withdrawal phase of alcohol abuse[25] and beta-blocker therapy.

Monoamine oxidase inhibitor use can be associated with a marked elevation in the systemic arterial blood pressure, if the patient consumes foods or medications containing tyramine or other sympathomimetic amines. Tyramine-containing foods include champagne, avocados, smoked or aged meats, and fermented cheeses. The monoamine oxidase inhibitor interferes with degradation of the tyramine in the intestine, leading to excess absorption and tyramine-induced catecholamine activity in the circulation. Other medications, including metoclopramide, a dopamine agonist; the calcineurin inhibitors cyclosporine and tacrolimus; and drugs of abuse, such as cocaine, phenylpropanolamine, phenylcyclidine, and methamphetamine, must be considered as possible factors in an ICU patient with elevated systemic arterial pressure.

After spinal cord injury, hypertensive states may occur particularly with stimulation of dermatomes and muscles below the level of the spinal cord injury. Patients with hypertension in this setting typically have lesions above the level of the thoracolumbar sympathetic neurons. Blood pressure elevation is believed to result from excess stimulation of sympathetic neurons. Hypertension is accompanied by bradycardia through stimulation of the baroreceptor reflex. Treatment is focused on minimizing stimulation and providing medical therapy as necessary. Patients with Guillain-Barré syndrome can manifest a similar syndrome.

MISCELLANEOUS CONDITIONS

PREECLAMPSIA/ECLAMPSIA

Preeclampsia/eclampsia is the second most common cause of maternal death in the United States after thromboembolic disease. Hypertension occurs as one manifestation of preeclampsia in a pregnant patient; the other key features are proteinuria and edema. Hypertension in pregnancy also can be seen secondary to chronic hypertension and transient or gestational hypertension. The new onset of hypertension after 20 weeks of gestation is most characteristic of a patient with preeclampsia.

When possible, the optimal treatment of preeclampsia is delivery of the fetus, an approach that prevents progression to eclampsia. Blood pressure should be regulated, however, to prevent end-organ damage. Hydralazine generally is considered the agent of choice in pregnant patients. Sodium nitroprusside (fetal defects), ACE inhibitors (renal dysfunction in fetus), and trimethaphan (meconium ileus) should be avoided because of associated toxicities in pregnant patients. In addition to hydralazine, alternative agents that can be used in this population include labetalol and nicardipine.

POSTOPERATIVE HYPERTENSION

Poorly controlled hypertension preoperatively and intraoperatively is associated with an increased rate of postoperative complications.[26,27] Hypertension in the postoperative period can be seen in 75% of patients, and the risk seems to be greater for vascular surgical procedures, including abdominal aortic aneurysm repair, carotid endarterectomy, and coronary artery revascularization.[28] Postoperative hypertension in these patients can lead to complications, including bleeding from suture lines, intracerebral hemorrhage, and left ventricular dysfunction. Postoperative hypertension can be caused by elevated systemic vascular resistance in response to circulating stress hormones, activation of the renin-angiotensin-aldosterone system, or altered baroreceptor function after certain types of surgery.

Patients with postoperative hypertension must be investigated thoroughly to rule out reversible causes before the institution of drug therapy. Factors such as pain, anxiety, hypervolemia, hypoxemia, hypercarbia, and nausea can contribute to postoperative hypertension. Postoperative hypertension often is limited in duration (i.e., 2 to 12 hours), and aggressive attempts to lower blood pressure acutely can lead to delayed hypotension.

Postoperative hypertension typically is treated by the administration of vasodilators, including sodium nitroprusside and nitroglycerin. Beta blockers can be added for additional control.

ANTIHYPERTENSIVE MEDICATIONS

The goal of antihypertensive therapy in the emergent situation is to lower blood pressure to a safe range as quickly as possible. In general, intravenous medications are preferred, allowing titration of dosing to minimize the risk of excessive hypotension. The precise level of blood pressure reduction necessary to reduce the risk of organ ischemia is not defined. A commonly proposed goal is to lower the mean arterial pressure by approximately 20%, or to reduce diastolic blood pressure to 100 to 110 mm Hg. To monitor carefully the effect of antihypertensive therapy, these patients are best monitored in the ICU.

For hypertensive urgencies, oral therapy generally can be used to lower the blood pressure to safer levels over a 24-hour interval. These patients in general do not require monitoring in an ICU.

TABLE 5–2. INTRAVENOUS ANTIHYPERTENSIVE THERAPY

Medication (Route)	Mechanism	Dosing	Indication	Contraindication
Nitroprusside (i.v. infusion)	Arteriolar and venous vasodilator	0.25-10 µg/kg/min i.v. infusion	Most hypertensive emergencies	Contraindicated in pregnancy. Caution with use in cerebral edema, acute coronary syndrome, or azotemia
Labetalol (i.v. infusion, oral)	Alpha/beta-adrenergic blocker	i.v. bolus 20 mg initially followed by 20-80 mg every 10 min Infusion: 0.5-2 mg/min	Most hypertensive emergencies	Contraindicated in acute heart failure or in patients nontolerant of beta blockers
Nicardipine (i.v. infusion)	Calcium channel blocker	Initial: 5 mg/h Maximum: 15 mg/h	Most hypertensive emergencies	Contraindicated in acute heart failure and caution with use in acute coronary syndrome
Fenoldopam (i.v. infusion)	Peripheral dopamine-1 antagonist	Initial: 0.1 µg/kg/min	Most hypertensive emergencies	Caution in patients with glaucoma
Nitroglycerin (i.v. infusion)	Venodilator	Initial: 0.25-0.5 µg/kg/min Maximum: 8-10 µg/kg/min	Acute coronary syndromes	
Phentolamine (i.v.)	Alpha-adrenergic blocker	5-10 mg every 5-15 min	Pheochromocytoma, catecholamine withdrawal, catecholamine excess	
Enalaprilat	Angiotensin-converting enzyme inhibitor	1.25-5 mg every 6 h	Scleroderma crisis and acute left ventricular dysfunction	Caution with use in acute coronary syndrome
Hydralazine (i.v., oral)	Arteriolar vasodilator	Initial: 10 mg every 20-30 min Maximum: 20 mg	Pregnancy	

Medications available for the treatment of elevated systemic arterial pressure are summarized in Table 5-2. Sodium nitroprusside has been the gold standard for the treatment of hypertensive emergencies because of its short duration of action allowing careful titration. Sodium nitroprusside acts as a direct vasodilator of arterioles and veins. The blood pressure response to nitroprusside infusion is rapid and mandates the use of this medication in a well-monitored environment. The infusion must be provided by a calibrated pump with frequent blood pressure recording. Typically, intra-arterial blood pressure recording is preferred owing to the need for rapid and frequent monitoring, particularly during the initial titration. An accurate noninvasive system may offer equal efficacy, however.

The major concern with sodium nitroprusside is the rare risk of cyanide, or thiocyanate, toxicity. Cyanide intoxication is manifested by alterations in mental status, gastrointestinal complaints, arrhythmias, seizures, or lactic acidosis. The last finding occurs in the setting of a reduced systemic oxygen uptake and a narrow arterial-venous oxygen gradient. Cyanide is liberated during the combination of nitroprusside with sulfhydryl groups in red blood cells and tissues. The circulating cyanide is converted rapidly in the liver to thiocyanate with subsequent excretion by the kidney. Cyanide toxicity from nitroprusside is uncommon and occurs primarily in patients receiving infusions for greater than 24 to 48 hours, in patients with underlying renal insufficiency, and in patients in whom the dose used exceeds the capacity of the body to detoxify cyanide (>2 µg/kg/min increases the risk of cyanide accumulation).

The treatment of cyanide intoxication involves the administration of sodium thiosulfate. Sodium thiosulfate donates its sulfane sulfur atom in a reaction catalyzed by the enzyme rhodanese to convert cyanide to the much less toxic thiocyanate ion, which is excreted in the urine. For severe cases, sodium nitrite also may be administered. The nitrites exert their effect by oxidizing hemoglobin to methemoglobin, with attraction of the cyanide molecule to the ferric ion; this results in displacement of the cyanide from the cytochrome aa_3 to form a ferricyanide complex. The onset of action of sodium nitrite is rapid, but the induction of methemoglobinemia decreases the oxygen-carrying capacity of blood and may be harmful in patients with anemia or significant carboxyhemoglobinemia.

Hydroxocobalamin (vitamin B_{12a}) is another safe and effective antidote for cyanide intoxication that does not effect oxygen-carrying capacity. This compound reacts with circulating cyanide to form cyanocobalamin, with subsequent urinary excretion. Hydroxocobalamin has been shown to minimize the risk of cyanide accumulation during nitroprusside use in surgery.[29]

Thiocyanate toxicity in association with nitroprusside infusion also is rare. Clinical manifestations include fatigue, gastrointestinal complaints, and mental status changes. The symptoms most typically appear with plasma thiocyanate levels that exceed 5 to 10 ng/dL and occur with higher dose nitroprusside infusion in renal impairment.

Intravenous fenoldopam is a postsynaptic dopamine-1 receptor antagonist with short-acting vasodilator properties. In contrast to sodium nitroprusside, fenoldopam administration is not associated with a risk of toxic metabolite accumulation. Similar to sodium nitroprusside, fenoldopam lowers blood pressure by decreasing peripheral vascular resistance. The medication causes slight elevation in heart rate and an increase in renal blood flow. The preservation of renal blood flow is attributed to the drug's mechanism as a dopamine-1 receptor agonist.

The hemodynamic effects of fenoldopam have been compared with nitroprusside in a multicenter investigation of patients with acute hypertension.[30] This prospective, randomized trial in 153 patients at 24 centers showed that fenoldopam was as effective as nitroprusside in controlling acute systemic hypertension. The average decreases in systolic and diastolic blood pressure at 6 hours of infusion were similar in the two study groups. The average maintenance infusion rate of fenoldopam was 0.41 µg/kg/min (range 0.1 to 1.62 µg/kg/min), and the average maintenance infusion rate of nitroprusside was 1.67 µg/kg/min (range 0.3

to 8 μg/kg/min) when target blood pressure control was achieved. The time required to reach the maintenance infusion rate also was similar in the two groups (85 minutes for patients who received fenoldopam and 94 minutes for patients who received nitroprusside). In a subset of the population studied, renal indices, including creatinine clearance, urinary output, and sodium excretion, were better in the group randomized to fenoldopam treatment. The study sample is too small to draw definitive conclusions, however. Both drugs were equally well tolerated.

The use of fenoldopam in patients with hypertensive emergencies was evaluated in 107 patients with a diastolic blood pressure greater than 120 mm Hg and clinical evidence of acute vasculopathy.[31] Infusion rates of 0.01 μg/kg/min, 0.03 μg/kg/min, 0.1 μg/kg/min, or 0.3 μg/kg/min for 24 hours were compared. The time required to reduce diastolic blood pressure by 20 mm Hg ranged from an average of 55 minutes among the patients given the highest dose to 133 minutes among the patients given the lowest dose. Within this range of doses, fenoldopam was safe and found to provide a flexible dose-titration regimen that is effective when the blood pressure must be reduced rapidly.

Labetalol is an oral and parenteral agent that acts as an alpha-adrenergic and nonselective beta-adrenergic blocker. The blood pressure–lowering effect is produced through a reduction in systemic vascular resistance without a compensatory increase in heart rate. The drug has been used effectively in patients with end-organ dysfunction and acute neurologic injury, pheochromocytoma, cocaine intoxication, dissecting aneurysm, and eclampsia. The primary contraindication to the use of labetalol relates to its nonselective beta-blocking properties. Labetalol is approximately one fifth as potent as propranolol as a nonselective beta blocker. Despite this knowledge, the drug should be used cautiously in patients with reactive airways disease, heart block, or decompensated left ventricular failure.

Nitroglycerin is a direct vasodilator that is known to promote coronary vascular dilation. When administered intravenously, the medication has a relatively short duration of action. Nitroglycerin has favorable effects for patients with acute coronary syndromes, including reducing myocardial oxygen demand via its effects on preload and afterload and augmenting myocardial oxygen delivery through its effects on the coronary circulation.

Nicardipine hydrochloride is a calcium channel blocker that acts primarily as a systemic and coronary artery vasodilator. The greater water solubility of this drug compared with other calcium channel blockers (e.g., nifedipine) allows intravenous administration with a short onset and duration of action and easy titration of therapeutic effect. The medication has no significant effect on cardiac inotropy and promotes afterload reduction. The medication has been reported most extensively in the preoperative and postoperative patient environments.

Comparative investigations of nicardipine and nitroprusside for postoperative hypertension have suggested the agents are equally effective.[32-34] Nicardipine offers the advantage of avoiding the issues related to cyanide and thiocyanate intoxication. Nicardipine is metabolized by the liver, and excretion can be impaired in these patients.

Enalapril is an intravenously administered ACE inhibitor. The medication reduces renin-dependent vasopressor activity and reduces aldosterone production. Similar to other ACE inhibitors, the medication is effective in patients with low-to-normal renin levels and hypertension.

Phentolamine is a rapid-acting, alpha-adrenergic blocker. Phentolamine is the drug of choice for hypertensive emergencies secondary to pheochromocytoma, monoamine oxidase–tyramine interactions, and clonidine rebound hypertension.

SUMMARY

The treatment of high systemic arterial blood pressure in the ICU must be incorporated into a comprehensive assessment of the patient. Clinical situations that are associated with progressive end-organ damage require urgent intervention, most frequently with a titratable medication and careful ongoing monitoring. In contrast, aggressive antihypertensive therapy in asymptomatic patients without immediate risk of organ dysfunction can be harmful. The intensivist is routinely challenged to recognize this distinction in a hypertensive patient.

Chapter 6

LOW SYSTEMIC ARTERIAL BLOOD PRESSURE

Kyle J. Gunnerson

When initially assessing a critically ill patient, it is essential to perform a rapid, focused physical examination (the ABCs of resuscitation). After ensuring that the patient has a patent airway (A) and is effectively breathing (B), the next step is to assess the adequacy of the circulation (C).

INITIAL EVALUATION

The initial evaluation should be a global assessment (Fig. 6–1). When walking into a patient's room, the clinician should think, "What do I see?" Quickly determine whether the patient is in distress or has problems related to the airway or breathing. Look for obvious evidence of external hemorrhage, and assess the adequacy of intravenous access. Look for evidence of hypoperfusion. Do not rely only on blood pressure readings, as there is no "normal" blood pressure applicable to every patient, and a blood pressure value in the normal range does not always equate with adequate tissue perfusion. A patient with a history of poorly controlled chronic hypertension may have signs of hypoperfusion even when the blood pressure is within the normal range (for nonhypertensive patients). Conversely, a patient with cirrhosis may be adequately perfused despite having a lower-than-normal blood pressure. A quick assessment of perfusion should include evaluation of mental status, urine output, and skin findings (temperature plus presence or absence of diaphoresis, mottling, and adequate capillary refill). If any of these parameters are abnormal, a more urgent approach to treatment must be taken.

A focused cardiac and pulmonary examination is essential. The examiner should seek evidence of jugular venous distention, presence of an S_3 or S_4 heart sound, new or worsening murmurs, or muffled heart sounds. The examiner should check for the presence of rales. It is also important to note whether there are absent breath sounds, a finding suggestive of pneumothorax.

During the initial evaluation, pay close attention to pulse pressure, diastolic pressure, and surrogates of systemic vascular resistance (SVR), such as capillary refill. These basic concepts of cardiac physiology will be useful in determining the cause and devising a treatment plan.

WHAT IS THE CAUSE?

To help focus the differential diagnosis of a hypotensive patient, it is important to review basic cardiovascular physiology. The first concept to remember is that *pressure = flow × resistance*, where flow is cardiac output and resistance is SVR. Because cardiac output is determined by stroke volume (SV) × heart rate, the presence of hypotension means that at least one of these parameters (i.e., SV, SVR, or heart rate) is abnormal.[1] Disturbances in heart rate are discussed in Chapter 7 and should be obvious by feeling the peripheral pulse or looking at the electrocardiogram monitor; the focus here is on conditions associated with decreased SV or SVR. By properly measuring pulse pressure and diastolic pressure, the clinician can determine whether the cause is a change in SVR or SV.

During systole, the SV is ejected into the proximal arterial conduits. Because more blood is being ejected than the peripheral circulation can accommodate in the arterioles, the arterial walls distend, increasing systolic blood pressure (SBP) in a way that is directly proportional to the SV and indirectly proportional to the capacitance (C) of the arterial wall. This relationship is represented by the formula $SBP = SV \div C$.[1] That is, for a fixed SV, if capacitance is higher, the SBP is lower.

During diastole, the portion of the SV that was "stored" by the distention of the arterial walls during systole fills the peripheral arterioles, leading to a progressive decrease in blood pressure until the next systolic phase. This is the diastolic pressure, a parameter that is directly related to the SVR and capacitance (i.e., low diastolic pressure = low SVR and/or capacitance).[1] When using these basic cardiovascular principles to understand the cause of hypotension, it is important to remember the following: (1) capacitance does not change from heartbeat to heartbeat, and (2) SV depends on preload, afterload, and contractility.

Numerous problems can be associated with low SVR, including sepsis (see Chapter 147), adrenal insufficiency (see Chapter 176), vasodilating medications (see Section XII), neurogenic shock (see Section III), and severe liver dysfunction (see Chapter 120). Decreased SVR is suggested by the presence of a widened pulse pressure and low diastolic pressure.[2,3]

Reduced SV can be due to decreased preload, decreased contractility, or increased afterload. The most common cause of inadequate preload is hypovolemia (see Chapter 229). Other causes of inadequate preload include increased intrathoracic pressure due to dynamic hyperinflation in mechanically ventilated patients (see Chapter 64)[4,5] or tension pneumothorax, pulmonary embolism,[6] mitral valve stenosis,[7,8] cardiac tamponade,[9] and right ventricular failure.[10] Decreased contractility can be caused by myocardial ischemia or infarction, cardiomyopathy, myocarditis, negative inotropic drugs, and direct myocyte toxins such as chemotherapeutic agents and inflammatory mediators (tumor necrosis factor and interleukin-1 beta).[11] A reduction in SV can be identified by decreased systolic blood pressure and normal or narrow pulse pressure.

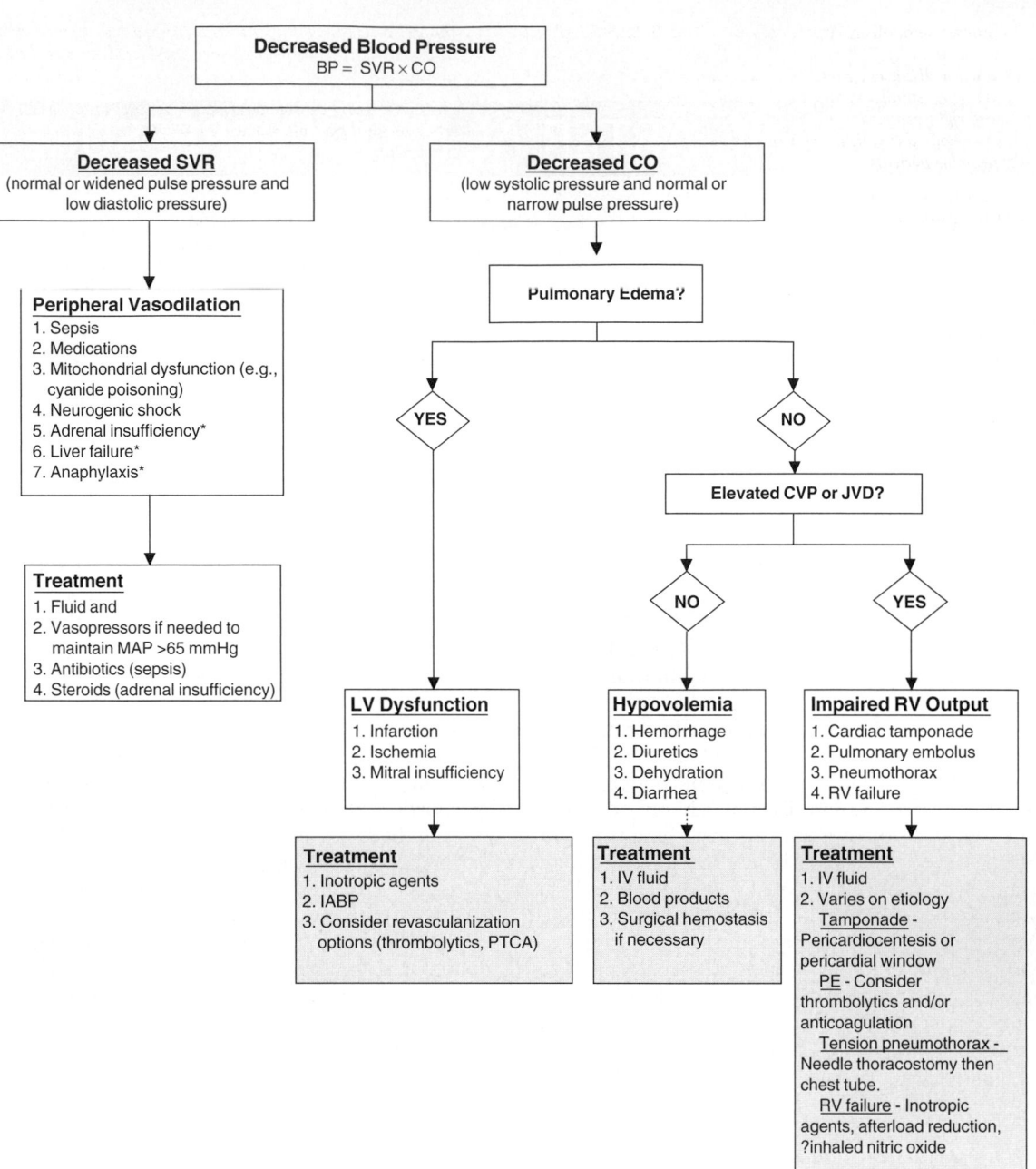

FIGURE 6–1. Initial approach to a patient with low systemic arterial blood pressure. *Adrenal insufficiency, liver failure, and anaphylaxis are sometimes listed as vasodilatory shock; however, data are inconclusive. BP, blood pressure; CO, cardiac output; CVP, central venous pressure; IABP, intra-aortic balloon pump; IV, intravenous; JVD, jugular venous distention; LV, left ventricle; MAP, mean arterial pressure; PE, pulmonary embolism; PTCA, percutaneous transluminal coronary angioplasty; RV, right ventricle; SVR, systemic vascular resistance.

TREATMENT

Until proved otherwise, hypotension should be considered synonymous with hypoperfusion and thus treated aggressively. This initial treatment includes monitoring *and* therapeutic measures. All patients should have adequate intravenous access, preferably two patent 18-gauge or larger catheters. The patient should be monitored using a standard electrocardiogram monitor and pulse oximetry, and a 12-lead electrocardiogram should be performed to look for evidence of myocardial ischemia. Supplemental oxygen should be given as needed to keep oxygen saturation greater than 92%. A 1-L fluid bolus of an isotonic crystalloid solution should be infused as rapidly as possible while data are being gathered.

The history, focused examination, and assessment of pulse pressure and diastolic pressure will aid in the formulation of a more specific treatment strategy.

ANNOTATED REFERENCES

Kumar A, Haery C, Parrillo JE: Myocardial dysfunction in septic shock. Part I. Clinical manifestation of cardiovascular dysfunction. J Cardiothorac Vasc Anesth 2001;15:364-376.

A superb review of myocardial dysfunction in sepsis from authors with extensive experience on the topic.

Landry DW, Oliver JA: The pathogenesis of vasodilatory shock. N Engl J Med 2001;345:588-595.

An excellent basic science review of the physiology of vasodilatory shock.

Olin JW: Pulmonary embolism. Rev Cardiovasc Med 2002;3(Suppl 2): S67-S74.

This review article discusses current diagnostic strategies, such as magnetic resonance imaging, spiral computed tomography, and echocardiography, for evaluating right ventricular dilatation, along with treatment options, including low-molecular-weight heparin and thrombolytics in hemodynamically unstable patients.

Pinsky MR: The hemodynamic consequences of mechanical ventilation: An evolving story. Intensive Care Med 1997;23:493-503.

An excellent review by an international expert in the field of heart-lung interactions, specifically discussing the hemodynamics of positive pressure ventilation.

Spodick DH: Acute cardiac tamponade. N Engl J Med 2003;349:684-690.

A thorough review of cardiac tamponade that covers cause, diagnosis, and treatment.

Arthur Boujoukos

Bradycardia (heart rate <60 beats/min) and tachycardia (heart rate >100 beats/min) are encountered frequently in the intensive care unit (ICU). Evaluation and management should proceed concurrently.

Bradycardia with or without hypotension should prompt a consideration of metabolic disturbances, drug effects, and myocardial ischemia. If bradycardia is of abrupt onset, hypoxemia or acidosis can be quickly excluded by obtaining an arterial blood gas measurement. If the patient is unresponsive, intubate him or her and institute mechanical ventilation. If the patient is already intubated, disconnect the ventilator and manually ventilate the patient (using an Ambu bag) to ensure adequate ventilation and oxygenation. Mucous plugging of the endotracheal tube or airways should be excluded in an acutely hypoxemic patient. Once these conditions are excluded, evaluate the electrocardiogram (ECG) for evidence of second- or third-degree heart block or ischemic changes. Aminophylline (100 mg i.v.) has been reported to correct ischemic heart block.[1] Insertion of a temporary transvenous pacemaker may be indicated in the setting of ischemic heart block, because further deterioration can occur unpredictably. Medications that can cause bradycardia include beta-adrenergic blockers, amiodarone, diltiazem, verapamil, digoxin, and propofol. Severe toxicity due to overdose with a beta-adrenergic antagonist leading to bradycardia, hypotension, and shock can be treated with glucagon (5 to 10 mg i.v., followed by an infusion of 1 to 10 mg/h diluted in D5W). Moderate drug-induced bradycardia (heart rate >40 beats/min) can be observed until the offending drug is metabolized, as long as peripheral perfusion appears to be adequate. Dopamine (starting at 3 µg/kg/min and titrated upward as needed) can be used to provide temporary support for bradycardic hypotensive patients. Atropine (1-mg i.v. bolus; repeat × 1 as necessary) is occasionally beneficial. Bradycardia in the setting of pre-existing shock and refractory acidosis is an ominous sign, and transcutaneous or transvenous pacing is generally futile.

When acute-onset tachycardia occurs, the degree of resulting hemodynamic instability must be assessed. It is critical to differentiate hypotension leading to tachycardia (e.g., rapid atrial fibrillation due to increasing dopamine titration in sepsis or hypovolemic shock causing sinus tachycardia) from hypotension caused by tachycardia (e.g., ventricular tachycardia after myocardial infarction). In the former situation, intravascular volume loading or decreasing the dose of a beta-adrenergic agonist is indicated. In the latter circumstance, rapid conversion of the rhythm should bring about hemodynamic stability.

Sustained regular tachycardia (heart rate >160 beats/min) associated with a narrow QRS complex on the ECG is often reentrant. These dysrhythmias can often be converted with carotid sinus massage. Adenosine can be administered (6 mg i.v., followed by 12 mg i.v. if no response to the lower dose) if sequential carotid sinus massage fails or is contraindicated. Patients presenting with reentrant supraventricular tachycardia in the ICU often have a past history of this dysrhythmia. Beta-adrenergic blockers or calcium channel blockers are reasonable choices for both acute conversion and maintenance therapy. Specific beta blockers include metoprolol 5 mg i.v. every 5 minutes or an esmolol infusion of 500 µg/kg/min over 1 minute, then a 50 µg/kg/min infusion. Esmolol can be rebolused and the drip titrated to a maximum of 400 µg/kg/min. For diltiazem, use 5- to 10-mg boluses titrated upward if the patient's blood pressure tolerates the increase.

Sinus tachycardia is probably the most common dysrhythmia encountered in the ICU. Its meaning, importance, and management vary, depending on the clinical circumstances. In trauma and postsurgical patients, tachycardia can be a sign of bleeding and hypovolemia. It is usually reasonable to administer an intravascular volume challenge (e.g., 500 mL of colloid solution in adults) and check the hemoglobin concentration. Sinus tachycardia and hypertension can be manifestations of opioid withdrawal, failure of a ventilator weaning trial, or inadequate sedation. Most patients at high risk for coronary disease warrant prophylactic treatment with a beta-adrenergic blocker to prevent myocardial ischemia secondary to a high "rate-pressure product" and high myocardial oxygen demand.[2,3] In particular, perioperative patients with significant cardiac risk should have titrated therapy with a beta-adrenergic blocker to maintain the heart rate at less than 80 beats/min unless significant contraindications exist.[4]

Sustained tachycardia associated with hemodynamic instability (i.e., arterial hypotension) and a wide QRS complex on the ECG should be treated as ventricular tachycardia (Fig. 7–1). Unsynchronized cardioversion should proceed expeditiously. Sustained and nonsustained ventricular tachycardia without hemodynamic instability typically occurs in patients with cardiomyopathy or acute myocardial infarction. Initial interventions should include correction of hypokalemia or hypomagnesemia (if present), reduction in the dose of beta-adrenergic agonists (if being infused), and removal of physical stimuli such as pulmonary artery catheters. Amiodarone (150-mg i.v. bolus, then 1 mg/min infusion for 6 hours, then infusion at a rate of 0.5 mg/min) is the preferred therapy in this setting. Consider myocardial ischemia as the cause of monomorphic ventricular tachycardia, and perform the appropriate diagnostic workup. Polymorphic ventricular tachycardia should prompt a

Wide Complex Tachycardia

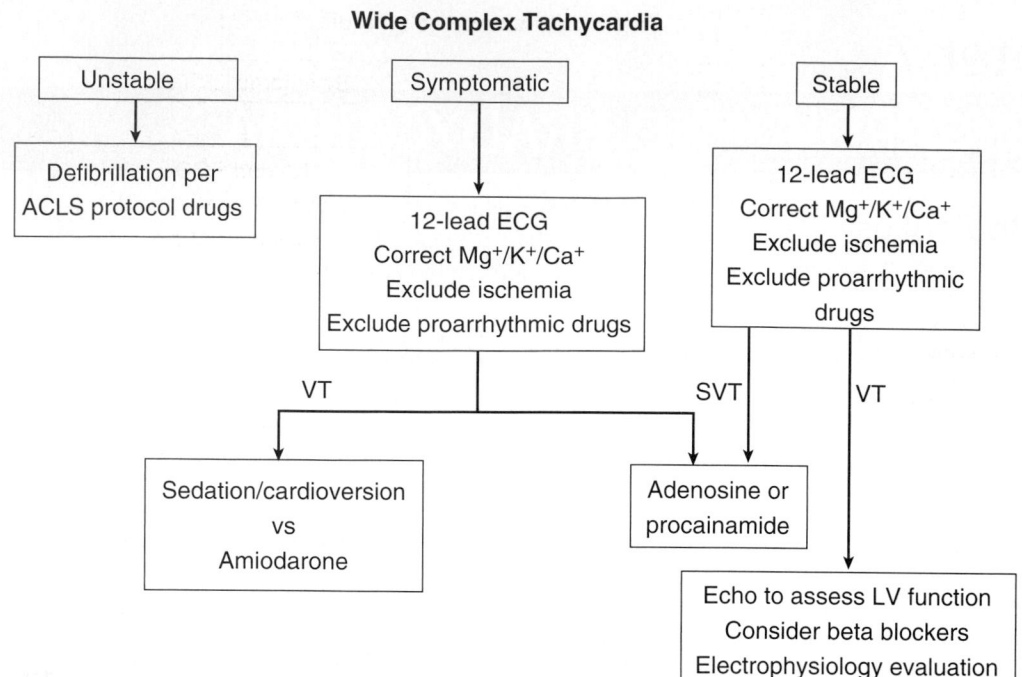

FIGURE 7–1. Algorithm for the diagnosis and testing of wide-complex tachycardia. ACLS, advanced cardiac life support; ECG, electrocardiogram; LV, left ventricle; SVT, supraventricular tachycardia; VT, ventricular tachycardia.

thorough evaluation of the medication list, searching for agents that prolong the QTc (Table 7–1).

Atrial fibrillation with rapid ventricular response can cause significant hemodynamic instability requiring emergent electrical cardioversion. The initial attempt should be synchronized, using 100 J of energy. If unsuccessful, subsequent cardioversion attempts should use escalating energy levels (i.e., 200, 300, 360 J). Atrial fibrillation with rapid

ventricular response in the absence of hemodynamic instability can be managed initially by using drugs or other interventions to provide rate control. The goal should be to reduce heart rate to less than 120 beats/min. First, minimize adrenergic stimulation by instituting mechanical ventilation, if high work of breathing and respiratory failure appear to be contributing factors. Reduce the rate of catecholamine (epinephrine, dobutamine, dopamine) infusions, if possible. If the patient is not currently receiving treatment with inotropes or vasopressors, consider beta-adrenergic blockade as the first-line therapy. Metoprolol (5 mg i.v. every 5 minutes) or esmolol (500 μg/kg over 1 minute, then 50 μg/kg/min infusion) is a reasonable choice. If the patient requires treatment with inotropic agents to support cardiac output, a trial of diltiazem (5- to 10-mg i.v. bolus, followed by an infusion of 5 to 20 mg/h) is warranted. Amiodarone (see previous dosing recommendations) is a reasonable choice for both rate control and conversion therapy. There have been multiple reports about amiodarone lung toxicity, even with short-term therapy, so caution is warranted, particularly in critically ill patients with underlying lung pathology.[5] Digoxin is the least effective option acutely; it is relatively ineffective for controlling ventricular rate when endogenous or exogenous adrenergic tone is high.[6] With new-onset atrial fibrillation, conversion to sinus rhythm is desirable in patients who are poor candidates for anticoagulation. Conversion to sinus rhythm is also beneficial for patients with profound left ventricular dysfunction, because coordinated atrial contraction can contribute substantially to cardiac output under these conditions. In other patients, the primary goal should be to achieve rate control.[7,8] Conversion is significantly more likely to occur during rate control with beta blockers (e.g., esmolol) than diltiazem, but this may actually reflect a reduction in the spontaneous conversion rate when diltiazem is used.[9,10]

TABLE 7–1. COMMON MEDICATIONS THAT MAY PROLONG THE QTc

Antibiotics
Ciprofloxacin
Clarithromycin
Erythromycin
Ketoconazole
Itraconazole
Antiarrhythmics
Procainamide
Amiodarone
Sotalol
Ibutilide
Dofetilide
Quinidine
Flecainide
Propafenone
Psychiatric
Tricyclic antidepressants
Tetracyclic antidepressants
Ziprasidone
Droperidol
Haloperidol
Phenothiazines
Other
Methadone
Bepridil

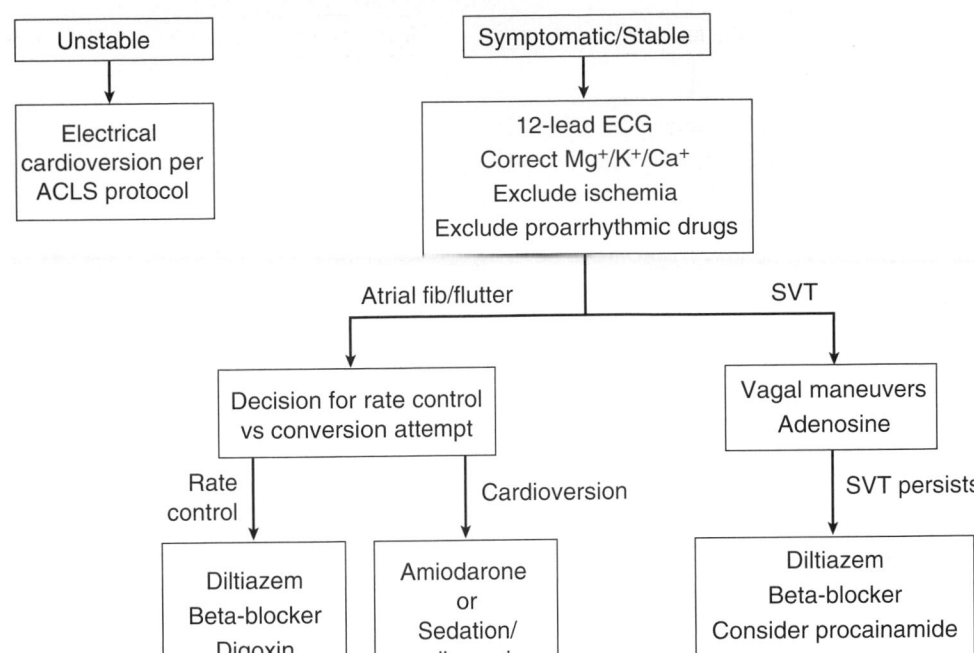

Narrow Complex Tachycardia

FIGURE 7–2. Algorithm for the diagnosis and testing of narrow-complex tachycardia. ACLS, advanced cardiac life support; ECG, electrocardiogram; fib, fibrillation; SVT, supraventricular tachycardia.

Amiodarone, particularly in patients with impaired ventricular function, is generally the drug of choice to achieve conversion.

Regular narrow-complex tachycardia with a heart rate between 145 and 155 beats/min is typically due to atrial flutter. Carotid sinus massage or adenosine can unmask this diagnosis, if it is in doubt from the 12-lead ECG (Fig. 7–2). Ventricular rate control is difficult to achieve pharmacologically when the dysrhythmia is atrial flutter; accordingly, conversion to sinus rhythm is the goal. Synchronized cardioversion should be tried starting at 50 J, using appropriate conscious sedation. If cardioversion converts the rhythm to atrial fibrillation, use synchronized electrical cardioversion again, starting with 100 J. If atrial fibrillation persists, treat with a rate-controlling agent and anticoagulation. If refractory or recurrent atrial flutter is the problem, attempt rate control with beta-adrenergic blockers or diltiazem, as for atrial fibrillation.

Chapter 8
RESPIRATORY DISTRESS WITH ARTERIAL HYPOXEMIA

Paul Rogers

Respiratory distress with hypoxemia is a common reason for patients to be admitted to the ICU. Because a patient's arterial oxygen saturation can be monitored easily using a continuous pulse oximeter, nurses and physicians are alerted immediately to changes in a patient's oxygen saturation. For these reasons, it is important for health care providers to understand the meaning of this measurement, recognize its limitations, and outline a plan for diagnosing and managing patients with hypoxemia.

Arterial hypoxemia is defined as a partial pressure of oxygen in arterial blood (PaO_2) less than 80 mm Hg while breathing room air. The PaO_2 represents the amount of oxygen in physical solution, whereas the oxygen saturation represents the fractional amount of oxyhemoglobin relative to total hemoglobin concentration. Oxygen saturation varies with the PaO_2 in a nonlinear relationship and is affected by temperature, partial pressure of carbon dioxide in arterial blood ($PaCO_2$), pH, and 2,3-diphosphoglycerate concentration (Fig. 8-1).

Falsely low saturations can be recorded if there is a poor waveform or if the light absorption is decreased by dark blue or black nail polish. Patients with methemoglobinemia may have a falsely low oxygen saturation, whereas patients with carboxyhemoglobinemia may have a falsely elevated oxygen saturation because the pulse oximeter cannot differentiate carboxyhemoglobin from oxyhemoglobin.[1] Finally, because the oxygen hemoglobin dissociation curve is affected by temperature, pH, partial pressure of carbon dioxide (PCO_2), and 2,3-diphosphoglycerate concentration, patients may have a higher or lower saturation for a given PaO_2.

Patients who have significant decreases in oxygen saturation attempt to maintain oxygen delivery by increasing cardiac output. Although patients with normal left ventricular function and normal coronary vasculature can tolerate lower oxygen saturation, patients with coronary artery disease or decreased contractility may not be able to tolerate the compensatory tachycardia. The decision to begin mechanical or noninvasive ventilation should be based on the patient's cardiopulmonary physiology and not a specific oxygen saturation. A PaO_2 less than 40 mm Hg or an oxygen saturation less than 75% results in tissue hypoxemia, however, even if cardiac output increases. Generally, saturations in the low 90s on escalating levels of inspired oxygen concentration indicate impending respiratory failure, and invasive or noninvasive mechanical ventilation is necessary.

Etiologies for hypoxemia are best understood if approached from a physiologic point of view rather than by referring to a list of possible differential diagnoses. Simply stated, hypoxemia results from an imbalance between pulmonary ventilation and pulmonary capillary blood flow.[2] There is inadequate oxygen tension in the alveoli, the oxygen is unable to get to the alveoli because of reduced ventilation, or there is a diffusion abnormality preventing oxygen from entering the capillaries.

REDUCED ALVEOLAR OXYGENATION

Alveolar oxygenation is defined by the equation: $PalvO_2 = FiO_2 (BP - BP_{H_2O}) - PaCO_2/RQ$, where FiO_2 is the concentration of inspired oxygen, BP is the barometric pressure, BP_{H_2O} is the partial pressure of water, and RQ is the respiratory quotient. The respiratory quotient represents the amount of oxygen consumed relative to the amount of carbon dioxide produced when nutrients are metabolized and is generally assumed to be 0.8. The normal alveolar oxygenation is 100 mm Hg. According to the equation, factors that contribute to lower alveolar oxygenation are a reduction in barometric pressure or an increase in $PaCO_2$. Clinically, significant increases in $PaCO_2$ are explained by the relationship: $PaCO_2$ = carbon dioxide production/respiratory rate (tidal volume – dead space). Accordingly, the $PaCO_2$ increases with either an increase in production or a decrease in alveolar ventilation.

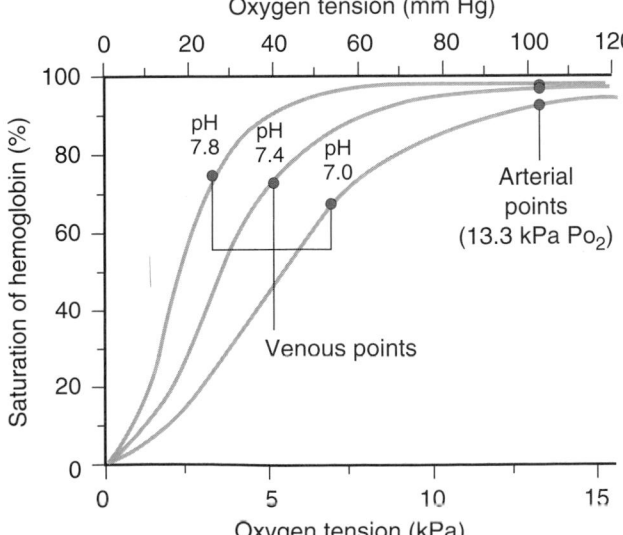

FIGURE 8-1. Oxygen saturation varies with the PaO_2 in a nonlinear relationship and is affected by temperature, $PaCO_2$, pH, and 2,3-diphosphoglycerate (2,3-DPG) concentration.

Alveolar ventilation represents that portion of the minute ventilation undergoing blood-gas exchange and is represented by the product of respiratory rate and tidal volume minus dead space.

Medications, such as narcotics and sedatives, and processes that reduce tidal volume, such as neuromotor weakness, are common causes of hypercarbia. If the alveolar oxygen tension is reduced, the arterial hypoxemia is due to factors that reduce the alveolar oxygen tension. If alveolar oxygen tension is normal, the hypoxemia is the result of either a ventilation/perfusion imbalance or a diffusion abnormality.

DIFFUSION ABNORMALITIES

Diffusion abnormalities are the least likely cause of hypoxemia in the ICU, but can occur as a result of an increase in the thickness of the capillary membrane, a reduction in total alveolar surface area, or a reduction in the capillary transit time. Increases in sympathetic tone because of fever, anemia, work of breathing, or sepsis can increase cardiac output and heart rate, resulting in faster transit times. With less opportunity for alveolar oxygen to diffuse into red blood cells, diffusing capacity is reduced. When capillary transit time is faster, the mean capillary arterial oxygen partial pressure decreases, and the diffusing capacity is reduced.

VENTILATION/DIFFUSION MISMATCH

The most common cause of hypoxemia is ventilation/perfusion mismatch. When perfusion is reduced as a result of a decrease in cardiac output or obstruction from pulmonary emboli, the percent of alveoli with adequate blood flow is reduced, increasing the dead space. If minute ventilation remains constant, the primary blood gas abnormality is an increase in carbon dioxide (PCO_2 = carbon dioxide production/respiratory rate × tidal volume – dead space).

When ventilation is reduced relative to perfusion, alveolar oxygenation decreases and results in arterial hypoxemia. This problem occasionally occurs with bronchospasm or bronchitis. Patients with ventilation/perfusion abnormalities generally respond to increasing the FIO_2. When there is no ventilation (as opposed to reduced ventilation), increasing the FIO_2 is not beneficial.

The portion of cardiac output that does not participate in gas exchange is called the *shunt fraction*. The normal shunt fraction is approximately 3% and is due to the bronchial arterial circulation. When alveoli are not ventilated, such as occurs with pulmonary edema, pneumonia, or atelectasis, the shunt fraction increases. As the shunt fraction increases, PaO_2 decreases (Fig. 8-2), and there is a blunted response to increasing the FIO_2, such that a patient with a shunt fraction greater than 50% has little response to increasing FIO_2 (Fig. 8-3).

Patients with refractory hypoxemia and a clear chest radiograph are often evaluated for a pulmonary embolus. In patients with otherwise previously normal lungs, pulmonary emboli are associated with modest decreases in arterial oxygenation; however, the major pathophysiology is an increase in dead space, which results in hypercarbia unless minute ventilation increases. The hypoxemia caused by pulmonary emboli is due to regional ventilation/perfusion abnormalities and responds to supplemental oxygen. If a patient with a pulmonary embolus has refractory hypoxemia unresponsive

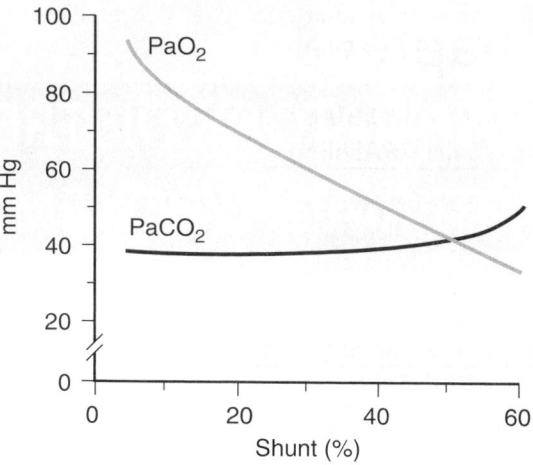

FIGURE 8–2. Decrease in PaO_2 with increasing shunt fraction.

to supplemental oxygenation, an echocardiogram should be performed to rule out a patent foramen ovale, which creates a right-to-left intracardiac shunt in response to the acute increase in pulmonary artery pressure.

Other causes of refractory hypoxemia with a clear chest radiograph are intracardiac shunts and intrapulmonary shunts resulting from either arterial-venous malformations or end-stage liver disease. Often the cause of refractory hypoxemia without radiographic findings on the plain chest film is atelectasis, which is not seen on the typical anteroposterior portable study obtained in the ICU.

It also is relatively common for patients to develop significant hypoxemia when they are started on an intravenous vasodilator, such as sodium nitroprusside. Infusion of sodium nitroprusside interferes with normal hypoxic vasoconstriction, leading to increased perfusion of poorly ventilated areas of the lung. As a result, shunt fraction increases.

Because calculating the shunt fraction, $QsCQ_t = CcO_2/C_{CO_2} – CV_{O_2}$, requires arterial and mixed venous blood gases for calculation of C_{CaO_2} (arterial) and C_{VO_2} (venous) oxygen contents, and because capillary oxygen cannot be directly measured, other indices have been used to estimate the extent of pulmonary gas exchange abnormality. These indices

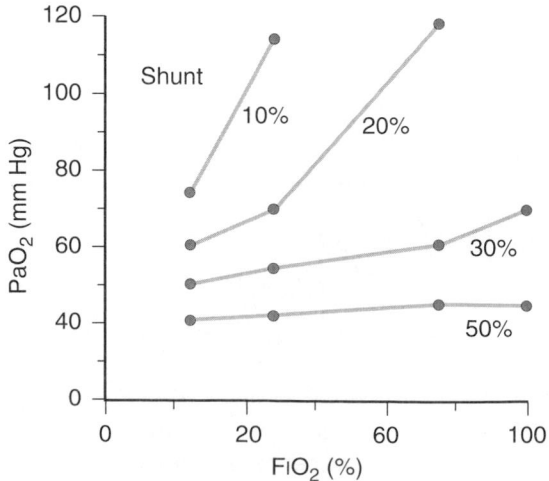

FIGURE 8–3. Blunted response to increasing the inspired oxygen concentration. A patient with a shunt greater than 50% has little response to increasing FIO_2.

include the alveolar-to-arterial (A-a) PO_2 gradient and the arterial/alveolar PO_2 ratio.

ALVEOLAR-ARTERIAL PARTIAL PRESSURE OF OXYGEN GRADIENT

The difference between the alveolar PO_2 and the arterial PO_2 (i.e., the A-a gradient) often is used to estimate the extent of pulmonary pathophysiology and to rule out hypoxemia due to low alveolar PO_2 as the cause of arterial hypoxemia.[3,4] A patient with a reduced alveolar PO_2 (e.g., secondary to breathing room air at high altitude) would have a normal A-a gradient, whereas a patient with ventilation/perfusion mismatching would have a widened A-a gradient. A patient with a PaO_2 of 48 mm Hg and a $PaCO_2$ of 80 mm Hg would have an alveolar PO_2 on room air of 50 mm Hg; the normal A-a gradient of 2 mm Hg is consistent with reduced alveolar PO_2, and causes of hypercarbia need to be ruled out and reversed.

The A-a gradient increases with age or increasing FIO_2, making it an unreliable predictor of the degree of pulmonary dysfunction.[4,5] The PaO_2/FIO_2 ratio also correlates with shunt fraction, but is influenced by increasing FIO_2.[3] The arterial/alveolar ratio is not influenced by FIO_2.[5]

These gradients and ratios are not a substitute for thorough bedside assessment. If a patient has low arterial oxygen saturation by pulse oximetry and is tolerating the reduced saturation without tachycardia or chest pain, adding supplemental oxygen and observing for an appropriate response is reasonable. If there is no increase in saturation, the patient has at least a 40% to 50% shunt and requires intubation or noninvasive ventilation to improve ventilation. Additional oxygen would not increase saturation. If the saturation responds to increasing the FIO_2, the patient has a shunt fraction less than 0.4 or ventilation/perfusion mismatching, and there is time to obtain a chest radiograph and arterial blood gas measurements. If the patient has low saturation and is unstable, immediate bag-and-mask ventilation and securing the airway take precedence over establishing a diagnosis.

REDUCED MIXED VENOUS OXYGEN

A final contribution to hypoxemia may be a reduced mixed venous oxygen content ($CmvO_2$) or saturation. In patients with normal lung function, reducing $CmvO_2$ has little influence on arterial oxygenation; however, in patients with a significant shunt fraction, reducing $CmvO_2$ contributes to arterial hypoxemia.[6] In patients with a widened A-a gradient and abnormally low $CmvO_2$, oxygenation can be improved by increasing venous saturation either by increasing oxygen delivery (increased hemoglobin concentration or cardiac output or both) or reducing oxygen consumption (e.g., induction of hypothermia or using neuromuscular blocking agents).

Chapter 9
ACUTE RESPIRATORY FAILURE

Lakshmipathi Chelluri

Acute respiratory failure is one of the leading causes of admission to an intensive care unit (ICU). In a recent study of cases in the United States, the reported incidence of acute respiratory failure requiring hospitalization was 137 in 100,000 population and the median age of the patients was 69 years.[1] Acute respiratory failure is secondary either to a failure of oxygenation (hypoxic respiratory failure) or to a failure of elimination of carbon dioxide (hypercarbic respiratory [ventilatory] failure). Chronic obstructive pulmonary disease (COPD) with acute exacerbation is the most common cause of ventilatory failure requiring ICU admission.

PATHOPHYSIOLOGY

Oxygenation and elimination of carbon dioxide are the primary gas exchange functions of the lung, and a failure of either one results in acute respiratory failure.[2]

CAUSES OF HYPOXIC RESPIRATORY FAILURE

HYPOVENTILATION

Arterial partial pressure of carbon dioxide ($PaCO_2$) increases with decrease in minute ventilation. An increase in $PaCO_2$ decreases alveolar partial pressure of oxygen (PaO_2) because the carbon dioxide displaces oxygen in the alveoli. Narcotics, anesthetics, and other medications that induce respiratory depression are the usual causes of primary hypoventilation.

VENTILATION-PERFUSION MISMATCH

Gas exchange is optimal when ventilation and perfusion in the lung are matched. A decrease in perfusion relative to ventilation (dead space) or a decrease in ventilation relative to perfusion (shunt) results in ventilation-perfusion ($\dot{V}/\dot{Q}$) mismatch. Hypoxia occurs as a result of $\dot{V}/\dot{Q}$ mismatch because of admixture of venous and arterial blood at the capillary level. $\dot{V}/\dot{Q}$ mismatch is the most common cause of hypoxia in hospitalized patients. In contrast to hypoxemia caused by an anatomic shunt, hypoxemia caused by $\dot{V}/\dot{Q}$ mismatching can be improved by administration of supplemental oxygen.

SHUNT

Hypoxia secondary to shunt occurs as a result of a direct mixture of venous and arterial blood in patients with a right-to-left shunt secondary to congenital cardiac disease or trauma. Oxygenation cannot be improved with supplemental oxygen in patients with an anatomic shunt.

DIFFUSION IMPAIRMENT

Thickening of the alveolar endothelial barrier or a decrease in transit time in the pulmonary capillary bed impairs diffusion of oxygen from the alveoli into the blood.

HIGH ALTITUDE

Barometric pressure decreases with increasing altitude, and, as a result, the partial pressure of oxygen in the ambient atmosphere decreases as well. Consequently, unless supplemental oxygen is provided, hypoxia is an inevitable consequence of respiration at high altitude.

IMPAIRED TISSUE PERFUSION

When tissue perfusion is impaired, the cells attempt to maintain normal oxygen consumption by extracting more oxygen from the available blood supply. As a consequence, venous oxygen tension decreases. Unless fractional pulmonary shunt flow is zero, decreased mixed venous oxygen tension inevitably decreases arterial oxygen tension. Although low tissue cardiac output or impaired blood flow to tissues can cause hypoxia, hypoperfusion is rarely a primary cause of clinically significant hypoxia. Nevertheless, hypoperfusion is a common factor exacerbating the degree of hypoxia caused by other problems.

If the circulating concentration of carboxyhemoglobin or methemoglobin increases, then the oxygen-carrying capacity of the blood decreases. Although arterial oxygen tension may be normal, arterial oxygen saturation is abnormally low because of the presence of hemoglobin derivatives that are incapable of transporting oxygen.

HYPERCARBIC RESPIRATORY FAILURE

Partial pressure of carbon dioxide in the arterial blood ($PaCO_2$) is inversely proportional to alveolar ventilation. $PaCO_2$ increases when the elimination of carbon dioxide is decreased because of a decrease in minute ventilation. $PaCO_2$ also increases if minute ventilation remains constant but carbon dioxide production increases. Primary pulmonary diseases are the most common cause of hypercarbia, although nonpulmonary causes contribute to hypoventilation, increased $PaCO_2$, and the need for mechanical ventilatory support.

Minute ventilation can be decreased due to pulmonary or nonpulmonary factors. Pulmonary causes of impaired minute ventilation include large airway obstruction (e.g., due to the presence of a foreign body or laryngeal spasm), small airway obstruction (e.g., bronchospasm), and destruction of lung parenchyma (e.g., emphysema). Extrapulmonary causes of hypercarbia include neurologic and muscular problems. Neurologic problems include depression of central respiratory drive due to the pharmacological effects of narcotics or sedatives; depression of respiratory drive as a consequence of stroke, intracranial hemorrhage, or head trauma (i.e., central alveolar hypoventilation); and impaired neuromuscular transmission to phrenic nerve injury or spinal cord injury (C5 or higher), Guillain-Barré syndrome, myasthenia gravis and the multifactorial syndrome, polyneuropathy of critical illness. Muscular weakness or skeletal abnormalities can cause a decrease in tidal volume and minute ventilation. The following are some causes of hypoventilation secondary to musculoskeletal abnormalities: prolonged use of neuromuscular blocking agents, malnutrition, hypomagnesemia, hypokalemia, hypophosphatemia, kyphoscoliosis, rib fractures, and flail chest.

Causes of hypercarbia secondary to increased carbon dioxide production and relative hypoventilation include overfeeding, since fat synthesis increases the ratio of carbon dioxide production relative to oxygen consumption (respiratory quotient), and fever and other hypercatabolic states.

CLINICAL PRESENTATION

Dyspnea is the most common symptom associated with acute respiratory failure. Dyspnea is usually associated with rapid shallow breathing and the use of accessory respiratory muscles.

The investigations to evaluate the causes of respiratory failure depend on the suspected mechanism of acute respiratory failure and the primary disease process. Pulse oximetry is a useful monitoring tool and should be carried out in virtually all cases. Other worthwhile diagnostic studies include the following:

Analysis of arterial blood gases will permit diagnosis of a widened alveolar-arterial PO_2 gradient and/or hypercarbia.

Examination of the chest radiograph is useful in almost all cases. If the chest film is clear, then the differential diagnosis should include pulmonary embolism, anatomic right-to-left shunt, pneumothorax, cirrhosis, and COPD. If the chest radiograph shows unilateral infiltrates or effusion, then the differential diagnosis should include pleural effusion, aspiration, lobar pneumonia, atelectasis, and infarction. If bilateral infiltrates are present, then the differential diagnosis should include pulmonary edema (cardiac and noncardiac causes), pneumonia, and pulmonary hemorrhage.[3]

Other more specialized tests, such as computed tomography and cultures, are needed based on the differential diagnosis for the suspected primary disease.

MANAGEMENT

The goal is to maintain adequate oxygenation and ventilation and treat the primary cause of respiratory failure. For hypoxic respiratory failure, the primary goal is to improve arterial oxygenation and maintain PaO_2 of 65 to 70 mm Hg and an arterial blood oxygen saturation (SaO_2) of greater than 93%. Administration of supplemental oxygen improves oxygenation in most clinical situations except for anatomic shunts. Low-flow oxygen can be delivered using a nasal canula or a face mask. The maximum fraction of inspired oxygen (FiO_2) that can be delivered using these approaches is about 0.4. This level of oxygen supplementation is not adequate when the alveolar-arterial (A-a) gradient is very wide. The FiO_2 delivered using a nasal canula or face mask also is dependent on minute ventilation. Accordingly, low-flow methods of providing supplemental oxygen should be used cautiously in patients who are dependent on hypoxic drive or have very high minute ventilation. A higher FiO_2 can be provided if a face mask is combined with a reservoir bag, because admixture of the supplemental oxygen with room air is minimized.

Noninvasive positive pressure ventilation and mechanical ventilation via an endotracheal tube are two approaches for providing supplemental oxygen and, at the same time, providing partial or total support for minute ventilation. In hemodynamically stable patients with mild or moderate respiratory failure, noninvasive positive pressure ventilation may decrease the need for intubation and mechanical ventilation and decrease the patient's length of stay in the ICU.[4,5] Noninvasive positive pressure ventilation should not be used in patients with altered mental status who are unable to protect the airway. Noninvasive positive pressure ventilation should not be used for patients who are unable to clear secretions adequately. For some patients, tolerance for noninvasive positive pressure ventilation can be improved by using a nasal mask and starting at a lower level of inspiratory pressure (5 cm H_2O).

In cases of hypercarbic respiratory failure, the primary goal of treatment is to maintain arterial pH at greater than 7.32 with a $PaCO_2$ appropriate for the pH.[6] Bronchodilators can be delivered as metered dose inhalers or nebulizers. Patients with tachypnea and respiratory distress may not be able to use metered dose inhalers. The bronchodilating effects of β-adrenergic agonists and anticholinergic drugs are synergistic. Long-acting β-adrenergic agonists should not be used to treat acute exacerbations of chronic bronchospasm. Corticosteroids are often used to treat acute exacerbations of diseases associated with airway inflammation and bronchospasm (e.g., asthma and COPD). The reported dosing range is wide. Intravenous methylprednisolone (40 mg i.v. every 12 h to 125 mg i.v. every 6 h) is often employed, if the response is inadequate to initial efforts using bronchodilator treatments with β-adrenergic agonists and anticholinergic agents. Aerosolized steroids may not improve bronchospasm during the acute episode but are useful for maintenance treatment. Although systemic absorption of aerosol steroids is not significant, they may cause adrenal suppression.

Patients who experience changes in the nature of the sputum and signs of infection may benefit from a short course (7-10 days) of antibiotic therapy.

The use of noninvasive positive pressure ventilation in hemodynamically stable patients with mild to moderate ventilatory failure may decrease the need for mechanical ventilatory support and length of stay. The precautions while using noninvasive positive pressure ventilation are the same as listed previously.

INTUBATION AND MECHANICAL VENTILATION

The need for mechanical ventilatory support is a clinical decision based on increased work of breathing (i.e., respiratory rate >35), inability to clear secretions and maintain an adequate airway. The clinician has only two basic maneuvers for improving PaO_2 using mechanical ventilation. The first is to increase FiO_2. The second is to increase mean airway pressure. The latter goal can be achieved in two main ways: (1) application of positive end-expiratory pressure; or (2) changing the duty cycle so that the duration of inspiration is longer (in the extreme, this maneuver is called inverse ratio ventilation). In patients with acute lung injury, tidal volume should be limited to 6 mL/kg (ideal body weight). Prone positioning, inhaled nitric oxide, and transtracheal gas insufflation are some of the other methods used to improve oxygenation in patients with profound hypoxemia due to acute lung injury, but none of these approaches have been shown to improve survival.

Ventilation should be adjusted to maintain pH and $PaCO_2$ at levels that are appropriate for the patient, particularly in patients with COPD and chronic respiratory acidosis. Hyperventilation and excessive correction of $PaCO_2$ in patients with chronic respiratory acidosis results in secondary metabolic alkalosis and delay in weaning from mechanical ventilation. Alveolar air trapping (so-called auto-positive end-expiratory pressure) and hypotension (due to impaired venous return) may develop in patients with inadequate exhalation time, and caution should be used when increasing minute ventilation by increasing either ventilator-delivered respiratory rate or tidal volume in patients with severe airway obstruction.

PROGNOSIS

Mortality in patients with respiratory failure requiring positive pressure ventilatory support is dependent on the primary cause. The hospital mortality rate is 30% to 40% and the 1-year mortality rate is 50% to 70%. Functional status deteriorates immediately after the illness and improves to baseline by 6 to 12 months in survivors.[7]

Chapter 10

POLYURIA

Ramesh Venkataraman • John A. Kellum

Although polyuria in the critically ill is less common than oliguria, it is an important manifestation of a number of clinical conditions. Unless recognized and appropriately managed, polyuria can rapidly lead to the development of hypovolemia, severe hypernatremia, or both. Generally, urine flow varies, depending on the fluid intake, insensible losses (e.g., perspiration), and renal function. The average person excretes about 600 to 800 mOsm of solutes per day, and the average urine output is about 1.5 to 2.5 L/day.

Polyuria has been defined variably in the literature. The most commonly used definition is based entirely on absolute urine volume and arbitrarily defines polyuria as urine volume of greater than 3 L/day. However, some authors prefer to define polyuria as "inappropriately high urine volume in relation to the prevailing pathophysiologic state," regardless of the actual volume of urine.[1,2]

CLASSIFICATION

Polyuria is broadly classified into water diuresis or solute diuresis, depending on whether water or solute is the primary driving force for the increased urine output. However, some patients have a mixed water and solute diuresis.

WATER DIURESIS

DEFINITION AND PATHOPHYSIOLOGY

If the urine output is greater than 3 L/day and the urine is dilute (urine osmolality <250 mOsm/L), total solute excretion is relatively normal, and the polyuria is due to excessive excretion of water. In general, diuresis is marked, and urine osmolality is often less than 100 mOsm/L. Water diuresis is usually secondary to excess water intake, as in primary polydipsia, or to the inability of the renal tubules to reabsorb free water, as in central or nephrogenic diabetes insipidus. A good understanding of water homeostasis is critical in recognizing and managing water diuresis.

The normal plasma osmolality is 275 to 285 mOsm/L. To maintain this steady state, water intake must equal water excretion. The primary stimulus for water ingestion is thirst, mediated by either an increase in effective osmolality or a decrease in blood pressure or effective circulating volume. Under normal circumstances, water intake generally exceeds physiologic requirements.

Unlike water intake, water excretion is tightly regulated by multiple factors. The most dominant regulating factor affecting water secretion is arginine vasopressin, a polypeptide synthesized in the hypothalamus and secreted by the posterior pituitary gland. Once released, arginine vasopressin binds to vasopressin-2 receptors located on the basolateral membranes of renal epithelial cells lining the collecting ducts. Binding of arginine vasopressin to vasopressin-2 receptors initiates a sequence of cellular events, ultimately resulting in the insertion of water channels into the luminal cell membrane. The presence of these water channels permits passive diffusion of water (and hence its reabsorption) across the collecting duct. Any derangement in this process results in a lack of or inadequate water reabsorption by the collecting duct, resulting in water diuresis. The major stimulus for the release of arginine vasopressin is plasma hypertonicity. Its release is also affected by other nonosmotic factors such as effective circulating volume, hypoglycemia, and drugs. In summary, water diuresis occurs because of either excessive water intake sufficient to overwhelm the renal excretory capacity (primary polydipsia) or impairment of renal water reabsorption (central or nephrogenic diabetes insipidus). Impaired renal water reabsorptive capacity (leading to water diuresis) can occur due to failure of arginine vasopressin release in response to normal physiologic stimuli (central or neurogenic diabetes insipidus) or failure of the kidney to respond to arginine vasopressin (nephrogenic diabetes insipidus). In most patients, the degree of polyuria is determined primarily by the degree of arginine vasopressin lack or resistance.

PRIMARY POLYDIPSIA

Primary polydipsia can be recognized clinically based on the history of the patient. Usually, there is a history of psychiatric illness along with a history of excessive water intake. Many patients with chronic psychiatric illnesses have a moderate to marked increase in water intake (up to 40 L/day).[3,4] It is presumed that a central defect in thirst regulation plays an important role in the pathogenesis of polydipsia. In some cases, the osmotic threshold for thirst is reduced below the threshold for the release of arginine vasopressin. The mechanism responsible for abnormal thirst regulation in this setting is unclear. There is evidence that these patients have other defects in central neurohumoral control as well.[5] The diagnosis of primary polydipsia is usually evident from low urine and plasma osmolalities in the face of polyuria. Hyponatremia, when present, also points to the diagnosis of primary polydipsia. Hypothalamic diseases, such as sarcoidosis; trauma; and certain drugs, such as the phenothiazines, can lead to primary polydipsia (Table 10–1). There is no proven treatment for psychogenic polydipsia. Free water restriction is the mainstay of therapy.

TABLE 10–1. CAUSES OF POLYURIA

Polyuria secondary to water diuresis
  Excessive intake of water
    Psychogenic polydipsia
    Drugs—anticholinergic drugs, thioridazine
    Hypothalamic diseases—surgery, sarcoidosis
  Defective water reabsorption by the kidney
    Central diabetes insipidus (vasopressin deficiency)
    Renal tubular resistance to arginine vasopressin
      Congenital nephrogenic diabetes insipidus
      Acquired nephrogenic diabetes insipidus
        Hypercalcemia
        Hypokalemia
        Drugs—lithium, demeclocycline
        Chronic renal diseases—postobstructive diuresis, polyuric
          phase of acute tubular necrosis
        Other systemic diseases—amyloidosis, sickle cell anemia
Polyuria secondary to solute diuresis
  Electrolyte-induced solute diuresis
    Iatrogenic—excessive sodium chloride load, loop diuretic use
    Salt-wasting nephropathy (rarely causes polyuria)
  Nonelectrolyte-induced solute diuresis
    Glucosuria—diabetic ketoacidosis, hyperosmolar coma
    Urea diuresis—high-protein diet, acute tubular necrosis
    Iatrogenic—mannitol

CENTRAL DIABETES INSIPIDUS

Lack of arginine vasopressin (central diabetes insipidus) can be caused by disorders that act at one or more of the sites involved in its secretion, interfering with the physiologic chain of events that lead to hormone release. The common causes of central diabetes insipidus, accounting for the vast majority of cases, include neurosurgery, head trauma, brain death, primary or secondary tumors of the hypothalamus, and infiltrative diseases (such as Langerhans cell histiocytosis).

NEPHROGENIC DIABETES INSIPIDUS

Nephrogenic diabetes insipidus refers to a decrease in urinary concentrating ability that results from renal resistance to the action of arginine vasopressin. The collecting duct cells may fail to respond to the actions of arginine vasopressin. Other factors that can cause renal resistance to arginine vasopressin involve interference with the countercurrent concentrating mechanism, such as medullary injury or decreased sodium chloride reabsorption in the medullary aspect of the thick ascending limb of the loop of Henle. In children, nephrogenic diabetes insipidus is usually hereditary. Congenital or hereditary nephrogenic diabetes insipidus is an X-linked recessive disorder resulting from mutations in the vasopressin-2 arginine vasopressin receptor gene.[6] The X-linked inheritance pattern means that males tend to have marked polyuria. Female carriers are usually asymptomatic but occasionally have severe polyuria. In addition, different mutations are associated with different degrees of arginine vasopressin resistance. Nephrogenic diabetes insipidus can also be inherited as an autosomal recessive disorder due to mutations in the acquaporin gene that result in absent or defective water channels, thereby causing resistance to the action of arginine vasopressin.[7]

The most common cause of nephrogenic diabetes insipidus in adults is chronic lithium ingestion. Polyuria occurs in about 20% to 30% of patients on chronic lithium therapy. The impairment in the nephron's concentrating ability is thought to be due to decreased density of vasopressin-2 receptors or to decreased expression of aquaporin-2, a water channel protein. Other secondary causes of nephrogenic diabetes insipidus include hypercalcemia, hypokalemia, sicke cell disease, and other drugs (see Table 10–1). A water diuresis also can follow relief of obstructive nephropathy. Hypercalcemia-induced nephrogenic diabetes insipidus occurs when the plasma calcium concentration is persistently above 11 mg/dL (2.75 mmol/L). This defect is generally reversible with correction of the hypercalcemia. The mechanisms responsible for hypercalcemia-induced nephrogenic diabetes insipidus are incompletely understood. Compared with hypercalcemia-induced diabetes insipidus, hypokalemia-induced nephrogenic diabetes insipidus is less severe and often asymptomatic. A rare form of nephrogenic diabetes insipidus can occur during the second half of pregnancy (gestational diabetes insipidus). This condition is thought to be caused by release of a vasopressinase from the placenta, leading to rapid degradation of endogenous or exogenous arginine vasopressin.[8]

DIAGNOSIS OF HYPOTONIC POLYURIA (WATER DIURESIS)

The correct diagnosis is often suggested by the plasma sodium concentration and the history. When the problem is primary polydipsia, the plasma sodium concentration is usually low (dilutional), whereas when the problem is central or nephrogenic diabetes insipidus, the plasma sodium concentration is typically normal or high (related to intravascular volume depletion). The rate of onset of polyuria sometimes provides a clue to the diagnosis; with central diabetes insipidus, the onset of polyuria is generally abrupt, whereas with nephrogenic diabetes insipidus or primary polydipsia, the onset of polyuria tends to be more gradual. Even if the history or plasma sodium concentration is helpful, the diagnosis of central versus nephrogenic diabetes insipidus should be confirmed by determining the urinary response to an acute increase in plasma osmolality induced by either water restriction or, less commonly, the administration of hypertonic saline (Fig. 10–1).

Comparing urine osmolality after dehydration with that after vasopressin administration can help differentiate diabetes insipidus due to vasopressin deficiency from other causes of water diuresis (see Fig. 10–1). In this test, fluids are withheld long enough to result in stable hourly urine osmolalities (<30 mmol/kg rise in urine osmolality for 3 consecutive hours). Plasma osmolality and urine osmolality are measured at this point; then the patient is given 5 units of aqueous vasopressin intravenously. The clinician measures the osmolality of a urine sample collected 30 to 60 minutes after the administration of vasopressin. In subjects with normal pituitary function, urine osmolality does not rise by more than 9% after vasopressin injection; however, in central diabetes insipidus, the increase in urine osmolality after vasopressin administration exceeds 9%. To ensure adequate dehydration, plasma osmolality before vasopressin administration should be greater than 288 mmol/kg. There is little or no increase in urine osmolality with dehydration in patients with nephrogenic diabetes insipidus, and there is no further change after vasopressin injection. In the future, a novel method to confirm the results of the water restriction test will be to measure the urinary excretion of aquaporin-2, the collecting tubule water channel that normally fuses with the

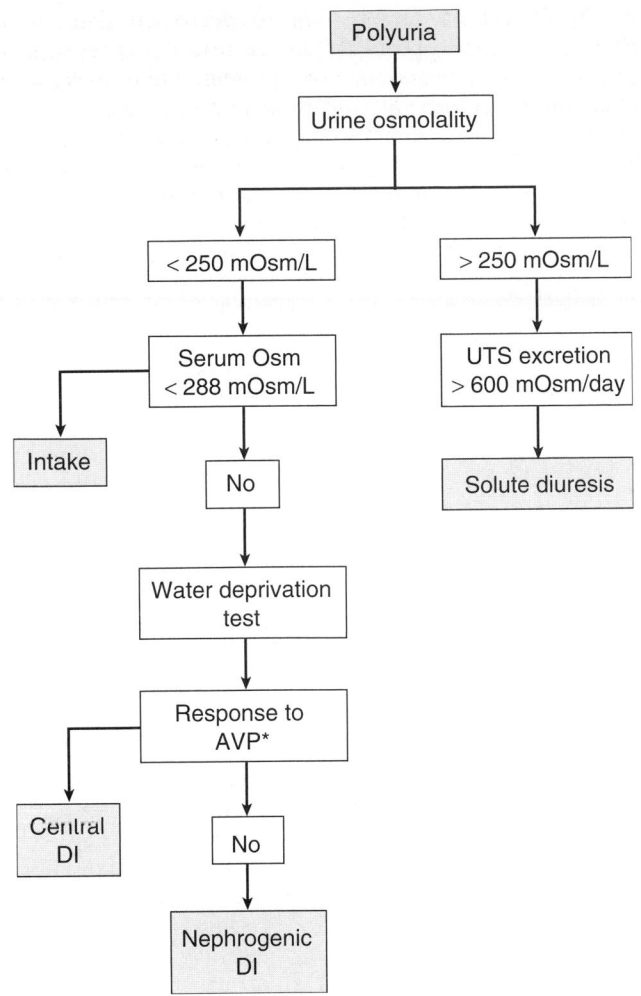

FIGURE 10–1. Approach to polyuria. *Response to arginine vasopressin (AVP) is defined as a greater than 9% increase in urine osmolality 30 to 60 minutes after vasopressin administration (see text for details). DI, diabetes insipidus; UTS, urine total solute concentration.

The mainstay of treatment of nephrogenic diabetes insipidus is solute restriction and diuretics. Thiazide diuretics in combination with a low-salt diet can diminish the degree of polyuria in patients with persistent and symptomatic nephrogenic diabetes insipidus. Thiazide diuretics (hydrochlorothiazide) act by inducing mild volume depletion. Hypovolemia induces an increase in proximal sodium and water reabsorption, thereby diminishing water delivery to the arginine vasopressin–sensitive sites in the collecting tubules and reducing the urine output. The potassium-sparing diuretic amiloride also may be helpful.[10]

SOLUTE DIURESIS

Solute diuresis causing polyuria is due to solute excretion in excess of the usual excretory rate.[11] Total urinary solute excretion varies widely among patients with different ethnicities, cultures, and dietary habits. The average urinary solute excretion in a healthy American adult is between 500 and 1000 mOsm/day. Solute diureses can be severe and can be caused by more than one solute concurrently. Solute diuresis is a relatively common clinical condition with important clinical implications. Unless there is adequate replacement of solute and water, a persistent solute diuresis contracts extracellular volume, leading to severe dehydration and hypernatremia. Although glucosuria is the major cause of an osmotic diuresis in outpatients, other conditions are often responsible when polyuria develops in the hospital. These conditions include administration of a high-protein diet, in which case urea acts as the osmotic agent, and volume expansion due to saline loading or the release of bilateral urinary tract obstruction. Multiplying urine osmolality by the 24-hour urine volume gives an estimate of total urinary solute concentration. If the total urinary solute concentration is abnormally large, a solute diuresis is present.

Solute diuresis can be due to either excessive electrolyte excretion or excessive nonelectrolyte solute excretion. If the total urinary electrolyte excretion exceeds 600 mOsm/day, an electrolyte diuresis is present. The total urinary electrolyte excretion (in mOsm/day) can be estimated as $2 \times$ (urine $[Na^+]$ + urine $[K^+]$) $\times$ total urine volume.[1,12]

An electrolyte diuresis is usually driven by a sodium salt, usually sodium chloride (NaCl).[13] Common causes of NaCl-induced diuresis are iatrogenic administration of excessive normal saline solution, excessive salt ingestion, and repetitive administration of loop diuretics. Most often, NaCl-induced diuresis is accompanied by water diuresis, causing a mixed solute-water diuresis. Also, more than one electrolyte may be responsible for the diuresis.

A clearly excessive value for urine nonelectrolyte excretion (>600 mOsm/day) implies that nonelectrolytes are the predominant solutes contributing to the diuresis. The urinary nonelectrolyte excretion can be calculated by subtracting urine electrolyte excretion from the total urinary solute excretion. The urine osmolality in these disorders is usually above 300 mOsm/kg; the high osmolality contrasts with the dilute urine typically found with a water diuresis. Further, total solute excretion (calculated as the product of urine osmolality and the urine output over a 24-hour urine collection period) is normal with a water diuresis (600 to 900 mOsm/day) but markedly increased with an osmotic diuresis. The most common nonelectrolyte solute causing excessive diuresis is glucose. Conditions associated with glucose-induced diuresis include diabetic ketoacidosis and

luminal membrane of the collecting tubule cells under the influence of arginine vasopressin. In one study, urinary aquaporin-2 excretion increased substantially and to a similar extent after the administration of vasopressin in normal subjects and in those with central diabetes insipidus.[9] However, in patients with hereditary nephrogenic diabetes insipidus, urinary aquaporin-2 excretion was unchanged after vasopressin administration.

TREATMENT OF WATER DIURESIS

Central diabetes insipidus can be treated by replacing arginine vasopressin. The agent of choice is desmopressin because it has prolonged antidiuretic activity and a minimal vasopressor effect. It is usually administered intranasally at doses of 10 to 20 µg once or twice per day. Patients with central diabetes insipidus with some residual releasable arginine vasopressin can be treated with drugs such as carbamazepine (100 to 300 mg twice daily), clofibrate (500 mg every 6 hours), or chlorpropamide (125 to 250 mg once or twice per day), which stimulate arginine vasopressin release.

Primary polydipsia can be treated only by eliminating the underlying problem. In patients with schizophrenia and polydipsia, clozapine has been shown to have a beneficial effect.

hyperosmolar coma.[14] Excessive excretion of urea is another important cause of solute diuresis. This problem can occur with enteral nutrition using a high-protein tube feeding formula, following relief of urinary tract obstruction, or during recovery from acute tubular necrosis.[15] Mannitol administration (e.g., as a therapy for intracranial hypertension) also can lead to significant solute diuresis. This issue is pertinent because mannitol is often administered to patients with head trauma, who are at risk for the development of nephrogenic diabetes insipidus.

The correct diagnosis of solute diuresis depends on a clear systematic approach (see Fig. 10–1). Management usually involves treatment of the underlying disorder and repletion of extracellular volume by hydration. Because solute diuresis is often accompanied by hypernatremia, and because rapid correction of hypernatremia can have disastrous consequences (e.g., cerebral herniation), it is crucial to carefully monitor serum $[Na^+]$. The serum $[Na^+]$ should not be permitted to decrease more than 0.5 to 1 mEq/L per hour.

Chapter 11

OLIGURIA

Sanjay Subramanian • Ramesh Venkataraman • John A. Kellum

Oliguria is a common diagnostic challenge facing the critical care practitioner. This chapter provides a practical, physiology-based approach to diagnosing and treating oliguria.

DEFINITIONS AND EPIDEMIOLOGY

Many definitions for oliguria can be found in the literature. In general, *oliguria* is defined as urine output less than 200 to 500 mL/24 h. To standardize the use of the term across different studies and populations, the Acute Dialysis Quality Initiative (www.ADQI.net) adopted a definition of oliguria as urine output less than 0.3 mL/kg/h for at least 24 hours.

Given the lack of consensus over definitions until now, it is difficult to determine the incidence of oliguria. Some studies estimated that 18% of medical-surgical ICU patients with intact renal function exhibit episodes of oliguria.[1] Of ICU patients who develop acute renal failure, 69% are oliguric.[2] Overall, acute renal failure in the ICU has a poor prognosis; the mortality rates ranges from 30% to 70%. Oliguric acute renal failure compared with nonoliguric acute renal failure carries a higher risk of death. It is essential to understand the physiologic derangements leading to this exceedingly common problem.

PATHOPHYSIOLOGY

Urine output is a function of glomerular filtration rate and tubular secretion and reabsorption. Glomerular filtration rate is directly dependent on renal perfusion. Renal perfusion is a function of arterial pressure and renal vascular resistance. The intrarenal vasculature is capable of preserving glomerular filtration rate in the face of varying systemic pressure through important neurohumoral autoregulating mechanisms that affect tone in the afferent and efferent arterioles. Of these mechanisms, the renin-angiotensin-aldosterone system is perhaps the most important (Fig. 11-1). Oliguria indicates either a marked reduction in glomerular filtration rate or a mechanical obstruction to urine flow.

REDUCTION IN GLOMERULAR FILTRATION RATE

Oliguria secondary to a decrease in glomerular filtration rate usually is related to one of the following conditions:

1. Absolute decrease in intravascular volume. Causes include trauma, hemorrhage, burns, diarrhea, or sequestration of extravascular fluid, as in pancreatitis or after major abdominal surgery.

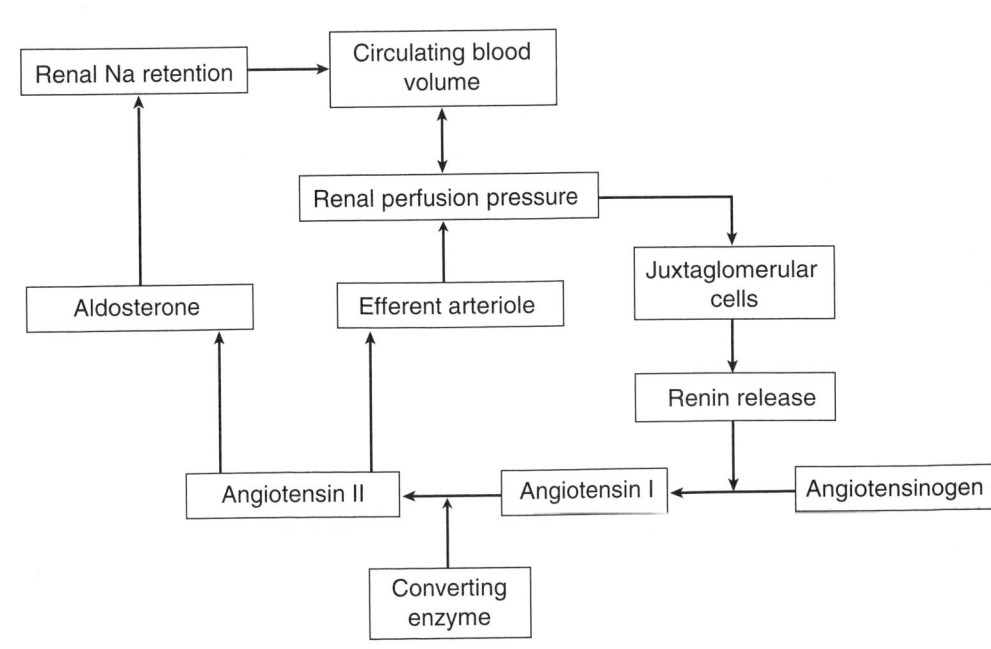

FIGURE 11–1. Network of effects and feedback loop for the renin-angiotensin-aldosterone system. As circulating blood volume or renal perfusion changes, renin secretion changes, resulting in downstream effects that ultimately influence renal resistance and sodium handling by the kidney. Changes in urine output are a direct result of these changes.

2. A relative decrease in blood volume. The primary disturbance is increased capacitance of the vasculature due to vasodilation. This abnormality is encountered commonly in patients with sepsis, hepatic failure, or nephrotic syndrome. Another cause of this abnormality is administration of vasodilating drugs, a category that includes many anesthetic agents.

3. Decreased renal perfusion. Factors that can reduce renal blood flow include structural causes, such as thromboembolism, atherosclerosis, dissection, and inflammation (vasculitis, especially scleroderma) affecting either the intrarenal or the extrarenal circulation. Although renal artery stenosis presents as subacute or chronic renal insufficiency, renal atheroembolic disease can present as acute renal failure with acute oliguria. Renal atheroembolization usually affects older patients with diffuse erosive atherosclerotic disease. Atheromatous embolization is seen most often after manipulation of the aorta or other large arteries during arteriography, angioplasty, or surgery.[3] This condition also may occur spontaneously or after treatment with heparin, warfarin, or thrombolytic agents. Certain drugs, such as cyclosporine, tacrolimus, and angiotensin-converting enzyme inhibitors, cause intrarenal vasoconstriction and reduce renal plasma flow, leading to oliguria. Rarely, decreased renal perfusion can be due to an outflow problem, such as renal vein thrombosis or abdominal compartment syndrome.

4. Acute tubular necrosis. Although acute tubular necrosis is often the result of the above-listed factors, it also can be due to direct nephrotoxic effects of agents such as antibiotics, heavy metals, solvents, contrast agents, or crystals (uric acid or oxalate).

MECHANICAL OBSTRUCTION

Oliguria secondary to mechanical obstruction can be subclassified further according to the anatomic site of the obstruction:

1. Tubular—ureteral obstruction, which can be caused by stones, papillary sloughing, crystals, or pigment.
2. Urethral or bladder neck obstruction—typically due to prostatic hypertrophy or malignancy.
3. A malpositioned or obstructed urinary catheter.

DIAGNOSTIC APPROACH TO OLIGURIA

Oliguria is associated with considerable morbidity and mortality. Merely reversing oliguria, particularly by administering diuretics, does not improve outcome. Rapidly determining the cause of oliguria is essential.

RULE OUT URINARY OBSTRUCTION

The initial step in diagnosis is to rule out urinary obstruction before embarking on a lengthy workup for prerenal or intrarenal causes of renal insufficiency. A prior history of prostatic hypertrophy may provide some clues to the presence of distal obstruction. In the ICU, distal obstruction presenting as oliguria is commonly due to obstruction of the urinary catheter (especially in male patients). In patients with new-onset oliguria, the urinary catheter must be flushed or

changed to rule out obstruction. Although uncommon in the acute setting, complete or severe partial bilateral ureteral obstruction also can lead to acute, "acute-on-chronic," or chronic renal failure. Early diagnosis of urinary tract obstruction is important because many causes can be corrected, and a delay in therapy can lead to irreversible renal injury. Renal ultrasonography is usually the test of choice to exclude urinary tract obstruction.[4] It is noninvasive and can be performed at the bedside. Ultrasonography also obviates the potential allergic and toxic complications of radiocontrast media. In almost all cases, ultrasonography successfully diagnoses hydronephrosis and establishes its cause. Ultrasonography also can detect other causes of renal disease, such as polycystic kidney disease. Under some circumstances, however, renal ultrasound may not yield good results. In early obstruction or obstruction associated with severe dehydration, hydronephrosis may not be visualized at the time of the initial ultrasound examination, but may appear on a study done later in the course of the disease. Computed tomography should be performed if the ultrasound results are equivocal, if the kidneys are not well visualized, or if the cause of the obstruction cannot be identified.

LABORATORY INDICES

Some authorities advocate examining the urine sediment, whereas others do not. Although hyaline and fine granular casts are common in prerenal disease, acute tubular necrosis usually is associated with coarse granular casts and tubular epithelial casts. These findings lack discriminating power, however, and are of limited practical value. The main reason to examine the urinary sediment is to detect red blood cell casts, which indicate glomerular disease. The urinary sediment in post–renal failure is often bland, lacking casts or sediments. Occasionally a few red blood cells and white blood cells may be seen. Eosinophilia, eosinophiluria, and hypocomplementemia, if present, suggest that atheroembolization may be the cause of acute oliguria.[5]

Table 11-1 lists laboratory values useful in distinguishing prerenal from intrarenal causes of acute renal failure. A fractional excretion of sodium less than 1 traditionally has been used as evidence for a prerenal cause of oliguria. These indices are unreliable when the patient has received diuretic or natriuretic agents (including dopamine and mannitol)

TABLE 11–1. BIOCHEMICAL INDICES USED TO DISTINGUISH PRERENAL FROM INTRARENAL ACUTE RENAL FAILURE

	Prerenal	Renal
Osmolality$_U$ (mOsm/kg)*	>500	<400
[Na$^+$]$_U$ (mmol/L or mEq/L)	<20	>40
[urea]$_S$/[creatinine]$_S$	>0.1	<0.05
[creatinine]$_U$/[creatinine]$_S$	>40	<20
Osmolality$_U$/osmolality$_S$	>1.5	>1
FE$_{Na}$ (%)	<1	>2
FE$_{urea}$ (%)	<25	>25

Osmolality$_U$, urine osmolality; [Na$^+$]$_U$, urinary sodium ion concentration; [urea]$_S$/[creatinine]$_S$, ratio of serum urea to serum creatinine concentration; [creatinine]$_U$/[creatinine]$_S$, ratio of urine creatinine concentration to serum creatinine concentration; osmolality$_U$/osmolality$_S$, ratio of urine osmolality to serum osmolality; FE$_{Na}$, fractional excretion of filtered sodium; FE$_{urea}$, fractional excretion of filtered urea. FE$_{Na}$ = [Na$^+$]$_U$ × [creatinine]$_S$/[Na$^+$]$_S$ × [creatinine]$_U$ × 100.

and may be confounded by endogenous osmolar substances (e.g., glucose or urea).

CLINICAL PARAMETERS

Traditional indicators of hydration status and tissue perfusion, such as systemic blood pressure, heart rate, body weight, presence or absence of jugular-venous pulsation, and presence or absence of peripheral edema, are of some utility. In the ICU, however, some of these indicators are less useful for a variety of reasons.

Presence or absence of jugular-venous pulsation is not an accurate way to assess right ventricular filling pressure when patients are receiving positive-pressure ventilation and positive end-expiratory pressure. Similarly, peripheral edema is often due to hypoalbuminemia and decreased oncotic pressure in critically ill patients. Patients may have a total body excess of salt and water and yet be intravascularly volume depleted. Blood pressure and heart rate are affected by numerous physiologic and treatment variables in the ICU and are unreliable measures of volume status.

In the ICU, it is common to assume that one can obtain a more accurate assessment of preload by measuring the central venous pressure or pulmonary artery occlusion pressure. These measurements provide unambiguous data, however, only when the pressures are low (<10 mm Hg). If central venous pressure or pulmonary artery occlusion pressure is increased, it does not ensure that filling pressures are adequate. Response to a single fluid challenge or even multiple fluid challenges may not detect hypovolemia depending on the degree of intravascular volume depletion. The presence of a cardiac index greater than 3 L/min/m^2 generally suggests *adequate* preload, but may not reflect *optimal* preload. The mixed venous oxygen saturation can serve as a surrogate for cardiac output, but does not define optimal filling. For patients receiving positive-pressure mechanical ventilation, the absence of arterial pulse-pressure variation provides robust evidence that intravascular volume is adequate. In other cases, echocardiography may provide the only reliable way to assess intravascular volume status.

ABDOMINAL COMPARTMENT SYNDROME

Another important and often overlooked reason for acute oliguria is abdominal compartment syndrome. *Abdominal compartment syndrome* is defined as symptomatic organ dysfunction that results from an increase in intra-abdominal pressure. Although this condition initially was described in trauma patients, abdominal compartment syndrome occurs in a wide variety of medical and surgical patients. Abdominal compartment syndrome is seen sometimes after major abdominal operations that are associated with massive resuscitation or tight abdominal wall closure. Abdominal compartment syndrome leads to acute renal failure and acute oliguria mainly by increasing renal outflow pressure and reducing renal perfusion. Other mechanisms include direct parenchymal compression and decreased venous return to the heart, leading to embarrassment of cardiac output and stimulation of the sympathetic nervous and renin-angiotensin systems on this basis. These factors lead to decreased renal and glomerular perfusion and manifest as acute oliguria. Intra-abdominal pressure greater than 15 mm Hg can lead to oliguria, and intra-abdominal pressure greater than 30 mm Hg can cause anuria.[6]

Abdominal compartment syndrome should be suspected in any patient with a tensely distended abdomen, progressive oliguria, and increased airway pressure (transmitted across the diaphragm). The mainstay of diagnosis is measurement of intra-abdominal pressure. The most common way to assess intra-abdominal pressure is to measure the pressure in the urinary bladder because it is easily performed. Bladder pressure has been shown to correlate well with intra-abdominal pressure over a wide range of pressures. Decompression of the abdomen with laparotomy, sometimes requiring that the abdomen be left open for a time, is the only definitive treatment for oliguria from abdominal compartment syndrome.

TREATMENT OF OLIGURIA

ENSURING ADEQUATE RENAL PERFUSION

The management of oliguria is based on identification and correction of precipitating factors. In addition, nephrotoxic drugs should be avoided, if possible, and doses of all renally excreted drugs should be adjusted appropriately. Efforts should be made to optimize renal perfusion by correcting hypotension and providing appropriate intravascular volume expansion. Correction of hypotension is especially crucial because in cases of acute renal failure secondary to sepsis and ischemia some of the important autoregulating mechanisms that help preserve glomerular filtration rate in the face of fluctuating blood pressure are disrupted. In these patients, renal blood flow is directly related to systemic arterial pressure. Vasoactive drugs may be necessary to increase the mean arterial pressures to more than usual values to maintain adequate renal perfusion urine output.[7] In patients with chronic hypertension and renal vascular disease, renal autoregulation curves (i.e., plots of renal perfusion as a function of blood pressure) are shifted to the right. A higher mean arterial pressure may be required to ensure adequate renal perfusion. Before starting treatment with a vasoactive drug, however, it is imperative to ensure that the patient is adequately volume resuscitated. The blood pressure target must be individualized based on numerous factors, such as the premorbid blood pressure and presence or absence of vascular disease. Hemodynamic monitoring devices may enable a more streamlined, "goal-directed" approach to therapy.

ROLE OF DIURETIC AGENTS

The use of diuretic agents in oliguric renal failure is widespread, despite a paucity of evidence supporting their efficacy. Traditionally, diuretics have been used in the early phases of oliguria to "jump start" the kidney and establish urine flow. Presumably the absence of oliguria makes it easier to regulate volume status, and given that nonoliguric renal failure generally has a better prognosis, clinicians frequently use diuretics in this setting.[8] A study by Anderson and coworkers[9] in 1977 claimed a reduction in mortality from 50% to 26% by using high doses of a loop diuretic to convert oliguric to nonoliguric renal failure. This study excluded patients with shock and perioperative renal failure. These results have not been reproduced in more recent trials. A study in 1997 by Shilliday and colleagues[10] examined the effect of treating acute renal failure patients with loop diuretics. Although administration of loop diuretics increased urine flow, there was no difference in the incidence of renal recovery, dialysis, or death among patients randomized to diuretic therapy or placebo. Two other randomized controlled trials by Brown and coworkers[11] and Kleinknecht and associates[12] also failed to show any improvement in survival when loop diuretics were used in patients with oliguric renal failure. The PICARD study group reported the results of a large cohort study of critically ill patients with acute renal failure from 1989 through 1995.[13] The study showed that diuretic use was associated with an increased risk of death or nonrecovery of renal function. Accordingly, it is unlikely that the use of diuretics in patients with oliguric acute renal failure affords any benefit to the kidney. The use of diuretics in this setting should be restricted to the treatment of volume overload, and even then caution is advised.

VASOACTIVE AGENTS

Other agents have been used to "treat" oliguria, including dopamine and related compounds. Because urine output often increases with the addition of "low-dose" dopamine, many intensivists assume that it has a beneficial effect. Low-dose dopamine has been advocated since the 1970s as therapy for oliguria on the basis of its action on dopamine-1 receptors in doses less than 5 μg/kg/min. There is abundant evidence, however, that low-dose dopamine does not afford any renal protection in oliguria. Most evidence in favor of low-dose dopamine comes from uncontrolled trials or anecdotal studies. A comprehensive meta-analysis of dopamine in critically ill patients by Kellum and Decker[14] showed that dopamine did not prevent the onset of acute renal failure or decrease mortality or the need for dialysis.

There are important physiologic considerations that argue against a protective role for dopamine or any other dopamine receptor agonists, such as fenoldopam or dopexamine, in the oliguric state. First, the effect of dopamine agonists on urine output may be merely the natriuretic response mediated by inhibition of Na^+,K^+-ATPase in tubular epithelial cells.[15] Dopamine increases urine output because it is a diuretic. Second, treatment with dopaminergic antagonists, such as metoclopramide, has not been shown to affect renal function adversely. Third, the effect of dopamine may be counteracted by increased plasma renin activity in critically ill patients. A significant hysteresis effect has been shown for the action of dopamine on renal blood flow. Finally, although dopamine increases renal blood flow, it does not increase medullary oxygenation,[16] and by increasing solute delivery to the distal tubule, dopamine agonists actually worsen medullary oxygen balance.[17] Despite claims to the contrary, newer dopamine agonists, such as fenoldopam and dopexamine, not only have these limitations, but also can induce hypotension and further increase the risk of renal injury.

CONCLUSION

The presence of oliguria should alert the clinician to undertake a diligent search for any correctable underlying causes. The mainstay of treatment is to ensure adequate renal perfusion by optimizing blood pressure, cardiac output, and intravascular volume status. The use of diuretics and vasoactive agents, although still fairly common, is not supported by the evidence, and emerging data actually suggest harm.

Chapter 12

ACID-BASE DISORDERS

John A. Kellum

Conventional wisdom posits that acid-base disorders are more important for what they tell the clinician about the patient than for any harm that happens to the patient as a direct consequence of abnormal blood (or tissue) pH. This view is reasonable because most acid-base disorders are mild and well tolerated, but they allow the astute clinician to recognize underlying disorders that might be difficult to diagnose or even suspect otherwise. However, there are certain circumstances in which acid-base derangements are themselves dangerous, such as when the disorders are extreme (e.g., pH <7.0 or >7.7), especially when the acid-base derangement develops quickly. Such severe abnormalities can be the direct cause of organ dysfunction and can manifest as cerebral edema, seizures, decreased myocardial contractility, pulmonary vasoconstriction, and systemic vasodilation. Even less extreme derangements can produce harm because of the patient's response to the abnormality. For example, a spontaneously breathing patient with metabolic acidosis will attempt to compensate by increasing minute ventilation. The workload imposed by increasing minute ventilation can lead to respiratory muscle fatigue with respiratory failure or diversion of blood flow from vital organs to the respiratory muscles, resulting in organ injury. Acidemia can promote the development of cardiac dysrhythmias in critically ill patients or increase myocardial oxygen demand in patients with myocardial ischemia. In such cases, one must treat the underlying disorder and also provide treatment for the acid-base disorder itself. Finally, emerging evidence suggests that changes in acid-base status influence immune effector cell function. Thus, avoiding acid-base derangements could influence outcome by modulating systemic inflammation and/or host defenses against infection.

GENERAL PRINCIPLES

Three widely accepted methods are used to analyze and classify acid-base disorders, yielding mutually compatible results. The approaches differ only in assessment of the metabolic component (i.e., all three treat P_{CO_2} as an independent variable): (1) HCO_3^- concentration ($[HCO_3^-]$); (2) standard base-excess; (3) strong ion difference. All three yield virtually identical results when used to quantify the acid-base status of a given blood sample.[1-4] For the most part, the differences among these three approaches are conceptual; in other words, they differ in how they approach the understanding of mechanism.[5-7]

There are three mathematically independent determinants of blood pH:

1. The difference between the sum of the concentrations of strong cations (e.g., Na^+ and K^+) and the sum of the concentrations of strong anions (e.g., Cl^-, lactate); this difference is called the strong ion difference.
2. The total weak acid "buffers" concentration (A_{TOT}), which is mostly composed of the concentrations of albumin and phosphate.
3. P_{CO_2}.

Only these three variables (strong ion difference, A_{TOT}, and P_{CO_2}) can independently affect blood pH. $[H^+]$ and $[HCO_3^-]$ are dependent variables, being functions of strong ion difference, A_{TOT}, and P_{CO_2}. Changes in plasma $[H^+]$ occur as a result of changes in the dissociation of water and A_{TOT} brought about by the electrochemical forces produced by changes in strong ion difference and P_{CO_2}. The standard base-excess is mathematically equivalent to the change in strong ion difference required to restore pH to 7.4 given a P_{CO_2} of 40 mm Hg and the prevailing A_{TOT}. Thus, a standard base-excess of −10 mEq/L means that the strong ion difference is 10 mEq/L less than the strong ion difference that is associated with a pH of 7.4 when P_{CO_2} is 40 mm Hg.

ASSESSING ACID-BASE BALANCE

Acid-base homeostasis is defined by the pH of blood plasma and by the conditions of the acid-base pairs that determine it. Because blood plasma is an aqueous solution containing both volatile (carbon dioxide) and fixed acids, its pH will be determined by the net effects of all these components on the dissociation of water. The determinants of blood pH can be grouped into two broad categories, respiratory and metabolic. Respiratory acid-base disorders are disorders of carbon dioxide (CO_2) tension, and metabolic acid-base disorders comprise all other conditions affecting the pH. This latter category includes disorders of both weak acids (often referred to as "buffers," although the term is imprecise) and strong acids and bases (including both organic and inorganic acids). Acid-base disorders can be recognized by any of the following:

1. An alteration in the pH of the arterial blood (normally 7.35 to 7.45). If the pH is less than 7.35, then acidemia is said to be present; if the pH is greater than 7.45, then alkalemia is said to be present.
2. An arterial partial pressure of CO_2 (Pa_{CO_2}) outside the normal range (35 to 45 mm Hg).
3. A plasma bicarbonate concentration outside the normal range (22-26 mEq/L).
4. An arterial standard base-excess of 3 or −3 mEq/L.

Although these criteria are useful in identifying an acid-base disorder, the absence of all four cannot exclude a mixed acid-base disorder, alkalosis plus acidosis, which is completely matched. Fortunately, such conditions are quite rare.

METABOLIC ACID-BASE DISORDERS

Metabolic acid-base derangements are associated with a greater number of underlying conditions than are respiratory acid-base disorders and tend to be more difficult to treat. Metabolic acidosis is produced by a decrease in the strong ion difference, which, in turn, generates an electrochemical force that increases $[H^+]$. The strong ion difference decreases when the concentration of organic anions (e.g., lactate or β-hydroxybutyrate) increases. The strong ion difference also decreases when there is a loss of sodium bicarbonate (e.g., due to diarrhea or renal tubular acidosis) or there is a gain of exogenous anions (e.g., iatrogenic acidosis or poisonings). Metabolic alkaloses occur when the strong ion difference is inappropriately wide, although it need not be greater than the "normal" 40 to 42 mEq/L. Widening of the strong ion difference can be brought about by the loss of strong anions in excess of strong cations (e.g., vomiting, diuretics), or, rarely, by administration of strong cations in excess of strong anions (e.g., transfusion of large volumes of banked blood containing sodium citrate).

Similarly, the treatment of metabolic acid-base disorders requires a change in the strong ion difference. Metabolic acidoses are repaired by increasing plasma Na^+ concentration more than plasma Cl^- concentration (e.g., by infusing $NaHCO_3$) and metabolic alkaloses are repaired by replacing Cl^- either as NaCl (large volumes), KCl, or even HCl. Note that so-called "chloride-resistant" metabolic alkaloses are resistant to chloride only because of ongoing renal losses that increase in response to increased Cl^- replacement (e.g., hyperaldosteronism).

Pathophysiology of Metabolic Acid-Base Disorders

Disorders of metabolic acid-base balance occur as a result of

1. Dysfunction of the primary regulating organs.
2. Exogenous administration of drugs or fluids that alter the body's ability to maintain normal acid-base balance.
3. Abnormal metabolism that overwhelms the normal defense mechanisms.

The organs responsible for regulating the strong ion difference in both health and disease are the kidneys and, to a lesser extent, the gastrointestinal tract.

The Kidneys

Plasma flow to the kidneys is approximately 600 mL/min. The glomeruli filter the plasma to yield 120 mL/min of filtrate. Normally, more than 99% of the filtrate is reabsorbed and returned to the plasma. Thus, the kidney can only excrete a very small amount of strong ions into the urine each minute, and several minutes to hours are required to achieve a significant impact on the strong ion difference. The handling of strong ions by the kidney is extremely important, because every Cl^- ion that is filtered but not reabsorbed decreases the strong ion difference. Accordingly, "acid handling" by the kidney is generally mediated through Cl^- balance. The purpose of renal ammoniagenesis is to allow the excretion of Cl^- without Na^+ or K^+. Viewed this way, renal tubular acidosis can be regarded as an abnormality of Cl^- handling rather than of H^+ or HCO_3^- handling.[3]

Renal-Hepatic Interaction

Ammonium ion (NH_4^+) is important to systemic acid-base balance not because it stores H^+ or has a direct action in the plasma (normal plasma NH_4^+ concentration is <0.01 mEq/L). NH_4^+ is important because it is "co-excreted" with Cl^-. Of course, NH_4^+ is not only produced in the kidney. Hepatic ammoniagenesis (and, as we shall see, glutaminogenesis) is also important for systemic acid-base balance and is tightly controlled by mechanisms sensitive to plasma pH.[8] This reinterpretation of the role of NH_4^+ in acid-base balance is supported by the evidence that hepatic glutaminogenesis is stimulated by acidosis.[9] Glutamine is used by the kidney to generate NH_4^+ and thus facilitates the excretion of Cl^-. The production of glutamine therefore can be seen as having an alkalinizing effect on plasma pH because of the way the kidney utilizes it.

The Gastrointestinal Tract

Different parts of the gastrointestinal tract handle strong ions in distinct ways. In the stomach, Cl^- is pumped out of the plasma and into the lumen, thereby reducing the strong ion difference and pH of gastric juice. The pumping action of the gastric parietal cells increases the strong ion difference of the plasma by promoting the loss of Cl^-; this effect produces the so-called "alkaline tide" at the beginning of a meal when gastric acid secretion is maximal.[10] In the duodenum, Cl^- is reabsorbed and the plasma pH is restored. Normally, only slight changes in plasma pH are evident because Cl^- is returned to the circulation almost as soon as it is being removed. However, if gastric secretions are removed from the patient, either through a suction catheter or as a result of vomiting, Cl^- is lost and the strong ion difference increases. It is important to realize that it is the Cl^- loss, not the H^+ loss, that is the cause for widening of the strong ion difference and the development of metabolic alkalosis. Although H^+ is "lost" as HCl, it is also lost with every molecule of water removed from the body.

In contrast to the stomach, the pancreas secretes fluid into the small intestine that has a strong ion difference much greater than that of plasma; the $[Cl^-]$ of pancreatic secretions is quite low. Thus, the strong ion difference in the plasma perfusing the pancreas decreases, a phenomenon that peaks about an hour after a meal and helps counteract the alkaline tide. If large amounts of pancreatic fluid are lost, for example from surgical drainage, acidosis develops as a consequence of the decreased plasma strong ion difference. Fluid in the lumen of the large intestine has a wide strong ion difference because most of the Cl^- has been removed in the small intestine and the remaining electrolytes are mostly Na^+ and K^+ and HCO_3^-. The body normally reabsorbs much of the water and electrolytes from this fluid but when there is severe diarrhea, large amounts of this HCO_3^--rich and Cl^--poor fluid can be lost. If these losses are persistent, the plasma strong ion difference decreases and acidosis results.

In addition, the small intestine may contribute strong ions to the plasma. This effect is most apparent when mesenteric blood flow is compromised and lactate is produced, sometimes in large quantities, by the tissues of the small intestine.

METABOLIC ACIDOSIS

Traditionally, metabolic acidoses are categorized according to the presence or absence of unmeasured anions. The presence of unmeasured anions is routinely inferred by measuring the

TABLE 12–1. CAUSES OF AN INCREASED ANION GAP (AG)

Common Causes

Renal failure
Ketoacidosis
   Diabetic
   Alcoholic
   Starvation
   Metabolic errors
Lactic acidosis
Toxins
   Methanol
   Ethylene glycol
   Salicylates
   Paraldehyde
   Toluene

Rare Causes

Dehydration
Sodium salts
   Sodium lactate
   Sodium citrate
   Sodium acetate
   Sodium PCN (>50 m units/day)
   Carbenicillin (>30 g/day)
Decreased unmeasured cation
   Hypomagnesemia
   Hypokalemia
   Hypocalcemia
Alkalemia

TABLE 12–2. POTENTIAL CLINICAL EFFECTS OF METABOLIC ACID-BASE DISORDERS

Metabolic Acidosis	Metabolic Alkalosis
Cardiovascular	*Cardiovascular*
Decreased inotropy	Decreased inotropy (Ca^{++} entry)
Conduction defects	Altered coronary blood flow*
Arterial vasodilatation	Digoxin toxicity
Venous vasoconstriction	
Oxygen Delivery	*Neuromuscular*
Decreased oxy-Hb binding	Neuromuscular excitability
Decreased 2,3-DPG (late)	Encephalopathy seizures
Neuromuscular	*Metabolic Effects*
Respiratory depression	Hypokalemia
Decreased sensorium	Hypocalcemia
	Hypophosphatemia
	Impaired enzyme function
Metabolism	*Oxygen Delivery*
Protein wasting	Increased oxy-Hb affinity
Bone demineralization	Increased 2,3-DPG (delayed)
Catecholamine, PTH, and aldosterone stimulation	
Insulin resistance	
Free radical formation	
Gastrointestinal	
Emesis	
Gut barrier dysfunction	
Electrolytes	
Hyperkalemia	
Hypercalcemia	
Hyperuricemia	

*Animal studies have shown both increased and decreased coronary artery blood flow.

53

concentrations of electrolytes in plasma and calculating the anion gap, as described later. The differential diagnosis for a positive-anion gap acidosis is shown in Table 12-1. Non-anion gap acidoses can be divided into three types: renal, gastrointestinal, and iatrogenic (Fig. 12-1). In the intensive care unit (ICU), the most common types of metabolic acidosis include lactic acidosis, ketoacidosis, iatrogenic acidosis, and acidosis secondary to toxins.

The potential effects of metabolic acidosis and alkalosis on vital organ function are shown in Table 12-2. Metabolic and respiratory acidosis may have different implications with respect to survival, an observation that suggests that the underlying disorder is perhaps more important than the absolute degree of acidemia.[11]

If metabolic acidemia is to be treated, consideration should be given to the likely duration of the disorder. If it is expected to be short lived (e.g., diabetic ketoacidosis), maximizing respiratory compensation is usually the safest approach. Once the disorder resolves, ventilation can be quickly reduced to normal and there will be no lingering effects of therapy. However, if the disorder is likely to be more chronic (e.g., renal failure), therapy aimed at restoring the strong ion difference is indicated. In all cases, the therapeutic target can be quite accurately determined from the standard base-excess. As discussed, the standard base-excess corresponds to the amount the strong ion difference must change in order to restore the pH to 7.4, assuming a P_{CO_2} of 40 mm Hg. Thus, if the strong ion difference is 30 mEq/L and the standard base-excess is –10 mEq/L, the target strong ion difference would be 40 mEq/L. Accordingly, the plasma Na$^+$ concentration would have to increase by 10 mEq/L for NaHCO$_3$ administration to completely repair the acidosis. If increasing the plasma Na$^+$ concentration is inadvisable for other reasons (e.g., hypernatremia), then NaHCO$_3$ administration is also inadvisable. Importantly, NaHCO$_3$ administration has not been shown to improve outcome in patients with lactic acidosis.[12]

In addition, NaHCO$_3$ administration is associated with certain disadvantages. Large (hypertonic) doses given rapidly can lead to hypotension[13] and have the potential to cause a sudden, marked increase in Pa_{CO_2}.[14] Accordingly, it is important to assess the patient's ventilatory status before NaHCO$_3$ is administered, particularly in the absence of mechanical ventilation. NaHCO$_3$ infusion also affects circulating [K$^+$] and [Ca^{++}] concentrations, which need to be monitored closely.

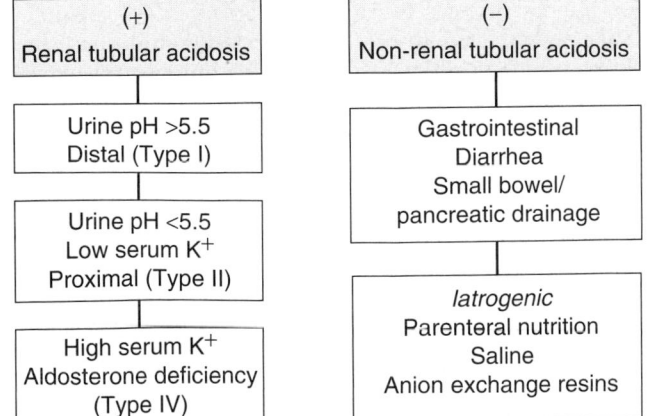

Urine SID (Na + K − Cl)

FIGURE 12–1. Differential diagnosis for a hyperchloremic metabolic acidosis. (SID, strong ion difference.)

Tromethamine (Tris-buffer or Tham) is an organic buffer that readily penetrates cells.[15] It is a weak base (pK = 7.9) that does not alter the strong ion difference and does not affect plasma [Na$^+$]. Accordingly, it is often used when administration of NaHCO$_3$ is contraindicated because of hypernatremia. This agent has been available since the 1960s, but limited data are available on its use in humans with acid-base disorders. In small uncontrolled studies, tromethamine appears to be effective in reversing metabolic acidosis secondary to ketoacidosis or renal failure without obvious toxicity.[16] However, adverse reactions have been reported, including hypoglycemia, respiratory depression, and even fatal hepatic necrosis when concentrations exceeding 0.3 *M* are used. In Europe, a mixture of tromethamine, acetate, NaHCO$_3$, and disodium phosphate is available (Tribonate). This mixture seems to have fewer side effects than tromethamine alone, but experience with Tribonate is still quite limited.

The Anion Gap and the Strong Ion Gap

For more than 30 years, the anion gap has been used by clinicians and it has evolved into a major tool to evaluate acid-base disorders.[17] The anion gap is estimated from the differences between the routinely measured concentrations of serum cations (Na$^+$ and K$^+$) and anions (Cl$^-$ and HCO$_3$). Normally, this difference, or "gap," is made up by albumin, and, to a lesser extent, by phosphate. Sulfate and lactate also contribute a small amount, normally less than 2 mEq/L. However, there are also unmeasured cations, such as Ca^{++} and Mg^{++}, and these tend to offset the effects of sulfate and lactate except when the concentration of sulfate or lactate is abnormally increased (Fig. 12-2). Plasma proteins other than albumin can be positively or negatively charged but in the aggregate tend to be neutral, except in rare cases of abnormal paraproteins such as in cases of multiple myeloma.[18] In practice, the anion gap (AG) is calculated as follows:

$$AG = ([Na^+] + [K^+]) - ([Cl^-] + [HCO_3^-])$$

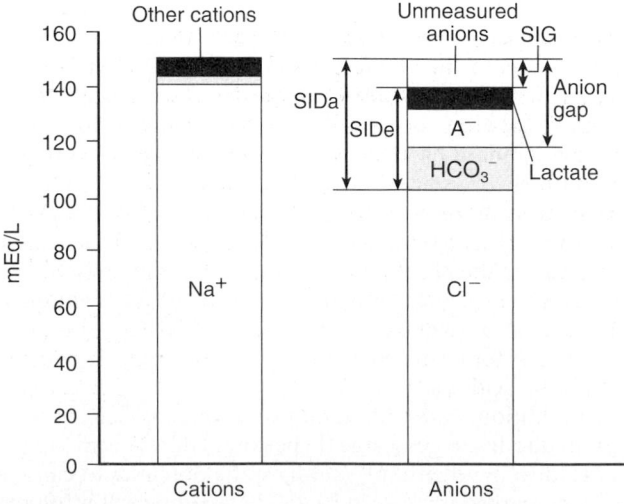

FIGURE 12–2. Charge balance in blood plasma. "Other cations" include Ca^{++} and Mg^{++}. The strong ion difference (SID) is always positive (in plasma) and SID – SIDe (effective) must equal zero. Any difference between SID apparent (SIDa) and SIDe is the strong ion gap (SIG) and must represent unmeasured anions.

Because of its low and narrow extracellular concentration range, K$^+$ is often omitted from the calculation. The normal value for anion gap is 12 ± 4 (if [K$^+$] is considered) or 8 ± 4 mEq/L (if [K$^+$] is not considered). The normal range has decreased in recent years following the introduction of more accurate methods for measuring Cl$^-$ concentration.[19,20] However, the various measurement techniques available mandate that each institution reports its own expected "normal anion gap."

The anion gap is useful because this parameter can limit the differential diagnosis for patients with metabolic acidosis. If the anion gap is increased, the explanation almost invariably will be found among five disorders: ketosis, lactic acidosis, poisoning, renal failure, or sepsis.[21] However, several conditions can alter the accuracy of anion gap estimation, and these conditions are particularly prevalent among patients with critical illness.[22,23] Dehydration can widen the apparent anion gap by increasing the concentration of all the ions used for the calculation. Hypoalbuminemia decreases the anion gap and has been recommended to "correct" the anion gap for changes in albumin concentration, because for every 1 g/dL decrease in serum albumin concentration, the apparent anion gap narrows by 2.5 to 3 mEq/L.[24] Respiratory and metabolic alkaloses are associated with an increase of up to 3 to 10 mEq/L in the apparent anion gap. The basis for this effect is enhanced lactate production (from stimulated phosphofructokinase enzymatic activity), reduction in the concentration of ionized weak acids (A$^-$), and, possibly, the additional effect of dehydration.

Other factors that can increase the anion gap are low Mg^{++} concentration and administration of the sodium salts of poorly reabsorbable anions (such as beta-lactam antibiotics).[25] Certain parenteral nutrition formulations, such as those containing acetate, may increase the anion gap. Citrate-based anticoagulants rarely can have the same effect after administration of multiple blood transfusions.[26] None of these rare causes, however, increases the anion gap significantly,[27] and they are usually easily identified. In recent years, some additional causes of an increased anion gap have been reported. It is sometimes widened in patients in non-ketotic hyperosmolar states induced by diabetes mellitus; the biochemical basis for this effect remains unexplained.[28] In recent years, unmeasured anions have been reported in the blood of patients with sepsis[29,30] and liver disease[31,32] and in experimental animals injected with endotoxin.[33] These anions may be the source of much of the unexplained acidosis seen in patients with critical illness.[34]

Additional doubt has been cast on the diagnostic value of the anion gap in certain situations, however.[22,30] Salem and Mujais[22] found routine reliance on the anion gap to be "fraught with numerous pitfalls." The primary problem with the anion gap is its reliance on the use of a "normal" range that depends on normal circulating levels of albumin and to a lesser extent phosphate, as discussed earlier. Plasma concentrations of albumin or phosphate are often grossly abnormal in patients with critical illness, leading to change in the "normal" range for the anion gap. Moreover, because these anions are not strong anions, their charge is affected by pH. These considerations have prompted some authors to adjust the "normal range" for the anion gap according to the albumin concentration[24] or phosphate concentration.[6] Each g/dL of albumin has a charge of 2.8 mEq/L at pH 7.4 (2.3 mEq/L at pH 7.0 and 3.0 mEq/L at pH 7.6). Each mg/dL of phosphate has a charge of 0.59 mEq/L at pH 7.4

(0.55 mEq/L at pH 7.0 and 0.61 mEq/L at pH 7.6). Thus, the "normal" anion gap can be estimated using this formula[6]:

$$\text{"normal" anion gap} = 2 \times [\text{albumin}] \text{ (g/dL)} + 0.5 \times [\text{phosphate}] \text{ (mg/dL)}$$

Or for international units:

$$\text{"normal" anion gap} = 0.2 \times [\text{albumin}] \text{ (g/L)} + 1.5 \times [\text{phosphate}] \text{ (mmol/L)}$$

These formulas only should be used when the pH is less than 7.35, and even then they are only accurate within 5 mEq/L. When more accuracy is needed, a slightly more complicated method of estimating [A⁻] is required.[31,35]

Another alternative to using the traditional anion gap is to use the strong ion difference. By definition, the strong ion difference must be equal and opposite to the negative charges contributed by [A⁻] and total CO_2. The sum of the charges from [A⁻] and total CO_2 concentration has been termed *strong ion difference effective*.[18] The *apparent strong ion difference* is obtained by measurement of each individual ion. Both the apparent strong ion difference and the strong ion difference effective should equal the true strong ion difference. If the apparent strong ion difference and strong ion difference effective differ, unmeasured ions must exist. If the apparent strong ion difference is greater than strong ion difference effective, these ions are anions and if the apparent strong ion difference is less than strong ion difference effective, the unmeasured ions are cations. This difference has been termed the strong ion gap to distinguish it from the anion gap.[31] Unlike the anion gap, the strong ion gap is normally zero and does not change with changes in pH or albumin concentration.

Positive Anion Gap Acidoses
Lactic Acidosis
In many forms of critical illness, lactate is the most important cause of metabolic acidosis.[36] Blood lactate concentration has been shown to correlate with outcome in patients with hemorrhagic[37] and septic shock.[38] Lactic acid has been viewed as the predominant source of metabolic acidosis due to sepsis.[39] In this view, lactic acid is released primarily from the musculature and the gut as a consequence of tissue hypoxia. Moreover, the amount of lactate produced is believed to correlate with the total oxygen debt, the magnitude of the hypoperfusion, and the severity of shock.[36] In recent years, this view has been challenged by the observation that during sepsis, even with profound shock, resting muscle does not produce lactate. Indeed, studies by various investigators have shown that the musculature actually may consume lactate during endotoxemia.[40-42] Data concerning the gut are less clear. There is little question that underperfused gut can release lactate; however, it does not appear that the gut releases lactate during sepsis if mesenteric perfusion is maintained. Under such conditions, the mesentery circulation can even become a net consumer of lactate.[40,41] Perfusion is likely to be a major determinant of mesenteric lactate metabolism. In a canine model of sepsis, gut lactate production could not be shown when flow was maintained with dopexamine hydrochloride.[42]

Studies in animals as well as humans have shown that the lung may be a prominent source of lactate in the setting of acute lung injury.[40,43-45] While studies such as these do not address the underlying pathophysiologic mechanisms of hyperlactatemia in sepsis, they suggest that using blood lactate concentration as evidence for tissue dysoxia is an oversimplification at best. Indeed, many investigators have begun to offer alternative interpretations of hyperlactatemia in this setting.[44-48] Table 12-3 lists several alternative sources of hyperlactatemia. In particular, pyruvate dehydrogenase, the enzyme responsible for moving pyruvate into the Krebs cycle, is inhibited by endotoxin.[49] However, data from recent studies suggest that increased aerobic metabolism may be more important than metabolic defects or anaerobic metabolism.[50] Finally, administration of epinephrine promotes lactic acidosis, presumably by stimulating cellular metabolism (e.g., increased hepatic glycolysis).

Administration of epinephrine may be a common cause of lactic acidosis in patients with critical illness.[51,52] Interestingly, this phenomenon does not occur when dobutamine or norepinephrine is infused[53] and does not appear to be related to decreased tissue perfusion.

Although controversy exists as to the source and interpretation of lactic acidosis in critically ill patients, there is no question about the ability of lactate accumulation to produce acidemia. Lactate is a strong ion by virtue of the fact that at a pH within the physiologic range, it is almost completely dissociated; for instance, the pKa for lactic acid is 3.9. Thus, at pH 7.4, 3162 lactic acid molecules are dissociated for every one that is not. Because the body can produce and dispose of lactate rapidly, it functions as one of the most dynamic components of the strong ion difference.

Plasma lactate concentration may be increased without an increase in [H⁺]. There are two possible explanations for this phenomenon. First, if lactate is added to the plasma, not as lactic acid but rather as the salt of a strong acid (e.g., sodium lactate), there will be little change in the strong ion difference. The strong ion difference does not change because a strong cation (Na⁺) is being added along with a strong anion. However, only if a very large amount of lactate is infused rapidly will there be an appreciable increase in the plasma lactate concentration. For example, the use of lactate-based hemofiltration fluid can result in hyperlactatemia with an *increased* plasma HCO_3^- concentration and pH.

TABLE 12–3. MECHANISMS ASSOCIATED WITH INCREASED SERUM LACTATE CONCENTRATION

Tissue Hypoxia

Hypodynamic shock
Organ ischemia

Hypermetabolism

Increased aerobic glycolysis
Increased protein catabolism
Hematologic malignancies

Decreased Clearance of Lactate

Liver failure
Shock

Inhibition of Pyruvate Dehydrogenase

Thiamine deficiency
Endotoxin?

Activation of Inflammatory Cells?

A more important mechanism whereby hyperlactatemia exists without acidemia (or with less acidemia than expected) is when the strong ion difference is corrected by the elimination of another strong anion from the plasma.[54] In the setting of sustained lactic acidosis induced by lactic acid infusion, Cl^- moves out of the plasma space, thus normalizing pH. Under these conditions, hyperlactatemia may persist but base-excess may be normalized by compensatory mechanisms to restore the strong ion difference.

Traditionally, lactic acidosis is subdivided into type A, in which the mechanism is tissue hypoxia, and type B, in which there is no hypoxia.[55] However, this distinction may be artificial. Some disorders, such as sepsis, may be associated with lactic acidosis due to a variety of mechanisms (Table 12-3), some of the "A" type and some of the "B" type. A potentially useful method of distinguishing anaerobically produced lactate from other sources is to measure the blood pyruvate concentration. The normal lactate to pyruvate ratio is 10:1.[56] A lactate-to-pyruvate ratio greater than 25:1 is considered to be evidence of anaerobic metabolism.[48] This approach makes biochemical sense, because pyruvate is reduced to lactate during anaerobic metabolism, thereby increasing the lactate-to-pyruvate ratio. Unfortunately, pyruvate is very unstable in solution and therefore is difficult to measure accurately in the clinical setting, greatly reducing the clinical utility of lactate/pyruvate determinations.

Treatment of lactic acidosis remains controversial. The only noncontroversial approach is to treat the underlying cause. The use of sodium bicarbonate ($NaHCO_3$) is equally controversial and remains of unproven value.[12]

Ketoacidosis

Another common cause of a metabolic acidosis with a positive anion gap is ketoacidosis. Ketones are formed by beta-oxidation of fatty acids, a process that is inhibited by insulin. In insulin-deficient states, ketone formation increases substantially. The accumulation of ketone bodies (acetone, β-hydroxybutyrate, and acetoacetate) in the plasma is exacerbated because elevated blood glucose concentrations promote an osmotic diuresis, leading to intravascular volume contraction. This state is associated with elevated circulating cortisol and catecholamine levels, which further stimulates free fatty acid production.[57] In addition, increased glucagon levels, relative to insulin levels, decreases intracellular concentrations of malonyl co-enzyme A and increases the activity of carnitine palmityl acyl transferase, effects that promote ketogenesis.

Both acetoacetate and β-hydroxybutyrate are strong anions (pKa 3.8 and 4.8, respectively).[58] Thus, like lactate, the presence of these ions decreases the strong ion difference and increases the $[H^+]$. Ketoacidosis may result from diabetes (diabetic ketoacidosis) or excessive alcohol consumption (alcoholic ketoacidosis). The diagnosis is established by measuring serum ketone levels. However, it is important to understand that the nitroprusside reaction only measures acetone and acetoacetate, and not β-hydroxybutyrate. Thus, the state of measured ketosis is dependent on the ratio of acetoacetate to β-hydroxybutyrate. This ratio is low when lactic acidosis coexists with ketoacidosis because the reduced redox state of lactic acidosis favors production of β-hydroxybutyrate.[59] In this circumstance, the apparent level of ketosis is small relative to the amount of acidosis and the elevation of the anion gap. There is also a risk of confusion during treatment of ketoacidosis because ketones as measured by the nitroprusside reaction can increase despite resolving

acidosis. This effect occurs as a result of rapid clearance of β-hydroxybutyrate, improving acid-base balance without changing the measured level of ketosis. Furthermore, circulating ketone levels can even appear to increase as β-hydroxybutyrate is converted to acetoacetate. Hence, it is better to monitor therapy by measuring blood pH and anion gap than by assaying levels of serum ketones.

Treatment of diabetic ketoacidosis includes infusing insulin and large amounts of fluid; 0.9% saline is usually recommended. Potassium replacement is often required as well. Fluid resuscitation reverses the hormonal stimuli for ketone body formation, as discussed earlier, and insulin promotes metabolism of ketones and glucose. Administration of $NaHCO_3$ may produce a more rapid rise in the pH by increasing the strong ion difference, but there is little evidence that this effect is desirable. Furthermore, because increasing the plasma Na^+ concentration increases the strong ion difference, the strong ion difference will be too high once the ketosis is cleared ("overshoot" alkalosis). In any case, administration of $NaHCO_3$ is rarely necessary and should be avoided except in extreme cases.[60]

A more common problem in the treatment of diabetic ketoacidosis is persistence of acidemia after resolution of ketosis. This hyperchloremic metabolic acidosis occurs as Cl^- replaces ketoacids, thus maintaining decreases in strong ion difference and pH. This effect appears to occur for two reasons. First, exogenous Cl^- is often provided in the form of 0.9% saline, which, if given in large enough quantities, results in a so-called dilutional acidosis (see later). Second, renal Cl^- reabsorption increases as ketones are excreted in the urine. Increases in the tubular Na^+ load produce electrical-chemical forces favoring Cl^- reabsorption.[61]

The acidosis seen in patients with alcoholic ketoacidosis is usually less severe. Treatment consists of intravenous fluid administration and infusion of glucose, instead of insulin, as would be the case with diabetic ketoacidosis.[62] Indeed, insulin is contraindicated, because it may cause precipitous hypoglycemia.[63] Thiamine also must be given to avoid precipitating Wernicke's encephalopathy.

Renal Failure

Renal failure, especially when chronic, leads to accumulation of sulfates and other acids, widening the anion gap, although this increase usually is not large.[64] Similarly, uncomplicated renal failure rarely produces severe acidosis, except when it is accompanied by a high rate of acid generation, such as occurs during hypermetabolism.[65] In all cases, the strong ion difference is decreased and remains so unless some therapy is provided. Hemodialysis removes sulfate and other ions and allows normal Na^+ and Cl^- balance to be restored, thus returning the strong ion difference to normal (or near normal). However, patients not yet requiring dialysis and those who are between treatments often require some other therapy to increase the strong ion difference. $NaHCO_3$ is used as long as the plasma Na^+ concentration is not already elevated.

Toxins

Metabolic acidosis with an increased anion gap is a major feature of various types of drug and substance intoxications (see Table 12-1).

Other and Unknown Causes

In the nonketotic hyperosmolar state associated with poorly controlled diabetes, the anion gap widens for unexplained reasons.[28] Even when very careful methods are applied, using the strong ion gap or similar strategies, unmeasured anions have been detected in the blood of patients with sepsis[29,30] and liver disease[31] and in experimental animals given endotoxin.[32] Furthermore, unknown cations also appear in the blood of some critically ill patients.[30] The significance of these findings remains to be determined.

Non-Anion Gap (Hyperchloremic) Acidoses

Hyperchloremic metabolic acidosis occurs as a result of either the increase in [Cl⁻] relative to strong cations, especially Na⁺, or the loss of cations with retention of Cl⁻. As seen in Figure 12-1, these disorders can be separated by history and by measurement of urinary Cl⁻ concentration. When acidosis occurs, the normal response by the kidney is to increase Cl⁻ excretion. Failure to do so identifies the kidney as the problem. Extrarenal causes of hyperchloremic acidosis are exogenous Cl⁻ loads (iatrogenic acidosis) or loss of cations from the lower gastrointestinal tract without proportional losses of Cl⁻.

Renal Tubular Acidosis

Examination of the urine and plasma electrolytes and pH and calculation of the urine apparent strong ion difference allow one to correctly diagnose most cases of renal tubular acidosis (see Fig. 12-1).[66] However, caution must be exercised when the plasma pH is greater than 7.35, because urinary Cl⁻ excretion is normally decreased when pH is this high. In such circumstances, it may be necessary to infuse sodium sulfate or furosemide. These agents stimulate Cl⁻ and K⁺ excretion and can be used to unmask the defect and probe K⁺ secretory capacity.

The defect in all types of renal tubular acidosis is an inability to excrete Cl⁻ in proportion to Na⁺, although the reasons vary by type. Treatment largely depends on whether the kidney responds to mineralocorticoid replacement or whether there are losses of Na⁺ that can be replaced as NaHCO₃.

Classic distal (type I) renal tubular acidosis responds to NaHCO₃ replacement; typically, only 50 to 100 mEq/day are required. Defects in K⁺ reabsorption are also common in this type of renal tubular acidosis and K⁺ replacement is also required. A variant of the classic distal renal tubular acidosis is a hyperkalemic form that actually is more common than the classic type. The central defect here appears to be impaired Na⁺ transport in the cortical collecting duct. These patients also respond to NaHCO₃ replacement. Proximal (type II) renal tubular acidosis is characterized by both Na⁺ and K⁺ reabsorption defects. The disorder is uncommon and usually appears as a component of Fanconi's syndrome, which also is characterized by defects in the reabsorption of glucose, phosphate, urate, and amino acids.

Treatment of this disorder with NaHCO₃ is ineffective because increased ion delivery merely results in increased excretion. Thiazide diuretics have been used to treat this disorder, with varying success.

Type IV renal tubular acidosis is caused by aldosterone deficiency or resistance. These disorders are diagnosed by the presence of high serum [K⁺] concentration and low urine pH (<5.5). Treatment is usually most effective if the cause can be removed; most commonly, drugs, such as nonsteroidal anti-inflammatory agents, heparin, or potassium-sparing diuretics, are responsible. Occasionally, mineralo-corticoid replacement is required.

Gastrointestinal Acidosis

Fluid secreted into the gut lumen contains higher amounts of Na⁺ than Cl⁻. Large losses of these fluids, particularly if volume is replaced with fluids containing equal amounts of Na⁺ and Cl⁻, results in a decrease in the plasma Na⁺ concentration relative to the Cl⁻ concentration and a decrease in strong ion difference. Such a scenario can be avoided if formulations such as lactated Ringer's solution are used instead of normal saline to replace gastrointestinal losses.

Iatrogenic Acidosis

Two of the most common causes of a hyperchloremic metabolic acidosis are iatrogenic and both are due to administration of Cl⁻. Modern parenteral nutrition formulas contain weak anions, such as acetate, in addition to Cl⁻. The proportions of each anion can be adjusted depending on the acid-base status of the patient. If an insufficient amount of weak anions is provided, the plasma Cl⁻ concentration increases, decreasing the strong ion difference and resulting in acidosis. A similar condition can arise when normal saline is used for fluid resuscitation, resulting in the development of "dilutional acidosis." Dilutional acidosis was first described more than 40 years ago,[67,68] although some authors have argued that this problem is rarely clinically significant.[69] This view pertains because large doses of NaCl produce only minor degrees of hyperchloremic acidosis in healthy animals.[70] This line of reasoning cannot be applied to critically ill patients, who often require infusion of a very large volume of resuscitation fluid. Furthermore, acid-base balance is often already deranged in critically ill patients, and these patients may not be able to compensate normally by increasing ventilation or may have abnormal buffer capacity due to hypoalbuminemia. In intensive care unit and surgical patients[71-73] as well as in animals with experimental sepsis,[74] saline-induced acidosis clearly occurs.

Administration of normal saline causes acidosis because this solution contains equal amounts of Na⁺ and Cl⁻, whereas the normal Na⁺ concentration in plasma is 35 to 45 mEq/L greater than the normal Cl⁻ concentration. Administration of 0.9% saline increases the Cl⁻ concentration relatively more than the Na⁺ concentration. Many critically ill patients have a significantly lower strong ion difference than do healthy individuals, even when there is no evidence of a metabolic acid-base derangement.[75] The lower strong ion difference in critical illness is not surprising given that the positive charge of the strong ion difference is balanced by the negative charges of A⁻ and total CO₂. Since many critically ill patients are hypoalbuminemic, A⁻ tends to be reduced. Because the body defends PCO₂ for other reasons, a reduction in A⁻ leads to a reduction in strong ion difference to maintain normal pH. Thus, a typical intensive care unit patient might have a strong ion difference of 30 mEq/L rather than 40 to 42 mEq/L. If this same patient then develops a metabolic acidosis (e.g., lactic acidosis), the strong ion difference decreases further. If the patient is resuscitated with a large volume of 0.9% saline, metabolic acidosis is exacerbated. This relationship is illustrated in Figure 12-3, which shows that a patient with a lower baseline strong ion difference is more susceptible to a subsequent acid load.

One alternative to using normal saline to resuscitate patients is to use Ringer's lactate solution. This fluid contains a more physiologic difference between [Na⁺] and [Cl⁻] and thus its strong ion difference is closer to normal (28 mEq/L as compared to 0 mEq/L for normal saline). Morgan and

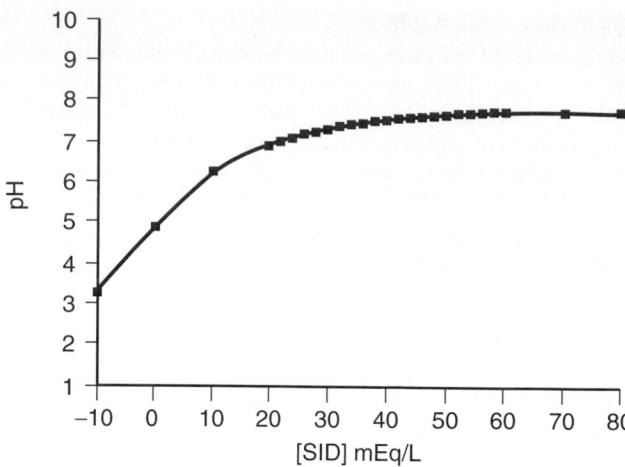

FIGURE 12–3. Plot of pH versus strong ion difference (SID). For this plot, A_{TOT} and P_{CO_2} were held constant at 18 mEq/L and 40 mm Hg, respectively. This plot assumes a water dissociation constant for blood of 4.4×10^{-14} (Eq/L). Note how steep the pH curve becomes at SID < 20 mEq/L.

TABLE 12–4. DIFFERENTIAL DIAGNOSIS OF A METABOLIC ALKALOSIS (INCREASED STRONG ION DIFFERENCE)

Chloride Loss < Sodium

Chloride-responsive (urine Cl⁻ concentration <10 mmol/L)
  Gastrointestinal losses
  Vomiting
  Gastric drainage
  Chloride wasting diarrhea (villous adenoma)
  Post-diuretic use
  Post-hypercapnea
Chloride-unresponsive (urine Cl⁻ concentration >20 mmol/L)
  Mineralocorticoid excess
  Primary hyperaldosteronism (Conn's syndrome)
  Secondary hyperaldosteronism
Cushing's syndrome
Liddle's syndrome
Bartter's syndrome
  Exogenous corticoids
  Excessive licorice intake
  Ongoing diuretic use

Exogenous Sodium Load (>Chloride)

Sodium salt administration (acetate, citrate)
  Massive blood transfusions
  Parenteral nutrition
  Plasma volume expanders
  Sodium lactate (Ringer's solution)

Other

Severe deficiency of intracellular cations
  Magnesium, potassium

colleagues recently showed that a solution with a strong ion difference of approximately 24 mEq/L results in a neutral effect on the pH as blood is progressively diluted.[76]

Unexplained Hyperchloremic Acidosis

Critically ill patients sometimes manifest hyperchloremic metabolic acidosis for unclear reasons. Often these patients have other coexisting types of metabolic acidosis, making the precise diagnosis difficult. Patients with sepsis and acidosis frequently have normal circulating lactate levels.[77] Often, unexplained anions are the cause,[29-31] but hyperchloremic acidosis also can be a contributing factor.

METABOLIC ALKALOSIS

Metabolic alkalosis occurs as a result of an increase in strong ion difference or a decrease in A_{TOT}. These changes can occur secondary to the loss of anions (e.g., Cl⁻ from the stomach, albumin from the plasma) or the retention of cations (rare). Sometimes the loss of Cl⁻ is temporary and can be treated effectively by replacing the anion; metabolic alkalosis in this category is said to be "chloride responsive." In other cases, hormonal mechanisms produce ongoing losses of Cl⁻. Thus, at best, the Cl⁻ deficit can be offset only temporarily by Cl⁻ administration; this form of metabolic alkalosis is said to be "chloride resistant" (Table 12-4). Similar to hyperchloremic acidosis, these disorders can be distinguished by measurement of the urine Cl⁻ concentration.

Chloride-Responsive Disorders

The chloride-responsive disorders usually occur as a result of Cl⁻ losses from the stomach, such as from vomiting or gastric drainage. The treatment is to replace the Cl⁻, which can be achieved slowly with NaCl or more rapidly with KCl or even HCl. Saline plus KCl is the treatment of choice because volume depletion and K⁺ usually coexist with the acid-base disturbance in patients with chloride-responsive metabolic alkalosis. Dehydration in turn stimulates aldosterone secretion, leading to increased tubular Na⁺ reabsorption and increased urinary losses of K⁺. Administration of normal saline is effective because the administration of equal amounts of Na⁺ and Cl⁻ result in larger relative increases in Cl⁻ concentration

compared to Na⁺ concentration. In rare circumstances, when neither K⁺ nor intravascular volume depletion is a problem, it may be desirable to give back Cl⁻ as HCl.

Diuretics and other forms of volume contraction produce metabolic alkalosis predominantly by stimulating aldosterone secretion, as discussed earlier. However, diuretics also induce K⁺ and Cl⁻ excretion directly, further complicating the problem and inducing metabolic alkalosis more rapidly.

Chloride-Resistant Disorders

The chloride-resistant disorders (see Table 12-4) are characterized by an increased urine Cl⁻ concentration (>20 mEq/L) and are said to be "chloride resistant" because of ongoing Cl⁻ losses. Most commonly, excessive chloride occurs as a result of excessive mineralocorticoid activity. Treatment requires that the underlying disorder be addressed (Table 12-5).

Other Causes of Metabolic Alkalosis

Rarely, an increased strong ion difference and therefore metabolic alkalosis occurs secondary to cation administration rather than anion depletion. Examples of these disorders include milk-alkali syndrome and intravenous administration of strong cations without strong anions. The latter occurs with massive blood transfusion because Na⁺ is given with citrate (a weak anion) instead of Cl⁻. Similar results occur when parenteral nutrition formulations contain too much acetate and not enough Cl⁻ to balance the Na⁺ load.

RESPIRATORY ACID-BASE DISORDERS

Respiratory disorders are far easier to diagnose and treat than metabolic disorders because the mechanism is always the same, although the underlying disease process may vary.

TABLE 12–5. TREATMENT OF METABOLIC ALKALOSIS

Condition	Treatment
Primary aldosteronism	Spironolactone or other agents that block distal tubular sodium reabsorption improve alkalosis, hyokalemia, and hypertension. Large doses may be necessary. Restriction of sodium intake and potassium supplementation may be necessary. When an adenoma can be identified, surgery is curative. When the cause is bilateral adrenal cortical hyperplasia, therapy is medical. Dexamethasone is effective in long-term therapy of familial dexamethasone-responsive aldosteronism.
Secondary aldosteronism	Angiotensin-converting enzyme inhibitors are usually effective. Repair of the underlying lesion, if feasible, may be required.
Cushing's syndrome	Due to pituitary oversecretion of ACTH: surgery or radiation Due to adrenal adenoma or carcinoma: adrenalectomy Due to secondary or ectopic ACTH production: address the underlying malignancy
Liddle's syndrome	Triamterene may be effective.
Bartter's syndrome	Treatment often unsatisfactory long-term. Potassium-sparing diuretics, potassium and magnesium supplementation, angiotensin-converting enzyme inhibitors, cyclooxygenase inhibitors are partially effective.
Exogenous corticoids	Discontinuation of the offending agent(s) and vigorous initial potassium replacement.
Severe K or Mg depletion	Replacement of these electrolytes (may require very large amounts).

From Spital and Garella[23] with permission.

CO_2 is produced by cellular metabolism or by the titration of HCO_3^- by metabolic acids. Normally, alveolar ventilation is adjusted to maintain the arterial $PaCO_2$ between 35 and 45 mm Hg. When alveolar ventilation is increased or decreased out of proportion to $PaCO_2$ production, a respiratory acid-base disorder exists.

Pathophysiology of Respiratory Acid-Base Disorders

Normal CO_2 production by the body (about 220 mL/min) is equivalent to 15,000 mM/day of carbonic acid.[78] This amount compares to less than 500 mM/day for all nonrespiratory acids that are handled by the kidney and gut. Pulmonary ventilation is adjusted by the respiratory center in response to changes in $PaCO_2$, blood pH, and PaO_2 as well as other factors (e.g., exercise, anxiety, wakefulness). Normal $PaCO_2$ (40 mm Hg) is maintained by precise matching of alveolar minute ventilation to metabolic CO_2 production. $PaCO_2$ changes in compensation for alterations in arterial pH produced by metabolic acidosis or alkalosis in predictable ways (Table 12-6).

Respiratory Acidosis

When CO_2 elimination is inadequate relative to the rate of tissue production, $PaCO_2$ increases to a new steady state determined by the new relationship between alveolar ventilation and CO_2 production. Acutely, the increase in $PaCO_2$ increases both the $[H^+]$ and the $[HCO_3^-]$ in blood according to the carbonic acid equilibrium equation. Thus, the change in $[HCO_3^-]$ is mediated simply by the dissociation of H_2CO_3 into H^+ and HCO_3^-, not by an active physiologic adaptation response. Similarly, the increase in $[HCO_3^-]$ does not "buffer" the increase in $[H^+]$. There is no change in the strong ion difference and hence no change in standard base-excess. Cellular acidosis always occurs in respiratory acidosis, since CO_2 builds up in the tissues. If the $PaCO_2$ remains increased, active compensatory mechanisms are activated and the strong ion difference increases to restore $[H^+]$ toward normal.

Primarily, compensation is accomplished by removal of Cl^- from the plasma space. Since movement of Cl^- into the tissues or red blood cells results in intracellular acidosis, Cl^- must be removed from the body to achieve a lasting effect on the strong ion difference. The kidney is the primary organ for Cl^- removal, although the adaptive capacity of the gastrointestinal tract for Cl^- elimination has not been fully explored. Accordingly, patients with renal disease have a difficult time adapting to chronic respiratory acidosis. When renal function is intact, Cl^- is eliminated in the urine and, after a few days, the strong ion difference increases to the level necessary to return blood pH to about 7.35. It is unclear whether this amount of time is required by the physiologic constraints of the system or to avoid being overly sensitive to transient changes in alveolar ventilation. In any case, this adaptation results in an increased pH for any degree of hypercarbia. According to the Henderson-Hasselbalch equation, the increased pH will result in an increased $[HCO_3^-]$

TABLE 12–6. OBSERVATIONAL ACID-BASE PATTERNS

Disorder	HCO₃⁻ (mEq/L)	Pco₂ (mm Hg)	SBE (mEq/L)
Metabolic acidosis	<22	$= (1.5 \times HCO_3^-) + 8$ $= 40 + SBE$	< -5
Metabolic alkalosis	>26	$= (0.7 \times HCO_3^-) + 21$ $= 40 + (0.6 \times SBE)$	$> +5$
Acute respiratory acidosis	$= [(P_{CO_2} - 40)/10] + 24$	>45	$= 0$
Chronic respiratory acidosis	$= [(P_{CO_2} - 40)/3] + 24$	>45	$= 0.4 \times (P_{CO_2} - 40)$
Acute respiratory alkalosis	$= [(40 - P_{CO_2})/5] + 24$	<35	$= 0$
Chronic respiratory alkalosis	$= [(40 - P_{CO_2})/2] + 24$	<35	$= 0.4 \times (P_{CO_2} - 40)$

From Kellum,[6] with permission.

for a given P_{CO_2}. Thus, the "adaptive" increase in $[HCO_3^-]$ *results from* the increase in pH and is not the *cause for* the increase in pH.

Although the change in HCO_3^- concentration is a convenient and reliable marker for the metabolic compensation, it is not the mechanism. This point is more than semantic because only changes in the independent variables of acid base balance (P_{CO_2}, A_{TOT}, strong ion difference) can affect the plasma $[H^+]$, and $[HCO_3^-]$ is not an independent variable.

Diseases of Ventilatory Impairment

As for virtually all acid-base disorders, treatment begins with addressing the underlying disorder. Acute respiratory acidosis can be caused by central nervous system suppression, neuromuscular disease or impairment (e.g., myasthenia gravis, hypophosphatemia, hypokalemia), or airway and parenchymal lung disease (e.g., asthma, acute respiratory distress syndrome). This last category of conditions also produces primary hypoxia, not just alveolar hypoventilation. The two can be distinguished by the alveolar gas equation:

$$P_{AO_2} = P_{IO_2} - P_{aCO_2}/R$$

where R is the respiratory exchange coefficient (generally assumed to be 0.8) and P_{IO_2} is the inspired oxygen tension (room air is approximately 150). Thus, as P_{aCO_2} increases, the P_{AO_2} will decrease in a predictable fashion. If the P_{AO_2} is reduced further, there is a defect in gas exchange.

Chronic respiratory acidosis is most often caused by chronic lung disease (e.g., chronic obstructive lung disease) or chest wall disease (e.g., kyphoscoliosis). Rarely, its cause is central hypoventilation or chronic neuromuscular disease.

When and How to Treat

The primary threat to life in cases of respiratory acidosis comes not from acidosis but from hypoxemia. If the patient is breathing room air, P_{aCO_2} cannot exceed 80 mm Hg before life-threatening hypoxemia results. Accordingly, supplemental oxygen is always required, although, unfortunately, oxygen administration alone is almost never sufficient treatment, and the defect in ventilation must be addressed directly. When the underlying cause can be addressed quickly (e.g., reversal of narcotics with naloxone), it may be possible to avoid endotracheal intubation. More often, however, mechanical ventilation must be initiated. Mechanical support is indicated when the patient is unstable or at risk for instability or when central nervous system function deteriorates. Furthermore, in patients who are exhibiting signs of respiratory muscle fatigue, mechanical ventilation should be instituted before overt respiratory failure occurs. Thus, it is not the absolute P_{aCO_2} value that is important but rather the clinical condition of the patient.

Chronic hypercapnia requires treatment when there is an acute deterioration. In this setting, it is important to recognize that the goal of therapy is not a normal value for P_{aCO_2} (35-45 mm Hg) but rather restoration of the patient's baseline P_{aCO_2} (if known). If the baseline P_{aCO_2} is not known, a target P_{aCO_2} of 60 mm Hg is reasonable. Overventilation has two undesirable consequences. First, life-threatening alkalemia can occur if the P_{aCO_2} is rapidly normalized in a patient with chronic respiratory acidosis and an appropriately large strong ion difference. Second, even if the P_{aCO_2} is corrected slowly, the patient will reduce the plasma strong ion difference over time, making it impossible to wean the patient from mechanical ventilation.

Noninvasive ventilation is another treatment option that is useful in selected patients, particularly those with normal sensorium.[79] Rapid infusion of $NaHCO_3$ in patients with respiratory acidosis can induce acute respiratory failure if alveolar ventilation is not increased to adjust for the increased CO_2 load. Thus, if $NaHCO_3$ is used, it must be administered slowly and alveolar ventilation adjusted appropriately. Furthermore, as discussed previously, $NaHCO_3$ works by increasing the plasma $[Na^+]$. If this is not possible or not desirable, $NaHCO_3$ should be avoided.

Occasionally, it is useful to reduce CO_2 production, which can be achieved by reducing the carbohydrate load in the nutritional support regimen, lowering the temperature in febrile patients, and providing adequate sedation for anxious or combative patients. Treatment of shivering in the postoperative period can reduce CO_2 production. However, it is unusual to control hypercarbia with these techniques alone.

Permissive Hypercapnia

In recent years, there has been increased recognition of ventilator-associated lung injury. Accordingly, a strategy designed to reduce minute ventilation and hence increase P_{aCO_2}, so-called permissive hypercapnia or controlled hypoventilation, has been increasingly employed.[11] However, permissive hypercapnia is not without risks. Sedation is mandatory and the use of neuromuscular blocking agents is frequently required. Hypercapnia is associated with increased intracranial pressure and pulmonary hypertension, making this technique unusable in patients with brain injury or right ventricular dysfunction. Controversy exists as to how low to allow the pH to go. While some authors have reported good results with pH values less than 7.0,[11] most authors advocate more modest pH reductions (>7.25).

Respiratory Alkalosis

Respiratory alkalosis may be the most frequently encountered acid-base disorder. It occurs in a number of pathologic conditions, including salicylate intoxication, early sepsis, hepatic failure, and hypoxic respiratory disorders. Respiratory alkalosis also occurs with pregnancy and with pain or anxiety. Hypocapnia appears to be a particularly bad prognostic indicator in patients with critical illness.[80] As in acute respiratory acidosis, acute respiratory alkalosis results in a small change in $[HCO_3^-]$ as dictated by the Henderson-Hasselbalch equation. If hypocapnia persists, the strong ion difference will begin to decrease as a result of renal Cl^- reabsorption. After 2 to 3 days, the strong ion difference assumes a new, lower, steady state.[81] Severe alkalemia is unusual in patients with respiratory alkalosis, and management is therefore directed to the underlying cause. Typically, these mild acid-base changes are clinically more important for what they can alert the clinician to, in terms of underlying disease, than for any threat they pose to the patient. In rare cases, respiratory depression with narcotics is necessary.

Pseudorespiratory Alkalosis

The presence of arterial hypocapnia in patients with profound circulatory shock has been termed *pseudorespiratory alkalosis*.[82] This condition can be seen when alveolar ventilation is supported but the circulation is grossly inadequate. In such conditions, the mixed venous P_{CO_2} is significantly elevated but the arterial P_{CO_2} is normal or even decreased secondary to decreased CO_2 delivery to the lungs and increased pulmonary transit time. Overall CO_2 clearance is markedly decreased and there is marked tissue acidosis, usually involving both metabolic and respiratory components. The metabolic component comes from tissue hypoperfusion and hyperlactatemia. Arterial oxygen saturation also may appear to be adequate despite tissue hypoxemia. This condition is rapidly fatal unless cardiac output is rapidly corrected.

UNIFIED APPROACH TO THE PATIENT WITH ACID-BASE IMBALANCE

CHARACTERIZING THE DISORDER

The first step in the approach to a patient with an acid-base imbalance is to characterize the disorder. Acid-base imbalances are usually recognized by abnormalities in the venous plasma electrolyte concentrations, so it is useful to start there. Measurement of venous $[HCO_3^-]$ is the easiest way to screen for acid-base disorders. However, a normal $[HCO_3^-]$ does not exclude the possibility of an acid-base derangement, even a serious one. Therefore, if the history and physical examination findings lead one to suspect a disease process that results in an acid-base imbalance, more investigation is required. The normal $[HCO_3^-]$ is 22 to 26 mEq/L. Increases in $[HCO_3^-]$ occur with primary and compensatory metabolic alkaloses and decreases occur with primary or compensatory metabolic acidoses. Unfortunately, in mixed disorders, $[HCO_3^-]$ may be misleading and the presence of any abnormality in $[HCO_3^-]$ requires further investigation. In addition to examining the $[HCO_3^-]$, venous blood can be used to calculate the anion gap: $([Na^+] + [K^+]) - ([Cl^-] - [HCO_3^-])$. If $[HCO_3^-]$ or the anion gap are abnormal or if there is clinical suspicion for a mixed disorder, arterial blood should be sampled for blood gas analysis. This test will provide information on the pH, Pa_{CO_2}, and standard base-excess. Although simple disorders will conform to the equations presented in Table 12-6, "mixed" disorders are quite common.

In patients with acidemia, the next step is to examine the anion gap. The anion gap should also be examined when there is suspicion of an occult metabolic acidosis even in a patient with alkalemia. However, severe alkalemia will increase the anion gap by 2 to 4 mEq/L and hence wider "tolerance limits" should be used. If the anion gap is calculated from an alkalemic blood sample, only significant abnormalities (>8-10 mEq/L above normal) should be considered important. More often, however, it is not excessive sensitivity but rather insensitivity that plagues the anion gap calculation. The accuracy of the anion gap can be improved easily by using a patient-specific normal range, rather than a standard one. If unmeasured anions are detected, it is a good idea to compare their amounts to the abnormality in standard base-excess. For example, if the calculated anion gap is 5 mEq/L greater than expected and the standard base-excess is −15 mEq/L, a mixed metabolic acidosis is present. The unmeasured anions (e.g., ketones) are accounting for a standard base-excess of −5 mEq/L while some other process is responsible for another 10 mEq/L. This sort of abnormality can occur if very large amounts of 0.9% saline are used to treat a patient with diabetic ketoacidosis. As the ketosis resolves, the acidosis persists because the strong ion difference has been decreased due to excessive Cl^- administration.

DETERMINING THE CAUSE

Once the disorder has been characterized, the clinician must integrate the information obtained from the history and physical examination to arrive at an accurate diagnosis. Mixed disorders continue to be problematic, as any acid-base disorder that fails to fit into the classification scheme shown in Table 12-5 can be considered a mixed disorder, but some mixed disorders appear to be simple disorders when first encountered. For example, a patient with chronic respiratory acidosis and a Pa_{CO_2} of 60 mm Hg would be expected to have a standard base-excess of +8 mEq/L (see Table 12-6). If this patient develops a metabolic acidosis, the standard base-excess will decrease and may be 0 mEq/L. At this point, it may appear that the patient has a pure, acute respiratory acidosis rather that a mixed disorder. If the metabolic acidosis causes an increase in the anion gap, this abnormality may provide a clue. Another useful method is to obtain at least two blood gas analyses to examine for trends. In general, however, it is only by careful attention to history and physical examination that the true diagnosis can be made.

Chapter 13

HYPERNATREMIA AND HYPONATREMIA

John K. McIlwaine • Howard L. Corwin

Disorders of plasma sodium concentration—hyponatremia and hypernatremia—are among the most common clinical problems observed in the critically ill. These disorders are often asymptomatic; however, in some patients, they may result in symptoms ranging from minor to life threatening. The approach to treating these disorders in individual patients involves balancing the risk of treatment versus the risk of the disorder itself.

HYPERNATREMIA

Hypernatremia is a common clinical problem, being observed in up to 2% of the general hospital population and 15% of patients admitted to the intensive care unit.[1-4] In the outpatient setting, hypernatremia is most prevalent in the geriatric patient population; however, hypernatremia in hospitalized patients is observed in all age groups.[1,5] Mortality rates in patients with hypernatremia can range as high as 70%.[1-6] Although this high mortality rate no doubt reflects the severity of underlying disease in these patients, there is significant morbidity related to hypernatremia itself. Neurologic sequelae from hypernatremia are common, particularly in the pediatric population.[6]

The maintenance of a normal serum sodium concentration (135 to 145 mEq/L) is dependent on the balance between water intake and water excretion. Hypernatremia results from a deficit of free water that leads to an increase in serum tonicity. The usual mechanism underlying the development of hypernatremia is inadequate water intake and increased free water loss. However, hypernatremia also can result from the intake of hypertonic sodium solutions. Hypernatremia may be associated with volume depletion, euvolemia, or hypervolemia, depending on the balance of salt and water loss and intake. Sodium content is low, normal, or high, respectively, in each of these circumstances. Relative sodium and volume status has important implications for the treatment of patients with hypernatremia.

The brain is particularly susceptible to the effects of hypernatremia. The acute increase in extracellular tonicity as a result of the hypernatremia results in intracellular dehydration as water moves across the cell membrane to maintain osmotic equilibrium. The net result is a loss of brain volume, which in turn places mechanical stress on cerebral vessels. This mechanical stress can result in bleeding. With chronic hypernatremia, cellular adaptation occurs. So-called idiogenic osmoles accumulate in brain cells, which minimizes cellular dehydration. However, the presence of these idiogenic osmoles presents a risk for the development of cerebral edema during the treatment of hypernatremia.

The symptoms of hypernatremia are nonspecific and often difficult to separate from those of the underlying illness in hospitalized patients. Central nervous system abnormalities are most common. These symptoms can include confusion, weakness, and lethargy in the early stages and progress to seizures, coma, and death in the later stages. The symptoms result from the movement of water out of the brain cells rather than the hypernatremia per se. Neurologic deterioration can be seen during treatment as a result of the development of cerebral edema. Signs of volume depletion or volume overload may be present, depending on the cause of the hypernatremia.

The treatment of hypernatremia is water repletion (Table 13–1). The water deficit may be estimated as follows: Water deficit = [0.6 × Total body weight] × [(Serum sodium concentration/140) − 1]. Total body water is assumed to be 60% of body weight. However, the percentage of water relative to total body weight is closer to 50% in women and in the elderly of both genders. Treatment should be instituted at a rate that balances the risk of hypernatremia with the risk of too rapid correction, particularly in cases of chronic hypernatremia. Half the calculated deficit should be replaced within the first 12 to 24 hours at a rate of sodium concentration correction no greater than 2 mEq/L per hour. The remainder of the water deficit can be replaced over the next 48 hours. The rapidity of replacement should be determined by the acuteness of onset and the severity of symptoms. Neurologic status needs to be closely monitored during replacement for evidence of the development of cerebral edema. Ongoing fluid and electrolyte losses also need to be replaced during treatment. In patients with hypernatremia associated with volume depletion and hemodynamic instability, volume replacement with isotonic saline is indicated initially. Once hemodynamic stability is achieved, water replacement can be initiated. Hypotonic saline (e.g., 0.45 saline) may be preferable to water as the replacement fluid

---

TABLE 13–1. TREATMENT OF HYPERNATREMIA

Calculate water deficit
Replace half the deficit over 12–24 h
Do not correct more rapidly than 2 mEq/L/h
Replace the remaining deficit over 48 h
If hemodynamic instability is present, give isotonic saline until stable before replacing water deficit with hypotonic saline
If volume overload is present, treat with diuretic and 5% dextrose
Dialysis may be indicated if renal failure is present
Ongoing fluid and electrolyte losses should be replaced
Neurologic status should be closely monitored

for these patients. If hypernatremia is associated with hypervolemia (e.g., intake of hypertonic saline or sodium bicarbonate), treatment should be directed toward reducing sodium intake and inducing its loss. In these patients, diuretics can be used along with free water (5% dextrose) infusion. However, if renal failure is present, dialysis may be necessary.

HYPONATREMIA

Hyponatremia is one of the most common electrolyte abnormalities seen in hospitalized patients. It occurs in 2% to 4% of hospitalized patients and up to 30% of patients in intensive care units.[7-10] Mortality for patients with acute hyponatremia is reportedly as high as 50%, whereas mortality for those with chronic hyponatremia is 10% to 20%.[7-11]

Hyponatremia is a water problem, not a sodium problem; there is always an excess of water relative to sodium when hyponatremia is present. In hyponatremia, water excretion by the kidney is impaired. Patients who are hyponatremic may be volume depleted, or hypovolemic (water deficit and sodium deficit), euvolemic (water excess and normal sodium content), or hypervolemic (water excess and sodium excess). As with hypernatremia, the patient's volume status has implications for the treatment of hyponatremia.

In the presence of hyponatremia, there is a decrease in extracellular tonicity relative to the intracellular space. The osmolar gap causes movement of water from the extracellular space into the intracellular space and results in cell swelling. In the central nervous system, cellular swelling manifests as cerebral edema and results in the symptoms associated with hyponatremia. The degree of cerebral cell swelling correlates with the severity of symptoms observed. The central nervous system adapts to hyponatremia in two ways. First, cerebral edema causes an increase in interstitial hydrostatic pressure and results in the movement of fluid from the interstitial space into the cerebrospinal fluid, leading to some amelioration of cerebral edema. Second, solutes are lost from cells, resulting in a decrease in intracellular osmolarity and thus water movement out of cells. The solutes lost are initially sodium and potassium, followed by organic solutes over the next several days. Because of cerebral adaptation, the severity of neurologic symptoms is related to the acuteness and magnitude of the hyponatremia. If hyponatremia develops gradually, brain cells can compensate by decreasing intracellular osmolarity through the loss of osmolytes, thereby limiting the degree of cerebral edema and resultant neurologic dysfunction. However, with the correction of chronic hyponatremia, the regeneration of these osmolytes lags behind, and cerebral dehydration can occur with rapid correction.

In acute hyponatremia, nausea, vomiting, lethargy, and confusion can progress to coma, seizures, and eventual herniation and death.[11,12] The elderly and the young are more likely to be symptomatic from hyponatremia.[9] Menstruating women also tend to be more symptomatic and are at greater risk for neurologic complications from acute hyponatremia.[11] Early in the development of hyponatremia, the symptoms are difficult to separate from those related to the underlying disease process.

Treatment of hyponatremia is dependent on the acuteness of the hyponatremia and the presence and severity of symptoms (Table 13–2). Acute (<48 hours) or chronic (>48 hours) symptomatic hyponatremia (e.g., seizures) requires immediate therapy. However, the optimal approach for the treatment of these patients is controversial.[12-14] The controversy results

TABLE 13–2. TREATMENT OF HYPONATREMIA

Acute Symptomatic Hyponatremia

3% hypertonic saline with loop diuretic
Correct no more than 2 mEq/L/h
Correct no more than 12–15 mEq/L/h over first 24 h

Chronic Symptomatic Hyponatremia (>48 h, or unknown duration)

3% hypertonic saline with loop diuretic
Correct no more than 1.5 mEq/L/h initially
Correct to resolution of symptoms or 10% correction of serum sodium
Correct no more than 12 mEq/L/24 h
Close monitoring of electrolytes and neurologic status

Asymptomatic Hyponatremia

Euvolemia
  Treat underlying cause
  Water restriction
  Occasionally loop diuretic or demeclocycline to lower urine osmolarity
  Hypertonic saline rarely indicated
Hypovolemia
  Treat underlying cause of fluid loss
  Normal saline
Hypervolemia
  Treat underlying cause of decreased effective circulating volume
  Salt and water restriction
  Loop diuretics for some patients

from reports of the occurrence of a central demyelination syndrome associated with the correction of hyponatremia in some patients.[15-22] This syndrome appears to be more common with chronic hyponatremia (>48 hours), overcorrection of hyponatremia, large corrections (>12 to 25 mEq/L per 24 hours), and rapid correction (>1 to 2 mEq/L per hour).[19-22]

The approach to the treatment of acute symptomatic hyponatremia is infusion of hypertonic saline (3%). Therapy is targeted toward resolution of symptoms or a 10% to 15% increase in serum sodium concentration. In patients with a high urine osmolarity, the addition of a loop diuretic facilitates correction of the hyponatremia by decreasing urine osmolarity. The rate of correction should be less than 2 mEq/L per hour and less than 15 mEq/L total over 24 hours. The amount of hypertonic saline necessary to correct the serum sodium concentration to a safe level (e.g., 120 mEq/L) can be estimated by calculating the sodium deficit:

$$\text{Sodium deficit} = 0.5 \times \text{Lean body weight} \times (120 - \text{Observed serum sodium concentration})$$

The amount of hypertonic saline required to replace the deficit is then infused at a rate that permits correction within the parameters noted earlier. Frequent checking of electrolytes is necessary to ensure that correction is not too rapid.

In treating patients with chronic (>48 hours, or of unknown duration) symptomatic hyponatremia, the higher risk of neurologic complications related to therapy mandates a more cautious approach. As with acute hyponatemia, neurologic symptoms predominate in the clinical presentation of these patients. Initial treatment with 3% sodium chloride should be directed toward the resolution of symptoms or a 10% increase in serum sodium concentration. The increase in serum sodium concentration should be at a rate less than

1.5 mEq/L per hour initially, and the total correction should not exceed 12 mEq/L per 24 hours. Close monitoring of serum electrolytes and neurologic status is mandatory. The resolution of symptoms allows for a decrease in the rate of correction. Calculation of sodium deficit can be used to estimate the volume of hypertonic saline necessary for correction, as noted earlier.

Most patients with hyponatremia are asymptomatic. Aggressive correction of serum sodium in these patients is not indicated. Treatment in asymptomatic patients is based on the underlying cause of the hyponatremia and the patient's volume status: euvolemic, hypovolemic, or hypervolemic (edema).

The majority of hyponatremic patients are euvolemic. In this group, the syndrome of inappropriate antidiuretic hormone is the most common diagnosis. The inappropriate (nonosmotic) presence of antidiuretic hormone impairs free water excretion by the kidney; impaired water excretion coupled with water intake results in hyponatremia. Water restriction is the mainstay of therapy for these patients. The amount of water restriction must be sufficient to achieve negative water balance (i.e., the difference between the total intake and excretion of water), or correction of hyponatremia will not occur. Therefore, all water losses (insensible losses, urinary losses, and gastrointestinal losses) must be considered when deciding on the degree of water restriction. If urine osmolarity is high, it may be necessary to decrease it to achieve a negative water balance. This can be achieved by adding a loop diuretic; however, salt intake must be increased to correct for losses resulting from the increased natriuresis with diuresis. Less commonly, demeclocycline (300 to 600 mg twice a day), which interferes with the action of antidiuretic hormone, is used to decrease urine osmolarity. In patients with more pronounced hyponatremia, the combination of normal saline and a loop diuretic can be used to correct hyponatremia. The use of hypertonic saline is rarely, if ever, indicated in these asymptomatic patients.

Hyponatremia associated with volume depletion is a result of the loss of both sodium and water, combined with the simultaneous intake of water or hypotonic fluids. The release of antidiuretic hormone stimulated by hypovolemia inhibits the kidney's ability to excrete water. The net result is positive water balance and hyponatremia. The treatment of hyponatremia in this setting is infusion of normal saline to correct the volume depletion. As volume status is corrected, antidiuretic hormone excretion is switched off, and the kidney excretes the excess water, correcting the serum sodium concentration. The cause of the initial sodium and water loss should also be identified and treated.

Hyponatremia associated with hypervolemia is very common. Clinical conditions associated with hyponatremia and hypervolemia include heart failure, cirrhosis, and nephrotic syndrome. The hallmark of these conditions is the presence of edema. The mechanism for the development of hyponatremia in these settings is diminished effective circulating volume leading to sodium and water retention. The water retention is a result of nonosmotic antidiuretic hormone release impairing the kidney's ability to excrete water. In this respect, the mechanism is similar to that responsible for hyponatremia associated with volume depletion. Therapy is directed toward correcting the primary disease process responsible for the decrease in effective circulating volume. Specific treatment of the hyponatremia consists of sodium and water restriction. The use of loop diuretics may facilitate free water excretion and correction of the hyponatremia; however, thiazide diuretics may exacerbate hyponatremia and should be avoided.

ANNOTATED REFERENCES

Ayus JC, Wheeler JM, Arieff AI: Postoperative hyponatremic encephalopathy in menstruant women. Ann Intern Med 1992;117:891–897.
This case-controlled and cohort study to determine the risk factors for hyponatremic encephalopathy and the clinical course of patients with encephalopathy found a correlation between poor neurologic outcomes and menstruant women in the setting of acute postoperative hyponatremia.

Karp BI, Laureno R: Pontine and extrapontine myelinolysis: A neurologic disorder following rapid correction of hyponatremia. Medicine 1993;72:359–373.
In this retrospective study of patients who developed neurologic dysfunction after correction of hyponatremia, there appeared to be a correlation between the rate of sodium correction and neurologic dysfunction.

Palevsky PM, Bhagrath R, Greenberg A: Hypernatremia in hospitalized patients. Ann Intern Med 1996;124:197–203.
This well-done prospective cohort study identifying the epidemiology and causes of hypernatremia in a hospitalized patient population found that hospitalized patients of any age may develop hypernatremia.

Snyder NA, Feigal DW, Arieff AI: Hypernatremia in elderly patients: A heterogeneous, morbid, and iatrogenic entity. Ann Intern Med 1987;107:309–319.
These investigators followed a prospective cohort of hospitalized elderly patients (older than 60 years) and determined that hospitalized patients often develop hypernatremia secondary to inappropriate fluid management. These patients had a longer length of stay and slightly increased mortality, although there was no control for severity of illness.

Sterns RH, Cappuccio JD, Silver SM, et al: Neurologic sequelae after treatment of severe hyponatremia: A multicenter perspective. J Am Soc Nephrol 1994;4:1522–1530.
This multicenter retrospective study evaluated the effect of correction rates of severe hyponatremia (<106 mEq/L) on outcome. Patients who were chronically hyponatremic and corrected to a normal serum sodium concentration at a rate of less than 12 mEq/day or 0.55 mEq/h did not develop postcorrection neurologic sequelae.

Chapter 14
HYPERKALEMIA AND HYPOKALEMIA

Sergio Zanotti-Cavazzoni • R. Phillip Dellinger

Hyperkalemia and hypokalemia are the most common electrolyte abnormalities found in hospitalized patients.[1] Data regarding their precise prevalence in intensive care unit (ICU) patients are not available. However, the high incidence of abnormalities in serum potassium concentration undoubtedly reflects both physiologic abnormalities that are common in ICU patients and the effects of therapeutic interventions that are commonly used in the care of critically ill patients. Because of comorbid conditions, critically ill patients are also at a higher risk of developing complications from altered serum potassium levels. Timely recognition and intervention are essential for minimizing morbidity and mortality due to abnormal serum potassium levels.

HYPERKALEMIA

Hyperkalemia is defined as a serum potassium concentration (serum $[K^+]$) greater than 5.0 mEq/L. Hyperkalemia is less frequent than hypokalemia but is more likely to cause serious complications in critically ill patients. Severe hyperkalemia requires rapid correction to prevent serious cardiovascular complications. The measured value for serum $[K^+]$ can be elevated as a result of in vitro phenomena, usually the release of K^+ from cells during the clotting process. Pseudohyperkalemia should be recognized and considered in patients with marked elevations of white blood cells or platelets.[2] Simultaneous measurements of plasma (unclotted) and serum (clotted) $[K^+]$ should identify this problem. A serum $[K^+]$ that is 0.2 to 0.3 mEq/L greater than plasma $[K^+]$ is indicative of pseudohyperkalemia. Pseudohyperkalemia may also result from hemolysis of a blood specimen after collection; this event is usually identified in the laboratory and reported.

True hyperkalemia occurs by two mechanisms: (1) impaired K^+ excretion, and (2) shifts in intracellular and extracellular K^+ (Table 14–1). Renal insufficiency is the most common cause of altered K^+ excretion. With acute oliguric renal failure, elevated potassium levels, if not treated, are life threatening. In most patients with nonoliguric chronic renal failure, mild hyperkalemia is evident.[3] With some causes of chronic renal failure, such as diabetes mellitus and tubulointerstitial diseases, hyperkalemia is more pronounced and is probably related to low circulating renin and aldosterone levels.[4] Decreased aldosterone production promotes the development of hyperkalemia. Patients with acquired adrenal insufficiency develop hyperkalemia despite normal renal function. Various drugs used in the ICU can produce hyperkalemia by impairing K^+ excretion. Patients with abnormal renal function are more susceptible to drug-induced hyperkalemia, and potassium supplements are the most common cause.[5] Potassium-sparing diuretics (spironolactone, amiloride, and triamterene) inhibit K^+ excretion and can produce severe hyperkalemia.[6,7] Spironolactone is the most dangerous of these drugs with respect to impaired K^+ excretion, and it has prolonged effects even after discontinuation. Its use has increased significantly after reports of improved mortality in patients with congestive heart failure.[8] Angiotensin-converting enzyme inhibitors reduce circulating aldosterone levels and are associated with hyperkalemia in patients with renal insufficiency.[9] Angiotensin receptor blockers have less impact on circulating aldosterone levels and are less likely to produce hyperkalemia.[9] Nonsteroidal anti-inflammatory drugs and cyclooxygenase-2 inhibitors block prostaglandin synthesis, causing indirect suppression of renin release and aldosterone secretion. Nonsteroidal anti-inflammatory drugs and cyclooxygenase-2 inhibitors also reduce renal blood flow and glomerular filtration rate, particularly in patients with prerenal azotemia (due to decreased intravascular volume or heart failure). These compounds may produce hyperkalemia by these mechanisms in patients with or without renal dysfunction.[10,11] Heparin inhibits aldosterone synthesis and can cause significant hyperkalemia in patients with altered renal function.[12–14] Other drugs that may cause hyperkalemia by decreasing glomerular filtration rate and aldosterone secretion include cyclosporine and tacrolimus.[15] Trimethoprim and pentamidine inhibit renal K^+ excretion and can cause hyperkalemia in patients with renal insufficiency.[15] Patients undergoing ureterojejunostomy may develop hyperkalemia in the immediate postoperative period, presumably from increased jejunal absorption of urinary K^+.[16]

TABLE 14–1. CAUSES OF HYPERKALEMIA

Impaired K^+ Excretion

Renal failure
Mineralocorticoid deficiency
  Addison's disease
  Renal tubular acidosis (type 4)
  Heparin-induced inhibition of aldosterone synthesis
  Hereditary enzyme deficiencies
Pseudohypoaldosteronism
Drugs: potassium-sparing diuretics, angiotensin-converting enzyme inhibitors, nonsteroidal anti-inflammatory drugs, trimethaphan, cyclosporine, tacrolimus, pentamidine

Shifts of K^+ out of Cells

Hypertonicity
Tissue breakdown: rhabdomyolysis, burns, trauma
Drugs: beta blockers, digoxin, succinylcholine, arginine, lysine
Familial hyperkalemic periodic paralysis
Insulin deficiency or resistance

Alterations in the relationship between intracellular and extracellular [K⁺] may lead to severe hyperkalemia in critically ill patients, either by increased release of intracellular K⁺ or by inhibition of extracellular-to-intracellular K⁺ movement. The effects of acidosis on serum [K⁺] are complicated and are not fully understood. The traditional teaching that acidosis produces a shift of K⁺ from the intracellular to the extracellular space, thus causing hyperkalemia, was based on observations of hyperkalemia in patients with diabetic ketoacidosis and renal failure.[17] Based on these data, an inverse relationship with serum pH and serum [K⁺] was described. This relationship has since been disproved, and changes in serum [K⁺] in relation to acid-base disorders are more complex than initially thought. Most forms of acute acidosis do not present with hyperkalemia. The most common forms of acute metabolic acidosis in critically ill patients, diabetic ketoacidosis and lactic acidosis, are not associated with K⁺ shifts out of cells.[18] Hyperkalemia seen with diabetic ketoacidosis is most likely caused by increased release of intracellular K⁺ due to the breakdown of muscle cells.[16] Hypertonicity of the extracellular fluid causes water to exit cells, and K⁺ follows. Unless renal function is adequate to eliminate the excess K⁺, hyperkalemia develops. This situation may occur in patients with uncontrolled diabetes and can lead to severe hyperkalemia in the presence of renal failure and hypoaldosteronism.[19] Massive tissue breakdown can occur with trauma, burns, and rhabdomyolysis, leading to release of K⁺ into the extracellular space. If renal mechanisms for K⁺ excretion are impaired, severe hyperkalemia may develop. Drugs can affect the transmembrane balance of K⁺. Beta-adrenergic blockers inhibit the entry of K⁺ into cells and, in combination with renal failure, can promote the development of hyperkalemia.[20] Succinylcholine blocks normal reentry of K⁺ into cells after depolarization and causes a transitory increase in serum [K⁺]. In patients with severe burns or extensive trauma, the transient hyperkalemia induced by succinylcholine can be more prolonged and severe.[21,22] Digoxin impairs K⁺ entry into cells by inhibiting the cell membrane Na⁺, K⁺-ATPase. It does not produce hyperkalemia in therapeutic doses but may cause hyperkalemia with toxic levels.[23,24] Familial hyperkalemic periodic paralysis is a rare congenital disease that causes a mutation in cell membrane Na⁺ channels, producing transient episodes of severe hyperkalemia secondary to paroxysmal shifts in K⁺ from cells to the extracellular compartment.[25]

CLINICAL EFFECTS

Most of the clinical consequences of potassium abnormalities are related to the effect on the transmembrane resting cell potential. Cardiac and neuromuscular cells are particularly sensitive to changes in serum [K⁺]. Most often, hyperkalemia is asymptomatic. However, it affects the cardiac conduction system, as evidenced by characteristic changes in the electrocardiogram (ECG) that serve as indicators of potential life-threatening arrhythmias (Table 14–2). The first sign of increased serum [K⁺] is tenting of the T wave. Changes associated with progressive increases in serum [K⁺] include widening of the QRS complex, the progressive development of atrioventricular conduction blocks, a slow idioventricular rhythm, an ECG tracing that looks like a sine wave, ventricular fibrillation, and finally asystole.[26] There is no absolute level of serum [K⁺] associated with a particular

TABLE 14–2. ELECTROCARDIOGRAM CHANGES CAUSED BY ABNORMAL [K⁺]

Hyperkalemia	Hypokalemia
Peaked T waves	Broad, flat T waves
Loss of P waves	ST depression
Widening QRS complexes	U wave
Sine wave	QT interval prolongation
Ventricular arrhythmias	Ventricular arrhythmias
Asystole	

ECG abnormality, but rapid rises seem to be more dangerous, particularly in patients without a history of chronic renal insufficiency.[27,28] Hyperkalemia can cause paresthesias and weakness in the arms and legs, followed by a symmetrical flaccid paralysis of the extremities that ascends toward the trunk, finally involving the respiratory muscles. The cranial nerves are usually not affected by hyperkalemia.

TREATMENT

The primary goal of treating hyperkalemia is to prevent adverse cardiac complications. Treatment modalities are aimed at one of three mechanisms to prevent or decrease these complications: (1) direct antagonism of hyperkalemic effect on the cell membrane polarization, (2) movement of extracellular K⁺ into the intracellular compartment, and (3) removal of K⁺ from the body. Patients with a serum [K⁺] greater than 6.5 mEq/L or ECG signs suggestive of hyperkalemia should be treated emergently.

Direct Antagonism of Hyperkalemic Effect on Cell Membrane Polarization. The intravenous infusion of calcium gluconate antagonizes the effects of hyperkalemia on the heart. This effect occurs within minutes and lasts 30 to 60 minutes. If a salutary effect is noted, repeat doses may be used. The recommended dose is 10 mL of 10% calcium gluconate or chloride. Extreme caution must be used in patients with hyperkalemia and digitalis toxicity, because the administration of ionized calcium may potentiate the effects of digoxin on the conduction system.[15,29] Calcium should be avoided in the setting of digoxin toxicity.

Movement of Extracellular K⁺ into the Intracellular Compartment. Administration of insulin shifts K⁺ into cells; this effect occurs in 15 to 30 minutes and lasts approximately 2 to 4 hours.[30] The recommended dose is 10 units of regular insulin intravenously; dextrose (50 g) should be added to avoid hypoglycemia. This dose will decrease serum [K⁺] by 0.5 to 1.5 mEq/L. Patients without intravenous access can be treated with inhaled beta₂-adrenergic agonists such as albuterol. Albuterol drives K⁺ into cells by increasing Na⁺, K⁺-ATPase activity. Albuterol (10 to 20 mg in 4 mL of saline by nasal inhalation over 10 minutes) can lower the serum [K⁺] by 0.5 to 1.5 mEq/L.[31] Sodium bicarbonate is much less effective than either insulin or albuterol but may produce shifting of [K⁺] into cells.[32] The use of sodium bicarbonate should be limited to situations in which it is indicated for the treatment of concurrent acidosis.

Removal of K⁺ from the Body. Finally, removal of K⁺ is necessary to prevent a recurrence of hyperkalemia once the effects of the preceding measures have waned. Loop diuretics can be helpful in patients with sufficient renal function (dosing depends on medication and renal function); however,

TABLE 14–3. TREATMENT OF HYPERKALEMIA

Treatment	Mechanism	Dosage/Comment	Onset	Duration
Calcium	Cardiac cell stabilizer	10 mL of 10% solution (calcium gluconate or calcium chloride)	Seconds	30–60 min
Insulin (regular)	Shifts K⁺ into cells	10 U i.v. + glucose (50 g)	15–30 min	2–4 h
Albuterol	Shifts K⁺ into cells	10–20 mg by inhaler over 10 min	20–30 min	2–3 h
Sodium bicarbonate	Shifts K⁺ into cells	In cases of acidosis	Delayed	—
Kayexalate with sorbitol	Removes K⁺ from body	Oral: 15–30 g	4–6 h	—
		Retention enema: 30–50 g	1 h	—
Loop diuretics	Removes K⁺ from body	Intravenous, varies by drug and renal function	1 h	—
Hemodialysis	Removes K⁺ from body	Preferred over peritoneal dialysis in acute cases	15–30 min	—

most often, other measures are needed. Sodium polystyrene sulfonate (Kayexalate) binds to K⁺ secreted in the colon. Each gram of resin removes 0.5 to 1 mEq of K⁺. The usual dose of Kayexalate is 15 to 30 g orally. Because the resin causes constipation, sorbitol (15 mL of a 70% solution) should be administered to induce osmotic diarrhea. If oral administration is not feasible, Kayexalate can be given as a retention enema, consisting of 30 to 50 g of the resin in 70% sorbitol solution. It is important, however, that the enema be retained for at least 30 to 60 minutes to obtain the desired therapeutic effect. The effects of Kayexalate on serum [K⁺] occur in 4 to 6 hours when the agent is given orally and in 1 to 2 hours when it is given as an enema. Serious side effects of Kayexalate and sorbitol include bowel necrosis and perforation. These complications seem to be more likely in severely immunocompromised patients or shortly after operation; accordingly, Kayexalate should be avoided in these circumstances.[33–35] Both peritoneal dialysis and hemodialysis are very effective in removing K⁺ from the body. In acute cases when serum [K⁺] needs to be corrected rapidly, hemodialysis is preferred. Hemodialysis can quickly remove 50 to 125 mEq of K⁺ and should be used as definitive treatment when other treatments fail. Peritoneal dialysis is also effective in removing K⁺ from the body, but its effects are slower than those achieved with hemodialysis or cation exchange resins. In addition to the implementation of rapid treatment, the causes of hyperkalemia should be sought and corrected, and offending drugs should be discontinued when possible. See Table 14–3 for a summary of the treatment for hyperkalemia.

HYPOKALEMIA

Hypokalemia is more common than hyperkalemia and is defined as serum [K⁺] less than 3.6 mEq/L. Severe hypokalemia can lead to significant complications; more important, understanding its causes and how to treat it may reduce complications from the treatment itself. Low serum [K⁺] reflects a disbalance of normal K⁺ homeostasis, with one rare exception. In patients with leukemia and markedly elevated white cell counts, K⁺ can be taken up by the abnormal cells in the test tube and produce pseudohypokalemia.[36] However, as noted earlier, in vitro changes in [K⁺] more commonly produce pseudohyperkalemia. Hypokalemia usually occurs as a consequence of K⁺ depletion due to either increased excretion or inadequate intake. Shifts in extracellular and intracellular [K⁺] also can cause hypokalemia (Table 14–4).

In critically ill patients, increased losses are more commonly responsible for K⁺ depletion than is inadequate ingestion. The use of diuretics is the most common cause of

hypokalemia in hospitalized patients. Both loop and thiazide diuretics cause increased delivery of Na⁺ and Cl⁻ to the collecting duct, promoting the secretion of K⁺ and causing hypokalemia. Diuretics are often used in high doses or administered by continuous infusion in critically ill patients, increasing the risk of hypokalemia. K⁺ losses can also occur from increased stool output. Because K⁺ is secreted into the colon, patients with high outputs from ileal or jejunal ostomies do not develop hypokalemia. Upper gastrointestinal losses such as vomiting or nasogastric suctioning contain small amounts of K⁺. However, these losses are associated with hypochloremia and metabolic alkalosis, both of which may cause increased renal K⁺ excretion, exacerbating the resultant hypokalemia. Large doses of laxatives or repeated enemas lead to excessive K⁺ losses and hypokalemia. Magnesium depletion and some forms of renal tubular acidosis (type 1 and some forms of type 2) can cause renal K⁺ wasting. Other drugs also can lead to hypokalemia. For example, fludrocortisone and hydrocortisone increase K⁺ excretion. Aminoglycosides, amphotericin B, cisplatin, and foscarnet

TABLE 14–4. CAUSES OF HYPOKALEMIA

Increased Excretion

Diarrhea, laxative or enema abuse
Renal losses
    Diuretics (loop and thiazides)
    Metabolic alkalosis
    Osmotic diuresis (uncontrolled hyperglycemia)
    Nonreabsorbable anions
    Mineralocorticoid excess
        Primary hyperaldosteronism
        Congenital adrenal hyperplasia
        Glucocorticoid-responsive aldosteronism
    Other causes
        Liddle's disease
        Enzyme deficiencies
        Bartter's syndrome
    Magnesium depletion
    High-dose glucocorticoids

Shifts of K⁺ into Cells

Drugs
    Beta-adrenergic agonists
    Insulin
    Theophylline
    Caffeine
Delirium tremens
Hyperthyroidism
Familial hypokalemic periodic paralysis
Barium poisoning

cause magnesium depletion and increased K$^+$ renal losses.[37] Penicillin and its synthetic derivatives, when given intravenously, cause increased Na$^+$ delivery to the distal nephron, promoting K$^+$ secretion and potentially causing hypokalemia.[37]

Alkalosis can cause movement of K$^+$ into cells. This effect is seen with both metabolic and respiratory alkalosis and occurs as a consequence of hydrogen ions leaving the cell to minimize changes in extracellular pH, and K$^+$ moving into the cells to maintain electroneutrality. The direct effects of alkalosis on serum [K$^+$] are small, and the hypokalemia seen with metabolic alkalosis is more often caused by chloride losses producing increased delivery of Na$^+$ to the distal nephron, which stimulates K$^+$ losses. A number of beta$_2$-adrenergic agonist drugs, including bronchodilators, decongestants, and tocolytics, can cause K$^+$ shifts into cells and transient hypokalemia.[37] Theophylline stimulates cell membrane Na$^+$, K$^+$-ATPase and promotes K$^+$ entry into cells; hypokalemia is commonly seen with theophylline toxicity.[38] Barium can block the exit of K$^+$ from cells and cause hypokalemia.[39] Thyroid hormone can stimulate Na$^+$, K$^+$-ATPase, and hypokalemia is sometimes seen with hyperthyroidism. Increased endogenous beta-adrenergic stimulation occurs with delirium tremens, producing intracellular movement of K$^+$ and hypokalemia.[40] Familial hypokalemic periodic paralysis, a rare hereditary disease, is associated with a mutation in cell membrane calcium channels and causes episodes of severe hypokalemia triggered by high sodium intake or exercise.[41] These patients can present with severe muscle weakness and respiratory failure from hypoventilation.

CLINICAL EFFECTS

It is estimated that approximately 20% of hospitalized patients have a serum [K$^+$] less than 3.6 mEq/L; most are asymptomatic. As discussed earlier, the consequences of changes in serum [K$^+$] occur as a result of alterations in the resting membrane potential, making cardiac and neuromuscular cells the most susceptible targets. The most serious and potentially fatal effects of hypokalemia are related to disturbances in cardiac electrical activity that can lead to cardiac arrest. However, cardiac arrest caused by hypokalemia occurs almost exclusively in patients with underlying cardiac disease or patients taking digitalis.[42] Hypokalemia is also associated with characteristic ECG changes (see Table 14–2). Progressive decreases in serum [K$^+$] produce broad, flat T waves; ST depression; and the appearance of U waves, QT interval prolongation, and finally ventricular arrhythmias, leading to cardiac arrest.[26] When serum [K$^+$] is less than 3.0 mEq/L, generalized weakness can develop. When serum [K$^+$] decreases to less than 2.5 mEq/L, muscle necrosis and rhabdomyolysis can occur. With progression of hypokalemia, an ascending muscle paralysis develops, leading to respiratory failure and arrest.

TREATMENT

The immediate goal of treatment in hypokalemia is to prevent or correct cardiac electrical disturbances and serious neuromuscular weakness. The long-term goal of treatment is to achieve repletion of total body potassium to normal levels. Supplementation of [K$^+$] is the principal treatment for hypokalemia and is achieved with the administration of potassium chloride or potassium phosphate. In general, plasma [K$^+$] decreases by approximately 0.3 mEq/L for each 100 mEq decrease in total body K$^+$. This relationship is more difficult to estimate when serum [K$^+$] is less than 2 mEq/L.[37] K$^+$ replacement should be given orally except when severe hypokalemia is associated with respiratory or cardiac instability, in which case the intravenous route is recommended. Intravenous administration of K$^+$ should not exceed 20 mEq/h, to minimize possible iatrogenic hyperkalemia. For infusion of K$^+$, an infusion pump and continuous cardiac monitoring are mandatory.[15] In the case of life-threatening arrhythmias due to severe hypokalemia, more rapid infusion into a central vein may be appropriate. In these rare circumstances, KCl should be diluted to 10 mEq per 100 mL of infusion fluid. In most cases, oral supplementation of K$^+$ is preferred, because this route is safer and produces a more gradual increase in serum [K$^+$]. Because supplementation of K$^+$ is usually not an emergency, it is best accomplished using moderate doses of KCl (20 to 40 mEq once or twice a day) over several days. Potassium phosphate is used when hypophosphatemia is also present (as in diabetic ketoacidosis); occasionally, potassium bicarbonate is used in the setting of metabolic acidosis and hypokalemia. However, for most cases of hypokalemia, KCl is the salt of choice for replacement of K$^+$. Serum [K$^+$] should be followed closely, especially when using intravenous or higher doses, to prevent the development of hyperkalemia. If magnesium levels are low, they should be corrected, because hypomagnesemia promotes renal loss of K$^+$, making correction of hypokalemia more difficult. Finally, prevention of further episodes should be addressed with proper K$^+$ intake and supplementation in patients with a continuous cause for hypokalemia. The use of potassium-sparing diuretics may be helpful in certain clinical situations, but caution must be exercised, because the development of hyperkalemia can have severe consequences.

Chapter 15

HYPOPHOSPHATEMIA AND HYPERPHOSPHATEMIA

Stephen Trzeciak • R. Phillip Dellinger

PHOSPHATE HOMEOSTASIS

Derangements in the metabolism of phosphate are common in the intensive care unit and can be clinically significant. One of the keys to understanding phosphate homeostasis is an appreciation of the fact that serum phosphate measurements may not reflect total body phosphorus stores because (1) the vast majority of total body phosphorus is found in the bones (in the form of hydroxyapatite); (2) the majority of phosphate is intracellular, and extracellular phosphate accounts for only a small fraction of total body phosphorus stores; and (3) shifts between the intracellular and extracellular compartments occur. There is no common laboratory test to accurately measure total body phosphate stores. Low serum phosphate concentration is referred to as *hypophosphatemia*, whereas a state of low total body phosphorus stores is referred to as *phosphate depletion*.

Phosphate serves a number of crucial functions. It is an essential component of the main energy "currency" of the cell: adenosine triphosphate. Phosphate is also a component of phospholipids in cell membranes and of hydroxyapatite, the structural matrix of bone. Phosphate also serves as a buffer against acid-base derangements.

Phosphate homeostasis is a function of bone metabolism, intestinal absorption, and kidney resorption. Bone metabolism is linked to calcium homeostasis. In the setting of hypocalcemia, increased parathyroid hormone levels cause phosphate and calcium to be released from the bone. Intestinal absorption of phosphate occurs in the small bowel, mostly in the jejunum. Vitamin D, produced by the kidney in increased amounts when serum phosphate levels are low, increases the intestinal absorption of both calcium and phosphate. Phosphate is excreted from the kidneys, but most of the excreted phosphate load undergoes resorption in the proximal tubule. Parathyroid hormone increases phosphate excretion by inhibiting phosphate resorption in the kidney. Resorption increases in the setting of phosphate deficiency.

HYPOPHOSPHATEMIA

Hypophosphatemia is typically classified as mild (serum phosphate concentration 2.5 to 3 mg/dL), moderate (1 to 2.5 mg/dL), or severe (<1 mg/dL). Although mild to moderate hypophosphatemia may be subclinical, severe hypophosphatemia may be associated with significant morbidity. The all-cause mortality rate in patients with serum phosphate concentrations less than 1 mg/dL has been reported to be as high as 30%.[1]

Common causes of hypophosphatemia are summarized in Table 15-1. Respiratory alkalosis (of any cause) may induce a transcellular shift of phosphate and cause hypophosphatemia. Other causes of hypophosphatemia include renal phosphate losses, inadequate intestinal absorption of phosphate, and extreme catabolic states. Renal losses of phosphate occur with osmotic diuresis or excessive diuretic therapy. Hyperparathyroidism (either primary or secondary) causes hypophosphatemia by decreasing urinary resorption of phosphate. Proximal renal tubular disorders also impair phosphate resorption and cause hypophosphatemia. Total body phosphate depletion also occurs in extreme catabolic states, such as burns or sepsis.

Hypophosphatemia should be anticipated when nutritional support is initiated in a chronically malnourished patient. When a carbohydrate load is administered in the setting of chronic malnutrition, there is a spike in insulin release that increases cellular phosphate uptake and can induce a precipitous decrease in serum phosphate concentration. This phenomenon has been termed the *refeeding syndrome*. A common example is the initiation of enteral or parenteral nutrition in an alcoholic patient who suffers from chronic hypophosphatemia due to malnutrition.[2] Profound hypophosphatemia in the refeeding syndrome can produce severe clinical manifestations, and death has been reported.[3] Concurrent hypokalemia and hypomagnesemia are common. In chronically malnourished patients, the refeeding syndrome can be avoided with a cautious introduction of nutritional

TABLE 15-1. COMMON CAUSES OF HYPOPHOSPHATEMIA

Transcellular shift
  Refeeding syndrome
  Respiratory alkalosis
  Insulin administration
Renal losses
  Diuretic therapy
  Osmotic diuresis
  Hyperparathyroidism (primary or secondary)
  Proximal renal tubular dysfunction
    Fanconi's syndrome
Insufficient intestinal absorption
  Malnutrition
  Phosphate-binding antacids
  Vitamin D deficiency
  Chronic diarrhea
  Nasogastric suctioning
  Malabsorption syndromes
Extreme catabolic states
  Burns
  Trauma
  Sepsis

support (especially carbohydrates), careful monitoring of serum phosphorus levels, and appropriate phosphate supplementation when indicated.[3]

Patients with diabetic ketoacidosis typically have phosphate depletion because hyperglycemia induces increased urinary losses of phosphate via an osmotic diuresis. However, the serum phosphate concentration may be normal in the initial phase of therapy, because severe acidosis causes a shift of phosphate into the extracellular space from the intracellular compartment. As the acidosis is corrected, however, phosphate shifts back to the intracellular compartment, leading to a precipitous decrease in serum phosphate levels.[4] Although common, the clinical significance of moderate hypophosphatemia in diabetic ketoacidosis is unclear. Therapy for hypophosphatemia in diabetic ketoacidosis is typically warranted only if the serum phosphate level is less than 1.0 mg/dL or if hypophosphatemia is associated with severe clinical manifestations, such as central nervous system or left ventricular dysfunction.[5]

Clinical manifestations due to hypophosphatemia are rare unless the serum phosphate concentration is less than 1 mg/dL. The clinical findings are summarized in Table 15–2. Diffuse skeletal muscle weakness may be profound.[6] Respiratory failure secondary to diaphragmatic weakness may occur.[7,8] Respiratory failure may be primary, or it may manifest as an inability to wean from mechanical ventilation. Central nervous system dysfunction may include confusion, lethargy, and gait disturbance. Hematologic manifestations, including acute hemolytic anemia and leukocyte dysfunction (impaired phagocytosis and chemotaxis), have been reported. Cardiovascular manifestations may include acute left ventricular dysfunction and a reversible dilated cardiomyopathy that typically responds only to phosphate repletion. Rhabdomyolysis also may occur.[9]

Hypophosphatemia also may cause disorders of oxygen transport. Profound hypophosphatemia can impair oxygen delivery to the tissues because of decreased production of 2,3-diphosphoglycerate, a key molecule in erythrocytes that facilitates the release of oxygen from hemoglobin. Decreased intracellular levels of 2,3-diphosphoglycerate cause a leftward shift of the oxyhemoglobin dissociation curve.

Because phosphate serves as a buffer in acid-base derangements, hypophosphatemia may be clinically significant in the interpretation of acid-base status. Phosphate and proteins (albumin) are measured anions. Unmeasured anions are accounted for in acid-base interpretation by calculation of the anion gap. Although there is no true "normal" value for the anion gap, the value is typically lower for a patient with low measurable anions (i.e., either hypophosphatemia or hypoalbuminemia, or both). Therefore, a "normal" value for the calculated anion gap in the setting of profound hypophosphatemia may actually represent the presence of unmeasured anions. As a rule, the expected anion gap (in mEq/L) equals twice the serum albumin concentration (in g/dL) plus one half of the serum phosphate concentration (in mM/L). Thus, a patient with hypophosphatemia and hypoalbuminemia may have an elevated anion gap even if the measured anion gap is less than the commonly used threshold of 10 to 12.

Severe hypophosphatemia (phosphate concentration <1 mg/dL) mandates intravenous phosphate replacement. Phosphate should not be administered by the intravenous route to patients with renal failure; it should also be avoided in patients with hypercalcemia, because metastatic calcification can occur. For moderate hypophosphatemia (phosphate concentration 1 to 2.5 mg/dL), oral supplementation may be adequate for a patient who is able to take medications by mouth or nasogastric tube. The degree of true phosphate depletion is difficult to assess because most phosphate is intracellular; therefore, it is impossible to accurately predict the exact amount of phosphate supplementation required to replenish phosphate stores.

HYPERPHOSPHATEMIA

Hyperphosphatemia is defined as a serum phosphate level greater than 4.5 mg/dL; it may be clinically significant at levels greater than 5 mg/dL. The most common cause of hyperphosphatemia is renal failure. Renal insufficiency causes hyperphosphatemia because phosphate excretion by the kidneys is impaired. The serum phosphate level is usually normal until the creatinine clearance falls below 30 mL/min. Other causes of hyperphosphatemia include rhabdomyolysis, hemolysis, and tumor lysis syndrome[10]; any insult causing extensive cell damage releases phosphorus into the extracellular space. Hyperphosphatemia has also been reported in patients using bisphosphonate medications (decreased renal phosphate clearance) and patients abusing phosphate-containing laxatives. Causes of hyperphosphatemia are summarized in Table 15–3.

The most frequent clinical findings in acute hyperphosphatemia are signs and symptoms of hypocalcemia.

TABLE 15–2. CLINICAL MANIFESTATIONS OF SEVERE HYPOPHOSPHATEMIA

Respiratory
  Acute respiratory failure
  Ventilator dependence
Musculoskeletal
  Muscle weakness
  Rhabdomyolysis
  Bone demineralization
Hematologic
  Hemolysis
  Disorders of leukocyte phagocytosis or chemotaxis
Neurologic
  Altered mental status
  Gait disturbance
  Paresthesias
Cardiovascular
  Cardiomyopathy
  Decreased inotropy

TABLE 15–3. COMMON CAUSES OF HYPERPHOSPHATEMIA

Renal
  Acute or chronic renal failure
  Increased renal resorption
    Hypoparathyroidism
    Thyrotoxicosis
Cellular injury
  Rhabdomyolysis
  Tumor lysis syndrome
  Hemolysis
Medication related
  Abuse of phosphate-containing laxatives
  Excessive (iatrogenic) phosphate administration
  Bisphosphonate therapy

Hyperphosphatemia produces hypocalcemia by three mechanisms: (1) precipitating calcium (formation of calcium-phosphorus complexes), (2) interfering with parathyroid hormone–mediated resorption of bone, and (3) decreasing vitamin D levels.[11] Clinical signs and symptoms of hypocalcemia, such as muscle cramping, tetany, hyperreflexia, and seizures, as well as cardiovascular manifestations, may be evident.

Management of acute hyperphosphatemia includes limiting phosphate intake and enhancing urinary phosphate excretion. In the absence of end-stage renal disease, phosphate excretion can be optimized with saline infusion (volume diuresis) and diuretic administration. Diuretics that work on the proximal tubule, such as acetazolamide, are especially effective for enhancing phosphate excretion. Any patient with life-threatening hyperphosphatemia should be considered for dialysis.

Oral phosphate binders decrease the absorption of phosphate in the gut and are a mainstay for preventing and treating hyperphosphatemia in patients with chronic renal failure. Calcium and aluminum salts are widely used. However, calcium salts can produce hypercalcemia and metastatic calcification from a high calcium-phosphorus $(Ca \times PO_4)$ product, and aluminum salts may be toxic. In dialysis patients, chronic management of hyperphosphatemia with calcium-free phosphate binders, such as sevelamer hydrochloride (Renagel), may reduce long-term mortality by preventing cardiovascular complications associated with a high calcium-phosphorus product.[12] Sevelamer is highly effective in increasing fecal elimination of phosphate without producing hypercalcemia or aluminum toxicity.[13] In the acute management of patients with hyperphosphatemia accompanied by hypocalcemia, the likelihood (and clinical significance) of metastatic calcification with acute calcium administration is unclear.

Chapter 16
HYPOMAGNESEMIA

D. Patrick Bryant • Robert N. Cooney

Magnesium (Mg++) is an important ion that participates in more than 300 enzymatic reactions, especially those involving adenosine triphosphate (ATP) as a cofactor. Although the relationship between hypomagnesemia and intracellular magnesium deficiency remains unclear, hypomagnesemia is common in critically ill patients and is associated with increased mortality.[1,2]

CELLULAR PHYSIOLOGY AND METABOLISM OF MAGNESIUM

Magnesium is a divalent cation that is localized predominantly to the intracellular compartment. It is the second most abundant intracellular cation after potassium and plays an important role in cellular metabolism and homeostasis. At the cellular level, magnesium influences membrane function by regulating ion transport. Magnesium is required for Na+, K+-ATPase activity, which maintains transmembrane gradients for sodium (Na+) and potassium (K+).[3,4] Magnesium also regulates intracellular calcium (Ca++) flux by competing for Ca++ binding sites and influencing intracellular Ca++ transport.[3,4] Magnesium is an essential cofactor for most processes that require ATP. It acts by neutralizing the negative charge on the phosphate anion of ATP to facilitate enzyme binding and hydrolysis of the phosphate moiety. Intracellular Mg++ is required for numerous critical biochemical processes, including DNA synthesis, activation of gene transcription, initiation of protein synthesis, and regulation of energy metabolism via glycolysis and the tricarboxylic acid cycle.[3-6]

Total body magnesium (21 to 28 g) is distributed in bone (53%), muscle (27%), soft tissue (19%), and blood (0.8%).[3] The normal concentration of total magnesium in serum is 1.5 to 2.3 mg/dL. Approximately 19% of circulating magnesium is bound to protein (predominantly albumin), whereas 14% is complexed to serum anions (citrate, phosphate, and bicarbonate). The majority of magnesium in serum exists as an ionized species (67%), which represents the physiologically active form.[3,7] Consequently, measurements of total serum Mg++ may not accurately reflect the relative abundance of circulating Mg++.[1-3]

Magnesium homeostasis is maintained by the small intestine, kidney, and bone.[3,8] The average dietary intake of magnesium is approximately 300 mg/day. Normally, only one third of dietary Mg++ is absorbed.[8,9] However, intestinal Mg++ uptake increases to compensate for dietary or total body Mg++ deficiency.[3,8,9] Unlike calcium, there are no hormonal mechanisms for regulating Mg++. Consequently, normal renal filtration and reabsorption of Mg++ are important regulatory

mechanisms for Mg++ homeostasis.[3,8] Non–protein-bound Mg++ is filtered by the glomerulus. Under normal conditions, up to 95% of filtered Mg++ is reabsorbed in either the proximal tubule (35%) or the thick ascending loop of Henle (60%).[3,8] Magnesium reabsorption in the loop of Henle is linked to sodium chloride transport and is inversely related to flow. Consequently, diuretic use and other conditions associated with increased tubular flow result in decreased Mg++ reabsorption.[3,8] Under conditions of persistent Mg++ deficiency, mobilization of Mg++ from bone also represents a potential homeostatic mechanism.[3]

PREVALENCE AND CAUSE OF HYPOMAGNESEMIA

The reported prevalence of hypomagnesemia in adult patients admitted to the intensive care unit ranges from 15% to 60%, depending on whether total or ionized magnesium is measured.[1,2,10,11] A recent study found that severe ionized hypomagnesemia is most common after liver transplantation and in patients with severe sepsis.[2] Magnesium deficiency in critically ill patients may be caused by inadequate Mg++ intake, increased renal or gastrointestinal losses, acute intracellular shifts of Mg++, and other medical conditions (e.g., burn injury, massive blood transfusion, cardiopulmonary bypass). Increased renal losses of Mg++ are associated with alcohol abuse, diabetes, acute tubular necrosis, diuretics, aminoglycosides, amphotericin, cyclosporine, cisplatin, digoxin, and other medications.[2,3,8,10,12] Vomiting, diarrhea, nasogastric tube losses, and pancreatitis are associated with increased gastrointestinal losses of Mg++.[2,3,8,10,12] Acute extracellular-to-intracellular shifts of magnesium caused by refeeding with glucose or amino acids, insulin, catecholamines, or metabolic acidosis may also result in hypomagnesemia.[2,3,8,10,12] Hypoalbuminemia is associated with a reduction in total Mg++ in plasma, but the ionized fraction may remain normal. Critically ill patients are at increased risk for hypomagnesemia, and the development of hypomagnesemia is associated with an increased risk of mortality.[1,2]

CLINICAL SIGNS AND SYMPTOMS OF HYPOMAGNESEMIA

Hypomagnesemia is frequently asymptomatic in critically ill patients and is commonly identified through routine blood work or when hypomagnesemia is suspected clinically.[8,10-12] However, the relationship between systemic and cytoplasmic hypomagnesemia is unclear, and it has not been established whether changes in enzymatic function caused by cytoplasmic

TABLE 16–1. CLINICAL SIGNS AND SYMPTOMS OF MAGNESIUM DEFICIENCY

Cardiovascular
  Atrial fibrillation, flutter
  Ventricular tachycardia, especially torsades de pointes
  Supraventricular tachycardia
  Electrocardiogram changes ($\uparrow$ PR, wide QRS, $\uparrow$ QT)
  Hypertension
  Risk of digitalis toxicity
Metabolic
  Hypokalemia
  Hypocalcemia
  Hypophosphatemia
  Insulin resistance
Neurologic
  Seizures
  Nystagmus
  Delirium
  Coma
  Athetoid movements
Neuromuscular
  Chvostek's sign
  Muscle cramps
  Carpopedal spasm
  Muscle weakness
  Muscle fasciculations

Mg^{++} depletion can lead to clinically significant problems. Hypomagnesemia is most commonly seen in conjunction with hypokalemia, hypocalcemia, and other electrolyte abnormalities. Consequently, it is difficult to assess the clinical consequences of isolated hypomagnesemia. In most instances, symptoms are attributed to Mg^{++} deficiency only after other electrolyte abnormalities are corrected.[3,8,10–12] As summarized in Table 16–1, the clinical sequelae of magnesium deficiency most commonly affect the cardiovascular, metabolic, and neuromuscular systems.

CLINICAL USES OF MAGNESIUM

Hypomagnesemia is associated with electrocardiographic changes that are similar to those found in hypokalemia; these include flattened T waves, U waves, and prolonged QT interval. Magnesium is a cofactor for Na^+, K^+-ATPase in cardiac tissue.[3,8,11,12] Reductions in intracellular K^+ result in cell depolarization and can lower the threshold for generation of an action potential, as well as decrease the time for repolarization. Consequently, hypomagnesemia is associated with atrial (premature atrial contractions, atrial fibrillation, multifocal atrial tachycardia), digoxin-related, and ventricular (ventricular tachycardia, torsades de pointes) dysrhythmias.[8,11,12] Magnesium is currently recommended as the initial therapy for torsades de pointes and as an adjunct for refractory ventricular dysrhythmias.[3,8,11,12] Magnesium administration during acute myocardial infarction was associated with reduced mortality in the second Leicester Intravenous Magnesium Intervention Trial (LIMIT-2)[13] but not the fourth International Study of Infarct Survival (ISIS-4).[14] However, in the ISIS trial, magnesium replacement was performed following coronary reperfusion. So at present, there are no conclusive data to support routine magnesium administration in patients with acute myocardial infarction. However, based on the LIMIT-2 study, there

is some evidence that magnesium may be beneficial if given before coronary reperfusion.[15]

Hypomagnesemia is commonly associated with both hypokalemia and hypocalcemia.[8] This association is related in part to the fact that medications and homeostatic changes that affect magnesium often affect potassium as well. In addition, renal losses of potassium are increased in hypomagnesemia and are refractory to supplementation unless the magnesium deficiency is corrected first.[3,8] A somewhat similar condition exists for hypocalcemia, in that hypomagnesemia suppresses parathyroid hormone release and activity.[16] Consequently, hypocalcemia is refractory to Ca^{++} replacement unless the magnesium deficiency is corrected as well.[3,8]

Magnesium can have a depressant effect on the nervous system due to its ability to cause presynaptic inhibition.[3,8,12] It depresses the seizure threshold by competitively inhibiting N-methyl-D-asparate receptors.[3,8,11,12] The neurologic and neuromuscular manifestations of hypomagnesemia include coma, seizures, weakness, and signs of muscular irritability.[3,8,11,12] Hypomagnesemic patients may have a positive Chvostek's sign even with normal ionized calcium and may develop nystagmus, tetany, or seizures followed by rhabdomyolysis.[3,8,11,12] Consequently, Mg^{++} replacement is indicated in this setting and is also commonly used in patients with preeclampsia (blood pressure >140/90 with proteinuria) or eclampsia (associated seizures) during late pregnancy.[11,12]

Magnesium replacement has been used to treat bronchospasm in patients with asthma.[11,12] The proposed mechanism of action for the therapeutic benefit of Mg^{++} in bronchospasm involves its relaxant effects on smooth muscle.[11,12] Several studies have shown improved FEV_1 following intravenous magnesium or improved peak flow rates with nebulized magnesium, while others have not.[11,12] Consequently, additional studies are needed to adequately define the role of magnesium in patients with asthma.

TREATMENT OF HYPOMAGNESEMIA

The initial step in managing hypomagnesemia is to identify and eliminate factors contributing to the development of magnesium deficiency. This may involve interventions to minimize gastrointestinal losses or reevaluating the need for medications that cause renal magnesium wasting (e.g., aminoglycosides, diuretics). The severity of hypomagnesemia, urgency of clinical symptoms (dysrhythmias, muscle cramps.), associated electrolyte abnormalities (K^+ and Ca^{++}), and renal function should be assessed before initiating Mg^{++} therapy.

In general, intravenous administration of Mg^{++} is preferred in symptomatic critically ill patients. However, caution must be used with Mg^{++} replacement when renal dysfunction is present, because severe hypermagnesemia may result. Current recommendations for magnesium replacement therapies are of limited value, owing to the lack of controlled studies examining time-matched controls and the use of total serum versus ionized magnesium concentration for monitoring. Magnesium can be administered intravenously as magnesium sulfate ($MgSO_4$; 1 g = 4 mmol) or magnesium chloride ($MgCl_2$; 1 g = 4.5 mmol) and orally as magnesium gluconate (500 mg = 1.2 mmol) or magnesium oxide (400 mg = 6 mmol). When intravenous magnesium replacement is used, a bolus followed by continuous infusion or infusion alone is preferred, because renal filtration and excretion may limit Mg^{++} retention. For torsades de pointes, 1 to 2 g of intravenous MgSO$_4$ over 5 minutes is recommended. For urgent hypomagnesemia, an intravenous bolus of 8 to 12 mmol of Mg^{++} (2 to 3 g MgSO$_4$), followed by an infusion of 40 mmol Mg^{++} (10 g MgSO$_4$) over the next 5 hours, should be considered. For routine treatment of hypomagnesemia, an infusion of 40 mmol Mg^{++} should be given over a 24-hour period. For outpatients on diuretics with chronic magnesium losses, oral magnesium therapy with 2 to 3 g (12 to 24 mmol) per day is recommended. Orally, magnesium oxide is more easily absorbed than other formulations.

Chapter 17

HYPOCALCEMIA AND HYPERCALCEMIA

Richard J. King • Robert N. Cooney

Abnormal serum calcium is a common finding in critically ill patients. The prevalence of hypocalcemia in intensive care unit (ICU) patients ranges from 70% to 90% when total serum calcium is measured and from 15% to 50% when ionized calcium is measured.[1] Hypercalcemia occurs less frequently; the reported incidence is less than 15% in critically ill patients.[2] Hypocalcemia is associated with injury severity and mortality in critically ill patients.[1,3-6] However, it is not known whether a low serum calcium concentration is protective, harmful, or simply prognostic in critical illness. Therefore, in most instances, the management of hypocalcemia involves treating the underlying medical condition, except when patients are symptomatic or hemodynamically unstable. This chapter provides a brief overview of calcium physiology, the regulation of serum calcium concentration, potential causes and symptoms of hypocalcemia, conditions associated with hypocalcemia, and guidelines for treating hypo- and hypercalcemia in critically ill patients.

CALCIUM PHYSIOLOGY AND METABOLISM

Calcium is a divalent ion (Ca^{++}) involved in critical biologic processes such as muscle contraction, blood coagulation, neuronal conduction, hormone secretion, and the activity of various enzymes.[3,7] Therefore, it is not surprising that intra- and extracellular calcium concentrations are tightly regulated. A normal adult has approximately 1 to 2 kg of total body calcium, localized primarily in bone (99%) as hydroxyapatite.[1,3,4] Skeletal stores of calcium represent a virtually unlimited reservoir. Release of calcium from this reservoir is regulated predominantly by extracellular Ca^{++} concentration, parathyroid hormone (PTH), and calcitonin. Extracellular concentrations of Ca^{++} are typically 10,000 times greater than cytoplasmic Ca^{++} levels.[1,3] Similarly, the majority of intracellular calcium (>90%) is found in subcellular organelles (mitochondria, microsomes, endoplasmic or sarcoplasmic reticulum) as opposed to the cytoplasmic compartment. Ca^{++}-mediated cell signaling involves rapid changes in cytoplasmic Ca^{++} concentration secondary to movement of the ion from both internal and external stores.[8,9] Cytoplasmic Ca^{++} influx occurs through cell membranes by receptor-activated, G protein–linked channels. The release of internal Ca^{++} from endoplasmic or sarcoplasmic reticulum is stimulated by second messengers.[8] The efflux of cytoplasmic Ca^{++} involves transport of Ca^{++} across the cell membrane and into the endoplasmic or sarcoplasmic reticulum by specific transporters.[8-10] Alterations in Ca^{++}-dependent signaling have been identified in muscle, hepatocytes, neutrophils, and T lymphocytes during sepsis and may contribute to the development of organ dysfunction during catabolic illness (for review see reference 9).

Extracellular calcium homeostasis is maintained by the coordinated actions of the gastrointestinal tract, kidneys, and bone.[1,3] Levels of extracellular Ca^{++} are detected by calcium-sensing receptors on parathyroid cells.[10] In response to low serum Ca^{++} concentrations, the parathyroid glands secrete PTH. This hormone reduces renal reabsorption of phosphate, increases renal calcium reabsorption, and stimulates renal hydroxylation of vitamin D.[1,3] PTH and 1,25-dihydroxy-vitamin D (calcitriol) promote the release of calcium from bone by activating osteoclasts.[1,3] Calcitriol also stimulates intestinal absorption of dietary calcium and regulates PTH secretion by inhibiting PTH gene transcription. PTH secretion is also influenced by serum phosphate concentration. Increases in circulating phosphate concentration stimulate PTH secretion by lowering the extracellular Ca^{++} concentration. Magnesium is required for the release of PTH from parathyroid cells, which may explain why hypocalcemia is common in patients with magnesium deficiency. Calcitonin is a calcium-regulating hormone secreted by the parafollicular C cells of the parathyroid glands during hypercalcemia. Although calcitonin inhibits bone resorption and stimulates urinary excretion of calcium, its does not appear to play a major role in calcium homeostasis in humans.[1,3]

The normal concentration of Ca^{++} in the extracellular space (plasma and interstitium) is 1.2 mmol/L and represents 50% of the total extracellular calcium; of the remaining 50%, 40% is bound to plasma proteins and 10% is combined with citrate, phosphate, or other anions. Total serum calcium normally ranges from 9.4 to 10.0 mg/dL (2.4 mmol). The distribution of ionized and bound calcium may be altered in critically ill patients. Chelating substances such as citrate and phosphate can influence the abundance of ionized Ca^{++}. An increased free fatty acid concentration caused by lipolysis or parenteral nutrition results in increased binding of calcium to albumin.[11] Protein-bound calcium is also increased during alkalosis and reduced during acidosis.[1,3] Correcting total serum calcium for albumin and pH does not accurately estimate ionized Ca^{++}.[12,13] Therefore, most ICU laboratories measure ionized calcium. Hypocalcemia is defined as an ionized Ca^{++} level less than 1.0 mmol/L or a total level less than 8.5 mg/dL.[13]

HYPOCALCEMIA IN CRITICALLY ILL PATIENTS

Ionized hypocalcemia is frequently seen in critically ill patients with sepsis, pancreatitis, or severe traumatic injuries or following major surgery. The incidence ranges from 15% to 50%.[3] The degree of hypocalcemia correlates with illness severity as measured by the Acute Physiology and Chronic

TABLE 17–1. CAUSES OF HYPOCALCEMIA

Impaired parathyroid hormone secretion or action
  Primary hypoparathyroidism
  Secondary hypoparathyroidism
Impaired vitamin D synthesis or action
  Poor intake
  Malabsorption
  Liver disease
  Renal disease
  Hypomagnesemia
  Sepsis
Calcium chelation or precipitation
  Hyperphosphatemia
  Citrate
  Pancreatitis
  Rhabdomyolysis
  Ethylene glycol
Decreased bone turnover
  Hypothyroidism
  Calcitonin
  Cis-platinum
  Diphosphonates
  Mithramycin
  Phosphates

From Zaloga GP: Hypocalcemia in critically ill patients. Crit Care Med 1992;20:251-261.

Health Evaluation (APACHE) II score and is associated with increased mortality in critically ill patients.[6] In particular, the degree of systemic inflammation as assessed by circulating cytokine or procalcitonin levels appears to correlate with hypocalcemia in ICU patients.[14] Potential causes for the hypocalcemia of critical illness include impaired PTH secretion or action, vitamin D deficiency or resistance, calcium sequestration or chelation, or impaired mobilization of Ca^{++} from bone (Table 17–1).

Hypocalcemia in the ICU is rarely caused by primary hypoparathyroidism. However, sepsis and systemic inflammatory response syndrome are commonly associated with hypocalcemia, which is caused in part by impaired secretion and action of PTH and failure to synthesize calcitriol.[1,3,14] Hypomagnesemia can contribute to hypocalcemia during critical illness by inhibiting PTH secretion and target organ responsiveness.[1,3,7] However, hypomagnesemia correlates with hypocalcemia in ICU patients only weakly.[6] In many instances, the cause of hypocalcemia of critical illness is multifactorial. Elderly patients are at increased risk for vitamin D deficiency owing to malnutrition, poor absorption, and hepatic or renal dysfunction.[3] Renal failure can precipitate hypocalcemia by impairing the formation of calcitrol and promoting hyperphosphatemia; phosphate chelates ionized calcium.[1,3] Other potential causes of ionized hypocalcemia in critically ill patients include alkalosis (increased binding of Ca^{++} to albumin), medications (anticonvulsants, antibiotics, diphosphonates, radiocontrast agents), massive blood transfusion, sepsis, and pancreatitis.[1,3,6,7]

Patients receiving blood transfusions can develop hypocalcemia as a consequence of Ca^{++} chelation by citrate, which is used as an anticoagulant in banked blood.[15–17] The incidence of transfusion-related hypocalcemia is related to both the rate and the volume of blood transfusion.[15,16] When blood transfusions are administered at a rate of 30 mL/kg per hour (2 L/h in a 70-kg patient) and hemodynamic stability is maintained, ionized Ca^{++} levels are preserved by physiologic compensatory mechanisms.[17] Transient hypocalcemia can be observed during rapid transfusion and can be prolonged or exacerbated by hypothermia or renal or hepatic failure.[15–17] Consequently, ionized calcium should be monitored and calcium replaced when clinically indicated during massive transfusion.

HYPOCALCEMIA IN SEPSIS AND PANCREATITIS

Hypocalcemia is especially common in critically ill patients with systemic infection and pancreatitis.[1,3,6,9,14] Animal models of sepsis demonstrate reductions in serum calcium concentration following endotoxin infusion.[9,14,18,19] When septic patients with hypocalcemia were compared with nonseptic controls, increased tumor necrosis factor and interleukin-6 levels were inversely correlated with ionized Ca^{++}.[20] Septic patients with hypocalcemia can have increased or decreased PTH levels; however, urinary excretion of calcium and bone resorption are preserved when compared with controls.[14,20] Procalcitonin levels appear to be increased during sepsis-induced hypocalcemia, but mature calcitonin exerts only a weak and transient effect on calcium levels.[20,21] The collective results from studies of animal models and patients suggest that the cause of hypocalcemia during severe infection is multifactorial, but the effects of inflammatory cytokines, impaired activation of vitamin D, and elevated procalcitonin levels are all contributory.

It is unclear whether sepsis-induced hypocalcemia is pathologic or protective. Calcium administration in experimental sepsis has been shown to increase or have no effect on mortality.[18,19] Similarly, investigations of the effects of Ca^{++} channel blockade on septic mortality demonstrate conflicting results.[22,23] Therefore, although sepsis-induced hypocalcemia is common in critically ill patients, neither routine replacement of calcium nor the use of calcium channel blockers is supported by the existing literature. As with most situations, sepsis-induced hypocalcemia should be treated if patients are symptomatic.

Pancreatitis represents another inflammatory condition that is associated with hypocalcemia in critically ill patients.[1,3,23–25] Saponification of retroperitoneal fat contributes to the development of hypocalcemia in patients with pancreatitis.[3,23–25] In experimental pancreatitis, injection of free fatty acids into the peritoneum induces hypocalcemia in rats.[23] However, the amount of calcium chelated is relatively small compared with the amount available for exchange from calcium stores in the bone reservoir. Interestingly, elevated levels of PTH seen in pancreatitis, as in sepsis, do not result in normalized ionized calcium levels.[25] Although resistance of bone and kidney to PTH may be a factor, it is likely that inflammatory pathways identical to those in sepsis are responsible. In pancreatitis, as in sepsis, hypocalcemia is an indicator of disease severity. As with most clinical conditions, calcium replacement during pancreatitis should be reserved for symptomatic or hemodynamically unstable patients.

SIGNS AND SYMPTOMS OF HYPOCALCEMIA

Hypocalcemia is frequently asymptomatic, and attributable signs or symptoms may be difficult to elucidate in critically ill patients. In general, the signs and symptoms of hypocalcemia correlate with both the magnitude of the condition and the rapidity of its onset. Neurologic (paresthesias, seizures, dementia) and cardiovascular (hypotension, impaired cardiac contractility, dysrhythmias) signs can be seen with ionized hypocalcemia when Ca++ is less than 1.0 mmol/L.[3,7] Neuromuscular symptoms of hypocalcemia include muscle spasms and tetany, when severe. Psychiatric disturbances (dementia, psychosis, depression) also may be attributable to hypocalcemia.[3,7]

Classic signs of hypocalcemia include Chvostek's and Trousseau's signs, which test for latent tetany. Chvostek's sign is an involuntary twitching of facial muscles in response to light tapping of the facial nerve. It is nonspecific and is present in 10% to 25% of normal adults, and it may be completely absent in chronic hypocalcemia. Trousseau's sign is carpopedal spasm induced by reduced blood flow to the hand when a blood pressure cuff is inflated to 20 mm Hg for 3 minutes. Trousseau's sign is also nonspecific and may be absent in a third of patients with hypocalcemia.

Cardiac dysrhythmias such as ventricular tachycardia, prolonged QT interval, and heart block are more serious complications of hypocalcemia.[3,7] In addition, decreased cardiac output and hypotension, especially when refractory to vasopressors and volume infusion, should prompt calcium replacement when hypocalcemia is present.[3,7]

TREATMENT OF HYPOCALCEMIA

Critical thresholds for calcium replacement vary, but severe ionized hypocalcemia (<0.8 mmol/L) and symptomatic hypocalcemia should be replaced in critically ill patients.[1,3,7,26] Calcium treatment of asymptomatic ionized hypocalcemia (>0.8 mmol/L) is usually unnecessary and may be potentially harmful in conditions such as sepsis and cellular hypoxia.[1,3,7,26]

Treatment of hypocalcemia requires intravenous calcium replacement. The two solutions most commonly used are 10% calcium chloride and 10% calcium gluconate. Each solution contains 100 mg/mL of calcium salt and is available in 10-mL ampules. Ten percent calcium chloride contains 27 mg/mL (1.36 mEq) of elemental calcium; 10% calcium gluconate contains 9 mg/mL (0.46 mEq). Typically, 10 mL of 10% calcium gluconate solution is infused over 10 minutes. A total of 200 mg of elemental calcium may be necessary to raise the total serum calcium by 1 mg/dL. Because the effect of calcium infusion is usually brief, a continuous infusion may be necessary. Calcium chloride should not be infused peripherally if calcium gluconate is available; the former can produce tissue necrosis and thrombophlebitis if extravasation occurs.

Hemodynamically unstable patients in the ICU who are hypocalcemic may show a transient increase in blood pressure or cardiac output with calcium administration. This is probably due to increased cardiac performance.[26] However, in the presence of tissue hypoxia, calcium administration may aggravate the cellular injury.[9,13,22] Nonetheless, calcium administration is probably warranted in hypocalcemic, hemodynamically unstable patients, especially those requiring adrenergic support.

HYPERCALCEMIA

Hypercalcemia is rare in critically ill patients, estimated to occur in 1% to 15% of ICU patients.[2] Defined as an increase in serum calcium above 10.4 mg/dL (2.60 mmol/L), hypercalcemia is usually caused by excessive bone resorption. Hyperparathyroidism and humoral hypercalcemia of malignancy are the most common causes of hypercalcemia in hospitalized patients.[2,7,27] Less common causes of hypercalcemia include sarcoidosis, prolonged immobilization, and medications such as thiazide diuretics.

Mild hypercalcemia is usually asymptomatic. However, patients with circulating Ca++ concentrations above 12 mg/dL may manifest symptoms of confusion, delirium, psychosis, and coma.[2,7,27] Patients with hypercalcemia may also experience nausea, vomiting, constipation, abdominal pain, and ileus. Cardiovascular effects of hypercalcemia include hypotension, hypovolemia, and shortened QT interval. Profound skeletal muscle weakness may result. Seizures, however, are rare.

Treatment of hypercalcemia should be directed at the underlying medical condition. Saline infusion and diuresis are indicated in symptomatic patients and when the serum calcium level rises above 14 mg/dL (3.5 mmol/L). For patients with underlying malignancy, treatment with salmon calcitonin, pamidronate, or plicamycin may be necessary. These agents act to inhibit bone resorption. Salmon calcitonin should be started at 4 IU/kg every 12 hours via subcutaneous or intramuscular injection. If the response is inadequate after 2 days, the dose may be increased to 8 IU/kg every 12 hours to a maximum of 8 IU/kg every 6 hours. Hydrocortisone can also be used in combination with calcitonin to treat hypercalcemia associated with multiple myeloma. Dosing of pamidronate depends on the severity of hypercalcemia. For a corrected serum calcium level of 12 to 13.5 mg/dL, pamidronate should be given as a single intravenous dose of 60 to 90 mg over 4 to 24 hours. For higher calcium levels, a single 90-mg dose should be given over 24 hours. Longer infusion times (i.e., >4 hours) may reduce renal toxicity. If necessary, retreatment should be initiated only after 7 days have elapsed, to allow time for a complete response to the initial dose. The dose and manner of treatment are the same as for initial therapy. The recommended dose of plicamycin for hypercalcemia is 25 µg/kg daily for 3 to 4 days. Additional treatments may be given at 1-week intervals. Usual maintenance regimens are two to three doses per week.

Chapter 18

HYPOGLYCEMIA

Greet Van den Berghe

DEFINITION AND DIAGNOSIS

Hypoglycemia is the most common endocrine emergency, the most frequent complication of insulin-requiring diabetes, and the principal factor limiting optimization of glycemic control. When unrecognized and not treated appropriately, significant morbidity, including permanent neurologic deficits and death, may ensue. Hypoglycemia is generally defined arbitrarily as a blood glucose concentration less than 50 mg/dL (2.8 mmol/L) with neuroglycopenic symptoms or less than 40 mg/dL (2.2 mmol/L) in the absence of symptoms. Clinically significant hypoglycemia is characterized by Whipple's triad: (1) symptoms of neuroglycopenia, (2) simultaneous blood glucose concentration less than 40 mg/dL (2.2 mmol/L), and (3) relief of symptoms with the administration of glucose. This blood glucose concentration cutoff corresponds to a plasma glucose concentration of 45 mg/dL (2.5 mmol/L). All three criteria should be met to establish a diagnosis of hypoglycemia, at least outside the intensive care unit (ICU), because a precipitous fall from hyperglycemia to euglycemia in a patient with diabetes can produce hypoglycemic symptoms,[1] and because asymptomatic hypoglycemia with glucose levels as low as 30 mg/dL (1.7 mmol/L) can occur during fasting in normal women and during pregnancy.[2] In the ICU, however, sedation can mask symptoms of neuroglycopenia and counterregulatory responses may be impaired, which complicates the diagnosis of hypoglycemia in this setting. Further, asymptomatic patients can have artifactual hypoglycemia due to in vitro consumption of glucose by blood cells (especially when the blood leukocyte count is very high).

A hypoglycemic disorder should be suspected whenever the blood glucose reading is low. However, most reflectance glucometers in home and hospital use have poor precision at low levels of blood glucose.[3] Caution should be exercised with alternative-site capillary blood glucose testing, which has been demonstrated to have a 30-minute lag time compared with finger-stick testing for the detection of hypoglycemia.[4] The recently developed continuous interstitial glucose monitoring system[5] and the noninvasive Glucowatch Biographer[6] are less effective at detecting low blood glucose levels and can have a delayed response to low blood glucose concentrations. Therefore, the laboratory measurement of a low plasma glucose concentration, in the presence of appropriate symptoms, remains the most reliable way to diagnose severe hypoglycemia. In the ICU, the measurement of arterial blood glucose concentration using modern blood gas analyzers approaches the accuracy of conventional laboratory methods.[7]

INCIDENCE OF SEVERE HYPOGLYCEMIA

Although the frequency of severe hypoglycemia in diabetes is well documented, there is little information on the incidence of serious hypoglycemia in nondiabetic subjects or in the general population. A retrospective study of adults requiring hospitalization indicated that 0.4% of acute medical admissions per year are hypoglycemia related.[8] In a prospective study of 130 hospital admissions due to adverse drug reactions, hypoglycemia was the fourth most common disorder.[9] A review of 54,850 autopsies in a large medical center revealed 123 deaths (0.2%) due to hypoglycemic coma.[10] Because of the difficulty of postmortem diagnosis and frequent associated comorbidities, severe hypoglycemia is often unrecognized, particularly in nondiabetic individuals.

Severe hypoglycemia occurs commonly in patients with diabetes, even if the stringent definition of the Diabetes Control and Complications Trial is employed (i.e., symptoms severe enough to require assistance for treatment). Hypoglycemia occurs at least once a year in up to 30% of patients with type 1 diabetes.[11] In type 2 diabetes, even with intensive therapy, the risk is probably 100-fold less. Over 6 years of observation in the United Kingdom Prospective Diabetes Study, severe hypoglycemia was reported in 2.4% of patients treated with metformin, 3.3% of those treated with a sulfonylurea, and 11.2% of those treated with insulin.[12] However, when matched for duration of insulin therapy and circulating levels of HbA_{1c}, the frequency of severe hypoglycemia was similar in type 1 and type 2 diabetes.[13] As insulin usage among patients with type 2 diabetes increases, it is inevitable that severe hypoglycemia will become more common in daily practice.

With the introduction of tight blood glucose control in the surgical ICU, the incidence of blood glucose values below 40 mg/dL (2.2 mmol/L) has been reported to range from 0.8% to 5.2% of patients, depending on the targeted level of blood glucose control.[7] With the use of algorithms advising frequent blood glucose measurements (i.e., every 1 to 4 hours), brief episodes of such low blood glucose levels do not impose a major risk of sequelae.

PATHOPHYSIOLOGY

The central nervous system relies primarily on glucose for the generation of cellular energy. Cells in the central nervous system have endogenous glucose reserves that are sufficient for only minutes if the supply of glucose from the bloodstream is inadequate. In addition, neurons are unable to synthesize glucose. Finally, the brain cannot use fuels other than glucose during acute hypoglycemia.[14] Hence, when the brain is acutely deprived of glucose, serious neurologic dysfunction occurs. Therefore, the body has several mechanisms to maintain the plasma glucose concentration within the narrow range of 60 to 140 mg/dL (3.3 to 7.7 mmol/L) in both the fed and fasting states. When glucose use exceeds glucose production, the brain senses decreasing glucose levels and activates counterregulatory pathways. The glucose threshold for activation of these mechanisms is approximately 67 mg/dL (3.6 mmol/L), but this setpoint can be altered by recent hyperglycemia or antecedent hypoglycemia. The important components of the endocrine defense against hypoglycemia were identified in the 1980s.[15] As glucose levels decline, the first counterregulatory mechanism is the suppression of endogenous insulin secretion. Next in the hierarchy of responses is the release of two hormones, glucagon and epinephrine, that antagonize the action of insulin. These hormones activate glycogenolysis and gluconeogenesis and stimulate fatty acid oxidation and protein breakdown to provide substrates for gluconeogenesis. With more severe or prolonged hypoglycemia (>3 hours), increases in growth hormone and cortisol release raise the blood glucose level.

The physiologic responses to hypoglycemia and the glucose threshold at which they occur can be modulated in normal and diabetic humans. In type 1 diabetes, the glucagon response to hypoglycemia is lost within 3 years after diagnosis, rendering patients dependent on epinephrine-mediated counterregulation and making them more vulnerable to prolonged episodes of severe hypoglycemia. Exposure to antecedent hypoglycemia diminishes the counterregulatory response to a subsequent episode. The brain adapts to antecedent hypoglycemia by increasing glucose uptake so that a more profound hypoglycemic stimulus is required to trigger sympathoadrenal activation and autonomic symptoms.[16] Also, the level of glycemic control affects counterregulatory thresholds. With strict glycemic control, epinephrine release is not triggered until a lower glucose level is reached.[17,18] Conversely, diabetic patients with poor glycemic control can experience hypoglycemic symptoms when the blood glucose concentration decreases to lower values within the normal or even hyperglycemic range.[19]

There are four pathophysiologic mechanisms capable of exceeding the body's counterregulatory capacity and causing severe hypoglycemia: (1) excessive insulin effect, (2) diffuse hepatic dysfunction, (3) limited substrate for gluconeogenesis, and, rarely, (4) excessive glucose consumption. More than one mechanism can be operative in critically ill patients.

DIFFERENTIAL DIAGNOSIS

Hypoglycemia is commonly classified as (1) drug or toxin induced, (2) fasting induced, or (3) postprandial. An alternative clinical classification of hypoglycemic disorders separates patients who appear healthy (with or without coexistent disease) from those who appear ill (including those with a predisposing illness and those who are hospitalized). For otherwise healthy patients, the most important causes of fasting hypoglycemia are accidental or factitious drug ingestion and insulinoma. The differential diagnosis in ill or hospitalized patients includes predisposing illness, drug interactions, and other iatrogenic factors (Table 18–1).[20]

Insulin treatment of diabetes is the most common cause of hypoglycemia in adults. Risk factors for frequent severe hypoglycemia in type 1 diabetes include lower HbA$_{1C}$ levels, higher daily insulin dose, longer duration of diabetes, absence of residual C peptide, and a prior history of severe hypoglycemia.[11] Hypoglycemia unawareness is the loss of autonomic warning symptoms of developing hypoglycemia. It affects approximately 25% of subjects with type 1 diabetes and is an important predictor of severe hypoglycemia. Insulin-treated type 2 diabetics are also vulnerable to severe hypoglycemia, especially if their disease is well controlled and they have been on insulin for many years.[13] Whether intensive insulin therapy increases the incidence of severe hypoglycemia is controversial.[21-23] Switching from animal to human insulin does not result in an increased incidence of severe hypoglycemia,[24] and newer insulin analogs, such as glargine and lispro, as well as continuous delivery systems, may lessen the risk of fasting or postprandial severe hypoglycemia.[25-27]

Sulfonylureas are a common cause of severe hypoglycemia.[28] The incidence is higher in the elderly and with the use of long-acting agents, such as chlorpropamide and glyburide (glibenclamide),[29] although the latter remains controversial.[19] Liver dysfunction prolongs the hypoglycemic

TABLE 18–1. DIFFERENTIAL DIAGNOSIS OF HYPOGLYCEMIA

	Increased Insulin Effect	Hepatic Dysfunction	Decreased Substrate	Increased Glucose Consumption
Drug/toxin	Insulin overdose Sulfonylureas Rodenticide Vacor Pentamidine Quinine Angiotensin-converting enzyme inhibitors	Ethanol Nonselective beta blockers	Chronic renal insufficiency	Exercise
Fasting	Insulinoma Autoimmune disease Insulin-like growth factor-II–secreting tumor	Congestive heart failure Septic shock Combined endocrine deficiencies	Uremia Severe wasting	Large tumors Prolonged exercise
Postprandial	Upper gastrointestinal surgery (e.g., Bilroth II) Ethanol Noninsulinoma Pancreatogenous hypoglycemia	Unripe akee fruit (*Blighia sapida*) (hypoglycin)		

activity of tolbutamide, acetohexamide, glyburide, and glipizide. Renal insufficiency especially prolongs the activity of chlorpropamide and glyburide. A crude rate of serious hypoglycemia of 1.23 per 100 person-years has been reported in elderly users of sulfonylureas.[30] Sulfonylurea-induced hypoglycemia can be prolonged (up to 27 days), with recurrences after initial normalization of glucose levels.[31] Discovery of inadvertent or factitious sulfonylurea overdose may avoid an exhaustive search for insulinoma in patients presenting with hyperinsulinemic hypoglycemia.[32]

The metabolism of ethanol depletes hepatocellular levels of nicotinamide-adenine dinucleotide, which is a cofactor critical for the entry of substrates into gluconeogenesis pathways.[33] Ethanol also inhibits cortisol and growth hormone responses and delays the epinephrine response to hypoglycemia.[34] However, ethanol does not inhibit glycogenolysis. Therefore, ethanol-induced hypoglycemia does not occur until hepatic glycogen stores have been depleted (after 8 to 12 hours of fasting).[35] There is no correlation between blood ethanol levels (although alcohol is usually detected) and the degree of hypoglycemia, and severe hypoglycemia can occur with ethanol levels as low as 45 mg/dL. The incidence of alcohol-induced hypoglycemia is generally less than 1% in adults, but hypoglycemic coma is commonly related to ethanol ingestion.[36]

In the absence of a drug or toxic cause, adults with severe fasting hypoglycemia should be evaluated for insulinoma, insulin-secreting tumor of the islets of Langerhans,[37] or unusual causes, such as excessive production of insulin-like growth factor II or rapid glucose consumption by tumors, diffuse hepatic dysfunction, septic shock, panhypopituitarism, polyglandular endocrine deficiency syndromes, and autoimmune hypoglycemia. The diagnosis of postprandial (reactive) hypoglycemia remains controversial.[38]

CLINICAL PRESENTATION

The symptoms of hypoglycemia can be divided into autonomic and neuroglycopenic. Autonomic symptoms such as sweating, palpitations, tremor, and hunger are due to the effects of increased activation of the sympathetic nervous system in response to blood glucose levels of approximately 55 mg/dL (3.7 mmol/L). Elderly patients report fewer autonomic symptoms.[39] Neuroglycopenic symptoms are due to impairment of cerebral functioning and include confusion, odd behavior, drowsiness, difficulty with speech, blurred vision, hemiplegia (Todd's palsy), seizure, and coma. Neuroglycopenic symptoms occur at blood glucose levels of approximately 45 mg/dL (2.5 mmol/L). Symptoms of hypoglycemia appear to be similar in type 1 and type 2 diabetes[13] and whether they are induced by sulfonylureas, insulin, or its analogs.[24,40,41]

Patients with hypoglycemia unawareness have a sevenfold increased risk of severe hypoglycemia, and episodes of hypoglycemia in these patients can be recurrent and unpredictable.[42] Likely pathogenic mechanisms for hypoglycemia unawareness include recurrent exposure to hypoglycemia, with subsequent increases in brain glucose uptake and possibly reduced beta-adrenergic sensitivity.[43,44] Fortunately, scrupulous avoidance of hypoglycemia for a period of weeks to months restores hypoglycemia awareness.[45,46] Surgical removal of an insulinoma also restores autonomic symptoms of hypoglycemia.[47]

EVALUATION

The first step in the evaluation of a patient with suspected hypoglycemia is documentation of low plasma glucose concentration in the presence of neuroglycopenic symptoms (Fig. 18–1). Unless there is an obvious medication-related cause for severe hypoglycemia, blood should be drawn for the measurement of glucose, insulin, and C peptide before the administration of glucose and, when indicated, for the diagnosis of thyroid hormone and cortisol deficiency or uremia. In cases of fasting hypoglycemia, intentional, accidental, or surreptitious ingestion of glucose-lowering medications should be investigated to avoid the lengthy workup for insulinoma.[37] Sulfonylurea ingestion causes elevated insulin and C peptide levels, which mimics the findings associated with an insulinoma. Confirmation of the diagnosis of sulfonylurea ingestion can be made using high-pressure liquid chromatography or radioimmunoassay to detect sulfonylureas in blood or urine. The results of these tests are extremely important for further management.

MANAGEMENT

In all cases of suspected severe hypoglycemia, a patent airway and hemodynamic stability should be secured while a rapid bedside estimation of blood glucose is performed. In cases of suspected overdose, emesis should not be induced in a hypoglycemic patient. When alcohol abuse is suspected, thiamine (100 mg i.v. or i.m. per day until the patient is consuming a complete diet) should be given to avoid acute Wernicke's encephalopathy. Administration of glucose is the fundamental remedy. In an awake patient with a protected airway, an initial dose of 20 g of glucose orally works. Examples of oral carbohydrates suitable for the correction of hypoglycemia are flavored glucose tablets and juices and sodas high in sugar content. A response should occur within 10 to 15 minutes and typically lasts 1 to 2 hours. Hence, a snack is advisable to avoid recurrent hypoglycemia.

When patients are unwilling or unable to take oral carbohydrates, intravenous dextrose (glucose) should be given. The recommended initial dose of 50 mL of 50% dextrose provides 25 g dextrose and, within 5 minutes, produces a mean rise in blood glucose to 220 mg/dL (12.5 mmol/L) from nadir values as low as 20 mg/dL (1.1 mmol/L).[48] In ICU patients receiving insulin by continuous intravenous infusion and also receiving a baseline enteral or intravenous glucose load, an additional 10-g glucose bolus is usually sufficient to correct hypoglycemia, and the smaller glucose load avoids the need to greatly modify the insulin dosing regimen.[7,49] For prolonged hypoglycemia (e.g., caused by sulfonylurea overdose), prolonged dextrose infusion plus octreotide may be required.[50]

Parenteral glucagon directly stimulates hepatic glycogenolysis. Glucagon is effective in restoring consciousness if given soon after the onset of hypoglycemic coma. Glucagon is particularly effective in pancreatectomized patients but is much less useful in type 2 diabetes because it stimulates insulin secretion as well as glycogenolysis. Patients with depleted glycogen stores, such as those with alcohol-induced hypoglycemia, may not respond to glucagon. Adverse reactions to glucagon administration include nausea and vomiting, delaying carbohydrate ingestion.

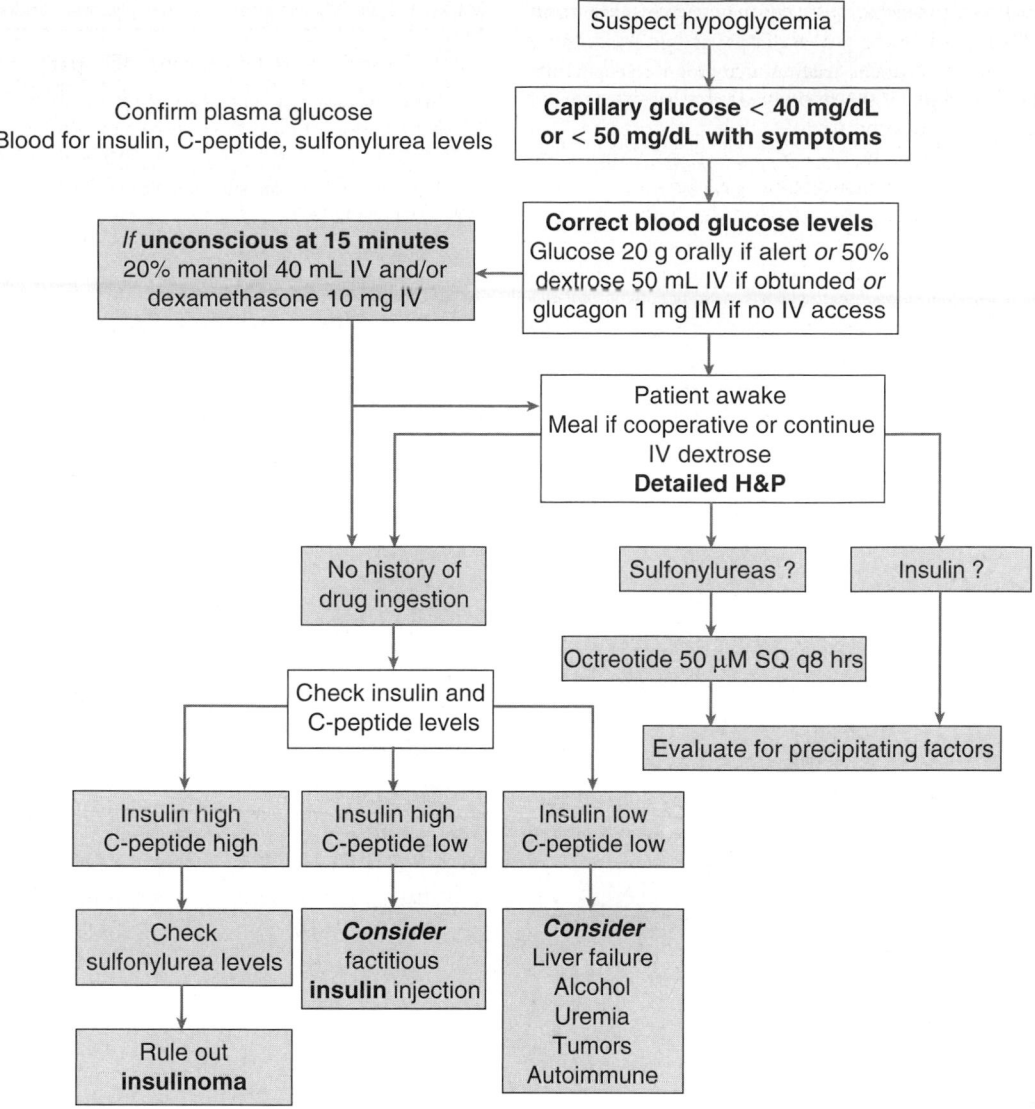

FIGURE 18–1. Approach to severe hypoglycemia in adults. H & P, history and physical examination.

In cases of sulfonylurea overdose, octreotide is more effective than diazoxide for reversing hyperinsulinemia, reducing dextrose requirements, and preventing recurrent hypoglycemia.[50] The recommended dose of octreotide as an antidote for sulfonylurea overdose is 50 μg subcutaneously, repeated every 8 hours if necessary. Activated charcoal binds sulfonylureas and can be administered in cases of suspected overdose.

Cerebral edema can complicate severe hypoglycemia and should be suspected when unconsciousness lasts more than 30 minutes following normalization of blood glucose. Treatment with intravenous mannitol (40 mL of a 20% solution) and glucocorticoids (10 mg of dexamethasone) in addition to intravenous dextrose is advised.

SEQUELAE

Although severe hypoglycemia induces marked cognitive dysfunction,[51] most patients recover rapidly and completely.[52] The effect of repeated severe hypoglycemia on cognitive function in adults is controversial.[53,54] Although focal neurologic symptoms secondary to severe hypoglycemia occur occasionally, severe and permanent cognitive impairment is usually the result of protracted hypoglycemia, often in association with excess alcohol consumption.

The overall mortality from severe hypoglycemia is unknown. The mortality rate from alcohol-induced hypoglycemia may be as high as 10% in adults.[36] An estimated 2% to 4% of deaths in patients with type 1 diabetes have been attributed to hypoglycemia. Severe hypoglycemia is the cause of unexpected overnight death in young diabetic patients,[55] which is explained by the impairment of hormonal responses to hypoglycemia during sleep in normal and diabetic patients.[47,56]

ANNOTATED REFERENCES

Boyle PJ, Kempers SF, O'Connor AM, Nagy RJ: Brain glucose uptake and unawareness of hypoglycemia in patients with insulin-dependent diabetes mellitus. N Engl J Med 1995;333:1726-1731.
This paper reports the results of a clinical study in which it was shown that in patients with diabetes and good blood glucose control, brain blood glucose uptake is normal, which preserves cerebral metabolism but reduces

the counterregulatory hormonal responses; this, in turn, evokes unawareness of hypoglycemia.

Diabetes Control and Complications Trial research group: Hypoglycemia in the Diabetes Control and Complications Trial. Diabetes 1997;46: 271-286.

This paper reports on the incidence of hypoglycemia in a multicenter, randomized, controlled clinical trial (N = 1441) of intensive versus conventional diabetes therapy, with an average follow-up of 6.5 years.

Jones TW, Porter P, Sherwin RS, et al: Decreased epinephrine responses to hypoglycemia during sleep. N Engl J Med 1998;338:1657-1662.

This paper reports the results of a clinical study showing that sleep impairs counterregulatory hormone responses to hypoglycemia in both normal and type 1 diabetic adolescents.

Marks V, Teale JD: Drug-induced hypoglycemia. Endocrinol Metab Clin North Am 1999;28:555-577.

Therapeutically administered antidiabetic drugs—notably, insulin and sulfonylureas—are the most common causes of hypoglycemia in clinical practice. Nevertheless, an impressive list of other drugs can produce hypoglycemia, as discussed in this review paper.

Wang PH, Lau J, Chalmers TC: Meta-analysis of effects of intensive blood-glucose control on late complications of type 1 diabetes. Lancet 1993;341:1306-1309.

This paper reports the results of a meta-analysis of 16 randomized trials of intensive therapy to estimate its impact on the progression of diabetic retinopathy and nephropathy and the risk of severe hypoglycemia.

Chapter 19
ANEMIA OF CRITICAL ILLNESS

Ali Hallal • Carl Schulman • Stephen Cohn

Anemia is a common clinical problem in the ICU. In the United States, 12.4 million units of blood were transfused into 4.5 million patients in 1999, with about 25% given to the critically ill.[1] Approximately 85% of patients spending more than 1 week in the ICU receive 1 or more units of packed red blood cells (RBCs) in their first week and continue to require 2 to 3 units of blood per week thereafter.[2] A recent multicenter European study showed that 37% of patients in the ICU are transfused.[3] Similarly, a multicenter observational study in the United States evaluated 4992 patients from 284 different ICUs and found that 44% of patients received at least one transfusion during their ICU stay.[4]

Blood is an increasingly scarce resource. The National Blood Data Resource Center suggests that the need for blood transfusion in the United States will exceed its availability in the near future. Patients have historically been transfused at a hemoglobin (Hb) threshold of 10 g/dL. Over the last decade, several studies have shown that packed RBC transfusion is independently associated with worse clinical outcomes, independent of the degree of anemia or the severity of illness. The scarcity of blood and the considerable economic impact of blood transfusion (about $500 per unit) have prompted new approaches for the management of anemia in the ICU.

There are three major classes of anemia: (1) hypoproliferative anemia secondary to marrow production defects, (2) ineffective erythropoiesis caused by red cell maturation defects, and (3) decreased survival of red cells secondary to blood loss, hemolysis, or both (Fig. 19-1). The majority of anemia cases (75%) are hypoproliferative. The pathogenesis of this type of anemia is explained by a form of marrow dysfunction characterized by inadequate erythropoiesis in response to the degree of anemia. Most cases of anemia encountered in critically ill patients are of the hypoproliferative type, although other causes may play a role.

BASIC LABORATORY PARAMETERS

The complete laboratory evaluation of anemia is beyond the scope of this chapter; only the pertinent iron studies that aid in understanding the pathogenesis of anemia of the critically ill are discussed. Of these, the most important laboratory tests are measurements of serum iron concentration, serum transferrin and transferrin receptor protein concentrations, total iron binding capacity, and serum ferritin concentration.

Iron absorbed from food or released from stores circulates in plasma bound to transferrin, the iron transport protein. The iron-transferrin complex interacts with a specific transferrin receptor protein on the surface of early erythroid cells. Subsequently, the complex is internalized, and iron is released intracellularly. Within erythroid cells, iron in excess of the amount needed for hemoglobin synthesis binds to the storage protein apoferritin, forming ferritin. Iron in the ferritin pool can be released and reused in the iron metabolism pathway. The serum ferritin level correlates with the total body iron stores and, therefore, is the most suitable laboratory estimate of iron stores.[5] During the maturation of reticulocytes to erythrocytes, the cells lose all activities of the components of the hemoglobin-synthesizing system, including transferrin receptor proteins, which are released into the circulation.[6] The level of transferrin receptor protein in the circulation provides a quantitative measure of total erythropoiesis and can be used to measure the expansion of the erythroid marrow in response to recombinant erythropoietin therapy. The serum iron level represents the amount of circulating iron bound to transferrin. The total iron binding capacity is an indirect measure of the circulating transferrin. Once the iron binding capacity of transferrin is exceeded, the expression of transferrin receptor protein decreases, limiting further access of iron into the cells. The normal range for serum iron is 50 to 150 µg/dL; the normal range for total iron binding capacity is 300 to 360 µg/dL, and transferrin saturation is normally 25% to 50%. Iron deficiency states are associated with a transferrin saturation of less than 18%. The normal values of ferritin vary with age and gender. Adult men have ferritin levels averaging approximately 100 µg/dL, whereas adult women have levels around 30 µg/dL. Normal values for transferrin receptor protein concentration are 4 to 9 µg/L.[5] Because the anemia of critical illness is caused by impaired iron release and a blunted response to erythropoietin, the laboratory findings in this syndrome are characterized by a low serum iron concentration, low total iron binding capacity and transferrin saturation, normal transferrin receptor protein level, and normal to high ferritin level.

CAUSE AND PATHOGENESIS

Anemia in critically ill patients is the result of multiple factors, including (1) blood loss secondary to phlebotomy, gastrointestinal bleeding, coagulation disorders, or surgical procedures; (2) bone marrow depression secondary to renal failure or chronic diseases; (3) nutritional deficiencies; and (4) immunologically mediated iron deficiency in combination with a blunted response to erythropoietin.

Blood loss due to phlebotomy is an often unrecognized yet significant cause of anemia in the ICU. A recent study

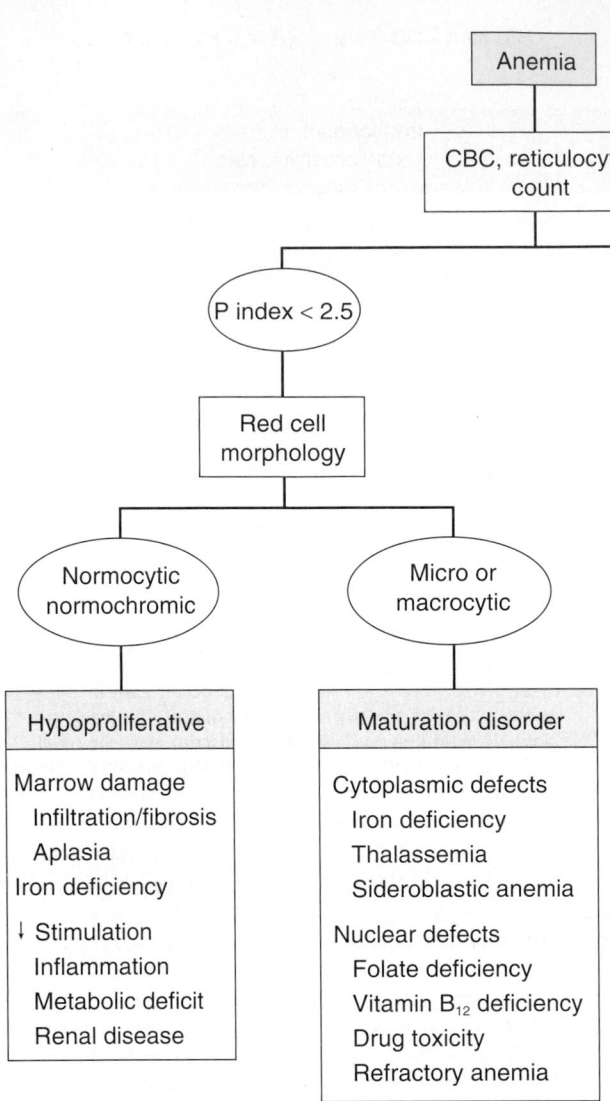

FIGURE 19–1. Physiologic classification of anemia. The reticulocyte production index (P index) is a correction of the reticulocyte count based on the level of anemia and the circulatory life span of a prematurely released reticulocyte. CBC, complete blood count. (From Adams JW, Longo DL: Anemia and polycythemia. In Braunwald E, Fauci AS, Kasper DL, et al: Harrison's Principles of Internal Medicine, 15th ed. New York, McGraw-Hill, 2001, p 352.)

showed that patients admitted to the ICU are phlebotomized an average of 4.6 times a day, for an average total volume of 41.1 mL.[3] Patients with arterial catheters have blood drawn four times a day, for a mean of 944 mL over the course of an ICU stay.[7] Approximately half of patients are transfused as a direct result of excessive phlebotomy.[2]

Although rare since the advent of effective gastrointestinal prophylaxis, gastrointestinal bleeding can be a serious problem in the ICU. The overwhelming majority of critically ill patients demonstrate evidence of mucosal damage within the first 24 hours of their admission to the ICU. Overt anemia occurs in 5% of patients with stress-related gastrointestinal bleeding. Clinically important bleeding necessitating transfusion is observed in only 1% to 4% of critically ill patients.[8] Stress gastritis occurs predominantly in critically ill patients on mechanical ventilation and those with coagulopathy.[9]

Anemia of critical illness is a distinct multifactorial entity, although it is similar in many respects to the anemia of chronic disease. Inflammation appears to be a major factor, causing an alteration in the metabolism of intracellular iron. In addition, these patients have a blunted response to erythropoietin, which leads to a decrease in RBC production.[10,11] In anemia related to critical illness, there is also a decrease in iron availability, secondary to a decrease in both iron reutilization and iron absorption.[12,13]

When iron availability is reduced, critically ill patients who are anemic fail to respond with an appropriate increase in circulating erythropoietin levels. In addition, their reticulocytes are unable to respond suitably to endogenous erythropoietin.[10] Erythropoietin is a glycoprotein with a molecular weight of approximately 34,000 daltons; it is produced mainly in the kidney and, to a lesser extent, in the liver. The primary role of erythropoietin is to regulate RBC production. It also is required for the survival and differentiation of erythroid progenitors in the bone marrow, but it is not responsible for the commitment of stem cells to the erythroid lineage.[14] Erythropoietin production is regulated by hypoxia, which leads to an increase in its gene transcription; it then exerts its action in the bone marrow by stimulating the expression of erythroid colony-forming units that become mature erythrocytes. As tissue oxygenation improves, receptors in the kidney act to down-regulate the production of erythropoietin through a negative feedback mechanism.

The erythropoietin response observed in critically ill patients appears to result from inhibition of the erythropoietin gene by inflammatory mediators. Interleukin-1 beta and tumor necrosis factor are known to suppress gene expression and erythropoietin production in isolated, perfused rat kidneys and in human hepatoma cell cultures.[15] Interleukin-6 is also an inhibitor of erythropoietin production in the kidney.[15]

The clinical data demonstrate that critically ill patients fail to produce the appropriate amount of endogenous erythropoietin in response to anemia and also have a markedly blunted response to exogenously administered erythropoietin. Rogiers and coworkers compared erythropoietin concentrations in critically ill patients and in those with iron deficiency anemia.[16] Serum erythropoietin concentrations were serially determined by enzyme-linked immunosorbent assay in 36 critically ill, nonhypoxemic patients who stayed more than 7 days in the ICU. Eighteen ambulatory patients with iron deficiency anemia served as the control group. Although erythropoietin concentrations in the critically ill patients were somewhat greater than those in adults without anemia, they were significantly lower than those measured in the control group at similar hematocrits. Whether the critically ill patient is a trauma victim[17] or a surgical, medical,[18] or pediatric patient,[19] the anemia encountered in the ICU appears to be the result of both a blunted response to erythropoietin and abnormalities in iron metabolism (Fig. 19-2). The cascade of events contributing to anemia in the critically ill is summarized in Figure 19-3.

MANAGEMENT

BLOOD TRANSFUSION

Blood transfusion is the standard management of anemia in the critically ill. Among the issues being reevaluated are the identification of patients who might benefit from conservative treatment of anemia and the threshold for transfusion at which the benefits outweigh the risks. These risks include infectious disease transmission, immune-mediated reactions (acute or delayed hemolytic reactions, febrile allergic reactions, anaphylaxis, and graft-versus-host disease), and non–immune-related complications (fluid overload, hypothermia, electrolyte toxicity, and iron overload).

Current estimates of the risk of infection per unit of blood are approximately 1 in 2 million for human immunodeficiency virus, 1 in 1 million for hepatitis C virus, and 1 in 100,000 for hepatitis B virus.[20] The most common transfusion-related infections are secondary to bacterial contamination, which occurs 12.6 times per 1 million units of allogeneic blood components transfused.[21] The risk of bacterial contamination is higher for packed cells than for whole blood. With RBC transfusion, gram-positive cocci (staphylococcal and streptococcal species) represent 58% of cases, gram-negative bacteria (*Yersinia enterocolitica*) represent 32%, and other bacteria represent 10%. In one study, 26.5% of cases of infection (49 of 185) were considered a serious threat, and 9.7% (18 of 185) had a fatal outcome. Overall, bacterial contamination accounted for 22% of all transfusion-related deaths.[21]

The incidence of major ABO mismatching is estimated at 1 in 138,673 RBC units.[21] Surprisingly, there is no significant difference in the incidence of major ABO mismatching between patients receiving allogeneic and autologous transfusion. The incidence of ABO mismatch-related death

is around 1 per 2 million units transfused.[21] Despite advances in the understanding of red cell antigens, fatal acute hemolytic reactions still occur in 1 of every 250,000 to 1 million transfusions.[22]

Half of all deaths from acute hemolytic reactions are caused by ABO incompatibility. One in 1000 patients

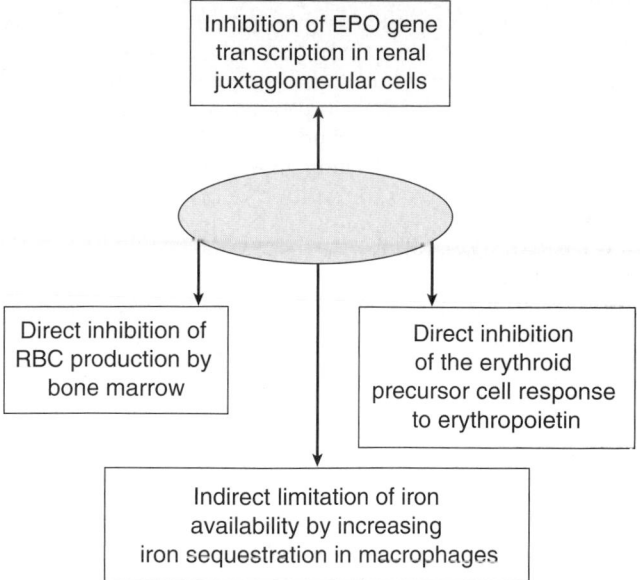

Blunted EPO Response in Critically III

FIGURE 19–2. The inflammatory response that occurs early in injury is related to the release of proinflammatory mediators. This leads to the inhibition of erythropoietin (EPO) gene transcription in the renal juxtaglomerular cells. The inflammatory response has a direct inhibitory effect on red blood cell (RBC) production in the bone marrow and also inhibits the erythroid precursor cell response to erythropoietin. The availability of iron is limited due to decreased iron absorption and increased iron sequestration. IFN, interferon; IL, interleukin; TGF, transforming growth factor; TNF, tumor necrosis factor. (Adapted from Advancement in Critical Care Education (ACCE): Managing Anemia in the Surgical Patient. Princeton, NJ, DesignWrite, 2003, p 28, fig 1.)

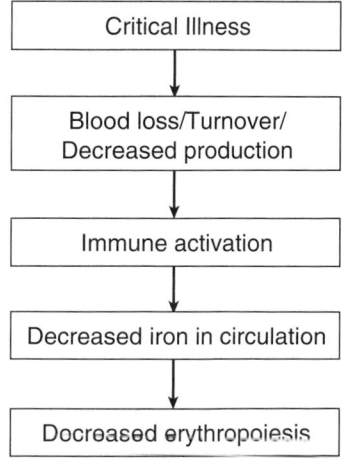

Cascade of Events Contributing to Anemia in the Critically III

FIGURE 19–3. Summary of the cascade of events leading to anemia in the critically ill. (Adapted from Advancement in Critical Care Education (ACCE): Managing Anemia in the Surgical Patient. Princeton, NJ, DesignWrite, 2003, p 7, fig 1.)

demonstrates clinical manifestations of a delayed hemolytic transfusion reaction.[22] Hemolytic transfusion reaction occurs as a result of antigens that are not routinely detected by antibody assays before transfusion.

Transfusion-related acute lung injury is a serious complication with clinical symptoms similar to those of acute respiratory distress syndrome.[23] It is estimated that transfusion-related acute lung injury occurs in 1 of 5000 transfusions and has a mortality rate of 5% to 10%.[23] The pathogenesis of transfusion-related acute lung injury is still not well understood, but a two-hit hypothesis has been advanced to explain why some blood transfusion recipients develop the condition and others do not. The first hit is thought to be the priming of neutrophils, and the second hit is postulated to involve the transfusion of a lipid cytokine or an antibody that activates the primed neutrophils, leading to an inflammatory process.[23] Unfortunately, treatment is currently limited to supportive measures.

Transfused blood appears to be an immunosuppressive agent. Numerous clinical studies have examined the association of perioperative allogeneic blood transfusion with either cancer recurrence or postoperative bacterial infection,[24-32] as well as organ dysfunction. Clinical evidence of transfusion-associated immunomodulation was initially suggested by Opelz and colleagues in 1973, when improved renal allograft survival was demonstrated in patients transfused before transplantation.[25] Although several theories have been postulated to explain transfusion-associated immunomodulation, both animal and human data suggest that it is most likely secondary to the effect of transfused white blood cells (WBCs).

Seven randomized, controlled trials designed to investigate the impact of allogeneic blood transfusion on the incidence of postoperative infection have yielded contradictory findings.[26-32] Van de Watering and colleagues looked at the effect of leukocyte-depleted versus buffy coat–reduced blood transfusion in cardiac surgery patients.[29] Their study detected an association between WBC-containing allogeneic blood transfusion and postoperative mortality from causes other than postoperative infection. Multivariate regression analysis showed that the number of RBC units transfused was the most significant predictor of postoperative mortality. Patients who received leukocyte-depleted blood transfusion had a significantly reduced mortality. Jensen and colleagues, studying patients undergoing colorectal surgery, observed a 71% reduction in the incidence of postoperative infection in recipients of poststorage leukocyte-depleted transfusions.[28] Houbiers and colleagues, in a similar study, found no difference in the incidence of postoperative infection between the two groups.[31] The existing data from the various studies, although not compelling, justify a high degree of suspicion that an adverse transfusion-associated immunomodulation effect does exist. Because the evidence implicates allogeneic WBCs in the production of transfusion-associated immunomodulation, several western European countries and Canada have instituted the universal reduction of WBCs in all transfused blood components. Appropriately designed clinical studies are still needed to confirm the benefit of leukocyte-depleted blood transfusions.

Vamvakas and Carven reported that patients who received allogeneic transfusions perioperatively had significantly longer hospital stays.[33] These observations concur with the data collected by Taylor and coworkers, who reviewed the relationship between transfusion and infections in a medical-surgical-trauma ICU.[34] The nosocomial infection rate for the entire cohort was 6%. The nosocomial infection rates for the transfusion and nontransfusion groups were 15% and 3%, respectively ($P < 0.005$). The chance of infection increased 1.5-fold with each unit of packed RBCs transfused. After adjusting for age and the probability of survival, nosocomial infection still occurred at a consistently higher rate in patients who were transfused. Certainly, the fact that patients requiring transfusion are likely more ill remains a confounding factor in these studies.

TRANSFUSION OF THE CRITICALLY ILL

The overuse of transfusion is a significant problem. In 1995 Corwin and colleagues reported that 40% of transfusion events in the ICU had no clinical indication.[2] More recently, a large multicenter U.S. trial showed that patients who were transfused did not differ significantly with respect to their mean pretransfusion hemoglobin, admitting diagnosis, or indication for transfusion.[3] Thus, it appears that the hemoglobin value is still the major determinant in the decision to transfuse. Several questions need to be answered when we consider transfusing critically ill anemic patients: (1) Is a low hematocrit harmful to the critically ill patient? (2) What is the lowest tolerable hemoglobin concentration? (3) Will RBC transfusion benefit the anemic critically ill patient?[35]

A reasonable indication for the transfusion of RBCs is to augment the oxygen carrying capacity of the blood. Unfortunately, there is a lack of data defining the hemoglobin concentration in humans that hinders adequate oxygen delivery and initiates tissue hypoxia.[36] Studies in animals and humans show that the oxygen extraction ratio (O_2 consumption/O_2 delivery) progressively increases as a compensatory response to hemodilution. However, isovolemic hemodilution to a hemoglobin concentration of 5 g/dL in resting humans does not produce evidence of inadequate systemic oxygen delivery or adverse clinical effects.[36] This finding is consistent with data obtained by studying anemic patients who refuse transfusion.[37] Recently a Canadian trial demonstrated that a restrictive transfusion strategy (transfusion trigger: hemoglobin concentration of 7 to 9 g/dL) was at least equivalent if not superior to a liberal transfusion strategy (transfusion trigger: hemoglobin concentration of 10 to 12 g/dL).[38]

The optimal hemoglobin concentration in critical illness is unknown. Nelson and colleagues observed that postoperative anemia of less than 28% is associated with a significant increase in myocardial ischemia and morbid cardiac events among high-risk patients undergoing infrainguinal arterial bypass procedures.[39] Fang and colleagues reported that the lowest hematocrit during cardiopulmonary bypass (<14% for low-risk patients and <17% for high-risk patients) was an independent risk factor for mortality among patients undergoing coronary artery bypass grafting.[40] Similarly, Carson and colleagues studied the effect of anemia in Jehovah's Witnesses undergoing surgery.[41] They demonstrated that a low preoperative hemoglobin or a substantial operative blood loss was associated with an increase in the risk of death or serious morbidity only in patients with cardiovascular disease. Gould and colleagues investigated the impact of anemia on surgical mortality in a historical control group who refused blood for religious reasons.[42] Their study showed a rise in mortality in perioperative

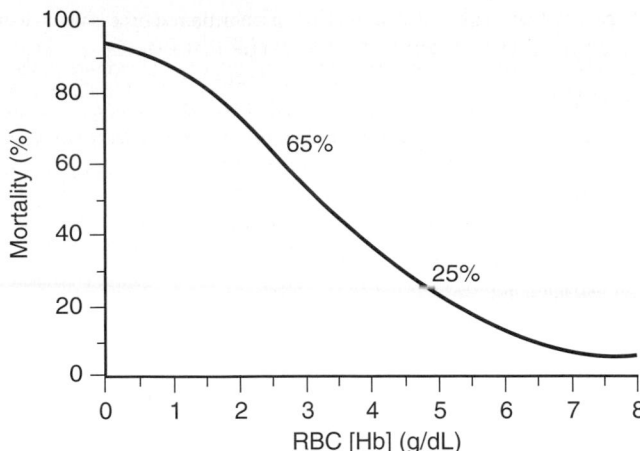

FIGURE 19–4. Mortality and hemoglobin levels in historical controls who refused blood for religious reasons. Note the sharp rise in mortality at hemoglobin levels less than 5 g/dL. RBC, red blood cell. (Adapted from Gould SA, Moore EE, Hoyt DB, et al: The life-sustaining capacity of human polymerized hemoglobin when red cells might be unavailable. J Am Coll Surg 2002;195:445-452, fig 4.)

patients as the hemoglobin level decreased below 5 g/dL (Fig. 19-4). The treatment of anemia in elderly patients (older than 65 years) is not as well defined as in other populations. Wu and colleagues demonstrated that blood transfusion is associated with a lower short-term mortality rate in elderly patients with acute myocardial infarction and a hematocrit less than 30.[43] Clearly, transfusion practices must be individualized to consider all disease processes and existing comorbidities.

Typically, blood is administered to improve oxygen delivery to the tissues. Although blood transfusion might acutely increase oxygen delivery, a matching improvement in tissue oxygen consumption is not necessarily seen, particularly in sepsis. For example, Dietrich and coworkers demonstrated that increasing oxygen carrying capacity with blood transfusion did not improve tissue oxygenation or decrease lactate levels in patients with shock.[44] The same conclusion was reached by Silverman and colleagues in a study evaluating the efficacy of dobutamine or packed RBC transfusion on splanchnic tissue oxygen utilization.[45] Indeed, blood transfusion may have an unfavorable impact on oxygen delivery in sepsis. Fitzgerald and coworkers concluded that storing rat RBCs for 28 days impairs their ability to improve tissue oxygenation when transfused into either control or septic rats.[46] This contrasted with an observation that transfusion of fresh blood acutely increases systemic oxygen uptake in this animal model. Marik and Sibbald showed that old blood (>15 days) transfused into septic patients was accompanied by splanchnic ischemia, as shown by gastric tonometry.[47] It is known that during storage, the concentration of 2,3-diphosphoglycerate (2,3-DPG) in RBCs progressively decreases. In addition, the adenosine triphosphate content of stored RBCs decreases, and the cells become less deformable. The microcirculation in septic patients is not normal, and old, poorly deformable RBCs may become entrapped in capillaries, promoting the development of tissue ischemia. Martin and colleagues observed a statistically significant association between the transfusion of old blood (>14 days) and increased duration of ICU stay.[48] The age of transfused RBCs was the only predictor of the length of ICU stay in patients who received transfusions. The implications

of this association between adverse outcomes and the infusion of aged RBCs is worrisome, given that a typical unit of transfused blood in ICUs is between 16 (Europe) and 21 (U.S.) days old.[3,4] Finally, blood transfusion has been shown in several studies to be an independent predictor of multiorgan failure, even after correction for other indices of shock.[3,49]

To elucidate the possible advantages of transfusion in critically ill patients, Hebert and colleagues in Canada conducted a randomized, controlled clinical trial (the TRICC study) to determine whether a restrictive approach to red cell transfusion (transfusion trigger: hemoglobin concentration between 7 and 9 g/dL) was equivalent to a more liberal transfusion strategy (transfusion trigger: hemoglobin concentration between 10 and 12 g/dL) in critically ill patients.[38] The average number of transfusions was reduced by 54% when the lower threshold was used, and 33% of the patients in the restrictive group did not require transfusion. The 30-day mortality rate was similar in both groups. However, the death rate was significantly lower with the restrictive strategy among typical ICU patients (Acute Physiology and Chronic Health Evaluation [APACHE] II score = 20) and among patients younger than 55 years. A subsequent subgroup analysis of patients with cardiovascular disease found no significant mortality differences between the two transfusion strategies.[50] There was a trend, however, toward decreased survival with the restrictive strategy in patients with active or severe ischemic heart disease. Finally, there appears to be no difference in the duration of mechanical ventilation between the two transfusion policies.[51] Therefore, the TRICC study provides convincing evidence that restricting transfusion to critically ill patients with a hemoglobin concentration of 7 g/dL or less is safe and conserves this precious resource. Use of a restrictive transfusion approach at our busy trauma center reduced our yearly consumption of packed cells by about 25% (absent changes in the use of platelets or clotting factors), with no discernible impact on outcome.

Despite a restrictive strategy, 60% of ICU patients are still transfused. Based on the growing body of evidence suggesting the detrimental clinical effect of blood transfusion, new therapies that can increase hemoglobin levels in critically ill patients have emerged. Recombinant human erythropoietin may assist in augmenting red cell production in this population. Recently, Corwin and colleagues demonstrated a 19% reduction in blood transfusion among a group of critically ill patients who received high weekly doses of recombinant human erythropoietin compared with those receiving a placebo.[52] There were no significant differences in the frequency of adverse events or in mortality between the two groups. The effect of erythropoietin translated into only 0.6 unit per patient over 28 days.

ANNOTATED REFERENCES

Corwin HL, Gettinger A, Pearl RG, et al: Efficacy of recombinant human erythropoietin in critically ill patients: A randomized controlled trial. JAMA 2002;288:2827-2835.

> The use of recombinant human erythropoietin is one of the new therapies that can increase hemoglobin levels in critically ill patients. In this randomized, prospective, multicenter trial, the authors showed a 19% reduction in the total units of RBCs transfused to critically ill patients receiving erythropoietin versus those receiving placebo.

Hebert PC, Wells G, Blajchman MA, et al: A multicenter, randomized, controlled clinical trial of transfusion requirement in critical care. N Engl J Med 1999;340:409-417.

To elucidate the possible advantages of transfusion in critically ill patients, these Canadian investigators conducted a randomized, controlled clinical trial that showed that a restrictive approach to red cell transfusion (transfusing at a hemoglobin of 7 to 9 g/dL) is equivalent to a more liberal transfusion strategy (transfusing at 10 to 12 g/dL).

Marik PE, Sibbald WJ: Effect of stored-blood transfusion on oxygen delivery in patients with sepsis. JAMA 1993;269:3024-3029.

Although blood transfusion might acutely increase oxygen delivery, a matching improvement in tissue oxygen consumption is not necessarily seen, especially in sepsis. These authors showed that transfusing old blood (>15 days) in septic patients is accompanied by splanchnic ischemia, as shown by gastric tonometry.

Rogiers P, Zhang H, Leeman M, et al: Erythropoietin response is blunted in critically ill patients. Intensive Care Med 1997;23:159-162.

This study used enzyme-linked immunosorbent aassay to measure erythropoietin levels in critically ill patients with no renal failure and compare them with levels in ambulatory patients with iron deficiency anemia. It showed that erythropoietin is inappropriately low in critically ill patients with sepsis.

Vincent JL, Baron JF, Reinhart K, et al: Anemia and blood transfusion in critically ill patients. JAMA 2002;288.

This trial, one of the largest prospective observational studies, showed that 37% of patients admitted to the ICU are transfused. In addition, it provided evidence of an association among transfusion, diminished organ function, and mortality.

Chapter 20
THROMBOCYTOPENIA

William C. Aird

INCIDENCE

Thrombocytopenia is often classified according to whether platelets are being consumed, sequestered, or underproduced in the bone marrow. However, a more practical classification takes into account the clinical setting (Table 20-1).[1] In the ICU, thrombocytopenia occurs in up to 20% of medical and 35% of surgical admissions.[2] Although there are many causes of thrombocytopenia in this setting, the two most important ones are sepsis and heparin. Sepsis is a major risk factor, being associated with thrombocytopenia in 35% to 59% of cases.[2] The incidence of heparin-induced thrombocytopenia is influenced by the dose and type of heparin preparation, as well as the patient population receiving it. It is estimated that 2% of cardiac medical patients and 15% of orthopedic patients develop heparin-induced thrombocytopenia antibodies following exposure to unfractionated heparin, and up to one half of patients who undergo cardiac bypass surgery develop such antibodies. Only a minority of patients who form heparin-induced thrombocytopenia antibodies develop thrombocytopenia, and an even smaller fraction develop the clinical complication of thrombosis (reviewed in reference 1).

PATHOPHYSIOLOGY

Patients with sepsis may develop de novo ethylenediamine-tetraacetic acid (EDTA)–dependent antibodies that cause platelet clumping in the test tube, with resultant pseudothrombocytopenia.[3] Immune mechanisms rarely contribute to sepsis-induced thrombocytopenia.[4] Nonspecific platelet-associated antibodies can be detected in up to 30% of ICU patients.[4] In these cases, nonpathogenic immunoglobulin G (IgG) presumably binds to bacterial products on the surface of platelets, to an altered platelet surface, or as immune complexes. A subset of patients with platelet-associated antibodies has autoantibodies directed against the integrin glycoprotein IIb/IIIa.[4] These antibodies have been implicated in the pathogenesis of immune thrombocytopenic purpura and, although not proved, may play a role in mediating sepsis-induced thrombocytopenia. Nonimmune platelet destruction is the most important cause of thrombocytopenia in severe sepsis. There is increased binding of platelets to the activated endothelium, resulting in their sequestration, activation, and destruction. Less commonly, thrombocytopenia is associated with underlying disseminated intravascular coagulation. Bone marrow specimens have demonstrated a high incidence of hematophagocytosis in patients with sepsis and thrombocytopenia.[5] The degree to which this pathologic process is a cause or simply a marker of sepsis-related thrombocytopenia is not clear.

Heparin-induced thrombocytopenia is a clinicopathologic syndrome that is diagnosed by the detection of circulating antibodies, usually of the IgG1 subclass, and thrombocytopenia with or without thrombosis. Heparin-induced thrombocytopenia antibodies, which recognize a cryptic autoantigen composed of multimolecular complexes of the chemokine platelet factor 4 (PF4) and heparin, may be detected by antigen assays or activation assays. Seroconversion occurs 5 to 10 days following initiation of heparin therapy. An important exception to this rule is that patients who have been treated with heparin in the past 100 days are at risk for developing rapid-onset heparin-induced thrombocytopenia promptly on re-exposure to heparin.[6] Heparin-induced thrombocytopenia occurs when platelet-bound PF4-heparin-IgG complexes interact with the Fcγ receptor type IIa (FcγRIIA), leading to platelet activation and aggregation.

In addition to sepsis and heparin-related mechanisms, other causes of thrombocytopenia should be considered in

TABLE 20–1. DIFFERENTIAL DIAGNOSIS OF THROMBOCYTOPENIA

Outpatients

Pregnancy
Immune thrombocytopenic purpura
Myelodysplastic syndrome
Hypersplenism
Antiphospholipid antibody syndrome
Hereditary thrombocytopenia

Non–ICU and MICU Inpatients

Drugs, including heparin
Sepsis
Disseminated intravascular coagulation
Dilutional thrombocytopenia
Post-transfusion purpura
Folate deficiency

Coronary Care Unit Inpatients

Heparin
Glycoprotein IIb/IIIa antagonists
Adenosine diphosphate receptor antagonists
Coronary artery bypass surgery
Intra-aortic balloon pump

Emergency Room Patients

Acute alcohol toxicity
Thrombocytopenic thrombotic purpura/hemolytic uremic syndrome
Immune thrombocytopenic purpura
Drugs

critically ill patients, including other drugs, dilutional thrombocytopenia following trauma or complicated surgery and multiple transfusions, acute folate deficiency,[7] and preexisting underlying disease (e.g., cancer, hypersplenism, immune thrombocytopenic purpura).

CLINICAL MANIFESTATIONS AND DIAGNOSIS

Patients with thrombocytopenia may develop petechiae, purpura, bruising, or frank bleeding. The diagnosis of thrombocytopenia is made from the complete blood count. It is important to examine the peripheral blood smear to rule out platelet clumping. If such a phenomenon is observed, the platelet count should be repeated in blood drawn into a tube that contains an anticoagulant other than EDTA. If thrombocytopenia is associated with consumptive coagulopathy, any or all of the following laboratory tests may be abnormal: International Normalized Ratio, partial thromboplastin time, thrombin time, circulating concentration of D-dimer, plasma fibrinogen level, concentration of thrombin-antithrombin complexes, and plasma concentration of prothrombin fragment 1.2. The peripheral smear may show schistocytes. Although patients with sepsis may have increased platelet-associated IgG, this test is nonspecific and does not help in guiding therapy.

It is important to recognize that thrombocytopenia associated with sepsis, and particularly heparin-induced thrombocytopenia, can coexist with an underlying hypercoagulable state. Indeed, patients with heparin-induced thrombocytopenia are at far greater risk for thrombosis than for bleeding. These patients typically have mild to moderate reductions in platelet counts (median, 60,000/μL). Only 5% of cases are associated with platelet counts less than 15,000/μL.[8] It is important to recognize that thrombotic complications may occur with a "normal" platelet count (i.e., >150,000/μL). Findings suggestive of the diagnosis of heparin-induced thrombocytopenia in these patients is a 30% to 50% or greater fall in the platelet count within the normal range, or the presence of erythematous or necrotic skin lesions at subcutaneous heparin injection sites.

PROGNOSIS

Thrombocytopenia is a predictor of mortality in ICU patients and in patients with severe sepsis.[9,10] The degree and duration of thrombocytopenia, as well as the net change in the platelet count, are important determinants of survival.[10-12]

TREATMENT

Treatment of thrombocytopenia depends on the underlying mechanism. As a general rule, when thrombocytopenia is associated with an increased risk for bleeding and is not attributable to immune mechanisms, patients should be transfused with platelets to maintain a minimal platelet count. Although guidelines for prophylactic transfusions in patients with chemotherapy-induced thrombocytopenia have been

established,[13] the threshold for transfusing in the ICU is not clear. This caveat notwithstanding (and in the absence of evidence-based guidelines), most patients are transfused to achieve a platelet count of 10,000/μL or greater. If the patient has concomitant coagulopathy (e.g., due to disseminated intravascular coagulation or liver disease), active bleeding, or platelet dysfunction (e.g., due to uremia), it may be prudent to employ a more liberal transfusion strategy with the goal of maintaining an even higher platelet count.

Patients with sepsis have an underlying shift in the hemostatic balance toward the procoagulant side. Indeed, platelets are activated in the setting of sepsis and likely contribute in important ways to the pathogenesis of the syndrome. Therefore, when considering the cost-effectiveness of platelet transfusion, it is important to consider the theoretic risk of accelerating the underlying pathophysiology (i.e., "adding fuel to the fire"). The best approach for treating sepsis associated thrombocytopenia is to target the host response. Indeed, as long as the low platelet count is causally related to the host response, optimal therapy consists of some combination of low tidal volume ventilation,[14] activated protein C,[15] low-dose glucocorticoids,[16] intensive insulin therapy,[17] and early goal-directed therapy.[18]

The treatment of choice in heparin-induced thrombocytopenia is to discontinue all heparin, including heparin flushes, and to institute therapy with an alternative rapid-acting anticoagulant that either inhibits thrombin or reduces thrombin generation. Warfarin, low-molecular-weight heparin, ε-aminocaproic acid (ancrod), and, as a general rule, platelet transfusions should be avoided, because they may exacerbate the underlying prothrombotic state. Two direct thrombin inhibitors, lepirudin and argatroban, have been evaluated and approved by the Food and Drug Administration for the treatment of heparin-induced thrombocytopenia–related thrombosis.[19] Lepirudin may be given with or without a 0.4 mg/kg i.v. bolus, followed by 0.15 mg/kg/h adjusted to 1.5 to 2.5 times the patient's baseline activated partial thromboplastin time or the mean of the laboratory range. Argatroban is given at 2 μg/kg/min i.v. adjusted to 1.5 to 3 times the patient's baseline activated partial thromboplastin time or the mean of the laboratory range. The dose of lepirudin and argatroban should be reduced in renal insufficiency and hepatobiliary disease, respectively. Selected patients with life- or limb-threatening thrombosis may benefit from adjuvant therapies, including thrombolytic drugs, surgical thromboembolectomy, intravenous gammaglobulin, plasmapheresis and antiplatelet agents.

ANNOTATED REFERENCES

Aird WC: The hematologic system as a marker of organ dysfunction in sepsis. Mayo Clin Proc 2003;78:869-881.

This review places sepsis-associated thrombocytopenia in context with other hematologic changes and makes a distinction between adaptive and nonadaptive host responses.

Warkentin TE, Aird WC, Rand JH: Platelet-endothelial interactions: Sepsis, HIT, and antiphospholipid syndrome. Hematology (Am Soc Hematol Educ Program) 2003;497-519.

This review summarizes both thrombocytopenia in sepsis and heparin-induced thrombocytopenia. Figure 5 provides specific treatment recommendations for heparin-induced thrombocytopenia.

Chapter 21

COAGULOPATHY

William C. Aird

Hemostasis is typically divided into two components: primary and secondary. Primary hemostasis refers to the cellular (or platelet) response, whereas secondary hemostasis refers to the protein response (clotting cascade). In reality, both primary and secondary hemostasis are tightly interconnected, feed back on each other, and operate in unison. Nevertheless, from a conceptual standpoint, it is helpful to consider each limb of hemostasis separately. In this chapter, we review the clotting mechanism. The reader is referred to Chapter 20 for a discussion of the most common platelet disorder in the ICU: thrombocytopenia.

GENERAL PRINCIPLES

The blood clotting cascade is highly complex, consisting of a series of linked reactions in which a serine protease, once it is activated, is capable of activating its downstream substrate. For purposes of this chapter, the scheme can be simplified according to the following themes: (1) the final step in the clotting cascade is the conversion of fibrinogen to fibrin, a process that is mediated by a serine protease called thrombin; (2) fibrin is the "glue" that holds platelet plugs together and contributes to the host defense against pathogens; (3) there are two pathways—extrinsic and intrinsic—that converge to induce thrombin generation and fibrin formation; (4) blood coagulation is always initiated by the extrinsic pathway (via tissue factor) and is amplified through the intrinsic pathway; (5) the prothrombin time (PT) measures the integrity of the extrinsic (and common) pathways, and the activated partial thromboplastin time (aPTT) measures the integrity of the intrinsic (and common) pathways; and (6) every procoagulant step is balanced by a natural anticoagulant. Tissue factor pathway inhibitor neutralizes the extrinsic pathway; heparin is a cofactor for antithrombin III, which serves to inhibit serine proteases (most notably, factor Xa and thrombin) in the cascade; activated protein C functions with its cofactor protein S to inactivate the cofactors of the procoagulant response (factors Va and VIIIa); and the fibrinolytic pathway degrades preformed fibrin. In the final analysis, hemostasis represents a balance between anticoagulant and procoagulant forces.[1,2]

Disorders in hemostasis occur when the hemostatic balance shifts toward one side or the other, resulting in one of two clinical phenotypes: bleeding or thrombosis. The myriad causes, diagnostic workup, and treatment of coagulation disorders are beyond the scope of this chapter. In the sections that follow, we consider the coagulopathy that occurs in patients with sepsis. The reasons for choosing sepsis as the case study are several-fold: (1) sepsis is common in the ICU and accounts for the preponderance of coagulopathy; (2) a consideration of the mechanisms, diagnosis, and therapy of coagulopathy in this setting may be widely applicable to conditions in which the innate immune response is activated (e.g., sepsis, trauma, burns, postoperative systemic inflammatory response syndrome); and (3) recent therapeutic breakthroughs emphasize the importance of targeting the host response rather than the clotting cascade per se.

INCIDENCE

Previous studies demonstrated that the coagulation system is activated in the vast majority of patients with severe sepsis.[3] For example, circulating levels of D-dimers are elevated in virtually all patients with severe sepsis,[4] and protein C levels are decreased in up to 90% of such patients.[4,5] Acquired antithrombin III deficiency is also common in the setting of sepsis, with levels below 60% occurring in more than half of patients.[6,7] Although the operational definition varies among studies, disseminated intravascular coagulation (DIC) is estimated to occur in 15% to 30% of patients with severe sepsis, including those with septic shock.[8-13]

MECHANISMS

In sepsis, the clotting cascade is initiated through the upregulation of tissue factor expression on circulating monocytes, tissue macrophages, and possibly subsets of endothelial cells.[14] At the same time, sepsis attenuates many of the natural anticoagulant mechanisms. For example, circulating levels of protein C and antithrombin III are reduced, and the fibrinolytic pathway is suppressed.[15,16] Moreover, sepsis-mediated down-regulation of thrombomodulin on the endothelial cell surface may impair the activation of protein C.[17] Together, these changes further tilt the balance toward the procoagulant side, resulting in thrombin generation, fibrin deposition, and clotting factor consumption. DIC represents the extreme in the pathophysiologic continuum. In addition to these systemic effects, sepsis results in local activation of the endothelium through the release of a number of inflammatory mediators. Once activated, the endothelium expresses a procoagulant phenotype. The nature and degree of this response vary among different sites of the vascular tree.[2,18,19] The systemic consumption of clotting factors may be accompanied by thrombocytopenia, and when sufficiently advanced, these processes may ultimately result in bleeding. Other factors that may contribute to sepsis-associated bleeding include trauma-related coagulopathy secondary to hypothermia, metabolic acidosis, or massive transfusions; vitamin K deficiency; liver dysfunction; and heparin treatment.[20]

Local activation of the coagulation system in sepsis is an integral component of the innate immune response and may play a protective role in walling off infection.[21] However, in patients with severe sepsis, systemic activation of coagulation is harmful to the patient and is associated with increased mortality.

CLINICAL MANIFESTATIONS AND DIAGNOSIS

Severe sepsis is usually associated with a net procoagulant state, as evidenced by local or diffuse microvascular thrombi. These changes occasionally manifest as skin lesions, as occurs in purpura fulminans. More commonly, the coagulation cascade interacts with the inflammatory pathway to induce endothelial cell activation and secondary dysfunction of internal organs, including the liver, kidneys, lungs, and brain. Patients are at risk for bleeding when the consumption of clotting factors outstrips the production.[22,23] Bleeding is more common when the coagulopathy is exacerbated by concomitant thrombocytopenia, liver disease, heparin use, and invasive procedures. In large prospective studies, the incidence of serious bleeding in patients with severe sepsis varies between 2% and 6%.[7,24] The most sensitive laboratory markers of sepsis-associated coagulopathy include reduced circulating protein C levels and increased circulating D-dimer levels. However, protein C levels are not routinely measured, and elevated D-dimers are nonspecific. In general, coagulation factor levels are inversely correlated with the severity of sepsis.[76] One exception is factor VIII, an acute phase protein. Fibrinogen, another acute phase protein, may be elevated in the early stages of sepsis but is reduced in up to 50% of patients with severe sepsis.[3,5,25]

Marked activation of coagulation and secondary consumption of clotting factors may lead to DIC. No single test is sufficiently sensitive or specific to make the diagnosis of DIC. Recently, a scoring system was proposed that employs simple laboratory tests, including platelet count, elevated fibrin-related marker (e.g., soluble fibrin monomers, fibrin degradation products), prolonged PT (or International Normalized Ratio), and fibrinogen level.[26,27] Other markers of coagulation activation, such as thrombin-antithrombin complexes, fibrinopeptides and $F_{1.2}$, are considered investigational in this setting.

The PT or aPTT may be elevated for reasons other than sepsis-associated consumption of clotting factors (Table 21-1). As a general rule, increased clotting times are caused by inhibitors against one or more clotting factors or a congenital or acquired deficiency state. In the ICU, prolongation of the PT or aPTT is almost always related to an acquired deficiency state. An isolated increase in PT indicates factor VII (extrinsic pathway) deficiency and may be seen in early liver failure or during the initial stages of warfarin (Coumadin) therapy. An isolated increase in the aPTT points to a defect in the intrinsic pathway, namely, factor XII, XI, IX, or VIII. An increase in both PT and aPTT reflects an abnormality in the common pathway (factors X or V, prothrombin, or fibrinogen) or a combined deficiency in the extrinsic and intrinsic pathways. The latter occurs with heparin therapy, long-term warfarin treatment, vitamin K deficiency, advanced liver disease, DIC, or dilutional coagulopathy.

PROGNOSIS

Certain markers of coagulation activation have been correlated with negative outcome in patients with sepsis.[28] For example, low antithrombin III levels in patients with sepsis

TABLE 21-1. CAUSES OF INCREASED PROTHROMBIN TIME (PT) OR ACTIVATED PARTIAL THROMBOPLASTIN TIME (APTT)

Increased PT—Defect in Extrinsic Pathway

Deficiency or inhibitor of factor VII
Early warfarin (Coumadin) therapy
Early liver disease

Increased aPTT—Defect in Intrinsic Pathway

Deficiency or inhibitor of factor XII, XI, IX, or VIII
Heparin (though usually affects PT as well)
Liver disease (though usually affects PT as well)
Lupus anticoagulant (may affect PT as well)

Increased PT and aPTT—Defect in Common Pathway or Combined Defect in Extrinsic and Intrinsic Pathways

Heparin (all serine proteases affected, especially II and X)
Disseminated intravascular coagulation (all factors, including pro- and anticoagulants, affected)
Liver disease (all factors except VIII affected)
Warfarin (factors II, VII, IX, and X affected)
Vitamin K deficiency (factors II, VII, IX, and X affected)
Direct thrombin inhibitors
Lupus anticoagulant

are predictive of poor survival.[25] Decreased protein C levels in severe sepsis have been shown to correlate with mortality, presence of shock, length of ICU stay, and ventilator dependence.[5] In clinical studies of multiple organ dysfunction, maximum PT and aPTT were shown to be longer in nonsurvivors than in survivors.[29] DIC is an independent predictor for mortality in patients with sepsis.[30]

TREATMENT

The consumption of clotting factors with or without secondary DIC is rarely associated with a bleeding diathesis in patients with sepsis. Rather, the underlying coagulopathy reflects a procoagulant state and is associated with increased fibrin deposition in the microvasculature. Thus, transfusion therapy with platelets, fresh frozen plasma, or plasma components is indicated only in patients with active bleeding or in those with a high risk for this complication (e.g., other types of coagulopathy, trauma, surgery, or other invasive procedures).[23,27]

Based on an understanding of the underlying pathophysiology, there has been a shift in emphasis from procoagulant replacement to anticoagulant therapy. Initial studies with thrombin inhibitors were disappointing. Although these drugs clearly inhibit thrombin generation and fibrin formation, they do not appear to have an impact on organ dysfunction and survival.[31] In contrast, preclinical and early-phase clinical studies employing recombinant human protein C, antithrombin III, and tissue factor pathway inhibitor resulted in not only decreased thrombin generation but also improved survival.[8,32-35] One possible explanation for these findings is that the natural anticoagulants have a dual function: inhibition of coagulation and suppression of inflammation. Activated protein C, antithrombin III, and tissue factor pathway inhibitor have each been shown to modulate the inflammatory response under in vitro and in vivo conditions.[36-38]

Unfortunately, in phase 3 studies, infusions with antithrombin III or tissue factor pathway inhibitor failed to improve 28-day all-cause mortality in patients with severe sepsis.[7] In contrast, the Protein C Worldwide Evaluation in Severe Sepsis trial, a large phase 3 study, confirmed the anticoagulant and anti-inflammatory properties of recombinant human activated protein C (drotrecogin alfa [activated]).[4] Most important, these effects translated into a survival advantage for patients with high-risk severe sepsis. At present, we do not know whether the different outcomes in the phase 3 trials of antithrombin III, tissue factor pathway inhibitor, and activated protein C are explained by differences in study design or whether they reflect important differences at the mechanistic level.

CONCLUSIONS

Most patients in the ICU have activation of the clotting cascade. This would be more apparent if we routinely tested patients with a sensitive assay of clotting activation, for example, protein C levels, markers of thrombin activation, or D-dimers. In the face of unrelenting coagulation activation, the clotting factors may become sufficiently consumed to create a bleeding diathesis. Important challenges for the intensivist are to (1) delineate and track a patient's position on the hemostatic scale (prothrombotic versus hemorrhagic), (2) understand that both phenotypes may occur concomitantly (e.g., microthrombi within internal organs and mucosal bleeding), and (3) target each component separately—that is, replenish the clotting factors in the face of severe of bleeding (e.g., plasma products) while attenuating the underlying host response (e.g., low tidal volume ventilation, activated protein C, low-dose glucocorticoids, intensive insulin therapy, and early goal-directed therapy).

ANNOTATED REFERENCES

Aird WC: Vascular bed–specific hemostasis: Role of endothelium in sepsis pathogenesis. Crit Care Med 2001;29:S28-S35.

This review emphasizes the notion of hemostasis as a balance between procoagulants and anticoagulants and applies the principle to an understanding of hemostatic changes in sepsis.

Bernard GR, Vincent JL, Laterre PF, et al: Efficacy and safety of recombinant human activated protein C for severe sepsis. N Engl J Med 2001;344:699-709.

This landmark study was the first to demonstrate a survival benefit of a drug in patients with severe sepsis. Clinicians who are involved in the care of patients with severe sepsis should be familiar with the inclusion and exclusion criteria that were used in this phase 3 clinical trial.

Faust SN, Levin M, Harrison OB, et al: Dysfunction of endothelial protein C activation in severe meningococcal sepsis. N Engl J Med 2001;345:408-416.

For those interested in the role of the endothelium in sepsis and the potential for bridging bench to bedside, this article is a must-read. It was previously shown that activated endothelial cells express lower levels of the natural anticoagulant thrombomodulin. In this study, the investigators demonstrated that a similar phenomenon occurs in the intact vasculature in patients with sepsis.

Levi M, Ten Cate H: Disseminated intravascular coagulation. N Engl J Med 1999;341:586-592.

This is an excellent and still timely review of DIC.

Taylor FB Jr, Toh CH, Hoots WK, et al: Towards definition, clinical and laboratory criteria, and a scoring system for disseminated intravascular coagulation. Thromb Haemost 2001;86:1327-1330.

There has been little consensus on the definition or diagnostic criteria of DIC. This paper represents an important first attempt to establish a set of criteria that may be tested prospectively in clinical trials.

Chapter 22
HYPERBILIRUBINEMIA

Mitchell P. Fink

Bilirubin is a byproduct of heme metabolism. Heme, which is largely derived from the hemoglobin in senescent red blood cells, is oxidized in the spleen, liver, and other organs by two isoforms of the enzyme heme oxygenase, in the presence of nicotinamide adenine dinucleotide phosphate (NADPH) and molecular oxygen, to form biliverdin, carbon monoxide, and iron.[1] Subsequently, biliverdin is converted into bilirubin by the phosphoprotein biliverdin reductase, which also uses NADPH as a cofactor. Bilirubin is lipophilic molecule. To be excreted, bilirubin that is produced in extrahepatic organs is bound to albumin and transported to the liver. The liver takes up the bilirubin-albumin complex through an albumin receptor. Bilirubin, but not albumin, is transferred across the hepatocyte membrane and transported through the cytoplasm to the smooth endoplasmic reticulum bound primarily to ligandin or Y protein, a member of the glutathione S-transferase gene family of proteins. Within hepatocytes, bilirubin is converted to water-soluble derivatives, bilirubin monoglucuronide and bilirubin diglucuronide, by the enzyme uridine diphosphate-glucuronosyl transferase. These conjugated forms of bilirubin are secreted across the canalicular membrane into bile via an energy-dependent process. Conjugated bilirubin is excreted in the bile into the intestine, where it is broken down by gut flora to urobilinogen and stercobilin.

Total serum bilirubin consists of an unconjugated fraction and a conjugated fraction. The conjugated forms of bilirubin exist both free in the serum and bound covalently to albumin; the latter is known as delta-bilirubin.[2] Conjugated bilirubin is water soluble and reacts directly when certain dyes are added to the serum specimen. The unconjugated bilirubin does not react with the colorometric reagents until a solvent is added. Accordingly, the conjugated and unconjugated forms of bilirubin are often referred to as "direct" and "indirect" bilirubin. The sum of these two measurements is "total" bilirubin. The normal total bilirubin concentration in adults is less than 18 μmol/L (1.0 mg/dL). Although any total bilirubin concentration that is higher than the upper limit of normal constitutes hyperbilirubinemia, jaundice (i.e., yellow discoloration of the sclerae, mucous membranes, and skin) is usually not clinically apparent unless the serum total bilirubin level is greater than 50 μmol/L (2.8 mg/dL). Unconjugated or indirect hyperbilirubinemia is present when the total serum bilirubin concentration is above the upper limit of normal and less than 15% of the total is in the direct or conjugated form.

DIFFERENTIAL DIAGNOSIS

The long list of diagnoses depicted in Table 22-1 divides the causes of hyperbilirubinemia into two large groups, according to whether the predominant abnormality is an increase in the circulating concentration of unconjugated (indirect) bilirubin or an increase in the concentration of conjugated (direct) bilirubin. Although this classification scheme is useful under some circumstances, many of the diagnoses listed in Table 22-1 are extremely rare and very unlikely to be

---

TABLE 22–1. DIFFERENTIAL DIAGNOSIS OF HYPERBILIRUBINEMIA

A. Unconjugated hyperbilirubinemia
1. Overproduction of bilirubin
   a. Hemolysis, intravascular: disseminated intravascular coagulation
   b. Hemolysis, extravascular
      (1) Hemoglobinopathies
      (2) Enzyme deficiencies such as glucose-6-phosphate dehydrogenase deficiency
      (3) Autoimmune hemolytic anemias
   c. Ineffective erythropoiesis
   d. Resorption of hematoma
   e. Massive transfusion
2. Hereditary unconjugated hyperbilirubinemia
   a. Gilbert's syndrome (autosomal dominant)
   b. Crigler-Najjar syndrome type I (autosomal recessive)
   c. Crigler-Najjar syndrome type II (autosomal dominant)
3. Drugs
   a. Chloramphenicol: neonatal hyperbilirubinemia
   b. Vitamin K: neonatal hyperbilirubinemia
   c. 5β-Pregnane-3α, 20α-diol: cause of breast milk jaundice
B. Conjugated hyperbilirubinemia
1. Inherited disorders
   a. Dubin-Johnson syndrome (autosomal recessive)
   b. Rotor syndrome (autosomal recessive)
2. Hepatocellular diseases and intrahepatic causes
   a. Viral hepatitis
   b. Alcoholic hepatitis
   c. Drug-induced hepatitis (e.g., due to isoniazid, nonsteroidal anti-inflammatory drugs, zidovudine)
   d. Cirrhosis
   e. Drug-induced cholestasis (e.g., due to prochlorperazine, haloperidol [Haldol], estrogens)
   f. Sepsis
   g. Postoperative jaundice
   h. Infiltrative liver disease: tumor, abscesses (pyogenic, amebic), tuberculosis, parasites (Toxoplasma), Pneumocystis jirovecii pneumonia, Echinococcus
   i. Primary biliary cirrhosis
   j. Primary sclerosing cholangitis
3. Extrahepatic causes
   a. Gallstone disease
   b. Pancreatitis-related stricture
   c. Pancreatic head tumor
   d. Cholangiocarcinoma
   e. Primary sclerosing cholangitis

Adapted from Bernstein MD: Hyperbilirubinemia. In Rakel RE (ed): Saunders Manual of Medical Practice. Philadelphia, WB Saunders 1996, pp 371-373, with permission.

TABLE 22–2. CLASSIFICATION FOR ACUTE JAUNDICE ASSOCIATED WITH CRITICAL ILLNESS

I. Extrahepatic Bile Duct Obstruction
   A. Choledocholithiasis
   B. Common bile duct stricture
   C. Traumatic or iatrogenic common bile duct injury
   D. Acute pancreatitis
   E. Malignancy (e.g., ampullary carcinoma)
II. Increased Bilirubin Production
   A. Massive transfusion
   B. Resorption of blood collections (e.g., hematomas, hemoperitoneum)
   C. Acute hemolysis
      1. Disseminated intravascular coagulation
      2. Immune-mediated
III. Impaired Excretion due to Hepatocellular Dysfunction, Hepatitis, or Intrahepatic Cholestasis
   A. Drug- or alcohol-induced hepatitis
   B. Drug-induced intrahepatic cholestasis
   C. Drug-induced hepatocellular necrosis
   D. Gilbert's syndrome
   E. Sepsis and other causes of systemic inflammation
   F. Total parenteral nutrition
   G. Viral hepatitis

encountered by the intensivist caring for critically ill (adult) patients. A more useful classification scheme is depicted in Table 22-2. In this scheme, the causes of jaundice are lumped into three primary categories: extrahepatic obstruction to bile flow; increased bilirubin production; or impaired excretion secondary to hepatocellular necrosis and/or intrahepatic cholestasis and/or hepatitis. Often multiple mechanisms are involved at once.

The incidence of hyperbilirubinemia among critically ill patients is quite variable. Jaundice is present in more than 50% of patients with intra-abdominal sepsis, 33% of victims of severe polysystemic trauma, and from 3% to more than 20% of ICU patients recovering from cardiac surgery.[3–6] Determining the cause of hyperbilirubinemia of new onset is important when managing ICU patients, because some problems can be corrected. Exclusion of a mechanical cause for jaundice (e.g., obstruction of the common bile duct due to choledocholithiasis or stricture) assumes the highest priority because failure to correct this problem in a timely fashion can lead to serious morbidity or even mortality.

Iatrogenic injuries to the common bile duct are fortunately quite rare, although the incidence of this complication is greater after laparoscopic cholecystectomy than after open excision of the gallbladder.[7] Damage to the biliary tree, stricture of biliary anastomoses, or retained stones after cholecystectomy or common bile duct exploration present as hyperbilirubinemia and elevated circulating levels of alkaline phosphatase or gamma-glutamyl transpeptidase. Most often the diagnosis is made by detecting dilation of intrahepatic and extrahepatic bile ducts using ultrasonography.

By exceeding the capacity of the liver to conjugate and excrete bilirubin into the bile, hemolysis can produce jaundice.

However, the liver can excrete about 300 mg/day of bilirubin,[8] so clinically significant hyperbilirubinemia is only apparent if the rate of hemolysis (i.e., number of red blood cells lysed per unit time) is fairly rapid. Approximately 10% of the erythrocytes in an appropriately crossmatched unit of packed red blood cells undergo rapid hemolysis, yielding about 250 mg of bilirubin.[9] Accordingly, transfusion of a single unit of packed red blood cells is not likely to increase serum total bilirubin concentration. However, transfusion of multiple units of blood over a short period almost inevitably leads to some degree of hyperbilirubinemia, particularly if hepatic function is already impaired. Other reasonably common causes of acute hemolysis in ICU patients include sickle cell disease and immune-mediated hemolytic anemia and disseminated intravascular coagulation.

Any condition that leads to extensive hepatocellular damage will increase circulating total bilirubin concentration. Conditions in this category that are commonly encountered in ICU patients include viral hepatitis, "shock liver," alcoholic hepatitis, and hepatocellular injury induced by drugs, especially acetaminophen.[10] In most forms of jaundice due to hepatic inflammation or hepatocellular damage, circulating levels of transaminases are elevated to a greater extent than is total bilirubin concentration. Making a diagnosis of acetaminophen overdose early is very important, because specific therapy using N-acetylcysteine can be lifesaving.[10]

Two other conditions that are commonly associated with jaundice in ICU patients are sepsis and total parenteral nutrition (TPN). Both are associated with the development of intrahepatic cholestasis. Hyperbilirubinemia is a common occurrence in patients with extrahepatic infections leading to the development of severe sepsis.[11,12] Persistent hyperbilirubinemia in septic patients is associated with a significantly increased risk of mortality.[12] Efforts to understand the pathophysiologic mechanisms responsible for cholestatic jaundice due to sepsis have largely focused on lipopolysaccharide (LPS)-induced alterations in the function and expression of various bile acid transporters.[13–16] Nevertheless, another factor that probably contributes to the development of intrahepatic cholestasis is back-leakage of bile from the canalicular spaces into the sinusoids.[17–19]

The basis for TPN-induced cholestasis is also probably multifactorial. Prolonged bowel rest and ileus may promote bacterial overgrowth and increased translocation of LPS into the portal vein on this basis. Phytosterols are present in the lipid emulsions used for TPN and have been associated with cholestasis, especially in premature infants.[20] Results from two retrospective studies suggest that administration of more than 1 g/kg/day of lipid emulsion is associated with increased incidence of hepatocellular dysfunction.[21,22] These data, however, were derived by studying patients receiving TPN at home for very prolonged periods and may not be applicable to ICU patients. In any case, TPN is associated with the development of jaundice and hepatocellular damage. Accordingly, except in rare cases, most ICU patients are better served by receiving enteral rather than parenteral nutrition.

Chapter 23

THE MANAGEMENT OF GASTROINTESTINAL BLEEDING

Omer Bajwa • Paul E. Marik

The cornerstone of management of gastrointestinal bleeding involves volume resuscitation, correction of coagulation disorders, and protection of the airway while initiating diagnostic procedures to determine the site of bleeding. Management is multidisciplinary, involving the emergency room physician, the gastroenterologist, the surgeon, and frequently the intensivist and interventional radiologist.

Upper gastrointestinal bleeding is twice as common in males as in females and its incidence increases with age.[1] The mortality rate for patients with upper gastrointestinal bleeding has remained relatively stable over the past 40 years, ranging from 6% to 10%.[2-4]

Significant improvements in the management of patients with gastrointestinal bleeding has been offset by the increasing number of cases in older patients, who frequently have significant comorbidities.[5-7] The risk of death depends on the patient's age, the presence of shock, comorbid medical conditions, the presence of major stigma of recent hemorrhage, and the underlying cause of the hemorrhage (Table 23-1). Scoring systems to predict mortality and risk of rebleeding are based on host factors, the patient clinical course, and endoscopic findings,[8] and the mortality rate is largely dependent on the cause. Variceal hemorrhage is associated with very high mortality rate: up to 30% of initial bleeding episodes are fatal, and as many as 70% of survivors have recurrent bleeding after a first variceal hemorrhage.[7,9] In contrast, bleeding peptic ulcer disease has a mortality rate of approximately 0.5% in patients younger than 60 years and 10.0% in patients older than 60 years.

CAUSES OF UPPER GASTROINTESTINAL BLEEDING

The source of upper gastrointestinal bleeding can be anywhere above the ligament of Treitz. Occasionally, it can arise outside the gastrointestinal tract. Significant bleeding from the nose, oropharynx, mouth, or lungs can be manifestation of upper gastrointestinal bleeding. Upper gastrointestinal bleeding can be classified into several broad categories based on anatomic and pathophysiologic factors:

1. Erosive or ulcerative
2. Portal hypertension
3. Arteriovenous malformation
4. Traumatic or post-surgical
5. Tumors

CAUSES OF LOWER GASTROINTESTINAL BLEEDING

Lower gastrointestinal bleeding refers to blood loss of recent onset originating from a site distal to the ligament of Treitz that results in hemodynamic instability, anemia, or the need for blood transfusion.[10] Causes can be grouped into several categories:

1. Anatomic
2. Vascular
3. Inflammatory
4. Neoplastic

In patients younger than 50 years of age, hemorrhoids are the most common cause of rectal bleeding.[11]

The reported incidence and differential diagnosis of lower gastrointestinal bleeding varies depending on a number of factors, including patient age and diagnostic method used. Although there are many reports on lower gastrointestinal bleeding, most are small studies from single institutions that may be biased by referral patterns and diagnostic methods used. Vernava and associates[12] analyzed the Department of Veterans Affairs databases over a 4-year period and reported that lower gastrointestinal bleeding was present in 17,941 patients or 0.7% of all discharges during that time period.

MAJOR CAUSES OF GASTROINTESTINAL BLEEDING

PEPTIC ULCER DISEASE

Peptic ulcer disease accounts for 50% of cases of upper gastrointestinal bleeding[10] and remains the most common cause of bleeding in patients with portal hypertension and varices.[13] Bleeding results from the development of a mucosal ulceration adjacent to a vessel, which can result from factors such as *Helicobacter pylori* infection, use of nonsteroidal anti-inflammatory drugs, and critical illness. Concurrent aspirin and oral anticoagulation use increases the risk of bleeding further.[14,15] Bleeding resulting from aspirin and nonsteroidal anti-inflammatory drug use is dependent on dose and duration of use.[16,17] The current practice of acid suppression with medical therapy (H_2-antagonists, proton-pump inhibitors) has not affected the predominance of peptic ulcer bleeding as the cause of acute hemorrhage.[18]

TABLE 23–1. RISK FACTORS FOR DEATH AFTER HOSPITAL ADMISSION FOR ACUTE UPPER GASTROINTESTINAL HEMORRHAGE

Advanced age
Shock on admission (pulse rate >100 beats/min; systolic blood pressure <100 mm Hg)
Comorbidity (particularly hepatic or renal failure and disseminated cancer)
Diagnosis (worst prognosis for advanced upper gastrointestinal malignancy)
Endoscopic findings (active, spurting hemorrhage from peptic ulcer; nonbleeding, visible blood vessel; large varices with red spots)
Rebleeding (increases mortality 10-fold)

STRESS ULCERS

Stress-related gastric ulcers were previously a common cause of acute upper gastrointestinal bleeding in patients who were hospitalized for life-threatening nonbleeding illnesses.[19] With more aggressive resuscitation and early enteral nutrition, bleeding from stress ulceration has become an uncommon problem.

ESOPHAGEAL VARICES

Gastroesophageal variceal hemorrhage is a major complication of portal hypertension resulting from cirrhosis and accounting for 10% to 30% of all cases of bleeding from the upper gastrointestinal tract.[20] The distal 2 to 5 cm of the esophagus contains superficial veins that lack support from surrounding tissues, and this is the most common site of varices (Fig. 23-1).[21] The dilation of distal esophageal varices depends on a threshold pressure gradient, which is most commonly measured by the hepatic venous pressure gradient, defined as the gradient between the wedged, or occluded, hepatic venous pressure and the free hepatic venous pressure (normal gradient <5 mm Hg). At a hepatic venous pressure gradient of less than 12 mm Hg, varices do not form.[22,23] Varices do not invariably develop in patients with gradients of 12 mm Hg or more; thus, this pressure gradient is necessary but not sufficient.[22,23] Gastroesophageal varices are present in 40% to 60% of patients with cirrhosis; their presence and size are related to the underlying cause, duration, and severity of cirrhosis.[24]

ESOPHAGITIS

Significant bleeding from esophagitis occurs in up to 8% of patients with upper gastrointestinal hemorrhage.[20,25-28] It more commonly causes occult blood loss rather than acute bleeding. Clinically obvious bleeding is most likely in patients with extensive ulcerative disease or with an underlying coagulopathy.

MALLORY-WEISS TEAR

Mallory-Weiss tears occur in gastric mucosa, although 10% to 20% can occur in esophageal mucosa. They account for approximately 5% to 10% of cases of upper gastrointestinal hemorrhage.[22,27-29] Although they are thought to be caused

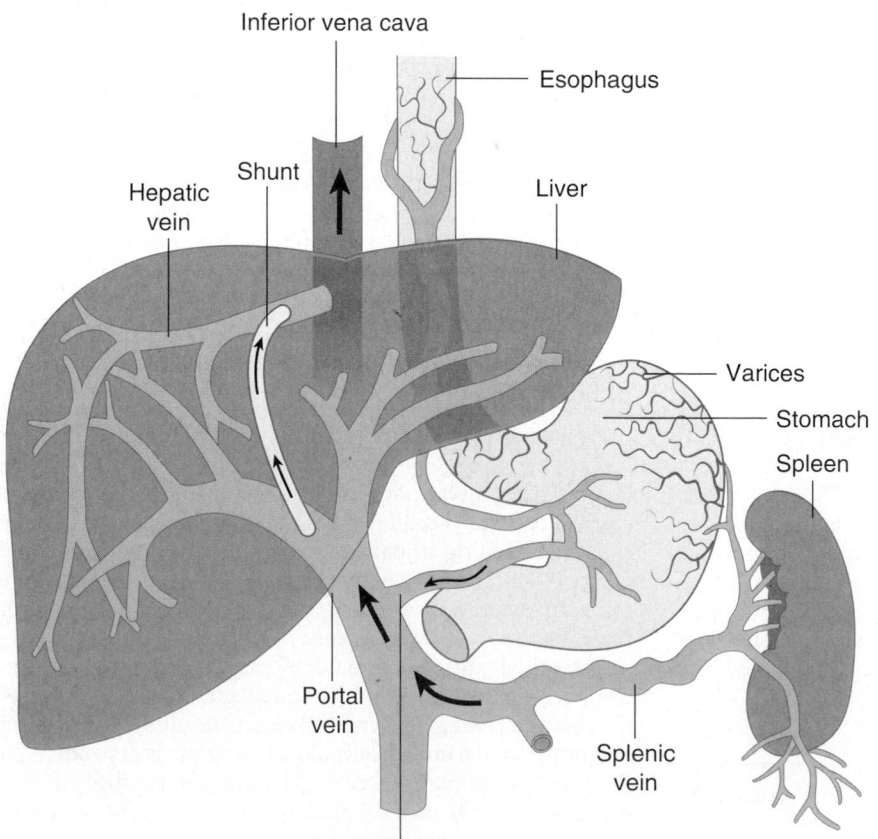

FIGURE 23–1. Transjugular intrahepatic portosystemic shunt (TIPS).

by retching, this history is obtained in less than one-third of patients.[27] Bleeding from Mallory-Weiss tears stops spontaneously in 80% to 90% of patients, and less than 5% of patients experience rebleeding, most often those with an underlying bleeding diathesis.[29,30]

ANGIODYSPLASIA

Angiodysplasia of the gastrointestinal tract is a common source of bleeding. The cause of these lesions is not clear. These lesions also occur in patients with Osler-Weber-Rendu syndrome. They are usually multiple and can occur anywhere from the stomach to the colon, although they are much more common in the colon.

DIVERTICULOSIS

The prevalence of diverticular disease is age-dependent, increasing from less than 5% at age 40, to 30% by age 60, to 65% by age 85. The high prevalence of the disease explains why diverticulosis is the most common cause of lower gastrointestinal bleeding even though less than 15% of patients with diverticulosis develop significant diverticular bleeding. Diverticular bleeding typically occurs in the absence of diverticulitis, and the risk of bleeding is not further increased if diverticulitis is present.[31] Risk factors for diverticular bleeding include[32]

1. Lack of dietary fiber
2. Aspirin and nonsteroidal anti-inflammatory drug use
3. Advanced age
4. Constipation

COLITIS

Infectious, ischemic, and idiopathic colitis (inflammatory bowel disease) can all manifest initially with hematochezia. Mucosal inflammation (colitis) is the common response to acute injury, resulting in activation of the immune system and inflammatory cascade. Establishing a specific diagnosis is paramount in the treatment of acute colitis, since therapy is dependent on the underlying disease process. The diagnosis requires an interpretation of the histologic and gross findings within its clinical context.

NEOPLASMS

Colon cancer is a relatively less common but serious cause of hematochezia. Neoplasm is responsible for approximately 10% of cases of rectal bleeding in patients older than 50 years of age but is rare in younger individuals.[33] Bleeding occurs as the result of overlying erosion or ulceration. The bleeding tends to be low grade and recurrent. Bright red blood suggests left-sided lesions; right-sided lesions can manifest with maroon blood or melena.

HEMORRHOIDS

Hemorrhoids are dilated submucosal veins in the anus located above (internal) or below (external) the dentate line. They are usually asymptomatic but can manifest with hematochezia, thrombosis, strangulation, or pruritus. Hematochezia results from rupture of internal hemorrhoids that are supplied by the superior and middle hemorrhoidal arteries. Hemorrhoidal bleeding is almost always painless. Bright red blood typically coats the stool at the end of defecation. Blood may also drip into the toilet or stain toilet paper. Occasionally, bleeding can be copious, causing great distress to the patient.

INITIAL MANAGEMENT OF GASTROINTESTINAL BLEEDING

Bleeding stops spontaneously in most patients, but aggressive management is required when bleeding does not quickly resolve or when patients are at high risk for rebleeding.[32] Priorities include achieving hemodynamic stability and the prevention of complications such as pulmonary aspiration.[34] The rate of bleeding dictates the urgency of management:

1. Patients with trace heme-positive stools and without severe anemia can be managed as outpatients.
2. Visible blood requires hospitalization and inpatient evaluation.
3. Persistent bleeding or rebleeding with hemodynamic instability necessitates admission to the intensive care unit (ICU).
4. Massive bleeding, defined as loss of 30% or more of estimated blood volume or bleeding requiring blood transfusion of 6 or more units in 24 hours, requires aggressive diagnostic and resuscitative methods in the ICU and the involvement of the intensivist, the gastroenterologist, and, frequently, the gastrointestinal surgeon.

In patients with upper gastrointestinal bleeding, the amount of blood loss can be estimated by measuring the return from a nasogastric tube. An approximate estimate of blood loss can be made by the hemodynamic response to a 2 L crystalloid fluid challenge:

1. If blood pressure returns to normal and stabilizes, blood loss of 15% to 30% has occurred.
2. If blood pressure rises but falls again, blood volume loss of 30% to 40% has occurred.
3. If blood pressure continues to fall, blood volume loss of greater than 40% has probably occurred.

The degree of blood loss can also be estimated clinically by an evaluation of the heart rate, blood pressure, respiratory rate, urine output, and mental status (Table 23-2). The clinical estimation of blood loss is somewhat more difficult in patients with cirrhosis who at baseline have a hyperdynamic circulation with a lower than normal systolic blood pressure and a widened pulse pressure.

History and Examination

A careful baseline cardiopulmonary evaluation is essential; this includes measurement of blood pressure and postural changes, heart rate, chest auscultation, and the ability of the patient to protect his or her airway. A digital rectal examination is always indicated to evaluate the quality of stool and look for the presence of blood, a mass, hemorrhoids, fissure, or fistula. Presence of significant comorbid disease must be determined.

The clinical features of the gastrointestinal bleeding provide clues to the probable source of bleeding within the gastrointestinal tract (Table 23-3). When small amounts of bright red blood are passed per rectum, the lower gastrointestinal tract

TABLE 23–2. CLINICAL INDICATORS AS TO DEGREE OF BLOOD LOSS

Blood loss (mL)	<750	750–1500	1500–2000	>2000
Blood loss (%bv)	<15%	15–30%	30–40%	>40%
Blood pressure	Normal	Normal	Decreased	Decreased
Pulse pressure*	Normal	Decreased	Decreased	Decreased
Pulse rate	<100	>100	>120	>140
Respiratory rate	14–20	20–30	>30	>35
Urine output (mL/hr)	>30	20–30	<20	<10
Mental status	Anxious	Anxious	Anxious and confused	Confused and lethargic
Fluid replacement	Crystalloid	Crystalloid	Crystalloid + blood	Crystalloid + blood

*Pulse pressure may be widened in patients with cirrhosis.

can be assumed to be the source. In patients with large-volume maroon stools, nasogastric tube aspiration should be performed to exclude upper gastrointestinal bleeding, although in approximately 15% of patients with upper gastrointestinal bleeding, nasogastric aspirate fails to reveals blood or "coffee ground" material. Concern that placement of a nasogastric tube may induce bleeding in patients with coagulopathies is outweighed by the benefits of the information obtained. A nasogastric tube should be inserted in *all* patients with upper gastrointestinal bleeding to monitor ongoing bleeding and to decompress the stomach. There are no data to suggest that nasogastric tube placement initiates or potentiates bleeding in patients with esophageal varices. Although there are no published reports of nasogastric tubes causing band dislodgment or variceal bleeding, cautious placement of a small nasogastric tube is recommended after variceal banding.

Iced-saline lavage does not prevent or decrease upper gastrointestinal bleeding.[35] Gastric lavage with lukewarm tap water is as safe as lavage with saline and considerably cheaper.[36] Coffee-ground material or a frankly bloody gastric aspirate confirms an upper gastrointestinal source of bleeding, while a non-bloody yellow-green nasogastric aspirate that contains duodenal secretions suggests the absence of bleeding proximal to the ligament of Treitz.[37] However, in up to 50% of patients with a bleeding duodenal ulcer, a nonbloody gastric aspirate is obtained,[35,36] possibly because of insufficient reflux of blood from the duodenum through the pylorus. Similarly, an intermittently bleeding upper gastrointestinal lesion may result in a nonbloody gastric aspirate. The color of the gastric aspirate is of prognostic significance. Patients with coffee-ground or black gastric aspirates and whose stool is melanotic have a reported mortality rate of 9%.[38] However, patients who have bright red blood per gastric aspirate and red blood per rectum have a 30% mortality

rate.[38] Red blood per rectum from an upper gastrointestinal source usually signifies rapid bleeding.[39]

After the gastric contents have been aspirated, the nasogastric tube should be left in place. The nasogastric tube allows monitoring of ongoing bleeding and is essential to prevent pulmonary aspiration. Once there is no longer any evidence of bleeding, the nasogastric tube can be removed. Maintaining this tube for a prolonged period, especially when the tube is attached to suction, may injure gastric mucosa and exacerbate the gastrointestinal hemorrhage.[40]

INITIAL RESUSCITATION

The first priority in the management of any patient with gastrointestinal bleeding is volume resuscitation. Two large-bore peripheral intravenous lines or a large-bore central line is essential. Volume resuscitation should be initiated with normal saline (a 2-L volume challenge) followed by lactated Ringer's solution. Large-volume resuscitation with normal saline alone will cause a hyperchloremic metabolic acidosis and is associated with coagulation abnormalities. Colloidal solutions have a limited role in patients with acute gastrointestinal bleeding. Patients with an estimated blood loss in excess of 15% to 30% (about 1 L) require blood transfusion (see Table 23-2). In addition, patients with a preexistent coagulopathy (due to liver disease or use of anticoagulants) require transfusion with fresh frozen plasma. Platelet transfusion is indicated if the platelet count is less than 50,000/mm³. Therefore, a complete blood count including platelet count, blood typing, a prothrombin time and partial thromboplastin time, in addition to blood chemistries and liver function tests should be obtained at the time of line placement. In patients with massive ongoing bleeding, type O blood can be used until cross-matched blood is obtained.

The end-points of resuscitation include normalization of the patient's blood pressure and pulse and indices of end-organ perfusion (mentation, urine output, skin perfusion). Vasopressor agents should be avoided (at least initially) because pressor-mediated vasoconstriction in a hypovolemic patient can cause severe end-organ ischemia.[41] Patients with a history of congestive heart failure, renal failure, or cirrhosis require close monitoring during volume resuscitation; overly aggressive volume resuscitation may precipitate acute pulmonary edema and respiratory failure. A pulmonary artery catheter may help titrate volume expansion in these patients.[42]

Once venous access has been established, a nasogastric or orogastric tube should be placed. Gastric lavage should be performed in all patients with upper gastrointestinal bleeding to remove particulate matter, fresh blood, and clots to facilitate

TABLE 23–3. CLINICAL INDICATORS OF GASTROINTESTINAL BLEEDING AND THE PROBABLE SOURCE LOCATION WITHIN THE GASTROINTESTINAL TRACT

Clinical Indicator	Probability of Upper Gastrointestinal Source	Probability of Lower Gastrointestinal Source
Hematemesis	Almost certain	Rare
Melena	Probable	Rare
Hematochezia	Possible	Probable
Blood-streaked stool	Rare	Almost certain
Occult blood in stool	Possible	Possible

endoscopy and to decrease the risk of massive aspiration. The risk of aspiration is especially high in patients with massive bleeding or those who have an altered mental status. Endotracheal intubation is recommended in these patients. In addition, endotracheal intubation facilitates endoscopy. In patients with severe upper gastrointestinal bleeding and clinical evidence or a history of advanced liver disease or a history of previous variceal bleeding, an octreotide infusion should be commenced prior to endoscopy (see treatment of variceal hemorrhage).

TRIAGE: WHO TO ADMIT TO THE INTENSIVE CARE UNIT?

At the time of presentation to hospital, patients should be stratified into a high risk (high risk of rebleeding, requiring surgery, and dying) or low risk group. Patients with one or more of the following criteria are stratified as high risk:

1. Systolic blood pressure of less than 100 mm Hg on presentation
2. Severe comorbid disease (e.g., cardiac, pulmonary, renal)
3. Evidence of active, ongoing gastrointestinal hemorrhage
4. Prothrombin time greater than 1.5 times normal

The rate of rebleeding is approximately 3% in the low-risk group and 25% in the high-risk group. Patients in the low-risk group therefore do not require admission to an ICU and can be adequately managed on a general medical floor. The decision regarding ICU admission should, however, be individualized based on the patient's risk stratification, age, comorbid diseases, clinical presentation, and endoscopic findings.[43] Patients with active bleeding and two or more comorbidities have a greater than 10% mortality rate and should be observed in the ICU.[44] Patients with coronary artery disease, regardless of the severity of the gastrointestinal bleeding, are best managed in the ICU because hypovolemia and hypoperfusion from gastrointestinal bleeding can precipitate myocardial ischemia.[45] Admission to the ICU should be considered when endoscopic stigmata of recent hemorrhage, particularly visible vessels, are noted.

FURTHER MANAGEMENT OF UPPER GASTROINTESTINAL BLEEDING

Over the past 20 years, endoscopy has developed as the modality of choice for determining diagnosis, prognosis, and therapy for upper gastrointestinal bleeding. Endoscopy should be performed only after the patient has received adequate volume resuscitation and has achieved a degree of hemodynamic stability but within 6 to 12 hours of presentation. In patients who have had relatively minor bleeding, endoscopy can be performed on a semi-elective basis.

Nonvariceal Bleeds. A meta-analysis of a large number of studies of nonvariceal bleeds demonstrated that endoscopic intervention decreased the mortality rate.[46] The main techniques are injection therapy and thermocoagulation. Employed as the sole therapy in the past, injection therapy is currently followed by thermocoagulation. Although sclerosing agents have been used, epinephrine-containing solutions are now preferred.[47]

Variceal Bleeding. Variceal bleeding stops spontaneously in more than 50% of patients; however, in those who continue

to bleed, the mortality rate approaches 70% to 80%. Sclerotherapy is effective for controlling acute bleeding but is associated with a high complication rate, including the risk of ulceration and stricture formation.[48] The risk of secondary ulceration and rebleeding following endoscopic injection sclerotherapy of gastric varices has been reported to be much higher than for esophageal varices.[49] Therefore, treatment of gastric varices without active bleeding or adherent clots should be avoided.

Without treatment to obliterate the varices, there is a 60% to 70% risk of rebleeding. The risk for acute recurrent bleeding is highest within the first 24 to 72 hours of the initial bleed and decreases with time, similar to peptic ulcer hemorrhage.[50,51] Another option is variceal band ligation[51-53]; advantages over injection sclerotherapy include fewer local and systemic complications, lower rebleeding rates, fewer endoscopic treatment sessions to obliterate varices, and lower mortality rate.[54-58]

The diagnostic and therapeutic value of endoscopy in patients with upper gastrointestinal bleeding is often limited by the presence of residual blood or clots. Failure to identify the cause of bleeding at the initial endoscopy examination due to residual blood often necessitates a second endoscopy within several hours with a resultant delay in diagnosis that can increase morbidity and mortality.[59] To avoid this problem, gastric lavage is usually performed with a large-diameter nasogastric tube just before endoscopy.[60] Erythromycin induces rapid gastric emptying in healthy subjects and in patients with diabetic gastroparesis.[60-62] An infusion of 250 mg erythromycin prior to endoscopy improves esophagogastroduodenal cleansing and enhances the quality of the endoscopic findings.[61]

FURTHER MANAGEMENT OF BLEEDING PEPTIC ULCERS

PHARMACOLOGIC THERAPY

Gastric acid-suppressing agents such as histamine receptor-2 blockers (H_2 blockers) have long been available as treatment options for patients with peptic ulcer disease. In acutely bleeding patients, these agents have not been shown to reduce the number of transfusions, episodes of further bleeding or rebleeding, or the need for surgery.[63]

During the past 10 years, proton pump inhibitors have been widely used to suppress gastric acid secretion in patients with a variety of acid-related disorders.[64] Data from a number of studies[65-71] suggest that intravenous proton pump inhibitors reduce the risk of recurrent upper gastrointestinal bleeding; however, they may not affect other outcome variables. Somatostatin is effective for controlling hemorrhage from esophageal varices,[72,73] but its efficacy in the setting of nonvariceal upper gastrointestinal hemorrhage has not been demonstrated.[74]

ROLE OF SURGERY

Although surgical intervention for peptic ulcer bleeding has become less commonplace than in the past, the indications for operation remain unchanged, including severe hemorrhage unresponsive to initial resuscitative measures; unavailability or failure of endoscopic or other nonsurgical therapies to control persistent or recurrent bleeding; and a coexisting second indication for operation, such as perforation, obstruction, or suspicion of malignancy.[75,76]

Patients in a trial randomized to endoscopic retreatment had significantly fewer complications and tended to have decreased transfusion requirements, 30-day mortality rate, and use of the ICU compared with patients randomized to surgery.[77] Nevertheless, 10% to 12% of patients with acute ulcer hemorrhage still require operative intervention for adequate hemostasis.[78]

FURTHER MANAGEMENT OF ESOPHAGEAL VARICES

PHARMACOLOGIC INTERVENTIONS

Vasopressin causes direct splanchnic and systemic vasoconstriction mediated via the V_1 receptor on vascular smooth muscle and thereby decreases portal venous flow and portal pressure.[79] Vasopressin may also compress esophageal submucosal vessels and decrease esophagogastric collateral blood flow by contracting esophageal smooth muscle and increasing lower esophageal sphincter tone.[79,80] Vasopressin can be administered either intravenously or directly into the superior mesenteric artery; the simpler route is preferred.[81] As with other potent vasoconstrictors, vasopressin must be administered via a central venous line. It is infused continuously, at an initial dose of 0.4 U/min, with gradual increments to a maximum of 1.0 U/min.[82] Higher doses are associated with increased toxicity without further benefit. Vasopressin achieves hemostasis in about 55% of patients.[83] Systemic side effects occur in 20% to 30% of patients. Ischemic side effects include myocardial ischemia, cerebral ischemia, and acrocyanosis.[82] Vasopressin is also associated with congestive heart failure, cardiac arrhythmias, hyponatremia, hypertension, and phlebitis at the venous infusion site. Vasopressin should be used extremely cautiously in patients with coronary artery disease or prior congestive heart failure. Concomitant administration of nitroglycerin, either intravenously or sublingually, improves vasopressin safety and efficacy.[84] The combination of vasopressin and nitroglycerin more effectively controls bleeding and reduces toxicity but does not reduce mortality as compared with vasopressin alone.[85] Vasopressin should not be administered for longer than 24 hours. Terlipressin, a synthetic vasopressin analog, has been used instead of vasopressin to attempt to reduce the toxicity.[86] Terlipressin is as effective as vasopressin in achieving hemostasis and may be associated with a lower incidence of adverse side effects.[82,87]

Somatostatin causes splanchnic vasoconstriction, reduces azygos blood flow, reduces portal collateral circulation, and decreases portal pressure.[88] Somatostatin has been successfully used as an alternative to vasopressin to control variceal bleeding.[89] Octreotide, a synthetic somatostatin analog, is more commonly used than somatostatin. Randomized, controlled trials have shown greater control of variceal bleeding with octreotide, as compared with control, but no improvement in survival.[90] Octreotide produces modest systemic hemodynamic effects and few cardiovascular complications.[89] Octreotide is administered as a 50-μg bolus, followed by infusion at 50 μg/h. If bleeding is controlled, the infusion is continued for 5 days, then discontinued without tapering. Several studies have shown that somatostatin and octreotide are as effective as endoscopic sclerotherapy.[89,91,92]

BALLOON TAMPONADE

Variceal hemorrhage that is unresponsive to combination therapy with octreotide and endoscopic therapy should be temporarily controlled by balloon tamponade. Balloon tamponade initially controls the hemorrhage in 60% to 90% of cases.[93,94] Rebleeding occurs in approximately 50% of cases after balloon deflation, when balloon tamponade is used alone.[95] Balloon tamponade should be only a temporizing measure, before more definitive therapy is instituted (transjugular intrahepatic portosystemic shunt or surgery). Endotracheal intubation and adequate sedation is essential before placement of the balloon.[96,97] Balloon tamponade is associated with significant morbidity, particularly when used by inexperienced clinicians. Relative contraindications to balloon tamponade include an esophageal stricture, recent caustic ingestion, recent esophageal surgery, large hiatal hernia, recent sclerotherapy, an unproven variceal source of bleeding, and an improperly trained support staff.[98,99] Esophageal rupture occurs in about 3% of cases. Other complications include pulmonary aspiration, alar necrosis, nasopharyngeal bleeding, and balloon impaction.[95,98,99]

TRANSJUGULAR INTRAHEPATIC PORTOSYSTEMIC SHUNT

Transjugular intrahepatic portosystemic shunt (TIPS) is an intrahepatic shunt between the hepatic and portal veins created by angiographic methods (see Fig. 23-1). The shunt is kept patent by a fenestrated metal stent. This low-resistance channel between the portal and hepatic (systemic) veins decompresses the portal vein, similar to a surgical side-to-side portacaval shunt, but avoids the need for general anesthesia and laparotomy.

Approximately 10% to 20% of patients fail to stop bleeding with endoscopic treatment combined with somatostatin infusion.[100-103] Others rebleed in the first few days after cessation of the index bleed. A second attempt at endoscopic hemostasis is sometimes effective and is generally recommended.[104] When two attempts at hemostasis fail, however, the risk of mortality rises exponentially.[105-107] Even though emergency surgery is highly effective in arresting hemorrhage

TABLE 23–4. COMPLICATIONS OF TRANSJUGULAR INTRAHEPATIC PORTOSYSTEMIC SHUNT (TIPS)		
Technique-Related Complications	**Complications Related to Portosystemic Shunting**	**Stent-Related Complications**
Neck hematoma	Hepatic encephalopathy	TIPS-associated hemolysis
Cardiac arrhythmias	Increased risk of bacteremia	Infection of stent
Perihepatic hematoma	Liver failure	Stent stenosis or ruptured liver
Extrahepatic puncture of portal vein		capsule malfunction

and preventing rebleeding, it is associated with a mortality rate of approximately 50%.[108-112] A recent study enrolled patients who were actively bleeding and who were considered to be poor-risk candidates for surgery.[113] Patients were initially stabilized with balloon tamponade, and a TIPS was placed within 12 hours. The balloon was deflated within 12 to 24 hours after TIPS placement. TIPS was placed successfully in all but one patient. The 5-week survival rate among this extremely high risk group of patients was 60%, compared with 10% for historical control subjects. Patients without pulmonary aspiration had a 90% survival rate at 5 weeks. These data have been corroborated by smaller series and provide the basis for the use of TIPS for esophageal variceal hemorrhage refractory to emergency endoscopic treatment and pharmacologic treatment in patients who are poor surgical candidates.[114-117]

The role of TIPS in treating active hemorrhage uncontrolled by first-line therapy in patients who are good surgical candidates (i.e., with well-preserved liver function and absence of complications of bleeding) remains controversial. In the absence of well-defined clinical guidelines, the choice of therapy is often dictated by the available expertise.

NONSELECTIVE BETA-BLOCKERS

Nonselective beta blockers (propranolol, nadolol) have been used to prevent recurrent bleeding. Treatment with these agents can reduce the risk of recurrent bleeding and death from bleeding by about 40%. Sympathetic adrenergic activity regulates splanchnic arteriolar resistance.[118] Alpha-adrenergic agents, acting locally, cause vasoconstriction, whereas beta-adrenergic agents cause vasodilation. Blockade of beta-adrenergic receptors allows unrestricted alpha-adrenergic activity, producing splanchnic arteriolar vasoconstriction and decreasing portal venous inflow. Propranolol is the prototypic nonselective beta blocker.[119]

After an oral or intravenous dose of propranolol, portal pressure decreases by 9% to 31%,[120-127] as measured by the hepatic venous pressure gradient. This decrease is primarily due to a decrease in hepatic wedge pressures, with a small contribution from increased systemic venous pressures.[123,128] It has been suggested that a decrease in heart rate and cardiac output also contributes to the decrease in portal venous inflow.[121-124] Findings suggest that the portal decompressive effect of propranolol is a specific splanchnic effect rather than a consequence of its systemic effects.[129] In the long term, tachyphylaxis occurs in 50% to 70% of patients,[144] which is clinically important because only those with a sustained decrease in portal pressures can benefit from beta blockade.[130,131] Patients whose hepatic venous pressure gradient increases above 12 mm Hg lose the protective benefit of beta blockade and are at an increased risk of bleeding. The underlying reason for this problem, in large part, is a concomitant increase in portocolateral venous resistance. In principle, the latter could be prevented by adding a venodilator after starting beta-blocker therapy. Nitrates such as isosorbide mononitrate have been shown to act synergistically with beta blockers in reducing hepatic venous pressure gradient. The cumulative risk of hemorrhage was decreased from 29% in those receiving nadolol alone to 12% in those who received the combination of nadolol and isosorbide mononitrate.[132] Nitrates, however, may worsen the vasodilation of cirrhosis and may impair tissue oxygenation, presumably by dilation of arteriovenous channels in the peripheral circulation.

Restriction of combination therapy to patients selected on the basis of a failure of beta blockers therefore seems prudent.

Several other nonselective beta blockers have also been used, including nadolol, sotalol, betaxolol, and mepindolol. Nadolol has a longer half-life of biologic activity[132,133] and can be administered once a day. It is more hydrophilic than propranolol; this hydrophilicity limits its intestinal absorption after oral administration as well as its ability to cross the blood-brain barrier.[134,135] Propranolol is administered orally twice a day. The dose should be increased slowly until the heart rate decreases by 25% from baseline but not below 55 beats/minute. Once a stable dose is achieved, propranolol can be changed to a once-a-day, sustained-release form[136] that is equally effective.[137-143]

SURGICAL MANAGEMENT

Surgery for bleeding esophagogastric varices continues to be the most reliable method to control acute hemorrhage and prevent its recurrence. Operative approaches generally consist of either decompression of the high-pressure portal venous system into the low-pressure systemic venous system by creation of a shunt or devascularization of the distal esophagus and proximal stomach with or without disconnection of the portal and azygous venous systems. In most instances, surgical procedures are used for prevention of recurrent hemorrhage rather than treatment of the initial bleeding episode. Because of the effectiveness of endoscopic therapies, emergency surgery for variceal hemorrhage in most centers is reserved for patients who have failed initial nonsurgical treatment and have reasonable hepatic function.[144]

ANTIBIOTICS IN VARICEAL BLEEDING

Bacterial infections are common in patients with cirrhosis. The overall incidence of bacterial infections in cirrhotic patients admitted with gastrointestinal hemorrhage is 44%. Spontaneous bacterial peritonitis is the most common manifestation of infection, which is usually caused by enteric Gram-negative bacteria (mainly *Escherichia coli*). Mortality has been shown to be higher in these patients than in noninfected patients.[145,146] It has also been shown that infections also predispose to recurrent variceal hemorrhage.[147] A meta-analysis of five trials of short-term antibiotic prophylaxis in patients with variceal bleeding showed both a decrease in the number of infections in treated patients and improved survival.[148] The current recommendation is oral administration of either levofloxacin (500 mg every day) or ciprofloxacin (500 mg q12h) for 7 days in all patients with cirrhosis admitted with an upper gastrointestinal bleed.

FURTHER MANAGEMENT OF LOWER INTESTINAL BLEEDING

The management of acute lower gastrointestinal hemorrhage is a challenging task that requires an efficient, disciplined, and orderly evaluation, choosing among several sophisticated diagnostic tools, while concurrently stabilizing the patient and planning definitive therapy. The source of the bleeding lesion can be extremely difficult to ascertain, as even massive hemorrhage can spontaneously stop, thereby thwarting even the most sophisticated and carefully planned efforts at localization. Eliciting a medical history and identifying pertinent risk factors help in determining the cause of lower intestinal bleeding. Use of aspirin or nonsteroidal anti-inflammatory drugs use is strongly associated with diverticular bleeding. Bleeding associated with antecedent hypovolemia should raise the possibility of ischemic colitis, whereas prior radiation therapy for prostate or pelvic cancer suggests radiation proctitis, which can appear months or years after radiation. A history of severe constipation should raise the possibility of a stercoral ulcer, and a recent colonoscopic polypectomy suggests post-polypectomy bleeding.

A careful digital rectal examination and sigmoidoscopy should be done to exclude anorectal pathology and to confirm the patient's description of the symptoms. Of rectal carcinomas diagnosed by proctoscopy, 40% are palpable on digital rectal examination.[149]

COLONOSCOPY

The role of colonoscopy in the evaluation and management of lower gastrointestinal bleeding has evolved over the past two decades. The practice of early and rapid diagnosis and treatment of bleeding by colonoscopy has gained widespread support, in part because of evidence that total colonic preparation with an oral purge is safe, even in elderly patients.[150-152] Elderly patients generally prefer colonoscopy to double-contrast barium enemas, and the yield and value of colonoscopy are well justified.[153] Endoscopic therapy is applied to lower gastrointestinal bleeding in 12% to 27% of cases.[154,155] Modes of endoscopic therapy for acute lower intestinal bleeding, in particular for angiodysplasia and diverticular disease, include thermal contact probes, laser, monopolar electrocautery (hot biopsy forceps), injection sclerotherapy, and band ligation.

SCINTIGRAPHY AND ANGIOGRAPHY

If the source of bleeding is not detected on colonoscopy, a bleeding scan followed by angiography should be considered if bleeding is severe. Although not as precise in identifying the site of bleeding as angiography, scintigraphy is safe and more sensitive, detecting active bleeding reliably at rates less than 0.1 mL/min.[156,157] Angiographic extravasation of contrast material can be seen with bleeding rates as low as 0.5 mL/min. Angiographic demonstration of a tumor, neovascularization, or vascular lesions may identify a presumed source of bleeding in the absence of extravasation. The rate of localizing the site of lower intestinal bleeding ranges from 28% to 77%.[158] A major limitation of diagnostic and therapeutic angiography is the risk of renal failure from intravenous contrast material.

Angiography may permit transcatheter administration of vasoconstrictor therapy for lower gastrointestinal bleeding.[159] Rates of initial hemostasis range from 62% to 100% with this technique, although bleeding can recur in 16% to 50% of patients in the short term. Efficacy rates in controlling colonic bleeding are somewhat higher (83%) compared with small bowel bleeding (71%). In one series, 41% of patients had complications from intra-arterial vasopressin, including fluid retention, hyponatremia, transient hypertension, sinus bradycardia, and transient arrhythmias (premature contractions and atrial fibrillation). Major complications occurred in 9% to 21% of patients and included pulmonary edema, serious arrhythmias, myocardial ischemia, and hypertension requiring treatment.[160]

Transcatheter embolization with various embolic agents, including surgical gelatin sponges, microcoils, polyvinyl alcohol particle, and detachable balloons, has been used to control massive lower intestinal bleeding. This technique has been associated with abdominal pain, fever, and mesenteric infarction. Ischemic complications appear to be more common when embolization is performed for colonic than for upper gastrointestinal hemorrhage because of the relatively sparse colonic collateral circulation. Embolic therapy may have utility in patients with coronary artery disease or in other situations in which vasopressin is relatively contraindicated or has failed and may be an alternative to emergency surgery in high-risk patients.

SURGERY

Age, probably by association with increased comorbidity, is an important risk factor for postoperative mortality. The postoperative mortality rate in patients undergoing surgery for colorectal cancer is 3.7% in patients aged 70 to 79 years, 9.8% in those aged 80 to 89 years, and 12.9% in those older than 90.[161] Surgery is generally considered in patients with acute lower intestinal bleeding, when the blood transfusion requirement is greater than 4 U during 24 hours, or when bleeding recurs. Accurate preoperative localization of the bleeding site is essential for successful segmental colonic resection. Blind segmental resection of the colon or segmental resection based solely on tagged red blood cell scan localization is associated with substantial risk of rebleeding and morbidity.[162] High morbidity and mortality rates are associated with blind limited resection and emergency total abdominal colectomy. The rebleeding rate for blind limited resection is 33%.[162] The mortality rate for total abdominal colectomy ranges from 5% to 33%, whereas the mortality rate for blind limited resection can be 57%.[154,155]

ANNOTATED REFERENCES

Bernard B, Grange JD, Khac EN, et al: Antibiotic prophylaxis for the prevention of bacterial infections in cirrhotic patients with gastrointestinal bleeding: A meta-analysis. Hepatology 1999;29:1655-1661.
This meta-analysis demonstrates the value of antibiotic prophylaxis in patients who have had a variceal bleeding episode.

Khuroo MS, Yattoo GN, Javid G, et al: A comparison of omeprazole and placebo for bleeding peptic ulcer. N Engl J Med 1997;336:1054-1058.
This is an important study that, for the first time, demonstrated the role of acid suppressive therapy in the management of acute bleeding peptic ulcers.

Laine L, Cook D: Endoscopic ligation compared with sclerotherapy for treatment of esophageal variceal bleeding: A meta-analysis. Ann Intern Med 1995;123:280-287.
This meta-analysis compares the success rate of sclerotherapy versus band ligation for the control of acute variceal bleeds.

Lau JYW, Sung JJY, Lam Y, et al: Endoscopic retreatment compared with surgery in patients with recurrent bleeding after initial endoscopic control of bleeding ulcers. N Engl J Med 1999;340:751-756.
This important study compared endoscopic retreatment in patients with peptic ulcer who bleed after initial endoscopic therapy as compared with surgery.

Pascal JP, Cales P, and the Multicenter Study Group: Propranolol in the prevention of first upper gastrointestinal hemorrhage in patients with cirrhosis of the liver and esophageal varices. N Engl J Med 1998;317:856-861.
This randomized placebo-controlled trial investigated the risk of recurrent bleeding after a variceal bleeding episode in patients treated with propranolol.

Chapter 24

ILEUS

Vishal Bansal • Juan B. Ochoa

DEFINITION

Ileus is defined as the absence of physiologic motility of the bowel leading to a disturbance in the progression of bowel contents through the gastrointestinal tract.

Ileus must be distinguished from mechanical bowel obstruction, which is defined as the presence of anatomic barriers, either extrinsic or intrinsic, that prevent the normal progression of bowel contents through the gastrointestinal tract.

PATHOPHYSIOLOGY

NORMAL GASTROINTESTINAL MOTILITY

During fasting states, the coordinated contractions of the gastrointestinal tract are called migrating motor complexes and are divided into three phases[1]:

1. Resting phase
2. Intermittent contractions of moderate amplitude
3. High-pressure waves

When a food bolus is introduced into the intestine, organized migrating motor complexes disappear and digested food (chyme) is propelled through the gastrointestinal tract by spikes in the contraction of smooth muscle in the wall of the gut. Longitudinal progression of intestinal contents (made up by food and secretions) occurs through the integration of several complex processes. Specifically, activation of the sympathetic nervous system decreases gastrointestinal motility. Activation of the parasympathetic nervous system increases gastrointestinal motility.[2] The interstitial cells of Cajal are distributed throughout the tunica muscularis and are electrically coupled with one another. These cells are responsible for the pacemaker activity of the gastrointestinal tract.[1] Myenteric and submucosal nerve plexi integrate with the autonomic nervous system. Nitric oxide produced by neuronal nitric oxide synthase produces smooth muscle relaxation and decreases gastrointestinal motility. Multiple endocrine substances affect gastrointestinal motility. Some of these substances, including motilin, gastrin, and cholecystokinin, increase gastrointestinal motility. Other hormones, notably somatostatin and glucagon, decrease gastrointestinal motility. Activation of the innate immune system can impair gastrointestinal motility in patients with sepsis or after surgical manipulation of the small bowel and colon. Inflammatory mediators, such as nitric oxide and prostaglandins, have direct inhibitory effects on normal contractile activity.[3]

CLINICAL CONSEQUENCES OF ILEUS

Ileus results in the inability to tolerate enteral feeding, nausea, vomiting, constipation, and obstipation. Accumulation of fluid and air in the bowel results in abdominal distention. Symptoms and consequences of ileus can range from minimal to life-threatening. Serious consequences of ileus include intestinal ischemia, intestinal perforation, and abdominal compartment syndrome. Intolerance of enteral feeding compromises the ability to provide adequate nutritional support to critically ill patients.

DIAGNOSIS

Tools to aid clinicians in identifying and diagnosing gastrointestinal dysfunction are poorly developed. Ileus is suggested by the presence of the following signs and symptoms: abdominal distention, nausea, vomiting, high output from a nasogastric (Salem sump) tube, high gastric residual volumes during enteral tube feeding, abdominal pain, absent bowel sounds, constipation, or obstipation. No clear guidelines exist to determine what is an abnormal degree of abdominal distention or an excessive amount of nasogastric output. The true incidence of ileus in cases of critical illness is unknown. Radiologic findings suggestive of ileus are increased air in the small intestine, bowel distention, and presence of air-fluid levels.

Ileus is often diagnosed by challenging the patient with an enteral diet. Gastric ileus (i.e., absence of normal gastric emptying) is observed in as many as one third of all critically ill patients and is more common in hemodynamically unstable patients. Thus, clinicians often attempt to place feeding tubes into the small bowel, where success in achieving nutritional goals is more common.

Three types of clinical ileus are observed:

1. Adynamic ileus
2. Spastic ileus observed rarely in diseases such as porphyria or lead poisoning
3. Ischemic ileus, identified in hemodynamically unstable patients with low flow states and classified as nonocclusive mesenteric ischemia

TREATMENT

1. *Adequate hemodynamic resuscitation* helps to ensure adequate organ blood flow. It is especially important to reduce infusion of exogenous catecholamines, if at all

possible, because these agents promote development of ileus.

2. *Judicious administration of intravenous fluids.* Excessive fluid resuscitation can promote bowel edema, decreasing intestinal blood flow and increasing intra-abdominal pressure.

3. *Maintaining or restoring normal circulating electrolyte levels is crucial.* Hypokalemia, in particular, inhibits normal muscle contraction and nerve depolarization.

4. *Avoiding narcotics.* Morphine and other opioids decrease coordinated contractions of the gut and decrease forward propulsion of chyme. These effects may be especially important in postoperative patients.

5. *Avoiding prolonged starvation.* Starvation is associated with mucosal atrophy. Early use of the gastrointestinal tract (within the first 24 to 48 hours of the onset of critical illness) is associated with achieving caloric goals earlier, earlier time to bowel movements, and overall shorter lengths of hospital stay. The initial goal of early enteral nutrition is to prevent development of intestinal mucosal atrophy, and thus a low rate (10-20 mL/h) of enteral feeding is all that is necessary.

6. *Do not assume that a patient has ileus and should not be fed enterally.* Passage of flatus and the presence of bowel sounds are not reliable indicators of normal gastrointestinal motility.[4] Virtually all hemodynamically stable postoperative patients should be fed enterally as soon as hemodynamic stability and resuscitation are achieved.

7. *Total parenteral nutrition (TPN) is not an adequate substitute for enteral nutrition.* TPN rarely achieves adequate nitrogen retention in patients with critical illness. There are no data to support indiscriminate use of TPN in patients with ileus.[5]

8. *Use of nonsteroidal anti-inflammatory agents.* In surgical patients, the use of systemic ketorolac is associated with early bowel movements, increased tolerance to oral diet, and a significant decrease in narcotic use. In animals subjected to surgical manipulation of the gastrointestinal tract, ketorolac is associated with faster gastric emptying and restoration of normal migrating motor complexes.[6]

9. *In the intensive care unit, the use of metoclopramide has not been shown to provide clinical benefit.* Erythromycin, used because of its molecular similarity to motilin, can be used in some cases, but its efficacy is disappointing.

10. *Newer agents are being tested for clinical use to aid in the prevention of or to hasten the resolution of ileus.* These agents include narcotic antagonists, nitric oxide synthase inhibitors, and protein tyrosine kinase inhibitors.

CONCLUSION

Ileus can lead to significant clinical adverse consequences and mortality, especially if the problem is not recognized and adequately treated. The criteria and tools for the diagnosis of ileus are poorly developed, and this fact hinders progress in this area. Inappropriately diagnosing ileus often leads to unnecessary, prolonged starvation of patients or inappropriate use of TPN. Significant progress in the understanding of the mechanisms that lead to the development of ileus will permit the implementation of logical treatments.

Chapter 25
DIARRHEA

Juan B. Ochoa • Vishal Bansal

Diarrhea is one of the most common abnormal manifestations of gastrointestinal dysfunction in the intensive care unit (ICU). The reported incidence ranges from 2% to 63% of cases.[1] Although many definitions exist in the literature, diarrhea is best defined as bowel movements that, because of increased frequency, abnormal consistency, or increased volume, are deleterious to the well-being of the patient.

CRITERIA

Several criteria are used to diagnose diarrhea[1]:

1. *Abnormal frequency.* Normal frequency is described as one or two bowel movements per day. Three or more bowel movements per day is abnormal.
2. *Abnormal consistency.* Stool that is either nonformed or contains excessive fluid content is abnormal. The normal water content of stool is 60% to 85% of total weight.
3. *Volume.* Stool volume varies according to the amount and type of food intake. Insoluble fiber adds bulk. Normal volume is approximately 200 g per bowel movement. Volumes greater than 500 g are abnormal.

PATHOPHYSIOLOGY

There are several classification systems for diarrhea, a situation that suggests that no classification system is ideal for helping clinicians care for patients. Perhaps the most useful approach is to classify diarrhea based on pathophysiology.

1. *Increased mucosal secretion that overwhelms mucosal absorption.* On average, up to 9 L of fluid is secreted into the gastrointestinal lumen. To this volume must be added the normal oral intake. Less than 1% of the total fluid volume is normally excreted as stool. Thus, the small and large intestine have an amazing capacity to absorb fluid. In the intestinal mucosa, passive and active transport of sodium determines the absorption of water. Increased formation of cyclic adenosine monophosphate within enterocytes inhibits absorption of sodium and promotes the active secretion of fluids into the lumen.[2] Thus, diarrhea caused by excessive secretion of fluids is called "secretory" diarrhea. Secretory diarrhea characteristically contains large amounts of fluid and is described as "watery." Secretory diarrhea is observed in patients with cholera or rotavirus infections and can also be observed in endocrine disorders, such as carcinoid syndrome or the syndrome associated with vasoactive intestinal peptide–secreting tumors.

2. *Increased mucus secretion from the large bowel.* Production of large amounts of mucus and other secretions from the large bowel characteristically leads to a different type of diarrhea. This form of diarrhea is observed in patients with colonic infections, such as *Clostridium difficile* colitis and amebiasis.[3]

3. *Diarrhea due to increased osmotic load.* Many substances that are taken orally and are not fully absorbed can exert a significant osmotic force overwhelming the physiologic absorptive capacity of the mucosa. Many patients with diarrhea in the ICU fall into this category. Subclassifications of osmotic diarrhea exist.

   a. *Osmotic diarrhea caused by medications.* Sorbitol, a poorly absorbed sugar alcohol, is used in the formulation of many orally administered drugs. Thus, sorbitol is frequently and inadvertently given to patients in the ICU when medications are administered via a feeding tube. Sorbitol often is overlooked as a causative factor leading to diarrhea.[4] Other osmotic agents include GoLYTELY solution and magnesium-containing medications.

   b. *Incomplete digestion and malabsorption.* The incidence of malabsorption among patients in the ICU is unknown. However, malabsorption may play an important role in ICU-acquired diarrhea in a variety of circumstances. Incomplete protein digestion (azotorrhea) is one cause of malabsorption leading to diarrhea. A key step in protein breakdown occurs in the stomach, catalyzed by the digestive enzyme pepsin. This enzyme is active only at low pH. In the ICU, virtually all patients receive medications (H_2 blockers and proton pump inhibitors) to increase gastric pH.[5] In addition, feeding tubes frequently bypass the stomach, delivering nutrients directly into the proximal small intestine. Poor digestion of carbohydrates can also contribute to diarrhea in the ICU. In addition to sorbitol, other enterally administered carbohydrates, including glucose, lactose, or fructose, can overwhelm the absorptive capacity of the small bowel causing an osmotic influx of fluid into the gut lumen. Inadequate digestion of fats is a third factor that promotes diarrhea on the basis of malabsorption. Steatorrhea (diarrhea caused by undigested fats) is characteristically observed in patients with pancreatic insufficiency. Inadvertent lack of mixing pancreatic enzymes with the food bolus can occur in patients with intestinal bypass or pancreatic fistulas or in patients that have undergone a pancreatectomy. Steatorrhea is also observed in patients with biliary diversion. Diarrhea due to an excessive load (overfeeding) of any of the above components (protein, carbohydrate, or fat) can be observed in the ICU.

Iatrogenic overfeeding occurs in up to 33% of patients in the ICU and is a result of inappropriate estimation of caloric and protein needs or inadequate metabolic surveillance.[6] Administration of an excessive load of any of these substances also can occur with specialized formulas that contain altered amounts of one or more of these components.

4. *Atrophy of the gastrointestinal tract.* Atrophy of the brush border is associated with decreased capacity for digestion and absorption. Atrophy is observed in malnourished patients; thus, diarrhea is often observed in patients with hypoalbuminemia. Mucosal atrophy also occurs when oral intake of food is discontinued for days or weeks. This cause of mucosal atrophy is a particular problem in surgical patients because prolonged periods of "bowel rest" are still frequently ordered.

5. *Abnormal motility.* Intestinal dysmotility (ileus) is a frequent problem in the ICU. The use of promotility agents (e.g., erythromycin) can inadvertently cause diarrhea in these patients.

6. *Abnormal gut flora.* The normal colonic flora is essential for the proper functioning of the large bowel. Systemic administration of antibiotics markedly alters the microbial ecology of the colonic lumen, possibly leading the development of diarrhea.

DIAGNOSIS

Careful and complete evaluation of diarrhea is necessary for good patient care. Unfortunately, diarrhea is often ignored or hastily treated. Diagnostic laboratory tests are inadequate, making it more difficult to properly diagnose and treat diarrhea. The following questions constitute a useful approach for managing patients with suspected diarrhea:

- Does the patient really have diarrhea? Clinicians rarely will question the diagnosis of diarrhea. Most often, the diagnosis is made by the nurse at the bedside.
  A concerted effort at defining diarrhea is essential:
- Can an iatrogenic cause explain the presence of diarrhea? Is the patient receiving a promotility agent or a stool softener? Is the patient receiving medications with a high concentration of sorbitol?
- Is the patient being fed excessively?
- Is the patient intolerant to any of the components of the diet?
- Is a specialized diet providing an excessive amount of a substance, such as fat, that the patient is having difficulty digesting?
- Is bypassing the stomach or inhibiting HCl secretion affecting the digestion of protein?
- Is the patient on any medications that can cause diarrhea?

Seek to determine whether diarrhea is caused by altered absorptive capacity:

- Could the patient have gut atrophy due to prolonged bowel rest?
- Is the patient malnourished?
- Does the patient have a condition (e.g., pancreatitis) that alters secretion of digestive enzymes?
- Does the patient have a chronic disease process (e.g., short gut syndrome) that alters absorption?

Seek to determine whether the patient might have an infectious cause of diarrhea:

- Is there any evidence of contamination of tube feeds?
- Are the tube feedings being administered via a closed system?
- Has the patient tested positive for *C. difficile* toxin?
- Has the patient been treated with multiple antibiotics, possibly leading to derangements in the colonic microbial ecology?

TREATMENT

Treatment depends on identification of the underlying cause or causes. Once identified, the causes of diarrhea should be eliminated, modified, or treated. This is particularly important when iatrogenic causes of diarrhea are identified. For example, antibiotics that are not needed (e.g., prophylactic antibiotics) should be discontinued.[7] Modification of the diet may be important, especially if the absorptive capacity is being overwhelmed by excessive quantities of a nutrient (often fat). Digestive aids, such as pancreatic enzymes or bile substitutes, should be administered to patients with a disease process (or treatment) that is associated with decreased production of these factors.

Agents that inhibit gastrointestinal motility, such as loperamide, should be used with caution. These agents are often ordered empirically but can worsen the underlying problem, especially when the problem causing diarrhea is an infection.

Bulk-forming agents are sometimes given to patients to improve the consistency of the fecal bolus. The proper amount of these agents must be prescribed, since bulk-forming therapeutics can also be a cause of diarrhea.[8]

Antibiotics to treat infectious diarrhea should be used with caution. If the diarrhea is causing minimal discomfort and is of no physiologic consequence, waiting for results from tests for *C. difficile* toxi may be prudent, rather than starting treatment for this infection empirically.[9]

Restoring normal colonic flora has become an increasingly frequent practice in the ICU. The administration of prebiotics and probiotics has been suggested by a number of different authors.[10,11] The side effects and complications associated with this new form of therapy are not clear at this point. The use of soluble fiber may have a role in restoring normal colonic function and flora.

When dealing with diarrhea, clinicians often stop administration of enteral nutrition or decrease the rate of enteral feeding. This strategy is reasonable only if the patient is being overfed or if the patient exhibits intolerance to the diet. Only very rarely is it appropriate to stop oral intake and start total parenteral nutrition as a treatment for diarrhea.

CONCLUSION

Diarrhea is a poorly studied clinical manifestation of gastrointestinal dysfunction in the ICU. The incidence of diarrhea is unknown due to lack of consistent definitions and a concerted effort to study the problem. We also have little understanding of the pathophysiology of diarrhea in the ICU. Despite these limitations, the cause of diarrhea often becomes obvious with a careful clinical evaluation of the patient.

Chapter 26
RASH AND FEVER

Burke A. Cunha

GENERAL CONCEPTS

The diagnostic approach to an ICU patient with a rash depends on whether the patient was admitted with the rash or acquired it in the hospital. Rashes are seldom the primary cause for an ICU admission. The best clinical approach to a patient ill enough to be admitted to the ICU with a rash acquired in the community is to analyze features of the rash. Its distribution and nature—maculopapular, vesicular, bullous, or petechial-purpuric—determine the range of diagnostic possibilities. Rashes are the dermatologic manifestation of an underlying infectious or noninfectious process, and patients admitted to the ICU with rash usually also have fever. Epidemiologic factors, patient age, and associated physical and laboratory findings all help narrow the diagnosis.[1-5]

Rashes acquired after hospitalization, either on the ward (requiring transfer to the ICU) or de novo in the ICU, represent a different set of diagnostic possibilities. The clinician must decide whether the rash is part of the basic underlying process that prompted the ICU admission or is the result of an unrelated process superimposed on the basic problem. For example, a patient in the ICU with an acute myocardial infarction may develop a rash on the basis of contact dermatitis or due to a hypersensitivity reaction to an antiarrhythmic medication.[6] Rash and fever in the ICU should always prompt an infectious disease consultation; in the absence of critical illness, patients with rash may also be referred for dermatologic consultation. As with community-acquired rashes, a patient who develops a rash in the ICU should be approached syndromically. In addition to the distribution of the rash, laboratory features and pulse-temperature relationships are of diagnostic importance. A history focusing on recent surgical procedures and medications is essential.[1,4]

COMMUNITY-ACQUIRED RASHES

Patients with rash who are ill enough to be hospitalized or transferred to the ICU are best approached diagnostically by analyzing the nature and distribution of the exanthem.

MACULOPAPULAR RASHES

Important causes of maculopapular rashes associated with serious illness include systemic lupus erythematosus (SLE), toxic shock syndrome (TSS), overwhelming staphylococcal bacteremia or sepsis, overwhelming pneumococcal bacteremia or sepsis, and drug reactions superimposed on an underlying disorder (e.g., myocardial infarction, pulmonary edema, acute pancreatitis, gastrointestinal hemorrhage,

adrenal insufficiency, overzealous diuresis). SLE can be a particularly vexing problem, because acute exacerbations of SLE can produce symptoms and signs that clinically mimic bacteremia, community-acquired pneumonia, acute bacterial meningitis, or acute peritonitis. Blood cultures and radiology findings differentiate uninfected SLE flare from SLE flare with infection. TSS can occur in any patient colonized or infected with a TSS-1 producing strain of *Staphylococcus aureus*. TSS is an obvious component of the differential diagnosis in the presence of staphylococcal infection but may not come to mind when there are no signs of clinical infection (e.g., staphylococcal colonization of the nares).[5,7,8]

VESICULAR RASHES

Vesicular eruptions limit the diagnostic possibilities. A vesicular rash can represent chickenpox or reactivation of varicella-zoster virus manifesting as herpes zoster (shingles). Herpes zoster can be localized or disseminated. Disseminated shingles may resemble chickenpox, but patients with herpes zoster have a prior history of chickenpox. Before the appearance of the rash, localized herpes zoster can be a difficult diagnostic problem, presenting with acute thoracic or abdominal pain, depending on the dermatomal distribution. The appearance of vesicles in the same dermatomal distribution as the preceding pain confirms the diagnosis.[7,8]

BULLOUS RASHES

Bullous lesions can be caused by *Vibrio vulnificus* or gas gangrene (clostridial myonecrosis). Patients with either of these bullous disorders are critically ill. Bullous lesions are painful and tense, and the lesions are accompanied by diarrhea. Establishing their cause depends on obtaining a proper history. Patients with *V. vulnificus* have ingested undercooked shellfish, usually originating from the Gulf of Mexico. Clostridial myonecrosis occasionally presents after a crush injury or trauma to an extremity, when previously embedded clostridial spores become activated.[1,5,7]

PETECHIAL-PURPURIC RASHES

Petechial-purpuric rashes are associated with some of the most virulent and lethal infectious diseases. Petechiae can also accompany benign viral infections (e.g., enteroviral infections) and noninfectious disorders (e.g., drug fever). The presence of a petechial or purpuric rash requires evaluation by an experienced infectious disease consultant. Meningococcemia with or without meningitis,

Rocky Mountain spotted fever, dengue fever, dengue hemorrhagic fever, dengue shock syndrome, and arbovirally transmitted hemorrhagic fevers are all potentially lethal infections. Dengue fever can have hemorrhagic manifestations, but such findings are not synonymous with dengue hemorrhagic fever or dengue shock syndrome. Dengue fever should be considered in the differential diagnosis if the patient has lived in or visited an area where the disease is endemic. A history of recent travel to Latin America, Asia, or Africa should prompt the clinician to consider arboviral hemorrhagic fevers.

The two potentially fatal infectious diseases that are most likely to be confused are meningococcemia and Rocky Mountain spotted fever (Table 26-1).[1,7,9-12] Rocky Mountain spotted fever is diagnosed on the basis of the rash distribution and a history of recent tick exposure. Meningococcemia is suggested by rapid onset of disease, asymmetrical distribution of lesions, and irregularly shaped petechial-purpuric lesions. Overwhelming pneumococcal sepsis can also resemble meningococcemia. The former does not occur in normal hosts, however, and is invariably related to impaired splenic function. Therefore, in a patient with fever, rash, hypotension, and an obvious splenectomy scar, diagnosis is not a problem. Making the correct diagnosis in a timely fashion can be more challenging in patients with diminished splenic function or with congenital asplenia. Clinicians should be familiar with the disorders associated with diminished splenic function, which predispose to pneumococcal bacteremia or sepsis (Table 26-2).[5,7,8]

TABLE 26-1. DIFFERENTIAL DIAGNOSIS OF MENINGOCOCCEMIA AND ROCKY MOUNTAIN SPOTTED FEVER

Key Diagnostic Findings	Meningococcemia	Rocky Mountain Spotted Fever
Clinical Features		
Onset of rash ≤12 h into illness	+	–*
Nontender macular/ petechial rash	–	+
Tender petechial rash	+	–
Relative bradycardia	–	+
Hypotension on admission	–†	–‡
Severe headache	–	+§
Conjunctival suffusion	–	+
Periorbital edema	–	+
Deafness	–	+
Abdominal pain	–	+
Splenomegaly	–	+
Edema of dorsum of hands/feet	–	+
Leg/muscle tenderness	–	+
Laboratory Features		
Thrombocytopenia	+	+
Leukopenia	–	+¶
Leukocytosis	–	+
↑ Erythrocyte sedimentation rate	–	+
↑ SGOT/SGPT	–	+

* Usually day 3 to 5.
† Only with Waterhouse-Friderichsen syndrome.
‡ Later, following excessive fluids or myocarditis.
§ Frontal or retro-orbital.
¶ Generalized.
SGOT/SGPT, aspartate transaminase/alanine transaminase.
Adapted from Woodward TE, Cunha BA: Rocky Mountain spotted fever. In Cunha BA (ed): Tickborne Infectious Diseases. New York, Marcel Dekker, 2000, pp 121-137.

TABLE 26-2. DISORDERS ASSOCIATED WITH DECREASED SPLENIC FUNCTION

Chronic alcoholism	Congenital asplenia
Chronic active hepatitis	Sickle cell trait/disease
Myeloproliferative disorders	Splenic infarct
Waldenström's macroglobulinemia	Systemic mastocytosis
Non-Hodgkin's lymphoma	Rheumatoid arthritis
Sézary syndrome	Necrotizing vasculitis
Celiac disease	Thyroiditis
Regional enteritis	Steroid therapy
Ulcerative colitis	Gammaglobulin therapy
Immunoglobulin A deficiency	Amyloidosis
Intestinal lymphangiectasia	Splenectomy
	Hyposplenism of the elderly
	Disorders that decrease splenic artery flow

Adapted from Cunha BA: Severe community-acquired pneumonia. J Crit Illness 1997;12:711-721.

Table 26-3 presents the differential diagnostic features of community-acquired rashes that accompany conditions warranting ICU admission. It is important to remember that arthropod-borne hemorrhagic fevers may resemble meningococcemia.[13-15]

HOSPITAL-ACQUIRED RASHES

Two types of rashes are commonly seen in the ICU: vesicular-bullous and maculopapular.

VESICULAR-BULLOUS RASHES

Vesicular-bullous eruptions can be drug related, but gas gangrene is a diagnosis that should not be overlooked. Patients with severe drug reactions have multiple bullous lesions or can develop Stevens-Johnson syndrome; in either case, the rash is not rapidly progressive. In contrast, in patients with gas gangrene, the vesicular or bullous eruptions spread rapidly (over hours). Gas gangrene in the ICU is likely to be a complication of gastrointestinal surgery performed during the past few days. Skin near the bullous lesions is extremely tender; patients with gas gangrene have little fever but often experience watery diarrhea. Rapidly progressive hemolytic anemia due to lysis of red blood cells by clostridial lethicinases completes the clinical syndrome of gas gangrene. Despite the terminology, gas in tissues is not a prominent feature of gas gangrene. There is no gross crepitus or gas visible on radiographs. Small gas bubbles present in the muscle fascicles usually are not clinically obvious. Copious amounts of gas in the soft tissues or on radiographs should suggest a mixed aerobic-anaerobic infection by gas-producing organisms (e.g., necrotizing fasciitis)—an entity that is clinically distinct from gas gangrene. Mixed aerobic-anaerobic soft tissue infections occur most often in diabetes; although these infections are serious, they are not as rapidly progressive as gas gangrene. Mixed aerobic-anaerobic soft tissue infections do not involve primarily the muscle, as does clostridial myonecrosis.[1,4,5,7,8]

MACULOPAPULAR RASHES

Maculopapular rash as a result of surgical TSS is uncommon but occasionally occurs in the ICU setting. The typical surgical TSS patient develops a wound infection days after an operation.

TABLE 26–3. COMMUNITY-ACQUIRED RASHES IN THE ICU

Type of Rash	Central > Peripheral	Peripheral > Central	Palms and Soles	Appearance of Rash after Fever	Clinical Features	Comments
Petechial-Purpuric Rash						
Meningococcemia	+	+	−	1-2 h	Irregular distribution of painful, irregular petechial lesions Early, spares palms and soles Generalized headache Hypotension (if Waterhouse-Friderichsen syndrome) Leukocytosis Thrombocytopenia	History of recent mild upper respiratory tract infection common in late winter–early spring May present alone or with meningococcal meningitis
Rocky Mountain spotted fever	−	+	+	3-5 days	Painless macular-petechial rash begins in wrists, ankles Conjunctival suffusion Severe frontal headache Periorbital edema Bilateral relative bradycardia Edema of dorsum of hands, feet Splenomegaly in some Hypotension late (due to excessive i.v. fluids, myocarditis) Leukocytosis Thrombocytopenia	Late spring–early fall Recent history of tick exposure No lung involvement unless CHF (late)
Hemorrhagic/toxic smallpox	+		−	1-3 days	Fever, headache, and vomiting precede the appearance of petechial hemorrhage in a "swimming trunk" distribution	Hemorrhagic smallpox presents with petechial lesions and profound toxemia Patients may expire before vesicular lesions develop
Overwhelming pneumococcal bacteremia	−	+	+	1-2 days	Diffuse asymmetrical purpuric lesions Hypotension, shock early Leukopenia Thrombocytopenia Howell-Jolly bodies on peripheral smear	Occurs in asplenic patients (e.g., trauma, staging procedures for lymphoma, sickle cell anemia) Source of pneumococcal pneumonia may not be clinically apparent
Dengue hemorrhagic fever, dengue shock syndrome	+	−	+	3-4 days	Rash begins on thorax Palpable pinpoint petechiae on trunk Pain on eye movement Severe headache, myalgias Generalized adenopathy may be present "Camel-back" fever curve Leukopenia Thrombocytopenia	Recent travel history to Caribbean, Latin America, Asia
Arboviral hemorrhagic fevers	+	−	+	3-4 days	Acute onset with prominent hemorrhagic manifestations Severe headache, myalgias "Camel-back" fever curve Possibly abdominal pain, generalized adenopathy Encephalopathy, lethargy common Sore throat, cough Conjunctivitis Nausea, vomiting, diarrhea Abdominal pain ↑ SGOT/SGPT Leukopenia Thrombocytopenia Generalized adenopathy may be present	History of recent travel to Africa, Latin America, or Asia Rapidly fatal
Overwhelming staphylococcal bacteremia	−	+	+	3-5 days	Asymmetrical hemorrhagic lesions or infarcts in distal extremities	Usually obvious staphylococcal focus or S. aureus ABE

Continued

TABLE 26–3. COMMUNITY-ACQUIRED RASHES IN THE ICU—CONT'D

Type of Rash	Central > Peripheral	Peripheral > Central	Palms and Soles	Appearance of Rash after Fever	Clinical Features	Comments
					Leukopenia Thrombocytopenia No relative bradycardia Heart murmur if source is ABE	
Maculopapular Rashes						
Toxic shock syndrome (TSS)	+	−	+	1-2 days	Conjunctivitis Scarlatiniform maculopapular rash Bilateral periorbital edema Edema of the dorsum of hands, feet Oral, vaginal erythema Leukocytosis Thrombocytopenia ↑ SGOT/SGPT ↑ BUN/creatinine	Recent or current history of tampon use, menses May have only streptococcal colonization with TSS-1 strain Severe cases may have persistent hypotension despite fluid replacement
Systemic lupus erythematosus (SLE)	+	+	−	With flare	Rash usually facial, but may involve extremities Possibly severe abdominal pain On SPEP, α_2-globulins ↑ in SLE flare, but not in infection LFTs normal in SLE flare; if SGOT/SGPT elevated, test for CMV Leukopenia, lymphopenia, thrombocytopenia suggest SLE flare Microscopic hematuria, ↑ serum creatinine also indicative of SLE flare	Flare usually occurs when steroids tapered CMV may induce SLE flare Associated signs of cerebritis, pneumonitis, peritonitis, or serositis with SLE flare Migratory pulmonary infiltrates with effusion characteristic of SLE pneumonitis Rule out infection to diagnose SLE flare Infections common in SLE, but not during SLE flare
Cutaneous anthrax	−	+	±		Circular, raised lesions may initially be pruritic before ulcerating Painless lesions may be accompanied by painful regional adenopathy	Well-developed anthrax lesion is surrounded by a raised "gelatinous halo" Initial painless ulcer has central necrosis and evolves into an eschar
Drug rash	+	−	+	Days to weeks	Erythema multiforme, Stevens-Johnson syndrome in severe cases ↑ ESR Eosinophils usually present; eosinophilia less uncommon Mildly ↑ SGOT/SGPT ↑ WBC (with left shift) Relative bradycardia Negative blood cultures (excluding contaminants)	"Sensitizing" medication, usually not an antibiotic
Measles	+	−	−	2-3 days	Toxic appearance Intense red or purple confluent rash begins on face (3 days head to feet) Cough prominent Conjunctivitis (Giant cell) pneumonia Leukopenia ± Thrombocytopenia ± ↑ SGOT/SGPT Pseudoappendicitis	Occurs in spring Koplik's spots present before rash
Vesicular Rashes						
Chickenpox	+	+	+	2-3 days	Lesions appear in crops for first 3 days, then stop Vesicles are in different stages of development Vesicles lying on skin surface have "dew drop on rose petal" appearance	Critically ill adults usually have varicella pneumonia

TABLE 26–3. COMMUNITY-ACQUIRED RASHES IN THE ICU—CONT'D

Type of Rash	Central > Peripheral	Peripheral > Central	Palms and Soles	Appearance of Rash after Fever	Clinical Features	Comments
					Vesicles surrounded by "red halo" are pruritic ↑ Basophils No leukopenia No thrombocytopenia ± ↑ SGOT/SGPT	
Typical smallpox	–	+	±	5-7 days	Macular lesions start at hairline, followed by papules, vesicles, and pustules that rapidly cover the face and spread to the extremities Relative sparing of the trunk	Pustules in each anatomic region are in same stage of development, but stage differs from region to region Pustule of smallpox is umbilicated and deep in the dermis
Herpes zoster (shingles)				3-4 days		Before the appearance of the rash, the pain of dermatomal zoster may mimic an acute abdomen, pneumonia, pulmonary edema, or myocardial infection Acutely ill adults usually have disseminated varicella-zoster virus
Bullous Lesions *Vibrio vulnificus*	+	–	–	1-3 h	Painful hemorrhagic, bullous rash on trunk, buttocks Watery, profuse diarrhea Abdominal pain No muscle involvement No anemia	Primary septicemia from ingestion in patients with liver disease or severe wound infection from water containing "halophilic vibrios"

ABE, acute bacterial endocarditis; BUN, blood urea nitrogen; CHF, congestive heart failure; CMV, cytomegalovirus; ESR, erythrocyte sedimentation rate; LFT, liver function test; SGOT/SGPT, aspartate transaminase/alanine transaminase; SPEP, serum protein electrophoresis; WBC, white blood cell.

Adapted from Cunha BA: Approach to the patient with fever. In Samiy AH, Douglas RG Jr, Barondess JA (eds): Textbook of Diagnostic Medicine. Philadelphia, Lea & Febiger, 1987, pp 132-141.

Drainage from the wound is serosanguineous rather than purulent.

Staphylococcal sepsis is usually related to an intravascular device or source. Staphylococcal acute bacterial endocarditis may present initially with maculopapular lesions that become hemorrhagic or gangrenous. The diagnosis should be suggested by a peripheral location of lesions with an irregular outline in the setting of staphylococcal bacteremia.

Cholesterol emboli can be released into the systemic circulation during cardiopulmonary bypass. Thus, after open-heart surgery a patient may develop cholesterol emboli syndrome, which presents as a maculopapular rash with a livedo reticularis–like appearance. The rash occurs on the extremities and can be accompanied by myocardial infarction, acute pancreatitis, acute renal failure, or stroke due to organ ischemia caused by cholesterol emboli. Excluding drug rashes, cholesterol emboli syndrome is the only rash in the ICU associated with peripheral eosinophilia.

Drug rash is a drug hypersensitivity reaction associated with a skin rash. Most patients who develop drug rash do so after receiving new medications in the hospital. Drug-induced rashes are usually maculopapular, generalized, and pruritic and can involve the palms and soles; fever is almost always present. Mild transaminasemia and peripheral eosinophilia complete the clinical presentation. The clinical problem is that drug rash is often superimposed on one or more underlying medical disorders that brought the patient to the ICU in the first place. Even after discontinuing therapy with the offending drug, the rash and fever can take days to weeks to resolve.[16]

Many patients develop contact dermatitis while in the ICU. This condition is very common and must be differentiated from a drug rash. Patients with contact dermatitis do not have fever; in addition, the rash of contact dermatitis is limited to a localized area (e.g., the back), whereas a drug rash is never asymmetrical or limited to only one extremity or anatomic region. Contact dermatitis is not accompanied by eosinophilia or increased serum transaminase levels.

The types of hospital-acquired rashes and their differential diagnoses are presented in Tables 26-4 and 26-5.

TABLE 26–4. HOSPITAL-ACQUIRED RASHES IN THE ICU

Type of Rash	Central > Peripheral	Peripheral > Central	Palms and Soles	Appearance of Rash after Fever	Clinical Features	Comments
Maculopapular Rashes						
Overwhelming staphylococcal sepsis	–	+	+	3-5 days	Asymmetrical hemorrhagic lesions or infarcts in distal extremities Positive blood cultures Leukopenia ± thrombocytopenia	Usually obvious staphylococcal focus or *S. aureus* acute bacterial endocarditis
Surgical toxic shock syndrome	+	–	+	1-2 days	Surgical wound nonpurulent with serosanguineous discharge Scarlatiniform, maculopapular rash Extremity edema Oral, vaginal erythema Watery diarrhea Liver, renal dysfunction Negative blood cultures, leukocytosis ± thrombocytopenia	Recent history of surgical wound infection Severe cases may have persistent hypotension despite fluid replacement
Cholesterol emboli syndrome	–	+	–	Hours-days	"Livedo reticularis" rash on extremities Multisystem organ dysfunction: myocardial infarction, pancreatitis, CVA, intestinal ischemia Eosinophilia a key diagnostic clue Negative blood cultures Leukocytosis No thrombocytopenia	Recent cardiothoracic or carotid surgical procedure
"Surgical" scarlet fever	+	–	–	1-2 days	Diffuse sunburn-like rash "Sandpaper" skin Rash subsides in 6-9 days "Strawberry" tongue Leukocytosis ± thrombocytopenia Eosinophilia Group A streptococci in wound cultures ↑ ASO/anti-DNAse titers	Group A streptococcal wound infection due to erythrotoxin-producing strains
Drug rash	+	–	+	Days to weeks	↓ Platelets common Relative bradycardia Erythema multiforme, Stevens-Johnson syndrome in severe cases Mildly ↑ serum transaminases ↑ ESR Eosinophils usually present; eosinophilia less uncommon, may be pruritic Thrombocytopenia common Negative blood cultures (excluding skin contaminants)	"Sensitizing" medication, usually not an antibiotic ↑ WBC with left shift common, mimicking infection
Bullous Lesions						
Gas gangrene (clostridial myonecrosis)	–	–	–	Hours to days	Low-grade or no fever Patients very apprehensive Intense local pain Relative tachycardia Little or no gas on auscultation Bullous, hemorrhagic rash Leukocytosis No thrombocytopenia Rapidly progressive hemolytic anemia Watery diarrhea Radiograph shows small bubbles in muscle	Related to recently fecally contaminated wound Gross gas on auscultation or radiograph argues against diagnosis of clostridial myonecrosis

ASO, antistreptolysin O; CVA, cerebrovascular accident; ESR, erythrocyte sedimentation rate; WBC, white blood cell.
Adapted from Cunha BA: Approach to the patient with fever. In Samiy AH, Douglas RG Jr, Barondess JA (eds): Textbook of Diagnostic Medicine. Philadelphia, Lea & Febiger, 1987, pp 132-141.

TABLE 26–5. DIFFERENTIAL DIAGNOSTIC FEATURES IN ACUTELY ILL PATIENTS WITH RASH AND FEVER

Rash and Shock
TSS
MC
Fulminant pneumococcal sepsis in an asplenic patient
Overwhelming *S. aureus* bacteremia
Arboviral hemorrhagic fevers
Hemorrhagic smallpox
ABE
DHF
DSS

Rash and Periorbital Edema
RMSF

Rash and Conjunctival Suffusion
RMSF
DHF, DSS
Arboviral hemorrhagic fevers
TSS

Rash and Abdominal Pain
V. vulnificus
Cholesterol emboli syndrome
RMSF
SLE
DHF, DSS
Arboviral hemorrhagic fevers

Rash and Diarrhea
V. vulnificus
Gas gangrene
TSS
DHF, DSS
Arboviral hemorrhagic fever

Rash and CVA
SLE
Cholesterol emboli syndrome
S. aureus ABE

Rash and Mental Status Changes
SLE (if cerebritis)
RMSF
MC
S. aureus ABE

Rash and Pulmonary Infiltrates
RMSF
SLE

Rash and Relative Bradycardia
RMSF
Arboviral hemorrhagic fevers

Rash on Palms and Soles
RMSF
DF
TSS

Rash and Vesicular Lesions
Chickenpox
Typical smallpox
VZV (localized/disseminated)

Rash and Bullous Lesions
V. vulnificus
Gas gangrene

Livedo Reticularis–Like Rash
SLE
Cholesterol emboli syndrome

Hemorrhagic Rash
MC
RMSF
Cholesterol emboli syndrome
DHF, DSS
Arboviral hemorrhagic fevers
Hemorrhagic smallpox

Rash and Edema of Hands, Feet
TSS
RMSF

ABE, acute bacterial endocarditis; CVA, cerebrovascular accident; DF, dengue fever; DHF, dengue hemorrhagic fever; DSS, dengue shock syndrome; RMSF, Rocky Mountain spotted fever; SLE, systemic lupus erythematosus; TSS, toxic shock syndrome; VZV, varicella-zoster virus.

Chapter 27

CHEST PAIN

David T. Huang

Chest pain in the ICU is a common complaint that demands urgent evaluation. It is also a somewhat different entity from chest pain seen in the office, ward, or emergency department (ED). Although ICU patients typically are sicker and their problems more complex, management is expedited. ICU patients have already been identified as being critically ill, and they are already in the most resource-rich area of the hospital. The keys to proper management of chest pain in the ICU are a rapid and focused assessment of immediate problems, a careful consideration of the differential diagnosis, a logical evaluation plan, and empirical treatment while awaiting a definitive diagnosis.

INITIAL APPROACH

An ICU patient with chest pain should be seen as soon as possible. When performing the initial evaluation (Fig. 27-1), a good policy is to obtain a fresh set of vital signs and determine whether anything else has changed. First, ensure the adequacy of the basic ABCs: airway, breathing, and circulation. Ensure that the patient has intravenous access and is on a cardiac monitor. Next, take a moment to note the patient's cardiac rhythm and arterial oxygen saturation (pulse oximetry). Check the ventilator settings and, if an arterial catheter or pulmonary artery catheter is in place, the systemic arterial or pulmonary arterial pressure waveforms, respectively. Determine whether the patient appears obtunded, dyspneic, mottled, cool, or diaphoretic. Auscultate the chest and precordium, listening for heart murmurs, friction rubs, and the presence and quality of breath sounds. Seek to identify immediate life-threatening problems, such as tension pneumothorax, ventricular arrhythmias, or arterial hypoxemia, before moving on to perform a more detailed assessment. If life-threatening problems are suspected, evaluation and treatment must be performed almost concurrently. Other chapters in this textbook discuss these time-urgent conditions in greater detail.

HISTORY

If the patient is stable after the initial evaluation, obtain a more detailed history. If the patient can communicate, start with an open-ended question, such as "What's going on, Mr. Jones?" Physicians typically interrupt their patients after about 23 seconds,[1] so force yourself to simply listen for at least 1 minute before saying anything else. The most pertinent information will usually come out during those 60 seconds. Next, fully characterize the chest pain. In one study, only 42% of patients with confirmed thoracic aortic

dissections were asked even basic questions about their pain.[2] Omitting one or more of these basic questions during the initial evaluation was associated with a delayed diagnosis. The mnemonic OLDCAAR can help clinicians avoid this mistake (Table 27-1).

The patient's bedside nurse should also be queried about recent changes in the patient's status (e.g., mental status, respiratory pattern, cardiac rate and rhythm). Last, a quick "chart dissection" should be performed, focusing on the initial history and physical examination, past medical history (paying special attention to cardiac risk factors and prior surgical procedures), reason for ICU admission, and the last few progress notes. Do not waste time asking the patient or nurse questions that can be answered by reading the medical record.

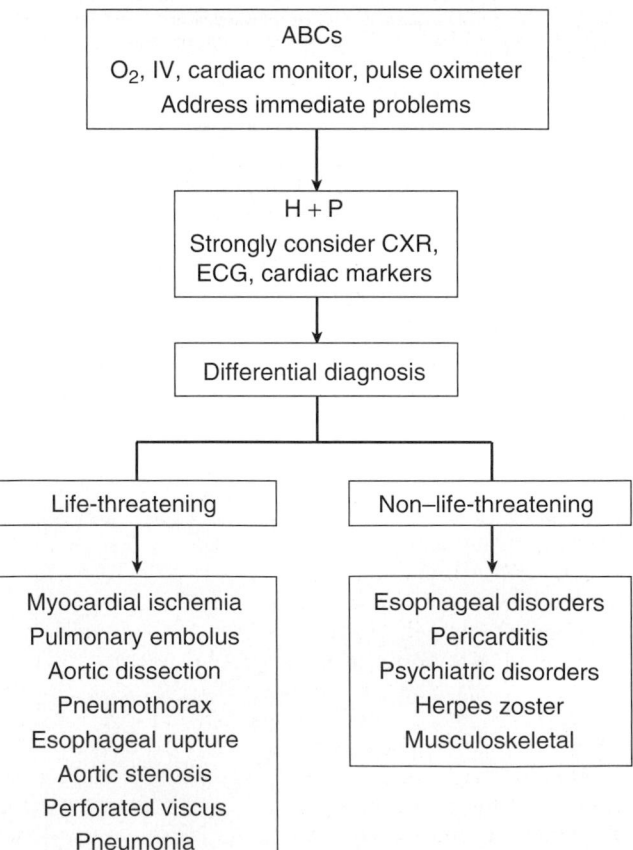

FIGURE 27–1. Approach to chest pain in the ICU. ABC, airway, breathing, circulation; CXR, chest x-ray; ECG, electrocardiogram; H + P, history and physical examination; IV, intravenous access.

TABLE 27–1. OLDCAAR MNEMONIC FOR EVALUATING PAIN

Domain	Suggested Questions
Onset	Sudden vs gradual? Maximal pain at onset?
Location	Generalized or localized? Can you point with one finger to where it hurts?
Duration	When did it start? Just now, or did the pain occur earlier, but you didn't want to bother anyone? Is it constant or intermittent? If intermittent, is there a trigger, or is it random?
Character	Sharp? Dull? Ache? Indigestion? Pressure? Tearing? Ripping?
Associated symptoms	"Dizzy"—vertiginous or presyncopal? Diaphoresis? Palpitations? Dyspnea? Nausea or vomiting?
Alleviating/ **A**ggravating	Position? Belching? Exertion? Deep breathing? Coughing?
Radiation	To the back? Jaw? Throat? Arm? Neck? Abdomen?

PHYSICAL EXAMINATION

Disrobe the patient to ensure optimal visualization, looking particularly for obvious chest wall asymmetry or deformities. Seek to identify areas of point tenderness or crepitus. Next, focus on the cardiac, pulmonary, and abdominal examinations. Check the blood pressure in both arms as you talk to the patient. Assess for asymmetry in pulse quality of the carotid, femoral, and radial pulses. There is a difference in the blood pressure recorded from the right and left upper extremities in about one third of patients with aortic dissection.[3] Check for pulsus paradoxus and jugular venous distention. Listen for asymmetry and quality of breath sounds in conjunction with a review of ventilator settings, if applicable. Evaluate the heart for diminished heart sounds, new murmurs, friction rubs, or gallops. Examine the abdomen for tenderness, pulsatile masses, and absent or abnormal (i.e., high-pitched) bowel sounds. Last, palpate and inspect the lower extremities for tenderness or size differential. Unfortunately, the physical examination is relatively insensitive, and supplemental tests are frequently necessary.[3]

DIAGNOSTIC ADJUNCTS

Unless the cause of new chest pain is obvious (e.g., tension pneumothorax, herpes zoster with visible lesions), a portable chest x-ray (CXR) and 12-lead electrocardiogram (ECG) and rhythm strip should almost always be obtained. In addition, serial measurements of circulating levels of creatinine phosphokinase MB or, preferably, troponin T or troponin I should be strongly considered to exclude a myocardial infarction (MI).

The CXR should be examined for pneumothorax; a widened mediastinum; new infiltrates; effusions; free subdiaphragmatic air; rib fractures; subcutaneous emphysema; malpositioned endotracheal, nasogastric, orogastric, or chest tube; and aortic silhouette abnormalities. Both the ECG and the CXR should be compared with the most recent study before the onset of chest pain.

The ECG and rhythm strip should be evaluated principally for arrhythmias and signs of ischemia, such as inverted T waves, ST segment depression or elevation, and new Q waves. More subtle ECG findings relevant to specific causes of chest pain are discussed in the next section.

An intravenous contrast–enhanced spiral computed tomography (CT) scan is helpful for excluding the diagnosis of pulmonary embolism and may detect other pathologic findings as well. In many centers, it is the diagnostic test of choice for pulmonary embolism. The ventilation-perfusion ($\dot{V}/\dot{Q}$) radionuclide lung scan is an alternative method of diagnosing pulmonary embolism. The $\dot{V}/\dot{Q}$ scan can be a useful alternative to spiral CT in patients with a history of allergic reaction to intravenous contrast material or those at high risk for contrast-induced nephropathy. Pulmonary angiography remains the gold standard for detecting pulmonary embolism, but it is an invasive procedure with a low but real risk of iatrogenic complications.

Echocardiography can be useful for assessing not only left and right ventricular function but also regional wall motion abnormalities, pulmonary hypertension, valvular disease, pericardial effusion, cardiac tamponade, and aortic dissection. Transthoracic echocardiography is usually the first step, followed by transesophageal echocardiography, if necessary. However, transthoracic echocardiography does not visualize the aorta well and can be limited by obesity, emphysema, and chest deformity. For patients in urgent need of aortic visualization, transesophageal echocardiography may be indicated as the initial choice.

DIFFERENTIAL DIAGNOSES

There are three rules to live by:

1. Do not assume that the admission diagnosis is necessarily correct or inclusive. MI can present as gastrointestinal complaints, especially among African Americans.[4] Conversely, the actual diagnosis among patients admitted with presumed (but unconfirmed) MI includes pneumonia, perforated duodenal ulcer, or acute cholecystitis, among myriad other possibilities.
2. Do not be biased by the type of ICU the patient happens to be in. For example, aortic dissection can present as a stroke, prompting admission to a neurologic ICU. Acute serious abdominal problems can occur in medical ICU patients. Indeed, a recent retrospective review of abdominal catastrophes in a medical ICU concluded, "delays in surgical evaluation and intervention are critical contributors to mortality rate in patients who develop acute abdominal complications in a medical ICU."[5]
3. Do not close your mind to alternative diagnoses, even if the diagnosis seems obvious.

ACUTE LIFE-THREATENING PROBLEMS

Myocardial Ischemia

The spectrum of myocardial ischemia ranges from angina to frank MI. Because coronary artery disease is highly prevalent in ICU patients, whether previously diagnosed or occult, a high index of suspicion for ischemia is mandatory. Enumeration of the patient's risk factors (hypercholesterolemia, hypertension, smoking history, family history, age, diabetes mellitus) is useful. The classic signs of myocardial ischemia include chest pain, diaphoresis, palpitations, nausea, syncope or near syncope, vomiting, and dyspnea. Pain often radiates to the neck, arm, or jaw. Unfortunately, myocardial ischemia can also present in much more subtle ways. The type of chest pain is variable and has been described as sharp, dull, tearing, or crushing. Many patients do not even report pain but describe only pressure or simply an odd feeling. Importantly, MI can often present as gastrointestinal symptoms alone, such as "gas," "heartburn," or simply nausea. A retrospective review of 434,877 patients with confirmed MI found that 33% did not have chest pain.[6] Further, patients without chest pain had higher in-hospital mortality rates, possibly due to delays in care. These atypical presentations are more common in patients with heart failure, a previous stroke, or diabetes and in the elderly, women, and minorities.[4,6]

An ECG should be obtained, and supplemental oxygen and pain relief should be provided, if myocardial ischemia is deemed possible. Unless contraindicated, antiplatelet therapy in the form of aspirin 162 to 325 mg p.o or clopidogrel 75 mg p.o. (if aspirin allergy is present) should also be administered. The ECG should be compared with the most recent previous one and examined for ST segment elevation or depression, new Q waves, and T wave inversion. Unfortunately, many MIs are associated with equivocal ECG findings,[7] in which case serial cardiac enzymes and serial ECGs are necessary for diagnosis. Nitroglycerin and morphine should be used to relieve pain, checking the blood pressure before and after each dose. If pain is not relieved with these measures, alternative diagnoses such as aortic dissection should be considered. However, if the diagnosis of MI is strongly suspected, an interventional cardiology consultation should be obtained because persistent chest pain is an indication for urgent cardiac catheterization.[8]

Pulmonary Embolus

Most ICU patients have at least one risk factor for pulmonary embolus (prolonged bed rest, postoperative state, hypercoagulable state, trauma, burns, heart failure); therefore, pulmonary embolus, like MI, should be strongly considered in this population. Pulmonary embolus can present in multiple ways, but most frequently as pleuritic chest pain and dyspnea or tachypnea. Other presentations include syncope, hemoptysis, diaphoresis, cough, and hypoxia. Although pulmonary embolus is often associated with a widened alveolar-arterial (A-a) gradient, this finding is not very useful among ICU patients because it is neither specific (ICU patients often have many other reasons for hypoxia) nor sensitive (the A-a gradient is normal in approximately 25% of patients with pulmonary embolus).[9] Large pulmonary emboli that significantly occlude the pulmonary circulation present with obstructive cardiogenic shock, hypotension, and a sudden rise in central venous, right ventricular, and pulmonary arterial pressures. Echocardiography can be useful in this setting to confirm the diagnosis by demonstrating right heart failure and right ventricular dilatation with septal shift and subsequent left ventricular outflow obstruction.

The CXR is insensitive for diagnosing pulmonary embolus, so more advanced studies are typically required (CT, $\dot{V}/\dot{Q}$ scan, pulmonary angiography). For each test, the risks of iatrogenic complications and complications during transport must be taken into account.

Aortic Dissection

The risk factors for aortic dissection overlap considerably with those for myocardial ischemia; therefore, this entity should always be considered among "rule out MI" patients (Table 27-2). Persistent chest pain without ECG changes is a potential clue that aortic dissection may be present.

The basic pathophysiology involves a tear of the aortic intima, leading to a false lumen between the intima

TABLE 27–2. AORTIC DISSECTION RISK FACTORS

Atherosclerosis risk factors (hypertension, diabetes, smoking, age, hypercholesterolemia)
Connective tissue disorders (Marfan's syndrome, Ehlers-Danlos syndrome)
Cocaine
Bicuspid aortic valve
Coarctation of the aorta
Trauma
Previous cardiac surgery (especially aortic valve replacement)
Intra-aortic catheterization
Giant cell arteritis

and adventitia. A recent systematic review noted that the vast majority of patients complain of severe chest pain (90%) of sudden onset (84%).[3] The review also noted that 28% have a diastolic murmur (due to aortic regurgitation), 31% have a pulse deficit or blood pressure differential (>20 mm Hg), and 17% have focal neurologic deficits. The physical examination should search for these findings.

Patients with aortic dissection were once thought to experience a tearing or ripping sensation. However, the International Registry of Acute Aortic Dissection reported in its series of 464 patients that pain was most commonly described as "sharp."[10] Further, only about half the patients described back pain. Therefore, the absence of tearing or ripping pain radiating to the back should not exclude the diagnosis of aortic dissection.

Although a normal CXR does not rule out aortic dissection, the presence of certain findings can be helpful. These findings include a wide mediastinum, separation of intimal calcification from the outer border of the aortic knob by 1 cm or greater, deviation of the trachea to the right, and blurring of the aortic margin. Comparison to the most recent CXR is key. Contrast-enhanced spiral CT is usually the best confirmatory test, but if the risk of transport is too high, bedside transesophageal echocardiography should be performed. Immediate management should focus on blood pressure control, ideally using beta-adrenergic blockade with or without a vasodilator, such as sodium nitroprusside.

Pneumothorax

ICU patients are at high risk for pneumothorax due to iatrogenic complications from central venous catheterization and thoracentesis; preexisting and acquired pulmonary disease, particularly emphysema, asthma, and acute respiratory distress syndrome; and barotrauma secondary to mechanical ventilation. It is absolutely critical to diagnose pneumothorax in patients receiving positive pressure mechanical ventilation, because positive airway pressure can transform a simple pneumothorax into a tension pneumothorax. The cardinal signs of tension pneumothorax are hypotension, jugular venous distention, absence of breath sounds and hyperresonance to percussion on the affected side, and tracheal deviation (away from the affected side). Treatment is immediate needle (14 gauge) decompression, followed by chest tube placement. Needle decompression is quickly accomplished by inserting a large-bore (16 or 18 gauge) needle through the second or third anterior interspace in the midclavicular line of the involved hemithorax.

Simple pneumothorax presents similarly but less dramatically with hypoxia, dyspnea or tachypnea, pleuritic chest pain, decreased breath sounds with hyperresonance, and increased peak airway pressure. An upright, expiratory CXR should be obtained in cases of suspected pneumothorax. If only a supine film is possible, the deep sulcus sign (hyperlucent, lowered hemidiaphragm with an unusually sharp cardiac border) can help make the diagnosis. Loculated pneumothoraces due to underlying pulmonary adhesions can be difficult to visualize on a CXR. In such cases, chest CT should be obtained promptly; left undiagnosed and untreated, simple pneumothorax can lead to tension pneumothorax. Communication with the radiologist is essential. If the diagnosis of a loculated pneumothorax is confirmed, CT-guided placement of a chest tube or pigtail catheter should be undertaken.

Esophageal Rupture

Prompt recognition is required, because esophageal rupture can lead to potentially lethal mediastinitis. Although usually suggested by a clear history of caustic substance ingestion, forceful vomiting, or iatrogenic trauma (secondary to orogastric lavage, esophageal stricture dilatation, nasogastric tube placement, esophageal intubation, endoscopy), less obvious causes can lead to a delay in diagnosis. Any sudden increase in intra-abdominal pressure can lead to esophageal rupture, and seizures and blunt abdominal trauma have been reported as inciting events. Patients with esophageal disease such as cancer, Barrett's esophagus, and varices are especially vulnerable to rupture.

Physical examination may reveal subcutaneous emphysema or the classic finding of mediastinal crackling on auscultation (Hamman's crunch). CXR may show pneumothorax, pneumomediastinum or pneumoperitoneum, pleural effusion, or subcutaneous emphysema. In victims of blunt abdominal trauma, several findings should increase the suspicion of esophageal rupture: left pneumothorax without associated rib fractures, pain or shock out of proportion to the injury, and particulate matter in the chest tube.[11] A water-soluble contrast study or esophagoscopy confirms the diagnosis.

Aortic Stenosis

The main physiologic effect of aortic stenosis is to impede left ventricular ejection, leading ultimately to left ventricular hypertrophy. Critical aortic stenosis results when this compensatory mechanism can no longer overcome the valvular stenosis or when the hypertrophy itself causes diastolic failure or excessive myocardial oxygen demand. The classic symptoms of angina, syncope, and dyspnea result. Clues suggesting critical aortic stenosis on physical examination include narrow pulse pressure, systolic murmur radiating to the carotid, S_4 gallop, and an aortic ejection click. CXR and ECG may show signs of left ventricular hypertrophy, but the definitive test is a Doppler echocardiogram. If positive, cardiac catheterization should be performed to look for concomitant coronary artery disease and to confirm the echo results. The urgency of these tests is determined by the severity of symptoms; once angina, heart failure, or syncope occurs, a prompt workup is required. Aortic valve replacement is the definitive therapy. Temporizing medical management focuses on cautiously decreasing afterload and treating angina with the careful administration of nitrates, angiotensin-converting enzyme inhibitors, and diuretics. Close hemodynamic monitoring is essential if these drugs are given, because decreases in diastolic pressure can worsen myocardial ischemia.

Miscellaneous

A perforated viscus sometimes presents as chest pain, but fortunately, this is usually easily picked up as free subdiaphragmatic air on an upright CXR. However, retroperitoneal perforations do not show up as free air under the diaphragm on CXR.

Pneumonia is often accompanied by pleuritic chest pain. Referred shoulder pain can result from diaphragmatic irritation by lower lobe pneumonia.

NON–LIFE-THREATENING PROBLEMS

All the following entities should be considered diagnoses of exclusion and should be considered only after life-threatening causes have been ruled out.

Esophageal Disorders

Owing to the shared innervation of the heart and esophagus, visceral pain originating from these two organs can be similar in character. Thus, it can be difficult to differentiate between myocardial ischemia and relatively benign esophageal disorders such as gastroesophageal reflux disease and esophageal dysmotility syndromes. The diagnosis of esophageal disease is supported by a history of pain precipitated by lying flat or the ingestion of hot or cold liquids or food. The diagnosis of an esophageal disorder is also supported if the pain is relieved by antacids. Nitroglycerin can relieve pain due to myocardial ischemia or esophageal spasm, so response to this drug it is not useful as a diagnostic tool. Confirmatory tests include esophageal manometry and esophageal pH monitoring. Alternatively, an empirical trial of a proton pump inhibitor can be tried first. Last, sometimes a nasogastric tube with the distal tip in the esophagus can produce pain, especially when left on suction.

Musculoskeletal Disorders

Chest wall pain is diagnosed with direct palpation or by asking the patient to press with his or her arms against resistance. Usually these maneuvers elicit pain from the affected area. Costochondritis and myofascial syndromes often have specific trigger points that can stimulate pain. Occult rib fractures should be sought carefully by examining the CXR. According to some reports, up to 15% of patients with MI also have chest wall pain, so unless a very specific, localized, and reproducible area of pain can be found, a cardiac workup should be performed.[12] The insertion points for each chest tube and central line should also be inspected. If chest pain is elicited on physical examination, the clinician should specifically ask the patient whether the pain is the same as the spontaneously occurring pain. A negative reply demands further workup.

Pericarditis

Although pericarditis itself is rarely life-threatening, other entities in the differential diagnosis, such as MI and cardiac tamponade, can be. Pain due to pericarditis is typically pleuritic, sharp or stabbing, and retrosternal or precordial, with radiation to the back, neck, shoulders, or arms. Pain is often relieved by leaning forward and worsened by lying flat. More useful in differentiating pericarditis from ischemia is the presence of a pathognomonic but often transitory triphasic (systole, early diastole, and presystole) friction rub. A pericardial rub sounds similar to hair being rubbed together and has been described as high-pitched. It is best heard with the diaphragm of the stethoscope at the cardiac apex, with the patient seated and leaning forward.

Characteristic ECG findings also help differentiate pericarditis from MI. Both entities demonstrate ST segment elevation, but with pericarditis, ST segment depression is absent in the reciprocal leads, except occasionally in aV_R and V_1. Absence of Q waves, concave (instead of convex) ST segment elevation, PR depression, and upright T waves also strongly favor pericarditis.[13] Careful ECG review, auscultation, and history are the key to distinguishing between these two disorders and avoiding potentially fatal complications of contraindicated therapy (administration of a thrombolytic agent to patients with pericarditis can precipitate hemotamponade) or missing a diagnosis of life-threatening MI.

Pericarditis can lead to pericardial effusion. If it is large or acute, pericardial effusion can lead to cardiac tamponade. Pericardial effusion can present similarly to pulmonary embolus with dyspnea or tachypnea, tachycardia, and chest pain or pressure. ECG findings of electrical alternans and low voltage, coupled with cardiomegaly on CXR, strongly favor pericardial effusion. Pulsus paradoxus may also be present. Beck's triad (jugular venous distention, hypotension, muffled heart tones) points to a more emergent condition. Note that cardiac tamponade and tension pneumothorax share the first two components of Beck's triad, but the latter condition is characterized by normal heart tones, decreased breath sounds, and hyperresonance of the involved hemithorax. Beck's triad is not always present in patients with tamponade. For instance, if the patient is hypovolemic, jugular venous distention may not be apparent. Tamponade should be suspected when the clinical condition looks like congestive heart failure but breath sounds are clear. The ECG and CXR findings discussed for pericardial effusion are useful, but urgent echocardiography should be ordered to confirm the diagnosis. If the patient is in extremis and the clinical picture strongly suggests tamponade, pericardiocentesis should be performed. Volume loading should be done concurrently, because it can partially overcome the hemodynamic effects of tamponade.

Last, it is important to determine the underlying cause of the pericarditis. Possibilities include infection, malignancy, trauma, autoimmune disorders, and connective tissue disorders; it can also be idiopathic.

Psychiatric Disorders

Anxiety disorders, somatization, and panic attacks can all present with chest pain. Panic attacks, in particular, can be associated with symptoms that closely mimic those of MI. Both conditions are commonly associated with diaphoresis, tachypnea, dyspnea, palpitations, presyncope, and a sense of impending doom. Many patients with panic attacks have had extensive cardiac and gastrointestinal workups in the past, and obtaining these reports is helpful. Nonetheless, the dictum that "psychiatric patients get sick too" should be remembered. Psychiatric patients with real cardiac or pulmonary disease can be especially challenging to diagnose, and a thorough, empathic history is essential. Depression is often a comorbid psychiatric condition and should be appropriately treated.

Herpes Zoster

Inspection of the patient's thorax usually makes the diagnosis of herpes zoster, although pain precedes skin manifestations by 1 to 3 days. The lesions are limited to a single dermatome and start as a maculopapular rash that quickly changes to the characteristic vesicular lesions. Acyclovir is the treatment.

CONCLUSION

Attention to immediate problems, a thorough history and physical examination, and consideration of each life-threatening possibility are the key steps to managing chest pain in the ICU. The test battery of a CXR, ECG, and serial cardiac enzymes should be used liberally but intelligently. A high index of suspicion for occult disease is necessary for complex ICU patients.

ANNOTATED REFERENCES

Canto JG, Shlipak MG, Rogers WJ, et al: Prevalence, clinical characteristics, and mortality among patients with myocardial infarction presenting without chest pain. JAMA 2000;283:3223-3229.

This study of 434,877 patients with confirmed MIs found that fully one third of MI patients do not complain of chest pain at presentation. These atypical patients tended to be older, female, and diabetic and to have prior heart failure. Most important, the in-hospital mortality for these patients was more than double that of patients who presented with chest pain.

Gajic O, Urrutia LE, Sewani H, et al: Acute abdomen in the medical intensive care unit. Crit Care Med 2002;30:1187-1190.

This retrospective cohort study found that delays in surgical evaluation and intervention were independent, statistically significant correlates of mortality. Interestingly, it also found that risk factors for surgical delay included opioid use, mechanical ventilation, no peritoneal signs, antibiotics, and altered mental state. This suggests that a heightened index of suspicion for an acute abdomen may be necessary in ICU patients with these risk factors.

Hagan PG, Nienaber CA, Isselbacher EM, et al: The International Registry of Acute Aortic Dissection (IRAAD): New insights into an old disease. JAMA 2000;283:897-903.

The IRAAD is composed of 12 international referral centers, from which 3 years of data and 464 patients were analyzed. A key finding was that classic presentations such as tearing or ripping chest pain (50.6%), aortic regurgitation (31.6%), and pulse deficit (15.1%) were frequently absent, leading the authors to urge clinicians to maintain a high index of suspicion.

Klinger D, Green-Weir R, Nerenz D, et al: Perceptions of chest pain differ by race. Am Heart J 2002;144:51–59.

In this study of 215 patients with confirmed MI, African-American patients attributed their initial symptoms to a gastrointestinal cause 61% of the time, versus 26% in white patients.

Marvel MK, Epstein RM, Flowers K, Beckman HB: Soliciting the patient's agenda: Have we improved? JAMA 1999;281:283-287.

Although this study was conducted in primary care offices and not in an ICU, it emphasizes the importance of the basic history-taking process and listening to patients. It found that physicians interrupted their patients after a mean of only 23.1 seconds and that late-arising patient concerns were more common when physicians did not solicit questions during the interview.

Section II

BASIC SCIENCE

Section II
BASIC SCIENCE

Chapter 28

REGULATION OF GENE EXPRESSION

Edward Abraham

KEY POINTS

1. Effective transcription requires assembly of a transcriptional apparatus that consists of RNA polymerase (Pol II), the enzyme that translates DNA sequences into RNA, with activator and coactivator proteins.

2. The stability of messenger RNA (mRNA) plays an important role in determining the final levels of gene products.

3. Cellular activation results in a sequence of signaling events, in which the initially activated kinases become capable of phosphorylating serine or tyrosine residues in downstream kinases or regulatory proteins. As a result of such kinase activity, transcriptional factors, nuclear coactivator proteins, and other regulatory molecules become phosphorylated, inducing enhanced transcriptional activity.

4. Dephosphorylation of regulatory proteins is an important negative regulatory event, resulting in down-regulation of transcriptional events, leading to a return to baseline levels of transcriptional activity.

5. The transcriptional regulatory factor nuclear factor-κB (NF-κB) is a central participant in modulating the expression of many of the immunoregulatory mediators involved in sepsis, acute lung injury, acute renal failure, and other organ system dysfunctions associated with critical illness and other inflammatory conditions, such as rheumatoid arthritis and inflammatory bowel disease.

6. The regulation of gene transcription is modulated positively by transcriptional activators and negatively by transcriptional repressors.

7. Interactions between transcriptional factors and chromatin structure determine that genes are transcribed at appropriate times and levels in response to cellular activation.

The expression of gene products is regulated at multiple steps. The initial events involve activation of intracellular kinases that phosphorylate transcriptional factors, regulatory cytoplasmic and nuclear proteins, resulting in enhanced gene transcription and messenger RNA (mRNA) production. Examples of such cascades are the phosphorylation of the p65 subunit of the transcriptional factor nuclear factor-κB (NF-κB), which increases transcriptional activity,[1,2] or of the inhibitory protein IκB-α,[3,4] which facilitates the degradation of IκB-α and nuclear translocation of NF-κB. Similarly, phosphorylation of the transcriptional factor cyclic adenosine monophosphate (cAMP) responsive element binding (CREB) protein on serine 133 by phosphokinase A, calmodulin kinases, or extracellular regulated kinases or through other kinase-mediated events enhances its transcriptional activity.[5,6] In the case of NF-κB, liberation from IκB-α allows NF-κB dimers to translocate to the nucleus, where they can interact with specific sequences in the promoter regions of genes and help initiate transcription.[7,8] CREB is normally bound to promoter sequences, but is not transcriptionally active unless phosphorylated on serine 133.[5,6]

Although availability in the nucleus of specific transcriptional factors is necessary for their interaction with binding sequences of the promoters and subsequent gene transcription, it is not sufficient. Evidence indicates that the presence of transcriptional factors in different locations in the nucleus is associated with different transcriptional activity.[9] Such information shows that it is not enough for a transcriptional factor simply to reach the nucleus to initiate transcription, but rather that there are differences between nuclear locations and that the transcriptional factor must find its way to the correct site before it can participate in gene expression.

Effective transcription requires assembly of a transcriptional apparatus that consists of RNA polymerase (Pol II), the enzyme that translates DNA sequences into RNA, with activator and coactivator proteins (Fig. 28-1). Pol II, when in the appropriate configuration with additional scaffolding, activator, and coactivator proteins, is required for transcription of genes from the 5′ end of their coding sequence. The transcriptional machinery cannot gain access to relevant promoter sites and initiate transcription unless chromatin surrounding the DNA is modified through acetylation, methylation, and association with many proteins, of which one of the most important seems to be ubiquitin.[10] Ubiquitin is a highly conserved 76-amino acid protein that is linked covalently to lysine residues in other proteins, including histones associated with DNA. Modifications in histones accomplished by addition of methyl and acetyl groups and of ubiquitin are required to expose DNA and allow access of the transcriptional apparatus to relevant promoter sequences, where it can initiate transcription.[11-13]

When mRNA is produced, its stability plays an important role in determining the final levels of gene products.[14-16] mRNA that remains available for translation for longer periods generally is associated with greater amounts of translated proteins. Post-translational events, including modification of protein length and structure, also are involved, in

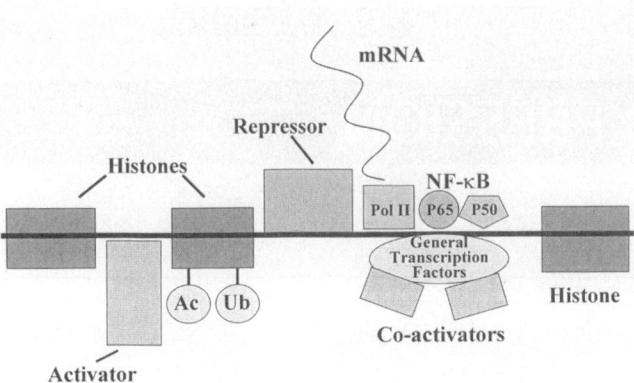

FIGURE 28–1. Regulation of gene transcription involves an interplay of histones, DNA, activators, repressors, and transcriptional machinery, primarily to allow RNA polymerase (Pol II) to produce mRNA. For transcription to occur, histones are acetylated and ubiquitylated, and a transcriptional apparatus, consisting of RNA polymerase, transcriptional factors (e.g., NF-κB), activators, and coactivators is assembled. The modifications of histones allow RNA polymerase to have access to relevant sequences in the promoter regions of genes and to initiate transcription from the 5′ end of the gene's coding sequence.

modifying intracellular and extracellular protein levels. An example of such post-translational regulation concerns the activity of caspase-1 in cleaving pro-interleukin (IL)-1β or pro-IL-18 to the mature extracellularly secreted forms of IL-1β and IL-18.[17-19]

KINASE-INDUCED PHOSPHORYLATION EVENTS AND GENE ACTIVATION

Phosphorylation of proteins by kinases often leads to their participation in signaling events that result in modified cellular activity. Kinase cascades become activated through receptor occupancy with their specific ligands, such as the interaction of lipopolysaccharide with the type 4 Toll-like receptor (TLR4) (Fig. 28-2).[17,20-22] Alterations in the intracellular milieu, including changes in oxidation state induced by increased concentrations of reactive oxygen intermediates in or around cells, also can result in the activation of kinases. Exposure of cell populations to hydrogen peroxide can produce increased activity of the inhibitor of NF-κB kinase (IKK) complex, resulting in enhanced nuclear concentrations of the NF-κB transcriptional factor.[23]

Cellular activation results in a sequence of signaling events, where the initially activated kinases become capable of phosphorylating serine or tyrosine residues in downstream kinases or regulatory proteins. As a result of such kinase activity, transcriptional factors, nuclear coactivator proteins, and other regulatory molecules become phosphorylated, inducing enhanced transcriptional activity. An example of such a cascade is the phosphorylation of the transcriptional coactivator TATA Box binding protein (TBP), a nuclear coactivator that participates in the transcriptional apparatus. Phosphorylation of TBP through activation of p38-related kinases allows enhanced association with NF-κB and increased transcription of NF-κB-dependent genes.[24]

In the same way that phosphorylation of regulatory proteins leads to increased transcriptional activity, dephosphorylation is an important negative regulatory event, resulting in down-regulation of transcriptional events, leading to a return to baseline levels of transcriptional activity. An example of the

importance of dephosphorylation in modulating transcription is provided by data showing that the serine/threonine protein phosphatase 2A (PP2A) participates in regulating the activity of the activating protein 1 (AP-1) transcriptional complex.[25] In particular, AP-1 is formed and becomes transcriptionally active when phosphorylated c-Jun associates with c-Fos. Phosphorylation of c-Jun is under the regulatory control of the c-Jun N-terminal kinase (JNK). PP2A is a key regulator of JNK through its ability to dephosphorylate JNK, decreasing JNK's activity and ability to phosphorylate c-Jun. Activation of PP2A can also down-regulate AP-1-dependent transcription through its effects in dephosphorylating c-Jun.

Kinase-mediated phosphorylation is involved in enhancing nuclear accumulation of transcriptional factors, a necessary event for the initiation and enhancement of transcription. Nuclear translocation of the transcriptional factor NF-κB depends on IKK-mediated phosphorylation of inhibitory IκB cytoplasmic molecules, which leads to their destruction in the 26S proteosome and liberation of NF-κB to move into the nucleus.[4,26,27] This issue is discussed in more detail in the next section of this chapter.

NUCLEAR FACTOR κB

NF-κB is a prototypical transcription factor involved in acute inflammatory responses associated with critical illness. The transcriptional regulatory factor NF-κB is a central participant in modulating the expression of many of the immunoregulatory mediators involved in sepsis, acute lung injury, acute renal failure, and other organ system dysfunctions associated with critical illness and other inflammatory conditions, such as rheumatoid arthritis and inflammatory

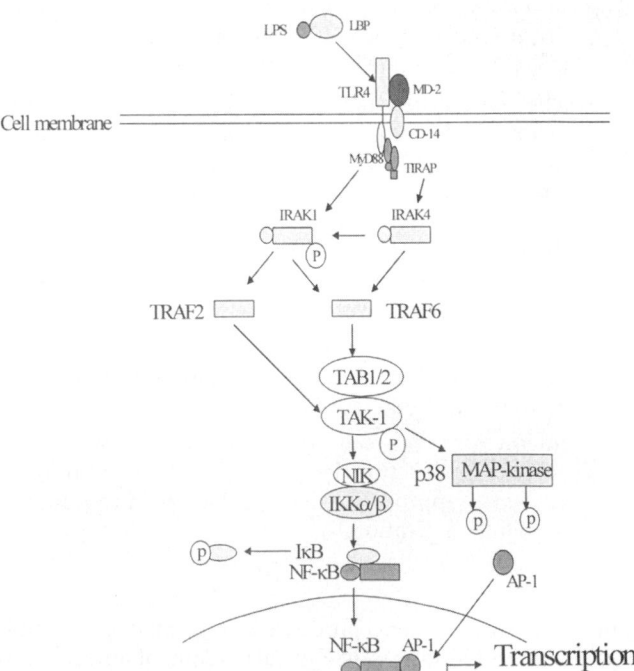

FIGURE 28–2. Interaction of lipopolysaccharide (LPS) and the LPS binding protein (LBP) with the type 4 Toll-like receptor (TLR 4) initiates a sequence of intracellular signaling events, involving activation of kinases that associate with scaffolding proteins, which ultimately leads to gene transcription through the activation of transcriptional regulatory factors, such as NF-κB and AP-1.

bowel disease. Signaling pathways initiated by engagement of TLRs, such as TLR 2 and TLR 4, by bacterial products or of cytokine receptors, including those for tumor necrosis factor (TNF)-α and IL-1, lead to nuclear accumulation of NF-κB and enhanced transcription of genes responsible for the expression of cytokines, chemokines, adhesion molecules, apoptotic factors, and other mediators of the acute inflammatory response associated with multiple organ system dysfunction in sepsis, acute lung injury, pancreatitis, burns, and other ICU conditions.[7,8,26,28,29]

In the active DNA binding form present in the nucleus and involved in transcriptional events, NF-κB is a dimer composed of members of the Rel family. Five mammalian members of this family have been identified: NF-κB1 (p50 and its precursor p105), NF-κB2 (p52 and its precursor p100), c-Rel, Rel A (p65), and Rel B. All of these proteins share a highly conserved Rel homology domain of approximately 300 amino acids composed of two immunoglobulin-like sequences. The Rel homology domain is responsible for dimerization of the NF-κB subunits, interaction with inhibitory IκB molecules, and DNA binding.

Various combinations of NF-κB have different transcriptional efficiency. The p50:p65 heterodimer promotes transcription, whereas p50:p50 homodimers suppress gene activation through preventing access to gene promoters by the transcriptionally active p50:p65 heterodimers.[30] Additionally, there is evidence that phosphorylation of the NF-κB subunits, particularly of p65, is important in optimizing transcriptional potential.[1]

NF-κB dimers normally are retained in the cytoplasm through interaction with inhibitors of the IκB family. Seven IκB molecules have been identified: IκB-α, IκB-β, IκB-γ, IκB-ε, Bcl-3, p100, and p105. Through their association with NF-κB cytoplasmic heterodimers and homodimers, IκB molecules mask the nuclear localization sequence of NF-κB and prevent its movement to the nucleus. Although IκB molecules initially were thought to reside only in the cytoplasm, more recent evidence shows that they shuttle in and out of the nucleus and have important roles in regulating the presence and activity of NF-κB dimers in the nucleus and the cytoplasm (Fig. 28-3).[31]

Cellular activation that leads to nuclear translocation of NF-κB and enhanced transcription of NF-κB-dependent genes can be induced by multiple stimuli, including LPS, peptidoglycans, and lipotechoic acid (from gram-positive bacteria); cytokines (e.g., TNF-α, IL-8, and IL-1β); T-cell and B-cell mitogens; complement fragments (e.g., C5a); reactive oxygen species; G-protein coupled receptor agonists; and other mediators associated with infection, ischemia, and stress responses. In a critically ill patient, in whom such proinflammatory stimuli are present at increased levels, the degree of NF-κB activation has been shown to correlate with patient outcome. In particular, nuclear concentrations of NF-κB in peripheral blood mononuclear cells from septic patients are higher in patients who subsequently die than in survivors.[32,33] Similar patterns of NF-κB activation, with greater nuclear accumulation being associated with a worse clinical outcome, specifically mortality or prolonged time on the ventilator, have been shown to be present among neutrophils from patients with acute lung injury.[34] These associations between enhanced nuclear levels of NF-κB and worse clinical outcome are not surprising because increased levels of many of the proinflammatory mediators under the regulatory control of NF-κB, such as TNF-α or IL-8, have

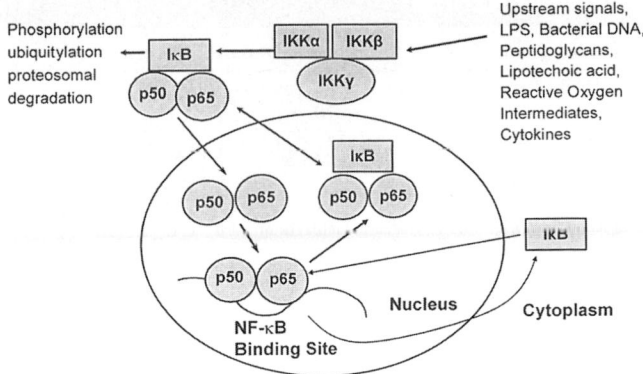

NF-κB Activation

FIGURE 28–3. Multiple mediators associated with critical illness lead to activation of the IKK complex, which then phosphorylates IκBs, such as IκB-α, resulting in degradation of IκB and liberation of NF-κB dimers to move into the nucleus. The IKK complex consists of the kinases IKKα and IKKβ and the scaffolding protein IKKγ. In the nucleus, NF-κB binds to specific sites in promoter regions, where it can initiate transcription, including that of IκB-α. IκBs are primarily present in the cytoplasm, but are able to enter the nucleus, where they can facilitate the disassociation of NF-κB from binding to promoter sites and facilitate movement of NF-κB to the cytoplasm.

been shown to participate in acute inflammatory responses and organ dysfunction in sepsis, acute lung injury, and many other critical illnesses.

After cellular activation by appropriate stimuli, IκB molecules associated with NF-κB in the cytoplasm (particularly IκB-α) are phosphorylated, linked to the protein ubiquitin (i.e., ubiquitylated), and degraded by the 26S proteosome. Degradation of IκB molecules permits nuclear translocation of NF-κB, where it binds to specific sequences in the promoter regions of genes, participates in the formation of a transcriptional apparatus consisting of activator and coactivator proteins (including CREB binding protein (CBP) and RNA polymerase), and initiates transcription (see Fig. 28-3).

Phosphorylation of IκB occurs through activation of IKK.[4,26,29] Three components of IKK have been identified: the serine/threonine kinases IKKα and IKKβ and a regulatory subunit called IKKγ or NEMO. Many different protein kinases activate IKK, including Akt, PKCζ, MEKK1, MEKK2, MEKK3, NIK, COT/TPL-2, and TAK1. Although p38 has been shown to increase NF-κB-dependent transcription, it is unclear if this kinase has a role in enhancing nuclear translocation of NF-κB or whether its activity is primarily due to phosphorylation of NF-κB-associated coactivator proteins, such as TBP, or to enhancing phosphorylation of NF-κB subunits, such as p65. TAB1, an adapter protein that associates with p38α, is able to activate the kinase TAK1, leading to downstream phosphorylation and enhancement of activity of the IKK complex.[21,24,35,36]

Many of the genes regulated by NF-κB participate in inflammatory reactions leading to organ dysfunction and death in critically ill patients with conditions such as sepsis, acute lung injury, hemorrhage, burns, and pancreatitis.[7,8,26,28,37-40] A partial list of NF-κB inducible genes is provided in Table 28-1. Several of the cytokines under the regulatory control of NF-κB, such as IL-1 and TNF-α, also are able to induce further activation of this transcriptional factor, leading to potentiation of inflammatory responses

TABLE 28–1. NF-κB INDUCIBLE GENES INVOLVED IN CRITICAL ILLNESS

Class	NF-κB-Dependent Genes
Cytokines	IL-1α and IL-1β
	TNF-α
	G-CSF
	GM-CSF
	IL-6
	IFN-β
Chemokines	MIP-1α
	MIP-2
	IL-8
Adhesion molecules	ICAM-1
	VCAM-1
	E-selectin
	ELAM-1
Coagulation factors	Tissue factor
	Tissue factor pathway inhibitor
Others	Inducible nitric oxide synthase
	Cyclooxygenase-2
	IκB-α
	C3 complement
	Complement factor B

in the critically ill patient and further enhancement of NF-κB-dependent gene expression.

ROLES OF UBIQUITIN AND CHROMATIN IN MODULATING TRANSCRIPTION

The regulation of gene transcription is modulated positively by transcriptional activators and negatively by transcriptional repressors. Transcriptional activators function through facilitating direct contact of components of the general transcriptional apparatus, such as TBP, with histone-modifying moieties, such as histone acetyl transferases, and activator and coactivator proteins, such as CBP. These interactions result in modifications of chromatin structure, allowing direct access of the transcriptional complex, which includes RNA polymerase, to DNA, where the gene then can be transcribed (see Fig. 28-1). Transcriptional repressors antagonize many of these steps by deacetylating histones, blocking the recruitment or assembly of the transcriptional apparatus, or interacting with transcriptional co-repressors.

Interactions between transcriptional factors and chromatin structure determine that genes are transcribed at appropriate times and levels in response to cellular activation. The ubiquitin system is composed of a family of proteins that are capable of linking covalently to target proteins.[10,21,41] *Ubiquitylation* is the process by which ubiquitin is conjugated to a substrate protein and is essential for regulating transcription and facilitating access of transcriptional factors to relevant promoter sites. After phosphorylation on serines 32 and 36, IκB-α is ubiquitylated, an essential step that facilitates its recognition and breakdown in the 26S proteosome, allowing NF-κB to move to the nucleus and initiate transcription.[20,21,41] Modification of chromatin through covalent association with ubiquitin influences other chromatin modifications, such as acetylation and methylation, involved in transcriptional control.

Ubiquitylated forms of histones H1, H2A, and H2B are associated specifically with actively transcribed genes, providing a marker of transcriptionally active chromatin. Ubiquitylation of H2B is required for methylation of the histone H3 at lysine residues 4 and 79, which is required for telomeric gene silencing, the transcriptional down-regulation of the expression of genes proximal to the telomere.[10] It also is likely that histone ubiquitylation is involved in the activation of genes. Ubiquitylation of the linker histone H1 seems to be involved in enhancing activity of the general transcription factor TFIID complex.[10]

COORDINATION OF STEPS INVOLVED IN GENE EXPRESSION

The final step in the transcriptional regulatory process is initiation of transcription at the 5′ end of a gene by RNA polymerase II (Pol II), resulting in production of mRNA, which, after migrating to the cytoplasm, is translated to protein.[42,43] As described earlier, access of RNA polymerase to relevant gene sequences is a highly regulated event, involving a balance between stimulatory events initiated by cellular activation through receptor-ligand interaction, kinase activation, phosphorylation of regulatory proteins, modification of histones, and down-regulatory processes that occur through phosphatases and other kinases able to modulate the phosphorylation, acetylation, and ubiquitylation that lead to gene expression. Exquisite control of gene expression is achieved through the interplay of these multiple regulatory processes. Additional fine-tuning of protein production is accomplished through post-transcriptional events, involving control of mRNA stability, translational rates, and post-translocation modification of proteins.

Despite the regulatory processes that are available to modulate gene expression, critical illness often is associated with altered and pathologic production of immunoregulatory and other molecules that induce the development of organ dysfunction. Gene polymorphisms that lead to overexpression of regulatory molecules, such as plasminogen activator inhibitor-1 (PAI-1), which is involved in coagulation cascades, or of proinflammatory or anti-inflammatory mediators, such as TNF-α or IL-1ra, are associated with outcome from severe infections.[44-48] Similarly, increased activation of kinases, such as Akt, or of transcriptional factors, such as NF-κB, in neutrophils or other cell populations correlates with worse outcome from acute lung injury.[34] Future use of gene expression arrays and proteomics, which would permit identification of genes and proteins whose expression is altered in cell populations from patients at risk for or with a critical illness, are likely to help not only in early diagnosis, but, more importantly, also should permit therapies to be tailored to correct the alterations in gene and protein expression that contribute to organ system dysfunction and death in critically ill patients.

ANNOTATED REFERENCES

Abraham E: Nuclear factor-kappaB and its role in sepsis-associated organ failure. J Infect Dis 2003;187(Suppl 2):S364-369.
  This article is an overview of NF-κB activation in sepsis and acute lung injury.

Dunne A, O'Neill LA: The interleukin-1 receptor/Toll-like receptor super-family: Signal transduction during inflammation and host defense. Sci STKE 2003;2003:re3.
  This article provides an excellent overview of signaling pathways associated with the Toll-like/interleukin-1 receptor (TIR) family, which includes the TLR (TLR1-11) and the IL-1R groups.

Muratani M, Tansey WP: How the ubiquitin-proteasome system controls transcription. Nat Rev Mol Cell Biol 2003;4:192-201.

This is an excellent review of the role of ubiquitination and proteosomal degradation in modulating transcriptional activity.

O'Connell MA, Bennett BL, Mercurio F, et al: Role of IKK1 and IKK2 in lipopolysaccharide signaling in human monocytic cells. J Biol Chem 1998;273:30410-30414.

Experiments presented in this article indicate that IKK2 (IKKβ) is the primary form of IKK responsible for activation of NF-κB in proinflammatory conditions, such as those initiated by lipopolysaccharide.

Saccani S, Pantano S, Natoli G: p38-Dependent marking of inflammatory genes for increased NF-kappa B recruitment. Nat Immunol 2002;3:69-75.

The p38 kinase pathway is known to be important in initiating inflammatory responses. The mechanisms through which p38 participates in inflammation are less clear. This article shows that p38 participates in inducing NF-κB transcription of inflammatory genes not through directly affecting nuclear translocation of NF-κB, but rather through altering histone-related acetylation, allowing increased NF-κB recruitment to such altered genes.

Shim J, Karin M: The control of mRNA stability in response to extracellular stimuli. Mol Cells 2002;14:323-331.

This article reviews mechanisms involved in regulating the stability of transcribed mRNA and how such mechanisms affect cellular responses to extracellular stimuli.

Zhong H, May MJ, Jimi E, Ghosh S: The phosphorylation status of nuclear NF-kappa B determines its association with CBP/p300 or HDAC-1. Mol Cell 2002;9:625-636.

This article provides experimental information showing that the transcriptional activity of NF-κB and association of NF-κB with coactivator proteins involved in transcription depend on phosphorylation of the NF-κB subunits. Nuclear translocation of NF-κB, although necessary for transcriptional activity, is not sufficient.

Chapter 29

THE NEUTROPHIL: BALANCING ANTIMICROBIAL EFFECTIVENESS AND THE POTENTIAL FOR DAMAGE TO THE HOST

Theo J. Morales • Tomoko Suzuki • Gregory P. Downey

KEY POINTS

1. Neutrophils are key cells in the innate immune system serving in host defense.

2. The importance of each step in neutrophil functioning is demonstrated by a variety of disease states that result from deficiencies in these specific functions.

3. "Excessive" or unregulated neutrophil activation may contribute to the host cell damage seen in a variety of inflammatory based diseases such as acute respiratory disease syndrome (ARDS).

4. Proteases, reactive oxygen and nitrogen species, and lipid metabolites from activated neutrophils may all contribute to the host damage seen in ARDS.

5. Signal transduction pathways involving the enzyme PI3 kinase, various mitogen-activated protein kinases, especially the p38 pathway, and ultimately the transcription factor NF-κB have been implicated in contributing to the increased neutrophil activity seen in ARDS.

6. Modification of neutrophil function to achieve the optimal balance between adequate host defense and minimal host damage remains on the horizon.

Neutrophils contribute to host defense primarily through the recognition and destruction of pathogenic microorganisms, a functional role that is achieved through a series of rapid and coordinated responses, including chemotaxis, phagocytosis, and release of cytotoxic products. These responses are initiated by the interaction of cell surface receptors with specific ligands found on microbial targets or in the inflammatory milieu and the consequent induction of intracellular signaling pathways that couple such activating stimuli to physiologic antimicrobial responses. Paradoxically, these cellular and biochemical events may also result in damage to host tissues in inflammatory conditions, including ischemia-reperfusion injury, sepsis, acute lung injury (ALI), and the acute respiratory distress syndrome (ARDS). Therefore, to maximize host defense capabilities while

minimizing damage to host tissues ("collateral damage"), neutrophil microbicidal responses must be tightly regulated. Notwithstanding the potential role of the neutrophil in inflammatory injury, it is important that the primary function of this "professional phagocyte" in host defense and in resolution of inflammation and tissue remodeling by clearance of debris is not eclipsed. In this chapter we briefly focus on the functions of neutrophils and then discuss the evidence implicating neutrophils in ARDS and ALI with ramifications for potential treatment options on the horizon.

NEUTROPHIL PRODUCTION

Neutrophils, so named because they stain in a neutral manner with Wright's stain, are crucial players in inflammation and the innate immune response. Formed in the bone marrow, the neutrophil progresses through defined stages of development from the myeloblast, promyelocyte, myelocyte, metamyelocyte, and band cell eventually to the mature polymorphonuclear neutrophil (PMN) (Fig. 29-1). This progression takes about 9 days. It is generally accepted that only the myeloblast, promyelocyte, and myelocyte are capable of cell division. Studies suggest approximately 100 billion neutrophils are produced in an adult per day. This can increase 1000-fold in times of need through the action of cytokines such as granulocyte-macrophage colony-stimulating factor. Once in the bloodstream neutrophils have a half life of approximately 7 hours.[1] A large group of mature neutrophils remain in the bone marrow for up to 2 days and outnumber circulating neutrophils 20 to 1. In addition, a portion of mature neutrophils marginate preferentially in the pulmonary vasculature. The reasons for this include the relatively large size of neutrophils compared with pulmonary capillaries, the organization of the pulmonary capillary bed, the lower pressure and shear stress of the pulmonary as compared with the systemic circulation, the less deformable nature of neutrophils as compared with red blood cells, and the fact that the pulmonary vasculature receives the entire cardiac output.[3]

The importance of the neutrophil in immune function is emphasized by various congenital and acquired conditions that result in neutropenia.[4] These patients are at risk for severe skin, lung, and other invasive bacterial and fungal infections.

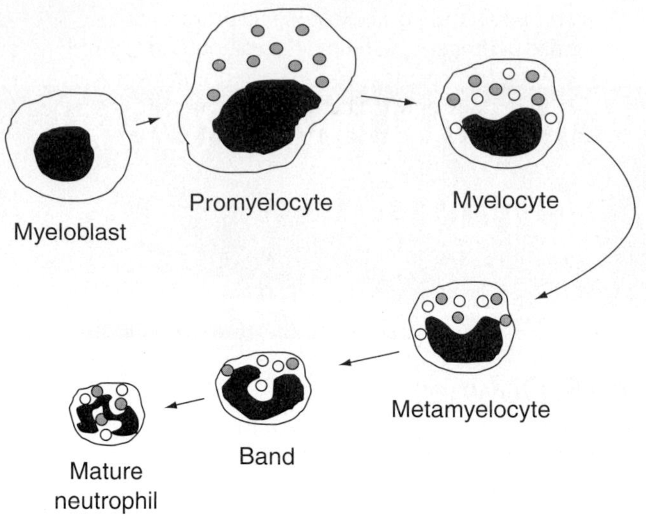

Myeloblast

Promyelocyte

Myelocyte

Metamyelocyte

Band

Mature neutrophil

FIGURE 29–1. Progression from myeloblast to myelocyte takes 4 to 6 days. Promyelocytes develop azurophilic granules and myelocytes develop specific granules. Maturation from myelocyte to mature neutrophil takes 5 to 7 days. (Adapted from Skubitz KM: Neutrophilic leukocytes. In Lee FJ et al [eds]: Wintrobe's Clinical Hematology. Philadelphia, Lippincott Williams & Wilkins, 1000, pp 300-350; and Abramson SL, Malech HL, Gallin JI: Neutrophils. In Crystal WJ [ed]: The Lung: Scientific Foundations. New York, Raven, 1991, pp 553-563.)

BASIC NEUTROPHIL FUNCTION

The physiologic functions of neutrophils that are involved in their antimicrobial role are described individually.

ADHESION

To eradicate microorganisms, circulating neutrophils must move out of the vasculature into the infected tissues. Adhesion of neutrophils to vascular endothelium is the first step in this process.[1,5] Neutrophils and endothelial cells express a variety of cognate adhesion molecules on their respective surfaces (Table 29-1), the expression of which is regulated by various stimuli present in an inflammatory milieu. Selectins mediate the initial rolling and tethering of a circulating neutrophil to the vascular endothelium. L-selectin is expressed on neutrophils whereas P- and E-selectin are found on endothelial cells. The interaction between selectins and their cognate ligands serves to tether neutrophils, slowing them in their journey through the microvasculature, where they sense chemoattractants and other inflammatory agonists, leading to firm adhesion mediated by integrins interacting with endothelial ligands. The major integrins expressed by neutrophils are β_2 integrins (CD11/CD18), although recent studies have indicated that activated neutrophils also express $\alpha_4\beta_1$ integrins.[6] Endothelial cells express intercellular adhesion molecules (ICAMs), which are members of the IgG superfamily and are ligands for β_2 integrins and mediate firm adhesion. After adhering to the endothelium, neutrophils spread and then move between or through endothelial cells and migrate along chemoattractant gradients toward the invading pathogens. Gap junctions form between neutrophils and endothelial cells and serve to facilitate cell communication to assist in transmigration.[7]

The importance of adhesion molecules in innate immunity is illustrated by the propensity to infections in congenital diseases where these molecules are deficient or absent. Leukocyte adhesion deficiency (LAD) type I is the result of a deficiency of β_2 integrins.[4,8] As a consequence, neutrophils cannot adhere and migrate to sites of infection, resulting in a predisposition to recurrent, severe infections, despite a high neutrophil count, and delayed umbilical stump separation in the newborn. LAD type II, secondary to defective selectins,[4] is an autosomal recessive condition with characteristic physical features, short stature, and a predisposition to recurrent infections as well.

TABLE 29–1. SELECTED NEUTROPHIL AND ENDOTHELIAL ADHESION MOLECULES

	Other Names		Ligands
Neutrophil Integrins			
$\alpha_2\beta_1$			Collagen, laminin
$\alpha_3\beta_1$			Collagen, laminin, fibronectin, tenascin
$\alpha_4\beta_1$	VLA-4	CD49d/CD29	VCAM-1, fibronectin
$\alpha_5\beta_1$	VLA-5	CD49e/CD29	Fibronectin
$\alpha_6\beta_1$	VLA-6	CD49f/CD29	Laminin
$\alpha_9\beta_1$			VCAM-1, tenascin
$\alpha_L\beta_2$	LFA-1	CD11a/CD18	ICAM-1 to 3
$\alpha_M\beta_2$	Mac-1	CD11b/CD18	ICAM-1, C3bi, fibrinogen, factor x
$\alpha_X\beta_2$	P150,95	CD11c/CD18	Fibrinogen, C3bi
$\alpha_V\beta_3$			Vitronectin
Neutrophil Selectins			
L-selectin	LAM-1	CD62L	Sialylated carbohydrates
Endothelial Selectins			
E-selectin	ELAM-1	CD62E	Sialylated carbohydrates
P-selectin	GMP-140, PADGEM	CD62P	Sialylated carbohydrates
Endothelial Ig Family			
ICAM-1		CD54	LFA-1, Mac-1
ICAM-2		CD-102	LFA-1

Data from references 1, 27, and 79.

CHEMOTAXIS

Once out of the vasculature, neutrophils must be able to find their way rapidly to areas of inflammation and infection. This process of directional motility along a chemoattractant gradient is known as chemotaxis. Many chemoattractants bind to G-protein–coupled 7 transmembrane spanning domain receptors (e.g., receptors for fMLP, C5a, platelet-activating factor, leukotriene B$_4$, interleukin [IL]-8), leading to dissociation of the G-protein complex and activation of signal transduction cascades,[9] Ultimately, polymerization and reorganization of the actin cytoskeleton occurs, driving extension of a pseudopodia or lamellipodia, which are sheet-like protrusions of membrane rich in actin filaments.[10] Adenosine triphosphate–dependent contraction mediated by myosin then contracts the cytoskeleton toward the leading pseudopodium.[1] Cycles of protrusion, adhesion, contraction, and de-adhesion are repeated, allowing the neutrophil to move through the extracellular membrane. Defective actin polymerization is one cause of a primary chemotactic disorder manifest clinically as recurrent infections, typically of fungal origin.[8]

PHAGOCYTOSIS

The process of phagocytosis, or engulfment of particles greater than 3 μm, is important both for removal of dead cells and for microbial killing.[11] Importantly, most microbial killing occurs inside the neutrophil. Phagocytosis occurs when the neutrophil internalizes microscopic particles through extensions of the plasma membrane that surround the particle and fuse around it, isolating the particle in a nascent phagosome (Fig. 29-2).[12,13] This serves to compartmentalize both the pathogen and the leukocyte-derived cytotoxic products that are destined to kill and digest the pathogen.

Neutrophils can recognize invading microbial pathogens by virtue of specific membrane receptors that recognize highly conserved motifs on pathogens not normally present on higher-order eukaryotic cells (e.g., specific carbohydrates, glycolipids such as lipopolysaccharide, glycoproteins, and proteins).[11] Collectively, these receptors are termed *pathogen-associated molecular pattern (PAMP) receptors.*[14] Phagocytes also express receptors that recognize specific host proteins such as antibodies or complement that coat ("opsonize") the pathogen. These "phagocytic receptors" include receptors for the Fc fragment of antibodies (Fc receptors) and complement receptors such as CR3 that recognize pathogens coated with antibodies or complement, respectively. Importantly, opsonization improves phagocytic efficiency dramatically.[12] There is no known specific inherited disorder resulting in a primary phagocytic defect.[8]

MICROBIAL KILLING

As previously stated, most microbial killing occurs inside the neutrophil in specialized compartments (phagosome, phagolysosome). In this way, potentially damaging effects of neutrophil products on host cells are minimized. The neutrophil can effectively kill microbes by releasing various molecules and compounds into the phagosome. Stimulated neutrophils, through the action of NAPDH oxidase, produce potent oxidants, including superoxide (O_2^-) and hydrogen peroxide (H_2O_2). These reactive oxygen species can be converted by myeloperoxidase to generate the hypohalous acids such as HOCl (bleach) that are extremely potent antimicrobial products. Nonoxidative killing mechanisms include acidification of the phagosome (pH 3.5 to 6), lysozyme (hydrolyses cell walls), lactoferrin (binds iron), various proteases (including elastase, collagenase, gelatinase, cathepsin G, and proteinase-3), and defensins (small microbicidal cationic peptides).[1,15]

Neutrophils contain four types of intracellular granules: azurophilic (primary), specific (secondary), and gelatinase (tertiary) granules and secretory vesicles.[1] The compounds contained in these granules aid in microbial killing and facilitate cell adhesion and locomotion by delivery of granule-associated proteins to the phagosome or to the cell surface (Table 29-2).

The Chédiak-Higashi syndrome is an autosomal recessive disorder of dysfunctional granules. Its molecular basis is not completely understood, but giant primary granules are seen in neutrophils, and those affected suffer recurrent skin and pulmonary infections, typified by delayed *Staphylococcus* killing. Rarely, specific granule deficiencies are seen in which neutrophils are missing secondary granules, resulting in a poor inflammatory response and recurrent infections.[4,8] MPO deficiency, especially in combination with diabetes, leads to a predisposition to *Candida* infections. Chronic granulomatous disease, caused by defects in the phagocyte NADPH oxidase, results in recurrent infections with catalase-positive organisms such as *Staphylococcus aureus* and granuloma formation.[4,8]

SECRETION OF INFLAMMATORY MEDIATORS

Although for many years the primary function of neutrophils was viewed as responding to signals derived from other host cells and invading pathogens, it is now appreciated that these cells also play an active role in regulating inflammation though production and release of the cytokines IL-1, IL-6, IL-8, and tumor necrosis factor-alpha (TNF-α).[1,16] In addition, leukocyte-derived proteases participate in substrate processing that can result in the formation and release of chemotactic peptides from surface- or matrix-bound precursors.

APOPTOSIS

Although not classically considered a neutrophil antimicrobial function, apoptosis serves an important purpose. Once the

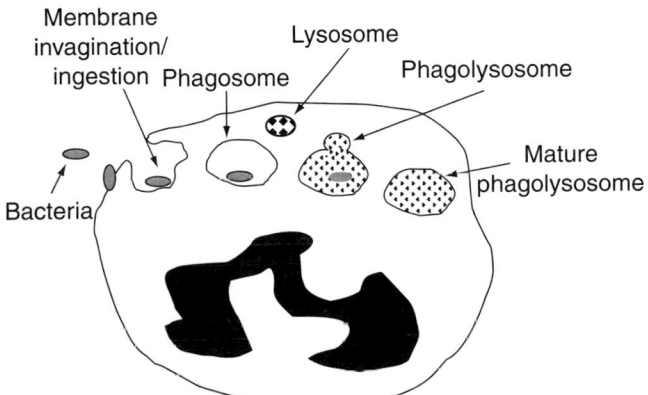

FIGURE 29–2. Process of phagocytosis.

TABLE 29–2. COMPOSITION OF HUMAN NEUTROPHIL GRANULES

	Azurophil (Primary)	Specific (Secondary)	Gelatinase (Tertiary)	Secretory
Membrane Proteins	CD66c, CD63, CD68	CD11b (Mac-1), CD15, CD66a, CD66b FMLP receptor Fibronectin receptor G-protein α subunit Laminin receptor Cytochrome b_{558} NB 1 antigen Rap 1 & 2 Thrombospondin receptor TNF receptor Vitronectin receptor u-PA receptor	CD11b FMLP receptor Cytochrome b_{558} Laminin receptor Diacylglycerol deacylating enzyme	CD10, CD11b, CD13, CD16, CD35 (CR1), CD45 Alkaline phosphatase Cytochrome b_{558} FMLP receptor DAF u-PA receptor
Serine Proteases	Elastase Cathepsin G Proteinase 3 Esterase N			
Microbicidal Enzymes	Myeloperoxidase Lysozyme Azurocidin Neuraminidase (sialidase)	Lysozyme Neuraminidase	Lysozyme	
Metalloproteinases	Collagenase	Collagenase Gelatinase	Gelatinase	
Acid Hydrolyases	N-Acetyl-β-glucosaminidase Cathepsin B Cathepsin D β-Galactosidase β-Glucuronidase β-Glycerophosphatase α-Mannosidase			
Inhibitors	α_1-Antitrypsin Heparin binding protein	Apolactoferrin Vitamin B_{12}–binding protein Protein kinase C inhibitor Histaminase Heparinase		
Other	Defensins Bactericidal permeability increasing protein (BPI) Acid mucopolysaccharide Ubiquitin	Plasminogen activator hCAP-18 SGP28 β_2-Microglobulin Lipocalin	Acetyltransferase	Albumin Tetranectin pro-u-PA/u-PA

Adapted from Skubitz KM: Neutrophilic leukocytes. In Lee GR, Lukens J, Paraskevas F, et al (eds): Wintrobe's Clinical Hematology. Philadelphia, Lippincott Williams & Wilkins, 1999, pp 300-350; and Abramson SL, Malech HL, Gallin JI: Neutrophils. In Crystal RG, West JB (eds): The Lung: Scientific Foundations. New York, Raven, 1991, pp 553-563.

threat of microbial invasion or tissue injury is over, inflammation must be rapidly down-regulated and neutrophils eventually disposed of in a manner that will not result in release of cytotoxic products with consequent host cell injury. One noninflammatory way of disposal of effete (spent) neutrophils is through apoptosis, also known as programmed cell death.[17] There are many signals for this process involving a variety of signal transduction pathways, and this subject is beyond the scope of this chapter, but interested readers are referred to recent reviews of this important subject.[17]

NEUTROPHILS AND INFLAMMATORY TISSUE INJURY

Although neutrophils primarily serve a protective role in the body, it is apparent that as part of the exuberant inflammatory response, neutrophils and their products can contribute to the tissue injury and dysfunction seen in sepsis and ALI and ARDS. Normally, unstimulated neutrophils pass through the pulmonary vasculature and are retained in the pulmonary capillary for seconds to minutes. This transit time can be affected by hemodynamic and soluble factors but no damage to the lungs typically occurs under physiologic circumstances. However, under pathologic conditions such as in ALI and ARDS, large numbers of neutrophils are sequestered in the microvasculature of the lung and other organs. In these strategic locations, the neutrophils become activated and may release cytotoxic products outside the cell that are capable of damaging host tissues. Under such circumstances, neutrophils are no longer innocuous. In experimental models of lung injury, there is evidence that direct activation of neutrophils, for example by preincubation with agonists such as lipopolysaccharide, can cause lung injury when re-injected into animals[18] and, conversely, that depletion of neutrophils can attenuate lung injury.[16,19,20] Despite this apparent propensity for host damage, neutrophil depletion is not a practical strategy for the treatment of ARDS for two reasons. First, there is evidence that ARDS can occur in neutropenic patients,[21,22] implying that neutrophil-independent mechanisms of lung injury may still be sufficient to engender acute lung injury. Second, and perhaps most importantly, is that neutrophil depletion undoubtedly predisposes the patient to infection, which is the most common cause of death in patients with ARDS.

MICROVASCULAR SEQUESTRATION AND ADHESION OF LEUKOCYTES

One of the earliest changes in ALI is increased neutrophil sequestration in the pulmonary capillaries that is reflected clinically by a transient leukopenia preceding respiratory deterioration.[23] The reasons for this remain incompletely understood but are likely related in part to an alteration in cellular biophysical properties (cell stiffening) as a consequence of polymerization and redistribution of the actin cytoskeleton.[74] This makes the 8-μm neutrophil less deformable and more likely to be unable to negotiate the 5.5-μm-wide pulmonary capillaries. Various signals, including IL-1, IL-6, IL-8, and TNF-α, mainly from alveolar macrophages and leukocytes, and bacterial products such as formyl peptides and lipopolysaccharide, can stimulate neutrophils and contribute to microvascular sequestration.[25] Alternatively, increased sequestration may be related to marrow release of neutrophils; in a rabbit model, therapy with granulocyte colony-stimulating factor (G-CSF) caused the bone marrow to release increased numbers of neutrophils that preferentially sequestered in the lungs.[26] It is noteworthy that production of G-CSF, a potent cytokine that mobilizes bone marrow neutrophils, is stimulated by bacterial products as well as host-derived cytokines such as TNF-α and IL-1.

Stimulation of neutrophils will induce the up-regulation of the number and function of cell surface adhesion molecules, leading to enhanced adhesivity.[24,27] In addition, mechanical deformation of the neutrophil, especially once activated, as occurs with passage through the pulmonary vasculature, leads to increased integrin/ICAM-1 binding.[28] Adhesion not only prolongs neutrophil sequestration and allows for transmigration but also activates various signaling cascades and thus impacts on many aspects of neutrophil function, including phagocytosis and the respiratory burst.[29]

Strategies to reduce leukocyte microvascular sequestration and adhesion with the goal of diminishing tissue injury are not always successful. In sheep, for example, blockage of P-selectin did not protect against lung injury in a burn model.[30] By contrast, in a murine "two-hit" model of endotoxemia combined with hemorrhagic shock, aggressive fluid resuscitation combined with reduced neutrophil endothelial adherence ameliorated the subsequent development of ALI.[31]

Once the neutrophil has adhered to the endothelial cell, it can then transmigrate across the endothelial barrier and into the interstitium after a chemotactic gradient.[32] In this extravascular location, neutrophil activation can lead to tissue damage. However, it is important to bear in mind that the process of transmigration from the vascular space into the alveolus per se does not necessarily lead to alterations in endothelial or epithelial permeability or injury.[33,34] Rather, damage may be mediated by extracellular release of proteases and other cytotoxic compounds during transmigration if the neutrophil is also subject to unregulated activation.[35]

ROS AND PROTEASES

There is a substantial body of evidence implicating neutrophil proteases in the pathogenesis of ALI.[36-41] Indeed, mice that are genetically deficient in both granulocyte elastase and cathepsin G are protected from LPS-induced lung injury.[42] Elastase, cathepsin G, proteinase 3, and various matrix metalloproteinases may injure the lung directly through proteolytic action on cells. Alternatively, proteases can enhance the inflammatory response by stimulating production of cytokines[43,44] and contribute to pathology through enhanced transcription of mucin genes.[45,46] In addition, proteases can cleave proteins in the airway and lead to the production of chemotactic peptides.[43,47] Evidence for benefit of protease inhibitors is limited to controlled animal studies[48] and a few small clinical trials. However, despite the purported role of proteases in ALI, the inflammatory milieu is sufficiently complex that simply delivering antiproteases to the lung may not ameliorate lung injury (hence the failure of the body's own natural antiproteases to prevent lung injury). Antiproteases can be inactivated by oxidation or by direct proteolytic cleavage rendering them ineffective. An additional consideration is the "protected space" between the neutrophil and the adjacent target cell in which a localized area of high protease concentration can exist that is isolated from high-molecular-weight antiproteases such as α_1-antitrypsin.[49]

Oxygen and nitrogen reactive species generated by neutrophils can contribute to pulmonary cell damage and the pathology of ALI.[50] Free radical formation can be secondary to the action of NADPH oxidase resulting in the formation of superoxide. Superoxide can then reduce iron, form hydrogen peroxide, and, through the action of myeloperoxidase, form oxidized halogens, such as hypochlorous acid. Alternatively, free radicals can be generated through inducible nitric oxide synthase (iNOS), leading to the formation of peroxynitrite (ONOO$^-$). Inhibition of either of these enzymes, in specific animal models, results in attenuation of ALI.[51-53]

PHOSPHOLIPASE A$_2$ METABOLITES

Although still uncertain, the neutrophil is believed to be a key cellular source of phospholipase A$_2$ (PLA$_2$) in the setting of ALI. This enzyme results in the formation of arachidonic acid from plasma membrane phospholipids and has been implicated in the pathogenesis of ALI. Bronchoalveolar lavage fluid PLA$_2$ activity is increased in humans with ARDS.[54] In animal models, delivery of PLA$_2$ intravenously[55] or by direct intratracheal instillation[56] can result in lung injury. Additionally, pharmacologic inhibition of PLA$_2$ attenuated ALI associated with intestinal ischemia reperfusion in rats[57] and targeted gene disruption of PLA$_2$ can attenuate ALI associated with sepsis and acid aspiration in mice.[58] PLA$_2$ may influence lung injury through the production of various arachidonic acid metabolites, including platelet-activating factor, lysophosphatidylcholine, and prostaglandins.[25] Inhibition of PLA$_2$ has not been attempted in humans with ALI/ARDS, but selective inhibition of specific PLA$_2$ isoforms may represent a therapeutic approach to ALI/ARDS, especially as more specific inhibitors are developed.

APOPTOSIS

Evidence exists that neutrophil apoptosis is delayed early in the course of ARDS by the presence of various proinflammatory cytokines such as GM-CSF.[17] This may result in a prolonged inflammatory process and contribute to further lung injury. In addition, delayed clearance of apoptotic neutrophils by alveolar macrophages may result in greater inflammatory injury. Mice deficient in caspase-1, a deficiency that resulted in delayed apoptosis, demonstrated prolonged pulmonary inflammation in response to intratracheal LPS administration.[59] However, the precise relationship between prolonged neutrophil survival in ALI remains to be defined, and given the potential untoward effects on the innate immune system of reducing neutrophil survival, further study is needed before this can be a suggested therapeutic approach.[17]

SIGNAL TRANSDUCTION PATHWAYS AS POTENTIAL THERAPEUTIC TARGETS

Research is uncovering the basic mechanisms regulating neutrophil function, and it is clear that specific cell signaling molecules fulfill important actions that allow the neutrophil to assume its role in inflammation and ALI. As our understanding of these processes increases, these molecules will become potential targets for pharmacologic modification in hopes of attenuating ALI and ARDS.

NF-κB

The transcription factor NF-κB binds to specific sequences in the promoter region of the genes for inflammatory cytokines such as IL-1β, IL-6, TNF-α, IL-8, and macrophage inflammatory protein as well as in other immunoregulatory molecules such as the endothelial adhesion molecules ICAM-1 and E-selectin that relate to the development and progression of lung injury.[60,61] NF-κB is normally composed of three components that bind to and form a complex (heterotrimer) that is retained in the cytoplasm through its association with the inhibitory molecule IκB. Phosphorylation, ubiquination, and proteolysis of IκB allows NF-κB to translocate to the nucleus and induce gene transcription.

The active form of NF-κB is a dimer composed of members of the Rel family in the active DNA-binding form. Five mammalian members of this family have been described: p50, p52, p65, c-Rel, and Rel B.[62,63] Various combinations of NF-κB have different transactivation abilities; for example, p50/p65 heterodimers are able to strongly promote transcription whereas p50/p50 homodimers produce important suppressive activities on gene activation.[60]

Hemorrhage or endotoxemia induces activation of NF-κB in lungs.[16,64] In this study, induced neutropenia significantly reduced the amount of NF-κB that accumulated in the nuclei of lung cell populations.[16] These observations indicate that neutrophils are important in modulating NF-κB activation in the lungs. Inhibition of NF-κB activation with antioxidants decreased edema, diminished neutrophil infiltration, and suppressed proinflammatory cytokine expression in the lungs.[64,65] As mentioned in the preceding section on apoptosis, apoptosis is thought to be a major mechanism for the clearance of effete neutrophils and especially important in the clearance of neutrophils from the injured lung.[66] NF-κB is considered to have both antiapoptotic and proapoptotic effects. Activation of the PI3-kinase/Akt pathway has potent antiapoptotic effects and NF-κB is a target of Akt. Activation of NF-κB results in enhanced transcription of antiapoptotic genes.[67-69] On the other hand, NF-κB may also have a proapoptotic role in p53-induced cell death.[70] Thus, NF-κB activation in the setting of acute lung injury may regulate not only the expression of proinflammatory mediators but also the numbers of activated neutrophils within the lung. Therefore, regulation of NF-κB is a logical target for potential therapeutic intervention for the prevention or minimization of ALI.

PHOSPHATIDYLINOSITOL-3-KINASE

Phosphatidylinositol-3-kinases (PI3K), a group of heterodimeric enzymes, catalyze the conversion of membrane phosphatidylinositol-3,4-biphosphate (PIP_2) to PIP_3 in response to various growth factors, hormones, chemokines, and chemoattractants.[71,72] PIP_3 can then lead to the activation of other cellular signaling pathways and thus impact on many aspects of neutrophil functioning, including chemotaxis, adhesion, and apoptosis. There are four isoforms of the catalytic subunit of PI3K, with PI3K-γ found exclusively in leukocytes. PI3K-α and PI3K-β knockout mice are not viable; however, PI3K-γ –/– mice, when exposed to LPS, have reduced lung edema, neutrophil accumulation, and pulmonary cytokine levels when compared with wild-type mice.[73] Although the precise mechanism by which PI3K inhibition modulates neutrophil-mediated lung injury is not clear, PI3K may contribute to ALI through its effects on NF-κB translocation, chemotaxis, or apoptosis.[60] There are currently no pharmacologic inhibitors specific to the γ isoform of PI3K, but with time PI3K-γ inhibition may be possible. Caution must be exercised, however, given the wide-ranging effects of PI3K.

MITOGEN-ACTIVATED PROTEIN KINASE

Three distinct mitogen-activated protein kinase (MAPK) pathways have been described in neutrophils: p38, extracellular signal-regulated kinase (ERK), and c-Jun NH2-terminal kinase (JNK). These signaling pathways, composed of a cascade of kinases that are activated by phosphorylation, function to transmit signals from the cell surface to the cytoplasm and nucleus.

The p38 pathway is important in neutrophil adhesion, chemotaxis, respiratory burst, and apoptosis.[74-76] Selective p38 inhibition, even up to 4 hours after aerosolized administration of lipopolysaccharide to mice, resulted in reduced neutrophil accumulation in the alveolar airspaces as compared with the findings in control animals.[74] Although promising, this result contrasts with observations in endotoxemia and hemorrhage-induced ALI in which p38 inhibition had no effect on neutrophil accumulation or other markers of ALI.[77] It may be that p38 activity is specific to neutrophil migration to the airspaces or in response to airway LPS.[60]

The ERK pathway has important roles in cytokine production and chemotaxis to fMLP, LTB4, C5a, and IL-8, but because ERK inhibitors are toxic, little information exists pertaining to inhibition of this pathway in modulation of lung injury.

The JNK pathway is important in cell proliferation and apoptosis and is activated in response to cellular stress. JNK-1 knockout mice have increased susceptibility to hyperoxia-induced ALI.[78] Interestingly, BAL neutrophil counts were lower in knockout compared with wild-type mice. The reason for this is not clear but may be due to decreased adhesion and migration or to increased neutrophil apoptosis. In this model it is difficult to determine the specific effects of neutrophil JNK inhibition because all cells were affected and increased epithelial cell apoptosis contributed significantly to the overall pathology. Inhibition of MAPK pathways in cell culture and controlled animal models may help distinguish the relative importance of these pathways in different cell types. However as a potential tool in humans, unless cell specific inhibitors are developed, generalized MAPK inhibition may prove to be an unrealistic therapeutic approach.

CONCLUSION

In this chapter, we have focused initially on the essential role of neutrophils in the innate immune response to invading microbial pathogens. The importance of this function is underscored by disease states resulting from the absence (neutropenia) or dysfunction (leukocyte adhesion deficiency and chronic granulomatous disease) where affected individuals have an enhanced susceptibility to infection. It remains a paradox that these essential antimicrobial processes can apparently turn against the host and result in tissue and organ injury. It must be emphasized that inflammation is an inherently beneficial process and that only when it becomes excessive or otherwise unregulated does host damage occur. Throughout this chapter we have indicated potential therapeutic targets that might be selected in an attempt to mitigate inflammatory injury while preserving the host defense functions of these essential phagocytes. It is clear, however, that given the complexities and redundancies

of this system, successful therapeutic intervention will not be an easy task.

ANNOTATED REFERENCES

Aderem A: How to eat something bigger than your head. Cell 2002;110:5-8.
  Brief review outlining importance of phagocytosis in innate immunity with discussion of role of endoplasmic reticulum recruitment to plasma membrane during phagocytosis.

Campbell EJ, Campbell MA: Pericellular proteolysis by neutrophils in the presence of proteinase inhibitors: Effects of substrate opsonization. J Cell Biol 1988;106:667-676.
  In vitro experiments illustrate concept of neutrophil-mediated proteolytic activity in pericellular microenvironments despite high concentrations of protease inhibitors.

Donnelly SC, et al: Plasma elastase levels and the development of the adult respiratory distress syndrome. Am J Respir Crit Care Med 1995;151: 1428-1433.
  Study in trauma patients reveals early elevation in serum neutrophil elastase level is associated with subsequent development of ARDS. This study implicates neutrophil activation in early stage of ARDS pathogenesis.

Janeway CAJ, Medzhitov R: Innate immune recognition. Annu Rev Immunol 2002;20:197-216.
  Well-referenced, salient review of innate immune system with special emphasis on the role of Toll-like receptors.

Ware LB, Matthay MA: The acute respiratory distress syndrome. N Engl J Med 2000;342:1334-1349.
  Recent overview of ARDS with attention to both the basic science and clinical perspectives.

Chapter 30
MACROPHAGE FUNCTION

Donna M. Paulnock • Stefanie N. Vogel

KEY POINTS

1. **Macrophages are present in blood (monocytes) and all tissues of the body.** At these sites they provide a critical first line of host defense, through recognition and elimination of entering pathogens.

2. **Macrophages throughout the body express a wide range of functional activities,** including phagocytosis, secretory activity, and microbial killing. Macrophages in individual tissues express a unique spectrum of these properties that is regulated at and characteristic of that tissue site.

3. **Macrophages are the central cells in the process of inflammation,** the classic innate immune response to microbial infection. Macrophages at the site of inflammation are activated by host and microbial factors to express enhanced functional activities.

4. In addition to their roles in innate immunity, **macrophages and dendritic cells serve a critical function in the initiation of adaptive immune responses,** through their ability to serve as antigen-presenting cells (APCs) for the activation of T lymphocytes.

MACROPHAGE DEVELOPMENT AND IDENTIFICATION

Cells of the mononuclear phagocyte system are ubiquitously distributed throughout the body, present in essentially all tissues, in peripheral blood and bone marrow, and in body cavities.[1] Immature progenitor populations begin the developmental process in the bone marrow, ultimately giving rise to monocytes that enter the circulation. Blood monocytes then migrate into the peripheral tissues, where they differentiate further into resident tissue macrophages.[1,2] The network of fixed tissue macrophage populations present throughout the body thus is ideally positioned to serve as a first line of defense at the major portals of microbial entry in the body. In addition, this system of cells serves critical roles in maintaining tissue homeostasis and regeneration.[3]

Cytokines present in the bone marrow stromal milieu, including in particular granulocyte-macrophage colony-stimulating factor (GM-CSF) and colony-stimulating factor-1 (originally termed macrophage-colony-stimulating factor),

control early macrophage progenitor cell commitment and differentiation.[4,5] Additional stimuli provided in each tissue, including both endogenous factors from other cells within the tissue and microbial factors resulting from the presence of circulating or commensal organisms, subsequently shape the functional and phenotypic attributes of resident macrophages present at that site, giving rise to cells adapted to perform specific functions within this local environment.[6-8] For example, in the liver, the fixed macrophage population, the Kupffer cells, provides key detoxification functions whereas microglia, specialized brain macrophages, are believed to provide cytokines and other growth and differentiation factors essential for other brain cells. Thus, a given macrophage population will have phenotypic and functional characteristics both in common with and distinct from macrophages found at other defined locations.

These aspects of macrophage development and anatomic location have made it difficult to identify markers that unequivocally define macrophages at various developmental stages or in various tissue sites. Few, if any, of the available monoclonal antibodies against macrophage surface antigens are either fully macrophage specific or identify all macrophage subpopulations. Nonetheless, recent characterizations have provided information on some molecules expressed solely by cells within the mononuclear phagocyte lineage. The antibody F4/80, although still functionally ambiguous, detects a cell surface glycoprotein that is expressed by mature mouse macrophages and often is used to identify these cells in tissue samples and preparations of isolated cells.[9] Similarly, the MAC-1 antibody detects the C3bi receptor, a critical member of the array of surface proteins expressed by macrophages, but also is expressed by granulocytic cells in the myeloid lineage.[10] The receptor for the differentiation factor CSF-1 serves as an alternative macrophage-specific marker, reflecting the critical role of CSF-1 in macrophage differentiation, and can aid in the identification of earlier developmental stages.[11]

A number of additional functionally associated surface molecules have been used to identify these cells in tissue and blood samples, although these clearly are not macrophage specific. Such molecules include cell surface receptors for the Fc portion of immunoglobulin G, for complement-coated particles, and for acute phase response proteins normally produced during the early stages of infection.[12-14] More recently, receptors for "pathogen-associated molecular patterns" (PAMPs) have been recognized as critical components of macrophage functional activities and thus useful as markers of these and other innate immune system cells. These include the Toll-like receptors (TLR) that play a major role in pathogen recognition and initiation of inflammatory responses and other endocytic receptors, such as type A scavenger receptors and C-type lectin family molecules.[15] However, this category of molecules again is not strictly confined to macrophages. Thus, unlike the situation for T and B lymphocytes, it has not been possible to define phenotypically distinct markers for various stages of macrophage differentiation. However, the presence of subsets of cells that belong to the mononuclear phagocyte system in mice and humans can be assessed using combinations of antibodies against sets of cell surface proteins and such reagents can be used effectively to isolate/characterize these cells.

One final issue regarding macrophage identification is the recent recognition that differentiation into mature, tissue-specific macrophages is not the only developmental option for a cell within the myeloid lineage. These cells also may give rise to dendritic cell (DC) populations. DCs and macrophages share a number of functional attributes, including internalization of pathogenic microorganisms, secretion of cytokines, and antigen presentation to T cells, although DCs clearly are recognized as the most potent professional APC for naive T cells.[16] DCs are now recognized to be descended from both lymphoid and myeloid progenitor cells, deriving from hematopoietic progenitors of those lineages as well as from blood monocytes.[17,18] The re-direction of less-mature macrophages toward DC development is driven by a variety of diverse stimuli, including multiple cytokine mediators produced during the development of immune response.[19] These observations support the idea that early in their differentiation process, macrophages retain some degree of developmental plasticity. This may contribute to the enrichment of DC populations, and therefore antigen presentation and lymphocyte activation, during immune responses but also may pose some challenges for the process of macrophage versus DC identification.

MACROPHAGE FUNCTIONAL ACTIVITIES

Functionally, macrophages are the quintessential "multi-tasking" cells of the immune response. Although a full review of macrophage functional activities is beyond the scope of this brief discussion, macrophages generally do express a variety of shared functional characteristics, including phagocytic capability, cytokine production, processing and presentation of antigens to lymphocytes, and killing of microbes and tumor cells.[20] These activities reflect the participation of macrophages in the process of pathogen elimination at all levels, including microbial detection, microbial engulfment and cellular destruction, and the activation of downstream immune response cellular elements. Through these activities, macrophages both act directly as antimicrobial effector cells and bridge the early innate immune response with the more antigen-specific adaptive immune response.

The ability of macrophages to phagocytose particles represents the first step in a series of events that ultimately lead to the elimination of intruding microorganisms, tumor cells, and cellular debris. Internalization of different substances is mediated through multiple distinct surface receptors. These include complement receptors, vitronectin, and other specialized receptors that recognize apoptotic cells and altered self molecules.[21] Phagocytosis can be dramatically enhanced through the use of receptors for the Fc region of immunoglobulins bound to target cells such as tumor cells and parasites.[22] Finally, as noted in the preceding section on macrophage

development, a large family of pattern recognition receptors (PRR) recognize various conserved motifs (mannans, lipopolysaccharides, polyanionic molecules, formylated peptides, and others) expressed by microbes but absent in their vertebrate hosts.[23] These evolutionarily conserved receptors are critical recognition receptors for initiation of multiple innate immune functions, and aspects of their structure and function are receiving considerable attention. Although phagocytosis is not a prerequisite for PRR-mediated signaling, the uptake of organisms after sensing through PRRs couples phagocytosis and intracellular signaling in many cases.[24,25] The specific molecular events that follow PRR engagement remain to be fully characterized for each receptor; however, activation of the NF-κB pathway of signal transduction and expression of genes transcribed after activation of this transcription factor family have emerged as prominent outcomes of innate recognition.[26]

Phagocytosis of microorganisms generally is followed by two outcomes in a macrophage population: the production of biologically active secreted products and the elimination of the phagocytosed target organisms. Two independent biochemical pathways principally contribute to the ability of macrophages to eliminate intracellular pathogens and extracellular targets. Synthesis of nitric oxide (NO) appears to be responsible for much of the antimicrobial activity of macrophages against certain pathogens.[27] This simple but strikingly effective molecule, along with additional reactive nitrogen intermediates, plays an essential role in the immune response to a number of intracellular pathogens, including *Mycobacterium tuberculosis*, the protozoan parasite *Toxoplasma gondii*, and the fungus *Cryptococcus neoformans*.[28-30] Reactive oxygen metabolites also are associated with the potent antimicrobial and antitumor activity of macrophages, including, most importantly, hydrogen peroxide and superoxide anion, which are directly toxic to microorganisms.[27] Toxic oxygen-derived products are produced as a result of the action of lysosomal enzymes, including NADPH oxidases, which on fusion of the phagosome and lysosome following organism internalization act to destroy the pathogen directly.[31,32] Additional microbicidal molecules derived from macrophages, including a large class of secreted antimicrobial peptides called defensins, various enzymes such as lysozyme, and diverse competitors for essential nutrients, such as lactoferrin, provide antimicrobial action for both intracellular and extracellular microbes.[33]

A second important outcome of the interaction between pathogens and macrophages is activation of these cells to release cytokines and other soluble mediators. Macrophages produce a vast array of secreted products after antigen interaction.[34] Many of these products result from induction of new gene expression as an outcome of PRR (and other receptor) engagement and the ensuing downstream signal transduction events. Recent studies using functional genomic analyses to dissect macrophage and DC innate responses have identified three broad classes of secreted products produced by macrophages after activation: (1) cytokines and chemokines, responsible for proinflammatory and anti-inflammatory effects, cell recruitment, and cell growth; (2) non–cytokine-secretory products, including enzymes that contribute to the inflammatory response (e.g., cyclooxygenase-2), hormones, and other molecules involved in basic cellular processes; and (3) products of inducible metabolic pathways, for example, NO and H_2O_2, the downstream products of inducible enzymes.[35-37] Some molecules within this spectrum of responses are likely to represent pathogen-specific responses, whereas others can be induced by multiple organisms or nonmicrobial activating ligands. This is, in part, regulated by the particular PRR engaged. For example, it is clear that the differential gene expression observed in response to engagement of distinct TLRs is related to differential utilization of adapter proteins on extracellular activation by microbial agonists.[38] Thus, while the ability to produce immunoregulatory factors is a defining function of activated macrophages, the diversity of cytokines or other products induced will, again, be influenced by the nature of the inducing stimulus and the local microenvironment of the cells.

CURRENT PARADIGMS OF MACROPHAGE ACTIVATION

Although newly arrived tissue macrophages constitutively display some of their characteristic functions, such as phagocytosis, essentially all macrophage functions are induced or enhanced by cellular activation. The notion of an "activated macrophage" was originally proposed by Mackaness, and extended by Russell, Hibbs, and others, to describe a cell that had developed increased microbicidal or tumoricidal capacities as a function of stepwise signaling.[39-42] This definition still is valuable in emphasizing that there are substantial changes in macrophage activity and function during the evolution of an immune response that have beneficial outcomes for the host. Within the context of modern immunology, the concept of an activated macrophage can be expanded to define a cell that has responded to cell-derived and/or environmental factors with specific molecular changes that allow an enhanced functional response specific for the inciting stimulus.

Multiple studies have confirmed that the underlying basis of the activation process is the induction of new gene expression in response to host and microbial ligands. These ligands are almost limitless in their number and include such diverse mediators as the cytokines interferon-gamma (a potent macrophage activating agent) and interleukin (IL)-12; arachidonic acid metabolites; and microbial products such as bacterial lipopolysaccharide, lipoteichoic acid, and CpG oligonucleotides, to name a few. Studies of the response of isolated mouse macrophage populations have demonstrated that each agonist has distinct effects and induces a unique pattern of induced genes.[35-37] In addition, the activation response of any macrophage will be influenced by the nature of the microenvironment of that particular population of macrophages and whether multiple stimuli are used, such as is commonly the case in the stepwise activation treatments used in in-vitro studies of macrophage function.[42] The genetic background of the mouse strain (and presumably of human cells) and the source of macrophage progenitors also influence the level of activation achieved.[43] These considerations suggest that, again, there is no single characteristic, metabolic or genetic, that can be used universally to define an activated macrophage. Instead, the nature of the activation response will be linked to the nature of the inducing stimulus/stimuli and environment.

Recent studies have proposed that two subsets of activated macrophages can be identified that preferentially promote or dampen inflammatory and antimicrobial responses, labeled classically activated versus alternatively activated macrophages, respectively. These populations are defined largely on the basis of the immunopotentiating (e.g., IL-12, IL-18) versus immunosuppressive (e.g., IL-10, transforming growth factor-beta) cytokines produced.[44,45] Given the nature of macrophage heterogeneity discussed earlier, it seems likely that these functionally based distinctions represent examples of macrophages at different points along the continuum of the activation process or as a function of specific types or combinations of stimuli. Nonetheless, the importance of identifying macrophages that display functional polarization during infection or tumor development may be important for understanding how these situations modulate innate and acquired immune responses.

CENTRAL ROLE OF MACROPHAGES IN INFLAMMATION

The inflammatory response serves as perhaps the best showcase of the array of macrophage functional activities. Innate immune recognition underlies most inflammatory responses, and this is set in motion by pathogen recognition. As noted previously, macrophages located in peripheral tissues serve as an effective surveillance system for pathogen entry or other alterations in the cellular environment, and the decision to respond or not respond to a particular ligand is largely made by phagocytic cells at these sites.

The presence of changes in the tissue environment both stimulates the macrophages already present in the tissue and induces the rapid recruitment of additional macrophages to that site. Macrophage influx into a site of injury or infection is part of the process of inflammation and is recognized as a central component of the innate immune response.[46] Macrophages active during the early stages of inflammatory responses and at the initiation of wound healing produce the soluble inflammatory mediators such as IL-1, tumor necrosis factor-alpha, and IL-6 that stimulate a systemic response to infection.[47] Similarly, production of chemokines, including IL-8 (CXCL8), is an important outcome of microbial recognition. These chemotactic mediators enhance the recruitment and entry of phagocytes and lymphocytes to the inflammatory site and mediate changes in the local expression of adhesion molecules on endothelial cells, promoting the migration of circulating cells to the inflammatory site.[48] Finally, as discussed more fully later, the APC functions of macrophages and DCs require the increased expression of co-stimulatory molecules, as well as production of cytokines such as IL-12 and IL-18, for effective T-cell activation to proceed. The exact profile of cytokines induced by microbial recognition and produced by macrophages is determined by the nature of the stimulatory agonist and the cell surface receptor(s) engaged. In turn, these molecules both promote the functional activities of neighboring phagocytic cells and influence the character of the adaptive immune response that develops in their presence.

In the final analysis, it is somewhat difficult to separate the concept of inflammation from the process of macrophage activation, because the cells participating in the initiation of an inflammatory response clearly become activated during the development of this response. Analysis of the global response of these cells to microorganisms has suggested that a large portion of the activation-specific gene products induced in macrophages following ligand recognition are involved in regulating the subsequent inflammatory process.[35,36] In many cases, the inflammatory response, and the activities of macrophages activated during that process, are sufficient to limit and even to clear an infection, occasionally without significant systemic effects in the infected host. Thus, this early macrophage response to infection is an effective host defense mechanism.

ROLE OF MACROPHAGES IN BRIDGING INNATE AND ADAPTIVE IMMUNE RESPONSES

If the innate immune response is not sufficient to contain infection, the ability of macrophages and DC to activate CD4+ T lymphocytes provides a critical bridge to the development of the adaptive response.[49] Much information is available concerning the events of T-cell stimulation by these professional APCs, and only a brief overview of this process is presented here. The stimulation of naive CD4+ T cells, or T helper cells, is the prototypical example of APC function, because activation of these cells is the cornerstone event in the development of adaptive immune responses.

The first stage of APC function is broadly referred to as antigen presentation and consists of antigen uptake, degradation, and loading onto major histocompatibility complex (MHC) molecules.[50,51] As noted previously, the ability of macrophages to phagocytose particles via both nonspecific and receptor-mediated uptake is a critical aspect of their presentation capacity. Antigen uptake, or in the case of intracellular pathogens the accessibility of microbial antigens within the cell, leads to the processing of these antigens into proteolytic peptides and their loading onto MHC class I or class II molecules.

Once effective peptide:MHC complexes are displayed by the APC, T-cell stimulation can follow. The process of T-cell priming (or the activation of naive cells) involves physical interaction with those cells in the T-cell zones of secondary lymphoid organs.[52] Cytokines and chemokines expressed by the macrophage after antigen uptake play a critical role in attracting and retaining naive T cells that are capable of responding to specific antigens, as noted in the previous section. T cells recognizing their cognate antigen on macrophages at these peripheral sites respond by binding the antigen:MHC complex via the T-cell receptor and binding co-stimulatory molecules such as B7.1 and B7.2 (CD80, 86) via the CD28 molecule. Increased expression of such co-stimulatory molecules is one consequence of macrophage-pathogen interaction, thus creating a reciprocal relationship between microbial recognition and T-cell stimulation. Additional engagement of adhesion molecules promotes formation of the T-cell synapse, thought to be critical for effective T-cell activation.[53] T-lymphocyte signaling through the T-cell receptor and co-stimulatory molecules then leads to T-cell activation, broadly defined as the induction of the new gene expression required for T-cell proliferation and differentiation. Effective activation requires that both the antigen:MHC complex and the co-stimulatory molecule(s) be expressed on the same APC and both must be recognized

within a specific time span to lead to effective activation in the T cell.[54]

The final stage of T-cell activation by APC is the polarization of the CD4+ T-cell response toward a specific functional pathway, termed *type 1 or type 2 differentiation pathways.* Differential maturation of these responses is regulated by the nature of the cytokines produced by the APC and is thought to be influenced both by the nature of the microbial pathogen or altered cell initially recognized as well as aspects of antigen processing and presentation.[55] In this way, the APC helps to shape the character of the adaptive response, through modulation of the initial T-cell response.

CONCLUSION

Since their initial description as "big eaters" more than 100 years ago, macrophages have been recognized as scavenger cells in both invertebrates and higher organisms.[56] It is now recognized that this ubiquitously distributed population of fixed and circulating mononuclear phagocytes can express tremendous functional, morphologic, and metabolic diversity that is shaped by both the anatomic location and the differentiation or activation stage of each cell. By providing both a first line of host defense against microorganisms and altered host cells and the capacity to stimulate an adaptive immune response, the macrophage plays a central role in the regulation of host immunity.

ANNOTATED REFERENCES

Gordon S: Alternative activation of macrophages. Nat Rev Immunol 2003;3:23-35.

> This paper highlights the current paradigm of how macrophages may provide both immune-enhancing and immune-suppressing modulatory functions as part of innate immune responses and host defense, contradictory effects long observed during the course of many infectious diseases.

Hume DA, Ross IL, Himes SR, et al: The mononuclear phagocyte system revisited. J Leuk Biol 2002;72:621-627; and Nau GJ, Richmond JFL, Schlesinger A, et al: Human macrophage activation programs induced by bacterial pathogens. Proc Natl Acad Sci U S A 2002;99:1503-1508.

> These two manuscripts bring consideration of macrophage biology into the molecular age. Using a genomic approach for analysis of changes in gene expression after pathogen recognition, these studies provide novel information about and a new view of macrophage activation that ultimately may be useful for effective manipulation of the consequences of microbial recognition, including inflammation.

Janeway CA Jr, Medzhitov R: Innate immune recognition. Ann Rev Immunol 2002;20:197-216.

> This review provides an overview of newly emerging information concerning the molecular mechanisms of microbial recognition by macrophages including the receptors involved in microbial recognition. Current efforts are devoted to understanding the interplay between microbial uptake and the signaling responses that both result from microbial detection.

Mackaness GB: Cellular immunity. J Exp Med 1962;116:381-406.

> This paper is a classic in the field of macrophage biology. It provides the first description of an activated or "angry" macrophage, a concept that remains central to our understanding of the host defense aspects of macrophage functions.

Chapter 31

ENDOTHELIAL FUNCTION

Larry W. Kraiss • Mark L. Martinez • Stephen M. Prescott • Guy A. Zimmerman

KEY POINTS

1. **Endothelial cells,** once thought to be inert vascular lining cells, **respond to signals from the environment with functional and phenotypic changes in physiologic conditions and in critical illness.** This process is termed *endothelial activation.*

2. **Endothelial activation** is induced by a variety of agonists that act via receptors of diverse classes. Endothelial receptors are linked to intracellular signaling cascades that regulate functional responses. Endothelial responses to hemodynamic and other mechanical forces and in injury also trigger intracellular signaling pathways.

3. **Endothelial responses triggered by activation or injury** influence vasoregulation, vascular permeability, hemostasis, acute and chronic inflammation, wound surveillance and repair, and other critical events, and they affect every organ.

4. **Endothelial function is dysregulated or becomes unregulated in human diseases,** including sepsis, ischemia-reperfusion syndromes, injury by oxidants or toxins, and other conditions. Endothelial cell dysfunction is a key pathophysiologic mechanism in **organ-specific syndromes** and in **systemic responses to injury.**

5. **Endothelial cell activation responses** provide molecular targets that may ultimately be useful for **therapeutic intervention** in syndromes of critical illness and other diseases. **Endothelial cell markers** may be useful in establishing the natural history of disease states and for following the course of specific syndromes.

INTRODUCTION

The vascular system of an adult human has a surface area of several square meters and is lined by 1×10^{13} or more endothelial cells,[1] which influence the function of every organ. Endothelial cells were once thought to be passive structural units with little or no capacity to respond to activating signals with changes in phenotype and function. Electron microscopic observations documenting that endothelial cells contain secretory granules and physiologic experiments suggesting that they are not passive in interactions with leukocytes, both of which were accomplished in the 1950s, indicated otherwise.[1] The studies of leukocyte–endothelial cell interactions built on earlier observations that the endothelium has particular roles in the response to injury[2] and in inflammation.[3] Multiple subsequent studies clearly demonstrated that endothelial cells respond to signals from the environment with diverse *activation* responses that are critical for vasoregulation, hemostasis, inflammation, wound repair, and organ-specific activities.[4,5] This is perhaps the most important conceptual advance in vascular biology in recent history. A corollary is that endothelial dysfunction contributes to a variety of human diseases and syndromes,[1,4] including critical illnesses.

The endothelium itself is now considered by many investigators and physicians to be an extended and complex organ with the capacity for local, regional, and systemic activation, depending on the physiologic or pathologic stimulus and concurrent modifying features.[1,6,7] In sepsis, trauma, ischemia-reperfusion, and other conditions that are common in critical illness, multiple biochemical and physical signals are generated that can be transmitted to intracellular transduction cascades in endothelial cells, mediating acute or more protracted functional changes. These activation events,[4,5] which are triggered by physical injury, microbial products, toxins, and other stimuli, were apparently conserved after a continuous endothelium appeared as part of a closed vascular system when vertebrate species emerged,[8] and they evolved to establish and preserve vascular integrity, maintain intravascular volume and oxygen and nutrient delivery, and recruit leukocytes and platelets for local defense and repair. Critical phenotypic changes of activated endothelium include rapid transformation to a vasoconstrictive, procoagulant, and proinflammatory state that can then be further modified in a time-dependent fashion.[1] Although these responses are required for homeostasis and defense, they can contribute to tissue damage if dysregulated (Fig. 31–1). In critically ill patients, endothelial cell activity varies, depending on the nature of the illness or injury. Endothelial responses have a critical influence on the complications of organ-specific or systemic illnesses such as acute respiratory distress syndrome (ARDS) and multiple organ failure (see Fig. 31–1).[9,10]

Vasculogenesis and *angiogenesis* are not reviewed in detail here but are fundamental processes with intricate molecular regulation that are important in neoplasia, chronic inflammation, responses of hypoxic tissues, and other pathologic processes, in addition to vascular and organ development.[1,11–16] Recent observations demonstrate novel mechanisms that regulate vascular guidance in developing tissues.[16,17] In critically ill patients, pro- and antiangiogenic signaling molecules are released by platelets and myeloid

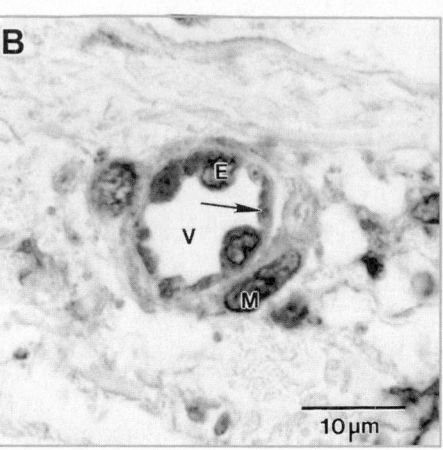
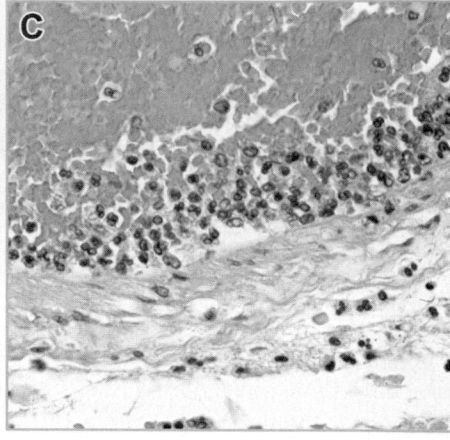

FIGURE 31–1. Endothelial cells are activated in human diseases and critical illness. *A,* Autologous radiolabeled leukocyte scanning in a patient early after the onset of acute respiratory distress syndrome secondary to Gram-negative sepsis demonstrates diffuse accumulation of polymorphonuclear leukocytes and monocytes in the lungs *(arrows),* an event mediated in part by endothelial cell activation. There is also significant uptake of radiolabeled leukocytes in the liver and spleen. (See text for details; also reference 74.) *B,* Endothelial cells in a systemic venule in tissue removed during surgical exploration for an abdominal aortic aneurysm stain intensely for the CXC chemokine epithelial neutrophil-activating peptide-78 (ENA-78). ENA-78 is not expressed by unactivated endothelial cells at baseline. A variety of other new gene products are also expressed by activated endothelial cells. (See text for details; also references 4 and 62.) *C,* Autopsy sample from a subject dying of Gram-positive sepsis demonstrates dramatic accumulation of neutrophils, monocytes, and platelets in a systemic venule. A variety of clinical and experimental observations indicate that systemic endothelial cells are activated in septic syndromes caused by Gram-positive as well as Gram-negative bacteria, contributing to the accumulation and activation of leukocytes and platelets. V, venule; E, endothelial cell; M, macrophage. (*A,* From Zimmerman GA, Albertine KH, McIntyre TM: Pathogenesis of sepsis and septic-induced injury. In Matthay MA [ed]: Lung Biology in Health and Disease, vol 179. New York, Marcel Dekker, 2003, pp 245-287. *B,* From Imaizumi T, Albertine KH, Jicha DL, et al: Human endothelial cells synthesize ENA-78: Relationship to IL-8 and to signaling of PMN adhesion. Am J Respir Cell Mol Biol 1997;17:181-192.)

leukocytes and are generated by other mechanisms.[10,11] Certain of these mediators, such as the vascular endothelial growth factor family of polypeptides and sphingosine-1-phosphate, influence vascular permeability and other functions in addition to angiogenesis.[18–22] Angiogenic responses of endothelial cells may influence organ dysfunction and repair in specific syndromes of critical illness, but these issues are largely unexplored.

Endothelial cells at different sites in the vasculature may be more similar than dissimilar.[23] However, there is evidence of endothelial cell *heterogeneity* both between and within specific tissues and organs and between macrovascular and microvascular sources.[1,24] The genetic determinants of endothelial cell subtypes and the developmental and signaling pathways that influence their phenotypic fates after initial vasculogenic and angiogenic cues remain to be completely characterized.[1] These variables are critical to approaches that involve therapeutic delivery of stem or vascular progenitor cells to injured or terminally diseased tissues,[25] where microenvironments and selective cell-cell and cell-matrix interactions may differentially influence cell fates.[1] Endothelial cell heterogeneity and local microenvironments also are determinants of these cells' participation in gene therapy protocols and approaches.[1]

A pivotal advance in the study of endothelial cell phenotype and function occurred when methodology was developed that allows the cultivation and analysis of isolated endothelial cells from humans and experimental animals in culture and, in some models, in coculture conditions with other vascular cells.[23,26, 27] Although isolated and cultured endothelial cells are not perfect replicas of the in vivo state, they have been remarkably informative (Fig. 31–2). For example, virtually all the adhesion and signaling molecules involved in endothelial interactions with leukocytes (see later) were identified using human endothelial cells in primary or early passage culture, and many additional activation events have been identified

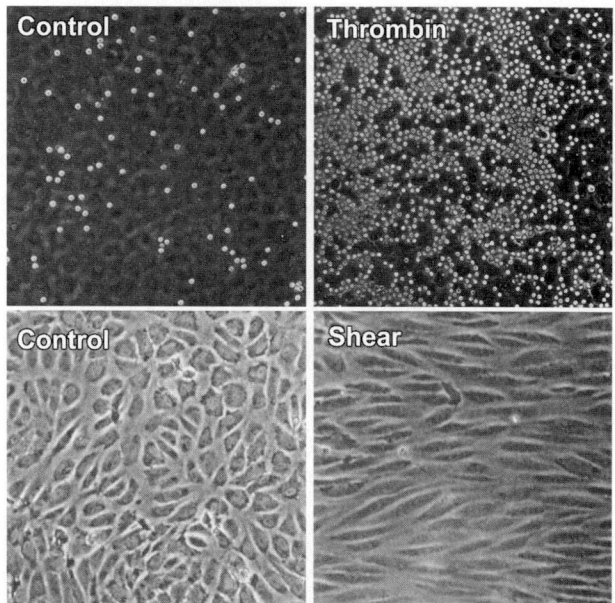

FIGURE 31–2. Cultured human endothelial cells are activated by diverse signals from the environment. *Top panels,* Human neutrophils (refractile white spheres) adhere dramatically to a monolayer of cultured human endothelial cells pretreated with nanomolar concentrations of thrombin for 5 minutes (right), compared with a control monolayer (left). Thrombin triggers endothelial cell activation, leading to neutrophil adhesion. The molecular mechanism for endothelial cell–dependent leukocyte adhesion under these conditions is shown in Figure 31–3A, and other relevant events are illustrated in Figure 31–4. (See text for details; also references 38, 40, and 41.) *Bottom panels,* A primary culture of human endothelial cells developed elongate morphology when subjected to shear (right), compared with a control monolayer incubated under static conditions (left) (L. W. Kraiss, unpublished experiment). As outlined in the text, cultured human endothelial cells undergo multiple additional activation events and phenotypic changes in response to clinically relevant signals from the environment. (*Top,* From Zimmerman GA, McIntyre TM, Prescott SM: Thrombin stimulates the adherence of neutrophils to human endothelial cells in vitro. J Clin Invest 1985;76:2235-2246.)

using this approach and validated in vivo (see Fig. 31–2). Strategies using isolated endothelial cells continue to be useful in defining characteristics relevant to critical illness. In addition, "in vivo cell biologic" approaches[10] are evolving and are likely to be informative in experimental models of critical illness and in clinical research involving human subjects in the intensive care unit. In animal models, endothelial-specific knockout and transgenic approaches now provide unique surrogate systems[28–30] that complement observations in in vitro and in vivo human systems and will expand our concepts of endothelial function and dysfunction.

The following sections outline specific aspects of endothelial cell function and pathobiology. Each topic is the subject of detailed discussions in vascular biology monographs and, because of space limitations, cannot be comprehensively discussed here. Therefore, the references include substantive reviews as well as illustrative archival reports.

ENDOTHELIAL RECEPTORS, INTRACELLULAR TRANSDUCTION CASCADES, AND ACTIVATION RESPONSES

Human endothelial cells display multiple surface receptors that transmit outside-in signals to intracellular transduction cascades, which then alter their functions and phenotypic characteristics. Certain endothelial adhesion molecules can also transmit outside-in signals. The diversity of endothelial signaling systems is evidence of the complexity of this cell type and its ability to mediate both physiologic responses and vascular alterations in critical illness and other pathologic conditions.

G protein–coupled pathways are major transduction mechanisms linked to surface *heptahelical receptors* and are ubiquitous in human cell signaling paradigms.[31] Human endothelial cells display heptahelical receptors (also called seven-membrane-spanning G protein–coupled receptors or serpentine receptors) that recognize thrombin, histamine, bradykinin, sphingosine-1-phosphate, and other hemostatic and inflammatory agonists. These surface receptors are differentially coupled to intracellular adapter proteins and enzymes that trigger phospholipase activation, calcium (Ca^{++}) transients, mitogen-activated protein kinase pathways, cyclic nucleotide turnover, and other intermediary events.[32] The resulting phenotypic changes and effector responses include surface translocation (degranulation) of intracellular storage granules (Weibel-Palade bodies), with von Willebrand factor release and P-selectin display on the cell surface; rapid platelet-activating factor (PAF) and prostacyclin (PGI_2) synthesis; cytoskeletal reorganization; altered permeability; altered gene expression; and others.

Human and murine endothelial cells constitutively express surface protease-activated receptors (PARs), a family of heptahelical G protein–coupled receptors that recognize thrombin and certain other proteases and transmit outside-in signals via a unique mechanism involving proteolytic release of a cryptic internal ligand.[29,33] Human endothelial cells also display PAR2, which recognizes mast cell tryptase, trypsin, and coagulation factors VIIa and Xa and is up-regulated by cytokines and lipopolysaccharide (LPS).[33–35] There is also evidence that PAR3 and PAR4 are expressed by endothelial cells and that expression of PAR4, like PAR2, is altered by inflammatory agonists.[36,37] Signaling via PARs provides regulated mechanisms by which endothelial cells respond to local thrombin generation and mast cell degranulation—two acute

responses that are central in tissue injury and physiologic host defense.[33,38,39] Thrombin-induced signaling and PAR activation are also pathways for dysregulated vascular responses in syndromes of critical illness.[32,38,40] Stimulation of endothelial cell monolayers with thrombin provided the first evidence of endothelial cell–dependent adhesion of neutrophils (Figs. 31–2 and 31–3; also see later).[38,41,42] These and a variety of other studies demonstrated that thrombin induces endothelial cell activation by receptor-mediated mechanisms.[32,33,38,41] In more recent experiments, thrombin activation of cultured macro- and microvascular endothelial cells influenced intercellular gap formation by a mechanism dependent on intracellular Ca^{++} transients and a subtype of adenyl cyclase.[43] It was also reported that PAR1 and PAR2 differentially trigger exocytosis and alter permeability in human endothelial cell monolayers by influencing Rho–guanosine triphosphatase activity.[44] These and a variety of other observations document multiple thrombin-activated functional changes in endothelial cells that are relevant to endothelial behavior in critical illness. There is also evidence for thrombin signaling in vascular development and angiogenesis.[45] These findings, together with earlier observations of degranulation, endothelial cell–dependent leukocyte adhesion, and mitogenesis,[33,34,38,40,41] illustrate the diverse changes in endothelial cell phenotype triggered by PAR-mediated pathways.

Human endothelial cells display histamine H1 and bradykinin B2 receptors that mediate vasoactive and inflammatory signaling when engaged.[46,47] Histamine induces many of the same activation responses as thrombin does, including degranulation, translocation of P-selectin to the surface, rapid synthesis of PGI_2 and PAF, and endothelial cell–dependent neutrophil adhesion, and it can trigger the release of preformed chemokines in models of chronic inflammation.[46,48,49] Many of these events, which were first identified in cultured human endothelial cell systems, have been documented in vivo.[50] By using H1 and PAR2 receptors, endothelial cells respond to histamine and tryptase, which are key inflammatory agonists that are released locally in response to tissue trauma.[39] When PAR1 or other PARs that recognize thrombin are engaged in parallel with histamine stimulation, as frequently occurs in tissue injury in vivo, complex intracellular signaling responses result.[47,51,52] Although receptors for thrombin and histamine trigger many parallel and convergent signaling cascades and functional activities in endothelial cells, they also have distinct effects on gene regulation pathways in this cell type (D. Schmid, L. W. Kraiss, unpublished observations).

Receptor tyrosine kinases are expressed by human and murine endothelial cells and play critical roles in the maintenance of vascular structure and the adaptation to tissue injury and remodeling. In addition, they have developmental roles in vasculogenesis and angiogenesis. Endothelial-specific receptor tyrosine kinases include three members of the vascular endothelial growth factor receptor family and two structurally related receptors with immunoglobulin and epidermal growth factor homology domains, Tie1 and Tie2, which recognize members of the angiopoietin family and other ligands.[1,20] In development, these receptors and their ligands act in concert with other angiogenic and guidance receptors and pathways.[1,13,16,17] In addition to mediating angiogenesis and lymphangiogenesis, engagement of vascular endothelial growth factor and Tie receptors on endothelial cells transmits signals to endothelial nitric oxide synthase (eNOS), vasopermeability regulatory mechanisms, and inflammatory

FIGURE 31–3. Human endothelial cells are activated by outside-in signals delivered by diverse inflammatory and thrombotic agonists and mechanisms. *A,* Human endothelial cells activated by thrombin via heptahelical protease-activated receptors (PARs) acutely translocate P-selectin from storage granules, rapidly synthesize platelet-activating factor (PAF), and use these factors as a juxtacrine adhesion and signaling system for neutrophils. (See text for details; also references 38, 40, and 41.) Human endothelial cells activated by thrombin via PAR pathways undergo additional changes that mediate inflammatory and thrombotic responses. *B,* Cytokines released by macrophages and other extravascular cells are recognized by receptors on endothelial cells, inducing multiple activation responses. Bacterial products, including lipopolysaccharide (LPS) and other endotoxins, bind to specific members of the Toll-like receptor family expressed by endothelial cells, also triggering activation events. *C,* Interleukin (IL)-1ß synthesized and released by stimulated platelets activates human endothelial cells, resulting in endothelial cell–dependent neutrophil adhesion. This illustrates a mechanism by which intravascular blood cells can initiate or amplify endothelial cell activation. ENA, epithelial neutrophil-activating peptide; OSM, oncostatin M; PMN, polymorphonuclear leukocyte; TNF, tumor necrosis factor. *(See also Color Figure 31–1.)* (*C,* Modified from Zimmerman GA, Albertine KH, McIntyre TM: Pathogenesis of sepsis and septic-induced injury. In Matthay MA [ed]: Lung Biology in Health and Disease, vol 179. New York, Marcel Dekker, 2003, pp 245-287.)

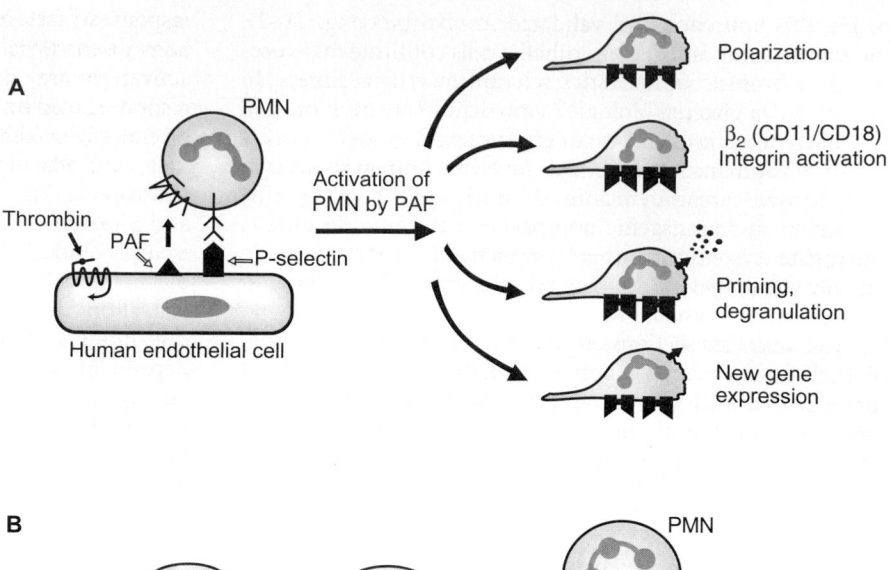

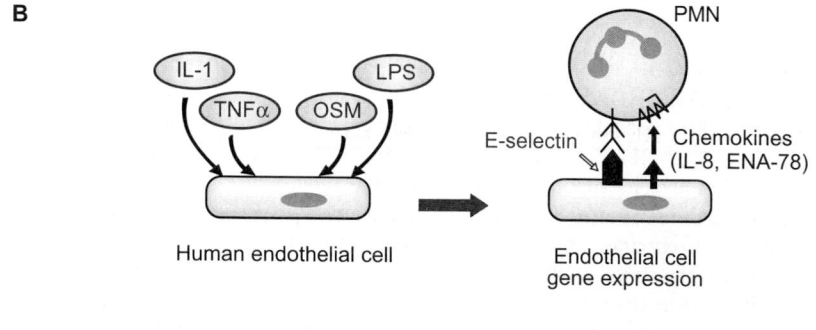

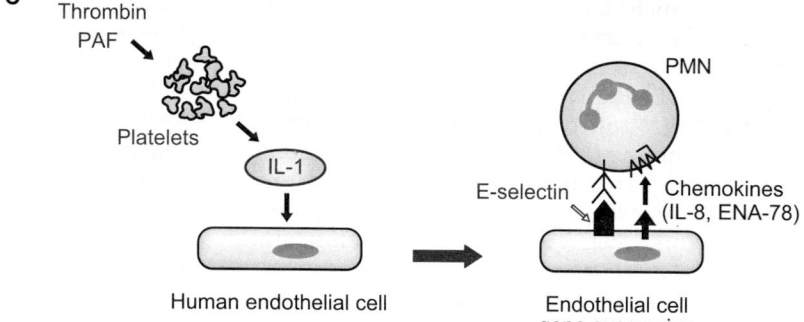

pathways.[20–22] Recent observations indicate that Tie2 expression is regulated by hypoxia and inflammatory cytokines in human endothelial cells.[15]

Cytokine receptors are regulators of endothelial cell phenotype and function in innate immune and acute inflammatory responses, hemostasis and thrombosis, acquired immunity and chronic inflammation, vascular remodeling, and other functions relevant to human disease (see Fig. 31–3). Endothelial cells constitutively express receptors for more than a dozen cytokines[53–55] and use them to transmit outside-in signals to mitogen-activated protein kinase cascades, ceramide turnover mechanisms, nuclear signaling pathways that involve nuclear factor kappa-B (NF-κB) and JAK/STAT activation, and other intracellular transduction circuits.[53–57] Endothelial responses to newly identified cytokines, such as high mobility group protein B1 (HMGB1), continue to be reported.[58,59] The most extensively characterized cytokine signaling events in human endothelial cells involve activation by tumor necrosis factor (TNF), interleukin-1alpha (IL-1α), and interleukin-1beta (IL-1β), which induce expression of genes that code for E-selectin and other adhesion molecules, interleukin-8 (IL-8), epithelial neutrophil-activating peptide-78 (ENA-78) and other chemokines, the inducible form of cyclooxygenase (COX-2), endothelial degranulating factors for neutrophils, and a variety of other inflammatory and thrombotic proteins and peptides.[53-56,60–64] The IL-1 signaling system, including recently identified IL-1 receptor-associated proteins, is conserved across evolutionary lines, is central to the responses of a variety of cells to infection and injury, and has both homologous features and molecular interfaces with Toll receptor signaling (see later).[65] Endothelial cells express the type I but not the type II ("decoy") IL-1 receptor—an unusual feature, because most cells display both.[53]

IL-1, TNF, IL-6, and other cytokines recognized by endothelial cell receptors are produced by macrophages and other extravascular cells in response to thrombotic or inflammatory stimuli (see Fig. 31–3).[53,54] In addition, some cytokines—for example, IL-1 and IL-6—are *endogenously* produced by inflamed endothelial cells themselves, providing the basis for autocrine signaling loops.[53,54] Alternatively, cytokine agonists for endothelial cells can be produced by intravascular platelets or leukocytes, providing mechanisms that link thrombosis and inflammation and amplify inflammatory responses.[5,54,66,67] For example, human platelets synthesize IL-1β from constitutive messenger RNA (mRNA) transcripts in response to thrombin, PAF, and other agonists and release it in sufficient concentrations to trigger endothelial cell–dependent polymorphonuclear leukocyte (PMN) adhesion in in vitro assays (see Fig. 31–3).[67] Signal-dependent translation of IL-1β is one of many inflammatory activities of stimulated platelets[68] and provides a novel mechanism that explains earlier observations that platelets release IL-1 activity.[54,67] Activated platelets can also signal endothelium locally by releasing or displaying ligands recognized by heptahelical, growth factor, and other receptor classes, triggering key functional changes.[18,19,66] In a second example of endothelial signaling by blood cells, human neutrophils were recently found to release the alpha subunit of the IL-6 receptor (IL-6Rα), which can then associate with homodimers of glycoprotein 130 that are basally present on human endothelial cells.[54,69,70] In contrast, IL-6Rα is not constitutively expressed by endothelium.[54,69,70] The association of soluble IL-6Rα with transmembrane glycoprotein 130 homodimers constitutes a competent heterotrimeric receptor that confers to endothelial cells a new responsiveness to endogenously or exogenously synthesized IL-6, inducing the expression of inflammatory and thrombotic genes.[69,70] One consequence of new gene expression is a "switch" from neutrophil to mononuclear leukocyte accumulation, an event that is required for the resolution of acute inflammatory responses but is also a central mechanism in the transition to chronic inflammation if it is pathologically dysregulated.[71,72] This novel mechanism of retrograde or *trans*-signaling of endothelial cells by PMNs[69,70,72] may mediate a variety of pathologic activities of IL-6, together with other complex regulatory features of the system.[73]

Endothelial cells respond to local or systemic microbial invasion and to activation by LPS and other bacterial products with complex changes in inflammatory phenotype and, in some cases, by triggering apoptotic programs.[74–78] Recent characterization of the *Toll-like family of transmembrane receptors* (TLRs), which are conserved, innate immune sensors, provides insights into endothelial and leukocyte signaling by LPS and other endotoxins and microbial products.[74,79,80] The TLR system is composed of specific receptors that recognize pathogen-associated molecular patterns with ligand-dependent specificity.[79] TLRs act together with cell surface–associated modifying proteins (CD14, MD-2) and use a cytoplasmic transduction system linked to gene regulatory pathways and other effector mechanisms.[79,80] As previously noted, conserved IL-1 receptor-associated kinases are central intermediaries.[65,80,81] Human macrovascular and microvascular endothelial cells express TLR2 and TLR4 and use them to differentially recognize and respond to LPS and to bacterial endotoxic lipoproteins, including the Braun lipoprotein of *Escherichia coli* and other microbes.[82–85] Expression of TLR2 and TLR4 on cultured endothelial cells and endothelial cell lines can be modulated by LPS, interferon gamma, and reactive oxygen species.[83,85] Experimental studies in murine models demonstrate important differences in leukocyte-endothelial interactions, depending on the specific bacterial product injected, systemic versus local challenge, and the TLR and CD14 phenotype.[86,87]

Previous studies in an in vitro model involving cultured human endothelial cells and whole blood demonstrated an indirect pathway of LPS-induced activation of endothelium that is mediated by monocytes and that dramatically amplifies endothelial sensitivity and response to this microbial product.[88] These and other studies indicate that in clinical sepsis and other vascular responses to pathogens, changes in endothelial phenotype and function likely involve both direct TLR signaling and indirect activation mediated by leukocyte and platelet products.[74]

Nuclear receptors recognize cell-permeant hormones, lipids, and therapeutic drugs.[89] A major nuclear hormone receptor in diverse cell types recognizes endogenous and synthetic glucocorticoids and mediates their regulatory effects on transcriptional programs.[89] The glucocorticoid receptor is present in nuclei of in situ human arterial endothelial cells, and its nuclear localization is influenced by shear stress in cultured bovine endothelial cells,[90] suggesting that nuclear receptor pathways may respond to endothelial activation or injury in a variety of conditions. Estrogen receptors, a second class of nuclear hormone receptors, are present in bovine and human endothelial cells.[91] Human endothelial cells also respond to activators of the peroxisome proliferators–activated receptor family under some conditions.[92]

In syndromes of critical illness, multiple endothelial cell surface and nuclear receptors are likely engaged in parallel and in sequence, generating complex phenotypic changes and functional responses. Sepsis is a sentinel example in which endothelial activation via several receptor pathways may be key to essential vascular and tissue responses,[74,77,78] as illustrated in this section.

ENDOTHELIAL RESPONSES TO HEMODYNAMIC FORCES

In vivo, endothelial cells are continuously subjected to hemodynamic forces. These forces include vascular wall distention induced by cyclic changes in transmural pressure and shear, which is the frictional force applied by blood flow.[93,94] Acute changes in shear induce phenotypic modulation and altered gene expression in cultured endothelial cells (see Fig. 31–2) and cellular remodeling in vessels and vascular grafts; both acute *increases* and *decreases* in shear induce phenotypic responses.[93–95] Alterations induced by shear and other hemodynamic forces are often similar to those triggered by inflammatory agonists.

Abrupt changes in shear induce rapid cytoskeletal remodeling and activation of intracellular signaling pathways in endothelial cells, including modulation of potassium channels, induction of calcium transients, alterations in inositol phosphates and diacylglycerol, generation of reactive oxygen intermediates, activation of mitogen-activated protein kinases, activation of Rho– and Rac–guanosine triphosphatases, and nuclear signaling and altered gene expression.[90,93–101] Functional consequences of shear-induced changes in endothelial cell phenotype include acute generation of nitric oxide (NO) and PGI₂, cytoskeletal and microtubular reorganization, changes in synthesis of inflammatory and thrombotic gene products, and altered DNA synthesis.[93,94,102–104] Endothelial cells also adapt to chronic changes in shear with structural alterations.[93] The mechanosensors that transmit hemodynamic outside-in signals to endothelial cells remain incompletely characterized.[93,105,106]

ENDOTHELIAL JUNCTIONS, PERMEABILITY, AND SELECTIVE BARRIER FUNCTIONS

Highly specialized junctional structures that link adjacent cells in interconnected monolayers of endothelial cells that line vascular channels regulate paracellular permeability and macromolecular transport and influence the transmigration of leukocytes from the intravascular space to the extravascular milieu.[107,108] Endothelial cell–matrix interactions mediated by basolateral integrins also influence permeability,[1,105] providing both cellular attachment and outside-in signals that modify specialized intercellular junctions. Junctional transfer of small molecules between adjacent endothelial cells occurs, potentially resulting in an additional mechanism of intercellular signaling.[109] As many as four types of junctions may mediate interactions between endothelial cells.[107] Adherens junctions and tight junctions are critical in regulating permeability and cell polarity and are modified by inflammatory and thrombotic signals,[107,110] including thrombin, sphingosine-1-phosphate, and other receptor-mediated agonists.[18,19,32,43] Thus, these multimolecular junctional structures and their interacting cytoskeletal elements are likely key sites of dysregulation in increased systemic and pulmonary vascular permeability in syndromes of critical illness.

Endothelial-specific cadherin 5, or vascular endothelial cadherin, is a central component of endothelial cell adherens junctions, contributes to the barrier function of endothelial cell monolayers, and is modified by receptor-mediated signals and leukocyte-endothelial interactions.[107,108,111] Vascular endothelial cadherin may signal through β-catenin, which influences vascular pattern and fragility in murine models,[30] and there is evidence for additional cadherin-catenin interactions.[112] Additional endothelial cell junctional molecules are involved in interactions between endothelial cells.[107] Recent observations indicate that S-ENDO 1–associated antigen (CD146), a transmembrane glycoprotein constitutively expressed by endothelial cells regardless of anatomic site or vessel size, is localized to intercellular boundaries and is coupled to a tyrosine kinase–mediated pathway that triggers intracellular Ca^{++} transients.[110,113] Cytoplasmic Ca^{++} levels regulate the activity of adenyl cyclase isoenzymes and interendothelial gap formation in cultured endothelial cell models,[43] suggesting that CD146 may have important influences on permeability via these mechanisms. These examples illustrate the concept that endothelial cell junctional molecules perform both adhesive and signaling functions and can be dysregulated in vascular injury.

The intricate mechanisms by which endothelial cell junctions are altered in leukocyte transmigration (Fig. 31–4) remain incompletely characterized and involve both adherens and tight junctions.[103,111] Vascular endothelial cadherin distribution is rapidly and dynamically modified during transmigration of PMNs and monocytes, providing a potential mechanism for interendothelial gap opening, leukocyte passage, and rapid gap closure.[111] Additional endothelial cell junctional molecules play specific roles in targeting leukocyte subclasses to intercellular sites of transmigration and stepwise emigration (see Fig. 31–4).[5] Platelet leukocyte adhesion molecule-1 is the best known of these.[5,114] Junctional adhesion molecule-1, also an immuglobulin superfamily protein, was recently reported to be a binding partner for $\alpha_L\beta_2$ integrin on PMNs, monocytes, and T lymphocytes that is expressed predominantly at tight junctions of resting endothelial and epithelial cells.[115] CD99, a recently characterized O-glycosylated protein, is localized to endothelial cell junctions and mediates the transmigration of monocytes across cultured endothelial cell monolayers.[116] These findings indicate that endothelial cell junctional complexes and specific proteins localized to endothelial cell–endothelial cell contact domains regulate selective barrier functions involving both macromolecules and emigrating leukocytes, key functions that can be disrupted in

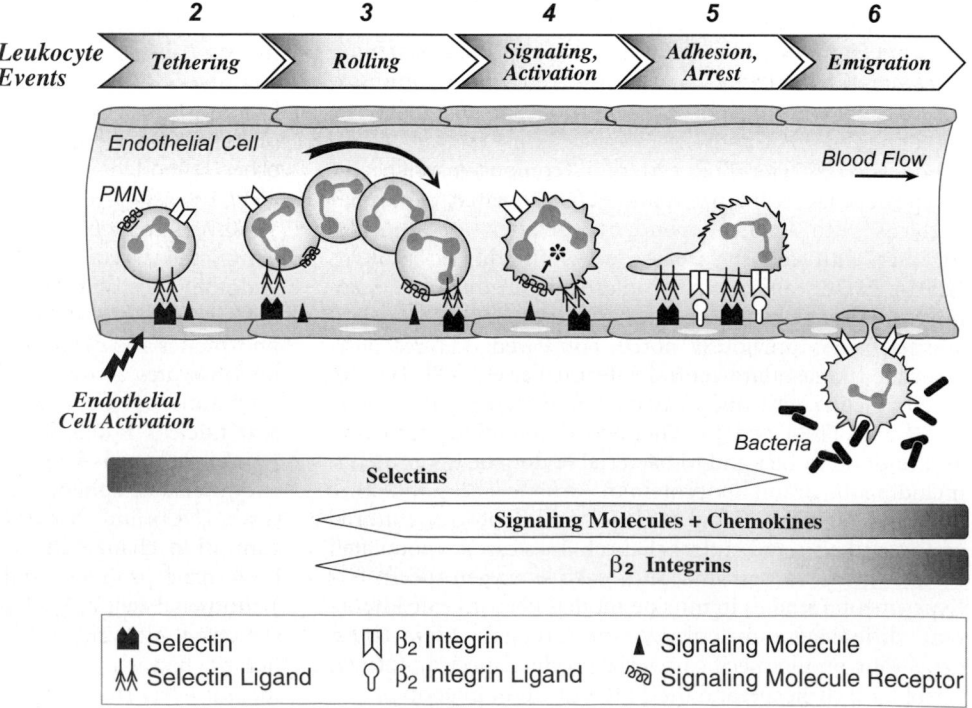

FIGURE 31–4. Activation of endothelial cells and multistep interactions control leukocyte targeting and function in inflammation. This multistep paradigm details key events in neutrophil (PMN) adhesion, localized activation, and transmigration in a postcapillary venule under conditions of flow. Each step (see text for details) is critical for PMN adhesion and emigration in dysregulated vascular injury. Initial activation of endothelial cells is key in this sequence of events. (From McIntyre TM, Prescott SM, Weyrich AS, Zimmerman GA: Cell-cell interactions: Leukocyte-endothelial interactions. Curr Opin Hematol 2003;10:150-158.)

inflammatory vascular injury involving dysregulated neutrophil accumulation and activation.[117–119]

ENDOTHELIAL CONTRIBUTIONS TO VASOREGULATION

Blood flow is partially regulated by the generation of vasoactive signaling factors by endothelium that act locally to modify vascular tone, caliber, responses to other stimuli, and hemodynamic variables.[1] NO and PGI$_2$ are key endothelial-derived vasodilators that also modify platelet responses and in some cases alter leukocyte-endothelial interactions.[1] Thus, they have both direct and indirect vasoactive features. In addition, endothelial cells synthesize vasoconstrictor substances, including endothelins and a number of other vasoactive factors, in response to signals delivered by surface receptors and hemodynamic forces.[1,120]

Endothelial cells generate NO in an enzymatic process catalyzed by nitric oxide synthase (NOS) in which L-arginine is converted to L-citrulline in the presence of oxygen and nicotinamide adenine dinucleotide phosphate (reduced form).[1] NO, a cell-permeant gas with a half-life of approximately 6 seconds, mediates intercellular interactions in a paracrine fashion and binds to the heme prosthetic group of guanyl cyclase in vascular smooth muscle cells, maintaining basal vascular tone and inducing vasorelaxation.[1] A parallel mechanism inhibits platelet activation responses and also leukocyte activities and smooth muscle migration and proliferation in some studies.[6,120] NO production is catalyzed by a family of NOS, including constitutive and inducible isoforms.[120] One isoform, eNOS (or NOS3), is basally active in endothelial cells, but its activity can be further increased by receptor-mediated agonists.[1] The effect of cytokines on eNOS activity and expression has species-specific characteristics, and these features may vary in individual vascular beds within a species.[1,6,54] Expression and activity of eNOS are increased in response to shear, in part secondary to transcriptional activation and a cis-acting shear response sequence in the promoter region of the gene,[1] and there is evidence for regulation by hypoxia.[121] eNOS activity can also be increased by Akt-dependent phosphorylation.[21,122] Additional features of the regulation of eNOS and inducible NOS isoforms have recently been reviewed.[120]

Activation of NOS in endothelial and other cell types influences hemodynamic events in sepsis and other syndromes of critical illness, although precise measures to modify these enzymes are not yet in general clinical practice.[123] Myeloperoxidase, a key PMN enzyme that is released by degranulation,[64] consumed NO and impaired endothelial-dependent vasodilatation in a rodent model of endotoxemia,[124] pointing to mechanisms that may contribute to pathologic hemodynamic responses in inflammatory vascular injury.

PGI$_2$, the first endothelial cell–derived relaxing factor to be identified, is also a major inhibitor of platelet activation and aggregation.[1,6,120] PGI$_2$ is synthesized by the microsomal enzyme cyclooxygenase (prostaglandin H synthase) acting on substrate arachidonic acid released from membrane phospholipids in response to cellular stimulation. The COX-1 isoform is constitutively expressed in endothelial cells, and PGI$_2$ generated by this enzyme is important in physiologic vasoregulation and as a local antithrombotic signal.[6,125,126] The inducible isoform, COX-2, is expressed in endothelial cells in response to stimulation with IL-1, TNF, LPS, and other inflammatory and thrombotic agonists and contributes PGI$_2$ and prostaglandin E$_2$ to the local inflammatory milieu.[6,60,61,125,126] The factors that regulate COX-2 expression in stimulated and inflamed endothelial cells are complex and continue to be dissected.[6,120,127,128]

ENDOTHELIAL REGULATION OF HEMOSTASIS

In the basal state, endothelial cells present an antithrombotic and anticoagulant surface, a critical phenotypic feature required for blood flow that acts in concert with mechanical forces and soluble factors.[1,6] In response to injury, the endothelium becomes prothrombotic and antifibrinolytic, providing a mechanism that facilitates hemostasis and wound repair and generates molecular links that couple endothelial activation to local myeloid leukocyte accumulation and other defensive inflammatory responses.[1,5,6,68,74] Endothelial procoagulant mechanisms that interface with inflammatory networks are part of an evolutionarily conserved innate defense system.[68,129,130] When dysregulated, however, this remarkable switch in endothelial phenotype initiates or amplifies pathologic thrombosis, a central mechanism of disease in critical illness.[5,74,77,129,130]

Anticoagulant and antithrombotic features of resting endothelial cells include pericellular heparin sulfate, glycosaminoglycans, and dermatan sulfate, which facilitate the activity of antithrombin III and heparin cofactor II, the expression of thrombomodulin and tissue factor pathway inhibitor (see later), and the release of PGI$_2$ and NO (see earlier). Each of these is dysregulated in specific syndromes of vascular injury and disease.[1,7,130]

The expression and activity of tissue factor are critical in hemostasis and in pathologic thrombosis. Tissue factor is a primary initiator of the coagulation cascade, a process that has been extensively reviewed.[130–134] Tissue factor potently accelerates factor VIIa–dependent activation of factors IX and X.[1] Thrombin generated by sequential protease-dependent steps in the tissue factor pathway subsequently cleaves fibrinogen to fibrin, the central component of the platelet-fibrin mesh that constitutes clots.[131–134] When endothelial cells that express tissue factor are exposed to plasma, thrombin is generated and fibrin is deposited on the endothelial cell surface.[1] Expression of tissue factor activity on endothelial cells is induced by a variety of pathophysiologically relevant stimuli in vitro, but factors that trigger its regional expression by endothelium in vivo remain in question.[1,6] Tissue factor is also synthesized by human monocytes and macrophages in response to LPS and other stimuli and is deposited on cell surfaces and shed into the blood in microparticles released by monocytes or neutrophils.[74,131,135] Tissue factor pathway inhibitor, a 42-kDa serine protease inhibitor with three tandem kunitz domains, is associated with endothelial granules and surfaces and is found to a lesser extent in association with platelets and in soluble form.[6,129,130,136] Tissue factor pathway inhibitor has anticoagulant effects by direct inhibition of factor Xa and by an indirect mechanism involving factor Xa–dependent inhibition of the tissue factor–factor VIIa complex.[130,137] In vivo, tissue factor pathway inhibitor expression is restricted to microvessels.[6] LPS and cytokines have only a slight effect on tissue factor pathway inhibitor expression by cultured endothelial cells in vitro, but during infusion of LPS in rodents, its expression on pulmonary capillaries is reduced by a mechanism yet to be defined.[6]

Thrombomodulin, an integral membrane protein, is basally expressed by macro- and microvascular endothelial cells in vitro and in vivo and has profound effects on the regulation of hemostasis.[133,134] When thrombin is locally generated, it is recognized by thrombomodulin and binds to it, inhibiting the procoagulant activities of thrombin while facilitating its ability to cleave circulating protein C to activated protein C.[6,74,133,134] Activated protein C interacts with a cofactor that is synthesized by endothelial and other cell types—protein S—and this complex then inactivates factors Va and VIIa, inhibiting further thrombin generation and providing an endogenous "brake" on the procoagulant cascade that is proportional to the magnitude of the hemostatic stimulus under regulated physiologic conditions.[1,133,134] Thus, endothelial cells express key molecules that regulate coagulation. There is also evidence that activated protein C inhibits proinflammatory as well as prothrombotic cascades.[74,130,134,138] Activation of protein C by the thrombin-thrombomodulin complex is further enhanced by its high-affinity binding to an additional endothelial cell plasma membrane factor, the endothelial cell protein C receptor.[133,134,139,140] Thrombomodulin has additional regulatory effects, including enhancement of inactivation of thrombin by antithrombin III and protein C inhibitor and activation of thrombin-activatable fibrinolysis inhibitor (procarboxypeptidase B).[6]

Factors that regulate endothelial expression of thrombomodulin and endothelial cell protein C receptor continue to be defined and have regional features that may reflect endothelial cell specialization.[6,133,134] Thrombomodulin is differentially expressed by endothelial cells in specific vascular beds and is absent from brain endothelium.[6,133] It is reduced on the plasma membranes of endothelial cells in response to LPS challenge in in vitro models and in histologic analysis of biopsies from patients with meningococcemia.[74] Endothelial cell protein C receptor expression is highly specific for macrovascular endothelial cells, with the exception of hepatic sinusoids, a property influenced in part by sequence information in the promoter region of its gene.[6,140,141] LPS infusion in rodents is accompanied by an increase in endothelial cell protein C receptor mRNA but not protein,[140] indicating post-transcriptional regulation. The increased plasma levels of soluble thrombomodulin and endothelial cell protein C receptor that are reported in sepsis and other conditions appear to result from shedding of the surface proteins.[6,74]

Endothelial cells also have a major role in the regulation of fibrinolysis and synthesize a complex group of plasminogen activators, plasminogen activator inhibitors, and receptors for fibrinolytic factors.[1,6] There is evidence for differential expression of tissue plasminogen activator and other fibrinolytic regulatory molecules in specific vascular beds and for dysregulation of this system in response to pathologic stimuli.[1,6]

The balance between anticoagulant and prothrombotic features of endothelium is altered in many, and perhaps all, syndromes of critical illness. Sepsis is an intensely studied example.[74,77,129,130,137,140] Dysregulation of endothelial control of hemostasis contributed extensively to the preclinical and clinical rationales for recent trials of recombinant activated protein C and tissue factor pathway inhibitor in patients with septic syndromes.[129,130,137]

ENDOTHELIAL INTERACTIONS WITH LEUKOCYTES AND OTHER BLOOD CELLS

Endothelial cells were previously thought to be passive in interactions with leukocytes, but observations in the last 2 decades have clearly demonstrated *endothelial cell–dependent mechanisms of leukocyte adhesion and signaling* (see Figs. 31–2 to 31–4).[4,5,38,40,41] This facet of endothelial biology has been extensively reviewed.[1,4–6,53,54,64,72,142–144] Leukocyte-endothelial interactions are early and critical events in defense against infection and in wound surveillance and repair, but dysregulated adhesion and signaling of leukocytes is a central pathogenetic mechanism in vascular injury and a variety of human inflammatory diseases.[5,38,39] Similarly, dysregulated interactions between the vessel wall and circulating platelets or erythrocytes contribute to specific vascular pathologies.[1,5]

A multistep paradigm involving the tethering of leukocytes to stimulated endothelial cells, followed by rolling, localized signaling, consequent tight adhesion, arrest of activated leukocytes, and subsequent emigration between endothelial junctions (see previous section), characterizes the targeting of myeloid cells and lymphocytes in inflammation (see Fig. 31–4).[5] Fundamental aspects of this sequence of events were initially worked out in human cell models and from clinical observations of patients with leukocyte adhesion deficiency syndromes, and they have been validated and refined using animal models and further clinical observations.[5,143]

The central paradigm can be illustrated using interactions of inflamed endothelial cells and neutrophils (PMNs), although it is important to emphasize that there are cell- and context-specific variations, depending on the leukocyte subtype being considered and whether the situation involves acute or chronic inflammation or injury.[5] An overview of the multistep paradigm[5,143,144] is illustrated in Figure 31–4 and summarized here. Under basal conditions, endothelial cells and circulating PMNs are not adhesive to each other. Stimulation of endothelial cells with inflammatory agonists induces their activation and differential expression of specific selectins on their plasma membranes, which then mediates the capture, tethering, and rolling of quiescent unactivated PMNs. In the first step, endothelial cell activation by thrombin, histamine, and certain other rapidly acting agonists induces translocation of P-selectin, which is constitutively present in Weibel-Palade storage granules, to the endothelial cell plasma membrane. In contrast, LPS, IL-1, TNF, and additional cytokines signal transcriptionally regulated synthesis of a different selectin, E-selectin, which is not basally present in most endothelial cells. After synthesis, E-selectin is also displayed on the endothelial cell surface and, like P-selectin, captures and tethers PMNs (step 2). In this step, selectin ligands on the PMN are engaged by P-selectin or E-selectin displayed on the inflamed endothelial cell surface. P-selectin glycoprotein ligand-1 is the dominant selectin ligand on human and murine PMNs and has been shown in in vitro and in vivo experiments to mediate both tethering and rolling (step 3). L-selectin on the PMN surface also mediates tethering and rolling by interacting with ligands on inflamed endothelial cells and acts as an adhesion molecule for cell-cell interactions with other PMNs that accumulate locally. After tethering and rolling, endothelial cell–dependent signaling of PMNs triggers their activation (step 4). When endothelial cells are stimulated by thrombin or histamine, PAF is rapidly synthesized and is translocated

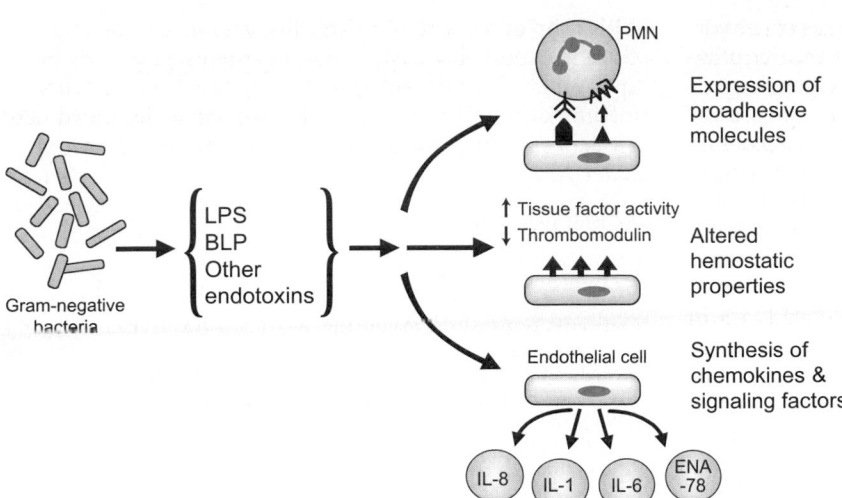

FIGURE 31–5. Endothelial cell activation and functional responses contribute to inflammatory vascular injury and thrombosis in septic syndromes. Lipopolysaccharide (LPS) and other endotoxins, such as Braun lipoprotein (BLP), activate human endothelial cells via Toll-like receptors and induce multiple phenotypic changes in experimental sepsis and clinical septic syndromes. ENA, epithelial neutrophil-activating peptide; IL, interleukin; PMN, polymorphonuclear leukocyte. (From Zimmerman GA, Albertine KH, McIntyre TM: Pathogenesis of sepsis and septic-induced injury. In Matthay MA [ed]: Lung Biology in Health and Disease, vol 179. New York, Marcel Dekker, 2003, pp 245-287.)

to the cell surface, where it acts as a signaling molecule that triggers PMN activation of PMNs tethered by P-selectin. Alternatively, in endothelial cells stimulated with LPS, IL-1, or TNF, IL-8 and ENA-78 are synthesized under transcriptional control and mediate the activation of PMNs in concert with tethering by E-selectin. Activation of PMNs by signaling molecules (e.g., PAF, IL-8, ENA-78) displayed in a juxtacrine fashion at the endothelial cell surface or when locally released induces stimulation-dependent changes in affinity and avidity of β_2 integrins on the leukocyte surface. Activated β_2 integrins then recognize intercellular adhesion molecule-1 and other ligands on the endothelial cell plasma membrane (step 5). Engagement of P-selectin glycoprotein ligand-1 enhances the activation of β_2 integrins on human PMNs signaled by PAF or IL-8. Binding of β_2 integrins to endothelial cells counterligands and then mediates tight adhesion and arrest of the PMNs (step 5), events that are essential to prevent the dislodgment of leukocytes by shear forces and for their subsequent emigration across endothelial cell junctions (step 6).

Activation of endothelial cells resulting in the display of selectins and the synthesis of PAF, IL-8, and other signaling molecules for neutrophils is critical for the sequence of events outlined in Figure 31–4 in host defense.[4,5,38,143] Similarly, constitutive and regulated expression of endothelial ligands for neutrophil β_2 integrins and expression of junctional proteins that participate in PMN emigration are essential determinants for orderly neutrophil targeting in physiologic inflammation.[5,111,115,116,143,144] Activation of endothelial cells is also central to targeting and spatially localized signaling of other classes of leukocytes in host defense.[5] In syndromes of inflammatory vascular injury, one or more of these critical steps can become disordered or unregulated, leading to pathologic accumulation and activation of leukocytes and consequent vessel and tissue damage (see Figs. 31–1 and 31–5).[5] Similarly, dysregulated accumulation and activation of platelets resulting from disruption at one or more molecular control points are central mechanisms in acute and subacute vascular injury.[5,144] These pathologic mechanisms are features of sepsis,[74] ischemia-reperfusion injury,[145,146] and other syndromes of vascular damage.

GENE EXPRESSION BY ACTIVATED ENDOTHELIAL CELLS: MECHANISTIC DIVERSITY

When appropriately stimulated, endothelial cells express or alter the expression of multiple genes. As with other responses outlined in this chapter, this was not predicted by earlier interpretations of endothelial cells as passive lining cells.[1] Patterns of transcript expression by endothelial cells may be markers of particular phenotypes in disease, such as neoplasia.[147]

Mechanisms of gene regulation in endothelial cells illustrate considerable diversity. Depending on the stimulus and time after activation, phenotypes of activated endothelial cells reflect transcriptional induction of new gene programs,[4,148–151] including genes controlled by transcription factors of the NF-κB and AP-1 families.[53,152–156] *Transcriptional regulation* is critical for new expression of E-selectin and certain other adhesion molecules by activated endothelial cells[153] and for altered expression of COX-2, chemokines, degranulating factors, and a variety of other endothelial cell gene products that are synthesized in response to injury or infection and in repair.[4,53,54,60–64,76,84,150]

In addition to transcriptional regulation, there is emerging evidence that endothelial cells have diverse *post-transcriptional mechanisms*, although these are largely uncharacterized. Individual examples that together indicate that post-transcriptional control is a key fact of gene expression in endothelial cells include shear-induced stabilization of granulocyte-macrophage colony-stimulating factor and COX-2 mRNAs,[97,128] differential expression of endothelial cell protein C receptor mRNA and protein in response to LPS,[140] and attenuation of the amount of E-selectin mRNA present in the actively translated polyribosome-associated fraction of transcripts when shear is applied to TNF-stimulated monolayers.[157] Post-transcriptional regulation provides important biologic advantages in gene regulation, including precise modulation of levels of specific proteins when acting in concert with transcriptional control.[158,159] Thus, cells with the complex functions subserved by endothelial cells would be expected to use these mechanisms.

Translational control, including signal-dependent translation of constitutive mRNAs,[5,68] is an important facet of post-transcriptional regulation.[160] Rapid synthesis of the corresponding protein without a requirement for transcription or nuclear export of the message is one advantage of signal-dependent translation of specific transcripts that are present in the basal state.[5,68] Translational control mechanisms in stimulated endothelial cells and their phenotypic consequences are now being characterized.[102,157,161–165] Human endothelial cells have p70S6 kinase and other key components of the mammalian target of rapamycin specialized translation control pathway[163,164] and use this mechanism to regulate expression of the NF-κB family member Bcl-3 in endothelial cell monolayers subjected to shear.[164] Rapamycin, an immunosuppressant and antiangiogenic agent, inhibits Bcl-3 translation under these conditions.[164] Tumstatin, an endothelial cell–specific inhibitor of protein synthesis, inhibits mammalian target of rapamycin and angiogenesis by an integrin signaling mechanism.[165] In addition, preliminary analysis of the "translational state" of multiple mRNA transcripts in activated endothelial cells indicates differential effects by specific inflammatory and thrombotic agonists and that multiple translational control mechanisms may be used.[166] Our preliminary studies also indicate that human endothelial cells have a portfolio of RNA binding proteins and other key regulatory components in post-transcriptional regulatory and translational control pathways (M. Martinez, A. S. Weyrich, G. A. Zimmerman, unpublished studies).

ENDOTHELIAL RESPONSES IN DISEASE

As outlined throughout this chapter, changes in endothelial phenotype and function are central mechanisms in acute and subacute responses to disease, including syndromes of critical illness that are considered in detail elsewhere in this text. Endothelial cell responses in sepsis (see Figs. 31–1 and 31–5) are particularly profound and illustrative examples. Endothelial alterations in septic syndromes have recently been reviewed.[74,77,78,130,137,140] Dysregulated endothelial mechanisms are also central to systemic manifestations in ARDS, to multiple organ failure, and to localized and systemic ischemia-reperfusion syndromes, including traumatic and hemorrhagic shock and resuscitation.[10,145,146,167,168] There is evidence for quantitative and qualitative differences in endothelial responses in trauma and hemorrhagic shock compared with sepsis.[169–174] Patterns of endothelial phenotype that result from the superimposition of sepsis, trauma,

ARDS, or other acute critical illnesses on the substrate of chronic endothelial dysfunction in atherosclerosis, diabetes, and other diseases of vascular dysfunction or chronic inflammation[1,175] remain to be precisely described and mechanistically characterized.

ACKNOWLEDGMENTS

We thank our colleagues and collaborators at the University of Utah and elsewhere for contributions to work cited. Mary Madsen and Michele Czerwinski prepared the manuscript, and Diana Lim drafted the figures. This contribution was supported in part by National Heart, Lung, and Blood Institute (NHLBI) awards HLO4151 (LWK) and HL44525 (GAZ), an NHLBI SCOR in ARDS (SMP, GAZ), a Lifeline Foundation Faculty Award (LWK), and the University of Utah Fellowship-to-Faculty transition program (LWK), which is funded by a Biomedical Support Grant to Medical Schools from the Howard Hughes Medical Institute.

ANNOTATED REFERENCES

Aird WC: Endothelial cell dynamics and complexity theory. Crit Care Med 2002;30:S180-S185.
Aspects of endothelial activity in hemostasis, coagulation, and thrombosis are discussed, and the complexity of endothelial responses and phenotypes is underscored. These issues are outlined in the context of infectious syndromes and sepsis.

Cines DB, Pollak ES, Buck CA, et al: Endothelial cells in physiology and in the pathophysiology of vascular disorders. Blood 1998;91:3527-3561.
Physiologic and pathophysiologic characteristics of endothelial cells are reviewed in detail and discussed in the context of human vascular diseases. This review is extensively referenced.

Mantovani A, Bussolina F, Introna M: Cytokine regulation of endothelial cell function: From molecular level to the bedside. Immunol Today 1997;18:231-240.
As discussed in this article, endothelial cells both respond to and synthesize cytokines, a feature that generates multiple activation events and molecular responses in inflammation, thrombosis, and disease.

McIntyre TM, Prescott SM, Weyrich AS, Zimmerman GA: Cell-cell interactions: Leukocyte-endothelial interactions. Curr Opin Hematol 2003;10:150-158.
This review summarizes recent observations on endothelial-leukocyte interactions and endothelial activation in response to inflammatory and pathologic signals.

Zimmerman GA, Albertine KH, Carveth HJ, et al: Endothelial activation in ARDS. Chest 1999;116:18S-24S.
The concept of endothelial cell activation and its relationship to endothelial injury are discussed, particularly with respect to acute lung injury syndromes. Endothelial gene expression and rapid responses that do not require changes in gene expression are outlined.

Chapter 32

LUNG EPITHELIAL FUNCTION

Michael A. Matthay

KEY POINTS

1. The **pulmonary epithelium is morphologically diverse** from the airway epithelium to the alveolar epithelium to subserve the specific functions required at each level of the lung epithelium.

2. The **alveolar epithelium provides a tight barrier** to the passive movement of solutes and protein to keep the airspaces dry so that they can carry out the main function of the lung: to excrete carbon dioxide and absorb oxygen.

3. The **alveolar epithelium contains sodium and chloride ion channels** that are responsible for the vectorial transport of alveolar fluid from the airspaces to the lung interstitium.

4. The **active ion transporting capacity of the alveolar epithelium** is responsible for the resolution of alveolar edema.

5. The **process of alveolar fluid reabsorption** can be up-regulated by cyclic adenosine monophosphate agonists.

This chapter first considers the morphologic characteristics of the proximal, distal, and alveolar epithelium, with particular reference to the pathophysiology of acute critical illnesses. The next section considers the abnormalities of the airway epithelium in acute and chronic obstructive lung diseases and how these may contribute to acute respiratory failure in critically ill patients. The final section focuses on the role of the alveolar epithelium in lung fluid balance in patients with pulmonary edema.

MORPHOLOGY OF THE PULMONARY EPITHELIUM

There are major differences in the morphologic features of the pulmonary epithelium from the proximal airway epithelium to the alveolar epithelium. Some of these differences and their relationship to the regional function of the lung epithelium are considered here.

AIRWAY EPITHELIUM

Overall, the conducting airways form the connection between the outside world and the terminal respiratory units where gas exchange occurs. There are three major groups of intrapulmonary airways: bronchi, membranous bronchioles and respiratory bronchioles, and gas exchange ducts. Bronchi, by definition, have cartilage in their walls. Respiratory bronchi serve a dual function—as conducting airways and as part of the alveolar volume for gas exchange.[1] Overall, the conducting airways occupy the first 16 generations of airways, but ultimately they end blindly in the alveoli. Gas exchange occurs primarily in the branches that make up the last seven generations, including the respiratory bronchioles, alveolar ducts, alveolar sacs, and alveoli (Fig. 32–1). The distal airway epithelium is composed of terminal respiratory bronchial units with polarized epithelial cells that have the capacity to transport sodium and chloride, including ciliated Clara cells and nonciliated cuboidal cells.

In reference to the pathophysiology of acute and chronic obstructive airway disease, it should be emphasized that most airway resistance resides in the upper airways in the bronchi. There are glands in the submucosa in the bronchi that secrete water, electrolytes, and mucins into the lumen. Studies of the regulation of secretion in vivo and by explant cultural systems in vitro have demonstrated that release can be modulated by neurotransmitters, including cholinergic, adrenergic, and inflammatory mediators. Goblet cells, which are mucin-secreting epithelial cells, are present at most airway levels (Fig. 32–2). Several other cells are associated with the airways, including basal cells, lymphocytes, smooth muscle cells, and mast cells. Lymphocytes are frequently found between airway epithelial cells. There are also circular bands of smooth muscle around the airway epithelium as far peripherally as the respiratory bronchioles. The tone in the smooth muscles is altered by the autonomic nervous system and by local mediators released from a variety of cells. Abnormalities of several of these structural and cellular components contribute to the pathophysiology of acute and chronic obstructive lung disease.[1]

ALVEOLAR EPITHELIUM

The alveoli are composed of a thin alveolar epithelium (0.1 to 0.2 µm) that covers 99% of the airspace surface area in the lung and contains thin, squamous type I cells and cuboidal type II cells (Fig. 32–3). Alveolar type I cells cover 95% of the alveolar surface.[1,2] The close apposition between the alveolar epithelium and the vascular endothelium facilitates the efficient exchange of gases, but it also forms a tight barrier to the movement of liquids and proteins from the interstitial and vascular spaces, thus assisting in maintaining relatively dry alveoli.

At the alveolar level, the tight junctions that bind the alveolar epithelium are critical for maintaining apical and

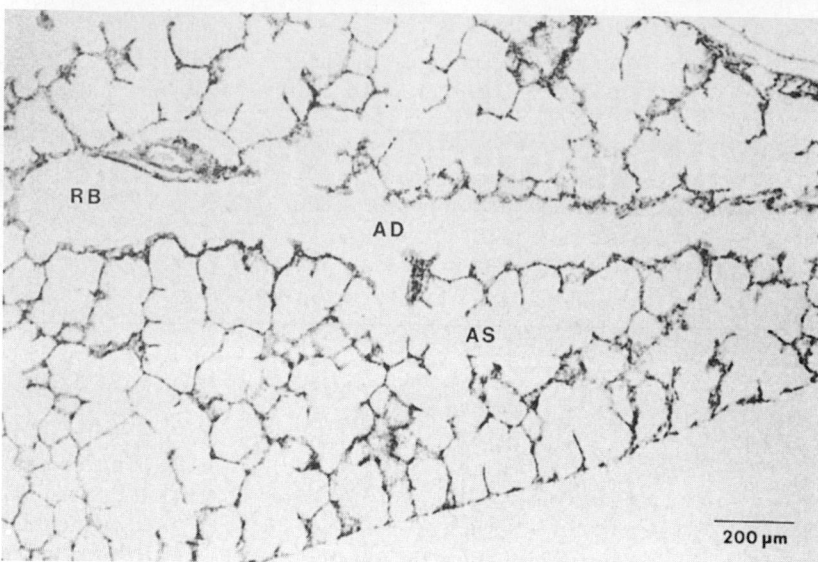

FIGURE 32–1. Longitudinal section of a gas exchange duct showing that its diameter remains relatively constant along the respiratory bronchiole (RB) and alveolar duct (AD). Alveolar sacs (AS) communicate with the gas exchange duct. (Human surgical specimen, 10-μm-thick paraffin section, light microscopy.) (From Albertine KH, Williams MC, Hyde DM: Anatomy of the lungs. In Murray JF, Nadel JA [eds]: Textbook of Respiratory Medicine, vol 1. Philadelphia, WB Saunders, 2000, pp 3-33.)

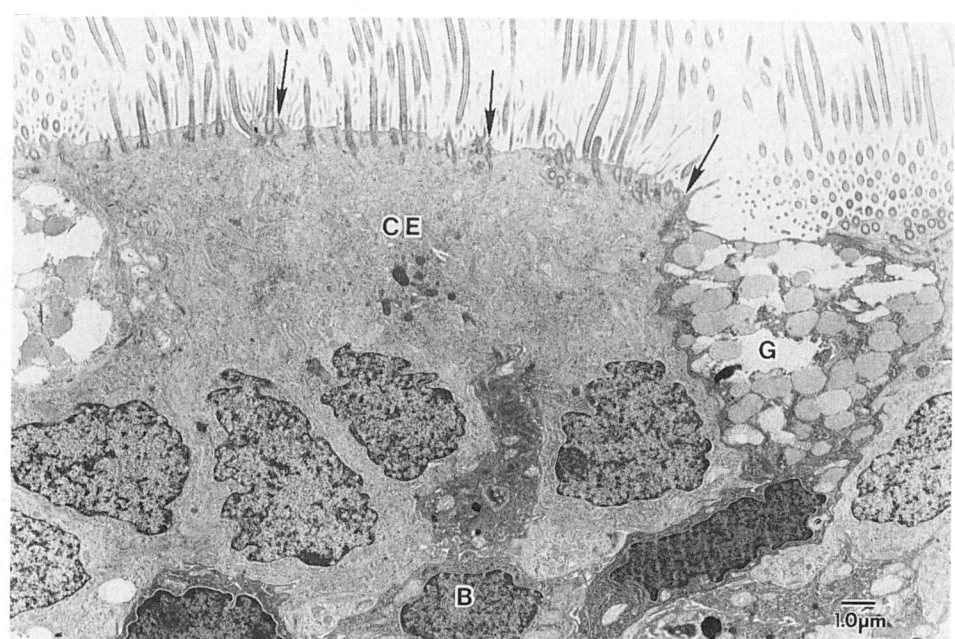

FIGURE 32–2. Cells comprising the bronchial epithelium are ciliated epithelial cells (CE), goblet cells (G), and basal cells (B). Goblet cells have abundant mucous granules in the cytoplasm, and their apical surface is devoid of cilia. Basal cells, as their name indicates, are located along the abluminal portion of the lining epithelium, adjacent to the basal lamina. The arrows at the apical surface of the airway cells indicate the location of junctional complexes between contiguous epithelial cells. (Human lung surgical specimen, transmission electron microscopy.) (From Albertine KH, Williams MC, Hyde DM: Anatomy of the lungs. In Murray JF, Nadel JA [eds]: Textbook of Respiratory Medicine, vol 1. Philadelphia, WB Saunders, 2000, pp 3-33.)

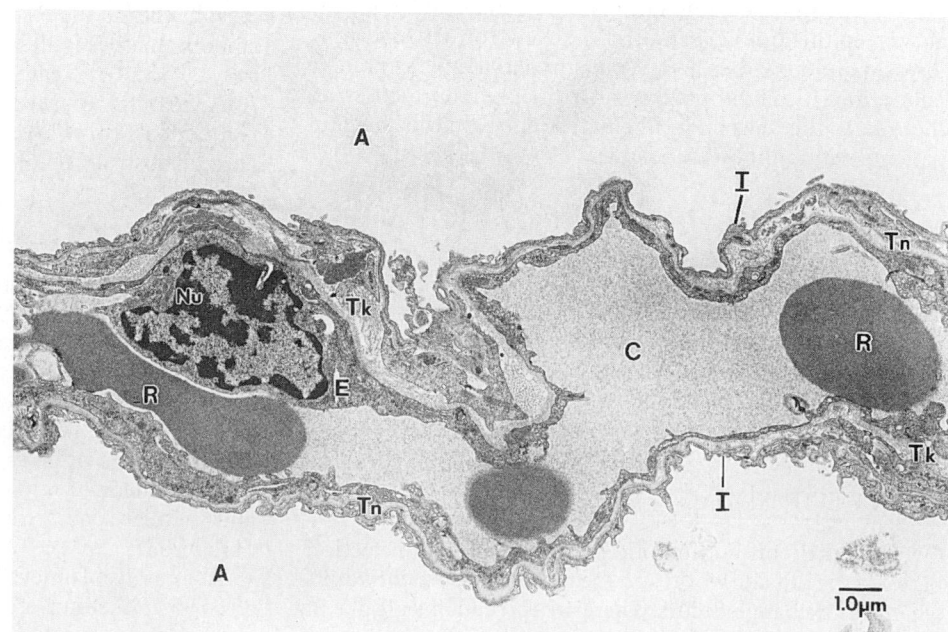

FIGURE 32–3. The thick (Tk) and thin (Tn) sides of an alveolar capillary (C) change as the capillary courses between alveoli (A). The basal laminae of the capillary endothelium and alveolar epithelium fuse in the thin regions. The nucleus (Nu) of an endothelial cell (E) is visible above a red blood cell (R). I, type I pneumonocyte. (Human lung surgical specimen, transmission electron microscopy.) (From Albertine KH, Williams MC, Hyde DM: Anatomy of the lungs. In Murray JF, Nadel JA [eds]: Textbook of Respiratory Medicine, vol 1. Philadelphia, WB Saunders, 2000, pp 3-33.)

basolateral polarity. Ion transporters and other membrane proteins are asymmetrically distributed on opposing cell surfaces, conferring vectorial transport properties to the alveolar epithelium. Based on a variety of physiologic studies, the distal alveolar epithelium is much tighter than the capillary endothelium, with an effective pore radius of 0.5 to 0.9 nm, versus 6.5 to 7.5 nm.[2]

The most extensively studied cell in the distal pulmonary epithelium is the alveolar type II cell (Fig. 32–4A), partly because it can be readily isolated from the lung and studied in vitro.[2-4] The alveolar type II cell is responsible for the secretion of surfactant, as well as for the vectorial transport of sodium and chloride from the apical to the basolateral surface. When the lung is injured, type II cells proliferate to provide a new alveolar epithelial barrier (see Fig. 32–4B). After the repair process is complete, the alveolar epithelium returns to its more normal appearance (see Fig. 32–4C). The active vectorial transport of ions by alveolar epithelial type II cells provides a major driving force for the removal of fluid from the alveolar space. Sodium uptake occurs on the apical surface, partly through amiloride-sensitive and amiloride-insensitive channels. Subsequently, Na^+, K^+-ATPase pumps sodium actively from the basolateral surface into the lung interstitium.[4] The epithelial sodium channel (ENaC), cloned in 1994, participates in sodium movement across the membrane. There is new evidence that cystic fibrosis transmembrane conductance regulator (CFTR), the product of the cystic fibrosis gene, plays an important role in cyclic adenosine monophosphate (cAMP) up-regulated fluid transport across alveolar type II cells and the alveolar epithelium in vivo.[5] The role of the alveolar type I cell and vectorial fluid transport in the lung is less certain, although some investigators recently found that type I cells express sodium channels.[6,7] Type I cells also express aquaporin-5 on the apical surface, although vectorial fluid transport does not seem to depend on the function of this water channel.[3]

AIRWAY EPITHELIUM IN ACUTE AND CHRONIC LUNG DISEASE

The contribution of abnormalities in the proximal and distal airway epithelium to several acute and chronic lung diseases has been explored in depth in recent years. This section focuses on abnormalities of pulmonary epithelium that occur in asthma, chronic obstructive pulmonary disease (COPD), and cystic fibrosis.

ASTHMA

Asthma is a disease of the airways characterized by airway narrowing with spontaneous and pharmacologic reversibility.[1] In patients who die of acute asthma, it is recognized that the airways are edematous and the blood vessels congested, and there are usually cellular infiltrates, including neutrophils and eosinophils. Mucous plugs frequently fill the peripheral airways, and there is desquamation of epithelial cells. In patients with asthma, there is evidence of abnormalities in airway cell growth and differentiation that are similar to those of chronic inflammatory diseases such as chronic bronchitis and cystic fibrosis. These abnormalities include metaplasia of the lining epithelium from ciliated cells to squamous and goblet cells. The basement membrane is often thickened. Anatomic studies of surviving patients with asthma also demonstrate some inflammatory changes,

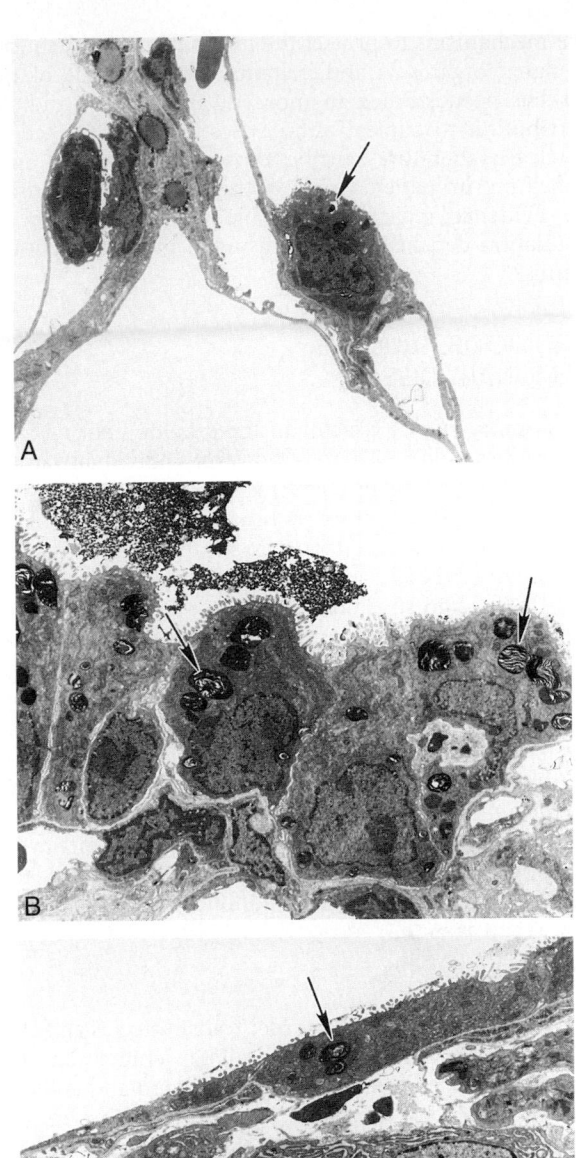

FIGURE 32–4. Ultrastructural appearance of normal rat lungs and rat lungs after the intratracheal instillation of bleomycin. *A*, Control lung (saline instilled). *B*, Ten days after instillation of bleomycin. *C*, Sixty days after instillation of bleomycin. Compared with the appearance of normal alveolar epithelial type II cells *(A, arrow)*, bleomycin-exposed alveolar type II cells *(B, arrow)* have more microvilli and larger lamellar bodies; these type II cells are hyperplastic and hypertrophied, apparently as a response to the bleomycin injury. Type II cell proliferation is the first stage of repair after injury has caused the death of type I cells, the thin cells that line most of the alveolar surface (see *A*). *C* shows recovery toward a more normal alveolar epithelial type II cell, which is flatter. (From Folkesson HG, et al: Upregulation of alveolar epithelial fluid transport after subacute lung injury in rats from bleomycin. Am J Physiol Lung Cell Mol Physiol 1998;275:L478-L490.)

including epithelial cell desquamation, squamous cell transformation, and neutrophil infiltration, as well as an increase in goblet cells.[1] It has generally been assumed that the airway epithelium exists as an interface between the body and the external environment; therefore, the airway epithelium must have mechanisms to protect the internal environment from damaging organisms and irritants. The response of these cells has been studied in more detail recently, and their contribution to clinical asthma is still being worked out, but clearly there are specific abnormalities in the airway epithelium in patients with asthma. There is considerable evidence regarding the role of inflammation and coagulation-dependent mechanisms in the pathogenesis of asthma.[8,9]

CHRONIC OBSTRUCTIVE PULMONARY DISEASE

The primary etiologic factor in the development of COPD is cigarette smoking. There is, however, individual variation in susceptibility. The mechanisms by which cigarette smoke causes emphysema, chronic bronchitis, and COPD are incompletely understood. In chronic bronchitis, there are inflammatory changes in airway epithelium. Ciliated epithelial cells undergo squamous metaplasia, and there is goblet cell proliferation, along with an increase in the volume of smooth muscle and glands. In emphysema, there is a loss of alveoli, resulting in what is commonly known as panlobular emphysema. Loss of alveoli and distal airspaces is a characteristic feature of emphysema resulting in ventilation and perfusion mismatch.[1] Recent evidence indicates that progression of COPD is associated with the accumulation of inflammatory mucous exudates in the lumen of small airways and infiltration of the airway walls with innate and adaptive immune cells that form lymphoid follicles.[10]

CYSTIC FIBROSIS

Cystic fibrosis is a genetic disorder transmitted as an autosomal recessive trait. In brief, the airway epithelium shows progressive evidence of inflammation, gland and goblet cell hypertrophy, and obstruction by secretions. The relationship between the genetic defect in cystic fibrosis and the actual clinical disease is not well understood. The abnormality in cystic fibrosis involves a failure to correctly encode CFTR, the integral protein of epithelial cells. This protein is a chloride channel that must have several other important effects, because abnormalities in transport do not explain all the abnormalities in patients with cystic fibrosis. CFTR is expressed in airway epithelium, although recent work indicates that it is also expressed highly in alveolar epithelium and has an important role in vectorial fluid transport (see next section). The mechanism by which pulmonary epithelium and airways are damaged in cystic fibrosis has been the subject of intense study. Abnormalities in ion transport, the airway surface liquid, and various innate immune responses to infection have all been implicated.[11]

ALVEOLAR EPITHELIUM

This section considers the role of the alveolar epithelial barrier in preventing alveolar flooding, as well as the role of the alveolar epithelium in resolving alveolar edema. On balance, considerable progress has been made in the last 2 decades in understanding the role of the alveolar epithelium in regulating lung fluid balance under normal and pathologic conditions.

FORMATION OF ALVEOLAR EDEMA

As described earlier, the alveolar epithelial barrier is a typical tight epithelium that resists the passive movement of macromolecules and even small solutes. This tight barrier facilitates the primary function of the alveolar epithelium—mainly, to maintain dry airspaces that can facilitate gas exchange. The epithelial barrier is also responsible for the secretion of surface-active material by alveolar epithelial type II cells.

Under normal conditions, the tight epithelial barrier prevents alveolar flooding, even in the presence of mild or moderate interstitial pulmonary edema. Several studies have demonstrated that the interstitial space of the lung can accommodate up to 500 mL of edema fluid before alveolar flooding occurs.[1] Therefore, patients may develop hydrostatic or increased permeability edema with interstitial pulmonary edema without flooding of the airspaces. From a radiographic perspective, this can be appreciated with radiographic signs of interstitial pulmonary edema and Kerley's B lines. In the presence of interstitial edema in the lung, gas exchange is minimally impaired. Once alveolar flooding occurs, pulmonary edema is associated with progressive arterial hypoxemia. The mechanisms of alveolar flooding are related primarily to a progressive rise in interstitial pressure that results in a breakdown of the epithelial barrier. The exact site of airspace flooding may be proximal to the alveolus under conditions of hydrostatic edema. In patients with acute lung injury, there may be injury to alveolar epithelial cells that facilitates the translocation of interstitial edema fluid into the distal airspaces of the lung. The active ion transport properties of the alveolar epithelium—specifically, the ability to transport fluid from the apical to the basal surface of distal lung epithelium—also helps prevent or minimize alveolar flooding. Once alveolar flooding does occur, active vectorial ion transport mechanisms are responsible for the removal of edema fluid from the distal airspaces of the lung (see next section).

RESOLUTION OF ALVEOLAR EDEMA

The distal airway and alveolar epithelium have ion transporters with the capacity to actively transport sodium and chloride, resulting in a mini-osmotic gradient that reabsorbs the water fraction of the edema fluid (Fig. 32–5). The first in vivo evidence that active ion transport in the mature lung accounted for the removal of alveolar edema fluid was obtained in studies of anesthetized, ventilated sheep.[12] In those studies, the critical discovery was that isosmolar fluid clearance of salt and water occurred in the face of a rising concentration of protein in the distal airspaces of the lung. The initial protein concentration of the instilled protein solution was the same as that of the circulating plasma. After 4 hours, the concentration of the protein increased from 6.5 to 8.4 g/100 mL, while the plasma protein concentration was unchanged. In longer-term studies in anesthetized, spontaneously breathing sheep, alveolar protein concentrations increased to even higher levels. After 12 and 24 hours, the alveolar protein concentration increased to 10.2 and 12.9 g/100 mL, respectively.[13] These data provided evidence that active ion transport must be responsible for the fluid clearance in the mature lung, especially in the face of a rising alveolar protein osmotic pressure. Additional studies in the intact lung supported the hypothesis that removal of alveolar

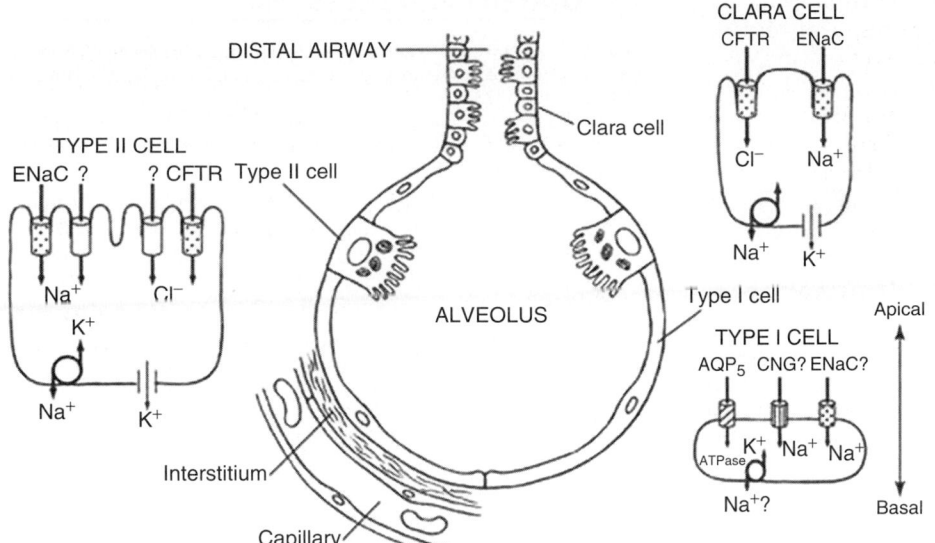

FIGURE 32–5. Schematic diagram of the distal pulmonary epithelium that is relevant for salt and water transport. AQP, aquaporin; CFTR, cystic fibrosis transmembrane conductance regulator; ENaC, epithelial sodium channel. (From Matthay MA: Lung epithelial fluid transport and the resolution of pulmonary edema. Physiol Rev 2002;82:569-600.)

fluid requires active transport processes. For example, elimination of ventilation to one lung did not alter the rate of fluid clearance in sheep, thus ruling out changes in transpulmonary airway pressure as a major determinant of fluid clearance, at least in the uninjured lung. Further, if active ion transport were responsible for fluid clearance, then fluid clearance should be temperature dependent. Studies in an in situ perfused goat lung preparation showed that the rate of fluid clearance progressively declined as temperature was lowered from 37° C to 18° C.[3] Additional evidence for active ion transport was obtained in intact animals with the use of amiloride, an inhibitor of sodium uptake by the apical membrane of alveolar epithelium and distal airway epithelium. Amiloride inhibited 40% to 70% of basal fluid clearance in most species, including the human lung. Studies were also done that used ouabain to inhibit Na+, K+-ATPase. The results showed that ouabain inhibited 90% of fluid clearance in isolated lung preparations.[2]

Interestingly, an early discovery from intact adult animal studies, as well as from earlier studies of fetal sheep, demonstrated that the rate of alveolar fluid clearance could be up-regulated by cAMP agonists.[3] Some species do not increase their fluid clearance with cAMP agonist therapy, but the majority of species double the rate of alveolar fluid clearance with beta-adrenergics, including the human lung.[2,3]

Several catecholamine-dependent mechanisms have the capacity to up-regulate alveolar fluid transport.[3] Both exogenous and endogenous catecholamine release can substantially up-regulate fluid clearance. For example, in the presence of hypovolemic or septic shock, the rapid rise in plasma catecholamines is sufficient to enhance alveolar epithelial fluid transport, thus preventing or limiting the formation of alveolar edema. In addition, several studies have demonstrated that aerosolized adrenergic therapy can increase the rate of fluid clearance in hydrostatic or increased permeability edema in a variety of experimental preparations.[2,3] From a clinical perspective, it is possible that administration of an aerosolized beta2 agonist might be effective in up-regulating alveolar fluid transport and enhancing the resolution of pulmonary edema in patients. Clinical trials are needed to test this possibility.

There are several catecholamine-independent factors that can regulate fluid clearance as well. For example, hormonal factors, such as glucocorticoids, can up-regulate transport by transcriptional mechanisms, and thyroid hormone may work by a post-translational mechanism. Some growth factors can work by either transcriptional or direct membrane effects, or by enhancing the number of alveolar epithelial type II cells. There is also evidence that a proinflammatory cytokine, tumor necrosis factor, can up-regulate sodium uptake and fluid transport by novel mechanisms.[3]

Recent research has identified mechanisms that can impair vectorial alveolar fluid transport under pathologic conditions. For example, the halogenated anesthetics can decrease fluid clearance by inhibition of the amiloride-sensitive component. The effect is rapidly reversible after exposure to the inhaled anesthetic; the effect can also be overcome through the administration of a beta2 agonist.[2] Lidocaine has been recognized as another anesthetic that can decrease alveolar fluid clearance, whether instilled directly into the lung or given intravenously in clinically relevant concentrations.[3] There is a growing body of literature demonstrating that alveolar hypoxia decreases alveolar fluid clearance by approximately 50% in the normal lung. The effect of hypoxia appears to be primarily at the membrane level, resulting in a decreased availability of ion transporters at both the apical and the basolateral membranes. Interestingly, beta2 agonists can also overcome the depressant effects of hypoxia.[14]

Overall, several new insights have been obtained regarding the role of alveolar epithelium in regulating lung fluid balance. The resolution of alveolar edema depends on an intact alveolar epithelium that can transport sodium and chloride, creating an osmotic gradient for the reabsorption of water from the distal airspaces of the lung. In clinical studies, the resolution of alveolar edema is rapid in patients with resolving hydrostatic edema. In the presence of acute lung injury, there is considerable heterogeneity in the capacity of the alveolar epithelium to reabsorb pulmonary edema fluid. Patients with impaired alveolar fluid transport have a worse clinical course and a higher mortality, suggesting that alveolar epithelial injury is a major determinant of outcome

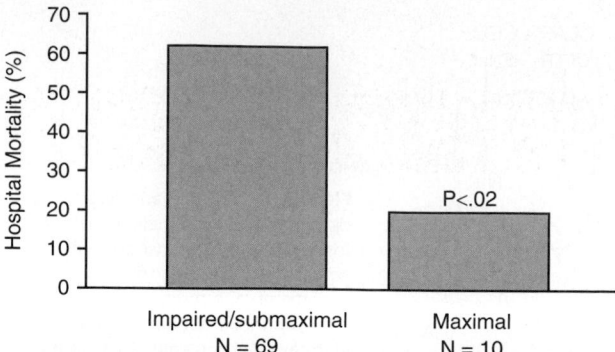

FIGURE 32–6. Hospital mortality (*y*-axis) plotted against two groups of patients with acute lung injury or acute respiratory distress syndrome—those with maximal fluid clearance (>14%/h), and those with impaired or submaximal fluid clearance (<14%/h). The columns represent present hospital mortality in each group (N = number of patients). Hospital mortality of patients with maximal fluid clearance was significantly less (*P* < 0.02). (From Ware LB, Matthay MA: Alveolar fluid clearance is impaired in the majority of patients with acute lung injury and the acute respiratory distress syndrome. Am J Respir Crit Care Med 2001;163:1376-1383.)

in patients with acute lung injury (Fig. 32–6).[15] Conceivably, the rate of alveolar fluid transport could be up-regulated in patients with acute lung injury by the administration of aerosolized beta$_2$-adrenergic agonists, but this hypothesis requires a clinical trial to test its efficacy.

ANNOTATED REFERENCES

Boucher RC, Knowles MR, Yanaskas JR: Cystic fibrosis. In Murray JF, Nadel JA (eds): Textbook of Respiratory Medicine, vol 1. Philadelphia, WB Saunders, 2000, pp 1291-1323.
> *Excellent chapter that summarizes what is known about cystic fibrosis clinically and the link between the genetic defects in cystic fibrosis and the clinical phenotypes.*

Fang X, Fukuda N, Barbry P, et al: Novel role for CFTR in fluid absorption from the distal airspaces of the lung. J Gen Physiol 2002;119:199-207.
> *This article presents evidence that CFTR plays a critical role in the alveolar epithelium in terms of up-regulatory cAMP-dependent alveolar fluid clearance.*

Johnson M, Widdicombe J, Allen L, et al: Alveolar epithelial type I cells contain transport proteins and transport sodium, supporting an active role for type I cells in regulation of lung liquid homeostasis. Proc Natl Acad Sci U S A 2002;99:1966-1971.
> *This study, as well as reference 6, provides evidence that alveolar epithelial type I cells may participate in the resolution of alveolar edema because they possess the necessary ion transporters.*

Matthay MA: Lung epithelial fluid transport and the resolution of pulmonary edema. Physiol Rev 2002;82:569-600.
> *This review summarizes 2 decades of research that has established the basic and clinical importance of active ion transport as the primary mechanism for the resolution of alveolar edema in the mature lung.*

Ware LB, Matthay MA: Alveolar fluid clearance is impaired in the majority of patients with acute lung injury and the acute respiratory distress syndrome. Am J Respir Crit Care Med 2001;163:1376-1383.
> *This clinical study found that alveolar fluid clearance is impaired in most patients with acute lung injury and that impaired fluid clearance is associated with a higher mortality.*

Chapter 33

LYMPHOCYTE FUNCTION AFTER INJURY

John A. Mannick • James A. Lederer

KEY POINTS

1. The initial immune response to serious injury is one of inflammation.

2. Multiple organ dysfunction syndrome is clearly recognized as a major cause of mortality after serious injury and is associated with perturbations of both innate and adaptive immunity.

3. The pivotal cell in the adaptive immune system is the T-helper lymphocyte, which through cytokine production and cognate interaction sets in motion both antigen-specific cell-mediated immune responses and antibody formation.

4. Serious injury in humans and in experimental animals results in impairment of immune functions mediated by T cells. Impairments include delayed hypersensitivity responses, rejection of skin allografts, and tumor immunity.

5. A variety of agents that increase T-helper-1 function have been shown to be effective in reducing mortality from a septic challenge in various animal models of injury. These agents include IFN-γ, GM-CSF, anti-IL-6 monoclonal antibody, anti-IL-10 antibody, IL-18, and IL-12. Treatments other than cytokines and their inhibitory antibodies have also proven effective, including prolactin, melatonin, cyclooxygenase II inhibitors, and hypertonic saline.

6. Proestrus female animals are less affected immunologically than males after serious injury and a testosterone receptor antagonist can improve T-helper-1 function and resistance to sepsis in injured male animals.

Most investigators now agree that the initial immune response to serious injury is one of inflammation, usually termed the *systemic inflammatory response syndrome* (SIRS).[1-3] In patients or experimental animals with major traumatic or thermal injury, SIRS is evident shortly after initial resuscitation; and in a significant minority of patients (25% to 35%) SIRS persists without respite and may lead directly to the multiple organ dysfunction syndrome (MODS), particularly if infection supervenes.[4] MODS is clearly recognized as a major cause of mortality after serious injury and infection.[1-3] Because cells of the innate immune system are the chief source of inflammatory mediators after injury, and cellular and molecular components of innate immunity are major effectors in the early defense against invading microorganisms, it is not surprising that the majority of research on the immune consequences of injury has focused on the innate immune system.[5-9]

The T and B lymphocytes of the adaptive immune system by contrast ordinarily respond only when activated by antigen-presenting cells of the innate immune system; and although T-cell receptors and antibodies produced by B cells demonstrate remarkable diversity and exquisite precision for individual antigenic epitopes, several days of clonal expansion after initial activation are ordinarily required for a significant adaptive response to become evident.[3] Thus, at first glance, the adaptive immune system appears to be ill suited to play a role in host defense early after injury, although later participation might be anticipated. And, in fact, in the majority of injured patients the SIRS response remits after several days without progression to early MODS[4] but the patient is often left with an increased susceptibility to nosocomial infection, which is associated with production of anti-inflammatory mediators by the adaptive immune system, referred to as the compensatory anti-inflammatory response syndrome (CARS).[4,10,11] Invasive infection occurring during this period of adaptive immune depression may again induce systemic inflammation, which in turn may lead to late MODS.[4]

DECREASED T-LYMPHOCYTE FUNCTION AFTER INJURY—HISTORICAL EVIDENCE

The pivotal cell in the adaptive immune system is the T-helper lymphocyte, which through cytokine production and cognate interaction sets in motion both antigen-specific cell-mediated immune responses and antibody formation.[3] For more than 3 decades it has been evident that serious injury in humans and in experimental animals resulted in impairment of immune functions mediated by T cells. These include delayed hypersensitivity responses, rejection of skin allografts, and tumor immunity.[12-16] Moreover, a number of reports indicated that the proliferative response to T-cell mitogens by peripheral blood mononuclear cells (PBMCs) was significantly impaired in patients after traumatic or thermal injury.[17,18] These early reports were followed by studies demonstrating that diminished T-cell mitogen–induced proliferation by PBMCs was associated with decreased production of interleukin (IL)-2 and interferon-gamma (IFN-γ) by the same cells.[19,20] Decreased production of these cytokines appeared to be associated with subsequent infectious complications although a causal relationship was not established.[19,20]

T-LYMPHOCYTE PHENOTYPE CHANGES IN INJURED PATIENTS

Following the report by Mosmann and coworkers[21] that mature T-helper cells expressed at least two phenotypes, it became clear that serious injury induced decreased production of cytokines typical of T-helper-1 (Th1) cells (e.g., IL-2 and IFN-γ). It was not certain whether this represented a generalized depression of T-helper cell function or whether the synthesis of T-helper-2 (Th2) cytokines was maintained or even increased after injury. Several groups including our own studied this question in injured patients and found that the production of the Th2 cytokine IL-4 was increased several days after injury, as revealed by mitogen stimulation of circulating T cells and by direct measurement of plasma cytokines.[22,23] Our laboratory and Sherry and colleagues[24,25] reported similar findings for IL-10, although there is at least one clinical study reporting no increase in IL-10 production after injury.[26] From these studies it appeared likely that Th1 cytokine production was inhibited after injury whereas Th2 cytokine production was maintained or perhaps increased. The vigorous IL-4 production noted several days after injury offered an explanation for the previously puzzling observation that injured patients frequently had elevated levels of immunoglobulin E (IgE) in their plasma,[27] because IL-4 is the principal inducer of this immunoglobulin isotype.

ANIMAL MODELS RELEVANT TO INJURED PATIENTS

To study these and other aspects of the immune response to injury more systematically, many investigators have turned to animal models of injury and sepsis. The clinical relevance of this animal research obviously depends on how closely the animal model(s) resemble populations of injured patients. Models that appear to mimic clinical injury include full-thickness burn models (of 25% to 60% body surface area) in mice and rats, models of hemorrhage and soft tissue trauma, and models of hemorrhage and skeletal trauma in the same species. Appropriate septic challenges used in these models include direct burn wound contamination with pathogenic bacteria, intratracheal administration of pathogenic organisms, and cecal ligation and puncture (CLP), which induces a localized peritonitis with mixed gut flora. These models have allowed a number of groups of investigators to confirm and expand observations made in seriously injured patients. Rodents, especially mice, are also available with multiple genetic modifications, which allow clear-cut answers to questions concerning the importance of specific cell types or mediators in the phenomena observed.

EVIDENCE THAT NORMAL RESISTANCE TO INFECTION REQUIRES A FUNCTIONAL ADAPTIVE IMMUNE SYSTEM

For example, by using the recombinase activating gene (Rag)–deficient mouse (which lacks an adaptive immune system) Hotchkiss and coworkers[28] were able to demonstrate convincingly that adaptive immunity, more specifically adaptively transferred, syngeneic T cells are essential for survival after CLP. In these experiments the T cells were genetically altered to overexpress the antiapoptotic protein Bcl-2, thus ensuring their protracted survival in the Rag hosts.

Similar experiments in our own laboratory have shown that the administration of wild-type splenocytes to the Rag animals will reconstitute T cells and B cells in the spleen and lymph nodes and will restore normal resistance to CLP.[29] Reconstitution of adaptive immune cells also reduces the excessive production of proinflammatory cytokines noted after burn injury in unmodified Rag animals.[29] The cell type responsible for the latter effect appears to be the CD4+ T-helper cell and, more specifically, the CD25+ CD4+ T-helper cell now known to have immunoregulatory properties in a variety of experimental systems.[30]

By using animal models it was also possible, beginning nearly 15 years ago, to confirm the clinical impression that serious injury induces lowered resistance to infection at predictable time points. For example, Moss and associates[31] from our laboratory showed that in a mouse burn model mortality versus sham burn animals after CLP was similar early after injury (15% to 20%) but that there was a nearly 80% mortality at 10 days in the burn mice, which then gradually returned to control (sham burn) levels over the ensuing 10 to 15 days. Similar time dependent susceptibility to infectious challenge has also been noted in animal models of hemorrhage and trauma by Ayala and Chaudry and their coworkers[32] and by Strong and coworkers.[33]

In several animal models the loss of resistance to an infectious challenge after serious injury was coincident with decreased production of T-helper-1 cytokines and increased production of Th2 cytokines by T cells undergoing polyclonal activation in vitro.[31,32,34-38] On the other hand, in some instances, loss of resistance to infection occurred at a time when cells of the innate immune system were shown to respond with greater than normal production of inflammatory mediators on exposure to molecules associated with pathogenic organisms (e.g., endotoxin or peptidoglycan).[33,39,40] Considered together these results suggest that after serious injury, when adaptive immunity manifests a maximal anti-inflammatory response associated with decreased resistance to infection, the innate immune system is capable of supranormal and possibly destructive proinflammatory mediator production when it encounters products of the microorganisms that might be expected to be present in a supervening infection. In other words, sepsis that follows CARS in seriously injured patients may induce an exaggerated and destructive SIRS response; thus, SIRS and CARS may coexist. These findings also may begin to provide a cellular and molecular explanation for the "second hit" phenomenon,[1,4,41] which has been defined by several investigators as an exaggerated inflammatory response to a second stressful event occurring several hours to several days after an initial injury (first hit). The second-hit phenomenon is believed by many clinicians to play a significant role in the induction of MODS in a sizeable number of patients.[1,4,41]

ALTERED T-HELPER CELL PHENOTYPE AFTER INJURY, IN VIVO EFFECTS, AND POSSIBLE MECHANISMS

Thus, animal studies in the aggregate demonstrate that serious injury, both thermal and traumatic, is followed in several days by loss of Th1 function and production of cytokines stimulatory of host defenses (i.e., IL-2 and IFN-γ), whereas there is normal or increased production of Th2 cytokines, which can be inhibitory of innate and adaptive immune responses.

Using the mouse burn model, we[42] also explored the question of whether loss of Th1 cytokine production in vitro by lymphocytes from injured animals was accompanied by a loss of Th1 function in vivo as indicated by production of Th1-dependent antibody isotypes. These studies showed that when mice were immunized with a conventional antigen at the time of injury, Th1-dependent IgG2a production by B cells was markedly inhibited at 10 days while production of the Th2-dependent isotypes IgG1 and IgE was unaffected. At the same time burn but not sham-burn animals demonstrated loss of antigen specific T-cell proliferation and marked diminution in antigen specific IL-2 and IFN-γ production.

To define some of the molecular mechanisms involved in the diminished Th1 cytokine production after injury we first determined that IL-2 and IFN-γ messenger RNA (mRNA) expression in Th cells were diminished after burn as compared with sham-burn injury in the mouse whereas IL-4 mRNA was increased.[43] We further showed that decreased IL-2 mRNA expression was associated with markedly lower expression of the transcription factors activator protein-1 (AP-1) and nuclear factor-kappa B (NF-κB) heterodimer, but not nuclear factor of activated T cells (NFAT), in the nuclei of Th cells from burn versus sham-burn animals.[44] AP-1 and NF-κB are known to be essential for IL-2 gene transcription. Similar, but not identical findings have been reported by Choudhry and colleagues[45] in a rat burn model.

An important question remaining is whether the diminished production of protective Th1 cytokines several days after injury is a compensatory reaction to stimulation of Th cells early after injury or whether it simply represents a response to down-regulatory signals from the innate immune system. Monocytes/macrophages of the innate immune system are known to express lower levels of antigen-presenting major histocompatibility complex class II molecules by several days after injury[46] and to be primed for increased production of potentially inhibitory mediators, including prostaglandin E_2 (PGE$_2$),[6,47-49] transforming growth factor-beta (TGF-β),[50] and perhaps IL-10.[51] At the same time these cells have diminished capacity to produce IL-12, the cytokine ordinarily required for induction of the Th1 phenotype.[49,51]

To shed further light on this issue, we have explored the possibility that T cells early after injury may be activated to make a vigorous Th1-type response. We[52] initially used two strains of T-cell–receptor transgenic mice for this purpose. Seventy-five percent of the Th cells in these animals respond only to a specific peptide antigen, which they would not be expected to encounter at the time of injury. In these animals it was found that the Th cells responded to the cognate antigen in vitro with increased rather than decreased IFN-γ production for as long as 7 days after injury when compared with sham-burn controls. The injection of the relevant antigen in vivo at the time of injury produced death in 100% of the burn animals and in none of the sham animals. These studies suggested that burn injury initially induced a state of increased and potentially harmful Th1 activity in these two transgenic strains.

To confirm these findings in wild-type animals, we turned to a bacterial superantigen, staphylococcal enterotoxin B (SEB), which activates approximately 20% of the Th cell population expressing the Vβ chain of the T-cell receptor to which the superantigen binds.[53] Thus, immediate evidence of T-cell reactivity could be obtained at the time of injury without the necessity for clonal expansion, which is a prerequisite for a detectable response to a conventional antigen. These studies again showed that superantigen administration at the time of burn injury caused death of burn, but not sham-burn, animals in a dose-dependent manner and that mortality could be prevented by anti–IFN-γ antibody and soluble TNF-α receptor (thus confirming the importance of these cytokines in the fatal response) and by blockade of T-cell co-stimulation through the use of cytotoxic lymphocyte–associated protein-4 bound to immunoglobulin (CTLA4-Ig), which binds to co-stimulatory molecules on antigen presenting cells. Abrogation of mortality by CTLA4-Ig further established that death by superantigen administration at the time of injury was, indeed, a T cell–mediated phenomenon.

The two experiments just described strongly suggested that the loss of Th1 function and cytokine production with the dominance of Th2-type cytokine production, noted at about a week after injury in several human and animal studies described earlier, represented a regulatory response to activation of T cells at the time of serious injury.

This proposition could be tested most easily in the T cell–receptor transgenic mouse model. As noted previously, when burn, but not sham-burn, animals were immunized with cognate antigen at the time of injury, 100% mortality ensued. However, we found that the administration of small amounts of the same cognate antigen at the time of injury permitted survival of the majority of the immunized T cell–transgenic animals. Splenic and lymph node T cells harvested from un-immunized burn animals 7 days after injury produced large quantities of IFN-γ in comparison with sham-burn controls when cultured with the cognate antigen. In contrast, the same cell population harvested at day 7 after injury from immunized burn, but not sham-burn, animals produced large quantities of IL-4 and IL-10 on antigen stimulation in vitro.[54] In wild-type animals there is an early spontaneous proliferation of Th cells but not T cytotoxic or B cells in vivo within the first 12 hours after burn, but not sham-burn, injury. The proliferative response ceases by 24 hours. There is evidence of selective Vβ chain expression by the proliferating T-helper cell population, thus suggesting, but certainly not proving, that endogenous superantigen may be involved in this process.[55]

THERAPEUTIC RESTORATION OF T-HELPER CELL FUNCTION AFTER INJURY

Can restoration of Th1 function restore normal resistance to infection after serious injury? A variety of agents have been shown to be effective in reducing mortality from a septic challenge in various animal models of injury. These include IFN-γ,[56] GM-CSF,[57] anti–IL-6 monoclonal antibody,[58] anti–IL-10 antibody,[59] IL-18,[60] and IL-12.[43,51] Agents other than cytokines and their inhibitory antibodies have also proven effective. These include prolactin,[61] melatonin,[62] cyclooxygenase II inhibitors,[6,33] and hypertonic saline.[63] Of considerable interest recently has been the demonstration that sex differences play a role in the loss of Th1 function after injury.[64-66] Female proestrus mice are far less affected than male mice, and the use of the testosterone receptor antagonist, flutamide, after hemorrhage or trauma/hemorrhage restored Th1 cytokine production and proliferative capacity in injured as compared with sham-injured male mice and also increased survival after CLP.

Among the therapeutic agents mentioned earlier, one which is known to affect Th1 function directly is IL-12, which induces the Th1 phenotype. The administration of low doses of recombinant IL-12 beginning shortly after injury in the mouse model of burn injury in our laboratory reduced mortality from subsequent CLP to that of sham-injured controls.[51] Whereas the effect of IL-12 was dependent on IFN-γ production, the results obtained with IL-12 were superior to those achieved with IFN-γ itself in the same model.[43] IL-12 therapy was similarly shown to be protective against death from infection in burn mice by Kobayashi and colleagues.[36] IL-12 therapy was further shown to restore production of Th1-dependent antibody isotypes.[42] However, the clinical use of IL-12 to attempt to reduce the incidence of infection and septic death after serious injury is not particularly attractive because of IL-12 toxicity as demonstrated in clinical cancer trials.[67]

In summary, it appears likely that T-helper cells are programmed for a proinflammatory Th1-like response early after serious injury, which is followed in several days by the emergence of a Th2-like regulatory phenotype. The appearance of the latter phenotype is associated with diminished resistance to infection in a number of animal models and some clinical studies. B cells of the adaptive immune system are deficient in production of certain complement fixing antibodies, notably those of the IgG2 family, which appears to result from loss of effective Th1 function. Increased production of the Th2-dependent antibody IgE has been commonly observed in both injured humans and in animal models.

The fact that restoration of Th1 function by a variety of interventions is associated with improved resistance to infection in the postinjury period in animal models suggests that one or more of these approaches could prove useful clinically in preventing the onset of nosocomial infection with its attendant risk of death from MODS in seriously injured patients.

ANNOTATED REFERENCES

Faist E, Kupper TS, Baker CC, et al: Depression of cellular immunity after major injury. Its association with posttraumatic complications and its reversal with immunomodulation. Arch Surg 1986;121:1000-1005.

The data presented in this manuscript indicate that major injury can lead to depression of the T cell responses, which correlates with the subsequent development of infectious complications. Inhibition of cyclooxygenase pathways was able to reverse or decrease this immunologic defect.

Goebel A, Kavanagh EG, Lyons A, et al: Injury induces deficient interleukin-12 (IL-12) production while IL-12 therapy after injury restores resistance to infection. Ann Surg 2000;231:253-261.

Serious injury is associated with loss of function of the Th1 lymphocyte phenotype and decreased IL-12 production. In this manuscript, IL-12 production was shown to be reduced in peripheral blood mononuclear cells from severely injured patients. In humans, there is a reciprocal relation between diminished IL-12 production and increased IL-10 production at approximately 1 week after injury. Low-dose IL-12 therapy in the mouse burn model markedly increased survival after a septic challenge, even when treatment was carried beyond the onset of sepsis. Low-dose IL-12 treatment in the mouse increased production of proinflammatory mediators important in host defense and at the same time maintained or increased production of IL-10, an important antiinflammatory cytokine.

Hotchkiss RS, Chang KC, Swanson PE, et al: Caspase inhibitors improve survival in sepsis: A crucial role of the lymphocyte. Nat Immunol 2000;1:496-501.

Sepsis induces lymphocyte apoptosis, and prevention of lymphocyte death may improve the chances of surviving this disorder. This study demonstrated that inhibition of caspase 3 in mice resulted in decreased lymphocyte apoptosis and improved resistance to infection. Such results indicate that caspase inhibitors enhance immunity by preventing lymphocyte apoptosis and also that lymphocyte apoptosis is involved in the control of infection during sepsis.

O'Sullivan ST, Lederer JA, Horgan AF, et al: Major injury leads to predominance of the T-helper-2 lymphocyte phenotype and diminished interleukin-12 production associated with decreased resistance to infection. Ann Surg 1995;222:482-492.

This paper shows that major burn and traumatic injury led to increased Th2 cell responses, and decreased IL-12 production. Such changes in T lymphocyte functions were associated with decreased resistance to infection.

Wichmann MW, Zellweger R, DeMaso CM, et al: Mechanism of immunosuppression in males following trauma-hemorrhage: Critical role of testosterone. Arch Surg 1996;131:1186-1192.

Male sex hormones appear to be associated with worsened outcome from sepsis and hemorrhage. In these experiments, castration of male mice before soft tissue trauma and hemorrhagic shock maintains normal immune function, whereas sham-castrated male mice show significant immunodepression. The maintenance of immune function by androgen deficiency was not related to changes in the release of corticosterone. Such results suggest that the use of testosterone-blocking agents after trauma/hemorrhage could prevent the depression of immune functions and decrease the susceptibility to sepsis under those conditions.

Chapter 34
COAGULATION

Charles T. Esmon

KEY POINTS

1. Inflammation promotes blood coagulation.
2. Blood clotting enzymes promote inflammation.
3. Proteolytic products of clotting factors (fragment 1-2) can be used to assess intravascular coagulation and fibrin formation or degradation (D-dimer).
4. Natural anticoagulants inhibit coagulation and dampen inflammation.
5. Natural anticoagulant mechanisms are impaired by inflammatory mediators.
6. Microparticles released from cells by potent agonists contribute to thrombosis.
7. Platelet activation promotes inflammation.

OVERVIEW OF BLOOD COAGULATION

Thrombosis and disseminated intravascular coagulation are relatively common complications in critically ill patients. Recent studies have shown that inflammation is a major driving force in initiating and amplifying the blood clotting process. Under normal circumstances, blood clotting is limited to the site of injury. This regulation is due in large part to natural anticoagulant pathways. Inflammation can down-regulate these pathways, leading to a tilt in the hemostatic balance favoring clot formation. Further, the blood clotting enzymes can amplify the inflammatory response, and several of the natural anticoagulant pathways exhibit anti-inflammatory activity. Thus, the change in the hemostatic balance impacts inflammation as well as favoring clot formation. Finally, normal circulation of the blood is important in preventing thrombosis. In large part, this is due to the presence of potent anticoagulant mechanisms that are concentrated in the microcirculation. Thus, when blood has little or no flow in the large blood vessels, the clotting process proceeds in the absence of adequate negative regulatory mechanisms.

The goal of this chapter is to provide a framework for understanding the regulation of the blood coagulation process. Biochemical details are presented only when they are deemed to be important for understanding the process. For a more complete biochemical description of the blood clotting process, see reference 1.

Triggering the innate immune system has long been recognized to result in potential stimulation of the blood coagulation system. More recently, the highly integrated interactions of these two systems have become apparent. Inflammation triggered by the innate immune system initiates not only the blood clotting process but also the natural anticoagulant pathways, components of which are consumed or down-regulated by the inflammatory mediators. The anticoagulant components play an important role in limiting the inflammatory response. This chapter summarizes current information on the linkage between the regulation of the coagulation and inflammatory responses to infection.

BLOOD COAGULATION PATHWAYS

The main pathways of blood coagulation are shown in Figure 34-1. All the reactions involved in generating thrombin, the enzyme responsible for blood clotting, require negatively charged phospholipid membranes to proceed at physiologically relevant rates. Functional membrane phospholipid expression (phosphatidylserine, phosphatidylethanolamine) requires exposure of the cells to potent activators such as collagen together with thrombin (for platelets) or the membrane attack complex (C5b9) of the complement system to achieve full activity.[2]

Tissue factor triggers the blood clotting process. Under normal circumstances, tissue factor is found primarily on cells lining the outside of the blood vessel,[3] where it is strategically placed to trigger hemostasis when the blood vessels are injured or severed. Once an inflammatory challenge occurs, tissue factor expression is induced on macrophage-monocytes.[4,5] Recently, it has been shown that circulating tissue factor is present in blood, albeit at low levels, where it appears to augment hemostasis and the growth of thrombi.[6] When tissue factor is exposed to blood, it binds factor VII. Factor VII is converted to the active serine protease, factor VIIa, by thrombin, factor Xa, or factor VIIa, processes that are accelerated by factor VII and factor VIIa binding to tissue factor.[7] The tissue factor–factor VIIa complex can convert either factor IX or factor X to their proteolytically active forms, factors IXa and Xa.[8] Factors V and VIII circulate as inactive high-molecular-weight proteins. They must be proteolytically activated by thrombin or factor Xa to participate effectively in the coagulation cascade. In the case of factor VIII, it circulates in complex with another very high molecular weight protein, von Willebrand's factor, a protein involved in platelet adherence to the vessel wall at wound sites. The von Willebrand's factor–factor VIII interaction helps stabilize factor VIII, a protein that is normally relatively unstable. Upon activation of factor VIII, von Willebrand's factor dissociates, leaving a relatively unstable factor VIIIa molecule. Factors Va and VIIIa are not proteases

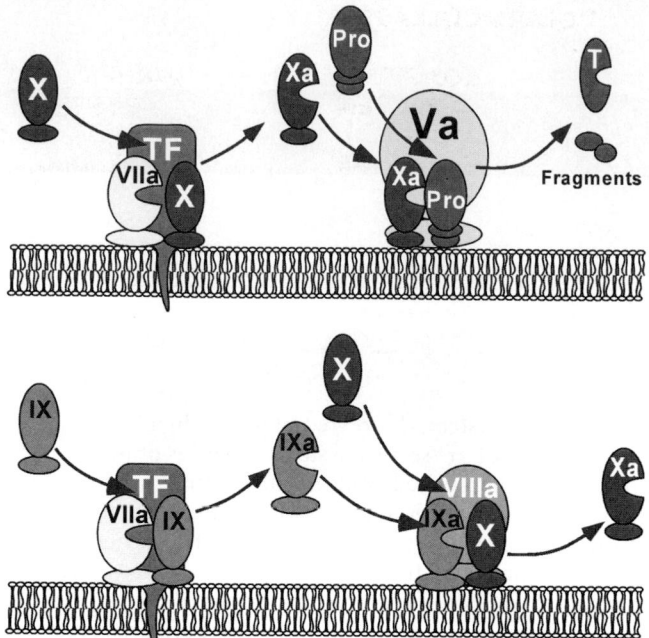

FIGURE 34–1. Initiation of the coagulation cascade. Tissue factor (TF) on extravascular cells is exposed to blood at a wound site. Factor VII (not shown) is activated by thrombin (T), factor Xa, or factor VIIa (when bound to tissue factor). The tissue factor–factor VIIa complex then cleaves factor X to generate the serine protease factor Xa. This binds to factor Va, and the complex converts prothrombin (Pro) to thrombin. Roughly half of the prothrombin molecule is released as activation fragment 1-2 (Fragments). Circulating levels of this fragment are used to determine the degree of intravascular coagulation. Alternatively, the tissue factor–factor VIIa complex can activate factor IX. Factor IXa binds to factor VIIIa to activate factor X. At this point, the different pathways converge. Factors VII, IX, and X and prothrombin need vitamin K for their synthesis. The vitamin generates γ-carboxyglutamic acid from glutamic acid residues located toward the amino terminus. These residues are required for calcium-dependent binding to negatively charged phospholipids.

but serve as cofactors that bind to both the substrates and the enzymes to accelerate the coagulation process. Factor IXa binds to factor VIIIa, and this complex also converts factor X to factor Xa. Factor Xa in complex with factor Va converts prothrombin to thrombin.[9] Nearly half the prothrombin, including the domain responsible for binding to negatively charged phospholipids, is released during activation. This activation fragment (fragment 1-2) can be detected in the circulation using immunoassays and is a monitor of intravascular coagulation (Table 34-1).

In addition to clotting blood, thrombin activates many cells, altering their phenotype by leading to tissue factor, leukocyte adhesion molecule, and cytokine expression.[10] Therefore, thrombin generation has the potential to amplify the inflammatory pathways.

TABLE 34–1. ASSAYS USED TO DETECT INTRAVASCULAR COAGULATION

Assay	Activity Measured
Fibrinopeptide A	Fibrin formation
Thrombin-antithrombin complex	Thrombin formation
D-dimer	Fibrin degradation
Prothrombin fragment 1-2	Prothrombin activation

Traditionally, blood coagulation was thought to occur via one of two pathways: the extrinsic pathway (described earlier), and the intrinsic pathway triggered by the activation of factor XII. Factor XII is activated on surfaces such as glass or collagen. Factor XIIa activates factor XI in vitro, and factor XIa in turn activates factor IX. From that point on, the pathways converge. The physiologic importance of the intrinsic pathway to coagulation is questionable, however, because patients with factor XII deficiency do not have bleeding problems. In contrast, patients with factor IX deficiency exhibit a variable and usually mild bleeding diathesis. Why factor XI deficiency, but not factor XII deficiency, is associated with increased bleeding risk remained unclear until it was shown that thrombin could feed back to activate factor XI, thereby bypassing the factor XII requirement.[11,12] Subsequently, it was shown that binding of factor XI to activated platelet receptors further enhanced this thrombin activation of factor XI.[13] This pathway is involved in bradykinin formation and has weak profibrinolytic activity (Fig. 34-2).

Once thrombin is formed, it clots fibrinogen, a process that requires the release of small peptides from fibrinogen, allowing the newly revealed N-termini to participate in fibrin formation. Fibrinogen is a complex molecule with two copies of three independently coded chains: α, β, and γ. These small fragments, referred to as fibrinopeptides A and B, are derived from the N-termini of the α and β chains (Fig. 34-3). Immunoassays designed to detect fibrinopeptides have been used to monitor intravascular coagulation (see Table 34-1).

The fibrin formed initially is somewhat fragile. Very rapidly during clot formation, factor XIII is activated by thrombin and crosslinks the clot (Fig. 34-3). Six transamidation reactions occur between the fibrin chains, each involving crosslinking between glutamine and lysine residues. The new amide bond is very stable. The resultant clot is more resistant to clot lysis and mechanical forces.[1,14]

FIBRINOLYSIS

Once the thrombus forms, it can be removed by the fibrinolytic system. The primary mechanism is initiated when tissue plasminogen activator (t-PA) binds to fibrin. The fibrin–t-PA complex rapidly converts plasminogen into the fibrinolytic enzyme plasmin. The process is facilitated by plasminogen binding to the fibrin clot and concentrating the enzyme and substrate in close proximity.[14] Fibrin is then degraded into fibrin degradation products, including D-dimer (see Fig. 34-3). D-dimer levels in the circulation are often used as a measure of intravascular coagulation (see Table 34-1). This is somewhat indirect, however, because it is a simultaneous measure of clot formation and lysis. If the fibrinolytic system is severely impaired, intravascular clot formation could be occurring without a concomitant increase in fibrinolysis and a subsequent increase in D-dimer levels.

Plasmin and t-PA are rapidly inactivated by α_2-antiplasmin and plasminogen activator inhibitor-1 (PAI-1). PAI-1 levels are elevated in inflammatory diseases and can result in impaired fibrinolysis.[15]

A weaker fibrinolytic system is initiated by another protease, urokinase. Urokinase can activate plasminogen without strong requirements for binding to fibrin. It is generally believed that the primary function of urokinase involves binding to a urokinase receptor, at which time it is involved

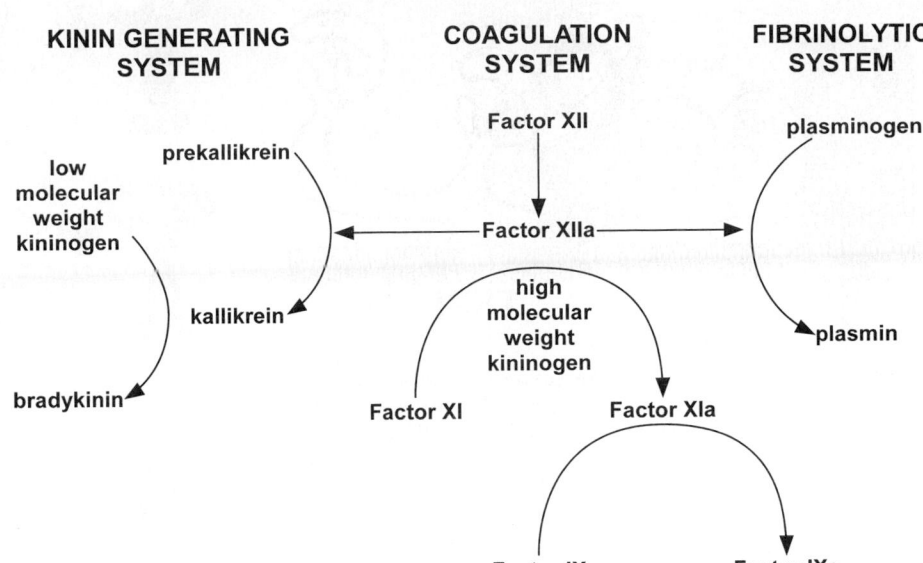

FIGURE 34–2. Intrinsic coagulation system. When blood contacts foreign surfaces such as glass, certain soils, or collagen, factor XII is activated. In the presence of high-molecular-weight kininogen, factor XIIa activates factor XI, which in turn activates factor IX. The pathway can also generate bradykinin. Factor XIIa activation of prekallikrein leads to the formation of bradykinin. Alternatively, factor XIIa can activate plasminogen, stimulating fibrinolysis.

in cellular migration, tumor growth, and development, in part mediated through cell surface activation of plasminogen.[14,16]

An obvious question is why there is so much complexity. In part, this seems to be due to the vast array of insults to which the coagulation system must respond—everything from minor nicks to severe trauma. A simple system could easily seal the wound, regardless of magnitude, but it would most likely lack the control mechanisms required to generate a hemostatic response without occlusive thrombosis. The potential thrombin that can be generated from prothrombin is more than 100 times enough to clot blood. Unchecked, these pathways would make more than enough thrombin to clot all the blood within seconds, making it essential to have

potent negative regulatory mechanisms in place. This is the function of the natural anticoagulant pathways described later in this chapter.

NATURAL ANTICOAGULANT PATHWAYS

INHIBITION OF TISSUE FACTOR–FACTOR VIIa COMPLEX

Two major mechanisms regulate tissue factor–factor VIIa activity: tissue factor pathway inhibitor (TFPI) and antithrombin-heparin. Both function by inhibiting the protease factor VIIa bound to tissue factor. TFPI has an unusual

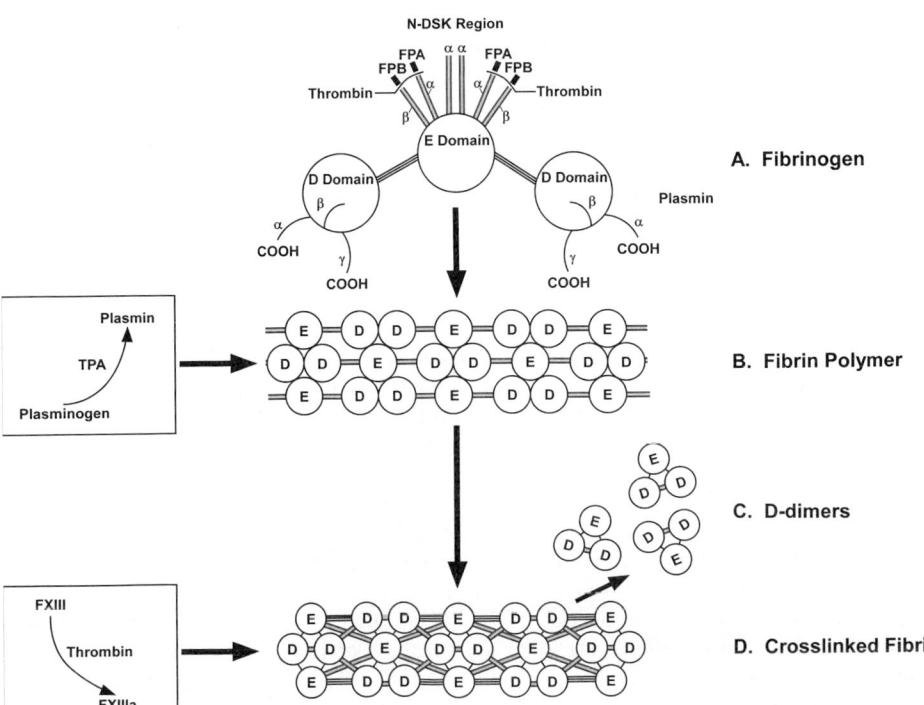

FIGURE 34–3. Formation and lysis of fibrin. Fibrinogen (A) has three globular domains. When thrombin releases small peptides from fibrinogen, a polymer forms (B). Plasmin cleaves the polymer to release fibrin degradation products, including D-dimers (C). Thrombin also activates factor XIII to cause fibrin crosslinking (D). This helps stabilize the clot. FPA, fibrinopeptide A; FPB, fibrinopeptide B; N-DSK, amino-terminal disulfide knot; TPA, tissue plasminogen activator.

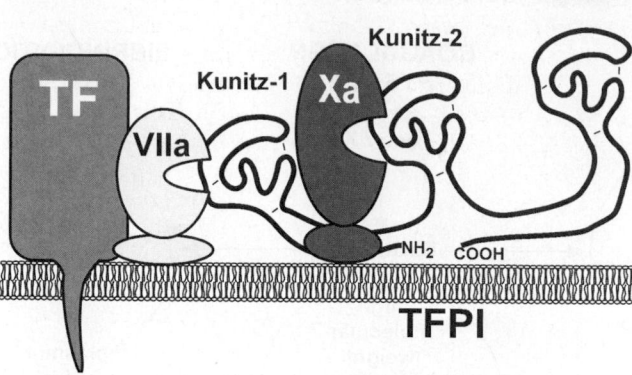

FIGURE 34–4. Proposed mechanism for tissue factor pathway inhibitor (TFPI) inhibition of the factor VIIa–tissue factor (TF) complex. Factor Xa first binds to the second Kunitz domain of the inhibitor. The complex then binds to the membrane surface. This concentrates the first Kunitz domain near factor VIIa and leads to factor VIIa inhibition. The process is reversed by removing calcium.

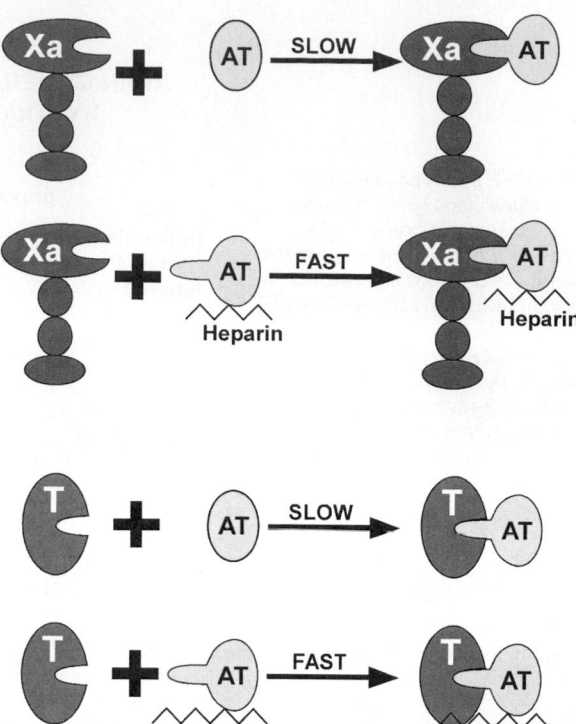

FIGURE 34–5. Heparin involvement in antithrombin function. Antithrombin (AT) undergoes a conformational change when bound to heparin, making the "bait" site more accessible. In the case of factor Xa, this is sufficient to stimulate inactivation. In the case of thrombin (T), longer heparin molecules are needed. This is the basis for some of the differences between low- and high-molecular-weight (unfractionated) heparin.

mechanism of action (Fig. 34-4).[17] Structurally, TFPI is composed of three Kunitz inhibitory domains. TFPI binds to factor Xa through the Kunitz 2 protease inhibitory domain. The factor Xa–TFPI complex then binds to negatively charged membrane surfaces in the presence of calcium, increasing the local concentration and favoring relatively stable, reversible inhibition of factor VIIa bound to tissue factor by the Kunitz 1 domain of TFPI.[17] Gene deletion of TFPI in mice results in an embryonic consumptive coagulopathy leading to embryonic lethality.[18] It is difficult to assess the impact of inflammation on TFPI function because the majority of TFPI is vessel associated,[17] and much of this is stored in agonist releasable endothelial cell granules.[19] Heparin also causes the release of TFPI from the vessel.[17]

Antithrombin can also inhibit the tissue factor–factor VIIa complex (see later). Although the relative importance of antithrombin versus TFPI inhibition of tissue factor–factor VIIa is uncertain, it is clear that antithrombin activity decreases markedly during severe sepsis, often dropping below 50%.[20] This decreased level of antithrombin is associated with thrombosis in thrombophilic patients.[21] Because the rate of inhibition is strongly dependent on the inhibitor concentration, a decrease in antithrombin would contribute to increased stability of the tissue factor–factor VIIa complex and hence favor intravascular coagulation.

ANTITHROMBIN REGULATION OF AMPLIFICATION REACTIONS

Antithrombin inhibition of the factor VIIa–tissue factor complex, factor IXa, factor Xa, and thrombin are all thought to be accelerated by vascular heparin-like proteoglycans. Antithrombin forms a tight, apparently covalent 1:1 complex with these enzymes (Fig. 34-5). Heparin is a highly sulfated sugar polymer that varies in size, sugar composition, and degree of sulfation. There is a relatively specific sugar sequence that determines high-affinity interaction with antithrombin.[22] Low-molecular-weight heparins are often used therapeutically. These have reduced activity toward thrombin because they cannot effectively form the bridge that is shown in Figure 34-5, but they retain a high activity toward factor Xa. Once the enzyme complex forms, heparin dissociates

due to major conformational changes in both the enzyme and the antithrombin or related inhibitors.[23] The vascular heparin-like molecules may be inactivated during severe sepsis,[24] further reducing the effectiveness of the natural anticoagulants. This is likely to be even more important when the antithrombin level has been reduced by consumption.

PROTEIN Z–PROTEIN Z PROTEASE INHIBITOR COMPLEX REGULATION OF FACTOR Xa

Protein Z, a vitamin K–dependent anticoagulant protein, plays a significant role in the inhibition of factor Xa. Protein Z binds tightly to protein Z protease inhibitor. The protein Z protease inhibitor–protein Z complex binds to negatively charged membrane surfaces due to direct protein Z interaction with the membrane. This complex then inactivates factor Xa.[25] Deletion of the protein Z gene in mice exacerbates the thrombotic response caused by other coagulation abnormalities,[26] but alone, it is not sufficient to cause thrombosis. Low protein Z levels in humans appear to be associated with an increased risk of stroke.[27] Because protein Z appears to be a negative acute-phase reactant,[28] inflammation may reduce the effectiveness of this system also.

INHIBITION OF FACTOR Va AND VIIIa BY ACTIVATED PROTEIN C: THE PROTEIN C ANTICOAGULANT PATHWAY

The protein C anticoagulant pathway is the most complex of the natural anticoagulant mechanisms and is also the most sensitive to down-regulation by acute inflammatory responses.

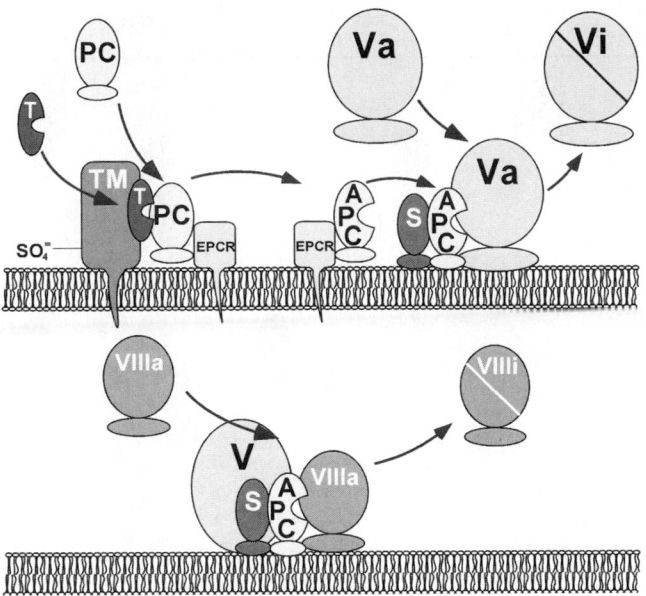

FIGURE 34–6. Protein C anticoagulant pathway. Thrombin (T) binds to thrombomodulin (TM) and activates protein C (PC). The activation is augmented by protein C binding to the endothelial cell protein C receptor (EPCR). Both protein C and activated protein C (APC) bind reversibly to EPCR. When APC dissociates from EPCR, it binds to protein S (S), and this complex inactivates factors Va (Va and Vi) and VIIIa (VIIIa and VIIIi). In the case of factor VIIIa, factor V (V) also increases the inactivation rate.

The pathway is illustrated in Figure 34-6. Protein C circulates as an inactive vitamin K–dependent zymogen at about 4 μg/mL in plasma. It is activated proteolytically on the surface of the endothelium by a complex between thrombin and thrombomodulin. Protein C activation rates are increased when protein C is bound to the endothelial cell protein C receptor (EPCR).[29] EPCR may be particularly important in preventing large vessel thrombosis[30] because it is most abundant on large blood vessels. Protein C and activated protein C (APC) bind to EPCR with comparable affinity (30 nM). The APC-EPCR complex does not appear to inactivate factor Va.[31] It is likely that this complex cleaves an alternative substrate or receptor.[32,33] This would be consistent with in vivo observations that APC infusion dampens cellular responses to inflammatory agents and decreases the generation of inflammatory cytokines.[34,35] When APC dissociates from EPCR, it can bind to protein S and catalyze the selective proteolytic inactivation of factors Va and VIIIa.[36] A common dimorphism exists in factor V in which the Arg residue at residue 506 is replaced by Gln, resulting in a factor Va that is more resistant to inactivation by APC. This condition, referred to as factor V Leiden or APC resistance, is associated with an increased risk of thrombosis.[21,37] It is found in approximately 5% of whites but is rare in other races.

APC also enhances fibrinolysis by forming a tight 1:1 complex with PAI-1 and thereby inactivating this major inhibitor of fibrinolysis. APC normally reacts slowly with PAI-1, but recently it has been shown that the reaction becomes quite rapid in the presence of vitronectin,[38] suggesting a dominant role for this reaction around platelets that release vitronectin.

Compared with other serine proteases or clotting factors, APC has a relatively long half-life in the blood of about 15 minutes before it becomes inactivated by α₁-antitrypsin (sometimes called α₁-proteinase inhibitor), protein C inhibitor or α₂-macroglobulin.[39] The APC-inhibitor complex is then cleared relatively rapidly from the circulation. Because of the relatively slow inactivation of APC, it is possible to detect circulating levels of it. This allows direct evaluation of APC levels in patients,[40,41] which in turn allows evaluation of the functionality of the protein C activation complex in vivo.

Thrombin binding to thrombomodulin not only augments protein C activation but also results in inhibition of fibrinogen clotting, platelet and endothelial cell activation, and factor V activation.[36] In addition, thrombin bound to thrombomodulin is inactivated much more rapidly than free thrombin is. Antithrombin and protein C inhibitor contribute similarly to the rapid inactivation of thrombin bound to thrombomodulin, resulting in an estimated half-life of 1 to 2 seconds for thrombomodulin bound to thrombin.[42] In severe sepsis, down-regulation of thrombomodulin would result in both decreased protein C activation and decreased thrombin clearance. It is apparent from studies of APC levels in septic patients that protein C activation can be severely impaired in a subset of patients with severe sepsis.[41,43] The modulation of thrombin functions, and the regulation resulting from thrombin-thrombomodulin interaction, allows thrombomodulin to serve as a molecular switch in the control of hemostasis and thrombosis.

IMPACT OF INFLAMMATION ON COAGULATION

Some of the changes in the vessel wall and the hemostatic balance that are caused by inflammation are illustrated in Figure 34-7. Bacteria and other pathogens can lead to the formation of inflammatory cytokines such as tumor necrosis factor (TNF) and interleukin-1 beta (IL-1β). These mediators, or endotoxin itself, induce synthesis and expression of tissue factor, primarily on monocytes and macrophages.[4,5] Because the monocytes and macrophages are in contact with the blood, they initiate intravascular coagulation when stimulated by these inflammatory mediators.

Complement activation as a result of inflammation can also augment the coagulant response. As mentioned previously, complement C5b9 (the membrane attack complex of complement) is a very effective cell agonist, leading to expression of negatively charged phospholipids on the surface of cells that can propagate the coagulation reaction.[44] During bacterial infections, complement activation occurs not only due to recognition of the infectious agent but also due to the increase in the acute-phase protein, C-reactive protein, which appears to augment complement activation during sepsis.[45] Cell surface expression of negatively charged lipids is a major regulatory event controlling physiologic and pathologic clotting. For instance, infusion of factor Xa at relatively high concentrations has little thrombotic effect unless coinfused with negatively charged phospholipids. These lipids are a surrogate for the activated cell surface or cellular microparticles released following treatment with potent cell agonists.[46] Further, when only an inflammatory cytokine such as TNF is infused into experimental animals, there is little fibrin formation unless appropriate lipids are also infused (and blood flow is impaired).[47] Thus, available evidence suggests that inflammation can contribute directly to two critical events in intravascular coagulation: the synthesis and expression of intravascular tissue factor and the generation

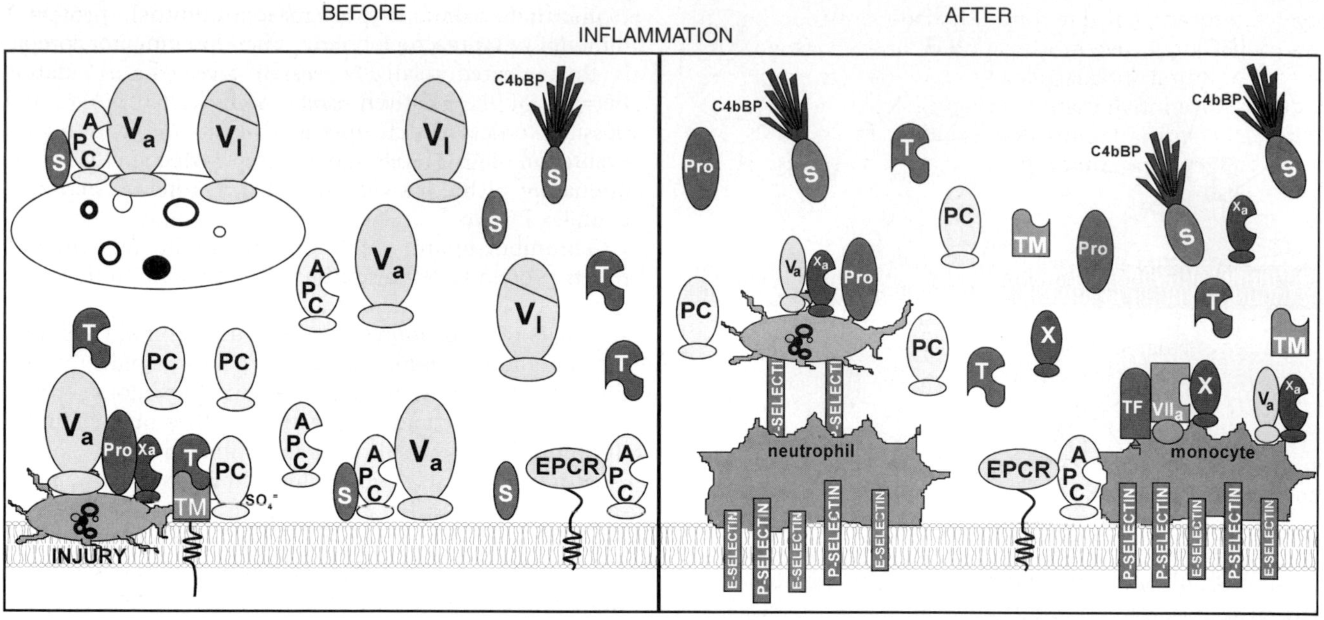

FIGURE 34–7. Impact of inflammation on the regulation of coagulation. Under normal circumstances, strong anticoagulant properties are associated with the endothelium. Inflammation causes leukocytes to adhere, thrombomodulin (TM) to be shed, and the endothelial cell protein C receptor (EPCR) to be down-regulated. Tissue factor (TF) is induced on leukocytes. Protein C (PC) is consumed, and free (active) protein S (S) decreases. Active lipid surface becomes exposed, propagating the coagulant response. APC, activated protein C; Pro, prothrombin; T, thrombin.

of membrane surfaces capable of augmenting the initiation and propagation of the coagulant response.

Thrombin impacts both its own generation and the inflammatory response. In addition to clotting fibrinogen and activating platelets, thrombin plays a major role in leukocyte activation by causing the expression of the leukocyte adhesion molecule P-selectin on platelets and endothelial cells.[48] Thrombin is a potent agonist for endothelial cell platelet-activating factor formation, a potent neutrophil agonist.[49] Neutrophil activation is potentiated by adhesion to P-selectin, further augmenting the inflammatory response. P-selectin appears to play an important role in thrombus formation. Blocking P-selectin binding to its ligand, the P-selectin glycoprotein ligand-1, decreases thrombus formation under both flow[50] and stasis conditions.[51]

Inflammatory mediators can also impact platelet function. For instance, interleukin-6 (IL-6) not only increases platelet production but also creates a population of platelets that are more thrombogenic. IL-6–induced platelets are more readily activated by platelet agonists such as thrombin.[52] Activated platelets are a rich source of the proinflammatory mediator CD40 ligand. CD40 ligand induces tissue factor formation[53,54] and increases inflammatory cytokines such as IL-6 and interleukin-8 (IL-8).[55,56]

IMPACT OF INFLAMMATION ON NATURAL ANTICOAGULANT PATHWAYS

Natural anticoagulant pathways play key roles in preventing excessive inflammation induced by augmentation of the coagulation response. In addition to preventing excess clotting, these pathways feed back to dampen the inflammatory response. However, in severe acute inflammatory diseases, some of the key negative regulatory pathways are down-regulated.

Both thrombomodulin and EPCR are down-regulated by inflammatory cytokines such as TNF at the transcriptional level.[57,58] In cell culture, about half the activity disappears in 8 hours. A single exposure of the endothelium to the cytokine reduces the protein and messenger RNA levels more than 90%, and these low levels are maintained for at least 24 hours. Neutrophil adhesion and activation on the endothelium can reduce thrombomodulin activity further, both through oxidation of a sensitive methionine residue[59] and by elastase-mediated release of soluble thrombomodulin,[60] a form with reduced activity. Decreased protein C activation is particularly important, because factors Xa and IXa are resistant to inactivation by antithrombin when they are complexed with factors Va and VIIIa, respectively.[61,62]

The protein C pathway seems to be particularly important in the prevention of microvascular thrombosis, as demonstrated by the purpura fulminans that develops in neonates with protein C deficiency.[63] Down-regulation of thrombomodulin, with the loss of thrombin clearance and decreased protein C activation, would therefore be expected to have a major effect on clotting in the microcirculation, a major site of thrombotic complications in sepsis.

ANTI-INFLAMMATORY ACTIVITIES OF NATURAL ANTICOAGULANT PATHWAYS

Natural anticoagulants have anti-inflammatory activities as well as anticoagulant functions. Antithrombin, TFPI, and APC have all been shown to protect baboons from *Escherichia coli* sepsis when given before the challenge.[64] In the baboon and several rodent models,[65] neither synthetic factor Xa inhibitors[65] nor active site-blocked factor Xa, an effective, high-affinity, competitive inhibitor of prothrombin activation in vivo,[66] protected the animals from death or organ failure and failed to diminish cytokine elaboration. In contrast to ineffective synthetic coagulation inhibitors, the ability of natural anticoagulants to both protect from sepsis and minimize inflammation-mediated injury suggests that cellular and anti-inflammatory activities of the natural anticoagulants may be important aspects of their physiologic functions.

ANTITHROMBIN

Antithrombin can protect experimental animals from endotoxin-mediated septic shock.[67] Heparin prevents this protection, despite increasing the antithrombotic activity. A negative effect of heparin and antithrombin coadministration was observed in clinical trials.[68] High levels of antithrombin in vitro have been shown to inhibit endotoxin-induced IL-6 formation by mononuclear cells and endothelium.[67,69] Antithrombin stimulates prostacyclin release from endothelial cells in culture,[70] a process that appears to be protective in lung injury models.[71] Antithrombin-mediated signaling probably occurs through syndecan-4.[69] Antithrombin binding to cell surface receptors has also been shown to block nuclear factor kappa-B (NF-κB) translocation.[72] This prevents the subsequent release of cytokines and the induction of adhesion molecules.

TISSUE FACTOR PATHWAY INHIBITOR

TFPI infusion can reduce leukocyte activation and decrease TNF in vivo.[65] Although inhibition of cytokine elaboration appears to be independent of blood coagulation, the mechanism responsible for TFPI-mediated cellular effects remains unknown.

PROTEIN C PATHWAY

APC has been shown to protect nonhuman primates from E. coli–induced sepsis whether given before or after the E. coli challenge.[73] Recently, this observation was confirmed and extended in clinical studies demonstrating that APC infusion can reduce the relative risk of all-cause 28-day mortality from severe sepsis by 19.4%.[74] One feature of critically ill patients is the relatively high frequency of antiphospholipid antibodies.[75] Some antiphospholipid antibodies inhibit APC anticoagulant activity extremely effectively,[36] but whether this is the case in critical care patients remains to be examined.

The protective effects of APC appear to be receptor mediated. APC binding to monocytic cells can block agonist-induced calcium transients[76] and inhibit NF-κB–mediated signaling.[34,77-79] In cultured endothelium, APC reduces NF-κB messenger RNA levels, reduces the expression of cell surface adhesion molecules and cytokine formation, and elevates molecules involved in preventing apoptosis.[35] On the monocytic cell line U937, APC has been shown to dampen both basal levels and the phorbol-induced expression of tissue factor in an EPCR-dependent fashion.[32] Under appropriate conditions, APC can also cleave protease-activated receptors,[33] which are normally cleaved by coagulation enzymes, particularly thrombin.[10] The role of cleavage of the protease-activated receptors in APC function remains to be fully elucidated. Most of the downstream events following activation of these receptors enhance inflammation.[80] It is possible that activation of the protease-activated receptors is a negative side reaction occurring under in vitro conditions.

Conway and coworkers[81] recently revealed a novel anti-inflammatory activity of thrombomodulin. The N-terminal lectin-like domain[82,83] dampened activation of the mitogen-activated protein kinase and NF-κB signaling systems in endothelium. This anti-inflammatory activity was imparted by either cellular thrombomodulin or the soluble lectin-like domain. Infusion of the lectin-like domain, which does not participate in protein C activation, resulted in decreased leukocyte adhesion to the endothelium. These observations have important implications. Thrombomodulin is down-regulated on endothelium overlying atherosclerotic plaques, on vein bypass grafts, in diabetes, and by acute inflammatory insults such as bacterial infection.[84] Loss of thrombomodulin would not only reduce protein C activation but also increase the endothelium's sensitivity to leukocyte-mediated injury. Important roles for thrombomodulin in vascular protection were demonstrated earlier when its overexpression was found to reduce thrombosis, restenosis, and leukocyte infiltration in rabbits with deep arterial injury.[85,86]

Thrombomodulin also accelerates thrombin activation of a plasma procarboxypeptidase B called thrombin-activatable fibrinolysis inhibitor (TAFI).[87] TAFI removes terminal lysine residues in fibrin. Lysine residues facilitate binding of plasminogen or plasmin and t-PA. Removal of these lysine residues decreases the rate of clot lysis about fourfold.[87] Initially, TAFI was considered a prothrombotic molecule. More recently, it was found that TAFI can remove terminal Arg residues very effectively from vasoactive substances such as the anaphylotoxin C5a, generated during complement activation; this inactivates C5a. Recent studies found that TAFI is the major enzyme responsible for the inactivation of C5a.[88,89] Activation of TAFI by the thrombin-thrombomodulin complex appears to be important in preventing vascular toxicity due to C5a in conditions in which complement activation is intense. Thus, thrombomodulin may play multiple roles in the regulation of clotting, inflammation, and complement-mediated cell injury.

EPCR was recently found to be important in controlling the inflammatory response to bacterial infusion. Specifically, when protein C binding to EPCR was blocked and the animals were challenged with a low dose of E. coli, both the coagulant and cytokine responses were elevated dramatically, and more leukocytes migrated into the tissues compared with controls.[90] A possible mechanism involved in diminishing leukocyte migration was suggested by the recent finding that soluble EPCR, released by a metalloproteinase in endothelium,[91] binds to activated neutrophils. Soluble EPCR binds to proteinase 3, a cytosolic protein of the neutrophil that is released upon activation. Proteinase 3 binds to neutrophil integrins, particularly Mac-1 (CD11b/CD18),[92] whether or not it is bound to EPCR. In vivo data suggest that this interaction reduces tight binding of neutrophils to activated endothelium.

EPCR is also a candidate for immune modulatory functions. The crystal structure of EPCR[93] reveals that it is closely related to the major histocompatibility complex (MHC) class 1/CD1 family of proteins, most of which are involved in inflammation. The crystal structure demonstrated that EPCR has a tightly bound phospholipid in the "antigen presenting groove."[93] CD1 family members serve as glycolipid antigen-presenting molecules. For instance, CD1c seems to present a lipid antigen derived from tuberculosis.[94] The CD1 family of proteins then instructs T cells to modulate the cellular and humoral response to inflammation.[95] Further, these proteins appear likely candidates for involvement in autoimmunity.[95] Whether EPCR plays similar roles should become clear through the analysis of genetically modified mice.[96]

STRUCTURES LINKING THE COAGULATION PATHWAY AND INFLAMMATION

Coagulation and inflammatory pathways share many conserved structures, suggesting parallel evolution. In addition to the EPCR–MHC class 1 similarities, tissue factor and the cytokine receptors share structural similarities,[97] and the selectins involved in leukocyte adhesion and the lectin domain of thrombomodulin are homologous.[98] The complement and coagulation systems also have functional interactions. Protein S and a complement regulatory protein, C4 binding protein, bind tightly. When binding occurs, protein S anticoagulant activity is lost, but this allows C4 binding protein to interact with membrane surfaces, probably protecting mammalian cells from complement activation–mediated damage.[99] These findings suggest that the coagulation and inflammatory pathways evolved in parallel.

SUMMARY

It is clear that coagulation and inflammation are involved in mutual regulation. Considering these interactions, it is apparent that inflammation can contribute to a hypercoagulable state by many discrete mechanisms. Likewise, natural anticoagulants can decrease the inflammatory process. The ability of natural anticoagulants to down-regulate the inflammatory process may provide new therapeutic strategies for the treatment of acute inflammatory disease.

ANNOTATED REFERENCES

Bernard GR, Vincent JL, Laterre PF, et al: Efficacy and safety of recombinant human activated protein C for severe sepsis. N Engl J Med 2001;344:699-709.
This study demonstrates that activated protein C improves survival in patients with severe sepsis.

Conway EM, Van de Wouwer M, Pollefeyt S, et al: The lectin-like domain of thrombomodulin confers protection from neutrophil-mediated tissue damage by suppressing adhesion molecule expression via nuclear factor κB and mitogen-activated protein kinase pathways. J Exp Med 2002;196:565-577.
This paper demonstrates that thrombomodulin is a constitutive anti-inflammatory protein on the endothelium. It is important, because thrombomodulin is down-regulated in many diseases.

Coughlin SR: Thrombin signalling and protease-activated receptors. Nature 2000;407:258-264.
This paper reviews the mechanisms by which coagulation factors activate cells.

Faust SN, Levin M, Harrison OB, et al: Dysfunction of endothelial protein C activation in severe meningococcal sepsis. N Engl J Med 2001;345:408-416.
This paper demonstrates that some septic patients have impaired protein C activation.

Peter L, Giesen A, Rauch U, et al: Blood-borne tissue factor: Another view of thrombosis. Proc Natl Acad Sci U S A 1999;96:2311-2315.
This paper demonstrates that circulating tissue factor contributes to thrombosis.

Chapter 35
COMPLEMENT

Niels C. Riedemann • Peter A. Ward

KEY POINTS

PATHWAYS OF ACTIVATION

1. The **complement system can be activated** by one of three separate pathways: the classic, lectin, and alternative pathways.

2. Typically, the **classic pathway is activated by immunoglobulin G immune complexes or C-reactive protein**. The lectin pathway is activated by mannose residues on surfaces of bacteria. The alternative pathway is activated by lipopolysaccharide from Gram-negative bacteria.

3. Regardless of the activation pathway, **the most important products of activation are the anaphylatoxins C3a and C5a and the membrane attack complex C5b-9**, which cause lysis of Gram-negative bacteria. C3a induces histamine release from mast cells and causes smooth muscle contraction. C5a reacts with receptors (C5aR) on neutrophils and macrophages to cause cell signaling, chemotactic movement, enzyme release, and generation of superoxide anion ($O_2^{\bullet}$) and H_2O_2, which are involved in the myeloperoxidase-dependent killing of bacteria.

COMPLEMENT RECEPTORS AND THEIR FUNCTIONS

1. **Complement receptors exist on a variety** of myeloid and nonmyeloid cells and induce signaling responses in the presence of the ligand (complement activation product).

2. **Receptors of C1q (C1qR)** exist on a variety of cell types and often work synergistically with Fc receptors to enhance the inflammatory response.

3. **Receptors for C3a (C3aR) and C5a (C5aR)** are abundant on myeloid cells. In mast cells, the presence of C3a induces granule secretion and histamine release. Engagement of C3aR on smooth muscle cells results in smooth muscle contraction, especially in the airways. Engagement of C5aR on phagocytic cells causes mitogen-activated protein kinase signaling cascades, resulting in chemotaxis, enzyme release, and generation of superoxide anion ($O_2^{\bullet}$) and H_2O_2. Engagement of C5aR on endothelial cells causes P-selectin and tissue factor expression on the endothelium and release of von Willebrand's factor, a procoagulant protein.

GENETICALLY BASED COMPLEMENT DEFICIENCIES

1. **Deficiencies of early complement components (C1q, C1r, C1s, C2, C4)** are associated with manifestations of systemic lupus erythematosus (SLE), glomerulonephritis, and susceptibility to streptococcal pneumonia. Deficiencies of C3 are often life-threatening owing to loss of innate immune defenses to bacteria. Deficiencies of C5, C6, C7, C8, or C9 cause increased susceptibility to infection by *Neisseria* species.

2. **Deficiency of C1 inhibitor** causes hereditary angioedema, and **deficiency of a glycoprotein I–anchored protein** prevents the functioning of complement regulatory proteins, resulting in paroxysmal nocturnal hemoglobinuria.

IN VIVO BIOLOGIC FUNCTIONS OF COMPLEMENT

1. **Ischemia-reperfusion injury in animals** undergoing gut or myocardial ischemia has been shown to be complement and neutrophil dependent.[1] Infusion of C1 inhibitor can ameliorate the injury. Complement activation products also play an important role in hyperacute rejection following organ transplantation.

2. **In the setting of sepsis in animals and humans**, there is clear evidence of complement activation. In animals with sepsis, blockade of C5a or its receptor (C5aR) is protective. There are also suggestions that complement activation occurs in acute respiratory distress syndrome and that C5a can also be generated by activated phagocytic cells.[2]

3. **In SLE, rheumatoid arthritis (RA), and many cases of glomerulonephritis**, there is evidence of complement activation in synovial tissues and in the kidney, as demonstrated by deposition of C3 or its activation products in these locations.

4. **In acute thermal injury and acute trauma**, including cases of closed head injury, there is evidence that complement activation has occurred.

COMPLEMENT INHIBITORS

Several mechanisms exist to prevent uncontrolled activation of the complement system (Fig. 35-1). Such inhibitors of complement activation either exist in plasma or are bound to the cell membrane. As explained later, genetic deficiency of such inhibitors is often associated with human disease.

The natural fluid phase inhibitors occur accordingly: C1 inhibitor inhibits activation of C1s and C1r and, thereby, the classic pathway, but it has also been shown to inhibit activation of the mannose-binding lectin (MBL) pathway. Heterozygous deficiency of C1 inhibitor manifests clinically as life-threatening angioedema. Factor H and C4 binding protein are large plasma proteins that inhibit C3 and C4

activation (in part, as cofactors for other inhibitors), thus inhibiting all pathways of complement activation. Factor I is a serum protease that inactivates C3b and C4b and, therefore, C3 and C5 convertases. It needs cofactors to elicit its effect. Carboxypeptidase N is another serum protein that greatly reduces the biologic activities of C3a and C5a. S protein, fibronectin, and clusterin are present in the plasma and disable the insertion of C5b-9 into the cell membrane.

The membrane-bound inhibitors elicit their effects at different points of the complement system as well. CD59 is a glycoprotein I (GPI)–linked protein that blocks the insertion of C9 into the membrane-bound C5b-9 and also prevents the polymerization of C9, which effectively inhibits the ability of C5b-9 to cause cell lysis.[3] Membrane cofactor protein and

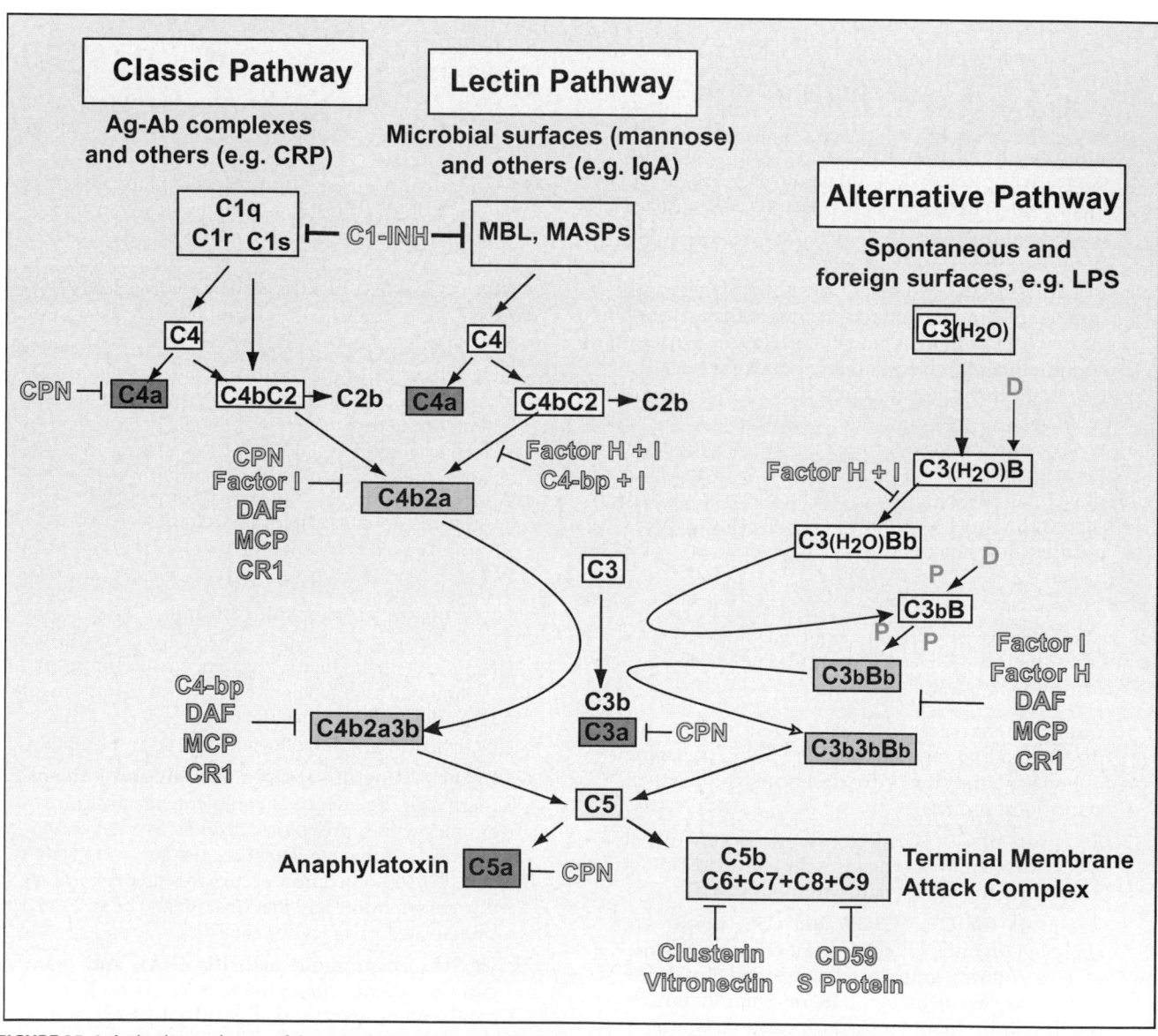

FIGURE 35–1. Activation pathways of the complement system. Complement components C1 to C9 are depicted in square boxes, as well as mannose-binding lectin (MBL) and the MBL-associated serine proteases (MASP). C3 and C5 convertases (classic and alternative) are depicted. The complement split products and anaphylatoxins C3a, C4a, and C5a are depicted. Cofactors of activation are factor D (D) and properdin (P). Inhibitor function is depicted with the symbol (⊥). Membrane-bound inhibitors are CD59, decay-accelerating factor (DAF), complement receptor 1 (CR1), and membrane cofactor protein (MCP). Fluid phase inhibitors are C1 esterase inhibitor (C1-INH), factor H, factor I, clusterin, vitronectin, S protein, and carboxypeptidase N (CPN). IgA, immunoglobulin A; LPS, lipopolysaccharide.

decay-accelerating factor act, either directly or as cofactors for factor I, to deactivate C3 and C5 convertases of all pathways, as well as to cleave C3b and C4b.

COMPLEMENT RECEPTORS

Many of the effects associated with complement activation are achieved by the binding of activated complement products (the anaphylatoxins and opsonic factors such as C3b) to specific receptors. A broad variety of complement receptors exists, although the function of some of them is not yet well established. Often, complement receptors bind various complement activation products with different affinities and thereby elicit a wide range of effects on different cell types (Table 35-1). In general, complement receptors may function as signaling units (transmembrane receptors) for various cell types or as inhibitors of complement activation, especially in their soluble form.

The C1q receptor is present on myeloid cells, endothelial cells, and platelets and can bind C1q as well as MBL. C1qR enhances the phagocytic activity of neutrophils, especially when initiated by Fc receptor activation (binding of immunoglobulin G [IgG] to the cell surface) or by complement receptor 1 (CR1) activation (see later). C1qR may be involved in the up-regulation of cell adhesion molecules on endothelial cells (see Table 35-1). CR1 exists on most blood cell types, as well as on dendritic cells, podocytes in renal glomeruli, and liver Kupffer cells, and also exists in a soluble form. CR1 binds C3b (and the derivative iC3b), as well as C4b and C1q, with high affinity. Many functions have been assigned to CR1.[4] CR1 elicits complement regulatory functions by facilitating, in concert with cofactor I (similar to decay-accelerating factor or membrane cofactor protein), cleavage of C3b and C4b, thereby inactivating C3 and C5 convertases. CR1 is believed to be involved in the clearance of C3b-bound immune complexes in the serum to promote phagocytosis activity and to activate T cells (see Table 35-1).

Complement receptor 2 (CR2) binds iC3b and C3d (cleavage products of C3b) and interacts less effectively with C3b. CR2 is also the receptor that binds Epstein-Barr virus. CR2 is present on B cells, some subtypes of T cells, thymocytes, and a variety of epithelial cells. CR2 is believed to be responsible for a variety of effects, especially activation of B cells and T cells and their adherence when bound to immune complexes.[5]

Complement receptors 3 and 4 (CR3, CR4) are members of the integrin family and are expressed on most myeloid cells. Both receptors bind iC3b and C3b but have affinities to many other ligands (e.g., fibrinogen, intercellular adhesion molecule-1). Besides many other effects elicited by these receptors, they are believed to enhance the phagocytic activity of neutrophils and macrophages.[6]

Whereas some complement receptors interact with a variety of C3 and C3b cleavage products (CR1–4), as well as with C1q (C1qR), other complement receptors specifically recognize the cleavage products C3a (C3aR) and C5a (C5aR). Both receptors are widely expressed on almost all cell types and operate through G-protein activation, leading to phosphorylation of various intracellular signaling pathways, such as the mitogen-activated protein kinase pathways. Most of the known biologic effects of complement ligation are associated with activation of C3aR or C5aR. Recent work suggests that C5aR plays a role in the onset of experimental sepsis and the development of multiorgan failure[7] and that it may be induced in various organs during sepsis by interleukin-6 (IL-6).[8] Similarly, it has been suggested that C3aR plays an important role in the lung during endotoxic shock.[9,10] Blockade of C5aR in experimental sepsis greatly improves survival.[7,11]

BIOLOGIC FUNCTIONS OF THE COMPLEMENT SYSTEM

Obviously, an important and already mentioned biologic effect of the complement system is its opsonic function (C3b), which marks invading microorganisms as "foreign," leading to a targeted host defense response. Ultimately, the formation of C5b-9 leads to the lysis of Gram-negative bacteria, another important defense mechanism of innate immunity. But besides these prominent functions, there are numerous other biologic effects elicited by activation of the complement system (Table 35-2). An important function with broad implications is the regulation of immune complex processing and solubility. Immune complexes often activate complement and bind C3b, resulting in clearance from the circulation via binding with CR1.[12] In addition, complement factors (especially C3b) are responsible for inducing the solubility of immune complexes, and thereby their size.[13] Similarly, the clearance of circulating necrotic or apoptotic

TABLE 35–1. COMPLEMENT RECEPTORS

Receptor	Molecular Weight	Biologic Functions
C1qR	126,000	Enhances Fc-receptor and CR1-mediated phagocytosis, induces adhesion molecule expression on endothelial cells
C5aR (CD88)	50,000	Induces C5a-dependent chemotactic responses of neutrophils, release of granular enzymes and production of superoxide anions in phagocytic cells, vasodilatation, increases in vascular permeability, increases in adhesion molecule expression on endothelial cells, procoagulatory and antifibrinolytic effects, increased expression of various cytokines in different cell types
C3aR	60,000	Similar to C5aR
CR1 (CD35)	190,000-250,000	Binds C3b (and iC3b), C4b, and C1q and facilitates, together with factor I, cleavage of C3 and C5 convertases, clearance of C3b-bound immune complexes in serum; promotes phagocytosis, activation of T cells
CR2 (CD21)	145,000	Binds iC3b and C3d and stimulates B cells (antibody production), Epstein-Barr virus receptor, maintenance of self-tolerance
CR3 (CD11b/CD18)	170,000	Binds iC3b and C3b as well as other molecules (e.g., fibrinogen, intercellular adhesion molecule), integrin-adhesion function, enhances phagocytosis activity of neutrophils, facilitates antibody-mediated phagocytosis
CR4 (CD11c/CD18)	150,000	Similar to CR3

TABLE 35–2. BIOLOGIC ACTIVITIES OF COMPLEMENT ACTIVATION PRODUCTS

Product	Biologic Functions
C1q	Clearance of immune complexes, enhancement of antibody-dependent cellular cytotoxicity, enhancement of phagocytosis in monocytic cells, increase in reactive oxygen species production in neutrophils, adhesive function in fibroblasts
C5a > C3a (>C4a) Anaphylatoxins	Chemotaxis of neutrophils, release of granular enzymes and superoxide anion production in phagocytic cells, increased vascular permeability and vascular dilatation, regulation of cytokine and chemokine production during sepsis, procoagulative and antifibrinolytic effects, pro- and antiapoptotic effects dependent on cell type
C3b	Opsonizing function for bacteria and other invading microorganisms leading to targeted phagocytosis, clearance of immune complexes and circulating apoptotic cells or cell debris, enhancement of antibody production by B cells, regulation of immune tolerance
C5b-9 (MAC)	Permeation of membranes and lysis of bacteria and other invading microorganisms, enhancement of cytokine and adhesion molecule production in various cell types, mediation of tissue injury during ischemia-reperfusion, regulation of cell apoptosis and cell cycle activity, increase in prothrombinase activity on platelets

MAC, membrane attack complex.

cells is believed to be strongly dependent on complement activation and interaction with C1q.[14,15] If, in the presence of complement deficiencies, such clearance becomes inefficient, circulating debris (including immune complexes and dead cells) could act as an autoantigen and possibly initiate the development of autoantibodies, resulting in autoimmune disease.[16] This may explain why most of the deficiencies in the classic complement pathway are associated with the development of SLE.

C5b-9 (membrane attack complex) in sublytic concentrations is involved in the regulation of apoptosis and cell cycle activity.[17] Besides this, membrane attack complex plays a role in the activation of various immune cells via signaling-induced gene transcription, leading to the generation of proinflammatory mediators in nucleated cells and to the generation of reactive oxygen species.[18] C5b-9 has also been demonstrated to make a major contribution to complement-mediated tissue injury after ischemia-reperfusion,[19,20] and it causes relaxation of coronary arteries.[21]

More recently, the biologic effects elicited by the anaphylatoxins C5a and C3a have generated a lot of attention because of their numerous, mostly proinflammatory effects. C5a facilitates a strong chemotactic effect on neutrophils,[22] the release of granular enzymes from phagocytic cells,[23] the production of superoxide anion in neutrophils,[24] and vasodilatation and increases in vascular permeability,[25] as well as expression of adhesion molecules, in endothelial cells.

Recent studies provide evidence of "cross-talk" between the complement system and the coagulation system, suggesting that C5a may be involved in procoagulant effects and antifibrinolytic effects during the onset of sepsis.[26] C5a and C5b-9 have been shown to increase the expression of tissue factor on endothelial cells and monocytes, and C5b-9 has been demonstrated to increase prothrombinase activity on endothelial cells. These observations provide a possible explanation for the described cross-talk.

Even though the complement system is regarded as one of the most powerful defense functions of innate immunity, it also plays an important role in the activation of the adaptive immune system in terms of antigen presentation and antibody production.[27,28] Complement activation (especially C3b deposition) is believed to enhance the antibody production of B cells[29] and to increase the survival time of B cells in various settings of inflammatory disease.

In addition to its affiliation with inflammatory responses, recent studies provide evidence that the complement system plays a role in modulating cellular responses and cell-cell interactions that are crucial to early development and cell differentiation.[30]

GENETIC DEFICIENCIES IN THE COMPLEMENT SYSTEM

Genetically based deficiencies in complement proteins or cofactors of complement activation are rare and, in many cases, are compatible with human life only in the heterozygous state,[31] because most of these defects are inherited in an autosomal recessive manner. Clinically, most patients with deficiencies in complement proteins or cofactors of complement activation have an increased risk of infection (Table 35-3), with meningococcus being the predominant bacterial infection in the case of complete deficiency of C5.[32,33] Generally, there is a distinction among deficiencies of the classic and MBL pathways (C1q, C1r, C1s, C2, C4, MBL), deficiencies of the alternative pathway (factors D and B, properdin), deficiencies of factor C3 together with factors H and I (all resulting in low C3 concentrations), and deficiencies of late-acting complement components (C5, C6, C7, C8, C9). Each of these groups of deficiencies presents with a distinctive pattern of bacterial infection, as described in detail elsewhere.[34] Deficiencies in the classic pathway group are all associated with an increased occurrence of SLE. Infections that occur in the presence of deficiencies involving classic pathway proteins, as well as in deficiencies in C3 and in alternative pathway proteins, are often severe and life threatening (see Table 35-3). Deficiencies in the terminal, late-acting complement components are associated with meningococcal meningitis, but individuals with one of the distal pathway deficiencies are often asymptomatic during their lifetimes. In general, the treatment for complement deficiencies is linked to prophylactic immunization, especially with tetravalent meningococcal vaccine and *Haemophilus influenzae* vaccine. Assessment for complement deficiencies usually is not done during routine screenings.

Deficiencies for the receptors CR1 and CR2 have not been reported, but defective CR3 or CR4 (heterodimeric β_2 integrins) due to mutations in the CD18 β chain results in so-called leukocyte adhesion deficiency, which is linked to frequent and severe bacterial infections.

In contrast to the rarity of deficiencies in complement components, deficiencies in inhibitory proteins of the

TABLE 35–3. GENETICALLY DETERMINED DEFICIENCIES IN THE COMPLEMENT SYSTEM AND RELATED CLINICAL SYMPTOMS

Deficient Component	Clinical Manifestations
Classic pathway (C1q, C1r, C1s, C2, C4)	SLE, glomerulonephritis, recurrent severe infections starting in early childhood (streptococcal pneumonia predominant)
Alternative pathway (factors B, D, P)	Reduced complement activation ability; infection (predominantly meningococcal) starting in adolescence—for factor D especially, often life-threatening
C3, factors H and I	Life-threatening recurrent bacterial infections (especially oropharynx, pulmonary, meninges), often leading to sepsis starting in early childhood; reduced clearance of immune complexes
C5-C9	Predominantly meningococcal infections or gonococcal sepsis, usually in adolescence; approximately 50% recurrent infections; rarely life-threatening. SLE associated in some cases
CR4, CR3 (integrins)	Leukocyte adhesion deficiency syndrome, bacterial infections rarely recurrent
C1-INH	Hereditary or acquired angioedema; also associated with SLE and autoimmune glomerulonephritis
GPI-anchoring protein (affecting CD59 and DAF function)	Paroxysmal nocturnal hemoglobinuria accompanied by thrombosis, iron deficiency anemia (manifestation in young adulthood)

DAF, decay-accelerating factor; GPI, glycoprotein I; INH, inhibitor; SLE, systemic lupus erythematosus.

complement system are more common. C1-esterase inhibitor deficiency can be either inherited (by autosomal dominant mutations) or acquired (formation of autoantibodies).[35] Both forms lead to the clinical picture of angioedema, which is associated with recurrent episodes of edema of the subcutaneous tissue and gastrointestinal tract and often life-threatening edema of the upper airways.[34] Experimental evidence suggests that both complement activation and kallikrein activation (generating bradykinin) are linked to edema in patients with hereditary or acquired angioedema.[36]

Another well-known clinical symptom associated with defects in the inhibitory part of the complement system is paroxysmal nocturnal hemoglobinuria.[37,38] Patients with this disorder develop recurrent hemolytic episodes involving all types of bone marrow–derived blood cells. The defect is a genetic deficiency in a GPI anchoring protein, which is necessary for the proper function of the GPI-linked membrane-bound complement inhibitors CD59 and decay-accelerating factor.[39] This defect results in a high rate of membrane buildup of C5b-9, which is usually controlled by CD59 and decay-accelerating factor. This results in a high rate of lysis of red blood cells especially, as well as other cell types such as granulocytes, lymphocytes, and monocytes. Patients with paroxysmal nocturnal hemoglobinuria often experience an increased incidence of thrombosis and related complications.

SEPSIS

The complement system has been demonstrated to play a key and harmful role in the onset of sepsis in rodents. Microorganisms in the bloodstream or their products, such as lipopolysaccharide, can cause complement activation. Given the well-known variety of proinflammatory effects of complement activation, it is not surprising that sudden "overactivation" of this powerful system can result in serious, harmful consequences in the host. Conversely, experimental data involving C3 and C4 knockout animals suggest that an intact complement system (at least involving C3 and C4) may be required to a certain extent to clear endotoxin and bacteria.[40,41] The harmful effects of complement activation in the context of sepsis have been ascribed to excessive generation of the potent anaphylatoxin C5a. Various clinical studies indicate that complement activation occurs during human sepsis, as exemplified by elevated serum levels of C3a and C5a. In some studies, these levels were significantly higher in nonsurviving septic patients and in those with multiorgan failure than in those with less severe sepsis and survivors.[42-44] Experimental studies in primates suggested some time ago that blockade of C5a by antibodies could significantly attenuate Escherichia coli–induced septic shock and acute respiratory distress syndrome (ARDS) in monkeys.[45,46] Studies in rats suggested that lipopolysaccharide-induced shock could be mimicked by the injection of C5a, whereas blockade of C5a with antibody attenuated lipopolysaccharide-induced responses.[47] Blockade of C5a during experimental sepsis was found to be protective in rats,[48] and in another study, the protective effects of C5a blockade during sepsis were associated with the prevention of multiorgan failure.[49] In these studies, C5a generation had to be inhibited early in the course of sepsis to protect against multiorgan failure and death. The exact role of C5a at the onset of sepsis has yet to be determined, but experimental evidence suggests that when C5a is generated in excessive amounts, it may be involved in the shutdown of crucial innate immune functions of neutrophils (generation of reactive oxygen species, release of granular enzymes, phagocytosis, chemotaxis), increasing the susceptibility for infection in the later stages of sepsis. Production of IL-6 and adhesion molecules is also linked to C5a. C5a can interact directly with endothelial cells and myeloid cells. C5aR has been shown to be up-regulated in an IL-6–dependent manner on various cell types (endothelial, epithelial) during experimental sepsis, potentially intensifying the effects of circulating C5a.[7] It remains to be determined whether such findings can be extrapolated to humans with sepsis and whether potential therapeutic targets can be derived from such findings.

The naturally occurring inhibitor of the classic complement and lectin pathways, C1-esterase inhibitor, also inhibits clotting factor XIIa–mediated contact activation of the coagulation system. It has been shown to be decreased in humans with sepsis.[50] Initial pilot clinical trials involved the infusion of C1 inhibitor into septic patients, with some suggestion of benefit in these patients.[51,52] A randomized, double-blind trial suggested that the administration of C1 inhibitor attenuated renal impairment in patients with severe sepsis or septic shock.[53] Larger phase II and III clinical trials will have to be conducted to confirm such findings.

ACUTE RESPIRATORY DISTRESS SYNDROME

A role for the complement system in ARDS has been suggested, based on elevated plasma levels of C3a and C5a in patients with ARDS. These levels were correlated with neutrophil aggregation and lung dysfunction.[54,55] Treatment with anti-C5a antibodies in an animal (primate) model of ARDS resulted in improved oxygenation and circulatory parameters.[45] Serum levels of C5a and C3a in humans with ARDS may reflect the severity of lung injury and might be useful for predicting clinical outcome.[56] Based on these and other findings, a phase I clinical trial used recombinant soluble CR1 in patients with ARDS,[57] but phase II trials will be necessary to determine the potential benefits of such treatment.

ISCHEMIA-REPERFUSION AND ORGAN TRANSPLANTATION

Clinical settings of ischemia-reperfusion, such as myocardial infarction, artery stenosis, thrombosis, and dissecting aortic aneurysm, as well as solid organ transplantation and heart surgery, are accompanied by rapid changes in cell homeostasis, leading to perturbations in signaling pathways and surface molecule expression. Depending on the time and severity of ischemia-reperfusion, toxic products accumulate intracellularly, leading to apoptosis and necrosis, causing loss of organ function. Depending on the duration and severity of ischemia-reperfusion, the injury may be completely or partially reversible. After the reestablishment of blood flow to the organ, oxygenation occurs, and repair mechanisms may be set into motion. During reperfusion, activation of the complement system and incoming neutrophils contribute to further cell injury; such injury appears to be dependent on the amount of complement and neutrophil activation. Experimental data suggest that complement products of the classic pathway are associated with ischemia-reperfusion cardiac injury in rats,[58] rabbits,[59] and humans,[60] and that complement depletion reduces infarct size.[61] Different strategies to block complement activation in experimental settings of ischemia-reperfusion have been successful in terms of reducing organ damage and impairing function. In experimental models of acute myocardial ischemia-reperfusion, successful strategies include the application of soluble CR1 (sCR1),[62] C1 inhibitor,[63-65] blocking antibodies to C5[66] or C5a,[67,68] a small molecular inhibitor of C1s,[69] and antibodies to MBL.[70] These and other findings led to the first successful use of C1 inhibitors in patients receiving emergency surgery for failed percutaneous transluminal coronary angioplasty in 1998. In another study, C1 inhibitor was administered to neonates undergoing transposition of the large arteries, with the beneficial effect of less inflammatory response in the treated group.[71] These preliminary data have not been confirmed in larger clinical trials. Another promising strategy is the use of monoclonal antibodies to C5, which may benefit patients undergoing cardiopulmonary bypass procedures.[72] In these studies, patients treated with anti-C5 showed significantly reduced postoperative myocardial injury, fewer cognitive defects, and less blood loss, suggesting a range of benefits. These findings need to be replicated in large phase II clinical trials.

It has also been suggested that complement activation is a major mediator of hyperacute organ rejection after transplantation. In an experimental model of lung allotransplantation, the administration of sCR1 significantly limited the amount of acute and subacute rejection.[73] No clinical data exist demonstrating the potential benefits of such a strategy in organ transplantation in humans, however. It is not clear to what extent the different complement pathways contribute to ischemia-reperfusion–related injury (reviewed in reference 74).

AUTOIMMUNE DISEASES

Various autoimmune diseases are associated with circulating immune complexes and evidence of complement activation. A possible role of complement activation in the development and progression of autoimmune diseases has been suggested. C1q, C4, C3, and C5b-9 have been found in association with tissue damage in SLE, RA, Sjögren's syndrome, Behçet's syndrome, bullous pemphigoid, dermatomyositis, myasthenia gravis, Alzheimer's disease, multiple sclerosis, and other neurologic diseases. Tissues often affected by complement activation in these autoimmune diseases are skin, kidney, choroid plexus, blood vessels (endothelial cells), and skeletal muscle. A strategy to target complement activation in these diseases in a clinical setting has not yet been developed. A few prominent examples are discussed here.

SYSTEMIC LUPUS ERYTHEMATOSUS

As mentioned earlier, complement deficiencies, especially in the classic pathway, are often associated with SLE. Indeed, C4 serum levels in SLE patients are often reduced (consumptive hypocomplementemia) and may be a useful monitor of disease progression.[34] About one third of SLE patients also have autoantibodies to C1q. In addition, in SLE nephritis, C3 deposition often occurs in kidney glomerular mesangial cells and is strongly associated with the severity of the nephritis. Blockade of C5 in a rodent model of SLE resulted in improved survival and reduced proteinuria and glomerular damage.[75] SLE mice that were deficient in factor B (alternative complement pathway) also showed less renal disease progression.[76]

RHEUMATOID ARTHRITIS

In the synovial fluid of RA patients, elevated levels of C5b-9 are frequent.[77,78] Interaction of C5b-9 with synovial fibroblasts in RA has been demonstrated.[79] In an experimental model of RA in rodents, blockade of the late complement components with monoclonal antibodies to C5 resulted in amelioration of disease activity and partial reversal of joint destruction.[80] Similar results were found in rodents treated with recombinant sCR1.[81] Genetic deficiency of C3, C5, or factor B significantly decreased joint destruction in RA models in rodents.[82-84] Accordingly, it has been suggested that the alternative complement pathway plays a critical role, in contrast to the classic pathway.[84] Recent studies demonstrated that C5a and its receptor, C5aR, are important mediators in experimental RA settings; blockade of C5aR with an oral antagonist or C5aR gene knockout resulted in greatly reduced joint destruction in such studies.[85,86] The complement system, therefore, appears to play a major role in the induction and progression of RA. The occurrence of C-reactive protein may be important for complement activation in RA in humans.[87]

IMMUNE COMPLEX GLOMERULONEPHRITIS

Circulating immune complex (deposited in a subepithelial location) and locally formed immune complex (deposited subendothelially or mesangially) are the cause of various types of glomerular diseases (reviewed in detail elsewhere).[34] A pathogenetic role for complement activation in immune complex–induced glomerulonephritis can be assumed from experimental Heymann glomerulonephritis models in which inhibition of complement activation resulted in attenuated acute and chronic renal injury. Genetic knockout of C3 as well as C4 in mice also resulted in beneficial effects in a glomerulonephritis model.[88,89] Similar results were obtained when various C3 inhibitors were overexpressed.[90,91]

ALZHEIMER'S DISEASE

This degenerative disease is characterized by "senile plaques," consisting of neurofibrillary tangles and interstitial deposition of β-amyloid in the brain tissue and cerebral blood vessels. In Alzheimer's disease, the presence of C1q, C3, C4, and C5b-9 has been demonstrated in senile plaques, suggesting a pathogenetic role for the complement system.[92,93] Other studies demonstrated that β-amyloid (peptides 39-43) effectively activates the classic complement pathway via C1q.[94] In addition, it was demonstrated that the production of C1 inhibitor in brain cells is reduced in senile plaques from Alzheimer's patients.[95] A recent study suggested a prominent role for C5aR in Alzheimer's disease progression,[96] and activation of the complement system may also be a key factor.[97] Recent studies provide evidence of the potential beneficial role of the complement product C3 in a mouse model of Alzheimer's disease; overexpression of a soluble complement receptor-related protein y (sCrry), which initiates C3 activation, caused increased deposition of β-amyloid, suggesting a possible regulatory role for C3.[98] Even though the complement system appears to be involved in the progression of Alzheimer's disease, it is not clear to what extent therapeutic strategies targeting activation of the complement system might be beneficial.

ACUTE BURN INJURY

Evidence of activation of the complement system in patients with acute burn injuries was found in the 1970s.[99] Subsequent studies demonstrated early consumptive depletion of C1q, C3, C4, and C5 after burn injury[100,101] and the generation of C3a.[102] Neutrophil activation is related to increased expression of CR1 and CR3 on neutrophils in burn patients.[103] In rodent models of burn injury, complement activation and deposition at the site of tissue injury were also noted,[104,105] and the generation of hydroxyl radicals was suggested as an initiating mechanism.[106] Additional activation of the alternative complement pathway in a murine model of burn injury worsened the outcome.[107] The vascular injury in the lungs of mice following thermal skin injury revealed a strict dependency on the generation of C5a, suggesting that this anaphylatoxin is a major player in burn-associated tissue injury.[108] In subsequent studies, complement inhibition with sCR1 in a rodent model of thermal injury demonstrated significant reduction in associated lung injury (reduced vascular lack of albumin and reduced hemorrhage).[109] In a thermal injury model in pigs, complement inhibition with C1 inhibitor was also reported to be beneficial,[110] perhaps related to reduced bacterial translocation in the gut barrier after skin burn injury[111] and significant reduction in vascular leak.[112] Clinical trials to confirm these findings have yet to be done.

ACUTE TRAUMA

Trauma patients often show elevated levels of inflammatory mediators in the blood. Tissue injury is believed to trigger an acute inflammatory response, especially by activation of the complement system. Although the exact mechanisms of such activation are not yet understood, it has been reported that patients with traumatic brain injury show elevated levels of the complement components C3 and factor B in cerebrospinal fluid.[113] An important role of the complement system has also been suggested in patients with multiple trauma, in whom elevated levels of complement activation products have been found. Elevated C3a levels reportedly correlate with outcome.[114,115] The complement system's role in organ dysfunction has been suggested in animal models of closed head injury.[116] One study reported that C5aR was induced on neurons after closed head injury in mice, mediated by tumor necrosis factor and lymphotoxin-α.[117] Recent studies suggest that in patients with head injury, elevated levels of C3b and C5b-9 are present,[113,118] the latter correlating with blood-brain barrier dysfunction.[119] Despite the strong evidence for the role of complement activation in trauma-related tissue injury, only one study exists demonstrating the beneficial effects of complement inhibition (using C1 inhibitor) in a murine model of acute trauma.[120] Whether therapeutic intervention (complement inhibition) in patients with acute trauma would be beneficial remains speculative. If so, the timing of drug administration would be crucial for achieving maximal clinical success.

CONCLUSION

Activation of the complement system appears to be a double-edged sword. Although complement activation is a crucial defensive function of the innate immune system in combating invading microorganisms, it also appears to be responsible for a variety of harmful effects. A broad spectrum of stimuli can activate the complement system, leading to the production of powerful proinflammatory and potentially harmful mediators such as the anaphylatoxin C5a and C5b-9. The complement system is clearly involved in the progression of autoimmune diseases and plays a role in acute inflammatory conditions such as sepsis, burn injury, trauma, and ischemia-reperfusion–related injury (e.g., myocardial ischemia and organ transplantation). In all these disorders, inhibition of complement activation has been demonstrated to have beneficial effects in experimental settings. Only preliminary data from clinical studies of complement inhibition in acute inflammatory disorders are available. In these studies, C1 inhibitor (in sepsis trials) and sCR1 and monoclonal antibodies against C5 (in trials of cardiopulmonary bypass) have been used and suggest potential benefits. However, larger clinical trials employing these interventions are needed.

Because the complement system is involved in so many different physiologic systems and defense mechanisms, each acute inflammatory disorder likely requires a specific target in the complement system for optimal beneficial effects. More research is needed to understand the precise contribution of the various complement activation pathways and the specific complement activation products involved in clinical disorders. General problems of drug discovery (half-life, side effects, safety, costs) and the potential problem of increased susceptibility to infection are important considerations if complement activation is to be inhibited (discussed in detail in reference 121).

Recent experimental data suggest the benefits of inhibiting C5a or C5aR with antibodies or with small molecular chemical inhibitors (especially for ischemia-reperfusion injury, sepsis, and RA). Because this approach does not target complement activation in general (as does C1 inhibitor or sCR1) but rather targets a more specific activation product downstream, this strategy appears to be promising and needs to be evaluated in a clinical setting.

Given the impressive experimental evidence of the beneficial effects of complement inhibition in various acute inflammatory (and other) disorders, it seems likely that successful therapeutic strategies will be developed in clinical settings in humans in the near future.

ANNOTATED REFERENCES

Barrington R, Zhang M, Fischer M, et al: The role of complement in inflammation and adaptive immunity. Immunol Rev 2001;180:5-15.
This paper describes the role of complement in both innate and adaptive immunity.

Czermak BJ, Sarma V, Pierson CL, et al: Protective effects of C5a blockade in sepsis. Nat Med 1999;5:788-792.
This study set the stage for defining the detrimental role of C5a in experimental sepsis.

Nakae H, Endo S, Inada K, et al: Serum complement levels and severity of sepsis. Res Commun Chem Pathol Pharmacol 1994;84:189-195.
This report stresses the finding of complement activation products in the sera from humans with sepsis.

Stahl G, Xu Y, Hau L, et al: Role of the alternative pathway in ischemia/reperfusion injury. Am J Pathol 2003;162:449-455; and Vakeva AP, Agah A, Rollins SA, et al: Myocardial infarction and apoptosis after myocardial ischemia and reperfusion: Role of the terminal complement components and inhibition by anti-C5 therapy. Circulation 1998;97:2259-2267.
These reports present evidence of the important role of complement in ischemia-reperfusion injury involving the gut and the myocardium (in animals and humans).

Volanakis JE, Frank MM: The Human Complement System in Health and Disease, 1st ed. New York, Marcel Dekker, 1998.
This is an excellent and extensive review of the protective functions of complement and its role in various inflammatory diseases.

Chapter 36

CYTOPATHIC HYPOXIA: MITOCHONDRIAL DYSFUNCTION IN SEPSIS

Mitchell P. Fink

KEY POINTS

1. Adenosine triphosphate (ATP) is the **energy currency of the cell.**

2. **Aerobic generation of ATP** by a process termed oxidative phosphorylation is carried out in cells by specialized organelles, the mitochondria.

3. Data from studies using animal models of sepsis or biopsies of human skeletal muscle support the view that **severe sepsis is associated with derangements in cellular respiration and mitochondrial dysfunction**; this phenomenon has been termed cytopathic hypoxia.

4. Although it is now well established that mitochondrial function is impaired in sepsis, **it remains to be determined whether cytopathic hypoxia is an epiphenomenon or one that actually contributes to organ dysfunction and mortality.**

According to the first law of thermodynamics, the total amount of energy in a system remains constant before and after any sort of transforming event. The second law of thermodynamics holds that even though the total amount of energy does not change after a transforming event, the total amount of usable energy—the Gibbs free energy (G)—always decreases. In accordance with the second law, all reversible chemical reactions proceed in a direction that results in a net decrease in the Gibbs free energy for the system; in other words, the change in G (ΔG) is always less than zero. When cells in living systems need to carry out a reaction for which ΔG is positive, they couple the reaction to another reaction that is energetically favorable (i.e., characterized by $\Delta G < 0$). If the algebraic sum of the ΔGs for the two coupled reactions is negative, formation of the desired product can proceed. Within cells, the exergonic reaction that drives the formation of the desired product is almost always the hydrolysis of the terminal pyrophosphate ester linkage of adenosine triphosphate (ATP) to yield adenosine diphosphate (ADP) and inorganic phosphate anion (Pi). The hydrolysis of ATP also drives other energy-requiring processes in cells, such as the active pumping of solutes against a concentration gradient across a membrane barrier. Thus, for proper functioning, all cells need a steady supply of ATP. Stated another way, ATP is the energy currency of the cell.

ATP can be generated in cells as a result of both aerobic and anaerobic processes. Anaerobic generation of ATP, or of the energetically equivalent compound guanosine triphosphate (GTP), occurs in both the cytosol and the mitochondria as a result of the phosphorylation reactions that are catalyzed by the enzymes phosphoglycerate kinase, pyruvate kinase, and succinyl coenzyme A synthase. Aerobic generation of ATP occurs in the mitochondria as a result of a carefully orchestrated series of reactions that effectively couple the oxidation of substrates by molecular oxygen (O_2) to the phosphorylation of ADP to form ATP.

Good "reducing agents" are elements or compounds that have a strong propensity to donate electrons to another element or compound. Conversely, good "oxidizing agents" are elements or compounds that avidly accept electrons. Molecular oxygen is a very potent oxidizing agent. Two strong reducing agents—the reduced forms of nicotinamide adenine dinucleotide (NADH) and flavin adenine dinucleotide ($FADH_2$)—are produced in cells during certain enzymatic reactions that occur during glycolysis and the citric acid cycle. In mitochondria, these two reducing agents are oxidized by O_2, and the energy released during this process is used to drive the formation of ATP.

The reaction of a strong reducing agent, such as NADH, with a powerful oxidizing agent, such as O_2, releases a large amount of energy (i.e., ΔG is very negative). To take optimal advantage of this highly exergonic redox reaction and capture as much of the energy released as possible in a usable form (i.e., the high-energy terminal pyrophosphate bond of ATP), mitochondria "step down" the reducing potential of NADH (and $FADH_2$) in stages. Thus, the electrons are not transferred from NADH to O_2 all at once; rather, they are transferred through a series of intermediate compounds, called electron carriers, that have progressively lower reducing potentials. Several of the electron carriers involved in the mitochondrial respiratory chain are organized as complexes (called complexes I to IV) located within the inner mitochondrial membrane (Fig. 36-1). These complexes use the energy released during electron transfer to actively pump hydrogen ions from the mitochondrial matrix into the intermembrane space, thereby generating an electrochemical gradient across the inner mitochondrial membrane. The presence of this gradient drives hydrogen ions through a mitochondrial enzyme, F_oF_1-ATPase, that catalyzes the formation of ATP from ADP and Pi.

For each mole of glucose metabolized to carbon dioxide and water, the net yield of ATP from substrate-level (anaerobic) phosphorylation reactions is 4 moles of ATP, whereas

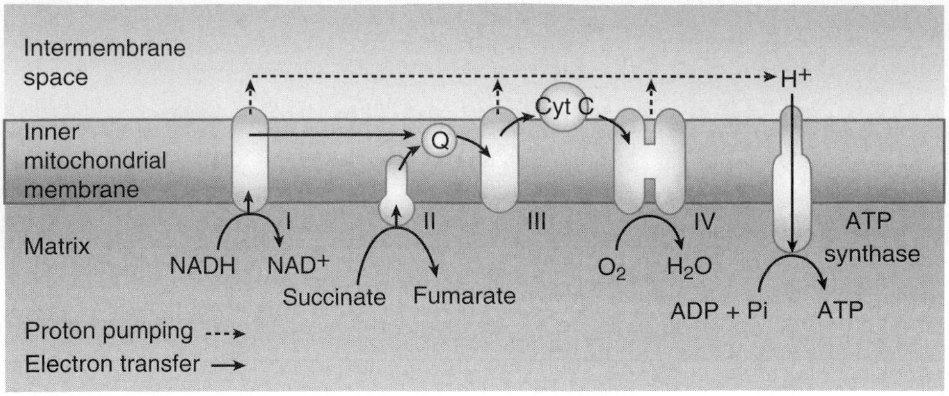

FIGURE 36–1. Diagrammatic representation of mitochondrial electron transport and proton pumping across the inner mitochondrial membrane. Oxidation or conversion of succinate to fumarate requires reducing equivalents supplied by flavin adenine dinucleotide (FADH$_2$). ADP, adenosine diphosphate; ATP, adenosine triphosphate; Cyt C, cytochrome *c*; NAD, nicotinamide adenine dinucleotide; NADH, reduced form of NAD; Pi, inorganic phosphate; Q, ubiquinone. (Adapted from Brealey D, Singer M: Mitochondrial dysfunction in sepsis. Curr Inf Dis Rpt 2003;5:365-371.)

the net yield of ATP from oxidative phosphorylation reactions is 32 moles of ATP. Thus, oxidative metabolism in normally functioning mitochondria is far more efficient at producing ATP than is anaerobic metabolism, and many cell types, such as hepatocytes, neurons, and cardiac myocytes, are dependent on a steady supply of O$_2$.

EVIDENCE FOR IMPAIRED MITOCHONDRIAL RESPIRATION IN SEPSIS

Convincing data support the view that early, aggressive efforts to improve systemic O$_2$ delivery by administering intravenous fluids, packed red blood cells, and inotropic agents can improve outcome for patients with septic shock.[1] By the same token, however, efforts to improve systemic O$_2$ delivery later in the course of sepsis are at best ineffective[2,3] and at worst deleterious.[4] If improving perfusion and O$_2$ delivery in patients with established sepsis fails to improve survival or prevent organ system dysfunction, one might wonder whether alterations in energy metabolism are important at all in the pathogenesis of the syndrome.[5] Alternatively, one could hypothesize that cellular energetics are deranged in sepsis not just because O$_2$ delivery is impaired but also because the cells' ability to use available O$_2$ is compromised. The term *cytopathic hypoxia* has been used to describe such an acquired intrinsic derangement in cellular respiration.[6,7] Although the clinical significance of this phenomenon has not been established with certainty, accumulated evidence supports the notion that cytopathic hypoxia occurs when certain cell types are exposed to proinflammatory cytokines or sera from septic patients in vitro.[8-10] Further, it is fairly clear that mitochondrial function is impaired in experimental animals with sepsis or endotoxemia.[11-15]

Measurements of Tissue Oxygen Partial Pressure and Cytochrome a,a_3 Redox State. Tissue hypoxia is an expected correlate of any of the three classic causes of impaired cellular aerobic metabolism identified by Barcroft more than 80 years ago.[16] Thus, when the delivery of O$_2$ decreases on the basis of low arterial oxygen tension (PO$_2$), anemia, or hypoperfusion, cells extract a greater fraction of the available O$_2$ in an effort to defend aerobic ATP production. As a consequence, the distribution of tissue PO$_2$ values shifts to the left (i.e., closer to 0). In contrast, when ATP production is impaired as a result of an intrinsic derangement in cellular respiration, cells extract less O$_2$ per unit time from the available supply. The expected consequence of this change in O$_2$ extraction is a rightward shift in the tissue PO$_2$ distribution (i.e., toward higher values).

One line of evidence that supports the concept of cytopathic hypoxia comes from studies measuring tissue PO$_2$ in patients or experimental animals. If tissue hypoperfusion is a major factor contributing to cellular dysfunction in sepsis, septic shock, or endotoxemia, one would predict the detection of abnormally low tissue PO$_2$ values in these conditions. However, if classic tissue hypoxia is not important, or if the main problem is an intrinsic derangement in cellular O$_2$ use, one would predict normal or even supranormal tissue PO$_2$ values in animals or patients with sepsis. Indeed, observations of this sort have been reported.

Astiz and colleagues used cecal ligation and puncture (CLP) in a rat model of sepsis and showed that mean skeletal muscle PO$_2$ was similar in septic animals and normal controls, provided that the rats with peritonitis were infused with albumin solution to expand intravascular volume.[17] In a conceptually similar study, Hotchkiss and coworkers used a novel approach to determine whether tissue hypoxia occurs after the induction of sepsis in rats.[18] Tissue PO$_2$ was not measured directly but was estimated by measuring the retention of [18F]-fluoroisonidazole, a lipophilic 2-nitroimidazole derivative that is irreversibly bound to intracellular macromolecules under hypoxic, but not normoxic, conditions. Retention of [18F]-fluoroisonidazole in a variety of tissues, such as skeletal muscle and liver, was similar in septic rats and nonseptic controls. These data provide very strong evidence that sepsis in rats is not associated with tissue hypoxia.

Some data support the even more remarkable conclusion that tissue PO$_2$ actually increases in sepsis relative to normal values. For example, VanderMeer and colleagues used a porcine model to investigate the effects of endotoxemia on intestinal mucosal PO$_2$.[19] When anesthetized pigs were infused with lipopolysaccharide (LPS) and simultaneously resuscitated to maintain normal cardiac output, mean mucosal PO$_2$ increased significantly. Similarly, Rosser and coworkers reported that bladder mucosal PO$_2$ increased in rats challenged with LPS.[12] The same pattern has been observed in humans. Boekstegers and colleagues showed that the distribution of PO$_2$ values in skeletal muscle was shifted to the left in patients with cardiogenic shock, as expected, but was shifted to the right (i.e., to supranormal values) in patients with septic shock.[20] Similar findings were reported by Sair and associates.[21] These data are consistent with the view that cellular utilization of O$_2$ is impaired in patients with sepsis and septic shock.

This same idea is supported by another related study. Simonsen and colleagues used near-infrared spectroscopy to monitor the redox state of the terminal element of the mitochondrial respiratory chain, cytochrome oxidase, in skeletal muscle cells of baboons rendered septic by an infusion of viable *Escherichia coli*.[22] The functional status of cytochrome oxidase was monitored by periodically causing temporary skeletal muscle ischemia using a proximally placed tourniquet. Inflating the tourniquet caused a decrease in the spectroscopic signal from oxidized cytochrome oxidase, whereas deflating the tourniquet resulted in an increase in the signal from the oxidized enzyme. Early in the sepsis protocol (i.e., at 6 hours), the rate of cytochrome oxidase reduction following tourniquet ischemia was the same as at baseline, although the rate of reoxidation following the release of ischemia was slowed. These data are consistent with the notion that delivery of O_2 to the tissue is decreased early in sepsis. Later in the sepsis protocol (e.g., at 18 hours), the rate of cytochrome oxidase reduction during tourniquet ischemia was markedly slowed, a finding that was thought to be consistent with either a defect in the enzyme's ability to accept electrons from O_2 or a limitation in the availability of reducing equivalents (i.e., NADH, $FADH_2$, or both). These data are particularly interesting because they suggest that cytopathic hypoxia is not present early in sepsis but develops after the septic process has evolved for many hours. These temporal considerations might explain the positive results obtained in a clinical trial of early, goal-directed hemodynamic support by Rivers and associates[1] and the negative results obtained in similar trials that included patients with more established critical illnesses.[3,4]

Not all studies of sepsis have obtained data showing that tissue PO_2 values are normal or increased. Indeed, contrary findings have been reported by a number of investigators. For example, two studies showed that intestinal mucosal PO_2 decreased when experimental animals were infused with LPS to a sepsis-like state.[23,24] Similarly, Sair and colleagues reported that skeletal muscle PO_2 decreased markedly in a rat model of endotoxemia.[25] Differences in the timing of the measurements (i.e., early versus late sepsis) or in the adequacy of resuscitation might explain the discordant findings regarding tissue PO_2 levels in different studies.

Measurements of Mitochondrial Respiration. The colorless compound 3-(4,5-dimethylthiazol-2-yl)-2,5-diphenyl tetrazolium bromide (MTT) is reduced by functioning mitochondria to a blue dye (MTT-formazan). Concentration of the blue product can be determined spectrophotometrically. Thus, reduction of MTT is a convenient, albeit indirect, way to assess mitochondrial function. In 1974, Bankey and coworkers used this approach to assess mitochondrial function in cocultures of rat hepatoctyes and rat liver macrophages.[26] Sequential stimulation of the cultures with a proinflammatory cytokine, interleukin-6 (IL-6), and then LPS decreased MTT reduction by about 50%. Similar results were reported more recently by Zingarelli and colleagues, who showed that MTT reduction is decreased in cultured macrophages and vascular smooth muscle cells after incubation with a proinflammatory cytokine, interferon gamma (IFN-γ), plus LPS.[27]

Unno and coworkers used the reduction of MTT to MTT-formazan to assess mitochondrial function in vivo.[28] In this study, rats were injected with saline or a low dose of LPS that caused neither hypotension nor mortality. Twenty-four hours later, the lumen of the intestine was loaded with a solution of MTT. After a 30-minute incubation period, the epithelial layer was scraped off the intestine, and the concentration of MTT-formazan in enterocytes was determined spectrophotometrically. MTT reduction was significantly lower in enterocytes from endotoxemic rats than in those from normal controls. When the endotoxemic rats were

treated with aminoguanidine, a drug that blocks inducible nitric oxide synthase (iNOS), MTT reduction was restored to normal levels. This latter finding suggests that impaired mitochondrial respiration in sepsis is mediated, at least in part, by a mechanism that depends on increased production of the mediator, nitric oxide (NO), due to up-regulated expression of the enzyme, iNOS.

The MTT assay reflects the activity of a number of different dehydrogenases, particularly succinate dehydrogenase,[29] and is not a direct measure of mitochondrial O_2 consumption per se. Several studies have obtained more direct evidence that cellular or mitochondrial respiration is impaired in animals with sepsis or endotoxemia. For example, Kantrow and associates showed that hepatocytes isolated from septic rats consumed significantly less O_2 than did hepatocytes from nonseptic control rats.[30] Later, King and colleagues showed that ileal mucosal O_2 consumption is impaired in endotoxemic rats.[11] In these studies, rats were injected with either LPS or a similar volume of the saline vehicle. Eight hours later, a strip of ileal mucosa was obtained from the animals and mounted in a polarographic chamber to determine the rate of O_2 consumption (Fig. 36-2). The decrease in the rate of ileal mucosal O_2 consumption induced by LPS injection was not due to decreased delivery, because the measurements were made ex vivo with the tissue suspended in a well-oxygenated buffer. If the endotoxemic rats were treated with aminoguanidine to block iNOS activity, normal ileal mucosal O_2 consumption was preserved. Thus, these findings support the notion that the development of cytopathic hypoxia in LPS-challenged rats requires iNOS-dependent NO production.

Chen and coworkers evaluated cardiac muscle mitochondrial function in rats with sepsis induced by CLP.[31] As in some previous studies, these investigators evaluated mitochondrial function both early after the onset of sepsis (9 hours after CLP) and later (18 hours after CLP). Rather than measuring cellular or mitochondrial O_2 consumption, these investigators used standard enzymatic assays to determine the activities of

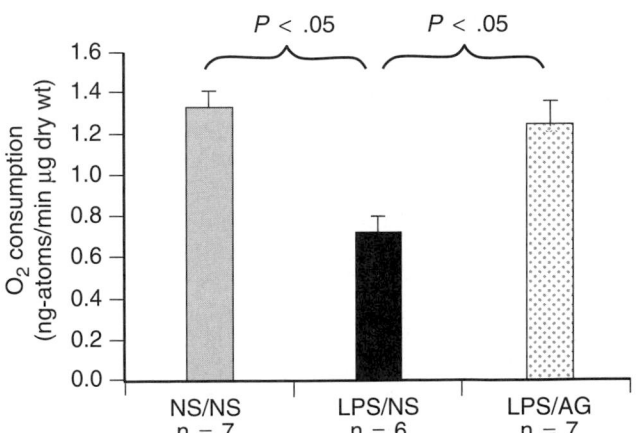

FIGURE 36–2. Effect of lipopolysaccharide (LPS) on ileal mucosal oxygen (O_2) consumption. Rats in the NS/NS group were injected at 0 hours with normal saline (NS) and treated with NS. Rats in the LPS/NS group were injected with LPS (5 mg/kg) at 0 hours and treated with NS. Rats in the LPS/AG group were challenged with the same dose of LPS and treated with aminoguanidine (AG; 30 mg/kg per dose at 1, 3, and 6 hours). Ex vivo O_2 consumption was measured at 8 hours. (Adapted from King CJ, Tytgat S, Delude RL, Fink MP: Ileal mucosal oxygen consumption is decreased in endotoxemic rats but is restored toward normal by treatment with aminoguanidine. Crit Care Med 1999;27:2518-2524.)

key mitochondrial enzymes (NADH cytochrome *c* reductase, succinate cytochrome *c* reductase, cytochrome *c* oxidase). Early after the induction of sepsis, these enzymatic activities were normal, as was expression of the four mitochondrial enzyme complexes involved in electron transport and respiration (complexes I to IV), as assessed by Western blotting. In contrast, in samples of cardiac tissue obtained 18 hours after the onset of sepsis, the function of all three mitochondrial enzymes was significantly decreased, as was the expression of complexes II and IV.

In addition to the results from animal studies, there are now data from clinical studies that support the idea that mitochondrial function is impaired in human sepsis as well. Brealey and coworkers assessed mitochondrial function in skeletal muscle biopsies obtained from 28 critically ill septic patients within 24 hours of admission to an ICU, as well as in biopsies obtained from 9 control patients undergoing elective hip surgery.[32] Using standard polarographic methods, these investigators assessed the activity of the four mitochondrial enzyme complexes responsible for electron transport and respiration (complexes I to IV). The biopsy specimens were also analyzed with respect to several other relevant biochemical parameters, including ATP concentration and nitrite-nitrate concentration (an index of NO production). Of the 28 patients with sepsis, 16 survived and 12 died. Complex I activity was significantly lower in septic nonsurvivors than controls. Skeletal muscle ATP concentrations were significantly lower in the 12 patients with sepsis who died than in the 16 septic patients who survived ($P = 0.0003$) and in controls ($P = 0.05$). Complex I activity was inversely correlated with tissue nitrite-nitrate concentration ($P = 0.0004$), suggesting that increased NO production and sepsis-induced cytopathic hypoxia are linked phenomena.

POTENTIAL MECHANISMS OF CYTOPATHIC HYPOXIA IN SEPSIS

INHIBITION OF PYRUVATE DEHYDROGENASE

The end product of glycolysis is pyruvic acid, a three-carbon alpha-keto acid. Pyruvic acid can either be reduced to lactic acid or enter the tricarboxylic acid (TCA) cycle, ultimately to be oxidized to water and carbon dioxide. The rate-limiting step for entry of pyruvate into the TCA cycle is the reaction catalyzed by the enzyme complex pyruvate dehydrogenase (PDH). In the presence of NAD^+ (the oxidized form of nicotinamide adenine dinucleotide) and coenzyme A, PDH converts pyruvate into acetyl coenzyme A. Because of its pivotal role in the regulation of intermediary metabolism, the activity of PDH is tightly regulated by both end-product inhibition and reversible phosphorylation. A group of isoenzymes, the PDH kinase family, catalyzes the phosphorylation of PDH to its inactive form (PDH_i). A PDH phosphatase catalyzes the dephosphorylation of PDH_i to the active form of the enzyme complex (PDH_a). Vary and coworkers showed that the PDH_i/PDH_a ratio in skeletal muscle tissue increases during chronic sepsis in rats.[33,34] The mechanism responsible for this effect is increased PDH kinase activity rather than decreased PDH phosphatase activity.[35,36] Because inactivation of PDH limits the flux of substrate through the TCA cycle, excess pyruvate accumulates in cells, leading to increased production of lactate. Thus, according to the data obtained by Vary and coworkers, hyperlactatemia in sepsis is not necessarily evidence of impaired O_2 delivery but may be the result of the combined effects of PDH inhibition and accelerated glucose transport into cells.[34] Some clinical data support this notion.[37]

NITRIC OXIDE–MEDIATED INHIBITION OF CYTOCHROME OXIDASE

Sepsis is associated with iNOS induction and increased production of the pluripotent signaling and effector molecule NO.[38] At physiologically relevant concentrations (~1 μM), NO rapidly, but reversibly, inhibits the activity of cytochrome oxidase, the terminal enzyme complex of the mitochondrial electron transport chain.[39-42] NO-mediated inhibition of mitochondrial O_2 consumption is the result of competition by the two gases (O_2 and NO) for the same binding site on the enzyme complex.[43,44] Accordingly, the inhibitory effect of NO tends to be more pronounced when PO_2 is relatively low.[40-42] Although much of the work related to this mechanism has been done using NO derived from an exogenous source (i.e., authentic NO gas or a chemical compound that releases NO in solution), it is clear that endogenously produced NO is also capable of causing reversible inhibition of cytochrome oxidase, leading to reduced cellular respiration.[45]

PEROXYNITRITE-MEDIATED INHIBITION OF MITOCHONDRIAL ENZYMES

Under the right conditions, NO reacts rapidly with a partially reduced form of O_2, superoxide radical anion (O_2^-), to form peroxynitrite ($ONOO^-$), a molecular species that is a potent oxidizing, nitrosating, and nitrating agent.[46-49] Appropriate conditions for the production of $ONOO^-$, namely, biosynthesis of approximately equimolar levels of NO and O_2^- in close proximity, are present in many cell types during sepsis. In addition, small quantities of O_2^- are continually being produced by mitochondria. Under certain conditions, such as when O_2 availability is limited[50] or cytochrome oxidase is inhibited by NO,[51] mitochondria generate increased quantities of O_2^- by this mechanism. Moreover, a calcium-dependent NOS isoform that is either identical or very similar to neuronal NOS is present in mitochondria.[52-56] Thus, within the confines of the organelle itself, mitochondria are capable of generating both NO and O_2^- and, under appropriate conditions, large quantities of the potentially toxic moiety $ONOO^-$.[54,57]

Incubating mitochondria with authentic $ONOO^-$ causes irreversible inhibition of mitochondrial respiration. The deleterious effects of $ONOO^-$ on mitochondrial function are potentiated by increases in the concentration of ionized calcium (Ca^{++}).[58,59] The synergistic effects of $ONOO^-$ and Ca^{++} are likely important in a number of pathophysiologic conditions relevant to critical care medicine (e.g., inflammation, tissue ischemia followed by reperfusion), because these conditions are known to increase intramitochondrial concentrations of both species.

Several mechanisms have been implicated as being important in this phenomenon. Specifically, $ONOO^-$ has been shown to inhibit the mitochondrial F_oF_1-ATPase that phosphorylates ADP to form ATP.[60] In addition, $ONOO^-$ inhibits two of the mitochondrial enzyme complexes (I and II) that are involved in electron transport.[60] Finally, $ONOO^-$ inhibits the activity of aconitase, the TCA cycle enzyme that converts citrate into isocitrate.[61] Endogenous production of

ONOO⁻ secondary to iNOS induction plus O_2^- generation has been implicated as the major factor in impaired mitochondrial respiration in some tissues, such as rat diaphragm, following in vivo challenge with LPS.[15] Data obtained by Brealey and colleagues support the view that complex I activity is impaired in skeletal muscle biopsy samples from patients with lethal septic shock, probably as a result of increased production of NO or a related compound, such as ONOO⁻.[32]

THE PARP HYPOTHESIS

PARP-1 is a nuclear enzyme that participates in a variety of cellular functions, including the repair of single-strand breaks in nuclear DNA,[62,63] DNA replication,[64] and apoptosis.[64] PARP-1 is activated by single-strand breaks in nuclear DNA and then catalyzes the cleavage of NAD⁺ into ADP-ribose and nicotinamide and the polymerization of the resultant ADP-ribose units into branching poly(ADP-ribose) homopolymers.[65,66] The poly(ADP ribose) generated by this process is degraded by various nuclear enzymes, most notably poly(ADP-ribose) glycohydrolase.[66,67] The concurrent actions of PARP-1 and poly(ADP-ribose) glycohydrolase constitute the functional equivalent of an NADase. In states of acute inflammation, reactive oxygen species, including ONOO⁻ (and related oxidants), cause single-strand breaks in nuclear DNA and thereby activate PARP-1. Activation of PARP-1 has also been identified within mitochondria following oxidant stress,[68] suggesting that damage to mitochondrial DNA induced by reactive oxygen species might be another mechanism leading to activation of the PARP pathway. Activation of PARP-1 leads to intracellular depletion of NAD⁺ and its reduced form, NADH. Because NADH is the main reducing equivalent used to support oxidative phosphorylation, activation of PARP-1 can lead to a marked impairment in the cells' ability to use O_2 to support ATP synthesis—in other words, cytopathic hypoxia.

The notion that redox stress can lead to PARP-1 activation and hence metabolic inhibition was first proposed by Schraufstatter and associates.[69,70] More recently, Szabó and coworkers showed that exposure of cultured cells to physiologically relevant concentrations of ONOO⁻ activates PARP-1 and thereby impairs mitochondrial respiration.[71] They further showed that endogenously generated ONOO⁻ was capable of activating PARP-1 and thereby inhibiting mitochondrial respiration in cultured immunostimulated macrophages[72] and vascular smooth muscle cells.[73]

Recent in vitro studies by Khan and colleagues support the importance of PARP-1–dependent NAD⁺/NADH depletion as a mechanism for cytopathic hypoxia caused by inflammatory mediators.[8] The consumption of O_2 by human Caco-2 enterocyte-like cells was measured using an O_2-sensitive optode. Incubation of the cells with cytomix—a cocktail of three proinflammatory cytokines (tumor necrosis factor, IL-1β, and IFN-γ)—decreased cellular O_2 consumption by more than 50%. This phenomenon was entirely reversible; if the cells were washed free of the cytokine cocktail and then incubated for a short period in normal culture medium, the normal rate of O_2 consumption was restored. Thus, the cytokine-induced decrease in O_2 consumption was caused not by cell death but by a sublethal process that impaired normal cellular respiration. The decrease in O_2 consumption induced by incubation with cytomix was significantly ameliorated by pharmacologically blocking NO or ONOO⁻

production, providing further support for the role of NO and related compounds in the pathogenesis of cytopathic hypoxia. Moreover, pharmacologic inhibition of PARP-1 also ameliorated the development of cytopathic hypoxia, providing support for the PARP hypothesis. The decrease in O_2 uptake induced by cytomix was associated with significantly decreased cellular levels of NAD⁺/NADH. Interestingly, incubating the cytomix-stimulated Caco-2 cells with NAD⁺ encapsulated in liposomes partially restored cellular NAD⁺/NADH levels and prevented the development of cytopathic hypoxia.

In addition to the findings just described, other data support the view that PARP-1 activation is a major factor in the pathogenesis of sepsis. For example, using pharmacologic agents to block PARP-1 activity can prevent LPS-induced vascular contractile dysfunction in rodents.[74,75] Moreover, in comparison to wild-type controls, mice with a genetic defect in the PARP-1 enzyme (i.e., PARP-1 knockout mice) are relatively resistant to the lethal effects of LPS.[76,77] Treatment with a potent PARP-1 inhibitor, PJ34, significantly improves survival in a porcine model of lethal bacterial peritonitis.[78]

The notion that NO-dependent activation of PARP-1 contributes to the pathogenesis of cytopathic hypoxia is also supported by clinical data. Specifically, Boulos and colleagues showed that serum samples from patients with septic shock inhibited the reduction of MTT by cultured human umbilical vein endothelial cells, whereas sera from control subjects did not have this effect. When the endothelial cells were treated with a PARP-1 inhibitor, 3-aminobenzamide, or with an NOS inhibitor, N-methyl-L-arginine, the impairment in mitochondrial respiration (as assessed by MTT assay) induced by sera from septic patients was significantly ameliorated.[9]

Despite the findings cited here, the PARP-1 story is more complicated than originally envisioned. It is now recognized that PARP-1 participates in activation of the proinflammatory transcription factor nuclear factor kappa-B (NF-κB). PARP-1 participates in NF-κB–dependent signaling by binding directly to the transcription factor,[79,80] binding to another coactivating molecule (the protein p300),[81] or poly(ADP-ribosyl)ating NF-κB.[82] These effects are not dependent on PARP-1–induced alterations in intracellular energy metabolism but can nonetheless explain why a genetic deficiency in PARP-1 or treatment with a PARP-1 inhibitor can alter responses to a proinflammatory stimulus such as LPS (see earlier). To further complicate matters, activation of PARP-1 conceivably can alter energy metabolism independent of any direct effects on mitochondrial function; recent data indicate that activation of PARP-1 can promote poly(ADP-ribosyl)ation of glyceraldehyde phosphate-3-dehydrogenase, a key enzyme in the glycolytic pathway.[83]

CYTOPATHIC HYPOXIA AS A CAUSE OF ORGAN DYSFUNCTION DUE TO SEPSIS

A decade ago, the notion that sepsis is associated with mitochondrial dysfunction was controversial. Indeed, a number of studies suggested that acute sepsis or endotoxemia in animal models caused an *increase* in mitochondrial function.[84,85] Today, few dispute that sepsis is associated with an acquired intrinsic derangement in cellular respiration (cytopathic hypoxia). It remains unclear, however, whether cytopathic hypoxia is an epiphenomenon or a pathophysiologic mechanism that actually contributes to organ dysfunction and, ultimately, mortality in patients with sepsis or septic shock.

For cytopathic hypoxia to impact the function or viability of cells (and hence the function of organs), the impairment in mitochondrial function has to be severe enough to cause a decrease in the cellular phosphorylation potential, the rate of ATP turnover, or both. The phosphorylation potential is determined by the relative concentrations of ATP, ADP, and Pi: phosphorylation potential = [ATP]/[ADP][Pi]. In many in vitro studies, the function or viability of cells is not markedly altered unless the ATP concentration or phosphorylation potential is substantially reduced ($\leq 70\%$ of normal).[86-89]

In animal models, the effects of sepsis on cellular ATP content are variable, depending on myriad factors, including the method of inducing sepsis (or systemic inflammation), the timing of the ATP measurements with respect to the onset of the inflammatory process, the tissue or organ studied, and the assay used to assess ATP concentration. When rodents are injected with LPS, ATP levels in a variety of organs typically decrease significantly,[90,91] although ATP levels in skeletal muscle are typically unchanged.[91-93] If skeletal muscle is stimulated to induce repetitive contraction, however, it is possible to detect impaired synthesis of ATP.[93] It is unclear whether LPS-induced depletion of cellular ATP concentration in rodent models of septic shock is due to impaired perfusion, mitochondrial dysfunction, or some combination of the two.

Despite the findings just cited, it is important to recognize that acute endotoxemia in rodents is probably not a good animal model for sepsis-induced multiple organ dysfunction in humans. Accordingly, it is pertinent that several studies have failed to detect evidence of cellular ATP depletion in animal models of sepsis characterized by the presence of a true focus of infection (e.g., CLP in rats).[94-97] Contrary results have been reported, however, possibly because of differences between early and late sepsis.[98] Further, in the clinical study by Brealey and colleagues cited previously, ATP levels were significantly lower in skeletal muscle biopsy samples from patients with lethal sepsis than in samples from sepsis survivors or control subjects.[32] Thus, the question of whether sepsis leads to ATP depletion must be regarded as open and worthy of further study.

Steady-state levels of ATP (or even phosphorylation potential) may not be the most important parameter. The rate at which ATP is consumed and synthesized (i.e., the ATP turnover rate) may be more important, because it is conceivable that cells could defend ATP concentration in the setting of either classic hypoxia or cytopathic hypoxia by decreasing the rate at which ATP is used; this phenomenon has been termed metabolic suppression.[99,100]

To investigate this issue, Berg and coworkers used an in vitro "reductionist" model of sepsis to test the hypothesis that ATP turnover rate is modulated by the presence of a proinflammatory milieu. Nontransformed rat enterocytes were studied under control conditions or following incubation for 24 or 48 hours with cytomix, a mixture of the proinflammatory cytokines tumor necrosis factor, IL-1β, and IFN-γ. To measure ATP turnover rate, ATP synthesis was acutely blocked by adding to the cells a mixture containing 2-deoxyglucose (to block glycolysis), potassium cyanide, and antimycin A (to inhibit oxidative phosphorylation). ATP content was measured at baseline (before metabolic inhibition) and 0.5, 1, 2, 5, and 10 minutes later. Log-linear ATP decay curves were generated, and the kinetics of ATP utilization

were calculated. Remarkably, the ATP consumption rate was higher in cytomix-stimulated cells than in control cells. In contrast, the rate of ATP disappearance was similar in cytokine-naïve and immunostimulated IEC-6 cells when protein and nucleic acid synthesis was inhibited, suggesting that the increased rate of ATP synthesis following incubation with cytomix was used to support increased protein synthesis. The rates of glucose consumption and lactate production were significantly greater in cytomix-stimulated cells, suggesting that the increased rate of ATP turnover was supported by enhanced (aerobic) glycolysis. Other investigators have shown that experimental sepsis is associated with accelerated aerobic glycolysis,[101] and clinical data are available to support this view as well.[102] It is noteworthy, therefore, that Scharte and coworkers showed that proinflammatory cytokines increase the expression of glycolytic genes in cultured epithelial cells, even in the absence of hypoxia.[103]

CONCLUSION

Several lines of evidence support the notion that cellular respiration is deranged in established sepsis, not just on the basis of inadequate tissue perfusion but also on the basis of impaired mitochondrial function. If this concept is correct, a promising approach will be to develop pharmacologic strategies—for example, administration of potent and selective PARP-1 inhibitors—to restore normal mitochondrial function. Further research is needed to determine whether altered cellular respiration during sepsis truly contributes to cellular and organ dysfunction or is simply an epiphenomenon.

ANNOTATED REFERENCES

Boulos M, Astiz ME, Barua RS, Osman M: Impaired mitochondrial function induced by serum from septic shock patients is attenuated by inhibition of nitric oxide synthase and poly(ADP-ribose) synthase. Crit Care Med 2003;31:353-358.

When human endothelial cells are incubated in vitro with sera from patients with septic shock, mitochondrial function is impaired via a process that appears to depend on nitric oxide formation and activation of poly(ADP-ribosyl) polymerase.

Brealey D, Brand M, Hargreaves I, et al: Association between mitochondrial dysfunction and severity and outcome of septic shock. Lancet 2002; 360:219-223.

This study provided the first direct evidence that lethal septic shock in humans is associated with impaired mitochondrial function.

Fink MP: Cytopathic hypoxia in sepsis. Acta Anaesthesiol Scand 1997;41(Suppl 100):87-95.

This review paper was the first to introduce the term cytopathic hypoxia.

Khan AU, Delude RL, Han YH, et al: Liposomal NAD⁺ prevents diminished O₂ consumption by immunostimulated Caco-2 cells. Am J Physiol Lung Cell Mol Physiol 2002;282:L1082-L1091.

The authors of this paper used a "reductionist" in vitro model to provide convincing evidence that depletion of nicotinamide adenine dinucleotide, mediated by activation of the enzyme poly(ADP-ribosyl) polymerase, is a key factor in impaired cellular respiration following exposure of cultured enterocytes to a cocktail of proinflammatory cytokines.

King CJ, Tytgat S, Delude RL, Fink MP: Ileal mucosal oxygen consumption is decreased in endotoxemic rats but is restored toward normal by treatment with aminoguanidine. Crit Care Med 1999;27:2518-2524.

This study showed that ileal mucosal oxygen consumption (assessed ex vivo) is impaired in rats injected 8 hours earlier with lipopolysaccharide, but this effect is abrogated if the animals are treated with a drug that blocks the enzymatic activity of inducible nitric oxide synthase.

Chapter 37

OXIDATIVE LUNG INJURY

Todd L. Astor • David Weill

KEY POINTS

1. In pulmonary tissue, smooth muscle cells, endothelial cells, alveolar cells, and leukocytes have all been shown to **produce free radicals.**

2. **Superoxide** may have the most central role in oxidative lung injury because of its dual ability to directly alter cellular proteins and to form other highly reactive radical species.

3. The **most significant sources of free radicals** in lung tissue cells are the mitochondria and endoplasmic reticulum.

4. **Nitric oxide** is highly radical as a result of an odd number of electrons and through a variety of reactions produces reactive nitrogen species.

5. The **most rapid formation of reactive nitrogen species** occurs as a result of a radical-radical reaction between nitric oxide and various free radicals.

6. **Three enzyme systems** are primarily responsible for the enzymatic component of the antioxidant defenses: (1) superoxide dismutase (SOD); (2) catalase; and (3) the glutathione system.

7. **Several nonenzymatic antioxidants contribute to the cellular defenses** by acting as scavengers of toxic radicals.

8. **Reactive oxygen and nitrogen pulmonary cytotoxicity** is primarily mediated by two mechanisms: (1) lipid peroxidation and (2) damage to DNA.

9. **A variety of pulmonary cell types are susceptible to oxidant toxicity.**

10. **Reactive oxygen and nitrogen species** can affect pulmonary artery smooth muscle contractility and endothelial cell proliferation.

11. A **combination of necrosis and apoptosis** is likely involved in **oxidant-induced lung injury.**

12. **Animal and human studies demonstrate mixed results** concerning the sensitivity of healthy lungs to hyperoxic exposure.

13. **Results of animal studies** show that oxidative lung injury plays a major role in hyperoxia-induced lung injury.

14. The antioxidant response to hyperoxia-induced free radical formation is a complex process that is dependent on changes in expression of a variety of enzymes and nonenzymatic scavenger compounds.

15. There is now substantial evidence that generation of oxidative and nitrosative species is a major contributor to inflammatory lung injury in ARDS.

16. Certain antioxidants that function well under normal physiologic conditions may become overwhelmed in ARDS, whereas others demonstrate increased expression and activity.

17. Ischemia-reperfusion lung injury continues to be a significant cause of early morbidity after lung transplantation.

18. Generation of reactive oxygen species occurs as a direct result of both anoxia-reoxygenation and ischemia-reperfusion that occurs during the procurement-storage-transplantation period.

19. Elevated levels of free iron, calcium, and activated leukocytes increase the generation of free radicals during ischemia-reperfusion of the allograft.

20. Paraquat, bleomycin, and nitrofurantoin are examples of agents with the potential for inducing oxidative lung injury.

21. Hyperoxic therapy has been implicated as the principal inciting factor in the development of bronchopulmonary dysplasia in infants.

22. Oxidative lung injury in bronchopulmonary dysplasia is primarily a result of the oxidation of surfactants, lipids, and proteins.

23. The antioxidant response in newborns with bronchopulmonary dysplasia is variable and is in large part dependent on the stage of development of the infant (i.e., preterm vs. term).

24. Limited data on the use of oxygen therapy suggest minimizing the length of exposure to an FiO_2 higher than 0.6, utilizing oxygen-sparing interventions, and avoiding oxygen therapy in patients with lung injury secondary to specific toxins.

25. Mechanical ventilation with a low tidal volume strategy (6 mL/kg) should be utilized in patients with possible oxidant lung injury.

26. Although several studies demonstrate a potential benefit for exogenous antioxidant administration, there are not yet enough conclusive data to support its routine use in the clinical setting.

Since the discovery of oxygen in 1775 we have marveled at the life-sustaining power that it possesses. However, we have also realized that oxygen holds the potential for the spoliation of life. Early scientists such as Priestley, Scheele, Lavoisier, Laplace, and Bert all recognized this "two-faced" nature of oxygen and conducted studies to better understand its destructive nature.[1-4] These studies were the preface to the understanding that we now have of the toxic effects of oxygen and its reactive metabolites, collectively known as oxidant injury. Oxidant injury can occur throughout the body, but the lung is the most susceptible organ, and lung injury induced by reactive oxygen species is often devastating and irreversible.

GENERATION OF REACTIVE OXYGEN SPECIES

In pulmonary tissue, smooth muscle cells, endothelial cells, alveolar cells, and leukocytes have all been shown to produce free radicals.[5-8] Superoxide may have the most central role in oxidative lung injury because of its dual ability to directly alter cellular proteins and to form other highly reactive radical species. Superoxide radicals are produced by both cellular enzymatic and nonenzymatic (auto-oxidation) reactions. Enzymes capable of forming superoxide include xanthine oxidase (by the oxidation of purines and of NADH), arachidonic acid peroxidases, nitric oxide synthase, NADPH oxidase, and NADH oxidase.[9-12] Phagocytic cells in the lung can form large amounts of superoxide during bursts of respiratory activity.[13]

The most significant sources of free radicals in lung tissue cells are the mitochondria and endoplasmic reticulum.[14-16] Formation of free radicals requires the presence of molecular oxygen and is a constant process occurring in normal cellular metabolism. Molecular oxygen is reduced by the sequential addition of electrons to form the highly reactive free radicals superoxide radical (O_2^-), hydrogen peroxide (H_2O_2), and hydroxyl radical ($OH\cdot$):

$$O_2 \rightarrow O_2^- \rightarrow H_2O_2 \rightarrow OH\cdot \rightarrow H_2O$$

Two molecules of water are produced in the reduction of molecular oxygen in a reaction catalyzed by cytochrome oxidase in the electron transport chain in the mitochondria. Cytochrome oxidase, which contains cytochrome a and cytochrome a3, acts as the terminal electron receptor. Under normal conditions there exists a small loss of electron flow (1% to 2%) along the proximal portion of the electron transport chain. Electron loss first occurs during the reduction of NADH dehydrogenase to form a flavin semiquinone free radical, which then reacts with O_2 to form O_2^- (auto-oxidation). Ubiquinone is the second site of electron loss, and the reduction of ubiquinone forms the ubisemiquinone free radical by auto-oxidation. Another important source of O_2^- is the electron transport chain of the endoplasmic reticulum.[16] In the endoplasmic reticulum O_2^- is most likely produced from the auto-oxidation of reduced NADPH cytochrome P_{450} reductase and the reduced cytochrome P_{450}.

Regardless of its source of production, O_2^- is relatively unstable. It can react with proteins that contain transition metal groups (e.g., heme, iron-sulfur), resulting in alteration of cellular function.[17-19] The majority of O_2^- produced,

however, is converted to H_2O_2 in a reaction catalyzed by superoxide dismutase[20]:

$$O_2^- + O_2^- + 2H^+ \rightarrow H_2O_2 + O_2^-$$

H_2O_2 is a more stable, nonradical compound. Most of the cellular damage by H_2O_2 results from its further reduction to form hydroxyl radicals by a series of iron catalyzed reactions. Iron is first reduced by O_2^- in the Haber-Weiss reaction, and the reduced form of iron in turn reduces H_2O_2 to form $OH\cdot$ in the Fenton reaction.[21] $OH\cdot$ is also produced directly from O_2^- in a reaction involving hypohalous acids.[22,23] Hypohalous acids are potent oxidants formed when H_2O_2 is oxidized by eosinophil-specific peroxidase and neutrophil-specific peroxidase in the presence of a halide.

GENERATION OF REACTIVE NITROGEN SPECIES

Nitric oxide (NO) is a cytotoxic agent present in many types of environmental pollutants, including cigarette smoke.[24] NO has also been shown to be produced endogenously throughout the body and serves a variety of significant regulatory functions. Nitric oxide synthase (NOS) catalyzes the formation of NO from L-arginine.[25,26] There are constitutive (NOS I, NOS III) and inducible (NOS II) forms of NOS. The constitutive forms are Ca^{++} and calmodulin dependent and synthesize small amounts of NO for brief periods. The inducible form produces large amounts of NO for extended periods.[27,28]

Nitric oxide is highly radical as a result of an odd number of electrons and through a variety of reactions produces reactive nitrogen species. In the presence of molecular oxygen, NO can be oxidized to nitrite (NO_2^-). The formation of NO_2^- leads to the oxidation of various biologic substrates in a reaction catalyzed by heme peroxidases such as MPO and EPO.[29-31] NO_2^- itself is oxidized to nitrogen dioxide radical ($NO_2\cdot$), as well as to nitrate (NO_3^-). Oxidation of NO by oxyhemoglobin (HbO_2) may lead to the formation of methemoglobin (Hb^{3+}) and NO_3^-.[32]

Potentially the most rapid formation of reactive nitrogen species occurs as a result of a radical-radical reaction between NO and various free radicals. For example, $ONOO^-$ is formed by the reaction on NO with O_2^-. $ONOO^-$ can be protonated to form peroxynitrous acid (ONOOH), a highly unstable and reactive compound capable of both oxidizing and nitrating reactions involving a variety of biochemical substrates (e.g., lipids, amino acids).[33]

ANTIOXIDANT MECHANISMS

During normal aerobic metabolism in lung cells, reactive oxygen and nitrogen species are produced that, at low levels, serve a variety of important biologic functions. However, these reactive metabolites are potentially very damaging to biologic substrates such as lipids, proteins, and carbohydrates. A system of enzymatic and nonenzymatic antioxidants exists in the lung to prevent the formation and facilitate the removal of these reactive species.

Three enzyme systems are primarily responsible for the enzymatic component of the antioxidant defenses: (1) superoxide dismutase (SOD); (2) catalase; and (3) the glutathione system. SOD is both an intracellular and extracellular enzyme, located in the cytosol, in the mitochondria, and on the outside of the plasma membrane.[34-36] The cytosolic form of SOD contains copper and zinc and is associated with pulmonary and endothelial vascular smooth muscle cells. The mitochondrial form contains manganese and is abundant in pulmonary artery smooth muscle and endothelium.[35] During times of oxidative stress, SOD has a significant role in protecting lung cells by catalyzing the dismutation of O_2^- to H_2O_2.[37]

Catalase and the glutathione system are the central mechanisms for the reduction of H_2O_2. Catalase is a hemoprotein found in peroxisomes. It has an iron-heme active site that undergoes divalent oxidation and reduction in catalyzing the reduction of H_2O_2.[38] The glutathione system is likely more important than catalase in the reduction of H_2O_2 and is also responsible for the elimination of lipid peroxidases formed from the free radical altered lipid membranes.[39] The glutathione system is actually a redox cycle in which the key enzyme is glutathione peroxidase. Glutathione peroxidase catalyzes the reduction of H_2O_2 and lipid peroxidases by using reduced glutathione as a cosubstrate. This reaction forms glutathione disulfide, which is subsequently reduced back to glutathione by glutathione reductase.[40] Glutathione reductase activity is dependent on NADPH generated from the hexose monophosphate shunt.[41]

Several nonenzymatic antioxidants contribute to the cellular defenses by acting as scavengers of toxic radicals. Vitamin E, the most important of these compounds, protects against oxidant-induced membrane injury by scavenging lipid peroxide radicals.[42] Thioredoxins, a newly described family of proteins located in the inner mitochondrial membrane of airway epithelial cells, respond to oxidative stress by scavenging reactive species and activating other antioxidant systems such as Mn-SOD.[43] Metallothionein, a metalloprotein expressed in pulmonary endothelial cells, is thought to have an important function in intracellular iron homeostasis and as a free radical scavenger of superoxide radicals.[44] Other free radical scavengers include vitamin C, uric acid, beta carotene, taurine, albumin, and bilirubin.

PATHOPHYSIOLOGY OF OXIDATIVE LUNG INJURY

Reactive oxygen and nitrogen species are cytotoxic to virtually all types of pulmonary cells. This toxicity is primarily mediated by two mechanisms: (1) lipid peroxidation and (2) damage to DNA.

All cell membranes are made up of polyunsaturated fatty acids. The hydroxyl free radical is particularly destructive to these fatty acids by removing a hydrogen atom from the fatty acid, resulting in the formation of peroxides and peroxyradicals. These radical intermediates may then remove another hydrogen atom from a different fatty acid, leading to a chain reaction resulting in the rapid destruction of the cellular membrane.[45] In addition, membrane phospholipase A_2 may be activated during lipid peroxidation, potentially contributing to the breakdown of the lipid bilayer.[46]

Cellular DNA is also a susceptible target for reactive oxygen species. The hydroxyl radical has been shown to directly hydroxylate guanine.[47] Reactive lipid species formed during lipid peroxidation are able to cross-link DNA proteins and cause strand breaks.[48] It has been suggested that this results

in the activation of poly (adenosine diphosphate-ribosyl) polymerase (PARP), resulting in excessive consumption of adenosine triphosphate (ATP) and cell death.[49] Some environmental toxins and drugs cause DNA damage through the formation of active complexes with DNA in the presence of oxygen (see section on bleomycin-induced lung injury).[50] Reactive oxygen species have also been implicated in the modulation of gene transcription. Schreck and coworkers have proposed a role for superoxide in the activation of nuclear factor-kappa B (NF-κB), a potent regulator of gene transcription.[51] Demple and associates demonstrated a superoxide effect on gene transcription that may protect the host in which superoxide activates a system (soxRS system) of transcription/translation that leads to the expression of superoxide dismutase.[52]

Oxygen free radicals also have a profound effect on pulmonary artery smooth muscle contractility and can cause vasoconstriction through several mechanisms. Superoxide radical destroys the NO that is produced in the vascular endothelium, thus blocking the vasodilatatory effect induced by NO.[53] Superoxide, in the presence of xanthine oxidase, can also directly stimulate the contraction of pulmonary artery rings, most likely through a mechanism involving protein kinase C.[54] Superoxide is also capable of stimulating the release of calcium from the sarcoplasmic reticulum, as well as increasing the microsomal ATP-dependent calcium uptake in pulmonary vascular smooth muscle cells.[55]

All pulmonary cell types are susceptible to oxidant toxicity. Pulmonary artery endothelial cells initially proliferate in response to superoxide exposure and are stimulated to release higher concentrations of superoxide than quiescent cells. Continued superoxide exposure results in DNA strand breakage resulting in the depletion of ATP and also causes membrane lipid peroxidation. Both mechanisms contribute to an inhibition of endothelial cell proliferation.[56] Bronchial and type I alveolar epithelial cell death occurs in the early stages of oxidant injury and is likely due to a pattern of necrosis rather than apoptosis.[57] Type I alveolar cells are then replaced by hyperplasia of type II alveolar epithelial cells, resulting in a thicker alveolar epithelium.[58] Clara cells, nonciliated epithelial cells distributed throughout the respiratory tree, are extremely rich in cytochrome P_{450} and thus are very sensitive to oxidant stress.[59] Naphthalene exerts its toxic effects primarily through selective damage to Clara cells.[60] Finally, although oxidant lung injury may indeed stimulate inflammatory cells to proliferate and further generate reactive oxygen species, there is some evidence that oxidants may impair the antibacterial function of these inflammatory cells. For example, O'Reilly and colleagues demonstrated impaired phagocytic function due to actin polymerization in mouse alveolar macrophages during hyperoxic exposure.[61] This process appears to be due to NO and the nitration of actin and does not occur in the absence of inducible NOS.

The mode of cell death in oxidant-induced lung cell injury and death is controversial and has been attributed to both necrosis and apoptosis. Animal studies have suggested that although apoptosis may play a key role in programmed lung cell death, necrosis is the predominant mode of death occurring in oxidant lung injury.[49] However, it has been postulated that apoptosis may play a role in limiting the extent of oxidative lung injury and in the remodeling of lung tissue during the repair phase.[62]

OXIDATIVE LUNG INJURY IN THE ICU

The specific pathology and natural history of oxidative lung injury varies with specific disease states. The cascade of events usually involves an acute phase in which cell injury results from the initial generation of reactive oxygen species. This is followed by an inflammatory phase, in which cell death occurs from the response of mononuclear cells and alveoli become obliterated with exudate and hyaline membrane formation. Finally, in extensive disease a proliferative phase usually occurs, leading to proliferation of type II alveolar cells and fibroblasts. Ultimately, fibrosis in the lung interstitium may occur.[63]

We will examine the specific mechanisms of oxidative lung injury in five specific pathologic lung conditions frequently encountered in the ICU: (1) hyperoxia-induced lung injury; (2) ARDS; (3) ischemia/reperfusion injury; (4) lung injury from exposure to toxins; and (5) bronchopulmonary dysplasia. Oxidant lung injury has been implicated in many other lung diseases, including asthma, sarcoidosis, idiopathic pulmonary fibrosis, and radiation pneumonitis. Discussion of these pulmonary disorders is beyond the scope of this chapter.

HYPEROXIA

Treatment with high concentrations of oxygen is often necessary to treat acute and chronic hypoxemia in patients with lung disease. Hyperoxia has been shown to damage alveolar epithelial cells and pulmonary vascular endothelial cells in several animal models. However, studies in humans have demonstrated mixed results concerning the ability of hyperoxic exposure to cause significant lung injury in the absence of underlying lung disease.

Results of early studies analyzing changes in vital capacity with hyperoxic exposure suggested that the safe threshold of PiO_2 is close to 0.6 atm.[64] This estimation was supported later by data from the U.S. Navy's shallow habitat air diving (SHAD) program studying long-term survival in a compressed air environment.[65,66] During several stages of this study men underwent shallow habitat dives with a PiO_2 of 0.51 atm and 0.57 atm for a period of 29.5 days and 28 days, respectively. All men tolerated the protocol well and there was no evidence of decreased pulmonary function. In the final arm of this study men were exposed to cycles of 0.51 atm and 0.81 atm, with a mean of 0.61 atm. These subjects demonstrated chest discomfort as well as decreases in the vital capacity that correlated with the exposure to the PiO_2 of 0.81 atm.

Determining the threshold for oxygen toxicity in actual patients is even more difficult. Patients requiring acute oxygen therapy usually have severe parenchymal lung injury, and therefore interpretation of worsening lung injury while receiving oxygen therapy can be obscured. However, there are several reports in the literature examining the effects of hyperoxic therapy on patients receiving mechanical ventilation for reasons other than primary lung disease. Singer and associates reported that post–cardiac surgical patients exposed to 100% FiO_2 for a mean of 24 hours demonstrated no adverse effects when compared with a similar group receiving a mean FiO_2 of 0.32.[67] Smith and coworkers analyzed pulmonary function, radiographs, and pathology in 41 patients treated with high-frequency jet ventilation using a mean FiO_2 of 0.92 for a mean of 4.1 days and did not find any evidence of oxygen toxicity.[68] Kobayashi described a

32-year old patient with myasthenia gravis who, because of technical limitations of a ventilator, was ventilated with an FiO_2 of 0.80 for 150 days.[69] Despite developing blindness secondary to systemic oxygen toxicity, this patient developed no evidence of pulmonary oxygen toxicity.

In contrast to these reports demonstrating an absence of pulmonary oxygen toxicity in patients receiving hyperoxic therapy, Barber and colleagues reported adverse pulmonary effects of hyperoxic ventilation in patients with cerebral trauma.[70] Patients ventilated with an FiO_2 of 100% for a mean of 2 days had a lower mean PaO_2, increased deadspace, and worsening of chest radiographs when compared with a similar group ventilated with room air. However, at autopsy there were no histopathologic differences discovered between the two groups, suggesting that hyperoxia-induced atelectasis may have played a greater role than direct parenchymal lung injury in explaining the clinical differences.

Therefore, the degree of sensitivity of healthy lungs to hyperoxia remains unclear. In addition, the specific underlying pathophysiologic phenomena causing the observed clinical sequelae are not known. For example, a decrease in vital capacity may result from an acute tracheobronchitis and hypoxemia could be a manifestation of absorption atelectasis. Also, as previously mentioned, patients receiving hyperoxic therapy usually have underlying lung disease and distinguishing the etiology of their lung physiology and histopathology is impossible.

Because of these difficulties in studying a human lung model of hyperoxia, there has been a strong reliance on animal studies to help elucidate the mechanisms of hyperoxic lung injury. There is now significant evidence that oxidant injury plays a principal role in hyperoxia-induced lung injury. Gerschman and colleagues first suggested that hyperoxia-induced tissue injury results from the generation of oxygen-derived free radicals.[71] Freeman and associates[14] demonstrated that hyperoxia increases oxygen free radical production in rat lungs. The cellular enzymatic and nonenzymatic (auto-oxidation) reactions generating free radicals during normoxia were previously discussed. Production from each of these sources is increased during hyperoxia, but the nonenzymatic formation of free radicals (auto-oxidation) appears to play a much more significant role.[14]

As previously described, several enzymes play important roles in the generation of O_2^- and other reactive species. These enzymes demonstrate low Michaelis-Menten kinetics. They are saturated with molecular oxygen during normoxia, and therefore their rates of reaction are not increased with higher concentrations of oxygen.[14] In addition, there appear to be negative feedback mechanisms that may lower enzyme activity during hyperoxia. For example, Elsayed and coworkers showed that hyperoxia decreases the activity of xanthine oxidase both in rat lungs and in cultured lung endothelial cells.[72] The decreased activity was reproduced with purified enzyme in the presence of oxygen free radicals, supporting the theory of a feedback mechanism.

The most important source of increased free radical production during hyperoxia is the auto-oxidation of flavins and quinones in the electron transport chains of the mitochondria and endoplasmic reticulum.[73] These reactions demonstrate first-order kinetics, and therefore the rate of formation of free radicals is proportional to the concentrations of molecular oxygen and the oxidizable substrate.[14] Grisham and coworkers estimated that during hyperoxia with 100% oxygen, 85% of the free radicals produced by lung cells are produced in the electron transport system of the endoplasmic reticulum and the remaining 15% are generated in the mitochondria.[74]

The antioxidant response to hyperoxia-induced free radical formation is a complex process that is dependent on changes in expression of a variety of enzymes and nonenzymatic scavenger compounds. Studies of gene expression in wild-type and knockout mice have better elucidated antioxidant expression during hyperoxia.[75] Perkowski and associates demonstrated no change in the gene expression of the antioxidant enzymes catalase, manganese SOD, and copperzinc SOD in mice exposed to greater than 95% oxygen. However, there was a moderate increase in the expression of glutathione peroxidase and heme oxygenase-1, as well as a 7-fold increase in the expression of the heavy metal binding protein metallothionein.

ACUTE RESPIRATORY DISTRESS SYNDROME

ARDS is a lung disease characterized by a diffuse, patchy pattern of inflammation in the lung parenchyma. The pathogenesis of ARDS involves a complicated cascade of humoral and cellular responses.[76] After an initial insult (i.e., infection, sepsis, trauma, severe burns) there is a massive release of inflammatory cytokines such as tumor necrosis factor-alpha, IL-1, and IL-6, leading to the activation of lung epithelial, endothelial, and mononuclear cells. There is an increase in the expression of various adhesion molecules, selectins, and integrins that induces the extravasation and adhesion of neutrophils and eosinophils to lung tissue. The ensuing lung injury results from the inflammatory response by these activated cells. Until recently the mechanisms by which lung injury occurs have not been well understood.

There is now substantial evidence that generation of oxidative and nitrosative species is a major contributor to inflammatory lung injury in ARDS.[77] Oxidant free radicals are produced by activated neutrophils and macrophages, as well as by lung endothelial, epithelial, and alveolar cells. Similarly, synthesis of NO and other reactive nitrogen species is increased in lung inflammation.[78]

Cochrane and colleagues were the first to demonstrate evidence of oxidant activity in ARDS.[77] Alpha$_1$-proteinase inhibitor (PI), an inhibitor of elastase found in the lung, was found to be inactivated in the bronchoalveolar lavage (BAL) fluid, but not the plasma, from patients with ARDS. In addition, the activity of the inactivated alpha$_1$-PI was restored with a reducing agent. Later studies showed an increased level of H_2O_2 in the expired breath condensates from patients with acute lung injury/ARDS as compared with patients with healthy lungs.[79] Weiland and Laurent found increased superoxide levels in leukocytes isolated from the blood from patients with ARDS.[80] Evidence of accelerated superoxide generation in ARDS has been demonstrated in several recent human and experimental animal studies. Quinlan and coworkers demonstrated increased levels of hypoxanthine and xanthine, substrates for xanthine oxidase, in the plasma from patients with ARDS.[81] In an experimental in-situ lung model of endotoxin-induced ARDS in rats, increased levels of superoxide were observed by use of chemiluminescence.[82]

Nitric oxide has also been shown to possess a significant role in ARDS. NO can be produced by airway epithelial cells, endothelial cells, and type II alveolar cells, as well as by activated neutrophils and macrophages.[83,84] There is evidence that synthesis of NO and other reactive nitrogen species is increased during lung inflammation in ARDS. Sittipunt and colleagues measured increased levels of nitrate and nitrite, breakdown products of NO, in the BAL fluid from patients with or at risk for ARDS.[85] The levels of nitrate and nitrite decreased to near-normal levels several weeks after the onset of ARDS. These results were supported in a similar study by Zhu and coworkers demonstrating significantly higher levels of nitrate in pulmonary edema fluid collected with a wedged suction catheter from patients with ARDS.[86] Other studies have addressed the toxic effects of these reactive intermediates by measuring the byproducts of nitration reactions involving a variety of functionally important lung proteins. Nitrotyrosine, the end product of the nitration of the tyrosine residues of many proteins, has been found in tissues during acute inflammation.[85] Increased levels of nitrotyrosine have been shown both in pulmonary edema and BAL fluid from patients with ARDS.[85,86] Nitrated ceruloplasmin, transferrin, alpha$_1$-PI, and alpha$_1$-antichymotrypsin have all been detected in the plasma from patients with ARDS.[87] Nitrated surfactant protein A has been discovered in the edema fluid from patients with ARDS.[86] Because it has been previously suggested that surfactant protein A may play a role in the removal of infectious pathogens from the alveolar space, it has been hypothesized that the nitration of this protein may alter its function and render the patient with ARDS more susceptible to secondary infections.[88]

Together these results support a significant role for oxidant-mediated lung injury in ARDS. Therefore, antioxidant expression and activity would seem to be a principal factor in moderating damage to lung tissue. Several studies have demonstrated a decrease in the level of several antioxidants in patients with ARDS. For example, levels of glutathione, an antioxidant with the significant role of reducing H_2O_2, were found to be decreased in the BAL fluid of patients with ARDS.[89] However, levels of catalase, another antioxidant responsible for the reduction of H_2O_2, were actually increased.[90] Other studies have demonstrated an increase in the response of some antioxidants and a decrease in others in both plasma and BAL fluid from patients with acute lung injury. These results suggest that whereas certain antioxidants that function well under normal physiologic conditions may become overwhelmed in ARDS, others demonstrate increased expression and activity.

ISCHEMIA-REPERFUSION LUNG INJURY

Since 1983 lung transplantation has become the definitive therapy for patients with end-stage lung disease. However, despite improvements in the selection of donors, preservation of donor lungs, surgical techniques, and perioperative care, ischemia-reperfusion lung injury continues to be a significant cause of early morbidity after lung transplantation. Ischemia-reperfusion lung injury is characterized by a pattern of alveolar damage, pulmonary edema, and hypoxemia that occurs within the first 72 hours after transplantation.[91] Several factors likely contribute to the extent of injury, including donor lung injury, hypothermic storage, and increased organ ischemia time. Although several mechanisms for ischemia-reperfusion injury have been proposed, generation of reactive oxidative species appears to play a principal role. Oxidative stress occurs as a direct result of both anoxia-reoxygenation and ischemia-reperfusion that occurs during the procurement-storage-transplantation period.[91]

During the period in which the donor lung is not ventilated, hypoxia/anoxia results in a significant decrease in the level of ATP and a subsequent increase in the degradation product hypoxanthine.[92] Hypoxanthine is oxidized to form superoxide radicals in a reaction catalyzed by xanthine oxidase, an enzyme found in abundance in the pulmonary vascular endothelium.[9,27,97] This reaction cannot occur in the absence of oxygen, and therefore a buildup of hypoxanthine takes place during the anoxic period. On ventilation/reoxygenation with transplantation, the hypoxanthine generates high concentrations of superoxide. Zhao and colleagues demonstrated that this process is disrupted with allopurinol, an inhibitor of xanthine oxidase.[93]

Storage of the donor lung is characterized by a period of ischemia in which there is no blood flow into the lung. Oxidant generation from ischemia occurs primarily in the endothelial cells and is not dependent on hypoxia.[96] In response to the absence of the mechanical component of blood flow during ischemia, the endothelial cell membrane is depolarized, activating NADPH oxidase, nitric oxide synthase, and NF-κB.[97,98] As previously discussed, these enzymes catalyze the reactions generating reactive oxygen and nitrogen species.

Free radical–induced lung damage is influenced by other processes occurring during ischemia-reperfusion injury. Levels of free iron are increased during ischemia as a result of its release from ferritin and cytochrome P_{450}.[99,100] Iron undergoes reduction and oxidation and is responsible for catalyzing the production of hydroxyl radical from superoxide and hydrogen peroxide in the Haber-Weiss and Fenton reactions. Iron may also contribute to oxidant stress by enhancing the oxidation of glutathione and the peroxidation of lipids.[101] Iron chelators such as deferoxamine have been shown to be effective in moderating ischemia-reperfusion injury in animal models.[102] Other factors that may influence or contribute to oxidant injury include elevated levels of cytosolic calcium (increases conversion of xanthine dehydrogenase to xanthine oxidase) and leukocyte activation (increases free radical production through membrane bound NADPH oxidase system).[103,104]

TOXIN-INDUCED OXIDANT LUNG DAMAGE

Many environmental and pharmacologic compounds can cause significant lung injury. These compounds can inflict toxic effects through a variety of mechanisms and are associated with a spectrum of disease patterns.

Paraquat can cause toxic effects in the kidney, liver, and thymus, but the lung is the most common site of toxicity.[105] Animal studies have demonstrated that paraquat lung toxicity is characterized by a morphologic pattern of inflammatory cell infiltration, necrosis of type I and II alveolar cells, fibroblast infiltration and proliferation and, finally, synthesis of large quantities of collagen. This cascade of events results in severe pulmonary fibrosis and can follow exposure by both parenteral and inhalational routes.[105-109]

The mechanisms of paraquat-induced lung injury have been well studied. Paraquat is a basic amine that, when taken up by the lung, results in significant increases in oxygen uptake and subsequent NADPH oxidation.[110] This is the first step of a redox cycle occurring in the endoplasmic reticulum of alveolar epithelial cells. Paraquat is reduced to a free radical in this reaction catalyzed by NADPH cytochrome c reductase. This free radical then immediately transfers its electron to molecular oxygen to form superoxide radical, and in the process it regenerates the original paraquat cation. The superoxide radical can then exert its direct toxicity or continue to react to form the equally dangerous hydrogen peroxide and/or hydroxyl radical. The regenerated paraquat cation is then free to restart the redox cycle, resulting in the generation of tremendous quantities of superoxide radicals.[110,111] Paraquat-induced lung injury has also been associated with increased NO synthesis, demonstrated by a decrease in injury with administration of inhibitors of NOS.[112]

With an understanding of these mechanisms of paraquat lung toxicity, one can predict the exogenous and endogenous factors that may influence the extent of lung damage. For example, Smith and Rose demonstrated that hyperoxia increases paraquat toxicity but hypoxia decreases it.[113] The host antioxidant response to paraquat toxicity is directed at the overwhelming production of superoxide. Animal studies have specifically identified important functions for glutathione, SOD, catalase, α-tocopherol, vitamin E, and selenium in counteracting paraquat-induced oxidant toxicity.[111]

Bleomycin is an antineoplastic drug used to treat various types of squamous cell cancers and lymphomas. Despite being a very effective cancer drug, its use is often limited by lung toxicity, initially manifesting as a pneumonitis and later progressing to pulmonary fibrosis.[114] The morphologic pattern of bleomycin-induced lung injury has been well studied in mice.[115] The initial stage of injury occurs within the first 4 weeks and is characterized first by vascular endothelial cell injury, followed by necrosis of type I alveolar epithelial cells, and finally by deposition of fibrin in the alveolar spaces. The second stage, typically occurring within 8 to 12 weeks, is characterized by metaplasia of type II alveolar epithelial cells, fibroblast organization and collagen deposition, and subsequent interstitial fibrosis.

The mechanisms of bleomycin-induced lung injury are not completely understood, but evidence strongly supports a role for reactive oxygen species. Scheulen and coworkers showed that cell destruction is a result of cleavage of both single- and double-stranded DNA and that this cleavage was dependent on oxygen, iron, and NADPH cytochrome P450 reductase.[116] In addition, bleomycin was found to significantly increase NADPH oxidation.[116] In response to these results, an active complex of bleomycin, iron, and oxygen has been implicated in the DNA damage associated with bleomycin lung injury, and three-dimensional models for this complex have been proposed.[117] Extracellular superoxide dismutase has been shown to play an important role in the antioxidant response to bleomycin-induced oxidative stress.[118]

Many other pharmaceutical and nonpharmaceutical agents are associated with oxidant-induced lung injury. Nitrofurantoin, an antibiotic used to treat urinary tract infections, causes lung toxicity by generation of superoxide, hydrogen peroxide, and hydroxyl radical by a mechanism similar to that of paraquat.[119] Naphthalene exposure can result in selective necrosis of pulmonary Clara cells and is likely mediated by reactive metabolites dependent on cytochrome P_{450}.[120] Vinylidine chloride (used in the plastics industry), malathion (insecticide), and 4-ipomeanol (produced by fungus in sweet potatoes) are all thought to induce oxidant-mediated lung injury through a variety of mechanisms.[121,122] Certain trace metals such as vanadium have been shown to cause lung injury through the induction of inflammation and apoptosis by reactive oxygen species.[123] Chronic exposure to ethanol renders the lung susceptible to acute lung injury by decreasing glutathione levels and therefore indirectly increasing levels of oxygen free radicals.[124] Reactive intermediates have even been implicated in certain types of lung malignancies resulting from exposures to carcinogens, as in the case of many polycyclic aromatic hydrocarbons.[125]

BRONCHOPULMONARY DYSPLASIA

Bronchopulmonary dysplasia (BPD) is a lung disease in preterm infants that occurs usually as a complication of the respiratory distress syndrome. It is characterized by a histologic pattern of obliterative changes in the bronchioles with the formation of cysts.[126] Hyperoxic therapy has been implicated as the principal inciting factor, and in the past it has been suggested that the generation of reactive oxygen and nitrogen species is the major contributor to lung injury in BPD.[127,128] In fact, preterm infants are at particular risk for oxidative lung injury for several reasons: (1) deficiency in pulmonary surfactant; (2) decreased levels and function of antioxidant enzymes; (3) increased exposure to infections with subsequent inflammatory cytokine release; and (4) increased levels of free iron in the plasma.[129]

Recent evidence has strongly supported a role for oxidative lung damage in BPD. Oxidative lung injury in BPD is primarily a result of the oxidation of surfactants, lipids, and proteins. Several studies have demonstrated increased levels of oxidized ascorbic acid, uric acid, and o-tyrosine, all markers of peroxidation, in tracheal lavage fluid from preterm infants who later developed BPD.[130,131] Nogee and associates showed that superoxide, hydrogen peroxide, nitric oxide, and peroxynitrite all inactivate surfactant protein.[132] The oxidation of surfactant protein A results in a loss in its surfactant function and possibly its ability to augment the alveolar immune response to infection.[133] Pitkanen and colleagues measured an increased level of pentane and ethane, products of lipid peroxidation, in exhaled gas from preterm infants who later developed BPD.[134] Varsila and coworkers detected higher concentrations of carbonyl groups, side chains formed during the oxidation of proteins, in tracheal aspirates from newborns with BPD.[135]

The antioxidant response in newborns with BPD is variable and is in large part dependent on the stage of development of the infant (i.e., preterm vs. term). Animal studies of preterm newborns have demonstrated a lower level of intracellular enzymatic antioxidants such as glutathione when compared with term newborns.[136,137] In addition, in preterm newborns expression of antioxidant enzymes is not increased during times of oxidative stress.[138] The diminished antioxidant defenses in the newborn coupled with the increased oxidant production associated with early infection, inflammation, and oxygen therapy contribute to the lung injury associated with BPD.

EFFECTS OF ICU THERAPEUTIC INTERVENTIONS ON OXIDANT LUNG INJURY

OXYGEN THERAPY

Oxygen is the most common "drug" administered in the intensive care setting. The detrimental effects of oxygen and its reactive metabolites have been presented in detail.

Oxygen toxicity can be viewed in a dose-response curve manner, with the dose equal to the product of the PIO_2 and the duration of exposure. Therefore, as with all drugs, the minimum dose should be used that is necessary to induce the anticipated therapeutic benefit. As previously discussed, the determination of that threshold dose has been very difficult because of a number of confounding variables inherent in any human study of hyperoxic lung injury. However, from the data available the following recommendations can be made:

- Minimizing the length of exposure to elevated FIO_2
- Utilizing oxygen-sparing interventions such as the application of positive end-expiratory pressure during mechanical ventilation and ensuring adequate oxygen delivery to organ tissues through the maintenance of cardiac output
- Avoiding oxygen therapy in patients with lung injury secondary to specific toxins (i.e., bleomycin, paraquat, and nitrofurantoin)

MECHANICAL VENTILATION

Ventilator management has been recognized as one of the most significant factors in determining clinical outcome in acute lung injury. Mechanical ventilation itself has been shown to induce a pattern of lung injury characterized by neutrophil infiltration of the interstitium and alveolar space and subsequent diffuse epithelial and endothelial cell injury.[139] These pathophysiologic effects are similar to those observed in ARDS and likely result from mechanical stress of alveolar overdistention and high transpulmonary pressures.[140] The ARDS Network published a landmark study in 2000 demonstrating that mechanical ventilation with low tidal volumes decreases mortality in patients with ARDS.[141] Several studies have suggested that a reduction in cytokine release is in part responsible for the protective effect of low tidal volume ventilation.[142] Hammerschmidt and associates demonstrated that mechanical ventilation with a low tidal volume (6 mL/kg) strategy attenuates increases in vascular permeability in a rabbit model of hypochlorite-induced oxidant lung injury. It has been further postulated that because mechanical ventilation may influence cellular metabolism, intrinsic antioxidant enzyme expression and function may be affected by ventilation strategy.[143] This limited evidence together with the results of the ARDS Network study support a recommendation of mechanical ventilation with a low tidal volume strategy (6 mL/kg) in patients with possible oxidant lung injury. In addition, adequate extrinsic positive end-expiratory pressure should be implemented in an attempt to reduce the FIO_2 and minimize the potential for hyperoxia-induced oxidant injury.

ANTIOXIDANTS

A better understanding of the endogenous antioxidant response to oxidant stress has generated interest in the therapeutic potential for exogenous antioxidant administration. Studies of antioxidant therapy have focused on administration of both enzymatic and nonenzymatic antioxidants in a variety of lung diseases. Robbins and coworkers demonstrated a reduction in hyperoxia-induced lung injury with the use of recombinant human superoxide dismutase.[144] Gadek and associates administered enteral nutrition supplemented with a variety of enzymatic and nonenzymatic antioxidants to patients with ARDS and observed a decrease in oxidant production and neutrophil count in BAL fluid.[145] Overexpression of extracellular superoxide dismutase has been shown to attenuate bleomycin-induced lung pulmonary fibrosis in mice.[118] Addition of reduced glutathione to preservation solutions for transplanted organs has been shown to reduce subsequent ischemia-reperfusion injury.[146] However, although these studies demonstrate a potential benefit for exogenous antioxidant administration, there are not yet enough conclusive data to support its routine use in the clinical setting.

FUTURE THERAPY

A variety of potential strategies to prevent and treat oxidative lung injury are being studied. The results of several animal studies have suggested that sublethal endotoxin injection may confer a protective effect against oxidative lung injury.[147] Studies of exogenous antioxidants targeted at specific oxidant mechanisms continue to demonstrate potential therapeutic benefit. A good example is the potential use of heme oxygenase-1 in protecting against oxidant-induced ischemia-reperfusion injury.[148,149] Attempts at improving delivery of antioxidants to lung tissue have yielded successful results. For example, Nakamura and coworkers used intratracheal administration of copper-zinc superoxide dismutase to prevent hyperoxia and ventilator-induced lung injury in newborn piglets.[150] Gene therapy techniques are also being studied in various animal models. Danel and colleagues showed that intratracheal administration of an adenovirus vector encoding copper-zinc superoxide dismutase improves survival of rats exposed to prolonged hyperoxia.[151]

ANNOTATED REFERENCES

Gram TE: Chemically reactive intermediates and pulmonary xenobiotic toxicity. Pharm Rev 1997;49:297-342.
This is a comprehensive review of pulmonary xenobiotic toxicity. The microscopic and ultrastructural effects of hyperoxic lung injury are first reviewed, followed by a summary of the enzymatic processes involved in oxygen toxicity. The author next reviews the mechanisms and pathologic changes associated with a variety of xenobiotic agents.

Nanavaty UB, et al: Oxidant-induced cell death in respiratory epithelial cells is due to DNA damage and loss of ATP. Exp Lung Res 2002;28:591-607.
In this study, Dr. Nanavaty and colleagues address the question of whether DNA damage or apoptosis is responsible for oxidant-induced lung injury. Using a model of hydrogen peroxide induced cytotoxicity in BEAS-2B and A549 cells, they demonstrate a decrease in cellular ATP and an absence of markers of apoptosis in response to injury. These results suggest that DNA damage is one of the primary reasons for oxidant-induced cell death.

Perkowski S, et al: Gene expression profiling of the early pulmonary response to hyperoxia in mice. Am J Respir Cell Mol Biol 2003;28:682-696.
The authors measure changes in total lung gene expression in C57BL/6 mice during hyperoxic exposure. Although no changes were noted in the expression of catalase, MnSOD, and Cu-Zn SOD in response to hyperoxia, glutathione peroxidase, glutathione-S-transferase, heme oxygenase-1, and metallothionein showed moderate increases. The expression of a variety of other lung genes in response to hyperoxia is also examined.

Perrot MD, Liu M, Waddell T, Keshavjee S: Ischemia-reperfusion-induced lung injury. Am J Respir Crit Care Med 2003;167:490-511.
The authors review the current evidence concerning the development of ischemia-reperfusion-induced injury in the lung allograft. The review first examines the role of donor lung assessment and management, including the effects of cold storage. The authors then look at the technique of lung preservation and review the current strategies for the prevention and treatment of ischemia-reperfusion-induced lung injury.

Saugstad OD: Bronchopulmonary dysplasia—oxidative stress and antioxidants. Semin Neonatol 2003;8:39-49.
In this review of BPD, Saugstad summarizes the role of oxidative stress in cellular and mitochondrial processes, leading to the inflammation and fibrosis observed in BPD. He also examines the host antioxidant responses in BPD and reviews the current and future therapeutic approaches to prevent oxidative injury in BPD.

Chapter 38

APOPTOSIS IN THE CRITICALLY ILL

Patricia S. Grutkoski • Chun-Shiang Chung • Jorge Albina • Walter Biffl •
Alfred Ayala

KEY POINTS

1. **Apoptotic cell death** results from one of three major pathways: cell death receptor driven (extrinsic), the mitochondrial pathway (intrinsic), or an endoplasmic reticular stress-induced process.

2. **Blood neutrophil (polymorphonuclear leukocyte [PMN]) constitutive apoptosis** is dysregulated in patients with systemic inflammatory response syndrome, acute respiratory distress syndrome (ARDS), sepsis, trauma, and severe burns. A similar response has been reported in patients with ARDS with respect to PMNs in bronchoalveolar lavage fluids.

3. **Circulating lymphocytes from patients suffering from severe burns, blunt trauma, and sepsis**, as well as from patients who have had major elective surgery (nonseptic), exhibit significantly more apoptosis (approximately 20% to 60% apoptotic) than do peripheral lymphocytes from healthy donors. Similarly, increased lymphocyte apoptosis has been detected in the spleen and gut of patients with sepsis and multiple organ dysfunction syndrome, as well as in trauma and shock patients.

4. Although alterations in apoptosis are most evident in the critically ill, and most experimental models are most obvious in tissues of immune system origin, **a variety of epithelial cells, as well as select parenchymal cells and possibly endothelial cells, may be affected by changes in this pathway.**

5. **The mediators of the apoptotic changes in critically ill patients are as different as the cell type examined.** Nonetheless, data from several experimental models suggest that selective targeting of apoptotic proteins such as caspases and death receptors may provide novel therapeutic avenues in the future.

One of the central components in the control of inflammation is the ability to sustain or to shut down or eliminate cells by regulating their cellular suicide program (apoptosis). Apoptosis is a method by which cells are eliminated from the body in a controlled manner, resulting in clearance of cells without damage to the surrounding environment. The process by which a cell undergoes apoptosis has been reviewed extensively.[1-3] Initially, apoptosis was thought to be a process by which selected cell populations could be actively deleted from specific tissues during morphogenesis and tissue remodeling[4]; it has since been extended to include a variety of roles in immune response resolution and clonal deletion.

Apoptotic cell death results from one of three major pathways: cell death receptor driven (extrinsic), the mitochondrial pathway (intrinsic), or an endoplasmic reticular stress-induced process.[1,5-7] A description of some of the more salient features of these processes is provided as an orientation to the studies discussed here (Fig. 38-1).

The extrinsic death receptor pathway is mediated by the interaction of a trimeric tumor necrosis factor (TNF) receptor (TNF-R)–like family of membrane receptors and their associated ligands, including Fas ligand (FasL), TNF, and TNF-related apoptosis-inducing ligand (see Fig. 38-1). The most studied and the best understood are the TNF–TNF-R and FasL-Fas systems. In this respect, recent studies suggest that Fas-driven apoptosis appears to go through one of two nonexclusive processes, depending on whether it takes place in a type I or type II cell.[8] Type I cells appear to use signaling via Fas-associated death domain–mediated death-inducing signaling complex formation through the activation of caspase-8, driving primarily caspase-3 activation and culminating in the activation of downstream proteases that induce nuclear apoptosis. Alternatively, in type II cells, FasL-Fas–induced cell death appears to be mediated through the subsequent activation of Bid, a cytoplasmic proapoptotic protein. Once Bid is cleaved by caspase-8, it translocates to the mitochondrial membrane, where it interacts with proapoptotic agents such as Bax protein, which in turn deactivates antiapoptotic agents such as Bcl-2, leading to mitochondrial release of cytochrome c and Apaf-1/caspase-9, as well as decreased mitochondrial membrane potential (organelle dysfunction). These events lead to the intrinsic apoptotic pathway, also known as the mitochondrial-driven cell death pathway.

Although much is understood about the components of the mitochondrial apoptotic transition and the consequences of activating this intrinsic pathway (protein release leading to apoptosome formation), its initiation and regulation are less clearly and less directly defined. In this respect, a wide variety of exogenous stressors, such as steroids, reactive oxygen intermediates, nitric oxide, peroxynitrite, and chemokines and cytokines (via activation or inhibition of signaling through phosphatidylinositol-3-kinase-AKT (PI3K-AKT), protein kinase (PKC), mitogen-activated protein kinase (MAPK), and other kinases), as well as the loss of essential growth factors such as interleukin (IL)-2, IL-4, and granulocyte-macrophage colony-stimulating factor (GM-CSF), can result in the induction of apoptosis through this intrinsic pathway (see Fig. 38-1). Finally, endoplasmic

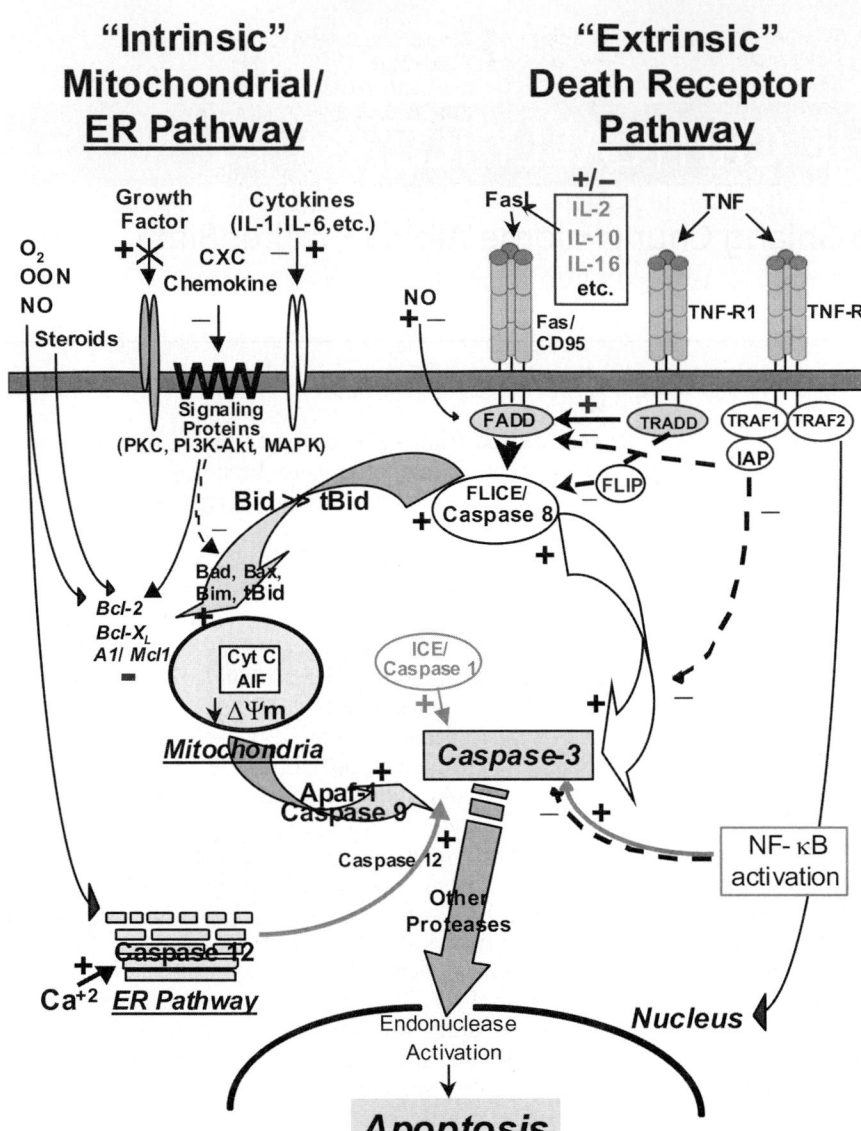

FIGURE 38–1. Central components in the mammalian apoptotic response mediated by either "extrinsic" death receptor or "intrinsic" mitochondrial or endoplasmic reticular (ER) pathways. AIF, apoptosis-inducing factor; CXC, family of alpha-chemokine; FADD, Fas-associated death domain; FLICE, FADD-like ICE; FLIP, FADD-like ICE inhibitory protein; IAP, inhibitor of apoptosis protein; ICE, interleukin-1β converting enzyme; IL, interleukin; MAPK, mitogen-activated protein kinase; NF-κB, nuclear factor kappa; NO, nitric oxide; PKC, protein kinase C; TNF, tumor necrosis factor; TRADD, TNF receptor-associated death domain; TRAF, TNF receptor-associated factor.

reticular stress-driven apoptosis is the least well understood. This pathway is mediated by the release and activation of caspase-12. However, little is known beyond the potential role of oxidant stress and Ca⁺⁺ as an activator of this process.

As alluded to earlier, the very process of macrophage or lymphocyte activation required to mount a competent inflammatory or adaptive immune response to a foreign pathogen sets in motion, for most cells, processes involved in mediating their own demise.[9,10] In this respect, the process by which a mature T cell is activated, via concordant T-cell receptor complex stimulation and costimulatory molecule engagement, simultaneously induces the up-regulation of death receptors (such as Fas) that make the activated T cells more susceptible to ligands that induce apoptosis.[10-12] With respect to the resolution of inflammation or local tissue injury, lymphocyte Fas-FasL–mediated fratricide is also a potentially important process, with numerous examples of lymphocyte-lymphocyte induction of cell death being documented.[13,14] Macrophages and monocytes may also use such a mechanism, with granulocytes encountered at sites of inflammation.[15]

POLYMORPHONUCLEAR LEUKOCYTE APOPTOSIS

SUPPRESSION

Polymorphonuclear leukocytes (PMNs, neutrophils) play a crucial role in the primary immunologic defense against infectious agents, and they use the apoptotic program not only for resolution but also as a means of natural cell turnover. Although the primary role for PMNs is to eliminate pathogens, they can also be detrimental, being major contributors to organ damage induced by ischemia-reperfusion, trauma, and sepsis. The importance of PMNs in organ damage and mortality has been demonstrated using anti-PMN therapies to block lung and liver damage after sepsis induced by cecal ligation and puncture (CLP),[16] anti–IL-8 therapy to block PMN infiltration into the lung after lipopolysaccharide (LPS) treatment,[17] and anti-macrophage inflammatory protein-2 (anti-MIP2) treatment to block PMN infiltration into the peritoneum after the induction

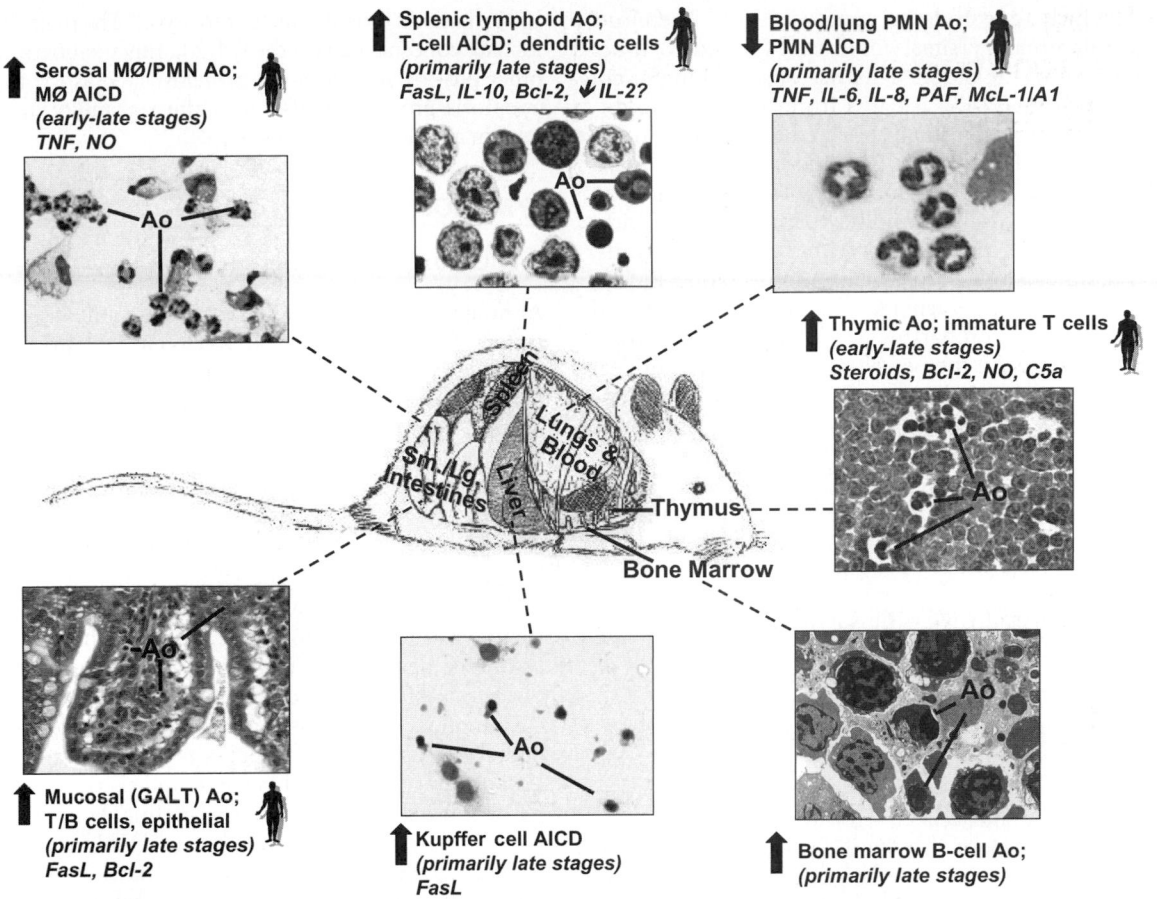

↑ Serosal MØ/PMN Ao;
MØ AICD
(early-late stages)
TNF, NO

↑ Splenic lymphoid Ao;
T-cell AICD; dendritic cells
(primarily late stages)
FasL, IL-10, Bcl-2, ↓*IL-2?*

↓ Blood/lung PMN Ao;
PMN AICD
(primarily late stages)
TNF, IL-6, IL-8, PAF, McL-1/A1

↑ Thymic Ao; immature T cells
(early-late stages)
Steroids, Bcl-2, NO, C5a

↑ Mucosal (GALT) Ao;
T/B cells, epithelial
(primarily late stages)
FasL, Bcl-2

↑ Kupffer cell AICD
(primarily late stages)
FasL

↑ Bone marrow B-cell Ao;
(primarily late stages)

FIGURE 38–2. The frequency of apoptosis (A$_o$), the immune cell populations affected, the onset or expression of apoptotic changes, and the agents that mediate these cell death effects vary in mice subject to experimental sepsis and in patients (♦) with multiple organ failure due to trauma or sepsis. General increases (↑) or decreases (↓) in apoptosis in the septic mouse model are indicated either for in vivo or ex vivo cells or tissues or for activation-induced cell death (AICD) seen in vitro for a given cell population. (♦) indicates that a comparable observation has been made in humans. The stage (time period) during experimental sepsis when such apoptotic changes typically become evident is italicized in parentheses, and the mediators reported to affect apoptosis are listed last in italics. GALT, gut-associated lymphoid tissue; IL, interleukin; MØ, macrophage; NO, nitric oxide; PAF, platelet-activating factor; PMN, polymorphonuclear leukocyte; TNF, tumor necrosis factor.

of sepsis.[18] In each situation, tissue or organ damage was significantly reduced, and survival was improved.

It has been established that once PMNs are released into circulation, their apoptotic program has already been activated, and the typical half-life of an unstimulated PMN is 6 to 12 hours.[19] Because clearance of PMNs would limit the damage they could induce, it is not unexpected that peripheral blood as well as bronchoalveolar lavage PMN apoptosis is dysregulated in patients with systemic inflammatory response syndrome, acute respiratory distress syndrome, sepsis, trauma, and severe burns (Fig. 38-2).[20-25] It is also of interest to note that PMN apoptosis can be suppressed by surgery alone (elective, non–trauma related) at time points (<24 hours) that preclude the possible development of the clinical situations listed.[26]

REGULATION BY INFLAMMATORY MEDIATORS

PMNs recruited to sites of inflammation are exposed to factors that can influence apoptosis, such as bacterial products, lipids, cytokines, and changes in oxygen tension.[27] Elevated levels of cytokines such as granulocyte colony-stimulating factor (G-CSF), GM-CSF, IL-1, IL-6, IL-8, and TNF are often found

in peritoneal fluid, bronchoalveolar lavage, and serum of trauma patients or experimental animals,[17,18,25,26,28-31] and each has been found, in vitro, to suppress apoptosis of PMNs from healthy volunteers.[19,25,32-34] Additionally, transmigration, bacterial products (e.g., LPS), and hypoxia have been found to suppress PMN apoptosis in vitro.[32,35,36] Similarly, when PMNs from healthy volunteers are incubated in bronchoalveloar lavage or serum from patients with burns,[23] acute respiratory distress syndrome,[29,37] or sepsis,[24] a significant reduction in apoptosis is observed. Although endothelial cells or macrophages are thought to produce a majority of these cytokines, PMNs have the ability to suppress their own apoptosis in an autocrine or paracrine manner through the production and secretion of antiapoptotic factors.[23,33,38-41]

EXTRACELLULAR MILIEU

Although the studies mentioned earlier demonstrate that inhibition of PMNs or their recruitment significantly improves the outcome of a septic insult, PMN apoptosis was not examined. In vitro experiments indicate that blood PMNs that were stimulated with various inflammatory stimuli, were subjected to in vitro migration, were exposed to various adhesins, or ingested microbes exhibit differences in the rate at which they undergo apoptosis.[32,35,42] Therefore, PMNs in inflammatory sites would be expected to differ from those seen in the blood. This was observed in patient studies in which the PMNs isolated from the lung had different characteristics from those purified from the blood of the same patient.[43,44] Using the CLP model of sepsis, Ayala and colleagues assessed the extent of apoptosis in phagocytes expressing Gr1 (the mouse granulocyte marker) from three separate tissue sites.[45] In agreement with findings in patients, decreased apoptosis was seen in CLP mouse blood PMNs, while no change in the percentage of apoptosis was detected in the myelopoietic compartment of the bone marrow.[46] However, an increase in the percentage of Gr1[+] cells undergoing apoptosis was evident in cells taken from the peritoneum of the CLP mice, and the extent of apoptosis in these cells appears to be regulated by TNF.[45] Whether other death receptor or non–death receptor pathways are also involved in regulating apoptosis at this or other sites of PMN accumulation in traumatized or septic animals is unknown.

ROLE OF Bcl-2 FAMILY MEMBERS

The mechanism by which inflammatory agents suppress PMN apoptosis remains an active area of study, but numerous agents have been found that regulate members of the Bcl-2 family, which can inhibit spontaneous (mitochondrial-driven) and induced (Fas- or TNF-R–driven) apoptosis (Table 38-1). PMNs, unlike lymphoid cells, do not express Bcl-2 but do express other members of this family, such as Bcl-w, Mcl-1, Bak, Bcl-X$_L$, and A1,[42,44,47-51] and changes in their expression in response to stimulation are specific for the agent used. Studies by Leuenroth and associates indicate that in the hypoxic environments (mimicked in vitro) encountered in hemorrhaged animals or trauma patients, the suppression of apoptosis, at least in human PMNs, is regulated by the induction of Mcl-1.[42] Mcl-1 is also up-regulated upon stimulation with G-CSF, GM-CSF, IL-1ß, TNF, and LPS,[48,49] while these same agents have no effect on Bcl-X expression.[48] Chuang and coworkers demonstrated that messenger RNA for A1 was increased in response to G-CSF, GM-CSF, and LPS, but not IL-1ß or TNF.[49] And finally, Bax expression was down-regulated by G-CSF and GM-CSF, but not IL-8, LPS, or TNF.[44,51] Although patient data are limited, Dibbert and colleagues reported that PMNs isolated from patients with inflammatory diseases express reduced amounts of Bax, suggesting that changes observed

in vitro mimic those that occur in vivo.[44] The majority of studies have concentrated on the Bcl-2 family members; changes in other pro- or antiapoptotic proteins, such as the inhibitor of apoptosis proteins (IAPs), that affect granulocyte cell death remain an area of active research.[52]

LYMPHOCYTE APOPTOSIS

IMMUNOSUPPRESSION

Although PMNs make up a large part of the innate immune system, lymphocytes (B and T cells) are the primary players in the adaptive immune response to an inflammatory challenge. This adaptive immune response involves the rapid expansion of these cells in response to cytokine and antigen stimulation. Apoptosis was initially proposed as a mechanism whereby autoreactive lymphocytes could be removed (deselected) or as a process by which the extent of immune cell activation could be contained (resolved).[1,53] However, it is apparent that this same process can contribute to the pathophysiology of disease states such as human immunodeficiency virus (HIV) immune depression, cancer, autoimmune disorders, neurodegenerative diseases, inflammatory bowel disease, and ischemic injury.[1,5,53]

Lymphocyte apoptosis is a major concern in the ICU, because many critically ill patients exhibit immunosuppression as a result of lymphocyte apoptosis from several compartments (see Fig. 38-2). Circulating lymphocytes from patients suffering from severe burns,[54,55] blunt trauma,[55] and sepsis,[56] as well as from those who have undergone major elective surgery (nonseptic),[56,57] exhibit significantly more apoptosis (approximately 20% to 60% apoptotic) than do peripheral lymphocytes from healthy donors. Hotchkiss and colleagues detected lymphocyte apoptosis in the spleen and gut of trauma and shock patients,[58-60] and Middleton and associates found a significant amount of thymocyte apoptosis in patients who died more than 3 hours after an initial trauma.[61] The loss of lymphocytes from all three compartments is thought to be directly associated with the decreased number of lymphocytes in the circulation. Unfortunately, this immunosuppression leaves patients vulnerable to infection or unable to fight existing sepsis and may result in organ failure. Until recently, the contribution of the process of apoptosis to the pathophysiology of multiple organ dysfunction in critically ill patients had not been examined.[19] As with human lymphocytes, lymphocytes from rodents subjected to burn injury[62] and sepsis (CLP)[63,64] also exhibit pronounced immunosuppression, accompanied by increased lymphocyte apoptosis. This is the model of sepsis that has provided most of our current knowledge about the role of apoptosis in the critically ill (see Fig. 38-2).

THYMOCYTE APOPTOSIS

The initial experimental studies of trauma- and sepsis-induced changes in lymphoid apoptosis focused on the thymus because it is readily accessible and highly susceptible to stress-induced apoptosis. Studies involving various trauma, burn, sepsis, and shock models all consistently reported that thymic apoptosis increases in these settings (see Fig. 38-2).[46,65-68] In the CLP model of sepsis and in burn injury, it was observed that a rise in thymic apoptosis could be detected as early as 4 hours after injury and increased through 24 hours.[46,66] This increased apoptosis in the mouse

TABLE 38–1. POLYMORPHONUCLEAR LEUKOCYTE APOPTOSIS—MEDIATORS AND THE Bcl-2 FAMILY OF PROTEINS

Mediator	Mcl-1	A1	Bcl-X	Bax
G-CSF	↑	↑	↔	↓
GM-CSF	↑	↑	↔	↓
IL-1β	↑	↔	↔	nd
IL-8	↑	nd	nd	↔
TNF	↑	↔	↔	↔
LPS	↑	↑	↔	↔
Hypoxia	↑	nd	nd	nd

Arrows indicate the ability of each mediator to alter the expression of the Bcl-2 family members listed: ↑, increased expression; ↓, decreased expression; ↔, no effect.
G-CSF, granulocyte colony-stimulating factor; GM-CSF, granulocyte-macrophage colony-stimulating factor; IL, interleukin; LPS, lipopolysaccharide; nd, no data (the proteins were not examined); TNF, tumor necrosis factor.

TABLE 38–2. AGENTS INVOLVED IN LYMPHOCYTE APOPTOSIS

	Agents
Thymocyte apoptosis	
Mediators	Glucocorticoids (+), NO (+), C5a (+), TNF (↔), endotoxin (↔), Fas/FasL (↔), IL-10 (–)
Protein expression after injury	Bcl-X$_L$ (↓), Bcl-2 (↓)
Splenocyte apoptosis—mediators	TGF-β (+), IL-10 (+), Fas/FasL (+)
GALT mediators	Fas/FasL (+), endotoxin (↔)

+, ability to promote lymphocyte apoptosis; –, ability to suppress lymphocyte apoptosis; ↔, no effect on lymphocyte apoptosis; ↓, decreased protein expression.
GALT, gut-associated lymphoid tissue; IL, interleukin; NO, nitric oxide; TGF, transforming growth factor; TNF, tumor necrosis factor.

thymus appears to be primarily a response to glucocorticoids, and possibly nitric oxide (NO), rather than to endotoxin or death receptors such as Fas and TNF-R. Treatment with mifepristone, a glucocorticoid receptor antagonist, but not the neutralizing Fas-fusion protein, blocked thymic apoptosis (Table 38-2).[46,66] Support for a putative role of NO in thymic apoptosis comes from in vitro data in which thymocytes cultured with LPS-activated endothelial cells, which produce NO, or with NO donors exhibited increased apoptosis.[69] Another putative mediator of thymocyte apoptosis, either directly or indirectly, is the complement anaphylatoxin C5a; blocking its activity with anti-C5a therapy inhibited thymic apoptosis after CLP in rats.[67] Additionally, because cytokines play a prominent role in lymphocyte activation and apoptosis, Oberholzer and coworkers were able to inhibit thymocyte apoptosis during sepsis by using targeted expression of IL-10, resulting in reduced blood bacteremia and improved mortality.[70] This is of interest because IL-10 is generally regarded as an anti-inflammatory cytokine, and it has been found to have a proapoptotic effect on the circulating lymphocytes of trauma patients.[57]

SPLENOCYTE APOPTOSIS

In addition to thymic apoptosis, apoptosis in the spleen has been documented after burn injury and trauma and in cases of sepsis (see Fig. 38-2).[58,65,71-73] Just as the degree of lymphocyte apoptosis correlates with disease severity in patients, splenic apoptosis is correlated with the severity of burns; no apoptosis could be detected in the spleens of mice subjected to burns covering 18% of their total body surface area,[68] but it could be detected in mice subjected to burns covering 25% and 40%, with the level of apoptosis higher in the 40% group.[71] Similarly, Guan and associates demonstrated that in rats subjected to multitrauma events (hemorrhage ± multiple fractures), apoptosis rates were directly correlated with trauma severity.[65] Studies by Hiramatsu and Hotchkiss and their colleagues showed evidence of increased splenic lymphocyte apoptosis in septic mice, associated with increased mortality.[72,73] Histologic analysis of spleens from septic human patients, but not from nonseptic patients, demonstrated that apoptosis in the spleen involves primarily B cells and CD4+ T cells.[58] Interestingly, in Rag-1 mice, which are deficient in B and T cells, apoptosis was still detected in thymic and splenic cell populations.[73] In vitro experiments to determine whether the increased lymphoid apoptosis in these tissues is associated with immune

hyporesponsiveness indicated that mitogenic stimulation of splenocytes isolated from mice 24 hours after CLP causes a significant increase in the rate of activation-induced cell death (AICD).[64] This increase in AICD also appears to be restricted to T cells of the helper (CD4+) lineage.[64]

APOPTOSIS IN THE GUT

A number of other lymphoid tissues also appear to actively undergo increased apoptosis following the onset of sepsis or shock (see Fig. 38-2). However, unlike in the thymus, where apoptosis is evident as early as 4 hours after CLP, apoptosis in other tissues typically does not appear until later (>12 hours). Mixed bone marrow cells showed an increase in apoptosis at 24 hours, but not at 4 hours, following CLP.[46] Although phenotypic and morphologic assessment indicated that most of the increase in apoptosis in the thymus was in the immature T-cell population (CD4+CD8+ and CD8-D4- cells), the increase in bone marrow cell apoptosis was associated with only the B-lymphocyte population. Gut-associated lymphoid tissues, such as Peyer's patches, also exhibit increased apoptosis in response to polymicrobial sepsis.[72,74] As with the bone marrow, these changes were restricted to the B-cell population, which exhibited an increase of Fas antigen expression; this therefore appears to be an example of AICD in sepsis.[1] Chung and coworkers reported similar findings following traumatic shock.[46] The functional aspect of this increased in vivo apoptosis appears to be related to the endogenous stimulation of immunoglobulin A production by B lymphocytes and increased nuclear c-Rel expression.[75]

These findings are not restricted to the Peyer's patches; similar findings have been observed in the B-lymphocyte subset of the lamina propria (see Fig. 38-2).[46] Assessment of lamina propria mononuclear cell (LPMC) preparations from septic mice indicates that there are increases in the percentage of apoptosis in CD4+ and CD8+ cells, as well as macrophages, at both 4 hours (except for CD4+) and 24 hours.[46] This is associated with a significant increase in the mixed LPMC IL-2, -10, and -15 gene expression observed at 24 hours, but not at 4 hours, after CLP. These findings correlate well with the in situ observations by Hiramatsu and colleagues, who reported evidence of increased apoptosis in Peyer's patches and in lymphoid cells lining the small and large intestines in mice 24 hours after CLP.[72] Hotchkiss and coworkers also documented that increased intestinal lymphoid apoptosis is a common finding in patients undergoing surgery after major trauma.[59] Intriguingly, it has been reported that the phenotypically distinct intestinal intraepithelial lymphocyte population also exhibits changes associated with increased apoptosis.[46] This appears to be a FasL-Fas antigen-mediated process independent of endotoxin sensitivity and may be a reflection of localized immune cell activation in response to sepsis (see Table 38-2).

CYTOKINES

One of the common effects of burn, trauma, and sepsis in both patients and animal models is a significant change in the expression of a number of pro- and anti-inflammatory cytokines, including TNF, IL-1, IL-4, IL-6, IL-10, IL-12, and IFN-γ.[76-79] The plasma concentration of several of these cytokines has been correlated with disease severity and levels of lymphocyte apoptosis in both patients and experimental animals.[57,76,77,80] Two cytokines that are prominent in burn injury, trauma, and sepsis are TNF and IL-1β, and modulation of their activity in animal models led to several clinical trials, but without success.

One cytokine that has been shown to have a direct effect on lymphocyte apoptosis is transforming growth factor beta, which induces lymphocyte apoptosis and is expressed at high levels that correlate with increased splenic lymphocyte apoptosis after burn injury.[71] In contrast, the roles of the other cytokines in lymphocyte apoptosis are vague but nevertheless important to survival. Because the balance between pro- and anti-inflammatory cytokines is crucial to survival, the importance of IL-10 and IL-13 as regulatory molecules has been demonstrated. Through the use of neutralizing antibodies, IL-13 has been shown to have a protective effect on organ damage (i.e., liver, lung, kidney) and ultimately on survival, primarily by limiting the expression of cytokines such as TNF, MIP-2, and keratinocyte-derived cytokine (KC).[81] Similarly, Hasko and associates showed that mice deficient in IL-10 (IL10–/–) had higher levels of TNF, IL-1β, IL-2, IL-6, IL-12, and IFN-γ than did wild-type controls during sepsis, and that this deficiency resulted in increased apoptosis in the thymus.[82] In support of this, Ayala and coworkers demonstrated that splenocytes isolated from septic IL10–/– mice or wild-type splenocytes cultured with antibodies to IL-10 had reduced AICD.[64] The proapoptotic effect of IL-10 on increased AICD in the circulating lymphocytes of surgical trauma patients has also been reported.[57] Finally, O'Sullivan and colleagues found that patients and mice with trauma or burn injuries had suppressed IL-12 levels, and mice receiving IL-12 had decreased mortality after CLP.[78] Taken together, these data implicate several pro- and anti-inflammatory cytokines present in the critically ill that can directly or indirectly affect the apoptotic changes in immune cells.

MONOCYTE-MACROPHAGE AND DENDRITIC CELL APOPTOSIS

Regarding macrophages, the majority of work has assessed the in vitro response to stimuli such as LPS, TNF, IL-1, IL-10, IFN-γ, FasL, and NO.[83,84] As with the other immune cells mentioned earlier, the response of macrophages to apoptotic stimuli also appears to be time dependent.[84] Although most of the components of the FasL-Fas and TNF pathways are evident, it is less clear whether a comparable series of anti-apoptotic gene products is present. The macrophage response to polymicrobial sepsis appears to be tissue specific. Evidence of ex vivo apoptosis can be seen in peritoneal (serosal) macrophages isolated as early as 4 hours after CLP, and it increases over time; however, a small but significant decrease in the basal apoptosis frequency is evident in liver macrophages.[85] Interestingly, if they are subsequently challenged in vitro with an inflammatory stimulus such as LPS, both these macrophage populations become considerably more apoptotic than do comparative sham-CLP animal cells.[85,86] This is associated with a functional disability in their capacity to release proinflammatory cytokines, such as IL-1 and IL-6, and with decreased caspase-1 but increased caspase-3, -8, and -9 activity.[84] The role of FasL-Fas signaling in these changes also appears to be tissue specific. In peritoneal macrophages, apoptosis and cytokine release do not appear to be affected by FasL-Fas activation, but in liver macrophages, changes are seen.[87] To the extent that such changes in macrophage apoptosis and function may be just

an aberration seen in mice, it is worth noting that Williams and coworkers reported similar observations in circulating monocytes derived from the blood of septic patients.[88] Finally, Hotchkiss and associates found that dendritic cells in patients who succumbed to sepsis also appear to exhibit increased evidence of apoptosis[89]; however, the mechanisms responsible for this are not clear. Studies examining dendritic cell apoptosis suggest that although they contribute to the fratricide of other cells, they may not be affected by FasL-Fas signaling themselves.[90] This remains to be determined in sepsis.

EFFECTS OF APOPTOTIC CELLS

Although we have discussed the potential direct pathologic effects of the apoptotic process on various cell lineages of the immune system, it is important to appreciate that the interaction with and clearance of apoptotic cells can have a significant effect on the host's immune response. The process of apoptotic cell clearance is primarily, but not exclusively, regulated by macrophages.[91] This process is mediated by the recognition of a variety of ligands expressed on apoptotic cells by receptors, primarily on macrophages, used to mediate the apoptotic cells' removal (Fig. 38-3). Through a pinocytotic mechanism, fibroblasts and epithelial cells may also contribute to apoptotic cell clearance.[92] The interaction of macrophages with apoptotic cells induces the expression of an anti-inflammatory phenotype in the macrophages. Until recently, there were few supportive data, but one could speculate that this might contribute to the anergy seen in macrophages isolated from septic mice or patients.[93] In this respect, Hotchkiss and colleagues recently showed that the administration or adoptive transfer of apoptotic lymphocytes derived from septic mice could suppress T helper 1 cytokine responsiveness while preserving the T helper 2 anti-inflammatory response associated with the immune-suppressive phenotype seen in experimental sepsis.[94]

Alternatively, the documented inability of monocytes or macrophages from septic, shocked, or traumatized animals to phagocytize materials at normal levels may contribute to the inadvertent accumulation of apoptotic cells in various hematopoietic, lymphatic, and immune tissues (see Fig. 38-3). In turn, the inability to appropriately clear these dying cells may allow them to progress to a state of secondary necrosis, producing localized bystander injury in the tissue. Such a scenario has been suggested by Vandivier and coworkers as a possible mechanism for tissue inflammation and the enhanced susceptibility to infection seen in cystic fibrosis patients.[95,96] It remains to be determined whether such defects in the macrophage-mediated clearance of apoptotic cells contribute to the changes seen in septic mice.

ANTIAPOPTOSIS THERAPIES

The importance of lymphocyte apoptosis in the development of multiple organ failure and subsequent death has been clearly demonstrated by the use of therapies to block the process at several steps in the apoptosis pathway. Starting at the cell surface, Chung and associates demonstrated that the use of Fas-fusion protein, which blocks FasL binding to cell surface Fas, preserves organ function and blood flow in mice subjected to CLP and reduces septic mortality (Fig. 38-4).[97] Hotchkiss and colleagues used several methodologies to inhibit apoptosis after CLP to assess its importance

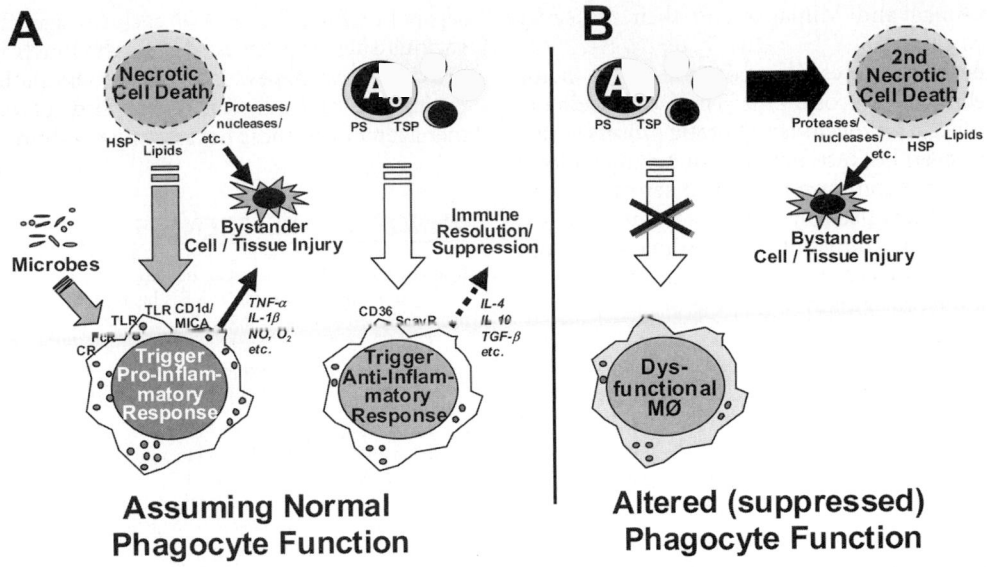

**Assuming Normal
Phagocyte Function**

**Altered (suppressed)
Phagocyte Function**

FIGURE 38–3. *A,* Depiction of the clearance of necrotic and apoptotic cell materials, as well as the effect of this process on the macrophage phenotype (proinflammatory versus anti-inflammatory), when phagocytic function is normal. *B,* The scheme in which phagocytic function is compromised, blocking apoptotic cell clearance and subsequently allowing apoptotic cells to move into secondary necrosis; this, in turn, produces bystander tissue injury. CD1d/MICA, nonvariant major histocompatibility class 1–like antigen family; CD36, cell differentiation antigen 36; CR, complement receptor; FcR, immunoglobulin constant region receptor; HSP, heat shock protein; IL, interleukin; MØ, macrophage; NO, nitric oxide; PS, phosphatidylserine; ScavR, scavenger receptor that binds PS; TGF, transforming growth factor; TLR, Toll-like receptor; TNF, tumor necrosis factor; TSP, thrombospondin.

in the pathology of sepsis (see Fig. 38-4).[98,99] Because caspase activity, particularly caspase-3, is crucial to all forms of apoptosis, they were able to use several pharmacologic caspase inhibitors to block lymphocyte apoptosis, which resulted in decreased apoptosis and increased survival. Similarly, sepsis did not induce lymphocyte apoptosis in caspase-3 –/– mice when compared with their background controls.[98] Finally, similar to the regulation of apoptosis in

PMNs, expression of members of the Bcl-2 family of proteins has been found to be altered in lymphocytes either stimulated in vitro or isolated from animals subjected to trauma or sepsis (see Table 38-2). Lee and coworkers demonstrated that CD40 can inhibit Fas-mediated apoptosis in a B-cell lymphoma cell line through the induction of Bcl-X and A1.[100] Thymocytes isolated from protein kinase B transgenic mice were found to have resistance to a variety of apoptotic stimuli, and this correlated with elevated levels of Bcl-X$_L$.[101] Bcl-X$_L$ was found to be significantly reduced in thymocytes after CLP,[67,102] and thymic apoptosis in response to sepsis was associated with decreased Bcl-2[102]; therapies that blocked apoptosis and improved survival either restored or increased Bcl-2 expression.[70,102] In light of this, it is no surprise that mice overexpressing Bcl-2 in T cells had improved survival in sepsis, which correlated with a lack of lymphocyte apoptosis in both the thymus and the spleen (see Fig. 38-4).[103]

NON–IMMUNE CELL APOPTOSIS

At this point, it should be clear that a significant amount of experimental as well as clinical evidence exists for the presence of marked apoptotic changes and potential pathologic sequelae in both animals and patients with sepsis and multiple organ failure syndrome. Surprisingly, demonstration of apoptosis in nonimmune tissues and cells has been substantially more difficult in the clinical setting.

For example, although apoptosis in the vascular endothelium has been proffered as an explanation for the frequently observed loss of hemodynamic responsiveness in critically ill patients and certain septic animal models, there is a paucity of direct evidence for such an event.[104] This is due in large part to the difficulty of assessing this process directly in experimental animals, let alone patients. Nonetheless, some indirect evidence of apoptosis-induced shedding of CD34+ cells into the bloodstream of critically ill patients has been

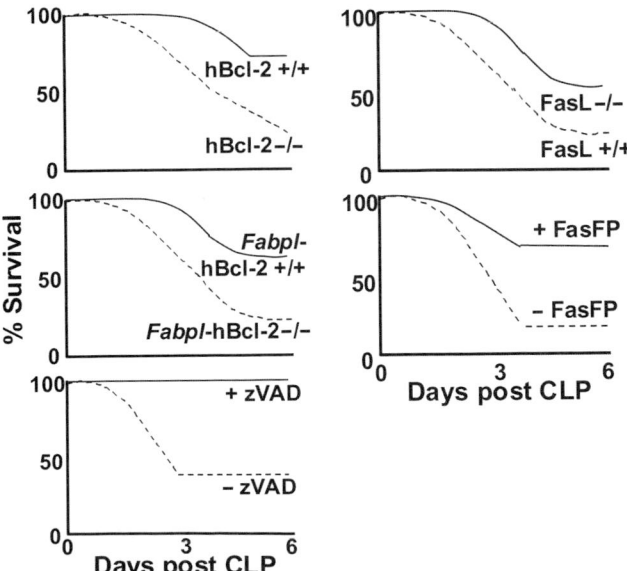

FIGURE 38–4. Results of survival studies illustrating the efficacy of directly inhibiting aspects of apoptosis in sepsis using the transgenic overexpression of the human Bcl-2 gene (under either a lymphoid restricted promoter [hBcl-2] or an intestinal epithelial cell restricted promoter [fabpl-hBcl-2]), pan-specific caspase inhibition (zVAD),[98] and death receptor inhibition in animals deficient in FasL (FasL–/–)[46] or administered Fas-fusion protein (FasFP) 12 hours after cecal ligation and puncture (CLP).

observed by Mutunga and Miniagar and their respective colleagues.[105,106]

Another potentially interesting apoptotic target is the surface of epithelial and mucosal cells. These cells, being at the mucosal interface, turn over via apoptotic processes on a regular basis. However, because mucosal sloughing and gut barrier dysfunction are common aspects of sepsis, trauma, and critical illness, it has been hypothesized that increased apoptotic cell death may contribute in a pathologic fashion to organ dysfunction in the gut[107,108] and in the lungs.[109] Experimental support for a pathologic role of gut epithelial cell apoptosis has been provided by Coopersmith and associates, who showed that septic mortality could be reduced in mice expressing the epithelial cell restricted overexpression of the human Bcl-2 gene (see Fig. 38-4).[107,110] Hotchkiss and colleagues also documented that, along with the predominance of lymphoid apoptosis seen in septic patients succumbing to their illness, there was consistent evidence of intestinal epithelial cell apoptosis; a similar but more transient observation was made in trauma patients undergoing bowel resection.[60] Epithelial cell injury in the lung has also been observed experimentally,[109,111,112] but its clinical contribution to chronic or acute lung injury remains to be clearly established. Further, the degree of interaction between immune cell subpopulations undergoing apoptosis and the extent of changes in epithelial cell apoptosis is unknown at present.

Beyond these observations and the substantial data provided by various experimental situations in vitro or in vivo,[113-120] there is little evidence of changes in the apoptotic process in the liver parenchyma, heart, kidney, or brain in the clinical setting of sepsis or multiple organ failure. This does not mean that apoptosis is not playing a role, but merely that it is not overt, or that the form of cell death induced in these organs, tissues, and cells is not solely apoptotic.

CONCLUSION

Our understanding of the mechanisms by which multicellular organisms regulate cell life and death via apoptosis has grown tremendously over the past few years. It is now clear that septic or traumatized animals and patients exhibit alterations in the apoptosis of cells in both the innate (PMNs) and the adaptive (lymphocytes) arms of the immune system. Even though PMN apoptosis is suppressed under similar conditions in which lymphocytes undergo increased apoptosis, the consequence of each appears to contribute to significant pathologic alterations in host cell function, which is associated with an increase in organ damage and mortality. However, we are just beginning to understand the mechanisms and mediators (e.g., FasL, TNF, IL-8, Bcl-2, Mcl-1, NO, steroids) that regulate these changes. The data clearly show the complexity of the apoptotic response, thus justifying the need to increase our understanding of apoptosis in the critically ill. This will require the use of complex and clinically comparable models of shock, trauma, burn, and sepsis in which the cells of each lineage can be assessed at various sites and times after insult. Such information will provide us with new insight into the pathobiology of the critically ill and may offer better therapeutic targets for the management of these devastating conditions.

ANNOTATED REFERENCES

Ayala A, Xu YX, Ayala CA, et al: Increased mucosal B-lymphocyte apoptosis during polymicrobial sepsis is a Fas ligand but not an endotoxin mediated process. Blood 1998;91:1362-1372.
This prospective animal modeling study illustrates that gut lymphoid apoptosis observed during experimental sepsis may be an effect of extrinsic, death receptor–driven apoptosis as well as intrinsic processes.

Coopersmith CM, Stromberg PE, Dunne WM, et al: Inhibition of intestinal epithelial apoptosis and survival in a murine model of pneumonia-induced sepsis. JAMA 2002;287:1716-1721.
This prospective, randomized experimental animal study demonstrates the contribution of increased intestinal epithelial cell apoptosis to the morbidity and mortality from pneumonia-induced sepsis using gut epithelial cell restricted overexpression of the antiapoptotic gene Bcl-2.

Hotchkiss RS, Chang KC, Grayson MH, et al: Adoptive transfer of apoptotic splenocytes worsens survival, whereas adoptive transfer of necrotic splenocytes improves survival in sepsis. Proc Natl Acad Sci U S A 2003;100:6724-6729.
This study documents a potential link (in the experimental setting of mouse polymicrobial sepsis) between the development or presence of increased lymphocyte apoptosis and the subsequent capacity of these cells (through their phagocytosis or clearance) to induce an immune-suppressive state in mice. The state of immune suppression is a hallmark of morbidity in this system in both the experimental setting and the clinical condition.

Hotchkiss RS, Swanson PE, Freeman BD, et al: Apoptotic cell death in patients with sepsis, shock and multiple organ dysfunction. Crit Care Med 1999;27:1230-1251.
This prospective study of patients dying from sepsis and multiple organ failure demonstrates a strong association between the development of significant lymphocyte and intestinal epithelial cell apoptosis and septic mortality.

Hotchkiss RS, Tinsley KW, Swanson PE, Karl IE: Endothelial cell apoptosis in sepsis. Crit Care Med 2002;30:S225-S228.
This article summarizes the understanding of the apoptotic process in endothelial cells and the difficulties encountered in demonstrating this form of cell death in vivo, both in experimental models of infection, sepsis, and inflammation and in the critically ill.

Hotchkiss RS, Tinsley KW, Swanson PE, et al: Prevention of lymphocyte cell death in sepsis improves survival in mice. Proc Natl Acad Sci U S A 1999;96:14541-14546.
This was one of the first prospective, randomized animal studies to document the potential of an antiapoptotic therapy (caspase inhibition) to block mortality in a model of polymicrobial sepsis.

Jimenez MF, Watson WG, Parodo J, et al: Dysregulated expression of neutrophil apoptosis in the systemic inflammatory response syndrome. Arch Surg 1997;132:1263-1270.
This study was one of the first to demonstrate that peripheral blood neutrophils obtained from septic patients exhibit a substantially depressed ability to undergo spontaneous apoptosis.

Kim Y-M, Kim T-H, Chung H-T, et al: Nitric oxide prevents tumor necrosis factor α–induced rat hepatocyte apoptosis by the interruption of mitochondrial apoptotic signaling through S-nitrosylation of caspase-8. Hepatology 2000;32:770-778.
This is one of several studies from this laboratory that illustrates the capacity of nitric oxide, like several other inflammatory agents present in critically ill patients, to be either antiapoptotic or proapoptotic.

Chapter 39

CELLULAR SIGNALING

Michael B. Fessler • Jerry A. Nick

KEY POINTS

1. **Intracellular signal transduction** describes mechanisms that allow an individual cell to coordinate responses to extracellular stimuli.

2. Intracellular signaling occurs primarily through **sequential phosphorylation of proteins.**

3. Although highly conserved, **signaling mechanisms are often adapted** for different uses by different cell types.

4. **Central signaling pathways** participate in multiple responses to a variety of receptors and stimuli.

5. Signaling pathways represent **potential targets to modify specific cellular responses.**

Signal transduction refers to sequential molecular interactions triggered within the cell in response to external conditions (e.g., ultraviolet radiation, heat, osmotic stress) or ligands (e.g., bacterial lipopolysaccharides, cytokines) that lead, in turn, to induction of specific cellular responses (e.g., transcription/translation, adhesion, chemotaxis). Intracellular signaling involves precisely timed, compartmentalized, specific, and reversible interactions between proteins and underlies biologic phenomena of health and disease alike, ranging from cellular proliferation to immunity to sepsis. Increasingly, the potential of cellular signaling molecules as diagnostic markers and therapeutic targets is being realized. A basic understanding of the principles of signal transduction and of the important cellular signaling cascades is necessary to evaluate current research in critical care medicine and may be of increasing use to the clinician.

BASIC PRINCIPLES OF SIGNAL TRANSDUCTION

PHOSPHORYLATION CASCADES AND ACTIVATION OF KINASES

Virtually all cellular signaling pathways described to date are regulated by protein phosphorylation. The phosphorylation of a target protein by a protein *kinase*—an enzyme that covalently attaches phosphate to the side chain of either serine, threonine, or tyrosine—can have multiple effects on the protein, including modulation of its enzymatic activity, stability, subcellular localization, and interaction with other proteins. Many signaling pathways involve *cascades* of two or more kinases in series in which an "upstream" kinase is phosphorylated, resulting in activation of the enzyme, with subsequent phosphorylation of a "downstream" kinase, which in turn is activated and able to phosphorylate specific substrates or additional kinases. Rare examples exist of inactivation of a target enzyme by phosphorylation (e.g., phosphorylation of glycogen synthase kinase 3 by protein kinase B).[1]

SIGNAL AMPLIFICATION AND REDUNDANCY

Fundamental principles determining the sensitivity of a signaling pathway to a stimulus are signal *amplification* and *redundancy*. Whereas a single-step phosphorylation pathway would yield an inefficient 1:1 molecular communication between external cellular ligand and cellular effector, multiple-step phosphorylation cascades utilizing kinases of increasing abundance in series permit multiplicative *signal amplification*. In a related fashion, an arrangement involving isolated, parallel signaling pathways with completely distinct stimuli and downstream functions would permit neither flexibility nor responsiveness to combinations of stimuli. This is avoided by the common phenomenon of *signal redundancy*: stimuli may activate more than one cascade, cascades may be activated by multiple different stimuli, and effector kinases may have overlapping substrate specificities.

REGULATION AND SPECIFICITY OF SIGNAL TRANSDUCTION

Many signaling molecules ubiquitous to human cells are co-localized in the cytoplasm and have overlapping or redundant downstream effects. Several sophisticated strategies have been identified that result in the pathway regulation and specificity necessary for effective, stimulus-appropriate signal transduction to occur. Considerable specificity may occur simply through maintenance in the cell of low "copy numbers" of particular kinases and their respective substrates. Because of this, research strategies that use transfection to investigate the functional role of signaling molecules (e.g., overexpression at nonphysiologic levels in cell lines) may unfortunately induce artifactual protein interactions. Larger-scale pathway regulation is made possible by counter-regulatory *phosphatases* and by interpathway signaling *crosstalk*. In addition to the specificity of receptor-ligand docking interactions, specific signaling protein-protein interactions are made possible by *scaffolding/anchoring/adaptor proteins* and by *protein interaction domains*.

PROTEIN INTERACTION DOMAINS

Virtually all signaling proteins described to date are constructed in a modular fashion from a combination of catalytic and interaction domains. Paired interaction domains in different proteins couple them into multi-protein complexes, thereby orchestrating complex signaling events. The extensive list of protein interaction domains described to date can be grouped into separate families characterized by their ligand specificity (Table 39-1). Prototypical examples include SH2 and PTB domains (recognizing phosphotyrosine motifs); 14-3-3, FHA, and WD40 domains (recognizing phosphoserine/ threonine motifs); and PH and FYVE domains (recognizing specific phospholipids to allow for membrane targeting). Further layers of complexity are imparted by the preference of certain interaction domains for particular flanking amino acids in the ligand, thereby permitting differential localization of protein isoforms within the cell. The inclusion of multiple interaction domains of varying ligand specificity in a single protein results in extensive combinatorial possibilities, as well as intraprotein interactions through folding.

SCAFFOLD, ANCHORING, AND ADAPTOR PROTEINS

In addition to specific motif recognition of ligands by kinases, specific kinase-substrate interactions are facilitated by co-localization of proteins on scaffold, anchoring, or adaptor proteins at specific subcellular sites. In this manner, efficient kinase-kinase information flow may be facilitated or, alternatively, signaling molecules may be sequestered in a latent state in proximity to their upstream activating receptor. A prototypical example of such a scaffolding protein is that of the JIP proteins, which regulate JNK activation via possessing separate binding sites for both JNK and its upstream kinases, MKK7, MLK3, and HPK1.[2] Furthermore, JIP1/2 can form large cytoplasmic protein complexes through their ability to homo- and hetero-oligomerize and have SH3 and PTB domains, presumably facilitating complex regulatory protein-protein interactions. A second prototypical example of a scaffolding protein is that of the A kinase anchoring proteins (AKAPs), which are thought to co-localize protein kinase A (PKA) in an inactive form with its substrates and regulators at specific subcellular sites, presumably poising PKA to respond to local fluxes in cyclic adenosine monophosphate concentration.[3]

KINASE INACTIVATION BY PHOSPHATASES

The regulatory counterpart to phosphorylation by kinases is dephosphorylation by phosphatases. In addition to signal transduction, numerous cellular processes ranging from metabolism to RNA splicing are regulated by phosphatases.[4]

TABLE 39–1. COMMON PROTEIN INTERACTION DOMAINS AND THEIR ASSOCIATED RECOGNITION MOTIFS

Protein Interaction Domain	Binding Specificity
SH2, PTB	Phosphotyrosine
14-3-3, FHA	Phosphoserine/threonine
PH, FERM, FYVE, C1, C2	Phospholipid
WW, GYF, SH3, EVH1	Proline-rich sequences
EF-hand	Calcium binding

Although it is estimated that greater than 1000 phosphatase genes exist in the human genome, the complex variety of these mediators can be simplified down into three functional families: (1) those targeting phosphoserine and/or threonine residues, (2) those targeting phosphotyrosine residues, and (3) dual-specificity phosphatases targeting phosphotyrosine and/or threonine residues. While some degree of substrate specificity is intrinsic to all phosphatases, an additional layer of specificity is imparted by the combinatorial effects of regulatory molecules included in larger functional phosphatase complexes.

CROSSTALK

Although most signaling pathways were initially conceptualized as completely independent and parallel, it is now evident that signaling often involves a network of more than one pathway. For example, the three MAPK subfamilies can regulate one another both at upstream and downstream levels. Tumor necrosis factor-alpha (TNF-α) activates the guanosine triphosphatase p21rac, in turn activating the MKKK p65PAK, which activates MKK3, 4, 6, and 7, and thereby both the p38 and JNK pathways. Downstream, in the TNF-α–stimulated human neutrophil, p38 regulates the JNK pathway via protein phosphatase-2A.[5] Examples also exist of crosstalk between MAPK and non-MAPK pathways; for example, ERK has been reported to inhibit transforming growth factor-beta (TGF-β) signaling via phosphorylation of Smad2/3, which inhibits its nuclear retention.[6]

PROTOTYPICAL INTRACELLULAR SIGNALING CASCADES

MITOGEN-ACTIVATED PROTEIN KINASES

The MAPK superfamily, which includes the extracellular-regulated kinase 1 and 2 (ERK1/2 or p42/p44), p38, and c-jun NH₂-terminal kinase (JNK) families, is a highly conserved signaling system that regulates biologic functions ranging from embryogenesis to acute hormonal responses. MAPKs are serine/threonine kinases regulating an array of specific substrates (e.g., transcription factors, cytoskeletal proteins, other kinases) and are the final kinase in a three-kinase cascade (Fig. 39-1). Specifically, MAPK activation requires phosphorylation of both a threonine and tyrosine residue by a specific MAPK kinase (MKK), which requires activation by a serine/threonine MAPK kinase kinase (MKKK). This canonical understanding of a three-kinase pathway for the MAPKs has been challenged by reports that p38α can be activated by TAB1, which is not an MKK but rather an adaptor protein.[7] Moreover, new members continue to be added to the MAPK superfamily (e.g., ERK3, ERK5, ERK7), with over 20 MAPK isoforms described to date. For the sake of brevity, only the three classic, well-described MAPK families are discussed. MAPKs are examples of signaling molecules that can phosphorylate substrates within the cytosol but can also enter the nucleus to regulate transcription via activation of transcription factors. MAPKs are of particular interest in defining mechanisms of cellular response in the context of critical care medicine.

p42/44 (ERK 1/2) MAPK

The ERK subfamily has two MAPK isoforms, ERK 1 and 2, and follows the characteristic three-tiered design of the

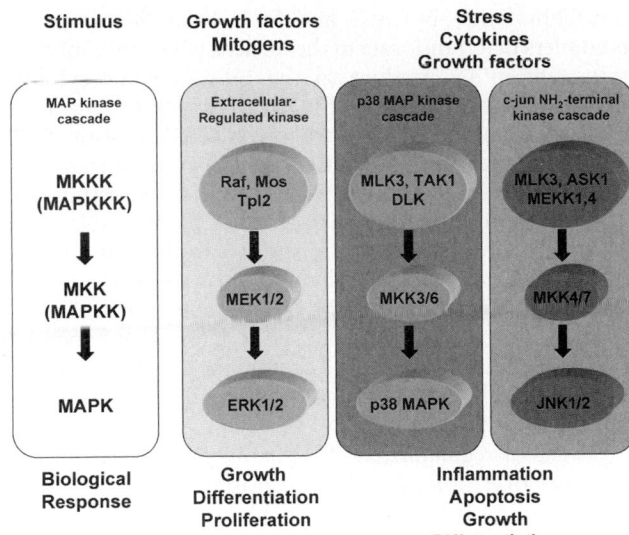

FIGURE 39–1. Mitogen-activated protein kinase (MAPK) cascades. The three major MAPK pathways are parallel signaling cascades, which include a MAPK kinase kinase (MKKK), a MAPK kinase (MKK), and a MAPK. After exposure of the cell to external stimuli, a variety of signaling mechanisms ultimately result in the phosphorylation (and activation) of serine/threonine kinases serving as MKKKs. The activated MKKK, in turn, phosphorylates one or more MKK-family members, which are then capable of phosphorylating both a threonine and tyrosine residue on one or more MAPKs. Once activated, the MAPKs serve as serine/threonine kinases, which phosphorylate an array of specific substrates within the cytosol (e.g., cytoskeletal proteins and other kinases) and nucleus (i.e., transcription factors).

MAPK superfamily, proceeding from raf kinase (MKKK) to MEK1/2 (MKK) to ERK1/2 (MAPK) (see Fig. 39-1). Raf, itself a proto-oncogene, is, in turn, activated at the plasma membrane by the proto-oncogenic G-protein ras. The ERK pathway is activated by several mitogens, including platelet-derived growth factor, epidermal growth factor, angiotensin II, TGF, insulin, and thromboxane A_2, and is generally considered to be a proliferation, transformation, and differentiation pathway. Nevertheless, the ERK1/2 pathway also plays a role in inflammation, because it may be activated in monocytes by both lipopolysaccharide and cellular adherence and is involved in monocytic production of proinflammatory cytokines (e.g., TNF-α).[8] Downstream substrates of ERK1/2 include MNK-1, Elk-1, and SAP-1.

p38 MAPK

The p38 subfamily has five known isoforms: p38α (also known as stress-activated protein kinase 2, or SAPK2), p38β, p38β2, p38δ (SAPK3), and p38γ. Each p38 isoform is characterized to varying extent by differences in tissue localization, preferred upstream activator, and potential substrates. The two major upstream activators of p38 are MKK3 and MKK6, although MKK6 is less abundant in leukocytes. In the neutrophil, MKK3 activates p38α.[9] Several diverse proteins appear capable of acting as MKKKs for the p38 pathway, including TAK1 and ASK-1. The p38 pathway is a major regulator of the inflammatory response, because it is activated by a broad range of proinflammatory stimuli (e.g., tumor necrosis factor, interleukin-1, platelet-activating factor, heat shock) and microbial stimuli (e.g., lipopolysaccharide, peptidoglycan) and plays a central role in many proinflammatory cellular responses[9] (e.g., production of TNF, interleukin [IL]-1, IL-6,

and IL-8 by monocytes and neutrophils; oxidative burst, degranulation, chemotaxis, and adhesion in neutrophils; and E-selectin expression in endothelium). Other roles include regulation of T-helper-1 (Th1) differentiation and cytokine production by lymphocytes. Important p38 substrates include the serine kinases MAPK-activated protein kinase-2 (MAPKAP-K2) and MAPKAP-K3, pro-inflammatory transcription factors (e.g., ATF-2, NFκB),[9] phospholipase A_2, MAPK-interacting kinase-1 (MNK-1), myocyte enhancer factor 2, CHOP, SAP-1, and Elk-1. Studies suggest a selective role for p38 MAPK in cellular regulation at both the transcriptional and translational levels.[10]

C-jun NH₂-Terminal Kinase (JNK)

JNK is encoded by three different genes, yielding 10 isoforms with differing tissue expression (e.g., *JNK1* and *JNK2* are ubiquitous, whereas *JNK3* is limited to brain, heart, and testis). JNK is activated by two MKKs—MKK4 and MKK7, which, in turn, can be activated by at least 13 different MKKKs. Most proximally, it is thought that the JNK pathway can also be activated by the rho family small G-protein axis of cdc42/rac/p21-activated kinase. Like p38 MAPK, JNK can be activated by a number of stress-related stimuli (e.g., TNF, IL-1, ultraviolet radiation). Because of only very recent development of a chemical inhibitor for JNK, its role in the inflammatory response remains less clear than that of p38. Nevertheless, studies in a variety of cell types indicate a role in apoptosis,[11] TNF expression,[12] T-cell proliferation and differentiation,[13] and endothelial E-selectin expression.[14] JNK substrates include transcription factors such as ATF-2, Elk-1, and C-jun (a component of the proinflammatory AP-1 transcription complex regulating multiple cytokine genes).

PROTEIN TYROSINE KINASES

Protein tyrosine kinases (PTKs) are classified into two distinct categories: receptor tyrosine kinases and cytoplasmic kinases. The former, typified by such mitogen receptors as the insulin receptor and epidermal growth factor receptor, have autophosphorylating activity, thereby creating recognition motifs on the cytoplasmic domain of the receptor for SH2-containing proteins, such as the adaptor protein GRB2. By contrast, cytoplasmic PTKs, typified by the SRC, JAK, SYK, and ABL families, play an important upstream role in multiple signaling cascades by either phosphorylating receptor endodomains or activating other signaling proteins. For example, SRC has been reported to play a role upstream of raf activation in the ERK1/2 pathway whereas SYK and LYN have been reported in B-cell receptor signaling.

JAK-STAT CASCADES

Chemokines and cytokines are two distinct classes of small (i.e., 8 to 30 kDa) mediators that play a wide spectrum of roles in the activation, maturation, and homing of leukocytes to sites of inflammation. The Janus kinase (JAK)-signal transducer and activator of transcription (STAT) pathway represents one of the initial signaling pathways that mediates the response of cells to cytokines and chemokines (Fig. 39-2). In this pathway, ligand-induced receptor subunit dimerization allows recruitment and activation of tyrosine kinase JAKs, which phosphorylate tyrosine residues on the cytoplasmic domain of the receptor. The phosphorylated receptor subunits

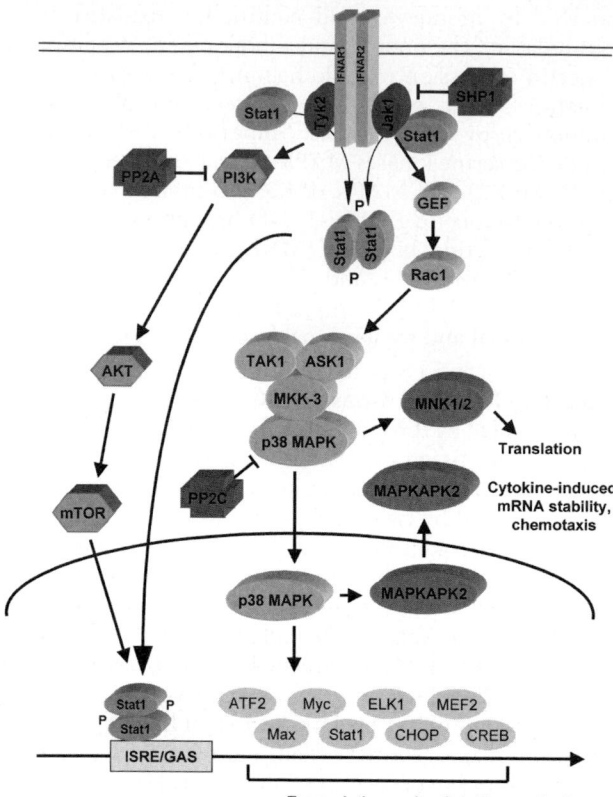

FIGURE 39–2. Potential relationship of major signaling pathways. Signal transduction by interferon-alfa (IFN-α) represents one of the best defined pathways to date and serves well as a backdrop to illustrate the potential regulatory interactions that exist between distinct signaling pathways (e.g., JAK/STAT, MAPK, PI3K, phosphatases) in coordinating the cellular response to an external stimulus. Signaling relationships depicted in this diagram are compiled from studies in a variety of cell types under a broad range of conditions and may well not be applicable to every human cell. Janus-family tyrosine kinase/signal transducer and activator of transcription (JAK/STAT) signaling: IFN-α binds to a type I IFN receptor (composed of subunits IFNAR1 and IFNAR2), which is associated with JAK-family members Tyk-2 and Jak-1. The receptor subunits provide docking sites for specific STATs, which are phosphorylated by JAKs, dissociate from the receptor, form dimers, and then translocate into the nucleus where they modulate transcription by binding to the promoters of cytokine-regulated genes. MAPK signaling: Crosstalk with the MAPK pathways may also occur as JAKs can regulate activation of small G-proteins such as rac1 via activation of guanine exchange factors (GEFs), and rac1, in turn, can activate the p38 MAPK cascade. p38 MAPK phosphorylates cytosolic proteins such as MAPK interacting kinase (MNK1/2) and also translocates to the nucleus, where it enhances cytokine transcription via activation of a broad array of transcription factors, and regulates stability of cytokine mRNAs via phosphorylation of the kinase MAPK activated protein kinase-2 (MAPKAPK-2). Phosphoinositol 3-kinase (PI3K) signaling: Activation of JAKs has also been linked to PI3K activation, which can then serve to activate AKT (protein kinase B). AKT is central to a wide range of signaling pathways, including activation of STATs via mammalian target of rapamycin (mTOR). Regulation by phosphatases: An important mechanism for limiting signal transduction is dephosphorylation (resulting in deactivation) of kinases by phosphatases. Protein tyrosine phosphatases (PTPs) such as SH2-containing phosphatase 1 (SHP1) dephosphorylate JAKs and MAPKs. JAK activates SHP2, which, in turn, dephosphorylates Tyk-2 and Jak-1. Protein serine/threonine phosphatases such as phosphoprotein phosphatase 2A and 2C (PP2A and PP2C) serve to dephosphorylate AKT and p38 MAPK, respectively.

then provide docking sites for specific members of a family of latent cytoplasmic transcription factors termed the *signal transducers and activators of transcription* (STATs) via their SH2 domains. Recruited STATs are activated via tyrosine phosphorylation by JAKs and form homodimers or heterodimers that translocate to the nucleus where they modulate transcription by binding to the promoters of cytokine-regulated genes. Specificity of JAK-STAT signaling is generated by the existence of four JAK and seven STAT isoforms. STAT4 and STAT6 have been described to play an important regulatory role in a murine model of sepsis.[15] Crosstalk with other signaling pathways exists since JAKs can regulate Rac1 phosphorylation via activation of a substrate-protein that functions as a guanine exchange factor for Rac1. In turn, Rac1 can activate the p38 MAPk cascade and the ERK1/2 cascade and the ERKs can phosphorylate and enhance activation of STAT.[16] In addition, chemokine-induced activation of JAKs results in activation of phosphoinositol-3-kinase (PI3K).

Negative regulation of JAK activity occurs in part by dephosphorylation of a critical tyrosine residue by protein tyrosine phosphatases (PTPs) such as SHP-1 and -2, which also bind to receptors via their SH2 domains, or by binding JAKs directly.

CLINICAL SIGNIFICANCE OF SIGNAL TRANSDUCTION

SIGNALING MOLECULES AS POTENTIAL DIAGNOSTIC MARKERS

The number of reports of signaling molecule modification in human disease continues to grow and, with it, the potential for harvesting new diagnostic and prognostic information from patient specimens. For example, in one clinical study, the quantity of p38 MAPK activation in alveolar macrophages proved to be a superior predictor of patients at risk for acute respiratory distress syndrome and for multiple organ dysfunction syndrome compared with a panel of standardized clinical parameters.[17] In inflammatory bowel disease, p38α expression is increased in intestinal lamina propria macrophages and neutrophils.[18] In acute respiratory distress syndrome, increased activation of the downstream proinflammatory transcription factor nuclear factor-kappa B (NF-κB) is detected in alveolar macrophages,[19] whereas decreased NF-κB or Akt activation in peripheral leukocytes predicts improved survival.[20]

SIGNALING PATHWAYS AS THERAPEUTIC TARGETS

Because of the ubiquitous expression of signaling molecules, and the differing role of particular molecules in various tissue types, systemic inhibition of signaling events carries with it the potential for uncertain side effects and even antagonism. For example, whereas endothelial p38 MAPK activation inhibits platelet aggregation by inducing prostacyclin production,[21] platelet p38 activation promotes platelet aggregation.[22] Moreover, specific signaling molecules may function in widely different roles in different cell types (e.g., ERKs regulate proliferation in many cell types but play a role in adhesion in neutrophils). Nevertheless, under certain conditions, specific cell types may be targeted. For example, the IC_{50} of p38-regulated TNF-α release by murine alveolar macrophages is 3 logs greater than that by murine neutrophils.[23]

Despite the aforementioned challenges, multiple chemical inhibitors of different MAPK family members have been developed in recent years. A MEK1/2 inhibitor has shown promise in pancreatic carcinoma. Inhibitors of p38 MAPK have shown promise in multiple animal models of arthritis, endotoxic shock, pancreatitis, ischemia-reperfusion injury, and acute pulmonary inflammation,[23,24] and clinical trials are underway for the treatment of rheumatoid arthritis and psoriasis. A recently developed JNK inhibitor appeared beneficial in a rat model of arthritis,[25] whereas a dual p38/JNK inhibitor has shown promise in Crohn's disease.[26] Furthermore, recent studies suggest that even *post-injury* treatment with a p38 MAPK inhibitor, as would occur in patient care, is effective in inhibiting ongoing inflammation.[74]

CONCLUSION

Significant progress has been made over the past decade in our understanding of the intracellular events that couple receptor-ligand binding to subsequent inflammatory and immune responses of the cell. Because proinflammatory events regulated by the MAPK, JAK-STAT, and other signaling cascades have been implicated in the pathogenesis of both acute respiratory distress syndrome and multiple organ dysfunction syndrome, it is probable that in upcoming years such signaling mediators will enter common parlance in the intensive care unit as both diagnostic biomarkers and therapeutic targets.

ACKNOWLEDGMENT

This work was supported by grants from the National Institutes of Health (HL068743) and American Heart Association (0275035N).

ANNOTATED REFERENCES

Arbabi S, Maier RV: Mitogen-activated protein kinases. Crit Care Med 2002;30(1 Suppl):S74-S79.
This review article, published within a helpful supplement of Critical Care Medicine composed of review articles on the signaling of critical illness, discusses the activation and functional role of the three MAPK cascades in the context of critical illness. Emerging evidence of their potential role as diagnostic biomarkers and therapeutic targets is also described.

Chen D, Davis RJ, Flavell RA: MAP kinases in the immune response. Annu Rev Immunol 2002;20:55-72.
This review presents the current understanding of how MAP kinases regulate cells of innate and adaptive immunity, as well as cell death, which is of particular interest in understanding signaling mechanisms in diseases common to critical care medicine.

Platanias LC: The p38 mitogen-activated protein kinase pathway and its role in interferon signaling. Pharmacol Ther 2003;98:129-142.
This encyclopedic reference serves well to illustrate the complexity of interactions between many of the signaling pathways described in this chapter (e.g., MAPKs, JAK/STAT, PI3K) in the context of interferon signaling. The biomedical functional relevance of the pathways is also illustrated.

Rane SG, Reddy EP: Janus kinases: Components of multiple signaling pathways. Oncogene 2000;19:5662-5679.
This detailed reference exhaustively covers the topic of cytokine-induced JAK/STAT signaling, including nomenclature, protein interaction domains, substrates, regulation, and putative roles in human disease.

Strassheim D, Park JS, Abraham E: Sepsis: Current concepts in intracellular signaling. Int J Biochem Cell Biol 2002;31:1527-1533.
In this review, the authors discuss current concepts of the interplay of endothelium and primary immune cells in generating the pathophysiology of sepsis syndrome, as well as of the interdependent role of signaling pathways and the transcription factors they activate.

Chapter 40

RECEPTOR PHYSIOLOGY

Frederick J. Ehlert

KEY POINTS

1. Physiologic receptors can be divided into four families, based on structural and functional properties: nuclear receptors (ligand-activated gene regulatory proteins), ligand-regulated enzymes, ligand-gated ion channels, and G protein–linked receptors.

2. There are five classes within the ligand-regulated enzyme family: receptor tyrosine kinases, which phosphorylate signaling proteins on tyrosine residues; tyrosine kinase–associated receptors, which associate with enzymes having tyrosine kinase activity; receptor tyrosine phosphatases, which cleave phosphotyrosine ester groups on signaling proteins; receptor serine-threonine kinases, which phosphorylate signaling proteins containing serine and threonine residues; and receptor guanylyl cyclases, which catalyze the formation of cyclic guanosine-3′,5′-monophosphate within the cytosol.

3. Hydropathy analysis of the primary sequences reveals at least three families of ligand-gated ion channels: the four transmembrane receptors, which include nicotinic acetylcholine receptors, 5-HT$_3$ receptors, glycine receptors, and GABA$_A$ receptors; the excitatory amino acid receptors; and the P2X purinergic receptors.

4. The GTPase cycle is set in motion when an agonist activates a G protein–linked receptor.

The idea of a "receptor" was first introduced by Ehrlich and Langley around the turn of the 20th century in an attempt to explain the remarkably selective and potent effects that some natural and synthetic chemicals had on biologic tissues. They argued that pharmacologic agents must interact specifically with macromolecular components in tissue to produce physiologic effects. This idea, of course, is now a readily demonstrable fact. Researchers have identified hundreds of receptors and determined the primary sequence of many of these proteins through gene cloning. The precision of our knowledge about receptors is perhaps most spectacularly illustrated by the nicotinic acetylcholine receptor. Electron micrographic analysis of crystallized nicotinic acetylcholine receptors from *Torpedo* has produced high-resolution pictures showing a channel-like structure with a central pore, presumably representing the microscopic tunnel through which positive cations flow when the receptor binds its neurotransmitter, acetylcholine.[1]

The identification of receptors as the target for many drugs has an important corollary. It implies that drugs do not create new responses in tissues; rather, they start, stop, or modulate natural physiologic functions. For example, synthetic muscarinic agonists are able to elicit contractions of intestinal smooth muscle because they bind with muscarinic receptors and trigger a signaling cascade that results in the mobilization of calcium and the activation of contractile proteins in the muscle. Obviously, this signaling pathway evolved to respond not to synthetic drugs but to the neurotransmitter acetylcholine. The idea that drugs use physiologic mechanisms also applies to responses that are somewhat more complex than the readily quantifiable responses in peripheral tissues. For instance, the sensation of euphoria and well-being produced by opiate drugs, such as morphine and heroin, implies the existence of reward pathways in the brain whose natural function is to provide positive reinforcement to the organism under appropriate conditions.[2]

Within this general context, one can define many classes or types of receptors. There are the so-called physiologic receptors, which mediate the effects of a variety of neurotransmitters, peptide and steroid hormones, biogenic amines, and eicosanoids. In addition, enzymes, transport proteins, and ion channels are important receptors for a variety of drugs that usually, but not always, block the function of these proteins. Finally, the cytoskeleton and DNA itself may constitute the "receptor" for some agents.

This chapter reviews some of the quantitative aspects of drug-receptor interactions and provides a brief survey of the major families of physiologic receptors and their signaling mechanisms.

RELATIONSHIP BETWEEN RECEPTOR OCCUPANCY AND RESPONSE

RECEPTOR THEORY

The binding of a reversible drug to a receptor usually obeys the following scheme:

$$D + R \leftrightarrow DR \qquad \text{[Equation 1]}$$

in which D denotes the drug concentration, R denotes the receptor concentration, and DR denotes the drug-receptor complex. At equilibrium, the relationship between the drug-receptor complex and the drug concentration is:

$$[DR] = \frac{[D] \cdot R_T}{[D] - K_D} \qquad \text{[Equation 2]}$$

in which R_T denotes the total concentration of receptors and K_D denotes the equilibrium dissociation constant of the drug-receptor complex. The K_D has units of concentration (e.g., molar) and is equivalent to the concentration of drug required for half-maximal receptor occupancy. The K_D is a measure of the observed affinity of a drug for a receptor. The lower the K_D, the higher the affinity. This scheme is usually called the law of mass action. Its consequences adequately reflect the manner in which a variety of drugs bind with receptors under physiologic conditions.

The size of the response elicited by a drug depends on its intrinsic efficacy and the percentage of receptors that it occupies. It is easier to understand the property of intrinsic efficacy if we consider how the drug-receptor complex behaves in the absence of other ligands or endogenous neurotransmitters. In the absence of drugs, most native receptors are silent. An agonist is a drug that binds to the receptor, turns it on, and triggers a response. The property that enables the agonist to turn on the receptor is called *intrinsic efficacy*. An antagonist is a drug that lacks intrinsic efficacy but is capable of binding to the receptor. Such agents have no effect by themselves but are capable of antagonizing the action of an agonist, whether it is an exogenous drug or an endogenous neurotransmitter. The amount of intrinsic efficacy can vary widely among different drugs, and drugs with small or intermediate levels of intrinsic efficacy are called *partial agonists*.

INVERSE AGONISTS

This general framework may not be sufficient to account for the behavior of all receptor systems. For example, the guanosine triphosphatase (GTPase) activity elicited by opiate receptors is already active in the absence of agonists when this function is measured in brain homogenate in a hypotonic buffer.[3] Under these conditions, the addition of agonists causes a further increase in the GTPase activity, whereas antagonists either have no effect or inhibit the ongoing basal GTPase activity. In other words, if the receptor is already turned on in the absence of agonists, some antagonists can actually turn off the receptor. Most of the few native receptors that behave in this fashion have been shown to do so under nonphysiologic conditions. However, some mutated

forms of receptors have been shown to be constitutively active.[4]

SPARE RECEPTORS CONCEPT

Figure 40-1 shows the relationship between occupancy and response for a highly efficacious agonist (Fig. 40-1*A*), a less efficacious agonist (Fig. 40-1*B*), and a partial agonist (Fig. 40-1*C*). In Figure 40-1*A*, the concentration-response curve for the agonist lies to the left of the occupancy curve, indicating that it requires only a low level of receptor occupancy to produce a maximal response. This behavior is typical for a highly efficacious agonist. In Figure 40-1*B*, there is closer agreement between the two curves, so that the response is proportional to receptor occupancy. Although this less efficacious agonist is capable of eliciting a maximal response, it can do so only at a much higher level of receptor occupancy compared with the more efficacious agonist shown in Figure 40-1*A*. In Figure 40-1*C*, the agonist has little intrinsic efficacy, so it is incapable of eliciting a maximal response even when the receptors are fully occupied. Consequently, the agonist is designated a partial agonist.

When an agonist is capable of eliciting a maximal response at a submaximal level of receptor occupancy (e.g., Fig. 40-1*A*), the situation is referred to as *spare receptors*. Unfortunately, this term has created considerable confusion in the pharmacologic literature. The term does not imply that some of the receptors are extra or unnecessary; rather, it means that only a small fraction of the total functional receptor population needs to be occupied by the agonist to elicit a maximal response. The presence of spare receptors enhances the potency of the agonist because lower concentrations of the agonist can produce effective responses. The functional activity of the total receptor population can be appreciated by considering what happens when some of the receptors are inactivated. After partial receptor inactivation, the concentration-response curve of a highly efficacious agonist shifts to the right without a decrease in the maximal response. The loss in potency associated with inactivation of some of the receptors illustrates that spare receptors are functional and maintain the sensitivity of the receptor system. Another important point is

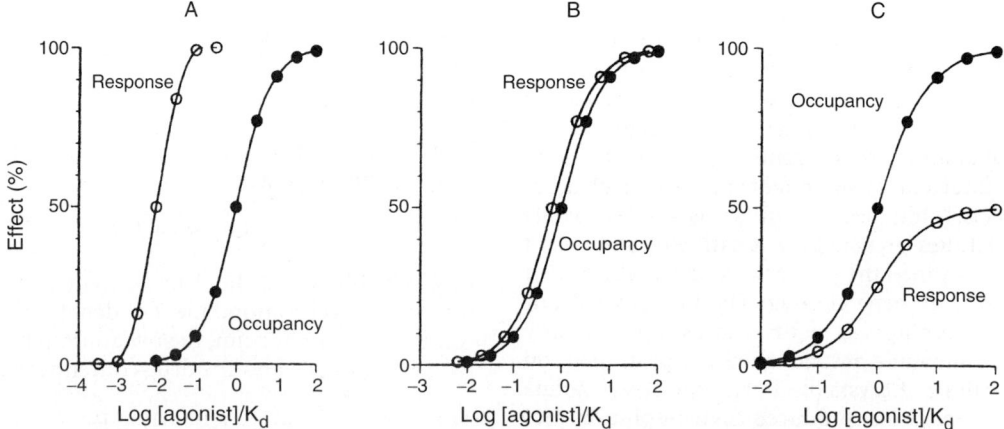

FIGURE 40–1. Relationship between receptor occupancy (●) and response (○) for a highly efficacious agonist *(A)*, a less efficacious agonist *(B)*, and a partial agonist *(C)*. Both occupancy and response are expressed as percentages of their maximum values and are plotted on the ordinate scale. The concentration of the agonist is expressed on the abscissa as a log of the ratio of the agonist concentration divided by the equilibrium dissociation constant of the drug-receptor complex (K_d).

that the presence of spare receptors does not imply that there are excess receptors relative to effectors. In fact, the converse is usually the case. In many signaling cascades, there is divergence along every step in the pathway. That is, one receptor may interact with several effector molecules, and each effector generates several second messenger molecules, and so forth. This divergence leads to amplification and thereby enables a relatively small number of agonist-receptor complexes to generate a significant physiologic response.

ANTAGONIST DISSOCIATION CONSTANT

Because antagonists lack intrinsic efficacy, all that is necessary to describe their interaction with a receptor at equilibrium is the K_D. This parameter can be estimated by measuring an agonist concentration-response curve in the absence and presence of the competitive antagonist. A competitive antagonist will shift the log concentration-response curve of an agonist to the right in a parallel fashion without causing a decrease in the maximal response. The K_D of the antagonist can be estimated from the shift in the dose-response curve using the following equation:

$$CR - 1 = [A]/K_D \qquad \text{[Equation 3]}$$

in which CR (concentration ratio) denotes the EC_{50} value of the agonist (concentration of agonist causing a half-maximal response) in the presence of the antagonist divided by that measured in its absence, and $[A]$ denotes the concentration of the antagonist.

SECONDARY ALLOSTERIC SITES

The relationships described earlier are adequate to account for the interactions of agonists and antagonists with the primary recognition site of a receptor. Some receptors have secondary allosteric sites where drugs can also bind and modify the ability of primary ligands to activate the receptor. One such example is the gamma-aminobutyric acid-A (GABA$_A$) receptor.[5] This receptor is a chloride channel that is regulated by the neurotransmitter GABA. When GABA binds to its site on the GABA$_A$ receptor, it causes the chloride channel to open. In addition to the GABA recognition site, there are other allosteric sites, including one for benzodiazepine-like drugs. A tranquilizing benzodiazepine, such as diazepam, binds to the allosteric site and increases the affinity of GABA for its site on the channel, thereby enhancing the effects of GABA. This allosteric effect can account for the pharmacologic properties of benzodiazepines, which include relief from anxiety, sedation, and protection against seizures. In contrast, some β-carboline derivatives bind to the allosteric site and inhibit the binding of GABA. These compounds have been called inverse agonists because they elicit responses that are opposite to those of benzodiazepines (i.e., anxiety, convulsions). However, they are more appropriately referred to as allosteric GABA antagonists because they produce their effects by antagonizing GABA. In addition, there are some compounds that bind to the allosteric site and have no effect on the binding of GABA. These compounds (e.g., Ro 151788) are called benzodiazepine antagonists, and although they have no effects by themselves, they antagonize both the tranquilizing effects of benzodiazepines and the convulsant effects of β-carbolines.

RECEPTOR FAMILIES

Physiologic receptors can be divided into four families, based on structural and functional properties[6]:

1. Nuclear receptors (ligand-activated gene regulatory proteins)
2. Ligand-regulated enzymes
3. Ligand-gated ion channels
4. G protein–linked receptors

Each family has a distinct overall structure and general function that are shared by all its members. Within each family, there is usually, but not always, a considerable amount of sequence homology. Previously, regions of high homology within a given family enabled molecular biologists to use low-stringency hybridization techniques to identify additional members of the same family; today, genome databases can be queried to identify potentially new members. In some instances, the endogenous ligands for the cloned receptor protein have not been identified, leading to their designation as orphan receptors. A cursory survey of the four receptor families follows.

NUCLEAR RECEPTORS

The nuclear receptors function as ligand-activated gene regulatory proteins that bind to DNA and regulate the activity of specific genes in a ligand-dependent manner.[7] This family includes receptors for thyroid hormone, retinoids, vitamin D, and the various steroid hormones, including glucocorticoids, mineralocorticoids, androgens, progesterone, and estrogen. Most of these receptors are located in the nucleus. Not surprisingly, the ligands for these receptors can readily penetrate the plasma membrane, and their access to the receptor is controlled by hormone binding proteins and by enzymatic processing of the ligand itself.

Receptors belonging to the nuclear receptor superfamily all share a similar structure having three major domains.[7] Near the center of the sequence is a highly conserved domain of 66 to 68 amino acids that constitutes the DNA binding region of the receptor. In this domain, the sequence forms two loops that are held in place by a zinc atom that interacts with cysteine residues on opposite sides of the loop. Each of the two loops is called a zinc finger, and many proteins that bind with DNA have a zinc finger–like structure. The second major domain of this family of receptors is the carboxy-terminal region, which functions as the ligand binding domain. This region of the receptor also shows considerable sequence homology, particularly among the androgen, glucocorticoid, mineralocorticoid, and progesterone receptors, which have structurally similar ligands (i.e., steroids). The third major domain is the amino-terminal region, which shows the greatest variation in size and the least conservation in sequence. This domain of the receptor is thought to mediate transcriptional activation.

A variety of evidence supports the existence of these distinct functional domains on steroid receptors. Perhaps the most dramatic evidence comes from studies of chimeric receptors in which a domain from one receptor is replaced with the corresponding domain from another. For example, when the 66–amino acid DNA binding region of the estrogen receptor is replaced with that of the glucocorticoid receptor, a chimeric receptor is formed that turns on a glucocorticoid-inducible gene in the presence of estradiol.[8] Truncated receptors have also yielded clues about functional domains, as well as the mechanism of ligand-induced activation. For example, glucocorticoid receptor mutants lacking most of the ligand binding domain demonstrate constitutive activity.[9] That is, the truncated receptor binds to DNA and causes transcriptional activation in the absence of hormone. Apparently, the ligand binding domain of the glucocorticoid receptor normally prevents DNA binding and transcriptional activation, whereas the binding of the hormone relieves this tonic inhibition. Finally, several cases of hormonal resistance have been attributed to point mutations in the ligand binding domain resulting in diminished hormone binding.[7]

Although the details are unclear, the binding of hormone to its receptor triggers the formation of receptor dimers that subsequently bind to DNA.[7] The site on DNA where binding occurs is called the *hormone response element*. These sites are located in the regulatory regions of steroid-induced genes, and several have been identified. The consensus sequences of hormone response elements exhibit dyad symmetry, which is consistent with the idea that a receptor dimer interacts with the hormone response element.

LIGAND-REGULATED ENZYMES

The ligand-regulated enzymes represent a huge family of cell surface receptors. The unifying structural feature of these receptors is the presence of an extracellular ligand binding domain that regulates an intracellular domain that either has intrinsic enzymatic activity or associates with an enzyme. In most instances, the two domains of the receptor are connected by a single transmembrane-spanning region. There are five classes within the ligand-regulated enzyme family:

1. Receptor tyrosine kinases (RTKs), which phosphorylate signaling proteins on tyrosine residues
2. Tyrosine kinase–associated receptors, which associate with enzymes having tyrosine kinase activity
3. Receptor tyrosine phosphatases, which cleave phosphotyrosine ester groups on signaling proteins

4. Receptor serine-threonine kinases, which phosphorylate signaling proteins containing serine and threonine residues
5. Receptor guanylyl cyclases, which catalyze the formation of cyclic guanosine-3′,5′-monophosphate (GMP) within the cytosol

Receptor Tyrosine Kinases

The RTK family includes receptors for numerous growth factors, including insulin, fibroblast growth factor, epidermal growth factor, and platelet-derived growth factor. The structural and functional properties of these receptors have been reviewed.[10,11] As mentioned earlier, members of this family have an extracellular ligand binding domain, an intracellular tyrosine kinase domain, and a transmembrane-spanning domain (Fig. 40-2). Most growth factor receptors are formed from a single polypeptide chain; however, the class II RTKs, which include receptors for insulin and insulin-like growth factor, are heterotetrameric, consisting of two α and two β subunits connected by disulfide bonds (see Fig. 40-2). The two α subunits contribute to the ligand binding domain, whereas the two β subunits traverse the membrane and possess the tyrosine kinase activity. The class I and II RTKs, which include the epidermal growth factor receptor and the insulin receptor, have cysteine-rich regions in their extracellular ligand binding domains. Another class, which includes the fibroblast growth factor receptor, has three immunoglobulin-like domains in the extracellular ligand binding portion of the receptor. The tyrosine kinase domain is the most highly conserved domain among the different classes of RTKs. This domain contains an adenosine triphosphate binding site and a tyrosine acceptor site. In the class III RTKs, these two functional regions of the kinase domain are separated by a hydrophilic, proline-rich sequence of 77 to 107 amino acids. The results of studies of chimeric receptors constructed from heterologous ligand binding and kinase domains provide further support for the existence of autonomous functional domains. In each case, the hybrid receptors displayed the appropriate ligand specificity and kinase activity.

Ligand binding to monomeric RTKs results in dimerization, which is a prerequisite for growth factor–dependent

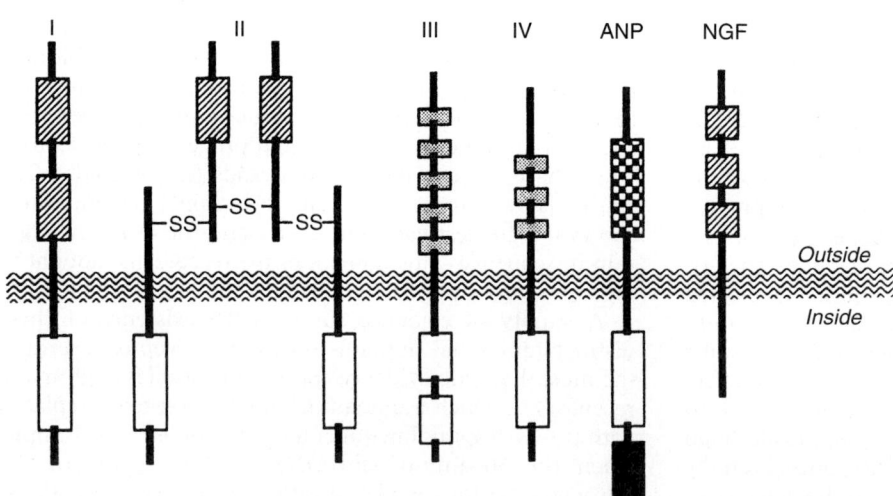

FIGURE 40–2. Structure of different members of the ligand-regulated enzyme superfamily of receptors. The figure shows the transmembrane topography of the primary sequences of the receptor tyrosine kinases (I, II, III, and IV), the receptor for atrial natriuretic peptide (ANP), and the receptor for nerve growth factor (NGF). The boxes indicate the various functional domains of the receptor, which are shaded according to the following scheme: diagonal lines, cysteine-rich domain; shaded, immunoglobulin domain; checkered, ANP binding domain; open, tyrosine kinase domain; and black, guanylyl cyclase domain.

kinase activation. Interestingly, the kinase activity of the tetrameric insulin receptor, which is analogous to an epidermal growth factor receptor dimer, is much greater than that of the dimeric αβ form of the insulin receptor. The results of ligand binding studies have demonstrated that growth factors bind to dimeric receptors with a higher affinity compared with monomers, suggesting that the tighter binding of the growth factor to the dimer provides the drive for receptor aggregation. Once made active by their respective ligands, all growth factor receptors autophosphorylate on several tyrosine residues. This autophosphorylation triggers a complex signaling pathway that is characterized by a series of protein-protein interactions and the phosphorylation of signaling proteins on tyrosine residues. The details of the signaling pathway can vary, depending on the receptor and the cell type.

When a growth factor triggers the autophosphorylation of its receptor, various signaling proteins bind to the receptor and become activated. These signaling proteins typically contain SH-2 domains that have high affinity for specific phosphotyrosine residues on the receptor. Myriad intracellular signaling proteins contain SH-2 domains, and these proteins are thought to mediate the effects of growth factors by binding to specific phosphotyrosine residues on the receptor.[12] These target proteins include the phosphoinositide-specific phospholipase Cγ (PLCγ), GTPase-activating protein, and members of the Src family of tyrosine kinases. In addition, several adapter proteins have been identified that lack enzymatic activity but contain both SH-2 and SH-3 domains. These adapter proteins are thought to bind to phosphotyrosine on the receptor via their SH-2 domains and to other signaling proteins via their SH-3 domains. Examples of adapter proteins are Grb2 and SHC, which enable mSOS to associate with the growth factor–receptor complex. The docking of mSOS to the receptor via adapter proteins enables mSOS to interact with the intracellular guanosine triphosphate (GTP) binding protein, Ras, and cause it to give up its bound guanosine diphosphate (GDP) and take up GTP. Once bound with GTP, Ras initiates a protein kinase signaling cascade that results in the activation of mitogen-activated protein kinase. This kinase triggers a variety of events associated with cellular growth and differentiation. The activity of Ras is inhibited by GTPase activating protein, which increases the intrinsic GTPase activity of Ras, thereby converting it from the active GTP bound form to the inactive GDP bound form.

Receptor Guanylyl Cyclases

Another member of the ligand-regulated enzyme superfamily is the receptor for atrial natriuretic peptide (ANP).[13,14] This receptor contains an extracellular ligand binding domain for ANP, a single transmembrane-spanning domain, and an intracellular domain that has guanylyl cyclase activity (see Fig. 40-2). The binding of ANP to this receptor causes an increase in the concentration of cyclic GMP inside the cell. This second messenger activates a cyclic GMP-dependent protein kinase, which ultimately triggers a variety of responses, including diuresis, natriuresis, and vasorelaxation. Interestingly, the extracellular domain of the ANP receptor is homologous with an ANP binding protein that is thought to have a role in the clearance of ANP from the circulation. The proximal portion of the intracellular domain is homologous to the kinase domain of RTKs, although no ANP-induced kinase activity has been detected. The most distal portion of the intracellular domain represents the catalytic domain, and it is homologous to the soluble form of guanylyl cyclase.

LIGAND-GATED ION CHANNELS

The ligand-gated ion channels represent a large superfamily that includes receptors for acetylcholine (nicotinic acetylcholine receptor), GABA (GABA$_A$ receptor), glycine, and various excitatory amino acids (e.g., glutamate, aspartate).[6] As the name implies, members of this superfamily are ion channels that open up and conduct an ionic current when an agonist binds on them. They share some homology with voltage-gated ion channels. In the case of the nicotinic acetylcholine receptor of the neuromuscular junction and the *Torpedo* electric organ, the ionic current is carried by positive monovalent cations, primarily sodium, whereas neuronal nicotinic receptors carry a rapidly desensitizing current of primarily calcium.[15] In the case of excitatory amino acid receptors, the ionic current is carried by both sodium and calcium, whereas inhibitory amino acid receptors (i.e., GABA and glycine receptors) carry a chloride current. The ligand-gated ion channels have a characteristic oligomeric structure consisting of different proteins (subunits) that come together to form the channel. Molecular cloning has revealed the existence of different structural groups of ligand-gated ions channels that are categorized on the basis of how many times the chain of amino acids composing their subunits crosses the membrane. Thus, hydropathy analysis of the primary sequences reveals at least three families:

1. The four transmembrane (4TM) receptors, which include nicotinic acetylcholine receptors, 5-HT$_3$ receptors, glycine receptors, and GABA$_A$ receptors
2. The excitatory amino acid (3TM) receptors
3. The P2X purinergic (2TM) receptors

The overall structure of the ligand-gated ion channels shows homology with many of the voltage-regulated ion channels, such as the sodium channel and the L-type calcium channel.[6] Although the ligand-gated ion channels are primarily chemosensitive, their gating characteristics are modified by the potential of the membrane. Conversely, although the voltage-gated ion channels are primarily potential sensitive, they are also modified by a variety of agonistic and antagonistic ligands that bind at different sites on the channel and are often allosterically linked to one another. When considered from this viewpoint, the ligand- and voltage-gated ion channels form a large superfamily of receptors.

The 4TM receptors are pentameric complexes composed of at least two α subunits, which have been shown to contain the binding site for the endogenous ligand. These binding sites are thought to exist at the interface between one side of the α subunit and its adjacent subunit. As mentioned at the outset, precise information about nicotinic acetylcholine receptors has been obtained through analysis of its crystal structure. Accordingly, the nicotinic acetylcholine receptor of the neuromuscular junction has a pentameric structure consisting of two α$_1$ subunits and one β$_1$, one γ, and one δ subunit. These subunits are arranged like the staves in a barrel-like structure, with a central pore that is thought to be the channel of the receptor.[1] Although the precise subunit structure of neuronal nicotinic receptors and the other ligand-gated ion channels has not been determined unequivocally, it is thought to be analogous to that of the neuromuscular nicotinic acetylcholine receptor, in that they are both pentameric with two α subunits. An approach that has been useful for drawing inferences about the subunit structure of other members of the 4TM family involves injecting the messenger RNA (mRNA) for different subunits into *Xenopus* oocytes and examining the functional activity of the expressed subunits pharmacologically.[16,17] For example, when an α subunit from the group α$_2$, α$_3$, and α$_4$ is expressed in combination with a β$_2$ subunit in *Xenopus* oocytes, functional receptors are formed, which presumably have a pentameric structure composed of two α and three β subunits. Similar results are obtained when an α subunit from the same group (i.e., α$_2$, α$_3$, or α$_4$) is expressed in combination with β$_4$ subunits. Also, α$_5$ subunit channels are thought to form in combination with α$_3$ and β$_4$ subunits. In most instances, the pharmacologic properties of each of the receptors exhibit different profiles from nicotinic agonists as well as some antagonists. It has also been shown that α$_7$, α$_8$, and α$_9$ subunits form functional homomeric channels in *Xenopus* oocytes, presumably consisting of five identical subunits. Moreover, recombinant homomeric GABA$_A$ receptors have been formed by injecting only mRNA for the α subunit into *Xenopus* oocytes, indicating that functional GABA-regulated ion channels can be formed from only α subunits.[18] However, these homomeric channels do not retain all the complex allosteric interactions characteristic of native GABA$_A$ receptors, and it is entirely possible that homomeric channels do not occur naturally. It is thought that the GABA binding sites form at the interface between α and β subunits of GABA$_A$ receptors and that benzodiazepine binding sites occur at the interface between α and γ subunits.[19] Several different subtypes of the individual subunits have been cloned for both the nicotinic and GABA$_A$ receptors, which raises the theoretical possibility of a large number of channel subtypes based on different combinations of the known subunits. However, functional studies in which the different mRNA subunits are expressed in *Xenopus* oocytes suggest a much smaller number of subtypes. These different subtypes of channels have different pharmacologic properties and sometimes unique developmental profiles.

Ligand-gated ion channels are widespread throughout the central and peripheral nervous systems and are responsible for rapid synaptic neurotransmission, characterized by synaptic delays of less than half a millisecond. The nicotinic acetylcholine receptor is present at the neuromuscular junction, where it is responsible for eliciting skeletal muscle contraction in response to impulse flow from motor neurons. These receptors are the targets for the neuromuscular blocking agents used as adjuncts to general anesthesia.[20] The GABA$_A$ receptor represents the major inhibitory neurotransmitter receptor in the brain, and it is an important target for a variety of drugs used to treat anxiety, convulsions, and insomnia.[21] Excitatory amino acid receptors are also abundant in the brain, and inhibitors of these ion channels may have a role in preventing the neuronal damage associated with brain ischemia following stroke.

G PROTEIN–LINKED RECEPTORS

Structure
The G protein–linked family of receptors is the largest, and it includes receptors for light, odorants, and a variety of endogenous neurotransmitters and signaling molecules,

including acetylcholine (muscarinic acetylcholine receptor), catecholamines, histamine, serotonin, eicosanoids, lipids, amino acids, proteins, peptides, chemokines, nucleotides, and hormones.[6] These receptors trigger responses by binding with heterotrimeric G proteins, which in turn activate various effectors, including ion channels and enzymes that generate second messengers (see later discussion). Besides being involved in neurotransmission at a variety of synapses and junctions throughout the brain and peripheral autonomic nervous system, members of this family are also involved in the special sensory functions of vision, taste, and olfaction.[22] The light receptor in the retina, rhodopsin, consists of a tightly bound complex between a protein called opsin and a photoactive ligand called 11-*cis*-retinal.[23,24] When light shines on 11-*cis*-retinal, it isomerizes to the *trans* isomer, which induces a conformational change in rhodopsin, causing it to activate a G protein called transducin. Ultimately, transducin initiates a cascade of events leading to a hyperpolarizing response in the retinal ganglion cell. This signaling pathway is so highly amplified that a single photon of light has a 50% probability of triggering a response in the retinal ganglion cell. G protein–linked receptors are also involved in olfaction to a remarkable extent. The results of searches of genomic databases indicate that there may be approximately 400 to 500 types of genes for odorant receptors in the nose, each of which may be receptive to a different spectrum of odorants.[25] These searches also suggest the presence of about 400 nonolfactory G protein–coupled receptors.

Receptors belonging to the G protein–linked class all share a similar structure consisting of seven highly conserved, transmembrane-spanning domains of α helix that are connected to the less conserved amino-terminal, carboxy-terminal, and intra- and extracellular loops. Previously, it had been assumed that the three-dimensional structure of G protein–linked receptors conformed to that of bacteriorhodopsin, which had been determined by x-ray diffraction.[26] More recently, the x-ray structure of bovine rhodopsin was determined.[27] In bovine and bacteriorhodopsin, the transmembrane domains run perpendicular to the plane of the membrane and circumscribe a central pore. Retinal neurotransmitters and the neurotransmitters for muscarinic and catecholamine receptors are thought to bind at a site within the pore. Accordingly, point mutations in a highly conserved aspartic acid residue in the third transmembrane segment cause a loss in agonist binding at muscarinic[28] and beta-adrenergic receptors.[29] Not surprisingly, the part of the receptor involved in G protein coupling is a relatively large, hydrophilic domain that projects into the cytoplasm—namely, the third cytoplasmic (i3) loop. The strongest evidence for the coupling role of the i3 loop comes from studies of chimeric receptors in which the i3 loop of one receptor is replaced with that from another. For example, when the i3 loop of the muscarinic receptor was switched with that of the beta-adrenergic receptor, the chimeric receptor triggered beta-adrenergic effects in response to muscarinic agonists.[30,31] Analogous results have been observed in studies of chimeras constructed from a variety of other G protein–linked receptors. Interestingly, the i3 loops of several receptors are constitutively active by themselves.[32] Thus, the ligand binding domain (seven transmembrane segments) of G protein–linked receptors probably exerts a tonic inhibitory effect on the i3 loop, and the binding of neurotransmitter relieves this inhibition.

G Proteins

The G proteins involved in receptor signaling are heterotrimeric, consisting of α, β, and γ subunits.[33,34] The $\beta\gamma$ subunits form a tightly bound complex that functions as a unit. The α subunits of heterotrimeric G protein are close relatives of many other low-molecular-weight G proteins that lack $\beta\gamma$ subunits, such as the Ras protein mentioned earlier. These small G proteins participate in numerous metabolic processes within the cell, including some that have little to do with transmembrane signaling at the cell surface. The basic function that G proteins accomplish at the expense of GTP hydrolysis is transportation between two destinations. In the case of the low-molecular-weight G protein elongation factor Tu, there is a transport of transfer RNA complexes on the ribosome, whereas in the case of heterotrimeric G proteins, the G protein shuttles between the receptor and its effector. Thus, nature uses G proteins for a variety of roles, and the involvement of heterotrimeric G proteins in receptor signaling at the cell membrane probably represents a highly specialized function.

The α subunit of heterotrimeric G proteins shows the greatest diversity, and more than 20 different types of α subunits have been cloned.[22] By contrast, the $\beta\gamma$ subunits seem to have fewer subtypes, and it appears that more than one type of α subunit can associate with the same dimer of $\beta\gamma$ subunits. The α subunit confers selectivity for different receptors as well as effectors; however, the degree of selectivity is not absolute (see later discussion). For example, the M_2 subtype of the muscarinic receptor can interact with more than one type of G protein (e.g., G_o and G_{i1-3}[32]), and a single G protein of the G_i family can interact with more than one type of receptor (e.g., M_2 muscarinic and D_2 dopamine). However, receptors that interact with G_i and G_o are usually ineffective at interacting with G_s, and vice versa.[35] Generally, a given receptor usually, but not always, exhibits selectivity for one of three G protein families–$G_{i/o}$, G_s, or G_q. There is also selectivity at the level of the G protein–effector interaction. For example, members of the G_i family can mediate an inhibition of adenylyl cyclase activity; however, these G proteins are much less effective at coupling receptors to phospholipase

Cβ (PLCβ). The α subunit of G proteins binds GTP, resulting in activation and a dissociation of the GTP-α complex from the $\beta\gamma$ subunits. In addition, the α subunit has GTPase activity that hydrolyzes GTP to GDP, causing the inactive GDP-α complex to coalesce with the $\beta\gamma$ subunits. The α subunits of some G proteins are also substrates for bacterial toxins that catalyze the adenosine diphosphate (ADP) ribosylation of the α subunit. For example, cholera toxin causes an ADP ribosylation of the α subunit of G_s, the G protein that stimulates adenylyl cyclase activity. This ADP ribosylation causes an inhibition of GTPase activity, resulting in an irreversible activation of G_s and, consequently, adenylyl cyclase. In contrast, pertussis toxin causes the ADP ribosylation of G_i and G_o, which prevents receptor-mediated activation of G_i and G_o. Transducin is a substrate for both cholera toxin and pertussis toxin.

GTPase Cycle

Figure 40-3 shows what happens inside the cell when an agonist activates a G protein–linked receptor:

1. Initially, the G protein is in its trimeric form, with GDP tightly bound to it. This inactive form of the G protein is a prerequisite for receptor interaction because the agonist-receptor complex cannot interact with free α or $\beta\gamma$ subunits, only with the trimeric complex. Although the cell contains high concentrations (approximately 0.1 mM) of GTP, this nucleotide cannot compete GDP off the G protein because the dissociation rate of GDP from the α subunit is negligible.
2. The binding of agonist to its receptor causes a conformational change so that the i3 loop can interact with the G protein. This interaction allows the agonist to increase the rate of dissociation of GDP so that GTP can now bind to the G protein.
3. The binding of GTP causes a dissociation of the GTP α subunit from both the $\beta\gamma$ subunits and the receptor, resulting in activation.
4. The GTP–α subunit complex and the free $\beta\gamma$ subunits then turn on their respective effectors and ultimately trigger the cell's response to the agonist (Table 40-1).

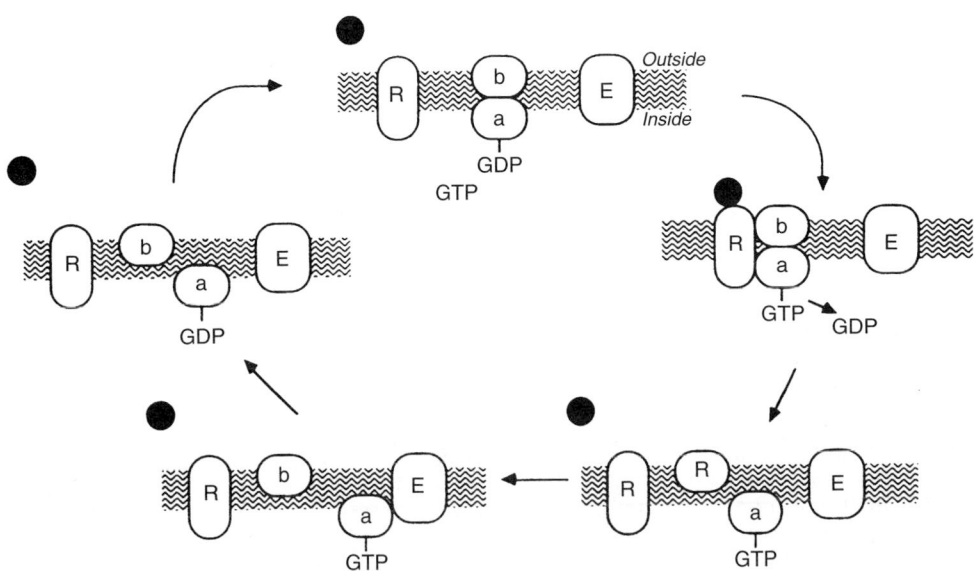

FIGURE 40–3. Receptor-activated GTPase cycle. Diagram of the interaction of an agonist *(black filled circle)* with its receptor (R) and the α (a) and $\beta\gamma$ (b) subunits of a G protein. E, effector; GDP, guanosine diphosphate; GTP, guanosine triphosphate.

TABLE 40–1. SIGNALING MECHANISMS OF G PROTEIN–LINKED RECEPTORS

G Protein Family	Representative Receptors	Effect of G Protein Subunits on Enzymes and Ion Channels
G_s	β-adrenergic D_1 dopamine H_2 histamine	$G_{s\alpha}$ stimulates adenylyl cyclases (I to IX), opens calcium channels
G_i/G_o	M_2 and M_4 muscarinic D_2 dopamine α_2-Adrenergic	$G_{i\alpha}$ inhibits adenylyl cyclases (I, V, VI) $G_{i\beta\gamma}$ stimulates adenylyl cyclases (II, IV, VII), opens potassium channels $G_{o\beta\gamma}$ closes calcium channels
$G_{q/11}$	M_1, M_3, and M_5 muscarinic α_2-Adrenergic Angiotensin II	$G_{q\alpha}$ stimulates PLCβ $G_{11\alpha}$ stimulates PLCβ
G_T	Mammalian rhodopsin	Stimulates cGMP phosphodiesterase

cGMP, cyclic guanosine monophosphate; PLCβ, phospholipase Cβ.
Data from Hepler JR, Gilman AG: G-Proteins. Trends Biochem Sci 1992;17:383-387; and Tang WJ, Hurley JH: Catalytic mechanism and regulation of mammalian adenylyl cyclases. Mol Pharmacol 1998;54:231-240.

5. The turn-off mechanism is the GTPase activity of the α subunit, which hydrolyzes GTP. The resulting GDP α subunit then coalesces with the βγ subunits to form the trimeric complex, which is inactive.

6. The cycle can repeat itself, provided that agonist is occupying the receptor.

7. Another important protein, RGS (regulator of G protein signaling), increases the GTPase activity of the G protein (not shown in the figure).[36]

Several experimental observations support the scheme described, and a few of these are mentioned here. Muscarinic agonists cause the M_2 receptor to form a stable complex with G_i that can be identified on Western blots with antibodies to G_i or the M_2 receptor.[35] In contrast, antagonists do not promote the formation of a receptor–G protein complex. Moreover, the ability of the ligand to promote the ternary (agonist–receptor–G protein) complex is proportional to the intrinsic efficacy of the agonist.[37] This relationship is shown in Figure 40-4 for M_2 muscarinic receptors in the heart. The propensity of the agonist to generate the ternary complex can be measured in a binding assay; this parameter is denoted by "Receptor-Gi Cooperativity" in Figure 40-4A. It can be seen that the cooperativity is proportional to intrinsic efficacy for a number of agonists. Another conspicuous feature of most G protein–linked receptors is that the binding of ligands to the receptor is modified by GTP in manner that is proportional to the intrinsic efficacy of the ligand. Both GTP and GDP cause a reduction in agonist binding affinity, but not antagonist affinity. The relationship between intrinsic efficacy and the inhibitory effect of GTP (GTP shift) on ligand binding to M_2 muscarinic receptors in the heart is shown in Figure 40-4B for a number of ligands. The proportional relationship between the negatively cooperative effects of GTP on agonist binding and the intrinsic efficacy of the agonist is readily apparent from the plot.

The relationships shown in Figure 40-4 provide insight into how the receptor works. In considering the figure, it is important to note that both GDP and GTP inhibit agonist affinity, but not antagonist affinity. This effect is allosteric because the agonist and the guanine nucleotide act at different sites. Therefore, the nature of the interaction between the two types of ligands is called *negative heterotropic cooperativity*. One of the properties of allosteric interactions is that they are reciprocal; that is, if GDP or GTP reduces the affinity of the agonist, then the agonist must reduce the affinity of the guanine nucleotide to precisely the same extent.[38] This agonist-mediated reduction in the affinity of GDP causes it to dissociate from the G protein more rapidly, allowing GTP to compete it off the G protein. Although this increase in the dissociation kinetics of GDP is achieved at the cost of reducing the affinity of GTP, it does not result in a decrease in the binding of GTP, because GTP is maintained at saturating concentrations inside the cell. For example, the K_D of GTP analogs for the G protein is in the nanomolar (10^{-9} M) range, whereas the concentration of GTP inside the cell is in the millimolar (10^{-3} M) range. Thus, it can be seen that the agonist-receptor complex works by increasing the dissociation kinetics of GDP from the G protein and that this effect is mediated by negative heterotropic cooperativity.

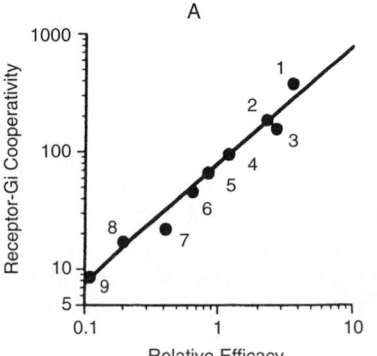

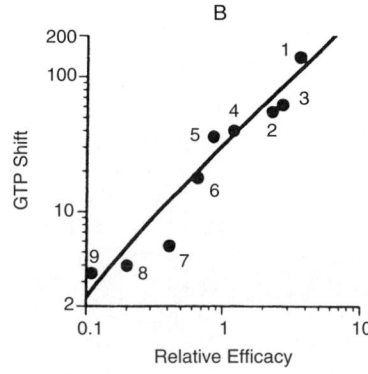

FIGURE 40–4. Correlation between relative efficacy and agonist binding properties at M_2 muscarinic receptors. *A,* The positive heterotropic cooperativity between the binding of the agonist and G_i is plotted against the relative efficacy of the agonist as determined by inhibition of adenylyl cyclase activity. *B,* The ratio of the concentration of the agonist in the presence and absence of guanosine triphosphate (GTP) is plotted against the relative efficacy of the agonist. 1, oxotremorine-M; 2, carbachol; 3, *cis*-dioxolane; 4, oxotremorine; 5, (+)-aceclidine; 6, (–)-aceclidine; 7, *N*-methylaceclidine; 8, BM5; 9, BOK1. (Data from Ehlert FJ: The relationship between muscarinic receptor occupancy and adenylate cyclase inhibition in the rabbit myocardium. Mol Pharmacol 1985;28:410-421.)

SIGNALING MECHANISMS OF G PROTEIN–LINKED RECEPTORS

G protein–linked receptors mediate myriad responses at the level of the whole tissue; however, at the subcellular level, these responses seem to be triggered by a relatively small number of transduction mechanisms. This situation illustrates that diversity is achieved through divergence in the signaling pathway, and that the factors that determine the intermediate and distal parts of the signaling mechanism are tissue specific. Thus, calcium mobilization resulting from activation of a PLCβ-linked receptor in smooth muscle may cause contraction,[39] whereas in an exocrine gland, the same transduction mechanism may cause secretion. Some of the major transduction mechanisms of G protein–linked receptors are summarized here and listed in Table 40-1.

CALCIUM MOBILIZATION

Perhaps the most universal mechanism for triggering a response is to increase the concentration of calcium within the cell.[40] Not surprisingly, several different signaling mechanisms ultimately affect the level of calcium within the cytoplasm. One common mechanism for elevating calcium is through activation of PLCβ, an enzyme that hydrolyzes the phospholipid phosphatidylinositol-4,5-bisphosphate (PIP$_2$) into inositol-1,4,5-trisphosphate (IP$_3$) and diacylglycerol (DAG).[41,42] This membrane-bound enzyme is activated by numerous receptors that signal through the G$_q$ family of G proteins (see Table 40-1). The two hydrolysis products, IP$_3$ and DAG, act as second messengers within the cell.[42] IP$_3$ causes a release of calcium from the endoplasmic reticulum, and DAG activates protein kinase C. IP$_3$ is phosphorylated in some cells to inositol-1,3,4,5-tetrakisphosphate (IP$_4$), which appears to have a role in assisting IP$_3$ to mobilize calcium.[43] Both IP$_3$ and IP$_4$ are unstable and are sequentially hydrolyzed by phosphatases back to inositol, which is then recycled for synthesis of new PIP$_2$. The final phosphatase in the sequence, myoinositol-1-phosphatase, is inhibited by lithium. Ultimately, this inhibition leads to an accumulation of inositol-1-phosphate and a depletion in inositol and inositol-containing phospholipids (e.g., PIP$_2$) within the brain. This depletion can lead to a dampening in receptor signaling through the PLCβ pathway, and it has been suggested that this dampening is the mechanism by which lithium attenuates the symptoms of manic-depressive psychosis.[44] Once calcium is elevated in the cell, it can mediate a variety of effects by binding to calmodulin and activating a variety of kinases and phosphatases. The protein kinase C that is activated by DAG also mediates numerous effects, and it is the target for some tumor-promoting phorbol ester derivatives.

ADENYLYL CYCLASE

Another important signaling mechanism within the cell is the regulation of adenylyl cyclase (see Table 40-1). G protein–linked receptors that affect adenylyl cyclase can be divided into two categories, depending on whether they stimulate or inhibit the enzyme.[22] G$_s$ mediates the stimulation, whereas in most instances, G$_i$ mediates inhibition through a distinct group of receptors. Nine different isoforms of adenylyl cyclase (AC1 to AC9) have been identified, and all these are activated by the α subunit of G$_s$ (i.e., α$_s$).[45,46] The α$_i$ subunit inhibits AC1, AC3, AC5, AC6, AC8, and AC9, whereas βγ subunits increase the activity of AC2, AC4, and AC7 in a manner dependent on activation by α$_s$. Once cyclic adenosine monophosphate (cAMP) rises within the cell, it can mediate a variety of effects through activation of cAMP-dependent protein kinase (protein kinase A). The turn-off mechanism for cAMP is phosphodiesterase, which rapidly hydrolyzes cAMP into AMP.

RECEPTOR CROSS-TALK

There are several possibilities for cross-talk between receptors that stimulate adenylyl cyclase and those that activate PLCβ. For example, AC1 (abundant in brain), AC3, and AC8 are activated by calcium.[47] Also, calcium stimulates phosphodiesterase in some tissues. Moreover, the stimulation of adenylyl cyclase caused by G$_s$-linked receptors is enhanced by activation of protein kinase C in some tissues. Finally, α$_s$-mediated stimulation of AC2 and AC4 has been shown to be greatly potentiated by the βγ subunits, which provides yet another mechanism for receptor cross-talk.

In addition to the second messenger systems described earlier, G protein–linked receptors can affect a variety of ionic conductances.[48] In several instances, these effects are mediated indirectly by second messengers, whereas in other cases, there is direct coupling of G proteins to ion channels. One such example is in the heart, where muscarinic receptors and beta-adrenergic receptors cause reciprocal changes in the conductivity of inwardly rectified potassium channels. These effects are mediated by G$_i$ and G$_s$, respectively, and represent the mechanisms by which the vagus nerve slows heart rate and the cardiac sympathetic nerves increase heart rate.

CELLULAR SIGNALING AND CANCER

Most cancer cells contain mutations in their DNA that presumably cause tumorigenesis.[49] These mutations are of two general forms: *recessive*, which result in a loss of function of tumor suppressor genes, and *dominant*, which result in a gain in function. The genes that contain these dominant mutations are designated oncogenes, and their normal counterparts are referred to as proto-oncogenes. Invariably, proto-oncogenes code for proteins that are part of normal receptor signaling cascades within the body. For example, truncated forms of the epidermal growth factor receptor lacking the ligand binding domain are constitutively active and cause tumorigenesis.[10] Relatively small changes in signaling proteins are oncogenic in numerous instances. For example, point mutations in G$_i$ have been implicated in carcinoma of the ovary and adrenal gland, whereas point mutations in G$_s$ are present in adenomas of the pituitary gland and carcinoma of the thyroid.[50] Interestingly, these point mutations result in a loss of the GTPase activity of these G proteins, causing them to become constitutively active. There are numerous other examples of oncogene products that are mutated signaling proteins, including ligand-regulated gene regulatory proteins, RTKs, G protein–linked receptors, and low-molecular-weight G proteins, including Ras. Thus, in numerous instances, tumorigenesis is caused by overactive, unregulated receptor signaling.

DIVERSITY AND REDUNDANCY

In considering the diverse mechanisms by which information is transmitted throughout the body by way of receptor signaling, one is struck by two seemingly opposite principles of nature: diversity and redundancy.[51] Nature is redundant in the sense that only four different types of mechanisms can account for the function of what may turn out to be more than a thousand different types of physiologic and sensory receptors. Also, the same general GTPase cycle is harnessed for innumerable functions within the cell, including protein synthesis, secretion, neurotransmission, taste, olfaction, and vision. To accomplish these diverse tasks, nature modifies a given mechanism in an extraordinary number of ways. An appreciation of the diversity and redundancy of nature will aid in the future unraveling of biologic mechanisms and in the development of therapeutic agents to treat disease.

ACKNOWLEDGMENTS

Portions of the author's work cited in this chapter were supported by National Institutes of Health grants NS30882 and NS26511.

ANNOTATED REFERENCES

Bourne HR, Sanders DA, McCormick F: The GTPase superfamily: A conserved switch for diverse cell functions. Nature 1990;348:125-132.
> *This review article describes the role that G proteins play in a variety of physiologic processes. It focuses on the mechanisms by which G protein–coupled receptors trigger physiologic responses.*

Fuller PJ: The steroid receptor superfamily: Mechanisms of diversity. FASEB J 1991;5:3092.
> *This review article describes the structure and function of nuclear receptors.*

Palczewski K, Kumasaka T, Hori T, et al: Crystal structure of rhodopsin: A G protein–coupled receptor. Science 2000;289:739-745.
> *This article describes the crystal structure of bovine rhodopsin, a prototypic G protein–coupled receptor.*

Stryer L: The molecules of visual excitation. Sci Am 1987;257:42-50.
> *This article describes the mechanisms by which light activation of rhodopsin in the eye ultimately triggers responses in the ganglion cells of the retina.*

van der Geer P, Hunter T, Lindberg RA: Receptor protein-tyrosine kinases and their signal transduction pathways. Annu Rev Cell Biol 1994;10:251-337.
> *This review article describes the structure, function, and signaling pathways of receptor tyrosine kinases.*

Chapter 41

PROSTAGLANDINS, THROMBOXANES, LEUKOTRIENES, AND OTHER PRODUCTS OF ARACHIDONIC ACID

James A. Cook • Hongkuan Fan • Perry V. Halushka

KEY POINTS

1. **Eicosanoids include a broad range of arachidonic acid metabolites,** including the cyclooxygenase products thromboxane B_2, prostaglandin E_2, prostacyclin, and 15-deoxy-$\Delta^{12,14}$-prostaglandin J_2, and the lipoxygenase products leukotriene B_4, C_4, D_4, and E_4 and lipoxin A_4.

2. **Eicosanoid synthesis and action can be inhibited by a variety of receptor antagonists and synthesis inhibitors,** the most recently developed of which are the cyclooxygenase 2 inhibitors.

3. **Both cyclooxygenase products and lipoxygenase products are increased** in animal models of endotoxemia, sepsis, and lung injury.

4. **Employment of specific cyclooxygenase or lipoxygenase synthesis inhibitors or specific arachidonic acid metabolite receptor antagonists** attenuates the sequelae or improves survival in animal models of endotoxemia, sepsis, and lung injury.

5. **Lipoxin A_4 and the J series of prostaglandins (cyclopentenone prostaglandins) are anti-inflammatory** and may play a role in inflammation resolution.

6. **Studies demonstrate increased synthesis** of thromboxane, prostacyclin, and leukotriene in patients with septic trauma or acute respiratory distress syndrome and suggest a deleterious role for thromboxane.

7. **Clinical trials with the nonsteroidal anti-inflammatory drug ibuprofen in severely septic patients** did not improve survival but reduced the febrile response and tachycardia and increased oxygen consumption and lactic acidosis.

8. **Combination drug therapy** with eicosanoid synthesis inhibitors, receptor antagonists, or anti-inflammatory eicosanoids may be more effective in sepsis or acute respiratory distress syndrome.

The first report of the biologic activity of what were subsequently identified as prostaglandins (PGs) was published in 1930, when it was found that extracts of seminal fluid contracted uterine tissue.[1] Von Euler attributed the activity of the extract to lipid substances that he named *prostaglandins*, because he thought they came from the prostate.[2] The structures of two of the prostaglandins (PGE_2 and $PGF_{1\alpha}$) were subsequently elucidated by the use of gas chromatography–mass spectrometry, and with this discovery, research in the field grew rapidly.[3] Thromboxane B_2 (TXB_2) was isolated by Samuelsson and colleagues in 1978 from human platelets.[4] It is the stable metabolite of TXA_2, whose structure was deduced at the time and was later proved to be correct. The name *thromboxane* was chosen because the substance causes platelet aggregation (thrombosis) and has an oxane ring system. It was ultimately shown that a rabbit aorta-contracting substance was TXA_2.[5] Prostacyclin (PGI_2) was discovered in 1976.[6]

The next major group of arachidonic acid metabolites to be discovered and characterized was the leukotrienes (LTs). Their name derives from the observation that they are made by leukocytes and have triene structures.[7] The sulfidopeptide leukotrienes were shown to be the active principals of the slow-reacting substance of anaphylaxis, released from mast cells and neutrophils.[7] Arachidonic acid, dihomo-γ-linolenic acid, and eicosapentaenoic acid are precursors of prostaglandins, thromboxanes, and leukotrienes. The first two are also known as *eicosatetraenoic acid* and *eicosatrienoic acid*, respectively; thus, the name *eicosanoids* is used generically for the products of these fatty acids.

The products of fatty acid cyclooxygenase and lipoxygenase pathways are named with letters and numbers. The letters for the cyclooxygenase pathway metabolites refer to substitutions on the cyclopentane ring; for the leukotriene pathway, the letters refer to the amino acids coupled with the fatty acid.[7] The numbers refer to the number of double bonds present on the side chains.

SITES OF SYNTHESIS AND PHARMACOLOGIC ACTIVITY OF THE EICOSANOIDS

FATTY ACID CYCLOOXYGENASE PRODUCTS

The pathway for the metabolism of arachidonic acid is shown in Figure 41-1. PGA, PGB, and PGC are nonenzymatic

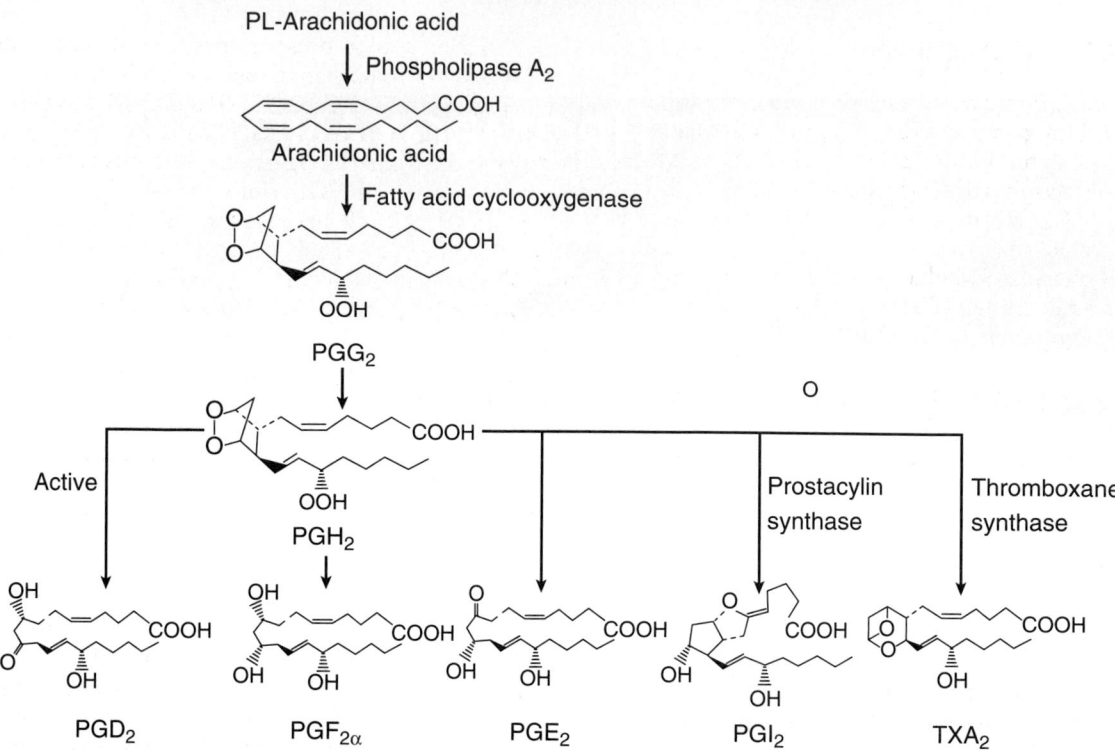

PL-Arachidonic acid

Phospholipase A_2

Arachidonic acid

Fatty acid cyclooxygenase

PGG_2

PGH_2

Active

Prostacylin synthase

Thromboxane synthase

PGD_2 $PGF_{2\alpha}$ PGE_2 PGI_2 TXA_2

FIGURE 41-1. Metabolism of arachidonic acid. PG, prostaglandin; PGI_2, prostacyclin; PL, phospholipase; TXA_2, thromboxane A_2. (From Wagner TR, Halushka PV, Cook JA: Cyclooxygenase products in septic endotoxic shock. In Neugebauer EA, Holaday JW [eds]: Handbook of Mediators in Septic Shock. Boca Raton, Fla, CRC Press, 1993, pp 395-418.)

dehydration products of PGE_2 and are considered artifacts of the extraction procedure. However, PGA is a vasodilator. PGD_2 is synthesized in large quantities by mast cells, being the major cyclooxygenase metabolite in this cell. It and its major metabolite, 9α, 11β, $PGF_{2\alpha}$, are potent bronchoconstrictors and are overproduced in mastocytosis.[8] Depending on the vascular bed, it may be either a vasoconstrictor or a vasodilator. Vasodilatation usually occurs at lower doses; however, PGD_2 also constricts the pulmonary artery. It is synthesized by platelets and inhibits platelet aggregation by increasing intraplatelet cyclic adenosine monophosphate (cAMP) levels. It has yet to be determined whether its synthesis is increased in shock.

PGE_2 is synthesized mainly by the kidneys, platelets, and blood vessels, but it is also synthesized by many other tissues in smaller amounts. It is a vasodilator, natriuretic, and diuretic; inhibits gastric acid secretion; and contracts uterine tissue. Depending on the tissue, PGE_2 can bind to four subtypes of receptors, designated EP_1, EP_2, EP_3, and EP_4. Seven EP_3 splice variants have been identified in humans.[9] The EP receptors are classic heptahelical G protein–coupled receptors.[10] EP_1 is coupled to Gq and activates phospholipase C. EP_2 and EP_4 couple to G_s and stimulate the synthesis of cAMP, whereas EP_3 is coupled to G_i, which inhibits cAMP formation. The EP_1, EP_3, and EP_4 receptors have also been shown to be expressed on nuclear membranes of endothelial cells, suggesting a potential level of control in nuclear events.[11] PGE_2 synthesis is significantly increased in shock syndromes (discussed later).

$PGF_{2\alpha}$ is synthesized in many tissues in variable amounts and is increased in sepsis. It is a bronchoconstrictor and venoconstrictor, and it contracts uterine smooth muscle. All these actions are mediated by $PGF_{2\alpha}$ receptors (FP).[10,12]

PGI_2 is synthesized by endothelial cells, macrophages, lungs, and kidneys. It is a vasodilator and antiaggregatory substance with a half-life of about 10 minutes; it spontaneously hydrolyzes to form the stable but inactive metabolite 6-keto-$PGF_{1\alpha}$. The major urinary metabolite of 6-keto-$PGF_{1\alpha}$ is 2,3-dinor-6-keto-$PGF_{1\alpha}$. The major biochemical action of PGI_2 is to stimulate adenylate cyclase. To date, only one class of PGI_2 receptors (IP) has been identified.[10,12]

TXA_2 is synthesized in large quantities by platelets, macrophages, monocytes, and lungs. It is unstable and has a half-life of only 30 seconds; it spontaneously hydrolyzes to form the stable but inactive TXB_2. The major plasma metabolite of TXB_2 is 11-dehydro-TXB_2. The major urinary metabolites are 11-dehydro-TXB_2 and 2,3-dinor-TXB_2. TXA_2 is a potent vasoconstrictor, bronchoconstrictor, and proaggregatory substance. Based on pharmacologic criteria, two subtypes of receptors have been identified for TXA_2. One is associated with platelet aggregation, and the other is associated with vascular smooth muscle cell contraction.[8,10,12] There is also a splice variant of the platelet receptor, which was first discovered in endothelial cells. Platelet aggregation and TXA_2 synthesis are markedly increased in shock syndromes.

Leukotriene B_4 (LTB_4) is synthesized by white blood cells, macrophages, and synoviocytes.[13] It is a potent chemotactic substance for white blood cells.

LTC_4 is synthesized by white blood cells, lung parenchymal tissue, and macrophages. It is converted to LTD_4, an active metabolite of LTC_4. It is a vasoconstrictor and bronchoconstrictor and increases capillary permeability and bronchial mucus secretion. Its synthesis is increased during sepsis and acute respiratory distress syndrome (ARDS).[14] The urinary excretion of N-acetyl LTE_4, a metabolite of LTD_4, is increased in ARDS and shock.[15]

ARACHIDONIC ACID RELEASE

Release of arachidonic acid from membrane phospholipids is the rate-limiting step in the formation of eicosanoids in nonpathologic states.[16] Stimulation of cells by hormonal and nonhormonal agonists results in activation of phospholipase (PL) A$_2$, C, or D. Activation of PLA$_2$ results in the release of arachidonic acid from the *sn2* position of phosphatidylcholine and phosphatidylethanolamine.[17] Isozymes of PLA$_2$ have demonstrated a specificity for catalyzing the release of arachidonic acid preferentially from either phosphatidyl choline or phosphatidylethanolamine.[18] PLA$_2$ has several subtypes. There is cytosolic PLA$_2$, which is Ca^{++} dependent, and secretory forms of PLA$_2$ designated PLA$_2$-I and PLA$_2$-II.[14] PLA$_2$-I is secreted by pancreatic acinar cells and is important in phospholipid digestion in the diet. PLA$_2$-II is secreted by inflammatory cells and has been shown to increase in plasma in response to a variety of inflammatory conditions such as sepsis, trauma, and pancreatitis.[19-22] Cytosolic PLA$_2$ is intracellular and is activated by a number of stimuli, including tumor necrosis factor (TNF), interleukin (IL)-β, bradykinin, and many other inflammatory stimuli.[23,24] PLC cleaves phosphatidylinositol 4,5-bisphosphate, resulting in inositol-1,4,5-trisphosphate and 1,2-diacylglycerol, both of which function as intracellular second messengers.[25-28] Diglyceride lipase then releases the arachidonic acid from the diacylglycerol.[29,30] The metabolite 1,2-diacylglycerol stimulates protein kinase C.

A variety of agonists can stimulate PLD.[31] Both guanine nucleotide regulatory proteins and kinases are coupled to receptor-mediated regulation of PLD. PLD activation requires a cofactor, phosphatidylinositol 4,5-bisphosphate. The metabolite phosphatidic acid produced by PLD may play a role in growth regulation, activation of Ca^{++}-independent forms of protein kinase C, neutrophil respiratory burst activity, stimulation of lysophosphatide acid receptors, and vesicle trafficking.[32]

The particular phospholipid substrate providing arachidonic acid in response to a specific stimulus may influence whether lipoxygenase or fatty acid cyclooxygenase products are formed. Resident murine macrophages, in response to stimuli that activate the lipoxygenase pathway, demonstrate dependence on the PLC–diglyceride lipase pathway,[33] whereas endotoxin- or phorbol myristate acetate–induced prostaglandin formation is independent of the PLC–diglyceride lipase pathway.

FATTY ACID CYCLOOXYGENASE (PROSTAGLANDIN H SYNTHASE)

Fatty acid cyclooxygenase (PGH synthase) catalyzes the committed step in the conversion of arachidonic acid to the prostaglandin endoperoxides PGG$_2$ and PGH$_2$.[34] PGH$_2$ is the direct precursor for primary prostaglandins and TXA$_2$. Fatty acid cyclooxygenase has been found in most of the organs of all mammalian species but not in all cell types.[33] Subcellular studies demonstrate that cyclooxygenase is an integral membrane protein concentrated in the endoplasmic reticulum, as well as in the nuclear envelope and the plasma membrane.[35,36] Cyclooxygenase is approximately 68 kDa; species variations are attributed to different amounts of *N*-glycosylation and mannose carbohydrate side chains.[37] Two sites of enzymatic activity have been proposed,[38] and heme-binding sites are conserved.[39]

Cyclooxygenase possesses two enzymatic activities.[40] The first activity cyclizes an oxygen molecule in a bis-dioxygenase configuration at carbon (C)-9 and C-11, converting arachidonic acid to PGG$_2$. PGH synthase then uses another oxygen molecule to peroxidize this unstable metabolite at C-15, converting PGG$_2$ into PGH$_2$. The bound heme of cyclooxygenase is believed to act as the electron transfer site in these reactions. PGH$_2$ is the substrate for the enzymes responsible for the synthesis of PGD$_2$, PGE$_2$, PGF$_{2\alpha}$, PGI$_2$, and TXA$_2$. The final product profile is dependent on the specific cell type.

Many fatty acids are substrates for cyclooxygenase, but arachidonic acid is the most common in vivo.[32] Cyclooxygenase is inhibited by aspirin and all the nonsteroidal anti-inflammatory drugs (NSAIDs). Aspirin irreversibly inhibits the enzyme by covalently acetylating a serine residue. In platelets, the inhibition lasts for the life of the platelet (7 to 10 days), because platelets are not capable of synthesizing new enzyme.

In the early 1990s, two isoforms of cyclooxygenase were identified: COX-1 and COX-2. These two isoforms have been extensively characterized. COX-1 is the constitutive, continuously expressed form that is thought to play a role in normal homeostatic processes in platelets, the kidneys, and the gastrointestinal tract. COX-2 is the inducible form.[41] Its synthesis is stimulated by inflammatory stimuli such as lipopolysaccharide and IL-1 and by growth factors.[41,42] Both enzymes are inhibited by aspirin, indomethacin, and other NSAIDs.

Pharmacologic studies led to the development of a new generation of COX-2 inhibitors (e.g., celecoxib [Celebrex], rofecoxib [Vioxx]). The COX-2 inhibitors retain the anti-inflammatory properties of traditional nonselective NSAIDs, but without the gastrointestinal bleeding side effects. The widespread use of COX-2 inhibitors proved that they are as active as traditional NSAIDs in reducing pain and fever.[43,44] It became apparent, however, that although COX-2 inhibitors have a better profile in terms of gastrointestinal mucosal protection, they still have renal side effects.[45] They may also produce a prothrombotic state, but this is controversial. Studies suggest that COX-2 also has a physiologic role, particularly in the kidney. The COX-1–COX-2 model does not accommodate acetaminophen, which has antipyretic and analgesic properties but no anti-inflammatory effects. Because acetaminophen is not an anti-inflammatory drug, this suggests that its pharmacologic effects cannot be explained by COX-2 inhibition.[46] Recent studies by Chandrasekharan and coworkers suggest that COX-3, a COX-1 variant, is inhibited by acetaminophen and other analgesic and antipyretic drugs.[47]

LIPOXYGENASE

The lipoxygenase pathways of arachidonic acid metabolism involve three species of lipoxygenases: 5-lipoxygenase, 12-lipoxygenase, and 15-lipoxygenase.[48-50] These enzymes insert a molecule of oxygen into arachidonic acid at C-5, C-12, and C-15, respectively, forming the 5-, 12-, and 15-hydroxyeicosatetraenoic acids (HETEs).

5-Lipoxygenase demonstrates several unique characteristics compared with the other human lipoxygenases. It is dependent on adenosine triphosphate and Ca^{++} for activation, as well as three additional components.[51,52] One of these components is an 18-kDa protein, called 5-lipoxygenase-activating protein (FLAP), that is required for both the translocation and the activation of 5-lipoxygenase.[51,53] 5-Lipoxygenase metabolizes arachidonic acid to 5-hydroperoxyeicosatetraenoic acid

(5-HPETE). 5-HPETE is further metabolized to 5-HETE and LTA$_4$. LTA$_4$ is an unstable intermediate that is rapidly metabolized to LTB$_4$ by LTA$_4$ hydrolase or to LTC$_4$ by LTC$_4$ synthase. LTC$_4$ consists of glutathione covalently bound to arachidonic acid at the C-6 position (a sulfidopeptide leukotriene). The glutamic acid moiety of glutathione is cleaved by a γ-glutamyltranspeptidase to produce LTD$_4$. LTD$_4$ is further metabolized by a peptidase or a cysteinyl-glycinase to form LTE$_4$. LTE$_4$ can be N-acetylated and subsequently excreted in the urine.

12-Lipoxygenase metabolizes arachidonic acid to 12-HPETE and the metabolites di-HETE and tri-HETE. 12-Lipoxygenase is found in platelets and is the predominant lipoxygenase in brain tissue.

15-Lipoxygenase is approximately 70 kDa in size.[54] Its activity is preferentially expressed only in certain cells,[55] but the biologic role of 15-lipoxygenase in these cell types is not fully understood.[56] Recent evidence suggests that lipoxins (LX) that are generated by 15-lipoxygenase may be involved in inflammation resolution. Polymorphonuclear leukocytes (PMNs) and tissue resident cells can generate LXs, which appear to regulate leukocyte function. LXA$_4$ and its metabolically stable analogs can inhibit PMN-mediated inflammation in vivo in a variety of tissues.[57] The LXs can augment monocyte chemotaxis and phagocytosis of apoptotic leukocytes and can modulate the expression of chemokines and cytokines.[58] It has been proposed that peripheral blood PMNs exposed to PGE$_2$ (produced in inflammatory exudates) switch eicosanoid biosynthesis from the predominantly 5-lipoxygenase pathway leading to LTB$_4$ production to the 15-lipoxygenase pathway producing LXA$_4$. The latter may function as a "stop signal" for inflammation.[59]

OTHER METABOLITES

The J series of prostaglandins (cyclopentenone PGs) is formed by progressive nonenzymatic dehydration of PGD$_2$ (Fig. 41-2). What makes the cyclopentenone PGJ$_2$ family unique is that, unlike other prostaglandins, it has no known membrane receptor. Instead, PGJ$_2$ and its metabolites interact with a class of nuclear receptors that comprise the peroxisome proliferator-activating receptor (PPAR) family (specifically, PPAR-γ). The PPAR family is ligand-activated by nuclear transcription factors, which form a heterodimer with retinoid X receptor, and binds to a PPAR-responsive element, the promoter region of specific inflammatory genes.[60] The 15-deoxy-Δ^{12,14}-PGJ$_2$ metabolite is the most potent ligand for PPAR-γ. Activation of PPAR-γ can transrepress the activation of many transcription factors, including nuclear factor kappa-B (NF-κB), activator protein-1, signal transducers of transcription, and nuclear factor of activated T cells. PPAR-γ is found in a variety of cells, including macrophages, dendritic cells, and B and T lymphocytes.[61-65] There is a rapidly expanding literature that PPAR-γ may play a role in regulating inflammation and immunomodulation.[66] However, many studies have shown that PPAR-γ ligands have anti-inflammatory effects only at concentrations that far exceed those required for activation of PPAR-γ.[67] It has been shown that these ligands (e.g., 15-deoxy-Δ^{12,14}-PGJ$_2$) clearly have PPAR-γ–independent activities through the covalent modification of critical cysteine residues in the inhibitor of NF-κB, the p50 NF-κB subunit, and extracellular signal-regulated kinase (ERK).[68-70]

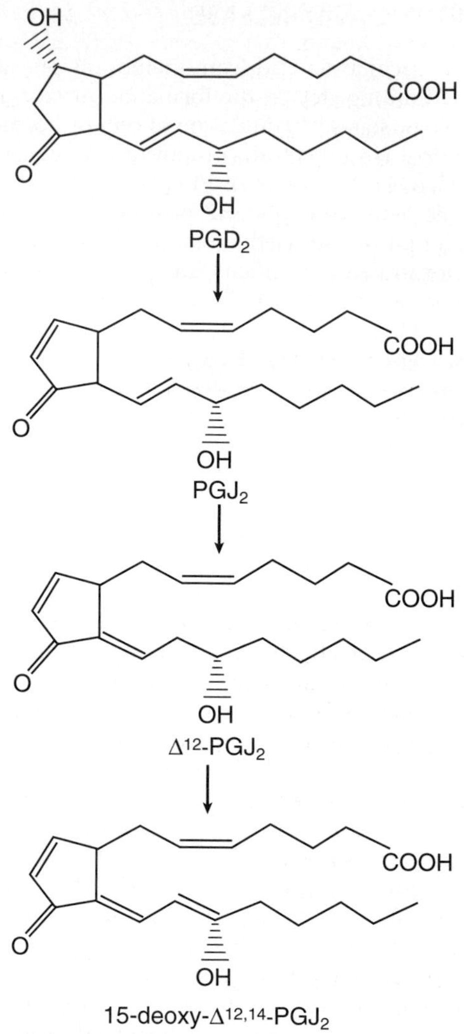

FIGURE 41–2. Metabolism of PGD$_2$ to 15-deoxy-Δ^{12,14}-PGJ$_2$. PG, prostaglandin.

Cytochrome P$_{450}$ can also oxygenate arachidonic acid at various sites.[71] This results in the production of a multitude of epoxides that have diverse biologic properties. These metabolites are usually synthesized in large quantities by the liver and kidneys. Whether these products are increased in sepsis remains unknown.

Isoprostanes are a novel group of nonenzymatically generated arachidonic acid metabolites.[72] They are formed directly by free radical oxidation of arachidonic acid while still esterified to the two positions of membrane phospholipids. Isoprostanes are structurally similar to prostaglandins and may exert some of their effects through the activation of TXA$_2$ receptors. They cause vasoconstriction, change in platelet shape, and increased pulmonary permeability.[73] Although they are generated under oxidative stress, the potential role of isoprostanes in ARDS and sepsis remains to be determined.

INCREASED SYNTHESIS OF EICOSANOIDS IN ENDOTOXEMIA AND SEPSIS

The seminal observation that eicosanoids may be involved in the pathogenesis of endotoxic shock was made by Northover and Subramanian in 1962.[74] They demonstrated that dogs treated with aspirin before exposure to endotoxin had an improved survival compared with control animals. At that time, it was not known that aspirin inhibited prostaglandin synthesis. In 1976, Herman and Vane demonstrated increased levels of PGE-like material in the renal veins of dogs given endotoxin.[75] Taken together, these two observations suggested that eicosanoids were important in the pathogenesis of septic shock.

Increased synthesis of eicosanoids in response to endotoxemia and sepsis occurs in several animal species and in humans. Increased plasma levels of TXB_2 and 6-keto-$PGF_{1\alpha}$ can be demonstrated in rats with experimental endotoxemia and sepsis.[48,76-78] Similar profiles of TXB_2 and 6-keto-$PGF_{1\alpha}$ in plasma are observed in endotoxemic or septic sheep,[79,80] pigs,[76,81-85] and baboons.[86,87] The relative amounts of TXB_2 and 6-keto-$PGF_{2\alpha}$ are influenced by the experimental route and frequency of endotoxin administration.[88,89]

5-Lipoxygenase products are also increased in endotoxemic animals and in patients with sepsis and ARDS.[90] In endotoxemic rats, Hagman and colleagues reported increases in biliary N-acetyl LTE_4, a stable metabolite of sulfidopeptide leukotrienes.[91] LTC_4 levels are increased in the lungs of rats with experimental endotoxemia.[92] Increased LTB_4 levels are found in bronchoalveolar lavage fluid of endotoxemic pigs[93] and in lung lymph in endotoxemic sheep.[94] Induction of cecal ligation and puncture (CLP) in mice was associated with eightfold higher levels of LTB_4 in peritoneal exudate compared with the sham group.[95] Slotman and coworkers compared the effect of sepsis and hemorrhagic shock on eicosanoid protection in a porcine model.[96] In sepsis-induced by Aeromonas hydrophila, there was an early peak in plasma TNF (at 60 minutes), followed by a rise in peak LTB_4 and LTC_4/D_4 levels (180 minutes). TXB_2 and 6-keto-$PGF_{1\alpha}$ continued to increase over the 4-hour duration of the study. In contrast, there was no increase in eicosanoids or TNF in the hemorrhagic group. These studies have implications for the development of therapies for these pathologic insults. Indeed, increases in sulfidopeptide leukotrienes and LTB_4 have been demonstrated in the bronchoalveolar lavage fluid of patients with ARDS, a complication associated with sepsis.[15,97-101]

EFFECT OF EICOSANOID SYNTHESIS INHIBITORS, RECEPTOR ANTAGONISTS, AND ANTI-INFLAMMATORY EICOSANOIDS

More direct evidence that eicosanoids mediate endotoxin-induced sequelae is provided by observations that the inhibition of eicosanoid synthesis or the blockade of specific receptors protects animals from shock sequelae (Fig. 41-3). Because PLA_2-II is increased in sepsis,[20] some studies examined the potential beneficial effect of inhibitors of PLA_2-II. The putative selective PLA_2-II inhibitor SB203347 and eucalyptus bioflavonoids (Quercetin), which alter neutrophil PLA_2-II release, improved survival in murine endotoxic shock.[102] PLA_2-II enzyme-deficient mice exhibited prolonged survival and reduced plasma cytokine in response to endotoxemia compared with wild-type subjects. PLA_2-II may, in part, potentiate lipopolysaccharide (LPS) shock by augmenting cellular responses to LPS. PLA_2-II potentiated LPS-induced IL-6 production in whole blood and binding of LPS to PMNs.[103]

Numerous NSAIDs have been evaluated for potential therapeutic benefit in endotoxemia and sepsis in animal models.[48] These compounds, when used in experimental sepsis or endotoxemia, have generally been found to improve survival or survival time and to reduce cardiopulmonary dysfunction and indices of tissue injury.[48,76-78] Among the most extensively studied prototype NSAID is ibuprofen. In various species with endotoxemia and sepsis, ibuprofen has been shown to improve systemic hypotension, pulmonary hypertension, protein and fluid extravasation, lung water flux, airway resistance, and oxygen delivery.[48,78,83,88,104-106] In some studies, however, ibuprofen did not improve shock sequelae.[106] Ibuprofen also alters neutrophil function, including inhibition of neutrophil aggregation, organ infiltration, and adherence.[104,106] As with

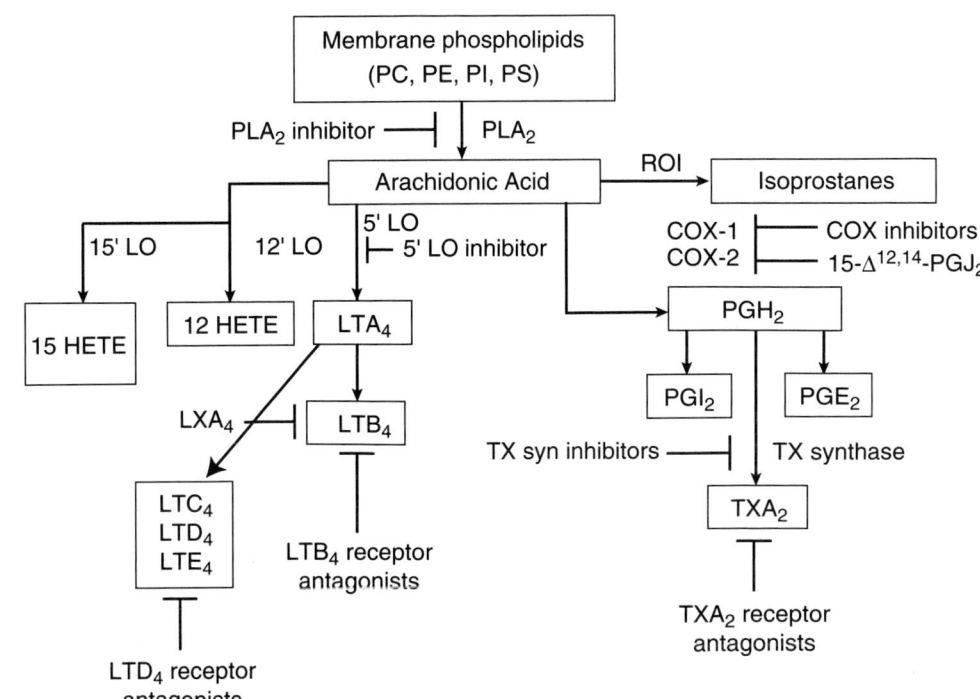

FIGURE 41-3. Metabolism of membrane phospholipids. COX, cyclooxygenase; HETE, hydroxyeicosatetraenoic acid; LO, lipoxygenase; LT, leukotriene; LXA_4, lipoxin A_4; PC, phosphatidylcholine; PE, phosphatidylethanolamine; PG, prostaglandin; PI, phosphatidylinositol; PLA_2, phospholipase A_2; PS, phosphatidylserine; ROI, reactive oxygen intermediates; TXA_2, thromboxane A_2.

other NSAIDs, it is likely that some of these salutary effects are the result of pharmacologic actions of ibuprofen other than inhibition of fatty acid cyclooxygenase. These actions include potential inhibition of LTB_4 production,[106] superoxide anion production,[106] scavenging of hydroxyl radicals,[107] and burn-induced inhibition of fibrinolysis.[108]

A major concern in the use of NSAIDs is their renal and gastrointestinal side effects. By inhibiting COX-1–dependent prostaglandin synthesis in those organs, NSAIDs can render septic animals more susceptible to renal failure[109,110] and gastrointestinal ulceration. The renal effects of NSAIDs can be reversed, at least in part, by the use of dopamine.[111] These side effects are due to the fact that NSAIDs inhibit both COX-1, the enzyme responsible for homeostasis in the kidneys and gastrointestinal tract, and COX-2, which is induced by LPS and probably mediates the increase in prostaglandin synthesis in sepsis. COX-2–selective drugs are currently approved for the treatment of arthritis and pain, and they may prove to have some benefit in the treatment of sepsis. NS-398, a selective COX-2 inhibitor, blocks inflammatory prostaglandin synthesis but does not inhibit gastric prostaglandin production and does not produce gastric erosion.[112] L-745,337, also a COX-2–selective inhibitor, has been found to reduce the core body temperature increase induced by LPS in rats.[113] However, selective inhibition of COX-2 with NS-398 did not provide long-term protection to mice subjected to endotoxin shock or sepsis induced by CLP.[114] In another study, the effect of selective COX-2 inhibitors (DFU and NS-398) or nonselective COX inhibitors (diclofenac and proquazone) on survival in murine endotoxemia was assessed.[115] Only specific dosages of DFU, NS-398, and proquazone prevented endotoxin-induced lethality. The investigators concluded that the effect of COX inhibitors on endotoxin shock is highly dose- and compound-dependent. Other studies with multiple injury models have shown that treatment with NS-398 in mice subjected to burns and *Pseudomonas aeruginosa* infections improved survival and absolute neutrophil count and reduced macrophage PGE_2 production.[116] The survival of mice traumatized by femur fracture and hemorrhage was improved by N-398.[117] Increases in in vivo IL-6 and in vitro Kupffer cell IL-6 production were inhibited in mice subjected to hemorrhage and subsequent CLP-induced sepsis.[118] Recent studies in COX-2–deficient mice suggest that COX-2–derived eicosanoids are deleterious in endotoxemia. Compared with endotoxemic wild types, COX-2–deficient mice exhibited improved survival, blunted inflammatory cell infiltration of tissues, suppressed NF-κB activation, and increases in the anti-inflammatory cytokine IL-10.[119] As even more selective COX-2 inhibitory drugs become available, more definitive assessment of COX-2 involvement in trauma and sepsis may be ascertained.

Pretreatment with TXA_2 synthase inhibitors or TXA_2 receptor antagonists improves survival time or attenuates certain shock sequelae in endotoxemic animals. The pathophysiologic events ameliorated by these pharmacologic agents include pulmonary hypertension,[120,121] reduced cardiac output, hypotension,[122,123] decreased renal blood flow, decreased glomerular filtration rate,[121,123,124] thrombocytopenia,[120-125] renal glomerular fibrin deposition,[126] and renal glomerular microthrombi.[123] Most studies have shown that the beneficial effects of these drugs are not obtained if they are given after endotoxin. However, in a porcine study, the TXA_2 synthase inhibitor dazmegrel, when administered 3 hours after endotoxin infusion in a chronically instrumented

young piglet model, was shown to reduce pulmonary hypertension and hypoxemia.[127] Other studies have not demonstrated improved outcome in sepsis and endotoxic shock.[128] Presumably, in these experiments, mediators other than TXA_2 dominate to produce pathophysiologic sequelae contributing to the development of shock and mortality. Use of TXA_2 receptor antagonists in endotoxemia may have several advantages over the use of TXA_2 synthase inhibitors. TXA_2 receptor antagonists block the effects of both PGH_2 and TXA_2 to activate TXA_2 receptors and do not produce shunting of PGH_2 to PGE_2 synthesis.

The 5-lipoxygenase inhibitor diethylcarbamazine improved the survival of mice in endotoxic shock,[93] and CGS8515 attenuated endotoxin-induced hemoconcentration and hypotension in rats.[129] AA-861, another 5-lipoxygenase inhibitor, attenuated endotoxin-induced neutropenia and concomitant oxygen radical synthesis in rats[130] and improved survival in endotoxemic mice.[131] L-651,392 blocked endotoxin-induced pulmonary hypertension and bronchoconstriction and increased arterial-alveolar oxygen difference and lung microvascular permeability in sheep.[94] Inhibition of 5-lipoxygenase by MK-886 attenuated hypotension and partially reversed the impaired vascular responsiveness to phenylephrine and acetylcholine.[132] MK-886 also inhibited coronary vasoconstriction and loss of myocardial contractility induced by *Escherichia coli* hemolysin in perfused rat hearts.[133]

Further evidence for the role of lipoxygenase products in endotoxin-induced shock sequelae is provided by studies using specific leukotriene receptor antagonists in experimental endotoxemia. The sulfidopeptide leukotriene receptor antagonist FPL57231 attenuated endotoxin-induced bronchoconstriction and pulmonary hypertension in sheep and cats.[134,135] The LTD_4 receptor antagonist SKF104353 prevented endotoxin-induced hemoconcentration and thrombocytopenia and improved survival time in rats.[136] The LTD_4/E_4 receptor antagonist LY171883 improved endotoxin-induced hypotension, hemoconcentration, and leukopenia in rats. SKF104353 and LY171883 were shown to prevent acute splanchnic permeability changes induced by endotoxin in rats[137] and mesenteric ischemia in pigs.[76] The LTB_4 receptor antagonist LY233978 has been shown to attenuate endotoxin-induced leukopenia, hemoconcentration, and hypotension in rats.[138] The LTB_4 antagonist LY306669 attenuated lung injury in a porcine endotoxemic model.[139] However, the protective effect of inhibitors of leukotriene biosynthesis or receptor antagonists may depend on the experimental model. MK-886 and an LTB_4 receptor antagonist, CP-105,696, reduced neutrophil infiltration into the peritoneal cavity, increased the peritoneal bacterial count, and reduced the survival rate in rats rendered septic by CLP.[95]

Some studies used combination therapy with cyclooxygenase inhibitors and leukotriene receptor antagonists or lipoxygenase inhibitors. Young and Passmore examined the effect of combined therapy with ibuprofen and LY171883 in canine endotoxic shock.[140] Combined blockade was more effective in maintaining blood pressure and cardiac output but provided no greater protection of renal blood flow or glomerular filtration rate. Turner and colleagues demonstrated good protection with a combined cyclooxygenase and lipoxygenase inhibitor (SKF86002) in a rat model of endotoxin-induced ARDS.[141] The inhibitor blocked the increase in lung wet-dry ratio, total bronchoalveolar lavage protein, hemoconcentration, and thrombocytopenia.

In contrast to the deleterious effects of certain eicosanoids (e.g., TXA_2), other prostanoids (e.g., PGE_1, PGI_2, 15-deoxy-$\Delta^{12,14}$-PGJ_2) may be beneficial in shock. PGI_2 infusion has been shown to be protective in canine endotoxic shock.[142] Prolonged PGE_1 infusion also had beneficial hemodynamic effects in hemorrhagic shock.[143] The cyclopentenone prostaglandin 15-deoxy-$\Delta^{12,14}$-PGJ_2 has been shown to be beneficial in several in vivo models of inflammation.[144-146] Although 15-deoxy-$\Delta^{12,14}$-PGJ_2 has been touted as the endogenous ligand for PPAR-γ, it is clear that it has PPAR-γ–independent effects that may be anti-inflammatory. The latter include inhibition of ERK1/2 and NF-κB signaling in response to microbial stimuli.[68,70,147,148] Recently, 15-deoxy-$\Delta^{12,14}$-PGJ_2 was found to improve the survival of rats subjected to polymicrobial sepsis induced by CLP and to inhibit tissue NF-κB and activator protein-1 signaling, tissue neutrophil infiltration, and cytokine production.[149]

SIGNIFICANCE OF EICOSANOIDS IN CRITICALLY ILL PATIENTS

Several studies have reported increased PLA$_2$-II, TXB_2, 6-keto-$PGF_{1\alpha}$, PGE_2, and $PGF_{2\alpha}$ levels in patients with septic shock.[150-152] Plasma PLA$_2$-II levels have been shown to correlate with hypotensive episodes and mortality in patients with acute sepsis and multiple organ failure. Oettinger and colleagues evaluated the relationship between plasma TXB_2 and 6-keto-$PGF_{2\alpha}$ levels and the severity of organ dysfunction in 106 patients with Gram-negative septic shock.[152] As in other studies, TXB_2 and 6-keto-$PGF_{1\alpha}$ levels were elevated throughout the course of sepsis but were highest during the early phase. TXB_2 levels were higher in hypodynamic patients than in hyperdynamic patients, whereas the opposite was observed for 6-keto-$PGF_{1\alpha}$. Patients in the hyperdynamic group had improved lung and kidney function, as determined by alveolar-arterial PO_2 gradient and creatinine clearance. In patients who underwent esophagectomy, which is associated with a high incidence of ARDS, there was a significant postoperative increase in postpulmonary TXB_2 levels only in patients who developed ARDS.[153] In patients with traumatic head injury, there was an increase in the TXB_2/6-keto-$PGF_{1\alpha}$ ratio in plasma, which positively correlated with the severity of injury and death.[154] Collectively, these studies demonstrate increased thromboxane and prostacyclin synthesis in patients with sepsis, trauma, or ARDS and suggest a deleterious role for thromboxane.

Leukotriene levels were also increased in several clinical situations. Seeger and coworkers reported increased LTB_4 metabolites in the bronchoalveolar lavage fluid of patients with ARDS.[101] Elevated sulfidopeptide leukotriene levels have also been reported in the bronchoalveolar lavage fluid, blood, and urine of patients with trauma or ARDS.[97,99,155] Higher leukotriene levels correlated with poor prognosis. Acutely ill patients with elevated plasma LTB_4 levels had a greater risk of developing ARDS than did those with lower levels.[100] Urinary excretion of LTE_4 was higher in trauma patients who developed ARDS than in those who did not have ARDS.[155]

There have been some clinical trials with eicosanoid inhibitors. Despite the association between increased plasma PLA$_2$-II concentration and sepsis severity, a human phase II trial in severe sepsis demonstrated that PLA$_2$-II inhibition was of no benefit.[156] The NSAIDs may have beneficial effects in the treatment of patients with trauma or sepsis. Faist and coworkers studied the effect of indomethacin in a randomized,

prospective study of 43 patients undergoing major surgical trauma.[157] The cellular immune status was evaluated preoperatively and up to a week after surgery. In contrast to untreated patients, patients receiving indomethacin exhibited an improvement in delayed-type hypersensitivity responses and mitogen-induced lymphocyte transformation and a lower rate of opportunistic infection. These results suggest that NSAIDs, by preventing the impairment of cell-mediated immunity, may reduce susceptibility to sepsis after surgery.

Bernard and associates conducted a double-blind, placebo-controlled trial of intravenous ibuprofen (10 mg/kg; maximum dose, 800 mg) given every 6 hours for eight doses in 455 patients with a diagnosis of sepsis.[158] The ibuprofen-treated group did not experience any increased incidence of renal dysfunction, gastrointestinal bleeding, or other adverse effects. Short-term treatment with ibuprofen did not significantly affect the duration of shock or the 30-day survival rate. However, ibuprofen did produce significant declines in urinary 6-keto-$PGF_{1\alpha}$ and TXB_2 excretion, temperature, heart rate, oxygen consumption, and lactic acidosis. In a subsequent analysis of a subset of hypothermic septic patients in this study, ibuprofen treatment was demonstrated to improve 30-day survival.[159]

In contrast to studies with eicosanoid inhibitors, certain eicosanoids may have beneficial hemodynamic or anti-inflammatory effects. Liposomal encapsulated PGE_1 was shown to reduce hypoxemia and to improve lung compliance and survival in a study of 25 ARDS patients.[160] However, in a subsequent phase III clinical trial with a total of 350 ARDS patients, intravenous liposomal PGE_1 was shown to improve indices of oxygenation but did not decrease the duration of mechanical ventilation or improve 28-day survival.[161] Aerosolized PGI_2 has also been tested in ARDS patients. The effect of PGI_2 was similar to that of inhaled nitric oxide, in that it induced pulmonary vasodilatation and improved ventilation perfusion.[162-164] This treatment approach also prevented hypoxemia in ARDS patients with respiratory failure caused by pneumonia.[165]

These studies provide the impetus for more extensive studies of eicosanoids and eicosanoid-altering drugs in trauma, sepsis, and ARDS. Also, the new generation of COX-2 inhibitors, with fewer side effects than traditional NSAIDs in critically ill patients, remains to be tested. Experimentally, combinations of drugs have been more effective than single-drug treatments.[166-171] Of particular interest, in view of the demonstrated increase of lipoxygenase products in patients with ARDS, is the potential application of lipoxygenase inhibitors or leukotriene receptor antagonists. The potential beneficial effect of certain eicosanoids (e.g., PGI_2) in ARDS suggests that complete inhibition of eicosanoid synthesis may not be desirable. Finally, the new and evolving concept that specific eicosanoids play pivotal roles in inflammation resolution[59,67] may direct future therapeutic interventions.

ACKNOWLEDGMENTS

This work was supported in part by NIH GM27673.

ANNOTATED REFERENCES

Arndt P, Abraham E: Immunological therapy of sepsis: Experimental therapies. Intensive Care Med 2001;27(Suppl 1):S104-S115.
 This review covers previous studies and recent experimental approaches for immunologic therapies for sepsis. Problems associated with entry criteria and definitions of sepsis are discussed, as are future recommendations.

Bernard GR, Wheeler AP, Russell JA, et al: The effects of ibuprofen on the physiology and survival of patients with sepsis: The Ibuprofen in Sepsis Study Group. N Engl J Med 1997;336:912-918.

The effect of ibuprofen on sepsis severity was examined in a large randomized, double-blinded, placebo-controlled trial. Ibuprofen reduced eicosanoid synthesis, fever, tachycardia, oxygen consumption, and lactic acidosis but did not prevent shock or improve survival.

Breyer RM, Bagdassarian CK, Myers SA, Breyer MD: Prostanoid receptors: Subtypes and signaling. Annu Rev Pharmacol Toxicol 2001;41:661-690.

This review examines the up-to-date literature characterizing prostanoid receptors, their subtypes, and the signaling pathway activated by the receptors.

Chandrasekharan NV, Dai H, Roos KL, et al: COX-3, a cyclooxygenase-1 variant inhibited by acetaminophen and other analgesic/antipyretic drugs: Cloning, structure, and expression. Proc Natl Acad Sci U S A 2002;99: 13926-13931.

This study provides evidence for a third distinct cyclooxygenase isoenzyme, COX-3, which is inhibited by acetaminophen. Inhibition of COX-3 may be a mechanism whereby drugs decrease pain and fever.

Lawrence T, Willoughby DA, Gilroy DW: Anti-inflammatory lipid mediators and insights into the resolution of inflammation. Nat Rev Immunol 2002;2:787-795.

This review examines lipid mediators that switch off inflammation. Endogenous mediators such as lipoxins and cyclopentenone prostaglandins suppress inflammatory gene expression, cell trafficking, inflammatory cell apoptosis, and phagocytosis, which are determinants of successful resolution of inflammation.

Chapter 42
NITRIC OXIDE

Sabah Hussain

KEY POINTS

1. **Nitric oxide (NO) has both direct and indirect modes of action.** Direct actions usually occur at relatively low levels of NO and include reaction with transition metals, including iron and copper. Activation of guanylate cyclase by NO is a prime example of a direct NO action. Indirect actions involve the reaction of NO with oxygen radicals and the formation of reactive nitrogen species, including the highly reactive peroxynitrite.

2. **NO is synthesized by three isoforms of nitric oxide synthase (NOS).** Neuronal NOS is constitutively expressed in central neurons, skeletal muscles, pulmonary epithelial cells, and nerve fibers supplying the lungs and intestinal system. Endothelial NOS is constitutively expressed mainly in endothelial cells. Inducible NOS has limited expression in normal cells; however, its expression is highly induced in response to proinflammatory cytokines and bacterial lipopolysaccharides.

3. **Activity of the human inducible NOS promoter** is less responsive to proinflammatory cytokines than is that of the murine promoter. Induction of inducible NOS expression in human cells is dependent on multiple transcription factors, including nuclear factor kappa-B and activator protein-1, and interferon regulatory factors.

4. **The gene of human neuronal NOS** is very complex, and both tissue-specific promoter activities and tissue-specific alternative splicing regulate its expression. Changes in gene expression of endothelial NOS have been documented in response to inflammatory mediators, changes in tissue PO_2, and alterations in regional blood flow.

5. **NOS activity can be inhibited in vivo** by many commercially available compounds, the majority of which are non–isoform selective. This category of nonselective inhibitors includes L-arginine analogs, aminoguanidine, and thiourea compounds. Highly selective inhibitors of inducible NOS have recently become available, including 1400W, GW273639, and GW274150.

6. **In normal vessels,** constitutive NO production by endothelial NOS localized in endothelial cells provides an important dilator mechanism that opposes the local myogenic response. This effect is mediated by activation of soluble guanylate cyclase and increased production of cyclic guanosine monophosphate in vascular smooth muscles. Inhibition of endothelial NO release induces a reduction in blood flow in various organs as a result of unmasking of the local myogenic tone.

7. **Basal NO production by endothelial cells** is sensitive to changes in shear stress and promotes higher local blood flow during increased metabolic demands (active hyperemia) and in response to transient interruptions of blood flow (reactive hyperemia).

8. **In septic patients,** many reports have documented high levels of plasma NO in adult patients with septic shock or severe sepsis and in pediatric patients with severe sepsis. The rise in plasma NO levels correlates negatively with patient survival. The exact isoform responsible for increased vascular NO production in septic humans remains to be documented.

9. **Infusion of nonselective NOS inhibitors in septic patients** restores arterial pressure and peripheral vascular resistance but significantly reduces cardiac output in septic patients. In one clinical trial, infusion of a nonselective NOS inhibitor in septic patients augmented mortality and resulted in early termination of the trial, leading to the conclusion that selective inhibitors of inducible NOS rather than nonselective NOS inhibitors should be administered to septic patients.

10. **Augmented NO production** has been documented in the livers of animals with severe sepsis or in hepatocytes exposed to proinflammatory cytokines. Administration of nonselective NOS inhibitors worsened liver injury in septic animals due to inhibition of constitutive endothelial NOS activity in hepatocytes and hepatic endothelial cells. Contradictory results have been reported in terms of whether inducible NOS plays a detrimental or a beneficial role in preventing hepatic injury in septic animals.

Nitric oxide (NO) may be the most intensively studied molecule over the past 20 years, by virtue of its functional centrality in almost every mammalian biologic system. It is most closely associated with the cardiovascular system, although thousands of publications have implicated NO in the regulation of many other physiologic processes as well. Detailing all the biologic functions of NO is beyond the scope of this chapter. What is presented is a brief discussion of the basic chemistry of NO, the structure and biochemical characteristics of the enzymes that synthesize it, how they are regulated, and NO's role in regulating vascular tone and hepatic function under normal conditions and in humans with severe sepsis or inflammatory liver injury.

BASIC CHEMISTRY

NO is a signaling and effector molecule with a wide range of biologic functions, including the regulation of blood pressure, neurotransmission, and tissue metabolism. Although it is considered a free radical, NO is not highly reactive per se. It mediates biologic functions through direct and indirect effects. Direct effects are mediated by physiologic (nonmolar) concentrations that help maintain homeostasis in most systems. Direct actions include reactions with transition metal centers (particularly iron and copper) in proteins, with the result being either protein activation or inhibition.[1] However, the most well-known direct effect of NO is its activation of soluble guanylate cyclase, which results in an increase in intracellular cyclic guanosine monophosphate (cGMP), an important regulator of smooth muscle contractility, platelet aggregation, and leukocyte adhesion.[2]

Direct effects of NO also include its reaction with cysteine redox centers, a process known as S-nitrosylation.[1] Several proteins have recently been identified as undergoing S-nitrosylation by NO, resulting in either activation or inhibition of activity. These proteins include nuclear factor kappa-B (NF-κB), Ca^{++}-dependent K$^+$ channels, ryanodine receptors, and caspase-3. Finally, NO also diffuses into red blood cells and reacts with oxyhemoglobin, forming NO$_2$ and methemoglobin.

Indirect effects of NO are mediated through its interactions with O$_2$ and O$_2^-$ and are usually elicited by relatively high (micromolar) concentrations of NO. In aqueous solutions, NO reacts with O$_2$ to form NO$_2$ and N$_2$O$_3$ (a potent S-nitrosylating agent), a reaction that is biologically relevant only at high concentrations of NO.[3] The most important indirect effect of NO is its near diffusion-limited reaction with O$_2^-$ anions to generate peroxynitrite (ONOO$^-$), a highly reactive radical with a very short in vivo half-life (1 sec).[4] Peroxynitrite rapidly dissociates to peroxynitrous acid or a carbonate adduct, which in turn rapidly generates carbonate and NO$_2$ radicals.[4] Peroxynitrite is a major contributor to cellular oxidative stress as a result of enhancement of thiol oxidation and lipid peroxidation and inhibition and inactivation of major antioxidant defenses such as reduced gluathione and superoxide dismutases (SODs).[5] It also targets specific tyrosine residues in several proteins and generates 3-nitrotyrosine. The range of tyrosine-nitrated proteins so affected includes those involved in apoptosis, glycolysis, mitochondrial respiration, structural support, and antioxidant defenses.[6] Tyrosine nitration of even a single residue, as in the case of Mn-SOD, may result in drastic inhibition of protein activity.

Formation of 3-nitrotyrosine has also been linked to several human pathologies, including acute lung injury and severe sepsis. It should be emphasized that the formation of peroxynitrite is usually restricted to specific conditions in which the local levels of both NO and O$_2^-$ are substantially elevated. Under normal conditions, however, O$_2^-$ anions are converted to H$_2$O$_2$ by SODs without significant peroxynitrite formation. It is also noteworthy that despite the possibility of peroxynitrite formation under special circumstances,

physiologic NO production is considered an antioxidant pathway because of the direct antioxidant actions of NO, which consist of reduction of toxic oxidants such as ferryl cations, inhibition of Fe^{+++}-catalyzed generation of hydroxyl radicals, and termination of lipid peroxidation.[7] Indirect antioxidant actions of NO include the induction of ferritin synthesis, which helps reduce free Fe^{++} levels. In addition, NO promotes the expression of heme oxygenase I, an important antioxidant enzyme by virtue of its products, carbon monoxide and bilirubin.[8] Finally, NO induces the expression of extracellular SOD, a key antioxidant enzyme responsible for dismutation of O$_2^-$ anions in the vascular system.[9]

NITRIC OXIDE SYNTHASES

NO is produced by NO synthases (NOSs) from the terminal guanidine nitrogen of L-arginine through a reaction that requires two molecules of O$_2$ and 1.5 mol of the reduced form of nicotinamide adenine dinucleotide phosphate (NADPH). Three distinct isoforms of NOS have been identified, each of which is a product of different genes and has different localization, regulation, catalytic properties, and inhibitor sensitivities. These isoforms are neuronal NOS (nNOS), which is expressed predominantly in neuronal tissue; inducible NOS (iNOS), which is inducible in a wide range of cells; and endothelial NOS (eNOS), which is expressed mainly in endothelial cells. NOS isoforms have also been classified on the basis of their constitutive (eNOS and nNOS) or inducible (iNOS) expression and their Ca^{++} dependence (eNOS and nNOS) or independence (iNOS). The nNOS gene (chromosome 12) has a complex structural organization with 29 exons and 28 introns and codes for a 1434–amino acid protein, whereas both the iNOS (chromosome 17) and eNOS (chromosome 7) genes consist of 26 exons and 25 introns, coding for 1153 and 1203 amino acids, respectively.[10]

All NOS isoforms consist of two domains—an N-terminal oxygenase domain that binds to heme, tetrahydrobiopterin (BH$_4$), and L-arginine, and a C-terminal reductase domain that binds to flavins (flavin adenine dinucleotide [FAD], flavin mononucleotide [FMN]) and NADPH (Fig. 42-1). NOSs are active only when they are homodimers, and they require an electron transfer from NADPH, which is catalyzed by bound FMN and FAD. BH$_4$ is required for dimerization, for coupling of NADPH oxidation to NO synthesis, and for protection against oxidation and autoinactivation. NOS proteins undergo autoinhibition when NO reacts with Fe^{++} atoms of the NOS-bound heme group, resulting in inhibition of NOS activity. The nNOS isoform is the most susceptible of the three to autoinhibition, with 95% of its activity being inhibited by self-derived NO.[11]

REGULATION OF NITRIC OXIDE SYNTHASES

The rate of NO production by NOS isoforms is regulated at several levels, including transcriptional and post-transcriptional regulation of NOS expression and pharmacologic regulation of NOS protein activity and localization.

TRANSCRIPTIONAL REGULATION

Human promoters of the three NOS isoforms have been cloned and characterized. With respect to iNOS, it has been well established that stimuli such as bacterial lipopolysaccharide

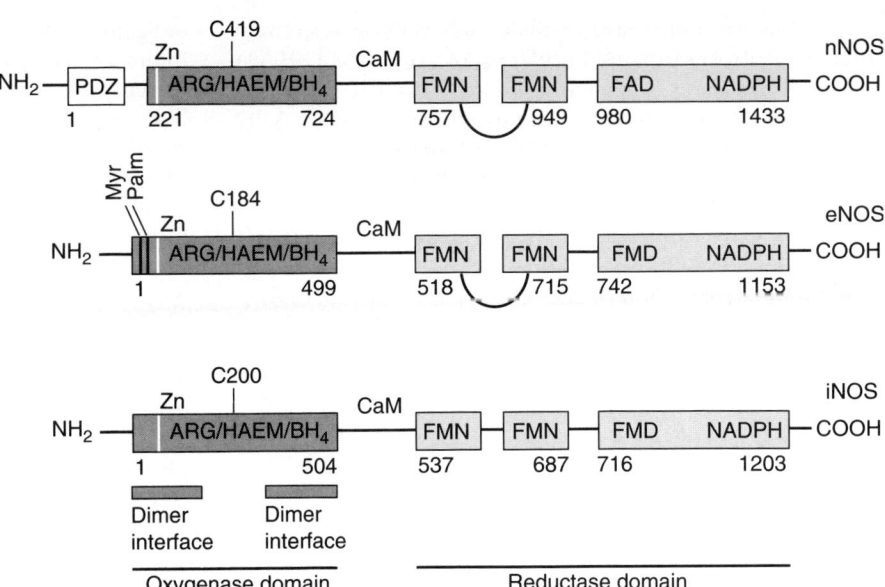

FIGURE 42–1. Domain structure of human neuronal nitric oxide synthase (nNOS), endothelial nitric oxide synthase (eNOS), and inducible nitric oxide synthase (iNOS). Oxygenase, reductase, and PDZ domains are denoted by solid boxes, and the amino acid residue number at the start or end of each domain is shown. The cysteine residue, which ligates the heme and the calmodulin binding site, is indicated for each isoform. Myristoylation (Myr) and palmitoylation (Palm) sites on eNOS are shown, as is the location of the zinc-ligating cysteines (Zn). The autoinhibitory loop within the flavin mononucleotide (FMN) regions of nNOS and eNOS is also shown, and gray bars indicate the dimer interface in the oxygenase domain. ARG, arginine; BH₄, tetrahydrobiopterin; NADPH, reduced form of nicotinamide adenine dinucleotide phosphate. (Adapted from Alderton WK, Cooper CE, Knowles RG: Nitric oxide synthases: Structure, function and inhibition. Biochem J 2001;357:593-615.)

(LPS) and cytokines, including tumor necrosis factor (TNF), interleukin (IL)-1, and interferon (IFN)-γ, are capable of inducing iNOS messenger RNA (mRNA) and protein in many human cells, including macrophages, hepatocytes, smooth muscles, and chondrocytes. In normal humans, iNOS mRNA expression is present in a few cell types, for example, airway epithelial cells. Cloning and expression of 8.3 and 16 kilobases (kb) of the human iNOS promoter revealed the following characteristics[12,13]: (1) Human promoter activity is only modestly induced in response to exposure of cultured cells to an LPS and cytokine mixture, compared with murine iNOS promoter activity. This difference has been attributed to the presence of multiple inactivating nucleotide substitutions in the enhancing elements responsible for LPS- and cytokine-induced expression in the human iNOS promoter. (2) Sequences conferring LPS and cytokine inducibility of the human iNOS promoter reside at upstream locations from the transcription initiation site (>4 kb). (3) Multiple transcription factors are involved in activating the human iNOS promoter, including the NF-κB family of transcription factors, activator protein-1 transcription factors, STAT-1α (signal transducer and activator of transcription) and INF regulatory factor-1. (4) Synergism between these transcription factors is required for enhancing iNOS promoter activity.

The expression of iNOS is also regulated by changes in mRNA stability and protein translation. The presence of several ATTTA sequence motifs (involved in protein-mRNA interactions) at the 3′ untranslated region (UTR) of human iNOS mRNA suggests that its stability may undergo significant regulation. Expression of iNOS mRNA is also regulated by alternative splicing within both 5′ UTR and the coding sequence.[14]

The human eNOS promoter possesses several binding sites for Sp1, GATA, activator proteins (AP-1, AP-2), E₂6 transformation specific (ETS), NF-κB, nuclear factor-1, NF-IL-6, shear stress, cyclic adenosine monophosphate response, acute-phase response, and IFN-induced transcription factors.[15] In vivo analysis of transgenic mice expressing 5200 base pairs of murine eNOS promoter elicited a robust expression in large and medium blood vessels, whereas small arterioles, capillaries, and venules showed very little transcriptional activity. In addition, many stimuli, including estrogens, angiotensin II,

proinflammatory cytokines, and hypoxia, alter eNOS mRNA expression through changes in its half-life.

The nNOS gene is the most complex human gene yet described in terms of promoter diversity and alternative splicing. Wang and colleagues described nine unique exon 1 variants of nNOS (exons 1a through 1i) that are associated with transcript initiation in various tissues.[16] Exons 1a, 1b, and 1c are abundantly expressed in skeletal muscles, whereas exons 1f, 1g, and 1i are present mainly in the brain. All nine exons are expressed in the testis. Analysis of alternative splicing of nNOS mRNA uncovered two main variants, nNOSβ and nNOSγ, which have 136- and 125-kDa molecular masses and are capable of producing 80% and 3% of nNOSα activity, respectively. Another splice variant of nNOS is nNOSμ, which has an additional 34 amino acids inserted between exons 16 and 17. It is abundantly expressed in skeletal muscle and in penile and urethral tissues.[17] This variant has similar enzyme kinetics to those of nNOSα.[17]

POST-TRANSLATIONAL REGULATION

One of the most important regulators of NOS activity is calmodulin binding, which increases the rate of electron transfer from NADPH to the flavins and heme group. It is triggered by a rise in intracellular Ca⁺⁺ and is inhibited by a motif of 40 to 50 amino acids localized in the FMN binding site. The absence of this motif in iNOS results in tight binding of calmodulin to the iNOS protein, rendering its activity insensitive to intracellular Ca⁺⁺ fluxes (hence the term Ca⁺⁺- and calmodulin-independent). NOS activity is also regulated through interactions with specific proteins such as protein inhibitor of nNOS, which inhibits nNOS activity by preventing monomer dimerization.[18]

Another regulator of NOS activity is heat shock protein 90, which interacts directly with eNOS and augments its activity by promoting calmodulin binding.[19] Other eNOS protein modifications include dual acetylation by myristate and palmitate, which are required for localization of eNOS at the caveolae. Myristoylation is an irreversible process that involves a single N-terminus glycine, whereas palmitoylation is reversible and develops at Cys-5 and Cys-26 and is modulated by intracellular Ca⁺⁺ levels.

NOS expression is also regulated when iNOS selectively interacts with two separate proteins, kalirin and a 110-kDa NOS-associated protein (NAP110).[20,21] Kalirin associates with iNOS in vitro and in vivo and inhibits its activity by preventing monomer dimerization. Similarly, NAP110 selectively interacts with the N-terminal portion of iNOS and inhibits its activity by about 90% in cultured cells.[21]

Finally, NOS activities are also mediated by phosphorylation of serine, threonine, and tyrosine residues. Increased shear stress and activation of protein kinase B induces eNOS phosphorylation at Ser-1177, which in turn activates this enzyme.[22] By contrast, phosphorylation of eNOS at Thr-495 inhibits its activity.[23] The nNOS protein is phosphorylated by Ca^{++} calmodulin-dependent kinases at Ser-847, thereby reducing nNOS activity.[24] There are also published reports of tyrosine phosphorylation of iNOS, which results in its activation.[25]

PHARMACOLOGIC REGULATION

Various biologic roles of NO have been uncovered as a result of the availability of pharmacologic inhibitors. However, many investigators have not been sufficiently careful in verifying the selectivity of these inhibitors, and a few have assigned in vivo isoform selectivity to inhibitors for which only in vitro selectivity has been established. Many NOS inhibitors, including L-arginine analogs such as N^G-monomethyl L-arginine (LNMMA), N^G-nitro-L-arginine (L-NA) and its methyl ester (L-NAME), thiocitrullines, 1400W, aminoguanidine, S-ethylisothiourea, N^5-iminoethyl-L-ornithine (L-NIO), N^6-iminoethyl-L-lysine (L-NIL), GW273629, and GW274150, bind NOSs at L-arginine binding sites and inhibit substrate binding. All these inhibitors require active enzyme activity and the presence of NADPH for their binding.[26] Aminoguanidine also inhibits NOS activity by forming complex covalent bonds with NOS proteins without interfering with NOS dimerization.[27]

Another class of inhibitors, including 4-amino BH_4 and BH_2, inhibit NOS activity by targeting the BH_4 binding site, whereas 7-nitroindazole and its related compounds compete for binding at both the L-arginine and BH_4 binding sites.[28] Additionally, the antifungal imidazoles hinder iNOS activity by binding to the heme group and competing with calmodulin binding.

Table 42-1 lists the selectivity and effective concentrations of various NOS inhibitors measured in vitro. Inhibitors with 10- to 50-fold selectivity are considered partially selective inhibitors. For example, S-ethyl- and S-methyl-L-thiocitrullines and ARL17477 are considered partially selective nNOS inhibitors. L-NIO and L-NIL are considered partially selective iNOS inhibitors. Recently, highly selective iNOS inhibitors have become available, such as 1400W, GW273639, and GW274150, which have enabled investigators to evaluate the functional roles of iNOS in a variety of physiologic contexts. It should be emphasized, though, that aminoguanidine, the most widely used iNOS inhibitor, has only about a 10-fold selectivity for iNOS relative to eNOS and has virtually no selectivity relative to nNOS. This inhibitor also attenuates catalase, diamine oxidase, and polyamine metabolism.

BIOLOGIC FUNCTIONS OF NITRIC OXIDE

NORMAL VASCULAR TONE

Vasodilatation is the earliest discovered and most widely studied action of NO in the cardiovascular system. In a 1980 landmark study, Furchgott and Zawadzki described the obligatory role of endothelium-derived relaxing factor in inducing vascular smooth muscle relaxation of large conduit vessels.[29] Two studies in 1986 and 1988 identified endothelium-derived relaxing factor as NO and proposed the presence of an NO synthesizing protein in endothelial cells.[2,30] The most important NOS isoform in the regulation of normal vascular tone is certainly eNOS. Although the nNOS isoform is expressed in perivascular nerves, cardiac conduction pathways, and myocardial sarcoplasmic reticulum, it is less important than eNOS in regulating vascular tone.

It is well established that eNOS-derived NO production by the endothelial cells is activated very rapidly by longitudinal shear forces acting on the endothelium and generated by blood flow and by the pulsatile stretch of the vasculature. This flow-dependent NO release provides a crucial mechanism for the dynamic coupling of tissue metabolic demands and upstream vascular resistance and has been documented in conduit arteries, resistance arteries, arterioles, and venules.[31] Because shear stress in blood vessels is determined by flow velocity, flow pulsatility, blood viscosity, and vessel diameter, these variables have significant effects on endothelial NO release both in vitro and in vivo (Fig. 42-2). Basal endothelial NO release in normal vessels is in dynamic equilibrium with the local constrictor provided by the intrinsic myogenic tone of smooth muscles and by sympathetic vasoconstrictor drive. When eNOS-derived NO synthesis is inhibited in vivo, the local myogenic tone becomes unmasked and causes a reduction in vessel diameter and a rise in vascular resistance in almost all vascular beds.[32] The dilator effect of NO on smooth muscles is triggered by soluble guanylate cyclase activation, which results in increased production of the second messenger cGMP. In turn, cGMP activates two cGMP-dependent protein kinases (PKGI and II), which regulate smooth muscle intracellular Ca^{++} levels and hence contractility by increasing Ca^{++} sequestration in and inhibiting Ca^{++} release from the sarcoplasmic reticulum.[33] In certain vascular beds, NO evokes smooth muscle relaxation by hyperpolarizing membrane potential, an effect that is mediated by the activation of Ca^{++}-dependent K^+ channels. Finally, NO-mediated smooth muscle relaxation can also be the result of a prejunctional effect on adrenergic nerve fibers, leading to inhibition of local catecholamine release.[34]

Increased shear stress also up-regulates eNOS expression when maintained for relatively long periods. Indeed, significant induction of eNOS mRNA and protein has been documented in cultured endothelial cell preparations in which shear stress was artificially maintained and in in vivo settings in which organ blood flow and shear stress were chronically elevated in response to exercise training or the result of arteriovenous fistulas.[35]

Vascular NO production is also acutely activated in response to agonist stimulation of endothelial membrane receptors by acetylcholine, adenosine triphosphate, bradykinin, and substance P. These agonists are synthesized and released by endothelial cells in response to shear stress and mechanical perturbations and act in an autocrine fashion to stimulate their prospective receptors. Activation of these receptors elicits a rise in intracellular Ca^{++} concentrations and thereby activates eNOS. Agonist-induced endothelial NO release, especially by adenosine triphosphate and bradykinin, provides another mechanism through which tissue metabolic demands are matched to local blood flow, as in human heart and forearm vasculatures.[36]

TABLE 42–1. SELECTIVITY OF NITRIC OXIDE SYNTHASE INHIBITORS

Inhibitor	IC$_{50}$ (μM)			Selectivity (Fold)		
	iNOS	nNOS	eNOS	iNOS	nNOS	eNOS
L-NA*	3.1	0.29	0.35	0.09	0.11	1.2
LNMMA	6.6	4.9	3.5	0.7	0.5	0.7
7-NI*	9.7	8.3	11.8	0.9	1.2	1.4
ARL17477	0.33	0.07	1.6	0.2	5.0	23†
AG*	31	170	330	5.5	11†	1.9
L-NIL	1.6	37	49	23†	49†	1.3
1400W	0.23	7.3	1000	32†	>4000‡	>130‡
GW273629	8.0	630	1000	78‡	>125‡	>1.6
GW274150	1.4	145	466	104‡	333‡	3.2

Results shown are for human NOS isoforms expressed in a baculovirus expression system. Activity assays were performed on cell lysates in the presence of 30 μM at 37°C for 15 minutes. NOS inhibitors were pre-exposed to inhibitors for a 15-minute period.
* Data obtained from J. Dawson and R. G. Knowles, unpublished results.
† Partially selective.
‡ Highly selective.
AG, aminoguanidine; eNOS, endothelial NOS; iNOS, inducible NOS; L-NA, N^G-nitro-L-arginine; L-NIL, N^6-iminoethyl-L-lysine; LNMMA, N^G-monomethyl-L-arginine; nNOS, neuronal NOS; NOS, nitric oxide synthase.
Adapted from Alderton WK, Cooper CE, Knowles RG: Nitric oxide synthases: Structure, function and inhibition. Biochem J 2001;357:593-615. Data from Young et al, except as otherwise noted.

In addition to the regulation of basal blood flow, endothelial NO contributes to the vasodilatory response to elevated metabolic demands (active hyperemia). The degree of this contribution, however, differs among vasculatures. For instance, Hussain and coworkers reported that endothelial NO contributes between 20% and 40% of the total active hyperemia of the in situ diaphragm in dogs,[37] whereas up to 50% of human myocardial active hyperemia induced by cardiac pacing was mediated by endothelial NO release.[38] Endothelial NO also participates in the reactive hyperemic response, which is the dilatation that follows transient vascular occlusion. This contribution is much more pronounced in tissues with high metabolic demands and manifests as prolongation of reactive hyperemia duration, with no influence on peak reactive hyperemic flow.[39] Another vascular phenomenon that is partly regulated by endothelial NO is autoregulation, defined as the ability of tissues to maintain their perfusion independent of changes in arterial pressure. It has been reported that inhibition of endothelial NO production and the subsequent augmentation of local myogenic tone lead to an improvement in flow autoregulation. However, this improvement is dependent on local metabolic rate and is more pronounced in tissues with relatively low metabolic rates, such as the mesenteric vasculature, than in tissues with high metabolic rates, such as the heart, kidneys, and brain; in the latter tissues, NOS inhibition only lowers blood flow levels, with no effect on the autoregulatory range.[40]

In addition to its role in the regulation of blood flow, NO has important functional significance for tissue metabolism, by virtue of its effect on mitochondrial respiration. It has been well established that NO donors or endogenous NO production inhibits, albeit reversibly, the activities of cytochrome

FIGURE 42–2. Key mechanisms involved in the regulation of perfusion by nitric oxide (NO). *A*, Endothelial NO production increases monotonically with time-averaged shear stress, reaching a plateau at 10 to 30 dynes/cm². *B*, NO release from the endothelium is sensitive to flow pulsatility, being maximal at pulse frequencies of about 5 Hz. *C*, In isolated vessels, acute increases in transmural pressure (ΔP) promote a myogenic constrictor response, normally attenuated by NO. Loss of NO activity also elevates basal constrictor tone. *D*, The amplitude of spontaneous oscillations in vascular caliber (vasomotion) is damped by NO. (Adapted from Griffith TM: Role of nitric oxide in the regulation of blood flow. In Ignarro LJ [ed]: nitric oxide Biology and Pathobiology. San Diego, Academic Press, 2000, pp 483-502.)

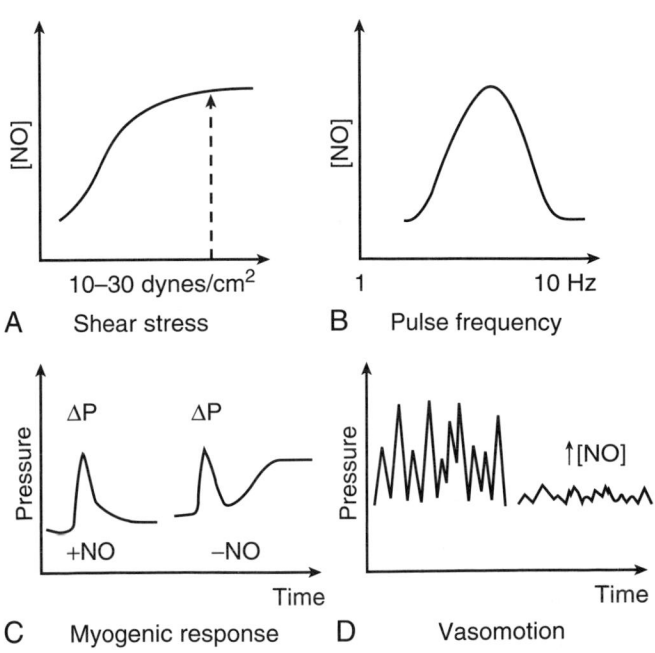

oxidase (the terminal enzyme of the mitochondrial respiratory chain) and aconitase (an important enzyme in the citric acid cycle).[41,42] Removal of this inhibition has been proposed as the mechanism behind the rise in whole body or organ oxygen consumption when NOS inhibitors are infused in vivo.[43]

Another vascular function of NO is the prevention of platelet aggregation. Many reports have confirmed that NO stimulates cGMP production inside the platelets and inhibits agonist-induced platelet aggregation through the regulation of intracellular Ca^{++} levels.[44] In addition, endothelial NO production has an important antiatherosclerotic function and protects against the early phase of atherosclerosis by inhibiting leukocyte adhesion to and migration through the endothelial cells. Both effects are achieved by reducing the expression of intercellular adhesion molecule-1, vascular cell adhesion molecule-1, and P-selectin.[45] The late stages of atherosclerosis are also inhibited by NO as a result of attenuation of endothelial permeability, reduction of lipoprotein influx into the vascular wall, and inhibition of oxidation of low-density lipoproteins.[46]

VASCULAR FAILURE DUE TO SEPSIS

The cardiovascular abnormalities associated with severe sepsis are characterized by low peripheral vascular resistance, hypotension, high cardiac output, maldistribution of blood flow, increased microvascular permeability, disseminated intravascular coagulation, and microthrombosis.[47] Many factors have been implicated in these dysfunctions, such as proinflammatory cytokines (TNF, IL-1, IFN-γ), reactive oxygen species, and prostaglandins that disrupt the normal balance between vasodilators (NO and prostacyclin) and vasoconstrictors (endothelins, catecholamines, angiotensin II). Numerous studies have also implicated excessive NO production by iNOS in the vascular dysfunction accompanying sepsis. The majority of these studies used models in which *Escherichia coli* LPS was administered as a bolus dose in mice or rats. In these models, arterial pressure declined within minutes of LPS injection, followed by partial recovery, then a sustained decline in pressure 3 to 4 hours later. It has now been well established that plasma concentrations of NO and its related products (NO_2^- and NO_3^-) rise severalfold in a progressive fashion a few hours after LPS injection. Moreover, many authors have documented iNOS mRNA and protein in endothelial cells, smooth muscles, cardiac myocytes, skeletal muscles, hepatocytes, and renal cells in LPS-injected rodents.[48] However, it should be emphasized that LPS rodent models of sepsis have limited clinical relevance, primarily because both rats and mice are less sensitive to LPS than humans are; thus, relatively large doses of LPS are required to elicit sepsis in these animals. A less dramatic rise or no change in NO production has been reported in rodent peritonitis models and in nonrodent models of sepsis. For instance, no significant changes in plasma NO levels were observed after short (<5 hours) or prolonged (9 to 18 hours) periods of endotoxemia in pigs. Moreover, only a 50% rise in plasma NO concentration was reported in endotoxemic dogs.[49]

Studies of humans with severe sepsis have also shown a significant increase in vascular NO production, but to a much lower degree than that observed in LPS rodent models. Ochoa and associates were the first to report that plasma NO_2^- and NO_3^- levels were higher in hyperdynamic septic patients than in trauma patients.[50] This finding was confirmed

by Arnalich and colleagues, who also found that plasma NO_2^- and NO_3^- levels were higher in patients with septic shock than in those with only severe sepsis.[51] Moreover, plasma NO_x (combined NO, NO_2^-, and NO_3^-) concentrations were significantly greater in patients who died of postoperative sepsis compared with septic patients who survived.[52] In 53 pediatric patients with severe sepsis, Doughty and coworkers reported that plasma NO_2^- and NO_3^- concentrations measured on day 1 of admission predicted persistent failure of three or more organs and sequential organ failure, but not mortality.[53] This has prodded investigators to question whether the rise in plasma NO_x levels in septic patients is the result of iNOS expression or poor renal excretion of NO_x compounds. This question has not yet been answered; however, evidence is emerging that iNOS mRNA and protein are induced in many cells of septic patients, including neutrophils, alveolar macrophages, and skeletal muscles.[54-56] Whether this expression is sufficient to cause an increase in circulating plasma NO_x levels remains unclear.

Despite extensive documentation of elevated NO production in the vessels of septic animals and humans, the contribution of individual NOS isoforms to the pathogenesis of sepsis-induced vascular failure remains the focus of many investigators. In early studies published in 1990, the administration of nonselective NOS inhibitors (LNMMA, L-NA, L-NAME) in rodent LPS models of sepsis reversed early hypotension and improved vascular reactivity to vasoactive agents.[57,58] The initial euphoria triggered by these observations was dampened when severe reduction in cardiac output; worsening of cardiac function; exacerbated microvascular leakage; amplification of inflammation in the liver, kidney, and intestine; and augmented animal mortality were observed after several hours of LNMMA, L-NA, or L-NAME infusion in septic rodents. These findings led to the conclusion that nonselective NOS inhibitors are not beneficial for septic animals because they inhibit important homeostatic functions of eNOS. Subsequent studies using highly selective iNOS inhibitors revealed that selective elimination of iNOS activity in various animal models of sepsis reverses hypotension, restores vascular reactivity, improves myocardial function, attenuates acute lung injury, and partially restores mitochondrial function.[59-61]

Petros and coworkers were the first to report, in 1991, that the injection of nonselective NOS inhibitors (LNMMA and L-NAME) in septic human patients restored arterial pressure and peripheral vascular resistance.[62] Schilling and colleagues confirmed these findings but also reported that these inhibitors reduced cardiac output to 66% of initial values.[63] Restoration of vascular response to vasoactive agents, restoration of arterial pressure, and a significant decline in cardiac index have also been observed after L-NA injection in septic patients (Fig. 42-3).[64,65] Three subsequent prospective, uncontrolled trials used continuous infusion of either L-NAME (1 to 3 mg/kg/h for 12 to 24 hours) or LNMMA (up to 20 mg/kg/h for 8 hours) and reported sustained elevation of arterial pressure and peripheral vascular resistance, coupled with a significant decline in cardiac output.[66-68] Despite the restoration of arterial pressure, the effect of NOS inhibition on the outcome of septic patients is still being debated. A phase III prospective, randomized, double-blinded, placebo-controlled trial was conducted to treat septic patients with LNMMA, along with dobutamine to maintain cardiac output. This trial was recently terminated because of a statistically significant higher mortality in the treatment group.[69]

In addition to nonselective NOS inhibitors, investigators have used methylene blue (inhibitor of soluble guanylate cyclase) to counteract the effects of excessive NO production. Short-term infusion and bolus injection of this compound in septic patients raised mean arterial pressure by 10 mm Hg without affecting cardiac output.[70,71] Neither patient mortality nor the possibility that methylene blue might have effects other than inhibition of soluble guanylate cyclase was addressed.

In summary, it is apparent from animal and human studies that the use of nonselective NOS inhibitors to treat vascular failure due to sepsis is not warranted because of eNOS inhibition and elimination of the possible beneficial effects of iNOS, which include anti-inflammatory and anti–platelet aggregation effects. Future trials using highly selective iNOS inhibitors in patients with sepsis should aid in elucidating the extent to which overproduction of NO by this isoform contributes to sepsis-induced vascular failure.

LIVER FUNCTION

Under normal conditions, the eNOS isoform is the main source of NO in hepatic cells and is involved in the regulation of hepatic blood flow and the prevention of leukocyte infiltration and platelet adhesion.[72] Hepatic nNOS expression is limited to the nerve fibers supplying large hepatic vessels. All human liver cells are capable of expressing iNOS when exposed to LPS; cytokines such as TNF, IL-1β, and IFN; activators of protein kinase C; arachidonic acid metabolites; and platelet-activating factor.[73] Hepatic iNOS expression is strongly inhibited by glucocorticoids, NO or NO donors, and hepatocyte, epidermal, and transforming growth factors.[74] Hepatocyte NO synthesis is involved in many processes, such as protein synthesis, glucose synthesis from pyruvate and lactate, glucagon-stimulated glycogenolysis, and activity of cytochrome P_{450} enzymes, which are involved in drug metabolism.[75]

INFLAMMATORY LIVER INJURY

The involvement of NO in hepatic dysfunction has been investigated extensively in various models of liver injury. In LPS-induced models of sepsis, liver injury is characterized by the presence of neutrophil, lymphocyte, and macrophage infiltration and by hypertrophy, vacuolization, and chromosomal margination of hepatocytes. Moreover, elevated serum levels of aspartate transaminase (AST) and alanine transaminase (ALT) have been used extensively as an index of hepatic injury. It has been well established that in vivo LPS injection elicits a substantial rise in hepatic NO production, iNOS mRNA, and protein induction in hepatocytes and endothelial, Kupffer, and bile duct cells.[76]

Early studies in which nonselective NOS inhibitors (LNMMA and L-NAME) were used revealed that inhibition of all NOS isoforms worsens hepatic injury, causes a further rise in serum AST and ALT levels, increases hepatocyte necrosis and leukocyte infiltration, and enhances lipid peroxidation and oxidative DNA damage.[77] These changes have been attributed to interference with hepatic microcirculation and a severe reduction in sinusoidal blood flow as a result of the elimination of endothelial eNOS production. Similar worsening of liver injury with the use of nonspecific NOS inhibitors has been reported in hemorrhagic shock-induced hepatocyte injury[78] and alcoholic hepatitis.[79] Although these findings confirm a beneficial role for eNOS, the nature of iNOS involvement in liver injury is controversial, with deleterious, beneficial, or minimal roles being proposed.

Authors who have compared the in vivo effects of nonselective versus highly selective iNOS inhibitors in LPS models have concluded that iNOS promotes liver injury through the formation of peroxynitrite.[80] This is supported by Szabo and colleagues, who used S-methylisothiourea to inhibit iNOS activity and reported significant attenuation in serum AST, ALT, and bilirubin levels in septic mice.[81] By comparison, MacMicking and associates reported that the degree of LPS-induced liver injury in iNOS knockout mice was similar to that elicited in wild-type mice, suggesting that iNOS is not a major contributor to this injury.[82] It should be emphasized, however, that the degree of liver dysfunction in this study was mild, because relatively low doses of LPS were used. Alternatively, several authors have concluded that iNOS activity protects liver cells against injury and oxidative stress elicited by exposure to LPS or proinflammatory cytokines.

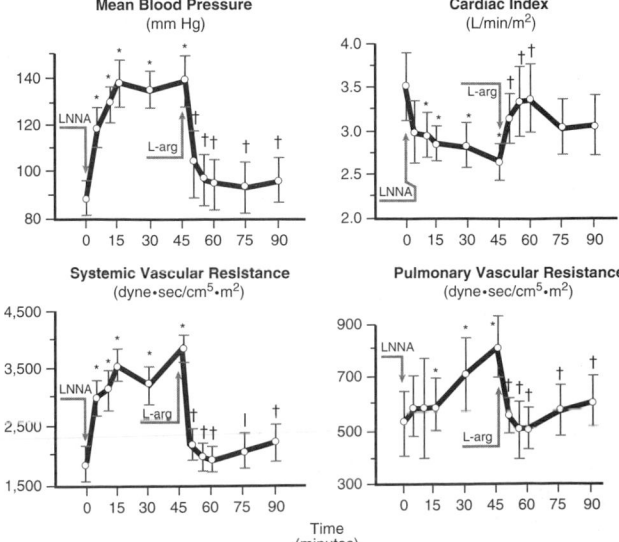

FIGURE 42–3. Hemodynamic changes induced by intravenous administration of Ng-nitro-L-arginine (LNNA) at minute 0 and L-arginine (L-arg) at minute 45 (mean ± standard error of the mean). *$P < 0.05$ for the comparison with minute 0; +$P < 0.05$ for the comparison with minute 45. (Adapted from Lorente JA, Landin L, De Pablo R, et al: L-Arginine pathway in the sepsis syndrome. Crit Care Med 1993;21:1287-1295.)

This proposal is supported by the observation that when iNOS mRNA was selectively expressed in the liver of transgenic mice, LPS-induced liver injury was attenuated by more than 50%, and the rise in plasma TNF and IL-1β levels was reduced as a result of NF-κB inhibition by iNOS activity.[83]

One possible mechanism by which iNOS activity may attenuate liver injury is through the inhibition of apoptosis. Ou and coworkers confirmed that continuous infusion of nonspecific NOS inhibitors into the portal vein significantly reduced serum AST and ALT levels and attenuated hepatic neutrophil infiltration 16 hours after LPS injection.[84] By comparison, selective iNOS inhibition with L-N-(1-iminoethyl)lysine did not alter AST and ALT levels or leukocyte infiltration; rather, it induced apoptosis of hepatocytes and endothelial cells, suggesting that hepatic iNOS activity may play an important antiapoptotic role. In summary, the contradictory conclusions regarding the role of iNOS in inflammation-induced liver injury are likely due to differences in the degree of liver damage, the rate of NO production, iNOS cellular localization, and the redox status of hepatic cells in various models of sepsis. Moreover, differences in the type, isoform selectivity, dosage, route, and timing of administration of NOS inhibitors should be taken into consideration when the role of iNOS is evaluated.

ANNOTATED REFERENCES

Aulak KS, Miyagi M, Yan L, et al: Proteomic method identifies proteins nitrated in vivo during inflammatory challenge. Proc Natl Acad Sci U S A 2001;98:12056-12061.

A proteomic approach was used for the first time to identify tyrosine-nitrated proteins in the lung and liver of septic animals. This study showed that nitration of tyrosine residues occurs in a wide variety of proteins, including glycolytic enzymes, protein involved in the regulation of apoptosis, and several important mitochondrial enzymes.

Furchgott RF, Zawadzki JW: The obligatory rule of endothelial cells in the relaxation of vascular smooth muscle by acetylcholine. Nature 1980;286:373-376.

This landmark study described the presence of endothelium-derived relaxing factor (EDRF), which is an important regulator of smooth muscle relaxation. In 1998, the first author was awarded the Nobel Prize for medicine for his discovery that EDRF is actually NO.

Jaffrey SR, Snyder SH: PIN: An associated protein inhibitor of neuronal nitric oxide synthase. Science 1996;274:774-777.

Protein inhibitor of nNOS (PIN), a subunit of the molecular motor dynein, was found to inhibit the activity of nNOS by preventing the dimerization of NOS monomers. The existence and tissue distribution of PIN were described for the first time.

Kilbourn RG, Gross SS, Adams J, et al: L-N^G-Methylarginine inhibits tumor necrosis factor–induced hypotension: Implications for the involvement of nitric oxide. Proc Natl Acad Sci U S A 1990;87:3629-3632.

This was one of the earliest studies to suggest that excessive NO production contributes to sepsis-induced hypotension. The authors found that infusion of TNF in dogs elicits systemic hypotension and that treatment with the NOS inhibitor L-NG-methylarginine reverses it.

Petros AJ, Bennett D, Vallance P: Effect of nitric oxide synthase inhibitors on hypotension in patients with septic shock. Lancet 1991;338:1557-1558.

The effect of NOS inhibition on the hemodynamics of patients with septic shock was described for the first time. In two septic patients whose blood pressure could not be restored by conventional therapy, administration of NG-monomethyl-l-arginine resulted in significant increases in blood pressure and systemic vascular resistance.

Chapter 43

CARBON MONOXIDE AND HEME OXYGENASE-1

Augustine M. K. Choi • Jigme Sethi

KEY POINTS

1. Heme oxygenase-1 (HO-1) is a unique enzyme with **dual roles in the cell—heme catabolism** and potent **cytoprotection**—and with antioxidant, antiapoptotic, antiproliferative, and anti-inflammatory activities.

2. HO-1 is **vigorously induced by** hypoxia, hyperoxia, heat shock, and a plethora of **oxidative and inflammatory stimuli**.

3. Increased activity of **HO-1** has been demonstrated to be **strongly protective** in a variety of models of oxidative stress and inflammation, including **acute lung injury, acute liver injury, acute renal failure, and cardiac xenotransplantation**.

4. All the **byproducts** of the reaction catalyzed by HO-1 (ferritin, carbon monoxide) **have major antioxidant and cytoprotective properties**.

5. **Carbon monoxide** has vasodilatory and bronchodilatory properties, functions as a neurotransmitter, and inhibits platelet and monocyte activation. It also demonstrates the cytoprotective properties attributed to HO-1 and **may be the major effector of the beneficial effects of HO-1 induction**.

6. **Carbon monoxide binds to heme proteins** such as **cytochrome P$_{450}$**, which it inactivates, and **soluble guanylate cyclase**, which it activates, thus modulating cellular function.

7. **Carbon monoxide** also **can modulate signaling through the mitogen-activated protein kinase pathways,** thereby down-regulating inflammation.

8. **These beneficial effects of exogenous inhaled carbon monoxide** are noted at doses that are only a fraction of toxic levels—as low as 100 to 250 parts per million.

HISTORICAL PERSPECTIVE

Humans, like other obligate aerobes, are dependent on oxygen as the "molecule of life," but at a price—the potential for oxidative damage caused by free oxygen radicals. The introduction of molecular oxygen into the atmosphere forced adaptive changes in all existing forms of life, specifically to guard against oxidative damage. One such adaptation was the chelation of free iron, another essential molecule, into

protoporphyrin complexes to prevent precipitation of the relatively insoluble oxidized ferric iron and the generation of toxic oxidant radicals by the reduction of ferric to ferrous iron. Recycling this sequestered iron between substrates in numerous biologic processes required the controlled catabolism of these protoporphyrin-iron, or heme, moieties. Thus it was no surprise when Tenhunen and associates identified heme oxygenase (HO) as the enzyme responsible for this reaction.[1] This enzyme uses the reduced form of nicotinamide adenine dinucleotide phosphate (NADPH) and three molecules of oxygen to cleave the alpha-methenyl bridges between pyrroles I and II of the heme porphyrin ring, producing biliverdin and liberating free iron and carbon monoxide (CO) in equimolar amounts (Fig. 43-1).[2] The free iron thus released is liberated for the synthesis of other iron-containing proteins or sequestered for transport or storage in transferrin or apoferritin, respectively. Understandably, initial research focused on this important but less than exciting role of HO in heme catabolism, until Applegate and colleagues showed that HO could be vigorously induced not just by its substrate heme but also by a variety of agents that shared the ability to generate reactive oxygen species (ROS) in the cell.[3] Examples of such agents are lipopolysaccharide (LPS), phorbol esters, sodium arsenite, sulfhydryl reagents, hydrogen peroxide, and heavy metals, as well as hyperthermia, hyperoxia, heat shock, and ultraviolet radiation. This extraordinary diversity of inducers for an enzyme that seemingly functioned only in heme turnover was very surprising and fueled speculation that it also served a powerful role in protecting the cell against oxidative stress. The seminal observation, by Nath and coworkers in 1992,[4] that prior induction of HO could protect rats from renal failure caused by glycerol-induced rhabdomyolysis triggered a wave of research into the role of HO in oxidant-mediated cellular and tissue injury. This enzyme has now been firmly established as a crucial and potent cytoprotective molecule with strong anti-inflammatory, antiapoptotic, and antiproliferative properties. Just how remarkable this enzyme really is, is evident from its ubiquitous distribution in nature, not merely in mammalian and lower eukaryotic systems but also in plants, algae, fungi, and bacteria. It has been extraordinarily conserved through evolution, with approximately 80% identity between rat and human HO isoforms and nearly 70% homology between human HO-1 and that derived from the pathogen *Corynebacterium diphtheriae*.[5] Not surprisingly, targeted deletions of the HO-1 gene in mice result in HO-1 null mice that usually do not survive to term.[6] No known mutant forms of HO have been discovered, despite the near universal distribution of this enzyme in nature.

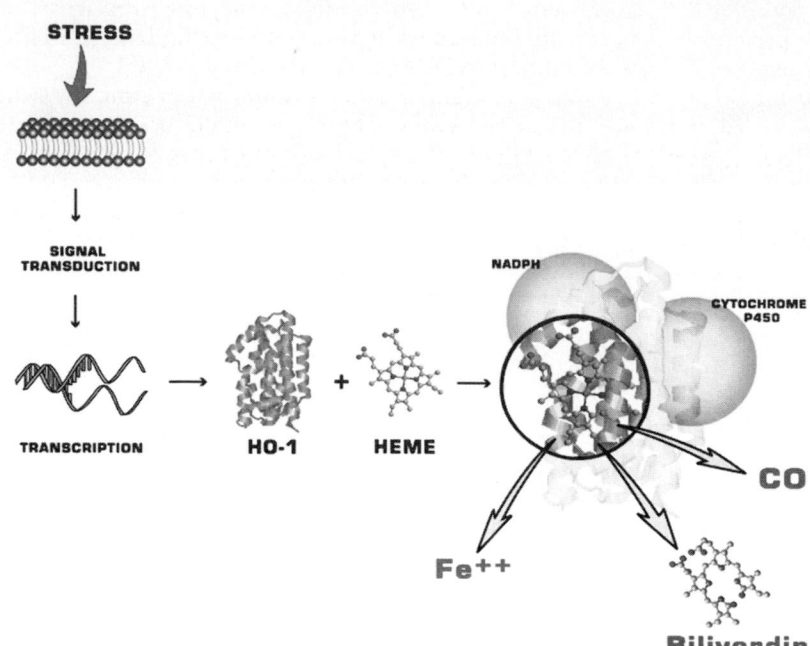

FIGURE 43–1. Reaction catalyzed by heme oxygenase-1. (See color section in this text.) (From Otterbein LE, et al: Heme oxygenase-1: Unleashing the protective properties of heme. Trends Immunol 2003;24:449-455.)

ENZYME STRUCTURE AND FUNCTION

Crystal analyses of the HO structure reveal the heme pocket to be sandwiched between two helices—the proximal and distal helices; histidine residues at positions 25 and 132 are critical for heme binding to each of these helices, respectively (Fig. 43-2).[7] The distal helix is most closely associated with heme and has the highest sequence identity between HO proteins derived from various species. Laboratory mutations that distort the structure of the distal helix decrease the efficiency of catalysis,[7] indicating that the distal helix might serve as a fingerprint motif for the HO proteins. There are several unique aspects of the HO protein that further its physiologic role. First, HO has an affinity for oxygen that is 30 to 90 times that of myoglobin, ensuring a steady supply of oxygen for substrate catalysis.[8] Second, the bound heme serves both as a cofactor for the enzyme and as its substrate.[9]

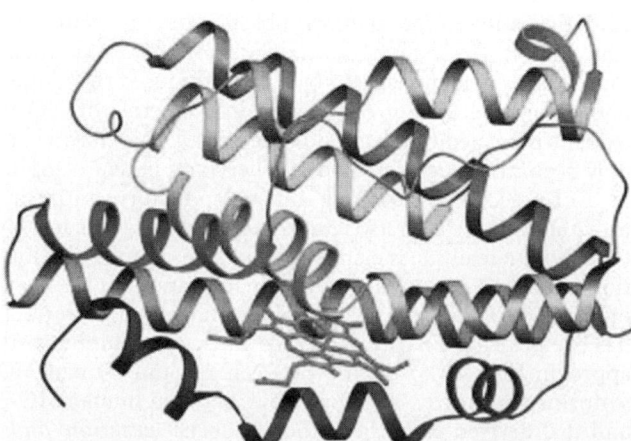

FIGURE 43–2. Structure of human heme oxygenase-1. The N-terminus is blue and the C-terminus is red, with green in the middle. The position of the heme ring is shown in pink. (See color section in this text.) (From Schuller DJ, et al: Crystal structure of human heme oxygenase-1. Nat Struct Biol 1999;6:860-867.)

Third, HO-1 is devoid of cysteine residues, making it insensitive to inactivation by reactive nitrogen and oxygen species, a critical property for a protein that serves as an antioxidant defense.

GENE STRUCTURE AND REGULATION

There are three distinct isoforms of human HO, coded for by three distinct genes.[10,11] HO-1 (inducible) and HO-2 (constitutively expressed) share 42% identical residues; HO-3 is 90% homologous with HO-2 but is not known to be functional.[11] HO-1 is widely distributed throughout the body; HO-2 is highly concentrated in the brain and testes; and HO-3 is localized to the prostate, liver, and kidney. Whereas HO-1 is induced to serve a protective role in pathophysiologic states, HO-2 may have a more routine physiologic function, such as control of blood pressure or neurotransmission (see later).[12]

The structure of the mouse HO-1 gene is best characterized, and the deduced amino acid sequence of mouse HO-1 exhibits 93.4% and 82.3% homology with rat and human sequences, respectively. It has five exons, the relative positions of which are similar in all three species.

Heme-dependent stimulation of HO activity can be inhibited by prior treatment with the RNA synthesis inhibitor actinomycin D, suggesting that enzymatic activation is regulated at the level of gene transcription.[13] This appears to be true not just for heme but for most other inducing agents as well, although it has been suggested that increased expression of HO-1 by nitric oxide may, in part, be due to increased HO-1 messenger RNA (mRNA) stability.[14] This increased stability has also been invoked as the mechanism for hypoxic induction of HO-1 in human skin fibroblasts.[15] The *cis*-acting DNA elements of the gene that interact with their cognate-inducing proteins are becoming better understood through experiments that mutate the potential binding sites and observe the effects on the induction of the HO-1 protein by various inducers. In the case of the mouse gene, the regulatory elements in the 5′ flanking region are arranged into three distinct areas: the proximal promoter region and two distal enhancers, DE 1 and 2, located 4 and 10 kilobase pairs upstream of the transcription initiation site, respectively.[16,17]

Although the promoter region has motifs that are variations of well-known transcription factor binding sites, the functionality of these transcription binding sites is not clearly understood.[18] However, the human gene promoter region, but not that of the mouse or rat, has a $(GT)_n$ repeat that is highly polymorphic, called a microsatellite polymorphism, with n varying from 15 to 40. These repeats may serve to modulate promoter activity or induction. In fact, promoter activity may decrease with increasing n.[19] Cigarette smokers with long repeats ($n > 31$) have a greater risk of developing emphysema than do those with shorter repeats ($n < 31$), perhaps because reduced HO-1 expression may be unable to protect against the oxidative stress of smoking.[19]

The dominant functional sequence motif in the enhancers is the stress response element (StRE). It is 10 base pairs in length; occurs repeatedly in the two distal enhancers; and, at least in the mouse, is required for the induction of HO-1 by all agents tested, except for hypoxia. In particular, induction by heme requires the entire 10 base pairs of the StRE.[20] Most likely, the DNA binding transcription factors v-Maf, NF-E2, and Nrf 1 and 2 are all involved in mediating the response to heme.[21] To respond to hypoxia, however, the hypoxia-inducible factor (HIF-1) that activates transcription of erythropoietin and vascular endothelial growth factor must bind to distinct hypoxia response elements that reside in DE 2.[22]

The first three residues of the StRE are the antioxidant-electrophile response elements, necessary for induction by oxidants and electrophiles.[23] The StRE also contains the heptad that recognizes the fos/jun (activator protein-1 [AP-1]) family of DNA-binding, transcription-activating proteins. Mutation of this site results in loss of activation by heavy metals, hydrogen peroxide, arsenite, and LPS.[17,24] Many potent antioxidant chemicals, including pyrrolidine dithiocarbamate and diphenylene iodonium, also activate HO-1 by activating AP-1 binding.[25] Another pathway of HO-1 activation during oxidative stress involves thioredoxin, a protein that keeps disulfide bonds in the reduced state, protecting intracellular proteins against oxidation.[26] Thioredoxin is induced by oxidative stress, translocates into the nucleus, and binds to intranuclear redox factor 1, which in turn reduces and activates the DNA binding activity of AP-1. This can lead to HO-1 induction.[27]

A unique situation pertains to the activation of HO-1 by interleukin (IL)-6 or interferon, both of which use the JAK-STAT pathway to induce gene transcription. When IL-6 binds to a surface receptor, a JAK factor is activated, which in turn phosphorylates and dimerizes a STAT factor, which then binds to the IL-6 response element in the PE locus of the mouse HO-1 gene.[28] In some unknown manner, a protein bound to the StREs located 4 kilobase pairs away is also needed for IL-6 induction of HO-1.[29] The mechanism of this "cooperativity" is not fully understood.

Hyperoxia also strongly induces HO-1 via the IL-6 response element.[30] Because IL-6 mRNA is induced by hyperoxia in 4 to 8 hours, well before the peak induction of HO-1 at 24 to 48 hours, it may simply be that IL-6 acts on the IL-6 response element to induce HO-1. However, both c-jun and c-fos, components of the AP-1 transcription factor, are induced by hyperoxia and could directly induce STAT binding to DNA via this site.

When organisms are exposed to hyperthermia or heat shock, a specific family of heat shock proteins is induced that confers cytoprotection against the oxidative and inflammatory stress resulting from hyperthermia. HO-1 is also known as heat shock protein 32, because it is involved in the heat shock response. Although the rat HO-1 gene is induced by heat shock, mediated by two heat shock elements in the PE region, human HO-1 heat shock induction is observed only in HeLa cells, skin fibroblasts, and the Hep3B hepatoma cell line. This is because the single heat shock element in the human HO-1 gene is constitutively repressed in vivo by a flanking sequence and the silencing action of $(GT)_n$ repeats.[31] A similar phenomenon of HO-1 repression has been demonstrated in cultured human astrocytes and coronary artery endothelial cells in response to hypoxia,[32] the significance of which is unknown. It has been suggested, however, that hypoxic repression of HO-1 may benefit some hypoxic cell types by conserving energy (given the high utilization of molecular oxygen by this enzyme), thereby protecting mitochondrial cytochrome oxidase against inhibition by CO.[33]

HO-1 AND CELLULAR PROTECTION

ANTIOXIDANT PROPERTIES

The realization that the wide variety of inducers of HO-1 all serve to generate oxidant stress led investigators to explore the potential beneficial effects of HO-1 induction in disease models characterized by overwhelming oxidant injury. One such condition, acute lung injury, involves widespread inflammatory damage to the alveoli of the lung caused by infectious pathogens, inhaled environmental toxins, trauma to nonpulmonary organs, blood transfusions, noxious gases, near drowning, or drug exposure. It is well known that many injurious agents, such as LPS derived from Gram-negative bacteria; drugs, such as bleomycin; exposure to 100% oxygen; or even host-derived tumor necrosis factor (TNF) all lead to the generation of ROS, generated from the oxidative burst of infiltrating inflammatory cells. These ROS are thought to initiate the damage to the alveolar epithelium in acute lung injury. Similarly, acute renal failure can result from many different insults, including glycerol-induced acute rhabdomyolysis, in which free heme is the nephrotoxic agent, or exposure to the nephrotoxic agent cisplatin. Again, ROS mediate the extensive tissue injury that occurs in this condition. Not surprisingly, HO-1 is intensely up-regulated in inflamed tissues in both these conditions.

Acute Lung Injury

Rats exposed to greater than 95% oxygen or sublethal injections of LPS develop acute lung injury that is remarkably similar to the human disease. Lung edema and particularly pleural effusions develop within 48 to 60 hours of exposure to greater than 95% oxygen, and rats uniformly die after 60 to 72 hours of continuous exposure. Intraperitoneal injections of LPS stimulate intense neutrophilic infiltration of the alveoli, together with hemorrhagic edema. Increased immunohistochemical staining for HO-1 protein is seen diffusely throughout the alveolar and bronchiolar epithelium and the infiltrating cells, accompanied by marked increases in HO-1 activity in the lung homogenates.[24,34]

The functional significance of this induction of HO-1 has been elucidated by experiments in which rats were pretreated with inhibitors of HO-1 activity. Pretreatment with tin protoporphyrin (SnPP) abrogated the induction of lung HO-1 in LPS-treated rats and increased susceptibility to a lethal dose of LPS; conversely, pretreatment with hemoglobin (a potent inducer of HO-1) conferred marked protection against neutrophilic alveolitis and hemorrhagic edema resulting from sublethal doses of LPS.[35] When an adenoviral vector containing the coding region of the HO-1 gene was instilled into rat lungs, it was taken up by the bronchiolar epithelium and resulted in increased protein expression of HO-1 in this region. These rats, when subsequently exposed to hyperoxia, exhibited a greater than 90% reduction in pleural effusions and survived longer than their control counterparts, which had received instillations of the adenoviral vector without the HO-1 gene insert.[36]

Acute Renal Failure

In models of acute renal failure, increased HO-1 mRNA and protein expression are noted along the tubules,[4,37] whereas in acute renal transplant rejection, the staining is localized to the infiltrating inflammatory cells.[38] As with acute lung injury, pretreatment with SnPP led to increased renal injury and death in rats undergoing rhabdomyolysis-initiated, heme-mediated acute renal failure, whereas prior treatment with hemoglobin unequivocally reduced mortality and renal damage in the same model.[4] A similar result was seen in cisplatin-induced acute renal injury,[37] implying that the benefit of HO-1 induction goes beyond protection against heme-induced injury alone.

These fundamental observations of the beneficial effects of HO-1 induction in states of oxidant injury have been extended with the availability of the HO-1[−/−] knockout mouse. (Normally, HO-1 knockout mice die in utero, so in vitro fertilization techniques were used to salvage the homozygous knockout mice.) As expected, fibroblasts derived from these mice were more sensitive to oxidant injury, and the mice exhibited increased mortality and increased liver damage resulting from LPS administration.[39] In the model of glycerol-induced rhabdomyolysis and acute renal failure, knockout mice demonstrated 100% mortality and increased tubular injury compared with their wild-type controls.[40] Similarly, administration of cisplatin to HO-1[−/−] mice resulted in more severe nephron damage than that seen in HO-1[+/+] mice.[41]

Acute Liver Injury

There is a unique topographic distribution of HO in the liver: HO-1 is prominent in Kupffer cells, and HO-2 predominates in hepatocytes.[42] This could explain the ability of HO-1, via CO, to regulate both biliary flow[43] and sinusoidal pressure (see later). Once again, it appears that ischemic stress, which liberates oxidant radicals, can be ameliorated by the induction of HO-1. Partial ligation of the portal vein in rats with portal hypertension strongly induced HO-1 in the liver.[44] Mice deficient in HO-1 demonstrated increased susceptibility to injury by endotoxin,[6] and in a model of compensated hemorrhagic shock, blockade of HO-1 was shown to increase centrilobular necrosis.[45]

Effects in the Brain

Mice lacking the HO-2 gene suffer a larger brain infarct than do controls after temporary occlusion of the middle cerebral artery, but this effect is not seen with deletion of HO-1.[46]

Inhibition of HO with SnPP increases the size of the infarct in wild-type mice, again suggesting a role for HO-2 in cerebral protection against transient ischemia.[47] HO protects neurons from hydrogen peroxide–mediated injury and limits neuronal apoptosis in cell culture, indicating the potential to limit neuronal cell death in the ischemic penumbra.[47]

Oxidative stress plays a central role in the pathogenesis of Alzheimer's disease and Parkinson's disease. HO-1 protein is greatly increased in the senile plaques and neurofibrillary tangles that are characteristic of Alzheimer's disease.[48] *Tau* protein, which forms the neurofibrillary tangles, is greatly reduced in cells that overexpress HO-1.[49] Amyloid precursor protein, which is believed to be the neurotoxic agent in Alzheimer's disease, may bind to and inhibit HO, leading to more oxidative neurotoxicity,[50] but HO-1 induction can reduce both the protein and the cytotoxicity from hydrogen peroxide in neuronal cells.[51] It appears that subjects who develop Alzheimer's disease have lower levels of protective HO-1 in plasma and cerebrospinal fluid and lower lymphocyte HO-1 mRNA than do healthy elderly controls.[52] HO-1 immunoreactivity is also enhanced in the substantia nigra of patients with Parkinson's disease[48] and even in mouse brains infected with the scrapie prion,[53] which induces HO-1.[54]

Atherosclerosis

HO-1 can be induced in both endothelial and vascular smooth muscle cells by proatherogenic stimuli, such as oxidized low-density lipoprotein (LDL), lipid metabolites, shear stress, and angiotension II, among others.[55] HO-1 is highly up-regulated in the endothelium and in the foam cells of intimal lesions from humans and apolipoprotein E–deficient mice.[56] The induction of HO-1 reduces atherosclerotic lesions in LDL receptor knockout mice.[57] HO-1 can also protect against atherosclerosis by producing CO, which is known to inhibit platelet aggregation.

Clearly, these observations implicate HO-1 as a potent antioxidant protein, but the beneficial effects of its induction seem to extend beyond this antioxidant role. Astonishingly, accumulating evidence suggests that this protein can also function in an antiapoptotic role, as a regulator of cell growth and proliferation, and as an anti-inflammatory agent; it may even modulate the immune system.

ANTIAPOPTOTIC PROPERTIES

Apoptosis, or programmed noninflammatory cell death, plays an important role in human disease. For example, in acute lung injury in both humans and rodents, soluble Fas ligand mediates the apoptotic cell death of distal airway epithelium, which expresses the receptor for this so-called death ligand. Soluble Fas ligand is present in the bronchoalveolar lavage fluid from humans with early acute lung injury, but not in those at risk for the development of this disease; high levels of this ligand are associated with increased mortality.[58] Overexpression of HO-1 has been shown to protect both cultured fibroblasts from TNF-induced apoptosis[59] and bovine aortic endothelial cells from peroxynitrite-mediated apoptotic cell death.[60] Exogenous transfer of adenoviral vector–encoded HO-1 into mouse lungs attenuates the degree of hyperoxia-induced lung cell apoptosis in vivo.[61]

Bleomycin, a chemotherapeutic agent, causes acute pulmonary inflammation in humans, but when given to mice, it results in lung fibrosis that is used as a model of the human disease idiopathic pulmonary fibrosis. Cellular apoptosis in the lung is a characteristic feature of this model, so a recent report that adenoviral-mediated overexpression of HO-1 in the lungs protected against pulmonary fibrosis caused by bleomycin is not surprising.[62]

CELL GROWTH AND PROLIFERATION

In vitro, HO-1 modulates cell growth. If pulmonary epithelial cells grown in culture are transfected with adenoviral vectors encoding the HO-1 gene, the resulting overexpression of HO-1 protein is associated with decreased cell proliferation, increased numbers of cells in the G_0/G_1 phase of the cell cycle, and reduced entry into the S phase, compared with cells transfected with the adenoviral vector alone, without the HO-1 insert. Cells that overexpress HO-1 are blocked in the G_2/M phase and are unable to progress through the cell cycle, despite serum stimulation. When SnPP is added, these effects are reversed, proving that growth arrest results from the actions of HO-1.[63] Similar growth slowing is seen in vascular smooth muscle cells transfected with HO-1,[64] and because pulmonary hypertension is associated with pronounced hypertrophy of smooth muscle in the media of the pulmonary arteries, this might well be the mechanism by which chemical preinduction of HO-1 protects rats against pulmonary hypertension from chronic hypoxia.[65] Transgenic mice overexpressing HO-1 in the lungs also develop less pulmonary hypertension in response to hypoxia.[66] HO-1 appears to regulate vascular remodeling in systemic vessels as well. In vivo, induction of HO-1 by hemin reduces neointimal thickness and medial wall thickness in the balloon-injured carotid arteries of rats.[67]

Not surprisingly, this antigrowth effect of HO-1 is applicable to tumor biology as well. A549 pulmonary epithelial cells injected into immunodeficient mice form tumors that grow rapidly. If, however, the cells are made to overexpress HO-1 before transfer to the mice, the tumors formed are half the size, and survival is improved by greater than 90%.[68] Expression of HO-1 in oral squamous cell carcinoma may be a marker for a low risk of regional lymph node metastases.[69]

THE IMMUNE SYSTEM

Increases in HO-1 protein are seen in alveolar macrophages obtained by sputum induction in humans with asthma, but not in healthy subjects.[70] In mice that develop an asthmatic phenotype brought about by prior sensitization and then challenge with inhaled ovalbumin aerosols, HO-1 induction in lung tissue can be readily demonstrated.[71] Higher HO-1 expression is seen in alveolar macrophages from humans who have acute or chronic graft rejection after lung allotransplantation, compared with those without overt rejection.[72] HO-1 is induced in the transplanted kidney after the development of acute rejection,[73] and adenoviral transfer of HO-1 dramatically protects rat liver transplants against rejection,[74] perhaps by modulating the T helper 1–T helper 2 cytokine balance.[75] HO-1 induction can protect islet cell transplants from apoptosis[76] and ameliorate the severity of graft-versus-host disease.[77] Dramatic proof of the immunomodulatory role of HO-1 comes from a mouse-to-rat cardiac xenotransplantation model.[78] Normally, mouse hearts survive indefinitely when they are transplanted under the skin of immunosuppressed rats, but pretreatment with SnPP to block HO-1 leads to rapid rejection. Transplantation of mouse hearts from HO-1$^{-/-}$ knockout mice also leads to rapid rejection. Together, these experiments prove that despite immunosuppression, HO-1 is necessary for xenograft survival.

ANTI-INFLAMMATORY EFFECTS

The mitogen-activated protein kinases (MAPKs) constitute hierarchic phosphorylation cascades responsible for transducing inflammatory signals from the cell surface to the nucleus, resulting in cellular activation and the production of cytokines that amplify inflammation. Thus, for example, when human neutrophils are stimulated by the peptide nFMLP, the ERK family of MAPKs transduces the inflammatory signals to the nucleus, resulting in a broad array of activation responses, including calcium influx, superoxide production, granule release, and chemotaxis. Similarly, LPS stimulates the p38 MAPK, resulting in TNF release. In vivo, selective chemical inhibition of p38 abrogates TNF release, and hence acute lung injury, in a rat model of pancreatitis-associated lung injury. Phosphorylation of the ERK 1/2 kinase cascade results in induction of the transcription factors AP-1 and nuclear factor kappa-B, both of which induce the expression adhesion molecules on endothelium and induce the production of IL-8 from endothelial cells.

HO-1 can modulate inflammation by changing signal transduction through the ubiquitous MAPK pathways. For example, HO-1 suppresses the phosphorylation of ERK 1/2 by TNF in rat pulmonary artery endothelial cells, providing a mechanism for the down-regulation of TNF-induced inflammation.[79] Stimulation of macrophages with LPS causes them to produce TNF, but if the macrophages are treated to overexpress HO-1 before stimulation with LPS, the production of TNF declines and the production of IL-10 (an anti-inflammatory cytokine) increases. Again, in a lethal endotoxic shock mouse model, the protective effects of IL-10 require the induction of HO-1.[80] On an organ system level, this translates to reduced inflammation and injury. For example, in a model of pleural inflammation, HO-1 up-regulation reduced inflammatory exudates and cellular infiltration, and these effects were reversed by HO-1 inhibition.[81] The protective effect of HO-1 in changing the T helper 1–T helper 2 balance in organ transplantation was alluded to earlier.

ISCHEMIA-REPERFUSION INJURY

HO-1 mRNA, protein, and activity are strongly induced in models of ischemia-reperfusion injury, both in the rat kidney[82] and in ischemic myocardium.[83] Preinduction of HO-1 can result in ischemic conditioning, ameliorating the injury caused by subsequent ischemia and reperfusion, as noted in guinea pig lung transplants[84] and in rats undergoing liver transplantation.[85]

MEDIATORS AND END PRODUCTS OF HO-1 INDUCTION

The heme moiety, despite being the cofactor for numerous enzymes and a critical component of hemoglobin, is highly toxic and can cause renal injury, as noted earlier. In addition, free heme is a potent pro-oxidant molecule, capable of oxidizing and damaging almost all the constituents of a cell, such as the lipid membranes, mitochondria, cytoskeleton, and even nucleus.[86] It would be reasonable to suppose that all the protective effects of HO-1 induction could be explained by the degradation of this toxic free heme moiety, but a closer look at the products of the enzymatic reaction catalyzed by HO-1 shows that they too may subserve antioxidant functions directly.

FERRITIN

Ferritin, which stores free iron, has been suggested to mediate the beneficial effects of HO-1. Ferrous iron, if left free in the cytoplasm, can donate an electron to hydrogen peroxide and thus generate, via the Fenton reaction, the highly reactive hydroxyl radical. Free iron can also stimulate lipid peroxidation. However, induction of HO-1 is associated with a simultaneous increase in ferritin, which immediately sequesters the free heme and thus resolves the paradox whereby an antioxidant protein such as HO-1 generates a potentially toxic free iron radical. For example, heme-mediated induction of HO-1 results in increased transcription of ferritin,[87] and in human skin fibroblasts, oxidative injury produced by ultraviolet radiation results in HO-1–dependent induction of ferritin and thereby protection from oxidative injury.[88] In addition, HO-1 can repress the expression of a highly active ferrous iron–adenosine triphosphatase transporter involved in iron efflux from cells.[89] This transporter is colocalized with HO-1 in the microsomal fraction of the cell, and it is notable that mice with a genomic deletion of HO-1 display increased tissue accumulation of iron. This coregulation of ferritin, the iron transporter, and HO-1 may partially explain the protective effects of HO-1 induction, but in an elegant experiment, Otterbein and colleagues provided evidence of additional mechanisms.[90] In their experiments, rats pretreated with both heme to induce HO-1 and with desferrioxamine to bind ferritin were fully protected against LPS-mediated lethal endotoxic shock; conversely, pretreatment of rats with inorganic iron alone, to induce ferritin but not HO-1, could not protect the animals against endotoxic shock. Exogenous apoferritin did not confer any protection in this model.[90]

CARBON MONOXIDE

A wealth of evidence now suggest that CO, the final byproduct of the heme catabolism pathway, is the main mediator of the cytoprotection exhibited by HO-1 induction. Sjostrand first discovered endogenous production of this gas in 1949,[91] 19 years before the discovery of HO itself. This gas was known to be a poison, with the initial description of CO poisoning attributed to Aristotle. In 1857, Bernard first noted its high affinity for hemoglobin. The toxicity of this gas in exogenously inhaled concentrations results from its ability to impair the oxygen-carrying capacity of hemoglobin in two ways. First, it binds to hemoglobin with an affinity 245 times that of oxygen (at pH 7.4), competitively inhibiting oxygen binding. Second, it causes an allosteric conformational change, from sigmoid to hyperbolic, in the hemoglobin molecule, such that the oxygen molecules bound to hemoglobin are less easily released, effectively left-shifting the hemoglobin dissociation curve and reducing tissue oxygen extraction from hemoglobin. It also binds to and inactivates the reduced form of cytochrome a_3, impairing tissue respiration.

CO is a colorless and odorless gas. Its solubility in water is about 30% less than that of oxygen (O_2). Given this low solubility and its high affinity for heme moieties, CO may be shuttled from heme moiety to moiety, based on the reaction constants within the different heme groups. Because O_2 also binds to heme moieties, it competes with these reactions; the relationship is defined in terms of the Warburg coefficient (K),

$$K = (n/1 - n) (CO/O_2),$$

where n is the fraction of heme moiety bound to CO. Thus, the Warburg coefficient is the ratio of the concentration of CO to that of O_2 required for 50% saturation of the heme compound (i.e., when n = 0.5). Because the Warburg coefficient is 0.4 for myoglobin, it follows that CO binds readily to myoglobin and that hemoglobin shuttles its CO content to myoglobin when the O_2 concentration in muscle drops to low levels during exercise.[92,93] In the case of cytochrome a_3, however, for which K ranges from 5 to 15, it does so only when present in high concentrations (estimated at >20%)[94] or in the presence of severe O_2 depletion (e.g., in the mitochondria of asphyxiated tissues). As excellently reviewed by Piantadosi,[95] CO *has* been shown to bind to cytochrome a, a_3 in vivo (e.g., in the brains of rats perfused with perfluorocarbons instead of blood, while exposed to CO).[96] Despite the fact that these ratios are defined from in vitro experiments, they help explain how a gas that is apparently toxic can be readily formed endogenously and how the reaction was retained through millions of years of evolution, without adverse effects to the organism.

CO is produced endogenously at a rate of about 0.42 ± 0.07 mL/h, or approximately 10 mL/day.[97] Nearly all the CO produced endogenously results from the catabolism of heme—about 85% from the erythron, and the remainder from nonhemoglobin heme. Minute amounts can be generated by NADPH- or iron ascorbate–dependent lipid peroxidation.[98] The cytochrome P_{450} system can metabolize dihalomethanes to CO in vivo,[99] which may be significant in cases of toxic inhalation of these compounds. The majority of CO produced in the body is excreted by exhalation, although, intriguingly, CO can also be oxidized to carbon dioxide by cytochrome a_3, the cellular target of CO.[100] The importance of this reaction as a pathway of elimination of CO from the body is unknown.

The first suggestion that CO could exert physiologic effects came in 1991, around the time that gaseous nitric oxide (NO) was recognized as a physiologic effector molecule.[101] Experiments in which exogenous CO has the same effects as up-regulation of HO-1, or in which CO can "rescue" the effects of HO-1 blockade, provide evidence for its role as a mediator of HO-1 cytoprotection. For example, pretreatment of rats with 250 parts per million (ppm) of CO protects against hyperoxia (Fig. 43-3) and LPS-induced injury in a manner comparable to overexpression of HO-1.[61] Likewise, CO inhibits lung cell apoptosis in hyperoxia-injured animals.[61] Exogenous CO in the same low doses can protect against TNF-induced apoptosis to the same extent as overexpression of HO-1.[59,102] In vitro, low-dose CO reduces TNF-induced ERK 1/2 phosphorylation in rat pulmonary artery endothelial cells in the same manner as does overexpression of HO-1.[79] In this system, p38 phosphorylation is increased by HO-1 overexpression and by CO, while the other MAPK pathway, JNK, is unaffected. This argues against these effects being the result of the general cellular toxicity of CO. Exposure of

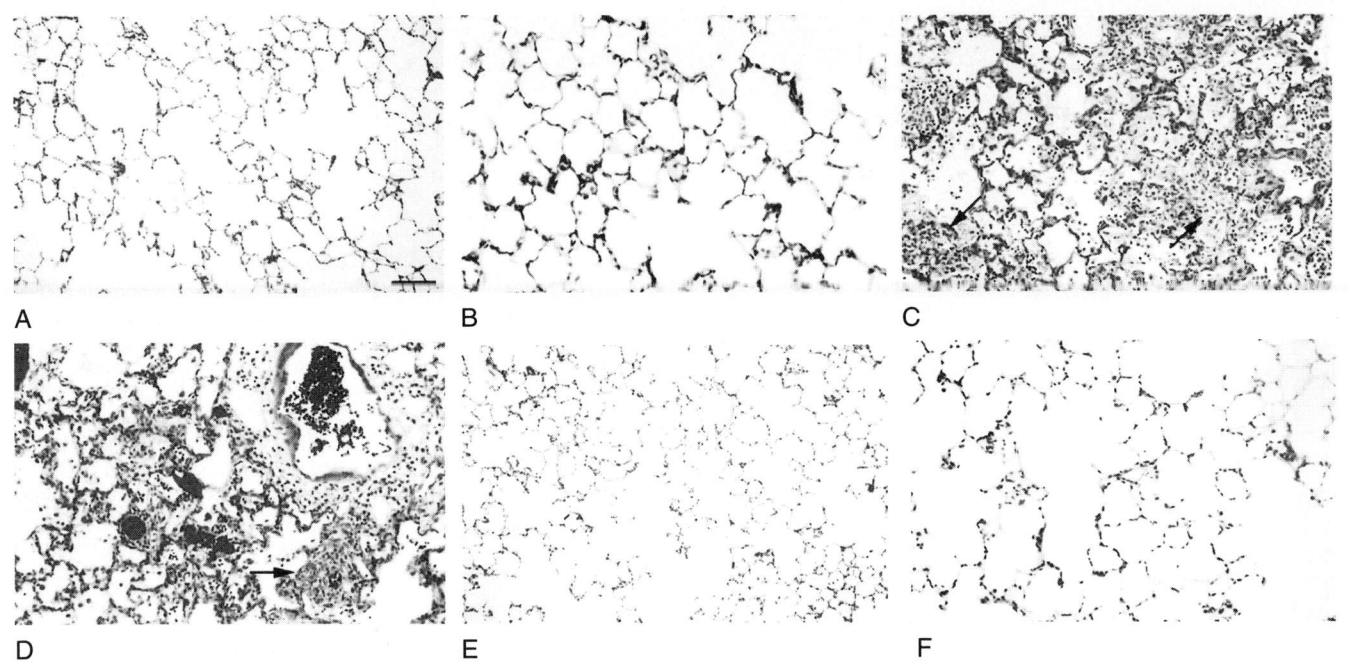

FIGURE 43–3. Protective effect of exogenous carbon monoxide (CO; 250 ppm) on hyperoxia-induced lung injury in rats. Histologic sections of rat lungs: *A*, normoxia control; *B*, CO control (256 ppm × 56 h); *C* and *D*, hyperoxia (× 56 h); *E* and *F*, hyperoxia (250 ppm CO × 56 h). (See color section in this text.) (From Otterbein LE, Mantell LL, Choi AM: Carbon monoxide provides protection against hyperoxic lung injury. Am J Physiol 1999;276:L688-L694.)

LPS-stimulated macrophages to low-dose CO results in the same constellation of reduced TNF generation and enhanced IL-10 production as seen with overexpression of HO-1 in these cells.[103] Low-dose CO retards the growth of tumors in vivo, just as is noted with HO-1 overexpression in A549 tumor cells injected into mice.[68] In mice sensitized and then challenged with aeroallergen, inhaled CO can selectively reduce the production of the eosinophil chemoattractant IL-5 and, consequently, eosinophil accumulation in the lung.[104] In the mouse-to-rat cardiac xenotransplantation model described earlier, treatment of both donor and recipient with exogenous CO results in indefinite survival of the xenotransplant, even in the face of inhibition of HO-1 by SnPP, exemplifying the ability of CO to substitute for HO-1.[105] Similar to the effects of HO-1 induction in preventing neointimal hyperplasia after balloon injury in rat carotid arteries, inhalation of low-dose CO for just 1 hour also virtually ablates neointimal hyperplasia (Fig. 43-4).[106]

Clearly, CO must be a major effector of the protection imparted by HO-1 induction. Nevertheless, CO has other physiologic roles of its own that might protect the body in a variety of disease states.

Vasodilator. Exogenous CO in high concentrations (10%) causes a reversible increase in coronary blood flow in isolated perfused rat hearts.[107] Although this may be an effect of hypoxia rather than a physiologic effect of CO, direct relaxation of vascular smooth muscle by CO has been shown in isolated porcine coronary arteries and veins[108] and in rabbit[109] and rat[110] aortas. In isolated perfused rat livers, inhibition of HO activity increased hepatic vascular resistance, but this effect was reversed by exogenous low-dose CO (1 µM).[111] CO generated by the induction of HO-1 lowers blood pressure in spontaneously hypertensive rats,[112] whereas inhibition of HO-1 raises blood pressure and total peripheral resistance in rats.[113] In the kidney, CO can attenuate the effect of vasoconstrictors on renal arterioles, and CO can reverse phenylephrine-induced vasoconstriction in

rat tail arteries.[114] Some of the vasodilator effects of CO may be mediated centrally, through the nucleus tractus solitarius.

Bronchodilator. Exogenous CO can reverse the bronchoconstriction due to histamine in anesthetized, ventilated guinea pigs, albeit at a high concentration (100%).[115] Inhibition of HO-1 with ZnPP also inhibits hypoxia-associated bronchoconstriction in vivo.[116] Recently, even low-dose exogenous CO has been shown to reverse the bronchoconstriction produced by methacholine in ventilated mice[117] and in guinea pig tracheal muscle ex vivo.[118]

Inhibitor of Platelet Function. CO inhibits the activation and aggregation responses of platelets,[119] which might explain the cardioprotective effect of CO in the mouse-to-rat xenotransplant described earlier. The surviving transplants had markedly reduced vascular thromboses.[105]

Neurotransmitter. In the myenteric plexus of the intestine, CO exhibits effects identical to those of NO, another gas molecule that functions as a neurotransmitter. Intestines of HO-2–deficient mice have impaired relaxation, and HO inhibitors cause intestinal contractions in NO synthase–deficient mice.[120] In the brain, intraventricular injection of HO inhibitors blocks the production of adrenocorticotropic hormone in response to electroshock; this action appears to be localized to the brain, not the pituitary.[121] There is evidence too that CO functions in long-term potentiation in the hippocampus,[122,123] and chemical inhibition of HO-1 activity can block glutamate receptor activation in the rat nucleus tractus solitarius.[124] In endotoxin-induced injury, CO inhibits the release of vasopressin.[125] CO regulates the nerve output of the carotid body, suppressing sensory discharge under basal conditions. During hypoxia, sensory discharge from the carotid body increases because of reduced CO generation.[126] Taken together, these effects are remarkably similar to those of the other diatomic gaseous neurotransmitter, NO.

Mechanism of Action. In the body, CO undergoes two types of reactions that have special significance (Fig. 43-5).

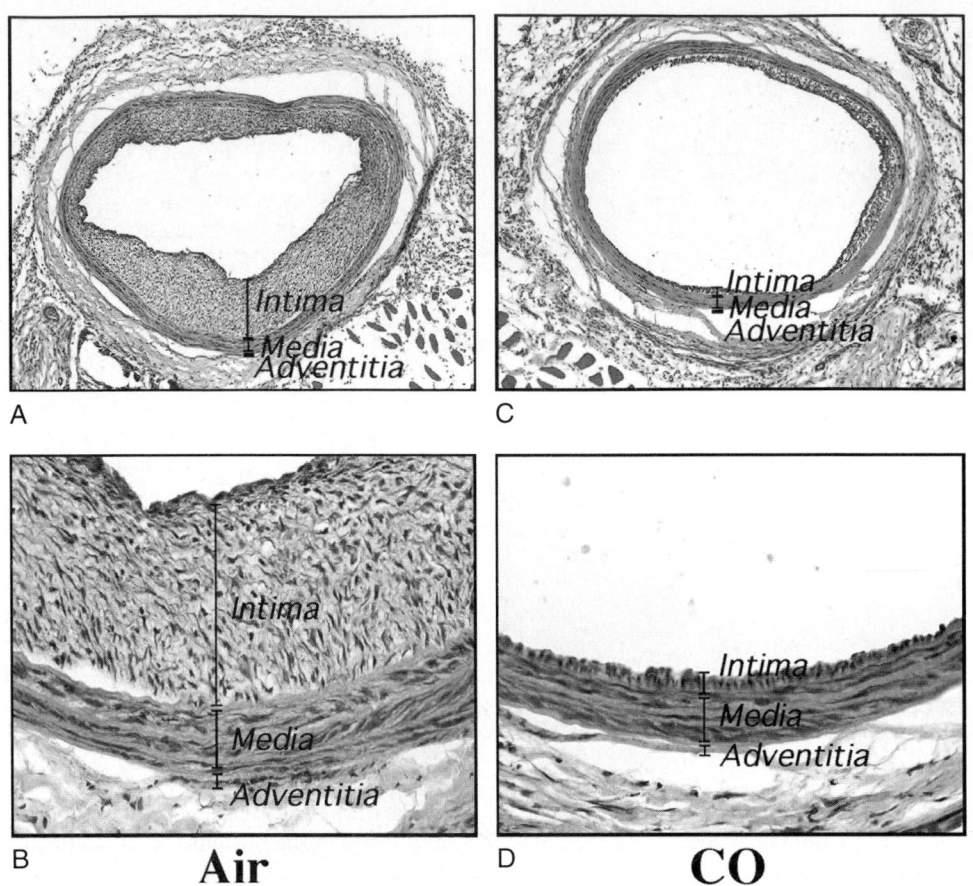

FIGURE 43–4. Pretreatment with exogenous carbon monoxide (CO; 250 ppm) greatly reduces the intimal proliferation after balloon injury in rat arteries. Rats were exposed to air (A and B) or exogenous CO for 1 h (C and D). Magnification is ×10 in the upper panels (A and C) and ×50 in the lower panels (B and D). (From Otterbein LE, Zuckerbraun BS, Haga M, et al: Carbon monoxide suppresses arteriosclerotic lesions associated with chronic graft rejection and with balloon injury. Nat Med 2003;9: 183-190.)

There are undoubtedly other reactions that may account for some of the biologic properties of CO, but these are not yet well delineated.

First, CO readily reacts with transitional metals to form metal carbonyls, and these may act as stores of CO in the body. Under some conditions, such as exposure to light, interaction with other ligands, or interaction with molecular oxygen, these metal carbonyls may gradually release CO. Motterlini and coworkers recently demonstrated the ability of synthetic metal carbonyls to deliver CO in vivo, and the actions of these chemicals mimic those of endogenously produced CO.[127]

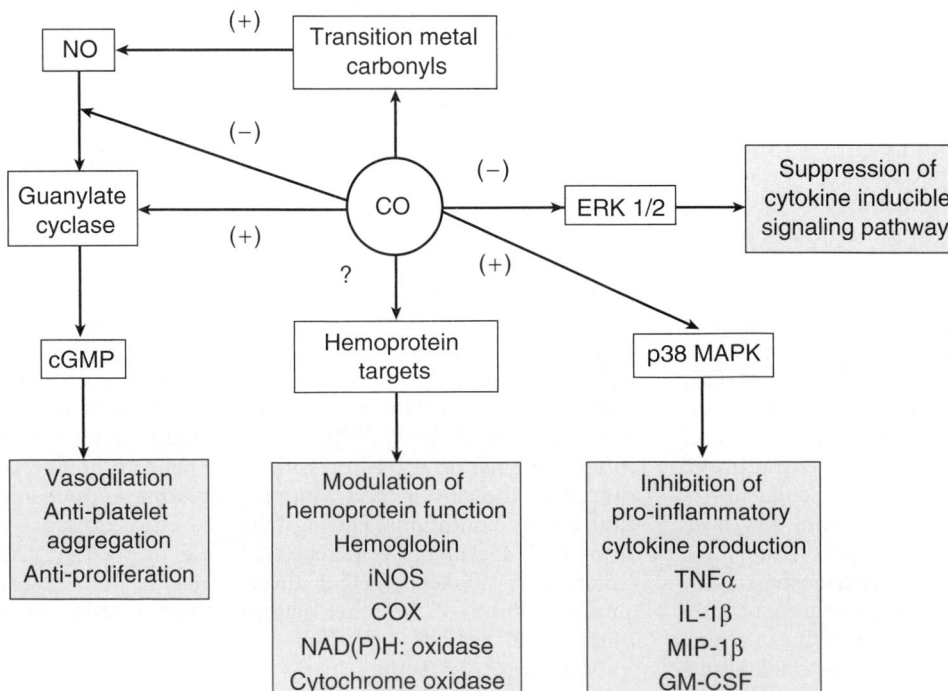

FIGURE 43–5. Mechanism of action of carbon monoxide (CO). cGMP, cyclic guanosine monophosphate; COX, cyclooxygenase; GM-CSF, granulocyte-macrophage colony-stimulating factor; IL, interleukin; iNOS, inducible nitric oxide synthase; MAPK, mitogen-activated protein kinase; NO, nitric oxide; TNF, tumor necrosis factor. (Adapted from Slebos DJ, Ryter SW, Choi AMK: Heme oxygenase-1 and carbon monoxide in pulmonary medicine. Respir Res 2003;4:7.)

Second, CO binds to the ferrous heme moieties of hemo-proteins but does not bind to ferric heme, unlike NO, which binds in both redox configurations. NO has an extremely high affinity for ferrous heme in comparison to CO, but the dissociation constant for CO bound to ferrous heme is much longer than that for NO,[128] resulting in the gradual dissociation of NO from ferrous hemoproteins in the presence of CO.[129] Thus, CO could exert some of its effects indirectly, through NO. Such effects have been described in the endothelium. For example, nitrotyrosine levels (the "footprint" or "signa-ture" of NO release) increase in aortic endothelium within 1 hour of ventilating rats with 50 ppm of CO,[129] and cultured endothelial cells release peroxynitrite upon exposure to 100 ppm of CO.[130]

The binding of CO to the hemoprotein cytochrome P_{450} (Warburg coefficient = 1) inactivates the enzyme, decreasing the metabolism of drugs such as barbiturates. Inactivation of cytochrome P_{450}–dependent synthesis of endogenous vaso-constrictors has been proposed to explain the vasodilatation induced by CO, but it is unclear whether oxygen concentra-tions are low enough in organs such as the liver to allow such reactions to proceed physiologically.

The binding of CO to the heme moiety of soluble guanylate cyclase (sGC), and the consequent activation of sGC, is a major mechanism by which CO exerts many biologic effects. The effects of CO on platelets and neutrophils, and the vasodilating effects of CO described earlier, are all mediated by sGC and can be abrogated by chemical inhibition of sGC. In the brain, HO-1 and HO-2 are colocalized with sGC, sug-gesting that many of the putative neurotransmitter effects of CO are also sGC mediated. CO exerts these effects even though it is, at best, a weak activator of sGC and produces a minimum of the conformational change that activates sGC, at least in comparison to the tremendously more potent NO. Curiously, a synthetic compound, YC-1, has been discovered that increases the activation of sGC by CO by an astounding 4000%, secondary to stabilization of the conformational change that accompanies sGC activation.[131] Similar endoge-nous compounds may bring about more marked activation of sGC by CO than is seen in vitro.

Another interesting feature of the relatively weak interac-tion between CO and sGC explains how CO can either facil-itate or antagonize the activation of sGC by NO. In the absence of NO, CO would activate sGC. Low concentrations of CO bound to sGC might actually inhibit NO binding and thereby inhibit activation of sGC by NO. In high concentra-tions, it is possible that CO would act much like an NO and amplify the effect of NO on sGC activation. For example, transgenic mice that have HO-1 overexpression targeted specifically to the endothelium actually show a significant increase in blood pressure, and aortic rings from these mice demonstrate impaired vasodilatation in response to NO, despite intact sGC activity. Because nitrovasodilatory activity is restored by the inhibition of CO, it appears that, in this context, CO is acting as a partial antagonist of NO.[132] This concentration-dependent ability of CO to function as a poten-tiator or partial inhibitor of NO-mediated sGC activation has been demonstrated in vitro.[133]

Not all the biologic activity of CO can be attributed to hemoprotein binding, however. The effect of exogenous low dose CO on the MAPKs is not mediated by sGC, and the kinases do not have heme groups. The TNF-mediated ERK 1/2 phosphorylation in rat pulmonary artery endothelial cells, described earlier, is also inhibited by n-acetylcysteine, a scavenger of oxidant species, suggesting that CO can exert indirect effects on the MAPK system by reducing free radical generation.[79] Similarly, CO can block vasoconstriction in rat tail arteries by both stimulating sGC and increasing the open probability of large-conductance, calcium-activated potassium channels.[114] Piglet pial arterioles vasodilate in response to infusions of heme, which stimulate HO-1 and lead to the local production of CO. These effects are blocked by HO-1 inhibition, as well as by blockade of the calcium-activated potassium channels described earlier. It is postulated that there is an interaction between CO and the histidine residues of the channel.[134]

CONCLUSION

Heme oxygenase's rise to fame—from a lowly enzyme serving to "recycle" hemoglobin to one of the most powerful cyto-protective proteins in nature—makes for fascinating reading. Equally exciting is the saga of carbon monoxide, as investi-gators around the world struggle to rehabilitate its image from poisonous gas to astoundingly multifunctional physiologic mediator. But these two biologic entities also underline how the relentless process of scientific discovery can overturn entrenched paradigms. HO was discovered in 1968, but it took another 23 years for its role beyond heme catabolism to be uncovered. And if not for the discovery of the remarkable physiologic role of NO, research into CO may have been stalled by those convinced only of its poisonous properties.

Although knowledge of the physiologic role of this HO-1–CO system is burgeoning, some experiments suggest that much more research is required before it can be fully understood and its power harnessed in pharmacology. For example, in contrast with the beneficial effects of HO-1 induction in protecting against heme- or cisplatin-induced renal failure, HO-1 is up-regulated in experimental gentamicin nephrotoxicity, but in this case, inhibition of the enzyme by SnPP does not modify the resulting renal injury.[37] Although moderate overexpression of HO-1 in fibroblasts confers protection against hyperoxic injury, higher levels of HO-1 overexpression lead to increased susceptibility to hyperoxia, suggesting a dosing threshold.[135] Similarly, CO in low concentrations (100 ppm) can generate oxidant radicals in vascular endothelium. Clearly, the preponderance of evidence favors the view that HO-1 and CO are vital to the organism's defense against injury, but much still needs to be learned. With more research into dosing and delivery, inhaled low-dose CO may well become a pharmacologic agent in the not-so-distant future.

ANNOTATED REFERENCES

Applegate LA, Luscher P, Tyrrell RM: Induction of heme oxygenase: A gen-eral response to oxidant stress in cultured mammalian cells. Cancer Res 1991;51:974-978.

> In this seminal paper, the authors detected increases in HO-1 mRNA in a human fibroblast cell line in response to a variety of oxidants and agents that alter cellular glutathione levels. This induction of HO-1 by oxidants led the authors to propose a secondary cytoprotective role for this enzyme, previously thought to function only in heme catabolism.

Nath KA, Balla G, Vercellotti GM, et al: Induction of heme oxygenase is a rapid, protective response in rhabdomyolysis in the rat. J Clin Invest 1992;90:267-270.

> This paper provided the first in vivo evidence of the protective effect of HO-1 induction against acute renal failure in a rat rhabdomyolysis model. Conversely, chemical inhibition of HO-1 exacerbated kidney dysfunction.

Otterbein L, Chin BY, Otterbein SL, et al: Mechanism of hemoglobin-induced protection against endotoxemia in rats: A ferritin-independent pathway. Am J Physiol 1997;272:L268-L275.

In this elegant study, the authors studied whether the protective effect of HO-1 on LPS-induced multiorgan failure in rats was mediated by ferritin. Rats pretreated with hemoglobin and desferoxamine (which induced HO-1 but blocked ferritin) were protected against LPS-induced organ failure and death, whereas rats pretreated with iron dextran (which induced ferritin but not HO-1) died.

Otterbein LE, Mantell LL, Choi AM: Carbon monoxide provides protection against hyperoxic lung injury. Am J Physiol 1999;276:L688-L694.

In this paper, the authors showed that exogenous gaseous CO in low doses (50 to 500 ppm) markedly attenuates the acute lung injury, inflammatory cell infiltration, cellular apoptosis, and pleural effusions that result when rats are exposed to hyperoxia. Survival was also improved, and this benefit was evident even when endogenous HO-1 was chemically inhibited, proving that CO may mediate or replace the benefits of HO-1 induction in oxidant-induced tissue injury.

Sato K, Balla J, Otterbein L, et al: Carbon monoxide generated by heme oxygenase-1 suppresses the rejection of mouse-to-rat cardiac transplants. J Immunol 2001;166:4185-4194.

It was known that HO-1 expression in the graft vasculature was critical to the survival of mouse-to-rat cardiac transplants by preventing platelet aggregation, endothelial cell apoptosis, and vascular thrombosis. In this study, HO-1 was chemically inhibited, but exogenous CO restored long-term graft survival, replicating the effects of HO-1 induction.

Chapter 44

MOLECULAR AND BIOCHEMICAL MONITORING

J. Perren Cobb • T. Philip Chung

KEY POINTS

1. The term **molecular monitoring** refers to the evaluation of patient status and disease using measurement methods derived from applied molecular biology.

2. The term **biochemical monitoring** usually refers to the use of sensitive protein detection methods to measure biomarkers to aid in establishing a diagnosis and prognosis.

3. Molecular biologic techniques, recently expanded by **technologic breakthroughs that span the entire genome**, promise to transform diagnostics in all fields of medicine, especially critical care.

4. The **sequences of the human and mouse genomes have been reported**, and efforts are under way to make the sequencing of each person's genome practical by means of readily available, high-throughput, automated DNA sequencing.

5. There are common, heritable genetic variations that contribute to susceptibility or resistance to disease. These common variants most frequently take the form of **single-nucleotide polymorphisms**.

6. The term **transcriptome** refers to the complete set of messenger RNAs (mRNAs) encoded by the genome for a particular cell type.

7. By varying the source of the target mRNA, investigators can compare relative levels of mRNA abundance using **DNA microarrays**, in practice generating a genome-wide expression profile—the *transcriptome*—for the cell or tissue of interest.

8. The term *proteome* was coined to describe the set of proteins encoded by the genome, and it defines the entire protein complement in a given cell or tissue.

9. The technology necessary to make protein "chips"—the tools needed to readily generate **genome-wide "snapshots" of the proteome**—is still emerging, some 5 years behind its DNA microarray cousin.

10. **The analytic process of classification** refers to the ability to distinguish between samples based on inherent, measurable features. Ideally, these features are easily quantitated, stable, and widely divergent between classes.

11. The overarching strategy for **molecular classification** includes the description of informational features in a training data set associated with the phenotype of interest—in essence, defining a molecular profile of the phenotype. Application of these features to unknown samples in a test data set determines the accuracy with which the features can classify unknown samples.

12. Although comprehensive reviews of **gene association studies** indicate that the majority of reported associations are not robust, meta-analysis indicates that larger, appropriately powered studies will likely find many single-nucleotide polymorphisms that are convincingly informational.

13. **Microarray gene expression analysis** has been used experimentally in the field of cancer to classify samples, addressing important clinical issues such as response to chemotherapy and propensity to metastasize. It is logical to assume that these same techniques will be widely applicable to many complex human diseases, including critical illness and injury.

14. Circulating leukocyte mRNA and protein abundance is a dynamic that varies as patients move along various **clinical trajectories (phenotypes) during sepsis**. Preliminary data in animals and human patients suggest that these trajectories can be characterized, monitored, and ultimately used to recognize infection in patients in whom sepsis is particularly difficult to diagnose. Important clinical advances in sepsis diagnostics are anticipated.

This chapter describes the current state of molecular monitoring and highlights recent advances in high-throughput genomic technology. The latter, when coupled with robust computational approaches, promises to yield more accurate diagnoses, improved understanding of underlying molecular mechanisms, and better therapeutic targets. Because of its central role as a determinant of organ dysfunction and mortality in ICUs, monitoring of systemic inflammation and infection is used as a case example.

MOLECULAR AND BIOCHEMICAL MONITORING IN CRITICAL CARE

The term *molecular monitoring* refers to the evaluation of patient status and disease using measurement methods derived from applied molecular biology. This is different from simply monitoring molecules (e.g., serum electrolytes, urinalysis, complete blood counts), as reviewed elsewhere. The term initially was used to describe the detection of minimal disease or tumor recurrence in patients with cancer using sensitive DNA or RNA detection methods[1,2]; more recently, applications in infectious disease have been reported.[3-5] These techniques are based on the polymerase chain reaction, an in vitro technique introduced in 1985 that can amplify by several orders of magnitude the abundance of a short stretch of DNA (typically <3000 base pairs) using a thermostable polymerase and sequence-specific primers. RNA can be used as the polymerase template for the chain reaction if reverse transcriptase is applied first to convert the RNA to DNA; this is called reverse transcription polymerase chain reaction. A more detailed description of these standard molecular techniques is beyond the scope of this chapter; interested readers are referred to several recent reviews for additional information (see also Chapter 28).[6-8]

The term *biochemical monitoring* usually refers to the use of sensitive protein-detection methods to measure biomarkers that can aid in diagnosis and prognosis (e.g., prostate-specific antigen).[9] There has been great interest in the past decade in pursuing markers for a number of conditions, including acute cardiac injury and sepsis. Regarding the former, the success of monitoring troponin I has revolutionized the workup and diagnosis of acute myocardial syndromes (see Chapter 95 for additional information).[10,11] The search for an accurate marker of sepsis, however, has largely failed, as evidenced by the report of a recent consensus conference.[12] Although the reasons for this failure are complex and incompletely understood, several lessons have been learned. The first is that a set of rigorous, specific, objective, measurable diagnostic criteria to use as a "gold standard" significantly aids the search for biochemical markers. This is characteristic of acute myocardial infarction but remains elusive for sepsis. Second, whereas acute myocardial syndromes involve a single, relatively homogeneous type of specialized tissue (myocardial cells) in a critical mass that carries out two readily observed functions (contraction and relaxation), sepsis involves an overwhelmingly complex interaction of multiple cell types (infecting agent, leukocytes, endothelial cells) in multiple compartments (blood, spleen, liver) that are in constant flux. In this context, the lack of success in the field of sepsis can be more readily understood. Examples of marker proteins that continue to generate interest are interleukin-6 and procalcitonin. Both reportedly serve as markers of systemic inflammation and the severity of the host response to sepsis.[12] However, insufficient and conflicting data confound the discussions supporting their use as sepsis biomarkers. It is to this end that molecular biologic techniques, recently expanded by technologic breakthroughs that span the entire genome, promise to transform diagnostics in all fields of medicine, especially critical care.

MONITORING IN THE GENOMIC ERA

It remains exceedingly difficult to gauge the clinical trajectory and response to therapy in any given patient. There are a host of probabilistic tools available (e.g., Acute Physiology and Chronic Health Evaluation [APACHE] III), based on clinical examination and physiologic parameters. What the current tools lack is an ability to measure or gauge a heritable predisposition to a given clinical trajectory and a patient's response to current therapy. Today, however, it is possible to both gauge heredity and measure the response to therapy at the molecular, whole-genome level. The biologic assumptions underlying these efforts are that (1) predisposition is determined to a greater or lesser degree by our genetics, and (2) response to therapy can be measured, predicted, and individualized at the level of RNA and protein. The promise of molecular monitoring is that it will be possible in the near future to get preliminary data when patients are admitted and, with a few repeated measures, to answer the questions "what is going on?" and "how are they going to do?" This will be important to families in terms of offering hope (or not) for the patient's recovery. It will be important to physicians because it will provide guidance for optimal and individualized therapy for the critically ill or injured.

THE GENOME (DNA)

The sequence of the human genome has been reported,[13-15] and efforts are under way to make the sequencing of each person's genome practical by means of readily available, high-throughput, automated DNA sequencing (e.g., dideoxynucleotide chain termination, or Sanger, method). Despite the overwhelming similarity in sequences among individuals (99.9%), there are common, heritable genetic variations that contribute to susceptibility or resistance to disease. These common variants most frequently take the form of single-nucleotide polymorphisms. Technically, single-nucleotide polymorphisms refer to DNA sequence variations that are present in at least 1% of the population. It is important to recognize that the approximately 10 million single-nucleotide polymorphisms in the human genome occur frequently because they have been conserved in our species, ostensibly because they provide an adaptive advantage to the organism under specific circumstances. Thus, single-nucleotide polymorphisms do not cause disease but likely influence the risk of developing a disease or the outcome from a disease (e.g., death from sepsis). Single-nucleotide and other polymorphisms exist in nonrandom patterns, or haplotypes (variant alleles located together along portions of individual chromosomes). In light of recent reports,[16,17] it has been argued that accurate characterization of genotype-phenotype associations will require the definition of haplotypes rather than the examination of individual single-nucleotide polymorphisms.[18] Thus, many in the field of functional genomics are awaiting the results of the HapMap (www.hapmap.org) efforts and are simply collecting DNA samples from at-risk patients for later analysis.[19] It is expected that successful mapping of human haplotypes will provide a critical resource for biomedical researchers who study health, disease, and variations in drug response based on genotypic differences (pharmacogenomics).

THE TRANSCRIPTOME (mRNA)

The term *transcriptome* refers to the complete set of messenger RNAs (mRNAs) encoded by the genome for a particular cell type. Unlike the genome, the transcriptome and the proteome (see later) are dynamic, characteristic of a particular cell type in a particular cell state at a specific time. For example, changes in the relative abundance of RNA and protein are what cause the dramatic changes induced by pregnancy, not the underlying maternal DNA "blueprint" that has been present since conception. Until recently, polymerase chain reaction technology was the mainstay for detecting RNA. In particular, real-time polymerase chain reaction is a popular method of quantitating changes in relative mRNA abundance between samples, usually on the order of a handful of genes. Although most genes have coding sequences that are hundreds of nucleotides in length, only a relatively short sequence (<100 nucleotides) is required to uniquely identify each gene. Advances in robotic and miniaturization technology have made it possible to study simultaneously the relative abundance of several thousand RNA species. Developers exploited these advances by fashioning glass slides ("chips") with minute quantities of short, gene-specific nucleotides. These gene-specific "probe" nucleotides—ideally, one for each gene in the genome—are arrayed on the chip surface to produce a DNA *microarray*. From cells or tissue of interest, mRNA can be isolated and labeled to produce "target" nucleotides. Hybridization of the microarray probes with the complementary-labeled targets results in the formation of a labeled heteroduplex. With the aid of a laser scanner and computational software, the relative degree of label signal intensity, correlating to the relative mRNA abundance for each gene, can be calculated. By varying the source of the target mRNA, investigators can compare relative levels of mRNA abundance, in practice, generating an expression profile—the *transcriptome*—for the cell or tissue of interest. It is now possible to profile the entire human and mouse transcriptomes using the latest-generation microarrays.

THE PROTEOME (PROTEIN)

The term *proteome* was coined to describe the set of proteins encoded by the genome, and it defines the entire protein complement in a given cell or tissue.[20] Comprehensive mechanistic insight into cellular behavior depends on detailed knowledge of protein interactions. Thus, although gene expression "snapshots" have been enormously helpful in providing our first glimpses of molecular systems, genome-wide proteomics will be required to take our understanding to the next level and facilitate the application of systems analysis. Unlike their oligonucleotide counterparts, peptides are more difficult to study for several reasons (see the accompanying box).[21-24] As a result, the technology necessary to make protein "chips"—the tools needed to readily generate genome-wide "snapshots" of the proteome—is still emerging, some 5 years behind its DNA microarray cousin. Thus, even though there are technologic hurdles to overcome, the promise of the proteome continues to engage the imagination of investigators and speculators alike, especially for clinical diagnostics and drug development.

To monitor and later identify different proteins in a given sample, they must be separated into relatively homogeneous fractions. Two-dimensional gel electrophoresis and mass spectrometry are mainstay technologies for proteomics.[21,23-26] Two recent advances are discussed here: two-dimensional differential gel electrophoresis and isotopic-coded affinity tagging. Single-dimensional gel electrophoresis has been used for decades to separate and study small numbers of proteins (e.g., Western immunoblot analysis). The technique exploits the negatively charged nature of proteins, which move in an electric field toward the cathode, with the rate of movement determined largely by size. Two-dimensional gel electrophoresis separates in the first dimension based on isoelectric point, and then orthogonally based on size. Fluorescent two-dimensional differential gel electrophoresis

is a new multiplexed method that enables the comparison of up to three experimental conditions in the same physical gel.[27] Two-dimensional differential gel electrophoresis is used to determine changes in the level of protein expression from arrays of approximately 2000 proteins (i.e., ~2000 gel spots are usually observed from plasma). The resulting differential protein expression profiles can be interpreted with greater confidence, with far fewer replicates, than with conventional two-dimensional gels. This methodology has been successfully applied in diverse systems.[28-33] The advantages of this method are that it is quantitative and allows image analysis; the disadvantage is that it poorly resolves proteins that are very high or low molecular weight, very alkaline, or hydrophobic.[34]

Isotopic-coded affinity tagging is a complementary technique that has significant advantages over two-dimensional differential gel electrophoresis for the identification of membrane proteins, proteins of lower abundance, and highly basic proteins (pI > 10).[24,35,36] Its disadvantages are that it poorly resolves proteins that are cysteine-poor and very acidic.[34] Typically, both two-dimensional differential gel electrophoresis and isotopic-coded affinity tagging are linked to subsequent analysis and identification by mass spectrometry, which measures mass-to-charge ratios of ionized analytes in the gas phase.[37] Mass spectrometry has demonstrated an ability to identify molecular signatures of peptides ("peptide-mass fingerprinting") that are diagnostic in cancer case-control studies.[22,38,39] It is expected that the proven utility of proteomics in cancer will be extended to the field of critical illness and injury, analogous to efforts in transcriptomics using DNA microarrays. Again, the expectation is that genes and pathways that are useful for diagnostics, this time at the protein level, will provide important molecular insight into regulation of the host response to critical illness and injury.

CLASSIFICATION USING MOLECULAR PROFILES

The analytic process of classification refers to the ability to distinguish between samples based on inherent, measurable features. Ideally, these features are easily quantitated, stable, and widely divergent between classes. The clinical application of classification strategies spans diagnosis, prognosis, and gauging the response to therapy. Although traditional statistics provides many robust classification tools using high-dimensional data in the fields of physics and economics, the application of classification strategies to functional genomic data is as new as the technology itself; both are evolving rapidly. Moreover, direct application of traditional computational strategies to high-dimensional biologic data can be hazardous, given that these strategies were not designed to account for the many limitations of biologic systems, such as nongaussian distributions and saturation (nonlinear) properties of probe-target interactions (microarray hybridizations). Despite these limitations, however, the power of molecular classification using genome, transcriptome, and proteome data is evident, as described later. The overarching strategy involves the description of informational features in a training data set associated with the phenotype of interest—in essence, defining a molecular profile of the phenotype. Application of these features to samples in a test data set determines the accuracy with which the features can classify unknown samples. The test data samples can be added to the training data set, typically improving the predictive ability of the model; then, new unknowns are tested in an iterative manner. Classification is based on recognition of a defined "fingerprint" characteristic of a particular phenotype; it is not necessary to know the identity or function of the features or genes that determine it. Application of these classification strategies in the ICU promises improved diagnostics and prognostics based on real-time monitoring of changes in relative RNA or protein abundance, in the context of predisposition data from DNA sequences (single-nucleotide polymorphisms). A more detailed description of the computational strategies used to analyze data from high-throughput technologies can be found in several recent reviews.[40-46]

CLASSIFICATION USING DNA SEQUENCE VARIATIONS

There is an established association between genetics and predisposition to infection, although the mechanisms are unknown. In a seminal paper, Sorensen and colleagues calculated the heritable predisposition for early death from several complex diseases in adoptees compared with their biologic or adoptive parents.[47] These investigators found that premature death in adults has a strong genetic correlation, especially death from infectious causes, suggesting a significant underlying genetic basis. The search for genetic clues to this predisposition for critical illness from infection and other causes has been accelerated dramatically by sequencing of the human and mouse genomes and identification of informational single-nucleotide polymorphisms.[13,48] A number of reports suggest a role for single-nucleotide polymorphisms as markers of sepsis severity and outcome after injury (reviewed in reference 49). For example, association studies have linked single-nucleotide polymorphisms in innate immunity genes (e.g., Toll-like receptors, CD14), cytokine genes (e.g., tumor necrosis factor, interleukin-1 beta), and endothelial genes (plasminogen activator inhibitor-1) with important clinical phenotypes, such as increased disease susceptibility and poor outcome.[49] The exact role of any given single-nucleotide polymorphism in determining outcome in critical illness and injury, however, remains controversial, primarily because of inadequate study design (underpowered studies).[17,50] Although comprehensive reviews of association studies indicate that the majority of reported associations are not robust (<5% were consistently replicated when three or more reports existed),[16] meta-analysis indicates that larger, appropriately powered studies will likely find many single-nucleotide polymorphisms that are convincingly informational.[17] Even when confirmed, these associations are unlikely to be causal, and additional research will be required to determine the reason for the association and its molecular link to disease pathophysiology.

CLASSIFICATION USING RELATIVE RNA ABUNDANCE

Microarrays have been touted as the divining rods of the 21st century,[51] given that transcriptome characterization using DNA microarrays has the potential to revolutionize molecular diagnostics. Notably, microarray analysis has been used experimentally in the field of cancer to classify samples, addressing important clinical issues such as response to chemotherapy and propensity to metastasize.[52] It has been suggested that expression profile typing for some tumors

may be significantly better than traditional diagnostic methods. With the appropriate confirmatory studies and attention to study design, it is expected that gene expression profiles will move from the bench to clinical reality shortly.[53] These studies can also be designed to couple sample classification (diagnosis, recovery trajectory, and response to therapy) with a study of gene function, discovery, interaction, and coregulation—in other words, making genomics "functional." It is logical to assume that these same techniques will be widely applicable to many complex human diseases, including critical illness and injury.[54-56]

To illustrate the power of this approach for cells of the immune system, Figure 44-1 depicts the classification of gene expression profiles of normal blood leukocytes, isolated T cells, and isolated monocytes. What differences in gene expression contribute to the differences observed among T cells, monocytes, and mixed cell populations? Shown at the right in Figure 44-1 is one version of the transforming growth factor-beta signaling pathway, arbitrarily chosen from one of the pathway discovery tools for microarray data, GenMAPP (www.genmapp.org). These data are consistent with a recent report indicating that human leukocyte expression profiles are cell specific.[57] Once a robust training data set has been collected describing the responses of isolated leukocytes in critically ill or injured patients, gene expression profiles will likely be monitored in the ICU to classify response to therapy and gauge clinical trajectories.[58]

CLASSIFICATION USING RELATIVE PROTEIN ABUNDANCE

Although DNA microarrays provide a molecular fingerprint that is useful in understanding the regulation of gene transcription, less than half the changes at the mRNA level are translated into changes at the protein level in the majority of systems. Thus, analyses of both the circulating transcriptome and proteome are indicated. Moreover, full mechanistic insight requires that changes in the transcriptome be linked to changes in the proteome, because the correlation between changes in relative mRNA and protein abundance varies, depending on the cellular role of the pathways studied.[59-61] This is irrelevant to the use of gene expression profiles for class prediction or modeling of gene coregulation, but it *is* relevant to understanding the biology of the host response. For example, close correlation was found between mRNA and protein abundance ratios for glycolysis genes in yeast, whereas abundance ratios for mitochondrial and protein synthesis genes were discordant, suggesting novel regulatory mechanisms.[61]

There are approximately 500 known (annotated) proteins in the circulating plasma proteome in humans.[22] Ideally, it would be desirable to employ "protein chips" in tandem studies to discover genome-wide protein expression profiles to complement our gene expression profiles. The combined data would allow us to find not only informational changes in blood that correlate with clinical trajectory and phenotype but also key regulatory information regarding control of gene and protein expression. However, this is not yet possible, because genome-wide proteomic technology is years behind transcriptomic technology. Despite the technologic challenges, however, recent reports highlight the potential of high-throughput proteomics. For example, simultaneous comparison of the proteome and transcriptome of human

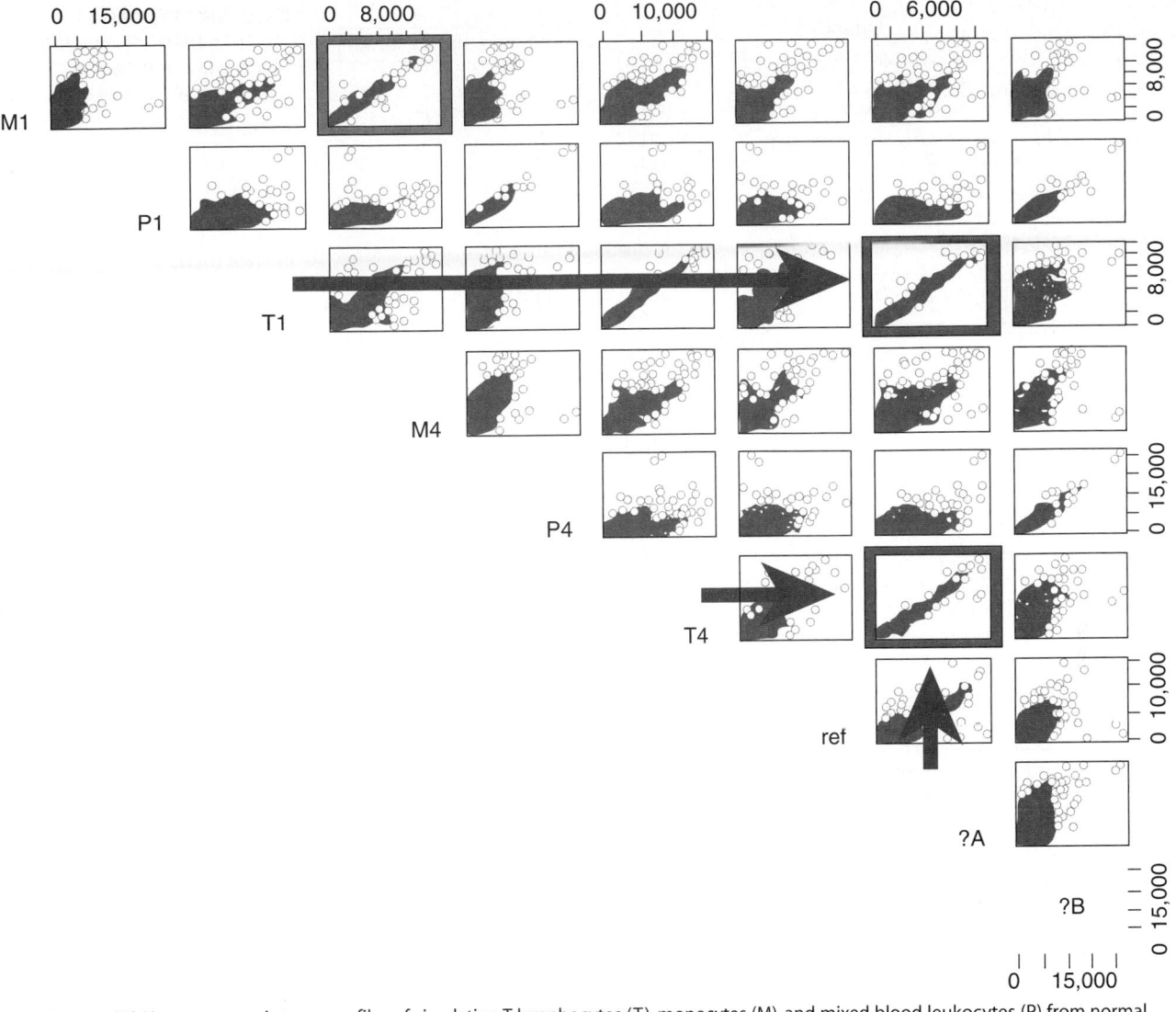

FIGURE 44–1. (A) Human transcriptome profiles of circulating T lymphocytes (T), monocytes (M), and mixed blood leukocytes (P) from normal volunteers (#1 and #4), compared with reference human RNA and two unknown samples (?A and ?B). At left, pair-wise comparisons of U95Av2 GeneChip expression signal for approximately 12,000 genes and expressed sequence tags show good pair-wise correlations between profiles of like cell types but not between different cell types in the same individual (e.g., compare good M1 to M4 correlation [yellow box] with poor M1 to T1 or P1 correlations). Moreover, assigning a cell type to the unknown samples A and B is easily accomplished, as shown by the orange arrows (?A to T cells, and ?B to mixed leukocytes). At right, the GenMAPP transforming growth factor-beta (TGF-β) pathway indicates differences in gene expression among T cell (red), monocyte (green), and PAXgene (blue). This program allows one to visually compare apparent levels of gene expression by color-coding genes that have increased expression in a given data set. In this example comparing blood leukocyte, isolated T cell, and isolated monocyte GeneChip signals, apparent gene expression for the type III TGF-β receptor (betaglycan) was greatest in T cells (red box); stress-induced protein 1 (SIP1) and c-FOS were greatest in monocytes (green boxes); and STAT3 was greatest in blood (mixed) leukocytes (blue box). The other genes shown (uncolored) were not changed. Thus, this figure indicates that apparent gene expression for the type III accessory receptor for TGF-β was greater in T cells, whereas apparent gene expression for SIP1 repressor and c-FOS cofactor was higher in monocytes. In contrast, there was higher apparent gene expression in blood (mixed) leukocytes only for the STAT3 cofactor. (See color section of this text.)

Continued on next page

neutrophils stimulated with lipopolysaccharide ex vivo indicated that isolated neutrophils have a much more complex and dynamic transcriptional response than previously appreciated.[60] Importantly, this study also highlighted the poor concordance between mRNA transcription and protein translation in a human neutrophil model of innate immune activation.

THE PROMISE OF MOLECULAR MONITORING IN THE ICU: SEPSIS

MH is a 74-year-old woman with a 3-day history of progressive dyspnea associated with crampy abdominal pain, nausea, and vomiting. Her past medical history is significant for childhood tuberculosis (left pneumonectomy) and dysfunctional uterine bleeding (open hysterectomy 3 years previously). In the triage area, her whole-body computed tomography scan was most consistent with partial small bowel obstruction and a mild basilar infiltrate in the remaining lung. The absence of a uterus and left lung was confirmed. Her peripheral leukocyte count was 11,000; the gene expression profile was consistent with inflammation. Plasma markers of infection were absent. She was admitted to the hospital with a working diagnosis of partial small bowel obstruction and treated with i.v. fluid hydration and nasogastric tube decompression. Her symptoms and signs of abdominal distention improved. On hospital day 2, however,

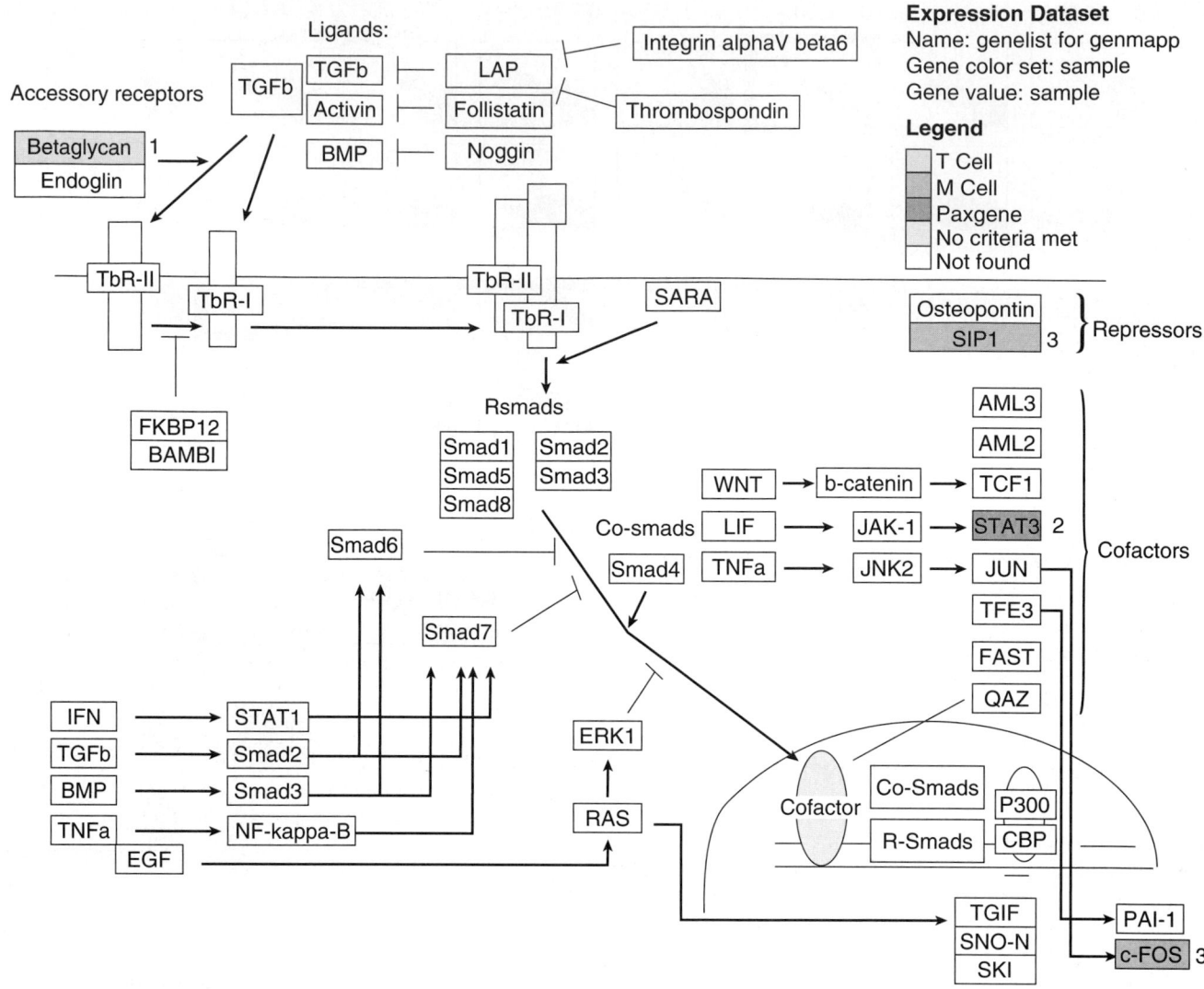

FIGURE 44–1—cont'd. (B)

her respiratory insufficiency worsened, requiring endotracheal tube insertion, mechanical ventilatory support, and admission to the ICU. Repeat leukocyte studies showed that her count had fallen to 6000, but the circulating gene expression patterns remained consistent with inflammation, and plasma markers of systemic infection were absent. On hospital day 5, the leukocyte count rose to 9000, and the pattern of sepsis molecular markers changed, indicating an expression profile consistent with Gram-positive infection. A diagnosis of Gram-positive bacterial pneumonia was made, and the patient was started on a narrow-spectrum antibiotic to treat Gram-positive organisms. The patient's abdominal examination and scans improved, and she was extubated with signs of resolving bowel obstruction and pneumonia on day 9.

As noted earlier, sepsis in the ICU presents several common diagnostic dilemmas. The hypothetical case just presented provides an example of how the advanced molecular diagnostics described herein will help discriminate between systemic infection and inflammation in the future. The assumption is that circulating leukocyte mRNA and protein abundance is a dynamic that varies as patients move along various clinical trajectories (phenotypes) during sepsis. We also anticipate that these trajectories can be characterized,

monitored, and ultimately used to recognize infection in patients in whom sepsis is particularly difficult to diagnose.[55] The promise of this line of investigation is that these patterns of change in gene expression and protein abundance will become, in effect, new genomic "vital signs."[62] The human tissue that is most easily accessible for such longitudinal profiling is peripheral (circulating) blood. Further, it has been hypothesized that this systematic approach, using genome-wide gene and protein expression profiling, can be used to identify molecular classification schemes that provide novel insight into the adaptive response to inflammation and infection.[54,55]

Sepsis is particularly appropriate for this type of diagnostic approach. Although still controversial, modifications of sepsis criteria continue to be useful, as evidenced by a recent randomized, prospective, controlled clinical trial testing the only agent reported to increase the survival of patients with severe sepsis.[63] The authors of that study noted that the resulting pool of "septic" patients had a wide range of clinical features and were heterogeneous with regard to a number of biochemical inflammatory classifiers, including serum plasma D-dimer, interleukin-6, and protein C. More important, the inability to reliably distinguish between different degrees of septic injury continues to frustrate

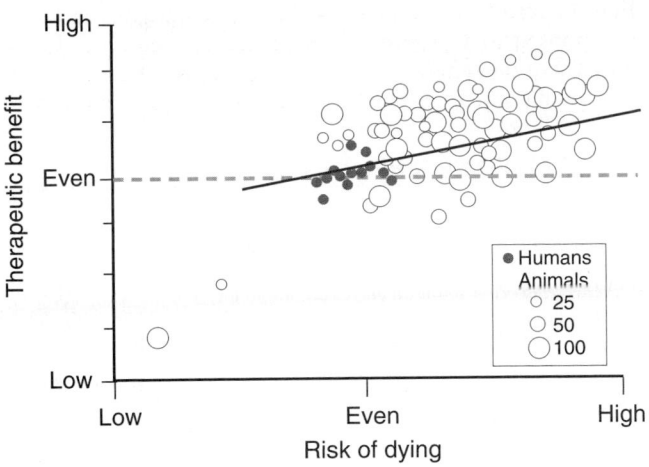

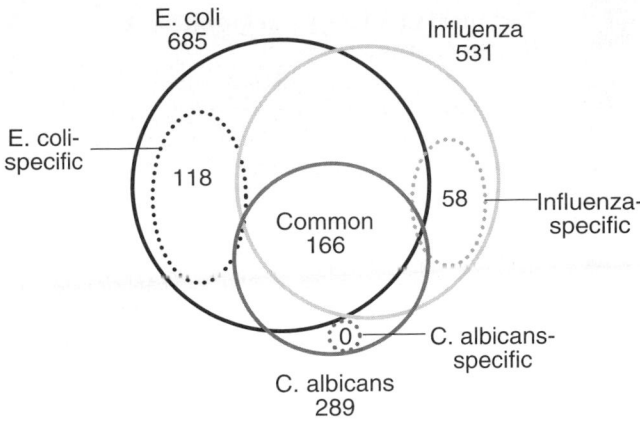

FIGURE 44–2. Relationship between the effect of anti-inflammatory treatment and the odds of the control group dying in animal and human sepsis trials. There is a significant correlation between the severity of illness and the likelihood of beneficial effect with treatment. Note that current enrollment in human studies centers around the point where therapies have no effect in animal models (in other words, the results of preclinical trials suggest that the human studies are unlikely to show benefit, given the current odds of dying in the human control groups). These data suggest that the ability to identify subpopulations of sicker patients would probably increase the likelihood of efficacy of anti-inflammatory agents. The technology needed to better classify septic patients is described in the text. (From Minneci PC, Deans KJ, Banks SM, et al: Should we continue to target the platelet-activating factor pathway in septic patients? Crit Care Med 2004;32:585-588.)

FIGURE 44–3. Overlapping sets of genes identified by DNA microarray analysis applied to human dendritic cells stimulated ex vivo with *Escherichia coli*, influenza virus, or *Candida albicans*.[67] Note that there were 166 genes in common, suggesting that there are both generic and stimulus-specific genes activated by infectious or inflammatory stimuli.

investigators and slow the development of sepsis therapeutics. For example, the efficacy of anti-inflammatory agents in treating sepsis is dependent on the severity of illness, with sicker patients and animals appearing to benefit the most from anti-inflammatory agents (Fig. 44-2).[64,65] Moreover, investigators must not only identify the infectious organism (e.g., Gram-positive bacteria versus fungi) to optimize outcome but also distinguish temporally among potential host responses to the invading organism, including the systemic inflammatory versus counterregulatory anti-inflammatory response syndromes. These tasks remain exceedingly difficult, despite ongoing improvements in diagnostic technology, and are still based largely on history, physical examination, and the results of common laboratory tests. As an example, recent evidence indicates that patients with ventilator-associated pneumonia are frequently misdiagnosed, based on an examination of postmortem specimens, radiographic findings, and clinical criteria.[66] Clearly, the ability to classify patients rapidly based on presence of infection, type of organism, and temporal phase of the host's adaptive response would increase the likelihood of therapeutic success. Thus, new strategies and tools are needed to correctly identify those who are most ill with sepsis, and thereby those who are most likely to benefit in clinical trials of sepsis therapeutics.

Recent reports using DNA microarray analysis indicate that inflammatory and infectious insults produce distinct molecular signatures. For example, microarray analysis of dendritic cells stimulated ex vivo exhibit both common and pathogen-specific immune responses.[67] Specifically, there were 166 genes expressed in response to bacterial, fungal, and viral stimulation, consistent with a common cluster of genes expressed in response to infection (Fig. 44-3).[67]

Interestingly, yeasts were found to respond similarly to diverse insults, expressing a so-called common stress response cluster.[68] In another study, gene expression profiles of human whole blood stimulated ex vivo with heat-killed *Staphylococcus aureus* or *Escherichia coli* lipopolysaccharide had both generic and bacteria-specific features.[69] It follows, then, that it may be possible to define clusters of mammalian genes that are commonly up-regulated or, conversely, down-regulated in response to sepsis—what could be called a "common sepsis response" cluster.[70] Finally, recent data from animal models of abdominal and pulmonary sepsis suggest that measurements of RNA relative abundance in blood can be used to predict not only whether a mouse is infected but also the type of infecting organism.[70,71] It is expected that proteomic data will be equally or even more revealing.[72] These preliminary data suggest that important advances in sepsis diagnostics can be anticipated in the near future based on analysis of blood transcriptomes and proteomes.

CONCLUSION

Critically ill and injured patients have suffered from clinicians' inability to accurately classify and gauge clinical trajectory and response to therapy. Coincident with the sequencing of the human and mouse genomes, the technology has become available to move critical care monitoring and diagnostics into the genomic era. This will be characterized by the appearance of novel tools capable of profiling DNA, RNA, and protein in a search for molecular fingerprints associated with clinically important phenotypes and, more important, individualized response to therapy. To realize the full potential of this technology, support for ongoing, large-scale, collaborative research projects using genomic and proteomic technology to define the immunoinflammatory phenotypes in response to critical illness and injury will be essential.* As described earlier, diagnosing sepsis and

*These include National Institutes of Health research projects currently funded by the National Institute of General Medical Sciences (http://www.nigms.nih.gov/funding/gluegrants.html); National Heart, Lung, and Blood Institute (http://www.nhlbi.nih.gov/resources/pga/); and National Institute of Allergy and Infectious Diseases (http://www.immunetolerance.org/ and http://www.septicshock.org/).

Technical Challenges to Monitoring the Proteome

At least 35% of proteins exist in multiple isoforms, secondary to alternative splicing and post-translational modification, a "seemingly infinite universe of post-transcriptional complexities."[22]

Proteomic analysis is substrate limited, as there is no means to amplify product (i.e., there is no polymerase chain reaction–equivalent for proteins).

Protein concentrations cover a huge dynamic range (10^6 in cells and 10^9 in plasma), yet current proteomic technology can measure changes over a range of only three to four orders of magnitude.

Only a portion of a given proteome (i.e., a subproteome) can be interrogated at one time, owing to limited substrate in the sample and limited dynamic range of the technology. Therefore, subtraction and enrichment strategies, and their limitations, are commonly encountered.

Current proteomic technology is primarily qualitative and inherently more complex than DNA or RNA technology, resulting in lower throughput.

monitoring the response to antibiotic therapy are prime examples. Annotated databases linking these data, with free access to the public, are sorely needed. Using gene and protein expression profile analysis, novel strategies for sepsis recognition, pathogen identification, and modeling of the leukocyte response are being tested. Industry reports suggest that the results of such tests will soon be available in hours, as opposed to the several days currently required. In the absence of new therapies, such a strategy will be essential to improving outcomes among the critically ill and injured.

ANNOTATED REFERENCES

Eichacker PQ, Parent C, Kalil A, et al: Risk and the efficacy of antiinflammatory agents: Retrospective and confirmatory studies of sepsis. Am J Respir Crit Care Med 2002;166:1197-1205.
This report contributes to our understanding of why the vast majority of anti-inflammatory therapies have failed in human sepsis trials. It also points out why it is critical to develop improved diagnostics in sepsis.

Eisen MB, Spellman PT, Brown PO, Botstein D: Cluster analysis and display of genome-wide expression patterns. Proc Natl Acad Sci U S A 1998;95:14863-14868.
This early report on the use of gene expression profiles to create molecular fingerprints characteristic of a given cell type (yeast) demonstrates the power of microarray technology coupled with systematic analysis.

Fessler MB, Malcolm KC, Duncan MW, Worthen GS: A genomic and proteomic analysis of activation of the human neutrophil by lipopolysaccharide and its mediation by p38 mitogen-activated protein kinase. J Biol Chem 2002;277:31291-31302.
These authors report on the simultaneous comparison of changes in gene and protein expression induced in human neutrophils by endotoxin.

Lander ES, Linton LM, Birren B, et al: Initial sequencing and analysis of the human genome. Nature 2001;409:860-921.
This is the first report of sequencing of the human genome.

Sorensen TI, Nielsen GG, Andersen PK, Teasdale TW: Genetic and environmental influences on premature death in adult adoptees. N Engl J Med 1988;318:727-732.
This landmark twin study made the association between genotype and risk of death from infection.

Chapter 45

GENETICS OF CRITICAL ILLNESS

Richard G. Wunderink

KEY POINTS

1. **Association studies**, comparing the frequency of polymorphisms in patients with a disease or a complication to that in a control population, are most likely to determine the genetic components of complex critical illnesses.

2. **The risk of dying from infection is familial**, and a good family history of infection should be obtained in all patients.

3. **The genetic predisposition to a disease**, such as septic shock, **may be different from the genetic predisposition to a specific manifestation**, such as acute respiratory distress syndrome or disseminated intravascular coagulation.

4. **Large databases and multivariate analyses are required** to tease out the relative contributions of genetic factors to infection, within the context of underlying diseases, the variable pathogenicity of microorganisms, treatment factors, and so forth.

5. **Establishing the genetic risk of developing a disease** will be clinically relevant when the genetic variability allows risk stratification of patients and leads to differences in management, and when diagnostic or screening tests are readily available.

6. The great hope of **pharmacogenomics**—use of genetic information to individualize drug therapy— is not only to identify the right dose of medication to use safely but also to individualize the choice of drug in specific circumstances and specific patients.

Understanding the genetic variability in the response to critical illness, with its implications for individualization of therapy, is likely to be a focus of research in the next few decades. Recent technologic advances have made routine genotyping in a clinically relevant time frame feasible. Unfortunately, knowledge about the clinical implications of individual genetic variation on the course or risk of critical illness lags far behind.

Genetic variability is likely to affect many aspects of the care of critically ill patients. The initial focus is on three main areas—the host immune response to infection, the risk of coagulation or thrombosis, and the effects on drug metabolism. Although research interest in other areas will undoubtedly develop, these three topics illustrate the importance of unraveling the role of genetic variability in the outcome of critical illness.

GENETIC PRINCIPLES

Variability is incredibly common in the human genome. A variant allele occurs in approximately 1 of every 300 to 500 bases in human DNA. Although new mutations can cause isolated disease, the majority of genetic variation is in the form of polymorphisms. Polymorphisms are allelic variations that exist stably in a population at a frequency (generally $\geq 1\%$) that cannot be accounted for by new mutations alone. The implication is that these mutations do not confer a strong selective disadvantage and may even be associated with a beneficial effect in specific circumstances.

Genetic polymorphisms can occur in a variety of forms. The most common is a single-nucleotide polymorphism (SNP), which is a variation in a single nucleotide. This can be a substitution of one base for another, a deletion, or an addition of a base pair. Larger sections of the chromosome can also be deleted. Variable tandem repeats are sections of the chromosome (minisatellites) that contain multiple copies of a segment of DNA. These usually occur in the large stretches of the chromosome that do not encode a gene. Multiple two, three, or four base pair repeats (microsatellites) are also common. The number of repeats in these microsatellites is highly variable, a fact that is useful in forensic medicine. Large chromosomal mutations can be seen in critically ill patients and are common causes of neonatal ICU admissions.

The area where a SNP occurs determines the resultant effect. If a mutation occurs in an exon of the gene, an abnormal protein is more likely. Because of the redundancy of codons coding for specific amino acids, the polymorphic allele may not result in a different amino acid sequence—a silent mutation. Association of disease or disease severity with a silent mutation most likely indicates that it is a marker for a different functional polymorphism. Mutations that change the codon to one that signals the end of gene transcription can occur but are rare, because of their generally deleterious effect. The area of chromosome before the first gene sequence, called the promoter region, is critical in initiating gene transcription. Mutations in the promoter region are therefore more likely to affect the amount of gene product produced as a result of differential binding of nuclear transcription factors, such as nuclear factor kappa-B. The variable amount of messenger RNA (mRNA) still codes for a normal protein. Mutations in introns, areas within the gene that code for sections of mRNA but are clipped off before translation into the final protein, are less likely to result in a functional difference in the amount of protein or a structural difference in the protein itself. However, a biologic effect from polymorphisms in these areas is possible.

Genetic Terminology

Allele: One of the variant forms of a gene at a particular locus, or location, on a chromosome.

Codon: Three bases in a DNA or RNA sequence that specify a single amino acid.

Exon: Region of a gene that contains the code for producing the gene's protein. Each exon codes for a specific portion of the complete protein.

Haplotype: Set of genetic markers on the same chromosome linked closely enough to be inherited as a unit.

Heterozygous: Possessing two different forms of a particular gene, one inherited from each parent.

Homozygous: Possessing two identical forms of a particular gene, one inherited from each parent.

Intron: Noncoding sequence of DNA that is initially copied into RNA but is cut out of the final RNA transcript.

Linkage: Association of genes or markers that lie near one another on a chromosome. Linked genes and markers tend to be inherited together.

Linkage disequilibrium: Two alleles at different loci that occur together in an individual more often than would be predicted by random chance.

Locus: Place on a chromosome where a specific gene is located—a kind of address for the gene. (The plural is loci.)

Lod score: Statistical estimate of whether two loci are likely to lie near each other on a chromosome and are therefore likely to be inherited together. A lod score of three or more generally indicates that the two loci are close.

Marker: Segment of DNA with an identifiable physical location on a chromosome whose inheritance can be followed. Because DNA segments that lie near each other on a chromosome tend to be inherited together, markers are an indirect way of tracking the inheritance pattern of genes that have not yet been identified but whose approximate locations are known.

Microsatellite: Repetitive DNA sequence with a repeat unit of 2 to 4 base pairs.

Minisatellite: Repetitive DNA sequence with a repeat unit of 5 to 30 base pairs.

Penetrance: The frequency of expression of genotype.

Polymorphism: A common variation in the sequence of DNA among individuals.

Promoter: The part of a gene that contains the information to turn the gene on or off. The process of transcription is initiated at the promoter.

Single-nucleotide polymorphism (SNP): Common but minute variations that occur in human DNA at a frequency of 1 every 1000 bases. (SNP is pronounced "snip.")

Variable number tandem repeats: Generic term for mini- and microsatellites. Often used as genetic markers to track inheritance in families.

From http://www.genome.gov/glossary.cfm.

Micro- and minisatellites can cause disease, such as the fragile X syndrome and Huntington's disease, but they are more likely to be markers for other functional polymorphisms.

DEMONSTRATION OF GENETIC RISK

A variety of methods are available for demonstrating the genetic component of critical illness. The two main methods are linkage analysis and association studies. Each type of analysis is appropriate or advantageous in different situations (Fig. 45-1).

LINKAGE ANALYSIS

Traditional family studies and pedigrees are powerful techniques to find rare mutations that consistently result in clinical disease (high penetrance). This type of genetic pattern is usually studied with linkage analysis. Linkage analysis involves genotyping specimens for multiple polymorphisms to determine which polymorphic alleles are transmitted together in affected individuals. The strength of the association can be described by the lod (logarithm of the odds) score—an estimate of whether the observed data are due to linkage or to random variation. Generally, a lod score of three or more is evidence of linkage between the marker and the causative gene.

Linkage analysis is less helpful in illnesses requiring ICU care because of the impact of environmental exposure, the frequent variability in gene penetrance, and the multiple-loci nature of complex illnesses. For these and other reasons, critical illness does not appear to occur in a familial pattern. Therefore, the only way linkage studies can be performed is to compare unrelated affected and unaffected individuals. The additional variability introduced by this factor precludes finding all but the strongest associations. Newer molecular technologies, including the use of gene array chips, hold great promise for future studies but are still both difficult to interpret and very expensive.

ASSOCIATION STUDIES

The most common type of study supporting a role for genetic variability in the complex diseases affecting the critically ill is the association study. Association studies essentially look for a different frequency of specific alleles in patients with a disease or complication compared with the frequency in a control population.

Association studies have a variety of problems.[1] The initial assumption of the association study is that the gene of interest is involved in the illness being studied. A strong physiologic rationale for the candidate gene is required to ensure that associations are not spurious. Association studies therefore are dependent on basic research and animal studies to identify

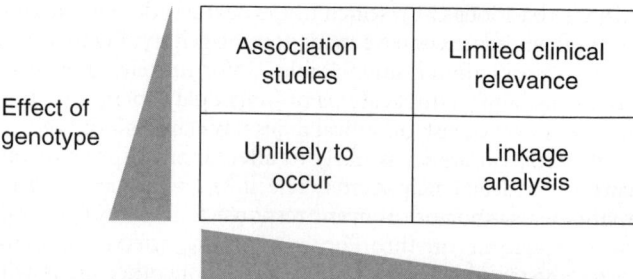

FIGURE 45–1. Approaches to determining genetic predisposition.

appropriate or novel candidate genes. Gene expression arrays are increasingly important as a method to identify unknown genes or genes with previously unrecognized importance.

In addition, the specific polymorphism studied may not be the causative locus. Genes are not inherited independently; they are inherited as whole chromosomes. Multiple mutations may occur in the gene of interest or in adjacent genes on the same chromosome, each of which may or may not affect either the actual protein structure or the amount of protein produced. For example, at least 10 mutations occur in the tumor necrosis factor (TNF) promoter region, several of which are known to affect the TNF response to a standard stimulus. Many of these mutations are in linkage disequilibrium with each other. An association between a specific mutation and an outcome, predisposition, or even physiologic response does not prove that the mutation causes the response. Therefore, any polymorphism associated with a clinical condition or outcome should be considered a marker for genetic risk until more extensive studies confirm that the mutation leads to a change in biologic function and that the change induced produces the outcome observed.

For complex diseases, the mutation must be common enough to affect a significant portion of the population. Although rare mutations can cause unique infection syndromes, such as disseminated bacille Calmette-Guérin infection after immunization, the majority of patients with a common infection such as community-acquired pneumonia are unlikely to carry these rare mutations. The known genetic mutations that have an impact on immunity, such as immunoglobulin deficiencies or cilia dysfunction, clearly do not explain the majority of cases of pneumonia or sepsis. Therefore, most association studies have examined polymorphisms.

Complex medical illnesses, such as those that present to the ICU, are likely to be polygenic, with multiple genes on different chromosomes interacting to cause the effect. Teasing out these interactions with association studies is difficult and requires large populations. Many published association studies are underpowered.

The appropriate comparison population is critical to association studies.[2] Ethnicity, age, gender, and exposure are important factors, but they do not guarantee a valid control group. Choosing the appropriate control population for critically ill patients is even more difficult and controversial. The appropriate controls for the development of an illness may be different from the controls for a specific manifestation once that illness has occurred. Simple tests, such as Hardy-Weinberg equilibrium (i.e., the genotype frequencies should equal that predicted by allele frequencies in the population), in the control population are needed to ensure selection bias. Newer statistical techniques of genomic controls may help exclude a spurious association based on nonrandom sampling.

Specific phenotypes are also difficult to define for the critically ill. The physiologic response to sepsis may be different based on whether the cause is Gram-negative bacteria, Gram-positive bacteria, fungi, or viruses; however, the distinction is often difficult to make clinically. Similarly, the risk for simple deep venous thrombosis may be different from that for pulmonary emboli, even though they are combined in many clinical studies. Many studies have focused on more objective outcomes, such as death, septic shock, or bacteremia, because of the difficulties in defining other phenotypic presentations.

Finally, environmental or nongenetic host factors complicate the interpretation of association studies. The host response (and therefore the genes involved) is very different for *Mycoplasma* pneumonia than for pneumococcal pneumonia. The effect of active alcohol ingestion can lead to a phenotypic change (increased risk of septic shock, neutropenia, or acute respiratory distress syndrome [ARDS]) that is not genetically based. Therefore, association studies should include multivariate analysis, with inclusion of known clinical risk factors (as well as other genetic risks) as part of the analysis.

The statistical analysis of association studies is not necessarily less complex than that of linkage analysis. Many studies examine several SNPs in the same population. The usual statistical correction for multiple comparisons may be too conservative and is probably inappropriate, because it assumes the comparison of independent factors when, in fact, multiple SNPs in the same or adjacent genes do not sort independently. Haplotype analysis may overcome this statistical issue, but it introduces greater complexity in other ways.

Despite these limitations, association studies are presently the most commonly used genetic study for complex multifactorial diseases, and most of the subsequent information presented in this chapter is derived from association studies. The genetic influence on complex illnesses continues to be a difficult area of research. Knowledge of the role of genetics in critical illness will continue to expand, and any discussion of specific genetic factors will likely be quickly outdated. However, reviewing the data currently available illustrates some of the principles that are important in evaluating future studies of genetic risk.

GENETIC INFLUENCE ON THE HOST IMMUNE RESPONSE

The strongest support for the role of genetics in infection is the adoptee study by Sorenson and colleagues.[3] They linked cause of death in adoptees to cause of death in both the natural parents and the adoptive parents. The risk of dying of infection if either natural parent died of infection by age 50 years was nearly six times greater than if neither died of infection. The increased risk exceeded the genetic risk of early death from cardiovascular disease or cancer (Fig. 45-2). In addition, the excess genetic risk for death from infection

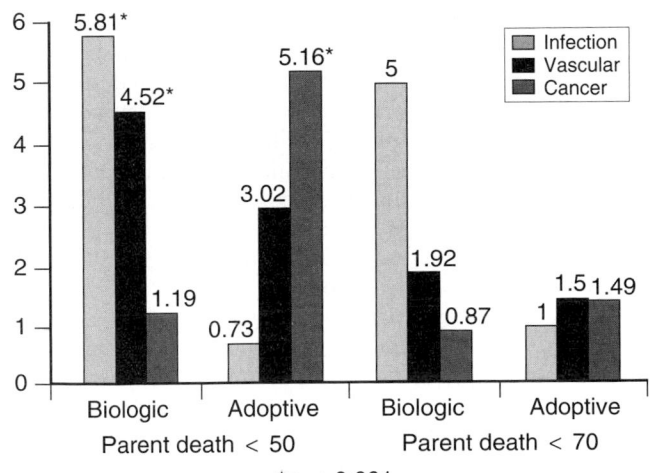

FIGURE 45–2. Relative risk of early death in adoptees based on identical cause of death in either natural or adoptive parents. (From Sorensen TI, Nielsen GG, Andersen PK, et al: Genetic and environmental influences on premature death in adult adoptees. N Engl J Med 1988;318:727-732.)

extended to parental death any time in the first 70 years of life. Despite well-documented genetic factors, familial risk of death from cardiovascular disease and malignancy is negligible when parental death occurs between ages 50 and 70 years.

Although these findings strongly support the role of genetic factors in infectious mortality, neither the type of infection nor the specific genetic factors can be determined from this type of study. Epidemiologic data suggest that pneumonia and bacteremia are the major causes of septic deaths in the United States. More unusual causes of severe sepsis, such as meningitis and endocarditis, also have high fatality rates. Although some of the earliest and strongest evidence for a genetic influence on response to infectious disease came from malaria studies, many studies of genetic risk focus on severe sepsis, pneumonia, and meningitis.

Ethnic and racial differences in mortality from infectious diseases have been known for centuries and provide additional evidence of the influence of genetic factors. Even accounting for socioeconomic differences, racial differences in death rates from pneumonia are consistently found. However, the type and degree of differences are not consistent. In many past studies, African Americans had higher mortality rates than white Americans, and Asian Americans had lower rates. However, recent data demonstrate that, for bacteremic pneumococcal pneumonia, mortality rates for Asian Americans are significantly greater than those for black and white Americans.[4] Several explanations for these contradictory findings are possible. For instance, different genetic backgrounds may be more important for bacteremic pneumococcal pneumonia than for pneumonia in general. However, the more likely explanation is that different subpopulations with different genetic backgrounds were sampled and that the statistical lumping of ethnically diverse populations into broad "races" confuses the issue. Other studies have demonstrated that the risk of death from pneumonia varies widely among different ethnic groups categorized as Hispanic American or Asian American. This variability within demographic groups actually supports the importance of genetic factors in the outcome of severe infection.

Because the genetic risk for severe infection likely involves multiple gene loci (many of which demonstrate variable penetrance), and because there is clearly a major environmental component (i.e., exposure to an infectious agent), several authors have suggested that family studies of infection cannot be done. However, classic family studies, such as triad studies (sampling the affected child and both parents), are possible if a careful and comprehensive family history is obtained.[5] Figure. 45-3 illustrates a family pedigree demonstrating a type of familial infection syndrome. Certain key features allow the recognition of a genetic predisposition to infection. Index cases of death from infection at an age younger than age 50 to 60 years, especially when no underlying systemic disease confuses the issue, are critical to recognize. Awareness that the genetic risk for infection may be generic in terms of site, such that different family members may be affected by a variety of infections, is also important.

From a practical standpoint, one of the more important reasons to take a complete and comprehensive family history is to increase suspicion of the myriad rare genetic causes of altered immunity. Although too extensive to discuss in this chapter, genetic defects in neutrophil or lymphocyte function, immunoglobulin deficiencies, cilia dysfunction, and the like can be seen (rarely) in the critically ill. In adults, the first manifestation is unlikely to be a critical illness; however,

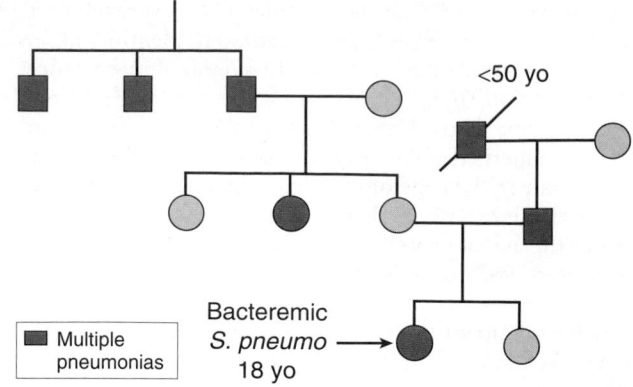

FIGURE 45–3. Pedigree of familial infection syndrome.

this may be the initial presentation in neonatal and pediatric ICUs. Simply because of their higher frequency, polymorphisms in the innate response are likely to affect a greater proportion of the critically ill.[6]

INNATE IMMUNE RESPONSE

Because of the rapidity and severity of onset, the types of illness precipitating ICU admission, especially infection, likely involve the innate immune response more often than the acquired immune response. The three main components of the innate immune response are pattern recognition molecules, inflammatory response mediators, and the important counterregulatory anti-inflammatory response mediators.

Pattern Recognition Molecules

Key to the innate immune response is the recognition of invading microorganisms. Pattern recognition molecules are inherited through the germ line; therefore, though common to all cells, their number is more limited than the remarkable diversity of receptors possible on individual lymphocytes involved in the acquired immune response. Because of this limited repertoire, pattern recognition receptors are usually focused on highly conserved structures present in large classes of microorganisms. These pathogen-associated molecular patterns are unique to microbial pathogens, without human homologues. In addition, the structures recognized are usually essential for either survival or pathogenicity of the microorganism.

Pattern recognition molecules can be secreted into the circulation and function by binding to microorganisms and facilitating recognition by phagocytes or the complement system. Mannose-binding lectin not only activates the complement system when bound to bacteria but also regulates inflammatory mediators. Several mutations in the gene or promoter region can lead to little or no serum mannose-binding lectin. The incidence of homozygous variant coding alleles appears to be almost twice as common in pneumococcal bacteremia as in noninvasive disease.[7] Mannose-binding lectin is phylogenetically related to surfactant proteins, rare mutations of which have also been associated with infection and lung disease.

Lipopolysaccharide-binding protein is another secreted pattern recognition molecule. Rare alleles of lipopolysaccharide-binding protein have been found to be increased in septic patients, and all septic patients homozygous for these alleles died.[8] No associations between sepsis and polymorphisms in the related bactericidal permeability increasing protein gene were found in the same population. Interestingly, the frequency of rare alleles was more common in males in one study; in another, it was more common in African Americans of both genders. The site may therefore be a marker for an as yet unidentified adjacent SNP that is important in sepsis. Support for this possibility comes from the finding that the originally described restriction length polymorphism cleavage site is actually at an adjacent nucleotide, resulting in a silent mutation.[9]

Pattern recognition molecules can also be located on cell surfaces, where they function either by mediating uptake into lysosomes for destruction and antigen processing or by activating signaling pathways to induce the expression of a variety of host response genes, especially inflammatory cytokines. Toll-like receptors (TLRs) are important examples. At least 10 different TLRs exist, with different affinities for various microorganisms. TLR4 appears to be essential for the recognition of endotoxin, whereas TLR2 is more important for the recognition of Gram-positive bacteria. Two polymorphisms, TLR4 Asp299Gly and Thr399Ile, were examined in a French cohort of 91 patients with septic shock and 73 healthy controls.[10] Both polymorphisms were uncommon, but carriage of 299Gly was found only in the shock cohort. This SNP did not appear to increase the risk or severity of meningococcal meningitis.

Increased levels of soluble CD14, a component of the endotoxin-lipopolysaccharide recognition pathway, may be an important risk factor for septic shock. A polymorphism at the −159 site has been associated with higher circulating levels of soluble CD14 and greater TNF production in peripheral blood mononuclear cells after stimulation with lipopolysaccharide or *Escherichia coli*. The CD14 −159 TT genotype was more common in patients with septic shock than in controls (71% versus 48%; $P = 0.008$).[11] In addition, mortality from shock was significantly higher in patients who carried a T allele.

Theoretically, functional polymorphisms in pattern recognition receptors should increase susceptibility to infection, but so far, the majority of data has found associations with indices of severity. This may be a function of study design. One of the few longitudinal studies in this literature found that TLR4 mutations increased the risk of serious bacterial infections.[12] The greatest risk appeared to be in patients with the 299Gly mutation in the absence of the 399Ile mutation. Although susceptibility to infection was not the primary focus of this particular study, longitudinal studies are a better design than cross-sectional studies to demonstrate such susceptibility.

Proinflammatory Mediators

Not surprisingly, much of the initial research into the role of genetic variability in infectious disease focused on the gene for TNF, a key mediator initiating the inflammatory cascade.[13-16] The TNF locus, especially the promoter region, is highly polymorphic. Several polymorphisms appear to be functional, with variable levels of TNF release in response to either infection in vivo or stimulation in vitro. Carriage of the A allele of TNF-308 SNP has been associated with an increased risk of septic shock, especially in surgical and trauma populations. The risk of septic shock appears to be less if the cause of infection is community-acquired pneumonia.[16,17] This discrepancy may relate to a differential effect in predominantly Gram-negative versus Gram-positive infections.

A SNP in the adjacent lymphotoxin alpha (LTA) gene has also been associated with increased TNF levels. Carriage of this LTA+250 AA genotype was associated with a substantially greater risk of septic shock and death from septic shock,[18] including in patients with community-acquired pneumonia.[16] Interestingly, respiratory failure in the absence of shock in community-acquired pneumonia strongly correlated with the opposite GG genotype (Fig. 45-4). This finding has important implications for the clinical definitions of severe sepsis and the systemic inflammatory response syndrome. Genetic predisposition to septic shock may be different from that to one manifestation of severe sepsis—hypoxemia. Similarly, the coagulation abnormalities of severe sepsis may be associated with polymorphisms in different genes, such as plasminogen activator inhibitor-1.[19]

The discrepancies in association studies of the TNF-308 SNP may be explained by significant linkage disequilibrium with the LTA SNP.[16] Linkage disequilibrium occurs when polymorphisms within the same or different genes are usually inherited together, resulting in a more frequent association than would be expected by chance of one allele in one gene with a specific allele in a nearby SNP. For example, the LTA+250 A allele is nearly always associated with a G allele at the TNF-308 site. Because the LTA+250 A allele is much more common than the TNF-308 A allele, provided that the degree of influence of each of these polymorphic sites is roughly equivalent, the LTA effect is much easier to observe when both sites are examined in the same population.

In addition to the very important HLA loci, the TNF and LTA genes are in close proximity to other immunologically important genes on chromosome 6, such as complement components and heat shock protein (HSP). The association between one HSP70 gene SNP and septic shock in a cohort of patients with community-acquired pneumonia was even stronger than that of the LTA+250 site mentioned earlier.[20] However, the two sites are in linkage disequilibrium, and haplotype analysis suggests that chromosomes containing an adenine at both the LTA+250 and the HSP70 loci are associated with the greatest risk of septic shock. These data suggest that

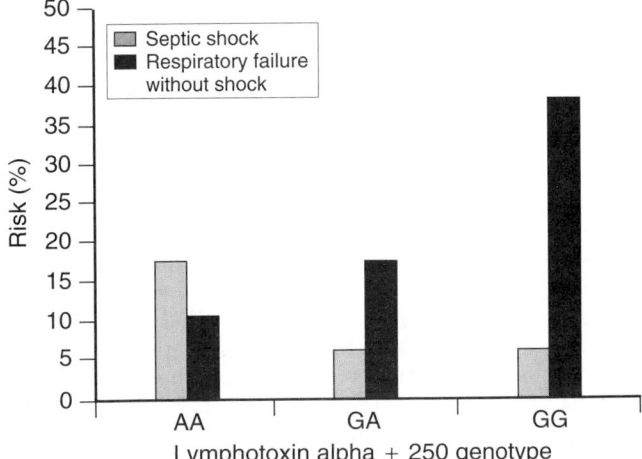

FIGURE 45–4. Relative risk of septic shock and hypoxemia without shock in different genotypes of the LTA+250 single-nucleotide polymorphism in a community-acquired pneumonia cohort. (From Waterer GW, Quasney MW, Cantor RM, et al: Septic shock and respiratory failure in community-acquired pneumonia have different TNF polymorphism associations. Am J Respir Crit Care Med 2001;163: 1599-1604.)

neither site is the true causative mutation; instead, they may be markers for some other important mutation in this area, which is rich in genes that are important in the inflammatory response.

Interleukin (IL)-6 levels are a marker of the severity and outcome of sepsis. Carriage of the low IL-6 secretor phenotype of the –174 SNP was associated with improved survival in those with severe sepsis. However, the in vitro IL-6 response is affected more by levels of TNF, IL-10, and IL-1 (and possibly gender) than it is by this polymorphism, casting doubt on the clinical importance of this SNP and emphasizing the importance of multivariate analysis in association studies.[17]

Anti-inflammatory Mediators

The ability to modulate the proinflammatory response is important for avoiding persistent inflammation and organ failure. An association study from a large cohort of meningitis patients illustrates the importance of this balance, as well as other issues involved in genetic association studies.[21] The IL-1 family includes the agonists IL-1α and IL-1ß and the IL-1 receptor antagonist IL-1RN, with genes located in a cluster on chromosome 2. IL-1β and IL-1RN SNPs were examined concurrently in 1106 patients with meningococcal meningitis. The investigators consciously chose SNPs that were not likely to be causative mutations but were known to be in tight linkage disequilibrium with functional genetic variants in the same gene. Mortality was independently related to age, serogroup of the infecting microorganism, and both genotypes. This study illustrates the ability of multivariate analysis in association studies to determine the effect of genotype independent of nongenetic host factors and the variable pathogenicity of the infecting microorganism.

The IL-1RN polymorphism considered most likely to be causative is a variable 86–base pair tandem repeat, which contains at least three sites for DNA-binding proteins. Alleles are designated A1, A2, A3, A4, and A5, based on their relative frequencies in healthy populations. Although the results regarding the risk of infection with the A2 allele have been inconsistent, an increased risk of death from infection (up to 6.47-fold higher) has been found for IL-1RN A2 carriers in several studies.[14,22] Similar to the findings in meningitis patients, the combination of proinflammatory gene polymorphisms (IL-1α, IL-1β, or LTA+250) and the IL-1RN A2 polymorphism was associated with an even greater risk of death.

Another major anti-inflammatory protein is IL-10. Like TNF, IL-10 is highly polymorphic. Family members of children who died from meningococcemia had significantly greater IL-10 production after lipopolysaccharide stimulation than did family members of children who survived.[5] A specific IL-10 SNP (–1082) was not randomly distributed in first-degree relatives of patients with meningococcal disease.[23] These family studies suggest that genetic differences in IL-10 production may be important in the outcome of severe sepsis, and they are supported by population-based association studies. Homozygotes for the G allele of the IL-10 –1082 SNP had an increased risk of septic shock (odds ratio, 6.1) among patients with pneumococcal bacteremia.[24] The –592 SNP A allele was associated with death in a cohort of critically ill patients. Interestingly, the excess deaths occurred both in patients who developed sepsis and in critically ill patients without sepsis. Generally, the IL-10 association studies suggest that polymorphisms may play a role in disease severity while not predisposing to infection.

ACQUIRED IMMUNE RESPONSE

Because the acquired immune response does not occur immediately, its role in critically ill patients is not as well studied as the innate response. Genetic variation may still play a role in illnesses requiring ICU care.

Infection

Attachment of immunoglobulin bound to specific bacterial antigens occurs via their receptors on the surface of leukocytes. Several polymorphisms in immunoglobulin receptors lead to reduced binding affinity. The most well studied is the CD32 (FcγRII) subclass polymorphism associated with decreased binding of the immunoglobulin G2 subclass, important for encapsulated microorganisms as well as C-reactive protein.

Homozygosity for the lower-affinity allele was more common in patients with bacteremic pneumococcal pneumonia than in either nonbacteremic or control populations, with all early deaths in homozygotes.[25] Complicating the association is the fact that the Fcγ receptor genes are located on chromosome 1, near other immunologically important genes, especially IL-10. Although not clearly in linkage disequilibrium with known IL-10 SNPs, the SNP combinations were not randomly distributed in first-degree relatives of patients with meningococcal disease.[23]

Autoimmune Disease

The acquired immune response can result in autoimmune disease if it is directed at antigens similar to host antigens. Autoimmune diseases such as systemic lupus erythematosus or Wegener's granulomatosis are common causes of ICU admission. The extremely variable responses and presentations of these diseases strongly suggest a genetic component, and associations with multiple polymorphisms have been suggested. The risk of complications, such as renal failure with lupus, may be increased in certain genotypes. In addition, many of the chronic inflammatory disorders, such as rheumatoid arthritis and inflammatory bowel disease, have been associated with the same inflammatory response polymorphisms studied in sepsis and other infections. Although the increased risk of infectious complications is usually ascribed to the use of immune-modulating agents, the genetic risk may also play a role.

Organ Transplant Immunology

Although the importance of matching donor and recipient for HLA and other tissue antigens is well known, evidence is accumulating that genetic variation in the inflammatory response may play a role in both acute and chronic graft rejection. For example, a hypersecretory polymorphism in the transforming growth factor-ß gene results in a significantly increased risk of bronchiolitis obliterans after lung transplantation.[26] This is a rapidly expanding area of research. Once again, the increased risk of infection in these patients may reflect a genetic predisposition, in addition to the effect of immunosuppressants.

Specific Organ Failure Modulators

With severe infection, a variety of organs can fail. Most of the attention has focused on the risk of septic shock. However, not every patient with septic shock experiences failure of the same organs. Differences in resuscitation are probably the major explanation, but genetic variability probably plays a role as well.

One of the worst complications is the development of ARDS. An insertion-deletion polymorphism in the angiotensin-converting enzyme gene has been associated with an increased risk for the development of ARDS, as well as increased mortality once ARDS had occurred.[27] This fact illustrates the importance of appropriate control groups. As seen in Figure 45-5, ICU patients without ARDS have a slightly lower incidence of the DD genotype than do normal controls or cardiac surgery patients. If the difference in incidence were smaller, a statistically significant difference might have been seen only if compared with a control group of non-ARDS ICU patients, whereas a nonsignificant difference would have been found if healthy controls or post–cardiac surgery patients were chosen as the control group. Use of three control groups adds to the reliability of the association found. A SNP in the surfactant protein B gene has also been associated with a 2.4-fold increase in the odds of developing ARDS, particularly ARDS due to pneumonia.

The coagulation abnormalities of sepsis are also likely to have a genetic component. The prototypical coagulation abnormality with sepsis is meningococcemia, and several cohorts have been studied. This disease is more common in children, facilitating family-based association studies. The relatively common factor V Leiden mutation has been associated with an increased risk of complications in heterozygotes.[28] The plasminogen activator inhibitor-1 insertion-deletion polymorphism is also associated with an increased risk of shock and other complications.[19] The availability of drotrecogin alfa for the treatment of sepsis will undoubtedly increase interest in the variability in coagulation pathways in sepsis and inflammation.

RISK OF COAGULATION OR THROMBOSIS

Genetic hypercoagulability syndromes play a role in many disorders leading to ICU admission. Chief among these are deep venous thrombosis, pulmonary emboli, myocardial infarction, cerebrovascular disease, and complications of pregnancy. Because of the frequency of these diseases, large-scale studies can be performed, allowing highly significant statistical associations to be found despite a very small attributable risk. These associations tend to be more apparent in younger patients, in whom the effect of comorbid illnesses

and environmental factors cause less interference with the genetic risk signal.

Deficiencies in protein C, protein S, or antithrombin are the classic examples of genetic risk factors for deep venous thrombosis and pulmonary emboli.[29] However, the genetic basis of these deficiencies is the combination of more than 120 specific mutations for each factor. Screening based on genotyping is therefore impractical, and the diagnosis of these genetic diseases relies on the measurement of blood levels. With the discovery of the factor V Leiden and prothrombin G20210A polymorphisms, the percentage of patients (especially whites) with venous thromboemboli who can be documented to have a hypercoagulable state increased from less than 10% to approximately 30%. In patients with a family or personal history suggesting an increased risk, the proportion diagnosed may reach 70%. A functional assay, activated protein C resistance, screens for factor V Leiden and several less common polymorphisms. However, genotyping is routinely available.

Factor V Leiden in thromboembolic disease illustrates the goal for most gene association studies in common clinical illnesses. This SNP impacts clinical management in that homozygous patients or heterozygotes with other concomitant causes of thrombophilia warrant prolonged treatment with anticoagulants. Clinical suspicion can lead to a high frequency of confirmed diagnoses, and a screening test is readily available. A definite diagnosis has implications for the individual, as well as family members. The role of this polymorphism is unquestioned, despite interactions with other genes and environmental factors. In spite of large studies, the clinical utility of diagnosing genetic variations in patients with myocardial infarction or stroke is poor compared with that in the hypercoagulable model.

PHARMACOGENOMICS

Pharmacogenomics is the use of genetic information to individualize drug therapy. It has been heralded as one of the most likely immediate benefits of the Human Genome Project. This is clearly another area in which genetics will have an impact on critical care medicine. The genetic influence will be seen in two main areas—effects on drug metabolism and individualized therapy.

DRUG METABOLISM

Interindividual differences in drug metabolism are well known. These differences commonly are responsible for adverse drug reactions. It is logical to assume that functional genetic polymorphisms may be a major component of these interindividual differences and, by extension, the adverse drug reactions associated with them.[30] Polymorphisms most often result in poor drug metabolism, but occasionally they can cause ultrarapid metabolism.

One of the more extensively studied metabolic pathways is the cytochrome P_{450} (CYP) enzyme superfamily. More than 30 CYP enzymes are known, with functional polymorphisms described in most of the common ones. Table 45-1 lists such enzymes that alter the metabolism of drugs commonly used in the ICU. At least 55% of the drugs cited in studies of acute drug reactions are metabolized by enzymes with variant alleles. Interestingly, simply altering drug metabolism may not increase the number of acute drug

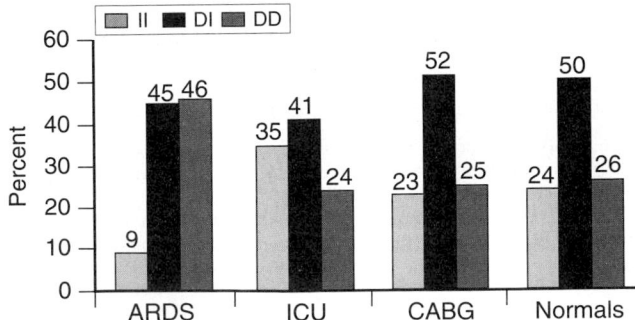

FIGURE 45–5. Comparison of angiotensin-converting enzyme (ACE) gene insertion-deletion polymorphism frequencies in acute respiratory distress syndrome (ARDS) patients versus other comparison populations. CABG, coronary artery bypass graft. (From Marshall RP, Webb S, Bellingan GJ, et al: Angiotensin converting enzyme insertion/deletion polymorphism is associated with susceptibility and outcome in acute respiratory distress syndrome. Am J Respir Crit Care Med 2002;166:646-650.)

TABLE 45–1. COMMON ICU DRUGS METABOLIZED BY ENZYMES WITH VARIANT ALLELES

Enzyme	Drugs
CYP1A2	**Verapamil, isoniazid, acetaminophen, haloperidol,** theophylline, diltiazem, erythromycin, imipramine, phenytoin, rifampin, fluoxetine
CYP2C9	**Warfarin, rifampin, ibuprofen, imipramine,** phenytoin, tolbutamide, fluoxetine, naproxen, isoniazid, verapamil
CYP2C18	Fluoxetine, imipramine, rifampin
CYP2C19	**Isoniazid,** omeprazole, diazepam, cyclophosphamide, nortriptyline, S-mephenytoin, rifampin, warfarin, fluoxetine
CYP2D6	**Metoprolol, imipramine, nortriptyline, codeine, encainide, flecainide,** dextromethorphan, fluoxetine, theophylline, diltiazem
CYP2E1	Theophylline, isoniazid, verapamil, fluoxetine
NAT2	**Isoniazid**

CYP, cytochrome P_{450}; NAT, N-acetyltransferase.
Bold indicates a major metabolic pathway.

reactions directly. Although CYP1A2 is the metabolic pathway for only 5% of all prescribed drugs, it is at least partially involved in the metabolism of 75% of the drugs that are associated with adverse reactions and metabolized by enzymes with variant alleles.[30]

One of the better examples of the clinical application of genetically determined drug metabolism is in the dosing of warfarin (Coumadin). Warfarin is metabolized by the CYP2C9 enzyme, and variant alleles of this enzyme lead to poor metabolism. Patients who carry these alleles (6% to 9% of whites) require significantly lower doses of warfarin. However, the risk of adverse drug reactions has not been shown conclusively to be greater. The genetic effect is partially offset by the individualization of dose and is clearly affected by environmental factors (diet) and other medical conditions (liver disease, cor pulmonale). However, time to therapeutic dosing, an important cost issue, may be optimized if the genotype is known. Lack of a commercially available assay limits the clinical use of individualized dosing regimens based on genotyping.

In addition to drug metabolism, drug receptor polymorphisms may play a role in therapeutic response. Polymorphisms in genes coding for a variety of common drug receptors are known, such as the beta-adrenergic agonist or glucocorticoid receptors.

INDIVIDUALIZED THERAPY

Although the polymorphisms involved in drug metabolism may be able to determine the appropriate individual dose, one of the nebulous goals of pharmacogenomics is individualizing drug choice in a specific clinical scenario. In the ICU, these decisions are increasingly important because of the availability of expensive drugs with low therapeutic ratios, such as drotrecogin alfa.

One concern is that not accounting for genetic variability may have sidetracked the development of effective agents. For example, would use of anti-TNF strategies or therapeutic use of IL-10 be beneficial in septic patients with TNF hypersecretor genotypes? Many of the novel agents studied in sepsis trials had good theoretical, experimental, and animal study support for their efficacy. The failure to document any benefit in large human trials may reflect the inability to choose appropriate patient groups rather than the agents' ineffectiveness.

The ultimate goals of genetic studies in critically ill patients revolve around two issues: to better understand the pathogenesis of the disease (in order to design better treatment interventions) and to better define the patient group at increased risk (in order to choose the appropriate patients for treatment). In future editions of this textbook, discussions of genetics will no doubt be incorporated into individual chapters on the risks and treatment options of specific diseases.

ANNOTATED REFERENCES

Kiechl S, Lorenz E, Reindl M, et al: Toll-like receptor 4 polymorphisms and atherogenesis. N Engl J Med 2002;347:185-192.
  This is one of the few long-term studies that provided data on the risk of infection based on genetic predisposition, although this was not a primary focus of the study.

Marshall RP, Webb S, Bellingan GJ, et al: Angiotensin converting enzyme insertion/deletion polymorphism is associated with susceptibility and outcome in acute respiratory distress syndrome. Am J Respir Crit Care Med 2002;166:646-650.
  This large study documented the association between the angiotensin-converting enzyme genotype and the risk and severity of ARDS. It also illustrated the potential risk of choosing different comparison populations.

Read RC, Cannings C, Naylor SC, et al: Variations within genes encoding interleukin-1 and the interleukin-1 receptor antagonist influence the severity of meningococcal disease. Ann Intern Med 2003;138:534-541.
  This large study from a referral center demonstrated interactions among pathogen (serotype), host (age), two genetic factors, and outcome. A combination of excess inflammatory and anti-inflammatory polymorphisms was associated with the worst outcome.

Sorensen TI, Nielsen GG, Andersen PK, et al: Genetic and environmental influences on premature death in adult adoptees. N Engl J Med 1988;318:727-732.
  This landmark study of adoptees demonstrated an increased risk of death from infection if one natural parent died of infection.

Stuber F, Petersen M, Bokelmann F, et al: A genomic polymorphism within the tumor necrosis factor locus influences plasma tumor necrosis factor-alpha concentrations and outcome of patients with severe sepsis. Crit Care Med 1996;24:381-384.
  This seminal article outlines the genetic influence on sepsis and critical illness.

Waterer GW, Quasney MW, Cantor RM, et al: Septic shock and respiratory failure in community-acquired pneumonia have different TNF polymorphism associations. Am J Respir Crit Care Med 2001;163:1599-1604.
  The authors document that different manifestations of severe community-acquired pneumonia are associated with different LTA genotypes.

Section III

CENTRAL NERVOUS SYSTEM

Chapter 46

BIOCHEMICAL, CELLULAR, AND MOLECULAR MECHANISMS OF NEURONAL DEATH AND SECONDARY BRAIN INJURY IN CRITICAL CARE

Robert S.B. Clark • Larry Jenkins • Yi-Chen Lai • Xiaopeng Zhang • Patrick M. Kochanek

KEY POINTS

1. Many of the biochemical, cellular, and molecular mechanisms that are important to the evolution of secondary damage after insults in neurointensive care, including cardiopulmonary arrest, stroke, traumatic brain injury, subarachnoid hemorrhage, status epilepticus, and hypoglycemia, share cerebral ischemia and/or energy failure as a critical initiator of damage.

2. Global cerebral ischemic insults, such as those that result from cardiopulmonary arrest, are generally brief in cases of patients who can be resuscitated successfully. The pathobiologic condition that results is characterized by delayed neuronal death in selectively vulnerable brain regions, and the biochemical and molecular cascades in these cases involve components of programmed cell death. However, classic apoptosis has not been observed.

3. Focal cerebral ischemic insults, such as those that result from stroke and subarachnoid hemorrhage, generally include an ischemic focus surrounded by peri-ischemic penumbral regions. The biochemical and molecular cascades involve necrosis and/or infarct expansion into the penumbra. Cell death in the penumbra can include phenotypes that span the continuum from necrosis to apoptosis.

4. In cases of traumatic brain injury, the biochemical and molecular mechanisms involved depend on the specific type of insult, ranging from focal contusion (in which local osmolar swelling and excitotoxicity predominate) to diffuse axonal injury (in which secondary axotomy from proteolysis predominates).

5. Excitotoxicity, resulting from increases in brain interstitial concentrations of a number of excitatory amino acids, is a common mediator of secondary injury across insults.

6. Programmed cell death, or apoptosis, involves several distinct pathways, including an extrinsic pathway triggered by external cell signals such as death receptor-ligand interaction; an intrinsic pathway triggered by signals from mitochondrial or endoplasmic reticulum; and a caspase-independent pathway involving mitochondrial dysfunction. However, delayed neuronal death in patients with critical central nervous system insults in the intensive care unit does not demonstrate classic apoptotic features but rather commonly exhibits a mixed phenotype.

7. Cerebral swelling can result from a variety of cellular mechanisms, including vasogenic edema, astrocyte swelling, increased tissue osmolar load, or vascular dysregulation with increased cerebral blood volume.

8. Inflammation appears to have a dichotomous role after cerebral ischemia or traumatic brain injury, including early exacerbation of damage by inflammatory mediators but secondary benefit through the link between inflammation and regeneration.

In this chapter, we provide a general discussion of the biochemical, cellular, and molecular mechanism of neuronal death and secondary brain injury that are germane to the central nervous system (CNS) insults that require neurointensive care, highlighting the important shared mechanisms in these conditions. In the chapter that follows, Dr. Kofke builds upon the biochemical and molecular mechanisms to address general pathophysiologic principles in neurointensive care, focusing on intracranial dynamics and the cerebral circulation. Finally, the chapters that follow address other important facets of neurointensive care, such as monitoring and coma, along with the specific pathophysiology and treatment of the key disease processes central to neurointensive care in both adults and children. This includes traumatic brain injury (TBI), cardiopulmonary arrest, stroke, subarachnoid hemorrhage (SAH), and seizures, among other insults.

A thumbnail sketch of the most important mechanisms of secondary injury involved in the brain after a traumatic or ischemic insult is provided in Figure 46-1. Central to all brain insults relevant to neurointensive care is the occurrence of cerebral ischemia and/or cerebral energy failure. Indeed, for cardiopulmonary arrest and stroke, global or focal brain

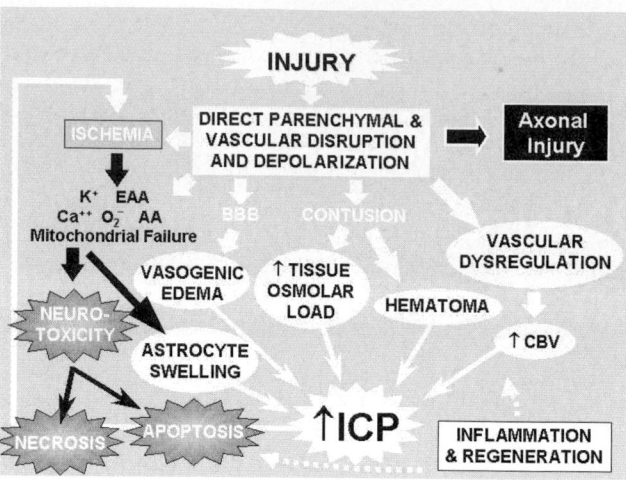

FIGURE 46–1. Categories of biochemical, cellular, and molecular mechanisms proposed to be involved in the evolution of secondary damage after ischemic or traumatic brain injury. Three major categories for these secondary mechanisms include (1) ischemia, excitotoxicity, energy failure, and cell death cascades; (2) cerebral swelling; and (3) axonal injury. A fourth category, inflammation and regeneration, contributes to each of these cascades.

ischemia, respectively, energy failure defines the insult. In cases of TBI, direct parenchymal or vascular disruption or vasospasm often leads to cerebral ischemia, although tissue deformation such as axonal and vascular stretching and shearing along with hemorrhage and dendritic injury also are involved. In cases of SAH, hemorrhage is often followed by delayed vasospasm, with subsequent secondary cerebral ischemia. Finally, seizures and hypoglycemia can lead to neuronal death and represent situations in which relative ischemia is produced, either from enhanced metabolic demands that are greater than supply or from reduced substrate delivery, respectively. Energy failure ensues, and if the insult is sufficient in duration, cellular injury or death can occur. Clearly, ischemia and energy failure are key culprits in producing the pathophysiology of neurointensive care insults.

The principal consequence of ischemic injury and/or energy failure is neuronal death. The two principal forms of ischemia in neurointensive care are global and focal, as seen in cases of cardiopulmonary arrest and stroke, respectively.

GLOBAL CEREBRAL ISCHEMIA

In patients with global cerebral ischemia, insults are dense and often square-wave in nature.[1] The classic example of a global cerebral ischemic insult in neurointensive care is ventricular fibrillation cardiopulmonary arrest (see Chapter 50). Using conventional approaches, patients can be successfully resuscitated from these insults only if they are brief in nature; that is, circulation must be restored in approximately 5 to 12 minutes, although the maximal duration compatible with intact neurologic outcome can depend on a variety of factors, such as temperature. In cases of complete global cerebral ischemia, adenosine triphosphate (ATP) and phosphocreatine levels in brain are depleted in less than 2 minutes.[1-3] Membrane failure ensues, with loss of ion homeostasis that includes cellular release of K^+ and uptake of Ca^{++}, Na^+, and Cl^-.[2,3] Upon reperfusion, a complex sequence of events is set into motion that depends on the duration of the insult. Disturbances in lipid metabolism such as free fatty acid release

and DNA damage result, along with a series of deleterious cascades including oxidative and nitrosative stress, excitotoxicity, poly-ADP-ribose polymerase (PARP) activation, mitochondrial and endoplasmic reticulum (ER) dysfunction, and a host of cell-signaling abnormalities. A number of endogenous neuroprotectant responses are also initiated. The specific biochemical, cellular, and molecular events are discussed later. The aforementioned increases in intracellular calcium level are believed to play a critical role in initiating many of these events. In situations in which there is potential salvage of the patient, such as with threshold insults, reperfusion results in transient hyperemia (minutes) followed by delayed hypoperfusion (hours).[1,4,5] The pattern of neuronal damage that is seen after global cerebral ischemia is classically termed *selective vulnerability*. This is often delayed and primarily neuronal in nature, and it is believed to result from complex biologic cascades involving some features of programmed cell death (discussed later).

A number of brain regions are specifically vulnerable to ischemia, including the CA1 region of the hippocampus, cortical layers 3, 5, and 6, portions of the amygdaloid nucleus, and cerebellar Purkinje cells, among others.[2,3,5] Global ischemic insults from cardiopulmonary arrest from which there is some potential for recovery are generally believed to be devoid of important increases in intracranial pressure, since, based on studies in animal models, it has been shown that the threshold for producing poor outcome in patients with global ischemic insults is less than that needed to generate clinically significant intracranial hypertension.[6] Thus, brain edema and vascular injury are not believed to represent important therapeutic targets after global cerebral ischemia. Two relevant but atypical global insults in neurointensive care are asphyxial cardiopulmonary arrest (particularly important in children and discussed in Chapter 59), and near-hanging episodes. In the latter, obstruction of cerebral venous drainage during the asphyxial insult compounds the ischemic insult.

FOCAL CEREBRAL ISCHEMIA

Focal ischemic insults in neurointensive care are produced by thrombotic or embolic events and generally produce a dense ischemic focus that is surrounded by a peri-ischemic penumbral region with intermediate cerebral blood flow (CBF) values.[2] The ischemic focus is generally believed to be unsalvageable unless reperfused almost immediately. In contrast, the ischemic penumbra is a region with some collateral flow and represents a therapeutic target for reperfusion with thrombolytics and/or pharmacological therapy. In cases of focal cerebral ischemia, a hierarchy of CBF thresholds has been demonstrated in experimental studies, with inhibition of protein synthesis being the most sensitive to CBF reductions, followed by loss of electrical activity (evoked potentials and electroencephalogram), and eventually membrane failure.[7,8] Unlike the selective vulnerability seen in global ischemic insults, focal cerebral ischemia produces pan-necrosis of the vasculature and astrocytes, resulting in infarction. However, cell death in the penumbra can demonstrate necrotic, apoptotic, and mixed phenotypes. Again, however, classic apoptosis is not seen. Astrocyte swelling and blood-brain barrier injury, with focal cerebral edema, can play important roles. In the penumbra, spreading depression waves resulting in depolarization can enhance excitotoxic damage with expansion of the lesion core. Reperfusion can occur spontaneously or with the administration of thrombolytics and can produce a microcosm of the aforementioned oxidative and nitrosative stress, mitochondrial and ER damage, and cell signaling abnormalities seen in global cerebral ischemia. In patients with focal cerebral ischemia, with large infarcts, brain swelling can be substantial enough that secondary ischemia can result from intracranial hypertension. Dr. Kofke discusses these concepts in greater detail in Chapter 47. Focal cerebral ischemia from delayed vasospasm is also the most common critical complication of SAH and is discussed in Chapter 52.

TRAUMATIC BRAIN INJURY

In cases of severe TBI, the biochemical and molecular mechanisms involved depend on the specific type of injury. In cases of focal contusion, direct disruption of parenchyma with local necrosis and hemorrhage results in superimposed vascular disruption, blood-brain barrier permeability, and local ischemia. This sets the stage for excitotoxicity and necrotizing cascades in the contusion penumbra, including oxidative and nitrosative stress, and calpain-mediated proteolysis, among other mechanisms.[9,10] Local axonal injury is also seen in patients with contusions. Focal contusions are commonly complicated by marked local swelling and often by intracranial hypertension with the potential for secondary focal or global ischemic insults or herniation syndromes. In contrast, in diffuse injury, a constellation of diffuse axonal and vascular disruption can be seen with characteristic findings of petechial hemorrhages in the white matter.[11] This insult can be devastating even in the absence of intracranial hypertension.[12] The biochemical and molecular events involved in axonal injury are discussed later. In cases of severe TBI, combined insults that include both multiple contusions and diffuse injury are also common. Finally, in addition to secondary ischemia from refractory intracranial hypertension, secondary extracerebral insults such as hypotension and hypoxemia can also negatively affect outcome and, importantly, complicate the biochemical and molecular response to severe TBI, markedly enhancing delayed neuronal death in brain regions that might otherwise have recovered.[13,14]

KEY BIOCHEMICAL AND MOLECULAR MECHANISMS OF NEURONAL SECONDARY DAMAGE

A number of pathologic cascades are shared by these important insults in neurointensive care, including excitotoxicity, programmed cell death, axonal injury, and inflammation, along with a spectrum of endogenous neuroprotectant responses.

EXCITOTOXICITY

Excitotoxicity describes the process by which glutamate and other excitatory amino acids cause neuronal damage. Lucas and Newhouse[15] first described the toxicity of glutamate. Olney[16] subsequently reported that intraperitoneal administration of glutamate produces brain injury in experimental animals. Although glutamate is the most abundant neurotransmitter in the brain, exposure to toxic levels produces neuronal death.[17] Glutamate exposure produces neuronal injury in two phases. Minutes after exposure, sodium-dependent neuronal swelling occurs.[18] This is followed by delayed, calcium-dependent degeneration. These effects are

mediated through both ionophore-linked receptors, labeled according to specific agonists (N-methyl-D-aspartate [NMDA], kainite, and α-amino-3-hydroxy-5-methyl-4-isoxazolepropionic acid [AMPA]), and receptors linked to second messenger systems, called metabotropic receptors. Activation of these receptors leads to calcium influx through receptor-gated or voltage-gated channels, or through the release of intracellular calcium stores. Increased intracellular calcium concentration is the trigger for a number of processes that can lead to cellular injury or death (Fig. 46-2). One mechanism involves activation of neuronal nitric oxide (NO) synthase, leading to NO production, peroxynitrite formation, and resultant DNA damage. PARP is an enzyme operative in DNA repair, and in the face of DNA damage, PARP activation leads to ATP depletion, metabolic failure, and cell death.[19-21] This may be important, since PARP knockout mice exhibit improved outcome versus controls after experimental stroke or TBI.[20,22]

There is considerable evidence in experimental laboratory models supporting an important contribution of excitotoxicity to the evolution of secondary damage in cases of global and focal cerebral ischemia, severe TBI, SAH, and status epilepticus.[23-30] Evidence supporting an important role for excitotoxicity in humans has similarly been provided in cases of severe TBI, stroke, and SAH. Persson and Hillered[31] reported increases in brain interstitial levels of glutamate in a patient with SAH as early as 1992. Palmer and associates[32] first demonstrated increased concentrations of excitatory amino acids in ventricular cerebrospinal fluid (CSF) from adult patients with TBI. Glutamate concentrations were about fivefold greater than in control patients (up to 7 μM)—levels sufficient to cause neuronal death in cell culture.[33] Bullock and associates[34] characterized patterns of glutamate release by measuring excitatory amino acids by microdialysis in patients after TBI. Patients with a normal head computed tomography scan and no secondary ischemic events had interstitial concentrations of glutamate that were increased early in their course, then returned to normal. In contrast, patients with a progressively rising level of glutamate died. Similarly, in cases of human stroke, Bullock and associates[35] reported massive increases in the excitatory amino acids glutamate and aspartate in a patient who required decompressive craniectomy to prevent brainstem herniation.

Despite these and many other clinical reports, clinical trials with anti-excitotoxic therapies have been unsuccessful in patients with either stroke or TBI. This may be due to problems with patient selection, side effects of the anti-excitotoxic agents that were tested, and the likelihood that treatment was initiated too late.[36] Inhibition of plasticity by anti-excitotoxic therapies may also limit their efficacy, especially at the interface between the acute and subacute periods after injury.[37]

APOPTOSIS/PROGRAMMED CELL DEATH CASCADES

It is now increasingly clear from experimental models and human data that cells dying after global or focal cerebral ischemia or TBI can be categorized on a morphologic continuum ranging from necrosis to apoptosis.[38,39] Apoptosis is a morphologic description of cell death defined by cell shrinkage and nuclear condensation, internucleosomal DNA fragmentation, and the formation of apoptotic bodies.[40] In contrast, cells dying of necrosis display cellular and nuclear swelling with dissolution of membranes. Apoptosis requires

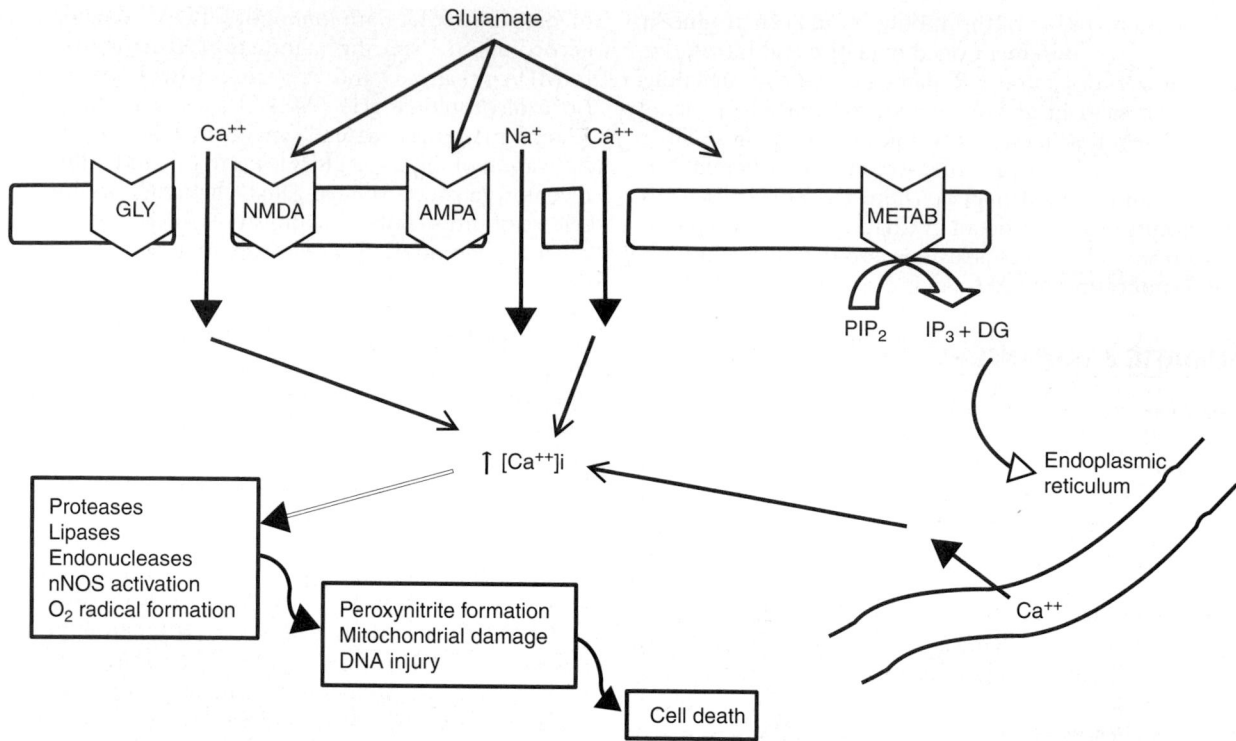

FIGURE 46–2. Mechanisms involved in excitotoxicity. Glutamate causes an increase in intracellular calcium concentration through stimulation of (1) the NMDA receptor with opening of the receptor-linked calcium ionophore, (2) the AMPA receptor with opening of the voltage-gated calcium channels, and (3) the metabotropic receptor, with the release of intracellular calcium stores via the second messengers inositol triphosphate and diacylglycerol. Increased intracellular calcium concentration leads to activation of proteases, lipases, and endonucleases, along with neuronal NOS (nNOS) stimulation and production of oxygen radicals. This results in peroxynitrite formation, mitochondrial damage, and DNA injury with subsequent cellular injury and death. AMPA, α-amino-3-hydroxy-5-methylisoxazole-4-propionic acid receptor; DG, diacylglycerol; GLY, glycine co-agonist site; IP$_3$, inositol triphosphate; METAB, glutamate metabotropic receptor; NMDA, N-methyl-D-aspartate receptor; PIP$_2$, phosphoinositide.

a cascade of intracellular events for completion of cell death; thus, *programmed cell death* is the currently accepted term for the process of cell death that leads to apoptosis.[41] In diseases with complex and multiple mechanisms, such as stroke and TBI, it is typically difficult to distinguish clinical apoptotic from necrotic cell death as classically defined.[42] Some cells may display DNA fragmentation and activation of proteases involved in programmed cell death, despite having nuclear and cellular swelling. Dying cells with mixed phenotypes are very common and may represent particularly difficult therapeutic targets.

Biochemical Pathways in Delayed Neuronal Death

Programmed cell death is an evolutionarily conserved process required for selective cell elimination during development, and it occurs in all tissues, including brain. Execution of programmed cell death requires novel gene expression and protein synthesis.[43-45] Programmed cell death is an intricate and critical mechanism for balancing cell proliferation, remodeling of tissues during development, and maintenance of tissues with a high rate of cell turnover. Programmed cell death can be thought of as "molecular débridement," delicately eliminating unwanted cells with minimal disturbance of neighboring cells. Programmed cell death is cybernetic and may occur via multiple pathways that can be independent (Fig. 46-3); however, cross-talk between these pathways also may occur.[46] At present, neuronal programmed cell death can be segregated into two

pathways, one involving the activation of a family of cysteine proteases termed *caspases*, and one that is caspase independent.[47]

Caspase family proteases include 14 currently identified members that are synthesized as pro-enzymes,[48] which for the most part are proteolytically activated.[49] Initiator caspases, including caspase-8, -9, and -10, are activated by autocleavage and aggregation. Executioner caspases, including caspase-3, -6, and -7, are cleaved and activated by initiator caspases. The proteolytic cleavage of caspase substrates produces the phenotypic changes characteristic of programmed cell death, including cytoskeletal disintegration, DNA fragmentation, and disruption of cellular and DNA repair processes (Fig. 46-4). Cytoskeletal caspase targets include spectrin and nuclear lamin[50]; in addition, caspase-3 activates the enzyme gelsolin, which cleaves actin.[51] Active caspase-3 can also cleave the inhibitor of caspase-dependent deoxyribonuclease, permitting caspase-dependent deoxyribonuclease to digest DNA into small oligonucleosomal fragments.[52] These small DNA fragments (multiples of approximately 180 base pairs) can be seen on a DNA gel as a ladder and are a hallmark of caspase-dependent programmed cell death. Caspase-3 also inhibits DNA repair by proteolytically inactivating many DNA repair proteins, including PARP.[53-55] This combination of features—silencing of the genome and incapacitation of DNA repair processes, and destruction of key cytoskeletal components, all with surgical-like precision and ultimately leading to cell death—illustrates why programmed cell death has been referred to as "cell suicide."

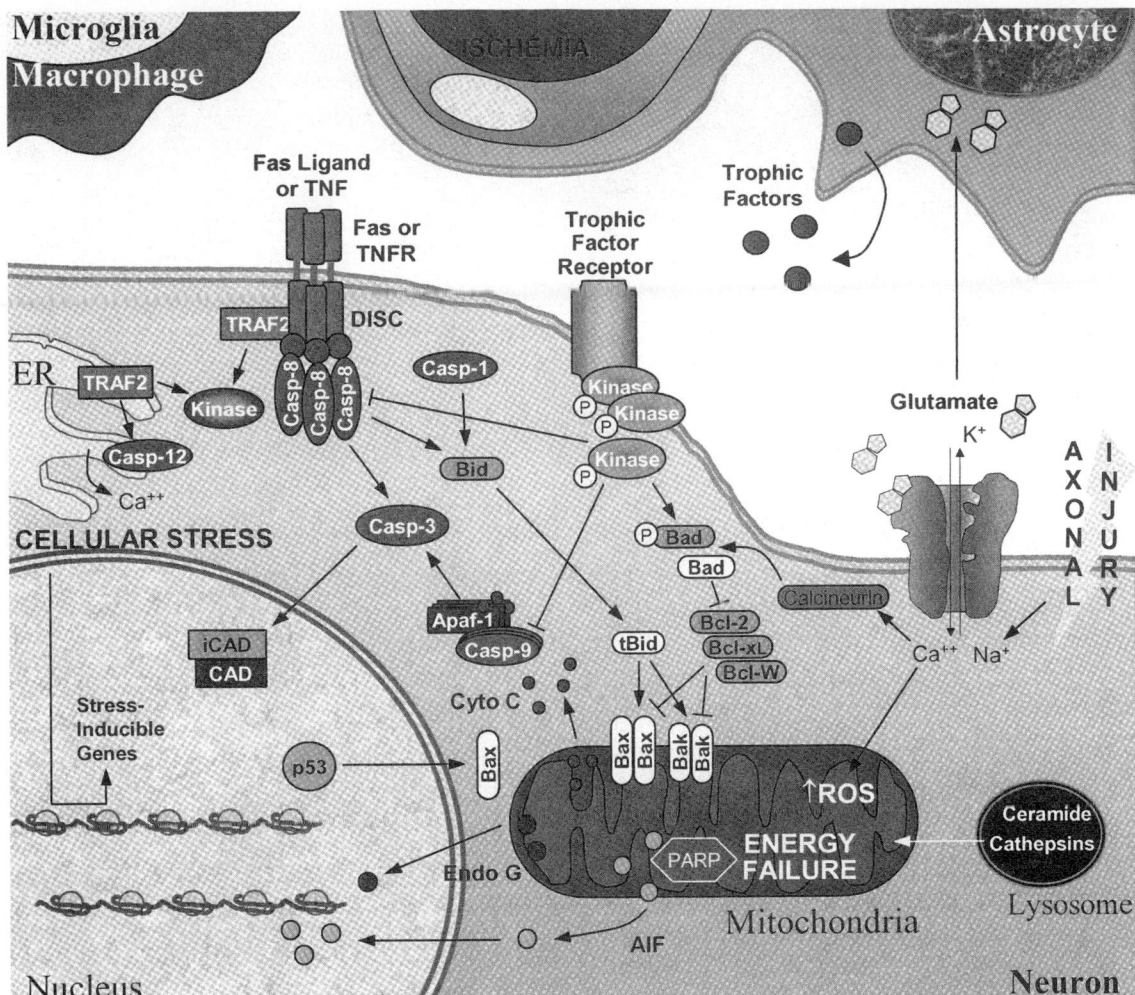

FIGURE 46–3. A simplified schematic representation of the initiation and regulation of neuronal programmed cell death after brain injury. Pathologic mechanisms triggering programmed cell death after brain injury include ischemia, oxidative stress, energy failure, excitotoxicity (primarily excess glutamate), axonal injury, trophic factor withdrawal, ER stress, and death receptor-ligand binding (e.g., TNF, Fas). Regulation of programmed cell death occurs via multiple pathways, including kinase-dependent intracellular signaling pathways and Bcl-2 family proteins. AIF, apoptosis inducing factor; Apaf-1, apoptotic protease activating factor-1; Bcl, B-cell lymphoma; CAD, caspase-activated deoxyribonuclease; casp, caspase; cyto c, cytochrome c; DISC, death-inducing signaling complex; Endo G, endonuclease G; ER, endoplasmic reticulum; iCAD, inhibitor of CAD; ROS, reactive oxygen species; tBid, truncated Bid; TNF, tumor necrosis factor; TNFR, TNF receptor; TRAF2, TNF receptor associated factor.

Extrinsic Pathways of Programmed Cell Death

Programmed cell death can be initiated by extrinsic or intrinsic signals. Extrinsic signals include cell surface death receptor-ligand interactions and cell signaling pathways. The most prominent cell death receptor family is the tumor necrosis factor (TNF) receptor superfamily, which includes TNF-α and Fas.[56] The coupling of cell surface TNF or Fas receptors with extracellular TNF-α or Fas ligand induces trimerization of the receptors that leads to the formation of submembrane complexes with intracellular death domain-signaling molecules. This death-inducing signaling complex then activates caspase-8[57] or -10.[58] Caspase-3 is then cleaved and activated, perpetuating the cascade. The extrinsic pathway can also be regulated by multiple intracellular signal transduction pathways that are initiated by G-protein coupled cell surface receptors, which can be either activated by neurotransmitters (e.g., cyclic nucleotides) or inactivated by interruption of trophic factors (e.g., nerve growth factor) after injury.[59] Perturbations in neurotransmitters and trophic factors controlling these pathways occur after ischemia

and TBI. Multiple interrelated pro-death or pro-survival kinase pathways have been identified, including those involving mitogen-activated protein kinases, and protein kinase B and protein kinase C.[60,61]

Intrinsic Pathways of Programmed Cell Death

The intrinsic programmed cell death pathway is triggered by stress on cellular organelles, notably mitochondria and ER. Mitochondrial stress can lead to caspase-dependent programmed cell death via mitochondrial release of cytochrome C induced upon mitochondrial membrane depolarization. Egress of cytochrome C into the cytosol enables interaction with apoptotic protease activating factor-1 (Apaf-1), dATP, and pro-caspase-9 to form a complex termed an *apoptosome*. Apaf-1 activates caspase-9 and subsequently caspase-3.[62] Several mitochondrial proteins are capable of inducing programmed cell death without direct activation of the caspase cascade, thus exemplifying pathways that are caspase-independent. Apoptosis-inducing factor (AIF) within the mitochondria serves as an antioxidant[63]; however, upon

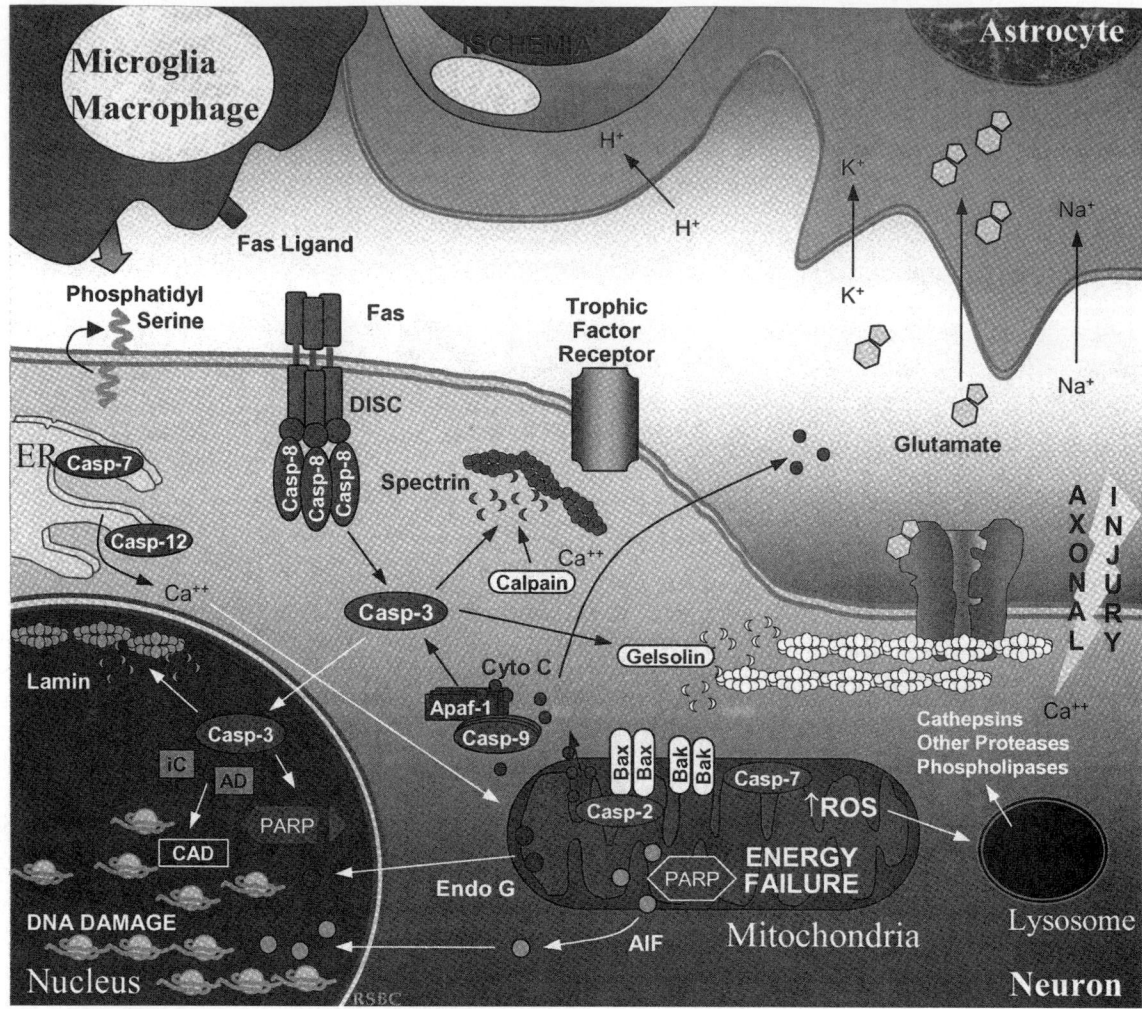

FIGURE 46–4. A simplified schematic representation of the execution of neuronal programmed cell death after brain injury. Execution of programmed cell death involves the caspase cascade and/or release of apoptogenic factors from organelles such as mitochondria. Ultimately, DNA fragmentation, cytoskeletal disintegration, and externalization of membrane phosphatidyl serine occur, signaling macrophages and microglia to engulf cellular debris. AIF, apoptosis inducing factor; Apaf-1, apoptotic protease activating factor-1; Bcl, B-cell lymphoma; CAD, caspase-activated deoxyribonuclease; casp, caspase; cyto c, cytochrome c; DISC, death-inducing signaling complex; Endo G, endonuclease G; ER, endoplasmic reticulum; iCAD, inhibitor of CAD; ROS, reactive oxygen species.

mitochondrial membrane depolarization, it can translocate from the mitochondria to the nucleus, where it is sufficient to induce programmed cell death.[64] Translocation of AIF into the nuclei induces the formation of large-scale DNA fragmentation (>50 kilobase pairs), in contrast to cytochrome C-mediated, caspase-dependent programmed cell death, which leads to oligonucleosomal DNA fragmentation (180-1200 base pairs). AIF-mediated programmed cell death occurs in neurons under conditions of experimental TBI[65] and cerebral ischemia.[66] Other mitochondrial proteins related to programmed cell death include endonuclease G,[67] Htr2A/Omi,[68] and Smac/Diablo[69]; however, their roles in neuronal death after brain injury remain unexplored. Disruption of ER calcium homeostasis and/or accumulation of excess proteins can lead to ER stress, which in turn can trigger programmed cell death via activation of ER-localized caspase-12, an upstream initiator caspase. ER stress–related activation of caspase-12 has been detected in experimental models of cerebral ischemia[70] and TBI.[71]

Regulation of Programmed Cell Death by the Bcl-2 Protein Family

Both caspase-dependent and caspase-independent programmed cell death are regulated by the B-cell lymphoma-2 (Bcl-2) family of proteins. The Bcl-2 family contains both pro-death and pro-survival members.[72] Bcl-2 family proteins regulate changes in permeability of the mitochondrial outer membrane independent of permeability transition pore formation. Bcl-2 family proteins contain highly conserved Bcl-2 homology domains (BH 1-4) essential for homo- and hetero-complex formation.[73] Complexes formed between proteins containing BH-3 domains such as Bax, truncated Bid, and Bad can facilitate mitochondrial cytochrome C release.[74,75] The anti-apoptotic members Bcl-2, Bcl-xL, and Mcl-1L prevent the release of mitochondrial proteins by inhibiting the pore formation.[76] Bax expression is associated with neuronal cell death after cardiac arrest in dogs.[77] Transgenic mice overexpressing Bcl-2 are partially protected from the neuropathologic sequelae of TBI versus wild-type mice.[78] Overexpression of Bcl-xL also inhibits neuronal cell death after focal cerebral ischemia.[79]

Programmed Cell Death in Human Brain Injury

Phenotypic descriptions of programmed cell death occurring after brain injury in humans date back to the 1940s.[80,81] However, biochemical evidence of programmed cell death after brain injury in humans has been reported only within the last decade and has now been reported after TBI,[82-84] stroke,[85] and epilepsy.[86] Brain tissue samples from TBI patients requiring decompressive craniectomy for the treatment of life-threatening intracranial hypertension were found to have evidence of DNA fragmentation by terminal deoxynucleotidyl transferase-mediated nick-end labeling (TUNEL) and cleavage of caspase-1 and -3, suggesting activation of the programmed cell death cascade.[82] Recently, the up-regulation of caspase-8 in human brain after TBI at both transcriptional and translational levels has been reported.[84] Caspase-8 was found predominantly in neurons and was associated with relative levels of the death receptor Fas, providing evidence of the extrinsic programmed cell death pathway within neurons. Increases in Fas and Fas ligand have also been reported in cerebrospinal fluid from TBI patients, with Fas levels correlating with intracranial pressure.[87,88] Activation of the intrinsic pathway also occurs after TBI. Alteration of Bcl-2 family proteins has been reported in human brain from adults and in CSF from infants and children after TBI.[82,83,89] In pediatric patients, lower concentrations of Bcl-2 were detected in patients who died than in those who survived, supporting a pro-survival role for Bcl-2.[83] After TBI in adults, the presence of pro-death Bcl-2 family protein Bax in patients in whom Bcl-2 was also detectable represented a more favorable outcome as compared with patients in whom Bax but not Bcl-2 was detectable.[90] In contrast to TBI patients, patients after stroke demonstrate reductions in soluble Bcl-2 and soluble Fas within CSF,[85] suggesting dysregulation of programmed cell death after stroke. In adolescents and young adults with refractory seizures, increases in Bcl-2 and Bcl-xL, as well as increases in expression and proteolysis of caspase-1 and -3, occur in resected temporal lobe.[86] These patients have had medically refractory seizures for several years, implying protracted as well as acute programmed cell death within the brain. Protracted programmed cell death after TBI also occurs. Cells with apoptotic morphologies and DNA damage detected by TUNEL have been reported in autopsy specimens from patients dying up to 12 months after injury,[91] perhaps implying that a relatively wide therapeutic window exists for the administration of treatments aimed at reducing programmed cell death.

Several notes of caution are in order. First, it is unclear what the quantitative contribution of programmed cell death is in clinical cases of cerebral ischemia or TBI.[92] It is likely that dying cells demonstrate some biochemical and phenotypic features of programmed cell death, but that the actual deathblow to the cell is not dependent on an active process.[92,93] In addition, even if programmed cell death mechanism plays a key role, it is not clear whether inhibiting neuronal death after injury is entirely beneficial, since programmed cell death is a vital mechanism for biologic systems to eliminate abnormal or aging cells. In other words, quiet elimination, via "cell suicide" of damaged or dysfunctional cells may lead to overall benefit of the patient, in essence "molecular débridement." Only clinical trials of novel therapies targeting programmed cell death will be able to determine whether this mechanism represents an important target in neurointensive care. Recent studies of the efficacy of mild hypothermia after experimental and clinical cardiopulmonary, however, suggest that the success of this intervention may be derived from its effects on programmed cell death.[94-96]

AXONAL INJURY

White matter damage is important in infarction that results from stroke but probably plays only a limited role in the pathology of reversible global cerebral ischemia. In contrast, axonal injury is of paramount importance in patients with TBI. This has been demonstrated both clinically[97-100] and in experimental models.[101-103] The extent and distribution of traumatic axonal injury depends on injury severity and category (focal versus diffuse).[104] The classic view that traumatic axonal injury occurs because of immediate physical shearing is represented primarily in cases of severe injury in which frank axonal tears occur.[97,98,105,106] However, recent experimental studies suggest that axonal damage predominantly occurs by a delayed process termed *secondary axotomy*.[102,107,108] Two hypothetical sequences have attempted to explain secondary axotomy, one attributing axolemmal permeability and calcium influx as the initiating event (Fig. 46-5), and the other a direct cytoskeletal abnormality impairing axoplasmic flow.[102,108,109] It has been posited that both forms of reactive axonal swelling take place but in different proportions depending on the severity of injury. Superimposed on these theories is the finding that hypoxic/ischemic insults can also produce axonal swelling. As a result, differing as well as unifying theories for axonal injuries in patients with brain injury have been proposed.[102,108-111] Common mechanistic features include focal ion flux, calcium dysregulation, and mitochondrial and cytoskeletal dysfunction.

Traumatic axonal injury contributes to the morbidity after TBI.[102,104-106] Until recently, the contributions of axonal injury to morbidity have remained speculative, since traumatic axonal injury has remained refractory to treatment even in the laboratory. However, recent studies in experimental TBI models have shown that hypothermia or cyclosporin-A can both reduce white matter damage.[112,113] These therapeutic advances should help determine more definitively the contributions of traumatic axonal injury to secondary damage. Recent application of magnetic resonance imaging (MRI) to the study of traumatic axonal injury[114,115] and axonal connectivity[116,117] may improve our understanding of both this injury mechanism and axonal regeneration.

CEREBRAL SWELLING

In addition to cascades of neuronal death and axonal damage, brain swelling is a hallmark finding in cases of focal cerebral ischemia, severe TBI, and severe global cerebral ischemia from prolonged cardiopulmonary arrest. Brain swelling often results in the development of intracranial hypertension. Cerebral swelling and accompanying intracranial hypertension contribute to secondary damage in two ways. Intracranial hypertension can compromise cerebral perfusion, leading to secondary ischemia. It can also produce the devastating consequences of brain deformation and vascular compression through herniation syndromes. Intracranial hypertension results from increases in intracranial volume

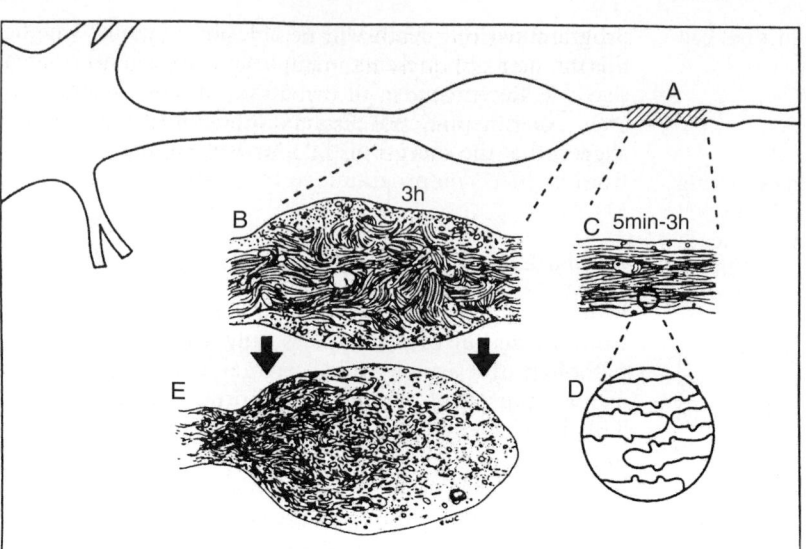

FIGURE 46–5. Reactive axonal swellings have been proposed to result from focal axolemmal disruption, ionic shifts, and neurofilamentous compaction at site *A* results in a reactive swelling at site *B* in an upstream region of the axon. At the site of ionic influx, neurofilamentous compaction and mitochondrial swelling is seen (*C*). Neurofilament compaction is associated with neurofilament sidearm loss (*D*). Obstructed axonal transport results in upstream axonal enlargement, neurofilament misalignment, organelle accumulation, and formation of the typical reactive axonal swelling (*E*).

from a variety of sources, which are outlined in Figure 46-1. In some cases of TBI or spontaneous intracranial hemorrhage, such as with epidural, subdural, or parenchymal hematoma formation, an extra-axial or parenchymal blood collection is the key culprit and can be addressed by surgical evacuation.[118] However, there are several important mechanisms that are more uniformly involved in the development of intracranial hypertension. These are related to either brain swelling from vasogenic edema, astrocyte swelling, and an increase in tissue osmolar load, or vascular dysregulation with swelling secondary to an increase in cerebral blood volume (CBV).

Most of the mechanistic work in this area has come from studies in the field of TBI. Recent data suggest that brain swelling after severe TBI results from edema rather than increased CBV. Marmarou and colleagues[119] measured both CBV and brain water in adults with TBI. Using a dye indicator technique (coupled to computed tomography) to measure CBV and MRI to quantify brain water, increases in brain water were commonly observed but were generally associated with reduced (not increased) CBV (see Fig. 46-6).

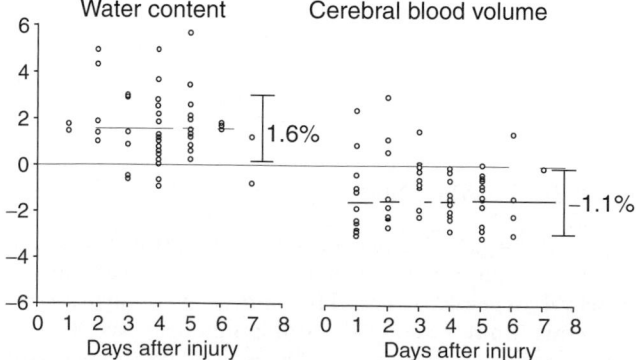

FIGURE 46–6. The percentage change in brain water content as assessed by magnetic resonance imaging and cerebral blood volume (CBV) as measured by computed tomography and indicatory dilution technique in 109 studies of adults with traumatic brain injury (TBI). Brain water is increased and CBV is reduced in adults with severe TBI. (From Marmarou A, Barzo P, Fatouros P, et al: Traumatic brain swelling in head injured patients: Brain edema or vascular engorgement? Acta Neurochir Suppl [Wien] 1997;70:68-70.)

Thus, edema rather than increased CBV appears to be the predominant contributor to cerebral swelling after TBI. Both cytotoxic and vasogenic edema may play important roles in cerebral swelling. However, the biochemical and molecular pathways involved in our traditional concept of cytotoxic and vasogenic edema are evolving. There appear to be four putative mechanisms for edema formation in the injured brain. First, vasogenic edema may form in the extracellular space as a result of disruption of the blood-brain barrier. Second, cellular swelling can be produced in two ways. Astrocyte swelling can occur as part of the homeostatic uptake of substances such as glutamate. Glutamate uptake is coupled to glucose utilization via a sodium/potassium ATPase, with sodium and water accumulation in astrocytes. Astrocyte swelling appears to be importantly linked to water movement through the aquaporin-4 channel found in the astrocyte foot processes near capillaries.[120-123] Recent studies have demonstrated reduced cerebral edema in mice genetically deficient in this channel.[124] Swelling of both neurons and other cells in the neuropil can also result from ischemia- or trauma-induced ionic pump failure. This can be important in the penumbral regions of focal cerebral ischemia and around cerebral contusions. Finally, osmolar swelling may also contribute to edema formation in the extracellular space, particularly in maturing cerebral contusions. Osmolar swelling, however, is actually dependent on an intact blood-brain barrier or an alternative solute barrier.

In both ischemic and traumatic brain injury, cellular swelling may be of greatest importance. Using a model of diffuse TBI in rats, Barzo and colleagues[125] applied diffusion-weighted MRI to localize the increase in brain water. A decrease in the apparent diffuse coefficient after injury suggested predominantly cellular swelling, rather than vasogenic edema, in the development of intracranial hypertension. Cellular swelling may be of even greater importance in the setting of TBI with a secondary hypoxemic-ischemic insult.[126] Katayama and colleagues[127] also suggested that the role of blood-brain barrier in the development of post-traumatic edema might have been overstated, even in the setting of cerebral contusion. One intriguing possibility is that as macromolecules are degraded within injured brain regions, the osmolar load in the contused tissue or infarcts increases. As the blood-brain barrier reconstitutes (or as other osmolar

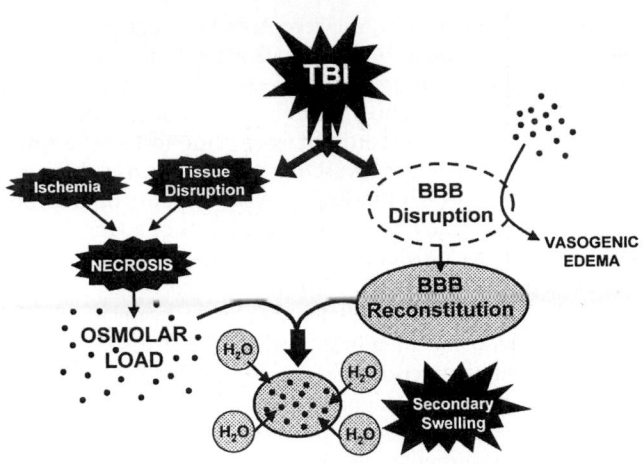

FIGURE 46–7. Schematic based on hypothesis of Katayama and colleagues[127] suggesting that as the osmolar load increases (breakdown of macromolecules in the region of contusion necrosis), a considerable driving force develops for the accumulation of water, resulting in the secondary swelling so often seen in and around cerebral contusions.

barriers are formed), a considerable osmolar driving force for the local accumulation of water develops, resulting in the marked swelling so often seen in and around cerebral contusions (Fig. 46-7). This has been supported by recent clinical studies of human cerebral contusion.[128]

In some cases, increases in CBV can be seen after TBI and contribute to intracranial hypertension. When an increase in CBV is seen, it may result from local increases in cerebral glycolysis, "hyperglycolysis" as described by Bergsneider and colleagues.[129] In regions with increases in glutamate levels, such as in contusions, increases in glycolysis are observed because astrocyte uptake of glutamate is coupled to glycolysis rather than oxidative metabolism. Recall that oxidative metabolism is generally depressed by approximately 50% in comatose victims of severe TBI in the intensive care unit.[130] Hyperglycolysis results in a marked local increase in cerebral glucose utilization with a coupled increase in CBF and CBV and resultant local brain swelling. A detailed discussion of this topic is beyond the scope of this chapter, but an expanded discussion of intracranial dynamics and vascular dysregulation in neurointensive care is provided in the next chapter.

As MRI and magnetic resonance-spectroscopic methods continue to develop and become applied to critically ill patients,[131] our knowledge of the mechanisms involved in

cerebral swelling should greatly advance. It must be remembered that although neuronal and axonal injury are key downstream events in the evolution of damage after severe TBI, brain swelling and resultant intracranial hypertension is still the principal target for titration of therapy in the intensive care unit.

INFLAMMATION AND REGENERATION

There appear to be both acute detrimental and subacute/chronic beneficial aspects of inflammation in cerebral ischemia and TBI. Inflammatory mechanisms in the evolution of secondary injury and repair have the greatest support in stroke and TBI, although some support for a role of inflammation in the regulation of neuronal death has been suggested even in cases of transient global ischemic insults.[132-135] There is robust acute inflammation after stroke and TBI.[136,137] This has been shown in experimental models and in patients.[138-146] Nuclear factor-κB,[147] TNF-α,[85,148-151] interleukin (IL)-1β,[152,153] eicosanoids,[154] neutrophils,[139,155,156] and macrophages[157,158] contribute to both secondary damage and repair.

Markers of inflammation after TBI have been assessed in humans using two general strategies, (1) examination of inflammation in contused brain tissue or cerebral infarcts resected from patients with refractory intracranial hypertension, and (2) study of mediator levels in CSF. Consistent with a role for IL-1β in the evolution of tissue damage in cases of human TBI, Clark and associates[39] performed Western analysis of brain samples resected from adults with refractory intracranial hypertension secondary to severe contusion. Interleukin-1-converting enzyme (ICE) was activated, as evidenced by specific cleavage in patients with TBI. ICE activation is critical to the production of IL-1β. ICE activation was not detected in patients who died of non-CNS causes (Fig. 46-8). This supports the production of IL-1β, a pivotal proinflammatory mediator, in the traumatically injured brain in humans. Similar support for increases in a variety of inflammatory mediators exists in human stroke.[85,145,146,150,151,156]

Studies of CSF further support a role for inflammation in TBI. Marion and associates[142] demonstrated increases in IL-1β in CSF after severe TBI in adults. These increases were attenuated by the use of moderate therapeutic hypothermia. Similarly, there are increases of a number of cytokines in CSF after severe TBI and stroke, including IL-6 and IL-8.[85,144,150,151,159] Contusion and local tissue necrosis

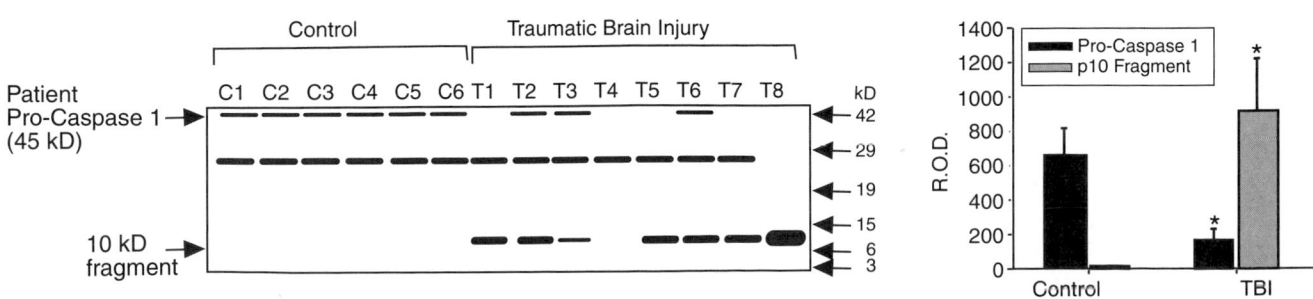

FIGURE 46–8. Evidence for activation of interleukin-1β converting enzyme (ICE) activation in cerebral contusions resected from adult patients with severe traumatic brain injury (TBI) and refractory intracranial hypertension. Western analysis demonstrating cleavage of the intact 45 kD pro-caspase-1 to the 10 kD fragment in each of eight victims of severe TBI but in none of six control brain samples from patients who died of non-central nervous system causes. (From Clark RS, Kochanek PM, Chen M, et al: Increases in Bcl-2 and cleavage of caspase-1 and caspase-3 in human brain after head injury. FASEB J 1999;13:813-821.)

appear to be important to trigger neutrophil influx with resultant secondary tissue damage.[139] Neutrophil influx is accompanied by increases in inducible nitric oxide synthase (iNOS) in brain[140,146] and is followed by macrophage infiltration, which peaks between 24 and 72 hours after injury.[160] Macrophage infiltration and the differentiation of endogenous microglia into resident macrophages may signal the link between inflammation and regeneration, with elaboration of a number of trophic factors (i.e., nerve growth factor [NGF], nitrosothiols, vascular endothelial growth factor).[153,159,161,162] Kossmann and associates[159] reported a link between IL-6 production and the production of neurotrophins, such as NGF in human head injury. Cultured astrocytes treated with either IL-6 or IL-8 in CSF from brain-injured adults produced NGF. Cytokine production after cerebral ischemia and TBI may be important to neuronal plasticity and repair, as discussed later.

Studies in models of TBI[149,163] suggest early detrimental effects of a number of inflammatory mediators but beneficial effects of inflammation on long-term outcome. Mice deficient in TNF-α exhibit improved functional outcome (versus wildtype) early after TBI. However, the long-term consequences of TNF-α deficiency on outcome are detrimental.[149] Similarly, despite a detrimental role for iNOS in the initial 72 hours after trauma,[165] iNOS-deficient mice demonstrated impaired long-term outcome versus controls.[164] iNOS is important in wound healing, and iNOS-derived nitrosylation of proteins may play a role.[162,165] Regeneration and plasticity play important roles in mediating beneficial long-term effects on recovery, and these responses are linked to inflammation. Analogs of these beneficial consequences of inflammation are anticipated in humans but remain to be demonstrated.

The contribution of the inflammatory response to cerebral ischemia and TBI remains to be determined. Although there are a few promising reports in models of the use of anti-inflammatory therapies in TBI and ischemia (targeting IL-1β, ICE, and TNF-α), it is unclear whether anti-inflammatory therapies will improve outcome after stroke or TBI in humans. Some of the initial trials have not been promising.[156] Finally, the consequences of anti-inflammatory therapies on the incidence of sepsis or secondary infectious complications must also be considered.[166] Similarly, the potential deleterious (or beneficial) CNS consequences of novel immunostimulatory therapies (such as GCSF or GMCSF) for the treatment of sepsis and multiple organ failure must also be carefully considered when these agents are used in patients with multisystem disease that includes CNS injury.[167]

ENDOGENOUS NEUROPROTECTANTS

Ischemia, excitotoxicity, or their combination, are a key facet of secondary injury. These mechanisms are linked to calcium overload, oxidative stress, and mitochondrial failure. There is, however, a coupled endogenous retaliatory response to these ischemic and excitotoxic insults. Two important components of this cascade are adenosine and heat shock protein 70 (HSP-70). Adenosine is an endogenous neuroprotectant produced in response to both ischemia and excitotoxicity. It antagonizes a number of events thought to mediate neuronal death.[168] Breakdown of ATP leads to formation of adenosine, a purine nucleoside that decreases neuronal metabolism and increases CBF, among other mechanisms. Adenosine binding to A1 receptors decreases metabolism by increasing K^+ and Cl^- and decreasing Ca^{++} conductances in the neuronal membrane. A1 receptors bind adenosine with high affinity and are located on neurons in brain regions that are susceptible to injury and are spatially associated with NMDA receptors.[169] Thus, locally released adenosine minimizes excitotoxicity. Binding of adenosine to lower affinity A2 receptors (on cerebrovascular smooth muscle) causes vasodilation, although binding to A2a receptors on neurons may be detrimental. Brain interstitial levels of adenosine are increased 50- to 100-fold early after experimental cerebral ischemia or TBI.[170-173]

In clinical studies, marked increases in brain interstitial levels of adenosine in adults with TBI were seen during episodes of jugular venous desaturation (secondary insults), supporting a role of adenosine as a "retaliatory" defense metabolite.[174] Surprisingly, increases in CSF levels of the commonly consumed adenosine receptor antagonist caffeine were associated with favorable outcome after severe TBI in humans, a finding that may be explained by up-regulation of A1 receptors by chronic caffeine exposure.[175,176] Another endogenous neuroprotectant that plays a role after cerebral ischemia, severe TBI, and SAH is HSP-70. HSP-70 optimizes protein folding as a molecular chaperone. It also inhibits proinflammatory signaling.[177] HSP-70 is induced as part of the preconditioning response in brain and has been shown to be increased in both CSF and brain tissue after severe TBI in humans.[178-180] Thus, the brain mounts an important endogenous defense response to TBI. Therapies designed to augment these pathways have not been examined adequately.

SUMMARY

Biochemical, cellular, and molecular mechanisms involved in the evolution of secondary brain injury after global and focal ischemia and TBI have been reviewed with particular attention to clinical studies relevant to neurointensive care. Our understanding of the biochemical, cellular, and molecular responses has progressed, particularly with the application of molecular biology methods to human materials. Future investigation should integrate these findings with bedside physiology and an improved assessment of outcome. Finally, novel imaging and diagnostic methods, particularly MRI, magnetic resonance spectroscopy, and positron emission tomography must be coupled with biochemical and molecular methods to clarify the mechanisms involved in secondary damage and the local effects of novel therapies, including the study of brain pharmacodynamics.

SELECTED BIBLIOGRAPHY

Barone FC, Feuerstein GZ: Inflammatory mediators and stroke: New opportunities for novel therapeutics. J Cereb Blood Flow Metab 1999; 19:819-834.
  A superb review article describing the molecular components and temporal sequence of events in the inflammatory cascade that is set into motion in cases of ischemic brain injury.

Bullock R, Zauner A, Woodward JJ, et al: Factors affecting excitatory amino acid release following severe human head injury. J Neurosurg 1998;89:507-518.
  A superb clinical report on excitotoxicity that used cerebral microdialysis to assess levels of glutamate in 80 consecutive severely head-injured patients. Four patterns of brain interstitial levels of excitatory amino acids were described, and increases in glutamate were as much as 50 times normal in 30% of the patients. This manuscript raises the important point that mechanisms such as excitotoxicity appear to vary greatly depending on the type of traumatic injury, time after injury, and presence of secondary insults such as hypoxemia or intracranial hypertension.

Clark RS, Kochanek PM, Chen M, et al: Increases in Bcl-2 and cleavage of caspase-1 and caspase-3 in human brain after head injury. FASEB J 1999; 13:813-821.

This is a bench-to-bedside study of a number of key molecular events in cases of secondary damage in human cerebral contusions including activation caspase-1 and caspase-3. These two processes are central to inflammation and programmed cell death. This was the first report of caspase activation in either ischemic or traumatic brain injury in humans.

Povlishock JT: Traumatically induced axonal injury: Pathogenesis and pathobiological implications. Brain Pathol 1992;2:1-12.

This is an outstanding review on the biochemical and molecular events that are involved in the evolution of axonal damage after severe traumatic brain injury. This article discusses the evidence supporting the now accepted concept of secondary axotomy and its consequences.

Siesjo BK: Cell damage in the brain: A speculative synthesis. J Cereb Blood Flow Metab 1981;1:155-185.

Highly quoted classic reference discussing a number of speculative biochemical mechanisms involved in the evolution of secondary damage after cerebral ischemia, epilepsy, and hypoglycemia. Despite being written before the molecular explosion, many of these hypotheses have shown merit as research in this area has progressed over the subsequent 25 years.

Siesjo BK, Katsura K, Zhao Q, et al: Mechanisms of secondary brain damage in global and focal ischemia: A speculative synthesis. J Neurotrauma 1995; 12:943-956.

This is an outstanding review article that contrasts the biochemical and molecular alterations seen in focal versus global cerebral ischemia. The discussion is based on studies done in experimental models but is germane to the clinical conditions of cardiopulmonary arrest and stroke.

Snyder JV, Nemoto EM, Carroll RG, Safar P: Global ischemia in dogs: Intracranial pressures, brain blood flow and metabolism. Stroke 1975;6:21-27.

Experimental animal study that constituted the first description of the development of early postischemic hypoperfusion after complete global cerebral ischemia, a fundamental finding in cardiopulmonary arrest and resuscitation that has withstood the test of time.

Chapter 47

CRITICAL NEUROPATHOPHYSIOLOGY

W. Andrew Kofke

KEY POINTS

1. The contributors to intracranial hypertension are defined by the contents of the brain: brain tissue, cerebrospinal fluid, blood, and masses. Brain tissue becomes important in the presence of edema, cerebrospinal fluid in the presence of hydrocephalus, blood volume in the presence of vasodilating or vasoconstricting conditions, and masses when of an unacceptable size. In clinical practice, physiologic and pharmacologic manipulations have the most impact on blood volume.

2. There are two types of intracranial hypertension, categorized according to cerebral blood flow as hyperemic or oligemic. Abrupt noxious stimuli briefly increase intracranial pressure (ICP) in the setting of decreased intracranial compliance. Such situations are associated with hyperemia, strongly suggesting that brief hyperemic intracranial hypertension is not a dangerous situation. However, it is reasonable to be concerned about such hyperemia related to herniation risk. In contrast, oligemic intracranial hypertension is associated with compromised cerebral perfusion and is clearly deleterious.

3. One category of pressure waves has been identified as plateau waves, which are known to be associated with increased cerebral blood volume (CBV). CBV increases exponentially as perfusion pressure decreases to levels of 80 mm Hg and below. A small decrease in blood pressure produces exponential increases in CBV in a setting of abnormal intracranial compliance with the ICP at the elbow of the ICP-intracranial volume curve.

4. Positive end-expiratory pressure can increase ICP in two ways. The first is through impedance of venous return, increasing cerebral venous pressure and ICP. The second is through decreased blood pressure and reflex increase of CBV increasing ICP.

5. Intracranial pressure can also be influenced by antihypertensive drugs. In general, vasodilator drugs such as nitroprusside, nitroglycerin, and nifedipine can be expected to increase ICP. Conversely, nonvasodilator antihypertensive drugs, generally sympatholytic drugs such as trimethaphan or beta-adrenergic blocking drugs such as esmolol or labetalol, can be expected to have little or no effect on ICP.

6. Temperature management can be critical in neurointensive care. In animal models, hyperthermia has been shown to have deleterious effects on outcome after cerebral ischemia, head trauma, and seizure. Conversely, mild hypothermia (32-36°C) has been shown to be protective.

7. Cerebrovascular reserve is compromised in many intracranial pathologic processes. Normally, the brain compensates for decrements in supply of oxygen and substrates by vasodilating to maintain or increase flow. Clinical examples of attenuated cerebrovascular reserve include cerebral edema, hypoxemia, carotid artery stenosis, peri-infarct penumbra, and anemia. In each of these situations, although not easy to quantitate, it is clear that added situations of compromised O_2 supply to the brain will risk neuronal injury.

8. Hyperglycemia is clearly deleterious in the context of global cerebral ischemia. Clinical studies suggest a deleterious effect in head trauma and stroke. It seems most appropriate to maintain blood glucose levels as close to normal as possible and feasible.

9. Ample laboratory and clinical evidence supports the notion that endogenous and exogenously administered catecholamines can be deleterious with compromised cerebral perfusion.

Neural function is essential to human existence. Thus, loss of any neural element in the course of a critical illness represents a major loss to a given individual. Neurons or supporting elements can be lost in a small, virtually unnoticeable manner, or there can be widespread selective neuronal loss or tissue infarction. Based on the notion that neural function is the essence of acceptable survival from critical illness, it is crucial for critical care management to include considerations of neural viability and the impact and interactions of the primary diseases and therapeutics on the nervous system.

There are numerous clinical scenarios in which a critically ill patient may present with a primary neurologic illness. In a general sense, these scenarios often involve ischemia, trauma, or neuroexcitation. Each of these may include a period of decreased cerebral perfusion pressure (CPP), usually due to elevated intracranial pressure, eventually compromising cerebral blood flow (CBF) sufficiently to produce permanent neuronal loss, infarction, and possibly brain death. In this chapter, I review the physiologic factors and intracranial

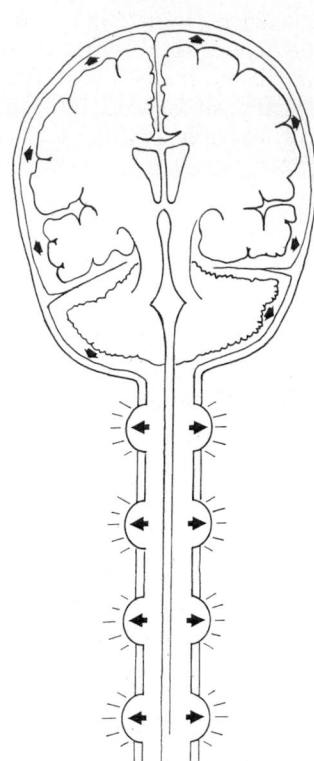

FIGURE 47–1. The brain, spinal cord, and blood are encased in the skull and vertebral canal, thus constituting a nearly incompressible system. System capacitance is thought to be provided via intervertebral spaces. (From Kofke W, et al: Neurologic intensive care. In Albin M [ed]: Textbook of Neuroanesthesia. New York, McGraw-Hill, 1997.)

pressure (ICP) considerations critical to contemporary neurointensive care.

ELEVATED INTRACRANIAL PRESSURE

PHYSIOLOGY

The brain, spinal cord, cerebrospinal fluid (CSF), and blood are encased in the protecting but noncompliant skull and vertebral canal, constituting a nearly incompressible system (Fig. 47-1). In a totally incompressible system, pressure would rise linearly with increased volume. However, there is capacitance in the system, thought to be provided by the intervertebral spaces. Once this capacitance is exhausted, the ICP increases dramatically with increased intracranial volume.

Based on the following relationship:

$$CBF = (MAP - ICP)/CVR,$$

the concern is raised mathematically that increasing ICP is associated with decrements in CBF. However, the effect of increasing ICP on CBF is not straightforward, as mean arterial pressure (MAP) may increase with ICP elevations,[1] and cerebral vascular resistance (CVR) adjusts with decreasing CPP (increasing cerebral vessel diameter) to maintain CBF until maximal vasodilatation occurs.[2,3] This results in an increase in cerebral blood volume (CBV). This is thought to occur at a CPP less than 50 mm Hg, although considerable individual heterogeneity in this value exists. Thus, increasing ICP initially is often associated with vasodilatation and/or increasing MAP to maintain CBF without a nutritive decrement.

Normal ICP is less than 10 mm Hg. ICP greater than 20 mm Hg is generally treated with ICP-reducing agents.[4] However, this is an epidemiologically derived action. Head trauma studies have indicated that patients with ICP greater than 20 mm Hg generally do poorly,[4] although simply elevating ICP to greater than 20 mm Hg (in experimental animals) is not necessarily associated with decrements in CBF or permanent sequelae, provided the above-noted compensatory mechanisms occur.[5]

Nonetheless, increasing ICP due to mass lesions or obstruction of CSF outflow can exhaust compensatory mechanisms with compromise of CBF. Initially, distal runoff of the cerebral circulation increases. As the process continues, the normally continuous (through systole and diastole) cerebral perfusion becomes discontinuous (systolic perfusion only) (Fig. 47-2).[6] Further compromise of CPP results in further oxygen extraction progressing to anaerobic metabolism, exacerbation of edema, and ultimately intracranial circulatory arrest.[6] Thus, when ICP increases, early recognition is important to determine whether a deleterious sequence of events is starting.

CONTRIBUTORS TO INTRACRANIAL HYPERTENSION

Brain. The brain normally occupies about 80% of the contents of the skull, but its volume can be increased by edema. There are two types of edema, cytotoxic and vasogenic, referring to swelling produced by cellular or vascular processes, respectively.[7] Any edema can increase ICP. It can be heterogeneously distributed such that pressure gradients occur, leading to a variety of herniation syndromes.

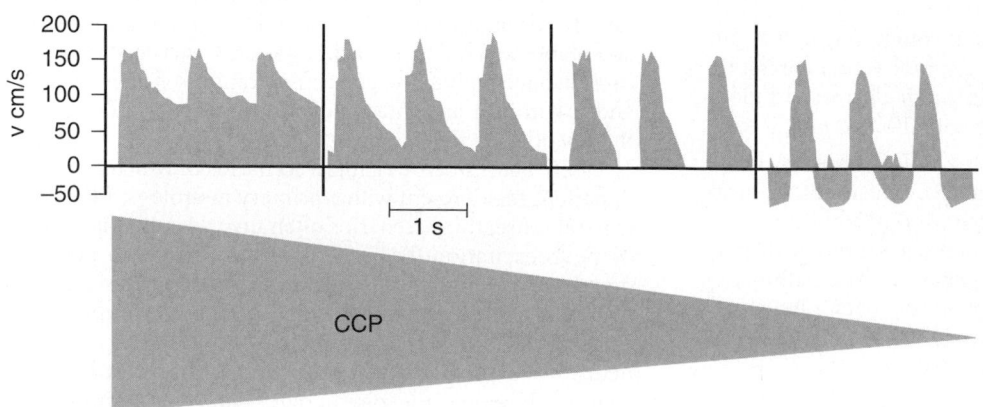

FIGURE 47–2. Progression of transcranial Doppler waveforms with decreasing cerebral perfusion pressure after head injury. Progression is apparent from a normal-appearing transcranial Doppler waveform to intracranial hypertension sufficient to induce intracerebral circulatory arrest. (From Hassler W, Steinmetz H, Gawlowski J: Transcranial Doppler ultrasonography in raised intracranial pressure and in intracranial circulatory arrest. J Neurosurg 1988;68:745.)

Cerebrospinal Fluid. CSF is generated in the choroid plexus and absorbed in the arachnoid villi. An equilibrium normally exists between production and absorption. Disruption of this equilibrium can lead to increased ICP with hydrocephalus, the condition wherein there is an excess of fluid in all or part of the CSF in the brain. Hydrocephalus is generally categorized as communicating or noncommunicating. In communicating hydrocephalus, the CSF circulation between the site of CSF production and absorption is intact. However, abnormally decreased absorption or increased production results in increased CSF accumulation. In noncommunicating hydrocephalus, the pathways are blocked such that CSF cannot circulate to the convexity of the brain to be absorbed. This results in accumulation of CSF in the ventricles, producing distension.[8]

Blood. CBV is an important contributor to variations in ICP, in part due to the wide variations in CBV that can occur with normal physiologic homeostasis and with the effects of drugs and disordered physiology. When CBV increases due to increased CBF, this can produce a dramatic increase in ICP, if intracranial compliance is abnormal. However, unlike ICP elevation due to increased CSF volume, edema, or a tumor, in which decreased CBF is expected, this variety of ICP increase is often produced by increased CBF, making the significance of the ICP elevation unclear. This is discussed later.

Another mechanism of increased CBV occurs with obstruction of venous outflow. This results in brain engorgement and CBV-mediated increased ICP, but without increased CBF.[9]

Masses. The fourth cause of increased ICP is pathologic masses. These can be in the form of hematoma or neoplastic tumors. In both cases, the faster the onset of the mass effect is, the more acute the rise in ICP. Evidently, there are compensatory mechanisms in intracranial compliance that can allow quite large slow-growing masses to arise in the brain without elevated ICP. On the other hand, similarly sized masses, arising acutely, are associated with symptomatic increases in ICP.

TYPES OF INTRACRANIAL HYPERTENSION

There are two types of intracranial hypertension, categorized according to CBF as hyperemic or oligemic (Fig. 47-3).

In the normal state, increases in CBF are not associated with increased ICP, because capacitive mechanisms compensate for the CBV-mediated increased intracranial volume. However, in the situation of disturbed intracranial compliance, small increases in intracranial volume produce significant increases in ICP.[2,3]

This suggests an important issue: raised ICP has traditionally been considered to be a concern because it indicates that cerebral perfusion might be jeopardized. It is unclear whether it is appropriate to be concerned about the potential for ICP-induced intracranial oligemia when the cause of the high ICP is intracranial hyperemia with associated increased CBV. There have been no detailed examinations of this question, although there have been some studies that allow reasonable inferences about the significance of hyperemic intracranial hypertension.

For many years it has been known that abrupt noxious stimuli briefly increase ICP in the setting of decreased intracranial compliance. Recent studies have revealed that such situations are associated with hyperemia, strongly suggesting that brief hyperemic intracranial hypertension is not a dangerous situation.[10] However, it is reasonable to be concerned about such hyperemia for three reasons. First, elevated ICP due to hyperemia in one portion of the brain may increase ICP to compromise CBF in other areas of the brain in which CBF is marginal. Secondly, increased pressure in one area of the brain may produce gradients that might lead to a herniation syndrome. Thirdly, there is theoretical concern that inappropriate hyperemia predisposes the brain to worsened edema or hemorrhage as occurs with hyperperfusion syndromes. Thus, hyperemic intracranial hypertension has a theoretical potential to be deleterious, although this has yet to be demonstrated in a systematic fashion. For brief periods, as may occur during intubation or other limited exposure to noxious stimuli, it is suggested (but not proven) that it may not be problematic.[11] An example of this conundrum is illustrated in Figure 47-4.

In contrast, oligemic intracranial hypertension is associated with compromised cerebral perfusion and is clearly deleterious.[6] This is supported by the high mortality rate observed in head trauma patients in whom ICP rises due to brain edema with decrements in CBF.[6,12] Transcranial Doppler echography and CBF studies on these patients have demonstrated that CBF is low and perfusion is discontinuous

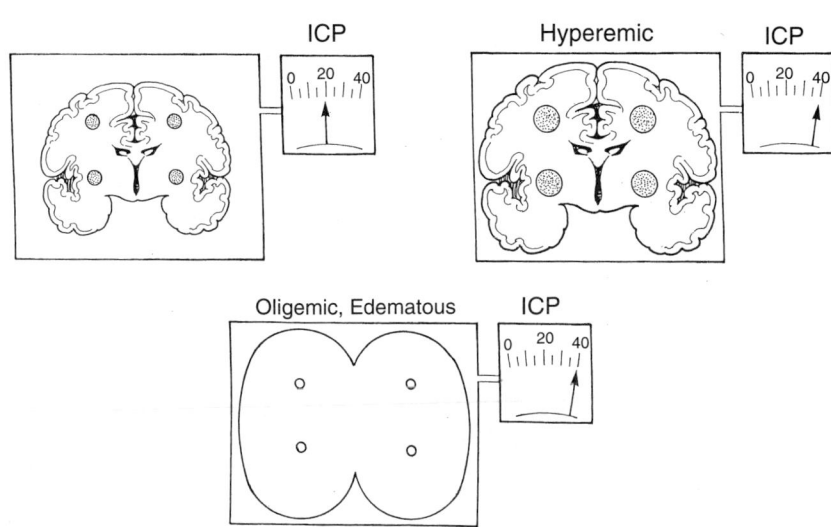

FIGURE 47–3. Two types of intracranial hypertension. From a baseline condition, ICP can increase in two ways. One is via an increase in cerebral blood volume associated with reflex vasodilation due to moderate blood pressure decreases. The second is via malignant brain edema or other expanding masses encroaching on the vascular bed to produce intracranial ischemia. The stippled circles in each coronal brain section represent the cerebral vasculature/blood volume. (From Kofke W, et al: Neurologic intensive care. In Albin M [ed]: Textbook of Neuroanesthesia. New York, McGraw-Hill, 1997.)

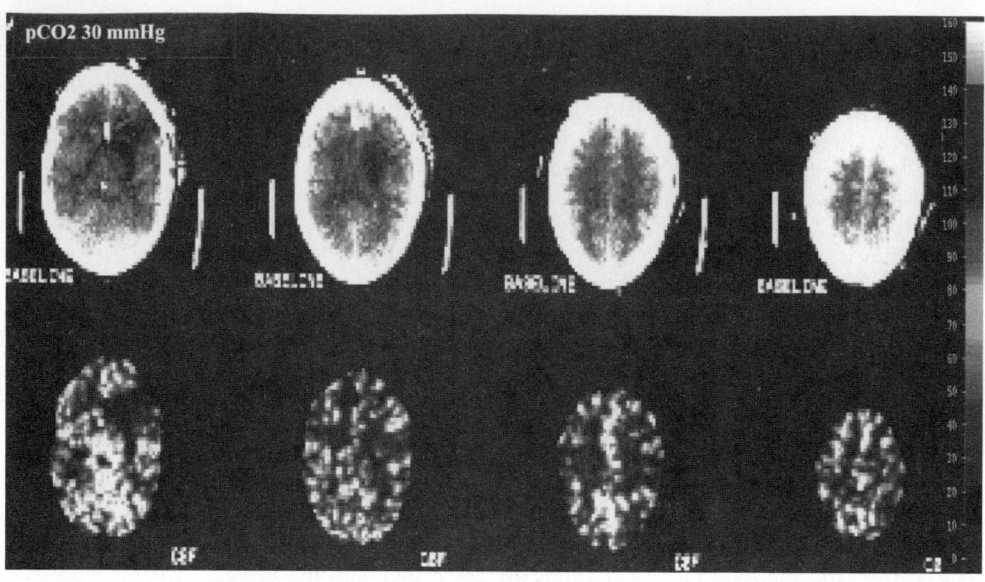

FIGURE 47–4. Computed tomography scans of a head-injury patient with an intracranial pressure (ICP) of 70 mm Hg and $Paco_2$ of 30 mm Hg but diffusely normal to hyperemic cerebral blood flows. (See color section in this text.) (Courtesy of Howard Yonas, University of Pittsburgh.)

during the cardiac cycle (see Fig. 47-2).[6,13] Moreover, jugular venous bulb data indicate that oxygen extraction is markedly increased, suggesting loss of reserve with occurrence of anaerobic metabolism.[13] In this setting, noxious stimuli can further increase the ICP, thus producing the situation of hyperemic, added to oligemic, intracranial hypertension. Presumably, in this setting, the hyperemic rise in ICP acts to further reduce regional CBF in compromised areas with brain edema and may contribute to vasogenic edema.

BLOOD PRESSURE EFFECTS ON INTRACRANIAL PRESSURE: PLATEAU WAVES

Lundberg, in a pioneering 1960 study,[13] monitored ICP in hundreds of patients, identifying characteristic pressure waves. One category of these waves has been identified as *plateau waves*, which are known to be associated with increased CBV (Fig. 47-5).[2] Such waves occur when the ICP abruptly increases to systemic blood pressure levels for about 15 to

30 minutes, occasionally accompanied by neurologic deterioration. Rosner[3] had synthesized the data and convincingly suggests that intracranial blood volume dysautoregulation is responsible for plateau waves. He induced mild head trauma in cats and subsequently intensively monitored the animals after the insult. With normal fluctuations in blood pressure, while in the normal range, he observed that mild blood pressure decrements to a mean of approximately 70 to 80 mm Hg preceded the development of plateau waves (Fig. 47-6). Cerebral blood volume in normally autoregulating brain tissue increases with decreasing blood pressure. However, the increase in CBV is nonlinear. There is an exponential increase in CBV as CPP decreases to levels of 80 mm Hg and below (Fig. 47-7).[3] A small decrease in blood pressure, although in the normotensive range, produces exponential increases in CBV in a setting of abnormal intracranial compliance with the ICP at the elbow of the ICP-intracranial volume curve. Thus, a small decrease in blood pressure introduces an exponential CBV change upon an exponential

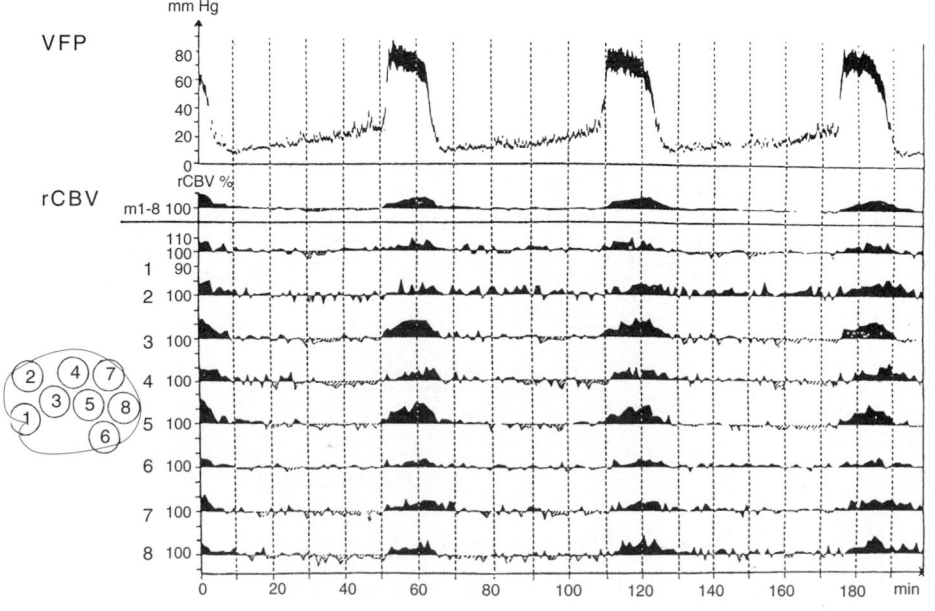

FIGURE 47–5. Plateau waves. Simultaneous recordings of regional cerebral blood volume (rCBV) and ventricular fluid pressure (VFP) during three consecutive plateau waves. The rCBV was measured in eight regions over the left hemisphere. The mean changes in the eight regions are shown in the uppermost curve of the rCBV diagram. Note that the rCBV and VFP curves show a very similar course during the three waves. (From Risberg J, Lundberg N, Ingvar DH: Regional cerebral blood volume during acute transient rises in the intracranial pressure (plateau waves). J Neurosurg 1969;31:303.)

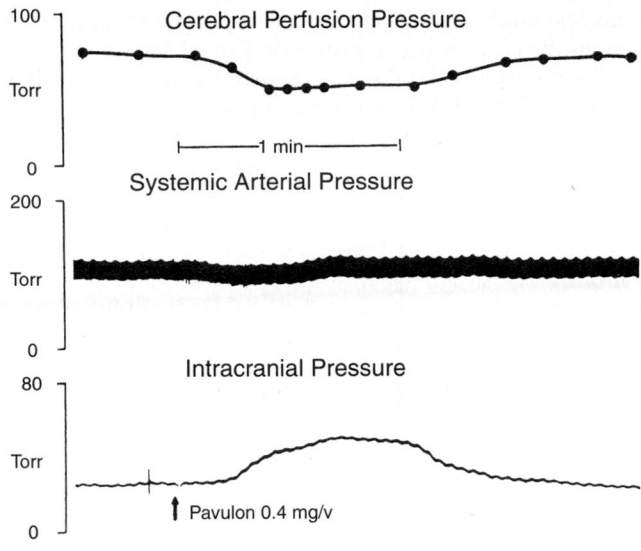

FIGURE 47–6. In an animal head trauma model, a trivial-appearing and transient decrease in systemic arterial blood pressure in the setting of borderline cerebral perfusion pressure precipitates sufficient cerebral vasodilatation to markedly increase the intracranial pressure. Restoration of cerebral perfusion pressure is associated with abolition of the plateau wave. (From Rosner MJ, Becker DP: Origin and evolution of plateau waves: Experimental observations and a theoretical model. J Neurosurg 1984;50:312.)

ICP relationship such that ICP will increase abruptly and to a significant extent.

Plateau waves spontaneously resolve with a hypertensive response or with hyperventilation that will act to oppose the increase in CBV. Clearly, to develop a plateau wave there must be a portion of the brain with normally reactive vasculature in the presence of other brain areas with a mass effect and raised ICP, a situation of *heterogeneous autoregulation*. In addition to preventing and treating plateau waves, data indicate that it is probably important to maintain MAP in the 80 to 100 mm Hg range in patients with high ICP.

Conversely, hypertension can also increase ICP, with animal models showing increased brain water with dopamine-induced increased blood pressure.[14] Typically, within the normal autoregulatory range, changes in blood pressure have no effect on ICP. However, with brain injury and associated vasoparalysis, blood pressure increases mechanically produce cerebral vasodilatation, increasing ICP (Fig. 47-8).[15]

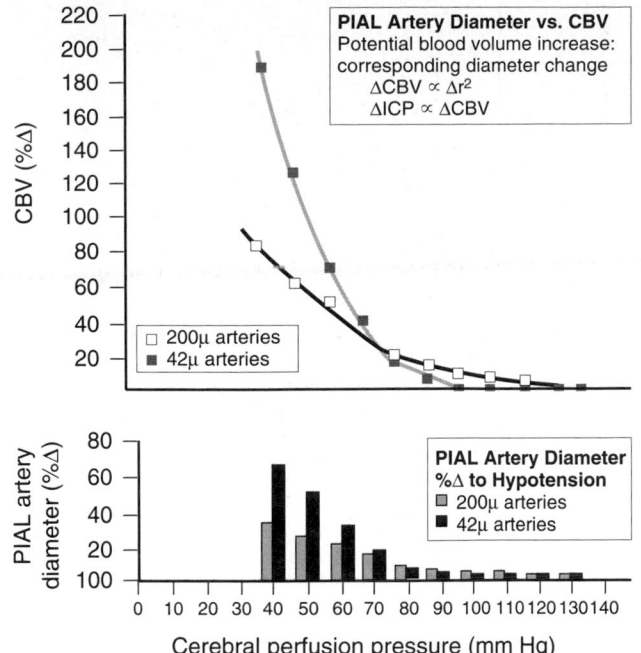

FIGURE 47–7. Cerebral vasodilatation occurs exponentially as cerebral perfusion pressure is reduced. (From Rosner MJ, Becker DP: The etiology of plateau waves: A theoretical model and experimental observations. In Ishii S, Nagai H, Brock M [eds]: Intracranial Pressure V. New York, Springer-Verlag, 1983, p 301.)

It appears that both increasing and decreasing blood pressure can increase ICP, suggesting the presence of a CPP optimum for ICP, probably 80 to 100 mm Hg, although this has not been definitively determined experimentally (Figs. 47-9 and 47-10).

POSITIVE END-EXPIRATORY PRESSURE AND INTRACRANIAL HYPERTENSION

Positive end-expiratory pressure (PEEP) can increase ICP in two ways. The first is through impedance of venous return, increasing cerebral venous pressure and ICP. The second is through decreased blood pressure and reflex increase of CBV, increasing ICP (Fig. 47-11). The latter is likely the most

FIGURE 47–8. Blood pressure changes within the normal autoregulatory range have no effect on intracranial pressure (ICP). However, with brain injury, increases in mean arterial pressure (MAP) produce increases in ICP with this effect more pronounced with more severe injury. Presumably, this effect is due to distention of vasoparalyzed blood vessels with a consequent increase in cerebral blood volume. (From Kofke W, et al: Neurologic intensive care. In Albin M [ed]: Textbook of Neuroanesthesia. New York, McGraw-Hill, 1997.)

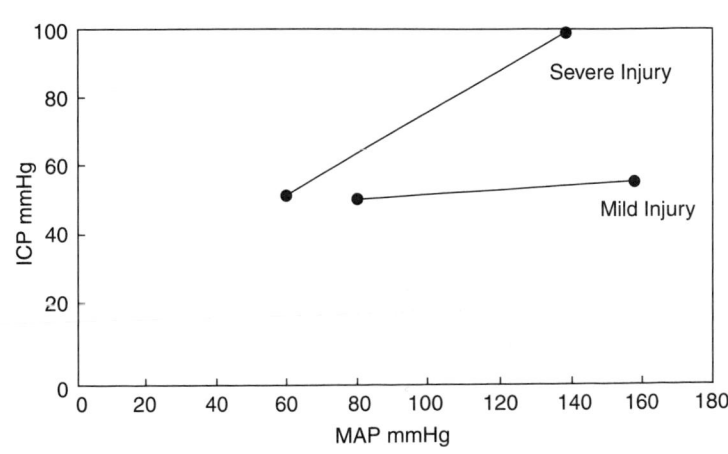

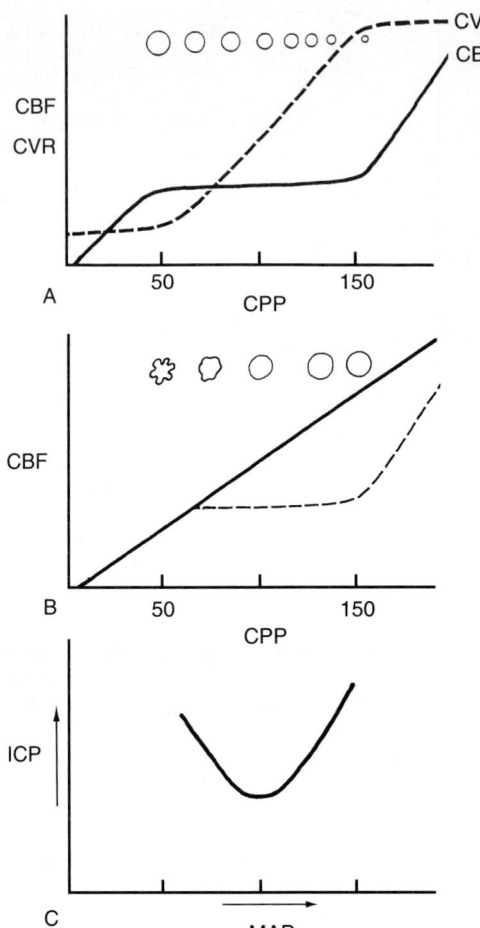

FIGURE 47–9. Cerebral perfusion pressure (CPP) versus cerebral blood flow (CBF) and cerebrovascular resistance (CVR). (**A**) Blood flow is normally maintained constant through changes in CVR, depicted as changes in vascular diameter (and therefore cerebral blood volume [CBV]) in the figure. CBV varies inversely with CPP. (**B**) With vasoparalysis due to injury, CVR does not change with CPP variations, such that CBF and CBV vary directly with CPP. (**C**) In the situation of decreased intracranial compliance, both of the factors illustrated in parts **A** and **B** may interact to increase ICP. Normally autoregulating tissue as in part **A** will predispose to CBV-mediated ICP elevation with decreasing blood pressure, whereas vasoparalyzed tissue (**B**) will predispose to CBV-mediated ICP elevations with increasing blood pressure, leading to the notion of an ICP optima (probably approximately 80 to 100 mm Hg) with varying CPP. (From Kofke W, et al: Neurologic Intensive Care. In Albin M [ed]: Textbook of Neuroanesthesia. New York, McGraw-Hill, 1997.)

common mechanism, as Huseby's data[16] suggest that cerebral venous effects only occur with very high PEEP.

Shapiro and colleagues[17] demonstrated increases in ICP in head-injured humans during intracranial hypertension with application of PEEP (Fig. 47-12). Examination of their data suggests that the most profound decreases in CPP occurred in patients with PEEP-induced decrements in MAP. This is consistent with the notion put forth by Rosner[3] that decreases in blood pressure increase CBV and ICP. Aidinis and colleagues,[18] in studies on cats, confirmed these observations in a more controlled setting. In addition, they assessed the role of pulmonary compliance, finding that decreased pulmonary compliance induced by oleic acid injections results in less effect of PEEP to increase ICP. In situations in which PEEP is likely to be needed, with decrements in pulmonary compliance, such observations indicate that any adverse effects on ICP are less likely to be manifest. This may be related to observations that hemodynamic effects of PEEP are less apparent with noncompliant lungs,[18,19] such that hypotensive-mediated increases in CBV do not occur.

The intuitive notion that PEEP increases cerebral venous pressure to increase ICP is not as straightforward as it initially may seem. For PEEP to increase cerebral venous pressure to levels that will increase ICP, the cerebral venous pressure must at least equal the ICP. Thus, the higher the ICP, the higher PEEP must be to have such a direct hydraulic effect on ICP. This concept was nicely proved by Huseby and colleagues[16] in dog studies in which PEEP was increased progressively with different starting levels of ICP (Fig. 47-13). It is important to note that they prevented PEEP-induced decrements in blood pressure, thus avoiding any reflex increases in cerebral blood volume. They suggested a hydraulic model to better conceptualize this (Fig. 47-14). For example, if all of a 10 cm H_2O PEEP application were transmitted to the cerebral vasculature, which is unlikely given the decreased pulmonary compliance associated with the need for such PEEP, ICP will only be affected if it is less than 10 cm H_2O (7.7 mm Hg), increasing to a level no higher than the applied PEEP. This presupposes no PEEP-induced arterial pressure decrement.

ANTIHYPERTENSIVE THERAPY EFFECTS ON INTRACRANIAL PRESSURE

Intracranial pressure can also be influenced by antihypertensive drugs. In general, vasodilator drugs such as nitroprusside,[20-22] nitroglycerin,[23] and nifedipine[24] can be expected to increase

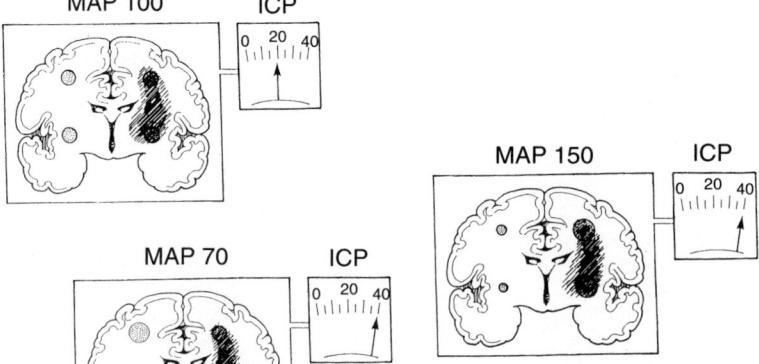

FIGURE 47–10. In the setting of heterogeneous autoregulation in the brain, conditions may predispose to cerebral blood volume (CBV)–mediated increases in intracranial pressure (ICP) with both increases or decreases in blood pressure. The stippled circles in each coronal brain section represent the cerebral vasculature/blood volume.

$$\text{Low PEEP} \rightarrow \downarrow CO \rightarrow \downarrow BP \rightarrow \uparrow CBV \rightarrow \uparrow ICP$$

$$\text{High PEEP} \rightarrow \uparrow CVP \rightarrow \uparrow P_{SS} > ICP \rightarrow \uparrow ICP$$

FIGURE 47–11. Two mechanisms of positive end-expiratory pressure (PEEP)–mediated increases in intracranial pressure (ICP). The addition of PEEP decreases cardiac output (CO) and blood pressure (BP), leading to a reflex increase in cerebral blood volume (CBV). If cerebral perfusion pressure is marginal with heterogeneous autoregulation, this can lead to further increases in ICP. Conversely, to increase sagittal sinus pressure to an extent sufficient to further increase ICP, which is already elevated, PEEP levels at or greater than the ICP must be applied. Pss, sagittal sinus pressure.

ICP. Conversely, nonvasodilator antihypertensive drugs, generally sympatholytic drugs such as trimethaphan, or beta-adrenergic blocking drugs such as esmolol or labetalol,[25] can be expected to have little or no effect on ICP. These observations suggest that the rise in ICP due to vasodilators is caused by increased CBF with attendant increase in CBV. The increase in ICP thus does not threaten ischemia, although herniation and hyperperfusion syndromes may occur and might be problematic. There has been a report of neurologic deterioration with nitroprusside use despite no change in blood pressure.[22] Another consideration in the use of vasodilators is the propensity to reflexively increase plasma catecholamines.[26] Such increases in plasma catecholamines may be deleterious to the marginally perfused injured brain.[27-29]

HYPERPERFUSION SYNDROMES

In a variety of clinical situations, CBF may be inappropriately increased for a given blood pressure. In the extreme case of

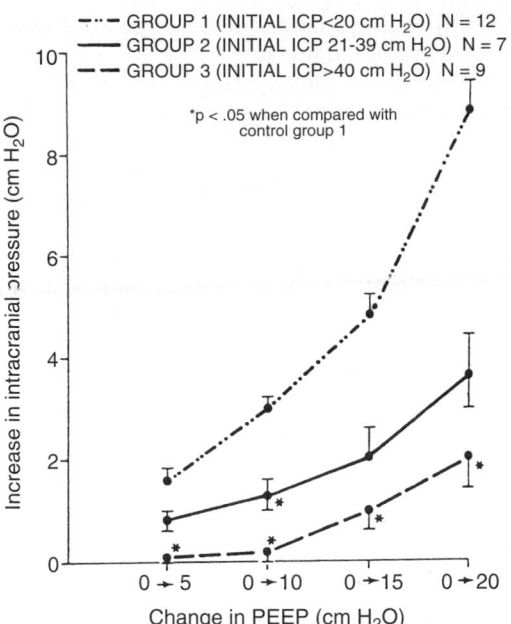

FIGURE 47–13. Increases in intracranial pressure (ICP) with positive end-expiratory pressure (PEEP) in dogs. Values are mean ± standard error of the mean. Group 1 included 12 animals with initial ICP less than 20 cm H_2O; group 2 included seven animals with initial ICP of 21 to 39 cm H_2O; group 3 included nine animals with initial ICP greater than 40 cm H_2O. Blood pressure was maintained constant in all animals. Note that with blood pressure maintained constant, the most significant increases in PEEP occur in the animals with the lowest starting PEEP level. (From Huseby JS, Luce JM, Cary JM, et al: Effects of positive end-expiratory pressure on intracranial pressure in dogs with intracranial hypertension. J Neurosurg 1981;55:704.)

such situations, vasoparalysis is present and CBF becomes more or less a linear function of blood pressure. Such hyperperfusion syndromes may occur early in cases of severe hepatic encephalopathy,[30] 2 to 3 days after severe head injury,[13] after resection of large arteriovenous malformations (AVMs),[31-33] after carotid endarterectomy of severely stenotic lesions with poor collaterals,[34] probably after cerebral arterial thrombolysis,

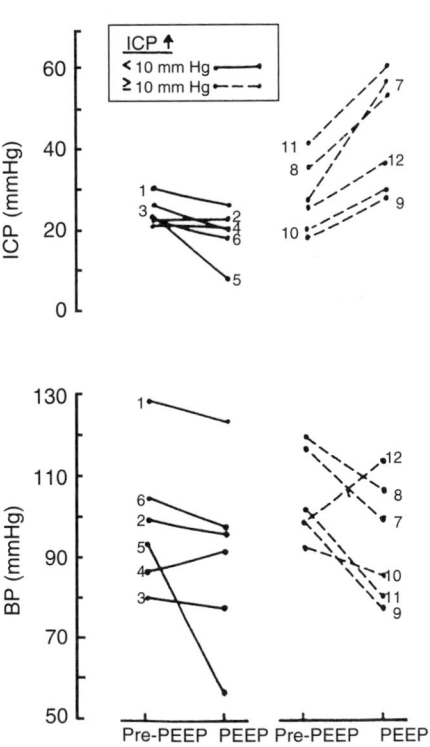

FIGURE 47–12. Intracranial pressure (ICP) and arterial blood pressure (BP) before and with the application of positive end-expiratory pressure (PEEP) (4-8 cm H_2O) in severely head-injured patients. The patients are arbitrarily divided into two groups: those with an ICP increase of 10 mm Hg or greater and those with ICP gains below 10 mm Hg. Note that PEEP-induced blood pressure decreases appear to be more marked in patients sustaining larger ICP increases. (From Shapiro HM, Marshall LF: Intracranial pressure responses to PEEP in head-injured patients. J Trauma 1978;18:254.)

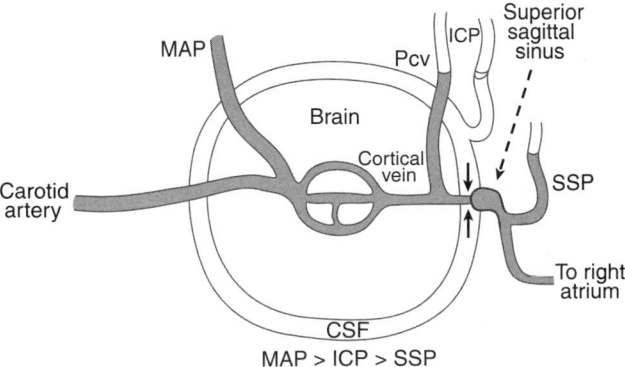

FIGURE 47–14. Schematic illustration of the intracranial space during raised intracranial pressure (ICP). The arrows indicate the position of the hypothesized Starling resistor. Here, the mean arterial pressure (MAP) is greater than ICP, which is greater than sagittal sinus pressure (SSP). Cortical vein pressure (Pcv) cannot fall below ICP, and thus flow is dependent on MAP minus ICP and independent of small changes in SSP. (From Huseby JS, Luce JM, Cary JM, et al: Effects of positive end-expiratory pressure on intracranial pressure in dogs with intracranial hypertension. J Neurosurg 1981;55:704.)

and possibly during administration of cerebral vasodilators at high systemic blood pressure.

Fulminant hepatic failure produces widespread physiologic changes, including altered cerebral physiology.[30] Aggarwal and coworkers[30] systematically examined cerebral hemodynamics and metabolism in severe hepatic encephalopathy and during recovery after hepatic transplantation. They have identified phases that are traversed in the course of going from normal cerebral physiology to brain death. Patients initially demonstrate elevated CBF at normotension. This is usually followed by hyperemic (high CBF and/or CBV) intracranial hypertension, then edema with oligemic intracranial hypertension, and finally intracranial circulatory arrest and brain death. The data clearly suggest that the hyperemia may be deleterious, possibly contributing to the development of subsequent cerebral edema. This is supported by observations that the cerebral edema seems to be prevented through the use of barbiturates and hyperventilation during the hyperemic phase.

Several investigators, in the course of examining cerebrovascular physiology after head trauma, have observed that patients with severe head injury initially have normal or low CBF. This is followed a few days later by increased CBF, which is associated with intracranial hypertension.[12] This may contribute to subsequent oligemic intracranial hypertension.

The concept of normal perfusion pressure breakthrough indicates hyperperfusion at normal blood pressure, such as after resection of a large AVM, when the remaining blood vessels lack the ability to constrict normally and regulate blood flow, resulting in abnormally high regional CBF. The pathogenesis is thought to be related to chronic arterial hypotension proximal to the AVM. The larger the AVM, the lower the intracranial blood pressure to which the patient is acclimated (i.e., the cerebral vasculature locally down-regulates the CBF-MAP autoregulatory relationship). Removing the AVM abruptly exposes the cerebral arterial vessels and arterioles to pressure never before experienced.[32] Thus, despite the blood pressure being within normal limits, the pressure-naive vasculature is unable to autoregulate and the physiology of malignant hypertension may ensue to cause cerebral edema and/or hemorrhage. This is an attractive hypothesis that makes physiologic sense. However, Young and coworkers[33] report that autoregulation of the vascular bed after AVM resection is generally intact, indicating that vasoparalysis due to chronic hypotension may not be the most important contributor to normal perfusion pressure breakthrough.

One cause of neurologic deterioration after carotid endarterectomy is cerebral edema and/or hemorrhage. This is rather unusual, but the presence postoperatively of a unilateral throbbing headache suggests that it may be present. Blood flow studies reveal such patients to have cerebral hyperemia associated with removal of a large proximal obstruction. While normotension is usually well tolerated, hypertension probably increases the risk of hemorrhage, especially if there was a preoperative cerebral infarction. Similar to the AVM situation, described earlier, vasculature that has acclimated to low proximal pressure now is presented with arterial pressure that is much higher, although within the epidemiologic norm.[34]

After thrombolysis of a cerebral artery, one important source of morbidity is edema or hemorrhage of the reperfused territory. With reperfusion of the ischemic tissue, hyperemia occurs for a period of time. If sustained, this suggests that irreversible endothelial damage has occurred and that the patient is at risk for secondary edema or hemorrhage, particularly if the depth of ischemia is sufficient to produce early changes on a computed tomography scan.[35]

Vasodilators such as nitroprusside are frequently used in patients with severe arterial hypertension. When CBF is measured, it is noted that nitroprusside has minimal CBF effect with induced hypotension.[36] However, data are not available on its CBF-CBV effects with treatment of hypertension. Such vasodilators are known to cause an increase in ICP,[22,37] suggesting an element of cerebral hyperemia. This is supported by reports of cerebral dysautoregulation induced by nitroprusside.[38] This ICP elevation and hyperemia[36,39] appear to decrease as blood pressure is lowered. This notion is supported by observations during neurosurgery with cerebral swelling present when nitroprusside is administered.[40] With its use for induced hypotension during neurosurgery, the brain is noted to be flaccid with no hyperemia evident. Thus, cerebral vasodilators can produce a cerebral dysautoregulation/hyperperfusion syndrome, the extent of which is likely dependent on blood pressure. Their use has not yet been reported to be associated with exacerbation of cerebral edema/hemorrhage.

All of the above syndromes describe a clinical course in humans consisting of inappropriate hyperemia for a given blood pressure followed by cerebral edema or hemorrhage. This suggests that the failure to autoregulate at normal pressure results in exposure of arterioles and capillaries to unacceptably high pressure. This then results in disruption of the blood-brain barrier with consequent transudation of fluid or frank bleeding.

HYPERTHERMIA

Temperature management can be critical in neurointensive care. In animal models, hyperthermia has been shown to have deleterious effects on outcome after cerebral ischemia,[41] head trauma,[41] and seizure.[42] Conversely, mild hypothermia has been shown to be protective.[43] It is of interest that the extent of hypothermia required to produce protection is modest (32-36°C). The extent of protection is not adequately explained by reduction in cerebral metabolic rate,[44] suggesting that hypothermia has additional beneficial effects, such as decreased free radical production or reduction in neurotransmitter neurotoxicity.[45]

Preliminary reports from a multicenter trial of head trauma indicate that moderate hypothermia confers cerebral protection when applied within 6 hours of insult and maintained for 24 to 48 hours.[43] This observation was not confirmed in a subsequent multi-institutional trial, although head-injured patients who presented with hypothermia had a better outcome.[46] In addition, two recent reports of hypothermia after cardiac arrest provide strong support for the notion that mild hypothermia is protective after cerebral ischemia.[47,48] Based on these reports, the American Heart Association has adopted hypothermia as a recommended therapy after resuscitation from cardiopulmonary arrest.[49]

Further complicating the role of hypothermia, however, are the recent results of the IHAST2 trial showing no protection from mild hypothermia during cerebral aneurysm surgery.

GAS EXCHANGE

Cerebrovascular reserve is compromised in many intracranial pathologic processes. Normally, the brain compensates for decrements in supply of oxygen and substrates by vasodilating to maintain or increase flow.[50] Animal experiments indicate that it is possible to produce a condition in which cerebrovascular reserve is compromised with increased tendency to cerebral infarction. For example, occlusion of one carotid artery or inducing moderate hypoxemia does not produce symptoms as cerebral vasodilatation occurs to compensate. Indeed, some investigators contend that arterial hypoxemia occurring with normal cerebral vascular compensatory mechanisms does not cause brain damage. Of course, one contributing factor to this notion is that hypoxic myocardial dysfunction produces circulatory collapse and death such that isolated post-hypoxic (without ischemia) neuronal injury cannot occur. However, if hypoxemia is added to carotid occlusion, or vice versa, a stroke can occur because compensatory mechanisms, already fully utilized, cannot accommodate the further decrease in oxygen supply.[51,52] Examples of variants of this situation abound clinically.[53] Such examples of attenuated cerebrovascular reserve include cerebral edema, hypoxemia, carotid artery stenosis, peri-infarct penumbra, and anemia. In each of these situations, although not easy to quantitate, it is clear that added situations of compromised oxygen supply to the brain will risk neuronal injury.

Changes in $PaCO_2$ have a profound impact on CBF. Normally, CBF varies linearly with $PaCO_2$ between 20 and 60 mm Hg.[53] $PaCO_2$-mediated changes in CBF occur with corresponding changes in CBV. Thus, in situations of abnormal intracranial compliance in which small changes in intracranial volume have large ICP effects, decreasing $PaCO_2$ reduces ICP and increasing $PaCO_2$ raises ICP.

The primary concern with raised ICP is that it may be associated with cerebral oligemia. Thus, these effects of $PaCO_2$ on ICP are paradoxical. That is, decreasing $PaCO_2$ reduces ICP, but at the expense of CBF (Fig. 47-15).[54] Minhas and colleagues[55] report that mild hyperventilation in brain-injured patients produces dangerous perilesional CBF decrements. However, Gupta and colleagues,[56] using tissue measures of brain-injured humans, reported sequential increases in $PtiO_2$ with decreasing $PaCO_2$ with an optimum at 26 to 30 mm Hg. Nonetheless, data from head trauma studies indicate that routine use of hyperventilation can worsen outcome.[57]

Conversely, allowing hypercapnia to occur, although leading to increased ICP, is associated with increased CBF. These observations pertain to normally autoregulating tissue. The CBF effects in injured brain tissue can be unpredictable. For example, allowing $PaCO_2$ to increase CBF in autoregulating brain areas, by increasing ICP, may compromise flow in other injured, already fully vasodilated regions.

Related to these concerns is the growing practice of permissive hypercapnia in some types of respiratory failure, performed to reduce the risk of ventilator-mediated lung injury. Reports are somewhat conflicting regarding its safety in the brain-injured patient. In a non-trauma porcine model, van Huls and colleagues[58] found that hypercapnia to 90 mm Hg increased tissue pO_2 while increasing ICP from 20 to 30 mm Hg. Their data and those of others suggest no harmful effects in the noninjured brain, but, theoretically, it seems this hyperemic elevation still might introduce a risk of hyperemia-mediated herniation. A recent report by Tasker and Peters,[59] however, suggests that the negative hyperemic effects associated with hypercapnia resolve over a day or so such that the pulmonary benefits of the hypercapnia can be gained as the adverse neurologic effects subside. This does raise the possibility of an unacceptable respiratory alkalosis on cessation of the permissive hypercapnia. Moreover, in neonates, hypercapnia increases CBF[60] that may lead to cerebral edema, increased ICP, and intraventricular hemorrhage.[61-64] Concerns are also raised by a pediatric case report of nonaneurysmal subarachnoid hemorrhage associated with and seemingly caused by permissive hypercapnia.[65]

The possibility of a neuroprotective effect of respiratory acidosis has also been reported.[66] Brain homogenates develop far fewer free radicals and less lipid peroxidation when pH is lowered by carbon dioxide than when it is lowered by hydrochloric acid,[67] and greater inhibition of tissue lactate production occurs when lowered pH is due to carbon dioxide than when it is due to hydrochloric acid.[68] Vanucci and colleagues[69] report a protective effect of modest hypercapnia in an in vivo model of neuronal hypoxia. In trauma patients with multiple organ dysfunction, Gentiello and colleagues[70] found permissive hypercapnia to increase ICP but adjusted the level of hypercapnia if ICP rises occurred. Similar problematic ICP

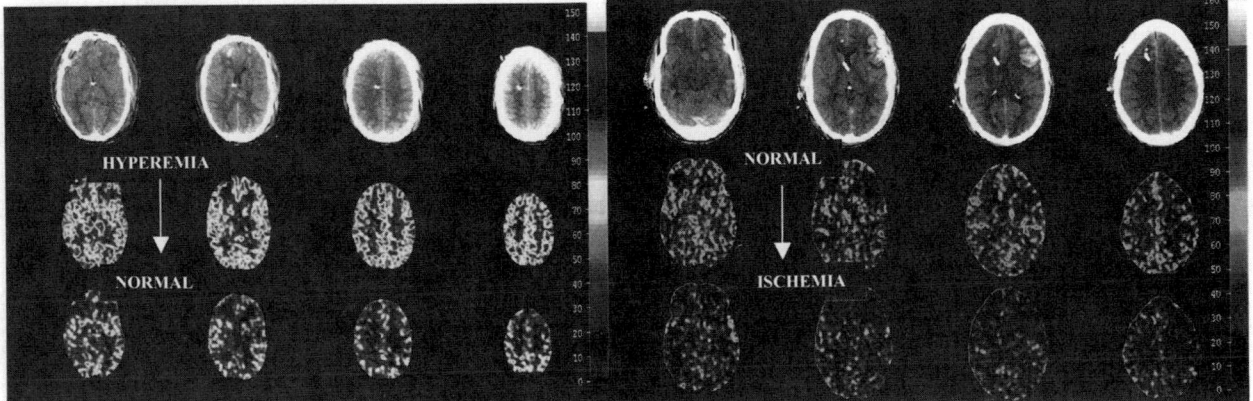

FIGURE 47–15. Effects of $PaCO_2$ changes on cerebral blood flow (CBF). Two examples of disparate effects of hyperventilation on CBF. Both figures are stable xenon CBF scans in head trauma patients with and without hyperventilation. CBF scale is indicated on the right in mL/100 g/min and PCO_2 is indicated above each study. Computed tomography images are indicated in the upper figures and CBF maps in the lower figures. In the left figure, $PaCO_2$ was decreased from 40 to 30 mm Hg. The baseline scan shows hyperemia and the hyperventilated scan shows CBFs of approximately 60 to 70 mL/100 g/min, probably acceptable flows. In the right figure, $PaCO_2$ was decreased from 38 to 30 mm Hg. The baseline CBFs were acceptable. The effect of this modest extent of hyperventilation was to produce widespread areas of CBF less than 20 mL/100 g/min, probably unacceptable flows. (See color section in this text.) (Courtesy of Howard Yonas, University of Pittsburgh.)

increases were also observed in two head-injured patients by Levy and colleagues,[71] which they managed through the use of tracheal gas insufflation, which may be a compromise solution in this conundrum of conflicting physiology and no outcome data. In summary, the data are not conclusive regarding the safety of permissive hypercapnia in the presence of brain injury. It seems that the optimal approach would be to cautiously apply it and adjust according to the ICP response. If unacceptable ICP elevations arise, then the options would include abandoning permissive hypercapnia, treating the ICP to allow normalization of the CBF response to the CO_2 elevation over a few days, and possibly adding tracheal insufflation to the ventilator strategy.

HYPERGLYCEMIA

Hyperglycemia has been associated with exacerbation of brain damage with both head trauma and cerebral ischemia,[72-74] but it is not a straightforward issue. Clearly, neuronal damage after global cerebral ischemia is exacerbated by hyperglycemia.[75] Some studies have suggested that a blood glucose level over 120 mg% is deleterious in stroke patients.[72] However, subsequent studies with subhuman primates subjected to global ischemia have suggested a threshold of around 180 mg%.[58] Clearly, a blood glucose concentration greater than 400 mg% causes striking worsening of neurologic outcome with global ischemia.[73,76]

With focal cerebral ischemia, the situation is less clear. There have been animal and human studies showing that brain damage is worsened, not affected, or lessened with hyperglycemia.[77-81] One report by Prado and colleagues[81] in rats suggested that the discriminating factor regarding worsened brain damage with hyperglycemia is whether there is collateral flow. Areas of the brain with minimal or absent collateral vessels were not affected or were improved with hyperglycemia. Brain areas with a continued trickle of flow sustained worse damage. Presumably, the continued substrate supply in oligemic (not ischemic) areas allowed greater accumulation of organic acids in the cells, leading to worsening brain damage.[77,82] Unfortunately, these observations are difficult to apply clinically to individual patients with focal ischemia.

Hyperglycemia has not been shown to have either deleterious or protective effects in two animal models of status epilepticus.[83,84] The model used in Swan's report[84] produced limbic system damage, whereas Kofke and colleagues[83] used a model producing substantia nigra damage. Seizure-induced nigral damage in rats is associated with hypermetabolic lactic acidosis,[85] which was not exacerbated with hyperglycemia. The fact that nigral damage was not exacerbated with hyperglycemia suggests that metabolic acidosis may not be the sole factor in the development of brain damage after seizure.

SEPSIS

Sepsis is known, in animal models, to decrease CBF while increasing cerebral metabolic rate and disrupting the blood-brain barrier.[86] In addition, it can decrease blood pressure in a manner that may not be well tolerated by the brain with abnormal cerebrovascular reserve. Sepsis-induced decreases in blood pressure can turn an area of cerebral oligemia into an area of ischemic cerebral infarction; however, specific study of this is limited.

SODIUM

Hypernatremia. Hypernatremia can occur in neurologic intensive care unit patients because of nonketotic diabetic coma, dehydration from lack of fluid intake or diuretic use, hypertonic fluid administration, diabetes insipidus, or panhypopituitarism.[87] It can be associated with thirst, irritability, seizures, intracranial hemorrhage, or coma, although the rate of increase in sodium concentration is thought to be an important factor in the clinical presentation. For example, a sodium level of 170 mEq/L can be associated with little neurologic symptomatology if the rise occurs over a prolonged period. Indeed, hypertonic saline is occasionally used as a primary therapy for raised ICP,[88,89] in which case the elevation in sodium should be considered desirable, with desirable ICP, vasoregulatory, and neurochemical effects. Moreover, treating it could precipitate a rebound increase in ICP.

Diabetes insipidus can occur when disease processes affect the pituitary gland or its vascular supply. It should be suspected when urine output is inappropriately increased. Typically, urine output can increase abruptly to greater than 1 L per hour and be associated with severe hypernatremia and hypovolemic hypotension. Diagnosis of diabetes insipidus is based on continued output of dilute urine in the context of hypertonic serum. The specific gravity of urine will be close to 1.001 with osmolarity less than 200 mOsm/L despite serum osmolarity that may be greater than 320 mOsm/L.[90]

Hyponatremia. Hyponatremia can occur because of the syndrome of inappropriate secretion of antidiuretic hormone, so-called cerebral salt wasting, or excessive free water administration. Syndrome of inappropriate secretion of antidiuretic hormone is generally associated with hypervolemia and cerebral salt wasting with hypovolemia. Both syndromes can be associated with elevated urinary sodium concentrations, making differentiation between the two syndromes difficult in routine clinical practice.[91] Rapidly increasing the sodium concentration can produce permanent neurologic damage due to central pontine myelinolysis.[92] When the sodium level achieved with such overcorrection is extreme (i.e., 168 to 195 mMol/L), then extrapontine myelinolysis has also been reported.[93]

CATECHOLAMINES

Subarachnoid hemorrhage (SAH) is an entity particularly notable for catecholamine effects, some of which are described elsewhere in this book. However, catecholamine effects also occur with increased ICP, stroke, head trauma, or any situation of compromised midbrain-hindbrain oxygen delivery.

Serum catecholamine levels increase dramatically after SAH, notably peaking at the same time as the peak incidence of post-SAH vasospasm with symptom development corresponding to serum catecholamine levels.[94-98] This leads to the notion that hypothalamic injury with excess catecholamine release may be an important factor in the genesis of post-SAH spasm and stroke.[95] Several lines of evidence further support this hypothesis:

1. The cerebral vasculature is invested somewhat with adrenergic nerves. With SAH, the adrenergic receptors in the cerebral vessels decrease in quantity.[98,99] This suggests that denervation hypersensitivity may be occurring such that the increase in humoral catecholamines with SAH produces spasm in hyperreacting vessels.

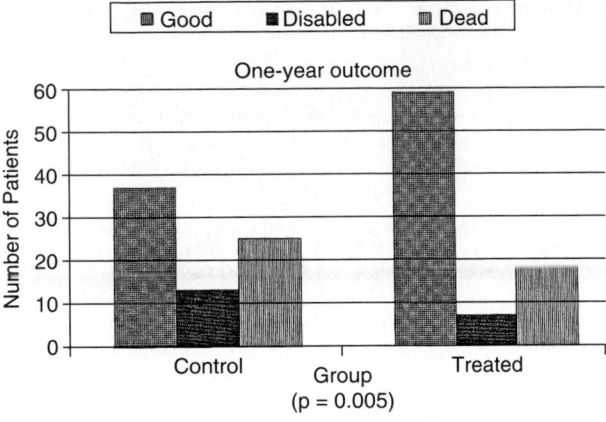

FIGURE 47–16. Subarachnoid hemorrhage patients were randomly treated with propranolol or placebo. Neurologic outcome was better in patients undergoing beta-blockade. (Data from Neil-Dwyer G, Walter P, Cruickshank JM: Beta-blockade benefits patients following a subarachnoid hemorrhage. Eur J Clin Pharmacol 1985;28[suppl]:25.)

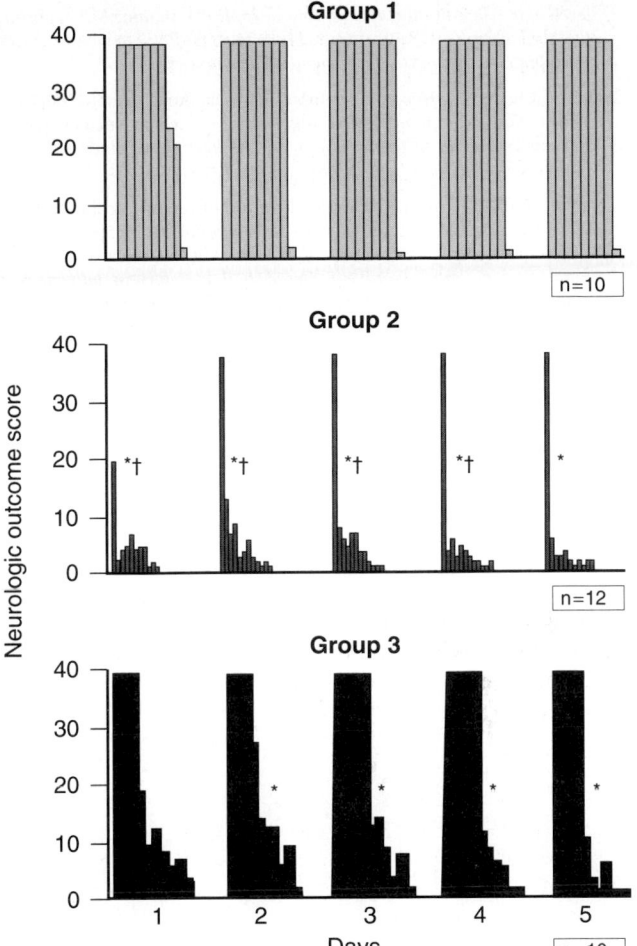

FIGURE 47–17. Neurologic deficit scores after incomplete focal cerebral ischemia in rats over a 5-day examination period. Each bar represents the neurologic score for each rat (*$P < .05$ vs. group 1; $P < .05$ vs. group 3). The rats are ranked according to total outcome score in descending order (0 = normal). Cerebral ischemia was induced with occlusion of one carotid artery with hemorrhagic hypotension. Group 1 rats received no vasoactive drugs; group 2 rats received preischemic hexamethonium; and group 3 rats received hexamethonium plus intravenous epinephrine and norepinephrine. Protection was conferred by hexamethonium in a catecholamine-reversible manner. (From Werner C, Hoffman WE, Thomas C, et al: Ganglionic blockade improves neurologic outcome from incomplete ischemia in rats: Partial reversal by exogenous catecholamines. Anesthesiology 1990;73:923.)

2. Catecholamine release after SAH is sufficient to produce electrocardiographic changes[94,96,100,101] with ventricular wall motion abnormalities[102] and myocardial injury.[103,104]
3. Treatment of humans with SAH with beta- and alpha-adrenergic antagonists is associated with an improvement in neurologic outcome (Fig. 47-16)[28] and electrocardiographic abnormalities.[101]
4. In animal models, selective destruction of hindbrain adrenergic nuclei with cephalad projections prevents the development of vasospasm.[104] Moreover, laboratory studies indicate an important role for vasopressin in cases of vasospasm, because vasospasm cannot be produced in vasopressin-deficient rats.[105]
5. Studies in cerebral ischemia models provide strong support for the notion that catecholamines can exacerbate ischemic injury. Compared with hemorrhage-induced hypotension, ischemic damage was decreased with hypotension induced through the use of ganglionic blockade with hexamethonium,[27] central adrenergic blockade with alpha-2 agonists,[29] and angiotensin converting enzyme inhibition.[106] Hemorrhaged control rats were noted to sustain an increase in exogenous catecholamine concentrations. To test the hypothesis that these catecholamines contributed to brain damage, some of the animals treated with hexamethonium also received intravenous catecholamine infusions. Reversal of the hexamethonium brain protective effect was observed in these animals (Fig. 47-17).[27]
6. Brain protection has been observed in laboratory studies with preischemic[107] and preseizure[108] treatment using reserpine, a drug that depletes presynaptic catecholamine stores.
7. Application of catecholamines directly to nonischemic cortical tissue has also been observed to have neurotoxic potential.[109] In addition, intravenous administration can exacerbate brain swelling after head trauma, although this is most likely a direct effect of blood pressure on a dysautoregulating brain (see Fig. 47-8) rather than a manifestation of biochemical neurotoxicity.[14]

SUMMARY

Brain damage can arise from a variety of seemingly disparate neurologic disease states. Such conditions, discussed in subsequent chapters, include ischemia, seizures, trauma, or other adverse processes. Raised ICP typically occurs as these types of conditions progress. When episodes of intracranial hypertension occur, it is important to distinguish hyperemic (with high CBV) from oligemic causes. Any brain injury is significantly impaired by the extracranial environment. Such extracranial factors include temperature, gas exchange, glucose, sepsis, sodium, and catecholamines. Optimal physiology-guided therapy is essential to optimize outcomes in neurointensive care.

ANNOTATED REFERENCES

Huseby JS, Luce JM, Cary JM, et al: Effects of positive end-expiratory pressure on intracranial pressure in dogs with intracranial hypertension. J Neurosurg 1981;55:704.

This study in dogs identified the role of hydraulic issues in the genesis of PEEP-induced increases, or lack of increases, in the presence of varying levels of ICP. The authors nicely showed, while maintaining MAP constant, that the higher the ICP was, the less likely it was for PEEP to increase sagittal sinus pressure to an extent sufficient to increase ICP.

Levine S: Anoxic-ischemic encephalopathy in rats. Am J Pathol 1960;36:1.
This article demonstrated the importance of cerebrovascular reserve. Rodents exposed to either hypoxia or carotid ligation sustained no deficits. However, induction of both insults reproducibly caused a stroke.

Lundberg N: Continuous recording and control of ventricular fluid pressure in neurosurgical practice. Acta Psychiatr Neurol Scand 1960;36(suppl 149):1.
This is the original paper, now a classic, describing plateau waves in a large number of patients. Lundberg placed ICP monitors in patients with nontraumatic intracranial hypertension and recorded his observations, identifying three types of plateau waves.

Neil-Dwyer G, Walter P, Cruickshank JM: Beta-blockade benefits patients following a subarachnoid hemorrhage. Eur J Clin Pharmacol 1985; 28(suppl):25.
This paper in humans with SAH showed an improvement in neurologic outcome when sympatholytic drugs were employed.

Rosner MJ, Becker DP: Origin and evolution of plateau waves: Experimental observations and a theoretical model. J Neurosurg 1984;50:312.
This important paper identified the relationship between blood pressure variations and plateau waves, then synthesized it with work of others to suggest an important role for changes in cerebral blood volume in still autoregulating brain to produce plateau waves.

Werner C, Hoffman WE, Thomas C, et al: Ganglionic blockade improves neurologic outcome from incomplete ischemia in rats: Partial reversal by exogenous catecholamines. Anesthesiology 1990;73:923.
This paper (and that of Hoffman et al[29]) on rodents provides excellent support for the notion that catecholamines can worsen the results of brain ischemia.

Chapter 48

ADVANCED BEDSIDE NEUROMONITORING

Roman Hlatky • Claudia Robertson

KEY POINTS

1. Evaluation of **neurologic** and mental **status** should be included in the monitoring protocol whenever possible.

2. **Intracranial pressure (ICP)** cannot be reliably estimated from any clinical feature in critically ill patients. On computed tomography (CT) scans, signs of brain swelling, such as midline shift and compressed basal cisterns, are predictive of raised ICP, but intracranial hypertension can occur without these findings.

3. Patients with traumatic brain injury who are at particular **risk for developing elevated ICP** include those with Glasgow coma scale (GCS) scores of 8 or less after resuscitation and abnormal CT scans, as well as those with GCS scores of 8 or less, normal CT scans, but adverse features such as age older than 40 years, systolic blood pressure of 90 mm Hg or less, and motor deficit.

4. The **ventriculostomy catheter** remains the preferred device for monitoring ICP and is the standard against which all new monitors are compared.

5. The two major **complications of ICP monitoring** are ventriculitis (1% to 10% of cases) and intracranial hemorrhage (1% to 2%).

6. **Normal** resting **ICP** is less than 10 mm Hg. Transient elevations of ICP occur normally with straining, coughing, or the Trendelenburg position. A sustained ICP greater than 20 mm Hg is clearly abnormal. An ICP greater than 40 mm Hg represents severe, usually life-threatening, **intracranial hypertension**.

7. The simplest measure of cerebral perfusion is **cerebral perfusion pressure** (CPP). For equivalent levels of CPP, cerebral perfusion is impaired more by reductions in blood pressure than by increases in ICP.

8. In head-injured patients, the average **jugular venous oxygen saturation (SjvO$_2$)** is higher than normal (55% to 71%), and the range for SjvO$_2$ is considerably wider than it is in normal subjects. If the strategy is to use SjvO$_2$ as a monitor of global oxygenation, cannulating the **dominant jugular vein** is logical, because it is the most representative of the whole brain.

9. Transcranial **Doppler ultrasonography** is a non-invasive monitor that provides indirect information about cerebral blood flow in one of the major arteries at the base of the brain. In the absence of vessel stenosis or vasospasm or changes in arterial blood pressure or blood rheology, the **pulsatility** reflects the distal cerebrovascular resistance.

10. The **Lindegaard (hemispheric) index** is a ratio of flow velocity in the middle cerebral artery and internal cerebral artery. The mean hemispheric index in normal individuals is 1.76 ± 0.1, and pathologic values suggestive of vasospasm are generally above 3.

11. The major limitation of SjvO$_2$ as a monitor of the adequacy of cerebral blood flow is that regional ischemia is not identified. In situations in which regional differences in cerebral blood flow may occur, such as brain trauma, **brain tissue oxygen partial pressure (PbtO$_2$)** as a monitor of cerebral oxygenation may have an important advantage.

12. **Normal values for PbtO$_2$** are 20 to 40 mm Hg, and critical reductions are 8 to 10 mm Hg.

13. **Microdialysis** is a technique for sampling the extracellular space of a tissue. It is based on the diffusion of water-soluble substances through a semipermeable membrane and allows continuous and on-line monitoring of changes in brain tissue chemistry.

14. The use of **electroencephalograms (EEGs)** in the ICU to detect early subclinical seizures may help reduce mortality and morbidity in status epilepticus. Continuous EEG monitoring is also useful in detecting ischemic cerebral events, including vasospasm following subarachnoid hemorrhage and intracranial hypertension after head injury.

Currently, little can be done to reverse the primary brain damage caused by an insult; however, one of the major factors influencing outcome in patients with acute brain injury is the additional brain damage that occurs from secondary injury processes. Intracranial hypertension and cerebral ischemia are the most significant secondary injury processes that can be monitored and treated in the ICU. In addition, secondary ischemic insults of extracerebral origin (e.g., arterial hypotension, hypocapnia) can be prevented or treated before they become severe enough to injure the brain. The purpose of continuous monitoring of the brain in the ICU is to detect these secondary insults, allowing for a more informed, individualized approach to treatment.

MONITORING OF NEUROLOGIC STATUS

Evaluation of neurologic and mental status should be included in the monitoring protocol whenever possible. Glasgow coma scale (GCS) score, motor function, status of cranial nerves, and any trend in neurologic status changes should be easily obtainable from the records. A 24-hour record of the patient's neurologic evaluation should be available on one sheet, together with information about vital signs and laboratory values. Computerized information systems are becoming more widespread in ICUs and can markedly reduce the burden of such record keeping. In critically ill patients, however, the neurologic examination is often obscured by the need to use sedation or neuromuscular blocking agents in the treatment of intracranial hypertension or other associated injuries or disorders.

One relatively new addition to the neurologic examination, which may reduce observer variability, is the hand-held pupillometer. A recent technical note reported good reliability in measuring pupillary diameter using the pupillometer; in addition, this device provides a quantitative measure of the velocity of the pupillary response to light.[1] Studies are needed to determine whether changes in the velocity of the pupillary response might be a sensitive measure of worsening neurologic status.

MONITORING OF INTRACRANIAL PRESSURE

Intracranial pressure (ICP) cannot be reliably estimated from any clinical feature in critically ill patients. Clinical symptoms of raised ICP, such as headache, nausea, and vomiting, are impossible to elicit in comatose patients. Papilledema is not a reliable sign of raised ICP in acute disorders. In one study of 426 patients with traumatic brain injury, only 3.5% had papilledema on funduscopic examination, although 54% of patients had increased ICP.[2] Other neurologic signs, including pupillary dilatation and decerebrate posturing, can occur in the absence of intracranial hypertension. On computed tomography (CT) scans, signs of brain swelling, such as midline shift and compressed basal cisterns, are predictive of raised ICP, but intracranial hypertension can occur without these findings.[3]

Because intracranial hypertension cannot be reliably determined clinically, the direct monitoring of ICP plays an important role in guiding therapy and assessing prognosis in patients with acute neurologic disorders. The ideal ICP monitor would be noninvasive; would provide an accurate, stable measure of pressure; and would provide continuously updated information. A number of noninvasive technologies have been explored as possible replacements or even adjuncts for the ICP monitor. These techniques include tissue resonance,[4] measurements of skull movement associated with ICP pulsations,[5] measurement of venous outflow pressure by ophthalmodynamometry,[6] measurement of tympanic membrane displacement,[7] and monitoring of visual evoked responses.[8] None of these tests is sufficiently reliable to replace the ventriculostomy catheter in the management of critically ill patients.

INDICATIONS

Monitoring of ICP can result in serious complications and is therefore indicated only in patients at significant risk of developing intracranial hypertension. In patients with traumatic brain injury, ICP has been systemically studied by many investigators, and there is a general consensus on the indications for invasive monitoring. Patients with traumatic brain injury who are at particular risk for developing raised ICP include those with GCS scores of 8 or less after resuscitation and abnormal CT scans, as well as those with GCS scores of 8 or less, normal CT scans, but adverse features such as age older than 40 years, systolic blood pressure of 90 mm Hg or less, and motor deficit.[9] More recent studies have shown that comatose patients without these adverse features may also have transiently elevated ICP, suggesting that all patients with GCS scores of 8 or less should have ICP monitoring.[10] Patients with GCS scores greater than 8 might be considered for ICP monitoring if they require treatment that would not allow serial neurologic examinations.[11] A severe coagulopathy is the only major contraindication to ICP monitoring. For critically ill patients with other, nontraumatic neurologic disorders, the indications for ICP monitoring are less clear, but the same general guidelines are often used.

TECHNIQUES

Although several new types of monitors have recently been marketed, the ventriculostomy catheter remains the preferred device for monitoring ICP and is the standard against which all new monitors are compared (Table 48-1).

TABLE 48–1. MONITORING OF INTRACRANIAL PRESSURE AND CEREBRAL PERFUSION

Monitoring Domain	Attributes of Ideal Monitor	Current Strategy of Choice		Current Alternatives
Intracranial pressure	Accurate, noninvasive	Ventriculostomy: most accurate, highest rate of complications		Parenchymal devices: cannot rezero, lower rate of complications
				Spiegelberg catheter: accurate pressure, also monitors intracranial compliance
Cerebral perfusion	Continuous or frequent serial bedside imaging of regional CBF	Early CBF imaging (xenon CT or perfusion CT) to determine nature of neurologic disorder		Plain CT imaging could substitute for CBF imaging by suggesting the likely nature of the disorder
		If diffuse: $Pbto_2$ or $Sjvo_2$ to monitor for secondary insults	If focal: $Pbto_2$ in area of hypoperfusion and $Sjvo_2$ as global monitor	Local CBF probes (laser Doppler or thermal diffusion) could substitute for $Pbto_2$
				Global measures (CPP, flow volume) could substitute for $Sjvo_2$

CBF, cerebral blood flow; CPP, cerebral perfusion pressure; CT, computed tomography; $Pbto_2$, brain tissue oxygen partial pressure; $Sjvo_2$, jugular venous oxygen saturation.

The ventriculostomy catheter is positioned with its tip in the frontal horn of the lateral ventricle and is coupled by fluid-filled tubing to an external pressure transducer that can be reset to zero and recalibrated against an external standard. The ventriculostomy ICP monitor allows intracranial hypertension to be treated by the intermittent drainage of cerebrospinal fluid. However, the risk of ventriculitis and of intracranial hemorrhage is high with ventriculostomy,[9] and proper placement of the catheter tip in the lateral ventricle can be difficult in patients with small, compressed ventricles.

When the ventricle cannot be cannulated, alternative devices can be used. The microsensor transducer[12] and the fiberoptic transducer[13] are the most widely available. These miniature transducer-tipped catheters can be inserted in the subdural space or directly into brain tissue. The main advantage of these monitors is their ease of insertion, especially in patients with compressed ventricles; however, the transducers cannot be reset to zero after they are inserted into the skull, and they exhibit drift over time.[14] Another ventricular catheter, employing an air pouch balloon catheter technology, allows automated monitoring of the intraventricular volume-pressure relationship, in addition to the intraventricular pressure.[15] Investigations are needed to determine whether intracranial compliance can provide an earlier indication of a developing mass lesion or worsening brain swelling than does the simple measurement of ICP.

COMPLICATIONS

The two major complications of ICP monitoring are ventriculitis and intracranial hemorrhage. Infection may be confined to the skin wound, but in 1% to 10% of cases, ventriculitis occurs. Most studies have found a higher rate of infection in ventriculostomy-monitored patients than in those monitored with subarachnoid bolts or subdural catheters.[9,16] An analysis of data from the Traumatic Coma Data Bank study also suggests that there is no benefit in changing ventriculostomy catheters at 5-day intervals.[17] The best strategy for reducing the risk of ventriculitis associated with ICP monitoring is to minimize the duration of monitoring. No controlled studies have demonstrated that prophylactic antibiotics can reduce the incidence of ventriculostomy-related infections. A randomized trial of ventriculostomy catheters impregnated with minocycline and rifampin demonstrated that the impregnated catheters were half as likely to become colonized as the control catheters were (17.9% and 36.7%, respectively, $P < .0012$).[18] Positive cerebrospinal fluid cultures were seven times less frequent in patients with antibiotic-impregnated catheters compared with those in the control group (1.3% and 9.4%, respectively, $P = .002$).

The second major complication of ICP monitoring is intracerebral hemorrhage. Although the risk of hemorrhage is low (1% to 2%), it is an important complication to recognize and treat.[9] Patients with coagulopathies have a greater risk of developing this complication.

NORMAL VALUES

Normally, resting ICP is less than 10 mm Hg. Transient increases in ICP occur normally with straining, coughing, or the Trendelenburg position. A sustained ICP greater than 20 mm Hg is clearly abnormal; an ICP between 20 and 40 mm Hg is considered moderate intracranial hypertension;

and an ICP greater than 40 mm Hg represents severe, usually life-threatening, intracranial hypertension.[19] These guidelines for determining the severity of intracranial hypertension assume a normal blood pressure. When a temporal mass lesion is present, however, herniation can occur at ICP values less than 20 mm Hg.[20] Both the American and European head injury guidelines recommend treatment of ICP that is greater than 20 to 25 mm Hg.[21,22]

MONITORING OF CEREBRAL PERFUSION AND OXYGENATION

The ideal neuromonitor for ischemia would provide continuously updated information about regional cerebral blood flow (CBF) and metabolism throughout the brain (see Table 48-1). Continuously updated information is needed because acute neurologic disorders evolve over time, and early intervention provides the best chance for a successful outcome. Regional information is required because neurologic disorders tend to develop regionally in the brain, especially early in the course.

An ideal monitor for ischemia does not currently exist. High-resolution maps of regional CBF are available with current imaging techniques; however, this type of study generally required that patients be taken out of the ICU to the radiology department. High-quality CT imaging, including of CBF, can now be obtained in the ICU. Reports suggest that this arrangement is safer for critically ill patients and is cost-effective.[23] It is likely that in the future, such imaging will be used in the ICU similar to a bedside monitor. The best monitoring strategy at present is the use of a monitor of global cerebral perfusion and a monitor of local cerebral perfusion placed strategically in the area of the brain considered most vulnerable to the development of ischemia.

There are several choices for measuring global and local cerebral perfusion. These monitors fall into two categories: those that measure CBF directly, and those that provide indirect information about CBF by measuring oxygen extraction. Measures of cerebral oxygenation, such as jugular venous oxygen saturation ($SjvO_2$) or brain tissue oxygen partial pressure ($PbtO_2$), are widely used in place of quantitative CBF measurements in critically ill patients because they indicate the adequacy of CBF relative to cerebral metabolic requirements. Because cerebral metabolic requirements may be reduced after traumatic brain injury, normal CBF values may not be optimal. For instance, when CBF is low (25 to 30 mL/100 g per minute), it can be difficult to decide whether this is an appropriate response to lower cerebral metabolic requirements or whether the brain is hypoperfused. A measure of cerebral oxygenation can be helpful in making this distinction. If the brain is hypoperfused, oxygen extraction will be increased, and $SjvO_2$ will be reduced. If CBF is appropriate for the brain's metabolic requirement, $SjvO_2$ will be normal. This information is often more clinically useful than are absolute CBF values.

GLOBAL MONITORS

Cerebral Perfusion Pressure

The simplest measure of cerebral perfusion is cerebral perfusion pressure (CPP), which is calculated by subtracting the ICP from the mean arterial blood pressure. The normal lower limit of autoregulation for CPP is 50 mm Hg. In severely head-injured patients, the ability to autoregulate

TABLE 48–2. NORMAL VALUES FOR NEUROPHYSIOLOGIC PARAMETERS

Parameter	Normal Values	Critical Values
Cerebral blood flow		
Global	52 ± 12 mL/100 g/min[67]	18-20 mL/100 g/min
Cortical	80 mL/100 g/min[68]	
Flow volume	268 ± 60 mL/min[69]	
Cerebral oxygenation		
$Pjvo_2$	40 mm Hg[68]	20-30 mm Hg
$Sjvo_2$	55-71%[39]	50%[39]
$Pbto_2$	20-40 mm Hg[70]	8.5-10 mm Hg[70]
$AVDo_2$	4.5-8.5 mL/100 mL[67]	
Cerebral metabolism		
$CMRO_2$	3.4 mL/100 g/min[32]	0.6 µmol/g/min
CMRG	0.325 µmol/g/min[32]	
CMRL	–0.02 µmol/g/min[32]	
MD-glucose	1.7 ± 0.9 µmol/L[71]	
MD-lactate	2.9 ± 0.9 mmol/L[71]	
MD-pyruvate	166 ± 47 mmol/L[71]	
MD-glutamate	16 ± 16 µmol/L[71]	

AVDo₂, arteriovenous oxygen difference; CMRG, cerebral metabolic rate of glucose; CMRL, cerebral metabolic rate of lactate; CMRO₂, cerebral metabolic rate of oxygen; MD, microdialysate; Pbto₂, brain tissue oxygen partial pressure; Pjvo₂, jugular venous oxygen partial pressure; Sjvo₂, jugular venous oxygen saturation.

may be impaired, and CBF may be inadequate even with CPP values greater than 50 mm Hg. CPP can be reduced through either decreases in blood pressure or increases in ICP. For equivalent levels of CPP, cerebral perfusion is impaired more by reductions in blood pressure than by increases in ICP.[24] As a monitor for cerebral perfusion, CPP is widely available and convenient; its limitation is that only ischemia caused by increased ICP or decreased blood pressure is assessed. A normal CPP does not confirm that CBF is adequate.

Kety-Schmidt Technique

Measurement of global CBF by the classic Kety-Schmidt technique (based on the Fick principle) uses nitrous oxide as the diffusible indicator. It can be performed at the bedside with a minimum of expense and equipment. Instruments for measuring regional CBF using the stable xenon-enhanced CT technique are also commercially available.[25-27] However, both these measurements of CBF are intermittent and require the patient to be hemodynamically stable during the time required for the measurements. Therefore, transient CBF reductions or CBF reductions in an acutely unstable patient are difficult to document with these technologies.

Jugular Venous Oxygen Saturation

Placement of an internal jugular vein catheter, similar to the type used for central venous pressure monitoring but directed cephalad into the jugular bulb, allows repetitive sampling of Sjvo₂ without repeated needle punctures.[28-32] More recently, the development of in vivo reflectance oximetry using fiberoptic catheters has allowed continuous monitoring of Sjvo₂ without the need to sample blood, except for calibration purposes.[33-35]

Side of Catheterization. Studies comparing bilateral measurements of Sjvo₂ or comparing Sjvo₂ to oxygen saturation in the confluence of the cerebral sinuses clearly indicate that when there are focal lesions after traumatic brain injury, there may be significant differences in oxygen saturation measured in the left and right jugular bulbs.[36,37] If the strategy is to use Sjvo₂ as a monitor of global oxygenation, cannulating the dominant jugular vein is logical, because it is most representative of the whole brain. However, if the strategy is to

identify the most abnormal oxygen saturation, the recommendations of Metz and colleagues should be followed.[37]

Normal Sjvo₂. Gibbs and coworkers studied 50 normal young males and observed that their Sjvo₂ ranged from 55% to 71% (mean, 61.8%; Table 48-2).[38] In head-injured patients, the average Sjvo₂ is higher than normal, and the range for Sjvo₂ is considerably wider than it is in normal subjects. In a series of 116 patients with continuous measurement of Sjvo₂ for the first 5 to 10 days after severe head injury,[39] Sjvo₂ averaged $68.1 \pm 9.7\%$ (range, 32% to 96%) in 1329 measurements. Pjvo₂ averaged 37 ± 7 mm Hg (range, 22 to 85 mm Hg).

Experimental studies have extensively examined the ischemic thresholds for CBF. Only a few studies have examined the Sjvo₂ threshold associated with the depletion of energy stores in animals and with loss of consciousness or electroencephalogram (EEG) changes during anoxia in normal humans.[40-42] From these studies, it appears that normal brain metabolism can be altered at Sjvo₂ values less than 50%, but that values less than 20% are required for irreversible ischemic injury.

LOCAL OR REGIONAL MONITORS

Transcranial Doppler Flow Velocity and Flow Volume

Transcranial Doppler ultrasonography is a noninvasive monitor that provides indirect information about CBF in one of the major arteries at the base of the brain. A 2-MHz pulsed ultrasound signal is transmitted through the skull (usually through the temporal bone) and, using the Doppler shift principle, measures red cell flow velocity. Flow volume is directly proportional to flow velocity and can be calculated by multiplying the velocity by the cross-sectional area of the vessel insonated.

Several studies have assessed the relationship between peak flow velocity and changes in CBF, suggesting that changes in middle cerebral artery flow velocity can be used as an indicator of relative changes in blood flow. Kofke and associates, investigating the relationship between middle cerebral artery flow velocity and CBF assessed by stable xenon CT during balloon test occlusion of the carotid artery in 31 patients, found a significant correlation in the alteration of flow detected by the two methods.[43] More recently, changes in middle cerebral artery flow velocity and changes in CBF assessed by stable xenon CT in patients with various intracranial pathologies, including eight with closed-head injuries, showed a close correlation.[44]

In the absence of vessel stenosis or vasospasm or changes in arterial blood pressure or blood rheology, pulsatility reflects the distal cerebrovascular resistance. This resistance is usually quantified by the pulsatility (or Gosling) index, which is calculated as follows: (systolic flow velocity – diastolic flow velocity)/mean flow velocity. The pulsatility index (normal, 0.6 to 1.1) has been shown to correlate better with CPP than with ICP.

During arterial spasm, flow velocity increases through the narrowed segment proportional to the reduction in the vessel's diameter. Severe vasospasm, with a greater than 50% reduction in vessel diameter, is associated with a flow velocity greater than 200 cm/sec.[45] However, an increase in flow velocity may also reflect hyperemia, which often occurs as a post-traumatic event. To differentiate between these two hemodynamic phenomena in the absence of direct CBF measurements, the middle cerebral artery–extracranial internal carotid artery flow velocity ratio, also known as the Lindegaard or hemispheric index, can be measured. In the presence of hyperemia, a raised flow velocity in both extracranial and intracranial vessels does not alter the ratio; however, in vasospasm, flow velocity is high only in the intracranial vessels, resulting in a high hemispheric index. The mean hemispheric index in normal individuals is 1.76 ± 0.1, and pathologic values suggestive of vasospasm are generally above 3.[46]

Doppler devices that are capable of measuring the diameter of the vessel being insonated may be a better way to differentiate between these two hemodynamic causes of increased flow velocity by calculating flow volume. Flow volume of the internal carotid artery has a close correlation to hemispheric CBF measured by the [133]xenon clearance technique[47] and may be useful as a bedside estimation of hemispheric CBF.

Thermal Diffusion and Laser Doppler Methods

Two methods for continuously measuring local CBF are now commercially available: thermal diffusion and laser Doppler. Both methods are invasive, requiring that the probe be placed on the surface of the brain or in the brain parenchyma. Both methods measure CBF in only a small volume of brain, which may or may not be representative of the whole brain. However, the continuous nature of the measurements provides a dynamic picture of brain perfusion. Although there is extensive documentation of the reliability of these methods in the laboratory, there is limited experience in the ICU.[48-50] Especially for patients undergoing craniotomy, these may become practical methods for monitoring CBF postoperatively.

Thermal diffusion flowmetry uses heat transfer as a tracer in the measurement of blood flow. The sensor consists of two gold disks embedded in a 3-mm Silastic leaf. One disk is heated to slightly greater than brain temperature (to a maximum of 44° C), and the other is neutral. The probe is laid on the surface of the brain. The temperature difference between the two disks is monitored and converted to blood flow in milliliters/100 g per minute by the monitor, using a digital display. Carter and Atkinson[51] modified a thermal sensor described by Brawley[52] and were able to quantify the flow

measured by the thermal sensor. They derived a mathematical formula by comparing thermal diffusion CBF with [133]xenon CBF[53] and confirmed the reliability through a comparison with hydrogen clearance.[54]

Gopinath and colleagues compared thermal diffusion CBF with global CBF values measured using the nitrous oxide saturation technique in a group of 35 patients with severe head injury.[55] As expected, the thermal diffusion CBF, which measures cortical flow, was significantly higher than the global CBF, which is a mixture of gray and white matter flow. However, there was a close temporal correlation between the two measures of CBF, and changes in thermal diffusion CBF reliably predicted a change in global CBF. These studies suggest that thermal diffusion CBF provides an accurate measure of local CBF under the probe and is a reasonable estimate of trend changes in global CBF.

Laser Doppler flowmetry is a technique whereby CBF is measured indirectly, based on the magnitude of frequency shift of monochromatic light by a moving column of blood. The laser light is directed at the region of interest through a small probe that illuminates about 1 mm^3 of tissue. With this high spatial resolution, it is designed primarily for measuring flow in capillaries.[56]

Brain Tissue Oxygen Partial Pressure

The major limitation of $SjvO_2$ as a monitor of CBF adequacy is that regional ischemia is not identified. In cases of brain trauma, regional differences in CBF may occur, giving $PbtO_2$ an important advantage as a monitor of cerebral oxygenation.[57,58] Figure 48-1 illustrates the changes in $PbtO_2$ in a focal area of evolving ischemia. $SjvO_2$ remains well preserved until the brain swelling from the infarction causes severe intracranial hypertension.

With recent technologic advances, two commercially available sensors have been produced. One sensor measures only brain tissue oxygen tension using a polarographic Clarke-type electrode; the other multiparameter sensor measures brain tissue oxygen, carbon dioxide, and pH using fiberoptic technology. Both these methods have the ability to measure brain temperature using a thermocouple. Both sensors are approximately 0.5 mm in diameter and can be inserted through a craniotomy intraoperatively or through a specially designed bolt that allows insertion and fixation to the skull in the ICU.

Normal values for $PbtO_2$ are 20 to 40 mm Hg, and critical levels are 8 to 10 mm Hg (see Table 48-2). Hoffman and coworkers, using single photon emission computed tomography, found that $PbtO_2$ in patients with ischemia averaged 10 ± 5 mm Hg, compared with 37 ± 12 mm Hg in normal brain.[59] Valadka and associates found that the likelihood of death following a severe head injury increased the longer the $PbtO_2$ remained at less than 15 mm Hg, and with any occurrence of $PbtO_2$ less than 6 mm Hg.[60] Kiening and colleagues correlated serial measurements of both $SjvO_2$ and $PbtO_2$ and found that an $SjvO_2$ of 50% generally correlates with a $PbtO_2$ of 8.5 mm Hg.[61]

Near-Infrared Spectroscopy

The principle of near-infrared spectroscopy is based on the fact that light in the near-infrared range (700 to 1000 nm) can pass through skin, bone, and other tissues relatively easily. Oxygenated hemoglobin, deoxygenated hemoglobin, and cytochrome aa_3 have different absorption spectra, depending on their oxygenation status. Changes in the concentration of

Admission CT

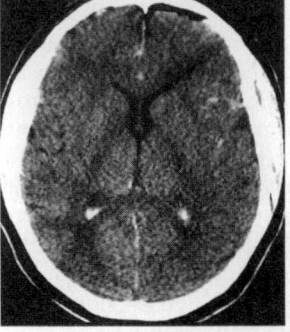

CT 12hr after admission

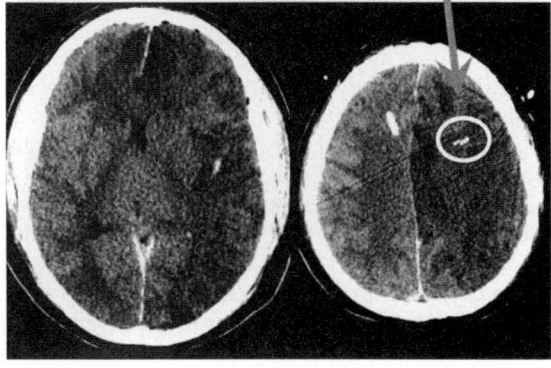

**probes placed in
left frontal lobe**

FIGURE 48–1. Monitoring in a patient with severe traumatic brain injury. Brain tissue oxygen partial pressure (Pbto$_2$) and microdialysis probes were placed in the left frontal lobe, where subarachnoid hemorrhage was present on the admission computed tomography (CT) scan. The Pbto$_2$ decreased, followed shortly by the microdialysate glucose and pyruvate. A follow-up CT scan showed a stroke developing in the brain surrounding the local probes. Cerebral perfusion pressure (CPP) and jugular venous oxygen saturation (Sjvo$_2$) provide measures of global cerebral perfusion, which is fairly well preserved until intracranial hypertension becomes severe and refractory to treatment. ICP, intracranial pressure; MAP, mean arterial pressure.

A

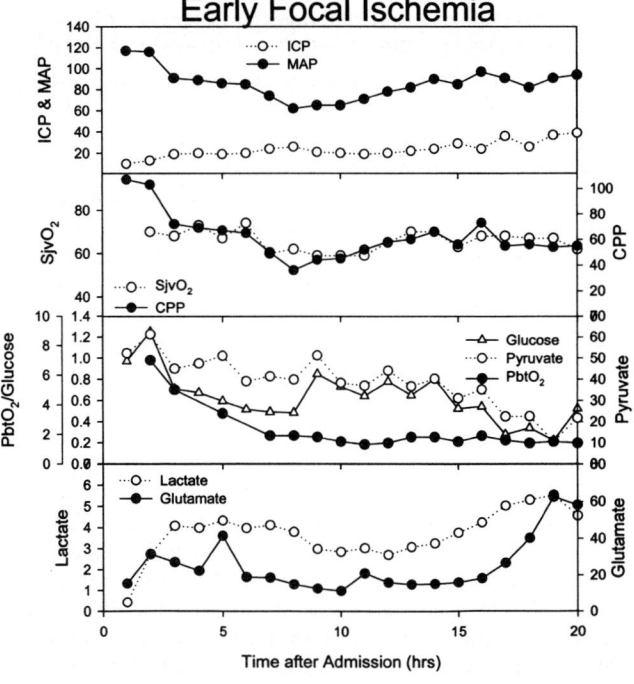

B

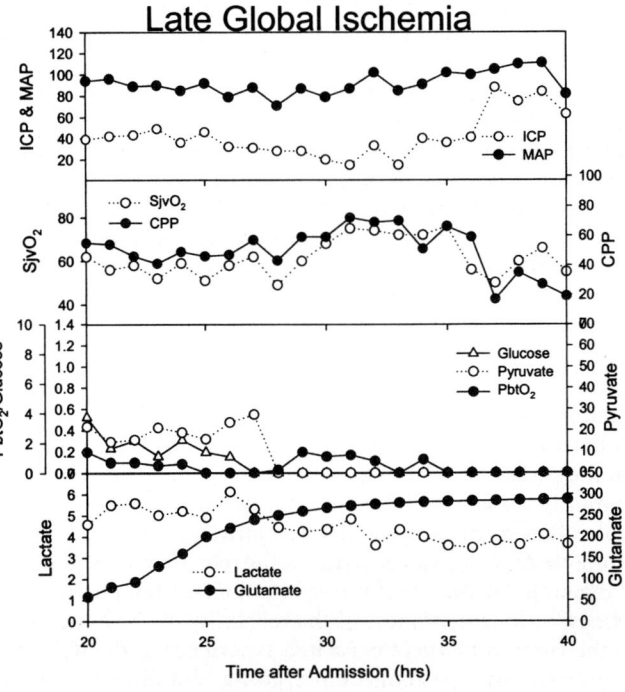

C

near-infrared light as it passes through these compounds can be quantified using a modified Beer-Lambert law, which describes optical attenuation. The main advantage of near-infrared spectroscopy is that it is a noninvasive method of estimating regional changes in cerebral oxygenation. However, its clinical use is limited by an inability to differentiate between intracranial and extracranial changes in blood flow and oxygenation, which adversely affects the reliability of the readings.[62]

MONITORING OF BRAIN METABOLISM

GLOBAL CEREBRAL METABOLIC RATE OF SUBSTRATES

The cerebral metabolic rate (CMR) of a substrate can be calculated by multiplying the arterial-jugular venous difference of the substrate by the global CBF. Measuring the CMR of oxygen, glucose, and lactate gives a comprehensive picture of the brain's overall metabolism. However, the measurements are not continuous, and regional abnormalities may not be reflected.

Glucose is the major energy substrate for the brain. The average CMR of glucose in adults is 0.325 µmol/g per minute, and the gray matter has higher metabolic requirements than the white matter does. More than 90% of the normal brain's metabolic demands are met by aerobic metabolism of glucose through the glycolytic pathway, citric acid cycle, and respiratory chain, providing 38 moles of adenosine triphosphate per mole of glucose.

In the resting state, anaerobic glycolysis represents less than 10% of the total glucose usage, yielding only 2 moles of adenosine triphosphate and lactate per mole of glucose metabolized. Neuronal stimulation results in an increase in glucose metabolism compared with oxygen consumption, signifying the importance of glycolytic metabolism in electrical activation. Normally, there is a small production of lactate by the brain, and the mean CMR of lactate is −0.02 µmol/g per minute.

The normal CMR of oxygen in the healthy adult brain averages 3.4 mL/100 g per minute (1.5 µmol/g per minute) but may range from 1.8 to 3.9 mL/100 g per minute without neurologic sequelae. The CMR of oxygen increases minimally during changes in mental activity, with the increased energy expenditure being provided by the anaerobic metabolism of glucose. In acute neurologic disorders resulting in coma, the CMR of oxygen is typically reduced by about 50%. A CMR of oxygen less than 0.6 µmol/g per minute is insufficient to maintain normal cellular function.

MICRODIALYSIS

Microdialysis is a technique of sampling the extracellular space of a tissue. It is based on the diffusion of water-soluble substances through a semipermeable membrane. Small molecules (<20,000 Da) from the extracellular fluid can diffuse across the membrane and enter the perfusate. Conversely, substances that have been added to the perfusate can diffuse across the membrane to gain entry to the tissue. The degree of permeability of the membrane determines the molecular weight of the substances that cross it.

The concentration of substances in the dialysate depends on the flow rate and chemical composition of the perfusate, the length of the dialysis membrane, the type of dialysis membrane, and the diffusion coefficient or "tortuosity" of the tissue. The recovery of a particular substance is defined as the concentration in the dialysate divided by the concentration in the interstitial fluid. If the membrane is long enough and the flow slow enough, the concentration in the perfusate will be the same as that in the interstitial fluid (i.e., 100%). The parameters that are commonly used in clinical studies (i.e., 10-mm membrane, perfusion with Ringer's solution, and flow rate of 0.3 µL/min) provide an in vivo recovery rate (extrapolation to zero flow method) of approximately 70%.[63]

The technique of cerebral microdialysis allows continuous and on-line monitoring of changes in brain tissue chemistry. In common with brain tissue oxygenation monitoring, microdialysis involves inserting a fine catheter (diameter 0.62 mm) into the brain. The catheter has a polyamide dialysis membrane at the tip and is perfused with a physiologic solution (e.g., Ringer's) at ultra-low-flow rates (0.1 to 2.0 µL/min) using a precision pump. This allows measurement of the concentration of chemicals in the extracellular space of

the brain. Molecules below the cutoff size of the semipermeable membrane (approximately 20,000 Da) diffuse from the extracellular space into the perfusion fluid, which is collected in vials that are changed every 10 to 60 minutes. The collected dialysate is then analyzed by sensitive assays.

In theory, any substance small enough to diffuse through the dialysis membrane can be measured,[63] but the key substances can be categorized as follows:

1. Energy-related metabolites (glucose, lactate, pyruvate, adenosine, xanthine)
2. Neurotransmitters (glutamate, aspartate)
3. Markers of tissue damage and inflammation (glycerol)
4. Exogenous substances (administered drugs)

Continuous on-line measurements of glucose, lactate, pyruvate, glutamate, and glycerol can be achieved using a bedside CMA600 microdialysis analyzer (CMA Microdialysis, Stockholm, Sweden). Cerebral microdialysis has been applied to patients in many different clinical situations, including those with head injury, subarachnoid hemorrhage, epilepsy, ischemic stroke, and tumor, as well as during neurosurgery.[64] Figure 48-1 illustrates the changes in these parameters that can be seen with evolving ischemia. Although the role of microdialysis as a reliable clinical tool in the ICU is not yet established, its usefulness as a research tool is undeniable.

MONITORING OF ELECTROENCEPHALOGRAPHIC ACTIVITY

An EEG represents spontaneous electrical activity of the cerebral cortex and is generated mainly by the summation of excitatory and inhibitory postsynaptic potentials of cortical neurons. It does not reflect activity in subcortical levels, cranial nerves, or the spinal cord. The electrical signal is amplified, filtered, and then displayed as either 8 or 16 channels (8 channels per hemisphere) to give an accurate representation of electrical activity throughout the cortex. EEG activity is usually interpreted in terms of frequency, amplitude, and location (focal or generalized activity).

To facilitate continuous EEG monitoring, several automated EEG processing systems have been developed. Power spectral analysis allows fast Fourier transformation of small intervals of an EEG to provide a graphic representation of the relative power content of the various frequency bands in each segment of the EEG. These spectral diagrams are then stacked to show how the frequency of the EEG alters with time to produce a compressed spectral array. This spectral analysis can also provide a single number (either the mean frequency or the frequency below which 95% of the signal lies) that can be tracked over time.

Cerebral function monitoring provides a single trace of total power that varies with both the amplitude and the frequency of raw EEG data. The cerebral function analyzing monitor is a similar method that produces displays of both amplitude and frequency and avoids the loss of information when these are processed together.

Use of EEGs in the ICU to detect early subclinical seizures may help reduce mortality and morbidity in status epilepticus.[65] Continuous EEG monitoring is also useful in detecting ischemic cerebral events, including vasospasm following subarachnoid hemorrhage and intracranial hypertension after head injury.[66] In sedated patients, EEGs may help detect focal neurologic disease, especially in those who cannot be fully examined and in those who are too unstable to undergo neuroradiographic imaging. Metabolic suppression using intravenous anesthetic agents can be monitored using cerebral function monitoring, where burst suppression or isoelectricity is a useful endpoint to titrate suppression of cortical electrical activity.

CONCLUSION

Many tools are currently available for monitoring cerebral physiology. Some of these methods, such as ICP monitoring, have established roles in the management of critically ill patients. For other methods, such as microdialysis, their roles have yet to be determined. Clearly, the use of these advanced monitoring tools must be based on an understanding of the nature of the patient's neurologic disorder and a knowledge of the type of secondary injury processes that are likely to complicate the patient's course.

ANNOTATED REFERENCES

Bullock RM, Chesnut R, Clifton GL, et al: Management and prognosis of severe traumatic brain injury. Part 1. Guidelines for the management of severe traumatic brain injury. J Neurotrauma 2000;17:451-553.

Most recent version of the guidelines for managing severe traumatic brain injury.

Dings J, Meixensberger J, Roosen K: Brain tissue pO₂-monitoring: Catheter stability and complications. Neurol Res 1997;19:241-245.

Detailed description of the technical principles, limitations, and possible complications of brain tissue oxygen tension monitoring.

Gopinath SP, Robertson CS, Contant CF, et al: Jugular venous desaturation and outcome after head injury. J Neurol Neurosurg Psychiatry 1994;57:717-723.

This study demonstrates a correlation between the occurrence of jugular venous desaturation and outcome following severe head injury.

Maas AIR, Dearden M, Teasdale GM, et al: EBIC guidelines for management of severe head injury in adults. Acta Neurochir (Wien) 1997;139:286-294.

European version of the guidelines for managing severe traumatic brain injury.

Reinstrup P, Stahl N, Mellergard P, et al: Intracerebral microdialysis in clinical practice: Baseline values for chemical markers during wakefulness, anesthesia, and neurosurgery. Neurosurgery 2000;47:701-709.

The study provides the physiologic extracellular levels of the most often measured parameters.

Chapter 49

COMA

Joerg-Patrick Stübgen • Fred Plum

KEY POINTS

1. **Altered arousal** is due to an acute or subacute brain insult and reflects either diffuse and bilateral cerebral dysfunction, failure of the brainstemthalamic ascending reticular activating system, or both.

2. **Coma is not a permanent state.** Patients who survive evolve through and into altered behavioral states that reflect various degrees of recovery.

3. **Urgent steps are required to minimize additional brain damage** often before the cause of coma is definitely established.

4. The initial assessment must focus on vital signs to determine the appropriate resuscitation measures (**airway/breathing/circulation**).

5. When the patient's condition is stable, **clues to the cause of coma** must be sought from informative sources.

6. A **systematic, detailed examination** is necessary of the comatose patient, who is in no condition to describe past or current medical history.

7. The correct interpretation is required of neurologic signs that reflect the **integrity or impairment of brain functional levels** to determine the cause and evolution of coma.

8. The **categorization of coma** (supratentorial or infratentorial structural lesions, metabolic-toxic encephalopathy, or psychogenic unresponsiveness) is important in deciding the sequence of diagnostic and therapeutic steps that ensure the best possible patient outcome.

9. **CT is the most expedient imaging technique** to give rapid information about a brain structural lesion and its consequences.

10. Although the outcome of a comatose patient cannot be absolutely predicted, **a highly probable poor prognosis should be made within 24 hours after admission** to ration ICU services and protect families from false hope.

11. As a rule, patients in coma due to exogenous agents carry a favorable prognosis and patients in post-traumatic coma fare better than those in a medical coma.

Altered states of consciousness are a common reason for visits to the emergency department and admission to ICUs. Few problems are more difficult to manage than the unconscious patient because there are many potential causes of an altered mental status and the time for diagnosis and effective intervention is short. *Consciousness* is defined as the state of awareness of the self and the environment. The phenomenon of consciousness requires two intact and interdependent physiologic and anatomic components: (1) arousal (or wakefulness) and its underlying neural substrate, the ascending reticular activating system (ARAS) and diencephalon, and (2) awareness, which requires the functioning cerebral cortex of both hemispheres. Most disorders that acutely disturb consciousness are, in fact, impairments of arousal that create circumstances under which the brain's capacity for consciousness cannot be accurately assessed; in other words, failure of arousal renders it impossible to test awareness.

Alterations of arousal may be transient, lasting only several seconds or minutes (after seizures, syncope, and cardiac dysrhythmia), or sustained, lasting hours or longer. Four terms describe disturbed arousal of a patient. *Alert* refers to a normal state of arousal. *Stupor* describes a state of unarousability in which strong external stimuli can transiently restore wakefulness. Stupor implies at least a limited degree of cognitive activity accompanies the arousal, even if transient. *Coma* is characterized by an uninterrupted loss of the capacity for arousal. The eyes are closed, sleep-wake cycles disappear, and even vigorous stimulation elicits at best only reflex responses. *Lethargy* describes a range of behavior between arousal and stupor. Only the terms *alert* and *coma* have enough precision to be used without further qualification; possibly *coma* has gradations in depth, but this cannot be accurately assessed once the patient no longer responds to external stimuli. *Stupor* and *coma* imply an acute or subacute brain insult. The cerebral reserve capacity is large; therefore, altered consciousness reflects either diffuse and bilateral cerebral dysfunction, failure of the brainstem/thalamic ARAS, or both. All alterations in arousal should be regarded as acute and potentially life-threatening emergencies.

The evaluation of a comatose patient demands a systematic approach with appropriate, directed diagnostic and therapeutic endeavors; time should not be wasted on irrelevant considerations. Urgent steps are required to prevent or minimize permanent brain damage from reversible causes. Patient evaluation and treatment must necessarily occur simultaneously. Such a systematic approach demands an understanding of the pathophysiology of consciousness and mechanisms by which it may be deranged.

ANATOMY, PATHOLOGY, PATHOPHYSIOLOGY

Consciousness depends on an intact ARAS in the brainstem and adjacent thalamus that acts as the alerting or awakening element of consciousness together with a functioning cerebral cortex of both hemispheres that determines the content of that consciousness.[1,2] The ARAS lies within a more or less isodendritic core that extends from the medulla through the tegmentum of the pons to the midbrain and paramedian thalamus. The system is continuous caudally with the reticular intermediate gray matter of the spinal cord and rostrally with the subthalamus, the hypothalamus, the anterior thalamus, and the basal forebrain.[3] The ARAS itself arises within the rostral pontine tegmentum and extends across the mesencephalic tegmentum and its adjacent intrathalamic nuclei. ARAS functions and interconnections are considerable and likely contribute more than only a cortical arousal system. The specific role of the various links from the reticular formation to the thalamus has yet to be fully identified.[4] Furthermore, the cortex feeds back on the thalamic nuclei to contribute an important loop that amplifies arousal mechanisms.[5,6]

The ascending arousal system contains cholinergic, monoaminergic, and γ-aminobutyric acid (GABA) systems, none of which has been identified as the arousal neurotransmitter.[2,7,8] Acute structural damage to, or metabolic-chemical disturbance of, either the ascending brainstem/thalamic activating system or the thalamocorticothalamic loop can alter the aroused, attentive state. Consciousness depends on the continuous interaction between the mechanisms that provide arousal and awareness. The brainstem and thalamus provide the activating mechanism, and the cerebrum provides full cognition and self-excitation. Content of consciousness is best regarded as the amalgam and integration of all cognitive function that resides in the thalamocortical circuits of both hemispheres. Altered awareness is due to disruption of this cortical activity by diffuse pathology. Focal lesions of the cerebrum can produce profound deficits, such as aphasia, alexia, amnesia, and hemianopsia, but only diffuse bilateral damage, sparing the ARAS and diencephalon, can lead to wakeful unawareness. Thus, there are two kinds of altered consciousness: (1) altered arousal due to dysfunction of the ARAS-diencephalon and (2) altered awareness due to bilateral diffuse cerebral hemisphere dysfunction.

Four major pathologic processes can cause such severe, global, acute reductions of consciousness.[1,9] In the presence of diffuse or extensive multifocal bilateral dysfunction of the cerebral cortex, the cortical gray matter is diffusely and acutely depressed or destroyed. Concurrently, cortical-subcortical physiologic feedback excitatory loops are impaired, with the result that brainstem autonomic mechanisms become temporarily, profoundly inhibited, producing the equivalent of acute "reticular shock" below the level of the lesion.[2] Direct damage to a paramedian upper brainstem and posteroinferior diencephalic ascending arousal system blocks normal cortical activation.[3] Widespread disconnection between the cortex and subcortical activating mechanisms acts to produce effects similar to both these conditions.[4] Diffuse disorders, usually metabolic in origin, concurrently affect both the cortical and subcortical arousal mechanisms, although to a different degree according to the cause.

STRUCTURAL LESIONS CAUSING COMA

Intracranial mass lesions that cause coma may be located in the supratentorial or infratentorial compartments. From either location, impaired arousal or coma is caused by compression of the brainstem/hypothalamic activating mechanisms secondary to swelling and displacement of deep lying intracranial contents; the ultimate event occurs either by halting axoplasmic flow or by sustained neuronal depolarization because of ischemia or hemorrhage. Factors important to the degree of loss of arousal are the rate of development, the location, and the ultimate size of the lesion. Cerebral mass lesions distort the intracranial anatomy and thereby alter the cerebrospinal fluid (CSF) circulation and brain blood supply. These changes result in increased bulk of the injured tissue and a reduction in intracranial compliance.

Intercompartmental pressure gradients result in herniation syndromes that are not necessarily associated with large increases in intracranial pressure (ICP). Recently sustained or evolving mass lesions can disturb cerebrovascular autoregulation that results in abrupt, briefly lasting vasodilatation. This, in turn, causes recurrent increases in ICP (pressure waves), with additional compromise of cerebral blood supply to injured regions.

Two herniation syndromes demonstrate the mechanism by which *supratentorial lesions* produce coma. The rate of evolution of a mass dictates whether the anatomic distortion precedes (in slowly evolving lesions) or parallels the patient's deterioration of wakefulness. Transtentorial herniation can be central or predominantly unilateral. *Central herniation* results from caudal displacement by deep midline supratentorial masses, large space-occupying hemisphere lesions, or large unilateral or bilateral compressive extra-axial lesions, with compression of the ARAS. The progressive rostrocaudal clinical and pathologic stages of this herniation syndrome have been outlined.[1] Pathologically, bilateral symmetrical displacement of the supratentorial contents occurs through the tentorial notch into the posterior fossa. Alertness is impaired early, pupils become small (to 3 mm) and reactive, and bilateral upper motor neuron signs develop. Cheyne-Stokes breathing, grasp reflexes, roving eye movements, or depressed escape of oculocephalic reflexes are the clinical manifestations. In the absence of effective therapy at this diencephalic stage, herniation progresses caudally to compress the midbrain, leading to a deep coma and fixed, midposition (3 to 5 mm) pupils, signifying both sympathetic and parasympathetic interruption. Spontaneous eye movements cease and oculovestibular and oculocephalic reflexes become difficult to elicit. Spontaneous extensor posturing may occur. Once this stage is reached, full recovery becomes unlikely. As the caudal compression-ischemia process advances, pontine and medullary function becomes destroyed, with variable breathing patterns and absent reflex eye movements. Finally, autonomic cardiovascular and respiratory functions cease as medullary centers fail.

Uncus herniation results from laterally placed hemisphere lesions, particularly of the temporal lobes, which cause side-to-side cerebral displacement as well as transtentorial herniation. Focal hemisphere dysfunction (hemiparesis, aphasia, seizures) precedes unilateral (usually ipsilateral) compression paralysis of the third cranial nerve. An early sign of uncus herniation is an ipsilateral (rarely contralateral) enlarged pupil that responds sluggishly to light followed by a fixed, dilated pupil and an oculomotor palsy (eye turned downward and outward).[1] The ipsilateral posterior cerebral artery can become compressed as it crosses the tentorium and causes ipsilateral occipital lobe ischemia. Progressively, the temporal lobe compresses the midbrain, with loss of arousal and bilateral or contralateral extensor posturing. Ipsilateral to the intracranial lesion, a hemiparesis may develop if the opposite cerebral peduncle becomes compressed against the contralateral tentorial edge (Kernohan's notch). Abnormal brainstem signs become symmetrical, and herniation proceeds in the same pattern seen with central herniation, as rostrocaudal brainstem displacement progresses.

Infratentorial lesions cause coma by displacement, compression, or direct destruction of the pontomesencephalic tegmental activating system. Displacement of the medulla downward sufficient to push the brainstem and cerebellar tonsils into the foramen magnum causes cardiorespiratory collapse. Acute intrinsic lesions of the brainstem, usually hemorrhagic or ischemic, cause abrupt onset of coma and are associated with abnormal neuro-ophthalmologic findings. Pupils are pinpoint, owing to disruption of pontine sympathetic pathways, or they are dilated, owing to destruction of the third cranial nerve nuclei or intra-axial exiting fibers. Dysconjugate eye movements and nystagmus occur, whereas vertical eye movements are relatively spared. Ocular bobbing signifies pontine damage. Upper motor neuron signs develop and patients can become quadriplegic; flaccidity in the upper extremities and flexor withdrawal responses in the lower extremities often accompany midbrain-pontine damage. Pathologically, *basilar artery occlusion* leads to asymmetric ischemia of the brainstem, with involvement of the ARAS, the neighboring densely packed neuropil, as well as the descending and ascending motor and sensory tracts. Thrombosis of the rostral basilar artery leads to infarction of the midline thalamic nuclei and brief coma without other obvious brainstem signs. Hemorrhage into the ventral pons sometimes spares consciousness but produces neuro-ophthalmologic signs and motor dysfunction. Extension of the hemorrhage into the rostral pontine tegmentum results in stupor, coma, or death. *Basilar artery migraine* can produce altered consciousness possibly by interfering with arterial blood flow in the basilar artery system. Rapidly developing, extensive central pontine myelinolysis may cause coma by extension into the pontine tegmentum. Other intrinsic brainstem lesions (e.g., tumor, abscess, granuloma, demyelination) tend to progress slowly and usually spare arousal mechanisms; however, they may reduce attention and other cognitive functions, leading to severe psychomotor retardation.

Extra-axial posterior fossa lesions cause coma by direct compression of the ARAS in the brainstem and in the diencephalon by upward transtentorial herniation. Compression of the pons may be difficult to distinguish from intrinsic lesions but is often accompanied by headache, vomiting, and hypertension due to a Cushing reflex. Upward herniation at the midbrain level is initially characterized by coma, reactive miotic pupils, asymmetric or absent caloric eye responses, and decerebrate posturing; caudal-rostral brainstem dysfunction then occurs, with midbrain failure and midposition, fixed pupils.[10] Causes of brainstem compression include cerebellar hemorrhage, infarction, and abscess; rapidly expanding cerebellar or fourth ventricle tumors; or, less commonly, infratentorial epidural or subdural hematomas. Drainage of the lateral ventricles to relieve obstructive hydrocephalus due to posterior fossa masses can potentially precipitate acute upward transtentorial herniation.[11,12]

Downward herniation of the cerebellar tonsils through the foramen magnum causes acute medullary dysfunction and abrupt respiratory and circulatory collapse. Less severe impaction of the tonsils in the foramen magnum can lead to obstructive hydrocephalus and consequent bihemispheric dysfunction with altered arousal. Clinical manifestations include headache, nausea, vomiting, lower cranial nerve signs, vertical nystagmus, ataxia, and irregular breathing. Lumbar puncture in this setting carries a risk of catastrophic consequences.[11]

NONSTRUCTURAL CAUSES OF COMA

Nonstructural disorders, such as metabolic or toxic disturbances, produce coma by diffusely depressing the function of the brainstem and cerebral arousal mechanisms. The anatomic locus of metabolic brain diseases has not been clearly defined. The onset of coma can be abrupt, as with toxic drug ingestion, general anesthesia, or cardiac arrest, or it may evolve slowly after a period of confusion and inattention. The chief manifestations of metabolic encephalopathy are disturbances in arousal and cognitive function. Other findings include abnormalities of the sleep-wake cycle, autonomic disturbances, and abnormal breathing variations.

A helpful distinguishing clinical feature of a diffuse encephalopathy is the preservation of the pupillary light response; the only exceptions are overdose of anticholinergic agents, near-fatal anoxia, or malingering. Usually, lack of pupillary reactivity requires a search for an underlying structural lesion. The neurologic examination shows a decreased level of arousal and a widespread cognitive decline. Deeply comatose patients without brainstem or hemisphere function and no known cause for coma must be assumed to have suffered accidental or intentional poisoning. Metabolic disturbances of arousal and cognition particularly affect elderly patients who suffer serious systemic illnesses or who have undergone complicated surgery.

Metabolic encephalopathy is clinically characterized by multilevel CNS dysfunction. At onset, abnormalities in cognition are at least as severe as the disturbance of arousal. Misperception, disorientation, hallucinations, concentration, and memory deficits, and, occasionally, hypervigilance, may progress to profound stupor and coma. The patient's level of arousal and consciousness often fluctuates between examinations. Motor abnormalities, if present, usually are symmetrical and bilateral. Patients often suffer tremor, asterixis, and multifocal myoclonus. Spontaneous motor activity may range from hypoactivity (in cases of sedating drug or endogenous metabolic disturbances) to hyperactivity (after drug withdrawal or overdose of stimulants, such as cocaine and phencyclidine). Seizures occasionally occur, particularly after alcohol or drug withdrawal, and in patients with established cortical pathology. Focal seizures may occur even without structural disease during hypoglycemia, hepatic encephalopathy, uremia, abnormal calcium levels, or toxin ingestion. Autonomic dysfunction can manifest as hypothermia due to hypoglycemia, myxedema, or sedative drug overdose. Hyperthermia can occur in withdrawal states, particularly delirium tremens, anticholinergic drug overdose, infection, neuroleptic malignant syndrome, or malignant hyperthermia.

The metabolic needs of the brain depend largely on the oxidation of glucose to carbon dioxide and water. Certain fatty acids and ketone bodies can supply part of the metabolic needs in emergency circumstances, but these alternate fuels never provide an entirely sufficient substrate to meet all energy requirements. Normal cerebral blood flow (CBF) is around 55 mL/100 g tissue/min. With a CBF of less than 20 mL/100 g/min oxygen delivery becomes insufficient for normal levels of oxidative metabolism and cerebral glycolytic rate increases. Patients lose consciousness and the electroencephalogram (EEG) is suppressed owing to synaptic failure at CBF levels between 16 and 20 mL/100 g/min. The cortical evoked response is abolished below about 15 mL/100 g/min. At CBF around 8 mL/100 g/min the energy-dependent membrane pump fails and the membrane potential collapses. Unless CBF is restored promptly, irreversible neuronal injury will ensue. However, the threshold for ischemic neuronal injury is time dependent. Complete cessation of CBF leads to loss of consciousness in 8 seconds, and EEG suppression occurs at 10 to 12 seconds. Adenosine triphosphate exhaustion and ionic pump failure occurs in 120 seconds. Selective neuronal damage starts after periods as brief as 5 minutes, and severe neuronal damage occurs after 20 to 30 minutes. Brain necrosis or infarction starts in 1 to 2 hours.

Under physiologic conditions, glucose is the brain's only substrate and crosses the blood-brain barrier by facilitated transport. The normal brain uses about 55 mg glucose/100 g/min. If there is *hypoglycemia,* defined in adults as blood glucose concentration less than 40 mg/dL, signs and symptoms of encephalopathy result from dysfunction of the cerebral cortex before the brainstem. Neurologic presentation of hypoglycemia can vary from focal motor or sensory deficits to coma. Acute symptoms of hypoglycemia are better correlated with the rate at which blood glucose levels decrease than with the degree of hypoglycemia. The blood glucose level at which cerebral metabolism fails and symptoms develop varies among individuals, but, in general, confusion occurs at levels less than 30 mg/dL and coma at less than 10 mg/dL. The brain stores about 2 g of glucose and glycogen. Thus, a patient in hypoglycemic coma may survive 90 minutes without suffering irreversible brain damage. The pathophysiology of coma from hypoglycemia is not well understood. The disorder cannot solely be attributed to glucose starvation of neurons. Rather than such an internal catabolic death, evidence suggests than neurons are killed from without. Around the time the EEG becomes isoelectric, endogenous neurotoxins are produced and released by the brain into tissue and CSF. The distribution of necrotic neurons is unlike that of ischemia and is related to white matter and CSF pathways. The toxins act by first disrupting dendritic trees, sparing the intermediate axons, an indication of excitotoxic neuronal injury. The exact mechanism of excitotoxic neuronal necrosis is now becoming clear and involves hyperexcitation culminating in cell membrane rupture. Also, during hypoglycemia, the synthesis is suppressed of amino acids such as GABA, glutamate, glutamine, and alanine, as well as acetylcholine. Whether reduction of these molecules or alteration in nerve synaptic transmission significantly contributes to the onset of coma associated with severe hypoglycemia is not established.

The pathophysiology of other metabolic encephalopathies is less well established and is extensively discussed elsewhere.[1] *Hepatic encephalopathy* is caused not merely by ammonia intoxication but likely also involves accumulation of neurotoxins such as short- and medium-chain fatty acids, mercaptans,

and phenols. Altered neurotransmission may play a role with accumulation of benzodiazepine-like substances, imbalance of serotonergic and glutaminergic neurotransmission, and the accumulation of false neurotransmitters. The identity of the neurotoxin in *uremic encephalopathy* is uncertain and includes urea itself, guanidine and related compounds, phenols, aromatic hydroxy acids, amines, various peptide "middle-molecules," myoinositol, parathormone, and amino acid imbalance. The cause of the dysequilibrium syndrome may entail more than osmotic water shifts from plasma into brain cells, and reduction is reported in cortical potassium, with intracellular acidosis due to increased production of organic acids in the brain. The pathogenesis of *pancreatic encephalopathy* may involve patchy demyelination of brain white matter owing to liberated enzymes from a damaged pancreas, disseminated intravascular coagulation, or fat embolism.

The mechanism of action of exogenous toxins or drugs depends partly on the structure and partly on the dose. As well as can be determined, none of the sedatives taken acutely produces permanent damage to the nervous system, making prompt diagnosis and effective treatment particularly important.

DIFFERENTIAL DIAGNOSIS

Several different behavioral states appear similar to, and can be confused with, coma. Differentiation of such states from true coma has important diagnostic, therapeutic, and prognostic implications. Moreover, coma is not a permanent state; patients who survive initial coma may evolve through and into these altered behavioral states. All patients who survive beyond the stage of acute, systemic complications reawaken and either proceed to recovery (with no or varying degrees of disability) or remain in a vegetative state.

The vegetative state can be defined as wakefulness without awareness and is the consequence of various diffuse brain insults.[1,13] It may be a transient phase through which patients in coma pass as the cerebral cortex recovers more slowly than the brainstem. Clinically, vegetative patients appear to be awake and to have cyclical sleep patterns; however, such individuals do not show evidence of cognitive function or learned behavioral responses to external stimuli. Vegetative patients may feature spontaneous eye opening and eye movements and stereotypic facial and limb movements; however, they are unable to speak or comprehend and they lack purposeful activity. Vegetative patients generate normal body temperature, usually have normally functioning cardiovascular, respiratory, and digestive systems, but are doubly incontinent. The vegetative state should be termed persistent at 1 month after injury and permanent at 3 months after nontraumatic injury or 12 months after a traumatic injury.[14,15] Extended observation of the patient is required to assess behavioral responses to external stimulation and to demonstrate cognitive unawareness. The EEG is never isoelectric but shows various patterns of rhythm and amplitude, inconsistent from one patient to the next. Normal EEG sleep-wake patterns are absent.

In *the locked-in syndrome,* patients retain or regain arousability and self-awareness but because of extensive bilateral paralysis (i.e., de-efferentation) can no longer communicate except in severely limited ways. Such patients suffer bilateral ventral pontine lesions with quadriplegia, horizontal gaze palsies, and lower cranial nerve palsies. Voluntarily, they are capable only of vertical eye movements and/or blinking.[1]

Sleep may be abnormal with marked reduction in non-rapid-eye-movement and rapid-eye-movement sleep phases. The most common cause is pontine infarction due to basilar artery thrombosis, but other causes are pontine hemorrhage, central pontine myelinolysis, and brainstem mass lesions. Neuromuscular causes of locked-in syndrome include severe, acute inflammatory demyelinating polyradiculoneuropathies, myasthenia gravis, botulism, and neuromuscular blocking agents. In these peripheral disorders, upward gaze is not selectively spared.

Akinetic mutism describes a rare subacute or chronic state of altered behavior in which an alert-appearing patient is both silent and immobile but not paralyzed.[16] External evidence of mental activity is unobtainable. The patient usually lies with eyes opened and retains cycles of self-sustained arousal, giving the appearance of vigilance. Skeletal muscle tone can be normal or hypertonic but usually not spastic. Movements are rudimentary even in response to unpleasant stimuli. Affected patients are usually doubly incontinent. Lesions that cause akinetic mutism may vary widely. One pattern consists of bilateral damage to frontal lobe or limbic-cortical integration with relative sparing of motor pathways. Vulnerable areas involve both basal medial frontal areas. Somewhat similar behavior also can follow incomplete lesions of the deep gray matter (paramedian reticular formation of the posterior diencephalon and adjacent midbrain), but such patients usually suffer double hemiplegia and act slowly yet are not completely akinetic or noncommunicative.

Catatonia is a symptom complex associated most often with psychiatric disease. This behavioral disturbance is characterized by stupor or excitement and variable mutism, posturing, rigidity, grimacing, and catalepsy. Catatonia can be caused by a variety of illnesses, both psychiatric (affective more than psychotic) disorders and structural or metabolic diseases (toxic- and drug-induced psychosis, encephalitis, and alcoholic degeneration). Psychiatric catatonia may be difficult to distinguish from organic disease because patients often appear lethargic or stuporous rather than totally unresponsive. Such patients also may have a variety of endocrine or autonomic abnormalities. Patients in catatonic stupor do not move spontaneously and appear unresponsive to the environment despite what appears to be a normal level of arousal and consciousness. This impression is supported by a normal neurologic examination and a subsequent recall of most events that took place during the unresponsive period. Patients usually lie with eyes opened and may not blink to visual threat, but one can usually elicit optokinetic responses. The pupils are semi-dilated and reactive to light, oculocephalic reflexes are absent, and vestibulo-ocular testing evokes normal nystagmus. Patients may hypersalivate and be doubly incontinent. Passive movement of the limbs meets with waxy flexibility, and catalepsy is seen in 30% of patients. Choreiform jerks of the extremities and facial grimaces are common. The EEG, both of catatonic excitement and stupor, most often shows a reactive, low-voltage, fast-normal record rather than the slow record of a comatose patient.

APPROACH TO COMA

The initial approach to stupor and coma is based on the principle that all alterations in arousal are acute, life-threatening emergencies. Urgent steps are required to prevent or minimize permanent brain damage from reversible causes often before the cause of coma is definitely established.

Patient evaluation and treatment must necessarily occur simultaneously. Serial examinations are needed with accurate documentation to determine a change in state of the patient. Accordingly, management decisions (therapeutic and diagnostic) must be made. The clinical approach to an unconscious patient logically entails the following steps: (1) emergency treatment; (2) history (from relatives, friends, and emergency medical personnel); (3) general physical examination; (4) neurologic profile, the key to categorizing the nature of coma; and (5) specific management.

EMERGENCY MANAGEMENT

The initial assessment must focus on the vital signs to determine the appropriate resuscitation measures; the diagnostic process begins later. Urgent, and sometimes empirical, therapy must be given to avoid additional brain insult.

Oxygenation must be ensured by the establishment of an airway and ventilation of the lungs. The threshold for intubation should be low in the comatose patient, even if respiratory function is sufficient for proper ventilation and oxygenation: the level of consciousness may deteriorate and breathing may decompensate suddenly and unexpectedly. An open airway must be ensured and protected from aspiration of vomitus and blood. While preparing for intubation, maximal oxygenation can be ensured by suction of the upper airway, gentle extension of the neck, elevation of the jaw, and manual ventilation with oxygen using a mask and bag. Bag-valve mask ventilation with 100% oxygen and 1 mg of atropine given intravenously helps prevent cardiac dysrhythmias. If a severe neck injury is a possibility, or has not been excluded, intubation should be performed by the most skilled practitioner with cervical spine precautions. A brief neurologic examination is mandatory before sedation required for intubation.

The key points of the "rapid neurologic examination" are hand drop from over the head (to assess for malingering or hysterical loss of consciousness); pupillary size and response to light; abnormal eye movements (active dysconjugate, unilaterally paralytic, passively induced, or absent); grimacing and withdrawal from noxious stimulation; and abnormal plantar response (unilateral or bilateral Babinski's sign).[17] Assisted ventilation should continue during the examination if necessary. Neuromuscular blockade required for patient management and care should be deferred, if possible, until the neurologic examination is completed (3 to 5 minutes). Signs of arousal or inadequate sedation include dilated, reactive pupils, copious tears, diaphoresis, tachycardia, systemic hypertension, and increased pulmonary artery pressure. Thereafter, monitoring patients neurologically may require head CT more frequently.

Evaluate *respiratory excursions:* arterial blood gas measurement is the only certain method to determine adequate ventilation and oxygenation. Pulse oximetry is useful, however, because it provides immediate, continuous information regarding arterial oxygen saturation. The comatose patient ideally should maintain a PaO_2 greater than 100 mm Hg and a $PaCO_2$ between 34 and 37 mm Hg. Hyperventilation ($PaCO_2 < 35$ mm Hg) should be avoided unless herniation is suspected. Positive end-expiratory pressure (PEEP) should be avoided if increased ICP is suspected, unless hypoxemia is not responsive to supplemental oxygen. Place a nasogastric tube to facilitate gastric lavage and prevent regurgitation.

Maintain *circulation* to ensure adequate cerebral perfusion. Appropriate resuscitation fluid is lactated Ringer's solution;

normal saline is also used when intracranial hypertension is suspected. A mean arterial pressure at about 100 mm Hg is adequate and safe for most patients. While obtaining venous access, collect blood samples for anticipated tests (Table 49-1). Treat hypotension by replacing any blood volume loss, and use vasoactive agents (preferably dopamine). Judiciously manage systemic hypertension with hypotensive agents that do not substantially raise ICP by their vasodilating effect (labetalol, hydralazine, or a titrated nitroprusside infusion are the favored agents for managing uncontrollable hypertension). For most situations systolic blood pressure should not be treated unless it is greater than 160 mm Hg. Maintain urine output at at least 0.5 mL/kg/h; accurate measurement requires bladder catheterization.

Glucose (and *thiamine*) levels need to be determined. Hypoglycemia is a frequent cause of altered consciousness; administer glucose (25 g as a 50% solution i.v.) immediately after drawing blood for baseline values. Empirical glucose treatment will prevent hypoglycemic brain damage and outweighs the theoretical risks of additional harm to the brain in hyperglycemic, hyperosmolar, or anoxic coma. Thiamine (100 mg) must be given with the glucose infusion to prevent precipitation of Wernicke's encephalopathy in malnourished, thiamine-depleted patients. Rarely, an established thiamine deficiency can cause coma.

Repeated generalized *seizures* damage the brain and must be stopped. Initial treatment should include intravenous

TABLE 49–1. EMERGENCY LABORATORY TESTS OF METABOLIC COMA

Immediate Tests

Venous Blood
Glucose
Electrolytes (Na^+, K^+, Cl^-) and CO_2, PO_4
Urea and creatinine
Osmolality

Arterial Blood (check color)
pH
Po_2
Pco_2
HCO_3^-
HbCO (if available)

Cerebrospinal Fluid
Gram stain
Cell count
Glucose

Electrocardiogram

Deferred Tests (initial sample, process later)

Venous Blood
Sedative and toxic drugs
Liver function tests
Coagulation studies
Thyroid and adrenal function
Blood cultures
Viral titers

Urine
Sedative and toxic drugs
Culture

Cerebrospinal Fluid
Protein
Culture
Viral and fungal titers

benzodiazepines, lorazepam (2 to 4 mg), or diazepam (5 to 10 mg). Seizure control can be maintained with phenytoin (18 mg/kg i.v. at a rate of 25 mg/min). Seizure breakthrough requires additional benzodiazepines.

Careful and mild *sedation* should be given to the agitated, hyperactive patient to prevent self-injury. Sedation facilitates ventilator support and diagnostic procedures. Small doses of intravenous benzodiazepines, intramuscular haloperidol (1 mg as often as hourly until desired effect), or morphine (2 to 4 mg, i.v.) are appropriate.

Consider specific *antidotes*. Drug overdose is the largest single cause (30%) of coma in the emergency department. Most drug overdoses can be treated by supportive measures alone. However, certain antagonists specifically reverse the effects of coma-producing drugs. Naloxone (0.4 to 2 mg i.v.) is the antidote for opiate coma. The reversal of narcotic effect, however, may precipitate acute withdrawal in an opiate addict. In suspected opiate coma the minimal amount of naloxone should be administered to establish the diagnosis by pupillary dilatation and to reverse respiratory depression and coma. Do not attempt to reverse completely all drug effects with the first dose. Intravenous flumazenil reverses all benzodiazepine-induced coma. Coma unresponsive to 5 mg of flumazenil in divided doses given over 5 minutes is not due to benzodiazepine overdose. Recurrent sedation can be prevented with flumazenil (1 mg i.v.) every 20 minutes.[18] The sedative effects of drugs with anticholinergic properties, particularly tricyclic antidepressants, can be reversed with physostigmine (1 to 2 mg i.v.). Pretreatment with 0.5 mg of atropine will prevent bradycardia. Only full awakening is characteristic of an anticholinergic drug overdose, because physostigmine has nonspecific arousal properties. Physostigmine has a short duration of action (45 to 60 minutes), and doses may have to be repeated.

Adjust *body temperature*. Hyperthermia is dangerous because it increases brain metabolic demand and, at extreme levels, denatures brain proteins.[19] Hyperthermia greater than 40° C requires nonspecific cooling measures, even before the underlying etiology is determined and treated. Hyperthermia most often indicates infection, but it may be due to intracranial hemorrhage, anticholinergic drug intoxication, or heat exposure. A body temperature of less than 34° C should be slowly increased to greater than 35° C to prevent cardiac dysrhythmia. Hypothermia accompanies profound sepsis, sedative-hypnotic drug overdose, near-drowning, hypoglycemia, or Wernicke's encephalopathy.

HISTORY

Once vital functions have been protected and the patient's condition is stable, clues to the cause of coma must be sought by interviewing relatives, friends, bystanders, or medical personnel who may have observed the patient before or during the decline in consciousness. The history should include:

- Witnessed events—head injury; seizure; details of a motor vehicle accident; circumstances under which the patient was found.
- Evolution of coma—abrupt or gradual; headache; progressive or recurrent weakness; vertigo; nausea and vomiting.
- Recent medical history—surgical procedures; infections; current medication.
- Past medical history—epilepsy; head injury; drug or alcohol abuse; stroke; hypertension; diabetes; heart disease; cancer; uremia.

- Previous psychiatric history—depression; suicide attempts; social stresses.
- Access to drugs—sedatives; psychotropic drugs; narcotics; illicit drugs; drug paraphernalia; empty medicine bottles.

GENERAL PHYSICAL EXAMINATION

A systematic, detailed examination is helpful and necessary in the approach to the comatose patient who is in no condition to describe prior or current medical problems. This examination is an extension of the initial evaluation and includes the following:

- The repeated assessment of vital signs to determine efficacy of resuscitation measures
- External evidence of trauma
- Evidence of acute or chronic medical illnesses
- Evidence of ingestion or self-administration of drugs (needle marks, alcohol on breath)
- Evaluation for nuchal rigidity. Care is required if severe neck injury is possible or has not been excluded. (Nuchal rigidity may disappear in deeply comatose patients with meningeal infection/inflammation.)

NEUROLOGIC PROFILE

The establishment of the nature of coma is critical for appropriate management and requires the following:

- The correct interpretation of neurologic signs that reflect the integrity, or impairment, of various functional levels of the brain
- Determination whether the pattern and evolution of these signs are best explained by a supratentorial or infratentorial structural lesion, a metabolic-toxic encephalopathy, or a psychiatric cause (Tables 49-2 and 49-3)

The clinical neurologic functions that provide the most useful information in making a categorical diagnosis are outlined in Table 49-4. These indices are easily and quickly obtained. Furthermore, they have a high degree of interexaminer consistency and, when applied serially, they accurately reflect the patient's clinical course. Once the cause of coma can be assigned to one of these categories, specific radiographic, electrophysiologic, or chemical laboratory studies can be used to make a disease-specific diagnosis and to detect existing or potential complications.

SPECIFIC MANAGEMENT

Supratentorial Mass Lesions

If the cause of coma is a presumed supratentorial mass, determine the severity and rate of evolution of signs. A stabilized patient next requires an emergency head CT or MRI. Carotid angiography is considerably less informative; a skull radiograph is a waste of time. The priority in deep coma or established/threatening transtentorial herniation is to apply successfully medical treatment of intracranial hypertension. Brief hyperventilation to a PaCO$_2$ between 25 and 30 mm Hg is the most rapid method to reduce intracranial hypertension. This is achieved by adjusting the ventilation rate to 10 to 16 breaths/min and tidal volume to 12 to 14 mL/kg.

TABLE 49–2. NEUROLOGIC PROFILE (A MODIFIED GLASGOW COMA SCALE)

Verbal Response

Oriented speech
Confused conversation
Inappropriate speech
Incomprehensible speech
No speech

Eye Opening

Spontaneous
Response to verbal stimuli
Response to noxious stimuli
None

Motor Response

Obeys
Localizes
Withdraws (flexion)
Abnormal flexion
Abnormal extension
None

Pupillary Reaction

Present
Absent

Spontaneous Eye Movement

Orienting
Roving conjugate
Roving dysconjugate
Miscellaneous abnormal movements
None

Oculocephalic Response

Normal (unpredictable)
Full
Minimal
None

Oculovestibular Response

Normal (nystagmus)
Tonic conjugate
Minimal or dysconjugate
None

Deep Tendon Reflexes

Normal
Increased
Absent

An osmotic agent must be administered concurrently. Sustained hyperventilation at less than 30 to 35 mm Hg removes all future value of this procedure. The preferred osmotic agent is a 20% mannitol solution as a 1g/kg intravenous bolus. Maximum reduction in ICP occurs within 20 to 60 minutes, and the effect of a single bolus lasts about 6 hours. Corticosteroids are not indicated in the emergent, empirical management of increased ICP, because full effects are observed only after a few hours. Furthermore, because corticosteroids are effective only for certain lesions (e.g., edema around a brain tumor or abscess), use can be delayed until a diagnosis has been made by head CT. After such initial ICP management, a head CT or MRI is required. The scan will demonstrate the nature of the supratentorial lesion and associated mass effect. Arrangements must be made to evacuate promptly an epidural or subdural hematoma. Intraparenchymal masses that acutely

TABLE 49–3. CORRELATION BETWEEN LEVELS OF BRAIN FUNCTION AND CLINICAL SIGNS

Structure	Function	Clinical Sign

Cerebral cortex	Conscious behavior	Speech (including any sounds)
		Purposeful movement
		  Spontaneous
		  To command
		  To pain

Brainstem activating and sensory (reticular activating system) pathways	Sleep/wake cycle	Eye opening
		  Spontaneous
		  To command
		  To pain

Brainstem motor pathways	Reflex limb movements	Flexor posturing (decorticate) Extensor posturing (decerebrate)
Midbrain CN III	Innervation of ciliary muscle and certain extraocular muscles	Pupillary reactivity
Pontomesencephalic MLF	Connects pontine gaze center with CN III nucleus	Internuclear ophthalmoplegia

Upper pons
  CN V
  CN VII
	Facial and corneal
	Facial muscle innervation
		Corneal reflex-sensory
		Corneal reflex-motor response
		  Blink
		  Grimace

Lower pons CN VIII (vestibular portion) connects by brainstem pathways with CN III, IV, and VI	Reflex eye movements	Doll's eyes Caloric responses
Pontomedullary junction	Spontaneous breathing Maintained blood pressure	Breathing and blood pressure do not require mechanical or chemical support
Spinal cord	Primitive protective responses	Deep tendon reflexes Babinski response

CN, cranial nerve.

produce deep stupor or coma initially are best managed non-surgically. When corticosteroids are indicated for severe vaso-genic edema, a dexamethasone bolus should be given (up to 100 mg i.v.), followed by 6 to 24 mg every 6 hours. Once signs

TABLE 49–4. CHARACTERISTICS OF CATEGORIES OF COMA

Supratentorial Mass Lesion Affecting the Diencephalon/Brainstem

Initial focal cerebral dysfunction
Dysfunction progresses rostral to caudal
Signs reflect dysfunction at one level
Signs often asymmetric

Infratentorial Structural Lesion

Symptoms of brainstem dysfunction or sudden-onset coma
Brainstem signs precede/accompany coma
Cranial nerve and oculovestibular dysfunction
Early onset of abnormal respiratory patterns

Metabolic-Toxic Coma

Confusion/stupor precede motor signs
Motor signs usually symmetrical
Pupil responses generally preserved
Myoclonus, asterixis, tremulousness, and generalized seizures common
Acid-base imbalance common with compensatory ventilatory changes

Psychogenic Coma

Eyelids squeezed shut
Pupils reactive or dilated, unreactive (cycloplegics)
Oculocephalic reflex unpredictable; nystagmus on caloric tests
Motor tone normal or inconsistent
No pathologic reflexes
(Awake-pattern EEG)

of herniation have abated, the ventilator rate should be carefully reduced to achieve a $PaCO_2$ of 34 to 37 mm Hg.

The patient's vital signs and neurologic condition require repeated examination. The head should be kept slightly elevated (15 degrees). Mannitol may be repeated, if necessary, every 4 to 6 hours; serum electrolytes and fluid balance must be monitored.

When patients with presumed increased ICP do not respond clinically as expected to medical management, or when obstructive hydrocephalus complicates a supratentorial mass lesion, we favor placement of a ventriculostomy into the lateral ventricle. The ventriculostomy allows accurate measurement of intraventricular ICP and provides a method for CSF drainage, if necessary. The placement of a ventriculostomy allows calculation of cerebral perfusion pressure (CPP) (mean systemic arterial pressure minus ICP), a critical determinant of CBF and, therefore, of oxygen and substrate delivery. Monitoring of ICP also allows adjustment of therapeutic intervention before clinical deterioration occurs in patients with diminished intracranial compliance. Drainage of CSF aims to relieve raised ICP to maintain CPP (greater than 60 mm Hg) and to improve intracranial compliance. After increased ICP has responded to emergency management and the patient's condition has stabilized, definitive treatment of the mass lesion is required as deemed appropriate.

Infratentorial Lesions

The evolution of neurologic symptoms and signs and the neurologic examination generally give sufficient information to localize the lesion to the posterior fossa; the lesions themselves may be intrinsic or extrinsic to the brainstem.

Rapid neurologic deterioration of a patient suspected of harboring an infratentorial lesion sometimes demands emergency treatment before CT of the head is performed.

Treatment of a presumed extrinsic compressive lesion of the brainstem entails measures that decrease ICP as outlined earlier. Patients who are stuporous or showing signs of progressive brainstem compression from a cerebellar hemorrhage or infarction require urgent evacuation of the lesion. Intrinsic brainstem lesions are best treated conservatively; an incompleted stroke may benefit from thrombolysis and/or heparin anticoagulation. Posterior fossa tumors are managed initially with osmotic agents and corticosteroids; definitive treatment includes surgery and/or radiation. The placement of a ventricular catheter for acute hydrocephalus must be considered cautiously and in consultation with a neurosurgeon; the danger exists of potentially fatal upward transtentorial herniation.[12]

Metabolic Toxic Coma

The task of the physician in first contact with the patient in metabolic coma is to preserve and protect the brain from permanent damage. Metabolic and toxicologic studies must be performed on the first blood sample drawn (see Table 49-1). There are several treatable conditions that quickly and irreversibly damage the brain.

Hypoglycemia. As noted earlier, glucose (50 mL of a 50% solution i.v.) should be administered during emergency treatment before blood results return. Prolonged hypoglycemic coma that has considerably damaged the brain will not be reversed by a glucose load; a glucose bolus may transiently worsen hyperglycemic, hyperosmolar coma. In contrast, the osmolar load of intravenous glucose may transiently decrease elevated ICP and lighten nonhypoglycemic coma. A glucose infusion is needed to prevent recurrent hypoglycemia.

Acid-Base Imbalance. The hyperventilating comatose patient with acute, severe metabolic acidosis and threatening cardiovascular collapse requires emergency treatment. For accurate assessment an arterial blood gas is required. Administration of sodium bicarbonate (1 mEq/kg i.v.) can be life saving; simultaneously, a search for, and specific treatment of, the cause must be conducted.

Hypoxia. Carbon monoxide poisoning requires hyperoxygenation with 100% oxygen to facilitate excretion of this toxin. Closely monitor and correct blood pressure and cardiac rhythm abnormalities. Idiopathic and drug-induced methemoglobinemia is treated with methylene blue (1 to 2 mg/kg i.v. over a few minutes; repeat dose after 1 hour if needed). Anemia alone does not cause coma but exacerbates other forms of hypoxemia. Transfusion of packed red cells is appropriate for severe anemia (hematocrit < 25%). Cyanide poisoning causes histotoxic hypoxia of the brain. Treatment entails amyl nitrite (vapor or crushed ampule inhaled every minute), sodium nitrite (300 mg i.v.) followed by sodium thiosulfate (12.5 g i.v.).

Acute Bacterial Meningitis. A lumbar puncture must be considered in any unconscious patient with fever and/or signs of meningeal irritation. If possible, an emergency head CT should be performed before lumbar puncture on a comatose patient to rule out unexpected mass lesions. Increased ICP is present in all cases of bacterial meningitis, but a lumbar puncture is not contraindicated when this diagnosis is suspected. Cerebral herniation seldom, if ever, occurs except in small children.[20] Clinical correlates of impending herniation demand a more cautious approach to lumbar puncture: coma or rapidly deteriorating level of arousal, focal neurologic signs, and tonic or prolonged seizures. Papilledema is rare in acute bacterial meningitis. Should unexpected herniation occur after lumbar puncture, treatment with hyperventilation and intravenous mannitol is indicated. Appropriate antibiotic treatment can usually await the results of CSF Gram stain. If the Gram stain is negative yet a bacterial cause is suspected, empirical, broad-spectrum antibiotic treatment with a third-generation cephalosporin and vancomycin is appropriate.

Drug Overdose. Certain general principles apply to all patients suspected of having ingested sedative drugs.[21,22] Most drug overdose is treated by emergent and supportive measures (see Table 49-5). Once vital signs are stable, attempts should be made to remove, neutralize, or reverse the effects of the drug. Patients in coma from recent drug ingestion require gastric lavage after endotracheal intubation. A large, preferably double-lumen, gastric tube must be placed orally. The lavage is performed in the head-down position on the left side. Lavage is performed with 200 to 300 mL bolus of tap water or 0.45% saline and continued until the return is clear. After lavage, 1 or 2 tablespoons of activated charcoal is passed down the lavage tube. With meticulous supportive measures, patients with uncomplicated drug-induced coma should recover without neurologic deficit. The recovery from coma due to massive doses of barbiturates or glutethimide can be hastened by hemodialysis.

Constant vigilance and attention to the patient's condition, with timely and appropriate diagnostic and therapeutic evaluation, ensures the best possible outcome of metabolic coma. Effective care demands meticulous attention to the maintenance of tissue perfusion and oxygenation, the documentation and anticipation of acute neurologic events (particularly diminished cerebral perfusion, herniation, or seizures), aggressive, rapid treatment of initial or subsequent infections, and prevention of agitation. Deep venous thrombosis can be prevented with either subcutaneous heparin (5000 units q 12h) or full-length leg pneumatic compression boots. Enteral or parenteral feeding within 36 to 48 hours is required to satisfy nutritional needs. Corneal injury can be prevented by protecting the eyes with lubricants and taping the lids shut.

THE ROLE OF SPECIAL INVESTIGATIONS

NEURODIAGNOSTIC IMAGING

Once the patient with an altered mental status is appropriately resuscitated and stabilized, further investigation may be necessary to document the location and type of the lesion and to provide guidance for therapeutic intervention. CT and MRI provide an anatomic and/or functional assessment of the central nervous system (CNS) and provide helpful information for defining the localization of lesions that produce coma. For details on the use of these modalities in neurointensive care, see Chapter 48.

Cranial CT is currently the most expedient imaging technique in the comatose patient and gives the most rapid information about possible structural lesions with the least risk. The value of CT to demonstrate mass lesions, hemorrhage, and hydrocephalus is well established. CT shows tissue shifts due to intracranial intercompartmental pressure gradients but compared with MRI may underestimate the anatomy of herniation.[11] Certain lesions such as early infarction (less than 12 hours' duration), encephalitis, and isodense subdural hemorrhage may be difficult to visualize. Posterior fossa pathology may be somewhat obscured by bone artifact

TABLE 49–5. NEUROLOGIC MANIFESTATIONS OF COMMON DRUG POISONING

Drug	Signs and Symptoms	Diagnostic Test	Treatment
Carbon monoxide	Confusion, agitation, headache, convulsions, coma, respiratory failure, cardiovascular collapse	History Carboxyhemoglobin level	Remove patient from area; administer 100% oxygen until carboxyhemoglobin levels fall to < 5%. Administer hyperbaric oxygen if central nervous system affected. Treat cerebral edema with hyperventilation, diuretics, and cerebrospinal fluid drainage, if necessary.
Salicylate	Tinnitus, hyperpnea, confusion, convulsions, coma, hyperthermia	Blood	Provide supportive care, gastric lavage, charcoal, systemic alkalinization, hemodialysis for coma or seizures.
Cyanide	Agitation, confusion, headache, vertigo, hypertension, hypotension, seizures, paralysis, apnea, coma	Blood	Use amyl nitrate, sodium nitrate, sodium thiosulfate, 100% oxygen, or hyperbaric oxygen for refractory signs. Vitamin B12 injection.
Anticonvulsants: Phenytoin Carbamazepine Phenobarbital (see Barbiturates) Valproic acid Primidone Ethosuximide Felbamate Clonazepam (see Benzodiazepines)	Drowsiness, ataxia, nystagmus, tremulousness, coma. Dysrhythmias with carbamazepine or phenytoin overdose.	Blood Ammonia level in patients taking valproic acid.	Provide supportive care, gastric lavage, charcoal. Watch for withdrawal seizures.
Sedative hypnotics: Benzodiazepines Barbiturates Chloral hydrate Meprobamate Ethchlorvynol (Placidyl)	Confusion, lethargy, ataxia, nystagmus, hypothermia, dysarthria, respiratory depression, coma. Pupillary reactions preserved except in instances of deep barbiturate coma. Possible withdrawal seizures.	Blood	Provide supportive care, gastric lavage, flumazenil for benzodiazepine overdose, hemoperfusion for extreme barbiturate intoxication.
Methaqualone	Agitation, hypertonic, hyperreflexia, ataxia, hallucinations, convulsions	Blood	As above
Ethanol	Confusion, agitation, delirium, ataxia, nystagmus, dysarthria, coma	Blood, breath	Provide supportive care, lavage if within 1 hour of ingestion, thiamine, glucose.
Opioids	Lethargy; small reactive pupils; hypothermia; hypotension; urinary retention; shallow, irregular respirations; convulsions	Urine Response to naloxone	Administer naloxone, 0.4 mg IV or IM; continuous naloxone infusion, if necessary. Provide supportive care with intubation as necessary. Lavage if overdose is by ingestion.
Stimulants: Amphetamine Methylphenidate Cocaine	Hypervigilance, paranoia, violent behavior, tremulousness, dilated pupils, hyperthermia, tachycardia or arrhythmia, focal neurologic signs secondary to CNS stroke or hemorrhage, seizures	Blood, urine	Provide supportive care; sedation with benzodiazepines. Watch for rhabdomyolysis.
Psychedelics (LSD, mescaline, phencyclidine)	Delirium, delusions, marked agitation, hallucinations, hyperactivity, dilated pupils, hyperreflexia, nystagmus	Blood Measure phencyclidine levels in gastric juice.	Use gastric lavage, charcoal. Give benzodiazepines and haloperidol for sedation.
Antidepressants: Tricyclic antidepressants	Anticholinergic effects: dry mouth, agitation, restlessness, ataxia, tachycardia or arrhythmias, hyperthermia, hysteria, convulsions, mydriasis	Blood, urine	Use cardiac monitoring, gastric lavage, charcoal, mild systemic alkalinization. Administer physostigmine for refractory arrhythmias and anticonvulsants for seizures.
Monoamine oxidase inhibitors	Drowsiness, ataxia, seizures, hypertensive crisis; hypotension with severe overdose		Provide symptomatic care, gastric lavage; avoid narcotics.
Neuroleptics	Dystonia, drowsiness, coma, convulsions, hypotension, miosis, tremor, hypothermia, neuroleptic malignant syndrome	Urine	Use gastric lavage. Treat extrapyramidal signs with diphenhydramine or benztropine mesylate.
Lithium	Lethargy, tremulousness, weakness, polyuria, polydipsia, ataxia, seizures, coma	Blood	Perform hemodialysis for delirium, seizures, or coma.
Methanol, ethylene glycol	Drunkenness, hyperventilation, stupor, convulsions, coma. Blindness with methanol use.	Blood	Provide symptomatic care, gastric lavage, ethanol infusion, hemodialysis. For methanol intoxication, 4-methylpyrazole is under investigation.
Antihistamines	Anticholinergic effects: dry		Provide supportive care, gastric lavage;

TABLE 49-5. NEUROLOGIC MANIFESTATIONS OF COMMON DRUG POISONING—CONT'D

	mucosa, flushed skin, hyperthermia, dilated pupils, delirium, hallucinations, seizures, coma		control seizures with benzodiazepines; use physostigmine for life-threatening anticholinergic effects.
Organophosphates	Cholinergic crisis: cramps, excessive secretions, diarrhea, bronchoconstriction. Later tremulousness, fasciculations, weakness, convulsions, hypertension, tachycardia, confusion, anxiety, and coma.	RBC cholinesterase level	Provide symptomatic care, decontamination, atropine, and pralidoxime.

inherent in the CT technique. Raised ICP is suggested by effacement of cortical sulci, a narrow third ventricle, and obliteration of the suprasellar or quadrigeminal cisterns but cannot be otherwise quantified. MRI can be performed, depending on the clinical setting and the stability of the patient's condition. The use of MRI is limited in the urgent setting of coma evaluation because of the length of time required to perform the imaging, image degradation by even a slight movement of the patient, and the relative inaccessibility of the patient for emergencies that may occur during the imaging process. Nevertheless, MRI provides superb visualization of posterior fossa structures that is useful when intrinsic brainstem lesions are suspected as the cause of coma.[11] MRI images anatomic lesions, such as those resulting from acute stroke, encephalitis, central pontine myelinolysis, and traumatic shear injury with greater resolution and at an earlier time than CT. The injection of the paramagnetic substance, gadolinium, helps delineate areas of blood-brain barrier breakdown and may augment the sensitivity of this scanning technique. Diffusion-weighted imaging can demonstrate ischemic brain virtually immediately. Sagittal MRI views are particularly useful in the documentation of the degree of supratentorial or infratentorial herniations and may enable intervention before clinical deterioration (Fig. 49-1).[11] Newer MRI techniques allow functional imaging of the CNS by measurement of CBF to a particular region. Future application of this technique may allow rapid determination of diminished CBF, such as occurs in stroke or vasospasm, and will probably be useful in assessing the effect of therapeutic interventions.

ELECTROENCEPHALOGRAPHY

The EEG can sometimes gives useful additional information in the evaluation of the unresponsive patient. With metabolic and toxic disorders, the EEG changes generally reflect the degree and severity of altered arousal or delirium characterized by a decreased frequency of the background rhythm and the appearance of diffuse slow activity in the theta (4 to 7 Hz) and/or delta (1 to 3 Hz) range. Bilaterally synchronous and symmetrical, medium to high-voltage broad triphasic waves are seen in various metabolic encephalopathies, most often in hepatic coma. Rapid beta activity (greater than 13 Hz) in a comatose patient suggests the ingestion of sedative hypnotics, such as barbiturates and benzodiazepines. Acute, focally destructive lesions show focal slow activity; when periodic lateralized epileptiform discharges appear in one or both temporal lobes, herpes

simplex encephalitis must be strongly considered. A nonreactive, diffuse alpha pattern in a comatose patient usually implies a poor prognosis and is most often seen after anoxic insults to the brain or acute, destructive pontine tegmentum damage.[23,24] A normally reactive EEG in an unresponsive patient suggests psychiatric disease; however, a relatively normal EEG can accompany the locked-in syndrome, some examples of akinetic mutism, and catatonia, all of which can be caused by structural brain lesions. Attempts to correlate the pattern and frequency spectra of a post-resuscitative EEG with neurologic outcome have been unsatisfactory because its predictive value is at best 88% accurate.[25] At present, the most useful information regarding patient prognosis is still obtained by the correct interpretation of physical signs.

Nonconvulsive generalized status epilepticus and repeated complex partial seizures may produce altered levels of awareness or arousal; the EEG is an indispensable tool in the diagnosis and management of both these disorders. Continuous EEG monitoring optimizes management of status epilepticus because clinical assessment is insufficiently sensitive to detect continued electrographic seizures. Furthermore, continuous EEG monitoring in the ICU has shown an unsuspected high incidence of electrographic seizure activity in critically ill neurologic patients.[26,27]

JUGULAR VENOUS OXIMETRY

Changes in jugular venous oxygen saturation measure the relationship between cerebral metabolic rate and CBF, and this monitoring tool is discussed in Chapter 48.[28] This form of monitoring offers the potential to minimize secondary insults after traumatic brain injury by providing warning of cerebral ischemia. It should be considered in comatose patients in conjunction with ICP monitoring (discussed later) to provide a logical approach to the treatment of brain injury.

TRANSCRANIAL DOPPLER ULTRASONOGRAPHY

Transcranial Doppler imaging (see Chapter 48) allows noninvasive measurement of blood flow velocity in basal cerebral arteries.[29] The high dynamic resolution provided, and confirmed correlation with other hemodynamic modalities, encourages increasing numbers of neurointensivists to adopt the technique. Its importance in coma is in early detection of vasospasm in subarachnoid hemorrhage and at the time of brain death,[30] where an oscillating reverberatory

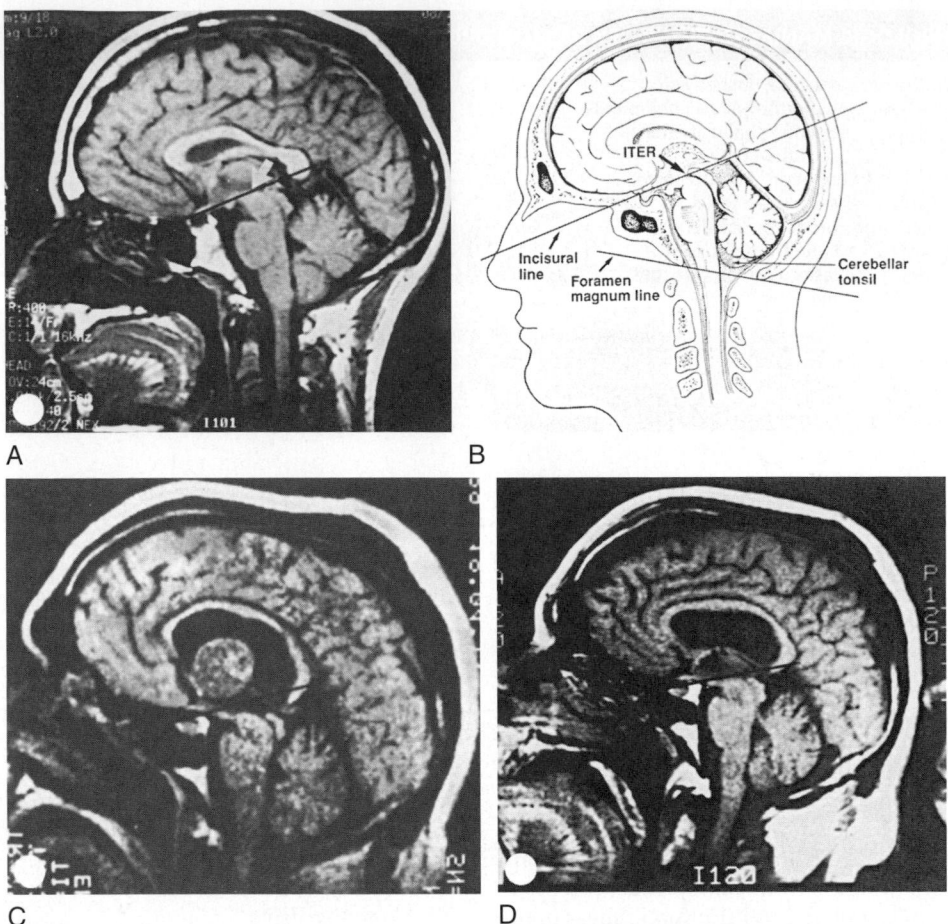

FIGURE 49–1. Midsagittal MRI views of a normal adult brain and of a brain with reversible downward transtentorial herniation. **A** and **B,** MRI view of a normal adult male brain and accompanying diagram. The opening of the tentorium of the cerebellum or anterior cerebellar notch lies along a line (incisural line) defined anteriorly by the anterior tubercle of the sella turcica and posteriorly by the junction of Galen's vein, the inferior sagittal sinus, and the confluence of the straight sinus. The proximal opening of the aqueduct of Sylvius, the iter ad infundibulum *(arrow),* lies within 2 mm of the incisural line. The foramen magnum line is defined between the inferior tip of the clivus anteriorly and the bony base of the posterior lip of the foramen magnum. **C,** A 47-year-old man who experienced 1 week of headache, nausea, vomiting, and gait ataxia presented with abrupt-onset coma, palsy of cranial nerve III, hyperreflexia, and bilateral extensor plantar responses. MRI revealed a third ventricular mass, obstructive hydrocephalus, and displacement of the iter ad infundibulum inferiorly by 6.5 mm. The cerebellar tonsils were not displaced. **D,** Subsequent MRI view in the patient in **C** at 2 weeks after surgical removal of a colloid cyst. The iter ad infundibulum is 1.2 mm below the incisural line. The patient had full neurologic recovery. (A, C, and D from Reich JB, Sierra J, Camp W, et al: Magnetic resonance imaging measurements and clinical changes accompanying transtentorial and foramen magnum brain herniation. Ann Neurol 1993;33:159-170.)

movement has been noted in the flow velocity waveforms. The diagnosis is suspected based on the finding of the reflux phenomenon during late systole after anterograde injection of blood into the vascular tree.

EVOKED POTENTIALS

Evoked potentials (EPs) are used to follow the level of CNS function in comatose patients.[31] Clinical use of brainstem auditory evoked potential (BAEP) and short latency somatosensory evoked potential (SEP) responses stem from the correlation between EP waveform and presumed generators within certain CNS structures. The SEP shows special promise in the ICU field because EP components generated supratentorially in the thalamus and primary sensory cortex can be identified and followed over time. Shifts of intracranial structures that lead to herniation syndromes are reflected in abnormalities in SEPs, whereas BAEPs are generated entirely at or below the lower midbrain and are less often affected. EPs are less affected than EEG readings by sedative

medications and septic or metabolic encephalopathies, factors that frequently confound interpretations in comatose patients. Anatomic specificity and physiologic and metabolic immutability are the basis of clinical utility of EPs. Abnormal test results, however, are etiologically nonspecific and must be carefully integrated into the clinical situation by a physician familiar with their clinical use. Caution is needed in the interpretation of SEPs to ensure that absent responses are not due to technical problems. Repeat SEPs are useful in following patients' progress. A progressive decline in response amplitude appears to be associated with worsening prognosis. Studies have shown that all patients with anoxic coma and bilaterally absent SEPs had died or remained in persistent vegetative state.[32] In traumatic coma, absent SEPs may be a less definitive prognostic indicator, because recovery of consciousness has been reported in some patients.[33] Furthermore, comatose patients, especially those with motor response of flexor posture or better, with an initial poor prognostic EEG pattern but normal SEPs, may have the potential for recovery and should be supported until the patient's condition has changed to a more prognostically definitive category.[34] BAEPs and median SEPs obtained within 24 hours of coma onset had a 3-month predictive outcome (compared with Glasgow outcome score) in patients with head injury, brain hemorrhage, or neoplasm.[35] Diagnostic sensitivity for an unfavorable outcome was low for both parameters, although specificity and positive predictive value was equally high for abnormal wave VI of BAEPs and median SEPs.

MONITORING OF INTRACRANIAL PRESSURE

Monitoring of ICP in neurointensive care is discussed in detail in Chapter 47. A review of published randomized controlled studies of real-time ICP monitoring by invasive or semi-invasive means in acute coma (traumatic or nontraumatic etiology) versus no ICP monitoring (i.e., clinical assessment of ICP) looked at outcome measures of all-cause mortality and severe disability at the end of a given follow-up period.[36] The conclusion drawn is that there are insufficient data to clarify the role of routine ICP monitoring in all severe cases of acute coma. However, it is of value in traumatic brain injury and should be considered on a case-by-case basis in other cases of coma.

PROGNOSIS

A complete evaluation of the comatose patient must include an estimate of prognosis. The outcome in a given comatose patient cannot be predicted with absolute certainty. Available serial data are not sufficiently specific or selective to help in establishing the prognosis in an individual patient. Guidelines on the outcome of coma have been compiled based on serial examinations. Although the status of the comatose patient on admission is valuable in providing early, informed discussion with relatives of patients and medical colleagues, that moment in most instances does not provide sufficient information to withhold immediate therapy. However, the early establishment of a highly probable poor outcome ideally should be made within 24 hours after hospital admission to ration intensive care services and protect families from false hope in futile cases. A logical and sensible approach to prognostication includes an etiologic subcategorization into medical, drug-induced, and traumatic coma.

Numerous prehospital descriptive scoring systems are used in an attempt to assess the severity of illness and predict outcome of patients. A 2-year prospective study compared severity of illness scoring systems (Acute Physiology and Chronic Health Evaluation [APACHE] II and Mainz Emergency Evaluation System [MEES]) to mental status measurement (Glasgow Coma Score [GCS]) in predicting outcome of 286 consecutive adult patients hospitalized for nontraumatic coma.[37] There were no statistically significant differences among the scoring systems to correctly predict outcome. APACHE II and MEES should not replace GCS. For the prediction of mortality, the GCS score provides the best indicator also in nontraumatic comatose patients (it is simple, less time consuming, and accurate in an emergency situation). Factors that are useful in determining the outcome of medical coma include the cause, the depth, and the duration of coma. Clinical signs reflecting brainstem, motor, and verbal function are the most helpful and best validated predictors (confidence interval 0.95).[38-41] Overall, only 15% of patients in established medical coma for 6 hours will make a good or moderate

recovery; others will die (61%), remain vegetative (12%), or become permanently dependent on others for daily living (11%). Prognosis depends on etiology of medical coma. Patients in coma due to a stroke, subarachnoid hemorrhage, or cardiorespiratory arrest have only about a 10% chance of achieving independent function. Thirty-five percent of patients will achieve moderate to good recovery if coma is due to other metabolic reasons, including infection, organ failure, and biochemical disturbances. As noted earlier, almost all patients who reach hospital after sedative overdose or other exogenous agents will recover moderately or completely. The depth of coma affects the individual prognosis. Patients who open their eyes in response to noxious stimuli after 6 hours of coma have a 20% chance of making a good recovery versus 10% if the eyes remain closed. The longer coma persists, the less likely are the chances for recovery; 15% of patients in coma for 6 hours make a good or moderate recovery compared with only 3% who remain unconscious at 1 week.[38,39] Coma after head trauma has a somewhat better prognosis (see later).

The severity of signs of brainstem dysfunction on admission inversely correlates with the chance of good recovery in medical coma. Absent pupillary responses at any time after onset and absent caloric-vestibular reflexes 1 day after onset indicate a poor prognosis (<2% recovery except in barbiturate or phenytoin poisoning). Except for sedative drug poisoning, no patient with absent pupillary light reflexes, corneal reflexes, oculocephalic or caloric responses, or lack of a motor response to noxious stimulation at 3 days after onset is likely to ever regain independent function. In a prospective study of 500 patients in medical coma, a uniform group of 210 patients suffered anoxic injury: 52 of these had no pupillary reflex at 24 hours, all of whom died. By the third day, 70 were left with a motor response worse than withdrawal and all died. By the seventh day, the absence of roving eye movements was seen in 16 patients, all of whom died.[38,39]

Patients likely to recover to functional independence will within 1 to 3 days speak words, open their eyes to noise, show nystagmus on caloric testing, or have spontaneous eye movements. More than 25% of patients with anoxic injury who show roving conjugate eye movements within 6 hours of the onset of coma or who show withdrawal responses to pain or eye opening to pain will recover independence and make a moderate or good recovery. The use of combinations of clinical signs helps to improve the accuracy of prognosis: at 24 hours the absence of a corneal response, pupillary light reaction, or caloric or doll's eye response is not compatible with recovery to independence.

Postanoxic convulsive status epilepticus and/or myoclonic status epilepticus reflect a poor prognosis. Occasional patients recover consciousness but remain handicapped. Most die or become vegetative.[42,43] Associated clinical findings, such as loss of brainstem reflexes or eye opening at the onset of myoclonic jerks, and sinister EEG patterns, such as suppression or burst-suppression, confirm a grim neurologic outcome in this group. Autopsy studies show that cerebral and cerebellar damage can be ascribed to the initial ischemic hypoxic event; there is no evidence that status epilepticus further contributes to this damage. We initially treat patients with an intravenous loading dose of a major anticonvulsant (phenytoin, 13 to 18 mg/kg at 25 mg/min, and/or phenobarbitol, 20 mg/kg at 50 mg/min). Myoclonic status epilepticus is generally resistant to therapy; we give intermittent doses of benzodiazepines (lorazepam, 2 to 4 mg, or clonazepam, 0.5 mg i.v.) as needed to suppress particularly severe myoclonus that interferes with ventilatory support. Anesthetic agents are rarely indicated and are unlikely to alter outcome.

A meta-analysis of prognostic studies in anoxic-ischemic coma examined the value of biochemical markers of brain damage in CSF or serum.[44] Only concentrations of CSF markers (creatine kinase brain isoenzyme, neuron-specific enolase, lactate dehydrogenase, and glutamate oxaloacetate) reached 0% false-positive rate. Because of small numbers of patients involved in studies (wide confidence levels) and methodologic limitations of studies the results available are not sufficiently accurate to provide a solid basis for management decisions of patients in coma.

The most accurate prediction of outcome in a patient in medical coma is obtained from the use of a combination of clinical signs and there is little to be added by more sophisticated testing other than in identifying the cause of the coma.[38,39] Within the first week, it is hard to justify the withdrawal of therapy from patients in medical coma unless they are already brain dead or lack all signs of brainstem function. After that, the probability of being able to predict the quality of life increases steadily. A multisociety task force of neurologists and neurosurgeons obtained a large number of data concerning the persistent vegetative state that provides guidelines to outcomes in patients remaining vegetative 1 month after severe head trauma or coma-producing medical illness (mostly anoxic).[15]

Among adults with head trauma who were in a vegetative state at 1 month (n = 434), 33% died, 15% remained vegetative, and 28% suffered severe disability at 1 year. Among children vegetative for 1 month after trauma (n = 106), 9% died, 29% remained in a persistent vegetative state, and 35% were severely disabled at 1 year; only 27% attained moderate/good recovery.

Nontraumatic (medical) coma results were even worse. Among 169 adults with nontraumatic brain injury and vegetative at 1 month, 53% died within a year, 32% remained vegetative, and only 14% made a moderate/good recovery. Outcome of 45 children in similar circumstances showed 22% dead, 65% still vegetative, and only 6% who made a moderate/good recovery at 1 year.

It is possible in a fraction of patients to predict within the first week those who will recover, those who will die in coma or enter a vegetative state, and those who will survive with severe disability. It is well established that patients in anoxic coma who are in a vegetative state at 1 month will never recover their full preanoxic physical or cognitive function.

Patients in coma due to *exogenous agents* (except carbon monoxide poisoning) carry an overall good prognosis provided that circulation and respiration are protected by avoiding or correcting cardiac dysrhythmia, aspiration pneumonia, and respiratory arrest. Despite absent brainstem reflexes (electrocerebral silence on EEG), patients with deep sedative drug intoxication have the potential for complete recovery. Therefore, in the emergent situation, patients in coma of uncertain etiology should be supported vigorously until the precise cause of coma has been fully established.

The outcome of *traumatic coma* is generally better than that of medical coma, and prognostic criteria are somewhat different[15,33,45]:

1. Many patients with head injury are young.
2. Prolonged, post-traumatic unconsciousness of up to several months does not always preclude a satisfactory outcome.

3. Compared with the initial degree of neurologic abnormality, patients in traumatic coma improve more than patients in medical coma. Patients in coma for longer than 6 hours after traumatic brain injury have a 40% chance to recover to moderate disability or better at 6 months.

The most reliable predictors of outcome at 6 months are:

1. Patient age (worse outcome especially after 60 years).
2. Depth and duration of coma (an inverse correlation with GCS score).
3. Pupil reaction and eye movements (absence at 24 hours predicts death or a vegetative state in 90%).
4. Motor response in the first week of injury (Table 49-6).

An independent poor prognostic indicator is sustained, uncontrollably increased ICP (greater than 20 mm Hg). Additional factors play a role in the eventual outcome from traumatic coma. Specific lesions, such as subdural hematoma, that result in coma can have a less than 10% recovery rate.[46] In studies with blunt trauma, comatose patients with increased plasma glucose, hypokalemia, or elevated blood leukocyte counts were associated with lower GCS scores and an increased probability of death.[47] There are some reports of patients who have suffered coma as a result of traumatic brain injury in whom an improvement from the vegetative state has been recognized after months, but these anecdotal cases of recovery are difficult to validate, and it seems possible that such patients were not truly vegetative, rather in a

TABLE 49–6. TRAUMA SCALE: TOTAL TRAUMA SCORE (SUM OF INDIVIDUAL SCORES)*

Glasgow Coma Scale	
14-15	5
11-13	4
8-10	3
5-7	2
3-4	1
Respiratory Rate	
10-24/min	4
25-35/min	3
>35/min	2
1-9/min	1
None	0
Respiratory Expansion	
Normal	1
None	0
Systolic Blood Pressure	
>89 mm Hg	4
70-89 mm Hg	3
50-69 mm Hg	2
0-49 mm Hg	1
No pulse	0
Peripheral Perfusion (Capillary Refill)	
Normal	2
Delayed	1
None	0

*Scores less than 10 represent less than 60% chance of survival.

state of profound disability but with cognition, at the beginning of the observation.[48]

A systematic review of trials reporting on multisensory stimulation programs in patients with traumatic brain injury in coma or the vegetative state found no reliable evidence of the effectiveness of such techniques when compared with standard rehabilitation.[49] Outcome measures included duration of unconsciousness (time between injury and response to verbal commands), level of consciousness (GCS), level of cognitive functioning, functional outcomes (GCS), or disability rating scale. The overall methodologic quality was poor, and studies differed widely in design and conduct. Because of the diversity in reporting of outcome measures a meta-analysis was not possible.

The prognostic guidelines for medical and traumatic coma should be applied with care. One must be sure that evaluation and interpretation of clinical signs are correct. The prognostic signs, however, predict general outcomes in large patient groups and cannot be applied with absolute precision to every individual comatose patient. In addition, the effect of anticholinergic agents, used during resuscitation, on pupillary reactivity and the effect of paralytic agents on motor response must be excluded.

The ability to predict prognosis after coma can benefit the patient, family, and physician. Families can be spared both the emotional and financial burdens of caring for individuals with an insignificant chance of independent function and quality life. Physicians can then properly allocate limited resources to patients with the potential to benefit from advanced medical care.

There are recognized difficulties in interpreting the outcome of studies of coma prognosis: the lack of prospective studies, failure to state confidence intervals, and the fact that patients in coma may die of a non-neurologic disease. The self-fulfilling nature of poor prognoses is difficult to eliminate: the care of a patient will reflect the treating physicians' impressions and opinions on patient outcome. Ideally, prognostic studies should only be performed on patients who will receive maximal life support for as long as possible, but this is inconsistent with the humane and sensitive management of patients and their relatives.

A recent analysis used data from the SUPPORT (Study to Understand the Prognoses and Preferences for Outcomes and Risks of Treatments) trial to estimate the cost-effectiveness of aggressive care for patients in nontraumatic coma.[50,51] Patients with reversible metabolic causes of coma were excluded. The incremental cost-effectiveness was calculated for aggressive care versus withholding cardiopulmonary resuscitation and ventilatory support after day 3 of coma. The incremental cost-effectiveness of the more aggressive strategy was $140,000 (1998 dollars) per quality-adjusted life year for high-risk patients and $87,000/quality-adjusted life year for low-risk patients (five risk factors were age older than 70 years, absent verbal response, absent withdrawal to pain, abnormal brainstem response, and serum creatinine value greater than 1.5 mg/dL). Earlier decisions to withhold life-sustaining treatments for patients with very poor prognoses may yield considerable cost savings. On moral and ethical grounds physicians may object to consideration of the cost factor when it comes to treatment decisions of more-or-less sick patients. Financial constraints imposed on the medical fraternity from "top down" by politicians and the business culture may no longer afford such "luxury" even in a country as wealthy as the United States.

ANNOTATED REFERENCES

Hund EF, Lehman-Horn F: Life-threatening hyperthermic syndromes. In Hacke W (ed): Neurocritical Care. Berlin, Springer-Verlag, 1994, pp 888-896.
  This textbook on neurocritical care gives concise access to causes and treatment of medical and neurologic coma. It is easy to access because topics are discussed in short, easy to read chapters with a short list of references.

Jennett B, Teasdale G, Braakman R, et al: Prognosis of patients with severe head injury. Neurosurgery 1979;4:283-301.
  This article helps guide physicians to focus on the important clinical prognostic factors when managing severely head-injured patients. Because the prognosis of traumatic coma is better than medical coma, these guidelines potentially minimize management errors in patients with other severe injuries.

Levy DE, Bates D, Caronna JJ, et al: Prognosis in non-traumatic coma. Ann Intern Med 1981;94:293-301; and Levy DE, Caronna JJ, Singer BH, et al: Predicting outcome from hypoxic-ischemic coma. JAMA 1985;253: 1420-1426.
  These two articles recognize the value/importance of the bedside evaluation in the prediction of outcome of medical (hypoxic-ischemic) coma. This bedside knowledge helps clinicians orient patient care in an increasingly high-tech hospital environment.

Plum F, Posner JB: The Diagnosis of Stupor and Coma. Philadelphia, FA Davis, 1980.
  This book is a convenient "one-stop" reference to stupor/coma. It is an excellent source of information about the pathophysiology and etiology of altered consciousness.

Synek VM: Prognostically important EEG coma patterns in diffuse anoxic and traumatic encephalopathies in adults. J Clin Neurophysiol 1988;5:161-174.
  The EEG is often used by clinicians (and requested by family) to help establish cause and prognosis of stupor and coma. This article usefully categorized EEG patterns according to a severity scale that can be incorporated into the bedside evaluation of a patient with altered consciousness.

Chapter 50

CARDIOPULMONARY-CEREBRAL RESUSCITATION

Clifton W. Callaway

Cardiopulmonary arrest may occur as the endpoint or consequence of many diseases. Examples include acute dysrhythmias, cardiac pump failure, hypoxemia, sepsis, hemorrhage, drug toxicity, and metabolic disturbances. Often the mechanism is unknown when treatment is initiated, and an algorithmic approach titrated to real-time monitoring (electrocardiography, capnometry, oximetry, blood pressure) is used. When the cause is known or suspected, therapy may be individualized and directed at that cause. In all cases, management has two priorities: (1) rapid restoration of cardiopulmonary function and (2) minimization of ischemic damage to end organs, primarily the brain. Restoration of circulation is composed largely of mechanical and electrical treatment. In contrast, brain injury involves primarily cellular and molecular events that are treated with specific and detailed intensive care. Meaningful survival is unlikely without attention to both heart and brain.

Previously, there has been little consensus on intensive care management of the patient resuscitated from cardiac arrest, but there is increasing evidence that differences in post-resuscitation management influence final outcomes.[1,2] Despite decades of attention to acute cardiac resuscitation, there has been little or no change in long-term survival.[3,4] Meaningful improvements in outcome will require an integrated approach to the patient that includes not only immediate resuscitation but also intensive care management after restoration of circulation (Fig. 50-1). The epidemiology of cardiac arrest, the initial approach for reversing cardiopulmonary arrest, modifications of this approach appropriate for specific disease states, and post-resuscitation care designed to minimize brain injury are reviewed.

EPIDEMIOLOGY

In the United States, heart disease is the overall leading cause of death. Cardiopulmonary arrest outside the hospital has an age-adjusted incidence of 100 to 120 events per 100,000 people per year.[5,6] Overall survival after out-of-hospital cardiac arrest in the United States is estimated at 6.4%,[7] with several large U.S. cities reporting a survival rate less than 2%.[8,9] The incidence of cardiac arrest in the hospital is about 0.17 event per hospital bed per year.[10] For inpatients experiencing cardiac arrest, survival to hospital discharge is estimated at 17%. Fewer than one half of cardiac arrests occur in an intensive care unit (ICU) setting, and survival does not appear to be related to the location of collapse.[11]

Demographic features of sudden cardiac death are similar to the characteristics of cardiovascular disease. Sudden cardiac death is more common in males than females both outside of the hospital[6] and in the hospital.[10] However, the incidence of cardiac arrest is higher in women (6.0%) than in men (4.4%) who are admitted to the hospital for acute myocardial infarction.[12] Cardiac arrest outside the hospital affects blacks more than whites or Asians.[6,8] Whereas sudden death can affect patients of all ages, the mean age for sudden cardiac arrest is between 65 and 70 years in most studies.[6,10]

Two temporally and mechanistically separate processes contribute to mortality: (1) cardiopulmonary collapse and (2) neurologic injury. In evidence of the first process, only one third of patients who collapse outside the hospital have

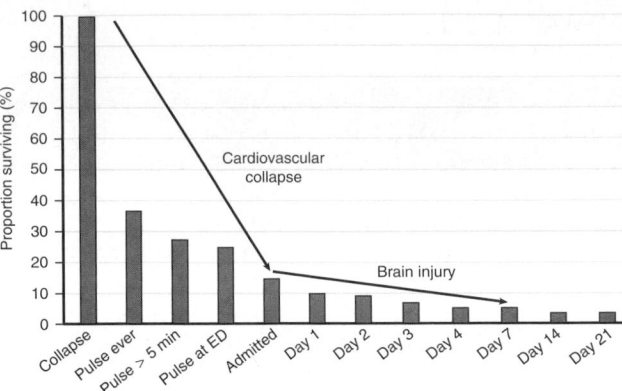

FIGURE 50–1. The survival curve for patients treated for out-of-hospital cardiac arrest in one city illustrates that risk of death occurs in two phases. Early death after cardiac arrest results from irreversible cardiopulmonary collapse, precluding survival to hospital admission for 70% to 80% of patients. Death during the first few days after hospital admission is usually related to brain injury and failure to awaken, precluding long-term survival for an additional 10% to 15% of patients. (Unpublished data from City of Pittsburgh.)

restoration of circulation long enough to be admitted to the hospital (see Fig. 50-1). Likewise, only 44% of patients who collapse in the hospital have return of circulation.[10] In evidence of the second process, two thirds of patients admitted to the hospital after out-of-hospital collapse die before discharge from the hospital.[13] Likewise, over 60% of patients initially resuscitated from cardiac arrest in the hospital do not survive to hospital discharge.[10] The most common reason for death among patients after restoration of circulation is post-ischemic brain injury. Failure to awaken leads to withdrawal of care and in-hospital death for as many as 44% to 68% of subjects after initial restoration of circulation.[10,14]

RESTORING CIRCULATION

Acute treatment of cardiac arrest consists of two essential, goal-directed activities: (1) artificial circulation (usually chest compressions augmented by peripheral vasoconstrictors) to circulate oxygenated blood to heart and brain and (2) electrical shock to terminate ventricular fibrillation (VF) and unstable tachyarrhythmias. Of these two procedures, artificial circulation (including ventilation) occupies most of the time and electrical rescue shock is invoked only when appropriate. Rescue shock is the only procedure for which interruption of artificial circulation is absolutely necessary and justified.

The recommended division of time and prioritization of activities is depicted in Figure 50-2. All other activities, including antidysrhythmic medications and advanced airway maneuvers, are designed to supplement these two core activities. Optimization of resuscitation requires that any interruption in the two core activities, especially artificial circulation, be minimized. In addition, continuous reassessment of the patient can be reduced to constant awareness of two parameters (Fig. 50-3). The organization of the electrocardiogram (ECG) and the presence of pulses will prompt appropriate selection of therapy.

The American Heart Association (AHA) and European Resuscitation Council provide consensus scientific statements about the acute management of cardiac arrest.[15] Those

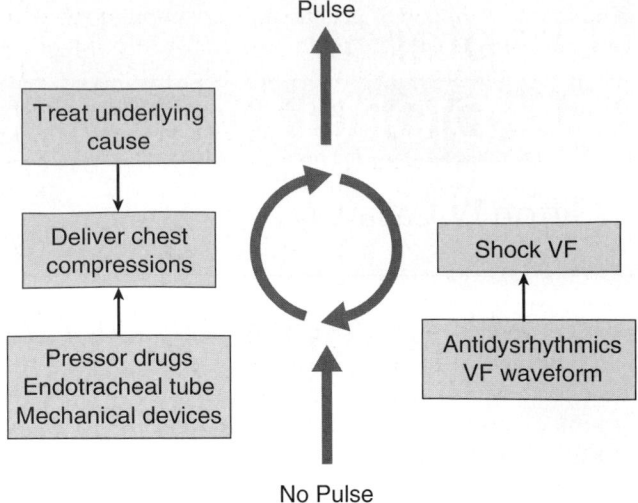

FIGURE 50–2. Prioritization of activities must occur during cardiac resuscitation. The central circle emphasizes that the core activity of artificial perfusion should be interrupted only to provide rescue shocks when appropriate. All drugs, airway devices, and other interventions are designed to augment either artificial circulation or defibrillation. None of these adjuncts should interrupt or detract from performing the two core activities.

guidelines have a detailed review of specific drugs and procedures. The following section provides an overview of airway management, circulation support, rescue shock for defibrillation, and drug therapy during cardiac arrest.

AIRWAY AND VENTILATION

Obstruction of the airway can occur in any patient with impaired consciousness, including cardiac arrest.[16] If uncorrected, this obstruction prevents oxygenation and

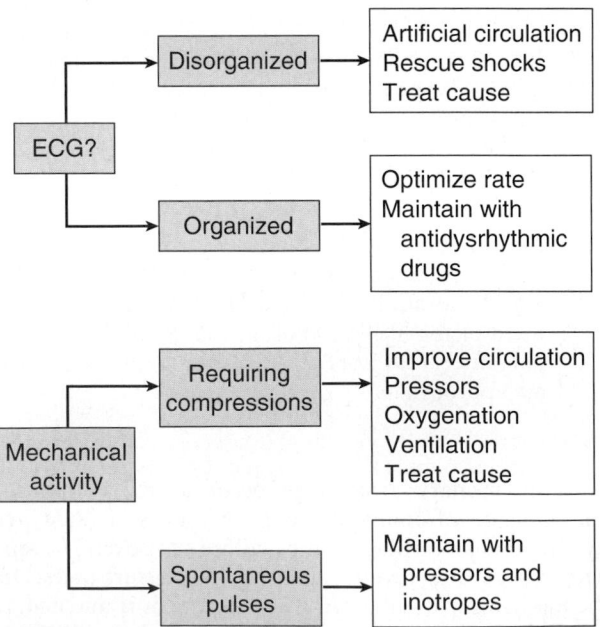

FIGURE 50–3. Continuous reassessment of the patient during cardiac resuscitation can focus on the electrocardiogram (ECG) and on the presence of cardiac activity (pulses). If an organized ECG is not present, interventions should be undertaken to restore an organized ECG. If mechanical cardiac activity is not present, interventions should be undertaken to improve mechanical cardiac activity.

ventilation, leading to or perpetuating cardiopulmonary collapse. In patients who are comatose because of primary cardiac arrest, the airway usually is not patent. Animal models typically do not mimic ventilation through the human airway because the most common research animals (dogs and swine) have straight orotracheal passages.

Agonal respirations occur after acute cardiac arrest for an additional 1 to 2 minutes.[17] These respirations may confuse lay people, delaying recognition of cardiac arrest. It is unclear whether these agonal respirations can generate sufficient ventilation to support life. The presence of gasping is associated with survival, but it also may be a surrogate marker for brief collapse-to-resuscitation intervals.[18] Regardless, the amplitude and frequency of agonal respirations declines over 1 to 2 minutes, necessitating artificial ventilation for all patients requiring more than momentary resuscitation efforts.

Simple maneuvers can establish patency of the human airway. Extension of the neck (head tilt) and forward displacement of the mandible (chin lift) straightens and opens the pharynx. The tongue can be displaced from the posterior pharynx by insertion of an oropharyngeal airway. With these steps, positive-pressure ventilation can be provided using mouth-to-mouth or bag-valve-mask ventilation. A positive-pressure breath of 10 to 15 mL/kg delivered over 2 to 3 seconds will fill the lungs. Ventilation with as little as 400 mL in adults (6 to 7 mL/kg) will cause the chest to rise.[19] While that volume is inadequate for conscious subjects, it is unclear what tidal volume is necessary to provide adequate gas exchange during cardiac arrest.

The minute ventilation required to accomplish resuscitation in humans has not been established. The need for gas exchange must be balanced against the fact that interrupting chest compressions lowers coronary perfusion (Fig. 50-4).[20] Comparison of different ratios of chest compressions to ventilation in swine suggests that two breaths per 50 chest compressions or more may be optimal for resuscitation.[21] An extreme point of view is that chest compressions without any artificial ventilation may be sufficient to accomplish resuscitation in certain individuals.[22] This position is contrary to early work demonstrating that the human airway collapses in most unconscious subjects and that compressions alone are unable to provide ventilation.[16] Therefore, the optimal ratio of chest compressions to ventilations remains to be established but may be greater than the 15:2 currently recommended in the AHA guidelines.

Ventilation can be confirmed with capnometry. During cardiac arrest, end-tidal CO_2 measurement is related to cardiac output and pulmonary blood flow.[23] Therefore, CO_2 levels may be very low (<10 mm Hg) at the onset of resuscitation. Adequate artificial circulation will cause CO_2 levels to increase, and these levels may be used as a feedback to improve or modify chest compressions. Data from emergency department patients suggest that an end-tidal CO_2 level greater than 15 to 16 mm Hg is associated with successful cardiac resuscitation.[24,25] Conversely, end-tidal CO_2 less than 10 mm Hg after 20 minutes of resuscitative efforts predicts nonsurvival.[26] However, drugs commonly used during resuscitation can disrupt the association between capnography readings and pulmonary blood flow. For example, epinephrine infusion reduces CO_2 levels and sodium bicarbonate infusion produces a transient, but profound, elevation of CO_2 levels. An abrupt increase in end-tidal CO_2 levels, usually to levels greater than 35 mm Hg, accompanies the return of spontaneous circulation.

AIRWAY DEVICES

The most common ventilation device used by rescue personnel, paramedics, and other health care providers is a self-inflating bag attached to a facemask (bag-valve-mask), which has several pitfalls. First, it is difficult to maintain an air-tight seal between the mask and the face of the patient, particularly when simultaneously performing head-tilt, chin-lift maneuvers. Adequate training and practice increases ventilation success by a single provider, but two providers achieve more reliable airway management. One provider squeezes the bag, while the second provider uses two hands to hold the mask on the face and position the head.

A second difficulty with bag-valve-mask ventilation is insufflation of the stomach.[27] Excessive air in the stomach can promote emesis, and the abdominal distention may impair venous return and lung compliance.[28] The esophagus prevents air entry into the stomach unless upper airway pressures exceed 15 to 20 cm H_2O.[29] However, during cardiac arrest, esophageal muscle tone declines, and air will enter the stomach with upper airway pressures greater than 5 to 8 cm H_2O.[30] If the upper airway is not patent, providers may try to ventilate with increased pressure to achieve chest rise. Furthermore, rapid squeezing of the bag during the excitement of the situation results in too high upper airway pressures. By avoiding these problems, mechanical ventilators with regulated flow rates and peak pressures may perform better than bag-valve-mask during resuscitation.

Endotracheal intubation can secure the airway definitively. A cuffed endotracheal tube protects from emesis and maintains airway patency. However, laryngoscopy requires an interruption in chest compressions and the endotracheal tube by itself does not correct cardiac arrest. Therefore, endotracheal intubation must be considered an adjunct to initial resuscitation that should not delay or interrupt more definitive interventions. Obviously, any patient with restoration of circulation and subsequent coma will require endotracheal intubation, but the interruption in artificial circulation required for this procedure should be carefully considered.

Alternative airway adjuncts, such as double-lumen, combination endotracheal-esophageal tubes (Combitube) or laryngeal mask airways can be used to temporarily manage the airway during resuscitation.[31,32] The Combitube and laryngeal mask airways have the advantage that they can be inserted blindly in seconds without laryngoscopy, thereby minimizing any interruption of chest compressions.[27] The degree to which these devices can protect from aspiration is debated.

ARTIFICIAL CIRCULATION

In the patient without pulses, circulation of blood can be accomplished by mechanical compression of the heart and chest. The critical parameter for restoring spontaneous circulation is the development of adequate coronary perfusion pressure (CPP). The CPP is quantified by the pressure gradient between the aorta and the inside of the ventricles (usually approximated by the pressure in the right atrium or the central venous pressure [CVP]). Measurement of CPP in clinical practice is difficult unless the patient has invasive monitoring before cardiopulmonary collapse. CVP can be estimated from a central line, and peripheral arterial pressures can be developed from approximate aortic pressures. In the spontaneously beating heart, most blood flows through the ventricular walls

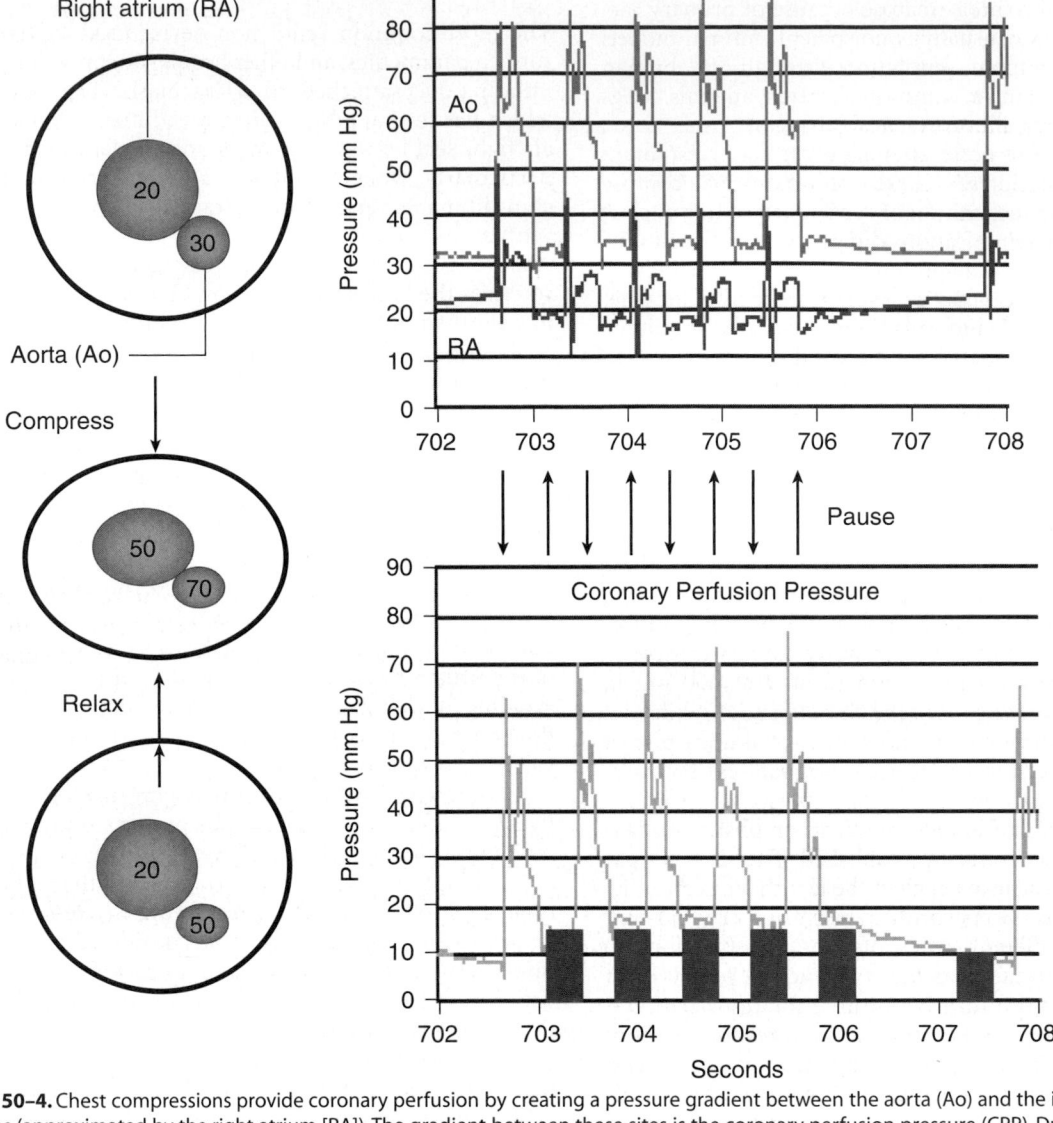

FIGURE 50–4. Chest compressions provide coronary perfusion by creating a pressure gradient between the aorta (Ao) and the inside of the ventricles (approximated by the right atrium [RA]). The gradient between these sites is the coronary perfusion pressure (CPP). During chest compression *(down arrows)* pressure increases in both Ao and RA. During relaxation *(up arrows),* pressure persists in Ao more than RA. Thus, myocardial blood flow is most related to CPP during the relaxation phase of chest compressions. Note that the CPP declines within 1 to 2 seconds when compressions are interrupted for ventilation. (Unpublished laboratory data.)

during diastole, when the ventricular pressure is lowest. With mechanical compression of the heart and chest during resuscitation, the primary perfusion of the heart occurs during the relaxation phase (see Fig. 50-4).

CPP is highly correlated with myocardial perfusion, and consequently with the likelihood of resuscitation.[33] In humans, return of circulation requires that the developed CPP exceeds 15 to 20 mm Hg. It is likely that with CPP less than 15 mm Hg, perfusion is inadequate to replete the energy state of the myocardium during cardiac arrest. It is important to recognize that peak arterial pressure or palpable pulses measured during chest compressions do not necessarily represent CPP because ventricular pressures are simultaneously elevated. Consequently, it is more useful to follow the "diastolic" or relaxation phase arterial pressure. If unable to follow these pressures, the clinician must rely on indirect evidence of myocardial perfusion, such as improved electrical and mechanical activity or increased pulmonary CO_2 excretion.

Direct cardiac compression via a thoracotomy is more effective than external chest compressions, producing roughly threefold increases in CPP.[34] This approach also allows recognition of cardiac tamponade and treatment by pericardiotomy. Mechanical activity and fibrillation are immediately visible, and electrical rescue shocks or pacing can be applied directly to the heart. In the setting of cardiopulmonary collapse due to exsanguination, thoracotomy also allows aortic compression to shunt blood to heart and brain, as well as the potential for direct control of intrathoracic bleeding. Until the 1960s, thoracotomy was the standard approach for treatment of sudden cardiac arrest, but this procedure has now been supplanted by closed-chest compressions. Case series describe how cardiac massage continues to be successful, and its use should be considered when closed-chest compressions are ineffective.[34] Open-chest cardiac massage is most likely to succeed if initiated early during resuscitation.[35]

Delivery of chest compressions is often inadequate, and uninterrupted chest compressions are critical for restoration of circulation.[20,36,37] A variety of mechanical devices have been developed to provide more consistent and continuous chest compressions.[38] Some of these devices exploit circumferential compression or active compression-decompression of the chest to increase the efficiency of artificial circulation. However, none has gained widespread use because of their weight and cost. Whereas no current device is poised to solve this challenge, the constant attention of industry to this area illustrates the need for strategies to improve delivery of chest compressions.

Extracorporeal perfusion for restoration of circulation is highly effective and can be used to resuscitate subjects for whom chest compressions have failed.[39,40] With extracorporeal support, more time becomes available to address the primary cause for cardiac arrest. However, this approach requires specialized technical skill and has increased cost and increased risk. Logistical issues include limited availability of perfusion equipment, increased set-up time for circuit priming, and delays in establishing adequate venous and arterial access. Development of portable cardiopulmonary bypass devices that can be primed quickly along with improved techniques for rapid vascular access could broaden the use of this technology.

ECG MONITORING

Continuous three-lead ECG monitoring provides information that can be used to titrate resuscitation. A practical division of the ECG is to divide rhythms into organized and not organized. Organized rhythms include supraventricular rhythms or ventricular tachycardia. Disorganized rhythms include VF and asystole. Disorganized rhythms cannot support the pumping of blood, regardless of volume status, cardiac muscle state, and vascular integrity. Therefore, restoring cardiac electrical activity to an organized rhythm is an essential step in resuscitation. Organized rhythms can support pumping of blood unless they are too slow (<30 to 40 complexes per minute) or too fast (>170 to 180 complexes per minute). An organized rhythm in the absence of pulses is termed *pulseless electrical activity* (PEA).

Any organized complex that is not associated with perfusion should be considered PEA. The absence of perfusion in the presence of organized electrical activity may result from damage to heart muscle (as in massive myocardial infarction) or from uncoupling of electrical and mechanical activity (as in prolonged circulatory arrest). Perfusion may be so poor that pulses are absent in ventricular tachycardia, supraventricular tachycardia, and atrial fibrillation with rapid ventricular response that are unresponsive to the filling of the heart. These tachyarrhythmias should be corrected by electrical cardioversion. Outside of these tachyarrhythmias, the rate of complexes in PEA is related to the ischemic state of the heart and may be used to monitor resuscitation efforts. With increasing ischemia, energy depletion will occur in the electrical system and the rate of PEA will slow. If resuscitation is improving the energy state of the heart, the rate of PEA will accelerate. Anecdotally, narrow complexes reaching rates of 80 to 100 beats/min often herald the return of pulses. Falling rates of complexes in PEA reflect unsuccessful resuscitation efforts, probably because of inadequate perfusion of the cardiac conduction system.

VF and asystole lie along a continuum of disorganized ECG. Arbitrary peak-to-peak amplitude of the ECG is usually used to distinguish asystole (amplitude < 0.1 to 0.2 mV) from VF (amplitude > 0.2 mV).[41] However, VF also exhibits temporal structure that may be absent in asystole.[42] VF is a chaotic electrical activity formed by multiple interacting waves

of activation within the heart.[43] VF emerges from broken wave fronts that result from an area of ischemia (as in myocardial infarction), an area of prolonged refractoriness (as in drug-induced or inherited prolonged QT intervals), or too rapid succession of activation potentials (as in tachycardia or an R-on-T premature beat). As the organization and amplitude of these waves decline, because of ischemia or hypoxemia, the amplitude of the ECG also declines. Reperfusion of the heart in asystole may restore VF. Furthermore, the amplitude and organization of the VF increase with reperfusion, providing a marker of adequate artificial perfusion.

RATIONAL USE OF RESCUE SHOCKS FOR DEFIBRILLATION

Delivery of immediate transthoracic electrical (rescue) shocks to patients in VF can convert it into an organized cardiac rhythm (Fig. 50-5). Rescue shocks are highly effective when VF is of very brief duration (<1 to 2 minutes). These shocks may work by depolarizing the heart, canceling the original wave fronts, or by prolonging the refractory periods.[43] Although rescue shocks can successfully restore an organized rhythm, repeated shocks may directly damage the myocardium. The precise magnitude of this damage is still unclear.[44] Nevertheless, optimal therapy should provide rescue shocks at the lowest effective energy while minimizing the number of unsuccessful rescue shocks.

Rescue shocks are more likely to fail when cardiac arrest has lasted more than a few minutes. In the out-of-hospital setting, only 9% of rescue shocks restore an organized ECG if the collapse was not witnessed by the paramedic.[45] Furthermore, resuscitation is less likely after rescue shocks that convert VF into asystole.[46] In one model for defibrillation, a "critical mass" of the heart must be depolarized by

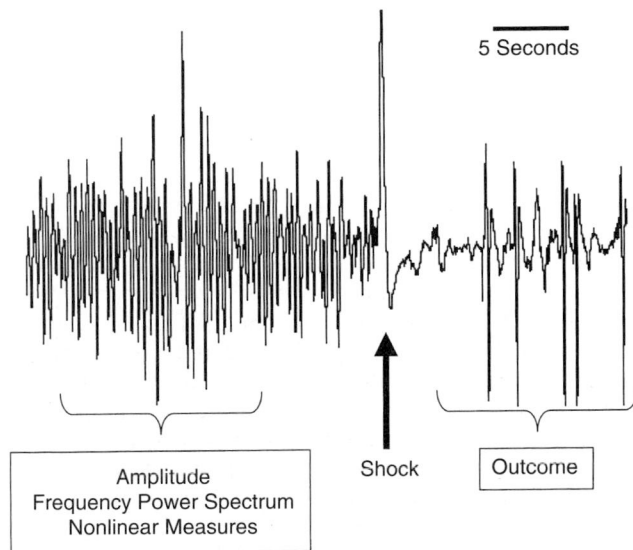

FIGURE 50–5. Rescue shock converts ventricular fibrillation into an organized rhythm. Note that several seconds pass between the rescue shock and the first appearance of complexes. Quantification of the waveform of ventricular fibrillation before shock using amplitude, frequency components, or nonlinear measures can predict the likelihood that the outcome will be an organized rhythm. The appearance of an organized rhythm does not guarantee pulses, and continued reevaluation is essential. (Unpublished data from City of Pittsburgh.)

a rescue shock to ensure that VF activation potentials are extinguished.[43] If a critical mass is not defibrillated, chaotic activity in the remaining regions will spread throughout the heart, rekindling VF. However, even when the entire heart is depolarized by the shock, VF may recur, perhaps because of heterogeneous areas of refractoriness or persistent foci.[47] Regardless, shocks must be of sufficient intensity to deliver depolarizing current to the majority of the heart.

Several maneuvers can facilitate electrical defibrillation. Increased pressure of paddles from 0.5 to 8.0 kg on the chest will decrease transthoracic impedance by as much as 14%, increasing delivery of current to the heart.[48,49] This advantage of paddles must be weighed against the increased safety and convenience afforded by hands-free adhesive defibrillation pads. Multiphasic shock waveforms that produce more effective depolarization of individual myocytes (e.g., biphasic waveforms) tend to accomplish defibrillation with less energy.[43] In the past, multiple shocks would be delivered in rapid succession to decrease chest impedance. However, repetitive shocks decrease chest impedance only about 8% in actual patients.[48] Rescue shock energy can be increased by much greater amounts, and this modest decrease in impedance afforded by repetitive shocks probably does not justify prolonging the interruption of artificial circulation. Together, these data suggest that rescue shocks of sufficient energy with multiphasic waveforms should be delivered singly to the patient in VF using firm paddle pressure on the chest.

For VF that has lasted more than 3 to 4 minutes, delaying rescue shocks until after a few minutes of chest compressions can improve the rescue shock success. In animals, reperfusion before rescue shocks appears to be preferable to immediate rescue shock after more than 5 minutes of untreated VF.[50-53] Researchers in two clinical studies have found that either 90 seconds or 3 minutes of chest compressions before delivery of the initial rescue shock improved resuscitation rates for subjects with VF outside the hospital, particularly when rescuer response intervals are longer than 4 minutes.[4,54] Thus, defibrillation should be provided immediately for VF shortly after a witnessed collapse, but a brief period of artificial circulation should precede any shock delivery to VF that has lasted longer.

Quantitative analysis of the VF waveform can distinguish early VF from late VF and may be useful for estimating the likelihood of rescue shock success (see Fig. 50-5).[55] Larger amplitude of VF suggests early VF and is associated with more successful resuscitation.[56] However, amplitude can be affected by body habitus and other recording conditions. Frequency-based measures, as well as nonlinear dynamic measures, also can be used to quantify VF and to estimate the probability of rescue shock success and are less dependent on recording conditions.[57-60] All of these measures, or some combination of these measures, are likely to be implemented in future generations of defibrillators. These devices will provide real-time, semi-quantitative estimates of the probability that a rescue shock will succeed in restoring an organized rhythm. Using this information, the clinician will be able to choose to shock VF when the probability of shock success is high or to concentrate on improving the situation with artificial perfusion when the probability of shock success is low.

DRUG THERAPY

All drug therapy in cardiac arrest can be divided into three categories: pressors, antidysrhythmics, and metabolic drugs.

There is good evidence that pressors improve artificial circulation, making resuscitation more likely. Antidysrhythmic drugs are effective for preventing dysrhythmias and therefore have a role in stabilizing the heart once circulation is restored. The value of an antidysrhythmic drug for terminating VF or reversing asystole is less clear. Metabolic drugs, primarily bicarbonate, can be used to reverse acidosis or other electrolyte problems when they are recognized. However, there are no data to support the routine use of these drugs for all patients.

Pressors used during resuscitation include epinephrine and vasopressin. Both of these drugs can increase CPP through actions on alpha-adrenergic (epinephrine) or vasopressin receptors (Fig. 50-6).[61,62] Epinephrine is usually administered in 1 mg (~0.015 mg/kg) increments. In laboratory studies, the pressor effects of epinephrine during cardiac arrest are brief (~5 minutes). Vasopressin has been administered as 40-unit boluses (~0.5 unit/kg) and produces a longer-lasting increase in CPP (~10 minutes). Both drugs should be titrated to improvement in clinical indicators (ECG waveform, mechanical activity, changes in end-tidal CO_2 or coronary perfusion pressure).

The 1-mg dose of epinephrine is widely believed to be subtherapeutic in the setting of circulatory arrest lasting more than a few minutes. Trials in out-of-hospital patients comparing higher initial boluses of epinephrine (15 mg vs. 1 mg) found a higher rate of restoration of pulses (13% vs. 8%) and admission to the hospital (18% vs. 10%).[63] However, overall survival was not different. Comparison of a lower dose (7 mg vs. 1 mg) of epinephrine in both in-hospital and out-of-hospital cardiac arrest found no change in restoration of pulses or survival.[64] Likewise, comparison of 0.02 mg/kg versus 0.2 mg/kg epinephrine found no change in restoration of pulses or survival.[65]

It is possible that the beta-adrenergic effect of these higher doses of epinephrine produces toxicity that limits long-term survival. Post-resuscitation impairment of cardiac index and oxygen delivery has been related to epinephrine dose.[66] No trial has completed a direct comparison of epinephrine with more selective alpha-adrenergic agents such as phenylephrine. However, one trial found no advantage from administration of 11 mg of norepinephrine.[63]

Vasopressin can increase coronary perfusion pressure without complicating beta-adrenergic effects. Resuscitation rates and survival are identical for inpatients resuscitated with vasopressin and standard doses of epinephrine.[67] For out-of-hospital cardiac arrest, vasopressin appears to be superior for resuscitation and survival of patients whose first ECG rhythm is asystole.[68] Post hoc analyses suggest that vasopressin may be superior for those subjects requiring multiple doses of vasopressors. At present, use of either drug is justified in the setting of cardiac arrest. None of the studies on these pressors standardized post-resuscitation care, and therefore all are limited in their ability to define drug effects on neurologic recovery.

The role of antidysrhythmic drugs during cardiac arrest is equivocal.[69,70] Atropine may relieve bradycardia when it is vagally mediated. However, nervous system influences on the heart are largely eliminated after more than 1 to 2 minutes of circulatory arrest. Lidocaine, procainamide, and bretylium have a long history of use in the treatment of VF. The basis for this use is principally the observation that these drugs can suppress dysrhythmias before cardiac arrest. Once VF is established, lidocaine can actually increase the electrical energy required

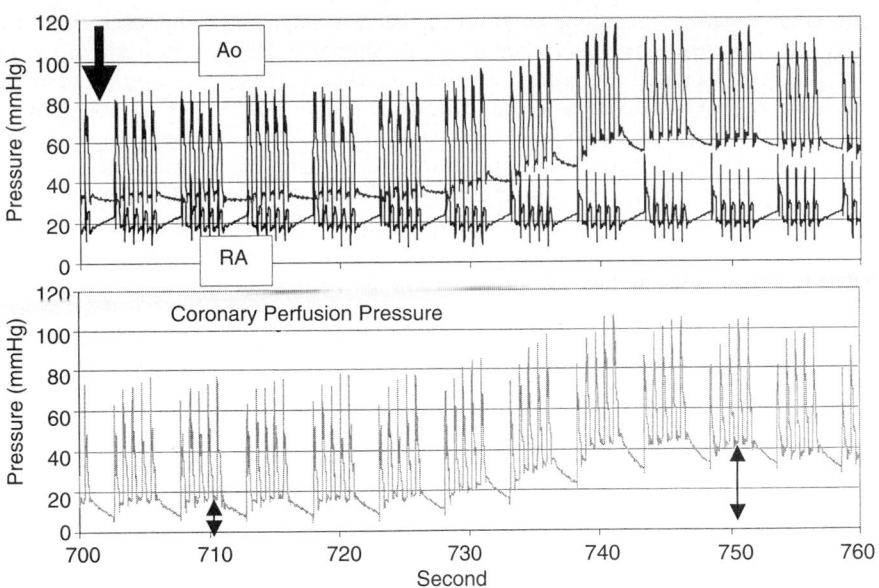

FIGURE 50–6. Administration of a pressor drug *(arrow)*, in this case vasopressin, can increase coronary perfusion pressure (CPP) produced by chest compressions. Note that the CPP generated by chest compressions alone (at ~710 seconds) is below the 15 to 20 mm Hg believed necessary for restoration of circulation. However, at 40 to 60 seconds after drug administration (at ~750 seconds) CPP increases above this threshold *(long, double-headed arrow)*. When treating cardiac arrest, it is unreasonable to expect physiologic responses to pressor drug administration until after at least 60 more seconds of chest compressions. (Unpublished laboratory data.)

to defibrillate by more than 50%.[71] This effect is not true for agents that are less potent as sodium channel antagonists. For example, administration of amiodarone (5 mg/kg) is superior to placebo[72] and to lidocaine[73] for restoration of pulses in out-of-hospital patients with VF that is not terminated by three rescue shocks. These studies did not control subsequent critical care and are thus not designed to determine any effect on long-term survival. In summary, antidysrhythmic drugs are commonly used during resuscitation, but only amiodarone use has supporting human data.

Empirical treatments of metabolic disturbances during cardiac arrest are not supported by prospective human data. Bicarbonate or other buffers may improve acidemia resulting from ischemia, but no efficacy study of human administration is available.[74] Aminophylline has been proposed as an antagonist of adenosine released during ischemia. Adenosine is hypothesized to suppress cardiac electrical activity. Two prospective studies of aminophylline administration to subjects with PEA or asystole failed to demonstrate any improvement in resuscitation.[75,76] Use of dextrose-containing fluids versus dextrose-free fluids did not alter outcome for out-of-hospital cardiac arrest.[77] Other metabolic therapies including calcium and magnesium also lack supporting data.[78,79] However, specific use of these agents for specific causes of cardiac arrest, such as known hyperkalemia, calcium channel blocker overdose, torsades, or hypomagnesemia remains appropriate.

Taken together, data support a simple pharmacologic approach to treatment of cardiac arrest. First, the vasopressors epinephrine and vasopressin are useful for augmenting CPP generated during chest compressions. Other vasopressors should also be useful but lack prospective data. Second, antidysrhythmic drugs are useful for maintaining organized rhythms but not for terminating VF. Only amiodarone has clinical data supporting its use during VF that persists after rescue shocks. All other drug therapy should be based on the clinical situation and the response of the patient.

ASPECTS OF CARDIAC ARREST IN SPECIFIC SITUATIONS

The original cause of cardiac arrest may not be known during acute resuscitation. However, if this information is available, treatment and prognosis can be individualized to the specific patient. Among out-of-hospital patients, as many as 66% have primary cardiac disturbances.[80] For in-hospital patients experiencing cardiac arrest, dysrhythmia and cardiac ischemia account for 59% of events.[10] This section reviews unique features of cardiac arrest resulting from both cardiac and noncardiac causes.

PRIMARY CARDIAC EVENTS

Cardiac arrest is most commonly attributable to cardiac disease. A primary dysrhythmia or cardiogenic shock is the most common proximate cause of cardiac arrest.[80,81] Patients undergoing angioplasty have 1.3% incidence of cardiac arrest, and survival in these patients resembles survival in other populations.[82] Among patients admitted to the hospital with acute myocardial infarction, cardiac arrest occurs in 4.8%.[12] Dysrhythmias are common during the hours after reperfusion therapy,[82] although reperfusion therapy reduces the overall risk of cardiac arrest.[83] During acute myocardial infarction, cardiac arrest is most likely in patients with lower serum potassium levels, more than 20 mm of total ST segment elevation, and a prolonged QTc interval during the first 2 hours of their event.[83] With a mean follow-up of 43 months, 3.3% of subjects surviving acute myocardial infarction suffered sudden cardiac death.[84] Abnormalities of the heart are present in most cases of cardiac arrest, with coronary artery disease present in at least 65% of autopsies.[85] Taken together, these data suggest that most patients with cardiac arrest will have contributing cardiovascular disease.

An acute coronary syndrome is present in more than one half of patients presenting with primary cardiac arrest outside the hospital. When angiography was performed on consecutive patients resuscitated from cardiac arrest, coronary artery occlusion was identified in 48%.[86] Similarly, 51% of initially resuscitated outpatients exhibited cardiac enzyme elevation or ECG evidence of acute myocardial infarction.[87] In one series, troponin T was elevated in 40% of out-of-hospital patients undergoing cardiopulmonary resuscitation (CPR), regardless of whether circulation was restored.[88] The direct myocardial injury from defibrillation and CPR may cause spurious elevations of creatine kinase that are unrelated to cardiovascular disease.[89] However, cardiac troponin elevations are believed to reflect acute myocardial infarction rather than injury from electrical shocks.[90] Thus, the 40% of subjects undergoing CPR with elevated troponin probably suffered myocardial injury before collapse.

The high likelihood of an acute coronary syndrome in the patient suffering cardiac arrest should prompt consideration of antiplatelet therapy, anticoagulation, beta blockade, and nitrates during the post-resuscitation care. Unless a clearly noncardiac etiology for cardiac arrest is evident, acute coronary angiography may reveal an indication for angioplasty, thrombolysis, or other reperfusion therapy. Early angioplasty or reperfusion therapy is associated with improved survival and outcome.[12,86,91]

Primary ventricular tachyarrhythmias are rapidly reversible and may be more likely than PEA or asystole for patients with a primary cardiac cause of collapse. Ventricular tachyarrhythmias are the initially recorded rhythm in 38% to 41% of out-of-hospital cardiac arrests[6,92] and in 25% of in-hospital cardiac arrests.[10] Because VF is rapidly reversible, patients with this rhythm comprise the majority of survivors of cardiac arrest. Data collected over three decades in one city noted that the prevalence of VF in out-of-hospital cardiac arrest has declined since 1978.[10] This trend may reflect a change in preventive medicine or in the epidemiology of cardiovascular disease over time. Once defibrillation is accomplished, short-term suppression of ventricular dysrhythmias with infusions of lidocaine, amiodarone, procainamide, or other antidysrhythmics is reasonable for these patients.

For subjects who survive sudden cardiac arrest and have decreased left ventricular function, long-term antidysrhythmia treatment should be considered.[93] Subjects surviving a life-threatening ventricular dysrhythmia had a 15% to 20% risk of death during a mean of 16 months of follow-up, even when a reversible cause of the dysrhythmia, such as electrolyte disturbance or hypoxemia, could be identified.[94] Implantable defibrillators have been found to be superior to antidysrhythmic drugs for reducing this risk of subsequent death.[95] This benefit is primarily in subjects with a left ventricular ejection fraction less than 0.35.[96] Implantable defibrillators were not better than antidysrhythmic drugs in a European trial that enrolled subjects resuscitated from cardiac arrest secondary to ventricular dysrhythmia without regard to left ventricular ejection fraction.[97] Nevertheless, these devices offer significant hope of preventing sudden cardiac death, and identification of patients whom they may benefit is an active area of research. At present, implantable defibrillators should be discussed for patients with left ventricular ejection fraction less than 0.35 and prior evidence of ventricular arrhythmias, particularly after acute myocardial infarction.

ASPHYXIA

Asphyxia-induced cardiac arrest can result from drowning, choking, asthma, progressive respiratory failure with hypoxemia, or traumatic coma with hypoventilation. Acute asphyxia causes transient tachycardia and hypertension, followed by bradycardia and hypotension, progressing to PEA or asystole. This period of blood flow with severe hypoxemia before cardiac arrest may make asphyxiation a more severe injury than VF or other rapid causes of circulatory arrest.[98] Brain edema was more common on computed tomography after resuscitation when cardiac arrest was caused by pulmonary rather than cardiac causes.[99]

During cardiac arrest, pulmonary edema develops from redistribution of blood into the pulmonary vasculature.[100] Thus, oxygenation is only worsened in the asphyxiated patient. Attention to the primary cause of asphyxia, as well as to maneuvers that will increase oxygenation, such as increased end-expiratory pressure or increased inspiration to expiration time ratios may be necessary.

PULMONARY EMBOLISM

Pulmonary emboli may occur in the postsurgical patient, as well as in medical patients with impaired mobility.[101] In one series, pulmonary emboli were present in 10% of in-hospital deaths,[102] and the prevalence among out-of-hospital deaths was similar.[103] Pulmonary emboli can result in rapid cardiopulmonary collapse and should be considered as a possible cause of cardiac arrest in the proper clinical setting or when collapse is preceded by sudden shortness of breath, hypoxemia, and/or pleuritic chest pain.

Physiologically, pulmonary emboli can result in cardiac arrest if a large thrombus obstructs right ventricular outflow into the pulmonary arteries. This situation results in a dilated, distended right ventricle and an empty left ventricle. Right ventricular dilation is sufficiently profound that it can be seen on transthoracic echocardiogram. Circulation cannot be restored unless this obstruction is relieved. Because the primary disturbance is hypoxemia and decreased cardiac output, cardiac arrest from pulmonary embolism should present as an initial rhythm of PEA or asystole.

Administration of bolus fibrinolytic drugs (tissue plasminogen activator, streptokinase, or urokinase) may help acutely during resuscitation of a patient with a suspected pulmonary embolism. Smaller pulmonary emboli can lead to cardiac arrest because of hypoxemia, and resuscitation may be possible before fibrinolysis if adequate oxygen exchange can be restored. Thrombolytic drugs have been used in a nonrandomized trial during resuscitation of undifferentiated patients with some success.[104] However, a randomized clinical trial of tissue plasminogen activator to patients with out-of-hospital cardiac arrest and an initial rhythm of PEA failed to demonstrate any benefit, although drug administration was late during resuscitation.[105]

ELECTROLYTE DISTURBANCES

Potassium disturbances are the most likely electrolyte disturbance to result in cardiac arrest. In cardiac patients, hypokalemia has been linked to the incidence of VF after myocardial infarction.[83,106] Hypokalemia also may account for the increased incidence of sudden death in patients taking large doses of diuretics. VF is rare in patients where the serum potassium concentration is maintained greater than 4.5 mEq/L. Conversely, hyperkalemia can prolong repolarization, increasing the likelihood of VF initiation. Hyperkalemia may also suppress automaticity in the myocardial electrical system, leading to bradycardic PEA or asystole. Cardiac arrest occurring during hemodialysis is not associated with high or low potassium levels but is more common when patients are dialyzed against a low (0 or 1.0 mEq/L) potassium dialysate.[107] These data suggest that rapid changes in potassium rather than the absolute value are important triggers of cardiac arrest in this population. Derangements of calcium and magnesium may produce similar or synergistic changes in cardiac conduction.

The clinical setting of cardiac arrest may suggest a primary electrolyte disturbance. Heavy diuretic use or intestinal fluid loss, for example, suggests potassium depletion. Suspected hypokalemia will not change acute resuscitation but must be addressed promptly in the post-resuscitation stabilization of the patient. Cardiac arrest in a patient with renal failure or during potassium infusion suggests hyperkalemia. Widened ventricular complexes with repolarization abnormalities on ECG would heighten this suspicion. If hyperkalemia is suspected, the usual acute resuscitation maneuvers can be supplemented by bolus injection of calcium carbonate (1 mg), bicarbonate (1 mEq/kg), and perhaps insulin (0.1 units/kg) with glucose (0.5 to 1 g/kg). These drugs may improve cardiac electrical stability, facilitating restoration of circulation.

POISONING

Cardiac arrest can result from drug overdose. Therapy does not change except when specific antidotes or countermeasures to the poison are available. For example, calcium channel blocker overdose may be countered by administration of intravenous calcium.[108] Beta-blocker toxicity may require large doses of inotropic agents[109] or may respond to glucagon.[110] Digoxin overdose may respond to digoxin-binding antibodies.[111] In the case of narcotic-induced respiratory depression, subsequent cardiac arrest is a specific result of asphyxia. One principle of poisonings is that the patient was often healthy before the event and may recover well once the poison is eliminated. This potential for a better outcome may justify longer and more aggressive efforts at resuscitation.

SEPSIS

Cardiac arrest can develop from sepsis for several reasons. Direct myocardial depression occurs, probably owing to humoral factors.[112,113] Vasodilation results in apparent hypovolemia. Finally, impaired oxygen extraction, shunting, and mitochondrial depression can produce cellular hypoxia. Because pump and vascular failure are the principal physiologic derangements, the most common initial ECG rhythm would be expected to be a rapid PEA that slows to asystole with ischemia. When these processes have progressed to cardiac arrest, large doses of inotropes, vasoconstrictors, and volume may be needed to restore circulation. Because the underlying sepsis physiology will still be present if pulses are restored, these patients may prove exceedingly unstable during the subacute recovery period and have a reduced chance for survival.[18,114-116]

TRAUMA/HEMORRHAGE

Hypovolemic cardiac arrest occurs after severe trauma, gastrointestinal hemorrhage, or other blood loss. Absence of venous return results in an empty heart, which cannot produce cardiac output despite normal inotropic state and normal or increased vascular tone. As with sepsis, this situation would most likely present with a rapid PEA that slows to asystole, but VF can develop in response to the global ischemia. Because cardiac function and vascular function are initially normal, inotropes and vasoconstrictors are unlikely to benefit hypovolemic cardiac arrest. Rapid replacement of volume with crystalloid infusion is indicated. Colloid or blood infusion should correct the situation more rapidly.[117] After restoration of circulation, patients with hemorrhagic cardiac arrest are likely to develop multisystem organ failure.[117]

During hypovolemic cardiac arrest the empty cardiac ventricles render external chest compressions ineffective. If blood loss is ongoing or if massive volume replacement cannot be instituted rapidly, thoracotomy allows clamping or compression of the aorta, perhaps retaining sufficient blood in the proximal aorta to perfuse the coronary and cerebral arteries. This procedure has produced success in the treatment of penetrating traumatic injuries[118] but not in blunt trauma.[119] Survival is better if thoracotomy occurs in the operating room after brief loss of pulses and best if the penetrating injury has created cardiac tamponade that is directly relieved by pericardotomy. Restoration of circulation must be accompanied by repair of the site of hemorrhage.

HYPOTHERMIA

Hypothermia represents an important situation in which prolonged resuscitative efforts are justified. If hypothermia develops before circulatory arrest, the tolerance of the heart and brain to ischemia is greatly prolonged. Survival with favorable neurologic recovery has been reported after cold-water submersion or exposure with cardiac arrest and resuscitation efforts lasting several hours.[120,121] Although all data are retrospective, subjects in whom circulatory arrest occurs because of hypothermia appear to be more salvageable than subjects who asphyxiate or have circulatory arrest before becoming cold.[122]

Treatment should be based on the initial temperature of the patient. Between 32°C and 37°C, no change in drug or electrical treatment is required, and this level of hypothermia may be beneficial for resuscitation of both brain and heart.[123,124] Between 29°C and 32°C, cardiac activity may be preserved, and external warming (warm air, heating lights, warm blankets) and warm intravenous fluids should accompany usual resuscitation efforts. The likelihood of generating sufficient perfusion to rewarm the body declines as temperature decreases from 32°C to 29°C, and more invasive warming should be considered if there is not a rapid response with external warming. More invasive and aggressive treatment will almost certainly be required for cooler patients, because both mechanical and electrical activity of the heart are disrupted at temperatures below 28°C. Patients below this temperature may exhibit PEA, VF that is refractory to defibrillation attempts, or asystole. Repetitive rescue shocks in such patients are not justified and may be detrimental. Efficacy of most resuscitation drugs may be impaired.

Several techniques for active rewarming during resuscitation of victims of severe hypothermia are available. Given the potentially prolonged tolerance of the cold patient to ischemia, there may be sufficient time to establish arterial and venous access for partial or complete cardiopulmonary bypass. Extracorporeal circulation is particularly useful in these subjects because it can provide artificial circulation at the same time as rewarming.[122,125,126] In the absence of extracorporeal circulation, placement of thoracostomy tubes and lavage of the chest with warm fluids is an option.[127] Thoracostomy is intuitively preferable to peritoneal lavage because the heart will be directly warmed. Warm air forced over the body surface can rewarm a patient, although this technique may provide the least heat exchange.[128] In any case, it is difficult to determine whether circulation can be reestablished in the profoundly hypothermic patient until near physiologic core temperatures (33°C to 37°C) are restored.

OTHER MEDICAL CONDITIONS

Comorbidities have a tremendous influence on the outcome from cardiac arrest.[81,129,130] In some cases, cardiac arrest may be an expected progression of the patient's disease but guidelines about limiting resuscitation were not defined. For example, no survivors were reported among cancer patients with expected cardiac arrest.[130] Therefore, it may be appropriate to set limits on resuscitation efforts in certain medical conditions before cardiopulmonary collapse. Ideally, discussion about the expectations for resuscitative efforts should be held with the patient, the family, or the patient representatives before cardiac arrest. If those discussions did not occur before the first cardiac arrest, they should follow promptly any initially successful resuscitation.

POST-RESUSCITATION CARE TO MINIMIZE BRAIN INJURY

Management of the patient after restoration of circulation affects ultimate outcome. For example, long-term survival differed for comparable patients treated by a single ambulance service but delivered to separate hospitals.[1,2] Institutional differences in in-hospital management, particularly in the permitted frequency of hyperthermia and hyperglycemia, were identified that may have accounted for these differences. Despite the apparent importance of post-resuscitation critical care, there are few guidelines for treatment.

Brain injury appears not to be acute neuronal necrosis during ischemia but instead to be an active process that develops over hours to days after resuscitation. Multiple cellular and molecular mechanisms contribute to neurologic injury after global brain ischemia.[131] These are discussed in greater detail in Chapter 46. Germane to cardiac arrest, during brain ischemia and immediately after reperfusion, studies have detected increased release of excitatory amino acids, free radicals, and energy failure. Protein synthesis is inhibited at the level of translation initiation for several hours.[132] There are focal disturbances of cerebral blood flow.[133] Specific intracellular and extracellular signaling pathways are activated for several hours after brain ischemia,[134,135] which may lead to specific changes in gene transcription. Finally, activation of specific proteases between 24 and 72 hours after reperfusion is associated with appearance of histologic signs of neuronal death.[136] The relative contribution of each of these processes to neuronal injury is unknown, and all may contribute synergistically to brain injury. All represent potential targets for therapeutic intervention.

Despite detailed knowledge of the mechanisms involved with brain ischemia, drugs that target specific pathways provide modest effects in laboratory studies, and no drug to date has demonstrated clear benefit in human trials.

Randomized clinical trials have examined thiopental, the calcium-channel blocker lidoflazine, magnesium, and diazepam.[137-139] One explanation for this failure is that multiple mechanisms contribute simultaneously to the process of ischemic neuronal death. Antagonizing one pathway leading to neuronal death may leave other mechanisms unaffected. Less-specific therapies or multifaceted therapies that affect multiple pathways may prove more effective.

In support of this idea, prospective randomized clinical trials confirm that induction of mild hypothermia (33°C to 34°C) for 12 to 24 hours after resuscitation improves survival and neurologic recovery.[123,140] Observational data also support avoidance of fever, hypotension, and hyperglycemia.[1,141-143] Therefore, systematic brain-oriented intensive care rather than a single therapeutic drug or intervention is required to improve outcome (Table 50-1).

TABLE 50–1. POST-RESUSCITATION INTENSIVE CARE

Temperature

Avoid fever for 48 hours
Induce mild hypothermia of 33°C to 34°C for 12-24 hours
Rewarm slowly (<1°C/hr)

Cardiovascular

Mean arterial pressure > 100 mm Hg for first day
   Inotropic and vasopressor support as needed
   Invasive monitoring as needed
   Must be balanced by concern for injured heart
Suppress dysrhythmias
Reperfusion therapy for acute myocardial infarction
Medical management for acute coronary syndromes
   Beta blockade, antiplatelet drugs, anticoagulation
   Nitrates as tolerated

Pulmonary

Usual care
Pneumonia common

Gastrointestinal

Usual care
Consider early refeeding to reduce translocation

Fluids/Electrolytes

Monitor central venous pressure and urine output with
   hypothermia/rewarming
Monitor potassium/electrolytes during temperature changes
Keep potassium ≥4.5 mEq/L
Monitor glucose concentration frequently, and avoid hyperglycemia

Hematologic

Prothrombotic state is common
Anticoagulation is of unproven benefit but reasonable

Infection

Bacteremia and pneumonia are common
Prophylactic antibiotics are of unproven benefit
Antipyretics are reasonable

Neurologic

Sedation as needed for hypothermia induction
Most clinical improvement occurs over first 72 hours
Clinical examination for prognosis
Electroencephalography and evoked potentials may add to clinical
   examination for selected patients

TEMPERATURE CONTROL

Meticulous avoidance of fever is important during the first 24 to 48 hours after ischemic brain injury. Temperature control after cardiac arrest may be confounded by the fact that the occurrence of bacteremia and spontaneous fever is common in the resuscitated patient.[144,145] The benefit of lower temperatures for injured brain tissue has been demonstrated after traumatic brain injury, stroke, and cardiac arrest.[141,146,147] Mechanistically, temperature probably affects more than brain metabolic rate. For example, manipulations of temperature that improve neurologic recovery in laboratory studies produce no effect on jugular venous lactate or oxygen uptake.[148] Recent laboratory investigations suggest that a variety of signaling pathways and cellular responses are sensitive to relatively small (1°C to 2°C) changes in brain temperature.[134,135]

Induction of mild hypothermia for resuscitated patients produces a 24% to 30% relative risk reduction for death or poor neurologic outcome (Fig. 50-7).[149] Mild hypothermia (33°C to 34°C) maintained for 12 or 24 hours significantly improved the odds of survival and good neurologic outcome for subjects resuscitated from VF cardiac arrest.[123,140] There is no reason to believe that this neurologic benefit of induced hypothermia is specific to patients with one type of cardiac rhythm, and use in all post-resuscitation patients seems reasonable. At the time of resuscitation, many patients are already mildly hypothermic with core temperatures between 35°C and 35.5°C.[123,140,150] This spontaneous cooling may result from equilibration of core and peripheral blood compartments during circulatory arrest. Subsequent to restoration of circulation, patients will rewarm within a few hours unless specific interventions are instituted.[141]

The optimal duration of cooling, the maximum delay in achieving target temperatures, the optimal target temperature, and the preferred rate of rewarming are unknown. Laboratory studies suggest that cooling to between 32°C and 35°C for 12 to 24 hours is beneficial, particularly if cooling is achieved within 6 hours after resuscitation. These studies also suggest that temperature is less important more than 48 hours after resuscitation and that rewarming should be performed slowly (<1°C/hr). Clinical data to answer these practical questions are likely to become available over the next few years as the use of therapeutic hypothermia becomes widespread.

After cardiac arrest, mild hypothermia can be induced by a variety of techniques. Surface cooling with ice packs and cooling blankets is tolerated by the comatose patient.[140,151] Neuromuscular blockade and sedation can help prevent shivering or other compensatory reflexes. However, surface cooling alone is slow and may require 4 to 6 hours to reach 34°C.[123,146,152] Lavage of the stomach with ice-cold water can accelerate cooling but is labor intensive. Local cooling of the head is unlikely to produce brain hypothermia when there is adequate perfusion by warm core blood,[150] although the head can be an effective site for removing heat from the body.[153] Intravascular devices can provide direct cooling of blood in the vena cava, but these devices are expensive and invasive.[124] Rapid infusion of 30 mL/kg cold (4°C) crystalloid produces a rapid decrease in core temperature and is tolerated by the post-resuscitation patient.[154] The volume required may limit this intervention to those patients without renal failure or pulmonary edema. Taken together, these data support the rapid induction of mild hypothermia by surface cooling and bolus

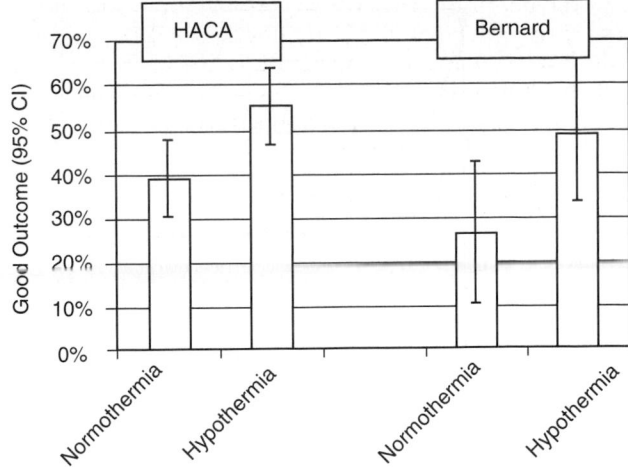

FIGURE 50–7. Improvement in good neurologic outcome was reported in two randomized clinical trials of therapeutic hypothermia. HACA[123] studied 275 subjects, with 137 receiving 24 hours of cooling to 32°C to 34°C. Bernard and colleagues[140] studied 77 subjects, with 43 receiving 12 hours of cooling to 33°C.

infusion of cold intravenous fluids (unless contraindicated), followed by maintenance of hypothermia by surface cooling, neuromuscular blockade, and sedation (Fig. 50-8.)

Fluid and electrolyte shifts are the primary management concerns during induction of hypothermia. Induction of cooling can result in peripheral vasoconstriction, with an apparent reduction in vascular volume.[155] CVP will increase, followed by diuresis. Conversely, at the time of rewarming, vessels will dilate, CVP will decrease, and the patient may become relatively hypovolemic. Volume status should be followed closely, and a need for additional volume infusion to maintain blood pressure and urine output should be anticipated at the time of rewarming. Inattention to this fluid shift was cited as a pitfall in trials of therapeutic hypothermia for traumatic brain injury.[155] The initial diuresis, along with shifts between intracellular and extracellular compartments, can result in hypokalemia, hypophosphatemia, and hypomagnesemia at cooling, followed by hyperkalemia at rewarming.[156,157] Frequent monitoring and correction of electrolytes during these transitions is warranted.

Cardiovascular complications of hypothermia are rare with temperatures greater than 30°C. Cooling from 37°C to 31°C actually has a positive inotropic effect, increasing stroke volume to a greater extent than it decreases heart rate.[158] Systemic vascular resistance does not appear to change greatly. Clinical data report a transient 18% decline in cardiac index with cooling to 33°C.[159] Conscious patients undergoing angioplasty for acute myocardial infarction tolerate mild hypothermia.[124] In these patients, cooling did not interfere with defibrillation when it was required.

Other complications of mild hypothermia are few when the cooling period lasts less than 24 hours. Infections do become more common if cooling is prolonged for more than 24 hours. There is a suggestion that infections were slightly more common in post-resuscitation patients cooled for 24 hours,[123] but not in those cooled for 12 hours.[140] Although mild hypothermia can inhibit platelet function and coagulation,[160] these changes are of small magnitude, leading to no bleeding complications in studies to date. These studies included subjects with concurrent trauma or administration of heparinoids

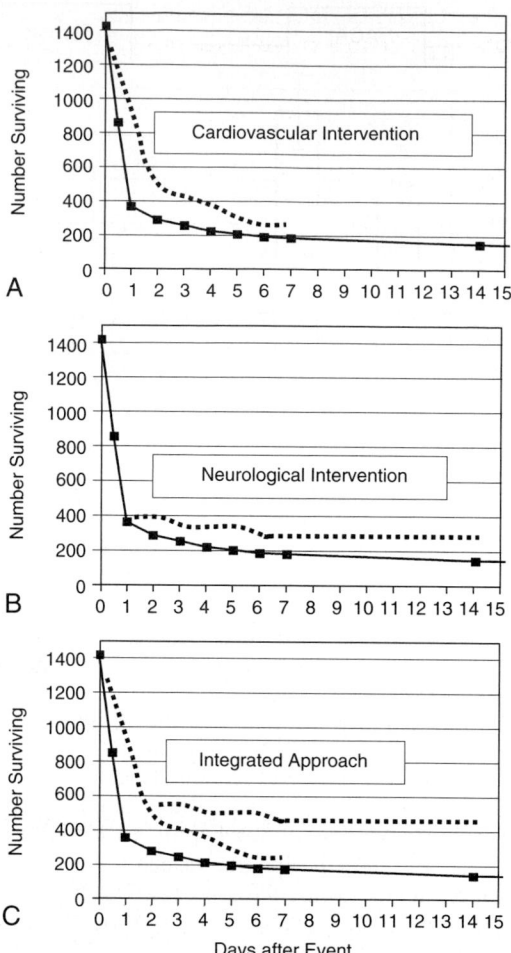

FIGURE 50–8. An integrated approach to cardiopulmonary-cerebral resuscitation is most likely to generate significant changes in patient survival after cardiac arrest. Hypothesized benefits are superimposed on recent survival curves from one city. **A,** Compared with current care, an intervention that improves cardiovascular resuscitation may increase admission to the hospital without preventing later death due to brain injury. **B,** An intervention that improves neurologic recovery may improve the proportion of subjects who awaken from coma, but the magnitude of this benefit for the population is obscured by the large number of deaths due to cardiopulmonary collapse. **C,** Combined care directed at both cardiopulmonary and neurologic injury may provide more than additive increases in meaningful survival.

and glycoprotein IIb/IIIa inhibitors.[124,146] Elevations of pancreatic enzymes have been reported in cooled patients, but these changes resolve with rewarming.[123,159] Creatinine clearance and platelet count may decrease during cooling, but both parameters normalize with rewarming.[159]

BLOOD PRESSURE AND CEREBRAL BLOOD FLOW

After cardiac arrest, the heart experiences a reversible period of decreased mechanical function.[161] The biochemical basis for this dysfunction is an active area of study. Moreover, reperfusion at the time of resuscitation includes oxidative stress or other triggers that can lead to myocyte death.[162] From a clinical standpoint, inotropic support will almost certainly be necessary for any patient resuscitated from cardiac arrest lasting more than 3 or 4 minutes.

This dependence on inotropes should decline over the subsequent 24 to 48 hours.

Autoregulation of cerebral blood flow is disturbed after cardiac arrest. Measurement of oxygen saturation in the jugular bulb venous blood allows calculation of brain oxygen extraction. Furthermore, cerebral blood flow can be estimated using transcranial Doppler ultrasound or nuclear imaging. During the first day after resuscitation from cardiac arrest, patients exhibit increased cerebral vascular resistance[163] and impaired cerebral autoregulation.[164,165] When autoregulation is present, it is right shifted such that brain perfusion declines when mean arterial pressure declines below 80 to 120 mm Hg. When blood pressure is maintained, clinical PET studies suggest that regional perfusion remains matched to metabolic activity after cardiac arrest.[166]

Therefore, after cardiac arrest, relative hypertension (mean arterial pressure greater than 100 to 110 mm Hg) should be maintained to prevent brain hypoperfusion. Maintaining this level of hypertension will require infusions of inotropes and/or pressors. In support of this recommendation, hypotension during the first 3 hours after resuscitation is associated with poor neurologic recovery in patients admitted to the hospital after cardiac arrest.[142] Future research is needed to develop hemodynamic support strategies that optimize both cerebral and cardiac perfusion and metabolism during ICU care after cardiac arrest.

GLUCOSE CONTROL

Elevated serum glucose is associated with poor outcome after cardiac arrest[77] and may be a marker of prolonged or difficult resuscitation. Both epinephrine and physiologic stress can elevate serum glucose levels. However, multivariate models that accounted for resuscitation time and medication usage still show an effect of serum glucose on admission and during the first 48 hours of intensive care on long-term outcome.[1,167] Despite this association, both studies noted that monitoring of glucose in nondiabetic patients was infrequent. Because no randomized clinical trial has been performed, it remains unclear whether aggressive management of serum glucose concentration will improve outcome.

HEMATOLOGIC CHANGES

Cardiac arrest is associated with activation of coagulation that is not balanced by fibrinolysis. This hematologic profile is reminiscent of DIC and may contribute to subsequent end-organ dysfunction. Markers of thrombogenesis that have been reported include increased thrombin-antithrombin complexes and fibrinopeptide A.[168,169] These increases are not balanced by fibrinolytic factors for at least 24 hours. The cause of these changes is unknown and may be related to ischemic injury to the endothelium.

At present, use of anticoagulation is variable and there are no prospective trials evaluating the effect of anticoagulation after resuscitation. Anticoagulation and even fibrinolytic drugs are safe after CPR.[169,170] A retrospective series noted a univariate relationship between anticoagulation and 6-month survival that was not significant in a multivariate model.[167] In a series of patients with cardiac arrest related to VF and cardiac ischemia, administration of thrombolytic drugs was associated with better neurologic outcome.[171] Given the hematologic evidence of active thrombogenesis, these data suggest that at least anticoagulation should be considered immediately after resuscitation.

INFECTION

The physiology of the post-resuscitation patient resembles that of systemic inflammatory response syndrome. Bacteremia has been noted in 39% of patients during the first 12 hours after resuscitation.[144] Fever is common in patients within 48 hours after resuscitation from cardiac arrest. Potential causes include contamination during emergent line placement, aspiration or transient bacteremia during airway management, and mesenteric ischemia contributing to bacterial translocation from the gut. Endotoxin and various cytokines are increased in serum after resuscitation.[172] Whereas an intestinal origin of endotoxin was suspected, pulmonary infections were more common than bacteremia. When they develop, severe infections are associated with mortality.[145] Despite these observations, the role of routine antibiotics and antipyretics has not been examined.

PREDICTING NEUROLOGIC RECOVERY

The goal of clinical practice always is to restore the patient to full consciousness and function.[173] All subjects with circulatory arrest of more than a 1 or 2 minutes will be comatose at initial presentation, but some of these same patients can recover and awaken. Therefore, signs of neurologic activity immediately after restoration of circulation are encouraging, but their absence does not preclude eventual recovery. Unfortunately, many cardiac arrest survivors fail to completely awaken and may meet criteria for a persistent vegetative state.[174,175] The status of patients who do not quite meet these criteria but are not awake has been described as a minimally conscious state.[176] Assessment of neurologic prognosis after resuscitation becomes increasingly reliable over the first 3 days of recovery.[177-179]

Several clinical signs have been used to assess awakening after cardiac arrest. A classic case series found that pupillary reaction to light, corneal reflexes, and motor activity can change over the first 72 hours after resuscitation.[179] By 72 hours, absence of eye reflexes and failure to have a localizing response to pain are highly predictive of permanent coma. A systematic review of literature since that initial report confirms the value of these clinical findings.[177] For individual patients who remain in coma, these series show how specific clinical signs can provide quantitative estimates of the probability of awakening.

NEUROPHYSIOLOGY

It is common for electroencephalography (EEG) to be done for prognostic purposes. However, the predictive value of EEG after resuscitation from cardiac arrest is unclear, and the timing of this test in relation to the ischemic event is rarely standardized. A burst-suppression pattern or an isoelectric electroencephalogram during the first week after resuscitation is associated with poor neurologic prognosis.[177] Recovery of longer-latency event-related potentials or evoked potentials (EPs) is associated with awakening.[180-182] Absence of early somatosensory EPs is very specific for poor neurologic outcome.[177] Both EEG and EPs vary with the elapsed time since resuscitation.[182] There are no data about the influence of induced hypothermia or other treatments on EEG and EPs.

BLOOD MARKERS

Several neuronal peptides appear in the blood after injury to the brain, including neuron-specific enolase (NSE) and S-100B. After cardiac arrest, NSE reaches a maximum level in serum at 72 hours. High NSE levels at 48 to 72 hours after resuscitation are associated with poor outcome.[181,183,184] Serial NSE levels that continue to rise over the first 72 hours also predict poor outcome.[184] In contrast to NSE, peak levels of S-100B in serum occur during the first 24 hours after resuscitation.[183] Higher S-100B levels are also associated with poor neurologic outcome.[183,185]

These data suggest that initial S-100B levels and the change in NSE over the first 72 hours after resuscitation may provide blood markers to follow brain injury. For example, in subjects treated with induced hypothermia, S-100B levels were not altered but decreasing NSE levels were more common.[186] More research is necessary to determine whether initial S-100B can be used to select patients for specific therapies or whether those therapies could be titrated to the changes in NSE.

IMAGING STUDIES

Imaging of the brain is important to exclude injury incurred at the time of collapse and to exclude intracranial causes of collapse. Cranial CT to exclude hemorrhage may be prudent in the comatose resuscitated patient before beginning anticoagulation or fibrinolytic therapy. Experience with more advanced imaging for making neurologic prognoses is limited. Cortical abnormalities on fluid-attenuated inversion recovery (FLAIR) MRI are associated with poor neurologic outcome.[187] In the long-term, cognitive deficits are associated with global brain volume loss after cardiac arrest.[188] At present, use of brain imaging beyond the cranial CT scan remains largely investigational.

WITHDRAWAL OF SUPPORT AND REHABILITATION

For adults who are neurologically devastated after cardiac arrest in North America, it is more common to die in the hospital than to receive long-term care. An estimated 44% of patients who are initially resuscitated from cardiac arrest in the hospital have withdrawal of care later during their hospitalization.[10] For patients resuscitated from out-of-hospital cardiac arrest, 68% have do not resuscitate (DNR) status established in the hospital, perhaps representing a comparable outcome.[14] These decisions are often based on the neurologic prognosis of the patient, and these decisions limit the number of neurologically impaired individuals who are discharged from the hospital. Quality of life for those patients who do leave the hospital is generally high.[13,189,190]

The role of rehabilitation or other therapy in recovery from neurologic impairment after cardiac arrest is relatively unstudied. It is clear that both patients and their caregivers have complex needs if neurologic injury is severe.[191] Unfortunately, long-term improvement is less common when neurologic devastation follows a medical cause, like cardiac arrest, than when it results from traumatic brain injury.[175] Popular reports of awakening after long coma may cause inappropriate optimism for families of patients or surrogate decision makers. Partial awakening of the patient into a persistent vegetative state or minimally conscious state can further confuse their expectations. These individuals should receive information about these syndromes, expectations of recovery, and any specific considerations for the patient. Religious, cultural, and personal beliefs will contribute to their decisions, and appropriate social service and pastoral support should be provided.

ANNOTATED REFERENCES

HACA—Hypothermia after Cardiac Arrest Study Group: Mild therapeutic hypothermia to improve the neurologic outcome after cardiac arrest. N Engl J Med 2002;346:549-556.

This prospective multicenter trial found that induction of mild hypothermia (33°C to 34°C) for 24 hours after restoration of circulation improved survival and neurologic recovery. Mild hypothermia reduced the relative risk of poor outcome by 26%.

Langhelle A, Tyvold SS, Lexow K, et al: In-hospital factors associated with improved outcome after out-of-hospital cardiac arrest: A comparison between four regions in Norway. Resuscitation 2003;56:247-263.

This cohort study examined survival of patients in the hospital after initial resuscitation from out-of-hospital cardiac arrest. Survival varied between regions, and survival was independently associated with lower temperature and lower serum glucose. While not a prospective trial, these data suggest that control of these parameters may be important.

Paradis NA, Martin GB, Rivers EP, et al: Coronary perfusion pressure and the return of spontaneous circulation in human cardiopulmonary resuscitation. JAMA 1990;263:1106-1113.

This prospective study placed central monitors in 100 subjects during chest compressions. Failure to develop coronary perfusion pressures of more than 15 mm Hg guaranteed the failure of resuscitation.

Wik L, Hansen TB, Fylling F, et al: Delaying defibrillation to give basic cardiopulmonary resuscitation to patients with out-of-hospital ventricular fibrillation. JAMA 2003;289:1389-1395.

In this prospective, randomized trial, subjects with ventricular fibrillation outside the hospital received either immediate rescue shocks or 3 minutes of chest compressions before rescue shocks. The subgroup of subjects for whom response intervals were longer than 5 minutes had better outcomes if chest compressions were performed first. Immediate rescue shocks may be appropriate for brief ventricular fibrillation, but reperfusion first may be better for prolonged ventricular fibrillation.

Zandbergen EG, de Haan RJ, Stoutenbeek CP, et al: Systematic review of early prediction of poor outcome in anoxic-ischaemic coma. Lancet 1998;352:1808-1812.

This paper reviews studies of prognostic tests for predicting neurologic outcome after cardiac arrest. The literature suggests that by the third day of recovery, pupillary response and motor response to pain are predictive of outcome and that, during the first week of recovery, somatosensory evoked potentials are also predictive. Other diagnostic tests are less specific.

Chapter 51

MANAGEMENT OF ACUTE ISCHEMIC STROKE

Lawrence R. Wechsler • Carol A. Barch

KEY POINTS

1. The success of acute stroke management begins with a patient's family member or bystander recognizing the symptoms of stroke (see Table 51-1) and calling 911 immediately.

2. On arrival, the prehospital team should complete a quick assessment. The assessment includes following the basics of the *ABCs-N: a*irway, *b*reathing, *c*irculation, and *n*eurology evaluation. Oxygen saturation should be maintained at least 96% to provide adequate oxygenation to the brain tissue. Continuous monitoring of the electrocardiogram is recommended because almost 30% of ischemic stroke patients have arrhythmias (e.g., atrial fibrillation). Blood pressure should be determined, but treatment should be considered only if blood pressure is greater than 220/120 mm Hg.

3. A stroke team consists of individuals from multiple disciplines with specialized knowledge and interest in acute stroke care. The team approach brings together the necessary skills to administer emergently whatever care is best suited to the situation and divides the workload so that tasks can be performed simultaneously rather than sequentially.

4. Studies do not support a reduced recurrence rate or improved outcome with anticoagulation when administered within 24 to 48 hours of stroke onset. There is little value in anticoagulating all patients with acute stroke.

5. In June 1996, the U.S. Food and Drug Administration (FDA) approved intravenous tissue plasminogen activator (tPA) for treatment of stroke within 3 hours of onset.

6. A growing body of evidence suggests a small benefit of intravenous tPA up to 4.5 hours after stroke onset, but the earlier treatment is initiated, the greater the likelihood of a good clinical outcome.

7. Patients receiving antiplatelet therapy usually are not excluded from thrombolytic therapy, although additional studies are needed to clarify the relative risk of thrombolysis in these patients.

8. Good outcomes have been reported with intra-arterial thrombolysis of basilar thrombosis well beyond the usual 6-hour time limit. Intravenous tPA also may result in improvement, but the large clot burden favors the intra-arterial approach.

9. Surgical decompression for hemispheric infarction should be considered for younger patients with a greater potential for recovery from massive stroke and particularly for nondominant strokes.

10. The availability of effective treatment to alter outcome within the first few hours after stroke onset necessitates dramatic changes in the evaluation of stroke. Patients with symptoms suggesting cerebral ischemia must be treated emergently from the prehospital encounter to the emergency department and the treating physicians. Imaging must be performed rapidly and provide useful information for the decision-making process.

Stroke is a medical emergency. The rationale for acute stroke treatment is based on the concepts of the ischemic penumbra. When an arterial occlusion occurs, an area of infarcted brain is surrounded by a region that has reduced blood flow impairing function, but not sufficiently severe to result in irreversible infarction. If adequate blood flow can be restored within a critical time frame, this area at risk may return to normal function. Experimental models of stroke indicate that lower levels of blood flow are tolerated for brief periods, whereas slightly higher blood flow can be maintained for several hours without developing infarction.[1] The precise relationships between blood flow levels and duration for human stroke are not known, but the more quickly flow is restored, the greater the likelihood that the tissue will be spared.

In 1995, the National Institute of Neurological Disorders and Stroke (NINDS) tPA study[2] was published showing for the first time in a randomized controlled trial a reduction in stroke morbidity with acute treatment. Other treatments, such as intra-arterial thrombolytics, clot disruptive devices, and neuroprotective agents, continue to be investigated. At present, intravenous tPA is approved by the FDA for treatment of acute stroke within 3 hours of onset.

New medical-surgical advances in stroke led to the development of acute stroke teams and stroke centers. The NINDS Stroke Group initiated the conceptual groundwork during the NINDS Stroke Trial to facilitate recruitment. The Brain Attack Coalition[3] published recommendations for the organization of these teams and health care delivery systems to facilitate a rapid response. The American Heart Association and the Joint Commission of Health Organizations support disease-specific stroke certification to measure the standards necessary to deliver high-quality stroke care. Stroke specialists, stroke centers, and future clinical trials will continue to drive advances in acute stroke management.

STROKE MECHANISMS

Appropriate treatment of ischemic stroke depends on identification of the mechanism of stroke. The duration of symptoms and the time course are not as important as the underlying etiology of the ischemic syndrome. Ischemic strokes generally are classified as large vessel thrombotic, small vessel thrombotic, or embolic. An embolic occlusion of a major intracranial artery may require a different therapeutic approach than an atherosclerotic occlusion. Similarly, small vessel thrombosis has different implications for treatment and a better prognosis than large vessel thrombosis.

In the first few hours after stroke, identification of stroke mechanisms may be difficult or impossible. Even distinguishing ischemic from hemorrhagic stroke may be hazardous based on clinical evaluation alone. Information obtained from history and rapid examination provides clues to pathophysiology,[3] but definitive diagnosis usually requires additional testing, such as ultrasound and imaging. Large vessel thrombotic strokes are often preceded by transient ischemic attacks or a stepwise progression of deficits. Risk factors include hypertension, smoking, diabetes, and elevated serum cholesterol level. Clinical deficits typically correspond to the territory of major cerebral arteries or their border zones. In embolic strokes, the onset is usually sudden, although in occasional cases a stepwise progression occurs in the first few hours. The presence of atrial fibrillation, rheumatic heart disease, or a recent myocardial infarction increases the probability of embolism. Several clinical syndromes are attributable to small vessel thrombotic or lacunar stroke, including pure motor stroke involving the face, arm, and leg; pure sensory stroke; ataxia hemiparesis; and dysarthria–clumsy hand syndrome. Other syndromes also may be due to lacunar strokes, but in such cases the mechanism is less certain, illustrating the hazards of deciding on stroke mechanism from clinical findings alone.

Pathophysiologic diagnosis is enhanced greatly by imaging modalities, including computed tomography (CT) and magnetic resonance imaging (MRI). These studies take time to complete, delaying administration of acute stroke therapy and potentially leading to irreversible brain injury before the diagnosis can be established. The time needed for imaging studies must be weighed against the benefit of the information obtained. Studies need to be performed rapidly with minimal delay, and the results must be used to decide on optimal treatment. Acute stroke treatment is likely to differ depending on stroke mechanism, and rapid imaging modalities should become increasingly important in acute stroke management.

PREHOSPITAL EVALUATION OF STROKE

The success of acute stroke management begins with a patient's family member or bystander recognizing the symptoms of stroke (Table 51-1) and calling 911 immediately. When there was no acute treatment for stroke, only primary and secondary preventive measures, health care professionals did little to educate the public on recognizing stroke, identifying risk factors, or promoting stroke prevention.

TABLE 51–1. STROKE RECOGNITION

Sudden onset of:
Numbness or weakness of the face, arm, or leg
Slurred speech or difficulty with speech
Blurred or loss of vision in one or both eyes
Onset of severe headache
Onset of clumsiness or loss of balance

On average, across the United States, stroke patients arrive at the hospital 24 hours after symptom onset. A huge effort is under way to educate the public at large of the warning signs of stroke, especially in individuals at risk and their family members (Table 51-2). The key message is how to recognize stroke, to take action, and to get to the hospital immediately.

In recent years, prehospital systems across the United States have begun to implement an acute stroke protocol. The protocol is published in the American Heart Association's *Advanced Cardiac Life Support 1997-1999* manual.[4] An algorithm for acute stroke was developed from the experience of conducting acute stroke trials.[5-7] Similar to the concept of time-focused field management of myocardial infarction, acute stroke now is being approached as a medical emergency. Rapid identification of the problem as a stroke, determining onset to be less than 6 hours, appropriate field assessment and management, rapid transport, and prenotification of the incoming stroke patient to the receiving emergency department are the key elements for prehospital personnel.

The process begins at dispatch. Any calls with complaints of "weakness, numbness, changes in speech, headache, confusion, found down, or unconscious," are considered a possible stroke. A crew is sent immediately to the scene.

On arrival, the prehospital team should complete a quick assessment, which includes following the basics of the *ABCs-N: a*irway, *b*reathing, *c*irculation, and *n*eurology evaluation. Oxygen saturation should be maintained at least 96% to provide adequate oxygenation to the brain tissue. Continuous monitoring of the electrocardiogram is recommended because almost 30% of ischemic patients have arrhythmias (e.g., atrial fibrillation). Blood pressure should be determined, but treatment should be considered only if it is greater than 220/120 mm Hg. Intravenous access should be established if this does not delay transport to the emergency department. If administering intravenous fluids, only isotonic solutions, such as normal saline or lactated Ringer's solution, should be used. Glucose should be avoided in intravenous fluids because it may be detrimental to ischemic brain tissue and can lead to unnecessary cerebral edema. Hypoglycemia can mimic stroke symptoms, and serum glucose should be checked. Glucose should be administered if hypoglycemia is found. Hyperglycemia needs to be treated on arrival to the emergency department.

TABLE 51–2. RESOURCES FOR PUBLIC STROKE EDUCATION

National Stroke Association (NSA)	1-800-STROKES
American Heart Association (AHA)	1-800-AHA-USA1
National Institute of Neurological Disorders and Stroke (NINDS)	www.nih.gov

TABLE 51–3. CINCINNATI PRE-HOSPITAL STROKE SCALE

Facial droop—have patient show teeth or smile	Normal—both sides of face move equally
	Abnormal—one side of the face does not move as well as the other side
Arm drift—patient closes eyes and holds both arms out	Normal—both arms move the same or both arms do not move at all
	Abnormal—one arm does not move or one arm drifts down compared with the other
Speech—have patient say "you can't teach an old dog new tricks"	Normal—patient uses correct words with no slurring
	Abnormal—patient slurs words, uses inappropriate words, or is unable to speak

It is important for the prehospital personnel to gather information about the onset of stroke symptoms. First, it is crucial to determine the time of onset of the symptoms; this is important because the emergency department may not have access to individuals who were present at the onset. Time of onset is determined by when the patient was last seen without a neurologic defect. When the deficit is present on awakening, the time of onset is considered the previous night before going to bed. If thrombolytic treatment is considered, it is important to obtain a history of trauma or falling when the symptoms occurred. The examiner should check for any signs of ecchymosis or laceration. Also, a history of seizure activity after the onset of symptoms should be obtained. Todd's paralysis, a syndrome that occurs after a seizure, often is confused with stroke symptoms.

To assess the patient's neurologic status, the best tool to use in the field is the Pre-hospital Stroke Scale developed by the University of Cincinnati (Table 51-3). This quick screen allows for uniformity in assessing stroke deficits that clarify communication of the results to the receiving team at the hospital.

Information that should be communicated to the receiving hospital includes age, sex, past medical history, current medications, presenting problem, onset time, neurologic status, vital signs, estimated time of arrival to hospital, and any concerns while in transport. Fieldwork can save precious minutes of additional work in the emergency department. The importance of care given by paramedics should not be underemphasized.

EMERGENT STROKE EVALUATION

GENERAL ASSESSMENT

Emergent assessment of the stroke patient begins immediately on arrival at the emergency department. If prenotification is obtained from emergency medical services, a physician should meet the patient at triage and begin the evaluation. Initial concerns include assessment of respiratory function, cardiovascular stability, and level of consciousness. An adequate airway must be established to ensure proper ventilation, particularly in obtunded or comatose patients. Aspiration is a serious concern and leads to subsequent pneumonia and is a major cause of morbidity and mortality during hospitalization.[8] Supplemental oxygen is often administered, but the benefit is uncertain when oxygenation is already adequate. Hypoxemia should be corrected immediately, however, and its source aggressively investigated. Arrhythmias are common in acute stroke. Bradycardia may signal underlying increased intracranial pressure or cardiac ischemia. Atrial fibrillation associated with rapid ventricular response often impairs cardiac output

requiring immediate treatment. Atrial fibrillation also may be an embolic source for stroke. Ventricular tachycardia or fibrillation rarely occurs with stroke[9] and when present usually is due to coexistent myocardial infarction. Hypotension should be corrected with intravenous fluids. Seizures should be controlled with anticonvulsants. The initial physician evaluation should be completed within 15 minutes.

BLOOD PRESSURE MANAGEMENT

Hypertension commonly accompanies ischemic and hemorrhagic stroke.[10] In most cases of ischemic stroke, abrupt lowering of blood pressure is not advised because of the risk of causing further impairment of perfusion in the ischemic region.[11] When a systemic or cardiac reason for reducing blood pressure is present, such as aortic dissection or acute myocardial infarction, the relative importance of the systemic and neurologic issues must be considered. Hypertensive encephalopathy is a syndrome of extreme hypertension, papilledema, altered mental status, microangiopathic hemolytic anemia, and renal insufficiency that responds to lowering blood pressure. In the absence of papilledema or systemic features, it is unlikely that acute neurologic deficits are due to hypertensive encephalopathy, and acutely lowering blood pressure is more likely to worsen deficits rather than improve them.

When thrombolytic therapy is considered, reducing blood pressure within limits is necessary. Before thrombolytic therapy is administered, systolic blood pressure should be less than 185 mm Hg and diastolic less than 110 mm Hg.[12] Labetalol typically is administered in increasing doses every 5 to 10 minutes to control blood pressure. If beta blockers cannot be used, enalapril is a reasonable alternative. Sublingual nifedipine should be avoided because of the potential to lower blood pressure precipitously. If these agents do not provide adequate control, thrombolytic therapy probably should be avoided. Although some authors recommend limiting treatment to one or two doses of labetalol before excluding the patient from thrombolytics, we generally proceed with treatment as long as the blood pressure is controlled within the time frame for treatment with thrombolytic therapy.

TRIAGE AND LABORATORY STUDIES

The immediate concern for the emergency department evaluation after initial cardiovascular stabilization is confirming the diagnosis of stroke, excluding stroke mimics, and establishing whether acute stroke intervention is appropriate for the patient. It is crucial to establish the time of onset with certainty. The time of onset should be considered the time the patient was last seen without a neurologic deficit, rather than the time the patient was found with a deficit. If deficits were present on awakening, the onset time should be considered the previous night when the patient was last seen neurologically normal. This time of onset may exclude some patients who otherwise would benefit, but it avoids the risk of causing hemorrhages in patients with long established infarction. For intravenous tPA, the window for treatment is currently 3 hours. The evaluating physician must allow for time needed for CT scanning and interpretation and preparing and administering tPA. Completion of CT scanning should take no more than 25 minutes from arrival, and interpretation should be completed within 45 minutes. tPA treatment should be initiated within 1 hour of arrival in the emergency department.

Conditions other than stroke that cause acute neurologic deficits must be considered before proceeding with acute stroke treatment. Occasionally, intracranial mass lesions present with acute deficits. Migraine, seizures, and metabolic aberrations such as hypoglycemia may present with focal neurologic signs. A brief history obtained from the patient or family usually excludes these possibilities. Two intravenous catheters should be established as soon as possible. Blood glucose should be checked and corrected if needed. Additional blood tests obtained immediately include coagulation studies, complete blood count, and electrolytes.

GLUCOSE

Evidence from animal models of stroke suggests that hyperglycemia increases the severity of ischemic injury.[13] Increased glucose concentration in the area of ischemia causes higher lactate concentrations and local acidosis; this increases generation of oxygen free radicals damaging neurons. Hyperglycemia also may increase ischemic edema, release excitatory amino acid neurotransmitters, and weaken blood vessels in the ischemic area.

Studies of stroke in humans show an inconsistent association between stroke outcome and initial blood glucose; however, admission glucose concentration correlates with initial stroke severity. Initial hyperglycemia also has been associated with higher mortality rates after stroke. Some authors have suggested that hyperglycemia in acute stroke is a stress reaction, but the relationship between initial blood glucose concentration and outcome is independent of initial stroke severity, arguing against a stress phenomenon.

Although a relationship exists between hyperglycemia and stroke outcome, no study has examined the effect of lowering glucose acutely on outcome. At least one randomized trial is currently in progress,[14] and others are planned.[15] In the absence of such data, it seems prudent to lower blood glucose in the first few hours after stroke when it is markedly elevated. Glucose levels greater than 200 mg/dL should be treated with insulin on a sliding scale to keep the level less than 200 mg/dL (ideally <150 mg/dL).

TEMPERATURE

Fever also has been associated with worse outcomes after stroke.[16] It is unclear, however, whether fever is a response to the stroke or a cause of neurologic worsening. Hypothermia reduces stroke severity in animal models of stroke,[17] but no randomized trials have been completed in humans with stroke to test the benefits of this therapy. Despite the uncertainty of benefit, maintenance of normothermia is advised after stroke. Cooling blankets and antipyretics should be used to treat temperature elevations. Intravascular cooling devices currently are being tested. These devices rapidly reduce body temperature and allow the temperature to be maintained within a narrow range.

Although "central" fever occasionally occurs after stroke, most temperature elevations are due to infection. A thorough search for the cause of fever is paramount. Appropriate antibiotic treatment must be instituted as quickly as possible.

FLUID MANAGEMENT

Most patients with acute stroke are volume depleted. Intravenous fluids should be replaced with either normal saline or lactated Ringer's solution. In patients with large strokes in danger of developing brain edema, fluid administration should be titrated carefully, and free water must be limited. Mild hyponatremia need not be treated acutely. More severe hyponatremia should be corrected slowly and usually reverses with infusion of normal saline.

STROKE TEAM

A stroke team consists of individuals from multiple disciplines with specialized knowledge and interest in acute stroke care. The team approach brings together the necessary skills to administer emergently the care best suited to the situation and divides the workload so that tasks can be performed simultaneously rather than sequentially. Ideally, a stroke team consists of a neurologist, neuroradiologist, nurse coordinator, and neurosurgeon. Not all hospitals have the resources necessary to provide a complete stroke team at all times, but at least one individual should be available with the ability to evaluate acutely the neurologic status of a stroke patient, interpret the CT scan, and institute acute stroke therapy in appropriate cases. The more components of the team involved in acute stroke care, the more rapidly treatment can be initiated. The stroke team is usually responsible for confirming the onset time, evaluating the CT scan, establishing the diagnosis, reviewing the inclusion/exclusion criteria for thrombolytic therapy, and making the final decision to proceed with treatment.

IMAGING OF ACUTE STROKE

Evaluation of patients with acute stroke depends heavily on imaging. Although CT and MRI of stroke is a component of standard stroke care, emergent imaging of stroke raises several new issues. For additional details on neuroimaging in intensive care, see Chapter 48. It is paramount to differentiate ischemic from hemorrhagic stroke before deciding on the use of thrombolytics. In the future, selection of appropriate neuroprotective agents also may depend on the presence of hemorrhage. Although still investigational, it is likely that identification of an arterial occlusion and information about cerebral blood flow would help triage acute stroke patients to a treatment regimen most likely to produce benefit, while limiting the potential for complications.

At present, selection of patients for thrombolytics or other acute stroke therapy is based entirely on clinical evaluation and historical time of onset. It is likely, however, that some patients within the 3-hour time window already have established infarction that would not reverse with thrombolysis and may result in hemorrhage owing to reperfusion of infarcted brain. In contrast, others may have salvageable brain tissue despite a greater than 3-hour interval since onset. A physiologic estimate of tissue viability would be preferable to a fixed time interval, if a study were found that reliably predicted viability of brain after stroke.[18] CT and MRI have the potential to provide this measurement.

COMPUTED TOMOGRAPHY

CT has been the imaging procedure of choice for patients with recent stroke to exclude hemorrhage as the etiology. CT has the potential to provide a great deal more information, however, in an acute stroke patient. Subtle parenchymal abnormalities show evidence of early edema or infarction. Spiral CT allows CT angiography and imaging of the intracranial and extracranial circulation. Cerebral perfusion can be examined with stable xenon CT and mapped to the arterial distribution of the major cerebral arteries. This battery of tests is performed without moving the patient from the CT scanner, minimizing the time delay before deciding on optimal treatment.

Not all patients can complete the entire battery of tests. CT angiography requires contrast administration and cannot be performed in patients with renal failure or contrast allergies. There is a potential problem in patients undergoing angiography for possible intra-arterial therapy after CT angiography because the dye load is increased by the combination of procedures. If digital angiography is used and arterial injections of contrast material are minimized, however, the contrast load should not be prohibitive. Xenon CT has few limitations, but excessive movement reduces the accuracy of the acquired blood flow information. Blood flow data may not be reliable in agitated patients. Vomiting occasionally occurs after xenon inhalation, and care must be taken to avoid aspiration.

Early Computed Tomography Changes

It previously was thought that parenchymal changes did not occur on CT for at least 6 hours after ischemic stroke. More recent studies indicate, however, that early changes of ischemia frequently occur within a few hours of stroke onset and have been seen 1 hour after stroke.[19] These changes include reduced attenuation in the basal ganglia,[1] loss of gray-white differentiation particularly in the insular region,[20] low density in the cortex and subcortical white matter, and loss of sulcal markings suggesting early mass effect and edema (Fig. 51-1A and B).[21] A hyperdense middle cerebral artery occurs in 20% to 37%,[22] indicating acute thrombus within the artery, but rarely occurs without at least one other early CT abnormality. Hyperdensity in the basilar artery associated with thrombosis also has been reported.[23] In 100 patients studied within 14 hours of stroke onset (mean 6.4 hours), multiple early CT abnormalities correlated with size of subsequent infarct and poor outcome.[22] In the ECASS trial of tPA for acute stroke (see later), early CT changes correlated with larger subsequent infarct volume[24] and a greater likelihood of hemorrhagic conversion after tPA.[25] Based on these results, some experts recommend withholding thrombolytic therapy in patients with extensive

early CT changes[26]; however, whether these abnormalities represent irreversible brain infarction is controversial. A report of a patient with hypodensity in 60% of the middle cerebral artery territory and clinical and CT resolution after reperfusion with intra-arterial urokinase suggests this is not always the case.[27] In the NINDS recombinant tPA trial of intravenous treatment within 3 hours of stroke onset, early ischemic changes did not predict symptomatic hemorrhage or response to treatment.[28] CT scanners used in this study from the early 1990s are likely less sensitive than modern-day scanners. In addition, the association of early CT changes with infarction, and risk of hemorrhage may be greater with longer intervals from stroke onset. Half of the patients in the NINDS trial were treated within 90 minutes. Extensive hypodensity may have greater predictive value than other early ischemic changes.

Computed Tomography Angiography

CT angiography can be performed using spiral CT technology adding only 15 to 20 minutes to the routine CT examination. Either the intracranial or the extracranial circulation may be imaged. In a patient with acute stroke, the intracranial study may be sufficient to diagnose proximal arterial occlusion. When extracranial carotid disease is suspected, both parts of the circulation can be studied. A single bolus of contrast material similar to that used for a contrast CT scan is given for this examination, limiting use in patients with renal failure or contrast hypersensitivity. In acute stroke, CT angiography has been shown to be highly reliable for diagnosis of intracranial occlusions and correlates with other imaging modalities (Fig. 51-1C and D).[29,30] Examination of the carotid bifurcation with CT angiography provides a three-dimensional view of carotid lesions and shows eccentric lesions or ulceration not seen by conventional angiography.[31] When used in combination with conventional CT and xenon CT, the major limitation is tube heating. The studies must be sequenced properly and the area of interest on CT angiography selected carefully to minimize the number of slices needed to obtain the necessary anatomic information. CT angiography in acute stroke patients provides important information about arterial occlusions and possibly collateral blood flow[32] and may be useful to triage patients with large proximal occlusions to thrombolytic therapy and avoid interventions in patients without demonstrable arterial occlusions. It is hoped that future acute stroke trials will incorporate these imaging modalities to assess the value of triaging patients based on anatomic evidence of occlusion.

Computed Tomography Perfusion

In addition to imaging the parenchyma with CT and the cerebral vasculature with CT angiography, CT perfusion adds assessment of cerebral blood flow and blood volume. Using a helical scanner during a bolus of intravenous contrast, the time-dependent concentration curve of contrast in each pixel can be acquired (see Chapter 48). Mean transit time and subsequently cerebral blood flow can be calculated. In patients with acute stroke, perfusion-weighted CT images, similar to cerebral blood volume, correlate with final infarct size and outcome, particularly after recanalization.[33] CT perfusion maps combining cerebral blood flow and cerebral blood volume information identify tissue that progresses to infarction if not reperfused, consistent with ischemic penumbra.[34]

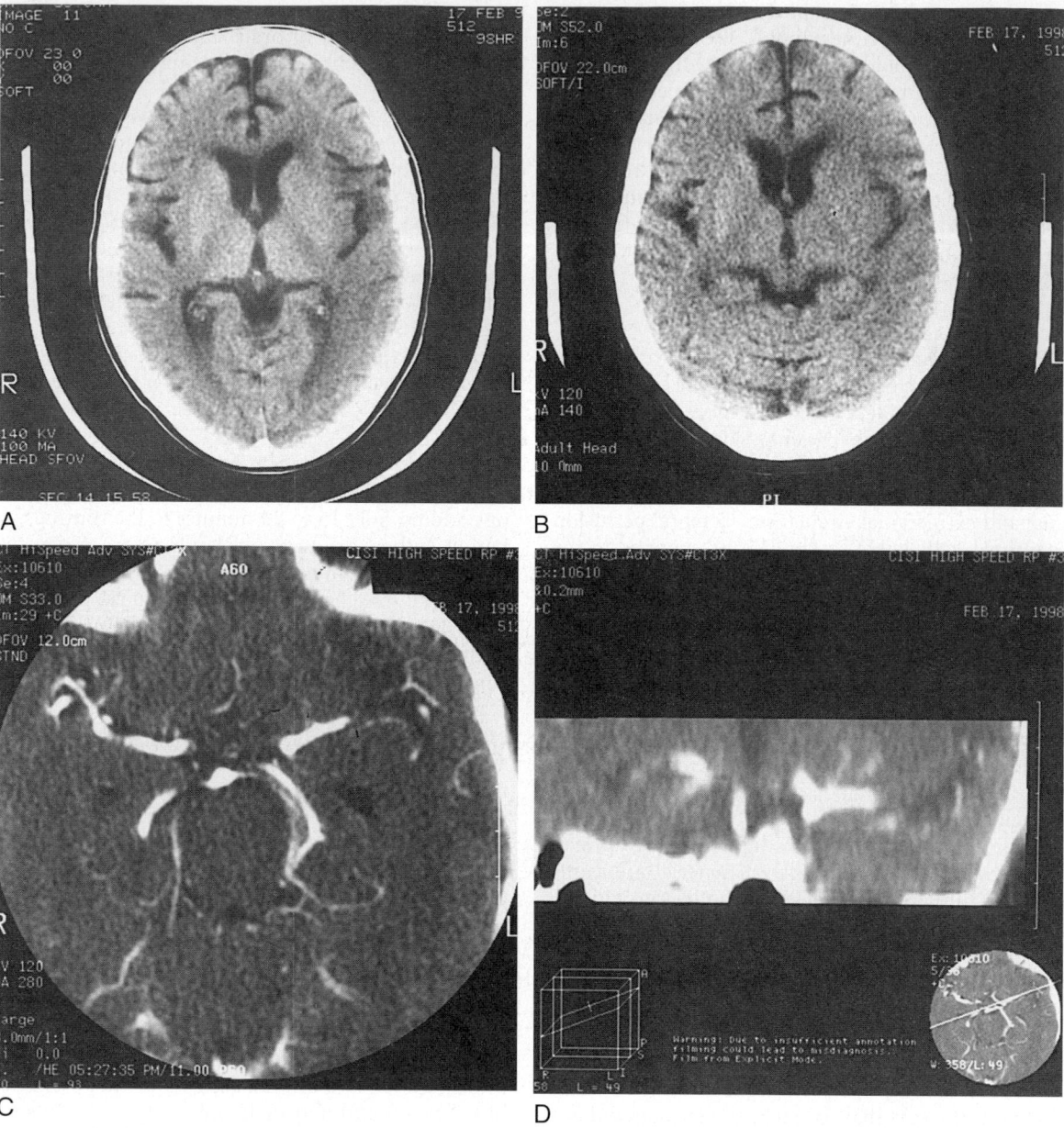

FIGURE 51–1. A, Normal computed tomography (CT) scan of brain 2 hours after onset of aphasia and left hemiparesis. **B,** Repeat CT scan at 5 hours after stroke onset shows early CT changes, including basal ganglia hypodensity, loss of the insular ribbon, and slight effacement of the sulci on the left. **C,** CT angiogram at 5 hours after stroke onset shows complete occlusion of the left middle cerebral artery. **D,** Rapid reconstruction of the CT angiogram again shows occlusion of the left middle cerebral artery.

Xenon Computed Tomography

Measurement of brain perfusion should be particularly beneficial in patients with stroke. Several methods of measuring cerebral blood flow are available; however, quantitative blood flow can be obtained only with xenon CT or positron emission tomography. Positron emission tomography has the advantage of providing corresponding metabolism data, but is more difficult to perform, particularly in acutely ill patients with stroke.

Stable xenon is an inert gas that is inhaled as a mixture of 27% xenon and 73% oxygen. During a 4-minute inhalation, rapid scanning is performed, and pixel-by-pixel blood flow values are calculated at three brain levels. Corresponding brain CT sections allow anatomic correlation. Xenon CT cerebral blood flow studies require about 15 minutes for completion. Reconstruction of images is accomplished within 5 minutes. In acute stroke patients, xenon CT identifies ischemic regions in patients without acute changes on CT. Patients with occlusion of the proximal middle cerebral artery have significantly lower cerebral blood flow in the middle cerebral artery distribution than patients with more distal occlusion (Fig. 51-2).[35] In addition, normal cerebral blood flow in a patient with an acute ischemic deficit is associated with rapid clinical improvement.[36] In a series of patients with middle cerebral artery occlusion studied with xenon CT, penumbral values of cerebral blood flow were present in all patients, and the percentage of middle cerebral artery territory in the penumbral range (cerebral blood flow 8 to 20 mL/100 g/min) remained relatively constant across the group. In contrast, the percentage of middle cerebral artery territory with cerebral blood flow values representing infarcted tissue (cerebral blood flow <8 mL/100 g/min) varied greatly.[37] Outcome was highly correlated with the area of infracted middle cerebral artery territory, not the amount

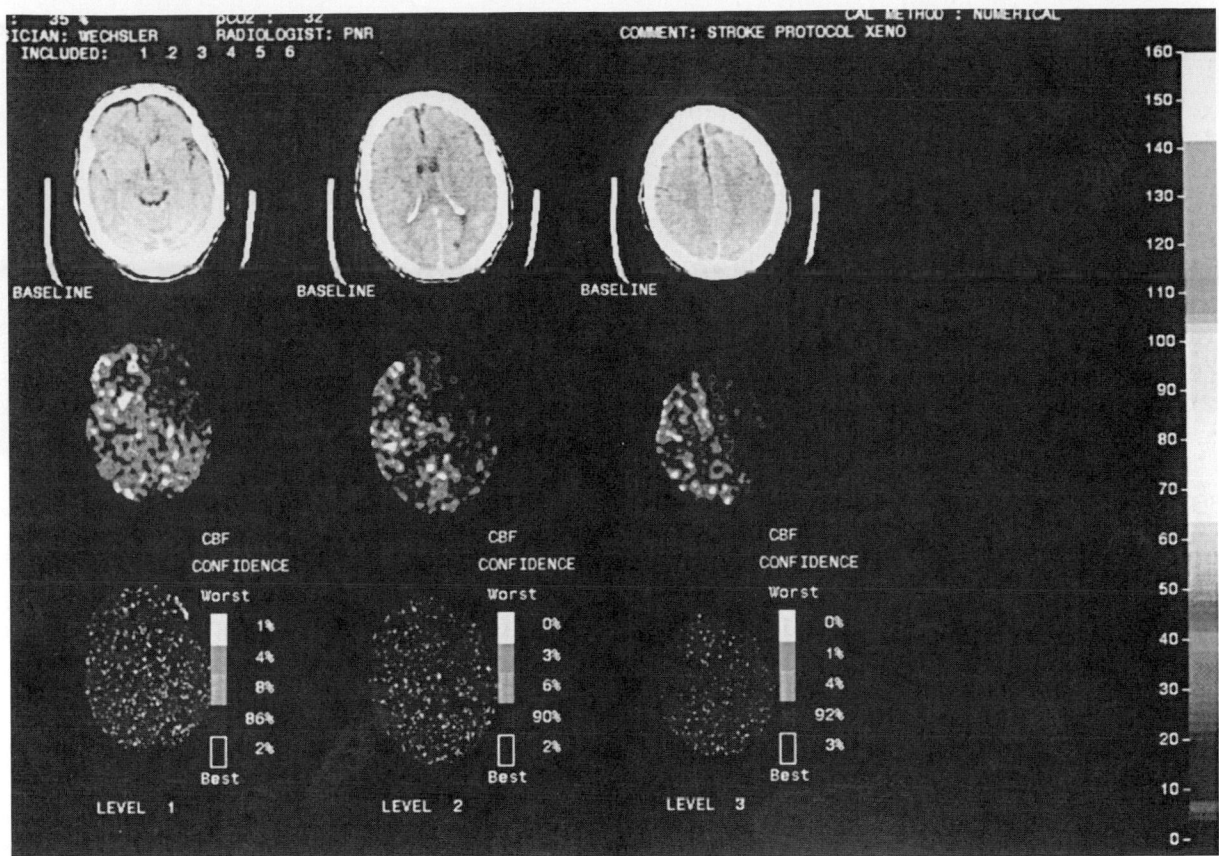

FIGURE 51–2. Xenon computed tomography blood flow study from a patient with large left hemisphere stroke 3 hours after onset of symptoms. Flow is nearly absent throughout the middle cerebral artery territory on the left.

of penumbra. These results suggest that after the first few hours, the size of the already infarcted tissue, not the amount of penumbra, may be the most important imaging parameter to determine suitability for acute stroke therapy.

The combination of CT, CT angiography, and CT perfusion or xenon CT represents a battery of tests easily and rapidly performed with the CT scanner and capable of providing important data for decision making regarding acute stroke interventions.[38] Patients with large vessel occlusion on CT angiography, minimal early CT changes, and the presence of penumbra with small areas of cerebral blood flow in the infarction range should be optimal candidates for reperfusion therapy.

MAGNETIC RESONANCE IMAGING

In many hospitals, MRI is available on an emergent basis and reliably identifies cerebral ischemia. Compared with CT, MRI is more sensitive to cerebral infarction, particularly in the brainstem and deep white matter.[39-41] Most comparisons preceded the recognition of early CT changes, however, and may favor MRI unfairly for diagnosis of cortical infarction. Absence of flow void in major cerebral arteries suggests occlusion or slow flow in that artery; this provides important information about arterial occlusion even without angiography that may be valuable particularly in the setting of acute stroke. The major drawback of MRI is the difficulty identifying hemorrhage. MRI signal abnormalities vary depending on the age of the hemorrhage.[42] Knowledge of the signal characteristics of hemorrhage of varying ages on specific imaging sequences is necessary for accurate diagnosis.

More knowledge, experience, and skill are needed for MRI interpretation of hemorrhage compared with CT. There is uncertainty about the reliability of MRI for detection of hyperacute hemorrhage and subarachnoid hemorrhage, although it is likely that experienced readers would make few mistakes.[43,44] Results of studies comparing modalities suggest that MRI is at least as sensitive as CT for detection of hemorrhage in patients with acute stroke. As MRI is more commonly used for multimodality imaging in acute stroke, the need for CT to detect hemorrhage should diminish.

Diffusion Weighted Imaging and Perfusion Imaging

Diffusion weighted imaging (DWI) shows parenchymal abnormalities earlier than conventional T2-weighted images in patients with acute stroke.[45] Perfusion imaging is based on transit times for contrast material through brain parenchyma. DWI detects the diffusion of water in the brain and shows hyperintensity in areas of reduced diffusion (Fig. 51-3). As water moves from the extracellular to the intracellular space, there is less movement of water and loss of signal resulting in hyperintensity.[46] DWI has potential advantages in the evaluation of acute stroke. First, early detection of lesions helps differentiate cerebral ischemia from other conditions that mimic stroke, such as seizures or toxic-metabolic states.[47] Hyperintensity on DWI may not be entirely specific for ischemia,[48] however, and at least one false-negative DWI scan has been reported (although a perfusion abnormality was present).[49] Second, combining DWI with perfusion imaging may identify reversibly ischemic tissue. In some cases, the area of perfusion abnormality is larger than the

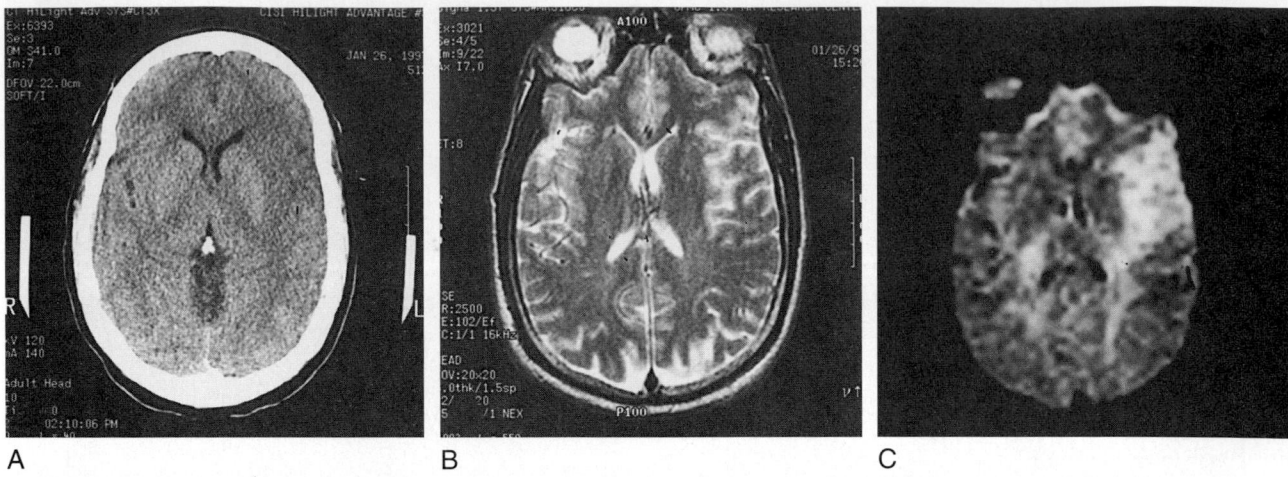

FIGURE 51–3. A, Computed tomography scan of the brain in a patient with sudden onset of expressive speech difficulty and right arm weakness 2.5 hours after onset of symptoms. There is early low density and sulcal effacement in the perisylvian region. **B,** T2-weighted magnetic resonance imaging study of the same patient 5 hours after stroke onset. Subtle increased signal intensity is seen in the perisylvian region. **C,** Diffusion-weighted image also at 5 hours after stroke onset. A larger area of signal abnormality is present in the left hemisphere.

DWI abnormality, indicating a region of brain that has impaired flow but has not yet become ischemic. Expansion of DWI abnormalities between the first few hours after stroke and repeat studies many hours later also suggests the existence of tissue at risk.[50] Several studies found that the size of DWI abnormalities correlated with clinical outcome.[51] Abnormal DWI does not always represent irreversible ischemia, however. In animal models of stroke, reduction in the size of DWI abnormalities after treatment has been shown,[52,53] and similar findings have been reported in humans after treatment with intra-arterial thrombolysis[54] and neuroprotective agents.[55] Progression to infarction is a complex phenomenon that depends on many factors in addition to cerebral blood flow.[56] The total DWI abnormality seen in the first few hours after stroke likely represents the core infarction and a portion of the penumbra.

In patients with stroke, the size of the diffusion abnormality and the growth of areas of abnormal DWI are strong predictors of outcome. Lesion growth may be an effective surrogate marker to be used in clinical trials of acute stroke therapy, particularly neuroprotective agents.[57] In acute stroke, a marker of tissue viability is needed, and some authors have suggested that the extent of mismatch between perfusion and diffusion abnormality can be used in this manner. Patients with a large mismatch might be more likely to respond to reperfusion therapy, whereas patients without mismatch have little to gain.[58] Patients without mismatch and with large areas of DWI abnormality may be at greater risk for hemorrhage. These concepts currently are undergoing testing in clinical trials. In some trials, only patients with DWI/perfusion imaging mismatch are selected for treatment expecting that they are most likely to respond. In others, after MRI all patients are treated to compare the response to treatment between patients with and without mismatch at baseline. These trials should add to understanding of the ability of a mismatch to select patients for acute stroke therapy.

Magnetic resonance angiography provides a noninvasive method of imaging the intracranial and extracranial circulation. Several techniques are available; most require no contrast and are based on time-of-flight techniques.[59] The arteries comprising the circle of Willis and the extracranial

vertebral and carotid arteries can be examined, allowing detection of occlusions in acute stroke. Occlusions of small peripheral branch arteries may not be detected by magnetic resonance angiography. Gadolinium-enhanced magnetic resonance angiography allows visualization of the intracranial and the extracranial circulation. Patients with claustrophobia or implanted metal devices, such as pacemakers, cannot undergo magnetic resonance angiography. Artifacts in some cases obscure proper identification of arterial pathology. Signal dropout may occur at the site of arterial stenosis owing to the effects of turbulent flow. If an artery is tortuous, it may extend out of the imaging section and appear occluded. In addition, construction of maximal intensity projections is subject to a variety of errors.[60] Experience and careful examination of studies typically avoids these pitfalls. In patients with stroke, magnetic resonance angiography correlates well with angiographic evidence of stenosis or occlusion of arteries in the intracranial[61,62] and the extracranial circulation.[63,64] In patients undergoing MRI and particularly DWI and perfusion imaging, the addition of magnetic resonance angiography to the battery provides evidence of arterial pathology and may add important diagnostic information when considering treatment options.

TREATMENT OF ACUTE STROKE

ANTICOAGULATION

The use of anticoagulants in acute stroke is controversial, although several randomized clinical trials provide information regarding its efficacy. Retrospective data previously suggested a significant incidence of early recurrences after ischemic stroke with reported rates of 20%. These studies also suggested that anticoagulation with heparin reduced recurrences. Hemorrhagic complications were acceptably low, particularly when patients with large strokes and uncontrolled hypertension were excluded from treatment. The results of more recent randomized clinical trials have challenged these findings and call into question the value of anticoagulation for treatment of acute stroke.[65]

The randomized studies completed to date include trials of low-molecular-weight heparin, heparinoid, and subcutaneous heparin. All have serious flaws in design that limit the ability to make definitive conclusions. The major results of these studies are summarized in Table 51-4. The studies do not support a reduced recurrence rate or improved outcome with anticoagulation when administered within 24 to 48 hours of stroke onset. Hemorrhage rates ranged from 1% to 2.5%. These results suggest that there is little value in anticoagulation for all patients with acute stroke, but it remains possible that some subgroups benefit. The TOAST study suggested that patients with large vessel disease may achieve better functional outcome.[66] The relatively high hemorrhage rate in some studies also may have obscured some benefit. In the International Stroke Trial (IST), a significant reduction in recurrent strokes from 3.8% in the control group to 2.9% in patients treated with subcutaneous heparin ($P < .01$) was offset by an increase in hemorrhagic stroke from 0.4% in controls to 1.2% in patients receiving heparin ($P < .00001$).[67] Even in patients with atrial fibrillation, the value of early anticoagulation is uncertain with studies showing benefit and lack of benefit in reducing recurrent stroke.[65]

Antiplatelet Therapy

There is less uncertainty about the benefit of aspirin in acute stroke. Two large randomized controlled trials, the Chinese Aspirin Stroke Trial (CAST)[68] and the IST,[67] showed a small but significant improvement in outcome in patients treated with aspirin. In the IST, patients received 300 mg of aspirin daily for 14 days. There was a significant reduction in stroke recurrence within 14 days in the aspirin group (2.8%) versus avoid-aspirin groups (3.9%) and a significant decrease in the risk of death or nonfatal recurrent stroke in the aspirin group (11.3%) versus avoid-aspirin groups (12.4%). In the CAST trial, 160 mg of aspirin was given per day for 4 weeks or until hospital discharge. In the aspirin group, there was a significant reduction in death within 4 weeks (3.3%) versus placebo (3.9%) and a significant reduction in death or nonfatal stroke during hospitalization. There also was a significant reduction in recurrent ischemic strokes in the aspirin group (1.6%) versus placebo (2.1%), which was offset only by a nonsignificant trend of excess of hemorrhagic strokes (aspirin 1.1% versus placebo 0.9%).

The CAST and IST were designed to be considered together and include more than 40,000 patients. Combining the results of both studies shows a significant reduction in recurrent stroke of 7 per 1000 ($P < .000001$) and reduction of death or dependency of 12 per 1000 ($P = .01$).[69] The risk of aspirin in the absence of thrombolytics is minimal, and the small but significant benefit argues in favor of routine treatment.

INTRAVENOUS THROMBOLYSIS

Trials of intravenous thrombolytic agents in acute stroke date back to the early 1960s. At that time, several trials of streptokinase,[70] fibrinolysin,[71] and urokinase[72] were performed and showed either no effect or higher mortality in patients treated with thrombolysis. These studies preceded CT scanning, and patients with hemorrhage were not excluded. The discouraging results inhibited further acute stroke trials until the 1980s, when several reports appeared showing favorable outcomes with intra-arterial thrombolytic therapy within a few hours of stroke onset.[73,74] These reports led to small randomized trials and feasibility studies of intravenous thrombolytics.[75,76] The results of two multicenter randomized controlled trials of intravenous tPA for acute ischemic stroke have been published more recently, with one showing for the first time a beneficial effect of acute stroke treatment when given within 3 hours of onset.

Tissue Plasminogen Activator within 3 Hours

The NINDS acute stroke study showed the benefit of intravenous tPA for patients within 3 hours of onset of stroke. This study was performed in two parts and included more than 600 patients with acute ischemic stroke.[77] All patients were treated within 3 hours, and half were treated within 90 minutes. Patients were randomly assigned to receive either intravenous tPA, 0.9 mg/kg to a maximum of 90 mg, or intravenous placebo. Primary outcome measures were favorable outcomes at 90 days measured by the National Institutes of Health stroke scale, Barthel index, Glasgow outcome scale, and Rankin scale. By all four measures, significantly more patients had a favorable outcome at 90 days in the tPA group compared with placebo. Treatment with tPA resulted in an 11% to 13% absolute increase in good outcomes and a slight, nonsignificant decrease in mortality at 3 months. The benefit was sustained at 12 months.[78] Intracerebral hemorrhage with clinical deterioration occurred in 6.4% of tPA-treated patients but only 0.6% of placebo patients. Despite the increase in hemorrhages, there was no significant increase in mortality or severe disability in the tPA group compared with placebo. The relationship between benefit and time from onset suggested there was little to be gained by treatment beyond 3 hours and possibly beyond 2.5 hours.

When strokes were classified according to initial impression of stroke subtype, all types of strokes had more favorable outcomes with tPA. There were no clear factors that predicted response to tPA.[79] Patients with large strokes as measured by the National Institutes of Health Stroke Scale (NIHSS, >20) and evidence of early low density or edema on CT had a higher rate of hemorrhage after tPA.[80]

TABLE 51–4. RANDOMIZED TRIALS OF ANTICOAGULATION IN ACUTE STROKE

Study	Treatment	Patients	Recurrence: Treatment Versus Control	Favorable Outcome: Treatment Versus Control	Hemorrhage: Treatment Versus Control
FISS	Nadroparin	308	1% vs. 4.7%	48% vs. 35%	0% vs. 1%
IST	Subcutaneous heparin	19,435	1.6% vs. 2.2%	17% vs. 17%	1.8% vs. 0.3%
TOAST	Danaparoid	1281	1.1% vs. 1.1%	49% vs. 47%	2.9% vs. 0.9%
HAEST	Daleparin	449	8.5% vs. 7.5%	23% vs. 21%	2.8% vs. 1.8%
TAIST	Tinzaparin	1486	3.3% vs. 3.1%	38% vs. 43%	1.4% vs. 0.2%

On the strength of the NINDS study results, in June 1996 the FDA approved intravenous tPA for treatment of stroke within 3 hours of onset. Since then, reports of small groups of patients suggest similar efficacy can be obtained at community hospitals without an increase in hemorrhages as long as the NINDS protocol is used for patient selection.[81] Not all patients respond to intravenous tPA. In a dose escalation trial of intravenous tPA (Duteplase, Burrows-Welcome), angiography was performed before thrombolysis in all patients documenting the site of arterial occlusion and repeated 2 hours later.[82] Only 31% of arterial occlusions recanalized. Proximal occlusions in the middle cerebral artery opened less frequently than distal branch occlusions, and only 8% of carotid occlusions recanalized. The resistance of carotid occlusion to intravenous thrombolysis also has been noted by others.[83]

Tissue Plasminogen Activator beyond 3 Hours

Several other tPA trials attempted to extend the window for treatment beyond 3 hours (Table 51-5). ECASS I and II[84,85] and the ATLANTIS study[86,87] treated patients with intravenous tPA 6 hours after stroke onset but failed to show a significant benefit compared with placebo. Several design differences between these studies and the NINDS trial could have contributed to the different results, but the major factor was likely the longer time to treatment. In these studies, few patients were treated within 3 hours, and most were 4 to 6 hours from onset of stroke.

Combined Analysis

Although no individual trial showed a statistically significant benefit of intravenous tPA beyond 3 hours based on the primary prespecified analysis, several post-hoc analyses suggest that a small benefit might exist. ECASS II did not find a significant benefit based on the prespecified endpoint of modified Rankin score 0 to 1 at 90 days; however, a significant benefit would have been shown had the endpoint of modified Rankin score 0 to 2 been used,[88] similar to the Prolyse in Acute Cerebral Thromboembolism (PROACT) II study of intra-arterial thrombolysis.[89] The latter endpoint encompasses independent functioning rather than normal or near-normal neurologic status. For studies with moderate-to-severe strokes and longer time windows, functional independence may be a more appropriate endpoint. In addition, a meta-analysis of eight intravenous tPA trials including more than 2800 patients found a significant reduction in death and disability (modified Rankin score 3 to 6) in patients treated 6 hours after stroke onset.[90] This finding translates into 57 fewer patients dead or disabled for every 1000 treated.

More recently, a combined analysis of intravenous tPA trials has been performed, including NINDS, ECASS I and II, and ATLANTIS A and B.[91] In contrast to a meta-analysis, the combined study pooled original patient information from all trials into a single database. A total of 2776 patients were analyzed for outcomes and hemorrhage rates. The odds ratio for good outcome (modified Rankin score 0 to 1) was greatest for treatment within 90 minutes but remained significant for treatment between 91 and 180 minutes (Table 51-6). In contrast to the individual trials, the combined analysis also showed a statistically significant benefit for treatment between 181 and 270 minutes. The odds ratio was only slightly lower than for between 91 and 180 minutes. No treatment effect was observed beyond 270 minutes. It is likely that the greater number of patients in the later time-to-treatment group allowed detection of a small but significant benefit between 3 and 4.5 hours. In patients treated between 3 and 4.5 hours, 37% reached the endpoint of modified Rankin score 0 to 1 at 90 days, whereas only 32% of controls achieved this outcome. There was no difference in mortality for treatment up to 4.5 hours, although mortality was increased beyond 4.5 hours in the tPA group. Overall symptomatic hemorrhage rate was 5.8%, and there was no relationship between time to treatment and the rate of symptomatic hemorrhage 6 hours after stroke onset. A growing body of evidence suggests a small benefit of intravenous tPA 4.5 hours after stroke onset, but the earlier treatment is initiated, the greater the likelihood of a good clinical outcome.

SITS-MOST and ECASS III

Approval for intravenous tPA (Actilyse) was granted in Europe for treatment within 3 hours, but was conditional on review of a safety monitoring study (Safe Implementation of Thrombolysis in Stroke [SITS-MOST]) of patients treated and a new randomized controlled trial of patients treated 3 to 4 hours after stroke onset (ECASS III). SITS-MOST is a mandatory registry of patients treated in Europe with intravenous tPA under the conditional approval. The goal of the registry is to confirm the rate of symptomatic intracerebral hemorrhage, mortality, and independence at 3 months equal or better than the data from randomized controlled trials. All patients treated throughout Europe will be entered into this registry for future analysis.

In addition to SITS-MOST, the European authorities mandated a randomized controlled trial of intravenous tPA for patients 3 to 4 hours from stroke onset. This placebo-controlled trial is expected to enroll 800 patients at 110 sites in 15 European countries and help settle the issue of benefit for intravenous tPA 4 hours after stroke onset. Patients with NIHSS greater than 24 are excluded. The primary efficacy endpoint is modified Rankin score 0 to 1 at 90 days.

TABLE 51–5. INTRAVENOUS TISSUE PLASMINOGEN ACTIVATOR TRIALS BEYOND 3 HOURS

Study	Design	Time To Treatment (h)	Symptoms On Hemorrhage: tPA/PL (%)	Good Outcome: tPA/PL (%)	Results
ECASS I	Intravenous tPA vs. PL	6	19.8/6.5	41/29	No benefit
ECASS II	Intravenous tPA vs. PL	6	8.8/3.4	40/36	No benefit
ATLANTIS A	Intravenous tPA vs. PL	6	11.3/0	47/49	No benefit
ATLANTIS B	Intravenous tPA vs. PL	3-5	7/1.1	34/32	No benefit

PL, placebo; tPA, tissue plasminogen activator.

TABLE 51–6. ODDS RATIOS FOR MODIFIED RANKIN SCORE 0-1 IN THE COMBINED TPA ANALYSIS

Time	N	Odds Ratio	95% CI
0-90	311	2.83	1.77, 4.53
91-180	618	1.53	1.11, 2.11
181-270	801	1.40	1.06, 1.85
271-360	1046	1.16	0.91, 1.49

CI, confidence interval.
Data from The ATLANTIS, ECASS and NINDS rt-PA Study Group Investigators: Association of outcome with early stroke treatment: Pooled analysis of ATLANTIS, ECASS and NINDS rt-PA stroke trials. Lancet 2004;363:768-774.

Other Thrombolytic Agents

At present, only tPA is approved by the FDA for treatment of acute stroke. Many other thrombolytic agents are in various stages of investigation, however. These alternative treatments offer the potential for greater efficacy with lower hemorrhage rates and improved convenience of administration. Whether these advantages are clinically relevant and sufficient to replace tPA for stroke therapy awaits the results of future clinical trials.

Desmoteplase is a plasminogen activator with higher selectivity and far greater specificity for fibrin than tPA. Additional advantages over tPA include a long half-life that allows bolus administration and the lack of hypofibrinogenemia. Desmoteplase is currently in phase 2 clinical trials. Tenecteplase is a modification of human tPA designed to achieve more effective thrombolysis. The half-life of tenecteplase is significantly longer, allowing administration as a single bolus. Similar to desmoteplase, tenecteplase has greater fibrin specificity and less fibrinogen depletion than tPA.[92] A pilot safety study of tenecteplase for acute ischemic stroke is currently in progress.[93] Reteplase is another genetically modified form of human tPA. It also has been shown to be effective in treatment of acute myocardial infarction. Because of a longer half-life, reteplase is administered as two bolus injections 30 minutes apart. A small trial of intra-arterial reteplase for acute ischemic stroke was reported.[94] Sixteen patients were treated 9 hours after stroke onset with complete recanalization in 88% and clinical improvement in 44% at 24 hours. Only one symptomatic hemorrhage occurred. An ongoing study (ROSIE) combines abciximab and intravenous reteplase treatments in patients 24 hours after stroke onset with an endpoint of MRI-based reperfusion at 24 hours. Abciximab alone has been studied in a phase 2b trial.[95] A glycoprotein IIb and IIIa inhibitor, abciximab may improve outcome through its powerful antiplatelet effects or by direct thrombolytic activity. The AbBEST study included 400 patients randomized to treatment with intravenous abciximab or placebo 6 hours after stroke onset. Based on a responder analysis, outcomes at 3 months were improved with abciximab in patients with mild or moderate strokes but not in patients with NIHSS greater than 15. The effect also was greater in patients treated within 5 hours of symptom onset. Symptomatic hemorrhage occurred in 3.6% of patients treated with abciximab. A larger phase 3 randomized controlled trial is under way.

Tissue Plasminogen Activator in Specific Subgroups

Further analysis of the results of the NINDS study did not identify any specific subgroups of patients with a greater or lesser likelihood of responding to tPA. The number of patients treated in many subgroups was quite small, however. Clinical experience has raised questions about treatment of several patient subgroups with conflicting evidence concerning the advisability of treatment with thrombolytics.

Age and Risk of Thrombolysis

One group of concern is elderly patients, in whom the incidence of cerebral amyloid angiopathy is greater and might predispose to hemorrhage after tPA. Some studies of anticoagulation with warfarin indicate a higher rate of intracerebral hemorrhage in the elderly.[96] In the NINDS study, older patients were less likely to have a favorable outcome but fared better with tPA than without.[97] In ECASS II, older patients had a greater risk of severe hemorrhagic transformation.[98] In contrast, a retrospective survey of patients treated with intravenous tPA at multiple centers did not find any difference in outcome or hemorrhage rate in 30 patients older than age 80 compared with 159 younger patients.[99] Advanced age should not be considered a contraindication to thrombolysis, but requires consideration of a lower probability of good outcome after treatment and possibly a higher rate of intracerebral hemorrhage.

Computed Tomography Findings on Baseline Scan

Another point of controversy is the significance of early CT abnormalities as a predictor of hemorrhage after thrombolysis for acute stroke. Before the randomized controlled tPA trials, several studies suggested that the presence of early changes in CT predicted a greater likelihood of hemorrhagic transformation.[100,101] In ECASS I, hypodensity greater than one third of the middle cerebral artery territory was an exclusion; however, many patients were entered despite such findings on CT. These patients had an increased mortality and showed no benefit from tPA.[84] In ECASS II, additional training of investigators reduced the number of protocol violations; however, in a subsequent analysis, the extent of hypodensity on baseline CT was found to be an independent risk factor for intracerebral hemorrhage.[98] The STARS study, a multicenter registry of 389 consecutive patients treated with intravenous tPA, found that the absence of extensive hypodensity on initial CT predicted a favorable outcome.[102,103] Quantitative assessment of CT changes using the ASPECTS scoring system in patients treated with intravenous tPA also showed a relationship between early CT hypodensity (ASPECTS <8) and hemorrhage.[104]

The NINDS group examined the association between early CT changes and hemorrhage and arrived at a different conclusion. Although outcomes were worse in patients with mass effect or edema on initial CT scan, more such patients had good outcomes if treated with tPA. The odds ratio of symptomatic hemorrhage was increased (2.9 versus 1.5) with hypodensity greater than one third of the middle cerebral artery territory. Few patients had this finding on baseline CT scan, however, and the difference did not reach significance.[105] Analysis of the Australian Streptokinase study including patients treated within 4 hours of stroke onset also failed to show any significant relationship between early ischemic changes and intracerebral hemorrhage.[106] The significance of early CT changes as a risk for hemorrhage and poor outcome after intravenous tPA therapy is unclear. At present, most tPA protocols continue to exclude patients from treatment with extensive low density on initial CT. In the future, MRI or cerebral blood flow measurement might allow more appropriate exclusion of patients with high risk of hemorrhage.

Stroke on Awakening

Frequently, patients arrive in the emergency department after awakening with a new neurologic deficit due to stroke. Because the time of onset cannot be established with certainty, these patients usually are excluded from thrombolytic therapy. Some of these patients may be within the time window for acute stroke treatment, however, and might benefit from thrombolysis.[107,108] Stroke-on-awakening patients may be an ideal group to undergo physiologic imaging studies to select patients appropriate for acute stroke treatment.

Aspirin Pretreatment

Many individuals at risk for stroke are treated with aspirin or other antiplatelet agents. Others take aspirin on the way to the hospital after onset of stroke symptoms. Whether aspirin pretreatment increases the risk of thrombolytic therapy is unclear. In the MAST-I study, patients treated with aspirin and streptokinase had a higher incidence of death from intracranial hemorrhage.[109,110] In ECASS II, there was a higher incidence of symptomatic hemorrhage in patients pretreated with aspirin. In the multicenter recombinant tPA Acute Stroke Survey, aspirin therapy was associated with a higher risk of symptomatic hemorrhage, but did not remain significant after adjustment for other factors. In contrast, a report of 300 patients treated with intravenous tPA failed to find any association between pretreatment with aspirin and hemorrhagic complications.[111] Aspirin pretreatment also was not associated with intracerebral hemorrhage in the NINDS intravenous tPA trial.[112] Patients receiving antiplatelet therapy usually are not excluded from thrombolytic therapy, although additional studies are needed to clarify the relative risk of thrombolysis in these patients.

Severe Stroke

In most studies of thrombolysis, prognosis and risk of hemorrhage are strongly related to initial severity of stroke as measured by the NIHSS score. In the NINDS trial, at 3 months 48% of patients with NIHSS greater than 20 were dead, and 21% were severely disabled. Symptomatic hemorrhage occurred in 17% compared with 6% in the entire cohort.[112] Despite the poor outcomes and increased hemorrhage rate, more patients had good outcomes with tPA than without (10% tPA versus 4% placebo). Severe stroke should not be considered a contraindication to thrombolytic therapy, although the overall poor prognosis and increased hemorrhage rate must be considered in deciding on treatment in individual cases.

INTRA-ARTERIAL THROMBOLYSIS

An alternative approach to intravenous thrombolysis is direct delivery of thrombolytic agents by a microcatheter embedded in the clot (Fig. 51-4).[113] The advantage of the intra-arterial approach is direct visualization of the occluded artery and knowledge of the recanalization status as thrombolysis proceeds. Delivery of the thrombolytic agent to the site of the clot should be more effective than intravenous infusion. The disadvantage is the additional time needed to bring the patient to angiography, prepare the groin, catheterize the femoral artery, and guide the catheter from the femoral artery to the intracranial circulation. Start of thrombolytic therapy typically is delayed by 45 to 60 minutes. Urokinase was used in most early studies of intra-arterial thrombolysis but is no longer available. Prourokinase (recombinant prourokinase) was used in clinical trials, but has not been approved by the FDA. Most intra-arterial thrombolysis is now done with tPA. Doses of 20 to 50 mg have been infused over 1 to 2 hours, but no systematic dose escalation studies have been completed. Some interventionalists advocate extremely small doses of intra-arterial tPA (e.g., 0.1 to 0.2 mg), but most use higher doses. A few reports of intra-arterial therapy with reteplase (Retavase) have appeared, and small pilot studies of intra-arterial Retavase are now in progress. Other issues with intra-arterial thrombolysis include whether to use mechanical catheter manipulation in conjunction with thrombolysis, the optimal dose of heparin, and the use of boluses of thrombolytic agents beyond and within the thrombus before starting an infusion. Most protocols include a small bolus (e.g., 2 mg of tPA) beyond the thrombus followed by 2 mg within, then an infusion over 1 to 2 hours. Progress is assessed every 15 to 30 minutes with an injection of contrast material, and the catheter is repositioned if the thrombus is partially dissolved. When recanalization is achieved, infusion of the thrombolytic agent can be discontinued.

The PROACT trial was the first randomized controlled trial of intra-arterial thrombolysis. PROACT I randomized 40 patients with occlusion of the M1 or M2 segment of the middle cerebral artery to either 6 mg of intra-arterial recombinant prourokinase infused over 2 hours or direct intra-arterial injection of saline within 6 hours of stroke onset.[114] Both groups also received intravenous heparin. In this small pilot study, there was a trend toward improved outcome in the recombinant prourokinase group, but the difference did not reach statistical significance. Based on these encouraging findings, PROACT II was initiated. Over 2.5 years, 180 patients were randomized in a 2:1 ratio to 9 mg of intra-arterial recombinant prourokinase in addition to heparin or to heparin alone.[115] More than 12,000 patients were screened at 50 centers to enter these trials. The primary endpoint of modified Rankin scale 2 at 90 days was achieved by 40% of the recombinant prourokinase group and only 15% of controls ($P = .043$). At least partial recanalization at 2 hours occurred in 67% of recombinant prourokinase patients. Complete recanalization was found in 20%. Symptomatic hemorrhage occurred in 10% of patients treated with recombinant prourokinase and in 2% of controls. Although the hemorrhage rate was higher than previous intravenous thrombolytic studies, the median NIHSS score of 17 indicates that the patients in the PROACT study had more severe strokes treated at a later time interval. A higher hemorrhage rate is expected. Based on factors predicting outcome in this group of patients, the treatment and control groups can be stratified according to risk. There was no differential effect of recombinant prourokinase across risk strata, indicating that all patients, regardless of risk, benefit equally from recombinant prourokinase.[116]

The PROACT study is the only acute stroke trial to show a statistically significant improvement of outcome when given 6 hours after stroke onset. The median time to treatment was 5.5 hours, and most patients were treated after 5 hours from stroke onset.[115] The clinical benefit was apparent despite this late time to treatment, and possibly a greater benefit would have been found had patients been treated earlier.

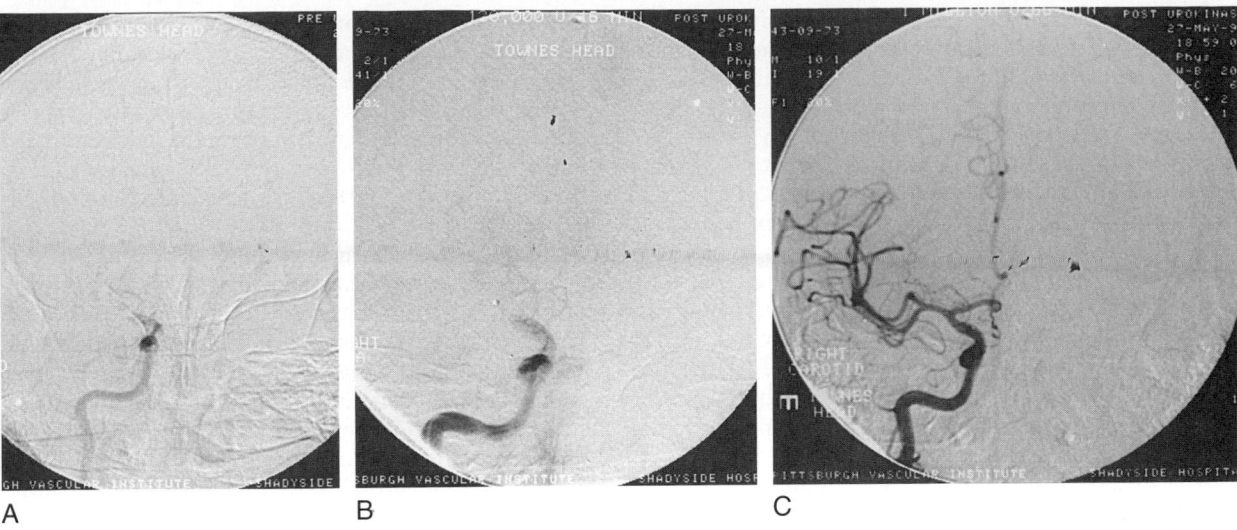

FIGURE 51–4. A, Right carotid angiogram from a patient with embolic occlusion of the right middle cerebral artery 4 hours after onset of symptoms. **B,** Angiogram from the same patient after placement of a microcatheter into the middle cerebral artery clot and infusion of 120,000 U of urokinase. There is no recanalization. **C,** Angiogram after infusion of 1 million U of urokinase directly into the clot, showing complete recanalization of the middle cerebral artery.

Several other factors may have limited the effectiveness of thrombolysis in this study. Infusion of the thrombolytic agent extended over 2 hours, and mechanical manipulation was not allowed. The thrombolytic regimen used in the PROACT study may not represent the optimal parameters, leaving considerable room for future improvement.

Basilar artery thrombosis carries a high morbidity and mortality[117] and may be particularly amenable to intra-arterial thrombolysis. Anecdotal reports indicate successful recanalization of the basilar artery is associated with good outcomes in 25% to 50% of patients,[118-120] a considerable improvement on the reported natural history. Good outcomes have been reported with intra-arterial thrombolysis of basilar thrombosis well beyond the usual 6-hour time limit.[121] Intravenous tPA also may result in improvement, but the large clot burden favors the intra-arterial approach.

Combination Therapy

The major problem with intra-arterial thrombolysis is the additional time necessary to place a catheter into the intracranial arteries; this requires 45 to 60 minutes beyond the time intravenous therapy could be given. If transport to a tertiary care center is needed, the delay may be longer. Combined therapy offers the prospect of beginning intravenous therapy, then proceeding to intra-arterial therapy if needed. If the patient presents within 3 hours of stroke onset, therapy is begun with intravenous tPA in a reduced dose of 0.6 mg/kg over 30 minutes. While the intravenous tPA is infusing, the patient is transported to angiography, and a catheter is placed in the intracranial circulation. If thrombus is present despite intravenous therapy, additional tPA is given intra-arterially in an attempt to clear the thrombus. This approach was used in a small group of patients randomized to either intravenous followed by intra-arterial tPA or placebo followed by intra-arterial tPA.[122] There was a greater recanalization rate in the combined group (partial or complete 81% combined versus 50% intra-arterial alone). Bleeding complications were slightly more common in the combined treatment group.

Mechanical Devices

Although most thrombolytic studies concentrate on time to treatment, the most important factor is probably time to recanalization. When infusion of thrombolytic agents requires 1 to 2 hours for complete thrombus dissolution, time to recanalization can be quite long. Mechanical devices offer the possibility of considerably shortening time to recanalization. In contrast to thrombolytic infusions, devices may be able to clear thrombus from large arteries within a few minutes. Thrombolytic agents may not have to be used, possibly reducing the rate of intracranial hemorrhage. Several devices are now being tested. Catheters capable of reaching the middle cerebral artery or basilar artery use lasers, ultrasound, or high-speed saline jets to agitate or emulsify thrombus. Simple snares to capture thrombotic material also are under development. These devices are now undergoing initial clinical trials but hold great promise for reducing time to recanalization and improving outcomes in acute stroke.

NEUROPROTECTIVE AGENTS

The extent of ischemic injury in the brain depends on the level of cerebral blood flow in the effected territory. Cerebral blood flows less than 10 mL/100 g/min are probably tolerated only for minutes, whereas intermediate levels of blood flow of 20 to 30 mL/100 g/min may be tolerated for several hours before irreversible changes occur.[123] During ischemia, there is insufficient energy for maintenance of normal membrane pump activity. Sodium diffuses into the cell across its gradient causing neuronal depolarization and impairing the ability of the neuron to generate an action potential. In addition, there is a tremendous outpouring of excitatory neurotransmitters, particularly glutamate.[124] Glutamate activates *N*-methyl-D-aspartate and non–*N*-methyl-D-aspartate receptors causing influx of calcium into neurons.[125] This influx results in production of toxic products, including nitric oxide, free radicals, and activation of phospholipases. The duration of this reversible ischemic state is uncertain, but animal models of focal stroke suggest it is only a few hours.[126]

Neuroprotective therapy is designed to interfere with the cascade of cellular events that results in cell death. Blocking any of the events involved in ischemic cell death may preserve function or prolong the time window for restoration of blood flow by other means, such as thrombolysis. Phase 3 randomized controlled trials of neuroprotective agents that are effective in animal models failed to show a clinical benefit in patients with stroke (Table 51-7). There are many potential reasons for the failure of animal trials to translate to the clinical setting. Aspects of the animal studies, such as the time window, dose equivalent, stroke subtype, and mode of administration, frequently were modified in clinical trials to maximize patient entry and to minimize side effects. The expected benefit from treatment often was overly optimistic, and in some cases outcomes in the control group were better than expected, making it more difficult to show a benefit from therapy. Neuroprotective agents may improve certain neurologic functions, such as cognitive activity, which is poorly measured by most commonly used stroke scales. It is also possible that what works in animals simply does not work in humans.

Despite these failures, several new neuroprotective agents are currently in phase 3 trials. NXY-059 is a nitrone spin-trap agent that has been shown to improve outcomes in rodent and primate models of acute stroke. Two randomized controlled trials are in progress to assess the efficacy of this drug for stroke within 6 hours of onset. A phase 3 trial of the serotonin agonist, repinotan, also is in progress for patients with hemispheric stroke. ONO-2506 is a neuroprotectant that modulates the uptake capacity of glutamate transporters and expression of gamma-aminobutyric acid receptors. A phase 3 trial using this agent is currently in progress. Magnesium is undergoing testing in a randomized controlled trial including patients 12 hours from stroke onset. Another study is examining hyperacute prehospital administration of magnesium. Finally, hypothermia is a promising neuroprotective therapy, and clinical trials of mild hypothermia in acute stroke are under way.

STROKECTOMY

Cerebral edema and herniation is the most frequent cause of death from stroke in the first few days.[127] Cerebral edema usually gradually increases and peaks 2 to 3 days after stroke onset. Steroids, do not effectively reduce edema due to stroke, and antiedema measures, such as mannitol or hyperventilation, are of limited benefit. Control of intracranial pressure is associated with improved outcome, but whether intracranial pressure monitoring to guide therapy is helpful is uncertain.

Surgical decompression of large hemispheric infarcts causing edema and increased intracranial pressure is a logical method of treatment because the edema is usually self-limited. If herniation can be avoided, recovery may occur similar to stroke without severe edema. Several different approaches to decompression have been proposed. Rengachary and colleagues[128] reported a marked reduction in mortality with hemicraniectomy in patients with severe edema after stroke. In a group of 32 patients with large nondominant hemisphere stroke, mortality was reduced to 40%, and long-term disability was only moderate after hemicraniectomy.[129] Kalia and Yonas[130] reported the results of strokectomy based on results of xenon CT cerebral blood flow studies in four patients with cerebral edema after stroke and impending herniation. Blood flow studies identify areas of nearly absent flow. This is a more reliable indicator than CT changes of irreversibly damaged brain and helps guide surgical removal avoiding areas of intact cortex. This procedure prevents fatal herniation, but whether long-term outcome is truly improved must be determined by randomized clinical trials. Until then, surgical decompression for hemispheric infarction should be considered for younger patients with a greater potential for recovery from massive stroke and particularly for nondominant strokes. The optimal timing of decompression is uncertain. If herniation is already in progress, irreversible brainstem damage may occur limiting the benefit of the procedure. Early edema may not progress to herniation, and surgery could be performed unnecessarily. Xenon CT findings of extensive areas of near-absent cerebral blood flow may help identify patients liable to have massive edema and herniation[131] and help select patients most likely to require surgical decompression.

Cerebellar infarction is a special case that clearly requires urgent surgical intervention.[132] Compression of the brainstem and fourth ventricle leading to hydrocephalus or severe pontomedullary compromise can be reversed by rapid surgical decompression of the infarcted cerebellum. The clinical syndrome of inferior cerebellar infarction, including vertigo and imbalance, may be mistaken for a vestibulopathy, and CT changes may be subtle or nonexistent. It is critical to suspect this diagnosis in patients at risk for cerebrovascular disease because surgical intervention may be lifesaving with little residual deficit.

SUMMARY

The availability of effective treatment to alter outcome within the first few hours after stroke onset necessitates dramatic changes in the evaluation of stroke. Patients with symptoms suggesting cerebral ischemia must be treated emergently from the prehospital encounter to the emergency department and the treating physicians. Imaging must be performed rapidly and provide useful information for the decision-making process. Therapy for acute stroke includes much more than thrombolysis. Appropriate management of blood pressure, glucose, intravenous fluids, and temperature all contribute to the overall outcome from acute stroke. Understanding of the benefits and hazards of thrombolysis continues to evolve with greater experience and additional studies. Neuroprotection holds great promise for further improvement of outcomes and possibly enhancement of effectiveness of thrombolysis or extension of the time window for reperfusion. At present, only

TABLE 51-7. FAILED NEUROPROTECTIVE TRIALS

Study	Type	Time to Treatment (h)	Results
Lubeluzole	Phase 3	8	No benefit
Cerestat	Phase 3	6	No benefit
Selfotel	Phase 3	6	No benefit
Enlimomab	Phase 3	6	Treatment worse
Cervene	Phase 3	6	No benefit
GM1 Ganglioside	Phase 3	12	No benefit
Nimodipine	Phase 3	24	No benefit
Fosphenytoin	Phase 3	6	No benefit
Citicoline	Phase 3	24	No benefit
GV150526	Phase 3	6	No benefit

a small percentage of patients with stroke arrive at an emergency department in time for acute stroke therapy.[133,134] Development of new acute stroke therapies and improvements in outcome with lower hemorrhage rates should encourage the medical system further to treat a greater number of stroke patients earlier. Rapid advancements in acute stroke therapy may necessitate a system of stroke centers similar to the trauma system to ensure that all stroke patients receive the optimal available therapy in the shortest time possible.

ANNOTATED REFERENCES

Chen ZM, Sandercock P, Pan HC, et al: Indications for early aspirin use in acute ischemic stroke: A combined analysis of 40,000 randomized patients from the Chinese Acute Stroke Trial and the International Stroke Trial. On behalf of the CAST and IST collaborative groups. Stroke 2000;31:1240-1249.
This article represents a combined analysis of two clinical trials, each with 20,000 patients, showing a significant reduction of recurrent stroke and death with aspirin treatment. There was a highly significant reduction of 7 per 1000 in recurrent ischemic stroke in patients treated with aspirin versus control, and a significant reduction of 4 per 1000 in death with aspirin treatment. The authors concluded that early aspirin treatment is of benefit for a wide range of patients and its prompt use should be widely considered for all patients with suspected acute ischemic stroke to reduce the risk of early occurrence.

Furlan A, Higashida R, Wechsler L, et al: Intra-arterial prourokinase for acute ischemic stroke. The PROACT II study: A randomized controlled trial. JAMA 1999;282:2003-2011.
Randomized controlled clinical trial of the use of intra-arterial thrombolytics in 180 patients at 50 centers showing significant improvement in outcome with treatment given up to 6 hours from stroke onset. Patients were randomized to receive 9 mg of IA r-pro UK plus heparin (n=121) or heparin only (n = 59). The primary outcome was based on the proportion of patients with slight or no neurologic disability at 90 days as defined by a modified Rankin score of 2 or less.

National Institutes of Neurological Disorders and Stroke. In Rapid Identification and Treatment of Acute Stroke. Pre-hospital Emergency Medical Care Systems, pp 17-48. NIH publication #97-4239. August 1997.
This publication provides the National Institutes of Health algorithm for the pre-hospital and emergency management of acute stroke that was developed from the experience of conducting acute stroke trials.

Rieke K, Krieger D, von Kummer R, et al: Decompressive surgery in space occupying hemispheric infarction. Crit Care Med 1995;73:1576-1587.
Clinical report of reduced mortality rate and favorable long-term outcome in 32 patients with large nondominant hemisphere stroke treated with hemicraniectomy. At follow-up in surgically treated patients, the Barthel Index showed an excellent level of daily activity in one patient, minimal assistance in 15 patients, and dependency in five patients. The Oxford Handicap Scale indicated no handicap in one patient, moderate handicaps in 15 patients, and moderately severe handicaps in five patients. In the control group, all five surviving patients needed assistance, and all but one patient demonstrated a moderately severe handicap.

The ATLANTIS, ECASS and NINDS rt-PA Study Group Investigators: Association of outcome with early stroke treatment: Pooled analysis of ATLANTIS, ECASS and NINDS rt-PA stroke trials. Lancet 2004;363:768-774.
This article represents a combined analysis of five clinical studies in 2775 patients randomly allocated to rt-PA or placebo. The study addresses the use of intravenous rt-PA and provides specific insight into its use beyond three hours of the onset of stroke. The authors concluded that the sooner that rt-PA is given to stroke patients, the greater the benefit, especially if started within 90 minutes. Their findings also suggested a potential benefit from this therapy applied beyond 3 hours, but this potential might come with some risks.

The National Institute of Neurological Disorders and Stroke rt-PA Stroke Study Group: Tissue plasminogen activator for acute ischemic stroke. N Engl J Med 1995;333:1581-1587.
A key clinical report in the field of stroke that showed, for the first time in a randomized controlled trial, a reduction in stroke morbidity with acute treatment. In June 1996, the FDA approved intravenous tPA for the treatment of stroke within 3 hours of onset.

Chapter 52

NONTRAUMATIC INTRACEREBRAL AND SUBARACHNOID HEMORRHAGE

Allyson R. Zazulia • Michael N. Diringer

KEY POINTS

INTRACEREBRAL HEMORRHAGE

1. **Intracerebral hemorrhage (ICH) injures the brain not only through direct mechanical compression** but also through secondary mechanisms such as ischemia and edema.

2. **Hematoma expansion occurs within the first few hours after symptom onset** in approximately one third of patients.

3. **In-hospital neurologic deterioration may occur in as many of two thirds of patients;** among these patients, one quarter will be found to have increased hematoma size.

4. **There appears to be no compelling reason to reduce blood pressure in the acute period after ICH.** If there are systemic concerns, modest reduction (15% to 20%) in patients with severe hypertension (mean arterial pressure >130 to 140) using short-acting agents with minimal cerebrovascular effects (e.g., labetalol, nicardipine, enalapril) appears to be safe.

5. **Randomized trials of surgical hematoma evacuation and corticosteroid treatment have failed to show a consistent benefit in the management of ICH.** The efficacy of osmotic agents has not been evaluated in a randomized trial.

6. **The most common cause of death after ICH is withdrawal of care,** followed by transtentorial herniation and medical complications of immobility.

SUBARACHNOID HEMORRHAGE

1. **Subarachnoid hemorrhage (SAH) typically presents as the sudden onset of a severe headache,** often associated with nausea, vomiting, and syncope. Focal neurologic deficits are uncommon.

2. **Rebleeding, which is often fatal, occurs most commonly within the first 24 hours** and is heralded by a sudden worsening of headache, vomiting, new neurologic deficit, or arrhythmia.

3. **Hydrocephalus may develop acutely within hours of SAH or gradually up to weeks later** and usually manifests as an insidious decline in mental status.

4. **Delayed vasospasm occurs in more than two thirds of patients, especially those with large amounts of subarachnoid blood,** and produces a new focal neurologic deficit in more than one third. Management options include nimodipine, hemodynamic augmentation, and endovascular maneuvers.

5. **Management of SAH-associated "cerebral salt wasting" often requires the administration of large volumes of fluid replacement** to prevent intravascular volume contraction and restriction of free water to treat hyponatremia.

6. **Cardiac abnormalities, including electrocardiographic changes, mildly elevated cardiac enzymes, and arrhythmias, are common after SAH** and are thought to be related to elevated catecholamine levels rather than myocardial ischemia.

INTRACEREBRAL HEMORRHAGE

Spontaneous (nontraumatic) intracerebral hemorrhage (ICH) accounts for approximately 10% of all strokes in North America and about 20% to 30% in East Asia. It is associated with greater mortality and more severe neurologic deficits than any other stroke subtype.[1-3] Nearly half of all patients die within the first 30 days; survivors often have significant residual disability.[4,5]

PATHOPHYSIOLOGY

The pathophysiologic mechanisms of brain injury due to ICH are complex. The primary injury is one of local tissue destruction as rupture of a cerebral blood vessel introduces a sudden stream of blood into the brain parenchyma. In more than one third of patients, continued bleeding or rebleeding results in hematoma enlargement and further mechanical injury within the first few hours after onset.[6] The mass of blood produces tissue shifts within the intracranial cavity.

In addition to the primary mechanical injury, further damage is believed to occur after the bleeding stops.

The mechanisms underlying this secondary injury are unknown, but ischemia and edema have been implicated. Experimental models of ICH suggest that ischemia is an important part of its pathophysiology.[7,8] Periclot and ipsilateral hemispheric hypoperfusion has been demonstrated almost uniformly in clinical studies,[9-11] but the importance of ischemia in patients with ICH has not been settled.[12,13] Positron emission tomography studies in humans performed 10 to 22 hours after symptom onset showed that both cerebral blood flow (CBF) and metabolism are reduced around the clot, suggesting that the hypoperfusion reflects the reduced metabolic demand of the damaged tissue surrounding the hematoma rather than ongoing ischemia.[13]

Cerebral edema occurs within hours of experimental ICH, variably thought to result from the toxic effects of blood-derived enzymes, from increased osmotic pressure exerted by clot-derived serum proteins, or from ischemia.[14-16] The presence, time course, and importance of edema in humans are debated. Part of the difficulty stems from the inability to unequivocally quantify edema in humans. Signal changes on radiographic studies after ICH indicate increased water content in the area surrounding the clot, but the clinical and pathophysiologic significance of this is not known.

Hemostasis after hemorrhage is initially achieved at the site of vascular injury by the formation of a platelet-fibrin plug. After several days, red blood cells within the clot begin to lyse, cellular infiltrates appear, and the process of reabsorption begins. Months later, a residual collapsed cavity is all that remains.

CAUSES AND RISK FACTORS

The leading risk factor for ICH, occurring in more than half of all cases, is chronic hypertension.[17,18] Long-term adequate treatment of chronic hypertension significantly reduces this risk.[19] Increasing age is another risk factor, with a doubling of the rate of hemorrhage with each decade of life until age 80, when the incidence plateaus at nearly 25 times that of the previous decade.[20]

Other risk factors include black race[21] and alcohol abuse.[22] The relationship of ICH to smoking[22,23] and low serum cholesterol[24,25] has not been convincingly established. Similarly, the impact of diabetes on the risk of ICH is disputed.[26,27]

Hypertensive Hemorrhage

Hypertensive ICH occurs predominantly deep in the cerebral hemispheres, most often in the putamen (Fig. 52-1).[17] Other frequently involved sites include the thalamus, lobar white matter, cerebellum, and pons. The common link among these sites is that they are all supplied by small penetrating arteries,[28] perpendicular branches directly off major arteries that are subject to high sheer stress and that have no collaterals. These features make them vulnerable to the effects of increased blood pressure. Chronic hypertension damages the tunica media, resulting in lipohyalinosis, fibrinoid necrosis, and microaneurysms (Charcot-Bouchard aneurysms). Although Charcot-Bouchard aneurysms have been demonstrated in the weakened vessel walls of patients with ICH, their pathogenetic role in vascular rupture is uncertain.[29] The occurrence of ICH in an atypical location, in multiple locations, or in association with subarachnoid hemorrhage raises the suspicion of a nonhypertensive cause, such as a cerebral vascular anomaly, blood dyscrasia, or trauma.

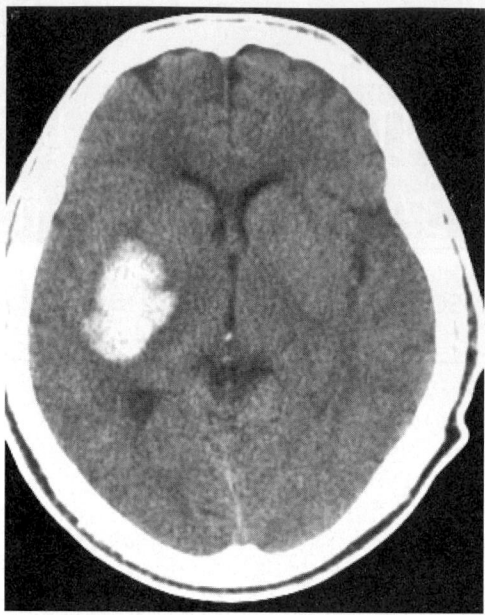

FIGURE 52–1. Typical moderate-sized putaminal hemorrhage. (From Diringer MN, Pucllicino P, Chan R: Intracerebral hemorrhage. Continuum 2003;9:170.)

Intracranial Aneurysms and Vascular Malformations

Up to one quarter of hemorrhages are due to bleeding from rupture of an intracranial aneurysm (fusiform and saccular) or vascular malformation (arteriovenous malformation [AVM] or angioma). Rupture of a saccular berry aneurysm produces ICH in 5% to 25% of cases. Although aneurysmal rupture is most commonly associated with hemorrhage in the subarachnoid space, the blood may also be directed into the substance of the brain if the aneurysm is adherent to the brain parenchyma. Rarely, aneurysms located at the middle cerebral artery bifurcation produce hemorrhages that appear identical to hypertensive hemorrhages into the basal ganglia, and anterior communicating artery aneurysms can produce flame-shaped hemorrhages in the base of the frontal lobes.

Approximately half of intracranial AVMs in adults present with hemorrhage.[30] In 60% of cases, the hemorrhage is parenchymal, involving virtually any location within the cerebrum, brainstem, or cerebellum.[31] The majority of AVMs become symptomatic by age 40; thus, hemorrhage due to AVMs occurs in a younger population than that due to aneurysms or hypertension. Multiple calcified vascular channels may be seen within the hematoma on computed tomography (CT) scans, suggesting the presence of an AVM. Magnetic resonance imaging (MRI) and four-vessel cerebral angiography are useful adjuncts in the diagnosis of these lesions.

Other Causes

Cerebral amyloid angiopathy is an important cause of predominantly lobar, often recurrent ICH in the elderly. Histopathologic studies demonstrate the deposition of β-amyloid protein in the media and adventitia of small meningeal and cortical vessels; deposition in the typical sites for hypertensive hemorrhage is rare, but it has been reported in the cerebellum.[32] The prevalence of amyloid in cerebral vessels increases dramatically with age[33,34] and may partially account for the exponential rise in the risk of ICH with increasing age. There is an overrepresentation of the apolipoprotein E ε2 and ε4 genotypes in hemorrhages related to cerebral amyloid angiopathy, and these alleles are associated with a younger age at hemorrhage onset and a higher risk of early recurrence.[35,36] Although there is no radiographic technique for diagnosing cerebral amyloid angiopathy, the finding of recurrent lobar ICH in an elderly nonhypertensive patient strongly suggests the diagnosis.

Approximately 10% of ICHs are due to hematologic causes.[37] Coagulopathy related ICH most often results from warfarin therapy[38] but may also be associated with the use of other antithrombotic and thrombolytic agents, as well as with systemic diseases (e.g., thrombocytopenia, leukemia, hepatic and renal failure) or congenital or acquired factor deficiencies.

Hemorrhage from an underlying neoplasm is rare; however, it occasionally occurs with malignant primary central nervous system tumors such as glioblastoma multiforme and lymphoma and with metastatic tumors such as melanoma, choriocarcinoma, renal cell carcinoma, and bronchogenic carcinoma.[39] Benign tumors are almost never associated with ICH.

ICH may also occur in association with infection (e.g., infiltration of vessel wall by fungal organisms),[40] necrotizing hemorrhagic encephalitis with herpes simplex virus,[41] vasculitis,[42] venous sinus occlusion,[43] in a delayed fashion after head trauma,[44] following reperfusion (e.g., after carotid endarterectomy or acute thrombolysis),[45] and with the use of various drugs, particularly sympathomimetics (e.g., cocaine, amphetamines, pseudoephedrine, phenylpropanolamine).[46,47] Finally, some degree of hemorrhagic transformation of acute cerebral infarcts is common,[48,49] although symptomatic ICH in this setting is rare in the absence of anticoagulation or thrombolytic therapy.[50,51]

CLINICAL FEATURES

The clinical presentation of ICH is often indistinguishable from that of ischemic stroke but more commonly includes altered level of consciousness, headache, and vomiting, reflecting the presence of increased intracranial pressure (ICP).[17] Blood pressure is elevated in the majority of patients (see later). Seizures occur in 15% to 25% of patients within the first 48 hours and are nearly always associated with lobar hemorrhages or underlying vascular or neoplastic lesions.[52,53] Symptoms are maximal at onset or develop over minutes to hours. Neurologic deterioration after hospital admission has been reported to occur in 33% to 61% of patients with ICH.[54,55] The cause for clinical worsening is not always evident, but increased hematoma size is found in more than 25% of cases.[54] The role of edema in clinical deterioration is much more elusive.

DIAGNOSTIC STUDIES

Noncontrast CT scanning remains the gold standard for the diagnosis of acute ICH. The typical CT appearance of an acute hematoma consists of a well-defined area of increased density surrounded by a rim of decreased density. Over time, the borders of both the high- and low-attenuation regions become increasingly indistinct, such that the hematoma is isodense with adjacent brain parenchyma by 2 to 6 weeks.[56,57]

Peripheral contrast enhancement can often be seen at this time.[58] By 2 to 6 months, there may be no CT evidence of previous hemorrhage, or there may be an area of hypodensity or a slitlike scar.[59]

Although the ability of MRI to reliably detect acute hemorrhage is controversial,[60] MRI is better than CT for determining the approximate age of a hematoma. This is because each hemoglobin oxidation state during the evolution of the hematoma produces a predictable pattern of signal intensity.[61] In addition, gradient-echo sequences may be useful in demonstrating the iron-containing deposits of previous asymptomatic hemorrhages.[62,63]

MRI and conventional angiography can be useful in evaluating the cause of ICH if an underlying aneurysm, vascular malformation, or neoplasm is suspected, but the yield of such studies is extremely low when the patient has chronic hypertension and the hemorrhage is in one of the typical sites associated with hypertensive hemorrhage.[64]

TREATMENT

Initial Stabilization

Acute ICH is a medical emergency requiring attention to airway and respiratory management, hemodynamic status, and correction of any underlying coagulopathy. As many as half of all patients with ICH undergo mechanical ventilation.[65] Blood pressure is often elevated at presentation, sometimes markedly so. Recent evidence indicates that the majority of hematomas enlarge over the first few hours, suggesting that aggressive correction of coagulopathies might be helpful.

Airway and Respiratory Management

Airway obstruction in ICH may occur for two reasons. First, there may be diminished consciousness, resulting in relaxation of the pharyngeal musculature and tongue and suppression of the cough and gag reflexes. Second, in ICH involving the posterior fossa, there may be complete loss of pharyngeal tone and absent cough, swallow, and gag reflexes.

Initial airway management includes proper positioning, frequent suctioning, and placement of an oral or nasal airway. Frequent assessments for sonorous respiration, inability to manage oral secretions, or decreased oxygen saturation are necessary. If conservative measures are ineffective, intubation may be necessary. Intubation of patients with ICH requires adequate sedation and jaw relaxation, as well as prevention of ICP elevation. Several factors may conspire to raise ICP during intubation, including hypoxemia, hypercarbia, and direct tracheal stimulation. Intravenous lidocaine (1 to 1.5 mg/kg) has been recommended to block this response,[66] although data supporting its use are lacking.[67] Short-acting intravenous anesthetic agents (thiopental 1 to 5 mg/kg or etomidate 0.1 to 0.5 mg/kg) also block this response[68] and additionally suppress brain metabolic rate,[68a] theoretically improving tolerance of a transient fall in cerebral perfusion pressure (CPP), should it occur. Etomidate is generally preferred over thiopental because it is less likely to lower blood pressure. Paralytic agents are usually unnecessary, but if needed, short-acting agents should be used. Intubated patients are at high risk for pneumonia via colonization of the oropharynx, sinuses, trachea, and gastrointestinal tract or contamination from hospital personnel or equipment. Appropriate measures should be taken to minimize this risk.

Hemodynamics

Arterial blood pressure is elevated on admission in the majority of patients with ICH, even in the absence of a history of hypertension.[17] Mean arterial pressure (MAP) is greater than 120 mm Hg in more than two thirds of patients and greater than 140 mm Hg in more than one third.[69] Although this acute increase in blood pressure is often implicated as the cause of the hemorrhage, it may simply be a reflection of chronic hypertension, the brain's attempt to maintain CPP in response to the sudden increase in ICP, pain and anxiety, and sympathetic activation. Even without pharmacologic intervention, blood pressure tends to decline to premorbid levels during the first 7 to 10 days after hemorrhage.[70]

There is substantial controversy over whether and when to lower blood pressure after acute ICH and how aggressive any intervention should be.[71,72] Proponents of rapid treatment of acute hypertension argue that high blood pressure may predispose to hematoma enlargement and may exacerbate vasogenic edema by increasing capillary hydrostatic pressure, especially in areas with a damaged blood-brain barrier. Yet an association between hypertension and edema has never been demonstrated, and data on the effect of hypertension on hematoma enlargement are inconsistent.[6,73,74] Another potential reason to lower blood pressure is that hypertension during the acute phase of ICH has been shown to correlate with a poor prognosis in some studies.[75,76] Causality has not been established, however, so it does not necessarily follow that lowering blood pressure will improve outcome. In fact, other studies have found no relationship between admission blood pressure and mortality.[55] In one report, patients whose mean blood pressure could be lowered to less than 125 mm Hg had a better outcome,[72] but it is unknown whether lowering the blood pressure improved the outcome or whether patients who respond to antihypertensive medications have less severe injury. Perhaps the most compelling reason to consider lowering blood pressure in ICH patients with moderate to severe hypertension is the potential for end-organ damage. Such patients are at risk for systemic complications of elevated blood pressure, including myocardial ischemia, congestive heart failure, and acute renal failure. Therefore, if hypertension is not treated, monitoring for such end-organ dysfunction is necessary.

The major argument against the treatment of elevated blood pressure is that lowering blood pressure might exacerbate ischemic damage in the tissue surrounding the hematoma by impairing CBF.[71] Chronic hypertension shifts the cerebral autoregulatory curve to the right, such that a higher CPP is required to maintain adequate CBF.[77,78] Thus, lowering the blood pressure to "normal" levels in these patients could lead to inadequate CBF. Similarly, because CPP is equal to the difference between MAP and ICP, lowering blood pressure may reduce CPP below the autoregulatory limit in patients with elevated ICP due to a large space-occupying clot or hydrocephalus.

Seeking to determine whether lowering blood pressure produces cerebral ischemia in acute ICH, several studies of CBF autoregulation in patients with recent ICH and elevated blood pressure (MAP >130 to 140 mm Hg) have been carried out.[79-81] Taken together, these studies demonstrate that regional and global autoregulation is preserved after ICH, down to a lower MAP limit that averages 110 mm Hg, or about 20% of the admission MAP, but there is substantial individual variation. MAP reductions in excess of 20%, or below approximately 85 mm Hg, may reduce CBF. None of

these studies provided data on ICP, and, with the exception of one in which hematoma size was not specified, all were carried out on patients with small to moderate hematomas. Although these data do not address the issue of whether early pharmacologic reduction in blood pressure is beneficial, they do challenge the assumption that such reductions are harmful and may provide useful guidelines when blood pressure treatment is deemed necessary in patients with acute ICH.

In summary, unless there are signs of systemic complications, there appears to be no compelling need to aggressively treat hypertension in the early period after ICH, especially in the setting of large hemorrhages and raised ICP. However, modest blood pressure reductions (15% to 20%) in very hypertensive patients (MAP >130 to 140 mm Hg) with small- to moderate-sized hemorrhages appear to be safe.

If the decision is made to treat hypertension in the setting of acute ICH, the most appropriate antihypertensive agent would have a short half-life and minimal cerebrovascular effects, and it would be administered in such a way as to avoid sudden large reductions in blood pressure. Vasodilators, especially those that dilate veins, can raise ICP by increasing cerebral blood volume and hence should be avoided. Sodium nitroprusside and nitroglycerin increase ICP and lower CBF in patients with reduced intracranial compliance. Ganglionic blockers may also lower CBF. Calcium channel blockers, beta blockers, and angiotensin-converting enzyme (ACE) inhibitors have minimal effects on CBF within the autoregulatory range of MAP and do not alter ICP. Therefore, popular agents in the setting of acute ICH include the combined alpha and beta blocker labetalol, the calcium channel blocker nicardipine, and the ACE inhibitor enalapril. It should be noted that large doses of labetalol may be required to counteract the sympathetic nervous system stimulation associated with ICH. Another useful agent is hydralazine.

Prevention of Hemorrhage Extension

Because hemorrhage extension is known to occur within the first few hours after symptom onset in approximately one third of patients (Fig. 52-2),[6] any coagulopathy should be corrected as rapidly as possible. Patients taking warfarin should receive intravenous vitamin K and enough fresh frozen plasma to normalize the coagulation profile. Cryoprecipitate may be a useful alternative. Care must be taken not to precipitate congestive heart failure, however, and diuretics may be required to maintain an appropriate fluid balance. Additionally, the administration of fresh frozen plasma carries the risk of transfusion-related acute lung injury, which can complicate the process considerably. Correcting coagulopathy associated with thrombolytic-induced ICH is discussed later.

Even in those patients without coagulopathy, promoting early hemostasis might limit ongoing bleeding and decrease hematoma volume. Factor VIIa is a coagulation factor that interacts with tissue factor exposed in the wall of a damaged blood vessel to drive a burst of thrombin that initiates platelet aggregation and accelerates formation of a stable fibrin clot. A recently completed international phase IIb placebo-controlled dose-ranging proof-of-concept study found that treatment with recombinant factor VIIa (rVIIa) given as a single i.v. bolus within four hours of ICH onset decreases hematoma growth and improves clinical outcome despite a small increase in thromboembolic events. The percent increase in ICH volume at 24 hours was significantly

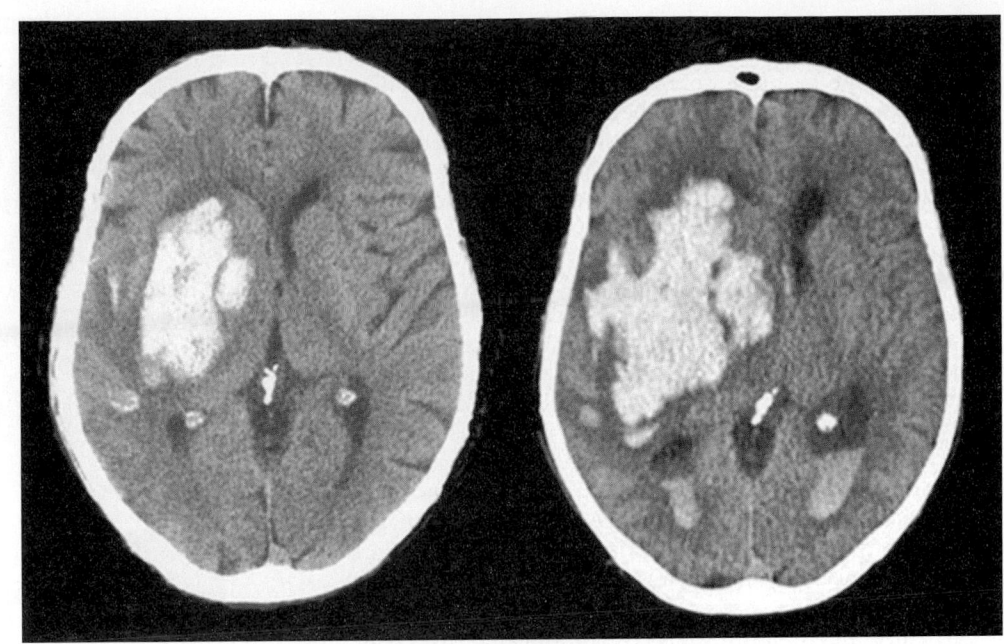

FIGURE 52–2. Hematoma enlargement with intraventricular extension. CT scan on the left was obtained 2 hours after symptom onset. CT scan on the right was obtained 2 hours later.

lower in the highest rVIIa dose group (160 μg/kg; 11%) compared with the placebo group (29%).[81a]

Intraventricular Hemorrhage and Hydrocephalus

In approximately 40% of patients with ICH, blood extends into the ventricular system (intraventricular hemorrhage).[82] Mortality in these patients is high.[83,84] Intraventricular hemorrhage may contribute to poor outcome by blocking cerebrospinal fluid pathways, with resultant hydrocephalus and increased ICP. In addition, intraventricular blood or its breakdown products may exert direct chemical irritative effects on periventricular structures.

Hydrocephalus may develop after ICH either in association with intraventricular hemorrhage or because of direct mass effect on a ventricle (e.g., on the third ventricle with a thalamic hemorrhage) (Fig. 52-3). External ventricular drainage (ventriculostomy) is frequently used to treat hydrocephalus and

intraventricular hemorrhage, but its efficacy has never been established, and retrospective data suggest that it does not improve outcome.[85] Ventriculostomy in the setting of intraventricular hemorrhage is difficult to manage because the catheter frequently becomes obstructed with thrombus, interrupting drainage and raising ICP. Flushing the system helps remove thrombus from the catheter but increases the risk of ventriculitis. Recently, investigators attempted to facilitate the removal of blood from the ventricles by the direct intraventricular administration of thrombolytic agents. A preliminary study using urokinase (which is no longer available) showed no increase in complications and a trend toward reduced mortality in the group receiving the thrombolytic.[86] A multicenter randomized study is currently under way to investigate the efficacy of this promising therapy.

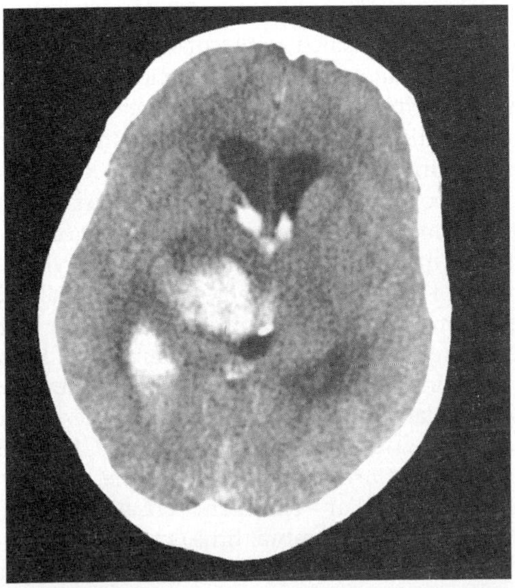

Intracranial Hypertension

The incidence, impact, and appropriate management of intracranial hypertension in ICH are not well understood. Factors likely to contribute to elevated ICP in this population include large hematoma size, minimal degree of underlying cerebral atrophy, and hydrocephalus, but the true incidence of intracranial hypertension is unclear because routine ICP monitoring is not performed. Because the hematoma is localized and the increase in volume it produces can be partially compensated for by the reduction in the size of the ventricles and subarachnoid space, a global increase in ICP may not be seen unless the hemorrhage is massive or is associated with marked hydrocephalus. In addition, mass effect with local tissue shifts can compress the brainstem or result in herniation in the absence of a global increase in ICP.[87,88]

Invasive ICP monitoring devices can be placed in extradural, subdural, intraparenchymal, intraventricular, or intraspinal locations, but ventricular catheters have the additional capacity to manage hydrocephalus. If ICP is elevated or there are clinical signs of herniation, treatment options include hyperventilation, diuretics, osmotic agents (mannitol, hypertonic saline), and, if the ventricles are enlarged, cerebrospinal fluid drainage. A recent case series suggested that the rapid reversal of clinical transtentorial herniation

FIGURE 52–3. Small thalamic hemorrhage with blood obstructing the foramina of Monro, causing hydrocephalus.

(decreased level of consciousness and dilated pupil) with hyperventilation and osmotic agents improved long-term outcome,[89] but the efficacy of these approaches in controlling ICP or altering outcome has not been evaluated in a randomized trial. Corticosteroids have no role in the management of increased ICP associated with ICH because they do not provide any benefit and increase the rate of complications.[90]

Surgical Evacuation

The rationale for surgical evacuation of a hematoma is that reducing mass effect and removing neurotoxic clot constituents should minimize injury to adjacent brain tissue and hence improve outcome. Unfortunately, several randomized, controlled trials of surgery for supratentorial ICH dating back to 1961 all failed to show a benefit.[91-94] A meta-analysis of three of these trials reported that patients undergoing surgical evacuation via open craniotomy had a higher rate of death or dependency at 6 months compared with those managed medically (83% versus 70%).[95] Criticisms of these trials are that the surgical techniques are outdated, patient selection was inadequate, and surgery was delayed too long.

Because open craniotomy is complicated by tissue damage sustained during the approach to the hematoma, a variety of new techniques for clot removal have been proposed, including an Archimedes screw, ultrasonic aspirator, modified endoscope, modified nucleotome, double-track aspirator, intraoperative CT monitoring, and instillation of thrombolytics. However, the recurrence of bleeding due to loss of the tamponade effect on adjacent tissue, which occurs in 10% of patients treated with open craniotomy, remains an issue with these techniques. In addition, because the new techniques involve limited surgical exposure, there is concern that rebleeding will be more difficult to control than with open craniotomy. One study comparing endoscopic aspiration to medical management found a better outcome in the surgical group (74% death or disability, compared with 90%), but the benefit was limited to patients with lobar hematomas.[94] Another study comparing stereotactic hematoma evacuation to conservative treatment in a select group of patients with putaminal hemorrhage found that surgery within 24 hours resulted in reduced mortality (11.8% vs. 23.5%) and greater likelihood of independent functional outcome (47.1% vs. 21.6%) in those patients who on admission had closed eyes that opened in response to strong stimuli. Of note, however, the authors provided no information regarding medical management or surgical technique.[95a] Three studies addressed the feasibility of early craniotomy for ICH. In one, 34 patients were treated within 12 hours of ICH.[96] Mortality was 18% in the surgical group and 23% in the medical group. In another study, 20 patients were randomized, with a median time to surgery of 8.5 hours from onset.[97] Good outcomes (Glasgow outcome scale score >3) were achieved in 56% of the surgical group and 36% of the medically treated group (P = NS). The third, a study of ultra-early surgery (<4 hours), found a disturbingly high rate of postoperative rebleeding.[98]

A lack of benefit of surgery in ICH was also shown in a recently completed multicenter trial in which 1033 patients were randomized within 72 hours of ICH onset to surgical hematoma evacuation (open craniotomy or stereotactic aspiration, at surgeon's discretion) or initial conservative management. Favorable outcome occurred in 26.1% in the surgery group and 23.8% in the initial conservative treatment group, a nonsignificant difference (odds ratio 0.89; 95% confidence interval 0.66 to 1.19). There was also no difference in

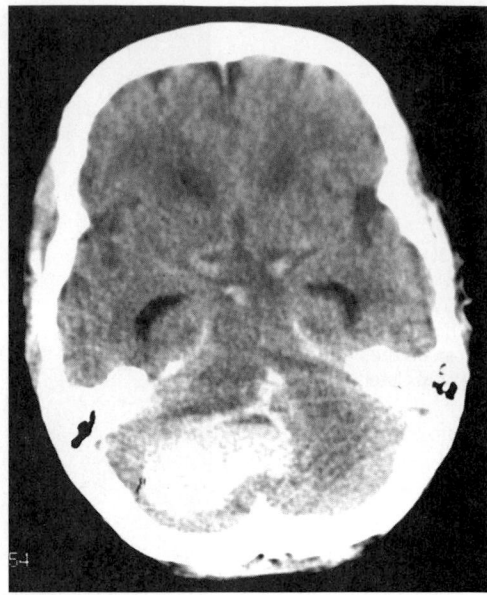

FIGURE 52–4. Typical cerebellar hemorrhage with early hydrocephalus evident by enlargement of the temporal horns of the lateral ventricles.

mortality (surgery 62.6% vs. conservative treatment 63.7%). Subgroup analysis suggested a possible benefit of surgery in patients with superficial hematomas (less than 1 cm from cortical surface).[98a]

Whether cerebellar hemorrhage represents a unique case with regard to the role of surgery is unclear. In the pre-CT era, urgent surgery was advocated for all patients with cerebellar hemorrhage because of the perceived likelihood of severe disability or death.[99,100] With the advent of CT, however, it became evident that many patients had a benign outcome without surgery.[101-104] Proposed criteria for when to evacuate a cerebellar hematoma include diminished level of consciousness, large hematoma size (>3 cm³), midline location, compression of basal cisterns or brainstem, and hydrocephalus (Fig. 52-4),[105-107] but whether these criteria select for patients who will benefit from surgery remains to be demonstrated in a randomized trial.

Thrombolytic-Induced Hemorrhage

Symptomatic ICH is a feared complication of thrombolytic therapy and is associated with considerable morbidity and mortality. It occurs after thrombolytic treatment of acute ischemic stroke in 3% to 20% of patients.[51,108-110] Symptomatic ICH is substantially less common after thrombolytic treatment of extracerebral thrombosis (myocardial infarction, pulmonary embolism, deep venous thrombosis, arterial and graft occlusion)[111] but results in a similarly poor outcome.[112] Factors that increase the risk of symptomatic ICH include higher dose of thrombolytic agent,[113] intra-arterial rather than intravenous route of administration,[114] elevated blood pressure before treatment,[115] and concomitant use of heparin.[116]

In the setting of thrombolytic therapy, any new neurologic deficit, especially a decline in consciousness, should be assumed to be due to hemorrhage. When ICH is suspected, the thrombolytic infusion is stopped, the patient's airway is reassessed, and an emergent CT scan is obtained. Blood studies (prothrombin time, partial thromboplastin time, thrombin and fibrinogen levels) should be performed to assess fibrinolytic state. At the first suspicion of hemorrhage, preparations should be made for giving fresh frozen plasma, cryoprecipitate, and platelets if needed. The National Institute of Neurological Disorders and Stroke (NINDS) study of tissue plasminogen activator stipulated 6 to 8 units of cryoprecipitate or fresh frozen plasma and 6 to 8 units of platelets, but only rarely was this amount of blood product given to an individual patient during the study.[51] Although neurosurgical consultation was frequently obtained in patients with symptomatic ICH in the NINDS trial, only one patient in the study underwent surgery, and that patient died.

PROGNOSTIC FACTORS AND CAUSES OF MORTALITY

Mortality following ICH is high (25% to 50%), with more than half of the deaths occurring in the first 48 hours. Although patients who have small hemorrhages and mild deficits may recover completely, the majority of ICH survivors have significant residual disability.[4,5,117] Many clinical and radiographic prognostic indicators have been identified, but they are not consistently recognized across studies. Clinical factors reported to predict poor prognosis include older age, reduced level of consciousness on admission, elevated blood pressure on admission, and in-hospital neurologic deterioration. Radiographic features include large initial hematoma size, intraventricular spread of the hemorrhage, midline shift, hydrocephalus, and hematoma growth.[6,54,55,75,82,118-120] It has been demonstrated, however, that withdrawal of support in patients thought likely to have a poor outcome biases predictive models in ICH and negates the predictive value of all other variables.[121] Thus, the most frequent cause of death after ICH is withdrawal of care, followed by early (within 48 hours) transtentorial herniation and progression to brain death. Medical complications of immobility (pulmonary embolism, pneumonia, sepsis) account for most of the other deaths.[117] For survivors of ICH, the risk of recurrent stroke is approximately 4% per year. Recurrent ICH occurs about twice as often as ischemic stroke, especially in those with previous lobar hemorrhage.[122]

SUBARACHNOID HEMORRHAGE

Although it is the least common form of stroke, subarachnoid hemorrhage (SAH) has a great impact on its sufferers. One quarter of patients die before reaching medical attention,[123] and because of the consequences of secondary insults—rebleeding, hydrocephalus, and delayed ischemia due to vasospasm—more than half of those who reach medical attention either die or are left with neurologic deficits.

PATHOPHYSIOLOGY

In SAH, the primary site of bleeding is within the subarachnoid space, but depending on the cause, it may also involve hemorrhage into the brain parenchyma, ventricular system, or subdural space. Rupture of an intracranial saccular aneurysm is by far the most common cause of spontaneous SAH. Saccular or berry aneurysms are small, rounded protrusions of the arterial wall occurring predominantly at arterial bifurcations of the circle of Willis at the base of the brain. The most common sites of ruptured aneurysms are the internal carotid artery, including the posterior communicating artery junction (41%); anterior communicating artery–anterior cerebral artery (34%);

middle cerebral artery (20%); and vertebrobasilar arteries (4%).[124] About 20% of patients have multiple aneurysms.[125]

Aneurysmal pathogenesis remains controversial, with the importance of developmental versus acquired factors in dispute. Proponents of the congenital theory suggest that aneurysms arise at sites of faulty fusion between muscular segments within the arterial wall. Supporters of the acquired-degenerative theory focus on the role of vascular damage caused by hemodynamic stress.[126] Citing the age-dependent occurrence of arterial defects and aneurysms' predilection for arterial bifurcations (sites of maximal hemodynamic stress), those favoring the importance of acquired features postulate that degenerative changes within the internal elastic lamina and media result in a local weakness that allows for aneurysm formation. The obvious third possibility is that aneurysms develop at sites harboring congenital defects with superimposed degenerative changes.

What leads to aneurysm growth and rupture is also debated. Hemodynamic stress and other factors intrinsic to the involved vessels may play a role. The time course over which aneurysms grow and subsequently rupture is unknown, although some aneurysms appear to grow rapidly, over weeks, whereas others grow slowly, over years.

The site of rupture of most aneurysms is the dome, where the wall may be as thin as 0.3 mm. Aneurysm rupture may cause local tissue damage due to the jet of blood under high pressure, as well as cause a global increase in ICP. Tension on the aneurysm wall is determined by the radius of the aneurysm and the pressure gradient across the wall (Laplace's law). The probability of rupture is related to size; aneurysms less than 7 to 10 mm in diameter have a very low rate of rupture.

CAUSES AND RISK FACTORS

Rupture of a saccular cerebral aneurysm is the cause of hemorrhage in more than three quarters of patients with nontraumatic SAH. Thus, genetic conditions that predispose to aneurysm formation, such as polycystic kidney disease, connective tissue disorders, and coarctation of the aorta, also predispose to SAH.[126] Other types of aneurysms that less commonly cause SAH include atherosclerotic, mycotic, and traumatic aneurysms. Among the causes of nonaneurysmal SAH, trauma is the most common. Arteriovenous malformations, cocaine and stimulant abuse, neoplasia, and vasculitis account for the bulk of the remainder. In a significant number of cases, no source of bleeding is identified.

The risk of SAH increases with age, peaking at 55 to 60 years. There is a slight male predominance in younger age groups and a slight female predominance among older patients.[127] Potentially reversible risk factors for SAH include cigarette smoking, oral contraceptive use, alcohol abuse, and hypertension.[128] Prospective cohort studies reported a relative risk of SAH as high as 5.7 for female and 4.7 for male smokers,[129] but no increased risk in former smokers. Oral contraceptive use, in addition to being an independent risk factor for SAH, dramatically increases the risk among smokers.[130] A dose-response relationship exists between alcohol consumption and incidence of SAH.[131,132] Finally, hypertension appears to be a risk factor[133] and may be the mechanism by which conditions such as polycystic kidney disease and stimulant drug use increase the risk for SAH.

Recently it has become clear that, in some patient populations, genetic factors play a role in aneurysm formation.[134,135] Individuals with two first-degree relatives with cerebral aneurysms should undergo diagnostic evaluation for an aneurysm. Conventional angiography remains, at present, the appropriate test.

CLINICAL FEATURES

Presentation

The most common initial symptom of SAH, occurring in more than 90% of patients, is sudden severe headache. Less severe "sentinel" headaches[136] may precede the presenting event in as many as half of patients and are thought to represent minor leaks. In 45% of patients, transient or persistent loss of consciousness accompanies the headache.[137] The mechanism responsible for this acute loss of consciousness is that, at the moment of hemorrhage, the sudden surge in ICP approaches systemic arterial pressure, resulting in inadequate cerebral perfusion. Vomiting can be prominent in awake patients. Seizure activity may be reported.[138] In some cases, it is unclear whether this represents true epileptic seizures or reflex posturing related to the sudden rise in ICP. Focal deficits at the onset of hemorrhage occur in less than 10% of cases but, when present, may point to the location of a thick extra-axial or intraparenchymal blood clot. After a few hours, a stiff neck can develop, reflecting the sterile meningeal inflammation induced by the presence of blood in the subarachnoid space.

Complications

A worsening neurologic status following stabilization or improvement of symptoms often indicates one of the three major complications of SAH: rebleeding, hydrocephalus, or vasospasm. An understanding of the timing and nature of the deterioration facilitates rapid diagnosis and treatment. It must be emphasized that systemic perturbations, such as infection, disturbance in serum sodium levels, fever, hypoxemia, and hypotension, may produce similar symptoms and should be sought and corrected as part of the evaluation process.

Early Complications

Rebleeding. Rebleeding is heralded by a sudden worsening of headache, vomiting, development of a new neurologic deficit, or arrhythmia. It occurs in up to one third of patients and is often fatal. The risk of rebleeding is greatest during the first 24 hours and declines rapidly over the next 2 weeks.[139] Rates of rebleeding are highest in women, those with a poor clinical grade, those in poor medical condition, and those with elevated systolic blood pressure.

Hydrocephalus. Hydrocephalus occurs after SAH because of disturbances in cerebrospinal fluid flow or reabsorption; subarachnoid blood may impair cerebrospinal fluid reabsorption at the arachnoid granulations, and ventricular blood may obstruct its flow. Acute hydrocephalus can develop within hours of SAH,[140] often in the absence of intraventricular blood. Hydrocephalus may also develop gradually at any time, even weeks later. It usually manifests as an insidious decline in level of responsiveness and must be distinguished from metabolic derangements, infection, and vasospasm. CT scan is essential in making the diagnosis. The natural history of untreated acute hydrocephalus is that about one third of patients progress, one third spontaneously improve, and one third remain static.[141]

Cardiac Abnormalities. Cardiac abnormalities are common in the first 48 hours after SAH. Electrocardiographic

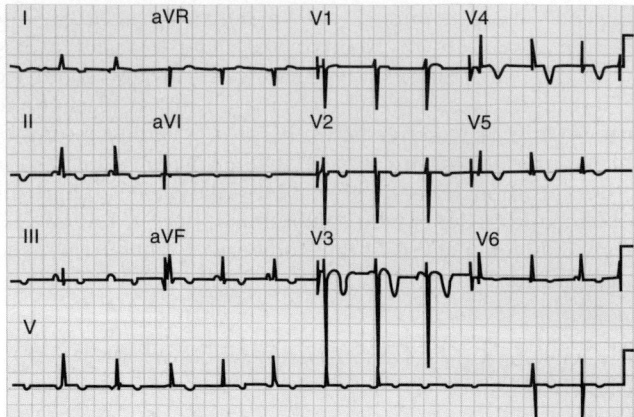

FIGURE 52–5. Electrocardiographic abnormalities following subarachnoid hemorrhage. (From Diringer MN: Subarachnoid hemorrhage. Continuum 2003;9:188.)

changes (Fig. 52-5), including tall peaked T waves ("cerebral T waves"), ST segment depression, and prolonged QT segments,[142] are frequent and have been linked to elevated levels of circulating catecholamines. It appears that these changes do not represent true myocardial ischemia; the myocardial lesions reported are pathologically distinct from ischemia. Cardiac enzymes may be mildly elevated.[143] Arrhythmias are typically benign but can be severe or fatal. In rare cases, "stunned myocardium" may occur, with impairment of myocardial contractility leading to a fall in cardiac output, hypotension, and pulmonary edema.[144] This phenomenon is transient, usually lasting 2 to 3 days, after which cardiac function returns to baseline.[145]

Delayed Complications

Vasospasm. Defined as segmental or diffuse narrowing of intracerebral arteries, vasospasm is a leading cause of morbidity and mortality following SAH. It can be detected angiographically (Fig. 52-6) in up to 70% of patients,[146] almost half of whom become symptomatic. The pathogenesis of vasospasm is complex and is not fully understood, but sustained exposure of vessels to extraluminal blood constituents and catecholamines is thought to play a role. It involves structural changes in the vessel walls and in adrenergic nerve fibers. The onset of vasospasm is delayed, most commonly developing in the latter half of the first week after the initial hemorrhage, and it may persist for up to 3 weeks. The strongest predictor of vasospasm is the amount and distribution of subarachnoid blood on the initial CT scan, with the greatest risk occurring in those having subarachnoid clots larger than 5 by 3 mm in the basal cisterns or layers of blood 1 mm thick or greater in the cerebral fissures (Fisher grade 3).[147] Focal neurologic deficits resulting from vasospasm reflect the territory of the involved arteries. They may appear abruptly or gradually and may fluctuate, exacerbated by hypovolemia or hypotension. Infarction may occur.

Serial transcranial Doppler studies have been used to screen for vasospasm. Criteria for vasospasm use an absolute linear blood flow velocity to define mild (>120 cm/sec), moderate (>160 cm/sec), or severe (>200 cm/sec) vasospasm.[148-150] Alternatively, the rate of rise in the linear blood flow velocity is used to define the onset of vasospasm. The sensitivity of transcranial Doppler in detecting vasospasm is about 80% when compared with angiography, at

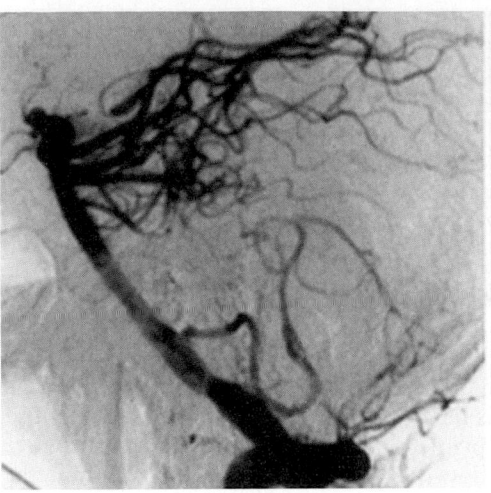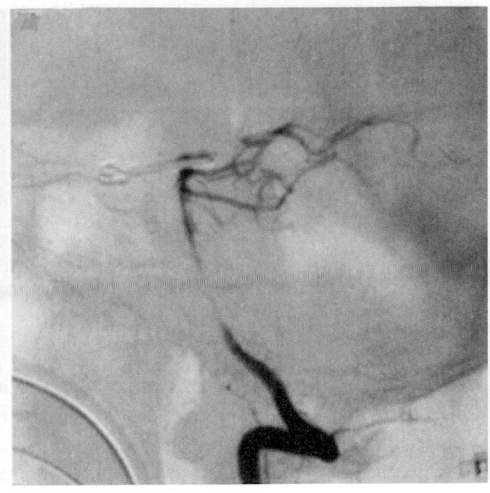

FIGURE 52–6. Baseline angiogram after subarachnoid hemorrhage (left) showing normal basilar artery caliber and distal flow, and repeat angiogram after 1 week (right) showing severe vasospasm of the basilar artery, with reduced distal flow. (From Diringer MN: Subarachnoid hemorrhage. Continuum 2003;9:191.)

least partly due to the fact that it samples only a small segment of the vasculature.[151]

Medical Complications

Blood pressure is often elevated after SAH and is associated with a greater risk of rebleeding and vasospasm, as well as higher mortality. Multiple factors may underlie the rise in blood pressure, including increased catecholamine production induced by hypothalamic dysfunction, agitation, and pain. Early on, the management of blood pressure focuses on preventing rerupture of the aneurysm. Following surgical or endovascular repair, the risk of rebleeding is virtually eliminated, and spontaneous elevations in blood pressure should be allowed to occur without intervention, because the risk of exacerbating vasospasm with hypotension is now the predominant concern.

Disturbances in sodium and water balance occur in approximately one third of patients, and hyponatremia and volume depletion after SAH are correlated with an increased risk of symptomatic vasospasm and poor outcome.[152,153] Although hyponatremia was once attributed to inappropriate secretion of antidiuretic hormone and was therefore treated with fluid restriction, later evidence suggested that both sodium and water are lost. In fact, when administered in normal "maintenance" volumes of fluid (2 to 3 L/day), as many as half of patients develop intravascular volume contraction.[154-158] The mechanisms underlying the volume contraction and the inability to conserve sodium ("cerebral salt wasting") are unknown.

Cardiac rhythm disturbances occur in about 30% to 40% of patients, although life-threatening cardiac arrhythmias occur in only about 5%.[159,160] Cardiac arrhythmias are most common on the day of hemorrhage and in the perioperative period. Although pulmonary edema has been reported in up to one quarter of patients,[161,162] its incidence is lower with careful monitoring of hemodynamic treatment for vasospasm.[163]

In a review of more than 450 patients with SAH, Solenski and colleagues reported some degree of hepatic dysfunction in 24%.[161] The majority had only mild abnormalities of hepatic enzymes, but severe hepatic dysfunction occurred in 4%. Thrombocytopenia was found in 4% of patients, usually in the setting of sepsis. Renal dysfunction occurred in 7% of patients and was considered life threatening in about 15% of those.

DIAGNOSTIC STUDIES

CT is the imaging modality of choice in screening for SAH, having a sensitivity of greater than 90%.[164] Blood appears as high attenuation within the perimesencephalic and interpeduncular cisterns surrounding the brainstem, basal cisterns, sylvian fissure, and sulci (Fig. 52-7). Certain bleeding patterns are associated with specific aneurysm locations; for example, blood in the anterior interhemispheric fissure commonly occurs with anterior communicating artery aneurysms. When blood is spread diffusely throughout the cerebrospinal fluid spaces, its site of origin may be difficult to detect.

The amount of subarachnoid blood on CT is graded using the Fisher scale (Table 52-1).[147] The risk of vasospasm is proportional to the Fisher grade. Early hydrocephalus is suggested by enlargement of the third ventricle and of the temporal horns of the lateral ventricles.

CT may fail to demonstrate SAH if the volume of blood is small, if the hemorrhage occurred several days before the CT scan, or if the hematocrit is extremely low.[164] If CT is negative and clinical suspicion is high, lumbar puncture is indicated for cerebrospinal fluid analysis. Following SAH,

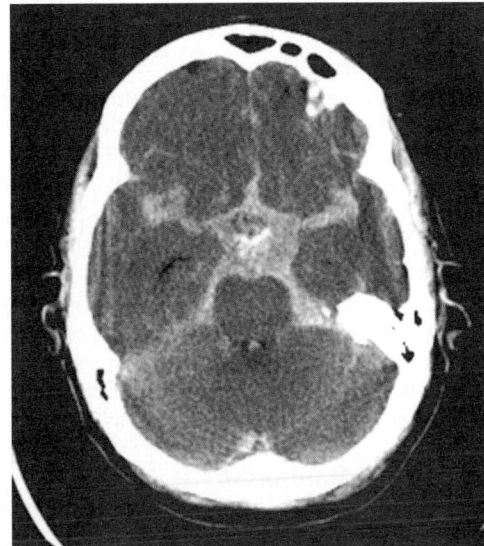

FIGURE 52–7. Subarachnoid hemorrhage with a thick layer of hyperdense blood filling the basal cisterns.

TABLE 52–1. FISHER GRADE OF SUBARACHNOID HEMORRHAGE ON INITIAL COMPUTED TOMOGRAPHY SCAN

Grade	Description
1	No blood detected
2	Diffuse or vertical layers <1 mm thick
3	Localized subarachnoid clot and/or vertical layers ≥1 mm thick
4	Intraparenchymal or intraventricular clot with diffuse or no subarachnoid hemorrhage

TABLE 52–2. HUNT AND HESS CLINICAL CLASSIFICATION OF SUBARACHNOID HEMORRHAGE

Grade	Description
I	Asymptomatic or mild headache and neck stiffness
II	Moderate to severe headache and neck stiffness ± cranial nerve palsy
III	Mild focal deficit, lethargy or confusion
IV	Stupor, moderate to severe hemiparesis
V	Deep coma, extensor posturing

cerebrospinal fluid contains red blood cells indicative of the hemorrhage, as well as a few white blood cells reflecting the secondary inflammatory response. A yellow pigment (xanthochromia), resulting from red cell breakdown, can be detected in the centrifuged fluid 2 to 6 hours after hemorrhage, allowing differentiation from a traumatic spinal puncture.[165] The common technique of comparing cell counts in the first and last tubes collected is not reliable in making this distinction. Xanthochromia persists for 1 to 4 weeks after SAH.

Once SAH has been diagnosed, cerebral angiography is performed to identify the responsible vascular lesion, search for other lesions (multiple aneurysms are found in 20% to 30% of patients with aneurysmal SAH), and assist in operative management. Angiography is negative in 10% to 15% of patients with nontraumatic SAH. In some cases, this may be due to vasospasm or inadequate views to detect a subtle aneurysm, especially in the region of the anterior communicating artery or in the posterior circulation. Repeat angiography in 1 to 2 weeks is therefore often recommended.[166] If the blood on CT is localized to the perimesencephalic cisterns and angiography is negative, the prognosis is excellent, and repeat angiography is almost always negative.[167]

MRI is not as sensitive as CT for the detection of SAH, and magnetic resonance angiography and CT angiography are not sufficiently sensitive to replace conventional angiography, because they tend to miss smaller aneurysms. Magnetic resonance angiography and CT angiography may be of assistance in planning surgical or endovascular approaches to aneurysm treatment, however.

TREATMENT

Initial Stabilization

The initial steps in the evaluation of a patient with suspected SAH should include assessment of ability to protect the airway and level of neurologic function. The Hunt and Hess scale[168] and the more recently developed World Federation of Neurological Surgeons scale[169] provide standardized measures of the patient's clinical condition (Tables 52-2 and 52-3).

As in ICH, some patients with SAH may not be able to protect the airway because of diminished consciousness. If the patient is lethargic or agitated, elective intubation should be considered before angiography. Sedation is often necessary for angiography, and in lethargic patients or those with mild early hydrocephalus, this can lead to airway obstruction.

Routine Care and Monitoring

The routine monitoring of all patients with acute SAH should include serial neurologic examinations, continuous electrocardiogram monitoring, and frequent determinations of blood pressure, electrolytes, body weight, and fluid balance.

Because seizures can increase the risk of rebleeding, anticonvulsants are indicated if seizures occur. The value of prophylactic anticonvulsants in patients who have not had a seizure is unknown. Dexamethasone is widely used to reduce meningeal irritation and intra- and postoperative edema, but there is no convincing evidence documenting its efficacy.

Fluid Management

A stable intravascular volume should be maintained by the use of hydration with isotonic saline and daily monitoring of fluid balance, body weight, and hematocrit. In some patients with severe cerebral salt wasting, large volumes of fluid are required to prevent intravascular volume contraction.[152] Hyponatremia can often be managed with the restriction of all *free* water by administering only isotonic intravenous fluids, minimizing oral liquids, and using concentrated enteral feedings. It is important to adjust the *tonicity*, not the *volume*, of fluids administered.[153] Fludrocortisone is of marginal benefit in treating salt wasting.[154,170] Persistent hyponatremia can be treated by using mildly hypertonic solutions (1.25% to 2% saline) as the sole intravenous fluid.

Hypertension

Initial attempts to treat hypertension should consist of analgesics and nimodipine; other antihypertensive agents should follow if needed. Useful medications include beta blockers (often in higher-than-usual doses to block the high level of sympathetic nervous system activity), hydralazine, nicardipine, and nitroprusside. When significant hydrocephalus is present, hypertension should not be treated until after the hydrocephalus is addressed. This is because the hypertension may be acting to maintain adequate cerebral perfusion in the face of elevated ICP.

Surgical and Endovascular Treatment

In aneurysmal SAH, the definitive way to prevent rebleeding is to obliterate the aneurysm by surgically clipping its neck. The optimal timing of surgery is controversial, but in patients

TABLE 52–3. WORLD FEDERATION OF NEUROLOGICAL SURGEONS CLINICAL CLASSIFICATION OF SUBARACHNOID HEMORRHAGE

Grade	Glasgow Coma Scale Score	Motor Deficits
I	15	Absent
II	13-14	Absent
III	13-14	Present
IV	7-12	Present or absent
V	3-6	Present or absent

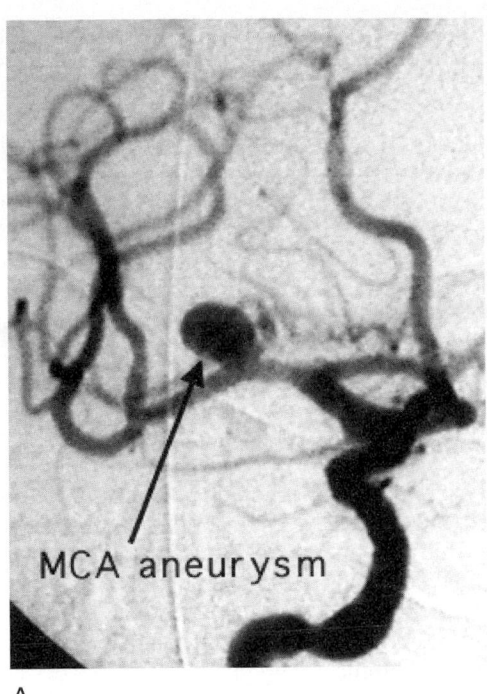
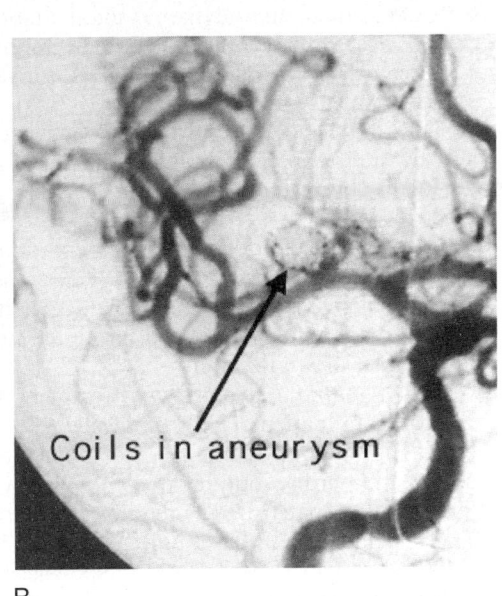

FIGURE 52–8. Angiography of middle cerebral artery (MCA) aneurysm before (*A*) and after (*B*) placement of detachable coils thrombosing the aneurysm. (From Diringer MN: Subarachnoid hemorrhage. Continuum 2003;9:190.)

MCA aneurysm

Coils in aneurysm

A

B

with a good clinical grade (Hunt-Hess grades I to III), favorable neurologic outcome is more common when surgery is performed early (within 72 hours).[171] Clipping of aneurysms has the additional advantage of permitting a safe elevation of blood pressure to treat vasospasm.

Endovascular techniques, using either detachable balloons that trap the aneurysm or electrolytically detachable coils that thrombose the aneurysm,[172] have been used to repair acutely ruptured aneurysms (Fig. 52-8). Initial experience was limited to patients who were considered poor surgical candidates owing to aneurysm configuration or poor medical condition.[173] Subsequent reports in which surgical considerations did not heavily influence the selection of patients for endovascular procedures suggest a similar outcome for the two treatments. A recent, somewhat controversial study suggested that for acutely ruptured aneurysms that were deemed equally amenable to surgical or endovascular repair, morbidity and mortality were lower with coiling.[174]

Management of Secondary Complications
Rebleeding
Multiple clinical trials have demonstrated that antifibrinolytic agents such as ε-aminocaproic acid and tranexamic acid reduce the risk of rebleeding, but this benefit is offset by an increased incidence of vasospasm and hydrocephalus.[175,176] With the advent of early surgery and endovascular treatment, the use of these agents has declined dramatically. A shorter course of antifibrinolytic therapy while awaiting surgery or endovascular treatment (before the risk period for vasospasm begins) has been suggested, but it appears that the negative effects persist.[177]

Initial management directed at the prevention of rebleeding includes avoiding situations that produce sudden changes in the transmural pressure across the wall of the aneurysm (i.e., sudden increases in arterial or venous pressure or decreases in ICP). Patients are placed on bed rest with minimal stimulation. In an agitated patient, sedation is indicated, though care must be taken to preserve the ability to assess the patient's responsiveness to stimulation. Opiates are a good choice for sedation because they also provide analgesia for headache. Because of the risk of impairing the ability to evaluate for clinical deterioration, long-acting sedative agents such as phenobarbital should be avoided. Measures should be taken to minimize cough and Valsalva's maneuvers. In intubated patients, repositioning of the endotracheal tube, suctioning, and antitussive agents (codeine, lidocaine) may be needed. Stool softeners are administered to avoid straining. If lumbar puncture or ventriculostomy is performed, rapid drainage of a large volume of cerebrospinal fluid should be avoided so as not to induce sudden changes in the transmural pressure.

Definitive prevention of rebleeding is accomplished by obliteration of the aneurysm, as described earlier. This should be performed as soon as possible.

Hydrocephalus
The decision to treat hydrocephalus is usually based on the CT appearance of enlarging ventricles in a patient whose level of consciousness is deteriorating to the point of obtundation. Upon placement of a ventriculostomy, the cerebrospinal fluid pressure is reduced slowly to lessen the risk of aneurysm rerupture. Cerebrospinal fluid drainage via ventriculostomy may be needed for many days to clear intraventricular blood before it can be determined whether a permanent shunt is required.

Vasospasm
Prevention. Routine measures to prevent or ameliorate the effects of vasospasm include mechanical removal of subarachnoid blood at the time of aneurysm surgery, administration of the centrally acting calcium channel antagonist nimodipine, and avoidance of intravascular volume contraction (see earlier) and hypotension. Nimodipine treatment (60 mg orally every 4 hours) for 3 weeks after SAH reduces the impact of symptomatic vasospasm and improves outcome.[178-181] It is not clear whether this beneficial effect is due to action on the cerebral vessels or prevention of calcium influx into ischemic

neurons. Hypotension that develops with nimodipine administration can usually be managed with fluids or by adjusting the dosage schedule to 30 mg every 2 hours. In patients receiving hemodynamic augmentation for symptomatic vasospasm, it may be difficult to maintain blood pressure goals following nimodipine administration.

Treatment of Delayed Ischemic Deficits. Because of the disparity in the incidence of vasospasm detected angiographically, by transcranial Doppler, and clinically, there is disagreement about the management of vasospasm when it is detected. Although the aggressive management of clinical vasospasm with hemodynamic augmentation and endovascular maneuvers to open constricted vessels is widely accepted, there is dispute over how aggressive to be in an asymptomatic patient with vasospasm detected by transcranial Doppler or angiography.

Hemodynamic Augmentation. Treatment of symptomatic vasospasm in patients with surgically clipped aneurysms begins with hemodynamic augmentation, in which blood volume and cardiac output are optimized with fluids, and blood pressure is increased by the administration of vasoactive agents to enhance CBF and prevent cerebral infarction.[182,183] The initial step is to rapidly correct hypovolemia with isotonic crystalloid or colloid. No data exist to indicate that hypervolemia is more beneficial than euvolemia,[184-186] but the potential complications of hypovolemia are clear. Some degree of volume expansion may be helpful in improving cardiac output, but this effect may plateau at pulmonary capillary wedge pressures greater than 14 mm Hg.[187] If there is no immediate response to fluid administration, vasoactive agents are required—either inotropes (dobutamine, dopamine) to improve cardiac output or vasopressors (phenylephrine, norepinephrine) to raise MAP.

It is unclear whether augmenting volume, cardiac output, or MAP is the most efficacious intervention.[185] One approach is to measure pulmonary capillary wedge pressure, cardiac output, and systemic vascular resistance with a Swan-Ganz catheter to titrate hemodynamic management. Use of a Swan-Ganz catheter is also beneficial in patients with cardiac disease to help guide therapy and prevent the congestive heart failure and myocardial ischemia that may complicate hemodynamic augmentation.

Goals for intravascular volume and blood pressure should be defined as a percent change from baseline (beginning with about a 15% change), rather than prespecified levels. Although defining such goals is useful to guide therapy, the degree of hemodynamic augmentation should be titrated continuously to the patient's neurologic status; thus, if a goal is reached but there is no neurologic improvement, the goal should be reassessed. Hemodynamic augmentation is weaned gradually over several days, guided by neurologic status.

Endovascular Treatment. The second strategy involves endovascular treatment of constricted vessels with either balloon angioplasty or intra-arterial infusion of vasodilating agents such as papaverine or nicardipine. Angioplasty on the proximal segments of vasospastic cerebral vessels yields impressive angiographic changes (Fig. 52-9) that appear to be long lasting,[188-191] but clear clinical efficacy has been difficult to establish because the procedure is typically used in conjunction with hemodynamic augmentation. One study suggested that "prophylactic" angioplasty in high-risk patients might reduce the incidence of symptomatic vasospasm.[192] The direct infusion of papaverine and nicardipine into vasospastic vessels has also been used to treat vasospasm. Papaverine produces clear vasodilatation and improvement in global blood flow, but the response is often transient, with

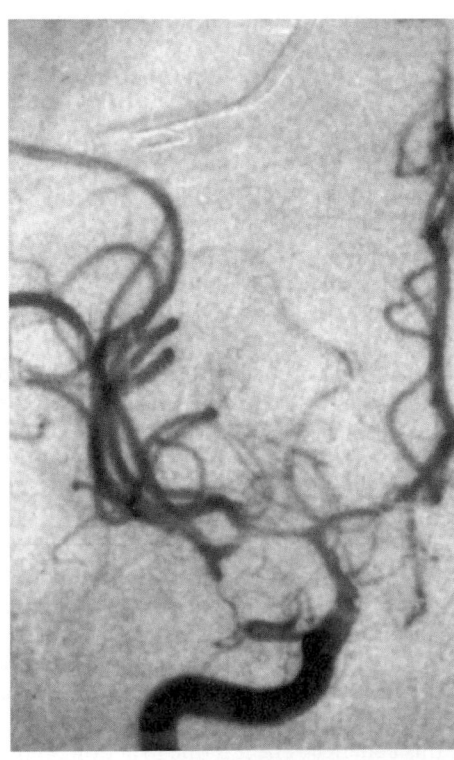 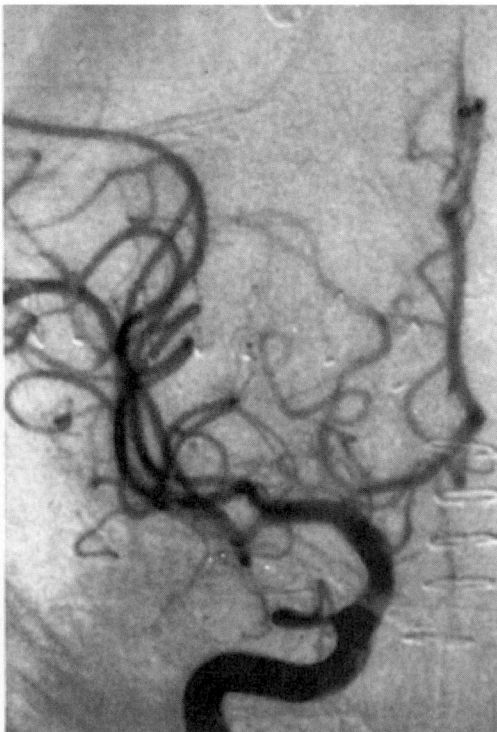

A B

FIGURE 52–9. Severe distal internal carotid and proximal middle cerebral artery vasospasm before (A) and after (B) angioplasty.

vasospasm returning after 24 to 48 hours.[193-195] Multiple treatments are frequently necessary to yield a sustained angiographic effect.

The timing of when to initiate endovascular therapy is debated. It is generally used if, after a few hours, the response to hemodynamic augmentation is inadequate, but it may be the initial therapy in patients with poor cardiac function who are at high risk of complications of hemodynamic augmentation. Potential complications of endovascular treatments include arterial perforation, cerebral infarction, and rebleeding of unprotected aneurysms.

PROGNOSTIC FACTORS AND CAUSES OF MORTALITY

Aneurysmal SAH carries a poor prognosis, with death occurring in 20% to 40% of those who reach medical care. Causes of death are about equally distributed among direct effects of the initial hemorrhage, rebleeding, vasospasm, and medical complications.[161] Overall, less than one third of patients achieve good neurologic recovery. Predictors of poor prognosis include loss of consciousness or poor neurologic condition (i.e., high Hunt-Hess grade) on admission, older age, hypertension, preexisting medical illness, subarachnoid blood 1 mm thick or greater on CT scan (Fisher grade 3), seizures, cerebral edema, aneurysm in the basilar artery, and symptomatic vasospasm.[196-200]

ACKNOWLEDGMENTS

This work was supported by grants from the American Heart Association (96006620) and the National Institutes of Health (NS35966 and 1K23NS044885).

ANNOTATED REFERENCES

Allen GS, Ahn HS, Preziosi TJ, et al: Cerebral arterial spasm—a controlled trial of nimodipine in patients with subarachnoid hemorrhage. N Engl J Med 1983;308:619-624.

This prospective, multicenter, randomized trial demonstrated that administration of the calcium channel blocker nimodipine within 96 hours of SAH was well tolerated and reduced the severity of ischemic neurologic deficits associated with vasospasm.

Brott T, Broderick J, Kothari R, et al: Early hemorrhage growth in patients with intracerebral hemorrhage. Stroke 1997;28:1-5.

This prospective observational study demonstrated that hematoma growth occurs in more than one third of patients with ICH within the first few hours of symptom onset and is associated with clinical deterioration.

Hankey GJ, Hon C: Surgery for primary intracerebral hemorrhage: Is it safe and effective? A systematic review of case series and randomized trials. Stroke 1997;28:2126-2132.

This meta-analysis of randomized controlled trials of surgical hematoma evacuation in primary ICH found a nonsignificant increase in the odds of death or dependency in patients treated surgically relative to those managed medically.

Kassell NF, Sasaki T, Colohan AR, Nazar G: Cerebral vasospasm following aneurysmal subarachnoid hemorrhage. Stroke 1985;16:562-572.

This review article summarizes the available data on the diagnosis, theories of pathogenesis, pathophysiology, and treatment of SAH-induced cerebral vasospasm.

Molyneux A, Kerr R, Stratton I, et al: International Subarachnoid Aneurysm Trial (ISAT) of neurosurgical clipping versus endovascular coiling in 2143 patients with ruptured intracranial aneurysms: A randomised trial. Lancet 2002;360:1267-1274.

This prospective, multicenter, randomized trial evaluated the efficacy of surgical aneurysm clipping versus endovascular treatment by detachable platinum coils in patients with acutely ruptured intracranial aneurysms deemed equally amenable to either treatment. In this carefully selected population, with follow-up limited to 1 year, treatment with coils resulted in better outcome.

III

353

Chapter 53

SEIZURES IN THE CRITICALLY ILL

Sarice L. Bassin • Thomas P. Bleck

KEY POINTS

1. Although conventional definitions of status epilepticus have used a cutoff of 30 or 60 minutes of sustained seizure duration, or discrete seizures without recovery, clinicians should recognize that most seizures will terminate spontaneously within a few minutes. Therefore, seizures that persist longer than 5 to 7 minutes should probably be treated as status epilepticus.

2. Patients begin to awaken within 15 to 20 minutes after the successful termination of status epilepticus; many regain consciousness much faster. Patients who do not start to awaken after 20 minutes should be assumed to have entered nonconvulsive status epilepticus. Nonconvulsive status epilepticus demands emergency treatment guided by electroencephalographic monitoring to prevent further cerebral damage, since there are no clinical criteria to indicate whether therapy is effective.

3. Observation is the most important activity to perform when a patient has a single seizure. This is the time to collect evidence of a partial onset to implicate structural brain disease. The postictal examination is similarly valuable; language, motor, sensory, or reflex abnormalities after an apparently generalized seizure are evidence of focal pathology.

4. In contrast to the patient with a single or a few seizures, the status epilepticus patient requires concomitant diagnostic and therapeutic efforts. Although 30 minutes of continuous or recurrent seizure activity usually define status epilepticus, one should not stand by waiting for this period to pass to start treatment. Since most seizures in critically ill patients stop within 2 to 3 minutes, it is reasonable to start treatment after 5 minutes of continuous seizure activity or after the second or third seizure occurs without recovery between the spells.

5. Electroencephalographic monitoring after control of convulsive status epilepticus can be essential in directing the course of treatment.

6. The intensive care unit patient with central nervous system disease who has even one seizure should usually be given chronic anticonvulsant therapy, and this approach should be reviewed before the patient is discharged. Initiating this treatment after the first *unprovoked* seizure may help prevent subsequent epilepsy. In the intensive care unit setting, phenytoin is frequently selected because of its ease of administration and lack of sedative effects.

7. The conventional agents used in the first-line of treatment of status epilepticus are the benzodiazepines (especially lorazepam, diazepam, and midazolam), phenytoin, and phenobarbital. Status epilepticus that is refractory to the traditional agents is treated with continuous infusions of the short-acting barbiturates, midazolam, or propofol.

Seizures complicate the course of about 3% of adult intensive care unit (ICU) patients admitted for non-neurologic conditions. The medical and economic impact of these seizures confers importance on them out of proportion to their incidence. A seizure is often the first indication of a central nervous system (CNS) complication, and delay in recognition and treatment of seizure is associated with an increased risk of mortality[2]; thus, the rapid diagnosis of this disorder is mandatory. In addition, since epilepsy affects 2% of the population, patients with preexisting seizures occasionally enter the ICU for treatment of other problems. Since the initial treatment of these patients is the province of the intensivist, he or she must be familiar with seizure management as it affects the critically ill patient. Patients developing status epilepticus often require a critical care specialist in addition to a neurologist.

Seizures have been recognized at least since Hippocratic times, but their relatively high rate of occurrence in critically ill patients has only recently been appreciated. Seizures complicating critical care treatments (e.g., lidocaine use) are also a recent phenomenon. Early attempts at treatment included bromides[3] and morphine[4] as well as ice applications. Barbiturates were first employed in 1912, and phenytoin in 1937.[5] Paraldehyde was popular in the next two decades.[6] More recently, emphasis has shifted to the benzodiazepines, which were pioneered in the 1960s.[7] Newer agents for treatment of seizures in critically ill patients include the phenytoin prodrug fosphenytoin, the anesthetic agent propofol, and the water-soluble benzodiazepine midazolam.

Status epilepticus refers to prolonged seizure episodes. Status epilepticus may be the primary indication for admission to the ICU or it may occur in any ICU patient with CNS disease. The definitions employed in studies of status epilepticus have varied substantially. Although conventional definitions of status epilepticus have used a cutoff of 30 or

60 minutes of sustained seizure duration, or discrete seizures without recovery, clinicians should recognize that most seizures terminate spontaneously within a few minutes. Recent data suggest that in only half of patients with seizure episodes lasting 10 to 29 minutes will the seizure self-terminate.[8] Therefore, seizures that persist longer than 5 to 7 minutes should probably be treated as status epilepticus.[9]

EPIDEMIOLOGY

Limited data are available on the epidemiology of seizures in the ICU. A 10-year retrospective study of all ICU patients with seizures at the Mayo Clinic revealed that 7 patients had seizures per 1000 ICU admissions.[10] Our 2-year prospective study of medical ICU patients identified 35 with seizures per 1000 admissions.[11] These two studies are not exactly comparable, as the patient populations and methods of detection differed. A recent series found 8% of comatose patients without clinical signs of seizure activity to be in electrographic status epilepticus.[12]

Up to 34% of hospital in-patients experiencing a seizure die during their hospitalization.[10] Our prospective study of neurologic complications in medical ICU patients showed that having even one seizure while in the ICU for a non-neurologic reason doubled in-hospital mortality.[12] Incidence estimates for generalized convulsive status epilepticus in the United States vary from 50,000 cases per year[13] to 195,000 cases per year.[14] Some portion of this difference can be accounted for by different definitions; however, the latter estimate represents the only population-based data available and may be more accurate. Mortality estimates similarly vary from 1% to 2% in the former study to 22% in the latter. This disagreement follows from a conceptual discordance: the smaller number describes mortality that the authors directly attribute to status epilepticus, whereas the larger figure estimates the overall mortality rate, even though death was frequently caused by the underlying disease rather than by status epilepticus itself. The elderly have an incidence of status epilepticus almost twice that of the general population and the highest associated mortality rate of any age group at 38%.[15]

Table 53-1 summarizes the most common causes of status epilepticus in adults in the community. Almost 50% of the cases were attributed to cerebral vascular disease.[13] Garzon and colleagues[16] found anti-epileptic drug noncompliance

TABLE 53–1. CAUSES OF STATUS EPILEPTICUS IN ADULTS PRESENTING FROM THE COMMUNITY

Prior Seizures	No Prior Seizures
Common	
Subtherapeutic anticonvulsant	Ethanol-related
Ethanol-related	Drug toxicity
Intractable epilepsy	CNS infection
	Head trauma
	CNS tumor
Less Common	
CNS infection	Metabolic aberration
Metabolic aberration	Stroke
Drug toxicity	
Stroke	
CNS tumor	
Head trauma	

CNS, central nervous system.

as the main cause of status epilepticus in patients with a prior history of epilepsy, and CNS infection, stroke, and metabolic disturbances predominated in the group without previous seizures.

Three major factors determine outcome in patients with status epilepticus: the type of status epilepticus, its cause, and its duration. Generalized convulsive status epilepticus has the worst prognosis for neurologic recovery; myoclonic status epilepticus following an anoxic episode carries a very poor prognosis for survival. Complex partial status epilepticus can produce limbic system damage, usually manifested as a memory disturbance. Causes associated with increased mortality included anoxia, intracranial hemorrhages, tumors, infections, and trauma. The mortality of patients with nonconvulsive status epilepticus has been reported as high as 33%[17] and correlates with the underlying cause, severe impairment of mental status, and the development of acute complications, especially respiratory failure and infection.[18] Data strongly suggest that prolonged seizure duration is a negative prognostic factor. A study of 253 adult status epilepticus patients demonstrated a 30-day mortality rate of 2.7% in patients with seizures lasting 30 to 59 minutes, compared with 32% in those with seizures of 60 minutes or longer.[19]

Limited data are available concerning the functional abilities of generalized convulsive status epilepticus survivors, and no data reliably permit a distinction between the effects of status epilepticus and effects of its causes. One review concluded that intellectual ability declined as a consequence of status epilepticus.[20] Survivors of status epilepticus frequently seem to have memory and behavioral disorders out of proportion to the structural damage produced by the cause of their seizures. Case reports of severe memory deficits following prolonged complex partial status epilepticus have been published.[21] Conversely, one prospective study of 180 children with febrile status epilepticus demonstrated no deaths and no cases of new cognitive or motor handicap.[22] Experimental animal[23] and human epidemiologic[24] studies suggest that status epilepticus may be a risk factor in the development of future seizures. Whether treatment of prolonged seizures reduces the risk of subsequent epilepsy remains uncertain.

CLASSIFICATION

The most frequently used classification scheme is that of the International League Against Epilepsy (Table 53-2).[25] This scheme allows classification on clinical criteria without inferring cause. *Simple partial seizures* start focally in the cerebral cortex, without invading other structures. The patient is aware throughout the episode and appears otherwise unchanged. Bilateral limbic dysfunction produces a *complex partial seizure*; awareness and ability to interact are diminished (but may not be completely abolished). *Automatisms* (movements that a patient makes without awareness) may occur. *Secondary generalization* results from invasion by epileptic electrical activity of the other hemisphere or subcortical structures.

Primary generalized seizures arise from the cerebral cortex and diencephalon at the same time; no focal phenomena are visible, and consciousness is lost at the onset. *Absence seizures* are frequently confined to childhood; they consist of the abrupt onset of a blank stare that usually lasts 5 to 15 seconds, after which the patient abruptly returns to normal. *Atypical absence seizures* occur in children with the Lennox-Gastaut

TABLE 53–2. INTERNATIONAL CLASSIFICATION OF EPILEPTIC SEIZURES

I. Partial seizures (seizures beginning locally)
  A. Simple partial seizures (consciousness not impaired; simple partial seizures)
    1. with motor symptoms
    2. with somatosensory or special sensory symptoms
    3. with autonomic symptoms
    4. with psychic symptoms
  B. Complex partial seizures (with impairment of consciousness; complex partial seizures)
    1. beginning as simple partial seizures and progressing to impairment of consciousness
      a. without automatisms
      b. with automatisms
    2. with impairment of consciousness at onset
      a. with no other features
      b. with features of simple partial seizures
      c. with automatisms
  C. Partial seizures (simple or complex), secondarily generalized
II. Primary generalized seizures (bilaterally symmetric, without localized onset)
  A. Absence seizures
    1. true absence ("petit mal")
    2. atypical absence
  B. Myoclonic seizures
  C. Clonic seizures
  D. Tonic seizures
  E. Tonic-clonic seizures ("grand mal")
  F. Atonic seizures
III. Unclassified seizures

Adapted from Bleck TP: Status epilepticus. In Klawans HL, Goetz CG, Tanner CM (eds): Textbook of Clinical Neuropharmacology, 2nd ed. New York, Raven Press, 1992, pp 65-73.

TABLE 53–3. CLINICAL CLASSIFICATION OF STATUS EPILEPTICUS

I. Generalized seizures
  A. Generalized convulsive status epilepticus
    1. Primary generalized status epilepticus
      a. tonic-clonic status epilepticus
      b. myoclonic status epilepticus
      c. clonic-tonic-clonic status epilepticus
    2. Secondarily generalized status epilepticus
      a. partial seizure with secondary generalization
      b. tonic status epilepticus
  B. Nonconvulsive status epilepticus
    1. absence status epilepticus (petit mal status)
    2. atypical absence status epilepticus (e.g., in the Lennox-Gastaut syndrome)
    3. atonic status epilepticus
    4. nonconvulsive status epilepticus as a sequel of partially treated generalized convulsive status epilepticus
II. Partial status epilepticus
  A. Simple partial status epilepticus
    1. typical
    2. epilepsia partialis continua
  B. Complex partial status epilepticus
III. Neonatal status epilepticus

Adapted from Lothman EW: The biochemical basis and pathophysiology of status epilepticus. Neurology 1990;40(Suppl 2):13-23.

syndrome. *Myoclonic seizures* start with brief synchronous jerks, without alteration of consciousness initially followed by a generalized convulsion. They frequently occur in patients with genetic epilepsy; in the ICU, they commonly follow anoxia or metabolic disturbances.[26] *Tonic-clonic seizures* start with tonic extension, evolve to bilaterally synchronous clonus, and conclude with a postictal phase. Clinical judgment is required to apply this system in the ICU. In patients in whom consciousness has already been altered by drugs, hypotension, sepsis, or intracranial pathologic lesion, the nature of partial seizures may be difficult to classify.

Status epilepticus is classified by a similar system that has been altered to match observable clinical phenomena (Table 53–3).[27] Generalized convulsive status epilepticus is the most common type encountered in the ICU and poses the greatest risk to the patient. It may either be primarily generalized, as in the drug-intoxicated patient, or secondarily generalized, as in the brain abscess patient who develops generalized convulsive status epilepticus. *Nonconvulsive status epilepticus* in the ICU frequently follows partially treated generalized convulsive status epilepticus. Some practitioners use the term for all cases of status epilepticus that involve altered consciousness without convulsive movements; this blurs the distinctions among absence status epilepticus, partially treated generalized convulsive status epilepticus, and complex partial status epilepticus, which have different causes and treatments. *Epilepsia partialis continua* (a special form of partial status epilepticus in which repetitive movements affect a small area of the body) sometimes continues for months or years.

The International League Against Epilepsy continues to work toward revising and updating the current classification system. The goal is a multi-axis diagnostic scheme that incorporates anatomic, etiologic, therapeutic, and prognostic implications. For the most recent information regarding this ongoing project, refer to *www.epilepsy.org.*[28]

PATHOGENESIS AND PATHOPHYSIOLOGY

The causes and effects of status epilepticus at the cellular, brain, and systemic levels are interrelated, but their individual analysis is useful for understanding them and their therapeutic implications. The ionic events of a seizure follow the opening of ion channels coupled to excitatory amino acid receptors. From the standpoint of the intensivist, three channels are particularly important because their activation may raise intracellular free calcium to toxic concentrations: alpha-amino-3-hydroxy-5-methyl-4-isoxazole propionic acid (AMPA), *N*-methyl-D-aspartate (NMDA), and metabotropic channels. These excitatory amino acid systems are crucial for learning and memory. Many drugs that block these systems are available but are too toxic for chronic use. Counter-regulatory ionic events are triggered by the epileptiform discharge as well, such as the activation of inhibitory interneurons, which suppress excited neurons via GABA$_A$ synapses.

The cellular effects of excessive excitatory amino acid channel activity include (1) the generation of toxic concentrations of intracellular free calcium; (2) activation of autolytic enzyme systems; (3) production of oxygen free radicals; (4) generation of nitric oxide, which both enhances subsequent excitation and serves as a toxin; (5) phosphorylation of enzyme and receptor systems, making seizures more likely; and (6) an increase in intracellular osmolality, which produces neuronal swelling. If adenosine triphosphate production fails, then membrane ion-exchange ceases and neurons swell further. These events produce the neuronal damage associated with status epilepticus. Longer status epilepticus duration produces more profound alterations and an increasing likelihood of permanence and of becoming refractory to treatment.[29] The processes involved in a single seizure and the transition to status epilepticus have been reviewed.[30]

Many other biophysical and biochemical alterations occur during and after status epilepticus. The intense neuronal activity activates immediate-early genes and produces heat shock proteins, providing indications of the deleterious effects of status epilepticus and insight into the mechanisms of neuronal protection.[31] The mechanisms by which status epilepticus damages the nervous system have been reviewed.[32] Absence status epilepticus is an exception among these conditions; it consists of rhythmically increased inhibition and does not produce clinical or pathologic abnormalities.

The electrical phenomena of status epilepticus at the whole brain level, as seen in the scalp electroencephalogram (EEG), reflect the seizure type that initiates status epilepticus (e.g., absence status epilepticus begins with a 3-Hz wave-and-spike pattern). During status epilepticus, this rhythm slows, but the wave-and-spike characteristic remains. Generalized convulsive status epilepticus goes through a sequence of electrographic changes (Table 53-4).[33] The initial discharge becomes less well formed, implying that neuronal firing loses synchrony. The sustained depolarizations that characterize status epilepticus alter the extracellular milieu, most importantly by raising extracellular potassium. The excess potassium ejected during status epilepticus exceeds the buffering ability of astrocytes.

The increased cellular activity of status epilepticus elevates demand for oxygen and glucose, and cerebral blood flow initially increases. After approximately 20 minutes, however, energy supplies are exhausted, causing local catabolism to support ion pumps (in an attempt to restore the internal milieu); this is a major cause of epileptic brain damage. In addition to damaging the CNS, generalized convulsive status epilepticus produces life-threatening systemic effects.[34] Excess secretion of epinephrine and cortisol cause systemic and pulmonary arterial pressures to rise dramatically at seizure onset and also produce hyperglycemia. Muscular work raises blood lactate levels. Both airway obstruction and abnormal diaphragmatic contractions impair respiration. Carbon dioxide excretion falls while its production increases markedly. Muscular work accelerates heat production, raising core body temperature.

The combined respiratory and metabolic acidoses frequently reduce the arterial blood pH to 6.9 or lower. The acidemia may produce hyperkalemia; in addition to its deleterious effects on cardiac electrophysiology, the elevated extracellular potassium level helps propagate seizure activity. Coupled with hypoxemia and the elevation of circulating catecholamine concentrations, these conditions rarely can produce cardiac arrest. This sequence probably accounts for some cases of epileptic sudden death; neurogenic pulmonary edema is the likely cause of many others. The severity of the acidosis may prompt consideration of bicarbonate administration. When this is attempted, however, the likelihood of the occurrence of pulmonary edema is inordinately high. Rapid termination of seizure activity is the most appropriate treatment; the restitution of ventilation and the metabolism of lactate quickly restore a normal pH.

After approximately 30 minutes of continuous convulsions, motor activity may diminish while electrographic seizures persist. Hypotension and hyperthermia ensue, and gluconeogenesis can fail, resulting in hypoglycemia. Generalized convulsive status epilepticus patients often aspirate oral or gastric contents, producing chemical pneumonitis or bacterial pneumonia. Rhabdomyolysis is common and may lead to renal failure. Compression fractures, joint dislocations, and tendon avulsions are other serious sequelae.

The mechanisms that terminate seizure activity are poorly understood. The leading candidates are inhibitory mechanisms, primarily GABA-ergic interneurons and inhibitory thalamic neurons.

CLINICAL MANIFESTATIONS

Three problems complicate seizure recognition: (1) the occurrence of complex partial seizures in the setting of impaired awareness, (2) the occurrence of seizures in patients receiving pharmacologically induced paralysis and/or sedation, and (3) misinterpretation of other abnormal movements as seizures. ICU patients often have depressed consciousness in the absence of seizures owing to their disease, its complications (such as hepatic[35] or septic[36] encephalopathy), or drug administration. A further decline in alertness may reflect a seizure; an EEG is required to confirm that one has occurred.

Patients receiving neuromuscular junction blocking agents do not manifest the usual signs of seizures. Patients with increased intracranial pressure (ICP) from primary brain injury, hepatic encephalopathy, or other critical illnesses may be both paralyzed and sedated, making identification of seizures particularly challenging. Tachycardia, tachypnea, and hypertension are signs of seizure that can be misinterpreted as evidence of inadequate sedation. Continuous EEG monitoring is warranted in this population if seizures are suspected.

Patients with metabolic disturbances, anoxia, and other types of nervous system injury may demonstrate abnormal movements that can be confused with seizure. Asterixis is a brief asynchronous loss of tone at the wrist or hip joints that

Stage	Typical Clinical Manifestations*	Electroencephalographic Features
1	Tonic-clonic convulsions; hypertension and hyperglycemia common	Discrete seizures with interictal slowing
2	Low or medium amplitude clonic activity, with rare convulsions	Waxing and waning of ictal discharges
3	Slight but frequent clonic activity, often confined to the eyes, face, or hands	Continuous ictal discharges
4	Rare episodes of slight clonic activity; hypotension and hypoglycemia become manifest	Continuous ictal discharges punctuated by flat periods
5	Coma without other manifestations of seizure activity	Periodic epileptiform discharges on a flat background

TABLE 53–4. ELECTROGRAPHIC-CLINICAL CORRELATIONS IN GENERALIZED CONVULSIVE STATUS EPILEPTICUS

*The clinical manifestations may vary considerably, depending on the underlying neuropathophysiologic process (and its anatomy), systemic diseases, and medications. In particular, stages of the electrographic progression may be sufficiently brief to be overlooked. Partially treating status epilepticus may dissociate the clinical and electrographic features.
Data from Treiman DM: Generalized convulsive status epilepticus in the adult. Epilepsia 1993;34(Suppl 1):S2-S11.

can appear in the setting of hepatic dysfunction. Stimulus-sensitive massive myoclonus after anoxia can be dramatic but usually self-abates in a few days. Controversy exists as to the epileptic origin of this disorder, and post-anoxic myoclonus has been reported in the presence of almost total cortical suppression.[37] Brain-injured patients may manifest paroxysmal episodes of sympathetic hyperactivity and associated rigidity or decerebrate posturing. These "hypothalamic seizures" can sometimes be distinguished from epileptic seizures with observation. Patients with tetanus are awake during their spasms and flex rather than extend their arms as seizure patients do. Psychiatric disturbances in the ICU occasionally resemble complex partial seizures. If doubt about the nature of abnormal movements persists, an EEG should be obtained.

The manifestations of status epilepticus depend on the type and, for partial status epilepticus, the cortical area of abnormality. Table 53-3 presents the types of status epilepticus encountered and focuses on those seen most frequently in the ICU.

Primary generalized convulsive status epilepticus begins as tonic extension of the trunk and extremities without preceding focal activity. No aura is reported and consciousness is immediately lost. After several seconds of tonic extension, the extremities start to vibrate; clonic (rhythmic) extension of the extremities quickly follows. This phase wanes in intensity over a few minutes. The patient may then repeat the cycle of tonus followed by clonic movements, or continue to have intermittent bursts of clonic activity without recovery. *Myoclonic status epilepticus* (bursts of myoclonic jerks that increase in intensity and lead to a generalized convulsion) is a less common form of generalized convulsive status epilepticus that is usually associated with anoxic coma.

Secondarily generalized status epilepticus begins with a partial seizure and progresses to a convulsive activity. The initial focal clinical activity may be overlooked. This seizure type implies a structural lesion, so care must be taken to elicit evidence of lateralized movements.

Of the several forms of generalized nonconvulsive status epilepticus, the one of greatest importance to intensivists is nonconvulsive status epilepticus as a sequela of inadequately treated generalized convulsive status epilepticus. When a patient with generalized convulsive status epilepticus is treated with anticonvulsants in inadequate doses, visible convulsive activity may stop, but the electrochemical seizure continues. Patients begin to awaken within 15 to 20 minutes after the successful termination of status epilepticus; many regain consciousness much faster. Patients who do not start to awaken after 20 minutes should be assumed to have entered nonconvulsive status epilepticus. Careful observation may disclose slight clonic activity. Nonconvulsive status epilepticus is an extremely dangerous problem because the destructive effects of status epilepticus continue even without obvious motor activity. Nonconvulsive status epilepticus demands emergency treatment guided by EEG monitoring to prevent further cerebral damage since there are no clinical criteria to indicate whether therapy is effective.

Failure to recognize nonconvulsive status epilepticus is common in patients presenting with nonspecific neurobehavioral abnormalities, such as delirium, lethargy, bizarre behavior, cataplexy, or mutism.[38] Patients may present in nonconvulsive status epilepticus without an inciting episode of generalized convulsive status epilepticus. A high suspicion for this disorder should be maintained in patients with unexplained alteration in level of consciousness or cognition admitted to the ICU.

Partial status epilepticus in ICU patients often follows a stroke or occurs with the rapid expansion of brain masses. Clonic motor activity is most easily recognized, but the seizure takes on the characteristics of adjacent functional tissue. Therefore, somatosensory or special sensory manifestations occur, and the ICU patient may be unable to report such symptoms. *Aphasic status epilepticus* occurs when a seizure begins in a language area and may resemble a stroke. *Epilepsia partialis continua* involves repetitive movements confined to a small region of the body. It may be seen with nonketotic hyperglycemia[39] or with focal brain disease; anticonvulsant treatment is seldom useful. *Complex partial status epilepticus* manifests with diminished awareness. The diagnosis often comes as a surprise when an EEG is obtained.

DIAGNOSTIC APPROACH

When an ICU patient has a seizure, one has a natural tendency to try to stop the event. This leads to both diagnostic obscuration and iatrogenic complications. Beyond protecting the patient from harm, very little can be done rapidly to influence the course of the seizure. Padded tongue blades, or similar items, should not be placed in the mouth; they are more likely to obstruct the airway than to preserve it. The seizures of most patients stop before any medication can reach the brain in an effective concentration.

Observation is the most important activity to perform when a patient has a single seizure. This is the time to collect evidence of a partial onset to implicate structural brain disease. The postictal examination is similarly valuable; language, motor, sensory, or reflex abnormalities after an apparently generalized seizure are evidence of focal pathology.

Seizures in ICU patients have several potential causes that must be investigated. Drugs are a major cause of ICU seizures, especially in the setting of diminished renal or hepatic function or when the blood-brain barrier is breached. Theophylline frequently produces seizures or status epilepticus if it has been rapidly loaded or if high concentrations of the drug occur; occasionally, however, these complications arise at "therapeutic" levels. Imipenem-cilastatin[40] and fluoroquinolones[41] have substantial potential to lower the seizure threshold, especially in patients with renal dysfunction. They should be avoided if possible in patients already at risk for seizure. Other antibiotics, especially beta-lactams, are occasionally implicated.[42] Sevoflurane, a volatile anesthetic agent, is dose-dependently epileptogenic in patients with no predisposition to seizures.[43]

Recreational drugs are frequently overlooked offenders in patients presenting to the ICU. Acute cocaine or methamphetamine intoxication is characterized by a state of hypersympathetic activity followed by seizures.[44] Although ethanol withdrawal is a common cause of seizures, discontinuing any hypnosedative agent may prompt convulsions 1 to 3 days later. One report suggests that narcotic withdrawal may produce seizures in the critically ill.[10] In the absence of other clear causes for seizure, complete toxicologic screening should be performed.

Serum glucose, electrolyte concentrations, and serum osmolality should also be measured. Nonketotic hyperglycemia[45,46] and hyponatremia can precipitate both focal and generalized seizures. Seizure activity may infrequently be the first presenting sign of diabetes mellitus. However, hypocalcemia rarely causes seizures beyond the neonatal period; its identification on analysis must *not* signal the end of the diagnostic work-up. Hypomagnesemia has an equally unwarranted reputation as the cause of seizures in malnourished alcoholic patients.

The physical examination should emphasize assessment for both global and focal abnormalities of the CNS. Evidence of cardiovascular disease or systemic infection should be sought and the skin and fundi examined closely.

The need for imaging studies in these patients has been an area of uncertainty. A prospective study of neurologic complications in medical ICU patients determined that 38 of 61 patients (62%) had a vascular, infectious, or neoplastic explanation for their seizures.[11] Hence, head computed

tomography or magnetic resonance imaging should be performed on ICU patients with new seizures. With current technology, there are almost no patients who cannot undergo computed tomography scanning. Magnetic resonance imaging is particularly helpful in detecting evidence of acute ischemic stroke and encephalitis. Magnetic resonance imaging cannot be performed on patients with pacemakers. Many ICP monitor catheters are compatible with magnetic resonance imaging, provided the device is not coiled when it is secured to the scalp. Patients who need cerebrospinal fluid analysis always require imaging of the brain first. When CNS infection is suspected, empirical antibiotic treatment should be started while these studies are being performed.

Electroencephalography is a vital diagnostic tool for evaluating the seizure patient. Partial seizures usually show EEG

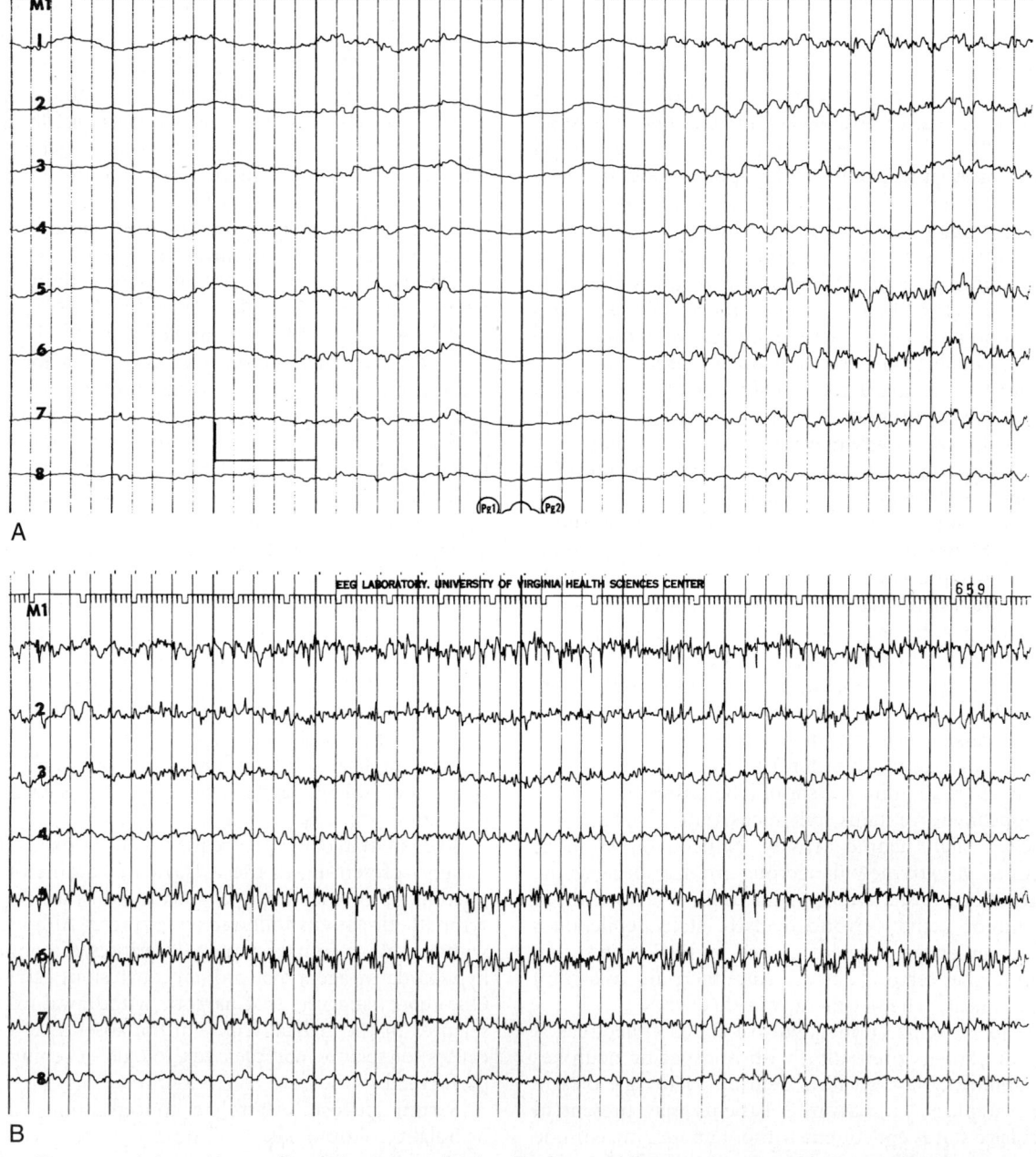

FIGURE 53–1. Electroencephalographic recording during status epilepticus. The first panel illustrates the onset of the seizure; the subsequent panels show its evolution. Montage: longitudinal bipolar; channels 1-4, left temporal, and channels 5-8, left parasagittal. Calibration: vertical, 50 μv; horizontal, 1 sec.

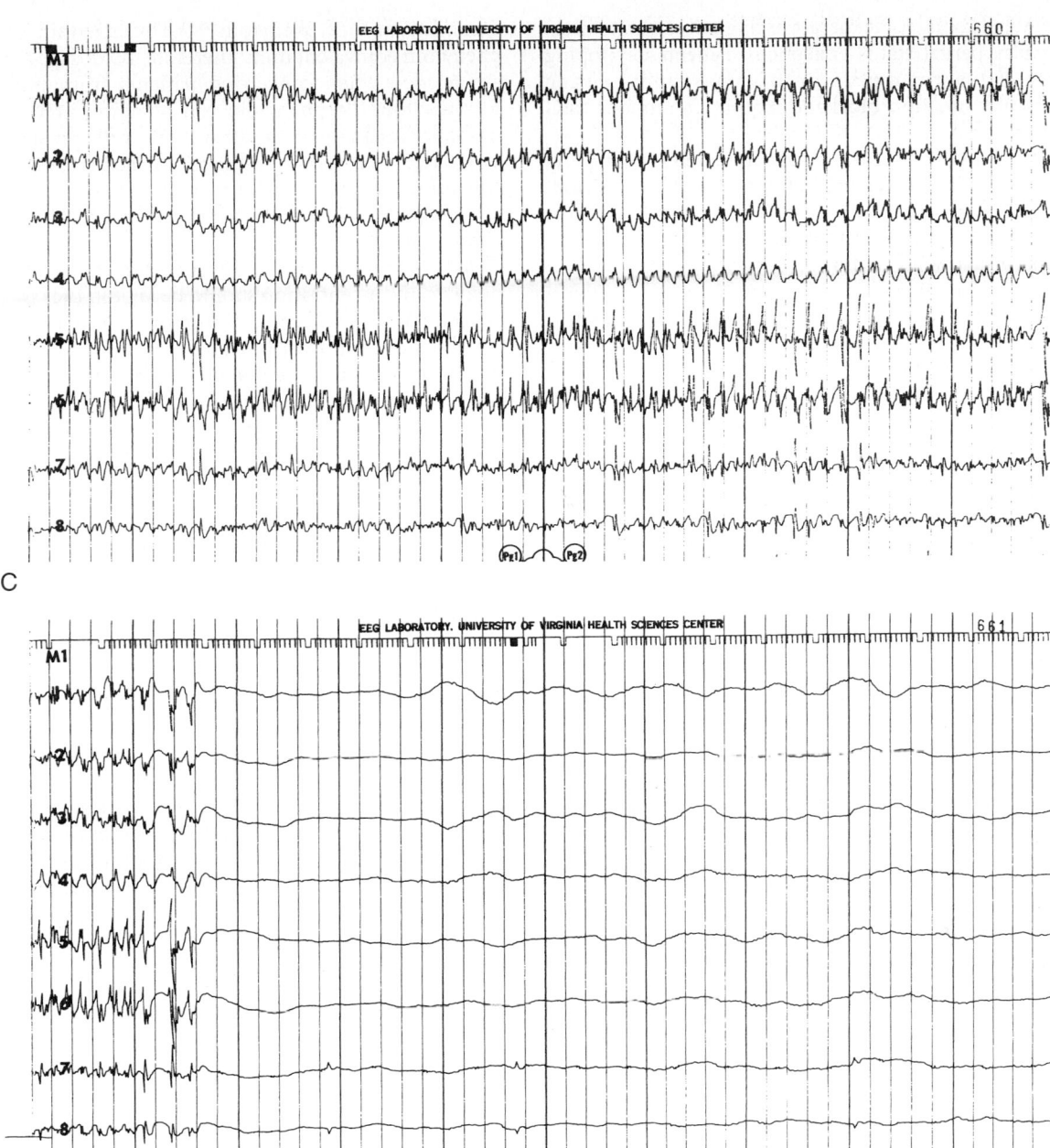

C

D

FIGURE 53–1.—cont'd

abnormalities that begin in the area of cortex that produces seizures. Primary generalized seizures appear to start over the entire cortex simultaneously. Postictal slowing or depressed amplitude provides clues as to the focal cause of the seizures, and epileptiform activity helps to classify the type of seizure and to guide treatment. An emergency EEG is necessary to exclude nonconvulsive status epilepticus in those patients who do not begin to awaken soon after seizures have apparently been controlled (Fig. 53-1).

In contrast to the patient with a single or a few seizures, the status epilepticus patient requires concomitant diagnostic and therapeutic efforts. Although 30 minutes of continuous or recurrent seizure activity usually define status epilepticus, one should not stand by waiting for this period to pass to start treatment. Since most seizures in critically ill patients stop within 2 to 3 minutes, it is reasonable to start treatment after 5 minutes of continuous seizure activity or after the second or third seizure occurs without recovery between the spells.

Treatment for status epilepticus should not be delayed to obtain an EEG. However, a prospective evaluation of 164 patients demonstrated that nearly half manifested persistent electrographic seizures in the 24 hours after clinical control of convulsive status epilepticus.[47] These data suggest that EEG monitoring after control of convulsive status epilepticus can be essential in directing the course of treatment. A variety of findings may be present on the EEG, depending on the type of status epilepticus and its duration (see Table 53-4). Complex partial status epilepticus patients are often without such organized discharges of generalized convulsive status epilepticus; instead, they have waxing and waning rhythmic activity in one or several brain regions. A diagnostic trial of intravenous benzodiazepine therapy is often necessary to diagnose complex partial status epilepticus. Patients developing refractory status epilepticus or having seizures during neuromuscular junction blockade require continuous EEG monitoring.

The availability of continuous paperless EEG monitoring allows for detection of seizure activity over a long period. Subclinical seizures have been observed to occur in patients receiving aggressive treatment for status epilepticus and even in patients treated with barbiturates to a burst-suppression EEG pattern. The clinical significance of these subclinical seizures, and their effect on prognosis, remains uncertain.

MANAGEMENT APPROACH

TREATING ISOLATED SEIZURES

Making the decision to administer anticonvulsants to an ICU patient who experiences one or a few seizures requires consideration of a provisional cause, estimation of the likelihood of recurrence, and recognition of the utility and limitations of anticonvulsants. For example, the occurrence of seizures during ethanol withdrawal does not indicate the need for chronic treatment, and giving phenytoin does not prevent further withdrawal convulsions. The patient may need prophylaxis against delirium tremens, but the few seizures themselves seldom require treatment. Patients with convulsions during barbiturate or benzodiazepine withdrawal, in contrast, should usually receive short-term treatment with lorazepam to prevent status epilepticus. Prolonged or frequent seizures caused by metabolic disturbances can be treated temporarily with benzodiazepines while the abnormality is being corrected. Seizures in these settings are notoriously resistant to treatment with phenytoin. In particular, treatment of patients with partial seizures related to nonketotic hyperglycemia should be directed at correction of the hyperglycemia and hypovolemia rather than anticonvulsant therapy.[46]

The ICU patient with CNS disease who has even one seizure should be given chronic anticonvulsant therapy, and this approach should be reviewed before the patient is discharged. Initiating this treatment after the first *unprovoked* seizure may help prevent subsequent epilepsy,[48] although there is considerable difference of opinion regarding this concept.[49] Starting therapy after the first seizure in a critically ill patient at risk for seizure recurrence may be even more important, especially if the patient's condition would be seriously complicated by a convulsion.

In the ICU setting, phenytoin is frequently selected owing to its ease of administration and lack of sedative effects. Hypotension and arrhythmias may complicate intravenous administration and can usually be prevented by slowing the infusion to less than 25 mg/min. Because of the rare occurrence of third-degree atrioventricular block, an external cardiac pacemaker should be available when patients with conduction abnormalities receive intravenous phenytoin. Propylene glycol in the parenteral formulation of phenytoin is the probable cause of these effects. Additionally, the parenteral formulation of phenytoin is alkaline, and this is thought to contribute to pain, burning, and redness at the injection site.

The phenytoin prodrug fosphenytoin is water soluble and its vehicle does not contain propylene glycol; adverse effects are less common with fosphenytoin than with intravenous administration of phenytoin.[50,51] Fosphenytoin is dosed by phenytoin equivalent units; therefore, no dosage adjustments are needed when converting patients from phenytoin to fosphenytoin. Fosphenytoin can be administered by intramuscular injection or by intravenous infusion at a rate of up to 150 mg phenytoin equivalents/min. Fosphenytoin is rapidly converted to phenytoin in vivo, and free phenytoin levels after fosphenytoin administration are not markedly different compared with phenytoin.

Whether phenytoin or fosphenytoin is used, the serum phenytoin concentration should be kept in the "therapeutic" range of 10 to 20 µg/mL (corresponding to an unbound or "free" concentration of 1 to 2 µg/mL), unless further seizures occur; the level can then be increased until signs of toxicity occur. Failure to prevent seizures at a concentration of 25 µg/mL is usually an indication to add phenobarbital to the regimen. When fosphenytoin is administered, phenytoin concentrations should not be measured until the biologic conversion to phenytoin is complete: 2 hours after an intravenous infusion or 4 hours after an intramuscular injection of fosphenytoin.

Phenytoin is approximately 90% protein bound in normal hosts. Patients with renal dysfunction have lower total phenytoin levels at a given dose because the drug is displaced from binding sites, but the unbound level is not affected. Thus, renal failure patients, and perhaps others who are receiving highly protein-bound drugs (which compete for binding), may benefit from determination of free phenytoin level. Only the free fraction is metabolized, so the dose is not altered with changes in renal function. The clearance half-time with normal liver function varies from about 12 to 20 hours (intravenous form) to more than 24 hours (extended-release capsules), so that a new steady-state serum concentration occurs in 3 to 6 days. Phenytoin need not be given more frequently than every 12 hours. Hepatic dysfunction mandates a decrease in the maintenance dose. Hypersensitivity is the major adverse effect of concern to the intensivist. This may manifest itself solely as fever but commonly includes rash and eosinophilia. Adverse reactions to phenytoin and other anticonvulsants have been reviewed elsewhere.[52]

Phenobarbital remains a useful anticonvulsant for patients who are intolerant to phenytoin or who have persistent seizures after adequate phenytoin administration. The target for phenobarbital in the ICU should be a serum concentration of 20 to 40 µg/mL. Hepatic and renal dysfunction alter phenobarbital metabolism. Since its usual clearance half-time is about 96 hours, maintenance doses of this agent should be given once a day. A steady-state level takes about 3 weeks to become established. Sedation is the major adverse effect; allergy to the drug occurs rarely.

Carbamazepine therapy is seldom started in the ICU because its insolubility precludes parenteral formulation. Oral loading in conscious patients may produce coma that lasts several days. This drug also causes hyponatremia in patients who receive it chronically.

TREATING STATUS EPILEPTICUS

Generalized convulsive status epilepticus obviously constitutes a medical emergency; however, nonconvulsive status epilepticus and complex partial status epilepticus are also emergencies but are more difficult to recognize. In each circumstance, one must act quickly to prevent additional cerebral damage.

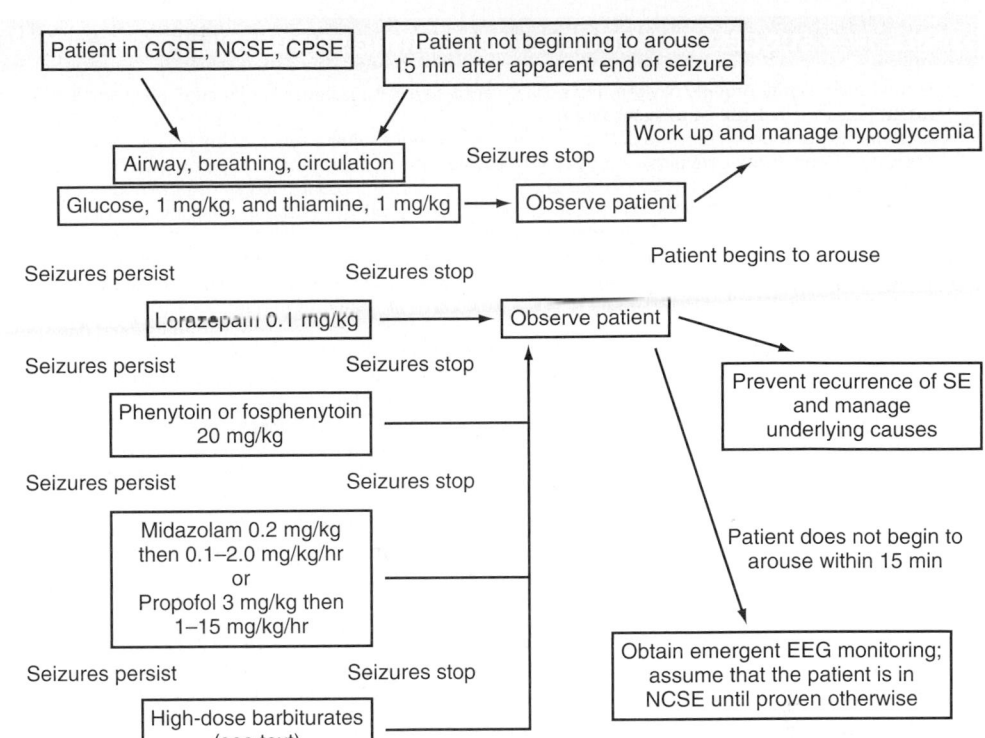

FIGURE 53–2. Management algorithm for status epilepticus. CPSE, complex partial status epilepticus; GSCE, generalized convulsive status epilepticus; NCSE, nonconvulsive status epilepticus; SE, status epilepticus.

Figure 53-2 shows a management algorithm for status epilepticus and Table 53-5 presents a sample management protocol for drug administration.[53] Patients with simple partial status epilepticus or epilepsia partialis continua are at less risk for the development of widespread cerebral damage and are also less likely to respond to the aggressive approach outlined in Table 53-5. In these patients, correcting underlying problems, such as nonketotic hyperosmolar hyperglycemia, is crucial. Errors in terminating status epilepticus include inadequate dosing of effective drugs and continued use of drugs that are ineffective in the patient being treated.

The conventional agents used in the first line of treatment of status epilepticus are the benzodiazepines (especially lorazepam, diazepam, and midazolam), phenytoin, and phenobarbital. Status epilepticus that is refractory to the traditional agents is treated with continuous infusions of the short-acting barbiturates, midazolam, or propofol. A recent multicenter clinical trial comparing lorazepam alone, phenytoin alone, diazepam followed by phenytoin, and phenobarbital alone as the initial drug treatment for generalized convulsive status epilepticus has been reported.[54] In this study, the highest rate of successful treatment of "overt" generalized convulsive status epilepticus was achieved with lorazepam. There was no demonstrable difference among these four drug regimens in the initial treatment of "subtle" generalized convulsive status epilepticus. Lorazepam has been our agent of first choice for terminating status epilepticus for many years and remains so with support from this study.

Advantages of lorazepam over diazepam are its duration of action against status epilepticus (4 to 14 hours as opposed to 20 minutes) and its higher initial response rate. European practitioners often use midazolam or clonazepam initially. In patients in whom intravenous access is difficult to attain, 0.2 mg/kg of midazolam administered intramuscularly will be rapidly and reliably absorbed. The use of midazolam in refractory status will be discussed later. Respiratory depression is the major adverse effect of the benzodiazepines, especially when they are given together with barbiturates or paraldehyde.

Phenytoin is an effective agent in the treatment of status epilepticus; however, the constraint on the rate of intravenous administration is of concern. Phenytoin has a long duration of action when an adequate dose is given (a 20 mg/kg dose produces a serum level above 20 μg/mL for 24 hours). Adding 5 mg/kg if the first 20 mg/kg load fails to stop status epilepticus may be useful. Fosphenytoin can be administered by a more rapid intravenous infusion and has fewer cardiovascular side- effects than phenytoin. Free phenytoin levels reach a therapeutic range 10 to 20 minutes after an infusion of fosphenytoin is started.[55,56] Intramuscular injection of fosphenytoin in patients with status epilepticus may be supported by the known pharmacokinetics of this route, but it should not be considered to be acceptable therapy for status epilepticus and should be reserved for only those rare circumstances in which intravenous access cannot be obtained.

Some practitioners advocate the use of phenobarbital as a first-line drug,[57] but it has typically been used as a third-line agent, after administration of a benzodiazepine and phenytoin.[58] Although this approach has been widely accepted by the neurologic community, we rarely use phenobarbital for two reasons. First, only a small percentage of patients who have failed treatment with two anticonvulsant drugs respond to a third conventional agent[59]; second, at least an additional 20 minutes are required to obtain control in the few patients who do respond. Phenobarbital remains an important drug in the management of simple partial status epilepticus and for those patients who are being weaned from high-dose midazolam or anesthetic barbiturates.

Pentobarbital and thiopental infusions are usually reserved for refractory status epilepticus.[55] Although these drugs are effective in sufficiently large doses, their side effects

TABLE 53–5. SUGGESTED PROTOCOL FOR TREATING STATUS EPILEPTICUS

I. Establish an airway, provide oxygen, and ensure ventilation. If neuromuscular junction blockade is required for intubation, use a short-acting agent (e.g., succinylcholine or vecuronium).

II. Determine blood pressure. If the patient is hypotensive, begin volume replacement or administration of vasoactive agents (or both), as indicated. Generalized convulsive status epilepticus patients who present with hypotension will usually require admission to a critical care unit. Hypertension should not be treated until status epilepticus is controlled, since terminating status epilepticus usually substantially corrects it, and many of the agents used to terminate status epilepticus can produce hypotension.

III. Unless the patient is known to be normo- or hyperglycemic, administer dextrose (1 g/kg) and thiamine (1 mg/kg).

IV. Terminate status epilepticus. The following sequence is recommended (see text for details); be cognizant of the potential of these drugs to eliminate the visible convulsive movements of generalized convulsive status epilepticus when leaving the patient in nonconvulsive status epilepticus. Patients who do not begin to respond to external stimuli 15 minutes after the apparent termination of generalized convulsive status epilepticus should be considered at risk for nonconvulsive status epilepticus and should undergo emergent EEG monitoring.

    A. Give lorazepam, 0.1 mg/kg at a rate of 0.04 mg/kg per min. This drug should be diluted in an equal volume of the solution being used for intravenous infusion, as it is quite viscous. Most adult patients who respond do so by a total administered dose of 8 mg. The latency of effect is debated, but lack of response after 5 minutes should indicate failure.

    B. If status epilepticus persists after lorazepam administration, consider phenytoin at up to 50 mg/min or fosphenytoin 20 mg/kg at up to 150 mg/min (dosed by phenytoin equivalent). Many investigators believe that an additional 5 mg/kg dose of phenytoin equivalent should be administered before the next line of therapy is attempted. However, this step may have more value for the prevention of status epilepticus recurrence than for its initial control.

    C. If status epilepticus persists, administer midazolam 0.2 mg/kg as a bolus, followed by an infusion of 0.1-2.0 mg/kg per hour to achieve seizure control (as determined by EEG monitoring). Intubate the patient at this stage if this has not already been accomplished. A patient reaching this stage should be treated in a critical care unit.

    E. Should the patient's condition not be controlled with midazolam, administer propofol or pentobarbital. Propofol is given as a continuous infusion at a rate of 1-15 mg/kg per hour to achieve seizure control (as determined by EEG monitoring). A bolus dose of propofol (3.0 mg/kg) is often given but may increase the occurrence of hypotension. Pentobarbital is given as a bolus dose of 12 mg/kg at a rate of 0.2-0.4 mg/kg per minute as tolerated, followed by an infusion of 0.25-2.0 mg/kg per hour, as determined by EEG monitoring (with an initial goal of burst-suppression; in some cases, an isoelectric electroencephalogram may be required to eliminate all electrical seizures). Most patients require systemic and pulmonary arterial catheterization, with fluid and vasoactive drug therapy as indicated to maintain blood pressure. Other complications of this treatment are discussed in the text.

V. Prevent recurrence of status epilepticus. The choice of drugs depends greatly on the cause of status epilepticus and the patient's medical and social situation. In general, patients not previously receiving anticonvulsants whose status epilepticus is easily controlled often respond well to chronic treatment with phenytoin or carbamazepine. In contrast, others (e.g., patients with acute encephalitis) will require two or three anticonvulsants at 'toxic' levels (e.g., phenobarbital at greater than 100 µg/mL) to be weaned from midazolam or pentobarbital and may still have occasional seizures.

VI. Treat complications.

    A. Rhabdomyolysis should be treated with a vigorous saline diuresis to prevent acute renal failure; urinary alkalinization may be a useful adjunct. If definitive treatment of generalized convulsive status epilepticus takes longer than expected because of hypotension or arrhythmias, neuromuscular junction blockade under EEG monitoring might be considered.

    B. Hyperthermia usually remits rapidly after termination of status epilepticus. External cooling usually suffices if the core temperature remains elevated. In rare instances, cool peritoneal lavage or extracorporeal blood cooling may be required. High-dose pentobarbital generally produces poikilothermia.

    C. The treatment of cerebral edema occurring secondary to status epilepticus has not been well studied. When substantial edema is present, one should suspect that status epilepticus and cerebral edema are both manifestations of the same underlying condition. Mannitol and mild hyperventilation may be valuable if edema is life threatening. If substantial cerebral edema is present, ICP monitoring should be strongly considered. Edema due to status epilepticus is vasogenic in origin; thus, steroids may be useful as well, but they have not been studied in this setting.

can limit their use and may be fatal.[60] However, they are important when other modalities have failed (see Table 53-5). Endotracheal intubation and mechanical ventilation are mandatory when high-dose barbiturates are used, and both continuous EEG and invasive hemodynamic monitoring are highly recommended. Severe hypotension is the most frequent side effect of pentobarbital therapy, and its occurrence is associated with increased mortality.[61] An increased occurrence of nosocomial respiratory tract infection has been reported in patients treated with pentobarbital infusion.[62] An inhibitory effect on leukocyte chemotaxis and paralysis of respiratory cilia by the barbiturates have been postulated. Despite these side-effects, barbiturate anesthesia should not be rapidly discontinued if it is successful in terminating refractory status epilepticus; rather, continuing therapy for at least 48 hours, gradual tapering of the infusion dose, and the administration of phenobarbital during the drug taper are recommended.[63]

Midazolam is a water soluble benzodiazepine that has demonstrated high efficacy in refractory status in adults and children.[64,65] At our institution, this agent is used as a second-line drug, after lorazepam has failed to control status epilepticus. Clinically significant hypotension is rare even at very high doses that are often required to address tachyphylaxis. Respiratory depression is uncommon after a loading dose, but should be anticipated with infusions of any duration. Sedation is quickly reversed after short-term infusions are discontinued. However, terminal half-lives of three to eight times normal have been reported with extended administration.[66] In addition, prolonged elimination times have been associated with critical illness and hepatorenal dysfunction. Others have recently discussed its use in this setting.[67]

Although intravenous paraldehyde has been abandoned, this agent is still useful. The current formulation is licensed only for enteral use. It can be given every 3 hours through a Teflon-coated nasogastric tube or rectally via a rubber catheter. The enteral form can be filtered for intramuscular injection; it should be given deeply into the lateral gluteal muscles, with special care taken to avoid the sciatic nerves. This route of administration should be confined to a few doses, when rectal or oral treatment is not feasible.

Isoflurane, an inhaled anesthetic, controls refractory status epilepticus; however, it is difficult to deliver such a gas outside of the operating suite or the recovery area. It has no known advantage over intravenous anticonvulsants and can raise ICP.

Propofol has been reported to be effective in the treatment of refractory status epilepticus, but direct comparisons with other agents have shown mixed results.[68,69] It may offer a lower risk of ventilatory depression and promote more rapid awakening compared with other drugs when it is discontinued. Early fears of a possible proconvulsant effect appear to be unfounded, although withdrawal convulsions may occur if the drug is abruptly terminated. A dosage range of 1 to 15 mg/kg/hr has been studied,[70] although the actual upper limit is not known. Acidosis and oxygenation difficulties have been reported in children.[71] Mortality with its use appears to be greater than with midazolam.[72] Careful monitoring of creatine kinase and oxygen saturation would be prudent.[73]

The role of the newer anticonvulsant agents has yet to be determined. Intravenous valproate may emerge as an important drug for the treatment of several forms of status epilepticus.[74] Topiramate may also be useful for refractory status epilepticus,[75] especially when an intravenous form becomes available.

ACKNOWLEDGMENT

The authors would like to recognize the contributions of Christopher Dunatov, MD, to the previous edition of this chapter.

ANNOTATED REFERENCES

Fountain NB, Adams RE: Midazolam treatment of acute and refractory status epilepticus. Clin Neuropharmacol 1999;22:261-267.

This thorough review discusses both the pharmacology of and the data supporting midazolam use in patients with status epilepticus. Practical clinical hints are conveyed regarding specific advantages and potential disadvantages of midazolam.

Lothman E: The biochemical basis and pathophysiology of status epilepticus. Neurology 1990;40(suppl 2):13-23.

A classic, comprehensive summary of clinical and experimental evidence explaining the alterations in systemic physiology and brain metabolism that occur during prolonged seizures.

Shneker BF, Fountain NB: Assessment of acute morbidity and mortality in nonconvulsive status epilepticus. Neurology 1996;47:83-89,

A retrospective review of 100 patients with nonconvulsive status epilepticus found a mortality rate of 18% that correlated with the underlying cause, severe impairment of mental status, and development of acute complications. Generalized spike-and-wave discharges did not correlate with mortality. This is the largest series to date.

Towne AR, Waterhouse EJ, Boggs JG, et al: Prevalence of nonconvulsive status epilepticus in comatose patients. Neurology 2000;54:340-345.

A retrospective review of the EEG recordings of 236 comatose ICU patients without clinical signs of status epilepticus found that nonconvulsive status epilepticus occurred in 18%. These findings suggest that EEG is an essential part of the coma evaluation.

Treiman DM, Meyers PD, Walton NY, et al: A comparison of four treatments for generalized convulsive status epilepticus. N Engl J Med 1998;339: 792-798.

This 5-year randomized, double-blind, multicenter trial of four intravenous regimens in the first-line treatment of generalized convulsive status epilepticus demonstrated that lorazepam is more effective than phenytoin. Although lorazepam was not found to be more efficacious than phenobarbital or diazepam and phenytoin, it was easier to use and therefore recommended for initial intravenous treatment. There were no significant differences in side effects among the four treatment groups.

Chapter 54

NEUROMUSCULAR DISORDERS IN THE ICU

Vern C. Juel • Thomas P. Bleck

KEY POINTS

1. Respiratory dysfunction due to neuromuscular disease typically presents with a combination of **upper airway dysfunction and diminished tidal volume (VT).**

2. Along with vital capacity, **trended measurement of the maximum inspiratory pressure** (PImax or negative inspiratory force [NIF]) is a useful index of ventilatory capacity. Inability to maintain a PImax greater than 20 to 25 cm H_2O usually indicates a need for mechanical ventilatory assistance.

3. **Autonomic failure and pulmonary embolism** are now the major causes of mortality in Guillain-Barré syndrome.

4. **Evidence-based guidelines for Guillain-Barré syndrome immunotherapy** have been published by the Quality Standards Subcommittee of the American Academy of Neurology. Plasma exchange is recommended for adult patients who cannot walk within 4 weeks of symptom onset. Intravenous immune globulin (IVIg) is recommended in these patients within 2 or possibly 4 weeks of symptom onset. Plasma exchange and IVIg are considered equivalent in efficacy, and no additional benefit is conferred by combining these treatments. In light of the therapeutic equivalence, the decision whether to employ plasma exchange or IVIg in treating acute Guillain-Barré syndrome may be determined by resource availability and by avoiding potential side effects related to a patient's medical comorbidities.

5. **In the initial North American outbreak of West Nile virus,** about 10% of infected patients experienced flaccid weakness with clinical features resembling Guillain-Barré syndrome.

6. Approximately 20% of patients with myasthenia gravis develop myasthenic crisis with **respiratory failure requiring mechanical ventilation.**

7. **Critical illness polyneuropathy** is a widespread axonal peripheral neuropathy that develops in the context of multiple organ failure and sepsis. Critical illness polyneuropathy is possibly the most common neuromuscular cause of prolonged ventilator dependency in patients without prior known neuromuscular disease.

8. **Acute quadriplegic myopathy** has developed most frequently in the setting of severe pulmonary disorders, in which neuromuscular blockade is used to facilitate mechanical ventilation and high-dose corticosteroids are concurrently administered. Given the growing recognition of acute quadriplegic myopathy, the use of high-dose corticosteroids should be avoided, if possible, when neuromuscular blockade is required.

Abnormal neuromuscular function may precipitate a patient's admission to an ICU or may develop as a consequence of another critical illness and its treatment. This chapter focuses primarily on respiratory failure as a consequence of neuromuscular disease but also addresses autonomic dysfunction occurring in this setting. To facilitate understanding of the concepts involved, a brief review of the motor unit and its physiology is provided and specific muscles critical to ventilation are identified.

THE MOTOR UNIT AND ITS PHYSIOLOGY

Central nervous system activity designated for motor output is ultimately conducted to lower motor neurons, also known as alpha motor neurons. A motor unit is composed of a lower motor neuron and its distal ramifications, its neuromuscular junctions, and the muscle fibers it innervates. The cell bodies of the lower motor neurons are located in the brainstem for cranial musculature and in the anterior horn of the spinal cord for somatic muscles. At the level of the brainstem or spinal cord, the motor neurons receive various excitatory and inhibitory inputs. Motor axons project through the subarachnoid space and penetrate the dura mater as nerve roots. They may join with other motor axons and with sensory and autonomic fibers in a plexus and then travel in peripheral nerves to the muscles they innervate. Alpha motor neurons are myelinated, a feature that accelerates nerve impulse propagation. The multiple terminal ramifications of the motor neuron synapse on individual muscle fibers.

The motor axon communicates with muscle via a specialized area termed the neuromuscular junction. On the presynaptic side of the neuromuscular junction the neurotransmitter acetylcholine is synthesized, packaged in vesicles, and stored for release. Depolarization of the axon opens presynaptic voltage-gated calcium channels, which activate the molecular machinery responsible for drawing the vesicles

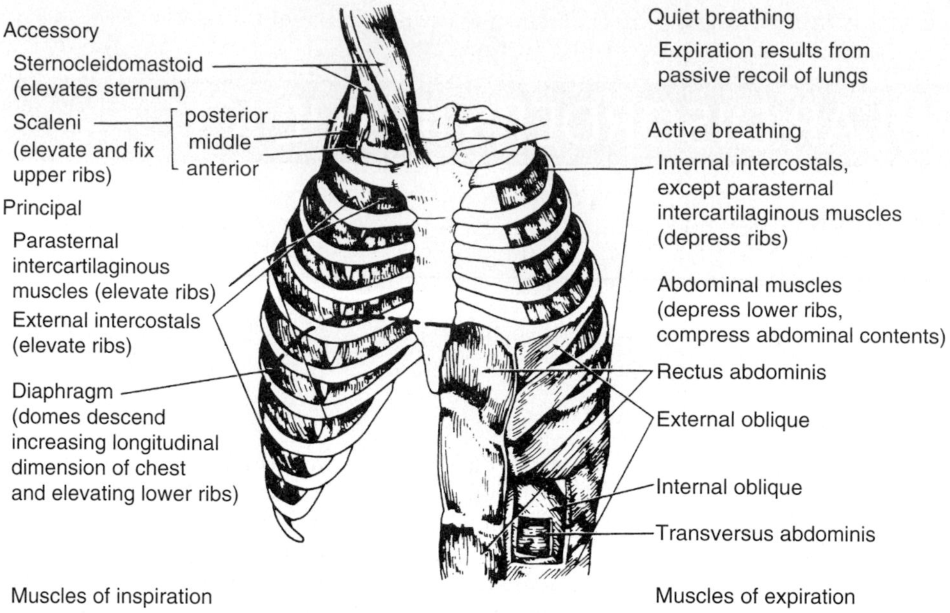

Muscles of inspiration

Accessory

Sternocleidomastoid (elevates sternum)

Scaleni (elevate and fix upper ribs) — posterior, middle, anterior

Principal

Parasternal intercartilaginous muscles (elevate ribs)

External intercostals (elevate ribs)

Diaphragm (domes descend increasing longitudinal dimension of chest and elevating lower ribs)

Muscles of expiration

Quiet breathing

Expiration results from passive recoil of lungs

Active breathing

Internal intercostals, except parasternal intercartilaginous muscles (depress ribs)

Abdominal muscles (depress lower ribs, compress abdominal contents)

Rectus abdominis

External oblique

Internal oblique

Transversus abdominis

FIGURE 54–1. Major respiratory muscles. Inspiratory muscles are indicated on the left and expiratory muscles are indicated on the right. (From Garrity ER: Respiratory failure due to disorders of the chest wall and respiratory muscles. In MacDonnell KF, Fahey PJ, Segal MS [eds]: Respiratory Intensive Care. Boston, Little, Brown, 1987, p 313.)

to the presynaptic membrane. The vesicles then fuse with the membrane and release acetylcholine into the synaptic cleft. Acetylcholine molecules bind to receptors on the postsynaptic membrane and cause an influx of sodium, which in turn increases the muscle end-plate potential. When the end-plate potential exceeds the threshold level, the muscle membrane becomes depolarized. This depolarization releases calcium ions from the sarcoplasmic reticulum, and muscle contraction occurs through a process known as excitation-contraction coupling. After activating the acetylcholine receptor complex, the acetylcholine molecule is degraded by cholinesterase; the choline released by this reaction is then recycled by the presynaptic neuron.

MUSCLES OF RESPIRATION

Three muscle groups may be defined based on their importance for respiration, as follows (Fig. 54-1):[1]

1. *Upper airway muscles:* palatal, pharyngeal, laryngeal, and lingual
2. *Inspiratory muscles:* sternomastoid, diaphragm, scalenes, and parasternal intercostals
3. *Expiratory muscles:* internal intercostal muscles (except for parasternals) and abdominal muscles

The upper airway muscles receive their innervation from the lower cranial nerves. Sternomastoid innervation arrives predominantly from cranial nerve XI, with a small contribution from C2. The phrenic nerve originates from cell bodies located between C3 and C5, with a maximum contribution from C4, and innervates the diaphragm. Innervation to the scalenes arises from C4 to C8, whereas that of the parasternal intercostals is from T1 to T7. The intercostal muscles receive innervation from T1 to T12, and the abdominal musculature receive it from T7 to L1. Reference to this innervation scheme is important in understanding the effects of spinal cord and nerve root injuries on respiration and for the differential diagnosis of disorders producing apparently diffuse weakness.

CLINICAL PRESENTATION OF NEUROMUSCULAR RESPIRATORY FAILURE

Patients experiencing respiratory dysfunction due to neuromuscular disease typically present with a combination of upper airway dysfunction and diminished tidal volume (VT). Difficulty with swallowing liquids, including respiratory secretions, is the most typical presentation of pharyngeal weakness, although some patients have an equal or greater degree of difficulty with solid food. A hoarse or nasal voice may also signal problems with the upper airway. These conditions are noted in patients who are at risk for aspiration and present with difficulty with attempts at negative-pressure ventilation (cuirass or iron lung), because the weakened muscles may not be able to keep the airway open as the pressure falls.[2] Paradoxical abdominal movement (inward movement of the abdomen during inspiration) is an important sign of diaphragmatic weakness.[3]

Loss of VT occurs most dramatically with diaphragmatic weakness but also follows insults that affect the ability of the parasternal intercostals to keep the chest wall expanded against negative intrapleural pressure. This is most apparent in lower cervical spinal cord injuries where atelectasis commonly develops despite preserved phrenic nerve function. This problem usually diminishes over weeks as the parasternal intercostal muscles develop spasticity.

Patients with progressive generalized weakness (e.g., with Guillain-Barré syndrome) commonly begin to lose VT before developing upper airway weakness. To maintain minute ventilation, and therefore carbon dioxide excretion, a patient's respiratory rate increases. Respiratory rate is thus one of the most important clinical parameters to monitor. As the vital capacity falls from the norm of about 65 to 30 mL/kg, a patient's cough weakens and clearing secretions becomes difficult. A further decrease of vital capacity to 20 to 25 mL/kg results in an impaired ability to sigh with progressive atelectasis. At this point hypoxemia may be present because of ventilation-perfusion mismatching and because an increasing percentage of VT is used to ventilate dead space. Before the vital capacity reaches 15 mL/kg, a patient should be in an ICU because respiratory failure is imminent and endotracheal intubation should be considered. The precise point at which mechanical ventilation is necessary varies with the patient, the underlying condition, and especially with the likelihood of a rapid response to treatment.

Regardless of the vital capacity, however, indications for intubation and mechanical ventilation include evidence of fatigue, hypoxemia despite supplemental oxygen administration, difficulty with secretions, and a rising $PaCO_2$. In the absence of hypercapnia, occasional patients (e.g., those with myasthenia gravis) can be managed under very close observation in an ICU with less invasive techniques (e.g., bilevel positive airway pressure [BiPAP]).[4]

In addition to vital capacity, trended measurements of the maximum inspiratory pressure (PImax, more typically recorded as negative inspiratory force [NIF]) are useful indicators of ventilatory capacity. Inability to maintain a PImax greater than 20 to 25 cm H_2O usually indicates a need for mechanical ventilation. Although the maximum expiratory pressure (PEmax) is a more sensitive indicator of weakness,[5] it has not proved to be as useful as an indicator of the need for mechanical ventilation. A more detailed discussion of these variables and their use may be found elsewhere.[6,7]

Because a patient with neuromuscular respiratory failure has intact ventilatory drive,[8] the fall in VT is initially matched by an increase in respiratory rate, keeping the $PaCO_2$ normal or low until the vital capacity becomes dangerously reduced. Many patients initially maintain their $PaCO_2$ in the range of 35 mm Hg because of either (1) a subjective sense of dyspnea at low VT or (2) hypoxia from atelectasis and increasing dead space. When the $PaCO_2$ begins to rise in this circumstance, abrupt respiratory failure may be imminent.

The modest degree of hypoxia in most of these patients worsens when the $PaCO_2$ begins to rise, displacing more oxygen from the alveolar gas. However, aspiration pneumonia and pulmonary embolism are also frequent causes of hypoxemia in these patients. To determine the relative contributions of these conditions to a patient's hypoxemia, one can use a simplified version of the alveolar gas equation as follows (derived elsewhere)[6,7]:

$$PAO_2 = PIO_2 - (PaCO_2/R)$$

where PAO_2 is the alveolar partial pressure of oxygen, PIO_2 is the partial pressure of inspired oxygen (in room air, 150 mm Hg), and R is the respiratory quotient (on most diets, about 0.8). This allows estimation of the alveolar-arterial oxygen difference ($PAO_2 - PaO_2$). Under ideal circumstances in young people breathing room air this value is about 10 mm Hg, but it rises to about 100 mm Hg when the fraction of inspired oxygen (FIO_2) is 1.0. The alveolar air equation allows one to factor out the contribution of hypercarbia to the decrease in arterial partial pressure of oxygen (PaO_2); it should be used to determine whether there is a cause of significant hypoxemia in addition to the displacement of oxygen by carbon dioxide.

Patients with orbicularis oris weakness may have artifactually low vital capacity and NIF measurements because they cannot form a tight seal around the spirometer mouthpiece. The need for nursing and respiratory therapy personnel who are experienced in the care of these patients is thus underscored. It is also important for physicians to observe these patients directly rather than relying solely on reported measurements. The physical findings associated with neuromuscular respiratory failure are reviewed elsewhere.[6,7] Among the most important findings are rapid, shallow breathing,[9] the recruitment of accessory muscles, and paradoxical movement of the abdomen during the respiratory cycle. Fluoroscopy of the diaphragm is occasionally valuable for the diagnosis of diaphragmatic dysfunction.[10]

Autonomic dysfunction commonly accompanies some of the neuromuscular disorders requiring critical care, such as Guillain-Barré syndrome, botulism, and porphyria (Table 54-1). In Guillain-Barré syndrome (discussed later) dysautonomia is common and may arise in parallel with weakness or may follow the onset of the motor disorder after a week or more.

NEUROMUSCULAR DISORDERS

Many chronic neuromuscular disorders and other central nervous system conditions affecting the suprasegmental innervation and control of respiratory muscles eventually compromise ventilation. In this chapter, however, we emphasize the more common acute and subacute neuromuscular disorders that precipitate or prolong critical illness due to ventilatory failure and autonomic dysfunction. A more complete listing of neuromuscular diseases appears in Table 54-1; reviews of this subject[11,12] or the references listed in Table 54-1 may be consulted for details of the more rare disorders. Some of the diseases listed (e.g., Lambert-Eaton myasthenic syndrome) rarely cause respiratory failure in isolation but may be contributing causes in the presence of other conditions,[13] such as neuromuscular junction blockade intended only for the duration of a surgical procedure.[14]

NEUROMUSCULAR DISEASES PRECIPITATING CRITICAL ILLNESS

Guillain-Barré Syndrome

Guillain-Barré syndrome, or acute inflammatory demyelinating polyradiculoneuropathy, is typically a motor greater than sensory peripheral neuropathy with subacute onset, monophasic course, and nadir within 4 weeks. Although the precise etiology is unknown, Guillain-Barré syndrome is immune mediated and related to antibodies directed against peripheral nerve components. Approximately 1.7 cases occur per 100,000 population per year.[28] Most patients suffer a demyelinating neuropathy, but in about 5% of cases the condition is a primary axonopathy.[29] Numerous antecedents have been implicated[30]; the more frequent ones are listed in Table 54-2. The association with antecedent infections suggests that certain agents may elicit immune responses involving antibodies that cross-react with peripheral nerve gangliosides. In particular, the development of ganglioside antibodies has been observed in Guillain-Barré syndrome after *Campylobacter jejuni* infections, such as GM_1 antibodies in axonal forms of Guillain-Barré syndrome[31] and GQ_{1b} antibodies in the Miller-Fisher variant of Guillain-Barré syndrome.[32]

The initial findings of patients with Guillain-Barré syndrome are subacute and progressive weakness, usually most marked in the legs, associated with sensory complaints but without objective signs of sensory dysfunction.[33] Deep tendon reflexes are often significantly reduced or absent at presentation, though this finding may take several days to develop.

TABLE 54–1. NEUROMUSCULAR CAUSES OF ACUTE RESPIRATORY FAILURE

Location	Disorder	Associated Autonomic Dysfunction?
Spinal cord	Tetanus[15]	Frequent
Anterior horn cell	Amyotrophic lateral sclerosis[16]	No
	Poliomyelitis	No
	Rabies	Frequent
	West Nile virus flaccid paralysis	No
Peripheral nerve	Guillain-Barré syndrome	Frequent
	Critical illness polyneuropathy	No
	Diphtheria	No, but cardiomyopathy and arrhythmias may occur
	Porphyria	Occasional
	Ciguatoxin (ciguatera poisoning)	Occasional
	Saxitoxin (paralytic shellfish poisoning)	No
	Tetrodotoxin (pufferfish poisoning)	No
	Thallium intoxication	No
	Arsenic intoxication[17,18]	No
	Lead intoxication	No
	Buckthorn neuropathy	No
Neuromuscular junction	Myasthenia gravis	No
	Botulism[19]	Frequent
	Lambert-Eaton myasthenic syndrome[20]	Yes, frequent dry mouth and postural hypotension
	Hypermagnesemia[21]	No
	Organophosphate poisoning	No
	Tick paralysis	No
	Snake bite	No
Muscle	Polymyositis/dermatomyositis	No
	Acute quadriplegic myopathy	No
	Eosinophilia-myalgia syndrome[22]	No
	Muscular dystrophies[23]	No, but cardiac rhythm disturbances may occur
	Carnitine palmitoyl transferase deficiency	No
	Nemaline myopathy[24]	No
	Acid maltase deficiency[25]	No
	Mitochondrial myopathy[26]	No
	Acute hypokalemic paralysis	No
	Stonefish myotoxin poisoning	No
	Rhabdomyolysis	No
	Hypophosphatemia[27]	No

The cerebrospinal fluid (CSF) typically reveals an albuminocytologic dissociation or elevated protein content without pleocytosis; this may not evolve until the second week of illness. The major reason to examine the CSF is to preclude other diagnoses. Although mild CSF lymphocytic pleocytosis (10 to 20 cells/mm^3) may suggest the possibility of associated human immunodeficiency virus (HIV) infection, in most patients, the nucleated cell count is less than 10 cells/mm^3.[34] Although they may be normal initially, results of electrodiagnostic studies (motor and sensory nerve conduction studies and needle electromyography) often reflect segmental nerve demyelination with multifocal conduction blocks, temporally dispersed compound muscle action potentials, slowed conduction velocity, and prolonged or absent F waves.[35] Differential diagnostic considerations for patients with suspected Guillain-Barré syndrome are primarily those listed in the "Peripheral Nerve" section of Table 54-1.

The components of treatment for patients with Guillain-Barré syndrome are as follows:

- Management of ventilatory failure
- Management of autonomic dysfunction
- Meticulous nursing care
- Psychologic support
- Physical and occupational therapy
- Prevention of deep venous thrombosis
- Nutritional support
- Early planning for rehabilitation
- Immunotherapy for the underlying autoimmune process

Patients with Guillain-Barré syndrome with evolving respiratory failure should generally be intubated when the vital capacity falls to about 15 mL/kg or when difficulty with secretions begins because the response to treatment is slow. If a patient has been immobile for several days before intubation and neuromuscular junction blockade is needed, a nondepolarizing agent should be used to avoid transient hyperkalemia. Oral intubation is again being viewed as preferable to the nasal route, because the endotracheal tube is frequently required for a week or longer, raising the risk of sinusitis with nasal intubation.

Many patients are too weak to trigger the ventilator; in such cases, the assist/control or intermittent mandatory ventilation mode is initiated. Weaning patients with Guillain-Barré syndrome from mechanical ventilation must wait for adequate improvement in strength. We usually shift to pressure support ventilation for weaning, although evidence of its superiority over intermittent mandatory ventilation or synchronized intermittent mandatory ventilation modes is only anecdotal. Although the majority of patients require mechanical ventilation for less than 4 weeks, as many as one fifth need 2 or more months of support before they can breathe without assistance. Improvement in vital capacity to greater than 15 mL/kg and in NIF to greater than 25 cm H$_2$O suggests that a patient has improved enough to begin

TABLE 54–2. MAJOR ANTECEDENTS OF GUILLAIN-BARRÉ SYNDROME

Frequent

Upper respiratory tract infections
Campylobacter jejuni enteritis
Cytomegalovirus (CMV) infection
Epstein-Barr virus (EBV) infection
Hepatitis A infection
Hepatitis B infection
Hepatitis C infection
HIV infection

Infrequent

Mycoplasma pneumoniae infection
Haemophilus influenzae infection
Leptospira icterohaemorrhagiae infection
Salmonellosis
Rabies vaccine
Tetanus toxoid
Bacille Calmette-Guérin immunization
Sarcoidosis
Systemic lupus erythematosus
Lymphoma
Trauma
Surgery

Questionable

Hepatitis B vaccine
Influenza vaccine
Hyperthermia
Epidural anesthesia

weaning from the ventilator. A formula using a combination of ventilatory and gas exchange variables may allow more accurate determination of a patient's ability to be weaned.[36]

Autonomic dysfunction related to Guillain-Barré syndrome most typically presents as a hypersympathetic state and is often heralded by unexplained sinus tachycardia. The blood pressure may fluctuate wildly. Patients may rarely experience bradycardic episodes, which may require temporary pacing. Autonomic surges during tracheal suctioning or due to a distended viscus may be very dramatic and should be minimized. Autonomic failure and pulmonary embolism are now the major causes of mortality in Guillain-Barré syndrome.

Nursing care for patients with Guillain-Barré syndrome is similar to that for other paralyzed and mechanically ventilated patients, but special care must be taken to remember that patients with Guillain-Barré syndrome are completely lucid. In addition to explaining any procedures carefully, arranging for distractions during the daytime (e.g., television, movies, conversation, visitors) and adequate sleep at night is very important. For the most severely affected patients, sedation should be considered. In concert with physical and occupational therapists, passive exercise should be performed frequently throughout the day.

Deep venous thrombosis is a significant danger for patients with Guillain-Barré syndrome. Episodic arterial desaturation is a common event, presumably owing to transient mucus plugging; submassive pulmonary emboli may therefore be overlooked. Adjusted-dose heparin (to slightly prolong the partial thromboplastin time) should be given, and sequential compression devices should be used on the legs; therapeutic anticoagulation may be considered. The risk of fatal pulmonary embolism extends through the initial period of improvement until patients are ambulatory.

Nutritional support should begin as soon as a patient is admitted, with appropriate concern for the risk of aspiration.[37] Most mechanically ventilated patients with Guillain-Barré syndrome can be fed via soft, small-caliber feeding tubes; autonomic dysfunction affecting the gut occasionally requires total parenteral nutrition.

Immunotherapy for Guillain-Barré syndrome includes removal of autoantibodies with plasma exchange or immune modulation with high-dose IVIg. The efficacy of plasma exchange has been evaluated in a Cochrane systematic review of six class II trials comparing plasma exchange alone with supportive care.[38] Most of the trials employed up to five plasma exchanges of 50 mL/kg over 2 weeks. In a large North American trial,[39] the time needed to improve one clinical grade (being weaned from the ventilator or being able to walk) was reduced by 50% in the plasma exchange group by comparison with the control group. There was no significant benefit when plasma exchange was begun later than 2 weeks after symptom onset. A meta-analysis demonstrated more rapid recovery in ventilated patients treated with plasma exchange within 4 weeks of onset.[38] The optimal number of plasma exchanges has been assessed in patients with mild (unable to run), moderate (unable to stand without assistance), and severe (requiring mechanical ventilation) Guillain-Barré syndrome by the French Cooperative Group.[40] On the basis of this trial, two exchanges are better than none in mild Guillain-Barré syndrome; four are better than two in moderate Guillain-Barré syndrome; and six are no better than four in severe Guillain-Barré syndrome. Albumin is the preferred replacement solution.[41] Treatment with IVIg for Guillain-Barré syndrome has also been examined in a Cochrane systematic review. Three randomized controlled trials demonstrated class I evidence that IVIg (2 g/kg over 2 to 5 days) is as effective as plasma exchange in Guillain-Barré syndrome patients with impaired walking.[42] Complication rates were somewhat higher in the plasma exchange groups. A large, international, multicenter, randomized trial compared plasma exchange (50 mL/kg × 5 exchanges over 8 to 13 days), IVIg (0.4 g/kg × 5 days), and plasma exchange followed by IVIg.[43] No significant outcome differences between these therapies were found with respect to functional improvement at 4 weeks or at 48 weeks.

Evidence-based guidelines for Guillain-Barré syndrome immunotherapy have been published by the Quality Standards Subcommittee of the American Academy of Neurology.[44] Plasma exchange is recommended for adult patients who cannot walk within 4 weeks of symptom onset. IVIg is recommended in these patients within 2 or possibly 4 weeks of symptom onset. Both treatments are deemed equivalent in efficacy, and no additional benefit is conferred by combining treatment with plasma exchange and IVIg. In light of their therapeutic equivalence, the decision whether to employ plasma exchange or IVIg in treating acute Guillain-Barré syndrome may be determined by resource availability and by avoiding potential side effects related to a patient's medical comorbidities. Patients with heart disease, renal insufficiency or failure, hyperviscosity, or IgA deficiency may be more susceptible to complications of treatment with IVIg, whereas plasma exchange may be complicated in patients with labile blood pressure, septicemia, and significant venous access problems.

Despite the autoimmune pathophysiology of Guillain-Barré syndrome and the efficacy of corticosteroids in more chronic forms of inflammatory neuropathy, corticosteroids have not demonstrated effectiveness in Guillain-Barré syndrome and are therefore not recommended for Guillain-Barré syndrome treatment.[44] A large, multicenter trial failed to demonstrate efficacy of high-dose intravenous methylprednisolone,[45] and another large, multicenter trial demonstrated no added clinical benefit in combined treatment with IVIg and methylprednisolone.[46]

West Nile Virus Acute
Flaccid Paralysis Syndrome

The large outbreak of West Nile virus encephalitis in the summer of 1999 in New York City marked the emergence of a relatively new cause for neuromuscular weakness with the potential for neuromuscular respiratory compromise. West Nile virus is a flavivirus transmitted between birds and mosquitoes. Humans may acquire West Nile virus from the bite of an infected *Culex* species mosquito, and a corresponding peak in human disease occurs in the late summer and fall. West Nile virus may also be transmitted to humans by organ transplantation,[47] blood and blood product transfusion,[48] transplacental exposure,[49] breast feeding,[50] and percutaneous laboratory injuries.[51] About 20% of humans experience a mild flulike illness lasting 3 to 6 days, and about 1 in 150 develop central nervous system disease, which usually presents as meningoencephalitis.[52]

In the initial North American outbreak of West Nile virus, about 10% of infected patients experienced flaccid weakness with clinical features resembling Guillain-Barré syndrome.[53] In one report from the original outbreak, a patient developed electromyographic evidence for segmental demyelination compatible with Guillain-Barré syndrome.[54] Although patients with West Nile virus infection exhibit a spectrum of clinical weakness,[55] the most prominent and distinctive syndrome documented in several subsequent reports of West Nile virus infection is an acute "poliomyelitis-like" or acute flaccid paralysis syndrome with pathology localizing to the ventral horns of the spinal cord and/or ventral roots.[56-62] These patients developed acute, asymmetrical, flaccid weakness in the absence of sensory abnormalities, diffuse areflexia, or bowel/bladder dysfunction. Some of the patients experienced concurrent meningoencephalitis, and a few required mechanical ventilation.[57,58] West Nile virus acute flaccid paralysis syndrome may occur in the absence of overt encephalitic signs (e.g., fever, confusion) or meningismus. Although the risk for West Nile virus encephalitis is significantly increased with age,[63] West Nile virus acute flaccid paralysis syndrome occurs in relatively younger patients.[56-62]

Electrodiagnostic studies in patients with West Nile virus acute flaccid paralysis syndrome demonstrate normal sensory potentials, the absence of findings suggesting segmental demyelination (e.g., motor conduction block, reduced conduction velocities, prolonged distal and F-wave latencies), low amplitude compound muscle action potentials in affected regions, and marked denervation changes in affected limb and in corresponding paraspinal muscles on needle electromyography. Corresponding MRI findings are sometimes observed and include abnormal signal in the spinal cord on T2-weighted images[60,61] and abnormal enhancement of the nerve roots and cauda equina.[59,60] CSF analysis usually demonstrates mild pleocytosis with lymphocytic predominance, mild to moderate protein elevation, and normal glucose.[64] Prognosis for recovery of strength in these patients appears poor.[65]

West Nile virus infection may be diagnosed by demonstrating West Nile virus RNA in serum, CSF, or other tissues by reverse-transcriptase polymerase chain reaction, although this is insensitive.[66] More commonly, a diagnosis is made by demonstration of West Nile virus IgM in CSF or serum by antibody-capture enzyme-linked immunosorbent assay. When serum West Nile virus IgM is present, diagnosis is confirmed by a fourfold increase in West Nile virus IgG titers between acute and convalescent sera obtained 4 weeks apart. Positive IgM and IgG antibody titers should be confirmed by plaque-reduction viral neutralization assay to exclude false-positive results related to other flaviviral infections such as St. Louis encephalitis. Serology may not become positive until 8 days after symptom onset.[52]

Particularly in the absence of a more typical encephalitic presentation of West Nile virus infection, a high index of clinical suspicion is needed to make a diagnosis of West Nile virus acute flaccid paralysis syndrome and to distinguish such cases from Guillain-Barré syndrome in patients presenting with acute weakness in the late summer or fall. Electrodiagnostic studies may help localize the pathology to the ventral horns of the spinal cord or ventral roots in West Nile virus cases and to exclude findings of segmental demyelination suggesting Guillain-Barré syndrome. CSF should also be evaluated to help discriminate between the albuminocytologic dissociation of Guillain-Barré syndrome and the lymphocytic pleocytosis observed in West Nile virus infection.

Although there is currently no specific treatment for West Nile virus acute flaccid paralysis syndrome, a multicenter study to evaluate the efficacy of Israeli IVIg in patients with West Nile virus meningoencephalitis or weakness began in the summer of 2003. The IVIg for this study contains high levels of West Nile virus antibodies because it was prepared from sera obtained after an Israeli West Nile virus epidemic in 2000.[67] Two candidate vaccines against West Nile virus are also being evaluated.[64]

Myasthenia Gravis

Myasthenia gravis is a consequence of autoimmune attack on the acetylcholine receptor complex at the postsynaptic membrane of the neuromuscular junction. This process results in clinical weakness with a fluctuating pattern that is most marked after prolonged muscle exertion. Myasthenia gravis occurs at a higher rate in early adulthood in women, but in later life the incidence rates for men and women become nearly equal. The reported prevalence is 14.2 cases per 100,000 population.[68] Myasthenia gravis typically involves ocular muscle weakness producing ptosis and diplopia, as well as bulbar muscle weakness resulting in dysphagia and dysarthria. This diagnosis should be considered in patients who have acute respiratory failure with these cranial nerve findings. A clinical diagnosis of myasthenia gravis may be supported by edrophonium testing, by electrophysiologic studies including repetitive nerve stimulation studies and single-fiber electromyography, and by acetylcholine receptor and muscle-specific receptor tyrosine kinase (MuSK) antibody testing.

Approximately 20% of patients with myasthenia gravis develop myasthenic crisis with respiratory failure requiring mechanical ventilation.[69] Intensivists may also encounter myasthenic patients for management of complications of immunomodulating treatment or for postoperative care after thymectomy. The most common precipitating factors for myasthenic crisis include bronchopulmonary infections

(29%) and aspiration (10%).[70] Other precipitating factors include sepsis, surgical procedures, rapid tapering of immune modulation, beginning treatment with corticosteroids, pregnancy, and exposure to drugs that may increase myasthenic weakness (Table 54-3).[71] Patients with myasthenia gravis are exceptionally sensitive to nondepolarizing neuromuscular blocking agents, but are resistant to depolarizing agents.[72] Thymomas are associated with more fulminant disease and have been identified in about one third of patients in myasthenic crisis.[70]

Although sometimes less appreciated than respiratory muscle weakness, upper airway muscle weakness is a common mechanism leading to myasthenic crisis.[73] Oropharyngeal and laryngeal muscle weakness may result in upper airway collapse with obstruction, along with inability to swallow secretions that may also obstruct the airway and become aspirated. Because direct assessment of oropharyngeal muscle strength is impractical, a focused history and examination to assess surrogate muscles in the head and neck region is important. Findings of bulbar myasthenia associated with upper airway compromise include flaccid dysarthria with hypernasal, staccato, or hoarse speech, dysphagia sometimes associated with nasal regurgitation, and chewing fatigue. Patients may exhibit facial weakness with difficulty holding air within the cheeks. Jaw closure is often weak and cannot be maintained against resistance. Patients with myasthenic tongue weakness may be unable to protrude the tongue into either cheek. Although neck flexors are often weaker, a dropped head syndrome due to neck extensor weakness may occur. Vocal cord abductor paralysis may produce laryngeal obstruction with associated stridor.[74,75]

Patients with features of impending myasthenic crisis including severe bulbar weakness, marginal vital capacity (less than 20 to 25 mL/kg), weak cough with difficulty clearing secretions from the airway, or paradoxical breathing while supine should be admitted to an ICU and made NPO to prevent aspiration.[76] Serial vital capacity and NIF measurements may be used to monitor ventilatory function in impending myasthenic crisis. However, with significant bulbar weakness, these measurements are often inaccurate, owing to difficulty sealing the lips around the spirometer mouthpiece and to inability to seal the nasopharynx. Vital capacity measurements may not reliably predict respiratory failure in myasthenia gravis, due to the fluctuating nature of myasthenic weakness.[77] The criteria for intubation and mechanical ventilation are similar to those discussed earlier for Guillain-Barré syndrome. If the upper airway is competent and there is no difficulty handling secretions or gross hypercapnia ($PaCO_2 > 50$ mm Hg), intermittent nasal BiPAP may be a useful temporizing measure.[4] The majority of patients who develop hypercapnia in myasthenic crisis require intubation, as do those who are becoming fatigued.

Plasma exchange is an effective short-term immunomodulating treatment for myasthenic crisis and for surgical preparation in symptomatic myasthenic patients. Significant strength improvement in myasthenic crisis is well documented in several series,[78-82] although there have been no controlled clinical trials. We perform a series of five to six exchanges of 2 to 3 L every other day. Onset of improved strength is variable but generally occurs after two to three exchanges.

IVIg may represent an alternative short-term treatment for myasthenic exacerbations or crises in patients who are poor candidates for plasma exchange owing to difficult vascular access or septicemia. Comparable efficacy for plasma exchange and IVIg was demonstrated in myasthenic exacerbations and crises in a relatively small randomized, controlled trial of IVIg at 1.2 and 2.0 g/kg over 2 to 5 days.[83] However, in a retrospective multicenter study of myasthenic crisis, plasma exchange proved more effective than IVIg in ability to extubate at 2 weeks and in 1-month functional outcome.[82] Treatment failures to IVIg subsequently responding to plasma exchange have also been reported.[84] Recent experience with preoperative IVIg for thymectomy in myasthenia gravis suggests that the time course of maximal response may be considerably delayed in some patients.[85]

Corticosteroids (e.g., prednisone, 1 mg/kg/day) are occasionally used in prolonged myasthenic crises that fail to respond to treatment with plasma exchange or IVIg. If begun early in the course of myasthenic crisis, the transient increase in myasthenic weakness associated with initiating corticosteroids may prolong mechanical ventilation. When preceded by unequivocal improvement in strength after plasma exchange or IVIg treatment, long-term treatment with corticosteroids may begin with reduced risk for corticosteroid-related exacerbations.

In the context of myasthenic crisis, excessive dosing of cholinesterase inhibitors may superimpose a cholinergic crisis owing to depolarization blockade and result in increased weakness. Other symptoms of cholinergic crisis include muscle fasciculations and prominent muscarinic symptoms, including miosis, excessive lacrimation and salivation, abdominal cramping, nausea, vomiting, diarrhea, thick bronchial secretions, diaphoresis, and bradycardia. Cholinergic crisis is rare in contemporary series of myasthenic crisis,[70] and it is now common practice to avoid repeated dose escalations of cholinesterase inhibitors in impending myasthenic crisis and to discontinue the use of cholinesterase inhibitors after intubation to reduce muscarinic complications. When there is a question of cholinergic excess contributing to respiratory insufficiency, it is most prudent to discontinue all cholinesterase inhibitors, protect the airway, and support respiration as necessary.

Thymectomy may result in long-term improvement in patients with a suspected thymoma or with a life expectancy of more than 10 years. However, a patient in acute respiratory failure is generally considered a poor operative risk, and thymectomy is generally delayed until the patient's condition has improved.[86] Post-thymectomy pain control and ventilatory function may be improved by postoperative administration of epidural morphine.[87]

TABLE 54-3. DRUGS THAT MAY INCREASE WEAKNESS IN MYASTHENIA GRAVIS

Neuromuscular blocking agents
Selected antibiotics
    Aminoglycosides, particularly gentamycin
    Macrolides, particularly erythromycin and azithromycin
Selected cardiovascular agents
    Beta-blockers
    Calcium channel blockers
    Procainamide
    Quinidine
Quinine
Corticosteroids
Magnesium salts
    Antacids, laxatives, intravenous tocolytics
Iodinated contrast agents
D-Penicillamine

NEUROMUSCULAR DISEASES SECONDARY TO CRITICAL ILLNESS AND ITS TREATMENT

Critical Illness Polyneuropathy

Critical illness polyneuropathy is a widespread axonal peripheral neuropathy that develops in the context of multiple organ failure and sepsis. This entity was recognized by several investigators in 1983[88-90] and has been further characterized in large part by Bolton and colleagues.[91,92] In a prospective series of 43 consecutive patients with sepsis and multiorgan failure, 70% developed electrophysiologic evidence of a sensorimotor axonal neuropathy and 15 patients developed difficulty weaning from mechanical ventilation as a consequence of the neuropathy.[93] Critical illness polyneuropathy is possibly the most common neuromuscular cause of prolonged ventilator dependency in patients without prior known neuromuscular disease.[94] Given the limitations to detailed clinical motor and sensory examinations in the setting of critical illness, the clinical features of critical illness polyneuropathy (extremity muscle weakness and wasting, distal sensory loss, and paresthesias) may not be recognized. Deep tendon reflexes are generally reduced or absent. In the setting of superimposed central nervous system insult with pyramidal tract dysfunction, however, deep tendon reflexes may be normal or increased.[95]

Electrodiagnostic studies are important in establishing a diagnosis of critical illness polyneuropathy, because the clinical findings may be unobtainable or indeterminate in this setting.[95] Nerve conduction findings include normal or near-normal conduction velocity and latency values and significantly reduced compound muscle action potential and sensory nerve action potential amplitudes. Needle electrode examination reveals denervation changes that are most marked in distal muscles, including fibrillation potentials, positive sharp waves, and reduced recruitment of motor unit potentials.[96] With recovery over time, the denervation potentials abate and the motor unit potentials become polyphasic and enlarged. Peripheral nerve histopathology has revealed widespread, primary axonal degeneration in distal motor and sensory fibers, and skeletal muscle has exhibited fiber-type grouping.[92]

Although the clinical history is usually adequate to distinguish between critical illness polyneuropathy and Guillain-Barré syndrome, the latter has developed in the context of recent surgery complicated by infection.[97] In some such instances, it may be necessary to differentiate between these two peripheral neuropathic disorders in a patient with extremity weakness and inability to wean from mechanical ventilation. Although only a few severe cases of critical illness polyneuropathy have been associated with facial weakness,[98] facial and oropharyngeal weakness are common in Guillain-Barré syndrome.[97] Dysautonomia and, occasionally, external ophthalmoplegia are also observed in Guillain-Barré syndrome but have virtually never been attributed to critical illness polyneuropathy.[98]

Electrophysiologic findings are also helpful in distinguishing these two disorders. Features of segmental demyelination may be observed in Guillain-Barré syndrome on nerve conduction studies (e.g., reduced conduction velocity, prolonged distal and F-wave latencies, conduction block, and temporal dispersion of compound muscle action potentials); these findings are not observed in critical illness polyneuropathy. Needle electromyographic findings may differ in that relatively less spontaneous activity is observed in clinically weak muscles within the first few days in Guillain-Barré syndrome.[96] Although electrophysiologic studies are quite helpful in demonstrating the classic, demyelinating form of Guillain-Barré syndrome, an electrophysiologic distinction between axonal forms of Guillain-Barré syndrome and critical illness polyneuropathy may not be reliable. The mean CSF protein level in Guillain-Barré syndrome is significantly higher than in critical illness polyneuropathy, although there is overlap between these populations.[96] Peripheral nerve histopathology may also distinguish between these two groups, because segmental demyelination and inflammatory changes may be observed in Guillain-Barré syndrome and are not seen in critical illness polyneuropathy.[92]

Although overall prognosis in critical illness polyneuropathy is dependent on recovery from the underlying critical illness, most patients who survive experience a functional recovery from the neuropathy within several months.[92] Critical illness polyneuropathy may prolong ventilator dependence, but it does not worsen long-term prognosis.[95] Proper positioning and padding are important to prevent compression neuropathies, because prognosis from superimposed compression neuropathies in the context of critical illness polyneuropathy is less favorable.[95]

The pathophysiology of critical illness polyneuropathy is unknown. No clear metabolic, drug, nutritional, or toxic factors have been identified,[92] although the severity of critical illness polyneuropathy has been correlated with the amount of time in the ICU, the number of invasive procedures, an increased glucose level, a reduced albumin level,[93] and the severity of multiple organ failure.[99] Given the common antecedents of multiple organ failure and sepsis in which significant release of various cytokines occurs, increased microvascular permeability has been postulated to ultimately result in axonal hypoxia and degeneration as a consequence of endoneurial edema.[100]

Prolonged Effects of Neuromuscular Blocking Agents

Prolonged neuromuscular blockade may occur with nondepolarizing agents, particularly when hepatic or renal function is impaired. In one study, administration of vecuronium for 2 or more consecutive days resulted in prolonged neuromuscular blockade and paralysis lasting from 6 hours to 7 days.[101] Although vecuronium is hepatically metabolized, patients with renal failure were susceptible to prolonged effects due to delayed excretion of the active 3-desacetyl metabolite. Acidosis and elevated serum magnesium levels were also associated with prolonged paralytic effects of vecuronium. A peripheral nerve stimulator may be used to monitor muscle twitch responses to a train of four stimuli during use of neuromuscular blocking agents. Drug dosage should be titrated to preserve one or two twitches to avoid overdosing. Two- to 3-hertz repetitive nerve stimulation studies may also be used to confirm neuromuscular blockade when it is suspected.

ACUTE QUADRIPLEGIC MYOPATHY

The syndrome known as acute quadriplegic myopathy[102] or acute myopathy of intensive care[103] was originally described in 1977 in a young woman who developed severe myopathy after treatment of status asthmaticus with high doses of corticosteroids and pancuronium.[104] Subsequent to that report, there have been numerous citations of an acute myopathy developing in critically ill patients without preexisting neuromuscular disease. Acute quadriplegic myopathy has developed most frequently in the setting of severe pulmonary disorders, in which neuromuscular blockade is used to facilitate mechanical ventilation and high doses of corticosteroids are concurrently administered. In a majority of reported cases, myopathy developed when nondepolarizing neuromuscular blocking agents were used for more than 2 days.[102-112] The development of acute, necrotizing myopathy with myosin loss also occurs in patients receiving high doses of corticosteroids and hypnotic doses of propofol and benzodiazepines to induce paralysis.[113] This observation highlights the significance of high-dose corticosteroid exposure in the development of this syndrome and suggests that paralyzed muscles may be generally susceptible to the toxic effects of corticosteroids. The occurrence of acute quadriplegic myopathy after organ transplantation may be caused by the use of high doses of corticosteroids to prevent graft rejection along with perioperative exposure to neuromuscular blocking agents.[114] Although most cases of acute quadriplegic myopathy have been associated with critical illness, high doses of corticosteroids, and paralytic agents, acute quadriplegic myopathy has developed after isolated corticosteroid exposure,[102,115-118] isolated nondepolarizing neuromuscular blocking agent use,[112,116,119] or neither.[120] Factors that may impair neuromuscular transmission (e.g., hypermagnesemia, aminoglycoside exposure), factors that may slow the elimination of nondepolarizing neuromuscular blocking agents (e.g., hepatic or renal failure), and factors associated with critical illness (e.g., sepsis and acidosis) have also been associated with acute quadriplegic myopathy.[105]

In typical cases, a diffuse, flaccid quadriparesis with involvement of respiratory muscles and muscle wasting evolves after several days of induced paralysis. External ophthalmoparesis has rarely been noted.[121] Sensation remains intact, but deep tendon reflexes are reduced or absent. The creatine kinase level is commonly elevated, but this may not be observed if creatine kinase is measured well after the myopathy has developed. Although the paralysis may be quite severe and may necessitate or prolong mechanical ventilation, the prognosis from the myopathy itself is good, with functional recovery over several weeks to months.[107] Electromyographic findings include reduced amplitude of compound motor action potentials with normal sensory nerve action potentials and normal nerve conduction velocities. M-wave amplitude improvement accompanies clinical recovery.[112] Repetitive nerve stimulation studies may yield significant decremental responses while residual effects of

nondepolarizing neuromuscular blocking agents or their active metabolites persist.[105,112] Needle electromyography often reveals small, low-amplitude, polyphasic motor unit potentials exhibiting early recruitment, sometimes along with positive sharp waves and fibrillation potentials.

A spectrum of muscle histologic changes may be observed, ranging from type II fiber atrophy and loss of adenosine triphosphatase (ATPase) reactivity in atrophic fibers to fiber necrosis in severe cases. However, the distinctive finding in most cases of acute quadriplegic myopathy is an extensive loss of thick filaments corresponding to myosin loss.[102,106,111,115,120] This finding may be demonstrated with immunohistochemical staining or electron microscopy. The increased expression of steroid receptors in denervated and immobilized muscle[122] may render these muscles susceptible to toxic catabolic effects of steroids.[102] Given the growing recognition of acute quadriplegic myopathy, the use of high doses of corticosteroids should be avoided, if possible, when neuromuscular blockade or induced paralysis is required.

ANNOTATED REFERENCES

Hughes RAC, Wijdicks EFM, Barohn R, et al: Practice parameter: Immunotherapy for Guillain-Barré syndrome. Report of the Quality Standards Subcommittee of the American Academy of Neurology. Neurology 2003;61:736-740.
   This contemporary report derives evidence-based guidelines for immunotherapy (plasma exchange, IVIg, corticosteroids) in Guillain-Barré syndrome based on a review of available literature.

Lacomis D, Giuliani MJ, Van Cott A, Kramer DJ: Acute myopathy of intensive care: Clinical, electromyographic, and pathological aspects. Ann Neurol 1996;40:645-654.
   The clinical, electrodiagnostic, and histopathologic features of acute quadriplegic myopathy/acute myopathy of intensive care are described.

Sejvar JJ, Haddad MB, Tierney BC, et al: Neurologic manifestations and outcome of West Nile virus infection. JAMA 2003;290:511-515.
   This community-based, prospective case series of patients with suspected West Nile virus infection in Louisiana documents a spectrum of neurologic presentations of acute West Nile virus infection, including a poliomyelitis-like syndrome of irreversible flaccid paralysis.

Thomas CE, Mayer SA, Gungor Y, et al: Myasthenic crisis: Clinical features, mortality, complications, and risk factors for prolonged intubation. Neurology 1997;48:1253-1260.
   This large series provides a contemporary review of myasthenic crisis including its antecedents, course, complications, and outcome subsequent to the widespread use of immunotherapy in myasthenia gravis.

Witt NJ, Zochodne DW, Bolton CF, et al: Peripheral nerve function in sepsis and multiple organ failure. Chest 1991;99:176-184.
   This prospective series identified a 70% incidence of polyneuropathy developing in patients with multiorgan failure and sepsis.

Chapter 55

TRAUMATIC BRAIN INJURY

Steven M. Cohen • Donald W. Marion

KEY POINTS

1. **Severe traumatic brain injuries** are the leading cause of morbidity and mortality for Americans between the ages of 1 and 45 years.

2. **Outcome following traumatic brain injury** is determined not only by the primary injury, such as skull fracture and subdural hematoma, but also by secondary injuries initiated by post-traumatic ischemia.

3. **Secondary brain injuries** are primarily responsible for the development of delayed intracranial hypertension.

4. The **goal of critical care management** of patients with severe traumatic brain injury is to enhance cerebral perfusion and avoid therapy that may cause regional cerebral ischemia.

5. **Early assessment and triage** of patients with severe traumatic brain injury should use the advanced trauma life support protocol prescribed by the American College of Surgeons Committee on Trauma.

6. **Patients with severe traumatic brain injury** are best managed at a level I trauma center with immediate neurosurgical availability.

7. **All patients with contusions or hematomas** visible on head computed tomography scans and Glasgow coma scale scores of 8 or less will benefit from intracranial pressure monitoring.

8. **A ventricular catheter coupled to an external strain-gauge transducer** is the optimal means of monitoring intracranial pressure because it provides accurate measurements and allows for CSF drainage—the most benign way of treating elevated intracranial pressure.

9. **Prophylactic hyperventilation therapy**, particularly when the intracranial pressure is less than 20 mm Hg, should be avoided.

10. **Patients with subdural hematomas or contusions** benefit from anticonvulsive prophylaxis for 7 days after injury.

11. **Early evaluation of brain-injured patients** by a physical therapist and rehabilitation specialist is highly recommended and allows for their rapid mobility.

12. **Patients with mild or moderate brain injuries**, particularly those with sports-related concussions, benefit from careful neuropsychological evaluation before returning to contact sports.

13. **Athletes who have persistent headaches and focal neurologic deficits** should not be allowed to return to play until these symptoms have subsided.

An estimated 5.3 million people in the United States currently live with permanent disabilities due to traumatic brain injury (TBI). In addition to the personal toll, the direct and indirect costs of these disabilities are estimated to exceed $4 billion annually.[1] Americans sustain an estimated 1.6 million TBIs each year. Approximately 270,000 require hospitalization; 52,000 die of their injuries, and 80,000 are left with severe neurologic impairments.[2] Another 760,000 are treated and released, and an additional 400,000 mild or moderate TBIs are thought to occur but never come to medical attention.[3]

TBI is the leading cause of morbidity and mortality for Americans between the ages of 1 and 45 years. Teenagers and the elderly are most at risk, although the primary causes vary demographically. Motor vehicle crashes are the main cause of head injuries in those 5 to 64 years old, whereas falls are most common in people aged 65 years and older. The primary cause of penetrating head injury is gunshot wounds. Males have twice the risk of TBI as females across all age groups.

TBI death rates in the United States fell 22% from 1979 to 1992, according to one study.[4] A substantial decline in motor vehicle–related fatalities was primarily responsible. At the same time, however, the incidence of gunshot wounds to the head rose, and in 1990, firearms surpassed motor vehicle crashes as the single largest cause of death due to TBI in some urban areas.

PATHOPHYSIOLOGY

Trauma to the head causes primary injury, such as skull fracture, cerebral contusion, and hemorrhage, that is a direct physical consequence of the impact. Hours or days after the traumatic incident, secondary injury usually occurs and may be a major determinant of the patient's ultimate neurologic outcome.

PRIMARY INJURY

Injury to the brain is caused by external forces to the head that strain the tissue beyond its structural tolerance.[5] These forces

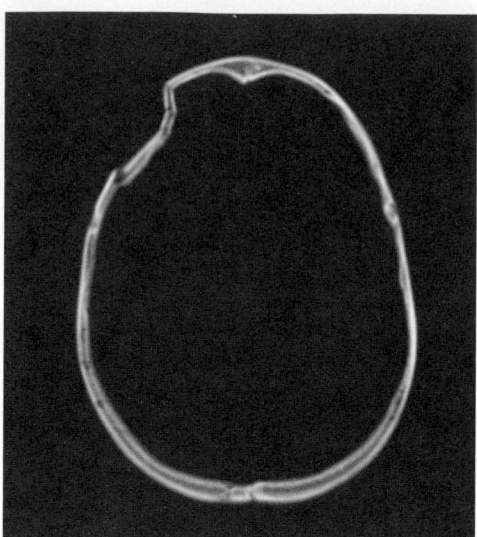

FIGURE 55–1. Right frontal depressed skull fracture caused by an assault with a hammer (axial CT scan, bone window).

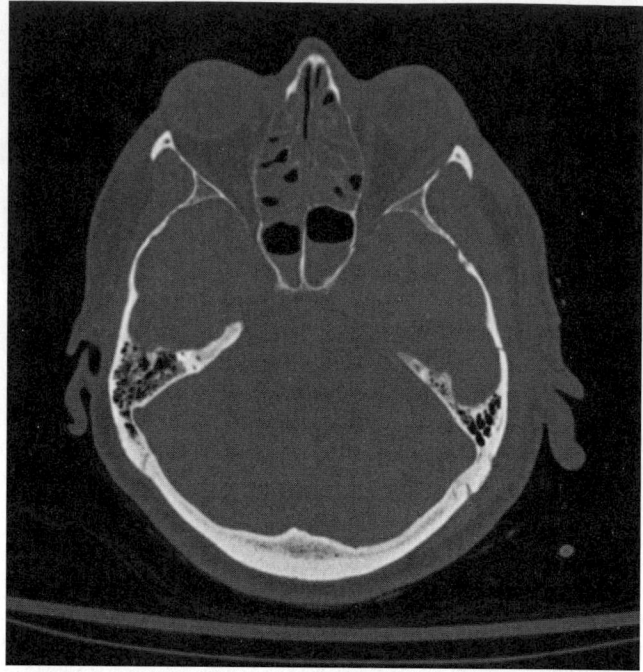

FIGURE 55–2. Basilar skull fractures through the anterior skull base typically cause cerebrospinal fluid rhinorrhea and tears in the adjacent dura. CT scans through the base of the skull may not show the fracture itself but often show fluid in the sphenoid sinus or the other paranasal sinuses (axial CT scan, bone window).

can be classified as contact or inertial.[6] Contact forces typically produce focal injuries such as skull fractures, contusions, and epidural or subdural hematomas. Inertial forces result from the brain undergoing acceleration or deceleration (translational, rotational, or both) and can occur without head impact. Inertial forces can cause focal or diffuse brain injuries: pure translational acceleration leads to focal injuries such as contrecoup contusions, intracerebral hematomas, and subdural hematomas, whereas rotational or angular acceleration, common with high-speed motor vehicle crashes, usually causes diffuse injuries. Although external signs of head injury, such as scalp abrasions, lacerations, and hematomas, are common with blunt-force trauma, the brain can also be severely injured solely by inertial forces, without accompanying scalp injuries.

Skull fracture results from a contact force to the head that is usually severe enough to cause at least brief loss of consciousness. Linear fractures are the most common type of skull fracture and typically occur over the lateral convexities of the skull. Most often, they are nondisplaced cracks in the skull, but a particularly intense impact can cause a gap (diastasis) between the edges of the fracture. A depressed skull fracture, in which skull fragments are pushed into the cranial vault, usually results from blunt force by an object with a relatively small surface area, such as a hammer (Fig. 55-1). The base of the skull can be fractured by severe blunt trauma to the forehead or the occiput. Basilar skull fractures are most common in the anterior skull base and often involve the cribriform plate, disrupting the olfactory nerves (Fig. 55-2). Posterior basilar skull fractures may extend through the petrous bone and internal auditory canal, thereby damaging the acoustic and the facial nerves.

Skull fractures per se are less detrimental than the associated damage to underlying tissues or vessels. For example, linear skull fractures that involve the squamous portion of the temporal bone are frequently accompanied by a tear of the middle meningeal artery, causing an epidural hematoma. Depressed skull fractures are often associated with contusions of the underlying brain tissue, and a scalp laceration overlying a depressed skull fragment can contaminate the fragment with bacteria from the scalp and hair. With a basilar skull fracture, the dura underlying the fracture is often disrupted, resulting in a cerebrospinal fluid fistula and leakage of cerebrospinal fluid from the nose or ear. Such fistulas allow bacteria to enter the intracranial space from the normally colonized nose, paranasal sinuses, or external auditory canal.

Common post-traumatic intracranial lesions are hemorrhage (epidural, subdural, and intraparenchymal), contusion, and diffuse brain injury. Subdural hematomas are seen in 20% to 25% of all comatose victims of TBI (Fig. 55-3). They develop between the surface of the brain and the inner surface of the dura and are believed to result from the tearing of bridging veins over the cortical surface or from disruption of major venous sinuses or their tributaries. The hematoma typically spreads over most of the cerebral convexity; the dural reflections of the falx cerebri prevent expansion to the contralateral hemisphere. Swelling of the cerebral hemisphere is common in those with subdural hematomas, given the associated damage to underlying brain tissue. Underlying cerebral contusions were found in 67% of patients with subdural hematomas in one series.[7] Subdural hematomas are classified as acute, subacute, or chronic, each having a characteristic appearance on computed tomography (CT): acute hematomas are bright white, subacute lesions are isodense with brain tissue and are therefore often overlooked, and chronic hematomas are hypodense relative to the brain.

Epidural hematomas develop between the inner table of the skull and the dura, usually when the middle meningeal artery or one of its branches is torn by a skull fracture. They occur in 8% to 10% of those rendered comatose by TBI.[8,9] The majority of epidural hematomas are located in the temporal or parietal regions, but they can also occur over the frontal or occipital lobes and, rarely, in the posterior fossa. They appear as hyperdense mass lesions on CT. Unlike subdural hematomas, their spread is limited by the suture lines of the skull, where the dura is very adherent. Because an

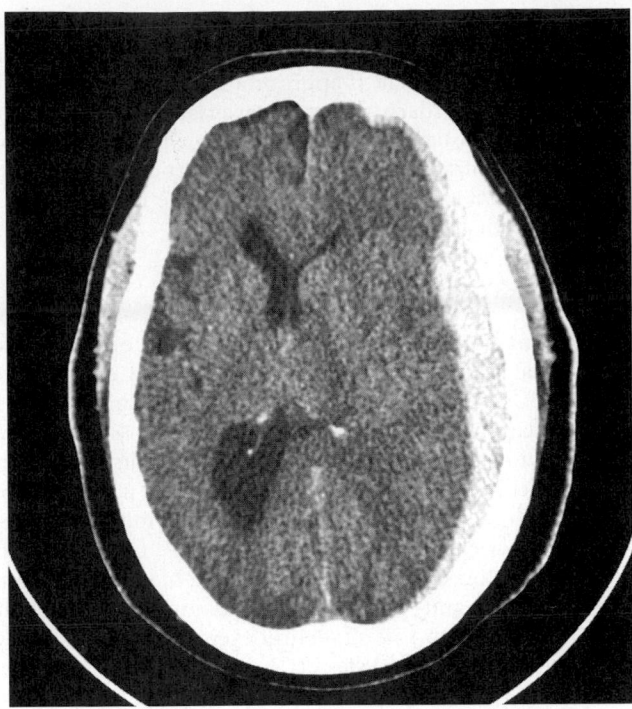

FIGURE 55–3. Acute subdural hematomas typically spread over the entire surface of the hemisphere.

epidural space normally does not exist, the clot must strip the dura from the inner table of the skull as it enlarges, resulting in its classic biconvex or lenticular shape (Fig. 55-4). Epidural hematomas are uncommon in infants and toddlers, presumably because their skulls are more deformable and less likely to fracture, and in TBI victims older than 60 years, because the dura is extremely adherent to the skull.

An intraparenchymal hematoma is a hemorrhage within the brain substance that occurs after a very severe TBI. It is usually associated with contusions of the surrounding tissue. Duret's hemorrhage, or hemorrhage into the base of the

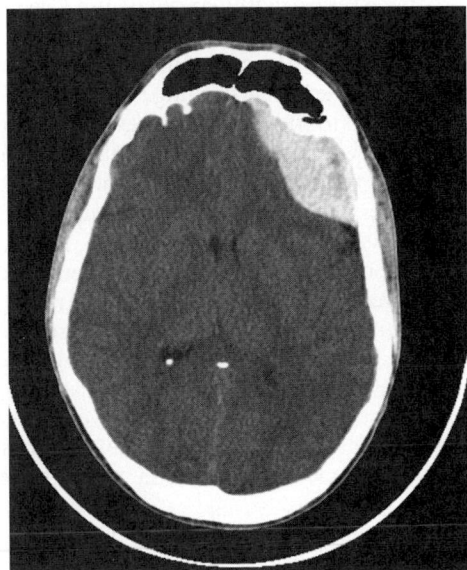

FIGURE 55–4. Epidural hematomas have a lens shape and a smooth inner border because they strip the dura from the inner table of the skull as they enlarge (axial CT scan).

pons or midbrain, is thought to result from disruption of the perforating arteries at the time of uncal herniation. Such brainstem hemorrhage almost always leads to death or vegetative survival.

Though common after severe TBI, subarachnoid hemorrhage does not produce a hematoma or mass effect.[10] However, it may be associated with an increased risk for post-traumatic vasospasm.[11]

Contusions are heterogeneous lesions comprising punctate hemorrhage, edema, and necrosis and are often associated with other intracranial lesions. One or more contusions occur in 20% to 25% of patients with severe TBI. Because they evolve over time, contusions may not be evident on the initial CT scan or may appear as small areas of punctate hyperdensities (hemorrhages) with surrounding hypodensity (edema) (Fig. 55-5). Local neuronal damage and hemorrhage lead to edema that may expand over the next 24 to 48 hours. With time, contusions may coalesce and look more like intracerebral hematomas. Depending on their size and location, they may cause significant mass effect, resulting in midline shift, subfalcine herniation, or transtentorial herniation. Contusions are most common in the inferior frontal cortex and the anterior temporal lobes,[12] where the surface of the inner table of the skull is very irregular; they result from shifting of the brain over this irregular surface at the time of impact. Direct blunt-force trauma to the head can produce a contusion in the tissue underlying the point of impact (coup contusion). If the head was in motion upon collision with a rigid surface, a contusion may occur in the brain contralateral to the point of impact (contrecoup contusion).

Diffuse axonal injury refers to lacerations or punctate contusions at the interface between the gray and white matter. Such punctate contusions are thought to result from the disparate densities of the gray and white matter and the

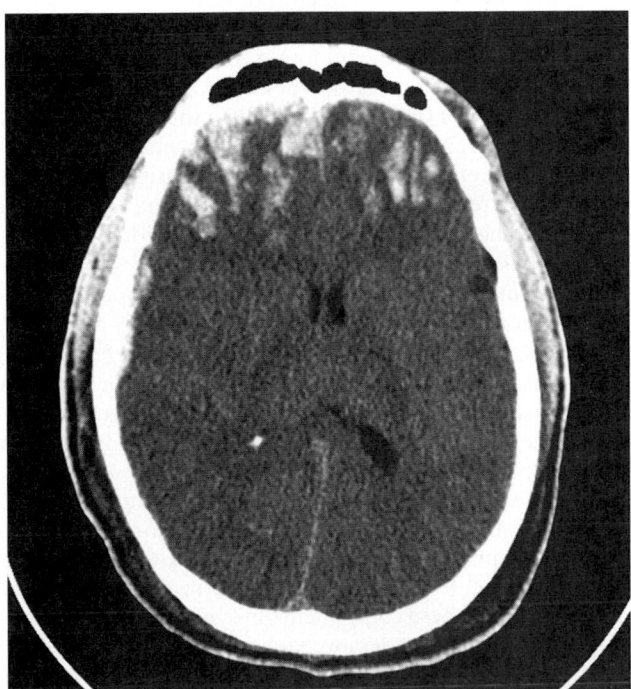

FIGURE 55–5. Contusions are most common in the inferior temporal and frontal lobes. In the first few hours after injury, they appear only as areas of hemorrhage mixed with edematous brain. Within 24 to 48 hours after injury, further hemorrhage may occur, causing significant enlargement of the contusion and hematoma (axial CT scan).

consequent difference in centripetal force associated with a rotational vector of injury.[13] Thus, diffuse axonal injury most often occurs after a high-speed motor vehicle crash, during which severe angular and rotational forces are applied to the head. Diffuse axonal injury was once thought to result solely from mechanical disruption at the time of impact; however, more recent research has identified cases in which the histologic footprints of diffuse axonal injury, such as fragmentation of axons and axonal swelling, do not appear until 24 to 48 hours after the incident, suggesting that some cases are a secondary manifestation of trauma.[14,15] Diffuse axonal injury is present in almost half of all patients with severe TBI and in one third of those who die, and it is a common cause of persistent vegetative state or prolonged coma.

Post-traumatic intracranial lesions cause neurologic dysfunction via direct and, in some cases, indirect mechanisms. By destroying brain tissue, contusions and intraparenchymal hemorrhage cause deficits directly related to the function of the damaged tissue. Uncal herniation is also an important mechanism of temporary or permanent neurologic deficits.[16,17] Semirigid dural reflections divide the intracranial contents into compartments. The tentorium cerebelli separates the anterior and middle cranial fossae from the posterior cranial fossa. The brainstem, specifically the midbrain, traverses an opening, the tentorial foramen, in the anterior central portion of this partition. The medial portion of the temporal lobe, the uncus, lies on both sides of the tentorial foramen. Because the most common TBIs, such as hematomas and contusions, are usually located over the lateral surfaces of the brain, and because the brain's extreme lateral surface is the rigid skull, such lesions tend to depress the brain medially. Therefore, a subdural hematoma over the surface of the temporal lobe or a hemorrhagic contusion of the temporal lobe itself is likely to displace the medial portion of the temporal lobe (uncus) into the tentorial foramen (i.e., uncal herniation). Such displacement compresses the midbrain, which contains neurons that are part of the reticular activating system. At the base of the midbrain is the crus cerebri, which contains pyramidal fibers from the cortex, and the third cranial nerve, which exits the midbrain through the interpeduncular cistern. Midbrain compression due to uncal herniation damages the reticular activating system, causing loss of consciousness; stretches the third cranial nerve and its associated parasympathetic fibers, causing pupil dilatation and loss of the light reflex; and injures the pyramidal fibers in the crus cerebri, causing abnormal posturing responses in the contralateral arm and leg.

Medial displacement of a cerebral hemisphere resulting from hemispheric swelling or a subdural or epidural hematoma also can cause herniation of the cingulate gyrus under the falx cerebri. Permanent neurologic dysfunction usually does not result, however.

Intracranial hypertension is a major cause of post-traumatic neurologic morbidity and mortality.[18] The intracranial pressure (ICP) is defined by the volume of cerebrospinal fluid, blood, and brain tissue in the cranial vault. The volume of these components is dynamic, and the brain can accommodate moderate changes in any of the three. For example, the blood volume can rise or fall by as much as 30% to 40%; cerebrospinal fluid absorption can increase to reduce the size of the ventricles by up to 90%; and brain tissue itself is compressible. Thus, the intracranial volume can gain 100 to 150 mL, equivalent to a moderate-sized subdural hematoma, without the ICP increasing significantly.

When these buffering mechanisms have been exhausted, however, even a small increase in the size of a hematoma will cause a rapid rise in ICP. If appropriate treatment is delayed, the ICP may approach the mean arterial pressure (MAP), causing a hydrostatic block of blood flow to the brain and brain death. Intracranial hypertension, particularly if refractory to medical or surgical treatment, is the most common cause of death after severe TBI.

SECONDARY INJURY

Post-traumatic ischemia initiates a cascade of metabolic events that lead to the surplus production of oxygen free radicals,[19-21] excitatory amino acids,[22,23] cytokines,[24,25] and other inflammatory agents.[26] Glutamate and aspartate are the excitatory amino acids most commonly implicated in excitotoxic injury,[27] which is mediated by activation of N-methyl-D-aspartate, α-amino-3-hydroxy-5-methylisoazole-4-proprionic acid, or kainic acid receptors.[23] Overactivation of these receptors causes an excessive influx of ionized calcium into the cytosol, and elevated amounts of ionized intracellular calcium play a key role in neurodegeneration after injury to the central nervous system (CNS).[28,29] In addition, post-traumatic nonischemic events, such as an increase in intracellular free Ca^{++} via receptor-gated or voltage-dependent ion channels, induce the release of oxygen free radicals from mitochondria.[30] Excessive levels of highly reactive oxygen free radicals cause lipid peroxidation of cell membranes, oxidation of intracellular proteins and nucleic acids, and activation of phospholipases A_2 and C, which hydrolyze membrane phospholipids, thereby releasing arachidonic acid. The liberation of arachidonic acid triggers the generation of free fatty acids, leukotrienes, and thromboxane B_2, all of which are associated with neurodegeneration and poor outcome after experimental TBI.[31-33] Inflammatory cytokines, particularly interleukin (IL)-1, IL-6, and tumor necrosis factor, also are overproduced after TBI.[34-36] In animal models, post-traumatic activation of microglia is a principal source of these cytokines.[25] IL-1 and IL-6 provoke an exuberant cellular inflammatory response believed to be responsible for astrogliosis, edema, and tissue destruction.[26,37]

TBI also increases extracellular potassium levels,[38] leading to an imbalance of intracellular and extracellular K^+, disruption of the Na^+,K^+-ATPase cell membrane regulatory mechanisms, and subsequent cell swelling.[39,40] Astrocyte swelling has been attributed to the clearance of excessive extracellular K^+.[41] High levels of extracellular K^+ have also been implicated as the cause of widespread neuronal depolarization and spreading depression seen after experimental TBI.[27,38,42] Moreover, potassium stimulates increased oxygen uptake in glial cells, potentially depriving adjacent neurons of oxygen.[43,44] Severe TBI also causes a substantial decrease in extracellular magnesium (Mg^{++}) levels, thereby impairing normal glycolysis, cellular respiration, oxidative phosphorylation, and the biosyntheses of DNA, RNA, and protein.[45-47] Because Mg^{++} competes with Ca^{++} at voltage-gated cell membrane–associated Ca^{++} channels, reduced levels of Mg^{++} will result in an abnormal influx of Ca^{++} into the cell.

PREHOSPITAL CARE

The acutely injured brain is vulnerable to further damage from systemic hypotension, cerebral hypoperfusion, hypercarbia, hypoxemia, and elevated ICP. Preventing these physiologic insults is crucial to limiting secondary brain injury. Care of the TBI victim always should begin with evaluating and securing a patent airway and restoring normal breathing and circulation. Early endotracheal intubation usually benefits comatose patients. Securing and maintaining an airway are essential to optimal oxygenation and ventilation, and early intubation has been found to reduce mortality after severe TBI.[48]

The airway is usually most easily and safely secured by orotracheal intubation, a method in which most emergency medical personnel are trained and experienced. Patients with severe maxillofacial trauma may require nasotracheal intubation, but this is less desirable because it is a relatively blind procedure; the nasal passageways can be irritated, causing blood pressure and ICP to surge; and, in those with severe anterior skull base fractures, the tube can inadvertently be passed into the brain. A third alternative for securing the airway is the laryngeal mask airway, an easily learned and rapidly applied device that has undergone successful field trials.[49] However, it does not protect against aspiration and cannot be used to achieve high airway pressures. A surgical airway (cricothyroidotomy) should be performed only after other attempts to secure an airway have failed, and only by an experienced provider.

The patient should be sedated and pharmacologically paralyzed before intubation, because irritation of the oropharynx typically causes transient hypertension, tachycardia, increased ICP, and agitation that can interfere with the procedure. Fentanyl, a short-acting opioid agonist that produces analgesia and sedation, is the most commonly used sedative. The usual dose is 3 to 5 μg/kg body weight, administered intravenously 3 minutes before intubation. Etomidate, an alternative to opioids, provides adequate sedation and is less likely to cause hypotension. Some prefer thiopental because it is an ultrashort-acting barbiturate and is thus less likely to conceal the neurologic status when the patient reaches the trauma center; however, it is more likely than other agents to cause hypotension. Neuromuscular blocking agents commonly used for endotracheal intubation include succinylcholine (1.5 mg/kg i.v.), which has the advantages of rapid onset, complete reliability, and very short duration of action. This last attribute is particularly important in the prehospital setting, where attempts at intubation sometimes fail. Vecuronium (0.01 mg/kg i.v.), an alternative paralytic agent, offers the theoretical advantage of being a nondepolarizing muscle relaxant. Because it has a relatively long duration of action (1 to 2 hours), however, it is less forgiving of failed intubation attempts. Table 55-1 shows a recommended rapid-sequence intubation pathway.

TABLE 55–1. RECOMMENDED RAPID-SEQUENCE INDUCTION FOR SEVERELY HEAD-INJURED PATIENTS

1. Preoxygenation
   100% oxygen for 5 min or four vital capacity breaths
2. Pretreatment
   Fentanyl (3 to 5 μg/kg i.v.)
3. Wait 2 to 3 min if possible
   Continue preoxygenation
4. Paralysis and sedation
   Succinylcholine (1.5 mg/kg i.v.)
5. Intubation with in-line cervical spine immobilization
6. Positive-pressure ventilation and possibly reparalysis with vecuronium if prolonged transport time is anticipated

Supplemental oxygen should be provided before and immediately after intubation. Ventilatory rates of 10 to 12 breaths per minute for adults, 20 breaths per minute for children, and 25 breaths per minute for infants should supply adequate oxygenation.[2] Therapeutic hyperventilation is inadvisable unless neurologic deterioration is clearly evident during evaluation and transport. Aggressive hyperventilation can cause cerebral vasoconstriction, reducing already low cerebral blood flow (CBF) and potentially causing or exacerbating cerebral ischemia.

Rapid fluid resuscitation and restoration of a normal blood pressure are critical in the prehospital setting, because hypotension has been associated with doubling of the mortality rate after severe TBI.[50] The most likely cause of hypotension is hemorrhage, usually in the abdomen or chest; therefore, hypovolemia should be assumed. Lactated Ringer's or normal saline solutions should be infused through a large-bore intravenous catheter as quickly as possible until normotension is achieved. Although preclinical studies suggest that hypertonic saline may be more effective than isotonic solutions for rapid volume resuscitation,[51,52] results of several small clinical trials have not been convincing.[53,54]

In all cases of severe TBI, defined as a Glasgow coma scale (GCS) score of 3 to 8 and an inability to follow commands, patients should be treated as if they have a spinal fracture until an adequate examination of the spine proves otherwise. Among those who survive long enough to reach the emergency department, the likelihood of a cervical spine fracture is 2% to 6%. More troubling, however, is that an estimated 10% to 25% of all post-traumatic spinal cord injuries are iatrogenic, occurring during transport to the hospital.[55] After respiratory and hemodynamic stabilization, the patient should be placed in a neutral position on a flat, hard surface. If the patient requires immediate endotracheal intubation, it should be performed while another person provides in-line cervical spine immobilization. A rigid cervical spine collar should be placed as soon as possible. Next, the patient should be placed on a backboard; the cervical spine can then be further immobilized with a buttress of foam or towels placed on both sides of the head. To prevent any movement during transport, the patient should be strapped to the board in several locations.

The organization of emergency medical services and regional trauma programs has improved outcomes for victims of trauma, particularly those with severe TBI.[56] Designation as a level I or II trauma center by the American College of Surgeons Committee on Trauma or a state health department ensures the availability of immediate neurosurgical care when the patient arrives. Therefore, every effort should be made to transport severely injured patients directly to a designated trauma center. Nonetheless, if an adequate airway or venous access cannot be obtained in the field, some patients may need to undergo respiratory or hemodynamic stabilization at a nearby emergency department en route to the trauma center.

EMERGENCY DEPARTMENT CARE

Upon arrival at the trauma center, the emergency medical personnel should concisely report their prehospital assessment and management, including mechanism of injury, stabilizing maneuvers, medications given, initial vital signs, GCS score, and hemodynamic stability during transport. A thorough physical and radiographic examination to identify all life-threatening injuries should then be performed. Most trauma centers follow the Advanced Trauma Life Support protocol, a comprehensive routine that has proved successful in quickly detecting all major injuries.[57] First, the airway is reassessed, and the need for endotracheal intubation is carefully reconsidered. For patients intubated in the field, proper placement of the endotracheal tube is verified both clinically and radiographically. When the airway is secure and adequate oxygenation is confirmed using a percutaneous oxygen saturation monitor or arterial blood gas analysis, two large-bore intravenous catheters are inserted to provide sufficient venous access for high-volume fluid resuscitation. An isotonic saline solution is infused to continue volume replacement, which probably began at the scene. Any life-threatening injuries, such as overt hemorrhage, tension pneumothorax, or cardiac tamponade, should be treated immediately upon discovery. A brief neurologic examination is performed, including assessment of the GCS score (Table 55-2), pupillary size and reaction to light, and symmetry and extent of extremity movements. The head is palpated to detect fractures, lacerations, or penetrating wounds, and lacerations are probed gently to ascertain the presence of a depressed skull fracture or foreign body. Large lacerations are compressed with pressure dressings or temporarily sutured to prevent further hemorrhage. Careful inspection of the head should reveal hemotympanum, periorbital or mastoid ecchymosis, and cerebrospinal fluid rhinorrhea or otorrhea.

Oxygen saturation is monitored continually, and blood pressure is measured frequently during this primary examination. A Foley catheter is placed to help monitor the fluid status, and an orogastric tube is inserted and connected to suction to decompress the stomach. Blood specimens are obtained and analyzed for glucose, electrolytes, complete blood count, platelets, prothrombin and partial thromboplastin times, and International Normalized Ratio. Type and crossmatch of a blood specimen should be considered, and an arterial blood gas obtained. Serum and urine toxicology screens are advisable if alcohol or substance abuse is suspected, and women of child-bearing age should undergo a pregnancy test.

The initial x-ray evaluation is usually performed in the trauma bay during the primary survey and includes chest, pelvis, and lateral cervical spine films. If the lower cervical spine is not visible on the lateral cervical spine film, a swimmer's view can be obtained, or this area can be imaged with axial CT.

After all life-threatening injuries have been identified and stabilized, the immediate concern is whether the patient requires a craniotomy to evacuate an intracranial mass lesion. A CT scan of the head should be performed, at intervals of 10 mm or less, from the C2 vertebra to the vertex. In addition to post-traumatic intracranial lesions, the scan should be examined for brain swelling, patency of the basal cisterns, and other characteristics that will guide subsequent treatment. If no surgical intracranial mass lesion is evident on the scan of the head, CT scans of the chest and abdomen can be performed to detect occult hemorrhage in these cavities. If a surgical mass lesion is seen on the head CT scan, however, it should be evacuated immediately, postponing any other imaging studies. Diagnostic peritoneal lavage is often performed during the craniotomy to detect abdominal bleeding. Conversely, if hemodynamic instability necessitates an emergent laparotomy or thoracotomy before a head CT scan can be obtained, several diagnostic procedures can be performed in the operating room to confirm a suspected intracranial injury. These procedures include an air ventriculogram or diagnostic burr holes and are most appropriate if the patient has lateralizing neurologic deficits, particularly a unilateral fixed and dilated pupil.

An air ventriculogram can detect most large hematomas. With the patient in the supine position, a right coronal ventriculostomy is inserted, and an anteroposterior radiograph of the skull is obtained. Just before the x-ray is performed, 3 mL of air is injected into the ventricles. The air outlines the ventricles on the film; a distorted or shifted outline suggests the presence and location of a hematoma.

An alternative to air ventriculography is the placement of diagnostic burr holes. The first burr hole should be placed over the temporal lobe ipsilateral to the dilated pupil. If no clot is detected, burr holes can be placed over the frontal and parietal lobes. If a hematoma is encountered, the burr hole is enlarged to a craniotomy, and the clot is evacuated.

DEFINITIVE TREATMENT

Critical to determining the severity of the brain injury and the appropriate treatment are CT findings combined with a reliable post-resuscitation GCS score and assessment of pupil size and reactivity. In the case of an acute subdural hematoma, for example, a patient with a moderate-sized lesion who has normal pupil size and reactivity and is able to follow commands might safely be treated nonoperatively. Conversely, surgery is unlikely to benefit an elderly patient with fixed and dilated pupils and a GCS score of 3 or 4, regardless of the CT findings. Other determining factors include the size and location of the hematoma, the presence and extent of an underlying contusion or brain swelling, and the results of the neurologic examination. Neurologic deterioration, particularly a decline in mental status, suggests enlargement of the hematoma, and a new CT scan should be obtained promptly. Hematomas less than 10 mm thick that cause a midline shift of less than 5 mm can usually be observed, especially if they do not involve the middle cranial fossa.[58] If nonoperative management is chosen for an intracranial hematoma, the

TABLE 55–2. GLASGOW COMA SCALE

Speech	Points
Alert, oriented, and conversant	5
Confused, disoriented, but conversant	4
Intelligible words, not conversant	3
Unintelligible sounds	2
No verbalization, even with painful stimulus	1

Eye Opening	
Spontaneous	4
To verbal stimuli	3
To painful stimuli	2
None, even with painful stimuli	1

Motor	
Follows commands	6
Localizes painful stimulus	5
Withdraws from painful stimulus	4
Flexor posturing with central pain	3
Extensor posturing with central pain	2
No response to painful stimulus	1

From Teasdale G, Jennett B: Assessment of coma and impaired consciousness: A practical scale. Lancet 1974;2:81-84.

patient should be monitored with frequent neurologic assessments in the ICU. If the patient cannot follow commands, ICP monitoring is recommended.

The classic presentation of a patient with an epidural hematoma is a period of unconsciousness immediately after impact to the head, followed by a so-called lucid interval in which consciousness returns for a few minutes to an hour or more before the patient lapses into a coma. This lucid interval actually occurs in less than one third of patients with epidural hematomas, however; most either remain conscious after the injury (smaller clots) or remain comatose.

A hematoma that compresses the temporal lobe is particularly ominous and can rapidly cause uncal herniation with minimal enlargement. Thus, such lesions warrant a lower threshold for evacuation compared with hematomas in other locations. If the clot is small enough not to require evacuation, it should be monitored with frequent CT scans during the first several days after injury. Enlarging middle fossa hematomas, even those large enough to cause herniation, do not always cause an increase in the ICP; therefore, ICP monitoring should not be relied on to follow their status.

The initial signs and symptoms of contusions vary greatly, depending on their size and location and the presence of other associated lesions. A small contusion may cause only a headache or no symptoms at all. If located in an eloquent area of the brain, such as the speech or motor areas, it may cause focal neurologic symptoms. Larger contusions, especially those involving the frontal lobes, typically cause elevated ICP and coma. Patients with small or deep-seated contusions without mass effect initially can be managed nonoperatively. The contusion should be followed closely with serial CT scans, however, because there is a 20% to 30% risk that the contusion will enlarge during the next 24 to 48 hours. The ICP should be monitored if the patient cannot follow commands. As with hematomas in the middle cranial fossa, contusions of the temporal lobes should be closely watched with CT scans. A temporal contusion can enlarge to the point of uncal herniation without a significant rise in ICP; thus, the threshold for evacuation of these lesions should be low (Fig. 55-6). Unilateral frontal or temporal lobectomies are usually well tolerated, do not cause measurable neurologic deficits, and provide space for further brain swelling.

In the ICU, the primary goal is to prevent cerebral ischemia and thereby limit secondary brain injury. The most common preventable causes of cerebral ischemia are hypotension, hypoxia, and intracranial hypertension. Thus, comprehensive physiologic monitoring should be performed so that these physiologic insults can be detected and treated promptly.

PHYSIOLOGIC MONITORING

Continual monitoring of the end-tidal partial pressure of carbon dioxide (PCO_2) and frequent analyses of arterial blood gases enable the early detection of deteriorating ventilatory status, which should prompt appropriate ventilator adjustments. Oxygen saturation should also be monitored continually with pulse oximetry. Blood pressure monitoring is best accomplished with an indwelling arterial catheter coupled to a pressure transducer. The catheter is usually inserted into the radial artery and can also be used to obtain arterial blood samples for blood gas analysis. Hypovolemia is a common cause of post-traumatic hypotension. It can result from overt hemorrhage, which is usually detected soon after injury;

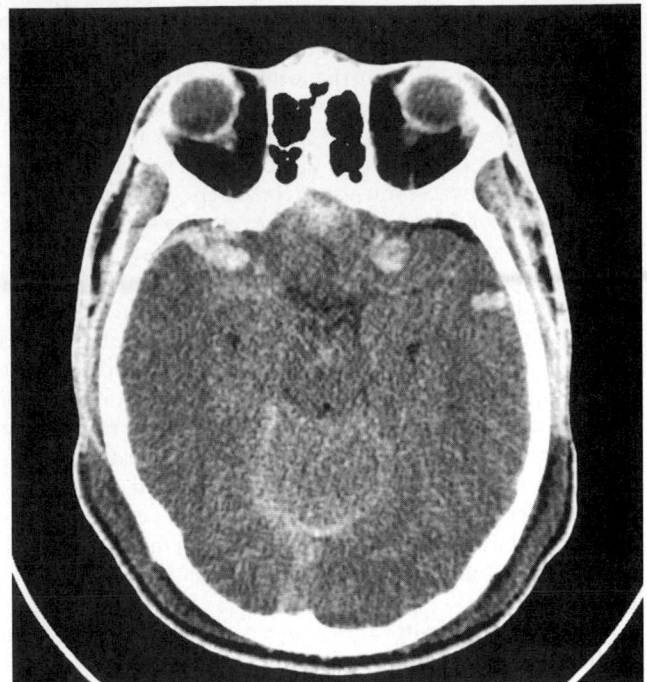

FIGURE 55–6. Temporal lobe contusions must be monitored closely, because even a slight enlargement can cause uncal herniation, often without an increase in intracranial pressure (axial CT scan).

from occult hemorrhage, which may not be recognized for several hours or days; or from soft tissue inflammation and swelling. Consequently, central venous pressure monitoring should be considered for patients with severe TBI, particularly those with significant non-CNS injuries. Indwelling subclavian or internal jugular venous catheters are used, coupled to pressure transducers. In elderly patients or those with severe pulmonary contusions, intravascular volume may be more accurately assessed by pulmonary artery catheterization with a Swan-Ganz catheter. Monitoring urine output with an indwelling Foley catheter is essential for determining the patient's fluid status.

Continuous ICP monitoring is essential for all patients who have severe TBI and abnormal CT findings, because intracranial hypertension develops in 53% to 63% of such patients.[59] ICP monitoring is also recommended for comatose patients who are older than 40 years and have unilateral or bilateral motor posturing or a systolic blood pressure less than 90 mm Hg, even if no abnormalities are seen on the initial CT scan.[60] The gold standard for ICP monitors is the ventricular catheter, coupled to an external strain-gauge transducer.[61] It is accurate, reliable, and far less expensive than newer self-contained pressure-sensing devices. In addition, ventricular pressure is considered more reflective of global ICP than is subdural, subarachnoid, or epidural pressure. Catheters placed in these extracerebral spaces are more prone to occlusion and, owing to the effects of compartmentalization, typically record a pressure that is lower than the global ICP. Other advantages of the ventriculostomy method of ICP monitoring are that the system can be rezeroed after insertion, which is not possible with most of the newer self-contained devices, and cerebrospinal fluid can be withdrawn to treat intracranial hypertension. The overall complication rate for ventricular ICP monitoring is 7.7% (infection, 6.3%; hemorrhage, 1.4%),[59] and some studies indicate that the infection rate increases significantly when a catheter remains in place for more than 5 days.[62]

Alternatives to the ventriculostomy technique have been developed that provide relatively accurate measurements of global ICP, are easier to insert, and may cause fewer complications. They include devices that contain a pressure-sensing transducer (either strain-gauge or fiber-optic technology) within the tip of the catheter.[61] These pressure sensors provide reliable ICP measurements even if they are inserted into the white matter and are often used when a ventricular catheter is difficult to insert because of small or collapsed ventricles. The primary disadvantage is that cerebrospinal fluid drainage is not possible. In addition, these devices can be calibrated only once, before insertion, and with some of them, measurement drift is as much as 1 to 2 mm Hg per day.

The cerebral perfusion pressure (CPP), defined as the difference between MAP and ICP, is a calculated physiologic measurement that is used to describe actual cerebral perfusion. Some have suggested that maintaining the CPP above a certain threshold is more important than any particular MAP or ICP.[63]

Devices that monitor the oxygen partial pressure (PO_2) of brain tissue can be used to determine whether cerebral oxygenation is adequate. These monitors continually measure the tissue PO_2 in the small region of brain into which they are inserted. The probes have been found to be very sensitive to changes in arterial PO_2 and PCO_2, as well as to medically induced or physiologic changes that may cause focal cerebral ischemia.[64] Although no methods are available for continuously monitoring global CBF, transcranial Doppler insonation of the middle cerebral arteries can provide indirect information. Positron emission tomography or CBF measurements with xenon, either as a radiolabeled agent or as a CT contrast medium, can provide periodic snapshots of the blood flow.

MEDICAL TREATMENT

Hypoxia is best avoided with the use of endotracheal intubation and mechanical ventilation. The fraction of inspired oxygen should be titrated to provide an arterial PO_2 of 100 mm Hg. Maintaining an arterial PCO_2 of approximately 35 mm Hg is advised to avoid the cerebral vasoconstriction associated with aggressive hyperventilation. A form of acute respiratory distress syndrome (ARDS) can develop in patients with severe chest injuries. In such cases, adequate oxygenation requires the use of positive end-expiratory pressure (PEEP). Concern has been raised that the use of PEEP in patients with TBI may increase the ICP. However, clinical studies have shown that, in the presence of ARDS, up to 14 to 15 cm H_2O of PEEP can be used without measurable changes in ICP, most likely because ARDS significantly reduces pulmonary compliance.

Hypotension, defined as a MAP of less than 90 mm Hg, should be treated aggressively. Normovolemia should be restored by infusing isotonic saline as needed to achieve a central venous pressure of 7 to 12 cm H_2O. Hypotonic intravenous solutions can exacerbate cerebral edema and should be avoided. If the patient is anemic, packed red blood cells should be transfused to restore the hematocrit to at least 30%. If hypotension is refractory to volume resuscitation, the patient should be given a continuous intravenous infusion of a vasopressor medication, with the dose titrated to raise the MAP above 90 mm Hg. Dopamine and norepinephrine are the preferred vasopressor agents.

Although some advocate the used of induced hypertension to raise the CPP above 70 mm Hg, particularly if the ICP is elevated and difficult to reduce,[65] others do not support this practice. A prospective, randomized clinical trial of patients with TBI compared a group whose CPP was kept above 70 mm Hg via induced hypertension with a group whose CPP was allowed to drift to 60 mm Hg.[66] Six-month clinical outcomes did not differ between the two groups. Moreover, the group whose CPP was kept above 70 mm Hg required more vasopressor agents and had a significantly higher incidence of ARDS and other pulmonary complications. Others have found that the brain tissue PO_2 in patients with TBI typically does not fall until the CPP drops below 60 mm Hg.[67] Based on these findings, the current recommendation is to maintain a CPP above 60 mm Hg.

Intracranial hypertension is defined as sustained ICP greater than 20 mm Hg. Several clinical studies have found that mortality and morbidity increase significantly when the ICP persistently remains above this threshold.[68] Based on this association and the widely accepted premise that elevated ICP can compromise cerebral perfusion and cause ischemia, the aggressive treatment of intracranial hypertension is almost uniformly endorsed. Before beginning therapy for intracranial hypertension, however, medical or physiologic conditions that can increase ICP should be considered and, if present, treated. These include seizures, fever, jugular venous outflow obstruction (e.g., poorly fitting cervical collars), and agitation.

Several medical and surgical options are available to reduce ICP. Depending on the type of brain injury, some may be more effective than others, and each is associated with potential adverse effects. A stepwise approach is usually followed, with the least toxic therapies being tried first and more toxic therapies added only if the initial treatment is unsuccessful. Sedation and pharmacologic paralysis are often an effective first treatment, particularly if the patient is agitated or posturing. A narcotic, such as morphine or fentanyl, is used for sedation, and vecuronium bromide is the paralytic agent. Narcotic-induced hypotension can be averted by using relatively low doses and ensuring that the patient is normovolemic before treatment. Because the ability to obtain an accurate GCS score is lost during this treatment, the pupil status, ICP, and CT scans must be closely monitored.

If intracranial hypertension is refractory to sedation and paralysis, intermittent ventricular cerebrospinal fluid drainage is used. Intermittent rather than continuous drainage enables reliable measurement of the ICP. If these measures fail to reduce the ICP, a bolus administration of mannitol is recommended (0.25 to 1 g/kg every 3 to 4 hours as needed). This osmotic diuretic lowers ICP and increases CPP by expanding the blood volume, reducing the blood viscosity, and increasing CBF and oxygen delivery to the tissues within a few minutes of infusion. Its duration of effect averages 3 to 5 hours. Continuous infusion is less desirable than bolus infusion, because the former is more likely to lead to extravasation of the drug into brain tissue, causing a reverse osmotic gradient and increased edema and ICP.[69] The serum osmolarity and sodium level should be monitored frequently during mannitol administration; to minimize the risk of acute tubular necrosis and renal failure, the drug should be discontinued if the serum sodium level exceeds 160 mg/dL or the osmolarity exceeds 320 mOsm. The intravascular volume should also be closely monitored to prevent dehydration.

If, despite these measures, the ICP remains above 20 mm Hg, the ventilatory rate can be adjusted to reduce the arterial PCO_2 to 30 mm Hg. Hyperventilation should be used cautiously during the first 24 to 48 hours after injury, however, because it will cause cerebral vasoconstriction at a time when CBF is already critically reduced. Recent evidence also suggests that even brief periods of hyperventilation can lead to secondary brain injury by causing an increase in extracellular lactate and glutamate levels.[70] Prophylactic hyperventilation is always contraindicated in the absence of elevated ICP.[71] If hyperventilation is used, the brain tissue PO_2 or jugular venous oxygen saturation should be monitored to detect any cerebral ischemia that the treatment might cause. The risk of tissue ischemia and poor outcome may increase if the brain tissue PO_2 falls below 10 mm Hg.[67]

If intracranial hypertension persists despite all these treatments, particularly if the ICP rises rapidly or if the patient's initial CT scan showed a small contusion or hematoma, another CT scan should be obtained immediately to determine whether there is a new mass lesion or a preexisting lesion has enlarged. Even if the lesion has enlarged only slightly, an emergent craniotomy and evacuation of the contusion or hematoma may be the best way to reduce the ICP quickly and effectively.

If the CT scan does not reveal an intracranial mass lesion requiring surgery, the next recommended treatment for intracranial hypertension is high-dose barbiturates. Barbiturates are thought to be effective by reducing cerebral metabolic demand and blood flow, and preclinical studies suggest significant cerebral protective effects.[72] Pentobarbital is the most commonly used drug for this purpose and is administered as an intravenous loading dose of 10 to 15 mg/kg over 1 to 2 hours, followed by a maintenance infusion of 1 to 2 mg/kg per hour. The dose can be increased until intracranial hypertension subsides or MAP begins to fall. Some recommend continuous electroencephalographic monitoring while increasing the dose until a burst suppression pattern is observed. Hypotension, the most common adverse effect of barbiturates, can usually be averted by ensuring a normal intravascular volume before administering the drug.

Only a few options remain when intracranial hypertension is recalcitrant to all these measures, and they are controversial and not uniformly embraced. Therapeutic moderate hypothermia has been used in several clinical trials over the past decade. The body temperature is lowered to 32°C to 33°C as soon as possible after injury and kept at that temperature for 24 to 48 hours using surface cooling techniques. Although some clinical trials have not found that this treatment improves neurologic outcome compared with normothermia, they have consistently shown that hypothermia significantly reduces ICP. Moreover, hypothermia does not cause significant medical complications when used for no longer than 48 hours.

Some advocate the use of decompressive craniectomies, such as large lateral or bifrontal bone flaps, with or without a generous temporal or frontal lobectomy. In one study of patients with severe TBI, 6-month outcomes were similar for a group that had large decompressive craniectomies and a group that did not, even though the craniectomy group had lower initial GCS scores and more severe radiographic injuries.[73] Importantly, the craniectomy group did not have a higher incidence of persistent vegetative state. Two studies reported good outcomes in 56% to 58% of patients whose refractory intracranial hypertension was treated with decompressive craniectomy as a last resort,[74,75] and another study suggested that decompressive temporal lobectomy, when performed soon after injury, improves the outcome for young patients.[76] However, others found that decompressive craniectomy does not improve ICP, CPP, or mortality rates.[77] The decision to perform decompressive surgery should take into account the patient's ultimate prognosis. Because age has such a profound impact on the likelihood of a meaningful recovery, these therapies are recommended only for patients who are younger than 40 years old.

Patients who have TBI, particularly those who are comatose or have significant non-CNS injuries, are at high risk for pneumonia and other infections, fever, malnutrition, seizures, deep venous thrombosis, pulmonary embolism, and other maladies endemic to the ICU. Most of these complications cause secondary brain injury and should be diagnosed and treated without delay. Fever is very common in the ICU and occurs in more than 90% of patients who are there for 10 days or more.[78] Preclinical studies have found that there is a log increase in neuronal death in ischemic brain regions for every degree of brain temperature above 39°C,[79,80] and this effect is observed for 24 hours or more after injury.[81] Clinical studies of TBI patients have shown that the brain temperature is often 1°C to 2°C higher than body temperature.[82] Consequently, the body temperature should be kept below 37°C at all times, and infectious or other causes of fever should be aggressively sought and treated.

Patients who are comatose, those being kept pharmacologically paralyzed, and those with pelvic or long bone fractures are at high risk for deep venous thrombosis and pulmonary embolism. They should receive early prophylaxis, which typically includes the use of lower extremity sequential compression devices as well as subcutaneous heparin or enoxaparin. The early (2 to 3 days after injury) use of mini-dose heparin or low-molecular-weight heparin is safe and has not been found to cause or worsen intracranial hemorrhage after TBI.[83,84]

Malnutrition is also common after severe TBI. The resting metabolic expenditure typically increases by 140% in a non-paralyzed patient with severe TBI.[85] Branched chain amino acids from muscle protein are used preferentially for energy metabolism, potentially compromising the effectiveness of physical therapy. Nitrogen wasting is also increased, with excretion of as much as 9 to 12 g/day. Thus, early enteral or parenteral feeding is advisable, with the aim of providing at least 140% of the daily basal metabolic caloric requirements by the third or fourth day after injury.[86] A normal-sized adult patient usually needs 2000 to 3000 kcal/day. Because parenteral feeding increases the risk of infection, enteral administration is preferable. For a patient expected to be in a prolonged coma, a surgical jejunostomy provides a convenient and well-tolerated route to administer tube feeding.

Post-traumatic contusions and subdural hematomas are well-known causes of generalized seizures. Anticonvulsant prophylaxis, usually with phenytoin, is therefore recommended for patients with these lesions. The drug should be given for the first 7 days after injury; a prospective clinical trial found no advantage to longer prophylactic treatment.[87] A common side effect of phenytoin is fever; this should be considered if infectious causes of fever have been ruled out. If a patient has seizures, especially if they are prolonged, the associated cerebral hypermetabolism will cause secondary brain injury; seizures should thus be treated aggressively, up to and including the use of general anesthesia if necessary. Seizures may not be readily evident in patients undergoing pharmacologic paralysis for the treatment of intracranial hypertension, because tonic-clonic extremity movements are absent. Such patients should receive anticonvulsant prophylaxis, and continuous electroencephalographic monitoring should be considered. Clinically silent seizures are a possible cause of abruptly deteriorating cerebral oxygenation or a sudden increase in ICP, but enlarging intracranial mass lesions remain the most likely cause.

PHYSICAL THERAPY AND REHABILITATION

The number of survivors of TBI is increasing due to greater success in understanding and treating the disease and improved motor vehicle safety devices. Accordingly, the demand for high-quality, well-organized TBI rehabilitation programs is also increasing. The primary goal of these programs is to reintegrate patients into their communities by either restoring normal or near-normal ability to function or teaching them alternative strategies to function well despite their disabilities. Such programs should involve a multidisciplinary team of physical, occupational, and speech therapists; neuropsychologists; and social workers, ideally coordinated by a physiatrist or a neurologist with special training in physical medicine and rehabilitation. The team should be experienced in TBI rehabilitation and thoroughly understand the special needs of these patients. Programs that focus exclusively on TBI rehabilitation are far preferable to those that mix patients with TBI, stroke, neurodegenerative diseases, and tumors, because the typical age groups are very different, as are their rehabilitative needs.

Rehabilitation of TBI patients should begin in the ICU during the first few days after injury, with the consultation of a physiatrist and passive range-of-motion exercises of the extremities. Mobilization helps prevent deep venous thrombosis, and studies indicate that early sitting of comatose patients may hasten the return of consciousness. Supplementing physical therapy with central neurostimulant medications is being investigated for those with more severe injuries and minimal responsiveness.[88] Rehabilitation after a TBI entails many other factors that are critical to optimizing outcome, but a thorough review is beyond the scope of this chapter.

PENETRATING INJURIES

Gunshot wounds to the head, the predominant cause of penetrating head injury, usually cause massive destruction of brain tissue, severe brain swelling, and death. The wounding potential of a bullet depends primarily on its velocity at impact and its mass, although the shape of the bullet and its lateral movements also play a role. The relationship of bullet mass and velocity to the energy imparted to the head is described by the equation $KE = \frac{1}{2}MV^2$, where KE is kinetic energy, M is the mass of the bullet, and V is the impact velocity of the bullet. According to this equation, the impact velocity is by far the most important determinant of a bullet's wounding potential. Consequently, high-velocity rifle wounds to the head are invariably fatal, whereas low-velocity open-chambered handgun wounds often are not. When a bullet enters the skull, it creates a variety of pressure waves within the brain, some of which can cause tissue pressures of nearly 100 atmospheres, resulting in further tissue injury. In addition to forward velocity, the bullet's lateral motion before and after impact affects the severity of tissue destruction. Such motion is described as yaw, or the angle between the bullet's path of flight and its long axis, and precession and nutation, which are circular rotations of the bullet around the center of its mass. These movements increase the bullet's relative surface area at the point of impact and enable it to pass more of its kinetic energy to the surrounding tissue. They increase the size of the entrance wound and cause greater cavitational injury. Bullets often fragment after they strike the skull, fracturing a portion of the skull into multiple fragments. Both the bullet and the bone fragments then become numerous secondary missiles that cause additional tissue damage.

Low-velocity missile wounds, such as those from knives, ice picks, or arrows, do not cause the massive brain injuries seen with bullets, as might be predicted by the kinetic energy equation. Usually, only the tissue in the immediate path of the missile is damaged, and patients often have a complete neurologic recovery after the missile is surgically extracted. Rarely, a missile injures a major intracranial artery or venous sinus, and these vascular injuries can result in large intracranial hematomas. Nonetheless, vascular injuries are always possible with high- or low-velocity missile injuries to the head, especially those in or near the skull base or the sylvian fissures.

The initial assessment and resuscitation of patients with penetrating head injuries are the same as for those with closed head injuries, as detailed earlier in this chapter. Prompt and aggressive cardiopulmonary resuscitation is critical. Knives or other missiles protruding from the head should never be removed in the field or emergency department; if they are tamponading a damaged intracranial vessel, removal could lead to massive intracranial hemorrhage. When a patient has a gunshot wound to the head, the neck, chest, and abdomen should be inspected carefully for other gunshot wounds, because wounds to the heart or great vessels in the chest or abdomen may be even more life threatening. A post-resuscitation GCS score should be obtained as soon as possible to guide future therapeutic decision-making. A CT scan of the head defines the intracranial path of the missile and related skull and tissue damage. More important, it identifies any large intracranial hematomas or contusions that may significantly affect outcome. If the missile trajectory is in or near the skull base or sylvian fissures and the patient is deemed salvageable, cerebral angiography should be performed.

Most patients who are expected to survive a penetrating head injury require at least limited operative treatment. Large intracranial hematomas should be evacuated promptly. A craniotomy is required for low-velocity missile wounds in which the object is still protruding from the head. After removing a segment of skull containing the missile and large enough to allow for intracerebral exploration, the surgeon can seek and immediately repair or occlude any vascular injuries caused by the missile. For gunshot wounds to the head, the surgeon should perform a limited debridement of the scalp and skull wound, removing scalp, bone, and bullet fragments penetrating the brain only if they lie near the surface. Easily accessible necrotic brain should be debrided, and meticulous hemostasis achieved. Dural closure is important because it reduces the risk of cerebrospinal fluid leak and infection, but it usually requires a pericranial graft. Artificial dural substitutes and allografts increase the risk of infection and therefore are not recommended.

Subsequent medical management of penetrating injuries is as described previously for closed head injuries. In addition, patients should receive prophylactic antibiotics for at least 14 days, because the missile usually carries skin and hair into the brain. Because a penetrating TBI, by definition, disrupts and contuses brain tissue, all patients with these injuries should also receive anticonvulsants for at least 7 days.

MILD AND MODERATE INJURY

A mild TBI is defined by an initial GCS score of 14 or 15; a moderate TBI, by a GCS score of 9 to 13. Often referred to as concussions, these injuries typically involve a brief loss of consciousness at the time of impact to the head and some degree of retrograde or post-traumatic amnesia; however, patients with such injuries can follow commands. They usually do not have the complex intracranial pathology associated with severe TBI and therefore are unlikely to die from the injury; mortality rates are near zero for those with mild TBI and approximately 4% for those with moderate TBI. Nonetheless, these injuries can cause long-term cognitive and neuropsychological impairment.[1] As many as 10% of those with mild injuries and 66% of those with moderate injuries suffer prolonged or permanent disabilities that prevent them from returning to work or school.

Rotational, acceleration, and deceleration forces are common causes of these injuries, particularly those that result in loss of consciousness. The impact usually is not intense enough to cause intracranial hematoma, cerebral contusion, skull fracture, or brain swelling. Although a small amount of subarachnoid hemorrhage may be present, usually in the sulci over the frontal or temporal lobes, CT findings are usually normal. Abnormal magnetic resonance imaging (MRI) findings have been reported in as many as 30% of these patients, most commonly diffuse hyperdense lesions on T2-weighted images. These lesions are thought to represent focal or punctate contusions.[89,90] Functional MRI often shows abnormal activation patterns, particularly if the patient has lost consciousness or is symptomatic at the time of the study.[90]

Several factors determine the appropriate level of medical evaluation and treatment after mild or moderate TBI. Any loss of consciousness at the time of impact or retrograde or antegrade amnesia of at least several minutes warrants a thorough medical assessment, as do persistent headache, confusion, dizziness, diplopia, weakness, or numbness. A formal examination in the emergency department is generally advisable. Patients who are neurologically normal and asymptomatic after at least an hour of observation and serial evaluations can usually be safely discharged, with clear instructions to return immediately if symptoms or signs of

TBI develop. Ideally, these instructions are given to both the patient and a responsible companion.

A patient with persistent symptoms or neurologic deficits should have a CT scan of the head and be admitted to the hospital for observation. This is particularly important for those with GCS scores of 13 or less, because the risk of an intracranial hematoma or contusion large enough to require emergent craniotomy increases as the GCS score decreases. Among patients whose initial GCS scores are 9 to 13, as many as 40% have CT abnormalities, and 8% require neurosurgical intervention.[91]

Athletes—especially those involved in contact sports such as boxing, football, soccer, wrestling, and field hockey—are at high risk for mild and moderate TBI. One report estimated the incidence of concussion to be 40,000 per year for high school football players.[92] Athletes also have an increased risk for multiple concussions, which are much more likely to cause prolonged or permanent neurologic disability than is a single concussion, particularly if they occur over a short time span. Second impact syndrome is a rare but potentially lethal problem first noted in athletes in 1973 and later implicated as the cause of sudden death in several high school football players.[93,94]

Because sports-related concussions are associated with such disabling and potentially life-threatening consequences, coaches and athletic trainers must carefully consider whether an athlete should be advised to return to play or retire from athletic competition after a concussion. Several groups have devised concussion grading scales to evaluate concussion severity and developed guidelines to determine when an athlete can safely resume play. The most widely adopted scales are those developed by Kelly and colleagues at the University of Colorado,[95] Cantu,[96] and the American Academy of Neurology[97] (Tables 55-3 and 55-4). Most authorities recommend that athletes abstain from play for at least one season if, during that season, they sustain three or more grade I or II concussions or two grade III concussions.[98] In addition, many athletic organizations at the high school, college, and professional levels have adopted neuropsychological testing as a means of objectively evaluating the cognitive and neuropsychological consequences of each concussion.[99] The comparison of postinjury and preseason scores is a powerful tool for guiding return-to-play decisions.

A common sequela of mild or moderate TBI is postconcussion syndrome, a constellation of symptoms that can be disabling for weeks or even months.[100] The most common symptoms are headache, irritability, dizziness, tinnitus, lethargy, and sleep disturbance.[101] One or more of these symptoms develop in approximately 30% of patients 1 week after a mild or moderate TBI, but they usually subside within 3 months.[102] After 1 year, only 7% of patients report

TABLE 55–3. GRADING SCALES FOR CONCUSSION

	Grade of Concussion		
Scale	I	II	III
Colorado[95]	Confusion; no LOC; PTA <30 min	LOC <5 min; confusion; PTA >30 min	LOC >5 min; PTA >24 h
Cantu[96]	PTA<30 min; no LOC	LOC <5 min; PTA 30 min to 24 h	LOC >5 min; PTA >24 h
AAN[97]	Transient confusion; symptoms <15 min; no LOC	No LOC; transient confusion; symptoms >15 min	Any LOC

AAN, American Academy of Neurology; LOC, loss of consciousness; PTA, post-traumatic amnesia.

TABLE 55–4. RECOMMENDATIONS FOR RETURN TO PLAY

Concussion Grade	Colorado Guidelines[95]	Cantu Guidelines[96]	AAN Guidelines[97]
I	Return after 20 min if normal examination	Return same day if normal at rest and exertion	Return same day if normal at rest and exertion
II	Return after 7 days if asymptomatic	Return after 2 wk if asymptomatic at rest and exertion for 7 days	Return after 7 days if asymptomatic
III	Evaluation by neurologist or neurosurgeon; return after 2 wk if asymptomatic and cleared by specialist	Return after 1 mo if asymptomatic at rest and exertion for 7 days	Evaluation by neurologist or neurosurgeon; return after 2 wk if neurologically cleared

AAN, American Academy of Neurology.

residual symptoms, most commonly persistent headache. Postconcussion syndrome is best treated by a primary care physician or neuropsychologist who thoroughly understands the disorder. Cognitive testing is recommended for patients whose symptoms last more than a few weeks, because symptoms such as frustration and irritability are often linked to an inability to resume normal daily activities. If such testing identifies specific deficits, cognitive rehabilitation is recommended.[103] Persistent headaches, dizziness, and tinnitus should be treated symptomatically after a CT scan of the head establishes the absence of intracranial lesions. Post-traumatic disturbances of the ossicles of the inner ear semicircular canals can cause severe positional vertigo, and patients with vertigo or tinnitus may benefit from evaluation by an otolaryngologist. Factors associated with an adverse long-term outcome after a concussion include old age,[104] prolonged post-traumatic amnesia,[105] and a below-normal premorbid intellectual capacity.[106]

PROGNOSIS

Predicting outcome soon after a TBI can help guide acute and chronic care and help prepare family members for the typically protracted recovery process. Equally important is that further treatment may be deemed futile, and expensive critical care or surgery can be reserved for those who are likely to benefit. Of course, early prognostication must be reliable, especially when withdrawal of life support is a consideration.

Several clinical and radiographic characteristics have proved useful for outcome prediction, but they must be used in concert.[107] Moreover, these criteria are more reliable for predicting death or vegetative survival than for accurately predicting mild or no dysfunction and a complete return to normalcy. The most powerful outcome predictors are age, initial GCS score (particularly the motor component), pupil size and reaction to light, ICP, and the nature and extent of intracranial injuries.

Old age correlates most consistently with a poor outcome after TBI. In the Traumatic Coma Data Bank study of more than 700 patients with severe TBI, the incidence of death, persistent vegetative state, or severe disability was 92% for those older than 60 years, 86% for those older than 56, and 50% for younger patients.[108] The older groups had a higher incidence of traumatic intracranial mass lesions, midline shift, and subarachnoid hemorrhage, and the presence of these insults correlated strongly with poor outcome. Subsequent studies confirmed the low probability of a good recovery for patients older than 60 years whose initial GCS scores are 8 or less.[109]

The second most important predictor of outcome is the initial post-resuscitation GCS score. Among patients with severe closed head injuries in the Traumatic Coma Data Bank study, good outcomes occurred in 4.1% of those with an initial GCS score of 3, in 6.3% whose score was 4, and in 12.2% whose score was 5. Again, later clinical studies corroborated the strong direct correlation between initial GCS score and outcome.[110]

Unilaterally or bilaterally dilated pupils that are unreactive to light usually reflect uncal herniation and significant brainstem compression and damage; thus, this sign is ominous. Several large clinical studies found that patients with bilaterally fixed and dilated pupils had a greater than 90% likelihood of death or vegetative survival.[111,112] Also, intracranial hypertension refractory to medication is associated with a 43% mortality rate and 0% chance of a functional outcome.[113]

Various studies have analyzed the effect of the type and size of post-traumatic intracranial lesions on outcome, in terms of both the specific lesions and the CT-defined characteristics of their mass effect. Subdural hematomas are associated with the worst prognosis. One study found that only 26% of patients with these clots had a functional recovery.[114] However, the prognosis for patients with subdural hematomas is also related to how soon after injury the clot is evacuated, with the best outcomes in those who have surgery within 2 hours.[7]

Epidural hematomas pose a much lower risk of mortality because, unlike subdural hematomas, they usually are not associated with underlying cerebral contusions or swelling. If left untreated, however, epidural hematomas can cause uncal herniation and death. One report noted an increase in mortality from 17% to 65% if an epidural hematoma was not evacuated within 2 hours after the onset of coma.[8]

The presence of traumatic subarachnoid hemorrhage is associated with a 50% greater risk of death.[10,115] The link between traumatic subarachnoid hemorrhage and worse outcomes is controversial, however. Many believe that this condition merely indicates a more severe TBI and has no direct association with outcome.

Marshall and colleagues devised a CT-based classification scheme that proved prognostically useful when applied to the patients in the Traumatic Coma Data Bank study (Tables 55-5 and 55-6).[116] The classification emphasizes the mass effect of post-traumatic intracranial lesions. Not surprisingly, these investigators found the worst outcomes among patients with large intracranial mass lesions and uncal herniation.

TABLE 55–5. COMPUTED TOMOGRAPHIC CLASSIFICATION OF TRAUMATIC BRAIN INJURY

Category	Definition
Diffuse injury I	No visible intracranial pathology
Diffuse injury II	Cisterns present, with midline shift 0 to 5 mm; no high-density lesion >25 mL
Diffuse injury III (swelling)	Cisterns compressed or absent, with midline shift 0 to 5 mm; no high-density lesion >25 mL
Diffuse injury IV (shift)	Midline shift >5 mm; no high-density lesion >25 mL
Evacuated mass lesion	Any lesion surgically evacuated
Nonevacuated mass lesion	High-density lesion >25 mL; not surgically evacuated

From Marshall LF, Marshall SB, Klauber MR, Clark M: A new classification of head injury based on computerized tomography. J Neurosurg 1991;75:Σ14-Σ20.

Based on these studies, one can say with certainty that an 80-year-old patient who presents with bilaterally fixed and dilated pupils, a GCS score of 3 or 4, and a large subdural hematoma will not have a functional outcome regardless of treatment. However, the prognosis is much better for young patients with higher GCS scores, and aggressive surgical and medical management is usually warranted.

The patient's salvageability and prognosis after a penetrating injury are far clearer than for those with closed head injuries. Most victims of gunshot wounds to the head die before or shortly after hospital admission. Among 314 patients with civilian craniocerebral gunshot wounds, 92% died; 73% of them were pronounced dead at the scene of the injury, and 12% died within 3 hours of injury.[117] In the Traumatic Coma Data Bank study, the mortality rate was 88% for the 151 patients with gunshot wounds to the head.[118] No patient with an initial GCS score of 8 or less regained normal neurologic function, and only three recovered to the level of moderate disability, suggesting that the initial GCS score is an even more powerful predictor of

TABLE 55–6. RELATIONSHIP OF COMPUTED TOMOGRAPHIC CLASSIFICATION TO OUTCOME AT DISCHARGE

Category	No. of Patients	Unfavorable Outcome* (%)	Favorable Outcome† (%)
Diffuse injury I	52	38	62
Diffuse injury II	177	65	35
Diffuse injury III	153	84	16
Diffuse injury IV	32	94	6
Evacuated mass	276	77	23
Nonevacuated mass	36	89	11

*Death, persistent vegetative state, or severe disability.
†Moderate disability or good recovery.
From Marshall LF, Marshall SB, Klauber MR, Clark M: A new classification of head injury based on computerized tomography. J Neurosurg 1991;75:Σ14-Σ20.

outcome for these patients than for those with closed TBI. A meta-analysis of recent clinical studies examining civilian gunshot wounds to the head found that favorable outcomes (Glasgow outcome scale scores of 4 or 5) occurred in only 5 of 490 patients with initial GCS scores of 3 to 5.[119] Mortality rates ranged from 51% to 87% for patients with scores of 8 or less. In contrast, those whose initial GCS scores were 13 to 15 all survived and had favorable outcomes. Other clinical signs associated with death or a poor outcome are fixed and dilated pupils, intracranial hypertension, and hypotension. Also, a gunshot wound is more likely to be lethal if self-inflicted.

The CT-defined extent of intracranial injury caused by the missile also has prognostic significance. Hyperdense lesions with a volume greater than 15 mL, midline shift of more than 3 mm, compressed or absent basal cisterns, subarachnoid hemorrhage, and intraventricular hemorrhage are all associated with mortality rates of 80% to 90%, as is a bullet trajectory that traverses both hemispheres, the basal ganglia, or the posterior fossa.[118,120]

ANNOTATED REFERENCES

Chestnut RM, Marshall SB, Piek J, et al: Early and late systemic hypotension as a frequent and fundamental source of cerebral ischemia following severe brain injury in the Traumatic Coma Data Bank. Acta Neurochir Suppl (Wien) 1993;59:121-125.

The authors reviewed blood pressure readings in a group of several hundred patients admitted to the Traumatic Coma Data Bank. They found that hypotension (systolic blood pressure <90 mm Hg) was associated with a twofold increase in the mortality rate compared with head-injury patients who did not have hypotension.

Dietrich WD: The importance of brain temperature in cerebral injury. J Neurotrauma 1992;9(Suppl 2):S475-S485.

This experimental study showed that in an ischemic rodent model, there was a log increase in the death of ischemic neurons for every degree centigrade the brain temperature exceeded 39°C. Subsequent studies from this laboratory showed that this effect is also observed 24 hours or more after injury.

Muizelaar JP, Marmarou A, Ward JD, et al: Adverse effects of prolonged hyperventilation in patients with severe head injury: A randomized clinical trial. J Neurosurg 1991;75:731-739.

This prospective, randomized, controlled clinical trial evaluated the effects of prophylactic hyperventilation therapy. Patients who had an initial GCS score of 5, 6, or 7 and were prophylactically hyperventilated to a mean PCO_2 of 25 mm Hg for the first 5 days after injury had a significantly worse outcome than patients who were kept at a mean PCO_2 of 35 mm Hg.

Narayan RK, Kishore PR, Becker DP, et al: Intracranial pressure: To monitor or not to monitor? A review of our experience with severe head injury. J Neurosurg 1982;56:650-659.

The authors reviewed their experience with more than 100 patients with severe TBI and identified indications for ICP monitoring. They found that patients who had GCS scores of 8 or less and abnormal CT scans were very likely to have problems with intracranial hypertension and would benefit from ICP monitoring.

Temkin NR, Dikmen SS, Wilensky AJ, et al: A randomized, double-blind study of phenytoin for the prevention of post-traumatic seizures. N Engl J Med 1990;323:497-502.

In this randomized, controlled, double-blind study of the benefit of prophylactic anticonvulsant therapy for patients with TBI, the authors found a significant reduction in the incidence of post-traumatic seizures during the first week of therapy, but no subsequent benefit was observed when therapy was continued longer than 7 days. This study has led most to discontinue the use of anticonvulsants 1 week after TBI, regardless of the nature of the injury.

Chapter 56

SPINAL CORD INJURY

Elizabeth A. Vitarbo • Allan D.O. Levi

KEY POINTS

1. Most spinal injuries result from high-speed motor vehicle accidents.

2. Suspected spinal cord injury alters the basics of the "ABCs" of resuscitation in several important ways.

3. The primary injury mechanism results from a mechanical insult that occurs at the time of impact and includes acute compression, impaction, distraction, laceration, and shear. Secondary injuries occur after the initial injury and account for some of the progressive pathologic changes associated with spinal cord injury.

4. Respiratory complications are a major source of morbidity and mortality after spinal cord injury.

5. In the elderly patient with a spinal cord injury, careful attention to volume replacement is required so as not to precipitate heart failure.

6. The prognosis for recovery from spinal cord trauma is inextricably linked to age, with the younger patients fairing much better than their older counterparts for regaining neurologic function.

Despite substantial improvements in emergency, diagnostic, and surgical care, spinal trauma continues to present a challenging spectrum of diseases for the neurosurgeon to manage. When spinal trauma results in a spinal cord injury, the emotional and financial toll inflicted on individuals and their families is enormous. Improvements in the quality of care delivered over the past few decades are partially reflected in the recognition that centers of excellence that focus on the acute treatment and the rehabilitation of the spinal cord injury patient are best equipped to deal with the magnitude of services these patients require.

EPIDEMIOLOGY

Spinal cord injury typically occurs in males at the peak of their productive lives. The incidence of traumatic spinal cord injury is approximately 10,000 new cases each year in the United States,[1] with a prevalence of 191,000. The prevalence of spinal cord injury patients is increasing steadily owing to improved survival in both the acute and chronic stages of the disease. The amount spent on the treatment of spinal cord injuries in the United States is approximately 5.6 billion dollars each year and rising annually.[2] The cost of caring for the individual spinal cord–injured patient is directly related to the injury level of the spinal cord and to the patient's age, with the highest costs associated with the older quadriplegic patients who are dependent on a ventilator.[2]

ETIOLOGY

Most spinal injuries result from high-speed motor vehicle accidents (Fig. 56-1). Falls and work-related injuries are other important contributors. Spinal cord injury that is due to violence is on a dramatic rise secondary to increased incidence of assaults. These injuries include both blunt and penetrating injuries, such as gun and knife wounds. Sports-related injuries, which include football, horseback riding, and hockey injuries, are relatively rare but have received recent media attention.[3,4] Finally, recreational injuries from jet skis, snowmobiles, snow skiing, snow boarding, and parachuting, to name but a few, appear to be on the rise, as "extreme sports" become more prevalent.

INITIAL MANAGEMENT

Suspected spinal cord injury alters the basics of the "ABCs" of resuscitation in several important ways. With respect to airway management, suspected spinal cord injury dictates in-line immobilization of the spine at all times. Therefore, hyperextension of the neck is contraindicated. A jaw thrust must be used to open the airway, and required intubation must be done with the head/neck in a neutral position. This is an important point to remember, because patients with a high spinal cord injury will have diminished or absent respiratory capacity and frequently require emergent intubation.

Aggressive resuscitation of spinal cord injury patients proceeds as with all trauma patients. As indicated earlier, however, upper spinal cord injury may be associated with neurogenic shock, requiring large volume fluid replacement. Although pressors are likely to be required in the setting of neurogenic shock, field management is commonly limited to fluid resuscitation. High incidence of associated head injury often requires use of colloid solutions in addition to normal saline/lactated Ringer's solution, in an effort to adequately resuscitate the patient while minimizing exacerbation of cerebral edema.

IMMOBILIZATION AND DIAGNOSTIC EVALUATION

Rigid immobilization is indicated if there is any doubt as to the presence of spinal cord injury. Presence of altered mental status in any way dictates the use of "spinal cord precautions."

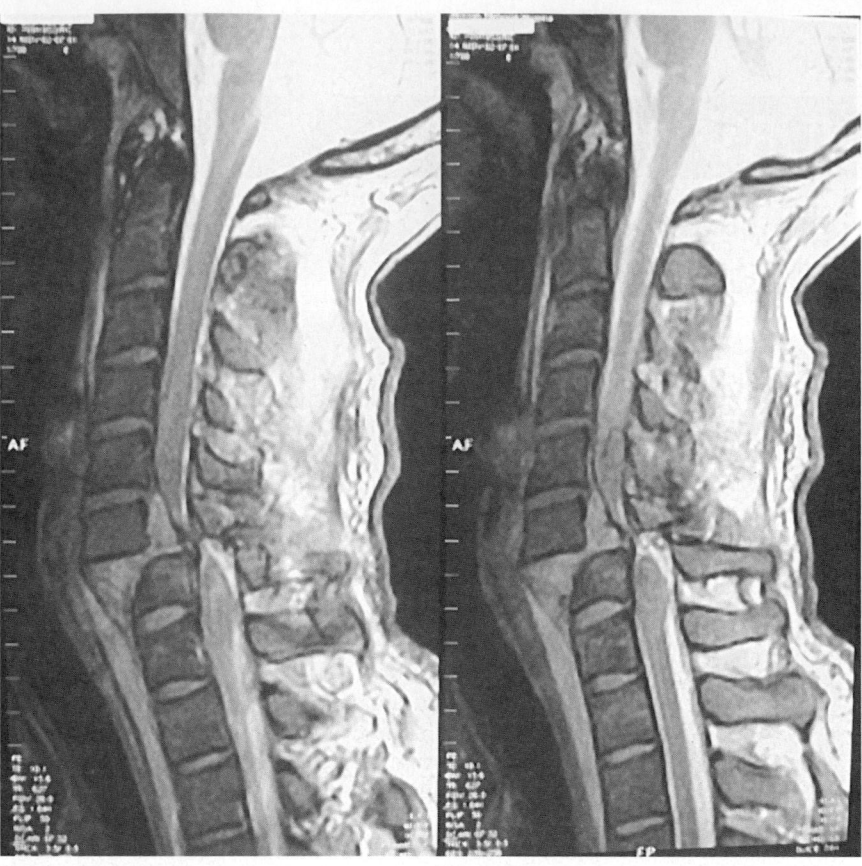

A   B

FIGURE 56–1. *A,* Sagittal T2-weighted MRI demonstrates a C6-C7 fracture-dislocation with severe cord compression in a patient who presented with complete C6 quadriplegia–ASIA. *B,* The patient was treated surgically to realign the spine and gained significant root recovery without any recovery of hand or lower extremity function.

These include use of in-line immobilization, maintenance of neutral position, cervical immobilization with a rigid collar, and use of backboards for transport.

After initial resuscitative efforts, diagnostic studies are undertaken. Initial studies must include lateral cervical spine radiographs clearly demonstrating the cervical spine down to the C7-T1 junction in patients with altered mental status and/or suspected cervical spine injury. Additional spine studies may be obtained after the patient has been stabilized and more emergent diagnostic studies have been undertaken. During this time, rigid cervical collar and backboard immobilization must be continued.

Further diagnostic studies will be dictated by the findings of the initial and secondary surveys, as well as findings of initial diagnostic studies. Several points are important to keep in mind. First, important information can be obtained from studies performed for other reasons. For example, routine chest and abdominal radiographs may provide important information regarding the presence of significant thoracic/lumbar spine injury. Although these do not replace subsequent "formal" spine studies, these are often obtained as part of the routine trauma work-up and provide early "clues" regarding the presence of spine trauma and may help prioritize subsequent imaging studies.

Whereas anteroposterior/lateral spine radiographs are tailored to complaints of spine pain and the neurologic examination, altered mental status dictates that cervical, thoracic, and lumbar anteroposterior and lateral films be obtained (Fig. 56-2). When abnormalities are identified, and/or studies are limited by body habitus, plain radiographs must be supplemented by CT to further characterize bony abnormalities. Sagittal reconstructions may be obtained and are often useful adjuncts to plain radiographs. The radiographs and particularly the CT are the most sensitive tools in detecting a fracture of the spine, but occasionally it is difficult to clear the spine—even in the absence of a fracture—because an unstable ligamentous injury without fracture may exist.

Patients with a suspected spinal column injury who are unconscious, uncooperative, or intoxicated, or who have associated traumatic injuries that distract from their assessment, will often require further radiographic study of the cervical spine before the discontinuation of cervical spine immobilization. Several options exist and include (1) maintenance of the collar and/or spine precautions until the patient becomes coherent and responsive, (2) dynamic imaging of the spine with physician monitoring, and (3) MRI of the spine to rule out a purely ligamentous injury. Of the three options, we frequently use MRI to clear the spine because a completely negative MR image in the setting of trauma indicates that there is no instability of the cervical spine (Fig. 56-3). Malalignment and evidence of spine trauma on these imaging studies frequently determines subsequent management and diagnostic decision making. Cervical subluxations often require the use of traction and/or manual reduction of the fracture-dislocation. Diazepam (Valium) or lorazepam (Ativan), along with careful neurologic monitoring, often in the ICU setting, is required because application of traction can realign the spine but can also result in neurologic deterioration.

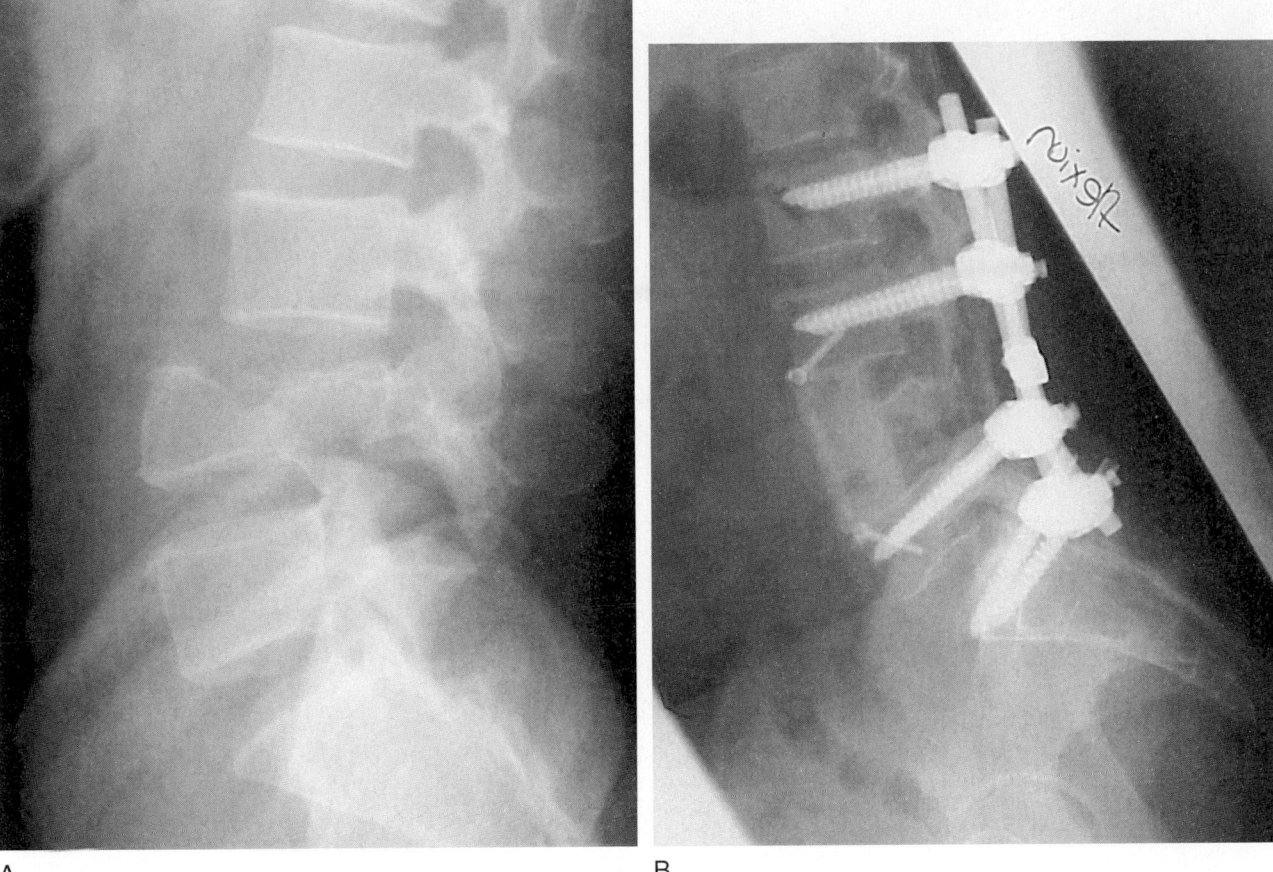

A   B

FIGURE 56–2. A 45-year-old man sustained a (*A*) L4 fracture-dislocation and presented with a dense footdrop and underwent a (*B*) anteroposterior reconstruction with instrumentation.

PEDIATRIC SPINAL CORD INJURY

Pediatric spine trauma is relatively uncommon, representing approximately 5% of all spinal cord injuries.[5] For a specific discussion of pediatric spinal cord injury, please see Chapter 248. In addition, guidelines have been published on this topic.[6]

PHARMACOTHERAPY

The concepts of primary and secondary spinal cord injury are important principles in understanding the pathophysiology and the role of pharmacotherapeutic agents in emergent treatment. The primary injury mechanism results from a mechanical insult that occurs at the time of impact and includes acute compression, impaction, distraction, laceration, and shear.[7] Secondary injuries occur after the initial injury and account for some of the progressive pathologic changes associated with spinal cord injury.[7] A number of drugs have been tested in the laboratory, but only a few of these agents have progressed to clinical trials to evaluate their efficacy. Five randomized controlled trials of pharmacotherapy for acute spinal cord injury have been conducted, focusing on the therapeutic effect of either corticosteroids or gangliosides.

CORTICOSTEROIDS

A number of studies have shown improved neurologic recovery in animals with spinal cord injuries that have received either dexamethasone or methylprednisolone.[8-12]

Corticosteroid treatment initially held promise as a potential therapeutic agent for its putative role in reducing white matter edema and inflammation. Current evidence, however, suggests that the major mechanism of action is by reducing the effects of secondary injury and, in particular, the destructive effects of lipid peroxidation on cell membranes.[2] Other actions include improving spinal cord blood flow, enhancing the postinjury activity of Na^+, K^+-ATPase, and facilitating the recovery of extracellular calcium ion.[8,13]

The first NASCIS investigator (NASCIS I) examined low- (100 mg) and high- (1000 mg) dose methylprednisolone given for 10 days. Unfortunately, this trial had no control group, and no significant difference in outcome was found except for an increased number of wound infections among patients in the high-dose group.[14]

The second NASCIS trial (NASCIS II) was a prospective, randomized, double-blind, multicenter trial that demonstrated improved neurologic outcomes after 6 weeks, 6 months, and 1 year in patients with nonpenetrating spinal cord injury who had received a regimen of methylprednisolone, which included a bolus dose of 30 mg/kg.[15] The improvement in motor and sensory scores associated with administration of methylprednisolone was only observed if the drug was given within 8 hours of injury when compared with naloxone or a placebo. The results of this study have been criticized.[16,17] Some of the criticisms relate to difficulties in randomization, reporting methods, analysis of benefit limited to small subgroups within the larger study, and lack of replication of results by a completely independent group of investigators,

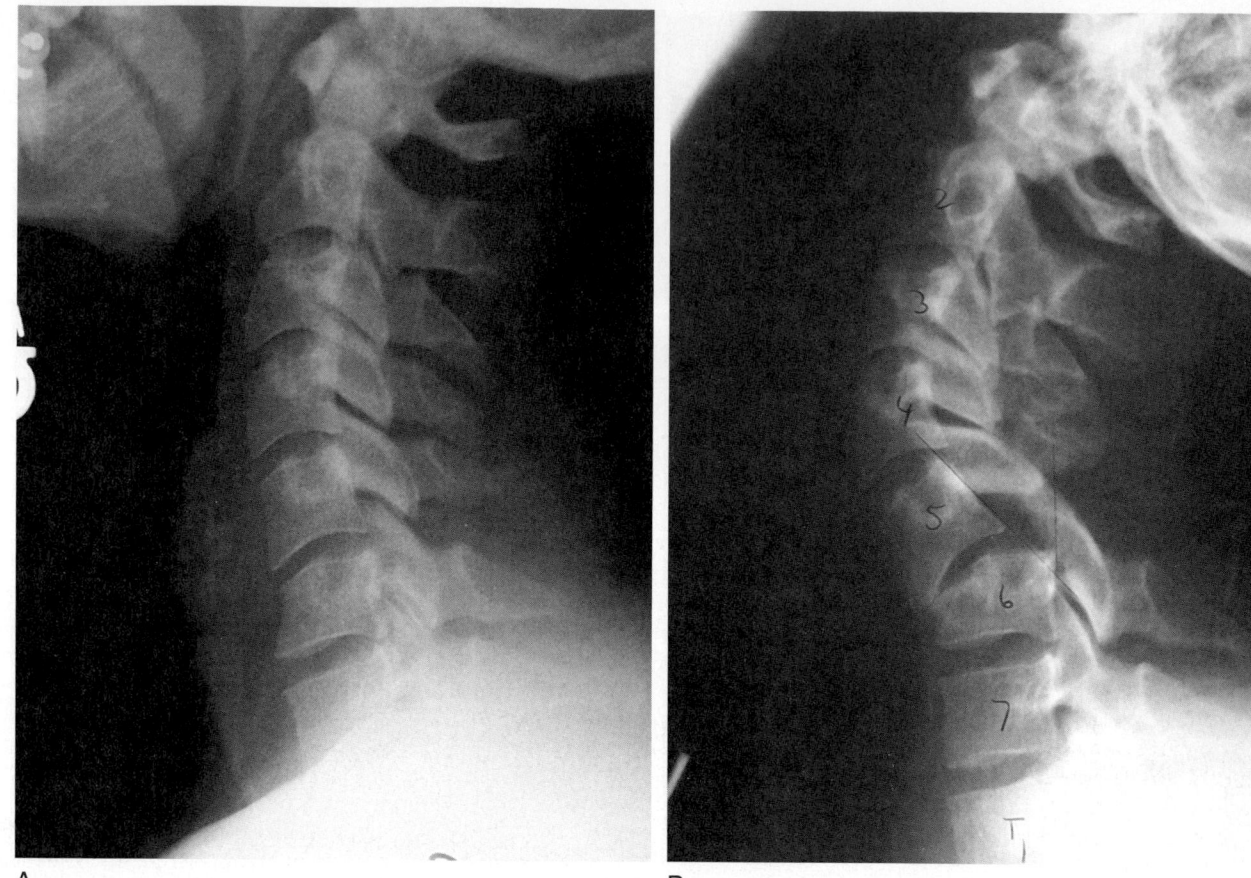

FIGURE 56–3. A, A 31-year-old man was "cleared" in the emergency department after cervical spine series and CT failed to demonstrate a fracture. The patient had a Glasgow Coma Scale score of 11 on admission with significant facial fractures. He presented 1 year post admission with increasing neck pain and was diagnosed with a severe cervical kyphotic deformity with bilateral perched facets at C5-C6. **B**, MRI (gradient-echo sequence) done on admission in this obtunded patient would have easily demonstrated the posterior ligamentous injury between the C5 and C6 spinous process, which is relatively subtle on the admission lateral radiograph seen in A.

among others. However, the administration of methylprednisolone is believed to reduce the amount of secondary injury that occurs after spinal cord injury and has become an important tool in the treatment of spinal cord injury in most North American centers.

The results of NASCIS III have been published and compared the dosage of methylprednisolone used in the NASCIS II protocol with a longer dosing regimen (48 hours) as well as with a 21-aminosteroid. The 21-aminosteroids (lazaroids), a new class of steroids that are potent inhibitors of lipid peroxidation, lack much of the glucocorticoid activity of many of the traditional steroid compounds. The results of the study suggested that when patients are seen within 3 hours of their injury, they should receive a bolus dose of methylprednisolone (30 mg/kg i.v.) followed by 23 hours of treatment (5.4 mg/kg/h i.v.). Patients seen between 3 and 8 hours should receive the same bolus followed by a longer dosing regimen (48 hours). The complications from 48 hours of treatment included a significant increase in severe sepsis and pneumonia.[18]

GANGLIOSIDES

Gangliosides are a complex sialic acid containing glycosphingolipids, which are present in high concentrations in neural membranes. These compounds are involved in a variety of cell surface phenomenon such as cell-substrate binding and receptor functions.[19] Basic research in the past 15 years has demonstrated that these compounds can (1) promote the survival of neurons in cell culture; (2) increase the number, length, and branching of neuronal processes in cell culture; and (3) improve functional recovery after a variety of traumatic and ischemic insults to the peripheral and central nervous system. A limited number of animal studies has examined the role of gangliosides after spinal cord injury and has shown only a modest effect on the regeneration of serotonergic neurons.[20] A recent prospective, randomized, double-blind, single center study found a beneficial effect in functional neurologic outcomes when the ganglioside GM_1 was administered within 72 hours of human spinal cord injury.[21] However, a multicenter trial demonstrated no statistically significant benefit with administration of this agent at 26 and 52 weeks after injury.[22]

ICU MANAGEMENT

Spinal cord injury is associated with profound effects on all vital systemic functions. Through primarily class III medical evidence, numerous reports indicate lower morbidity and mortality rates in patients with spinal cord injury managed with ICU monitoring and aggressive medical management of these changes.[23-31] At the least, these studies taken together indicate that a systematic approach must be taken to evaluate and treat each of the potential complications. Early and late complications will be seen, and the degree of involvement of each system is usually correlated with the level and severity of injury.

RESPIRATORY SYSTEM

Respiratory complications are a major source of morbidity and mortality after spinal cord injury, with an 18% to 30% mortality rate reported in patients with tetraplegia.[27,32] In a study by Hachen and associates,[23,25] most early deaths were related to pulmonary complications, with the likelihood of severe insufficiency related to spinal cord injury severity. Whereas most cervical spinal cord injuries occur below C4 with the phrenic nerves continuing to innervate the diaphragm, the respiratory system is frequently severely affected, particularly after cervical spinal cord injuries. Specifically, marked reductions in (forced) vital capacity, inspiratory capacity, and expiratory flow rates frequently result in a relative hypoxemia.[23,27,33-36] These changes may be attributed to variable paralysis of the intercostal muscles and accessory muscles of respiration. Loss of abdominal muscle tone and ileus also reduce the mechanical efficiency of breathing.

In general, there is a period of grace in which the patient with a cervical spinal cord injury will maintain his or her respiratory status. However, it is not uncommon for respiratory failure to ensue 24 to 48 hours after admission. Additional injuries such as rib fractures, hemathorax, and so on can accelerate this respiratory deterioration. Preparation for such events should be undertaken early so that if intubation is required it can be done with stabilization using in-line traction and often supplemented by fiberoptic technique using a bronchoscope. Measurements of arterial blood gases, negative inspiratory force, and forced vital capacity may provide a method of early detection of respiratory failure.

The most common respiratory complications include atelectasis, pneumonia, pulmonary embolus, pulmonary edema, and acute respiratory distress syndrome. In addition to difficulty with taking deep breaths and coughing, patients are often unable to clear airway secretions. Accumulation of secretions and/or mucus plugs can result in respiratory failure. Prevention includes respiratory treatment with bronchodilators, frequent pulmonary toilet, chest physiotherapy, increasing airway humidity, intubation, and mechanical ventilation including the use of continuous positive airway pressure. The use of the Roto-rest bed significantly decreases pulmonary complications associated with spinal cord injury[27,37] because it improves pulmonary blood flow and reduces the incidence of pulmonary emboli.

Pulmonary infections frequently complicate spinal cord injuries. Within days of admission, the normal flora of the oral cavity will contain increasing numbers of nosocomial organisms. Hospital-acquired pulmonary infections are heralded by fever, increased white blood cells both in the sputum and in the peripheral blood, and, lastly, by changes on the chest radiograph. After obtaining appropriate cultures, commencement of broad-spectrum antibiotics should be instituted.

Most patients can be discontinued or "weaned" from the ventilator after they have been medically stabilized, which usually means treatment of pulmonary infections, re-establishment of euvolemia, enhancement of respiratory muscle function, and nutritional supplementation to off-set the high caloric requirements of the trauma. Initially, weaning the intermittent mandatory ventilation rate is followed by weaning of the positive airway pressure (either continuous or end-expiratory). With prolonged periods of ventilation (greater than 2 weeks), and/or multiple failed extubations, one should consider a tracheostomy. The likelihood of requiring a tracheostomy increases after a high spinal cord injury, preexisting pulmonary disease, and the age of the patient. Tracheostomy effectively reduces the physiologic dead space. Northrup and colleagues[38] have demonstrated that a tracheostomy can be performed before anterior cervical instrumentation of the spine with a low risk of infection, but in our patient population early surgery for stabilization is advocated and, consequently, few patients undergo tracheostomy before anterior cervical stabilization surgery.

CARDIOVASCULAR SYSTEM

Significant confusion arises when the term *spinal shock* is used after spinal cord injury. The misunderstanding regarding its use stems from multiple causes. First, many physicians use the terms *spinal shock* and *neurogenic shock* interchangeably. Neurogenic shock, however, refers to a condition characterized by hypotension and bradycardia, resulting from interruption of the sympathetic nervous system pathways within the spinal cord. The incidence of significant neurogenic shock increases with injuries above the T6 level, because unopposed vagal tone slows the heart and reduces systemic vascular resistance, resulting in venous pooling. The condition responds to administration of fluids and/or colloids and occasionally requires the use of pressors. Neurogenic shock is distinct from hypovolemic shock, which may occasionally occur concomitantly in the multitrauma patient with a spinal cord injury who has evidence of either external or internal bleeding. Whereas isolated hypovolemic shock is characterized by hypotension with tachycardia, relative bradycardia (for a given degree of hypotension) is to be expected in the setting of multitrauma with spinal cord injury.

Spinal shock encompasses a number of different neurologic manifestations of spinal cord injury with varying time courses. Traumatic injuries to the spinal cord interrupt and/or temporarily damage a number of descending and ascending pathways. The most common initial presentation of a complete spinal cord injury with respect to reflex and autonomic function is a period of areflexia and flaccidity that is gradually replaced by hypertonia, exaggerated reflexes, and, in many cases, spasticity. The transition period may last from days to weeks. The immediate onset of hyperreflexia and spasticity is uncommon; and, when it occurs, it is a bad prognostic sign. The period of transition in reflex and autonomic function is often referred to as spinal shock. Concomitant changes in motor and sensory function are also common.

Animal studies indicate that ischemia underlies many of the secondary mechanisms of post-spinal cord injury, often dictating the resultant deficits.[23,39-41] Human studies suggest a direct correlation between the severity of spinal cord injury and the incidence and severity of cardiovascular problems.[23,42] Together, this suggests that reducing the magnitude of secondary injury should be at the forefront of medical management of spinal cord injury.

The typical patient with a spinal cord injury without associated vascular or visceral injury presents to the emergency department with a mean arterial blood pressure of 80 mm Hg and a heart rate of 65 beats/min.[30] Persistent bradycardia is a frequent finding and is often profound enough to produce hemodynamic compromise.[23,43] The patient's blood pressure may respond to volume resuscitation, but not uncommonly these patients require low dose pressors. Aggressive medical management, including volume expansion and maintenance of mean arterial blood pressure above 85 mm Hg, is believed to potentially enhance neurologic outcome by maximizing spinal cord perfusion at the injury site and thus reducing the likelihood of secondary injury.[7] Invasive hemodynamic monitoring will demonstrate a normal cardiac index with a low systemic vascular resistance. In the elderly patient with a spinal cord injury, careful attention to volume replacement is required so as not to precipitate heart failure.

GASTROINTESTINAL SYSTEM

Hypoactive bowel sounds and impaired peristalsis are a common accompaniment after spinal cord injury owing to the lack of sympathetic modulation. To avoid gastric and small bowel dilatation, it is wise to delay enteral feeding. In any patient in whom gastric distention impairs respiratory function, a nasogastric tube is indicated. Most cervical cord injuries require nasogastric suction because of impaired bowel motility, air swallowing producing gastric distention, and respiratory compromise due to paralysis of intercostal muscles.

Patients with spinal cord injuries are at a high risk of developing gastric and duodenal stress ulcers. The use of steroids compounds the risk of developing significant gastrointestinal hemorrhage. All patients with spinal cord injuries should receive at minimum an H_2 blocker to prevent this dreaded complication. The reported risk of gastrointestinal hemorrhage in NASCIS II for the control group was 3% and for the methylprednisolone group it was 4.5%.[15]

URINARY SYSTEM

During the period of spinal shock after a cervical or thoracic spinal cord injury, the urinary bladder is atonic and flaccid. Over time it becomes an upper motor neuron bladder with small capacity. An indwelling Foley catheter is initially placed. After 3 to 4 days this is switched to intermittent bladder catheterization to maintain urinary volumes below 500 mL. Urinary tract infections are common, and if any fevers occur, urine cultures must be obtained and antibiotics selected based on culture sensitivities. Patients with spinal injuries above T6 may also develop autonomic dysreflexia if the bladder becomes overdistended; or, sometimes, with catheterization, sympathetic overactivity and thus headaches, hypertension, sweating, and reduced body temperature result. Long-term complications include chronic infections, obstructive uropathy, and renal calculi; and, if left untreated, renal failure may develop.

INTEGUMENT

The spinal cord–injured patient is extremely susceptible to developing decubiti. Frequent log rolling is invaluable in preventing skin breakdown. Additionally, the Roto-Rest bed[37] can reduce the incidence of skin breakdown by preventing pressure on a single area from frequent turning. Early intervention for skin breakdown frequently involves application of the Duoderm patch (Convatel, Princeton, NJ) to prevent progression.

THROMBOEMBOLIC COMPLICATIONS

Patients with spinal cord injury are at high risk of lower extremity venous thromboembolism, which may manifest by deep vein thrombosis in the lower or upper extremities resulting in leg swelling and/or pulmonary embolism. Depending on injury severity, age, and diagnostic methods, an incidence of thromboembolic events ranges from 7% to 100%.[44] The majority of these events occur within the first 3 months after injury, except in patients who are elderly, obese, or who have had prior thromboembolic events.[44]

Numerous studies have addressed the issue of preventive measures. Prevention has traditionally included the administration of low doses of heparin (5000 units subcutaneously) twice daily or more. However, meta-analysis of available literature suggests that better alternatives include the combination of pneumatic compression stockings with low-molecular-weight heparin (Lovenox, Rorers, Collegeville, PA) or adjusted-dose heparin.[44]

Current recommendations for the evaluation of suspected thromboemboli include use of Doppler ultrasound for suspected deep venous thrombosis and venography if a strong clinical suspicion exists for deep venous thrombosis despite a negative ultrasound or if pulmonary embolism is suspected.[44,45] Treatment of pulmonary emboli or above-knee deep vein thrombosis requires heparinization. Should there be a contraindication to heparinization, an inferior vena cava filter should be placed. Prophylactic placement of inferior vena cava filters has been advocated,[44,46-49] but these procedures are not without risk and no study thus far compares success rates to the aforementioned conservative prevention modalities.[44]

PROGNOSTIC FACTORS FOR RECOVERY

The clinician uses the neurologic examination, age, and the appearance of the spinal cord on MRI, as well as other clinical data, to guide the patient and his or her family on the expected outcome for a specific injury. In any traumatic spinal cord injury, it is important to ascertain whether the patient has a functionally complete or incomplete neurologic deficit. The distinction is important because the prognosis for neurologic recovery differs for these two conditions. Patients with no evidence of motor or sensory function below their spinal column injury are considered to have functionally complete injuries. Patients with no voluntary motor control and only slight sensory preservation in their lowest sacral dermatomes or some anal tone are still considered to have incomplete injuries. Functionally, patients with complete cervical spinal cord injuries, who remain complete within the first 24 hours of admission, are unlikely to regain significant ambulatory function (1% to 3%).[50,51] However, most patients who enter the hospital with an incomplete neurologic injury obtain some degree of recovery. The level and degree of an incomplete injury also provides important prognostic information. Cervical injuries have a higher potential for recovery when compared with thoracic and/or thoracolumbar injuries. The less severe the spinal cord injury, the more likely for the patient to recover.[52]

The majority of injuries occur in males, with well over half the injuries occurring in the 16- to 30-year-old age group. The prognosis for recovery is inextricably linked to age, with the younger patients fairing much better than their older counterparts for regaining neurologic function after spinal cord injury.[53] The two most important potential neurologic explanations are the capacity of the "young" spinal cord to function with major deficiencies in the neural circuitry, as well as the possibility of some spontaneous regeneration of the central nervous system after injury.[54] The reverse also appears to be true. It is well recognized that patients with stable incomplete injuries who may age may lose function, and this may simply be the result of the loss of the last few functioning neurons or axons within the damaged region of spinal cord.[55] Neuronal loss is a normal part of the aging process for both the brain and the spinal cord, and the clinical deterioration observed after spinal cord injury may be likened to the postpolio syndrome.

MRI after spinal cord injury allows visualization of the spinal cord in a noninvasive manner. The images provide immediate feedback to the surgeon as to the degree of spinal cord compression, as well as information regarding the stability of the spinal column through an assessment of the integrity of the ligaments, disks, and surrounding soft tissues. In addition, intramedullary hemorrhage may be easily discerned, and it provides important prognostic information. Intramedullary hemorrhage is more commonly observed after neurologically complete injuries, and hemorrhage signifies a worse neurologic and functional outcome.[56,57] MRI of spinal cord injury is discussed in greater detail in Chapter 57.

RESEARCH

Spinal cord injury research is an absolute priority of the National Institutes of Health. Models of spinal cord injury, mechanisms of secondary injury, treatment of the acute phase of spinal cord injury, as well as the development of transplantation strategies to repair the damaged spinal cord are ongoing across North America and around the world. The treatment arms of the research can be divided into two categories: (1) agents that can be given during the acute phase of injury and that may limit secondary injury mechanisms or (2) strategies to promote regeneration. Two of the most promising drugs, methylprednisolone and ganglioside GM_1, have only yielded modest results. Methylprednisolone, which is used in almost all major spinal cord injury centers, is coming under closer scrutiny as to its effectiveness.[17] Drugs of the future include neurotrophins, which can promote the survival and regeneration of injured nerve cells, drugs that prevent the inflammatory response to spinal cord injury,[58] and drugs that prevent apoptotic cell death.[59] In the transplantation arena, cellular therapies to treat the chronic injury are important. Cells of interest include Schwann cells, olfactory ensheathing glia, embryonic spinal cord, and neural progenitor cells. Antibodies that neutralize the inhibitory proteins within myelin have also demonstrated promise. Strategies that combine a number of the aforementioned treatments are most likely to have a beneficial effect in the future.

CONCLUSION

It appears that despite the enormous advancements in the diagnosis and treatment of spinal fractures over the past three decades there exists a number of unanswered questions regarding the most appropriate management of patients with traumatic spinal fractures. Although only a few aspects of the surgical management of spine trauma are raised in this chapter, it is clear that a number of issues remain unresolved. Technologic advancements in spinal instrumentation and pharmacotherapeutics will continue in the 21st century. It will be critical that both neurosurgeons and orthopedic surgeons work together to test both the efficacy and cost effectiveness of some of the newer treatment modalities, because both the best possible treatment and cost containment will be part of management equation in the future. Outcome assessment should be at the forefront of all new ideas. Only through a critical and open-minded analysis of our treatment strategies will we be able to provide the best care for those patients who will often be changed for the remainder of their lives by their injuries and the rapid sequence of events that revolve around their acute hospitalization.

ANNOTATED REFERENCES

Deep venous thrombosis and thromboembolism in patients with cervical spinal cord injuries. Neurosurgery 2002;50:S73-S80.

Recommendations of the recent (2002) guidelines for the management of acute cervical spine and spinal cord injuries that are pertinent to prophylaxis for prevention of deep venous thrombosis.

Northrup BE, Vaccaro AR, Rosen JE, et al: Occurrence of infection in anterior cervical fusion for spinal cord injury after tracheostomy. Spine 1995;20:2449-2453.

A small clinical study in 11 patients found that tracheostomy was not associated with an increased infection risk in subsequent anterior cervical surgery in adults with cervical spine injury.

Schaefer DM, Flanders AE, Osterholm JL, et al: Prognostic significance of magnetic resonance imaging in the acute phase of cervical spine injury. J Neurosurg 1992;76:218-223.

Clinical study of 57 patients that suggests that the MR imaging pattern observed in the acutely injured human spinal cord has a prognostic significance in the final outcome of the motor system.

Tator CH, Fehlings MG: Review of the secondary injury theory of acute spinal cord trauma with emphasis on vascular mechanisms. J Neurosurg 1991;75:15-26.

Review article by two respected authorities in clinical spinal cord injury on the mechanisms involved in the evolution of secondary damage.

Vale FL, Burns J, Jackson AB, et al: Combined medical and surgical treatment after acute spinal cord injury: Results of a prospective pilot study to assess the merits of aggressive medical resuscitation and blood pressure management. J Neurosurg 1997;87:239-246.

Clinical trial in 77 patients with acute spinal cord injury in which aggressive ICU care, including optimized volume expansion and pressor support, was associated with favorable outcome.

Chapter 57
NEUROIMAGING

Fred J. Laine

KEY POINTS

METHODS

1. Computed tomography (CT) is rapid and accurate and is the most widely used imaging modality in the acute setting.
2. Constant improvements in CT and magnetic resonance imaging (MRI) techniques not only afford greater sensitivity and specificity but also allow the evaluation of metabolic and physiologic functions of the brain.
3. Other modalities, such as nuclear medicine studies and angiography, have more specific indications and are generally not used as primary screening modalities.

BRAIN

1. The three types of brain edema—vasogenic, cytotoxic, and interstitial—can usually be differentiated, which helps in determining the underlying lesion.
2. The MRI appearance of hemorrhage is dependent on the age of the hemorrhage because the blood breakdown products have varying paramagnetic properties that influence the MRI signal.
3. Herniation can be identified on CT and MRI directly, by visualizing portions of brain that cross dural membranes and bony ridges, or indirectly, by noting the mass effect on adjacent structures.
4. Acute head injury is best evaluated initially with CT to rapidly establish the presence of surgical lesions; MRI is used secondarily to establish the presence of more subtle lesions.
5. The imaging evaluation of a patient suspected of having a stroke should include an anatomic study to determine the presence and type of infarct, as well as a physiologic study to evaluate parameters such as brain perfusion, blood volume, and vasculature status.
6. The distinction between recurrent tumor and postradiation necrosis is difficult on standard imaging but can be greatly facilitated by magnetic resonance spectroscopy and positron emission tomography.

SPINE

1. The possible causes of spinal disease can be significantly narrowed if the lesion can be placed into one of the three spinal compartments: intramedullary, extramedullary intradural, and extradural.
2. In the evaluation of spinal injury, CT is useful for evaluating bony pathology such as fractures and subluxation, whereas MRI is useful in soft tissue injuries such as cord contusion or acute disc herniation.
3. MRI is the modality of choice when evaluating patients suspected of having discitis, cord compression, or metastatic disease.

METHODS

PLAIN RADIOGRAPHS

Plain radiographs are rapid, inexpensive, and accurate but are of limited value in studying the central nervous system (CNS). Although useful in evaluating soft tissue abnormalities of the chest, abdomen, and pelvis, plain radiographs are inadequate for evaluating the soft tissues of the head and spine. Their main usefulness, with respect to the CNS, lies in their ability to depict osseous integrity and alignment. Therefore, they are typically the first studies obtained when evaluating traumatic injuries of the spine. Radiographs of the skull following head injury can demonstrate fractures but fail to provide significant information about intracranial injury.

COMPUTED TOMOGRAPHY

Computed tomography (CT) is the most widely used imaging modality for evaluating critical care patients with CNS pathology. CT is widely available, rapid, and accurate and has virtually no contraindications in the acute setting. The clinical utility of CT is increased by multiple modifications, including contrast administration, window techniques, and various reconstruction techniques. Iodinated contrast agents are available for intravenous injection. With their use, lesions that cause a breakdown in the blood-brain barrier, as well as normal or abnormal vascular structures, enhance or "light up" on CT scans. Varying the gray scale "window level" permits the evaluation of osseous structures with a wide window and soft tissue structures with a narrow window.

Spiral or helical CT scanners are now widely available, and this form of CT has many advantages over standard scans. It allows rapid imaging through a large volume of the body, usually with a single breath-hold. Rapid, thin-section axial images can be obtained with very little artifact, and they can be merged and reproduced in any plane. Three-dimensional reconstructed CT images can also be produced and rotated in any plane. CT angiography is one example of a technique that is possible with helical CT. Thin-section axial images, contrast bolus tracking, and elimination of background tissue allow accurate visualization of vascular structures. Reconstruction of these images allows a noninvasive CT evaluation of vascular structures.

Xenon CT involves the inhalation of xenon gas over a period of time, with sequential CT cuts and subsequent calculations of xenon uptake. This technique is valuable for measuring cerebral blood flow. Spiral CT has also allowed the development of perfusion CT techniques. Dynamic intravenous administration of contrast material is tracked with rapid serial imaging during its first-pass circulation through the brain tissue capillary bed. Post-processing mathematic models for computing perfusion maps allow the measurement of cerebral blood volume, cerebral blood flow, and mean transit time. This technique is becoming more valuable in the physiologic assessment of brain tissue in patients with stroke, tumor, trauma, dementia, vasospasm, and epilepsy.[1]

MAGNETIC RESONANCE IMAGING

Magnetic resonance imaging (MRI) uses magnetic field gradients and radiofrequency pulses rather than ionizing radiation. Many sequences that vary the MRI signal parameters are obtained, allowing tissue characterization based on the tissue's inherent response to magnetic field and radiofrequency pulses. Continual refinements in MRI sequence techniques have drastically reduced imaging time and increased the conspicuity of pathologic changes. A gadolinium-based contrast agent can be injected intravenously, which allows better visualization of intracranial and intraspinal pathology. Magnetic resonance angiography (MRA) sequences use the property of flowing spins to create an angiographic image. These methods create greater signal intensity in flowing blood than in the surrounding stationary tissues. The background tissue is effectively subtracted from the tissue volume, and the resultant images can be "reconstructed" and simulate a standard angiogram.

A wide variety of MRI sequences are being investigated that are based on physiologic changes rather than anatomic changes. Functional MRI techniques are showing promise in the detection and assessment of cerebral pathophysiology and in the characterization and regional mapping of distinct human cognitive functions, such as vision, motor skills, language, and memory.[1] Diffusion-weighted MRI is based on the evaluation of free versus restricted movement of water molecules. Diffusion-weighted MRI is now considered a standard sequence in evaluating stroke, because it is more sensitive than standard MRI in identifying acute stroke and in differentiating stroke from other pathologies.[2,3] Magnetic resonance perfusion can be performed by different methods, but the final outcome allows the measurement of vascular supply to brain tissue. Perfusion can also be used to measure metabolic activity, because blood supply and tissue activity are related. Although evaluation of brain ischemia is the most common clinical application, perfusion studies are also proving useful in tumor characterization.[4]

Magnetic resonance spectroscopy can noninvasively measure numerous biochemicals in a small volume of brain tissue. Many nuclei can be detected, but phosphorous (^{31}P) and proton (^{1}H) spectroscopy have the most clinical utility. Phosphorous spectroscopy provides information concerning tissue energetics, phospholipid metabolism, and intracellular pH. Proton spectroscopy can provide information on neuronal density, membrane constituents, amino acid metabolism, and glycolysis. Current uses include characterizing tumors, differentiating recurrent tumor from radiation necrosis, and distinguishing intracranial tumor from infection.[5] However, many other disease processes are also being studied with spectroscopy.[6]

The disadvantages of performing MRI on critical care patients involve the preprocedural preparation and screening.[7] MRI is contraindicated in patients with pacemakers, certain cardiac valves, and intraocular metal fragments. Careful screening for the presence of cerebral aneurysm clips and other metallic devices, stents, and surgical implants is necessary. In addition, respirators and physiologic monitors must be MRI compatible. Only oxygen and nitrogen tanks composed of aluminum can enter the magnet suite. Frequently, patients must be switched from MRI-incompatible respirators to MRI-compatible ones before the procedure can take place. All these precautions and modifications can significantly delay imaging in the acute setting. In addition, such basic medical instruments as stethoscopes, hemostats, and scissors must remain outside the MRI suite.

NUCLEAR MEDICINE STUDIES

Evaluation of CNS pathology with nuclear medicine techniques is still undergoing investigation, but it is an area of rapid development because of its ability to provide physiologic imaging rather than standard anatomic imaging. Positron emission tomography (PET) generates cross-sectional images by quantitatively measuring administered compounds containing various cyclotron-generated positron emitters such as ^{18}F-fluorodeoxyglucose. PET can provide functional information such as glucose and oxygen utilization, as well as hemodynamic data about blood flow and blood volume.[8] Single photon emission computed tomography (SPECT), developed from PET, analyzes the distribution of radiopharmaceuticals that are incorporated into biologically active compounds. Cerebral blood flow, tissue metabolism, neuroreceptors, and glucose and amino acid metabolism can be evaluated with this technique.[9]

ANGIOGRAPHY

Percutaneous transfemoral catheterization is used to evaluate cerebral and spinal vascular anatomy and integrity. Cerebral angiography is an invasive procedure and imposes some risk. The overall complication rate is 2% to 4%, with the majority of complications being minor and transient, such as groin hematoma, subintimal injections, and minor allergic reactions.[10] More severe complications, such as cerebral infarction, seizure, and death, occur infrequently.

Although Doppler ultrasonography, CT angiography, and MRA have had a significant impact on the evaluation of cerebrovascular diseases, especially atherosclerotic disease, cerebral angiography is still considered the gold standard. In the acute setting, in cases of intracranial hemorrhage, angiography is necessary to establish the presence of vascular malformations or aneurysms. In trauma, angiography is used to evaluate vascular integrity.

Interventional neuroradiology has made great strides in the treatment of a variety of neurovascular lesions. Safer microcatheters and a wide variety of treatment options are now available that gain access to lesions through preexisting vascular paths. Therapeutic techniques include embolization of vascular tumors, aneurysms, and arteriovenous malformations; stent placement; angioplasty; and thrombolysis.

BRAIN

PATTERNS OF DISEASE

Edema

Cerebral edema or brain swelling is caused by a localized or diffuse abnormal accumulation of water and sodium. This differs from cerebral engorgement caused by vasodilatation or obstructed venous outflow. Both conditions lead to an increase in brain volume and are difficult to distinguish on routine imaging studies. Newer methods such as xenon CT and diffusion-weighted MRI are useful in this regard.

Three types of edema have been described:

1. *Vasogenic edema* is the result of increased capillary permeability and involves mainly the white matter. This type of edema is most often associated with tumor, abscess, or trauma but can also be seen with infarct and ischemia.
2. *Cytotoxic edema* is the result of cellular swelling and involves both gray and white matter. Ischemia, anoxia, and hypo-osmolar states are the primary considerations.
3. *Interstitial edema* is the result of cerebrospinal fluid migration into the periventricular white matter. This form of edema is secondary to conditions that impede cerebrospinal fluid absorption, such as hydrocephalus.

Except for location, the CT and MRI appearance of all types of edema is similar. On CT scans, increased water is seen as a decrease in density and appears dark. On MRI scans, an increase in water is seen as an area of decreased signal on T1-weighted images and an area of increased signal on T2-weighted images. The vasogenic form of edema extends along the fingers of white matter, interposed between normal gray matter (Fig. 57-1). This pattern has a nonvascular distribution and is often associated with mass effect. The cytotoxic form of edema involves gray and white matter, and the decreased density extends uniformly to the calvaria. Typically, this edema follows a vascular distribution and produces less mass effect for its size (Fig. 57-2). The interstitial form of edema involves the periventricular white matter and appears as a fairly symmetrical low-density rim in the periventricular region that masks the ventricular wall and gradually fades into the surrounding white matter.

Hemorrhage

Intracranial hemorrhage may be parenchymal or extra-axial (epidural, subdural, and subarachnoid spaces) in location. Parenchymal hemorrhage can be traumatic in origin but is more likely nontraumatic, from an underlying disease such as hypertension or neoplasm or from a vascular anomaly. Epidural and subdural extra-axial hemorrhage is most often a result of trauma. Subarachnoid hemorrhage is most often secondary to trauma but is also associated with ruptured congenital aneurysm.

The imaging appearance of hemorrhage is dependent on the age of the hemorrhagic event. On CT, acute hemorrhage typically appears hyperdense because of the high hematocrit and globin component (Fig. 57-3A). However, this pattern may vary in different clinical situations. Acute hematomas may be isodense to brain in anemic patients when the hemoglobin drops below 10 g/dL[11] or in patients with a coagulopathy who fail to produce clot retraction.[12] As the hemorrhage resolves, the CT appearance also changes. Initially, as the clot retracts, the CT density may rise for 2 to 3 days after the initial event. Thereafter, the clot begins to liquefy and then resorb. The CT appearance demonstrates gradually decreasing density through an isodense stage between 1 and 6 weeks (depending on size) and finally a hypodense stage. The final CT appearance of resolved hemorrhage may show no residual abnormality or demonstrate a focus of low attenuation or calcification.[13]

The appearance of hemorrhage on MRI is more complicated because of the varying paramagnetic properties of blood breakdown products. As hemorrhage resolves, fibrinolysis, leukocyte infiltration, hemoglobin denaturation, and changes in red blood cell morphology interact to alter the MRI appearance at different stages.[14] The progression of resolution represents a continuum of changing intensity values and is not an all-or-none phenomenon. It progresses through the following stages (during resolution, these stages may be present simultaneously):

1. During the first 24 hours after parenchymal hemorrhage, intact red blood cells containing oxyhemoglobin accumulate. The oxyhemoglobin is diamagnetic and appears slightly hypo- to isointense on T1-weighted images and iso- to hyperintense on T2-weighted images.
2. Within 3 to 5 days, the hemoglobin becomes deoxygenated. The deoxyhemoglobin is paramagnetic and appears similar to oxyhemoglobin on T1-weighted images but becomes hypointense to brain on T2-weighted images (see Fig. 57-3B and C).
3. Between 3 and 7 days, intracellular methemoglobin starts to accumulate, beginning peripherally and advancing toward the center of the clot. On T2-weighted images, the intracellular methemoglobin behaves similarly to deoxyhemoglobin and remains hypointense, but the T1 values begin to increase, causing the periphery of the clot to become hyperintense (see Fig. 57-3B and C).
4. Between 7 days and 2 to 3 months, the red blood cells lyse and release methemoglobin into the extracellular space. During this phase, signal intensities increase on both T1- and T2-weighted images. Hence, the hemorrhage appears bright on both sequences (see Fig. 57-3B and C).
5. During the final stage, which may begin within 2 weeks and last for years, conversion of methemoglobin to hemosiderin occurs as a result of phagocytic degradation. Iron is removed from the hematoma and deposited at the periphery. Signal intensities again decrease and give rise to hypointense signal on both T1- and T2-weighted images.

Most hematomas are associated with a surrounding area of edema that can be misinterpreted as an additional area of hemorrhage. Similar to oxyhemoglobin, edema is hypo- to isointense in comparison to brain on T1-weighted images

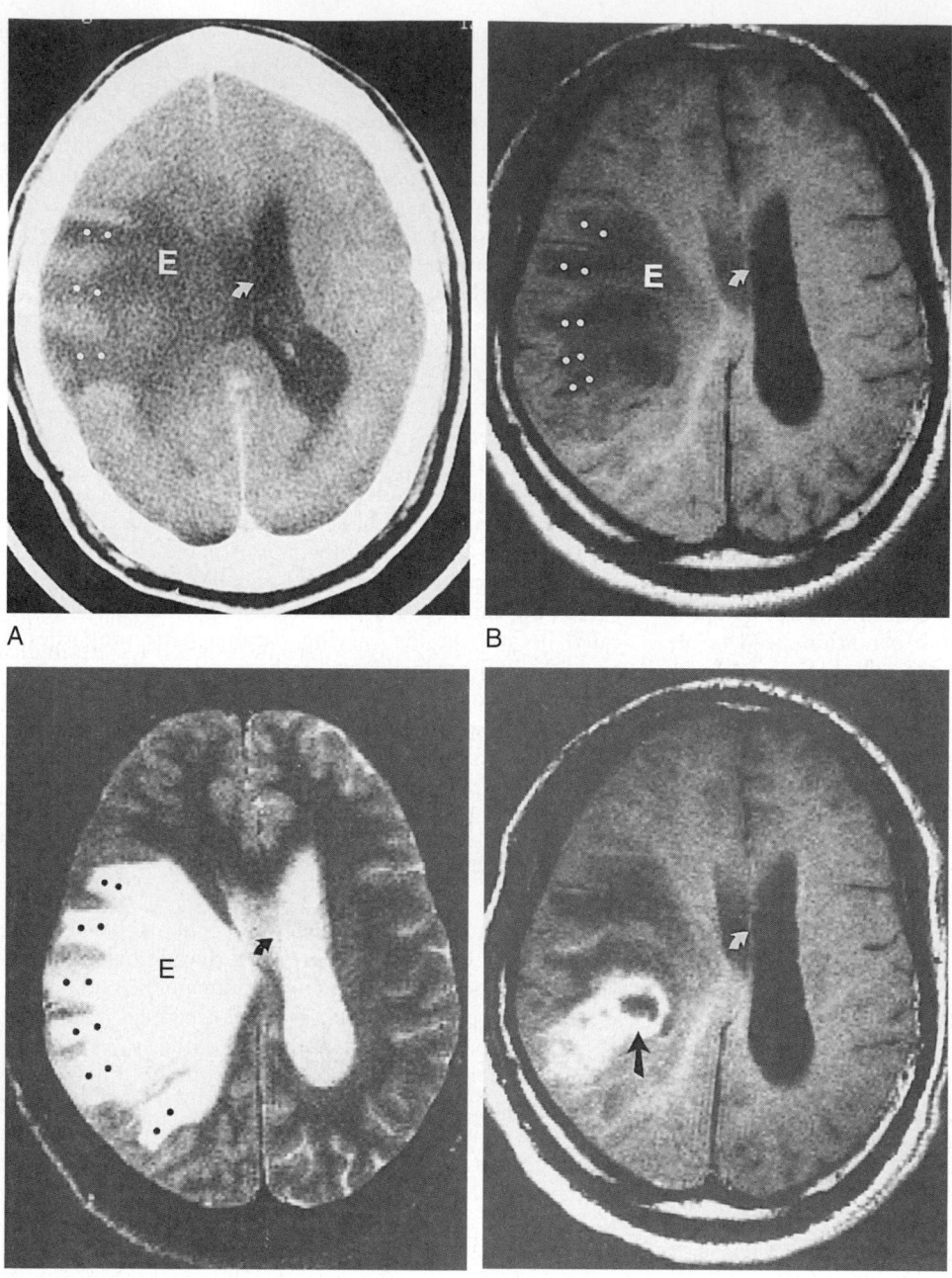

FIGURE 57–1. Vasogenic edema in glioblastoma. Non-contrast-enhanced axial CT scan *(A),* axial T1-weighted MRI scan *(B),* and axial T2-weighted MRI scan *(C)* all demonstrate an area of edema (E). The edema extends along the white matter fibers *(dots),* with normal gray matter interposed. Axial T1-weighted MRI scan following contrast enhancement *(D)* demonstrates the enhancing tumor nidus *(arrow),* distinct from the surrounding edema. Subfalcine herniation is also demonstrated on these images by displacement of the falx *(curved arrows).*

and hyperintense on T2-weighted images. However, the signal characteristics of edema remain constant, and it gradually fades over time. Extra-axial blood collections resolve in an identical fashion, although the time required to resolve is slightly longer between stages.

Mass Effect, Shift, and Herniation

Lesions that increase intracerebral mass may eventually cause brain herniation.[15] This may be the direct result of an enlarging lesion, such as a tumor, or the indirect result of a lesion, such as edema caused by a tumor. Two relatively fixed dural partitions are present within the skull and create compartments across which brain substance may herniate. The falx cerebri separates the cerebral hemispheres, and the tentorium separates the cerebral hemispheres from the posterior fossa structures. Herniation is described in terms of location.

Subfalcine herniation occurs when the medial surface of a hemisphere, usually the cingulate or supracingulate gyrus,

is compressed against or displaced beneath the falx. With CT or MRI, early signs may appear as compression or distortion of the lateral ventricles (see Fig. 57-1). Later stages are recognized by deviation of the falx and identification of the hemispheric structures that are crossing the midline.

Transalar herniation occurs when a mass, located in the frontal or temporal lobe, displaces brain tissue across the sphenoid ridge. When the mass arises in the temporal lobe and brain is displaced above the sphenoid ridge into the anterior cranial fossa, it is termed *ascending* transalar herniation. When the mass arises in the frontal lobe and displaces brain inferiorly into the middle cranial fossa, it is termed *descending* transalar herniation. With CT or MRI, displacement of the sylvian portion of the middle cerebral artery can identify the herniated brain directly or indirectly.

Transtentorial herniation occurs when a mass arising on either side of the tentorium results in brain herniation through the tentorial incisura. *Descending* transtentorial herniation is

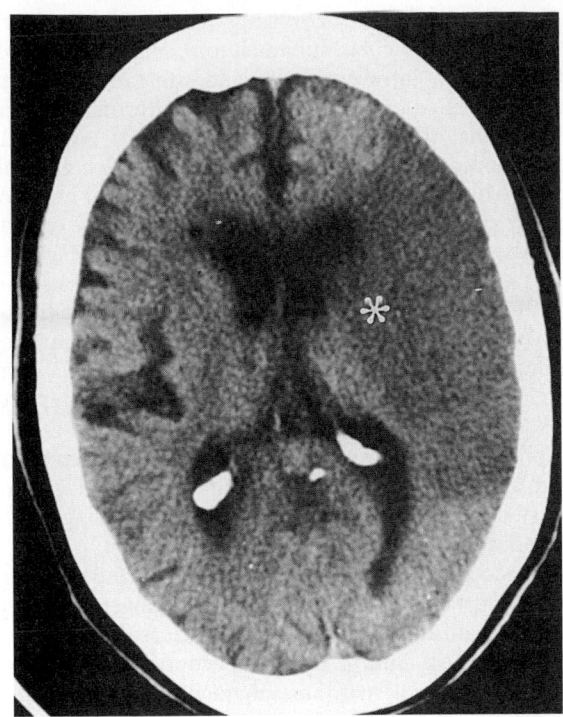

FIGURE 57–2. Cytotoxic edema and acute infarct. Axial non-contrast-enhanced CT scan demonstrates an area of decreased density *(asterisk)* involving the left middle cerebral artery territory. Gray and white matter structures are involved, and there is little mass effect.

caused by a supratentorial mass that displaces the medial temporal lobe through the incisura. On CT or MRI, the herniated brain pushes against and rotates the brainstem. This produces widening of the ipsilateral brainstem cistern and effacement of the contralateral cistern (Fig. 57-4). Associated findings may include dilatation of the contralateral temporal horn secondary to ventricular trapping. *Ascending* transtentorial herniation is caused by an infratentorial mass that displaces the pons, vermis, and adjacent portions of the cerebellar

hemispheres upward through the incisura. On CT and MRI, the brainstem cisterns are symmetrically effaced as the cerebellar vermis bulges up through the incisura. There is often associated acute hydrocephalus caused by compression of the sylvian aqueduct.

Tonsillar herniation occurs when the cerebellar tonsils are pushed through the foramen magnum. This results in medullary compression and dysfunction of the vital respiratory and cardiac control centers. Sagittal MRI is the primary modality for demonstrating tonsillar herniation and the secondary effects on the brainstem.

SPECIFIC DISEASE PROCESSES

Head Trauma

In patients with acute head injury, management decisions must be made quickly. The critical issue is rapid and accurate detection of potentially treatable or surgically correctable lesions. In this regard, CT continues to be the primary modality for the initial evaluation of patients with head injury.[16] Its advantages include fast examination time, wide availability, fracture detection, lack of contraindications, and high accuracy.[17] Although MRI is more sensitive in detecting intracranial traumatic lesions, it is limited by a longer examination time, less conspicuity of hyperacute hematomas, and difficulty in monitoring patients.[17] For the evaluation of chronic head injury, MRI is the modality of choice. It can identify small foci of old hemorrhage and gliosis and evaluate the presence and extent of diffuse axonal injury (shear injury) with greater sensitivity than CT scan.[18]

Injury to brain parenchyma may result in contusion, axonal (shear) injury, or hematoma. The imaging appearance of hematomas has been described previously. Contusions are caused by the direct impact of parenchyma against bone and are most common along the gyral surface of the frontal and temporal lobes. Shear injuries are secondary to rotational forces that produce tears in axonal fibers and are most common within white matter (subcortical white matter, corpus callosum, internal capsule, brainstem). Except for

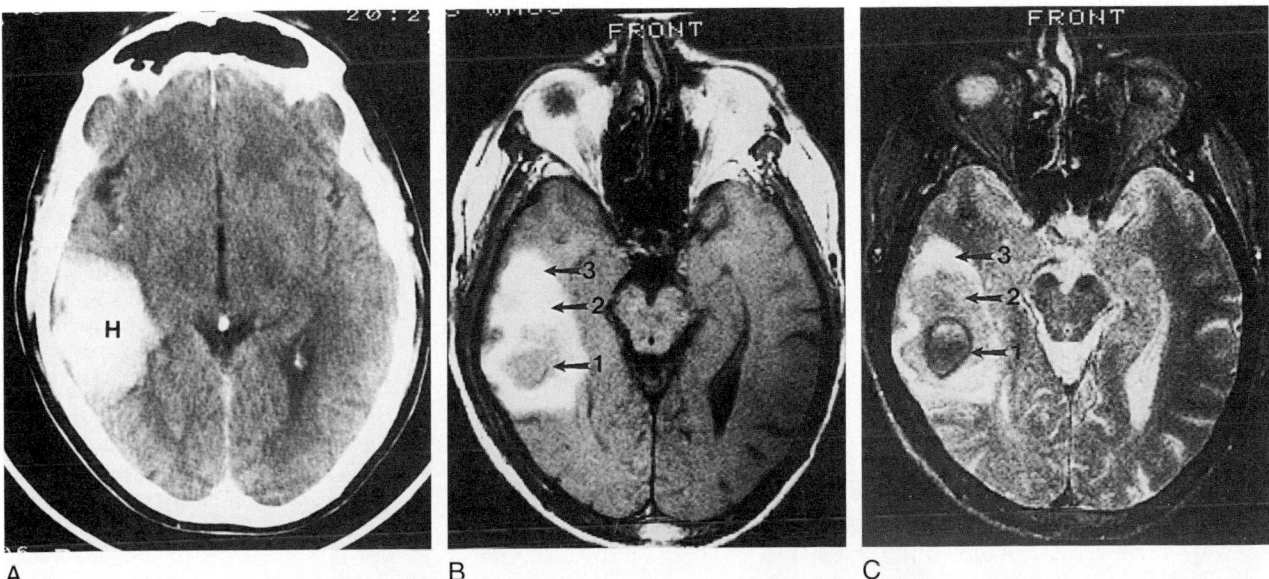

FIGURE 57–3. Hemorrhage. Axial CT image *(A)* demonstrates a large area of acute hemorrhage (H) in the right temporal lobe. T1-weighted *(B)* and T2-weighted *(C)* MRI scans demonstrate the hemorrhage in various stages of breakdown. The center of the lesion is dark on the T1- and T2-weighted images, indicating oxyhemoglobin (1). The intermediate zone is bright on the T1-weighted image and gray on the T2-weighted image, indicating intracellular methemoglobin (2). The outer rim is bright on both the T1- and T2-weighted images, indicating extracellular methemoglobin (3).

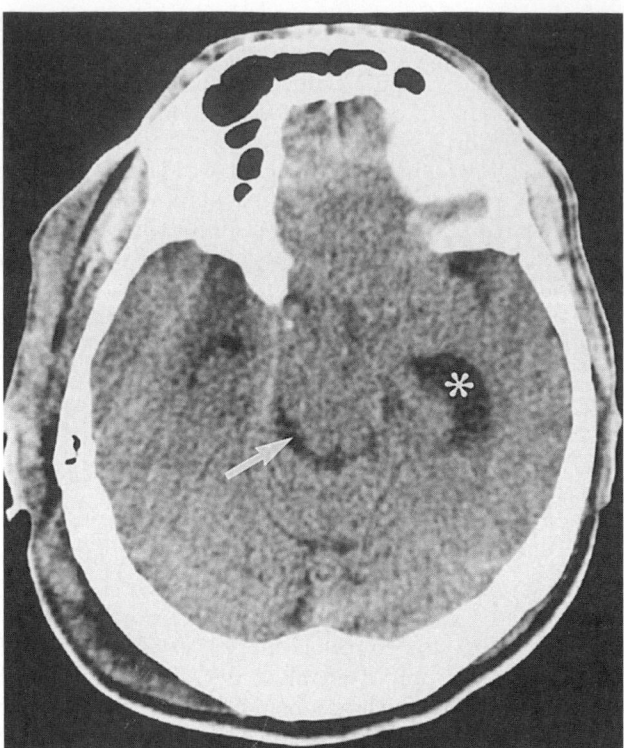

FIGURE 57–4. Right descending transtentorial herniation in a patient with a large right parietal subdural hematoma. Axial non-contrast-enhanced CT scan of the head at the level of the midbrain shows that the ipsilateral subarachnoid cistern is widened *(arrow)*, and the contralateral subarachnoid cistern is obliterated because of brainstem rotation. The left temporal horn is also dilated *(asterisk)*, indicating trapping of the left lateral ventricle.

location, the imaging characteristics of nonhemorrhagic contusions and shear injuries are similar. Initial studies may be normal or demonstrate small foci of edema. Shear injuries may remain nonvisible on CT but become more apparent on MRI. Larger contusions may contain petechial hemorrhage and appear as ill-defined heterogeneous lesions with little or no mass effect. Edema and mass effect may increase in the first 48 hours after trauma, making these lesions more evident on imaging studies.

Damage to the brain coverings may lead to hemorrhage into the intraventricular, subarachnoid, subdural, or epidural spaces. On CT, intraventricular and subarachnoid hemorrhage is identified by replacement of the normal low-density cerebrospinal fluid by high-density blood. When subtle, subarachnoid hemorrhage can be mistaken for generalized edema, with loss of the basal cisterns. Subdural hematomas typically appear as crescentic mixed or hyperdense collections that cross suture lines but not dural attachments (Fig. 57-5A). Epidural hematomas appear as biconvex, hyperdense collections that cross dural attachments but not suture lines (see Fig. 57-5B). With rapid accumulation of blood, unretracted semiliquid clot may be present. In this situation, CT demonstrates hypodense areas within the hyperdense hematoma, the so-called swirl sign.[19] Distinction between these two collections is important, because an epidural hematoma is due to arterial bleeding and is a surgical emergency. Without surgery, these lesions resolve by gradually decreasing in density and appear hypodense at about 3 weeks' time.

Nonaccidental head injury is the leading cause of morbidity and mortality in abused children younger than 2 years old.[20] Mechanisms include direct impact, asphyxia, and shaking or whiplash injury. Injuries encountered include skull fracture, subdural hematoma, subarachnoid hemorrhage, and shear injuries. Cerebral infarction can also be seen secondary to numerous mechanisms, including smothering, strangulation, and shaking. Subdural hematoma is regarded as one of the most characteristic CNS lesions encountered in "shaken baby" syndrome. In fact, subdural hematomas are more often associated with nonaccidental injury than with accidental trauma.[21] The CT appearance of nonaccidental injury in children is similar to that in adults. However, subdural hematoma is more common along the posterior interhemispheric fissure and appears as increased attenuation along the falx. Other common locations include the anterior interhemispheric, tentorial, and parieto-occipital regions. MRI can determine the age of the blood products and provide an accurate estimate of the time the hemorrhage occurred because of the stages of resolution, as discussed earlier. The blood clot resolves similar to a parenchymal hemorrhage but at a different rate. MRI can also determine the coexistence of blood products of different ages, indicating repeated abuse (Fig. 57-6).

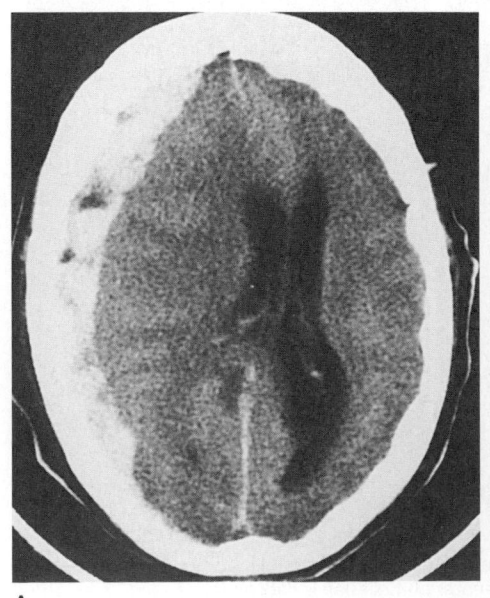

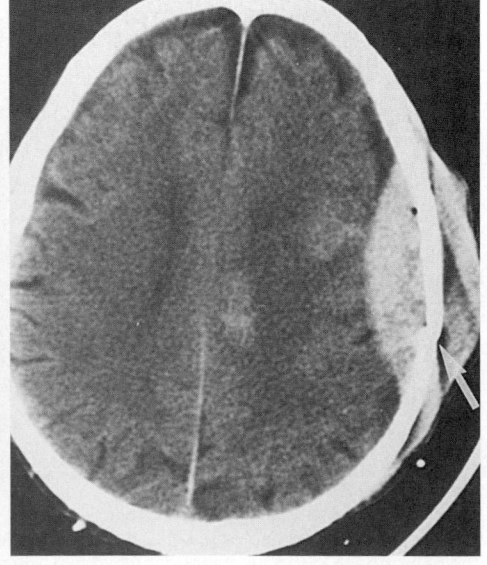

FIGURE 57–5. Subdural and epidural hematoma. *A,* Axial CT scan of the head demonstrates a mixed-density subdural hematoma along the right frontoparietal lobes. The mixed-density appearance is most likely due to the presence of unretracted, semiliquid clot. *B,* Axial CT scan of the head demonstrates a left biconvex hyperdense collection that is classic for epidural hematoma. A fracture *(arrow)* can also be identified.

A

B

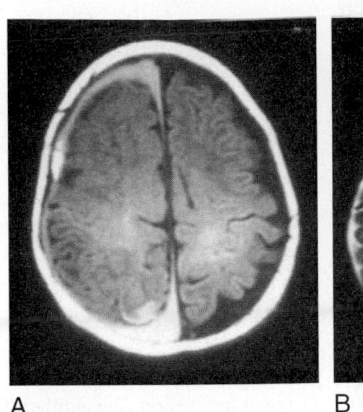 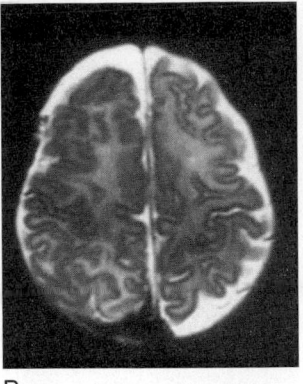

A   B

FIGURE 57–6. Nonaccidental head injury. Axial T1- *(A)* and T2-weighted *(B)* MRI scans of an infant reveal bilateral subdural blood collections of different ages. The right collection shows blood in the late subacute phase (2 to 4 weeks old), and the left shows blood in the chronic phase (>1 month). This finding is almost proof positive of repeated abuse.

Vascular Lesions

Ischemia, Hypoxia, and Infarct. Although CT demonstrates only about half of infarcts within the first 48 hours, it remains the imaging modality of choice in evaluating patients with symptoms of transient ischemic attack, reversible ischemic neurologic deficit, or completed stroke.[22] In the acute setting, CT can identify the location and extent of infarction; distinguish among ischemic stroke, hemorrhagic infarction, and primary intracerebral hemorrhage; and effectively exclude lesions that mimic stroke.

The CT appearance depends on the age of the infarct, as follows:

- In the hyperacute stage (first 24 hours), the CT scan may be normal or demonstrate a subtle decrease in density and loss of gray-white differentiation (Fig. 57-7).

- During the acute stage (within the first week), the infarct becomes more pronounced owing to the decreased density produced by cytotoxic edema (see Fig. 57-2). The infarct is better defined, involves both gray and white matter, and corresponds to a known vascular territory.

- The subacute stage may persist for 1 to 3 weeks, during which time the edema and mass effect begin to resolve.

- Chronic infarcts demonstrate parenchymal replacement, with well-defined, sharply marginated zones of cystic encephalomalacia and gliosis. The infarct behaves like a contracting, rather than an expanding, mass.

The MRI appearance reflects the changes of cytotoxic edema (Fig. 57-8). Nonhemorrhagic infarcts begin with subtle increased signal intensity on T2-weighted images and minimal changes on T1-weighted images. Subtle findings include stagnation of blood flow (arterial enhancement) and swelling of the involved gyri. Diffusion-weighted MRI has become a standard in the evaluation of acute ischemia (Fig. 57-9). Acute ischemia induces water influx into cells (cytotoxic edema), which results in an increased proportion of restricted water. The diffusion-weighted sequence is sensitive to this restricted water, which can be demonstrated on images as increased signal. The apparent diffusion coefficient values can be mapped and an additional image generated that confirms the acute nature of the infarct as an area of low signal.

CT and MRI perfusion techniques can demonstrate diminished blood perfusion within minutes of an insult. When MRI perfusion studies are coupled with diffusion images, a penumbra can be identified as a zone of decreased perfusion surrounding an area of absent perfusion. Only the central area shows the diffusion restriction. The penumbra represents viable tissue that is at risk for infarction but may still be salvageable.[23] Perfusion techniques can also demonstrate subtle areas of decreased perfusion without a completed infarct (Fig. 57-10).

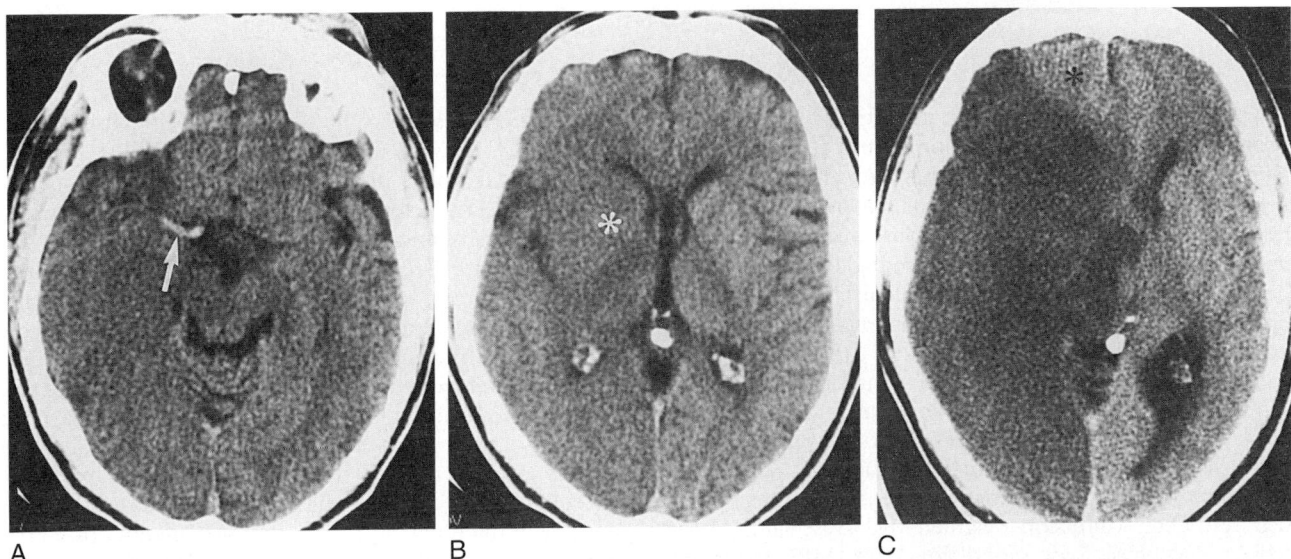

A   B   C

FIGURE 57–7. Acute infarct. Axial non-contrast-enhanced CT images obtained at the level of the temporal lobe *(A)* and through the level of the basal ganglia *(B)* demonstrate an area of low density involving the gray and white matter of the right hemisphere. There is loss of gray-white matter differentiation, especially noticeable in the region of the basal ganglia *(asterisk, B)*. Compare the right and left sides. High density is identified within the right middle cerebral artery *(arrow, A)*, representing clot. Axial non-contrast-enhanced CT scan obtained 48 hours later *(C)* demonstrates marked edema involving the territories of the right, middle, and posterior cerebral arteries. Note the sparing of the right anterior cerebral artery territory *(asterisk, C)*.

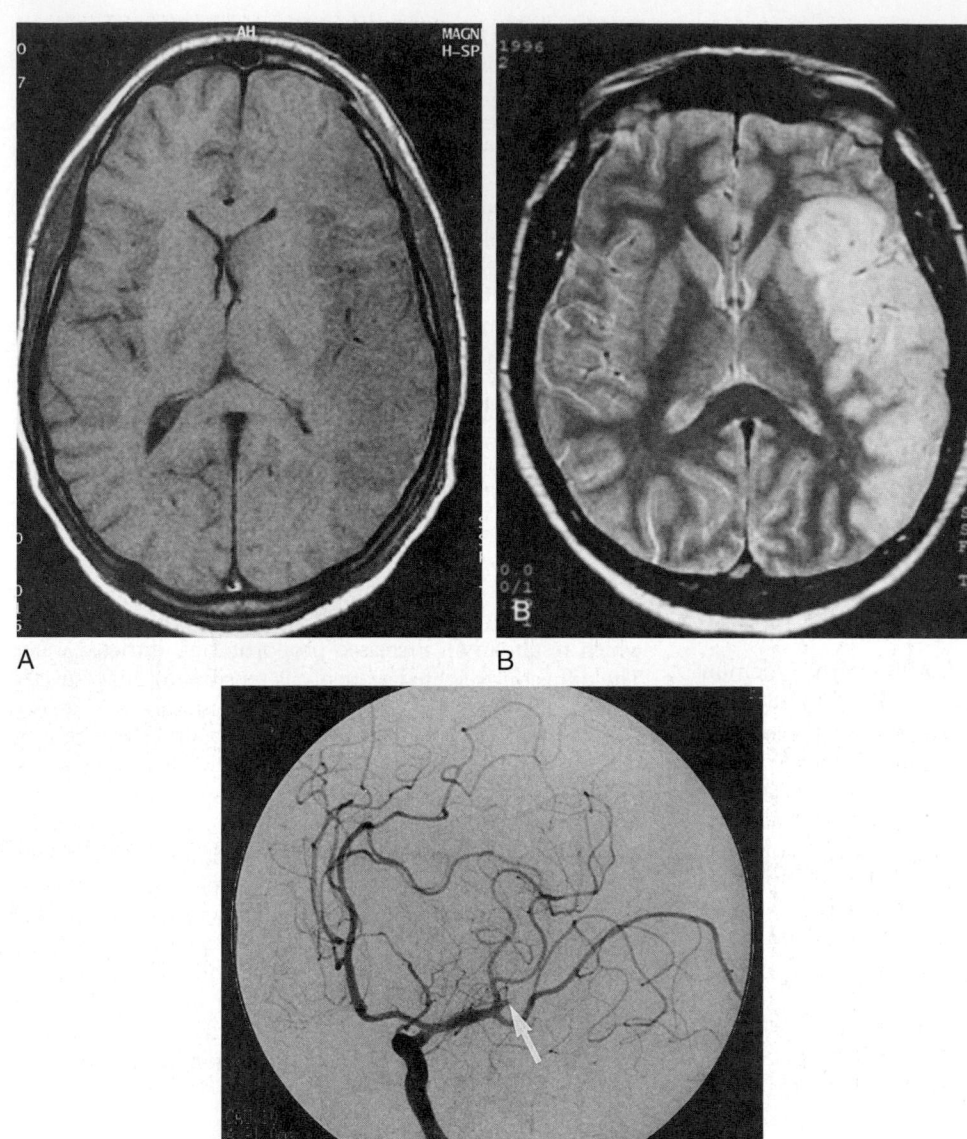

A

B

C

FIGURE 57–8. Infarct. Axial T1-weighted *(A)* and T2-weighted *(B)* MRI scans of a patient being evaluated for stroke. The initial CT scan (not shown) was normal. MRI demonstrates an area of cytotoxic edema involving the distal left middle cerebral artery territory. The edema is hypointense to brain on the T1-weighted image and hyperintense to brain on the T2-weighted image. Left internal carotid artery angiogram *(C)* demonstrates the occluded branch of the left middle cerebral artery *(arrow)*. Within the proper time frame, intra-arterial thrombolysis would be a method of management for this patient.

Treatment of acute embolic infarct with interarterial thrombolysis has been gaining momentum and is changing the role of imaging. Thrombolysis has a very narrow window (0 to 3 hours) for the initiation of treatment. Any delay decreases the positive outcome. Because of this time frame, many methods have been developed to replace routine CT as the initial imaging modality.[24] The goal is to increase the sensitivity for detecting early infarction and demarcating the area at risk. Standard CT coupled with CT perfusion and CT angiography is one alternative. MRI techniques can provide significant information regarding acute cerebral infarction.[24] Use of a series of MRI sequences, a "stroke protocol," can reveal changes in gross anatomy (standard MRI), metabolic alterations (magnetic resonance spectroscopy), water movement restrictions (diffusion-weighted MRI), vasculature status (MRA), and physiologic blood flow data (MRI perfusion) (see Fig. 57-10).[23] During the hyperacute and early acute stages, when CT is usually negative, MRI can readily demonstrate the zone of infarction. In addition, patterns of contrast enhancement in acute ischemia may have prognostic implications with regard to the completeness or reversibility of

the ischemic insult.[25] Other methods being used include xenon CT, SPECT, Doppler ultrasonography, and PET. The advantages and disadvantages of these techniques and their future roles in stroke therapy are still under investigation.

Hypertensive encephalopathy is a syndrome that occurs in patients with elevated blood pressure of any cause. Severe preeclampsia and eclampsia of pregnancy are the most common causes, and CNS involvement is common. Typical MRI findings include nonspecific white matter hyperintensities on T2-weighted images at the gray-white matter junction. Cortical and subcortical white matter edema occurs primarily in the occipital lobes. Characteristically, these lesions resolve completely with treatment. Hypotensive encephalopathy can occur in patients who have suffered an episode of hypotension such as that seen after cardiac arrest. Typically, this results in infarction in the watershed distribution, basal ganglia nuclei, thalamus, hippocampus, cerebellum, and brainstem.

Venous infarction can occur in isolation and is associated with thrombosis of a dural sinus or large draining vein. In contrast to arterial infarctions, venous infarctions are typically

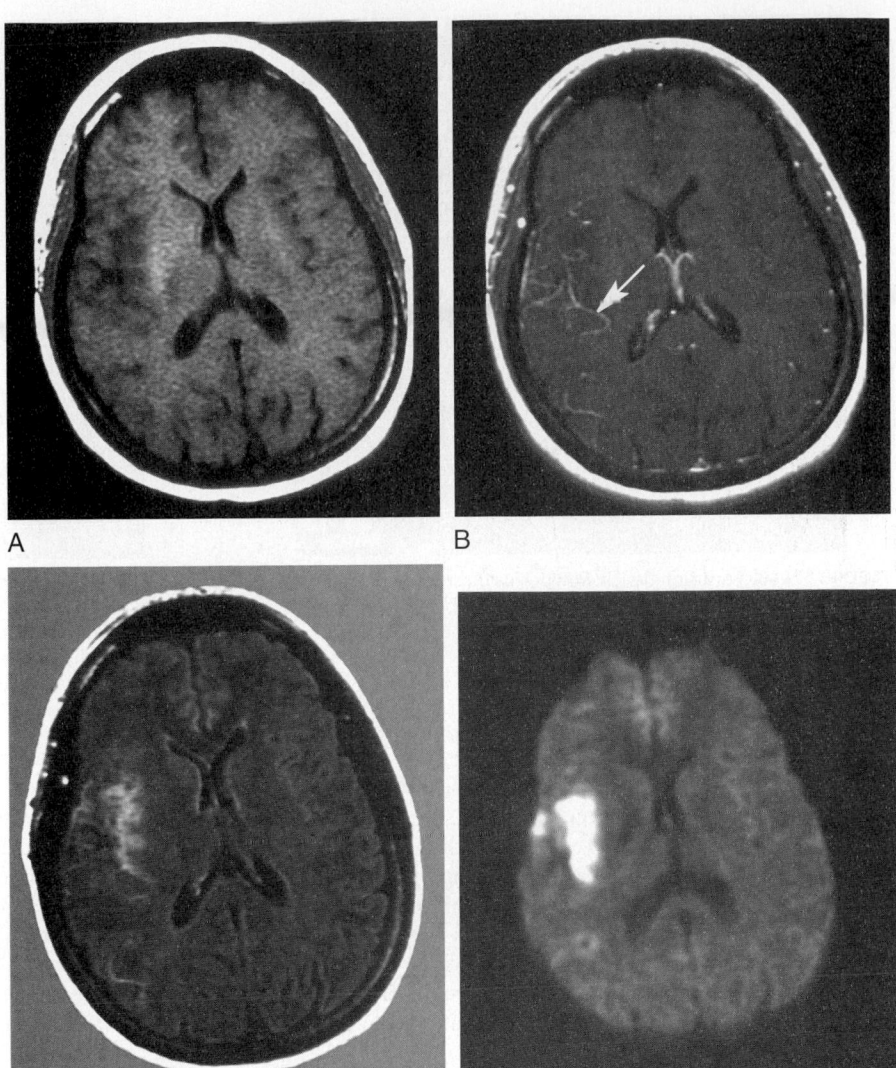

FIGURE 57–9. Hyperacute infarct. Axial T1-weighted images before (A) and after (B) contrast administration reveal subtle low intensity and arterial enhancement (arrow) in the right insular cortex. The fluid-attenuated inversion recovery (FLAIR) sequence (C) helps define the area of involvement. The diffusion-weighted sequence (D) shows the infarct to the best advantage. The acute phase is confirmed by the low signal on the apparent diffusion coefficient map (E).

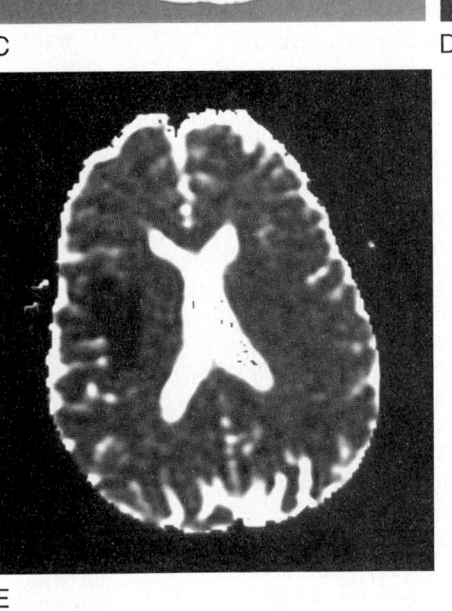

hemorrhagic and affect primarily the white matter. Pregnancy, dehydration, sepsis, and hypercoagulable states are common causes. CT can demonstrate the hemorrhagic infarct as well as the high-density clot in the venous sinus. MRI is very sensitive to the hemorrhagic foci and edema. Thrombosis of the venous sinus can be seen on routine MRI by identifying the clot in the vein. Magnetic resonance venography, performed similar to MRA, can also be helpful in identifying the occluded sinus.

Neonatal and pediatric stroke differs from adult stroke, and the imaging is more complex. The normal imaging appearance of the neonatal brain changes during development

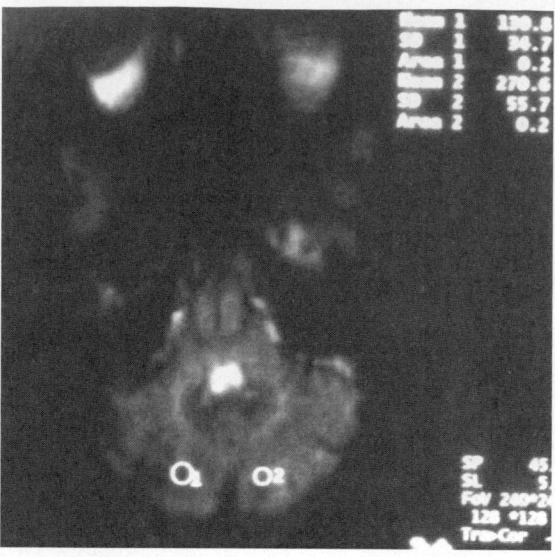

FIGURE 57–10. Perfusion deficit. MRI perfusion study shows hypoperfusion in the right posterior inferior cerebellar artery territory. The normal left side measured 270.6, and the abnormal right side measured 130.8.

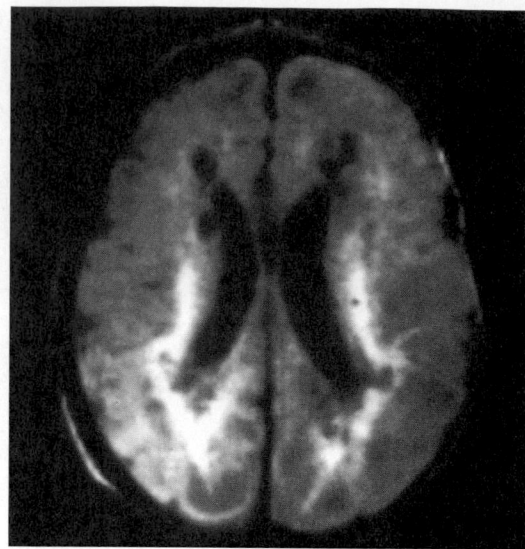

FIGURE 57–11. Periventricular leukomalacia. Axial fluid-attenuated inversion recovery (FLAIR) image obtained on a child with spastic diplegia and a history of prematurity and hypoxic episodes. Multifocal white matter hyperintensities, reduced white matter volume, irregular ventricular contours, and cystic changes are typical findings of periventricular leukomalacia.

because of the degree of myelination. In general, the brain of a term infant has myelinated fibers only in the brainstem and cerebellum. As the baby grows, myelination proceeds from inferior to superior and posterior to anterior. Myelination is typically complete at age 1 year. These changes create variable CT and MRI appearances, depending on the age of the baby. The differences among a preterm infant's brain, a term infant's brain, and an older child's brain are dependent on blood supply and metabolic demands, which differ at each stage. The imaging appearance is therefore dependent on the age of the child at the time of the insult and the duration of the insult.

In the preterm brain, the early imaging findings after an anoxic event include germinal matrix hemorrhage, periventricular venous infarction, and periventricular leukomalacia.[26] The germinal matrix is a rich vascular stroma in the subependymal caudothalamic groove that is very vulnerable to hemorrhage. When an insult occurs, the germinal matrix bursts, and blood leaks into the ventricles or parenchyma. Ultrasonography is used to stage the degree of hemorrhage. Venous infarctions are similar to those discussed earlier but occur in the periventricular region. These focal hemorrhages are readily seen with MRI and are frequently seen with CT. Periventricular leukomalacia represents areas of coagulation necrosis of the white matter, leading to reduction of the central white matter. CT and MRI demonstrate loss of white matter, primarily in the parietal and occipital regions, and enlargement of the ventricles, with ragged borders (Fig. 57-11). Cystic areas may be present, and the sulci extend almost to the ventricles.

In the term brain, diffuse or focal edema, basal ganglia necrosis, and lamina necrosis are the patterns typically seen. At this age, MRI is more sensitive to changes from ischemia than are other modalities. The earliest sign of infarct in the term infant is loss of the gray-white differentiation that is normally seen on T2-weighted images. Occasionally, subtle edematous changes, such as swollen gyri, are the only signs of an acute infarct. Diffuse high signal in the basal ganglia on T1-weighted images can be seen 7 to 10 days after the insult. Cortical lamina necrosis is identified as curvilinear high

signal intensity on T1-weighted images in the deeper layers of the cortex and bases of the sulci.

Mention should be made of total anoxia in preterm and term infants. The pattern of injury in total anoxia involves primarily the brainstem, basal ganglia, thalamus, and perirolandic areas. On CT and MRI, changes reflecting edema are seen in these regions. In older children, there is involvement of the cerebral hemispheres. On CT, the cerebral hemispheres are of low density, with loss of gray-white matter differentiation secondary to the accumulation of water (Fig. 57-12). The cerebellum is spared and has normal blood flow that results in a "bright cerebellar" sign. On MRI, the

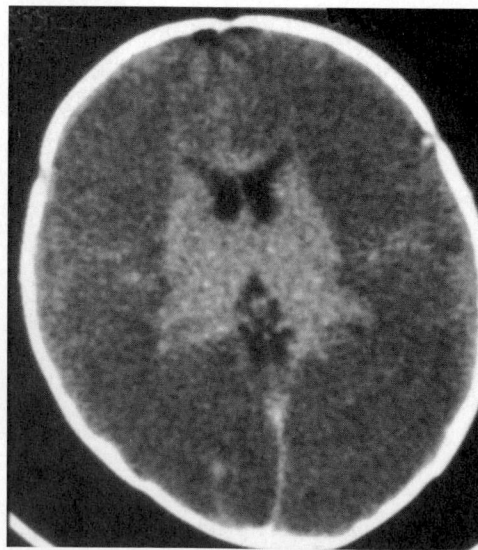

FIGURE 57–12. Global anoxia. Axial CT scan of a child following cardiac arrest. There is diffuse low density in the cerebral hemispheres and compression of the ventricles and sulci, reflecting the increased water accumulation (edema) and resultant mass effect. The basal ganglia and thalami appear bright, showing the "reversal" sign of global anoxia.

accumulation of water is reflected in the loss of gray-white matter differentiation, swollen gyri, and abnormal signal in the basal ganglia.

Congenital Aneurysm and Subarachnoid Hemorrhage. Evaluation of a patient with a suspected ruptured cerebral aneurysm should begin with a noncontrast-enhanced CT scan to demonstrate subarachnoid hemorrhage (Fig. 57-13). If the scan is positive and the patient is a surgical candidate, a cerebral angiogram is performed to identify the aneurysm, identify additional aneurysms, determine which aneurysm ruptured (when multiple aneurysms are present), and assess the presence or absence of associated vasospasm (see Fig. 57-13). MRI and MRA are increasingly important in the evaluation of aneurysms, but primarily in the nonacute setting to screen patients considered to be at high risk for aneurysms or those with focal cranial nerve deficits.[27]

Therapy of congenital aneurysms is undergoing significant changes. Intravascular techniques using detachable coils or balloons now play an important role in the management of certain ruptured and nonruptured aneurysms. Endovascular occlusion of intracranial aneurysms using detachable platinum coils provides a therapeutic alternative, especially in patients with aneurysms that are considered technically difficult or have a high surgical risk.[28,29]

For patients with suspected vasospasm, imaging modalities other than angiography have proved useful. Xenon CT can assess regional blood flow in patients symptomatic from vasospasm.[30] Transcranial Doppler ultrasonography provides an additional noninvasive method of measuring flow velocities and indirectly assessing vessel diameter.[31,32] Treatment of symptomatic vasospasm is also undergoing changes. Percutaneous transluminal balloon angioplasty and intra-arterial papaverine infusion have been effective in treating patients with vasospasm.[33]

Vascular Malformations. Four types of vascular malformations are described: (1) arteriovenous malformation (AVM), (2) capillary telangiectasia, (3) cavernous angioma, and (4) developmental venous anomaly (venous angioma).

AVMs are the most common type. An unruptured AVM may not be apparent on non-contrast-enhanced CT or may appear as a subtle hyperdense region. After contrast administration, large, linear, tortuous, high-density structures representing the serpentine vessels are identified (Fig. 57-14). On MRI, these abnormal vessels appear as areas of absent signal (flow void) caused by rapid blood flow through the normal vessels. Angiography is performed to evaluate these lesions because it demonstrates the feeding arteries and draining veins and can establish pial, dural, or mixed supply (see Fig. 57-14). Intravascular embolization of all or a portion of the AVM may also be performed as a treatment option.[34] When an AVM ruptures, the imaging characteristics are those of hemorrhage, as described previously.

Capillary telangiectasia and cavernous angioma are best evaluated by MRI, because angiography is typically normal and CT is insensitive. The MRI signal characteristics are variable because of the presence or absence of blood products.

Developmental venous anomalies (venous angiomas) are typically not apparent on non-contrast-enhanced CT, but the large transcortical vein can be identified after contrast administration. The caput medusae or smaller feeding veins are frequently seen and are diagnostic. On MRI, the large vein and caput are seen as linear flow voids. Angiography is not necessary for the evaluation of venous angiomas because of the classic CT and MRI appearance and the untreatable nature of these lesions.

Neoplasm

Neoplasms are typically grouped according to location. This method helps narrow the differential diagnosis, because the imaging characteristic of tumors vary widely, based on their internal components. Knowledge of the imaging characteristics of specific tumors, the age and sex of the patient,

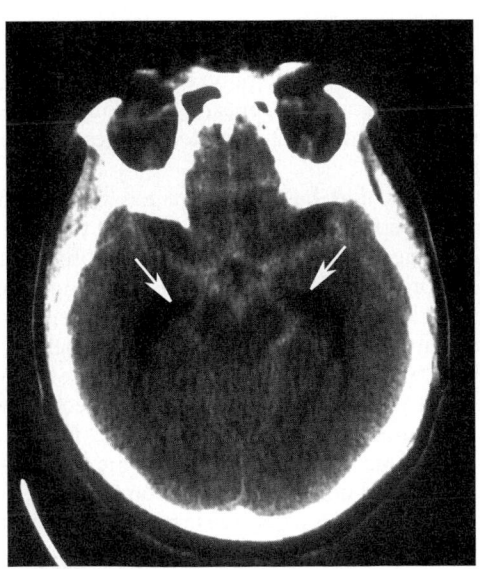
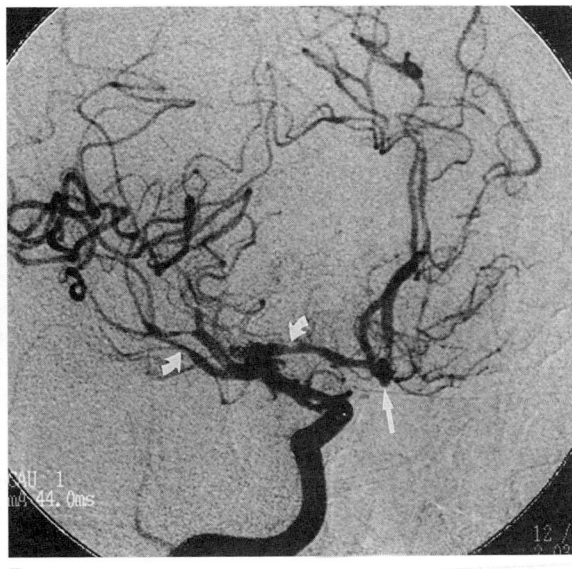

A   B

FIGURE 57–13. Subarachnoid hemorrhage and aneurysm. *A,* Axial non-contrast-enhanced CT scan of the head reveals high density (blood) replacing the normal low density of cerebrospinal fluid within the suprasellar cistern and subarachnoid spaces. This indicates subarachnoid hemorrhage. Note also the dilated temporal horns *(arrows),* indicating acute hydrocephalus. *B,* Right internal carotid artery angiogram demonstrates the presence of a congenital anterior communicating artery aneurysm *(arrow),* as well as vasospasm *(curved arrows).*

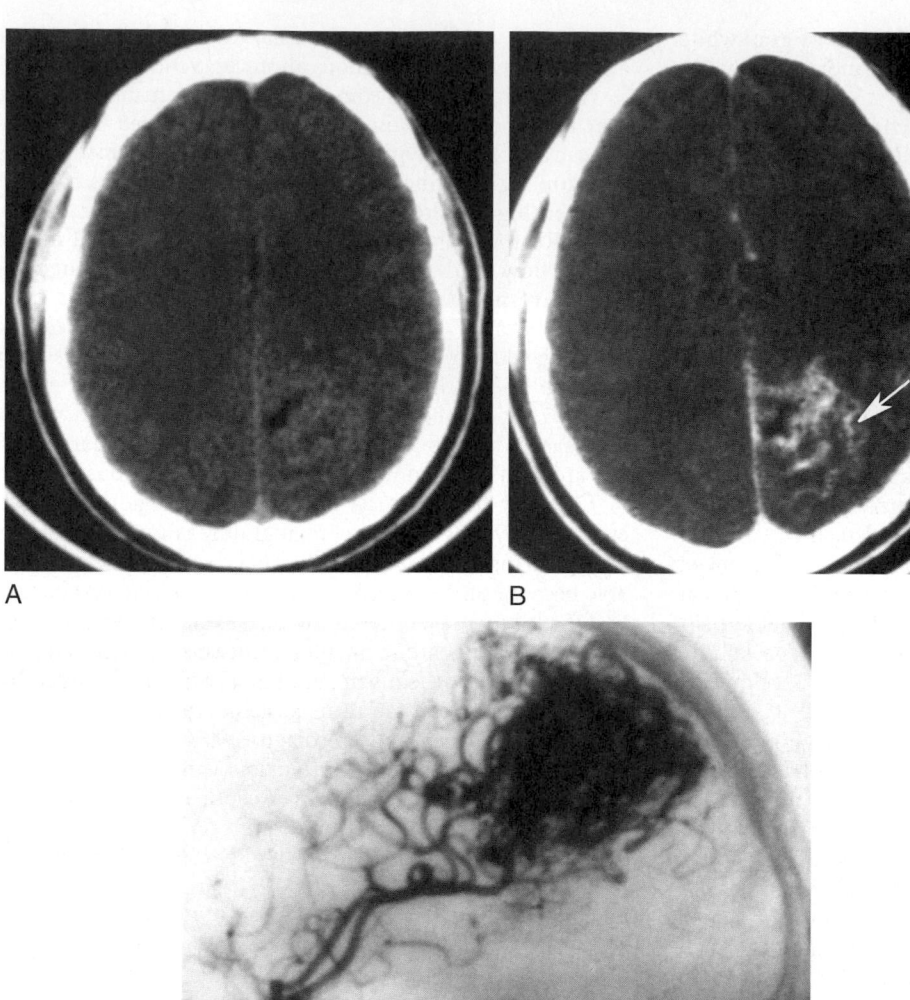

A

B

C

FIGURE 57–14. Arteriovenous malformation. *A,* Axial non-contrast-enhanced CT scan of the head reveals a vague area of hyperdensity in the posterior left parietal region. *B,* Contrast-enhanced CT scan demonstrates serpiginous enhancement of this lesion *(arrow). C,* Internal carotid artery angiogram demonstrates an arteriovenous malformation being fed by the middle cerebral artery.

the clinical presentation, and the lesion location can narrow the differential diagnosis further and often provides a specific diagnosis.[35] On CT, low-grade gliomas may appear as subtle nonenhancing masses, but higher-grade gliomas often demonstrate heterogeneous enhancement, with large areas of necrosis and vasogenic edema (see Fig. 57-1). Metastatic lesions may be low-density and enhancing masses, as seen with lung or breast carcinoma, or they may have high density secondary to hemorrhagic components, as seen with melanoma and thyroid and renal cell carcinomas (Fig. 57-15). Cystic tumors, such as cystic astrocytomas, may be composed of large cysts with the density of cerebrospinal fluid. Epidermoid and dermoid tumors frequently contain areas of fat density and therefore appear very hypodense (less dense than cerebrospinal fluid).

MRI has high sensitivity but low specificity in the evaluation of neoplasms, because most tumors appear similar. Tumors are typically of low intensity on T1-weighted images and high intensity on T2-weighted images (see Fig. 57-1). There are a few notable exceptions, however, because the signal characteristics reflect tumor composition. For example, meningiomas, because of their homogeneous cellular makeup,

tend to be isointense to brain on T1- and T2-weighted images. Epidermoid tumors appear bright on T1-weighted images and less bright on T2-weighted images, reflecting their high fat content.

Tumors that have been treated with radiation therapy present a special problem when trying to determine whether increasing mass effect and edema represent tumor recurrence or post-radiation necrosis. Routine imaging modalities are limited and are based on the observation of changes over time. This can delay further treatment or prematurely instigate unnecessary surgery. A variety of imaging modalities, including magnetic resonance spectroscopy and PET, are becoming increasingly important in this regard. With magnetic resonance spectroscopy, the diagnosis is based on the concentration of various metabolites. Recurrent tumors show an increase in choline levels and a decrease in *N*-acetyl aspartate, representing neuronal loss (Fig. 57-16), and radiation necrosis shows decreased levels of choline. Depending on the technique used, PET measures local glucose consumption, blood flow, or oxygen metabolism. These measurements are increased with recurrent tumor and decreased with radiation necrosis.

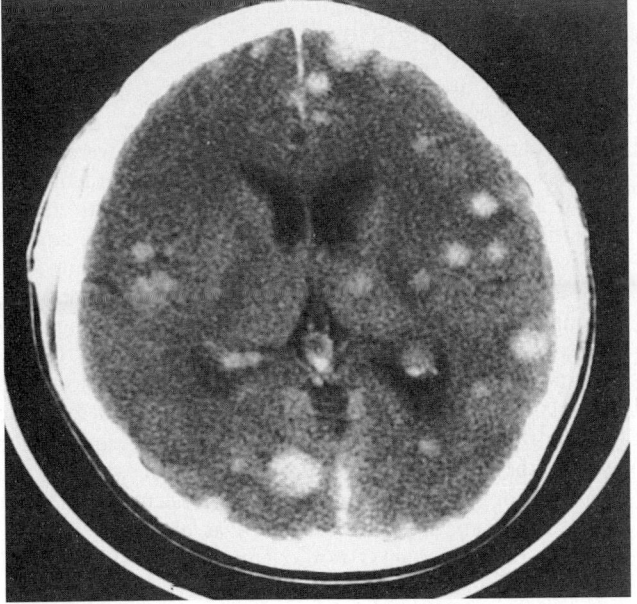

FIGURE 57–15. Intracranial metastatic disease. Axial contrast-enhanced CT scan of the head reveals multiple enhancing nodules throughout the gray and white matter structures, consistent with metastatic disease.

Infection and Inflammation

Infectious and inflammatory processes are considered according to their primary site of involvement: parenchymal or extra-axial.

Parenchymal Infection. Parenchymal infections include encephalitis, cerebritis, and abscess. Encephalitis, a diffuse inflammation of the brain, is often viral or toxic in origin. MRI is more sensitive than CT and demonstrates the changes earlier, making it the modality of choice when encephalitis is suspected clinically. On CT, there are vague areas of low density and subtle gyral enhancement after contrast administration. On MRI, affected brain typically appears hypointense on T1-weighted images and hyperintense on T2-weighted images, reflecting edematous changes. Herpes simplex virus (HSV) encephalitis is a common and specific form of encephalitis with fairly consistent imaging findings. HSV encephalitis is caused by HSV 2 in neonates and HSV 1 in children and adults. Imaging studies show gyral edema with a predilection for the temporal lobes, insular cortex, and cingulate gyri. Acute disseminated encephalomyelitis is an immune-related response to a previous viral infection or vaccination. MRI is the modality of choice and typically shows multifocal subcortical hyperintense lesions on T2-weighted images. Deep white matter can be affected, and lesions are typically bilateral and asymmetrical.

Cerebritis, an early phase of abscess formation, looks like encephalitis but is more focal in nature. Cerebral abscess results from liquefactive necrosis, producing a localized collection of pus or caseous material in a cavity surrounded by a fibrous capsule. On CT, an abscess cavity demonstrates central hypodensity (necrotic cavity); a thin, isodense wall (capsule); and surrounding low density (edema). Following contrast administration, there is enhancement of the capsule. Unlike the shaggy, irregular walls of a tumor, the walls of an abscess are typically smooth, well defined, and uniform in thickness; these are important differential features. MRI findings are similar to CT findings. The central cavity has variable signal characteristics, depending on the contents. The capsule is iso- to hyperintense on T1-weighted images,

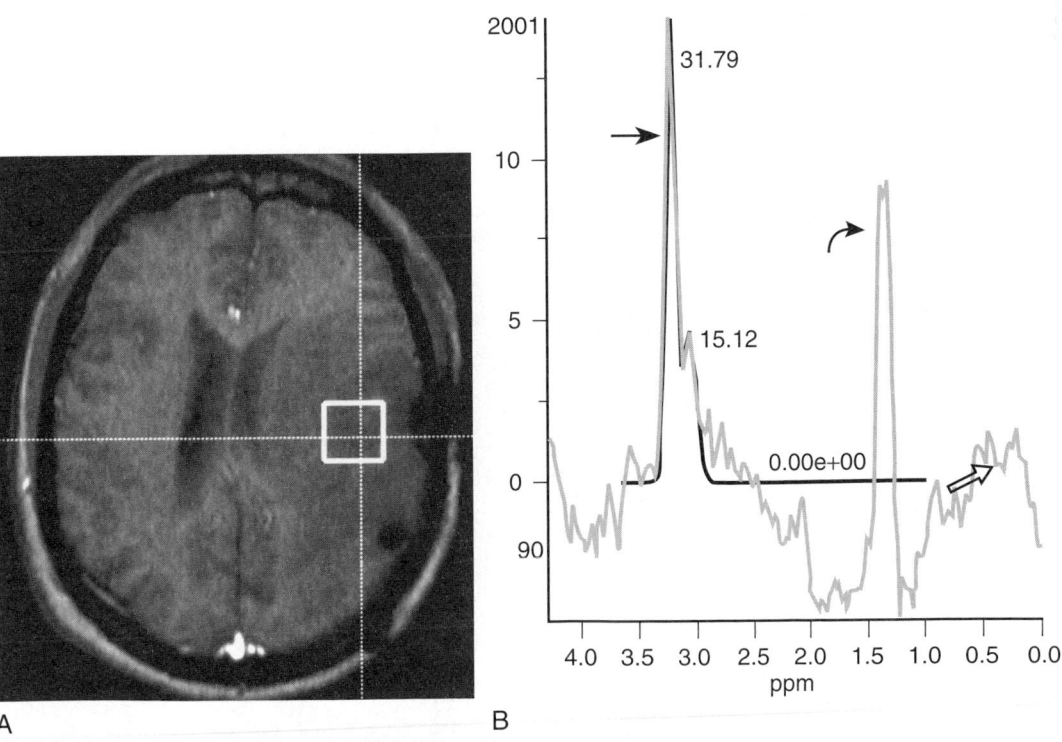

FIGURE 57–16. Recurrent high-grade astrocytoma. A study performed after radiation therapy (not shown) showed increased edema and mass effect, and the differential diagnosis included recurrent tumor and radiation necrosis. *A,* Axial MRI scan shows the volume of tissue *(box)* selected for spectroscopy. *B,* Proton spectroscopy reveals an increase in the choline peak *(arrow),* a decrease in the *N*-acetyl aspartate peak *(curved arrow),* and the appearance of a lactate peak *(open arrow).* This appearance is consistent with recurrent tumor, which was verified with repeat surgery and biopsy.

is hypointense on T2-weighted images, and enhances after contrast administration.

Extra-axial Infection. Extra-axial infections include ventriculitis, meningitis, and subdural or epidural empyemas. MRI is usually the modality of choice for extra-axial infections. In general, with both CT and MRI, contrast administration is necessary to establish the diagnosis of extra-axial infection. On CT and MRI, ventriculitis is characterized only by enhancement of the involved ventricular wall or walls. In meningitis, CT and MRI may be normal or demonstrate diffuse enhancement of the meningeal surfaces after contrast administration. The diagnosis of meningitis is made on clinical grounds and cerebrospinal fluid studies. Imaging is performed to exclude an associated abscess or empyema or to evaluate for complications, such as hydrocephalus and vascular thrombosis. Subdural and epidural empyemas are collections of pus that most often occur as complications of sinusitis, otitis, surgery, or trauma. On CT, the collections frequently have a density intermediate between cerebrospinal fluid and acute blood. On MRI, the collections are typically hypointense to brain on T1-weighted images and hyperintense on T2-weighted images.

White Matter Diseases

White matter diseases are classified as dysmyelinating (improper formation or maintenance of myelin) or demyelinating (normal myelin destroyed by exogenous or endogenous agents). Dysmyelinating disorders include the leukodystrophies and storage diseases. Demyelinating disorders can be idiopathic (multiple sclerosis), postinfectious (progressive multifocal leukoencephalopathy), toxic-degenerative, or vascular. MRI is much more sensitive than CT and is the study of choice for determining the presence and extent of white matter disease (Fig. 57–17). On T1-weighted images, these lesions appear as vague regions of low intensity. On T2-weighted images, white matter lesions appear hyperintense. Newer T2-weighted imaging sequences have the ability to suppress the bright signal produced by cerebrospinal fluid and increase the conspicuity of white matter lesions.[36] Although the majority of white matter diseases appear similar on imaging studies, occasionally the pattern of white matter involvement can lead to a more limited or specific diagnosis.

White matter diseases seldom present acutely; typically, they present as slow progression of neurologic deficits. When the presentation is acute, toxic and vascular diseases are the primary considerations (vascular disorders were already discussed). Toxic demyelination results from interaction of a chemical compound with the brain and may occur acutely. Radiation therapy or chemotherapeutic agents, such as cyclosporin A and methotrexate, may result in acute transient leukoencephalopathy. MRI demonstrates white matter lesions involving the deep white matter, with sparing of the cortex and underlying subcortical arcuate fibers.[37] Central pontine myelinolysis occurs in alcoholic or malnourished patients or in those who have undergone rapid correction of hyponatremia. On MRI, the white matter abnormalities are seen in the pons, with sparing of the corticospinal tracts. Acquired hepatocerebral degeneration occurs with many types of chronic liver disease, such as alcoholic cirrhosis, hepatitis, and portal systemic shunts.[38] MRI frequently demonstrates bilateral basal ganglia hyperintensities on T1-weighted images.

SPINE

PATTERNS OF DISEASE

It is often useful to classify spinal canal pathology according to the three spinal compartments, or spaces: intramedullary, extramedullary-intradural, and extradural (Fig. 57-18). Certain pathologic lesions occur with greater frequency in specific spaces; therefore, the diagnostic considerations can be significantly narrowed if a lesion can be localized to one of these spaces. In most instances, MRI is the modality of choice in evaluating spinal pathology, especially in the acute setting. The high degree of tissue contrast and spatial resolution can localize most lesions to a specific compartment, determine the extent of disease, and offer an accurate differential diagnosis. The only exception is acute trauma, in which case bony alignment and stability are best demonstrated by

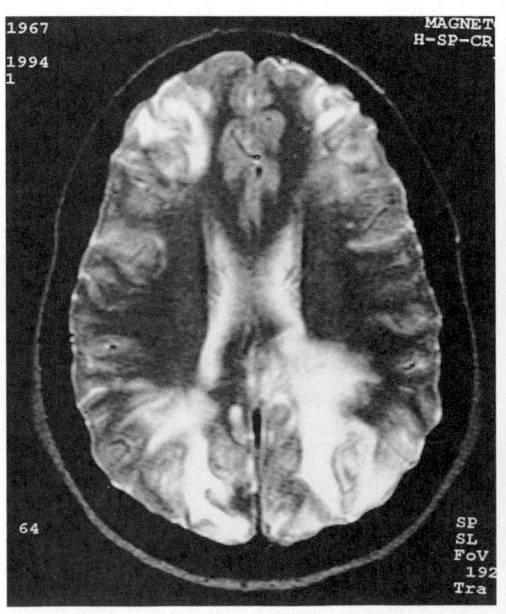

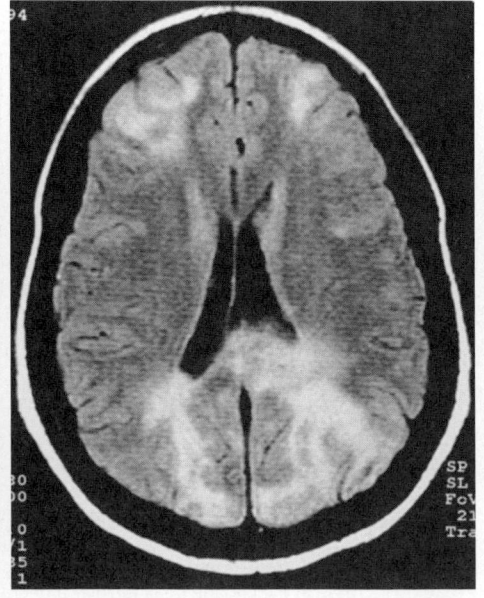

A   B

FIGURE 57–17. Progressive multifocal leukoencephalopathy. Axial T2-weighted *(A)* and fluid-attenuated inversion recovery (FLAIR) *(B)* images in a patient with human immunodeficiency virus (HIV). Multiple areas of white matter disease are identified; the FLAIR image increases their conspicuity. These findings in an HIV-positive patient indicate a postinfectious demyelinating process—progressive multifocal leukoencephalopathy.

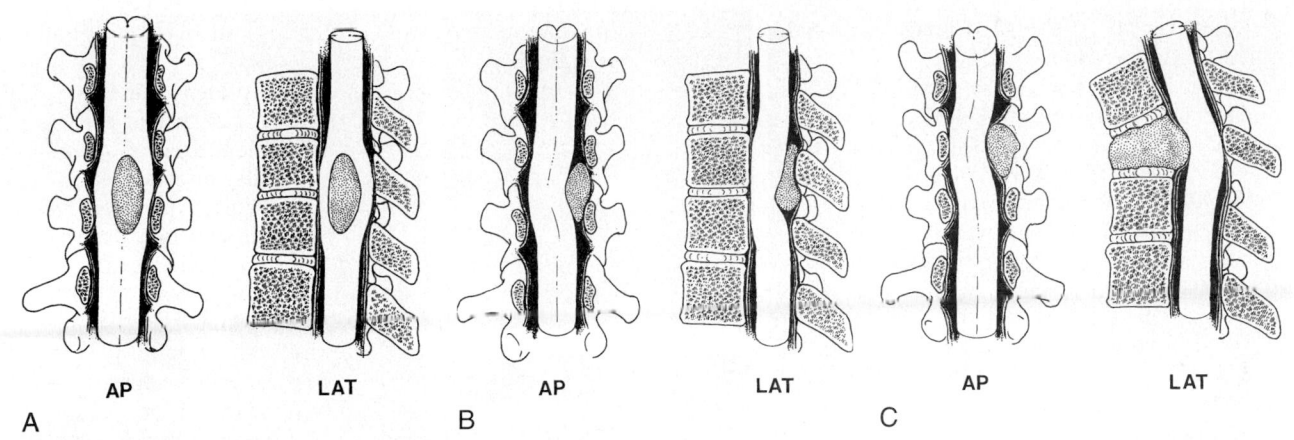

FIGURE 57–18. Spinal compartments. Anteroposterior (AP) and lateral (LAT) views of the spinal cord and canal demonstrate the appearance of an intramedullary lesion *(A)*, an extramedullary intradural lesion *(B)*, and an extradural lesion *(C)*.

plain films, and fracture evaluation and fragment displacements are best demonstrated with CT.

Intramedullary lesions expand the spinal cord as they enlarge, gradually thinning the subarachnoid space, usually symmetrically (see Fig. 57-18A). If of sufficient size, the intramedullary expansion may produce changes in the bony spinal canal, including posterior scalloping of the vertebral bodies, flattening of the spinous processes, widening of the interpeduncular distance, and overall widening of the canal. Intramedullary disease is usually secondary to a variety of neoplasms, most often gliomas (ependymoma, astrocytoma, glioblastoma). Other tumors include dermoid cysts, sarcomas, hemangioblastomas, and intramedullary metastases. In the acute setting, infectious processes such as transverse myelitis, granulomas (sarcoidosis, tuberculosis), and abscesses must be considered. Traumatic injuries such as cord contusion and hematomas can also produce an intramedullary pattern.

Extramedullary-intradural lesions are contained within the subarachnoid space but are external to the cord (see Fig. 57-18B). These lesions displace the arachnoid layer of the meninges but leave the dura in place. On imaging studies, the subarachnoid space flares out to form a "cap" at its interface with the lesion. Tumors, mostly benign, account for the majority of lesions in this space, particularly meningiomas and nerve sheath tumors. Less common lesions occurring in this space include arachnoid cysts, drop metastases, lymphomas, and dermoid and epidermoid tumors.

Extradural lesions lie outside the subarachnoid space. Except for the absence of the subarachnoid cap at the interface with the lesion, the imaging pattern of extradural lesions may be indistinguishable from that of extramedullary-intradural lesions. Extradural lesions typically produce a more gradual displacement of the subarachnoid space and spinal cord (see Fig. 57-18C). Excluding disc disease, the most common extradural pathology is metastatic disease with epidural extension. Pathologic fractures of the involved vertebrae occur frequently and are often associated with spinal cord compression. Primary tumors of the spine and direct extension from paraspinal neoplasms make up the other malignant lesions of the extradural compartment; these include lymphoma, myeloma-plasmacytoma, sarcoma, and vertebral body chordoma.[39] Benign lesions are uncommon in this compartment and include nerve sheath tumor, meningioma, lipoma, and primary bone lesions such as osteoblastoma, giant cell tumor, and aneurysmal bone cyst. Discitis-osteomyelitis with epidural abscess is an additional consideration.

SPECIFIC DISEASE PROCESSES

Spinal Cord Injury

The sequence of performing the various imaging studies to evaluate spine injury remains controversial and is usually based on their availability at the particular trauma center. Initial evaluation usually involves a plain film series. Plain radiographs are rapid, accurate, and widely available and provide a confident diagnosis of stable or unstable injuries. However, only bony injuries are seen directly with this technique; soft tissue injury can be inferred by identifying changes in bone alignment (Fig. 57-19A). With cervical spine injury, a single lateral view is often obtained. If alignment is normal, a complete series is obtained, including oblique and odontoid views. With suspected thoracic and lumbar injuries, lateral and anteroposterior films suffice, but oblique views can be added if questionable areas are identified.

Indications for CT include further evaluation of detected fractures, further evaluation of suspected fractures or confusing plain film findings, and evaluation of areas not well imaged on standard plain films.[40] The sensitivity of CT for fracture detection is between 78% and 100%.[40] Higher resolution and sagittal and coronal reformations aid in the sensitivity (see Fig. 57-19B and C). However, meticulous attention to technique is needed, because subtle alignment abnormalities that suggest ligamentous injury may be missed. Because of the high sensitivity of CT for most types of bony injury, some studies recommend that CT be the primary modality in patients with suspected cervical spine injury.[41,42]

MRI is the only method that can directly visualize intrinsic spinal cord and soft tissue injuries (see Fig. 57-19D). It can identify and distinguish between cord hematoma and contusion (edema), which affects the prognosis. Cord hematoma has a poor prognosis and indicates a complete lesion, whereas localized edema has a better prognosis for recovery of motor function.[43] Traumatic disc herniations can be readily identified. The presence of disc herniation with cord compression can change management from nonsurgical to surgical or change a posterior stabilization approach to a combined anterior and posterior approach.

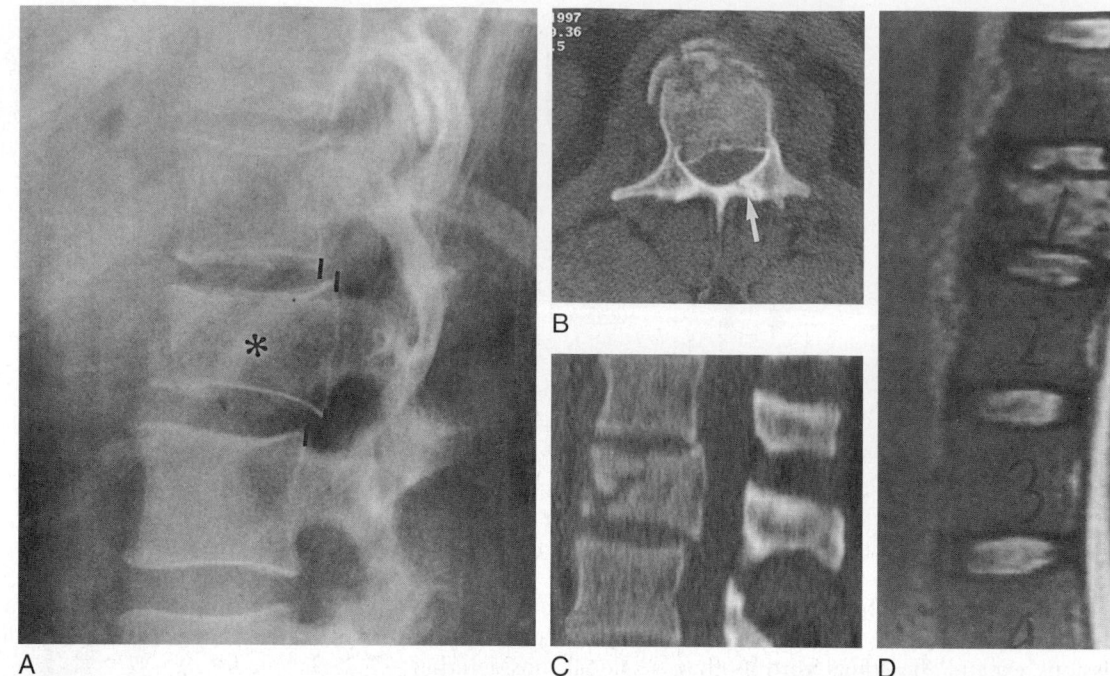

FIGURE 57–19. Post-traumatic vertebral body compression fracture. *A,* Lateral plain film of the thoracolumbar junction reveals a compression fracture involving the L1 vertebral body *(asterisk).* The decreased height of the vertebral body and the inferior anterior corner fracture are well seen. The retropulsed body can also be seen when the outline of the adjacent vertebral bodies *(lines)* are compared. *B* and *C,* Axial *(B)* and sagittal reconstructed *(C)* CT scans of the same patient add substantial detail to the degree of canal narrowing secondary to the retropulsed fragment. A left laminar fracture *(arrow, B)* is also seen, which was not apparent on the plain film. *D,* Sagittal T2-weighted MRI demonstrates the compression fracture of L1 and the retropulsed posterior body, as well as contusion and swelling of the conus *(arrows)* as a direct result of the compression fracture.

MRI is also useful in detecting ligamentous injury by showing edematous changes or discontinuity in the ligaments. Although these findings are usually secondary, detection of isolated ligamentous injury may identify patients at risk for delayed instability. Epidural hematoma and the extent to which it is compressing the cord are also identified with MRI. Finally, although fractures are difficult to detect with MRI, the effect of bony fragment displacement and

alignment abnormalities on the cord or nerve roots is elegantly seen with this modality (see Fig. 57-19*D*).

In summary, plain films are a useful screening tool to identify bony fractures and alignment abnormalities. CT further defines identified or suspected fractures and clarifies ambiguous areas on plain films. MRI is useful to identify intrinsic cord injuries and extrinsic soft tissue and bone abnormalities and their effect on the cord. Occasionally, all

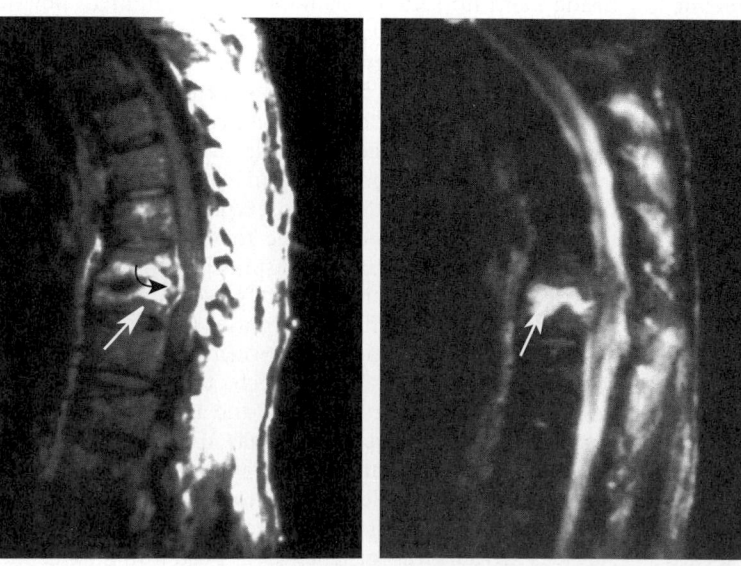

FIGURE 57–20. Discitis with epidural abscess. Sagittal post-contrast T1-weighted *(A)* and T2-weighted *(B)* MRI scans demonstrate features of discitis and adjacent osteomyelitis. The vertebral bodies and disc space are of low signal intensity on the T1-weighted image and bright signal intensity on the T2-weighted image *(straight arrows).* An epidural abscess surrounding and compressing the cord is also identified *(curved arrow).*

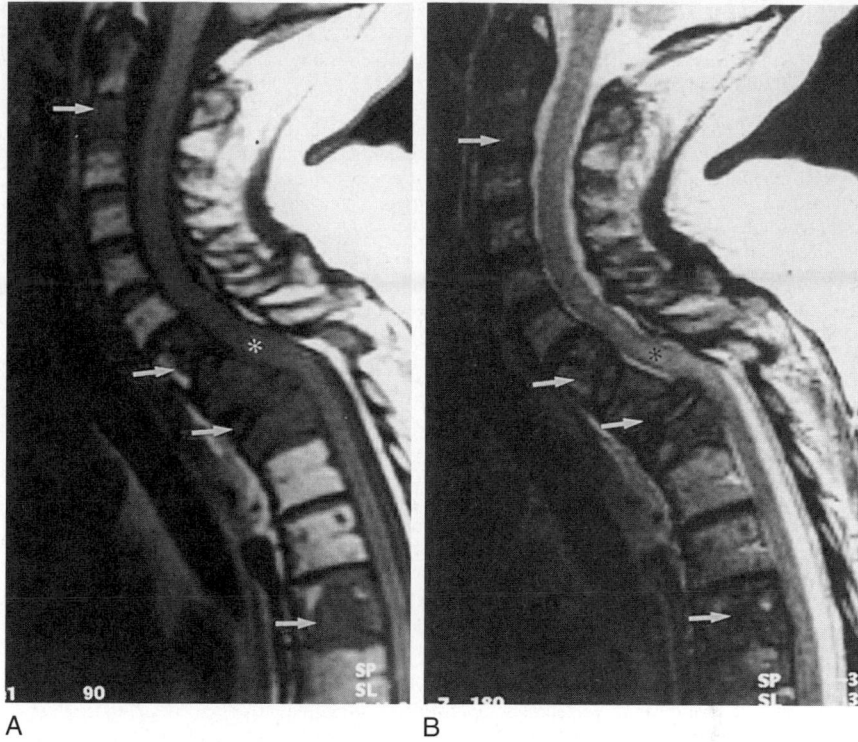

FIGURE 57–21. Metastatic disease. Sagittal T1-weighted *(A)* and T2-weighted *(B)* MRI scans of the spine show the metastatic lesions *(arrows)* as low intensity on the T1-weighted image, replacing the normal bright marrow. The high signal within the uninvolved vertebral bodies represents post-radiation changes. The hypointense lesions on the T2-weighted image (in contrast to the more typical hyperintensity) reflect the post-treatment appearance. Multiple compression fractures are identified within the upper thoracic spine, with collapse, retropulsed fragments, and cord compression. Edematous changes within the cord secondary to compression *(asterisk)* are also identified.

three modalities are necessary to establish the appropriate treatment plan.

Spinal Infection

Infections that involve the spine include discitis, epidural and subdural infections, myelitis, and cord abscess. In the management of spinal infections, delayed treatment can lead to increased morbidity and mortality,[44] making early diagnosis critical. MRI is the primary imaging modality in all types of spinal infection because of its higher sensitivity and its ability to detect changes earlier than plain films and CT. MRI findings with discitis are characteristic (Fig. 57-20). T1-weighted images show a narrowed disc space and hypointensity in the adjacent vertebral bodies. T2-weighted images show high signal in the affected disc space and vertebral bodies. Post-contrast studies show enhancement of the infected disc space and osteomyelitic bone. Paraspinal abscess, epidural extension, meningeal involvement, and cord compression are also readily seen with MRI.

Although MRI is sensitive in defining areas of myelitis, the findings are nonspecific and resemble those of other noninfectious and demyelinating disorders. Typically, focal or diffuse areas of hyperintensity are seen within the cord on T2-weighted images. Contrast enhancement is variable.

Neoplasm

Neoplasms involving the spinal axis typically present with progressive symptoms of myelopathy or cord compression. MRI is the primary modality for the evaluation of any suspected spinal tumor. It can demonstrate the location, extent, and nature of most tumors, regardless of the compartment of origin. Primary tumors of the bony elements and direct extension from paraspinal neoplasms are also easily identified with MRI.

In the evaluation of metastatic disease, MRI is more sensitive than bone scintigraphy.[45] Epidural and paraspinous soft tissue involvement and cord compression are also easily evaluated with MRI. Diffuse metastatic disease is recognized as heterogeneous or homogeneous hypointensity on T1-weighted images and hyperintensity on T2-weighted images (Fig. 57-21). MRI is valuable in identifying compression fractures and associated cord compression and is frequently able to distinguish between benign (osteoporotic) and pathologic (metastatic) fractures. Benign fractures have marrow intensity that is isointense with the marrow of uninvolved vertebral bodies on all sequences (Fig. 57-22), whereas pathologic fractures demonstrate the signal changes described earlier for metastatic disease.[46]

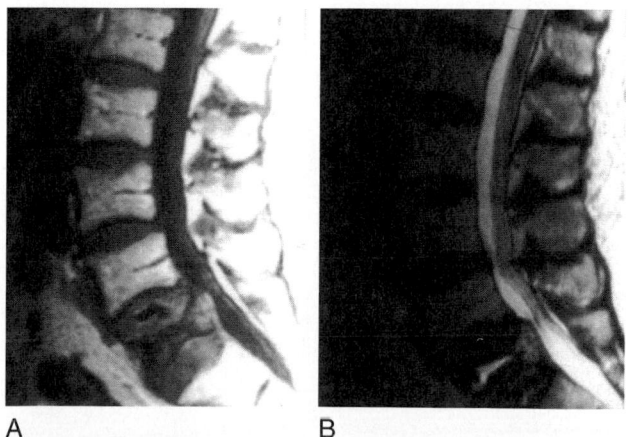

FIGURE 57–22. Benign compression fracture. Sagittal T1-weighted *(A)* and T2-weighted *(B)* MRI scans demonstrate a compression fracture of L5. Compare the signal characteristics of the remaining bony elements and pedicles with the signal of the normal bony structures.

ANNOTATED REFERENCES

Askoy FG, Lev MH: Dynamic contrast-enhanced brain perfusion imaging: Technique and clinical applications. Neuroimaging Clin N Am 2001;11: 485-500.

Brain perfusion studies are the next step in neuroimaging for many forms of pathology and, more important, for the evaluation of head injury and stroke. This article provides an easily understood overview of the different MRI and CT perfusion techniques used. In addition, there is a detailed discussion of the clinical applications of perfusion imaging, with an emphasis on patients with stroke.

Beauchamp NJ, Bryan RN: Acute cerebral infarction: A pathophysiologic review and radiologic perspective. AJR Am J Roentgenol 1998;171:73-84.

The first part of this article reviews the progression from ischemia to stroke, the role of blood flow, and the biochemical ischemic cascade. The second part discusses the shortcomings of the current imaging approach for the diagnosis and treatment of stroke and the use of advanced techniques to overcome these shortcomings.

Cornelius RS, Leah JL: Imaging evaluation of cervical spine trauma. Neuroimaging Clin N Am 1995;5:451-463.

This article summarizes the most appropriate techniques in the evaluation of patients with suspected cervical spine injury. Although other modalities are covered, CT and MRI are emphasized. The issue of the role of imaging in low-risk patients is also covered.

Kleinman PK, Barnes PD: Head trauma. In Kleinman PK (ed): Diagnostic Imaging of Child Abuse. St Louis, Mosby, 1998, pp 285-342.

This chapter covers all aspects of head injury in children in a detailed and illustrative manner. Examples of the imaging characteristics of all forms of head injury in the pediatric population are clearly demonstrated and discussed.

Romaro JM, Schaefer PW, Grant PE, et al: Diffusion MR imaging of acute ischemic stroke. Neuroimaging Clin N Am 2002;12:35-53.

This article presents the theory and practice of diffusion-weighted imaging. Although the beginning of the article involves physics and biophysics, the remainder of the article contains practical information for the evaluation of ischemia and stroke. The article also discusses the use of diffusion-weighted images with stroke mimics, as well as other pathologic entities.

Chapter 58

INTENSIVE CARE AFTER NEUROSURGERY

Andrew I.R. Maas • Nino Stocchetti

KEY POINTS

1. Successful care for the neurosurgical patient requires excellent collaboration between neurosurgeon and intensivist. The result of a technically perfect operation can be ruined by inadequate postoperative care, and a complicated operative procedure will necessitate expert intensive care to correct abnormalities in homeostatic mechanisms and restore brain function.

2. The principal goal of postoperative neurosurgical intensive care is early detection and treatment of post-surgery complications. The second goal is to prevent secondary insults, which may initiate or exacerbate secondary damage in a vulnerable central nervous system.

3. Specific care and monitoring of the postoperative neurosurgical patient requires accurate knowledge of the preoperative situation and the intraoperative procedure, including the surgery, anesthesiology, and any surgical complications or difficulties.

4. The goal of cardiopulmonary and respiratory monitoring is to ensure accurate control of systemic hemodynamic and respiratory function, essential for optimization of cerebral oxygenation. Invasive arterial blood pressure monitoring is recommended with the reference point set at the same level as intracranial pressure measurement to allow accurate calculation of cerebral perfusion pressure.

5. The development of cerebral herniation (tentorial herniation/cerebellar tonsillar herniation) constitutes a neurosurgical emergency. A rapid intervention is required prior to further investigations to determine the cause.

Appropriate neurocritical care is fundamental to the success of neurosurgical operations to the brain and spinal cord. The great technical advances in operative procedures over the past decade have made lesions previously considered inoperable now treatable, and the advances in anesthesia have led to an increased number of operative procedures in both elderly and critically ill patients. Consequently, the number of patients requiring postoperative intensive care treatment has increased.

Successful care for the neurosurgical patient requires excellent collaboration between neurosurgeon and intensivist. The result of a technically perfect operation can be ruined by inadequate postoperative care, and a complicated operative procedure will necessitate expert intensive care to correct abnormalities in homeostatic mechanisms and restore brain function. Understanding of the complex interaction between the central nervous system and systemic functioning requires intimate knowledge of both general intensive care and cerebral and spinal pathophysiology. It can be safely concluded that the best care for neurosurgical patients can be provided by dedicated specialists with knowledge of both fields and a large amount of experience in treating such patients. We do not wish to challenge the concept of a closed format intensive care unit (ICU) but believe that concentration of care in units with sufficient volume, experience, and knowledge of neurocritical care is essential to the success of neurosurgery. The benefits of concentration of care have been well established in different fields of intensive care medicine, including trauma[1,2] and neonatology.[3,4] Treatment of patients with spontaneous intracerebral hemorrhage in a neuro-ICU is associated with reduced mortality, when compared with patients admitted to a general ICU[5,6] and the rate of mortality after aneurysmal subarachnoid hemorrhage is lower in centers with a higher case volume.[7] Protocol-driven approaches also improve results.[8-10]

The admission policy for postoperative neurosurgical care to ICUs varies widely between countries and centers and even within centers. In some centers, all patients are admitted for a 24-hour observation period after intracranial procedures; this is motivated by the observation that some patients, although fully alert and neurologically intact initially, develop complications such as a postoperative hematoma with rapid neurologic deterioration necessitating prompt intervention.

In other centers, patients are only admitted to the ICU after intracranial complications have been detected. Some hospitals have dedicated neuro-ICUs and in others, patients are admitted to general intensive care, sometimes even to different ICUs within one hospital. In general, the scarcity of intensive care beds has led to a more restrictive admission policy for postoperative neurosurgical care. The institution of high care units, sometimes termed "step down units" may permit more rational allocation of scarce intensive care resources, while at the same time affording sufficient guarantees for adequate postoperative monitoring. Here again, however, care should be provided by personnel well experienced in the care of neurosurgical patients, thus permitting early detection of possible deterioration and prevention of secondary complications.

PRIORITIES AND GOALS OF POSTOPERATIVE NEUROSURGICAL CARE

The principal goal of postoperative neuro-ICU is early detection and treatment of post-surgery complications.

TABLE 58–1. POSTOPERATIVE COMPLICATIONS

Systemic Complications	Neurosurgical Complications
Thromboembolic (DVT, pulmonary embolism, myocardial infarction)	Postoperative hematoma (subgaleal, epidural, subdural, intraparenchymal)
Infection (pneumonia, urinary tract infection, catheter sepsis)	Brain swelling (edema, vasodilation)
Hypovolemia (insufficient pre- and perioperative hydration, blood loss)	Cerebral ischemia (subarachnoid hemorrhage, vasospasm, vessel occlusion)
Coagulation disorders (blood loss, disseminated intravascular coagulation)	Infection (meningitis, subdural empyema, cerebral abscess)
Air embolism (sitting position, opening of large cerebral veins during surgery)	Seizures (infection, depressed compound skull fracture, cortical lesions)
Pulmonary (atelectasis, pneumothorax)	Hydrocephalus (obstruction/resorption)
Metabolic (hyperglycemia [steroid induced], diabetes insipidus, hyponatremia)	Tension pneumocephalus
Pressure sores and decubitus ulcers (intraoperative positioning, cervical traction, paraplegia)	CSF fistula
	Inverse cerebellar herniation
	Cranial nerve lesions

The second goal is to prevent secondary insults, which may initiate or exacerbate secondary damage in a vulnerable central nervous system.

Consequently, priorities are to ensure adequate monitoring facilities, which, in the sedated and ventilated patient, may require further invasive monitoring of the intracranial system, and to ensure adequate oxygenation and perfusion of the brain.

POSTOPERATIVE COMPLICATIONS AND SECONDARY INSULTS

Postoperative complications may be systemic or neurosurgical (Table 58-1).

PREVENTION AND MANAGEMENT OF SYSTEMIC COMPLICATIONS AFTER NEUROSURGERY

The prevention and management of systemic complications after neurosurgical procedures follows general principles of "intensive care" medicine. It is important to realize, however, that systemic complications and secondary insults may initiate or aggravate cerebral damage. Aggressive treatment aimed at preventing and limiting secondary insults is of paramount importance. The main secondary insults, their causes, and adverse effects on brain homeostasis and function are summarized in Table 58-2, further illustrating the complex interactions between systemic events and central nervous system (CNS) function.

TABLE 58–2. SYSTEMIC SECONDARY INSULTS

Event	Main Causes	Adverse Effect
Hypoxemia	Hypoventilation Aspiration atelectasis Pneumothorax Pneumonia Anemia	Decrease in oxygen delivery and increased risk of ischemic damage
Hypotension	Hypovolemia Cardiac failure Sepsis, spinal cord injury	Decreased CPP, decrease in CBF, increased risk of ischemia
Anemia	Blood loss	Decrease in oxygen delivery and increased risk of ischemic damage
Hypercapnia	Respiratory depression	Increased cerebral blood volume (CBV), raised ICP
Hypocapnia	Hyperventilation, spontaneous or induced	Cerebral vasoconstriction with increased risk of ischemic damage
Hyperthermia	Hypermetabolism, stress response, infection Central dysregulation	Metabolic requirements may exceed substrate delivery, resulting in energy depletion
Hypothermia	Exposure, central dysregulation	May be neuroprotective, but can cause significant coagulopathy and electrolyte disturbances
Hyperglycemia	Hypothermia, IV infusion of dextrose, steroids, stress response	Acidosis, electrolyte disturbances
Hypoglycemia	Inadequate nutrition, insulin overdose, pituitary insufficiency	Energy depletion, seizures
Hyponatremia	Insufficient intake (hypotonic fluids) Excessive sodium loss (cerebral salt wasting) Inappropriate ADH syndrome	Increased edema, seizures
Hypernatremia	Diabetes Insipidus Osmotic agents (mannitol, hypertonic saline)	Lethargy, coma

Conversely, CNS events may induce systemic derangement. For example, in response to raised intracranial pressure, mean arterial blood pressure may increase. In such situations, treatment of hypertension is contraindicated because it may exacerbate cerebral ischemia. In other situations, however, arterial hypertension may aggravate the occurrence of cerebral edema, and the clinical dilemma is then to balance a desire to limit edema formation with a desire to maintain adequate perfusion. Electrocardiographic abnormalities, and cardiac arrhythmias may be caused by subarachnoid hemorrhage, traumatic brain injury (TBI), or raised intracranial pressure (ICP). Many drugs routinely used in neurosurgical patients (e.g., steroids, antiepileptic agents) can cause complications or side effects. CNS damage may lead to disturbance in temperature control, causing hypo- or hyperthermia. Release of factors from damaged brain tissue may further initiate acute respiratory distress syndrome (neurogenic pulmonary edema) or induce coagulopathy. Various studies have confirmed a transient hypercoagulopathy syndrome both in the immediate postoperative phase after brain surgery[11] and in patients with TBI.[12-16] Deep venous thrombosis has been reported to occur in 18% to 50% of neurosurgical cases[17] and pulmonary embolism in 0% to 25%. The incidence of deep venous thrombosis and pulmonary embolism incidence is particularly high in patients with brain tumor.[18] Nevertheless, neurosurgeons tend to underestimate the risk of deep venous thrombosis and pulmonary embolism[19] and remain reluctant to routinely prescribe anticoagulant prophylaxis for fear of increasing the risk of postoperative bleeding.[20,21]

Existing evidence, however, does not clearly show an increased risk of clinically significant hemorrhagic complications with anticoagulant prophylaxis but does show a beneficial effect in reducing deep venous thrombosis and pulmonary embolism.[22-26] This supports the administration of antithrombotic prophylaxis prior to neurosurgical procedures in all patients,[27] including those with intracranial hemorrhagic lesions,[28] those with closed TBI,[29] and high-risk trauma patients.[30] In addition, early mobilization in the postoperative phase, whenever possible, is recommended. More consensus exists concerning routine administration of anticoagulant therapy in patients with spinal cord injuries.

PREVENTION AND MANAGEMENT OF NEUROSURGICAL POSTOPERATIVE COMPLICATIONS

SUPRATENTORIAL PROCEDURES

Postoperative Subgaleal Hematoma
Postoperative subgaleal hematoma can occur in up to 11% of procedures.[31,32] These hematomas generally result from either inadvertent damage to the superficial temporal artery with inadequate hemostasis or from hemorrhage from the temporal muscle. If the superficial temporal artery is damaged during the operation, ligation is preferred over coagulation. The occurrence of subgaleal hematomas can be minimized by routine use of postoperative wound drainage for 24 hours. Reoperation for subgaleal hematomas is seldom necessary unless there is a communication with the intracranial compartment resulting in secondary compression of the brain.[33]

Intracranial Hemorrhage
Intracranial postoperative hemorrhage occurs in approximately 1% of procedures and mainly concerns intraparenchymal

hematomas (43-60%), epidural hematomas (28-33%), and subdural hematomas (5-7%).

After every supratentorial procedure, some blood may accumulate in the epidural space. Appropriate surgical technique aims to minimize this epidural space by circumferentially suturing the dura to the bone, periosteum, or galea. Inadequate hemostasis of meningeal arteries, blood loss from the temporal muscle, or blood loss from the bone may, however, induce a larger postoperative epidural hematoma. In cases of neurologic deterioration considered due to the postoperative epidural hematoma, surgical evacuation is indicated. Postoperative subdural hematomas occur less frequently and may result from delayed rupture of bridging veins after a large intracerebral decompression. On occasion, such subdural hematomas can occur distant from the primary site of operation.

Parenchymal hemorrhages are the most frequent cause of hematomas after supratentorial procedures and generally occur at the site of operation, particularly following partial tumor resection. An increase in systemic blood pressure at the end of surgery is another factor that may increase the risk of parenchymal hemorrhage. In rare cases, the hematoma may be located distant from the primary site of operation, and cerebellar hematomas have even been described after supratentorial surgery.[34] The possibility of a postoperative hematoma should be considered in all patients who are not fully alert after anesthesia as well as in those who exhibit secondary deterioration.

Postoperative Brain Swelling
Modern neuroanesthesiology techniques have diminished the incidence of peri- and postoperative brain swelling. Nevertheless, significant swelling may occur, causing surgical difficulties and possibly critical problems in the ICU. Predisposing factors are hypercapnia, arterial hypertension, and obstruction of venous drainage. In any patient with brain swelling during the surgical procedure, the possibility of a deep hematoma should be considered and urgent postoperative computed tomography (CT) should be performed. Brain swelling due to vasodilation can be corrected by hyperventilation and barbiturate administration. Brain swelling due to cerebral edema should be preferentially treated by osmotic agents and mild hyperventilation. Recently, a new syndrome has been described in which significant brain swelling after uneventful surgery was ascribed to intracranial hypotension caused by subgaleal suction.[35]

Tension Pneumocephalus
On postoperative CT scans, some air collection is generally observed.[36] In rare circumstances, the postoperative rewarming of air in the intracranial compartment or continuous air leakage, due to a cerebrospinal fluid fistula of the skull base, may lead to a tension pneumocephalus, with clinical symptomatology including a decreasing level of consciousness, signs of raised intracranial pressure, and occasionally seizures. Generally, postoperative air accumulations are self-limiting and do not require specific treatment.

Seizures
An epileptic seizure in the immediate postoperative period should be considered a serious complication that may cause significant deterioration due to vasodilation, increased cerebral oxygen consumption, and increased brain edema.

The benefits of prophylactic antiseizure medication should be balanced against risks. In some centers, routine prophylaxis is prescribed in all patients undergoing supratentorial brain surgery. In others, the indications are restricted to patients with a higher risk:

- Cerebrovascular surgery (arteriovenous malformation, aneurysm)
- Cerebral abscess and subdural empyema
- Convexity and parafalcial meningiomas
- Penetrating brain injury
- Compound depressed skull fracture

Opinions vary on the duration of prophylactic antiseizure therapy, with some centers recommending a treatment duration of 2 weeks and others continuing for at least 3 months.

INFRATENTORIAL SURGERY

The care for patients in the direct postoperative phase after infratentorial procedures poses specific problems: postoperative complications in the posterior fossa can lead to rapid deterioration due to the relatively small infratentorial reserve capacity and the immediate compression of the brainstem, resulting in respiratory insufficiency and acute herniation. Irritation of the brain stem may induce large swings in arterial blood pressure, increasing the risk of postoperative hemorrhage during hypertensive episodes. Cranial nerves are more susceptible to damage due to surgical manipulation than peripheral nerves.[37] Lesions of the lower cranial nerves may lead to a diminished gag reflex with increased risk of aspiration and pneumonia. After any infratentorial procedure, the risk of acute hydrocephalus due to obstruction at the level of the fourth ventricle is increased. Increased pressure in the infratentorial compartment may, in rare cases in which supratentorial cerebrospinal fluid drainage is performed, cause upward (inverse) herniation.

These aspects specific to the care of patients who have undergone posterior fossa surgery warrant the routine admission of all patients following such surgery for frequent monitoring in the ICU. Particular attention should be paid to the presence of the gag reflex before extubation and in the early stages after extubation, and even then frequent monitoring of the respiratory status is imperative.

After posterior fossa surgery, some patients develop a syndrome of aseptic meningitis.[38] This is characterized by meningeal symptoms, headaches, and an inflammatory response in the cerebrospinal fluid in the absence of evidence for infection. The origin of this syndrome has not been fully clarified, but symptoms may resolve sooner with intermittent cerebrospinal fluid drainage.

An infrequent transient complication observed after resection of large mid-line posterior fossa tumors is cerebellar mutism. The exact cause is poorly understood, but a vascular phenomenon has been hypothesized.[39-43] After surgery in the cerebellar pontine angle, specific attention should be paid to the function of the trigeminal and facial nerves, and prophylactic measures should be taken to prevent corneal damage.

For a discussion of aneurysmal subarachnoid hemorrhage, please see Chapter 52.

TABLE 58–3. POSTOPERATIVE INTAKE AFTER NEUROSURGICAL OPERATIONS

Preoperative situation	Neurologic deficit (level of consciousness, focal paresis, cranial nerve lesions, hormonal deficits)
	Preexisting disease (especially pulmonary and cardiac)
	Preoperative medication
	History of seizures
	Allergy
	Surgical position
Intraoperative details (anesthesia)	Narcotic agents and antagonists
	Blood loss and substitution
	Intraoperative laboratory values
	Intraoperative secondary insults, diabetes insipidus, etc.
	Indication, approach, and duration of surgery
Intraoperative course (surgical)	Surgical difficulties and complications (brain swelling, difficult hemostasis, temporary or definite vascular occlusion, opening of air sinus)
	Immobilization/positioning of patient.
Postoperative instructions (surgeon and anesthetist)	Postoperative medication (e.g., anticonvulsants, antibiotics, steroids, mannitol, antithrombosis prophylaxis)
	Instructions for postoperative care and monitoring
	Instructions for removal of drainage, tubes, and stitches
	Preferred duration of postoperative artificial ventilation.
	Instructions for follow-up computed tomography examination (if indicated)

ADMISSION EXAMINATION AND MONITORING IN THE INTENSIVE CARE UNIT

Specific care and monitoring of the postoperative neurosurgical patient requires accurate knowledge of the preoperative situation and the intraoperative procedure, including the surgery, anesthesiology, and any surgical complications or difficulties. Pertinent aspects are summarized in Table 58-3.

On admission, a full examination of the patient is required, including, whenever possible, assessment of level of consciousness and neurologic functioning. Medical care for the patient should be provided in joint collaboration between intensivist and neurosurgeon. Intensive care monitoring includes clinical surveillance, technical monitoring, and follow-up CT or magnetic resonance imaging (MRI). The various approaches to monitoring are summarized in Table 58-4. These are discussed in greater detail in Chapter 48.

CLINICAL SURVEILLANCE

Even in this era of sophisticated monitoring procedures, routine clinical examinations are essential. The clinical assessment has the purpose of disclosing major, life-threatening complications early after surgery, and of assessing neurologic deficits in the following hours to days that follow.

Early Evaluation

A simple check of consciousness, pupils, and the development of focal (mostly motor) deficits remains the most important

TABLE 58–4. POSTOPERATIVE MONITORING AFTER INTRACRANIAL PROCEDURES

Clinical surveillance	Level of consciousness (Glasgow Coma Scale), pupillary reactivity, focal deficits, cranial nerve lesions
Systemic monitoring	Electrocardiogram and heart rate, respiration, pulse oximetry, end tidal CO_2, blood pressure (invasive, noninvasive), temperature, central venous pressure
Brain specific monitoring	Intracranial pressure and cerebral perfusion pressure, jugular oximetry, brain oxygen tension monitoring, microdialysis, transcranial Doppler, electroencephalogram, evoked potentials
Accesses	Central or peripheral venous catheter, arterial catheter, urinary catheter, gastric tube
Laboratory examinations	Blood gases, hematology, electrolytes, on indication coagulation status
Imaging examinations	Chest radiograph (ventilated patients and after lung procedures) Computed tomography or magnetic resonance imaging follow-up (as required)

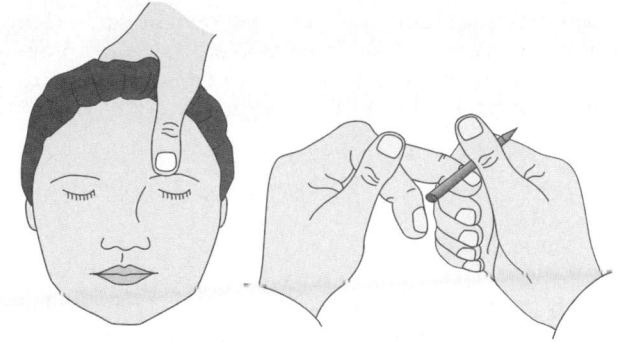

FIGURE 58–1. Supraorbital and nailbed pressure for assessment according to the Glasgow Coma Scale.

method for assessing patients in the neurosurgical ICU. Neurologic assessment should be repeated at regular intervals throughout the ICU course, as change in the examination findings is the most sensitive method for detecting neurologic deterioration.

The level of consciousness should be assessed by the Glasgow Coma Scale (GCS).[44] In this scale standardized assessment of three aspects of responsiveness is performed: the eye, motor, and verbal response (Table 58-5).

When administration of painful stimuli is required to assess the level of responsiveness, standardized administration is required: pressure on the nail bed and supraorbital pressure to test the localizing response of the motor scale (Fig. 58-1).

Accurate determination of the full GCS is not always possible because of sedation and paralysis, but, when possible, at least the best motor score should be recorded.

Some authors advocate separating the eye and verbal scores from the motor score in sedated and/or ventilated patients.[45] However, the motor score is the main predictor in unconscious patients and we would prefer an approach in which only the motor score is assessed when the level of sedation so permits. The development of pupillary abnormalities is a sensitive indicator for pressure on the midbrain (tentorial herniation). The pupillary reaction to light is mediated through parasympathetic fibers of the third cranial nerve (oculomotor nerve). Afferent light perception, conducted through the second cranial nerve (optic nerve) connects at the level of the internal eye muscle nuclei to the oculomotor

nerve supplying parasympathetic fibers to the sphincter pupillae muscle via the ciliary ganglia. Pressure on the oculomotor nerve leads to a loss of function of the parasympathetic fibers, causing a diminished pupillary response or absent pupillary reactivity, generally initially on the side of a lesion (Fig. 58-2). With progressive increases in pressure, both pupils become dilated and unresponsive to light. In patients with a lesion of the optic nerve, the consensual light reflex—that is, contraction of the pupil when a light is shone into the opposite eye—remains intact.

Further Evaluation

When major complications have been ruled out, it remains necessary to evaluate the persistence of previous deficits, their improvement after surgery, or the appearance of new signs attributable to surgery. It is expected, for example, that after the surgical removal of an eighth nerve neurinoma, some degree of damage of cranial nerve VII can occur. After surgical intervention on structures located in, or close to, the brainstem, deficits of the lower cranial nerves can occur as well. A careful, complete neurologic examination is required at this stage, since the simple check proposed in the previous section will not fully evaluate cranial nerve function. This evaluation is important because cranial nerve deficits can require immediate treatment, for example protection of the globe to prevent keratitis or avoidance of oral feeding if swallowing is impaired.

SYSTEMIC MONITORING: CARDIOPULMONARY, RESPIRATORY, AND TEMPERATURE

The goal of cardiopulmonary and respiratory monitoring is to ensure accurate control of systemic hemodynamic and respiratory function, essential for optimization of cerebral oxygenation. Invasive arterial blood pressure monitoring is recommended with the reference point set at the same level as ICP measurement to allow accurate calculation of cerebral perfusion pressure (CPP). Hypovolemic shock is common in the setting of multisystem injury or intraoperative blood loss with inadequate replacement. It is important to recognize that tachycardia and signs of peripheral vasoconstriction such as skin pallor and poor capillary refill can precede a drop in blood pressure. Treatment is rapid fluid resuscitation using isotonic crystalloid fluids, volume expanders, small volume resuscitation (hypertonic saline), and blood transfusions. Central venous pressure monitoring

TABLE 58–5. GLASGOW COMA SCALE

Eyes	Motor	Verbal
1: none	1: none	1: none
2: to pain	2: abnormal extension	2: incomprehensible (groaning)
3: to speech	3: abnormal flexion	3: inappropriate
4: spontaneous	4: flexion (withdrawal)	4: disoriented, confused
	5: localizing	5: oriented
	6: obeying commands	

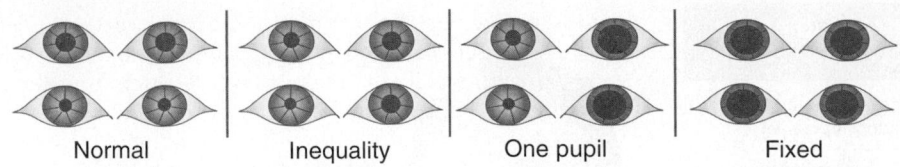

Normal pupils | Inequality of pupils | One pupil wide and dilated | Fixed and dilated

FIGURE 58–2. Pupillary reactivity and size.

can be used to guide volume resuscitation. After initial volume resuscitation, we suggest a hematocrit of approximately 30% to 33% as optimal in the acute postoperative period in patients in the neuro-ICU. After intracranial or spinal cord procedures we would advocate a more liberal use of blood transfusions than generally recommended in intensive care medicine, to promote adequate oxygenation of the central nervous system. This corresponds to the recommendations proposed by Goodnough and coworkers[46] in case of ischemia.

Cardiogenic shock due to primary loss of cardiac function is less common in neurosurgical patients but occurs in the elderly patient with either secondary cardiac ischemia or arrhythmias. These patients usually require the use of a pulmonary artery catheter to optimize volume status and cardiac output. Large pulmonary emboli, sepsis, or spinal paraplegia should also be considered in patients with systemic hypotension. In patients with spinal distributive shock, typically the hypotension is associated with bradycardia with a pulse 35 to 50. These patients should not be managed with excessive volume resuscitation but rather with vasopressors to restore alpha-adrenergic peripheral vasomotor tone. Central venous pressure monitoring or preferably pulmonary artery catheterization can guide the use of intravenous fluids and vasopressor therapy, with a goal of attaining a pulmonary artery wedge pressure of 12 to 14 mm Hg.

The combination of hypertension and bradycardia (Cushing response) should alert the physician to the potential of an expanding intracranial lesion and risk of brainstem herniation. In this situation, the use of antihypertensive agents is contraindicated and therapy should be aimed at the raised ICP.

Temperature monitoring is also important in the neuro-ICU, since hypothermia can depress neurologic function to the point of obtundation or coma. Conversely, fever, by increasing metabolic requirements, may exacerbate secondary injury. Core temperature should be kept lower than 38.0°C, using medications (e.g., acetaminophen, paracetamol, diclofenac) and external or intravascular cooling. Hypothermia may be due to adrenal or pituitary insufficiency, hypothalamic disorders, hypoglycemia, or intraoperative exposure. Deliberate hypothermia is sometimes used in complicated cerebrovascular procedures and as second tier therapy in patients with TBI to reduce ICP.

The possible benefits of hypothermia should be carefully balanced against potential risks (coagulation disorders, electrolyte shifts, fluid overload).

Brain specific monitoring, including the use of ICP monitoring, assessment of cerebral blood flow (CBF), cerebral oxygenation (using either a jugular venous bulb catheter or an oxygen-3 sensitive electrode), and electroencephalographic (EEG) monitoring can be helpful in postoperative patients in the neuro-ICU. These specific modalities are discussed in detail in Chapter 48.

Monitoring of ICP is indicated in trauma patients with severe brain injury (GCS score < 8), with abnormalities on the initial CT scan and further in patients with a normal admission CT scan if two or more of the following features are present: age greater than 40 years, unilateral or bilateral motor posturing, systolic blood pressure less than 90 mm Hg.

Routine ICP monitoring is not generally indicated in patients with mild or moderate head injury but may be considered when other severe extracranial injuries are present, necessitating anesthesia for surgery, or when the initial CT scan shows traumatic lesions with space-occupying effects. ICP monitoring is further indicated in poor grade patients with subarachnoid aneurysmal hemorrhage. Further, it may be considered in patients with other intracranial disorders, who are sedated and ventilated and in whom the risk of raised ICP is considered present (postoperative swelling, stroke, Reye syndrome). Relatively few data exist on routine ICP monitoring in the postoperative situation. In a series of 30 patients after severe head injury and elective craniectomy, 156 instances of ICP rise and/or drop in CPP were recorded.[47] These instances were only accompanied by clinical deterioration in 15 cases.

Telemetric ICP control has been proposed after posterior fossa surgery.[48] In a series of 514 patients after supra- and infratentorial surgery, Constantini and associates[49] described raised ICP in 13% to 18% of cases. Neurologic deterioration occurred in approximately half of the patients suffering ICP rise and was always preceded by the ICP increase. In a large series of 780 patients submitted to routine ICP monitoring after intracranial surgery, 47% required ICP-directed therapy.[50] In a report concerning 850 cases, Bullock and associates[51] concluded that ICP monitoring allows earlier identification of recurrent hematomas. These data would support a more routine application of ICP monitoring after intracranial surgery, particularly in more complex cases. In some institutions, ICP is routinely measured as part of the postoperative surveillance after major neurosurgical procedures, especially when there is the risk of postoperative bleeding. Figure 58-3 illustrates a case in which a substantial ICP rise was detected in the first postoperative hours. That was caused by an enlarging hemorrhage, which required re-intervention. Intracranial hemorrhages are a rare complication of ICP monitoring and are usually caused by multiple punctures in the presence of coagulopathies. This risk of infection is highest in the case of ventricular monitoring, and the rate of infection has been shown to be proportional to the duration of monitoring.

CEREBRAL BLOOD FLOW AND OXYGENATION

Intermittent measurements of CBF can be obtained with stable Xenon CT scanning or positron emission

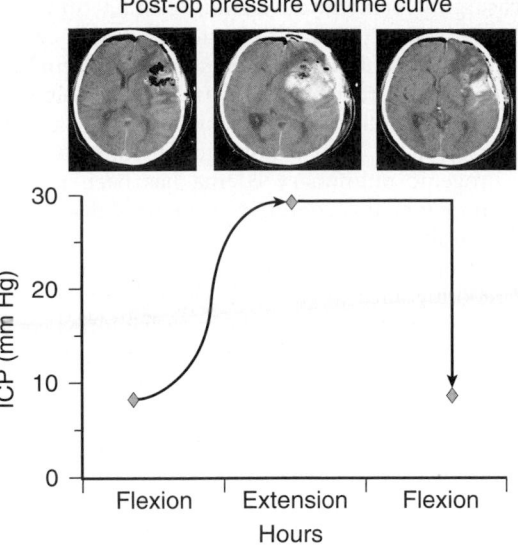

Post-op pressure volume curve

FIGURE 58–3. Raised intracranial pressure (ICP) as the first indication of a developing postoperative hematoma.

tomography studies. Techniques for continuously monitoring CBF at the bedside are currently being developed but are not routinely available. Transcranial Doppler echography provides a noninvasive assessment of blood flow velocity through the basal cerebral arteries. Transcranial Doppler echography is most useful for documenting the development of cerebral vasospasm. Global cerebral oxygenation can be assessed using jugular oximetry, which is discussed in Chapter 48. A decrease in jugular venous saturation of oxygen ($SjvO_2$) indicates that the brain is extracting more oxygen, suggesting that the oxygen supply is not adequate for metabolic demands. Interpretation of results of jugular oximetry require that systemic information, such as hemoglobin concentration and arterial saturation, and intracranial data, such as CPP, are combined. The technique has several limitations: first, continuous monitoring of $SjvO_2$ with fiberoptic devices is prone to artifact; and second, under conditions of anemia or arteriovenous shunting, hypoxia may be present at the tissue level despite normal values of $SjvO_2$.

Regional monitoring of brain tissue oxygen tension is possible by inserting an oxygen-sensitive electrode in the cerebral cortex or white matter. By definition, this concerns a regional technique, and there is still considerable debate about whether this technique should be employed in relatively undamaged parts of the brain—and as such be considered representative of more global oxygenation and metabolism—or preferably be employed in the penumbral zone of lesions, the aim being to limit secondary damage in potential viable regions. Increased hyperventilation has further been shown to reduce cerebral tissue PO_2. Experimental and clinical evidence suggests that CPP therapy may be targeted toward appropriate levels, based on results of tissue oxygen monitoring. Other techniques quantifying regional CBF by thermal diffusion or laser Doppler have been used mainly for research purposes but have not yet provided results on the basis of which therapeutic procedures can be targeted. Finally, the technique of microdialysis allows for the measurement of substrate and metabolites (glucose, lactate, pyruvate), amino acids (glutamate), and indicators of cerebral damage (glycerol) in the extracellular fluid of the brain. Dialysate fluid obtained after infusing saline through a semipermeable membrane reflects the composition of the extracellular fluids around the probe. Microdialysis is employed in various specialized neuro-ICUs, mainly for research purposes. Variable results and delays in obtaining real-time values have inhibited the application of results toward individualized targeted treatment.

ELECTRICAL MONITORING

Continuous EEG monitoring has the potential for detecting nonconvulsive status epilepticus in ICU patients. However, the value of this monitoring has been shown most often in the setting of stroke and TBI. As primary monitor of brain function, continuous EEG can be used to titrate continuous infusion of sedative agents, and the technique can further alert the physician to development of focal or global ischemia.[52,53] The sensitivity for detecting ischemia and hypoxia is high, but the specificity is low due to the effect of sedative medications. Continuous EEG may permit detection and treatment of such adverse events at an early stage, with a potential positive effect on outcome.[54] Measurement of evoked potentials,[55] assessing the integrity of sensor and motor pathways, may provide diagnostic and prognostic information but because of the complexity of the technique is not recommended for general use.

SPECIFIC THERAPEUTIC APPROACHES

TREATMENT OF CEREBRAL HERNIATION AND ELEVATED INTRACRANIAL PRESSURE

The development of cerebral herniation (tentorial herniation/cerebellar tonsillar herniation) constitutes a neurosurgical emergency. A rapid intervention is required prior to further investigations to determine the cause. According to the concept of the volume pressure curve (Fig. 58-4), a small reduction in intracranial volume will already significantly decrease raised intracranial pressure and reverse herniation. The emergency measures to be taken include the following:

- Ventricular cerebrospinal fluid drainage (if access is available)

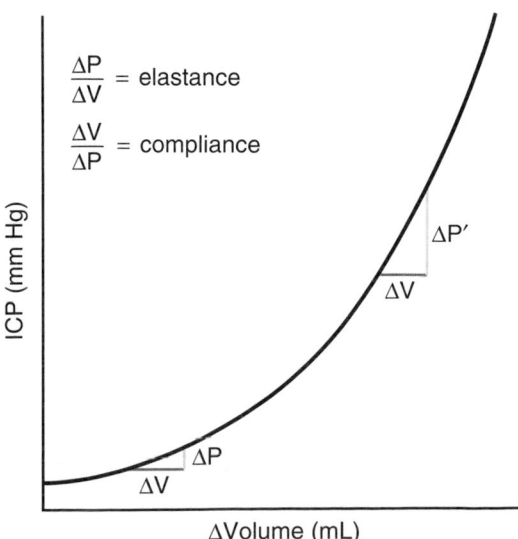

$$\frac{\Delta P}{\Delta V} = \text{elastance}$$

$$\frac{\Delta V}{\Delta P} = \text{compliance}$$

FIGURE 58–4. Intracranial pressure (ICP) volume curve.

- Administration of mannitol, 1 g/kg bodyweight
- Rapid sequence intubation with a neuroprotective strategy

Lumbar cerebrospinal fluid drainage should never be attempted, as this may increase herniation.

Following these emergency procedures, emergency head CT scan should be performed to detect the cause of raised ICP and permit targeted treatment, such as evacuation of a post-operative clot or further treatment of an acute obstructive hydrocephalus. In the absence of an acute cerebral herniation, elevated ICP is addressed first by ruling out treatable intracranial mass lesions and monitoring malfunction and remediable extracranial causes (Table 58-6).

The main intracranial causes of raised postoperative ICP are:

- Mass lesions (hematoma)
- Edema (vasogenic, cytotoxic, osmotic, hydrostatic)
- Increased cerebral blood volume (vasodilation)
- Disturbance of cerebrospinal fluid flow (hydrocephalus, benign intracranial hypertension)

Where appropriate, surgical intervention is indicated. Conservative therapy of raised ICP includes:

- Sedation, analgesia, and mild to moderate hyperventilation ($Paco_2$ 4-4.5 kPa [30-50 mm Hg])
- Osmotic therapy: preferably mannitol given repeatedly in bolus infusions (dose: 0.25-0.5 g/kg bodyweight, or as indicated by monitoring). Serum osmolarity should be maintained at less than 315 mOsm/L. If osmotherapy has insufficient effect, furosemide (Lasix) can also be administered.
- Cerebrospinal fluid drainage
- Volume expansion and inotropes or vasopressors when arterial blood pressure is insufficient to maintain CPP and CBF in a normovolemic patient

If these methods fail, second tier therapies for raised ICP include (1) more intensive hyperventilation (which should be used only with monitoring of cerebral oxygenation to detect cerebral ischemia); (2) administration of barbiturates; (3) mild or moderate hypothermia; and, alternatively, (4) decompressive surgery.

HEMODYNAMIC AND CEREBRAL PERFUSION MANAGEMENT

Neurogenic Pulmonary Edema
The development of neurogenic pulmonary edema has been described early in the postoperative period after a variety of neurosurgical procedures, including brain tumors (particularly those resected in the posterior fossa), cysts, hydrocephalus, intracranial hemorrhages, and brainstem lesions.[56-59] Although an infrequent event, this is a potentially life-threatening event that requires rapid evaluation and emergent therapy in the ICU. A 9% mortality rate directly attributable to neurogenic pulmonary edema has been reported in a recent review of this condition. Generally, this complication appears in the initial 4 hours after the neurologic event and is more common in women than in men, possibly related to the preponderance of cases in patients with subarachnoid hemorrhage.[59] The mechanism underlying this condition is generally believed to include central sympathetic discharge with pulmonary venoconstriction, although both low and high protein content have been reported in the edema fluid.[59,60] It is commonly associated with raised ICP, and, in addition to therapies directed at intracranial hypertension, therapeutic measures are mostly supportive. Supplemental oxygen is uniformly required and endotracheal intubation with mechanical ventilation and the application of positive end-expiratory pressure (PEEP) has been reported in about 75% of patients.[59] Most patients require vasoactive drugs.[60] Epinephrine has also been touted to have a direct beneficial effect on clearance of the alveolar fluid.[61] Remarkably, there do not appear to be any literature reports of the use of inhaled nitric oxide for this condition.

In some patients, the normal pressure autoregulatory mechanisms are disturbed and the risk exists that increased CPP may worsen cerebral edema. Careful observation of the change in ICP with respect to arterial blood pressure changes is required to determine whether the change in CBF in response to changes in blood pressure are consistent with disturbed or intact autoregulation. The general principles behind blood pressure manipulation in the injured brain are discussed in Chapter 47.

Vasopressor therapy may be needed in the postoperative care of patients in the neuro-ICU. Vasopressors are often required in the treatment of subarachnoid hemorrhage and severe traumatic brain injury (see Chapters 52 and 55). They may also be needed in the setting of the postoperative decompensation of a patient to maintain stability prior to reoperation and in the setting of neurogenic pulmonary edema. The vasopressors most frequently used in the care of the postoperative neurosurgical patient are listed in Table 58-7.

Neuroprotection
The original concept of neuroprotection depended on the initiation of treatment before the onset of an event leading to brain damage, and the methods employed aimed to minimize the intensity of an insult or its immediate effects upon the brain. Over the past two decades, the concept of neuroprotection has been extended to include treatment started

TABLE 58–6. REMEDIABLE EXTRACRANIAL CAUSES OF INTRACRANIAL HYPERTENSION

Calibration errors
Airway obstruction (kinked endotracheal tube, tongue, sputum retention, pneumothorax)
Hypoxia (FiO_2, lung disease/collapse)
Hypercapnia (hypoventilation)
Hypertension (pain, sedation, coughing/straining)
Hypotension (hypovolemia, sedation, cardiac)
Posture (Trendelenburg position, neck rotation)
Hyperpyrexia
Seizures
Hypo-osmolality (sodium, protein)

TABLE 58–7. VASOPRESSORS COMMONLY USED IN THE NEONATAL INTENSIVE CARE UNIT

Agent	Adrenergic Effect	Doses (µg/kg/min)
Dopamine	Primarily beta (low dose)	0.4-4
	Increasing alpha (higher dose)	5-8
Norepinephrine	Mainly alpha	0.04-0.1
Phenylephrine	Pure alpha	2-4

TABLE 58–8. MAIN APPROACHES IN NEUROPROTECTION

Strategies Aimed at Improving Metabolism and Micro-environment	Agents Acting on Specific Mechanisms	Pluripotent Agents Affecting Various Mechanisms	Strategies Promoting Cell Survival and Regeneration
Hypothermia	Alpha-adrenoceptor drugs	Barbiturates	Cellular replacement
Mannitol	Anti-inflammatory agents	Corticosteroids	Gene therapy
THAM	Apoptosis inhibitors, caspase inhibitors, and cyclosporine	Dexanabinol	Neurotrophic factors
	Arachidonic acid metabolism-modulators	Erythropoietin	
	Calcium channel antagonists	Magnesium	
	Calpain antagonists		
	Sex hormones		
	Ion channel modulators		
	Kappa opioid modulators		
	Kinin antagonists		
	Neurotransmitter-targeted agents		
	Nitric oxide modulators		
	Free radical scavengers and inhibitors of lipid peroxidation		

after the onset of an insult (i.e., resuscitation), reflecting our increased understanding of progressive pathophysiologic mechanisms causing and/or enhancing secondary brain damage. In neuroprotection, four main approaches can be discerned (Table 58-8). Although the agents used may have more utility in the specific settings of cardiopulmonary arrest, subarachnoid hemorrhage, TBI, and stroke (see Chapters 50, 51, 52, and 55), they may be useful in some post-operative neurosurgical patients, especially in cases with complications.

STRATEGIES AIMED AT IMPROVING METABOLISM AND MICROENVIRONMENT

Methods for improving metabolism and microenvironment include hypothermia to minimize the effects of energy failure, tris(hydroxymethyl)amino-methane (THAM) to correct brain acidosis, and mannitol to reduce ICP and improve CBF. Hypothermia decreases CBF by approximately 5.2% per degree of reduction in body temperature. The cerebral metabolic rate for oxygen ($CMRO_2$) and the arterial jugular venous oxygen difference ($AVDO_2$) fall after the institution of moderate hypothermia. This reflects a reduction in energy requirement and hence less energy loss in the injured brain. Stabilization of the cell membrane[62] and reduction of neurotransmitter turnover may also contribute to the benefit seen in models of ischemia.[63] Hypothermia has been associated with several complications, including cardiovascular instability (mainly arrhythmias), coagulopathy, electrolyte abnormalities,[64,65] and increased risk of infection and shivering. The use of hypothermia is therefore not without risks and requires high-level neuro-intensive care. Various approaches to cooling have been adopted, but the most frequently used employ surface cooling or gastric lavage with cold fluids. More recently, Marion[66] reported favorable results with the use of devices for intravascular cooling, and this technique can be expected to become standard for induction of hypothermia in the near future. Increased lactate acidosis in the cerebrospinal fluid was recognized in clinical investigations many years ago in the injured brain.[67,68] More recent studies, including magnetic resonance techniques and microdialysis, have confirmed earlier findings. The recognition of the occurrence of brain tissue and cerebrospinal fluid

acidosis has stimulated studies to investigate the use of alkalizing agents such as THAM (tromethamine). THAM is a biologically inert amino alcohol that buffers carbon dioxide and acids in vitro and in vivo. Clinical studies have not shown conclusive evidence of benefit in the use of THAM, but nevertheless it is still used in some centers. It has been postulated that a possible beneficial effect of THAM could be to counteract ischemia produced by marked hypocapnia in patients treated with intensive hyperventilation.[69]

Mannitol is widely used in neurosurgery to treat raised ICP and to decrease brain bulk during intracranial operations and to treat cerebral ischemia. Mannitol is considered to exert beneficial effects by two mechanisms:

1. An immediate plasma expanding effect, reducing hematocrit and blood viscosity and consequently increasing CBF and cerebral oxygen delivery.
2. An osmotic effect, which is delayed for 15 to 30 minutes, while gradients are established between plasma and cells. Mannitol can be given in acute emergency situations such as cerebral herniation or as part of a conservative approach to treatment of raised ICP. Mannitol is thought to be more effective when given in small, frequent doses rather than by continuous infusion.[70] Given in high doses, mannitol may induce hypernatremia, decrease hematocrit, and increase osmolarity. A serious potential side effect is acute renal failure, which can occur if serum osmolarity increases above 320 mmol/L.

AGENTS ACTING ON SPECIFIC MECHANISMS

The increased understanding of the existence of progressive pathophysiologic mechanisms causing or enhancing secondary brain damage has led to the development of a large range of specifically targeted neuroprotective agents aimed at ameliorating such mechanisms, often showing marked beneficial effect in experimental studies. Unfortunately, in various fields of neuro-intensive care, promising experimental results have not translated into clinical efficacy. Calcium channel antagonists have proven benefit in the prevention and treatment of delayed ischemic deficits following aneurysmal subarachnoid hemorrhage. By far the largest experience exists with the di-hydropyridine analogue nimodipine. In a meta-analysis performed by Barker and Ogilvy,[71] notable improvements in good and fair outcomes as well as reductions in death due to vasospasm and CT-detected infarcts were observed with nimodipine. Various studies on the use of calcium channel antagonists in the field of TBI have, however, yielded conflicting results, and current evidence does not support the use of these agents in patients with TBI, although the possibility of a small beneficial effect, particularly in patients with traumatic subarachnoid hemorrhage, cannot be definitely excluded.

PLURIPOTENT AGENTS AFFECTING VARIOUS MECHANISMS

The realization that various pathophysiologic mechanisms are frequently concurrently or sequentially active has increased interest in the use of agents with multiple mechanisms, and for such agents the term "dirty drugs" has been coined.[72]

Corticosteroids are widely used within neurosurgery to treat edema associated with brain tumors and to prevent brain edema associated with operative procedures. The presumed mechanisms of action include reduction of vascular permeability, reduction of cerebrospinal fluid production, attenuation of free radical production, inhibition of lipid peroxidation, reversal of intracellular calcium accumulation, and an anti-inflammatory effect. Despite the availability of many (small) studies, considerable uncertainty still remains concerning possible beneficial effects in patients with TBI.

Barbiturates are commonly used as second tier therapy for the treatment of raised ICP refractory to other treatment modalities. The main mechanisms by which barbiturates are neuroprotective has not been established.[73] The most important effects may relate to the coupling of CBF to regional metabolic demands, resulting in a decrease in CBF and related cerebral blood volume as a result of decreased metabolic requirements. Other possibilities include scavenging of oxygen free radicals and stabilization of cell membranes. The main complication of the use of barbiturates is arterial hypotension, which occurs in up to 58% of patients.[74] The decline in blood pressure may be greater than the reduction in ICP, risking a decrease in CPP, especially in patients with hypovolemia or cardiac disease. Other complications include hypoglycemia, hypernatremia, an increased risk of infection, liver and renal dysfunction, and cardiac failure.[74,75]

Dexanabinol, erythropoietin, and magnesium are agents with neuroprotective potential currently undergoing further clinical evaluation.

STRATEGIES PROMOTING CELL SURVIVAL AND REGENERATION

Strategies to promote cell survival and regeneration include cellular replacement, gene therapy, and administration of trophic factors. These futuristic approaches are aimed at promoting regeneration and neuroplasticity and may ultimately lead to improved functional recovery.[76,77] The potential of these novel therapies is strengthened by promising experimental and clinical results obtained in neurodegenerative diseases, including Parkinson disease, Huntington disease, and stroke.[77-80] This approach is currently the focus of large research efforts, which, it is hoped, will provide possibilities for further improving outcome in the subacute and chronic phases.

ANNOTATED REFERENCES

Constantini S, Cotev S, Rappaport ZH, et al: Intracranial pressure monitoring after elective intracranial surgery: A retrospective study of 514 consecutive patients. J Neurosurg 1988;69:540-544.

Study of 514 patients after supra- and infratentorial surgery demonstrating raised ICP (greater than 20 mmHg) in 18% of cases during the postoperative period. Of the 89 patients with elevated ICP, 47 (52.8%) had an associated clinical deterioration. It was concluded that ICP monitoring is advantageous in the immediate postoperative management after elective intracranial surgery and is almost risk-free. It should therefore be used liberally, especially when risk factors for ICP elevation can be identified prior to the end of surgery.

Constantini S, Kanner A, Friedman A, et al: Safety of perioperative minidose heparin in patients undergoing brain tumor surgery: A prospective, randomized, double-blind study. J Neurosurg 2001;94:918-921.

Prospective, randomized, double-blind trial that demonstrated the safety of the perioperative use of minidose heparin (5000 U) treatment in 103 patients undergoing craniotomy for supratentorial brain tumors. Treatment was started 2 hours before surgery and continued until full mobilization or for 7 days.

Diringer MN, Edwards DF: Admission to a neurologic/neurosurgical intensive care unit is associated with reduced mortality rate after intracerebral hemorrhage. Crit Care Med 2001;29:635-640.

Study using data prospectively collected from 36,986 patients listed in Project Impact demonstrating the benefits of focused neurointensive care in patients with spontaneous intracerebral hemorrhage when compared to care provided in a general ICU. Multivariate analysis of the data revealed that not being in a neuro-ICU was associated with an increase in hospital mortality rate (odds ratio, 3.4).

Fontes RB, Aguiar PH, Zanetti MV, et al: Acute neurogenic pulmonary edema: Case reports and literature review. J Neurosurg Anesthesiol 2003;15:144-150.

This article provides a review of the literature of case reports of neurogenic pulmonary edema, an uncommon but important post-neurosurgical complication that requires emergency ICU assessment and therapy. The most frequent underlying factor was subarachnoid hemorrhage (42.9%). Symptom onset occurred less than 4 hours after the neurologic event in 71.4% of cases. One third of the patients presented with pink frothy sputum. Chest radiography showed bilateral diffuse infiltrates in 90.5% of cases. Supportive measures included oxygen support and vasoactive drugs. Recovery was usually very rapid: 52.4% of patients recovered in less than 72 hours. However, almost 10% of patients died of neurogenic pulmonary edema.

Livingston BM, Mackenzie SJ, MacKirdy FN, Howie JC: Should the presedation Glasgow Coma Scale value be used when calculating Acute Physiology and Chronic Health Evaluation scores for sedated patients? Scottish Intensive Care Society Audit Group. Crit Care Med 2000;28:389-394.

Study in 13,291 consecutive admissions of the optimal application of the GCS score in the APACHE II and III scoring in the ICU. The GCS was found to be an important component of both APACHE II and APACHE III and should be assessed directly whenever possible. When patients are sedated, using the GCS score recorded before sedation was found to be preferable to the assumption of normality.

Mirski MA, Chang CW, Cowan R: Impact of a neuroscience intensive care unit on neurosurgical patient outcomes and cost of care: Evidence-based support for an intensivist-directed specialty ICU model of care. J Neurosurg Anesthesiol 2001;13:83-92.

Retrospective study that demonstrated reduced mortality rate, improved discharge disposition, and reduced length of hospital stay and cost when comparing similar cohorts of patients with intracranial hemorrhage treated in a neurosurgical ICU versus a general ICU.

Chapter 59

KEY ISSUES IN PEDIATRIC NEUROINTENSIVE CARE

Patrick M. Kochanek • Robert W. Hickey • Hülya Bayir • Ericka L. Fink
Randall A. Ruppel • Robert S. B. Clark

KEY POINTS

1. There are important **age-related differences** in both the CNS insults and the response to these insults in infants and children.

2. Neurointensive care for infants and children should focus on the **prevention of secondary extracerebral insults** and optimize brain-directed therapies. Optimization of cardiopulmonary physiology, maintenance of euglycemia, and prevention of hyperthermia and hyponatremia are important to optimize outcome.

3. Cardiopulmonary arrest in infants and children results from **asphyxia** in the majority of cases.

4. The **goals of treating status epilepticus** are to provide respiratory and cardiovascular support, terminate seizure activity, identify and treat the precipitating factors, and prevent systemic complications.

5. Congenital and acquired heart disease are the most important underlying causes of **embolic stroke** in infants and children.

6. The etiology and treatment of **bacterial meningitis** differ between neonates and older infants and children.

7. **Herpes simplex virus** is an important cause of severe encephalitis in children.

8. **Treatment of impending herniation** includes immediate airway control, mannitol or hypertonic saline administration, hyperventilation, cerebrospinal fluid drainage (if available), and emergent CT evaluation.

In this chapter we outline the epidemiology, presentation, course, and management of key disorders in pediatric neurointensive care. Critically ill infants and children with a compromised central nervous system (CNS) are complex patients and are often highly vulnerable to secondary brain injury. Minimizing physiologic derangements and optimizing therapy are essential from the scene through the pediatric ICU. In most cases, transport to a specialized pediatric facility is desirable. Trained specialists in pediatric critical care medicine, pediatric neurologic surgery, and child neurology should deliver the ICU care to these infants and children, with appropriate pediatric ancillary support. The information provided in this chapter is germane to practitioners involved in stabilization, emergency treatment, and transport and to pediatric subspecialists at the tertiary care centers.

Recommendations in the areas of pediatric trauma (head and spinal cord injury), procedures, and monitoring are addressed in Chapters 47, 228, and 248. Neurointensive care issues relevant to the field of neonatology are outside the scope of this chapter and specialized textbooks and/or reviews in this area should be sought for information in that field.

ISSUES UNIQUE TO PEDIATRICS

Two key factors contribute to the unique nature of the practice of pediatric neurointensive care: differences in the specific insults to the CNS in infants and children versus adults and age-related differences in the response to these insults.

CNS INSULTS IN INFANTS AND CHILDREN

Unlike in adults, atherosclerotic vascular disease, resulting in stroke, intracerebral hemorrhage, and cardiopulmonary arrest plays little role in pediatric neurointensive care. For example, cardiopulmonary arrest in infants and children results primarily from asphyxia rather than myocardial infarction. Similarly, traumatic brain injury in infants younger than 2 years of age is largely the result of inflicted childhood neurotrauma (shaken baby syndrome, child abuse). Unique issues in victims of child abuse, such as chronic injury or delay in presentation, contribute to important differences in diagnosis, treatment, and outcome. The specific CNS insults relevant to pediatric neurointensive care include traumatic brain injury and spinal cord injury, cardiopulmonary arrest, status epilepticus, stroke, critical CNS infections, postoperative neurosurgical conditions, and several other less common disorders; traumatic brain and spinal cord injury are addressed in Chapters 55 and 56.

AGE-RELATED DIFFERENCES IN THE RESPONSE TO CNS INSULTS

Brain Water and Blood-Brain Barrier

Many biochemical, physiologic, and physical factors exhibit large fluctuations during brain development. Although the magnitude of these changes are most dramatic during prenatal development, they may contribute to age-related differences in response to critical CNS disorders.[1,2] Large decreases in brain water content occur during postnatal development into adult life.[3-5] These changes are global and correlate with the amount of myelination. The impact of these changes on edema formation after brain injury is unclear; however, the rapid and diffuse cerebral swelling phenomenon described in many CNS insults in infants and children may be related to this high water content in the immature brain. This is suggested by studies showing that parenchymal injection of glutamate into the immature (but not adult) rat brain rapidly produces a large area of edema.[6] The rapidity of development and the great magnitude of edema may result, in part, from rapid diffusion of glutamate and other mediators through the immature brain. In contrast to the changes in brain water during development, there is little evidence to support similar changes in blood-brain barrier permeability.[7,8] However, studies in experimental models suggest that the immature blood-brain barrier is highly vulnerable to injury.[9-11] Blood-brain barrier permeability after CNS insults has received little study in pediatric patients.

Cerebral Blood Flow and Energy Metabolism

Postnatal changes in cerebral blood flow (CBF) and energy metabolism have been reported in numerous mammalian species including humans.[12-19] In all cases, CBF is quite low both before birth and during infancy, rapidly increases to a peak during childhood, and then decreases to a plateau with a gradual decline with increasing age during adulthood. In a study of 42 normal infants and children, cortical CBF in newborns was between 30 and 45 mL/100 g/min—lower than that reported in adults. In contrast, cortical flow in children between the ages of 5 and 6 years was between 50% and 85% higher than in adults. CBF decreased to adult values by about age 15 years (Fig. 59-1).[20,21] Increased CBF in children (vs. either adults or infants) corresponds to the period of maximal postnatal "brain growth," specifically, maximal increases in the number of synapses.[22-24] Similarly, cerebral metabolic rate for glucose is maximal in children between the ages of 3 and 9 years.[17] The impact of these factors in CNS injury is poorly understood. Hyperemia after injury has been implicated as an important facet of the pathophysiology of pediatric CNS injury. Because the level of CBF in the normal child is greater than in adults, the frequency of hyperemia in children is probably lower than has been suggested. Hyperemia in most gray matter structures, in children between the ages of 3 and 10 years, should probably be based on a flow value greater than about 70 mL/100 g/min[19-21,24] rather than the value of about 45 mL/100 g/min suggested for adults.[25] Alterations in metabolic demands after injury must also be considered.

Cerebral Perfusion Pressure

Cerebral perfusion pressure (CPP; mean arterial blood pressure–intracranial pressure [ICP]) is a critical determinant of CBF outside the limits of autoregulation or when autoregulation of blood pressure is disturbed. In adults, the normal range for CPP is generally accepted to be between 60 and 150 mm Hg.[26,27] Based on studies in normal immature animals, the lower limit for blood pressure autoregulation of CBF is directly related to age.[28-30] This is anticipated since CPP is a function of arterial blood pressure, which is dependent on age. Unfortunately, few data are available on normal values for CPP in infants and children. A mean value of 37.5 ± 4.9 mm Hg (± SD) was reported in normal preterm infants.[31] The lower limit of blood pressure autoregulation was not determined. This is well below the 60 mm Hg critical CPP value for the lower limit of CBF autoregulation in adults and highlights the problem in defining optimal CPP in pediatric neurointensive care—it is likely not a single number. There are also limited data available on the lower limit of blood pressure autoregulation of CBF in brain-injured infants and children. A study of 17 infants and children with meningitis and encephalitis showed a critical threshold for CPP of about 30 mm Hg.[32] However, survival, not CBF, was the outcome variable in that study. Muizelaar and coworkers[20,21] and Sharples and colleagues[33] examined CBF autoregulation after traumatic brain injury in children; however, normal values for blood pressure autoregulation of CBF for infants and children were not determined. Two recent studies suggest that the presence of mild hypertension after severe brain injury is associated with improved outcome in infants and children.[34,35] However, the impact of inducing mild hypertension in this setting on outcome remains to be studied.

Myelination

In humans, considerable myelination occurs during postnatal life.[23] The impact of this process on the age-related response in pediatric CNS injury is not known but has been suggested by many to contribute to enhanced plasticity in the pediatric brain.

Excitotoxicity

Increases in brain interstitial concentrations of excitatory amino acids such as glutamate are part of a fundamental

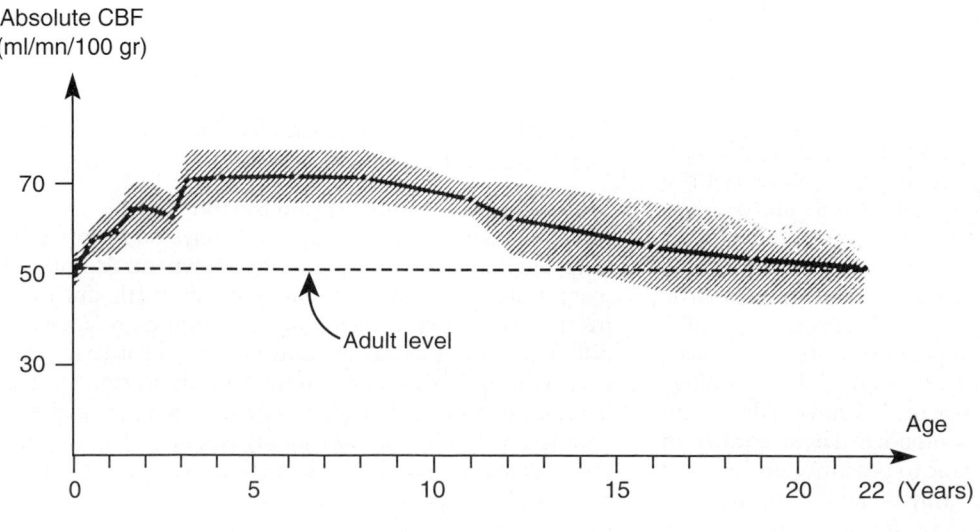

FIGURE 59–1. Mean *(the curve)* and ± 1 SD *(hatched area)* for normal cerebral blood flow in 42 children from 2 days to 19 years old compared with adult values *(dotted line)*. Compared with adult values, cerebral blood flow is lower in infancy, but thereafter values throughout childhood exceed those of adults. (From Chiron C, Raynaud C, Maziere B, et al: Changes in regional cerebral blood flow during brain maturation in children and adolescents. J Nucl Med 1992;33:696-703. Reprinted by permission of the Society of Nuclear Medicine.)

response to CNS insults across all ages.[36-45] Excitotoxicity-mediated damage after brain injury has been reported in laboratory models in mature and immature animals and is suggested in clinical reports in children.[37,41-45] There are, however, important age-dependent facets of excitotoxicity. At several periods in development large numbers of excitatory amino acid receptors are produced, and these periods correlate temporally with increased synaptic plasticity.[38-41] Experimental data strongly suggest that the immature brain is at great risk for excitotoxicity.[37-39] In hypoxia-ischemia models, studies in immature animals (particularly those modeling the newborn) suggest that glutamate receptor antagonists, such as MK-801, are potent neuroprotectants.[38,39,41] The results of clinical trials in adults of agents targeting this receptor may not predict their effectiveness in infants or children with critical CNS insults. Further study in children is warranted.

Apoptosis

Experimental models and human data have made it increasingly clear that cells dying after CNS insults can be categorized on a morphologic continuum from necrosis to apoptosis.[46-48] The event involved in the cascades of neuronal death after CNS insults is discussed in detail in Chapter 38. The importance of balanced apoptosis (or programmed cell death) in embryogenesis and recent reports examining apoptosis in experimental traumatic brain injury suggest that there may be important age-related differences in the cell death cascades in response to traumatic or ischemic brain injury.[49] For example, neurons in developing animals appear to be more vulnerable to apoptosis than in mature animals.[46,49] There are also data supporting the concept that physiologic levels of excitatory amino acids are necessary for neuronal survival in the developing brain.[50] The implications on these data in experimental animals must be assessed with caution; however, they raise concern about the ability of therapies such as barbiturates or inhibitors of excitatory amino acid receptors to actually induce neuronal death during development. The fetal alcohol syndrome is the prototypical condition cited in this regard.[51] What remains unclear, however, is if this enhanced apoptotic response to CNS injury is limited to prenatal development or if it is important during treatment of infants and children in the pediatric ICU. Nevertheless, an important role for apoptosis in pediatric brain injury is suggested by the fact that analysis of cerebrospinal fluid (CSF) in infants and children with severe traumatic brain injury has provided some of the most compelling molecular data for the participation of these pathways in humans.[2] These data include participation of death effectors such as cytochrome-c and Fas receptor/ligand interactions and failure of anti-apoptotic pathways in infants and children with poor outcome after severe brain injury.[2,52-55] How these findings will influence our therapies remains to be determined, but they suggest that apoptotic neuronal death may represent a particularly important therapeutic target in pediatric neurointensive care.

Extracerebral Factors

Many "extracerebral" factors play a role in the age-related differences in the response to critical CNS disorders, including age-related differences in (1) the response to hypoxemia-ischemia and hypotension, (2) atherosclerosis and other risk factors for stroke, and (3) acute and chronic ethanol consumption. These are rarely discussed in this context.

Hypotension and hypoxemia are the two most important secondary insults in patients with critical CNS disorders. Hypotension is the most important extracerebral factor associated with poor outcome after severe traumatic brain injury.[56] This may contribute to the high mortality rate (62%) in this condition in children younger than age 4 years.[57] Nearly 50% of these children present with shock, versus only 30% of adults.[57] The limited blood volume of infants and young children make relatively small amounts of blood loss from scalp lacerations or other foci important. In contrast, the immature brain and cardiovascular systems are resistant to hypoxic-ischemic insults compared with mature individuals.[58] The duration of asphyxia resulting in cardiac arrest is inversely related to age.[59-62] Resistance to asphyxia-induced cardiac arrest in the immature individual, however, could have complex effects. For example, children may survive protracted episodes of hypoxemia and hypotension that would be lethal in adults. Resistance of the immature myocardium to asphyxia does not preclude the development of cerebral damage from hypoxemia, because between 25% and 56% of children who suffer asphyxia without cardiac arrest have poor neurologic outcome.[63] This might also explain some of the severe pathology seen in infants after inflicted childhood neurotrauma, in which apnea, seizures, and agonal states occur.[64]

Unlike adults, atherosclerotic vascular changes are largely absent in children. This influences pathophysiology. Although normal aging produces a gradual decline in CBF, this decline is accentuated in adults by the presence of risk factors for stroke (e.g., diabetes, cigarette smoking, hypertension), which enhance incipient cerebrovascular disease.[65] Atherosclerosis also limits the ability of cerebral circulation to respond to a metabolic challenge.[66-69] Some adults may even have maximally dilated cerebral vessels in the resting state. The potential of these factors to unfavorably affect outcome in adults (vs. children) is obvious. Ethanol consumption is associated with severe traumatic brain injury in adults, with as high as 50% of patients having positive blood alcohol levels.[70-73] Chronic and acute alcohol consumption can have either detrimental or beneficial effects on brain injury.[73] Ethanol use or intoxication is uncommon in pediatric traumatic brain injury, particularly in infants and young children.

SPECIFIC DISEASES OR CONDITIONS

CARDIOPULMONARY ARREST

Cardiopulmonary arrest in adults is addressed in detail in Chapter 50. Although some of that chapter is germane to pediatric patients, the importance of asphyxia as the etiology in children mandates a separate discussion.

Epidemiology

The causes of cardiopulmonary arrest in childhood are heterogeneous. Causes of arrest in the prehospital setting include trauma, sudden infant death syndrome, poisoning, and respiratory distress secondary to drowning, choking, severe asthma, or pneumonia.[74] Traumatic arrest secondary to exsanguination, massive head injury, or airway compromise is the leading cause of death in childhood and young adulthood. Nontraumatic arrest typically occurs as a consequence of hypoxemia and hypercarbia, leading to respiratory arrest, bradycardia, and, ultimately, asystole or pulseless electrical activity.[74-76] Ventricular tachycardia or fibrillation occurs less commonly in children than adults, but it is not rare. Five to 15 percent of children with prehospital arrest have these rhythms.[77-79] The majority of arrests in the prehospital setting occur in previously healthy patients, whereas most in-hospital arrests occur in children with preexisting medical conditions.[80] Children with special health care needs are especially vulnerable to acute deterioration.

Outcome

The rate of survival from pediatric cardiopulmonary arrest is about 13%, with survival from in-hospital arrest greater than that from prehospital arrest (24% vs. 9%).[76] Asystolic patients have the lowest rate of survival (~5%) whereas patients with ventricular fibrillation or ventricular tachycardia have higher rates of survival (~30%). Patients presenting with isolated respiratory arrest have the highest rate of survival (~75%).[81,82] Witnessed arrest and bystander cardiopulmonary resuscitation (CPR) are associated with survival, whereas CPR of greater than 30 minutes and administration of more than two doses of epinephrine are associated with poor outcome.[74,77,83,84] About 60% of survivors will have good neurologic outcome, with the remainder showing severe disabilities. Intermediate outcomes are uncommon. Reported mortality rates for children remaining comatose after brain injury range between 34% and 73% dependent on whether traumatic brain injury is included.[85-90] Accurate prediction of poor outcome in this group can enable withdrawal of support and decrease the possibility of "rescuing" children to survival in a neurologically devastated state.[91,92] Predictors of poor outcome in children include remaining comatose at 24 hours, a Glasgow Coma Scale (GCS) score of less than 5, absence of spontaneous respirations, absence of pupillary reflex, and specific abnormalities found on electroencephalography (EEG) or after testing of somatosensory-evoked potentials. Predictors of poor outcome should be applied with caution to children suffering cardiopulmonary arrest caused by drug overdose or hypothermic exposure (ice cold water drowning) in which good outcomes have been reported in some cases after even prolonged durations of arrest.

Treatment

The optimal treatment of pediatric cardiopulmonary arrest is prevention. The use of child restraints in motor vehicles, bicycle helmets, pool fences, and fire alarms has contributed to important reductions in morbidity and mortality. Also, the number of cases of sudden infant death syndrome has decreased in the United States from 4900 infants in 1992 to 2600 infants in 1999 in association with the recognition that placing infants on their backs during sleep lowers the risk of this condition. For health care providers, the key to prevention is recognizing and treating *early* signs of cardiopulmonary compromise (tachycardia and increased work of breathing).

If cardiopulmonary arrest occurs, the most important first step is to provide immediate CPR. Many infants and children, especially in the prehospital setting, will be rescued solely by the administration of CPR.[74] The technique for children is similar to that used in adults except for delivery of chest compressions. Only one hand is used to deliver chest compressions to children younger than age 8 years. Two methods are approved for delivering chest compressions to infants. When two or more rescuers are available, one rescuer provides chest compressions by encircling the chest with two hands and depressing the sternum with both thumbs while

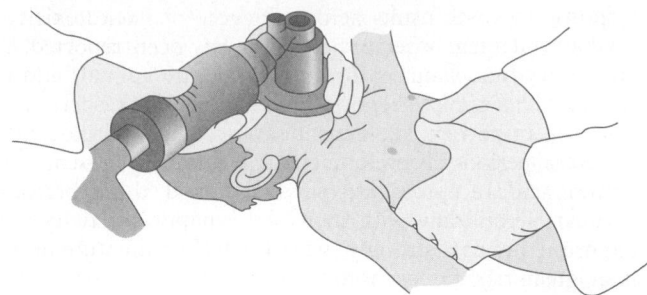

FIGURE 59–2. Two-person technique for cardiopulmonary resuscitation in infants and young children. (Reprinted from Pediatric Basic Life Support. Guidelines 2000 for Cardiopulmonary and Emergency Cardiovascular Care: International Consensus on Science. Circulation 2000;102(8)(Suppl):I253-I290.)

the other rescuer provides ventilation (Fig. 59-2). When only one rescuer is present, two fingers from one hand are used to provide chest compressions and the other hand is used to maintain the head-tilt. Providing adequate ventilation is especially important for children because most pediatric arrests are secondary to airway compromise. In contrast, adults frequently suffer from cardiac causes of arrest and require intensified efforts at providing chest compressions and early defibrillation. Thus, the recommended ratio of chest compressions to ventilations for young children is 5:1, compared with a ratio of 15:2 for older children and adults. Once the patient is intubated, ventilations should be asynchronous. Although ventricular fibrillation and ventricular tachycardia are uncommon in children, survival with this rhythm is high (about 30%) and thus cardiac rhythm should be ascertained as early as possible.[76] Automated external defibrillators that can deliver a 50-J dose are now available and are appropriate for use in children aged 1 to 8 years.[93]

Intubation of pediatric patients is a difficult task for inexperienced providers. Furthermore, the short length of the trachea combined with patient movement during transport and patient care can easily result in displacement of the endotracheal tube.[94] Thus, secondary confirmation of endotracheal tube placement is critical. End-tidal CO_2 detection is the method most commonly utilized for secondary confirmation of endotracheal tube placement in children. However, a false-negative reading can occur when circulatory collapse is so severe that CO_2 is not delivered to the alveolar space. If CO_2 is not detected during CPR, tube placement can be confirmed by visualizing the airway with a laryngoscope. Although no single confirmation technique is 100% reliable in all circumstances, some effort of secondary confirmation of tube placement should be performed after intubation of *all* children.

Patients are initially resuscitated using 100% oxygen. The rationale is that hypoxia often causes or contributes to the development of cardiac arrest, and an oxygen debt accumulates during cardiac arrest. However, there is increasing awareness that oxygen might contribute to reperfusion injury, and thus *prolonged* delivery of *unnecessarily* high concentrations of oxygen should be avoided.[95]

Adults resuscitated from cardiac arrest demonstrate intact cerebrovascular reactivity with evidence of hyperventilation-associated ischemia.[96] Although there is evidence that injured brain has diminished metabolism, which may offset the decrease in blood flow, it seems prudent to avoid decreasing CBF to injured brain. Therefore, hyperventilation should be reserved for patients with signs of cerebral herniation syndrome or suspected pulmonary hypertension. In addition to avoiding purposeful hyperventilation, it is prudent to guard against inadvertent hyperventilation during patient transport.[97] Increased use of quantitative continuous CO_2 monitors throughout the health care system would decrease the occurrence of inadvertent hyperventilation.

Establishing vascular access in children can be challenging. Fortunately, intraosseous access can be achieved within 30 to 60 seconds and provides a route for drug and fluid administration when intravascular access cannot be readily achieved. Drugs, including lidocaine, epinephrine, atropine, and naloxone (mnemonic "LEAN") can be administered through the endotracheal tube. Optimal doses for drugs given via the endotracheal tube are not established, but the recommended dose of epinephrine is 0.1 mg/kg (10 times the intravenous dose). A bedside glucose measurement should be obtained; and if hypoglycemia is present, it should be treated with 0.5 to 1.0 g/kg of glucose given intravenously. There is experimental evidence that hyperglycemia exacerbates ischemic injury in mature brain and hypoglycemia exacerbates ischemic injury in immature brain. Thus, euglycemia is desirable. Initial resuscitation fluids should be limited to isotonic crystalloid solutions, such as normal saline or lactated Ringer's solution.

The most commonly used drugs in pediatric resuscitation are epinephrine, atropine, and sodium bicarbonate (Table 59-1). Magnesium and calcium are reserved for specific indications such as torsades de pointes, hypocalcemia, and calcium channel blockade. Amiodarone has recently been added to the American Heart Association (AHA) pediatric algorithms based on extrapolation from adult experience.[98] Adults with ventricular fibrillation or ventricular tachycardia in the prehospital setting are more likely to be successfully defibrillated after intravenous administration of amiodarone compared with lidocaine.[99] Accordingly, amiodarone (5 mg/kg bolus) is a therapeutic option for children with pulseless arrest. Amiodarone (5 mg/kg infused over 20 to 60 min) is also an option for ventricular tachycardia with a pulse but should be used with extreme caution because of the risk for profound hypotension. Vasopressin has been added to the AHA adult algorithms as an alternative to epinephrine on the basis of its improved myocardial and CBF effects. However, subsequent clinical data in adults have not consistently yielded positive results and pediatric data are limited to small case series.[100,101] The optimal vasopressor for hemodynamic support after return of circulation in children is not known.

Extracorporeal membrane oxygenation (ECMO) has been used to successfully resuscitate children from selected causes of in-hospital cardiac arrest.[102-106] ECMO-CPR provides greater cerebral and myocardial blood flow than either closed- or open-chest CPR and facilitates titration of temperature, blood flow, and oxygen-carrying capacity. Good outcomes have been documented with the use of ECMO even when initiated after durations of conventional CPR typically associated with poor outcome. It is best reserved for patients with reversible conditions or as a bridge to cardiac transplantation.

Post-Resuscitative Care

Temperature control is a priority for patients who remain comatose after cardiac arrest. Adults cooled to 32°C to 34°C for 12 to 24 hours after resuscitation from ventricular fibrillation demonstrate improved survival and neurologic outcome.[107,108] In contrast, fever worsens outcome in experimental models of brain injury and has been associated with worse clinical outcome in adults with ischemic brain injury. Children resuscitated from cardiac arrest often develop mild hypothermia followed by delayed fever.[109] There is a consensus that initial hypothermia, if tolerated, should be permitted to continue and fever should be vigilantly avoided. The practice of inducing hypothermia in normothermic children is more controversial. Experimental models using either pediatric mechanisms of injury (asphyxia, hypovolemic shock) or examining the immature brain suggest a beneficial effect of induced hypothermia. However, clinical data are limited and there is a concern about hypothermia-impaired immune function and risk of pneumonia/sepsis. Clinical trials of induced hypothermia for neonatal asphyxia are ongoing.

During recovery from global ischemia there is a period of prolonged, multifocal, decreased CBF. Hypotension and hypoxia should be avoided during this period to prevent development of a secondary brain injury. As previously mentioned, the optimal regimen of oxygen and pressor therapy is not known and requires further study.

Sustained elevation of ICP may be more common after asphyxial arrests versus arrests of cardiac origin[110] and is a poor prognostic sign in children with drowning. ICP monitoring fell out of favor in the 1980s when it was found to not influence outcome in small case series.[111] However, studies using contemporary ICP-directed therapy (perhaps including induced hypothermia) deserve reevaluation.

TABLE 59–1. DRUGS COMMONLY USED IN ARREST OR PERI-ARREST CONDITIONS

Drug	Dose	Maximum Single Dose	Route
Adenosine*	0.1 mg/kg Repeat dose: 0.2 mg/kg	12 mg	i.v. (rapid push)
Atropine	0.2 mg/kg (0.1 mg/min)	Children: 0.5 mg Adolescents: 1 mg	i.v., i.o., e.t.
Amiodarone	5 mg/kg	300 mg	i.v., i.o. (bolus in pulseless arrest, otherwise give slowly)
Calcium chloride (10%)	20 mg/kg	500 mg	i.v., i.o. (slowly)
Dextrose	0.5-1 mg/kg	N/A	i.v., i.o.
Epinephrine	0.01 mg/kg (0.1 mg/kg if given e.t.)	5 mg	i.v., i.o., e.t.
Lidocaine	1 mg/kg	100 mg	i.v., i.o., e.t.
Narcan	0.1 mg/kg	2 mg	i.v., i.o., e.t.
Magnesium	25-50 mg/kg	2 g	i.v., i.o.
Sodium bicarbonate (8.4%)	1 mEq/kg	N/A	i.v./i.o.

i.v., intravenous; i.o., interosseous; e.t., endotracheal.
*For supraventricular tachycardia.

Miscellaneous

Most pediatric victims of cardiopulmonary arrest will not be successfully resuscitated. The difficulty of accepting this reality often results in prolonged attempts at resuscitation. The AHA 2000 Guidelines state, "In the absence of recurring or refractory ventricular fibrillation or ventricular tachycardia, history of a toxic drug exposure, or a primary hypothermic insult, resuscitative efforts may be discontinued if there is no return of spontaneous circulation despite advanced life support. In general, this requires no more than 30 minutes."[98] This acknowledges the futility of prolonged resuscitative efforts and empowers clinicians to feel *permitted to stop* resuscitative efforts. The guideline does not mandate stopping at a specific duration of CPR, but clinicians should recognize that the chance of survival with lifelong severe disabilities correlates with the duration of CPR.

Surveys indicate that most family members would like to be present during resuscitation attempts of a loved one.[112-115] Presence during resuscitation can help family members adjust to the death of a loved one.[116,117] Although allowing family presence during resuscitation requires planning and additional resources, when done properly it is worth the effort. Perhaps one of the most disheartening statistics in resuscitation research is the high divorce rate (up to 90%) of parents after the death of a child. Thus, pastoral and social services can be integral components of care during both the acute resuscitation event and long-term follow-up.

STATUS EPILEPTICUS

Status epilepticus is a pediatric emergency traditionally defined as either a continuous seizure of at least 30 minutes or more than two discrete seizures without complete recovery of consciousness. Refractory status epilepticus is defined as failure of two first-line antiepileptic medications to treat this condition for greater than 60 minutes. Many children with refractory status epilepticus have new or established CNS lesions.[118]

Epidemiology and Etiology

The incidence of pediatric status epilepticus from a prospective study is 40 cases/100,000 per year. Infants younger than 1 year of age have the highest incidence at 150 cases/100,000 per year.[119] More than 90% of cases are convulsive status epilepticus. The first episode of status epilepticus occurs at a mean age of 4.2 years.[120] There is a slight male predominance in status epilepticus.[119,121]

There are five etiologic categories of status epilepticus that have bearing on treatment and prognosis. A child with *idiopathic or cryptogenic* status epilepticus has no prior history of seizures and no known risk factors. *Atypical febrile* status epilepticus occurs during fever in children with no prior history of seizures without fever. Children with *acute symptomatic* status epilepticus have new CNS lesions such as encephalitis, trauma, tumor, stroke, or anoxia. Children with *remote symptomatic* status epilepticus have pre-existing CNS lesions and therefore a lowered seizure threshold. In these children status epilepticus can occur without provocation, sometimes even years after the initial insult. Finally some children have status epilepticus resulting from *progressive encephalopathy*, including neurodegenerative diseases, malignancies, and neurocutaneous syndromes (Table 59-2).[119,121,122]

In one study, status epilepticus accounted for 1.6% of total pediatric ICU admissions and etiology varied with age.

TABLE 59-2. ETIOLOGY OF STATUS EPILEPTICUS

Idiopathic/cryptogenic (24%)
Atypical febrile (24%)
  Previously normal
  Previously abnormal
Acute symptomatic (23%)
  CNS infection
  Anoxia
  Trauma
  Stroke/hemorrhage
  Intoxication
  Metabolic
  Anticonvulsant withdrawal
Remote symptomatic (23%)
Progressive encephalopathy (6%)
  Neurocutaneous syndrome
  Neoplasm
  Genetic/metabolic

In children younger than 2 years of age, *acute symptomatic* status epilepticus from meningitis and encephalitis accounted for 51% of cases whereas *remote symptomatic* status epilepticus in children with a prior diagnosis of epilepsy was seen in 16% of children. Older children were more likely than younger children to have a history of epilepsy.[121] Mortality rates for status epilepticus in children are between 3% and 6%.[119,122] Mortality is dependent on etiology, age, and duration of status epilepticus. Mortality rates of 0% and 12.5% were seen when patients were divided into either unprovoked/febrile status epilepticus or acute CNS insult/progressive encephalopathy groups, respectively.[121] Morbidity risk varies from between 11% and 25%. Infants are at great risk for morbidity because the etiology in this group is commonly *acute symptomatic* status epilepticus. Neurologic sequelae of status epilepticus include epilepsy, recurrence, mental retardation, and motor disorders. However, many of the morbidities can be attributed to the underlying disease and not status epilepticus per se. Risk of recurrence in the category of *idiopathic* status epilepticus is less than 5%. In contrast, recurrence of status epilepticus in children in the *acute symptomatic* groups can be as high as 60%.[119,123] Systemic complications occur, with increasing frequency, in proportion to the duration of status epilepticus, the most important being respiratory failure and cardiovascular compromise and autonomic and metabolic disturbances.[124]

Diagnosis

Status epilepticus can be convulsive or nonconvulsive, when comparing clinical events with electrographic information. Convulsive seizures either begin as generalized seizures or progress from partial seizures. Nonconvulsive seizures are characterized as having subtle clinical signs such as nystagmus, irregular clonic twitches along with decreased consciousness, and/or ictal discharges on EEG. Included under the subheading of nonconvulsive seizures are complex and simple partial and absence seizures.[125]

Treatment

The goals in treating status epilepticus are to provide respiratory and cardiovascular support, terminate clinical and electrical seizure activity, identify and treat precipitating factors, and prevent systemic complications.[125] Recognizing that a prolonged duration of seizure increases the risk of morbidity and mortality, the Epilepsy Foundation of America published a consensus view to initiate antiepileptic drugs for treatment 10 minutes after the onset of an episode of status epilepticus.[126] A timetable for treatment of status epilepticus in children is provided in Table 59-3.

History of present and past illness may be useful in determining the cause of status epilepticus and in choosing therapy, but it should not delay resuscitation efforts. Initial treatment includes basic life support—airway, breathing, and circulation (ABCs). The prevention of hypoxemia and hypotension, which exacerbate neuronal injury, is important. The airway should be kept open with simple maneuvers and 100% oxygen applied to the patient with a non-rebreathing mask. The airway should also be kept clear of airway secretions. Efficacy of oxygenation efforts should be monitored by pulse oximeter. Ventilation efforts are assessed clinically or by arterial blood gas determinations. If the patient is unable to maintain adequate oxygenation or ventilation, endotracheal intubation using rapid sequence intubation technique is indicated. Circulation is monitored by assessment of ECG, blood pressure, and perfusion. Ideally, a large-bore peripheral intravenous catheter should be placed for fluid and drug administration. A bedside blood glucose determination should be obtained. Serum electrolyte levels, renal and liver functions, and anticonvulsant levels should be assessed. Serum and urine toxicology screen should be obtained. Fever and hypoglycemia should be treated as quickly as possible to prevent CNS injury. The neurologic examination follows, focusing on GCS score, signs of raised ICP, focal deficits, and pupil size. In patients receiving neuromuscular blockade, electrical seizure activity should be monitored with continuous EEG. The ABCs should be reassessed throughout the resuscitation.

First-line antiepileptic drugs for pediatric status epilepticus include benzodiazepines, phenytoin or fosphenytoin, and phenobarbital. Drug choice depends on the route available (intravenous is preferred), the patient's maintenance anticonvulsants (a different class is recommended), and

patient characteristics. Evidence-based studies of anticonvulsants in children are rare. Recommendations are extrapolated from studies in adult. The optimal first-line treatment of status epilepticus in children is controversial.

Phenytoin/Fosphenytoin. In a study in adults comparing lorazepam, phenytoin, phenobarbital, and diazepam, phenytoin had the highest success rate in stopping status epilepticus.[127] Phenytoin is not commonly associated with respiratory depression and has less of an effect on the impairment of consciousness than either benzodiazepines or barbiturates. Fosphenytoin has the advantage of having a faster infusion rate, shorter onset of action, and less cardiovascular side effects than phenytoin but is more expensive.

Lorazepam. In the same study in adults, lorazepam had the second highest success rate in stopping status epilepticus.[127] Lorazepam can be administered rapidly, has a long duration of effect, and is effective even when administered rectally. Lorazepam produced less respiratory failure requiring intubation than diazepam in retrospective[128] and prospective studies.[129] Incidence of respiratory depression in these studies varied widely—between 3% and 76%.

Diazepam. Although the onset of action of diazepam is rapid (between 1 and 3 minutes after intravenous administration), it has a large volume of distribution; therefore, its duration of action is only 15 to 30 minutes. Thus, concomitant maintenance antiepileptic drugs are generally needed. Rectal diazepam has gained attention recently through its use as a first-line outpatient drug for use by parents or emergency services.

Phenobarbital. Phenobarbital is a very effective anticonvulsant, but it is often not the first choice in the treatment of status epilepticus because of side effects of respiratory depression and cardiovascular disorders, especially when it is used in combination with benzodiazepines. Infants metabolize phenobarbital more rapidly than older children and often require higher doses adjusted for body weight. Nevertheless, the pharmacokinetics of phenobarbital are more predictable than those of phenytoin in infants.

TABLE 59–3. SUGGESTED TIMETABLE FOR THE EMERGENCY DIAGNOSIS AND TREATMENT OF STATUS EPILEPTICUS

Time	Exam/Intervention	Testing
Initial presentation: *0 min*	Airway, breathing, circulation IV access, monitoring	Glucose, oxygenation via pulse oximetry ± blood gas analysis

Primary survey: *5 min*	Neurologic exam
	Administer antiepileptic drugs
	   Lorazepam, 0.1 mg/kg i.v.
	   Phenobarbital, 20 mg/kg i.v.
	Normal saline maintenance i.v.
	Reduce fever
		Electrolytes, renal and liver function, ammonia, anticonvulsant levels, toxicology, complete blood cell count, urinalysis

Secondary survey: *15-30 min*	Evaluate treatment results
	Second line antiepileptic drug if seizure persists
	   Phosphenytoin, 20 mg/kg i.v. or
	   phenytoin, 20 mg/kg i.v.
		Patient-specific: cranial imaging (CT vs. MRI), lumbar puncture, EEG, ECG

Status epilepticus: *>30 min*	Intubation and mechanical ventilation	

Refractory status epilepticus: *>60 min*	Titrate anti-epileptic drug to burst suppression.
	   Pentobarbital, 10 mg/kg i.v. given over 30 min, then 5 mg/kg every hour for 3 doses, then 1 mg/kg/h; titrate to effect
	   Midazolam, 0.15 mg/kg i.v. then 1-2 μg/kg/min titrate to effect
	   Phenobarbital, 5-10 mg/kg i.v. every 20 minutes to achieve burst suppression, then every 12 hours
	Evaluate need for vasopressors.
		Continuous EEG
		Neurologic consultation
		Consider anesthesia consultation for treatment with inhaled gas.

Additional Diagnostic Workup

Lumbar puncture is best performed early after presentation, but not in unstable patients or those who may have increased ICP. The decision to perform lumbar puncture should be guided by head CT. Otherwise, the type of neuroimaging used in infants and children with status epilepticus should be individualized, depending on history and physical findings. Both electrocardiography and EEG are useful to investigate cause of status epilepticus (i.e., long QT syndrome or identifiable EEG patterns). EEG is also useful in titrating therapy (see later).[125]

Drug Treatment for Refractory Status Epilepticus

Initiation of treatment for refractory status epilepticus should occur by 60 minutes, usually with neurologic consultation and with appropriate monitoring in a pediatric ICU or intermediate unit. These patients are mechanically ventilated, and seizures are typically treated with a variety of therapies, generally to induce burst suppression on continuous EEG. Most commonly, pentobarbital is used as a continuous infusion to treat refractory status epilepticus. Pentobarbital is given initially as a slow intravenous loading dose of 5 to 15 mg/kg, followed by an infusion rate of 1 mg/kg/hr titrated to effect. There are differing opinions on when to begin to wean therapy, but it is generally recommended that about 12 hours of seizure cessation be attained before weaning the infusion.[130] In children, placement of either a central venous pressure or pulmonary artery catheter is indicated to titrate fluid, inotropic, and/or pressor support. Pentobarbital use often requires the addition of inotropes or pressors. As an alternative to continuous barbiturate infusion, phenobarbital can be administered every 20 minutes (5 to 10 mg/kg i.v.) to achieve burst suppression, and then as a chronic therapy every 12 hours. A midazolam infusion has also been shown to be effective in refractory status epilepticus in some children (0.15 mg/kg IV bolus followed by infusion of 1 to 2 mg/kg/min). The infusion can be increased every 15 minutes if seizures are still present on continuous EEG or if burst suppression is not achieved. With this approach, in one series, inotropic support was not required.[131]

STROKE

Epidemiology

Stroke in children is becoming increasingly recognized and now exceeds an incidence of 8 cases per 100,000 children per

TABLE 59–4. MOST COMMON RISK FACTORS FOR CHILDHOOD ISCHEMIC STROKE

Vascular	Acquired Prothrombotic States
Arteriopathies	Prothrombotic medications
Transient cerebral arteriopathy of childhood	Pregnancy and the postpartum period
Postvaricella angiopathy	Lupus anticoagulant
Fibromuscular dysplasia	Anticardiolipin antibodies
Moyamoya syndrome	Lipoprotein abnormalities
Postradition vasculopathy	Hyperhomocysteinemia
Vasospastic Disorders	***Congenital Prothrombotic States***
Migraine	Antithrombin deficiency
Ergot poisoning	Protein S deficiency
Vasospasm with systemic arterial hypertension	Protein C deficiency
	Plasminogen deficiency
Vasculitis	Factor V Leiden
Meningitis	Prothrombin gene mutation
Systemic lupus erythematosus	Methylenetetrahydrofolate reductase
Polyarteritis nodosa	
Granulomatous angiitis	***Metabolic Disorders***
Takayasu's arteritis	Hyperhomocysteinemia
Dermatomyositis	Hyperlipidemia
Inflammatory bowel disease	
Drug abuse (cocaine, amphetamines)	**Embolic**
Systemic Vascular Disease	***Congenital Heart Disease***
Early atherosclerosis	Complex congenital heart defect
Diabetes	Ventricular/atrial septal defect
Ehlers-Danlos syndrome	Coarctation of the aorta
Pseudoxanthoma elasticum	Patent foramen ovale
Homocystinuria	Patent ductus arteriosus
Fabry's disease	
	Acquired Heart Disease
Trauma	Rheumatic heart disease
Brain herniation and arterial compression	Prosthetic heart valve
Posttraumatic dissection	Bacterial endocarditis
Intra-oral traumatic brain injury	Cardiomyopathy and myocarditis
Carotid ligation (e.g., extracorporeal membrane oxygenation)	Atrial myxoma
Arteriography	Cardiac rhabdomyoma
	Cardiac arrhythmia
Intravascular	
	Trauma
Hematologic Disorders	Amniotic fluid or placental embolism
Hemoglobinopathies (sickle cell anemia)	Fat or air embolism
Thrombocytosis	Foreign body embolism
Polycythemia	Cardiac catheterization
Leukemia or other hematologic neoplasms	

TABLE 59–5. DIAGNOSTIC WORKUP IN PEDIATRIC STROKE

There are no published consensus guidelines on the evaluation of stroke in children, but several systematic approaches have been recommended. The evaluation should include:

1. History of head trauma, neck trauma, recent infection, illness, unexplained fever or malaise, drug ingestion, developmental delay, family history of bleeding problems, and associated headache
2. Family history, with special attention to premature vascular disease, hematologic disease, and mental retardation
3. Physical examination including head circumference, skin abnormalities, cardiac evaluation, and carotid artery examination
4. MRI and MRA (CT if MR unavailable)

If the MRI and MRA reveal an infarct, with vascular distribution, then consider:

1. Echocardiogram, electrocardiogram
2. Blood studies including complete blood cell count, erythrocyte sedimentation rate, hemoglobin electrophoresis, protein S, protein C, antithrombin III, factor V Leiden, anticardiolipin antibodies, lupus anticoagulant, homocysteine, cholesterol, and varicella titer
3. Lumbar puncture
4. Transcranial Doppler with bubble study
5. Radiograph of cervical spine (posterior infarctions)

If the MRI and MRA reveal an infarct, with nonvascular distribution, then consider:

1. Cerebrospinal fluid lactate levels
2. Plasma ammonia and amino acids
3. Urine organic acids

If the MRI and MRA reveal a hemorrhage, then consider:

1. Coagulation studies
2. Conventional angiography

If the MRA is normal, then consider conventional angiography.

*Adapted from the Children's Hemiplegia and Stroke Association. Website: http://www.chasa.org/diagnosis.htm.

year.[132] Substantial advances in our knowledge of this condition in children have resulted from the work of the Canadian Pediatric Ischemic Stroke Registry. Neonates account for about 25% of these cases. The increasing incidence is believed to result from improvements in diagnostic tools (MRI, CT, MRA) applied to the pediatric population and to increasing survival rates in infants and children with stroke risk factors (e.g., complex congenital heart disease, malignancies).

Etiology

As discussed, atherosclerosis is a key risk factor for stroke in adults. In pediatric and neonatal stroke, extracerebral risk factors contribute to about 75% of cases; however, the spectrum of risk factors differs from those seen in adults. DeVeber[132] grouped the most common risk factors for childhood ischemic stroke into vascular, intravascular, and embolic categories (Table 59-4). The most common vascular risk factor has been reported to be transient cerebral arteriopathy.[133] Post-varicella arteriopathy, migraine, traumatic carotid dissection, and vasculitis, such as moyamoya, are also important examples in this category. In the intravascular category, sickle cell anemia, sinus thrombosis, leukemias, and both acquired and congenital prothrombotic states are important examples. Dehydration and intravascular volume depletion increase stroke risk in these settings, which are of special importance in the pediatric ICU. Recent data revealed an 84% incidence of an acute systemic illness and a 30% incidence of dehydration in cerebral sinovenous thrombosis in infants and children.[134] Congenital and acquired heart disease in infants and children are the most important underlying causes of embolic stroke.[132] The risk of stroke in children after surgery for congenital heart disease is about 1 in 250 cases.[135]

Diagnosis

The clinical presentation of stroke in infants and children is age related. Infants present typically with seizures and lethargy whereas older children may present with acute focal neurologic deficits or diffuse symptoms (headache, lethargy, or seizures).[132,136] In some cases, the duration of neurologic deficits in pediatric stroke may be shorter than the 24-hour deficits classically required to differentiate stroke from transient ischemic attack in adults.[137] It is often difficult to differentiate migraine, Todd's paralysis, and stroke in children. Complicating this problem, CT may be normal within the initial 12 hours.[132] MRI is a more sensitive technique for diagnosing stroke, and advanced MRI modalities such as perfusion, diffusion, and MRA are important adjuncts to making the diagnosis. These methods are discussed in Chapter 48. Because of the impact of making specific vascular diagnoses on the management strategy, angiography is often recommended in children with idiopathic stroke.[132]

In addition to the importance of echocardiography in the diagnostic work of stroke after cardiac surgery or catheterization, endocarditis, cardiomyopathy, and other occult cardiac abnormalities are also important risk factors for embolic stroke, thus recognizing the importance of echocardiography and the general diagnostic workup for stroke in children.[138,139] A general diagnostic approach to pediatric stroke is presented in Table 59-5.

Treatment

In the acute setting, antithrombotic therapy has been used increasingly in the therapy for pediatric stroke. Strater and colleagues[140] compared treatment with low-molecular-weight heparin versus aspirin in 135 children across a variety of causes (including idiopathic, cardiac, vascular, and infectious) and suggested safety when used to prevent stroke recurrence. This is a controversial area for which there is a lack of systematic study.[141] DeVeber[132] recommends that neonates do not require antithrombotic treatment because of negligible recurrence risk, whereas older children require aspirin (2 to 3 mg/kg/day).[142] In dissection, high-grade stenosis, or severe prothrombotic state, low-molecular-weight heparin or warfarin (Coumadin) is recommended for several months. In endocarditis, anticoagulation is not recommended because of the risk of rupture of occult mycotic aneurysms. Thrombolytic therapy has been subjected to very limited study in children. Cases describing the use of tissue plasminogen activator and cerebral balloon angioplasty in acute stroke in children with dramatic results are being reported.[143]

Supportive Care in the Pediatric ICU

An evidence-based approach for care in the pediatric ICU of children with stroke is lacking. Nevertheless, intensive care for the child with stroke must be at a level that is commensurate with that provided for other critical pediatric neurologic disorders, such as severe traumatic brain injury[144] and ruptured arteriovenous malformation.[145]

Careful attention to the ABCs with a neurointensive care approach is essential. If the GCS score is 8 or less and/or the airway or ventilation is compromised, intubation is indicated and should be performed using a neuroprotective rapid-sequence approach. Normal values for both $PaCO_2$ and PaO_2 should be ensured.

Arterial blood pressure must be adequate to optimize cerebral perfusion. The management of systemic hypertension in the setting of pediatric stroke can be complicated by the variety of underlying disorders (i.e., status post cardiac surgery, underlying hypertension) and the presence or absence of hemorrhage. In adults with thrombotic or hemorrhagic stroke and systemic hypertension, it is generally recommended that mean arterial blood pressure not be aggressively reduced below 130 mm Hg.[146] Age-appropriate guidelines for this question are not available for children. In the pediatric ICU, for acute stroke, it is a reasonable first approach to extrapolate from the adult recommendations.

In infants and children with severe stroke with infarction and cerebral swelling, signs and symptoms of raised ICP can develop. Standard protocols for monitoring ICP and treatment of raised ICP in stroke in infants and children have not been developed. Nevertheless, intracranial hypertension can develop; and even in the absence of controlled trials on the beneficial effects of ICP-directed therapy in severe pediatric stroke, ICP monitoring and ICP-directed therapy should be considered if signs and symptoms of intracranial hypertension develop. Anecdotal reports of successful treatment with a variety of therapies including mild hypothermia and decompressive craniectomy have been reported.[147,148] Plasticity in the pediatric brain, particularly in the recovery from focal lesions, should prompt the consideration of an aggressive approach.[149-151] However, long-term morbidity remains substantial after stroke in childhood.[152]

Other aspects of contemporary pediatric neurointensive care should include maintenance of euglycemia and careful fluid management to maintain both a euvolemic state and avoid hyponatremia. In children, normal saline or 5% dextrose in normal saline should be used in the initial 24 hours, carefully following blood glucose concentration, followed by the addition of dextrose or initiation of hyperalimentation after 24 hours. In infants, either 5% or 10% dextrose in normal saline should be used, with insulin titrated to treat hyperglycemia. The specific glucose level associated with the exacerbation of secondary damage in infants and children has not been determined. A value of 200 mg/dL is a reasonable threshold in the absence of clear-cut evidence. Appropriate nutritional support should also be instituted as soon as possible. Rehabilitation services should be consulted during the pediatric ICU admission.

CRITICAL CNS INFECTIONS

Any microbe may cause CNS infections; age and immune status of the host and epidemiology of the pathogen give evidence to the specific pathogens. Regardless of the etiology, most children with CNS infection present with nonspecific symptoms including fever, headache, nausea, vomiting, anorexia, and irritability. Photophobia, neck pain and rigidity, seizures, mental status change, and focal neurologic deficits are common signs that are determined by the specific pathogen and area of CNS infected.

Bacterial Meningitis
Epidemiology
The etiology of bacterial meningitis and its treatment differ in neonates (0 to 28 days of life) versus older infants and children.

During the first 2 months of life, the bacteria that cause meningitis in normal infants reflect the maternal flora and the environment to which the infant is exposed. The most common pathogens include groups B and D streptococci, gram-negative enteric bacilli, and *Listeria monocytogenes*. Occasionally, *Haemophilus influenzae* (both type B and non-encapsulated strains) and other pathogens—more typically found in older patients—can be the etiologic agent. Bacterial meningitis in children between 2 months and 12 years of age is usually caused by *Streptococcus pneumoniae*, *Neisseria meningitides*, or *H. influenzae* type b. After the implementation of immunization against *H. influenzae*, the incidence of *H. influenzae* meningitis decreased rapidly. Subsequent to the universal recommendation for the use of conjugated pneumococcal vaccine at 2 months of age in 2000, the incidence of meningitis caused by this pathogen is also decreasing. Anatomical abnormalities, surgical procedures, neurotrauma, or immune deficiency often underlie meningitis caused by other agents.[153]

Bacterial meningitis most commonly results from hematogenous dissemination of microorganisms from a distant site of infection; bacteremia usually precedes meningitis or occurs concomitantly. Colonization of the nasopharynx with a pathogenic microorganism is the usual source of bacteremia. Bacteria gain entry to the CSF through the choroid plexus of the lateral ventricles and the meninges and then circulate to the extracerebral CSF and the subarachnoid space. Bacterial cell wall lipopolysaccharide of gram-negative bacteria and pneumococcal cell wall components stimulate a marked inflammatory response, with local production of tumor necrosis factor-alpha, interleukin-1β, prostaglandin E, and other mediators, leading to neutrophil infiltration, increased vascular permeability, and thrombosis. Inflammation of spinal nerves and roots produces meningeal signs, and inflammation of the cranial nerves produces optic, oculomotor, facial, and auditory neuropathies. Intracranial hypertension can produce oculomotor and abducens nerve palsy. Intracranial hypertension in meningitis is believed to result from a combination of cell death (cytotoxic cerebral edema), cytokine-induced increased capillary vascular permeability (vasogenic edema), and increased hydrostatic pressure after obstruction of CSF reabsorption and/or flow. Rarely, meningitis may follow bacterial invasion from a contiguous focus of infection such as paranasal sinusitis, otitis media, mastoiditis, orbital cellulites, or cranial or vertebral osteomyelitis or may occur after introduction of bacteria via penetrating head trauma or meningomyelocele.[154]

Diagnosis
The clinical presentation may be as fulminant as rapidly progressing shock, purpura, disseminated intravascular coagulation, and altered consciousness, frequently resulting in death within 24 hours. More often, however, children present with several days of fever with upper respiratory tract or gastrointestinal symptoms, followed by nonspecific signs of CNS infection such as lethargy and irritability. The presence of headache, emesis, bulging fontanelle, widening of the sutures, oculomotor or abducens nerve paralysis, hypertension with bradycardia, apnea, or hyperventilation suggests intracranial hypertension. Papilledema is uncommon in uncomplicated meningitis and suggests a more chronic process, such as intracranial abscess, sinus thrombosis, or subdural empyema. Seizures can result from cerebritis, infarction, or electrolyte abnormalities and occur in between 20% and 30% of children with meningitis. Seizures that occur at presentation or

within first 4 days of onset are usually of no prognostic significance. Seizures that persist beyond the fourth day of illness and those that are difficult to treat are associated with poor prognosis.[155]

The diagnosis of acute bacterial meningitis is confirmed by analysis of CSF. Contraindications for an immediate lumbar puncture are (1) evidence of increased ICP (other than bulging fontanelle), (2) presence of severe cardiopulmonary compromise or likelihood that positioning for the procedure would significantly compromise cardiopulmonary function, (3) infection of the skin overlying the needle insertion site, and (4) coagulopathy. If lumbar puncture is delayed, then empirical antibiotic treatment should be started after a blood culture is obtained. Blood culture reveals the susceptible bacteria in 80% to 90% of cases of meningitis. The need for a cranial CT scan, for signs and symptoms of increased ICP or brain abscess, should not delay therapy. Table 59-6 summarizes the CSF findings in CNS infections. Pleocytosis with lymphocyte predominance may be seen early in bacterial meningitis; conversely, neutrophilic pleocytosis may be present in patients during the early stages of acute viral meningitis. The shift to lymphocytic-monocytic predominance in viral meningitis invariably occurs within 8 to 24 hours. A traumatic lumbar puncture complicates the diagnosis of meningitis. If the CSF is bloody, it should be collected in three or more tubes. If the CSF clears in successive tubes, it suggests a traumatic lumbar puncture. Blood that does not clear is more suggestive of intracranial bleeding. The CSF leukocyte to erythrocyte ratio in CSF from a traumatic lumbar puncture is generally similar to that in a concurrently obtained peripheral blood sample (usually 1:500 to 1:1000).[156]

The mortality rate of bacterial meningitis after the neonatal period is less than 10% secondary to appropriate recognition, prompt antibiotic treatment, and supportive care. Severe neurodevelopmental sequelae occur in between 10% and 20% of pediatric patients. The most common sequelae include hearing loss, mental retardation, epilepsy, delay in language acquisition, visual impairment, and behavioral problems. Sensorineural hearing loss occurs in 30%, 10%, and 5% to 10% of patients with pneumococcal, meningococcal, and *H. influenzae* type b meningitis, respectively.[157]

Treatment

The initial (empirical) choice of antibiotic treatment in immunocompetent infants and children is primarily determined by the antibiotic susceptibilities of *S.pneumoniae*. In the United States, between 25% and 50% of strains of *S. pneumoniae* are currently resistant to penicillin, and up to 25% of isolates are resistant to cefotaxime or ceftriaxone. Based on this, empirical therapy is with vancomycin (60 mg/kg/24 hr, divided q 6h) and cefotaxime (200 mg/kg/24 hr, divided q 6h) or ceftriaxone (100 mg/kg/24 hr, given either as a single daily dose or divided q 12h). Patients allergic to beta-lactam antibiotics can be treated with chloramphenicol (100 mg/kg/24 hr, divided q 6h). If *L. monocytogenes* infection is suspected, as in infants between 1 and 2 months of age or patients with T-lymphocyte deficiency, ampicillin (200 mg/kg/24 hr, divided q 6h) should be administered with either cefotaxime or ceftriaxone. If a patient is immunocompromised and gram-negative bacterial meningitis is suspected, ceftazidime and an aminoglycoside may be used as initial therapy. The duration of treatment should be either 10 or 14 days depending on the bacteria; gram-negative bacillary meningitis should be treated for 3 weeks or for at least 2 weeks after sterilization of CSF. Repeat lumbar puncture may be indicated in some neonates and in children with gram-negative or beta-lactam–resistant meningitis caused by *S. pneumoniae*. Of the adjunctive treatments that might limit CNS inflammation, only corticosteroids have been properly assessed in clinical trials. Adjuvant corticosteroid use was associated with lower case fatality and lower rates of both severe hearing loss and long-term neurologic sequelae in acute bacterial meningitis. Corticosteroids administered either before or with the first dose of antibiotic reduced severe hearing loss in bacterial meningitis caused by *H. influenzae* as well as in meningitis caused by *S. pneumoniae*.[159] The recommended dose of dexamethasone is 0.6 mg/kg/24 hr divided every 6 hours

TABLE 59–6. CEREBROSPINAL FLUID FINDINGS IN CNS INFECTIONS

Type of Infection	Pressure (cm H₂O)	Leukocytes (mm³)	Protein (mg/dL)	Glucose (mg/dL)
Normal	5-8	< 5, ≥ 75% lymphocytes < 30 for neonates	20-45 Up to 180 for neonates	>50 (or 75% serum glucose)
Acute bacterial	↑ (10-30)	300-2000 PMNs predominate	100-500	↓ (<40 or <50% serum glucose)
Partially treated bacterial meningitis	nl or ↑	5-10,000 Usually PMNs	100-500	nl or ↓
Viral meningitis or meningoencephalitis	nl or slightly ↑ (8-15)	Rarely >1000 PMNs early, then mononuclear cells	50-200	nl (decreased in some mumps cases)
Tuberculous meningitis	↑	10-500 PMNs early, lymphocytes predominate through most of the course	100-3000	<50
Fungal meningitis	↑	5-500 PMNs early, lymphocytes predominate through most of the course	25-500	<50
Syphilis	↑	50-500 Lymphocytes predominate	50-200	nl
Amebic (*Naegleria*) meningoencephalitis	↑	1000-10,000 or more PMNs predominate	50-500	nl or slightly ↓

for 4 days.[154] There are no data about the role of corticosteroids in newborns or in patients with nosocomial or CSF shunt–associated meningitis.

The patients who manifest signs of poor perfusion, cutaneous manifestations of disseminated intravascular coagulation (purpura, petechiae), irregular respiratory pattern, altered mental status, cranial nerve involvement, and other signs potentially indicative of raised ICP and the patients who have rapid clinical presentation, significant metabolic acidosis, hypoxemia, hypercapnia, neutropenia, hyponatremia, anemia, and abnormal liver or renal function should be admitted to the pediatric ICU—at least until (1) the course of illness can be determined, (2) the first several doses of antibiotics are administered, and (3) a tentative bacteriologic diagnosis is made. Early recognition of complications such as shock or raised ICP and initiation of treatments in a timely fashion may improve outcome in cases of fulminate meningitis.

Acute CNS complications during the treatment of meningitis include seizures, intracranial hypertension, cranial nerve palsies, stroke, herniation, and thrombosis of the dural venous sinuses (Fig. 59-3).[160] Subdural effusions develop in between 10% and 30% of pediatric patients and are more common in infants. They are asymptomatic in between 85% and 90% of the cases. Aspiration of subdural effusions is indicated in the presence of raised ICP; fever alone is not an indication for aspiration. SIADH with hyponatremia and reduced serum osmolality occurs in between 30% and 50% of children. Cerebral salt wasting can also be seen. Attention as to maintaining a normal serum sodium concentration using either normal saline or judicious titration of hypertonic saline is important to preventing exacerbation of brain edema. Prolonged fever (>10 days) occurs in 10% of the patients. It is usually due to intercurrent viral infection, secondary or nosocomial bacterial infection, thrombophlebitis, drug reaction, pericarditis, or arthritis. Thrombocytosis, eosinophilia, or anemia may also develop during treatment.[155]

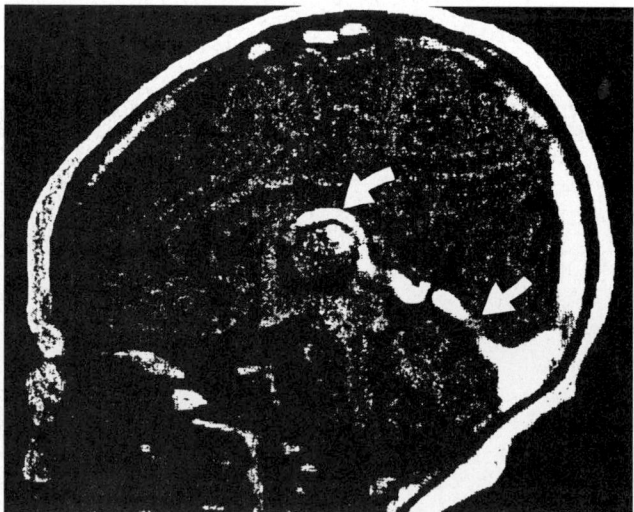

FIGURE 59–3. Sagittal T1-weighted MR image revealing thrombosis of the sagittal sinus (*high signal over the convexity of the hemisphere*), straight sinus (*arrow*), and internal cerebral veins (*curved arrow*) as a complication of bacterial meningitis in an infant. (From Connor SEJ, Jarosz JM: Magnetic resonance imaging of the cerebral venous sinus thrombosis. Clin Radiol 2002;57:449-461.)

Supportive Care in the Pediatric ICU

The issues in ICU care for infants and children with bacterial meningitis are similar to ones mentioned under encephalitis. The reader is referred to the following section for details.

Viral Encephalitis

Epidemiology

Enteroviruses are the most common etiologic agent for encephalitis in children. The severity of the disease ranges from mild illness to severe encephalitis with death or long-term morbidity. Enterovirus infections spread directly from person to person, with an incubation period of between 4 and 6 days. Most cases occur in summer and fall in temperate climates. Arboviruses are responsible for some cases of encephalitis in children. The most common arboviruses responsible for CNS infection in the United States are St. Louis and California encephalitis and the West Nile virus.[161]

Several members of the herpesvirus family can cause encephalitis. Herpes simplex virus type 1 is an important cause of severe encephalitis in children and adults. The cerebral cortex, especially the temporal lobe, is often severely affected by herpes simplex virus. Neonatal herpes infections are usually caused by herpes simplex virus-2 contracted at delivery via vertical transmission. Three forms of the disease develop in neonates: (1) skin, eye, mouth disease (seen in 45% of cases), (2) encephalitis (seen in 35% of cases), and (3) disseminated intravascular coagulation (seen in 20% of cases). The transmission rate from mother to infant is between 30% and 40% when genital infection is primary and 3% for reactivated herpes infection. The mean age at onset of cutaneous or systemic disease is 6 days after birth. In contrast, the mean age at onset of encephalitis is 11 days after birth. The diagnosis of herpes simplex virus infection in neonates can be difficult to make unless skin lesions are present. Cultures of conjunctiva, nasopharynx, and rectum at between 48 hours and 72 hours of age may identify early infection. In neonates, the mortality rates are approximately 50% and 14% for herpes simplex virus disseminated disease and encephalitis, respectively.[161]

A number of other viral causes are important in pediatric encephalitis. Varicella-zoster may cause CNS infection in close proximity to chickenpox. The most common manifestation of CNS infection by varicella-zoster is cerebellar ataxia. Cytomegalovirus infection of the CNS may be either part of congenital infection or disseminated disease in an immunocompromised host. CNS diseases caused by Epstein-Barr virus may present as perceptual distortions of sizes, shapes, and spatial relationships known as "Alice in Wonderland syndrome." There may be meningitis, seizures, ataxia, facial palsy, transverse myelitis, and encephalitis.[161]

Infectious agents can enter the brain via a hematogenous route or by neuronal tracts. Many hematogenous pathogens cause direct endothelial damage to arteries, arterioles, and capillaries, resulting in vasculitis, hemorrhage, and thrombosis. Postinfectious encephalitis is an autoimmune process characterized by a perivenulitis with demyelination. It is uncommon in children younger than 1 year of age.[162] The mortality rate in untreated cases of herpes simplex virus encephalitis is 70%, and fewer than 3% return to normal function. Early treatment with acyclovir reduces the mortality rate to 20% to 30%, but there is still substantial morbidity.[163]

Diagnosis

The onset of illness is generally acute and often preceded by a nonspecific febrile illness of few days' duration. The manifestations of viral encephalitis in older children are headache and hyperesthesia, whereas in infants, irritability and lethargy predominate. Adolescents frequently complain of retrobulbar pain. Fever, nausea, vomiting, photophobia, and pain in the legs, back, and neck are common. Exanthems often precede or accompany the CNS signs. Seizures occur in 60% of the cases during the course of herpes simplex virus encephalitis. The diagnosis of viral encephalitis is usually made on the basis of clinical presentation of nonspecific prodrome followed by progressive CNS symptoms. The CSF usually shows a mild mononuclear predominance. In the diagnostic workup, the CSF should be cultured for viruses, bacteria, fungi, and mycobacteria.[164] Detection of viral DNA or RNA by polymerase chain reaction is useful for diagnosis of herpes simplex virus, varicella-zoster, cytomegalovirus, Epstein-Barr virus, and enteroviral meningoencephalitis. Polymerase chain reaction of CSF is 100% specific and more than 90% sensitive for herpes simplex virus.[165] About 50% of patients with herpes simplex virus encephalitis have focal abnormalities on nonenhanced CT. MRI is the imaging modality of choice and should ideally be the first step after initial clinical examination. The EEG is abnormal in almost all cases of herpes simplex virus encephalitis and may show periodic lateralized epileptiform discharges (Fig. 59-4).[166]

Treatment

Antiviral therapy with acyclovir is indicated for herpes simplex virus encephalitis. Acyclovir has a relatively short half-life in plasma, and more than 80% is excreted unchanged in the urine; thus, renal impairment can exacerbate toxicity. The standard dose of acyclovir for herpes simplex virus encephalitis is 30 mg/kg/24 hr divided every 8 hours for 14 days. The dose in neonates is 60 mg/kg/day. The duration of treatment is 21 days for immunocompromised patients. Acyclovir is effective in encephalitis due to herpes simplex virus types 1 and 2 and varicella-zoster. The dose of acyclovir for varicella-zoster encephalitis is similar to that for herpes simplex encephalitis.[164]

Supportive Care in the Pediatric ICU

A substantial body of data supporting an evidence-based approach to care in the pediatric ICU of children with meningitis and encephalitis is lacking. Careful attention to the ABCs with a neurointensive care approach is essential. If the GCS score is less than 8 and/or the airway or ventilation is compromised, intubation is indicated and should be performed using a neuroprotective rapid-sequence approach. Normal values for both $PaCO_2$ and PaO_2 should be ensured. Bacterial meningitis and encephalitis can be associated with severe septic shock that should be approached and treated according to published guidelines.[167] Arterial blood pressure must be adequate to optimize cerebral perfusion.

In infants and children with meningitis and encephalitis, increased ICP may develop. The most important morbidity and mortality of CNS infections is herniation of brain tissue secondary to intracranial hypertension. No randomized controlled trial has been conducted to evaluate the effect ICP monitoring has on outcome in meningitis or encephalitis in children or adults. However, evidence supports the association of intracranial hypertension and poor neurologic outcome in infants and children.[168-170] In addition, ICP monitoring and

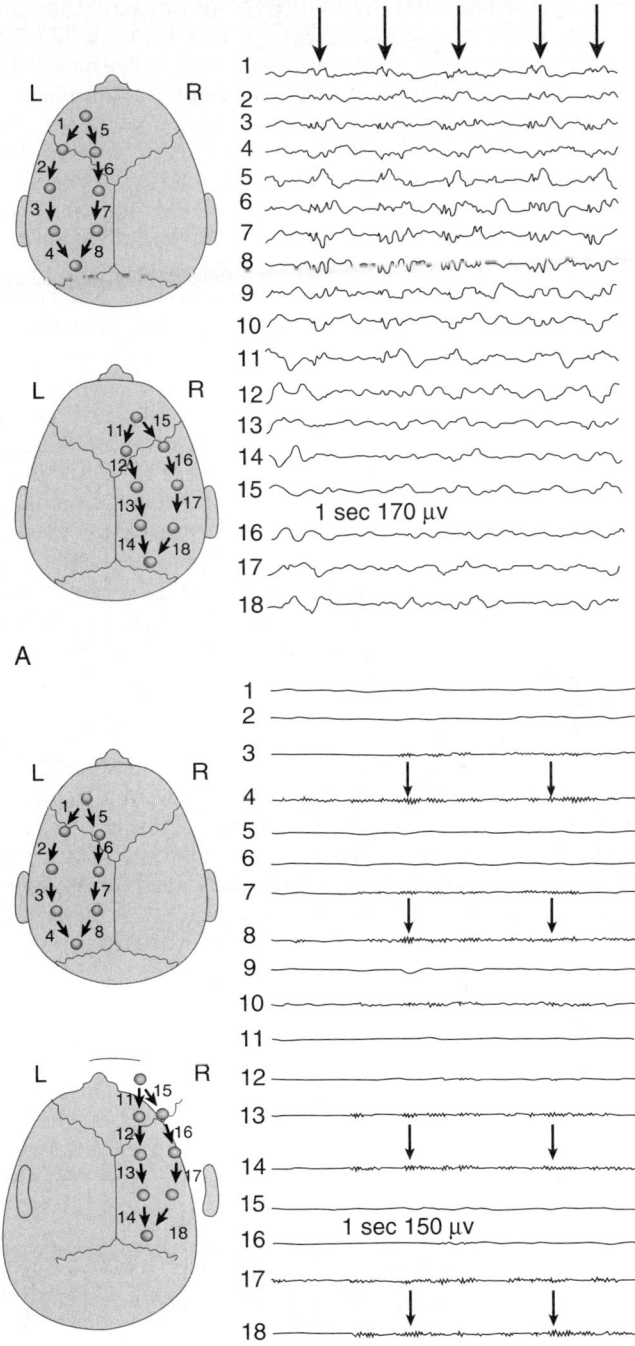

FIGURE 59–4. A, Electroencephalogram showing periodic lateralized epileptiform discharges (PLEDS) in a child with herpes simplex encephalitis. The discharges are seen diffusely in the left hemisphere (leads 1 to 10) occurring at intervals at about 2.5 seconds (arrows). B, Normal background activity in an awake subject for comparison. Arrows show normal alpha rhythm in posterior leads bilaterally. (From Watenberg N, Morton LD: Images in Clinical medicine: Periodic lateralized epileptiform discharges. N Engl J Med 1996;334(10):634.)

aggressive treatment of intracranial hypertension showed reductions in the expected mortality rate in pediatric and adult patients with meningitis and encephalitis.[171-174] ICP monitoring and ICP-directed therapy should be considered if signs and symptoms of intracranial hypertension develop in children with meningitis and encephalitis. ICP monitoring in patients with known or suspected CNS infection with a GCS score less than 8 may be considered at the discretion of the physician. An external ventricular drain is the preferred route of ICP monitoring if there is hydrocephalus or CSF is required for therapeutic or diagnostic drainage.

Other aspects of contemporary pediatric neurointensive care should be included in the treatment regimen, including maintenance of euglycemia and careful fluid management to maintain both a euvolemic state and avoid hyponatremia. This is particularly important because the syndrome of inappropriate secretion of antidiuretic hormone is common in these conditions. Appropriate nutritional support as outlined in Chapter 113 should also be instituted as soon as possible.

Brain Abscess

Epidemiology and Diagnosis

Brain abscesses are most common in children between the ages of 4 and 8 years. The underlying causes of brain abscess include chronic otitis media and sinusitis, orbital cellulitis, dental infections, penetrating head injury, infection of ventriculoperitoneal shunts, immunodeficiency states, embolization due to congenital heart disease with left-to-right shunts, and meningitis. About 80% of brain abscesses in children occur in frontotemporal and parietal lobes, and 30% have multiple sites of involvement. Table 59-7 summarizes the relationships between predisposing conditions and site of brain abscess, likely pathogens, and suggested initial empirical treatment. In the early stages, the clinical presentation of brain abscess includes low-grade fever, headache, and lethargy. Vomiting, papilledema, focal neurologic signs, and seizures may develop as the inflammation proceeds. Nystagmus, ipsilateral ataxia and dysmetria, headache, and vomiting are characteristic signs of cerebellar brain abscess. If the abscess ruptures into the ventricular cavity, severe shock may rapidly develop and death may result.[175]

Contrast medium–enhanced head CT and MRI are the most reliable methods of identifying brain abscess. An abscess cavity shows a ring-enhancing lesion with enhanced CT. MRI with gadolinium administration may reveal a capsule. Blood cultures are positive in roughly 10% of cases. Lumbar puncture should not be undertaken in a patient with suspected brain abscess because examination of CSF is seldom useful and this procedure may precipitate herniation.

Treatment

Treatment is initiated with an antibiotic regimen that is based on the probable pathogenesis and most likely organism. An encapsulated abscess should be treated by antibiotics and aspiration, which is also the most likely diagnostic approach. Surgery is indicated when the abscess (1) is larger than 2.5 cm in diameter, (2) contains gas, (3) is multiloculated, (4) is located in the posterior fossa, or (5) when fungus is identified. The duration of treatment depends on the organism and response but usually ranges between 4 and 6 weeks. Other aspects of neurointensive care in the pediatric ICU for infants and children with brain abscess should mirror those presented previously for meningitis and encephalitis.[176]

POSTOPERATIVE NEUROSURGICAL CASES

Epidemiology

Neurosurgical procedures for children vary widely in all aspects and include elective and emergent operations in all ages of children for a variety of illnesses, most commonly brain tumors, hydrocephalus, and arteriovenous malformations.

Diagnosis

The need for admission to a pediatric ICU is largely determined by the potential complications associated with the specific surgery involved. The most common complications that require intensive monitoring after neurosurgical procedures include hydrocephalus, airway compromise, bleeding, vascular complications, fluid and electrolyte abnormalities, and seizures. Hydrocephalus is an obvious concern in patients undergoing procedures for the treatment of hydrocephalus, either with shunting, ventriculostomy, or a decompressive procedure. Patients with congenital hydrocephalus require ICU monitoring, depending largely on their preoperative status. A child with slowly progressive hydrocephalus with few clinical symptoms may not require admission to the pediatric ICU, whereas preoperative symptoms that raise a

TABLE 59–7. PREDISPOSING CONDITIONS, ETIOLOGIC AGENTS, AND EMPIRICAL TREATMENT IN BRAIN ABSCESS

Predisposing Condition	Site of Abscess	Etiologic Agents	Treatment
Sinusitis Orbital cellulites Dental infection	Frontal lobe	Streptococci *Bacteroides* Enterobacteriaceae *Staphylococcus aureus* *Haemophilus* species	Vancomycin + third-generation cephalosporin + metronidazole
Otitis media Mastoiditis	Temporal lobe/cerebellum	Streptococci *Bacteroides* Enterobacteriaceae *S. aureus* *Haemophilus* species *Pseudomonas aeruginosa*	Vancomycin + third-generation cephalosporin + metronidazole
Head trauma Postsurgical infection	Site of the injury or surgery	*S. aureus* Streptococci Enterobacteriaceae *Clostridium*	Vancomycin + third-generation cephalosporin + metronidazole
Congenital cyanotic heart disease	Middle cerebral artery distribution	*Streptococcus viridans* Anaerobic and microphilic streptococci	Penicillin + metronidazole
Ventriculoperitoneal shunt	Site of the shunt	*P. aeruginosa* Streptococci Enterobacteriaceae	Vancomycin + ceftazidime

concern of potential herniation will require close observation and monitoring. Patients with Chiari malformations, tumors impinging on CSF drainage, or ventricular hemorrhages all carry a significant risk of developing postoperative hydrocephalus.

Airway compromise is a potentially life-threatening complication that is of particular concern after neurosurgical procedures involving the brainstem, because vocal cord paralysis or cranial nerve damage is possible. Patients with congenital facial abnormalities are also at risk for respiratory compromise. A third scenario that predisposes neurosurgical patients to airway problems is a procedure requiring prone positioning during surgery, because significant facial swelling can result.

Although the potential for bleeding is always a concern after surgical procedures, there are certain diseases that carry more than the typical risk for hemorrhage. In particular, surgical resection of a vascular malformation is of concern for bleeding if complete resection is incomplete or impossible. However, all procedures carry a risk for postoperative bleeding, including procedures that do not involve a craniotomy.

Surgical procedures near major arteries can cause vasospasm with resultant cerebral ischemia or infarct. Subarachnoid hemorrhage from aneurysmal or vascular malformation rupture is another well-known cause of vasospasm.

Electrolyte abnormalities can result from three disturbances in normal regulatory mechanisms: diabetes insipidus, the syndrome of inappropriate secretion of antidiuretic hormone, and cerebral salt wasting (see later for management). Other complications from neurosurgical procedures include CSF leak, aseptic meningitis, and pseudomeningocele.

Physical Examination

The immediate examination should include an evaluation of the ABCs. Specific to neurosurgical patients, however, a rapid neurologic examination is important to evaluate for baseline deficits after surgery. This is essential for evaluation of changes in neurologic status. For example, unequal pupillary size may be a result of surgical intervention and would be present immediately after the surgery. However, development of unequal pupils in a patient who previously had equal pupillary size may be the first sign of impending herniation. The initial neurologic examination should include a gross evaluation of mental status. Patients routinely have a depressed level of consciousness after anesthesia, but repeated examinations are necessary to ensure that mental status continues to improve. Measurement of the GCS score is one means of objectively quantifying a child's level of consciousness. Cranial nerve examination is limited by the child's ability to cooperate but should include pupillary response (cranial nerve II), observation of extraocular movements (cranial nerves III, IV, and VI), jaw deviation during sucking in an infant (cranial nerve V), facial asymmetry while crying or laughing (cranial nerve VII), gag reflex (cranial nerves IX and X), and shoulder droop (cranial nerve XI). The motor examination relies heavily on careful observation of movements, because few patients will be able to cooperate with a formal examination early after surgery. Similarly, the sensory examination involves observing gross responses to stimuli. A full evaluation of deep tendon reflexes is usually possible. Neurologic evaluation should be repeated frequently during the first 24 hours, evaluating for new or progressing neurologic deficits.

Treatment

All patients in the pediatric ICU should have cardiorespiratory monitoring. Respiratory monitoring should be designed to warn of impending airway compromise, including measurement of respiratory rate, pulse oximetry, and repeated examinations evaluating work of breathing, air entry, and evidence of stridor. Hemodynamic monitoring is useful for evaluating both hemodynamic and neurologic status. Increases in heart rate and blood pressure can be an indication of pain or of seizure activity. Increased blood pressure with a low heart rate is worrisome for raised ICP and impending herniation, although herniation is not always signaled by Cushing's triad in children. Tachycardia with prolonged capillary refill or hypotension may indicate excessive fluid losses, either from bleeding, third space losses, or excessive urine output. Tachycardia and hypotension can also result from loss of vasomotor tone, either from infection, medications, or loss of neurologic regulation after spinal surgery. Invasive blood pressure monitoring is necessary when patients are at high risk for any of the complications listed earlier. Strict measurement of fluid intake and output is essential to monitor fluid balance and interpret disturbances in fluid and electrolyte regulation. When the surgical procedure carries a high risk of a complicating fluid regulation abnormality, as in craniopharyngioma resections, serum and urine electrolytes should be tested every 4 to 6 hours, along with continuous urine measurement and central venous pressure monitoring.

Temperature control is important after neurosurgical procedures and should therefore be monitored closely. Aggressive measures to prevent hyperthermia are warranted because neurologic injury is exacerbated by high brain temperature.

Fluid management for the postoperative neurosurgical patient differs from other postoperative patients in a few key ways. Although maintenance of circulating volume is important, it is important to avoid excessive hydration to prevent exacerbating cerebral edema. In general, neurosurgical procedures do not result in the large third-space losses seen with other surgeries. Once adequate volume status is achieved to maintain perfusion, fluid requirements will usually be met with a maintenance fluid rate.

Euglycemia is important after neurologic surgery, because both hypoglycemia and hyperglycemia can exacerbate neurologic injury. Based on recommendations in adults, initial intravenous fluids in older children should generally be normal saline or 5% dextrose in normal saline and serum glucose levels should be monitored closely. The duration for the dextrose restriction in older children is controversial because ketosis develops even with euglycemia. Generally this is maintained for the initial 24 hours. Hyperglycemia, however, should probably be avoided throughout the entire acute period after CNS insults. Infants, on the other hand, do not have the same capacity for maintaining serum glucose levels if maintained with no source of carbohydrate intake. Initial dextrose concentration in the infant with a CNS insult should probably be 5% (in normal saline). When higher dextrose concentrations are used, such as with hyperalimentation, hyperglycemia should be carefully managed with insulin infusion. It must be recognized that the risk of exacerbation of brain injury by hyperglycemia in infants and children is likely but somewhat theoretical. In contrast, it is clear that hypoglycemia can be harmful to the injured brain and should be avoided.

Hyponatremia is of particular concern in neurosurgical patients because the osmotic effects can result in increasing cerebral edema. Normal saline is the preferred intravenous fluid to avoid this complication. When hyponatremia occurs in conjunction with a decreasing urine output, a high specific gravity, and a high sodium concentration in the urine, it is likely a result of the syndrome of inappropriate secretion of antidiuretic hormone. In this case, fluid restriction is indicated. Neurosurgical patients also have two unique possible sources for excessive sodium loss: CSF losses from extraventricular drainage and urine losses from cerebral salt wasting. Both require correction of sodium losses.

Mild hypernatremia is generally not detrimental and is usually a result of excessive intake or osmotic diuresis. A progressively increasing serum sodium concentration in the presence of increasing volume of hypo-osmolar urine, however, suggests diabetes insipidus. This complication is unusual except with surgeries that have the potential for pituitary injury. Management of diabetes insipidus requires careful titration of fluids, with a maintenance rate to cover insensible losses ($300 \text{ mL/m}^2/\text{day}$) plus total replacement of urine output with a fluid that matches the urine electrolyte concentrations. Vasopressin or desmopressin therapy may be required to control the free water loss.

A few medications should be considered for every neurosurgical patient. First, antiemetics are important to prevent postanesthesia nausea and vomiting, because vomiting can cause a dramatic increase in intracranial pressure. Ondansetron and droperidol are good choices for antiemetic therapy because they are minimally sedating.[177] Postoperative seizures can have serious consequences. Antiepileptics should be considered in all patients at risk for postoperative seizures. Typically, phenytoin is the least sedating drug for seizure prophylaxis. Patients on chronic anticonvulsants should have their usual regimen started as soon as possible after the surgery. Dexamethasone is used to reduce edema formation around brain tumors and reduce tumor size.[178] The use of corticosteroids is controversial in most other settings. However, patients who received corticosteroids preoperatively may require stress-dose corticosteroids during the postoperative period. Prophylaxis with H_2 blockers may reduce gastrointestinal hemorrhage in critically ill patients[179] but may also increase the risk of nosocomial infections.[180] Gastrointestinal bleeding is more common after resection of a posterior fossa tumor, and use of prophylaxis has been advocated in these patients.[181]

Emergency Intervention

The postoperative problem of most concern, and sometimes the most difficult to evaluate in a child, is an altered mental status. Although anesthetics or narcotics can produce an altered sensorium, emergent evaluation is indicated if reversal of these medications does not yield a reassuring examination. If the patient's GCS score is less than 8, intubation should be performed before any transport or testing. If an extraventricular drain is in place, it should be opened and low enough to allow CSF drainage. Mannitol should be given if signs of impending herniation exist and transient hyperventilation begun until a definitive surgical intervention is carried out. An emergent head CT should then be performed. Further action will be guided by the CT findings.

OTHER CRITICAL CNS DISORDERS IN INFANTS AND CHILDREN

There are other critical CNS disorders in infants and children including hepatic encephalopathy, hypertensive encephalopathy, and Reye's syndrome. Discussion of these less common disorders is beyond the scope of this chapter, and the reader is referred to the appropriate primary references or other textbooks focused on pediatric critical care medicine. Reye's syndrome was once a key disorder in the field of pediatric neurointensive care—reaching a peak of 555 cases in the United States in 1980. In the past decade fewer than 2 cases per year have been reported.[182]

ANNOTATED REFERENCES

Bonthius D, Karacay B: Meningitis and encephalitis in children: An update. Neurol Clin 2002;20.
  Contemporary and thorough review on the changing face of meningitis and encephalitis in pediatric neurointensive care, with over 100 relevant references.

Chiron C, Raynaud C, Maziere B, et al: Changes in regional cerebral blood flow during brain maturation in children and adolescents. J Nucl Med 1992;33:696-703.
  The most comprehensive study of normal CBF in infants and children.

deVeber G: Arterial ischemic strokes in infants and children: An overview of current approaches. Semin Thromb Hemost 2003;29:567-573.
  Recent review by one of the foremost authorities on ischemic stroke in infants and children that presents a contemporary discussion of the rising recognition and incidence of this condition and implications on therapy.

Kochanek PM, Clark RS, Ruppel RA, et al: Biochemical, cellular, and molecular mechanisms in the evolution of secondary damage after severe traumatic brain injury in infants and children: Lessons learned from the bedside. Pediatr Crit Care Med 2000;1:4-19.
  A comprehensive review of the current knowledge of the pathophysiology, biochemistry, and molecular biology of the secondary injury response to brain injury in infants and children.

Lacroix J, Deal C, Gauthier M, et al: Admissions to a pediatric intensive care unit for status epilepticus: A 10-year experience. Crit Care Med 1994;22:827-832.
  An excellent case series on status epilepticus in 147 children covering the spectrum of etiologies from the perspective of the PICU.

Raju TNK, Doshi UV, Vidyasagar D: Cerebral perfusion pressure studies in healthy preterm and term newborn infants. J Pediatr 1982;100:139-142.
  Seminal report on the age-related differences in CPP, with a specific focus on the newborn.

Reis AG, Nadkarni V, Perondi MB, et al: A prospective investigation into the epidemiology of in-hospital pediatric cardiopulmonary resuscitation using the international Utstein reporting style. Pediatrics 2002;109:200-209.
  Contemporary international report on resuscitation from in-hospital cardiac arrest in 176 infants and children outlining the differences in etiologies and outcomes in in-hospital vs. out-of-hospital arrests in children.

Schindler MB, Bohn D, Cox PN, et al: Outcome of out-of-hospital cardiac or respiratory arrest in children. N Engl J Med 1996;335:1473-1479.
  Classic report outlining the poor prognosis for out-of-hospital cardiac arrest in pediatric patients.

Zwienenberg M, Muizelaar JP: Severe pediatric head injury: The role of hyperemia revisited. J Neurotrauma 1999;16:937-943.
  An outstanding discussion of age-related differences in the cerebrovascular response of the injured brain.

Section IV

RESPIRATORY DISORDERS

Chapter 60

BEDSIDE MONITORING OF PULMONARY FUNCTION

Richard H. Kallet • Julin F. Tang

KEY POINTS

PULSE OXIMETRY

1. Because **pulse oximeters cannot be calibrated**, their accuracy is highly variable and dependent on both the calibration curve programmed into the monitor and the quality of signal processing.

2. **Carboxyhemoglobin** and oxyhemoglobin absorb equivalent amounts of red light, so that **carbon monoxide poisoning** results in a falsely elevated oxygen saturation as measured by pulse oximeter (SpO_2).

3. **Motion artifact and low perfusion** are the most common sources of SpO_2 inaccuracies.

4. **Falsely low SpO_2 readings** occur when even minor gaps exist between the probe and skin.

5. **Pulse oximeters** have greater bias and less precision in patients with dark pigmentation.

CAPNOMETRY

1. In **normal subjects**, the gradient of partial pressure of carbon dioxide in arterial blood to partial pressure of carbon dioxide in end-tidal exhaled gas ($PaCO_2$-$PETCO_2$ gradient) is 4 to 5 mm Hg, whereas in **critically ill patients**, the $PaCO_2$-$PETCO_2$ gradient can be markedly elevated, particularly in those with obstructive lung diseases (7 to 16 mm Hg).

2. **The $PaCO_2$-$PETCO_2$ gradient** is affected by changes in respiratory rate, tidal volume, CO_2 production, and mixed venous CO_2 content.

3. **At frequencies above 30,** capnometers tend to underreport the true $PETCO_2$.

4. **In some patients with acute respiratory distress syndrome,** the $PaCO_2$-$PETCO_2$ gradient may be an effective way to titrate positive end-expiratory pressure (PEEP).

5. **During precordial compressions,** $PETCO_2$ can distinguish between successful and unsuccessful resuscitation, with values greater than 10 mm Hg associated with successful resuscitation.

ASSESSMENT OF PULMONARY MECHANICS

1. **Distinguishing the resistive from the elastic recoil-related pressures** requires the introduction of an end-inspiratory circuit occlusion after tidal volume delivery.

2. In clinical practice, the **pause-time used for an end-inspiratory circuit occlusion** is set at 0.5 to 1 second, to limit any potential artifact from spontaneous breathing efforts that may falsely raise or lower the end-inspiratory plateau pressure.

3. The **driving pressure necessary to overcome resistance** increases disproportionately to changes in gas flow, so that resistance can be determined accurately only with a constant inspiratory flow (square wave) pattern.

4. **Intrinsic PEEP is measured** by occluding both limbs of the ventilator circuit for 3 to 5 seconds at end-expiration, thus allowing alveolar pressure to equilibrate with airway pressure. This pressure represents the average intrinsic PEEP throughout the lungs.

5. When using the **pressure-volume curve of the respiratory system** for lung-protective ventilation in patients with acute respiratory distress syndrome, PEEP is set 2 cm H_2O above the lower inflection point to ensure optimal lung recruitment, and tidal volume is set below the upper inflection point to prevent lung injury from excessive stretch.

ASSESSMENT OF BREATHING PATTERN, STRENGTH, AND CENTRAL DRIVE

1. A **threshold value of less than 105** for the respiratory rate–tidal volume ratio has both a high positive predictive value (0.78) and a negative

predictive value (0.95) for the ability to maintain unassisted breathing.

2. **In patients recovering from respiratory failure**, successful weaning is generally associated with a maximal inspiratory pressure greater than –30 cm H_2O.

3. During brief trials of unassisted breathing, an inspiratory occlusion pressure 100 msec after the onset of effort (P0.1) greater than 7 cm H_2O tends to describe patients requiring total ventilatory support and has been reported as a cutoff level in patients who ultimately fail a trial of extubation.

The safe and effective management of patients with acute respiratory failure requires accurate bedside monitoring of pulmonary function. This chapter focuses on the more common noninvasive techniques for monitoring pulmonary gas exchange, respiratory system mechanics, and breathing pattern.

PULSE OXIMETRY

Pulse oximetry is a microprocessor-based instrument that incorporates both oximetry and plethysmography to provide continuous noninvasive monitoring of the oxygen saturation of arterial blood (SaO_2). It is considered one of the most important technologic advances for monitoring patients during anesthesia and critical care.[1] Oximetry uses spectrophotography to determine SaO_2. According to the Beer-Lambert law, the concentration of a substance can be determined by its ability to transmit light.[2] Oxygenated hemoglobin (HbO_2) and deoxygenated or "reduced" hemoglobin (HbR) species absorb light differently, so that the ratio of their absorbencies can be used to calculate saturation. In addition, there are two minor hemoglobin species: carboxyhemoglobin (COHb) and methemoglobin (MetHb). Fractional SaO_2 is the proportion of oxygenated hemoglobin relative to the four hemoglobin species:

$$\frac{HbO_2}{HbO_2 + HbR + COHb + MetHb} \times 100$$

Measuring fractional hemoglobin requires a co-oximeter that incorporates four wavelengths to distinguish each species. In contrast, oxygen saturation as determined by pulse oximeter (SpO_2) uses two wavelengths, so that it measures functional SaO_2:

$$\frac{HbO_2}{HbO_2 + HbR} \times 100$$

The pulse oximeter probe is embedded into either a clip or an adhesive wrap and consists of two light-emitting diodes on one side, with a light-detecting photodiode on the opposite side. Either a finger or an earlobe serves as the sample "cuvette." The tissue bed is transilluminated, and the forward-scattered light is measured. Pulse oximetry targets the signal arising from the arterial bed as light absorbance fluctuates with changing blood volume. Arterial blood flow causes signal changes in light absorption (the pulsatile, or alternating current, component) that can be distinguished from venous and capillary blood in the surrounding tissues (the baseline, or direct current, component) (Fig. 60-1).[2] The ratio of absorbencies is calibrated empirically against SaO_2 measured by co-oximetry in normal volunteers subjected to various levels of oxygenation. Pulse oximeters are calibrated against measured SaO_2 down to 70% (saturations below this level are determined by extrapolation).[3] The resulting calibration curve is stored in the monitor's microprocessor to calculate SpO_2.[4]

ACCURACY AND PRECISION

Because pulse oximeters themselves cannot be calibrated, their accuracy is highly variable and dependent on both the calibration curve programmed into the monitor and the quality of signal processing.[3,4] The accuracy of the calibration curve depends on laboratory testing conditions (co-oximeter used, range of oxygenation studied, and characteristics of sample subjects). Most manufacturers report an accuracy of ±2% at an SaO_2 greater than 70% and ±3% when the SaO_2 is 50% to 70%.[2] In normal subjects tested at an SaO_2 between 99% and 83%, pulse oximetry has a bias and precision that are within 3% of co-oximetry.[5] However, under hypoxic conditions (SaO_2 78% to 55%), when the monitor must rely on extrapolated values, bias increases (8%) and precision deteriorates (5%).[5] Likewise, in critically ill patients, pulse oximeters historically perform well when the SaO_2 is greater than 90% (bias of 1.7%; precision of ±1.2%), but accuracy diminishes at an SaO_2 below 90% (bias of 5.1%; precision of ±2.7%).[6] Technologic advances over the past decade have apparently improved this performance; a recent study comparing pulse oximetry to co-oximetry reported a bias of 0.19% and a precision of

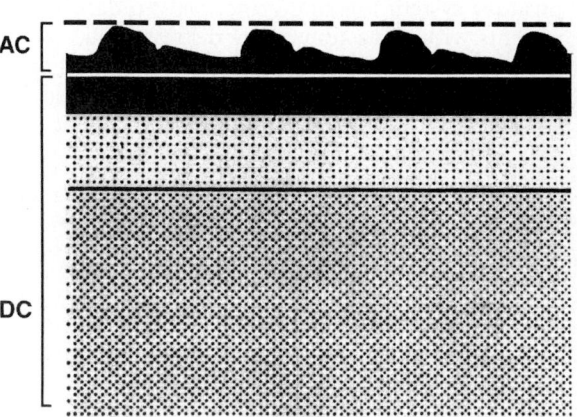

AC — pulsatile arterial blood absorption

non-pulsatile arterial blood absorption

venous and capillary blood absorption

tissue absorption

DC

TIME

FIGURE 60–1. Schematic depiction of the pulse oximeter light absorption signal, whereby the signal change caused by arterial blood flow (pulsatile, or alternating current, component) can be distinguished from that of the tissue and surrounding venous blood (baseline, or direct current, component). (Adapted with permission from Datex-Ohmeda Inc., Madison, Wis.)

±2.22% over an SaO_2 range of 60% to 100%.[7] The most significant sources of inaccuracy were finger thickness, hemoglobin level, skin color, and peripheral temperature.

DYNAMIC RESPONSE

Because pulse oximeters detect very small optical signals (and must reject a variety of artifacts), data must be averaged over several seconds, thus affecting response time.[3] Pulse oximeters may register a near-normal SpO_2 when the actual SaO_2 is less than 70%.[3] A prolonged lag time is more common with finger probes than ear probes[3,8,9] and is attributed to hypoxia-related peripheral vasoconstriction.[3] Bradycardia also is associated with a prolonged response time.[9]

SOURCES OF ERROR

Dyshemoglobins and Vascular Dyes. Significant amounts of carboxyhemoglobin or methemoglobin can cause errors in SpO_2. Carboxyhemoglobin and oxyhemoglobin absorb equivalent amounts of red light, so that carbon monoxide poisoning results in a falsely elevated SpO_2. In contrast, methemoglobin causes substantial absorption of both red and infrared light, so that the ratio approaches 1 (estimated SpO_2 of 85%).[2] Significant methemoglobin causes falsely low SpO_2 values when the actual SaO_2 is greater than 85% and falsely high values when the SaO_2 is less than 85%.[2] Administration of methylene blue or indocyanine green dyes for diagnostic tests causes a false, transient (1- to 2-minute) drop in SpO_2 to as low as 65%.[10,11]

Motion Artifact and Low Perfusion. Motion artifact and low perfusion are the most common sources of SpO_2 inaccuracies, because the photoplethysmographic pulse signal is very low compared with the total absorption signal.[12,13] The combination of motion artifact and low perfusion substantially lowers SpO_2 accuracy compared with either artifact alone.[14] Causes of motion artifact include shivering, twitching, agitation, intra-aortic balloon pump assistance, and patient transport.[15,16] Signs of motion artifact include a false or erratic pulse rate reading or an abnormal plethysmographic waveform. Peripheral hypoperfusion from hypothermia, low cardiac output, or vasoconstrictive drugs may increase bias, reduce precision, and prolong the detection time for a hypoxic event.[16]

Venous Pulsation and Cardiac Arrhythmia. Venous congestion and arteriovenous anastomoses cause the cutaneous veins to pulsate, resulting in a falsely low SpO_2.[17] Similar artifacts may occur during hypovolemia and high airway pressure ventilation.[18] Cardiac arrhythmias apparently do not affect SpO_2 accuracy.[19]

Nail Polish and Skin Pigmentation. Both dark skin pigmentation and dark nail polish interfere with the absorption of the wavelengths used by pulse oximetry. Pulse oximeters thus have greater bias and less precision in black patients.[6] Whereas an SpO_2 of 92% is sufficient to predict adequate oxygenation in white patients, a saturation of 95% is required in black patients.[6] Dark nail polish falsely lowers SpO_2, whereas red polish does not affect accuracy.[20] When nail polish cannot be removed, mounting the oximeter probe sideways on the finger produces an accurate reading.[21]

Ambient Light, Anemia, and Hyperbilirubinemia. Although pulse oximeters compensate for the presence of ambient light, the sensor should be shielded from intense light sources with an opaque material. Falsely low SpO_2 readings occur when even minor gaps exist between the probe and skin, allowing reflected light off the skin surface to "shunt" directly to the photodiode.[22] Xenon surgical lamps and fluorescent lighting can cause a falsely low SpO_2.[23] Under conditions of anemia (Hb 8 g/dL) and severe hypoxia (SaO_2 54%), SpO_2 bias is markedly increased (−14%).[24] Hyperbilirubinemia does not affect SpO_2 directly.[25] However, carbon monoxide is a byproduct of heme metabolism, and icteric patients tend to have higher levels of carboxyhemoglobin,[25] so that SpO_2 may be falsely elevated.

REFLECTANCE PULSE OXIMETRY

Reflectance pulse oximetry was designed to counter signal detection problems associated with finger probes during hypoperfusion. Whereas traditional probes work by transilluminating a tissue bed and measuring the forward-scattered light on the opposite side of the finger or earlobe, reflectance probes are constructed with the light-emitting diodes and the photodetector located on the same side. The photodetector measures the back-scattered light from the skin.[26] Reflectance pulse oximetry probes are usually placed on the forehead, which is less susceptible to vasconstriction.[26] In addition, the more liberal placement sites for reflectance pulse oximetry has allowed fetal monitoring during labor.[27] Intraesophageal SpO_2 monitoring is currently under investigation.[28] Anasarca, excessive head movement, and difficulty in securing the probe site are some of the problems encountered with reflectance pulse oximetry.[29] Light "shunting" from poor skin contact and direct sensor placement over a superficial artery are associated with artifacts.[30] Reflectance pulse oximetry is also limited by poor signal-to-noise ratio and variability among sites in the arrangement of blood vessels and tissue blood volume.[30]

TECHNOLOGIC ADVANCES

Recent advances in signal analysis and processing have markedly improved SpO_2 accuracy during low perfusion and have reduced the problem of motion artifact.[14,31] According to recent independent testing, these advances have been made by several manufacturers.[32] Durban and Rostow reported that new pulse oximeter technology can accurately detect SaO_2 in 92% of the cases in which traditional SpO_2 monitoring failed due to low perfusion and motion artifact.[33]

CAPNOMETRY

Capnometry consists of the measurement and numeric display of expired carbon dioxide (CO_2) at the patient's airway opening.[34] When a waveform plotting CO_2 against time or volume is also displayed, it is referred to as capnography, and the waveform is referred to as a capnogram.[34] Capnometry is most commonly measured by infrared light absorption. CO_2 absorbs infrared light at a peak wavelength of approximately 4.27 μm.[34,35] Because this is close to the peak absorbency wavelength for nitrous oxide (which can interfere with the partial pressure of CO_2 [PCO_2] signal),[34] capnometers can be adjusted for monitoring during general anesthesia. Capnometry works by passing infrared light through a sample chamber to a detector on the opposite side. More infrared light passing through the sample chamber (i.e., less CO_2) causes a larger signal in the detector relative to the infrared light passing through a reference cell. Either the sample chamber is attached directly to the Y-adapter of the ventilator circuit (mainstream), or a sampling line at the Y-adapter continuously aspirates gas into a sampling chamber located inside the monitor (sidestream).

CLINICAL APPLICATIONS

Capnometric determination of the partial pressure of CO_2 in end-tidal exhaled gas ($P_{ET}CO_2$) is used as a surrogate for the partial pressure of CO_2 in arterial blood ($PaCO_2$) during mechanical ventilation.[36,37] Capnometry is used for diverse purposes, such as the diagnosis of pulmonary embolism,[38] determination of lung recruitment response to positive end-expiratory pressure (PEEP),[39,40] detection of intrinsic PEEP,[41] evaluation of weaning,[42,43] indirect marker of elevated deadspace ventilation,[44,45] assessment of cardiopulmonary resuscitation,[46] indirect determination of cardiac output through partial CO_2 rebreathing,[47] verification of endotracheal cannulation,[48] detection of airway accidents,[49] and even verification of feeding tube placement.[50]

$PaCO_2$-$P_{ET}CO_2$ GRADIENT

Normal subjects have a $PaCO_2$-$P_{ET}CO_2$ gradient of 4 to 5 mm Hg.[36,38,42,51-55] In critically ill patients, the $PaCO_2$-$P_{ET}CO_2$ gradient can be markedly elevated, with a tendency toward wider gradients in obstructive lung diseases (7 to 16 mm Hg)[41,42,52] than in acute lung injury or cardiogenic pulmonary edema (4 to 12 mm Hg).[41,42,56-58] A strong correlation between $\Delta P_{ET}CO_2$ and $\Delta PaCO_2$ (r = 0.82), along with minor bias and reasonable precision between $P_{ET}CO_2$ and $PaCO_2$, suggests that arterial blood gas monitoring may not be needed to assess ventilation unless the $\Delta P_{ET}CO_2$ exceeds 5 mm Hg.[43] Yet several studies found that the $\Delta P_{ET}CO_2$ often falsely predicts the degree and direction of $\Delta PaCO_2$.[53-55,58] Therefore, despite $P_{ET}CO_2$ monitoring, routine arterial blood gas analysis is still required in critically ill patients.

Several factors determine the $PaCO_2$-$P_{ET}CO_2$ gradient. Whereas $PaCO_2$ reflects the mean partial pressure of CO_2 in alveolar gas (P_ACO_2), $P_{ET}CO_2$ approximates the peak P_ACO_2.[59] During expiration, lung regions with high ventilation-to-perfusion ratios dilute the mixed CO_2 concentration so that $P_{ET}CO_2$ is usually lower than $PaCO_2$.[60] However, when CO_2 production is elevated (or expiration is prolonged), $P_{ET}CO_2$ more closely resembles mixed venous PCO_2, as a higher amount of CO_2 diffuses into a progressively smaller lung volume.[59] Thus, the $PaCO_2$-$P_{ET}CO_2$ gradient can be affected by changes in respiratory rate and tidal volume (V_T), owing to alterations in expiratory time, and by CO_2 production and mixed venous CO_2 content.[59] In fact, it is not uncommon for $P_{ET}CO_2$ to exceed $PaCO_2$.[60] Inotropic or vasoactive drugs may affect the $PaCO_2$-$P_{ET}CO_2$ gradient in an unpredictable manner, either by increasing cardiac output and pulmonary perfusion (thereby reducing alveolar deadspace) or by reducing pulmonary vascular resistance and magnifying intrapulmonary shunt by countering hypoxic pulmonary vasoconstriction.[53]

In addition, mechanical factors can cause either inconsistencies or inaccuracies in $P_{ET}CO_2$. The sample tubing length and aspirating flow rates used in sidestream capnometers affect the time required to measure changes in tidal CO_2 concentration.[61] At frequencies above 30, capnometers tend to underreport the true $P_{ET}CO_2$.[62] This may occur because of gas mixing between adjacent breaths during transport down the sampling line and in the analysis chamber.[62] This problem can be avoided with mainstream analyzers, which provide near-instantaneous CO_2 measurement (<250 msec).[63]

$PaCO_2$-$P_{ET}CO_2$ GRADIENT, POSITIVE END-EXPIRATORY PRESSURE, AND LUNG RECRUITMENT

PEEP recruits collapsed alveoli, improves ventilation-perfusion matching, and reduces alveolar deadspace, although excessive levels cause overdistention and increased alveolar deadspace.[64] Because the $PaCO_2$-$P_{ET}CO_2$ gradient correlates strongly with the physiologic deadspace–to–tidal volume ratio (V_D/V_T),[44,45] it may be useful in titrating PEEP in acute respiratory distress syndrome (ARDS). An animal model of ARDS found that the stepwise application of PEEP progressively reduced the $PaCO_2$-$P_{ET}CO_2$ gradient and coincided with maximal or near-maximal improvements in oxygenation.[56] However, PEEP applied beyond the lowest $PaCO_2$-$P_{ET}CO_2$ gradient caused a secondary rise in the gradient, along with decreased cardiac output. Although a subsequent trial was unable to reproduce these findings in humans,[57] another study found that the $PaCO_2$-$P_{ET}CO_2$ gradient narrowed (14 to 8 mm Hg) and oxygenation improved when PEEP was set at the lower inflection point of the pressure-volume curve.[40] When PEEP was set 5 cm H_2O above the lower inflection point, the $PaCO_2$-$P_{ET}CO_2$ gradient rose to 11 mm Hg, and cardiac output trended downward. In patients without a lower inflection point, the $PaCO_2$-$P_{ET}CO_2$ gradient did not change in response to PEEP. Thus, in a subset of ARDS patients, the $PaCO_2$-$P_{ET}CO_2$ gradient may be an effective way to titrate PEEP.

$P_{ET}CO_2$ MONITORING DURING CARDIOPULMONARY RESUSCITATION

Monitoring end-tidal CO_2 concentration is a reliable method for evaluating the effectiveness of cardiopulmonary resuscitation.[65] In animal models, $P_{ET}CO_2$ is strongly correlated with coronary perfusion pressure and successful resuscitation,[66] whereas in humans, changes in $P_{ET}CO_2$ are directly proportional to changes in cardiac output.[67] $P_{ET}CO_2$ during precordial compressions can distinguish successful from unsuccessful resuscitation, with values greater than 10 mm Hg[68] or greater than 16 mm Hg[69] associated with successful resuscitation.

MEASUREMENT OF DEADSPACE VENTILATION

Ventilation-perfusion abnormalities are the primary physiologic disturbance in nearly all pulmonary diseases and the principal mechanism for elevated $PaCO_2$.[70] Deadspace ventilation (V_D), the portion of V_T that does not encounter perfused alveoli, directly impacts CO_2 excretion and is used as an indirect measure of ventilation-perfusion abnormalities. Physiologic V_D represents the summation of anatomic-(conducting airway) and nonperfused alveolar components. Clinically, physiologic V_D/V_T is used to assess the severity of pulmonary disease and the efficacy of ventilator manipulations.

Physiologic V_D/V_T typically is measured during a 3- to 5-minute exhaled gas collection into a 30- to 60-L Douglas bag. An arterial blood gas reading is obtained during the midpoint of the collection. V_D/V_T is calculated using the Enghoff modification of the Bohr equation, whereby the difference between $PaCO_2$ (a surrogate for the mean P_ACO_2)

and mean expired CO_2 tension ($PECO_2$) is divided by $PaCO_2$:

$$\frac{V_D}{V_T} = \frac{(PaCO_2 - PECO_2)}{PaCO_2}.$$

The deadspace volume per breath or per minute can be determined by multiplying V_D/V_T by the simultaneously measured average V_T or minute ventilation ($\dot{V}E$)[71]:

$$V_D = \frac{(PaCO_2 - PECO_2)}{PaCO_2} \times V_T \text{ or } \dot{V}_D = \frac{(PaCO_2 - PECO_2)}{PaCO_2} \times \dot{V}E$$

By subtracting the physiologic V_D per minute from the $\dot{V}E$, the alveolar minute ventilation ($\dot{V}A$) is obtained ($\dot{V}A = \dot{V}E - \dot{V}D$). $\dot{V}A$ also can be calculated as the volume production of CO_2 per minute ($\dot{V}CO_2$) divided by the $PaCO_2$[71]:

$$\dot{V}A = \frac{\dot{V}CO_2}{PaCO_2} \times 0.863$$

Expired gas collection with a Douglas bag is the classic method for measuring V_D/V_T. However, the gas collection system requires additional valving and connectors, making the procedure time-consuming and awkward. Metabolic monitors produce equally accurate, reliable results and are less cumbersome.[72,73] In addition, newer monitors incorporating capnography and pneumotachygraphy now provide accurate single-breath determinations of V_D/V_T.[74]

A significant source of measurement error is the contamination of expired gas with circuit compression volume.[75] During positive-pressure ventilation, part of the V_T is compressed in the circuit, and during expiration, this gas mixes with CO_2-laden gas from the lungs. The dilution of the expired CO_2 results in a falsely elevated V_D/V_T that is directly proportional to the peak inspiratory pressure and circuit compliance. Clinically, correcting V_D/V_T for compression volume is done by multiplying the measured $PECO_2$ by the ratio of the ventilator-set V_T to the V_T delivered to the patient.[76] This requires determination of the ventilator circuit compliance.

Clinically, V_D/V_T may assist in the management of pulmonary disease in terms of both ventilator adjustments and diagnostic testing. Suter and colleagues found that V_D/V_T decreased as the lung was recruited but increased with lung overdistention during PEEP titration in ARDS.[64] Fletcher and Jonson used V_D/V_T to optimize V_T and inspiratory time settings during general anesthesia.[77] Measuring V_D/V_T may assist in identifying patients who can be removed from mechanical ventilation. Hubble and coworkers found that values less than 0.50 predicted successful extubation, and values greater than 0.65 identified patients at risk for post-extubation respiratory failure.[74]

One of the main clinical uses of V_D/V_T is to aid in the diagnosis of acute pulmonary embolism. V_D/V_T is comparable to radioisotopic lung scanning in detecting acute pulmonary embolism, with a value less than 0.40 suggesting that a significant embolus is improbable.[78] Single-breath estimates of alveolar V_D are also capable of identifying patients with pulmonary embolus.[79] Recently, increased physiologic V_D/V_T (>0.60) was found to be significantly associated with mortality in patients with ARDS[80] and in neonates with congenital diaphragmatic hernia.[81] In particular, the findings that V_D/V_T is elevated early in the course of ARDS and is associated with increased mortality may be particularly useful. The efficacy of new therapies for ARDS may be judged, in part, by their ability to reduce V_D/V_T.

ASSESSMENT OF PULMONARY MECHANICS

Assessment of pulmonary mechanics is crucial to monitoring pulmonary function during artificial ventilation. It requires the measurement of V_T, peak inspiratory flow rate, and four pressures: peak airway pressure, end-inspiratory plateau pressure, end-expiratory pressure in the circuit, and any occult end-expiratory pressure measured during an end-expiratory pause maneuver. From these variables, the compliance and resistance of the respiratory system are determined.

COMPLIANCE

Under conditions of passive mechanical ventilation, peak airway pressure denotes the total force necessary to overcome the resistive and elastic recoil properties of the respiratory system (i.e., both lungs and chest wall). Distinguishing the resistive from the elastic recoil–related pressures requires introduction of an end-inspiratory circuit occlusion after V_T delivery (Fig. 60-2).[82] During the end-inspiratory pause, peak airway pressure dissipates down to a stable plateau pressure. After a 3-second pause-hold, "quasi-static" conditions usually exist, so that the corresponding plateau pressure represents the elastic recoil pressure. Dividing the V_T by the plateau pressure (Pplat) minus the PEEP yields the "quasi-static" compliance of the respiratory system (Crs-stat).[83] Even at moderate levels of $\dot{V}E$ (>10 L/min), dynamic gas trapping frequently occurs,[84] so that Crs-stat should be based on the total PEEP (PEEPtot) measured during an end-expiratory pause rather than the PEEP applied at the airway:

$$Crs\text{-}stat = \frac{V_T}{Pplat - PEEPtot}$$

During patient-triggered ventilation, the assessment of pulmonary mechanics becomes uncertain. Clinically, the pause time is decreased to 0.5 to 1 second, to limit any potential artifact from spontaneous breathing efforts that may falsely raise or lower the plateau pressure.

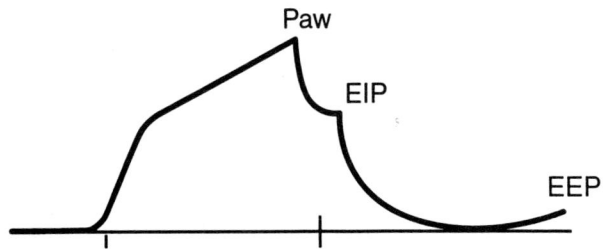

FIGURE 60–2. Depiction of a scalar (time) waveform of peak airway pressure (Paw) during constant volume mechanical ventilation with a square wave of inspiratory flow. As inspiration commences, the abrupt increase in flow against the resistance of the patient-ventilator circuit results in an immediate pressure step that is proportional to both the flow rate and the resistance. The slope in the pressure-time curve reflects the rate rise in alveolar pressure and provides qualitative information about the dynamic compliance of the respiratory system (lungs and chest wall). The introduction of an end-inspiratory pause-hold results in dissipation of Paw down to a stable end-inspiratory plateau pressure (EIP), which reflects the elastic recoil pressure of the respiratory system. Release of the pause-hold expels the tidal volume (V_T), and pressure is released down to the baseline end-expiratory pressure (EEP). Dividing V_T by EIP – EEP yields the quasi-static compliance of the respiratory system, whereas dividing the inspiratory flow rate by Paw – EIP yields the resistance of the respiratory system.

RESISTANCE

Respiratory system resistance (Rrs) is the ratio of driving pressure to flow[85] and is calculated as the difference between the peak airway pressure (Paw) and the end-inspiratory plateau pressure (Pplat) divided by the preocclusion peak inspiratory flow rate ($\dot{V}_I$) and expressed as cm H_2O/L per second[86]:

$$Rrs = \frac{Paw - Pplat}{\dot{V}_I}$$

Resistance is flow dependent, because the driving pressure necessary to overcome resistance increases disproportionately to changes in $\dot{V}_I$ (due to increased turbulence).[87] Therefore, respiratory system resistance can be accurately determined only with a constant inspiratory flow (square wave) pattern.[86] Because resistance is expressed as cm H_2O/L per second, a $\dot{V}_I$ of 60 L/min (1 L/sec) is a convenient setting to measure resistance, and it also happens to be a standard setting for patient comfort.

COMPLIANCE AND RESISTANCE IN NORMAL AND PATHOLOGIC CONDITIONS

In mechanically ventilated, normal patients, compliance is 57 to 85 mL/cm H_2O, and resistance is 1 to 8 cm H_2O/L per second.[88-90] Abnormalities in compliance and resistance in patients with acute respiratory failure are dependent on both the cause and the severity of the disease. Patients with ARDS or cardiogenic pulmonary edema tend to have a low compliance (35 or 44 mL/cm H_2O, respectively) and an elevated resistance (12 or 15 cm H_2O/L per second, respectively).[91] In contrast, patients with chronic airway obstruction tend to have both a higher compliance (66 mL/cm H_2O) and a higher resistance (26 cm H_2O/L per second).[91]

DYNAMIC GAS TRAPPING AND INTRINSIC POSITIVE END-EXPIRATORY PRESSURE

Dynamic gas trapping occurs whenever the expiratory time is less than 3.5 time constants (an exponential function defining the time required for volume or pressure equilibration across the respiratory system).[92] At end-expiration, if the respiratory system remains above its relaxed position, the elastic recoil pressure in the lung is positive. This is referred to as intrinsic PEEP.[93] Intrinsic PEEP is measured by an end-expiratory circuit occlusion whereby, after a normal expiratory time elapses, both the inspiratory and expiratory ventilator valves close for 3 to 5 seconds, allowing alveolar pressure to equilibrate with airway pressure (Fig. 60-3).[94,95] This pressure represents an average intrinsic PEEP throughout the lungs[94,96] and underestimates the peak end-expiratory alveolar pressure, because some volume egresses into the circuit.[94] Intrinsic PEEP is common in mechanically ventilated patients with various lung diseases. Patients with ARDS or cardiogenic pulmonary edema tend to have markedly lower levels of intrinsic PEEP (3 to 4 cm H_2O) compared with patients with chronic obstructive lung diseases (14 cm H_2O).[91]

Different degrees of intrinsic PEEP may coexist in the lungs because of regional variations in time constants.[95,96] Comparing dynamic measurements of intrinsic PEEP with static measurements provides a gross indication of time

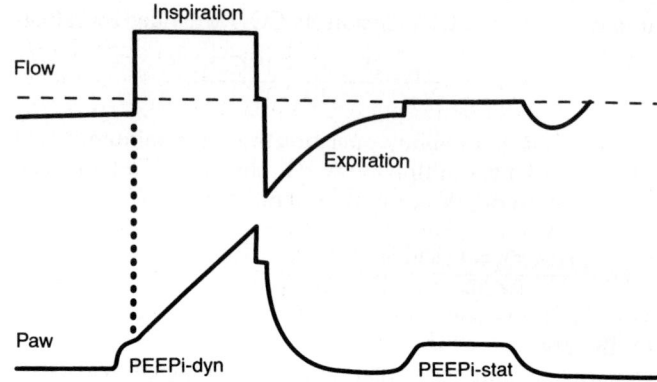

FIGURE 60–3. Simultaneous scalar waveforms of flow and peak airway pressure (Paw) illustrate the clinical measurement and separation of dynamic from static measurements of intrinsic positive end-expiratory pressure (PEEPi). Dynamic measurements reflect the lowest level of PEEPi in the respiratory system and are measured as the positive Paw just before inspiratory flow begins. The maximal level of PEEPi is the pressure plateau measured during an end-expiratory pause-hold.

constant inhomogeneity and intrinsic PEEP variation within the lungs.[95] Dynamic measurements are based on the fact that inspiratory flow does not begin until airway pressure exceeds total PEEP.[93,95] By using waveform graphics, the airway pressure above applied PEEP (just before inspiratory flow begins) represents the minimal level of total PEEP in the respiratory system (see Fig. 60-3).[95]

PRESSURE-VOLUME CURVES

The static pressure-volume relationship is used to analyze the elastic properties of the respiratory system and to guide mechanical ventilation in ARDS.[97] Pressure-volume (P-V) curves usually have a sigmoidal shape (Fig. 60-4). When inflation begins below functional residual capacity (FRC), there is relatively little volume change as transpulmonary pressure increases. This is referred to as the "starting compliance" and corresponds to the first 250 mL of volume change.[98] It reflects either the relatively high pressure required to overcome small airway closure in the dependent lung zones[99] or the relatively small area of aerated lung tissue as

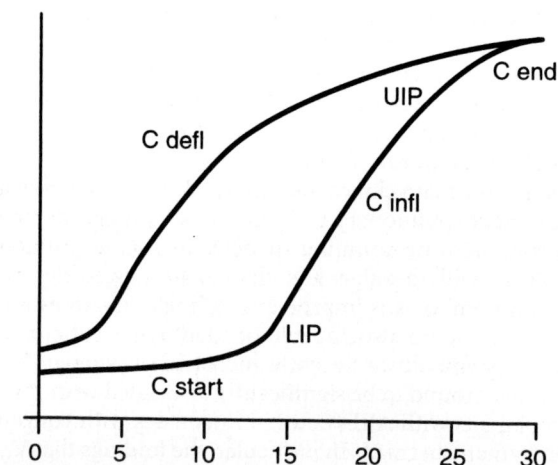

FIGURE 60–4. Static pressure-volume relationship (curve) of the respiratory system depicted from below functional residual capacity to total lung capacity. Cdefl, deflation compliance; Cend, end compliance; Cinfl, inflation compliance; Cstart, starting compliance; LIP, lower inflection point; UIP, upper inflection point.

inflation commences.[98] Typically, this low compliance segment in the P-V curve is followed by an abrupt slope change with a concave appearance that is termed the lower inflection point,[100] or "Pflex."[101] A common interpretation of the lower inflection point is that it signifies an abrupt reopening of collapsed peripheral airways and alveoli.[97,99-101] Above the lower inflection point, the P-V curve becomes linear and is referred to as the "inflation compliance."[102] As the total lung capacity is approached, compliance decreases and the P-V curve becomes convex (bow shaped). This is referred to as "end compliance"[102] and is thought to signify the loss of distensibility at maximal inflation.[99] The zone at which inflation compliance transforms to end compliance is referredto as the upper inflection point.[102] As the lung is deflated, the linear portion of the curve is referred to as the "deflation compliance," or "true physiologic compliance," as it represents the elastic properties of the lung after full recruitment.[103] As lung deflation proceeds below FRC, an inflection point often occurs that represents small airway closure.[103] On the deflation limb, airway closure occurs at a lower pressure because the minimal force necessary to maintain patent airways is less than the pressure needed to recruit collapsed ones.[104]

Pressure-Volume Curve Construction

There are two general approaches for measuring the P-V curve: the step method[102] and the pulse method.[105] In the step method, the chest is passively inflated (and then deflated) in small-volume steps with a calibrated supersyringe over a volume range of 1.5 to 2 L. P-V curve measurements require a short-acting neuromuscular blocking agent and sedation to ensure complete passive ventilation. Generally, the patient's lung volume history is standardized with several deep inflations. Afterward, the patient is disconnected from the ventilator for 5 seconds to ensure that the relaxed elastic recoil volume is reached. Then the patient is connected to a calibrated supersyringe filled with 100% oxygen and connected to a pressure manometer. Volume steps of 100 mL are used to inflate the chest, and the system pressure is measured after a 2- to 3-second pause, to allow for resistive pressure dissipation.[104] Inflation continues until either a volume of 1.5 to 2 L is delivered or a maximum pressure of 40 to 50 cm H_2O is reached.[102] Deflation of the chest is accomplished in the same stepwise fashion back to its relaxed volume. The entire procedure usually requires 60 to 90 seconds.[100] Volume steps are plotted against the corresponding static pressure points on graph paper to obtain the curve. Respiratory system compliance is the slope of the inflation and deflation curves between volumes of 0.5 and 1 L.[100]

The pulse method is based on the principle that when a low, constant flow of gas is injected into the lungs, volume change is proportional to time, so that direct volume measurement is unnecessary.[106] The technique requires either a calibrated oxygen flowmeter with sufficient pressure or ventilator manipulation. However, the inspiratory flow rate must be low enough (≤10 L/min) to minimize resistive pressures.[107] This may be problematic when a ventilator is used, because the rate, V_T, and inspiratory time adjustments required to achieve a flow of 10 L/min or less will be limited by the lowest preset rate and the longest inspiratory duty cycle.

Determination of Lower and Upper Inflection Points

In clinical practice, the lower inflection point of the inflation limb is usually determined by the graphic technique

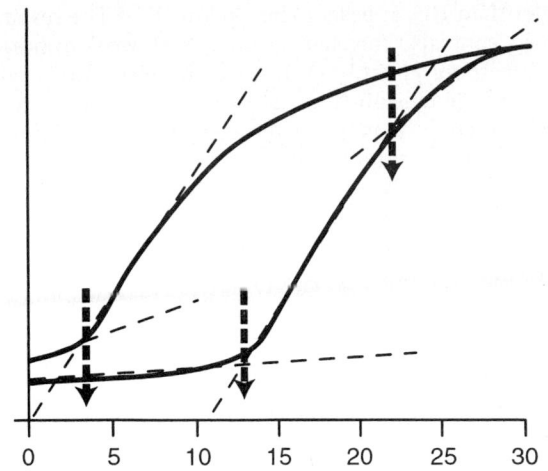

FIGURE 60–5. Graphic technique for determining the lower and upper inflection points of the pressure-volume curve. Tangents are drawn, extending the slopes of the various compliance segments of the curve. Where the tangents intersect, a third tangent is dropped down to the horizontal axis (arrows).

(Fig. 60-5).[97] First a tangent is drawn extending the slope of the starting compliance. Another tangent is drawn extending the slope of the inflation compliance down toward the horizontal axis. Where the two tangents intersect, a third tangent is drawn down to the horizontal axis, and this point is considered the lower inflection point. The same technique can be used to determine the upper inflection point on the inflation limb, as well as the deflation limb's lower inflection point. Typically, PEEP is set 2 cm H_2O above the lower inflection point to ensure optimal lung recruitment,[97] and V_T is set below the upper inflection point to prevent lung injury from excessive stretch.[108]

ASSESSMENT OF BREATHING PATTERN, STRENGTH, AND CENTRAL DRIVE

RATE AND TIDAL VOLUME

Basic assessment of the respiratory pattern includes the measurement of respiratory rate and V_T. A normal respiratory rate is 12 to 24 breaths/min, and mechanical ventilation is generally indicated when it exceeds 35.[109] A V_T of 5 mL/kg is considered sufficient to maintain unassisted breathing.[110] Tachypnea is often the earliest sign of impending respiratory failure, even when arterial blood gases remain within normal limits.[111] This may reflect the fact that muscle fatigue (which results from a mechanical workload that exceeds the power capacity of the ventilatory muscles) occurs before overt ventilatory pump failure.[112] Experimentally, adaptation of a rapid-shallow breathing pattern follows the onset of fatigue.[113]

Of particular interest is the utility of breathing pattern in assessing the feasibility of weaning from mechanical ventilation. Typically, patients who fail to wean are more tachypneic (respiratory rate >32) and have an abnormally low V_T (<200 mL).[114] The respiratory rate–V_T ratio is an elegant method to evaluate weaning. Using a threshold of less than 105, this ratio has both a high positive predictive value (0.78) and a negative predictive value (0.95) for the ability to maintain unassisted breathing.[115] Although the utility of the respiratory rate–V_T ratio has been confirmed by other studies,[116,117] the original negative predictive value, at a cutoff greater than 105, appears to be too low.[117,118] The respiratory rate–V_T ratio also correlates strongly with work of breathing and breathing effort.[119,120] In fact, the respiratory rate–V_T ratio and the tension-time index of the ventilatory muscles are considered the major pathophysiologic determinants of the successful transition from ventilator dependence to unassisted breathing. This suggests that, in general, sophisticated bedside work-of-breathing measurements are unnecessary for evaluating the feasibility of weaning. In fact, the efficacy of the respiratory rate–V_T ratio may obviate the need to routinely measure other weaning variables.

MAXIMAL INSPIRATORY PRESSURE

Maximal inspiratory pressure (MIP) reflects the force reserve of the inspiratory muscles. Normal subjects making voluntary inspiratory efforts against an occluded airway can generate a MIP of approximately –90 cm H_2O.[121] In patients recovering from respiratory failure, successful weaning has generally been associated with a MIP greater than –30 cm H_2O.[122] Although MIP is not as useful as the respiratory rate–V_T ratio in predicting weaning success (positive predictive value of 0.58), a value more positive than –20 cm H_2O has a negative predictive value of 1.[115] MIP is useful in determining whether a patient's inability to tolerate weaning trials can be explained by weakness. In particular, patients with suspected dynamic hyperinflation should have MIP measured over approximately 10 efforts (or 20 seconds) with directional values in place, so that each effort takes place from a lung volume at or below normal FRC.[123] This should improve the force-length relationship of the inspiratory muscles and help determine whether weakness can be attributed to a geometric disadvantage of muscles (secondary to hyperinflation) or whether there is a biochemical or histologic component. In particular, the clinician should observe whether the MIP can be sustained for several seconds or the pressure rapidly decays. We have observed that regardless of the value obtained, a MIP that quickly dissipates is common among ventilator-dependent patients and may be indicative of inadequate energy reserves.

CENTRAL VENTILATORY DRIVE

An important aspect of monitoring breathing pattern is the assessment of central ventilatory drive. Heightened drive increases the work of breathing during mechanical ventilation.[123] Next to respiratory rate, the most important clinical measure of central ventilatory drive is the inspiratory occlusion pressure 100 msec after the onset of effort ($P_{0.1}$). Briefly occluding the airway at the onset of inspiratory effort results in isometric contraction of the inspiratory muscles, so that $P_{0.1}$ is independent of respiratory system mechanics.[124] Measuring airway pressure at 100 msec indirectly reflects efferent motor neuron output. An increasing stimulus to the inspiratory muscles causes a more forceful contraction, with a proportional increase in pressure development. The selection of 100 msec is based on the fact that conscious or nonconscious perception of (and response to) sudden load changes requires approximately 250 msec.[125] It is convenient that during mechanical ventilation, the lag associated with the trigger phase provides sufficient time to measure $P_{0.1}$.[126]

Some ventilators[127] and pulmonary mechanics monitors[128] now measure $P_{0.1}$. Experimentally, $P_{0.1}$ has been used for closed-loop control of pressure support levels during weaning from mechanical ventilation.[129]

At rest, $P_{0.1}$ is normally 0.8 cm H_2O and varies directly with $\dot{V}_E$,[130] whereas in patients with respiratory failure, it ranges from 2 to 6 cm H_2O, depending on the level of ventilatory support.[126,128,131-133] $P_{0.1}$ correlates highly with patient work of breathing, and changes in $P_{0.1}$ (which occur with ventilator adjustments) show a high degree of sensitivity and specificity for corresponding changes in patient work.[134,135] $P_{0.1}$ has been used to predict weaning and extubation success in patients recovering from acute respiratory failure. Levels exceeding 6 cm H_2O may predict weaning failure in chronic obstructive lung disease,[136] whereas a $P_{0.1}$ greater than 4 cm H_2O may presage failure in ARDS.[137] During brief trials of unassisted breathing, a $P_{0.1}$ greater than 7 cm H_2O tends to describe patients requiring total ventilatory support and has been reported as a cutoff level in patients who ultimately fail a trial of extubation.[138] $P_{0.1}$ values between 4 and 7 cm H_2O may indicate patients who can be managed with partial ventilatory support, whereas a value less than 4 cm H_2O may indicate patients no longer in need of mechanical assistance.[137]

A limitation of $P_{0.1}$ is that it dissociates from ventilatory drive when muscle weakness is present or hyperinflation alters the force-length relationship of the inspiratory muscles. In these situations, relating $P_{0.1}$ to MIP may provide a more accurate assessment of a patient's ability to sustain unassisted breathing. Evidence suggests that $P_{0.1}$/MIP ratios exceeding 0.15 describe patients requiring ventilatory support.[137,138]

ANNOTATED REFERENCES

Alberti A, Gallo F, Fongaro A, et al: P0.1 is a useful parameter in setting the level of pressure support ventilation. Intensive Care Med 1995;21:547-553.
This paper describes the potential use of P0.1, an indirect measurement of central respiratory drive and inspiratory effort, as a simple method for both titrating the level of mechanical ventilatory support and assessing weaning tolerance.

Falk JL, Rackow EC, Weil MH: End-tidal carbon dioxide concentration during cardiopulmonary resuscitation. N Engl J Med 1988;318:607-611.
This landmark paper introduced one of most important clinical applications of capnography: the monitoring of spontaneous circulation and the effectiveness of precordial compressions in the setting of cardiac arrest. A sudden rise in end-tidal CO2 concentration from approximately 1% to 3% (7 to 20 mm Hg) coincides with the return of spontaneous circulation.

Nuckton TJ, Alonso JA, Kallet RH, et al: Pulmonary dead-space fraction as a risk factor for death in acute respiratory distress syndrome. N Engl J Med 2002;346:1281-1286.
This study provides the first evidence that a pulmonary-specific variable can independently predict the risk of death in patients with ARDS. Deadspace fraction may prove to be a useful measurement by which to judge the efficacy of future therapies for ARDS.

Pepe PE, Marini JJ: Occult positive end-expiratory pressure in mechanically ventilated patients with airflow obstruction. Am Rev Respir Dis 1982;126:166-170.
This case series report introduced one of the most crucial concepts and monitoring imperatives of invasive mechanical ventilation. This description of the mechanics and clinical implications of dynamic hyperinflation remains one of the most lucid in the critical care and pulmonary literature.

Tremper KK, Barker SJ: Pulse oximetry. Anesthesiology 1989;70:98-108.
This paper remains one of the best written on the subject of pulse oximetry. It provides clinicians with an elegant discussion of the history, physics, engineering, and clinical aspects of this technology.

Chapter 61

PRINCIPLES OF GAS EXCHANGE

John J. Marini

IV

453

KEY POINTS

1. The **quantity of oxygen loaded onto the arterial bloodstream** per unit time (O_2 delivery, DO_2) is the product of the cardiac output and the oxygen contained within each milliliter of blood. Thus, a deficiency of either cofactor can be partially offset by a compensatory increase of the other.

2. **Hypoxemia** due to a relatively small number of lung units with very low $\dot{V}/\dot{Q}$ characteristics may not respond noticeably to oxygen therapy unless a very high FIO_2 is employed; however, it is possible to convert very poorly ventilated lung units into airless, unventilated units with inspired gas having a very high FIO_2, owing to replacement of unabsorbable nitrogen with absorbable oxygen (absorption atelectasis). **In the presence of shunt or very low $\dot{V}/\dot{Q}$ units,** however, the influence of mixed venous oxygen content may be profound, owing to its admixture with well-oxygenated pulmonary venous blood.

3. Because of the **hyperbolic relationship of $PaCO_2$ to alveolar ventilation,** relatively small changes of effective ventilation can profoundly influence $PaCO_2$ and pH when alveolar ventilation is low and $PaCO_2$ is high. Once $PaCO_2$ has climbed to approximately double its normal value, fluctuations of pH and $PaCO_2$, with their attendant adverse effects on hemodynamics and pulmonary artery pressure, place the critically ill patient at risk of blunted ventilatory drive.

4. The **expiratory capnogram** offers data of considerable clinical value when PCO_2 is plotted along a volume axis: it provides estimates for the "anatomic" (Fowler) deadspace, as well as for the mixed expired CO_2 concentration used in calculations of deadspace fraction and CO_2 production.

The primary purpose of the lung is to allow the respiratory gases, oxygen (O_2) and carbon dioxide (CO_2), to exchange freely between gas and blood. Unless otherwise compensated by adjustments of blood flow and cardiac output, failure to maintain arterial values of O_2 and CO_2 within tolerated physiologic limits interferes with effective cellular energy production, upsets the body's chemical balance, and, when severe, may be the proximate cause of lasting disability or death. The objective of this chapter is to review the principles of respiratory gas exchange across the lungs, with special reference to the setting of critical illness.

OXYGEN EXCHANGE

Most O_2 carried in the blood is bound reversibly to hemoglobin, with only a small quantity dissolved in plasma. Whereas O_2 binding by hemoglobin is essentially complete at a partial pressure (PaO_2) less than 150 mm Hg, depending on pH, temperature, and innate hemoglobin affinity, the dissolved fraction continues to rise linearly with increasing PaO_2. The equation relating blood O_2 content, expressed as milliliters per deciliter, to hemoglobin concentration ([Hgb], in g/dL), to O_2 saturation (a decimal fraction), and to PaO_2 is:

$$CaO_2 = 1.31 \bullet [Hgb]\, SaO_2 + 0.0031 \bullet PaO_2.$$

Except in extreme conditions under which hemoglobin is unable to bind O_2 (e.g., carbon monoxide intoxication, methemoglobinemia) or under which very severe anemia limits the hemoglobin bound O_2 fraction, dissolved O_2 accounts for a very small percentage of the total.[1] In fact, hemoglobin is such an effective carrier for O_2 that the quest to develop an effective blood substitute for clinical use has been only partially successful. Intravascularly delivered products based on stroma-free hemoglobin (an avid O_2 binder) and perfluorocarbon (an efficient dissolver of O_2) are potentially effective but have encountered problems with stability, toxicity, and cost.[2] For the present, blood substitutes must be considered impractical for the clinical setting.

OXYGEN DELIVERY

Metabolizing tissues require an adequate supply of O_2 to efficiently produce the energy needed for cellular function. The quantity of O_2 loaded onto the arterial bloodstream per unit time (O_2 delivery, DO_2) is the product of the cardiac output and the O_2 contained within each milliliter of blood. Therefore, a deficiency of either cofactor can be partially offset by a compensatory increase of the other. Conversely, sluggish blood flow, whether caused by low cardiac output or high resistance through the tissues, can limit the O_2 actually delivered to the cell. Increased blood viscosity impedes the transit of erythrocytes through the capillary bed, thereby acting to limit oxygen consumption (VO_2).[3] For this reason, paraproteinemia, extreme leukocytosis, and polycythemia can pose life-threatening challenges to O_2 consumption that are only partially explained by their impact on cardiac output.[3] Studies performed in animal models demonstrate that hematocrit (Hct), a primary determinant of viscosity, bears a nonlinear relationship to Do_2 that varies somewhat with circulating blood volume.[4] At low values of Hct a rising hemoglobin concentration predictably adds to O_2 content. Above an Hct of 30% to 34%, however, it is difficult to demonstrate in critically ill patients additional O_2 consumption or outcome benefit from increases of O_2 content that arise from further increments of hemoglobin.[5] At an Hct of 55% to 57%, Do_2 reaches its maximum in normal subjects, falling sharply with each further rise (Fig. 61-1). Above an Hct of approximately 65% phlebotomy may be required to avert a hemodynamic crisis, because vital tissues may be deprived of delivered O_2. Viscosity, and therefore tolerance for higher Hct, is partially determined by the circulating blood volume; the polycythemia associated with intravascular volume contraction is much less well tolerated than that of polycythemia vera.[3] As might be expected, patients with vascular disease are less tolerant to the adverse rheologic effects of high Hct.

At the mitochondrial level, O_2 acts as the terminal acceptor in a chain of organic electron donors known as the cytochromes. The Po_2 within the mitochondrion needed to sustain this process is very low—estimated to be much less than 1 mm Hg.[6] To provide that needed level of Po_2, an appropriate O_2 diffusion gradient must be established from the arterial blood, across tissue and cellular boundaries, and into the cellular organelles. At sea level, normal levels of mitochondrial O_2 are achieved at a PaO_2 of about 95 mm Hg. The actual Po_2 within the mitochondrion, however, is affected by many factors other than arterial Po_2, such as tissue metabolic rate, microvascular control, tissue properties, and blood flow. Over time, varying degrees of accommodation occur to subnormal PaO_2 by adjustments of the cardiovascular system, hemoglobin concentration, capillary system, and mitochondrial density.[7] Although this adaptive phenomenon is commonly observed in patients with chronic lung diseases, the extent to which accommodation to hypoxemia can occur and should be encouraged in patients who are critically ill is a provocative and largely unexplored question.

OXYGEN TRANSFER ACROSS THE LUNG

Oxygen is driven from the airspace to the pulmonary capillary by a diffusion gradient determined by the Po_2 difference between them and the resistance to diffusion presented by the intervening tissues and fluids. To keep the alveolar O_2 tension adequate, the O_2 supplied to the alveolus must be replaced at a rate equal to or greater than that at which the O_2 is removed by the passing capillary blood. Classically, six mechanisms can account for hypoxemia:

1. Low FIO_2
2. Hypoventilation
3. Impaired pulmonary diffusion capacity
4. Ventilation-perfusion ($\dot{V}/\dot{Q}$) imbalance
5. Shunt
6. Desaturation of pulmonary arterial (mixed venous) blood

Low FIO_2 is an important mechanism of hypoxemia occurring at altitude and in fires that occur in confined spaces. Although the relationship is not a linear function, as a rough estimate, inspired O_2 declines approximately 15 mm Hg for each 1000 meters of altitude above sea level.[8] For practical purposes, however, a lack of inspired O_2 does not account for hypoxemia occurring in the setting of critical illness. Hypoventilation alters the alveolar oxygen tension (PaO_2) in proportion to the rise of $PaCO_2$ (and $PaCO_2$) and becomes an important factor when it occurs during breathing of room air (as in narcotic overdose) or of relatively low inspired concentrations of supplemental O_2 (e.g., via nasal cannulae). The importance of impaired diffusion as a hypoxemic mechanism is sometimes debated, because the transfer of O_2 from alveolus to hemoglobin usually requires only a brief time for completion—somewhat less than the normal transit time of the erythrocyte through the capillary.[9] Yet, under many conditions that are commonly encountered, the rate at which blood flows through the lung is accelerated, diffusion distances are lengthened, and the O_2 driving gradient is reduced by disease. For this reason, impaired diffusion is likely to contribute to hypoxemia occurring in the stressed patient with critical illness who receives near-normal FIO_2.

$\dot{V}/\dot{Q}$ imbalance is the most common contributor to clinical hypoxemia, and perhaps the mechanism least well understood among practitioners. Here, it is the relative *distribution* of ventilation and perfusion that is critical to effective oxygenation. Ventilation must take place where perfusion does, or else the same levels of each that normally allow oxygenation and alveolar ventilation may produce both hypoxemia and wasted ventilation (ventilatory deadspace). With respect to impaired oxygenation, this concept is perhaps best understood by considering the PaO_2 to fall as a result of regional alveolar hypoventilation. Owing to the sigmoidal shape of the oxyhemoglobin dissociation curve, excess ventilation of normal alveoli cannot fully compensate for regional desaturation elsewhere, so that the net PaO_2 declines after blood from these two types of unit admix in the pulmonary venous blood. Like hypoxemia due to low FIO_2, hypoventilation, and diffusion impairment, hypoxemia resulting from $\dot{V}/\dot{Q}$ imbalance responds to supplementation of inspired O_2. Poor ventilation of a given lung unit can be compensated for by raising the O_2 concentration of the inspired gas it receives.

Whereas the relationship of FIO_2 to PaO_2 is more or less linear for the first three O_2-responsive mechanisms already covered, the response to O_2 supplementation for $\dot{V}/\dot{Q}$ imbalance depends on the distribution of abnormal $\dot{V}/\dot{Q}$ units contributing to the problem.[10] Hypoxemia due to a relatively small number of lung units with very low $\dot{V}/\dot{Q}$ characteristics may not respond noticeably to O_2 therapy unless a very high FIO_2 is employed. Conversely, a lung characterized by a large

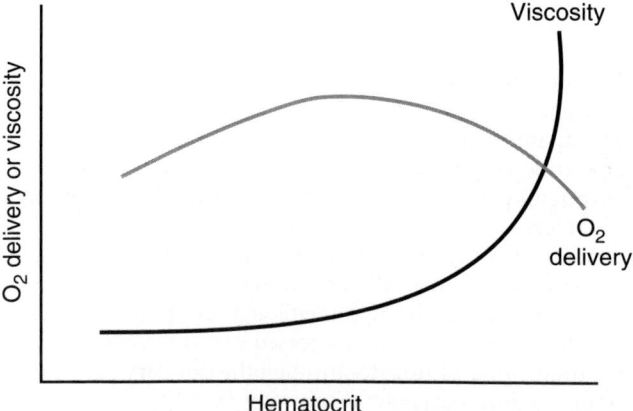

FIGURE 61-1. Effect of hematocrit on viscosity and oxygen delivery. Raising hematocrit simultaneously increases oxygen content and viscosity, which adversely affects blood rheology. Consequently, oxygen delivery reaches a maximum at hematocrit values in the upper mid range.

number of lung units with mild V̇/Q̇ impairment tends to respond in more linear fashion (Fig. 61-2). It is also possible to convert very poorly ventilated lung units into airless, unventilated units with inspired gas having a very high FiO₂, owing to replacement of unabsorbable nitrogen with absorbable O₂, leading to the unit's contraction and eventual collapse as this process continues below the closing volume of the compromised region (absorption atelectasis).[11] Unless compensation by hypoxic vasoconstriction is complete, raising FiO₂ can paradoxically increase shunt even as it improves O₂ transfer in units that remain patent.

Given the importance of matching blood flow to ventilation, it is not surprising that several mechanisms have developed to effect pulmonary microvascular regulation. Autonomic control, although less prominent and less precise than in the peripheral vasculature, is important nonetheless. Severe head injury, for example, can cause dysregulation and hypoxemia via this mechanism.[12] Local acidosis, such as that existing in poorly ventilated areas, tends to vasoconstrict the pulmonary arterial microvessels. The strength of this reflex, however, pales before that of hypoxic pulmonary vasoconstriction, which for most individuals is a well-developed protection against perfusing underventilated areas.[13] These mechanisms may be overpowered by pathologic processes or by pharmacologic interventions. For example, local release of inflammatory mediators or use of certain vasoactive drugs (e.g., nitroprusside) may counter these protective reflexes[14] and an abrupt rise of pulmonary artery pressure may overwhelm them.

Shunting occurs when venous blood is not brought into proximity with the inspired gas. Shunt can originate in the heart (e.g., through a patent communication at the atrial or ventricular level). Rarely, direct venous to arterial transfer occurs through microvascular or macrovascular defects known as pulmonary arteriovenous fistulas. Such communications are encountered in relatively common diseases, such as hepatic cirrhosis, as well as in other settings, exemplified by the heritable Osler-Weber-Rendu abnormality. Diseases that affect the lung parenchyma are much more common causes of shunt than these cardiovascular disorders. Filling of the airspaces with fluid (e.g., edema) or cellular infiltrate (e.g., pneumonia) prevents gas-blood contact. Inflammatory conditions may inhibit hypoxic vasoconstriction, worsening

arterial hypoxemia, as does hypocapnic alkalosis.[15] Collapse of lung units may occur at any anatomic scale, resulting in shunt through the affected regions. Causes for collapse vary from compression (e.g., by a pleural effusion), to disease-induced surfactant depletion or inactivation, to airway plugging by retained secretions. Sustained reversal of atelectasis requires attention to the inciting cause as well as recruitment of the problem area by deep lung expansion. Pure O₂ breathing will not improve hypoxemia due to shunting. Conversely, reduction of FiO₂ in that setting will not cause shunt-related hypoxemia to worsen and may spare ventilated areas exposure to potentially toxic concentrations of inspired O₂ (Fig. 61-3).

Under normal circumstances, variations in mixed venous O₂ content do not influence PaO₂ perceptibly, because recharging of desaturated hemoglobin with O₂ takes place at the alveolar-capillary junction, even during exercise. In the presence of shunt or very low V̇/Q̇ units, however, the influence of mixed venous O₂ content may be profound, owing to its admixture with well-oxygenated pulmonary venous blood. Because mixed venous O₂ content is influenced primarily by the ratio of O₂ consumption to DO₂, hypoxemia may be at least partially alleviated by reducing O₂ demand or improving DO₂. The equation relating these variables, which is easily derived by rearrangement of the Fick equation for O₂, is:

$$S\overline{v}O_2 \approx SaO_2 - \dot{V}O_2/([Hgb][SaO_2] \bullet Q).$$

Online measurements of Sv̄O₂ with a fiberoptic Swan-Ganz catheter enable venous desaturation to be detected and monitored without effort.

RELATIONSHIP OF PO₂ TO BLOOD O₂ CONTENT

Even though the oxyhemoglobin dissociation relationship is implicitly used for clinical decision making, many practitioners do not fully understand important nuances (Fig. 61-4). Over the clinically relevant range, the oxyhemoglobin dissociation

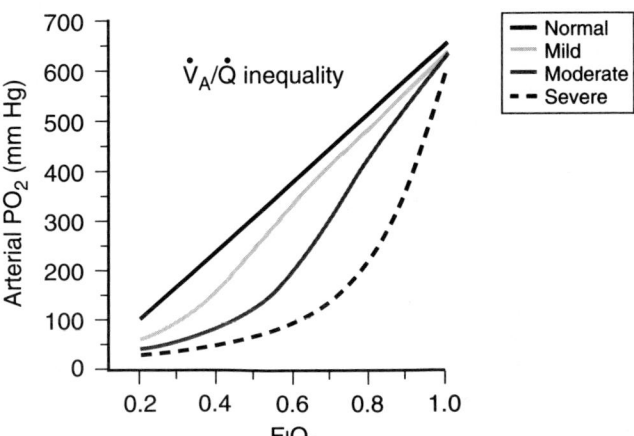

FIGURE 61-2. Influence of severity of V̇/Q̇ on the FiO₂ to arterial PO₂ relationship. Arterial PO₂ rises linearly in normal and mildly affected lungs, whereas very high inspired oxygen fractions may be necessary to raise arterial PO₂ when the V̇/Q̇ abnormality is severe.

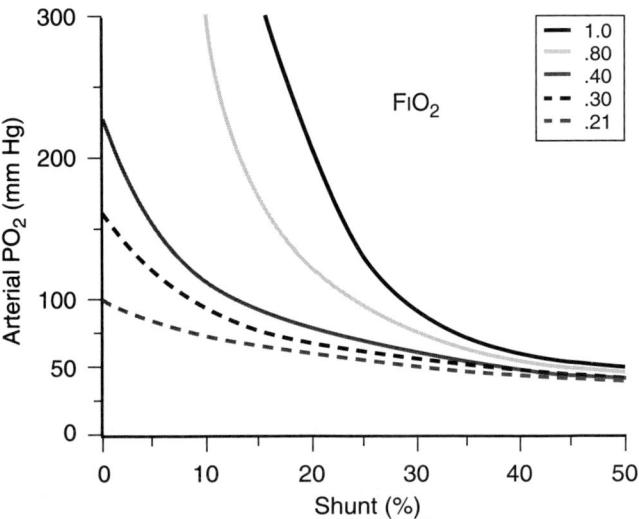

FIGURE 61-3. Effect of shunt percentage on arterial PO₂ for a range of FiO₂. When shunt percentage exceeds 35% to 40%, variations of FiO₂ only modestly affect arterial PO₂. Moreover, because the risk of oxygen toxicity rises hyperbolically with inspired oxygen concentration, reductions of FiO₂ from 1.0 to 0.8 may yield benefit with only marginal impact on arterial oxygenation.

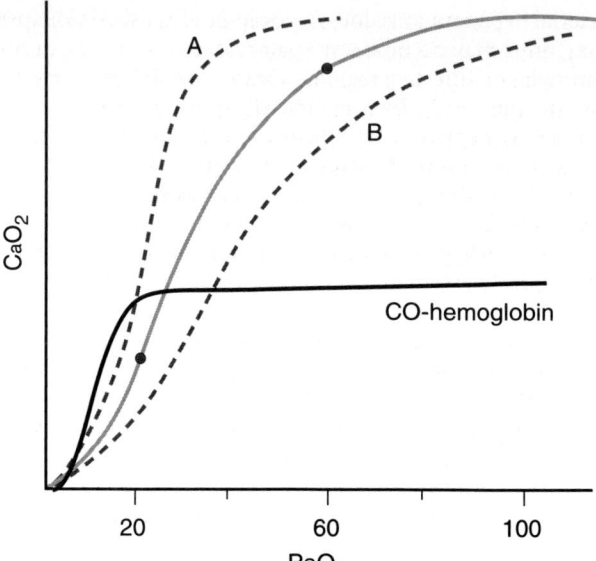

FIGURE 61–4. Relationship of PaO_2 to blood oxygen content (CaO_2). The oxyhemoglobin dissociation curve normally plateaus at a PO_2 of approximately 100 mm Hg *(upper solid line)*. Alkalosis and hyperthermia (A) shift the relationship up and to the left, whereas acidosis and hyperthermia (B) shift it downward to the right. Carbon monoxide causes tighter binding of oxygen to hemoglobin but reduces the capacity of hemoglobin to bind oxygen.

curve is highly nonlinear, so that a drop of a few percentage points in SaO_2 over the 95% to 100% interval reflects a much larger change in PaO_2 than does a similar decrement that occurs over the 80% to 85% interval. Pulse oximeters record the relative absorption of light by oxyhemoglobin and deoxyhemoglobin. Therefore, for a fixed value of viable hemoglobin, the saturation parallels its relative O_2 content, but a high saturation guarantees neither its total O_2 content nor the adequacy of tissue DO_2. For example, a patient may have a "full" SaO_2 after inhaling a high concentration of carbon monoxide and, yet, directly measuring arterial O_2 *content* per deciliter of blood (e.g, using a co-oximeter) may demonstrate profound arterial O_2 depletion (see Fig. 61-4). Moreover, a patient in circulatory shock may maintain a perfectly normal SaO_2 despite serious O_2 privation. Because cyanide blocks the uptake of O_2 by the tissues, O_2 consumption is low, even as arterial and mixed venous saturations remain normal or increased. It is occasionally forgotten that SaO_2 bears no direct relationship to the adequacy of ventilation; a patient breathing a high inspired concentration of O_2 will maintain a nearly normal SaO_2 for a brief period in the presence of a full respiratory arrest.

DELIVERY DEPENDENCE OF OXYGEN CONSUMPTION

Controversy has surrounded the concept of supply dependency of O_2 consumption for patients having sustained trauma, massive surgery, or sepsis. Prognosis in these conditions is somewhat better for critically ill patients in whom higher DO_2 is manifest. By inference, it has been suggested that in these settings supranormal DO_2 is needed to satisfy the O_2 demands of certain vital organs.[16] Whereas there is little doubt that prompt and vigorous resuscitation must be carried out[17] or that patients who do not spontaneously generate sufficient DO_2 or who cannot extract O_2 effectively have a worse

prognosis than other patients undergoing the same stress who do, it is highly questionable whether attempts to sustain DO_2 at supranormal values are well advised. Some data even suggest potential harm. Specific subgroups of surgical patients could, in fact, benefit, but there are no tightly controlled clinical trial data available to settle this question in either direction. Patients having sustained massive trauma or extensive surgery may represent a fundamentally different physiologic problem and respond more favorably than patients with medical crises. On the strength of a well-designed multicenter Italian trial,[18] it now seems clear that maintaining supranormal values for DO_2 confers no routine benefit for patients in the latter category. For nonmoribund patients with sepsis and/or acute respiratory distress syndrome (ARDS), supply dependency may not, in fact, exist. Without better evidence, therefore, maximizing VO_2 cannot be accepted as the primary target variable for circulatory support in patients admitted to the ICU. The data for patients with septic shock in the emergency department may be somewhat different, because there is evidence that they may benefit from therapies aimed at improving central $S\overline{v}O_2$ if applied in the period immediately after admission to the emergency department.[17]

ASSESSING THE EFFICIENCY OF OXYGEN EXCHANGE

Mean PAO_2 must first be computed to judge the efficiency of gas exchange across the lung. The ideal PAO_2 is obtained from the modified alveolar gas equation:

$$PAO_2 = PIO_2 - (PaCO_2/R) + [(PaCO_2 \times FIO_2 \times (1 - R)/R)]$$

where R is the respiratory exchange ratio and PIO_2 is the inspired O_2 tension, adjusted for FIO_2 and water vapor pressure at body temperature (47 mm Hg at 37°C).

Therefore,

$$PIO_2 = (barometric\ pressure - 47) \times FIO_2.$$

Under steady-state conditions, R normally varies from 0.7 to 1.0, depending on the mix of metabolic fuels (see later). When the same patient is monitored over time, R generally is assumed to be 0.8 or neglected entirely. Under most clinical conditions, the alveolar gas equation can be simplified to:

$$PAO_2 = PIO_2 - (1.25 \times PaCO_2)$$

For example, at sea level with a normally ventilated patient breathing room air:

$$PAO_2 = 0.21 \times (760 - 47) - 1.25 \times (PaCO_2)$$
$$= 150 - (1.25 \times 40)$$
$$\cong 100\ to\ 110\ mm\ Hg$$

Alveolar-Arterial Oxygen Tension Difference P(A-a)O₂

The difference between alveolar and arterial O_2 tensions, $P(A-a)O_2$, takes account of alveolar CO_2 tension, thereby eliminating hypoventilation and hypercapnia from consideration as the sole cause of hypoxemia. However, a single value of $P(A-a)O_2$ does not characterize the efficiency of gas exchange across all FIO_2 measurements, even in normal subjects. The $P(A-a)O_2$ normally ranges from ~10 mm Hg (on room air) to ~100 mm Hg (on an FIO_2 of 1.0). Moreover, PAO_2 changes nonlinearly with respect to FIO_2 as the extent of $\dot{V}/\dot{Q}$ mismatch increases. Thus, when the $\dot{V}/\dot{Q}$ abnormality is severe and nonhomogeneously distributed among gas exchanging units, the PAO_2 may vary little with FIO_2 until high fractions of inspired O_2 are given (see Fig. 61-2). Finally, the $P(A-a)O_2$ may be influenced by fluctuations in venous O_2 content.

Simplified Measures of Oxygen Exchange

Several pragmatic approaches have been taken to simplify bedside assessment of O_2 exchange efficiency. The first is to quantitate $P(A-a)O_2$ during the administration of pure O_2. After a suitable wash-in time (5 to 15 minutes depending on the severity of the disease), pure shunt accounts for the entire $P(A-a)O_2$. Furthermore, if hemoglobin is fully saturated with O_2, dividing the $P(A-a)O_2$ by 20 approximates shunt percentage (at $FIO_2 = 1$). As pure O_2 replaces alveolar nitrogen, some patent but poorly ventilated units may collapse—the process of absorption atelectasis.[11] Moreover, because shunt percentage is affected by changes in cardiac output and mixed $S\bar{v}O_2$, these simplified measures may give a misleading impression of changes within the lung itself.

The PaO_2/FIO_2 (or P/F) ratio is a convenient and widely used bedside index of O_2 exchange that attempts to adjust for fluctuating FIO_2. However, although simple to calculate, this ratio is affected by changes in $S\bar{v}O_2$ and does not remain equally sensitive across the entire range of FIO_2, especially when shunt is the major cause for admixture. Another easily calculated index of O_2 exchange properties, the PaO_2/PAO_2 (or "a/A") ratio, offers similar advantages and disadvantages as FIO_2 is varied. Like the P/F ratio, it is a useful bedside index that does not require blood sampling from the central circulation but loses reliability in proportion to the degree of shunting. Furthermore, in common with all measures that calculate an "ideal" PAO_2, even the a/A ratio can be misleading when fluctuations occur in the primary determinants of $S\bar{v}O_2$ (hemoglobin and the balance between O_2 consumption and delivery).

None of the indices discussed thus far accounts for changes in the functional status of the lung that result from alterations in positive end-expiratory pressure (PEEP), auto-PEEP, or other techniques for adjusting average lung volume (e.g., inverse ratio ventilation, lateral or prone positioning). If the objective is to categorize the severity of disease or to track the true O_2 exchanging status of the lung in the presence of such interventions, the P/F ratio falls short. The *oxygenation index* (OI) is shown as:

$$OI = PaO_2/(FIO_2 \times mean\ Paw).$$

This calculation takes the effects of PEEP and inspiratory time fraction into account, has gained widespread popularity in neonatal and pediatric practice, but has yet to catch hold in adult critical care. Although preferable, this index, too, is imperfect; mean airway pressure (Paw) and FIO_2 bear complex and alinear relationships to PaO_2 when considered across their entire ranges.

CO_2 EXCHANGE

PHYSIOLOGIC EFFECTS OF CO_2

For the major waste product of oxidative metabolism, CO_2 is a relatively innocuous gas. Apart from its key role in regulation of ventilation, the clinically important effects of CO_2 relate to changes in cerebral blood flow, pH, and adrenergic tone. Hypercapnia dilates the cerebral vessels and hypocapnia constricts them, a point of importance for patients with raised intracranial pressure. Acute increases in CO_2 depress consciousness probably as the result of intraneuronal acidosis. Slowly developing increases in CO_2 are well tolerated, presumably because buffering has time to occur. Nonetheless, a higher $PaCO_2$ signifies alveolar hypoventilation that tends to cause a decrease in alveolar and arterial PO_2. With hypoxemia and acidosis averted by supplemental O_2 and compensatory acidosis, some outpatients with $PaCO_2$ levels that chronically exceed 90 mm Hg continue to lead active lives. Conversely, patients with renal insufficiency lack the ability to buffer carbonic acid and tolerate hypercapnia poorly.

The adrenergic stimulation that accompanies acute hypercapnia causes cardiac output to rise and peripheral vascular resistance to increase. During acute respiratory acidosis these effects may have partially offset those of hydrogen ion on cardiovascular function, allowing better tolerance of pH than with metabolic acidosis of similar degree. Constriction of glomerular arterioles also occurs by adrenergic stimulation producing oliguria in some patients. Muscular twitching, asterixis, and seizures may be observed at extreme levels of hypercapnia in patients made susceptible by electrolyte or neural disorders. Prompted by a favorable experience with "permissive hypercapnia" (discussed elsewhere in this text) on important clinical outcomes of life-threatening asthma[19] and acute respiratory distress syndrome,[20] considerable attention has been directed toward the beneficial actions of CO_2 as an antioxidant and anti-inflammatory agent.[21,22] It is conceivable that in selected circumstances hypercapnia may not only be acceptable but also desirable.

The major cardiovascular effects of acute hypocapnia relate to alkalosis. Alkalosis adversely affects myocardial conduction, cellular energy kinetics, and neuronal function.[23] Abrupt lowering of $PaCO_2$ reduces cerebral blood flow and raises neuronal pH, altering cortical and peripheral nerve function. Lightheadedness, circumoral and fingertip paresthesia, and muscular tetany can result. Sudden major reductions of $PaCO_2$ (e.g., shortly after initiating mechanical ventilation) can produce life-threatening arrhythmias and seizures, albeit rarely. Because of the importance of adrenergic compensation for the vasodilatory effects of hypercapnic acidosis, hemodynamic manifestations of acute hypercapnia are more profound in the presence of beta- and/or alpha-adrenergic blockade.

CO_2 PRODUCTION AND STORAGE

The quantity of CO_2 produced for excretion is a function of O_2 consumption and any CO_2 that is liberated in the buffering of hydrogen ion. The metabolic exchange ratio, R, varies with the mix of metabolic fuels, with carbohydrate, protein, and fat associated with ratios of 1.0, 0.7, and 0.6, respectively. CO_2 is both more diffusible and more soluble than O_2, and most CO_2 carried in the blood is in dissolved form. A smaller but very significant proportion of CO_2 is bound within the erythrocyte as bicarbonate through the action of carbonic anhydrase. In passing through the lung it is evolved by the same enzyme.

Body stores of CO_2 are far greater than those of O_2. When breathing room air, only about 1.5 L of O_2 is stored (much of it in the lungs); and some of this stored O_2 remains unavailable for release until life-threatening hypoxemia is under way. Although breathing pure O_2 can fill the alveolar compartment with an additional 2 to 3 L of O_2 (a safety factor during apnea or asphyxia), these O_2 reserves are still much less than the approximately 120 L of CO_2 normally stored in body tissues. Because of limited O_2 reserves, PaO_2 and tissue PO_2 change rapidly during apnea, at a rate that is highly dependent on FIO_2.

CO_2 stores are held in several forms (dissolved, bound to protein, fixed as bicarbonate) and distributed in compartments that differ in their volumetric capacity and ability to exchange CO_2 rapidly with the blood.[24] Well-perfused organs constitute a small reservoir for CO_2 capable of quick turnover, skeletal muscle is a larger compartment with sluggish exchange, and bone and fat are high-capacity chambers with very slow filling and release. From a practical point of view, the existence of large CO_2 reservoirs with different capacities and time constants of filling and emptying means that equilibration to a new steady-state $PaCO_2$ after a step change in ventilation (assuming a constant rate of CO_2 production, VCO_2) takes longer than generally appreciated-especially for step *reductions* in alveolar ventilation (Fig. 61-5). With such a large capacity and only a modest rate of metabolic CO_2 production, the CO_2 reservoir fills rather slowly, so that $PaCO_2$ rises only 6 to 9 mm Hg during the first minute of apnea and 3 to 6 mm Hg each minute thereafter. Depletion of this reservoir can occur at a faster rate.

Measurement of CO_2 excretion is valuable for metabolic studies, computations of deadspace ventilation, and evaluation of hypercpnea. Estimates of CO_2 production are representative when the sample is collected carefully in the steady state over adequate time. The rate of CO_2 elimination is a product of minute ventilation (VE) and the expired fraction of CO_2 in the expelled gas. If gas collection is timed accurately and the sample is adequately mixed and analyzed, an accurate value for excreted CO_2 can be obtained. However, whether this value faithfully represents metabolic CO_2 production depends on the stability of the patient during the period of gas collection, not only with regard to VO_2 but also in terms of acid-base fluctuations, perfusion constancy, and ventilation status with respect to metabolic needs. During acute hyperventilation or rapidly developing metabolic acidosis, for example, the rate of CO_2 excretion overestimates metabolic

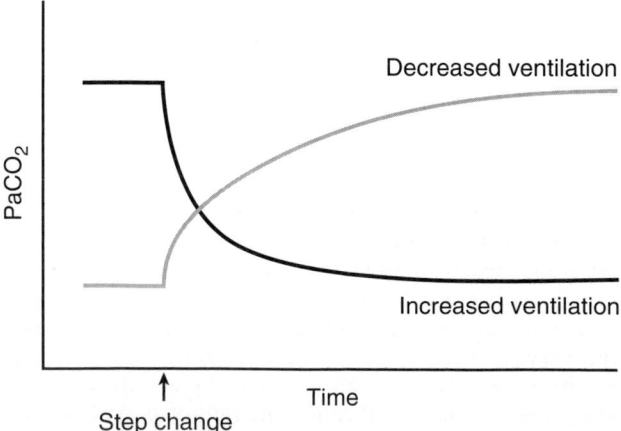

FIGURE 61–5. Effect of step changes of ventilation on $PaCO_2$. A stepped-increase in ventilation will cause $PaCO_2$ to fall in approximately exponential fashion. A stepped decrease in ventilation will cause $PaCO_2$ to approach equilibrium exponentially at a slower rate that is influenced by the magnitude of CO_2 storage capacity and CO_2 production.

rate until surplus body stores of CO_2 are washed out or bicarbonate stores reach equilibrium. The opposite obtains during abrupt hypoventilation or transient reduction in cardiac output.

EFFICIENCY OF CO_2 EXCHANGE

The volume of CO_2 produced by the body tissues varies with metabolic rate (e.g., fever, pain, agitation, sepsis). In the mechanically ventilated patient, many vagaries of CO_2 flux can be eliminated by controlling ventilation and quieting muscle activity with deep sedation with or without paralysis. $PaCO_2$ must be interpreted in conjunction with the VE. For example, the gas-exchanging ability of the lung may be unimpaired even though $PaCO_2$ rises when reduced alveolar ventilation is the result of diminished respiratory drive or marked neuromuscular weakness. As already noted, alveolar and arterial CO_2 concentrations respond quasi-exponentially after step changes in ventilation, with a half-time of about 3 minutes during hyperventilation but a slower half-time (16 minutes) during hypoventilation.[25] These differing time courses should be taken into account when sampling blood gases after making ventilator adjustments.

Deadspace

The physiologic deadspace (VD) refers to the "wasted" portion of the tidal breath that fails to participate in CO_2 exchange. A breath can fail to accomplish CO_2 elimination either because fresh (CO_2-free) gas is not brought to the alveoli or because fresh gas fails to contact systemic venous blood. Thus, tidal ventilation is wasted whenever CO_2-laden gas is recycled to the alveoli with the next tidal breath. Alternatively, a portion of the tidal volume is wasted if fresh gas distributes to inadequately perfused alveoli, so that CO_2-poor gas is exhausted during exhalation (Fig. 61-6). If this concept is understood, then it becomes clear why VD should not be considered as a composite of physical volumes. Nonetheless, wasted ventilation traditionally is characterized as the sum of the "anatomic" (or "series") dead space and the "alveolar" dead space. Because the airways fill with CO_2-containing alveolar gas at the end of the tidal breath, the physical volume of the airways corresponds rather closely to their contribution to wasted ventilation (the series or "anatomic" dead space), provided that mixed alveolar gas is similar in composition to the gas within a well-perfused alveolus. This is almost true for a quietly breathing normal subject, in whom the alveolar deadspace (poorly perfused alveolar volume) is negligible. When the parenchyma is well aerated and well perfused, the anatomic deadspace is relatively fixed at approximately 1 mL per pound (0.4 kg) of body weight.[26] (Patients with endotracheal tubes and tracheostomies have less series deadspace, whereas those with attached breathing apparatus may have more). Anatomic deadspace becomes an important concern at very low tidal volumes. For patients with lung disease that affects the lung parenchyma, and those ventilated at pressures that overinflate some lung units, alveolar deadspace predominates. Here, the lung is composed of well and poorly perfused units, so that the *mixed* alveolar gas within the airways at end exhalation has a CO_2 concentration lower than that of pulmonary arterial blood.

For normal subjects, deadspace increases with advancing age and body size and is reduced modestly by recumbency, extended breath holding, and decelerating inspiratory flow patterns. External apparatus attached to the airway that

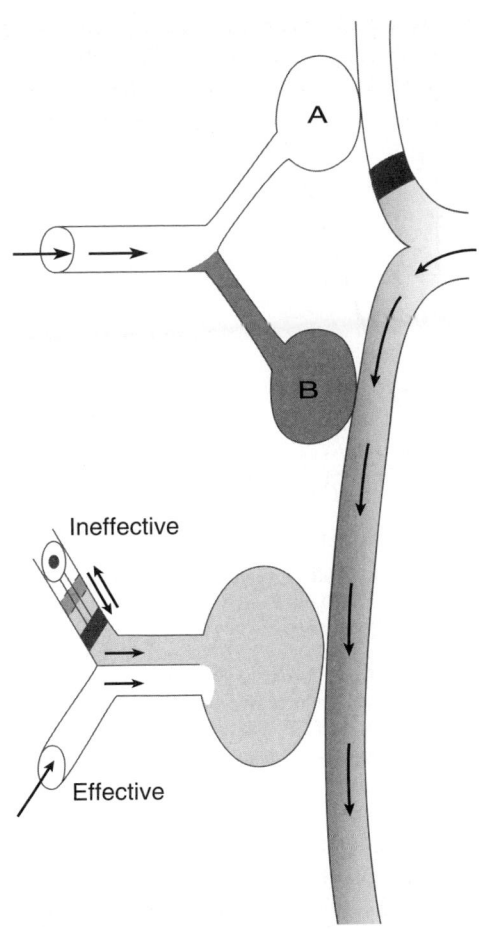

Ineffective

Effective

FIGURE 61–6. Concept of ventilatory deadspace. Wasted ventilation (deadspace) develops as the result of inadequate perfusion (alveolar compartment, A) or from the failure of ventilation to eliminate carbon dioxide from the conducting airways. In both instances efforts expended in ventilation do not result in effective CO_2 elimination from the affected lung units.

remains unflushed by fresh gas may add to the series deadspace, whereas tracheostomy reduces it. The supine position reduces deadspace by decreasing the average size of the lung and by increasing the number of well-perfused lung units.

Numerous diseases increase V_D. Destruction of alveolar septa, low output circulatory failure, pulmonary embolism, pulmonary vasoconstriction or vascular compression, and mechanical ventilation with high tidal volumes or PEEP are common mechanisms that often act in combination.

Deadspace Fraction

In the setting of parenchymal lung disease, deadspace varies in proportion to tidal volume over a remarkably wide range. Series deadspace tends to remain fixed but generally constitutes a small percentage of the total V_D, overwhelmed by the alveolar deadspace component. Therefore, except at very small tidal volumes, the *fraction* of wasted ventilation (V_D/V_T) tends to remain relatively constant as the depth of the breath varies. The deadspace fraction can be estimated from analyzed specimens of arterial blood and mixed expired ($P_{E}CO_2$) gas:

$$(V_D/V_T) = (PaCO_2 - P_{E}CO_2)/PaCO_2$$

where $P_{E}CO_2$ is the CO_2 concentration in mixed expired gas. (This expression is known as the Enghoff-modified Bohr

equation.) As already noted, $P_{E}CO_2$ can be determined on a breath-by-breath basis if exhaled volume is measured simultaneously. Alternatively, exhaled gas can be collected over a defined period. The P_{CO_2} of gas exiting a mixing chamber attached to the expiratory line provides a continuous "rolling average" value. In collecting the expired gas sample during pressurized ventilator cycles, an adjustment should be made for the volume of any sampled gas stored in the compressible portions of the ventilator circuit.

In healthy persons, the normal V_D/V_T during spontaneous breathing varies from 0.35 to 0.15, depending on the factors noted earlier (e.g., position, exercise, age, tidal volume, pulmonary capillary distention, breath holding). In the setting of critical illness, however, it is not uncommon for V_D/V_T to rise to values that exceed 0.7. Indeed, increased deadspace ventilation usually accounts for most of the increase in the V_E requirement and the CO_2 retention that occurs in the terminal phase of acute hypoxemic respiratory failure. High and increasing deadspace values may portend an adverse outcome in ARDS.[27] Conversely, improving deadspace has been reported as a propitious sign in prone positioning.[28] In addition to pathologic processes that increase deadspace, changes in V_D/V_T occur during periods of hypovolemia or overdistention by high airway pressures. This phenomenon often is apparent when progressive levels of PEEP are applied to support oxygenation. Conversely, recruitment of functioning lung tissue tends to reduce the deadspace fraction. Examination of the airway pressure tracing under conditions of controlled, constant inspiratory flow ventilation may demonstrate concavity or a clear point of upward inflection, indicating overdistention, accelerated deadspace formation, and escalating risk of barotrauma. Small reductions in PEEP or tidal volume may then dramatically reduce peak cycling pressure and V_D/V_T.

$PaCO_2$ is influenced by CO_2 production, minute ventilation, and the ventilatory deadspace according to the following equation:

$$PaCO_2 = (V_{CO_2}/V_A) \bullet 0.863.$$

In a different form:

$$PaCO_2 = P_B \times V_{CO_2}/[V_E(1 - V_D/V_T)].$$

where $PaCO_2$, V_A, and P_B refer to alveolar PCO_2, alveolar ventilation, and barometric pressure, respectively. In view of the hyperbolic relationship of $PaCO_2$ to alveolar ventilation (Fig. 61-7), it can be understood that relatively small changes of effective ventilation can profoundly influence $PaCO_2$ and pH when alveolar ventilation is low and $PaCO_2$ is high. Once $PaCO_2$ has climbed to approximately double its normal value, fluctuations of pH and $PaCO_2$, with their attendant adverse effects on hemodynamics and pulmonary artery pressure, place the critically ill patient at risk. Moreover, ventilatory drive is blunted when $PaCO_2$ values are increased. Conversely, small changes in ventilation may cause $PaCO_2$ to plummet. In this context it is interesting to consider tracheal gas insufflation, a novel technique in which fresh gas is injected near the carina during expiration so as to wash the proximal airway free of CO_2 and thereby improve ventilation efficiency.[29] In this setting of extreme hypercapnia, the improvement in alveolar ventilation proves valuable in reducing $PaCO_2$ and its attendant consequences.

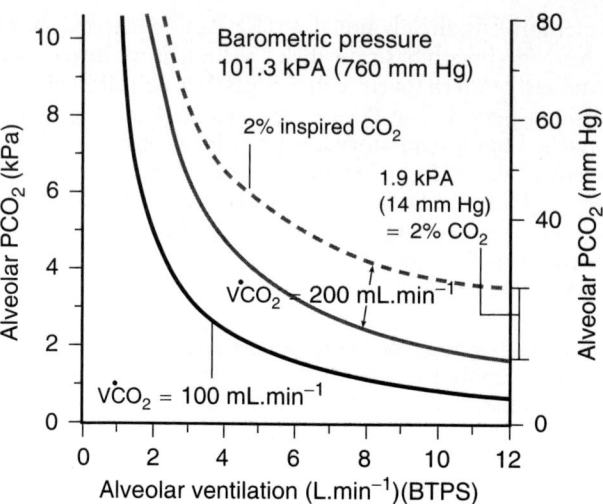

FIGURE 61–7. Relationship of alveolar ventilation and alveolar CO_2. Despite the varying conditions depicted, the hyperbolic function that relates them implies that small changes of effective ventilation translate into marked changes of alveolar PCO_2, and consequently of $PaCO_2$ and pH.

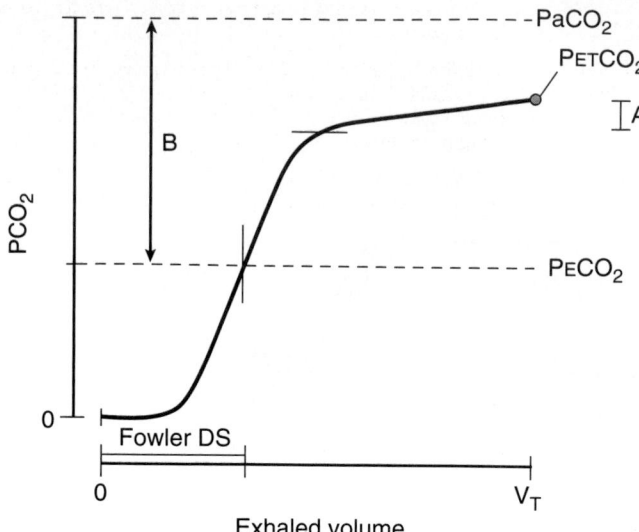

FIGURE 61–8. Capnogram with expired PCO_2 plotted against exhaled volume. Important data can be derived from the expired capnogram obtained under steady-state passive conditions: anatomic or "Fowler" deadspace; physiologic deadspace (the difference [B] between $PaCO_2$ and mixed expired CO_2 $PECO_2$, expressed as a fraction of $PaCO_2$); slope of the "alveolar plateau" (A), an indicator of the heterogeneity of ventilation; and an estimate of CO_2 production (obtained from the product of mixed expired CO_2 referenced to total barometric pressure and exhaled volume).

MONITORING OF EXHALED GAS

Capnography analyzes the CO_2 concentration of the expiratory air stream, plotting CO_2 concentration against time or, more usefully, against exhaled volume. After anatomic deadspace has been cleared, the CO_2 tension rises progressively to its maximal value at end exhalation, a number that reflects the CO_2 tension of mixed alveolar gas. For normal subjects, the transition between phases of the capnogram is sharp and, once achieved, the alveolar plateau rises only gently. Furthermore, when ventilation and perfusion are evenly distributed, as they are in healthy subjects, end-tidal PCO_2 ($PETCO_2$) closely approximates $PaCO_2$. ($PETCO_2$ normally underestimates $PaCO_2$ by 1 to 3 mm Hg.) This difference widens when ventilation and perfusion are matched suboptimally, so that alveolar deadspace gas admixes with CO_2-rich gas from well-perfused alveoli.

When plotted against a *volume* axis, as opposed to the more commonly encountered time axis, the capnogram offers data of considerable clinical value. Inspection of such tracings can yield estimates for the "anatomic" (Fowler) deadspace, as well as for the end-tidal and mixed expired CO_2 concentrations (Fig. 61-8). By knowing the barometric pressure, the mixed expired value can be expressed as a percentage of the exhaled volume, which is also immediately available from the tracing. If the VT remains constant, the product of the $PECO_2:PB$ ratio and VE is the VCO_2, and the mixed expired CO_2 concentration can be used in the Enghoff-modified Bohr equation to estimate the physiologic deadspace fraction.

As with other monitoring techniques, exhaled CO_2 values must be interpreted cautiously. The normal capnogram is composed of an ascending portion, a plateau, a descending portion, and a baseline. In disease, the sharp distinctions between phases of the capnogram, as well as the slopes of the composite segments, are blurred. Moreover, failure of the airway gas to equilibrate with gas from well-perfused alveoli invalidates $PETCO_2$ as a reflection of $PaCO_2$, especially as respiratory frequency fluctuates. (The $PECO_2$ per cycle, however,

remains valid.) End-tidal PCO_2 gives a low range estimate of $PaCO_2$ in virtually all clinical circumstances, so that a high $PETCO_2$ strongly suggests hypoventilation. Abrupt changes in $PETCO_2$ may reflect such acute processes as aspiration or pulmonary embolism, if the VE and breathing pattern (f, VT, and I:E ratio) remain unchanged. Although breath-to-breath fluctuations in $PETCO_2$ can be extreme, the trend of $PETCO_2$ over time helps identify underlying changes in CO_2 exchange.

CONCLUSION

Because effective exchange of respiratory gases is fundamental to cellular function, elaborate mechanisms have evolved to ensure its regulation. When the clinician confronts life-threatening disorder of the heart or lung, mastery of the underlying physiologic principles of gas exchange facilitates appropriate and timely intervention. Careful monitoring of the variables in play is fundamental to successful therapy.

ANNOTATED REFERENCES

Gattinoni L, Brazzi L, Pelosi P, et al: A trial of goal-oriented hemodynamic therapy in critically ill patients. SvO2 Collaborative Group. N Engl J Med 1995;333:1025-1032.
Increasing cardiac output toward greater than customary targeted values did not improve outcome. Many patients could not reach the therapeutic targets despite aggressive intravascular volume expansion and vasoactive drugs.

Laffey JG: Protective effects of acidosis. Anaesthsia 2001;56:1013-1014.
This provocative commentary reviews the experimental evidence and argues the benefit of hypercarbic acidosis on inflammation.

Nuckton TJ, Alonso JA, Kallet RH, et al: Pulmonary dead-space fraction as a risk factor for death in the acute respiratory distress syndrome. N Engl J Med 2002;346:1281-1286.

High levels of ventilatory deadspace were associated with greater risk for adverse or fatal outcomes.

Pontoppidan H, Geffin B, Lowenstein E: Acute respiratory failure in the adult (parts I-III). N Engl J Med 1972;287:690-698, 743-752, 799-806.

An ageless, comprehensive review of physiologic principles that guide management of acute respiratory failure.

Rivers E, Nguyen B, Havstad S, et al: Early goal-directed therapy in the treatment of severe sepsis and septic shock. N Engl J Med 2001;345:1368-1377.

An influential clinical trial that demonstrated the value of quickly reversing the hemodynamic compromise associated with sepsis.

West JB: Ventilation-perfusion relationships. Am Rev Respir Dis 1977;116:919-943.

An instructive overview of the complex interrelationships between the blood and gas flows to the lung.

Chapter 62

ARTERIAL BLOOD GAS INTERPRETATION

Robin L. Gross • R. Phillip Dellinger

INTERPRETATION OF ARTERIAL BLOOD GASES

INDICATION FOR ABG ANALYSIS

Arterial blood gas analysis became available approximately 50 years ago when techniques developed by Clark,[1] Stow and coworkers,[2] and Severinghaus and Bradley[3] permitted the measurement of the partial pressures of oxygen (PaO_2) and carbon dioxide ($PaCO_2$). ABGs have been demonstrated to be the most frequently ordered test in the ICU[4] and have become so essential to the management of critically ill patients that recent critical care guidelines[5] recommend 24-hour ABG availability.

In the appropriate clinical scenario, hypoxemia is suggested by tachypnea, tachycardia, or cyanosis, although these signs are not consistently reliable.[6] With the widespread availability of noninvasive techniques to measure oxygenation,

the primary role of ABG has evolved into the assessment of ventilatory and metabolic disturbances. However, when pulse oximetry (PO) cannot be obtained (profound hypotension or cardiac arrest) or would be predicted not to correlate with PaO_2 (known or suspected abnormal hemoglobin values), ABGs may indicate the presence of significant hypoxemia.[7] Clinical changes such as respiratory distress, deterioration in mental status, and shock are clear indications for ABG analysis.[8] Patients with refractory exacerbations of chronic obstructive pulmonary disease (COPD) require ABG analysis to detect hypercapnia and acidosis. However, ABGs are not routinely needed in acute exacerbations of asthma because CO_2 retention does not usually occur until FEV_1[9] or peak flow[10] falls to less than 25% predicted. Thus, oxygenation is assessed with SaO_2 and only those patients who decompensate require ABG to determine whether they are progressing to respiratory failure. In this setting, repeat ABG samples should be drawn to assess the adequacy of either invasive or noninvasive ventilatory support.

In the setting of severe metabolic derangement, ABGs identify the presence of inadequate respiratory compensation or a mixed acid-base disturbance. However, in certain settings, such as diabetic ketoacidosis, ABGs may not influence treatment.[11] Finally, when immediate hemoglobin and chemistry data are required for the management of surgical and unstable patients, the capability of some analyzers to measure these values along with ABGs provides faster results than most stat laboratories.

COMPLICATIONS

When drawing blood for ABG, efforts to properly position the patient facilitate the procedure and limit complications, which are rare.[12] Fleming and Bowen[13] reported a 0.58% incidence of hematoma after ABG analysis with a 5-minute compression time, which is shortened by using a smaller (25-gauge) needle.[14] Other complications include vasospasm,[15] arterial aneurysm, and fibrosis.[16] Infection is extremely rare.[13] Pain is usually not severe and may be minimized by local anesthesia without raising the level of difficulty or length of time required to complete the procedure.[17]

Arterial line placement is associated with more frequent ABGs,[4] and the catheter size and material may contribute to arterial thrombosis (less occlusion with Teflon than polyethylene), particularly in the setting of decreased perfusion.[18] Iatrogenic anemia[19] may be minimized by using the minimal necessary discard volume (twice the catheter deadspace or 1 mL of blood)[20] and collecting the smallest sample size necessary. Although newer instruments are capable of analyzing microliter sample sizes, the recommended minimum sample amount is 1 mL of blood.[21]

TECHNIQUE/EQUIPMENT

ABG analysis is typically performed on whole blood. PaO_2, $PaCO_2$, and pH are directly measured with standard electrodes and digital analyzers; oxygen saturation is calculated from standard O_2 dissociation curves and may be directly measured with a co-oximeter. Bicarbonate (HCO_3^-) concentration is calculated using the Henderson-Hasselbalch equation:

$$pH = pK_A + \log\{[HCO_3^-]/[CO_2]\}$$

where pK_A is the negative logarithm of the dissociation constant of carbonic acid.

Base excess (BE, the amount of base necessary to return pH to 7.4) is also calculated.

FACTORS THAT MAY ALTER RESULTS

Inconsistent results with ABGs occur owing to a number of factors. Intrasubject variability may affect PaO_2, $PaCO_2$,[22-24] and pH.[24] Severe hypotension[25] may require forceful aspiration of the sample, and results, particularly for PaO_2, may be falsely low.[26] Hyperventilation resulting from anxiety and/or pain may acutely alter results from baseline values.[15,27] Leukocytosis and thrombocytosis accelerate the decline of PaO_2 and pH and elevation of $PaCO_2$[28] within a stored sample. This PaO_2 decrease is more pronounced at higher PaO_2 levels, is attributable to cellular oxygen consumption, and may be attenuated when samples are stored at colder temperatures.[28-30] Red blood cell glycolysis may generate lactic acid[31] and change pH.

Significant increases in $PaCO_2$ and decreases in pH occur when samples are stored at room temperature for more than 20 minutes.[32] At lower temperatures, the pK′ for carbonic acid[33] and pH rise and $PaCO_2$[34] and PaO_2 fall.[35] Here, the solubility of O_2 increases and hemoglobin has greater affinity for O_2.[28] However, although measured PaO_2 is elevated, O_2 saturation remains constant.[36] Whereas temperature correction formulas and nomograms were previously applied to pH, $PaCO_2$, and PaO_2,[36-38] newer analyzers can automatically correct these values to patient temperature. However, temperature correction is not always performed for PaO_2[39] and is not required for pH and $PaCO_2$.[40]

Collection equipment and technique influence results. Increased deadspace in the syringe lowers $PaCO_2$ content,[41] and both $PaCO_2$[28] and PaO_2 (particularly at high O_2 tensions)[42] may diffuse out of plastic syringes.[43] Needle size rarely causes variability,[25] and the smaller (25 g) needle is recommended, because it causes less patient discomfort.[14] Heparin is usually added to prevent coagulation, and dilution with older liquid solutions caused spuriously low $PaCO_2$.[41,44,45] Today, dry (sodium or lithium) heparin in ABG kits may interfere with electrolyte measurement and, when concentrated, may lower pH.[46] Sample preparation is important[26] because air bubbles falsely elevate PaO_2.[32] Also, the timing of ABG collection relative to ventilator changes should permit equilibration of alveolar and arterial PO_2.[47] It has been suggested that PaO_2 values may equilibrate within 10 minutes after FiO_2 adjustment in stable patients,[48] although this may

not be the case with either PaO_2 or PCO_2 if changes in minute ventilation or positive end-expiratory pressure occur.[49] Also, patients with COPD require a longer equilibration period[50] before ABG draw.

Variation among ABG analyzers is assessed by using bias (the consistent variation of measurement from a standard) and precision (the standard deviation of this variation).[51,52] The accuracy (a combination of precision and bias) of blood gas analyzers for PaO_2 measurement may differ by 10% or more when tested against standard tonometer values.[53] Aside from interlaboratory variation, errors in calibration and electrode contamination with protein[8] or other fluids[54] may alter results.[55]

STANDARDS

Standards are recommended for sample collection[15,56] and analysis of ABG specimens. Blood gases should be drawn 20 to 30 minutes after ventilator setting changes.[15] The International Federation of Clinical Chemistry[31] recommends that ABG drawn in plastic syringes should be measured immediately to ensure accurate PaO_2 measurement; glass syringes (although rarely used) may allow more accurate measurement when PaO_2 is greater than 200 mm Hg. Either sodium or lithium heparinate should comprise less than 5% of the sample. The specimen should be collected anaerobically with immediate removal of air bubbles.[31] Universal precautions should be maintained at all times.[15] If the sample is stored, it should be on ice and remixed before analysis.[15]

The U.S. Department of Health and Human Services has published accepted parameters for limits of ABG error as ± 0.04 units for pH, ± 5.0 mm Hg (or 8%; whichever is greater) for $PaCO_2$, and ± 3.0 interlaboratory standard deviation of the ABG analyzer for PaO_2.[57] Laboratories should routinely practice quality control measures[58] and perform proficiency testing with fluorocarbon-based control solutions[59] or tonometry.[60] Newer electrodes have less drift and usually perform calibrations before measurement of each sample.[61]

ABG VALIDITY

Despite the adherence to collection and measurement standards, it is important to ascertain that the data are consistent before proceeding to interpretation of results. Kassirir and Bleich[62] demonstrated that this could be done using a modified Henderson-Hasselbalch equation by determining the proton concentration [H+]:

$$[H^+] = 24 \cdot \{[PaCO_2]/[HCO_3^-]\}$$

where 24 is a constant that reflects a combination of the solubility coefficient of CO_2 and the pK′. [H+] is used to estimate the pH; a divergence of 1 nmol/L from the baseline of 40 will cause the pH to change reciprocally by approximately 0.01 unit[62] within the range of pH 7.1 to 7.5. Data may not correlate owing to breach of collection procedure, specimen mislabeling, laboratory error, or inappropriate timing of chemistry and ABG sample collection after therapeutic interventions. If this is the case (i.e., the calculated pH differs from the measured pH) the specimens should be redrawn before proceeding with further calculations.

TABLE 62–1. NORMAL ARTERIAL BLOOD GAS VALUES ON ROOM AIR

	Normal Values
pH	7.35 to 7.45
$PaCO_2$	35 to 45 mm Hg
PaO_2	86 to 100 mm Hg
HCO_3^-	22 to 26 mmol/L
Base excess	0 mmol/L
O_2 saturation	94% to 100%

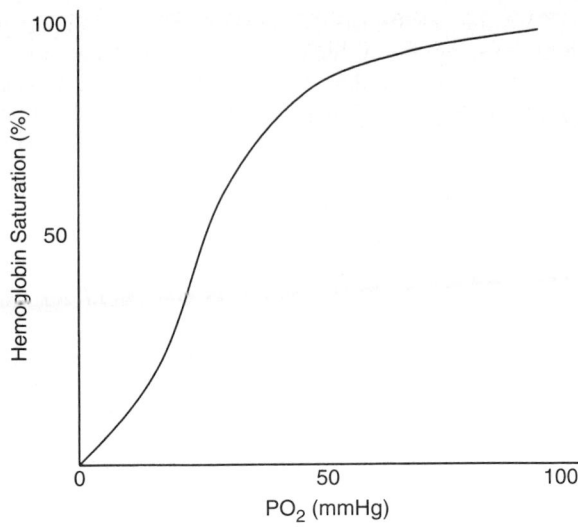

FIGURE 62–1. The oxygen-hemoglobin dissociation curve. Oxygen delivery to tissues is increased when the curve is shifted to the right by acidosis, increased temperature, and increased 2,3-diphosphoglycerate. On the higher portion of the curve, small variations in SaO_2 produce large variations in PaO_2.

NORMAL VALUES

Normal blood gas values are shown in Table 62-1. Although physiologic deadspace (the amount of ventilated air that does not participate in gas exchange)[63] increases with age, $PaCO_2$ usually does not decline.[64,65] Alveolar oxygen tension (PAO_2) remains constant, but PaO_2 decreases with age,[66] probably because of ventilation/perfusion ($\dot{V}/\dot{Q}$) inequalities.[67-69] Thus, several equations have been suggested to correct measurements,[67-69] and PaO_2 may be roughly estimated using 100 mm Hg − 0.3 × age (years). Recently, Crapo assessed values with newer ABG analyzers and demonstrated that PaO_2 generally declines by 0.245 mm Hg/yr after age 25 and should be corrected for atmospheric pressure.[40] Although weight may affect PaO_2 by altering $\dot{V}/\dot{Q}$ relationships in some age groups,[68] correction formulas are not necessary.

OXYGENATION

NORMAL RELATIONSHIPS AND DELIVERY

As mentioned, ABG permits the assessment of oxygenation, which is dependent on O_2 content, delivery, and utilization. O_2 content is calculated using the following equation:

$$O_2 \text{ content} = Hgb \text{ (g/dL)} \times O_2 \text{ saturation (%)} \times 1.39 + (PaO_2 \times 0.0031)$$

where Hgb is hemoglobin and 1.39 represents the amount of O_2 (mL) carried by hemoglobin (g). Oxygen delivery is:

$$\dot{V}DO_2 \text{ (mL/min/M}^2) = O_2 \text{ content} \times CO \text{ (L/min)}$$

where CO is cardiac output. Thus, O_2 saturation, and not PaO_2, is the parameter of oxygenation that contributes most to O_2 delivery.

The relationship between PaO_2 and SaO_2 is demonstrated by the oxygen-hemoglobin dissociation curve (Fig. 62-1),[70] which is "S" shaped owing to allosteric alterations in the O_2-hemoglobin complex.[71] Although SaO_2 reflects PaO_2 on the steep portion of the curve, small variations or errors in SaO_2 produce large variations in PaO_2 on the higher segment.[72] Factors that shift the curve to the right facilitate the release of O_2 into tissues by decreasing the affinity of hemoglobin for O_2 and include higher temperature, 2,3-diphosphoglycerate (DPG), [H+], and CO_2. Carbon monoxide alters both the position (left shift) and contour of the curve in that it competitively binds hemoglobin to displace O_2 from binding sites,[73] resulting in less available oxygen for tissue delivery.

HYPOXEMIA

Hypoxemia differs from hypoxia in that hypoxemia defines decreased PaO_2 whereas hypoxia defines inadequate cellular oxygen uptake or utilization. Hypoxemia results from decreased PIO_2 (secondary to high altitude or decreased FIO_2), shunt (intracardiac or intrapulmonary), low $\dot{V}/\dot{Q}$ ratio (typically called $\dot{V}/\dot{Q}$ mismatch), and diffusion abnormalities. Cellular hypoxia results from decreased cardiac output or decreased O_2 content, that is hypoxemia, decreased hemoglobin, or abnormal hemoglobin.[7] Hypoventilation also causes hypoxemia to a lesser degree. Some disease states have more than one cause of hypoxemia, such as acute respiratory distress syndrome (ARDS), in which aberrant $\dot{V}/\dot{Q}$ relationships[74] occur in addition to shunt. Abnormalities in $\dot{V}/\dot{Q}$ relationships account for most episodes of hypoxemia.[75] Arterial blood gases are particularly useful in assessing a shunt when results collected at room air are compared with those at 100% FIO_2. Several shunt equations have been proposed. The classic equation requires a pulmonary arterial (PA) catheter:

$$Qs/Qt = (CcO_2' - CaO_2)/(CcO_2' - CvO_2)$$

where Qs is blood flow through the shunt, Qt is total blood flow, CcO_2' is the oxygen content of pulmonary capillary blood, CaO_2 is the oxygen content of arterial blood, and CvO_2 is the oxygen content of mixed venous blood. The estimated shunt equation does not require a PA catheter and assumes a $C(a-v)O_2$ of 3.5 vol%[76]:

$$Qs/Qt = (CcO_2' - CaO_2)/3.5 + (CcO_2' - CaO_2)$$

and the modified equation makes the above assumption as well as a PaO_2 greater than or equal to 100 mm Hg:

$$Qs/Qt = [(PAO_2 - PaO_2) \times 0.003]/[3.5 + (PAO_2 - PaO_2) \times 0.003]$$

Despite little clinically significant difference between the results of these equations, the limits of agreement are wide, so a PA catheter with the classic shunt equation is preferred when assessing hemodynamically unstable patients.[77] It should be recognized that the presence of carbon monoxide may alter results, because the calculated shunt value may be erroneously high if a co-oximeter is not used to estimate O_2 content.[72]

PaO_2/FiO_2 RELATIONSHIP

Hypoxemia may be assessed using the PaO_2/FiO_2 ratio, which varies based on its point on the O_2-hemoglobin dissociation curve, lung $\dot{V}/\dot{Q}$ relationships,[78] and the degree of shunt.[75] For example, in the setting of a normal or high $\dot{V}/\dot{Q}$ ratio, as FiO_2 is raised, PaO_2/FiO_2 increases and then stabilizes. However, the same rise in FiO_2 in an alveolus with a low $\dot{V}/\dot{Q}$ ratio might initially decrease PaO_2/FiO_2, particularly on the steep portion of the curve.[78] In this alveolus, additional increases in FiO_2 cause absorption atelectasis[79] and subsequent alterations in $\dot{V}/\dot{Q}$ relationships due to vascular adaptation.[80] The result is a variable PaO_2/FiO_2 ratio that becomes a less reliable index of oxygenation if measured at only one point in time.[81]

ALVEOLAR-ARTERIAL OXYGEN TENSION DIFFERENCE

The alveolar-arterial difference ($AaDO_2$) considers the impact of the amount of CO_2 present in the blood and alveoli on O_2 exchange. The alveolar air equation is used to calculate the ideal alveolar oxygen tension (PAO_2):

$$PAO_2 = PIO_2 - PaCO_2 \times (FiO_2 + [1 - FiO_2]/RQ)$$

where RQ is the respiratory exchange ratio (the ratio of CO_2 production to O_2 consumption) and is assumed to be 0.8. Here,

$$PIO_2 = FiO_2 (PB - PH_2O)$$

where PB is barometric pressure and PH_2O is water vapor pressure. At sea level, ambient pressure is 760 mm Hg and $PH_2O = 47$ mm Hg.

A more simplified version is used in common practice:

$$PAO_2 = PIO_2 - PaCO_2/R$$

$AaDO_2$ is then calculated using the PAO_2 from the ABG:

$$AaDO_2 = PAO_2 - PaO_2$$

In the setting of increased $PaCO_2$ and normal oxygen exchange, the $AaDO_2$ should be normal. Thus, an elevated $AaDO_2$ warrants a search for a cause of hypoxemia other than hypoventilation.[82] The normal value is 3 to 16 mm Hg and increases with age because of $\dot{V}/\dot{Q}$ inequalities[40,64,66] and increased closing volumes.[65] Factors that influence $AaDO_2$ calculation include temperature (hypothermia may increase $AaDO_2$)[83] and changes in the respiratory exchange ratio (R). R may exhibit both intrasubject[84] and intersubject[85] variability and be significantly altered in the setting of hyperventilation.[27] Moreover, in COPD patients with significant hypercapnia, the $AaDO_2$ may be misleading because normal values may mask underlying sources of hypoxemia,

such as shunt.[86] Although $AaDO_2$ increases with higher FiO_2 levels, normal $AaDO_2$ values are not known for intermediate ranges of FiO_2[47] leading some investigators to suggest other methods for assessing hypoxemia.

OTHER INDICES OF OXYGENATION

The $a/APaO_2$ ratio may be used in the assessment of oxygenation:

$$a/APO_2 = 1 - AaDO_2/PAO_2$$

While some suggest that it is a better index of oxygenation than $AaDO_2$,[47] this value has limitations. a/APO_2 appears to be more stable than $AaDO_2$ in the setting of respiratory failure with a large shunt but is less accurate in the setting of low $\dot{V}/\dot{Q}$ ratio or when PaO_2 is greater than 100 mm Hg.[87] In some cases the a/APO_2 may be used to predict PaO_2[88] during FiO_2 adjustment (and thus obviate the need for additional ABG), but at times the ratio may overestimate PaO_2.[89]

Another value, the respiratory index, is occasionally used:

$$\text{Respiratory index} = P[A-a]O_2/PaO_2$$

Like $AaDO_2$ and a/APO_2, it incorporates the effect of $PaCO_2$ by including PAO_2. Although usually minimal, the effect of $PaCO_2$ may become important in the setting of permissive hypercapnia if FiO_2 is not adequate.[75,90] Because the relationship between PaO_2 and oxygen content is not linear, it has been suggested that a preferred index of oxygenation would be independent of FiO_2.[81]

ASSESSMENT OF ACID-BASE DISTURBANCES

NORMAL ACID-BASE RELATIONSHIPS

Interpretation of ABGs includes the assessment of acid-base status. Whereas acidosis and alkalosis reflect accumulation of acid or base, acidemia is defined as a pH less than 7.35 and alkalemia as a pH greater than 7.45. Detailed reviews of acid-base balance and metabolic disturbances are presented in Chapters 12 and 127, respectively. ABG reports often include the base excess (BE), which is not dependent on the respiratory physiology (i.e., $PaCO_2$)[91] and therefore provides information regarding the metabolic acid-base status of the patient. Siggaard-Anderson[92] first proposed evaluating BE in whole blood, defined as the quantity (mM) of strong acid needed to restore pH to 7.4 in a blood sample equilibrated at $PaCO_2 = 40$ mm Hg using the Van Slyke equation[91,93]:

$$BE = \{[HCO_3^-] - 24.4 + (2.3 \times [Hgb] + 7.7) \times (pH - 7.4)\} \times (1 - 0.023 \times [Hgb])$$

A negative BE is called a base deficit. The BE may be further adjusted to eliminate the effects of ventilation and $PaCO_2$ alterations on the value; thus the standard base excess (SBE) is usually reported by most ABG analyzers using Hgb = 3.1 mM (5 g/dL).[94] However, recently the original BE has been shown to be reliable, despite changes in $PaCO_2$ or Hgb.[91] The relationship between $PaCO_2$ and ΔSBE has been described[95]:

$$\text{Acute } PaCO_2 \, \Delta: \Delta SBE = 0 \times \Delta PaCO_2$$

$$\text{Chronic PaCO}_2 \ \Delta: \Delta\text{SBE} = 0.4 \times \Delta\text{PaCO}_2$$

$$\text{Metabolic acidosis: } \Delta\text{PaCO}_2 = 1.0 \times \Delta\text{SBE}$$

$$\text{Metabolic alkalosis: } \Delta\text{PaCO}_2 = 0.6 \times \Delta\text{SBE}$$

Acid-base relationships are affected by protein values, particularly albumin. Hypoproteinemia is associated with elevation of chloride[96] and low calculated anion gap[97] (see Chapter 127) as well as mild hyperventilation.[98] Thus, the protein state should be considered when using ABG and chemistry results to assess the acid-base status of a patient.

DISTURBANCES OF VENTILATION

Assessment of Normal Ventilation

Ventilation is controlled by the brainstem's response to chemoreceptor feedback. The central chemoreceptor is located near the medulla and responds to extracellular and cerebrospinal fluid pH[99]; variations in $PaCO_2$ therefore affect the central receptor through pH alterations, which then effect ventilatory changes through the medulla. The peripheral chemoreceptors include the carotid bodies, which respond to decreases in PaO_2 and pH and increases in $PaCO_2$, and the aortic bodies, which play a less active role in humans.[100] The ventilatory response to both hypoxia and hypercapnia varies among individuals and may be influenced by genetic factors.[101,102] Significance bands describing responses to respiratory acidosis[103] and alkalosis[104] are available for acid-base analysis, although they may not adequately detect mixed respiratory and metabolic disorders.[104]

Because the estimation of alveolar ventilation (V_A) by patient observation is extremely difficult, hypoventilation may go unnoticed.[105] Thus, the ABG analysis is essential because $PaCO_2$ is used for the calculation:

$$V_A = K \cdot V_{CO_2}/\text{PaCO}_2$$

where $K = 0.863$, V_{CO_2} is CO_2 production, and V_A is alveolar ventilation. $PaCO_2$ is assumed to be equal to $PaCO_2$ because CO_2 readily diffuses across the alveolar-capillary membrane.[84] However, in the presence of significant $\dot{V}/\dot{Q}$ abnormalities or shunt, $PaCO_2$ may be lower than $PaCO_2$.[63] V_A is influenced by several factors, as demonstrated by the following equation:

$$V_A = f\,(V_T - V_D)$$

where f is frequency, V_T is tidal volume, and V_D is deadspace volume. Thus, factors that decrease f or V_T will decrease V_A and increase $PaCO_2$. Physiologic deadspace consists of anatomic and alveolar deadspace and can be estimated with the Bohr equation:

$$V_D/V_T = [\text{PaCO}_2 - \text{PeCO}_2]/\text{PaCO}_2$$

where $PeCO_2$ is expired CO_2.

Ventilation usually increases with hypoxemia. Whereas the relationship between oxygen content (CaO_2) and ventilation is linear, that of ventilation and PaO_2 is hyperbolic (similar to the O_2-Hgb dissociation curve).[106] The ventilatory response to hypoxemia is increased in the setting of acute hypercapnia and decreased in the setting of acute hypocapnia,[106] when the inverse linear correlation between

TABLE 62–2. DISORDERS ASSOCIATED WITH RESPIRATORY ACIDOSIS

Central respiratory depression (drug overdose, obesity hypoventilation syndrome)
Neuromuscular disorders (Guillain-Barré, neuropathy, myopathy, malnutrition)
Parenchymal disorders progressing to respiratory failure (pneumonia, ARDS, pulmonary edema)
Metabolic disorders (hypophosphatemia)
Abnormalities of chest wall motion (kyphoscoliosis)
Disturbances in ventilation/perfusion
Airflow obstruction (asthma or COPD exacerbation)
Upper airway obstruction (foreign body, laryngospasm)
Iatrogenic (permissive hypercapnia or inadequate ventilator settings)
Increased CO_2 production (carbohydrate load, malignant hyperthermia)
Compensation for metabolic alkalosis

SaO_2 and ventilation becomes nonlinear.[107] The ventilatory response to hypoxemia is also decreased during chronic exposure to high altitude.[108] O_2 influences CO_2 through the Haldane effect[109] because hemoglobin collects H^+ ions easily after carbonic acid dissociation. Thus, in the setting of lower hemoglobin O_2 saturation, a particular $PaCO_2$ level will be associated with a higher CO_2 content.

Respiratory Acidosis

Causes of hypoventilation and subsequent respiratory acidosis are listed in Table 62-2. Patients with CO_2 retention may present with lethargy, confusion, and, in some cases, agitation. Elevated $PaCO_2$ is also associated with central nervous system (CNS) toxicity (seizures), cardiac arrhythmias, and pulmonary vasoconstriction.

In patients without COPD, acute respiratory failure may be defined as a state in which PaO_2 falls below the predicted normal range for the patient's age or $PaCO_2$ is above 50 mm Hg (in the absence of compensation for metabolic alkalemia).[110] When respiratory failure occurs secondary to $\dot{V}/\dot{Q}$ inequalities, eventual muscle fatigue often leads to respiratory muscle failure.[111] In patients with COPD during acute exacerbations, hypercapnia due to O_2 administration occurs because of several factors and not simply respiratory drive suppression. Although minute ventilation initially decreases, $\dot{V}/\dot{Q}$ inequality is a major factor.[112,113] Loss of pulmonary vasoconstriction occurs,[79] and alveolar deadspace increases.[114] Impaired respiratory muscle function secondary to hyperinflation also contributes to respiratory failure.[115]

Although deleterious effects may occur with acute hypercapnia, permissive hypercapnia[90] is used quite frequently in the treatment of mechanically ventilated patients with ARDS. Although shunt is increased,[116] there are usually few or no untoward effects. In fact, it is possible that hypercapnia, through the resulting acidosis, improves oxygen exchange in areas of $\dot{V}/\dot{Q}$ inequality by increasing vasoconstriction.[25] Also, acidosis may be protective in certain settings by decreasing inflammation.[117] Thus, treatment of respiratory acidosis should be individualized and, when appropriate, targeted to facilitate CO_2 elimination (e.g., intubation) or decrease CO_2 production.

Respiratory Alkalosis

Causes for respiratory alkalosis are listed in Table 62-3. During hyperventilation, equilibration of PaO_2 and $PaCO_2$ requires several minutes because of body stores, which are

TABLE 62–3. DISORDERS ASSOCIATED WITH RESPIRATORY ALKALOSIS

Central neurologic insults with high respiratory drive
   (intracranial hemorrhage, cerebrovascular accident, trauma)
Hypoxemia
Pain
Anxiety
Salicylate intoxication
Sepsis
Iatrogenic (hyperventilation on ventilator)
End-stage liver disease
Pregnancy
Fever
High altitude
Compensation for metabolic acidosis

larger for $PaCO_2$ due to blood and interstitial fluid bicarbonate.[118] The effect of hyperventilation on PaO_2 is usually small.[119] However, as mentioned, the ventilatory response to hypoxemia is blunted during hypocapnia, possibly owing to the effect of PCO_2 (and thus pH) on the central chemoreceptor.[119] The converse is also true.

Whether respiratory or metabolic, alkalosis is associated with increased mortality, particularly when the pH exceeds 7.65.[120] Very high pH levels are often due to mixed metabolic and respiratory disorders or high minute ventilation due to inappropriate ventilator settings. Severe alkalosis is associated with decreased hypoxic pulmonary vasoconstriction, abnormalities in cardiac contractility, and seizures. However, in the proper setting, alkalosis may simply represent a normal physiologic response and treatment is not always necessary. In fact, the cerebral vasoconstriction produced by lesser degrees of hypocapnia may be therapeutic in patients with neurologic injury and high intracranial pressures.

EXPECTED COMPENSATORY CHANGES IN RESPONSE TO METABOLIC AND RESPIRATORY ABNORMALITIES

Compensatory mechanisms are much stronger for acidosis than alkalosis.[121] The body's buffering systems include bicarbonate/carbonic acid, erythrocytes, tissues, and plasma proteins.[121,122]

Respiratory Acidosis

In acute hypercapnia, the relationship between $[H^+]$ and PCO_2 is linear.[103] Early metabolic buffering mechanisms are primarily extrarenal[103] with small changes in bicarbonate. This response is influenced by the underlying metabolic state. In the canine model,[123] chronic metabolic acidosis is associated with a larger increase in H^+ and HCO_3^- whereas chronic metabolic alkalosis is associated with a smaller increase. The underlying ventilatory state is also important. Chronic respiratory acidosis results in higher compensatory HCO_3^- levels and smaller alterations of pH at the central chemoreceptor, causing a reduced ventilatory response to acute hypercapnia.[63]

Although chronic hypercapnia is associated with a better compensatory response than acute hypercapnia, the pH does not completely normalize.[103] In the canine model,[124] chronic hypercapnia causes the bicarbonate concentration to rise initially and then reach a steady state within 3 to 5 days. The rise in H^+ concentration correlates linearly with the change in $PaCO_2$. In patients with lung disease, bicarbonate can rise

to a level of 65 $mmol/L$[122] and acidosis will develop after that point. Until HCO_3^- reaches this level, the pH may actually be alkalotic (possibly secondary to treatment). Thus, ABG interpretation of the primary process may be difficult (i.e., whether there is a primary metabolic alkalosis or primary respiratory acidosis with metabolic compensation).[122]

The expected compensatory changes of HCO_3^- and H^+ in response to acute respiratory acidosis are[125]:

$$10 \, \Delta[HCO_3^-] = \Delta PaCO_2 \text{ and } \Delta[H^+] = 0.8 \, \Delta PaCO_2 \text{[103]}$$

For chronic respiratory acidosis, the expected HCO_3^- and H^+ are:

$$10 \, \Delta[HCO_3^-] = 3.5 \, PaCO_2 \text{ and } \Delta[H^+] = 0.3 \, \Delta PaCO_2 \text{[124]}$$

Measured values that do not correlate with calculated values suggest the presence of an underlying metabolic acidosis or alkalosis.

Respiratory Alkalosis

In acute hypocapnia, HCO_3^- initially decreases, owing to buffering by hemoglobin and tissue,[104] followed by kidney buffering. Chronic hypocapnia reduces bicarbonate levels and decreases renal acid excretion, although patients initially remain alkalemic because the metabolic response is weaker than the respiratory response.[126] In recovery, as $PaCO_2$ normalizes there is an initial metabolic acidosis, followed by acid excretion that is associated with cation retention.[127] The underlying metabolic state may influence the compensatory response to chronic hypocapnia. For example, a preexisting metabolic acidosis inhibits the compensatory decrease in renal acid excretion[126] and a chronic metabolic alkalosis may result in a larger decline in HCO_3^- in response to hypocapia.[128] However, in the absence of an underlying metabolic disorder, the expected HCO_3^- and H^+ changes for acute respiratory alkalosis may be estimated[125]:

$$10 \, \Delta[HCO_3^-] = 2 \, \Delta PaCO_2 \text{ and } \Delta[H^+] = 0.8 \, \Delta PaCO_2 \text{[104]}$$

For chronic respiratory alkalosis, the compensatory changes are:

$$10 \, \Delta[HCO_3^-] = 5 \, \Delta PaCO_2 \text{ and } \Delta[H^+] = 0.17 \, \Delta PaCO_2 \text{[127]}$$

Results that differ from calculated values indicate the presence of an underlying metabolic disturbance, and a cause should be sought.

Metabolic Acidosis

Because respiratory compensation and the fall in $PaCO_2$ are rapid, determining whether a metabolic acidosis is acute or chronic is difficult.[95] The expected $PaCO_2$ may be estimated using Winter's formula[129]:

$$PaCO_2 = 1.5[HCO_3^-] + 8 \pm 2$$

Thus, a measured PCO_2 above or below the calculated $PaCO_2$ value indicates the presence of an additional respiratory acidosis or alkalosis, respectively.

Metabolic Alkalosis

The compensatory mechanism for metabolic alkalosis is hypoventilation, accomplished primarily by decreasing tidal volume.[130] This compensatory mechanism is the weakest of all because profound compensation is limited by hypoxemia. A suggested formula for estimation of $PaCO_2$ is:

$$PaCO_2 = 0.9[HCO_3^-] \pm 15$$

As discussed earlier, if measured $PaCO_2$ differs from the calculated value, an additional respiratory disturbance exists.

AN ALGORITHMIC APPROACH TO ABG INTERPRETATION

The Stewart approach[131] to acid-base disorders provides a rational method for the assessment of a patient's acid-base status and is discussed in Chapter 12. Here we present an alternative approach. When interpreting ABG data, one should ask the following questions:

1. Are the data internally consistent? Kassirer's[62] modified Henderson-Hasselbalch equation is used to predict pH by calculating the expected $[H^+]$ and pH.
2. What is the underlying acid-base abnormality? The pH will almost always reflect the primary abnormality, unless a respiratory alkalosis coexists with an underlying metabolic acidosis.[126]
3. Is the primary problem an acidosis? If yes, is it metabolic or respiratory?
4. If a metabolic acidosis is present, is there an anion gap (AG) (i.e., is the acidosis caused by unmeasured anions?)[132]

$$AG = ([Na^+] + [K^+]) - ([Cl^-] + [HCO_3^-])$$

Usually, the AG is calculated without K^+ and a normal value is 8 to 12 mEq/L. Causes of an AG acidosis are discussed in Chapter 127.

5. In the setting of an AG, is an additional metabolic disturbance present? Calculate the delta (Δ) gap, that is, the difference between this AG and a normal AG: Δ gap = AG − 12. The Δ gap, when added to the measured $[HCO_3^-]$ should equal 24. If the result is less than 24, a non-AG acidosis is present; and if it is greater than 24, a metabolic alkalosis exists.
6. Is the respiratory process purely compensatory, or is there an underlying respiratory acidosis or alkalosis? Use Winter's formula to calculate the expected $PaCO_2$ in the setting of pure compensation.
7. Is the primary problem an alkalosis? If so, is it respiratory and/or metabolic? The BE is helpful in this setting. Is it chronic or acute?
8. Determine the underlying causes for the metabolic and respiratory derangements.

OTHER ISSUES

VENOUS BLOOD ANALYSIS AS AN ALTERNATIVE TO ABG ANALYSIS

Mixed venous blood ($S\bar{v}O_2$) represents an admixture of blood from many tissues. Normal $S\bar{v}O_2$ is 65%, and lower values may represent decreased oxygen delivery or aberrant tissue oxygen uptake.[7] Mixed venous blood gases have been demonstrated to be superior to arterial blood gases for the diagnosis of early hemorrhagic shock[133] because the early low pH that is seen in mixed venous blood may not be apparent in arterial blood. During cardiac arrest,[134] an elevated $PaCO_2$ may be detected in mixed venous blood before being mixed in arterial blood. This is thought to be due to decreased pulmonary CO_2 clearance and possibly increased CO_2 production.[134] Continuous $S\bar{v}O_2$ may be used as a monitor of oxygen delivery. However, $S\bar{v}O_2$ monitors measure values on the steeper part of the HbO_2 dissociation curve, so a larger error in oxygen content will be introduced with small errors in $S\bar{v}O_2$ measurements.[72] Thus, if $S\bar{v}O_2$ results are questionable, a sample of blood should be drawn to directly measure mixed venous oxygen content.

Central venous blood (CVB) can be used for screening because normal CVB values usually reflect normal ABG values.[135] Generally, CVB pH is lower and PcO_2 is higher than arterial blood. Trends in venous pH measurements are also useful in the management of diabetic ketoacidosis when ABGs are not routinely ordered.

ARTERIAL-TONOMETRIC PCO_2 GAP

In shock states (particularly sepsis) gastric tonometry may signal early inadequate O_2 delivery before other hemodynamic parameters because splanchnic O_2 consumption rises. The gastric mucosa subsequently experiences regional hypoperfusion as blood flow is directed toward vital organs.[136] A nasogastric balloon with a saline- or air-filled tonometer measures the PCO_2 of the fluid in the gut lumen, which is believed to reflect the PCO_2 of the mucosa. The mucosal pH (pH_i) is then calculated using the blood bicarbonate value (assumed to be equal to mucosal bicarbonate) and a known time-dependent equilibration factor in the Henderson-Hasselbalch equation.[137]

A normal pHi is 7.35 or greater; decreased levels are associated with higher mortality.[136] It has been suggested that pHi-guided treatment may improve survival,[138] although this has not been consistently demonstrated. The pHi has limitations because it is altered by fluctuations in $PaCO_2$[139] and SBE[140]; although HCO_3^- is used to calculate the pHi, it is not localized to the gastric mucosa.[137] For these reasons, it has been suggested that the $PtCO_2$-$PaCO_2$ difference (the PCO_2 gap) may be a better indicator of gastric ischemia.[139-141] A high PCO_2 gap early in admission may predict multisystem organ failure and mortality,[142,143] although this has not been consistently demonstrated. The effect of vasoactive medication on tonometry parameters is also unpredictable and may vary based on disease severity.[144,145] Although gastric tonometry may facilitate the management of critically ill patients, it is expensive and has not gained widespread acceptance for clinical use.

VENOUS-ARTERIAL PCO_2 GRADIENT

As mentioned previously, during tissue hypoperfusion, the difference in pH and PCO_2 between venous and arterial blood may be significant.[134] The PCO_2 gradient ($VAPCO_2$) increases as cardiac index decreases secondary to decreased elimination of CO_2 at the tissue level,[146,147] resulting in venous hypercapnia and arterial hypocapnia.[148] In animal models, both $VAPCO_2$ and VApH increase as oxygen delivery (DO_2) declines, and this response is augmented as critical

DO_2 is reached.[147,149] In septic shock an elevated $VAPCO_2$ is seen in those patients with low cardiac output as well as those with pulmonary disease who cannot eliminate CO_2.[150] In patients with cardiogenic shock, $VAPCO_2$ decreases as hemodynamic variables improve with dobutamine.[151] This has led to the suggestion that this ratio be used to determine whether cardiac output is sufficient for the degree of oxygen demand[146,151] in the setting of hypoperfusion.

OTHER SURROGATE MONITORS

END-TIDAL CO_2 AS AN ESTIMATE OF $PaCO_2$

Whereas capnometry measures the CO_2 concentration in a gas, capnography is a graphic representation of CO_2 at the end of the alveolar plateau, or end-tidal CO_2 ($PetCO_2$).[152] Generally, this value correlates with $PaCO_2$.[152] However, changes in $PetCO_2$ do not always reflect those of $PaCO_2$ owing to the effects of $\dot{V}/\dot{Q}$ inequalities, breathing patterns,[153] and particularly deadspace; in low flow states,[154] when poorly perfused units are ventilated, the $PetCO_2$ may not adequately reflect the $PaCO_2$.

PULSE OXIMETRY AS AN ESTIMATE OF PaO_2

Pulse oximetry uses a photodetector and light source to measure SpO_2 by calculating the differential absorption of light by oxygenated and reduced capillary hemoglobin. Its use is associated with fewer ABGs[155,156] and may reduce cost when the assessment oxygenation is important and knowledge of ventilation and acid-base status is not necessary. Manufacturers usually recommend 95% of PO readings be within 5% of the co-oximeter reading. Inconsistency with ABG readings is usually due to motion artifact, hypothermia, or hypotension[157] with poor perfusion. With high PaO_2, just as with SaO_2, minimal SpO_2 error may be associated with large error in PaO_2, owing to the shape of the oxygen dissociation curve. Also, readings may be altered by the presence of carboxyhemoglobin and methemoglobin. In any of these settings where SpO_2 is thought not to correlate with ABG values, samples should be drawn for ABG analysis.

TRANSCUTANEOUS MONITORS

$PtcO_2$ and $PtcCO_2$ depend on arterial values, hemoglobin concentration, the oxygen-hemoglobin dissociation curve, skin thickness, and adequate blood flow.[158] Although TcO_2 correlates with PaO_2, wide variations have been reported,[159] leading some to suggest analysis of the $PtcO_2$ index $[P(a\text{-}tc)O_2/PO_2]$, because it may reflect decreased perfusion and cardiac output.[160] $Tc\text{-}CO_2$ has been shown to correlate with $PaCO_2$, but results vary at higher CO_2 levels.[161] It is thought that transcutaneous monitors generally reflect O_2 and CO_2 transport to and from skin electrodes and may not reflect arterial values.[158] Thus, transcutaneous monitoring is not routinely used in the ICU setting as a replacement for ABG analysis.

CONTINUOUS ABG MONITORS

Continuous ABG monitors intermittently or continuously display ABG results on a bedside screen and permit the observation of trends over time.[159] The newer ABG analyzers have sensors called optodes that detect variations of light and fluorescence.[61] The O_2 sensor uses a fluorescent die, and the H^+ and CO_2 sensors use fluorescent acids; fluorescent intensity is inversely proportional to the amount of substance being measured.[24] Some monitors have cartridges that permit measurements every 2 to 3 minutes; these closed systems minimize health care worker exposure to blood and do not require interruption of the arterial line for sample collection. Also, measured blood is returned to the patient and is thus conserved.[162]

Several limitations are associated with these monitors. Lower precision is more frequent with PaO_2 measurements,[162,163] and less accurate readings occur at higher PaO_2 and $PaCO_2$ levels.[164] Motion artifact affects values[163,165] and clot may form on the catheter tip. Finally, "wall effect" may alter PaO_2 readings; here, a sensor adjacent to the vessel wall may combine blood and tissue PaO_2 readings.[24,162,163] Although continuous ABG monitors are not used routinely, they may show promise in the future.

ANNOTATED REFERENCES

AARC clinical practice guideline. Sampling for arterial blood gas analysis. Respir Care 1992;32:913-917.

This review includes standards for the collection and processing of ABG samples.

Aubier M, Murciano D, Milic-Emili J, et al: Effects of the administration of O_2 on ventilation and blood gases in patients with chronic obstructive pulmonary disease during acute respiratory failure. Am Rev Respir Dis 1980;122:747-754.

This prospective study demonstrated that CO_2 retention due to O_2 administration during COPD exacerbation was not simply the result of a decreased "hypoxic drive to breathe" but most likely due to ventilation-perfusion inequalities.

Bakker J, Vincent JL, Gris P, et al: Veno-arterial carbon dioxide gradient in human septic shock. Chest 1992;101:509-515.

This observational study in patients with septic shock documented venoarterial CO_2 gradient elevations in patients with lower cardiac index, as well as those with pulmonary injury. Although not predictive of survival, nonsurvivors had a higher gradient than survivors.

Krapf R, Beeler I, Hertner D, Hulter HN: Chronic respiratory alkalosis: The effect of sustained hyperventilation on renal regulation of acid-base equilibrium. N Engl J Med 1991;324:1394-1401.

The effects of hypoxia-induced respiratory alkalosis were evaluated in normal subjects with and without an underlying induced metabolic acidosis. Regardless of the underlying metabolic state, both groups experienced an increase in pH, suggesting that the compensatory metabolic response was not as strong as the $PaCO_2$ decline.

Schmidt C, Müller-Plathe O: Stability of Po_2, Pco_2 and pH in heparinized whole blood samples: Influence of storage temperature with regard to leukocyte count and syringe material. Eur J Clin Chem Clin Biochem 1992;30;767-773.

The effects of both temperature and leukocytosis on ABG results were found to be significant. Because the permeability of plastic (vs. glass) syringes affected values, it was suggested that samples in plastic syringes be measured within 15 minutes of collection.

Chapter 63

RESPIRATORY SYSTEM MECHANICS AND RESPIRATORY MUSCLE FUNCTION

Sean M. Caples • Rolf D. Hubmayr

KEY POINTS

1. A simple model of the respiratory system is useful in assessing mechanics in the ICU. Mechanical ventilator models using linear one-compartment analogs are helpful in detecting the presence of lung disease or respiratory muscle activity and may assist in guiding disease-specific ventilatory strategies.

2. Pressures applied to the respiratory system are either stored as a function of elasticity or dissipated as resistive energy. A basic understanding of the mechanics and derivation of these pressures from mechanical ventilator output is useful during the bedside assessment of ICU patients.

3. Evidence supporting the use of the pressure-volume curve to determine specific ventilator settings is circumstantial. However, information about respiratory system mechanics derived from the pressure-volume curve can be helpful in identifying patients at risk for ventilator-associated lung injury.

4. Respiratory muscle fatigue is an important factor in respiratory failure. Current methods of quantifying muscle fatigue, based on surrogate measurements of muscle strength in the time domain, are limited by their low specificity and interaction with systemic disease, such as sepsis.

5. Critical illness polyneuropathy and myopathy are important causes of respiratory muscle dysfunction in the ICU and are associated with certain modifiable risk factors, including the use of neuromuscular blocking agents.

In its simplest form, the respiratory system can be modeled as a balloon connected to a tube. The balloon represents the elastic element (lungs and chest wall), and the tube represents the resistive element (conducting airways). To serve the purpose of ventilation, the respiratory pump (or a mechanical ventilator) must generate sufficient pressure to overcome both the elastic and flow-resistive properties of the respiratory system.

Classic respiratory mechanics are based on Newtonian physics, as expressed in the equation of motion. The respiratory system model is derived from an elementary monodimensional system, as depicted by a block with an attached spring, acted on by a unidirectional force (Fig. 63-1A).[1]

Upon application of the force, the response of the system can be characterized in terms of displacement, velocity, and acceleration of a block with a mass of M. The balance of forces acting on the block can be expressed as follows:

$$F_{appl(t)} = F_{el(t)} + F_{res(t)} + F_{in(t)} \qquad \text{(Equation 1)}$$

where the total force applied to the system (F_{appl}) at a given time (t) is equal to the sum of the elastic (F_{el}), resistive (F_{res}), and inertial (F_{in}) forces. The equation may be rewritten as

$$F = Kx + R(dx/dt) + M(d^2x/dt^2) \qquad \text{(Equation 2)}$$

where the elastic force originates in the spring and is the product of the spring constant (K) and the distance (x) that the block is displaced. The resistive force is constituted by friction between two surfaces and equals the cross-product of the resistance constant (R) and velocity (dx/dt), whereas inertance (I) is determined by mass (M) and acceleration (d^2x/dt^2). Accordingly, the equation of motion for a three-dimensional pneumatic system may be written as

$$P_{(t)} = E(V_{(t)}) + R\dot{V}_{(t)} + I\ddot{V}_{(t)} \qquad \text{(Equation 3)}$$

where $P_{(t)}$ is the pressure exerted on the system at a given time; E is the elastance (the reciprocal of compliance, i.e., 1/C), which relates pressure to volume (V); and R is the resistance constant, relating pressure to flow. The third term of the equation describes the pressure required to accelerate tissue and gas in the airway, which is an important factor under certain circumstances, such as coughing or high-frequency oscillatory ventilation. The inertance constant (I) relates pressure to linear acceleration ($\ddot{V}$). However, the third term is usually omitted in this model of the respiratory system, because inertive forces are negligible during quiet breathing and most forms of mechanical ventilation.[2] Thus, in most applications, the respiratory system derivative of the equation of motion considers only the elastic and flow-resistive elements that oppose an applied pressure at time (t).

$$P_{(t)} = E(V)_{(t)} + R\dot{V}_{(t)} \qquad \text{(Equation 4)}$$

which may also be expressed as

$$P_{(t)} = 1/C(V)_{(t)} + R\dot{V}_{(t)} \qquad \text{(Equation 5)}$$

Thus, in this model, any force applied to the respiratory system is either stored as elastic energy or dissipated as resistive

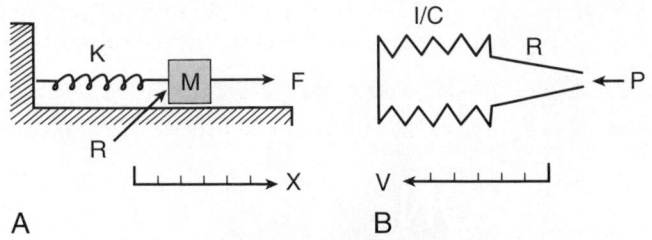

FIGURE 63–1. Mechanical analogs of the equation of motion. *A*, System with unidirectional motion. *B*, Three-dimensional system. (From Rodarte JR, Rehder K: Dynamics of respiration. In Macklem PT, Mead J [eds]: Handbook of Physiology, sec 3, The Respiratory System. Baltimore, Williams & Wilkins, 1986, pp 131-144.)

energy. Figure 63-1*B* shows a three-dimensional model of the respiratory system as it relates to the equation of motion.

This simple model of respiratory system mechanics is useful because, in the normal operating range, the relationships among airway pressure, volume, and flow can be approximated by straight lines. Linear one-compartment analogs are particularly well suited for modeling mechanical ventilation, because the pressure applied to lungs and chest wall can be readily measured and displayed. In turn, departures from linearity provide useful clues about concurrent respiratory muscle activity, alert the health care provider to the presence of lung disease, or serve as a warning that the lungs are being ventilated at inappropriately high or low volumes.

STATIC BEHAVIOR OF THE RESPIRATORY SYSTEM

In accordance with the model described in the preceding section, in the absence of gas flow, a pressure applied to the respiratory system is opposed by elastic forces (P_{el}). During flow, this pressure can be approximated by alveolar pressure (P_{alv}), which, upon interruption of airflow, equilibrates with airway opening pressure (P_{ao}).

The elastic element of the respiratory system (rs) consists of two component structures, the chest wall (w)—functionally, the thoracic cage and abdomen—and the lungs (l). The forces that act on these two structures can be summed, because the lungs and chest wall behave like springs in series.

$$P_{el,rs} = P_{el,w} + P_{el,l} \qquad \text{(Equation 6)}$$

The net distending pressure applied to the lung by contraction of the inspiratory muscles or by positive-pressure ventilation is represented by transmural forces, termed the transpulmonary pressure (P_L). Transpulmonary pressure is determined by the difference between alveolar pressure and pleural pressure (P_{pl}):

$$P_L = P_{alv} - P_{pl} \qquad \text{(Equation 7)}$$

The pressure across the chest wall (transthoracic pressure, P_w) is determined by the difference between pleural pressure and atmospheric pressure (P_{bs}).

$$P_w = P_{pl} - P_{bs} \qquad \text{(Equation 8)}$$

Because it is used as a reference to all other measured pressures, atmospheric pressure is considered to be zero, thus,

$$P_w = P_{pl} \qquad \text{(Equation 9)}$$

An esophageal balloon catheter can be used to approximate pleural pressure, keeping in mind that pleural pressure is nonuniform and that topographic gradients in pleural pressure vary with posture.[3] Particularly in the recumbent posture, there is no site in the esophagus at which local pressure approximates average lung surface pressure (i.e., average pleural pressure). However, at least in normal lungs, the average change in surface or pleural pressure can be inferred using esophageal manometry.

The static pressure across the entire respiratory system can be summarized as follows:

$$P_{rs} = P_l + P_w = (P_{ao} - P_{pl}) + (P_{pl} - P_{bs}) = P_{ao} \qquad \text{(Equation 10)}$$

The static respiratory system pressure-volume (P-V) curve is often measured in intubated, mechanically ventilated patients to make inferences about the mechanical properties of the lungs. Although the utility of P-V measurements in clinical decision-making remains to be established, the determinants of the P-V relationship should nevertheless be understood. The P-V curve is generated by inflating and deflating the relaxed respiratory system in a stepwise fashion between residual volume and total lung capacity. The airway occlusion pressure at each volume defines the corresponding elastic recoil pressures of the lungs and chest wall. Because the inflation and deflation relationships differ from each other, the resulting curve is often referred to as a P-V loop. The respiratory system P-V loop is the summation of individual lung and chest wall P-V loops, termed a Rahn diagram (Fig. 63-2).

As seen in Figure 63-2, during normal tidal volume breathing (30% to 70% vital capacity), the relationship between elastic pressure and volume is essentially linear, and the system's elastic properties can be defined by a constant, namely, elastance. The term *compliance* is more frequently

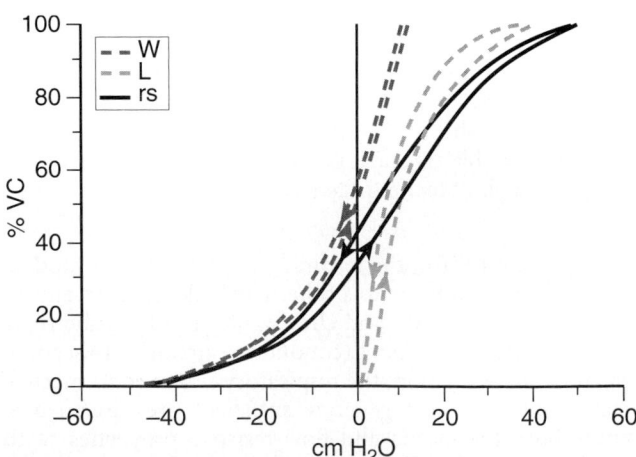

FIGURE 63–2. Pressure-volume (P-V) loop (Rahn diagram) of the respiratory system (rs), and summation of individual chest wall (W) and lung (L) loops. VC, vital capacity. (From Agostoni E, Hyatt RE: Static behavior of the respiratory system. In Fishman AP [ed]: Handbook of Physiology. Baltimore, Williams & Wilkins, 1986, pp 113-130.)

used and is simply the inverse of elastance, defined as the change in volume per unit change in applied pressure. Static respiratory system compliance can be determined by the slope of the P-V curve. In the quiet breathing range, the normal respiratory system elastance averages 8 to10 cm H_2O/L, corresponding to a static respiratory system compliance of 0.08 to 0.1 L/cm H_2O.

Figure 63-2 also shows the P-V curves of the respiratory system's component structures, the lung and chest wall. At high lung volumes, the total respiratory system compliance is reduced (the P-V curve is concave to the pressure axis), primarily because the lung reaches total capacity, its structural limit. In contrast, the P-V curve of the chest wall remains linear at high volumes (i.e., the chest wall offers much less resistance to further lung expansion). At low lung volumes, a decrease in chest wall compliance is the major contributor to the low respiratory system compliance. At relaxation volume (functional residual capacity), the inward recoil of the lung is equal to the outward recoil of the chest wall, so that alveolar pressure is atmospheric. At a volume of 60% of vital capacity, the chest wall reaches a "resting" position, that is, it exerts no force on the lungs, and the pleural pressure is atmospheric. In the normal tidal breathing range, the slopes of the lung and chest wall P-V curves are similar (i.e., lung and chest wall contribute about equally to overall respiratory system compliance). Figure 63-3 shows the volume dependence of the inwardly and outwardly directed forces of the respiratory system during inflation.[3]

Lung recoil is the collapse force of the lung that is in equilibrium with the transpulmonary distending pressure originating from the chest wall and inspiratory muscles. It is generated by:

1. Tension carried by lung parenchyma, including the collagen network that extends from the alveolar septae to the visceral pleura.
2. Surface forces originating from air-liquid interfaces in distal lung units.[4]

Surface forces (i.e., surface tension) are generated because liquid molecules, in contact with air, attempt to conserve energy by decreasing the area available for interaction. In the lung, the resulting force acts parallel to the alveolar septa and balances a helical fiber network that supports alveolar ducts and forms alveolar entrance rings.[5]

As demonstrated in Figure 63-4, the elimination of surface tension has two important consequences on lung mechanics:

1. There is an approximately 50% reduction in recoil pressure at all lung volumes.
2. The difference in isovolume recoil pressure between inflation and deflation (hysteresis) is largely abolished.

Findings indicate not only that surface tension is an important source of lung elastic recoil but also that recoil pressure varies with volume, volume history, and time. In the normal lung, hysteresis is caused by volume- and time-dependent changes in the molecular composition and hence the biophysical properties of surfactant. Surfactant is a protein-enriched lipid film that coats air-liquid interfaces in distal lung units and lowers surface tension. Hysteresis implies that energy added to the system during inflation is not fully recovered during deflation. The hysteretic loss of energy does not scale with frequency and flow the way a Newtonian viscous resistance does, underscoring one of the many limitations of linear resistance-compliance circuits in modeling lung mechanics.[6] Whereas interfacial phenomena are the

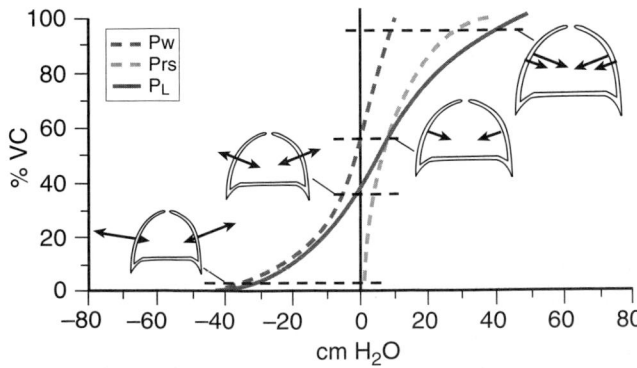

FIGURE 63-3. Static pressure-volume curves of the chest wall (P_w), lungs (P_L), and respiratory system (P_{rs}). Drawings of the thorax (from left to right) at residual volume, functional residual capacity, resting position (no force exerted by the chest wall), and total lung capacity. Arrows indicate the direction of elastic recoil. VC, vital capacity. (From Agostoni E, Hyatt RE: Static behavior of the respiratory system. In Fishman AP [ed]: Handbook of Physiology. Baltimore, Williams & Wilkins, 1986, pp 113-130.)

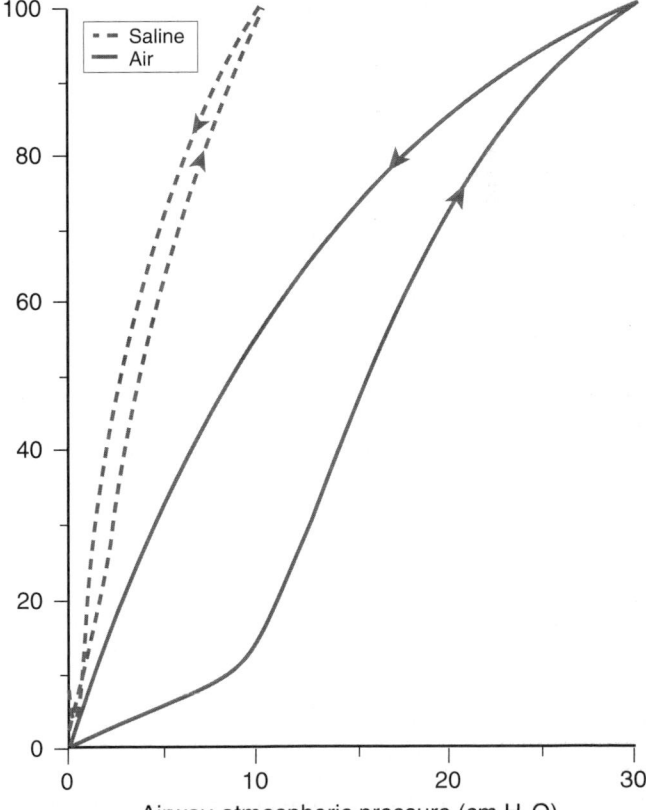

FIGURE 63-4. Plot of airway–atmospheric pressure gradient for an isolated lung inflated with air *(solid line)* and saline *(dashed line)*. The reduction in surface tension in the saline-filled lung results in increased compliance. (From Taylor A, Rehder K, Hyatt R, et al: Mechanics of breathing: Static. In Taylor AE [ed]: Clinical Respiratory Physiology. Philadelphia, WB Saunders, 1989, pp 89-105.)

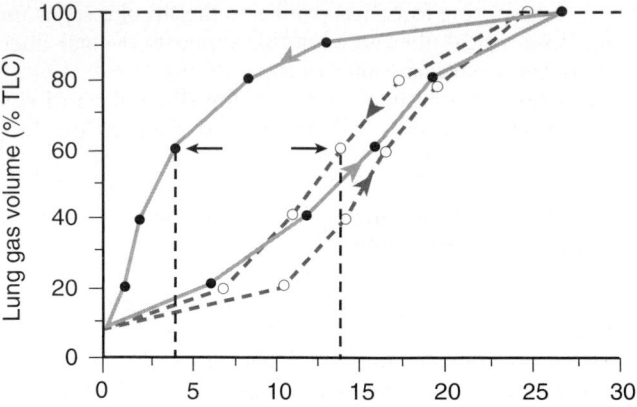

FIGURE 63–5. Pressure-volume loop of a normal lung *(solid line)* and a surfactant-depleted lung *(dashed line)*. TLC, total lung capacity. (From Taylor A, Rehder K, Hyatt R, et al: Mechanics of breathing: Static. In Taylor AE [ed]: Clinical Respiratory Physiology. Philadelphia, WB Saunders, 1989, pp 89-105.)

primary source of hysteresis in the normal lung, alveolar recruitment and derecruitment are important sources of hysteresis in disease.

According to the law of Laplace, the pressure (P) required to inflate a bubble is directly related to the surface tension (T) and is inversely proportional to the radius of curvature (r) (P = 4T/r). Applied to the lung, this means that changes in alveolar dimensions at low lung volumes would promote alveolar collapse were it not for surfactant's surface tension–lowering properties. A surfactant-depleted lung exhibits alveolar instability and collapse in the tidal breathing range.[7] Therefore, larger than normal transpulmonary pressures are required to keep the surfactant-depleted lung inflated, as illustrated in Figure 63-5.

DYNAMIC BEHAVIOR OF THE RESPIRATORY SYSTEM

The transpulmonary pressure generated by the respiratory pump must also overcome the resistive forces related to gas flow. The respiratory system resistance constant scales resistive pressure and flow in the equation of motion discussed previously. The reciprocal of resistance is conductance, which is proportional to lung volume as the airways, tethered to the entire connective tissue network, are pulled open with larger inflation volumes.

According to Ohm's law, resistance (R) can be calculated by dividing the driving pressure by flow:

$$R = (P_{alv} - P_{ao})/\dot{V} \qquad \text{(Equation 11)}$$

Total pulmonary resistance reflects the gas flow–dependent pressure dissipation in conducting airways (airway resistance) and the frequency-dependent loss of energy associated with parenchymal deformation (tissue resistance). Originally ignored as only a minor component of total pulmonary resistance, it is now appreciated that the so-called tissue resistance dominates the measurement, at least at low frequencies.[8] As elegantly outlined by Fredberg and Stamenovic,[6] tissue resistance and tissue hysteretic properties

are model-specific descriptors of energy loss, the structural and molecular basis of which remains uncertain.[9]

The physical laws governing fluid flow in tubes can be applied to gas flow in the airways. According to fluid mechanics, tube length and geometry and gas velocity and physical properties (i.e., density and viscosity) determine whether flow is laminar or turbulent. These determinants can be captured by the Reynold's number, a quantity that represents the ratio of inertial forces to viscous forces.[10] A low Reynold's number (<50) corresponds to laminar flow, and a Reynold's number greater than 2300 is associated with turbulent flow. Accordingly, the low gas velocity in peripheral airways favors laminar flow, and the acceleration associated with the decrease in total cross-sectional area in central airways promotes turbulence. In the presence of laminar flow, frictional pressure losses are linearly related to flow and viscosity and inversely proportional to tube radius to the fourth power (Poiseuille's equation). In contrast, turbulent flow is associated with nonlinear pressure-flow relationships that are gas-density dependent. The density dependence of turbulent flow is occasionally exploited in the medical use of heliox, a low-density helium-oxygen mixture given to patients with central airway lesions or asthma.[11]

The flow-dependent shift from laminar to turbulent flow is captured in the Rohrer equation:

$$P = K_1\dot{V} + K_2\dot{V} \qquad \text{(Equation 12)}$$

where K_1 and K_2 are constants that scale frictional pressure dissipation associated with laminar and turbulent flow, respectively.

A second mechanism of pressure loss during gas flow is related to the Bernoulli principle, which describes convective pressure dissipation. That is, as a gas flows from a large cross-sectional area to a smaller area, velocity must increase to maintain flow. This results in energy dissipation and a drop in pressure and correlates to expiratory flow of gas from the bronchioles to the central airways.

As mentioned previously, ohmic resistance can be computed by dividing resistive pressure by inspiratory flow (equation 11). In a mechanically ventilated patient, where endotracheal and ventilator tube resistance dominate measured total respiratory system resistance, the derived value of respiratory resistance must be interpreted with caution. Artificial tubing is not a truly ohmic resistor, and estimates of resistance are highly dependent on inspiratory flow rates. Even after correction for tube size, high inspiratory resistance may be confounded by inspissated secretions or "tube biting." When using inspiratory flow settings of less than 1 L/sec with an endotracheal tube greater than 7 mm internal diameter, resistive pressure is usually less than 10 cm H_2O. A resistive pressure exceeding this value, in the absence of obvious intrinsic airway disease, should prompt an investigation for a possible ventilator hardware problem. It should be kept in mind that a normal inspiratory resistance does not preclude the presence of severe airflow obstruction, as seen in chronic obstructive pulmonary disease (COPD).

The respiratory time constant (τ) is the time required for the lungs to fill or passively discharge approximately 63% of its contents. It can be determined from the slope of the passive expiratory flow-volume curve (Fig. 63-6) or calculated directly by the equation

$$\tau = R_{rs}/E_{rs} = R_{rs} \cdot C_{rs} \qquad \text{(Equation 13)}$$

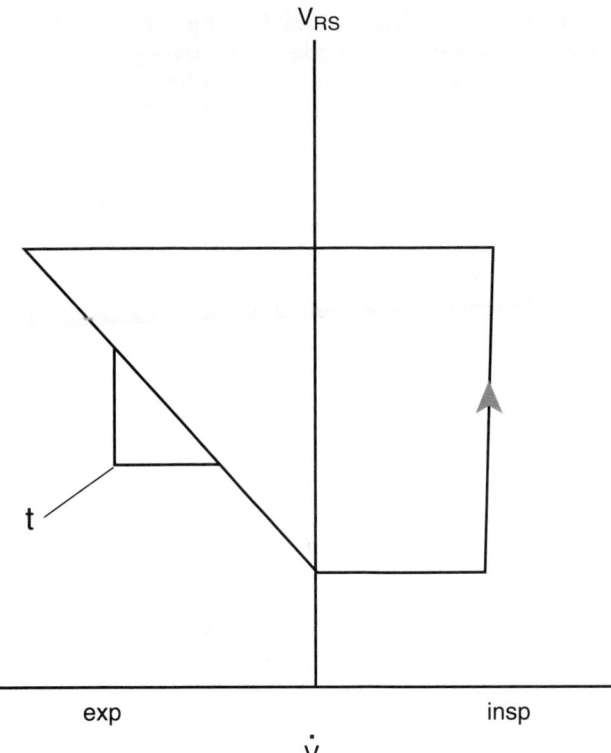

FIGURE 63–6. Flow-volume curve. The expiratory time constant (τ) is equal to the slope of the expiratory limb. $\dot{V}$, flow; V_{RS}, volume of respiratory system. (From Loring SH: Mechanics of the lung and chest wall. In Marini JJ, Slutsky AS [eds]: Physiological Basis of Ventilatory Support. New York, Marcel Dekker, 1998, pp 177-205.)

Because respiratory system resistance (R_{rs}) is expressed in units of pressure • time • volume^{-1} and respiratory system compliance (C_{rs}) is expressed in units of volume • pressure^{-1}, the product τ has the unit of time (E_{rs}, respiratory system elastance). The value of τ for a normal respiratory system is approximately 0.3 second.[2] As can be inferred from the equation, patients with high respiratory system resistance or compliance, such as those with COPD, have correspondingly large τ values. The added resistance of the artificial tubing in a mechanically ventilated patient increases τ to 1 second or more. Depending on the set expiratory time, patients with even minimally elevated τ values may not fully empty the lungs during mechanical ventilation. Consequently, the demand for expiratory flow is not met as the lungs near relaxation volume, resulting in dynamic hyperinflation.

Some basic concepts regarding flow limitation are helpful as a prelude to a discussion of bedside assessment in the ICU. The left side of Figure 63-7 shows an expiratory flow-volume plot for a normal subject, similar to that generated by a forced vital capacity maneuver in the pulmonary function lab. The right side of the figure shows three driving pressure–flow curves at progressively smaller lung volumes from A to C. The curves are nonlinear, and each has a driving pressure–dependent and –independent limb, separated by the critical driving pressure. In a classic set of experiments performed on normal subjects, Fry and Hyatt demonstrated that maximal expiratory flow is determined by lung volume.[12] That is, higher lung volumes (curve A) yield higher expiratory flow rates compared with the flow seen at lower lung volumes (curve C). They concluded that, on the basis of volume-related dynamic airway collapse, this expiratory flow plateau cannot be exceeded, irrespective of the magnitude of subject effort or applied transpulmonary pressure. Herein lies the value of the forced vital capacity maneuver as a reproducible measure of maximal expiratory flow. Although this seems most applicable to ambulatory outpatients, these general principles can help guide bedside decision-making in the ICU, as discussed later.

ASSESSMENT OF RESPIRATORY SYSTEM MECHANICS IN THE INTENSIVE CARE UNIT

The preceding sections defined the basics of respiratory system mechanics as they relate to volume, pressure, and flow. With this foundation, we can proceed to the correlation of mechanics with clinical conditions encountered in the ICU. To examine basic concepts, we use the example of expected waveforms generated by a volume-preset mechanical ventilator in a relaxed patient with otherwise normal respiratory system mechanics.

FIGURE 63–7. *Left,* maximal expiratory flow-volume curve. *Right,* three isovolume pressure-flow curves at different lung volumes (A, B, C). Note flow limitation associated with submaximal lung volumes B and C. TLC, total lung capacity. (From Hyatt RE: Forced expiration. In Macklem PT, Mead J [eds]: Handbook of Physiology, sec 3, The Respiratory System. Baltimore, Williams & Wilkins, 1986, pp 295-314.)

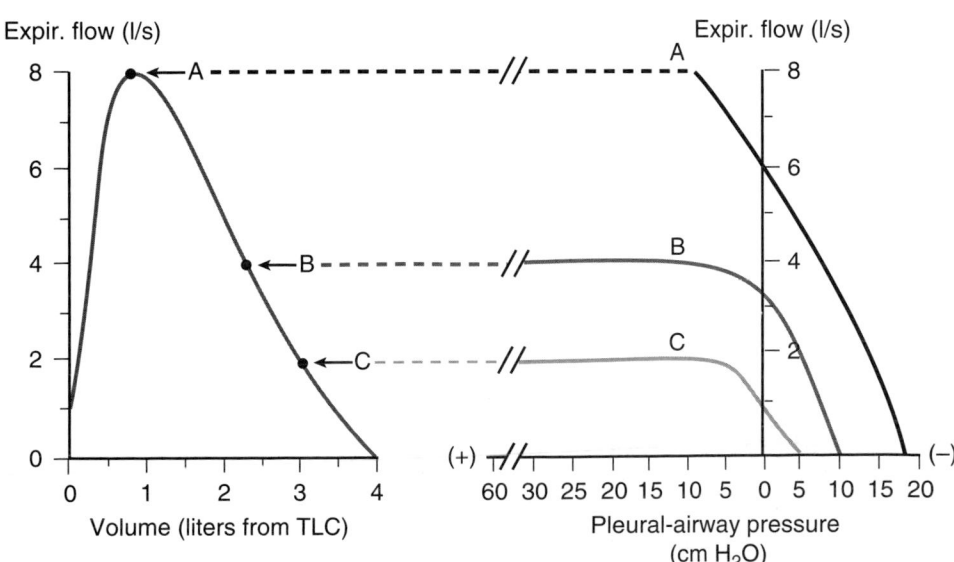

The typical waveform output is demonstrated by Figure 63-8, with a model of the system represented on the right. Pressures are measured at the ventilator inlet. Assuming inflation onset with a constant (square wave) flow, an initial step change in driving pressure is recorded, which precedes alveolar filling, and corresponds to resistive pressure related to gas flow in the airways. In the otherwise normal lung, an identical step-off in resistive pressure may be noted during an applied airway occlusion at end-inspiration, when gas flow falls to zero (see the arrow in Fig. 63-8). The resultant remaining value is referred to as the plateau pressure and represents the static summation of elastic recoil forces corresponding to the applied tidal volume. The purported significance of plateau pressure is discussed later.

Assuming constant flow in a relaxed or paralyzed patient without respiratory muscle contribution, pressure at the ventilator inlet increases linearly with time and volume to a peak airway pressure. (Inspiratory muscle activity would be represented by transient perturbations in the linearity of the airway opening pressure curve with a constant inspiratory flow rate). Peak airway pressures that deviate from the inspiratory occlusion pressure by more than 10 cm H_2O should prompt an investigation of an endotracheal tube resistance problem, such as tube kinking or inspissated secretions.

As previously mentioned, the elastic properties of the respiratory system can be determined from the slope of the P-V curve. Provided there is no contribution from respiratory muscles (as evidenced by a perfectly linear inspiratory P-V curve), the elastance (E_{rs}), or reciprocal of compliance, can be derived from time-based curves with the following equation:

$$E_{rs} = \Delta P_{el}/\Delta vol = dP/dt \times dt/dV = dP/dt \times 1/\dot{V} \qquad \text{(Equation 14)}$$

where dP = change in pressure; dt = change in time; and dV = change in volume.

Positive end-expiratory pressure (PEEP) can be applied to the system manually (extrinsic PEEP) or may be inadvertent, known as intrinsic or auto PEEP, related to dynamic hyperinflation. Intrinsic PEEP can occur in any mechanically ventilated patient, once a certain threshold of ventilation is reached. In patients with deranged respiratory system mechanics, particularly obstructive lung disease (with abnormally large τ values), the propensity to develop intrinsic PEEP is increased. PEEP (extrinsic or intrinsic) is represented on the pressure waveform by end-expiratory pressures exceeding zero.

Passive expiration of the respiratory system is driven by elastic recoil, as manifested by alveolar pressure at a corresponding lung volume. Expiratory flow is a function of the elastance and resistance and is demonstrated as

$$\dot{V}exp_{(t)} = P_{el(t)}/R_{rs} \qquad \text{(Equation 15)}$$

Because the elastic pressure is determined by elastance and the corresponding lung volume, the equation may be rewritten as

$$Vexp_{(t)} = [E \times V_{(t)}]/R = V_{(t)}/(\tau) \qquad \text{(Equation 16)}$$

As noted previously, τ is the product of resistance and compliance. It is possible to overwhelm the expiratory function of either a normal or a diseased lung during mechanical ventilation with a combination of relatively large tidal volume and relatively short expiratory time, leading to intrinsic PEEP. The volume of trapped gas that corresponds to the inadvertent PEEP can be calculated by the formula

$$V_{trapped} = \dot{V}T/(e^{Te/\tau} - 1) \qquad \text{(Equation 17)}$$

where Te is the expiratory time.

SPECIFIC APPLICATIONS

INJURED LUNGS

Acute lung injury (ALI) and acute respiratory distress syndrome (ARDS) are associated with impaired lung barrier function. Pulmonary capillary leak and overwhelming of the lungs' ability to clear water and solute from airspaces results in so-called noncardiogenic pulmonary edema.[13] Flooding of alveolar spaces leads to the functional loss of these units from effective ventilation, a process termed derecruitment, particularly in the dependent portions of the lungs.[14] This results in what has been termed the "baby lung," where gas flow is directed to aerated low-impedance units.[15] Because respiratory system elastance scales with lung size, injured lungs appear stiff.[16] Total respiratory system resistance is also increased, particularly in the dependent regions of the lungs.[17] Whether abnormal lung mechanics reflect the collapse of dependent units or are the consequence of alveolar flooding remains controversial.[18]

There is unimpeachable evidence that the injured lung is susceptible to further injury related to mechanical ventilation, termed ventilator-associated lung injury.[19] An understanding of respiratory mechanics provides some insight into the possible pathogenetic mechanisms of this injury. First, the number of recruitable alveoli, capable of expanding during inspiration, is reduced—the "baby lung" concept noted earlier. Thus, tidal volumes are distributed to fewer lung units and produce a greater local deformation. Second, the heterogeneous distribution of liquid and associated surface tension in distal airspaces results in adjacent units with vastly different mechanical properties (i.e., opening pressure). This invokes the theory of injury related to interdependence, whereby, during the opening of a flooded unit juxtaposed

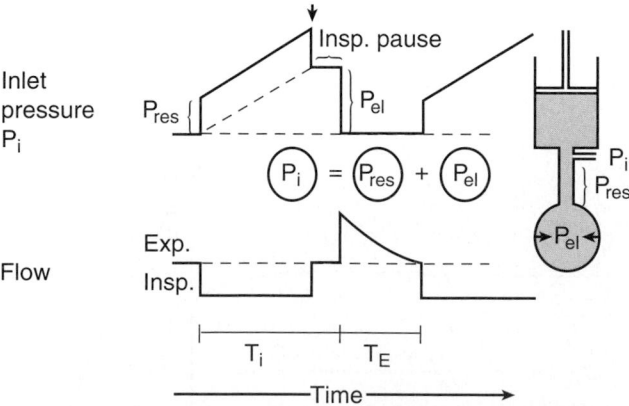

FIGURE 63–8. Airway pressure and flow wave patterns during volume-preset mechanical ventilation. Schematic of a linear one-compartment model is shown at the right. P_{el}, elastic pressure; P_i, pressure at ventilator inlet; P_{res}, resistive pressure; T_E, expiratory time; T_i, inspiratory time. (From Gay PC, Rodarte JR, Tayyab M, et al: The evaluation of bronchodilator responsiveness in mechanically ventilated patients. Am Rev Respir Dis 1987;136:880-885.)

with an open unit, a shear stress across the tissue attachment results that is substantially higher than the average transpulmonary pressure.[20]

Although there continues to be debate about the dominant pathogenetic mechanisms of ventilator-associated lung injury, it is clear that low tidal volume ventilation (~6 mL/kg ideal body weight) of ARDS patients translates to reduced mortality when compared with the traditional (≥10 mL/kg) tidal volume assignment.[19] Still, ARDS remains a devastating disease, with high mortality and morbidity. Although further efforts have been made to modify ventilatory strategies based on mechanical principles, as will be discussed later, no other interventions have been shown to affect clinical outcome.

Much attention has been focused on the pressure-volume relationship in injured lungs, as a means to both improve gas exchange and prevent ventilator-associated lung injury in predisposed lungs. Use of the P-V curve in clinical decision-making, however, has been the subject of much controversy.[18,21] First, there are technical limitations related to the numerous methods used to generate a P-V curve. The supersyringe method for static P-V curve recordings has been associated with spurious changes in lung volume, on account of gas absorption during measurement.[22] There are also issues related to user interpretation, such as difficulties in defining morphologic characteristics of the curve, and interobserver variability is often high.[23,24] Some have advocated inductive machine learning in an attempt to standardize interpretation.[25]

Compared with the static P-V curve shown in Figure 63-2, the P-V curve in ARDS and ALI (Fig. 63-9) has a number of distinguishing features. These include:

1. Sigmoidal shape with two "knees"—the upper and lower inflection points.
2. Increased recoil pressure at all lung volumes.
3. Reduced compliance defined by the slope of the inflation curve between the lower and upper inflection points.

Traditionally, the lower inflection point has been interpreted as the pressure at which previously underventilated or collapsed airways or alveoli are recruited, corresponding to the pressure at which "best PEEP" should be set. Similarly, the upper inflection point, where the inflation curve loses its linearity, is thought to be the pressure at which no further increases in lung recruitment occur, thereby representing the highest airway pressure safely administered before overdistention occurs. If these assumptions are correct, ventilator settings should be adjusted until lung expansion is restricted to the linear midrange of the inflation P-V curve. This hypothesis finds application in stress index monitoring,[26] which allows for breath-by-breath assessment of adherence to this treatment target.

Critical appraisal of the P-V curve has revealed low specificity for some derived parameters. For example, a prominent lower inflection point has been associated with conditions of high surface tension rather than actual closure or collapse of airways, such as with mineral oil rinses or air insufflation into saline-filled lungs.[27,28] Attention has been refocused on edema, airway liquid, and interfacial phenomena as causes of higher opening pressures and increased lung impedance.[18]

The lower inflection point may originate in the chest wall rather than the lung in some patients, particularly in those with low end-expired thoracic volumes (recall that the P-V curve of the chest wall is nonlinear at low lung volumes; see Fig. 64-2).[29] Because of concerns about chest wall–related P-V artifacts, esophageal manometry has been used to guide the ventilatory management of patients with injured lungs. Data from esophageal catheters may be misleading, however, because derecruited dependent lung units that appose the esophageal probe may fail to generate local pressure swings, thereby biasing the measurement.[30]

It is clear that adjustments in PEEP are helpful in optimizing gas exchange, with improvements noted in the ratio of arterial oxygen pressure to inspired oxygen fraction (PaO_2/FIO_2). However, PEEP adjustments via P-V loop guidance do not necessarily translate into improvements in outcome or survival. Indeed, in the ARDSnet trial, early improvements in arterial oxygenation were noted in patients who were ventilated with higher tidal volumes but turned out to have increased mortality.[19] A subsequent study by the same group showed no difference in mortality between ARDS patients randomized to higher "optimal" PEEP and "conventional" PEEP.[31]

Many clinicians have advocated using the upper inflection point as an analog of plateau pressure (end-inspiratory occlusion pressure), and recommendations not to exceed 30 to 35 cm H_2O are pervasive. Although some regions of the lungs may approach their maximal volume at pressures near the upper inflection point, the evidence is circumstantial that ventilating patients near these airway pressures (with relatively low tidal volume) causes injury.

It appears that respiratory mechanics in patients with injured lungs are helpful in identifying those at greatest risk for ventilator-associated lung injury, and reassessment of the ventilation strategy (applied PEEP, tidal volume) should be triggered when static airway pressures exceed 30 to 35 cm H_2O. Most experts agree that a routine PEEP setting of 5 cm H_2O is too low, although the use of specific P-V curve–generated indices has not proved beneficial.

OBSTRUCTIVE LUNG DISEASE

COPD and its bedside monitoring are reviewed extensively elsewhere in this text. Some points about the disease as it relates to the respiratory system's mechanical properties are warranted, however, particularly in mechanically ventilated patients.

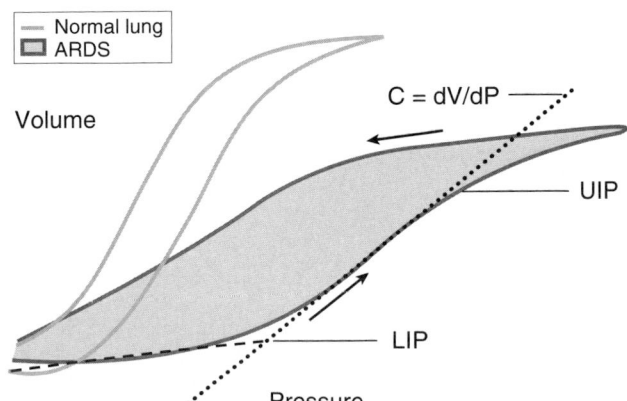

FIGURE 63–9. Pressure-volume curve in acute respiratory distress syndrome (ARDS) compared with the normal respiratory system. C, compliance; dV/dP, change in volume/change in pressure; LIP, lower inflection point; UIP, upper inflection point. (From de Chazal I, Hubmayr RD: Novel aspects of pulmonary mechanics in intensive care. Br J Anaesth 2003;91:81-91.)

A hallmark finding of all patients with obstructive lung disease is the inability to generate normal expiratory flows, which, in a mechanically ventilated patient, leads to dynamic hyperinflation. One of the most readily available means to detect hyperinflation is the measurement of intrinsic PEEP by the end-expiratory airway occlusion method. Intrinsic PEEP is defined as total PEEP minus applied or extrinsic PEEP, and it reflects the elastic recoil of the respiratory system at end-expiration.[32] It should be noted, however, that intrinsic PEEP is not a specific marker of airway obstruction. Patients with "normal" lungs can hyperinflate above a critical minute ventilation, as explained by equation 16. Moreover, the presence of intrinsic PEEP and dynamic hyperinflation does not necessarily indicate an absolute increase in end-expiratory volume. For example, on the basis of mass loading of the chest wall in the recumbent position, many patients with ascites or obesity breathe at lung volumes near residual volume.[33] It should also be noted that the reliability of the end-expiratory occlusion method is dependent on complete respiratory muscle inactivity and therefore may not be reliable in a patient who assists the ventilator.

In assessing for the presence of airflow limitation, the expiratory time constant, τ, can be determined by the slope of the flow-volume curve (see Fig. 63-6) or by the product of resistance and compliance (see equation 16). However, a more readily available tool for detecting airway obstruction is simple pattern recognition of ventilator-generated waveforms. Recall from Figure 63-8 that the initial step change in airway pressure during lung inflation should be equal to the recovery of pressure at the end of the tidal volume, that is, the difference between peak and plateau or airway occlusion pressure. The early step change is determined by any load that must be overcome to commence lung inflation. This includes resistive pressure as well as intrinsic PEEP, which drives expiratory flow. Thus, dynamic hyperinflation should be considered when the initial pressure step change significantly exceeds the terminal pressure recovery. This concept is also demonstrated in Figure 63-10, which shows an example of typical volume, airway pressure, and flow curves in an obstructed, dynamically hyperinflated patient.[34] The arrow pointing to the airway opening pressure curve denotes the intrinsic PEEP that must be counterbalanced before lung inflation begins. This method of assessing for hyperinflation

has the added advantage of being less susceptible to patient effort, because thoracic neuromechanical feedback mechanisms tend to blunt effort at end-inspiration. The initial flow spike, or transient, in Figure 64-10 represents the rapid expulsion of gas that occurs during dynamic airway collapse early in expiration. Following the initial spike, there is deterioration in expiratory flow, as opposed to the monoexponential reduction expected in normal lungs. Indeed, the persistence of flow during the shift from expiration to inspiration suggests that the lung has not completely emptied. The terminal portions of the curves in Figure 63-10 were recorded during stepwise lung deflation. At end-expiration, intrinsic PEEP is measured by airway occlusion pressure as 16 cm H_2O.

In the normal lung, expiratory driving pressure is determined by the difference between alveolar pressure and airway opening pressure. In the relaxed or paralyzed state, this driving pressure is the respiratory system recoil pressure at that particular end-inspiratory lung volume. In normal lungs, the net driving pressure may be reduced by the application of extrinsic PEEP, which serves as a load that must be overcome before volume can be expired. Consequently, in a volume-preset ventilatory mode, this would result in reduced expiratory flow, hyperinflation, and elevated peak airway pressures over subsequent breaths. As explained in Figure 64-7, if extrinsic PEEP does not affect expiratory flow, flow limitation is present. In other words, in patients with severe airway obstruction who are breathing in the tidal volume range, end-inspiratory recoil pressure far exceeds that required for maximal expiratory flow. These patients would not exhibit reductions in expiratory flow in response to the application of small levels of extrinsic PEEP.[35] Accordingly, as shown in Figure 63-11, the application of up to 5 cm H_2O of extrinsic PEEP in an obstructed patient fails to raise volume or peak pressure.

RESPIRATORY MUSCLE FUNCTION

The primary task of the respiratory muscles is to drive the respiratory pump. To do so, they must generate forces necessary to overcome the elastic and resistive elements of the respiratory system described in the preceding sections. The respiratory muscles are striated in nature and thus subscribe to Starling's law regarding length-tension relationships. As such, inspiratory muscles that act to expand the chest wall exert their greatest forces at low lung volumes (Fig. 63-12). Conversely, expiratory muscles, working to actively deflate the lungs, are most efficient at high lung volumes.[3]

Dynamic hyperinflation, as described earlier, is frequently encountered in mechanically ventilated patients and can lead to disruption of the optimal length-tension relationships of respiratory muscles, thereby contributing to respiratory failure.[36]

The muscles of respiration perform in a complex, integrated fashion to maximize breathing efficiency. Although the diaphragm is the primary muscle of respiration, it is known that muscles previously thought to have only an accessory role in breathing are actively taking part in quiet respiration to aid in movement of the chest wall.[37] These include the intercostal and scalene muscles. Relaxation allows passive recoil of the respiratory system to its resting functional residual capacity position. During exercise, phasic contraction of expiratory muscles drives the respiratory system below its resting position. Subsequent relaxation at end-expiration increases lung volume, thereby reducing

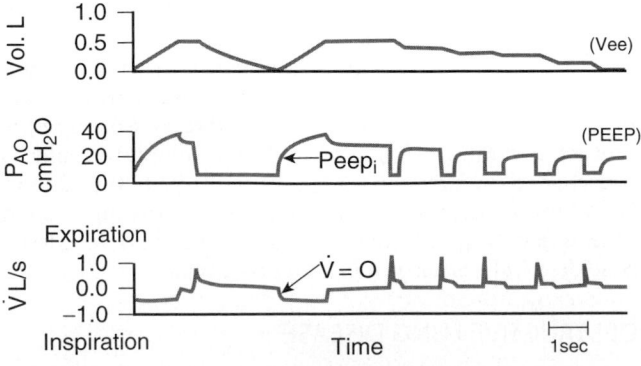

FIGURE 63–10. Volume, pressure (P_{AO}), and flow ($\dot{V}$) tracings during mechanical ventilation of an obstructed, dynamically hyperinflated patient. PEEP, positive end-expiratory pressure; PEEP$_i$, intrinsic PEEP; V_{ee}, end-expiratory volume. (From Gay PC, Rodarte JR, Tayyab M, et al: The evaluation of bronchodilator responsiveness in mechanically ventilated patients. Am Rev Respir Dis 1987;136:880-885.)

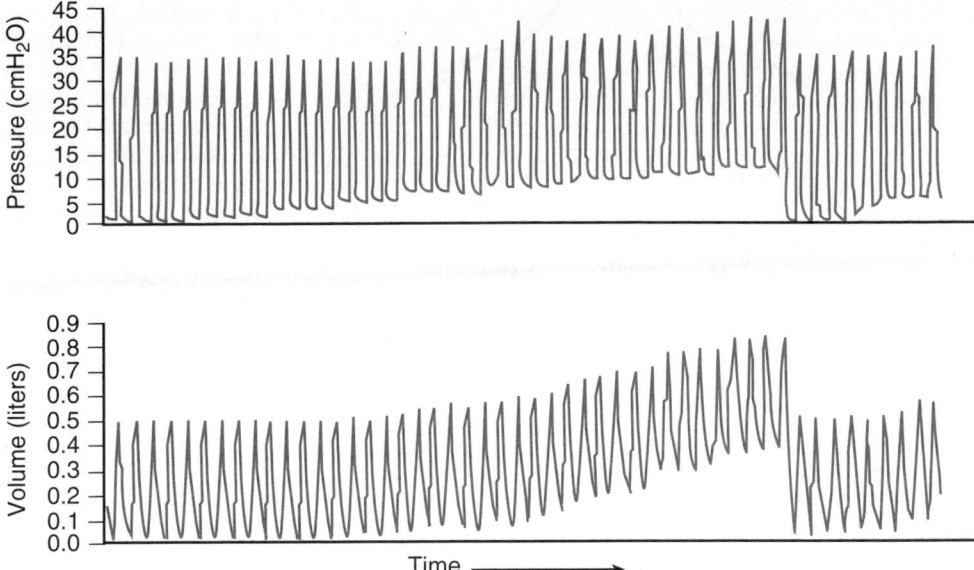

FIGURE 63–11. Response of airway pressure and volume to extrinsic positive end-expiratory pressure in a dynamically hyperinflated, mechanically ventilated patient with chronic obstructive pulmonary disease. (From Gay PC, Rodarte JR, Hubmayr RD: The effects of positive expiratory pressure on isovolume flow and dynamic hyperinflation in patients receiving mechanical ventilation. Am Rev Respir Dis 1989;139:621-626.)

the load on the inspiratory muscles for the next respiratory cycle.[2]

CHEST WALL

The chest wall collectively includes the thoracic cage and the abdominal compartment, which compose a parallel circuit. The rib cage is the most extensive portion of the chest wall and therefore contributes most to thoracic displacement during breathing. The ribs, during rest, are situated ventrally, with a downward slope. Because of their articulations with the sternum and spinal transverse processes, they are confined and move in a stereotypical manner during breathing. During inspiration, the ribs are displaced cranially to become more horizontal, so that both the anteroposterior and transverse diameters of the rib cage increase.

The intercostal muscles, innervated by the intercostal nerves, act directly on the ribs to effect movement. Three different intercostal muscle groups have varying effects on respiration, depending on their origin and insertion points, which dictate orientation. The external (and parasternal) intercostals serve as inspiratory muscles by raising the ribs during contraction. In contrast, the internal intercostal muscles, which run at right angles to the externals, serve an expiratory function by contracting during expiration to induce caudal motion of the lower ribs.

The scalene muscles, considered primary muscles of respiration, originate at the cervical spine transverse processes and insert on the first two ribs anteriorly. Their contraction aids inspiration by expanding the rib cage. A number of muscles serve an accessory role, facilitating the primary muscles' role during periods of increased effort (exercise, fatigue). These muscles include the sternocleidomastoids, pectoralis minor, and erector spinae, all of which elevate the ribs during contraction.[2]

DIAPHRAGM

The most important inspiratory muscle is the dome-shaped diaphragm. It is composed of muscle fibers that radiate from the central tendon to attach to the lower rib cage. The crural portion inserts on the anterior portions of lumbar vertebrae 1 through 3, and the costal portion inserts on the xiphoid process and the upper, inner margins of the lower six ribs. The majority of the muscular portion of the diaphragm lies directly beside the lower rib cage, referred to as the zone of apposition (Fig. 63-13). Also referred to as the costophrenic sulcus, the zone of apposition is 6 to 9 cm in height and occupies 25% to 30% of the total interior surface of the rib cage.[37]

The diaphragm exerts two types of forces upon contraction. First, there is an insertional force during contraction, related to the shortening of muscle fibers, to displace the dome caudally. This increases intra-abdominal pressure, which causes ventral displacement of the anterior abdominal wall. The net effect is the lowering of pleural pressure to effect lung expansion. In other words, diaphragmatic contraction increases transdiaphragmatic pressure (P_{di}), which is

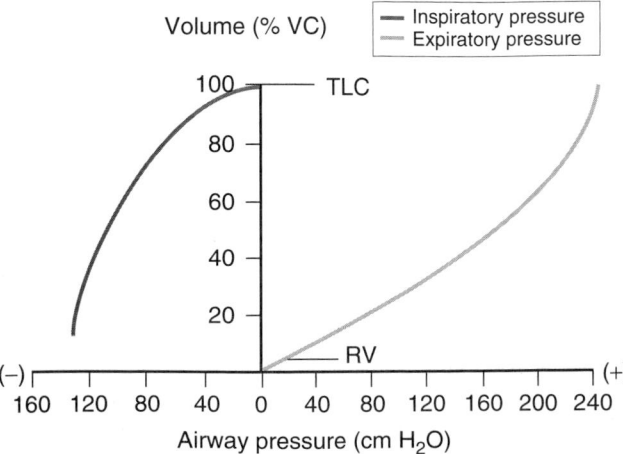

FIGURE 63–12. Plot of inspiratory and expiratory pressures as a function of lung volume. Note the higher pressures generated by expiratory muscles. TLC, total lung capacity; VC, vital capacity. (From Taylor A, Rehder K, Hyatt R, et al: Mechanics of breathing: Static. In Taylor AE [ed]: Clinical Respiratory Physiology. Philadelphia, WB Saunders, 1989, pp 89-105.)

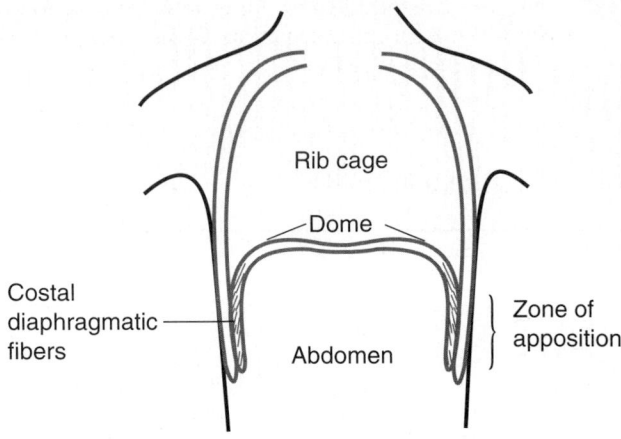

FIGURE 63–13. Chest wall, frontal section, at end-expiration. The costal diaphragmatic fibers are cranially oriented, resulting in apposition to the lower rib cage. (From De Troyer A: Respiratory muscle function. In Pinsky MR [ed]: Textbook of Critical Care. Philadelphia, WB Saunders, 2000, pp 1172-1184.)

partially dependent on abdominal pressure (P_{ab}), as shown in the equation

$$P_{di} = P_{pl} - P_{ab} = P_{ga} - P_{es} \qquad \text{(Equation 18)}$$

where P_{ga} is gastric pressure and P_{es} is esophageal pressure. Second, the contracting diaphragm exerts what is termed an appositional force. This is related to the configuration of the muscle fibers in the zone of apposition, which, in contrast to fibers in the dome, have a much larger radius of curvature (i.e., less of a curve). In accordance with the law of Laplace, less pressure is generated to move the diaphragm. Instead, the pleural space in the zone of apposition is exposed to approximate abdominal pressure, thereby acting directly to push the lower rib cage in an outward direction.[38] Thus, the rise in abdominal pressure caused by descent of the diaphragmatic dome is transmitted through the appositional portion of the diaphragm to expand the lower rib cage.[39] Accordingly, pressure in the pleural recess between the apposed diaphragm and the rib cage actually *increases* during inspiration.

It should be noted that diaphragmatic contraction can have inspiratory *or* expiratory effects on the thoracic cage, depending on several factors.[2] For example, mechanical properties of the abdominal compartment have a marked influence on diaphragmatic function. Low compliance (tense ascites) results in reduced dome excursion and decreased insertional force, whereas decrements in abdominal resistance (evisceration) cause loss of the zone of apposition, with resultant expiratory actions on the lower rib cage.[37] There are also important effects related to lung volume. The area of apposition increases as the lungs approach residual volume, causing a greater inspiratory effect on the lower rib cage. Conversely, near total lung capacity, the zone of apposition is nearly absent, resulting in an expiratory force. Studies of diaphragmatic contraction in subjects with cervical spinal cord transection have demonstrated expiratory effects on the upper rib cage and inspiratory effects on the lower rib cage.[40,41]

ABDOMINAL MUSCLES

The abdomen, with the exception of the diaphragm superiorly and the anterior abdominal wall (and small amounts of gas in the gastrointestinal tract), is an essentially incompressible compartment with fixed boundaries. As such, the movement of the diaphragm and thoracic cage is coupled with movement of the anterior abdominal wall. This is a clinically important relationship that should be assessed during a physical examination, because asynchronous and paradoxical motion of the rib cage and abdomen has been associated with an increased respiratory drive[42] and possible risk of ventilatory failure.[43]

The respiratory muscles of the abdominal wall, including the obliques, rectus abdominis, and transversus abdominis, are primarily expiratory in function, by virtue of the increase in abdominal pressure upon contraction. This becomes important when flow demands are not met by passive elastic recoil. As mentioned previously, they aid in unloading the inspiratory muscles during times of stress by their effects on lung volume. In addition, the tonic contraction of the abdominal muscles to help maintain posture in the upright position elongates the diaphragm, thus improving its length-tension relationship.

ASSESSMENT OF CHEST WALL FUNCTION

Pressure measurements across the chest wall can be readily obtained to assess the ability of the respiratory muscles to perform the work of breathing. As mentioned earlier with regard to the respiratory system, the chest wall can be studied during static as well as dynamic maneuvers to obtain important information about function. It should be noted that although these functional tests are of interest to physiologists and researchers, their clinical application is limited.

The Rahn diagram is a graphic representation of the relaxed respiratory system's P-V characteristics (see Fig. 63-2). It provides information on the passive elastic properties of the components of the respiratory system. For accurate chest wall measurements, complete respiratory muscle relaxation is required.

The function of the active chest wall can be assessed with the Campbell diagram (Fig. 63-14), which plots changes in lung volume against pleural pressure. Two curves are generated, one representing a passive inflation of the lungs similar to the Rahn tracing, and the other representing an active inspiration, correlating progressively negative pleural pressures with increasing volume. The work performed by the inspiratory muscles,

$$\int (Pmus\ \Delta V,) \qquad \text{(Equation 19)}$$

is represented by the hatched areas of the Campbell diagram. The sum of both areas gives the total work of breathing per inspired breath. The average total work of breathing has been found to be 2.2 ± 0.92 g * cm/mL at a frequency of 15 breaths per minute.[44] Muscle force reserve can be determined from a Campbell diagram that includes plots of maximal respiratory pressures. Here, the difference between the maximal static inspiratory pressures and actual peak pressure can provide an estimation of the likelihood of fatigue.

These methods are difficult to use in mechanically ventilated patients. In this setting, simple ventilator waveform analysis can be helpful. For example, deviation of the inspiratory flow waveform from the relaxed tracing indicates active patient effort as a result of flow deprivation—that is, the patient's demands are not being met by the set inspiratory flow.[45] Maximal inspiratory pressure is a commonly used measurement in the ICU, particularly in weaning protocols.

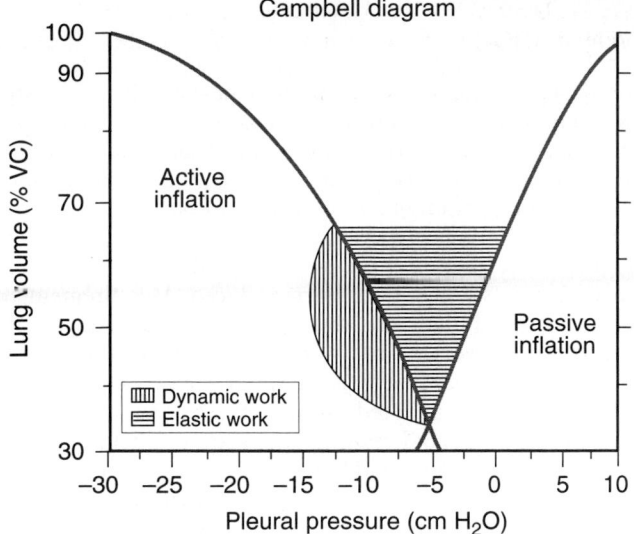

Campbell diagram

FIGURE 63–14. Campbell diagram, representing work performed by inspiratory muscles during a breathing cycle. *Vertical hatching,* Work done to overcome resistive pressures. *Horizontal hatching,* Work done to overcome respiratory system elastance. VC, vital capacity. (From American Thoracic Society/European Respiratory Society: ATS/ERS statement on respiratory muscle testing. Am J Respir Crit Care Med 2002;166:518-624.)

High generated pressures probably correlate with adequate muscle strength, but low values may be related to volitional factors. Moreover, standardized testing has shown poor reproducibility.[46]

RESPIRATORY MUSCLE FUNCTION IN DISEASE

Impairment or failure of the respiratory pump can occur at any of several levels. Dysfunctional central respiratory control, such as during coma or intoxication, alters neural output to the respiratory muscles. Neuromuscular diseases, such as myasthenia gravis or muscular dystrophy, result in primary muscle weakness, whereas metabolic abnormalities (malnutrition, thyroid disease) affect the muscle tension-generating machinery. Lung hyperinflation, such as occurs in COPD or asthma, puts the chest wall at a mechanical disadvantage because of alterations in the length-tension relationship.

Much attention has been given to the concept of respiratory muscle fatigue,[47] both in acute respiratory failure and in relation to chronic lung disease. Muscle fatigue is defined as a condition associated with loss of the capacity for developing force, velocity, or both resulting from muscle activity, which is reversible by rest.[48] This contrasts with the definition of muscle weakness, in which the rested muscle remains impaired. Fatigue can be induced in striated muscle when working against an increased load. This has been reproduced in normal human respiratory muscles forced to work against high inspiratory airflow resistance.[49] Fatigue can be classified as central fatigue, peripheral high-frequency fatigue, or peripheral low-frequency fatigue.[50] It is likely that all three play a role in respiratory muscle fatigue at any given time.

There is no single measurement of force that can adequately measure respiratory muscle fatigue. Rather, fatigue is implied by the deterioration of force during serial measurements over time. The factors important in respiratory

muscle fatigue—magnitude and duration of contraction—are incorporated into the calculation of the pressure-time index of the diaphragm (PT_{di}):

$$PT_{di} = (P_{di}/P_{di,max})(T_i/T_{tot}) \qquad \text{(Equation 20)}$$

where P_{di} denotes transdiaphragmatic pressure (a measure of magnitude), T_i is inspiratory time, and T_{tot} is total breath time. When breathing is accomplished primarily by diaphragmatic function, a critical pressure-time index is reached at values of 0.15 to 0.18, above which functional failure readily occurs.[51] Similar ranges have been obtained for rib cage muscles as well.[52] Unfortunately, because these values were experimentally obtained in normal subjects breathing against imposed loads, the true values that apply to patients with impending respiratory failure, in whom other factors (hypoxemia, hemodynamic instability) are in play, is not known.

RESPIRATORY MUSCLE FUNCTION IN ACUTE RESPIRATORY FAILURE

The inability of the respiratory pump to meet metabolic demands, resulting in acute respiratory failure, is a result of either increase in the ventilatory load above a critical level or inability of the respiratory muscles to generate sufficient force. Assessment of the breathing pattern may be helpful in patients with impending respiratory failure. For example, tachypnea and paradoxical motion of the thorax and abdomen are frequently encountered in this setting, but they are not specific or diagnostic of muscle fatigue.

Work of breathing is a global measure of respiratory pump activity and reflects the imposed respiratory load, which is often a result of abnormalities in respiratory mechanics. Most of the work of breathing, in both health and disease states, occurs during inspiration (W_i) and is related to the static elastance (E_{st}) of the respiratory system[53]:

$$W_{i,st} = 0.5 \, E_{st} \cdot \Delta V \qquad \text{(Equation 21)}$$

A linear relationship is assumed between elastance and the volumes measured. The contribution of dynamic factors to work of breathing, such as increases in airway resistance in COPD or asthma resulting in dynamic hyperinflation, must also be accounted for. In such cases, the equation becomes:

$$W_{i,st} = 0.5 \, E_{st} \cdot \Delta V + PEEP_i \cdot \Delta V \qquad \text{(Equation 22)}$$

Patients with acute respiratory failure related to COPD have been found to have increased inspiratory resistance, increased dynamic elastance, and up to twice the level of intrinsic PEEP ($PEEP_i$) compared with COPD patients not in acute respiratory failure.[54] Dynamic hyperinflation has secondary deleterious effects on respiratory muscle function, related primarily to Starling's law (suboptimal coupling of the tension-generating components of the muscle fibers). The increased work of breathing resulting from dynamic hyperinflation can be demonstrated graphically by the Campbell diagram (Fig. 63-15).[55]

Thus, relatively small insults leading to increased work of breathing and subsequent respiratory muscle fatigue could precipitate acute respiratory failure in patients with "compensated" COPD. Although impairment of inspiratory muscle function related to dynamic hyperinflation is classically

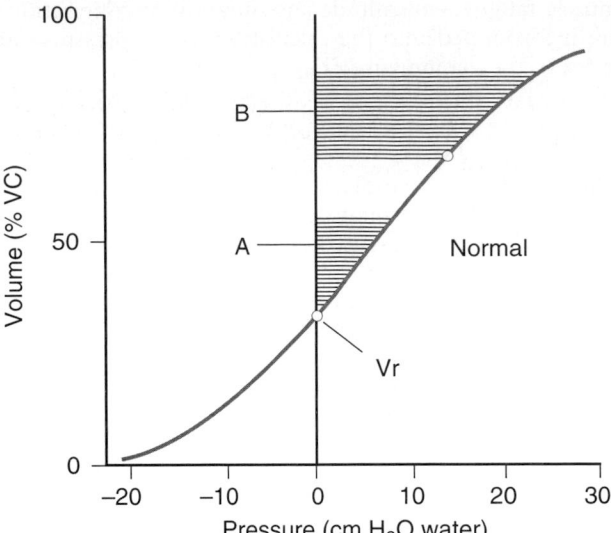

FIGURE 63–15. Volume-pressure (Campbell) diagram of the relaxed respiratory system of a dynamically hyperinflated subject. *Hatched area A,* Elastic work for a breath starting from relaxation volume (Vr). *Hatched area B,* Elastic work for a breath starting from a volume of 29% vital capacity (VC) above Vr. (From Eissa NT, Milic-Emili J: Modern concepts in monitoring and management of respiratory failure. Anesthesiol Clin 1991;9:199-218.)

associated with obstructive lung diseases, it is also seen in cases of pneumonia and chest trauma.[42]

A number of other disorders seen in critical illness have been associated with reduced respiratory muscle force generation. Sepsis, even in the absence of direct lung involvement, can cause respiratory failure related to increased metabolic demands as well as respiratory muscle dysfunction.[56] Direct effects on muscle function have been related to failure of neuromuscular contraction, derangements in excitation-contraction coupling, and direct cytotoxic effects.[56]

Critical illness polyneuropathy, associated with varying degrees of weakness and axonal degeneration on electromyography and denervation atrophy on muscle biopsy, has a reported incidence as high as 25%.[57] The causative role of critical illness polyneuropathy in respiratory failure is controversial, because it is often associated with other conditions that affect global muscle function, such as sepsis and multiorgan system failure.[58] It has, however, been documented in cases of respiratory failure independent of these risk factors.[59] Critical illness myopathy, which can coexist with polyneuropathy, is most commonly reported in cases of severe asthma and may be related to glucocorticoid and neuromuscular blocking agent administration.[60] Finally, there is mounting animal model data showing that mechanical ventilation has direct harmful effects on diaphragmatic structure and function.[61,62] Putative mechanisms include atrophy related to disuse (particularly with prolonged mechanical ventilation), tonic effects of PEEP, and confounding effects of anesthesia and neuromuscular blocking agents.

WEANING FROM MECHANICAL VENTILATION

Clinical assessment alone is insufficient to predict successful weaning from mechanical ventilation,[63] and respiratory muscle function is only one determinant of weaning ability. Unfortunately, the incorporation of many objective methods into weaning paradigms has not proved particularly useful. The shortcomings of breathing pattern assessment were mentioned earlier, and measurements of maximal inspiratory pressures are not easily reproduced. Measurement of pressure-time indices has not been readily adopted in ICU practice, and work-of-breathing determinations are cumbersome and seemingly restricted to the research setting. The most widely adopted and useful predictor of weaning success is the ratio of breathing frequency to tidal volume, as first reported by Yang and Tobin.[64] This involves the simple use of a spirometer attached to the endotracheal tube during a spontaneous breathing trial. A ratio of 105 breaths/min per liter provides the best separation between subjects who will succeed and fail at weaning.

ACKNOWLEDGMENTS

This work was supported by National Institutes of Health grants HL 57364 and HL 6317.

ANNOTATED REFERENCES

Fredberg JJ, Stamenovic D: On the imperfect elasticity of lung tissue. J Appl Physiol 1989;67:2408-2419.
  An elegant exploration of energy losses related to tissue resistance and hysteresis and the coupling of changes in elastic energy storage and dissipative energy loss, which appears to reside within the same stress-bearing element of the lung.

Fry DL, Hyatt RE: A unified analysis of the relationship between pressure, volume and gas flow in the lungs of normal and diseased human subjects. Am J Med 1960;29:672-689.
  Report of a classic set of human experiments that forms the physiologic basis of the forced vital capacity maneuver in modern pulmonary function testing.

Hubmayr RD: Perspective on lung injury and recruitment: A skeptical look at the opening and collapse story. Am J Respir Crit Care Med 2002;165:1647-1653.
  A discussion of current controversies about ventilation strategies, emphasizing the uncertainties of physiologic changes at the acinar level. The theory of alveolar collapse in derecruitment is questioned, and the interpretation of the P-V curve and the best PEEP is argued.

Laghi F, Tobin M: Disorders of the respiratory muscles. Am J Respir Crit Care Med 2003;168:10-48.
  A wide-ranging discussion of various diseases of respiratory muscles, including an explanation of the molecular mechanisms of clinically applicable disorders encountered in the ICU.

Loring S: Mechanics of the lung and chest wall. In Marini JJ (ed): Physiological Basis of Ventilatory Support. New York, Marcel Dekker, 1998, pp 177-205.
  A comprehensive review of the physiologic basis of classic respiratory system mechanics. Discusses lung and chest wall mechanical properties, as well as assessment of respiratory muscle function.

Chapter 64

HEART-LUNG INTERACTIONS

Michael R. Pinsky

KEY POINTS

1. **Spontaneous ventilation is exercise.**

2. In patients with cardiovascular insufficiency and increased work of breathing, initiation of mechanical ventilatory support improves oxygen (O_2) delivery to the remainder of the body by decreasing respiratory muscle O_2 demand. To the extent that mixed venous O_2 also increases (owing to reduced O_2 consumption), arterial O_2 partial pressure also increases, without any improvement in gas exchange.

3. The transition from mechanical ventilatory support to spontaneous ventilation is a cardiovascular stress test. Patients who fail to wean manifest cardiovascular insufficiency during the attempt. Myocardial ischemia, infarction, gut ischemia, and decreasing mixed venous O_2 are all manifestations of failure to wean. Improving cardiovascular reserve or supplementing support with inotropic therapy may allow a patient to bridge from mechanical to spontaneous ventilation.

4. **Changes in lung volume alter autonomic tone and pulmonary vascular resistance** and, at high lung volumes, compress the heart in the cardiac fossa in a fashion analogous to cardiac tamponade.

5. Small increases in lung volume induce vagal withdrawal and inspiration-associated cardiac acceleration. Loss of such respiratory sinus arrhythmia is a manifestation of dysautonomia in diabetics with peripheral neuropathy. Larger increases in lung volume induce withdrawal of sympathetic tone and may be a cause of cardiac depression in patients with acute lung injury, in whom ventilation hyperinflates the remaining aerated lung units.

6. Changes in lung volume are determined by changes in transpulmonary pressure and lung compliance. As lung volume increases, so does the pressure difference between airway and pleural pressure. When this pressure difference exceeds pulmonary artery pressure, pulmonary vessels collapse as they pass from the pulmonary arteries into the alveolar space, increasing pulmonary vascular resistance. Thus, increasing lung volume and hyperinflation may increase pulmonary vascular resistance, pulmonary artery pressure, and right ventricular afterload, impeding right ventricular ejection.

7. Decreases in lung volume below functional residual capacity, as occurs in patients with acute lung injury, are associated with collapse of terminal airways, resorption of alveolar O_2, and subsequent increased pulmonary vasomotor tone by the process of hypoxic pulmonary vasoconstriction. Recruitment maneuvers, positive end-expiratory pressure, and continuous positive airway pressure may all refresh collapsed alveoli, reversing hypoxic pulmonary vasoconstriction and reducing pulmonary artery pressure.

8. Overinflation of the lungs compresses the heart, decreasing biventricular volumes while increasing cardiac filling pressures. At the extreme, this can cause volume-unresponsive hypovolemic shock.

9. **Spontaneous inspiration and spontaneous inspiratory efforts decrease intrathoracic pressure,** and diaphragmatic descent increases intra-abdominal pressure. These combined effects cause right atrial pressure inside the thorax to decrease, but venous pressure in the abdomen to increase, markedly increasing the pressure gradient for systemic venous return.

10. The augmentation in venous return is constrained by the Starling resistor forces, limiting maximal venous flow as intrathoracic pressure becomes negative relative to atmosphere, and vascular compression in the liver from diaphragmatic descent. Right ventricular filling is limited by pericardial constraints that limit maximal biventricular volume.

11. The greater the decrease in intrathoracic pressure, the greater the increase in left ventricular ejection pressure for a constant arterial pressure. With obstructed inspiratory efforts, as occur with obstructive sleep apnea, upper airway obstruction, and bronchospasm, the increase in left ventricular afterload can precipitate acute left ventricular failure, pulmonary edema, and cardiovascular collapse. Mechanical ventilation, by abolishing the negative swings in intrathoracic pressure, selectively decreases left ventricular afterload, as long as the increases in lung volume and intrathoracic pressure are small.

12. Positive-pressure ventilation increases intrathoracic pressure, and diaphragmatic descent increases

intra-abdominal pressure. Thus, the decrease in the pressure gradient for venous return is less than would otherwise occur if the only change were an increase in right atrial pressure. However, in hypovolemic states, positive-pressure ventilation can induce profound decreases in venous return.

13. Increases in intrathoracic pressure decrease left ventricular afterload and augment left ventricular ejection. In patients with hypervolemic heart failure, this afterload-reducing effect can result in improved left ventricular ejection, increased cardiac output, and reduced myocardial O_2 demand.

Ventilation can profoundly alter cardiovascular function. The boundaries of the cardiovascular unit's responsiveness are defined by both cardiovascular and pulmonary factors. These limitations include the myocardial reserve, circulating blood volume, blood flow distribution, autonomic tone, endocrinologic responses, lung volume, intrathoracic pressure (ITP), and surrounding pressures for the remainder of the circulation.

RELATION AMONG AIRWAY PRESSURE, INTRATHORACIC PRESSURES, AND LUNG VOLUME

Since the introduction of positive-pressure ventilation, the concept of relating hemodynamic consequences to airway pressure has been widely accepted.[1,2] This gross simplification has been the source of much confusion in the clinical literature, largely because changes in airway pressure are often equated with changes in both pleural pressure and lung volume. However, the association between airway pressure and other hemodynamically relevant factors is highly variable as ventilatory patterns, airway resistance, and lung compliance change; does not accurately reflect changes in pericardial pressure, which is a primary determinant of transmural left ventricular (LV) pressure; and may mislead the caregiver into altering therapy based on these wrong assumptions. Numerous studies have demonstrated that the primary determinants of the hemodynamic responses to ventilation are due to changes in intrathoracic pressure and lung volume,[3] not airway pressure. We use the term *intrathoracic pressure (ITP)* to refer to a nonspecific intrathoracic surface pressure. When specific intrapleural surface pressures are meant, they are referred to as lateral chest wall, diaphragm, and juxtacardiac pleural pressures or pericardial pressure, as appropriate.

AIRWAY PRESSURE, LUNG VOLUME, AND REGIONAL PLEURAL PRESSURES

During positive-pressure inspiration, increases in airway pressure parallel increases in lung volume. In a sedated and paralyzed patient, only lung and thoracic compliance determines the relation between airway pressure and lung volume at end-inspiration. However, if a ventilated patient actively resists lung inflation or sustains expiratory muscle activity at end-inspiration, end-inspiratory airway pressure will exceed resting airway pressure for that lung volume. Similarly, if patient activity prevents full exhalation by expiratory braking,

for the same end-expiratory airway pressure (often measured as positive end-expiratory pressure [PEEP]), lung volume may be much higher than predicted from end-expiratory airway pressure values alone. Finally, even if inspiration is passive and no increased airway resistance is present, airway pressure may rapidly increase over minutes as chest wall compliance decreases. If intra-abdominal pressure increases, end-expiratory airway pressure must also increase for a constant tidal volume. During inspiration, airway pressure increases as a function of both total thoracic compliance and airway resistance. Thus, in subjects with marked bronchospasm, such as asthmatics, peak airway pressure greatly exceeds end-inspiratory plateau airway pressure.

Changes in airway pressure are related to changes in lung volume through the interaction of airway resistance and both lung and chest compliance, as manifested by the relative increase in ITP during inspiration. Several common clinical examples support this statement. If either lung or chest wall compliance changes, airway pressure may change without an actual change in the tidal breath. The two common clinical scenarios of this phenomenon are mucus plugging and fighting the ventilator. Similarly, if spontaneous breaths cause ITP to decrease during positive-pressure inspiration, both peak and mean airway pressures will decrease, whereas if bronchospasm causes airway resistance to increase, for a constant tidal breath, both peak and mean airway pressures will increase.

As the lung expands, it pushes on the surrounding structures, distorting them and causing their surface pressures to increase. This lung expansion induces an increase in lateral wall, diaphragmatic, and juxtacardiac pleural pressure, as well as pericardial pressure. The degree of increase in each of these surface pressures is a function of the compliance and inertance of their opposing structures. These interactions were described by Novak and colleagues, who demonstrated that the changes in pleural pressure induced by positive-pressure ventilation are not similar in all regions of the thorax and increase differently as inspiratory flow rate and frequency increase.[4] Pleural pressure on the diaphragm increases least during inspiration, and juxtacardiac pleural pressure increases most. Because the diaphragm is very compliant, it seems reasonable that diaphragmatic ITP should increase less than lateral chest wall pleural pressure in response to sudden increases in lung volume. However, if abdominal distention develops, the diaphragm becomes relatively noncompliant because of the increase in abdominal pressure. Under these conditions, ITP tends to increase similarly across the thorax.

A hydrostatic pressure gradient exists in the pleural space. Dependent regions have a higher baseline pressure than nondependent regions in proportion to their height above or below the heart (measured in centimeters), which equates with an equal pressure difference (measured in cm H_2O). In a supine subject, steady-state apneic pleural pressures along the horizontal plane from apex to diaphragm are similar, whereas anterior pleural pressure is less and posterior gutter pleural pressure is greater (Fig. 64-1).

Care must be taken to determine not only what types of ventilation are being compared but also how and where estimates of pleural pressure and pericardial pressure are made. For example, if estimates of transpulmonary pressure are needed to define lung compliance and its change with recruitment maneuvers, lateral chest wall pleural pressure more accurately reflects the pressure-volume characteristics of the intact lung.[4] Similarly, if diaphragmatic work is to be

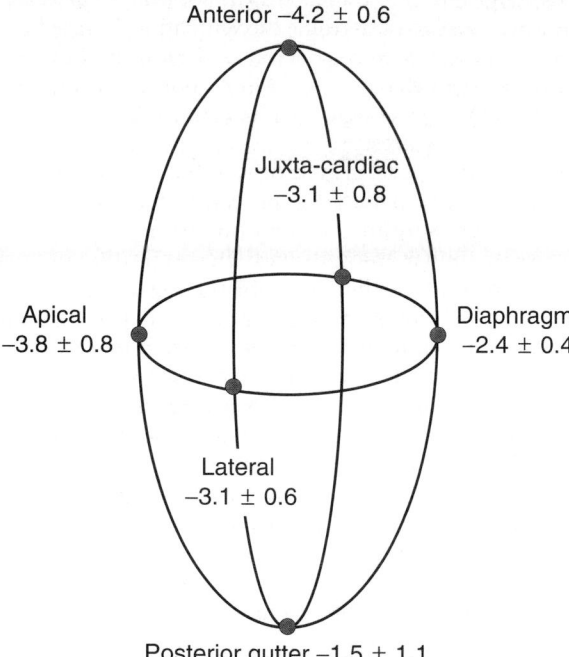

FIGURE 64–1. Apneic pleural pressure (Ppl) (mean ± standard error) in torr for six pleural regions of the right hemothorax of an intact supine canine model: anterior, apical, posterior gutter, diaphragmatic, juxtacardiac, and lateral. Ellipses represenst regional measurements defining three orthogonal planes. (From Novak RA, Matuschak GM, Pinsky MR: Effect of ventilatory frequency on regional pleural pressure. J Appl Physiol 1988;65:1314-1323.)

monitored, either esophageal or diaphragmatic pleural pressure should be used. Finally, if heart-lung interactions are being examined, juxtacardiac pleural pressure is the most accurate measure of pleural pressure; increases during positive-pressure inspiration will be underestimated by esophageal pressure. Because the heart is fixed within a cardiac fossa, juxtacardiac pleural pressure increases more than lateral chest wall or diaphragmatic pleural pressure does. If pericardial volume restraints exist, juxtacardiac pleural pressure will underestimate pericardial pressure. However, with sustained lung compression of the heart overriding tamponade, both juxtacardiac pleural pressure and pericardial pressure will be similar.

PLEURAL PRESSURE AND LUNG VOLUME IN ACUTE LUNG INJURY

The interaction of airway pressure, lung volume, and ITP in the setting of lung disease is complex and can differ in the same pathologic setting, depending on the tidal volume, inspiratory flow rate, ventilatory frequency, and body position. The presence of parenchymal disease, airflow obstruction, and extrapulmonary processes that directly alter chest wall–diaphragmatic contraction also profoundly alters these interactions. Static lung expansion occurs as airway pressure increases because the transpulmonary pressure (airway pressure relative to ITP) increases. If lung injury induces alveolar flooding or increased pulmonary parenchyma stiffness, greater increases in airway pressure will be required to distend the lungs to a constant end-inspiratory volume. Romand and coworkers demonstrated that airway pressure increased more during acute lung injury (ALI) than in control conditions for

a constant tidal volume, whereas lateral chest wall pleural pressure and pericardial pressure increased similarly between both conditions if tidal volume was held constant (Fig. 64-2).[5] These data agree with the studies of O'Quinn and associates, which found that the primary determinant of the increase in pleural pressure and pericardial pressure during positive-pressure ventilation is lung volume change, not airway pressure change.[6] Presumably, pericardial pressure does not increase as much as ITP because the increasing lung volume reduces the filling of the ventricles, decreasing their size inside the cardiac fossa. To summarize, for a constant increase in lung volume, ITP increases similarly, despite drastic changes in lung compliance and airway resistance.

AIRWAY, PLEURAL, AND PERICARDIAL PRESSURES

Because the distribution of alveolar collapse and lung compliance in acute respiratory distress syndrome (ARDS) and ALI is nonhomogeneous, lung distention during positive-pressure ventilation must reflect overdistention of some regions of the lung at the expense of noncompliant or poorly compliant regions. Accordingly, airway pressure reflects the distention of lung units that were aerated before inspiration but may

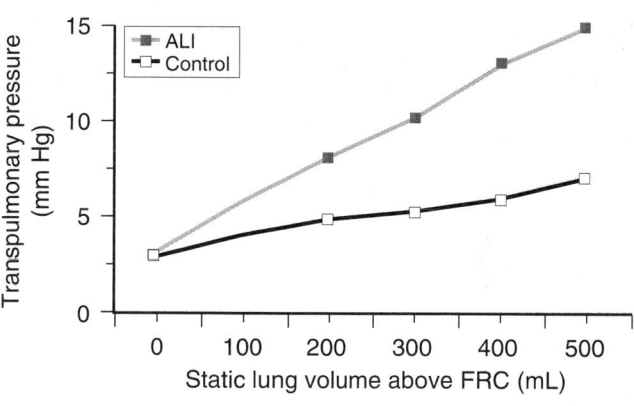

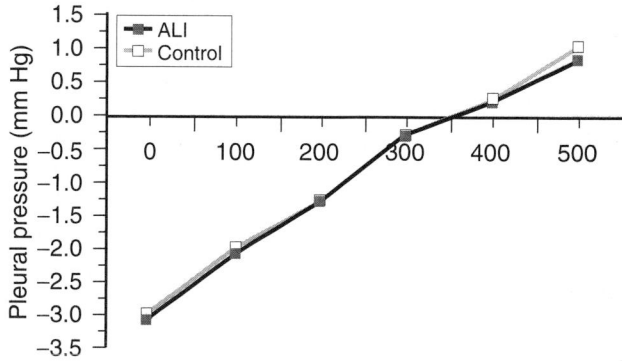

FIGURE 64–2. Relation between airway pressure (Paw) and tidal volume (Vt) and between pleural pressure (Ppl) and tidal volume (Vt) in a control group and in oleic acid–induced acute lung injury (ALI) in a canine model. Note that despite greater increases in airway pressure for the same tidal volume during ALI as compared with control conditions, pleural pressure and pericardial pressure increase similarly in both groups for the same increase in tidal volume. FRC, functional residual capacity. (From Romand JA, Shi W, Pinsky MR: Cardiopulmonary effects of positive pressure ventilation during acute lung injury. Chest 1995;108:1041-1048.)

not reflect the degree of lung inflation of nonaerated lung units. In an animal model of ALI, in which tidal volume was either kept constant at preinjury levels or reduced to match preinjury plateau airway pressure (pressure-limited ventilation), both pleural pressure and pericardial pressure increased less in comparison to both preinjury states and in ALI when tidal volume remained at preinjury levels.[5]

Because ALI is often nonhomogeneous, with aerated areas of the lung displaying normal specific compliance, large increases in airway pressure overdistend aerated lung units.[7] Vascular structures that are distended have a greater increase in their surrounding pressure than do collapsible structures that do not distend.[8] Romand and colleagues[5] and Scharf and Ingram[9] demonstrated that despite this nonhomogeneous alveolar distention, if tidal volume is kept constant, pleural pressure will increase equally, independent of the mechanical properties of the lung. Thus, under constant tidal volume conditions, changes in peak and mean airway pressures reflect changes in the mechanical properties of the lungs and patient coordination but may not reflect changes in ITP. Similarly, these changes in airway pressure may not alter global cardiovascular dynamics. Underscoring airway pressure's limited ability to reflect either ITP or pericardial pressure, Pinsky and coworkers demonstrated in postoperative patients that the percentage of airway pressure increase transmitted to the pericardial surface is not constant from one subject to the next as PEEP is increased (Fig. 64-3).[10] Thus, one cannot predict the amount of increase in pericardial pressure or pleural pressure that will occur in patients as PEEP is increased. Accordingly, assuming some constant fraction of airway pressure transmission to the pleural surface as a means of calculating the effect of increasing airway pressure on pleural pressure is inaccurate and potentially dangerous to patient management.

Although it may be difficult to know the actual pleural pressure, it is possible to determine the ventilation-induced change in pleural pressure. During airway occlusion maneuvers, lung volume does not change, and transpulmonary pressure is also constant; this means that the change in ITP is equal to the change in airway pressure.[11]

Two limitations to the use of intrathoracic vascular pressures to estimate pericardial pressure and ITP exist. First, pericardial pressure and ITP may not be similar and may not increase by similar amounts with the application of positive airway pressure if the pericardium becomes a limiting membrane.[12,13] Operationally, this equates to pericardial pressure exceeding juxtacardiac pleural pressure by the degree to which the pericardium limits biventricular dilatation. Thus, determinations of pericardial pressure using ITP measures may underestimate pericardial pressure and overestimate the increase in pericardial pressure as airway pressure is increased. Second, esophageal pressure is often used clinically to estimate swings in both pleural pressure and pericardial pressure. However, esophageal pressure changes underestimate both the positive swings in pleural pressure and the mean increase in pleural pressure seen with increases in lung volume during positive-pressure ventilation.

HEMODYNAMIC EFFECTS OF VENTILATION

Lung volume increases in a tidal fashion during both spontaneous and positive-pressure ventilation. However, ITP decreases during spontaneous inspiration and increases during positive-pressure inspiration. Thus, changes in ITP and in the metabolic requirements to create these changes represent the primary determinants of the hemodynamic differences between spontaneous and positive-pressure ventilation.[14,15]

Heart-lung interactions can be broadly grouped, based on three concepts that usually coexist in the clinical setting. First, spontaneous ventilatory efforts are exercise; they require oxygen (O_2) and blood flow, thus placing demands on cardiac output and producing carbon dioxide (CO_2), adding ventilatory stress on CO_2 excretion. Second, inspiration increases lung volume above resting end-expiratory volume. Thus, some of the hemodynamic effects of ventilation may be due to changes in lung volume and chest wall expansion. Third, spontaneous inspiration decreases ITP, whereas positive-pressure ventilation increases ITP; thus, the differences between spontaneous ventilation and positive-pressure ventilation reflect primarily the differences in ITP swings and the energy necessary to produce them.

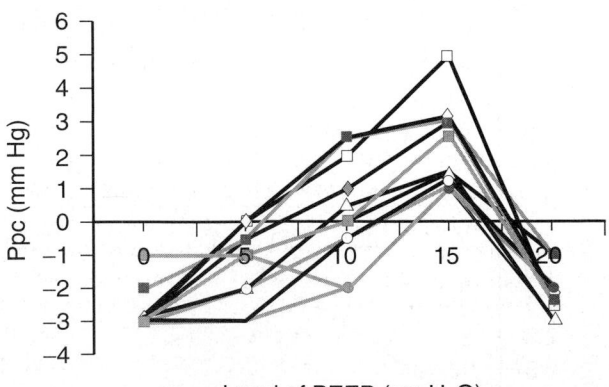

FIGURE 64–3. Relation between pericardial pressure (Ppc) and airway pressure as apneic levels of positive end-expiratory pressure (PEEP) are progressively increased from 0 to 15 cm H_2O and then back to 0 in increments of 5 cm H_2O in patients immediately following open heart surgery. Note that although pericardial pressure increases in all subjects as PEEP is increased from 0 to 15 cm H_2O, the initial pericardial pressure value and the proportional change in pericardial pressure with incremental increases in PEEP are quite different among subjects, such that no specific proportion of airway pressure transmission to the pericardial surface can be assumed to occur in all patients. (From Pinsky MR, Vincent JL, DeSmet JM: Estimating left ventricular filling pressure during positive end-expiratory pressure in humans. Am Rev Respir Dis 1991;143:25-31.)

VENTILATION AS EXERCISE

Spontaneous ventilatory efforts are induced by respiratory muscle contraction. Blood flow to these muscles is derived from several arterial circuits whose absolute flow is believed to exceed the highest metabolic demand of maximally exercising skeletal muscle.[16] Thus, under normal cardiovascular conditions, blood flow is not the limiting factor determining maximal ventilatory effort. Although ventilation normally requires less than 5% of total O_2 delivery to meet its demand,[16] in lung disease states in which the work of breathing is increased, such as pulmonary edema or bronchospasm, the work of breathing can increase metabolic demand for O_2 to

25% or 30% of total O_2 delivery.[16-19] Further, if cardiac output is limited, blood flow to other organs and to the respiratory muscles may be compromised, inducing both tissue hypoperfusion and lactic acidosis.[20-23] Starting mechanical ventilation may reduce metabolic demand, increasing venous O_2 saturation for a constant cardiac output and arterial oxygen content (CaO_2). Intubation and mechanical ventilation, when adjusted to the metabolic demands of the patient, may dramatically decrease the work of breathing, resulting in increased O_2 delivery to other vital organs and decreased serum lactic acid levels. These cardiovascular benefits can also be realized with the effective use of noninvasive continuous positive airway pressure (CPAP) by ventilation mask.[24] The obligatory increase in venous O_2 saturation will result in an increase in arterial O_2 partial pressure if fixed right-to-left shunts exist, even if mechanical ventilation does not alter the ratio of shunt blood flow to cardiac output. Finally, if cardiac output is severely limited, respiratory muscle failure will develop despite high central neuronal drive, such that many patients with heart failure die of respiratory failure before cardiovascular standstill.[25]

Ventilator-dependent patients who fail to wean from mechanical ventilation may occasionally have impaired baseline cardiovascular performance,[26] but during weaning attempts, they routinely develop overt signs of heart failure such as pulmonary edema,[26,27] myocardial ischemia,[28-31] tachycardia, and gut ischemia.[32] Jabran and associates demonstrated that although all subjects increase their cardiac output in response to a weaning trial, those who subsequently fail to wean demonstrate a reduction in mixed venous O_2 saturation, consistent with a failing cardiovascular response to increased metabolic demand.[33] Importantly, the increased work of breathing may come from endotracheal tube flow resistance.[34] Thus, weaning from mechanical ventilatory support can be considered a cardiovascular stress test. Investigators have documented weaning-associated signs of ischemia (on electrocardiogram and thallium cardiac blood flow scan) both in subjects with known coronary artery disease[30] and in otherwise normal patients.[29,31] Using this same logic, placing patients with severe heart failure or ischemia on ventilatory support by either intubation and ventilation[35] or noninvasive CPAP[36] can reverse myocardial ischemia.

CHANGES IN LUNG VOLUME

Changing lung volume alters autonomic tone and pulmonary vascular resistance. At high lung volumes, the enlarged lungs compress the heart in the cardiac fossa, limiting absolute cardiac volumes in a fashion analogous to tamponade. But unlike tamponade, wherein pericardial pressure selectively increases, with hyperinflation, both juxtacardiac pleural pressure and pericardial pressure increase together.

Autonomic Tone

The lungs are richly innervated with integrated somatic and autonomic fibers that originate in, traverse, and end in the thorax. Inflation induces immediate changes in autonomic output. The most commonly described inflation-chronotropic responses act through vagal-mediated reflex arcs.[37,38] Lung inflation to normal tidal volumes (<10 mL/kg) increases heart rate via parasympathetic tone withdrawal. Inspiration-associated cardioacceleration is referred to as respiratory sinus arrhythmia[39] and denotes normal autonomic tone.[40] Loss of respiratory sinus arrhythmia denotes dysautonomia.

However, some degree of respiratory-associated heart rate change is intrinsic to the heart itself. For example, in denervated human hearts (transplants), a small degree of ventilation-associated heart rate change persists,[41] suggesting that mechanoreceptors in the right atrium can alter sinoatrial tone.

Lung inflation to larger tidal volumes (>15 mL/kg) decreases heart rate. Pulmonary vasoconstriction also may occur through vagal reflex arcs[42] but does not appear to have significant hemodynamic effects. Reflex arterial vasodilatation can also occur with lung hyperinflation.[37,43-47] This inflation-vasodilatation response appears to be mediated by afferent vagal fibers, because it is abolished by selective vagotomy. Interestingly, blocking sympathetic afferent fibers also blocks this reflex,[45,48] presumably by withdrawing central sympathetic tone. Although this inflation-vasodilatation response induces expiration-associated reductions in LV contractility in healthy volunteers[49] and in ventilator-dependent patients with the initiation of high-frequency ventilation[37] or hyperinflation,[45] its clinical significance in other patient groups is unknown. Because patients with ALI often ventilate a small amount of lung, these patients may experience regional hyperinflation and develop reflex cardiovascular depression. Interestingly, several studies comparing larger tidal volume ventilation with pressure-limited ventilation documented better hemodynamic status with pressure-limited ventilation. Importantly, for the same decrease in cardiac output, the heart rate increases less with the application of PEEP than with hemorrhage.[42] The reasons for this difference are not known but may reflect PEEP-induced sympatholytic actions and increased arterial pressure minimizing baroreceptor stimulation.

Ventilation also alters the control of intravascular fluid balance via hormonal release. Both positive-pressure ventilation and sustained hyperinflation stimulate endocrinologic responses that induce fluid retention by means of right atrial stretch receptors. Plasma norepinephrine, plasma rennin activity,[50,51] and atrial natriuretic peptide[52] increase during positive-pressure ventilation with or without PEEP.

Determinants of Pulmonary Vascular Resistance

Changes in lung volume are caused by changes in transpulmonary distending pressure, the pressure difference between alveolar pressure and ITP. Because pulmonary tissue pressure and ITP are nearly identical, increasing lung volume increases the difference between alveolar and tissue pressures, making pulmonary vascular resistance increase independent of any effect of volume change on humeral or autonomic responses.[14,53-58] Lung inflation affects cardiac function and cardiac output primarily by altering right ventricular (RV) preload and afterload.[57]

RV afterload is the maximal RV systolic wall stress during contraction,[59] which, by Laplace's law, equals the product of the RV radius of curvature (a function of end-diastolic volume) and transmural pressure (a function of systolic RV pressure).[60] Changes in ITP that occur without changes in lung volume, as may occur with obstructive inspiratory efforts, do not alter the pressure gradient between the right ventricle and the pulmonary artery, so pulmonary vascular resistance is not changed.

Systolic RV pressure approximates transmural systolic pulmonary artery pressure when no pulmonary stenosis is present. Transmural pulmonary artery pressure can increase by one of two mechanisms: (1) an increase in pulmonary artery pressure without an increase in pulmonary vasomotor tone, as occurs with increases in blood flow (exercise) or passive increases in outflow pressure (LV failure), or (2) an increase in pulmonary vascular resistance. Usually any increase in transmural pulmonary artery pressure during positive-pressure ventilation is due to an increase in pulmonary vascular resistance, because neither instantaneous cardiac output[61] nor LV filling[11] increases. Increases in transmural pulmonary artery pressure impede RV ejection,[62] decreasing RV stroke volume[63] and causing RV dilatation and passive obstruction to venous return,[64,65] which can rapidly progress to acute cor pulmonale.[66] If RV dilatation and pressure overload persist, RV free wall ischemia and infarction may develop.[67] Importantly, rapid fluid challenges in the setting of acute cor pulmonale can precipitate profound cardiovascular collapse due to excessive RV dilatation, RV ischemia, and compromised LV filling through the process of ventricular interdependence (discussed later). During normal end-inspiration, mild hypoxemia (arterial O_2 partial pressure >65 mm Hg) and low levels of PEEP (<7.5 cm H_2O) should minimally increase transmural pulmonary artery pressure. If slight increases in transmural pulmonary artery pressure are sustained, however, fluid retention occurs, either by intrinsic humeral mechanisms (increased atrial natriuretic peptide secretion) or by therapeutic intravascular volume infusion,[68] resulting in an increase in RV end-diastolic volume and maintenance of cardiac output.[60,69]

The mechanism by which ventilation alters pulmonary vasomotor tone is complex. If regional partial pressure of O_2 in alveolar gas (P_AO_2) decreases below 60 mm Hg, local pulmonary vasomotor tone increases, reducing local blood flow.[70] This process of hypoxic pulmonary vasoconstriction is mediated, in part, by variations in the synthesis and release of nitric oxide by pulmonary vascular endothelial cells. Many pathologic pulmonary processes are associated with regional reductions in P_AO_2, such as atelectasis, airway obstruction, and ventilation-perfusion mismatching. Hypoxic pulmonary vasoconstriction optimizes ventilation-perfusion matching by reducing pulmonary blood flow to those hypoxic regions. However, if alveolar hypoxia occurs throughout the lungs, overall pulmonary vasomotor tone increases, increasing pulmonary vascular resistance and impeding RV ejection.[71] At low lung volumes, alveoli spontaneously collapse as a result of loss of interstitial traction and closure of the terminal airways, causing alveolar hypoxia. Patients with acute hypoxemic respiratory failure have small lung volumes.[72,73] Therefore, pulmonary vascular resistance is often increased in these patients, owing to alveolar collapse and the resultant hypoxic pulmonary vasoconstriction.

Mechanical Ventilation–Induced Changes in Pulmonary Vascular Resistance

Mechanical ventilation can reduce active pulmonary vasomotor tone by one of several related processes. Hypoxic pulmonary vasoconstrictor tone can be decreased by increasing global P_AO_2 by enriching alveolar gas O_2,[74-77] re-expanding collapsed alveolar units by increasing P_AO_2 in those local alveoli,[3,78-80] increasing alveolar ventilation and thus reversing acute respiratory acidosis,[76] or merely decreasing central sympathetic output by allowing patients with ALI to stop fighting for every breath.[81,82] These effects need not require positive-pressure breaths but merely the expansion of collapsed alveoli.[83] This is usually accomplished by the addition

of PEEP or CPAP. Thus, if PEEP opens collapsed lung units and replenishes alveolar gas with O_2, hypoxic pulmonary vasoconstriction will be reduced, pulmonary vascular resistance will decrease, and RV ejection will improve.

Changes in lung volume can also profoundly alter pulmonary vasomotor tone by passively compressing the alveolar vessels.[72,79,80] The pulmonary circulation can be separated into two groups of blood vessels, depending on the pressure that surrounds them (Fig. 64-4).[79] The small pulmonary arterioles, venules, and alveolar capillaries sense alveolar pressure as their surrounding pressure and are referred to as alveolar vessels. The large pulmonary arteries and veins, as well as the heart and intrathoracic great vessels of the systemic circulation, sense interstitial pressure or ITP as their surrounding pressure and can be called extra-alveolar vessels. Alveolar pressure minus ITP is the transpulmonary pressure. Increasing lung volume requires transpulmonary pressure to increase. Thus, this extravascular pressure gradient between alveolar and extra-alveolar vessels varies proportionally with changes in lung volume. Importantly, the radial interstitial forces of the lung that keep the airways patent[78,84,85] also act on the extra-alveolar vessels. As lung volume increases, the radial interstitial forces increase, increasing the diameter of both extra-alveolar vessels and airways. This results in a reduction in airway resistance at higher lung volumes and also greater extra-alveolar vessel diameter, increasing their capacitance.[86] This tethering effect is lost with lung deflation, thereby increasing pulmonary vascular resistance.[75,78] The collapse of small airways also induces alveolar hypoxia. Thus, at small lung volumes, pulmonary vascular resistance is increased owing to the combined effect of hypoxic pulmonary vasoconstriction and extra-alveolar vessel collapse.

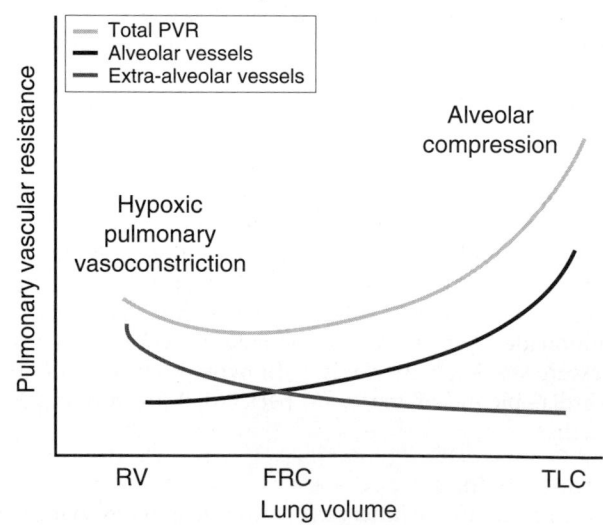

FIGURE 64-4. Schematic diagram of the relation between changes in lung volume and pulmonary vascular resistance (PVR), with the extra-alveolar and alveolar vascular components separated. Note that pulmonary vascular resistance is minimal at resting lung volume or functional residual capacity (FRC). As lung volume increases toward total lung capacity (TLC) or decreases toward residual volume (RV), pulmonary vascular resistance also increases. However, the increase in resistance with hyperinflation is due to increased alveolar vascular resistance, whereas the increase in resistance with lung collapse is due to increased extra-alveolar vessel tone.

Increases in lung volume progressively increase alveolar vessel resistance, becoming noticeable above resting lung volume or functional residual capacity.[75,87] There are two causes of this increased alveolar vessel resistance. First, the heart and extra-alveolar vessels sense ITP as their surrounding pressure, but the alveolar vessels sense alveolar pressure as their surrounding pressure. Thus, an extraluminal transpulmonary pressure gradient exists between these extra-alveolar and alveolar vessels. As lung volume increases, this extraluminal pressure difference increases as well. Because the intraluminal pressure in the pulmonary arteries is generated by RV ejection relative to ITP, but the outside pressure of the alveolar vessels is alveolar pressure, if transpulmonary pressure increases enough to exceed intraluminal vascular pressure, the pulmonary vasculature will collapse where extra-alveolar vessels pass into alveolar loci, reducing the vasculature cross-sectional area and increasing pulmonary vascular resistance. Similarly, increasing lung volume by stretching and distending the alveolar septa may also compress alveolar capillaries, although this mechanism is less well substantiated. Hyperinflation can create significant pulmonary hypertension and may precipitate acute RV failure (acute cor pulmonale)[88] and RV ischemia.[67] Thus, PEEP may increase pulmonary vascular resistance if it induces overdistention of the lung above its normal functional residual capacity. Recently, the effect of inflation on RV input impedance was validated in humans using echocardiographic techniques.[89] Similarly, if lung volumes are reduced, increasing lung volume back to baseline levels by the use of PEEP decreases pulmonary vascular resistance by reversing hypoxic pulmonary vasoconstriction.[90]

Ventricular Interdependence

Changes in RV output must invariably alter LV filling, because the two ventricles are serially linked through the pulmonary vasculature. However, LV preload can also be directly altered by changes in RV end-diastolic volume. If RV volume increases, LV diastolic compliance will decrease by the mechanism of ventricular interdependence.[91] Ventricular interdependence functions through two separate processes. First, increasing RV end-diastolic volume induces a shift of the intraventricular septum into the left ventricle, thereby decreasing LV diastolic compliance (Fig. 64-5).[92] Thus, for the same LV filling pressure, RV dilatation will decrease LV end-diastolic volume and, therefore, cardiac output. This interaction is believed to be the major determinant of the phasic changes in arterial pulse pressure and stroke volume seen in tamponade, referred to as pulsus paradoxus, which can be easily demonstrated during loaded spontaneous inspiration in normal subjects. Spontaneous inspiration increases venous return, causing RV dilatation and decreasing LV end-diastolic compliance. Maintaining a relatively constant rate of venous return, by either volume resuscitation[93] or vasopressor infusion,[1] minimizes this effect. Thus, the presence of pulsus paradoxus can be used as a marker of functional hypovolemia, even if the actual intravascular volume is not reduced.

Mechanical Heart-Lung Interactions

With hyperinflation, the heart may be compressed between the two expanding lungs,[94] increasing juxtacardiac ITP. Because the chest wall and diaphragm can move away from the expanding lungs, whereas the heart is trapped within its cardiac fossa, juxtacardiac ITP may increase more than lateral chest wall or diaphragmatic ITP does.[4,13] This compressive

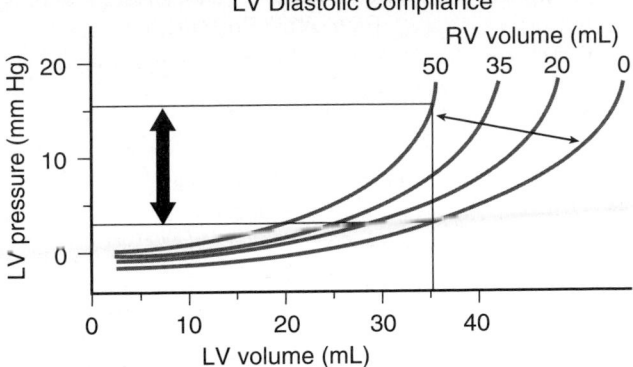

FIGURE 64–5. Schematic diagram of the effect of increasing right ventricular (RV) volumes on the left ventricular (LV) diastolic pressure-volume (filling) relationship. Note that greater RV volumes decrease LV diastolic compliance, such that a higher filling pressure is required to generate a constant end-diastolic volume. (After Taylor RR, Corell JW, Sonnenblick EH, Ross J Jr: Dependence of ventricular distensibility on filling the opposite ventricle. Am J Physiol 1967;213:711-718.)

effect of the inflated lung can be seen with either spontaneous[95] or positive-pressure–induced hyperinflation.[84,85] This decrease in "apparent" LV diastolic compliance[93] was previously misinterpreted as impaired LV contractility, because LV stroke work for a given LV end-diastolic pressure or pulmonary artery occlusion pressure is decreased.[96,97] However, numerous studies have shown that when patients are fluid-resuscitated to return LV end-diastolic volume to its original level, both LV stroke work and cardiac output also return to their original levels,[55,93] despite the continued application of PEEP.[98]

CHANGES IN INTRATHORACIC PRESSURE

The heart within the thorax is a pressure chamber within a pressure chamber. Therefore, changes in ITP affect the pressure gradients for both systemic venous return to the right ventricle and systemic outflow from the left ventricle, independent of the heart itself (Fig. 64-6). Increases in ITP, by increasing right atrial pressure and decreasing transmural LV systolic pressure, reduce the pressure gradients for

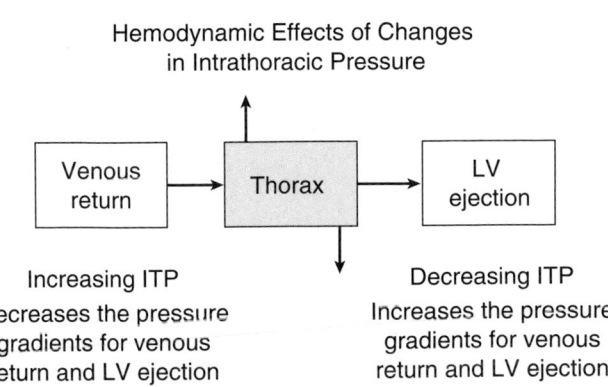

FIGURE 64–6. Schematic diagram of the effect of increasing or decreasing intrathoracic pressure (ITP) on the left ventricular (LV) filling (venous return) and ejection pressure.

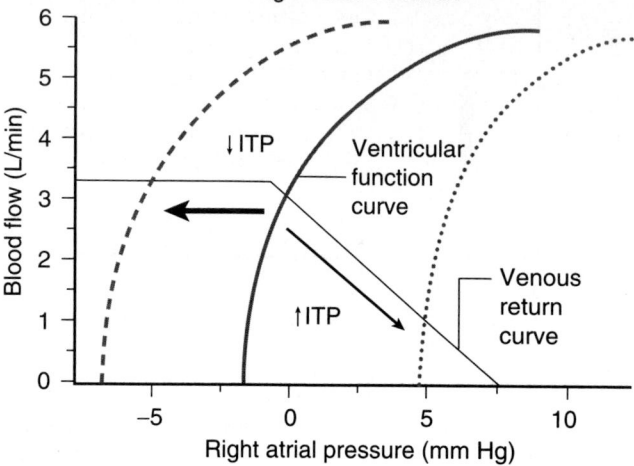

FIGURE 64–7. Schematic representation of the effects of increasing or decreasing intrathoracic pressure (ITP) on steady-state venous return. Note that decreases in ITP that decrease right atrial pressure to below 0 relative to atmospheric pressure increase venous return by only a limited amount, whereas increases in ITP progressively decrease venous return to a complete circulatory standstill.

venous return and LV ejection, decreasing intrathoracic blood volume. Using the same argument, decreases in ITP augment venous return and impede LV ejection and increase intrathoracic blood volume.

Systemic Venous Return

As downstream right atrial pressure varies (as occurs with ventilation), the rate of venous return inversely changes. Pressure in the upstream venous reservoirs is called mean systemic pressure, which is a function of blood volume, peripheral vasomotor tone, and the distribution of blood within the vasculature.[99] Mean systemic pressure does not change rapidly during the ventilatory cycle, whereas right atrial pressure does, owing to concomitant changes in ITP. Accordingly, variations in right atrial pressure are the major determining factor in fluctuations of the pressure gradient for systemic venous return during ventilation.[61,100] Positive-pressure inspiration increases ITP and right atrial pressure, decreasing the pressure gradient for venous return, which decreases venous blood flow,[63] RV filling, and, consequently, RV stroke volume.[61,63,101-108] These long-documented physiologic effects were recently validated in humans using minimally invasive echocardiographic techniques, wherein vena caval flow varies with the phase of the ventilatory cycle (Fig. 64-7).[109] During normal spontaneous inspiration, the converse occurs: with decreases in ITP, right atrial pressure decreases, accelerating venous blood flow and increasing RV filling and RV stroke volume (Fig. 64-8).[1,15,63,66,103,106,110,111]

The decrease in venous return during positive-pressure ventilation is often lower than one might expect based on the increase in right atrial pressure. Because a large proportion of venous blood is in the abdomen, the net effect of PEEP is to increase mean systemic pressure and right atrial pressure. Accordingly, the pressure gradient for venous return may not be reduced by PEEP, especially in patients with hypervolemia. In fact, abdominal pressurization by diaphragmatic descent may be the major mechanism by which the decrease in venous return is minimized during positive-pressure ventilation.[71,112-115] When cardiac output is restored to pre-PEEP levels by fluid resuscitation[71,116] and PEEP is maintained, liver clearance mechanisms increase above pre-PEEP levels.[116-119] These data are consistent with a PEEP-induced alteration in intrahepatic blood flow distribution. Thus, ventilation may have less of an effect on venous return than was originally postulated. Van den Berg and colleagues examined the effects of varying levels of CPAP on right atrial pressure, intra-abdominal pressure, and cardiac output in

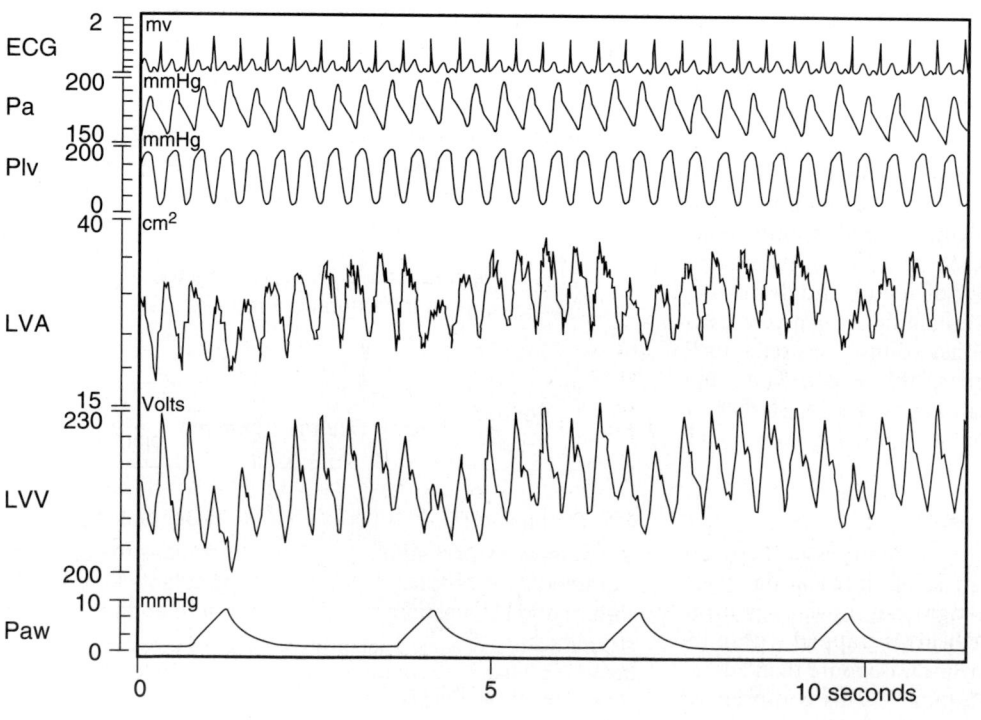

FIGURE 64–8. Effect of positive-pressure ventilation on left ventricular volume (LVV) and related hemodynamic measures in a perioperative intact patient. ECG, electrocardiogram; LVA, left ventricular area; Pa, arterial pressure; Paw, airway pressure; Plv, left ventricular pressure. (From Denault AY, Gasior TA, Gorcsan J 3rd, et al: Determinants of aortic pressure variation during positive-pressure ventilation in man. Chest 1999;116:176-186.)

42 postoperative cardiac surgery patients.[120] Up to 20 cm H_2O, CPAP did not significantly decrease cardiac output, as measured 30 seconds into an inspiratory hold maneuver. The reason for this apparent paradoxical effect became obvious when the investigators compared the associated changes in right atrial pressure, abdominal pressure, and RV end-diastolic volume (Fig. 64-9). They found that only 30% of the increased airway pressure was transmitted to the right atrium; however, and perhaps more important, most of the increase in right atrial pressure was realized by an increase in intra-abdominal pressure. Thus, it was not surprising that RV end-diastolic volume fell by less than 8% from pre-CPAP values. These data demonstrate that in fluid-resuscitated patients, institution of positive-pressure ventilation may not result in a decrease in blood flow. However, if intra-abdominal pressure is allowed to decrease, as would occur with an open laparotomy and decompression of tense ascites, a marked preload-responsive effect of positive-pressure ventilation should occur.

With exaggerated swings in ITP, as occur with obstructed inspiratory efforts, venous return behaves as if abdominal pressure is additive to mean systemic pressure in defining total venous blood flow.[121-124] Recent interest in inverse ratio ventilation has raised questions about its hemodynamic effect, because its application includes a large component of hyperinflation.

Right Ventricular Filling

When RV filling pressure, defined as right atrial pressure minus pericardial pressure, was directly measured in patients undergoing open chest operations, RV filling pressure was unaltered by acute volume loading.[125] Although right atrial pressure increased, pericardial pressure also increased, such that RV filling pressure remained unchanged. Similar data are seen when RV volumes are reduced by the application of PEEP in postoperative cardiac patients.[126] These data

suggest that under normal conditions, RV diastolic compliance is very high and that most of the increase in right atrial pressure seen during volume loading reflects pericardial compliance and cardiac fossa stiffness rather than changes in RV distending pressure. Accordingly, changes in right atrial pressure do not follow changes in RV end-diastolic volume.

When cardiac contractility is reduced and intravascular volume is expanded, RV filling pressure increases as a result of decreased RV diastolic compliance, increased pericardial compliance, increased end-diastolic volume, or a combination of all three. In support of this hypothesis, RV filling pressure does not increase until RV volume exceeds a certain threshold value.[179] In postoperative cardiac surgery patients,[10,18,127] PEEP and, by extension, lung expansion compress the heart within the cardiac fossa in a fashion analogous to pericardial tamponade.

Venous return is the primary determinant of cardiac output.[99] The closer right atrial pressure remains to zero relative to atmospheric pressure, the greater is the pressure gradient for systemic venous blood flow.[104,128] For this mechanism to operate efficiently, RV output must equal venous return; otherwise, sustained increases in venous blood flow would overdistend the right ventricle, increasing right atrial pressure. Fortunately, under normal conditions of spontaneous ventilation, the increase in venous return is in phase with inspiration, decreasing again during expiration as ITP increases.[61] Likewise, the pulmonary arterial inflow circuit is highly compliant and can accept large increases in RV stroke volume without changing pressures (Fig. 64-10).[63,69]

This compensatory system rapidly becomes dysfunctional if RV diastolic compliance decreases or if right atrial pressure increases independent of changes in RV end-diastolic volume. An example of decreased RV diastolic compliance is acute RV dilatation or cor pulmonale (pulmonary embolism, hyperinflation, and RV infarction), which induces profound decreases in cardiac output that are not responsive to fluid resuscitation. Dissociation between right atrial pressure and RV end-diastolic volume occurs during either tamponade or positive-pressure ventilation, because right atrial pressure is artificially increased by the increasing ITP. Accordingly, positive-pressure ventilation impairs normal circulatory adaptive processes. Further, even if one restores the coupling of right atrial pressure and RV volume by using partial ventilatory support modes, cardiac output will increase only if the right ventricle can transduce the associated increase in venous return to forward blood flow. Thus, during weaning from mechanical ventilation, occult RV failure may be exposed, manifested by a rapid rise in right atrial pressure and a fall in cardiac output. Because the primary effect of any form of ventilation on cardiovascular function in normal subjects is to alter RV preload by altering venous blood flow, the detrimental effect of positive-pressure ventilation on cardiac output can be minimized either by instituting fluid resuscitation to increase mean systemic pressure[1,101,120,121] or by keeping both mean ITP and swings in lung volume as low as possible. Accordingly, prolonging expiratory time, decreasing tidal volume, and avoiding PEEP all minimize this decrease in systemic venous return to the right ventricle.[17,61,103-107,129,130]

Because spontaneous inspiratory efforts increase lung volume by decreasing ITP, there is an increase in venous return with spontaneous inspiration, owing to the fall in right atrial pressure.[15,53,104-106] This augmentation of venous return is limited,[122,124] however, because if ITP decreases below atmospheric pressure, venous return becomes flow-limited

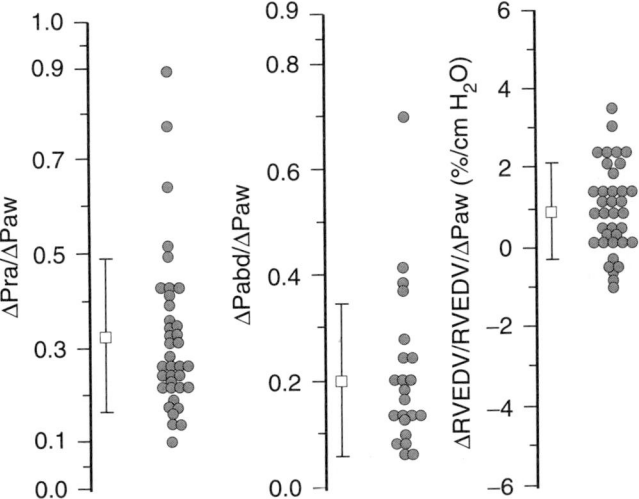

FIGURE 64–9. Effect of increasing levels of continuous positive airway pressure (CPAP) on the relationship between increasing airway pressure (Paw) and right atrial pressure (Pra) (left graph), airway pressure and intra-abdominal pressure (Pabd) (center graph), and airway pressure and changes in right ventricular end-diastolic volume (RVEDV) (right graph) in 43 postoperative fluid-resuscitated cardiac surgery patients. (From data in Van den Berg P, Jansen JRC, Pinsky MR: The effect of positive-pressure inspiration on venous return in volume loaded post-operative surgical patients. J Appl Physiol 2002;92:1223-1231.)

when the large systemic veins collapse as they enter the thorax.[128] This flow limitation is a safety valve for the heart, because ITP can decrease greatly with obstructive inspiratory efforts,[46] and in the absence of flow limitation, the right ventricle could become over distended and fail.[131] Still, in patients with decreased RV compliance, negative swings in ITP can augment RV filling.

Left Ventricular Preload and Ventricular Interdependence

Changes in venous return must eventually result in directionally similar changes in LV preload, because the two ventricles are linked in series. This phase delay in output adjustments from the right ventricle to the left ventricle is exaggerated if tidal volume or respiratory rate is increased and in the setting of hypovolemia.[17,56,58,93,96,97,108,129,132-136] Independent of this series interaction, direct ventricular interdependence can also occur and be clinically significant. Increasing RV volume shifts the intraventricular septum into the left ventricle and simultaneously decreases LV diastolic compliance. During positive-pressure ventilation, RV volumes are usually decreased, minimizing ventricular interdependence.[91,134-137] Echocardiographic studies document that although PEEP results in some degree of right-to-left intraventricular septal shift, the shift is small.[55,56] In fact, increases in lung volume during positive-pressure ventilation primarily compress the two ventricles into each other, decreasing biventricular volumes.[138] The decrease in cardiac output commonly seen during PEEP is due to a decrease in LV end-diastolic volume, and both LV end-diastolic volume and cardiac output are restored by fluid resuscitation,[139,140] without any measurable change in LV diastolic compliance.[93]

During spontaneous inspiration, RV volumes increase transiently, shifting the intraventricular septum into the left ventricle,[92] decreasing LV diastolic compliance and LV end-diastolic volume.[90,137,141] This transient RV dilatation-induced septal shift is the primary cause of inspiration-associated decreases in arterial pulse pressure, which, if greater than 10 mm Hg or 10% of the mean pulse pressure, are referred to as pulsus paradoxus.[15] Because spontaneous inspiratory efforts can occur during positive-pressure ventilation, and especially during partial ventilatory assist, pulsus paradoxus can also be seen in mechanically ventilated patients.

Left Ventricular Afterload

LV afterload can be equated to systolic wall tension, which, by the Laplace equation, is proportional to the product of transmural LV pressure and the radius of curvature of the left ventricle, which itself is proportional to LV volume. Maximal LV wall tension normally occurs at the end of isometric contraction, reflecting both a maximal product of the LV radius of curvature (end-diastolic volume) and aortic pressure (diastolic pressure). When LV dilatation exists, as in congestive heart failure, maximal LV wall stress occurs during LV ejection, because the maximal product of these two variables occurs at this time. Accordingly, LV afterload varies, based on the baseline level of cardiac contractility, arterial pressure, and intravascular volume. LV ejection pressure is the transmural LV systolic pressure, which can be approximated as transmural arterial pressure. Because normal baroreceptor mechanisms located in the carotid body tend to keep arterial pressure constant with respect to atmosphere, if arterial pressure were to remain constant as ITP increased, LV wall tension would decrease as well. Similarly, if transmural arterial pressure were to remain constant as ITP increased but LV end-diastolic volume were to decrease, because of the increased ITP-induced decrease in systemic venous return, LV wall tension would also

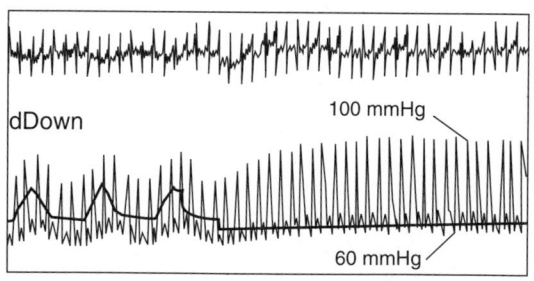

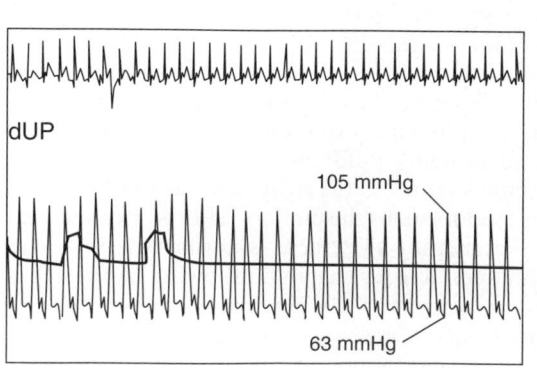

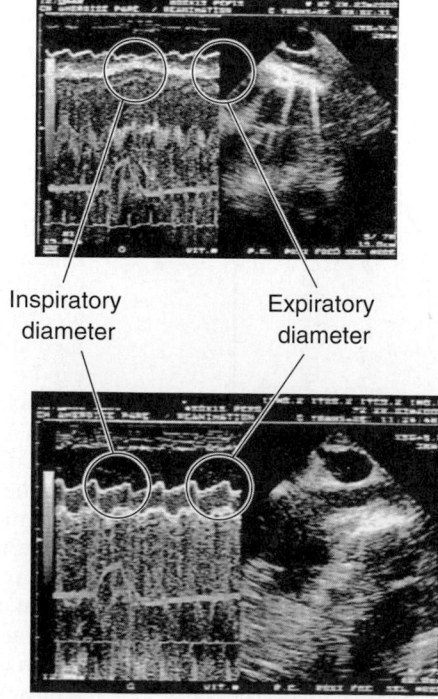

FIGURE 64–10.
Echocardiographic and pulse Doppler images of superior vena cava (SVC) flow patterns during positive-pressure ventilation. Note the inspiratory phase-dependent decrease in venous flow. (From Jardin F, Vieillard-Baron A: Right ventricular function and positive-pressure ventilation in clinical practice: From hemodynamic subsets to respirator settings. Intensive Care Med 2003;29:1426-1434.)

decrease.[142] Thus, by either mechanism, increases in ITP decrease LV afterload. Similarly, decreases in ITP with a constant arterial pressure increase LV transmural pressure, increasing LV afterload.[11,143] These two opposing effects of changes in ITP on LV afterload have profound clinical implications.

First, any process associated with marked decreases in ITP must also be associated with increased LV afterload and myocardial O_2 consumption. Because the transition from positive-pressure ventilation to spontaneous ventilation may result in dramatic ITP swings and changes in the energy requirements of the respiratory muscles, weaning from mechanical ventilation is a cardiovascular stress test.[142,144,145] Interestingly, Jabran and associates demonstrated that all ventilator-dependent patients had increased cardiac output during weaning, but in those who failed to be weaned from mechanical ventilation, venous O_2 saturation decreased, consistent with cardiovascular compromise.[33] A similar argument can be made for the observed improvement in LV systolic function in patients with severe LV failure who are placed on mechanical ventilation.[145]

Pulsus paradoxus occurs during spontaneous inspiration under conditions of marked pericardial restraint. This may occur because of pericardial limitations, such as tamponade and constrictive pericarditis, as well as during loaded spontaneous ventilatory efforts, when RV volumes swell and ITP decreases. In both cases, LV stroke volume decreases.[146-150] Perhaps the most prominent mechanism creating an inspiratory decrease in both LV stroke volume and systolic arterial pressure is the transient decrease in LV diastolic compliance induced by increased venous return, which decreases LV end-diastolic volume. The negative swings in ITP also increase LV ejection pressure (LV pressure minus ITP), increasing LV end-systolic volume.[11] Hypoxia directly reduces LV diastolic compliance, as well as decreasing myocardial contractile function.[151]

Sustained increases in ITP must eventually decrease aortic blood flow and arterial pressure, owing to the associated decrease in venous return.[11] Because normal baroreceptor-based homeostatic mechanisms tend to sustain a constant arterial pressure, to keep organ perfusion constant,[45] if ITP increased arterial pressure without changing transmural arterial pressure, the periphery would reflexively vasodilate to maintain a constant extrathoracic arterial pressure-flow relation.[132] Because coronary perfusion pressure reflects the ITP gradient for blood flow, it is not increased by ITP-induced increases in arterial pressure. However, compression of the coronaries by the expanding lungs may obstruct coronary blood flow. Thus, the combined decrease in coronary blood flow may induce myocardial ischemia.[152-154]

There is little difference in LV energetics between decreasing LV ejection pressure by increasing ITP above atmospheric pressure and increasing ITP from a negative value to atmosphere, if the absolute change in ITP is similar. In both cases, the LV ejection pressure will decrease in proportion to the relative increase in ITP. However, the effect of removing large negative levels of ITP is not similar to that of adding positive ITP on venous return. Relative increases in ITP from very negative values to zero, relative to atmosphere, minimally alter venous return, whereas increases in ITP above atmosphere impede venous return by increasing right atrial pressure. Thus, very negative swings in ITP, as seen with vigorous inspiratory efforts in the setting of airway obstruction (asthma, upper airway obstruction, vocal cord paralysis) or

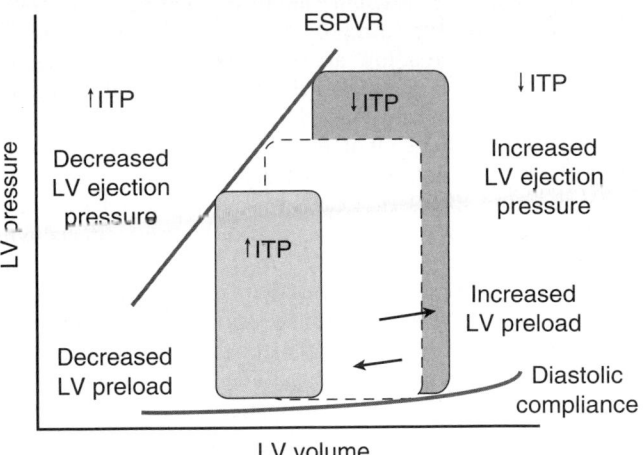

FIGURE 64–11. Schematic representation of the effects of changes in intrathoracic pressure (ITP) on left ventricular (LV) pressure-volume relations when cardiac contractility is normal. ESPVR, end-systolic pressure-volume relation.

stiff lungs (interstitial lung disease, pulmonary edema, ALI), selectively increase LV afterload. Such spontaneous inspiratory efforts may be the cause of the often observed LV failure and pulmonary edema seen in these conditions,[14,46,155,156] especially if LV systolic function is already compromised (see Fig. 64-7).[26,157] Similarly, removing large negative swings in ITP by either bypassing upper airway obstruction (endotracheal intubation) or instituting mechanical ventilation or PEEP-induced loss of spontaneous inspiratory efforts should selectively reduce LV afterload without significantly decreasing either venous return or cardiac output.[1,36,69,128,153,158,159] Reversing this argument, weaning from mechanical ventilation, with its associated increase in both metabolic demand and LV afterload, is a form of cardiac stress testing.[33]

Using Changes in Intrathoracic Pressure to Define Cardiovascular Performance

Sustained increases in airway pressure can be used to measure cardiac contractility, as defined by the end-systolic pressure-volume relation.[160] In a preload-dependent patient, passive inspiratory hold maneuvers that increase airway pressure to 5 to 10 cm H_2O (e.g., CPAP) selectively decrease venous return without greatly altering either pulmonary vascular resistance or LV afterload, because the changes in lung volume and ITP are relatively small. Denault and coworkers documented that, in mechanically ventilated patients undergoing cardiac surgery, LV performance could be measured during ventilation using combined estimates of LV volume and ejection pressure.[161] As shown in Figure 64-8, ventilation induces profound dynamic changes in LV volumes, consistent with rapid changes in LV filling.

HEMODYNAMIC EFFECTS OF VENTILATION BASED ON CARDIOPULMONARY STATUS

Spontaneous and positive-pressure ventilation can have profound hemodynamic consequences. Further, the same ventilatory maneuver (initiation of or withdrawal from mechanical ventilation) can have opposite effects on cardiovascular stability in different patient populations. Schematic examples of how increasing or decreasing ITP alters the LV pressure-volume relation are depicted for conditions in which LV function is normal (see Fig. 64-11) and depressed (Fig. 64-12). Because the hemodynamic responses to ventilation are highly dependent on the existing cardiovascular state, the specific responses to defined ventilatory maneuvers not only define the baseline cardiovascular state but also allow accurate predictions of what hemodynamic effects will occur.

In patients with cardiovascular insufficiency due to impaired LV ejection or volume overload, the institution of mechanical ventilatory support can be lifesaving because of its ability to support the cardiovascular system while decreasing global O_2 demand. In patients who are predominantly preload dependent or hypovolemic (hemorrhagic shock, loss of vasomotor tone) and in those who may develop RV failure with hyperinflation (anterior chest trauma, spinal cord shock, severe obstructive lung disease), positive-pressure ventilation must be instituted with caution, because profound cardiovascular insufficiency may develop rapidly during intubation and initiation of mechanical ventilation. Similarly, withdrawal of ventilatory support can be considered an exercise stress test, and patients with limited cardiovascular reserve may not be successfully weaned, even if their traditional weaning parameter values are acceptable.[26,157]

MECHANICAL VENTILATION

The hemodynamic differences between different modes of total mechanical ventilation at a constant airway pressure and PEEP can be explained by their differential effects on lung volume and ITP.[162] Importantly, when two different modes of total or partial ventilatory support cause similar changes in ITP and ventilatory effort, their hemodynamic effects are also similar, despite markedly different airway waveforms. Partial ventilatory support with either intermittent mandatory ventilation or pressure-support ventilation results in similar hemodynamic responses when matched for similar tidal volumes.[163] Of note, high-frequency jet ventilation, when delivered at low levels, results in a constant cardiac output in patients with heart failure.[112]

ACUTE LUNG INJURY

Patients with ALI often require PEEP to maintain alveolar distention and arterial oxygenation. Positive-pressure ventilation decreases intrathoracic blood volume,[104] and PEEP decreases it even more[125,126] without altering LV contractile function.[164] However, increases in airway pressure may not reflect increases in ITP, because patients with ALI have varying degrees of increased lung stiffness and decreased chest wall compliance. Further, it is the increase in lung volume, not airway pressure, that determines the degree of increase in ITP during positive-pressure ventilation.[5] Lessard and colleagues, in a study of nine patients with ARDS, found no significant hemodynamic differences among volume-controlled, pressure-controlled, and pressure-controlled inverse ratio ventilation adjusted to keep total PEEP and tidal volume consistent among treatment arms.[165] Davis and associates studied the hemodynamic effects of volume-controlled versus pressure-controlled ventilation in 25 patients with ALI.[166] When matched for the same mean airway pressure, both methods resulted in the same cardiac outputs. However, when airway pressure was increased during volume-controlled ventilation by sine wave to square wave flow pattern, cardiac output fell. Singer and coworkers showed in 18 ventilator-dependent but hemodynamically stable patients that the degree of hyperinflation, not the airway pressure, determined the decrease in cardiac output.[167]

Different modes of mechanical ventilation affect cardiac output to a similar extent for similar increases in lung volume.[112,168] Most of the decrement in cardiac output can be reversed by fluid resuscitation that restores intrathoracic blood volume to pre-PEEP levels.[164,169-171] That the PEEP-induced decrease in cardiac output is due to a decreased pressure gradient for venous return was elegantly shown by Gunter and colleagues,[172] who minimized the decrease in cardiac output in ventilator-dependent septic patients by lowering body compression. Importantly, if cardiac output does not increase with fluid resuscitation, other processes, such as cor pulmonale, increased pulmonary vascular resistance, or cardiac compression, may also be inducing cardiovascular depression.[173]

CONGESTIVE HEART FAILURE

Increases in cardiac output along with increases in airway pressure suggest the presence of congestive heart failure.[36,174] Grace and Greenbaum noted that adding PEEP did not decrease cardiac output in patients with heart failure, and it actually increased cardiac output if pulmonary artery occlusion pressure exceeded 18 mm Hg.[175] Similarly, Calvin and associates[176] noted that patients with cardiogenic pulmonary edema had no decrease in cardiac output when given PEEP.[177] Unfortunately, PEEP may be detrimental in patients with combined heart failure and ALI. Rasanen and coworkers

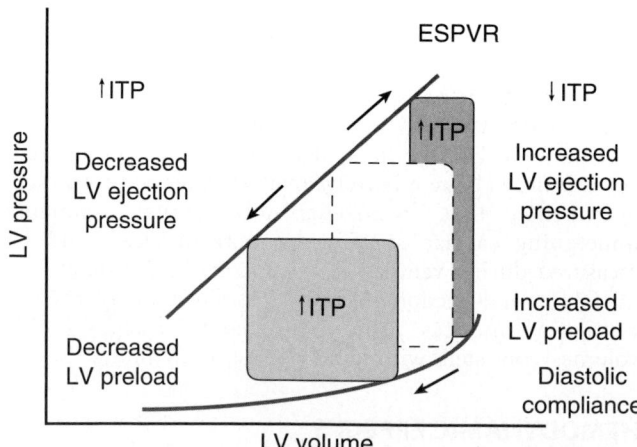

Effect of Changes in Intrathoracic Pressure in Congestive Heart Failure

ESPVR

↑ITP   ↓ITP

↑ITP

Decreased LV ejection pressure

Increased LV ejection pressure

↑ITP

Decreased LV preload

Increased LV preload

Diastolic compliance

LV pressure

LV volume

FIGURE 64–12. Schematic representation of the effects of changes in intrathoracic pressure (ITP) on left ventricular (LV) pressure-volume relations when cardiac contractility is impaired and intravascular volume status is expanded. ESPVR, end-systolic pressure-volume relation.

documented that decreasing levels of ventilatory support in patients with myocardial ischemia and acute LV failure worsened ischemia,[36,178] but this effect could be minimized by preventing spontaneous inspiratory effort–induced negative swings in ITP.[35] Because weaning from mechanical ventilatory support is a form of exercise stress test, withdrawal of ventilatory support can unmask cardiac failure in otherwise stable patients with acute respiratory failure.[26] Such patients may not be weanable from mechanical ventilatory support unless supplemented by positive inotropes.[157]

The cardiovascular benefits of positive airway pressure can be seen with the removal of negative swings in ITP, as created by increasing levels of CPAP.[179,180] Even CPAP levels as low as 5 cm H_2O can increase cardiac output in patients with congestive heart failure; cardiac output decreases with similar levels of CPAP in both normal subjects and those with heart failure without volume overload. Further, these hemodynamic effects of increased airway pressure do not require endotracheal intubation. Patients with congestive heart failure but in whom forced diuresis has induced a relative hypovolemic state, manifested by a pulmonary artery occlusion pressure of 12 mm Hg or less, will decrease their cardiac outputs equally whether they receive CPAP or bilevel positive airway pressure at the same mean airway pressure.[181]

If positive airway pressure augments LV ejection in heart failure states, then systolic arterial pressure should not decrease but should actually increase during inspiration—so-called reverse pulsus paradoxus. This was what Abel and coworkers found in 10 patients after cardiac surgery.[174] Other investigators suggested that the relation between ventilatory effort and systolic arterial pressure can be used to identify which patients may benefit from cardiac assist maneuvers.[182-184] Patients who increase their systolic arterial pressure during ventilation relative to an apneic baseline tend to have a greater degree of volume overload[183] and heart failure,[182] whereas those subjects in whom systolic arterial pressure decreases tend to be volume responsive. This logic has recently been applied to a hemodynamic test, with arterial pulse pressure substituted for systolic pressure. Michard and colleagues found in a series of ventilator-dependent septic patients that the greater the degree of arterial pulse pressure variation during positive-pressure ventilation, the greater the subsequent increase in cardiac output in response to volume expansion therapy.[185]

CHRONIC OBSTRUCTIVE PULMONARY DISEASE

The primary hemodynamic problem seen in patients with chronic obstructive pulmonary disease (COPD) is related to hyperinflation due to bronchospasm, loss of lung parenchyma, or dynamic hyperinflation. The lungs expand and compress the heart, increasing pulmonary vascular resistance and impeding RV filling. Dynamic hyperinflation is also referred to as intrinsic PEEP. Intrinsic PEEP alters hemodynamic function in a similar fashion to extrinsic PEEP. Matching intrinsic PEEP with externally applied PEEP has no measurable detrimental hemodynamic effect,[186-188] although such matching decreases the work cost of spontaneous breathing. Further, CPAP, like PEEP, has little detrimental effect in patients with COPD when delivered below the intrinsic PEEP level.[189]

Weaning of patients with COPD taxes the cardiovascular system. Patients with severe COPD but adequate ventilatory weaning parameters may go into cardiogenic pulmonary edema during weaning.[26] This probably reflects a combined volume overload and increased LV failure, because LV ejection fraction decreases during such trials[190]; following diuresis, many of these patients can be weaned. Jabran and associates demonstrated that although all ventilator-dependent COPD patients had increased cardiac output during weaning trials, those who failed to wean also had decreased venous O_2 saturation, consistent with an increased metabolic demand in excess of cardiovascular reserve.[33] Thus, occult cardiovascular insufficiency may play a major role in failure to wean in critically ill patients.[191] This theory, though attractive, has not been proved conclusively.

ACKNOWLEDGMENTS

This work was supported in part by National Institutes of Health grants NHLBI K-24 HL67181 and NRSA 2-T32 HL07820.

ANNOTATED REFERENCES

Buda AJ, Pinsky MR, Ingels NB, et al: Effect of intrathoracic pressure on left ventricular performance. N Engl J Med 1979;301:453-459.
    The first demonstration in humans that swings in ITP inversely alter LV afterload independent of any changes in venous return.

Calvin JE, Driedger AA, Sibbald WJ: Positive end-expiratory pressure (PEEP) does not depress left ventricular function in patients with pulmonary edema. Am Rev Respir Dis 1981;124:121-128.
    First study in humans to report improved LV function with the use of PEEP in patients with congestive heart failure.

Denault AY, Gorcsan J 3rd, Pinsky MR: Dynamic effects of positive-pressure ventilation on canine left ventricular pressure-volume relations. J Appl Physiol 2001;91:298-308.
    The definitive physiologic study showing the dynamic effects of ventilation on instantaneous LV pressure-volume relations, defining the influence of preload, ventricular interdependence, and LV afterload on LV performance.

Holt JP: The effect of positive and negative intrathoracic pressure on cardiac output and venous return in the dog. Am J Physiol 1944;142:594-603.
    One of the original papers showing the reciprocal and changing effects of cyclic breathing on venous return. In fact, all the hemodynamic effects were attributed to changes in venous return.

Jardin F, Farcot JC, Boisante L: Influence of positive end-expiratory pressure on left ventricular performance. N Engl J Med 1981;304:387-392.
    This study documented for the first time in humans that the cardiac depressive effects of PEEP were due to decreased venous return. When LV volumes were restored, cardiac output returned to baseline, despite continuing PEEP. This stopped the search for the PEEP-induced cardiac depressant.

Jardin F, Vieillard-Baron A: Right ventricular function and positive-pressure ventilation in clinical practice: From hemodynamic subsets to respirator settings. Intensive Care Med 2003;29:1426-1434.
    First study in humans to show dynamic and cycle-specific changes in venous return and RV stroke volume during positive-pressure ventilation, as predicted by earlier studies in animals. Although no new information is provided, the illustration are elegant, and there is a web-based video.

Kaneko Y, Floras JS, Usui K, et al: Cardiovascular effects of continuous positive airway pressure in patients with heart failure and obstructive sleep apnea. N Engl J Med 2003;348:1233-1241.
    Good clinical trial documenting the sustained improvement in LV function in patients with heart failure and obstructive sleep apnea who were given nighttime CPAP to relieve the repetitive negative swings in ITP and presumably LV afterload. Good discussion of the mechanisms of interaction in a large outpatient population.

Lemaire F, Teboul JL, Cinoti L, et al: Acute left ventricular dysfunction during unsuccessful weaning from mechanical ventilation. Anesthesiology 1988;69:171-179.
    The first study in humans to show that weaning to spontaneous ventilation could induce immediate and severe LV failure and pulmonary edema.

Marini JJ, Culver BN, Butler J: Mechanical effect of lung distention with positive pressure on cardiac function. Am Rev Respir Dis 1980;124:382-386.

Alerted clinicians to the cardiodepressive effects of hyperinflation and auto-PEEP by impeding both venous return and cardiac filling.

Pinsky MR, Matuschak GM, Klain M: Determinants of cardiac augmentation by increases in intrathoracic pressure. J Appl Physiol 1985;58:1189-1198.

The definitive physiologic study of the dynamic effects of positive-pressure ventilation on venous return and LV afterload. Excellent discussion of ventriculoarterial coupling.

Rasanen J, Nikki P, Heikkila J: Acute myocardial infarction complicated by respiratory failure: The effects of mechanical ventilation. Chest 1984;85:21-28.

First study in humans to report the association among negative swings in ITP, LV afterload, and myocardial ischemia, and the reversal of ischemia with the removal of negative swings in ITP. This concept altered the management of cardiogenic pulmonary edema in the setting of ongoing ischemia.

Sharpey-Schaffer EP: Effects of Valsalva maneuver on the normal and failing circulation. BMJ 1955;1:693-699.

Described the arterial pressure response to a Valsalva maneuver in patients with either normal cardiac function or heart failure. First to describe the square wave arterial pressure response of heart failure, now used as a diagnostic tool.

Van den Berg P, Jansen JRC, Pinsky MR: The effect of positive-pressure inspiration on venous return in volume loaded post-operative cardiac surgical patients. J Appl Physiol 2002;92:1223-1231.

The first study in humans to show that positive-pressure inspiration does not reduce the pressure gradient for venous return because it simultaneously increases intra-abdominal pressure. Good discussion of heart-lung interactions.

Chapter 65

ASSIST-CONTROL MECHANICAL VENTILATION

Neil R. MacIntyre

KEY POINTS

1. **Ventilator breath delivery** is characterized by the trigger, target, and cycle variables.

2. The **interaction of a positive-pressure breath and respiratory system mechanics** is summarized by the equation of motion: Driving pressure = (Flow × Resistance) + (Volume/System compliance).

3. **The goal of assist-control ventilation** is to provide adequate gas exchange while protecting the lung from overdistention and recruitment-derecruitment injury.

4. **Assist-control ventilation in obstructive lung disease** poses the additional risk of producing overdistention from air trapping.

5. **High-frequency ventilation** shows promise as a better lung-protective strategy in parenchymal lung injury.

Positive-pressure mechanical ventilatory support provides pressure and flow to the airway in order to effect oxygen (O_2) and carbon dioxide (CO_2) transport between the environment and the pulmonary capillary bed. The goal is to maintain appropriate levels of partial pressure of O_2 and CO_2 in arterial blood while unloading the ventilatory muscles. Conceptually, this mechanical ventilatory support can be either total or partial. With total support, the mechanical device completely unloads the ventilatory muscles and provides virtually all the work of breathing. With partial support, the mechanical device only partially unloads the ventilatory muscles, requiring the patient to provide the remainder of the work of breathing. In general, total support is used in acute respiratory failure when the patient's muscles are clearly overloaded or fatigued or when gas exchange is very unstable or unreliable. Partial support is generally used in less severe forms of respiratory failure (especially during the recovery or weaning phase). Partial support issues are discussed in Chapters 66 and 67. This chapter focuses on positive-pressure ventilation designed to provide total support.

DEVICE DESIGN FEATURES FOR TOTAL VENTILATORY SUPPORT

POSITIVE-PRESSURE BREATH CONTROLLER

Most modern ventilators use piston-bellows systems or high-pressure gas sources to drive gas flow.[1,2] Tidal breaths are generated by this gas flow and can be classified in terms of what initiates the breath (trigger variable), what controls gas delivery during the breath (target or limit variable), and what terminates the breath (cycle variable).[3,4] Trigger variables are either patient effort or a machine timer. During total support, breaths can be initiated by patient effort (assisted breaths) or by the machine timer (controlled breaths). Target or limit variables are generally either a set flow or a set inspiratory pressure. With flow targeting, the ventilator adjusts pressure to maintain a clinician-determined flow pattern; with pressure targeting, the ventilator adjusts flow to maintain a clinician-determined inspiratory pressure. Cycle variables are generally a set volume or a set inspiratory time. Breaths can also be cycled if pressure limits are exceeded.

MODE CONTROLLER

The availability and delivery logic of different breath types define the mode of mechanical ventilatory support.[3,4] The mode controller is an electronic, pneumatic- or microprocessor-based system designed to provide the proper combination of breaths according to set algorithms and feedback data (conditional variables). For total support, the most commonly used modes provide breaths that are either patient or machine initiated (i.e., assisted or controlled) and are either flow or pressure targeted. In addition, the flow-targeted breaths are generally volume cycled, and the pressure-targeted breaths are generally time cycled. Collectively, these approaches are referred to as assist-control modes and are generally divided into volume assist-control and pressure assist-control ventilation. Figure 65-1 depicts the four basic breath types used during assist-control ventilation.

New ventilator designs incorporate advanced monitoring and feedback functions into these controllers to allow continuous adjustments in mode algorithms as the patient's condition changes.[5] The most common of these new feedback designs is the addition of a volume target backup to pressure assist-control, termed pressure-regulated volume control. This feature adjusts the inspiratory pressure level above or below the clinician-set target to achieve the volume target. Other feedback systems adjust the mandatory rate (minimum minute ventilation) or the total minute ventilation being supplied (adaptive support ventilation), according to various criteria.

EFFORT (DEMAND) SENSORS

Assisted breaths require sensors to detect patient effort. These sensors are usually either pressure or flow transducers in the ventilatory circuitry and are characterized by their

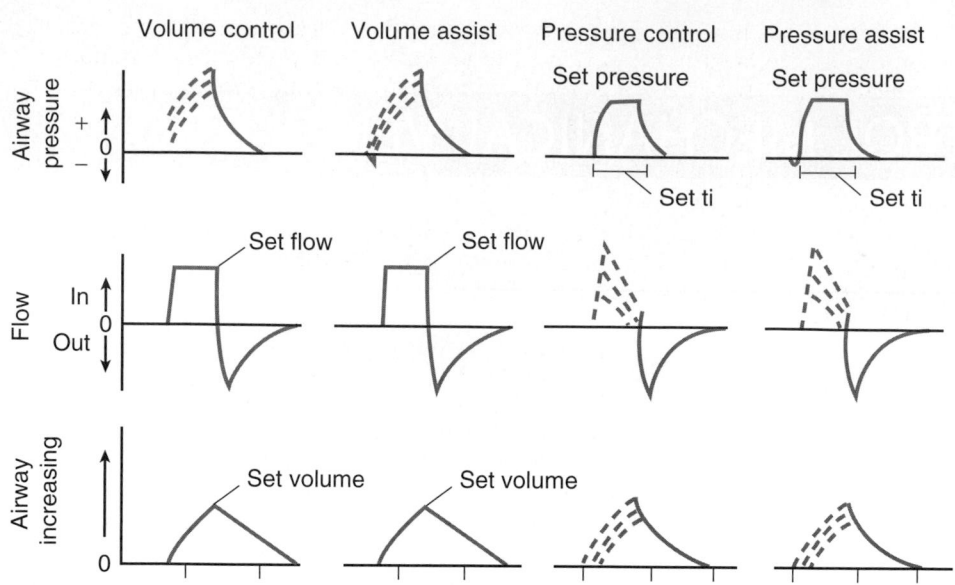

FIGURE 65–1. Airway pressure, flow, and volume tracings over time depicting the four basic breaths available for assist-control ventilation on most modern mechanical ventilators. Breaths are classified by their trigger, target or limit, and cycle variables. Patient-triggered assisted breaths are identified by the small drop in airway pressure before pressure and flow delivery; machine-triggered controlled breaths have no such drop. The target or limit is a clinician-set flow or inspiratory pressure. On most modern ventilators, flow-targeted assist-control breaths are volume cycled; pressure-targeted assist-control breaths are time (ti) cycled.

sensitivity (how much of a circuit pressure or flow change must be generated to initiate a ventilator response) and their responsiveness (the delay in providing this response).[6]

OTHER FEATURES

Blenders mix air and O_2 to produce a delivered inspired O_2 fraction (FIO_2) from 0.21 to 1.0. On newer systems, blenders are also available for other gases such as heliox, nitric oxide, and anesthetic agents. *Humidifiers* adjust blended gas mixtures to approximate body conditions using either passive heat-moisture exchangers in the circuitry or active systems that add heat and moisture directly. *Positive end-expiratory pressure (PEEP)* is usually applied by regulating pressure in the expiratory valve of the ventilator system, but a continuous flow of source gas during the expiratory phase can produce a similar effect. The *gas delivery circuit* consists of flexible tubing that often has pressure or flow sensors and an exhalation valve. It is important to remember that this tubing has measurable compliance (4 mL/cm H_2O is a representative figure), and significant amounts of delivered gas may only distend this circuitry rather than enter the patient's lungs when high airway pressures are encountered.

PHYSIOLOGIC EFFECTS OF POSITIVE-PRESSURE MECHANICAL VENTILATION

EQUATION OF MOTION

Lung inflation during mechanical ventilation occurs when pressure and flow are applied at the airway opening. These applied forces interact with respiratory system compliance (both lung and chest wall components), airway resistance, and, to a lesser extent, respiratory system inertance and lung tissue resistance to effect gas flow.[7,8] For simplicity's sake, because inertance and tissue resistance are relatively small, they can be ignored. Thus, the interactions of pressure, flow, and volume with respiratory system mechanics can be expressed by the simplified equation of motion:

$$\text{Driving pressure} = (\text{Flow} \times \text{Resistance}) + (\text{Volume/System compliance})$$

In a mechanically ventilated patient, this relationship is expressed as:

$$dPAO = (V' \times R) + (VT/CRS)$$

where dPAO is the change in pressure above baseline at the airway opening; V' is the flow into the patient's lungs; R is the resistance of the circuit, artificial airway, and natural airways; VT is the tidal volume; and CRS is the respiratory system compliance.

By performing an inspiratory hold at end-inspiration (i.e., no-flow conditions: $V' = 0$), the components of dPAO required for flow and for respiratory system distention can be separated. Specifically, when $V' = 0$ at end-inspiration, dPAO is referred to as a "plateau" pressure and reflects the static respiratory system compliance (CRS = VT/dPAOplateau). Adding dPAO to the baseline pressure gives the total respiratory system distending pressure at end-inspiration (dPAOplateau + baseline pressure = PAOplateau). Calculating the difference in dPAO during flow and during no-flow (the "peak to plateau difference") allows the calculation of inspiratory airway resistance (R = dPAOpeak – dPAOplateau/V').

Separating chest wall and lung compliance (CCW and CL, respectively) during a passive, machine-controlled positive-pressure breath requires an esophageal pressure measurement (Pes) to approximate pleural pressure. With this measurement, the inspiratory change in Pes (dPes) can be used in the following calculations: CCW = VT/dPes, and CL = VT/(dPAO – dPes). In clinical practice, because CCW is usually quite high and dPes is thus quite low, dPAOplateau and PAOplateau are often taken as an approximation of only lung distending pressure. However, in situations in which CCW is reduced (e.g., obesity, anasarca, ascites, surgical dressings), the stiff chest wall can have a significant effect on dPAOplateau and PAOplateau and must therefore be considered when using these measurements to assess lung stretch.

BREATH TARGET AND CYCLE CRITERIA

As noted earlier, there are two basic approaches to delivering positive-pressure breaths during assist-control ventilation: pressure targeting–time cycling and flow targeting–volume cycling. Although similar ranges of tidal volume and inspiratory time are available with either strategy, these breath characteristics interact differently with changing respiratory system mechanics and patient efforts. Changes in compliance or resistance cause a change in tidal volume (but not in pressure at the airway opening) with a pressure-targeted breath. In contrast, similar changes in compliance or resistance cause a change in pressure at the airway opening (but not in flow or volume) with a flow-targeted breath. Patient effort during a pressure-assist breath causes the ventilator to augment flow (and thus volume) to maintain the inspiratory pressure target; this same effort during a volume-assist breath does not affect delivered flow or volume but instead causes a fall in the measured circuit pressure.

INTRINSIC POSITIVE END-EXPIRATORY PRESSURE AND THE VENTILATORY PATTERN

Intrinsic PEEP develops within the alveoli because of inadequate expiratory time or collapsed airways during expiration (or both). Intrinsic PEEP depends on three factors: minute ventilation, the expiratory time fraction, and the respiratory system's expiratory time constant (the product of resistance and compliance).[9] As minute ventilation increases, expiratory time fraction decreases, or time constant lengthens (i.e., higher resistance or compliance values), the potential for intrinsic PEEP to develop increases.[9]

The development of intrinsic PEEP has different effects on volume assist-control and pressure assist-control ventilation. In volume assist-control, the constant delivered tidal volume (and thus the change in pressure at the airway opening) in the setting of a rising intrinsic PEEP increases both the peak airway opening pressure and the end-inspiratory plateau airway opening pressure. In contrast, in pressure assist-control, the limit on airway opening pressure, coupled with a rising intrinsic PEEP level, decreases the delta pressure at the airway opening and thus the delivered tidal volume (and minute ventilation).

In a passive patient, intrinsic PEEP can be assessed in two ways. First, when an inadequate expiratory time is producing intrinsic PEEP, analysis of the flow graphic will show that expiratory flow has not returned to zero before the next breath is given. Second, intrinsic PEEP in alveolar units with patent airways can be quantified during an expiratory hold maneuver that permits equilibration of the intrinsic PEEP throughout the ventilator circuitry.

DISTRIBUTION OF VENTILATION

A positive-pressure tidal breath must distribute itself among the millions of alveolar units in the lung.[10,11] Factors affecting this distribution include regional resistances, compliances, and functional residual capacities and the delivered flow pattern (including inspiratory pause). In general, positive-pressure breaths tend to distribute more to units with high compliance and low resistance and away from obstructed or stiff units (Fig. 65-2). This creates the potential for regional overdistention of healthier lung units, even in the face of "normal-sized" tidal volumes.

It should be noted that a more uniform ventilation distribution does not necessarily mean better ventilation-perfusion ($\dot{V}/\dot{Q}$) matching (e.g., a more uniform ventilation distribution may actually worsen ($\dot{V}/\dot{Q}$) matching in a lung with inhomogeneous perfusion). Because of all these considerations, predicting which flow pattern will optimize $\dot{V}/\dot{Q}$ matching is difficult and often an empirical trial-and-error exercise.

ALVEOLAR RECRUITMENT

Infiltrative lung disease produces severe ($\dot{V}/\dot{Q}$) mismatching through alveolar flooding and collapse.[12] In many (but not all) of these disease processes, the collapsed alveoli can be recruited during a positive-pressure ventilatory cycle.[13] Three specific techniques to optimize recruitment are the application of PEEP, the use of recruitment maneuvers, and the prolongation of inspiratory time.

PEEP is defined as an elevation of transpulmonary pressures at the end of expiration.[13,14] As noted earlier, PEEP can be produced either by expiratory circuit valves (applied PEEP) or as a consequence of ventilator settings interacting with respiratory system mechanics (intrinsic PEEP). Note that expiratory muscle contraction can also raise intrathoracic pressures at end-expiration; this should not be considered PEEP, however, because it is not a transpulmonary pressure (i.e., alveolar-pleural pressure).

Alveoli that are prevented from "derecruiting" by PEEP provide several potential benefits. First, recruited alveoli improve ($\dot{V}/\dot{Q}$) matching and gas exchange.[13-15] Second, as discussed in more detail later, patent alveoli throughout the ventilatory cycle are not exposed to the risk of injury from the shear stress of repeated opening and closing.[16] Third, PEEP prevents surfactant breakdown in collapsing alveoli and thus improves lung compliance.[17] PEEP, however, can also be detrimental. Because the tidal breath is delivered on top of the baseline PEEP, end-inspiratory pressures are raised by PEEP application. This must be considered if the lung is at risk for stretch injury (see Ventilator-Induced Lung Injury). Moreover, because alveolar injury is often quite heterogeneous, appropriate PEEP in one region may be suboptimal in another region and excessive in another. Optimizing PEEP is thus a balance between recruiting the recruitable alveoli in diseased regions without overdistending already recruited alveoli in healthier regions. Another potential detrimental effect of PEEP is that it raises mean intrathoracic pressure. This can compromise cardiac filling in susceptible patients (see Cardiac Effects).[18]

Recruitment maneuvers are based on the concept that alveolar recruitment occurs throughout a positive-pressure inflation—all the way to total lung capacity.[19] In practice, recruitment maneuvers are performed using sustained inflations (e.g., 30 to 40 cm H_2O for up to 2 minutes).[19,20] An alternative approach is to use frequent "sigh breaths" that briefly take the lung to near total capacity on a frequent basis.[21] It must be pointed out that recruitment maneuvers provide only initial alveolar recruitment; the duration of recruitment almost certainly depends on an appropriate setting of PEEP to prevent subsequent derecruitment.

Prolonging the inspiratory time (generally by adding a pause), often used in conjunction with a rapid decelerating-flow (i.e., pressure-targeted) breath, has several physiologic effects.[22] First, the longer inflation period may recruit more slowly recruitable alveoli. Second, increased gas mixing time may improve ($\dot{V}/\dot{Q}$) matching in infiltrative lung disease. Third, the development of intrinsic PEEP can have similar effects to that of applied PEEP (see earlier). Indeed, much of the improvement in gas exchange associated with long

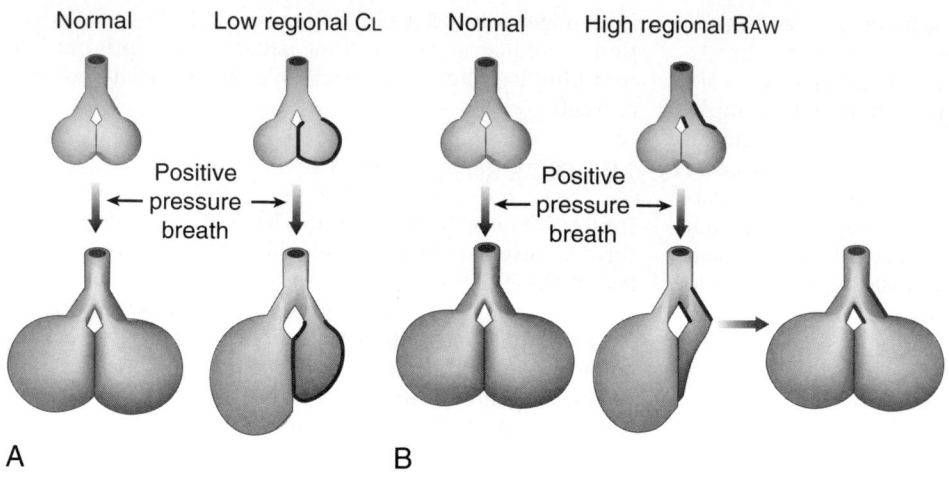

Normal   Low regional CL   Normal   High regional RAW

Positive pressure breath

Positive pressure breath

A

B

FIGURE 65-2. Schematic effects of the distribution of ventilation in two unit lung models with homogeneous mechanical properties, abnormal compliance distribution, and abnormal resistance distribution. Note that in situations involving inhomogeneous lung mechanics, positive-pressure breaths are preferentially distributed to "healthier" regions of the lung and can produce regional overdistention—even when a normal-sized global tidal volume is delivered. (From MacIntyre NR: Mechanical ventilatory support. In Dantzker D, MacIntyre NR, Bakow E [eds]: Comprehensive Respiratory Care. Philadelphia, WB Saunders, 1995.)

inspiratory time strategies may be merely a PEEP phenomenon.[23] It should be noted, however, that the distribution of intrinsic PEEP (most pronounced in lung units with long time constants) may be different from that of applied PEEP; thus, ($\dot{V}/\dot{Q}$) effects may also be different. Fourth, because these long inspiratory times significantly increase total intrathoracic pressures, cardiac output may be affected (see Cardiac Effects). Finally, inspiratory-expiratory ratios that exceed 1:1 (so-called inverse ratio ventilation [IRV]) are uncomfortable, and patient sedation or paralysis is often required unless a relief mechanism allows spontaneous breathing during the inflation period (airway pressure release ventilation, see below).

ADVERSE EFFECTS OF POSITIVE-PRESSURE VENTILATION

VENTILATOR-INDUCED LUNG INJURY

The lung can be injured when it is stretched excessively by positive-pressure ventilation. The most well-recognized injury is alveolar rupture, presenting as extra-alveolar air in the mediastinum (pneumomediastinum), pericardium (pneumopericardium), subcutaneous tissue (subcutaneous emphysema), pleura (pneumothorax), and vasculature (air emboli).[24] The risk for extra-alveolar air increases as a function of the magnitude and duration of alveolar overdistention. Thus, interactions of respiratory system mechanics and mechanical ventilation strategies (high regional tidal volume and PEEP—both applied and intrinsic) that produce regions of excessive alveolar stretch (i.e., transpulmonary distending pressures in excess of 40+ cm H_2O) for prolonged periods create alveolar units that are at risk for rupture.[24]

A parenchymal lung injury not associated with extra-alveolar air can also be produced by mechanical ventilation strategies that stretch the lungs beyond the normal maximum (i.e., transpulmonary distending pressures >30 to 35 cm H_2O). Pathologically, this manifests as diffuse alveolar damage[25-27] and is associated with cytokine release[28] and bacterial translocation.[29]

In addition to simple overstretching the lung, ventilator-induced lung injury (VILI) appears to be potentiated by a shear stress phenomenon that occurs when injured alveoli are repetitively opened and collapsed during the ventilatory cycle.[16,30,31] VILI may also be worsened by increasing the frequency of excessive lung tidal stretch and from acceleration forces associated with rapid initial gas flow into the lung.[32]

VILI occurs clinically when low resistance–high compliance units receive a disproportionately high regional tidal volume in the setting of high alveolar distending pressures (see Fig. 65-2). Concern about overdistention injury is the rationale for using "lung-protective" ventilator strategies that accept less than normal values for pH and O_2 partial pressure in exchange for lower (and safer) distending pressures.

CARDIAC EFFECTS

In addition to affecting ventilation and ventilation distribution, intrathoracic pressure changes resulting from positive-pressure ventilation can affect cardiovascular function.[18] In general, as mean intrathoracic pressure is increased, right ventricular filling is decreased. This is the rationale for using volume repletion to maintain cardiac output in the setting of high intrathoracic pressure. Conversely, elevations in intrathoracic pressure can actually improve left ventricular function because of an effective reduction in afterload.[33] Indeed, a sudden release of intrathoracic pressure (e.g., during a ventilator disconnect or spontaneous breathing trial) can sometimes precipitate flash pulmonary edema because of the acute increase in afterload coupled with an increased venous return.[34]

Intrathoracic pressures can also influence the distribution of perfusion. The relationship of alveolar pressures to perfusion pressures in the three-zone lung model can help explain this.[35] Specifically, the supine human lung is generally in a zone 3 (distention) state. As intra-alveolar pressures rise, however, zone 2 and zone 1 regions can appear, creating high $\dot{V}/\dot{Q}$ units. Indeed, increases in deadspace (i.e., zone 1 lung) can be a consequence of ventilatory strategies using high ventilatory pressures (e.g., IRV).

Positive-pressure mechanical ventilation can affect other aspects of cardiovascular function. Specifically, dyspnea, anxiety, and discomfort from inadequate ventilatory support can lead to stress-related catechol release, with subsequent increases in myocardial O_2 demands and risk of dysrhythmias. In addition, coronary blood vessel O_2 delivery can be compromised by inadequate gas exchange from the lung injury, coupled with low mixed venous O_2 partial pressure due to high O_2 consumption demands by the ventilatory muscles.

OTHER ADVERSE EFFECTS

Oxygen concentrations approaching 100% are known to cause oxidant injuries in airways and lung parenchyma.[36] Many of the data supporting this concept, however, have come from animal studies, and animals and humans often have different O_2 tolerances. It is thus not clear what the "safe" O_2 concentration or duration of exposure is in sick humans. Most consensus groups have argued that FIO_2 values less than 0.4 are safe for prolonged periods and that FIO_2 values greater than 0.8 should be avoided if possible.

Mechanically ventilated patients are at risk for pulmonary infections for several reasons.[37] First, the natural protective mechanism of glottic closure is compromised by an endotracheal tube. This permits continuous seepage of oropharyngeal material into the airways. Second, the endotracheal tube itself impairs the cough reflex and serves as a potential portal for pathogens to enter the lungs. This is particularly important if the circuit is contaminated. Third, airway and parenchymal injury from both the underlying disease and management complications make the lung prone to infections. Fourth, the ICU environment itself, with its heavy antibiotic use and the presence of very sick patients in close proximity, poses a risk for a variety of infections.

Preventing ventilator-associated pneumonias is critical, because length of stay and mortality are heavily influenced by their development.[37] Hand washing and carefully chosen antibiotic regimens for other infections can have important beneficial effects. Management strategies that avoid breaking the integrity of the circuit (e.g., circuit changes only when visibly contaminated) also appear to be helpful.[38] Finally, continuous drainage of subglottic secretions may be a simple way of reducing lung contamination with oropharyngeal material.[39]

APPLYING ASSIST-CONTROL MECHANICAL VENTILATORY SUPPORT

TRADEOFFS

To provide adequate support but minimize VILI, mechanical ventilation goals must involve tradeoffs. Specifically, the need for potentially injurious pressures, volumes, and supplemental O_2 must be weighed against the benefits of gas exchange support. To this end, a rethinking of gas exchange goals has occurred over the last decade; pH goals as low as 7.15 to 7.20 and O_2 partial pressure goals as low as 55 mm Hg are now considered acceptable if the lung can be protected from VILI.[40] Ventilator settings are thus selected to provide at least this level of gas exchange support while at the same time meeting two mechanical goals: (1) provision of enough PEEP to recruit the recruitable alveoli, and (2) avoidance of a PEEP–tidal volume combination that unnecessarily overdistends lung regions at end-inspiration. These goals embody the concept of a "lung-protective" mechanical ventilatory strategy, and these principles guide current recommendations for the specific management of parenchymal and obstructive lung disease.[40,41]

PARENCHYMAL LUNG INJURY

Parenchymal lung injury describes disease processes that involve the airspaces and the interstitium of the lung. In general, parenchymal injury produces stiff lungs and reduced lung volumes.[12] Functional residual capacity is thus reduced, and the compliance curve is shifted to the right. It is important to realize, however, that in all but the most diffuse diseases (e.g., diffuse cardiogenic edema), there are often marked regional differences in the degree of inflammation present and thus the degree of mechanical abnormalities that exist. This heterogeneity can have a significant impact on the effects of a particular mechanical ventilation strategy. This is because delivered gases will preferentially go to the regions with the highest compliance and lowest resistance (i.e., the more normal regions) rather than to sicker regions with low compliance (see Fig. 65-2). A "normal-sized" tidal volume may thus be distributed preferentially to the healthier regions, resulting in a much higher regional tidal volume and the potential for regional overdistention injury.

Parenchymal injury can also affect the airways, especially the bronchioles and alveolar ducts.[12] These narrowed and collapsible small airways can contribute to reduced regional ventilation to injured lung units. This can also lead to air trapping, and it may be a factor in subsequent cyst formation during the healing phase.

Gas exchange abnormalities in parenchymal lung injury are a consequence of alveolar flooding or collapse, coupled with a maldistribution of ventilation that results in $\dot{V}/\dot{Q}$ mismatching and shunts. Because deadspace ($\dot{V}/\dot{Q} = \infty$) is not a major manifestation of parenchymal lung disease unless there is severe or end-stage injury, hypoxemia tends to be more of a problem than CO_2 clearance is.

Frequency–tidal volume settings for supporting parenchymal lung injury must focus on limiting end-inspiratory stretch. The importance of this limitation in improving outcome has been suggested by several recent clinical trials[42] but was most convincingly demonstrated by the National Institutes of Health–sponsored trial, which showed a 10% absolute reduction in mortality with a ventilator strategy using a tidal volume of 6 mL/kg compared with 12 mL/kg.[41] Because of this, initial tidal volume settings should start at 6 mL/kg ideal body weight. Moreover, strong consideration should be given to further reducing this setting if end-inspiratory plateau pressures, adjusted for any effects of excessive chest wall stiffness, exceed 30 cm H_2O. Increases in tidal volume settings might be considered if there is marked patient discomfort or suboptimal gas exchange, provided that the subsequent plateau pressures do not exceed 30 cm H_2O. Respiratory rate settings are then adjusted to control pH. Unlike in obstructive diseases (see later), the potential for air trapping in parenchymal lung injury is low if the breathing frequency is less than 35 breaths per minute and may not develop even at frequencies exceeding 50 breaths per minute.

The choice of pressure-targeted or volume-targeted breaths often depends more on clinician familiarity with the two modes than on important clinical differences between them. As noted earlier, both modes provide a comparable range of tidal volumes and inspiratory times. In general, pressure-targeted breaths are preferable when an absolute pressure limit is desired in the circuit or when patient effort is very active, with variable flow demands. In contrast, volume-targeted breaths are preferable when it is critical to maintain a certain level of minute ventilation.

Setting the inspiratory time and the inspiratory-expiratory ratio in parenchymal injury involves several considerations. The normal ratio is roughly 1:2 to 1:4; this produces the most comfort and is the usual initial setting. Assessment of the flow graphic should also be done to ensure that an adequate expiratory time is present to avoid air trapping. As noted earlier, inspiratory-expiratory prolongation beyond the physiologic range of 1:1 (IRV) can be used as an alternative to increasing PEEP to improve $\dot{V}/\dot{Q}$ matching in severe respiratory failure.[22,23] A variation on IRV is airway pressure release ventilation (also known as biphasic or bilevel ventilation).[43] Airway pressure release ventilation incorporates the ability to spontaneously breathe during the long inflation period of a pressure-controlled breath—a feature that may enhance recruitment and comfort.[43]

Generally, IRV strategies are reserved for patients in whom the plateau pressure from the PEEP–tidal volume combination exceeds 30 cm H_2O and potentially toxic concentrations of FIO_2 are being used without meeting arterial O_2 saturation or O_2 delivery goals. It must be emphasized, however, that although IRV strategies have physiologic appeal, good outcome studies supporting their use do not exist.

There are both mechanical and gas exchange approaches to setting the PEEP-FIO_2 combination to support oxygenation. Mechanical approaches use either a static pressure-volume plot to set the PEEP–tidal volume combination between the upper and lower inflection points[44] or step increases in PEEP to determine the PEEP level that gives the best compliance.[45] With either of these approaches, a recruitment maneuver could be used to recruit the maximal number of recruitable alveoli before setting the PEEP. FIO_2 adjustments are then set as low as clinically acceptable. Gas exchange criteria to guide PEEP application generally involve algorithms designed to provide adequate values for arterial partial pressure of O_2 while minimizing FIO_2 (Table 65-1).[41] Note that constructing a PEEP-FIO_2 algorithm is usually an empirical exercise in balancing arterial O_2 saturation with FIO_2 and depends on the clinician's perception of the relative "toxicities" of high thoracic pressures, high FIO_2, and low arterial O_2 saturation.

OBSTRUCTIVE AIRWAY DISEASE

Respiratory failure from airflow obstruction is a direct consequence of increases in airway resistance. Airway narrowing and increased resistance lead to two important mechanical changes. First, the increased pressures required for airflow may overload ventilatory muscles, producing a "ventilatory pump failure," with spontaneous minute ventilation inadequate for gas exchange. Second, the narrowed airways create regions of lung that cannot properly empty and return to their normal resting volume, and intrinsic PEEP is produced.[9] These regions of overinflation create deadspace and put inspiratory muscles at a substantial mechanical disadvantage, which further worsens muscle function. Overinflated regions may also compress more healthy regions of the lung, impairing $\dot{V}/\dot{Q}$ matching. Regions of air trapping and intrinsic PEEP also function as a threshold load to trigger mechanical breaths.[46]

The gas exchange abnormalities that accompany worsening airflow obstruction are several. First, although there may be transient hyperventilation due to dyspnea in patients with asthma, worsening respiratory failure in those with obstructive lung disease is generally characterized by a falling minute ventilation as respiratory muscles become fatigued in the face of airflow obstruction. The result is termed hypercapneic respiratory failure. Second, as noted earlier, regional lung compression and regional hypoventilation produce $\dot{V}/\dot{Q}$ mismatch, which results in progressive hypoxemia. Alveolar inflammation and flooding, however, are not characteristic features of respiratory failure due to pure airflow obstruction; thus, shunts are less of an issue than in parenchymal lung injury. Third, overdistended regions of the lungs, coupled with underlying emphysematous changes in some patients, result in capillary loss and increasing deadspace. This wasted ventilation further compromises the inspiratory muscles' ability to supply adequate ventilation for alveolar gas exchange. These emphysematous regions also have reduced recoil properties that can worsen air trapping. Fourth, hypoxemic pulmonary vasoconstriction, coupled with chronic pulmonary vascular changes in some airway diseases, overloads the right ventricle, further decreasing blood flow to the lung and making the deadspace worse.

Setting the frequency–tidal volume pattern in obstructive lung disease involves many considerations that are similar to those in parenchymal lung injury. Specifically, tidal volumes should be sufficiently low (e.g., 6 mL/kg ideal body weight) to ensure that plateau pressure is less than 30 cm H_2O.[41] In obstructive disease, however, clinicians should be aware that high *peak* airway pressures, even in the presence of acceptable values for plateau pressure, may transiently subject regions of the lung to overdistention injury because of a pendelluft effect (see Fig. 65-2). As with parenchymal lung injury, tidal volume reductions should be considered to meet plateau pressure goals. Tidal volume increases can be considered for comfort or gas exchange, provided that plateau pressure values do not exceed 30 cm H_2O. The set rate is used to control pH. Unlike parenchymal disease, however, the elevated airway resistance (and often the low recoil pressures of emphysema) greatly increases the potential for air trapping, and this limits the range of breath rates available.

The inspiratory-expiratory ratio in obstructive lung disease is generally set as low as possible to minimize the development of air trapping. For the same reason, approaches using IRV strategies are almost always contraindicated.

Because alveolar recruitment is less of an issue in obstructive lung disease than in parenchymal lung injury, the

---

TABLE 65–1. PEEP-FIO_2 ALGORITHM

FIO_2	.30	.40	.40	.50	.50	.60	.70	.70	.70	.80	.90	.90	.90	1.0	1.0	1.0	1.0
PEEP	5	5	8	8	10	10	10	12	14	14	14	16	18	18	20	22	24

This table was used during the National Institutes of Health study.[41] The clinical target is an oxygen partial pressure of 55 to 80 mm Hg or SpO_2 of 88% to 95%. If the patient is below these target values, move up the table to the right. If the patient is above these targets, move down the table to the left.
FIO_2, inspired oxygen fraction; PEEP, positive end-expiratory pressure.

PEEP-FIO$_2$ steps in Table 65-1 should probably be shifted to emphasize FIO$_2$ for oxygenation support. A specific role for PEEP in an obstructed patient occurs when intrinsic PEEP serves as an inspiratory threshold load on the patient's attempting to trigger a breath. Under these conditions, judicious application of circuit PEEP (up to 75% to 85% of intrinsic PEEP) can "balance" expiratory pressure throughout the ventilator circuitry to reduce this triggering load and facilitate the triggering process.[46]

In severe airflow obstruction, use of the low-density gas helium can facilitate ventilator settings. Helium is available as 80:20, 70:30, or 60:40 helium-oxygen breathing gas mixtures and can both reduce patient inspiratory work and facilitate lung emptying (recall that driving pressure decreases and flow increases through a tube as gas density decreases). If using a helium-oxygen gas mixture, it must be remembered that many flow sensors must be recalibrated to account for the change in gas density.

NEUROMUSCULAR RESPIRATORY FAILURE

The risk of VILI is generally less in a patient with neuromuscular failure because lung mechanics are often near normal, making regional overdistension less likely. More "generous" tidal volumes can thus be used to improve comfort, maintain recruitment, and prevent atelectasis. At the same time, however, maximal distending pressures should be monitored and kept as low as possible while still being compatible with the other goals noted earlier. Certainly, plateau pressure should always be kept well below 30 cm H$_2$O. Low levels of PEEP are often beneficial in preventing derecruitment (atelectasis) in these patients, who are often supine and incapable of secretion clearance or spontaneous sigh breaths.

RECENT INNOVATIONS IN ASSIST-CONTROL MECHANICAL VENTILATORY SUPPORT

TRACHEAL GAS INSUFFLATION

Tracheal gas insufflation involves placing a catheter at the distal end of the endotracheal tube to provide fresh gas to flush the tube of CO$_2$ during exhalation.[47,48] The rationale is that the next delivered breath will effectively be free of endotracheal tube CO$_2$ and thus will have a reduced deadspace. This approach has particular appeal during lung-protective ventilatory strategies in which the arterial CO$_2$ partial pressure is rising. A number of studies have shown that the concept of tracheal gas insufflation accomplishes this physiologic goal (i.e., reduced deadspace), but there is the potential for an inadvertent PEEP buildup.

Tracheal gas insufflation catheters can deliver fresh gas either continuously or only during exhalation. The former approach is easier to implement, but the latter approach reduces the potential for excessive end-inspiratory overinflation. Catheters can also be designed to deliver gas directly into the lung or in a retrograde fashion back up the endotracheal tube. The former enhances gas mixing, but the latter reduces inadvertent PEEP buildup. At present, it is unclear what is the best way to deliver tracheal gas insufflation or whether it can significantly affect outcome. Clearly, however, such systems need to have safeguards to protect the lung from inadvertent overdistension.

HIGH-FREQUENCY VENTILATION

High-frequency ventilation uses very high breathing frequencies (120 to 300 breaths per minute in an adult), coupled with very small tidal volumes (often less than anatomic deadspace) to provide gas exchange in the lungs.[49] Gas transport under these seemingly unphysiologic conditions involves such mechanisms as Taylor dispersion, coaxial flows, and augmented diffusion.[50]

High-frequency ventilation can be supplied by either jets or oscillators. Jets inject high-frequency pulses of gas into the airways. Oscillators vibrate a fresh bias flow of gas delivered at the tip of the endotracheal tube.

The putative advantages to high-frequency ventilation are twofold. First, the high gas flow provides for considerable intrinsic PEEP and thus alveolar recruitment. This is particularly effective following recruitment maneuvers. Second, the very small tidal pressure swings keep the lung well below the overdistension threshold. Because of these features, high-frequency ventilation has sometimes been considered the "ultimate" lung protection strategy.[51]

Clinical experience with high-frequency ventilation has been most extensive in the neonatal and pediatric population. Recent studies suggest that in neonates at risk for overdistension injury, high-frequency ventilation improves outcome.[52] Adult experience is less extensive; only recently have devices become available to adequately support gas exchange in this setting.[53] However, a recent randomized trial comparing high-frequency ventilation with "conventional" ventilation in adults with acute respiratory distress syndrome showed a trend toward improved survival with high-frequency ventilation.[54]

CONCLUSION

Mechanical ventilatory support is a critical component in the management of patients with respiratory failure. It must be remembered, however, that this technology is supportive, not therapeutic; it cannot cure lung injury. Indeed, the best we can hope for is to "buy time" by supporting gas exchange without harming the lungs.

There are exciting innovations on the horizon, but they must be assessed properly. This is particularly important for innovations with significant risks or costs. Only with properly conducted studies of clinically relevant factors such as mortality, ventilator-free days, barotrauma, and cost can we properly assess the sometimes bewildering array of new approaches to this vital life-support technology.

ANNOTATED REFERENCES

American Association for Respiratory Care Consensus Group: Essentials of mechanical ventilators. Resp Care 1992;37:1000-1008.
  An excellent report examining mechanical ventilator design and application, including the major features of modern mechanical ventilators, breath delivery features, monitor and alarm strategies, and utility in various settings.

Dreyfuss D, Saumon G: Ventilator induced lung injury: Lessons from experimental studies. Am J Respir Crit Care Med 1998;157:294-323.
  An excellent review attempting to link important data from animal studies of ventilator-induced lung injury to the clinical setting, with an emphasis on how ventilator strategies can produce both lung and systemic injury.

NIH ARDS Network: Ventilation with lower tidal volumes as compared with traditional tidal volumes for acute lung injury and the acute respiratory distress syndrome. N Engl J Med 2000;342:1301-1308.
  This landmark study clearly established the link between excessive lung stretch during mechanical ventilation and worse survival in patients with

acute lung injury. *The message from this paper is very clear: even though large tidal volumes may improve gas exchange, they ultimately cause harm by overstretching healthier regions of the lung.*

Pinsky MR, Guimond JG: The effects of positive end-expiratory pressure on heart-lung interactions. J Crit Care 1991;6:1-15.

An excellent overview of the complex interactions of intrathoracic positive pressure and cardiac function. The fact that the twin effects of decreased right heart filling and decreased left ventricular afterload can have both positive and negative effects is carefully explained.

Slutsky AS: ACCP consensus conference: Mechanical ventilation. Chest 1993;104:1833-1859.

An excellent review of the application of mechanical ventilation, stressing the balance between providing respiratory support and not harming the patient.

Truwit JD, Marini JJ: Evaluation of thoracic mechanics in the ventilated patient. Part I. Primary measurements. J Crit Care 1988;3:133-150; Part II. Applied mechanics. J Crit Care 1988;3:192-213.

This two-part report comprehensively reviews all aspects of respiratory system mechanics as they apply to mechanical ventilation. Both theory and practical applicability are provided.

Chapter 66

PATIENT-VENTILATOR INTERACTION

Vincenzo Squadrone • Cesare Gregoretti • V. Marco Ranieri

KEY POINTS

1. **Patient-ventilator asynchrony is common**, is often unrecognized and underestimated, and is often inappropriately treated in the clinical setting.

2. **Patient-ventilator asynchrony takes place when the three physiologic variables** of the patient's breathing pattern—ventilatory drive, ventilatory requirements, and duration and ratio of inspiratory time to total breath cycle duration—do not match ventilator trigger, ventilator-delivered flow, and ventilator cycling criteria.

3. **Clinical optimization of patient-ventilator interactions** can be obtained only by continuously matching the triggering, flow delivering, and cycling functions of the ventilator with the patient's physiologic variables.

4. Optimization of patient-ventilator interactions implies **continuous measurement** of physiologic variables and **continuous adaptation** of the ventilator to the spontaneous variations in these physiologic variables.

5. **Future developments in ventilator technology** should be oriented toward a system with the capability to automatically interface between physiologic parameters and ventilator outputs. Such technology will be based on a closed-loop algorithm able to realize total patient-controlled mechanical support.

The clinical management of patients with acute respiratory failure is based on the assumption that significant abnormalities in respiratory mechanics, respiratory muscle performance, and control of breathing are the underlying mechanisms responsible for acute respiratory failure.[1] The effects of mechanical ventilation on gas exchange, respiratory muscle load, and dyspnea depend on the matching between the ventilator settings and the patient's respiratory physiology. However, mechanical ventilation is rarely optimized, which would require that ventilator settings be based on accurate and reproducible measurements of lung and chest wall mechanics, respiratory muscle function, and respiratory drive.[2-5]

RESPIRATORY PHYSIOLOGY

The goal of the ventilatory control system is to generate the timing and intensity of the phrenic nerve signal, integrating inputs from chemoreceptors, pulmonary stretch receptors, variations in metabolic demands, and so forth. Contraction of the respiratory muscles leads to the generation of flow and volume to provide adequate alveolar ventilation with minimal work of breathing.[6] During spontaneous breathing,[7] the respiratory muscles generate pressure (Pmus) to produce flow against the resistive properties (R_{RS}) and volume against the elastic properties (E_{RS}) of the respiratory system and to eventually overcome intrinsic positive end-expiratory pressure (PEEPi). Under these circumstances, the act of spontaneous breathing can be described at any instant as follows:

$$Pmus = Pres + Pel + PEEPi \qquad \text{(Equation 1)}$$

where Pres represents the resistive pressure and is a function of flow (Pres = Flow × R_{RS}), and Pel represents the elastic recoil pressure and is a function of volume (Pel = Volume × R_{RS}). Assuming that R_{RS} and E_{RS} are linear, the equation becomes:

$$Pmus = PEEPi + (Flow \times R_{RS}) + (Volume \times E_{RS})$$
$$\text{(Equation 2)}$$

In patients with acute respiratory failure requiring ventilatory support, pressure generated by the ventilator (Pappl) is added to the pressure generated by the contraction of the respiratory muscles, according to the following equation:

$$Pmus + Pappl = PEEPi + (Flow \times R_{RS}) + (Volume \times E_{RS})$$
$$\text{(Equation 3)}$$

The complex interaction among all the variables in equation 3 can be summarized with the concept of neuroventilatory coupling (Fig. 66-1).[8] Under normal conditions, as well as at the onset of acute respiratory failure, the spontaneous contraction of the respiratory muscles suddenly generates flow and volume; the slope of the relationship between effort and ventilatory output is conditioned by the contractile properties of the respiratory muscles and the impedance of the respiratory system. When positive pressure is applied to assist the action of breathing in most common modes of mechanical ventilation (pressure support or assist mandatory ventilation), the coupling between effort and output is compromised. During assist-mandatory ventilation, flow and volume remain constant, despite changes in muscle contraction; during pressure support ventilation, despite a sort of coupling between inspiratory effort and ventilatory output, any increase in respiratory

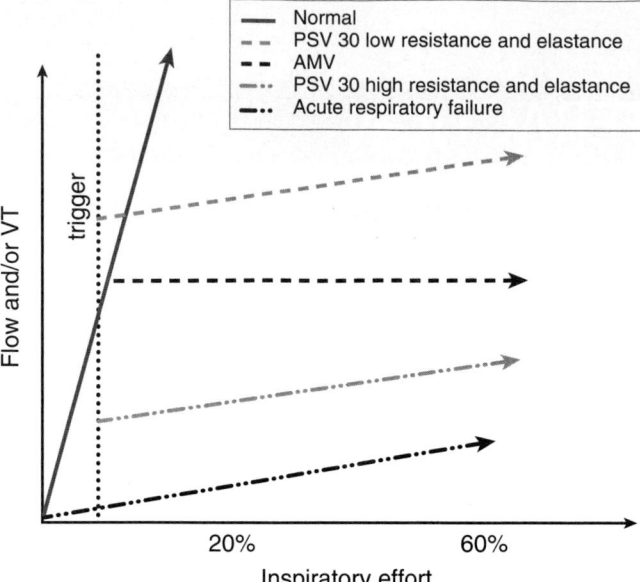

FIGURE 66–1. Neuroventilatory coupling. Under normal conditions, as well as at the onset of acute respiratory failure, the spontaneous contraction of the respiratory muscles suddenly generates flow and volume; the slope of the relationship between effort and ventilatory output is conditioned by the contractile properties of the respiratory muscles and the impedance of the respiratory system. When positive pressure is applied to assist the action of breathing in most common modes of mechanical ventilation, the coupling between effort and output is compromised. During assisted mandatory ventilation (AMV), flow and volume remain constant, despite changes in muscle contraction; during pressure support ventilation (PSV), despite a sort of coupling between inspiratory effort and ventilatory output, any increase in respiratory impedance decreases the amount of delivered flow and volume. VT, tidal volume.

impedance decreases the amount of delivered flow and volume.[8]

PATIENT AND VENTILATOR VARIABLES

PATIENT

The patient interacts with the ventilator based on three physiologic variables[2,9,10]:

1. Ventilatory drive, or when inspiration starts[11]
2. Ventilatory requirements, or how much flow and volume are necessary to satisfy metabolic demands[5]
3. Timing of the integrated circuits generating the respiratory rhythm, as measured by the duration and ratio of inspiratory time to total breath cycle duration[9]

VENTILATOR

The ventilator interfaces with the patient's physiology based on three technologic variables:

1. The inspiratory trigger, or when the ventilator starts to deliver flow, volume, and pressure[12,13]
2. The delivery mechanisms of gas—that is, the algorithm used by the ventilator to assist ventilation through the delivery of flow, volume, or pressure[14-19]
3. The cycling criteria, or when the ventilator stops assisting the inspiratory effort and lets the patient exhale spontaneously[20,21]

Intrinsic manufacturing features of ventilators, such as blowers and inspiratory, expiratory, and PEEP pressure valves, are also important in determining the interaction between patient and ventilator.[22-24]

To unload the respiratory muscles, restore sufficient gas exchange, and relieve the patient from dyspnea, the health care team must establish an interface between patient and ventilator. To do so, there are two options: total ventilator-controlled mechanical support, or partial patient-controlled support.

Total Ventilator-Controlled Mechanical Support. In this method, the patient's breathing pattern is totally controlled by the ventilator. The pressure generated by the respiratory muscles is abolished by paralysis or sedation. Flow, volume, and pressure are imposed by the ventilator, and the patient's breathing pattern is totally replaced by that of the ventilator. The risk of patient-ventilator asynchrony is therefore abolished, but there are potential risks associated with sedation and paralysis,[25] respiratory muscle atrophy,[26] lung damage due to overdistention,[27] patient discomfort,[28] and difficulty weaning after prolonged controlled mechanical ventilation.[1]

Partial Patient-Controlled Mechanical Support. With this method, spontaneous breathing activity is partially preserved.[29] The need for sedation and paralysis may be reduced, disuse atrophy of the respiratory muscles may be minimized, and the weaning process may be accelerated, provided the patient's ventilatory demand and ventilator settings are synchronized.[30] The ability to restore gas exchange, unload respiratory muscles, and relieve patient dyspnea with partial patient-controlled mechanical support therefore depends on the absence of patient-ventilator asynchrony.[31]

Although there are no well-accepted definitions, patient-ventilator asynchrony is common; it is often unrecognized, underestimated, and inappropriately treated.[3-5,19-21,31] The cause of patient-ventilator asynchrony can be described as occurring because of a mismatch between the three physiologic variables characterizing spontaneous breathing (ventilatory drive, ventilatory requirements, and duration and ratio of inspiratory time to total breath cycle duration) and the three technologic variables characterizing ventilator function (trigger function, gas delivery algorithm, and cycling criteria).

RESPIRATORY DRIVE–VENTILATOR TRIGGER ASYNCHRONY

The goal of the ventilator trigger is to track inspiratory effort in order to couple the patient's effort with the delivery of pressure, flow, or volume. The inspiratory effort necessary to trigger a breath may be a significant part of the total inspiratory effort, representing 17% and 12% of the total inspiratory effort during pressure and flow triggering, respectively.[12-22] Aslanian and coworkers found that even though the time required for triggering was 43% shorter and effort during the time of triggering was 62% less with flow triggering than with pressure triggering, effort during the post-triggering phase was equivalent for both pressure and flow triggering.[32] The clinical benefit of flow triggering therefore appears to be much less relevant than commonly stated.[3]

Inspiratory phase asynchrony may be due to problems with inspiratory triggering, and this can be correlated with

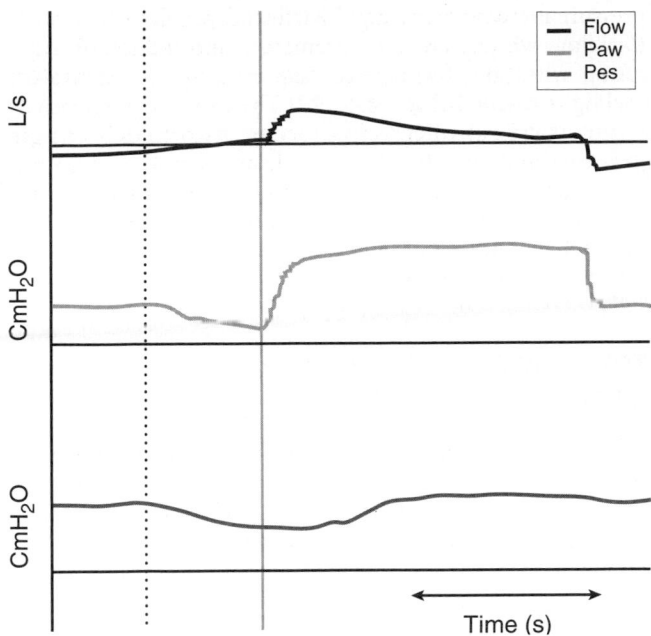

FIGURE 66–2. Representative tracings show the interaction between patient effort and triggering of the ventilator. The delay between the beginning of inspiratory muscle activity (*dotted line*) and the beginning of mechanical inflation (*solid line*) can cause an inspiratory phase asynchrony. Flow, flow generated at the airway opening; Paw, pressure applied at the airway opening; Pes, esophageal pressure.

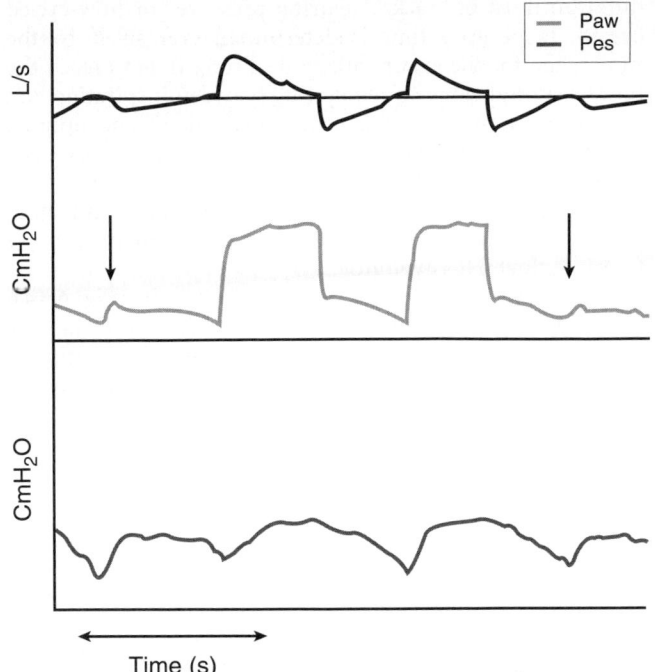

FIGURE 66–3. Representative tracings show ineffective triggering due to the ventilator's inability to detect the patient's "request" for an assisted breath. As indicated by the *arrows,* a substantial inspiratory effort generates only a bump in the flow and pressure tracings, instead of a mandatory assisted breath. Flow, flow generated at the airway opening; Paw, pressure applied at the airway opening; Pes, esophageal pressure.

respiratory drive. Phase lag quantifies the delay between the commencing of inspiratory muscle activity and the beginning of mechanical inflation (Fig. 66-2).[3,9,10] The presence of a threshold load, such as dynamic intrinsic PEEP, may further complicate patient-ventilator interaction during the triggering phase.[12] Giuliani and coworkers suggested that effort during triggering determines patient effort during the remaining portion of inspiration.[33] Leung and coworkers demonstrated that the higher the level of ventilator-applied pressure, the lower the respiratory drive but the longer the time required to trigger the ventilator; as a result, respiratory muscles generate smaller inspiratory swings in intrathoracic pressure, but over a longer inspiratory time.[2] Another problem is related to the fact that pressure is detected on the expiratory limb of the ventilator circuit; therefore, any resistive load (e.g., endotracheal tube or upper airways during non-invasive ventilation) reduces the responsiveness of the gas delivered by the ventilator in response to patient effort.[19]

Ineffective triggering is due to the ventilator's inability to detect the patient's "request" for an assisted breath, despite substantial inspiratory effort (Fig. 66-3). This phenomenon usually occurs with high levels of ventilator assistance and with short expiratory times. Mechanical characteristics that may induce ineffective triggering include low elastance, high resistance, and intrinsic PEEP; ineffective triggering is not correlated to an increase in the patient's inspiratory effort.[2] The application of external PEEP below the intrinsic PEEP level can reduce the patient's inspiratory effort required to trigger the ventilator.[34] Parthasarathy and coworkers demonstrated that prolonging mechanical inflation into neural expiration reduces the time available for unopposed exhalation, resulting in the need for a greater inspiratory effort to trigger the ventilator.[35] Younes and colleagues found that ineffective triggering in ventilator-dependent patients exacerbates dynamic hyperinflation.[36]

VENTILATORY REQUIREMENT–GAS DELIVERY ASYNCHRONY

Gas delivery asynchrony occurs when ventilator-delivered flow, volume, and pressure are insufficient to meet the patient's ventilatory demand. Ward and coworkers demonstrated that increasing the flow rate could be used as a means of reducing the patient's respiratory drive and active respiratory muscle work,[14] although doing so may exert an excitatory effect on respiratory rate and on the rate of rise of inspiratory muscle activity.[3,16,17,37-43] Laghi and colleagues demonstrated that the imposed inspiratory time during mechanical ventilation determines respiratory frequency independent of inspiratory flow and tidal volume.[17] Pressure-targeted breath may better match the patient's ventilatory requirements, because pressure is the independent variable; as a consequence, flow is continuously adjusted by the ventilator to maintain a constant pressure. In addition, the rapid pressurization of the airways is coupled with high inspiratory flow only at the beginning of inspiration, thus reproducing the physiologic flow profile.[44]

INSPIRATORY TIME–VENTILATOR CYCLING ASYNCHRONY

Ventilator-patient asynchrony occurs when the patient is trying to exhale but the ventilator is still delivering gas.[32,35,45] In patients ventilated with a time-cycled breath, expiratory phase asynchrony takes place when the patient's neural inspiratory time is shorter or longer than the ventilator inflation time. For proper cycling off of the ventilator and optimal patient-ventilator synchrony, the patient's inspiratory flow and ratio of inspiratory time to total breath cycle duration must be tracked. During pressure- or flow-cycled breath, inspiratory time is determined exclusively by the time taken for the exponentially declining flow to reach the flow threshold value (when cycling between inspiration and expiration occurs).[20,46] For proper cycling off and optimal patient-ventilator synchrony, the ventilator needs to track patient's inspiratory flow. The algorithm for the "expiratory trigger" depends on the manufacturer, but most ventilators use a percentage of a drop in inspiratory flow or a preset terminal flow. This expiratory sensitivity can be fixed or can vary from 5% to 90% or from 5 to 25 L/min (Fig. 66-4). Preset terminal flow algorithms can be problematic in patients with chronic obstructive pulmonary disease.[47] The setting of the pressure rise time (pressure slope) can also modify the expiratory threshold by modifying the inspiratory flow.[48,49]

Although there is some evidence that rapid pressure rise times might reduce the patient's work of breathing,[48] a fast

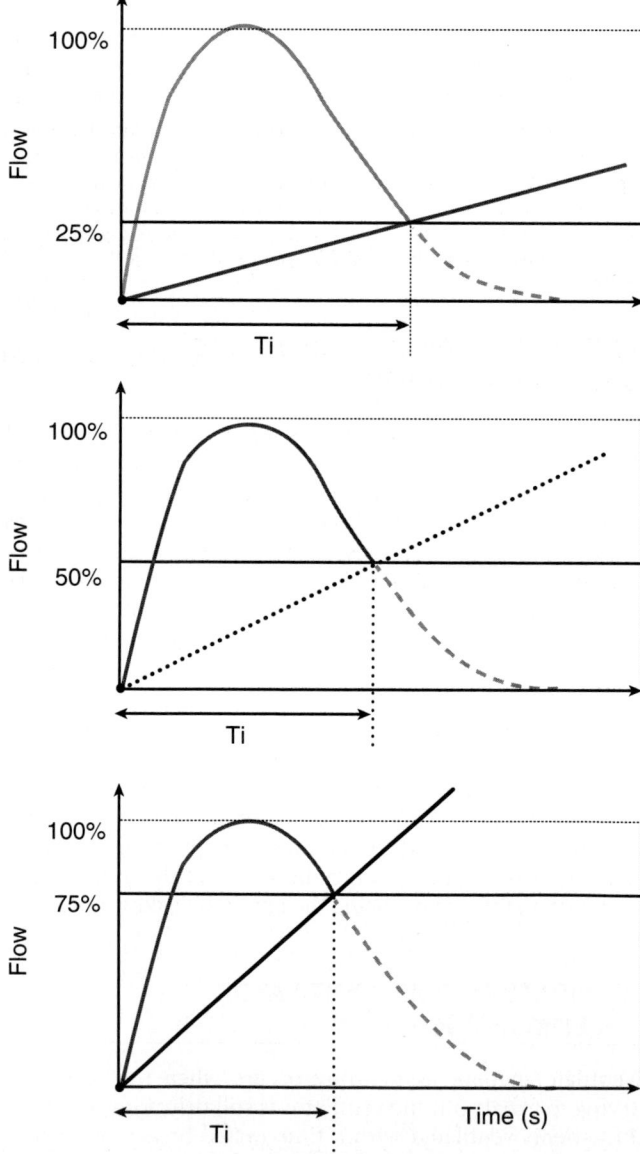

FIGURE 66–4. Representative tracings show different settings for expiratory trigger sensitivity on a flow-time plot. From top to bottom: expiratory trigger set at 25%, 50%, and 75% of peak flow. Ventilator inspiratory time is influenced by the preset flow expiratory trigger sensitivity, at which point the ventilator switches to expiration.

pressure increase may lead to particularly high peak inspiratory flow, which may cause premature termination of inspiration when the fixed percentage criterion for expiratory cycling is reached (Fig. 66-5).[19,50] The expiratory sensitivity setting is crucial when ventilators are used to deliver noninvasive ventilation, because air leaks may cause an abnormal prolongation of the inspiratory time; during this time, the patient may make several efforts to exhale against the machine or to inhale, without receiving any ventilatory support (inspiratory hang-up) (Fig. 66-6).[51-54]

TOTAL PATIENT-CONTROLLED MECHANICAL SUPPORT

Clinical optimization of patient-ventilator interactions can be obtained only by continuous matching between the triggering, flow delivering, and cycling functions of the ventilator and the patient's ventilatory drive, spontaneous inspiratory flow demand, and ratio of inspiratory time to total breath cycle. This implies continuous measurement of physiologic variables and continuous adaptation of the ventilator to the spontaneous variations in these variables. Future development in ventilator technology should be oriented toward systems with the capability to automatically interface between physiologic parameters and ventilator outputs. Such technology will be based on a closed-loop algorithm able to achieve total patient-controlled mechanical support.[4]

The design features of an automatic control system in a mechanical ventilator include (1) what activates the system (the input), (2) what the system produces (the output), (3) the protocol used to link input and output (the controlling algorithm). In a closed-loop system, the output will activate and condition the input. When changes in output are opposite to changes in input, the closed loop is said to be negative. The closed loop is positive when variations in output mirror variations in input. The most common example of a negative closed-loop control system in the clinical setting is the ventilator humidifier. In this case, the input is the temperature inside the chamber, and the output is the temperature of the gas being delivered to the patient. The controlling algorithm is designed to keep the latter constantly above a value set by the operator. If the output (i.e., the temperature of gas delivered to the patient) is lower than the preset level, the algorithm will increase the input (i.e., the temperature in the chamber); if the output is higher than the preset level, the algorithm will decrease the input. Closed-loop systems are hence able to stabilize and limit the performance of a mechanical system. In the case of acute respiratory failure, the patient is unable to provide sufficient output (i.e., minute ventilation). The ventilator should therefore be able to detect the input from the patient and continuously adapt the output to it. If the input is increasing (i.e., ventilatory requirements are increasing), the ventilator will increase the output (i.e., apply more positive pressure); if the input is decreasing (i.e., ventilatory requirements are decreasing), the ventilator will decrease the output (i.e., apply less positive pressure). The controlling closed loop eventually applied by the ventilator must therefore be positive. Positive closed-loop control systems are inherently unstable in the sense that they tend to (1) "run away" with ventilatory assistance—if the pressure generated by the ventilator is higher than the pressure required to offset the passive properties of the respiratory system, the ventilator will continue to deliver flow and volume while the

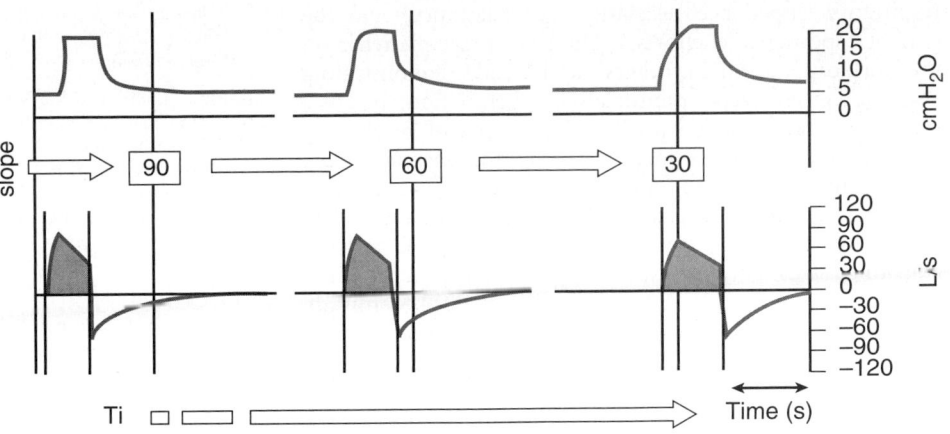

FIGURE 66–5. Representative tracings show different pressure-rise time sensitivities on a flow-time plot. From left to right: pressure-rise time set at 90%, 60%, and 30% of maximal pressurization time. Ventilator inspiratory time *(shaded area)* is influenced by the preset pressure-slope sensitivity that generates a different peak inspiratory flow. Paw, pressure applied at the airway opening.

patient stops his or her inspiratory effort and tries to initiate expiration; and (2) "extinguish" ventilatory assistance—if the patient does not produce any inspiratory effort, the ventilator will not produce any ventilatory support.

Based on a closed-loop algorithm, new modes of mechanical ventilation have been proposed. They represent modifications of pressure support ventilation and are characterized by the patient's ability to control the amount of assistance provided by the ventilator. They are differentiated by the patient-related variable used to close the loop.

PROPORTIONAL ASSISTED VENTILATION AND PROPORTIONAL PRESSURE SUPPORT

During proportional assisted ventilation and proportional pressure support, the ventilator generates pressure in proportion to patient-generated flow and volume; the ventilator amplifies patient effort without imposing any ventilatory or pressure targets. Ventilator-generated pressure rises as long as inspiratory muscle effort is produced by the patient. The preset parameter is not a target pressure but the proportion between pressure applied by the ventilator and flow and volume generated by the patient's inspiratory muscle effort.[55,56] During this type of mechanical support, the clinician adjusts the percentage of flow-assisted or volume-assisted ventilation, after determining the patient's resistance and elastance. In other words, the physician must determine how much to reduce the load imposed by the patient's elastance[57] and resistance.[58,59] Despite the exciting potential of this technique,[59-62] applied either invasively or noninvasively,[63-69] no large-scale studies have demonstrated an improvement in patient outcome compared with other modes of ventilation.

NEURAL-ADJUSTED VENTILATORY ASSISTANCE

With this method, electrical activity of the diaphragm is measured by means of an electrode array inserted into a nasogastric tube and placed in the lower esophagus; this information is then used to control the ventilator to generate flow, volume, and pressure.[8,70,71] Unlike with the proportional method described earlier, estimates of respiratory mechanics are not needed. With neural-adjusted ventilatory assistance, the patient's respiratory center controls the assisted positive breaths in all phases of the ventilation cycle, from triggering to cycling off of inspiration. Any change in patient ventilatory output is matched breath by breath by the ventilator, even in the presence of variations in respiratory mechanics. This system is not yet available, and a number of issues must be sorted out before it can be used routinely.

ADAPTIVE SUPPORT VENTILATION

Adaptive support ventilation is basically an assist time–limited, pressure-targeted mode of ventilation (pressure-controlled ventilation), relying on a negative closed-loop system of regulating ventilator settings in response to changes in both

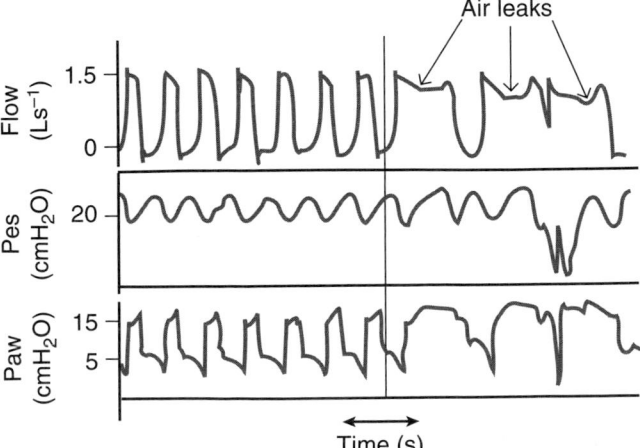

FIGURE 66–6. Representative record of air leaks during noninvasive facemask pressure support ventilation. The presence of air leaks causes a prolonged ventilator inspiratory time *(arrows)*. Flow, flow generated at the airway opening; Paw, pressure applied at the airway opening; Pes, esophageal pressure.

respiratory impedance (elastance and resistance) and the patient's spontaneous efforts.[72] The basic principle relies on the work of Otis and coworkers[73] and Mead,[6] demonstrating that, for a given level of minute alveolar ventilation, there is a respiratory rate that is least costly in terms of respiratory work. With adaptive support ventilation, the operator enters the patient's body weight and sets the desired percentage of minute ventilation. The expiratory time constant is determined by analysis of the expiratory flow-volume curve,[74] adjusting inspiratory pressure, inspiratory-expiratory time ratio, and respiratory rate to obtain the prescribed minute ventilation. Adaptive support ventilation thus adjusts inspiratory pressure, inspiratory-expiratory time ratio, and mandatory respiratory rate to maintain the target minute ventilation and respiratory rate, within a framework designed to avoid both rapid, shallow breathing and excessive inflation volumes. Spontaneous breathing triggers either a pressure-controlled or a spontaneous breath with inspiratory pressure support, the level of which is adjusted to meet the target respiratory rate–tidal volume combination.

ACKNOWLEDGMENTS

This work was supported by Ministero Università e Ricerca: COFIN 21544 (2002-2004).

ANNOTATED REFERENCES

Appendini L, Purro A, Gudjonsdottir M, et al: Physiologic response of ventilator-dependent patients with chronic obstructive pulmonary disease to proportional assist ventilation and continuous positive airway pressure. Am J Respir Crit Care Med 1999;159:1510-1517.

This study found that in difficult-to-wean patients with chronic obstructive pulmonary disease, proportional assisted ventilation improves ventilation and decreases inspiratory muscle effort. It also found that the combination of proportional assisted ventilation and continuous positive airway pressure can unload the inspiratory muscles to values close to those in normal subjects.

Beck J, Sinderby C, Lindström L: Effects of lung volume on diaphragm EMG signal strength during voluntary contractions. J Appl Physiol 1998;85:1123-1134.

These authors found that variations in end-expiratory lung volume between breaths can affect the transformation of respiratory muscle activation into mechanical output (neuromechanical coupling).

Calderini E, Confalonieri M, Puccio PG, et al: Patient-ventilator asynchrony during noninvasive ventilation: The role of the expiratory trigger. Intensive Care Med 1999;25:662-667.

This article describes the loose patient-ventilator synchrony in the presence of air leaks and noninvasive pressure support ventilation.

Laghi F, Karamchandani K, Tobin MJ: Influence of ventilator settings in determining respiratory frequency during mechanical ventilation. Am J Respir Crit Care Med 1999;160:1766-1770.

These authors found that during assist-control mode, ventilator inspiratory time can determine respiratory frequency independently of inspiratory flow and tidal volume.

Leung P, Jubran A, Tobin MJ: Comparison of assisted ventilator modes on triggering, patients' effort, and dyspnea. Am J Respir Crit Care Med 1997;155:1940-1948.

This study found that when receiving assist-control ventilation or high levels of pressure support, one quarter to one third of a patient's inspiratory efforts may fail to open the inspiratory valve triggering the machine. The number of ineffective triggering attempts increases in proportion to the level of ventilatory assistance and is not correlated to the magnitude of inspiratory effort at a given level of assistance.

Parthasarathy S, Jubran A, Tobin MJ: Cycling of inspiratory and expiratory muscle groups with the ventilator in airflow limitation. Am J Respir Crit Care Med 1998;158:1471-1478.

These authors found that the continuation of a mechanical mandatory breath into neural expiration is associated with a waste of inspiratory effort, defined as failure of the subsequent inspiratory attempt to trigger the ventilator.

Parthasarathy S, Tobin JM: Effect of ventilator mode on sleep quality in critically ill patients. Am J Respir Crit Care Med 2002;166:1423-1429.

These authors found that inspiratory assistance during pressure support causes hypocapnia, which, combined with the lack of a backup rate and wakefulness drive, can lead to central apneas and sleep fragmentation, especially in patients with heart failure. A backup rate, as during assist-control volume-targeted ventilation, prevents the development of apneas and perhaps decreases arousals.

Sinderby C, Navalesi P, Beck J, et al: Neural control of mechanical ventilation in respiratory failure. Nat Med 1999;5:1433-1436.

This article describes a completely new mode of detecting inspiratory effort, based on the measurement of electrical activity of the diaphragm by means of an electrode array inserted into a nasogastric tube and placed in the lower esophagus. Output generated from the electrodes, filtered out for, is used to control the ventilator that finally generates the respiratory ouput.

Tobert DG, Simon PM, Stroetz RW, Hubmayr RD: The determinants of respiratory rate during mechanical ventilation. Am J Respir Crit Care Med 1997;155:485-492.

The authors examined the rate response of eight normal volunteers during both quiet wakefulness and non–rapid-eye-movement (non-REM) sleep in the setting of mechanical ventilation through a nasal mask in an assist-control mode with a machine backup rate of 2 breaths per minute. They found that both tidal volume and inspiratory flow settings affect the respiratory rate and can affect carbon dioxide homeostasis. During non-REM sleep, hypocapnia resulted in wasted ventilator trigger efforts. Thus, ventilator settings appropriate for wakefulness may cause ventilatory instability during sleep.

Younes M, Webster K, Kun J, et al: A method for measuring passive elastance during proportional assist ventilation. Am J Respir Crit Care Med 2001;164:50-60.

A noninvasive method to continuously measure elastance of the respiratory system during proportional assisted ventilation is described.

Chapter 67

WEANING FROM MECHANICAL VENTILATION

Belén Cabello • Olga Rubio • Jordi Mancebo

IV

511

KEY POINTS

1. **Liberation from the ventilator is different from extubation.** They are different processes with different pathophysiologic mechanisms that may lead to failure.

2. **Cardiovascular dysfunction may complicate weaning** in a significant number of patients owing to the switch from positive intrathoracic pressure to spontaneous breathing, with a consequent increase in preload and afterload.

3. **The presence of undiagnosed illnesses at the time of extubation** may complicate the subsequent clinical course. Patients with extubation failure have an increased mortality rate that varies based on the specific cause of the failure.

4. **The implementation of weaning protocols improves outcome** in terms of duration of mechanical ventilation and length of stay in the ICU. This effect can be attributed mostly to the fact that patients are checked daily for the ability to maintain spontaneous breathing.

5. **Noninvasive ventilation** may prevent re-intubation and facilitate extubation.

Weaning from mechanical ventilation represents the period of transition from total ventilatory support to spontaneous breathing. The majority of intubated, mechanically ventilated patients (about 75%) are extubated after disconnection from the ventilator or after breathing at low levels of pressure support for a short time, generally 30 to 120 minutes.[1,2] The remaining patients (about 25%) need progressive withdrawal from artificial ventilatory support.

Early liberation from mechanical ventilation (weaning) and removal of the endotracheal tube (extubation) are clinically important. Unnecessary prolongation of mechanical ventilation increases the risk of complications, including infection (particularly of bronchopulmonary origin), barotrauma, cardiovascular compromise, tracheal injury, and muscle deconditioning. Clinicians should take steps to hasten the process that ultimately leads to endotracheal tube removal so as to maximize patient outcomes.[3]

Liberation and extubation are different issues. Once a patient has been weaned from mechanical ventilation and no longer requires ventilatory support, the clinician has to consider a different question: Is the patient able to breathe spontaneously without the endotracheal tube? Recent investigations have clearly determined that liberation and extubation are different entities and that the pathophysiologic mechanisms underlying weaning failure and extubation failure are not the same. In terms of magnitude, the extubation failure rate is variable and ranges from 5% to 20% of extubated patients.

MECHANISMS OF LIBERATION FAILURE

Weaning attempts that are unsuccessful usually indicate incomplete resolution of the illness that generated the need for mechanical ventilation.

RESPIRATORY PUMP FAILURE

The most common mechanism of weaning failure is respiratory pump insufficiency, which is caused by an imbalance between capability and demand.[4-6] During spontaneous breathing, the inspiratory muscles must generate sufficient force to overcome the elasticity of the lungs and chest wall (elastic load), as well as airway and tissue resistance (resistive load). This requires generation of a signal in the respiratory centers of the brainstem, anatomic and functional integrity of the nerves that conduct the signal, unimpaired neuromuscular transmission, and adequate respiratory muscle strength (the aggregate is termed neuromuscular competence). The ability of the respiratory muscles to sustain these loads without fatiguing is called endurance and is determined by the balance between energy supply and energy demand.

Jubran and Tobin investigated the progression of respiratory mechanics during spontaneous breathing trials in patients with chronic obstructive pulmonary disease (COPD).[7] At the beginning of the trials, patients who subsequently failed had slightly higher airway resistance, respiratory system elastance, and intrinsic positive end-expiratory pressure (PEEP) compared with those who succeeded. However, during the course of the trials, respiratory mechanics progressively worsened in patients who failed. They developed rapid, shallow breathing, and most developed an increase in partial pressure of carbon dioxide in arterial blood ($PaCO_2$). Together, these abnormalities resulted in increased inspiratory muscle effort, which in some patients was probably close to the threshold of muscle fatigue.

The issue of fatigue was recently revisited by Laghi and Tobin.[8] They studied 19 intubated patients during weaning from mechanical ventilation; 11 patients failed, and 8 succeeded. Several physiologic indices were measured before and 30 minutes after a spontaneous breathing trial. Before the trial, the transdiaphragmatic twitch pressure, elicited by magnetic bilateral phrenic stimulation, did not differ between those who failed and those who succeeded, and it did not decrease after the trial in either group. A fall in transdiaphragmatic twitch pressure is a physiologic index of low-frequency fatigue. Patients who failed the spontaneous breathing trial were reconnected to the ventilator because of clinical signs of intolerance. In this study, the ratio of swings in gastric pressure to swings in pleural pressure (an index of rib cage and expiratory muscle contribution to tidal breathing) was significantly higher in the failure group over the course of the trial. These alterations, together with the reinstitution of mechanical ventilation, might defend against the development of low-frequency fatigue. It was concluded that weaning failure was not accompanied by low-frequency diaphragmatic fatigue, although patients who failed to wean exhibited severe diaphragmatic weakness, because twitch pressures were always low.

Disorders That Alter the Balance of Capacity and Load

Reduced Neuromuscular Capacity

Reduced output of the respiratory control centers may occur after the administration of sedatives, narcotics, and anesthetic agents. Central nervous system and brainstem disorders are frequently accompanied by altered levels of consciousness. These disorders are often associated with attenuated cough and upper airway protection reflexes and depressed respiratory drive, all of which can contribute to difficult weaning and, eventually, unsuccessful extubation.

Phrenic nerve dysfunction can occur after traumatic injuries (e.g., high cervical spine lesions) and is also common after cardiac surgery.[9] Diaphragmatic dysfunction may occur after upper abdominal surgery.[10] Critical illness polyneuropathy and myopathy, which are frequent complications of sepsis and multiple organ system failure,[11,12] may impede weaning as well. Finally, neuromuscular blocking agents (with or without concomitant corticosteroids) and aminoglycosides may contribute to weaning failure.[13-17]

Intravenous corticosteroids and prolonged use of neuromuscular blockade have been implicated in ICU-acquired myopathy.[18] In a study of acute asthma requiring mechanical ventilation, Behbehani and colleagues found that the incidence of myopathy was 10.4% among all patients and 30% among patients who received neuromuscular blocking agents.[19] These authors found that the duration of muscle relaxation was the only independent predictor of the development of myopathy. In addition, malnutrition, deconditioning due to prolonged bed rest or mechanical ventilation, and increased muscle catabolism can induce severe muscle dysfunction.

In a multicenter study by De Jonghe and coworkers, a high incidence of ICU-acquired paresis was found in patients without preexisting neuromuscular disorders who had received mechanical ventilation for at least 7 days.[12] In this group of 95 patients, 25% were diagnosed with acquired paresis. The duration of mechanical ventilation after discontinuation of neuromuscular blockade was significantly longer in patients who had paresis compared with those who did not (18.2 versus 7.6 days; $P = 0.03$). In this investigation, the independent predictors of ICU-acquired paresis were female sex, number of days with dysfunction of two or more organs, duration of mechanical ventilation requiring neuromuscular blockade, and administration of corticosteroids.

Although the incidence of paresis was elevated, the mortality rate of these patients (4 of 24, 7%) did not significantly differ from the mortality observed in the control group (4 of 71, 6%).

Increased Muscle Load

Increased work of breathing results from increased mechanical loads (elastic, resistive, or both) or from processes that require higher minute ventilation. Increased ventilatory requirements are quite common in critically ill patients, particularly during periods of hyperthermia, overfeeding, and hyperventilation (related to anxiety or pain). An increase in the deadspace–tidal volume ratio is another source of increased ventilatory requirements.

Increased elastic workloads occur when lung or chest wall compliance is reduced (e.g., pulmonary edema, extreme hyperinflation during acute asthma attack, pulmonary fibrosis, abdominal distention, obesity, trauma, thoracic deformities). The presence of intrinsic PEEP is another example of increased elastic workload and is a relatively common phenomenon, especially in patients with COPD. Dynamic pulmonary hyperinflation, apart from generating an elastic threshold load, places the diaphragm in a mechanically disadvantageous position. If lung volume is increased above passive functional residual capacity, the diaphragm flattens and its radius of curvature increases. Consequently, the capacity to generate pressure decreases.

Resistive work of breathing during critical illness may increase because of bronchospasm, excessive secretions, endotracheal tube resistance (which increases with kinking and deposition of secretions), and ventilator valves, circuits, and humidifiers, especially when inspired gases are conditioned with heat and moisture exchangers. The latter also increase deadspace.

CARDIOVASCULAR DYSFUNCTION

The presence of cardiovascular dysfunction can contribute to weaning failure by augmenting loads and reducing neuromuscular capacity. A study by Epstein showed that as many as 33% of weaning failures resulted solely or partly from congestive heart failure,[20] whereas only 14% failed due to cardiovascular reasons in other studies.[21] Cardiovascular dysfunction may result from physiologic changes that occur during the resumption of spontaneous unassisted breathing.[22] When spontaneous breathing resumes, intrathoracic pressure swings during inspiration are negative, which increases left ventricular preload and afterload. Cardiac loading is thus expected to be most marked in patients with large mechanical respiratory muscle loads (e.g., those with severe obstructive or restrictive respiratory diseases), who require relatively large negative pleural pressure swings to inspire. A significant decrease in left ventricular ejection fraction has been described during spontaneous breathing trials in COPD patients without coronary artery disease.[23]

Increased myocardial loading may be sufficient, especially when coupled with left ventricular noncompliance, to precipitate congestive heart failure (which stiffens the lungs and further increases loads). Moreover, increased heart loads augment myocardial oxygen demand and may precipitate myocardial ischemia in patients with coronary artery disease.[24] Myocardial ischemia causes left ventricular dysfunction, which may induce overt acute pulmonary edema and arterial hypoxemia.

Jubran and colleagues examined hemodynamics and mixed venous saturation in patients during weaning trials.[25] Successfully weaned patients demonstrated increases in cardiac index and oxygen transport compared with values during mechanical ventilation. Patients who failed weaning also failed to increase oxygen delivery to the tissues, due in part to elevated right and left ventricular afterloads. Consequently, these abnormalities can jeopardize respiratory muscle function.

MECHANISMS OF EXTUBATION FAILURE

Extubation failure refers to patients who, once extubated, require the reinstitution of ventilatory assistance within 24 to 48 hours. Thus, the extubation failure rate is the number of patients requiring reinstitution of mechanical ventilation divided by the total number of extubated patients. Extubation is performed after the decision to disconnect the patient from mechanical ventilation has been made and after the patient has tolerated a spontaneous breathing trial. The duration of a spontaneous breathing trial is variable, usually 30 to 120 minutes. Patients are subsequently extubated if, during this period of spontaneous breathing, they do not exhibit signs or symptoms of poor clinical tolerance and also show that they are able to cough adequately.[26]

The re-intubation rate may differ according to the cause of respiratory failure. For instance, in a large study including 217 medical and surgical patients, Vallverdú and associates noted that the overall re-intubation rate was 15.5%, ranging from 35.7% (15 of 42) in neurologic patients to 0% (0 of 13) in COPD patients.[27] The re-intubation rate in patients who had acute respiratory failure due to other causes was 8.6% (8 of 93). Data from Esteban and coworkers indicate that good clinical tolerance of a 2-hour trial with low pressure support levels (7 cm H_2O) is as good at predicting extubation success as the classic 2-hour T-piece trial.[28] With this strategy, the re-intubation rate was 18.8% with T-piece and 18.5% with pressure support ventilation (PSV).[28] A study by the same group found that a trial of spontaneous breathing (T-piece) with a target duration of 30 minutes was as effective in identifying patients who could be safely extubated as a trial with a target duration of 120 minutes.[29] In this study, the 48-hour re-intubation rates were also similar (13.5% in the 30-minute group, and 13.4% in the 120-minute group).

Mechanisms explaining extubation failure include physiologic abnormalities not diagnosed at the time of extubation (e.g., pneumonia, ongoing cardiac failure) and an inability to keep the tracheobronchial tree free of copious secretions.[26,27] Finally, intubation can result in laryngotracheal injury, which may explain some episodes of extubation failure; this tends to occur more frequently with a longer duration of intubation and in females.[30]

The majority of investigations indicate that failed extubation is associated with increased hospital mortality.[27-29,31,32] Extubation failure also results in a marked increase in the duration of mechanical ventilation, length of ICU and hospital stay, and need for tracheostomy.[28,29,33] The cause of extubation failure also influences outcome, with mortality being lower for airway problems (upper airway obstruction, aspiration, excess pulmonary secretions) and higher when re-intubation is required for other reasons.[28,29,33,34] Patients requiring re-intubation because of respiratory failure had a mortality rate of 30%, whereas mortality in patients needing re-intubation because of upper airway obstruction was only

7%.[33] In a study by Epstein and Ciubotaru, mortality was lowest for those re-intubated within 12 hours; it increased as the time between extubation and resumption of ventilatory support increased.[33] After controlling for severity of illness, presence of comorbid conditions, organ failure, and cause of re-intubation, time to re-intubation was found to be an independent predictor of outcome. These data suggest that extubation failure is probably a marker of underlying disease severity.

INDICES TO PREDICT WEANING OUTCOME

Many indices have been proposed in an attempt to predict weaning outcome. There are those that assess simple ventilatory parameters, assess oxygenation, assess respiratory muscle strength, assess central respiratory drive, measure respiratory muscle reserve, assess work of breathing, integrate different variables of respiratory function (composite indices), and analyze the pattern of spontaneous breathing in terms of tidal volume (V_T) and respiratory rate (f). In general, except for the f/V_T ratio, these indices have relatively poor positive and negative predictive value. In addition, the performance of these indices is affected by a number of factors. For example, the duration of ventilatory support before weaning is attempted varies widely, and these indices tend to have better predictive capabilities if the duration of mechanical ventilation is short. The time at which the patients are studied is also important, because weaning outcome is likely to be influenced by the different clinician practices from unit to unit (including the use of sedatives, analgesics, and neuromuscular blocking agents). Last, differences in patient populations involving age and disease processes can also strongly influence weaning outcome. Indeed, weaning outcome and respiratory parameters used as weaning predictors vary considerably, depending on the underlying disease.[27]

Yang and Tobin studied the predictive power of several weaning indices and showed that the rapid, shallow breathing index (f/V_T) had the best predictive value.[35] In their study, 95% of patients with f/V_T ratios greater than 105 failed a test of spontaneous breathing. Other studies, however, did not confirm these results. For instance, Epstein and Ciubotaru found that between 27% and 40% of patients with f/V_T ratios greater than 100 could be successfully extubated.[20,30] They also showed that women, especially when breathing through small endotracheal tubes, have higher f/V_T ratios than men.

Vallverdú and associates studied 217 patients receiving mechanical ventilation (33 COPD, 46 neurologic, and 138 acute respiratory failure) who met standard weaning criteria and had undergone a 2-hour T-piece weaning trial.[27] Before starting the T-piece trial, functional respiratory parameters were measured. If the spontaneous breathing trial was clinically well tolerated, the patients were extubated. If clinical tolerance of the T-piece trial was poor, patients were reconnected to ventilatory support. Ventilatory support was resumed because of intolerance in 60.6% of COPD patients. In these patients, the best predictive indices of extubation success were f/V_T and airway occlusion pressure.

For routine care, simple clinical weaning parameters (e.g., the rapid, shallow breathing index) appear to be most useful at the bedside. However, one has to consider that some patients with negative weaning parameters can tolerate disconnection from the ventilator. From a practical standpoint, the information conveyed by weaning indices and clinical judgment needs to be combined in clinical decision-making.

INDICES TO PREDICT EXTUBATION OUTCOME

In contrast to the discontinuation of mechanical ventilation, indices that reliably predict extubation outcome have not been developed. In two large trials including more than 1000 patients, physiologic parameters such as respiratory rate, heart rate, and systolic blood pressure rapidly deteriorated, usually within the first 15 minutes of spontaneous breathing, in patients who failed the weaning trial.[2,28] However, none of these measurements could discriminate between patients who required re-intubation and those who tolerated extubation.

The frequency of re-intubation and its adverse impact on survival indicate that the accurate prediction of extubation outcome is important. The majority of clinicians assess patient readiness for both weaning and extubation by conducting a spontaneous breathing trial of variable duration. The importance of performing such a trial before deciding to extubate was proved by Zeggwagh and colleagues.[36] These authors proceeded directly to extubation (without performing a spontaneous breathing trial) after medical ICU patients had demonstrated clinical improvement. Of the 119 cases of extubation, 44 (37%) resulted in re-intubation. This rate is much higher than that reported for patients who are extubated after passing a spontaneous breathing test.

Patients incapable of protecting the airway and clearing secretions with an effective cough are at increased risk for extubation failure. Traditional assessment consists of demonstrating the presence of a cough reflex when stimulated with a suction catheter and the absence of excessive secretions, but these criteria have not been standardized. In intubated, mechanically ventilated subjects, a "sawtooth" pattern on the flow-volume curve indicates the presence of excess airway secretions but does not provide quantitative information.[37]

Although tolerance of a spontaneous breathing trial is a good predictor of successful extubation, Vallverdú and associates noted that a high percentage (35.7%) of neurologic patients who passed a 2-hour spontaneous breathing test and were extubated needed subsequent re-intubation.[27] Coplin and coworkers studied the variability in extubating brain-injured patients.[38] Their data provided no justification for delaying extubation in patients whose only indication for prolonged intubation is a depressed level of consciousness. They found that timely extubation of patients who met standard weaning criteria appeared to be safe (no increased risk of re-intubation or subsequent tracheotomy), potentially beneficial (associated with a lower incidence of pneumonia), and less expensive (shorter ICU stay and lower hospital costs). In this study, the re-intubation rate was 18% (24 of 136 patients). Re-intubation for airway or pulmonary dysfunction was not related to extubation delay or to coma at the time of extubation. Only two components of a semi-quantitative assessment of the need for airway care were associated with successful extubation: spontaneous cough ($P = 0.01$) and suctioning frequency ($P = 0.001$).

Namen and colleagues evaluated a respiratory-driven weaning protocol (daily screens and spontaneous breathing trial) in 100 neurosurgical patients.[39] Because of concerns about neurologic impairment, the implementation of this classic protocol was limited, and no differences were observed between intervention and control groups. The re-intubation rate was 16%, and multivariate analysis showed that a favorable Glasgow Coma Scale score and PaO_2/FiO_2 ratio were associated with extubation success.

Recently, Smina and coworkers studied a group of 95 patients admitted to a medical ICU who passed a spontaneous breathing test and were ready to be extubated.[40] They hypothesized that the strength of a patient's cough, measured by peak expiratory flow, and the volume of suctioned endotracheal secretions per hour could predict extubation outcome. They found that patients with peak expiratory flows of 60 L/min or lower were five times as likely to have an unsuccessful extubation. In addition, patients with neurologic problems were more likely to have a failed extubation than were those without neurologic problems (risk ratio, 2.7; 95% confidence interval, 1.0 to 7.3). These data emphasize that patients who are incapable of protecting the airways and clearing secretions are at increased risk for unsuccessful extubation.

In an attempt to avoid re-intubation after failed extubation, Keenan and coworkers undertook a randomized, controlled trial in 81 patients.[41] One group ($n = 42$) was allocated to receive standard treatment alone, and the other group ($n = 39$) received the same plus noninvasive ventilation via facemask. The re-intubation rates (69% versus 72%), ICU mortality rates (24% versus 15%), and hospital mortality rates (31% for both groups) were not significantly different. According to these data, noninvasive ventilation is not recommended in patients who require mechanical ventilation for more than 48 hours and who develop respiratory distress within 48 hours after planned extubation. Whether noninvasive ventilation might be useful to avoid re-intubation in certain subgroups of patients is not known.

There is little agreement on what constitutes an acceptable extubation failure rate. Centers reporting very low rates may be keeping patients on mechanical ventilation longer than necessary. In contrast, high failure rates may indicate insufficient assessment before extubation. At present, good clinical tolerance of a spontaneous breathing trial seems to be the best predictor of extubation success.

PROGRESSIVE WITHDRAWAL OF MECHANICAL VENTILATION

Weaning from mechanical ventilation represents the period of transition from total ventilatory support to spontaneous breathing. The most common techniques used to withdraw mechanical ventilation in patients who failed an initial weaning trial are PSV and breathing through a T-piece. Two prospective, multicenter, randomized clinical trials showed that synchronized intermittent mandatory ventilation (SIMV) is less efficacious than the other techniques.[1,2]

ROLE OF PROTOCOLS

A fundamental advance in recent years is the observation that routine screening of patients' ability to breathe spontaneously is the best approach to speeding extubation.[42,43] Saura and colleagues showed that implementation of a weaning protocol based on daily screening of simple clinical weaning parameters dramatically shortened weaning time.[42]

This was attributable mostly to the sharp fall in the number of patients undergoing progressive reduction in ventilatory support because they could be extubated sooner. With this approach, the incidence of re-intubation remained stable (between 14% and 17%), but the length of mechanical ventilation was shortened by an average of 4 days. These data were confirmed by the subsequent randomized, controlled trials of Ely[43] and Kollef[44] and their associates. Both trials focused on monitoring patients' ability to sustain spontaneous breathing. This approach was associated with faster extubation and shorter ICU stay, without increasing the re-intubation rate.

The use of sedative drugs, often administered via continuous intravenous infusion, is common in intubated, mechanically ventilated patients. An important study revealed that regular interruption of these drugs can significantly reduce the duration of mechanical ventilation.[45] Patients randomly allocated to daily interruption were ventilated for a median of 4.9 days, whereas patients treated with the usual approach (interruption of sedatives at the discretion of the clinician) were ventilated for a median of 7.3 days ($P = 0.004$). Moreover, the daily discontinuation strategy allowed for a better assessment of neurologic status, required less diagnostic testing, and was not associated with more complications compared with the usual strategy.

The major impact of protocols to hasten the weaning process was pointed out in a recent study of difficult-to-wean COPD patients requiring invasive mechanical ventilation for more than 15 days.[46] This multicenter study enrolled 26 patients who were weaned with PSV and 26 who were weaned with intermittent spontaneous breathing trials. Weaning success rates (73% versus 77%), duration of ventilatory assistance (180 versus 130 days), and mortality rates (11.5% versus 7.6%) did not differ significantly between the groups. However, when the data obtained in the randomized patients was compared with that from historical controls, it was observed that the weaning success rate was significantly greater (87% versus 70%), and the time spent on mechanical ventilation in surviving weaned patients was significantly shorter (103 versus 170 hours), in protocol patients than in historical controls.

PRESSURE SUPPORT VENTILATION

PSV is a patient-triggered, pressure-limited, flow-cycled mode in which airway pressure is maintained at near constant levels during inspiration. When inspiratory flow reaches a certain threshold level, cycling from inspiration to expiration occurs. This method of ventilatory assistance allows the patient to retain control over respiratory rate and timing, inspiratory flow rate, and tidal volume. During weaning, PSV levels are decreased according to the patient's clinical tolerance, usually by steps of 2 to 4 cm H_2O at least twice a day. In general, adequate clinical tolerance of a PSV level of around 8 cm H_2O is required before extubation is performed, although this level may vary according to individual patient characteristics.

The pressure level, which should be adjusted to begin weaning, is usually determined by letting the patient breathe in a "comfortable" way. However, both previous clinical experience[1,2] and data from clinical research[47,48] suggest that optimal initial levels are those that provide respiratory rates between 25 and 30 breaths per minute. The level of external PEEP to be used in patients with clinically suspected dynamic hyperinflation and dynamic airway collapse should be adjusted with great caution, because measurement of dynamic intrinsic PEEP in spontaneously breathing patients is not easy. To that end, it has been suggested that external PEEP can be titrated according to changes in airway occlusion pressure.[49]

SPONTANEOUS BREATHING WITH A T-TUBE

The T-tube system offers very little resistance to gas flow No additional work of breathing is imposed, because neither ventilator valves nor circuits are involved. Tolerance of the T-tube is a good way to evaluate a patient's capacity to maintain autonomous spontaneous breathing.[50,51] The optimal duration of the test is at least 30 minutes but no more than 120 minutes.

The main disadvantage of the T-piece trial is related to the lack of a connection to a mechanical ventilator; the patient is not monitored and therefore must be closely supervised, which places great demands on the nursing staff. Additionally, the transition between periods of muscular rest and periods of spontaneous unassisted breathing can be too abrupt for some patients, especially those who have panic reactions after disconnecting from the ventilator and those with latent left ventricular failure and myocardial ischemia.

NONINVASIVE VENTILATION

In Nava and coworkers' prospective randomized trial, patients with COPD who failed an initial spontaneous breathing trial and were extubated to noninvasive PSV were liberated from the ventilator more quickly (10.2 versus 16.6 days), spent less time in the ICU (15.1 versus 24 days), and were more likely to survive (92% versus 72%) than were patients weaned with PSV via endotracheal tube.[52] At 60 days, 88% of patients ventilated noninvasively were successfully weaned, compared with 68% of patients ventilated invasively.

Girault and colleagues prospectively studied 33 COPD patients who failed a 2-hour T-piece trial.[53] Sixteen patients were randomly assigned to conventional invasive PSV weaning, and 17 were randomly assigned to noninvasive PSV weaning immediately after extubation. Although weaning with noninvasive PSV significantly reduced the total duration of invasive mechanical ventilation and the probability of remaining intubated and mechanically ventilated, the total duration of ventilatory support related to weaning was greater in the noninvasive PSV group. The length of ICU and hospital stay and the mortality rate at 3 months were similar in both groups. The contrast between these findings and those in Nava's study may be due to differences in disease severity, selection of patients with regard to timing of extubation, PSV settings, and amount of experience in delivering PSV.

The usefulness of noninvasive ventilation to facilitate early extubation was reanalyzed in a recent randomized multicenter trial.[54] This study was conducted in 43 mechanically ventilated patients with persistent weaning failure. One group of patients ($n = 21$) was extubated and received noninvasive ventilation with pressure support and a full facemask. The other group ($n = 22$) remained intubated and followed a traditional weaning strategy with daily spontaneous breathing trials. The main results of this investigation were a shorter period of invasive ventilation, shorter ICU and hospital length of stay, and increased ICU and 90-day survival in patients extubated early and treated with noninvasive ventilation, compared with the control group. This study, performed in a nonselected population of ICU patients who met weaning criteria, suggests that early use of noninvasive ventilation may be effective in skilled hands. Another interpretation, however, is that the criteria used to determine failure of a spontaneous breathing trial were too strict and physicians were overzealous in interpreting clinical intolerance (or that some type of bias existed due to the unblinded nature of the study), and that these patients were kept on invasive mechanical ventilation for an unduly prolonged period.

NEW MODALITIES

Intubated and mechanically ventilated patients have varying ventilatory needs and exhibit changes in respiratory mechanics and breathing pattern. These occur during the weaning period as well. Consequently, fixed levels of ventilatory assistance (provided with either volume- or pressure-limited breaths) may be inappropriate when mechanics or demand changes. For this reason, manufacturers have developed new modes with the aim of improving tolerance of assisted ventilation, patient comfort, and patient-ventilator synchrony and avoiding excessive respiratory effort. Some of these modes are closed-loop systems, whereby the ventilator takes into account current physiologic information about the patient (e.g., respiratory rate, end-tidal PCO_2, tidal volume) and adapts its output according to predefined targets.

A number of these systems have been tested extensively, particularly those implementing closed-loop PSV,[55,56] and have the potential to reduce the total duration of mechanical ventilation by continuously adapting the ventilator's assistance to the patient's needs. Such permanent control and adaptation are not feasible even in the best current clinical environment, simply because of the lack of time and sufficient caregivers to undertake these tasks. Whether such systems may further decrease the duration of mechanical ventilation compared with traditional protocols is not known. That question will soon be answered, however, when the results of ongoing clinical trials are known.

UNPLANNED EXTUBATION DURING WEANING

Unexpected removal of the endotracheal tube (unplanned extubation) may be deliberate, as a result of patient agitation or lack of cooperation, or accidental, due to rupture of the endotracheal cuff, nursing procedures, coughing, or other unintentional events. Unplanned extubation is estimated to occur in 8.5% to 13% of intubated, mechanically ventilated patients.[57-63]

In a prospective study carried out during a 32-month period, 59 episodes of unplanned extubation were observed in 55 of 750 patients (frequency, 7.3 %) who required mechanical intubation for more than 48 hours.[61] The extubation was deliberate in 77.9% and accidental in 22.1% of cases. Twenty-seven episodes (45.8%) occurred in patients on full mechanical ventilatory support, and 32 episodes (54.2%) occurred during the weaning period. This parameter had not been studied previously, and it played an important role in determining the subsequent need for re-intubation. The results from this study indicate that the need for re-intubation after an episode of unplanned extubation is dependent on

whether the patient is in the weaning phase of mechanical ventilation. Patients who had unplanned extubations during weaning required significantly fewer re-intubations than did those who were not in the weaning phase (odds ratio, 6.6). Only 15.6% of patients (5 of 32) who were being weaned from mechanical ventilation needed re-intubation, whereas re-intubation was necessary in 81.5% of patients (22 of 27) receiving full mechanical ventilatory support ($P < 0.001$). In view of these results, it is conceivable that the process of weaning may be longer than necessary in some patients. Indeed, in this study, at least 15% of the patients being weaned from mechanical ventilation could have been extubated earlier, because they did not require re-intubation.

Epstein and colleagues performed a case-control study involving 75 patients with unplanned extubations and 150 controls matched for Acute Physiology and Chronic Health Evaluation (APACHE II) score, presence of comorbid conditions, age, indication for mechanical ventilation, and gender.[62] They observed that unplanned extubation was not associated with increased mortality, although they noted an increase in total duration of mechanical ventilation, length of ICU and hospital stay, and need for chronic care in the unplanned extubation group. A comparison of mortality between the group that needed re-intubation and the group that did not revealed a higher mortality rate in the former. Finally, these authors reported significant differences regarding re-intubation rates between patients who had an unplanned extubation during weaning trials and those who had one during full ventilatory support (44% in the former; 76% in the latter).

These studies suggest that the incidence of unplanned extubation can be used as an indicator of the quality of nursing and medical care in the ICU. In addition, a high incidence of unplanned extubation and a low incidence of re-intubation in these patients indicate that invasive ventilatory support is being provided for longer than necessary.

SUMMARY

Major advances have been made in the area of weaning from mechanical ventilation. The pathophysiologic mechanisms of weaning failure and extubation failure are better understood. It has been recognized that the vast majority of intubated, mechanically ventilated patients can be successfully liberated from the ventilator after passing a short spontaneous breathing test. Moreover, the best strategy to shorten the total time on mechanical ventilation is based on a simple protocol and a daily clinical approach that determines a patient's ability to sustain spontaneous unassisted breathing. When spontaneous breathing trials fail, techniques for progressive withdrawal of mechanical ventilation (PSV and volume-assisted mechanical ventilation with daily spontaneous breathing trials) seem to be equivalent. This is true as long as the use of these techniques is based on the same criteria used to evaluate tolerance. In the future, new semi-automated ventilatory modalities may be beneficial in difficult-to-wean patients. Noninvasive ventilation may be helpful to hasten weaning in selected populations and when used appropriately. Despite a better understanding of the mechanisms of extubation failure, it still occurs and is associated with increased mortality. Current data show that the employment of noninvasive ventilation in cases of impending extubation failure does not avoid re-intubation any better than a conventional approach does.

ANNOTATED REFERENCES

Brochard L, Rauss A, Benito S, et al: Comparison of three methods of gradual withdrawal from ventilatory support during weaning from mechanical ventilation. Am J Respir Crit Care Med 1994;150:896-903.

This was the first randomized trial comparing three different methods of weaning. The authors concluded that the outcome of weaning is influenced by the modality chosen. The weaning duration was shorter with PSV than with SIMV or T-piece used together.

Ely EW, Baker AM, Dunagan DP, et al: Effect on the duration of mechanical ventilation of identifying patients capable of breathing spontaneously. N Engl J Med 1996;335;1864-1869

This randomized, controlled trial demonstrated that daily screening for the ability to sustain spontaneous breathing, followed by a T-piece trial, reduces the duration of mechanical ventilation and ICU costs without increasing the number of complications.

Esteban A, Frutos F, Tobin MJ, et al: A comparison of four methods of weaning patients from mechanical ventilation. N Engl J Med 1995;332: 345-350.

In this randomized, multicenter study comparing four different methods of weaning, the authors found that weaning with a once-daily spontaneous breathing trial was twice as fast as with PSV and three times faster than SIMV. Multiple trials of spontaneous breathing did not reduce the time of weaning compared with a once-a-day trial.

Jubran A, Tobin MJ: Pathophysiologic basis of acute respiratory distress in patients who fail a trial of weaning from mechanical ventilation. Am J Respir Crit Care Med 1997;155:906-915.

This physiologic study determined the mechanisms of acute respiratory distress. COPD patients who failed a spontaneous breathing trial developed rapid, shallow breathing and worsening of pulmonary mechanics, which caused an increase in $PaCO_2$.

Kress J, Pohlman A, O'Connor M, et al: Daily interruption of sedative infusions in critically ill patients undergoing mechanical ventilation. N Engl J Med 2000;342:1471-1477.

This randomized, controlled trial demonstrated that a daily interruption of sedative drugs in intubated and mechanically ventilated patients reduces the duration of mechanical ventilation and length of stay in the ICU.

Chapter 68

NONINVASIVE POSITIVE-PRESSURE VENTILATION

Thomas Rajan • Nicholas S. Hill

KEY POINTS

1. The use of noninvasive positive-pressure ventilation in patients with acute respiratory failure is a recent phenomenon, mainly because of **advances in noninvasive interfaces and ventilator modes.**

2. **Noninvasive positive-pressure ventilation delivered by nasal or oronasal mask** reduces the need for endotracheal intubation, decreases the length of stay in the ICU and hospital, and reduces mortality when used in selected patients with exacerbations of chronic obstructive pulmonary disease (COPD).

3. **The efficacy of noninvasive positive-pressure ventilation has been demonstrated** for acute pulmonary edema, for respiratory failure in immunocompromised patients, and to facilitate extubation in COPD patients.

4. **Patients who develop respiratory failure or who refuse intubation** are potentially good candidates for noninvasive positive-pressure ventilation, but all patients must be selected carefully.

5. **Several factors are vital to the success of noninvasive positive-pressure ventilation:** careful patient selection; properly timed initiation; comfortable, well-fitting interface; coaching and encouragement; and careful monitoring.

6. **Noninvasive ventilation should be used to avert endotracheal intubation rather than as an alternative to it.** One should not persist in the use of noninvasive positive-pressure ventilation if it will lead to a delay in necessary intubation.

7. **A trial of noninvasive ventilation should be instituted in properly selected patients with acute respiratory failure** before respiratory arrest is imminent, to provide ventilatory assistance while the factors responsible for the respiratory failure are aggressively treated.

8. Noninvasive ventilation is an important addition to the methods available to assist patients with acute respiratory failure and, **if properly applied, improves patient outcome in the critical care setting.**

Noninvasive ventilation is defined as the provision of ventilatory assistance to the lungs without an invasive artificial airway. Noninvasive ventilators consist of a variety of devices, including negative- and positive-pressure ventilators.

Until the early 1960s, negative-pressure ventilation in the form of tank ventilators was the most common type of mechanical ventilation outside the anesthesia suite.[1] However, during the Copenhagen polio epidemic of 1952, it was observed that the survival rate improved when patients with respiratory paralysis were treated with invasive positive-pressure anesthesia devices. After that, invasive positive-pressure mechanical ventilation gradually became the preferred means of treating acute respiratory failure.[2] Negative-pressure and other so-called body ventilators were the mainstay of ventilatory support for patients with chronic respiratory failure until the mid-1980s.[1]

With the introduction of nasal continuous positive airway pressure (CPAP) to treat obstructive sleep apnea in the early 1980s,[3] and the discovery that nasal masks were a convenient conduit to assist ventilation,[1] noninvasive positive-pressure ventilation rapidly displaced negative-pressure ventilation as the treatment of choice for chronic respiratory failure in patients with neuromuscular and chest wall deformities. Over the past dozen years, noninvasive ventilation has moved from the outpatient to the inpatient setting, where it is used to treat acute respiratory failure. A 1997 survey of medical ICUs in France, Switzerland, and Spain demonstrated that noninvasive ventilation was used in 16% of cases in which mechanical ventilation was required for respiratory failure,[4] and a follow-up survey found that this rate was up to 23% in 2001.[5] This chapter discusses the rationale for the increasing use of noninvasive positive-pressure ventilation in critical care, as well as appropriate indications, practical applications, and monitoring.

RATIONALE

The most important advantage of noninvasive ventilation is the avoidance of complications associated with invasive mechanical ventilation. These include complications related to direct upper airway trauma, bypass of the upper airway defense mechanisms, increased risk of nosocomial pneumonia, and interference with upper airway functions, including the ability to eat and communicate normally.[6] By averting airway intubation, noninvasive ventilation leaves the upper airway intact, preserves airway defenses, and allows patients to eat orally, vocalize normally, and expectorate secretions. Compared with invasive mechanical ventilation, noninvasive ventilation reduces infectious complications, including pneumonia, sinusitis, and sepsis.[7-9] Strengthening the rationale for its use is evidence accumulated over the past decade that noninvasive ventilation lowers morbidity and mortality rates of selected patients with acute respiratory failure and may shorten hospital length of stay, thus reducing costs.

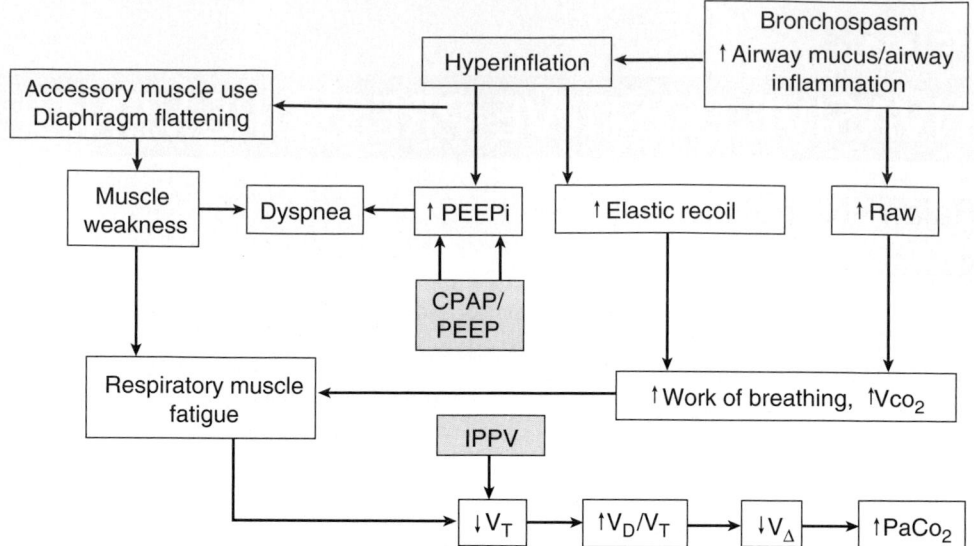

FIGURE 68–1. The pathophysiology of acute hypoxemic respiratory failure, and the points where positive-pressure and oxygen supplementation interrupt the process. Low ventilation-perfusion (V/Q) ratios, shunt, and alveolar hypoventilation cause hypoxemia. Hypoxemia is treated by increasing the inspired oxygen fraction (F_{IO_2}) (limited benefit with shunt) and by applying positive pressure (continuous positive airway pressure [CPAP] or positive end-expiratory pressure [PEEP]) to increase functional residual capacity, open collapsed alveoli and narrowed airways, and enhance compliance. An additional beneficial effect of CPAP may occur in patients with cardiogenic pulmonary edema, because it reduces both venous return and left ventricular (LV) afterload, which may enhance cardiovascular performance in patients with dilated, hypocontractile left ventricles.

The main indication for mechanical ventilatory assistance is to treat respiratory failure, either type 1 (hypoxemic), type 2 (hypercapnic), or both. Figure 68-1 shows that airspace collapse, surfactant abnormalities, and airway narrowing and closure contribute to ventilation-perfusion abnormalities and shunt, which cause hypoxemia. By opening collapsed airspaces and narrowed airways, positive airway pressure reduces shunt and improves ventilation-perfusion relationships, ameliorating hypoxemia. In addition, positive airway pressure can reduce the work of breathing by improving lung compliance as a consequence of opening collapsed airspaces. Another potential benefit of positive airway pressure is enhanced cardiovascular function via the afterload-reducing effect of increased intrathoracic pressure. Conversely, deleterious cardiovascular effects may occur if the preload-reducing effect outweighs the afterload-reducing effect, as may be seen in patients with reduced intravascular fluid volume.

MECHANISMS OF ACTION

Figure 68-2 shows the pathophysiologic mechanisms that contribute to ventilatory failure. Increased airway resistance, reduced respiratory system compliance, and intrinsic positive end-expiratory pressure (PEEP) contribute to increased work of breathing, predisposing to respiratory muscle fatigue. In patients with chronic obstructive pulmonary disease (COPD), the increased radius of the diaphragmatic curvature, which increases muscle tension and thereby increases impedance to blood flow, exacerbates the situation. By counterbalancing intrinsic PEEP with extrinsic PEEP, and by augmenting tidal volume with intermittent positive-pressure ventilation, noninvasive ventilation reduces the work of breathing and averts the vicious circle leading to respiratory failure. Work of breathing measurements, including trans-diaphragmatic pressure, diaphragmatic pressure-time product, and diaphragmatic electromyographic amplitude, are all

decreased when noninvasive ventilation is delivered to patients with exacerbations of COPD. In such patients, CPAP and pressure support ventilation (PSV) both reduce the work of breathing, but the combination of the two (PSV + PEEP) is more effective than either alone.[10]

INDICATIONS

A number of causes of acute respiratory failure are now considered appropriate for noninvasive ventilation therapy and are listed in Table 68-1. The evidence supporting these indications is rated in the table and briefly discussed here; guidelines for patient selection are discussed later.

AIRWAY OBSTRUCTION

Chronic Obstructive Pulmonary Disease
Starting in 1990, a historically controlled study,[11] a number of subsequent randomized, controlled trials,[12,13] and a meta-analysis[14] have consistently shown that compared with conventional therapy, noninvasive ventilation improves vital signs, gas exchange, and dyspnea scores; reduces the rates of intubation, morbidity, and mortality; and shortens hospital length of stay in patients with moderate to severe exacerbations of COPD. Thus, noninvasive ventilation is considered the ventilatory mode of choice in selected patients with acute exacerbations of COPD. Some studies suggest that the addition of heliox to noninvasive ventilation further improves the work of breathing and gas exchange during COPD exacerbations,[15] but a recent multicenter trial found no improvement in other outcomes compared with noninvasive ventilation alone.[16]

Asthma
Uncontrolled studies have reported improvements in gas exchange and low rates of intubation after the initiation of

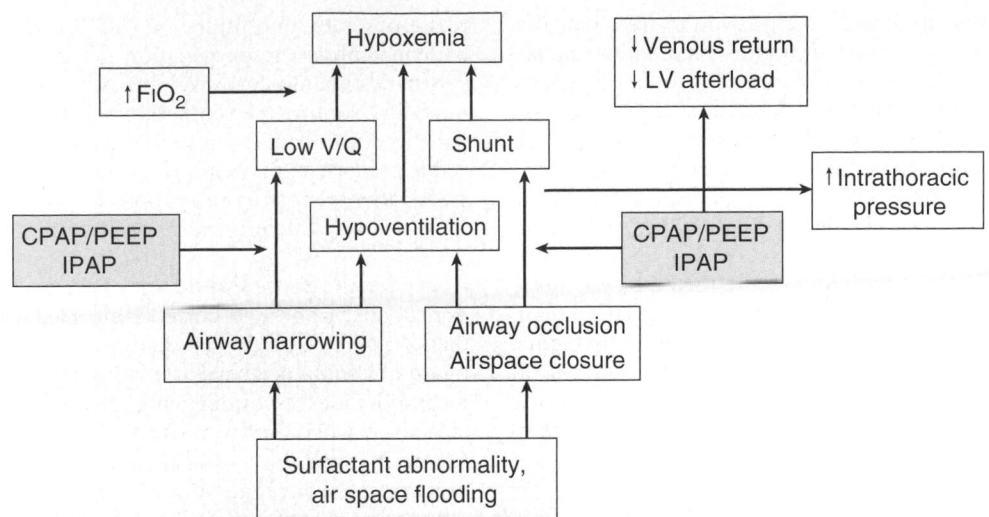

FIGURE 68–2. The pathophysiology of acute hypercapnia, and the points where continuous positive airway pressure (CPAP), positive end-expiratory pressure (PEEP), and pressure support (PS) interrupt the process *(large arrows)*. Hypercapnia (increased partial pressure of carbon dioxide in arterial blood [PaCO₂]) occurs when the respiratory muscles fail to adequately ventilate alveoli to maintain homeostasis with carbon dioxide production. Respiratory muscle failure occurs when the work of breathing is normal (e.g., acute or chronic neuromuscular disease) or increased (e.g., patients with chronic obstructive pulmonary disease, asthma, or the obesity hypoventilation syndrome), and presumably because of inadequate oxygen delivery to the respiratory muscles (e.g., approximately one third of patients presenting with cardiogenic pulmonary edema). Strategies to counter these pathophysiologic mechanisms include applying CPAP or PEEP to counterbalance intrinsic PEEP (PEEPi), increasing alveolar ventilation by augmenting tidal volume (V_T), using intermittent positive-pressure ventilation (IPPV), and reducing carbon dioxide production by decreasing the work of breathing.

noninvasive ventilation in patients with severe asthma attacks.[17] A recent controlled trial demonstrated a more rapid improvement in expiratory flow rates and a decreased hospitalization rate in acute asthma patients treated with noninvasive ventilation compared with a sham mask, but it is not clear that aerosolized bronchodilators were effectively delivered in the sham group.[18] Nonetheless, these data support a trial of noninvasive ventilation in asthmatics responding poorly to initial bronchodilator therapy. Noninvasive ventilation can be combined with continuous nebulization and heliox, although the added value of these latter therapies has not been established in controlled trials.

Cystic Fibrosis

Uncontrolled studies indicate that noninvasive ventilation is useful to stabilize gas exchange in the treatment of acute episodes of respiratory failure in end-stage cystic fibrosis patients and can serve as a bridge to transplantation.[19]

Upper Airway Obstruction

Anecdotally, noninvasive ventilation can be used to treat patients with upper airway obstruction such as that caused by glottic edema following extubation. In this situation, noninvasive ventilation can be combined with aerosolized medications or heliox, but no controlled trials have demonstrated the efficacy of this approach. If therapy with noninvasive ventilation is considered, patients should be selected with great caution and monitored closely, because upper airway obstruction can lead to precipitous deterioration. The use of noninvasive ventilation in patients with tight, fixed upper airway obstruction is inappropriate, because it delays the institution of definitive therapy.

HYPOXEMIC RESPIRATORY FAILURE

Hypoxemic respiratory failure is defined as severe hypoxemia (arterial oxygen partial pressure–inspired oxygen fraction ratio <200), combined with a respiratory rate greater than 35 breaths per minute and a non-COPD diagnosis, including acute pneumonia, acute lung injury, acute respiratory distress syndrome (ARDS), pulmonary edema, or trauma.

TABLE 68–1. INDICATIONS FOR THE USE OF NONINVASIVE VENTILATION IN THE ACUTE CARE SETTING

Airway Obstruction

COPD (A)*
Asthma (B)
Cystic fibrosis (C)
Obstructive sleep apnea or obesity hypoventilation (C)
Upper airway obstruction (C)
Facilitation of weaning in COPD (A)
Extubation failure in COPD (C)

Hypoxemic Respiratory Failure

ARDS (C)
Pneumonia (C)
Trauma or burns (C)
Acute pulmonary edema (use of CPAP) (A)
Immunocompromised patients (A)
Restrictive thoracic disorders (C)
Postoperative patients (B)
Do-not-intubate patients (C)
During bronchoscopy (C)

---

*Letters in parentheses indicate the level of evidence supporting the use of noninvasive ventilation: A, multiple randomized, controlled trials—recommended; B, at least one randomized, controlled trial—weaker recommendation; C, case series or reports—can be tried, but with close monitoring.
ARDS, acute respiratory distress syndrome; COPD, chronic obstructive pulmonary disease; CPAP, continuous positive airway pressure.

Controlled trials of noninvasive ventilation to treat patients with acute hypoxemic respiratory failure have shown statistically significant reductions in the rate of intubation, length of hospital stay, and incidence of infectious complications, and a trend toward lower mortality.[6,20] However, because of the heterogeneity of causes, these studies fail to demonstrate that all patient subgroups with hypoxemic respiratory failure benefit equally from noninvasive ventilation. Further, when patients are stratified according to acuity of illness, patients with a simplified acute physiologic score (SAPS II) less than 35 fare considerably better with noninvasive ventilation than do those with higher scores.[21] Thus, the selection of patients with less severe disease is likely to enhance the success of noninvasive ventilation in treating hypoxemic respiratory failure, and studies that examine individual subgroups within the larger category are likely to be more useful clinically.

Pneumonia

One controlled trial showed that noninvasive ventilation in patients with severe community-acquired pneumonia lowers the rate of endotracheal intubation and shortens the length of ICU stay compared with conventional therapy; however, a subgroup analysis revealed that the benefits occurred only in patients with underlying COPD.[22] No benefit was apparent in the non-COPD patients with severe pneumonia. A subsequent uncontrolled trial in non-COPD patients with severe pneumonia found that two thirds of such patients treated with noninvasive ventilation eventually required intubation.[23] Although the latter authors deemed a trial of noninvasive ventilation in non-COPD patients with severe pneumonia to be a reasonable approach, controlled data to support such a recommendation are currently lacking.

Immunocompromised States

The dismal prognosis of invasively ventilated immunocompromised patients makes noninvasive ventilation an appealing ventilatory mode, with its demonstrated ability to decrease the rate of nosocomial infection.[7] In a study of 51 patients undergoing solid organ transplantation who developed acute hypoxemic respiratory failure within 3 weeks, noninvasive ventilation reduced the rate of intubation, frequency of invasive procedures, rate of nosocomial infection, duration of ICU stay, and ICU mortality (but not hospital mortality) compared with conventional therapy.[24] In a subsequent randomized trial of neutropenic patients with pulmonary infiltrates and acute hypoxemic respiratory failure (most of whom had hematologic malignancies), noninvasive ventilation lowered the intubation rate, occurrence of nosocomial infections, and ICU and hospital mortality rates (the latter from 80% to 46%).[25] More recently, noninvasive ventilation has been reported to yield similar benefits in acquired immunodeficiency syndrome (AIDS) patients with *Pneumocystis carinii* pneumonia versus invasive mechanical ventilation in physiologically and demographically matched patients.[26] Thus, whenever possible, noninvasive ventilation should be tried first in immunocompromised patients with hypoxemic respiratory failure because of the potential to avoid the high morbidity and mortality rates associated with invasive mechanical ventilation in these patients.

Acute Respiratory Distress Syndrome

A small retrospective study reported that noninvasive ventilation averted intubation in 50% of patients during the early phase of acute lung injury or ARDS.[27] However, for ARDS patients with severe oxygenation defects and multiple organ system dysfunction, invasive ventilation remains the preferred modality. Noninvasive ventilation may be considered in ARDS patients with relatively mild oxygenation defects (P/F >100), stable hemodynamics, and no other organ involvement, but such patients must be monitored closely to avoid any delay in intubation if deterioration occurs.

Acute Cardiogenic Pulmonary Edema

A meta-analysis of randomized, controlled trials demonstrated that compared with oxygen therapy, CPAP (though not a true mode of ventilatory support) is highly effective at relieving respiratory distress, improving gas exchange, and averting intubation when used to treat patients with acute cardiogenic edema.[28] Inspiratory assistance combined with expiratory pressure can reduce the work of breathing and alleviate respiratory distress more effectively than CPAP alone, and several uncontrolled trials and two controlled trials found that noninvasive ventilation and CPAP are equally effective in improving vital signs and avoiding intubation. One controlled trial demonstrated that noninvasive ventilation lowers arterial carbon dioxide partial pressure ($PaCO_2$) and respiratory rate and improves oxygenation more rapidly than CPAP alone, but the noninvasive ventilation group had an increased rate of myocardial infarction, leading to premature termination of the study.[29] This was a small study, and there were concerns about adequate randomization. A recent preliminary report by the same group using a different "bilevel" ventilator at lower pressures (inspiratory positive airway pressure, 12 cm H_2O; expiratory positive airway pressure, 4 cm H_2O) for delivering noninvasive ventilation showed more rapid improvement in oxygenation and no increased risk of myocardial infarction when compared with CPAP alone.[30] The current recommendation is to use CPAP alone or noninvasive ventilation as initial therapy; if CPAP is used initially, inspiratory pressure support should be added if the patient has persistent hypercapnea or dyspnea.[31]

Postoperative Respiratory Failure

Noninvasive ventilation has been studied in postoperative patients who develop respiratory failure after various kinds of surgery. It reduces extravascular lung water and improves lung mechanics and gas exchange after coronary artery bypass surgery.[32] Controlled trials showed that noninvasive ventilation improves oxygenation, reduces the need for re-intubation, and lowers the mortality rate after lung resectional surgery[33,34] and enhances pulmonary function after gastroplasty.[35] Thus, noninvasive ventilation should be used in selected postoperative patients with respiratory failure, especially in the setting of underlying COPD or pulmonary edema.

Trauma and Burns

Trauma patients develop respiratory failure for a multitude of reasons, but some have chest wall injuries such as flail chest or mild acute lung injury that might respond favorably to noninvasive ventilation. In a retrospective survey of 46 trauma patients with respiratory insufficiency that had been treated with noninvasive ventilation, Beltrame and coworkers found rapid improvements in gas exchange and a 72% success rate; however, patients with burns responded poorly.[36] Despite these promising results, the uncontrolled design of the study limits the ability to draw conclusions or to make recommendations on the use of noninvasive ventilation in trauma patients.

Restrictive Lung Disease

The use of noninvasive ventilation in patients with underlying restrictive disease and acute deterioration of respiratory status has not been studied extensively because they constitute only a small portion of patients admitted to acute care hospitals. Patients with restriction related to an underlying neuromuscular disease and superimposed acute respiratory failure may benefit from a trial of noninvasive ventilation. Small case series have reported that using noninvasive ventilation in patients with myasthenic crises may avoid intubation.[37] In contrast, patients with end-stage pulmonary fibrosis in respiratory extremis have been reported to do poorly with mechanical ventilation.[38]

Do-Not-Intubate Patients

Although controversial, noninvasive ventilation may be a useful tool in patients with acute respiratory failure who do not wish to be intubated. There are several reports of good outcomes (>50% survival to discharge) with noninvasive ventilation in this subset of patients, especially those with COPD and congestive heart failure.[39] Noninvasive ventilation may also reduce dyspnea, preserve patient autonomy, and provide time for finalization of affairs for some terminal patients.[40] However, there is concern that this may merely prolong the dying process, and patients and their families must be informed that noninvasive ventilation is being used as a form of life support in this setting and should be given the option to refuse it.

Facilitation of Weaning and Extubation

Patients who require invasive mechanical ventilation initially and fail to wean promptly are potential candidates for noninvasive ventilation to facilitate extubation, thus reducing the complications related to prolonged intubation. Several randomized, controlled trials have demonstrated that noninvasive ventilation significantly shortens the duration of invasive mechanical ventilation, reduces the length of ICU stay, and improves survival compared with patients weaned in the routine fashion.[41-43] Another potential application of noninvasive ventilation in the weaning process is to avoid reintubation in patients with extubation failure, a complication of invasive mechanical ventilation associated with a high mortality rate. Earlier studies looking at the role of noninvasive ventilation in this situation showed promise, but more recent randomized studies failed to show improved outcomes.[44] One preliminary study even found that noninvasive ventilation may delay needed intubation in this setting, resulting in an increased mortality rate.[45] Thus, although the use of noninvasive ventilation to facilitate weaning and extubation appears to benefit patients with COPD, its overzealous application could lead to increased extubation failure rates and other adverse consequences.

Bronchoscopy

Both CPAP and noninvasive ventilation have been studied as ways of supporting oxygenation and ventilation during bronchoscopy. Using a specially designed open CPAP system during bronchoscopy in patients with marginal oxygenation, Maitre and colleagues observed maintenance of adequate gas exchange and avoidance of respiratory failure.[46] In a controlled trial, Antonelli and associates demonstrated equivalent oxygenation and complication rates in patients undergoing bronchoscopy and supported with either noninvasive or invasive mechanical ventilation.[47] Thus, noninvasive ventilation is an effective way of providing ventilatory support in patients undergoing bronchoscopy.[48]

PRACTICAL APPLICATION

PATIENT SELECTION

Noninvasive ventilation should be viewed as a "crutch" that assists patients through a period of acute respiratory failure while reversible factors are being treated, helping them avoid invasive mechanical ventilation and its attendant complications. To optimize the chance of success, noninvasive ventilation should be used early, when patients first develop signs of incipient respiratory failure. In addition, predictors of success are useful in identifying patients most likely to benefit (Table 68-2). The selection process might be viewed as taking advantage of a "window of opportunity": the window opens when the patient first needs ventilatory assistance and closes when the patient becomes too unstable.

Based on the predictors of success and criteria used in prior controlled trials, we recommend the following two-step selection process. The first step is to identify patients in need of ventilatory assistance by using clinical and blood gas criteria. Patients with mild respiratory distress and no more than mild gas exchange derangement are likely to do well without ventilatory assistance and should not be considered. Good candidates are those with moderate to severe dyspnea, tachypnea, and impending respiratory muscle fatigue, as indicated by the use of accessory muscles of breathing or abdominal paradox. The level of tachypnea used as a criterion depends on the underlying diagnosis. Those with COPD are considered candidates for noninvasive ventilation when the respiratory rate exceeds 24 breaths per minute; with hypoxemic respiratory failure, higher respiratory rates are used, in the range of 30 to 35 breaths per minute. The second step is to exclude patients for whom noninvasive ventilation would be unsafe. Those with frank or imminent respiratory arrest should be promptly intubated, because the successful initiation of noninvasive ventilation requires some time for adaptation. Patients who are medically unstable with hypotensive shock, uncontrolled upper gastrointestinal bleeding, unstable arrhythmias, or life-threatening ischemia are better managed with invasive mechanical ventilation. Additionally, noninvasive ventilation should not be used for patients who are uncooperative, unable to adequately protect their upper airway or clear

TABLE 68–2. PREDICTORS OF NONINVASIVE VENTILATION SUCCESS IN PATIENTS WITH ACUTE RESPIRATORY FAILURE

Lower acuity of illness (Acute Physiology and Chronic Health Evaluation [APACHE] score)
Ability to cooperate; better neurologic score
Ability to coordinate breathing with ventilator
Less air leakage; intact dentition
Hypercarbia, but not too severe ($PaCO_2$ between 45 and 92 mm Hg)
Acidemia, but not too severe (pH between 7.1 and 7.35)
Improvements in gas exchange and heart and respiratory rates within first 2 h

secretions, or intolerant of masks, or for recipients of recent upper gastrointestinal or airway surgery.

INITIATION OF NONINVASIVE VENTILATION

Once an appropriate candidate for noninvasive ventilation has been selected, a ventilator and interface must be chosen, initial settings must be selected, and the patient must be monitored closely in an appropriate location until stabilized. The roles of physicians, respiratory therapists, and nurses are of paramount importance in explaining the process to and gaining the confidence of the patient. Noninvasive ventilation can be initiated wherever the patient presents with acute respiratory distress, but he or she should be transferred to an ICU or step-down unit that offers adequate continuous monitoring until stabilized. During transfer, ventilatory assistance and monitoring should be continued.

VENTILATOR SELECTION

Selection of a ventilator is based largely on availability, practitioner experience, and patient comfort. Pressure-limited modes, including pressure support and pressure control, are available on most critical care ventilators. Pressure control ventilation delivers time-cycled, preset inspiratory and expiratory pressures, with adjustable inspiratory-expiratory ratios, at a controlled rate. Most such modes also permit patient triggering and selection of a backup rate. PSV delivers preset inspiratory and expiratory pressures to assist spontaneous breathing efforts. Nomenclature and the specific characteristics of these modes may differ among ventilators, and this must be taken into account to avoid errors. For example, with some ventilators, pressure support is the amount of inspiratory assistance added to the preset expiratory pressure. Others require independent selection of inspiratory and expiratory positive airway pressures, with the difference between the two determining the level of pressure support.

PSV is a flow-triggered and -cycled mode, and the patient's effort determines tidal volume and duration of inspiration. Thus, pressure support modes have the potential to match breathing pattern quite closely, and they have been rated by patients as more comfortable for noninvasive ventilation than volume-limited ventilation.[49] However, leaks during noninvasive ventilation can interfere with the detection of reduced inspiratory flow at the termination of inspiration, causing expiratory asynchrony. Noninvasive pressure-limited modes of ventilation are usually administered using either standard critical care ventilators or portable bilevel ventilators. Most bilevel devices have limited pressure-generating capability (≤ 30 cm H_2O) and lack oxygen blenders or sophisticated alarm or battery backup systems, precluding their use in patients who require high oxygen concentrations or inflation pressures. Newer versions are more appropriate for the acute setting, being equipped with sophisticated alarm and monitoring capabilities, graphic displays, and oxygen blenders. These devices are capable of enhancing synchrony by offering ways to limit inspiratory duration and an adjustable "rise time"—the time to reach the targeted inspiratory pressure. If desired, volume-limited ventilation can be delivered using critical care ventilators, but a higher tidal volume than that commonly used for invasive mechanical ventilation is recommended to compensate for air leakage.

Initial ventilator pressure settings are usually low to facilitate patient acceptance, but they can be set higher if necessary to alleviate respiratory distress. Typical starting pressures are an inspiratory positive airway pressure of 10 to 12 cm H_2O and a PEEP (or expiratory positive airway pressure) of 4 to 5 cm H_2O. For volume ventilation, initial tidal volumes range from 10 to 15 mL/kg. The ventilator is set in a spontaneously triggered mode, with or without a backup rate. Pressures commonly used to deliver CPAP in patients with acute respiratory distress range from 5 to 12.5 cm H_2O. CPAP can be applied using compressed air with a regulator system, blower-based CPAP devices, bilevel devices, or critical care ventilators.

INTERFACES

The major difference between invasive and noninvasive ventilation is that with the latter, pressurized gas is delivered to the airway via a mask rather than via an invasive conduit. The open breathing circuit of noninvasive ventilation permits air leaks around the mask or through the mouth, rendering the success of noninvasive ventilation dependent on ventilators designed to deal effectively with air leaks and to optimize patient comfort and acceptance. Interfaces—the devices that connect the ventilator tubing to the nose, mouth, or both—enable pressurized gas to enter the upper airway during noninvasive ventilation. Commonly used interfaces in the acute setting include nasal masks and full face (or oronasal) masks.

Nasal masks are widely used for the administration of CPAP or noninvasive ventilation, particularly for chronic applications. Nasal masks are usually better tolerated than full face masks for long-term applications, because they cause less claustrophobia and discomfort and allow eating, conversation, and expectoration. The standard nasal mask is a triangular or cone-shaped clear plastic device that fits over the nose and uses a soft cuff that forms an air seal over the skin. The mask exerts pressure over the nasal bridge, often causing skin irritation and redness and occasionally ulceration. Many modifications are available to avoid complications, such as the use of forehead spacers or masks with ultrathin silicon seals or heat-sensitive gels that minimize skin trauma.

Full facemasks cover both the nose and the mouth (Fig. 68-3) and are preferable to nasal masks in the acute setting. The efficacy of both nasal and oronasal masks in lowering $PaCO_2$ and avoiding intubation is similar in the acute setting, but in a recent randomized, controlled trial,[50] patients tolerated the full facemask better because of reduced air leakage through the mouth. Recently, a "total" facemask has become available; it seals around the perimeter of the face and resembles a hockey goalie's mask. Made of optical-grade plastic, it is easy to apply and causes no more claustrophobia than standard facemasks. Mouthpieces are seldom used to administer noninvasive ventilation in the acute setting but are occasionally used during initiation, when the patient holds the mouthpiece in place to adapt to the sensation of positive-pressure ventilation.

Selection of a comfortable mask that fits properly is key to the success of noninvasive ventilation. The full facemask should be tried first in the acute setting, and if possible, the patient should be allowed to hold the mask in place initially. The mask straps are then tightened with the least tension necessary to avoid excessive air leakage. Some leaking is acceptable and is even obligatory with bilevel ventilators, because of the need to flush carbon dioxide from the single-channel ventilator circuit. Bilevel ventilators compensate for air leakage better than critical care ventilators do, but

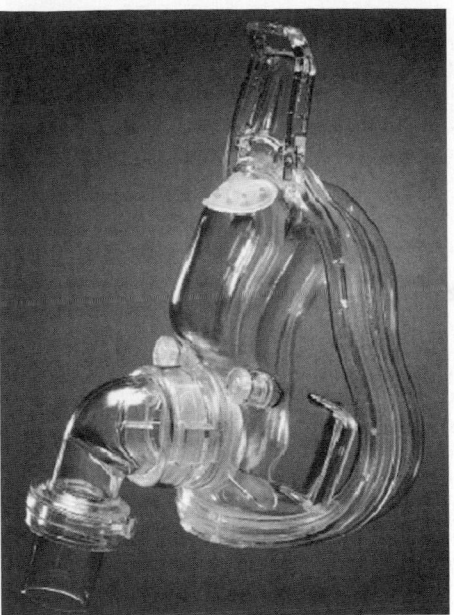

FIGURE 68–3. Full facemask with a soft silicon seal to minimize pressure on the nasal bridge. A disposable version of this mask is widely used in the acute care setting.

Location
    Critical care or step-down unit
    Medical or surgical ward if able to breathe unassisted
    for >20-30 min
"Eyeball" test
    Dyspnea
    Comfort (mask, air pressure)
    Anxiety
    Asynchrony
    Leaks
Vital signs
    Respiratory and heart rates
    Blood pressure
    Continuous electrocardiography
Gas exchange
    Continuous oximetry
    Arterial blood gases (baseline, after 1-2 h, and as clinically indicated)

excessive air leakage can lead to noninvasive ventilation failure with any ventilator.

Head straps hold the mask in place and are important for patient comfort. Straps attach at two to five points, depending on the type of mask. More points of attachment add to stability.

OXYGENATION AND HUMIDIFICATION

Oxygen is titrated to achieve a desired oxygen saturation, usually greater than 90% to 92%, either by using oxygen blenders on critical care and some bilevel ventilators or by adjusting liter flow (up to 15 L/min, as per manufacturer's recommendations), delivered via oxygen tubing connected directly to the mask or ventilator circuit. Bilevel ventilators have limited oxygenation capabilities (maximal inspired oxygen fraction, 0.45 to 0.5), so ventilators with oxygen blenders should be used for patients with hypoxemic respiratory failure. A heated humidifier should be used to prevent drying of the nasal passage and oropharynx when the duration of application is anticipated to be more than a few hours.

MONITORING

Once noninvasive ventilation is initiated, patients should be closely monitored in a critical care unit or a step-down unit until they are sufficiently stable to be moved to a regular medical floor. The aim of monitoring is to determine whether the main goals are being achieved, including relief of symptoms, reduced work of breathing, improved or stable gas exchange, good patient-ventilator synchrony, and patient comfort (Table 68-3). A drop in the respiratory rate with improved oxygen saturation or improving pH with a lower $PaCO_2$ within the first 1 to 2 hours portends a successful outcome.[51] Abdominal paradox, if present initially, subsides,

and the heart rate usually falls. The absence of these propitious signs indicates a poor response to noninvasive ventilation and the need to make further adjustments. Leaks should be sought and corrected, patient-ventilator synchrony should be optimized, and pressures may have to be adjusted upward to relieve respiratory distress and achieve a reduction in $PaCO_2$. If these adjustments fail to improve the response within a few hours, noninvasive ventilation should be considered a failure, and the patient should be promptly intubated if it is still clinically indicated. Excessive delay in intubation may precipitate a respiratory crisis and add to morbidity and mortality.

ADVERSE EFFECTS AND COMPLICATIONS

When applied by experienced caregivers to appropriately selected patients, noninvasive ventilation is usually well tolerated and is associated with minimal complications. The most frequent adverse effects and complications are related to the mask, ventilator airflow or pressure, patient-ventilator interaction, or airway secretions.

Common adverse effects related to the mask include discomfort and erythema or skin ulcers, usually on the nasal bridge, related to pressure from the mask seal. Proper fitting and attachment, consistent use of artificial skin over the nose, and newer masks with softer silicone seals help minimize these problems. Adverse effects related to airflow or pressure include conjunctival irritation caused by air leakage under the mask into the eyes and sinus, or ear pain related to excessive pressure. Refitting the mask or lowering inspiratory pressure may ameliorate these problems. Nasal or oral dryness caused by high airflow is usually indicative of air leaking through the mouth. Measures to minimize leakage may be useful, but nasal saline or emollients and heated humidifiers are often necessary to relieve these complaints. Nasal congestion and discharge are also frequent complaints and can be treated with topical decongestants or steroids and oral antihistamine-decongestant combinations. Gastric insufflation occurs commonly, may respond to simethicone, and is usually tolerated.

Patient-ventilator asynchrony is a common occurrence during noninvasive ventilation. Failure to adequately synchronize compromises the ventilator's ability to reduce the work of breathing and may contribute to noninvasive ventilation failure. The asynchrony may be related to patient agitation, which can be treated with the judicious use of sedatives. Failure to synchronize can also result from inadequate ventilator triggering or inability to sense the onset of patient expiration because of air leakage. This can be corrected by minimizing air leaks and by using ventilator modes that permit limitation of maximal inspiratory duration. Even with the best efforts to optimize settings and comfort, a minority of patients still fail. This may be partly due to progression of the underlying disease process or the patient's inability to tolerate noninvasive ventilation, but every effort should be made to ascertain that it is not due to technologic problems that could be corrected by mask or ventilator adjustments. Once again, intubation should not be delayed if improvement is not apparent within a few hours.

ANNOTATED REFERENCES

Antonelli M, Conti G, Rocco M, et al: A comparison of noninvasive positive-pressure ventilation and conventional mechanical ventilation in patients with acute respiratory failure. N Engl J Med 1998;329:429-435.

A prospective, randomized study comparing noninvasive positive-pressure ventilation delivered through a facemask with conventional endotracheal intubation and mechanical ventilation in patients with acute respiratory failure. Noninvasive ventilation was as effective as conventional ventilation in improving gas exchange and was associated with fewer serious complications and shorter stays in the ICU.

Brochard L, Isabey D, Piquet J, et al: Reversal of acute exacerbations of chronic obstructive lung disease by inspiratory assistance with a face mask. N Engl J Med 1990;323:1523-1530.

An early landmark study looking at the ability of noninvasive ventilation to provide inspiratory pressure support by means of a facemask in COPD exacerbations. Based on a comparison with historical controls, noninvasive ventilation shortened the duration of mechanical ventilation and ICU stay.

Girou E, Schortgen F, Delclaux C, et al: Association of noninvasive ventilation with nosocomial infections and survival in critically ill patients. JAMA 2000;284:2361-2367.

In this matched case-control study in patients with acute exacerbations of COPD or hypercapnic cardiogenic pulmonary edema, noninvasive ventilation was associated with a lower risk of nosocomial infection, less antibiotic use, shorter length of ICU stay, and lower mortality compared with invasive mechanical ventilation.

Hilbert G, Gruson D, Vargas F, et al: Noninvasive ventilation in immunosuppressed patients with pulmonary infiltrates, fever, and acute respiratory failure. N Engl J Med 2001;349:481-487.

This study shows that in 52 selected immunosuppressed patients with pneumonitis and acute respiratory failure, early initiation of intermittent noninvasive ventilation significantly reduced the rates of endotracheal intubation and serious complications and improved the likelihood of survival to hospital discharge.

Nava S, Ambrosino N, Clini E, et al: Noninvasive mechanical ventilation in the weaning of patients with respiratory failure due to chronic obstructive pulmonary disease: A randomized, controlled trial. Ann Intern Med 1998;128:721-728.

A multicenter, randomized trial to determine whether noninvasive ventilation improves the outcome of weaning from invasive mechanical ventilation when used to achieve early extubation in patients failing a T-piece trial after 48 hours of invasive ventilation. Patients extubated to noninvasive ventilation had higher 30-day weaning rates, shorter lengths of stay in the ICU, a trend toward decreased nosocomial pneumonia rates, and improved survival at 60 days.

Chapter 69

HIGH-FREQUENCY VENTILATION

Jeffrey M. Singh • Thomas E. Stewart

KEY POINTS

1. **High-frequency ventilation** is a method of mechanical ventilation that uses very small tidal volumes at high frequencies. The most commonly used modes include high-frequency jet ventilation and high-frequency oscillatory ventilation.

2. **Ventilator-induced lung injury** can be a clinically important consequence of mechanical ventilation in patients with respiratory failure, particularly those with underlying acute lung injury. **Volutrauma** from high transpulmonary pressures, **atelectrauma**, and **oxygen toxicity** may all contribute to lung injury, and mechanical ventilation strategies should attempt to mitigate these injurious forces.

3. Despite the recent **clinical success of conventional lung-protective ventilation strategies**, they do not completely prevent lung injury and may be associated with other clinical problems and sequelae, particularly respiratory acidosis.

4. Experimental models suggest that **high-frequency ventilation may mitigate ventilator-induced lung injury.**

5. **In pediatric patients with respiratory distress syndrome, high-frequency oscillatory ventilation is safe and effective** and may be slightly more beneficial than conventional mechanical ventilation when patient selection and clinical conditions are stringently controlled.

6. **In adults, high-frequency oscillatory ventilation has been shown to be safe and effective as salvage therapy** for patients with hypoxic respiratory failure deemed to be failing conventional mechanical ventilation.

7. Despite recent clinical validation of high-frequency ventilation in adults with respiratory distress, **significant research remains to be done to determine the best application of high-frequency ventilation modes**, particularly optimal settings, timing of initiation, and weaning from high-frequency ventilators to conventional ventilators.

High-frequency ventilation is a mode of mechanical ventilation in which small tidal volumes are delivered at high supraphysiologic frequencies. Various types of high-frequency ventilation have been developed over the last 3 decades, including high-frequency positive-pressure ventilation, high-frequency percussive ventilation, high-frequency jet ventilation, and high-frequency oscillatory ventilation. Initially, high-frequency ventilation was mainly of academic interest, with a limited role in rescue and neonatal therapy, but there has recently been renewed enthusiasm for its use as part of a lung-protective ventilation strategy for adult and pediatric patients with acute lung injury and acute respiratory distress syndrome (ARDS).

Over the last 20 years, our understanding of the potential harm of mechanical ventilation has evolved, especially in the case of an injured lung in which normal function is disturbed. Lung damage may occur through injurious mechanical forces generated during mechanical ventilation. This lung injury may contribute to increased systemic inflammation, possibly leading to multiple organ dysfunction and increased morbidity and mortality. Lung-protective mechanical ventilation strategies now aim to reduce these injurious forces and subsequent lung damage while providing adequate ventilation and oxygenation. The mechanics of high-frequency ventilation make it particularly well suited to protecting the lung, and there is growing clinical experience with the use of high-frequency ventilation as an alternative to conventional mechanical ventilation or as salvage therapy in patients failing conventional ventilation strategies.

DESCRIPTION AND CLASSIFICATION

Modes of high-frequency ventilation are characterized by high respiratory rates and lower tidal volumes than those used in conventional mechanical ventilation. Often, the tidal volume is less than anatomic deadspace, and gas exchange is maintained by increasing the respiratory rate to supra-physiologic frequencies. Gas exchange under these conditions may occur through a number of proposed contributory mechanisms (see Mechanisms of Gas Transport). High-frequency positive-pressure ventilation, high-frequency percussive ventilation, high-frequency jet ventilation and high-frequency oscillatory ventilation are described briefly here.

High-Frequency Positive-Pressure Ventilation. High-frequency positive-pressure ventilation delivers small volumes (approximately 3 to 4 mL/kg) of conditioned gas at high frequencies (60 to 100 breaths/min) using a conventional mechanical ventilator. Valves in the inspiratory and expiratory limbs of the ventilator circuit allow control of the inspiratory flow rate (which is generally high) and positive end-expiratory pressure (PEEP), respectively. Expiration is passive and relies on the elastic recoil of the patient's respiratory system. The clinician controls the respiratory rate, inspiratory flow rate, diving pressure, and PEEP. Because high respiratory rates leave little time for passive expiration, there is a risk of gas trapping, with hyperinflation and resultant overdistention injury.

High-Frequency Percussive Ventilation. High-frequency percussive ventilation is a hybrid that attempts to combine the principles of high-frequency and conventional ventilation using a proprietary mechanical ventilator.[1] A conventional ventilation circuit is fitted with a gas-driven piston at the end of the endotracheal tube. The reciprocating piston generates pressure oscillations at 3 to 15 Hz with short expiratory times, which are superimposed on the conventional inspiratory-expiratory pressure waves. The high-frequency beats are delivered in bursts to generate auto-PEEP through breath stacking, then stopped to allow alveolar pressure to fall back to baseline. It has been hypothesized that the auto-PEEP generated may improve alveolar recruitment without exposing the alveoli to the high peak airway pressures that would be generated with comparable conventional mechanical ventilation. The high-frequency percussion also provides some internal mucokinesis, improving pulmonary toilet and reducing endotracheal suctioning requirements. Although the high-frequency pressure oscillations are driven actively in both directions, the bulk of exhalation from the underlying conventional mechanical ventilation breaths is passive. Clinicians have control of all aspects of these underlying breaths, as well as the frequency and pressure of the high-frequency beats.

High-Frequency Jet Ventilation. High-frequency jet ventilation employs a small-aperture nozzle to direct a high-pressure stream of gas into the lung (Fig. 69-1). Flow of gas through the nozzle is controlled by a solenoid valve, allowing control of frequency and inspiratory time. During inspiration, a high-pressure jet streams into the proximal airways,

entraining air from the circuit. Tidal volumes are largely dependent on the momentum of the jet and the entrainment of gas from the surrounding circuit. Expiration is passive, relying on respiratory system recoil. PEEP is determined by changing the flow of fresh gas through the circuit and the resistance to flow through the expiratory limb. The small size of the injector nozzle (2 to 3 mm) allows it to be placed in the endotracheal tube or proximal trachea, which not only decreases deadspace but also allows better visualization and access during surgical procedures involving the upper airway.

The clinician has control over frequency, inspiratory time, jet drive pressure, and mean airway pressure applied through the ventilator circuit. Larger tidal volumes can be delivered by increasing jet drive pressure and inspiratory time. Larger jet catheters and endotracheal tubes also augment tidal volume by increasing jet flow and gas entrainment, respectively. Because expiration is passive, gas trapping with intrinsic PEEP may occur at high frequencies when expiration is limited by progressively shorter expiratory times.

Complications specific to high-frequency jet ventilation include traumatic upper airway injury. The high-velocity inspiratory jet may cause direct trauma to the proximal airways, and necrotizing tracheobronchitis is a well-established complication of high-frequency jet ventilation in both infants and adults.[2,3] Gas conditioning in high-frequency jet ventilation, particularly humidification and warming, is also problematic. Although the gas entrained from the proximal circuit is warmed and humidified, the gas projecting from the jet nozzle expands and cools, compromising the overall conditioning of the inspired gas. It has also been hypothesized that high gas flow rates and rapid increases in lung volume could cause lung injury through the generation of shear forces at the interface of adjacent compliant and atelectatic lung units.

High-Frequency Oscillatory Ventilation. In high-frequency oscillatory ventilation, an oscillating diaphragm creates pressure waves in the ventilator circuit (Fig. 69-2). Because the diaphragm is actively driven in both directions, the ventilator creates both inspiratory and expiratory pressure waves, meaning that expiration is active. This distinguishes high-frequency oscillatory ventilation from other forms of high-frequency ventilation, in which expiration is passive and dependent on the elastic recoil of the respiratory system. Active expiration may be advantageous in controlling lung volumes and preventing hyperinflation. Although all modes of high-frequency ventilation may generate some degree of auto-PEEP, which may be beneficial in increasing alveolar recruitment, high levels of auto-PEEP can cause hyperinflation and lung injury. High-frequency oscillatory ventilation has been shown to be associated with less gas trapping than other forms of high-frequency ventilation.[4] Mean airway pressure is determined by adjusting the resistance to the flow of fresh gas (bias flow) across the circuit.

Clinicians set the bias flow rate, mean airway pressure, frequency, inspiratory-expiratory ratio, and energy applied to the oscillating diaphragm. The generation of pressure oscillations is controlled in part by the frequency and the energy applied to the moving diaphragm (power). The excursion of the diaphragm (and presumably the delivered tidal volume) is inversely related to the frequency. High frequencies result in a short inspiratory period that limits the time during which the diaphragm can move. This can be overcome in part by increasing power, which increases its excursion at a given frequency.

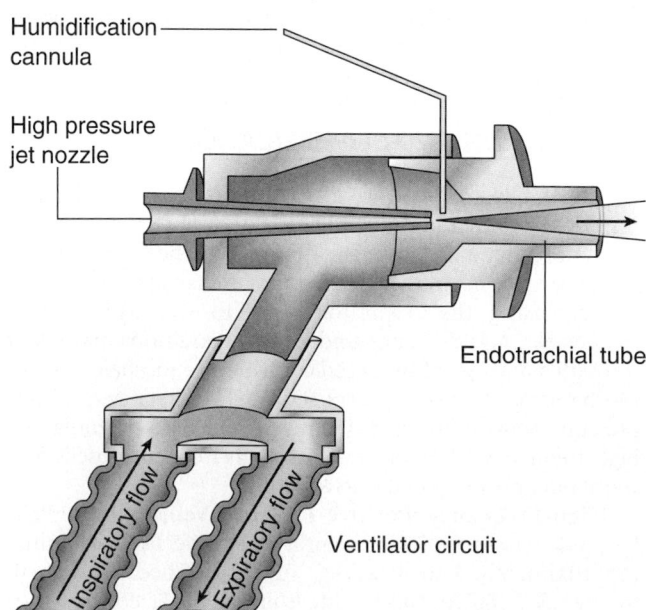

Humidification cannula

High pressure jet nozzle

Endotrachial tube

Inspiratory flow

Expiratory flow

Ventilator circuit

FIGURE 69–1. Typical high-pressure jet cannula and humidification system used in high-frequency jet ventilation. Note that the gas jet is directed down the endotracheal tube, entraining gas from the proximal ventilator circuit.

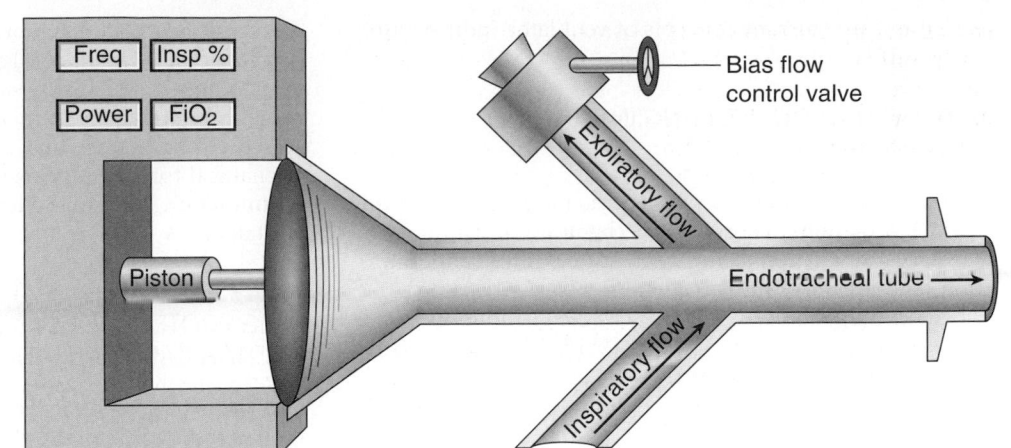

FIGURE 69–2. Schematic of high-frequency oscillatory ventilator. A computer allows precise control over the piston driving the oscillating diaphragm. Adjustment of the bias flow of conditioned gas allows control of mean airway pressure.

MECHANISMS OF GAS TRANSPORT

During conventional mechanical ventilation, when tidal volumes are larger than anatomic deadspace, gas exchange is largely related to bulk flow of gas to the alveoli. High-frequency ventilation is thought to generate tidal volumes smaller than anatomic deadspace, and adequate ventilation under these conditions must rely on alternative gas exchange mechanisms. A number of proposed mechanisms may contribute to gas transport during high-frequency ventilation.[5]

When tidal volume approximates anatomic deadspace, the leading edge of the gas front may actually reach a number of proximal alveoli and thus contribute to some gas exchange through bulk flow.[5] Although it is thought that high-frequency ventilation modes generally generate tidal volumes that are lower than anatomic deadspace, recent experimental data suggest that larger tidal volumes may be generated under some conditions. High-frequency oscillatory ventilation, which is usually considered to have the smallest tidal volumes among high-frequency modes, was found in one animal model to deliver tidal volumes significantly greater than anatomic deadspace when applied using settings similar to those traditionally used in adults (frequency, 3 to 6 Hz; ΔP, 60 to 90 cm H_2O).[6] The in vitro characteristics of pediatric high-frequency oscillatory ventilators have been studied, revealing a tidal volume of 3 to 11 mL.[7] Thus, bulk flow may still contribute to gas exchange during high-frequency ventilation, although to a much lesser degree than during conventional mechanical ventilation.

Pendelluft is a phenomenon of regional gas movement that occurs as a result of heterogeneity in alveolar filling rates. The filling rate of a lung unit is dependent on its time constant (τ), a property related to the product of compliance and resistance.[8] Adjacent lung units with different time constants may fill at different rates during inspiration. Following inspiration, there is redistribution of inspired gas from full, fast-filling units to slower-filling units, augmenting gas exchange.[9]

Convective streaming occurs as a result of the asymmetrical velocity profile of the inspired gas front as it moves through the bronchial tree. When inspired gas flows down the bifurcating bronchial tree, the gas front is skewed, such that inspired gas streams down the inside wall of distal airways. During exhalation, the velocity profile of the gas front is flat across the airway cross section. The asymmetry in gas velocity between the inspiratory and expiratory phases of breathing results in a net streaming of fresh gas down the inside walls of distal airways and of carbon dioxide (CO_2)–laden gas back along the outside walls.[10,11] The asymmetrical streaming of fresh gas down airways creates a radial concentration gradient (augmented diffusion), which may contribute significantly to gas mixing.[12] In addition, the beating heart may enhance gas exchange through agitation of surrounding lung tissue (cardiogenic mixing) in these lung units and molecular diffusion.

The extent to which each of these mechanisms contributes to gas exchange at any one moment in a given patient is unknown and may be of questionable clinical relevance, beyond the fact that adequate gas exchange can be achieved with high-frequency ventilation. Experimental models have shown that CO_2 elimination is a product of the frequency and the square of the tidal volume ($V_{CO_2} \alpha = f \times V_T^2$),[13] suggesting that adequate CO_2 elimination may become problematic as tidal volumes decrease, unless accompanied by proportionately larger increases in frequency. Regardless, clinical experience has demonstrated that adequate gas exchange can be achieved with mechanical ventilation using tidal volumes that are less than anatomic deadspace.

RATIONALE FOR HIGH-FREQUENCY VENTILATION

More than 3 decades after its first description, high-frequency ventilation remains an "alternative" mode of mechanical ventilation, with the exception of a few specialized indications (e.g., airway control during laryngeal surgery, ventilation of patients with bronchopleural fistula). The mechanical characteristics of high-frequency ventilation, however, make it well suited for use in the injured lung. There has recently been a resurgence of interest in high-frequency ventilation, particularly high-frequency oscillatory ventilation, as part of a lung-protective strategy in patients with severe lung injury and ARDS. Appreciation of the potential advantages of high-frequency ventilation, particularly with respect to lung protection, requires an understanding of the mechanics of high-frequency ventilation, the proposed mechanisms of gas exchange in high-frequency ventilation, and current concepts of ventilator-induced lung injury (VILI).

VENTILATOR-INDUCED LUNG INJURY AND LUNG PROTECTION

The last 20 years have witnessed a greater appreciation of the potential lung injury caused by mechanical ventilation itself. Mechanical ventilation using high inspired oxygen concentrations, high pressure, and large volumes is largely accepted as being harmful, but recent research has shed light on the some of the pathogenic mechanisms of VILI. The pathogenesis of VILI is complex and remains incompletely elucidated, although current data support several mechanisms, including volutrauma, atelectrauma, barotrauma, and biotrauma.

Mechanical ventilation with large tidal volumes can overdistend alveoli and result in lung injury. Animal studies suggest that high transpulmonary pressures (with resultant large lung volumes and overdistention), rather than high inflation pressures alone, are the cause of lung injury.[14-16] Supporting evidence shows that animals ventilated with large volumes develop pathologic abnormalities similar to those seen in ARDS, even using negative-pressure ventilators.[14] Mechanical restriction of lung volume in the same animal model mitigates this damage, even when extremely high inflation pressures are applied.[14] This understanding has led to adoption of the term "volutrauma." The exact mechanism by which large volumes cause lung injury is not clear but may be related to alveolar wall stretch, stress failure of the lung ultrastructure, and cellular mechanotransduction leading to the release of inflammatory mediators.[17]

Although high-volume ventilation can be harmful, mechanical ventilation at low end-expiratory volumes can also be injurious. "Atelectrauma" occurs when end-expiratory volume is insufficient to maintain inflation of lung units throughout the respiratory cycle. Under these conditions, lung units collapse at end-expiration, only to be forced open during inspiration. Shear forces generated during this cyclic collapse and re-inflation injure the alveolar walls, contributing to VILI.[18] Similar forces may also be generated at the interface between aerated and atelectatic lung units during the respiratory cycle, stressing the connecting alveolar walls.[19] Further, underlying lung pathology may predispose or exacerbate atelectrauma-type injury. Although cyclic collapse can be tolerated for short periods in healthy lungs,[20] the shear forces are intensified when lung mechanics are altered by surfactant depletion and underlying lung injury.[21]

The end-organ effects of VILI are not isolated to the lung. "Biotrauma" refers to the contribution of VILI to systemic inflammation.[22] Injurious mechanical ventilation is associated with increases in circulating inflammatory mediators, and this increase can be attenuated through the use of mechanical ventilation strategies that avoid these injurious forces.[23] The production of systemic inflammatory mediators may contribute to multiple organ dysfunction and mortality. The potential benefit of reducing biotrauma becomes more obvious when it is noted that the majority of deaths among patients with ARDS are due not to oxygenation failure but to multiple organ failure.

Mechanical ventilation strategies designed to reduce VILI have been termed "lung-protective." The current goals of lung protection are threefold: (1) prevention of overdistention-related lung injury through the reduction of tidal volumes and the avoidance of high transpulmonary pressures; (2) recruitment and maintenance of lung volume (the "open lung" concept), with the goal of preventing cyclic collapse and atelectrauma-type lung injury; and (3) reduction of inspired oxygen fraction requirements, thereby reducing oxygen toxicity.[24] The hope is that the reduction of these injurious mechanical forces will translate into a decrease in systemic inflammation and subsequent end-organ dysfunction and mortality.

SUCCESSES AND LIMITATIONS OF LUNG-PROTECTIVE CONVENTIONAL MECHANICAL VENTILATION

The principles of lung-protective ventilation have been applied successfully in the clinical setting using conventional mechanical ventilation. Approaches to minimize VILI include limiting tidal volumes to prevent volutrauma and using PEEP and recruitment maneuvers to maintain end-expiratory lung volume, thereby preventing cyclic collapse. One study evaluating a lung-protective strategy in adults with ARDS demonstrated improved survival at 28 days, although this benefit did not persist to hospital discharge.[25] Although criticized for a high mortality rate in the control arm, this study demonstrated conclusively that changes in ventilatory management can contribute to mortality. In another randomized clinical trial that evaluated a lung-protective strategy based on low tidal volumes and reduced airway pressures, a 9% absolute reduction in mortality was observed.[26] Lung-protective conventional mechanical ventilation is also associated with lower levels of circulating inflammatory mediators, supporting the hypothesis that mitigating the injurious forces during mechanical ventilation may help decrease biotrauma and its contribution to multisystem organ failure.[23,26]

The clinical application of these ventilation protocols, however, is often complicated by impaired ventilation. The use of lower tidal volumes may lead to a decrease in alveolar ventilation that may not be completely offset by increases in respiratory rate. Consequently, clinicians may be forced to accept hypoventilation and respiratory acidosis, so-called permissive hypercapnia, if they wish to maintain low tidal volumes. In addition, even the best possible lung-protective strategy may contribute to the injury of some lung units. Computed tomography studies have demonstrated that lung injury in ARDS is heterogeneous,[27] resulting in local differences in lung mechanics and variable susceptibility to VILI. Relatively healthy lung units may have higher compliance and lower time constants than their more severely injured neighbors, making them more prone to volutrauma-type injury. Conversely, relatively noncompliant lung units may be more prone to atelectrauma-type injury if allowed to collapse at end-expiration. Thus, even when conventional mechanical ventilation is applied with low, lung-protective tidal volumes (4 to 6 mL/kg), patients may still suffer atelectrauma-type injury in diseased, noncompliant lung units while adjacent healthy lung units are injured by overdistention. Further, determining the ideal level of PEEP to prevent end-expiratory collapse may be difficult. One study found that alveolar recruitment occurred progressively over the entire inflation limb of the pressure-volume curve, making reliable identification of the lower inflection point difficult.[28]

Thus, although lung-protective conventional mechanical ventilation has been found to decrease mortality in well-designed clinical trials, it may be possible to further optimize lung protection. Currently, other adjuncts and alternative ventilator modes, including high-frequency ventilation, are under investigation. Finally, despite the best use of conventional mechanical ventilation, some patients fail to be adequately oxygenated and ventilated, and alternative salvage therapies may be needed.

THEORETICAL ADVANTAGES TO HIGH-FREQUENCY VENTILATION

High-frequency ventilation may be well suited to accomplish all the goals of lung protection. By nature of its low tidal volumes, high-frequency ventilation may decrease the risk of overdistention injury, even to relatively healthy, compliant lung units. In addition, because these tidal volumes are delivered using relatively small pressure swings at high rates, mean airway pressure can be maintained at higher levels than are generally used during conventional mechanical ventilation (Fig. 69-3). This high mean airway pressure may optimize end-expiratory lung volume, leading to improved oxygenation and prevention of cyclic collapse and resultant atelectrauma.

The ideal application of high-frequency ventilation might involve "opening" the lung using sustained inflation maneuvers and appropriate levels of PEEP and mean airway pressure, pushing the lung onto the expiratory limb of the pressure-volume curve and optimizing oxygenation and lung compliance (Fig. 69-4). The open lung is then ventilated using small tidal volumes and pressure swings, minimizing alveolar overdistention and collapse throughout the respiratory cycle. In animal models comparing high-frequency oscillatory ventilation to lung-protective conventional mechanical ventilation, such a strategy has been found to decrease pulmonary inflammation and attenuate the increase in systemic inflammatory mediators observed during conventional mechanical ventilation.[29,30]

CLINICAL EXPERIENCE WITH HIGH-FREQUENCY VENTILATION

High-frequency ventilation is largely considered an alternative mode of mechanical ventilation and traditionally has been used only in specialized situations or as salvage therapy when conventional mechanical ventilation fails. Although clinical experience with high-frequency ventilation in pediatric

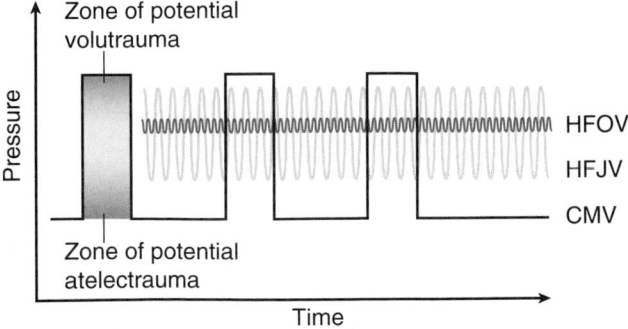

FIGURE 69–3. Comparative pressure-time diagram depicting the pressure-time swings for the most common modes of high-frequency ventilation compared with conventional mechanical ventilation (CMV). HFJV, high-frequency jet ventilation; HFOV, high-frequency oscillatory ventilation.

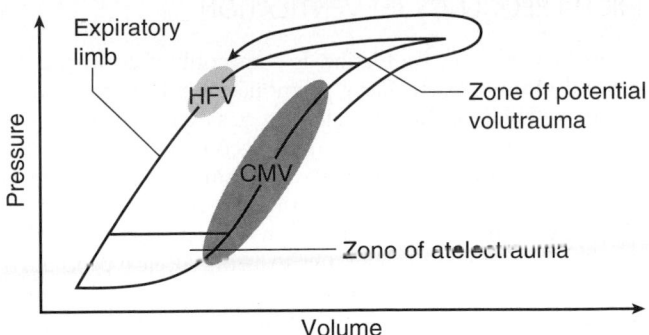

FIGURE 69–4. Pressure-volume curve depicting the "open lung" concept using high-frequency ventilation (HFV). Potential lung injury is reduced when ventilation of the lung is shifted onto the expiratory portion of the curve using aggressive lung recruitment. Lung volume is then maintained using high mean airway pressures and small tidal volumes. CMV, conventional mechanical ventilation.

and neonatal populations is sizable, published experience with high-frequency ventilation modes in adults remains modest, with the largest experience involving high-frequency oscillatory ventilation and high-frequency jet ventilation. There has been renewed interest in the use of high-frequency ventilation in adults, however, as greater understanding of VILI has spurred the search for more lung protective ventilation strategies. This section reviews the existing clinical experience with the various modes of high-frequency ventilation.

HIGH-FREQUENCY POSITIVE-PRESSURE VENTILATION

First described in 1969 as an experimental technique,[31] high-frequency positive-pressure ventilation has found limited clinical use in specialized upper airway surgical procedures and bronchoscopy.[32] Published clinical experience with high-frequency positive-pressure ventilation is largely limited to neonatal populations. One meta-analysis found that synchronized mechanical ventilation delivered as high-frequency positive-pressure ventilation was associated with decreased barotrauma and shorter length of hospital stay compared with conventional mechanical ventilation.[33] The effect of high-frequency positive-pressure ventilation on mortality and chronic oxygen dependency was not clear after analysis of the published studies. In adult patients, high-frequency positive-pressure ventilation has been used only in specialized applications.[34-36]

HIGH-FREQUENCY PERCUSSIVE VENTILATION

The existing literature evaluating high-frequency percussive ventilation in patients with acute respiratory failure is limited to one case series in pediatric patients[37] and several case reports and case series in adults.[38-43] In most of these series, the investigators observed improvements in oxygenation after switching from conventional mechanical ventilation to high-frequency percussive ventilation, without a significant rise in peak or mean airway pressure. These uncontrolled series were small, however, and did not detect differences in mortality or other clinical outcomes.

HIGH-FREQUENCY JET VENTILATION

High-frequency jet ventilation is commonly used in specific clinical settings, particularly pulmonary air leak syndromes, when the ability to achieve adequate gas exchange with lower peak airway pressures may be advantageous.[44] Additionally, the decreased reliance on bulk flow when using high-frequency jet ventilation may improve gas distribution and gas exchange in the presence of large air leaks. High-frequency jet ventilation has also been used intraoperatively during surgical procedures involving the airway and upper trachea; the small tidal volumes minimize movement of the proximal airways, and the small jet catheter and lack of a cuffed endotracheal tube improve visualization of the operative field. High-frequency jet ventilation has also been used in acute respiratory failure in both adults and infants, where it was generally found to improve gas exchange while decreasing peak airway pressures. The published clinical experience with high-frequency jet ventilation in acute respiratory failure remains small compared with that of conventional mechanical ventilation, and to date, the greatest clinical experience is in the neonatal and pediatric populations.

Several studies comparing high-frequency jet ventilation with conventional mechanical ventilation in premature infants with respiratory distress syndrome and pulmonary interstitial emphysema showed that the former is safe and provides improved ventilation at lower peak airway pressures. Although one study demonstrated improved outcomes (decreased incidence of bronchopulmonary dysplasia and home oxygen use at 36 weeks),[45] the majority of studies did not demonstrate a significant advantage of high-frequency jet ventilation over conventional mechanical ventilation with respect to long-term outcome or mortality, despite short-term improvements in gas exchange and respiratory parameters.[46-48] One study evaluating the early use of high-frequency jet ventilation in 73 premature infants found that infants receiving high-frequency jet ventilation were more likely to suffer adverse outcomes (cystic periventricular leukomalacia, intraventricular hemorrhage, death) than were infants receiving conventional mechanical ventilation.[49]

The published experience with high-frequency jet ventilation in adult respiratory failure is limited, although many ICUs have sizable anecdotal experience. Comparative clinical trials have shown that high-frequency jet ventilation is safe and offers improved oxygenation and ventilation compared with conventional mechanical ventilation, while improving respiratory parameters and decreasing required peak pressures.[50-52] None of these trials, however, demonstrated a significant clinical advantage.

HIGH-FREQUENCY OSCILLATORY VENTILATION

High-frequency oscillatory ventilation has recently been the subject of renewed interest for use in acute respiratory failure. It has the potential to achieve all the goals of lung protection; the small, high-frequency pressure oscillations allow the application of high mean airway pressures to optimize lung volume recruitment and prevent end-expiratory collapse, without exposing the lung to injurious peak airway pressures during inflation. In addition, the circuit allows optimal gas conditioning, reducing the likelihood of airway trauma and inspissation of secretions.

The most extensive published clinical evaluation of high-frequency oscillatory ventilation has been in the neonatal and pediatric populations.[53-62] In neonates, the safe and effective application of high-frequency oscillatory ventilation appears to require lung volume recruitment maneuvers and possibly exogenous surfactant. The majority of studies using high-frequency oscillatory ventilation in this manner have demonstrated that it is safe, improves oxygenation, and may reduce the risk of air leak and barotrauma.[54-58] Although the efficacy of high-frequency oscillatory ventilation in reducing infant mortality and morbidity is contentious, two studies suggest that in carefully controlled clinical settings, it is beneficial.[57,61]

A meta-analysis of the existing trials evaluating pediatric high-frequency oscillatory ventilation found no difference in mortality between it and conventional mechanical ventilation, although high-frequency oscillatory ventilation may have been associated with a modest reduction in chronic lung disease compared with conventional ventilation.[63]

Because the cause and pathophysiology of respiratory failure in preterm neonates and adults are different, the results of trials of neonatal high-frequency oscillatory ventilation are inadequately extrapolated to adult populations. Clinical application of high-frequency oscillatory ventilation in adult subjects was initially hampered by technical failures and a lack of adequately powered ventilators. With the development of more robust ventilators that could generate sufficient power to oscillate an adult patient, there has been a resurgence of interest in high-frequency oscillatory ventilation as part of a lung-protective strategy in patients with ARDS. Two published case series described patients with ARDS who were ventilated with high-frequency oscillatory ventilation after failing conventional mechanical ventilation and found improved oxygenation and decreased inspired oxygen fraction requirements.[64,65] The mortality rate in these uncontrolled series was high (32% to 53%), but this is not surprising, given that high-frequency oscillatory ventilation was used as salvage therapy, preselecting patients with high mortality rates. Other small case series have described the use of high-frequency oscillatory ventilation in burn and trauma patients, both with similar improvements in oxygenation.[66,67]

The best evidence for the use of high-frequency oscillatory ventilation in ARDS comes from two prospective series[68,69] and a prospective clinical trial.[70] Both Mehta and David and their respective colleagues reported experience with high-frequency oscillatory ventilation in patients failing conventional mechanical ventilation and found significant improvements in oxygenation compared with baseline.[68,69] High-frequency oscillatory ventilation was safe and well tolerated, without causing significant hemodynamic compromise. Although the series by Mehta and colleagues had a very high mortality rate, their patient population included very high-risk patients (hematologic malignancy and burn victims). Derdak and colleagues published the first prospective, randomized trial comparing high-frequency oscillatory ventilation with conventional mechanical ventilation in early ARDS and found that the former was safe and improved oxygenation.[70] Although not statistically significant, there was a trend toward decreased mortality in the patients receiving high-frequency oscillatory ventilation. Of interest, all three of these prospective studies found that a longer duration of conventional mechanical ventilation before instituting high-frequency oscillatory ventilation was predictive of a poor outcome, which led some investigators to propose early application of high-frequency oscillatory ventilation in an attempt to attenuate VILI and possible mortality.

In summary, high-frequency oscillatory ventilation is safe and effective in pediatric patients with hypoxic respiratory failure and in adult patients failing conventional mechanical ventilation. In carefully selected children, high-frequency oscillatory ventilation may be superior to conventional mechanical ventilation. Despite the paucity of published experience in adults, there is a suggestion that the early use of high-frequency oscillatory ventilation may be of additional benefit, although this has yet to be established by rigorous clinical trials.

FUTURE OF HIGH-FREQUENCY VENTILATION

Despite several decades of research into the principles and clinical application of high-frequency ventilation, many important issues remain unresolved, particularly regarding its use in adults. In fact, even the mechanical characteristics of high-frequency ventilation (tidal volumes, gas exchange mechanisms) are still incompletely understood. The optimal settings to maximize lung protection and gas exchange are not clear for many modes of high-frequency ventilation. It has been theorized that optimization of such modes would involve minimizing tidal volumes to reduce the risk of overdistention injury and cyclic lung unit collapse and maximizing alternative gas transport mechanisms. Further, the best time to initiate high-frequency ventilation is not clear; for example, do the benefits of early application outweigh the risks of the increased sedation and paralysis necessary?

These issues must be resolved, because the inappropriate use of high-frequency ventilation may be associated with increased morbidity. The early negative results in trials of high-frequency oscillatory ventilation in neonatal populations without the use of aggressive lung volume recruitment are testament to the importance of the proper ventilation protocol. It is important that these questions be answered before embarking on comparative trials, lest high-frequency ventilation be dismissed not because of lack of benefit but because of inappropriate application. Despite these unknowns, however, high-frequency ventilation possesses many theoretical advantages over conventional mechanical ventilation of the injured lung, especially in upholding the principles of lung protection.

CONCLUSION

All high-frequency ventilation modes are characterized by small tidal volumes delivered at high frequencies, and they take advantage of alternative mechanisms to achieve adequate gas exchange when tidal volumes are less than anatomic deadspace. Evolving understanding of VILI has prompted clinicians to apply mechanical ventilators in a way that minimizes such injury—so-called lung-protective ventilation. The mechanical characteristics of high-frequency ventilation make it well suited to use in the injured lung, because it may reduce volutrauma-type injury while achieving higher mean airway pressures and maintaining end-expiratory lung volume, reducing cyclic collapse. Clinical experience with high-frequency ventilation, particularly high-frequency oscillatory ventilation, has found it to be safe and effective for improving oxygenation in neonatal and adult populations failing conventional mechanical ventilation. It may also be advantageous to apply high-frequency oscillatory ventilation early in the course of ARDS to avoid VILI related to aggressive conventional mechanical ventilator settings. Despite these initial promising results, however, more research is needed to determine the optimal settings and timing of initiation of high-frequency ventilation, as well as its role in the evolving armamentarium of lung-protective ventilation strategies.

ANNOTATED REFERENCES

Courtney SE, Durand DJ, Asselin JM, et al: High-frequency oscillatory ventilation versus conventional mechanical ventilation for very-low-birth-weight Infants. N Engl J Med 2002;347:643-652.

This large, multicenter trial (along with that of Johnson and colleagues) represents the most recent evaluation of high-frequency oscillatory ventilation in neonates at high risk for bronchopulmonary dysplasia. These authors found a small but significant clinical benefit from high-frequency oscillatory ventilation when it was applied under rigorously controlled conditions.

Derdak S, Mehta S, Stewart TE, et al: High-frequency oscillatory ventilation for acute respiratory distress syndrome in adults: A randomized, controlled trial. Am J Respir Crit Care Med 2002;166:801-808.

This trial represents the first prospective, randomized clinical trial comparing conventional mechanical ventilation and high-frequency oscillatory ventilation early in the course of ARDS. It found high-frequency oscillatory ventilation to be effective and safe, with a trend toward decreased mortality in patients randomized to receive it. Of note, pre-enrollment conventional ventilation for more than 5 days was predictive of mortality.

Imai Y, Nakagawa S, Ito Y, et al: Comparison of lung protection strategies using conventional and high-frequency oscillatory ventilation. J Appl Physiol 2001;91:1836-1844.

This laboratory study suggested the superiority of high-frequency oscillatory ventilation over conventional mechanical ventilation in an animal model. The authors found decreased systemic and local inflammatory mediators and histologic lung damage in the animals ventilated with high-frequency oscillatory ventilation.

Johnson AH, Peacock JL, Greenough A, et al: High-frequency oscillatory ventilation for the prevention of chronic lung disease of prematurity. N Engl J Med 2002;347:633-642.

In contrast to the study by Courtney and colleagues, these authors found no advantage to high-frequency oscillatory ventilation over conventional mechanical ventilation.

Mehta S, Lapinsky SE, Hallett DC, et al: Prospective trial of high-frequency oscillation in adults with acute respiratory distress syndrome. Crit Care Med 2001;29:1360-1369.

This prospective clinical study established the safety and efficacy of high-frequency oscillatory ventilation as salvage therapy in adults with ARDS failing conventional mechanical ventilation. High-frequency oscillatory ventilation was safe and effective at improving oxygenation, and prolonged conventional ventilation before switching to the high-frequency mode was predictive of death, suggesting the need for further investigation into the timing of high-frequency ventilation.

Rotta AT, Gunnarsson B, Fuhrman BP, et al: Comparison of lung protective ventilation strategies in a rabbit model of acute lung injury. Crit Care Med 2001;29:2176-2184.

Like the report by Imai and colleagues, this laboratory study suggested the superiority of high-frequency oscillatory ventilation over conventional mechanical ventilation in an animal model.

Chapter 70

EXTRACORPOREAL LIFE SUPPORT

Stephen A. Rowe • Robert H. Bartlett

KEY POINTS

1. **Extracorporeal life support should be instituted early,** before significant ventilator trauma.

2. **The main complication of extracorporeal life support is hemorrhage.**

3. **Venovenous support is the primary mode for respiratory failure.** Venoarterial bypass provides full support for both respiratory and cardiovascular failure.

4. **Extracorporeal life support is not active treatment but allows time** for the native organs to regain function.

Extracorporeal life support, also known as extracorporeal membrane oxygenation, is the use of a cardiopulmonary bypass device to prolong the life of a critically ill patient who has inadequate pulmonary or cardiac function. Extracorporeal life support was first used successfully in 1972 in a patient who developed acute respiratory distress syndrome (ARDS) after a motorcycle crash.[1] The basis for extracorporeal life support was the development of cardiopulmonary bypass devices for open heart surgery. The original devices used a direct blood-gas interface and were used for only a few hours[2]; however, the development of membrane blood-gas interfaces by Kolobow and others initiated the laboratory study and clinical application of prolonged extracorporeal circulation.[3-5] In 1976, the first successful neonatal extracorporeal life support was reported.[6] Currently, extracorporeal life support is used for pulmonary and cardiac failure in all age groups, with an overall survival rate ranging from 30% in cardiac arrest to 90% in neonatal respiratory failure.

INDICATIONS

Extracorporeal life support is used for patients with severe (predicted mortality 80%) but potentially reversible cardiopulmonary failure. It is invasive and expensive and requires anticoagulation; therefore, it is reserved for patients who have failed simpler treatment regimens. Extracorporeal life support provides rest from high ventilator settings, high inspired oxygen fractions (FIO_2), and high doses of pressors. It is best used early in the treatment of cardiopulmonary failure rather than as a "rescue" treatment.[7]

Neonates must be at least 32 weeks' gestation and have an oxygenation index greater than 25. The presence of intraventricular hemorrhage or coagulopathy precludes extracorporeal life support. Major genetic abnormalities are also a relative contraindication. Common neonatal conditions for which extracorporeal life support is used are meconium aspiration syndrome, persistent pulmonary hypertension, congenital diaphragmatic hernia, pneumonia, and respiratory distress syndrome.[8,9]

Adult and pediatric patients have similar criteria. High mortality risk in adults and children with hypoxic respiratory failure is identified by a partial pressure of arterial oxygen (PaO_2)/FIO_2 ratio less than 100, compliance less than 0.5 mL/cm H_2O per kilogram, or shunt fraction greater than 30% in the setting of maximal medical therapy. High mortality risk in cardiac failure is identified by low cardiac index despite optimal pharmacologic support, increasing lactic acidosis, failure to wean from cardiopulmonary bypass postoperatively, and persistent hypotension.[10-14] Absolute contraindications are incurable disease, poor neurologic status, and active bleeding. Relative contraindications are advanced age and duration of positive-pressure ventilation. Pulmonary fibrosis increases with time on the ventilator and is usually irreversible when pulmonary artery pressures are two thirds of systolic pressures or if the patient has been on high ventilator settings for more than 7 days. Common diagnoses leading to extracorporeal life support are pneumonia; ARDS following surgery, trauma, or sepsis; status asthmaticus; aspiration; and pulmonary embolism.[15-17] Sepsis and septic shock were previously considered to be contraindications to extracorporeal life support; however, septic patients are now commonly treated successfully.[18,19]

Specific indications and contraindications for neonates and for children and adults are summarized in Tables 70-1 and 70-2, respectively.

TECHNIQUE

Extracorporeal life support involves the continuous drainage of venous blood to a pump and membrane oxygenator and re-infusion to a major vein or artery. Venoarterial bypass was originally the standard method of access but is now reserved for patients who require hemodynamic support or neonates whose veins are too small to accommodate an adequate double-lumen cannula. Cannulation and management techniques are described in detail elsewhere.[20]

Venoarterial bypass is performed by accessing the right atrium or inferior vena cava for venous drainage and infusion into the carotid or femoral artery. Access to all vessels except the carotid can usually be performed by percutaneous Seldinger technique.[21,22] Because arterial flow is antegrade and directed to the proximal aorta, there is hypothetically

TABLE 70–1. CRITERIA FOR NEONATAL EXTRACORPOREAL LIFE SUPPORT

Age >32 wk
Weight >1.5 kg
No intracranial hemorrhage (>grade 1); recent head
    ultrasonography needed
No coagulopathy
Ventilation <10-14 days
AaDO >605-620 for not more than 4-12 h
$AaDO_2 = 713$
Oxygenation index >25

TABLE 70–2. CRITERIA FOR ADULT AND PEDIATRIC EXTRACORPOREAL LIFE SUPPORT

Indications	Contraindications
Poor gas exchange	>7 days on high ventilator settings (adult)
	>14 days on high ventilator settings (pediatric)
Compliance <0.5 mL/cm H_2O/kg	Incurable disease (e.g., malignancy)
PaO_2/FIO_2 <100	
Shunt fraction >30%	Age >70 yr
	Pulmonary artery pressures >{2/3} systolic pressures
	Poor neurologic status
	Active bleeding or unresolved surgical issues

better perfusion to the brain, coronary vessels, and viscera. However, the incidence of cerebrovascular accident is as high as 15%. In children weighing less than 25 kg, cannulation through the neck is the only option for venoarterial bypass, because the femoral artery cannot be adequately cannulated. The advantage of cannulating the femoral vessels is that it can be performed completely percutaneously. The disadvantages of femoral artery cannulation are retrograde flow and the possibility of rendering the cannulated leg ischemic. However, the ischemia can be treated by placing a third cannula in the ipsilateral leg and "Y-ing" it to the arterial side of the extracorporeal life support circuit. Figure 70-1 displays a typical venoarterial extracorporeal life support setup.

Venovenous access is the most common route of extracorporeal support for respiratory failure.[23] In adults, the right atrium and inferior vena cava are cannulated via the internal jugular and femoral veins. In neonates and small children, double-lumen cannulas can be inserted into the internal jugular vein. Venovenous support has several advantages: percutaneous techniques can be used, the risk of cerebrovascular accident is greatly reduced, normal hemodynamics are maintained,

and there is no risk of ischemia to the lower extremity. A typical venovenous setup is displayed in Figure 70-2.

Once bypass is initiated, flow is begun at around 50 to 60 mL/kg per minute. The extracorporeal life support circuit provides the majority of support, and the ventilator settings are minimized to decrease pulmonary trauma.[24] Typical ventilator settings with extracorporeal life support are pressure of 30/10, frequency of 5, and FIO_2 of 0.40. Systemic heparinization is maintained and titrated to activated clotting time, which should range from 160 to 220 seconds. Extracorporeal life support provides full life support in the absence of cardiac or pulmonary function, but it is not active treatment. It affords time to treat the primary condition without reliance on native heart or lung function. Patients with respiratory failure undergo diuresis or hemofiltration to their dry weights and are benefited by intermittent prone positioning. Any underlying cause of ARDS, such as pneumonia or sepsis, is treated. The ventilator is gradually resumed until native lung function is adequate to wean the patient off of extracorporeal life support. Patients with cardiac failure may

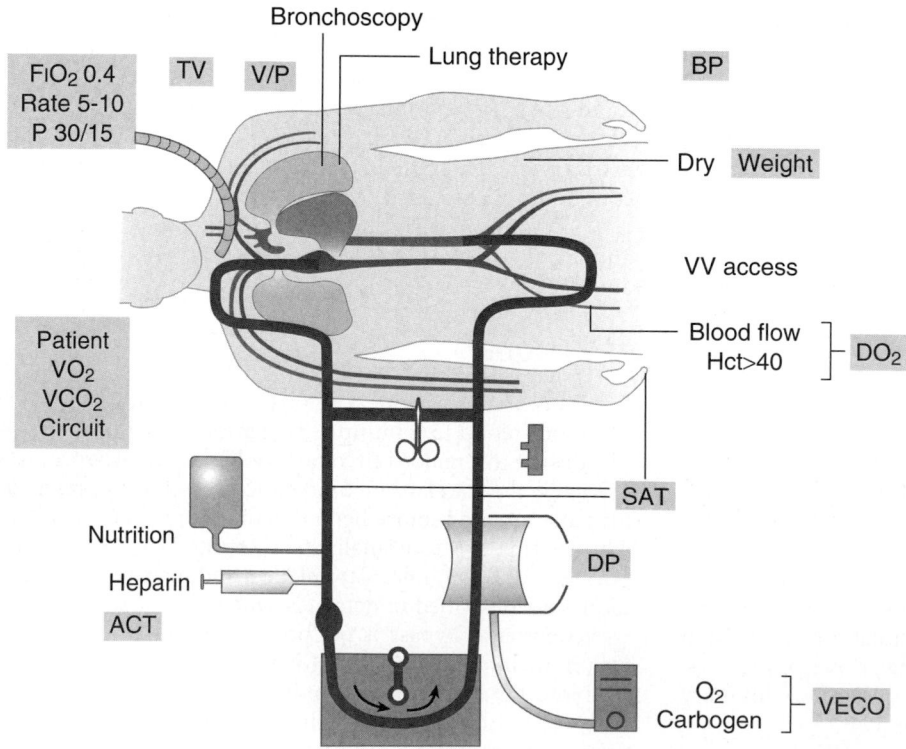

FIGURE 70–1. Typical venoarterial bypass setup. ACT, activated clotting time; BP, blood pressure; Hct, hematocrit.

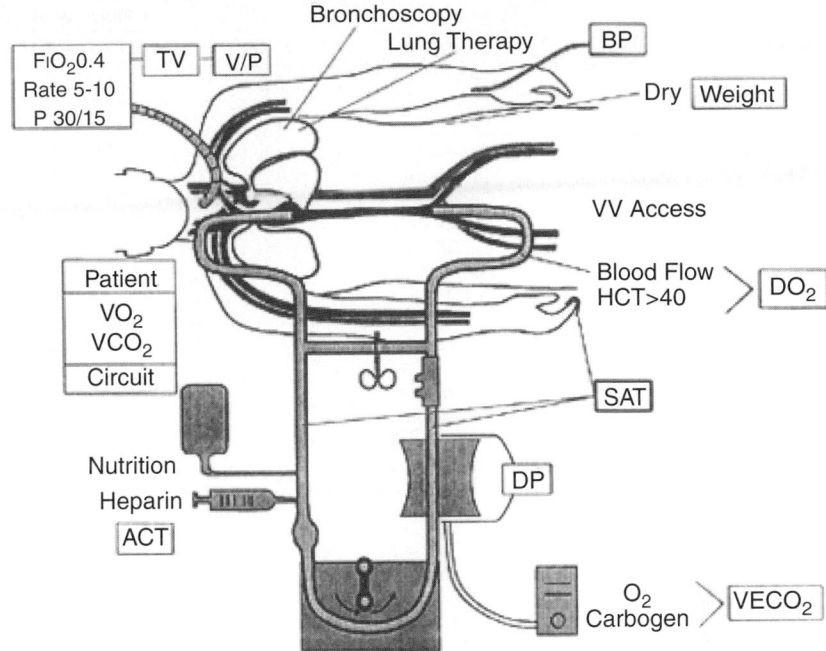

FIGURE 70–2. Typical venovenous bypass setup. ACT, activated clotting time; BP, blood pressure; Hct, hematocrit.

improve with time, but some cardiac patients require ventricular assist devices and transplant evaluations.

Because of the complexity of the extracorporeal life support circuit, a bedside specialist monitors the equipment at all times. In addition to titrating the heparin, the specialist maintains the circuit and repairs any malfunction, oxygenator failure, or tube rupture. The patient's dependence on the extracorporeal life support circuit dictates that these repairs occur within a few minutes. In experienced centers, extracorporeal life support can be maintained for weeks without major complications.

OUTCOME

Extracorporeal life support is a viable and effective treatment. Patients who are placed on extracorporeal life support typically have a 20% predicted survival rate without bypass. In the 1970s, trials failed to show improved survival with extracorporeal life support. However, since that time, there

have been improvements in technology, technique, and understanding of the involved pathophysiology. A randomized, controlled trial is currently under way in the United Kingdom to assess the outcome with current extracorporeal life support protocols.[25]

The Extracorporeal Life Support Organization maintains a registry of patients treated with extracorporeal life support. As of July 2003, 27,219 patients had undergone extracorporeal life support, with 76% surviving to decannulation and 67% surviving to discharge. Neonates cannulated for respiratory failure have by far the best success rate, with 77% surviving to discharge. A summary of survival outcomes is listed in Table 70-3.[26] Table 70-4 summarizes several major studies on survival of ARDS with and without extracorporeal life support.[11,24,27-39]

Given the complexity of extracorporeal life support, it should be no surprise that the complication rate is as high as 24%.[26] The most common complication is bleeding, which is reported in 15% to 20% of patients. Premature infants are at risk for intracranial bleeding; adults are

TABLE 70–3. SURVIVAL OUTCOME OF PATIENTS ENTERED IN THE EXTRACORPOREAL LIFE SUPPORT ORGANIZATION REGISTRY AS OF JULY 2003

	Group	Total	Number Surviving to Decannulation (%)	Number Surviving to Discharge (%)
Neonatal	Respiratory	18,283	15,644 (86)	14,156 (77)
	Cardiac	1,965	1,098 (56)	733 (37)
	ECPR	107	66 (62)	42 (39)
Pediatric	Respiratory	2,548	1,620 (64)	1,410 (55)
	Cardiac	2,684	1,505 (56)	1,130 (42)
	ECPR	218	105 (48)	85 (39)
Adult	Respiratory	891	518 (58)	462 (52)
	Cardiac	419	193 (46)	138 (33)
	ECPR	104	49 (47)	34 (33)

TABLE 70–4. SURVIVAL IN ACUTE RESPIRATORY DISTRESS SYNDROME WITH AND WITHOUT EXTRACORPOREAL LIFE SUPPORT

Author	Year	Treatment	Number of Patients (% Survived)			
			All ARDS	Severe ARDS	Severe ARDS with ECLS	ECLS Only
Zapol	1991	General	635 (58)	149 (15)	—	—
Artigas	1991	General	583 (41)	403 (31)	—	—
Sloane	1992	General	153 (46)	—	—	—
Vasilyev	1995	General	1426 (56)	311 (18)	—	—
Weg	1998	Surfactant	725 (55)	—	—	—
Luhr	1999	General	221 (58)	—	—	—
Zapol	1979	NIH-ECMO	686 (34)	48 (8)	—	42 (10)
Gattinoni	1986	ECCOR	—	—	—	43 (49)
Morris	1994	Randomized	—	19 (42)	—	21 (33)
Brunet	1993	ECCOR	—	—	—	23 (50)
Macha	1996	ECLS	—	—	—	33 (39)
Kolla	1997	ECLS	—	—	—	100 (54)
Peek	1997	ECLS	—	—	—	50 (66)
Lewandowski	1997	Algorithm & ECLS	—	—	122 (75)	49 (55)
Rich	1998	Algorithm & ECLS	—	—	141 (62)	100 (54)
Ullrich	1999	Algorithm & ECLS	84 (80)	—	—	13 (62)

ARDS, acute respiratory distress syndrome; ECLS, extracorporeal life support; ECMO, extracorporeal membrane oxygenation; NIH, National Institutes of Health.

susceptible to gastrointestinal hemorrhage. Bleeding on extracorporeal life support is managed by decreasing the activated clotting time to 160 to 180 seconds and correcting the platelet count to 150,000.[39] Mechanical complications include oxygenator failure, clotting, and rupture of the tubing. Mechanical complications are addressed immediately by the bedside specialist and are rarely fatal.

TRANSPORT ON EXTRACORPOREAL LIFE SUPPORT

In some cases, patients at referring facilities are too unstable to be transported on conventional ventilation. The University of Michigan recently reported 100 patients transported on extracorporeal life support. Overall survival to discharge was 66%, and the complication rate during transport was 17%, with no deaths in transit.[40,41] Currently, the technology exists to transport any patient by ground. Technical issues preclude the transport of patients weighing less than 10 kg by air. Although it is possible to transport patients on extracorporeal life support, it is preferable to refer severe cardiac or pulmonary failure patients to an extracorporeal life support center on conventional support.

SUMMARY

Extracorporeal life support provides a means of keeping patients alive following cardiopulmonary collapse that is refractory to conventional means of support. Additionally, these patients are afforded time for the treatment and improvement of native cardiopulmonary function while avoiding the detrimental effects of high ventilator settings. The last decade has seen improvements in extracorporeal life support technology and refinements in the techniques used to manage patients with severe cardiopulmonary failure. In children and neonates, the utility of extracorporeal life support has been proved by prospective, randomized trials. In adults, retrospective data suggest that survival might be increased with extracorporeal life support.

ANNOTATED REFERENCES

Bartlett RH, et al: Extracorporeal membrane oxygenation (ECMO) cardiopulmonary support in infancy. Trans Am Soc Artif Intern Organs 1976;22:80-93.
This is the first description of the use of extracorporeal life support in neonatal patients.

Bartlett RH, Roloff DW, Custer JR, et al: Extracorporeal life support: The University of Michigan experience. JAMA 2000;283:904-908.
The largest single-center report of extracorporeal life support.

Hill JD, O'Brien TG, Murray JJ, et al: Extracorporeal oxygenation for acute post-traumatic respiratory failure (shock-lung syndrome): Use of the Bramson membrane lung. N Engl J Med 1972; 286:629-634.
This is the first description of successful long-term use of extracorporeal life support.

Kolla S, et al: Extracorporeal life support for 100 adult patients with severe respiratory failure. Ann Surg 1997;226:544-564; discussion 565-566.
In addition to summarizing survival data in a large series of patients, this paper provides details on criteria for the use of extracorporeal life support.

Rich PB, Awad SS, Kolla S, et al: An approach to the treatment of severe adult respiratory failure. J Crit Care 1998;13:26-36.
Provides guidelines for the development of clinical protocols to treat patients with severe ARDS who are on extracorporeal life support.

Chapter 71

ADJUNCTIVE RESPIRATORY THERAPY

Sanjay Manocha • Keith R. Walley

IV

539

KEY POINTS

1. Inability to effectively clear secretions is common in critically ill patients, increasing the risk of aspiration, atelectasis, and pneumonia.

2. Chest physiotherapy and positional therapy should be considered in all critically ill patients.

3. Other adjunctive forms of respiratory therapy should be considered on an individual basis based on the underlying clinical condition.

4. Aerosolization of medications is an effective way of delivering medications directly to the lungs.

5. Metered-dose inhalers (MDIs) are preferred over nebulization for the delivery of bronchodilators in both the spontaneously breathing and mechanically ventilated patient.

6. Inhaled nitric oxide can be safely administered in the critically ill patient with proper monitoring.

7. Inhaled nitric oxide is associated with improved pulmonary and cardiac physiologic parameters when administered in a variety of clinical conditions encountered in the ICU.

Most critically ill patients are unable to effectively clear secretions that accumulate in the central and peripheral airways. This can be due to factors such as increased secretion production, impaired cough reflex, weakness, and pain. The presence of an endotracheal tube prevents closure of the glottis to generate the high expiratory pressures needed for an effective cough, thereby promoting the retention of secretions. In addition, in critically ill patients, cilia in the pulmonary tree are impaired in function and reduced in number.[1,2] This leads to an increased risk of aspiration, atelectasis, and pneumonia, which is detrimental in the critically ill patient.

Adjunctive respiratory therapy addresses many of these concerns to prevent and treat respiratory complications that are encountered in the critically ill patient. As highlighted in Table 71-1, they range from simple measures such as proper body positioning and suctioning to more complex interventions such as chest physiotherapy, bronchoscopy, and use of aerosolized/inhaled medications that act directly on the pulmonary system.

METHODS TO IMPROVE PULMONARY MUCOCILIARY CLEARANCE

PERCUSSION

Percussion of the chest can aid in secretion clearance. It is performed by clapping cupped hands over regions of the thorax that are affected in a rhythmic fashion or using mechanical devices that mimic the same action. The energy of the force generated by the cupped hands is transmitted through the thorax to dislodge secretions. When used in conjunction with postural drainage to maximize secretion movement, this is an effective method to mobilize secretions from the pulmonary tract. It is a technique often used in the daily management of cystic fibrosis patients[3] and those with severe bronchiectasis.

HIGH-FREQUENCY CHEST COMPRESSION

High-frequency chest compression (HFCC) relies on rapid pressure changes to the respiratory system during expiration to enhance movement of mucus in the peripheral airways to the central airways for clearance. This method employs a vest worn by the patient that is attached to an air-pulse generator. Small volumes of gas are introduced into the vest at a rapid rate ranging from 5 to 25 Hz producing pressures up to 50 cm H_2O. This technique is mainly used in cystic fibrosis patients and is equivalent to conventional chest physiotherapy techniques of percussion and postural drainage.[4-6] One study examined the use of HFCC in nine long-term mechanically ventilated patients.[7] In this observational study, the HFCC was compared with percussion and postural drainage. No difference was seen in the amount of sputum production, oxygen saturation, or patient comfort between the two methods. In this small study, HFCC was determined to be safe and believed to save staff time. It is difficult to apply this technique to most critically ill patients because the size of the vest covering the thorax may prevent adequate monitoring.

MANUAL HYPERINFLATION

Manual hyperinflation with a manual inflation bag using high tidal volumes involves disconnecting the patient from the ventilator. Typically, the lungs are inflated slowly to one and one-half to two times the tidal volume or peak airway pressures of 40 cm H_2O as measured by a manometer. It is held at end inspiration with an inspiratory pause to allow for filling of alveoli with slow time constants. This is followed by a quick release to allow for rapid expiration. The goal of

TABLE 71–1. ADJUNCTIVE RESPIRATORY THERAPIES

Methods to Improve Pulmonary Mucociliary Clearance

Chest physiotherapy
   Percussion
   Postural drainage
   Chest vibration
Suctioning
   Oropharyngeal suctioning
   Nasopharyngeal suctioning
   Endotracheal suctioning
Continuous lateral rotation
Positive expiratory pressure devices
Forced expiration
Closed chest oscillation
Bronchoscopy
Manual hyperinflation
Bronchodilators
Mucoactive agents

Methods to Improve Lung Expansion

Deep breathing
Incentive spirometry
Intermittent positive ventilation
Optimum body position

Methods to Improve Oxygenation and Ventilation

Inhaled vasodilators
   Nitric oxide
   Prostaglandins
Helium-oxygen (heliox)

manual hyperinflation is to recruit atelectatic lung regions to improve oxygenation and improve clearance of secretions. Similar to recruitment maneuvers described with mechanical ventilators, manual hyperinflation only leads to transient improvements in oxygenation without any long-term clinically significant improvement on outcomes.[8-11] It also has the disadvantage of requiring a ventilator disconnect, and this method can be mimicked by a mechanical ventilator.

Contraindications include hemodynamic compromise and high intracranial pressure. There is also a risk of barotrauma because of preferential inflation of open lung regions that are highly compliant compared with collapsed regions.

POSITIONING AND MOBILIZATION

Mobilization of patients in the ICU either through active or passive limb exercises may improve overall patient well-being and in the long term may lead to better patient outcomes. Positioning also plays an important role. Position of the patient with the head of the bed elevated at least 30 degrees significantly reduces the risk of aspiration and ventilator-associated pneumonia.[12] Upright positioning of patients in whom there is no contraindication improves lung volumes and therefore gas exchange and work of breathing, especially in those in whom the supine or semi-recumbent position leads to an increased work of breathing. Positioning of selected individuals with unilateral lung disease on their side with the affected side up can lead to improved ventilation-perfusion ($\dot{V}/\dot{Q}$) matching (by gravitational increased perfusion to the dependent "good" side).[13,14] If atelectasis secondary to retained secretions is the cause, having the affected side up leads to postural drainage.

Postural drainage involves positioning the body to allow gravity to assist in the movement of secretions. Postural drainage is indicated in patients with a sputum production of

more than 25 to 30 mL/day and in those who have difficulty clearing their secretions.[15] In cystic fibrosis, postural drainage with percussion is an effective method to clear pulmonary secretions and is associated with improved lung function.[16,17]

TRACHEAL SUCTION

Used in conjunction with other techniques to mobilize secretions from the peripheral airways to the central airways, suctioning is an effective way of removing secretions to improve bronchial hygiene. It can be performed using open methods where the patient is disconnected from the ventilator and a disposable suction catheter is placed. The closed system involves a closed circuit with the suction catheter placed in a protective sheath and directly connected to the ventilator circuit. No disconnect is required, and the risk of environmental cross contamination is less. Routine changes of in-line suction catheters are not required, and the procedure is cost-effective.[18,19] But, overall, the risk of nosocomial pneumonia between open and closed systems is not different.[20,21]

Because of the anatomic arrangement of the large central airways, the suction catheter most often enters the right mainstem bronchus compared with the left mainstem bronchus. Specially designed curved-tipped "left-sided" suction catheters increase the likelihood of suctioning from the left mainstem bronchus.

Nasotracheal suctioning has fallen out of favor over direct tracheal suctioning and should only be considered in patients who are able to protect their airway and used in conjunction with assisted coughs and other forms of chest physiotherapy.

Complications with suctioning include hypoxemia, especially in the setting of a ventilator disconnect, increased intracranial pressure with vigorous stimulation of the airways, mechanical trauma to the trachea, and bacterial contamination. All patients should be preoxygenated with 100% oxygen for 1 to 2 minutes before suctioning. To reduce the risk of agitation, the patient should be informed before tracheal suctioning is performed. The suctioning should be limited to 15 to 20 seconds. The suction port on the catheter should be opened and closed intermittently and not closed for more than 5 seconds at a time.

CONTINUOUS ROTATION THERAPY

Continuous rotational or kinetic therapy extends the practice of regular 2 hourly repositioning of patients from one side to the other by placing the patient on a bed that moves to pre-programmed angles on a more frequent basis or through the use of air mattresses that deflate alternatively from side to side to provide the continuous postural position changes. Most studies on various patient populations demonstrate a lower incidence of nosocomial pneumonia or atelectasis but no overall improvement in other clinically significant outcomes such as duration of mechanical ventilation, length of stay in the ICU, or mortality.[22-28]

COUGHING

Assisted coughing is often required in spontaneously breathing patients because of an ineffective cough for a variety of reasons, as previously highlighted. Techniques include "huffing" in the setting of an open glottis where in expiration the patient forcibly exhales quickly several times. Other maneuvers include abdominal or thoracic compression on expiration to generate high intrathoracic pressures mimicking a cough.

POSITIVE EXPIRATORY PRESSURE THERAPY

Positive expiratory pressure therapy (PEP) involves the use of a facemask or mouthpiece that provides a resistance to airflow of 10 to 20 cm H_2O on expiration. After repeating this maneuver a number of times, mucus in the peripheral airways is mobilized and moved toward the larger airways to be coughed or expelled with other techniques. Its use in critically ill patients who are spontaneously breathing is likely limited by the coordination required for slow expirations. Other methods may be easier to perform in this patient population to aid in secretion clearance.

BRONCHOSCOPY

Fiberoptic bronchoscopy has the advantage of providing direct visualization of the airways and permits suctioning of specific segments where secretions may be retained, causing problems such as atelectasis. Bronchoscopy can be considered as an adjunctive therapy for the treatment of atelectasis or removal of secretions. As highlighted in one review,[29] bronchoscopy is a moderately effective technique for the treatment of atelectasis in the critically ill patient, with success rates ranging from 19% to 89% depending on the extent of the atelectasis (lobar atelectasis responds better than subsegmental atelectasis). But when compared with aggressive multimodal chest physiotherapy, in the only randomized trial, no difference in the rate of resolution was seen between the two methods.[30] Being an invasive procedure, bronchoscopy is not without risks, including complications associated with sedation required for the procedure, transient increases in ICP, hypoxemia, and hemodynamic consequences/arrhythmias. Therefore, it cannot be recommended as first-line therapy except in certain situations such as extensive unilateral atelectasis leading to significant difficulties in oxygenating or ventilating that have not resolved with other methods such as suctioning.

CHEST PHYSIOTHERAPY

Chest physiotherapy is a multimodal therapy with the goals of improving pulmonary function (gas exchange, improved lung compliance, and improved pulmonary mucus clearance). Techniques include percussive therapies (manual or mechanical chest percussion), postural drainage, chest vibration, manual hyperinflation, mobilization, suctioning, and rotational therapy. Overall, chest physiotherapy provides transient improvements in oxygenation and lung compliance likely secondary to airway clearance and recruitment of atelectatic regions. Chest physiotherapy may, in specific situations, improve outcome and clinical course such as in the prevention of ventilator-associated pneumonia[31] or acute lobar atelectasis.[32]

AEROSOL THERAPIES

AEROSOLIZATION

The aerosolization of medications is an effective method for drug delivery directly to lungs. The two most common methods of delivery are via nebulization or via metered-dose inhalers (MDIs). The theoretical advantage of this form of therapy includes direct delivery and activity at the site of pathology and the ability to deliver high concentrations with minimal systemic absorption and toxicity. The most common aerosolized therapy is the administration of bronchodilators. Other medications that can be administered directly to the lungs include corticosteroids, antibiotics, antifungal agents, surfactant, mucolytic agents, and saline.

Nebulization is the process of using a high flow of gas (usually 6 to 8 L/min) to produce small respirable particles of the liquid medium containing the medication of interest. The most common nebulizer is the pneumatic (jet) nebulizer. In the spontaneously breathing patient, approximately 50% of the nebulized liquid is in the respirable range of a mass median aerodynamic diameter (MMAD) of 1 to 5 μm, with approximately 10% reaching the lower respiratory tract/small airways. In mechanically ventilated patients, 1% to 15% is delivered to the lower respiratory tract. Ultrasonic nebulization uses high-frequency ultrasonic waves on the surface of the liquid medium to generate respirable particles. Its use is limited by the expense of the equipment involved.

MDIs are pressurized canisters with the drug suspended in a mix of propellants, preservatives, and surfactants. On activation, particles ranging from 1 to 2 μm are produced. The MDI in conjunction with a chamber/spacer device significantly increases drug delivery in both spontaneously breathing patients and when attached to the ventilator circuit either directly to the endotracheal tube or as part of an in-line device in the inspiratory limb of the Y-piece.

Factors that influence the efficacy of aerosol delivery in the mechanically ventilated patient include[33]:

1. *Position of administration in the circuit:* the MDI should be closer to the endotracheal tube at the Y-piece with a chamber, compared with a pneumatic nebulizer, which should be at least 30 cm from the Y-piece.
2. *Humidification:* this can decrease aerosol delivery to the respiratory tract because of greater deposition in the ventilator circuit. Higher doses may be required to achieve the desired effect.
3. *Timing of delivery:* the aerosol should be delivered during the inspiratory phase to maximize drug delivery.
4. *Flow rates:* slower inspiratory flow rates (and therefore longer inspiratory time) increase delivery of nebulized medications. A decelerating flow pattern can also increase delivery to the lower airways.
5. *Tidal volumes:* larger tidal volumes greater than 500 mL ensure optimal delivery.
6. *Endotracheal tube size:* tube sizes less than 7.0 mm reduce delivery.
7. *Density of inhaled gas:* low-density gases such as helium-oxygen mixtures increase deposition to the lower airways by increasing laminar flow and producing smaller respirable particle size.

BRONCHODILATORS

Bronchodilators are the most frequently administered aerosolized therapy in the critically ill patient. Inhaled beta$_2$ agonists such as albuterol or fenoterol are generally well tolerated in the critically ill patient. Adverse effects such as arrhythmias and hypokalemia can occur in those receiving excessive doses in which significant systemic absorption is likely. Other bronchodilators such as ipratropium bromide are also effective, especially when used in conjunction with a beta$_2$ agonist. Bronchodilators administered via MDI are equally as effective as a nebulizer in spontaneously breathing patients.[33] In mechanically ventilated patients, the use of nebulization is either equally as good as[34] or less effective[35,36] than an MDI with a spacer. MDI administration has the advantage of easier use without the risk of bacterial contamination and need for adjustment of flow rates.[33]

ANTIBIOTICS

Aerosolization of antibiotics as a form of topical treatment for pulmonary infections has been studied for over 20 years. Theoretical advantages of aerosolized antibiotics include direct therapy at the site of infection at higher concentrations with a lower risk of systemic absorption and side effects. In chronic pulmonary infective states such as cystic fibrosis and severe bronchiectasis,[37-39] inhaled aerosolized antibiotics have a role in reducing bacterial concentration in the sputum but only provide a long-term clinical benefit in cystic fibrosis.[37] In the acute infective state with an exacerbation of the disease, they have no additional benefit to parenteral antibiotics.[40,41]

In the intubated or tracheostomy patient, colonization of the airway frequently occurs with a significant increase in the risk for nosocomial pneumonia. In an observational study of six chronically ventilated patients, aerosolized aminoglycosides (tobramycin or amikacin) eradicated the colonizing bacteria 67% of the time with a significant reduction in inflammatory markers within the sputum.[42] As a preventive measure for ventilator-associated pneumonia, one small randomized trial in a cohort of trauma patients showed a reduction in the frequency of pneumonia with aerosolized ceftazidime.[43] But as an adjuvant for treatment of ventilator-associated pneumonia, the instillation of tobramycin through the endotracheal tube, although eradicating the causative pathogen more frequently than did placebo, did not result in any clinically significant improvement in outcomes.[40] Concerns of bacterial resistance must be considered in any preventive form of therapy with antibiotics. Side effects reported in spontaneously breathing patients treated with inhaled tobramycin include increased cough, dyspnea, and chest pain.[38]

The role for aerosolized or instilled (via the endotracheal tube) antibiotics as an adjuvant for the prevention or treatment of pulmonary infections in the ICU remains to be defined with better clinical studies.

MUCOACTIVE AGENTS

In chronic inflammatory lung states (e.g., chronic obstructive pulmonary disease [COPD], cystic fibrosis, bronchiectasis, intubation/tracheostomy), overproduction of mucus and impaired clearance result in complications commonly encountered in critical care patients, such as airflow obstruction, atelectasis, and infection. The mucus is primarily composed of water, mucin glycoprotein, cellular debris, neutrophil-derived filamentous actin and DNA, and bacteria.[44] Mucoactive agents can help improve the clearance of mucus secretions.

Expectorant methods such as simple hydration and oral expectorant medications such as guaifenesin or bromhexine that act via the vagal-mediated increase in airway secretion to decrease mucus viscosity have not been shown to be effective

methods of clearance of secretions.[45,46] Oral iodine preparations (e.g., saturated solution of potassium iodine), although described as a mucoactive agent, similarly are not effective and may be associated with significant side effects such as hypothyroidism or hyperkalemia.[44]

Mucolytic agents reduce the viscosity by breaking down the mucin glycoprotein network or free DNA strands, thereby improving mucus rheology to improve clearance. Aerosolized N-acetylcysteine (NAC) breaks down the disulfide bonds of the mucin glycoprotein network and is associated with improved mucus clearance. However, because of the increased risk of bronchospasm, its use is limited, but it may be used in conjunction with an inhaled bronchodilator.[44] Free DNA can significantly increase the viscosity of mucus and therefore impede clearance from the airways. Recombinant human DNase (rhDNase, dornase alfa) improves pulmonary function in the chronic management of cystic fibrosis patients but without any significant effect in acute exacerbations of cystic fibrosis.[47,48] In non–cystic fibrosis bronchiectasis, rhDNase is not effective and may potentially be harmful.[49]

RACEMIC EPINEPHRINE

Racemic epinephrine has been used as a therapy for acute upper airway obstruction secondary to inflammation, corticosteroids, and surfactant.

METHODS TO IMPROVE LUNG EXPANSION

Atelectasis is a common complication encountered in the critically ill patient. This is often secondary to prolonged supine body position and retained secretions obstructing airways. Lung expansion techniques mimic normal sigh maneuvers to help reverse and prevent atelectasis. These techniques are often used in postoperative patients at high risk for pulmonary complications such as those undergoing thoracic and upper abdominal surgery and patients with neuromuscular or chest wall disorders.

Deep breathing and incentive spirometry involve coached inspiratory maneuvers to voluntarily increase lung volumes to greater than the vital capacity of the patient. It requires an awake, cooperative patient who is able to tolerate the maneuver. The only advantage of using an incentive spirometer is that it provides visual feedback and a reminder to the patient to continue these maneuvers. Both incentive spirometry and deep breathing are equally effective in reducing postoperative pulmonary complications compared with no forms of chest physiotherapy.[50]

Intermittent positive-pressure breathing is a method to improve lung expansion that has fallen out of favor as a preventive measure in postoperative patients because of the expense, lack of difference in outcomes compared with deep breathing or incentive spirometry, and complications such as abdominal distention.[50,51]

METHODS TO IMPROVE OXYGENATION AND VENTILATION

NITRIC OXIDE

The effects of nitric oxide (NO) have been known for over 20 years. Since the initial discovery of NO as the "endothelial derived relaxing factor," it has grown to a potential therapeutic agent in the care of the critically ill patient.

Nitric oxide was first described as a vascular-derived relaxing factor that caused vasodilation via vascular smooth muscle relaxation. It is a highly lipid-soluble gas that allows for rapid diffusion through the alveoli-blood barrier into the pulmonary circulation and smooth muscle cells of the vasculature. The main action of NO is mediated by activating guanylate cyclase and increasing intracellular cyclic guanylate monophosphate, thereby causing smooth muscle and subsequent vasomotor relaxation.[52] The beneficial effects observed with inhaled NO are mediated primarily through this action on the pulmonary vascular smooth muscle. Pulmonary blood flow is specifically increased in well-ventilated regions, which improves matching of perfusion to ventilation. A reduction in pulmonary vascular resistance from arteriolar and venous vasodilation leads to a reduced intravascular pressure at the level of the capillaries with the potential benefit of a reduced fluid leak into the alveolus. Additional benefits observed include a reduction in platelet aggregation and neutrophil adhesion/sequestration in the lungs.[53-55] NO is rapidly inactivated by binding to the heme moiety of hemoglobin. Because of this short half-life, it does not enter the systemic circulation, making it an ideal selective pulmonary vasodilator.

The most common use of NO in the ICU is in the setting of acute lung injury (ALI) and acute respiratory distress syndrome (ARDS). Numerous clinical observational studies in ALI/ARDS have demonstrated improvements in oxygenation by improving $\dot{V}/\dot{Q}$ mismatch as demonstrated by a 10% to 20% increase in PaO_2/FiO_2 ratio and a reduction on pulmonary vascular resistance and mean pulmonary arterial pressures by at least 5 to 8 mm Hg.[56]

These physiologic benefits from both animal and clinical observational studies suggest that clinical use will be beneficial. Randomized controlled trials of varying sample size and design had similar findings.[57-60] Typically, NO improved the PaO_2 and PaO_2/FiO_2 ratios acutely, but by 24 to 72 hours those in the control group achieved the same level of improvement. Similarly, although a reduction in mean pulmonary artery pressure was also observed in these trials with the use of NO, this did not translate into clinically meaningful outcomes of a decrease in mortality, less organ failure, or days free of mechanical ventilation. A trend toward a benefit was seen in a post-hoc analysis in one trial in the more severe forms of ARDS but further studies are needed.[57] Only 60% of ALI/ARDS patients respond to inhaled NO.[57] No clear predictors of who will respond to NO exist. Given that doses below 40 ppm were safe without any significant adverse effects, it can be considered a "rescue" therapy to possibly allow for more protective forms of ventilation with decreases in FiO_2 and mean airway pressures to maintain acceptable oxygenation or in situations in which secondary pulmonary hypertension leads to compromised hemodynamic function from right ventricular failure, especially in more severe cases.

Almitrine bismesylate enhances pulmonary vasoconstriction in areas of hypoxic vasoconstriction, thereby enhancing redistribution of blood flow from shunt areas to lung units with normal $\dot{V}/\dot{Q}$ ratios.[61,62] This therefore potentiates the response of gas exchange to inhaled NO. Almitrine is not readily available in North America and requires further study to define its role in combination with NO.

In addition to ALI/ARDS, other clinical conditions in which the use of NO may be beneficial are listed in Table 71-2.

TABLE 71-2. CLINICAL CONDITIONS IN WHICH INHALED NITRIC OXIDE MAY BE USED

Acute respiratory distress syndrome
Severe primary and secondary pulmonary hypertension[79]
Congenital cardiac syndromes[80,81]
Right ventricular failure in acute pulmonary embolism or after cardiac surgery[82-85]
Pulmonary ischemic-reperfusion injury after a heart-lung or lung transplant[63,85]
Sickle cell crisis[86,87]

Inhaled NO has been used after heart and lung transplants as a method to reduce right ventricular afterload in the setting of high pulmonary pressures.[63] In lung transplants, NO has been described to reduce the risk of ischemic-reperfusion injury, but this was not supported by one randomized clinical trial early in the course of lung transplants.[64] Further studies are necessary.

Inhaled NO is typically started at low doses ranging from 1 to 2 ppm and gradually increased until the desired effect is achieved. One method, as recommended from the U.K. Consensus conference on NO use, is to perform a dose response test starting at 20 ppm and reducing the doses to 10, 5, and 0 ppm to find the lowest effective dose.[65] A significant response should be considered as a 20% increase in the PaO_2/FiO_2 ratio or at least a 5 mm Hg decrease in the mean pulmonary artery pressure. The improvement in gas exchange is usually seen at lower doses. The dose required to reduce mean pulmonary artery pressure is usually higher. The usual dose ranges from 10 to 40 ppm. Doses greater than 80 ppm are associated with a higher risk for adverse effects. From the clinical trials, longer administration is generally safe with no evidence of the effect wearing off. However, the patient should be weaned from inhaled NO as soon as improvement occurs.

Adverse effects of NO include the formation of methemoglobin and the spontaneous oxidation to nitrogen dioxide (NO_2). NO_2 is known to be toxic to the respiratory system with maximal exposure limited to 5 ppm. Complications from NO_2 exposure include airway irritation and hyperreactivity with levels as low as 1.5 ppm, pulmonary edema, and pulmonary fibrosis when exposed to higher levels. Despite these adverse effects, the development of methemoglobinemia or other toxicities related to NO_2 during acute or prolonged NO inhalation has been unusual, especially when NO is administered at doses less than 80 ppm.[66]

To reduce the risk of exposure to NO_2, NO should be stored at concentrations no higher than 1000 ppm in a pure nitrogen environment and only exposed to oxygen at the time of administration. NO should be delivered into the ventilator circuit as close to the patient as possible. NO and NO_2 levels should be monitored closely on the inspiratory side of the Y-piece when using doses greater than 2 ppm. Care should be taken to prevent abrupt discontinuation of NO. Rebound pulmonary vasoconstriction can occur with sudden discontinuation leading to rapid worsening of $\dot{V}/\dot{Q}$ mismatch and pulmonary hypertension with significant hemodynamic collapse.[67] Backup supplies of NO and delivery systems should be readily available.

An absolute contraindication to NO therapy is methemoglobinemia reductase deficiency (congenital or acquired). Relative contraindications include bleeding diathesis (secondary to reports of alteration in platelet function and bleeding time with inhaled NO), intracranial hemorrhage, and severe left ventricular failure (New York Heart Association grade III or IV).[65]

INHALED PROSTAGLANDINS

Inhaled prostaglandins I_2 (PGI_2) and E_1 (PGE_1) are alternative medications that have effects similar to inhaled nitric oxide with minimal systemic effects. For PGI_2, doses ranging from 1 to 25 ng/kg/min are favorably tolerated with similar reductions in pulmonary artery pressures and improvements in oxygenation as inhaled NO.[68,69] PGE_1 has the advantage of a more rapid degradation by the pulmonary endothelial cells, providing a selective advantage over PGI_2 at higher doses.[70] Additional studies are required to define a role for these agents, but they can be considered as alternatives for rescue therapy for similar conditions treated with inhaled NO.

HELIOX

Helium is an inert gas with a significantly lower density than room air (1.42 g/L for oxygen versus 0.17 g/L for helium). By substituting helium for nitrogen in a helium-oxygen mix (heliox), the degree of reduction in density of the gas is directly proportional to the fraction of the inspired helium concentration in the mix. The higher the concentration of helium, the lower the density from 100% oxygen. Heliox reduces the Reynolds number and thereby results in more laminar flow, therefore reducing airflow resistance, work of breathing, and dynamic hyperinflation associated with a high resistance. Clinical situations in which heliox may be used include conditions with high airflow resistance such as severe acute exacerbations of asthma or COPD, bronchiolitis, bronchopulmonary dysplasia, and extrathoracic or tracheal obstruction. It may also be used during noninvasive ventilation in patients with exacerbations of COPD to improve compliance, reduce work of breathing, and avoid intubation[71,72] and to improve aerosolized drug delivery.[73] In the management of moderate-to-severe exacerbations of asthma, routine use is not supported by two systematic reviews of the literature but can be considered as an adjuvant in severe cases.[74,75] In COPD exacerbation, researchers in one multicenter trial did not find any difference in intubation rate or length of stay in the ICU with the addition of heliox but there was an overall cost benefit from a shorter hospital length of stay.[76] Heliox is generally well tolerated without any significant adverse effects. Disadvantages of using heliox in critically ill patients include the cost of therapy and the high concentrations of helium required. Most studies utilize helium:oxygen mixes of 80:20 or 70:30 to achieve a therapeutic benefit. At higher concentrations of oxygen, the effect of helium is less and therefore is limited in use to those not requiring high FIO_2. When used in conjunction with nebulized medications, higher flows may be required to ensure adequate delivery of the medication, although this may be offset by the smaller particle size generated in a heliox mixture.[73,77] Ventilators also require recalibration for measured FIO_2, flows, and tidal volumes when using heliox.[78]

CONCLUSION

Pulmonary disease and complications are common in the critically ill patient, especially those undergoing mechanical ventilation. It is important for the clinician to recognize these potential complications and the many forms of adjunctive respiratory therapies available to prevent further morbidity. Simple therapies such as chest physiotherapy, suctioning, and positioning should be utilized in most patients, whereas more advanced procedures and therapies should be used on a selective basis based on the underlying clinical condition.

ANNOTATED REFERENCES

Dellinger RP, Zimmerman JL, Taylor RW, et al: Effects of inhaled nitric oxide in patients with acute respiratory distress syndrome: Results of a randomized phase II trial. Inhaled Nitric Oxide in ARDS Study Group. Crit Care Med 1998;26:15-23.

A multicentered, randomized, blinded, controlled trial of 177 patients within 72 hours of developing acute respiratory distress syndrome. In this patient population, inhaled nitric oxide was associated with a transient improvement in oxygenation and mean pulmonary artery pressures but this did not translate into differences in 28-day mortality or days alive and free of mechanical ventilation.

Jolliet P, Tassaux D, Roeseler J, et al: Helium-oxygen versus air-oxygen noninvasive pressure support in decompensated chronic obstructive disease: A prospective, multicenter study. Crit Care Med 2003;31:878-884.

In this well-conducted, randomized, multicentered study, the addition of heliox to noninvasive positive-pressure ventilation in patients with acute exacerbations of COPD did not demonstrate a beneficial effect with respect to intubation rate, ICU length of stay, or mortality. The use of heliox was associated with a significantly lower post-ICU hospital length of stay and hospital costs.

Kollef MH, Prentice D, Shapiro SD, et al. Mechanical ventilation with or without daily changes of in-line suction catheters. Am J Respir Crit Care Med 1997;156(2 pt 1):466-472.

A randomized trial comparing daily versus as-needed in-line suction catheter change. This study demonstrated that the rate of ventilator-associated pneumonia and hospital mortality was not different between the two groups and that an "as-needed" approach was highly cost-effective. This provides good evidence that routine changes of in-line suction catheters are not necessary.

Meade MO, Granton JT, Matte-Martyn A, et al: A randomized trial of inhaled nitric oxide to prevent ischemia-reperfusion injury after lung transplantation. Am J Respir Crit Care Med 2003;167:1483-1489.

A small randomized, placebo-controlled trial that did not demonstrate a protective effect of inhaled nitric oxide therapy on the risk of developing ischemia-reperfusion injury after a lung transplantation when given soon after reperfusion of the transplanted lung.

Ntoumenopoulos G, Presneill JJ, McElholum M, Cade JF: Chest physiotherapy for the prevention of ventilator-associated pneumonia. Intensive Care Med 2002;28:850-856.

A small prospective clinical trial examined the benefit of a common adjunctive respiratory therapy—chest physiotherapy—on a common clinical complication of mechanical ventilation—ventilator-associated pneumonia (VAP). In this study, routine, twice-daily chest physiotherapy was associated with a lower occurrence of VAP compared with standard therapy, supporting its role as a simple preventive measure for VAP.

Chapter 72

INDICATIONS FOR AND MANAGEMENT OF TRACHEOSTOMY

Bradley D. Freeman • Timothy G. Buchman

KEY POINTS

1. Patients requiring prolonged mechanical ventilation should undergo tracheostomy in an effort to facilitate ventilator weaning, diminish the incidence of infectious complications, promote oral hygiene and pulmonary toilet, enhance patient comfort, provide airway security, and, in selected patients, allow oral nutrition and speech.

2. The presence of a "difficult airway" in a patient requiring prolonged mechanical ventilation is an absolute indication for tracheostomy.

3. The optimal timing of tracheostomy for most patients remains debated. General guidelines for timing of tracheostomy are as follows. For patients in whom the need for ventilatory support is anticipated to be less than 10 days, translaryngeal intubation is preferred. If the need for ventilatory support is anticipated to exceed 21 days, a tracheostomy is preferred. When the anticipated need for mechanical ventilation is unclear, daily assessment is required to determine when conversion to tracheostomy is indicated.

4. For appropriately selected patients, there may be advantages of percutaneous dilational tracheostomy compared with conventional surgical tracheostomies. These include cost savings, a lower incidence of selected perioperative and postoperative complications, and ease of performance. Percutaneous dilational tracheostomy should not be used on an emergent basis.

5. A variety of tracheostomy tube designs are commercially available, including cuffed tracheostomy tubes, cuffless tracheostomy tubes, fenestrated tracheostomy tubes, and metal tracheostomy tubes. Intensivists should have a working knowledge of the indications and rationales for these standard tracheostomy tube designs.

6. Tracheostomy cuff pressures should be monitored on a regular basis to prevent cuff-related complications such as tracheomalacia and tracheal stenosis.

7. Before tracheostomy tube removal (or decannulation), the patient should have tolerated liberation from mechanical ventilation for at least 24 to 48 hours and should be able to breathe without difficulty with an occluded and deflated tracheostomy tube in place. Inability to do this may indicate the presence of tracheal stenosis. Such patients should undergo further evaluation before decannulation.

8. Intensivists should be able to recognize and manage complications associated with tracheostomy use. These include cuff leak, tracheostomy tube occlusion, tracheostomy tube dislodgment, and tracheoinnominate artery fistula formation.

Tracheostomy is one of the most commonly performed surgical procedures in critically ill patients requiring prolonged mechanical ventilation.[1] Although a large body of literature has accumulated in recent years regarding benefits, risks, and technical aspects of this procedure, little consensus exists as to what constitutes optimal tracheostomy practice in the critically ill patient.[2] It is our goal in this chapter to review basic aspects of tracheostomy management in the intensive care setting, particularly focusing on indications, timing, techniques, and management of complications.

INDICATIONS FOR TRACHEOSTOMY

The presence of a "difficult airway" in a patient requiring prolonged mechanical ventilation is an absolute indication for tracheostomy. Patients with "difficult airways" include those with conditions such as significant maxillofacial trauma, angioedema, obstructing upper airway tumors, or other anatomic characteristics that would render translaryngeal intubation technically difficult to perform in the event of inadvertent airway loss. As a group, patients with difficult airways represent a small fraction of all patients undergoing tracheostomy in most ICUs. More commonly, patients requiring prolonged mechanical ventilation undergo this procedure in an effort to facilitate ventilator weaning, diminish the incidence of infectious complications, promote oral hygiene and pulmonary toilet, enhance patient comfort, provide airway security, and, in selected patients, allow oral nutrition and speech.[3] In most circumstances, tracheostomy is performed in an elective fashion. Accordingly, before undergoing this procedure, patients should be clinically optimized (e.g., minimal ventilatory support ($FiO_2 < 50\%$, positive end-expiratory pressure < 7.5 cm H_2O), hemodynamically stable, and have correction of metabolic and hemostatic derangements. Because many of the benefits of tracheostomy relative to prolonged translaryngeal intubation are either unproven or subjective, unambiguous criteria for selecting patients for tracheostomy are lacking.

TIMING OF TRACHEOSTOMY IN ACUTE RESPIRATORY FAILURE

In the formative era of critical care medicine, endotracheal tubes were composed of relatively inflexible material and used a low-volume, high-pressure cuff. Consequently, tracheostomy was performed "early"—within 48 hours of initiating mechanical ventilation—in an effort to minimize laryngeal injury resulting from translaryngeal intubation.[4] With advances in material sciences leading to the manufacture of less rigid endotracheal tubes, the trauma associated with prolonged translaryngeal intubation appeared to lessen.[4] Furthermore, a prospective study conducted by Stauffer and coworkers to examine risks associated with tracheostomy suggested a high rate of morbidity (e.g., stomal hemorrhage and infection rates exceeding 30%, rates of tracheal stenosis exceeding 50%) and mortality (e.g., 4%) accompanied this procedure.[5] Accordingly, enthusiasm for the routine performance of tracheostomy diminished. With refinement in tracheostomy techniques, perioperative complication rates associated with this procedure diminished. In addition, subsequent studies attempting to establish the relationship between prolonged translaryngeal intubation, prolonged tracheostomy, and laryngotracheal damage have been conflicting.[4] At present no data clearly establish that translaryngeal intubation should be limited to any specific duration or that tracheostomy should be performed at any specific point in a patient's course in an effort either to limit chronic laryngeal dysfunction or minimize tracheal injury.

While early studies focused on the risks and adverse consequences associated with tracheostomy, more recent clinical investigations have centered on the potential benefits associated with timing of tracheostomy, particularly with respect to the development of infectious complications, duration of mechanical ventilation, and other measures of resource expenditure (Table 72-1). There is no consensus as to what constitutes "early" and "late" tracheostomy. Rodriguez and coworkers assigned 106 patients who developed acute respiratory failure after major trauma to either undergoing tracheostomy within 7 days of ICU admission ("early" tracheostomy) or to undergoing tracheostomy at least 8 days after ICU admission ("late" tracheostomy). Compared with patients undergoing "late" tracheostomy, patients in the "early" tracheostomy group had a trend toward a lower incidence of pneumonia, as well as significant reductions in duration of mechanical ventilation, ICU length of stay, and hospital length of stay. The reported morbidity associated with performance of tracheostomy in this study was 4%.[6] Likewise, Lesnik and associates reported a retrospective analysis of 101 patients who developed acute respiratory failure after blunt trauma, comparing patients who underwent "early" tracheostomy creation (within 4 days of ICU admission) to "late" tracheostomy creation (more than 4 days after ICU admission). Compared with patients undergoing "late" tracheostomy creation, patients having tracheostomy established early had a significantly shorter duration of mechanical ventilation and lower incidence of pneumonia.[7] Finally, Brook and coworkers performed a prospective cohort study of patients requiring prolonged mechanical ventilation and reported that "early" tracheostomy (performed within 10 days of intubation) was associated with significant reductions in duration of mechanical ventilation, shorter ICU length of stay, and lower hospital costs.[8] In contrast, Blot and associates reported that neutropenic patients developing acute respiratory failure who underwent "early" tracheostomy (within 48 hours of intubation) had longer duration of mechanical ventilation and longer hospital length of stay than did patients who either underwent tracheostomy formation after 7 days or not at all.[9] Given the conflicting results, variability in study quality, heterogeneity in populations enrolled, and inconsistency in endpoints studied, it is difficult to draw on the conclusions of these and similar studies to ascertain the optimal timing of tracheostomy creation.[10,11]

TABLE 72–1. EFFECT OF TRACHEOSTOMY TIMING ON INFECTIOUS COMPLICATIONS AND MEASURES OF RESOURCE UTILIZATION

Authors	Design	Population	Tracheostomy Timing	Outcome
Rodriguez, et al.[6]	Prospective, nonrandomized	Multiple trauma (n = 106)	< 7 days vs. > 8 days after ICU admission	Trend towards decreased incidence of pneumonia Decreased duration of MV, ICU LOS, hospital LOS ($P < .05$).
Lesnik, et al.[7]	Retrospective	Multiple trauma (n = 111)	< 4 days vs. > 4 days after ICU admission	Trend towards decreased incidence of pneumonia Decreased duration of MV ($P < .001$)
Dunham, et al.[11]	Prospective, randomized	Multiple trauma (n = 74)	< 4 days vs. > 14 days after initiation of MV or no tracheostomy	No difference in incidence of laryngotracheal trauma or infectious complications
Blot, et al.[9]	Retrospective	Neutropenia (n = 53)	<2 days vs. > 7 days after initiation of MV or not at all	No difference in incidence of pneumonia or death Increased duration of MV and hospital LOS in early tracheostomy group ($P < .05$)
Brook, et al.[8]	Prospective, observational	Medical intensive care unit population (n = 90)	< 10 days vs. > 10 days after initiation of MV	Decreased duration of MV and ICU LOS in early tracheostomy group ($P < .05$)

MV, mechanical ventilation; LOS, length of stay.

There are several reasons why a tracheostomy may facilitate weaning from mechanical ventilation.[4] Resistance to airflow in an artificial airway is proportional to air turbulence, tube diameter, and tube length. Air turbulence is increased in the presence of extrinsic compression and inspissated secretions.[4] Because of its rigid design, shorter length, and removable inner cannula (to allow for evacuation of secretions), airflow resistance and associated work of breathing should theoretically be less with tracheostomies relative to endotracheal tubes. This, however, has not been demonstrated clinically. Furthermore, the presence of a tracheostomy may allow clinicians to be more aggressive about weaning patients from mechanical ventilation. Specifically, if a patient with a tracheostomy tube in place does not tolerate liberation from mechanical ventilation, he or she may be reconnected to the ventilator without difficulty. In contrast, if a patient who is translaryngeally intubated does not tolerate extubation, he or she must be sedated and re-intubated. This might represent a potential barrier to extubation in patients who are of a marginal pulmonary status. Finally, efforts to determine the relative advantages of tracheostomy and translaryngeal intubation with respect to aspiration are inconclusive.[12] However, if the presence of a tracheostomy does translate into earlier liberation from mechanical ventilation, one might expect the incidence of ventilator-associated pneumonia in this group to be lower.

A clinical study that adequately addresses the question as to optimal timing of tracheostomy in the setting of prolonged mechanical ventilation must have a homogeneous patient population, protocols in place for ventilator weaning and other facets of clinical management, and well-defined endpoints. Given the lack of evidence on which to base decision-making on this issue, the following guidelines have been formulated by a consensus conference of the American College of Chest Physicians[3]:

- For patients in whom the need for ventilatory support is anticipated to be less than 10 days, translaryngeal intubation is preferred.
- If the need for ventilatory support is anticipated to exceed 21 days, a tracheostomy is preferred.
- When the anticipated need for mechanical ventilation is unclear, daily assessment is required to determine when conversion to tracheostomy is indicated.

Once the decision to proceed with tracheostomy has been made, patients should undergo this procedure as quickly as practical to limit the duration of the translaryngeal airway.[13]

METHODOLOGY—SURGICAL VERSUS PERCUTANEOUS DILATIONAL TRACHEOSTOMY

Traditionally, tracheostomies have been performed in the operating room using standard surgical principles.[14] In 1985, Ciaglia and colleagues described percutaneous dilational tracheostomy (PDT) in which tracheostomy is accomplished via a modified Seldinger technique, typically with the aid of bronchoscopy.[15] Percutaneous dilational tracheostomy has subsequently gained wide acceptance and has become the predominant method of tracheostomy creation in many centers.[16-18] The technical aspects of percutaneous dilational tracheostomy are covered elsewhere in this text (see Chapter 219). In this section we discuss the potential benefits, indications, and limitations of this approach.

There are several potential advantages of PDT relative to surgically created tracheostomies (SCT). PDT may be performed at the bedside and thus avoids the inconvenience and risk of transporting a critically ill patient, as well as the expense of utilizing operating room resources. In a prospective randomized study comparing PDT and SCT, Freeman and associates found that PDT was associated with a reduction of approximately $1500 in patient charges per procedure.[19] Other investigators have reported comparable findings.[20,21] In addition, whereas studies comparing PDT and SCT vary with respect to quality and endpoints measured (Table 72-2),[21-29] a meta-analysis of prospective trials comparing PDT with SCT suggests that PDT may be associated with fewer complications, specifically postprocedure bleeding and peristomal infection (Fig. 72-1).[23] This may reflect that there is minimal deadspace between the tracheostomy tube and adjacent pretracheal tissues after PDT, which may have a tamponading effect on minor bleeding and serve as a barrier to infection.[23] Finally, PDT is relatively simple to learn. Individuals who have not received formal surgical training may become facile with this procedure and perform it safely and effectively.[12,17]

TABLE 72–2. SELECTED STUDIES COMPARING PERCUTANEOUS DILATIONAL TRACHEOSTOMY (PDT) AND SURGICALLY CREATED TRACHEOSTOMIES (SCT)

Authors	Design	Size (SCT/PDT)	Outcome
Crofts, et al.[22]	Prospective, randomized	28/25	No difference in complication rates comparing SCT and PDT
Freeman, et al.[19]	Prospective, randomized	40/40	PDT performed more quickly and associated with decreased patient charges
Friedman, et al.[24]	Prospective, randomized	26/27	PDT performed more quickly and associated with fewer postprocedural complications
Griggs, et al.[25]	Prospective, nonrandomized	153/74	SCT associated with higher perioperative complication rate
Gysin, et al.[26]	Prospective, randomized	35/35	Complication rate similar comparing techniques
Hazard, et al.[27]	Prospective, randomized	24/22	SCT associated with higher perioperative and postoperative complication rate
Heikkinen, et al.[21]	Prospective, randomized	30/26	PDT associated with lower costs but comparable complication rate
Holdgaard, et al.[28]	Prospective, randomized	30/30	PDT performed more quickly and associated with lower perioperative and postoperative complication rate
Porter, et al.[29]	Prospective, randomized	12/12	PDT performed more quickly; similar complication rate comparing techniques

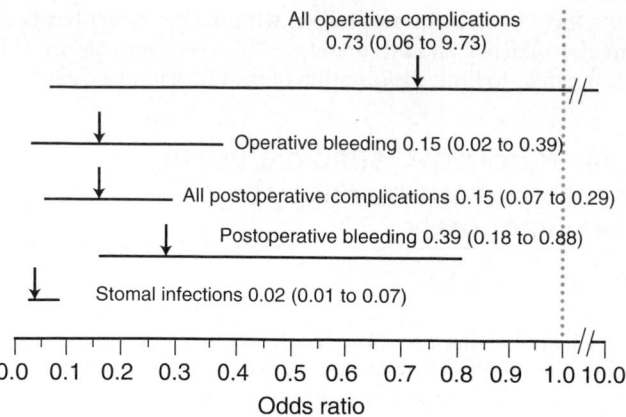

FIGURE 72–1. Rate of complications comparing surgically created tracheotomies (SCT) and percutaneous dilational tracheotomies (PDT). Odds ratios with 95% confidence intervals (represented by *arrows* and *horizontal bars,* respectively) for operative and postoperative complications comparing these two techniques. An odds ratio of 1.0 *(dashed line)* indicates no difference in complication rates comparing these procedures, an odds ratio less than 1 suggests a lower complication rate with PDT, and an odds ratio of greater than 1 suggests a lower complication rate with SCT. There was no difference comparing these two techniques with respect to overall operative complication rates (OR with 95% CI 0.73 [0.06 to 9.37]). However, relative to SCT, PDT was associated with less perioperative bleeding (0.15 [0.02 to 0.39]), a lower overall postoperative complication rate (0.15 [0.07 to 0.29]), as well as a lower postoperative incidence of bleeding (0.39 [0.18 to 0.88]), and stomal infection (0.02 [0.01 to 0.07]). This may reflect that there is minimal deadspace between the tracheostomy tube and adjacent pretracheal tissues after PDT, which may have a tamponading effect on minor bleeding and serve as a barrier to infection. (Used with permission from Freeman BD, Isabella K, Lin N, Buchman TG: A meta-analysis of prospective trials comparing percutaneous and surgical tracheostomy in critically ill patients. Chest 2000;118:1412-1418.)

Patient selection is essential to achieving satisfactory results with PDT. Candidates for PDT should be on low levels of ventilatory support (i.e., $FIO_2 < 50\%$, PEEP < 7.5 cm H_2O), have an intact coagulation system (international normalized ratio and platelet counts correctable to less than 1.3 and greater than $100,000/mm^3$, respectively), and have suitable neck anatomy such that external landmarks (cricoid cartilage, trachea, and sternal notch) are easily palpable with the neck fully extended. PDT is contraindicated in patients who are sufficiently obese so as to make identification of these landmarks difficult as well as in patients with unstable cervical spines precluding neck extension. Likewise, PDT is contraindicated in patients with "difficult airways," such as patients with maxillofacial trauma, glottic edema, poorly visualized vocal cords, or any condition that would make it difficult to reestablish translaryngeal intubation in the event of airway loss. Finally, PDT is an elective procedure and should not be used to establish an emergent airway.

Although there are many potential advantages of PDT, this procedure has been associated with a significant number of highly morbid complications, many of which, such as pretracheal insertion, tracheal laceration, esophageal perforation, pneumothorax, and loss of airway, are unusual in surgically created tracheostomies.[30-35] Accordingly, whereas PDT may be performed competently by those not trained in surgical techniques, persons who are expert at surgical airway management should be immediately available in the event complications arise.[12]

SELECTION, MAINTENANCE, AND CARE OF TRACHEOSTOMY TUBES

TRACHEOSTOMY TUBE SELECTION

While a detailed discussion of the various types and designs of tracheostomy tubes is beyond the scope of this text,[36,37] a working knowledge of tracheostomy tube features is essential to the competent care of patients who have undergone placement of these devices (Fig. 72-2). Briefly, most tracheostomy tubes are manufactured from polyvinyl chloride, silicone, a combination of these materials, or metal. They are available in either single-lumen (no removable inner cannula) or dual-lumen (removable inner cannula) configurations. The purpose of the removable inner cannula is to facilitate cleaning of inspissated secretions that may lead to tube occlusion. Because silicone is relatively secretion resistant, tubes manufactured from this material frequently do not have an inner cannula. Tracheostomy tubes are available with and without cuffs (the internal balloon surrounding the outer cannula). The purpose of the cuff is to maintain a seal between the tube and the trachea sufficient to prevent escape of air from around the tracheostomy tube during mechanical ventilation (e.g., cuff leak). Furthermore, the cuff minimizes but does not prevent aspiration. Tracheostomy tubes with foam cuffs conform to a patient's trachea and remain consistently inflated at low pressure. These tubes are indicated in patients who have sustained damage from excessive cuff pressure (e.g., tracheomalacia). Once a cuffed tracheostomy tube is no longer required, that is, the patient no longer requires mechanical ventilatory support and is not considered an aspiration risk, the cuffed tube is exchanged for a cuffless tube. Tracheostomy caps are generally provided with tracheostomy tubes for use in the decannulation process, as noted later. Fenestrated tubes are used to promote speech and are generally used in individuals who tolerate liberation from mechanical ventilation for varying periods. Fenestrated tubes have an opening or openings on their superior aspect such that when the inner cannula is removed, the cuff deflated, and the external orifice occluded (e.g., with a Passey-Muir type valve), air can pass the vocal cords allowing phonation.

EXCHANGING TRACHEOSTOMY TUBES

In general, tracheostomy tubes should be changed because of malfunction (e.g., pilot balloon rupture), inspissated secretions compromising luminal diameter, or when another tracheostomy tube design is desired.[38] We believe that "routine" changing of a tracheostomy tube (e.g., every 7 days) is neither indicated nor supported by available literature. Changing a tracheostomy tube is not a benign procedure, is frequently uncomfortable for the patient, and may be complicated by the inability to insert the replacement tube or by insertion of the replacement tube into a false passage in the pretracheal space. If indicated, it is desirable to postpone the initial tracheostomy tube exchange for at least 1 week after creation of the tracheostomy to allow the surgical track to sufficiently mature.

To accomplish tracheostomy tube exchange, the replacement tube should have the pilot balloon tested to ensure that there are no leaks. The tube should be lubricated with either sterile water or a small amount of water-soluble lubricant and inserted over a semi-rigid rubber catheter (e.g., a Robnel) or a

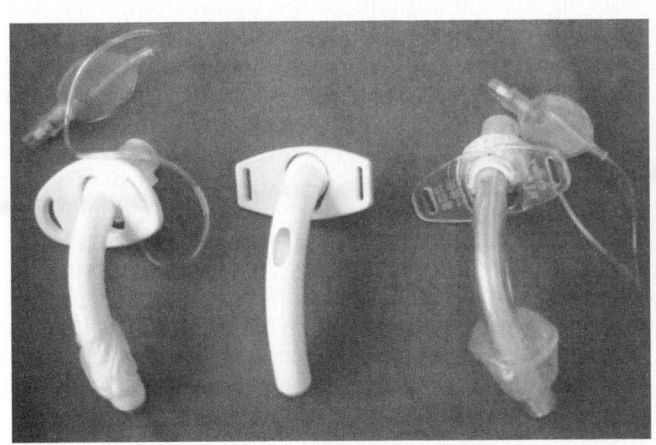

A

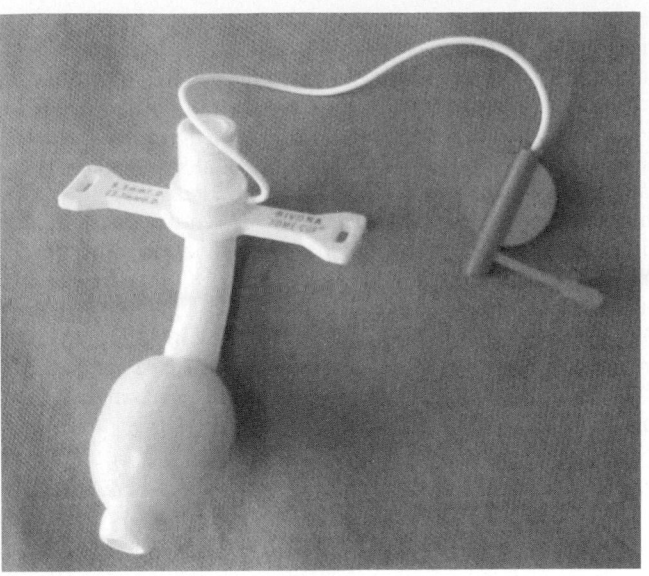

B

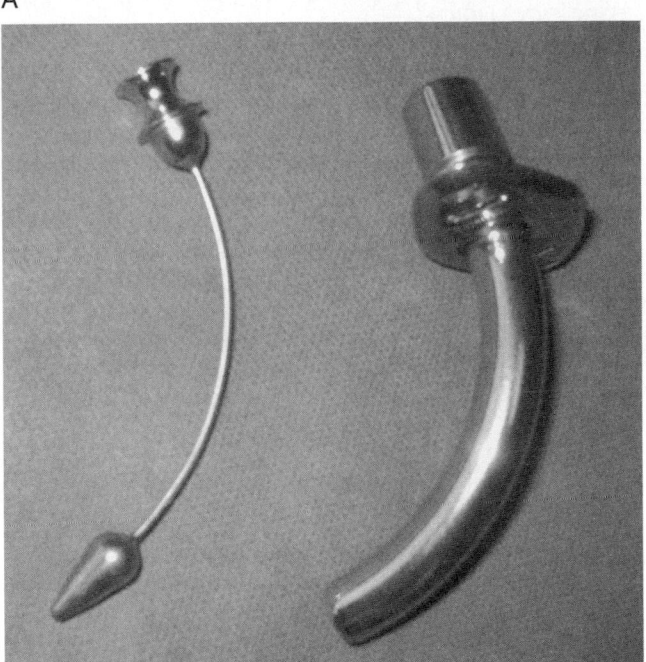

C

FIGURE 72–2. Standard tracheostomy tube designs. **A,** Pictured left to right are a standard cuffed tracheostomy tube, a cuffless fenestrated tube, and a cuffed tracheostomy tube with elongated "limbs" (portion of tube proximal and distal to curvature) to accommodate patients with variant neck anatomy. **B,** Tracheostomy tube with a foam cuff. These tubes are designed to provide a large-volume, low-pressure cuff and are particularly suited to patients with tracheomalacia or in patients who have sustained complications from tracheostomy tube or endotracheal tube cuffs. **C,** Cuffless metal tracheostomy tubes (shown with obturator on the left) are useful for decannulation or in patients who require a tracheostomy but without need for a cuff.

suctioning catheter to lessen the likelihood that the tracheostomy tube is inserted into a false passage. Gentle dilatation of the tracheostomy tract may be useful when exchanging a tracheostomy that has been placed by percutaneous technique.

MONITORING CUFF INFLATION PRESSURE

Tracheostomy tube cuffs require monitoring to maintain an inflation pressure of 20 to 25 mm Hg. Assuming that a tracheostomy tube is of appropriate size, an insufficiently inflated cuff may both result in a sizable amount of air leaking around the cuff ("cuff leak"), rendering mechanical ventilation difficult as well as providing poor protection against aspiration. Alternatively, excessive cuff pressures (exceeding 25 mm Hg) may result in compression of mucosal capillaries,

giving rise to mucosal ischemia and attendant complications such as tracheomalacia and tracheal stenosis. The most reliable method of monitoring cuff inflation pressure is through direct measurement. Maneuvers such as pilot balloon palpation to estimate cuff pressure or inflation of the cuff until end-inspiratory leaks are extinguished during positive-pressure ventilation are not recommended because of their inaccuracy.[38] Tracheal cuff inflation pressures should be measured and recorded on a regular basis for purposes of quality assurance.

ORAL NUTRITION

The presence of a tracheostomy both provides opportunity for oral nutrition in the mechanically ventilated patient with its attendant psychological benefits and complicates alimentation because of the interference of the tracheostomy tube with mechanisms of normal swallowing and airway control.[38] The presence of a tracheostomy inhibits physiologic upward movement of the larynx during deglutition, hinders glottic closure, and produces dysphagia due to mechanical compression of the esophagus. Furthermore, an inflated tracheostomy balloon does not protect from aspiration. Patients with tracheostomies who are candidates for oral nutrition should mentate normally, have adequate oxygenation with low inspired oxygen concentrations (e.g., 30% FiO_2), and possess sufficient ventilatory reserve such that they can physiologically tolerate an episode of aspiration during the introduction of oral feeding. Ideally, a speech therapist should assess aspiration risk before institution of an oral diet. Initial efforts at feeding should be carefully supervised.

DECANNULATION

Patients who remain stable for 24 to 48 hours after discontinuation of mechanical ventilation may be evaluated for decannulation. The patient's ability to protect the airway should be assessed for 24 hours by deflating the tracheostomy tube balloon and observing for signs of aspiration. If aspiration is present, laryngoscopic examination should be performed. Airway strictures and adequacy of the native airway can be assessed by deflating the tracheostomy tube balloon and occluding the tracheostomy tube. Patients who are able to breathe around a capped and deflated No. 8 tracheostomy tube most likely have adequate respiratory reserve and a sufficiently preserved native airway to tolerate decannulation. Patients who have difficulty breathing around a capped No. 8 tube should be reassessed with a capped No. 7 tracheostomy tube. Successful breathing with a capped and deflated No. 7 tube in place suggests that a patient will tolerate decannulation. Patients who fail breathing trials with capped tracheostomy tubes should undergo laryngoscopic evaluation to exclude the presence of tracheal stenosis. Many patients recovering from long-term mechanical ventilatory support may have normal airways but fail breathing around a capped No. 7 or No. 8 tracheostomy tube because of limited ventilatory reserve (e.g., neuromuscular disease or underlying chronic obstructive pulmonary disease). These patients may benefit from "downsizing" of the tracheostomy stoma using progressively smaller cuffless tracheostomy tubes with intermittent capping using stomal obturators. Tracheostomy tubes with foam cuffs should not be used for decannulation trials because these cuffs spontaneously reinflate, making the assessment of airway stenosis difficult.

COMPLICATIONS

A variety of complications resulting from tracheostomy placement have been described. A brief discussion of the more common complications occurring in the critical care setting and their management follows.

CUFF LEAKS

Cuff leak is a commonly encountered problem in patients with tracheostomies and may be manifest by either an audible leak around the tracheostomy tube or loss of returned volume in mechanically ventilated breaths. A mechanical problem with the tracheostomy tube should first be excluded

by determining that when the cuff is inflated it does not leak air. A malfunctioning tracheostomy tube requires exchange (see earlier). Once tracheostomy tube malfunction is excluded, the most common cause of cuff leak is tracheomalacia with resulting dilation adjacent to the tracheostomy tube cuff. This is particularly common in patients who have been maintained on mechanical ventilation for extended periods. It should *not* be treated by hyperinflating the tracheostomy tube cuff in an effort to achieve total occlusion, in that this will result in further dilation of the trachea and may lead to mucosal ischemia. If the cuff leak is well tolerated, such that the ability to ventilate the patient is not compromised, we recommend maintaining the tracheostomy tube in place at the appropriate inflation pressure (e.g., 20 to 25 mm Hg). Conversely, if the cuff leak is sufficient so as to impair gas exchange, consideration should be given to exchanging the tracheostomy tube for either a larger size or for a tracheostomy tube design that incorporates a large-volume, low-pressure cuff (e.g., a foam-cuffed tracheostomy tube).

TUBE OCCLUSION

A second frequently encountered problem in patients with tracheostomies is tracheostomy occlusion. This is typically manifest by either high airway pressures or inability to pass a suctioning catheter. Tracheostomy tube occlusion is frequently the result of inspissated secretions. Many commonly used tube designs have a removable inner cannula to facilitate cleaning of the inner portion of the tracheostomy tube. A second common cause of tracheostomy tube occlusion is tube malpositioning, such that the end of the tracheostomy tube abuts the tracheal wall or the tube has migrated such that its tip resides in the pretracheal tissues. If tracheostomy malpositioning is suspected, the operating surgeon should assist in assessing it for either reinsertion or use of another tube design.

TUBE DISLODGMENT

Although dislodgment of the tracheostomy tube may occur at any time after tracheostomy placement, this complication is most problematic in the immediate postoperative period, before the tracheostomy tract has matured.[39] Factors predisposing to tracheostomy tube dislodgment include an inadequately secured tube, excessive coughing, and patient agitation. Tracheostomy tube dislodgment should be suspected when a patient is able to speak immediately after tracheostomy placement, the airway becomes obstructed, or respiratory distress develops. Because it is generally technically difficult to reinsert the tracheostomy tube in this situation, the authors recommend that the airway be reestablished by means of translaryngeal intubation. The tracheostomy should then be reinserted in the operating room with appropriate anesthetic assistance, lighting, and instrumentation. If tracheostomy tube dislodgment occurs once the tracheostomy track is sufficiently mature (i.e., the tracheostomy track is at least 1 week old), it is generally technically feasible to reinsert the tracheostomy tube at the patient's bedside as noted above (see Exchanging Tracheostomy Tubes, earlier).

TRACHEOESOPHAGEAL FISTULA

The development of tracheoesophageal fistulas after tracheostomy is rare, occurring in fewer than 1% of patients, and is typically the result of pressure necrosis of the tracheal and esophageal mucosa from the tracheostomy cuff. A number of potential risk factors have been reported (e.g., high airway pressures, excessive cuff inflation pressures, the use of nasogastric tubes, excessive tracheostomy tube movement). Clinical manifestations are nonspecific and include excessive tracheal secretions, coughing, and gastric distention. The presence of a tracheoesophageal fistula can be demonstrated on fiberoptic examination after removal or retraction of the tracheostomy tube. Because the use of fiberoptic examination alone is insensitive, it should be combined with an enterally contrasted esophageal evaluation if clinical suspicion exists (e.g., water-soluble contrast swallow or computed tomography). Tracheoesophageal fistula requires surgical repair. Temporizing measures include positioning of an endotracheal tube cuff below the level of the fistula to limit aspiration, removal of nasogastric tubes, and placement of feeding gastrostomy tubes.[40]

TRACHEOINNOMINATE ARTERY FISTULA

Tracheoinnominate artery fistula likewise is a rare complication after tracheostomy formation and theoretically results from pressure necrosis or injury to the trachea adjacent to the course of the innominate artery.[39] A number of risk factors have been postulated, including excessive tube movement, aberrant innominate artery anatomy, use of an excessively long or curved tracheostomy tube that erodes through the tracheal wall, inferior positioning of the tracheostomy tube, tracheal infection, and corticosteroid therapy.[39] Tracheoinnominate artery fistula may become apparent as quickly as a few days or as late as several months after tracheostomy placement. The classic presentation is of a "sentinel hemorrhage" in which a large volume of blood emanates from the tracheostomy tube. Fiberoptic examination to evaluate for the presence of tracheoinnominate artery fistula should be performed in the operating room in the event that airway manipulation results in massive hemorrhage. Temporizing measures in patients who develop massive bleeding include hyperinflation of the tracheostomy cuff, insertion of an endotracheal tube through the tracheostomy stoma in an effort to tamponade bleeding, or translaryngeal intubation and digital compression of the bleeding site through the tracheostomy stoma. Definitive repair entails median sternotomy ligation of the innominate artery and generous drainage of the mediastinum.

ANNOTATED REFERENCES

Ciaglia P, Firsching R, Syniec C: Elective percutaneous dilational tracheostomy. Chest 1985;87:715-719.
One of the first articles to describe the technique of percutaneous dilational tracheostomy.

Consensus conference on artificial airways in patients receiving mechanical ventilation. Chest 1989;96:178-180.
The consensus recommendations regarding timing of tracheostomy form the basis of current practice for many intensivists.

Freeman BD, Isabella K, Cobb JP, et al: A prospective, randomized study comparing percutaneous with surgical tracheostomy in critically ill patients. Crit Care Med 2001;29:926-930.
A prospective study examining the cost-effectiveness of percutaneous dilational tracheostomies relative to surgically created tracheostomies in critically ill patients.

Freeman BD, Isabella K, Lin N, Buchman TG: A meta-analysis of prospective trials comparing percutaneous and surgical tracheostomy in critically ill patients. Chest 2000;118:1412-1418.
A meta-analysis of the relative risks and benefits of percutaneous dilational tracheostomies compared with tracheostomies performed by conventional surgical techniques.

Heffner JE, Hess D: Tracheostomy management in the chronically ventilated patient. Clin Chest Med 2001;22:55-69.
An excellent and practical review of virtually all facets of tracheostomy care.

Chapter 73

HYPERBARIC OXYGEN IN CRITICAL CARE

Stephen R. Thom

KEY POINTS

1. **Advances in research have led to identification of several therapeutic mechanisms of action** for hyperbaric oxygen therapy that stem from two fundamental effects: hyperoxygenation of perfused tissues and reduction of gas bubble volume.

2. **Safe treatment of critically ill patients** can be accomplished in either one-man, "monoplace" or larger, multiple-person hyperbaric chambers.

3. **Efficacy of hyperbaric oxygen therapy** has been documented by randomized clinical trials for a heterogeneous group of disorders.

Hyperbaric oxygen (HBO_2) treatment involves intermittent breathing of pure oxygen at greater than ambient pressure. There has been a progressive increase in interest with this treatment modality since the 1960s, when investigational treatment of clostridial myonecrosis (gas gangrene) suggested that HBO_2 may have applications in addition to treatment of gas bubble diseases, such as air embolism and decompression sickness.[1] Over the past 20 years HBO_2 has undergone a refinement, with clarification of mechanisms of action and clinical applications. Along with an expansion of the knowledge base, formalized education now exists for emergency, critical care/anesthesia, and surgically trained physicians, who may obtain special competency board certification through the American Board of Medical Specialists. This chapter will summarize existing literature on uses for hyperbaric oxygen therapy and some special issues related to care of critically ill patients.

APPLICATIONS

HBO_2 treatment is carried out in either a monoplace (single person) or multiplace (typically 2 to 14 patients) chamber. Pressures applied while in the chamber are usually 2 to 3 atmospheres absolute (ATA), the sum of the atmospheric pressure plus additional hydrostatic pressure equivalent to one or two atmospheres. Treatments usually are for 2 to 8 hours, depending on the indication, and may be performed from one to three times daily. Monoplace chambers are usually compressed with pure oxygen. Multiplace chambers are pressurized with air, and patients breathe pure oxygen through a tight-fitting facemask, a hood, or endotracheal tube. During treatment, the PaO_2 typically exceeds 2000 mm Hg and levels of 200 to 400 mm Hg occur in tissues.[2]

HBO_2 should be viewed as a drug and the hyperbaric chamber as a dosing device. Elevating tissue oxygen tension is a primary effect. Although this may alleviate physiologic stress to hypoxic tissues, lasting benefits of HBO_2 must relate to abatement of underlying pathophysiologic processes. The accepted indications[3] comprise a heterogeneous group of disorders (Table 73-1), thus implying that there are several mechanisms of action (Table 73-2).[4-21]

ARTERIAL GAS EMBOLISM (AGE) AND DECOMPRESSION SICKNESS (DCS)

Among the earliest applications of hyperbaric therapy was to treat disorders related to gas bubbles in the body. Compressed air construction work required exposure to elevated ambient pressure within compartments (caissons) for many hours to excavate tunnels or bridge foundations in muddy soil that otherwise would flood. In the 19th century, workers were noted to frequently experience joint pains, limb paralysis, or pulmonary compromise when they returned to ambient pressure. This condition—DCS, caisson disease, or bends—was later attributed to nitrogen bubbles in the body, and recompression was found to relieve symptoms.[22] The mechanism, based purely on Boyle's law with reduction of gas bubble volume due to pressure, was later improved by adding supplemental oxygen to hasten inert gas diffusion out of the body. Similar observations were made at later times for scuba divers, who are also prone to develop AGE due to pulmonary overpressurization on decompression.

Iatrogenic AGE has been reported in association with cardiovascular, obstetric/gynecologic, neurosurgical, and

TABLE 73–1. ACCEPTED INDICATIONS FOR HYPERBARIC OXYGEN THERAPY

- Air or gas embolism
- Carbon monoxide poisoning
- Clostridial myositis and myonecrosis
- Crush injury, compartment syndrome, acute traumatic ischemia
- Decompression sickness
- Enhancement of healing in selected wounds
- Exceptional blood loss anemia
- Necrotizing fasciitis
- Chronic refractory osteomyelitis
- Radiation necrosis
- Skin flap or graft compromise
- Thermal burns

From Hampson NB (ed): Hyperbaric Oxygen Therapy: Committee Report. Kensington, MD, Undersea and Hyperbaric Medical Society, 1999.

TABLE 73–2. MECHANISMS OF ACTION OF HYPERBARIC OXYGEN

Related to Hyperoxygenation of Tissues

- Angiogenesis in ischemic tissues[4-6] (mechanisms likely include O_2 behaving as intracellular signal transducer leading to augmentation of one or more growth factors[7-9])
- Bacteriostatic/bactericidal actions[10-12]
- Carboxyhemoglobin dissociation hastened[13]
- *Clostridium perfringens* α toxin synthesis inhibited[14,15]
- Phagocytic bacterial killing improved[16]
- Temporary inhibition of neutrophil β_2 integrin adhesion[17-19]
- Vasoconstriction[20,21]

Related to Pressurization

- Reduction of gas bubble volume (Boyle's law)

orthopedic procedures and generally whenever disruption of a vascular wall occurs. Nonsurgical processes reported to cause AGE include overexpansion during mechanical ventilation, hemodialysis, and after accidental opening of central venous catheters.

Treatment of gas bubble disorders includes standard support of airway, breathing, and circulation plus application of HBO_2. Recommendation is for referral as soon as possible, but even when treatments may be delayed for hours to days a trial of therapy is recommended. Gas bubbles have been reported to persist for several days, and many reports note success when HBO_2 is begun after long delays.[23-27] Controlled animal trials support efficacy of HBO_2, but randomized clinical trials have not been done.[28]

Mechanisms of action of HBO_2 in AGE and DCS treatment include the well-recognized reduction of gas volume to acutely reduce vascular compromise (Boyle's law), hyperoxygenation to hasten inert gas diffusion, and a hypothetical effect associated with leukocyte adherence to endothelium. Neutrophils have been implicated as exacerbating tissue injury in bubble-related disorders, presumably because of endothelial irritation that leads to perivascular adherence.[29,30] Animals depleted of leukocytes before experimental cerebral air embolism suffer less severe reduction of cerebral blood flow and better neurologic outcome.[31] A recent report demonstrated that efficacy of HBO_2 in a decompression sickness model was associated with inhibition of neutrophil β_2-integrin adhesion.[32] This action has been described in a number of animal models including skeletal muscle ischemia-reperfusion, cerebral ischemia-reperfusion, pulmonary smoke inhalation injury, and brain injury after carbon monoxide (CO) poisoning.[18,33-35] The mechanism appears to be related to impairment of cytoskeletal control of the adhesion molecules expressed on the cell surface, a process related to function of the membrane-bound guanylate cyclase.[17] The same mechanism has been described in human neutrophils, and exposure to HBO_2 has been shown to temporarily inhibit human β_2-integrin adhesion function.[19]

CARBON MONOXIDE POISONING

Carbon monoxide is the leading cause of injury and death by poisoning in the world.[36] The affinity of CO for hemoglobin, to form carboxyhemoglobin (COHb), is more than 200-fold greater than that of O_2. CO-mediated hypoxic stress is a primary insult, but COHb values correlate poorly with clinical outcome.[37-43] Therefore, alternative mechanisms to explain the toxicity of CO have been sought. Oxidative injury to brain after CO poisoning has been shown to occur in several animal models.[44,45] Excessive release of excitatory amino acids, such as glutamate, has been implicated as a component of CO-mediated brain injury.[46-48]

Survivors of acute CO poisoning are at risk for developing delayed neurologic sequelae (DNS) that include cognitive deficits, memory loss, dementia, parkinsonism, paralysis, chorea, cortical blindness, psychosis, personality changes, and peripheral neuropathy. DNS typically occur from 2 to 40 days after poisoning, and their incidence is from 25% to 50% after severe poisoning.

Administration of supplemental oxygen is the cornerstone of treatment of CO poisoning. Oxygen inhalation will hasten dissociation of CO from hemoglobin, as well as provide enhanced tissue oxygenation. HBO_2 causes carboxyhemoglobin dissociation to occur at a rate greater than that achievable by breathing pure oxygen at sea level.[12] Additionally, HBO_2, but not ambient pressure oxygen treatment, has several actions that have been demonstrated in animal models to be beneficial in ameliorating pathophysiologic events associated with central nervous system (CNS) injuries mediated by CO. These include an improvement in mitochondrial oxidative processes,[49] inhibition of lipid peroxidation,[50] and impairment of leukocyte adhesion to injured microvasculature.[18] Animals poisoned with CO and treated with HBO_2 have been found to have more rapid improvement in cardiovascular status,[51] lower mortality,[52] and lower incidence of neurologic sequelae.[53]

Five prospective, randomized trials have assessed clinical efficacy of HBO_2 for acute CO poisoning.[41-43,54,55] Several failed to find benefit,[41,55] but methodologic weaknesses as discussed by several authors[45,56] have diminished their clinical impact. The current consensus is that HBO_2 treatment significantly reduces the incidence of DNS and in retrospective comparisons appears to also diminish acute mortality.[56] As yet, however, there is no agreement among hyperbaric practitioners as to the length of delay from poisoning beyond which there is no chance for benefit from HBO_2.[57]

BLOOD LOSS ANEMIA

In rare instances when transfusion is not possible due to crossmatching incompatibilities or religious beliefs, intermittent use of HBO_2 has been applied to temporarily relieve physiologic stress from severe, acute anemia. Anecdotal reports describe using 2.5 to 3.0 ATA O_2 to raise PaO_2 in plasma to meet metabolic needs.[58-60] Treatments are often administered for only brief times, when physiologic decompensation occurs, because O_2 toxicity can be a problem (see later). Short-term treatments, applied many times over several days, have been used to support life until red cells become available or until adequate red cell mass is generated endogenously.

CLOSTRIDIAL MYONECROSIS (GAS GANGRENE)

Successful treatment of gas gangrene is highly dependent on prompt recognition and aggressive intervention. Mortality rates from 11% to 52% have been reported. There are four retrospective comparisons and 13 case series in the literature, and many were cited in a previous review.[2,61-65] Because of difficulties with comparison among patient groups, impartial assessment based on mortality or "tissue salvage" rates is difficult. Most authors comment on clinical benefit to treatment, and I share this opinion. Temporal improvement of vital signs in patients with gangrene can be among the most dramatic observations in day-to-day practice.

CRUSH INJURY

There is limited experience with HBO_2 for acute traumatic peripheral ischemia and suturing of severed limbs. A single randomized controlled trial (involving 36 patients) on this type of injury has been performed, which found HBO_2 to improve healing and reduce infection and wound dehiscence.[66] In a case series of 23 patients, HBO_2 was deemed to improve limb preservation and it was also observed that the change in transcutaneous tissue oxygen level from ambient to hyperbaric conditions may predict outcome.[67] The rationale for considering HBO_2 is to temporarily improve oxygenation to hypoperfused tissues and because arterial hyperoxia will cause vasoconstriction that can diminish edema formation.[20,21] This latter mechanism has been demonstrated most convincingly in the context of experimental compartment syndrome.[68]

PROGRESSIVE NECROTIZING INFECTIONS

The use of HBO_2 for treatment of necrotizing fasciitis and Fournier's gangrene, which are mixed aerobic-anaerobic infections, has been reported in six nonrandomized comparisons and three case series.[69-77] As with gas gangrene, variations in time of diagnosis and clinical status on admission compromise assessment of the existing literature. Riseman and coworkers reviewed their experience of 29 patients and found HBO_2 in addition to surgery and antibiotics reduced mortality versus surgery and antibiotics alone.[69] Most recently, Brown and associates reported a multicenter experience where 30 patients received HBO_2 and 24 received only surgery and antibiotics.[70] Although only a nonsignificant trend toward increased survival was seen in the HBO_2 group (30% with HBO_2 and 42% without), the authors state their support for continued use of HBO_2 because of apparent selection bias between groups. Animal trials have been difficult to assess, because synergistic bacterial processes are difficult to establish. One report has found HBO_2 to potentiate antibiotics in streptococcal myositis,[78] and several animal models of polymicrobial bacteremia and sepsis have reported increased survival with HBO_2.[79-81] Mechanisms of action may include suppressed growth of anaerobic microorganisms and improved bactericidal action of leukocytes (that function poorly in hypoxic conditions).[10-12,16]

THERMAL BURNS

Some burn centers employ adjunctive HBO_2 to severe burns, but as controversy persists this is not a universal practice. Animal models have documented benefits with HBO_2 in reducing partial to full-thickness skin loss, hastened epithelialization, and lower mortality.[2] Randomized clinical trials, albeit with small patient numbers, have reported improved rates of healing with shorter hospitalization stays and therefore reduced costs.[82-84] Uncontrolled series have also reported

efficacy, but some studies have failed to find benefit.[85-87] Rationale for treatment has been based on reducing tissue edema and increasing capillary angiogenesis. The latter mechanism has not been directly shown with thermal injuries but is a well-documented effect in chronic applications of HBO_2 for radiation injuries and microvascular deficient wounds as occur in many diabetics.[2,88-94]

CRITICAL CARE IN HYPERBARIC MEDICINE

Hyperbaric treatment centers typically have the ability to manage patients who require critical care support. This is accomplished with close cooperation among the treating physicians, nurses, and respiratory therapists and the presence of specialized equipment to manage and monitor the patients.

Plans for treatment begin while the patient is still in the ICU, before transport to the hyperbaric chamber is initiated. Issues to be addressed include informed consent, determination that all intravenous/arterial lines and nasogastric tubes/Foley catheters are secured, capping all unnecessary intravenous catheters, placing chest tubes to one-way Heimlich valves, and adequately sedating or paralyzing the patient as clinically indicated. During transport, emergency drugs for advanced life support resuscitation should be available.

The environment of the hyperbaric chamber imposes limitations on equipment, including space restrictions, fire codes, and the effect of pressure on equipment function. Electrical components of equipment are located outside the hyperbaric chamber. Cables penetrate the chamber bulkhead to make connection to the pneumatic portion of ventilators, internal cardiac pacer wires, electrocardiogram attachments, and arterial line transducers. The patient is attached to equipment at ambient pressure before treatment, and once the treatment pressure is achieved all settings are checked and transducers recalibrated. Among the items that must be checked is the cuff pressure of endotracheal tubes. The usual practice is to replace the air in these cuffs with an equivalent volume of sterile saline before treatment to avoid volume changes related to pressurization.

There are several intravenous infusion pumps that operate normally in the multiplace chamber environment. If glass bottles, pressure bags, or any other gas-filled equipment are used inside a hyperbaric chamber, they must be adequately vented and closely monitored during a treatment. IVAC Medsystem Infusion Pumps (IVAC Corporation, San Diego, CA) or the Abbott-Shaw Hyperbaric Pump are typically used with monoplace chamber operations. These pumps can remain on the outside of monoplace chambers and are capable of infusing despite the elevated pressure differential. The Abbott is a volumetric pump, so flow rate is a function of chamber pressure and must be closely monitored. The IVAC is a pulsatile pump and infusion volume is influenced by both the pump rate that is set and the drip chamber.

ADVERSE EFFECTS

HBO_2 therapy should never be considered unless proper supportive medical care can be delivered. Most chamber facilities today have equipment and treatment protocols analogous to an ICU. The inherent toxicity of O_2 and potential for injury due to elevations of ambient pressure must be addressed whenever HBO$_2$ is used therapeutically.

BAROTRAUMA

Middle ear barotrauma is the most common adverse effect of HBO$_2$ treatment.[95] As the ambient pressure within the hyperbaric chamber is increased, a patient must be able to equalize the pressure within the middle ear by autoinsufflation. If a pressure gradient develops across the tympanic membrane, pain followed by hemorrhage or serous effusion will develop. Standard protocols include instruction of patients on autoinsufflation techniques and adding oral or topical decongestants when needed. When autoinsufflation fails, tympanostomy tubes must be placed. The incidence of tube placement has been reported to be approximately 4% in one series.[96] Others report an overall incidence of aural barotraumas to be between 1.2% and 7%.[97,98]

Pulmonary barotrauma during HBO$_2$ treatment is extremely rare but should be suspected when any significant chest or hemodynamic symptoms occur during, or shortly after, decompression. Because the offending gas in virtually all cases will be pure O$_2$, absorption within the body may occur. If symptoms do develop, however, decompression should be stopped and the patient evaluated. If pneumothorax is suspected, placement of a chest tube is appropriate. Preexisting pneumothorax should be treated with chest tube drainage before initiating therapy.

OXYGEN TOXICITY

Biochemical toxicity due to O$_2$ can be manifested by injuries to lungs, central nervous system (CNS), and eyes. Pulmonary insults can impair mechanics (elasticity), vital capacity, and gas exchange.[2] These changes are typically observed only when treatment duration and pressures exceed typical therapeutic protocols. There is one report of reversible small airways changes in 4 of 21 patients treated daily for 90 minutes at 2.4 ATA for 21 days.[99] Most studies have failed to identify any adverse pulmonary effect from standard protocols.[100-102]

CNS O$_2$ toxicity is manifested as a grand mal seizure. This occurs at an incidence of approximately 1 to 4 in 10,000 patient treatments.[103-105] The risk is higher in hypercapnic patients, and possibly those who are acidotic or with compromise due to sepsis, because an incidence of 7% (23 in 322 patients) was reported in case series of HBO$_2$ treatment of gas gangrene.[61-65] Seizures are relatively easy to manage in most cases: simply reduce the inspired O$_2$ tension while leaving the patient at the same ambient pressure (to avoid pulmonary overexpansion injury when a patient is in tonic convulsion phase). Pathologic changes in association with isolated O$_2$-mediated seizures have not been found in studies with guinea pigs, rabbits, and humans.[106]

Progressive myopia has been reported in patients who undergo prolonged daily therapy, but this typically reverses within 6 weeks after termination of treatments.[107]

Development of nuclear cataracts has been reported with excessive treatments that exceed a total of 150 to 200 hours, and the change does not spontaneously reverse.[108] Although there is a theoretical risk for retrolental fibroplasia in neonates,[109] there are no reports of this having occurred. Currently, experimental and clinical evidence does not indicate that typical HBO$_2$ therapy protocols have detrimental effects on neonates or the unborn fetus.[110] This is likely due to the relatively short duration of hyperoxia.

OTHER RISKS

Confinement anxiety may occur and is typically managed with use of sedating agents. Any environment with an elevated concentration of O$_2$ presents a risk for fire. Scrupulous attention to avoiding an ignition source is standard in HBO$_2$ therapy programs. Over the past 20 years no fires resulting in injury have been reported in the United States; however, worldwide 52 deaths have been reported.[111] Virtually all these were preventable. In 10 incidents, fire resulted when banned substances such as cigarettes and lighters were taken into the chamber.

ANNOTATED REFERENCES

Bouachour G, Cronier P, Gouello, et al: Hyperbaric oxygen therapy in the management of crush injuries: A randomized double-blind placebo-controlled clinical trial. J Trauma 1996;41:333-339.

This blinded, randomized trial of 36 crush injury patients documented efficacy of hyperbaric oxygen therapy in improving wound healing and reducing repetitive surgery, particularly in those older than 40 years and with severe (grade III) injuries.

Faglia E, Favale F, Aldeghi A, et al: Adjunctive systemic hyperbaric oxygen therapy in treatment of severe prevalently ischemic diabetic foot ulcer. Diabetes Care 1996;19:1338-1343.

This prospective, randomized trial involving 70 consecutive diabetic patients with diabetic ulcers documented efficacy of hyperbaric oxygen therapy in improving limb salvage and wound healing for those with Wagner grade IV ulcers.

Marx RE, Johnson RP, Kline SN: Prevention of osteoradionecrosis: A randomized prospective clinical trial of hyperbaric oxygen versus penicillin. J Am Dental Assoc 1985;111:49-54.

This prospective, randomized trial of 74 patients who required dental extractions after receiving in excess of 6800 cGy external beam radiotherapy demonstrated efficacy of prophylactic hyperbaric oxygen therapy in reducing the incidence and severity of postoperative osteoradionecrosis.

Riseman JA, Zamboni WA, Curtis A, et al: Hyperbaric oxygen therapy for necrotizing fasciitis reduces mortality and the need for debridements. Surgery 1990;108:847-850.

This retrospective analysis of 29 patients with necrotizing fasciitis having similar age and illness severity describes the apparent efficacy of adjunctive hyperbaric oxygen therapy plus surgery and antibiotics in reducing mortality and wound morbidity.

Weaver LK, Hopkins RO, Chan KJ, et al: Hyperbaric oxygen for acute carbon monoxide poisoning. N Engl J Med 2002;2347:1057-1067.

This prospective, randomized, placebo controlled trial of 152 patients with carbon monoxide poisoning describes the efficacy of hyperbaric oxygen therapy in reducing neurologic morbidity among those with a history of unconsciousness, or with cerebellar dysfunction, or those with a carboxyhemoglobin level greater than 25%.

Chapter 74

IMAGING OF THE CHEST IN ICU

Nisa Thoongsuwan • Jeffrey P. Kanne • Eric J. Stern

KEY POINTS

1. Although **portable chest radiographs** are limited by both technical and patient factors, knowledge of complications of various diseases and therapies as well as their respective radiographic appearances can lead to improved patient care.

2. **Knowledge of the normal position of life support devices** on the chest radiograph is important so that malposition can be corrected and potential complications averted.

3. Even though many chest radiographs in the ICU setting may have a similar appearance, particularly with respect to parenchymal opacification, **understanding the diverse pathology** encountered in critical care and the specific clinical settings in which they are found provides a context for interpretation and may improve the diagnostic yield.

Chest imaging plays a central role in management of critically ill patients. Both bedside chest radiography and computed tomography (CT) aid in diagnosis as well as in evaluating response to therapy. In this chapter we review chest imaging in the ICU setting, focusing on radiography and CT, and discuss radiographic techniques used at the bedside and appropriate positioning of various monitoring and life support devices. In addition, imaging findings of common pathologic processes encountered in critically ill patients are described. A discussion of imaging of neonatal and pediatric ICU patients is beyond the scope of this chapter.

PRINCIPLES OF IMAGING IN THE ICU

Portable chest radiography plays a major role in patient care, especially in critically ill patients. In some hospitals, up to 50% of all chest radiographs are obtained at the bedside.[1] The benefit of obtaining routine daily chest radiographs in the ICU remains controversial. Some studies support the concept of routine chest radiographs in ICU patients[2] whereas others dispute the usefulness of obtaining chest radiographs in the ICU without a clear indication, arguing that a very small minority of examinations have any significant impact on patient management.[3-7] We believe that radiographs showing no new significant findings, even given their limitations, can be reassuring that no new serious abnormalities are present.

Interpretation of bedside chest radiographs can be quite challenging because of the degree of variation in quality from both technical and patient factors. The ill health of the patient and multiple cumbersome life support devices limit proper patient positioning while difficulty controlling respiratory and body motion can blur the radiographic images, all potentially leading to low-quality radiographs. The importance of having dedicated and competent radiology technologists and an effective quality assurance program cannot be overemphasized.

In addition to film quality issues, common pathologic processes such as pleural effusion or pneumothorax have different appearances on supine or semi-upright bedside examinations as compared with standard upright postero-anterior chest radiographs.[8] Understanding and accepting the limitations of bedside chest radiography allows for appropriate utilization of other imaging modalities such as CT.

CONVENTIONAL RADIOGRAPHY

By its very nature, conventional portable chest radiography suffers from several disadvantages, some technical and others related to patient factors. Bedside chest radiographs are obtained in the anteroposterior projection, ideally with the patient upright. However, supine and semi-upright positioning is often the rule and not the exception owing to the severity of these patients' illnesses. The combination of the anteroposterior projection and a shorter film-tube distance lead to geometric magnification of structures more anterior in the chest, such as the heart. The maximum tube current and voltage are limited on portable units, so exposure times are relatively long and image contrast may be excessive.[9]

DIGITAL RADIOGRAPHY

In addressing the technical and patient-related problems encountered in portable chest radiography, development of digital image technology has shown promising improvement over conventional radiography. Digital (or computed) radiography uses a phosphor plate in lieu of a film-screen combination to capture and store the radiographic image and has the advantages of consistent film density, flexible image processing, and lower radiation dose to the patient. The diagnostic accuracy of digital chest radiography systems is similar to that obtained with conventional film-screen radiography.[10]

Digital image processing identifies the portion of the dynamic range containing the diagnostic information and adjusts the final output for display at consistent and optimized contrast and density, obviating the need for repeated examinations because of errors in exposure. This also decreases the need to interpret radiographs of marginal diagnostic quality. These advantages, however, do not preclude the need for accurate positioning of the patient and alignment of the x-ray beam, and overall time required for obtaining the radiograph remains the same. Nevertheless, not only does computed radiography have the immediate advantages of improved image quality and flexibility but also it readily allows for placing images on a digital network.

COMPUTED TOMOGRAPHY

Computed tomography provides better anatomic detail and a higher degree of diagnostic accuracy than conventional chest radiography, but for critically ill patients, transportation and cumbersome monitoring devices limit access to CT. Appropriate use of CT in critically ill patients can aid in patient management.[11-13] A mobile CT scanner has been developed to image critically ill patients in the ICU and avoid the need for transportation, but these units have not been widely accepted because of their suboptimal image quality.[14]

PICTURE ARCHIVING AND COMMUNICATIONS SYSTEM (PACS)

Immediate access to bedside chest images is particularly useful in the ICU, where information is desired without delay. A picture archiving and communications system (PACS) permits transmission of medical images over a digital network for simultaneous display within minutes of their acquisition at multiple locations such as in the ICU, clinics, or operating rooms.[15] In addition, PACS allows for rapid retrieval of previous examinations for comparison and workstation tools enable accurate measuring and adjustment of digital image parameters such as window and level settings.

MONITORING AND SUPPORT DEVICES

ENDOTRACHEAL TUBES

Endotracheal tubes (ETTs) are placed in the setting of airway obstruction, failure to maintain adequate gas exchange, or inability of a patient to protect the airway from aspiration or obstruction.[16] On the chest radiograph, position of an ETT is determined by the location of the tube's tip in relation to the carina with respect to the position of the patient's chin.[17] With the chin in the neutral position, the tip of the ETT should be 3 to 7 cm above the carina (Fig. 74-1). When the carina is not visible, the tip of the ETT should project over the T3 or T4 vertebral body, because the carina is located between T5 and T7 on anteroposterior radiographs in about 92% of individuals.[18] Alternatively, carinal position can be ascertained by following the inferior margins of one or both of the main bronchi proximally.

When assessing ETT position, the position of the chin should also be assessed. Neck flexion and extension can result in 2 cm of downward and upward displacement, respectively, of the ETT.[19] Projection of the anterior portion of the mandible over the lower cervical spine indicates neck flexion whereas a nonobscured cervical spine denotes that the neck is in extension.

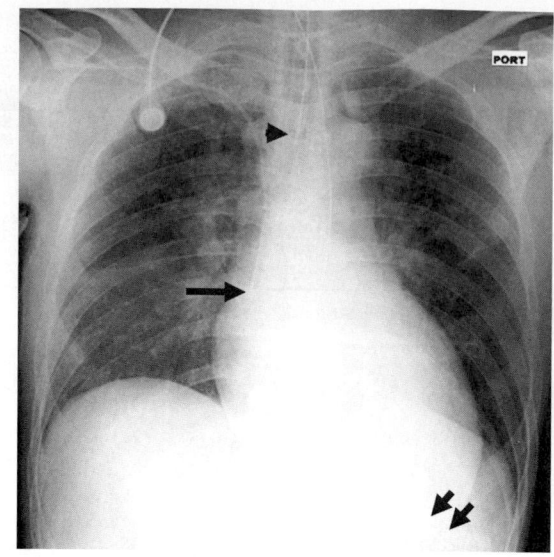

FIGURE 74–1. Typical normal line and tube positions. Note the expected positions of the ETT (superimposed over the T3 vertebral body [*arrowhead*]), a central venous catheter (in the origin of SVC [*arrow*]), and the nasogastric tube (in the stomach [*double arrows*]).

The most common complication of ETT placement is inadvertent intubation of the right main bronchus (Fig. 74-2) because of the smaller angle the right main bronchus has in relationship to the trachea as compared with the left main bronchus.[20] Additionally, esophageal placement of the ETT can occur, but this is usually detected on physical examination. However, when esophageal intubation is not appreciated clinically, the chest radiograph may identify the errant position of ETT. Radiographic findings of esophageal intubation include direct visualization of the ETT lateral to the tracheal wall, gaseous distention of the stomach, and displacement of the trachea by an overdistended balloon cuff.[21]

TRACHEOSTOMY TUBES

A tracheostomy tube is required in patients who need long-term assisted ventilation or tracheal suction or in whom

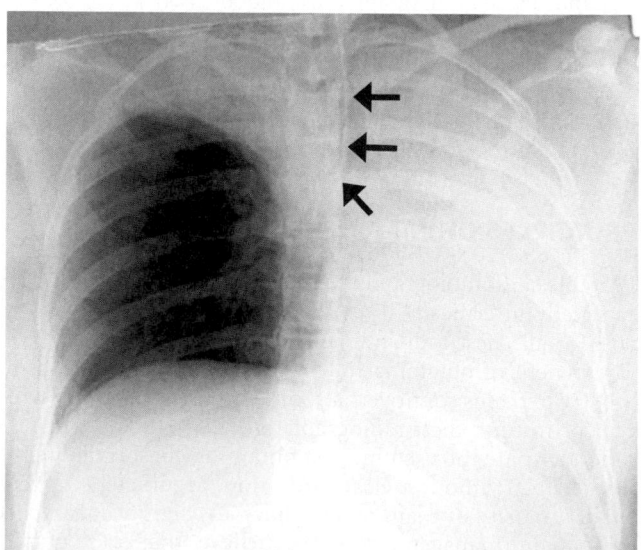

FIGURE 74–2. Anteroposterior chest radiograph shows the ETT (*arrows*) extending into the bronchus intermedius with resulting collapse of the left lung and right upper lobe from hypoventilation.

transoral or transnasal tracheal intubation is not possible. The tip of the tube should be several centimeters above the carina, and the tube's diameter should be approximately two-thirds that of the trachea.[22] Unlike with ETTs, chin position does not affect tracheostomy tube position. The presence of air in the subcutaneous tissue of the neck and upper mediastinum is usually an insignificant finding immediately after tracheostomy tube placement.[23] However, pneumothorax and mediastinal hematoma, the latter manifesting as a widened mediastinum, are complications of tracheostomy tube placement that can be identified on the chest radiograph.

CENTRAL VENOUS CATHETERS

Central venous catheters are used for monitoring central venous pressure, for venous access for fluid and medication administration, and for parenteral nutrition.[17] They are inserted from an internal jugular, subclavian, or femoral approach. The optimal location of the catheter tip is at the origin of the superior vena cava, distal to the central venous valves. On the anteroposterior chest radiograph, the origin of the superior vena cava usually lies to the right of midline at the level of the first intercostal space (see Fig. 74-1).[24] Catheters should ordinarily not be placed beyond the level of the azygos vein because the superior vena cava enters the pericardium at this location and unintentional vessel perforation may cause pericardial effusion or cardiac tamponade.[17]

Portable chest radiographs should be obtained immediately after central venous catheter placement to determine catheter position and identify any complications such as pneumothorax, vessel perforation (Fig. 74-3), cardiac perforation, retained or fragmented introducer or catheter, or a knotted catheter.

SWAN-GANZ CATHETERS

Swan-Ganz catheters are used for measuring the pulmonary capillary wedge pressure, which is an indirect assessment of both left atrial pressure and left ventricular end-diastolic volume. This catheter is typically used to distinguish cardiogenic from noncardiogenic pulmonary edema, particularly in patients who have underlying systemic or pulmonary disease in addition to left ventricular failure. The Swan-Ganz catheter has a small balloon near the tip and is introduced via a jugular, subclavian, or femoral venous approach. The ideal position for the catheter tip is within the left or right main pulmonary artery or in a proximal interlobar artery. If the tip extends beyond these larger arteries (Fig. 74-4), pulmonary infarction from occlusion of the pulmonary vessel or pseudoaneurysm can ensue.[17] The balloon should be inflated only when obtaining pressure measurements, so an inflated balloon should never be present on a portable chest radiograph. Complications are similar to those that occur with other central venous catheters but also include pulmonary vascular perforation and pulmonary hemorrhage when the catheter extends into the lung periphery.[25]

INTRA-AORTIC BALLOON PUMPS

An intra-aortic balloon pump (IABP) is used for assisting left ventricular function in patients with cardiac shock or serious left ventricular dysfunction, usually after myocardial infarction. The device consists of an inflatable balloon, about 16 cm in length, which is inflated during systole, thereby reducing afterload and augmenting coronary artery perfusion.[26] The IABP is advanced into the descending thoracic aorta through the common femoral artery. On the frontal chest radiograph, the tip of the balloon should be located within the descending thoracic aorta just distal to the origin of the left subclavian artery, typically at the level of aortic arch.[24] A more proximal location of the balloon can result in occlusion of the subclavian and vertebral arteries, whereas a more distal location can lead to occlusion of the mesenteric and renal arteries.[27] IABPs can migrate, so position should be reassessed on subsequent chest radiographs.

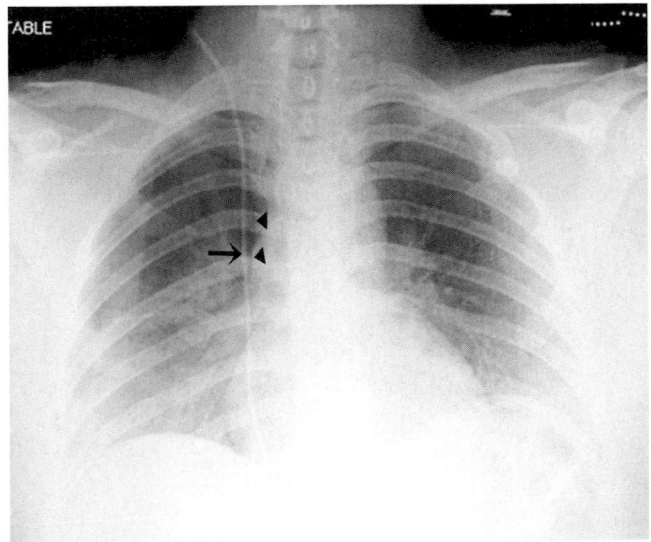
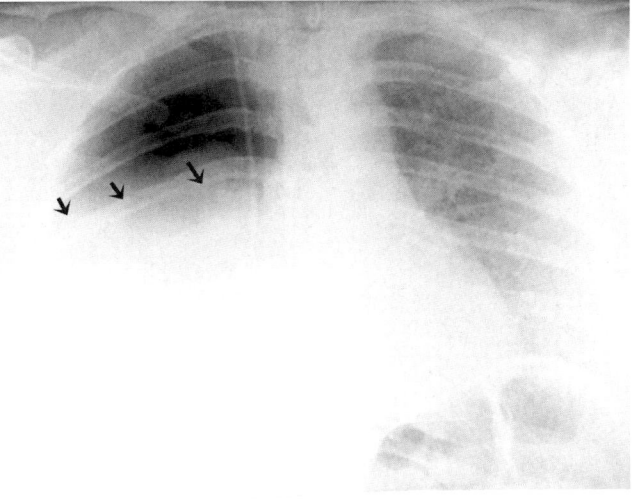

A   B

FIGURE 74–3. Complication of intravenous catheter placement. **A,** The right IJ catheter *(arrow)* is lateral to the right mediastinal margin *(arrowheads),* indicating that the catheter is extravascular. **B,** Twelve hours later, a pleural fluid collection has developed from inadvertent infusion of saline into the right pleural space *(arrows).* A CT scan *(not shown)* showed the catheter to be in the pleural space.

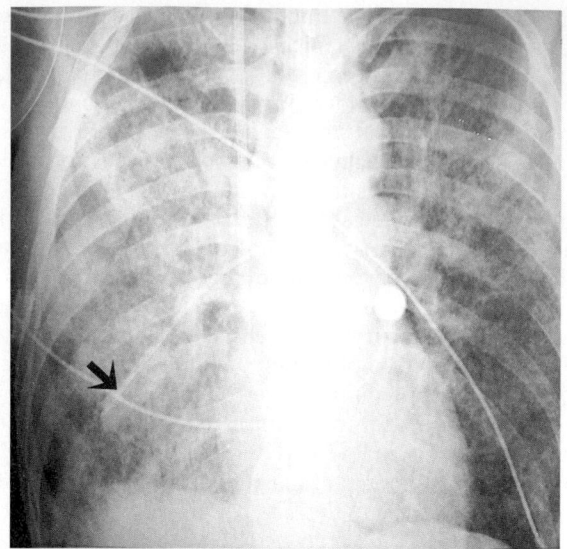

FIGURE 74–4. The tip of the Swan-Ganz catheter extends into the right lower lobe pulmonary artery. In this location, the risk of vessel injury increases.

PERIPHERALLY INSERTED CENTRAL CATHETERS

The peripherally inserted central catheter (PICC) is a relatively new device gaining widespread acceptance for long-term central venous access. PICCs allow for administration of medications, blood products, or intravenous alimentation. The catheter is small, with sizes ranging from 2 to 5 French, and is placed into the superior vena cava through a large upper extremity vein. Complication rates are low when compared with other central vascular catheters.

PICCs may be difficult to visualize on the bedside chest radiographs because of their small size and faint opacity. They, in particular, are more susceptible to displacement than other intravenous catheters owing to increased flexibility of the material.[28] As with all tubes, location should be reassessed on all subsequent radiographs.

THORACOSTOMY TUBES

Thoracostomy tubes are placed in the pleural space to drain unwanted fluid or gas, both of which are frequently encountered in critically ill patients. The position of the thoracostomy tube can usually be assessed on a chest radiograph. The side port, marked by the disruption in the radiographically opaque line, should be located medial to the inner margin of the ribs. However, thoracostomy tubes, particularly those placed at the bedside, can be malpositioned, with the tips residing in the subcutaneous soft tissues, pulmonary fissures, or, rarely, within the lung parenchyma. Poor positioning of the tube is suspected when the tube does not drain as expected.

In some instances, the precise location of the thoracostomy tube cannot be determined from the bedside chest radiograph.[17] Subcutaneous placement can be very difficult to ascertain, and a fissural location can only be suspected when the tube follows the course of one of the pulmonary fissures.[29] CT, because of its cross-sectional nature, is superior to chest radiography for accurately identifying the course of the thoracostomy tube[30] and its relationship to abnormal gas or fluid collections (Fig. 74-5).

ENTERIC TUBES

Enteric tubes are placed into the stomach or proximal small bowel through a transoral or transnasal approach and come in a variety of sizes and configurations (see Fig. 74-1). They are used for gastric decompression or lavage, medication administration, and providing nutrition.[31] These tubes are frequently placed in ICU patients, especially those with endotracheal intubation. Although the best position of tubes used for feeding is controversial, placement distal to the pylorus may decrease the risk of aspiration.[31] Position of enteric tubes is

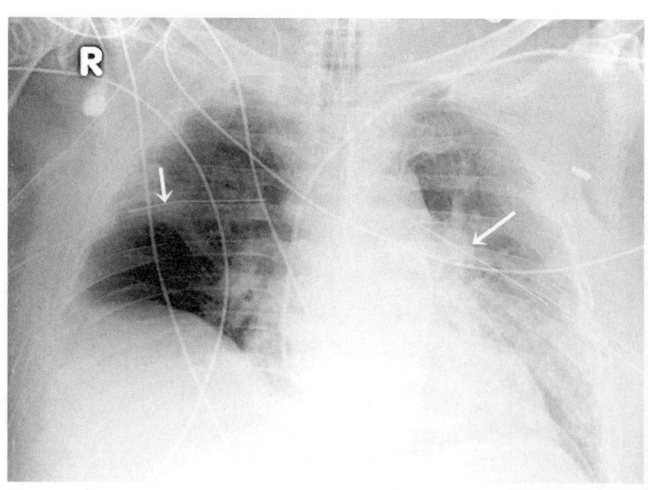
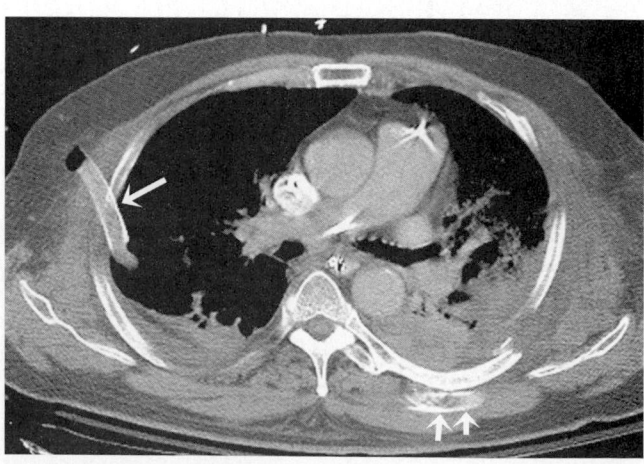

A B

FIGURE 74–5. Malpositioned thoracostomy tubes after bedside placement. **A,** Anteroposterior chest radiograph shows bilateral thoracostomy tubes *(arrows)* with tips and side ports projecting over the lungs. **B,** CT shows that the left thoracostomy tube *(double arrows)* is in the posterior chest wall. The right thoracostomy tube *(single arrow)* is in satisfactory position.

easily assessed from the chest or abdominal radiograph. The most common complication from insertion of these tubes is coiling in the pharynx or esophagus. However, inadvertent insertion into the tracheobronchial tree (Fig. 74-6), occurring in 0.2% to 0.3% of patients,[32,33] and esophageal perforation have more serious consequences.

APPROACH TO ICU CHEST IMAGING

In many large hospitals, the ICU has evolved from a single unit for patients requiring mechanical ventilation to system- or illness-specific units to provide the most effective patient care. Understanding the diversity of pathologic processes in critical care and the specific settings in which they are found provides a context for interpretation of radiographic abnormalities and may improve diagnostic accuracy.

CARDIAC ICU

The most common lung opacity found in the cardiac ICU setting is cardiogenic pulmonary edema. Other causes of parenchymal opacity include atelectasis, pneumonia, and, less commonly, noncardiogenic pulmonary edema from any cause. In the setting of cardiogenic pulmonary edema, lung opacity is almost always associated with an enlarged heart, engorgement of central pulmonary veins, interstitial edema, effusions, and altered distribution of pulmonary blood flow (Fig. 74-7). The classic pattern of bilateral perihilar fluffy opacity, referred to as the butterfly or bat-wing appearance, is seen in less than 10% of patients with pulmonary edema.[34] Asymmetry of pulmonary edema can also occur because of variations in patient position and underlying cardiopulmonary disease such as emphysema or mitral valve insufficiency.[35] The lung opacity associated with cardiogenic pulmonary edema can fluctuate rapidly, a clue to its diagnosis.

NEUROLOGIC ICU

Patients cared for in the neurologic ICU include both surgical and nonsurgical patients with conditions affecting

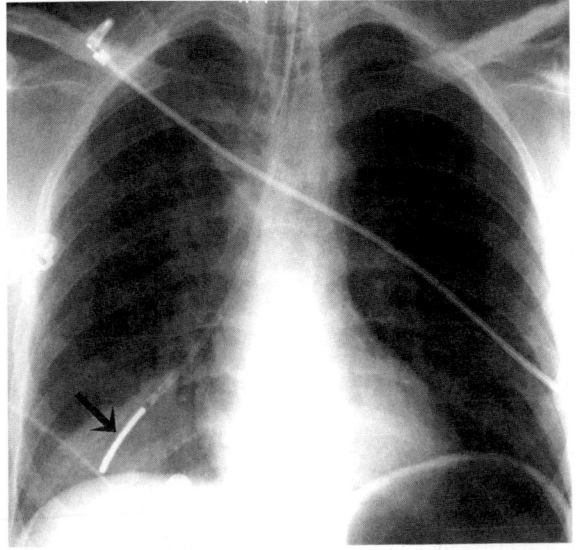

FIGURE 74-6. Distal-weighted enteric feeding tube *(arrow)* extending into the right lower lobe bronchus.

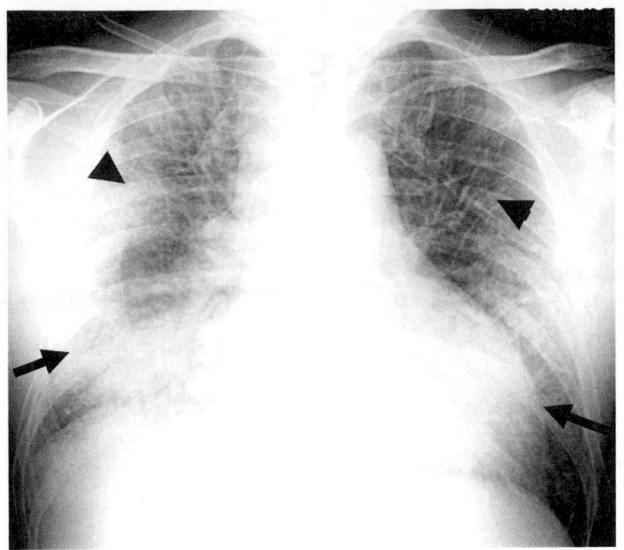

FIGURE 74–7. Cardiogenic pulmonary edema in a 54-year-old man with acute myocardial infarction. Chest radiograph shows cardiomegaly with bibasilar opacities and diffuse interlobar thickening in both lungs. Note Kerley's A *(arrowheads)* and Kerley's B lines *(arrows)*.

the nervous system such as intracranial hemorrhage, recent intracranial or spinal surgery, and seizure. The most common abnormalities encountered on the chest radiographs of these patients include hypervolemia, neurogenic pulmonary edema, and aspiration.

Neurogenic Pulmonary Edema

Neurogenic pulmonary edema occurs with many neurologic conditions that increase intracranial pressure, such as head trauma, intracranial hemorrhage, intracranial tumor, stroke, seizures, and infection.[36] Elevated microvascular pressure and increased vascular permeability in the lungs are thought to play a role in its development. Neurogenic pulmonary edema can develop immediately after the insult to the central nervous system, within minutes to hours, or several days later.[37]

On the chest radiograph, neurogenic pulmonary edema usually manifests as a homogeneous pulmonary opacity similar to that of cardiogenic pulmonary edema but without cardiomegaly or engorgement of the pulmonary vasculature and interstitium. The distribution of the opacity is usually diffuse,[38] but sometimes the opacity is focal.[39] Variability in the radiographic appearance of neurogenic pulmonary edema likely reflects gravity, patient position, and heterogeneity in pulmonary venous pressure.[40] Radiographic abnormalities may not develop until 24 hours after the onset of neurogenic pulmonary edema. Rapid clearing of the lungs several days after the insult to the central nervous system is removed is characteristic, in contrast to other forms of noncardiogenic pulmonary edema in which opacity can persist.[41]

In addition to neurogenic pulmonary edema, evidence of positive fluid balance is almost always found on radiographs of patients in the neurologic ICU, whether directly related to neurogenic pulmonary edema or as an indirect effect from treatment with large volumes of intravenous fluid. In other ICU settings, however, evidence of fluid volume overload may have different clinical implications.[42]

Aspiration

Patients with a decreased level of consciousness after stroke or head injury and those experiencing seizure are at high risk for aspiration.[42] The clinical severity and radiographic appearance depend on both the amount of fluid aspirated as well as its composition.[43] Radiographically, aspiration can result in development of bilateral, multilobar pulmonary opacities predominating in the dependent portions of the lungs, including the posterior segments of the upper lobes and the superior and posterior basilar segments of the lower lobes (Fig. 74-8). Aspirated particulate matter can obstruct the airways and add to volume loss.[42,44]

SURGICAL ICU

Patients in the surgical ICU can develop complications directly relating to recent thoracic surgery. Thoracotomy with or without pneumonectomy or lobectomy can alter the expected appearance of the intrathoracic structures, and knowledge of the normal expected changes after surgery allows for better identification of changes that may indicate a complication.

Pneumonectomy

Radiographs obtained immediately after pneumonectomy normally show midline position of the mediastinum and gas filling the pneumonectomy space. After several days, fluid begins to accumulate within the pneumonectomy space as the gas is resorbed. The rate of the fluid accumulation varies, but in most cases one half to two thirds of the hemithorax fills within the first week. However, this process can take up to 6 months in some patients.[45,46]

After pneumonectomy, the ipsilateral hemidiaphragm elevates and the mediastinum begins to shift toward the operative side as the remaining lung hyperinflates. The degree of mediastinal displacement depends primarily on the compliance and the degree of hyperinflation of the remaining lung.[46] Appropriate mediastinal displacement is the most reliable indicator of a normal course after pneumonectomy. Failure of the mediastinum to shift to the operative side almost always indicates an abnormality in the pneumonectomy cavity.[45] Complications of pneumonectomy, as described later,

are categorized as either acute or chronic, but most of those encountered in the ICU are acute.

Post-pneumonectomy Pulmonary Edema

Post-pneumonectomy pulmonary edema describes a fall in PO_2 with an increase in water content in the lung.[47] It is an uncommon condition[48,49] but carries a high mortality rate.[49] An increase in pulmonary capillary permeability is believed to be the central factor for developing post-pneumonectomy pulmonary edema.[48] Radiographic features include mild interstitial edema and ill-defined vascular structures. In more severe cases, the pattern of radiograph is identical to that of noncardiogenic pulmonary edema.[35]

Bronchopleural Fistula

Although an uncommon complication after pneumonectomy, bronchopleural fistula, with an incidence of 2% to 5%,[50,51] has a high morality rate ranging from 30% to 70%.[50,52,53] Clinical characteristics of bronchopleural fistula include sudden onset of dyspnea and bloody expectoration during the first 10 days after surgery.[53] The time at which the fistula develops reflects its cause, because leakage in the first week after pneumonectomy usually indicates inadequate closure of the bronchial stump whereas leakage developing during the second or third week is usually the result of poor healing.[46] Radiographic findings of bronchopleural fistula include an unexpected disappearance of fluid or abrupt decrease in the gas-fluid level in the pneumonectomy cavity (more than 2 cm in height)[54] and contralateral shift of the mediastinum (Fig. 74-9).[46]

Hemothorax, Chylothorax, and Empyema

The nature of fluid within the pneumonectomy cavity usually cannot be determined on the chest radiograph. However, hemothorax, chlyothorax, and empyema, as complications of pneumonectomy, differ in when they develop. Rapid opacification of the pneumonectomy cavity likely indicates hemorrhage, whereas chylothorax occurs with a delay up to 10 days. Empyema usually occurs several weeks after surgery.[46] On the chest radiograph, hemothorax, chylothorax,

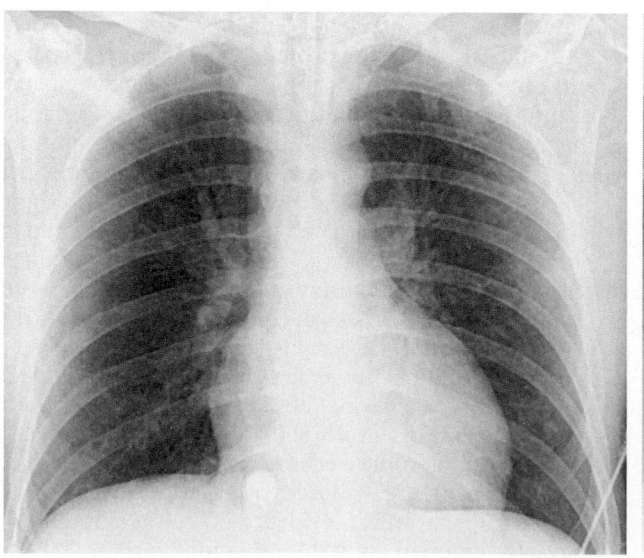
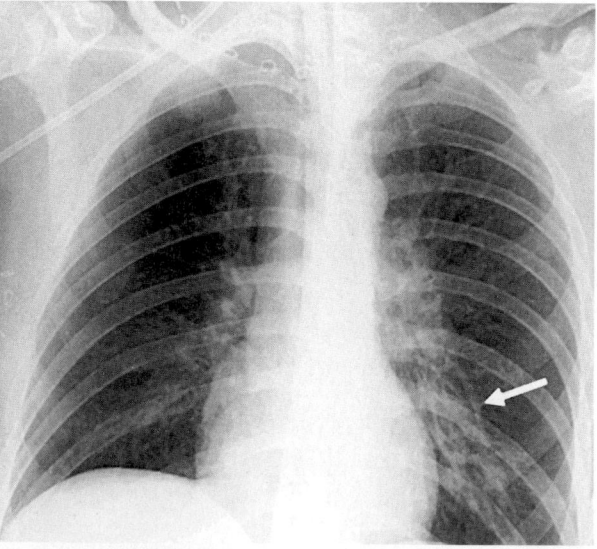

A

B

FIGURE 74–8. A 49-year-old man presented with seizure and witnessed aspiration. **A,** Initial anteroposterior chest radiograph is normal. **B,** Twenty-four hours later, patchy left lower lobe opacity *(arrow)* has developed, consistent with aspiration pneumonia. Note the increased opacity behind the heart.

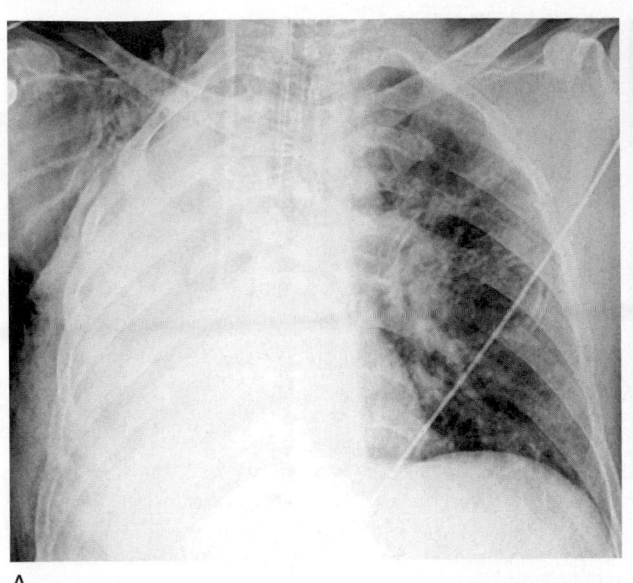

A

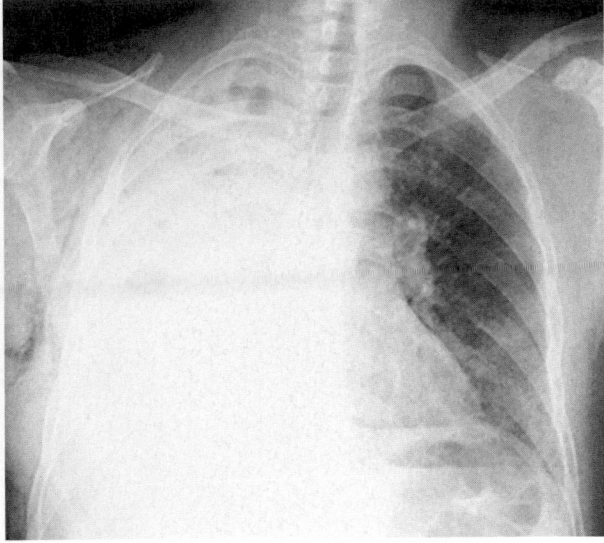

B

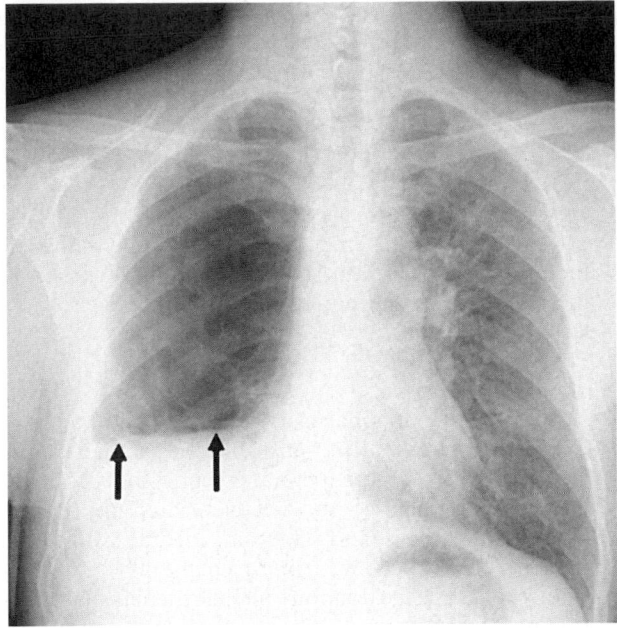

C

FIGURE 74–9. Serial chest radiographs after right pneumonectomy show development of a bronchopleural fistula. **A,** Supine view obtained the day after surgery shows fluid in the right hemithorax and rightward deviation of the mediastinum, as expected. Tube and line are in expected position. **B,** Four days later the mediastinum is now shifted to the left, and several lucencies have developed in the right hemithorax. **C,** Two weeks after pneumectomy, an upright posteroanterior radiograph shows gas-fluid level *(arrows)* and leftward mediastinal deviation, opposite of what is expected, consistent with bronchopleural fistula, typically from a stump leak.

and empyema opacify the hemithorax on the operative side with contralateral shift of the mediastinum in contrast to the ipsilateral shift seen with normal filling of the pneumonectomy space. In the case of empyema, gas may develop in the previously opacified pneumonectomy cavity.[46]

Lobectomy

After uncomplicated lobectomy, the chest radiograph can show rotation and hyperinflation of the remaining lobe(s),[55] change in the orientation of the remaining bronchovascular structures, as well as other subtle changes such as subsegmental atelectasis and development of pleural effusion. Reorientation of the remaining bronchovascular anatomy should not be confused with atelectasis. Complications of lobectomy occur with a lower frequency than with pneumonectomy but are similar. In addition, lung torsion, which has a high mortality rate, occurs rarely and manifests as rapid opacification of a lobe or lung associated with unusual configuration of the hilum.[56] Anastomotic suture lines are

evident when the fissure incompletely divides the lung into lobes.[57]

TRAUMA ICU

Patients in the trauma ICU usually have multiple injuries ranging from visceral lacerations to complex fractures of an extremity. Chest trauma, in particular, affects the morbidity and mortality of these patients owing to impairment of the cardiovascular and respiratory systems. Imaging of these patients focuses on identifying acute complications from the trauma as well as recognizing additional injuries that may have been obscured or overlooked on initial evaluation.

Mediastinal Injury

Acute Traumatic Aortic Injury

Tears of the thoracic aorta (Fig. 74-10) are caused by acute deceleration injury such as occurs with a high-speed motor vehicle crash or a fall or as a result of crush injury to the chest.

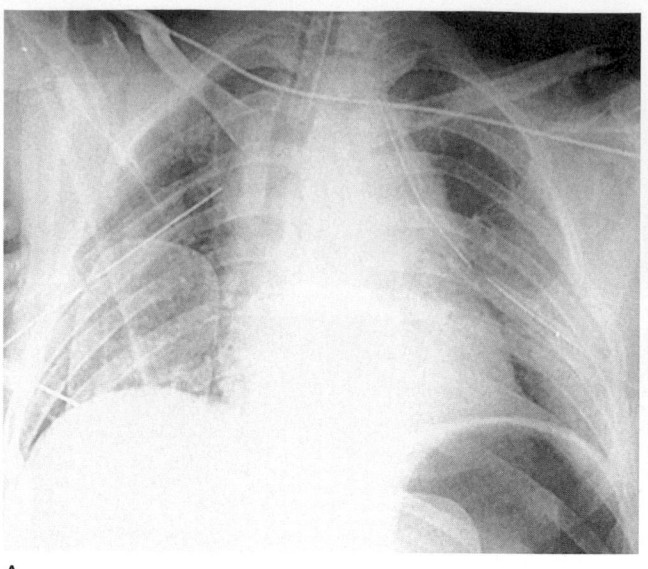

A

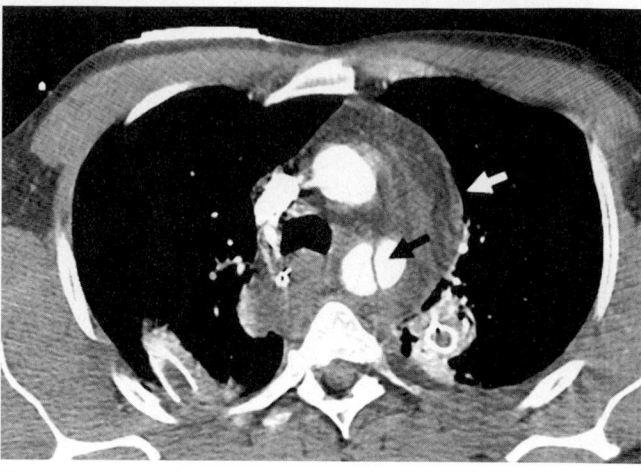

B

FIGURE 74–10. A 35-year-old man was involved in a high-speed motor vehicle crash. **A,** Anteroposterior chest radiograph shows abnormal contour of the mediastinum, obscuration of the aortic knob, and rightward displacement of the trachea, consistent with mediastinal injury. Note tubes are in satisfactory position. **B,** Axial CT image shows intimal flap within the aortic lumen *(black arrow),* representing aortic dissection, surrounded by mediastinal hematoma *(white arrow).*

A tear of the thoracic aorta almost always occurs in a transverse orientation, typically at the aortic isthmus,[58] with the adventitia remaining intact in 60% of cases.[59] Tears of the ascending aorta or complete transection are nearly universally fatal.

Many radiographic abnormalities suggest aortic injury in the acute setting. These include a widened mediastinum, indistinct aortic contour, rightward deviation of the trachea, downward displacement of the left main bronchus, and thickening of the right paratracheal stripe.[59,60] Of these, mediastinal widening and abnormal contour of the aortic arch are shown to be the most reliable.[61-63] Chest radiographs have great value in excluding traumatic aortic injury with a negative predictive value around 98%.[59,61]

In patients whose chest radiographs are equivocal or highly suspicious for aortic injury, contrast medium–enhanced CT is indicated.[64] CT findings of acute aortic injury include irregularity of the aortic wall, pseudoaneurysm, abrupt change in aortic caliber, intimal flap, extravasation of contrast material, and periaortic hematoma.[64-66] Digital subtraction aortography should follow abnormal or equivocal CT scans.

Tracheobronchial Tree Rupture

Rupture of the tracheobronchial tree is an uncommon result of blunt trauma, with bronchial rupture occurring more often than rupture of the trachea.[67] With bronchial rupture, the injury is usually located in the main bronchus 1 to 2 cm distal to the carina. Disruption of the trachea typically involves the membranous portion just proximal to the carina.[67] Associated vascular injury occurs more frequently with tracheal tear than with the bronchial injury.[68,69]

About 70% of chest radiographs show pneumomediastinum or pneumothorax in the setting of tracheobronchial disruption.[70] The "fallen lung" sign (Fig. 74-11), indicating complete bronchial disruption, describes the severed and collapsed lung lying against the posterolateral aspect of the chest wall or the diaphragm.[71-73] Other findings that strongly suggest tracheobronchial injury include a large pneumothorax not responding to percutaneous drainage, pneumothorax and pneumomediastinum in the absence of pleural effusion, and pneumomediastinum in patients not receiving positive-pressure ventilation.[74-76]

Esophageal Rupture

Rupture of the esophagus is an uncommon injury that occurs more frequently by iatrogenic means than from blunt chest trauma.[77] Mediastinitis and septic shock can rapidly ensue, accounting for the relatively high mortality rate. Typical clinical signs and symptoms include vomiting, chest pain, and subcutaneous emphysema.[78] The radiographic findings of esophageal rupture include mediastinal widening, pneumomediastinum, pleural effusion, pneumothorax, and hydropneumothorax.[70,79] Contrast esophagography is the standard approach for diagnosis esophageal rupture. On CT, the area of greatest esophageal thickening often represents the perforation site.[70] CT also provides more detailed information than radiography on developing complications.

Thoracic Duct Rupture

The most common cause of thoracic duct disruption is iatrogenic injury, reported in about 0.2% of patients undergoing thoracic surgery.[80] Thoracic duct injury from blunt chest injury is very rare[81] and is thought to occur with hyperextension of the thoracic spine.[82] Chylothorax, which usually develops several days to weeks after the trauma, is the typical radiographic finding. However, chylothorax and pleural effusion are radiographically indistinguishable. The delay in development of chylothorax, a clue to the diagnosis, occurs because chyle accumulating in the mediastinum needs sufficient pressure to rupture into the pleural space.[83] CT findings are usually the same as with other pleural effusions, and the injury site is best identified with lymphangiography.

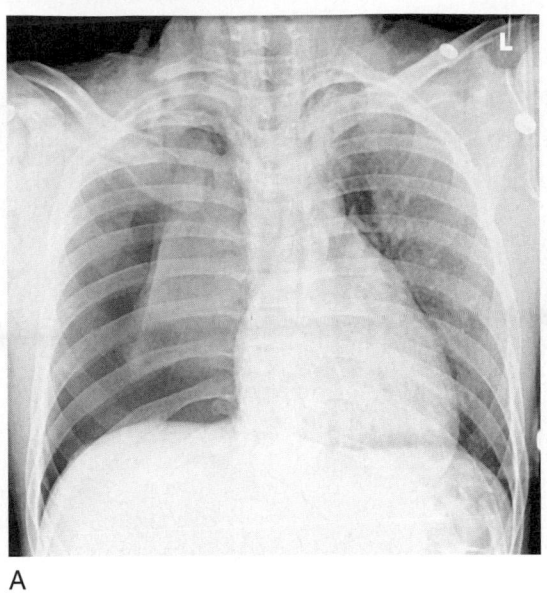

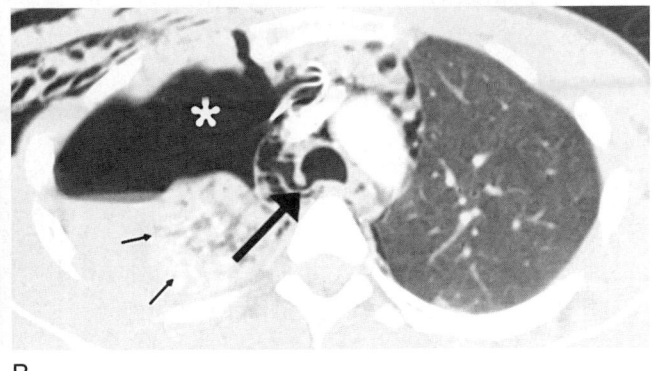

A   B

FIGURE 74–11. A 22-year-old man was involved in a high-speed motor vehicle crash. **A,** Anteroposterior chest radiograph shows right pneumothorax, pneumomediastinum, right lung collapse, and subcutaneous emphysema. **B,** Axial CT image shows tracheal laceration *(large arrow),* right pneumothorax *(asterisk),* and the collapsed right lung *(small arrows)* in the dependent portion of the chest (fallen lung sign).

Lung Parenchyma
Pulmonary Contusion

Pulmonary contusion is the most common pulmonary injury after blunt chest trauma.[84] It is characterized by leakage of blood into the pulmonary interstitium and alveolar spaces and clinically presents as dyspnea, tachycardia, and hypoxia after blunt injury to the chest. On chest radiographs, the contusion manifests as pulmonary opacity in a nonanatomic distribution,[85] in contrast to the usual segmental or lobar distribution of pneumonia or atelectasis. The contusion is usually found in the lung periphery deep to the site of chest wall impact (Fig. 74-12). Sometimes, however, contusion can occur opposite from the location of the chest wall injury due to a contrecoup effect.[86] Bilateral contusions usually occur from blast injuries.[86]

The timing of the developing opacity on the chest radiograph suggests the diagnosis in the setting of acute trauma, invariably presenting within 6 hours of injury.[87] Contusion usually resolves without sequelae within 3 to 10 days.[67] CT is more sensitive than conventional radiography for detecting pulmonary contusion[88,89] as well as associated chest wall injuries.[90]

Pulmonary Laceration

Pulmonary laceration is more severe than pulmonary contusion and is characterized by frank disruption of the lung parenchyma. Radiographic features of pulmonary laceration change over time and are usually masked by the surrounding contusion during the first few days. In the acute phase, the hematoma within the laceration appears as a well-circumscribed, homogeneous area of soft tissue attenuation. As the hematoma evolves, a round or elliptical gas collection, called a pneumatocele, becomes more obvious.[91] Most pneumatoceles appear within a few days, but some may develop over several weeks (Fig. 74-13). Diameters range from 2 to 5 cm but can be larger.[91] CT is more sensitive than conventional chest radiography in identifying pulmonary lacerations.[89]

Fat Embolism Syndrome

Fat embolism syndrome is a rare but serious complication characterized by pulmonary, cerebral, and cutaneous manifestation in the setting of recent severe fracture and usually occurs 12 to 72 hours after the injury.[92] Both mechanical obstruction from lipids and biochemical-mediated responses lead to the clinical manifestations of fat embolism syndrome.[93,94] In mild cases, the chest radiograph often shows no abnormality. In more severe cases, the initial chest radiograph may be normal but airspace and interstitial opacities resembling other causes of pulmonary edema (Fig. 74-14) can develop within 12 to 72 hours,[85] with

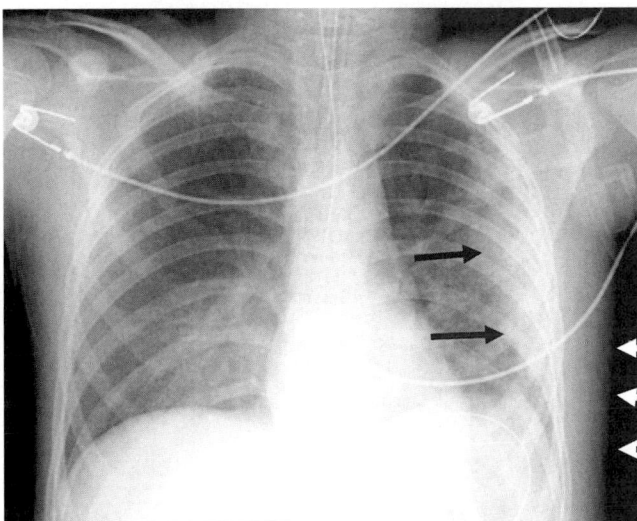

FIGURE 74–12. A 12-year-old boy presented with injuries sustained in a motor vehicle accident. Chest radiograph shows peripheral pulmonary contusion *(arrows).* Swelling of the soft tissue of the left chest wall adjacent to the area of pulmonary contusion is noted *(arrowheads).*

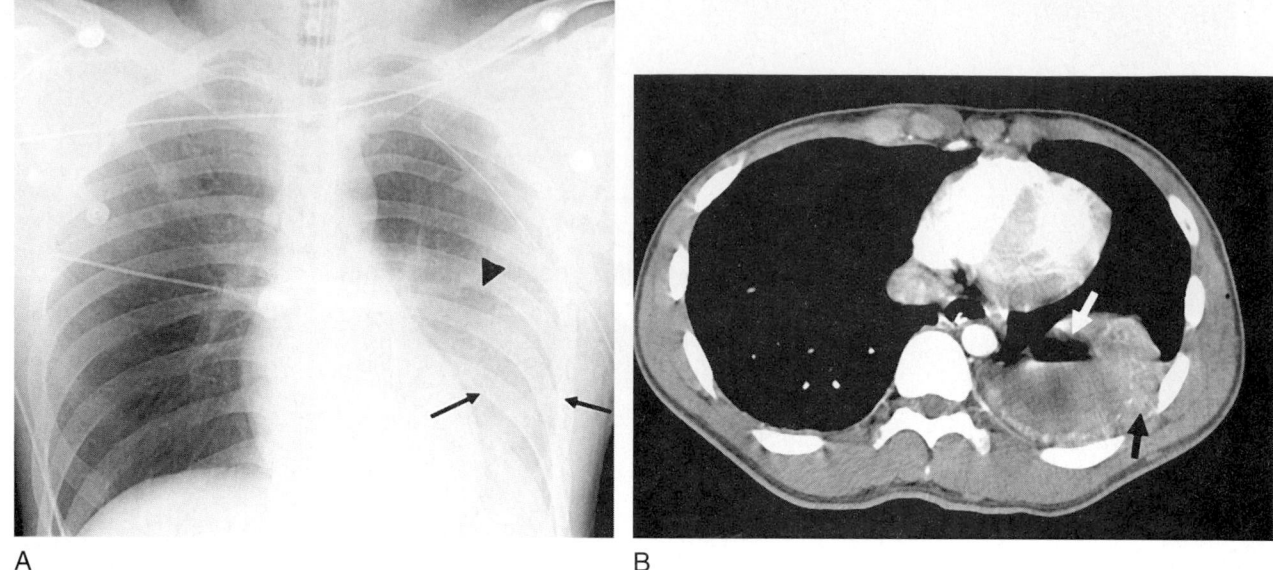

A

B

FIGURE 74–13. A 30-year-old man was involved in motor vehicle crash. **A,** Chest radiograph shows small lucent area *(arrowhead)* within area of the left lower lobe opacity *(arrows).* **B,** Axial CT image of the chest shows a "cavity" with an air-fluid level *(white arrow)* in the left lower lobe, representing a pulmonary laceration surrounded by pulmonary contusion and hemorrhage *(black arrow).*

resolution typically occurring in 10 to 14 days in the absence of superimposed disease. The delay in onset of abnormal opacities on the chest radiograph and the history of fracture are clues that can distinguish fat embolism syndrome from pulmonary contusion or pneumonia.

Pleura

Pneumothorax

Pneumothorax is more common with blunt chest trauma (15% to 38%) than with penetrating injuries to the chest (18% to 19%).[95,96] The clinical significance of pneumothorax depends on the patient's underlying cardiopulmonary function

and not on the physical size of the pneumothorax.[97] However, pneumothoraces in all trauma patients should be considered significant, regardless of the size, because they can rapidly become life threatening if positive-pressure mechanical ventilation is instituted.[98]

In the supine position free gas will localize in the nondependent caudal and anteromedial aspects of the pleural space. Evidence of pneumothorax on the supine chest radiograph is often indirect and includes a prominent costophrenic sulcus (deep sulcus sign), relative basilar hyperlucency, increased sharpness of the ipsilateral hemidiaphragm, increased sharpness of cardiac border, presence of gas in the minor fissure,

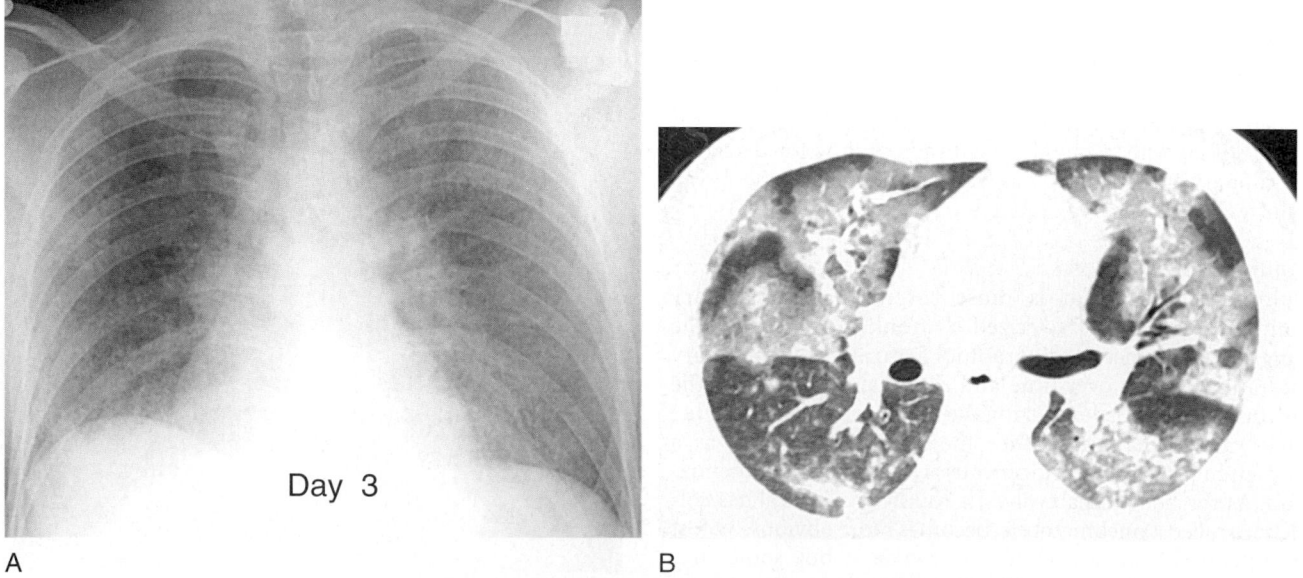

Day 3

A

B

FIGURE 74–14. A 33-year-old man presented with a left femur fracture and clinical fat embolism syndrome. The initial chest radiograph was normal. **A,** Seventy-two hours later, diffuse pulmonary opacity developed without cardiomegaly, coinciding with dyspnea, an altered level of consciousness, and diffuse petechiae. **B,** Axial CT image on the same day shows geographic appearance of ground-glass opacity in both lungs, consistent with noncardiogenic pulmonary edema.

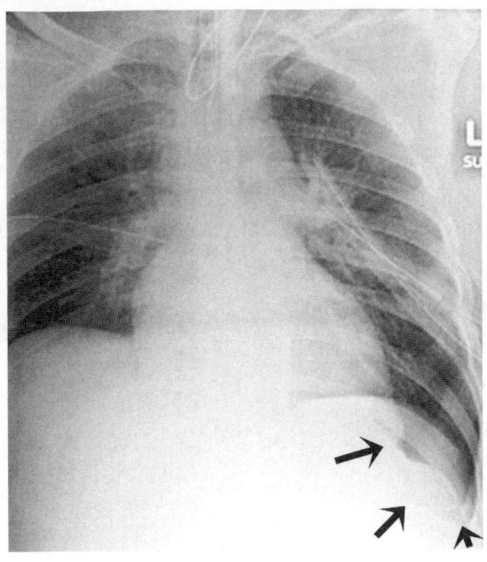

FIGURE 74–15. Bedside anteroposterior chest radiograph shows lucency without pulmonary vessels in the lower left lateral hemithorax expanding the costophrenic sulcus *(arrows)*, despite two left thoracostomy tubes, consistent with pneumothorax, reflecting the deep sulcus sign.

and caudal displacement of the ipsilateral hemidiaphragm (Fig. 74-15).[99-101] CT is more sensitive than chest radiography for detecting pneumothorax and is especially helpful in critically ill patients who cannot tolerate lateral decubitus positioning.

Hemothorax

In contrast to pneumothorax, hemothorax is more common with penetrating chest trauma (63.9% to 82.3%) than with blunt chest injuries (23.2% to 51%).[96,102] Clinical signs and symptoms include hypotension and decreased breath sounds with dullness to percussion over the affected hemithorax.

The supine chest radiograph shows findings identical to those seen with pleural effusion and include increased opacity on the affected hemithorax, a crescentic opacity interposed between the inner margin of ribs and the lung, and an apical cap.[97]

Diaphragmatic Rupture

Rupture of the diaphragm is a rare complication found in 0.8% to 1.6% of patients admitted with blunt trauma.[103] Radiographic findings of diaphragmatic rupture include a gas-filled viscus or the tip of a properly placed enteric tube above the diaphragm (the most strongly suggestive diagnosis sign),[104] irregularity of diaphragmatic contour, elevation of the affected hemidiaphragm without evidence of atelectasis, and contralateral shift of the mediastinum without pleural effusion or pneumothorax (Fig. 74-16).[97,104,105] However, the sensitivity of chest radiographs for detecting diaphragmatic rupture is quite low (46% for ruptures on the left and 17% for ruptures on the right).[104]

CT has proved to be more valuable in the detection of diaphragmatic injuries with a sensitivity of 71% (78% for injuries on the left and 50% for those on the right) and a specificity approaching 100%.[106,107] Findings of diaphragmatic rupture on CT include discontinuity of the diaphragm, visceral herniation, waist-like constriction of the bowel (the collar sign), and layering of the herniated viscus against the posterior ribs (the dependent viscera sign).[108-110] Delay in diagnosis is common, especially in patients receiving positive-pressure ventilation, because the injury is masked by the positive-pressure gradient between the thoracic and abdominal cavities.[111]

MEDICAL ICU

The medical ICU provides care for patients suffering from diseases requiring respiratory support, for patients with severe infections, and those who need close monitoring. This section will focus on patients with acute respiratory distress syndrome (ARDS), pulmonary infection, and pulmonary thromboembolic disease.

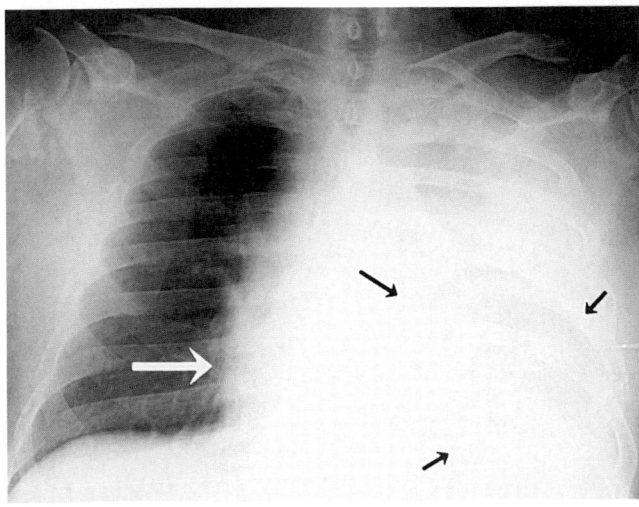

A

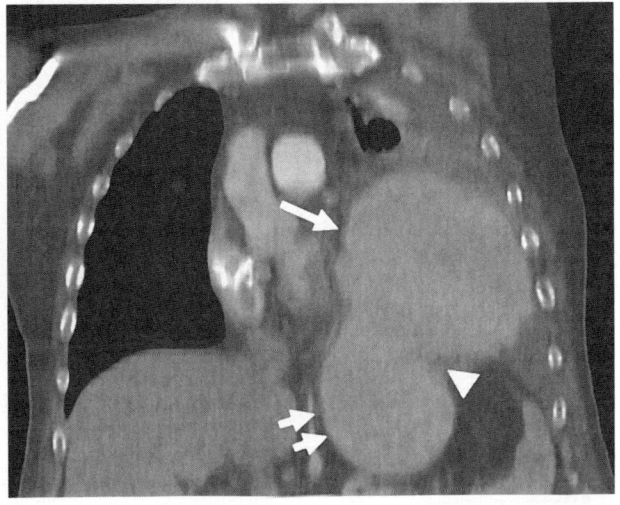

B

FIGURE 74–16. A 48-year-old man involved in a motor vehicle crash sustained a diaphragmatic injury. **A,** Bedside chest radiograph shows diffuse opacity in the left hemithorax and rightward mediastinal displacement *(white arrow)*. A round lucency representing the gastric bubble is present within the opacified left hemithorax *(black arrows)*. **B,** Coronal CT re-formation shows partial herniation of the stomach (gastric fundus [*single arrow*] and gastric body [*double arrows*]) into the chest through a large defect in the diaphragm *(arrowhead)*.

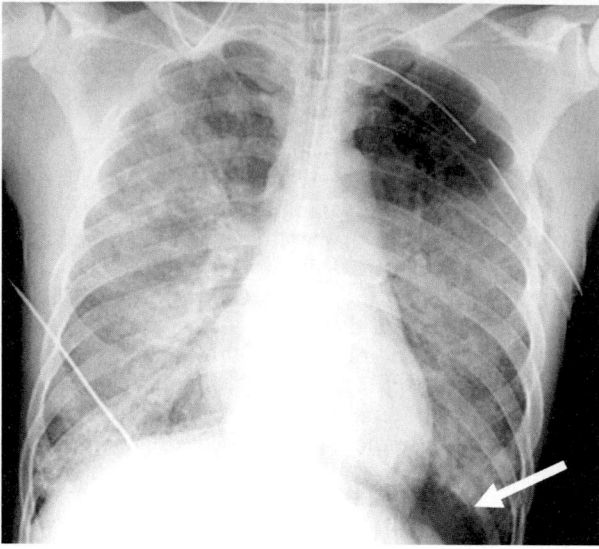

FIGURE 74–17. A 22-year-old man with clinical sepsis developed hypoxia 2 days after admission. An anteroposterior chest radiograph shows diffuse lung opacity with normal heart size, consistent with noncardiogenic pulmonary edema. Also note a pneumothorax in the left costophrenic angle *(arrow).*

Acute Respiratory Distress Syndrome

ARDS represents a massive inflammatory reaction in the lungs resulting from a variety of causes and is characterized by severe hypoxemia. The incidence of ARDS is difficult to determine, partly owing to the variety of causes, but it is a common problem in hospital ICUs. Various published estimates have ranged from 1.5 to 71 cases per 100,000 people. Earlier estimates suggest that approximately 150,000 Americans are affected each year.[112] The radiographic manifestations depend on the stage of the disease. In the acute phase, diffuse ill-defined opacities may be present. Initially, these opacities predominate in the periphery of the lungs[113] and, as the disease progresses, the entire lung can become opacified (Fig. 74-17).[114] During the subacute phase (5 to 10 days later), proliferation of endothelial cells and fibroblasts leads to a pattern of progressive lung destruction on the chest radiograph.

Some patients recover from ARDS without any residual deficit in pulmonary function whereas others progress to the chronic phase several weeks after the initial lung injury with permanent respiratory sequelae. Fibrosis and focal emphysema are usually evident on radiographs at this stage.[115] In contrast to cardiogenic pulmonary edema, ARDS progresses gradually over several days.

Infection
Pneumonia

Nosocomial pneumonias are a serious problem in all critical care units and can have a high mortality, especially in elderly patients and those with other coexistent illnesses.[116,117]

Ventilator-associated pneumonia is defined as the development of new and persistent pulmonary opacities in a patient at least 48 hours after initiation of mechanical ventilation in association with two of the following clinical criteria: fever, leukocytosis, and purulent proximal airway secretions. However, sensitivity and specificity of these criteria are low and blood and airway secretion cultures may be useful in the setting of diffuse lung injury.[118]

The radiographic hallmark of community-acquired pneumonia is airspace consolidation with air bronchograms in a segmental, lobar, or diffuse distribution.[115] The majority of patients with nosocomial pneumonia, however, have a pattern of bronchopneumonia on the chest radiograph characterized by patchy peribronchial opacities, volume loss, and bronchial wall thickening (Fig. 74-18). In mild disease, usually only bronchial wall thickening is evident, whereas in more advanced stages, heterogeneous areas of consolidation develop in several lobes.[119,120] Because of primary involvement of the airways, volume loss in the affected segments or

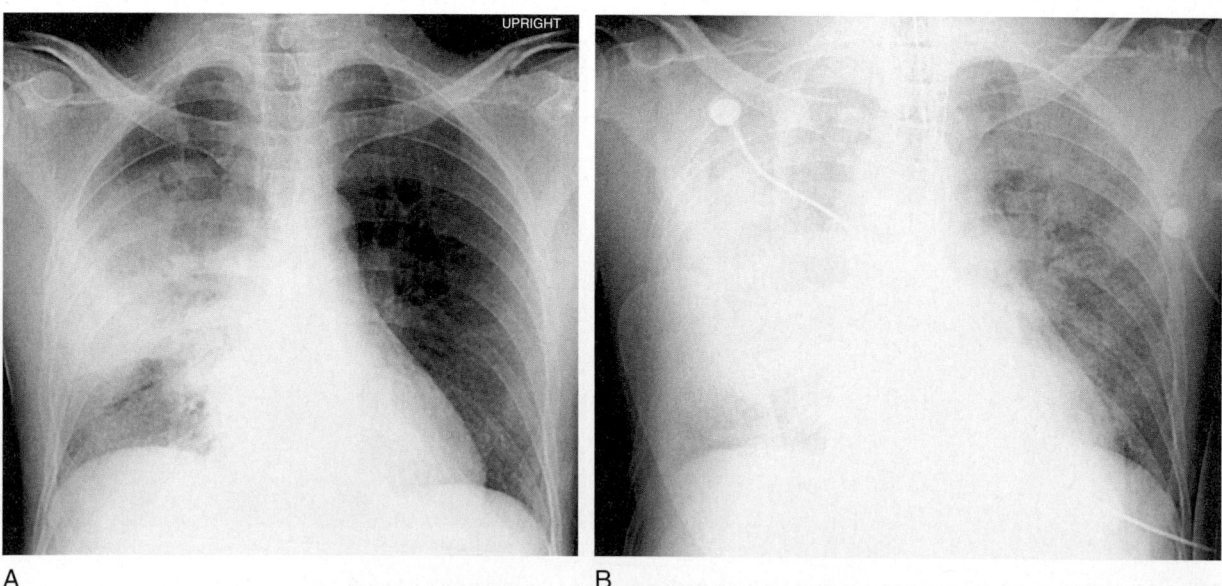

A   B

FIGURE 74–18. A 30-year-old man presented with *Klebsiella pneumoniae* infection. **A,** Initial chest radiograph shows right upper lobe opacity consistent with lobar pneumonia. **B,** Two days later, the right lung is nearly completely opacified, showing the rapid spread of infection. Tube and line are in expected location. Pacing pad is superimposing on the right chest.

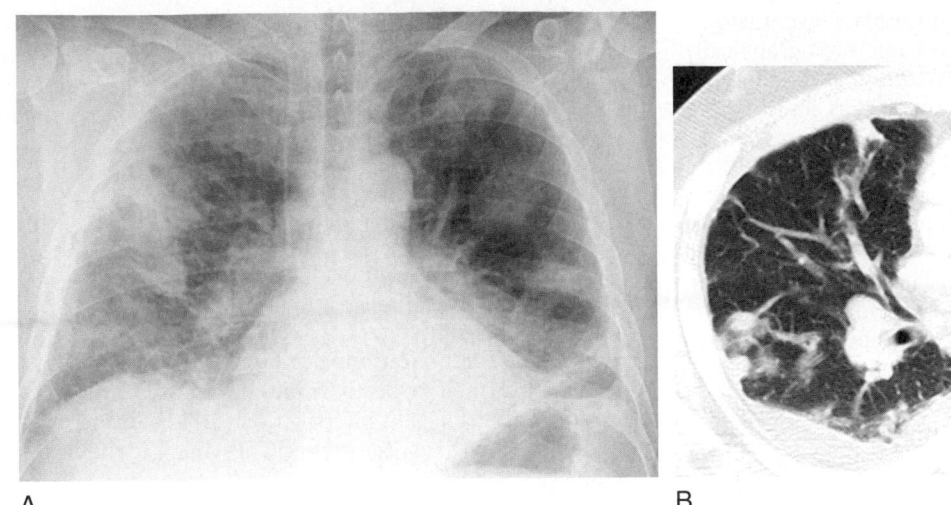

FIGURE 74–19. A 46-year-old intravenous drug abuser presented with septic emboli. **A,** Bedside chest radiograph shows multiple bilateral peripheral opacities, some of which are cavitating. **B,** Axial CT scan shows multiple peripheral well-defined pulmonary nodules with a pulmonary vessel terminating at one of the nodules *(arrow),* an example of the feeding vessel sign of septic embolism.

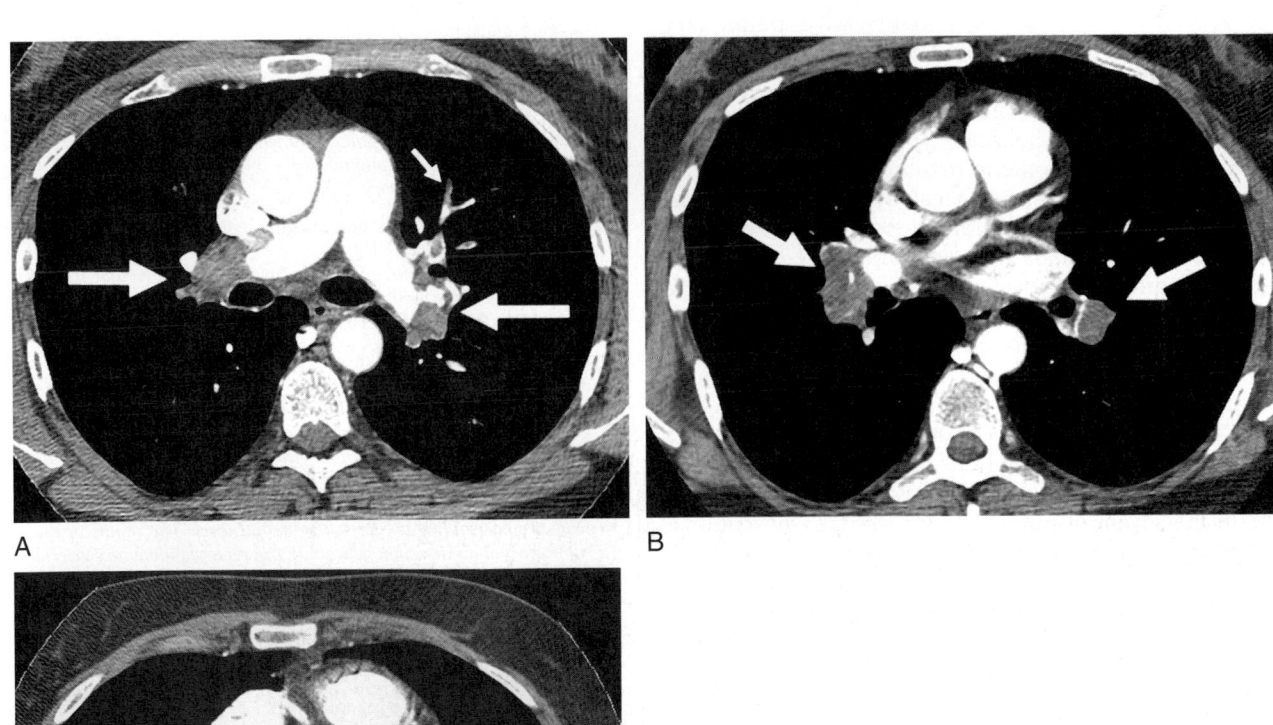

FIGURE 74–20. A 46-year-old woman presented with acute shortness of breath and hypoxia. Chest radiograph is normal. **A,** Axial CT scan of the chest shows evidence of low attenuation filling defect in the left and right main pulmonary arteries *(large arrows)* and left upper lobe segmental artery *(small arrow)* representing massive pulmonary embolism. The emboli extend to the left and right interlobar arteries *(arrows)* as well as left lower lobe segmental artery *(arrow)* as seen in **B** and **C,** respectively.

lobes may accompany bronchopneumonia.[120] Ventilatory-associated pneumonia is indistinguishable radiographically from other causes of nosocomial pneumonia. Radiographs may also show associated complications such as abscesses and pneumatoceles.

Septic Emboli

Septic emboli to the lungs come from a variety of sources, including infected right-sided heart valves, peripheral and pelvic thrombophlebitis, and infected intravenous catheters. The usual radiographic findings of septic emboli are bilateral ill-defined nodular opacities, with or without cavitation, in the lung periphery that develop at different times and show features of different stages of evolution.[121] On CT, multiple parenchymal nodules and wedge-shaped subpleural areas of consolidation are the usual findings. Location adjacent to the end of a pulmonary vessel (feeding vessel sign) often occurs (Fig. 74-19).[122]

Pulmonary Thromboembolic Disease

Acute pulmonary embolism is a potentially lethal condition that can be difficult to diagnose clinically because of the non-specific clinical presentation. Prompt diagnosis and treatment reduce morbidity and mortality.[123,124] The annual incidence of pulmonary embolism is 70 to 133 per 100,000 individuals, with approximately 12% of patients with pulmonary embolism dying within 30 days.[125] Although many imaging modalities including ventilation-perfusion scintigraphy and conventional pulmonary angiography have been used to diagnose pulmonary embolism, CT pulmonary angiography (CTPA) has emerged as the initial imaging study of choice given its high sensitivity and specificity and the additional advantage of evaluating the entire thorax for other explanations for cardiopulmonary signs and symptoms.[126,127]

Many findings on conventional chest radiographs have been described in patients with pulmonary embolism, but they are inconsistently present and are nonspecific. Features diagnostic for acute pulmonary embolism on CTPA include a partial or complete filling defect in the pulmonary arteries (Fig. 74-20).[126,127] Associated parenchymal abnormalities such as regional oligemia, volume loss, and a wedge-shaped pleural-based opacity may also be present.

With the advent of multi-detector row CT, conventional pulmonary angiography has been relegated to an infrequently used problem-solving tool in pulmonary thromboembolic disease. Pulmonary angiography may be indicated in cases in which clinical suspicion for pulmonary embolism remains high despite normal pulmonary vasculature on CTPA and no evidence of deep venous thrombosis on sonographic evaluation of the veins of the lower extremities.[128] In addition, pulmonary angiography may be the appropriate diagnostic examination when visualization of the peripheral pulmonary arteries is limited by technical factors. However, even conventional angiography may fail to detect small peripheral emboli,[129-131] particularly isolated subsegmental clots. The clinical significance of these isolated peripheral thrombi is still debated and likely depends on the patient's underlying cardiopulmonary function.[128]

CONCLUSION

Chest imaging is an important component in diagnostic evaluation of critically ill patients. Although bedside chest radiography is limited by both technical and patient factors, knowledge of complications of various diseases and therapies as well as their respective radiographic appearances can lead to improvement in patient care. CT is indicated when radiographic findings are equivocal or when the chest radiograph does not explain the patient's clinical picture.

ANNOTATED REFERENCES

Brainsky A, Fletcher RH, Glick HA, et al: Routine portable chest radiographs in the medical intensive care unit: Effects and costs. Crit Care Med 1997;25:801-805.

This paper examines the utility of daily chest radiographs in patients admitted to a medical ICU. Approximately a third of the routine radiographs had radiographic findings, 8% of which prompted clinical actions. These results indicate that obtaining routine chest radiograph in the medical ICU not only reveals important clinical findings but also results in net financial savings.

Gluecker T, Capasso P, Schnyder P, et al: Clinical and radiologic features of pulmonary edema. Radiographics 1999;19:1507-1531; discussion 1532-1533.

This paper provides a comprehensive overview of the radiologic findings associated with pulmonary edema.

Kazerooni EA, Cascade PN: Chest imaging in the cardiac intensive care unit. Respir Care 1999;44:1033-1043.

This review of the utility of chest radiographs in the cardiac ICU provides an overview of the ability of chest radiographs to evaluate clinically significant issues in this patient population.

Qanadli SD, Hajjam ME, Mesurolle B, et al: Pulmonary embolism detection: Prospective evaluation of dual-section helical CT versus selective pulmonary arteriography in 157 patients. Radiology 2000;217:447-455.

This study evaluated dual-section helical computed tomography and compared it to helical computed tomography in the evaluation of pulmonary embolism. Dual-section helical CT was found to be an improvement over helical CT that provided higher sensitivity and specificity for pulmonary embolism, including at the subsegmental level. The results of this study indicate that dual-section helical CT can replace pulmonary arteriography for the direct demonstration of pulmonary embolism in most patients.

Shanmuganathan K, Killeen K, Mirvis SE, White CS: Imaging of diaphragmatic injuries. J Thorac Imaging 2000;15:104-111.

This review provides an approach to imaging patients with presumed diaphragmatic injuries. It reviews the relative utility of chest radiographs, spiral CT, and MRI in such patients.

Zinck SE, Primack SL: Radiographic and CT findings in blunt chest trauma. J Thorac Imaging 2000;15:87-96.

This article is a review of the utility of chest radiographs, chest CT, and MRI in the evaluation of patients with blunt thoracic trauma.

Chapter 75

ACUTE LUNG INJURY AND ACUTE RESPIRATORY DISTRESS SYNDROME

Lorraine B. Ware • Gordon R. Bernard

KEY POINTS

1. **ALI/ARDS is very common in critically ill patients and is underdiagnosed.** It is important to make the diagnosis so that appropriate therapy including a lung protective ventilatory strategy can be initiated.

2. The **most common causes of ALI/ARDS** are sepsis, pneumonia, aspiration of gastric contents, and multiple trauma.

3. Despite numerous randomized controlled clinical trials, there is **no specific treatment for ALI/ARDS** that has been proven to be beneficial other than a lung protective ventilatory strategy.

4. Ventilation in volume control mode with a tidal volume of 6 mL/kg predicted body weight and plateau pressure less than 30 cm H_2O has been shown to **improve mortality in ALI/ARDS** compared with a larger tidal volume (12 mL/kg).

Acute lung injury (ALI) and the acute respiratory distress syndrome (ARDS) are common problems in the ICU and can complicate a wide spectrum of critical illnesses. First described by Ashbaugh and colleagues in 1967,[1] ARDS was initially termed the *adult respiratory distress syndrome* to distinguish it from the respiratory distress syndrome of neonates. However, with the recognition that ALI/ARDS can occur in children, the term *acute* has replaced *adult* in the nomenclature, in recognition of the typical acute onset that defines the syndrome. Although specific treatments for ALI/ARDS have been slow to emerge, the recent development of new modes of mechanical ventilation that improve mortality emphasizes the importance of identifying and treating all patients with ALI/ARDS. Although this point would seem to be straightforward, in practice both disorders remain largely underdiagnosed,[2] which perpetuates inappropriate or inadequate treatment.

The exact incidence of ALI/ARDS has been difficult to estimate for a variety of reasons. Until recently, variable definitions were used.[3] The wide variety of causes and coexisting disease processes has also made identification of cases difficult both at the clinical and at the administrative coding level.[4] The National Institutes of Health (NIH) first estimated the incidence at 75 per 100,000 population in 1977.[5]

A number of studies since then have reported lower incidences.[4] However, a recent study that utilized the enrollment logs from the National Heart, Lung and Blood Institute–sponsored ARDS Network of 20 hospitals estimated that the incidence could be as high as 64 cases per 100,000 population, not far off from the original NIH estimate. This dataset has the advantage of being prospectively collected from a large number of academic medical centers. Regardless of the exact incidence, it is clear that ALI/ARDS is a major public health problem that will be encountered frequently by all physicians who care for critically ill patients.

PATHOPHYSIOLOGY

The pathophysiology of ALI/ARDS is complex and remains incompletely understood. Microscopically, lungs from afflicted individuals in the early stages show diffuse alveolar damage with alveolar flooding by proteinaceous fluid, neutrophil influx into the alveolar space, loss of alveolar epithelial cells, deposition of hyaline membranes on the denuded basement membrane, and formation of microthrombi (Fig. 75-1).[6] The alveolar flooding occurs as a result of injury to the alveolar-capillary barrier and is a major determinant of the hypoxemia and altered lung mechanics that characterize early ALI/ARDS. The alveolar-capillary barrier is formed of two separate cell layers: the microvascular

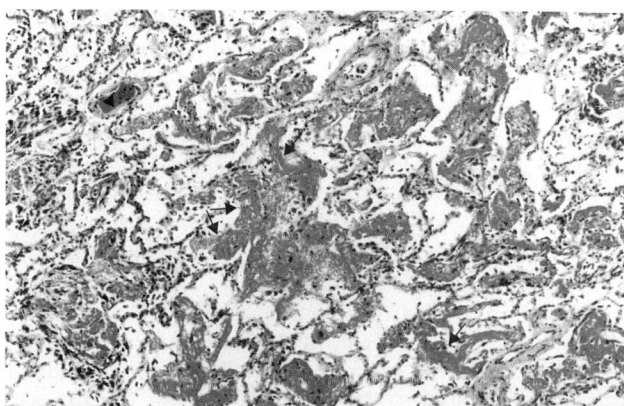

FIGURE 75–1. Low-power photomicrograph of a histologic section from the lung of a patient with the acute respiratory distress syndrome. Note the presence of hyaline membranes (*arrows*), neutrophilic inflammation, and presence of microthrombi (*arrowhead*).

endothelium and the alveolar epithelium. Injury to the alveolar epithelium is a prominent feature histologically with loss of alveolar epithelial barrier integrity and necrosis and sloughing of alveolar epithelial type I cells. Although endothelial injury is less obvious at the microscopic level, ultrastructural studies reveal that it is widespread.[7,8] Endothelial injury allows leakage of plasma from the capillaries into the interstitium and airspaces. The alveolar flooding in ALI/ARDS is characteristically with a protein-rich edema fluid, owing to the increased permeability of the alveolar capillary barrier, in contrast to the low protein pulmonary edema that results from hydrostatic causes such as congestive heart failure or acute myocardial infarction.[9-12]

The mechanisms by which the microvascular endothelium and alveolar epithelium are injured are probably multiple and may vary depending on the inciting event. Neutrophils appear to play an important role.[13] Early ALI/ARDS is characterized by migration of neutrophils into the alveolar compartment.[7,8] Neutrophils can release a variety of injurious substances, including proteases such as neutrophil elastase, collagenase, and gelatinases A and B and reactive nitrogen and oxygen species. In addition, they can elaborate proinflammatory cytokines and chemokines that serve to amplify the inflammatory response in the lung. Resident alveolar macrophages are also involved in initiating and sustaining a proinflammatory cytokine cascade that leads to recruitment of neutrophils into the lung.

In addition to acute neutrophilic inflammation and elaboration of a proinflammatory cytokine cascade, a variety of other abnormalities contribute to the pathogenesis of ALI/ARDS. Surfactant dysfunction is characteristic with abnormalities in both the protein and lipid components[14-17] and likely results from disruption of normal surfactant activity by the influx of plasma proteins into the airspaces, intra-alveolar proteolysis, and injury to the alveolar epithelial type II cells. Surfactant dysfunction may have important implications both for lung mechanics and for host defense.[18] Activation of the coagulation cascade and impaired fibrinolysis are also apparent in patients with ALI/ARDS[19,20] both in the lung and systemically.[21,22] An alteration in the balance of endogenous oxidants and antioxidants with a fall in endogenous antioxidants[23] despite the increased oxidant production has also been observed.[24]

Recently, the contribution of ventilator-associated lung injury to the pathogenesis of ALI/ARDS has been recognized. There are several mechanisms by which mechanical ventilation can injure the lung. Ventilation at very high volumes and pressures can injure even the normal lung, leading to increased permeability pulmonary edema likely due to capillary stress failure.[25] In the injured lung, even tidal volumes that are well tolerated in the normal lung can lead to alveolar overdistention in relatively uninjured areas because the lung available for distribution of the administered tidal volume is greatly reduced and because of uneven distribution of inspired gas.[26,27] In addition to alveolar overdistention, cyclic opening and closing of atelectatic alveoli can cause lung injury even in the absence of alveolar overdistention. The combination of alveolar overdistention with cyclic opening and closing of alveoli is particularly harmful and can initiate a proinflammatory cytokine cascade.[28] A ventilatory strategy that was designed to minimize alveolar overdistention and maximize alveolar recruitment ameliorated this proinflammatory cytokine release.[29] This fundamental insight into the pathogenesis of clinical ALI/ARDS has led to

TABLE 75–1. RISK FACTORS ASSOCIATED WITH DEVELOPMENT OF ACUTE LUNG INJURY AND ACUTE RESPIRATORY DISTRESS SYNDROME

Direct Lung Injury	Indirect Lung Injury
Pneumonia	Sepsis
Aspiration of gastric contents	Multiple trauma
Pulmonary contusion	Cardiopulmonary bypass
Fat, amniotic fluid, or air emboli	Drug overdose
Near-drowning	Acute pancreatitis
Inhalational injury	Transfusion of blood products
Reperfusion pulmonary edema	

multiple clinical trials of novel ventilatory strategies for patients with ALI/ARDS,[30-33] culminating in the landmark ARDS Network trial of 6 mL/kg versus 12 mL/kg tidal volume ventilation (see Treatment section below).

The clinical syndrome of ALI/ARDS appears to be a characteristic and nonspecific response of the lung to a wide variety of insults (Table 75-1). The commonly associated clinical disorders can be separated into those that directly injure the lung and those that indirectly injure the lung. Although it is not always feasible to determine the exact cause of ALI/ARDS in a given patient, direct causes appear to account for approximately one half of all cases of ALI/ARDS.[34] It is not clear whether the distinction between direct and indirect lung injury is clinically useful.[35] Some investigators have demonstrated reduced respiratory system compliance in patients with ARDS due to direct pulmonary injury compared with indirect causes,[36] although total respiratory system compliance (including the chest wall) is similar.[37] Patients with direct lung injury may be more likely to have improved lung mechanics with the application of positive end-expiratory pressure (PEEP). However, in the largest cohort of patients studied to date there was no difference in mortality between those with direct (pulmonary) and indirect (extrapulmonary) causes of lung injury.[34] Regardless of the underlying cause of ALI/ARDS, most patients with ALI/ARDS appear to have a systemic illness with inflammation and organ dysfunction that is not confined to the lung.[38]

Sepsis is the most common cause of indirect lung injury, with an overall risk of progression to ALI or ARDS of 30% to 40%.[39-42] Severe trauma with shock and multiple transfusions also can cause indirect lung injury. Although the other causes of indirect lung injury are less common, many, such as blood transfusions, are frequent events in the ICU setting. The most common cause of direct lung injury is pneumonia, which may be of bacterial, viral, or fungal origin. The risk of developing ALI/ARDS increases substantially in the presence of multiple predisposing disorders.[39] Secondary factors may also increase the risk. Such factors include chronic lung disease[40] and chronic alcohol abuse.[43] To some extent, every patient in the ICU is at risk for developing ALI/ARDS, and vigilance is required to recognize the diagnosis and treat appropriately.

DIAGNOSIS

In 1994, the American European Consensus Conference published new clinical definitions for ALI/ARDS (Table 75-2).[3] Prior to this time, a variety of definitions were used clinically, including the Murray Lung Injury Score.[44]

TABLE 75–2. AMERICAN EUROPEAN CONSENSUS CONFERENCE DEFINITIONS OF ACUTE LUNG INJURY AND THE ACUTE RESPIRATORY DISTRESS SYNDROME

Acute Lung Injury	Acute Respiratory Distress Syndrome
Acute onset	Acute onset
Bilateral infiltrates on chest radiograph consistent with pulmonary edema	Bilateral infiltrates on chest radiograph consistent with pulmonary edema
Absence of clinical evidence of left-sided heart failure (PAWP ≤ 18 mm Hg if measured)	Absence of clinical evidence of left-sided heart failure (PAWP ≤ 18 mm Hg if measured)
PaO_2/FiO_2 ratio ≤ 300	PaO_2/FiO_2 ratio ≤ 200

PAWP, pulmonary artery wedge pressure; PaO_2, arterial partial pressure of oxygen; FiO_2, fraction of inspired oxygen.
From Bernard GR, Artigas A, Brigham KL, et al: The American-European Consensus Conference on ARDS. Definitions, mechanisms, relevant outcomes, and clinical trial coordination. Am J Respir Crit Care Med 1994;149:818-824.

To meet the Consensus diagnostic criteria for either ALI or ARDS, the acute onset of bilateral radiographic infiltrates is required. There should be no clinical evidence of left atrial hypertension, with a pulmonary artery wedge pressure (PAWP) less than or equal to 18 mm Hg if measured. Although not strictly part of these definitions, an underlying cause of lung injury should be sought. In the absence of an identifiable underlying cause (see Table 75-1), particular attention should be given to the possibility of other causes of pulmonary infiltrates and hypoxemia, such as hydrostatic pulmonary edema. If not already in place, flotation of a pulmonary artery catheter may be useful in differentiating high-pressure (hydrostatic) pulmonary edema from the increased permeability pulmonary edema of ALI/ARDS, based on the pulmonary artery wedge pressure. Even this measurement is not foolproof, however, because ALI/ARDS can be complicated by volume overload, severe hypoproteinemia (e.g., as in cirrhosis), or heart failure with concomitant increases in left atrial pressure.

The standardization of definitions for ALI/ARDS has been helpful from several perspectives. For clinical research, it has been valuable in allowing the comparison of different studies and the rapid identification of patients for enrollment in clinical trials. Clinically, the new definitions are easy to apply and facilitate the rapid identification and appropriate treatment of patients with ALI/ARDS. However, it should be noted the nature of ALI/ARDS is such that any definition will have significant shortcomings. First, the definitions must be based solely on clinical criteria because currently there is no laboratory test that allows clinical assessment of the presence or absence of ALI/ARDS. Second, there is no reference to pathogenesis or underlying cause. This is because the list of potential causes of ALI/ARDS is so long, diverse, and common in the critically ill. Third, the presence or absence of multiorgan dysfunction, an important determinant of outcome, is not specified. Finally, although the presence of bilateral infiltrates has major prognostic significance and is clearly a hallmark of ALI/ARDS, the radiographic findings are not specific.[45,46]

In the majority of patients, the initial diagnosis of ALI/ARDS is made clinically. Invasive techniques for diagnosis are of limited clinical utility, and the benefits rarely outweigh the risks. In the past, open lung biopsy was obtained more frequently for diagnosis. Interestingly, the degree of histologic abnormality on lung biopsy does not correlate with ultimate outcome as measured by pulmonary function.[47] Open or thoracoscopic lung biopsy may still be useful in some cases where the diagnosis is uncertain and the underlying cause is not apparent. Occasionally, unsuspected diagnoses requiring specific therapy can be made, such as miliary tuberculosis, pulmonary blastomycosis, or bronchiolitis obliterans organizing pneumonia. Bronchoscopy also has a limited role in diagnosis and may be most useful in the immunocompromised host. Bronchoalveolar lavage for cultures and cytologic examination can identify the cause of pneumonia and is particularly useful in the diagnosis of opportunistic infections. Lavage fluid usually has a predominance of neutrophils, and there may be evidence of diffuse alveolar hemorrhage. Cytologic examination can be used to confirm the presence of diffuse alveolar damage.[48]

In addition to familiarity with the Consensus definitions of ALI and ARDS, the critical care clinician should be aware that ALI and ARDS also have been called by a variety of other terms, some of which are seen mainly in older literature but some that remain in clinical use. Some of the more common of these terms include *adult hyaline membrane disease, postperfusion lung or pump lung, shock lung, ventilator-associated lung injury,* and *adult respiratory insufficiency syndrome.* The term *primary graft failure* or *transplant lung* has been used to describe ALI/ARDS from reperfusion pulmonary edema occurring immediately after lung transplantation. Regardless of the name applied, ALI/ARDS may have prognostic and therapeutic implications above and apart from the underlying cause (e.g., infections, aspiration, trauma). This fact should not take away the imperative to identify these underlying causes, if present, and treat them aggressively.

CLINICAL COURSE

EARLY ALI/ARDS

The Consensus definitions are designed to identify ALI/ARDS patients early in their course, in the acute or exudative phase. Clinically, the acute phase is manifested by the acute onset of radiographic infiltrates consistent with pulmonary edema, hypoxemia, and increased work of breathing. Radiographic infiltrates are bilateral (by definition) but may be patchy or diffuse and fluffy or dense (Fig. 75-2), and pleural effusions may occur.[49] Chest computed tomographic (CT) imaging, although rarely of use clinically, has been employed as an investigative tool to better define the nature of the infiltrates in patients with ALI/ARDS. The distribution of infiltrates by CT is surprisingly patchy; areas of alveolar filling and consolidation occur predominantly in dependent zones, whereas nondependent regions can appear relatively spared.[50,51] Even areas that appear spared in radiographic images may have substantial inflammation when sampled using bronchoalveolar lavage.[52]

The hypoxemia that characterizes early ALI/ARDS is usually relatively refractory to supplemental oxygen. The increased work of breathing in the acute phase of ALI/ARDS is due to decreased lung compliance as a result of alveolar and interstitial edema combined with increased airflow resistance.[53] The combination of hypoxemia and increased work of breathing usually necessitates endotracheal intubation

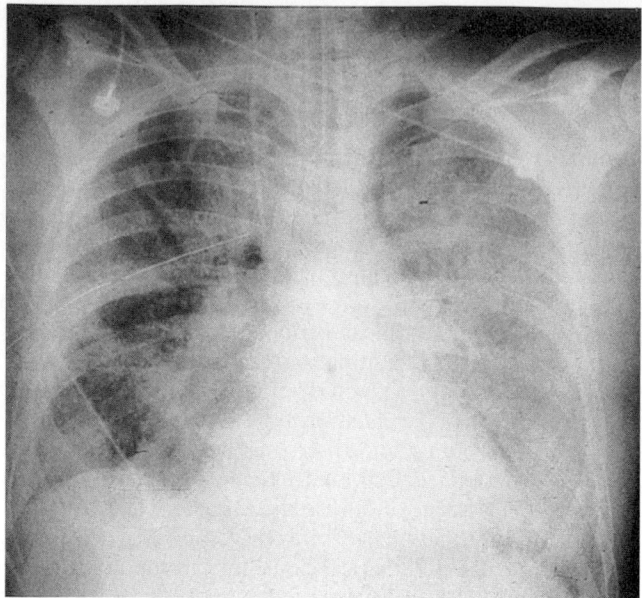

FIGURE 75–2. Portable anteroposterior chest radiograph from a patient with early acute respiratory distress syndrome. Note the diffuse bilateral infiltrates, normal heart size, endotracheal intubation, and the presence of a right-sided thoracostomy tube for drainage of pneumothorax.

and mechanical ventilation, although occasionally patients can be managed with noninvasive ventilation (see Treatment section).

LATE FIBROPROLIFERATIVE ALI/ARDS

In most patients, ALI/ARDS will substantially resolve after the acute phase. However, in others, a fibrosing alveolitis may become clinically apparent after 7 to 10 days, although evidence of deposition of extracellular matrix has been identified in alveolar lining fluid from patients as early as the first day after intubation.[54] Radiographically, linear opacities develop, consistent with the evolving fibrosis. Histologically, pulmonary edema and neutrophilic inflammation are less prominent. A severe fibroproliferative process fills the airspaces with granulation tissue that contains extracellular matrix rich in collagen and fibrin as well as new blood vessels and proliferating mesenchymal cells.[55,56]

Clinically, the late fibroproliferative phase of ALI/ARDS is characterized by continued need for mechanical ventilation, often with persistently high levels of PEEP and FiO_2. The lung compliance may fall even further, and pulmonary deadspace is elevated. Pulmonary hypertension may develop owing to obliteration of the pulmonary capillary bed, and right ventricular failure may occur.[57] This phase of the illness can be prolonged, lasting weeks, and can be very frustrating for the clinician, patient, and family because small gains in pulmonary function are frequently offset by new problems such as hospital-acquired infections, organ failures, or barotrauma. Progressive deconditioning can make eventual weaning from mechanical ventilation difficult if the fibrosing alveolitis stage is prolonged.

RESOLUTION OF ALI/ARDS

Lung biopsy samples from ALI/ARDS survivors typically show normal or near-normal lung histology. For such histologically complete resolution of ALI/ARDS to occur, a variety

of processes must be reversed. Alveolar edema is actively reabsorbed by the vectorial transport of sodium and chloride from the distal airway and alveolar spaces into the lung interstitium.[58] Water is passively absorbed along the osmotic gradient, probably through water channels, the aquaporins.[59] The majority of patients with early ALI/ARDS have impaired alveolar fluid transport; in those with intact alveolar fluid transport, faster rates of alveolar epithelial fluid transport are associated with better outcomes.[12] Soluble and insoluble protein must also be cleared from the airspaces. Soluble protein probably diffuses by a paracellular route into the interstitium, where it is cleared by lymphatics. Insoluble protein probably is cleared by macrophage phagocytosis or alveolar epithelial cell endocytosis and transcytosis.[60]

The denuded alveolar epithelium must be repaired. The alveolar epithelial type II cell serves as the progenitor cell for repopulating the alveolar epithelium. Type II cells proliferate, migrate, and differentiate to reconstitute a tight alveolar epithelial type I cell barrier. The inflammatory cell infiltrate must also resolve, but here the mechanisms are less clear. Resolution of neutrophilic inflammation may be predominantly via neutrophil apoptosis and phagocytosis by macrophages. However, one report suggests that neutrophil apoptosis is impaired in the lungs of patients with ALI/ARDS.[61] The resolution of fibrotic changes is also not well understood. Clearly, however, substantial remodeling is necessary to restore a normal or near-normal alveolar architecture. In patients with advanced fibrosis, this process likely takes place over many months, as pulmonary function abnormalities continue to improve, sometimes remarkably so, out to the first year in survivors of ALI/ARDS (see later).[62]

CLINICAL OUTCOMES

Reported mortality from ALI/ARDS appears to be gradually declining. Prior to the 1990s, mortality in clinical trials was 40% to 60%.[63] Several recent single center studies suggest that mortality rates measured in the same centers had declined over time.[64-67] In the recent ARDS Network study of 861 patients with ALI/ARDS, aggregate mortality to hospital discharge was 31% in the 6 mL/kg tidal volume arm and 40% in the 12 mL/kg tidal volume arm. However, mortality data from this study may significantly underestimate overall ALI/ARDS mortality because many severely ill patients were excluded, including those with advanced liver disease, bone marrow transplantation, severe chronic respiratory disease, burns greater than 30% body surface area, or any other underlying condition with a likelihood of death greater than 50% within 6 months. As has previously been observed in other studies, in this study, risk of in-hospital mortality was highest in those with sepsis (43%), intermediate in those with pneumonia (36%) or aspiration (37%), and lowest in those with multiple trauma (11%).[34] The low tidal volume strategy was effective at reducing mortality across all causes of ALI/ARDS.[34]

Several recent multicenter studies in France,[68] Sweden,[69] Australia,[70] and Argentina[71] attempted to define mortality and prognostic variables in observational population-based studies rather than from clinical trial participants. In these studies, mortality was variable, ranging from 32% for ALI to 58% to 60% for ARDS. The highest mortality observed in patients who met Consensus definitions of ARDS was reported from the French study (60%). Factors that were independently associated with mortality from ALI/ARDS varied from study to study and included age, Acute Physiology Score, PaO_2/FiO_2 ratio, organ failures or septic shock, immunosuppression, and chronic liver disease.[68-71] Two other U.S. studies of patients with ALI/ARDS predominantly from medical ICUs reported high overall mortality rates (58%).[72,73] Mortality was associated with chronic liver disease and other underlying disease such as HIV infection or cancer. In summary, these studies suggest that while some improvements in ALI/ARDS mortality have been made, mortality remains quite high in population-based studies.

In addition to high mortality rates, ALI/ARDS survivors frequently have long-term functional disability. Interestingly, pulmonary function frequently returns to normal or near normal in survivors. In a recent report of 1 year follow-up in 109 survivors of ARDS,[62] lung volumes and spirometry had returned to normal by 6 months. However, carbon monoxide diffusing capacity was persistently low throughout the year. Six-minute walk distances were persistently low at 12 months, largely owing to muscle wasting and weakness rather than pulmonary function abnormalities.[62] Treatment with any systemic corticosteroid, the presence of illness acquired during the ICU stay, and the rate of resolution of the lung injury and multiorgan dysfunction during the ICU stay were the most important determinants of the 6-minute walk distance during the first year of follow-up. In other studies, patients who survive ALI/ARDS have been reported to have both reduced health-related quality of life and reduced pulmonary-disease–specific health-related quality of life.[74-76]

TREATMENT

STANDARD SUPPORTIVE THERAPY

The gradual decline in mortality attributable to ALI/ARDS over time likely reflects improvements in standard supportive therapy. Although it is beyond the scope of this chapter to discuss all aspects of supportive therapy in detail, a few aspects are considered.

Treatment of Predisposing Factors
First and foremost, a search for the underlying cause of ALI/ARDS should be undertaken. Appropriate treatment for any precipitating infection such as pneumonia or sepsis is critical to enhance the chance of survival. In the immunocompromised host, invasive diagnostic evaluation including bronchoscopy may be warranted to look for evidence of opportunistic infections. In a patient with sepsis and ALI/ARDS of unknown source, an intra-abdominal process should be considered. Timely surgical management of intra-abdominal sepsis is associated with better outcomes.[77] In some patients, the cause of lung injury will not be specifically treatable (e.g., aspiration of gastric contents) or will not be readily identifiable.

Fluid and Hemodynamic Management
The appropriate goals for management of volume status and hemodynamics in patients with ALI/ARDS are controversial. A theoretical case can be made for aggressive diuresis, in an effort to reduce the formation of pulmonary edema. Indeed, in experimental lung injury, lower left atrial pressures are associated with less formation of pulmonary edema.[57,78] There is some clinical evidence to support this approach.[79-82] However, reductions in intravascular volume can have adverse effects on cardiac output and tissue perfusion, factors that

could contribute to multisystem organ failure. This is a legitimate concern, because mortality in ALI/ARDS is usually from nonpulmonary causes including other organ failures. In the study by Martin and coworkers, human serum albumin was used to support vascular volume while diuresis was simultaneously affected by furosemide to reduce lung edema.[82] In this pilot randomized clinical trial (n = 37), such treatment did produce transient improvements in oxygenation without compromising the circulation. However, additional studies will be needed to determine effects on ultimate outcome. Some investigators have proposed that clinical outcomes in ALI/ARDS can be improved by delivery of supranormal levels of oxygen using vigorous volume resuscitation and positive inotropes. However, no benefit to supranormal levels of oxygen delivery has been demonstrated in patients with ALI/ARDS.[83,84] One study suggested increased mortality with this approach.[85] Nevertheless, there continues to be a great deal of uncertainty about the appropriate goals for fluid and hemodynamic therapy in ALI/ARDS. While we await the results of ongoing randomized trials, a reasonable strategy is to aim to achieve the lowest intravascular volume that maintains adequate tissue perfusion as measured by urine output or other organ perfusion and metabolic acid-base status. If organ perfusion cannot be maintained in the setting of adequate intravascular volume, then administration of vasopressors and/or inotropes should be used to restore end-organ perfusion.[57] Available evidence does not support the use of one particular vasopressor or combination of vasopressors.

Nutrition
Standard supportive care for the patient with ALI/ARDS includes the provision of adequate nutrition. Although the provision of nutrition has never been studied in randomized controlled trials comparing feeding to withholding of feeding, the available evidence favors the provision of adequate nutrition in critically ill patients. The enteral route is preferred to the parenteral route and is associated with less infectious complications.[86] Enteral feeding may also have other beneficial effects. Experimentally, lack of enteral feeding promoted translocation of bacteria from the intestine.[87] In normal volunteers, administration of parenteral nutrition with bowel rest increased circulating levels of tumor necrosis factor-alpha, glucagon, and epinephrine and increased febrile responses, compared with volunteers who received enteral nutrition.[88]

The goals of nutritional support in any critically ill patient include the provision of adequate nutrients for the patient's level of metabolism and the treatment and prevention of any deficiencies in micronutrients or macronutrients.[89] Whether a particular dietary composition could be beneficial in patients with ALI/ARDS is unclear. Immunomodulation via dietary manipulation has been attempted by a number of investigators in critically ill patients using various combinations of omega-3 fatty acids, ribonucleotides, arginine, and glutamine. A meta-analysis of these trials suggested a beneficial effect on infection rate but not overall mortality.[90] In ALI/ARDS, only one randomized controlled trial of an immunomodulatory nutritional supplement has been published.[91] In that trial, a diet rich in fish oil, gamma-linoleic acid, and antioxidants was associated with a shorter duration of mechanical ventilation and fewer organ failures but no difference in mortality. This trial has yet to be duplicated in a larger patient population. Using a different approach, a high-fat, low-carbohydrate diet reduced the duration of mechanical ventilation in patients with acute respiratory failure.[92] Although the mechanism of this beneficial effect was postulated to be due to reduction of the respiratory quotient and a resultant fall in carbon dioxide production, the most common cause of a high respiratory quotient in critically ill patients is not dietary composition but simply overfeeding.[89] Overall, there is still no compelling evidence to support the use of anything other than standard (enteral) nutritional support, with avoidance of overfeeding, in patients with ALI/ARDS. How early to attempt institution of feeding remains an unanswered question.

MECHANICAL VENTILATION

Lung Protective Ventilation

Although historically a tidal volume of 12 to 15 mL/kg was recommended in patients with ALI/ARDS, it is now clear that a low tidal volume, protective ventilatory strategy reduces mortality. In 2000, the NIH ARDS Network published the findings of their first randomized, controlled,

multicenter clinical trial in 861 patients.[93] The trial was designed to compare a low tidal volume ventilatory strategy (6 mL/kg predicted body weight, plateau pressure less than 30 cm H_2O) with a higher tidal volume (12 mL/kg predicted body weight, plateau pressure less than 50 cm H_2O). The rationale for the clinical trial was the growing body of clinical and experimental evidence suggesting that ventilation with high tidal volumes and high plateau pressures might be harmful to the injured lung (see Pathophysiology earlier). In this trial, the in-hospital mortality rate was 40% in the 12 mL/kg group and 31% in the 6 mL/kg group, a 22% reduction. Ventilator-free days and organ-failure-free days were also significantly improved in the low tidal volume group. These findings were truly remarkable, because no prior large randomized clinical trial of any specific therapy for ALI/ARDS has ever demonstrated a mortality benefit.

The protocol for the ARDS Network low tidal volume ventilatory strategy is summarized in Table 75-3. Predicted body weight is calculated based on measured height, using the equations provided. This is a key point that is often overlooked by clinicians; use of actual rather than predicted body weight can result in the use of erroneously high and potentially

---

TABLE 75–3. SUMMARY OF THE NIH ARDS NETWORK LOWER TIDAL VOLUME STRATEGY

Calculate Predicted Body Weight (PBW):

- Males: PBW (kg) = 50 + 2.3[(height in inches) − 60] or 50 + 0.91[(height in cm) − 152.4]
- Females: PBW (kg) = 45.5 + 2.3[(height in inches) − 60] or 45.5 + 0.91[(height in cm) − 152.4]

Ventilator Mode:

- Volume assist/control until weaning

Tidal Volume (VT):

- Initial VT: adjust VT in steps of 1 mL/kg PBW q1-2h until VT = 6 mL/kg.
- Measure inspiratory plateau pressure (Pplat, 0.5 sec inspiratory pause) every 4 hours *and* after each change in PEEP or VT.
- If Pplat > 30 cm H_2O, decrease VT to 5 or to 4 mL/kg.
- If Pplat < 25 cm H_2O and VT < 6 mL/kg PBW, increase VT by 1 mL/kg PBW.

Respiratory Rate (RR):

- With initial change in VT, adjust RR to maintain minute ventilation.
- Make subsequent adjustments to RR to maintain pH 7.30-7.45, but do not exceed RR = 35/min and do not increase set rate if $PaCO_2$ < 25 mm Hg.

I:E Ratio:

- Acceptable range = 1:1 to 1:3 (no inverse ratio)

FIO2 , PEEP, and Arterial Oxygenation:

- Maintain PaO_2 = 55 to 80 mm Hg or SpO_2 = 88% to 95% using the following PEEP/FIO_2 combinations:

FIO2	0.3-0.4	0.4	0.5	0.5	0.6	0.7	0.7	0.7	0.8	0.9	0.9	1
PEEP	5	8	8	10	10	10	12	14	14	16	18	18-25

Acidosis Management:

- If pH < 7.30, increase RR until pH ≥ 7.30 or RR = 35 breaths/min.
- If pH remains < 7.30 with RR = 35, consider bicarbonate infusion.
- If pH < 7.15, VT may be increased (Pplat may exceed 30 cm H_2O).

Alkalosis Management:

- If pH >7.45 and patient is not triggering ventilator, decrease set RR but not below 6 breaths/min.

Weaning:

- Initiate weaning by Pressure Support when all of the following criteria are present:
  - FIO_2 < 0.40 and PEEP < 8 cm H_2O.
  - Not receiving neuromuscular blocking agents.
  - Inspiratory efforts apparent (ventilator rate may be decreased to 50% of baseline level for up to 5 minutes to detect inspiratory effort).
  - Systolic arterial pressure > 90 mm Hg without vasopressor support.

injurious tidal volumes. The tidal volume should initially be set at 6 mL/kg predicted body weight. Interestingly, a tidal volume of 6 mL/kg predicted body weight is similar to normal tidal volumes in spontaneously breathing adults at rest. So, although this size tidal volume is often referred to as low tidal volume, it is really *normal* tidal volume ventilation. *However*, if end-inspiratory plateau pressure (measured during a 0.5-second pause) is still greater than 30 cm H_2O, then tidal volume must be reduced in a stepwise fashion by 1 mL/kg to a minimum of 4 mL/kg. Ventilation with this size tidal volume is generally well tolerated. Some patients may have breath stacking or significant dyssynchrony with the ventilator. Increasing the inspiratory flow rate and, if necessary, the level of sedation is usually sufficient to manage these problems. As with any mode of ventilation in ALI/ARDS, occasionally patients will require neuromuscular blockade, but this should be used only as a last resort in patients with refractory hypoxemia because the use of paralytics may increase the risk of critical illness polyneuropathy and myopathy. Respiratory acidosis may develop but is usually not symptomatic. Raising the respiratory rate is usually sufficient to compensate for the decreased tidal volume; a rate as high as 35 breaths/min was used in the clinical trial.

In the ARDS Network protocol, the level of PEEP and FIO_2 is titrated according to a set of predetermined values (see Table 75-3). The optimal level of PEEP in ALI/ARDS has been controversial and has never been established. Various strategies for the application of PEEP have been used, including prophylactic PEEP (Table 75-4). The levels of PEEP in the ARDS Network protocol were arrived at by consensus of the ARDS Network investigators. As discussed earlier, recurrent opening and closing of atelectatic alveoli at end expiration may trigger a cytokine cascade and propagate lung injury. This concern has led some to propose that higher levels of PEEP be used to maintain alveolar recruitment. In a small trial, one investigator reported that a ventilator strategy that incorporated low tidal volume and titration

of the PEEP level to above the lower inflection point on each individual patient's pressure-volume curve improved mortality in ARDS.[30] However, measurement of the pressure-volume curve in any given patient is not practical clinically. To address the question of clinical utility of higher PEEP levels in ALI/ARDS, the ARDS Network has completed a large multicenter trial comparing the ARDS Network protocol (see Table 75-3) with a similar protocol that used higher PEEP levels for each level of FIO_2.[94] There was no difference in clinical outcomes between the two groups.

Other Modes of Mechanical Ventilation

A variety of other modes of mechanical ventilation have been used anecdotally or in small clinical trials. Some of these strategies are summarized in Table 75-4. Currently there are no data from large randomized multicenter clinical trials to support the use of any alternative ventilatory strategy. However, the clinician caring for patients with ALI/ARDS may occasionally be faced with severe refractory hypoxemia that is unresponsive even to FIO_2 of 1.0 and a PEEP level of 24 cm H_2O or more. In these situations, deeper sedation and neuromuscular blockade may be helpful. If hypoxemia persists, then alternative strategies might be considered as rescue therapies. Prone positioning and inhaled nitric oxide both can produce transient improvements in oxygenation. However, neither therapy has been shown to improve outcome from ALI/ARDS in large randomized clinical trials (see Table 75-4). More invasive strategies such as ECMO or ECCOR are not widely used outside of the pediatric setting, and there are no data to support their use. High-frequency ventilation and liquid or partial liquid ventilation remain experimental therapies in adults at this time.

Noninvasive Ventilation

Noninvasive positive-pressure ventilation delivered by nasal or full facemask has been highly successful in avoidance of intubation in patients with acute exacerbation of chronic

TABLE 75–4. SUMMARY OF ALTERNATIVE VENTILATOR STRATEGIES FOR ACUTE LUNG INJURY AND THE ACUTE RESPIRATORY DISTRESS SYNDROME

Ventilatory Strategy	Year	How Studied	No. of Patients	Comments	Study
High levels of PEEP	1975	Observational	28	Very high levels of PEEP may improve oxygenation but are associated with a high incidence of pneumothorax.	Kirby, et al.[127]
ECMO	1979	Phase III	90	In this relatively large, multicenter trial there was no benefit with the use of ECMO.	Zapol, et al.[128]
Prophylactic PEEP (8 cm H_2O)	1984	Phase III	92	Prophylactic PEEP did not decrease the incidence of ARDS in patients at risk in this study.	Pepe, et al.[129]
ECCOR	1994	Phase III	40	This newer form of extracorporeal therapy did not improve mortality in ALI/ARDS.	Morris, et al.[130]
Prone positioning	2001	Phase III	304	Although prone positioning improved oxygenation, there was no mortality benefit in this large multicenter trial.	Gattinoni, et al.[131]
Inhaled nitric oxide	1998 / 1999	Phase II / Phase III	177 / 203	Although some patients will have improvement in oxygenation with inhaled nitric oxide, there was no mortality benefit in either of these large studies.	Dellinger, et al.[132]; Payen, et al.[133]
Low tidal volume	1999	Phase III	861	Mortality was reduced by 22% with a 6 mL/kg predicted body weight tidal volume. This is the first large randomized multicenter controlled trial to show a mortality benefit from a specific therapy in ALI/ARDS.	ARDS Network[93]
Low tidal volume with high PEEP	2002	Phase III	549	There was no mortality benefit to increased levels of PEEP compared with the standard ARDS Network low tidal volume strategy.	ARDS Network[94]

PEEP, positive end-expiratory pressure, ECMO, extracorporeal membrane oxygenation, ECCOR, extracorporeal CO_2 removal.

obstructive pulmonary disease (COPD).[95] The role for non-invasive ventilation in ALI/ARDS is less clear. A growing number of small studies suggest that bilevel noninvasive ventilation with pressure support ventilation and PEEP may reduce the need for intubation and improve outcomes in selected patients with ALI/ARDS.[96] However, data from large randomized controlled trials are still lacking. Furthermore, it seems likely that the majority of patients with ALI/ARDS will still require invasive mechanical ventilation. In one large multicenter study of 354 of 2770 patients with acute hypoxemic respiratory failure *who were not already intubated*, noninvasive ventilation failed in 30% of patients but failed in 51% of patients with ARDS.[97] One group of patients in whom noninvasive ventilation is particularly appealing is those patients who are immunosuppressed for various reasons and are at highest risk for nosocomial infections. Encouraging results have now been reported in a variety of patients with acute respiratory failure and immunosuppression.[98-100] Pending data from larger randomized clinical trials, a trial of noninvasive mechanical ventilation could be considered in a patient with ALI/ARDS who does not have a severe oxygenation defect, hemodynamic instability, or altered mental status as long as the patient can be closely observed and readily intubated if noninvasive ventilation fails.

Pharmacologic Therapy

There is no specific pharmacologic therapy for ALI/ARDS. A variety of treatment strategies have been investigated in large randomized trials with a predominant focus on anti-inflammatory strategies. Agents that appeared promising in experimental and early clinical studies, but failed in large randomized trials, include early glucocorticoids,[101,102] alprostadil,[103,104] surfactant,[105,106] ketoconazole,[107] N-acetylcysteine,[108] procysteine,[108] and lisofylline.[109] Some investigators have suggested that glucocorticoid therapy, although not helpful for the acute phase of ALI/ARDS, might hasten the resolution of late fibroproliferative ALI/ARDS. In one very small randomized study (plagued by crossovers such that only four patients remained in the placebo arm) there was a suggestion that glucocorticoid therapy might be beneficial in late ARDS.[110] However, given the serious concern about safety of high doses of glucocorticoids in critically ill patients, including the possibility of increasing the risk of nosocomial infections or critical illness polyneuropathy/myopathy, routine use of glucocorticoids cannot be recommended. An ARDS Network randomized, double-blind study of late corticosteroids in ALI/ARDS is ongoing and results are expected soon.

Despite the dismal findings in the numerous studies of pharmacologic therapy for ALI/ARDS to date, new therapeutic strategies are under investigation and may yet be beneficial. One area that has been largely ignored in the therapeutic realm is modulation of coagulation. There is mounting evidence that, like sepsis, ALI/ARDS is a procoagulant, antifibrinolytic state.[19,20] The recent report of a significant mortality reduction in severe sepsis with intravenous drotecogin alfa activated, a recombinant activated protein C, raises the hope that therapies that modulate coagulation or fibrinolysis may also have efficacy in ALI/ARDS.[111] Another area that is actively under investigation is strategies to hasten or facilitate the resolution of ALI/ARDS. Such therapies might be targeted at enhancing the rate of alveolar fluid clearance or at modulating alveolar repair.

COMPLICATIONS

Complications are common in any critically ill patient population. Supportive care for all critically ill patients must include vigilance in both preventing and diagnosing common complications such as pulmonary embolus, acute myocardial infarction, gastrointestinal bleeding, and nosocomial infection. Certain complications are more common in ALI/ARDS patients and deserve special mention.

Barotrauma

Barotrauma occurs when air dissects out of the airways or alveolar space into surrounding tissues, leading to pneumothorax, pneumomediastinum, pneumatocele, or subcutaneous emphysema (Fig. 75-3). The exact incidence of pulmonary barotrauma in ALI/ARDS is unclear but appears to be declining. Data from two recent large randomized trials of protective ventilatory strategies suggest an incidence of early pneumothorax of 12% to 13%.[31,93] Higher incidences have been reported in the past, a finding that may have been the result of the use of mechanical ventilation with high tidal volumes and very high inspiratory plateau pressures.[112] In 861 patients enrolled in the NIH ARDS Network trial, approximately 10% of patients developed some form of barotrauma regardless of whether they were in the 6- or 12-mL/kg tidal volume arm. Furthermore, PEEP level was the only factor that predicted the development of barotrauma in a multivariate analysis.[113]

Treatment of barotrauma depends on the location of the extravasated air. Pneumothorax can be life threatening,

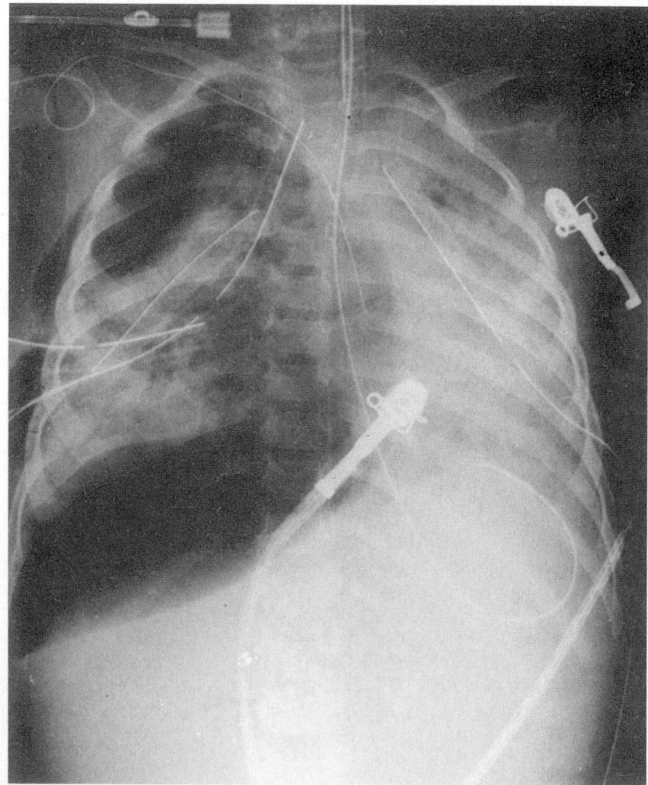

FIGURE 75–3. Portable anteroposterior chest radiograph from a patient with late fibroproliferative acute respiratory distress syndrome and large right sided tension pneumothorax. The patient had multiple episodes of tension pneumothorax due to pulmonary barotrauma and required multiple bilateral tube thoracostomies.

particularly if it is under tension, and immediate diagnosis and tube thoracostomy is essential. Pneumothorax should be considered in any mechanically ventilated patient with ALI/ARDS who develops sudden, unexplained worsening of hypoxemia, respiratory distress, or hemodynamic instability. A chest radiograph (preferably upright) is usually sufficient to make the diagnosis, but in many cases there may not be time to obtain one. Pneumomediastinum and subcutaneous emphysema can be painful but, other than analgesia, do not require specific therapy. Air embolus is a potentially fatal complication of positive-pressure mechanical ventilation that has been reported occasionally in patients with ALI/ARDS[114-116] and usually occurs in conjunction with other evidence of pulmonary barotrauma, many times simultaneously.

Nosocomial Pneumonia

The incidence of nosocomial pneumonia in patients with ALI/ARDS is difficult to quantify. Depending on the diagnostic definition and/or strategy employed, estimates range from 15% to 60% of patients.[117-119] There is yet no consensus regarding the appropriate way to diagnose nosocomial pneumonia in the mechanically ventilated patient. Because patients with ALI/ARDS frequently die of uncontrolled infection, recognition, although notably difficult, and treatment of nosocomial pneumonia is an important part of caring for the ALI/ARDS patient. Clinical criteria that are commonly used in the diagnosis include fever, elevated white blood cell count, purulent secretions, and pulmonary infiltrates. But these signs are often present in patients with ALI/ARDS, even in the absence of nosocomial pneumonia.[120] Autopsy studies of patients dying with ALI/ARDS show a high incidence of unsuspected pneumonia.[121-123] An in-depth discussion of diagnostic strategies is presented elsewhere in this text. Regardless of the methods used for diagnosis, early, appropriate empirical therapy is the mainstay of treatment for nosocomial pneumonia. The adequacy and timeliness of initial empirical therapy are important determinants of outcome. Knowledge of local resistance patterns is crucial, and a high index of suspicion is required.

Multiorgan System Dysfunction

Although ALI and ARDS are often thought of as primary pulmonary disorders, evidence is accumulating to suggest that they are systemic disorders with many similarities to sepsis or SIRS. Multiorgan system dysfunction is a common complication in ALI/ARDS. Organ dysfunction may result from the underlying cause of ALI/ARDS, such as sepsis, or occur independently. The exact incidence of multiorgan system dysfunction in ALI/ARDS is difficult to quantify. In the ARDS Network trial of low tidal volume ventilation, the mean number of nonpulmonary organ system failures was 1.8.[93] Given the simultaneous occurrence of multiple organ failures, it is often difficult to determine the exact cause of death in ALI/ARDS patients, and survival ultimately depends on the successful support of the failing organs.

Neuromuscular Weakness

Patients with ALI/ARDS are at high risk for developing prolonged muscle weakness that persists after resolution of pulmonary infiltrates and can complicate weaning from mechanical ventilation and rehabilitation. These clinical syndromes are commonly called critical illness polyneuropathy but actually have components of neuropathy and myopathy that can coexist or occur separately.[124] Although little prospective data are available, one study suggests that neuromuscular abnormalities are persistent in many survivors of critical illness, even when studied up to 5 years after ICU discharge.[125] Prolonged muscle weakness is most common in critically ill patients who are treated with glucocorticoids. In one study, use of corticosteroids was shown to be the best independent predictor of ICU-acquired paresis (odds ratio 14.9, 95% CI 3.2 to 69.8).[126] In other studies neuromuscular blockade has also been implicated, and for this reason the use of neuromuscular blockade should be reserved for those patients who are unable to be adequately oxygenated or who have problematic dyssynchrony with the mechanical ventilator despite deep sedation. In the absence of a compelling clinical indication such as underlying connective tissue disease, the use of glucocorticoids also should not be routine, unless new clinical evidence in support of their clinical utility in late ALI/ARDS becomes available.

ANNOTATED REFERENCES

Bernard GR, Artigas A, Brigham KL, et al: The American-European Consensus Conference on ARDS: Definitions, mechanisms, relevant outcomes, and clinical trial coordination. Am J Respir Crit Care Med 1994; 149:818-824.

This paper presents the findings of the American-European Consensus Conference on ARDS, including the new definitions for acute lung injury and the acute respiratory distress syndrome that are now widely used both clinically and in research studies.

Herridge MS, Cheung AM, Tansey CM, et al: One-year outcomes in survivors of the acute respiratory distress syndrome. N Engl J Med 2003;348:683-693.

In this multicenter study the authors evaluated 109 survivors of ARDS at 3, 6, and 12 months after discharge from the hospital. Notably, functional disability was very common even at 12 months and was largely caused by muscle wasting and weakness. By contrast, pulmonary function was normalized other than persistent decrements in the diffusing capacity for carbon monoxide.

Rubenfeld GD: Epidemiology of acute lung injury. Crit Care Med 2003;31:S276-S284.

This is a scholarly review of all the pertinent issues that hamper an accurate estimate of the incidence of ALI/ARDS.

The Acute Respiratory Distress Syndrome Network: Ventilation with lower tidal volumes as compared with traditional tidal volumes for acute lung injury and the acute respiratory distress syndrome. N Engl J Med 2000; 342:1301-1308.

This was a multicenter trial of 6 mL/kg compared with 12 mL/kg tidal volume in 861 mechanically ventilated patients with ALI or ARDS. The major finding was a reduction in hospital mortality in the 6 mL/kg group from 40% to 31%.

Ware LB, Matthay MA: Medical progress: The acute respiratory distress syndrome. N Engl J Med 2000;342:1334-1349.

This review article presents a comprehensive overview of the pathogenesis, clinical features, and treatment of ALI and ARDS.

Chapter 76

ASPIRATION PNEUMONITIS AND PNEUMONIA

Paul E. Marik

KEY POINTS

1. *Aspiration pneumonitis* is defined as acute lung injury following the aspiration of regurgitated gastric contents and results in a chemical burn of the tracheobronchial tree and pulmonary parenchyma with an intense parenchymal inflammatory reaction.

2. **The severity of lung injury after aspiration of gastric contents** increases significantly with the volume of the aspirate and indirectly with its pH, with a pH less than 2.5 and a volume of 20 mL being required to cause aspiration pneumonitis.

3. **The treatment of aspiration pneumonitis** is essentially supportive; corticosteroids and antibiotics have no proven benefit.

4. **Aspiration pneumonia develops after the aspiration of colonized oropharyngeal contents in patients with dysphagia.**

5. **The most common causes of dysphagia** leading to aspiration pneumonia include cerebrovascular and degenerative central nervous system disease.

6. **The treatment of aspiration pneumonia** includes antibiotics directed against the most likely pathogens (including aerobic gram-negative organisms), an evaluation by a speech and language pathologist, aggressive oral hygiene, and treatment with an angiotensin-converting enzyme (ACE) inhibitor.

Aspiration is defined as the misdirection of oropharyngeal or gastric contents into the larynx and lower respiratory tract.[1] An assortment of pulmonary syndromes may occur after aspiration depending on the quantity and nature of the aspirated material, the frequency of aspiration, as well as the nature of the host's defense mechanisms and the host's response to the aspirated material.[2] The most important syndromes include *aspiration pneumonitis* or Mendelson's syndrome, which is a chemical pneumonitis caused by the aspiration of gastric contents, and *aspiration pneumonia,* an infectious process caused by the aspiration of oropharyngeal secretions colonized by pathogenic bacteria. Although there is some overlap between these two syndromes, they are distinct clinical entities.

ASPIRATION PNEUMONITIS

Aspiration pneumonitis is best defined as acute lung injury after the aspiration of regurgitated gastric contents. This syndrome occurs in patients with a marked disturbance of consciousness, such as drug overdose, seizures, massive cerebrovascular accident, following head trauma, and anesthesia. Drug overdose is the most common cause of aspiration pneumonitis, occurring in approximately 10% of patients hospitalized after a drug overdosage.[3,4] Adnet and Baud demonstrated that the risk of aspiration increases with the degree of unconsciousness (as measured by the Glasgow Coma Scale).[5] Historically, the syndrome most commonly associated with aspiration pneumonitis is Mendelson's syndrome, reported in 1946 in obstetric patients who aspirated while receiving general anesthesia.[6] Mendelson's original report consisted of 44,016 nonfasted obstetric patients whom he studied between 1932 and 1945, of whom more than half received "operative intervention" with ether by mask without endotracheal intubation. He described aspiration in 66 patients (1:667). Although several of the patients were critically ill from their aspirations, "recovery was usually complete" within 24 to 36 hours and only two patients died (1:22; $P = .0008$).

Although aspiration is a widely feared complication of general anesthesia, clinically apparent aspiration in modern anesthesia practice is exceptionally rare, and in healthy patients the overall morbidity and mortality are low. The risk of aspiration with modern anesthesia is about 1 in 3,000 anesthetics, with a mortality of approximately 1:125,000, accounting for between 10% to 30% of all anesthetic deaths.[7-10] The risk of aspiration is greatly increased in patients intubated emergently in the field, emergency department, or ICU. In these patients every effort should be made to reduce the risk of aspiration; this includes removing dentures and clearing the airway and in certain circumstances placing a nasogastric tube to empty the stomach before intubation.[10] If there is an immediate risk of airway compromise, endotracheal intubation should be performed before placement of a nasogastric tube. However, if the patient is likely to have a full stomach (e.g., upper gastrointestinal hemorrhage, small bowel obstruction, ileus), it may be prudent to place a nasogastric tube before endotracheal intubation. When intubating emergently, suction equipment must be immediately available and rapid-sequence induction using cricoid pressure should be performed. Those factors that are reported to increase the risk of aspiration during endotracheal intubation are listed in Table 76-1.

Mendelson emphasized the importance of acid when he showed that unneutralized gastric contents introduced into the lungs of rabbits caused severe pneumonitis indistinguishable from that caused by an equal amount of 0.1 N hydrochloric acid.[6] However, if the pH of the vomitus was neutralized before aspiration, the pulmonary injury was minimal.[11]

TABLE 76–1. RISK FACTORS FOR ASPIRATION DURING ENDOTRACHEAL INTUBATION

Emergent situations
Upper gastrointestinal hemorrhage
Difficult intubation/multiple intubation attempts
Advanced age (>70 yr)
Seizures
Conditions predisposing to gastroesophageal reflux:
    Bowel obstruction
    Ileus
    Hiatal hernia
    Peptic ulcer disease
    Gastritis

Experimental studies have demonstrated that the severity of lung injury increases significantly with the volume of the aspirate and indirectly with its pH, with a pH of less than 2.5 being required to cause aspiration pneumonitis.[11-13] However, the stomach contains a variety of other substances in addition to acid. Several experimental studies have revealed that aspiration of small, particulate food matter from the stomach may cause severe pulmonary damage, even if the pH of the aspirate is above 2.5.[14,15]

Aspiration of gastric contents results in a chemical burn of the tracheobronchial tree and pulmonary parenchyma with an intense parenchymal inflammatory reaction. Experimental studies have shown a biphasic pattern of lung injury after acid aspiration.[16] The first phase peaks at 1 to 2 hours after aspiration and presumably results from the direct caustic effect of the low pH on the alveolar-capillary wall lining cells. The second phase, which peaks at 4 to 6 hours, is associated with infiltration of neutrophils into the alveoli and lung interstitium with a histologic picture of acute inflammation. The mechanisms causing the lung injury after gastric aspiration have been shown to involve a diverse spectrum of inflammatory mediators, inflammatory cells, adhesion molecules and enzymes, including tumor necrosis factor-alpha (TNF-α), interleukin (IL)-8, cyclooxygenase and lipoxygenase products, and reactive oxygen species.[17-21] However, neutrophils appear to play a key role in the development of lung injury after gastric aspiration. Experimental studies have demonstrated that neutropenia, inhibition of neutrophil function, and inactivation of IL-8 (a potent neutrophil chemoattractant) attenuates the acute lung injury induced by acid aspiration.[18,22,23] Intercellular adhesion molecule-1 (ICAM-1) may play a central role in the trafficking of neutrophils into the lung after acid aspiration. Bronchial epithelium expresses ICAM-1 constitutively, and this expression is increased with acid exposure.[24,25] In animal models anti–ICAM-1 antibodies reduce neutrophil infiltration after acid exposure.[21] Pentoxifylline inhibits surface expression of ICAM-1 on alveolar epithelial cells and has been demonstrated to decrease acid-induced lung injury.[26]

Gastric acid prevents the growth of bacteria, and thus the contents of the stomach are normally sterile. Bacterial infection, therefore, does not play a significant role in the early stages of acute lung injury after aspiration of gastric contents. Bacterial superinfection may occur at a later stage; however, the incidence of this complication has not been studied. Colonization of the gastric contents by potentially pathogenic organisms may occur when the gastric pH is increased by the use of antacids, H_2 blockers, or proton pump inhibitors.[27-29] In addition, gastric colonization by gram-negative bacteria

occurs in patients receiving gastric enteral feedings, as well as in patients with gastroparesis and small bowel obstruction.[30-32] In these circumstances the pulmonary inflammatory response is likely to result from both bacterial infection and the inflammatory response of the gastric particulate matter.

Aspiration of gastric contents can present dramatically with a full-blown picture that includes gastric contents in the oropharynx, wheezing, coughing, shortness of breath, cyanosis, pulmonary edema, hypotension, and hypoxemia, which may progress rapidly to severe acute respiratory distress syndrome (ARDS) and death.[33] Many patients may not develop signs or symptoms associated with aspiration, whereas others may develop a cough or wheeze. In some patients aspiration may be clinically silent, manifesting only as arterial desaturation with radiologic evidence of aspiration. Warner and colleagues studied 67 patients who aspirated while undergoing anesthesia.[8] Forty-two (64%) of these patients were totally asymptomatic, 13 required mechanical ventilatory support for more than 6 hours, and 4 died.

MANAGEMENT

The upper airway should be suctioned after a witnessed aspiration. Endotracheal intubation should be considered in patients who are unable to protect their airway. While common practice, the prophylactic use of antibiotics in patients with suspected or witnessed aspiration is not recommended. Similarly, the use of antibiotics shortly after an aspiration episode in a patient who develops a fever, leukocytosis, and a pulmonary infiltrate is discouraged because it may select for more resistant organisms in a patient with an uncomplicated chemical pneumonitis. However, empirical antimicrobial therapy is appropriate in patients who aspirate gastric contents in the setting of small bowel obstruction or in other circumstances associated with colonization of gastric contents. Antimicrobial therapy should be considered in patients with an aspiration pneumonitis that fails to resolve within 48 hours. Empirical therapy with broad-spectrum agents is recommended. Antimicrobials with anaerobic activity are not routinely required. Lower respiratory tract sampling (protected specimen brush/bronchoalveolar lavage) and quantitative culture in intubated patients may allow targeted antimicrobial therapy and the discontinuation of antibiotics in culture-negative patients.[34-36]

Corticosteroids have been used in the management of aspiration pneumonitis since 1955.[37] However, limited data exist on which to evaluate the role of these agents, with only a single prospective, placebo-controlled study having been performed. In this study, Sukumaran and colleagues reported that radiographic changes improved more quickly in the steroid group; however, these patients had a longer ICU stay and there was no significant difference in the incidence of complications or outcome.[38,39] In a case-controlled study, Wolfe and colleagues reported that the occurrence of gram-negative pneumonia after aspiration was more frequent in the patients treated with corticosteroids.[40] Similarly, animal models have failed to demonstrate a beneficial effect of corticosteroids on pulmonary function, lung injury, alveolar-capillary permeability, or outcome after acid aspiration.[41,42] Furthermore, considering the failure of two multicenter, randomized, controlled trials to demonstrate a benefit from high-dose corticosteroids in ARDS, corticosteroids cannot be recommended.[43,44]

ASPIRATION PNEUMONIA

Aspiration pneumonia develops after the aspiration of colonized oropharyngeal contents. Aspiration of pathogens from a previously colonized oropharynx is the primary pathway by which bacteria gain entrance to the lungs. Indeed, *Haemophilus influenzae* and *Streptococcus pneumoniae* first colonize the naso/oropharynx before being aspirated and causing community-acquired pneumonia (CAP).[45] Furthermore, nosocomial pneumonia and ventilator-associated pneumonia occur after the aspiration of colonized oropharyngeal material.[46] However, when the term *aspiration pneumonia* is used, it refers to the development of a radiographic infiltrate in the setting of patients with risk factors for increased oropharyngeal aspiration (dysphagia). The clinical setting in which pneumonia develops largely distinguishes aspiration pneumonia from other forms of pneumonia. However, there is much overlap. This is illustrated by the fact that otherwise healthy elderly patients with CAP have been demonstrated to have a significantly higher incidence of silent aspiration when compared with age-matched controls.[47]

Several studies list "aspiration pneumonia" as the cause of CAP in 5% to 15% of cases.[48-50] It has been estimated that in the United States approximately 500,000 people each year are affected by dysphagia resulting from neurologic disorders.[51] Aspiration pneumonia is the major cause of death in these patients.[52,53] Epidemiologic studies have demonstrated that the incidence of pneumonia increases with aging, with the risk being almost six times higher in those over age 75 years, compared with those younger than age 60 years.[54-57] The attack rate for pneumonia is highest among those in nursing homes.[56] Marrie found that 33 of 1,000 nursing home residents per year required hospitalization for treatment of pneumonia, compared with 1.14 of 1,000 elderly adults living in the community.[58] The high rate of pneumonia in inhabitants of nursing homes and other long-term care facilities that house the aged is largely related to an increased incidence of dysphagia in this group of patients.

Approximately one half of all healthy adults aspirate small amounts of oropharyngeal secretions during sleep.[59,60] Presumably the low virulent bacterial burden of normal pharyngeal secretions together with forceful coughing, active ciliary transport, and normal humoral and cellular immune mechanisms result in clearance of the inoculum, without sequelae. However, if the mechanical, humoral, or cellular mechanisms are impaired or if the aspirated inoculum is large enough, pneumonia may follow. Any condition that increases the volume and/or bacterial burden of oropharyngeal secretion in the setting of impaired host defense mechanism may lead to aspiration pneumonia. Indeed, in stroke patients undergoing swallow evaluation there is a strong correlation between the volume of the aspirate and the development of pneumonia.[61] Factors that increase oropharyngeal colonization with potentially pathogenic organisms and that increase the bacterial load may augment the risk of aspiration pneumonia. Terpenning and colleagues demonstrated that an edentulous patient had a lower risk of aspiration pneumonia than a dentate patient.[62] Furthermore, a number of studies have demonstrated that a program of aggressive oral care in elderly patients living in nursing homes reduces the incidence of aspiration pneumonia.[63-65]

RISK FACTOR FOR DYSPHAGIA

Dysphagia occurs commonly after a stroke. In patients with an acute stroke the incidence of dysphagia ranges from 40% to 70%, with approximately 500,000 patients per year in the United States developing neurologic dysphagia.[51,52,66-71] Forty to 50 percent of stroke patients with dysphagia aspirate. Dysphagic patients who aspirate are at an increased risk of developing pneumonia.[71,72] Specifically, the development of pneumonia is seven times greater in stroke patients who aspirate, as compared with those who do not.[52,71] Although dysphagia improves in most patients following a stroke, in many the swallowing difficulties follow a fluctuating course, with 10% to 30% continuing to have dysphagia with aspiration.[67,68] Nakajoh and colleagues evaluated the cough reflex and swallowing in 143 stroke patients whom they followed for 1 year.[70] Forty-three patients had a normal cough reflex and swallow; none of these patients developed pneumonia. However, 24 of the 100 patients with abnormal cough reflex and swallow function developed pneumonia. Elderly patients are at risk of silent cerebral infarction. Nakagawa and coworkers demonstrated that elderly patients with silent cerebral infarction have a fivefold higher risk of developing pneumonia than elderly patients with normal head computed tomographic (CT) scans.[73]

Almost all patients with degenerative diseases of the central nervous system develop dysphagia.[74-80] In patients with Alzheimer's disease, amyotrophic lateral sclerosis (ALS), and Parkinson's disease, dysphagia usually occurs early in the course of the disease and the severity of dysphagia does not necessarily relate to the overall severity of the neurologic disease. Considering the high incidence of cerebrovascular and degenerative neurologic diseases in nursing home residents it is not surprising that the reported incidence of dysphagia in this population is between 50% to 75% and explains the extremely high attack rate of pneumonia in these patients.[58,81-83]

While the presence of dysphagia and the volume of the aspirate are key factors that predispose elderly patients to aspiration pneumonia, a number of other factors play an important role.[61] Colonization of the oropharynx is an important step in the pathogenesis of aspiration pneumonia. The elderly have increased oropharyngeal colonization with pathogens such as *Staphylococcus aureus* and aerobic gram-negative bacilli (e.g., *Klebsiella pneumoniae* and *Escherichia coli*).[84-86] Although this increased colonization may be transient, lasting less than 3 weeks, it underlies the increased risk in the elderly of pneumonia with these pathogens. The defects in host defenses that predispose to enhanced colonization with these organisms are uncertain; however, dysphagia with a decrease in salivary clearance and poor oral hygiene may be major risk factors.[84]

In patients with aspiration pneumonia, unlike the case of aspiration pneumonitis, the episode of aspiration is generally not witnessed. The diagnosis is therefore inferred when a patient with known risk factors for aspiration has an infiltrate in a characteristic bronchopulmonary segment. In patients who aspirate in the recumbent position the most common sites of involvement are the posterior segments of the upper lobes and the apical segments of the lower lobes. In patients who aspirate in the upright or semi-recumbent position the basal segments of the lower lobes are favored. The usual picture is that of an acute pneumonic process, which runs a course similar to that of a typical CAP. If untreated, however, these patients appear to have a higher incidence of cavitation and lung abscess formation.[87]

BACTERIOLOGY

Despite extensive investigations, the diagnosis of the bacterial cause of CAP is made in 50% or less of patients overall; this is particularly so in the elderly, who may not be able to produce adequate sputum specimens for evaluation.[88,89] Oropharyngeal colonization with gram-negative pathogens and *S. aureus* with subsequent aspiration accounts for the greater prevalence of these pathogens in elderly patients with CAP. It is unclear, however, if patients with dysphagia are at an increased risk of developing pneumococcal pneumonia, because no study has specifically reported the microbiology of CAP in patients with oropharyngeal dysphagia and aspiration. However, Kikuchi and colleagues reported a high incidence of silent aspiration in otherwise healthy elderly ambulatory patients with no specific risk factors for gram-negative or *S. aureus* oropharyngeal colonization who developed CAP.[47] Unfortunately, in this study the microbial causes of CAP were not reported.

A number of studies performed in the early 1970s investigated the bacteriology of community-acquired "aspiration pneumonia."[87,90-92] Bacteriologic specimens were obtained by percutaneous transtracheal sampling and/or thoracocentesis. In all these studies anaerobic organisms were the predominant pathogens, isolated alone or together with aerobes. Based on these studies, antibiotics with anaerobic activity have became "the standard of care" for patients with aspiration pneumonia.[2,93] However, it is important to recognize that in all these studies the microbiologic specimens were obtained after a significant delay and frequently after complications such as abscesses, necrotizing pneumonia, or empyema had developed. Furthermore, many of the patients were chronic alcoholics, had been symptomatic for up to 90 days, and complained of having a putrid sputum. These patients are clearly distinct from the typical patients seen today with acute aspiration pneumonia. Furthermore, it is possible that the organisms recovered by transtracheal aspiration represent oropharyngeal flora that contaminated the trachea during the procedure (due to aspiration) or bacteria that colonized the trachea, rather than representing true pulmonary pathogens. This postulate is supported by Moser and colleagues, who demonstrated discrepancies between bacteria recovered by transtracheal aspiration and by transthoracic needle aspiration in dogs with experimental pneumonia.[94]

Recently, two studies have been reported in which invasive lower respiratory tract sampling (protected specimen brush) together with quantitative and anaerobic culture techniques were performed in the patients with acute aspiration syndromes.[95,96] Mier and colleagues studied 52 patients admitted to an ICU with "aspiration pneumonia."[95] Bacterial pathogens were isolated in significant concentrations ($\geq 10^3$ colony-forming units/mL) in only 19 patients, the spectrum of organism being determined by whether the aspiration was community or hospital acquired, with *S. pneumoniae*, *S. aureus*, *H. influenzae*, and Enterobacteriaceae predominant in patients with community-acquired aspiration and gram-negative organisms, including *Pseudomonas aeruginosa* in patients with hospital-acquired aspiration. No anaerobic organism was isolated in any of the patients. In a similar study, we performed blind protected specimen brush

sampling in 25 patients with gastric aspiration.[96] Bacterial pathogens were isolated in 12 patients. Risk factors for gastric colonization were present in 8 of the 12 patients (small bowel obstruction/ileus, tube feeding, H_2 blockers). The spectrum of pathogens was similar to that reported by Meir and colleagues.[95] Furthermore, we did not isolate any pathogenic anaerobic organisms.

MANAGEMENT

Antimicrobial therapy is unequivocally indicated in patients with aspiration pneumonia. The choice of antibiotics should depend on the setting in which the aspiration occurs (home, nursing home, or hospital) as well as on the patient's premorbid condition. However, antimicrobial agents with gram-negative activity such as fluoroquinolones, third-generation cephalosporins, piperacillin, or a carbapenem are usually required. Penicillin and clindamycin, the "standard" antimicrobial agents for aspiration pneumonia, provide inadequate activity in the majority of patients with aspiration pneumonia.[95] Antimicrobials with specific anaerobic activity are not routinely warranted and may be indicated only in patients with severe periodontal disease, patients expectorating putrid sputum, and patients with a necrotizing pneumonia or lung abscess on chest radiograph.[95,96]

All elderly patients with CAP and all patients with aspiration pneumonia require consultation by a speech and language pathologist to assess for the presence of dysphagia. Assessment of the cough and gag reflex is unreliable in screening for patients at risk of aspiration; a comprehensive swallowing evaluation performed by a specialized speech-language pathologist is, therefore, required. The speech-language pathologist can reliably identify those patients who aspirate by performing a bedside swallowing evaluation supplemented by either a videofluoroscopic swallow study or a fiberoptic endoscopic evaluation.[97-99] This evaluation identifies those patients who require further behavioral, dietary, and medical management to reduce the risk of aspiration.

The neurotransmitter substance P is believed to play a major role in both the cough and swallow sensory pathways. Angiotensin-converting enzyme (ACE) inhibitors prevent the breakdown of substance P and may theoretically be useful in the management of patients with aspiration pneumonia. Arai and associates measured serum substance P levels in hypertensive patients with cerebrovascular disease and symptomless dysphagia and control patients with no dysphagia.[100] The patients with symptomless dysphagia had significantly lower serum levels of substance P than the control subjects. In this study, dysphagia as assessed by technetium-tin colloid scanning improved in 62% of patients treated with an ACE inhibitor, this improvement being associated with a normalization of the serum substance P levels. Sekizawa and colleagues studied the incidence of pneumonia in 127 stroke patients treated with ACE inhibitors compared with 313 patients treated with other antihypertensive agents.[101] During a 2-year follow-up period, pneumonia was diagnosed in 7% of patients receiving an ACE inhibitor compared with 18% in patients taking other hypertensive agents (RR of 2.65; 95% CI 1.3 to 5.3, $P = .007$). Similarly, Arai and associates compared the risk of pneumonia in 576 elderly hypertensive patients who were treated with an ACE inhibitor or a calcium channel blocker.[102] The rate of pneumonia was 3.3% in the ACE group compared with 8.9% in the patients who were treated with a calcium channel blocker ($P = .025$).

In a follow-up study, Arai and colleagues demonstrated a significantly lower rate of pneumonia in elderly hypertensive patients randomized to an ACE inhibitor compared with an angiotensin-II receptor antagonist.[103] These studies provide compelling evidence that patients with oropharyngeal dysphagia should be considered for treatment with an ACE inhibitor (even if normotensive).

Sedative medication has been demonstrated to increase the risk of pneumonia in residents of long-term care facilities and should therefore be avoided.[104] The prescription of a phenothiazine and haloperidol should be very carefully considered, because they reduce oropharyngeal swallow coordination, causing dysphagia.[105,106] Medications that dry up secretions, including antihistamines and drugs with anticholinergic activity, make it more difficult for patients to swallow and should therefore also be avoided.[105,107]

Occupants of residential homes have been shown to have poor oral hygiene and rarely receive treatment from dentists and oral hygienists.[108,109] An aggressive protocol of oral care will reduce colonization with potentially pathogenic organisms and decrease the bacterial load. These measures have been demonstrated to reduce the risk of pneumonia.[63-65] In addition, aggressive oral care has been shown to increase salivary substance P.[110] The elevated substance P levels in the saliva may reflect enhanced activity of the afferent pathway of the swallow mechanism.

TUBE FEEDING

Nutritional supplementation, as determined by the clinical dietitian, may be required. Tube feeding is not essential in all patients who aspirate. Every attempt to encourage safe oral intake is recommended. The practice of tube feeding in the end stages of degenerative illnesses in the elderly should be carefully reconsidered. Finucane and colleagues found no data to suggest that tube feeding of patients with advanced dementia prevented aspiration pneumonia, prolonged survival, reduced the risk of pressure sores or infections, improved function, or provided palliation.[111]

Short-term tube feeding, however, may be indicated in elderly patients with severe dysphagia and aspiration in whom improvement of swallowing is likely to occur. Nakajoh and colleagues demonstrated that the incidence of pneumonia was significantly higher in stroke patients with dysphagia who were fed orally compared with those who received tube feeding (54.3 vs. 13.2%, $P < .001$), despite the fact that the orally fed patients had a higher functional status (higher Barthel index).[112]

Colonized oral secretions are a serious threat to dysphagic patients, and feeding tubes offer no clear protection. There are no data to suggest that patients fed with gastrostomy tubes have a lower incidence of pneumonia than patients fed with nasogastric tubes.[113,114] Similarly, the incidence of aspiration pneumonia has been shown to be similar in stroke patients with postpyloric as compared with intragastric feeding tubes.[115-117] Over the long term, aspiration pneumonia is the most common cause of death in gastrostomy tube–fed patients.[118,119] Patients who are likely to recover their ability to swallow within a few weeks are not candidates for gastrostomy tubes.

CONCLUSION

In the management of patients with aspiration syndromes, it is vitally important to distinguish aspiration pneumonitis from aspiration pneumonia. Although some overlap exists, these are distinct clinical syndromes. Antibiotics are not indicated (at least initially) in the majority of patients with aspiration pneumonitis, with corticosteroids having no proven benefit. Aspiration pneumonia should be considered in all elderly patients with CAP and in any patient with dysphagia and an infiltrate in a dependent bronchopulmonary segment. Broad-spectrum antibiotics are indicated in most patients with aspiration pneumonia.

ANNOTATED REFERENCES

Agency for Health Care Policy and Research: Diagnosis and Treatment of Swallowing Disorders (Dysphagia) in Acute Care Stroke. Patients Summary, 1999. Available at www.ahcpr.gov/clinic/dysphsum.htm.
> This is an excellent review on the diagnosis and treatment of swallowing disorders.

Finucane TE, Christmas C, Travis K: Tube feeding in patients with advanced dementia: A review of the evidence. JAMA 1999;282:1365-1370.
> This important position paper reviews the utility of placing feeding tubes in patients with advanced dementia.

Folkesson HG, Matthay MA, Hebert CA, Broaddus VC: Acid aspiration-induced lung injury in rabbits is mediated by interleukin-8–dependent mechanisms. J Clin Invest 1995;96:107-116.
> This experimental model highlights the role of neutrophils and IL-8 in the pathophysiology of aspiration pneumonitis.

Kikuchi R, Watabe N, Konno T, et al: High incidence of silent aspiration in elderly patients with community-acquired pneumonia. Am J Respir Crit Care Med 1994;150:251-253.
> This paper assesses the incidence of aspiration in patients who have recovered from community acquired pneumonia. They report a high incidence of "silent aspiration" in this group of patients as compared with age-matched controls.

Marik PE: Aspiration pneumonitis and pneumonia: A clinical review. N Engl J Med 2001;344:665-672.
> This is a comprehensive review on the epidemiology, pathophysiology, and treatment of aspiration pneumonia and aspiration pneumonitis.

Warner MA, Warner ME, Weber JG: Clinical significance of pulmonary aspiration during the perioperative period. Anesthesiology 1993;78:56-62.
> This paper evaluates the natural history and clinical course of patients who aspirate during anesthesia.

Chapter 77

SEVERE ASTHMA EXACERBATION

Thomas Corbridge • Susan J. Corbridge

KEY POINTS

1. **Any asthmatic** can develop a severe exacerbation, even one with mild disease.

2. **The general appearance of the patient** provides a guide to severity, response to therapy, and need for intubation. Measurement of peak flow helps to confirm the diagnosis, assess severity, and determine treatment response.

3. **Inhaled beta agonists, systemic corticosteroids, and low-flow oxygen** are first-line therapies in asthmatics with severe exacerbation. Alternate therapies include ipratropium bromide, magnesium sulfate, leukotriene modifiers, heliox, and noninvasive ventilation.

4. **Hypotension after intubation** may occur from an inadequate expiratory time resulting in dynamic lung hyperinflation and decreased preload to the right side of the heart. A trial of apnea or hypopnea is diagnostic and therapeutic in this setting.

5. **During mechanical ventilation**, prolong the expiratory phase by setting low minute ventilation and adequate inspiratory flow. Assess the degree of hyperinflation by checking the plateau pressure and, if necessary, accept moderate hypercapnia to limit dangerous hyperinflation.

6. **Avoid prolonged use of paralytics** to decrease risk of myopathy.

7. Education, environmental control measures, and anti-inflammatory medications help prevent future exacerbations.

DEFINITIONS

Each year in the United States acute asthma accounts for 2 million emergency department (ED) visits, 500,000 hospitalizations, 25,000 episodes of respiratory failure requiring intubation, and 5,000 deaths.[1,2] The total annual cost is 5 billion dollars. Acute attacks frequently reflect inadequate outpatient management—particularly in the subgroup of patients who depend on crisis-oriented ED management. These patients commonly reside in urban environments, have low incomes, and demonstrate inadequate understanding of asthma and use of controller agents.[3,4] Indeed only

between 28% and 42% of patients are taking inhaled corticosteroids before ED treatment for acute asthma.[5,6] Programs aimed at education and initiation of inhaled corticosteroids in the ED are crucial in this subgroup. These programs work[7]; so does referral to an asthma specialist.[8]

In most simple terms, asthma exacerbation is an acute deterioration in signs and symptoms of asthma, but there is considerable heterogeneity in the severity, tempo, and degree of inflammation and bronchospasm.[9] Severe asthma exacerbation (SAE) is defined by several, but not necessarily all, of the following features: dyspnea at rest, upright positioning, inability to speak in phrases or sentences, respiratory rate greater than 30 breaths/min, use of accessory muscles of respiration, pulse greater than 120 beats/min, pulsus paradoxus greater than 25 mm Hg, peak expiratory flow rate (PEFR) less than 50% predicted or personal best, hypoxemia, and eucapnia or hypercapnia.[10] Altered mental status, paradoxical respiration, bradycardia, a quiet chest, and absence of pulsus paradoxus from respiratory muscle fatigue are features of imminent respiratory arrest.

Insofar as it provides rationale for patient assessment and management, we begin this chapter with a review of pathophysiology. We then discuss clinical presentation, differential diagnosis, physical examination, and laboratory testing, followed by an update on pharmacologic therapy. Finally, we provide recommendations for ventilator management.

PATHOPHYSIOLOGY OF ACUTE AIRFLOW OBSTRUCTION

The speed with which SAE develops varies considerably.[11] Fewer than 15% of patients present with sudden-onset exacerbation in which severe airflow obstruction develops in less than 3 to 6 hours. These attacks represent a more pure form of smooth muscle–mediated bronchospasm with the potential to improve rapidly after use of bronchodilators.[12-15] Compared with attacks of slower progression, the airways have more neutrophils in the submucosa and fewer secretions.[16,17] Sudden attacks are triggered by allergen or irritant exposure, stress, inhalation of crack cocaine or heroin, or use of nonsteroidal anti-inflammatory agents or beta-adrenergic blockers in susceptible patients.[18-21] Respiratory tract infection is not a trigger; commonly, no cause is identified.[21]

Slower-onset attacks are triggered by a variety of infectious, allergic, and nonspecific irritant exposures. Airway wall inflammation, bronchospasm, and accumulations of intraluminal mucus are characteristic. Mucus plugs consisting of sloughed epithelial cells, eosinophils, fibrin, and other serum components that have leaked through the denuded airway epithelium obstruct large and small airways.[22] The tempo of these attacks provides a clear opportunity to increase anti-inflammatory medications in the outpatient setting.[23] However, only 13% to 22% of patients initiate oral corticosteroids before arrival at the ED.[5,24]

No matter the tempo, patients with SAE have critical airflow obstruction limiting exhalation. In severe cases, expiratory flow may not cease for as long as 60 seconds. Because expiratory time is shorter (1 to 5 seconds) during spontaneous or assisted breathing, there is incomplete emptying of gas and dynamic lung hyperinflation (DHI). Fortunately, DHI is self-limiting because as lung volume increases so do lung elastic recoil pressure and airway diameter—factors that favor expiratory flow. However, DHI places the diaphragm in a mechanically disadvantageous position at a time when hypoperfusion and respiratory acidosis may further decrease diaphragm force generation.[25]

At end exhalation, incomplete gas emptying elevates alveolar volume and pressure, a state referred to as auto–positive end-expiratory pressure (PEEP).[26] Auto-PEEP is a threshold pressure that must be overcome to initiate inspiratory flow. This combines with narrowed airways and variable degrees of hyperinflation-induced parenchymal noncompliance to increase the inspiratory work of breathing. The resulting imbalance between respiratory muscle strength and work of breathing predisposes to ventilatory failure.

Multiple inert gas elimination technique (MIGET) analysis demonstrates small areas of high ventilation ($\dot{V}$) relative to perfusion ($\dot{Q}$) and slightly increased dead space in acute asthma, presumably because hyperinflation limits blood flow.[27,28] An increase in the dead space to tidal volume ratio (V_D/V_T) favors the development of hypercapnia:

$$P_{CO_2} = V_{CO_2} \times 0.863/V_A$$
$$= V_{CO_2} \times 0.863/[V_E \times (1-V_D/V_T)]$$

where V_{CO_2} is carbon dioxide production, V_A is alveolar ventilation, V_E is minute ventilation, and V_D/V_T is the dead space to tidal volume ratio.

In mild acute asthma, V_E increases more than V_D/V_T, causing respiratory alkalosis. As the severity of airflow obstruction increases (particularly when FEV_1 is < 1.0 L),[29] $PaCO_2$ increases owing to inadequate V_A (reflecting a decrease in V_E and an increase in V_D/V_T as the patient nears respiratory arrest).

Airway obstruction decreases ventilation relative to perfusion in other lung units causing hypoxemia. Because this is not shunt (a $\dot{V}/\dot{Q}$ of zero), oxygen supplementation readily corrects hypoxemia.[27] There is a rough correlation between severity of airflow obstruction and hypoxemia.[30] For example, most patients with PaO_2 less than 60 mm Hg have a PEFR less than 200 L/min or an FEV_1 less than 1.0 L.[29] However, the vast majority of patients present with PaO_2 greater than 60 mm Hg and an SaO_2 greater than 90% while breathing room air at sea level.[31] In one study of over 1000 children with acute asthma, only 4% had an initial SaO_2 less than 88%.[32] In this study, mean SaO_2 was 95% on room air: 93% for children admitted to hospital and 96% for those discharged home ($P < .001$). Twenty-three percent of patients were admitted, but in the subgroup of patients with SaO_2 less than 88%, the admission rate was 73% compared with 8% when SaO_2 was 100%.

In recovering patients, MIGET analysis demonstrates that spirometry often improves before PaO_2 and $\dot{V}/\dot{Q}$ inequality.[33]

This may be because spirometry tracks large airway function, whereas gas exchange reflects the function of peripheral airways.[34]

Large swings in pleural pressure are responsible for the circulatory changes in SAE. Right heart preload decreases during expiration because of positive intrathoracic pressure, but during vigorous inspiration, intrathoracic pressure falls and blood flow increases. This fills the right ventricle early in inspiration and shifts the intraventricular septum leftward. Lung hyperinflation also increases pulmonary vascular resistance and right ventricular afterload.[35,36] The conformational change that occurs in the left ventricle causes diastolic dysfunction and incomplete left ventricular filling; furthermore, negative pleural pressures directly impair left ventricular emptying.[37,38] Rarely, diastolic dysfunction and increased left ventricular afterload cause pulmonary edema.[39] The net effect of these cyclical changes is to accentuate the normal drop in systolic blood pressure that occurs during inspiration, a phenomenon termed *pulsus paradoxus* (PP). The PP is a valuable indicator of asthma severity,[40] but the lack of a widened PP can also indicate fatigue and inability to generate large swings in pleural pressure.

CLINICAL ASSESSMENT

Analysis of several factors including the medical history, physical examination, measures of airflow obstruction, assessment of initial response to therapy, arterial blood gases, and occasionally the chest radiograph are necessary to assess severity, risk of deterioration, and differential diagnosis.[41] Imperative in the medical history are risk factors for asthma death (Table 77-1), of which prior intubation is the most important.[42-47]

"All that wheezes is not asthma" is a clinical saw worth considering during the initial evaluation. In older patients, an extensive smoking history suggests chronic obstructive pulmonary disease and the potential for compensated respiratory acidosis. Cardiac asthma refers to airway hyperreactivity and wheezing that may accompany congestive heart failure.[48] An enlarged cardiac silhouette, a left-sided third heart sound, and pulmonary edema suggest this diagnosis. Occasionally, distinguishing between heart failure and asthma is difficult because airflow obstruction can cause pulmonary edema (see earlier) and bronchodilators partially reverse cardiac asthma.[49] In the setting of coronary artery

---

TABLE 77–1. RISK FACTORS FOR FATAL OR NEAR-FATAL ASTHMA

Frequent emergency department visits
Frequent hospitalization
Intensive care unit admission
Prior intubation
Hypercapnia
Barotrauma
Psychiatric illness
Medical noncompliance
Illicit drug use
Low socioeconomic status
Inadequate access to medical care
Use of more than two canisters/month of inhaled beta agonist
Poor perception of airflow obstruction
Comorbidities such as coronary artery disease
Sensitivity to *Alternaria* species

disease, imbalance between oxygen supply and demand may cause myocardial ischemia.[50] Pulmonary embolism rarely causes wheeze; consider this diagnosis when dyspnea is out of proportion to signs and objective measures of expiratory flow.[51,52]

Vocal cord dysfunction (and other causes of upper airway obstruction) should be considered when there is stridor, normal oxygenation, or resolution of airflow obstruction after intubation.[53] In contrast to asthma, upper airway (extrathoracic) obstruction classically flattens the inspiratory portion of the flow-volume loop, leaving the expiratory loop intact. Fiberoptic laryngoscopy can confirm paradoxical vocal cord movement in a symptomatic individual. Response to breathing helium-oxygen mixtures (heliox) suggests upper airway obstruction, but heliox also may be of use in asthma and should not be used to distinguish upper from lower airway obstruction. In cases of suspected tracheal stenosis (e.g., from prior intubation), fiberoptic bronchoscopy or spiral computed tomography is indicated.

A foreign body should be considered in the very young and old, in individuals with altered mental status or neuromuscular disease, and when symptoms develop after eating or dental work. Localized wheeze and, rarely, asymmetrical hyperinflation on chest radiography are clues to foreign body aspiration.

Pneumonia complicating asthma is unusual, but it should be considered when there is fever, purulent sputum, localizing signs, and hypoxemia that does not correct with low-flow oxygen. Antibiotics are frequently prescribed for asthmatics with increased sputum. However, sputum that looks purulent in asthma may contain eosinophils, not neutrophils.

On physical examination, the general appearance of the patient (posture, speech, positioning, and alertness) provides a quick guide to severity, response to therapy, and need for intubation. Patients assuming the upright position have a higher heart rate, respiratory rate, and PP, and a significantly lower PaO$_2$ and PEFR than patients who are able to lie supine.[54] Diaphoresis is associated with an even lower PEFR. Accessory muscle use and a widened PP indicate severe asthma; however, their absence does not rule out a severe attack.[55]

Examination of the head and neck should focus on identifying barotrauma and upper airway obstruction. Prolonged inspiration, stridor, and suprasternal retractions suggest upper airway obstruction. The mouth and neck should be inspected for signs of previous surgery such as tracheostomy or thyroidectomy and angioedema. Tracheal deviation, asymmetrical breath sounds, "mediastinal crunch," and subcutaneous emphysema suggest pneumomediastinum or pneumothorax. Rarely, tracheal deviation is caused by atelectasis from mucus plugging, foreign body aspiration, or endobronchial tumor.

Chest auscultation reveals expiratory phase prolongation and wheeze. However, wheeze is not a reliable indicator of the severity of airflow obstruction.[56] A silent chest indicates that there is insufficient airflow for noise generation. Localized wheeze or crackles may represent mucus plugging and atelectasis but should prompt consideration of pneumonia, pneumothorax, and endobronchial obstruction.

Sinus tachycardia is common.[57] Supraventricular and ventricular arrhythmias are more common in the elderly[58] but rarely complicate management. Bradycardia is an ominous sign of impending respiratory arrest. PP greater than 20 mm Hg is common in SAE; PP less than 10 mm Hg suggests either a milder attack or respiratory muscle fatigue

and imminent respiratory arrest.[10] SAE can cause examination and electrocardiographic findings of right-sided heart strain and, less commonly, pulmonary edema.[59] Dynamic hyperinflation, forceful exhalation, and tension pneumothorax distend neck veins.

Measuring PEFR or FEV$_1$ helps assess the severity of airflow obstruction. A PEFR or FEV$_1$ less than 50% predicted or the patient's personal best defines SAE. Objective measurements are important because physician estimates are often inaccurate (whereas patients are more accurate in guessing PEFR).[60] Emerman and Cydulka demonstrated a modest correlation between pretreatment estimates of pulmonary function and the actual value.[61] Physicians underestimated the degree of obstruction and changed management 20% of the time after PEFR measurements. In general, it is easier to measure PEFR than FEV$_1$, although this maneuver is still difficult for sick patients. In severely dyspneic patients we defer peak flow determination because it rarely alters initial management and may worsen bronchospasm,[62] even to the point of respiratory arrest.[63]

Measurement of the change in PEFR or FEV$_1$ predicts the need for hospitalization. Several studies have demonstrated that failure of initial therapy to improve expiratory flow after 30 minutes predicts a more severe course and need for ongoing treatment in the ED or hospitalization.[64-67] Values before 30 minutes of treatment are not predictive.[68]

When FEV$_1$ is less than 1 L or PEFR is less than 200 L/min, we recommend an arterial blood gas analysis to assess the degree of hypoxemia and acid-base status. In the early stages of SAE, mild hypoxemia and respiratory alkalosis are common. As the severity of airflow obstruction increases, PaCO$_2$ increases. Hypercapnia denotes severe disease; however, hypercapnic patients may improve with pharmacologic therapy and do not always require intubation.[69] Conversely, the absence of hypercapnia does not rule out impending respiratory arrest.[70]

Patients who waste serum bicarbonate in response to respiratory alkalosis develop a metabolic acidosis with a normal anion gap. Metabolic acidosis with an elevated anion gap reflects excess serum lactate likely due to increased work of breathing. Lactic acidosis is more common in men, in the setting of severe obstruction and during treatment with parenteral beta agonists.[71-73]

Repeat blood gas sampling is generally not necessary to determine clinical course. In most cases, serial attention to patient posture, use of accessory muscles, diaphoresis, estimates of air movement during auscultation, pulse oximetry, and PEFRs allows for valid determinations. Patients whose condition deteriorates on these grounds should be considered for intubation. In mechanically ventilated patients, serial blood gas analysis helps guide ventilator management.

Chest radiographs influence treatment in 1% to 5% of cases.[74-76] In one study,[77] atelectasis may have been the explanation for radiographic findings in 34% of cases. These data suggest that chest radiographs are indicated only when there are localizing signs, concerns regarding barotrauma or pneumonia, or if it is not clear that asthma is the correct diagnosis. In mechanically ventilated patients, chest radiographs confirm proper endotracheal tube position.

ADMISSION CRITERIA

Patients demonstrating a good response to initial therapy may be discharged home with close follow-up. These patients should report no distress, have an essentially normal examination, and have an FEV_1 or PEFR of greater than or equal to 70% of predicted or personal best.[10] Observation for 60 minutes after the last dose of beta agonist helps ensure stability before discharge. Patients should receive written medication instructions, a written plan of action to be followed in the event of deterioration, and a follow-up appointment before discharge. In general, patients discharged home on oral corticosteroids do well, particularly if they had not been optimally treated before the ED visit.[78] An 8-day course of 40 mg/day of prednisone is as efficacious and safe as an 8-day tapering schedule.[79] Alternatively, a single intramuscular dose of 40 mg of triamcinolone diacetate has also been shown to be as effective as the 40 mg/day dose of prednisone for 5 days after ED treatment for asthma.[80]

Patients with mild cases with a good response to bronchodilators may be considered for inhaled corticosteroids alone. In children discharged from the ED, a short-term dose schedule of inhaled budesonide, starting at a high dose and then tapered over 1 week, was shown to be as effective as a tapering course of oral prednisolone.[81] Depending on the situation, inhaled steroids should be started, continued, or increased while the patient is in the ED.

Patients with SAE (PEFR < 50% predicted or personal best) who demonstrate a poor response to initial therapy (e.g., less than 10% increase in PEFR) or whose condition deteriorates during therapy should be admitted to an intensive care unit (ICU). ICU admission is also indicated for respiratory arrest, altered mental status, myocardial injury, and when there is need for frequent nebulizer treatments.

An incomplete response to treatment occurs when there is persistent dyspnea and a PEFR or FEV_1 between 50% and 70% predicted. Patients in this group require ongoing treatment either in the ED or on the general medical ward. Physicians should err on the side of admission when there is an undesirable home environment and when directly observed therapy is needed in noncompliant patients.

Contrary to the just described guidelines, in common practice half of patients with a final PEFR of less than 50% of predicted are discharged from the ED.[82] Interestingly, short-term relapse is uncommon in these patients and not associated with final PEFR, suggesting that strict adherence to PEFR cutoffs may be unnecessary.

PHARMACOLOGIC THERAPY

OXYGEN

Low-flow oxygen by nasal cannula is recommended to maintain arterial oxygen saturation greater than 90% (>95% in pregnancy and ischemic heart disease). This practice improves oxygen delivery to peripheral tissues (including respiratory muscles), reverses hypoxic pulmonary vasoconstriction, and may stimulate bronchodilation. Oxygen also protects against hypoxemia resulting from beta agonist–induced pulmonary vasodilation and increased blood flow to low $\dot{V}/\dot{Q}$ units.[28,83]

BETA AGONISTS

Beta agonists are central to treatment of bronchospasm and should be administered immediately, preferably by inhalation, regardless of prior use.[84] Approximately two thirds of asthmatics respond well enough to albuterol to be discharged

from the ED. In the study by Rodrigo and Rodrigo, 67% of patients were discharged from the ED after 2.4 mg of albuterol, with half meeting the discharge criteria after receiving only 12 puffs of albuterol (Fig. 77-1).[85] Similarly, Strauss and coworkers found that two thirds of patients with acute asthma could be discharged after three 2.5-mg doses of albuterol by nebulization every 20 minutes.[86] Patients with a blunted cumulative dose-response relationship require hospitalization (or extended treatment in an ED holding area). These patients may have extensive inflammation, architectural disruption of the airways, and intraluminal mucus, limiting their response to beta agonists.

The most widely used and studied beta agonist is albuterol. Albuterol is more $beta_2$ selective and longer acting than metaproterenol, although metaproterenol and isoetharine are occasionally used for initial therapy because of their faster onset of action, despite the potential for increased side effects.[87-89] Levalbuterol, the R-isomer of racemic albuterol, is a newer therapeutic option for patients with asthma. Racemic albuterol consists of a 50:50 mixture of R- and S-albuterol, with the R-isomer conferring bronchodilator effects. Emerging preclinical data suggest that the S-isomer, previously thought to be inert, is not only proinflammatory

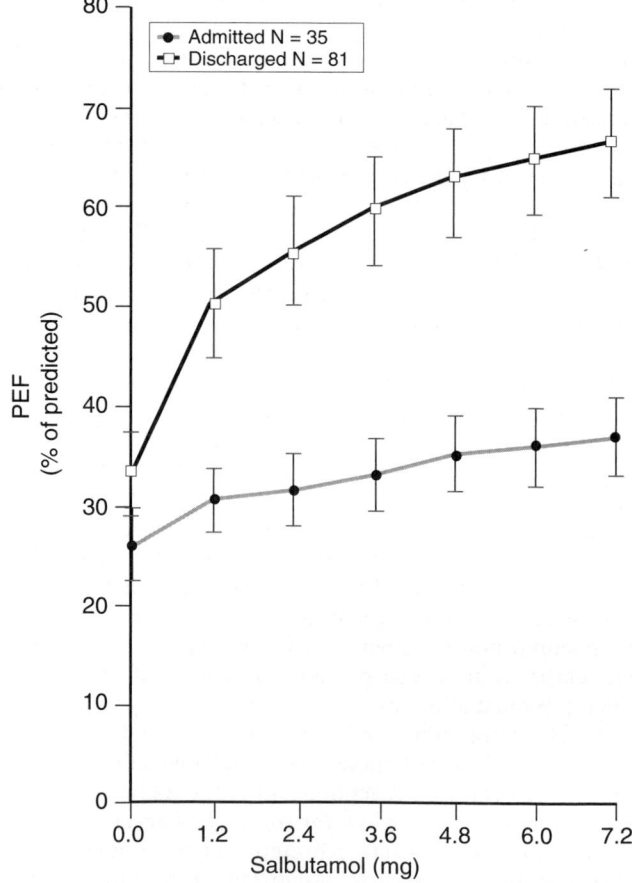

FIGURE 77–1. Dose-response relationship to albuterol 4 puffs (400 μg) every 10 minutes in 116 acute asthmatics. Sixty-seven percent of patients obtained discharge criteria after administration of 2.4 mg albuterol within 1 hour; half of responders met discharge criteria after 12 puffs. Patients with a blunted cumulative dose-response relationship were hospitalized. (Reproduced with permission from Rodrigo C, Rodrigo G: Therapeutic response patterns to high and cumulative doses of salbutamol in acute severe asthma. Chest 1998;113:593.)

but also preferentially retained in the lung.[90,91] These effects may help explain why levalbuterol, 1.25 mg, causes greater bronchodilation than the same amount of levalbuterol in a racemic mixture (2.5 mg) in stable asthmatics.[92] Fewer data are available in acute asthma. In an open-label study of 91 acutely ill patients with FEV_1 between 20% and 55% predicted, patients were stratified into cohorts receiving 0.63 to 5 mg of levalbuterol or 2.5 to 5 mg of albuterol (three treatments in 1 hour).[93] Patients receiving levalbuterol demonstrated faster onset of action and a greater degree of bronchodilation. Results of a large, multicenter trial are expected soon.

Long-acting beta agonists are not indicated in the initial treatment of SAE but may be considered for add-on therapy in hospitalized patients. In hospital, salmeterol added to albuterol results in greater improvements in FEV_1 after 48 hours without greater toxicity compared with placebo.[94] For maintenance, addition of a long-acting beta agonist to an inhaled corticosteroid results in fewer asthma exacerbations and exacerbations of lesser severity.[95]

Metered-dose inhalers (MDIs) or hand-held nebulizers deliver inhaled beta agonists equally well. Anywhere from 4 to 12 puffs by MDI with spacer achieves the same degree of bronchodilation as one 2.5-mg nebulized treatment of albuterol.[96-99] MDIs with spacers carry the advantage of lower cost and faster drug delivery times; hand-held nebulizers require fewer instructions, less supervision, and less coordination.

The recommended dose of albuterol is 2.5 mg by nebulization every 20 minutes during the first hour of treatment depending on clinical response and side effects.[10] Other dosing strategies have been studied. McFadden and colleagues compared two 5.0-mg treatments of albuterol by nebulization over 40 minutes to three 2.5-mg treatments with albuterol every 20 minutes in 160 ED patients.[5] Both treatment strategies were effective, but the 5-mg regimen increased peak flows more rapidly and to a greater extent than the standard 2.5-mg approach. Patients receiving 5-mg doses also reached discharge criteria quicker and left the ED with higher PEFRs. There was also a trend toward fewer hospitalizations in the high-dose group. Emerman and colleagues compared the effects of 2.5 to 7.5 mg albuterol every 20 minutes for a total of three doses in 160 acute asthmatics.[100] There was no difference in improvement in FEV_1 or admission rates between groups. In another study, a single high-dose treatment with albuterol (7.5 mg) was found to be no better (and more toxic) than three treatments with 2.5 mg every 20 minutes.[101] Dosing after the first hour of therapy depends on the clinical response and side effect profile. Fortunately, high-dose inhaled beta agonists are generally well tolerated. Tremor and tachycardia are common, but significant cardiovascular morbidity is not.[102,103]

Albuterol can be administered in a continuous or repetitive manner. Depending on the study, there is either no difference between continuous and repetitive dosing or there is a slight benefit to continuous administration (at the same total dose) in severely obstructed patients.[104-107]

There is no advantage to subcutaneous epinephrine or terbutaline over inhaled albuterol in the initial management of SAE, unless the patient is unable to comply with inhaled therapy because of an altered mental status or near-arrest situation.[108-110] However, if there is a poor response to several hours of inhaled therapy, subcutaneous epinephrine may be helpful.[111] Coronary artery disease is a relative contraindication to parenteral therapy.[112] Intravenous administration of beta agonists is not recommended. Several studies have demonstrated that inhaled therapy improves airflow greater with less toxicity compared with intravenous administration.[113-116] Combinations of inhaled and parenteral treatment have not been adequately evaluated.

IPRATROPIUM BROMIDE

Data generally support a benefit to adding ipratropium bromide to albuterol in the initial treatment of SAE.[117-119] Rodrigo and Rodrigo conducted a randomized trial of high and cumulative doses of ipratropium bromide and albuterol. In their study, combined albuterol, 120 µg, and ipratropium bromide, 21 µg per puff (in one inhaler), was compared to albuterol and placebo in 180 patients with acute asthma.[120] Four puffs were administered through an MDI with spacer every 10 minutes for 3 hours. Subjects who received combination therapy had 20.5% and 48.1% greater improvements in PEFR and FEV_1, respectively, compared with albuterol alone. The rate of hospitalization decreased significantly from 39% with albuterol alone to 20% with combination therapy. Subgroup analysis showed that patients most likely to benefit from high doses of ipratropium bromide were those with an FEV_1 less than 30% of predicted and symptoms for more than 24 hours before ED presentation. O'Driscoll and colleagues showed similar benefit to combination therapy, particularly in patients with PEFR less than 140 L/min at entry.[121] Garrett and colleagues randomized 338 asthmatics to a single nebulized dose of 0.5 mg of ipratropium bromide combined with 3.0 mg of salbutamol or to 3.0 mg of salbutamol alone.[122] Mean FEV_1 at 45 and 90 minutes was significantly higher with combined therapy. Karpel and colleagues studied 384 patients randomized to 2.5 mg of albuterol or to 2.5 mg albuterol mixed with 0.5 mg of ipratropium at entry and at 45 minutes.[123] At 45 minutes, there were significantly more responders in the ipratropium group; however, median change in FEV_1 from baseline did not differ between groups, and by 90 minutes there was no difference in the percentage of responders and median change in FEV_1 between groups and there was no difference in the number of patients requiring additional ED or hospital treatment. Lin and colleagues demonstrated that combination therapy resulted in greater improvement in PEFR than albuterol alone in 55 adult asthmatics.[124] In two other studies, combination therapy tended to improve outcome measures, but differences were not statistically significant.[125,126] In children, combination therapy decreases ED treatment time, albuterol dose requirements, and hospitalization rates.[119,127-129]

To the contrary, McFadden did not show benefit in PEFR, admission rate, or ED length of stay to combination ipratropium bromide and albuterol in the first hour of treatment.[130] Similarly, in children, Ducharme and Davis did not demonstrate benefit from combination therapy in their study of nearly 300 asthmatics with mild to moderate acute asthma.[131]

CORTICOSTEROIDS

The data are mixed regarding the benefits of systemic corticosteroids in the first few hours of treatment. Early data from McFadden and colleagues demonstrated no differences in physiologic or clinical variables in the first 6 hours in

38 patients receiving hydrocortisone hemisuccinate or placebo.[132] Similarly, Rodrigo and Rodrigo showed that early administration of corticosteroids does not improve pulmonary function in the first 6 hours of treatment.[133] These authors came to the same conclusion after an evidence-based evaluation of selected trials.[134] However, Littenberg and Gluck demonstrated that 125 mg of methylprednisolone given intravenously on arrival decreased admission rates compared with placebo.[135] Similarly, Lin and colleagues, studying the effects of 125 mg of methylprednisolone given intravenously on arrival in patients with a PEFR less than 50% predicted after albuterol, demonstrated improved PEFR after 1 and 2 hours.[136] A systematic review of 12 studies for the Cochrane database demonstrated that use of corticosteroids within 1 hour of arrival to the ED reduces the need for hospitalization and that benefits are greatest in patients with more severe asthma and those not previously taking corticosteroids.[137] Corticosteroids decrease the number of relapses in the first 7 to 10 days and the risk of asthma death.[138-141] In hospitalized patients, they speed the rate of recovery.[142,143]

Whether there is a dose-response relationship to systemic steroids in SAE is not clear. In one meta-analysis, Manser and colleagues found no therapeutic differences between low doses of corticosteroids (<80 mg/day of methylprednisolone or <400 mg/day hydrocortisone) and higher doses in the initial management of hospitalized asthmatics.[144] Emerman and Cydulka compared 500-mg and 100-mg doses of methylprednisolone in the ED, finding no benefit to higher-dose therapy.[145] Haskell and coworkers compared three doses of methylprednisolone (15 mg, 40 mg, and 125 mg) given intravenously every 6 hours for 3 days.[146] The high-dose group improved significantly by the end of the first day, the medium-dose group improved by the middle of the second day, and the low-dose group did not improve significantly by day 3. Bowler and colleagues found no difference between 50 mg of hydrocortisone given intravenously four times daily for 2 days followed by low-dose oral prednisone and 200 or 500 mg of hydrocortisone also administered four times daily for 2 days followed by higher doses of prednisone.[147]

The recommendation by the expert panel from the National Institutes of Health is to deliver 120 to 180 mg/day of either prednisone, methylprednisolone, or prednisolone in three or four divided doses for 48 hours and then 60 to 80 mg/day until the PEFR reaches 70% of predicted or the patient's personal best.[10] We recommend 60 mg of methylprednisolone (Solu-Medrol) (or its equivalent) every 6 hours by vein during initial management. Oral drug is as effective[148] but should be avoided in patients with gastrointestinal upset or in patients at risk for intubation.

Recent trials have demonstrated benefit to inhaled corticosteroids in acute asthma. Rodrigo and Rodrigo conducted a randomized, double-blind trial of 1 mg of flunisolide versus placebo combined with 400 μg of salbutamol every 10 minutes for 3 hours in 94 ED subjects.[149] They found that the PEFR and FEV_1 were approximately 20% higher in the flunisolide group, beginning at 90 minutes. This benefit may stem from steroid-induced vasoconstriction and decreases in airway wall edema, vascular congestion, and plasma exudation.[150] Rodrigo and Rodrigo also demonstrated therapeutic benefit from triple-drug therapy (flunisolide, albuterol, and ipratropium bromide) in high doses in patients not receiving systemic corticosteroids.[151]

To the contrary, Guttman and colleagues found no benefit from adding 7 mg of beclomethasone every 8 hours by MDI with spacer to nebulized salbutamol and systemic corticosteroids.[152] This group also demonstrated that beclomethasone (5 mg delivered by MDI) during the initial 4 hours of ED treatment did not confer added benefit to albuterol in adults with mild to moderately severe asthma.[153]

THEOPHYLLINE

Numerous studies have demonstrated that theophylline does not add to maximal doses of beta agonists in the first few hours of treatment and that theophylline increases the incidence of tremor, nausea, vomiting, and tachyarrhythmias.[154-160] In the meta-analysis by Parameswaran and colleagues, 15 studies in adults were analyzed demonstrating that intravenous therapy with aminophylline did not result in any additional bronchodilation compared with standard care with beta agonists, although there was a nonsignificant trend toward higher PEFRs in treated patients at 12 and 24 hours.[160]

Fewer studies demonstrate benefit to aminophylline use in SAE.[161-165] Some studies demonstrated that theophylline use in the ED resulted in fewer hospitalizations even though airflow rates were not different from placebo, raising the possibility that nonbronchodilating properties of theophylline may be important.[166,167] In one meta-analysis of aminophylline use in school-aged children, intravenous aminophylline was shown to improve FEV_1 by 6 to 8 hours, an effect that was maintained at 24 hours.[168]

MAGNESIUM SULFATE

Prospective trials have yielded conflicting results regarding the efficacy of magnesium sulfate ($MgSO_4$) as a bronchodilator in acute asthma. Several studies failed to show a benefit to the use of $MgSO_4$ added to standard therapies[169-173]; other studies have demonstrated that $MgSO_4$ improves spirometry or rates of admission.[174-176] In an attempt to shed further light on the use of $MgSO_4$, meta-analyses have been published,[177-179] but they reach different conclusions. One analysis by Rowe and colleagues of seven trials (five adult and two pediatric) involving 668 patients did not support routine intravenous use of $MgSO_4$ in all patients with acute asthma. However, $MgSO_4$ was found to be safe and effective in improving spirometry in asthmatics with severe acute exacerbations. Similarly, when 135 asthmatics were randomized to 2 g of intravenous $MgSO_4$ or placebo after 30 minutes and followed for 4 hours, hospital admission rates and FEV_1 were no different between treated patients and controls.[172] However, subgroup analysis showed that $MgSO_4$ decreased admission rates and improved spirometry in asthmatics with FEV_1 less than 25% predicted. Subsequently, a placebo-controlled, double-blind, randomized trial in 248 patients with FEV_1 less than 30% showed a small but statistically significant increase in FEV_1 after 240 minutes in the $MgSO_4$-treated group but no difference in hospitalization rates.[175] Additional evidence supporting benefit in severe disease comes from an uncontrolled study of five intubated asthmatics given magnesium.[180] In this study, patients were given high doses of $MgSO_4$ (10 to 20 g) over 1 hour, after which there was a significant decrease in peak airway pressure (43 to 32 cm H_2O) and in inspiratory flow resistance. $MgSO_4$ may also be of greater benefit in premenopausal women because estrogen augments the bronchodilating effect of magnesium.[181]

MgSO$_4$ can also be administered by nebulized solution. Nannini and colleagues evaluated the efficacy of MgSO$_4$ (225 mg) versus normal saline as a vehicle for nebulized salbutamol in a randomized, double-blind, controlled trial of 35 patients in an ED.[182] At 20 minutes, patients who received MgSO$_4$ and salbutamol had an absolute increase in PEFR of 134 ± 70 L/min versus 86 ± 64 L/min in the saline and salbutamol group, a 57% greater percentage increase. More recently, Hughes and colleagues enrolled 52 patients with SAE in a randomized controlled trial of salbutamol mixed with 2.5 mL of isotonic MgSO$_4$ or isotonic saline on three occasions 30 minutes apart.[183] At 90 minutes, mean FEV$_1$ in the MgSO$_4$ group was 1.96 L and 1.55 L in the saline group (difference 0.37 L, $P = .003$).

LEUKOTRIENE MODIFIERS

Cysteinyl leukotrienes are elevated in asthmatic sputum compared with controls and higher in subjects studied within 48 hours of exacerbation.[184] Preliminary data demonstrating efficacy of the leukotriene receptor antagonist zafirlukast in acute asthma are available from a double-blind, randomized trial.[185] Two doses of zafirlukast (20 mg and 160 mg) administered orally were compared with placebo in 641 asthmatics after 30 minutes of standard treatment. Zafirlukast, 160 mg, decreased admission rates, relapses, and treatment failures. In another double-blind, placebo study of 20 patients not receiving systemic steroids, oral montelukast, 10 mg, resulted in a trend toward a shorter duration of stay and higher peak flows and fewer patients requiring aminophylline or corticosteroids.[186] More recently, Camargo and colleagues conducted a randomized, double-blind, parallel group trial in 201 acute asthmatics receiving standard therapy plus 7 mg or 14 mg of montelukast intravenously or placebo.[187] Montelukast improved FEV$_1$ over the first 20 minutes (14.8% vs. 3.6% with placebo). Benefits were seen within 10 minutes and lasted for 2 hours; both treatment doses were equivalent. Montelukast also tended to result in less beta agonist use and fewer treatment failures.

HELIOX

Heliox is a gas consisting of 20% oxygen and 80% helium (30:70% and 40:60% mixtures are also available). As the percent of helium decreases, so does the benefit of breathing this gas blend. Concentrations of helium less than 60% are ineffective, precluding its use in patients requiring significant supplemental oxygen. Heliox is slightly more viscous than air, but significantly less dense, resulting in a more than threefold increase in kinematic viscosity (the ratio of gas viscosity to gas density) compared with air. Theoretically, this property decreases the driving pressure required for gas flow by two mechanisms. First, for any level of turbulent flow, breathing low-density gas decreases the pressure gradient required for flow. Second, heliox decreases the Reynolds number, favoring conversion of turbulent flow to laminar flow.[188] Heliox does not treat bronchospasm or airway wall inflammation.

Heliox improves dyspnea, work of breathing, and arterial blood gases in upper airway obstruction.[189] In adult asthmatics treated in an ED, an 80:20 mix increased PEFR and decreased PP, suggesting improved airway resistance and work of breathing.[190] Similar results have also been published in children.[191] Other studies have failed to demonstrate a benefit.[192-194] In a recent meta-analysis for the Cochrane database of four randomized trials including 288 patients, Rodrigo and colleagues concluded that the evidence does not support the use of heliox in nonintubated asthmatics.[195] However, methodologic differences between studies and failure to control for concurrent upper airway obstruction (e.g., vocal cord dysfunction) limit conclusions. If heliox is effective, it may "buy time" for concurrent therapies to work and thereby avert the need for intubation in some cases. Of theoretical concern is the potential for heliox to mask worsening airflow obstruction, so that there may be less time (and no margin for error) to control the airway.

Whether heliox augments the bronchodilator effect of inhaled beta agonists compared with delivery in air is also unclear. Data are available demonstrating a benefit to heliox as a driving gas,[196] but there are also data to the contrary.[197]

ANTIBIOTICS

In their 2002 update, the expert panel from the National Institutes of Health did not recommend the use of antibiotics in asthma exacerbation unless there was fever with purulent sputum, evidence for pneumonia, or suspected bacterial sinusitis.[198] In a separate review of the literature, Graham recently selected 2 of 128 possible studies adequate for review, concluding that the role of antibiotics is difficult to assess.[199]

MECHANICAL VENTILATION

Noninvasive Positive Pressure

Noninvasive positive pressure by facemask is potentially useful in refractory patients—who are not in need of immediate airway control. In one study of 21 acute asthmatics with a mean PEFR of 144 L/min, nasal CPAP of 5 or 7.5 cm H$_2$O significantly decreased respiratory rate and dyspnea compared with placebo.[200] This benefit presumably stems from help overcoming the inspiratory threshold load created by auto-PEEP (see earlier).[201] Meduri and colleagues reported their observational experience with bilevel positive airway pressure (BiPAP) during 17 episodes of SAE.[202] In all but one patient (who subsequently required intubation), BiPAP improved dyspnea. BiPAP improved blood gases, heart rate, and respiratory rate, and only 2 patients required intubation. Soroksky and colleagues' pilot study of BiPAP in 15 patients with acute asthma compared with 15 controls receiving sham BiPAP for 3 hours demonstrated that BiPAP improved lung function and reduced need for hospitalization.[203]

Intubation

Respiratory arrest and impending respiratory arrest (e.g., extreme exhaustion and changes in mental status) mandate intubation. Oral intubation is preferred because it allows for a large endotracheal tube—important to decrease airway resistance and remove tenacious mucus plugs. Nasal intubation may be attempted in an awake patient with a difficult airway (e.g., short, obese patients), but nasal intubation necessitates a smaller endotracheal tube and may be complicated by polyps and sinusitis.

Postintubation Hypotension

The time immediately after intubation can be difficult for the patient with severe airflow obstruction. Care must be taken to stabilize the patient during this period through the thoughtful use of sedatives, paralytics, bronchodilators, intravenous fluids, and positive-pressure ventilation.

Immediate concerns are hypotension and pneumothorax. Hypotension has been reported in 25% to 35% of patients after intubation.[204] It occurs from a loss of vascular tone due to sedation, hypovolemia, tension pneumothorax, or overzealous ventilation. The latter results in dangerous levels of DHI when adequate time is not provided for exhalation. Clues to DHI include excessive effort during manual inflation, decreased breath sounds, hypotension, and tachycardia. A trial of hypopnea (2 to 3 breaths/min) or apnea in a preoxygenated patient is both diagnostic and therapeutic for DHI. When successful, hypopnea improves cardiopulmonary status within 30 to 60 seconds. Irrespective of clinical improvement, tension pneumothorax should be considered. Close inspection of the chest radiograph is mandatory because DHI may limit lung collapse. Because it causes preferential ventilation to the contralateral lung, unilateral pneumothorax increases the risk of bilateral pneumothoraces. Management of pneumothorax consists of hypoventilation, volume resuscitation, and tube thoracostomy (unilateral or bilateral as required).

Initial Ventilator Settings

During mechanical ventilation, the expiratory time, tidal volume, and severity of airway obstruction determine the level of DHI (Fig. 77-2). Because treatment of airway obstruction has been maximized in most intubated patients, expiratory time and tidal volume become important variables during ventilator management. Minute ventilation and inspiratory flow rates determine exhalation time.[205,206] At a set inspiratory flow, a drop in minute ventilation prolongs expiratory time and decreases DHI. To avoid dangerous levels of DHI, initial minute ventilation should be less than 115 mL/kg/min or approximately 8 L/min in a 70-kg patient.[207] This can be achieved with a respiratory rate between 12 and 14 breaths/min combined and a tidal volume between 7 and 8 mL/kg. The use of a low tidal volume avoids undue peak lung inflation, which may occur even with acceptably low minute ventilation.

Shortening the inspiratory time by use of a high inspiratory flow rate also prolongs expiratory time. We favor an inspiratory flow rate of 80 L/min, using a square or constant flow regimen. High inspiratory flow rates increase peak airway pressure by elevating airway resistive pressure, but peak airway pressure does not correlate with morbidity or mortality (see later). Rather it is the state of lung hyperinflation that predicts outcome, and any ventilator strategy that lowers peak airway pressure shortens expiratory time and worsens DHI. One concern is that high inspiratory flow rates in patients breathing in the assist-control mode will increase the respiratory rate and thereby decrease the expiratory time.[208]

There is little consensus regarding ventilator mode in acute asthma. In paralyzed patients synchronized intermittent mandatory ventilation (SIMV) and assist-controlled ventilation (AC) are equivalent. In patients triggering the ventilator, AC may increase minute ventilation but SIMV may be associated with increased work of breathing.[209,210] Volume-controlled (VC) ventilation is recommended over pressure-controlled (PC) ventilation for several reasons, including staff familiarity with its use. PC ventilation offers

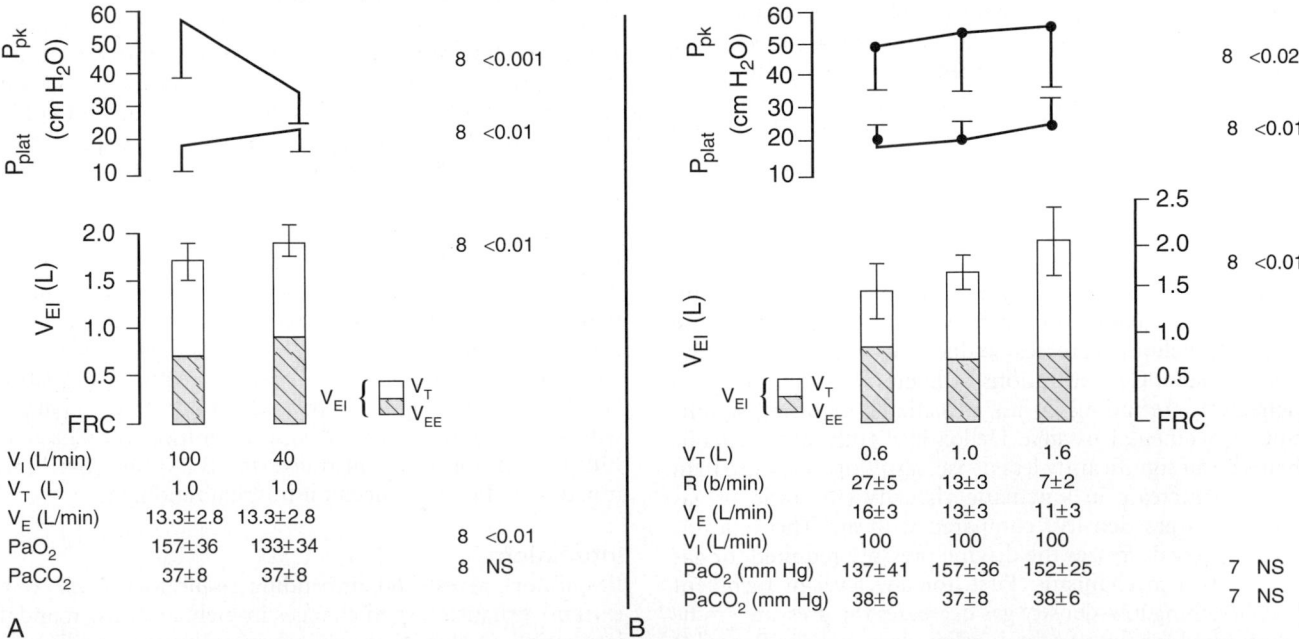

FIGURE 77–2. Effects of ventilator settings on airway pressures and lung volumes during normocapnic ventilation of eight paralyzed asthmatic patients. V_{EE}, lung volume at end expiration; V_{EI}, lung volume at end inspiration; Ppk, peak airway pressure; Pplat, end-inspiratory plateau pressure, V_E, minute ventilation, V_I, inspiratory flow. The numerals 7 and 8 are patient numbers. The numerals <0.001, <0.01, and <0.02 are p values. **A,** As inspiratory flow is decreased from 100 L/min to 40 L/min at the same V_E, Ppk falls but hyperinflation increases due to dynamic gas trapping. **B,** Dynamic hyperinflation is reduced by low respiratory rates and high tidal volumes (as long as V_E is decreased), but high tidal volumes result in high Pplat. (Reproduced with permission from Tuxen DV, Lane S: The effects of ventilatory pattern on hyperinflation, airway pressures, and circulation in mechanical ventilation of patients with severe air-flow obstruction. Am Rev Respir Dis 1987;136:872.)

the advantage of limiting peak airway pressure to a predetermined set value (e.g., 30 cm H$_2$O). However, during PC ventilation tidal volume is inversely related to auto-PEEP and minute ventilation is not guaranteed. Also, PC requires a decelerating inspiratory flow pattern, which may shorten the expiratory time.

Ventilator-applied PEEP is not recommended in sedated and paralyzed patients because it may increase lung volume if used excessively.[211] In spontaneously breathing patients, low levels of ventilator-applied PEEP (e.g., 5 cm H$_2$O) decrease inspiratory work of breathing by decreasing the pressure gradient required to overcome auto-PEEP.

Assessing Lung Inflation

Determination of the severity of DHI is central to risk management and adjustment of ventilator settings. Numerous methods have been proposed to measure DHI. The volume at end-inspiration, termed V$_{EI}$, is determined by collecting expired gas from total lung capacity to functional residual capacity during 40 to 60 seconds of apnea. A V$_{EI}$ greater than 20 mL/kg has been correlated with barotrauma.[207] Indeed, this is the only measure of DHI that has been shown to predict barotrauma (although it may underestimate air trapping if there are slowly emptying airspaces). The utility of this measure is limited by the need for paralysis and by staff who are unfamiliar with expiratory gas collection.

Alternate measures of DHI include the single-breath plateau pressure (Pplat) and auto-PEEP. Pplat is an estimate of average end-inspiratory alveolar pressures that is determined by stopping flow at end-inspiration. Auto-PEEP is the lowest average alveolar pressure achieved during the respiratory cycle. It is obtained by measuring airway-opening pressure during an end-expiratory hold maneuver. In the presence of auto-PEEP airway-opening pressure increases by the amount of auto-PEEP present. Persistence of expiratory gas flow at the beginning of inspiration (which can be detected by auscultation or flow tracings) also demonstrates auto-PEEP.[212]

Accurate measurement of Pplat and auto-PEEP requires patient-ventilator synchrony and absence of patient effort. Paralysis is generally not required for valid measurements. Unfortunately, neither measure has been validated as a predictor of complications. Pplat is affected by the entire respiratory system, including lung tissue and chest wall; thus, variations in DHI occur from patient to patient at the same pressure. Despite these limitations, experience suggests that when Pplat is less than 30 cm H$_2$O the outcome is generally good. Auto-PEEP can underestimate the severity of DHI possibly owing to poor communication between the alveoli and airway opening during mechanical ventilation.[213] In most cases, however, auto-PEEP less than 15 cm H$_2$O is acceptable.

Ventilator Adjustments

With the previous considerations in mind we offer an algorithm for the ventilator adjustments (Fig. 77-3). This algorithm relies on Pplat as the measure of lung hyperinflation and arterial pH as a marker of ventilation. If initial ventilator settings result in Pplat greater than 30 cm H$_2$O, respiratory rate should be decreased until this goal is achieved, even at the cost of hypercapnia. Fortunately, hypercapnia is well tolerated, even with arterial PCO$_2$ as high as 90 mm Hg, as long as a sudden rise in PaCO$_2$ does not occur.[214,215] Anoxic brain injury and myocardial dysfunction are contraindications to permissive hypercapnia because hypercapnia dilates cerebral vessels, decreases myocardial

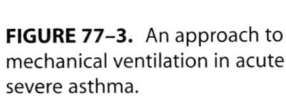

FIGURE 77–3. An approach to mechanical ventilation in acute severe asthma.

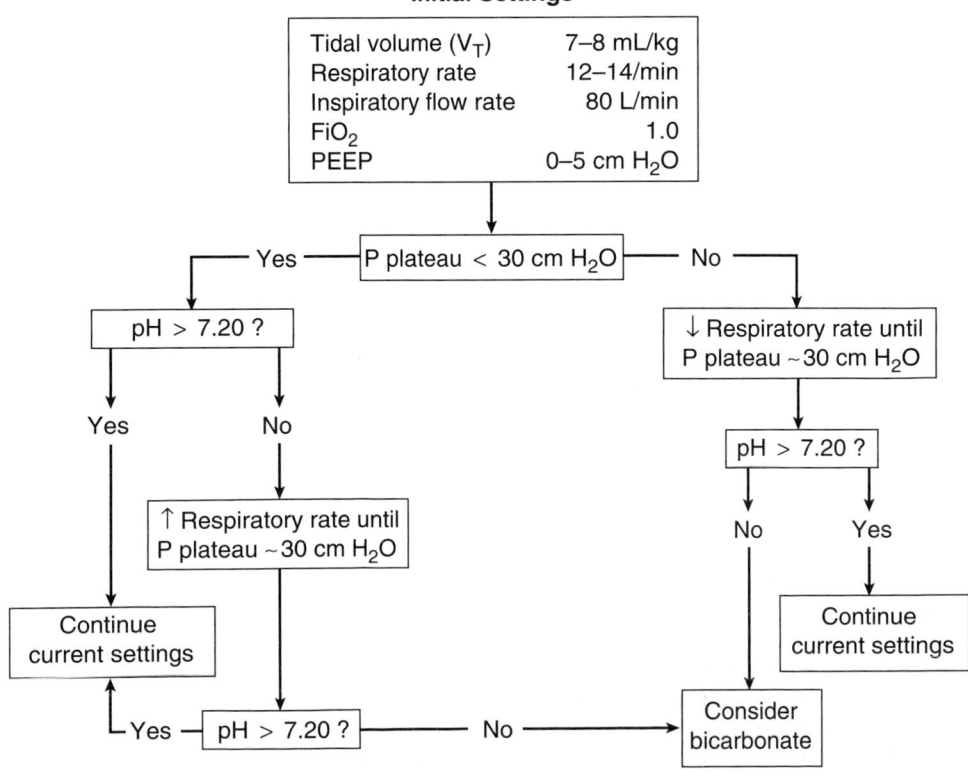

contractility, and constricts pulmonary vessels.[216] Lowering the respiratory rate may not increase $PaCO_2$ as expected if less DHI lowers dead space. If hypercapnia results in a blood pH of less than 7.20 and the respiratory rate cannot be increased because of the Pplat limit, we consider an infusion of sodium bicarbonate, although this has not been shown to improve outcome.[217] If Pplat is less than 30 cm H_2O and pH is less than 7.20, the respiratory rate is increased until Pplat nears 30 cm H_2O.

Sedation and Paralysis

Sedation improves comfort, safety, and patient-ventilator synchrony. This is particularly important when hypercapnia stimulates respiratory drive. In patients who can be extubated within hours (e.g., those with sudden-onset asthma), propofol is attractive because it can be titrated to a deep level of sedation and allow for rapid reversal after discontinuation.[218] Benzodiazepines, such as lorazepam and midazolam, are less expensive alternatives.[219] Time to awakening after discontinuation of these drugs is less predictable than with propofol.

To provide amnesia, sedation, analgesia, and suppression of respiratory drive, a narcotic can be added by continuous infusion to either propofol or a benzodiazepine.[220] Morphine and fentanyl are the two most commonly used narcotics. Fentanyl has a quicker onset of action and is slightly more expensive than morphine, although the magnitude of this difference is small. Daily interruption of sedatives avoids undue drug effects.[221]

Ketamine, an intravenously administered anesthetic with sedative, analgesic, and bronchodilating properties, is reserved for intubated patients with severe bronchospasm despite the use of standard therapies.[222-224] Ketamine must be used with caution because of its sympathomimetic effects and ability to cause delirium.

When safe and effective mechanical ventilation cannot be achieved by sedation alone, consideration should be given to short-term muscle paralysis. Short- to intermediate-acting agents include atracurium, *cis*-atracurium, and vecuronium. Pancuronium is a less expensive alternative, but it lasts longer and may cause unwanted tachycardia. Pancuronium and atracurium both release histamine, but the clinical significance of this property is doubtful.[225] In our ICU we prefer *cis*-atracurium because it is essentially free of cardiovascular effects, does not release histamine, and does not rely on hepatic and renal function for clearance.

Paralytics may be given intermittently by bolus or continuous intravenous infusion. If a continuous infusion is used, a nerve stimulator should be used or the drug should be withheld every 4 to 6 hours to avoid drug accumulation and prolonged paralysis. Paralytics should be stopped as soon as possible to decrease the risk of postparalytic myopathy.[226-228] Acute myopathy is rare in patients paralyzed for less than 24 hours. Most patients with postparalytic myopathy recover, but there may be significant disability.

Administration of Bronchodilators during Mechanical Ventilation

Data from controlled trials are needed to determine the efficacy of bronchodilators in intubated asthmatics and to provide evidence for or against current clinical recommendations.[229] One consistent observation is that intubated patients require higher drug dosages to achieve a clinical effect. Indeed in some intubated asthmatics a clinical effect may not be apparent at all. This may be because intubated patients are more likely albuterol nonresponders (see earlier) and because albuterol is delivered inadequately. In one study, only 2.9% of a radioactive aerosol delivered by nebulizer was deposited in the lungs of mechanically ventilated patients.[230] In another study, the efficacy of albuterol delivered by MDI via a simple inspiratory adapter (no spacer) was compared with nebulized albuterol in mechanically ventilated patients.[231] Using the peak-to-pause pressure gradient at a constant inspiratory flow to measure airway resistance, the authors found no effect (and no side effects) from the administration of 100 puffs (9.0 mg) of albuterol. However, albuterol delivered by nebulizer to a total dose of 2.5 mg reduced the inspiratory flow-resistive pressure 18%. Increasing the nebulized dose to a total of 7.5 mg further reduced airway resistance in 8 of 10 patients but caused side effects half the time.

When MDIs are used during mechanical ventilation, the use of a spacing device on the inspiratory limb of the ventilator improves drug delivery.[232] In general, nebulizers should be placed close to the ventilator and in-line humidifiers should be stopped during treatments. Inspiratory flow should be reduced to approximately 40 L/min during treatments to minimize turbulence, although this strategy may worsen DHI and should be time limited.[231] Patient-ventilator synchrony helps to optimize drug delivery.

Regardless of whether an MDI with spacer or nebulizer is used, higher drug dosages are required and the dosage should be titrated to achieve a fall in the peak-to-pause airway pressure gradient. When no measurable drop in airway resistance occurs, other causes of elevated airway resistance such as a kinked or plugged endotracheal tube should be excluded. Bronchodilator nonresponders should be considered for a drug holiday.

Other Considerations

Rarely, the aforementioned strategies are unable to stabilize the patient on the ventilator. In these situations, consideration should be given to other therapies. Halothane and enflurane are general anesthetic bronchodilators that can acutely reduce peak pressure and $PaCO_2$.[233,234] These agents are associated with myocardial depression, arterial vasodilation, and arrhythmias, and their benefits do not last after drug discontinuation. Heliox delivered through the ventilator circuit also decreases peak pressure and $PaCO_2$.[235] However, safe use of heliox requires significant institutional expertise and planning. Ventilator flowmeters (which are gas-density dependent) must be recalibrated to low density gas, and a spirometer should be placed on the expiratory port to measure tidal volume. A trial of heliox in a lung model is recommended before patient use.

Strategies to mobilize mucus such as chest physiotherapy, mucolytics, or expectorants have not proved to be efficacious in controlled trials. Bronchoalveolar lavage, on the other hand, using either saline or acetylcysteine may be useful in nonintubated patients.[236-238] This procedure is theoretically risky because the presence of a bronchoscope increases expiratory airway resistance and may provoke bronchospasm.

Extubation

Weaning and extubation criteria have not been validated for patients with acute asthma. One approach is to perform a spontaneous breathing trial once (1) $PaCO_2$ normalizes at a minute ventilation that achieves a safe level of DHI, (2) airway resistance is less than 20 cm H_2O, (3) the patient follows commands, and (4) neuromuscular weakness has not been identified. Patients with labile asthma may meet these criteria within hours of intubation, but more often 24 to 48 hours of treatment is required. We extubate as soon as possible because the endotracheal tube may aggravate bronchospasm. After extubation, observation in an ICU is recommended for an additional 12 to 24 hours. During this time the focus can switch to safe transfer to the ward and outpatient management.

ANNOTATED REFERENCES

Corbridge T, Hall JB: The assessment and management of status asthmaticus in adults. Am J Resp Crit Care Med 1995;151:1296-1316.

This manuscript provides a comprehensive review of the initial evaluation and treatment of patients with life-threatening asthma.

Nelson H, Bensch G, Pleskow WW, et al: Improved bronchodilation with levalbuterol compared with racemic albuterol in patients with asthma. J Allergy Clin Immunol 1998;102:943.

This manuscript demonstrates that bronchodilation is improved in patients who receive levalbuterol versus the standard racemic form of this inhaled bronchodilator.

Newhouse MT, Chapman KR, McCallum AL, et al: Cardiovascular safety of high doses of inhaled fenoterol and albuterol in acute severe asthma. Chest 1996;110:595.

Patients with severe asthma may respond to higher doses of bronchodilators than what are used in outpatient maintenance therapy. This paper shows that such doses do not have untoward cardiovascular effects.

Rodrigo GJ, Rodrigo C: First-line therapy for adult patients with acute severe asthma receiving a multiple-dose protocol of ipratropium bromide plus albuterol in the emergency department. Am J Resp Crit Care Med 2000;161:1862-1868.

Combination of ipratropium plus inhaled albuterol results in improved response in patients with severe asthma, as compared with albuterol alone. This article provides important evidence justifying the use of ipratropium in severe asthmatics.

Rowe BH, Spooner CH, Ducharme FM, et al: Early emergency department treatment of acute asthma with systemic corticosteroids (Cochrane Review). In The Cochrane Library, Issue 2. Oxford, Update Software, 2003.

A topical review of the utility of corticosteroids in patients with severe asthma.

Weber EJ, Silverman RA, Callaham ML, et al: A prospective multicenter study of factors associated with hospital admission among adults with acute asthma. Am J Med 2002;113:371-378.

In this study, the factors predicting admission of asthmatic patients to the hospital are reviewed. Whereas many of the factors, such as severity of airflow limitation, are not surprising, other more subtle findings on history and physical examination also have predictive value.

Chapter 78

CHRONIC OBSTRUCTIVE PULMONARY DISEASE

Peter M. A. Calverley

KEY POINTS

1. **The prognosis of patients with chronic obstructive pulmonary disease (COPD)** admitted to the ICU is better than commonly believed.
2. The **burden of symptomatic COPD** is likely to rise for several decades, despite an effective smoking cessation program.
3. **Small changes in forced expiratory flow** are associated with significant impairment in lung mechanics, particularly airway closure and dynamic hyperinflation, and worse gas exchange.
4. **Common upper respiratory tract pathogens and respiratory viruses precipitate most exacerbations of COPD.** Treatment aimed at these agents is useful, but it is not as important as improving lung emptying and maintaining gas exchange until the acute insult resolves.
5. **Oral and intravenous corticosteroids shorten the duration of an exacerbation and reduce the risk of relapse.** However, high-dose treatment beyond 2 weeks provides no advantage and actually poses a risk, especially in ventilated patients.
6. **Maintaining oxygenation is relatively easy, but there are risks** of carbon dioxide retention and acidosis if high-flow oxygen is administered. An oxygen saturation between 91% and 93% ensures adequate tissue oxygen delivery if the cardiac output is stable.
7. **Respiratory acidosis is a poor prognostic marker** in COPD exacerbations and a strong indicator of the need for assisted ventilation.
8. **Unless contraindicated, noninvasive ventilation is the safest and most effective way of managing acute respiratory failure.** More acidotic patients should be managed in an ICU facility with the option of intermittent positive-pressure ventilation if noninvasive ventilation fails.
9. **COPD patients meet conventional weaning criteria less frequently than other ICU patients do,** but they are more likely to wean successfully when they do meet the criteria.
10. **Seriously ill patients should be encouraged to make advance directives,** particularly after an ICU admission involving any form of ventilatory support.

Chronic obstructive pulmonary disease (COPD) is a major cause of death and disability worldwide and is one of the most common reasons for ICU admission. Several monographs review this complex disorder in some detail.[1,2] The intensivist's view of COPD is predominantly physiologic, focusing on the impact of disrupted function on the individual's normal homeostatic mechanisms. Although many important insights that have shaped our understanding of COPD have come from ICU studies, other aspects of this disorder must be considered if a rational approach to COPD management is to be developed.

Access to ICU care for sick COPD patients remains relatively inequitable among different health care systems. In North America and parts of western Europe, most patients are offered ICU care, but in other relatively developed health care systems, such as in the United Kingdom, this is not the case. Even physicians in the same health care system differ significantly in their selection of patients for ICU referral.[3] These choices may be influenced by local resource availability, but they are also conditioned by the generally pessimistic view of the outcome achievable with this treatment intervention. However, poor response to treatment is not universal, and extended periods of positive-pressure ventilation are not invariably required to successfully manage patients with COPD.[4] Nevertheless, intensivists often take a particularly bleak view of the prognosis of COPD patients compared with others entering their units. Inevitably, value judgments about the worth of an individual's life come into play, especially when resources are limited. However, such decisions should not be made in the emergency room without sufficient medical information or a proper discussion with the family. Supportive therapies should be offered until it is clear what the patient's wishes are and what the likely outcome of treatment will be.

This chapter reviews some of the relevant pathophysiology of COPD requiring ICU admission, considers the common reasons for such admissions, reviews the treatment options to support the patient and shorten the duration of the illness, and considers the role of assisted ventilation.

DEFINITION AND NATURAL HISTORY

Although the most appropriate definition of COPD has been debated in the wider pulmonary community, it has less of an impact in the context of ICU care, where acute hospitalization is usual only in cases of severe and well-established disease. The currently favored definition, developed by the global initiative for chronic obstructive lung disease, is as follows: "Chronic obstructive pulmonary disease (COPD) is a disease state characterised by airflow limitation that is not fully reversible. The airflow limitation is usually both progressive and associated with an abnormal inflammatory response of the lungs to noxious particles or gasses."[5]

The emphasis here is on incompletely reversible airflow obstruction that is persistent and progressive. Symptoms and disability usually parallel these processes, although some individuals can apparently cope with a severe degree of airflow limitation without seeking medical help. Such patients finally present to the emergency room when they develop a severe exacerbation of COPD. In this situation, it is wisest to offer ventilatory support until the patient has at least had a chance to improve with conventional medical therapy. More common is a patient whose progressive illness is accompanied by repeated exacerbations, events that identify an accelerated decline in both lung function and health status.[6,7] Such patients have often been hospitalized previously, and their response to treatment is usually clearly established.

The usual inhaled particles or gases that produce COPD are a complex mixture of hydrocarbons and particulates derived from tobacco smoke. These are the principal causes of COPD in the United States and western Europe,[8,9] although other factors, such as poor lung function during childhood, bronchial hyperresponsiveness, and low birth weight, may also be important. The associated inflammatory changes, which persist when smoking stops,[10] are thought to explain the airway and parenchymal destruction and fibrosis within the lung, although this has not been conclusively established as the only mechanism.

The natural history of COPD explains why the number of patients presenting for ICU care has not diminished in the last 3 decades, as might be expected given the overall reduction in tobacco consumption in Western countries. This is illustrated by the classic study of Fletcher and Peto (Fig. 78-1).[11] Although the rate of decline of lung function is reduced in individuals who stop smoking, the lung function already lost is never regained, and even if the rate of decline of lung function returns to normal, these patients are still more likely to experience disability as they age. Thus, in an aging population that contains many former smokers, a significant number

will still develop the complications of COPD that require ICU care. The situation is complicated by the steadily rising number of women who smoke, who appear to be at least as susceptible as men to the adverse effects of tobacco.[12] Thus, the initial reduction in new cases of COPD is partially offset by the increased incidence of women with significant symptoms.

PATHOLOGY

The pathologic features of COPD depend on the stage of the illness and the part of the lung examined.[13] Central airways show mucous gland hypertrophy and goblet cell metaplasia, whereas more peripheral airways show variable combinations of smooth muscle hypertrophy, peribronchial fibrosis, luminal occlusion by mucus, and enlarged lymphoid follicles.[14] Alveoli are often but not invariably enlarged by the loss of alveolar walls, with an attendant loss of support for the small non-cartilaginous airways in this region of the lung. There is evidence of persistent inflammation, with neutrophils in the airway lumen and macrophages in the airway wall. CD8[+] T lymphocytes are more prominent in this response than in bronchial inflammation of an asthmatic type, although intermediate states appear to exist.[15,16] Inflammatory cells are also present adjacent to breaks in the alveolar wall.[17] Overall, as the clinical and spirometric severity of the disease increases, so do the numbers of each cell involved in the inflammatory process.[18] Data on exacerbations, though limited, support an increased role for neutrophils and, surprisingly eosinophils.[19]

PHYSIOLOGY

The pathologic changes just described combine to produce the characteristic diagnostic finding of reduced forced expiratory flow at a given lung volume (FEV_1), which is usually assessed on a time base as an FEV_1/forced vital capacity (FVC) ratio of less than 0.7. Technically, this should be 70% of the age-adjusted normal value for this ratio, because lung elastic recoil declines with age, even in healthy individuals. Use of the uncorrected ratio tends to overdiagnose COPD among the very elderly.[20] In practice, however, this does not cause problems for COPD patients admitted for ICU care, because they are invariably more severely affected.

COPD affects all aspects of lung function, but its primary impact is a change in lung mechanics. This is traditionally analyzed in terms of the static (no flow) and dynamic (flow) properties of the respiratory system.[21] Because chest wall mechanics are believed to be normal in COPD (although they are seldom measured directly), changes in the pressure-volume characteristics of the respiratory system are determined by alterations in lung compliance, often attributed to the loss of elastic recoil due to emphysema. How large a role this plays in changes in tissue compliance is not known. The resulting steeper slope, early-onset inspiratory plateau, and increase in end-expiratory lung volume are typical of the pressure-volume relationships in patients with COPD. Changes in end-expiratory lung volume and increases in residual volume change chest wall geometry to favor a lower, flatter diaphragm and a more horizontal rib cage; these changes, in turn, impair the inspiratory muscles' ability to develop pressure, and increase the overall work of breathing.[22] Expiratory muscle activation is common in more severe COPD,[23,24] even at rest, and provides a useful clinical marker of respiratory distress. Flattening of the diaphragm redirects the axis of shortening of

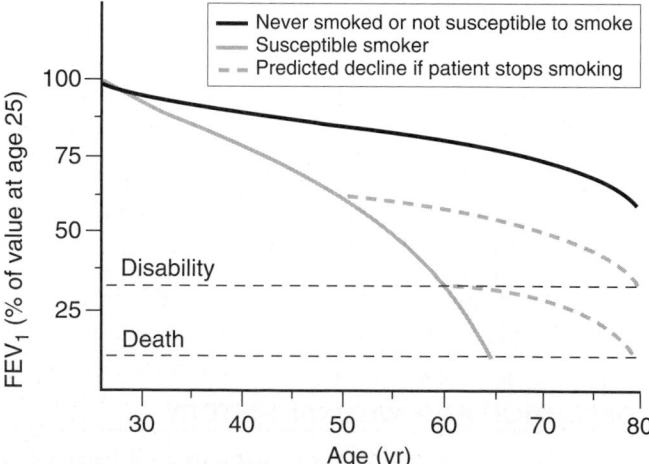

FIGURE 78–1. Natural history of chronic obstructive pulmonary disease and the effect of smoking cessation. Compared with lung function standardized to age 25, smokers show an accelerated rate of decline in forced expiratory volume (FEV_1), which returns to more normal values when they stop smoking. However, they are operating at a lower FEV_1 than that predicted for their age, and the physiologic decline continues. This explains why older ex-smokers can present to the ICU with severe disease despite years of abstinence. (Adapted from Fletcher C, Peto R: The natural history of chronic airway obstruction. BMJ 1977;1:1645-1648.)

the skeletal muscle and often produces paradoxical in-drawing of the lower thoracic rib cage (so-called Hoover's sign), which becomes more evident as pulmonary hyperinflation and respiratory drive to breathe rise.

The dynamics of the respiratory system are influenced by these static properties but also differ significantly between inspiration and expiration. Maximum inspiratory flow is affected by inspiratory resistance, as well as by the inspiratory muscles' ability to develop pressure (and thus indirectly by chest wall geometry). Maximum expiratory flow is influenced by expiratory pressure generation and, more importantly, by the onset of volume-related airflow limitation, best described by the maximum expiratory flow-volume loop. As lung volume falls during expiration, airways close or become flow limited; hence, the flow at a specific lung volume is reduced. Although an assessment of flow (FEV_1) relative to total volume change during expiration (FVC) is useful in defining COPD, an assessment of tidal flow limitation is more helpful in determining the degree of dyspnea experienced by the patient.[25] More attention is now being paid to the determination of expiratory flow limitation under tidal conditions. In the past, detection was difficult, involving invasive measurements or reliance on body plethysmography, which tended to overestimate the incidence of tidal expiratory flow limitation. The development of the negative expiratory pressure test and, more recently, within-breath variation in respiratory system impedance has changed this.[26] In general, the lower the FEV_1, the greater the likelihood that expiratory flow limitation is present. However, some COPD patients are not flow-limited on every breath and regulate their end-expiratory lung volume to try to minimize this. When respiratory drive rises (e.g., during exercise), during disease exacerbations, or when minute ventilation has to increase to maintain gas exchange during ventilator weaning, this resting variation in expiratory lung volume is likely to decrease. If expiratory flow and hence tidal volume are to increase, end-expiratory lung volume must rise; this further increases the work of breathing and the sensation of respiratory distress. This process, described as dynamic hyperinflation, has been clearly demonstrated during exercise[27] and can be lessened by bronchodilator treatment, which aids lung emptying.

In the ICU, where the first observations about dynamic hyperinflation were made,[28] the same constraints occur. Patients have a high respiratory drive during weaning and adopt a rapid, shallow breathing pattern (see later). Total respiratory muscle work increases, in part because of the increased operating lung volumes, but also because of the presence of intrinsic positive end-expiratory pressure (PEEPi). This represents the pressure that must be developed to overcome residual expiratory driving pressure before inspiratory flow can begin. Calculating the size of this variable is fraught with technical difficulties beyond the problems of accurate placement of the balloon catheter system in intubated patients. Several methods have been proposed that correct for the effects of coexisting abdominal muscle activation, with recent work favoring a correction based on the total decay of gastric pressure.[29] However, the need to compute this variable in clinical practice has been questioned.[30]

What is clear is that the overall impairment of mechanical function in COPD is substantial and that both static and dynamic properties interact—a concept best captured by the time constant of the respiratory system, which is the product of the total respiratory system resistance in compliance. This is greatly lengthened in COPD and helps explain why lung emptying is delayed and dynamic hyperinflation occurs. There is substantial evidence of regional inhomogeneity in more severe COPD. Differences in the regional time constants explain why COPD patients are prone to barotrauma during mechanical ventilation, despite seemingly acceptable peak inspiratory pressures, as well as why gas exchange can be quite disordered in this population (see later).

GAS EXCHANGE

Arterial hypoxemia is common in COPD but becomes clinically significant only when the partial pressure of oxygen in arterial blood (PaO_2) falls below 60 mm Hg, a problem largely confined to patients with an FEV_1 below 35% of their predicted value. It arises predominantly due to ventilation-perfusion mismatching, often worsens during exercise, and is readily corrected by a small increase in the inspired oxygen concentration, unless the situation is made worse by secretion retention or severe pneumonia.[31] Arterial hypercapnia is seen in some but not all hypoxemic patients who are clinically stable, but it is more frequent, at least temporarily, in hospitalized individuals.[32] A combination of ventilation-perfusion mismatching due to an increase in physiologic deadspace and a degree of effective alveolar hypoventilation explains this phenomenon (see later). Acute rises in the partial pressure of arterial carbon dioxide ($PaCO_2$) precipitate respiratory acidosis, a more reliable guide to prognosis and the need for ventilation than the $PaCO_2$ itself.[33,34]

CONTROL OF BREATHING

Despite years of study, there is no conclusive evidence that ventilatory control is abnormal in COPD patients. However, the response to sustained mechanical loading appears to be variable in healthy subjects[35] and may explain why some individuals adopt the breathing patterns they do. Traditional techniques of studying respiratory control, which involve stimulation with exogenous CO_2 or nitrogen, suggested that respiratory drive was reduced. However, studies using mouth occlusion pressure techniques or recording the electrical activation of inspiratory muscles suggest that respiratory drive is generally high, even in those who tolerate relatively high levels of CO_2.[36-38] Studies of breathing pattern have been more instructive. In general, the lower the tidal volume, the higher the $PaCO_2$.[39] This is because the ratio of deadspace (its fixed, predominantly anatomically determined volume) to tidal volume increases as the latter is reduced. Small tidal volumes are accompanied by an increased respiratory frequency, to maintain the somewhat higher than normal level of minute ventilation. The resulting shortening of inspiratory time is also associated with hypercapnia.[39] The system appears to be regulated to minimize peak inspiratory pressure generation, even at the cost of impaired gas exchange. There are theoretical reasons for believing that this is both energy efficient and likely to minimize the occurrence of inspiratory muscle fatigue.[40] This also explains the usefulness of rapid, shallow breathing as an index of weaning failure when neuromechanical coupling in the respiratory system is under considerable stress.[41]

PULMONARY CIRCULATION

In the past, considerable attention was paid to the determination of pulmonary artery pressure in COPD patients, but this is now thought to be less important. Undoubtedly, pulmonary artery pressure increases by day and at night[42] in hypoxemic COPD patients, reflecting a combination of hypoxic vasoconstriction and pulmonary vascular remodeling. How important this is in the daily limitation of exercise reported by these patients is not clear, but it is known that treatment with domiciliary oxygen prevents disease progression[43] and may even reduce pulmonary artery pressure. More specific attempts at therapy both inside and outside the ICU have been unsuccessful, usually resulting in worsening of ventilation-perfusion mismatching, which is thought to be clinically unacceptable.[44] In general, assessment of pulmonary hypertension has fallen out of favor as part of a routine evaluation in COPD patients, but its occurrence is important to note when interpreting changes in central venous pressure in instrumented patients.

SYSTEMIC EFFECTS

There is good evidence that systemic (extrapulmonary) factors are important in COPD. Patients with a reduced body mass index die sooner than better-nourished individuals with a similar degree of pulmonary function impairment, although those who can gain weight fare better.[45] There are data to show that peripheral muscle function is impaired,[46] fiber type is altered,[47] and exercise is associated with increased oxidative stress.[48] This has led to the concept of a specific COPD myopathy,[49] although how much of this reflects inactivity and the effects of impaired oxygen delivery during exercise has yet to be established. There are data suggesting altered oxidative metabolism in circulating lymphocytes[50] and increased concentrations of tumor necrosis factor, which may predispose to cachexia in some cases.[51] Whether one or several inflammatory pathways are involved in producing these diverse effects is not clear, but their presence is generally a marker of a poorer prognosis and can lead to specific problems in the ICU.

EXACERBATIONS

A recent consensus conference defined an exacerbation of COPD as a sustained worsening of the patient's condition from the stable state, beyond normal day-to-day variation, that is acute in onset and necessitates a change in regular medication.[52] The key feature here is the sustained change from usual daily symptoms. The operational requirement for a change in treatment is more arbitrary but is almost always present in patients referred for ICU care. Disease exacerbation is the principal cause of ICU admission with COPD, and patients commonly have or are at risk of developing significant respiratory failure, defined as a PaO_2 below 60 mm Hg with or without an increase in $PaCO_2$.[53] The most common causes of exacerbation are listed in Table 78-1. Viral and bacterial infections are both relevant,[54] with rhinoviruses commonly reported in most series; *Haemophilus influenzae* and *Streptococcus pneumoniae* are the principal microbial pathogens.[55] Some patients, particularly those with a regular cough and green sputum production, develop persistent lower respiratory tract colonization, making the interpretation of qualitative microbiology difficult.[56] Usually, there is an increase in the absolute number of colony-forming units of microorganisms in these patients during exacerbations, reflecting an increased burden of infection, although more

TABLE 78–1. CAUSES OF CHRONIC OBSTRUCTIVE PULMONARY DISEASE EXACERBATION

New infection
    Bacterial (*Haemophilus influenzae, Streptococcus pneumoniae, Moraxella haemophilus*)
    Change in an existing strain (e.g., *H. influenzae*)
    Viral (influenza, rhinovirus, respiratory syncytial virus)
Atmospheric pollution
    Sulfur dioxide, oxides of nitrogen
Temperature change
    Often related to pollution episodes
Intercurrent illness*
    Pneumonia, pulmonary embolus, pneumothorax
Postoperative
    Especially after upper abdominal surgery

*Clinical presentation is dominated by the primary illness, but respiratory failure can occur.

subtle changes have been reported involving the introduction of a different serotype of *H. influenzae*.[57] Not all exacerbations have an infectious precipitant, and changes in the degree of atmospheric pollution can precipitate events in some patients.[58] How frequently individuals develop exacerbations after exposure to a specific precipitating event is not clear, although the likelihood of meeting the consensus definition rises as spirometric impairment worsens.[59]

The physiologic consequences of increased airflow obstruction secondary to increased inflammation within the bronchial tree are summarized in Figure 78-2. Whatever the precipitant, the key event appears to be a change in lung mechanics. Previously, attention focused on alterations in respiratory system resistance, but more recent data emphasize that airway narrowing and closure may be more important, particularly by producing changes in operating lung volumes (see earlier). This may explain why the small changes in pulmonary function that accompany exacerbations can be associated with substantial deterioration in gas exchange and clinical well-being, leading to hospitalization.

CLINICAL FEATURES

Key clinical features of the acute presentation are summarized in Table 78-2. In addition to obtaining an appropriate history and performing a physical examination, it is necessary to assess the degree of abnormal gas exchange and the presence of acidosis by measuring the arterial blood gases. In the context of an exacerbation, more direct measurements of lung mechanics are usually impractical, and the severity of the mechanical problem is evaluated indirectly by its effect on gas exchange. An urgent chest x-ray is useful for identifying specific precipitating factors, particularly alveolar shadowing due to infection, the presence of a pneumothorax, or radiographic features of pulmonary edema. The last is especially important, because it is commonly associated with hypercapnic respiratory failure—the combination of an increased ventilatory drive and poor perfusion of respiratory muscles, together with further impairment of ventilation-perfusion matching favoring CO_2 retention. In this context, an electrocardiogram is invaluable to screen for both underlying ischemic heart disease and rhythm disturbances. If major thromboembolic events are suspected on clinical grounds, quantitative D-dimer and urgent helical computed tomography scans with intravenous contrast to visualize the pulmonary circulation are the best way to establish their

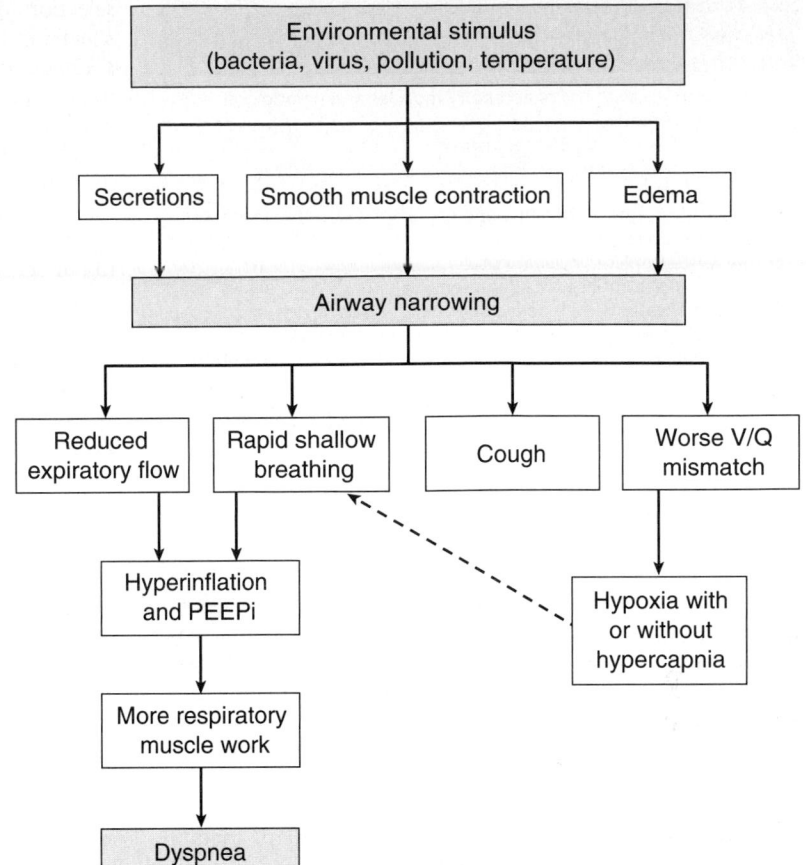

FIGURE 78–2. Schematic presentation of the principal physiologic changes that accompany an exacerbation of chronic obstructive pulmonary disease. Note that deterioration in one area tends to produce worsening in other areas and leads to a downward spiral in functional abnormality. PEEPi, intrinsic positive end-expiratory pressure; V/Q, ventilation-perfusion.

existence. Reliance on isotope ventilation-perfusion scanning is particularly prone to overdiagnosis in these patients and should be avoided. Simple laboratory tests such as the hemoglobin and white cell count can be valuable guides to the need for oxygenation and the likelihood of coexisting sepsis.

Exacerbation of airway inflammation is not the only reason for the deterioration of postoperative COPD patients, who are at significant risk after any type of surgery. This may reflect the consequences of anesthesia and impaired secretion clearance, the risks of lower respiratory tract infection after intubation, or the effects of surgery itself. Both pain and the drugs administered to relieve it are likely to depress ventilation in these patients. Thoracic and upper abdominal surgery impairs the function of the inspiratory and expiratory muscles, respectively. In those with severe COPD, abdominal muscle activation is an important involuntary technique to "share" the work of breathing between the inspiratory and expiratory muscles; impairment of abdominal muscle activation commonly increases the degree of breathlessness and may precipitate respiratory muscle fatigue. Persistent smoking before elective procedures should be discouraged, because this further compromises the already reduced compensatory mechanisms in COPD patients. In this setting, it is not surprising that respiratory failure develops in a significant number of individuals with severe disease, necessitating ICU care.

ICU REFERRAL

The need for mechanical ventilation is the primary reason for ICU referral among COPD patients. Although the various indications for mechanical ventilation (Table 78-3) vary in frequency from institution to institution, they represent the most common causes for ICU admission and have been acknowledged as such in a number of treatment guidelines.[5,60]

Before referring a patient for ICU care, and especially for any form of ventilatory support, it is important to determine what degree of intervention is appropriate. Advance

---

TABLE 78–2. CLINICAL FEATURES OF CHRONIC OBSTRUCTIVE PULMONARY DISEASE EXACERBATION

Sustained increase in dyspnea*
Increased cough (with or without sputum)*
Increased sputum volume or purulence*
Symptoms of upper respiratory tract infection (variable and should be accompanied by a major symptom)
Fever (infrequent in the absence of pneumonia)
Cyanosis (with advanced disease)
Tachypnea
Pursed lip breathing
Accessory muscle use (including abdominals)
Pulmonary overinflation (reduced cricoid distance, Hoover's sign, resonant percussion over the heart)
Tachycardia
Boundary pulse
Hypotension†
Flapping tremor†
Impaired level of consciousness†

*Major symptom.
†Severe illness.

TABLE 78–3. INDICATIONS FOR INVASIVE MECHANICAL VENTILATION

Severe dyspnea, with use of accessory muscles and paradoxical abdominal motion
Respiratory frequency >35 breaths/min
Life-threatening hypoxemia (PaO_2 <40 mm Hg or PaO_2/FIO_2 <200 mm Hg)
Severe acidosis (pH <7.25) and hypercapnia ($PaCO_2$ >60 mm Hg)
Respiratory arrest
Somnolence, impaired mental status
Cardiovascular complications (hypotension, shock, heart failure)
Other complications: metabolic abnormalities, sepsis, pneumonia, pulmonary embolism, barotrauma, massive pleural effusion
Noninvasive positive-pressure ventilation failure (or exclusion criteria)

FIO_2, inspired oxygen fraction; $PaCO_2$, partial pressure of carbon dioxide in arterial blood; PaO_2, partial pressure of oxygen in arterial blood.

directives are becoming increasingly common among COPD patients, particularly in the United States. These are specific orders about the level of intervention desired by the patient, informed by discussions with his or her physician. These difficult and potentially upsetting discussions are necessary when patients are approaching the terminal phase of an illness, and they should be encouraged as a routine practice, particularly in those who have already been admitted to an ICU and have a clear idea of what therapy involves. However, it is important to ensure that such interviews are conducted when the patient is clinically stable and capable of making rational judgments about what the future holds. We still have some way to go before this important aspect of care becomes a routine part of our clinical practice.

PRINCIPLES OF TREATMENT

Four general principles guide the management of COPD patients presenting acutely to the ICU, and each should contribute to shortening the duration of illness and stabilizing the patient physiologically until either the natural course of the disease or the effects of therapy lead to its resolution.

TREAT PRECIPITATING FACTORS

Bacterial infection is the most common reason for ICU admission in COPD patients. Infection confined to the airways can be managed with broad-spectrum antimicrobials, provided the patient is capable of swallowing and has reasonable gastrointestinal absorption. Otherwise, intravenous therapy is required; this is usually the case in patients sick enough to merit ICU admission. Radiographic evidence of pneumonia likely requires a broadening of the antibiotic spectrum, but whether the infection is confined to the airways or involves the alveoli, antibiotic therapy should follow locally established guidelines designed to minimize the development of resistance within the ICU and to address known patterns of drug resistance in the community and the hospital. Broad-spectrum penicillins or, more commonly, cephalosporins are usually recommended, often with an intravenous macrolide. Some advocate the prophylactic use of quinolone in COPD patients in the ICU,[61] but this practice requires confirmation before being accepted as universally effective. Colonization with methicillin-resistant *Staphylococcus aureus* is still a frequent problem and requires particular vigilance in the

selection of antibiotics. Likewise, excessive use of broad-spectrum agents can produce superinfection, such as *Clostridium difficile* diarrhea. This can be particularly distressing in a patient with severe COPD and a low body mass index and requires early identification and appropriate therapy.

The role of antiviral drugs, such as the neuraminidase inhibitors, in the management of acutely ill COPD patients remains to be determined. In some cases in which deterioration is extremely rapid, there may be some advantage in introducing these expensive agents, although the opportunity to maximize their ability to shorten the duration of the illness may have been lost by the time the patient reaches the hospital.

For those with postoperative pain, epidural anesthesia is frequently helpful, as it permits adequate analgesia without the unwanted ventilatory depressant effects noted earlier. Prophylaxis for pulmonary embolism should follow established guidelines in other high-risk groups managed in the ICU setting.

REDUCE LUNG VOLUME AND INCREASE EXPIRATORY FLOW

Agents that improve lung emptying, commonly by increasing airway caliber or preventing airway closure, interfere with the vicious circle of pulmonary hyperinflation described in Figure 78-2. This has been demonstrated in stable patients using exercise as a model of hyperinflation,[62] but the data in spontaneously breathing COPD patients during exacerbations are much less satisfactory. Nonetheless, treatment with regular but high doses of short-acting nebulized beta agonists, such as albuterol or ipratropium (2.5 to 5 mg or 250 to 500 µg, respectively), is usually recommended. There is no clear evidence that one drug is better than the other,[63] and combination therapy is commonly used. The outcomes of the few studies conducted in this setting were based on FEV_1 rather than symptoms or lung volume change. Intravenous theophylline, or one of its derivatives, is often added to these regimens, but there are few data to support doing so.[64]

REDUCE PULMONARY INFLAMMATION

Several randomized, controlled trials have shown that oral corticosteroids shorten the duration of hospitalization and accelerate improvement of post-bronchodilator FEV_1 during an exacerbation of COPD.[65,66] Patients randomized to treatment with oral corticosteroids were less likely to relapse during the subsequent month and showed a number of other benefits, although these did not always reach statistical significance.[67] There does not appear to be any additional benefit from using particularly high doses of corticosteroids or prolonging treatment beyond 10 days to 2 weeks. In the ICU, corticosteroid treatment is often given peremptorily to patients on ventilators; caution should be exercised, however, because these individuals are often at risk for relatively acute-onset corticosteroid myopathy.[68] If corticosteroid therapy has been maintained for a longer-than-normal period, or if courses of oral corticosteroids to treat less serious exacerbations have been given more frequently, a tapered dose-reduction plan should be introduced. Otherwise, treatment can be discontinued at the end of the normal 10 to 14 days. Patients given this therapy may benefit from subsequent treatment with inhaled corticosteroids,[69] but they should be evaluated for significant side effects. Osteoporosis is particularly common in COPD patients, whether they receive corticosteroid treatment or not, and it is probably worth identifying in any individual who requires ICU care.[70]

MANAGE GAS EXCHANGE

It is relatively easy to improve oxygenation in an uncomplicated exacerbation of COPD.[71] Raising the inspired oxygen concentration to 28% to 35% is usually sufficient to achieve a PaO_2 greater than 90 mm Hg. However, this is often accompanied by an undesirable increase in $PaCO_2$, with its accompanying respiratory acidosis. This impairs respiratory muscle function, at least during loaded breathing,[72] and often precedes more serious clinical deterioration, including impairment of consciousness. The reasons for this effect have been debated for many years, with some advocating a reduction in respiratory drive from the carotid chemoreceptors, and others citing a worsening ventilation-perfusion match as the cause.[71] Each view has evidence to support it, but the actual cause is likely a combination of both problems, with ventilation-perfusion mismatching being particularly important in severely ill patients, and hypoventilation playing a larger role in those not yet sick enough to require intubation.[73]

Although the phenomenon of oxygen-induced hypercapnia has been recognized for decades, it remains a real problem. In one large center in the United Kingdom, 34% of individuals showed evidence of oxygen-induced hypercapnia.[54] The use of high-flow oxygen in the emergency room is widespread, as is the false sense of security provided by a high pulse oxygen saturation. Many intensivists have legitimate concerns about the failure to adequately oxygenate COPD patients with compromised circulation, along with the attendant risk of unanticipated mortality. However, the solution is to carefully consider the risks of excessive or insufficient oxygen in a given individual, rather than to slavishly adhere to one view or the other. Patients whose problems are predominantly due to COPD and who have a normal hemoglobin and preserved cardiac output can maintain adequate tissue oxygen delivery with an oxygen saturation as low as 85%, and they will do quite well if an arterial oxygen saturation (SaO_2) of 90% to 93% is maintained. The modest increase in inspired oxygen needed to achieve this (often 24% to 28%) is accompanied by less hypercapnia and may avoid the need for ventilatory support. However, if cardiac output is impaired (reduced blood pressure, poor peripheral circulation) or the metabolic demands of the tissue are increased (e.g., in sepsis secondary to pneumonia), a higher SaO_2 will be required to ensure that there is sufficient oxygen delivery; in this case, the consequences of any resultant hypercapnia, including the need for ventilatory support, must be accepted.

Oxygen can be delivered accurately by facemask, using the Venturi principle of entraining room air into the mask. This is a precise method of giving a known inspired oxygen concentration to COPD patients,[74] but many patients dislodge facemasks and are unlikely to keep nasal prongs in place.[75] Nasal prongs allow the patients to speak and drink, but the inspired oxygen fraction (FIO_2) is more variable, and it may be necessary to monitor arterial blood gases more frequently. Institutions where nebulizers are used to deliver bronchodilator drugs should be cautious about nebulizing these drugs using wall oxygen, because this can produce severe hypercapnia. A better policy is to nebulize in air, with the patients keeping their nasal cannulas in place.

For many years, respiratory stimulants were used to waken semiconscious patients and permit physiotherapy and other forms of suction, but this approach was never tested scientifically and must be viewed with some skepticism today. There are data that continuous infusion of the nonspecific ventilatory stimulant doxapram can lower $PaCO_2$ values and allow a higher inspired oxygen to be delivered,[76] and groups have recommended this as a way of deferring the need for positive-pressure ventilation.[60] The advent of nasal positive-pressure ventilation has changed this approach, and the only study that directly compared the effects of doxapram and this modality in COPD concluded that patients did better with noninvasive ventilation and were less likely to deteriorate.[77] If chemical ventilatory stimulants are used, they should be considered a short-term means of sustaining the patient until a more appropriate method of ventilation can be instituted. Ultimately, some kind of mechanical ventilatory support is the best way to address the problems of hypercapnia.

NONINVASIVE VENTILATION

This topic is reviewed in detail in Chapter 68, but some key issues relevant to COPD are worth emphasizing. Many of the data supporting the use of noninvasive ventilation were obtained in patients with hypercapnic respiratory failure due to COPD exacerbation, and several excellent reviews have analyzed these data.[78,79]

Noninvasive ventilation has a number of potentially beneficial effects in COPD. Intuitively, it seems reasonable to expect that it would increase tidal volume, improve CO_2 elimination, and hence reduce respiratory drive. Studies of gas exchange using a multiple inert gas elimination methodology confirmed that CO_2 elimination is increased but overall ventilation-perfusion mismatch is not changed during noninvasive ventilation.[80] A more important effect is the unloading of the respiratory muscles, which are often close to fatigue conditions in severe episodes of respiratory failure. By assuming some of the additional work required to overcome intrinsic PEEP, noninvasive ventilation directly reduces the drive to breathe, and the respiratory rate falls, a good prognostic feature. Data from randomized, controlled trials suggest that there is a mean fall of 3.1 breaths per minute (95% confidence interval 4.3 to 1.9).[78] This allows more effective emptying of the lungs and less dynamic hyperinflation. The resulting improvement in the intensity of breathlessness is usually a much earlier sign of successful noninvasive ventilation treatment in COPD than are changes in blood gas tensions, which often lag behind evidence of clinical improvement.

Evidence-based reviews provide a reasonable series of recommendations based on the relative effectiveness of noninvasive ventilation. Key points, including the number of patients needed to be treated to prevent one significant event or complication, are shown in Table 78-4. Noninvasive ventilation is associated with less treatment failure, lower mortality, fewer complications, and a lower intubation rate compared with conventional medical treatment. It reduces the ICU or hospital stay by approximately 3 days and favorably influences gas exchange. Thus, pH increases by a mean value of 0.03 (0.02 to 0.04), $PaCO_2$ falls by 3 mm Hg (5.9 to 0.23 mm Hg), and PaO_2 rises by 2 mm Hg (−2 to +6 mm Hg). The lower rate of nosocomial pneumonia associated with noninvasive ventilation is a particular advantage.

These data support the use of noninvasive ventilation as a first-line treatment in patients with exacerbations of

TABLE 78–4. EFFICACY OF NONINVASIVE VENTILATION COMPARED WITH USUAL CARE

Outcome	Number of Patients Studied	Relative Risk (95% Confidence Interval)	NNT
Treatment failure	529	0.51 (0.38-0.67)	5
Death	523	0.41 (0.26-0.64)	8
Intubation	546	0.42 (0.31-0.59)	5
Complications	143	0.32 (0.18-0.56)	3

NNT, number needed to treat—the number of patients who must be treated to prevent this outcome in one individual.

COPD and moderate respiratory acidosis (pH <7.35) despite medical treatment. In general, most patients with pH in the range of 7.3 to 7.35 survive without noninvasive ventilation, although the number patients needed to prevent one exacerbation is still only 10.[81] As acidosis becomes more severe, the benefits of noninvasive ventilation become greater; this treatment should be encouraged in anyone with a pH less than 7.3. In patients with more severe acidosis (pH <7.25), the benefit is less clear, and results in different trials suggests that such patients have a better outcome if they are managed in the ICU with mechanical ventilation and intubation; however, these trials are influenced by selection bias. In clinical practice, it is reasonable to offer a trial of noninvasive ventilation unless the patient has some of the established contraindications to this treatment (Table 78-5). Even then, there are occasions when noninvasive ventilation is appropriate first-line therapy, for example, if a patient does not wish to be intubated (as indicated in an advance directive) or has a "ceiling of treatment" determined by his or her prior health status.

Treatment failure, which occurs in approximately 30% of cases,[82] reflects an inability to adapt to noninvasive ventilation or progression of the underlying disease. Although early failure may reflect rapid clinical deterioration, such as worsening of oxygenation toward progressive consolidation, it is more often due to the patient's inability to synchronize with the ventilator and thus effectively offload the respiratory muscles. Failure to trigger the machine or excess trigger sensitivity can lead to problems of coordination between patient and machine. Air leakage can be a problem when facemasks are used, the usual approach in patients with COPD. Reducing rather than increasing inspiratory positive airway pressure often lessens this complication and allows better patient-ventilator coordination. Some patients develop hypercapnia, occasionally due to rebreathing in the mask, but more often due to ineffective cough and retained secretions. Conversion to a nasal mask and chinstrap allows more effective cough,

TABLE 78–5. CONTRAINDICATIONS TO NONINVASIVE VENTILATION

Impaired consciousness (unless oxygen induced)
Confusion, agitation
Significant risk of vomiting
Profound hypoxemia
Excessive secretions
Facial or upper airway trauma or surgery

without loss of ventilator support. Late failure (after 48 hours or more of noninvasive ventilation), suggested by worsening acidosis, is a poor prognostic sign; it usually reflects deterioration caused by the underlying lung disease. If this occurs, the institution of invasive positive-pressure ventilation needs to be considered.[83] Patients treated in this way may have a better prognosis, although the interpretation of data is difficult, given the nonrandomized design of the relevant study.[83] What is clear is that extending the period of noninvasive ventilation in a patient with physiologic evidence of deterioration is not likely to produce a successful result.

In addition to its role in the acute phase of respiratory failure, noninvasive ventilation can be valuable as a "bridge" in helping patients wean from intermittent positive-pressure ventilation. In an important multicenter, prospective trial, Nava and colleagues randomized people who had failed a T-piece weaning trial to either noninvasive ventilation or further mechanical ventilation.[84] Noninvasive ventilation was associated with fewer days of ventilatory support (10.2 versus 16.6, respectively), shorter ICU stay (15.1 versus 24 days), less nosocomial pneumonia, and a better 60-day survival (92% versus 72%). These results were achieved in a unit with a lot of experience with noninvasive ventilation. As this technique is used more often, both inside and outside the ICU setting, it is likely that noninvasive ventilation will yield good results and will become a more standard approach than is currently the case.

MECHANICAL VENTILATION

Practical aspects of intermittent positive-pressure ventilation are reviewed in detail elsewhere in this book. This treatment should be considered when noninvasive ventilation is not appropriate (see Table 78-5) or has failed. Patients with a pH below 7.25 are more likely to require this therapy. Persistent significant hypoxemia despite treatment, hypotension, and impaired mental state are all predictors of imminent respiratory arrest and the need for intermittent positive-pressure ventilation.

The major risk during intubation is hypotension. This reflects a combination of problems, including reduced venous return secondary to positive intrathoracic pressures, direct vasodilatation, and reduced sympathetic tone produced by the anesthetic agents. Reoxygenation of the patient with rapid-sequence induction of anesthesia is recommended, and this is normally accompanied by cricoid pressure to reduce the risk of aspiration, although the benefits of this technique remain unclear.[85] Short-acting muscle relaxants are usually used. Because of concerns about the risk of hyperkalemia, nondepolarizing drugs are often preferred in this circumstance. Hypotension is normally combated with fluid replacement, and if it is persistent, it is sensible to disconnect the endotracheal tube from the ventilator and allow the patient to return to a true end-expiratory lung volume before resuming ventilation.

VENTILATION STRATEGIES

A wide range of ventilation strategies have been advocated for use in COPD, each with its own proponents; none has shown a clear advantage over its competitors, however. Familiarity with the equipment in the context of COPD patients is probably more important than the relatively

TABLE 78–6. MODES OF VENTILATION

Mode	Method	Comment
Assist-control	Preset tidal volume, patient triggered with backup rate	Patient still performs substantial work of breathing; dynamic hyperinflation worsens this
Spontaneous intermittent mandatory ventilation	Preset number of breaths of a preset volume—patient does the rest	Patient still makes an effort during part of machine breath—involves more patient work, especially at low respiratory rates
Pressure support ventilation	Pressure set to augment each inspiration—tidal volume depends on patient effort, pulmonary mechanics, and pressure applied	Basis of noninvasive ventilation therapy, pressure titrated to a respiratory rate below 27 breaths/min; asynchrony with machine breaths a problem at high pressures
Proportional assist ventilation	Flow and volume generated proportional to patient effort	Experimental technique; requires accurate measurement of elastance and resistance + an intact drive to breathe; proven effective in COPD patients

minor differences between ventilator modes. The most commonly used approaches, together with their proposed advantages, are summarized in Table 78-6.

SETTINGS

In general, a combination of a relatively low respiratory rate, prolongation of the expiratory time, and limited tidal volume increases the risks of barotrauma, reduces the degree of dynamic hyperinflation, and allows better synchronization between machine-delivered breaths and the patient's own lengthened respiratory time constants. In the United Kingdom, patients are commonly paralyzed for the first 12 to 24 hours of intermittent positive-pressure ventilation to heighten ventilator synchrony and stabilize gas exchange. Although a degree of permissive hypercapnia is usual with this regimen, it is generally well tolerated. Typical ventilator settings are a tidal volume of 8 to 12 mL/kg, a frequency of 10 to 14 breaths per minute, and an inspiratory-expiratory ratio of 1:2.5 or 1:3. Increasingly, pressure control ventilation is used; with this method, the respiratory flow more closely resembles the patient's own spontaneous breathing pattern, and there is more equal ventilation of all lung units rather than preferential ventilation of those with the highest compliance, as occurs during volume cycle ventilation. The optimal extrinsic PEEP remains contentious in this setting, as there is a risk of inducing hyperinflation if too much pressure is added. In general, 5 cm H_2O of PEEP is probably sufficient to overcome intrinsic load without risking passive hyperinflation. The difficulties of assessing this variable have already been considered.

ASSISTED VENTILATION AND WEANING

As acidosis resolves and oxygen requirements fall, it is possible to reduce the degree of sedation and allow the patient to make some contribution to ventilation before weaning. Several modes of ventilatory support are available in these circumstances, and again, there is no specific advantage of one over another.[86,87] There is an impression, however, that reliance on spontaneous intermittent mandatory ventilation prolongs subsequent weaning. Although not universally accepted, there are good data supporting the use of spontaneous breathing trials in patients who are clinically stable,

to determine when they are ready to wean.[87-89] The ability to sustain ventilation in the absence of increasing CO_2, worsening acidosis, or clinical distress (reflected by an increase in blood pressure, heart rate, or restlessness) is generally agreed to be a predictor of future weaning success. Although COPD patients are less likely to achieve these goals as early as other ICU patients, the re-intubation rate in those who do meet these criteria is low.[88,89] Unfortunately, breathing through the ventilator on a continuous positive airway pressure circuit may be associated with significant increases in inspiratory resistance,[90] and it is sensible to use pressure support to offset some of this additional respiratory work. This reflects the necessity of identifying patients who can be weaned using the ventilator alone and those who need more prolonged support. In the latter circumstance, weaning supported by noninvasive ventilation is particularly helpful.

A variety of predictors of weaning success have been developed to try to identify when successful weaning will occur. Unfortunately, none has proved entirely reliable, and relatively few have been assessed prospectively. An empirical approach based on the criteria listed in Table 78-7 is widely used. An aggressive policy toward weaning is justified in COPD patients, because an inability to wean is invariably associated with a worse prognosis and prolonged ventilation.

NONVENTILATORY ISSUES

Therapy employed in spontaneously breathing patients is still required in those undergoing mechanical ventilation. High-dose nebulized bronchodilators are commonly used, singly and in combination,[91,92] although it is important to pay attention to the details of drug delivery. Drug deposition within the ventilator circuit and endotracheal tube can lead to a significant loss of effective drug.[93] When using a nebulized drug, the nebulizer should be placed in the inspiratory line,

TABLE 78–7. CRITERIA FOR WEANING FAILURE

Increasing hypercapnia or worsening hypoxemia (<55 mm Hg)
pH <7.32
Increased respiratory rate, >35 breaths/min
Increase in heart rate or blood pressure by 20% of baseline
Agitation, sweating, or impaired consciousness

at least 30 cm from the endotracheal tube; this allows the tubing to act as a spacer device and increases the respirable fraction.[93] If a metered dose inhaler is used instead, it should always be given with some form of spacer device, for the same reason. Parenteral corticosteroids are commonly administered. This is not without hazard, particularly because of the real risk of myopathy (see earlier). As noted previously, there does not seem to be any advantage in giving high doses, nor should the period of treatment extend beyond 5 days.

Clearance of secretions is important in ventilated patients, and it is essential that the patient's hydration state be maintained. Whether specific mucolytic drugs such as N-acetylcysteine are helpful is unclear, and no good scientific studies to support or reject their use are available. Introduction of a mini-tracheostomy often facilitates secretion clearance without compromising subsequent weaning. For patients requiring longer periods of ventilation, a formal tracheostomy is needed; the introduction of a speaking valve or fenestrated tube permits speech and improves patient communication and morale.

The benefits of nutritional support are unclear, although it is obviously needed in patients who are catabolic and poorly nourished. However, concerns about providing an excessive metabolic CO_2 load are unfounded. Simple nursing measures are often surprisingly effective; in particular, keeping the patient's head elevated prevents nosocomial pneumonia and is more effective than other approaches, such as gut sterilization, in patients with COPD.

PROGNOSIS

The prognosis following an exacerbation of COPD is better than the gloomy outlook proposed by some physicians. Nonetheless, patients who experience exacerbations appear to have a more severe clinical course than those who do not, and they report a worse overall quality of life.[94] Mortality after an ICU admission is significant, at least in North American series.[95] Ten percent to 15% of such subjects die as inpatients; over the next 2 years, 30% to 60% of patients die. Patients with a low FEV_1, significant comorbidity, and a particularly poor performance status at home have the worst outlook.[96] These factors should be considered when decisions about the requirement for ventilatory support are made. It is important to discuss these issues with a patient who has recovered from a severe exacerbation so that he or she can make an informed judgment about future treatment. This is best done away from the immediate ICU environment, after the patient's normal performance status has been reestablished. Anecdotal

evidence suggests that some individuals deteriorate significantly after a major exacerbation and never regain their previous sense of well-being. Because it can take a number of months before this new stable state is achieved, it makes sense for these patients' long-term caregivers to review their ICU needs. In patients with severe disease—and certainly anyone who has required ICU admission or ventilation—this should be an essential part of their continuing care.

ANNOTATED REFERENCES

Aaron SD, Vandemheen KL, Hebert P, et al: Outpatient oral prednisone after emergency treatment of chronic obstructive pulmonary disease. N Engl J Med 2003;348:2618-2625.
  Davies L, Angus RM, Calverley PMA: Oral corticosteroids in patients admitted to hospital with exacerbations of chronic obstructive pulmonary disease: A prospective randomised controlled trial. Lancet 1999;354:456-460.

Niewoehner DE, Erbland ML, Deupree RH, et al: Effect of systemic glucocorticoids on exacerbations of chronic obstructive pulmonary disease. N Engl J Med 1999;340:1941-1947.
  These three papers defined the evidence base for the use of oral and intravenous corticosteroids in COPD exacerbations.

Calverley PMA, MacNee W, Pride NB, Rennard SI (eds): Chronic Obstructive Pulmonary Disease, 2nd ed. London, Arnold, 2003.
  Comprehensive and up-to-date overview of all aspects of COPD by a team of internationally respected authors.

Connors AFJ, Dawson NV, Thomas C, et al: Outcomes following acute exacerbation of severe chronic obstructive lung disease: The SUPPORT investigators (Study to Understand Prognoses and Preferences for Outcomes and Risks of Treatments). Am J Respir Crit Care Med 1996;154:959-967; erratum, Am J Respir Crit Care Med 1997;155:386.
  Still the major study of outcomes in COPD patients managed in the ICU.

Lightowler JV, Wedzicha JA, Elliott MW, et al: Non-invasive positive pressure ventilation to treat respiratory failure resulting from exacerbations of chronic obstructive pulmonary disease: Cochrane systematic review and meta-analysis. BMJ 2003;326:185.
  Valuable overview of the relative benefits of noninvasive ventilation in the management of acute respiratory failure in COPD.

Skeletal muscle dysfunction in chronic obstructive pulmonary disease: A statement of the American Thoracic Society and European Respiratory Society. Am J Respir Crit Care Med 1999;159:S1-S40.
  Excellent and comprehensive overview of current knowledge about the impact of COPD on skeletal muscle function.

Soler N, Torres A, Ewig S, et al: Bronchial microbial patterns in severe exacerbations of chronic obstructive pulmonary disease (COPD) requiring mechanical ventilation. Am J Respir Crit Care Med 1998;157:1498-1505.
  Important paper describing the role of lower respiratory tract colonization in the genesis of COPD exacerbations in an ICU population.

Younes M: Dynamic intrinsic PEEP (PEEP(i),dyn): Is it worth saving? Am J Respir Crit Care Med 2000;162:1608-1609.
  Thoughtful overview of a physiologically important but technically difficult measurement.

Chapter 79

PULMONARY EMBOLISM

Graham F. Pineo • Russell D. Hull

KEY POINTS

1. **The clinical diagnosis of deep venous thrombosis** (DVT) is highly nonspecific because none of the symptoms or signs is unique and each may be caused by nonthrombotic disorders.

2. **The clinical presentation of pulmonary embolism** (PE) depends on the size, location, and number of emboli and on the patient's underlying cardiorespiratory reserve.

3. There is evidence that the **prognosis for long-term survival and recurrent venous thromboembolism** (VTE) is worse with patients presenting with PE as opposed to DVT.

4. Multiple studies indicate that in more than one half of all patients with clinically suspected PE **the diagnosis is not confirmed by objective testing.**

5. **Determining the clinical probability of VTE** and the use of various forms of D-dimer to rule out VTE have been incorporated into diagnostic algorithms for the diagnosis and management of VTE.

6. Further studies are required to fully identify **the role of spiral CT in the diagnosis of PE.**

7. **Efficacy of heparin therapy** depends on achieving a critical therapeutic level of heparin within the first 24 hours of treatment.

8. **Low-molecular-weight heparin (LMWH) replaced intravenous unfractionated heparin** in the initial management of patients with VTE.

9. Safer and more effective anticoagulant therapy is required for the **treatment of VTE in patients with cancer.**

10. At this time, there is **no justification for the use of the lesser intensive warfarin program.**

11. Until the proper randomized clinical trials have been carried out, **thrombolytic therapy should only be used for patients with massive PE complicated by shock.**

12. **Routine insertion** of inferior vena cava filters in patients with free-floating thrombi cannot be supported.

Venous thromboembolism (deep venous thrombosis [DVT], pulmonary embolism [PE], or both [VTE]) usually complicates the course of sick, hospitalized patients but may also affect ambulant and otherwise apparently healthy individuals.[1-3] PE remains the most common preventable cause of hospital death and is responsible for 150,000 to 200,000 deaths per year in the United States. Most patients who die of PE succumb suddenly or within 2 hours of the acute event before therapy can be initiated or can take effect.[4] Effective prophylaxis against VTE is now available for most high-risk patients.[5-7] Prophylaxis is more effective in preventing death and morbidity from VTE than is treatment of the established disease.

PATHOPHYSIOLOGY

Venous thrombi are composed predominantly of fibrin and red cells and have a variable platelet and leukocyte component. The formation, growth, and dissolution of venous thromboemboli represent a balance between thrombogenic stimuli and protective mechanisms. The factors that predispose to the development of venous thromboemboli are venous stasis, activation of blood coagulation, and vascular damage. The protective mechanisms that counteract these thrombogenic stimuli include (1) the inactivation of activated coagulation factors by circulating inhibitors (e.g., antithrombin III, α_2-macroglobulin, α_1-antitrypsin, and activated protein C); (2) clearance of activated coagulation factors and soluble fibrin polymer complexes by the reticuloendothelial system and by the liver; and (3) dissolution of fibrin by fibrinolytic enzymes derived from plasma and endothelial cells and digestion of fibrin by leukocytes.

Various risk factors predispose to the development of venous thromboembolism (Table 79-1).[2,8,9]

PE originates from thrombi in the deep veins of the leg in 90% or more of patients.[10-14] Other, less common sources of PE include the deep pelvic veins, the renal veins, the inferior vena cava, the right ventricle, and the axillary veins. Most clinically important PE arise from thrombi in the popliteal or more proximal deep veins of the leg. PE occurs in 50% of patients with objectively documented proximal DVT; many of these emboli are asymptomatic.[10] Usually, only part of the thrombus embolizes, and 50% to 70% of patients with angiographically documented PE have detectable DVT of the legs at the time of presentation.[11] The clinical significance of PE depends on the size of the embolus and on the cardiorespiratory reserve of the patient.

TABLE 79–1. FACTORS PREDISPOSING TO VENOUS THROMBOEMBOLISM

Clinical Risk Factors	Inherited or Acquired Abnormalities
Surgical and nonsurgical trauma	Activated protein C resistance
Previous venous thromboembolism	Hyperhomocystinemia
	Prothrombin 20210A
Immobilization	Protein C deficiency
Malignant disease	Protein S deficiency
Heart disease	Antithrombin-III deficiency
Leg paralysis	Dysfibrinogenemia
Age > 40 years	Heparin-induced thrombocytopenia
Obesity	
Estrogens	

CLINICAL FEATURES

The clinical features of DVT include leg pain, tenderness and swelling, a palpable cord, discoloration, venous distention, prominence of the superficial veins, and cyanosis. The clinical diagnosis of DVT is highly nonspecific because none of the symptoms or signs is unique, and each may be caused by nonthrombotic disorders. Patients with relatively minor symptoms and signs may have extensive DVT, whereas those with florid leg pain and swelling, suggesting extensive DVT, may have negative results on objective testing. Thus, objective testing is mandatory to confirm or exclude a diagnosis of DVT.[12-15]

The location of the initial DVT has an impact on the incidence of recurrence; thus the presence of an iliofemoral vein thrombosis was shown to have a higher rate of recurrent VTE compared with popliteal vein thrombosis.[16,17] Also, there is a high correlation between venographic results as measured by the Marder score in recurrence of VTE.[18]

The clinical presentation of PE depends on the size, location, and number of emboli and on the patient's underlying cardiorespiratory reserve. The clinical manifestations of acute PE generally can be divided into several syndromes that overlap considerably: (1) transient dyspnea and tachypnea in the absence of other associated clinical manifestations; (2) pulmonary infarction or congestive atelectasis (also known as ischemic pneumonitis or incomplete infarction), which includes pleuritic chest pain, cough, hemoptysis, pleural effusion, and pulmonary infiltrates on the chest radiograph; (3) right ventricular failure associated with severe dyspnea and tachypnea; (4) cardiovascular collapse with hypotension, syncope, and coma (usually associated with massive PE); and (5) less common and highly nonspecific clinical features, including confusion and coma, pyrexia, wheezing, resistant cardiac failure, and unexplained arrhythmia.

There is evidence that the prognosis for long-term survival and recurrent VTE is worse with patients presenting with PE as opposed to DVT.[19] This may be reason to treat patients presenting with PE more aggressively in the future, but at the present time the anticoagulant management is identical. Various studies have attempted to identify risk factors for recurrent VTE, including fatal PE in patients presenting with an initial PE.[20-22]

Factors contributing to recurrent VTE include length of an initial hospitalization, presence of cancer, older age at hospitalization for multiple injuries, or surgery within 3 months.[20]

Risk factors for an adverse outcome include factors such as age older than 70, hypotension, congestive heart failure, chronic obstructive pulmonary disease, cancer, the presence of a DVT, and right ventricular hypokinesis on echocardiography. Evidence of right ventricular damage in the form of an elevated troponin-T level may also have prognostic significance.[23,24]

It is now widely accepted that the clinical diagnosis of PE is highly nonspecific. Multiple studies indicate that in more than half of all patients with clinically suspected PE the diagnosis is not confirmed by objective testing.[9,14-16] Therefore, objective testing is mandatory to confirm or exclude the presence of PE.[25-28]

DIAGNOSIS OF PULMONARY EMBOLISM

The differential diagnosis of PE is wide, depending on the clinical scenario, and includes pneumonia, pneumothorax, pulmonary edema, pericarditis, rib fracture, and myocardial infarction. Various ancillary tests, such as chest radiograph, arterial blood gas determination, electrocardiography, and laboratory tests such as serum lactate dehydrogenase have a role in the diagnosis of VTE, but they all lack sensitivity and specificity for PE. The main role of these tests is to rule out other conditions that may mimic PE, such as acute myocardial infarction or pneumothorax.[28] The key tests for the diagnosis of PE include ventilation-perfusion lung scanning, spiral computed tomography (spiral CT), pulmonary angiography, and objective tests for proximal DVT.[28] Echocardiography may be useful for both diagnosis and prognostication, and there is increasing evidence that magnetic resonance angiography (MRA) may also have a useful role in the diagnosis of PE.

In recent years, numerous studies have shown that use of standardized clinical assessments for determining the clinical probability of VTE and the use of various forms of D-dimer to rule out VTE have been incorporated into diagnostic algorithms for the diagnosis and management of VTE.[29-33] The most thoroughly validated clinical models are those of Wells[31] and Wicki[32] and their colleagues. It is now clear from prospective studies that clinical assessment can stratify the probability of PE in a wide spectrum of patients both in the emergency department and in hospital. Thus, the problem of PE is expected to be less than 10% in patients with a low clinical probability, around 25% for those with an intermediate probability, and greater than 60% for patients with a high clinical probability of PE.

Performance of a quantitative D-dimer alone or in conjunction with assessment of probability further enhances the diagnostic approach.[34,35] The D-dimer is formed when cross-linked fibrin undergoes lysis by plasmin. The elevated levels can be found in numerous conditions in addition to VTE. Thus, conditions such as infection, cancer, surgery, trauma, and increasing age will produce elevated levels of D-dimer. Therefore, this assay is only useful if the test is negative. In such circumstances it can be used to exclude VTE. Numerous assays for D-dimer have been tested, but quantitative tests with a rapid turnaround, such as enzyme-linked immunosorbent assays or latex agglutination assays, have proven to be the most useful.[34-38] These tests have been shown to have an extremely high negative predictive value and in conjunction with clinical probability assessment may be used to exclude further diagnostic testing in a large number of patients presenting with suspected VTE.[36,38]

OBJECTIVE TESTS FOR THE DIAGNOSIS OF PULMONARY EMBOLISM

Ventilation-Perfusion Lung Scanning

Perfusion lung scanning is the key diagnostic test for patients with suspected PE. A normal perfusion scan result excludes clinically important PE.[39-41] An abnormal perfusion scan result, however, is nonspecific and may occur in conditions that produce either increased radiographic density (e.g., pneumonia, atelectasis, and pleural effusion) or regional reduction in ventilation (e.g., chronic obstructive lung disease, acute asthma, bronchial mucus plugs, and bronchitis, all of which are frequently associated with normal radiographic results).

Ventilation imaging was introduced to improve the specificity of an abnormal perfusion scan result by differentiating embolic occlusion of the pulmonary vasculature from perfusion defects occurring secondary to a primary disorder of ventilation.[42-44] This basic premise that perfusion defects that ventilate normally [ventilation-perfusion mismatch] are due to PE, whereas matching ventilation-perfusion abnormalities are due to other conditions, has been shown to be incorrect by prospective clinical trials.[41,45]

Ventilation lung scanning is helpful only if the perfusion defect is segmental or greater and is associated with ventilation mismatch; such patients have a high probability (86%) of PE confirmed by pulmonary angiography.[11,41-45] Abnormal findings on lung scans, such as matching ventilation-perfusion defects (either segmental or subsegmental, so-called low-probability), subsegmental defects with ventilation mismatch, or perfusion defects that correspond to an area of increased density on chest radiography (indeterminate perfusion scan), are associated with a 20% to 40% frequency of PE.[11,41,45] These scan patterns are nondiagnostic. Further investigations, including pulmonary angiography and objective tests for DVT, are therefore required in patients who have nondiagnostic ventilation-perfusion scan findings.[11,27,41,45,46] Pulmonary angiography, or venography, or both should be used when other approaches are unavailable or inconclusive. The morbidity associated with these tests is substantially less than that arising from unnecessary anticoagulant therapy and inappropriate hospitalization.

Pulmonary Angiography

Pulmonary angiography is the accepted diagnostic reference standard for PE.[47-49] The diagnosis is established if an intraluminal filling defect is constant on multiple films or if abrupt termination (cut-off) of a vessel greater than 2 to 5 mm in diameter occurs and is constant on multiple films.[47,48] Other abnormalities, such as oligemia, vessel pruning, and loss of filling of small vessels, are nonspecific and occur in many conditions, including pneumonia, atelectasis, bronchiectasis, emphysema, and pulmonary carcinoma.[47,48]

In recent years, the diagnostic resolution of pulmonary angiography has markedly improved, and the risk to the patient decreased, by the use of selective catheterization and repeated injections of small volumes of dye. This technique is safe in the absence of severe chronic pulmonary hypertension or severe cardiac or respiratory decompensation.[50] Clinically significant complications, including tachyarrhythmias, endocardial or myocardial injury, cardiac perforation, cardiac arrest, and hypersensitivity reactions to contrast medium, occur in up to 3% to 4% of patients.[47,50]

Spiral CT

Spiral CT (also known as helico or continuous volume CT) has come into wide use for the diagnosis of PE. A single breath hold of 15 to 20 seconds allows a full lung examination to be carried out. Abnormalities other than PE (identified intraluminal filling defects) that may be causing the symptoms and signs suggestive of PE can also be identified, which is an advantage of spiral CT.[51,52] These conditions include malignancy, pleural disease, postoperative changes, pneumonia, cardiac disease, and pulmonary fibrosis. The technology for spiral CT is rapidly changing with its new multichannel equipment that permits full-lung scanning with a single breath hold of approximately 5 seconds.[51,52]

The use of spiral CT has gained popularity in clinical practice without adequate assessment. Two systematic reviews of the literature up to the year 2000 indicated that the sensitivity of spiral CT for isolated subsegmental PE was in the range of 30%.[53,54] Thus, although the sensitivity of spiral CT for large PE was acceptable, the authors recommended caution in using anticoagulant treatment in patients with negative results on spiral CT. Indeed, an initial prospective follow-up of patients with suspected PE with negative studies on spiral CT and negative venous ultrasound indicated that up to 5% may have VTE in follow-up, including fatal PE.[55]

The changing technology for spiral CT requires ongoing assessment. Indeed, two management studies in which more modern equipment for spiral CT was used in conjunction with bilateral leg ultrasound indicated it was safe to withhold anticoagulant therapy in the patients with negative studies, particularly if they had low or moderate pretest clinical probability.[56-59] One further advantage of spiral CT is that the venous system can be studied down to the popliteal veins with a single infusion of contrast medium. Studies comparing spiral CT venography and ultrasonography illustrate that the test has a high sensitivity and specificity.[60,61]

Further studies are required to fully identify the role of spiral CT in the diagnosis of PE. Indeed, the second Prospective Investigation of Pulmonary Embolism Diagnosis (PIOPED II) is designed to assess the role of spiral CT in comparison with ventilation-perfusion lung scanning, ultrasonography of the legs, pulmonary angiography, and venography in more than 1000 patients presenting with suspected PE. This multicenter study, which is funded by the National Institutes of Health, has completed enrollments and will be reported in the near future.[62]

Echocardiography

The value of echocardiography has been firmly established and has four main advantages:

1. It is noninvasive and easily available.
2. It can exclude other causes of cardiogenic shock (e.g., extensive left ventricular infarction, pericardial tamponade, or dissecting aortic aneurysm).
3. It allows an estimate of pulmonary artery pressure and so provides information on the severity of pulmonary artery obstruction.[63-69]
4. It can be used serially to assess response to treatment.

Echocardiographic findings are not specific and reflect the response of the right side of the heart to acute pulmonary artery hypertension. They consist of distention of the pulmonary artery trunk, right ventricular (RV) dilation and hypokinesis, reduced left ventricular (LV) size, an increased RV to LV diameter, diastolic and systolic flattening of the interventricular septum, and paradoxical systolic wall motion.[63] This pattern is mimicked, in particular, by RV infarction associated with LV dysfunction.

Scoring systems have been developed that correlate well with the angiographic severity index, and the value of serial echocardiography has been demonstrated in patients treated with thrombolytic agents. Rarely, RV thrombus may be visualized, a clinical situation associated with a high mortality rate, with 30% of such patients succumbing as a result of massive pulmonary thromboembolism.

There are several limitations to the applications of echocardiography. At least 40% of the pulmonary vascular bed needs to be obstructed to produce detectable features. Coexistent cardiorespiratory disease also limits its value because of the nonspecific nature of the abnormalities and because imaging via the transthoracic route may be difficult. Transesophageal echocardiography may be valuable in this situation, particularly in making a full hemodynamic assessment in the shocked, intubated patient.[67-69]

Magnetic Resonance Angiography

MRA has been compared with pulmonary angiography and spiral CT for the diagnosis of PE in patients in whom the diagnosis is suspected.[70,71] During one study, the sensitivity of 77% was found and this varied with the subsegmental, segmental, or central or lobar embolism on pulmonary angiography. Specificity, however, was 98%.[70] Oudkerk and coworkers suggest that MRA could become part of the diagnostic strategy for PE,[70] although this diagnostic modality requires further study. MRA may have obvious advantages for patients for whom the risk of pulmonary angiography is high or for the diagnosis of VTE in pregnancy.

DIAGNOSIS AND TREATMENT OF PULMONARY EMBOLISM BASED ON OBJECTIVE TESTING FOR PROXIMAL DEEP VEIN THROMBOSIS

At least 80% of patients with PE have thrombi originating in the lower leg veins.[10,11,13] Because of the diagnostic inaccuracy of noninvasive tests for PE, particularly in patients with nondiagnostic lung scan results, the concept of using objective tests for the detection of proximal DVT in the legs was developed in patients suspected of having PE.[25-27] This combined strategy for the diagnosis and treatment of PE or DVT (i.e., VTE) has been applied in prospective clinical trials.[72]

Noninvasive tests such as compression ultrasonography have advantages because they are free of morbidity and are readily repeatable. For patients presenting with acute PE, compression ultrasonography of the proximal veins is positive in approximately 50% of patients. Venography is positive in approximately 70% of patients. The fact that approximately 30% of such patients with angiographically documented PE have negative venography indicates that either the thrombosis that had been present in the legs has embolized to the lung or the PE may have originated from a source other than the deep veins in the legs.[11,36-38,73-76]

In patients with a nondiagnostic lung scan and a negative two-point compression ultrasound of both legs, particularly in the presence of a low to moderate pretest clinical probability

and a negative D-dimer, there is a very low likelihood of developing VTE in follow-up.[35-38] However, patients with a high clinical probability for pulmonary embolus or a previous history of VTE require further studies such as venography or pulmonary angiography.[36] As an alternative, repeat ultrasonography at 7 days may be performed.[74]

DIAGNOSTIC ALGORITHMS

In a typical algorithm, patients with a low or moderate clinical probability undergo D-dimer testing. If the test is negative no further studies are required. If the D-dimer test is positive, ventilation-perfusion scanning is carried out. Those with a normal ventilation-perfusion scan have no further studies and PE is excluded. Patients with a high-probability lung scan are treated. Patients with a nondiagnostic lung scan undergo ultrasound study of the legs: those who are positive are treated, whereas those who are negative have no further studies or have a repeat test in 1 week. Patients with low probability for PE who have a high probability lung scan should undergo spiral CT or pulmonary angiography. Patients with moderate pretest probability and negative ultrasound should have a repeat test in 1 week or undergo pulmonary angiography.[76]

Patients who have a high probability for PE go directly to ventilation-perfusion scanning as with the other group. For those with a nondiagnostic lung scan, ultrasound is carried out unless negative pulmonary angiography is indicated or the patient undergoes serial ultrasound. As an alternative, patients with nondiagnostic lung scan and a high clinical probability may go directly to spiral CT or pulmonary angiography.

These algorithms are modified for patients with prior PE or DVT, and D-dimer is not recommended for patients in whom it can be predicted that the test will be positive. The future role of spiral CT and MRA will undoubtedly be modified as further studies are carried out and may replace ventilation-perfusion scanning and pulmonary angiography in many patients suspected of having PE.

ANTICOAGULANT THERAPY FOR VENOUS THROMBOEMBOLISM

Anticoagulant drugs (heparin, low-molecular-weight heparin, and warfarin) are the mainstay of the management of venous thromboembolism.[76] As mentioned previously the treatment for DVT and/or PE is the same at the present time. Numerous new antithrombotic agents are under intensive investigation. The anti-Xa inhibitor fondaparinux (Arixtra, Sanofi-Synthelabo, New York, NY) or the antithrombin agent ximelagatran (Xanta, Astra Zeneca LP, Wilmington, DE) will be coming on the market in the near future and will modify the current approach to treatment of VTE.

Objectives of treatment in patients with VTE are to prevent death from PE, recurrent VTE, and post-thrombotic syndrome.

The use of graduated compression stockings has been shown to significantly decrease the incidence of the post-thrombotic syndrome. Furthermore, the incidence of the post-thrombotic syndrome is decreasing in recent years, suggesting that the more efficient treatment of VTE and the prevention of recurrent DVT are having a positive impact on this complication.

UNFRACTIONATED HEPARIN THERAPY

The anticoagulant activity of unfractionated heparin depends on a unique pentasaccharide that binds to antithrombin III (AT III) and potentiates the inhibition of thrombin and activated factor X (Xa) by AT III.[77-79] Approximately one third of all heparin molecules contain the unique pentasaccharide sequence, regardless of whether they are low- or high-molecular-weight fractions.[77-79] It is the pentasaccharide sequence that confers the molecular high affinity for AT III.[77-79] In addition, heparin catalyzes the inactivation of thrombin by another plasma cofactor (cofactor II), which acts independently of AT III.[79]

Heparin has a number of other effects. These include the release of tissue factor pathway inhibitor; binding to numerous plasma and platelet proteins, endothelial cells, and leukocytes[77]; suppression of platelet function; and an increase in vascular permeability.[79] The anticoagulant response to a standard dose of heparin varies widely between patients. This makes it necessary to monitor the anticoagulant response of heparin using either the activated partial thromboplastin time (aPTT) or heparin levels and to titrate the dose to the individual patient.[79]

The accepted anticoagulant therapy for VTE is a combination of continuous intravenous heparin and oral warfarin. The length of the initial intravenous heparin therapy has been reduced to 5 days, thus shortening the hospital stay and leading to significant savings.[80-81] The simultaneous use of initial heparin and warfarin has become clinical practice for all patients with VTE who are medically stable. Exceptions include patients who require immediate medical or surgical intervention, such as in thrombolysis or insertion of a vena cava filter, or patients at very high risk of bleeding. Heparin is continued until the International Normalized Ratio (INR) has been within the therapeutic range (2 to 3) for 2 consecutive days.[82]

It has been established from experimental studies and clinical trials that efficacy of heparin therapy depends on achieving a critical therapeutic level of heparin within the first 24 hours of treatment.[81,83,84] Data from three consecutive double-blind clinical trials indicate that failure to achieve the therapeutic aPTT threshold by 24 hours was associated with a 23.3% subsequent recurrent venous thromboembolism rate, compared with a rate of 4% to 6% for the patient group who were therapeutic at 24 hours.[83,84] The recurrences occurred throughout the 3-month follow-up period and could not be attributed to inadequate oral anticoagulant therapy.[83] The critical therapeutic level of heparin, as measured by the aPTT, is 1.5 times the mean of the control value or the upper limit of the normal aPTT range.[81,83] This corresponds to a heparin blood level of 0.2 to 0.4 U/mL by the protamine sulfate titration assay and 0.35 to 0.70 by the anti–factor Xa assay.

However, there is wide variability in the aPTT and heparin blood levels with different reagents and even with different batches of the same reagent. It is therefore vital for each laboratory to establish the minimal therapeutic level of heparin, as measured by the aPTT, that will provide a heparin blood level of at least 0.35 U/mL by the anti–factor Xa assay for each batch of thromboplastin reagent being used, particularly if the reagent is provided by a different manufacturer.[79]

Although there is a strong correlation between subtherapeutic aPTT values and recurrent thromboembolism, the relationship between supratherapeutic aPTT and bleeding (aPTT ratio 2.5 or more) is less definite.[83] Indeed, bleeding during heparin therapy is more closely related to underlying clinical risk factors than to aPTT elevation above the therapeutic range.[83] Recent studies confirm that weight and age older than 65 are independent risk factors for bleeding on heparin therapy.

Numerous audits of heparin therapy indicate that administration of intravenous heparin is fraught with difficulty and that the clinical practice of using an ad hoc approach to heparin dose titration frequently results in inadequate therapy. The use of a prescriptive approach or protocol for administering intravenous heparin therapy has been evaluated in two prospective studies in patients with venous thromboembolism.[83,85,86]

In one clinical trial for the treatment of DVT, patients were given either intravenous heparin alone followed by warfarin or intravenous heparin and simultaneous warfarin.[81] The heparin nomogram is summarized in Tables 79-2 and 79-3. Only 1% to 2% of the patients were undertreated for more than 24 hours in the heparin group and in the heparin and warfarin group, respectively. Recurrent VTE (objectively documented) occurred infrequently in both groups (7%), at rates similar to those previously reported. These findings demonstrated that subtherapy was avoided in most patients and that the heparin protocol resulted in effective delivery of heparin therapy in both groups.

In the other clinical trial, a weight-based heparin dosage nomogram was compared with a standard-care nomogram (Table 79-4).[85] Patients on the weight-adjusted heparin nomogram received a starting dose of 80 U/kg as a bolus and 18 U/kg/h as an infusion. The heparin dose was adjusted to maintain an aPTT of 1.5 to 2.3 times control. In the weight-adjusted group, 89% of patients achieved the therapeutic

---

TABLE 79–2. HEPARIN PROTOCOL

1. Administer initial intravenous heparin bolus: 5000 U.
2. Administer continuous intravenous heparin infusion: commence at 42 mL/h of 20,000 U (1680 U/h) in 500 mL of two thirds dextrose and one third saline (a 24-hour heparin dose of 40,320 U), except in the following patients, in whom heparin infusion is begun at a rate of 31 mL/h (1240 U/h, a 24-hour dose of 29,760 U):
   a. Patients who have undergone surgery within the previous 2 weeks
   b. Patients with a previous history of peptic ulcer disease or gastrointestinal or genitourinary bleeding
   c. Patients with recent stroke (i.e., thrombotic stroke within 2 weeks previously)
   d. Patients with a platelet count less than 150/L.
   e. Patients with miscellaneous reasons for a high risk of bleeding (e.g., hepatic failure, renal failure, or vitamin K deficiency)
3. Adjust heparin dose by use of the aPTT. The aPTT test is performed in all patients as follows:
   a. At 4 to 6 hours after commencing heparin, the heparin dose is then adjusted.
   b. At 4 to 6 hours after the first dosage adjustment
   c. Then as indicated by the nomogram for the first 24 hours of therapy
   d. Thereafter once daily, unless the patient is subtherapeutic,* in which case the aPTT test is repeated 4 to 6 hours after the heparin dose is increased.

*Subtherapeutic = aPTT less than 1.5 times the mean normal control value for the thromboplastin reagent being used.
aPTT, activated partial thromboplastin time.

TABLE 79–3. INTRAVENOUS HEPARIN DOSE TITRATION NOMOGRAM ACCORDING TO THE aPTT

aPTT (sec)	Rate Change (mL/h)	Dose Change (IU/24 h)*	Additional Action
≤45	+ 6	+ 5760	Repeated aPTT[†] in 4 to 6 hours
46-54	+ 3	+ 2880	Repeated aPTT in 4 to 6 hours
55-85	0	0	None[‡]
86-110	− 3	− 2880	Stop heparin sodium treatment for 1 hour; repeat aPTT 4 to 6 hours after restarting heparin treatment.
>110	− 6	− 5760	Stop heparin treatment for 1 hour; repeat aPTT 4 to 6 hours after restarting heparin treatment

*Heparin sodium concentration 20,000 IU in 500 mL = 40 IU/mL.
[†]With the use of Actin-FS thromboplastin reagent (Dade, Mississauga, Ontario, Canada)
[‡]During the first 24 hours, repeat aPTT in 4 to 6 hours. Thereafter, the aPTT will be determined once daily, unless subtherapeutic.
aPTT, activated partial thromboplastin time.
Adapted from Hull RD, Raksob GE, Rosenbloom DR, et al: Optimal therapeutic level of heparin therapy in patients with venous thrombosis. Arch Intern Med 1992;152:1589, with permission.

range within 24 hours compared with 75% in the standard-care group. The risk of recurrent VTE was more frequent in the standard-care group, supporting the previous observation that subtherapeutic heparin during the initial 24 hours is associated with a higher incidence of recurrences. This study included patients with unstable angina and arterial thromboembolism in addition to VTE, which suggests that the principles applied to a heparin nomogram for the treatment of VTE may be generalizable to other clinical conditions. Continued use of the weight-based nomogram has been similarly effective.

Complications of Heparin Therapy

The main adverse effects of heparin therapy include bleeding, thrombocytopenia, and osteoporosis. Patients at particular risk are those who have had recent surgery or trauma or who have other clinical factors that predispose to bleeding on heparin, such as peptic ulcer, occult malignancy, liver disease, hemostatic defects, weight, age older than 65 years, and female gender.[79]

The management of bleeding on heparin will depend on the location and severity of bleeding, the risk of recurrent VTE, and the aPTT. Heparin should be discontinued temporarily or permanently. Patients with recent VTE may be candidates for insertion of an inferior vena cava filter. If urgent reversal of heparin effect is required, protamine sulfate can be administered.[79]

Heparin-induced thrombocytopenia is a well-recognized complication of heparin therapy, usually occurring within

5 to 10 days after heparin treatment has started.[87-90] Approximately 1% to 2% of patients receiving unfractionated heparin will experience a fall in platelet count to less than the normal range or a 50% fall in the platelet count within the normal range. In the majority of cases, this mild to moderate thrombocytopenia appears to be a direct effect of heparin on platelets and is of no consequence. However, 0.1% to 0.2% of patients receiving heparin develop an immune thrombocytopenia mediated by IgG antibody directed against a complex of platelet factor 4 and heparin.[87]

The development of thrombocytopenia may be accompanied by arterial thrombosis or DVT, which may lead to serious consequences such as death or limb amputation.[90] The diagnosis of heparin-induced thrombocytopenia, with or without thrombosis, must be made on clinical grounds, because the assays with the highest sensitivity and specificity are not readily available and have a slow turnaround time.

When the diagnosis of heparin-induced thrombocytopenia is made, heparin in all forms must be stopped immediately. In those patients requiring ongoing anticoagulation, several alternatives exist.[88-90] The agents most extensively used recently include the heparinoid danaparoid,[88] hirudin,[89] and, most recently, the specific antithrombin argatroban.[90] Danaparoid is available for limited use on compassionate grounds, and hirudin and argatroban have been approved for use in the United States and Canada. Warfarin may be used but should not be started until one of the other agents has been used for 3 or 4 days to suppress thrombin generation. Insertion of an inferior vena cava filter is seldom indicated.

Osteoporosis has been reported in patients receiving unfractionated heparin in dosages of 20,000 U/day (or more) for more than 6 months. Demineralization can progress to the fracture of vertebral bodies or long bones, and the defect may not be entirely reversible.[79]

LOW-MOLECULAR-WEIGHT HEPARIN (LMWH)

Heparin currently in use clinically is polydispersed unmodified heparin, with a mean molecular weight ranging from 10 to 16 kDa. In recent years, low-molecular-weight derivatives of commercial heparin have been prepared that have a mean molecular weight of 4 to 5 kDa.[91,92]

The LMWHs commercially available are made by different processes (such as nitrous acid, alkaline, or enzymatic

TABLE 79–4. WEIGHT-BASED NOMOGRAM FOR INITIAL INTRAVENOUS HEPARIN THERAPY*

aPTT	Dose (IU/kg)
Initial dose	80 bolus, then 18/h
aPTT <35 sec (<1.2×)	80 bolus, then 4/h
aPTT 35-45 sec (1.2-1.5×)	40 bolus, then 2/h
aPTT 46-70 sec (1.5-2.3×)	No change
aPTT 71-90 sec (2.3-3.0×)	Decrease infusion rate by 2/h
aPTT > 90 sec (>3.0×)	Hold infusion 1 h, then decrease infusion rate by 3/h

*Figures in parentheses show comparison with control.
aPTT, activated partial thromboplastin time.
Adapted from Raschke RA, Reilly BM, Guidry JR, et al: The weight-based heparin dosing nomogram compared with a "standard care" nomogram. Ann Intern Med 1993;119:874, with permission.

depolymerization), and they differ chemically and pharmacokinetically.[91,92] The clinical significance of these differences, however, is unclear, and there have been very few studies comparing different LMWHs with respect to clinical outcomes.[92] The doses of the different LMWHs have been established empirically and are not necessarily interchangeable. Therefore, at this time, the effectiveness and safety of each of the LMWHs must be tested separately.[92]

The LMWHs differ from unfractionated heparin in numerous ways. Of particular importance are the following: increased bioavailability (>90% after subcutaneous injection), prolonged half-life and predictable clearance enabling once- or twice-daily injection, and predictable antithrombotic response based on body weight, permitting treatment without laboratory monitoring.[79,91,92] Other possible advantages are their ability to inactivate platelet-bound factor Xa, resistance to inhibition by platelet factor 4, and their decreased effect on platelet function and vascular permeability (possibly accounting for less hemorrhagic effects at comparable antithrombotic doses).

There has been a hope that the LMWHs will have fewer serious complications such as bleeding[91,92] and heparin-induced thrombocytopenia[87] when compared with unfractionated heparin. Evidence is accumulating that these complications are indeed less serious and less frequent with the use of LMWH. LMWH has been approved for the prevention and treatment of VTE in pregnancy. These drugs do not cross the placenta, and small case series suggest they may be both effective and safe. The LMWHs all cross react with unfractionated heparin, and they can therefore not be used as alternative therapy in patients who develop heparin-induced thrombocytopenia. The heparinoid danaparoid possesses a 10% to 20% cross-reactivity with heparin, and it can be safely used in patients who have no cross-reactivity.

Several different LMWHs are available for the prevention and treatment of VTE in various countries. Four LMWHs are approved for clinical use in Canada and three LMWHs have been approved for use in the United States.

In a number of early clinical trials (some of which were dose finding), LMWH given by subcutaneous or intravenous injection was compared with continuous intravenous unfractionated heparin, with repeat venography at day 7 to 10 being the primary endpoint. These studies demonstrated that LMWH was at least as effective as unfractionated heparin in preventing extension or increasing resolution of thrombi on repeat venography.

Subcutaneous unmonitored LMWH has been compared with continuous intravenous heparin in a number of clinical trials for the treatment of proximal DVT using long-term follow-up as an outcome measure.[18,94-99,101-103] These studies have shown that LMWH is at least as effective and safe as unfractionated heparin in the treatment of proximal DVT. Pooling of the most methodologically sound studies indicates a significant advantage for LMWH in the reduction of major bleeding and mortality.[98] More recent studies have indicated that LMWH used predominantly out of hospital was as effective and safe as intravenous unfractionated heparin given in hospital (Table 79-5).[101-103] Two clinical trials showed that LMWH was as effective as intravenous heparin in the treatment of patients presenting with PE.[100,104] Economic analysis of treatment with LMWH versus intravenous heparin demonstrated that LMWH was cost effective for treatment in hospital as well as out of hospital.[105] As these agents become more widely available for treatment, they have replaced intravenous unfractionated heparin in the initial management of patients with VTE.

Long-term LMWH has been compared with warfarin therapy in patients presenting with proximal DVT. Although these studies differ in design and doses of LMWH, they do indicate that LMWH is a useful alternative to warfarin therapy, particularly in patients who have recurrence of VTE while on therapeutic doses of warfarin (e.g., in the cancer population).[106,107]

COUMARIN THERAPY

Pharmacokinetics and Pharmacodynamics of Warfarin

There are two distinct chemical groups of oral anticoagulants: the 4-hydroxycoumarin derivatives (e.g., warfarin sodium) and the indane-1,3-dione derivatives (e.g., phenindione).[108] The coumarin derivatives are the oral anticoagulants of choice because they are associated with fewer nonhemorrhagic side effects than are the indanedione derivatives. In North America the most commonly used agent is coumarin (Coumadin, Bristol-Myers Squibb), but in recent years various generic forms of warfarin sodium have been introduced.

Warfarin is a racemic mixture of stereoisomers (R and S forms). Warfarin is highly water soluble and is highly bioavailable.[109] Peak absorption occurs around 90 minutes, and the half-life is between 36 and 42 hours. Warfarin is highly protein bound (primarily albumin), and only the non–protein-bound material is biologically active. Any drug or chemical that is also bound to albumin may displace warfarin from its protein binding sites and thereby increase the biologically active material.[109] Warfarin is metabolized in the liver by the p450 (CYP2C9) system of enzymes. Interference with the CYP2C9 enzymes by various drugs or a mutation in the gene coding for one of the common CYP2C9 enzymes can markedly interfere with the metabolism of warfarin.[110]

TABLE 79–5. PREDOMINANTLY OUTPATIENT TREATMENT OF PROXIMAL DEEP VEIN THROMBOSIS WITH LOW-MOLECULAR-WEIGHT HEPARIN VS. INPATIENT TREATMENT WITH INTRAVENOUS HEPARIN

Study	Treatment	Recurrent DVT	Major Bleeding
Koopman et al[101]	Nadroparin vs. heparin	14/202 (6.9%)	1/202 (0.5%)
		17/198 (8.6%)	4/198 (2.0%)
Levine et al[102]	Enoxaparin vs. heparin	13/247 (5.3%)	5/247 (2.0%)
		17/253 (6.7%)	3/253 (1.2%)
Columbus study[103]	Reviparin vs. heparin	27/510 (5.3%)	16/510 (3.1%)
		24/511 (4.9%)	12/511 (2.3%)

The anticoagulant effect of warfarin is mediated by the inhibition of the vitamin K–dependent gamma-carboxylation of coagulation factors II, VII, IX, and X.[108,109] This results in the synthesis of immunologically detectable but biologically inactive forms of these coagulation proteins. Warfarin also inhibits the vitamin K–dependent gamma-carboxylation of proteins C and S[110] and protein Z.[111] Protein C circulates as a proenzyme that is activated on endothelial cells by the thrombin/thrombomodulin complex to form activated protein C. Activated protein C in the presence of protein S inhibits activated factor VIII and activated factor V activity.[112] Therefore, vitamin K antagonists such as warfarin create a biochemical paradox by producing an anticoagulant effect due to the inhibition of procoagulants (factors II, VII, IX, and X) and a potentially thrombogenic effect by impairing the synthesis of naturally occurring inhibitors of coagulation (proteins C and S).[112] Heparin or LMWH and warfarin treatment should overlap by 4 to 5 days when warfarin treatment is initiated in patients with thrombotic disease. The role of protein Z in the coagulation process is less definite.

The anticoagulant effect of warfarin is delayed until the normal clotting factors are cleared from the circulation, and the peak effect does not occur until 36 to 72 hours after drug administration.[113] During the first few days of warfarin therapy, the prothrombin time (PT) reflects mainly the depression of factor VII, which has a half-life of 5 to 7 hours. Equilibrium levels of factors II, IX, and X are not reached until about 1 week after the initiation of therapy. The use of small initial daily doses (e.g., 5 mg) is the preferred approach for initiating warfarin treatment.[114] The dose-response relationship to warfarin therapy varies widely between individuals and, therefore, the dose must be carefully monitored to prevent overdosing or underdosing.

A number of factors influence the anticoagulant response of warfarin in individual patients; these include inaccuracies in laboratory testing and noncompliance of patients, but more importantly reflect the influence of dietary changes or the influence of drugs that interfere with the metabolism of warfarin. The availability of vitamin K can be influenced by dramatic changes in dietary intake or by drugs such as antibiotics, which interfere with the synthesis of vitamin K in the gastrointestinal tract. A wide variety of drugs may interact with warfarin. However, a critical appraisal of the literature reporting such interactions indicates that the evidence substantiating many of the claims is limited.[115] The interactions of drugs and food with warfarin are reviewed in detail in a recent publication.[8] Aspirin is particularly problematic because it interferes with platelet function and displaces warfarin from its protein binding, thus augmenting its biologic activities. Also, as with the nonsteroidal anti-inflammatory drugs (NSAIDs) it may cause gastric erosions, thus creating a site for bleeding. Nonetheless, in certain patients the use of aspirin and warfarin is indicated to improve efficacy even though bleeding may be somewhat increased. It is important that patients be warned against taking any new drugs without the knowledge of their attending physician, and it is prudent to monitor the INR more frequently when any drug (including natural compounds) is added or withdrawn from the regimen of the patient being treated with an oral anticoagulant.

Laboratory Monitoring and Therapeutic Range

The laboratory test most commonly used to measure the effects of warfarin is the one-stage prothrombin time.

The PT is sensitive to reduced activity of factors II, VII, and X but is insensitive to reduced activity of factor IX. Confusion about the appropriate therapeutic range has occurred because the different tissue thromboplastins used for measuring the PT vary considerably in sensitivity to the vitamin K–dependent clotting factors and in response to warfarin.[116,117]

To promote standardization of the PT for monitoring oral anticoagulant therapy, the World Health Organization (WHO) developed an international reference thromboplastin from human brain tissue and recommended that the PT ratio be expressed as the International Normalized Ratio.[109] The INR is the PT ratio obtained by testing a given sample using the WHO reference thromboplastin. For practical clinical purposes, the INR for a given plasma sample is equivalent to the PT ratio obtained using a standardized human brain thromboplastin known as the Manchester Comparative Reagent, which has been widely used in the United Kingdom.[109] In recent years thromboplastins with a high sensitivity have been commonly used. In fact, many centers have been using the recombinant tissue factor that has an International Sensitivity Index (ISI) value of 0.9 to 1.0, giving an INR equivalent to the PT ratio.

Warfarin is administered in an initial dose of 5 mg/day for the first 2 days, and the daily dose is then adjusted according to the INR. Heparin or LMWH therapy is discontinued on the fifth day after initiation of warfarin therapy, provided the INR is prolonged into the recommended therapeutic range (INR 2.0 to 3.0) for at least 2 consecutive days.[109] Frequent INR determinations are required initially to establish therapeutic anticoagulation.

Once the anticoagulant effect and patient's warfarin dose requirements are stable, the INR should be monitored every 1 to 3 weeks throughout the course of warfarin therapy. However, if there are factors that may produce an unpredictable response to warfarin (e.g., concomitant drug therapy),[109,114] the INR should be monitored more frequently to minimize the risk of complications due to poor anticoagulant control.

ADVERSE EFFECTS OF ORAL ANTICOAGULANTS

Bleeding

The major side effect of oral anticoagulant therapy is bleeding.[118] A number of risk factors have been identified which predispose to bleeding on oral anticoagulants.[119-121] The most important factor influencing bleeding risk is the intensity of the INR.[119-122] Other factors include a history of bleeding, previous history of stroke or myocardial infarction, hypertension, renal failure, diabetes, and a decreased hematocrit.[121] Efforts have been made to quantify the bleeding risk according to these underlying clinical factors.[121] Introduction of a multicomponent intervention combining patient education and alternative approaches to the maintenance of the INR resulted in a reduced frequency of major bleeding in the patients in this group.[120] Furthermore, patients in the intervention group were within the therapeutic INR a significantly greater amount of time than were patients in the standard care group.[120] In a retrospective cohort study of patients with an INR greater than 6.0, it was shown that a prolonged delay in the return of the INR to the therapeutic range was seen in patients who had an INR over 4.0 after two doses of warfarin were withheld; patients with an extreme elevation of the INR[121]; and older age patients, particularly those with decompensated congestive heart failure and active cancer. Numerous randomized clinical trials have demonstrated that clinically important bleeding is lower when the targeted INR is 2.0 to 3.0 and that bleeding increases exponentially when the INR increases above 4.5 or 5.0.[117,122,123] There is a strong negative relationship between the percentage of time that patients are within the targeted INR and both bleeding and recurrent thrombosis.

Oral anticoagulant therapy in elderly patients presents further problems.[124,125] Many of these patients require long-term anticoagulants because of their underlying clinical conditions that increase with age, while at the same time they are more likely to have underlying causes for bleeding, including the development of cancer, intestinal polyps, renal failure, and stroke and they are more prone to having frequent falls. The daily requirements for warfarin to maintain the therapeutic INR also decrease with age, presumably owing to decreased clearance of the drug.[126] Therefore, before initiating oral anticoagulant treatment in elderly patients, the risk/benefit ratio of treatment must be considered. If they are placed on oral anticoagulant therapy, careful attention to the INR is required.

Patients with cancer are more likely to bleed on oral anticoagulant treatment.[127] Compared with patients on oral anticoagulants who do not have cancer, patients with cancer have a higher incidence of both major and minor bleeding and anticoagulant withdrawal is more frequently due to bleeding. Patients with cancer have a higher thrombotic complication rate and a higher bleeding rate regardless of the INR, whereas bleeding in noncancer patients was seen only when the INR was greater than 4.5. Safer and more effective anticoagulant therapy is required for the treatment of VTE in patients with cancer.[127]

Management of Overanticoagulation

The approach to the patient with an elevated INR depends on the degree of elevation of the INR and the clinical circumstances.[114] Options available to the physician include temporary discontinuation of warfarin treatment, administration of vitamin K, or administration of blood products such as fresh frozen plasma or prothrombin concentrate to replace the vitamin K-dependent clotting factors. If the increase is mild and the patient is not bleeding, no specific treatment is necessary other than reduction in the warfarin dose. The INR can be expected to decrease during the next 24 hours with this approach. With more marked increase of the INR in patients who are not bleeding, treatment with small doses of vitamin K_1 (e.g., 1 mg), given either orally or by subcutaneous injection, could be considered.[114,128] With very marked increase of the INR, particularly in a patient who is either actively bleeding or at risk for bleeding, the coagulation defect should be corrected. Vitamin K can be given by the intravenous or subcutaneous route or by the oral route. Where possible the oral route is preferred.[128] If ongoing anticoagulation with warfarin is planned, then repeated small doses of vitamin K should be given so that there is no problem with warfarin resistance.[128,129]

Reported side effects of vitamin K include flushing, dizziness, tachycardia, hypotension, dyspnea, and sweating.[130] Intravenous administration of vitamin K_1 should be performed with caution to avoid inducing an anaphylactoid reaction. The risk of anaphylactoid reaction can be reduced by slow administration of vitamin K_1. In most patients, intravenous administration of vitamin K_1 produces a demonstrable effect on the INR within 6 to 8 hours and corrects the increased INR within 12 to 24 hours. Because the half-life of vitamin K_1 is less than that of warfarin sodium, a repeat course of vitamin K_1 may be necessary. If bleeding is very severe and life threatening, vitamin K therapy can be supplemented with concentrates of factors II, VII, IX, and X.

When bleeding occurs in a patient on oral anticoagulants it is important to consider the site of bleeding. Bleeding from the upper gastrointestinal tract is commonly seen in patients on oral anticoagulants, and the concomitant use of other medications is often an association. When the bleeding is controlled, it is important to carry out the necessary investigations to identify bleeding lesions in the gastrointestinal or genitourinary tract, which are often unsuspected.[114,131] The various protocols for the perioperative management of patients receiving oral anticoagulants were recently reviewed.[132]

CLINICAL USES OF ORAL ANTICOAGULANTS

Long-Term Treatment of VTE

Patients with established DVT or PE require long-term anticoagulant therapy to prevent recurrent disease.[82,133] Warfarin therapy is highly effective and is preferred in most patients. Adjusted dose subcutaneous heparin or LMWH are the treatments of choice where long-term oral anticoagulants are contraindicated, such as in pregnancy,[133] and for the long-term treatment of patients in whom oral anticoagulant therapy proves to be very difficult to control.[106] In patients with proximal DVT, long-term therapy with warfarin reduces the frequency of objectively documented recurrent VTE from 47% to 2%. The use of a less intense warfarin regimen (INR 2 to 3) markedly reduces the risk of bleeding from 20% to 4%, without loss of effectiveness in comparison with more intense warfarin.[117] With the improved safety of oral anticoagulant therapy using a less intense warfarin regimen, there has been renewed interest in evaluating the long-term treatment of thrombotic disorders.

OPTIMAL DURATION OF ORAL ANTICOAGULANTS AFTER A FIRST EPISODE OF VENOUS THROMBOEMBOLISM

It has been recommended that all patients with a first episode of VTE receive warfarin therapy for at least 3 to 6 months. Attempts to decrease the treatment to 4 weeks[134,135] or 6 weeks[136] resulted in higher rates of recurrent VTE in comparison with either 12 or 24 weeks of treatment (11% to 18% recurrent VTE in the following 1 to 2 years). Most of the recurrent thromboembolic events occurred in the 6 to 8 weeks immediately after anticoagulant treatment was stopped, and the incidence was higher in patients with continuing risk factors, such as cancer and immobilization.[136] Treatment with oral anticoagulants for 6 months reduced the incidence of recurrent thromboembolic events, but there was a cumulative incidence of recurrent events at 2 years (11%) and an ongoing risk of recurrent VTE of 5% to 6% per year.[136] In patients with a first episode of idiopathic VTE treated with intravenous heparin followed by warfarin for 3 months, continuation of warfarin for 24 months led to a significant reduction in the incidence of recurrent DVT when compared with placebo.[137] In a further recent trial comparing 3 months with 12 months of oral anticoagulant therapy after the occurrence of a first episode of idiopathic proximal DVT it was shown that patients treated with 3 months had a higher incidence of recurrence of VTE during the subsequent 12 months compared with those patients who were continued on anticoagulants for 12 months.[138] However, the cumulative hazard of recurrent VTE at 36 months was the same in both groups. The incidence of recurrence after discontinuation of treatment was 5.1% per patient-year in patients in whom oral anticoagulant therapy was discontinued after 3 months and 5.0% per patient-year in patients who received an additional 9 months of oral anticoagulant therapy. The recurrence occurred in the initially unaffected leg more than half the time. This suggests that the recurrences were related to a hypercoagulable state and the duration of anticoagulant therapy did not influence the ultimate recurrence rate.

VTE should be considered a chronic disease, with a continued risk of VTE often associated with minor provocation.[139] The continued risk of recurrent thromboembolism even with 12 months' treatment after a first episode of DVT has encouraged the development of clinical trials evaluating the effectiveness of long-term anticoagulant treatment beyond 6 months. In a recent trial, patients with documented proximal DVT with or without the diagnosis of thrombophilia who had received adequate anticoagulation were randomized to received Coumadin with a targeted INR of 1.5 to 2 compared with an identical placebo. This study showed that the lower intensity warfarin significantly decreased the incidence of recurrent VTE in follow-up with no added risk for major bleeding.[140] However, in a study reported in abstract form, warfarin with a targeted INR of 1.5 to 2 was compared with warfarin with a targeted INR of 2 to 3 in a similar patient population. This study indicated that the usual INR of 2 to 3 resulted in a significantly lower incidence of recurrent VTE with no added risk for bleeding.[141] Therefore, at this time there is no justification for the use of the lesser intensive warfarin program.

OPTIMAL DURATION OF ORAL ANTICOAGULANT TREATMENT IN PATIENTS WITH RECURRENT VTE

In a multicenter clinical trial, Schulman and associates randomized patients with a first recurrent episode of VTE to receive either 6 months or continued oral anticoagulants indefinitely, with a targeted INR of 2.0 to 2.85.[142] The analysis was reported at 4 years. In the patients receiving anticoagulants for 6 months, recurrent VTE occurred in 20.7%, compared with 2.6% of patients on the indefinite treatment ($P < .001$). However, the rates of major bleeding were 2.7% in the 6-month group compared with 8.6% in the indefinite group. In the indefinite group, two of the major hemorrhages were fatal, whereas there were no fatal hemorrhages in the 6-month group. This study showed that extending the duration of oral anticoagulants for approximately 4 years resulted in a significant decrease in the incidence of recurrent VTE, but with a higher incidence of major bleeding. Without a mortality difference, the risk of hemorrhage versus the benefit of decreased recurrent thromboembolism with the use of extended warfarin treatment remains uncertain and will require further clinical trials.

From the sixth American College of Chest Physicians Consensus Conference on Anti-thrombotic Therapy the following recommendations are made.[82] Oral anticoagulant therapy should be continued for at least 3 months to prolong the PT to a targeted INR of 2.5 (range: 2.0 to 3.0). Patients with reversible or time-limited risk factors can be treated for 3 to 6 months. Patients with a first episode of idiopathic VTE should be treated for at least 6 months. It should be noted that these recommendations antedated the results of the Agnelli study.[138] Patients with recurrent VTE or a continuing risk factor such as cancer, antithrombin deficiency, or the antiphospholipid syndrome, should be treated indefinitely. Patients with activated protein C resistance (factor V Leiden) should probably receive indefinite treatment if they have recurrent disease, are homozygous for the gene, or have multiple thrombophilic conditions. Accumulated evidence indicates that symptomatic isolated calf vein thrombosis should be treated with anticoagulants for at least 3 months.[82]

THROMBOLYTIC THERAPY

Several studies have demonstrated that the mortality from PE can be decreased by heparin. Treatment with intravenous heparin and oral anticoagulants reduces the mortality rate to less than 5%, and this may be further reduced with the use of LMWH. In the PIOPED trial,[41] only 10 of 399 (2.5%) patients who had angiographically confirmed PE died. However, patients who present with acute massive PE and hypotension have a mortality rate of approximately 20%. For such patients, the appropriate use of thrombolytic agents has a role.

Several trials have compared thrombolytic drugs with heparin.[143-148] Outcome measures for accelerated thrombolysis included quantitative measures on repeat pulmonary angiograms, quantitative scores on repeat pulmonary perfusion scans, and measures of pulmonary vascular resistance. Although all studies demonstrated superiority of thrombolysis (and in particular with tissue plasminogen activator) in radiographic and hemodynamic abnormalities within the first 24 hours, this advantage was short lived.[143] Repeat perfusion scans at 5 to 7 days revealed no significant difference between the patients treated with thrombolytic agents or with heparin. However, at 1 year, those receiving thrombolytic therapy had both high CO diffusion capacity and lung blood capillary volume compared with patients receiving heparin. Follow-up of 23 patients at 7 years showed that patients who had been treated with thrombolytic therapy had lower pulmonary artery pressure and pulmonary vascular resistance. There have been two recent systematic reviews comparing thrombolytic therapy to heparin treatments.[147,148] In one study the composite endpoint of death and recurrent PE was lower with the use of thrombolytic agents but the risk of major bleeding was higher.[147,148] Both of these studies and an accompanying editorial indicated that until the proper randomized clinical trials have been carried out, thrombolytic therapy should only be used for patients with massive PE complicated by shock.[147-149]

Two thrombolytic agents have been approved by the Food and Drug Administration (FDA) for the treatment of acute PE. The dosage schedules are as follows:

- Streptokinase 250,000 units over 30 minutes, followed by 100,000 U/h for 24 hours
- Recombinant tissue plasminogen activator (rt-PA), 100 mg, administered over 2 hours

Anticoagulation with heparin or LMWH is usually begun when the aPTT is less than two times the control.

INFERIOR VENA CAVAL INTERRUPTION

Early approaches to inferior vena caval interruption included ligation or plication using external clips. Both procedures were accompanied by an operative mortality rate of 12% to 14%, a recurrent pulmonary emboli rate of 4% to 6%, and an occlusion rate of 67% to 69%. These complications gave rise to the development of catheter-inserted intraluminal filters. An ideal filter is one that is easily and safely placed percutaneously, is biocompatible and mechanically stable, is able to trap emboli without causing occlusion of the vena cava, which does not require anticoagulation, and is not ferromagnetic (i.e., does not cause artifacts on MRI). Although there is as yet no ideal filter, several types are available. These include the Greenfield stainless-steel filter, titanium Greenfield filter, bird's nest filter, Vena Tech filter, and Simon-Nitinol filter. In experienced hands, these devices can be quickly and safely inserted under fluoroscopic control. One filter (e.g., Antheor TU 50-125, Medi-Tech, Boston Scientific Corp.) can be inserted temporarily in conjunction with thrombolytic therapy and then removed. The follow-up data available show that the Greenfield filter has had the best performance record and any future comparative studies should use this filter as the standard.[150]

The main indications for caval filters are contraindications to anticoagulants, recurrent PE despite adequate anticoagulation, and prophylactic placement in high-risk patients. In the last category are patients with cor pulmonale or a previous history of PE who are placed in high-risk situations such as acetabular fracture or patients who have cancer. More controversial indications for the prophylactic insertion of a filter include emergency surgery occurring within the first 4 weeks of beginning anticoagulant therapy after thrombolytic therapy.[150]

In the past, the detection of a free-floating thrombus by ultrasound examination has been considered as indication for either thrombectomy or insertion of an inferior vena cava filter.[151] An important study compared the clinical outcomes of patients who had either the presence or absence of a free-floating thrombus in a proximal leg vein.[152] There was no difference in the incidence of PE or death between the two groups. The authors conclude that the routine insertion of inferior vena cava filters in patients with free-floating thrombi cannot be supported.[152] This is in keeping with an earlier observation that free-floating thrombi become attached to the vein wall rather than embolizing. In a further study, patients with proximal DVT were randomized to receive an inferior vena cava filter or anticoagulant treatment alone.[153] All patients were treated with heparin, followed by oral anticoagulant therapy for 3 months. At 10 days, there was a significant difference in the incidence of PE but no difference in mortality. Extended follow-up at 1 to 2 years showed a nonsignificant increase in the incidence of PE in the control group but a higher incidence of recurrent DVT in the vena cava filter group and no difference in mortality.[153]

CONCLUSION

Over the past 20 years a large number of trials have been carried out on the diagnosis, prevention, and treatment of VTE. Clinical practice has dramatically changed in response. A number of studies are underway to explore new approaches to diagnosis and treatment. These include the use of pretest clinical probabilities and the D-dimer, the role of spiral CT, and trials to determine the optimal management using LMWH and newer anticoagulants such as pentasaccharide and specific antithrombin agents. Longer duration of anticoagulant therapy with LMWH or warfarin is aimed at decreasing recurrent DVT and PE and decreasing the incidence of the post-thrombotic syndrome. The role of thrombolytic therapy in patients with submassive or massive PE remains controversial, and further randomized clinical trials are needed.

ANNOTATED REFERENCES

Gould MK, Dembitzer AD, Doyle RL, et al: Low-molecular-weight heparins compared with unfractionated heparin for treatment of acute deep venous thrombosis: A meta-analysis of randomized, controlled trials. Ann Intern Med 1999;130:800.

Meta-analysis of randomized clinical trials comparing low molecular weight heparin with unfractionated heparin for the initial treatment of acute deep venous thrombosis. Based on these and subsequent studies, low-molecular-weight heparin has become the treatment of choice for the initial management of patients with deep vein thrombosis and/or pulmonary embolism.

Kelly J, Hunt BJ, Moody A: Magnetic resonance direct thrombus imaging: A novel technique for imaging venous thromboemboli. Thromb Haemost 2003;89:773.

Magnetic resonance angiography may have a useful role in the diagnosis of pulmonary embolism, particularly in patients at high risk of pulmonary angiography, in patients with significant renal insufficiency, and for the diagnosis of venous thromboembolism in pregnancy.

Palareti G, Legnani C, Lee A, et al: A comparison of the safety and efficacy of oral anticoagulation for the treatment of venous thromboembolic disease in patients with or without malignancy. Thromb Haemost 2000;84:805.

This paper highlights the difficulty of managing venous thromboembolism in patients with cancer.

PIOPED Investigators: Value of the ventilation/perfusion scan in acute pulmonary embolism: Results of the Prospective Investigation of Pulmonary Embolism Diagnosis (PIOPED). JAMA 1990;263:2753.

The PIOPED investigators established the role of the ventilation and perfusion scan in the diagnosis of acute pulmonary embolism. PIOPED II, evaluating the role of spiral CT in the diagnosis of acute pulmonary embolism, is to be reported in the fourth quarter of 2004.

Wells PS, Anderson DR, Rodger M, et al: Excluding pulmonary embolism at the bedside without diagnostic imaging: Management of patients with suspected pulmonary embolism presenting to the emergency department by using a simple clinical model and D-dimer. Ann Intern Med 2001;135:98.

Managing patients with suspected pulmonary embolism on the basis of a standardized pre-test probability and the result of a D-dimer test was proven to be safe and to decrease the need for further diagnostic imaging. See also Well PS, et al: Evaluation of D-dimer in the diagnosis of suspected deep vein thrombosis. N Engl J Med 2003;349:1227-1235.

Chapter 80

OTHER EMBOLIC SYNDROMES

Claus-Martin Muth • Erik S. Shank

KEY POINTS

GAS EMBOLISM

1. Any venous gas embolism may become an arterial embolism through intracardiac or extracardiac right-to-left shunting. Arterial gas embolus must be entertained early to rapidly initiate hyperbaric therapy.

2. Treatment of venous gas embolism is prevention of further air entry and cardiopulmonary support with emphasis on reestablishing stable hemodynamics. For arterial gas embolism, the definitive therapy is hyperbaric oxygen therapy.

FAT EMBOLISM SYNDROME

3. This syndrome presents as acute respiratory collapse. It is a diagnosis that should be entertained early in orthopedic surgeries and trauma to the long bones. It remains a diagnosis of exclusion.

AMNIOTIC FLUID EMBOLUS

4. This is managed initially with aggressive cardiopulmonary support. In the postresuscitation period it is vital to follow the coagulation profile and be prepared to treat disseminated intravascular coagulation (DIC).

5. It may strike any woman in the peripartum period. Risk factors often cited for amniotic fluid embolus such as tumultuous labor or multiparity in an older woman have not been demonstrated in recent reviews. It is a syndrome of peripartum cardiovascular collapse and coagulopathy.

The presentation, pathophysiology, and treatment of embolic disease other than thromboembolic processes are discussed in this chapter. Included are emboli associated with iatrogenic complications of medical diagnostic and therapeutic manipulations as well as sequelae from skeletal trauma and pregnancy.

AIR EMBOLISM

Air embolism, the entry of gas into vascular structures, is a largely iatrogenic clinical entity responsible for serious morbidity, and even mortality, in many varied medical specialties (Table 80-1).[1] Furthermore, it is one of the most serious problems in diving medicine.[2] The medical use of varied gases has created numerous other gas embolisms, including carbon dioxide, nitrous oxide, and nitrogen emboli.

There are two broad categories of gas embolism, venous and arterial, depending on the mechanism of gas entry and where the emboli ultimately lodge.

VENOUS GAS EMBOLISM

A venous gas embolism occurs by the entry of gas into the systemic venous system.[3] This gas is then transported to the lungs via the pulmonary arteries, causing interference in gas exchange, arrhythmias, pulmonary hypertension, right ventricular strain, and finally cardiac failure. Predispositions that allow the entry of gas into the venous system include incision of noncollapsed veins and the presence of subatmospheric pressure in these vessels. These conditions occur when the surgical field is above the level of the heart (for instance, during neurosurgical operations performed in the sitting position).[4] Other potential pathways include entry of air into central venous and hemodialysis catheters[1] and entry into the veins of the myometrium in the peripartum period.[1,5]

Pathophysiology

The most common scenario is insidious, where there is a continuous entry of small gas bubbles into the venous system. With rapid entry, or larger volumes of gas, increasing strain on the right ventricle follows because of the migration of the emboli to the pulmonary circulation. The pulmonary arterial pressure increases, while the increased resistance to right ventricle outflow causes diminished pulmonary venous return. This is reflected in decreased left ventricular preload, resulting in diminished cardiac output and, ultimately, systemic cardiovascular collapse.[6] Quite often tachyarrhythmias develop, but bradycardias are possible as well. When large quantities of gas/air (over 50 mL) are injected abruptly, acute cor pulmonale and/or asystole can occur.[3] These alterations of lung vessel resistance and ventilation-perfusion mismatch in the lung cause intrapulmonary right-to-left shunt with increased alveolar deadspace, leading to arterial hypoxia and hypercapnia.

Diagnosis

To diagnose venous gas embolism, clinical findings should be assessed. The so-called mill-wheel murmur is relatively typical and can be auscultated by a precordial or esophageal stethoscope. A capnometric decrease of end-tidal carbon

TABLE 80–1. MEDICAL SPECIALTIES WITH DOCUMENTED CASES OF GAS EMBOLISM

Specialty	Mechanism of Gas Embolism
All medical specialties	Inadvertent entry of air through peripheral intravenous circuits
All surgical specialties	Intraoperative use of hydrogen peroxide generating arterial and venous oxygen emboli
Anesthesiology	Entry of air through disconnected intravascular catheters, inadvertent infusion of air through intravascular catheters
Cardiac Surgery	Entry of air into extracorporeal bypass pump circuit, incomplete removal of air from heart post cardioplegic arrest, carbon dioxide–assisted harvesting of peripheral veins
Cardiology	Entry of air through intravascular catheters during angiographic studies and procedures
Critical Care/Pulmonology	Entry of air through disconnected intravascular catheters, pulmonary barotrauma, rupture of intra-aortic balloon pumps, entry of air in extracorporeal membrane oxygenator (ECMO) circuit
Diving Medicine and Hyperbaric Medicine	Pulmonary barotrauma, paradoxical embolism after decompression injury, entry of gas through disconnected intravascular catheters
Endoscopic/Laparoscopic Surgery	Entry of gas into veins or arteries during insufflation of body cavities
Gastroenterology	Entry of gas into veins during upper and lower endoscopies and endoscopic retrograde pancreatography (ERCP)
Neonatology/Pediatrics	Pulmonary barotrauma in treatment of infants with premature lungs
Nephrology	Inadvertent entry of air through hemodialysis catheter and circuit on hemodialysis machine
Neurosurgery	Entry of air through incised veins and calvarial bone especially during sitting craniotomies
Obstetrics/Gynecology	Cesarean sections, gas insufflation into veins during endoscopic surgery, intravaginal/intrauterine gas insufflation during pregnancy
Otolaryngology	Laser (Nd:YAG) surgery on the larynx and trachea/bronchi
Orthopedics	Gas insufflation into veins during arthroscopy, total hip arthroplasty, prone spine surgery
Radiology	Injected air/gas as contrast agent, inadvertent injection of air during angiographic studies
Thoracic Surgery	Entry of air into pulmonary vasculature during lung biopsies and video-assisted thoracoscopy (VATS), chest trauma (penetrating and blunt), lung transplants
Urology	Transurethral prostatectomy (TURP), radical prostatectomy
Vascular Surgery	Entry of air during carotid endarterectomies

dioxide suggests a change in the relation of ventilation and perfusion by the obstruction of the pulmonary arteries.[7] Precordial Doppler ultrasonography is a sensitive and practical monitor to detect intracardiac air and is often utilized in neurosurgical procedures[1,8] in the sitting position and in other procedures with a high risk for gas embolism. An even more sensitive and definitive monitor for detecting intracardiac gas is transesophageal echocardiography; however, this technique requires significant training in application and interpretation to be effective.[1,9]

Treatment (Table 80-2)

When a venous gas embolism is suggested, further entry of gas must be avoided. Catecholamine therapy and cardiopulmonary resuscitation should be initiated for cardiovascular collapse. Adequate oxygenation is often only possible with a significant increase in the oxygen concentration of the inspired gas (i.e., 100% oxygen). Supplemental oxygen also reduces the size of the gas embolism by increasing the gradient for nitrogen egress from the bubble.[10] Rapid volume resuscitation is recommended to elevate venous pressure, thus decreasing the continued entry of gas into the venous circulation. Some authors recommend attempting to evacuate air from the right ventricle by a central venous catheter (multi-orifice catheters may be more effective than a single lumen) or a pulmonary arterial catheter.[11] Hyperbaric oxygen therapy is not a first-line treatment but may be a useful adjunct in severe cases. It should certainly be considered if there are neurologic findings. If central nervous system symptoms are present, a paradoxical embolism should be presumed.

PARADOXICAL EMBOLISM

A paradoxical embolism arises when air/gas entrained in the venous circulation manages to enter the systemic arterial circulation causing symptoms of end-artery obstruction. There are a number of mechanisms by which this can occur. One of these is the passage of gas across a patent foramen ovale to the systemic circulation. A patent foramen ovale is detectable in about 30% of the population and makes right-to-left shunting of gas bubbles possible.[12] Elevated pulmonary arterial pressure due to a venous gas embolism may be reflected

TABLE 80–2. TREATMENT OF GAS EMBOLISM

	Venous Gas Embolism	Arterial Gas Embolism
Prevent Further Gas Entry	Increase venous pressure (e.g., Valsalva, IV fluids) Identify and disable entryway for gas	Identify and disable entryway for gas
Definitive Therapy	Supportive	Hyperbaric oxygen therapy as soon as patient stable for transfer to hyperbaric oxygen facility
Supportive Therapy	Oxygen, intravascular volume expansion, catecholamines	Oxygen, intravascular volume expansion, catecholamines
Positioning	Supine	Supine
Evacuation of Embolized Gas	Aspiration of multi-lumen central venous catheter; patient in left lateral decubitus position	Hyperbaric oxygen
Adjunctive Therapy	Hyperbaric oxygen	Lidocaine, antiepileptics

in elevated right atrial pressures predisposing to bubble transport across a patent foramen. In addition, the decrease in left atrial pressure caused by controlled ventilation and use of positive end-expiratory pressure may create a pressure gradient across the patent foramen ovale favoring passage of gas into the systemic circulation.[1]

In other situations, venous gas may enter the arterial circulation by overwhelming the filter capacity of the lungs normally in place to prevent arterial gas emboli. Clinical cases are documented in which a fatal cerebral arterial gas embolism developed, caused by a large venous gas embolism, although no intracardiac defects or shunt mechanisms could be demonstrated.[13] The filtration threshold of the pulmonary circulation for gas emboli can be affected by various anesthetic agents. In particular, volatile anesthetics have been shown to reduce the threshold for spillover of venous bubbles into systemic arteries in experimental studies.[14]

Treatment

Therapy of paradoxical embolism is identical to that of a primary arterial gas embolism (see Table 80-2). It should be stressed that every venous gas embolism has the potential to evolve into an arterial gas embolism.

ARTERIAL GAS EMBOLISM

Arterial gas embolism occurs by the entry of gas into the pulmonary veins or directly into the arteries of the systemic circulation. Mechanisms include the overexpansion of the lung through decompression barotraumas in diving, pulmonary barotraumas in the ventilatory therapy for critical care patients, and paradoxical embolism. Additionally, all cardiac surgical operations with extracorporal bypass are a potential mechanism for these events.[1] The entry of even small amounts of gas into the arterial system leads to a flow of gas bubbles into functional end arteries and occlusion of these vessels. Although possible in all arteries, the embolic obstruction of the coronary arteries or the nutritive arteries of the brain, termed a *cerebral arterial gas embolism*, are especially critical and can be fatal owing to the vulnerability of these organs to short periods of hypoxia.

Pathophysiology

Entry of gas into the aorta causes distribution of gas bubbles into nearly all organs. Small emboli in the vessels of the skeletal muscles or viscera are well tolerated, although organ dysfunctions such as rhabdomyolysis and/or renal insufficiency may occur as well.[15] Embolization to the cerebral or coronary circulation may result in severe morbidity or death.

Embolization into the coronary arteries can induce electrocardiographic changes typical of ischemia and infarction with dysrhythmias, myocardial depression, cardiac failure, and cardiac arrest. Circulatory responses may also be seen with embolization to the cerebral vessels.[16] Cerebral arterial gas embolization typically involves migration of gas to small arteries of the brain. The emboli generate pathology by two broad mechanisms: reduced perfusion distal to the obstruction and an inflammatory response to the bubble.[1]

Clinical Features

The signs and symptoms associated with cerebral arterial gas embolism can develop suddenly. The clinical presentation is determined by the absolute quantity of gas and the brain areas affected. Thus, a comparatively mild clinical picture with minor motor weakness, headache, or moderately marked confusion may be present. Conversely, complete disorientation, hemiparesis, convulsions, loss of consciousness, and coma may present. Additionally, asymmetry of pupils, hemianopsia, and impairment of respiratory and circulatory centers (bradypnea, Cheyne-Stokes breathing, cardiac arrhythmias, and circulatory failure) are all well-known complications. After surgeries with risks for the development of gas embolism, a delayed recovery from general anesthesia or a transitional stage of impaired consciousness can be a clue to a cerebral arterial gas embolism. The diagnosis in these cases is not easy because anesthesia complications such as central anticholinergic syndrome, residual anesthetic, or muscle relaxant can mimic a mild cerebral arterial gas embolism.

Diagnosis

The most important criterion is the patient's history, because the clinical suspicion of embolism is based on the initial neurologic symptoms and the direct temporal relation with an invasive medical therapy. The greatest risks for venous or arterial gas embolism are present in craniotomies performed in the sitting position, cesarean sections, hip replacements, and cardiac surgery using cardiopulmonary bypass. All these procedures have in common an incised vascular bed and a hydrostatic gradient favoring the intravascular entry of gas.

Differentiating a cerebral arterial gas embolism from a cerebral infarct or an intracerebral hemorrhage can sometimes be made using computed tomography (CT). However, pathologic changes are sometimes very subtle and not well visualized on CT, and the diagnosis of cerebral arterial gas embolism must be entertained early. Magnetic resonance imaging of the cerebrum can sometimes show local increase of water density concentrated in the injured tissue. But this method is not completely reliable and may fail when only mild symptomatology is present. Another nonspecific finding, but described in a number of cases, is hemoconcentration with increased hematocrit, possibly the direct consequence of the extravascular shift of fluid into the injured tissues.[17]

Treatment

Protection and maintenance of vital functions is the primary goal. If warranted, cardiopulmonary resuscitation must be performed, because not only venous but also primary arterial gas embolism may lead to serious impairment of the cardiovascular system. For somnolent or comatose patients, endotracheal intubation should be performed to maintain adequate oxygenation and ventilation. Additionally, oxygen should be administered in as high a concentration as possible.[1,18] This is important not only to treat hypoxia and hypoxemia but also for the elimination of the gas in the bubbles through a diffusion gradient favoring egress of gas from the bubble.

The current therapeutic recommendation is to maintain a flat supine position for these patients, because neither head-down positions nor an elevated head position provides any detectable cardiovascular benefits and may aggravate the cerebral insult.

Cerebral gas embolism may be associated with the development of generalized seizures that may resist management by benzodiazepines. In these cases it is advised to suppress the seizure activity with barbiturates. It must be stressed, however, that with sufficient doses of barbiturates, respiratory drive is depressed and the patient's ventilation must be supported.

The definite treatment of arterial gas embolism is hyperbaric oxygen therapy (HBO-T),[19,20] with best results reported when performed as early as possible. HBO-T involves the placement of the patient in an environment pressurized above sea level pressure while breathing 100% oxygen. This therapy causes a mechanical diminution of the gas bubble by both raising the ambient pressure and creating systemic hyperoxia. Hyperoxia produces a diffusion gradient for oxygen into the gas bubble, as well as for egress of nitrogen (or other gas) from the bubble. Hyperoxia also enables significantly larger quantities of oxygen to be dissolved in the plasma and also increases the diffusion distance of oxygen in tissues. The improved oxygen-carrying capacity and delivery is important to offset the embolic insult to the microvasculature.

Hyperbaric oxygen has other postulated benefits. These include anti-edema effects and reducing blood vessel permeability while supporting the integrity of the blood-brain barrier.[21] In addition, there are experimental studies indicating that hyperbaric oxygen diminishes the adherent properties of leukocytes to the damaged endothelium.[22]

The aforementioned benefits suggest that all patients with the clinical symptomatology of arterial gas embolism should receive treatment with hyperbaric oxygen. Although immediate institution of such therapy demonstrates the best response, treatment in a hyperbaric chamber is still indicated after a longer period of time and may result in amelioration of the patient's condition. Treatment of arterial gas emboli with hyperbaric oxygen is the first-line therapy of choice. Thus, once the patient is stabilized from a cardiopulmonary standpoint, transfer to a hyperbaric oxygen facility should be accomplished without delay.

Further Therapeutic Measures

As a consequence of a gas embolism, hemoconcentration may occur, resulting in increased blood viscosity and further impairing the already compromised microcirculation. One important maneuver to optimize the microcirculation is therefore to achieve euvolemia. In animal studies it has been demonstrated that a moderate hemodilution to a hematocrit of 30% leads to a reduction of the neurologic damage.[23] It is therefore acceptable to decrease the hematocrit within certain limits. The use of crystalloid solutions may exacerbate cerebral edema; thus, colloid solutions should be favored.

Placement of a central venous catheter is strongly recommended to properly assess central venous pressure (CVP). CVP should be kept around 12 mm Hg. As a further monitor of normovolemia, the urine output should be monitored by Foley catheter.

There is some evidence that heparin may be of use in the treatment of gas embolism.[24] Studies have shown that the clinical course of arterial gas embolism is less severe if the patient has been treated with heparin before the embolic event. The mechanism seems to be not only anticoagulative but also that heparin has an inhibitory effect on thromboinflammatory processes. Arguing against heparinization is the risk of hemorrhage into the infarcted tissue. At present, the use of heparin for the acute therapy of cerebral arterial gas embolism is not yet recommended.

The use of corticosteroids remains controversial. Some authors recommend the use of corticosteroids for arterial gas embolism to combat vasogenic brain edema, which results from a gas embolization in the cerebral arteries. Cerebral gas embolism initially induces a rapidly developing cytotoxic brain edema with diminished extracellular spaces and enlarged intracellular areas. This form of edema does not, in general, respond to corticosteroids. Other authors report the use of steroids aggravating ischemic injury post vessel occlusion.[25] Thus, because corticosteroids appear to be without benefit in cytotoxic edema and potentially may aggravate neuronal ischemic injury, they are not indicated in arterial gas embolism.

Although still experimental, there are suggestions that lidocaine may be beneficial.[26,27] In animals receiving prophylactic doses of lidocaine, the depressant effects of gas embolism on somatosensory evoked potentials and elevations in intracranial pressure could both be reduced. In a clinical trial, cerebral protection during cardiac operations was demonstrated.[27] Therefore, a strong argument can be made for the administration of lidocaine in therapeutic concentrations after severe arterial gas embolism.

FAT EMBOLISM SYNDROME

Fat embolism syndrome (FES) is a clinical entity first described over 150 years ago by Bergmann.[28] It is very important to differentiate FES, a complex with potentially catastrophic cardiopulmonary and cerebral dysfunction, from fat embolization, a far more common and often subclinical entity.[29]

FES is most frequently seen status post lower extremity and pelvic trauma, intramedullary nailing of long-bone fractures, hip arthroplasty, and knee arthroplasty.[30] However, FES has also been described in association with diverse diseases, such as sickle cell disease, acute pancreatitis, and diabetes mellitus and with liposuction procedures, burns, decompression sickness, and total parenteral nutrition infusion.[31-33] In a retrospective review of patients with fractures of the long bones from trauma, the incidence of FES was 0.9%.[34]

FES always involves pulmonary compromise. The presentation may range from subclinical shunting to fulminant pulmonary failure. In response to the lodging of fat particles in the pulmonary vasculature, the patient may present with right-sided heart failure, cardiovascular collapse, or severe hypoxia. Frequently there is cerebral involvement. Cerebral symptomatology may be due to paradoxical fat embolization to the central nervous system and/or a response to the severe hypoxia associated with this syndrome.

Intramedullary orthopedic surgeries are the most common iatrogenic cause of FES. In hip and knee arthroplasties, the manipulation of the femoral components can generate intramedullary pressures exceeding 800 mm Hg. Cementing the prosthesis has been implicated in raising the intramedullary pressure even further.[35] However, this may not be as straightforward as previously thought. One study has suggested that there is no additional risk of FES associated with cementing the prosthesis.[36]

The pathophysiology of FES is complex and probably has both a mechanical component as well as a secondary biochemical process. In the initial phase, fat and marrow are displaced from the bones, enter the venous system, and travel through the heart to enter the lungs. There the emboli may cause shunting, severe hypoxemia, and right ventricular dysfunction. Analogous to gas emboli, the fat may travel, paradoxically, to other organs via the systemic circulation either by transpulmonary passage or through an intracardiac shunt, most commonly through a patent foramen ovale. The secondary phase may involve inflammatory mediators responsible for the interstitial edema or acute respiratory distress syndrome that may ensue. Additionally, bone marrow contains thromboplastin that may activate coagulation cascades. These mechanisms may be responsible for the delayed petechial rash seen 24 to 48 hours after the initial event in approximately 50% of patients with FES.

The diagnosis of FES remains one of exclusion. A number of authors have suggested clinical criteria for diagnosing FES. The most notable are Gurd's,[37] Schonfeld's,[38] and Lindeque's.[39] All include acute respiratory collapse as a major criterion. Schonfeld and Gurd both stress the presence of petechiae in their criteria for FES. Petechiae, as mentioned earlier, are not a consistent sign of FES and present relatively late in the process. Laboratory tests that may help in making the diagnosis include arterial blood gases (hypoxia), electrocardiogram (right-sided heart strain), chest radiograph (diffuse bilateral infiltrates and opacities), magnetic resonance imaging (for signs of cerebral FES), and CT.[40] Bronchoalveolar lavage (BAL) may help confirm the diagnosis by demonstrating fat droplets in alveolar macrophages, although the sensitivity and specificity of this test are unclear.[41,42] Intraoperative transesophageal echocardiography (TEE) will demonstrate multiple echogenicities in the right heart chambers in the presence of fat embolization. It may also show paradoxical echogenic particles in the left heart chambers should a patent foramen ovale or other means for right-to-left intracardiac shunting be present.[43] A pulmonary arterial catheter may show elevations in right-sided heart pressures.[44] Urinalysis may show lipuria.[45]

Treatment of FES remains supportive. There are no specific drug regimens recommended for FES. Cardiovascular therapy including maintaining adequate preload and positive inotropy is necessary to preserve cardiac output. The severe hypoxemia associated with FES must be aggressively treated, usually with 100% oxygen via an endotracheal tube. Even with ideal pulmonary care, lung function may further deteriorate with a clinical picture resembling acute respiratory distress syndrome. Prophylactic corticosteroid therapy may minimize the incidence of FES,[46] but other therapeutic regimens used after the development of FES, including heparinization, dextran, and parenteral ethanol, cannot be recommended.

AMNIOTIC FLUID EMBOLISM

Amniotic fluid embolism is an entity first described by Meyer[47] in 1926 and involves the introduction of amniotic fluid containing fetal elements into the maternal circulation. In 1941, it was further characterized by two pathologists, Steiner and Lushbaugh, who reported the histologic findings in 42 women who died during the third trimester of pregnancy.[48] Nine of the women had squamous cells and eosinophilic material possibly of fetal origin. The pathologists suggested that this was a syndrome associated with tumultuous labor in multiparous older women. This group became the basis for the "classic" amniotic fluid embolism (AFE).

Estimates for the incidence of amniotic fluid embolism vary from 1 in 8000 to 1 in 80,000 pregnancies. It is currently the most common cause of peripartum deaths.[49] Clark and colleagues, reviewing the national registry of AFE, suggested the descriptive terminology "syndrome of acute peripartum cardiovascular collapse and coagulopathy" to describe AFE. They determined, in contrast to previously accepted notions, that no demographic variables, including maternal age, parity, race, or route of delivery of the infant, predicted elevated risk of AFE.[49] In 73% of the patients there were fetal elements in the pulmonary vasculature of the mothers. Interestingly, the syndrome was not associated more with vasopressin-induced labor, nor was cesarean section an apparent risk factor. The authors did note a strong temporal association to placement of intrauterine monitoring devices or artificial rupture of membranes and presentation of AFE symptoms. A significant association was made between AFE and male sex of the fetus.

Amniotic fluid embolism may present initially as seizures or seizure-like states or as cardiopulmonary symptoms.[50] These may include acute dyspnea, hypotension, fetal distress, pulmonary edema, or cardiac arrest. Cardiac events are relatively evenly distributed between pulseless electrical activity, severe bradycardias, ventricular tachycardias, and asystole.

Patients who survive the initial insult usually proceed to a consumption coagulopathy. This is associated with fibrinogen depletion (less than 100 mg/dL), increased fibrin split products, elevation of prothrombin and activated partial thromboplastin times, as well as decreased platelet levels.[51] In some cases, coagulopathy may be the presenting sign of an AFE.[51]

Amniotic fluid embolism appears due to an exposure of the maternal circulation to fetal products. However, unlike other embolic diseases discussed in this chapter, exposure to fetal products usually does not generate the AFE syndrome. In fact, it has been demonstrated that amniotic fluid infusion into the maternal circulation is generally innocuous.[52] This is fortunate because the outcome, over 50 years since the syndrome was described, remains dismal. Fewer than 15% of women who are stricken with AFE survive neurologically intact.

Even with ideal care, AFE remains a disease with an extremely poor outcome. In spite of rapid and aggressive resuscitation, neurologic sequelae are common in the survivors. That AFE should present often as seizures or a seizure-like state is relatively surprising. It may be due to profound hypoxia as well as hypotensive insults to the central nervous system.

Clark and colleagues[49] have suggested that AFE may share similar mechanisms to septic shock and other anaphylactoid responses. The premise is that fetal components in the amniotic fluid initiate a complex inflammatory cascade with resultant cardiopulmonary collapse. Nishio and colleagues presented data that support this hypothesis in a patient with presumed fatal AFE and elevation of serum mast cell tryptase levels indicating recent mast cell degranulation (a common denominator of anaphylactoid reactions).[53] The coagulopathy may be due to the activation of clotting cascades by amniotic fluid containing platelet factor III, factor X–like properties, as well as functionally active tissue factor.[54] Tissue factor when combined with maternal factor VII will activate the extrinsic coagulation pathway.[51]

The diagnosis of AFE is one mostly of exclusion. It should be entertained in any pregnant woman who experiences acute cardiovascular collapse or coagulopathy. It has been described in women undergoing first-trimester therapeutic abortions as well as during the peripartum period. There is no definitive diagnostic test for AFE. Demonstrating fetal matter in the pulmonary vasculature on autopsy supports the diagnosis but is nonspecific.[55] Fetal elements were found in only 73% of patients who died of presumed AFE. Aspirating from a wedged pulmonary artery catheter or sampling mixed venous blood for fetal elements may also help support the diagnosis,[56] although in one study only 50% of patients being resuscitated for presumed AFE had fetal elements aspirated by a wedged pulmonary artery catheter.

Treatment of AFE is largely supportive. Initial cardiopulmonary resuscitation should be performed with left lateral displacement to maintain uterine perfusion and venous return. Management should be directed toward maintaining oxygenation, usually with 100% oxygen through an endotracheal tube. Additional cardiovascular support should be initiated rapidly with volume and pressor support. If the fetus has not yet been delivered, this should be accomplished by emergent cesarean section.[57] An arterial line and pulmonary catheter may help guide therapy.[55] Epinephrine may be the first-line agent of choice, as it is in other anaphylactoid reactions. Corticosteroids may be helpful, but therapeutic heparinization to minimize consumption coagulopathies remains controversial.[55]

It is vital to aggressively follow the coagulation profile and treat the disseminated intravascular coagulation (DIC) that frequently ensues once the initial cardiovascular collapse has been addressed. The mortality from DIC may be as great as 75%, in spite of optimal therapy.[51] Treatment is usually with blood components, including red blood cells followed by platelets, fresh frozen plasma, and cryoprecipitate.[58]

ANNOTATED REFERENCES

Awad IT, Shorten GD: Amniotic fluid embolism and isolated coagulopathy: Atypical presentation of amniotic fluid embolism. Eur J Anaesth 2001;18:410-413.
> A report stressing the possibility of coagulopathy without prior cardiovascular collapse in a case of presumed amniotic fluid embolism.

Clark SL, Hankins GD, Dudley DA, et al: Amniotic fluid embolism: Analysis of the national registry. Am J Obstet Gynecol 1995;172:1158-1169.
> A retrospective review of the National Registry for Amniotic Fluid Embolism cases. This review discusses the presentation, outcome, and possible pathophysiology.

Georgopoulos D: Fat embolism syndrome: Clinical examination is still the preferable diagnostic method (editorial). Chest;123:982-983.
> A well-written and compelling discussion of the new diagnostic modalities to aid in the diagnosis of fat embolism syndrome and the reasons why clinical criteria remain the preferred method for diagnosing FES.

Kim YH, Oh SW, Kim JS: Prevalence of fat embolism following bilateral simultaneous and unilateral total hip arthroplasty performed with or without cement. J Bone Joint Surg Am 2002;8:1372-1379.
> A randomized prospective study comparing the incidence of fat emboli in femoral necks that were cemented versus those that were not cemented during hip arthroplasties.

Muth CM, Shank ES: Gas embolism. N Engl J Med 2000;342:476-482.
> This review article discusses the variety of iatrogenic mechanisms able to generate gas emboli as well as presenting up-to-date recommendations for treatment.

Chapter 81
PULMONARY HYPERTENSION

David B. Badesch • Lewis J. Rubin

KEY POINTS

1. **The evaluation of patients with pulmonary artery hypertension (PAH) is directed at the detection of underlying contributing factors and associated conditions,** such as left-sided cardiac dysfunction, underlying congenital heart disease, pulmonary thromboembolic disease, collagen vascular disease, parenchymal lung disease, obstructive sleep apnea, liver disease, amphetamine or appetite suppressant use, intravenous drug abuse, or human immunodeficiency virus (HIV) infection.

2. **Patients with severe PAH are particularly prone to vasovagal events,** and when these occur they can lead to severe consequences, including syncope, cardiopulmonary arrest, and death.

3. **Hypoxemia and hypercarbia are both pulmonary vasoconstrictors** and can contribute to the worsening of pulmonary hypertension.

4. **The induction of anesthesia and intubation for surgical procedures can be a particularly high-risk time for patients with PAH,** as they are at risk for vagal events, hypoxemia, hypercarbia, and shifts in intrathoracic pressure with associated changes in cardiac filling pressures.

Pulmonary hypertension is defined as a pulmonary artery mean pressure (PAPm) of 25 mm Hg or greater and may be precapillary or postcapillary in etiology. Postcapillary causes include processes affecting the left side of the heart (e.g., left ventricular systolic or diastolic dysfunction, mitral stenosis or regurgitation, aortic valvular disease) or, more rarely, the pulmonary veins (pulmonary veno-occlusive disease). Management of postcapillary pulmonary hypertension typically involves treating the underlying left-sided cardiac process. Medications used to treat precapillary pulmonary hypertension are often not only ineffective for postcapillary pulmonary hypertension but may, in fact, be harmful, potentially leading to the development of pulmonary edema.

Precapillary pulmonary hypertension, or pulmonary arterial hypertension (PAH), can be idiopathic (IPAH—previously known as primary pulmonary hypertension [PPH]) or may occur in association with a variety of underlying disease processes such as collagen vascular disease, portal hypertension, congenital systemic to pulmonary shunts, drug or toxin exposure, or HIV infection.[1] IPAH/PPH is principally a disease of young women, but it can affect all age groups and both sexes.

A genetic predisposition may underlie a substantial proportion of these cases.[2-8]

Initial therapy may be directed at an underlying cause or contributing factor, such as using continuous positive airway pressure (CPAP) and supplemental oxygen for PAH associated with obstructive sleep apnea. Following the identification and treatment of underlying associated disorders and contributing factors, specific therapy for PAH should be considered. IPAH/PPH carried a very poor prognosis (median survival approximately 2.8 years from the date of diagnosis) through the mid-1980s. Subsequently, a number of therapeutic options have been developed, and three have been approved by the U.S. Food and Drug Administration (FDA): epoprostenol, treprostinil, and bosentan. Other agents that are being studied for PAH include sitaxsenten, ambrisentan, sildenafil, and inhaled iloprost.

DIAGNOSIS

SYMPTOMS, SIGNS, AND CLINICAL HISTORY

Because of the insidious onset of symptoms, PAH is often advanced at the time of diagnosis. Dyspnea on exertion is a common presenting symptom, but it is sometimes attributed to deconditioning or other cardiorespiratory ailment. Chest pain, mimicking angina pectoris, may occur. Patients with advanced disease may present with syncope or signs and symptoms of right-sided heart failure, including lower extremity edema, jugular venous distention, and ascites.

The clinical history should focus initially on the exclusion of underlying causes of pulmonary hypertension. Important clues to an underlying condition might include a previous history of a heart murmur, deep venous thrombosis or pulmonary embolism, Raynaud's phenomenon, arthritis, arthralgias, rash, heavy alcohol consumption, hepatitis, heavy snoring, daytime hypersomnolence, morning headache, and morbid obesity. A careful family history should be taken. Medication exposures, particularly to appetite suppressants and amphetamines, should be noted. Cocaine is a powerful vasoconstrictor and may contribute to the development of pulmonary hypertension. Intravenous drug abuse has been associated with the development of PAH.

PHYSICAL EXAMINATION

Signs of PAH may not become apparent until late in the disease. Findings such as an accentuated second heart sound, a systolic murmur over the left sternal border, jugular venous distention, peripheral edema, and/or ascites might suggest the presence of pulmonary hypertension and right ventricular dysfunction. Associated systemic diseases, such as collagen vascular disease or liver disease, may also become apparent during routine examination.

LABORATORY EVALUATION

Laboratory evaluation can provide important information in detecting associated disorders and contributing factors. A collagen vascular screen, including antinuclear antibodies, rheumatoid factor, and erythrocyte sedimentation rate, is often helpful in detecting autoimmune disease, although some patients with IPAH/PPH will have a low titer positive antinuclear antibody test.[9] The scleroderma spectrum of disease, particularly limited scleroderma or the CREST syndrome, has been associated with an increased risk for the development of PAH.[10,11] Liver function tests (aspartate aminotransferase, alanine aminotransferase, alkaline phosphatase) may be elevated in patients with right ventricular failure and passive hepatic congestion but may also be associated with underlying liver disease. Liver disease with portal hypertension has been associated with the development of pulmonary hypertension. Thyroid disease may occur with increased frequency in patients with IPAH/PPH and should be excluded with thyroid function testing.[12] HIV testing and hepatitis serologic studies should be considered in patients at risk. Routine laboratory studies such as the complete blood cell count, complete metabolic panel, prothrombin time, and partial thromboplastin time are recommended during the initial evaluation and as indicated to monitor the patient's long-term clinical status.

ECHOCARDIOGRAPHY

Doppler echocardiography is useful in estimating the severity of pulmonary hypertension and detecting left-sided heart disease. Findings may include enlargement of the right ventricle, flattening of the interventricular septum, and compression of the left ventricle. Bubble contrast echocardiography may detect a right-to-left shunt, but exclusion of a left-to-right intracardiac shunt may require cardiac catheterization with an oximetry series. Echocardiography may be a useful noninvasive means of long-term follow-up,[13] although not all patients have suitable echocardiographic windows.

RADIOGRAPHIC EVALUATION AND EXCLUSION OF THROMBOEMBOLIC DISEASE

Chest radiography may reveal enlargement of the central pulmonary vessels and evidence of right ventricular enlargement. Evidence of parenchymal lung disease may be apparent. When parenchymal lung disease is suspected, pulmonary function testing and high-resolution computed tomography (CT) of the chest may be indicated. Ventilation-perfusion lung-scanning should be performed in an attempt to exclude chronic-recurrent pulmonary thromboembolic disease, which is among the most preventable and treatable causes of pulmonary hypertension. Diffuse mottled perfusion can be seen in IPAH/PPH, whereas larger segmental and subsegmental mismatched defects are suggestive of chronic recurrent pulmonary thromboembolic disease. Intermediate results on ventilation-perfusion lung scanning may require pulmonary arteriography to obtain a definitive diagnosis. Although contrast medium–enhanced CT has been popularized recently

for the diagnosis of acute pulmonary thromboembolic disease, there is limited experience with this technique in chronic thromboembolic disease. Accordingly, we recommend caution at present in using contrast-enhanced CT to exclude chronic recurrent thromboembolic disease.

PULMONARY FUNCTION TESTING

Pulmonary function testing is indicated to detect underlying parenchymal lung disease. The diffusing capacity is often reduced in pulmonary vascular disease, consistent with impaired gas exchange. Oximetry testing of patients at rest, with exertion, and nocturnally, is useful in detecting hypoxemia and the need for supplemental oxygen.

RIGHT-SIDED HEART CATHETERIZATION AND VASOREACTIVITY TESTING

Right-sided heart catheterization remains an important part of the evaluation. Left-sided heart dysfunction and intracardiac shunts can be excluded, the degree of pulmonary hypertension can be accurately quantified, and the cardiac output can be measured. Pulmonary vascular resistance can then be calculated. Acute pulmonary vasoreactivity can be assessed using a short-acting agent such as prostacyclin (epoprostenol), inhaled nitric oxide, or intravenous adenosine.[14,15] The European Society of Cardiology consensus definition of a positive acute vasodilator response in an IPAH/PPH patient is a fall of PAPm of at least 10 mm Hg to less than or equal to 40 mm Hg, with an increased or unchanged cardiac output. The primary objective of acute vasodilator testing in patients with IPAH/PPH is to identify patients who might be effectively treated with oral calcium channel blockers. The acute response to a short-acting agent, such as prostacyclin, has been shown to be predictive of the response to calcium channel blocker.[14] Unstable patients or those in severe right-sided heart failure, who would not be candidates for treatment with calcium channel blockers, need not undergo vasodilator testing.

TREATMENT

GENERAL CARE

Warfarin, Oxygen, Diuretics, Digoxin, and Vaccination

Improved survival has been reported with oral anticoagulation in IPAH/PPH.[16,17] The target International Normalized Ratio in these patients is 1.5 to 2.5. Anticoagulation of patients with PAH occurring in association with other underlying processes, such as scleroderma or congenital heart disease, is controversial. Generally, patients with PAH treated with chronic intravenous epoprostenol are anticoagulated in the absence of contraindications, owing in part to the additional risk of catheter-associated thrombosis.

Hypoxemia is a pulmonary vasoconstrictor and can contribute to the development or progression of PAH. It is generally considered important to maintain oxygen saturations at greater than 90% at all times. Supplemental oxygen use is more controversial in patients with Eisenmenger physiology but may decrease the need for phlebotomy and potentially reduce the occurrence of neurologic dysfunction and complications.

Diuretics are indicated in patients with evidence of right ventricular failure and volume overload (i.e., peripheral edema and/or ascites). Careful dietary restriction of sodium and fluid intake is important in the management of patients with PAH with right-sided heart failure. Rapid and excessive diuresis may produce systemic hypotension, renal insufficiency, and syncope. Serum electrolytes and measures of renal function should be followed closely in patients receiving diuretic therapy.

Although not extensively studied in PAH, digitalis is sometimes utilized in refractory right ventricular failure or atrial dysrhythmias. Drug levels should be followed closely, particularly in patients with impaired renal function.

Because of the potentially devastating effects of respiratory infections in PAH, immunization against influenza and pneumococcal pneumonia is recommended.

Calcium Channel Blockers

Patients with IPAH/PPH who respond to vasodilators and calcium channel blockers[16] generally have improved survival. Unfortunately, this tends to represent a relatively small proportion of patients, comprising fewer than 20% of IPAH/PPH patients and even fewer patients with other causes of PAH.

Prostanoids

Prostacyclin, a metabolite of arachidonic acid produced primarily in vascular endothelium, is a potent systemic and pulmonary vasodilator that also has antiplatelet aggregatory effects. A relative deficiency of prostacyclin may contribute to the pathogenesis of PAH.[18]

Epoprostenol

In a 12-week, prospective, multicenter, randomized, controlled, open-label trial, continuously intravenously infused epoprostenol plus conventional therapy (oral vasodilators and anticoagulation) improved exercise capacity and hemodynamics compared with conventional therapy alone.[19] Eight patients died during the study, all of whom had received conventional therapy. Serious complications included four episodes of catheter-related sepsis and one thrombotic event.

A similar multicenter, randomized, controlled, open-label study of chronic intravenous epoprostenol showed improvement in exercise capacity and hemodynamics in patients with PAH occurring in association with the scleroderma spectrum of disease.[20] Four patients in the epoprostenol group and five in the conventional therapy group died.

Epoprostenol therapy is complicated by the need for continuous intravenous infusion. The drug is unstable at room temperature and is generally best kept cold before and during infusion. It has a very short half-life in the bloodstream (<6 minutes), is unstable at acidic pH, and cannot be taken orally. Because of the short half-life, the risk of rebound worsening with abrupt/inadvertent interruption of the infusion, and its effects on peripheral veins, it should be administered through an indwelling central venous catheter. Common side effects of epoprostenol therapy include headache, flushing, jaw pain with initial mastication, diarrhea, nausea, a blotchy erythematous rash, and musculoskeletal aches and pain (predominantly involving the legs and feet). These tend to be dose dependent and often respond to a cautious reduction in dose. Severe side effects can occur with overdosage of the drug. Acutely, overdosage can lead to systemic hypotension. Chronic overdosage can

lead to the development of a hyperdynamic state and high output cardiac failure.[21] Abrupt or inadvertent interruption of the epoprostenol infusion should be avoided, because this may lead to a rebound worsening of pulmonary hypertension with symptomatic deterioration and even death. Other complications of chronic intravenous therapy with epoprostenol include line-related infections (which can range from small exit site reactions to tunnel infections and cellulitis to bacteremic infections with sepsis), catheter-associated venous thrombosis, systemic hypotension, thrombocytopenia, and ascites.

The beneficial effects of epoprostenol therapy appear to be sustained for years in many patients with IPAH/PPH. Barst and coworkers[22] reported long-term benefit in a small group of patients from several centers involved in the earliest clinical usage of epoprostenol. Shapiro and colleagues[23] and McLaughlin and associates[24] have described sustained benefit in larger numbers of patients. McLaughlin and associates have reported long-term epoprostenol therapy in 162 patients with IPAH/PPH followed for a mean of 36.3 months.[25] Observed survival with epoprostenol therapy at 1, 2, and 3 years was 87.8%, 76.3%, and 62.8% and was significantly greater than the expected survival of 58.9%, 46.3%, and 35.4% based on historical data.

Treprostinil

Treprostinil, a prostacyclin analog with a half-life of 3 hours, is stable at room temperature. An international, placebo-controlled, randomized trial demonstrated that treprostinil improved exercise tolerance, although the 16-meter median difference between treatment groups in 6-minute walk distance was relatively modest.[26] Treprostinil also improved hemodynamic parameters. Common side effects included headache, diarrhea, nausea, rash, and jaw pain. Side effects related to the infusion site were common (85% of patients complained of infusion site pain and 83% had erythema or induration at the infusion site).

Inhaled Iloprost

Iloprost is a chemically stable prostacyclin analog, with a serum half-life of 20 to 25 minutes.[27] In IPAH/PPH, acute inhalation of iloprost resulted in a more potent pulmonary vasodilator effect than acute nitric oxide inhalation.[28,29] In uncontrolled and controlled studies of iloprost for various forms of PAH,[30-32] inhaled iloprost at a total daily dose of 30 to 200 μg divided in 6 to 12 inhalations improved functional class, exercise capacity, and pulmonary hemodynamics for periods up to 1 year of follow-up. The treatment was generally well tolerated except for mild coughing, minor headache, and jaw pain in some patients. The most important drawback of inhaled iloprost is the relatively short duration of action, requiring the use of 6 to 9 inhalations a day.

Beraprost

Beraprost sodium is an orally active prostacyclin analog[33] that is absorbed rapidly in fasting conditions. It has been evaluated in peripheral vascular disorders such as intermittent claudication,[34] Raynaud's phenomenon, and digital necrosis in systemic sclerosis,[35] with variable results. Although several small open uncontrolled studies reported beneficial hemodynamic effects with beraprost in patients with IPAH/PPH,[33,36,37] two randomized, double-blind, placebo-controlled trials have shown only modest improvement and suggest that beneficial effects of beraprost may diminish with time.[38,39]

Endothelin Receptor Antagonists

Endothelin-1 is a vasoconstrictor and a smooth muscle mitogen that may contribute to the pathogenesis of PAH.[40] Endothelin-1 expression, production, and concentration in plasma[41,42] and lung tissue[43] are elevated in patients with PAH, and these levels are correlated with disease severity.[43]

Bosentan

Bosentan is a dual endothelin receptor blocker that has been shown to improve pulmonary hemodynamics and exercise tolerance and delay the time to clinical worsening in PAH patients falling into NYHA Classes III and IV.[44,45] The most frequent and potentially serious side effect with bosentan is dose-dependent abnormal hepatic function (as indicated by elevated levels of alanine aminotransferase and/or aspartate aminotransferase). Because of the risk of potential hepatoxicity, the FDA requires that liver function tests be performed at least monthly in patients receiving this drug. Bosentan may also be associated with the development of anemia, which is typically mild: hemoglobin/hematocrit should be checked regularly.

Phosphodiesterase Inhibitors

Phosphodiesterases (PDEs) are enzymes that hydrolyze the cyclic nucleotides, cyclic adenosine monophosphate (cAMP) and cyclic guanosine monophosphate (cGMP), and limit their intracellular signaling. Drugs that selectively inhibit cGMP-specific PDEs (or type 5, PDE5 inhibitors) augment the pulmonary vascular response to endogenous or inhaled nitric oxide in models of pulmonary hypertension.[46-52] PDE5 is strongly expressed in the lung, and *PDE5* gene expression and activity are increased in chronic pulmonary hypertension.[53,54]

Dipyridamole

Early studies demonstrated that dipyridamole can lower pulmonary vascular resistance (PVR), attenuate hypoxic pulmonary vasoconstriction, decrease pulmonary hypertension, and, at least in some cases, augment or prolong the effects of inhaled nitric oxide in children with pulmonary hypertension.[51,55] Some patients who failed to respond to inhaled nitric oxide responded to the combination of inhaled nitric oxide plus dipyridamole.[51]

Sildenafil

Sildenafil is a potent specific PDE5 inhibitor that is approved for erectile dysfunction. Recent reports have shown that sildenafil blocks acute hypoxic pulmonary vasoconstriction in healthy adult volunteers[56] and acutely reduces PAPm in patients with PAH.[57] In comparison with inhaled nitric oxide, sildenafil produced similar reductions in PAPm; but unlike nitric oxide, sildenafil also had apparent systemic hemodynamic effects.[57,58] When combined with inhaled nitric oxide, sildenafil appears to augment and prolong the effects of inhaled nitric oxide.[57,58] As observed with dipyridamole, sildenafil appears to prevent rebound pulmonary vasoconstriction after acute withdrawal of inhaled nitric oxide.[59] Several nonrandomized, single-center studies suggest promise in PAH with chronic sildenafil.[60-63] Appropriately designed randomized clinical trials are needed and are in progress. Sildenafil treatment in animal models with experimental lung injury reduced PAP, but gas exchange worsened owing to impaired ventilation-perfusion mismatch.[64,65] Accordingly, caution is advised when using sildenafil to treat pulmonary hypertension in patients with severe lung disease.

Nitric Oxide

Nitric oxide contributes to maintenance of normal vascular function and structure. It is particularly important in normal adaptation of the lung circulation at birth, and impaired nitric oxide production may contribute to the development of neonatal pulmonary hypertension.[66,67] L-Arginine is the sole substrate for nitric oxide synthase and thus is essential for nitric oxide production.

Inhaled Nitric Oxide

Inhaled nitric oxide has been shown to have potent and selective pulmonary vasodilator effects during brief treatment of adults with IPAH/PPH.[28] It is a potent pulmonary vasodilator in newborns with pulmonary hypertension (PPHN), children with congenital heart disease, and patients with postoperative pulmonary hypertension, acute respiratory distress syndrome, or undergoing lung transplantation.[68] It is of substantial benefit in PPHN, decreasing the need for support with extracorporeal membrane oxygenation (ECMO).[69,70] Although inhaled nitric oxide has been used in diverse clinical settings, especially in intensive care medicine, FDA approval for this therapy is limited to newborns with hypoxemic respiratory failure at this time.

In chronic PAH, the use of inhaled nitric oxide has been primarily for acute testing of pulmonary vasoreactivity during cardiac catheterization (see earlier) or for acute stabilization of patients during deterioration. Pulsed delivery of inhaled NO has been shown to lower PVR in some patients,[71] and experience with the use of chronic inhaled nitric oxide therapy in children and adults with PAH has been described[72] but is quite limited. Work is needed to determine whether chronic inhaled nitric oxide in the ambulatory setting is safe, acceptable, feasible, and effective.

LUNG TRANSPLANTATION

Lung transplantation for PAH is generally reserved for patients whose condition is failing despite the best available medical therapy. Whereas lung transplantation is challenging in general, it is even more so in the group of patients with PAH.[73] Worldwide, overall survival is approximately 77% at 1 year and 44% at 5 years.[74] Survival in PAH patients undergoing lung transplantation is 66% to 75% at 1 year (one center has reported 1- and 5-year actuarial survival of 75% and 57%, respectively).[75] The higher early mortality in PAH patients may be related to higher anesthetic and operative risks, the need for cardiopulmonary bypass,[76] and the increased occurrence of postoperative reperfusion pulmonary edema in patients with PAH undergoing single lung transplantation. In this situation, reperfusion pulmonary edema may be aggravated by the increased blood flow to the newly engrafted lung. In addition, ventilation-perfusion mismatching can be particularly severe.[77] Most centers therefore seem to prefer bilateral lung transplantation for patients with PAH.[78] The timing of transplantation in PAH is challenging. It is probably most useful in patients showing clear evidence of deterioration, such as decline in functional capacity and the development of right-sided heart failure, despite maximal medical therapy.

SPECIAL SITUATIONS IN THE ICU

DEEP VENOUS THROMBOSIS PROPHYLAXIS

Patients with PAH are likely at increased risk for the occurrence of deep venous thrombosis (DVT) and are certainly at increased risk for poor outcomes as a consequence of the development of DVT. Patients with PAH are prone to a more sedentary lifestyle and to chronic venous congestion of the lower extremities owing to increased right-sided cardiac filling pressures. Hospitalization in the ICU, often with discontinuation of anticoagulation in anticipation of invasive procedures, likely places these patients at even higher risk for DVT. For these reasons, meticulous attention must be paid to DVT prophylaxis.

PROCEDURES AND SURGERY

Procedures and surgery in patients with PAH can be associated with substantially increased operative and perioperative risks, and appropriate precautions should be undertaken to optimize outcomes. As always, careful consideration should be given to whether an invasive procedure is absolutely necessary.

Vasovagal Events

Patients with severe PAH are particularly prone to vasovagal events, which can lead to severe consequences, including syncope, cardiopulmonary arrest, and death. Pain, nausea, vomiting, or even a bowel movement can lead to a vasovagal event in patients with severe PAH. Cardiac output may be particularly dependent on heart rate in this situation, and the bradycardia and systemic vasodilatation that accompany a vasovagal event can therefore result in an abrupt decrease in systemic arterial pressure. Patients should therefore have close monitoring of their heart rate during invasive procedures, with ready availability of atropine or a similar agent.

Avoidance of Hypoxemia and Hypercarbia

Hypoxemia and hypercarbia are both pulmonary vasoconstrictors and can contribute to the worsening of pulmonary hypertension. Oversedation can lead to ventilatory insufficiency and precipitate clinical deterioration. Caution should be utilized in laparoscopic procedures in which carbon dioxide is used for abdominal insufflation, because absorption can lead to hypercarbia. The induction of anesthesia and intubation for surgical procedures can be a particularly high-risk time for patients with PAH, because they are at risk for vagal events, hypoxemia, hypercarbia, and shifts in intrathoracic pressure with associated changes in cardiac filling pressures.

PREGNANCY

The hemodynamic changes in pregnancy are substantial, and volume shifts occur immediately post partum, with cardiac filling pressures increasing as a result of decompression of the vena cava and the return of uterine blood into the systemic circulation. The changes induced by pregnancy impose a significant hemodynamic stress in women with IPAH/PPH, leading to an estimated 30% to 50% mortality rate.[79,80] A meta-analysis of the outcome of pulmonary vascular disease and pregnancy reported a maternal mortality rate of 36% in Eisenmenger's syndrome, 30% in IPAH/PPH,

and 56% in secondary pulmonary hypertension.[80] Because of high maternal and fetal morbidity and mortality rates, most experts recommend effective contraception and early fetal termination in the event of pregnancy.[81] There have been case reports of successful treatment of pregnant IPAH/PPH patients with chronic intravenous epoprostenol,[82-85] inhaled nitric oxide,[86-88] and oral calcium channel blockers.[89] In general, management includes early hospitalization for monitoring, supportive therapy with cautious fluid management, supplemental oxygen, diuretics, and dobutamine, as needed. The use of a pulmonary artery catheter for close hemodynamic monitoring and for titration of vasodilator and cardiotonic therapy has been recommended. Recommendations regarding mode of delivery remain controversial.

PORTOPULMONARY HYPERTENSION

Patients with chronic liver disease have an increased prevalence of pulmonary vascular disease.[90,91] Two forms of pulmonary vascular disease can complicate chronic liver disease: the hepatopulmonary syndrome and portopulmonary hypertension. Both tend to occur in patients with chronic, late-stage liver disease, and each may increase the risk associated with liver transplantation.

Hypoxemia and intrapulmonary shunting characterize the hepatopulmonary syndrome. Shunting may be manifest echocardiographically by the late appearance (after three to five cardiac cycles) of bubble contrast in the left side of the heart. Treatment is generally supportive, with supplemental oxygen. The syndrome may improve in some patients after liver transplantation. Severe hepatopulmonary syndrome may increase the risk associated with undergoing liver transplantation.

Portopulmonary hypertension occurs in patients with chronic, late-stage liver disease and/or portal hypertension.[92-98] Portopulmonary hypertension often differs hemodynamically from IPAH/PPH, and these differences may affect the approach to therapy. Patients with portopulmonary hypertension have lower pulmonary arterial diastolic and mean pressures, higher cardiac outputs, and lower pulmonary and systemic resistances.[92] Later-stage patients may develop hemodynamic findings more similar to those of patients with IPAH/PPH, and this group may have a poorer prognosis and be at higher risk with attempted liver transplantation. It is occasionally possible to make a borderline candidate for liver transplantation an acceptable one through aggressive treatment of the PAH. Supplemental oxygen should be used as needed to maintain saturations greater than or equal to 91% at times. Diuretic therapy should be utilized to control volume overload, edema, and ascites. Anticoagulant therapy has not been carefully studied in this population and should probably be avoided in patients with significant coagulopathy due to impaired hepatic synthetic capability and in patients at increased risk of bleeding due to gastroesophageal varices. There have been a number of case reports and small case series describing the use of intravenous epoprostenol for treatment of portopulmonary hypertension.[99-103] Interestingly, some patients may demonstrate improvement in their pulmonary hypertension after liver transplantation.[104] Other patients may develop worsening of their pulmonary hypertension well after transplantation. It may be possible to wean an occasional patient off epoprostenol after liver transplantation. This should probably be done very gradually, under close observation. The development of increasing dyspnea, fluid retention, or fatigue should prompt reevaluation and reinstitution of epoprostenol if necessary. Because of its potential for hepatoxicity, most experts would likely recommend avoiding the oral endothelin antagonist bosentan in this population.

ANNOTATED REFERENCES

Barst RJ, et al: A comparison of continuous intravenous epoprostenol (prostacyclin) with conventional therapy for primary pulmonary hypertension. The Primary Pulmonary Hypertension Study Group. N Engl J Med 1996;334:296-302.

This prospective, multicenter, randomized, and controlled trial showed that chronic therapy with intravenous epoprostenol improved exercise capacity, cardiopulmonary hemodynamics, and survival in patients with IPAH/PPH.

Fuster V, et al: Primary pulmonary hypertension: Natural history and the importance of thrombosis. Circulation 1984;70:580-587.

This early study suggested that anticoagulation with warfarin improved survival in patients with IPAH/PPH.

Lane KB, et al: Heterozygous germline mutations in *BMPR2*, encoding a TGF-beta receptor, cause familial primary pulmonary hypertension. The International PPH Consortium. Nat Genet 2000;26:81-84; and Deng Z, et al: Familial primary pulmonary hypertension (gene *PPH1*) is caused by mutations in the bone morphogenetic protein receptor-II gene. Am J Hum Genet 2000;67:737-744.

These seminal papers report that mutations in the BMPR2 gene, encoding a TGF-beta receptor, cause familial IPAH/PPH. This important discovery may provide critical insight into the mechanisms underlying the development of IPAH/PPH and ultimately lead to better-targeted and more effective therapy.

Rich S, Kaufmann E, Levy PS: The effect of high doses of calcium-channel blockers on survival in primary pulmonary hypertension. N Engl J Med 1992;327:76-81.

This study showed that a subset of patients with IPAH/PPH demonstrate vasoreactivity and will respond to chronic therapy with oral calcium channel blockers. It also supported the concept that anticoagulation with warfarin may improve survival in IPAH/PPH.

Rubin LJ, et al: Bosentan therapy for pulmonary arterial hypertension. N Engl J Med 2002;346:896-903.

This international, prospective, multicenter, randomized, placebo-controlled, double-blind trial showed that endothelin receptor blockade with bosentan improved exercise capacity in patients with IPAH/PPH and PAH occurring in association with collagen vascular disease.

Chapter 82

PLEURAL DISEASE IN THE INTENSIVE CARE UNIT

John T. Huggins • Dov Weissberg • Steven A. Sahn

KEY POINTS

1. Ultrasonography is an emerging diagnostic tool in the management of pleural complications in the ICU. Pleural ultrasound has a sensitivity of 84%, a specificity of 100%, and 94% accuracy in detecting a pleural effusion. **Use of ultrasonography during thoracentesis increased the rate of accurate site location in 26% of cases and prevented the possibility of accidental organ puncture in 10% of cases.**

2. Approximately 50% of patients develop small unilateral or bilateral pleural effusions 24 to 48 hours after abdominal surgery. These effusions generally resolve spontaneously and do not require diagnostic thoracentesis. Loculation and persistent fever may mandate a diagnostic thoracentesis to exclude infection.

3. **Congestive heart failure (CHF) is the most common cause of all transudative pleural effusions.** Increase in pulmonary venous pressure is the mechanism responsible for pleural fluid formation in CHF. Therapy for CHF-related pleural effusions consists of decreasing preload and afterload and improving cardiac output.

4. **Pleural effusions are commonly observed with pancreatitis.** The pathogenesis of pleural fluid formation in acute pancreatitis involves the transdiaphragmatic passage of amylase-rich fluid as well as increased capillary permeability mediated by the release of inflammatory cytokines. In acute pancreatitis, the pleural effusion is small to moderate and on the left side in 60%. Chronic pancreatic effusions result from pancreatic duct disruption and fistula formation into the pleural space. These are large to massive, unilateral, left-sided effusions that recur rapidly after therapeutic thoracentesis. Fifty percent will resolve spontaneously, whereas the other half require surgery.

5. **Small left-sided pleural effusions after coronary artery bypass surgery (CABG) are universally present in the immediate postoperative course.** Some patients after CABG may develop a moderate to large hemorrhagic pleural effusion associated with internal mammary artery harvesting. Infrequently, a trapped lung can develop months after CABG.

6. **Esophageal rupture carries a significant morbidity and mortality risk and requires a timely diagnosis** so that appropriate therapy can be instituted. Disruption of the mediastinal pleura in effect will create an anaerobic empyema. The presence of food particles and squamous epithelial cells on cytologic examination confirms the diagnosis of esophageal rupture. **When surgical closure is performed in the first 24 hours, survival exceeds 90%.**

7. **Hemothorax can be differentiated from a bloody pleural effusion by arbitrarily defining hemothorax with a hematocrit or red blood cell count that is 50% or more of the peripheral blood hematocrit or red blood cell count.** The treatment of a hemothorax involves volume expansion, correction of coagulopathy, and pleural space drainage with a large-bore chest tube. Guidelines for surgical management of a hemothorax include initial drainage exceeding 1500 mL, continued bleeding of more than 200 mL/h for 2 to 4 hours, or ongoing hemodynamic instability despite aggressive volume resuscitation.

8. **Pleural effusions occur in approximately 6% of patients with cirrhosis and clinical ascites.** Hepatic hydrothorax presents as a right-sided pleural effusion in 85% of patients. An important complication of a hepatic hydrothorax is the development of spontaneous bacterial empyema (SBE). The clinical criterion for the diagnosis of SBE is similar to that established for spontaneous bacterial peritonitis (SBP); however, it is important to exclude pneumonia before making the diagnosis of SBE. Antibiotic therapy alone is sufficient for treatment of SBE.

9. **Approximately 50% of patients with pulmonary embolism develop a pleural effusion.** Pleural fluid formation is the result of ischemia leading to increased pleural capillary permeability, pulmonary infarction, or atelectasis. With pulmonary infarction, more than 80% will have a hemorrhagic exudative pleural effusion. The presence of a bloody pleural effusion is not a contraindication to full dose anticoagulation.

10. **Postcardiac injury syndrome (PCIS) is characterized by fever, pleuropericarditis, and pulmonary**

infiltrates within days to weeks after traumatic insult to the pericardium or myocardium. The incidence of PCIS after myocardial infarction is 4% and is up to 30% after cardiac surgery. The detection of antimyocardial antibodies in the pleural fluid can assist in discriminating PCIS-related pleural effusion from other exudates.

11. **The radiographic sign of pneumothorax in the supine patient differs from an erect view in which the visceral pleural line is visualized.** In the supine patient, pneumothorax gas migrates along the anterior surface of the lung, requiring careful inspection of the base, lateral chest wall, and juxtacardiac areas.

12. **The detection of a pneumothorax in a patient receiving positive-pressure ventilation mandates placement of a chest tube to prevent the development of a tension pneumothorax.** A tension pneumothorax usually presents as an acute cardiopulmonary emergency, beginning with respiratory distress; and if unrecognized and untreated, it can lead to cardiovascular collapse and death.

Pleural disease as a primary reason for admission to the ICU is relatively uncommon. These instances include unilateral or bilateral large pleural effusions causing respiratory failure, hemothorax requiring intensive monitoring for rate of bleeding and hemodynamic status, empyema with associated sepsis, and secondary spontaneous pneumothorax causing respiratory insufficiency and tension physiology. Pleural complications of diseases and procedures performed in the ICU are common and may even be overlooked in the critically ill patient; they are often overshadowed by the major presenting illness that is the reason for admission to the ICU.

The detection of pleural effusion or pneumothorax in the critically ill patient is often a subtle finding on clinical examination and even on chest radiography. A pleural effusion may not be seen on the supine chest radiograph because a diffuse alveolar infiltrate may silhouette the posterior layering of pleural fluid; the effusion may be misinterpreted by the physician as an underexposed film or attributed to objects outside the chest. Pneumothorax may not be detected in the supine patient because pleural air is situated anteriorly and will not produce the diagnostic visceral pleural line seen on upright radiographs. When a pneumothorax develops in the setting of positive-pressure ventilation, it can be a life-threatening event, and appropriate action should be taken without delay to prevent a tension pneumothorax.

RADIOLOGIC SIGNS OF PLEURAL EFFUSION

STANDARD CHEST RADIOGRAPH

In the normal pleural space, air and fluid distribute according to gravitational effects. Air accumulates in the apex and superior portion of the lung, whereas fluid accumulates between the inferior margin of the lung and the diaphragm on erect radiographs. In the critically ill patient, radiographs are often taken in the supine or semi-erect positions, thereby changing the radiographic appearance of free pleural fluid and air.

In the supine position, the radiolucency of the lung base is equal to or greater than that of the lung apex owing to the anteroposterior diameter of the lung apex being greater than the lung base. Furthermore, lateral displacement of breast and pectoral tissue in the supine patient generates increased radiolucency. A pleural effusion is suspected on supine radiographs when there is an increased homogeneous density over the lower lung fields compared with the upper lung fields. This radiographic appearance can be mimicked by patient rotation, absent pectoral muscle, previous lobectomy or mastectomy, scoliosis, hypoplastic pulmonary artery, and pleural or chest wall mass.[1]

On an erect chest radiograph 175 to 525 mL of pleural fluid will produce blunting of the costophrenic angle.[2] This quantity of pleural fluid can be detected on a supine chest radiograph as a homogeneous density over the lower lung zone. An inability to visualize the hemidiaphragm and apical capping is likely to be seen in pleural effusions of at least 500 mL.[3] The major radiographic finding of a pleural effusion on supine radiographs is an increased homogeneous density in the lower lung zone; until the effusion is large, this density does not obliterate the normal bronchovascular markings, demonstrate air bronchograms, or produce hilar or mediastinal displacement (Fig. 82-1). Obtaining an erect or lateral decubitus radiograph may be helpful to confirm the presence of a suspected pleural effusion seen on a supine chest radiograph (Table 82-1).

A common and often problematic diagnostic dilemma is the differentiation of an empyema from a lung abscess. Radiographic clues that are helpful in making this differentiation include the following[4]:

- Bronchovascular markings are displaced by an empyema and obliterated by a lung abscess.
- An empyema crosses major lobar boundaries, whereas a lung abscess conforms to segmental or lobar boundaries.
- An empyema forms an obtuse angle and a lung abscess forms an acute angle with the chest wall.

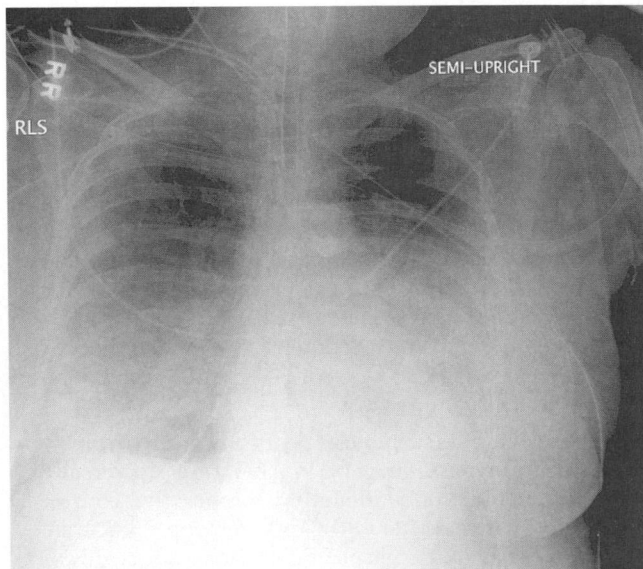

FIGURE 82–1. A semi-upright anteroposterior chest radiograph shows bilateral alveolar infiltrates and pleural fluid veiling consistent with pleural effusions.

TABLE 82–1. RADIOGRAPHIC SIGNS OF PLEURAL EFFUSION AND PNEUMOTHORAX IN THE SUPINE PATIENT

Pleural Effusion	Pneumothorax
<500 mL fluid (small)	Hyperlucency in anteromedial and subpulmonic recesses (64%)
Homogeneous density over lower lung zone	
Veil appearance to lung	Visualization of visceral pleural line (rare)
Lung markings not obliterated	Deep sulcus sign
Air bronchograms absent	*Tension pneumothorax*
500 to 1000 mL fluid (moderate)	Increased volume of hemithorax
Silhouetting of diaphragm	Depression of hemidiaphragm
Apical capping	Widening of intercostal spaces
1000 to 3000 mL fluid (large)	Contralateral tracheal deviation
Silhouetting of diaphragm	
(±) Contralateral mediastinal shift	
>3000 mL fluid (massive)	
Opacification of the hemithorax	
Contralateral mediastinal shift	

- A lung abscess has a spherical shape and equal length of the air-fluid level in both frontal and lateral views, whereas the air-fluid level of an empyema is longer in one of the two projections.
- The air-fluid level of an empyema extends to the periphery of the lung.
- The edge of a lung abscess tends to be indistinct from the surrounding lung, whereas the edge of an empyema is sharply defined.

Because of concomitant parenchymal lung disease in the critically ill patient, the identification of a pleural effusion can be problematic. Therefore, the utilization of more sensitive diagnostic modalities—ultrasonography and computed tomography (CT)—can confirm the presence of a pleural effusion.

COMPUTED TOMOGRAPHY

CT is helpful in assessing the pleural process in the critically ill patient and has several advantages over a standard chest radiograph. CT provides better resolution of both parenchymal abnormalities and evaluation of the cardiomediastinal structures and distinguishes pleural from parenchymal abnormalities.[1] On CT, free-flowing pleural fluid produces a sickle-shaped opacity in the most dependent portion of the thorax.[5] Loculated pleural fluid collections are seen as lenticular or round opacities in a fixed position. CT may also be helpful in the diagnosis and management of loculated pleural collections.[6,7] A reliable CT sign for an empyema is the "split pleura" sign.[6] After the administration of intravenous contrast medium, both the parietal and visceral pleura will be thickened and will demonstrate contrast medium enhancement around the fluid collection. The extrapleural fat between the empyema and the chest wall may be increased.[6-9] The "split pleura" sign is seen in up to 68% of patients presenting with an empyema and is usually identified during the organizing late phase.[7]

ULTRASONOGRAPHY

Pleural-based opacities on chest radiographs are often diagnostically problematic. If the opacity is free flowing on decubitus films, one can be certain of the presence of a pleural effusion. However, in the absence of mobility, the differential diagnosis includes a loculated pleural effusion, consolidated lung, pleural thickening, atelectasis, or consolidated lung. Real-time ultrasonography is a sensitive tool in distinguishing these diagnostic possibilities.

The advantages of chest sonography compared with CT are decreased time consumption, less expense, and greater convenience; for example, chest sonography allows critically ill patients to be evaluated at bedside rather than being transported to the CT scanner. The disadvantages of chest sonography include strong dependence on the operator expertise; inhibition of air artifact in the evaluation of thoracic structures being studied; inferior evaluation of the lung parenchyma compared with CT; and restricted field of view owing to the bony structures of the thoracic cage.[10]

Pleural ultrasound in the detection of pleural effusion has a sensitivity of 84%, a specificity of 100%, and 94% accuracy.[11] The diagnosis of pleural fluid on sonography can be made with certainty when any dynamic sign during respiration is visualized, such as change in shape of the collection, flapping movements of the edge of the lung, undulating movements of fibrinous strands, or swirling motion of debris within a hypoechoic space.

The value of chest ultrasonography to clinical examination for diagnostic thoracentesis has been studied: it prevented the possibility of accidental organ puncture in 10% of cases and increased the rate of accurate site location in 26% of cases. These findings were independent of physician experience in performing the physical examination.[12] It is clear that ultrasonography is an emerging diagnostic tool that can increase patient safety during invasive procedures, such as thoracentesis, and can positively affect patient management and outcome.[10]

PLEURAL EFFUSIONS

Refer to Table 82-2 for a list of the pleural effusions commonly seen in the ICU. Table 82-3 lists the differential diagnosis of pleural effusions in the ICU.

ABDOMINAL SURGERY

Approximately 50% of patients develop small unilateral or bilateral pleural effusions 24 to 48 hours after

TABLE 82–2. LIST OF COMMON CAUSES OF PLEURAL EFFUSIONS IN THE ICU

Medical ICU	Surgical ICU
Atelectasis	Atelectasis
Congestive heart failure	Congestive heart failure
Pneumonia	Duropleural fistula
Hypoalbuminemia	Pneumonia
Pancreatitis	Pancreatitis
ARDS	Hypoalbuminemia
Pulmonary embolism	Coronary artery bypass surgery
Hepatic hydrothorax	ARDS
Esophageal sclerotherapy	Pulmonary embolism
Postmyocardial infarction	Esophageal rupture
Iatrogenic	Hemothorax
	Chylothorax
	Abdominal surgery
	Iatrogenic

TABLE 82–3. DIFFERENTIAL DIAGNOSIS OF PLEURAL EFFUSIONS IN THE ICU

	Clinical Features	Chest Radiograph	Pleural Fluid Analysis	Diagnosis	Comments
Transudates					
CHF	Usual signs and symptoms plus I > O, weight gain, worsening $(P_A\text{-}a)O_2$, $\downarrow C_{ST}$	Bilateral effusions, R > L, cardiomegaly, extravascular lung water	Serous, nucleated cells < 1000/μL, lymphocytes, mesothelial cells, pH 7.45-7.55	Presumptive	Associated with $\uparrow$ PCWP, acute diuresis may result in an exudate
Atelectasis	Asymptomatic or dyspnea, worsening $(P_A\text{-}a)O_2$	Small unilateral or bilateral effusions, volume loss	Serous, nucleated cells < 1000/μL, lymphocytes, mesothelial cells, pH 7.45-7.55	Presumptive	Common after upper abdominal surgery, also with PE, mucus plug
Hepatic hydrothorax	Stigmata of liver disease, clinical ascites, asymptomatic or dyspnea, worsening $(P_A\text{-}a)O_2$, poor response to low-flow O_2	Unilateral R or bilateral effusions, small to massive, normal heart size, no other CXR abnormalities	Serous-serosanguineous nucleated cells < 1000/μL, lymphocytes, mesothelial cells, pH 7.40-7.55	Presumptive PF protein and LDH similar to ascitic fluid	6% of patients with clinical ascites, fluid movement from abdomen to chest via diaphragm defect
Hypo-albuminemia	Asymptomatic or dyspnea, anasarca	Small to moderate bilateral effusions, normal heart size, no other CXR abnormalities	Serous, nucleated cells < 1000/μL, lymphocytes, mesothelial cells, pH 7.45-7.55	Presumptive	Serous albumin < 1.5 g/dL, never have isolate pleural effusion
Iatrogenic: extravascular migration of central venous catheter	Chest pain, dyspnea	Abnormal position of catheter, widening of mediastinum, small to large unilateral effusion	Serous-hemorrhagic, may contain PMNs, chemistries similar to infusate, PF/S glucose > 1.0	Presumptive	Highest incidence with L external jugular vein placement, aspiration or retrograde flow of blood confirms intravascular placement
Exudates					
Para-pneumonic effusions: uncomplicated	Fever, chest pain, $\uparrow$WBC, purulent sputum	New alveolar infiltrate, moderate to large ipsilateral free-flowing effusion	Turbid, PMNs, glucose > 60 mg/dL, LDH < 700 IU/L, pH $\geq$ 7.30	Presumptive	Effusion resolves without sequelae on antibiotics only
Para-pneumonic effusion: complicated	Fever, chest pain, $\uparrow$WBC, purulent sputum	New alveolar infiltrate, moderate to large ipsilateral effusion with or without loculation	Pus, positive bacteriology, pH < 7.10, glucose < 40 mg/dL, LDH > 1000 IU/L	Based on PFA, positive bacteriology, aspiration of pus, loculation	Putrid odor, anaerobic empyema, requires pleural space drainage for resolution
Pancreatitis	Acute abdominal pain, nausea, vomiting, fever	Small, unilateral, L effusion (60%), atelectasis	Turbid, nucleated cells 10,000-50,000 /μL PMNs, pH 7.30-7.35, PF/S amylase > 1.0	PF/S amylase > 1.0 or > upper limits of normal for serum	Effusion resolves as pancreatitis resolves without need for pleural space drainage
Pulmonary embolism	Acute dyspnea, tachypnea, chest pain, $\uparrow$ $(P_A\text{-}a)O_2$	Unilateral, small to moderate effusion, peripheral infiltrate atelectasis	Serous-bloody nucleated cells 100-50,000/μL, PMNs or lymphocytes	Presumptive	20% transudates, effusion present on admission, reaches maximum by 72 h
Postcardiac injury syndrome	Chest pain, pericardial rub, fever, dyspnea 3 days to 3 wk after cardiac injury, $\uparrow$ WBC, $\uparrow$ ESR	L or bilateral small to moderate effusion, L lower lobe infiltrates	Serosanguineous-bloody, nucleated cells 500-39,000/μL, PMNs or lymphocytes, pH > 7.30	Presumptive	Effusion resolves in 1-3 wk, may require steroids
Esophageal sclerotherapy	Chest pain after sclerotherapy with large sclerosant volume, effusion appears by 48-72 h	Small, unilateral or bilateral effusion	Serous-sanguineous, nucleated cells 100-38,000/μL, PMNs or mononuclear, pH > 7.30	Presumptive	Requires no specific therapy, resolves over days to weeks
ARDS	Depends on cause	Bilateral alveolar infiltrates tend to mask small bilateral effusions	Serous-serosanguineous, PMNs	Presumptive	Requires no specific therapy, effusions resolve as ARDS resolves
Spontaneous esophageal rupture	Severe retching or vomiting followed by thoraco-abdominal pain, fever, subcutaneous air	Subcutaneous/mediastinal air; L pneumothorax, followed by L effusion	Early: serous, pH > 7.30; later: turbid-purulent effusion, PMNs, pH approaches 6.00, $\uparrow$ amylase	Pleural fluid pH < 7.00, with $\uparrow$ salivary amylase and positive bacteriology	With early diagnosis prognosis good with primary closure and drainage

TABLE 82–3. DIFFERENTIAL DIAGNOSIS OF PLEURAL EFFUSIONS IN THE ICU—CONT'D

	Clinical Features	Chest Radiograph	Pleural Fluid Analysis	Diagnosis	Comments
Hemothorax	After blunt and penetrating chest trauma, invasive procedures, malignancy, anticoagulation	Small to massive unilateral effusion, other abnormalities depending on cause of hemothorax	Gross blood, PF/blood Hct > 50%	PF/blood Hct > 50%	Often not appreciated on initial radiograph in setting of trauma; should be drained with chest tube
Coronary artery bypass graft	Asymptomatic, dyspnea	Small to moderate L effusion without parenchymal infiltrates, L lower lobe atelectasis, elevation of L hemidiaphragm	Hemorrhagic PF/blood Hct 5%, nucleated cells < 10,000/μL, pH > 7.40	Presumptive	May require weeks for resolution, rarely results in trapped lung
Abdominal surgery	Asymptomatic 48-72 h after upper abdominal surgery	Small bilateral effusions, atelectasis	Serous nucleated cells < 10,000/μL, pH usually > 7.40	Presumptive	Larger L effusions following splenectomy Most commonly found with atelectasis and diaphragmatic irritation, resolves spontaneously
Chylothorax (traumatic)	Asymptomatic or dyspnea after intrathoracic surgery, especially coarctation and esophagectomy	Small to massive L, R, or bilateral effusion	Milky, fluid, nucleated cells < 7,000/μL almost all lymphocytes, pH 7.40-7.80, ↑ triglycerides	Triglycerides > 110 mg/dL chylomicrons on lipoprotein electro-phoresis	Defect in thoracic duct frequently closes spontaneously with tube drainage, minimizing chyle formation

ARDS, acute respiratory distress syndrome; CXR, chest radiograph; ESR, erythrocyte sedimentation rate; I, input; L, left; LDH, lactate dehydrogenase; O, output; PCWP, pulmonary capillary wedge pressure; PF, pleural fluid; PFA, pleural fluid acidosis; PF/S, pleural fluid/serum; PMN, polymorphonuclear leukocyte; R, right; WBC, white blood cell.
Adapted from Sahn SA: Pleural disease in the critically ill patient. In Irwin RS, Cerra FB, Rippe JM (eds): Intensive Care Medicine, 4th ed. Philadelphia, Lippincott-Raven, 1999, pp 714-715.

abdominal surgery.[13-15] The incidence is higher with upper abdominal surgery, preexisting ascites, and concomitant atelectasis.[14] Large, left-sided pleural effusions can occur after splenectomy.[14] The effusions are exudative with normal glucose levels, pH greater than 7.40, and less than 10,000 nucleated cells/μL.[14] These pleural effusions generally resolve spontaneously and do not require diagnostic thoracentesis. Loculation and persistent fever may mandate a diagnostic thoracentesis to exclude the presence of an empyema.

ACUTE RESPIRATORY DISTRESS SYNDROME (ARDS)

The presence of pleural effusions in the setting of ARDS has not been well appreciated. In a retrospective study of 25 patients with ARDS, 36% were found to have pleural effusions.[16] All patients had extensive alveolar pulmonary edema and endotracheal fluid that was compatible with increased permeability pulmonary edema. Several experimental models of increased permeability pulmonary edema have been shown to produce pleural effusions.[17-19] Based on these animal models, it appears that the pleura acts as a reservoir for excess lung water in both increased capillary permeability and hydrostatic pulmonary edema. Pleural effusions in the setting of ARDS are clinically underdiagnosed because they are often masked by diffuse alveolar infiltrates. Experimentally, the effusion is serous to serosanguineous, with a predominance of neutrophils.[19] The effusions diminish as ARDS resolves and require no specific therapy.

ATELECTASIS

Atelectasis is a common cause of small pleural effusions in comatose, immobile patients in the ICU.[20] Other causes of atelectasis include abdominal surgery, bronchial obstruction from a mucus plug, malignancy, and foreign body. The mechanism by which atelectasis causes pleural fluid formation is related to decreased pleural pressure. With alveolar collapse, the lung and chest wall separate, creating local areas of decreased pleural pressure. A hydrostatic gradient is created, favoring the movement of fluid, presumably from the parietal pleural surface into the pleural space. The fluid accumulates until equilibrium is established between the parietal pleura, the interstitial space, and the intrapleural environment.[21]

Pleural fluid from atelectasis is a serous transudate; glucose concentration is equivalent to serum with a low number of mononuclear cells and a pH range from 7.45 to 7.55. Once the atelectasis resolves, the pleural fluid dissipates over several days.

CHYLOTHORAX

A chylothorax is defined by the accumulation of chyle in the pleural space. The three major mechanisms of chylothorax formation include disruption of the thoracic duct, extravasation from pleural lymphatics, or transdiaphragmatic flow from chylous ascites.[22,23] Lymphoma is the most common cause of chylothorax, accounting for 37% of chylothoraces in a series of 191 patients.[24] In this series, the second leading cause of chylothorax was trauma, accounting for 25%. Most of the traumatic chylothoraces were related to surgical procedures. The incidence of chylothorax after cardiothoracic surgery is reported to be 0.36% to 0.42%,[25,26] and after lower neck surgery it is 1.9%.[27] Postoperative chylothorax has been described after virtually every cardiothoracic procedure as well as neck surgery. The highest incidence (4%) of chylothorax has been associated with esophagectomy.[28] Nonsurgical trauma, including blunt or penetrating injuries, can lead to the formation of a chylous pleural effusion. Obstruction of the superior vena cava or left subclavian vein thrombosis from a central venous catheter can produce a chylothorax.[29] Esophageal varices, when treated by sclerotherapy, and translumbar aortography have been reported as rare causes of iatrogenic chylothorax.[30,31]

The patient may be asymptomatic if the effusion is small or dyspneic with a larger effusion. The pleural fluid is usually milky; however, it may be serous, serosanguineous, or even bloody.[32] The pleural fluid typically has less than 7000 nucleated cells/μL and greater than 80% lymphocytes. The pH is alkaline (7.40 to 7.80), and the triglyceride concentration in the pleural fluid exceeds that in serum.[21] Pleural triglyceride levels greater than 110 mg/dL virtually diagnose a chylothorax, whereas triglyceride levels less than 50 mg/dL are usually not chylous. If the pleural fluid triglyceride level is in the intermediate range (50 to 110 mg/dL), then a lipoprotein electrophoresis should be performed to evaluate for the presence of chylomicrons. The presence of chylomicrons establishes that the fluid is a chylothorax.[32]

Up to 2 to 3 L of chyle is produced daily. Severe nutritional depletion and immunodeficiency can result if the losses through the chest tube drainage are not addressed in a timely fashion. The optimal management of a chylothorax remains controversial. The underlying cause, volume, duration of the chylothorax, and the patient's underlying comorbid and nutritional state are important factors in determining the optimal management. Resolution of a chylothorax occurs in the majority of patients with a traumatic chylothorax in 10 to 14 days when managed by a nonsurgical approach, including chest tube drainage, bowel rest, and total parenteral nutrition.[33-35] If the chylothorax fails to resolve with conservative measures, there are several surgical options that can be effective in controlling the chylous leak. These options include pleuroperitoneal shunt, chemical pleurodesis, parietal pleurectomy, percutaneous transabdominal embolization of the thoracic duct, and thoracic duct ligation/repair.[24,36,37]

CONGESTIVE HEART FAILURE

CHF is the most common cause of all transudative pleural effusions; and in one study, it was the leading cause of pleural effusions seen in a medical ICU.[38] The mechanism by which pleural effusions form in CHF is attributed to an increase in pulmonary venous pressure.[39] In a study of 37 patients admitted for CHF, the mean pulmonary capillary wedge pressure was higher in those with pleural effusions compared with those without, 24.1 versus 17.2 mm Hg, respectively.[39] Isolated increases in systemic venous pressure and right atrial pressure are not associated with pleural effusions. Therefore, patients with chronic obstructive pulmonary disease (COPD) and cor pulmonale rarely develop pleural effusions in the absence of left ventricular dysfunction or other causes of transudates or exudates.

For virtually all patients presenting with pleural effusions secondary to CHF, signs and symptoms related to CHF will be present. The chest radiograph will typically demonstrate cardiomegaly with the presence of bilateral, small to moderate-sized pleural effusions. The right-sided pleural effusion is slightly greater than the left. Pulmonary edema is usually present in a perihilar distribution.

Pleural effusions from CHF are transudates with less than 1000 nucleated cells/μL. In up to 38% of patients receiving diuretics, the pleural effusion may develop classic exudative characteristics.[40,41] In the afebrile patient with clinical signs and symptoms of CHF, cardiomegaly, and bilateral pleural effusions (right > left), the diagnosis is secure and observation is warranted. However, in patients who present with fever, pleuritic chest pain, a unilateral effusion, effusions of disparate size, and a larger left-sided effusion, pleural fluid analysis to exclude other causes of the effusion is recommended.

Therapy for CHF-related pleural effusions consists of decreasing preload with diuretics, improving cardiac output with inotropes, and decreasing afterload with optimal blood pressure control. The pleural effusions resolve within days to a few weeks after resolution of the pulmonary edema.

CORONARY ARTERY BYPASS SURGERY

Immediately after CABG, a small left-sided (presumably transudative) pleural effusion is universally present and is associated with left hemidiaphragm elevation and left lower lobe atelectasis. Some patients after CABG may develop moderate to large hemorrhagic pleural effusions.[42] These effusions are associated with internal mammary artery harvesting.[43]

The pleural fluid is an exudate with a low nucleated cell count, glucose level similar to serum, and a pH greater than 7.40. Rarely, a loculated hemothorax may form after CABG and lead to a trapped lung that requires decortication.[44] In these patients with persistent, large bloody pleural effusions and pleural fluid/blood hematocrit less than 50%, a single therapeutic thoracentesis is usually curative if trapped lung is excluded.

Finally, patients undergoing CABG may develop a recurrent, neutrophil predominant, presumably immunologic mediated exudate that is secondary to a postcardiac injury (PCIS). Therapy for these patients consists of aspirin, nonsteroidal anti-inflammatory drugs (NSAIDs), and corticosteroids.[42] Postcardiac injury is discussed later in this chapter.

DUROPLEURAL FISTULA

Duropleural fistula (DPF) develops if there is disruption of the dural membrane and parietal pleura either from trauma or during surgery. Of the 33 reports of DPF documented in medical literature since 1959, 23 resulted from blunt or penetrating trauma, 6 followed thoracotomy, 1 case followed rupture of an intrathoracic meningocele, and 3 followed elective spinal surgery.[45-48]

The pleural fluid characteristics of a DPF vary depending on the cause (traumatic or nontraumatic). In a nontraumatic DPF, the pleural fluid is colorless with a low nucleated cell count, glucose values equivalent to serum, total protein (<1.0 g/dL), and LDH values in the transudative range. Previous authors have described both transudates and exudates with traumatic DPF.[47,48] Because concomitant pleural processes related to trauma (hemothorax) may be present, the diagnosis of DPF by pleural fluid analysis may be obscured.

Beta$_2$-transferrin is accepted as a specific marker for cerebrospinal fluid leaks. The detection of beta$_2$-transferrin in the pleural fluid establishes the diagnosis of DPF.[49] Confirmation with conventional or radionuclide myelograms to demonstrate a fistula between the subarachnoid and pleural space is advocated if surgery is contemplated.

ESOPHAGEAL RUPTURE

Esophageal rupture carries significant morbidity and a mortality risk and requires a timely diagnosis so that appropriate therapy can be instituted. Esophageal rupture most commonly occurs as a complication of endoscopy and can also be associated with nasogastric/orogastric tube placement, Minnesota tubes, and rarely blunt thoracic trauma. Spontaneous esophageal rupture (Boerhaave's syndrome) after severe retching and vomiting occurs rarely and may initially be clinically silent.[50]

The chest radiograph findings vary depending on the interval between the time of perforation and when the radiograph is obtained, the site of perforation, and the integrity of the mediastinal pleura.[51] Pneumothorax is present in 75% (70% on left, 20% on right, and 10% bilateral) of patients.[52] Pleural effusion with or without pneumothorax occurs in 75%, whereas mediastinal emphysema is seen in approximately 50% of cases.[53]

Pleural fluid characteristics depend on the timing and the integrity of the mediastinal pleura. With an intact mediastinal pleura, pleural fluid is a sterile, serous exudate with a predominance of neutrophils, pleural glucose level equivalent to that of serum glucose, and a pH greater than 7.30.[54] Disruption of the mediastinal pleura in effect will create an anaerobic empyema. Amylase of salivary origin will appear in high concentrations in the pleural fluid.[55] The pleural pH rapidly falls and may approach 6.00 owing to seeding of anaerobic bacteria and neutrophil influx.[54,56] The presence of food particles and squamous epithelial cells on cytologic examination confirms and may obviate the need for radiographic confirmation with an esophagogram.

Spontaneous esophageal rupture dictates early operative intervention. If a primary closure is accomplished in the first 24 hours, greater than 90% survival is noted. Survival is reduced if treatment is not begun until after 24 hours. In conjunction with surgical therapy, pleural and mediastinal drainage, antibiotics, and bowel rest should be promptly instituted.

ESOPHAGEAL SCLEROTHERAPY

Sodium morrhuate and absolute alcohol are sclerotherapeutic agents used in the treatment of esophageal varices and are common causes of pleural effusions. The reported incidence of pleural effusions with the use of sodium morrhuate is 40% to 50% and with absolute alcohol 19%.[57] Patients most commonly present with pleuritic chest pain. Pleural effusions associated with sclerotherapeutic agents occur mostly on the right side; however, they may occur on the left or bilaterally, depending on the site of injection. The proposed mechanism for pleural fluid formation after variceal injection with these chemicals involves a transmediastinal spread

of inflammation from the esophagus to the mediastinal pleura. Effusions are radiographically evident within 24 hours and spontaneously resolve by 7 days. Empyema is an infrequent complication.

EXTRAVASCULAR MIGRATION OF A CENTRAL VENOUS CATHETER

Insertion of a central venous catheter (CVC) and its extravascular migration can cause a pneumothorax, hemothorax, chylothorax, or transudative pleural effusions.[58-60] Extravascular migration of a CVC occurs in 0.4% to 1.0% of insertions and is more common with left subclavian and internal jugular vein approaches.[59] The proper placement of a CVC on a postprocedure chest radiograph is confirmed when the catheter is parallel to the long axis of the superior vena cava and the tip is positioned at the right tracheobronchial angle.[61]

In the conscious patient, infusion of fluid into an extravascular space, such as the mediastinum, may result in dyspnea and chest pain. Respiratory compromise and cardiac tamponade can occur with rapid and large volume infusions into the mediastinum. The pleural effusion will have similar biochemical properties to the infusate. If a glucose-containing solution is being infused, the pleural fluid to serum glucose ratio is greater than unity.[59] Protein and LDH values are in the transudative range with pleural fluid protein less than 1 g/dL.

If extravascular migration of CVC is suspected, the catheter should be removed immediately. Observation is sufficient if the effusion is small. Thoracentesis should be performed if the effusion is large or causes respiratory distress.

HEMOTHORAX

Hemothorax results most commonly from blunt, penetrating, or iatrogenic thoracic trauma. Spontaneous hemothorax may be a complication of anticoagulation therapy, and coagulopathy, pulmonary embolism with infarction, ruptured aortic aneurysm, and malignancy are rare causes of hemothorax.[62-64]

It is important to differentiate a hemothorax from a bloody, pleural effusion, because the latter can result from only a few drops of blood in a serous fluid collection. An arbitrary definition of a hemothorax is a bloody pleural effusion with a hematocrit or red blood cell count that is 50% or more of the peripheral blood hematocrit or red blood cell count.[65] A hemothorax should be suspected in any patient with a pleural effusion on a chest radiograph after blunt or penetrating trauma.

The treatment of a hemothorax involves volume expansion to correct hypovolemia and pleural space drainage. Pleural drainage is best accomplished with the placement of a chest tube (28 to 36 Fr. for adults). Pleural space drainage achieves the following goals in the treatment of hemothorax: (1) it allows the clinician to monitor the rate of bleeding; (2) it allows for apposition of the parietal and visceral pleurae, potentially tamponading the site of bleeding; and (3) it will decrease the risk of empyema and subsequent fibrothorax.[63,64]

The guidelines for surgical management of a hemothorax include hemodynamic instability despite aggressive resuscitation, initial drainage exceeding 1500 mL, continued bleeding of more than 200 mL/h for 2 to 4 hours, and a retained blood clot exceeding more than one third of the pleural space.[64] Likely sources of bleeding include intercostal vessels, major pulmonary vessels, great vessels, and the heart. The chest tube should never be clamped, because it will not provide a tamponade effect and can worsen gas exchange and hemodynamics.[66]

HEPATIC HYDROTHORAX

Pleural effusions occur in approximately 6% of patients with cirrhosis of the liver and clinical ascites.[67,68] The effusions result from movement of ascitic fluid through congenital or acquired diaphragmatic defects.[67] A patient with a hepatic hydrothorax usually has the classic stigmata of cirrhosis and clinically apparent ascites. Rarely, an hepatic hydrothorax may exist without clinically apparent ascites, implying the presence of a large diaphragmatic defect.

The chest radiograph usually demonstrates a normal cardiac silhouette and a right-sided pleural effusion in 85% of patients, which can vary from small to massive; effusions are less commonly isolated to the left pleural space (13%) or are found bilaterally (2%).[69] The right hemidiaphragm is more likely to have embryologic or acquired defects.[70] The pleural fluid is a serous transudate with a low nucleated cell count, a predominance of mononuclear cells, a pH greater than 7.40, a glucose level similar to the serum glucose level, and an amylase value less than the serum amylase level. If the diagnosis remains unclear, injection of a radionuclide into the ascitic fluid and detection of the radioisotope in the pleural space confirms the diagnosis.

A reported complication of a hepatic hydrothorax is SBE. SBE is comparable to spontaneous bacterial peritonitis (SBP), which can occur in patients who have hepatic hydrothorax with or without ascites.[71,72] *Spontaneous bacterial pleuritis* is a better descriptive term for this clinical entity. Nevertheless, the criteria for diagnosis of SBE are similar to that of SBP and include a positive pleural fluid culture or total neutrophil count exceeding 500 cells/μL; pleural effusion with a serum to pleural fluid albumin gradient greater than 1.1 is also seen with the absence of radiographic infiltrates. The formation of SBE is a result of either bacterial translocation from infected ascitic fluid or hematogenous spread. SBE can occur even in the absence of SBP.[72] Antibiotic therapy is sufficient for treatment of SBE. Chest tube drainage is not recommended unless an empyema is identified.

Treatment of hepatic hydrothorax is similar to the treatment of ascites and involves sodium restriction, diuretics, and paracentesis.[69,74] The management of hepatic hydrothorax is problematic and often does not respond to medical therapy. If the patient is acutely dyspneic and hypoxemic, therapeutic thoracentesis may be done as a temporizing measure. Chest tube drainage is contraindicated because it may lead to pleural space infection, lymphocyte depletion, and renal failure. Attempts to seal the pleural space with chemical pleurodesis are usually unsuccessful owing to rapid movement of ascitic fluid into the pleural space. Transjugular intrahepatic portosystemic shunt (TIPS) and video-assisted thoracoscopic surgery (VATS) to patch the diaphragmatic defect, followed by pleural abrasion procedure, have been used successfully to treat refractory cases of hepatic hydrothorax but are associated with significant morbidity and mortality.[74-76] Currently, the only definitive treatment of refractory hepatic hydrothorax associated with end-stage cirrhosis remains liver transplantation.

HYPOALBUMINEMIA

Most patients admitted to the medical ICU have underlying chronic illness and associated hypoalbuminemia. The true incidence of hypoalbuminemia-related pleural effusions remains unknown. When serum albumin levels are less than 1.8 g/dL, pleural effusions may be observed.[77] Because the pleural space has an effective lymphatic drainage system, it tends to be the final reservoir for extravascular fluid to collect in those with low oncotic pressure. Therefore, it is unusual to see an isolated pleural effusion due to hypoalbuminemia in a patient without anasarca. The chest radiograph usually shows small bilateral effusions. The cardiac silhouette is normal in size. The pleural fluid is a serous transudate with less than 1000 nucleated cells/μL, with glucose levels equivalent to serum. Diagnosis is presumptive when other causes of transudative effusions are excluded. Correction of hypoalbuminemia either by maximizing nutrition or by preventing protein loss results in resolution of the effusions.

PANCREATITIS

Pleural effusions are commonly observed with pancreatitis due to the close proximity of the pancreas to the diaphragm. There are striking differences between pleural effusions in acute versus chronic pancreatitis. In acute pancreatitis, the incidence of pleural effusions ranges from 3% to 17%,[78,79] whereas the incidence of pleural effusions due to chronic pancreatitis is unknown. The pathogenesis of pleural fluid formation in acute pancreatitis involves the transdiaphragmatic passage of amylase-rich fluid as well as increased capillary permeability due to inflammatory mediators. In chronic pancreatitis, the effusions are associated with pancreatic duct disruption with fistula formation and movement of fluid into the pleural space. In acute pancreatitis, the pleural effusions are small to moderate and are found on the left side in 60%; the effusions may be isolated to the right side in 30% or occur bilaterally in 10%.[80] Chronic pancreatic effusions are large to massive unilateral left effusions that recur rapidly after thoracentesis. Pleural fluid in acute pancreatitis is turbid to hemorrhagic; nucleated cell counts approach 50,000 cells/μL, with a predominance of neutrophils, pH ranges from 7.30 to 7.35, glucose level is similar to serum, and the pleural fluid to serum amylase ratio is greater than 1. A normal pleural fluid amylase may be seen in the acute presentation.[21] The pleural effusions in chronic pancreatitis tend to be serous or hemorrhagic exudates, with amylase levels exceeding 100,000 IU/L.

No specific therapy is necessary for pleural effusions associated with acute pancreatitis. The pleural effusions tend to resolve in 2 to 3 weeks after resolution of the pancreatic inflammation. Some studies suggest that there is an increased mortality in those who develop pleural effusions in acute pancreatitis.[81] The management of chronic pancreatitis-induced pleural effusions is more problematic. Conservative strategies consisting of bowel rest and pleural drainage are successful in only 50%, whereas the remainder will require surgical intervention or somatostatin.

PARAPNEUMONIC EFFUSIONS AND EMPYEMA

Parapneumonic effusions occur as a complication of pneumonia. Although most patients with community-acquired pneumonia do not develop pleural effusions, up to 60% of patients hospitalized for community-acquired pneumonia have radiographic evidence of pleural effusions.[82-85] Most of these effusions are uncomplicated and resolve with appropriate antibiotic therapy. However, in 5% to 10% of patients, these effusions follow a complicated course and will need pleural drainage for complete recovery. The end stage of a parapneumonic effusion is an empyema, which, by definition, is frank pus.

The pleural fluid protein, nucleated cell count, and percentage of neutrophils are not helpful in differentiating a complicated from an uncomplicated parapneumonic effusion. When the effusion is free flowing on a lateral decubitus chest radiograph or ultrasound and has a lactate dehydrogenase (LDH) level less than 1000 IU/L, a glucose level greater than 60 mg/dL, and a pH greater than 7.20, the patient has a high likelihood of pleural fluid resolution with antibiotics alone (uncomplicated parapneumonic effusion). If frank pus is aspirated during the thoracentesis, the diagnosis of empyema is established and pleural drainage is mandated. Most authorities would advocate pleural drainage if the Gram stain or culture is positive, regardless of the fluid biochemical properties. Most clinicians would also recommend drainage if the pH is less than 7.20, the LDH is greater than 1000 IU/L, the glucose level is less than 40 mg/dL, and the effusion occupies more than one third of a hemothorax or shows radiographic evidence of loculation. All of the above findings define the effusion as complicated. A recent meta-analysis examined the diagnostic utility of pleural fluid pH, LDH, and glucose in identifying patients who require pleural drainage. This report concluded that pleural fluid pH had a higher diagnostic accuracy compared with glucose or LDH for identifying the need for drainage.[88] This analysis suggested that a single pH cutoff point is not ideal for all patients with parapneumonic effusions because of the variability of host factors and the nature of the bacterial pathogen. The authors recommended draining fluid with pH less than 7.30 in high-risk patients and less than 7.20 in low-risk patients. A high-risk patient would have one or more of the following: a large or loculated pleural effusion, advanced age, underlying comorbid conditions, or virulent organism (*Staphylococcus aureus, Streptococcus pyogenes,* or gram-negative bacteria). Pleural fluid samples for pH should be handled similarly to blood gas specimens and measured in a blood gas analyzer to ensure accurate results.[82,90]

In nonloculated complicated parapneumonic effusions and empyemas, drainage can be accomplished by chest tube thoracostomy or image-guided percutaneous catheters. No prospective randomized trial exists to guide clinicians concerning the optimal treatment of multiloculated parapneumonic effusions. Nevertheless, potential strategies include image-guided catheters with instillation of fibrinolytic agents[91,92] or VATS.[93,94]

Percutaneous catheters are most effective in patients with nonviscous pleural fluid in the exudative or early fibrinopurulent phase of empyema.[95,96] However, in patients who have progressed to the late fibrinopurulent or organized stage of empyema formation, percutaneous drainage is usually ineffective and slows recovery for this subset of patients.

The options for surgical drainage are multiple. VATS is an effective and minimally invasive approach to drain the fibrinopurulent or early empyema stage. Conversion to open thoracotomy is required in 10% to 20% of patients undergoing VATS.[97-101] For some in the late fibrinopurulent and virtually all in the organized stage of empyema formation and who are deemed appropriate surgical candidates, the primary surgical drainage involves an open thoracotomy. Decortication may need to be performed to allow for lung expansions if there is a significant pleural peel.

PULMONARY EMBOLISM

Approximately 50% of patients with pulmonary embolism have a pleural effusion.[102] There are several pathogenic mechanisms by which pleural effusions form in this setting: ischemia and increased pleural capillary permeability, pulmonary infarction, and atelectasis.[102,103] In the setting of pulmonary infarction, more than 80% will have a hemorrhagic pleural effusion. Ipsilateral pleuritic chest pain occurs in most patients with pleural effusions complicating pulmonary embolism.[102] A coexistent pulmonary infiltrate is noted on a chest radiograph in up to 50% who have pulmonary embolism and pleural effusion.

Pleural fluid analysis is quite variable, and both transudative and exudative effusions can be present.[21] In the absence of chest trauma, recent cardiac surgery, asbestos exposure, and malignancy, the presence of a bloody pleural effusion should increase the suspicion of a pulmonary embolism.[104] In two of three patients, the gross appearance of pleural fluid is hemorrhagic. The number of red blood cells exceeding 100,000/μL is seen in less than 20%.[21]

The nucleated cell count ranges from less than 100 in the atelectatic transudate to 50,000 cells/μL in the setting of pulmonary infarction. Neutrophils predominate in the acute phase but are subsequently replaced with lymphocytes. Pleural fluid eosinophilia has also been described. Effusions from pulmonary embolism are apparent in more than 90% of patients on initial presentation, and they reach maximum volume in the first 72 hours.[102] Progression of the pleural effusion after 72 hours despite therapy would mandate evaluation for a recurrent embolism, a hemothorax secondary to anticoagulation, an infected infarct with empyema or parapneumonic fluid collection, or an alternate diagnosis. In the absence of an infiltrate on chest radiograph, effusions normally resolve in 1 week. With the presence of an infiltrate, presumably representing a pulmonary infarction, the resolution time is longer, typically 2 to 3 weeks.

The association of pleural effusion with pulmonary embolism does not alter therapy. The presence of a bloody effusion is not a contraindication to full dose anticoagulation therapy.[105] However, an enlarging pleural effusion on anticoagulation necessitates thoracentesis to exclude hemothorax, because hemothorax has been described as a rare complication of heparin therapy. The development of a hemothorax during therapy requires discontinuation of anticoagulation, drainage of the pleural space, and placement of an inferior vena caval filter.

POSTCARDIAC INJURY SYNDROME/DRESSLER'S SYNDROME

PCIS is characterized by the development of fever, pleuropericarditis, and pulmonary infiltrates in days to weeks after a traumatic insult to the pericardium or myocardium.[106-108] PCIS has been described after myocardial infarction, cardiac surgery, blunt chest trauma, percutaneous left ventricular puncture, and pacemaker implantation. The incidence of PCIS after myocardial infarction is estimated at 4%[109] and occurs at a greater frequency (up to 30%) after cardiac surgery.[110] The pathogenic mechanism is speculated to be an autoimmune process mediated by the development of antimyocardial antibodies.[111] Pleuropulmonary manifestations are the hallmark of PCIS. The most common presenting symptoms are pleuritic chest pain, fever, pericardial/pleural friction rub, dyspnea, and crackles.[111] Fifty percent of patients will have leukocytosis, and almost all will have an elevated erythrocyte sedimentation rate.[112]

The most common radiographic abnormality is a left-sided or bilateral pleural effusion; a unilateral right pleural effusion is unusual.[112] Pulmonary infiltrates are seen in 75% of patients and are most commonly evident in the left lower lobe. The pleural fluid is a serosanguineous or bloody exudate with a glucose level greater than 60 mg/dL and a pleural fluid pH greater than 7.30. Nucleated cell counts range from 500 to 39,000 cells/μL, with a predominance of neutrophils evident early in the course. The detection of high titer antimyocardial antibodies in the pleural fluid can assist in discriminating PCIS-related pleural effusion from other possible diagnoses, such as a parapneumonic effusion, early post-CABG surgery effusion, or pulmonary embolism.

PCIS is usually a self-limited illness and requires no therapy if symptoms are minimal. PCIS responds to aspirin or other NSAIDs; however, some patients may require systemic corticosteroids for resolution. In those who respond, the pleural effusion resolves in 1 to 3 weeks.

UREMIA

Uremic pleural effusions have been reported in 3% to 5% of patients receiving chronic dialysis.[113] In a study of 100 patients on long-term hemodialysis with pleural effusions, uremic pleurisy was thought to be the cause in 16% of cases.[114] Uremic pleurisy typically presents as fever, cough, dyspnea, chest pain, and pleural friction rub. The chest radiograph usually shows a moderate, unilateral pleural effusion, although massive and bilateral effusions have been reported.[113-115] The pleural fluid is a serosanguineous or bloody exudate, with less than 1500 nucleated cells/μL and a predominance of lymphocytes. Although the pleural fluid creatinine concentration is high, the pleural fluid to serum creatinine ratio is less than unity, in contrast to a urinothorax in which the pleural fluid to serum creatinine ratio is greater than 1 and is a transudate.[21] The effusion generally resolves over several weeks with continued dialysis. A late pleural sequela of uremic pleuritis is the development of a trapped lung.[116,117]

PNEUMOTHORAX

DEFINITIONS AND CLASSIFICATION

Pneumothorax is defined by the presence of air in the pleural space and represents one of several forms of extra-alveolar air. Other examples of extra-alveolar air include pneumomediastinum, pneumopericardium, pneumoperitoneum, pulmonary interstitial emphysema, systemic air embolism, and subcutaneous emphysema.

The classification of pneumothorax is shown in Table 82-4. Spontaneous pneumothorax occurs without an obvious inciting event. Primary spontaneous pneumothorax occurs without clinical evidence of underlying lung disease. Secondary spontaneous pneumothorax occurs as a consequence of clinically manifest lung disease. Traumatic pneumothorax results from penetrating or blunt chest injury. Iatrogenic pneumothorax occurs as a consequence of diagnostic or therapeutic procedures, which may include barotrauma secondary to mechanical ventilation, placement of central venous catheters, thoracentesis, pericardiocentesis, or placement of small-bore feeding tubes. Common causes of pneumothorax in the ICU are listed in Table 82-4.

PATHOPHYSIOLOGY

During normal breathing, airway presence exceeds intrapleural pressure during the entire respiratory cycle.[118] Airway pressures can be increased dramatically during coughing, Valsalva maneuvers, or strenuous exercise; however, pleural pressures rise concomitantly, such that the transpulmonary pressure gradient is changed minimally. With rapid fluctuations in intrathoracic pressures, a large transpulmonary pressure gradient can occur transiently.

TABLE 82–4. CLASSIFICATION AND CAUSES OF PNEUMOTHORAX

Spontaneous

Primary
No clinical lung disease

Secondary
Clinical presence of lung disease
Airway diseases
  COPD
  Status asthmaticus
  Cystic fibrosis
Interstitial lung diseases
  Langerhans' cell histiocytosis
  Usual interstitial pneumonitis
  Stage IV sarcoidosis
Pulmonary Infections
  Pneumocystis carinii
  Necrotizing pneumonia
  Tuberculosis
  Lung abscess
Diffuse alveolar damage
  ARDS

Iatrogenic

Barotrauma
  Mechanical ventilation
Procedure-related
  Central venous catheter placement
  Thoracentesis
  Endotracheal intubation
  Tracheostomy
  Cardiopulmonary resuscitation
  Bronchoscopy
  Nasogastric tube placement

Trauma

Blunt chest trauma
Penetrating chest trauma
Rib fractures
Esophageal rupture
Tracheobronchial injuries

This can surface in the setting of positive-pressure ventilation and bronchial obstruction, resulting in air trapping, inducing a large transpulmonary pressure gradient. When the transpulmonary pressure gradient is transiently increased, alveolar rupture can occur; air will enter the interstitial tissue of the lung and will either dissect through the visceral pleural, resulting in pneumothorax, or move toward the hilum, along with the bronchovascular bundle, creating a pneumothorax.[119,120] Mediastinal air may decompress into subcutaneous tissues or the retroperitoneum. With acute increase in mediastinal pressure, air can rupture the mediastinal parietal pleura, yielding a pneumothorax. it is by this mechanism, rather than by direct rupture of subpleural blebs, that a pneumothorax occurs.[119]

In the setting of a pneumothorax, the lung collapses due to its elasticity, and it continues to collapse until either the pleural defect seals or there is equalization between alveolar and pleural pressures. Occasionally, a ball-valve effect occurs at the pleural defect, allowing an excess of air into the pleural space. This results in an accelerated increase in pleural pressure, producing a tension pneumothorax. Tension pneumothorax compresses the mediastinal structures, causing a decrease in venous return, cardiac output, and, at times, hemodynamic collapse.[121,122]

Patients with primary spontaneous pneumothorax have a decreased vital capacity and an increased alveolar-arterial (A-a) gradient. The development of hypoxemia and increased A-a gradient is due to an intrapulmonary shunt and decreased ventilation-perfusion matching in the atelectatic lung.[123,124] The uninvolved lung can maintain the necessary alveolar ventilation to prevent hypercapnia. In contrast, patients with secondary spontaneous pneumothorax commonly develop hypercapnia in addition to hypoxemia.[125,126]

Because of the potential severity for gas exchange abnormality in secondary spontaneous pneumothorax, it is not uncommon to have these patients admitted to the ICU.

RADIOGRAPHIC EVALUATION

The radiographic signs of pneumothorax in the supine patient differ from an erect view in which the classic visceral pleural line is seen. In the supine patient, pneumothorax gas migrates along the anterior surface of the lung; therefore, careful inspection of the base, lateral chest wall, and juxtacardiac areas should be performed.[127] In a study of 88 critically ill patients with 112 pneumothoraces, the anteromedial and subpulmonic recesses were involved in 64% of patients in the supine and semi-erect position.[128] Thirty percent of the pneumothoraces in this study were not initially detected on standard chest radiography, whereas 50% of these patients progressed to tension pneumothorax (see Table 82-1). Therefore, a high clinical suspicion is essential in critically ill patients to avoid catastrophic complications.

Pneumothorax in supine patients can occur in subpulmonic and posteromedial locations (Fig. 82-2).[128] A subpulmonic pneumothorax may be recognized as a basilar hyperlucency.[129,130] Occasionally, a distinct pleural line may be visualized at the base of the lung. A subpulmonic pneumothorax may be present if there is a hyperlucency extending deep into the costophrenic sulcus (deep sulcus sign), depression of the hemidiaphragm, or visualization of a very distinct cardiac border (Fig. 82-3).[131,132]

Radiographic signs of a tension pneumothorax include an increase in the volume of the ipsilateral hemithorax,

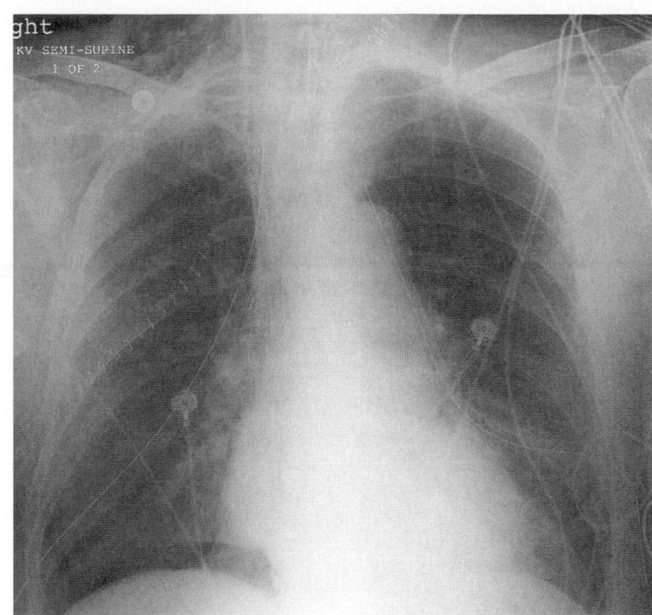

FIGURE 82–2. A semi-upright anteroposterior chest radiograph shows subcutaneous air and a hyperlucency along the right hemidiaphragm consistent with a basilar pneumothorax.

depression of the ipsilateral hemidiaphragm, contralateral displacement of the mediastinum, widening of the intercostal space due to increase in hemithorax volume, and compression of the contralateral lung. In patients with decreased lung compliance, a tension pneumothorax may be present with minimal mediastinal shift and only diaphragmatic depression (see Table 82-3).[133]

If possible, an erect or decubitus radiograph should be obtained to confirm or dismiss the presence of a pneumothorax. In problematic cases, CT or ultrasonography can be diagnostic. CT remains the gold standard for diagnosing pneumothorax, with numerous studies documenting the

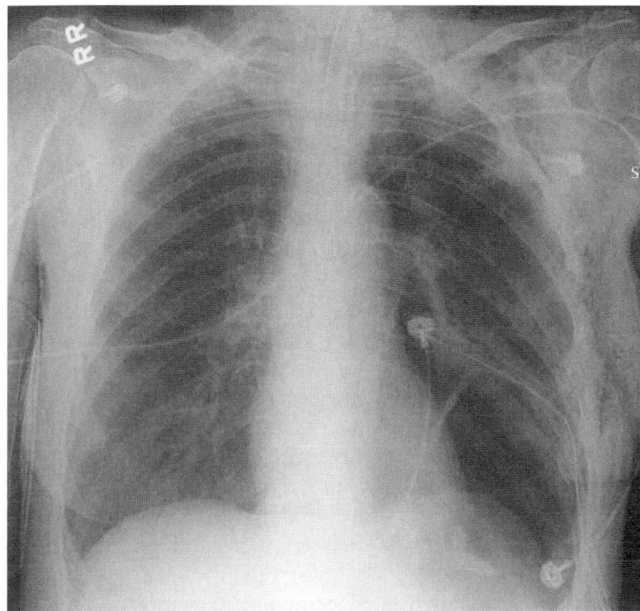

FIGURE 82–3. A supine chest radiograph shows evidence of a deep sulcus sign on the left consistent with the presence of a pneumothorax.

presence of pneumothorax on CT that was not apparent on chest radiography.[134-136] At times, a pneumothorax may be confused with large bulla in patients with COPD, and it may be helpful in making the diagnosis.[137]

Ultrasonography is an emerging diagnostic tool to evaluate the presence of a pneumothorax. Air cannot be visualized with ultrasound; therefore, a pneumothorax cannot be directly observed. On real-time ultrasonography, the absence of "lung sliding" is an indirect sign that establishes the diagnosis of pneumothorax. "Lung sliding" refers to lung movement relative to the chest wall and can be seen as a sliding motion synchronized to respiration. The disappearance of lung sliding was 95% sensitive for detecting a pneumothorax, although false-positive results did occur.[138-140] The specificity of "lung sliding" on ultrasonography is lower than CT or plain chest radiography.

PNEUMOTHORAX IN THE INTENSIVE CARE UNIT

The most common cause of pneumothoraces in ICU patients is barotrauma/volutrauma from mechanical ventilation and invasive procedures. Unlike patients with primary spontaneous pneumothorax, those with secondary spontaneous pneumothorax may be admitted to the ICU because they develop hypoxemic and occasionally hypercapnic respiratory failure. The mechanism of hypoxemia is thought to be a result of the development of anatomic shunts and low ventilation-perfusion defects in the atelectatic lung.[141,142]

In patients with primary spontaneous pneumothorax, the contralateral lung can maintain alveolar ventilation while the hypoxemia is managed with supplemental oxygen. In those who suffer a secondary spontaneous pneumothorax the contralateral lung cannot maintain the necessary ventilation to prevent severe gas exchange abnormalities.[143,144]

IATROGENIC PNEUMOTHORAX

The placement of CVCs is routinely done in the critically ill patient for aggressive volume resuscitation as well as drug and parenteral nutrition administration. The morbidity and mortality associated with CVC use are physician related and are, more importantly, associated with physician experience with placement.[145]

The reported incidence of iatrogenic pneumothorax after invasive procedures ranges from 6% to 52%.[146,147] The wide range in iatrogenic pneumothorax is multifactorial and may reflect institutional variability in the utilization of various invasive techniques, reporting biases, and, primarily, level of training by performing physicians at different medical centers.[148]

The pneumothorax occurrence rate also varies, depending on the type of invasive procedure performed. The estimated pneumothorax occurrence rates for transthoracic lung biopsy are less than 10% to 50% and are 5% to 20% for thoracentesis and less than 1% to 13% for central line placement.[149] The cannulation site for central line placement associated with higher risk of pneumothorax rests with the subclavian vein (13%) when compared with the internal jugular vein (<0.2%).[150,151] Most pneumothoraces occur at the time of central line placement and result from direct lung puncture. Delayed pneumothoraces have been reported; therefore, it is prudent to view a chest radiograph

12 to 24 hours after the procedure. Bilateral pneumothoraces have been reported after unilateral attempts, and death can occur if the diagnosis is delayed.

Cardiopulmonary resuscitation has been noted as a cause of iatrogenic pneumothorax. A pneumothorax may occur in this setting either from rib fractures sustained during resuscitation or from barotrauma as a consequence of bag ventilation.[152,153] Because of these observations, a chest radiograph should be obtained in all patients after successful resuscitation to evaluate for pneumothorax. Furthermore, if a patient becomes difficult to bag ventilate, if subcutaneous emphysema develops, or if electromechanical dissociation is present, the diagnosis of a tension pneumothorax should be suspected. Immediate steps should be undertaken to decompress, because this may be a lifesaving endeavor.

Pneumothorax has been reported after endotracheal intubation. The mechanism of pneumothorax in this setting is due to rupture of the membranous portion of the trachea.[154,155] The incidence of pneumothorax after endotracheal intubation is reported to be approximately 1%.[156] Pneumothorax has also been reported with open or bedside percutaneous dilational tracheostomy. The incidence of pneumothorax after tracheostomy ranges from less than 1% to 4%.[157-159]

Bronchoscopy in critically ill patients may also cause a pneumothorax. The risk is higher when transbronchial biopsies are performed compared with bronchoalveolar lavage (BAL). The degree of risk for pneumothorax in the setting of bronchoscopy for those on positive-pressure ventilation compared with nonventilated patients is unknown. Furthermore, the performance of BAL alone may produce a pneumothorax, and all ventilated patients undergoing BAL should have a chest radiograph to exclude pneumothorax.[160-162]

BAROTRAUMA

Because of the widespread use of mechanical ventilation, pulmonary barotrauma is recognized as a common clinical problem. In the 1970s, mechanical ventilation–related iatrogenic pneumothorax was the leading cause of pneumothoraces in the ICU.[148] Barotrauma is manifested by parenchymal interstitial gas, pneumomediastinum, subcutaneous emphysema, pneumoperitoneum, and pneumothorax.[163-165]

The form most clinically relevant is pneumothorax, occurring in 1% to 15% of all patients on positive-pressure ventilation. In patients with ARDS, pneumothorax may occur in 25% to 87%.[166,167] Important predictors in the development of a pneumothorax include the number of ventilator days, underlying lung disease (ARDS, necrotizing pneumonia, COPD), plateau pressures, and the use of positive end-expiratory pressure (PEEP).[163-165] When a pneumothorax develops in the setting of positive-pressure ventilation, 30% to 97% of patients develop tension pneumothorax.[167-169]

Currently, there is a decline in mechanical ventilation–related pneumothoraces. The decline may be attributed to newer ventilator modes and strategies.[170-171] Limiting the delivered tidal volume, utilizing permissive hypercapnia, and setting PEEP above the lower inflection point on static pressure-volume curves appear to have lowered the incidence of iatrogenic pneumothoraces in ARDS.

When evidence of barotrauma without pneumothorax is observed in a patient requiring mechanical ventilation, immediate attempts should be made to lower the plateau airway pressure. This can be accomplished by decreasing tidal volumes and allowing for controlled hypoventilation.[172,173] Decreases in inspiratory flow rates and attempts to minimize PEEP should be strongly considered. In situations in which ventilator-patient dyssynchrony is present, neuromuscular blockers and sedatives should be considered.[174] There is no evidence to support the use of prophylactic chest tubes for those with barotrauma without pneumothorax. However, this subgroup of patients should be monitored closely for the development of a tension pneumothorax and provisions made to perform an emergent bedside tube thoracostomy.

TENSION PNEUMOTHORAX

A tension pneumothorax occurs when intrapleural pressure exceeds atmospheric pressure throughout the respiratory cycle. Tension pneumothorax occurs when a one-way valve exists on either the visceral or mediastinal pleura, allowing air to enter the pleural space during inspiration and close during expiration, preventing the egress of air from the pleural space.[175]

A tension pneumothorax usually presents as an acute cardiopulmonary emergency, beginning with respiratory distress; if unrecognized and untreated, it progresses to cardiovascular collapse and subsequent death. Conscious patients with tension pneumothorax appear acutely ill with dyspnea, tachypnea, tachycardia, and cyanosis. The following are evident on physical examination: decreased ipsilateral breath sounds, hyperresonance to percussion, distended neck veins, tracheal deviation to the contralateral side, and hypotension. Hypoxemia may be one of the earlier signs of a tension pneumothorax in the unconscious or critically ill patient. For those on mechanical ventilation, increasing PEEP and plateau air pressures, decreasing static and dynamic lung compliance, and the development of auto-PEEP should alert the clinician of the possibility of a tension pneumothorax. Difficulty in bag ventilation in delivering adequate tidal volumes may be noted. Furthermore, it is paramount to consider a tension pneumothorax in the differential diagnosis of any patient who develops pulseless electrical activity (electromechanical disassociation).

When the clinical signs and symptoms are noted in mechanically ventilated patients, treatment should not be delayed to obtain radiographic confirmation. This point is illustrated in a report of 74 patients who developed mechanical ventilator-associated pneumothoraces. The diagnosis of pneumothorax was made clinically in 45 (61%) patients based on hypotension, hyperresonance, decreased breath sounds, and tachycardia.[176] The mortality rate was 7% in the patients diagnosed clinically. The diagnosis of the remaining 29 patients was delayed between 30 minutes to 8 hours, and 31% mortality secondary to tension pneumothorax was reported. In summary, the diagnosis of a tension pneumothorax is a clinical diagnosis, and radiographic findings of tension pneumothorax, such as contralateral mediastinal shift, tracheal deviation, and ipsilateral diaphragmatic depression, may be absent on chest radiographs.[133,177]

MANAGEMENT OF IATROGENIC AND TENSION PNEUMOTHORAX

Most critically ill patients in the ICU have poor underlying cardiopulmonary reserves and may be unable to tolerate even a minimal pneumothorax. In nonventilated patients who sustain an iatrogenic pneumothorax after placement of a CVC, close observation and supplemental oxygen are recommended in those who have minimal symptoms and a small (<15%) pneumothorax. If a patient is more symptomatic or has a larger pneumothorax (>15%), placement of a small-bore chest tube is recommended.[178,179] In the ACCP consensus statement, the distance between the chest wall and visceral pleural surface can be used in substitution of the percent of lung collapse. Based on these guidelines, observation is done for a pneumothorax of less than 3 cm and pleural drainage is required for 3 cm or greater of lung collapse.

Patients with iatrogenic pneumothoraces on mechanical ventilation, regardless of cause, are highly likely to develop a tension pneumothorax. All patients in this setting require placement of a chest tube; observation should not be considered.

TRAUMATIC PNEUMOTHORAX

Traumatic pneumothoraces can be either closed or open and are usually accompanied by additional injuries, such as pulmonary contusion, fractured ribs, flail chest, and ARDS. Diagnosis of pneumothorax by chest radiography may be difficult in this setting, and these patients may require chest CT. The management follows the same guidelines as for spontaneous pneumothorax, with modifications for concomitant injuries.

PERSISTENT PNEUMOTHORAX

Pneumothorax is defined as persistent when it lasts more than 10 days, while treated uninterruptedly by tube thoracostomy with underwater seal, with or without suction. The most common cause of persistence is bronchopleural fistula[8,27,180,181]; other causes include formation of fibrinous peel over the lung, pleural adhesions, bronchial or pulmonary tear due to trauma, and bronchial obstruction. The possibility of obstruction mandates bronchoscopy to rule out mucus plugs, tumor, or a foreign body. Extraction of the foreign body or aspiration of bronchial secretions will nearly always result in immediate expansion of the lung.[21,182] Other causes of persistence are best sought by inspection of the pleura at thoracoscopy. Thoracoscopy is also indicated for evaluation of patients with recurrent pneumothorax. Approximately 90% of patients with pneumothorax suffer either one or two episodes of pneumothorax on the same side, and only 10% have three or more ipsilateral episodes.[11,183] While those 90% do not usually need further investigation, thoracoscopy is indicated in the 10% who experience multiple recurrences. It enables direct inspection of the entire pleural surface and search for causes of recurrence.

The use of direct thoracoscopy in the management of pneumothorax was first suggested by Anton Sattler in 1937.[28,184] Using an instrument of his own device, he observed pleural changes in patients with pneumothorax, either recurrent or persistent, and suggested immediate treatment according to findings. It has been recommended that thoracoscopy be performed for persistence, or for second ipsilateral recurrence, when pneumothorax occupies at least 20% of the pleural space. If irregularly scattered adhesions are found, they are divided with diathermy, and then 2 g of asbestos-free sterile talc is lightly sprinkled over the entire pleural surface. If subpleural blebs are seen and the lung is fully expansible, the blebs are excised, talc is insufflated, and the pleural drain is attached to underwater seal with suction. Expansion is thus maintained, while adhesions form, preventing further episodes of recurrence. If there is a tear and the lung does not expand well, all blebs are resected and the tear is stapled. Finding a large emphysematous bulla makes resection mandatory. Presence of pleural fibrosis mandates decortication, either open or thoracoscopic. If no abnormalities are found, talc is insufflated, and a pleural drain is attached to underwater seal with suction.[29,182] ARDS after the use of talc has been reported by Rinaldo and associates.[30,186] This is apparently a dose-related phenomenon, and the amount of talc used per insufflation should be less than 2 g.[31,187]

Of other agents used to obliterate the pleural space, tetracycline, bleomycin, and quinacrine were used most commonly. However, the use of tetracycline results in much pain. Stephenson compared it to injecting scalding water through the pleural tube.[32,188] Therefore, it must be used with the patient under heavy sedation. In addition, the effectiveness of tetracycline is only about 50%, compared with 95% for talc.[33,34,189,190] Bleomycin and quinacrine are systemically absorbed, and both have a potential for systemic toxicity.[31,35-37,187,191-193] Alternatively, obliteration of the pleural cavity can be achieved without the use of any chemical agents, by surgical means only. It includes suture or stapling of air leaks, resection of all blebs and bullae, and either abrasion of the entire pleural surface using dry gauze or a limited apical pleurectomy.[38,194] Both procedures are highly effective and can be performed either through a small, muscle-sparing axillary thoracotomy[39,40,195,196] or with VATS.[41,197] Hemostasis must be meticulous and, at the end of the procedure, a large-bore pleural drain should be placed at the apex of the chest cavity.

ANNOTATED REFERENCES

Aberle DR, Wiener-Kronish JP, Webb WR, et al: Hydrostatic vs increased permeability pulmonary edema: Diagnosis based on radiographic criteria in critically ill patients. Radiology 1988;168:73-79.
  In a retrospective study of 25 patients with ARDS, 36% were found to have pleural effusions.

Baumann MH, Strange C: Treatment of spontaneous pneumothorax: A more aggressive approach? Chest 1997;112:789-804.
  An exhaustive review of all available approaches to pneumothorax.

Colt HG, Russack V, Chiu Y, et al: A comparison of thoracoscopic talc insufflation, slurry, and mechanical abrasion pleurodesis. Chest 1997;111:442-448.
  In this experimental work, four different methods of creating pleural adhesions are compared. Thoracoscopic talc insufflation was consistently effective and more reliable than other methods.

Deslauriers J, Piraux M: Diagnosis and management of spontaneous pneumothorax in the young adult: Role of parietal pleurectomy. In Deslauriers J, Laquet LK (eds): Thoracic surgery: Surgical management of pleural diseases. St. Louis, Mosby, 1990, pp 119-127.
  A strong case for apical parietal pleurectomy as the most reliable method to prevent recurrences of pneumothorax.

Duntley P, Siever J, Korwes ML, et al: Vascular erosion by central venous catheters: Clinical features and outcomes. Chest 1992;101:1633-1638.
  In this study, extravascular migration of a central venous catheter occurred in 0.4% to 1.0% of insertions and was more common with left subclavian and internal jugular vein approaches.

Jarratt MJ, Sahn SA: Pleural effusions in hospitalized patients receiving long-term hemodialysis. Chest 1995;108:470-474.
  In a study of 100 patients on long-term hemodialysis with pleural effusions, uremic pleurisy was thought to be the cause in 16% of cases.

Khan AH: The postcardiac injury syndromes. Clin Cardiol 1992;15:67-72.
  In this study, the incidence of postcardiac injury syndrome after myocardial infarction is estimated at 4%.

Rozycki GS, Pennington SD, Feliciano DV: Surgeon-performed ultrasound as an extension of the physical examination to detect pleural effusion. J Trauma 2001;50:636-642.
  In this study, the utilization of pleural ultrasound in detecting pleural effusion has a sensitivity of 84%, 100% specificity, and 94% accuracy.

Sattler A. Zur Behandlung des Spontanpneumothorax mit besonderer Berücksichtigung der Thorakoskopie. Beitr Klin Tuberk 1937;89:395-408.
  This is the first suggestion to use thoracoscopy in the management of pneumothorax. It is based on rich personal experience and is the basis of the present treatment of pneumothorax by VATS.

Tocino IM, Miller MH, Fairfax WR: Distribution of pneumothorax in the supine and semirecumbent critically ill adult. AJR Am J Roentgenol 1985;144:901-905.
  In a study of 88 patients with 112 pneumothoraces, the anteromedial and subpulmonic recesses were involved in 64% of patients in the supine and semi erect positions. Thirty percent of the pneumothoraces were not initially detected on standard chest radiography.

Valentine VG, Raffin TA: The management of chylothorax. Chest 1992;102:586-591.
  In a series of 191 patients with chylothorax, lymphoma was the most common cause, accounting for 37% of cases. The second leading cause of chylothorax was trauma (25% of cases) in this series.

Weissberg D, Refaely Y: Pneumothorax: Experience with 1199 patients. Chest 2000;117:1279-1285.
  Summary of experience with nearly 1200 patients with pneumothorax, all managed by one surgeon and his team over 18 years. It brings into account changes in management of pneumothorax that occurred during that time and supplies an algorithm of management.

Chapter 83

COMMUNITY-ACQUIRED PNEUMONIA

Michael S. Niederman

KEY POINTS

1. Community-acquired pneumonia (CAP) is a common illness, but only about 20% of all affected patients are admitted to the hospital and only 10% to 20% of admitted patients require ICU care.

2. Risk factors for CAP becoming severe include smoking, alcohol abuse, serious comorbid medical illnesses, and advanced age. Risk factors for CAP mortality include severe physiologic abnormalities, delays in the initiation of appropriate antibiotic therapy, advanced age, rapid radiographic progression, the development of respiratory failure, and the presence of certain high-risk pathogens.

3. Prognostic scoring systems are useful for predicting CAP mortality but are less accurate for identifying patients who require ICU care. ICU care is needed for patients with respiratory failure, septic shock, multilobar infiltrates, severe hypoxemia (PaO_2/FIO_2 ratio < 250), and systolic blood pressure less than 90 mm Hg. Early recognition of severe CAP may allow the ICU to be used in a fashion that can reduce the mortality of this illness.

4. The failure to localize infection to a single site in the lung, with excessive systemic and pulmonary inflammation, is a common feature in patients with severe forms of CAP.

5. Clinical features of pneumonia cannot help to predict the microbial etiology, especially in older patients with impaired immune response who commonly have less dramatic clinical findings than younger patients with a similar severity of illness.

6. The most common pathogens causing severe CAP include pneumococcus, atypical pathogens (*Legionella* species, *Mycobacterium pneumoniae*, and *Chlamydia pneumoniae*), enteric gram-negatives (including *Pseudomonas aeruginosa*), *Staphylococcus aureus*, and *Haemophilus influenzae*, but infection can also be the result of viral illness (influenza, SARS), bioterrorism (anthrax), and other miscellaneous organisms.

7. Antibiotic-resistant pneumococci are increasingly common and must be considered in the choice of initial antibiotic therapy for severe CAP, but the impact of resistance on the outcomes of patients is uncertain.

8. It is difficult to establish an exact etiologic diagnosis in patients with severe CAP, but diagnostic testing should always include a chest radiograph, oxygenation assessment, blood cultures, and, in selected patients, sputum Gram's stain and culture, bronchoscopic culture, and urinary antigen testing for *Legionella* and pneumococcus.

9. Therapy for severe CAP must be done promptly and empirically, using multiple antibiotics directed against pneumococcus, atypical pathogens, enteric gram-negative organisms, and, in some patients, *P. aeruginosa*. This usually requires the combination of a specific beta-lactam with either a macrolide or a quinolone and sometimes the addition of other agents. Quinolone monotherapy is not recommended for the empirical management of severe CAP.

10. Adjunctive therapies for severe CAP include chest physiotherapy, inhaled bronchodilators, and activated protein C, all used in carefully selected populations.

11. Nonresponse in severe CAP can be recognized as early as 24 to 48 hours and requires consideration of unusual or drug-resistant pathogens, noninfectious diseases that mimic pneumonia, and pneumonia complications.

12. Prevention of pneumonia can be accomplished by focusing on smoking cessation and immunization for pneumococcus and influenza, with consideration of a hospital-based immunization program.

Pneumonia is an infection of the gas exchanging units of the lung that is most commonly caused by bacteria but occasionally caused by viruses, fungi, parasites, and other infectious agents. It is the sixth leading cause of death in the United States and the number one cause of death from infectious diseases.[1] When this infection arises in patients who are residing out of the hospital, it is termed *community-acquired pneumonia* (CAP), although the population included in this definition is expanding. Currently, the "community" includes complex patients such as those who have recently been hospitalized, those in nursing homes, and those with chronic diseases who are commonly managed in such facilities as dialysis centers or nursing homes. This discussion includes pneumonia arising in immune-competent individuals and excludes discussion of patients with HIV infection or traditional immune suppression (cancer chemotherapy, immune suppressive medications).

INCIDENCE

In 1994, over 5.6 million people were diagnosed with CAP in the United States. The majority, 4.5 million, were treated out of the hospital, yet only a minority of hospitalized patients were cared for in the ICU.[1,2] Although the majority of CAP is managed in the outpatient setting, the morbidity, the mortality, and the overwhelming majority of the cost of treatment is focused on hospitalized patients, particularly those admitted to critical care units. In addition, those with comorbid illness and those of advanced age make up a large proportion of the hospitalized, critically ill population. In particular, the elderly have a higher mortality from CAP than younger patients, generally as a reflection of the fact that they more commonly have comorbid illness.[2]

Although CAP can vary from being a mild to a severe illness, very few hospitalized patients are severely ill enough to require ICU admission.[3-5] Torres specifically examined all ICU admissions over a 4-year period and found that 10% were related to CAP.[4] In that study, CAP patients who required ICU care were admitted directly to the ICU 42% of the time, after admission to another ward 37% of the time, or after transfer from another hospital in 21% of patients.[4] In another study, of 395 patients admitted to the hospital with CAP, only a total of 64 (approximately 15%) were admitted to the ICU.[3] Whereas the proportion of CAP patients admitted to the ICU will vary in relation to the types of patients who develop pneumonia, there still remains no exact definition of which patients have severe pneumonia and require ICU care.

Recently, Kaplan and colleagues evaluated the cost of care for elderly patients with CAP in the United States.[5] Using Medicare data, they evaluated all individuals age 65 or older admitted to nonfederal hospitals in 1997. A total of 623,718 patients were evaluated, with 86% being age 70 or older, and the mean age was 77 years. Underlying illness was present in two thirds, with congestive heart failure, the most common comorbidity, present in 32%. In this population, the use of ICU, mechanical ventilation, or both, was common, with 140,226 patients having complex courses of illness. The overall mortality rate was 10.6% but rose higher with advancing age, nursing home residence, and comorbid illness. The mean length of stay was 7.6 days, with a mean cost of $6949, but costs were greater for patients with complex illness and mechanical ventilation and less for those with simple pneumonia. Costs generally paralleled length of stay but were disproportionately high for those needing mechanical ventilation, where the mean length of stay was 15.7 days and the cost $23,961. Interestingly, there was little extra cost for nonsurvivors compared with survivors, except in the group with complex pneumonia as a whole but not in those requiring mechanical ventilation. The findings not only emphasize the high impact of CAP on costs and outcomes in the United States but also demonstrate the disproportionate increase in costs when patients are treated with mechanical ventilation, thereby raising for discussion the ethics and appropriateness of such care in the very elderly.

RISK FACTORS

In all studies of CAP, patients who are admitted to the hospital or ICU commonly have a number of coexisting illnesses,

TABLE 83–1. RISK FACTORS FOR DEVELOPING SEVERE COMMUNITY-ACQUIRED PNEUMONIA

Advanced age
Comorbid illness (e.g., chronic respiratory illness, cardiovascular disease, diabetes mellitus, neurologic illness, renal insufficiency, malignancy)
Cigarette smoking
Alcohol abuse
Absence of antibiotic therapy before hospitalization
Failure to contain infection to its initial site of entry
Immune suppression
Genetic polymorphisms in the immune response

suggesting that individuals who are chronically ill have an increased risk of developing severe illness (Table 83-1). In one study, the mean age of all CAP patients was 59 years, coexisting illness was present in 46%, whereas 74% had a history of prior cigarette smoking.[6] The most common chronic illnesses in these patients were respiratory disease, cardiovascular disease, and diabetes mellitus, findings that have been echoed in a number of studies.[4,6-8] In studies of severe CAP, serious coexisting illness is present in 46% to 66% of all patients.[4,5,9] The most common respiratory illness in CAP patients is chronic obstructive pulmonary disease (COPD), a finding that applies to those with either mild or severe forms of CAP.[4] Among those with severe CAP, cigarette smoking and alcohol abuse are also quite common, and cigarette smoking has been identified as a risk factor for bacteremic pneumococcal infection.[4,10] Other common illnesses in those with CAP include malignancy, neurologic illness (including seizures), as well as AIDS.[6-8] One recent study identified alcohol abuse as a risk factor, along with the failure to receive antibiotic therapy before hospital admission, a finding suggesting that a delay in therapy may convert milder forms of pneumonia into a more severe illness.[7,11] In addition, genetic differences in the immune response may predispose certain individuals to more severe forms of infection and adverse outcomes and may be reflected by a family history of severe pneumonia or adverse outcomes from infection.

PROGNOSTIC FACTORS

In a meta-analysis of 33,148 patients with CAP, the overall mortality rate (OR) was 13.7%, but those admitted to the ICU had a mortality rate of 36.5%, a finding that has been corroborated in a number of other studies.[12] Eleven prognostic factors were significantly associated with mortality:

1. Male sex (OR = 1.3)
2. Pleuritic chest pain (OR = 0.5)
3. Hypothermia (OR = 5.0)
4. Systolic hypotension (OR = 4.8)
5. Tachypnea (OR = 2.9)
6. Diabetes mellitus (OR = 1.3)
7. Neoplastic disease (OR = 2.8)
8. Neurologic disease (OR = 4.6)
9. Bacteremia (OR = 2.8)
10. Leukopenia (OR = 2.5)
11. Multilobar infiltrates (OR = 3.1)

In other studies, the clinical features that predict a poor outcome (Table 83-2)[13] include advanced age (>65 years), preexisting chronic illness of any type, the absence of fever

TABLE 83–2. RISK FACTORS FOR A POOR OUTCOME FROM COMMUNITY-ACQUIRED PNEUMONIA

Patient-Related Factors

Male sex
Absence of pleuritic chest pain
Nonclassic clinical presentation
Neoplastic illness
Neurologic illness
Age >65 years
Family history of severe pneumonia or death from sepsis

Abnormal Physical Findings

Respiratory rate >30 breaths/min on admission
Systolic (<90 mm Hg) or diastolic (<60 mm Hg) hypotension
Tachycardia (>125 beats/min)
High fever (>40°C) or afebrile
Confusion

Laboratory Abnormalities

Blood urea nitrogen >19.6 mg/dL
Leukocytosis or leukopenia
Multilobar radiographic abnormalities
Rapidly progressive radiographic abnormalities during therapy
Bacteremia
Hyponatremia (<130 mmol/L)
Multiple organ failure
Respiratory failure
Hypoalbuminemia
Arterial pH <7.35
Pleural effusion

Pathogen-Related Factors

High-risk organisms
Type III pneumococcus, *Staphylococcus aureus,* gram-negative bacilli
   (including *Pseudomonas aeruginosa*), aspiration organisms, severe
   acute respiratory syndrome (SARS)
Possibly high levels of penicillin resistance (minimal inhibitory
   concentration of at least 4 mg/L) in pneumococcus

Therapy-Related Factors

Delay in initial antibiotic therapy (more than 4 hours)
Initial therapy with inappropriate antibiotic therapy
Failure to have a clinical response to empirical therapy within
   72 hours

on admission, respiratory rate greater than 30 breaths/min, diastolic or systolic hypotension, elevated blood urea nitrogen (>19.6 mg/dL), profound leukopenia or leukocytosis, inadequate antibiotic therapy, need for mechanical ventilation, hypoalbuminemia, and the presence of certain "high risk" organisms (type III pneumococcus, *Staphylococcus aureus*, gram-negative bacilli, aspiration organisms, or postobstructive pneumonia). Other studies have found that when CAP patients have a delay in the initiation of appropriate antibiotic therapy, mortality is increased.[4,9,11,14]

When these findings are viewed together, they suggest some general principles. Mortality is more likely in CAP patients who have severe physiologic derangements, serious underlying illnesses, delay in the initiation of appropriate therapy, and the presence of atypical clinical features. This last factor suggests that an unusual clinical presentation (low fever, nondistinct respiratory symptoms) is associated with mortality, which may be the result of its reflecting an inadequate inflammatory response to infection and because it can also lead to a delay in the recognition of pneumonia and the institution of appropriate therapy.

One approach to evaluating CAP patients is to use a scoring system to define prognosis and predict the risk of death. The investigators in the Pneumonia Outcomes Research Team (PORT) study have developed a mortality prediction rule that classifies all patients into one of five groups (Pneumonia Severity Index [PSI] classes I to V), each with a different risk for death.[15] Patients in classes IV and V have a predicted mortality risk of 8.2% to 9.3% and 27% to 31.1%, respectively, whereas those in classes I and II have a mortality risk of 0.1% to 0.4% and 0.6% to 0.7%, respectively, and those in class III have a risk of death of 0.9% to 2.8%. To use this scoring system, patients have points calculated based on such factors as age, sex, the presence of comorbid medical disease, certain physical findings, and certain laboratory data.[15]

While the PORT scoring system has been shown to be accurate for predicting mortality and prognosis, it is important to realize that it does not directly measure severity of illness, since many points in the scoring system are for comorbid conditions, rather than features of illness. The investigators from the PORT study evaluated the use of ICU by patients with CAP, and the ability of the scoring system to predict need for ICU care. From the original database of the PORT study, 170 patients were admitted to the ICU and compared to 1169 who were managed out of the ICU.[16] Reasons for ICU admission included respiratory failure (57%), hemodynamic monitoring (32%), and shock (16%). While the PORT rule was useful for predicting mortality, there was a poor correlation between the need for ICU admission and the risk of death. In fact, 27% of the ICU patients were in PSI risk classes I to III, and this group, although needing intensive care, had a significantly lower mortality than patients in risk classes IV and V.[16] The findings are quite important for demonstrating that the need for ICU care is not the same as meaning that the patient has a high risk of death. In the American Thoracic Society (ATS) CAP guidelines, these limitations were discussed, including the fact that age and comorbidity are heavily weighted variables for defining mortality risk, tending to move all older patients into high PORT score classes.[1] On the other hand, in a young patient without comorbid illness, the pneumonia must be particularly severe to place the patient in a high mortality risk group, and certain vital sign thresholds must be exceeded to accumulate points toward a poor prognosis. These thresholds are heart rate greater than 125 beats/min, respiratory rate greater than 30 breaths/min, and systolic blood pressure less than 90 mm Hg.

Although prognostic scoring systems can be complex and difficult to apply in clinical practice, the PORT prediction rule has been promoted as a way to avoid overestimating severity of illness, and calculation of the score has been advocated as a way of keeping some patients out of the hospital who have a low risk of death. For the critical care physician, the opposite problem, underestimating severity of illness, is a more serious concern, and the use of the British Thoracic Society (BTS) rule, which is simple and easily applied, may help to avoid this problem. In one study, Farr and colleagues examined 245 patients with CAP and evaluated 42 prognostic factors using a stepwise logistic regression analysis.[13] With this approach, only three factors, the BTS rule, emerged as predictive of mortality in a multivariate analysis: respiratory rate greater than or equal to 30 breaths/min, diastolic blood pressure less than or equal to 60 mm Hg, and a blood urea nitrogen greater than 19.6 mg/dL.[13] If any two of these variables were present, the risk of dying was 9 to 21 times greater than if fewer than two of these variables were present. Overall, the positive predictive value for mortality of finding two of these abnormalities was 28.6%, while the negative predictive value of two abnormalities being absent was 96.9%. More recently, Neill and colleagues used a modified version of the BTS rule, adding a fourth criterion, confusion, to the other three findings and identified patients as having increased mortality risk if two of four criteria were present.[17] This rule was then applied prospectively and was able to identify, on admission, 19 of the 20 patients (of a group of 255) who died of CAP. Interestingly, of the 19 patients identified as severely ill by this rule, only 12 were identified by the clinicians, at the time of initial assessment, as being seriously ill. In this study, the BTS rule was a valuable way to accurately assess severity of illness, which was a problem for some clinicians who did not adequately evaluate respiratory rate and signs of reduced tissue perfusion. One other advantage to using the BTS rule is that the prognosis of CAP can be accurately determined using relatively simple assessments, all of which are immediately available when first evaluating a patient in the hospital setting.

Another modification of the BTS has been termed *CURB-65*, an acronym for the clinical features used to assess pneumonia severity and prognosis.[18] With this approach, the factors associated with 30-day mortality are each given 1 point, on a 5-point scale, including confusion, blood urea greater than 7 mmol/L, respiratory rate greater than or equal to 30 breaths/min, blood pressure of <90 mm Hg systolic or ≤60 mm Hg diastolic, and age greater than or equal to 65 years. In one study, when the score was 0 to 1, the mortality rate was 0%, whereas mortality was more than 20% for a score of 3 or higher, and those with a score of 2 had a mortality of 8.3%. The use of prediction rules is a particular problem in the elderly. Recently, Lim and associates have shown that the BTS rule does not work as well in the elderly as in younger patients, reflecting the altered clinical presentations of pneumonia in this population. In one study, the rule had a 66% sensitivity and a 73% specificity for predicting mortality in a population that included 48% who were at least 75 years of age.[19,20] Interestingly, although the BTS rule was not optimal in an elderly population and did not work as well as it did in other populations, it had a higher sensitivity for predicting mortality than the Prognostic Scoring Index (PSI), derived from the PORT study.[15,19]

PATHOGENESIS

Pneumonia results when host defenses are overwhelmed by an infectious pathogen. This may occur because the patient has an inadequate immune response, often as the result of underlying comorbid illness (congestive heart failure, diabetes, renal failure, COPD, malnutrition), because of anatomic abnormalities (endobronchial obstruction, bronchiectasis), as a result of acute illness-associated immune dysfunction (as can occur with certain viral infections) or because of therapy-induced dysfunction of the immune system (corticosteroids). Pneumonia can also occur in patients who have an adequate immune system if the host defense system is overwhelmed by a large inoculum of microorganisms or if the patient encounters a particularly virulent organism to which he or she has no preexisting immunity or to which the patient has an inability to form an adequate acute immune response.[21,22]

Most pneumonias result from microaspiration, but patients can also aspirate large volumes of bacteria if they have impaired neurologic protection of the upper airway (stroke, seizure) or if they have intestinal illnesses that predispose to vomiting. Other routes of entry include inhalation, which applies primarily to viruses, *Legionella pneumophila,* and *Mycobacterium tuberculosis;* hematogenous dissemination from extrapulmonary sites of infection (right-sided endocarditis); and direct extension from contiguous sites of infection (such as liver abscess).

With this paradigm in mind, it is easy to understand why previously healthy individuals develop infection with virulent pathogens such as viruses *L. pneumophila, Mycoplasma pneumoniae, Chlamydia pneumoniae,* and *Streptococcus pneumoniae.* On the other hand, chronically ill patients can be infected by these organisms, as well as by organisms that commonly colonize patients, but only cause infection when immune responses are inadequate. These organisms include enteric gram-negative bacteria (e.g., *Escherichia coli, Klebsiella pneumoniae, P. aeruginosa, Acinetobacter spp.*) and fungi.

Recent studies have evaluated the normal lung immune response to infection and have shown that in most patients with unilateral CAP the inflammatory response is limited to the site of infection, not spilling over to the uninvolved lung or the systemic circulation.[21] In patients with localized pneumonia, tumor necrosis factor (TNF), interleukin (IL)-6, and IL-8 levels were increased in the pneumonic lung and generally not increased in the uninvolved lung or in the serum.[23,24] In patients with severe pneumonia, the immune response is characterized by a "spillover" of the immune response into the systemic circulation, reflected by increases in serum levels of TNF and IL-6.[25] It remains uncertain why localization does not occur in all individuals and why some patients develop diffuse lung injury (e.g., acute respiratory distress syndrome [ARDS]) or systemic sepsis as a consequence of pneumonia. These complications may result from an inability to develop a brisk lung immune response, as a consequence of either specific bacterial virulence factors, inadequate or delayed therapy, or genetic polymorphisms in the immune response. In fact, one study suggested that if bacteria persisted in the lung in spite of therapy, then inflammation in the form of IL-1β was persistent, and at a high level, presumably being driven by the ongoing presence of the organisms.[26]

CLINICAL FEATURES

SYMPTOMS AND PHYSICAL FINDINGS

Patients with CAP and an intact immune system generally have respiratory symptoms such as cough, sputum production, and dyspnea, along with fever and other complaints. Cough is the most common finding and is present in up to 80% of all patients but is less common in those who are elderly, those with serious comorbidity, or patients coming from nursing homes.[27,28] The elderly generally have fewer respiratory symptoms than a younger population, and, as mentioned, the absence of clear-cut respiratory symptoms and an afebrile status have themselves been predictors of an increased risk of death.[29] Pleuritic chest pain is also common in patients with CAP, and in one study its absence was also identified as a poor prognostic finding.[30]

In the elderly patient, pneumonia can have a nonrespiratory presentation with symptoms of confusion, falling, failure to thrive, altered functional capacity, or deterioration in a preexisting medical illness, such as congestive heart failure.[27-31] In one study, delirium or acute confusion were significantly more frequent in the elderly patients with pneumonia than in age-matched controls who did not have pneumonia.[31] In that study there was no association between the type of isolated microorganisms and the clinical presentation of CAP, except for pleuritic chest pain, which was more common in pneumonia caused by bacterial pathogens such as *S. pneumoniae.* Approximately 16% of elderly patients with pneumonia were considered well nourished, compared with 47% of controls, with kwashiorkor-like malnutrition being the predominant type of nutritional defect and the one associated with delirium on initial presentation. Several other studies have examined the clinical presentation of pneumonia in the elderly and found that a nursing home elderly population had a substantially higher mortality rate than other individuals with CAP (32% vs. 14%).[28] These findings may be a reflection of the fact that those from the nursing home had a higher frequency of comorbid illness and dementia. In another study, Metlay and coworkers studied 1812 patients of all ages and found that with advancing age, patients tended to have a longer duration of symptoms such as cough, sputum production, dyspnea, fatigue, anorexia, myalgia, and abdominal pain.[27] In general, overall symptoms were less prominent in those older than age 65 than in those who were younger.

Another study evaluated 1474 patients with CAP of whom 305 were older than age 80 years.[32] The population excluded those in nursing homes and the population of severe immune suppression (neutropenia, AIDS, and transplant). Clinically, the very elderly had less pleuritic chest pain, headache, and myalgias and were more likely to be afebrile and to have altered mental status on admission. Overall mortality was higher in the older patients (15% vs. 6%), as were in-hospital complications and early mortality (within 48 hours). The PSI values, as expected, were higher in the older population, in part because comorbid illness and age itself add to the PSI score, but, still, the mortality rate for patients in PSI class V was 24% in the younger population versus 32% in the elderly.

Physical findings of pneumonia include tachypnea, crackles, rhonchi, and signs of consolidation (egophony, bronchial breath sounds, dullness to percussion). Patients should also be evaluated for signs of pleural effusion. In addition, extrapulmonary findings should be sought to rule out metastatic infection (arthritis, endocarditis, meningitis) or to add to the suspicion of an "atypical" pathogen such as *M. pneumoniae* or *C. pneumoniae,* which can lead to such complications as bullous myringitis, rash, pericarditis, hepatitis, hemolytic anemia, or meningoencephalitis. As already discussed, one of the most important ways to recognize severe CAP early in the course of illness is to carefully count the respiratory rate. In the elderly, an elevation of respiratory rate can be the initial presenting sign of pneumonia, preceding other clinical findings by as much as 1 to 2 days.[33] In fact, in one study, tachypnea was the most common finding in elderly patients with pneumonia, being present in over 60% of all patients and being present more often in the elderly than in younger patients with pneumonia.[27]

RADIOGRAPHIC FEATURES

The entry point into most algorithms for CAP is the presence of a new radiographic infiltrate, but not all patients with this illness will have this finding when first evaluated. Even when the radiograph is negative, if the patient has appropriate symptoms and focal physical findings, pneumonia may still be present. In one study, 47 patients with clinical signs and symptoms of CAP were evaluated with both chest radiography and high-resolution CT of the chest.[34] Eight patients were identified by CT to have pneumonia; they also had a negative chest radiograph, and many patients had more extensive disease on CT than on chest radiography.[34] The findings of this study confirm the need to repeat the chest film after 24 to 48 hours in certain symptomatic patients with an initially negative chest film. Although some studies have suggested that febrile and dehydrated patients can have a normal chest radiograph when first admitted with pneumonia, the idea of hydrating pneumonia is in the realm of "conventional wisdom" and anecdotal reports.[35]

The presence of alveolar densities (lobar or bronchopneumonic) has been associated with a high likelihood of a bacterial etiology, but there is strong evidence that it is extremely difficult to distinguish among specific pathogens by using patterns of radiographic abnormalities.[36] The chest radiograph may have prognostic value in patients with severe pneumonia, with multilobar infiltrates or rapid progression of infiltrates serving as poor prognostic signs, helping to identify patients who require intensive care.[4] Chest radiographs can be supplemented by CT, which can have value in the critically ill patient in situations when a noninfectious process is being considered, or when complications such as pneumothorax, empyema, or abscess are suspected. CT can suggest certain alternative noninfectious diagnoses such as Wegener's granulomatosis, acute eosinophilic pneumonia, and bronchiolitis obliterans with organizing pneumonia.

When a pleural effusion appears on the initial chest radiograph, it is necessary to distinguish an empyema from a simple parapneumonic effusion, which is best done by sampling the pleural fluid. In some studies, the presence of bilateral pleural effusion has been an independent predictor of short-term mortality in CAP.[37] Pneumococcal pneumonia is the infection most commonly complicated by effusion (36% to 57% of patients), but other pathogens causing effusion include *H. influenzae, M. pneumoniae, Legionella* species, and tuberculosis.[38]

TYPICAL VS. ATYPICAL PNEUMONIA SYNDROMES

In the past, the clinical and radiographic features of CAP have been organized into patterns of either "typical" or "atypical" pneumonia, with the idea being that specific patterns could suggest certain etiologic agents. The typical pneumonia syndrome is characterized by sudden onset of high fever, shaking chills, pleuritic chest pain, lobar consolidation, a toxic-appearing patient, and the production of purulent sputum. Although this pattern has been attributed to pneumococcus and other bacterial pathogens, these organisms do not always lead to such classic symptoms, particularly in the elderly. The atypical pneumonia syndrome, which is characterized by a subacute illness, nonproductive cough, headache, diarrhea, or other systemic complaints, is usually the result of infection with *M. pneumoniae, C. pneumoniae, Legionella* species, or viruses. However, patients with impaired immune responses may present in this fashion, even with bacterial pneumonia. Thus, the ability to use the features on clinical presentation to predict the likely etiologic agents is limited and often misleading.[1,36,39-41]

In one study examining the microbial etiology and clinical presentation of CAP, clinical features were no more than 42% accurate in differentiating pneumococcus, *M. pneumoniae,* and other pathogens from one another.[40] In another study of 359 patients with CAP, a comparison of patients with *S. pneumoniae, H. influenzae, L. pneumophila,* and *C. pneumoniae,* revealed no significant differences in their clinical presentations.[41] The limitations of clinical features in defining the microbial etiology also apply to evaluations of radiographic pattern.[36]

USING CLINICAL FEATURES TO DEFINE SEVERE COMMUNITY-ACQUIRED PNEUMONIA

Although there is no uniformly accepted definition for severe CAP, this term generally refers to any patient who is admitted to the ICU because of CAP. Most of these patients have "respiratory failure," which is defined by the presence of hypoxemia or hypercarbia, and not all such patients require mechanical ventilation. Bacteremia may not specifically correlate with more severe illness, and its presence alone is not always a predictor of a poor outcome, with most episodes of bacteremia being due to pneumococcus. However, in the elderly with pneumococcal pneumonia, bacteremia is present in one fourth of patients with CAP and is often associated with azotemia and multilobe involvement.[42] When an infection, such as pneumonia, is complicated by severe sepsis or septic shock (not just bacteremia), outcome is adversely affected, with increases in mortality, length of stay, and costs for survivors.[43]

In the 1993 ATS guidelines, 10 criteria from the literature were identified to define patients who needed ICU admission, with the presence of any one of these criteria defining severe illness.[3] However, subsequent studies showed that 65% of all admitted CAP patients (not needing ICU care) also had one of these criteria, and thus a more specific definition of the need for ICU admission was required.[3] To better define the need for ICU care in CAP, Ewig and colleagues applied the 10 ATS criteria to 64 patients who were admitted to the ICU and compared the findings to the features present in 331 patients admitted to the hospital but not the ICU.[3] With this approach, a better definition of severe CAP was derived, with a sensitivity of 78%, a specificity of 94%, a positive predictive value of 75%, and a negative predictive value of 95%. This definition required the presence of either two of three "minor criteria" present on admission or one of two "major criteria" present on admission or later in the hospital course. The minor criteria were systolic blood pressure less than 90 mm Hg, PaO_2/FIO_2 ratio less than 250, or multilobar infiltrates. The major criteria were need for mechanical ventilation or septic shock. As discussed earlier, another way to identify patients with more severe illness is to apply the BTS rule in its original or modified version. One study found that the use of the revised ATS criteria had a sensitivity of 70.7% and a specificity of 72.4% for predicting need for ICU admission.[16] The BTS criteria were much less sensitive, with similar specificity, whereas the PORT rule (class IV or V) had similar sensitivity but lower specificity (although this latter rule was very effective at predicting risk of death).

There is some debate about the benefit of ICU care for patients with CAP, but the benefit seems most certain if patients are admitted early in the course of severe illness, thus emphasizing the need for sensitive criteria to define severe illness.[44] The measurement of admission respiratory rate is a simple and reliable assessment, and in one study investigators observed a linear relationship between admission respiratory rate (once it rose >30 breaths/min) and mortality.[45] If patients are put in the ICU when they meet several "minor" criteria, or when they have an elevated respiratory rate, this type of expectant management may have benefits and may keep mortality rates in the 25% to 50% range. This is in marked contrast to the experience of Hook and coworkers, who observed a 76% mortality rate for pneumococcal bacteremia patients admitted to an ICU, leading the investigators to conclude that ICU care could not favorably affect the outcome of this illness.[44] However, in that study, 45 patients were admitted to the ICU and 42 required intubation, a marked contrast to other studies of severe CAP in which approximately 60% of all patients admitted to the ICU were intubated.[3,4] Comparing Hook's data to these experiences, it seems quite likely that if the critical care physician can rapidly identify a CAP patient with a poor prognosis, this can lead to the use of the ICU in an expectant fashion, and this type of early intervention may have a mortality benefit, compared with an approach that reserves ICU care only for patients with far-advanced pneumonia.

ETIOLOGIC PATHOGENS

LIKELY PATHOGENS

Even with extensive diagnostic testing, an etiologic agent is defined in only about half of all patients with CAP, pointing out the limited value of diagnostic testing and the possibility that we do not know all the organisms that can cause CAP.[1,41] In the past 3 decades, a variety of new pathogens for this illness have been identified, including *L. pneumophila, C. pneumoniae,* and hantavirus. In addition, antibiotic-resistant variants of common pathogens such as *S. pneumoniae* have become increasingly common. One of the ways that CAP leads to respiratory failure is when it is complicated by ARDS. All of the bacteria and viruses listed here, as well as pneumonia due to aspiration, have been reported to cause ARDS.

The likely pathogens for infection vary depending on patient risk factors for specific pathogens and the presence of certain comorbid illnesses, referred to in guidelines as "modifying factors," but for all patient groups, including those with severe CAP, pneumococcus is the most common pathogen.[1] In fact, in one recent study, this organism was even identified as being common in patients who had no diagnosis established by routine diagnostic testing.[46] In the past several years, the incidence of antibiotic-resistant pneumococci has increased, and up to 40% of these organisms can have reduced sensitivity to penicillin or other antibiotics.[1,47-51] Not every patient is at risk for infection with these organisms, but identified risk factors for drug-resistant *S. pneumoniae* (DRSP) include beta-lactam therapy in the past 3 months, alcoholism, age older than 65 years, immune suppression, multiple medical comorbidities, and contact with a child in day care.[1,51-53] Other common infecting organisms in those with severe CAP include viruses (e.g., influenza, respiratory syncytial virus, and the coronavirus illness of severe acute respiratory syndrome [SARS]), *L. pneumophila,*

M. pneumoniae, M. tuberculosis, and *H. influenzae* (especially in smokers). In the setting of severe pneumonia, patients can be infected with *S. aureus* or enteric gram-negatives and, rarely, anaerobes. In the elderly, and in those with underlying cardiopulmonary disease, enteric gram-negative organisms are often seen.

The frequency of gram-negative CAP is difficult to define, but in one study of 559 hospitalized patients with CAP, 60 patients had gram-negative enteric infections, including 39 with *P. aeruginosa.*[1,54] A definite etiologic diagnosis of bacterial pneumonia was made if one of the following was present: blood cultures were positive, pleural fluid was positive, or bacterial cultures were positive above a diagnostic threshold using bronchoscopic sampling. A presumptive diagnosis was made if there was a predominant organism on a valid sputum culture. Risk factors for gram negative organisms were probable aspiration (OR = 2.3), previous hospital admission within 30 days of admission (OR = 3.5), previous antibiotics within 30 days of admission (OR = 1.9), and presence of pulmonary comorbidity (OR = 2.8). Risk factors for *P. aeruginosa* were pulmonary comorbidity (OR = 5.8) and previous hospitalization (OR = 3.8). Infection with a gram-negative pathogen led to ICU admission and mechanical ventilation more often than infection with other organisms. The mortality rate of CAP due to *P. aeruginosa* was 28%.

Although aspiration has often been considered a risk factor for anaerobic infection, studies of severe CAP in elderly patients with aspiration risk factors suggested that this population is very likely to have gram-negative infection.[55,56] One study evaluated 95 residents of long-term care facilities who had pneumonia requiring ICU admission, in the presence of risk factors for oropharyngeal aspiration, such as swallowing disorders due to neurologic illness, disruption of the gastroesophageal junction, dysphagia, or anatomic abnormalities. Using protected bronchoalveolar lavage (BAL) sampling within 4 hours of admission, a total of 67 pathogens were identified, with enteric gram-negatives in 49%, anaerobes in 16%, and *S. aureus* in 12%. Fifty-five percent of the anaerobes were recovered along with aerobic gram-negative co-infection. The presence of anaerobes did not correlate with oral hygiene but did correlate with functional status, being more common in patients who were totally dependent. Of the seven patients who received inadequate therapy for anaerobes, six recovered, raising a question about whether these organisms really need to be treated. These findings suggest that anaerobes may not really be pathogens but could simply be colonizers in the institutionalized elderly, including those with aspiration risks.[55]

Primary pulmonary infection with atypical pathogens has been reported for patients with severe CAP for many years. In fact, in one ICU in Spain, atypical pathogens were present in almost 25% of all patients but the responsible organism varied over time. *Legionella* was the most common atypical pathogen leading to severe CAP in 14% of patients during one time period, but in the same hospital a decade later, it was seen in only 2%, having been replaced by *Mycoplasma* and *Chlamydia* infection, which were found in 17% of patients compared with only 6% a decade earlier.[11] Several studies have shown that even if bacterial pathogens lead to CAP, they can be accompanied by atypical pathogens, in the form of mixed infection.[57–59] Atypical pathogens can include *C. pneumoniae, M. pneumoniae,* and *L. pneumophila,* and some recent studies have shown that these infections are common in patients of all ages, not just young and healthy individuals; these organisms have even been reported among the elderly in nursing homes.[1,57,60] When mixed infection is present, it may lead to a more complex course and a longer length of stay than if a single pathogen is present, which may explain the increasing number of studies that show a reduction in CAP mortality, including those in the ICU, when initial therapy provides coverage for these organisms, compared with regimens that do not provide coverage for these organisms.[61,62] There may be a particular synergy between *C. pneumoniae* and pneumococcus, with either sequential, or mixed infection with *C. pneumoniae* leading to a more severe course for pneumococcus.[58] The frequency of atypical pathogens can be as high as 60%, in some series, with as many as 40% of all CAP patients having mixed infection.[59] These high incidence numbers have been derived with serologic testing, which is of uncertain accuracy.

Atypical organism pneumonia may not be a constant phenomenon, and the frequency of infection may vary over the course of time and with geography. In fact, one study showed that the benefit of providing empirical therapy directed at atypical pathogens was variable, being more important in some calendar years than in others.[62] The incidence of *Legionella* infection among admitted patients has varied from 1% to 15% or more and is also a reflection of geographic and seasonal variability in infection rates, as well as a reflection of the extent of diagnostic testing.

RISK FACTORS FOR SPECIFIC PATHOGENS

Table 83-3 summarizes the common pathogens causing CAP in hospitalized patients, including those admitted to the ICU. The classification is based on the presence of clinical risk factors for specific pathogens, referred to as "modifying factors." The modifying factors for DRSP are age older than 65 years, beta-lactam therapy within the past 3 months, alcoholism, immune suppressive illness (including therapy with corticosteroids), multiple medical comorbidities, and exposure to a child in day care.[1,52,63] The modifying factors for

---

TABLE 83–3. COMMON PATHOGENS CAUSING COMMUNITY-ACQUIRED PNEUMONIA

Inpatient, with no cardiopulmonary disease or modifying factors	*Streptococcus pneumoniae, Haemophilus influenzae, Mycoplasma pneumoniae, Chlamydia pneumoniae,* mixed infection (bacteria plus atypical pathogen), viruses, *Legionella* species, and others (*M. tuberculosis,* endemic fungi, *Pneumocystis carinii*)
Inpatient, with cardiopulmonary disease and/or modifying factors	All of the above, but drug-resistant *S. pneumoniae* (DRSP) and enteric gram-negative organisms are more of a concern
Severe community-acquired pneumonia, with no risks for *P. aeruginosa*	*S. pneumoniae* (including DRSP), *Legionella* species, *H. influenzae,* enteric gram-negative bacilli, *S. aureus, M. pneumoniae,* respiratory viruses, others (*C. pneumoniae, M. tuberculosis,* endemic fungi)
Severe CAP, with risks for *P. aeruginosa*	All of the pathogens above plus *P. aeruginosa.*

TABLE 83-4. CLINICAL ASSOCIATIONS WITH SPECIFIC PATHOGENS

Condition	Commonly Encountered Pathogens
Alcoholism	*Streptococcus pneumoniae* (including penicillin-resistant), anaerobes, gram-negative bacilli (possibly *Klebsiella pneumoniae*), tuberculosis
Chronic obstructive pulmonary disease/current or former smoker	*S. pneumoniae, Haemophilus influenzae, Moraxella catarrhalis*
Residence in nursing home	*S. pneumoniae*, gram-negative bacilli, *H. influenzae, S. aureus, Chlamydia pneumoniae;* consider *M. tuberculosis*. Consider anaerobes, but less common.
Poor dental hygiene	Anaerobes
Bat exposure	*Histoplasma capsulatum*
Bird exposure	*Chlamydia psittaci, Cryptococcus neoformans, H. capsulatum*
Rabbit exposure	*Francisella tularensis*
Travel to southwestern USA	*Coccidioidomycosis;* hantavirus in selected areas
Exposure to farm animals or parturient cats	*Coxiella burnetii* (Q fever)
Postinfluenza pneumonia	*S. pneumoniae, S. aureus, H. influenzae*
Structural disease of lung (e.g., bronchiectasis, cystic fibrosis)	*P. aeruginosa, P. cepacia,* or *Staphylococcus aureus*
Sickle cell disease, asplenia	Pneumococccus, *H. influenzae*
Suspected bioterrorism	Anthrax, tularemia, plague
Travel to Asia	Severe acute respiratory syndrome (SARS), tuberculosis, melioidosis

enteric gram-negatives include residence in a nursing home, underlying cardiopulmonary disease, multiple medical comorbidities, and recent antibiotic therapy. In predicting the likely etiologic pathogens for those admitted to the ICU, patients are divided into a population at risk for pseudomonal infection and a population without this organism being likely. The risk factors for *P. aeruginosa* infection are structural lung disease (bronchiectasis), corticosteroid therapy (>10 mg prednisone/day), broad-spectrum antibiotic therapy for more than 7 days in the past month, and malnutrition.[1]

Table 83-4 shows that certain clinical conditions are associated with specific pathogens, and these associations should be considered in all patients when obtaining a history. For example, if the presentation is subacute, following contact with birds, rats, or rabbits, then the possibility of psittacosis, leptospirosis, tularemia, or plague should be considered. Certain exposures should also raise concern about specific organisms. Thus, *Coxiella burnetii* (Q fever) is a concern with exposure to parturient cats, cattle, sheep, or goats; *Francisella tularensis* is a concern with rabbit exposure; hantavirus with exposure to mice droppings; *Chlamydia psittaci* with exposure to turkeys or infected birds; and *Legionella* with exposure to contaminated water sources (saunas). Following influenza, superinfection with pneumococcus, *S. aureus,* and *H. influenzae* should be considered. With travel to endemic areas in Asia, the onset of respiratory failure after a preceding viral illness should lead to suspicion of SARS. Endemic fungi (coccidioidomycosis, histoplasmosis, and blastomycosis) occur in well-defined geographic areas and may present acutely as symptoms that overlap with acute bacterial pneumonia.

Although a variety of radiographic patterns can be seen in pneumonia, specific findings cannot generally be used to predict the microbial etiology in CAP, but there are certain patterns to keep in mind.[35] Focal consolidation can be seen with infections caused by pneumococcus, *Klebsiella* species, aspiration (especially if in the lower lobes or other dependent segments), *S. aureus, H. influenzae, M. pneumoniae,* and *C. pneumoniae.* Interstitial infiltrates should suggest viral pneumonia as well as infection due to *M. pneumoniae, C. pneumoniae, C. psittaci,* and *P. carinii.* Lymphadenopathy with an interstitial pattern should raise concerns about anthrax, *F. tularensis,* and *C. psittaci,* whereas adenopathy can be seen with focal infiltrates in tuberculosis, fungal pneumonia,

anthrax, and bacterial pneumonia. Cavitation can be the result of an aspiration lung abscess, infection with *S. aureus* or aerobic gram-negatives (including *P. aeruginosa*), tuberculosis, fungal infection, nocardiosis, and actinomycosis.

FEATURES OF SPECIFIC PATHOGENS

Streptococcus pneumoniae

This is the most common pathogen for CAP and is a gram-positive, lancet-shaped diplococcus, of which there are 84 different serotypes, each with a distinct antigenic polysaccharide capsule. Eighty-five percent of all infections are caused by one of 23 serotypes, which are now included in a vaccine. Infection is most common in the winter and early spring, which may relate to the finding that up to 70% of patients have a preceding viral illness.[64] The organism spreads from person to person and commonly colonizes the oropharynx of patients before it leads to pneumonia. Pneumonia develops when colonizing organisms are aspirated into a lung that is unable to contain the aspirated inoculum. The classic radiographic pattern is a lobar consolidation, but bronchopneumonia can also occur, and in some series this is the most common pattern.[65] Bacteremia is present in up to 20% of hospitalized patients, and extrapulmonary complications include meningitis, empyema, arthritis, endocarditis, and brain abscess.

In the past decade, antibiotic resistance among pneumococci has become increasingly common, and penicillin resistance, along with resistance to other common antibiotics (macrolides, trimethoprim/sulfamethoxazole, selected cephalosporins), is present in over 40% of these organisms.[1,46,48,51] Fortunately, most penicillin resistance is of the "intermediate" type (penicillin minimal inhibitory concentration [MIC] of 0.1 to 1.0 mg/L) and not of the high level type (penicillin MIC of 2.0 or more). Although the clinical impact of in vitro resistance is uncertain, one large database has data showing that only organisms with a penicillin MIC of more than 4 mg/L can lead to an increased risk of death.[1,47,49]

Whereas early studies could not show an increased mortality rate, after adjusting for disease severity, in patients with resistance, more recent studies have not been so clear.[50,66,67] Turrett and colleagues studied a population of 462 patients with pneumococcal bacteremia, of which more than half were HIV positive and high-level resistance was a predictor of mortality.[66] Other investigators did not find an increased risk of death from infection with resistant organisms but did find an enhanced likelihood of suppurative complications (empyema) and a more prolonged hospital length of stay.[48,67] The conflicting data in earlier reports may have been the result of studying relatively few patients. Feikin and colleagues studied the impact of pneumococcal resistance in 5837 patients with bacteremic CAP.[49] They found an increased mortality for patients with a penicillin MIC of at least 4 mg/L or greater or with a cefotaxime MIC of 2.0 mg/L or more. However, this increased mortality was only present if patients who died in the first 4 days of therapy were excluded from analysis. Fortunately, very few organisms are currently at this level of resistance, but to prevent more organisms of this type from emerging it may be necessary to identify patients with risk factors for resistance and to target them with highly active antipneumococcal regimens. One limitation of the Feikin study was the failure to account for severity of illness or therapy choices. More recently, Moroney and associates used both cohort study and matched control methods and found that severity of illness, and not resistance or accuracy of therapy, was the most important predictor of mortality.[68] Interestingly, in the case-control part of the study, severity of illness was greater in patients without resistant organisms, implying a loss of virulence among organisms that become resistant, a finding echoed in another study that found absence of invasive illness to be a risk factor for pneumococcal resistance.[52]

The relationship of prior antibiotic use to subsequent pneumococcal resistance has been known, and prior therapy with macrolides, beta-lactams, and quinolones has been identified as a predisposing factor for subsequent resistance to the same class of antibiotic.[52,69-73] One recent study has tried to define if usage of certain specific antibiotic classes was more relevant than others in causing penicillin resistance and how long in the past the usage of antibiotics would predispose to resistance.[73] In this study, 303 patients with pneumococcal bacteremia were evaluated and 98 had penicillin-nonsusceptible strains. The use of penicillins, sulfonamides, and macrolides within either 1 or 6 months before infection was associated with an increased risk of bacteremia with penicillin-nonsusceptible *S. pneumoniae* (PNSP). The odds ratio of increased risk was from threefold to sixfold for beta-lactams and pneumococci. Interestingly, the risk was no lower for therapy in the past 6 months compared with therapy in the past 1 month. Although quinolones were associated with a slightly increased risk of infection with PNSP, this increase was not statistically significant, but other studies have shown that quinolone therapy can predispose to subsequent pneumococcal resistance to this class of antibiotics.[71,72] Prolonged and repeated courses of therapy may be particular risk factors for promoting pneumococcal resistance to beta-lactams, sulfonamides, and macrolides.[73]

Legionella pneumophila

This small, weakly staining, gram-negative bacillus was first characterized after an epidemic in 1976 and can occur either sporadically or in epidemic form. At present, 12 different serogroups of the species *L. pneumophila* have been described, and these account for 90% of all cases of legionnaires' disease, with serogroup 1 causing the most cases. The other species that commonly causes human illness is *L. micdadei*.

The organism is water-borne and can emanate from air-conditioning equipment, drinking water, lakes and river banks, water faucets, and shower heads.[74] Infection is generally caused by inhalation of an infected aerosol generated by a contaminated water source. When a water system becomes infected in an institution, endemic outbreaks may occur. In its sporadic form, *Legionella* may account for 7% to 15% of all cases of CAP, being a particular concern in patients with severe forms of illness.[1,11,74]

The classic *Legionella* syndrome is characterized by high fever, chills, headache, myalgias, and leukocytosis.[74] The diagnosis is also suggested by the presence of a pneumonia with preceding diarrhea, along with mental confusion, hyponatremia, relative bradycardia, and liver function abnormalities, but this syndrome is usually not present. Symptoms are rapidly progressive, and the patient may appear to be quite toxic, so this diagnosis should always be considered in patients admitted to the ICU with CAP and in those with rapidly progressive radiographic abnormalities.

Other Organisms

CAP can also be caused by *S. aureus*, which can lead to severe illness and to cavitary lung infection. This organism can also seed the lung hematogenously from a vegetation in the patient with right-sided endocarditis. The incidence of viral pneumonia is difficult to define; but during epidemic times, influenza should be considered. It can lead to a primary viral pneumonia or to secondary bacterial infection with pneumococcus, *S. aureus*, or *H. influenzae*.[75] Viral illness may be responsible for 5% to 15% of CAP cases, and viruses that can lead to respiratory failure, in addition to influenza, include respiratory syncytial virus (which can affect the elderly), varicella (a particular concern in pregnant females with chickenpox), and hantavirus (endemic in the Four Corners area of New Mexico.[75,76] Finally, it important to always consider the diagnosis of tuberculosis in patients with CAP and, in endemic areas, fungal infection with coccidioidomycosis and histoplasmosis, especially in HIV-infected persons.

Several rickettsiae can cause CAP, including Q fever (*Coxiella burnetii*), which occurs worldwide, Rocky Mountain spotted fever (RMSF), and scrub typhus (*Rickettsia tsutsugamushi*) in Asia and Australia.[77] Transmission typically involves an intermediate vector, often ticks (Q fever, RMSF) or mites (scrub typhus) but also sheep, cows, and contaminated milk (Q fever). These infections have a variable incubation period, ranging from days to a few weeks, and are characterized by a febrile syndrome that may have a pneumonic component and a maculopapular rash (Q fever and RMSF).

Severe Acute Respiratory Syndrome

In late 2003, a respiratory viral infection, caused by a coronavirus, emerged in parts of Asia and was termed *severe acute respiratory syndrome* (SARS). The illness affected people from a variety of endemic areas in Asia but was seen in North America when an outbreak occurred in Toronto, Canada. Importantly, worldwide as many as 20% of affected patients were health care workers, particularly those caring for patients admitted to the ICU. Transmission risk was greatest during emergent intubation and was also possible during noninvasive ventilation, making this latter modality of therapy contraindicated if SARS is suspected.[78] Infection control may be quite effective in preventing the spread of SARS to health care workers and includes the careful handling of respiratory secretions, ventilator circuits, the use of N-95 respirator masks, and careful gowning and gloving.[79] Even more elaborate infection control measures, including personal air exchange units, are needed for health care workers involved in high-risk procedures such as intubation.

Clinically, SARS patients present after a 2- to 11-day incubation period with fever, rigors, chills, dry cough, dyspnea, malaise, headache, and, frequently, pneumonia and ARDS. Laboratory data show not only hypoxemia but also elevated results of liver function tests. In the Toronto experience, about 20% of hospitalized patients were admitted to the ICU and 15% were mechanically ventilated. Respiratory involvement typically began on day 3 of the hospital stay, but respiratory failure was not until day 8.[79] The mortality rate for ICU-admitted SARS patients was over 30%; and when patients died it was generally from multiple system organ failure and sepsis. There is no specific therapy, but anecdotal reports have suggested a benefit to the use of pulse doses of corticosteroids and ribavirin.

Bioterrorism Considerations

Certain airborne pathogens can cause pneumonia as the result of deliberate dissemination by the aerosol route, in the form of a biologic weapon, and present a clinical syndrome of CAP. The pathogens that are most likely to be used in this fashion and that can lead to severe pulmonary infection are *Bacillus anthracis* (anthrax), *Yersinia pestis* (plague), and *F. tularensis* (tularemia).[51,80-84] The Centers for Disease Control and Prevention (CDC) has classified these agents as category A pathogens because of their high mortality rate and their potential impact on public health.[80] Other pneumonic pathogens could also serve as agents of biologic warfare but are potentially less serious and are categorized as category B and include *C. burnetii* and *Brucella* species. Certain emerging pathogens are categorized as category C agents and are not widely available as weapons but have the potential for high morbidity and mortality and include hantavirus and multi-drug–resistant tuberculosis.[81] Some agents of bioterrorism can be spread via the aerosol route but do not generally present as pneumonia and include smallpox and viral hemorrhagic fevers (Ebola, Marburg).

In the fall of 2001 in the United States a series of intentional attacks with anthrax led to 11 confirmed cases of inhalational illness.[82,83] Anthrax is an aerobic gram-positive, spore-forming bacillus that had rarely led to disease before 2001. Particle size is essential in determining the infectiousness of the spores, and a size of 1 to 5 μm is required for inhalation into the alveolar space, but generally infection requires an inoculum size of 8000 to 40,000 spores. The organisms initially enter alveolar macrophages and are transported to mediastinal lymph nodes, where they can persist and germinate and produce two toxins (lethal toxin and edema toxin). Illness follows rapidly after germination.[82,83] Although respiratory symptoms are often present, anthrax is not a typical pneumonic illness but rather a disease characterized by hemorrhagic thoracic lymphadenitis, hemorrhagic mediastinitis, and pleural effusion. Whereas the incubation period of anthrax has varied from 2 to 43 days in prior outbreaks, in the October 2001 series the incubation period was from 4 to 6 days.[82] In the U.S. experience, all patients had chills, fever, and sweats and most had nonproductive cough, dyspnea, nausea, vomiting, and chest pain. Chest radiographs were abnormal in all of the first 10 patients, 7 had mediastinal widening, 8 had pleural effusions (generally bloody), and 7 had pulmonary infiltrates.[82,83] Blood cultures were positive in all 8 patients in whom they were obtained before therapy, but sputum culture and Gram's stain are unlikely to be positive. Five of the 11 patients died.

Therapy for anthrax includes supportive management and antibiotics, with possibly some role for corticosteroids if meningeal involvement or mediastinal edema is present. Recommended therapy is ciprofloxacin (400 mg i.v. bid) or doxycycline (100 mg i.v. bid). Until the patient is clinically stable, one to two additional agents should be added, including clindamycin, vancomycin, imipenem, meropenem, chloramphenicol, penicillin, ampicillin, rifampin, and clarithromycin.[82] Therapy should be continued after an initial response, with either ciprofloxacin or doxycycline for at least 60 days.[82] Postexposure prophylaxis can be done with ciprofloxacin or, alternatively, doxycycline or amoxicillin for a total of 60 days.

DIAGNOSTIC EVALUATION

In the patient with severe CAP, diagnostic testing is done to define the presence of pneumonia, the severity of illness and its complications, and the etiologic pathogen. Most studies of severe CAP have not found that establishing an etiologic diagnosis can lead to improved outcome, and mortality is lowest when patients are given empirical therapy that is likely to be effective and that leads to a good clinical response within 48 to 72 hours.[14] As discussed, the diagnosis of CAP is suggested by the history and physical examination and confirmed by chest radiograph. The history may suggest certain pathogens on the basis of epidemiologic considerations (see Table 83-4), but the clinical features and chest radiograph cannot give an exact etiologic diagnosis. An etiologic diagnosis is best established if blood or pleural fluid cultures identify a pathogen, if bronchoscopic techniques demonstrate an organism in high concentrations, or if serologic testing confirms a fourfold rise in titers to specific pathogens (comparing acute and convalescent samples collected weeks apart).

Although defining a specific etiologic diagnosis of CAP allows for focused antibiotic therapy, most patients do not have a specific pathogen identified, and many who do, have this diagnosis made days or weeks later, as the results of cultures or serologic testing become available. In addition, recent studies have emphasized the mortality benefit of prompt administration of effective antibiotic therapy, with a goal of administering intravenous antibiotics within 4 to 8 hours of admission to the hospital for those with moderate to severe illness.[85] Thus, therapy should never be delayed for the purpose of diagnostic testing, and the diagnostic workup should be streamlined, with all patients receiving empirical therapy based on algorithms as soon as possible. With such empirical regimens, as many as 90% of admitted patients will have a prompt response to therapy.[86]

For admitted patients, after a chest radiograph defines the presence of pneumonia, testing should include an assessment of oxygenation (pulse oximetry or blood gas, the latter if retention of carbon dioxide is suspected), routine admission blood work, and two sets of blood cultures (Table 83-5).[1] If the patient has a pleural effusion, this should be tapped and the fluid sent for culture and biochemical analysis. Although blood cultures are positive in only 10% to 20% of CAP patients, they can be used to define a specific diagnosis and to define the presence of drug-resistant pneumococci.[1,47] Sputum culture should be limited to patients suspected of infection with a drug-resistant or unusual pathogen.[1] Urinary antigen testing for pneumococcus or *Legionella* has

TABLE 83–5. DIAGNOSTIC TESTING FOR COMMUNITY-ACQUIRED PNEUMONIA

Test	Sensitivity	Specificity	Comment
Chest radiograph	65%–85%	85%–95%	Computed tomography is more sensitive to infiltrates. Recommended for all patients.
Computed tomography	Gold standard	Not infection specific	Should not be done routinely but helpful to identify cavitation and loculated pleural fluid. Recommended in the evaluation of nonresponding patients.
Blood cultures	10%–20%	High when positive	Usually shows pneumococcus (in 50%-80% of positive samples) and defines antibiotic susceptibility. Recommended in patients with severe CAP.
Sputum Gram's stain	40%–100% depending on criteria	0–100% depending on criteria	Can correlate with sputum culture to define predominant organism and can use to identify unsuspected pathogens. Recommended if sputum culture obtained. May not be able to narrow empirical therapy choices.
Sputum culture			Use if suspect drug-resistant or unusual pathogen, but positive result cannot separate colonization from infection.
Oximetry or arterial blood gas			Both define severity of infection, need for oxygen; if hypercarbia is suspected, a blood gas sample is needed. Recommended in severe community-acquired pneumonia.
Serologic testing for Legionella, Chlamydia pneumoniae, Mycobacterium pneumoniae, viruses			Accurate, but usually requires acute and convalescent titers collected 4 to 6 weeks apart. Not routinely recommended.
Legionella urinary antigen	50%–80%		Specific to serogroup 1, but the best acute diagnostic test for Legionella
Pneumococcal urinary antigen	70%–100%	80%	False positives if recent pneumococcal infection. Can increase sensitivity with concentrated urine

some potential value for providing a rapid diagnosis. *Legionella* urinary antigen is specific to serogroup 1 infection and is positive in a little more than half of all infected patients, but it is the test that is most likely to be positive in the setting of acute illness.[87] Pneumococcal urinary antigen has a high sensitivity and specificity for diagnosing pneumococcal pneumonia, especially if concentrated urine is examined, but false-positive tests can occur in patients who have had recent pneumococcal infection.[88]

The role of Gram's stain of sputum to guide initial antibiotic therapy is controversial, but this test has its greatest value in guiding the interpretation of sputum culture and can be used to define the predominant organism present in the sample. The role of Gram's stain in focusing initial antibiotic therapy is uncertain because the accuracy of the test to predict the culture recovery of an organism such as pneumococcus depends on the criteria used. If the finding of any gram-positive diplococcus is used to define a positive test, then the test will be sensitive but not very specific. On the other hand, the finding of a predominance of gram-positive diplococci will be specific but not sensitive for predicting the culture recovery of pneumococcus.[1,89] In a recent study, the practical limitations of the test were clear: of 116 patients with CAP, only 42 could produce a sputum sample, of which 23 were valid and only 10 samples were diagnostic, with antibiotics directed to the diagnostic result in only 1 patient.[90] Even if Gram's stain findings were used to focus antibiotic therapy, this would not allow for empirical coverage of atypical pathogens that might be present with pneumococcus, as part of a mixed infection. In spite of these limitations, Gram's stain can be used to broaden initial empirical therapy by enhancing the suspicion for organisms that are not covered in routine empirical therapy (such as *S. aureus* being suggested by the presence of clusters of gram-positive cocci, especially during a time of epidemic influenza).[1]

Routine serologic testing is not recommended.[1,91] However, in patients with severe illness, the diagnosis of legionellosis can be made by urinary antigen testing, which is the test that is most likely to be positive at the time of admission but a test that is specific only for serogroup 1 infection.[87] Bronchoscopy is not indicated as a routine diagnostic test and should be restricted to immune compromised patients and to selected individuals with severe forms of CAP. In the patient admitted to the ICU with CAP, bronchoscopy with quantitative cultures is often done, to be sure that all efforts are being made to define the etiologic agent, but the benefit of this approach is unclear. As mentioned, several studies[9,14,86] have not shown any improvement in outcome when a specific etiologic diagnosis is made for patients with severe CAP. Rather, outcome is improved if the initial empirical therapy is accurate and the patient has a prompt clinical improvement.[14] However, patients who have rapidly progressive lung infection, in spite of therapy, may benefit from invasive diagnostic testing, but again a favorable impact of this testing on patient outcome has not been demonstrated. One population that should be considered for invasive testing is the corticosteroid-treated COPD patient who has a slowly responding or nonresponding pneumonia, because these individuals are at risk for infection with *Aspergillus* and this organism can be recovered from a bronchoscopic sample.[92] In addition, bronchoscopy may have value for the nonresponding patient or other immune-suppressed individuals; and in one study it provided diagnostically useful information for such patients.[93]

One recent study of severe CAP demonstrated the value of diagnostic testing for guiding modifications of antibiotic therapy, rather than focusing on the impact of these methods on initial therapy.[94] In this study, 214 patients with severe CAP were studied and a microbiologic diagnosis was established in 57.3%. When the yield of specific tests was examined, the investigators found that sputum or tracheal aspirate cultures had the highest yield of any microbiologic investigation, being positive in 44.4% of all patients in which a sample was collected. Blood cultures were positive in 21.1% of the 189 patients sampled, whereas bronchoscopic protected specimen brush was positive in 25% of the 62 patients who were sampled and bronchoalveolar lavage was positive in 34% of the 41 patients who were sampled. When diagnostic testing identified a cause, antibiotics were changed in 74.3% of patients, compared with 32.7% of patients without an etiologic diagnosis (P <.05). In most instances, the change in therapy was a simplification of the initial empirical antibiotic regimen that occurred in 65 patients.

THERAPY

Initial antibiotic therapy for severe CAP is necessarily empirical, with the goal of targeting the likely etiologic pathogens, based on the considerations in Tables 83-3 and Table 83-4, which categorize patients on the basis of severity of illness and risk factors for specific pathogens. The likelihood of organisms such as DRSP, enteric gram-negative organisms, and *P. aeruginosa* is determined by the presence of cardiopulmonary disease or "modifying factors."[1] Although a set of likely pathogens can be predicted for each patient (see Table 83-3), and this information can be used to guide initial empirical therapy, if diagnostic testing shows the presence of a specific pathogen, then therapy can be focused.

In choosing empirical therapy of CAP, certain principles and therapeutic approaches should be followed (Table 83-6). For the non-ICU inpatient, therapy can be with an intravenous macrolide (azithromycin) alone, provided that the patient has no underlying cardiopulmonary disease and no risk factors for infection with DRSP, enteric gram-negative organisms, or anaerobes. Although very few patients of this type are admitted to the hospital, macrolide monotherapy has been documented to be effective in this population.[95] The majority of admitted patients will have cardiopulmonary disease and/or modifying factors, and they can be treated with either a selected intravenous beta-lactam (ampicillin/sulbactam, cefotaxime, ceftriaxone, ertapenem, or high-dose ampicillin) combined with a macrolide, or they can receive an intravenous antipneumococcal quinolone (gatifloxacin,

levofloxacin, or moxifloxacin) alone.[1,47,51] From the available data, it appears that either regimen is therapeutically equivalent; and, although not proven, it may be useful to use these two types of regimens interchangeably, striving for "antibiotic heterogeneity" in the hospital, so that one regimen is not used exclusively in all patients.[1,51] The choice between these two options may best be determined by using a regimen that is different from what the patient has recently received.

In the ICU population, all individuals should be treated for DRSP and atypical pathogens but only those with appropriate risk factors (see earlier) should have coverage for *P. aeruginosa*.[1] Because the efficacy (especially for meningitis complicating pneumonia), effective dosing, and safety of quinolone monotherapy has not been established for ICU-admitted CAP patients, the therapy for such patients, in the absence of pseudomonal risk factors, should be with a selected intravenous beta-lactam (see earlier), combined with either an intravenous macrolide or an intravenous quinolone. For patients with pseudomonal risk factors, therapy can be with a two-drug regimen, using an antipseudomonal beta-lactam (cefepime, imipenem, meropenem, piperacillin/tazobactam) plus ciprofloxacin (the most active antipseudomonal quinolone) or, alternatively, with a three-drug regimen, using an antipseudomonal beta-lactam plus an aminoglycoside plus either an intravenous nonpseudomonal quinolone or a macrolide.[1]

Although they should not be used as monotherapy for ICU-admitted CAP patients, the antipneumococcal quinolones have assumed great importance because they can cover pneumococcus (including DRSP), nonpseudomonal gram-negative organisms, and atypical pathogens.[96] Quinolones penetrate well into respiratory secretions and are highly bioavailable, achieving the same serum levels with oral or intravenous therapy and thereby allowing rapid switch to oral therapy in responding patients. Among the antipneumococcal quinolones, there are differences in their intrinsic activity against pneumococcus.[1,96,97] On a MIC basis, the available intravenous agents can be ranked from most to least active as moxifloxacin, gatifloxacin, and levofloxacin. Some data suggest a lower likelihood of both clinical failures and the induction of pneumococcal resistance to quinolones, if the more active agents are used in place of the less active agents.[71,97,98] In addition, there are now reports of failures in pneumococcal pneumonia with levofloxacin, and these have occurred in patients who were infected with levofloxacin-resistant organisms, which arose either after a recent course of quinolone therapy or with the acquisition of resistance during therapy.[71,72]

In addition to the general approach to therapy outlined earlier, there are several other therapeutic issues in the management of CAP.

TIMELINESS OF INITIAL THERAPY OF HOSPITALIZED PATIENTS

For inpatients with CAP, the use of timely and accurate therapy is essential to reduce mortality. In patients with severe CAP, improved survival has occurred if initial empirical therapy is accurate and if it leads to a rapid clinical response.[14,61,85] In one study, if initial therapy led to a clinical response within 72 hours, mortality of severe CAP was approximately 10%, compared with a mortality rate of 60% in patients who had initially ineffective therapy.[14] Another recent finding is the need to provide initial intravenous

---

TABLE 83–6. EMPIRICAL THERAPY REGIMENS FOR SEVERE COMMUNITY-ACQUIRED PNEUMONIA

No Pseudomonal Risk Factors

Selected beta–lactam (cefotaxime, ceftriaxone)
plus
Intravenously administered macrolide *or* quinolone

Pseudomonal Risk Factors Present

Selected antipseudomonal beta-lactam (cefepime, piperacillin/tazobactam, imipenem, meropenem)
plus
Ciprofloxacin
or
Selected antipseudomonal beta-lactam
plus
Aminoglycoside
plus
Intravenously administered macrolide or antipneumococcal quinolone

antibiotic therapy within 8 hours of the patient's arrival to the hospital.[85] In a large Medicare study of 14,069 patients, mortality at 30 days was significantly reduced for the 75% of patients who received their first dose of therapy within 8 hours of coming to the hospital.[85] Although this has become a target time frame for initial therapy, there was additional benefit for therapy given even sooner, and the new standard is to provide initial therapy within 4 hours of arrival to the hospital.

THE NEED TO TREAT ALL POPULATIONS FOR ATYPICAL PATHOGEN INFECTION

Although the term *atypical* does not accurately describe a specific clinical pneumonia syndrome, the term can be used to refer to a group of pathogens that includes *M. pneumoniae*, *C. pneumoniae*, and *Legionella;* and this group of organisms cannot be reliably eradicated by beta-lactam therapy (penicillins and cephalosporins) but must be treated with a macrolide, tetracycline, or a quinolone. In the current North American CAP guidelines, initial empirical therapy for all patients requires therapy for the possibility of atypical pathogen infection, either as primary infection or as part of a mixed infection.[1,47,51] This recommendation is based on a number of studies, as mentioned earlier, that show a high frequency of these pathogens, when using serologic diagnosis, often in the form of mixed infection, coexisting with a bacterial pathogen.[57-59] In one study of inpatients in the United States, infection with atypical pathogens was more common in older individuals (65 to 79 years) than in those younger than 35 years, and other studies have shown these pathogens to be common in patients with severe CAP.[11,57]

In addition to these data, a number of studies of large populations of inpatients have shown that when therapy includes a macrolide or a quinolone, outcomes, including mortality, are improved, compared with when a beta-lactam is used by itself.[61,62] In the setting of severe CAP, Rello and colleagues evaluated 466 patients and found that when a macrolide was added to a beta-lactam, the mortality and length of stay were improved compared with therapy that did not provide coverage for atypical pathogens.[99] Although these findings are not definitive, they do suggest the need for routine therapy of atypical pathogens, a strategy that may even be needed in patients with bacteremic pneumococcal pneumonia. To date, two studies have suggested that when patients with this infection receive a beta-lactam alone, the mortality is higher than if they receive a beta-lactam combined with a macrolide.[100,101]

Legionella is a potentially important pathogen in patients with severe CAP, and there are many drugs available with in vitro activity against *L. pneumophila*, but there are limited prospective, comparative data on the role of therapy in the outcome of this infection.[74] Retrospective data and long clinical experience support the use of erythromycin at a dose of 4 g/day in the hospitalized patient with *L. pneumophila*. Rifampin should be added in patients with multilobar disease, organ failure, or severe immunosuppression and be administered for the first 3 to 5 days.[1,102] Other macrolides (clarithromycin and azithromycin) are also effective, and azithromycin is available in an intravenous form. Alternatives to the just presented regimen include quinolone antibiotics (ciprofloxacin , levofloxacin, gatifloxacin, and moxifloxacin) or doxycycline.[51] Quinolones are particularly effective in animal models of *Legionella* pneumonia.[102]

There is little information on the proper duration of therapy in patients with CAP, especially those with severe illness. Even in the presence of pneumococcal bacteremia, short durations of therapy may be possible, with a rapid switch from intravenous to oral therapy in responding patients.[103] Generally, *S. pneumoniae* can be treated for 5 to 7 days if the patient is responding rapidly and has received the correct dose of an accurate therapy. The presence of extrapulmonary infection (e.g., meningitis), and the identification of certain pathogens (such as bacteremic *S. aureus* and *P. aeruginosa*) may require longer durations of therapy. Identification of *L. pneumophila* pneumonia may require at least 14 days of therapy, depending on severity of illness and host defense impairments. Most therapy in the ICU will be given intravenously; however, recent studies, using a variety of antibiotics, have suggested that oral therapy may be instituted after as early as 2 to 3 days of parenteral therapy, assuming that the patient's condition has stabilized and is afebrile.[104,105] The switch to oral therapy, even in severely ill patients, may be facilitated by the use of quinolones that are highly bioavailable and achieve the same serum levels with oral therapy as with intravenous therapy.

ADJUNCTIVE THERAPY MEASURES

In addition to antibiotic therapy, the patient with severe CAP may require chest physiotherapy, especially if the patient has either an excessive volume of purulent sputum (>30 mL/day) or severe respiratory muscle weakness resulting in ineffective cough.[106] Aerosolized humidification has been used to reduce sputum viscosity, thereby enhancing clearance in patients who have generally ineffective cough. However, it is likely that much of the generated water vapor is deposited in the upper airway where it is likely to stimulate cough but unlikely to influence the rheologic properties of sputum. Bronchodilator therapy, which also enhances mucociliary clearance, and ciliary beat frequency, is most likely to be of benefit in patients with pneumonia complicating COPD. Activated protein C infusion has been shown to reduce 28-day mortality in patients with severe sepsis and an APACHE II score of more than 26, but in the original trial over half of the treated patients had pneumonia as the cause of sepsis, suggesting a role for this therapy in patients with severe CAP.[107] Adjunctive immune therapy with granulocyte colony-stimulating factor has also been used in severe CAP, with no benefit in mortality or in the course of illness resolution.[108]

EVALUATION OF RESPONSE TO THERAPY

The majority of patients will respond rapidly to accurate empirical therapy within 24 to 72 hours. Clinical response is defined as improvement in symptoms of cough, sputum production, and dyspnea, along with ability to take medications by mouth, declining white blood cell count, and an afebrile status for at least two occasions 8 hours apart.[103-105] In the critically ill patient, improvement in oxygenation may be one of the earliest signs of response to therapy, although few studies have examined mechanically ventilated patients. When a patient has met criteria for clinical response, it is appropriate to consider a switch to an oral therapy regimen, if the patient is otherwise medically and socially stable.[1,104,105] Radiographic improvement lags behind clinical improvement and, in a responding patient, a chest radiograph is not necessary until 2 to 4 weeks after starting therapy. In general, 50% of patients with pneumococcal pneumonia have radiographic clearing at 5 weeks, whereas the majority clear in 2 to 3 months. With bacteremic disease, 50% have a clear chest radiograph at 9 weeks and most are clear by 18 weeks.[109,110] Radiographic resolution is most influenced by the number of lobes involved and the age of the patient. Radiographic clearance of CAP decreases by 20% per decade after age 20, and patients with multilobar infiltrates take longer to clear than those with unilobar disease.[109]

If the patient fails to respond to appropriate therapy in the expected time interval, then it is necessary to consider infection with a drug-resistant or unusual pathogen (tuberculosis, *C. burnetii*, *Burkholderia pseudomallei*, *C. psittaci*, endemic fungi, or hantavirus); a pneumonic complication (lung abscess, endocarditis, empyema); or a noninfectious process that mimics pneumonia (bronchiolitis obliterans with organizing pneumonia, hypersensitivity pneumonitis, pulmonary vasculitis, bronchoalveolar cell carcinoma, lymphoma, pulmonary embolus).[1] The evaluation of the nonresponding patient should be individualized but may include CT of the chest, pulmonary angiography, bronchoscopy, and, occasionally, open lung biopsy.

PREVENTION

Prevention of CAP is important for all groups of the population but especially the elderly patient, who is at risk for both a higher frequency of infection and a more severe course of illness. Appropriate patients should be vaccinated with both pneumococcal and influenza vaccines, and cigarette smoking should be stopped in all at-risk patients. Even for the patient who is recovering from CAP, immunization while in the hospital is appropriate to prevent future episodes of infection and the evaluation of all patients for vaccination need and the provision of information about smoking cessation are now performance standards used to evaluate the hospital care of CAP patients.[51]

PNEUMOCOCCAL VACCINE

Pneumococcal capsular polysaccharide vaccine can prevent pneumonia in otherwise healthy populations, as was initially demonstrated in South African gold miners and American military recruits.[111-115] The benefits in those of advanced age or with underlying conditions in nonepidemic environments are less clearly defined. The vaccine efficacy has ranged from 65% to 84% in patients with diabetes mellitus, coronary artery disease, congestive heart failure, chronic pulmonary disease, and anatomic asplenia.[1,111-113] In immunocompetent patients over the age of 65, effectiveness has been documented to be 75%. In the immunocompromised patient, effectiveness has not been proven, and this includes patients with sickle cell disease, chronic renal failure, immunoglobulin deficiency, Hodgkin's disease, lymphoma, leukemia, and multiple myeloma. One recent retrospective cohort study evaluated 47,365 patients older than 65 years to determine the impact of pneumococcal vaccination on three different clinical events: hospitalization for CAP, outpatient therapy for CAP, and documented pneumococcal bacteremia.[116] The use of vaccination was associated with a significant reduction in the incidence of pneumococcal bacteremia (OR = 0.56) but no change in the frequency of pneumonia treated in or out of the hospital.

A single revaccination is indicated in a person who is older than age 65 years who initially received the vaccine more than 5 years earlier and was younger than age 65 on first vaccination.[1,51] If the initial vaccination was given at age 65 or older, repeat is not indicated unless the patient has anatomic or functional asplenia or has one of the immune compromising conditions listed earlier. In these patients, revaccination is indicated and the second dose is given at least 5 years after the original dose.

The available pneumococcal vaccine is widely underutilized, but the 23-valent pneumococcal vaccine contains 23 pneumococcal serotypes that cause 85% of all infections due to pneumococcus. A protein-conjugated pneumococcal vaccine has been licensed, and it appears more immunogenic than the older vaccine, but it contains only 7 serotypes, is recommended for healthy children, and has not yet been adequately tested in adults.[51,114] Hospital-based immunization could be highly effective, because over 60% of all patients with CAP have been admitted to the hospital, for some indication, in the preceding 4 years, and hospitalization could be defined as an appropriate time for vaccination.[115] Pneumococcal vaccine can be given simultaneously with other vaccines such as influenza vaccine, but each should be given at a separate site, and the vaccine can, and often should, be given before discharge in the patient admitted for CAP.

INFLUENZA VACCINATION

Influenza epidemics contribute to morbidity and mortality both by causing direct infection and by leading to postinfluenza complications. The influenza vaccine preparations are revised annually to account for changes in the antigenic nature of the virus (antigenic drift) that is present each season. Three strains are represented in each vaccine preparation: an influenza A strain (H3N2); an influenza A strain (H1N1); and one influenza B strain. Vaccination should be given to all patients older than age 65 and to those with chronic medical illness (including nursing home residents) and to those who provide health care to patients at risk for complicated influenza.[1,117] It is given yearly, usually between September and mid November. While the traditional influenza vaccine contains an inactivated virus, there is now an intranasal vaccine containing a live attenuated influenza virus. It is currently approved for individuals ages 5 to 49 years who are not immune suppressed or chronically ill and who do not have asthma.[51]

When the vaccine matches the circulating strain, it can prevent illness in 70% to 90% of healthy persons younger than age 65.[1,118] For older persons with chronic illness, the efficacy is less but the vaccine can still attenuate the influenza infection and lead to fewer lower respiratory tract infections and the associated morbidity and mortality that follow influenza. In many studies, the vaccine has been shown to be cost effective and able to prevent severe illness and death and it can reduce the occurrence of secondary pneumonia and hospitalization.[118]

ANNOTATED REFERENCES

El-Solh AA, Pietrantoni C, Bhat A, et al: Microbiology of severe aspiration pneumonia in institutionalized elderly. Am J Respir Crit Care Med 2003;167:1650-1654.
 Prospective microbiologic evaluation of elderly patients admitted to the ICU from a nursing home with severe CAP in the setting of risk factors

for aspiration. The predominant organisms were gram negative and not anaerobic; and even when anaerobes were identified, specific antibiotic therapy did not appear to be necessary.

Ewig S, Ruiz M, Mensa J, et al: Severe community-acquired pneumonia: Assessment of severity criteria. Am J Respir Crit Care Med 1998;158: 1102-1108.

Retrospective single-center study of patients hospitalized with CAP to identify what features were present in those admitted to the ICU. ICU care was best predicted by the presence of one of two major criteria (need for mechanical ventilation or septic shock) or two of three minor criteria (multilobar infiltrates, PaO$_2$/FIO$_2$ ratio <250, and systolic BP <90 mm Hg).

Niederman MS, Mandell LA, Anzueto A, et al: Guidelines for the management of adults with community-acquired lower respiratory tract infections: Diagnosis, assessment of severity, antimicrobial therapy and prevention. Am J Respir Crit Care Med 2001;163:1730-1754.

Evidence-based guideline of CAP, focusing on epidemiology, bacteriology and management. A definition of severe CAP is provided, along with a discussion of the limitation of available prognostic scoring systems. For patients with severe CAP, the likely etiologic pathogens are identified and accompanied by suggestions for initial empirical therapy.

Ruiz M, Ewig S, Torres A, et al: Severe community-acquired pneumonia: Risk factors and follow-up epidemiology. Am J Respir Crit Care Med 1999; 160:923-929.

In this single-center study of severe CAP, the etiologic pathogens were defined in two consecutive decades. In both time periods, pneumococcus was the most common pathogen, and atypical organisms were also identified in nearly 20% of all patients. However, the identity of the specific atypical pathogens varied over time, with Legionella species predominating in one period and being replaced by Mycoplasma and Chlamydia in the other period.

Waterer GW, Somes GW, Wunderink RG: Monotherapy may be suboptimal for severe bacteremic pneumococcal pneumonia. Arch Intern Med 2001; 161:1837-1842.

Retrospective study of patients with bacteremic pneumococcal pneumonia showing reduced mortality if patients received a dually effective antibiotic therapy regimen, compared with a single effective antimicrobial agent. The explanation for the benefit of combination therapy was unclear, but patients who received a second agent that provided for atypical pathogen coverage generally did better than patients who did not receive coverage for these organisms, a surprising finding because all patients had proven bacteremic pneumococcal infection.

Chapter 84
NOSOCOMIAL PNEUMONIA

Jean-Yves Fagon • Jean Chastre

KEY POINTS

1. **Nosocomial pneumonia is a common complication occurring in ICU patients.** The risk of nosocomial pneumonia is considerably higher in patients treated with mechanical ventilation.

2. **Etiologic agents differ** according to the population of ICU patients, duration of hospital stay, and prior antimicrobial therapy. Local microbiologic data must be considered when choosing and adapting treatment.

3. **Nosocomial pneumonia is associated with high mortality and morbidity,** particularly in case of infection due to high-risk pathogens such as *Pseudomonas aeruginosa* and *Acinetobacter* species and when initial antimicrobial therapy is inappropriate.

4. **Any strategy designed to manage patients suspected of nosocomial pneumonia** should be able to select appropriate therapy initiated at an early stage of infection and to avoid the overuse of antibiotics. Bronchoscopic techniques, when performed before introduction of new antibiotics, enable physicians to identify patients who need immediate treatment and help to select optimal therapy.

5. **Very simple, no-cost measures may have tremendous impact** on the frequency of nosocomial pneumonia.

Nosocomial pneumonia (NP) or hospital-acquired pneumonia (HAP) is defined as pneumonia occurring more than 48 hours after hospital admission and excluding any infection that is incubating at the time of hospital admission. NP is the second most frequent nosocomial infection and represents the leading cause of death from infection that is acquired in the hospital. ICU-acquired pneumonia is pneumonia that arises more than 48 hours after ICU admission. The term *ventilator-associated pneumonia* (VAP) refers to pneumonia that occurs in patients intubated and treated with mechanical ventilation. There are patients with severe NP who are transferred to the ICU and become intubated; similarities between the management of such patients and patients with VAP exist; they are, however, not included in the definition of VAP. Most studies cited in this chapter have examined VAP.

EPIDEMIOLOGY

INCIDENCE

The majority of studies have reported incidence rates of NP in general ICU populations varying between 8% and 20%.[1] The risk of pneumonia seems to be considerably higher in the subset of ICU patients treated with mechanical ventilation. Cross and Roup have published specific data on overall rates of nosocomial pneumonia in relation to the use of respiratory devices.[2] Pneumonia rates in patients with an endotracheal tube and mechanical ventilation were increased 10-fold over patients with no respiratory therapy devices. Prolonged mechanical ventilation is the most important factor associated with NP. However, VAP may occur within the first 48 hours after intubation.[3] It is usual to distinguish early-onset VAP, which occurs during the first 4 or 5 days of mechanical ventilation, from late-onset VAP, which develops 5 days or more after initiation of mechanical ventilation. Not only are the causative pathogens commonly different but the disease is usually less severe and the prognosis better in early-onset VAP.[4] By using an actuarial method, the cumulative risk of pneumonia in this context was estimated to be 6.5% at 10 days and 19% at 20 days after the onset of mechanical ventilation. Furthermore, the incremental risk of pneumonia was virtually constant throughout the entire ventilation period, with a mean rate of about 1% per day.[5] In contrast, Cook and colleagues demonstrated in a large series of 1014 mechanically ventilated patients that, although the cumulative risk for developing VAP increased over time, the daily hazard rate decreased after day 5.[6] The risk per day was evaluated at 3% on day 5, 2% on day 10, and 1% on day 15. However, the daily risk for developing VAP is highly dependent on the population being studied (including underlying illnesses, comorbid disease, severity of illness) and also on many other factors, including therapeutic interventions and particularly the number of patients in the given population who received antibiotics after their admission to the ICU.

VAP is thought to be a common complication of the acute respiratory distress syndrome (ARDS). Most clinical studies have found that pulmonary infection affects between 34% and 70% or more of patients with ARDS, often leading to the development of sepsis, multiple organ failure, and death.[1,7-11] In one study on 56 ARDS patients, protected specimen brush and bronchoalveolar lavage were used to define pneumonia and the VAP rate was 55%,[9] whereas it was only 28% for 187 non-ARDS patients diagnosed with the same criteria during the same period. It was specified that early-onset VAP was relatively rare in ARDS patients: only 10% of the first VAP episodes, as opposed to 40% in non-ARDS patients.

MORTALITY, MORBIDITY, AND COST

Crude ICU mortality rates of 24% to 76% have been reported for VAP at a variety of institutions. The results of several studies conducted between 1986 and 2001 have confirmed that observation: despite variations among studies that partly reflect the populations considered, overall mortality rates for patients with or without VAP were, respectively, 55% versus 25%,[12] 71% versus 28%,[13] 33% versus 19%,[14] 38% versus 9%,[15] and 44% versus 19%.[16] These rates correspond to increased risk ratios of mortality of VAP patients of 2.2, 2.5, 1.7, 4.4, and 2.3, respectively. They are increased by age, severity of illness, late onset, medical diagnosis, resistant pathogens, and inappropriateness of initial antimicrobial therapy. Studies evaluating the attributable mortality of VAP are difficult to interpret because they were conducted in different populations that used different diagnostic criteria to identify patients with infection and different methods to control for confounding factors.

The prognosis for aerobic, gram-negative bacilli VAP is considerably worse than that for infection with gram-positive pathogens, which are fully susceptible to antibiotics. Death rates associated with *Pseudomonas* pneumonia are particularly high, ranging from 70% to more than 80% in several studies.[13,17,18] Concerning gram-positive pathogens, in a study comparing VAP due to methicillin-resistant *Staphylococcus aureus* (MRSA) or methicillin-sensitive *S. aureus* (MSSA), mortality was found to be directly attributable to pneumonia for 86% of the former cases versus 12% of the latter, with a relative risk of death equal to 20.7 for MRSA pneumonia.[19]

Using multiple logistic regression analysis, Torres and coworkers emphasized the complex relationships among the severity of pneumonia itself, the severity of underlying disease leading to ICU admission and the adequacy of initial antimicrobial treatment.[14] The important prognostic role played by the appropriateness of the initial empirical antimicrobial therapy was analyzed by several other investigators.[20-24]

Thus, considering many different kinds of evidence, VAP seems indeed associated with a 20% to 30% higher risk of death than that due to the underlying disease alone.

It is impossible to accurately evaluate the morbidity and excess costs associated with nosocomial pneumonia. However, with respect to morbidity measures, the prolonged hospital stay as a direct consequence of pneumonia has been estimated in several studies; it ranges from 4 to 8 days in the majority of studies.[25,26] These prolonged hospitalizations underscore the considerable financial burden imposed by the development of VAP.[27]

ETIOLOGIC AGENTS

Nosocomial pneumonia may be caused by a variety of pathogens and, in many patients, more than one pathogen may be isolated. Microorganisms responsible for nosocomial pneumonia may differ according to the population of ICU patients, the durations of hospital and ICU stays, and the specific diagnostic method(s) used. Several studies have reported that greater than 60% of VAP are caused by aerobic, gram-negative bacilli, such as *Pseudomonas aeruginosa, Escherichia coli, Klebsiella pneumoniae,* or *Acinetobacter* species.[1,5,14,27-32] More recently, however, some investigators have reported that gram-positive bacteria have become increasingly more common in this setting, with *S. aureus* being the predominant gram-positive isolate. For example, *S. aureus* was responsible for most episodes of nosocomial pneumonia in the European Prevalence of Infection in Intensive Care (EPIC) study, accounting for 31% of the 836 cases with identified responsible pathogens.[33] The data from 24 investigations conducted on ventilated patients, for whom bacteriologic studies were restricted to uncontaminated specimens, confirmed those results: gram-negative bacilli represented 58% of recovered organisms, and a relatively high rate of gram-positive pneumonias was also reported in those studies, with *S. aureus* involved in 20% of the cases (Table 84-1).[1]

The high rate of polymicrobial infection in VAP has been emphasized repeatedly. In a study on 172 episodes of bacteremic nosocomial pneumonia, 13% of lung infections were caused by multiple pathogens.[34] Similarly, when the protected specimen brush (PSB) technique was used to identify the causative agents in 52 consecutive cases of VAP, a 40% polymicrobial infection rate was found,[5] a value similar to that observed in another study conducted at the same time on a comparable population of ventilated patients.[35]

Underlying diseases may predispose patients to infection with specific organisms. Patients with chronic obstructive pulmonary disease (COPD) are, for example, at increased risk for *Haemophilus influenzae, Moraxella catarrhalis,* or *S. pneumoniae* infections; cystic fibrosis increases the risk of *P. aeruginosa* and/or *S. aureus* infections, whereas trauma and neurologic patients are at increased risk for *S. aureus* infection.[4,19,27,36] Furthermore, the causative agent for pneumonia differs among ICU surgical populations,[37] with 18% of the nosocomial pneumonias being due to *Haemophilus* or pneumococci, particularly in trauma patients.

Despite somewhat different definitions of early-onset pneumonia, varying from less than 3 to less than 7 days,[4,32] high rates of *H. influenzae, S. pneumoniae,* MSSA, or susceptible Enterobacteriaceae were constantly found in early-onset VAP, whereas *P. aeruginosa, Acinetobacter* species, MRSA, and multiresistant gram-negative bacilli were significantly more frequent in late-onset VAP.[4,31,32] This different distribution pattern of etiologic agents between early- and late-onset VAP is also linked to the frequent administration

TABLE 84-1. ETIOLOGY OF VENTILATOR-ASSOCIATED PNEUMONIA AS DOCUMENTED BY BRONCHOSCOPIC TECHNIQUES IN 24 STUDIES FOR A TOTAL OF 1689 EPISODES AND 2490 PATHOGENS

Pathogen	Frequency (%)
Pseudomonas aeruginosa	24.4
Acinetobacter spp.	7.9
Stenotrophomonas maltophilia	1.7
Enterobacteriaceae*	14.1
Haemophilus spp.	9.8
Staphylococcus aureus†	20.4
Streptococcus spp.	8.0
Streptococcus pneumoniae	4.1
Coagulase-negative staphylococci	1.4
Neisseria spp.	2.6
Anaerobes	0.9
Fungi	0.9
Others (<1% each)‡	3.8

*Distribution when specified: *Klebsiella* spp., 15.6%; *Escherichia coli,* 24.1%; *Proteus* spp., 22.3%; *Enterobacter* spp., 18.8%; *Serratia* spp., 12.1%; *Citrobacter* spp., 5.0%; *Hafnia alvei,* 2.1%.
†Distribution when specified: MRSA, 55.7%; MSSA, 44.3%.
‡Including *Corynebacterium* spp., *Moraxella* spp., and *Enterococcus* spp.

of prior antimicrobial therapy in many patients with late-onset VAP. In a prospective study that included 129 episodes of nosocomial pneumonia documented by PSB specimens, the distributions of responsible pathogens were compared according to whether the patients had received antimicrobial therapy before pneumonia onset.[28] The most striking finding was that the rate of pneumonia caused by gram-positive cocci or *H. influenzae* was significantly lower ($P < .05$) in patients who had received antibiotics, whereas the rate of pneumonia caused by *P. aeruginosa* was significantly higher ($P < .01$). A stepwise logistic regression analysis retained only prior antibiotic use (OR = 9.2, $P < .0001$) as significantly influencing the risk of death from pneumonia.[28] Very similar results were obtained when multivariate analysis was used to determine risk factors for VAP caused by potentially drug-resistant bacteria such as MRSA, *P. aeruginosa*, *A. baumannii*, and/or *S. maltophilia* in 135 consecutive episodes of VAP.[32] Only three variables remained significant: duration of mechanical ventilation before VAP onset for 7 days or more (OR = 6.0), prior antibiotic use (OR = 13.5), and prior use of broad-spectrum drugs (third-generation cephalosporin, fluoroquinolone, and/or imipenem) (OR = 4.1).[32] Not all studies, however, have confirmed this distribution pattern. Their finding may, in part, be due to the prior hospitalization and use of antibiotics in many patients developing early-onset VAP before their transfer to the ICU.

The incidence of multiresistant pathogens is also closely linked to local factors and varies widely from one institution to another. Consequently, each ICU has to continuously collect meticulous epidemiologic data. With these aims, variations of VAP etiology among three Spanish ICUs were analyzed[31] and compared with data collected in Paris.[32] The authors concluded that VAP pathogens varied widely among these four treatment centers, with marked differences in all of the microorganisms isolated from VAP episodes in Spanish centers as compared with the French site. Clinicians must clearly be aware of the common microorganisms associated with both early-onset and late-onset VAP in their own hospitals to avoid the administration of initial inadequate antimicrobial therapy.

Legionella species,[38] anaerobes,[39] fungi,[40] viruses,[41] and even *Pneumocystis carinii* should be mentioned as potential causative agents but are not considered to be common in the context of pneumonia acquired during mechanical ventilation. However, several of these causative agents may be more common and potentially underreported because of difficulties involved with the diagnostic techniques used to identify them, including anaerobic bacteria and viruses.[39,41] By examining currently available data, the clinical significance of anaerobes in the pathogenesis and outcome of VAP remains unclear, except as etiologic agents in patients with necrotizing pneumonitis, lung abscess, or pleuropulmonary infections. *Legionella pneumophila* as a cause of nosocomial pneumonia is variable but probably more frequent in immunocompromised patients, particularly organ transplant recipients, and in hospitals with the organism present in the hospital water supply. Isolation of fungi, most frequently *Candida* species, at significant concentrations poses interpretative problems. Invasive disease has been reported in VAP but, more frequently, yeasts are isolated from respiratory tract specimens in the apparent absence of disease. One prospective study examined the relevance of isolating *Candida* species from 25 non-neutropenic patients who had been mechanically ventilated for at least 72 hours.[40] Just after death, multiple culture

and biopsy specimens were obtained with bronchoscopic techniques. Although 10 patients had at least one biopsy specimen positive for *Candida* species, only 2 had evidence of invasive pneumonia as demonstrated by histologic examination.

PREDISPOSING FACTORS

A number of factors have been suspected or identified to increase the risk of pneumonia in ICU, including those identified in the subset of mechanically ventilated patients. The data indicated specific high-risk populations (i.e., patients with COPD, ARDS, serum albumin level less than 2.2 g/dL, patients undergoing mechanical ventilation for more than 3 days, those requiring intracranial pressure monitoring, those with coma or impaired consciousness, burns, or trauma, and more generally those with severe underlying medical conditions as evaluated by a high APACHE II or APACHE III score or presence of organ failure) and specific treatment modalities or therapeutic intervention (i.e., use of H_2 blockers or antacids, previous antibiotics, use of drugs that are markers for severe underlying disease such as dopamine, dobutamine, or paralytic agents or continuous sedation, re-intubation, and frequent changes of ventilator circuits, bronchoscopy, or nasogastric tube) as being independently associated with nosocomial pneumonia.

SURGERY

Postsurgical patients are at increased risk for pneumonia.[15,37,42] A history of smoking, low albumin level, longer preoperative stays, longer surgical procedures, and thoracic or upper abdominal operative sites were significant risk factors for postoperative pneumonia. In their study comparing adult critical-care populations, Cunnion and colleagues demonstrated that surgical ICU patients were found to have consistently higher rates of nosocomial pneumonia than medical ICU patients with a risk ratio equal to 2.2.[26] The relative importance of the surgical procedure itself versus intubation, prophylactic antibiotics, and/or other variables therefore remains to be clearly elucidated in surgical patients.

MEDICATION

Antimicrobial Agents

The use of antibiotics in the hospital setting has been associated with an increased risk of nosocomial pneumonia and selection of resistant pathogens.[15,28,32,33,36,43] In a cohort study of 320 patients, prior antibiotic administration was identified by logistic regression analysis to be one of the four variables independently associated with VAP along with organ failure, age older than 60 years, and the patient's head positioning (i.e., flat on his back or supine vs. head and thorax raised 30 to 40 degrees or semirecumbent).[15] However, other investigators found that antibiotic administration during the first 8 days was associated with a lower risk of early-onset VAP.[44,45] For example, Sirvent and coworkers showed that a single dose of a first-generation cephalosporin given prophylactically was associated with a lower rate of early-onset VAP in patients with structural coma.[46] Finally, the results of the multicentric Canadian study on the incidence of and risk factors for VAP indicated that antibiotic treatment conferred protection against VAP.[6] This apparent protective effect of antibiotics disappears after 2 to 3 weeks, suggesting that a higher risk of VAP cannot be excluded beyond this point.

In contrast, prolonged antibiotic administration to ICU patients for primary infection is thought to favor selection and subsequent colonization with resistant pathogens responsible for superinfections.[5,32,43,47,48] According to our data on 567 ventilated patients, those who had received antimicrobial therapy within the 15 days preceding lung infection were not at higher risk for development of VAP[5] but 65% of the lung infections that occurred in patients who had received broad-spectrum antimicrobial drugs versus only 19% of those developing in patients who had not received antibiotics were caused by *Pseudomonas* or *Acinetobacter* species. Therefore, strong arguments suggest that the prophylactic use of antibiotics in the ICU increases the risk of superinfection with multiresistant pathogens while only delaying the occurrence of nosocomial infection.

Stress Ulcer Prophylaxis

According to meta-analyses of the efficacy of stress-ulcer prophylaxis in ICU patients, respiratory tract infections were significantly less frequent in patients treated with sucralfate than those receiving antacids or H_2 blockers.[49-52] However, this conclusion was not fully confirmed in a very large, multicenter, randomized, blinded, placebo-controlled trial that compared sucralfate suspension (1 g q6h) with the H_2-receptor antagonist ranitidine (50 mg q8h) for the prevention of upper gastrointestinal bleeding in 1200 patients who required mechanical ventilation.[53] Clinically relevant gastrointestinal bleeding developed in 10 of the 596 (1.7%) patients receiving ranitidine, as compared with 23 of the 604 (3.8%) receiving sucralfate (RR, 0.44; 95% CI, 0.21 to 0.92; $P = 0.02$). In the ranitidine group, 114 of 596 (19.1%) patients had VAP, as diagnosed by an adjudication committee using a modified version of the CDC criteria, versus 98 of 604 (16.2%) in the sucralfate group (RR, 1.18; 95% CI, 0.92 to 1.51; $P = 0.19$). Thus, although pneumonia rates were similar for the two groups, the relative risks suggest a trend toward a lower pneumonia rate for patients receiving sucralfate. Furthermore, VAP occurred significantly less frequently in patients receiving sucralfate when the diagnosis of pneumonia was based on Memphis VAP Consensus Conference criteria (if there was radiographic evidence of abscess and a positive needle aspirate, or histologic proof of pneumonia at biopsy or autopsy) ($P = .03$).[53]

Sucralfate appears to have a small protective effect against VAP because stress-ulcer prophylactic medications that raise the gastric pH might themselves increase the incidence of pneumonia. This contention is supported by direct comparisons of trials of H_2-receptor antagonists versus no prophylaxis, which showed a trend toward higher pneumonia rates among the patients receiving H_2-receptor antagonists (OR, 1.25; 95% CI, 0.78 to 2.00).[51] Furthermore, the comparative effects of sucralfate and no prophylaxis are unclear. Among 226 patients enrolled in two randomized trials, those receiving sucralfate tended to develop pneumonia more frequently than those given no prophylaxis (OR, 2.11; 95% CI, 0.82 to 5.44).[54,55]

ENDOTRACHEAL TUBE, RE-INTUBATION, AND TRACHEOSTOMY

The presence of an endotracheal tube by itself circumvents host defenses, causes local trauma and inflammation, and increases the probability of aspirating nosocomial pathogens from the oropharynx around the cuff. Clearly, the type of endotracheal tube may also influence the incidence of aspiration. With low-volume, high-pressure endotracheal cuffs, an incidence of 56% was reported, which decreased to 20% with the advent of high-volume, low-pressure cuffs.[56]

In addition to the presence of endotracheal tubes, re-intubation is, per se, a risk factor for nosocomial pneumonia, as indicated by Torres and colleagues.[57] This result is probably related to an increased risk of aspiration of colonized oropharyngeal secretions into the lower airways in patients with glottic dysfunction and/or impaired consciousness after several days of intubation. Another explanation is direct aspiration of gastric contents into the lower airways, particularly when a nasogastric tube is kept in place after extubation. In their case-control study, Torres and colleagues found a 47% pneumonia rate in reintubated patients as compared with 4% in controls matched for the duration of prior mechanical ventilation ($P = .0007$).

The role of early tracheotomy in VAP prevention remains controversial, with only a few studies that examined this issue.[58-60] Whereas some studies found a reduction in the rate of VAP in patients with early tracheotomy,[59] others could not demonstrate any benefit.[58,60] For example, in a randomized, prospective, multicenter trial on 112 patients who were thought to need prolonged mechanical ventilation, there were no differences, at least until day 14, between ICU length of stay, pneumonia rate, or mortality between the 53 patients who underwent early (day 3 to 5) tracheotomy and the 59 who were managed using translaryngeal intubation. In the absence of any meaningful data, until a properly constructed randomized trial is performed to define the timing and utility of tracheotomy in the ICU, its true impact on decreasing VAP will remain merely speculative.[61]

NASOGASTRIC TUBE, ENTERAL FEEDING, AND PATIENT POSITION

Nearly all patients receiving mechanical ventilation have a nasogastric tube inserted to manage gastric and enteral secretions, prevent gastric distention, or provide nutritional support. The nasogastric tube is not widely considered to be a potential risk factor for pneumonia, but it may increase oropharyngeal colonization, cause stagnation of oropharyngeal secretions, and increase reflux and the risk of aspiration. Using multivariate analysis, Joshi and colleagues identified the presence of a nasogastric tube as one of the three independent risk factors for nosocomial pneumonia in a series of 203 patients admitted to the ICU for 72 hours or more.[62]

Early initiation of enteral feeding is generally regarded as beneficial in critically ill patients, but it may increase the risk of gastric colonization, gastroesophageal reflux, aspiration, and pneumonia.[63] Winterbauer and colleagues described a 38% incidence of aspiration in enterally fed, critically ill patients with small-bore nasogastric tubes, but all patients were fed by the bolus technique.[64] Recent data suggest that aspiration is infrequent when small-bore feeding tubes and continuous infusion are used.[65,66] The aspiration rate generally varies as a function of differences in the patient population, neurologic function, type of feeding tube, location of the feeding port, and the method of evaluating aspiration.[67] Clinical impression and preliminary data suggest that postpyloric or jejunal feeding entails less risk of aspiration and may therefore be associated with fewer infectious complications than gastric feeding, although this point remains controversial.[68,69]

Maintaining mechanically ventilated patients with a nasogastric tube in place in the supine position is also a risk factor for aspiration of gastric contents into the lower airways. Torres and colleagues injected radioactive material via a nasogastric tube directly into the stomach of 19 mechanically ventilated patients and found that mean radioactive counts in endobronchial secretions were higher in a time-dependent fashion in samples obtained while patients were in the supine position than in those obtained while patients were in the semirecumbent position.[70] The same microorganisms were isolated from stomach, pharynx, and endobronchial samples in 32% of the specimens taken while patients were semirecumbent and in 68% of those taken while patients were in the supine position. These results suggest that placing mechanically ventilated patients in the semirecumbent position is a simple and effective means to minimize aspiration of gastric contents into lower airways and hence constitutes a recommendable, no-cost prophylactic measure for those who can tolerate this position. Such experimental results were indirectly confirmed by Kollef, who demonstrated that supine patient head positioning during the first 24 hours of mechanical ventilation was an independent risk factor for acquiring VAP.[15] However, another study published by the same group that demonstrated the effect of body position on gastric content aspiration reported disappointing results, strongly supporting that gastroesophageal reflux in mechanically ventilated patients with a nasogastric tube occurs irrespective of body position.[71] A randomized trial conducted by the same group was stopped after the planned interim analysis because the frequency and the risk of VAP were significantly lower for the semirecumbent group.[72]

RESPIRATORY EQUIPMENT

Respiratory equipment itself may act as a source of bacteria responsible for nosocomial pneumonia. In past years, the major risk of infection was associated with contaminated reservoir nebulizers, designed to deliver small-sized particles suspended in the effluent gas.[12] These observations led to the current trends in respiratory therapy with the use of cascade humidifiers, which do not generate microaerosols. Nevertheless, respiratory equipment continues to provide a source of bacterial contamination. For example, medication nebulizers inserted into the inspiratory phase tube of the mechanical ventilator circuit may produce bacterial aerosols after a single use.[73]

Mechanical ventilators with humidifying cascades often have high levels of tubing colonization and condensate formation that may also be risk factors for pneumonia. Craven and colleagues examined condensate colonization in 20 circuits and found a median level of 2.0×10^5 organisms/mL, and 73% of the 52 gram-negative isolates present in the patient's sputum were subsequently isolated from condensate.[74] As most of the tubing colonization was derived from the patient secretions, the highest bacterial counts were present near the endotracheal tube. Simple procedures such as turning the patient or raising the bed rail may accidentally wash contaminated condensate directly into the patient's tracheobronchial tree. Inoculation of large amounts of fluid with high bacterial concentrations is an excellent way of overwhelming pulmonary defense mechanisms and producing pneumonia. Heating ventilator tubing markedly reduces the rate of condensate formation, but heated circuits are often nondisposable and are expensive. To date, no scientific evidence confirms that heated circuits reduce the incidence of VAP. In-line devices with one-way valves to collect condensate are probably the easiest way to handle this problem. They should be correctly positioned into disposable circuits and emptied regularly.

Similarly, there is not sufficient evidence to suggest that heat and moisture exchangers (HME) are superior to cascade humidifiers in terms of the risk of VAP. Dreyfuss and colleagues reported similar rates of pneumonia in 61 patients allocated to humidification with a HME and 70 patients with a heated humidifier (10% vs. 11%, NS).[75] When HME was used, changing the HME every 48 hours did not affect ventilator circuit colonization, and the authors suggest that the cost of mechanical ventilation may be substantially reduced without any detriment to the patient by extending the time between HME changes from 24 to 48 hours.[76] In recent years, several authors have reported no difference in pneumonia rates with ventilator circuit changes at 48-hour and 7-day intervals or with no change.[77-79]

SINUSITIS

While many studies have compared the risk of nosocomial sinusitis as a function of the intubation method used and the associated risk of VAP,[80-84] only a few were adequately powered to give a clear answer. In one study on 300 patients who required mechanical ventilation for at least 7 days and were randomly assigned to undergo nasotracheal or orotracheal intubation, computed tomographic (CT) evidence of sinusitis was observed slightly more frequently in the nasal than oral endotracheal group ($P = .08$), but this difference disappeared when only bacteriologically confirmed sinusitis was considered.[85] The rate of infectious maxillary sinusitis and its clinical relevance were also prospectively studied in 162 consecutive critically ill patients, who had been intubated and mechanically ventilated for 1 hour to 12 days before enrollment.[84] All had a paranasal CT scan within 48 hours of admission that was used to divide them into three groups (no, moderate, or severe sinusitis), according to the radiologic appearance of the maxillary sinuses. Patients who had no sinusitis at admission (n = 40) were randomized to receive endotracheal and gastric tubes via the nasal or oral route and, based on radiologic images, respective sinusitis rates were 96% and 23% ($P < .03$); yet, no differences in the rates of infectious sinusitis were documented according to the intubation route. However, VAP was more common in patients with infectious sinusitis, with 67% of them developing lung infection in the days after the diagnosis of sinusitis.[84] Therefore, whereas it seems clear that infectious sinusitis is a risk factor for VAP, no studies have yet been able to definitively demonstrate that orotracheal intubation decreases the infectious sinusitis rate compared with nasotracheal intubation, and thus no firm recommendations on the best route of intubation to prevent VAP can be advanced.

INTRAHOSPITAL PATIENT TRANSPORT

A prospective cohort study conducted on 531 mechanically ventilated patients evaluated the impact of transporting the patient out of the ICU to other sites within the hospital.[86] Results showed that 52% of the patients had to be moved at least once for a total of 993 transports and that 24% of the transported patients developed VAP compared with 4% of the patients confined to the ICU ($P < .001$). Multiple logistic regression analysis confirmed that transport out of the ICU was independently associated with VAP (OR = 3.8; $P < .001$).

EPIDEMIOLOGY

Diagnosis of ventilator-associated pneumonia is a controversial subject.[87,88] This debate is the result of differences in the analysis of three important questions: interpretation of clinical signs and symptoms suggestive of lung infection, differentiation between colonization and infection of the lower respiratory tract, and use of antibiotics in the ICU.

The first major difficulty in diagnosing VAP is that the presence of signs suggestive of pneumonia in non-ICU patients are too nonspecific to be of diagnostic value for ventilated patients.[1,89,90] The systemic signs of infection, such as fever, tachycardia, and leukocytosis, are nonspecific findings and can be caused by any condition that releases cytokines.[91] In trauma and other surgical patients, fever and leukocytosis should prompt the physician to suspect infection, but during the early post-traumatic or postoperative period (i.e., during the first 72 hours), these findings usually are not conclusive. However, later, fever and leukocytosis are more likely to be caused by pulmonary or nonpulmonary (vascular catheter infection, gastrointestinal infection, urinary tract infection, sinusitis, or wound infection) infections, but even then, other events associated with an inflammatory response (e.g., devascularized tissue, open wounds, pulmonary edema, and/or infarction) can be responsible for these findings. Although the plain (usually portable) chest radiograph remains an important component in the evaluation of hospitalized patients with suspected pneumonia, it is most helpful when it is normal and rules out pneumonia. When infiltrates are evident, the particular pattern is of limited value for differentiating among cardiogenic pulmonary edema, noncardiogenic pulmonary edema, pulmonary contusion, atelectasis (or collapse), and pneumonia. Because atelectasis is common in ICU patients, the contribution of repeating the chest radiograph after vigorous pulmonary physiotherapy was emphasized to differentiate infiltrates caused by atelectasis from those due to infection.[92] Very few studies have examined the accuracy of the portable chest radiograph in the ICU.[90,92-95] In a review of 24 patients with autopsy-proven pneumonia who were receiving mechanical ventilation, no single radiographic sign had a diagnostic accuracy greater than 68%.[93] When the group was divided into patients with and without ARDS, however, a significant difference was noted. The presence of air bronchograms or alveolar opacities in patients without ARDS correlated with pneumonia, whereas no such correlation was found for patients with ARDS. A variety of causes other than pneumonia can explain asymmetrical consolidation in patients with ARDS, and marked asymmetry of radiographic abnormalities has also been reported in patients with uncomplicated ARDS.[96] Several clinical studies confirmed the poor correlation between clinical signs and bacteriologic demonstration of VAP. Meduri and associates demonstrated the presence of lung infection in only 42% of the patients with clinically suspected VAP and frequent occurrence of multiple infectious and noninfectious processes.[97] In 1991, a composite clinical score was proposed, based on seven variables (temperature, blood leukocyte count, volume and purulence of tracheal secretions, oxygenation,

pulmonary radiography, and semiquantitative culture of tracheal aspirate) accorded 0, 1, or 2 points.[98] That study on 28 patients requiring prolonged mechanical ventilation showed a good correlation (r = .84, $P < .0001$) between this clinical score and quantitative bacteriology of bronchoalveolar lavage (BAL) samples, with a threshold value of 6 enabling identification of patients with infection. However, this scoring system is quite tedious to calculate and difficult to use in clinical practice, because several variables, such as progression of pulmonary infiltrates and results of semiquantitative cultures of tracheal secretions, can lead to different calculations depending on the observer. Furthermore, its value remains to be validated in a large prospective study, especially in patients with bilateral pulmonary infiltrates.

The second major obstacle to be confronted for the diagnosis of VAP is that, unlike patients developing community-acquired pneumonia, the presence of bacteria in the lower airways of intubated patients is not sufficient to diagnose true lung infection. Most VAP seems to result from aspiration of potential pathogens that have colonized the oropharyngeal airways. Intubation facilitates the entry of bacteria into the lung by pooling and leakage of contaminated secretions around the endotracheal cuff.[99] The tracheobronchial tree and the oropharynx of mechanically ventilated patients are frequently colonized by enteric gram-negative bacilli.[4,100,101] Based on specimens simultaneously obtained from the deep trachea and lung for culture from 48 patients with respiratory failure undergoing open-lung biopsy, culture results agreed for only 40% of these paired samples.[102] For patients with histologically documented pneumonia, endotracheal aspirate sensitivity was 82%, but its specificity was only 27%. The relationship between tracheal colonization and lung infection, however, remains unclear. Johanson and associates demonstrated that only 23% of colonized patients subsequently developed nosocomial pneumonia.[100]

Whereas simple qualitative culture of endotracheal aspirates is a technique with a high percentage of false-positive results due to bacterial colonization of the proximal airways observed in most ICU patients, some recent studies using quantitative culture techniques suggest that endotracheal aspirate cultures may have an acceptable overall diagnostic accuracy, similar to that of several other more invasive techniques.[103-107] In one study, the operating characteristics of endotracheal aspirate quantitative cultures, using 10^6 colony-forming units (cfu)/mL of respiratory secretions as the interpretative cutoff point, compared favorably with those of the PSB technique, with slightly higher sensitivity (82% vs. 64%) and lower specificity (83% vs. 96%).[103] To assess the reliability of that method, fiberoptic bronchoscopy with protected specimen brush and bronchoalveolar lavage was used to study 57 episodes of suspected lung infection in 39 ventilator-dependent patients with no recent changes of antimicrobial therapy.[106] The operating characteristics of endotracheal aspirate cultures were calculated over a range of cutoff values (from 10^3 to 10^7 cfu/mL) and the threshold of 10^6 cfu/mL appeared to be the most accurate, with a sensitivity of 68% and a specificity of 84%. However, when this threshold was applied to the study population, almost one third of the patients with pneumonia were not identified. Furthermore, only 40% of microorganisms cultured in endotracheal aspirate samples coincided with those obtained from PSB specimens. Other authors have emphasized that, although quantitative endotracheal aspirate cultures can correctly identify patients with pneumonia, microbiologic results cannot be used to infer which microorganisms present in the trachea are really present in the lungs. In a study comparing quantitative endotracheal aspirate culture results with postmortem quantitative lung-biopsy cultures, only 53% of the microorganisms isolated from the former samples at concentrations greater than 10^7 cfu/mL were also found in the latter cultures.[108]

The third major problem with the management of patients suspected of having VAP concerns the use of antibiotics. Most epidemiologic investigations have clearly demonstrated that the indiscriminate administration of antimicrobial agents to patients in the ICU has immediate and long-term consequences, which contribute to the emergence of multiresistant pathogens and increase the risk of severe superinfections with potentially increased morbidity and mortality, in addition to antibiotic-related toxicity and higher cost.[15,109-111] On the other hand, patient survival may improve if pneumonia is treated correctly and rapidly.[1,112,113] Using multivariate analysis, it was demonstrated that inappropriate therapy was strongly associated with fatality.[14,114] More precisely, the prognostic importance of the appropriateness of initial antimicrobial therapy has been underlined in many, mostly recent, studies: an inadequate antibiotic regimen, initiated before obtaining the results of cultures from respiratory secretions, was associated with greater hospital mortality rate compared with an antibiotic regimen, which provided adequate antimicrobial coverage of all identified pathogens from obtained cultures.[20-24] Unfortunately, two factors seem to render the choice of antibiotics difficult in this setting. First, VAP is likely to result from highly resistant organisms, especially in patients who were previously treated with antibiotics[115] or in case of pneumonia occurring more than 7 days after initiation of mechanical ventilation.[32] Second, multiple organisms are frequently cultured from the pulmonary secretions of patients considered to have pneumonia, especially when the sampling technique is not specific enough to differentiate colonizing from infecting pathogens.[5,14,116]

Ideally, any diagnostic strategy intended to be used in patients clinically suspected of having developed hospital-acquired pneumonia should be able to reach the three following objectives:

1. Accurately identify patients with true pulmonary infection, and, in case of infection, isolate the causative microorganisms (to initiate immediate appropriate antimicrobial treatment and then to optimize therapy based on pathogen susceptibility patterns).
2. Identify patients with extrapulmonary sites of infection.
3. Withhold and/or withdraw antibiotics in patients without infection.

Two diagnostic algorithms can be used in cases in which HAP is suspected. One option is to treat every patient clinically suspected of having a pulmonary infection with new antibiotics even when the likelihood of infection is low. In this option, the selection of appropriate empirical therapy is based on risk factors and local resistance patterns and involves qualitative testing to identify possible pathogens, with antimicrobial therapy being adjusted according to culture results or clinical response (Fig. 84-1). This "clinical" approach has two potential advantages: (1) no specialized microbiologic techniques are required and (2) the risk of missing a patient who needs antimicrobial treatment is minimal, at least when all suspected patients are treated with new antibiotics.

However, such a strategy leads to overestimation of the incidence of HAP. Qualitative endotracheal aspirate cultures contribute indisputably to the diagnosis of HAP only when they are completely negative for a patient with no modification of prior antimicrobial treatment. In such a case, the negative-predictive value is very high and the probability of the patient having pneumonia is close to null.[24]

Concern about the inaccuracy of clinical approaches to HAP recognition had led numerous investigators to postulate that "specialized" diagnostic methods, including quantitative cultures of endotracheal aspirates or specimens obtained with bronchoscopic or nonbronchoscopic techniques including BAL and/or PSB, could improve identification of patients with true HAP and facilitate decisions whether to treat, and thus clinical outcome.[23,25-28] Using such a strategy, the decision algorithm is similar to the one described in Figure 84-1 except that therapeutic decisions are taken based on results of direct examination of distal pulmonary samples and results of quantitative cultures (Fig. 84-2).

EVALUATION OF DIAGNOSTIC STRATEGIES

Other than decision-analysis studies[117,118] and one retrospective study,[119] only four trials have so far assessed the impact of a diagnostic strategy on antibiotic use and outcome of patients suspected of having HAP using a randomized scheme.[23,120-122] No differences in mortality and morbidity were found when either invasive (PSB and/or BAL) or noninvasive (quantitative endotracheal aspirate cultures) techniques were used to diagnose HAP in three Spanish randomized studies.[23,120,122] However, those studies were based on relatively few patients (51, 76, and 88, respectively) and antibiotics were continued in all patients despite negative cultures, thereby neutralizing one of the potential advantages of any diagnostic test in patients clinically suspected of having HAP. Concerning the latter, several prospective studies have concluded that antibiotics can indeed be stopped in patients with negative quantitative cultures with no adverse effects on the recurrence of HAP and mortality.[21,119,123-125] One of the first studies to clearly demonstrate a benefit in favor of invasive techniques was a prospective, randomized trial that compared the two strategies in 413 patients suspected of having VAP.[121] Compared with patients managed clinically, those receiving invasive management had a lower mortality rate on day 14 (16% and 25%; $P = .02$), and lower mean sepsis-related organ failure assessment scores on days 3 and 7 ($P = 0.04$). At 28 days, the invasive-management group had significantly more antibiotic-free days (11 ± 9 vs. 7 ± 7; $P < 0.001$), and only multivariate analysis showed a significant difference in mortality (hazards ratio, 1.54 [CI, 1.10 to 2.16]; $P = 0.01$).[26] Thus, implementation of bronchoscopic techniques for the diagnosis of VAP may reduce antibiotic use and improve patient outcome.

The choice of procedure(s) may eventually depend on the preferences and experiences of individual physicians and the patient's underlying disease(s). Despite broad clinical experience with the PSB and BAL techniques, it remains, nonetheless, unclear which one should be used in clinical practice. Most investigators prefer to use BAL rather than PSB to diagnose bacterial pneumonia, because BAL (1) has a slightly higher sensitivity to identify HAP-causative microorganisms, (2) enables better selection of an empirical antimicrobial treatment before culture results are available, (3) is less dangerous for many critically ill patients, (4) is less

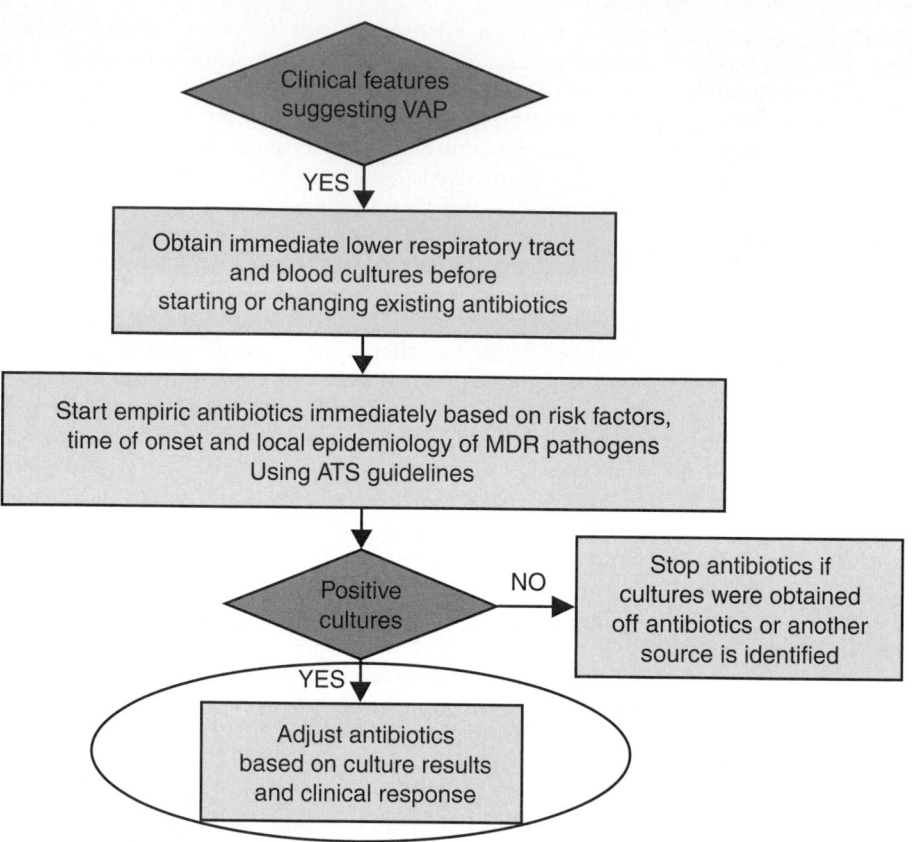

FIGURE 84–1. Clinical VAP strategy.

costly, and (5) may provide useful clues for the diagnosis of other types of infections. However, it must be acknowledged that a very small return on BAL may contain only diluted material from the bronchial rather than alveolar level and thus give rise to false-negative results, particularly for patients with very severe COPD. In these patients, the diagnostic value of BAL techniques is greatly diminished and the PSB technique should be preferred.[126]

Cultures of pulmonary secretions for diagnostic purposes after initiation of new antibiotic therapy in patients suspected of having developed HAP can clearly lead to a high number of false-negative results, regardless of the way in which these secretions are obtained. Using a lower threshold to define a positive quantitative result in such a setting may be inaccurate, because follow-up cultures can be completely negative in at least 40% of true cases of VAP.[127,128] Pulmonary secretions therefore need to be obtained before new antibiotics are administered, as is the case for all microbiologic samples.

The diagnosis of bacterial pneumonia in the severely ill, mechanically ventilated patient remains a difficult dilemma for the clinician. Our personal bias is that the use of bronchoscopic techniques to obtain PSB and/or BAL specimens from the affected area in the lung of ventilated patients with signs suggestive of pneumonia allows definition of a therapeutic strategy superior to that based exclusively on clinical evaluation (see Figs. 84–1 and 84–2). When performed before introduction of new antibiotics, these bronchoscopic techniques enable physicians to identify most patients who need immediate treatment and help to select optimal therapy, in a manner that is safe and well tolerated by patients. Furthermore, these techniques prevent resorting to broad-spectrum drug coverage in all patients who develop a clinically suspected infection. Although the true impact of this decision

tree on patient outcome remains controversial, available data clearly suggest that being able to withhold antimicrobial treatment from some patients without infection may constitute a distinct advantage in the long term, by minimizing the emergence of resistant microorganisms in the ICU and redirecting the search for another (the true) infection site.

In patients with clinical evidence of severe sepsis with rapidly deteriorating organ dysfunction, hypoperfusion, or hypotension, the initiation of antibiotic therapy should not be delayed while awaiting fiberoptic bronchoscopy, and patients should be treated immediately with antibiotics. It is probably in this latter situation that simplified nonbronchoscopic diagnostic procedures could be most justified, because distal pulmonary secretions can be obtained on a 24-hour basis, just before starting new antimicrobial therapy. Because several studies have indicated that delays in the administration of effective antibiotic therapy may impact on VAP outcome, antibiotic therapy should not be postponed for more than a few hours (<6 hours) pending performance of fiberoptic bronchoscopy, even when the patient is clinically stable.

When fiberoptic bronchoscopy is not available to physicians treating patients clinically suspected of having VAP, we recommend using either a simplified nonbronchoscopic diagnostic procedure, replacing fiberoptic bronchoscopy in the algorithm depicted in Figure 84-1 by one of these techniques, or following the strategy described by Singh and associates,[129] in which decisions regarding antibiotic therapy are based on a clinical score constructed from seven variables, the CPIS score. Such an approach avoids prolonged treatment of patients with a low likelihood of infection, while allowing immediate treatment of patients with VAP. However, two conditions must rigorously be respected when

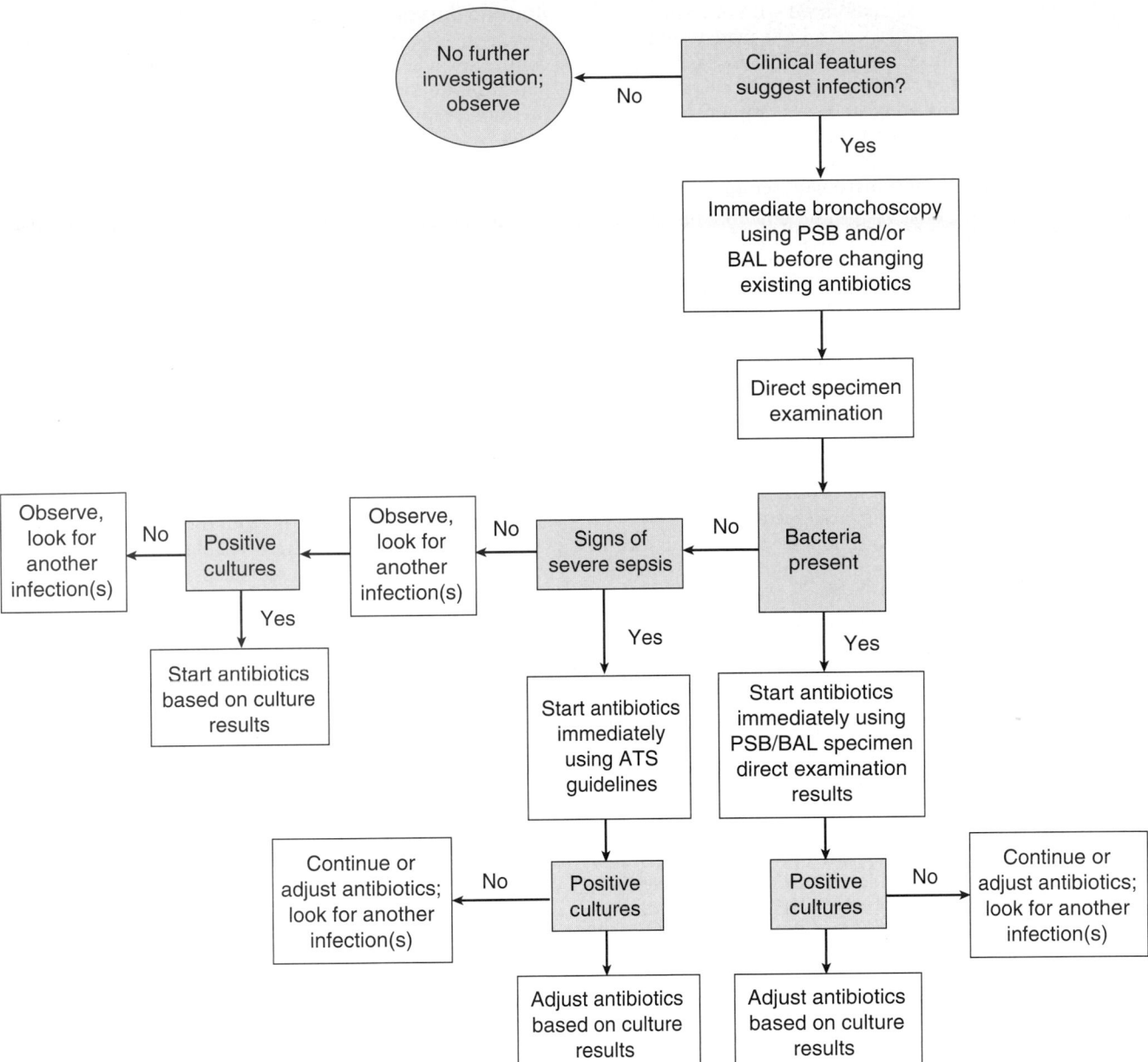

FIGURE 84–2. "Invasive" (microbiologic) strategy.

implementing this strategy. First, selection of the initial antimicrobial therapy should be based on predominant flora responsible for VAP at each institution. It is highly probable that ciprofloxacin would not be the right choice in numerous institutions due to the high prevalence of MRSA infections in many of them.[130] Second, it should be made clear to physicians that antimicrobial treatment should be reevaluated on day 3, when susceptibility patterns of the microorganism(s) considered to be VAP causative are available, in order to select treatment with a narrower spectrum.

TREATMENT

EVALUATION OF CURRENT ANTIMICROBIAL STRATEGIES

Despite many advances in antimicrobial therapy, successful treatment of patients with nosocomial pneumonia remains a difficult and complex undertaking. No consensus has been reached concerning issues as basic as the optimal antimicrobial regimen for therapy or duration of treatment. Although some investigators have recommended two-drug parenteral therapy for most cases, recent data have demonstrated the efficacy of a monotherapy for some patients. Similarly, the efficacy of endotracheal or aerosolized antibiotics as either the sole or adjunctive therapy for gram-negative pneumonia remains controversial. In fact, to date, evaluation of various antimicrobial strategies for the treatment of bacterial pneumonia in mechanically ventilated patients has been difficult for several reasons.

First, nearly all previous therapeutic investigations have relied solely on clinical diagnostic criteria and therefore have probably included patients who did not have pneumonia. Second, most of these studies used cultures of tracheal secretions as the major source of samples for microbiologic analysis despite the fact that the respiratory tract of most ventilated patients is usually colonized with multiple potential pathogens. Finally, the lack of an adequate technique to directly sample the infection site in the lung has hampered assessment of the ability or inability of antibiotics to eradicate the causative pathogens from the lower respiratory tract and therefore the ability to predict their bacteriologic efficacy.

Montravers and colleagues evaluated the bacteriologic and clinical efficacy of antimicrobial therapies, selected on the basis of the etiologic microorganisms identified by cultures of PSB samples obtained during bronchoscopy, for the treatment of nosocomial bacterial pneumonia in 76 patients receiving mechanical ventilation.[127] Using a follow-up PSB sample culture to directly assess the site of infection in the lung, their results demonstrated that the administration of an antimicrobial therapy combining, in most cases, two effective agents, was able to sterilize or control the lower respiratory tract infection after only 3 days of treatment in 67 (88%) of the patients included in the study. The only two bacteriologic failures were observed in patients who did not receive adequate treatment because of errors in the selection of antimicrobial drugs. Early superinfection caused by bacteria resistant to the initial antibiotics was, however, documented in 7 (9%) patients, emphasizing the need to carefully monitor the impact of treatment on the initial microbial flora for optimal management of such patients when the clinical response is suboptimal. Furthermore, results of cultures of follow-up PSB samples were well correlated with the clinical outcome noted during the 15-day observation period, making this test a good prognostic indicator in patients with VAP.

FACTORS CONTRIBUTING TO SELECTION OF INITIAL TREATMENT

Important factors to be considered for the optimal selection of initial antibiotic therapy include (1) putative causative pathogens and their patterns of antibiotic susceptibilities, based on the clinical setting and previous epidemiologic studies, (2) data obtained by surveillance cultures in the same patient, (3) information given by direct microscopic examination of pulmonary secretions, and (4) intrinsic antibacterial activities of antimicrobial agents and their pharmacokinetic characteristics.

Clinical Setting

Underlying diseases and specific risk factors may predispose patients to infection with specific organisms, as well as some intrinsic factors linked to each hospital or ICU.[4] Therefore, selection of initial antimicrobial therapy needs to be tailored to each institution's local patterns of antimicrobial resistance.[31,130] Based on the results of a French prospective study in which the responsible microorganisms for infection in 135 consecutive episodes of VAP observed in the ICU were documented using bronchoscopic specimens, the distribution of infecting pathogens was markedly influenced by prior duration of mechanical ventilation and prior antibiotic use.[32] Taking these epidemiologic characteristics into account allowed the authors to devise a rational decision-tree for selecting initial treatment in this setting that prevents using broad-spectrum drug coverage in all patients. A computerized decision-support program linked to computer-based patient records can facilitate the dissemination of such information to physicians for immediate use in therapy decision-making and improve the quality of care.[131,132]

Routine Surveillance Culture Results

Several investigators have recommended routine surveillance cultures of ICU patients because they may be predictive of patients who are at high risk of invasive disease and, furthermore, should invasive disease develop, empirical therapy can be selected based on the predominant pathogens identified by these cultures.[4,133] However, the accuracy of this approach for selecting initial antimicrobial treatment for ICU patients requiring new antibiotics for VAP has not yet been established. This hypothesis was recently retested in a prospective study conducted on 125 patients who required mechanical ventilation for more than 48 hours and for whom strict bronchoscopic criteria were applied to diagnose pneumonia and identify the causative pathogens.[134] Although a large number of various prior microbiologic specimen culture results were obtained before fiberoptic bronchoscopy for each HAP episode, only 33% of the 220 HAP-causative microorganisms were isolated by these routine analyses with susceptibility patterns available to guide initial antimicrobial treatment. When the analysis focused on HAP episodes for which prior (within 72 hours) respiratory secretion culture results were available, results were better but still disappointing because all causative pathogens were recovered for fewer than 60% of cases. Such a strategy may also considerably increase the workload of the microbiology laboratory without having any positive impact on patient management.

Colonization with potentially drug-resistant pathogens, such as MRSA or extended-spectrum β-lactamase–producing strains of *K. pneumoniae* or other Enterobacteriaceae, is associated with an increased risk of infection caused by the corresponding microorganism. These results were confirmed in the study by Hayon and associates, with positive-predictive values of recovering such a microorganism from a specimen of 62%, 52%, or 24% for VAP caused by MRSA, *P. aeruginosa,* or *A. baumannii,* respectively.[134] However, because the sensitivity of prior microbiologic culture results for identifying bacteria causing HAP do not exceed 70%, selection of initial antimicrobial therapy for patients with HAP can hardly be based only on these results, especially for deciding to use (or not to use) vancomycin and/or a broad-spectrum β-lactam effective against *P. aeruginosa* and/or *A. baumannii.*

Information Given by Direct Examination of Pulmonary Secretions

Direct microscopy of pulmonary secretions is extremely important not only to identify patients with true VAP but also to select appropriate treatment, especially when BAL specimens are used to prepare cytocentrifuged Gram-stained smears.[135] In patients with pneumonia, the morphology and Gram staining of bacteria are closely correlated to the results of bacterial cultures, enabling early formulation of a specific antimicrobial regimen before the culture results are available. In a study of 94 mechanically ventilated patients with suspected HAP who underwent fiberoptic bronchoscopy with BAL and PSB, direct BAL fluid examination results were available within 2 hours, BAL and PSB culture results were available after 24 hours, and antibiotic susceptibility was learned after 48 hours.[136] At each step in the strategy, the senior physician and the resident in charge of the patient were asked their diagnoses and their therapeutic plans based on the available data. Using a threshold of 1% infected cells, direct BAL examination discriminated well between patients with and those without VAP (sensitivity

94%, specificity 92%, area under the ROC curve 0.95). Therefore, a strategy based on bronchoscopy and direct examination of BAL fluid may lead to more rapid and appropriate treatment of HAP than a strategy based only on clinical evaluation.

Intrinsic Antibacterial Activities of Antimicrobial Agents

Effective antibiotic treatment of bacterial pneumonia depends on adequate delivery of antibacterial agents to the infection site; therefore, scrupulous attention must be given to optimal doses, routes of administration, and pharmacodynamic characteristics of each agent used to treat this infection. Owing to major methodologic problems, published data concerning the penetration of most antibiotics into the lung should probably be viewed with caution, and only general trends concerning concentrations achievable at the infected site in lung tissue can be derived from those studies.[137,138]

For penicillins and cephalosporins, the bronchial secretion-to-serum drug-concentration ratios range between 0.05 and 0.25. Fluoroquinolones have better penetration characteristics, and bronchial secretion concentrations are between 0.8 and 2 times those in serum. Aminoglycosides and tetracyclines have ratios of 0.2 to 0.6. Host-related as well as drug-related factors may, however, influence the penetration of antimicrobial drugs across the blood/bronchus and alveolar/capillary barriers. Thus, for those drugs, such as the β-lactams and glycopeptides, which do not cross membranes readily, penetration might increase in the presence of inflammation because of enhanced membrane permeability.[139]

Several published reports have demonstrated a relationship among serum concentrations of β-lactams or other antibiotics, the in vitro minimal inhibitory concentration (MIC) of the infecting organism, and the rate of bacterial eradication from respiratory secretions in patients with lung infection, thereby emphasizing that clinical and bacteriologic outcomes can be improved by optimizing the therapeutic regimen according to pharmacokinetic properties of the agent(s) selected for treatment.[140-144] Most investigators distinguish between antimicrobial agents that kill by a concentration-dependent mechanism (e.g., aminoglycosides and fluoroquinolones) from those that kill by a time-dependent mechanism (e.g., β-lactams and vancomycin).

Development of a priori dosing algorithms based on MIC, patient creatinine clearance and weight, and a clinician-specified pharmacokinetic-pharmacodynamic variable, such as the 24-hour area under the concentration/time curve divided by the MIC (AUIC), might therefore be a valid way to improve treatment of these patients, leading to a more precise approach than current guidelines for optimal use of antimicrobial agents.

DE-ESCALATION

Once the microbiologic data become available, it is also necessary to de-escalate therapy to avoid prolonged use of a broader spectrum of antibiotic therapy than is justified by the available information. For many patients, including those with late-onset infection, the culture data will not show the presence of highly resistant pathogens, and in these individuals therapy can be narrowed, or even reduced, to a single agent in light of the susceptibility pattern of the causative

pathogens without risking inappropriate treatment. While a de-escalating approach to antibiotic therapy (i.e., culture-guided treatment) may not help individual patients, it could benefit the ICU as a whole by reducing the selection pressure for resistance. Every possible effort should therefore be made to obtain, before new antibiotics are administered, reliable pulmonary specimens for direct microscope examination and cultures from each patient clinically suspected of having developed HAP.[145]

MONOTHERAPY VERSUS COMBINATION THERAPY

Several studies have examined the use of a single antibiotic (e.g., a third-generation cephalosporin, imipenem–cilastatin, or a fluoroquinolone) to treat HAP.[146-150] In general, monotherapy has proved to be a useful alternative to combination therapy, with the same success rate and no more superinfections or colonizations by multiresistant pathogens. Because those studies included nonhomogeneous populations of patients with different types of infections and given the potential inaccuracy of using only clinical criteria to diagnose lung infection, further trials are needed to clarify all these uncertainties. Furthermore, for patients with severe infection due to *P. aeruginosa* or other multiresistant bacteria, such as *Klebsiella* species or *Acinetobacter* species, combining an antipseudomonal β-lactam with an aminoglycoside or ciprofloxacin is likely to obtain a much better outcome than monotherapy, as previously shown. In a prospective clinical study on 200 patients with *P. aeruginosa* bacteremia, mortality rates for patients with pneumonia receiving monotherapy or combination therapy as the initial empirical treatment were 88% (7/8 patients) or 35% (7/20 patients), respectively (P = .03).[151] Similarly, for the subgroup of 55 patients who experienced hypotension within 72 hours prior to or on the day of the positive blood culture in a prospective observational study on 230 *Klebsiella* bacteremias, the mortality rate was significantly lower for those patients who received combination therapy (24%) than those given monotherapy (50%).[152] It should be noted, however, that the β-lactam agents used in those studies were older agents, with less potent activity than the advanced cephalosporins or the carbapenems available today.

Based on these data, it is probably safer to use a β-lactam antibiotic in combination with an aminoglycoside or a quinolone for patients with severe HAP, at least for the first days of therapy, while culture results of pulmonary secretions are pending. It may be that monodrug therapies for nosocomial pneumonia would best be reserved for infections in which *P. aeruginosa* or other multiresistant microorganisms, such as *Klebsiella, Enterobacter, Citrobacter, Serratia,* or *Acinetobacter* species, have been excluded as the etiologic agents.

DURATION OF ANTIMICROBIAL THERAPY

The optimal antimicrobial regimen and duration of therapy for patients who develop pneumonia has not been established. Most experts recommend that the duration be adapted to the severity of the disease, the time to clinical response, and the microorganism(s) responsible.[4] A "long" treatment, that is, a minimum of 14 to 21 days, is prescribed for the following situations: multilobular involvement, malnutrition, cavitation, gram-negative necrotizing pneumonia, and isolation of *P. aeruginosa* or *Acinetobacter* species, which correspond to the majority of pulmonary infections occurring in patients requiring mechanical ventilation. This duration is essentially justified by the high theoretical risk of relapse, especially in case of infection caused by *P. aeruginosa* and MRSA, which are particularly difficult to eradicate from the respiratory tract.[153] Thus, at present, a short-term regimen is rarely prescribed in patients who develop HAP, despite the potential major advantages it could have in terms of bacterial ecology and the prevention of the emergence of multiresistant bacteria. Lowering the amount of antibiotics administered to patients hospitalized in ICUs is indeed a primary objective of every strategy aimed at reducing the emergence and dissemination of such bacteria.[111,154]

A prospective, randomized, multicenter trial was recently conducted in France to compare the clinical efficacy of two predefined durations of antimicrobial treatment (an 8-day and a 15-day course of antibiotics) in patients with microbiologically proven VAP.[155] This trial was designed to demonstrate both the noninferiority of the effect of the short course regimen on mortality and recurrence of pulmonary infection, and its superiority in terms of antibiotic use, as assessed by the number of days alive and free of antibiotics. These outcome measures were all assessed 28 days after the onset of pneumonia. Of 401 patients enrolled, 197 were randomly assigned to receive a short (8-day) course of antibiotics and 204 to receive a long (15-day) course of therapy. Compared with patients who received a long course of therapy, patients who received a short course had neither excess mortality (18.8% vs. 17.2%; 90% CI for the difference, −3.7 to +6.9 percentage points) nor excess pulmonary infection recurrence (28.9% vs. 26.0%; 90% CI for the difference, −3.2 to +9.1 percentage points), but they had significantly more antibiotic-free days (13.1 ± 7.4 vs. 8.7 ± 5.2 days, $P < .0001$). Therefore, an 8-day regimen can probably be the standard for the duration of antibiotic therapy in patients with HAP. Such an approach might help to control health care costs and to contain the development of bacterial resistance in ICUs.

PREVENTION

Because VAP has been associated with increased morbidity, longer hospital stay, increased health care costs, and higher mortality rates, prevention of this infection is a major challenge for intensive care medicine. A number of recommendations published for the prevention of nosocomial pneumonia are empirical rather than based on controlled observations for several reasons that make evaluation of the impact of such interventions difficult:

1. The difficulty of obtaining an accurate diagnosis of VAP, that is, to distinguish patients with true infection from patients with tracheal colonization and/or other pathologic processes since only patients who develop true VAP are likely to benefit from preventive measures.
2. The difficulty of precisely determining the impact of a prophylactic measure on the overall mortality of a general ICU population, that is, to identify preventable deaths, directly attributable to VAP, among all deaths occurring in a population of ventilated ICU patients.
3. The difficulty of evaluating the effects of a preventive measure on a potentially pathogenic mechanism, for

example, to evaluate the exact role played by prevention or reduction of tracheal colonization in modifying the development of VAP.[156-161]

CONVENTIONAL INFECTION-CONTROL APPROACHES

These measures should be the first step taken in any prevention program.[162] The design of the ICU has a direct effect on the potential for nosocomial infections. Adequate space and lighting, proper functioning of ventilation systems, and facilities for hand washing lead to lower infection rates.[163] It should, however, be kept in mind that physical upgrading of the environment does not per se reduce the infection rate unless personnel attitude and practices are improved. In any ICU, one of the most important factors is probably the team that staffs it—the number, quality, and motivation of its medical, nursing, and ancillary members. The team should include a sufficient number of nurses to avoid having them move from one patient to another and to avoid working under constant pressure. The importance of personal cleanliness and attention to aseptic procedures must be emphasized at every possible opportunity. At the same time, unnecessarily rigid restrictions should be avoided. It is clear that careful monitoring, decontamination, and compliance with the usage guidelines of respiratory equipment decrease the incidence of nosocomial pneumonia.[164] In any case, hand washing or hand rubbing with alcohol-based solution remains uncontested as the most important infection control practice.[165,166]

A bacterial monitoring policy facilitates the early recognition of colonization and infection and has been associated with statistically significant reductions in nosocomial infection rates.[167] The focal point for infection control activities in the ICU is a surveillance system designed to establish and maintain a database that describes endemic rates of nosocomial infection. Awareness of the endemic rates enables the recognition of the onset of an epidemic when infection rates rise above a calculated threshold.

Preventing infection by modifying host risk has focused on treatment of underlying diseases and complications and control of antibiotic use. Adoption of an antibiotic policy restricting the prescription of broad-spectrum agents and useless antibiotics is of major importance.[168] Simple, safe, inexpensive, logical, but unproven measures, including the use of physiotherapy,[169] the judicious use and prompt removal of a useless nasogastric tube, and removal of tubing condensate, may have tremendous impact on the frequency of nosocomial pneumonia in mechanically ventilated patients.

SPECIFIC PROPHYLAXIS AGAINST VENTILATOR-ASSOCIATED PNEUMONIA

Because invasive mechanical ventilation is a risk factor for VAP, strategies that reduce its duration might reduce its incidence. Optimization of weaning protocols is a first way to reduce the duration of exposure to risk.[170,171] Noninvasive ventilation is an alternative approach to the use of artificial airways to avoid infectious complications and injury of the trachea in patients with acute respiratory failure. Many observations and studies, unfortunately small and not blinded, suggest that patients who tolerate noninvasive ventilation have a lower incidence of pneumonia than those tracheally intubated.[172-175] However, although seven randomized trials have compared noninvasive ventilation with conventional mechanical ventilation for prevention of pneumonia, only one could demonstrate a statistically significant benefit in favor of noninvasive ventilation.[171,176-181]

Apart from these protocols aiming at reducing the duration of mechanical ventilation, seven prophylactic approaches have been studied: semi-recumbent positioning, oscillating and rotating beds, continuous or intermittent aspiration of subglottic secretions, ventilator circuits management, methods of enteral feeding, stress ulcer prophylaxis, and antibiotic use including selective digestive decontamination.

Semi-Recumbent Positioning

Supine patient positioning has been shown to be independently associated with the development of VAP.[182] Placing ventilated patients in a semi-recumbent position to minimize reflux and aspiration of gastric contents is a simple measure, although some practical problems can occur in unstable patients. Three trials have evaluated the efficacy of semi-recumbent positioning,[183-185] but only one measured the incidence of VAP: Drakulovic and colleagues clearly indicated significantly lower rates of both clinically suspected and bacteriologically confirmed VAP and identified supine positioning as an independent risk factor for VAP with enteral nutrition, mechanical ventilation for 7 days or more, and a Glasgow Coma Scale score of less than 9 points. These results explained the higher risk of VAP observed in patients receiving enteral nutrition in the supine position. There was no difference in mortality in this study.[184] No adverse effects were observed in patients assigned to semi-recumbent positioning.

Oscillating and Rotating Bed

Immobility in critically ill patients treated with mechanical ventilation results in atelectasis and impaired secretions drainage, and potentially predisposes to pulmonary complications including VAP. Oscillating and rotating beds may help in preventing pneumonia.[186] Six randomized trials,[187-192] including mostly surgical and trauma patients, ventilated or not, summarized in a meta-analysis by Choi and Nelson[193] have compared continuous lateral rotational therapy with standard beds for the prevention of nosocomial pneumonia. The meta-analysis found a statistically significant reduction in the risk for pneumonia, principally concerning early-onset (<5 days) pneumonia and a decreased duration of ICU stay. Notably, the only randomized, controlled trial (not included in the meta-analysis) conducted on a general ICU population did not show any differences in pneumonia rates but showed a significantly shorter length of ICU stay.[194] Some adverse events have been described with these beds, including disconnection of catheters or pressure ulceration; in addition, nursing care is potentially complicated with oscillating beds. Finally, in spite of the cost of such beds, cost-benefit analyses performed in those studies suggested favorable results, mainly caused by the reduction of ICU length of stay.

Aspiration of Subglottic Secretions

Repeated microinhalations of colonized oropharyngeal (subglottic) secretions are the major well-documented mechanism resulting in the development of VAP. Continuous or intermittent aspiration of oropharyngeal secretions has been proposed to avoid chronic aspiration of secretions through the tracheal cuff of intubated patients. Aspiration of subglottic secretions requires the use of specially designed endotracheal tube with a separate lumen that opens into the subglottic region. Three randomized controlled trials have studied aspiration of subglottic secretions for the prevention of VAP.[195-197] Mahul and associates found that pneumonia was significantly less frequent in patients with an endotracheal tube having a separate dorsal lumen for hourly suctioning of stagnant secretions above the cuff than in others and that VAP development was delayed.[195] Similarly, in a 3-year prospective, randomized, controlled study, Valles and coworkers documented a lower VAP rate when continuous subglottic aspiration was performed.[196] However, this difference was fully explained by VAP occurring during the first week, whereas late-onset pneumonias were more frequent in the aspiration group. Furthermore, detailed microbiologic analysis demonstrated that this reduction concerned only pneumonia due to *H. influenzae* or gram-positive cocci. The incidence of VAP due to *P. aeruginosa* or Enterobacteriaceae did not differ between the two groups. Kollef and colleagues performed a randomized trial on 343 post-cardiac surgery patients to compare continuous subglottic aspiration and standard postoperative medical care.[197] Although those authors found similar rates of VAP in both groups, VAP episodes occurred significantly later in patients receiving subglottic aspiration than in those treated conventionally. No difference in mortality rates was observed in these three studies. No adverse events were reported with aspiration of subglottic secretions in studied patients; however, experimental data suggest the possibility of tracheal damages in sheep intubated with this type of tube.

Ventilator Circuit Management

Decreased frequency of ventilator-circuit change, replacement of heated humidifiers by heat and moisture exchangers, decreased frequency of heat and moisture exchanger change, and closed suctioning systems have been tested for preventing VAP. Four randomized trials of decreased frequency of ventilator circuit changes have been published[198-201] comparing changes every 2 days, 7 days, and no scheduled change and did not find significant difference in the rate of VAP as summarized in a recent meta-analysis.[202] One meta-analysis summarized the results of five randomized, controlled trials that compared the effects of heated humidifiers and heat and moisture exchangers on the risk of VAP.[161] Only one of these five studies found a significant reduction of VAP rate with the use of heat and moisture exchangers.[203] Efficacy of both humidification strategies seems comparable; however, two studies reported increased rates of endotracheal tube occlusion with the use of heat and moisture exchangers,[161] and increased resistive load resulting in difficulties in the ventilation and weaning process of patients with severe ARDS—related with larger dead space—has been reported in observational studies.[204] No other adverse effects were observed. No effect on mortality was reported. Finally, one study has evaluated the impact of less frequent changes (daily vs. every 5 days) in heat and moisture exchangers on the development of VAP.[205] No difference in the VAP rates was observed.

To avoid hypoxia, hypotension, and contamination of suction catheters entering the tracheal tube, investigators have examined closed suctioning systems.[206,207] They found a nonsignificantly lower prevalence rate of VAP for patients managed with the closed system compared with those with the open system without demonstrating any adverse effect[206] or not only failed to show a statistically significant protective effect of the closed system on the incidence of VAP but also observed an increased frequency of endotracheal colonization associated with the closed device.[207]

Methods of Enteral Feeding

Nearly all patients receiving mechanical ventilation have a nasogastric tube inserted to manage gastric and enteral secretions, prevent gastric distention, or provide nutritional support. The nasogastric tube may increase the risk for gastroesophageal reflux, aspiration, and VAP.[208]

Four randomized, controlled trials have evaluated methods of enteral feeding aimed at preventing VAP: postpyloric or jejunal feeding (vs. gastric feeding), the use of motility agents (metoclopramide vs. placebo), acidification of feeding (with addition of hydrochloric acid), and intermittent (vs. continuous) feeding.[209-212] These studies did not find differences in incidence of VAP and/or mortality rates. Potentially serious adverse affects have been observed in patients receiving acidified feeding (gastrointestinal bleeding) or intermittent enteral feeding (increased gastric volume and lower volumes of feeding). Thus, to date, methods of enteral feeding aimed to reduce the incidence of VAP cannot be recommended for routine use.

Stress Ulcer Prophylaxis

Gastric colonization by potentially pathogenic organisms has been shown to increase with decreasing gastric acidity.[213] Thus, medications that decrease gastric acidity (antacids, H_2 blockers) may increase organism counts and increase the risk for VAP. In contrast, medications that do not affect gastric acidity (sucralfate) may not increase this risk.

Seven meta-analyses of more than 20 randomized trials have evaluated the risk for VAP associated with the methods used to prevent gastrointestinal bleeding in critically ill patients.[214-220] These studies reported a significant reduction in four, or nonsignificant trends in reduction in three, of VAP incidence with sucralfate therapy compared with H_2 blockers. Three studies reported a statistically significant mortality benefit in patients given sucralfate.[215-217]

The relationships between prophylaxis of stress ulcer and prophylaxis of VAP are complex:

1. VAP is a possible indirect consequence of the use of drugs that raise the stomach pH.
2. Gastrointestinal bleeding is a serious complication in critically ill patients at high risk for stress ulcer (i.e., patients with coagulopathy or need for prolonged mechanical ventilation) but is extremely rare in patients at low to moderate risk.
3. The largest randomized trial comparing ranitidine to sucralfate showed ranitidine was superior in preventing gastrointestinal bleeding and did not increase the risk of VAP.[221]
4. The risk of VAP is unknown when accurate methods of enteral feeding or other preventive measures are used in combination with stress ulcer prophylaxis.

Clinicians must weigh the potential benefit of sucralfate (with potentially less VAP and more gastrointestinal bleeding) versus H_2 blockers (with potentially more VAP and less gastrointestinal bleeding) and probably limit stress ulcer prophylaxis to high-risk patients.

Antibiotic Use and Selective Digestive Decontamination

There is theoretical interest in using topical antibiotics to sterilize the oropharynx and stomach in mechanically ventilated patients, with the goal of reducing the incidence of VAP.[222] Several groups have used topical prophylactic antibiotics for selective decontamination of the oropharynx and digestive tract (SDD) in patients at high risk for nosocomial pneumonia. The SDD regimen usually includes a short course of systemic antibiotic therapy, such as cefotaxime, trimethoprim, or a fluoroquinolone, and nonabsorbable local antibiotic prophylaxis consisting of a combination of an aminoglycoside, polymyxin B, and amphotericin.[222] Since the original studies published by Stoutenbeek and coworkers in 1984,[223,224] which demonstrated a decrease of the overall infection rate in patients receiving the SDD regimen, more than 40 randomized, controlled trials and seven meta-analyses have been published.[225-231] All seven meta-analyses reported a significant reduction in the risk of VAP, and four reported a significant reduction in mortality.[227,228,230,231] No mortality benefit occurred with topical prophylaxis alone.[225,227,230,231] However, a clear consensus as to the effectiveness of SDD has not been established, owing to discordances among these meta-analyses related to limitations and methodologic deficiencies of analyzed studies, particularly the use of clinical diagnosis of pneumonia as a study endpoint; the heterogeneity of the populations studied; the wide variety of oral regimens; inconsistent addition of systemic administration of antibiotics (cefotaxime or ceftazidime); and differences in analytic methods.[232,233]

Conclusions drawn based on meta-analyses of SDD studies may be summarized as follows:

1. SDD reduces the incidence of VAP and, when a combined topical and systemic regimen is used, may reduce mortality.
2. An inverse relationship has been described between methodologic quality of the studies and benefits questioning the overall value of results reported in meta-analyses.
3. The long-term effects of SDD on emergence of resistance and risk of superinfections is unknown.
4. The impact of SDD on the duration of mechanical ventilation, ICU stay, and hospital stay appear to be limited.

Early attempts at systemic prophylaxis by using parenteral antibiotics alone against pneumonia were clearly unsuccessful.[234,235] In contrast, recent studies showed that a short-course of antibiotic regimen in patients with structural coma or severe burns was an effective prophylactic strategy to decrease the VAP rate.[236] In addition, indirect arguments from SDD studies, including systemic antibiotic therapy, and a recent study evaluating a short course of antibiotic therapy for patients with a low probability of developing VAP[129] suggest that antibiotic prophylaxis merits being more precisely investigated in this setting.

The influence of rotating of antibiotics (generally associated with restrictive use) in the ICU on VAP prevalence has been investigated by comparing successive periods during which one antibiotic was used in place of another for the empirical treatment of suspected gram-negative bacterial infections. Some investigators found that VAP occurred significantly less frequently during the after period compared with the before period.[168,237]

CONCLUSION

Effective antimicrobial therapy and adequate supportive measures remain the mainstay of treatment for VAP. More active and less toxic antibacterial agents are still needed, especially for some problematic pathogens, such as multiresistant nonfermenting gram-negative bacteria or MRSA. However, it should be emphasized that, in the event that one or several specific etiologic agents are identified by a reliable diagnostic technique, the choice of antimicrobial drugs is much easier, because the optimal treatment can be selected in light of the susceptibility pattern of the causative pathogens without resorting to broad-spectrum drugs or risking inappropriate treatment. Every possible effort should therefore be made to obtain, before new antibiotics are administered, reliable pulmonary specimens for direct microscope examination and cultures from each patient clinically suspected of having developed VAP.

ANNOTATED REFERENCES

Chastre J, Wolff M, Fagon JY, et al: Comparison of 8 vs 15 days of antibiotic therapy for ventilator-associated pneumonia in adults: A randomized trial. JAMA 2003;29:2588-2598.
Large prospective, multicenter, randomized trial comparing 8-day to 15-day antibiotic regimens for treating VAP; results suggest that a 8-day regimen reduces antibiotic use and decreases the emergence of multiresistant bacteria in the lung without modification of the prognosis.

Fagon JY, Chastre J, Wolff M, et al: Invasive and noninvasive strategies for management of suspected ventilator-associated pneumonia. A randomized trial. Ann Intern Med 2000; 132:621-630.
Large prospective, multicenter, randomized trial comparing clinical and "invasive" management in patients suspected of VAP; results suggest that implementation of bronchoscopic techniques may reduce antibiotic use and improve patient outcome.

Ibrahim EH, Ward S, Sherman G, et al: Experience with a clinical guideline for the treatment of ventilator-associated pneumonia. Crit Care Med 2001;29:1109-1115.
A prospective before-and-after study evaluating a clinical guideline for the treatment of VAP; results suggest that such clinical guideline increases the adequacy of initial treatment and decreases the overall duration of antibiotic therapy without deleterious consequences for the patients.

Sirvent JM, Torres A, El-Ebiary M, et al: Protective effect of intravenously administered cefuroxime against nosocomial pneumonia in patients with structural coma. Am J Respir Crit Care Med 1997;155:1729-1734.
The only study, conducted in patients with structural coma, demonstrating that antibiotic given prophylactically was associated with a lower rate of early-onset ventilator-associated pneumonia.

Trouillet JL, Chastre J, Vuagnat A, et al: Ventilator-associated pneumonia caused by potentially drug-resistant bacteria. Am J Respir Crit Care Med 1998;157:531-539.
The first study clearly identifying duration of mechanical ventilation and previous antibiotic usage as risk factors for multi-drug resistant pathogens in VAP.

Chapter 85

PULMONARY INFECTIONS IN THE IMMUNOCOMPROMISED PATIENT

Carlos Agustí • Ana Rañó • Antoni Torres

KEY POINTS

1. Pulmonary infections are the **most frequent complications** in immunocompromised patients and have **a high mortality,** especially when intubation and mechanical ventilation are required.

2. The evaluation of the **patient's net state of immunosuppression** is key for the proper management of the pulmonary complication. Particularly important is the specific type of underlying immune deficiency, the immunosuppressive therapy received, and the potential epidemiologic exposures.

3. **Bacteria** are the most frequent cause of pulmonary infections in the different groups of immunocompromised patients. However, **opportunistic fungi are emerging as a common cause of pneumonia** in neutropenic patients and are associated with an elevated mortality.

4. Periodic surveillance of **serum galactomannan** and early implementation of **thoracic CT** in patients at high risk for invasive pulmonary aspergillosis may improve outcome.

5. A **marked decrease in the incidence of *Pneumocystis carinii*** pneumonia has been observed over the past years owing to prescription of *P. carinii* prophylaxis in patients at risk. Similarly, with the introduction of highly active antiretroviral therapy (HAART), the incidence of **pulmonary tuberculosis** in HIV-infected patients has dropped significantly.

6. Major emphasis must be placed on the **prevention of CMV disease in high-risk patients. CMV antigenemia** based on the detection of the pp65CMV antigen in peripheral blood leukocytes and **quantitative PCR** for early detection of viral DNA/RNA in serum have been implemented for early detection of active infection. Both assays have a sensitivity and specificity for the diagnosis of active infection of greater than 80% and diagnose active infection 1 to 3 weeks before conventional tools.

7. A confident diagnosis can seldom be made based on clinical and conventional radiology in immunocompromised patients. **Fiberoptic bronchoscopy** needs to be considered early after the appearance of the pulmonary infiltrates. **Bronchoalveolar lavage** is a very reliable technique, can provide a specific diagnosis in 50% to 80% of cases, and can also give the diagnosis of alternative noninfectious causes.

8. **Early implementation of noninvasive ventilation** is indicated in early stages of hypoxemic acute respiratory failure, because it decreases the requirement of intubation and the incidence of nosocomial pneumonia.

9. **Empirical treatment of pneumonia** in immunocompromised patients will vary depending on factors influencing the net state of immunosuppression. The selection of antimicrobial agents must be adapted to local patterns of microbial resistance.

The number of immunocompromised patients has increased over the past decade.[1-3] Improvements in solid-organ transplant (SOT) and hematopoietic stem cell transplant (HSCT) techniques, the expanded use of chemotherapeutic treatments and glucocorticoids,[4] and the appearance of new immunomodulatory therapies are among the main reasons for this increase. The recognition and management of pulmonary complications, particularly infections that result from immunosuppression, is a challenging task for clinicians. Despite the introduction of potent broad-spectrum antimicrobial agents, complex supportive care modalities, and the use of preventive measures, pulmonary infections continue to be the most frequent complications in these patients and are associated with high mortality,[5-7] especially when intubation and mechanical ventilation are required. Early diagnosis and intervention are essential because they are associated with better outcome.

EVALUATING THE NET STATE OF IMMUNOSUPPRESSION

The proper assessment of factors involving the patient's state of immunosuppression is of paramount importance (Table 85-1). Most important are the specific type of underlying immune deficiency, the immunosuppressive therapy received, and the epidemiologic exposures the patients encounter (in both the community and the hospital). A timetable with intervals during which each type of infection and of noninfectious pulmonary complication tends to be most prevalent is shown in Table 85-2. A proper knowledge

TABLE 85–1. VARIABLES TO BE CONSIDERED IN EVALUATING THE NET STATE OF IMMUNOSUPPRESSION

Specific type of underlying immune deficiency:
  Neutrophil defect: aplasia, neutropenia, leukemia
  Immunoglobulin defect: multiple myeloma
  T-cell defect: AIDS, solid organ transplant, lymphoma
Type, dose, and duration of immunosuppressive therapy
Type of organ transplanted
Presence or absence of leukopenia
Integrity of the mucocutaneous barriers
Timing between transplantation and development of
  pulmonary infiltrates
Disturbances secondary to transplant: graft-vs.-host disease
Environmental exposures
Infection with immunomodulating viruses: cytomegalovirus,
  Epstein-Barr virus
Other metabolic conditions: uremia, diabetes

TABLE 85–2. TIMETABLE OF THE MOST LIKELY PULMONARY COMPLICATIONS IN IMMUNOCOMPROMISED TRANSPLANT PATIENTS

First 30 Days after Transplant

Bacterial and fungal infections
Herpesvirus, respiratory viruses
Noninfectious complications: pulmonary edema, diffuse
  alveolar hemorrhage

2 to 6 Months after Transplant

Bacterial and fungal infections
Immunomodulatory viruses: cytomegalovirus, Epstein-Barr virus
Opportunistic infections: *Pneumocystis carinii,
  Listeria monocytogenes*

More than 6 Months after Transplant

Community-acquired respiratory viruses and bacteria
In patients with poor allograft function: consider opportunistic
  infections.

of these temporal-related complications, as well as the particular considerations involving each patient, will help guide diagnostic tests and implement appropriate empirical therapy.

ETIOLOGY OF PNEUMONIA IN IMMUNOCOMPROMISED PATIENTS

BACTERIAL INFECTIONS

Bacteria are the most frequent cause of pulmonary infections in the different groups of immunocompromised patients. Encapsulated organisms such as *Streptococcus pneumoniae* and *Haemophilus influenzae* are particularly prevalent in patients with immunoglobulin defects, such as those suffering from multiple myeloma. In HIV-infected patients, bacteria are the most common cause of pulmonary infection, with the most common microorganisms being *S. pneumoniae, H. influenzae,* and *Staphylococcus aureus.* Many other bacteria must also be considered in ICU patients, particularly *Staphylococcus aureus* (including methicillin-resistant [MRSA]) and multi-resistant gram-negative bacilli (*Pseudomonas aeruginosa,*[8] *Acinetobacter* species,[9] and *Stenotrophomonas maltophilia*).[10] Epidemiologic studies have shown that *Legionella* pneumonia is nine times more prevalent in the immunocompromised host,[11] particularly among recipients of renal allografts.[12] Occasionally, uncommon opportunistic bacteria such as *Nocardia* must be considered in the differential diagnosis, especially in organ transplant patients (most notably, renal).[13]

FUNGAL INFECTIONS

Aspergillus species are among the most common microorganisms causing pneumonia in the immunocompromised patient.[14] A high clinical suspicion and the prompt institution of specific therapy are the only chances to control dissemination of disease. Because neutrophils are the key cells in the defense against *Aspergillus,* the neutropenic patient (e.g., HSCT patient) is at a highest risk for dissemination. In these patients, periodical surveillance of serum galactomannan[15] (a polysaccharide antigen of the wall of *A. fumigatus*) permits early detection of the infection. Early use of

thoracic CT in patients at high risk for invasive pulmonary aspergillosis may also improve outcome.[16]

Candida species colonize the respiratory tract and are often recovered from pulmonary specimens in immunocompromised patients, but they are only considered as truly pathogenic if fungemia occurs or lung tissue invasion can be demonstrated. With the expanded use of new antifungal therapies, a higher incidence of infections due to *C. krusei* and *C. glabrata* has been reported.[17] Other fungi expand rapidly in response to environmental exposures, causing lethal infections, such as those due to *Penicillium purpurogenum* and *Scedosporium prolificans.*[18-21] Mucormycosis occurs almost always in the presence of immunosuppression, most notably diabetes, and often causes tissue invasion and destruction requiring surgical resection. The deep-seated fungal infections due to *Histoplasma capsulatum, Coccidioides immitis,* and *Blastomyces dermatitidis* must be considered in endemic areas, mostly in the United States.

A marked decrease in the incidence of *P. carinii* pneumonia has been observed owing to the use of *P. carinii* prophylaxis in patients at risk and the use of highly active antiretroviral therapy (HAART) in HIV-infected patients.[22-24] A CD4+ count less than 200 cells/mm³ is associated with a markedly increased risk for *P. carinii* pneumonia. In SOT recipients, the risk for *P. carinii* is higher in the first 6 months after intense immunosuppression, particularly in heart-lung recipients but can appear later on in patients treated for rejection (HSCT patients with graft-versus-host disease). *P. carinii* pneumonia in patients with AIDS has a longer median duration of symptoms and a better outcome than in patients with SOT and HSCT. The chest radiograph can vary from normal to any type of infiltrates, although diffuse bilateral infiltrates is the most common presentation. An increase in serum lactate dehydrogenase and, particularly, the presence of pneumothorax raises the suspicion of *P. carinii* pneumonia.

MYCOBACTERIUM INFECTIONS

Pulmonary tuberculosis has experienced a marked decrease in HIV-infected patients with the introduction of HAART[25]; however, remarkable geographic differences are observed. A high level of suspicion is necessary to diagnose pulmonary tuberculosis in immunocompromised patients. It should be suspected in patients with a T-cell defect (see Table 85-1). The typical radiologic pattern is often replaced by diffuse, basal or miliary infiltrates as well as mediastinal lymph nodes. Although sputum is a good noninvasive test for *Mycobacterium* staining, most patients will undergo bronchoscopy with a diagnostic yield of more than 90%. Different polymerase chain reaction (PCR) techniques have been developed to try to circumvent the problem of diagnostic delay in tuberculosis, however, false-positive results in patients shedding nonviable microorganisms limit the clinical use of these techniques. Atypical mycobacterial infections, particularly *M. avium* complex, were common in HIV-infected patients with less than 50 CD4+ cells/mm^3. With the introduction of HAART, the incidence of these infections has dropped significantly. With the exception of lung transplant patients, atypical mycobacterial infections are rare in SOT recipients.

VIRUSES

Cytomegalovirus (CMV) is the most prevalent and lethal virus causing pneumonia in immunocompromised patients. The incidence of CMV infection will depend on several factors: (1) type of transplant (highest in allogeneic HSCT recipients), (2) degree of immunosuppression (highest when graft rejection is present and/or additional immunosuppressive treatment is required), and (3) previous serologic status. Thus, the incidence of CMV infection is as high as 60% to 70% during the first 3 months after allogeneic HSCT when graft donor or patients are pre-transplantation CMV seropositive. The incidence of CMV disease among SOT patients ranges from 8% to 35% in kidney, heart, and liver transplant recipients but is considerably higher in pancreas (50%) and lung or heart-lung recipients (50% to 80%). By contrast, introduction of HAART has resulted in a drastic decrease in the number of cases of CMV disease in HIV-infected patients and is extremely rare in patients with cancer.[26] Because one third of patients with evidence of CMV infection will develop CMV pneumonia, major emphasis must be placed on the prevention of CMV disease in high-risk patients. CMV also may contribute to the net state of immunosuppression, resulting in an increased susceptibility to other infectious agents. CMV antigenemia based on the detection of the pp65CMV antigen in peripheral blood leukocytes and quantitative PCR for early detection of viral DNA/RNA in serum have been implemented for early detection of active infection. Both assays have a sensitivity and specificity for the diagnosis of active infection of greater than 80% and diagnose active infection 1 to 3 weeks before conventional tools.[27] As a rule, symptomatic infection will not develop before 2 to 3 weeks after transplantation, and the peak incidence occurs between 4 and 8 weeks after the transplant. Although late symptomatic cases are well described, more than 90% of cases occur in the first 4 months after transplantation. The clinical and radiologic findings of CMV pneumonia are nonspecific. Occasionally, involvement of other organ systems with hepatitis, ulcerative gastroenteritis, hemorrhagic colitis, or retinitis may be a clue to the etiology of the pulmonary disease. Before the development of surveillance and prophylactic measures, CMV pneumonia had a high mortality that reached 85%. Currently, mortality is between 30% and 50%.

Recent developments in molecular-based diagnostic tools have shown that conventional respiratory viruses (influenza, parainfluenza, respiratory syncytial virus, adenoviruses, enteroviruses, and rhinoviruses) are frequent causes of respiratory illnesses and are associated with high rates of morbidity and mortality among immunocompromised patients.[28]

DIAGNOSTIC APPROACH

The evaluation of pulmonary infiltrates in the immunocompromised host is often a diagnostic challenge. Diagnosis can seldom be made based on clinical findings or conventional radiology in immunocompromised patients. Sputum cultures have a low sensitivity but are certainly indicated because organisms isolated in the upper respiratory tract are likely to be the cause of the pneumonia. Because immunocompromised patients with pulmonary infection are at risk for rapid dissemination of the disease with accompanying acute respiratory failure, fiberoptic bronchoscopy needs to be considered early after the appearance of the pulmonary infiltrates. The early use of fiberoptic bronchoscopy may add to the prompt identification of the specific etiologic agent, facilitating an etiology-guided treatment and avoiding unnecessary and potentially harmful additional treatment. In this sense, it has been shown that early diagnosis of both viral and fungal infections decreases mortality.[29,30] Fiberoptic bronchoscopy is a low-risk procedure that can be safely performed in most patients, including those with hypoxemia, with the application of supplemental oxygen. The use of fiberoptic bronchoscopy in immunocompromised patients provides a specific diagnosis in 50% to 80% of the cases.[31-33] Bronchoalveolar lavage (BAL) is a very reliable technique for detecting opportunistic infections such as *P. carinii*, CMV, and fungi but also bacteria, mycobacteria, and other pathogens.[34-36] BAL is particularly efficient in that it still recovers resistant pathogens after several days of empirical treatment, allowing modifications of the primary antimicrobial regimen. Bronchoscopy also provides material to diagnose alternative noninfectious causes, such as diffuse alveolar hemorrhage[37] or alveolar proteinosis,[38] which often afflict immunocompromised patients. The protected specimen brush (PSB) does not seem to add diagnostic information to BAL. By contrast, a simple, safe, and cost-effective technique such as tracheobronchial aspirate may constitute a good complement to BAL in the diagnosis of the etiology of pneumonia in immunocompromised patients.[32] Very rarely, an open lung biopsy will be needed for diagnostic purposes.[39] Although its diagnostic yield is high, and often leads to changes in therapy, the indications and proper moment must be selected carefully owing to potential morbidity and mortality.

Thoracic computed tomography (CT) is an important diagnostic tool in invasive pulmonary aspergillosis. The halo sign (hemorrhagic pulmonary nodule) and air-crescent sign (cavitation) are early radiologic signs typical of invasive pulmonary aspergillosis. This technique is also quite valuable in detecting pneumonic infiltrates in febrile neutropenic patients, particularly in transplant recipients, because it very often detects pulmonary infiltrates when a chest radiograph is normal.[40] Neutropenic patients with fever, showing a normal high-resolution CT scan, have a very low risk of pneumonia. A potential drawback of CT in the evaluation of pulmonary infiltrates in immunocompromised patients is the incapacity to detect polymicrobial infections. The possibility of more than one etiologic agent can be as high as 15% in some groups of immunocompromised patients.

TABLE 85–3. VARIABLES RELATED TO MORTALITY IN DIFFERENT GROUPS OF IMMUNOCOMPROMISED PATIENTS

APACHE II score > 20
Bilateral infiltrates in chest radiography
Mechanical ventilation requirement
Inadequate empirical treatment
Delay in diagnosis

PROGNOSTIC FACTORS OF PNEUMONIA IN IMMUNOCOMPROMISED PATIENTS

Pneumonia in immunocompromised patients is associated with high mortality irrespective of the factors leading to the altered immune status. Those with the highest mortality rate are recipients of an HSCT. Different factors have been identified that portend a poor prognosis.[41] Some of these factors are common to the different groups of the ICU patients whereas others relate to specific groups (Table 85-3). Particularly relevant is the requirement of mechanical ventilation. Needing mechanical ventilation bears a grim prognosis, particularly in HSCT recipients, where the mortality rate is >90% and very few survive 6 months after the onset of the pulmonary complication.[42] A prognostic factor that has a decisive influence on the clinical practice is the inadequacy of the empirical treatment. The difficulty of making an antibiotic selection in light of growing resistance and the wide spectrum of potential etiologic factors emphasizes the importance of designing strategies aimed at obtaining an early diagnosis. The impact of diagnostic delay on mortality is an important theme in the care of seriously ill patients, particularly as it affects the adequacy of initial therapy.[43] Early implementation of fiberoptic bronchoscopy may have prognostic implications.

THERAPEUTIC STRATEGIES

NONINVASIVE VENTILATION

The requirement of mechanical ventilation portends a poor prognosis in immunocompromised patients. Patients requiring mechanical ventilation may have a worse prognosis than similar patients matched for general severity-of-illness scoring systems such as Acute Physiology and Chronic Health Evaluation II (APACHE II), because mechanical ventilation may be directly injurious through increasing the risk for nosocomial pneumonia. Early implementation of noninvasive mechanical ventilation is indicated in immunocompromised patients because it decreases the requirement of intubation and the incidence of nosocomial pneumonia.[44-47]

EMPIRICAL TREATMENT OF SUSPECTED PNEUMONIA

Empirical treatment of pneumonia in immunocompromised patients will vary depending on factors influencing the net state of immunosuppression (see Tables 85-1 and 85-2). For neutropenic patients with fever, the administration of empirically chosen intravenous antibiotics is a widely accepted clinical practice.[48-51] The selection of antimicrobial agents must be adapted to local patterns of microbial resistance. Broad-spectrum antibiotics with activity against gram-negative bacilli, including *P. aeruginosa*, and gram-positive pathogens are indicated. Therapy must be modified to cover fungi based on identification or increased likelihood of this infection (long-term neutropenia), lack of response to initial antibiotics, or clinical worsening. Early performance of fiberoptic bronchoscopy must be always considered for a specific, etiologic-based therapy, avoiding unnecessary and potentially harmful additional treatments.

CONCLUSION

Pneumonia represents a serious challenge for clinicians caring for immunocompromised patients. Mortality in immunocompromised patients is high, particularly in patients undergoing HSCT and those requiring mechanical ventilation. A great diversity of diagnostic and laboratory procedures is available, and the clinician must determine the tests that should be performed based on the net state of immunosuppression. Early diagnosis is advantageous, and fiberoptic bronchoscopy substantially increases the diagnostic yield, causing changes in the empirical treatment in the majority of patients. Neutropenic patients with fever of unknown origin and normal chest radiographs should undergo high-resolution CT. Early application of noninvasive ventilation is warranted to avoid intubation and improve prognosis.

ANNOTATED REFERENCES

Heussel CP, Kauczor HU, Heussel GE, et al: Pneumonia in febrile neutropenic patients and in bone marrow and blood stem-cell transplant recipients: Use of high-resolution computed tomography. J Clin Oncol 1999;17:796-805.
This prospective study was performed in febrile neutropenic patients with unknown focus of infection with persisting fever for more than 48 hours despite empirical antibiotic treatment. The high frequency of inflammatory pulmonary disease after a suspicious high resolution CT scan (>50%) proved that pneumonia is not excluded by a normal chest radiograph. Patients with normal HRCT scan, particularly transplant recipients, have a very low risk of pneumonia during follow-up.

Hilbert G, Gruson D, Vargas F, et al: Noninvasive ventilation in immunocompromised patients with pulmonary infiltrates, fever, and acute respiratory failure. N Engl J Med 2001;95:358-364.
This is a prospective, randomized trial of intermittent noninvasive ventilation, as compared with standard treatment with supplemental oxygen, in a population of immunocompromised patients with pulmonary infiltrates, fever, and an early stage of hypoxemic acute respiratory failure. The study shows that early initiation of noninvasive ventilation was associated with significant reduction in the rate of endotracheal intubation and serious complications.

Huaringa AJ, Leyva FJ, Giralt SA: Outcome of bone marrow transplantation patients requiring mechanical ventilation. Crit Care Med 2000;28:1014-1017.
This retrospective study demonstrates that the ICU survival rate of bone marrow patients who develop pulmonary complications and require mechanical ventilation is less than 20%.

Stover DE, Zaman MB, Hajdu SI, et al: Bronchoalveolar lavage in diagnosis of diffuse pulmonary infiltrates in the immunocompromised host. Ann Intern Med 1984;101:1-7.
This is a classical prospective study that demonstrated that bronchoalveolar lavage is a valuable procedure for evaluation of pulmonary disease in the immunosuppressed host.

Pizzo PA: Fever in immunocompromised patients. N Engl J Med 1999; 341:893-900.
This review article focuses on some of the challenges clinicians face in the management of fever in immunocompromised patients.

Chapter 86

LUNG TRANSPLANTATION

David Weill

HISTORICAL PERSPECTIVE

Lung transplantation evolved from heart-lung transplantation as a method by which donor organs could be used more efficiently. Heart-lung transplantation was first performed in 1981[1] and was initially the procedure of choice for diseases that are now more commonly treated by transplant using either bilateral sequential lung transplantation or even single-lung transplantation. The appeal of developing the isolated lung transplant technique was the improvement in donor organ utilization. Specifically, by using each of the three thoracic organs available from a single donor (i.e., two lungs and a heart), donor organ utilization can be maximized while achieving acceptable outcomes.

The double-lung transplant procedure, originally accomplished by en bloc replacement using a tracheal anastomosis, was first performed in 1983 in Toronto. The bilateral procedure is now performed as a sequential transplant using bilateral bronchial anastomoses. The bilateral sequential technique, as compared with the en bloc tracheal anastomotic technique, has been associated with fewer airway anastomotic complications, likely as a result of the superior blood supply from retrograde pulmonary artery flow.

In a report by the Toronto Transplant Group, single-lung transplantation was first described in 1986.[2] The advantage of the procedure is that it has allowed maximal donor utilization while being associated with good patient outcomes. The single-lung procedure has historically been accepted as the procedure of choice for common transplant indications, such as emphysema and idiopathic pulmonary fibrosis, and is currently performed as commonly as the bilateral procedure.[3]

SURVIVAL AND DEMOGRAPHICS

Worldwide, 1200 to 1400 patients receive a lung transplant each year. Despite the yearly increase in patients on the transplant waiting list (recently nearly 4000 patients), the number of transplant procedures performed each year has been relatively stable over the past several years (Fig. 86-1).[3] Significant discussion and research regarding methods to expand the donor pool are ongoing,[4] but, until strategies to increase lung donor procurement are actually employed, the number of transplants performed each year will likely remain stable.

Long-term survival after lung transplantation is limited by the development of the bronchiolitis obliterans syndrome (BOS), which is commonly referred to as chronic rejection. BOS, defined by declining spirometry below the best postoperative level achieved, is variable in time to onset but increases in frequency as duration post transplant lengthens. Unfortunately, the etiology of BOS remains elusive, but it likely involves both immune and nonimmune mechanisms, including frequent early acute rejection episodes, infection with cytomegalovirus (CMV), severe early postoperative lung injury, and donor factors. Largely because the mechanism of BOS is unknown, satisfactory treatment is currently not available.

INDICATIONS AND PROCEDURE CHOICE

Indications for lung transplant are listed in Table 86-1 according to the generally accepted procedure choice. Although there are many end-stage lung diseases that can potentially be amenable to lung transplantation, four diseases compose the vast majority of lung transplant recipients: emphysema (both cigarette-induced and due to alpha$_1$-antitrypsin deficiency), cystic fibrosis, primary pulmonary hypertension, and idiopathic pulmonary fibrosis.[3] Contraindications to transplant include evidence of extrapulmonary disease such as significant kidney, liver, or cardiac disease; poor nutritional or rehabilitation status; recent or current malignancy; and a poor psychosocial profile.

Generally the procedure of choice is the one that can be performed safely while utilizing the available donor organs most efficiently. Emphysema is the most common lung transplant indication and has consistently been associated with the best survival post transplant.[3] While some controversy exists regarding the optimal procedure choice (single vs. double) in this group of patients,[5] most patients with emphysema who have undergone a lung transplant have received a single-lung transplant. Bilateral lung transplant has traditionally been reserved for suppurative lung diseases,

NUMBER OF LUNG TRANSPLANTS REPORTED BY YEAR

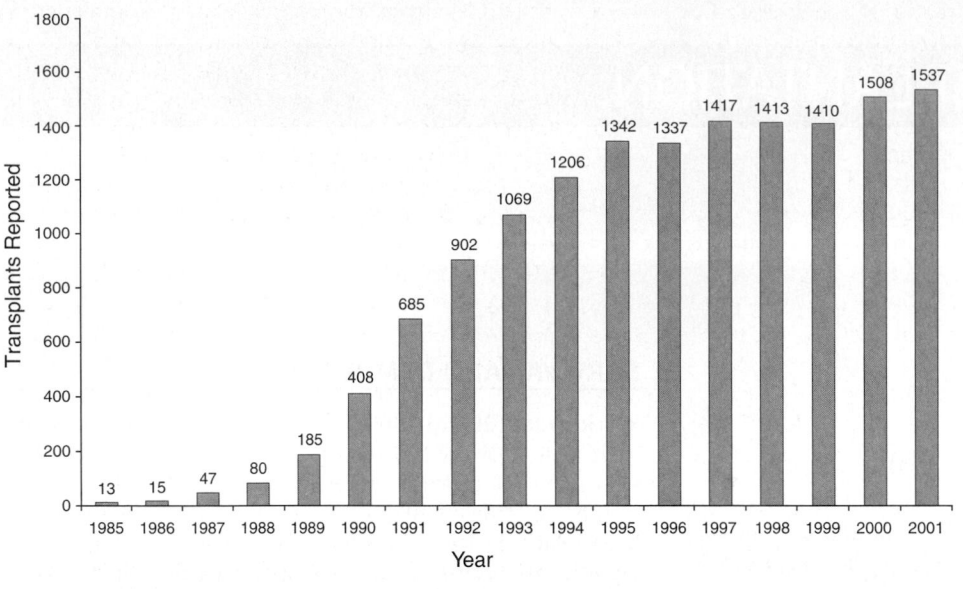

FIGURE 86-1. Number of lung transplants reported by year.

such as cystic fibrosis and other bronchiectatic diseases, where replacing as much infected lung tissue as possible is the primary goal. Also, patients with primary pulmonary hypertension generally receive a bilateral lung transplant, because this prevents the potentially life-threatening situation that occurs when, in performing a unilateral transplant, nearly all of the cardiac output flows to the allograft, given its relatively lower vascular resistance as compared with the native primary pulmonary hypertension lung. In the early transplant period when single lungs were transplanted for this indication, the result in most centers was profound unilateral pulmonary edema in the allograft.

CANDIDATE SELECTION

Because of the rigors of a major thoracic surgery, such as lung replacement, an extensive evaluation process occurs in all potential lung transplant recipients. The majority of the preoperative testing is directed toward excluding significant extrapulmonary disease, particularly those diseases that would lessen the chances of survival in the immediate postoperative period or make tolerance of the commonly used postoperative immunosuppression difficult. Occult coronary artery disease or malignancies are not uncommonly uncovered as the evaluation proceeds, particularly in those patients who have significant cigarette smoking histories. Other important goals of the evaluation process are to determine the likelihood of compliance with the complicated

postoperative medical regimen and the existence of a solid support system to help with medical care once the patient leaves the hospital.

WAITING LIST CONSIDERATIONS

TIME ON WAITING LIST

Waiting times for lung transplant recipients are highly unpredictable and vary considerably geographically. Waiting list priority is strictly according to time, or "seniority," on the list. Currently, there is no waiting list status system, although there likely will continue to be significant efforts to give priority to those on the waiting list who are more ill and who are most likely to do well post transplant. Unfortunately, devising such a system for lung allocation is problematic, primarily owing to the lack of compelling data correlating likelihood of waiting list mortality among the various disease groups with the highest probability of survival after transplantation. At most centers, as patients referred for transplant increase and patients on the waiting list increase, waiting times continue to increase and mortality on the waiting list will increase as well.

CARE OF PATIENTS ON WAITING LIST

Management of patients on the lung transplant waiting list involves close interaction with the referring physician. Treatment is directed toward the underlying disease process and is not generally affected by the patient's waiting list status. However, clinical activities that may affect transplant outcome should be a prominent aspect of the medical care plan. For instance, enrollment and participation in a cardiopulmonary rehabilitation program is of paramount importance so that waiting patients can develop or maintain the best cardiovascular fitness possible. Furthermore, weight management is often an important issue and regular exercise can help avoid excessive weight gain, which is associated with poor outcomes after transplantation. Conversely, in patients with cystic fibrosis, weight maintenance can be achieved by regular consultation with nutritional support

TABLE 86–1. LUNG TRANSPLANT BY PROCEDURE TYPE (IN ORDER OF FREQUENCY)	
Single Lung Transplant	**Double Lung Transplant**
Emphysema/COPD	Cystic fibrosis
Idiopathic pulmonary fibrosis	Emphysema/COPD
Alpha$_1$-antitrypsin deficiency	Alpha$_1$-antitrypsin deficiency
Re-transplant	Idiopathic pulmonary fibrosis
	Primary pulmonary hypertension
	Bronchiectasis

personnel familiar with patients in whom specific dietary needs exist. Other considerations requiring the attention of the transplant team include substantial increases in corticosteroid use, which, although never definitively linked to poor outcomes post transplant, remain a theoretical concern in terms of bronchial anastomotic and wound healing. As lung transplant waiting lists grow at most centers, regular outpatient clinic visits to monitor patients on the waiting list will likely become more important so that clinical issues that may affect transplant success can be detected and addressed.

DONOR ISSUES

DONOR CRITERIA

The expansion of lung transplantation as a therapy for end-stage lung disease is not limited by the number of potential recipients but rather by the availability of suitable donor organs. The standard, or "classic," lung donor criteria are well known, if not closely followed, among lung transplant practitioners. Although some of these criteria certainly make good sense (i.e., a clear chest radiograph, no bronchoscopic evidence of aspiration), nearly all the others are controversial, often ignored, and not based on convincing research data.[4] The standard or classic lung donor criteria are listed in Table 86-2. Whereas certain geographic regions of this country, some countries in Europe, and Australia have adopted more aggressive donor management strategies that have resulted in more donor lungs, many areas with lung transplant programs have fewer than expected lung donors.

POSTOPERATIVE CARE

The early postoperative care of lung transplant recipients can be divided into four general categories: (1) hemodynamic management, (2) respiratory management, (3) initiation of an immunosuppression regimen, and (4) infectious disease prophylaxis. Although many basic critical care principles apply to the care of lung transplant recipients, certain special considerations apply.

HEMODYNAMIC MANAGEMENT

Fluid Administration

In the early postoperative period, proper fluid management may be the most important aspect of lung transplant care. Because the lymphatic drainage is disrupted during surgery, the transplanted lung has a propensity toward pulmonary edema, and this tendency toward pulmonary edema is

TABLE 86–2. STANDARD LUNG TRANSPLANT DONOR CRITERIA

Age < 55 yr
ABO blood group compatibility
Clear chest radiograph
PaO_2 > 300 mm Hg on fractional inspired oxygen of 1.0 and positive end-expiratory pressure = 5 cm H_2O
Less than 20 pack-year smoking history
Absence of chest trauma
No aspiration or sepsis
Gram stain shows sputum sample free of bacteria, fungus, and significant number of white blood cells

exacerbated by several conditions. First, owing to the procurement and reimplantation process, lung allografts suffer a lung injury that is characterized by a diffuse capillary leak. The process, commonly referred to as ischemia-reperfusion injury or the reimplantation response, is usually mild and treated easily with supportive measures. This type of injury is characterized by diffuse pulmonary infiltrates radiographically and varying degrees of oxygenation impairment. In cases of severe injury, the pulmonary edema may be profound and require more aggressive measures, such as independent lung ventilation, inhaled nitric oxide, and, in extreme cases, extracorporeal membrane oxygenation (ECMO). Second, because intraoperative and early postoperative hypotension occurs commonly, overexuberant resuscitation with crystalloid solutions sometimes occurs and worsens the pulmonary edema. In some circumstances, hypotension or decreased urine output has been treated with starch solutions that, because of the large molecules in these solutions, results in passage of even greater amounts of fluids through the dilated capillary channels.

Especially in the first 72 hours after surgery, judicious use of intravenous fluids should be exercised and efforts should be made to minimize fluid administration while maintaining adequate urine output.

Use of pulmonary artery catheters is standard in the early postoperative care of transplant recipients and helps guide fluid management. Low central venous pressures (0 to 5 mm Hg) are the objective. Also, careful attention to input and output measurements provides additional information regarding volume status and is a reminder to administer only essential fluids. Generally, if renal function allows, a worthy goal is to keep the patient 1 L negative for the first 3 postoperative days. This is best achieved with the liberal use of loop diuretics and the limiting of extra fluid infusions.

Hypotension is common after lung transplantation. Not only is the patient, by design, intravascularly volume depleted but he or she is also receiving medications that cause hypotension, such as paralytics, sedatives, and analgesics. As a result, during the early postoperative period, patients typically will have episodes of hypotension that need to be addressed. Another important consideration is the effect of positive-pressure ventilation on the hemodynamics of a recent lung transplant recipient, particularly in those receiving a single-lung transplant for emphysema, owing to discrepancies in native lung and allograft compliance characteristics. These discrepancies, coupled with many recipients who not only have preoperative right ventricular dysfunction but also in whom postoperative intravascular volume depletion is intentionally achieved, can result in overinflation of the native lung. The concept of native lung hyperinflation is covered in more detail in the section on Ventilator and Respiratory Management, but one must consider whether early post-operative hypotension is best treated with ventilator management strategies that address overdistention of the native lung.

During periods where hypotension is found to be the result of profound intravascular volume depletion, fluid resuscitation should ideally include solutions that have the greatest tendency to remain in the vascular space and not simply migrate through the dilated pulmonary capillary channels. Colloid solutions, such as albumin, and packed red blood cells (RBCs), are ideal in this setting, as is replacement with clotting factors, particularly in the patient who has postsurgical consumption of these factors. Generally, in the hypotensive patients with hemoglobin less than 10 g, use of packed RBCs is the treatment of choice. If a patient has very little postoperative bleeding, albumin infusions provide a temporary solution to intravascular volume depletion and can be given in conjunction with a loop diuretic to achieve a more brisk diuresis by transiently increasing effective renal blood flow. This effect is likely short-lived but nonetheless provides a temporary increase in oncotic pressure that may lessen the development of pulmonary edema.

VENTILATOR AND RESPIRATORY MANAGEMENT

The initial care of early postoperative lung transplant recipients is directed toward ventilatory stability. Ventilator mode is generally dictated by the patient's level of consciousness in the early postoperative period. For example, patients who are deeply sedated and/or under the influence of paralytic agents will obviously require full control of their ventilation. The assist-control mode meets this requirement and is generally the preferred ventilatory mode in the immediate postoperative period. However, because an effort is made at many programs to extubate patients sooner after surgery, use of less sedation and the avoidance of paralytic agents are being employed. In this group of patients, less ventilatory control is required and patients usually do well with intermittent mandatory ventilation until early extubation is achieved. In patients with poor early graft function, for example those with primary graft failure, ventilatory strategies that limit barotrauma are most efficacious and usually include pressure-control modalities. Certainly, with pressure-control ventilation, the use of sedation and paralytics is warranted, recognizing the potential deleterious neurologic effects of the latter when used in combination with high doses of corticosteroids and, in some instances, aminoglycoside antibiotics.

The Use of Positive End-Expiratory Pressure

Positive end-expiratory pressure (PEEP) can be safely used in lung transplant recipients, especially those patients who have received a bilateral lung transplant. In the double-lung recipients, the compliance characteristics of the two allografts will be similar; therefore, the positive pressure exerted on each lung will be nearly evenly distributed. PEEP of +5 to +15 is safe in this patient population. In fact, some believe that PEEP has a beneficial effect in this group in decreasing postoperative bleeding by increasing intrathoracic pressure, which would lead to tamponade of the small blood vessels in the chest. This point, however, is not widely accepted and has not been supported by conclusive data.

In single-lung recipients, the use of PEEP can be more problematic. The differing compliance characteristics of the remaining native lung and the allograft lead to the potential for a majority of the positive pressure being directed at only one lung. This is particularly true in emphysema recipients who have a highly compliant native lung and a less compliant transplanted lung. In this situation, nearly all the positive pressure is exerted on the native lung, which leads to a situation known as acute native lung hyperinflation. The hyperinflated native lung can cause both cardiac tamponade, manifested as acute hypotension associated with a reduction in cardiac index, and allograft compression, manifested by hypoxemia and hypercarbia. Because of these potential problems, the avoidance of PEEP in patients with emphysema

undergoing single-lung transplantation is generally recommended. The use of PEEP in single-lung recipients with other disease processes is usually not problematic. A more complete review of the differences in ventilator management associated with single- and double-lung recipients is presented later in the chapter.

Chest Physiotherapy and Patient Positioning

Chest physiotherapy (CPT) is an essential part of postoperative respiratory management. Because the allograft is denervated, the cough reflex in lung transplant recipients is impaired. CPT therefore is imperative in the clearance of retained mucus and blood in the airway. As the postoperative recovery ensues, CPT is less important because patients learn to cough periodically, regardless of the impetus to do so. Before patients are trained to do this, aggressive CPT is used (i.e., usually every hour in the first few postoperative days while the patient is awake and every 2 hours during sleep) and includes vibratory percussion, intermittent positive-pressure ventilation, and patient-directed incentive spirometry. Whereas CPT devices that deliver excessive airway pressure are to be avoided due to concerns of potential anastomotic disruption, positive-pressure devices using less than 20 cm Hg airway pressure are generally safe.

Patient positioning in the bed can help minimize the development of pulmonary edema. The lung that is positioned toward the bed when the patient is in the lateral decubitus position receives relatively less blood flow than the upward positioned lung, primarily owing to the effects of gravity. This is especially important in single-lung transplant recipients because the vascular compliance characteristics differ between the native lung and the allograft with the newly transplanted lung receiving relatively more blood flow due to less vascular resistance. Of course, if the new lung experiences significant reperfusion injury after transplant, then the vascular resistance would likely be higher in the allograft. Regardless of the initial condition of the transplanted lung, the allograft side should be placed upward for the first 6 hours postoperatively while the patient is in the lateral decubitus position to diminish its blood flow and ideally its tendency to develop pulmonary edema. The single-lung recipient should then be positioned with the new lung down for 1 to 2 hours before being again placed with the allograft upward. Also of note, one can determine how well the allograft is functioning by comparing oxygenation when the native lung and allograft are receiving the majority of the blood flow. For instance, when the patient oxygenates better with the native lung downward (and therefore receiving the majority of the blood flow) than when the allograft is receiving most of the pulmonary blood flow, that is an indication that the new lung is not yet functioning well. In double-lung recipients, which side is positioned downward is less important and patients are simply turned from side to side periodically (e.g., every 2 hours).

Single-Lung vs. Double-Lung Issues

Management of the mechanical ventilator after lung transplant surgery is heavily influenced by the type of lung transplant procedure performed (i.e., a single- or double-lung transplant). In recipients who receive a bilateral transplant, the ventilator management is very similar to that for nontransplant recipients. However, in single-lung recipients, the compliance differences between the native lung and the allograft mandate different ventilator strategies. Different strategies are particularly important in single-lung recipients with emphysema rather than in single-lung recipients with fibrotic lung, owing to the tendency of the native emphysematous lung to hyperinflate under the influence of positive pressure. Because of this tendency, some programs have advocated double-lung transplants routinely for patients with emphysema owing to the potential for increased mortality in the single-lung recipients with emphysema.[6] Fortunately, proper ventilator management in the single-lung recipients can prevent most of the problems with native lung hyperinflation, and concerns about this phenomenon should not influence procedure choice.[7]

Ventilator management in patients with emphysema who receive a single-lung transplant should be directed toward limiting airway pressure and allowing maximal expiratory time. The avoidance of PEEP and the use of excessively large tidal volumes limit the degree of native lung hyperinflation because any degree of positive pressure will have a tendency to be directed to the highly compliant native emphysematous lung. Because some degree of native lung hyperinflation is unavoidable, strategies to allow maximal emptying of the native lung should be employed and include reducing the set respiratory rate and increasing inspiratory flow rate to allow a longer expiratory time. If the problems associated with acute native lung hyperinflation cannot be resolved with simple ventilator maneuvers and if the patient has not experienced significant ischemia-reperfusion injury, then extubation should be strongly considered because the removal of all positive pressure will resolve the problem. By using these management strategies and by clearly understanding the physiology involved with single-lung transplant recipients, one can usually avoid the untoward effects of native lung hyperinflation and its associated morbidity and mortality.

Native lung hyperinflation is more common when acute lung injury is present in the allograft, because the compliance discrepancy between the native lung and the allograft is even more pronounced. In this rare circumstance, independent lung ventilation using a double-lumen endotracheal tube can be initiated and can provide a means to ventilate the native lung and allograft according to the compliance characteristics of each.[8] Independent lung ventilation outside of the operating room setting is associated with difficulties, particularly relating to endotracheal tube malpositioning and subsequent acute lobar or total lung collapse. Unfortunately, prevention and recognition of tube dislodgment requires constant surveillance, generally endoscopically, and is difficult unless personnel skilled with endoscopic endotracheal tube management skills are available on a continuous basis. Under these circumstances, diligent nursing care is required, including the administration of appropriate sedation and/or paralytic agents as well as the avoidance of routine repositioning of the patient.

Extubation

The extubation criteria in a lung transplant recipient are similar to those for other types of ventilated patients, particularly postsurgical patients. The patient should certainly be free of any lingering effects of the anesthetic and able to meet standard extubation criteria published elsewhere.[9] As more experience with lung transplant management has developed, the decision to extubate is being made sooner; and some centers are even trying to extubate patients in the operating suite soon after surgery.[10] Other programs, however, are reluctant to extubate this quickly because of concerns about delayed ischemia-reperfusion injury that would compromise allograft function or uncertainty about whether anesthetic medications have been completely cleared. Regardless, the dogma about leaving patients ventilated for a predetermined amount of time is now being challenged.

Chest Tube Management

Lung transplant recipients generally have two chest tubes per transplanted lung after surgery. A posterior tube is positioned to drain surgical bleeding, while the anterior tube evacuates air from the pleural space. The anterior tube is usually the first tube to be removed given that, in the absence of a bronchial anastomosis dehiscence, prolonged air leaks into the chest tube are uncommon. In fact, much of what is often mistakenly regarded as an air leak coming from the thorax is often air being introduced via the skin incision at the chest tube site. The posterior tube is removed when total 24-hour drainage from it is less than 150 mL. In a bilateral lung transplant, one should be cognizant that there is communication between the two hemithoraces because the pleural space has been opened. Because of this, chest tubes in bilateral transplants should be removed one tube per side at a time with the anterior tubes being removed first followed by the posterior tubes.

Bronchoscopy after Lung Transplantation

The initial bronchoscopy after lung transplantation typically occurs in the operating room. The goal of the procedure is to assess the bronchial anastomoses and to clear retained blood and sputum from the airway. Once the patient returns to the ICU there is generally no need to bronchoscope the patient again in the first 24 postoperative hours unless complications develop. For instance, acute ventilatory insufficiency should prompt a bronchoscopic examination of the transplanted lung or lungs to make certain that acute mucus plugging of the airways is not accounting for the ventilatory insufficiency. Because of blood in the airway from the operation and caused by retained secretions from the native lung in single-lung recipients, mucus plugging happens not uncommonly. Serious complications from bronchoscopy early after surgery are rare. Transient oxygen desaturation during bronchoscopy is common but not generally harmful to the patient.

IMMUNOSUPPRESSIVE REGIMENS

Review of Commonly Used Agents

Different transplant centers use different immunosuppressive regimens. However, general comments can be made about the more commonly used medications. Some programs use an induction strategy that involves the early administration of antibody, either directed directly at the lymphocyte ("lymphocyte-depleting") or against interleukin receptor sites.[11] Most antibodies delivered are monoclonal and are more easily tolerated than the polyclonal antibodies used in the earlier transplant era. Regardless of which induction agent is preferred, a primary advantage of this strategy involves the early avoidance of nephrotoxic immunosuppressive agents (such as calcineurin inhibitors like cyclosporine or tacrolimus), while still providing adequate immunosuppression. This benefit is particularly important during the immediate postoperative period when renal insufficiency is common owing to purposeful intravascular volume depletion, use of nephrotoxic antibiotics and antiviral agents, and the effects of cardiopulmonary bypass (if used).

Although a thorough review of immunosuppressive medications is available elsewhere, a few basic comments about immunosuppressive strategies can be made. Most lung transplant programs use a three-drug immunosuppressive regimen. Corticosteroids are a central part of the early strategy, particularly during the period when adequate blood levels of the other immunosuppressive agents are not yet achieved. Because of the large corticosteroid doses used immediately after surgery, a variety of side effects can be expected. For example, fluid retention, systemic hypertension, and poor glucose control should be anticipated. Acute changes in mental status can also occur and clinically present as delirium or psychosis. Many of these effects can be eliminated by administrating the corticosteroids in a tapering fashion that aims to reduce the dosage as quickly as it is safe to do so.

Calcineurin inhibitors such as tacrolimus and cyclosporine-based medications comprise the second part of the three-drug strategy. These medications are typically administered intravenously early in the postoperative period for a number of reasons. First, lung transplant recipients are generally not able to take oral medications in the first 24 hours after surgery. Second, the intravenous absorption is more predictable and avoids the rapid absorption seen early after oral administration, which is highly desirable in lung recipients in whom one would like to avoid nephrotoxic effects that could impede good urine output. Finally, because the intravenous delivery is highly amenable to dose titration, turning off the intravenous drip in response to reduced urine output can quickly reestablish adequate urine output and helps achieve the goal of relative intravascular volume depletion that is critical in the early postoperative period. In the first 48 hours after surgery, a cyclosporine level equal to or less than 100 ng/mL and a tacrolimus level no greater than 5 is desirable. Once urine output is adequate and renal function is stable, drug dosage can be increased to achieve more therapeutic medication blood levels.

The third part of the immunosuppressive regimen involves the use of either azathioprine or mycophenolate mofetil. Azathioprine is generally well tolerated and is usually associated with mild, reversible side effects, such as leukopenia, anemia, thrombocytopenia, and liver function test abnormalities. Mycophenolate mofetil, a newer agent, can also cause leukopenia and anemia. Furthermore, in some circumstances, the drug can lead to nausea, vomiting, and abdominal pain, all of which can be ameliorated by reducing the dose or temporarily stopping the drug. The monitoring of mycophenolic acid blood levels is being performed in some solid organ recipients,[12,13] but the precise target levels in lung transplantation are unknown.

INFECTIOUS DISEASE PROPHYLAXIS

Infections after lung transplant are common and occur because of baseline immunosuppression, transmission from the donor, and ICU-related instrumentation (e.g., chest tubes, central venous catheters, endotracheal tubes). The antibiotic prophylactic regimen is directed toward preventing pneumonia, surgical site infections, and central line–related infections. Usually, this goal is achieved through the prophylactic use of late-generation cephalosporins and vancomycin. Because of their colonization with *Pseudomonas* species,

TABLE 86–3. CMV PROPHYLAXIS PROTOCOL

	Recipient Positive	Recipient Negative
Donor Positive	6 wk GCV* (2 wk i.v. and 4 wk p.o.) CMV-IG 3 doses (1 dose every 2 wk)	12 wk GCV* (6 wk i.v., p.o.) CMV-IG† 7 doses in 6 wk
Donor Negative	No prophylaxis used	

GCV, ganciclovir; CMV IG, CMV hyperimmune globulin.
*Intravenous dose 5 mg/kg q12h adjusted for creatinine clearance.
†150 mg/kg within 72 h post transplant, then every 2 weeks for 4 doses, then 100 mg/kg every 4 weeks for 2 additional doses.

patients with cystic fibrosis receive a third prophylactic antibiotic with good gram-negative coverage, such as an aminoglycoside.

Infection with CMV after transplant can lead to deleterious acute and chronic effects. Acutely, patients are at risk to develop CMV pneumonia, which in many instances leads to severe morbidity and mortality. Also, CMV syndrome, caused by CMV replication in the bloodstream, is heralded by the onset of malaise, fever, nausea, and vomiting. Furthermore, many believe that CMV infection (even asymptomatic) can lead to more long-term sequelae, such as chronic allograft dysfunction (BOS).[14]

To prevent both the acute and chronic consequences of CMV infection, many programs have adopted an aggressive CMV prophylactic protocol. The more aggressive protocols include combination therapy using both ganciclovir and CMV hyperimmune globulin.[15] The duration of therapy is dependent on CMV serology status of the donor and the recipient and is outlined in Table 86-3. Other less aggressive strategies are also used and, although less expensive and associated with less treatment-associated toxicity, likely lead to an increased incidence of CMV-related diseases.

The prophylactic use of antifungal agents is controversial and varies among centers.[16] There are single-center studies that have demonstrated a reduction in invasive fungal disease after instituting a fungal prophylactic regimen.[17] Those programs that do use antifungal prophylaxis generally use medications in the azole class or aerosolized amphotericin.[18,19] While there have been no conclusive studies in lung transplant to support an antifungal prophylactic strategy, some lung transplant physicians use these agents primarily for their ability to raise blood levels of the calcineurin inhibitors, which ultimately results in significant cost savings because the calcineurin inhibitor dose can be reduced.[20] One concern with this strategy, however, is the potential to select for resistant fungal infections, particularly candidal species.

INTENSIVE CARE UNIT ISSUES

In the early postoperative period, while the patient is mechanically ventilated, the use of sedative medications and paralytics is common. However, in most cases, when early allograft function is adequate, the routine use of paralytic medications can be avoided. The avoidance of these drugs is desirable given that paralyzing agents have been associated with prolonged paralysis, which in lung transplant recipients can impair ability to wean from mechanical ventilation and to participate fully in the postoperative physical therapy regimen. The deleterious effects of the paralytic agents can be exacerbated by the concomitant use of high-dose corticosteroids and aminoglycoside antibiotics,[21] both of which are commonly used in the early postoperative period in lung transplant recipients.

Strategies involving gastrointestinal prophylaxis and prophylaxis against deep vein thrombosis are similar to those employed in any thoracic surgical patients. Generally, gastrointestinal prophylaxis is achieved using H_2 blockers or a proton-pump inhibitor and is particularly important early postoperatively when the patient is exposed to high doses of corticosteroids. Most programs continue the gastrointestinal prophylactic measures indefinitely. Because of the risk of surgical bleeding, prophylaxis is initially achieved using antistasis devices to the lower extremities. As the risk of postoperative bleeding diminishes, standard prophylactic regimens for deep venous thrombosis using heparin-based drugs can be safely used until the patient is fully ambulatory.

EARLY POSTOPERATIVE COMPLICATIONS

HEMODYNAMIC INSTABILITY

As discussed earlier, the immediate hemodynamic goal in the lung transplant recipient is intravascular volume depletion. Although achieving the goal of reducing the tendency toward pulmonary edema, this strategy often results in hypotension. Furthermore, the combination of intravascular volume depletion, a poorly compliant right ventricle requiring higher filling pressures, the use of sedative and paralytic medications that cause hypotension, and positive pressure provided by the mechanical ventilator can result in exacerbation of blood pressure difficulties. Fortunately, the hypotension that occurs commonly under these circumstances can be readily reversed by a few different measures.

For example, gentle volume resuscitation with colloids such as albumin or red blood cell transfusion can reestablish an adequate blood pressure, while not contributing significantly to pulmonary edema development. Of course, in some patients with known preoperative right ventricular dysfunction, such as that seen in primary or secondary pulmonary hypertensives, maintaining adequate right ventricular filling pressures using volume expansion is important in ensuring adequate cardiac performance even in the presence of normal systemic blood pressures. The hemodynamic effect in certain situations of positive-pressure ventilation has been discussed previously. If the recipient experiences problems with positive-pressure–related hypotension, removal from the mechanical ventilator is the treatment of choice. Not only does this remove the hemodynamic effects of positive-pressure ventilation but it also obviates the need for administration of sedative and paralytic medications, all of which have hypotensive side effects. Rarely is there a need for ionotropic or cardiopressor support, except in instances of early postoperative hypothermia or profound hemorrhage.

VENTILATORY INSTABLITY

Ventilatory instability in the early postoperative period requires similar evaluation as any postsurgical patient. Initial efforts to determine the etiology of ventilatory problems should be directed at diagnosing mechanical problems related to the mechanical ventilator and the endotracheal tube. For instance, the acute onset of hypercarbia in the early postoperative setting should lead to investigation of the patency of the endotracheal tube specifically and the bronchial tree generally. Plugging of the airways, either with retained mucus or blood, is very common in this setting and can cause rapid ventilatory insufficiency. The development of this problem is suggested by acute increases in ventilatory pressure but is definitively diagnosed by bronchoscopic examination of the airways. Treatment involves the removal of mucus or blood blocking the airway. Of course, improper patient-ventilator synchrony can cause a similar clinical scenario and may result from inadequate patient sedation.

Problems with early allograft function also lead to inadequate ventilation and oxygenation. These problems are usually temporary and are best managed simply through supportive measures. However, in the case of primary graft failure, the oxygenation and ventilatory problems are more profound and require more complex management strategies. In the setting of a double-lung transplant, the management should include the application of increased levels of PEEP and, if necessary, alterations of inspiratory to expiratory ratios. In single-lung recipients, one can selectively ventilate the native lung while other measures are taken to improve allograft performance. This strategy can be accomplished through the use of double-lumen endotracheal tubes, which allow independent lung ventilation.[22] In cases of important allograft dysfunction, positioning the patient on the side with the native lung "down" can lead to increased perfusion to that side (i.e., the side with less pulmonary edema) and can lead to improvements in oxygenation.

EXTRACORPOREAL MEMBRANE OXYGENATION

In instances in which none of the measures described earlier results in hemodynamic and ventilatory stability, ECMO is an alternative treatment strategy.[23-25] Although associated with significant morbidity, ECMO can rapidly restore hemodynamic and ventilatory stability. Important morbidity as a result of this therapy includes bleeding complications secondary to the anticoagulation necessary to maintain the ECMO circuit. Bleeding can occur anywhere and is particularly evident at the cannula insertion site. However, intracranial hemorrhage is the most catastrophic complication and is the most common cause of death associated with ECMO.[26] The preferred ECMO method in lung transplant recipients is generally the venoarterial route, although the venovenous route has been used as well.[27] Insertion of the ECMO cannulas is best performed at the femoral site, because local control of bleeding can be achieved. Although associated with good hemodynamic stability, central cannulization often results in poorly controlled bleeding.

OPERATIVE COMPLICATIONS

Postoperative bleeding issues are similar to other thoracic surgical patients and are best handled by correction of coagulopathies and replacement of red blood cells. As in other thoracic patients, careful chest tube output monitoring is essential in detecting and, ultimately, treating excessive bleeding. Return to the operating room for exploration in the presence of excessive bleeding is not uncommon after lung transplantation. Bleeding complications are generally more common in patients in whom dissection to free the native lung is difficult, such as in cystic fibrosis patients or in patients with fibrotic lung diseases. There is also a tendency toward more bleeding in patients who have required cardiopulmonary bypass.[28]

As improvements in surgical technique have developed, a decrease in airway, venous, and pulmonary artery anastomotic complications has occurred.[29] Although uncommon, anastomotic complications in the immediate postoperative period generally involve the vascular connections rather than the bronchial anastomosis. Complications with the bronchial anastomosis, such as dehiscence or stricture, usually occur later in the postoperative period. Conversely, problems with the venous[30,31] or pulmonary artery anastomosis[32] manifest immediately postoperatively and are life threatening, particularly if not detected promptly.

Pulmonary artery stricture, or narrowing, is fortunately very uncommon. When it does occur, problems with oxygenation are seen and usually occur in the absence of radiographic abnormalities. The diagnosis is initially one of exclusion, where more common causes of poor oxygenation are investigated first. Once no evidence of other causes of poor allograft function can be found, evaluation of the pulmonary artery anastomosis should occur and usually is best accomplished via pulmonary angiography. Pulmonary perfusion scanning can in some instances be helpful and is noninvasive. However, nonspecific alterations in allograft blood flow do not distinguish among the usual causes of postoperative allograft dysfunction. Pulmonary angiography, on the other hand, can anatomically demonstrate pulmonary artery narrowing and provides the means to measure pressure gradients across the pulmonary artery anastomosis.[33] If a significant gradient across the pulmonary artery anastomosis were to exist, the suspicion of a pulmonary artery stricture would be high enough to warrant surgical re-exploration.

Of the complications associated with the vascular anastomoses, problems with the venous anastomosis are most common. Because of the technical challenges associated with it and the low-flow state of the venous system, the venous anastomosis is susceptible to kinking or clot formation. Both of these complications cause impedance of venous return and back flow of blood into the pulmonary vasculature. This results in immediate and profound pulmonary edema that is refractory to all supportive measures. A clinical scenario of this kind should prompt immediate investigation, ideally via visualization and Doppler measurement of the venous anastomosis using transesophageal echocardiography.[34,35]

TRANSFER FROM ICU

In uncomplicated cases, lung transplant recipients can generally be discharged from the ICU within 24 to 48 hours.

Once the respiratory status is stable, plans can be made to transfer patients to less intensive care settings. Aside from reducing the potential for ICU-related infections, discharge from an ICU setting allows more freedom of movement so that more effective pulmonary rehabilitation can occur. Additionally, from a psychosocial standpoint, patients feel less isolated and are able to visit more frequently with friends and family members in less acute care settings.

ANNOTATED REFERENCES

Garrity ER Jr, Villanueva J, Bhorade SM, et al: Low rate of acute lung allograft rejection after the use of daclizumab, an interleukin 2 receptor antibody. Transplantation 2001;71:773-777.

Garrity and his colleagues evaluated the impact of induction therapy using daclizumab on acute rejection incidence. They found that induction therapy with daclizumab significantly reduced the incidence of acute rejection and was not associated with a significantly increased incidence of infections.

Meyers BF, Sundt TM III, Henry S, et al: Selective use of extracorporeal membrane oxygenation is warranted after lung transplantation. J Thorac Cardiovasc Surg 2000;120:20-26.

The authors reviewed their experience using ECMO in post–lung transplant recipients. Although ECMO is associated with increased morbidity, it is a viable therapeutic option in patients with profound respiratory and hemodynamic embarrassment. The authors further explain the technical approach to ECMO therapy.

Weill D, Lock BJ, Wewers DL, et al: Combination prophylaxis with ganciclovir and cytomegalovirus (CMV) immune globulin after lung transplantation: Effective CMV prevention following daclizumab induction. Am J Transplant 2003;3:492-496.

The authors compared monotherapy using intravenous ganciclovir to combination therapy using intravenous ganciclovir and hyperimmune CMV globulin. Weill and colleagues found that a significant reduction in CMV disease and infection was observed in the combination therapy, as compared with using ganciclovir alone.

Weill D, Torres F, Hodges TN, et al: Acute native lung hyperinflation is not associated with poor outcomes after single lung transplant for emphysema. J Heart Lung Transplant 1999;18:1080-1087.

The authors report on the incidence and effect of acute native lung hyperinflation in the University of Colorado Lung Transplant Program. Acute native lung hyperinflation while radiographically common was not associated with increased morbidity or mortality. Consequently, aggressive measures to prevent acute native lung hyperinflation, such as dual lung ventilation, contralateral lung volume reduction surgery, or the routine use of double-lung transplant for emphysema patients are not warranted.

Yonan NA, el-Gamel A, Egan J, et al: Single lung transplantation for emphysema: Predictors for native lung hyperinflation. J Heart Lung Transplant 1998;17:192-201.

Yonan and colleagues discuss factors that predict the development of acute native lung hyperinflation. The authors conclude that acute native lung hyperinflation was common and led to increased morbidity and mortality. Yonan suggested that acute native lung hyperinflation could be avoided by the routine use of contralateral lung volume reduction surgery, double-lung transplant, or dual lung ventilation.

Chapter 87

BURNS AND INHALATION INJURY

Soman Sen • Richard L. Gamelli

KEY POINTS

1. **Careful and focused history and physical examination** including the extent of exposure and the nature of inhaled substance aid in the diagnosis and treatment of inhalation injury.

2. **Nature of the inhaled substance,** including physical properties and heat-carrying capacity, can give an indication of the level and extent of damage on the tracheobronchial tree.

3. **Pathologic changes of inhalation injury** include upper airway edema (glottic cartilage), necessitating mechanical ventilation, and damage to the epithelial lining of the tracheobronchial tree, resulting in increased recruitment of inflammatory mediators and further damage. Mortality of burn injury and inhalation injury is greater than either alone.

4. **Pulmonary complications from inhalation injury** are related to direct damage from thermal energy and toxins, infection from opportunistic organisms, damage caused by inflammatory mediators (alveolar macrophages, neutrophils), reduction in surfactant production, and mucociliary dysfunctions.

5. **Long-term complications from inhalation injury** include a persistence of symptoms such as cough, dyspnea, and symptoms of obstruction. Structural changes may include tracheal stenosis, bronchiectasis, and bronchiolitis obliterans.

6. Initial **medical management** includes adequate fluid resuscitation, maintenance of airway patency, and, when needed, effective mechanical ventilation. Regular pulmonary toilet and effective antibiotic therapy are important after the initial injury period.

7. **Mechanical ventilation** during inhalation injury involves both providing adequate oxygenation and ventilation and minimizing further damage to lung tissue. The use of high-frequency ventilation has been shown to provide some benefit in patients with acute lung injury.

Inhalation injury often occurs in combination with thermal injury and leads to serious complications that manifest at different points in the disease process. Inhalation injury alone carries a 5% to 8% mortality risk; however, when combined with burn injury the mortality can increase by 20% or more.[1]

These factors when combined with a complicated pathologic course make inhalation injury a potentially difficult and dangerous disease process.

CLASSIFICATION OF INJURY

Classifications of inhalation injury have been developed according to several different schemes. One of the first schemes was developed as a result of observations made at the Cocoanut Grove fire of 1942 and grouped patients according to outcomes and their initial symptoms. Early signs of hypoxia that were directly attributable to respiratory tract injury had the highest and most immediate mortality. Signs of cyanosis and dyspnea that occurred within a few hours of the insult could be attributable to development of pulmonary edema. At 24 hours, upper airway edema was found to be increased and necessitated establishment of an airway (tracheostomy, intubation). After 48 hours, the final group of patients developed worsening respiratory symptoms due to atelectasis and subsequent pneumonia.[2]

Other classification symptoms for inhalation injury were based on the anatomic location of injury. Upper airway injury involves the nasopharyngeal and oropharyngeal regions to the larynx. This damage results in massive edema and compromise of airway patency, often necessitating intubation or tracheostomy. Injury to the distal parts of the tracheobronchial tree manifests at a later time. Tracheal and major bronchi injuries result in direct mucosal damage and desquamation of the epithelial lining. Injury to the distal alveoli results in atelectasis and predisposes to pneumonia.[3]

THE INITIAL INHALATION INSULT

The initial manifestations of inhalation injury are due to direct damage to airway surfaces that result in inflammation and edema. This damage is more often than not due to the heat content of inhaled material. For example, smoke, which is dry and has a low specific heat, causes damage to upper airways whereas steam, which has 4000 times the heat-carrying capacity, can cause more extensive tracheobronchial damage.[4] The clinical symptoms that appear initially are stridor, hypoxia, and respiratory distress.[5]

Management of the initial insult incorporates a thorough physical examination as well as careful and specific history that provides details about extent of exposure to the inhaled substance and nature of the substance itself. Evaluation of physical symptoms should include examination of the oropharynx for direct damage and documentation of stridor, cyanosis, and confusion, but it is not unusual for there to be no obvious physical symptom of inhalation injury at the initial evaluation. Initial management includes providing adequate oxygenation as well re-evaluation and maintenance of airway patency.[6]

ENVIRONMENTAL VARIABLES THAT DETERMINE SEVERITY

The extent of inhalation injury is related to the duration of exposure and severity of trauma to the tracheobronchial tree. A major component of the degree of the initial inhalation energy is the amount of heat-carrying capacity of the inhaled substance. Dry heat has a lower heat-carrying capacity than steam and thus usually injures upper airway and supraglottic structures.[7] Thermal injury produces direct injury to the mucosa of upper airway structures. In rare occasions, the lower airway may be damaged. Clinically this manifests as upper airway edema within the first 24 hours.[3]

The level of injury produced by inhalation of particulate matter depends on the diameter of the matter. Large-diameter particles less than 100 μm enter the airway but usually do not travel beyond the upper respiratory tract. Particles less than 10 μm can reach the lower tracheobronchial tree and particles less than 5 μm can reach the terminal bronchus and alveolus. Particulate matter can cause direct mechanical damage and can also carry toxins beyond the level of the initial inhalation.[3]

The ability of gases and toxins to exert damage on the tracheobronchial tree depends on the capacity of the toxin to reach different areas of the airway.[5] Water solubility affects the location of deposit of gases and toxins. Mucous membranes line much of the upper respiratory tract, which allows gases that are highly water soluble to be absorbed in the upper tract and cause irritation to these structures. Because less soluble gases are not absorbed in the upper airway, they travel to the lower airway and cause irritation and damage to those structures.[3]

PATHOLOGY

UPPER AIRWAY INJURY

Upper airway structures that are in direct danger from inhalation injury include the mucous membranes of the nasopharynx, hypopharynx, epiglottis, glottis, and larynx. The mucous membranes of these structures can undergo a significant amount of inflammation due to direct injury. However, the cartilage of the glottis is not tolerant of edema, and damage to this structure can produce life-threatening compromise of airway patency.[7]

Injury to the upper airway occurs earliest and quickly manifests symptoms. Most of the early damage is due to direct thermal injury to mucous membranes of upper airway structures. Mucous membranes are damaged when the temperature of inhaled gases reaches 150°C. The resulting damage initiates an inflammatory cascade that leads to increased capillary permeability, histamine release, and inflow of transudative fluid, all of which results in edema. This process initiates over the course of the first 24 hours post exposure, and the resulting edema resolves in 4 to 5 days. Airway compromise occurs when edema and swelling cause the airway diameter to fall below 8 mm and mandates the need for a mechanical airway.[7]

LOWER AIRWAY INJURY

Thermal Injury. Direct thermal injury to lower airway structures is an uncommon occurrence (5%). This is due to the dissipation of heat during travel through the airway and to reflexive closing of the glottis at high temperatures (150°C). Small particulate matter (<5 μm) can travel to terminal bronchi and alveoli and cause damage to protective structures such as epithelial cells and alveolar macrophages.[8]

Tracheobronchial Injury. Cytoplasmic vacuolization and cytoplasmic blebbing are seen in epithelial cells of the bronchial tree 48 hours after severe smoke inhalation.[9] This is followed by epithelial necrosis, hemorrhage, and perivascular congestion. This damage initiates an inflammatory cascade that recruits inflammatory cells, neutrophils, and macrophages that cause further damage.[10] In addition, the congestion and increased lymphatic flow lead to obstruction of bronchial segments and impair gas exchange.

Parenchymal Damage. Direct damage to the lung epithelium causes the recruitment of inflammatory mediators that produce increased parenchymal damage. Neutrophils are among the first mediators recruited. In addition to growth factors and cytokines, neutrophils release reactive oxygen species and proteases that cause direct cellular damage. This damage triggers further inflammation and leads to pulmonary dysfunction.[11] This dysfunction begins at the cellular level with evidence of increased apoptosis of lung epithelial cells. This leads to a decrease in surfactant release and defective surfactant mechanisms, resulting in obstruction and collapse of lung segments.[12] In addition, alveolar macrophages release free radicals that cause further damage to pulmonary parenchyma.[13] With extensive destruction and inflammation, pulmonary compliance is reduced and gas exchange is impaired, leading to altered pulmonary blood flow patterns and ventilation-perfusion mismatches.[14]

DAMAGE FROM ASPHXIANTS

Smoke generates compounds—carbon monoxide (CO) and cyanide—that are absorbed systemically and impair oxygen utilization and delivery. These compounds directly interfere with oxygen uptake and delivery mechanisms, which results in cellular and local tissue hypoxia and eventually organ failure and death.

CO is an odorless nonirritating gas that is responsible for up to 600 accidental deaths per year. The pathology of CO poisoning is attributable to its ability to rapidly diffuse into the bloodstream and bind to the iron moiety of heme normally bound by oxygen. Because of higher affinity (240 times) for the heme-binding site, CO easily displaces oxygen and impairs the ability of hemoglobin to deliver oxygen. In addition, the stoichiometry of hemoglobin is altered, further impairing oxygen delivery by the other sites of hemoglobin. CO also binds to enzymes within mitochondria involved in the utilization of oxygen by cells and tissues. By binding to these enzymes, myoglobin, cytochromes, and NAPDH reductase, the cellular and local tissue acidosis increases, further impairing oxygen delivery. This results in progressive cellular dysfunction and, ultimately, organ failure.[15]

Neurologic symptoms are often the first manifestation of CO poisoning. Mild carboxyhemoglobin levels (5% to 10%) are usually well tolerated. When concentrations reach 10% to 30% symptoms begin to manifest. Headaches, nausea, and dizziness are common initial symptoms in mild to moderate CO poisoning. With severe poisoning (50% carboxyhemoglobin levels), more dangerous neurologic symptoms occur, such as syncope, seizures, and comas. The diagnosis is made based on a combination of physical symptoms along with elevated levels of systemic carboxyhemoglobin. Pulse oximetry values do not differentiate between carboxyhemoglobin and oxyhemoglobin and thus remain paradoxically elevated. Blood P_{O_2} level remains normal because it reflects oxygen dissolved in plasma that is not affected by CO.[16] Neurologic symptoms may persist in the form of delayed neuropsychiatric sequelae. The symptoms of this syndrome include a persistent vegetative state, parkinsonism, short-term memory loss, behavioral changes, hearing loss, and psychosis. These symptoms may manifest from 3 to 240 days after recovery, and 50% to 75% of patients with delayed neuropsychiatric sequelae recover fully in 1 year.[17]

The hallmark of treatment of CO poisoning involves maintaining adequate oxygenation. The CO half-life decreases from 6 to 8 hours to 40 to 80 minutes with 1 hour of treatment with 100% oxygen. When administered in a hyperbaric chamber the half-life decreases to 15 to 30 minutes.[18] Administration of 100% oxygen can be done via facemask or by mechanical ventilation. Hyperbaric oxygen treatment has been shown to have an advantage over normobaric oxygen treatment for CO poisoning. However, given the limited number of hyperbaric chambers available, the widespread use of hyperbaric therapy is limited.[17,19]

Cyanide inhalation is a potentially life-threatening occurrence that requires immediate intervention. Once inhaled, cyanide rapidly crosses into the blood and disrupts normal cellular utilization of oxygen by binding to cytochrome oxidase, thus interfering with cellular respiration. Like CO, cellular lactic acid production is increased and cellular dysfunction soon follows.[20]

Diagnosis is made by careful review of the history of inhalation and duration of exposure as well as by clinical symptoms. Physical manifestations of cyanide poisoning include headache and confusion, followed by coma, seizures, fixed pupils, bradycardia, hypotension, arrhythmias, heart block, and cardiac failure. Diagnostic tests include measurement of blood concentrations of cyanide, which are considered toxic at levels of 0.5 mg/L.[20]

Treatment of cyanide inhalation includes administration of oxygen as well as decontamination agents. When cyanide toxicity is suggested, 100% oxygen should be administered immediately This can be done under normobaric or hyperbaric conditions, but the use of hyperbaric chambers is yet to be proven to provide a benefit.[21] Amyl and sodium nitrates can be used as decontamination agents. These compounds induce the formation of methemoglobin to which cyanide has a high affinity. Methemoglobin thus acts as a scavenger for cyanide. Other compounds include sodium thiosulfate, which transfers a sulfur group to cyanide and converts it to thiocyanate, which is excreted by the kidneys, and hydroxycobalamin (not approved by the U.S. Food and Drug Administration), which detoxifies cyanide by binding to it, forming cyanocobalamin.[22,23]

FEATURES OF SPECIFIC IRRITANTS

Smoke produces a variety of compounds that have been shown to cause or initiate damage to the lung. The mechanism of damage for many of these compounds is unknown

TABLE 87–1. SPECIFIC LUNG IRRITANTS

Chemical Irritants	Properties	Mechanism of Toxicity
Smoke:		
Acrolein	Lipophilic	Direct epithelial damage
Industrial:		
Chlorine	Water soluble	Forms free radicals
Phosgene	Low solubility	Causes the release of arachidonic acid metabolites
Nitric oxide	Lipid soluble	Causes lipid peroxidation
Sulfur dioxide	Water soluble	Causes lipid peroxidation
Ammonia	Water soluble	Forms hydroxyl ions and causes liquefactive necrosis

but the location of damage within the respiratory tract is related to the ability of the compound to reach that location (Table 87-1).

Acrolein. Acrolein is a toxic compound found in the inhalation of several materials, including tobacco smoke, vehicle exhaust, and wood smoke. Acrolein is a lipophilic aldehyde carbonyl with an attached vinyl group. Its lipophilic nature allows it to pass by the upper airway and penetrate lower airway structures, where it is absorbed. Systemic acrolein is metabolized by the liver by reacting with glutathione, resulting in mercapturic acids that are renally excreted.[24] This transformation, however, does not occur as readily in the lung, and thus acrolein levels remain elevated in lung tissue and cause direct epithelial damage.[25,26]

Hydrogen Chloride. The toxicity of chlorine is related to its water solubility as well as duration of exposure. Chlorine is a moderately water-soluble gas that can penetrate deep into the lower lung structures. Within the upper airway, chlorine has a direct irritant effect that causes inflammation and edema. Within the lower airway hydrogen chloride forms reactive ions that create free radicals. These free radicals react with various compounds and lead to mucosal destruction, pulmonary edema, and parenchymal damage.[27,28]

Phosgene. Phosgene is an acylating agent found in plastics and aniline dyes. It is a low-soluble gas that when inhaled produces severe pathology within the bronchoalveolar spaces. Phosgene reacts with glutathionine and causes the release of arachidonic acid metabolites.[29-31]

Ammonia. The inhaled form of ammonia, anhydrous ammonia, is highly water soluble and is mostly absorbed in the upper airway. However, owing to its toxic nature, lower airway structures can also be affected. Ammonia exerts its effects by reacting with tissues, creating hydroxyl ions, which results in liquefactive necrosis.[32]

Nitrogen Oxide. Nitric oxides are highly lipid soluble compounds that are absorbed in the lower lung regions. Nitric oxides exert their toxic effects by the production of free radicals through lipid peroxidation, leading to parenchymal damage and pulmonary edema.[33,34]

Sulfur Dioxide. Sulfur dioxide is a highly water-soluble gas that is mainly absorbed in the upper airways. Sulfur dioxide, like nitric dioxide, reacts with tissues to produce free radicals via lipid peroxidation.[35]

THE ROLE OF A CUTANEOUS THERMAL INJURY

The combined effect of thermal injury and inhalation injury is synergistic on morbidity and mortality, creating increased pulmonary vascular changes and inflammation that lead to decreased pulmonary compliance and pulmonary functions. Burn injury alone increases vascular permeability and can result in pulmonary edema. When associated with inhalation injury this increase in pulmonary edema is exacerbated and results in a massive influx of inflammatory mediators, which increases damage to the lung parenchyma.[36] With increasing damage to lung parenchyma, pulmonary compliance decreases and ventilation-perfusion mismatches occur. With the resulting edema, atelectasis and consolidation of the lung from the increased vascular permeability and increased lymphatic flow set the stage for secondary bacterial infections.[37-39] In addition, the pulmonary edema and decreased pulmonary compliance result in increased intrathoracic pressure, which causes a left side–dominant myocardial depression and contributes to the altered hemodynamic profile observed in combined thermal and inhalation injury.[40]

POSTINHALATION PULMONARY COMPLICATIONS

Inhalation injury directly injures upper and lower airway structures through thermal energy, toxic irritants, and particulate matter deposition. This damage causes increased vascular permeability, leading to an influx of inflammatory mediators, all of which results in parenchymal damage. This parenchymal damage leads to further pulmonary dysfunctions, leading to decreased pulmonary compliance, infection, and the acute respiratory distress syndrome (ARDS). Burn injury also increases vascular permeability and causes release of inflammatory mediators.

LOCAL FACTORS

Ciliary Dysfunctions. Inhalation injury causes direct damage to mucosal and ciliary elements, leading to dysfunctions in ciliary motility. This damage is caused by several agents, including acrolein and other aldehydes.[26] In addition, inflammatory mediators such as thromboxane have been shown to decrease mucociliary activity. Thus, inhalation injury produces mucociliary dysfunction by both direct toxic injury as well as by causing the release of inflammatory mediators.[41] This allows particles and toxins to exert their effects on other local defense mechanisms as well as initiate a cascade of parenchymal damage and bacterial infection.[42]

The Pulmonary Alveolar Macrophage. Alveolar macrophage numbers increase in smoke inhalation injury as well as production of superoxide anions that can cause extensive tissue damage.[43] In addition, phagocytic function of macrophages is decreased, which leads to increased toxin and bacterial exposure to lung parenchyma.[13,44] This combined with extensive parenchymal damage caused by alveolar macrophages contributes to pulmonary dysfunctions, infectious complications, and development of ARDS.

Surfactant. Surfactant function and production are altered with severe inhalation injury. In lung injury models, surface tension generated by surfactant is reduced, leading to a loss of force that maintains alveolar patency and results in alveolar collapse. The changes in surfactant function are related to the level of inflammation because studies have shown that increased capillary permeability leads to reduced surfactant production.[12] In addition, there is reduction in surfactant protein levels as well (SP-A, SP-B) that could lead to reduced

lung defense mechanisms, further enhancing lung pathology during inhalation injury.[45]

Infections. Infectious complications are a common occurrence with burn injury, and pneumonia, in particular, can reach occurrence rates of up to 50% in severely burned patients, with the majority (65%) of these patients requiring mechanical ventilation.[46,47] Inhalation injury doubles the risk of pneumonia in these patients and leads to pulmonary complications. The mortality for the deadly duo of inhalation injury and nosocomial pneumonia can reach 50% to 86%.[48] The root cause of this synergistic effect has to do with both direct lung injury from inhalation as well as systemic inflammation and immune dysfunctions. This creates an environment that is susceptible to opportunistic hosts, such as *Pseudomonas aeruginosa* and *Acinetobacter*, and can lead to fulminant pneumonias.[49]

Pathogens. In thermal injury, pneumonias are a common complication of the clinical course.[50] With concomitant inhalation injury pulmonary infections can be a potentially devastating complication and lead to increased mortality rates.[49] Organisms that cause these infections in inhalation injury can be organized into groups according to the pathogens' exogenous/endogenous state or to the time from injury to infection. Organisms that are endogenous and cause infections are those that are present in the oral and respiratory tract or those in the gut at the time of admission. These include *Staphylococcus aureus, Streptococcus pneumoniae, Haemophilus influenzae, Proteus mirabilis,* and *Escherichia coli.* Those organisms that are exogenous are those acquired during the hospital course and were not present in either the gastrointestinal or respiratory tract. These include methicillin-resistant *S. aureus, Acinetobacter, Pseudomonas aeruginosa,* and other opportunistic organisms (e.g., *Candida*). Within these groupings, early infections tend to be from endogenous organisms whereas infections at a later time tend be from exogenous organisms. Another grouping scheme classifies organisms as occurring early or late in the clinical course. *S. pneumoniae* and *H. influenzae* commonly occur earlier in the clinical course, and *P. aeruginosa* and *S. aureus* occur late.[46] *P. aeruginosa* infection has been shown to significantly increase mortality rates in burn-injured patients. The emergence of *Acinetobacter* species has increased in burn injury and is an increasingly difficult and virulent organism due to its easy transmissibility and multi-drug resistance.[51] Like *P. aeruginosa*, infections by *Acinetobacter* tend to occur later in the time course of treatment and carry a high mortality rate.[52] Recognition and understanding of the pathogens involved in inhalation injury and the time course for the onset of infections are important to tailor effective antimicrobial therapy and avert serious complications.

The Acute Respiratory Distress Syndrome. ARDS is characterized by pulmonary edema not of cardiac origin and pulmonary inflammation leading to alterations in ventilation and perfusion.[53] During thermal injury, inflammatory mediators are released systemically and travel to the highly vascular lung tissue and increase vascular permeability, recruit immune cells, and reduce surfactant function.[10,54] This leads to alveolar collapse and ventilation-perfusion mismatches. This is further enhanced by inhalation injury, which causes direct lung damage and inflammation. Thus, burn and inhalation injury carry a significant risk in the development of ARDS, which results in a fairly high mortality rate (50% to 60%).[55]

THE ENDOGENOUS MEDIATORS OF LUNG INJURY

The Neutrophil. During inhalation injury there is a sequestration of neutrophils in the lungs mediated by direct lung damage. Neutrophils release oxygen radicals and proteases, which results in further damage to lung parenchyma and epithelia. This causes further release of inflammatory mediators that increase pulmonary vascular permeability, resulting in pulmonary edema.[11] Mucosal damage and pulmonary edema lead to collapse of bronchial segments, changes in pulmonary blood flow, and decreased gas exchange. The importance of neutrophil-mediated lung injury in the pathology of ARDS during inhalation injury is further corroborated by studies showing that the inhibition of neutrophil rolling reduces epithelial injury and vascular permeability and may lead to improved outcomes.[56]

Endothelium. Lung injury induces changes in endothelial function that increase vascular permeability and polymorphonuclear leukocyte recruitment, leading to increased inflammation and lung damage. These changes include a reduction of vascular endothelial growth factor that occurs during inflammation and sepsis, which may impair repair mechanisms and lead to further inflammation. In addition, endothelial damage causes release of thromboxanes that cause further inflammation and damage.[57]

Complement. In the lung, complement activation causes endothelial expression of P-selectin, a chemoattractant for neutrophils. P-selectin is up-regulated and augments the recruitment of neutrophils.[58] In addition, complement activation also causes the formation of cell lysing complexes that are activated by macrophages. These lysing complexes contribute to the damage to the lung caused by neutrophils and macrophages.[59]

Eicosanoids. Thromboxanes and leukotrienes are potent mediators of inflammation produced from the arachidonic acid pathway. Thromboxane A_2 increases permeability in the lung and results in interstitial as well as pulmonary edema. Leukotriene B_4 functions as a potent chemoattractant for neutrophils, further exacerbating the damage caused by these cells.[60] Together both thromboxanes and leukotrienes amplify the inflammatory process initiated by injury.[61,62]

Activation of the eicosanoid pathway is mediated by phospholipase A_2. Phospholipase A_2 causes the release of arachidonic acid from the phospholipids of cell membranes. Once released, arachidonic acid is metabolized by cyclooxygenases and lipoxygenases in the lung, which generates a large amount of eicosanoids. Phospholipase A_2 levels have been shown to be elevated after inhalation injury.[63] This activation pathway has been investigated as a potential therapy, and evidence shows that inhibition of phospholipase A_2 can attenuate lung injury in animal models.[64,65]

ONGOING PULMONARY DAMAGE AFTER INHALATION INJURY

Oxygen Toxicity. Oxygen toxicity can complicate the treatment of inhalation injury. After 48 hours of exposure to elevated oxygen levels (FiO_2 of 90%), damage to endothelial cells and an increase in interstitial edema occur.[66] After 72 hours of exposure, type I epithelial cells show evidence of damage. The mechanism by which this occurs is the generation of highly reactive oxygen radicals, which cause direct DNA damage and induce cells to undergo apoptosis, leading to necrosis of epithelial structures.[67,68]

Fluid Management. A key to the initial management of inhalation injury and burns is adequate fluid resuscitation.[6] The parameters used to determine adequate fluid management include urine output, blood pressure, and other hemodynamic parameters. Because inhalation injury causes destruction of mucosal barriers that results in tissue damage and increases in pulmonary vascular permeability, increased fluid requirements can cause a worsening of the pulmonary edema. Studies have shown that combined burn and inhalation injuries have an increased fluid requirement compared with burn injuries alone.[69] These factors combine to make fluid management of inhalation injury patients, especially those with burn injury, challenging. The management strategy incorporates providing minimal amounts of fluid to maintain adequate hemodynamic parameters and urine output.[70]

Long-Term Sequelae. Inhalation injury produces changes in pulmonary architecture that have complex long-term consequences. Long-term studies of survivors of inhalation injury may have symptoms similar to asthma such as cough, dyspnea, and symptoms of obstruction. The extent of obstruction is related to the extent of the inhalation injury and the amount of smoke inhaled. Residual inhaled toxins and irritants are thought to underlie continued long-term bronchial obstruction.

Studies have shown a persistence of inflammation in both bronchial lavage fluid as well as serum. Increased levels of cytokines and lymphocytic inflammation continue to persist up to 6 months after the initial injury. In addition, carbonaceous material has been found in alveolar macrophages months after smoke inhalation and may provide the irritants necessary to create increased levels of inflammatory mediators and bronchial hyper-responsiveness.[71,72]

Long-term structural abnormalities from inhalation injury affect about 10% of patients. These include tracheal stenosis, found only in patients who required intubation or tracheostomy. Bronchiectasis, a dilation of the bronchial tree, and bronchiolitis obliterans are both rare occurrences that lead to pulmonary dysfunctions and symptoms of obstruction. Bronchiolitis obliterans has been found after inhalation with toxic chemicals such as chlorine, phosgene, and ammonia and is thought to occur from residual toxins remaining in the lungs.[73]

TREATMENT

Medical Management. A burn injury with an inhalation injury initially necessitates stabilization and resuscitation of the patient. The cornerstones of management include adequate fluid resuscitation, maintenance of airway patency, adequate and effective mechanical ventilation when required, and vigilant surveillance for infectious complications. However, it is often noted that fluid needs may exceed calculated resuscitation in burn injury complicated by inhalation injury by over 50%.

Pulmonary Toilet. Endoscopic intervention has several roles in the evaluation and treatment of inhalation injury. In the initial injury period airway edema and mucosal sloughing can present in the first 12 to 24 hours. Laryngoscopy and bronchoscopy are used in this period to evaluate the extent of injury to tracheobronchial mucosa and provide predictive indicators for airway patency and collapse. During the clinical course of treatment, bronchoscopy is used for removal of debris and casts as well as surveillance for infectious events.[74] Other aspects of pulmonary toilet such as frequent endotracheal suctioning and chest physiotherapy are useful adjuncts in the prevention of pneumonia during treatment of inhalation injury.[75]

Antibiotics. Inhalation injury, especially with concomitant burn injury, predisposes the patient to nosocomial infections by opportunistic organisms. In an effort to reduce the rate of these infections prophylactic antibiotic coverage has been studied and has shown no benefit and may lead to increased antimicrobial resistance by these organisms. Currently, broad-spectrum antibiotics are used when infections or sepsis is suspected; they are not initiated prophylactically.[42] Once an infectious agent is identified by culture or Gram stain, the antibiotic therapy is directed at that source.[76]

Steroid Therapy. In burn injury complicated by inhalation injury, systemic corticosteroid therapy is detrimental except for the treatment of severe bronchospasm. However, with isolated inhalation injury corticosteroid therapy may be useful.[12] The use of corticosteroids early in the course of lung injury has shown confounding results and often results in deleterious outcomes. These studies have shown no improvement in outcome or mortality rates compared with control groups, and in some cases corticosteroid treatment leads to worse outcomes and complications. One meta-analysis of corticosteroid therapy for lung injury has shown that use of systemic corticosteroids should be considered only in patients with persistent ARDS who have no septic or infectious complications.[78,79]

Ventilator Management. The hallmark of ventilator management during the treatment of inhalation injury is to minimize further damage and inflammation to lung tissue and provide adequate ventilation and oxygenation.[80] This management strategy has led to several schemes of mechanical ventilation incorporating reduced barotrauma and improved pulmonary gas exchange.[55]

Positive End-Expiratory Pressure. During inhalation injury, injury to the lung increases the capillary permeability and results in influx of inflammatory mediators and edema. This causes an increase in the hydrostatic pressure across the alveolar regions of the lung, resulting in collapse. This coupled with changes in surfactant due to lung injury results in increased opening alveolar pressures and extensive atelectasis. Studies have shown that increasing positive endexpiratory pressure (PEEP) above that of the hydrostatic pressures can prevent collapse of these regions.[81] However, because hydrostatic pressures are not evenly distributed and atelectasis tends to occur in dependent lung regions, increasing PEEP to overcome the collapse in these regions could lead to overdistention of other regions, resulting in barotraumas.[82]

Inverse Ratio Ventilation. With severe lung injury, mechanical ventilation leads to increase in shear forces and changes in pulmonary blood flow. This coupled with a reduction in elasticity, which results in decreased lung compliance, leads to further injury to the lung and ventilationperfusion mismatches.[83,84] One way of counteracting the mechanical ventilation–induced damage to lung parenchyma and reducing the shearing forces is to change the inspiratory to expiratory ratio.[85] By reversing the ratio from increased expiratory time to an increased inspiratory time, the peak inspiratory pressure of the lung is reduced and oxygenation is improved.[86] This is possibly a result of the prolonged inspiratory phase of ventilation that dissipates the shearing forces on the lung, increases distal alveolar pressure as well as delivered tidal volume, and results in less damage from mechanical ventilation. In addition, owing to the shortened expiratory time, intrinsic PEEP increases, thus preventing alveolar collapse and increasing lung reruitment.[87] Despite the theoretical advantages of inverse ratio ventilation, studies have yet to consistently show an advantage over conventional ventilation.[88]

High-Frequency Ventilation. The high-frequency mode of ventilation uses rapid respiratory rates and small tidal volumes to achieve adequate oxygenation and ventilation while minimizing barotrauma.[89] There are three major types: high-frequency positive-pressure ventilation (HFPPV), high-frequency jet ventilation (HFJV), and high-frequency oscillation (HFOV). HFPPV and HFJV are the oldest forms of high-frequency ventilation and incorporate passive expiration dependent on chest wall elastic recoil. HFPPV delivers small tidal volumes (4 mL/kg) at high flow rates (250 L/min) and frequency (100 breaths/min). Because expiration within this mode is passive, there is an increased risk of air trapping and overdistention. HFJV also delivers small tidal volumes and high respiratory rates. The volume is determined by the jet velocity and duration of flow. Like HFPPV, tidal volumes are difficult to measure and manipulate with HFJV, and thus ventilation is adjusted empirically.[90] Also like HFPPV, expiration is passive and can result in air trapping. HFOV maintains open lung volumes by applying a constant airway pressure but does not allow for patient-triggered inspiratory flow. Thus, inspiration and expiration are active processes and air trapping is reduced. Oxygenation is maintained by increasing the mean airway pressure until an adequate oxygen level is reached. Ventilation is achieved by oscillating the airway pressure through electromagnetically driven pistons that deliver cyclic tidal volumes and facilitate ventilation. The oscillatory frequency determines the piston displacement, and thus reduced frequency increases tidal volume delivery and improves ventilation.[91] The therapeutic advantage of HFOV is due to the maintenance of mean airway pressure that reduces the opening and closing of alveolar spaces at low lung volumes and thus reduces the trauma due to the shearing forces created by the decreased compliance. In addition, the reduced tidal volumes and the high frequency of ventilation results in increased end-expiratory volumes, increasing recruitment of atelectatic segments and reducing lung injury due to overdistention and shearing forces.

Many of the recent studies investigating the usefulness of high-frequency ventilation have focused on HFOV because of this mode's theoretical protective advantage.[92] Several trials of HFOV in patients with acute lung injury and ARDS have shown improvements in oxygenation and ventilation. However, sample sizes for these studies have not been large enough to show a significant survival benefit.[93,94] In addition, more information is needed to refine algorithms for the use of HFOV in these settings.

Extracorporeal Membrane Oxygenation. Extracorporeal membrane oxygenation (ECMO) is used in situations in which mechanical ventilation fails to provide adequate oxygenation or elimination of carbon dioxide. The use of ECMO has shown variable results, and a few studies have shown some improvement of survival.[95] However, large trials on the use of ECMO are lacking.[96,97] As the ECMO technology improves, this alternative to mechanical ventilation in patients in pulmonary failure who do not respond to conventional interventions may become more widespread.

FUTURE DIRECTIONS

Burn and inhalation injuries pose difficult challenges for clinicians. In particular, interventions such as mechanical ventilation aimed at treating pulmonary failure from lung injury often cause further injury. Future avenues of investigation should include a larger assessment of different ventilation modes (inverse ratio ventilation, high-frequency ventilation) that reduce the damage inflicted on the lungs by mechanical ventilation. In addition, therapeutic interventions (surfactant replacement, antithrombolytic therapy) that are designed to attenuate the inflammatory response, which is responsible for much of the damage, also need further investigation.

ANNOTATED REFERENCES

Hollingsed TC, Saffle JR, Barton RG, et al: Etiology and consequence of respiratory failure in thermally injured patients. Am J Surg 1993;166:592-596.
Provides information on pathologic consequences of inhalation injury and also gives information on the possible causes of respiratory failure.

Monafo WW: Initial management of burns. N Engl J Med 1996;335:1581-1586.
Provides information about the evaluation and management of burn patients as well important clinical signs and symptoms.

Pruit BA Jr, Cioffi WG, Shimazu T, et al: Evaluation and management of patients with inhalation injury. J Trauma 1990;30:S63-S68.
Outlines evaluation and initial management issues of patients with severe inhalation injuries as well as provides valuable criteria for triage of inhalation injury.

Soejima K, Schmalstieg FC, Sakurai H, et al: Pathophysiological analysis of combined burn and smoke inhalation injuries in sheep. Am J Physiol Lung Cell Mol Physiol 2001;280:L1233-L1241.
In a sheep model, provides information on the early physiologic and cellular dysfunctions that occur with inhalation injury.

Tasaki O, Goodwin CW, Saioth D, et al: Effects of burns on inhalation injury. J Trauma 1997;43:603-607.
Evaluates the effect of burn injury on the pathology of inhalation injury as well as correlates outcomes of combined burn and inhalation injuries.

Chapter 88

DROWNING

David Szpilman • James P. Orlowski • Joost Bierens

KEY POINTS

1. Each year, **drowning is responsible for an estimated 500,000 deaths around the world.** The exact number is unknown because many deaths go unreported.

2. **Among those aged 5 to 14 years,** drowning is the leading cause of death worldwide for males and the fifth leading cause for females.

3. **Drowning is a process that begins when the airway goes below a liquid surface (usually water) and, if uninterrupted, may lead to death.** A patient can be rescued at any time during the process and given appropriate resuscitative measures.

4. Despite some pathophysiologic differences in experimental models, from a clinical and therapeutic view, **there are no important differences in humans between drowning in fresh water and drowning in salt water.**

5. **Prevention is the most powerful intervention.**

6. Hypoxia caused by submersion results first in cessation of breathing, leading to cardiac arrest in a short time if not corrected. **In-water resuscitation (ventilation only) provides the victim a 3.15 times better chance of surviving without sequelae.**

7. During resuscitation, **attempts at active drainage by placing the victim's head down increase the risk of vomiting more than fivefold** and lead to a small but significant increase in mortality (19%) when compared with keeping the victim in a horizontal position.

8. **Bringing the medical equipment to the victim (rather than vice versa) saves precious time.**

9. **Once a victim is intubated, oxygenation and ventilation can be achieved, even through copious pulmonary edema fluid.**

10. **In severe cases (grades 4 to 6), hospital care is feasible only if adequate and prompt prehospital care was given.** If this is not the case, the appropriate approach is to step back and follow accident site protocols.

11. **Pools and beaches usually do not have sufficient bacterial colonies to cause pneumonia immediately after the incident.** If the victim needs mechanical respiratory assistance, the incidence of secondary pneumonia increases from 34% to 52%

in the third or fourth day of hospitalization, when pulmonary edema is almost resolved.

12. Rarely, drowning victims who seem healthy on assessment in the emergency department, including having normal chest radiographs, can develop **fulminant pulmonary edema as long as 12 hours after the incident.**

13. **Grade 3 to 6 drownings have the potential to cause multisystem organ failure. With advances in intensive care therapy, prognosis is based primarily on neurologic outcome.** Grade 1 to 5 drowning victims return home without sequelae in 95% of cases.

Drowning is usually related to leisure situations that take a dramatically dangerous turn. Parents, friends, relatives, baby-sitters, or guardians may feel not only profound loss and grief but also guilt for failing to fulfill their responsibilities, or intense anger at others who did not provide adequate supervision or medical care. Drowning is a neglected public health problem.[1] Each year, drowning is responsible for an estimated 500,000 deaths around the world. The exact number is unknown because many deaths go unreported.[2] Age, gender, alcohol use, socioeconomic status (as measured by income or education), and lack of supervision are key risk factors for drowning. Considering all ages, males die five times more often from drowning than females do. An estimated 40% to 45% of drowning deaths happen during swimming.[3] Young children, teenagers, and older adults are at highest risk of drowning.[4] In those aged 5 to 14 years, drowning is the leading cause of death worldwide among males and the fifth leading cause among females.[4] The patterns of drowning are highly dependent on geographic factors. In the United States, drowning is the third most common cause of death related to unintentional injury for all ages, and it ranks second for people aged 5 to 44 years.[5] Considering all deaths from drowning in the United States (4390 in 1993), 53% drowned in swimming pools[3]; each year, 50,000 new pools are built, in addition to the 2.2 million residential pools and 2.3 million nonresidential pools already in existence. In Brazil, drowning is the second leading cause of death for those aged 5 to 14 years and the third leading cause of injury-associated death for all ages. Brazil has an average of 7210 deaths per year due to drowning (5.2 per 100,000 inhabitants).[6] Ironically, 90% of all drowning deaths occur within 10 meters of safety.[2] On Rio de Janeiro beaches, precipitant causes are discernible in 13% of all cases; the most common are alcohol (37%), convulsion (18%), trauma (including boating accidents; 16.3%), cardiopulmonary disease (14.1%), skin diving and scuba diving (3.7%), diving resulting in head or spinal cord injury, and others (e.g., homicide, suicide, syncope, cramps, immersion syndrome; 11.6%). It is important to recognize the cause to drowning, because it might guide specific approaches to rescue and resuscitation. In Brazil, freshwater drowning happens more commonly in rivers, lakes, and dams, accounting for half of the deaths by drowning.[7]

In contrast to the United States and Brazil, in the Netherlands, there are many more drowning deaths secondary to suicide than from accidental causes, a demonstration of geographic and cultural differences. In the Netherlands, children are most at risk, but less than 6% of all drownings occur at beaches. Each year in the Netherlands, some 300 persons die from drowning, and 450 are admitted to hospitals. The average hospital stay is 11 days, but 33% of patients are discharged within 48 hours; 10% die.

NEW DEFINITION

The lack of information about the impact of drowning on public health is partly due to a paucity of sound epidemiologic data in this field. Data collection has been hampered by the absence of a uniform and internationally accepted definition that includes both fatal and nonfatal cases. This lack of consensus is evident by the different definitions and terminology used by various water safety and health organizations, experts in the field, papers in the scientific medical literature, and laypersons.[8]

Within the framework of the first World Congress on Drowning, a definition was developed to provide a common basis for future epidemiologic studies worldwide. The Task Force on Epidemiology of Drowning was established in 1998, and in 1999, one task force member (David Szpilman) was invited to write a discussion paper on the definition of drowning and other water-related injuries. This was released on the World Congress's web site in 2000 and provoked a lively electronic discussion, with contributions from many experts around the world. Based on this discussion, the task force released a revised discussion paper on the web site at the beginning of 2002. At the task force's 2002 meeting, the following definition was adopted: "Drowning is the process of experiencing respiratory impairment from submersion or immersion in liquid." The drowning process is a continuum that begins when a person's airway goes below the surface of a liquid, usually water; if this process is uninterrupted, it can lead to death. A person can be rescued at any time during the process and given appropriate resuscitative measures, in which case the process is interrupted. Any submersion or immersion incident without evidence of liquid aspiration should be considered a water rescue (i.e., no respiratory impairment is evident, regardless of the presence of other injury or hypothermia). The term "near-drowning" has been abandoned, and confusing terms such as dry drowning and secondary drowning (delayed onset of respiratory distress) have been eliminated. The final and complete discussion of this new definition can be reviewed at www.drowning.nl.[9]

PATHOPHYSIOLOGY

Despite some pathophysiologic differences in experimental models between drowning in fresh water and drowning in salt water, from a clinical and therapeutic view, there are no important differences in humans. The most significant pathophysiologic alteration is hypoxia.[10] When there is no way to keep the airways out of water, breath holding is the first automatic response when there is no hypoxia and consciousness is preserved. Water in the mouth is spit out or actively swallowed. The initial involuntary aspiration of water produces coughing or, rarely, laryngospasm, leading to hypoxia. If laryngospasm occurs, it is short-lived, owing to worsening hypoxia. As more water is aspirated into the lungs, hypoxemia worsens, and consciousness is lost or deteriorates; progressive hypoxemia leads to irreversible apnea and then asystole (death). Respiratory disturbances depend less on water composition and more on the amount of water aspirated. The aspiration of either fresh or salt water produces surfactant destruction, alveolitis, and noncardiogenic pulmonary edema, resulting in an increased intrapulmonary shunt and hypoxia.[11] In animal research, aspiration of 2.2 mL of water per kilogram of body weight decreases the arterial partial pressure of oxygen (PaO_2) to approximately 60 mm Hg within 3 minutes.[12] In humans, aspiration of as little as 1 to 3 mL/kg of water produces profound alterations in pulmonary gas exchange and decreases pulmonary compliance by 10% to 40%.[11] Humans rarely aspirate sufficient water to cause significant electrolyte disturbances, and victims need no initial electrolyte correction.[13] Ventricular fibrillation in humans is related to hypoxia and acidosis, not hemolysis and hyperkalemia. Hypoxia produces a well-established sequence of cardiac deterioration: tachycardia, bradycardia, a pulseless phase of ineffective cardiac contractions (pulseless electrical activity), and finally complete loss of cardiac rhythm and electrical activity (asystole). Decreased cardiac output, arterial hypotension, and increased pulmonary arterial pressure and pulmonary vascular resistance are the results of hypoxia.[11] Also common is intense peripheral vasoconstriction caused by hypoxia, epinephrine release, and hypothermia.

A victim can be rescued at any time during the drowning process and may not require any intervention at all or may need appropriate resuscitative measures, in which case the drowning process is interrupted. The victim may recover after only the initial resuscitation or may need subsequent therapy aimed at eliminating hypoxia, hypercarbia, and acidosis and restoring normal organ function. In drowning, apnea occurs first, and if the victim is not ventilated soon enough, circulatory arrest will ensue and, in the absence of effective resuscitative efforts, death will result. It should be noted that the heart and brain are the two organs at greatest risk for permanent, detrimental changes from relatively brief periods of hypoxia. The development of posthypoxic encephalopathy, with or without cerebral edema, is the most common cause of death and morbidity in hospitalized drowning victims.

DROWNING CHAIN OF SURVIVAL: PREVENTION TO HOSPITAL

In 1996, the United States Lifesaving Association reported 62,747 rescues on the shores of U.S. beaches and estimated that there were eight cases of drowning for each reported death. On Rio de Janeiro beaches, approximately 290 rescues occurred for each reported death (0.34%), and there was 1 death for every 10 victims admitted for medical care at the Drowning Resuscitation Center. In 31 years of work, the lifeguards of the Rescue Service of Rio de Janeiro have made

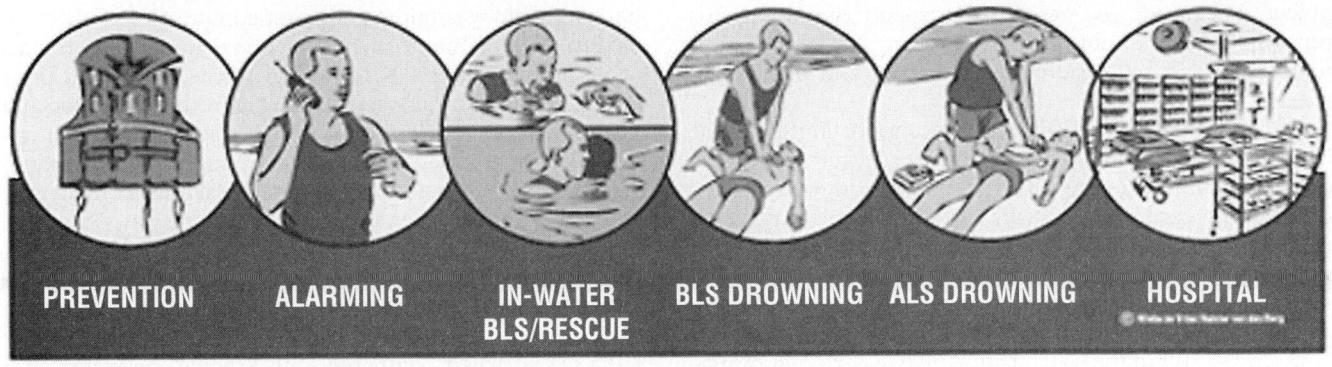

PREVENTION   **ALARMING**   **IN-WATER BLS/RESCUE**   **BLS DROWNING**   **ALS DROWNING**   **HOSPITAL**

FIGURE 88–1. Drowning chain of survival. ALS, advanced life support; BLS, basic life support. (From Szpilman D, Morizot-Leite L, Vries W, et al: First aid courses for the aquatic environment. In Handbook of Drowning. Netherlands, in press.)

approximately 166,000 rescues on beaches, and 8500 victims needed medical attention in the Drowning Resuscitation Center.[14] Rescue is an essential component of keeping the patient alive, and the first-aid evaluation is made in a hostile environment (water). It is essential for physicians to be aware of the complete drowning chain of survival,[15] from the prehospital to the hospital setting (Fig. 88-1).[15]

PREVENTION

Despite the emphasis on immediate treatment, the best approach to drowning is prevention (Table 88-1). Prevention could have been effective in more than 85% of drownings.

RECOGNITION OF THE DROWNING INCIDENT

Any attempt at rescue must be preceded by the recognition that someone is drowning. Contrary to popular belief, the victim does not wave or call for help.[16] The victim is typically in an upright posture with arms extended laterally, thrashing and slapping the water. Individuals close by may not recognize that the victim is struggling and may assume that the victim is just playing and splashing in the water. The victim may submerge and surface his or her head several times during this struggling activity. Children can struggle for only 10 to 20 seconds before final submersion, and adults can struggle for up to 60 seconds.[16] Because efforts at breathing take precedence, the drowning victim is usually unable to cry for help.

IN-WATER BASIC LIFE SUPPORT AND RESCUE

For non-lifeguards, the priority is to avoid becoming a second victim. If possible, potential rescuers should follow the advice to "throw before you go and reach (with long objects) before you assist." They can also advise the victim how to get out of the situation (e.g., choose a better way to escape, swim, float) and provide reassurance that assistance is coming.

The decision when to do basic water life support[15] is based on the victim's level of consciousness. If the victim is conscious, rescue to land without any further medical care is the protocol.[17] A panicked and struggling victim can be dangerous to a would-be rescuer. For this reason, it is always best to approach a struggling victim with an intermediary

TABLE 88–1. DROWNING: PREVENTIVE MEASURES

General

Watch children carefully; 84% of drownings occur because of inadequate adult supervision.
Begin swimming lessons beginning when children are 2 years old.
Avoid inflatable swimming aids such as "floaties"; they can give a false sense of security. Use a lifejacket!
Never try to rescue someone if you are not sure you can do it. Many people have died trying to save someone else.
Avoid drinking alcohol and eating heavily before swimming.
Do not dive in shallow water—cervical spine injury could occur.

Beaches	**Pools and Similar Places**
Always swim in a lifeguard-supervised area.	More than 65% of deaths occur in fresh water, even on the coast.
Ask the lifeguard to point out safe places to swim or play.	Fence off your pool, and include a gate. Fencing can decrease the chance of drowning by 50% to 70%.
Read and follow warning signs posted on the beach.	
Do not overestimate your swimming capability—46.6% of drowning victims thought they knew how to swim.	Whenever infants or toddlers are in or around water, be within arm's length, providing "touch supervision."
Swim away from piers, rocks, and stakes.	
Take lost children to the nearest lifeguard tower.	Use portable phones in pool areas, so you are not called away to answer.
More than 80% of drowning events occur in rip currents (the rip is usually the most falsely calm place between two sandbars). If caught in a rip, swim transversely to the sandbar, or let it take you away without fighting and wave for help.	Do not hyperventilate to increase submersion time.
If you are fishing on rocks, be cautious about waves that may sweep you into the ocean.	Learn CPR. More than 42% of pool owners are not aware of first-aid techniques.
Keep away from marine animals.	

object. Lifeguards use rescue or torpedo buoys for this purpose that can double as thorax and face flotation devices to keep the victim's head out of the water and the airways free.[16]

For an unconscious victim, the most important step is the immediate institution of resuscitative measures. Hypoxia caused by submersion results first in cessation of breathing, followed by cardiac arrest within a short time if not corrected. In-water resuscitation (ventilation only) provides the victim a 3.15 times better chance of surviving without sequelae. Rescuers should check ventilation and, if possible and if indicated, attempt to provide mouth-to-mouth ventilation while still in the water. Unfortunately, external cardiac compressions cannot be performed effectively in the water, so assessment for a pulse and chest compressions must be delayed until the victim is out of the water.[17]

A few studies have been done to determine how often in-water cervical spine injury occurs. In one study of sandy beaches, 46,060 water rescues were evaluated retrospectively, and it was determined that the incidence of cervical spine injury in this setting is very low (0.009%).[18] In another retrospective survey of more than 2400 drownings, only 11 patients (<0.5%) had cervical spine injuries, and all had a history of obvious trauma from diving, falling from height, or a motor vehicle accident.[19] Other water locations may have different rates of cervical spine injury, depending on a wide variety of factors. Any time spent immobilizing the cervical spine in an unconscious victim with no signs of trauma could lead to cardiopulmonary deterioration and even death; thus, routine cervical spine immobilization in water rescues is not recommended.[18,19] If a spinal cord injury is suspected, rescuers should float the victim supine into a horizontal position, allowing the airways to be out of the water, and check for spontaneous breathing. If there is no spontaneous breathing, protocols for in-water (mouth-to-mouth) resuscitation should be followed while maintaining the head in as neutral a position as possible. The jaw thrust without a head tilt or chin lift can be used to open the airway. If there is spontaneous breathing, rescuers should keep floating the victim, using their hands to stabilize his or her neck in a neutral position. If possible, a back support device should be used to move the victim to a dry place, maintaining the neck in a neutral position. The head, neck, chest, and body should be aligned and supported if the victim must be moved or turned.[10]

ON-LAND BASIC DROWNING LIFE SUPPORT

Level of consciousness determines how the victim is removed from the water, but a vertical position is preferred to avoid vomiting and further compromise of the airways.[20] If the victim is exhausted, confused, or unconscious, however, transport should be accomplished in a position as near horizontal possible, but with the head maintained above body level (keep the body horizontal in cases of prolonged immersion or cold water drowning).[20] Airways must be kept open at all times. The first procedure on land is to place the victim in a position parallel to the waterline,[20] as horizontal as possible and lying supine, far enough away from the water to avoid incoming waves. If the victim is conscious, reposition him or her supine with the head up. If the victim is breathing, use the recovery (lateral decubitus) position.[20]

In a 10-year study in Australia, vomiting occurred in more than 65% of victims who needed ventilatory support during the rescue period and in 86% of those who required both ventilatory support and chest compressions.[21] Even in victims who required no intervention after water rescue, vomiting occurred in 50% once they reached shore. The presence of vomit in the airway can result in further aspiration and impairment of oxygenation by obstructing the airways; it can also discourage rescuers from attempting mouth-to-mouth resuscitation.[21] The abdominal thrust (Heimlich) maneuver should never be used as a means of expelling water from the lungs—it is ineffective and carries significant risks. During resuscitation, attempts at active drainage by placing the victim head down increase the risk of vomiting more than fivefold and lead to a small but significant increase in mortality (19%) when compared with keeping the victim in a horizontal position.[20] If vomiting occurs, turn the victim's mouth to the side and remove the vomitus with a finger sweep, a cloth, or suction.

One of the most difficult medical decisions a lifeguard or an emergency medical technician must make is how to treat a drowning victim appropriately. Cardiopulmonary or isolated respiratory arrest is present in approximately 0.5% of all rescues. The most basic questions are whether the rescuer should administer oxygen, call an ambulance, transport the person to a hospital, or observe on site. Even hospital emergency physicians may be unsure of the appropriate treatment modalities, because the severity of injury varies in drowning victims. To address these issues, a classification system was developed in Rio de Janeiro in 1972 and updated in 1997 to assist lifeguards, ambulance personnel, and physicians who treat drowning victims.[22] It was based on an analysis of 41,279 rescues, of which 2304 (5.6%) needed medical attention. It was revalidated in 2001 by a 10-year study of 46,080 rescues.[23] This classification system (Fig. 88-2) covers support from the site of the accident to the hospital, recommends treatment, and predicts the likelihood of death based on injury severity. The severity can easily be assessed by an on-scene rescuer, emergency medical technician, or physician using only clinical variables.[22]

ADVANCED DROWNING LIFE SUPPORT ON SITE

Bringing medical equipment to the victim instead of carrying the victim to the ambulance saves precious time. Advanced medical treatment is given according to the drowning classification, described here from most to least severe.

Dead Body. Victim with submersion time greater than 1 hour or with obvious physical evidence of death (rigor mortis, putrefaction, dependent lividity). Do *not* start resuscitation—follow to the morgue.

Grade 6—Cardiopulmonary Arrest. Resuscitation started by a layperson or a lifeguard at the scene must be continued by advanced life support personnel until successful. If there is no way to warm the victim appropriately at the scene, the patient should be transported while receiving resuscitation to a hospital, where advanced warming measure can be accomplished. The first priority is adequate oxygenation and ventilation. Medical staff should continue cardiac compressions while starting artificial ventilation using a bag and facemask with 15 L of oxygen until an orotracheal tube can be inserted. Suctioning the airways to intubate is usually necessary. Once intubated, victims can be oxygenated and ventilated effectively, even though there may be copious pulmonary edema fluid. The Sellick maneuver should be used, if possible, during intubation to prevent

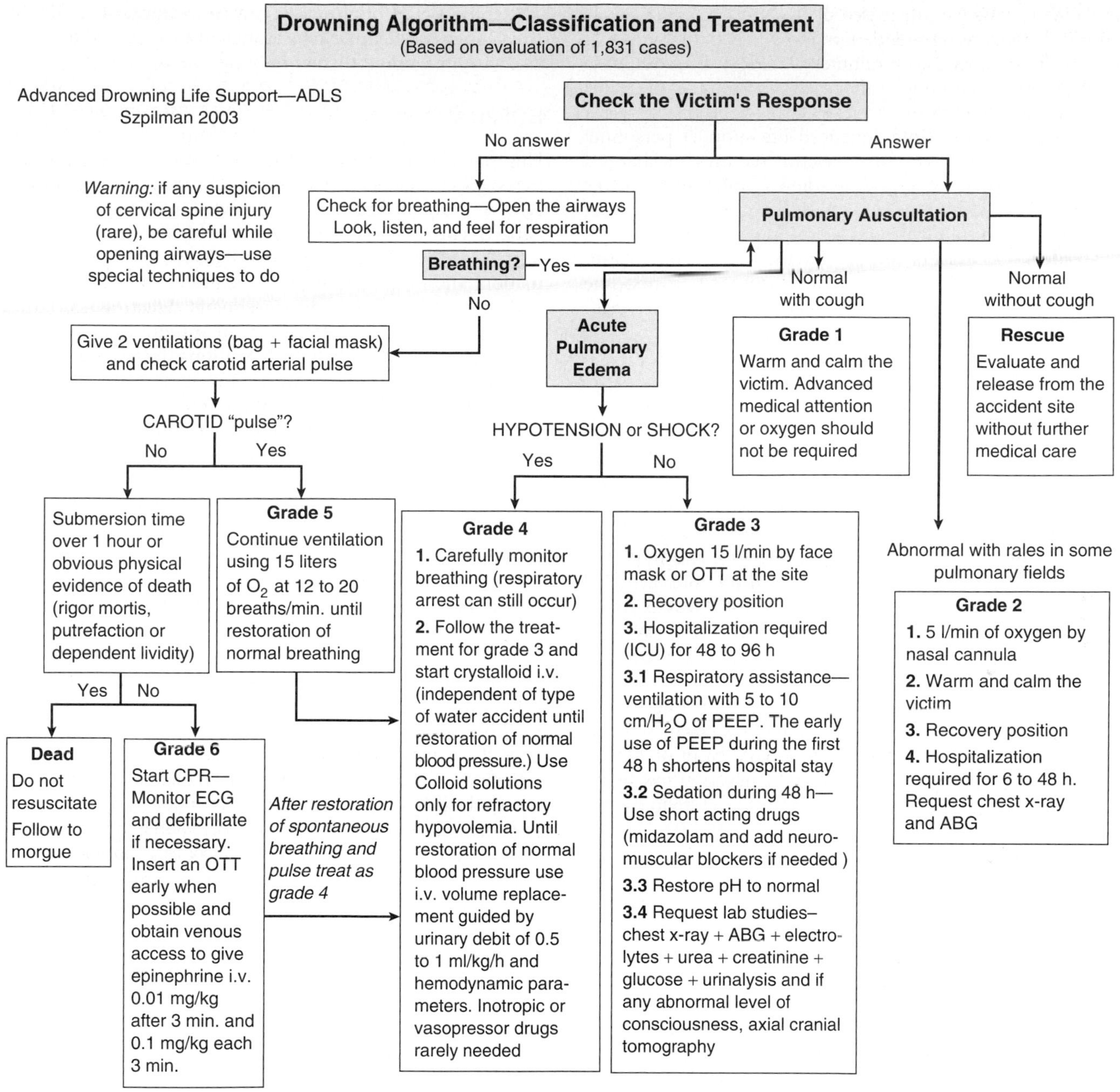

Drowning Algorithm—Classification and Treatment
(Based on evaluation of 1,831 cases)

Advanced Drowning Life Support—ADLS
Szpilman 2003

Check the Victim's Response

No answer — Answer

Warning: if any suspicion of cervical spine injury (rare), be careful while opening airways—use special techniques to do

Check for breathing—Open the airways
Look, listen, and feel for respiration

Pulmonary Auscultation

Breathing?—Yes

No

Normal with cough — Normal without cough

Give 2 ventilations (bag + facial mask) and check carotid arterial pulse

Acute Pulmonary Edema

Grade 1
Warm and calm the victim. Advanced medical attention or oxygen should not be required

Rescue
Evaluate and release from the accident site without further medical care

CAROTID "pulse"?
No — Yes

HYPOTENSION or SHOCK?
Yes — No

Submersion time over 1 hour or obvious physical evidence of death (rigor mortis, putrefaction or dependent lividity)
Yes — No

Grade 5
Continue ventilation using 15 liters of O_2 at 12 to 20 breaths/min. until restoration of normal breathing

Grade 4
1. Carefully monitor breathing (respiratory arrest can still occur)
2. Follow the treatment for grade 3 and start crystalloid i.v. (independent of type of water accident until restoration of normal blood pressure.) Use Colloid solutions only for refractory hypovolemia. Until restoration of normal blood pressure use i.v. volume replacement guided by urinary debit of 0.5 to 1 ml/kg/h and hemodynamic parameters. Inotropic or vasopressor drugs rarely needed

Grade 3
1. Oxygen 15 l/min by face mask or OTT at the site
2. Recovery position
3. Hospitalization required (ICU) for 48 to 96 h
3.1 Respiratory assistance—ventilation with 5 to 10 cm/H_2O of PEEP. The early use of PEEP during the first 48 h shortens hospital stay
3.2 Sedation during 48 h—Use short acting drugs (midazolam and add neuro-muscular blockers if needed)
3.3 Restore pH to normal
3.4 Request lab studies–chest x-ray + ABG + electro-lytes + urea + creatinine + glucose + urinalysis and if any abnormal level of consciousness, axial cranial tomography

Abnormal with rales in some pulmonary fields

Grade 2
1. 5 l/min of oxygen by nasal cannula
2. Warm and calm the victim
3. Recovery position
4. Hospitalization required for 6 to 48 h. Request chest x-ray and ABG

Dead
Do not resuscitate
Follow to morgue

Grade 6
Start CPR—Monitor ECG and defibrillate if necessary. Insert an OTT early when possible and obtain venous access to give epinephrine i.v. 0.01 mg/kg after 3 min. and 0.1 mg/kg each 3 min.

After restoration of spontaneous breathing and pulse treat as grade 4

FIGURE 88–2. Do not spend time trying to drain the water from lungs; this will only increase the occurrence of vomiting and complications. Do not enthusiastically aspirate foam while ventilating. Do not use diuretics or water restriction to treat pulmonary edema. Do not use antibiotics before 48 h except if the accident occurred in an area of high water bacterial colonization (CFU >10²⁰). Do not use steroids except in case of refractory bronchospasm. Always treat hypothermia. Do not stop CPR until body temperature rises to 34°C. There is no difference in ADLS support between different kinds of water. Drowning classification algorithm—advanced drowning life support (ADLS). ABG, arterial blood gas; CPR, cardiopulmonary resuscitation; ECG, electrocardiogram; ICU, intensive care unit; OTT, oro-tracheal tube; PEEP, positive end-expiratory pressure. (From Szpilman D: Near-drowning and drowning classification: A proposal to stratify mortality based on the analysis of 1831 cases. Chest 1997;112:660-665.)

regurgitation and aspiration. The orotracheal tube should be aspirated only when fluid interferes with effective ventilation.

External defibrillation patches may have a role in monitoring the cardiac rhythm. If the patient is pulseless and hypothermic (<34°C), cardiopulmonary resuscitation (CPR) must continue. Although ventricular fibrillation is uncommon, especially in pediatric victims, some adults may develop it, possibly as a consequence of coronary artery disease or the therapies administered, such as epinephrine. Peripheral venous access is the preferred route for drugs. Although some drugs can be administered endotracheally, despite copious fluid, the drug dosage and rate of absorption are unclear.[16] The dose of epinephrine for resuscitation in

drowning victims is controversial; in these patients, the time elapsed before initiation of resuscitation can be much longer and the outcome much different from that in other situations. Both beneficial and toxic physiologic effects of epinephrine administration during CPR have been shown in animal and human studies. Initial or escalating high-dose epinephrine occasionally results in the return of spontaneous circulation and early survival; however, higher doses of epinephrine do not improve long-term survival or neurologic outcome in nondrowning cardiac arrest when used as initial therapy. Therefore, high-dose epinephrine is not recommended for routine use, but it can be considered if 1-mg doses fail.[24] Nevertheless, in some studies, high doses of epinephrine in drowning victims have increased the rate of successful resuscitation.[22,25] Our recommendation is to use a first dose of 0.01 mg/kg i.v. after 3 to 5 minutes of CPR[26]; if no response occurs, increase to 0.1 mg/kg after each 3 to 5 minutes of CPR.[10]

Grade 5—Respiratory Arrest. Respiratory arrest is usually reversed by the time advanced life support personnel arrive at the scene. An apneic victim requires mechanical ventilatory support. Oxygenation and ventilation protocols for grade 6 should be followed until spontaneous breathing is restored; then follow protocols for grade 4.

Grade 4—Acute Pulmonary Edema with Hypotension. Oxygen with mechanical ventilatory support is first-line therapy. Initially, oxygen should be administered by facemask at 15 L/minute until an orotracheal tube can be inserted. In grade 4 drownings, early intubation is needed in 100% of cases, with provision of positive airway pressure. Mechanical ventilation is indicated by an arterial oxygen saturation (SaO_2) of less than 90%, an arterial partial pressure of carbon dioxide ($PaCO_2$) of more than 45 mm Hg, or an abnormally high respiratory rate or effort to maintain adequate arterial blood gases, such that the patient is consuming large amounts of energy breathing and is likely to tire.[16] Patients should be given sedatives, analgesics, and muscular blockers as needed to tolerate intubation and artificial mechanical ventilation with a tidal volume of at least 5 mL/kg body weight. The inspired oxygen fraction (FIO_2) can start at 1.0 but should be reduced to 0.45 or less as soon as possible to avoid adding oxygen toxicity to pulmonary injury. Positive end-expiratory pressure (PEEP) should be added initially at a level of 5 cm H_2O and then increased by increments of 2 to 3 cm H_2O until an intrapulmonary shunt of 20% or less or a PaO_2/FIO_2 of 250 or more is achieved. If low blood pressure is not corrected by oxygen, a rapid crystalloid infusion should be used before trying to reduce PEEP.[11,27]

Grade 3—Acute Pulmonary Edema without Hypotension. Victims with an SaO_2 greater than 90% with the use of 15 L of oxygen by facemask can tolerate noninvasive ventilatory support in only 27.6% of cases. The rest need intubation and mechanical ventilation, which should be instituted using the same protocols as for grade 4.

Grade 2—Abnormal Auscultation with Rales in Some Pulmonary Fields. Victims need oxygen by nasal cannula in 93.2% of cases; the rest need no oxygen assistance.

Grade 1—Coughing with Normal Lung Auscultation. Victims do not need any oxygen or respiratory assistance.

Rescue—No Coughing, Foamy Secretions, or Difficulty Breathing. The victim can be evaluated and released from the accident site without further medical care.

HOSPITAL

Hospital care is recommended for grades 2 to 6. Decision-making in the emergency department about admission to an ICU or hospital bed versus observation in the emergency department or discharge home should involve a thorough history of the accident and previous illnesses, a physical examination, and diagnostic studies, including chest radiographs and arterial blood gas measurements. Electrolytes, blood urea nitrogen, creatinine, and hemoglobin should be assessed serially, although perturbations in these laboratory tests are unusual. In some cases, a toxicologic screen for suspected alcohol or drug ingestion might be warranted. Patients classified as grades 3 to 6 should be admitted to an ICU for close observation and therapy. Grade 2 patients can be observed in the emergency room for 6 to 24 hours, and grade 1 and rescue cases with no complaints or associated illnesses can be released home. Table 88-2 shows the need for hospital admission and overall and hospital mortality rates for each grade of severity.

Except in rare situations, grade 4 to 6 patients arrive at the hospital mechanically ventilated with acceptable oxygenation. If not, the emergency physician should follow grade 4 ventilation protocols. Once the desired oxygenation is achieved at a given level of positive airway pressure, that level of PEEP should be maintained unchanged for 48 hours to permit adequate surfactant regeneration. During that time, if the level of consciousness allows the patient to breathe spontaneously, it is reasonable to use continuous positive airway pressure (CPAP) plus pressure support ventilation. In selected cases, CPAP may be provided by mask (e.g., in cooperative adolescents) or nasal cannula (e.g., in infants who are obligate nasal breathers). A clinical picture similar to that of acute respiratory distress syndrome (ARDS) is common after significant drowning episodes (grades 3 to 6), but with a more rapid recovery. Ventilatory management is similar to that of other patients with ARDS, including efforts to minimize volutrauma and barotrauma. However, permissive hypercapnia probably is not suitable for grade 6 drowning victims with significant hypoxic-ischemic brain injury. Instead, mild to moderate hyperventilation, aiming for a $PaCO_2$ in the

TABLE 88-2. RATES OF MORTALITY AND HOSPITAL ADMISSION FOR DROWNING, BY GRADE

Grade	No. of Patients	Overall Mortality (%)	Admitted to Hospital (%)	Hospital Mortality (%)
Rescued	38,976	0 (0)	0 (0)	0 (0)
1	1,189	0 (0)	35 (2.9)	0 (0)
2	338	2 (0.6)	50 (14.8)	2 (4.0)
3	58	3 (5.2)	26 (44.8)	3 (11.5)
4	36	7 (19.4)	32 (88.9)	7 (19.4)
5	25	11 (44)	21 (84)*	7 (33.3)
6	185	172 (93)	23 (12.4)†	10 (43.5)
Total	1,831‡	195 (10.6%) $P < 0.0001$	187 (10.2%)	29 (15.5%)

*Not included are 4 patients who were pronounced dead and taken directly to the morgue.
†Not included are162 patients who were pronounced dead and taken directly to the morgue.
‡Excluding the rescues cases.
From Szpilman D: Near-drowning classification: A proposal to stratify mortality based on the analysis is of 1831 cases. Chest 1997;112:660-665.

range of 30 to 35 mm Hg, is indicated, together with other therapeutic measures to control cerebral edema.

Despite aggressive management, neurologic injury and sequelae, including persistent vegetative state, can complicate the management of grade 6 drowning victims. In those who are hemodynamically unstable or have severe pulmonary dysfunction (grades 4 to 6), pulmonary artery catheterization may improve the ability to assess and treat the patient. No evidence exists to support the routine administration of hypertonic solutions and transfusions for freshwater drowning or hypotonic solutions for saltwater drowning.[11,27] Echocardiography to assess cardiac function and ejection fraction may help the clinician decide whether to use inotropic agents, vasopressors, or both if the patient remains hypotensive after volume resuscitation. Some studies have shown that cardiac dysfunction, with low cardiac output, is common in the period immediately after severe drowning (grades 4 to 6).[11] Supportive measures include Foley catheter placement to monitor urine output.

Metabolic acidosis is present in 70% of severe drowning patients when they arrive at the hospital.[13] Acidosis should be corrected when the pH is lower than 7.2 or the bicarbonate is less than 12 mEq/L, if the victim has adequate ventilatory support.[27] Significant depletion of bicarbonate is rarely present in the first 10 to 15 minutes of CPR, contraindicating bicarbonate replacement in the early resuscitative phase.[26]

Usually, pools and beaches do not have sufficient bacteria to cause pneumonia during the immediate postdrowning period.[28] If the patient needs mechanical respiratory assistance, the incidence of secondary pneumonia increases from 34% to 52% by the fourth day of hospitalization.[29] Prophylactic antibiotics are of doubtful value in the initial management of drowning victims and tend to select out more resistant and aggressive organisms. An altered chest radiograph should not be interpreted as pneumonia, because it is usually the result of pulmonary edema and aspirated water in the alveoli and bronchi. A preferable approach is daily monitoring of tracheal aspirates with Gram stain, culture, and sensitivity. At the first sign (usually after the first 48 to 72 hours of ICU care) of pulmonary infection—gauged by prolonged fever, sustained leukocytosis, persistent or new pulmonary infiltrates, and leukocytosis in the tracheal aspirate—antibiotic therapy should be selected based on the predominant organism and pattern of sensitivity. Fiber-optic bronchoscopy may be useful for obtaining quantitative cultures, for determining the extent and severity of airway injury in cases of solid aspiration, and, rarely, for therapeutic clearing of sand, gravel, and other solids. Corticosteroids are of doubtful value in pulmonary injury and should not be used, except for bronchospasm.

The clinician must be aware of and vigilant for potential complications of ventilatory therapy, such as volutrauma and barotrauma.[28] Spontaneous pneumothoraces are common (10%), secondary to positive-pressure ventilation and local areas of hyperinflation. Any sudden change in hemodynamic stability during mechanical ventilation should be evaluated to rule out pneumothorax or other barotrauma. Nasogastric tube placement reduces gastric distention and prevents further aspiration. Rarely, drowning victims who seem healthy on assessment in the emergency department, including having normal chest radiographs, develop fulminant pulmonary edema as long as 12 hours after the incident. Whether this late-onset pulmonary edema is delayed ARDS or neurogenic pulmonary edema secondary to hypoxia is unclear, but it is extremely unusual.

Renal insufficiency or renal failure is rare in drowning victims but can occur secondary to anoxia, shock, or hemoglobinuria.

Besides the reversible pulmonary injury, the most important complication is the anoxic-ischemic cerebral insult that may be present after resuscitation. Most late deaths and long-term sequelae of drowning are neurologic in origin.[28] Although the highest priority is restoration of spontaneous circulation, in the early stages after rescue, every effort should be made to resuscitate the brain and prevent further neurologic damage. These steps include the provision of adequate oxygenation (SaO_2 >92%) and cerebral perfusion (mean arterial pressure around 100 mm Hg). Any victim who remains comatose and unresponsive after successful CPR or deteriorates neurologically should be evaluated for the development of cerebral edema.

Continuous monitoring of core and brain (tympanic) temperature is mandatory in the emergency department and ICU (and in the prehospital setting, if possible). Drowning victims in whom adequate spontaneous circulation has been restored but who remain comatose should not be actively rewarmed to temperatures greater than 32°C to 34°C. If the core temperature exceeds 34°C in a comatose patient, hypothermia (32°C to 34°C) should be achieved as soon as possible and sustained for 12 to 24 hours. Hyperthermia should be prevented at all times in the acute recovery period.

Although there is insufficient evidence to support a specific target $PaCO_2$ or oxygen saturation during and after resuscitation, hypoxemia should be avoided. In select cases, the induction of barbiturate coma can control cerebral edema and intracranial hypertension when other therapies are unsuccessful. Unfortunately, studies evaluating the results of cerebral resuscitation measures in drowning victims failed to demonstrate that therapies directed at controlling intracranial hypertension and maintaining cerebral perfusion pressure improve outcome. These studies showed poor outcomes (i.e., death or moderate to profound neurologic sequelae) when the intracranial pressure was 20 mm Hg or more and the cerebral perfusion pressure was 60 mm Hg or less, even when therapies directed at controlling and improving these pressures were used.

New therapeutic interventions for drowning victims, such as extracorporeal membrane oxygenation, artificial surfactant, nitric oxide, and liquid lung ventilation, are still in the investigational stage.

OUTCOME AND SCORING SYSTEMS

Grade 3 to 6 drownings have the potential to cause multisystem organ failure.[16] Grade 1 to 5 drowning victims return home without sequelae in 95% of cases.[22] A major concern among researchers is grade 6 drowning. Several questions need to be answered: How do we know when to make the effort to resuscitate? How long we should continue? How different should the treatment be? What will the patient's quality of life be after successful resuscitation?[11] Both at the rescue site and in the hospital, no one indicator is reliable in predicting the outcome in grade 6 patients.[30] Based on the longest documented submersion time in cold water (66 minutes) with complete recovery,[16] resuscitation should be started without delay in every victim without a palpable carotid pulse who has been submerged for less than 1 hour or does not have obvious physical evidence of death (rigor mortis, putrefaction, dependent lividity).

TABLE 88–3. PROBABILITY OF DEATH OR SEVERE NEUROLOGIC IMPAIRMENT, BASED ON DURATION OF SUBMERSION

Duration of Submersion (min)	Probability of Death or Severe Neurologic Impairment (%)
0 to <5	10
5 to <10*	56
10 to <25	88
>25	100

*Note that the 5 additional minutes of submersion increases mortality almost 6 times.
From Cummins RO, Szpilman D: Submersion. In Cummins RO, Field JM, Hazinski MF (eds): ACLS—The Reference Textbook, vol 2, ACLS for Experienced Providers. Dallas, American Heart Association, 2003, pp 97-107.

Some clinical series claim that successful resuscitation after prolonged submersion is possible only in cold or icy water; however, there are anecdotal cases of prolonged warm water drowning and survival without sequelae.[22,31,32] Multiple studies have established that outcome is determined almost solely by one factor—duration of submersion (Table 88–3).[17,21,22,28,31-35] Based on a report of a drowning victim who was successfully resuscitated after 2 hours of CPR,[28] efforts should stop only if asystole persists after rewarming the victim above 34°C.

After successful CPR, it is crucial to stratify the severity of neurologic deficits, which allows the comparison of different therapeutic approaches. Various prognostic scoring systems have been developed to predict which patients will do well with standard therapy and which are likely to have significant cerebral anoxic encephalopathy requiring aggressive measures to protect the brain. One of the best measures is the Glasgow coma scale score in the period immediately (during the first hour) after resuscitation (Conn and Modell neurologic classification).[28,36] Because of the typical 2- to 6-hour delay between rescue and transfer from an outlying emergency facility to an ICU, many patients with severe anoxic-ischemic cerebral insults and coma have had multiple determinations of neurologic status before definitive therapy is begun. Data suggest that patients who remain profoundly comatose (i.e., decorticate, decerebrate, or flaccid)

2 to 6 hours after the drowning accident are brain dead or will have moderate to severe neurologic impairment. Patients who are improving but remain unresponsive have a 50% likelihood of a good outcome. Patients who are definitely improving and alert or are stuporous or obtunded but respond to stimuli 2 to 6 hours after the incident are likely to have normal or near-normal neurologic outcomes. These prognostic variables are important in counseling family members in the early stages after the accident and in deciding which patients are likely to have a good outcome with standard supportive therapy and which victims are candidates for experimental cerebral resuscitation therapies.[33]

ANNOTATED REFERENCES

Bierens JJLM, Velde EA, Berkel M, Zanten JJ: Submersion in the Netherlands: Prognostic indicators and results of resuscitation. Ann Emerg Med 1990;19:1390-1395.
This retrospective study revealed some important prognostic indicators and found that submersion time is the most important one. However, no one indicator can predict the final outcome of drowning.

Cummins RO, Szpilman D: Submersion. In Cummins RO, Field JM, Hazinski MF (eds): ACLS—The Reference Textbook, vol 2, ACLS for Experienced Providers. Dallas, American Heart Association, 2003, pp 97-107.
An excellent review article that highlights important issues such as in-water resuscitation, cervical trauma, and prognostic indicators in the prehospital setting.

Orlowski JP, Szpilman D: Drowning—rescue, resuscitation, and reanimation: Pediatric critical care: A new millennium. Pediatr Clin North Am 2001;48:627-646.
A very good review article that highlights issues such as prevention, physiopathology, basic life support, and treatment.

Special resuscitation situations: Guidelines for cardiopulmonary resuscitation and emergency cardiac care (ECC). Circulation 2000;102:122-153.
These guidelines deal with many different aspects of drowning, including modification of definitions, classification, and new approaches in advanced life support.

Szpilman D: Near-drowning and drowning classification: A proposal to stratify mortality based on the analysis of 1831 cases. Chest 1997;112:122-153.
This retrospective study reviewed 41,279 water rescues to establish a classification system for drowning according to severity, based on mortality rates. Using clinical parameters ranging from first-aid observations, presence of breathing, arterial pulse, pulmonary auscultation, and arterial blood pressure, six grades were developed, representing different mortality rates and treatment.

Chapter 89

ACUTE PARENCHYMAL DISEASE IN INFANTS AND CHILDREN

Kathleen M. Ventre • John H. Arnold

KEY POINTS

1. Whereas **inhaled bronchodilators and systemic corticosteroids are of proven benefit** in the management of asthma-induced bronchospasm, symptomatic medical therapies have not been shown to alter outcomes in critically ill children with airways obstruction due to bronchiolitis.

2. **In critically ill patients with lower airways disease,** noninvasive positive-pressure ventilation may be a feasible strategy to avoid intubation in select pediatric patients. Noninvasive respiratory support has been used successfully in the management of asthma and bronchiolitis.

3. **Noninvasive mechanical ventilatory support** may also obviate the need for intubation in pediatric patients with alveolar disease. This technique has been applied with success in a variety of alveolar diseases in pediatric patients.

4. A great deal of experimental data support the use of **lung-protective ventilation in pediatric alveolar disease.** Lung-protective ventilation involves the preservation of end-expiratory lung volume by judicious use of positive end-expiratory pressure (PEEP) and/or recruitment maneuvers, minimizing cyclic stretch, and avoidance of parenchymal overdistention at end inspiration by limiting tidal volume and transpulmonary pressure.

5. **High-frequency oscillatory ventilation** has theoretical advantage in providing a lung-protective strategy of ventilation by maintaining maximal recruitment throughout the respiratory cycle and achieving ventilation through use of very small phasic changes in pressure and volume.

6. **In pediatric patients, interstitial lung disease may develop** as a result of either congenital abnormalities of the alveolar-capillary unit or acquired pulmonary conditions. The potential causes for interstitial lung disease in children differ from those in adult patients.

7. **Bronchopulmonary dysplasia, or acquired chronic lung disease of infancy,** is believed to develop as a result of inflammatory response to lung injury. A strategy involving promotion and maintenance of alveolar recruitment and minimizing cyclic changes in lung volume is likely to limit excess lung injury in neonates.

8. Recent experience with the **supportive care of infants with congenital diaphragmatic hernia** seems to favor delaying surgical repair until physiologic stability is achieved as well as the judicious titration of mechanical ventilatory support to limit excess lung injury.

9. **Successfully separating the pediatric patient from mechanical ventilatory support** requires timely recognition of acceptable respiratory mechanics and gas exchange. A protocol for gradual weaning of mechanical ventilatory support may not be important for the majority of pediatric patients.

Pulmonary parenchymal processes in children whom the intensive care clinician may encounter include common and uncommon diseases of the lower airways, alveoli, and pulmonary interstitium. Among the more challenging conditions to manage in the ICU are those that include disease or dysfunction of all three of these components, such as bronchopulmonary dysplasia (BPD) and congenital diaphragmatic hernia (CDH). In this chapter we discuss the pathophysiology and management principles pertinent to each disease category, with emphasis given to common examples and conditions that are unique to the pediatric patient.

DISEASES OF THE AIRWAYS

STATUS ASTHMATICUS

Although unusual anatomic conditions of the lower airways can occur in pediatric patients (Table 89-1), status asthmaticus and bronchiolitis are probably the most common causes of lower airways disease in the pediatric ICU. Severe exacerbations of asthma in children present a common management challenge for the critical care clinician. Asthma is common in the industrialized world. Annual rates of hospitalization for the disease in infants and children up to 14 years of age have increased dramatically over the past decade, and pediatric patients continue to have the highest hospitalization rate of any age group.[1,2] Mortality rates for American children age 5 to 14 years with asthma seemed to peak in the early 1990s and have declined slightly since then.[1,2] Status asthmaticus is characterized by acute, severe airway obstruction due to bronchoconstriction that is refractory to initial management

TABLE 89–1. ANATOMIC CAUSES OF LOWER AIRWAYS DYSFUNCTION

Tracheomalacia, bronchomalacia
  Vascular anomaly
  Tracheoesophageal fistula
  Idiopathic
Bronchiectasis
Congenital lobar emphysema
Cystic adenomatoid malformation
Pulmonary sequestration
Bronchogenic cyst

with supplemental oxygen, inhaled bronchodilators, and corticosteroids. The pathophysiology of the condition begins with a precipitant that triggers contraction of hyper-responsive bronchial smooth muscle, mucus secretion, and mucosal edema, which result in obstruction of large and small airways. Hyperinflation from premature closure of lower airways in expiration leads to an increased functional residual capacity[3] and an increased respiratory workload that ultimately leads to alveolar hypoventilation and hypoxemia. An abrupt and profound acidosis can occur when respiratory compensation for accumulated inorganic acids no longer

occurs (Fig. 89-1).[3] On physical examination, the child with status asthmaticus will often appear anxious or lethargic, will often demonstrate accessory muscle use, and, depending on the quality of air entry, can demonstrate either cough with profound inspiratory and/or expiratory wheezing and prolongation of audible expiration, or a silent chest. Pulsus paradoxus, far in excess of normal, can often be demonstrated, reflecting the profoundly negative intrapleural pressures generated by these patients during spontaneous respiration.

Therapy

Supportive care in status asthmaticus begins with maintaining the airway, monitoring the quality of respirations, and maintenance of euvolemia. Standard medical therapies for these patients include bronchodilators and corticosteroids, and several adjunctive therapies have been investigated as possible rescue agents in difficult cases (Table 89-2). Short-acting beta-agonist agents, targeted to mediate airway smooth muscle relaxation via local beta$_2$ receptors,[3] are the most commonly used bronchodilators for status asthmaticus. Among these agents, albuterol is the most widely used. Unlike epinephrine and isoproterenol, it is relatively beta$_2$ selective[3] and it is most commonly administered by nebulization. It is typically given at 0.15 mg/kg/dose up to 5 mg on a frequent intermittent

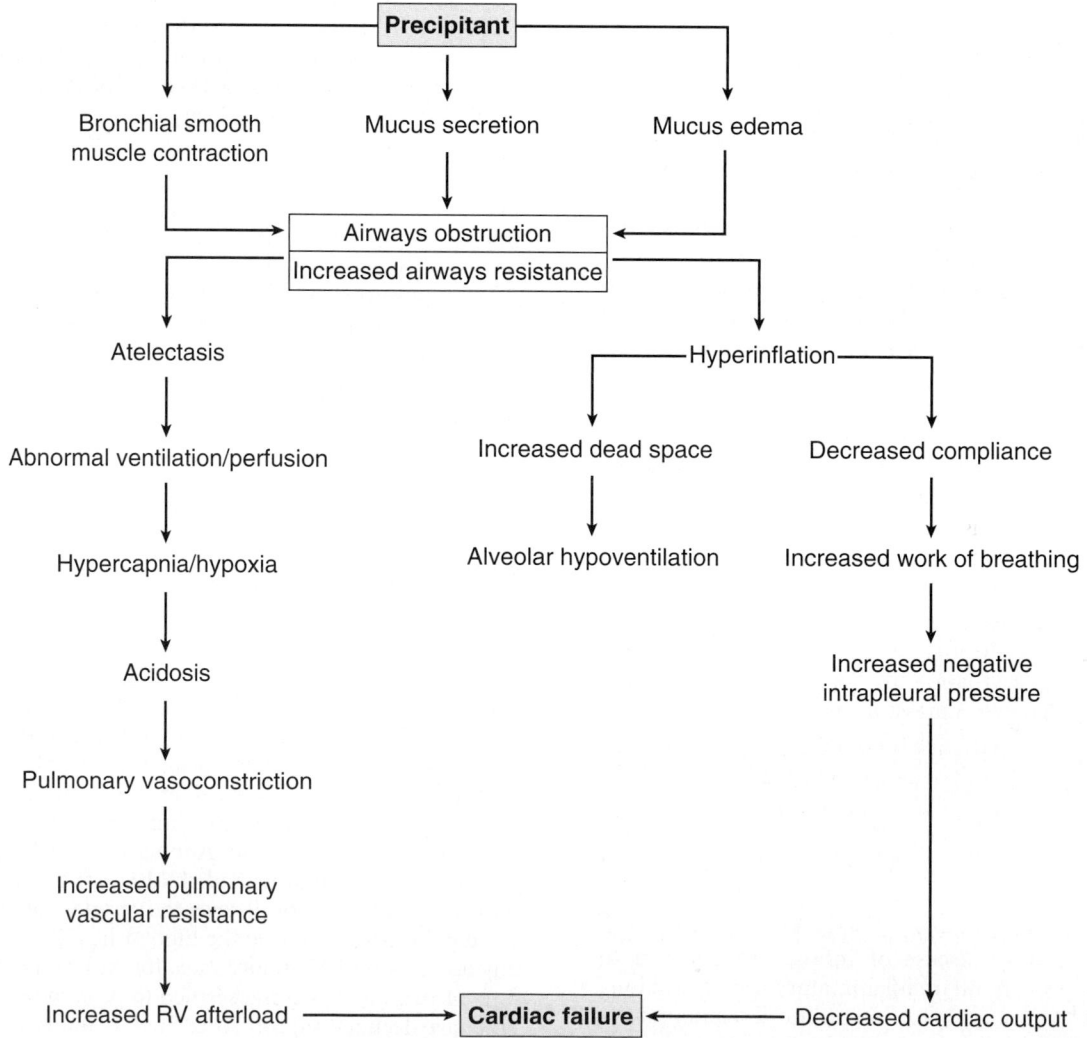

FIGURE 89–1. Pathophysiology in status asthmaticus. (Modified from Helfaer M, Nichols D, Rogers M: Lower airway disease: Bronchiolitis and asthma. In Rogers M [ed]: Textbook of Pediatric Intensive Care, 3rd ed. Baltimore, Williams & Wilkins, 1996, p 141.)

TABLE 89–2. SELECTED PHARMACOTHERAPIES FOR STATUS ASTHMATICUS

Nebulized Therapies

Albuterol (0.5%), 0.15 mg/kg/dose (0.03 mL/kg/dose) inhaled q1-6 h prn. Continuous inhalation 0.5 mg/kg/h
Ipratropium, 0.25-0.5 mg inhaled q4-6h
Racemic epinephrine (2.25%), 0.25-0.5 mL inhaled qh prn

Subcutaneous Therapies

Epinephrine (1:1000), 0.01 mg/kg/dose (0.01 mL/kg/dose) s.c. (max: 0.5 mL/dose)

Intravenous Therapies

Terbutaline, 10 μg/kg i.v. × 1, followed by 0.4-6 μg/kg/min i.v. infusion
Magnesium sulfate 25-50 mg/kg IV over 20 minutes (max 2 g/dose)
Methylprednisolone, 1 mg/kg/dose i.v. q6h

basis, but only a small fraction of the nebulized dose may actually be delivered to the lung, particularly in critically ill infants and children who are intubated with small endotracheal tubes.[4-6] Several studies have demonstrated that small doses of nebulized beta agonist given in rapid sequential fashion produce sustained improvements in forced expiratory volume more often than when larger doses are given less frequently,[7,8] and there is also evidence to suggest that continuous nebulization of the drug may actually lead to more rapid and sustained clinical improvement.[9]

A preparation of the therapeutically active isomer of albuterol (levalbuterol) has been proved effective when administered to children with stable asthma.[10] There are no controlled trials presently available to evaluate its use in children with acute exacerbations of the disease. Inhaled anticholinergic agents such as ipratropium also have a role in the management of severe bronchospasm in children with asthma. Addition of inhaled ipratropium to inhaled beta agonists has been demonstrated to result in significant patient improvement and pulmonary function, especially in children with severe asthma.[11,12] In the patient who does not respond to inhaled bronchodilators, it is possible to administer beta-agonist therapy by the parenteral route. In some countries, the intravenous preparation of albuterol is available, which allows for the parenteral administration of this beta$_2$-selective agent. In the United States where this agent is not available, terbutaline, which has some beta$_2$ selectivity, can be administered intravenously. Although terbutaline has not been associated with clinically significant cardiac toxicity in most pediatric patients,[3,13] it is advisable to monitor the electrocardiogram and serum troponin level during its administration.

The inflammatory basis for asthma has long been recognized, and corticosteroids have had an important role in the management of status asthmaticus. The use of corticosteroids has been demonstrated to significantly improve airways obstruction in patients with severe acute asthma.[14] The parenteral route is the method of choice for administering these agents to the critically ill child, and it is important to realize that fatal anaphylaxis to these drugs has been reported.[15,16] Methylprednisolone is one of the most commonly used agents for acute severe asthma. Because of its half life, steady-state levels can be achieved relatively quickly; and although dosing regimens vary, it is probably most appropriate to dose the drug every 6 hours. There does not seem to be any advantage to administering massive doses of glucocorticoids in status asthmaticus.[17] If methylprednisolone is not available, equipotent doses of another glucocorticoid may be used.

Magnesium has been investigated for use in status asthmaticus because of its potential to augment the effects of bronchodilators by causing relaxation of airway smooth muscle. A recent randomized controlled trial in adults demonstrated that intravenous administration of 2 g of magnesium sulfate improves pulmonary function when administered as an adjunct to nebulized beta agonists and intravenously administered corticosteroids in patients with especially low FEV$_1$ (<20% of predicted).[18] Although magnesium is occasionally added to standard therapy in pediatric status asthmaticus, the evidence supporting its use in this population is limited.[19]

Enthusiasm for the use of methylxanthines (theophylline, aminophylline) in pediatric asthma has fluctuated over time. These drugs are primarily phosphodiesterase inhibitors, but the mechanism of their effects in asthma is not well understood. A recent randomized controlled trial investigated the effects of aminophylline on 163 children in status asthmaticus to whom the drug was administered as an adjunct to nebulized beta agonists, nebulized anticholinergics, and parenteral corticosteroids.[20] Aminophylline appeared to improve pulmonary function and may have averted intubation in a portion of those patients who received it.[20] Although it may have a role as adjunct therapy in the treatment of severe status asthmaticus, its widespread use is limited by a narrow range of therapeutic serum levels that overlaps with levels that are associated with systemic toxicity.[3]

BRONCHIOLITIS

Bronchiolitis involves invasion of the large and small airway respiratory epithelium by inflammatory cells in the setting of acute respiratory illness. The primary cause of bronchiolitis is respiratory syncytial virus (RSV), which is responsible for 45% to 75% of cases, although parainfluenza viruses, rhinoviruses, adenoviruses, influenza viruses, enteroviruses, and *Mycoplasma pneumoniae* can produce the clinical syndrome as well. RSV dependably produces yearly epidemics, which occur during the winter and spring months. Infection with RSV is nearly universal among infants and children by age 2 years, but only 1% require hospitalization.[21] Among all hospitalized children, the percentage requiring intensive care has been reported as 7% to 9% among patients without comorbidity and as high as 20% to 37% in those with preceding cardiac disease, chronic lung disease, prematurity, age younger than 6 weeks, and immunocompromise.[22] These patients are also at increased risk of mortality from RSV[23] and have been identified as candidates to receive monthly prophylaxis with an RSV antigen-specific monoclonal antibody (palivizumab) each month during RSV season.

The mode of transmission may be either through direct contact with contagious secretions or by exposure to aerosolized particles from the respiratory mucosa.[21] The incubation period varies from 2 to 8 days,[21] symptoms tend to escalate over 3 to 5 days, and convalescence can be prolonged (up to several weeks in the most vulnerable small infants). On histologic examination, reappearance of ciliated respiratory epithelium commonly takes more than 2 weeks.[21] Viral shedding from the respiratory tract typically occurs over 3 to 8 days but may also continue for up to 4 to 6 weeks in small infants. Symptoms typically begin with signs of upper respiratory illness, including fever, coryza, and, possibly, otitis media. Small infants commonly present with lethargy and central apnea[24] early in the course of illness. Cough and tachypnea soon develop as the illness progresses to the lower airways, usually 1 to 3 days after incubation.[21] Wheezing, produced by flow limitation in peripheral airways, is a nearly universal finding and may be attributable in large part to intermittent obstruction of large and small airways with necrotic epithelial debris, edema, and mucus,[21] rather than to the bronchospasm more commonly seen in asthma. Radiographic findings are often nonspecific but commonly include hyperinflation, peribronchial thickening, subsegmental consolidation, and multiple areas of atelectasis or infiltration, involving most frequently the right middle and right upper lobes. A large prospective study of RSV-infected hospitalized children found that secondary bacterial infection occurred in only 1.2% of the study cohort, establishing that risk of bacterial disease is low in RSV bronchiolitis, despite potentially suggestive radiographic findings and the widespread use of broad-spectrum antimicrobial agents in these patients.[25]

Therapy

Treatment of the infant or child with bronchiolitis is primarily supportive. Many years of clinical experience with empirical use of symptomatic medical therapies have failed to determine a clear role for any of these agents in the management of this disease. Data on the use of medical therapies in critically ill children with bronchiolitis is especially scant. Aerosolized ribavirin, a synthetic guanosine analogue with broad-spectrum antiviral activity, is currently the only specific therapy approved for hospitalized infants with RSV bronchiolitis.[21] In general, it has been shown to improve oxygenation and clinical status scores and to reduce inflammatory mediators associated with ongoing wheezing in patients with RSV.[21] A meta-analysis of three studies on the use of ribavirin in ventilated patients showed a small but significant decrease in ventilator days associated with the use of this agent.[26] Nonetheless, prospects for widespread administration of this agent or even additional large-scale trials to further evaluate its role are limited by the technical challenges, cost, and occupational hazards associated with its use.[27-29]

Widespread use of bronchodilators and corticosteroids for the management of bronchiolitis is common despite the absence of evidence for improved clinical outcomes in critically ill children.[26] There are presently no randomized, controlled trials evaluating the effect of bronchodilators in critically ill children with bronchiolitis.[26] A recent large, randomized controlled trial[30] as well as a systematic review[31] have failed to establish that any bronchodilator produces a significant improvement in relevant outcome measures in less severely ill hospitalized children with bronchiolitis. A few small studies have associated some short-term physiologic benefit with the use of corticosteroids, immune globulin, and surfactant in critically ill infants and children with bronchiolitis, but effectiveness of these therapies in altering outcomes in this population has not been established.[26] Because future prospects for providing lasting immunity to RSV remain doubtful,[21] there is an ongoing need for large, multicenter studies to identify therapies that may benefit critically ill children with this disease.

Meanwhile, supportive care of the patient with bronchiolitis consists of an ongoing assessment of airway patency, the adequacy of respirations, and maintenance of adequate circulating volume. Supplemental oxygen is often required to reverse hypoxemia, and the clinician should be attentive to a change in neurologic status, which often heralds impending respiratory failure.

MECHANICAL VENTILATION

The need for mechanical ventilation in the patient with lower airways disease arises commonly from failure of ventilation and resulting hypercapnia. Hypoxemia and recurrent apnea, which are common in young infants with bronchiolitis, also frequently precipitate the institution of ventilatory support. Assuming adequate airway protection, oxygenation, and respiratory drive, it is probably best to avoid intubation in the patient with lower airways disease unless the overall clinical status of the child warrants the risk of augmenting airway hyperreactivity.[32] To this end, there are several adjunctive therapies that may obviate the need for intubation when added to aggressively applied conventional therapies. An inspired mixture of helium and oxygen (heliox) has been used to alleviate airway obstruction in pediatric patients. Because of its low density and reduced Reynolds number, helium is able to convert turbulent gas flow to laminar flow in airways, and its clinical effect is generally immediate. Because it is an inert gas, it can potentially lower airways resistance without toxicity. When given as 60% to 80% of the total inspired gas mixture, helium can produce more efficient delivery of oxygen as well as nebulized drugs.[33] In general, use of heliox in patients with lower airways disease has produced inconsistent results. A small randomized controlled trial in spontaneously breathing children with status asthmaticus demonstrated that administration of heliox improves respiratory mechanics by lowering the pulsus paradoxus, increasing peak flow, and decreasing the dyspnea index, which may decrease the need for mechanical ventilation.[34] In another small series, a 60:40 heliox mixture administered to 7 intubated patients resulted in a 15% to 50% reduction in peak inspiratory pressure and a 30% to 60% reduction in $PaCO_2$.[35] A recent literature review on the use of heliox in patients of all ages with acute asthma concluded that it may be useful in the short-term management of these patients but that clinical advantage attributable to its use diminishes over time.[36] There is little evidence available on the use of heliox in critically ill patients with bronchiolitis. This issue was prospectively investigated in a nonrandomized study of 38 nonintubated infants with RSV bronchiolitis admitted to an ICU.[37] The investigators were able to demonstrate favorable changes in respiratory status through the first 4 hours of heliox administration and a significant decrease in ICU length of stay among infants who received heliox therapy.[37] In a small randomized, crossover study of RSV-positive, nonintubated patients, clinical indicators of respiratory status improved during heliox administration, particularly among children with more severe disease.[38] However, many of the patients required another form of respiratory support and the study was not designed to evaluate outcomes such as ICU length of stay.[38]

The application of noninvasive forms of mechanical support such as continuous positive airway pressure (CPAP) or bilevel positive pressure using either a nasal or full facemask has potential advantage in the patient with adequate respiratory drive. Careful titration of applied CPAP (or PEEP) noninvasively may prevent premature airways closure during expiration and decrease gas trapping. The patient who develops high levels of intrinsic PEEP due to hyperinflation manifests an increased work of breathing and, ultimately, respiratory muscle fatigue that may precipitate dramatic and rapid clinical deterioration. Noninvasive respiratory support may allow unloading of the muscles of respiration without adding to airway reactivity and has been used with success in managing asthma as well as bronchiolitis.[39-41]

In the patient with respiratory failure for whom noninvasive mechanical support is not feasible, intubation and mechanical ventilation is warranted. Once tracheal intubation is performed in the patient with airways disease, the clinician should be watchful for complications of the transition to positive-pressure ventilation. In the spontaneously breathing child with severe airways obstruction, profoundly negative intrathoracic pressures develop to generate lung inflation. These conditions produce maximal venous return as right atrial pressure remains subatmospheric.[42] The transition to positive-pressure ventilation in this setting increases juxtacardiac pressures and right ventricular afterload, resulting in decreased venous return, decreased left ventricular end-diastolic volume, and decreased left ventricular compliance,[42] with risk of air leak, hypotension, and cardiac arrest.[3] Initial ventilator settings can be guided by auscultation, careful ventilator waveform analysis, and attention to inspiratory plateau pressure. It is generally preferable to allow the patient to breathe in a spontaneous ventilator mode, using a strategy of permissive hypercapnia. If controlled ventilation is necessary, it is preferable to apply the lowest minute ventilation that provides adequate gas exchange.[43] High-frequency oscillatory ventilation (see later) has been used to rescue a limited number of pediatric patients with asthma and bronchiolitis who demonstrate respiratory failure refractory to management with conventional ventilation.[44] One report recommends the use of high distending pressures to decrease airways resistance, low frequencies, longer expiratory times, and muscle relaxation to minimize gas trapping.[45,46]

Sedation and muscle relaxation to ensure compliance with the ventilator strategy may be necessary if the patient exhibits significant distress and dyssynchrony with the ventilator. Ketamine, a dissociative anesthetic with sympathomimetic and bronchodilatory properties, is often used for sedation in the intubated asthmatic child.[47] The inhalational anesthetic isoflurane may be a useful adjunct to the management of severe status asthmaticus in the intubated child who is difficult to sedate or who is unresponsive to other therapies because of its favorable effects on airways reactivity. The mechanism underlying its bronchodilatory properties is not well understood.[48] Although isoflurane has a better safety profile than halothane when used for this purpose, periodic monitoring of renal function may be advisable in the child who requires prolonged therapy with this agent.[48]

DISEASES OF THE ALVEOLI

PNEUMONIA

Defined as acute respiratory symptoms accompanied by parenchymal infiltrates on a chest radiograph, pneumonia is a common syndrome in children that may be caused by viral or bacterial pathogens.[49] Important viral pathogens responsible for pneumonia in infants and children include RSV, influenza, parainfluenza, and adenovirus. As previously discussed, each of these is agents is also capable of producing the clinical syndrome of "bronchiolitis" in infants and children. The precise infectious etiology may be suggested by the physical examination, the age of the patient, and seasonal incidence patterns. Virologic or bacteriologic confirmation by microbiologic analysis is generally sought to enhance therapeutic decisions as well as cohorting of similarly affected patients. RSV is the most common viral cause of lower respiratory tract infection in infancy,[50] although, as discussed earlier, RSV infection involves primarily the small airways. Influenza is another very important cause of pediatric pneumonia. Infection rates in healthy children are estimated at 10% to 40% each year, and approximately 1% of these children require hospitalization.[50] The course of up to 25% of infected children is complicated by lower respiratory tract disease.[50] Neonates and children up to 5 years of age, especially those with underlying lung disease, congenital heart disease, immunocompromise, and other chronic conditions, seem to be at special risk for influenza pneumonia.[50] Neonates are at risk for especially severe influenza syndromes, which may also include apnea and sepsis.[50] Infants and children older than 6 months of age, especially those in high-risk categories, are candidates for annual vaccination against influenza.[51] Antiviral therapy for A and B strains of influenza are now available and can be considered for patients of appropriate age who are at high risk of complicated or severe disease.[50] When administered within 48 hours of disease onset, amantadine, which is approved for use in children older than age 1 year, may decrease the severity of influenza A disease, but data in young patients are limited.[50] Oseltamivir, a neuraminidase inhibitor active against both A and B strains of influenza, has been demonstrated to decrease symptom duration when administered early in disease and is approved for use in children older than 1 year of age.[52] Unlike RSV, secondary bacterial pneumonia is common in influenza infection and is typically caused by *Streptococcus pneumoniae* or *Staphylococcus aureus,* making it especially important to consider appropriate empirical antimicrobial therapy in certain cases.[53,54] Parainfluenza viruses are also responsible for causing pneumonia in children, and seasonal epidemics commonly occur in autumn.[50] Primary infection tends to occur in young children 2 to 6 years of age, and recurrent infection is generally less severe, except perhaps in the immunocompromised.[50] Finally, adenoviruses have been reported to cause up to 20% of pneumonias in children younger than age 5 years and the mortality rate attributable to the disease in this population has been reported as high as 20%.[55] In neonates, adenovirus can produce an especially severe syndrome of disseminated disease and sepsis, which can present in the first 10 days of life.[55] The incubation period is generally 2 to 14 days,[50] and the virus can produce a profound and destructive lower respiratory process. Necrotizing bronchitis, purulent exudative alveolitis, and hyaline membrane formation have been identified on autopsy specimens of affected patients.[55] Survivors of severe adenoviral infections commonly demonstrate chronic sequelae, such as recurrent wheezing and bronchiolitis obliterans.[55]

Most commonly, bacterial presence is established in the lower respiratory tract as a result of oropharyngeal overgrowth of environmentally acquired pathogens and subsequent introduction of these secretions into the lower airways. Children with aspiration syndromes, immunodeficiencies, and malformations of the respiratory tract are at increased risk of bacterial lower respiratory infection.[56] Bacterial pathogens remain an important cause of potentially lethal pediatric pneumonias in the developing world, and they are the most important cause of severe and complex pneumonia in Europe and North America.[49] It is challenging to establish a causal role for specific bacteria when these agents are normally found in the upper airway secretions, which are most commonly obtained for diagnosis in children. The best data regarding etiology comes from lung puncture studies, which reveal that *Streptococcus pneumoniae*, *Haemophilus influenzae*, and *Staphylococcus aureus* are among the important causes of bacterial pneumonia in children.[49] In neonates and young infants up to about 3 months of age, group B *Streptococcus* (GBS), *Listeria monocytogenes*, and gram-negative enteric organisms are the major causes of pneumonia and sepsis.[50,56] Widespread maternal intrapartum antibiotic prophylaxis has influenced the incidence of perinatal GBS infection as well as its antimicrobial resistance patterns.[57] Incidence of GBS sepsis has declined among very low birth weight infants in the era of ampicillin prophylaxis, whereas the incidence of *Escherichia coli* sepsis (largely resistant to ampicillin) has increased in the same time period.[57] Perinatally acquired *Chlamydia trachomatis* is another important cause of lower respiratory tract infection in infants up to age 12 weeks.[56] Although uncommon, periodic epidemics of infection with *Bordetella pertussis* occur among incompletely immunized infants and children.[56] Apnea and intermittent cyanosis, which frequently accompany acute *B. pertussis* infection in young children, may warrant intensive care.

Since the introduction of a conjugate vaccine against *H. influenzae* type B (Hib) in 1988, the incidence of invasive disease in infants and young children attributable to this organism has declined by 99%.[50] Other serotypes of the organism, including nonencapsulated strains, may also cause pneumonia.[50] In recent years, the heptavalent pneumococcal conjugate vaccine has also become available, which has made it possible to provide immunity to relevant strains of *S. pneumoniae* in infants and young children, a subset of the pediatric population most susceptible to infection with this organism. Children with congenital or acquired immunodeficiency syndromes, absent or deficient splenic function, as well as African Americans and some Native American populations may be especially susceptible to infection with encapsulated organisms and stand to benefit considerably from aggressive immunization efforts.[50]

Therapy

In the clinical arena one is often faced with having to select empirical antimicrobial therapy before definitive viral or bacterial diagnosis. The presence of a focal alveolar process on chest radiographs, especially if accompanied by significant parapneumonic effusion, evidence of parenchymal necrosis and/or abnormal peripheral blood cell counts, and C-reactive protein, adds considerably to the predictive value for the presence of bacterial disease.[49] Before demonstrating evidence of localized infection, neonates and young infants may demonstrate nonspecific but potentially ominous signs of lethargy, hypothermia, and apnea. Infants younger than 3 months of age should be treated with both ampicillin and

gentamicin, and consideration should be given to adding a third-generation cephalosporin in severe cases.[49] Investigation and empirical coverage for infection with *B. pertussis* should also be considered in infants with severe respiratory disease that features profound peripheral lymphocytosis, paroxysmal cough, and/or apnea.

For the critically ill child with community-acquired bacterial pneumonia, reasonable coverage may be obtained with a third-generation cephalosporin.[49,56] A macrolide agent can be added in cases in which infection with atypical agents such as *M. pneumoniae* and *Chlamydia pneumoniae* is possible, particularly in patients with sickle cell disease.[49,58] Although emerging resistance to penicillins in *S. pneumoniae* is well known, high doses of cephalosporins are still appropriate in the majority of nonsusceptible strains if meningitis is not also suspected, but the addition of vancomycin may be warranted in some cases.[49,59] If infection with *S. aureus* is possible, an antistaphylococcal penicillin such as oxacillin should be added, unless local resistance patterns warrant the use of vancomycin.[49] In patients at risk for aspiration pneumonia and in immunocompromised children, special consideration should be given to administration of two antibiotics effective against gram-negative organisms (e.g., *Pseudomonas*) and to optimizing coverage for anaerobic organisms.

Management of pleural effusion is another important consideration in the care of the patient with bacterial pneumonia. Although drainage of parapneumonic effusions is indicated under certain circumstances, satisfactory recovery may occur in many cases without intervention.[60] Recently, an evidence-based clinical practice guideline was developed for the medical and surgical treatment of parapneumonic effusions in adults.[61] The panel issued management suggestions according to the underlying risk of poor clinical outcome based on effusion size and loculation, as well as on microbiologic and chemical analysis of the pleural fluid.[61] Pleural fluid drainage was recommended for large effusions occupying more than 50% of the hemithorax, whether or not loculation or pleural thickening is present. Drainage was also recommended for purulent effusions, those with positive culture or Gram stain, or those with pH less than 7.20 as measured by a blood gas analyzer.[61] In situations in which drainage is indicated, more complex or invasive options such as thoracoscopic or "open" procedures are likely to be necessary for sufficient control of the effusion.[61] Although much has been published on the management of parapneumonic effusion, there are few randomized, controlled trials in adult patients. It must be emphasized that the consensus panel's recommendations are based primarily on case series, historical controls, and expert opinion.[61]

The literature on parapneumonic effusion in children also does not presently provide robust evidence on which to base clinical intervention. The data do suggest that *S. pneumoniae* is a very important cause of pediatric pneumonia that is complicated by necrosis and/or effusion. In a recent review of 368 hospitalized children with pneumococcal pneumonia, there was an increased incidence of complications associated with the disease over the 6.5-year course of the study, and pneumococcal serotypes associated with these events tended to be ones not covered by the conjugate vaccine.[62] The effect of image-guided needle aspiration versus percutaneous pigtail catheter drainage was also examined in a 5-year retrospective study of pediatric parapneumonic effusions.[63] When comparing outcomes in the two groups, the authors found no difference in length of stay but did report a significant decrease in the need for second intervention in patients who received a chest drain.[63] Other independent predictors for second intervention in their study population included loculation of pleural fluid and pH less than 7.2. A combination of low glucose and low pH in the pleural fluid specimen was especially predictive of the need for re-intervention.[63]

The decision to perform thoracostomy drainage in pediatric patients with parapneumonic effusion may depend on the clinical context in which it occurs. In a small series of children with necrotizing pneumonia or lung abscess, bronchopleural fistula was associated with placement of chest drains in five of nine patients with necrotizing pneumonia,[64] whereas clinical experience with this disease in children suggests that complete resolution often takes place without the need for invasive procedures.[64,65] Other potentially promising therapies in children with parapneumonic effusions include video-assisted thoracic surgery (VATS)[66] and intrapleural thrombolysis.[67]

In summary, it is certainly important to drain large parapneumonic effusions when they are suspected of causing hemodynamic instability in the critically ill child. Pleural drainage may also be useful to relieve respiratory embarrassment that may contribute to respiratory failure or ongoing ventilator dependence. The best opportunity to achieve sufficient drainage is probably in the first 48 to 72 hours of disease, before organization of the effusion begins to take place. A randomized, controlled trial is necessary to resolve the issue of which pediatric patients with parapneumonic effusion would benefit from aggressive pleural drainage.

ACUTE RESPIRATORY DISTRESS SYNDROME

What was once known as the adult respiratory distress syndrome is now called the acute respiratory distress syndrome (ARDS) in an effort to acknowledge its prevalence in the pediatric population. A syndrome of lung injury featuring exudative pulmonary edema that leads to hypoxic respiratory failure had been described in adults for many years, but consensus criteria for the diagnosis of the syndrome did not enter the scientific literature until 1994. Acute lung injury, which often precedes ARDS, may arise as a consequence of primary pulmonary disease or as a feature of systemic pathophysiology that is nonpulmonary in origin. The incidence of the syndrome in children is believed to be similar to that in adults, and pediatric ARDS most commonly occurs in the setting of sepsis.[68] Among patients with the sepsis syndrome who go on to develop ARDS, the most frequent primary sources of infection are the bloodstream and the abdomen.[68] Pneumonia arising from infectious causes and noninfectious causes (e.g., aspiration events and thermal injury) as well as head trauma, chest trauma, and post-resuscitation syndromes are other important causes of ARDS in children.[68-71] On the basis of a series of small studies, mortality rate in pediatric ARDS averages 52% and has been reported to range from 28.5% to 90%.[68,71] Although consensus diagnostic criteria have been derived for adults,[72] accurate mortality prediction in the pediatric population remains problematic. At present, there are several multicenter efforts designed to investigate therapeutic interventions in pediatric ARDS, including prone positioning and surfactant administration. At this time, these trials have not been completed and preliminary results have not been published.

MECHANICAL VENTILATION

Mechanical ventilatory support of the patient with acute lung injury and ARDS is often necessary to provide adequate oxygenation. In relatively stable patients, noninvasive ventilation may be effective when instituted early in the disease process. This method has been used with success in the management of alveolar disease in immunocompromised adult patients and reduced rates of intubation and mortality.[73] Data on the use of noninvasive positive-pressure ventilation in pediatric patients are limited, but several case series report success with the application of this technique in children with alveolar disease.[74-76] In a recent investigation, noninvasive bilevel positive airway pressure was used to support pediatric patients with pneumonia, acute chest syndrome and sickle-cell disease, underlying chronic hypoventilation syndromes, and postoperative hypoventilation with atelectasis.[76] The authors report favorable changes in respiratory rate, heart rate, and oxygenation among all patients receiving noninvasive support, and 91% of respiratory failure episodes in their study were reversed without the need for intubation.[76]

When noninvasive techniques are not appropriate or have failed, endotracheal intubation is warranted. It has been well established in a number of animal and human studies that ventilatory strategy may have a profound influence on the course of disease and ultimately on clinical outcome.[77-81] In pediatric ARDS, in which duration of mechanical ventilation may commonly exceed 3 weeks,[68] it is especially important to maximize lung protective ventilatory strategies. Lung protective ventilation involves (1) preservation of end-expiratory lung volume by judicious use of PEEP and/or recruitment maneuvers to minimize atelectrauma; (2) minimization of cyclic stretch; and (3) avoidance of parenchymal overdistention at end inspiration by limiting tidal volume and transpulmonary pressure.[77-81]

When oxygenation failure is refractory to conventional ventilation, high-frequency oscillatory ventilation (HFOV) is a modality that is well established in the pediatric population. During HFOV, lung recruitment is maintained by application of a relatively high mean airway pressure with superimposed pressure oscillations at a frequency of 3 to 15 Hz.[80] Because maximal recruitment is maintained throughout the respiratory cycle and ventilation is achieved using very small phasic changes in pressure and volume, this technique allows the lung to be ventilated above the critical opening pressure of injured lung units while avoiding end-inspiratory overdistention of more compliant lung units (Fig. 89-2).[44,82,83] Such an "open lung" strategy of mechanical ventilation can capitalize on pulmonary hysteresis to achieve satisfactory gas exchange at lower alveolar pressures (Fig. 89-3). In 1994, a prospective multicenter, randomized clinical study compared HFOV and conventional mechanical ventilation in pediatric patients with diffuse alveolar disease or air leak syndromes.[84] Patients in the HFOV arm showed rapid and sustained improvements in oxygenation without suffering adverse effects on ventilation.[84] Ultimately these patients showed a decrease in barotrauma as evidenced by a decreased need for supplemental oxygen at 30 days and demonstrated improved outcomes compared with their cohorts in the conventional arm, particularly when HFOV was instituted within 72 hours of intubation.[84] The "oxygenation index" (OI), defined as $(MAP \times FIO_2 \times 100)/PaO_2$, used often in the pediatric literature to quantify oxygenation

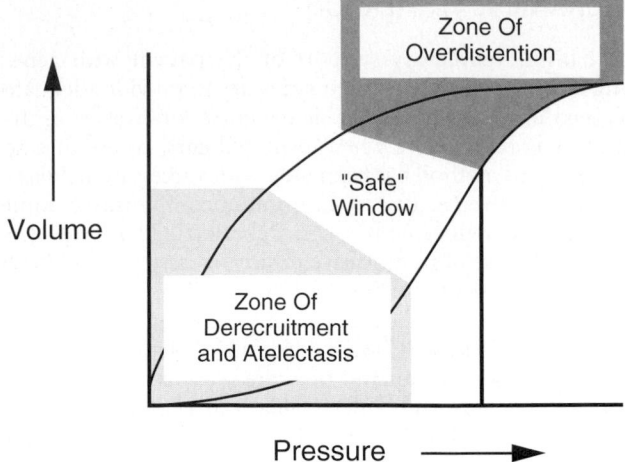

FIGURE 89–2. Pressure-volume relationships in acute lung injury. High end-expiratory pressures and small tidal volumes minimize the potential for derecruitment *(lower left)* and overdistention *(upper right).* (From Froese AB: High-frequency oscillatory ventilation for adult respiratory distress syndrome: Let's get it right this time! Crit Care Med 1997;25:906-908.)

failure, was shown to discriminate between survivors and nonsurvivors in the first 72 hours of therapy.[84] Furthermore, the time at which changes in the OI were found to occur seemed to influence the likelihood of survival: an OI = 42 at 24 hours predicted mortality with an odds ratio of 20.8, a sensitivity of 62%, and a specificity of 93%.[84] The OI may prove to be a time-sensitive predictor of survival in patients with hypoxic respiratory failure. Such an indicator would facilitate development of a stepwise approach to the mechanical support of these patients.[85]

Inhaled nitric oxide (iNO) has been credited with significantly decreasing the need for extracorporeal membrane oxygenation (ECMO) in neonates with hypoxic respiratory failure, especially when used in combination with HFOV in patients who have failed either therapy alone.[86,87] The idea that improved pulmonary recruitment offered by HFOV might enhance the effect of iNO seems to be applicable to older children as well.[88] However, as has been well established in a number of adult studies,[89-91] iNO produces short-term physiologic improvements in oxygenation without sustained clinical benefit or improvement in outcome in pediatric patients.[88,92,93] Risk of rebound pulmonary hypertension and profound deterioration of oxygenating efficiency after abrupt discontinuation of iNO warrants careful weaning of the dose when the drug is used in managing the neonate with pulmonary hypertension.[94]

DISEASES OF THE INTERSTITIUM

The interstitial lung diseases (ILD) in children are a diverse group of rare conditions that involve alteration of the alveolar wall, infiltration and fibrosis of the pulmonary interstitium, and loss of functional alveolar-capillary units.[95] The major clinical findings include abnormal gas exchange and both restrictive and obstructive pulmonary physiology. There are numerous potential causes, ranging from primary congenital abnormalities of the alveolar-capillary unit that present in early infancy to acquired syndromes of chronic interstitial disease referable to infection, recurrent aspiration, or symptomatic cardiovascular disease (Table 89-3).[95] In children, as

in adults, the morbidity and mortality of these diseases are high[96,97] but the frequency distribution of specific causes may be very different in the two populations. For example, a recent descriptive, prospective evaluation of 51 pediatric patients with ILD reported no cases of idiopathic pulmonary fibrosis or desquamative interstitial pneumonitis (DIP), and only one case of lymphocytic interstitial pneumonitis (LIP).[96] The rarity of these conditions among pediatric patients has been previously described.[97] Usual interstitial pneumonitis (UIP) is believed to be particularly rare in children.[98] In contrast, infectious causes may be much more common in the pediatric population, accounting for perhaps 20% of pediatric ILD in some series.[95,96] Given the wide variety of potential causes in ILD, a systematic approach to the diagnostic workup has been suggested.[96] Although history and physical examination may not be helpful in the majority of instances, noninvasive tests such as serologic studies, cultures, chest radiographs, chest computed tomography, barium swallow, pH studies, and echocardiograms will more often allow the clinician to arrive at a specific diagnosis.[96] In those children in whom an etiology still cannot be determined, invasive testing such as bronchoalveolar lavage, cardiac catheterization, and lung biopsy should be considered.[96] Results of biopsy specimens may be particularly important to guide decision making in critically ill children who are not responding to therapy.

Therapy

Because many of the causes for pediatric ILD may begin with an inflammatory response to lung injury, treatment of children with this condition commonly involves the use of anti-inflammatory agents such as corticosteroids. A favorable response to corticosteroids among children with ILD may be evident in only 40% of cases,[99] and this variability may reflect the diverse potential causes of the disease. Because of its anti-inflammatory properties, hydroxychloroquine has also been used in the management of pediatric ILD but it is associated with the development of hepatic toxicity and retinopathy in children who receive it.[99] Ultimately, identifying and controlling underlying causes and contributing issues are very important, when this is possible.

COMPLEX PARENCHYMAL DISEASES

BRONCHOPULMONARY DYSPLASIA

Bronchopulmonary dysplasia is a term that describes histopathologic changes in the lungs of infants who require mechanical ventilation in the neonatal period and who demonstrate radiologic abnormalities and supplemental oxygen dependence at 28 days of life.[100] These changes include heterogeneous alveolar consolidation, squamous metaplasia of airway epithelium, hyperplasia of mucous glands, peribronchial fibrosis, airway smooth muscle hypertrophy, and vascular lesions of pulmonary hypertension.[101,102] Clinically, the syndrome is associated with airway hyperreactivity and intermittent obstruction, leading to increased work of breathing, recurrent wheezing, chronic abnormalities of gas exchange, and pulmonary hypertension in some cases.[102] Focal airway collapse consistent with tracheomalacia and/or bronchomalacia (see Table 89-1) has also been documented in these infants,[103] and their pathogenesis in this context is not known. BPD is most likely to develop in premature infants with birth weight less than 1000 g.[101,102] These infants

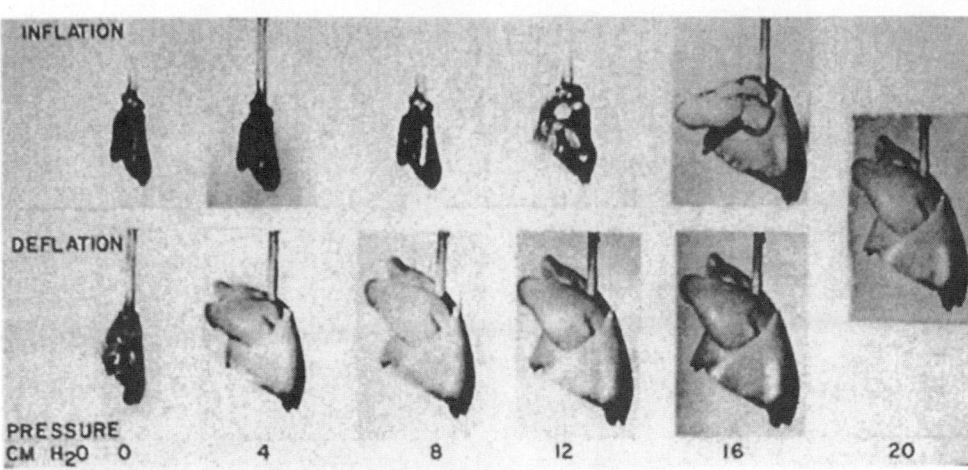

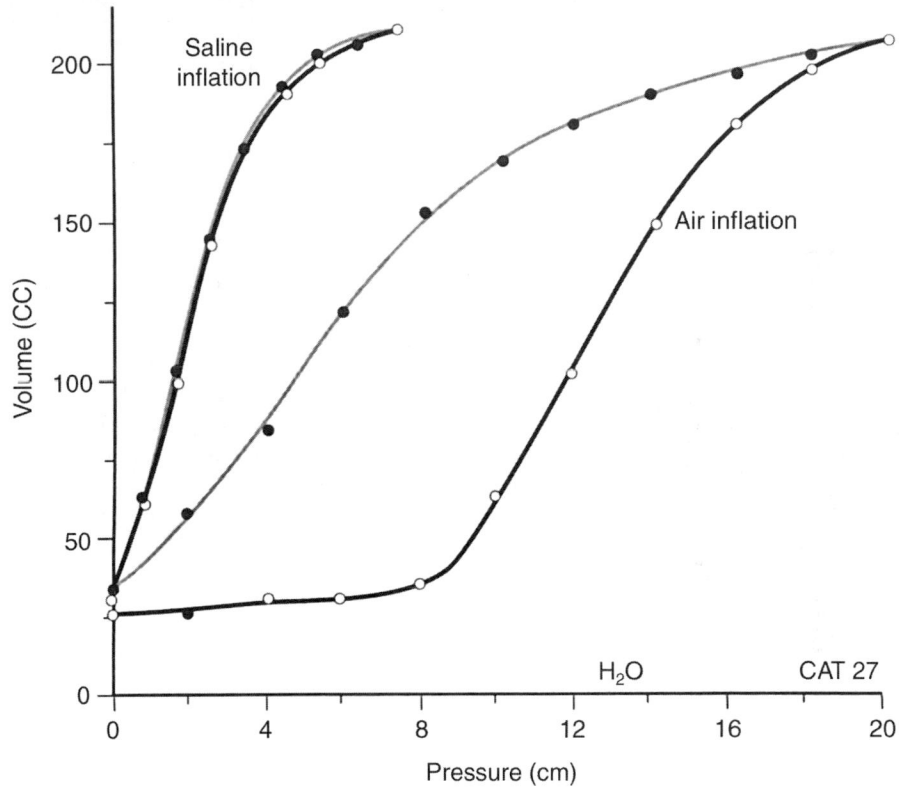

FIGURE 89–3. Static hysteresis. Pulmonary volume-pressure curve obtained by air inflation of excised cat lungs. As pressure is increased above 8 cm H_2O, volume recruitment occurs up to approximately 20 cm H_2O. During deflation (expiration), higher lung volumes are maintained at lower corresponding pressures. (Modified from Radford E: Static mechanical properties of mammalian lungs. In Fenn W, Rahn H [eds]: Handbook of Physiology: A Critical, Comprehensive Presentation of Physiological Knowledge and Concepts. Washington, DC, American Physiological Society, 1964, vol I, pp 434-435.)

may be born at a gestational age (24 to 26 weeks) at which alveolar development is not yet complete, so lung injury acquired at this time can result in structural derangement of the alveoli as well as enduring alveolar hypoplasia.[101]

The spectrum of pathology is believed to derive from an inflammatory response to lung injury, because numerous investigations have identified mediators of inflammation in the BAL fluid of infants with chronic lung disease.[104] The present understanding of the pathogenesis of lung injury in the neonate mirrors what has been learned from laboratory and clinical investigations of this process in adults. Neonates and young infants with respiratory failure, however, may be especially susceptible to ventilator-associated lung injury because surfactant deficiency, high chest wall compliance, and a dynamic functional residual capacity that is near closing capacity in this age group may potentiate a cycle of de-recruitment and re-inflation, which has been shown to promote lung injury in animal models and humans (including surfactant-deficient preterm animals).[77-79,105,106] Mechanical ventilatory techniques targeted to promote alveolar

recruitment and maintain lung volume have in fact decreased the incidence of ventilator-associated lung injury in neonates. Numerous large prospective, randomized, controlled trials have found favorable outcomes among high-risk infants supported with HFOV compared with cohorts who are supported with conventional phasic ventilation, with no apparent increase in the development of intracranial hemorrhage or other significant morbidities.[107-109]

Pulmonary edema from cardiogenic and noncardiogenic causes, infectious issues, and exposure to high concentrations of supplemental oxygen are other factors important in the pathogenesis of BPD. Premature infants may be at special risk from exposure to high concentrations of supplemental oxygen because they are deficient in antiproteases and antioxidant enzymes, which are necessary to limit lung injury from reactive oxygen species.[100] Improvements in neonatal supportive care, including the availability of surfactant therapy, have dramatically improved survival rates among premature infants, but chronic lung disease among survivors of prematurity remains an important clinical issue.[100]

TABLE 89–3. CAUSES OF INTERSTITIAL LUNG DISEASE IN PEDIATRICS

Known Etiology

Infection
    Viral
    Bacterial
    Fungal
    Parasitic
    Opportunistic
Bronchopulmonary dysplasia
Environmental/drug exposure
Lipid storage diseases
Aspiration syndromes
    Gastroesophageal reflux
    Swallowing disorders

Unknown Etiology

Usual interstitial pneumonitis
Desquamative interstitial pneumonitis
Lymphocytic interstitial pneumonitis
Pulmonary hemosiderosis
Pulmonary infiltrates with eosinophilia
Pulmonary vascular disorders
    Alveolar capillary dysplasia
    Hemangiomatosis
    Veno-occlusive disease
    Telangiectasia
    Lymphangiomatosis
    Lymphangiectasis
Bronchiolitis obliterans
Bronchiolitis obliterans with organizing pneumonia
Surfactant protein deficiency
Cellular interstitial pneumonitis

Etiologies Associated with Systemic Disease

Connective tissue disorders
Histiocytosis X
Metastatic malignancy
Neurocutaneous syndromes
Sarcoidosis

Adapted from Howenstine MS, Eigen H: Current concepts on interstitial lung disease in children. Curr Opin Pediatr 1999;11:200-204 and Fan LL, Langston C: Chronic interstitial lung disease in children. Pediatr Pulmonol 1993;16:184-196.

Therapy

Lower respiratory tract infection is one of the most common reasons for hospital readmission in the first year of life for infants with BPD and accounts for a significant fraction of these pulmonary exacerbations.[101] Other potential causes include aspiration syndromes, worsening pulmonary hypertension, and the evolution of clinically important systemic-to-pulmonary collateral vessels.[102] Therefore, the diagnostic approach to the infant with BPD who demonstrates unexplained deterioration may include dynamic airway studies as well as echocardiography and, in certain cases, cardiac catheterization.[102] Treatment of these episodes is supportive and often includes empirical antibiotic coverage for potential infectious causes. Among the medications that may be useful in producing short-term improvements in pulmonary mechanics are bronchodilators, corticosteroids, and diuretics (Table 89-4).[100,102,110] Aerosolized beta agonists may be useful in the management of smooth muscle–mediated bronchospasm in the infant with chronic lung disease, but the consequent decrease in airway smooth muscle tone may aggravate airway collapse in the infant with tracheomalacia or bronchomalacia.[103] Diuretics may be especially helpful in the management of these infants because many demonstrate

TABLE 89–4. PHARMACOTHERAPIES COMMONLY USED IN MANAGEMENT OF INFANTS WITH BRONCHOPULMONARY DYSPLASIA

Inhaled Therapies

Albuterol (0.5%), 0.15 mg/kg/dose inhaled q1-6h prn. Continuous
    nebulization 0.5 mg/kg/h
Ipratropium, 0.25-0.5 mg/dose inhaled q4-6h
Fluticasone, 44-88 μg bid (maintenance therapy) (max: 440 μg/day)

Diuretic Therapies

Furosemide, 1-2 mg/kg/dose i.v./p.o q6h
Chlorothiazide, 10-20 mg/kg/day i.v. divided q12h (max 1000 mg/day)
    < 6 months: 20-40 mg/kg/day p.o. divided q12h
    ≥ 6 months: 20 mg/kg/day p.o. divided q12h
Spironolactone, 1.5 mg/kg/dose p.o. q12h

Gastrointestinal Therapies

Metoclopramide, 0.1-0.2 mg/kg/dose i.v./p.o. q6h (max: 10 mg/dose)
Ranitidine, 1 mg/kg/dose i.v. q8h; 2-3 mg/kg/dose p.o. q12h

a tendency to accumulate fluid in the pulmonary interstitium on the basis of alterations in pulmonary vascular resistance, plasma oncotic pressure, and capillary permeability, as well as impaired lymphatic drainage.[104] Judicious use of diuretics can also facilitate the delivery of adequate nutrition to the infant with chronic lung disease.[104] iNO has also been studied for its potential role in treating refractory hypoxemia in infants with chronic lung disease. Case series have documented improvements in oxygenation with the use of iNO, including in infants with intercurrent infection, with a sustained response reported in some cases.[111,112]

CONGENITAL DIAPHRAGMATIC HERNIA

Management of the infant with CDH is one of the greatest clinical challenges that the intensive care clinician encounters. The Bochdalek hernia is the most severe form and occurs when herniation of abdominal contents occurs into the thoracic cavity through a posterolateral diaphragmatic defect, usually at around the 10th week of gestation. This phase of gestation concurrently includes the branching of bronchi and pulmonary arteries, and this crucial process may be interrupted by the growing mass of herniated viscera.[113] On the other hand, the discovery that administering the teratogen nitrogen to rats in mid-gestation results in diaphragmatic defects in the developing fetus as well as a spectrum of anomalies in other organ systems similar to that seen in humans with CDH suggests that the pathogenesis of this syndrome may originate from fetal exposure to an agent that causes generalized maldevelopment from that point forward.[114-117] The complex pathology associated with CDH in humans includes a hypoplastic and abnormally muscularized pulmonary arterial tree.[113] Other congenital anomalies are associated with CDH in up to 39% of cases. Congenital cardiac disease is the most commonly associated feature and most frequently involves some degree of cardiac hypoplasia, although a wide variety of structural cardiac anomalies may be associated with CDH.[118] Genitourinary, gastrointestinal, neurologic, and skeletal defects are also commonly described.[113] Adjunctive medical therapies have not managed to improve the dismal survival statistics of these infants, whose mortality rate is traditionally reported in the range of 50%. Nonetheless, there are experienced centers that have

TABLE 89-5. THERAPEUTIC HISTORY AND OUTCOMES FOR CONGENITAL DIAPHRAGMATIC HERNIA, CHIILDREN'S HOSPITAL, BOSTON

	1981-1984	1984-1987	1987-1991	1991-1994	P Value
ECMO	N/A	Postop	Preop	Preop	
Surgery	Immediate	Immediate	Delayed	Delayed	
Ventilation	Hyper	Hyper	Hyper	Permissive hypercapnia	
Paralysis	Yes	Yes	Yes	No	
Analgesia	High-dose fentanyl	High-dose fentanyl	High-dose fentanyl	Epidural	
Monitoring	Postductal	Postductal	Postductal	Preductal	
Survival, Isolated CDH					
ECMO	N/A	50%	48%	71%	NS
CMV	73%	67%	80%	100%	0.02
Overall	73%	61%	57%	84%	0.02

CMV, conventional mechanical ventilation.
From Wilson JM, Lund DP, Lillehei CW, Vacanti JP: Congenital diaphragmatic hernia—a tale of two cities: The Boston experience. J Pediatr Surg 1997;32:401-405.

reported encouraging results in recent years by adopting strategic forms of mechanical support in these patients that incorporate much of what has been learned about minimizing pulmonary and hemodynamic consequences of mechanical ventilation.

Therapy

In infants with CDH, as in those with BPD, intensive care management targets lower airways disease, alveolar disease, and pulmonary vascular dysfunction. Initial medical stabilization of the infant with CDH includes endotracheal intubation and nasogastric decompression. It is preferable to obtain preductal (i.e., right radial) arterial access, when possible. Information from preductal blood gases should guide clinical intervention because it reflects the oxygenation, ventilation, and acid-base status of the cerebral circulation. Initially, echocardiography is suggested to rule out structural cardiac disease, and it may be repeated as necessary throughout the clinical course to determine evidence of ongoing right-to-left shunting as well as estimates of right ventricular pressure and function in response to therapy.[113] iNO has been used in infants with CDH with varying results, and a role for the drug in reducing the need for ECMO or in improving survival among these patients was not established by a large, randomized controlled trial on the use of iNO in neonates with pulmonary hypertension.[119] In general, data supporting the use of iNO in the management of infants with CDH is limited to small case series and individual case studies.[120-122] In CDH, as in BPD, deficient alveolar development may explain the limited potential benefit from iNO.[112] Finally, recommendations for the optimal timing of surgical repair in these infants have evolved over time. It was once considered appropriate to refer infants with CDH for immediate repair. Growing experience with the mechanical support of these patients, along with the observation that pulmonary vascular resistance and reactivity as well as pulmonary compliance could become more favorable for successful repair within days after birth, have since favored delaying surgical repair until a satisfactory level of stability can be achieved.[113,123]

MECHANICAL VENTILATION

Given what is presently known about ventilator-associated lung injury, it is logical to apply lung protective ventilation strategies to infants with chronic lung disease as well as to infants with CDH. Although the technique has not been traditionally applied to neonates, permissive hypercapnia is, in

fact, well tolerated by most infants.[124-126] Because of the heterogeneity of airspace involvement in these diseases, regional hyperinflation can easily occur. Therefore, it makes sense to maintain end-expiratory lung volume with a careful titration of PEEP and limit tidal volume to 4 to 6 mL/kg to ventilate at the area of maximal compliance on the pressure-volume curve.[127] While managing these patients, monitoring of tidal volume at the endotracheal tube is important because compressible volume losses in the ventilator circuit can be significant. Judicious use of sedation and the use of spontaneous ventilation (e.g., flow-triggered pressure support) may improve matching of ventilation to perfusion and may allow optimal patient-ventilator synchrony.

A review of all infants with CDH managed at Children's Hospital in Boston revealed a significant increase in survival from 44% to 69% during the period in which permissive hypercapnia was used to manage these infants, with even higher survival rates noted in infants without coexisting heart disease (Table 89-5).[128] Of note, neither the introduction of ECMO nor delaying surgical repair was associated with significant increases in survival in this single-center historical experience.[128] Other case series have also reported favorable results using "kinder, gentler" ventilatory strategies, rather than more aggressive techniques that attempt to control pulmonary vascular resistance.[123,129,130] These observations suggest that ventilator-associated lung injury may greatly contribute to excess mortality in infants with CDH,[123,128] and it is possible that a survival benefit attributable to ECMO may emerge as lung-sparing mechanical ventilation is more widely applied.[128] At least one single-center experience suggests that epidural analgesia in the postoperative period maximizes spontaneous ventilation and may further improve pulmonary outcomes in these infants.[128] In some infants with CDH who develop refractory hypoxemia and hypercarbia, one center has reported successful use of high-frequency oscillatory ventilation.[123]

WEANING THE PEDIATRIC PATIENT FROM MECHANICAL VENTILATION

Although it is clear that it is best to discontinue mechanical ventilatory support as soon as this is feasible, a great deal of controversy surrounds ventilator mode selection, the pace of weaning, and timing of separation from mechanical support in children. In the largest pediatric study presently available in the literature, the use of specific weaning modes and ventilator weaning protocols was evaluated against standard care (no defined protocol) for mechanically ventilated infants and children.[131] Patients with alveolar disease as well as lower airways disease were included, whereas those older than 2 years of age with status asthmaticus and those with CDH were excluded. In this study, 182 intubated, spontaneously breathing children who met standardized bedside criteria for extubation readiness were randomized to application of pressure support ventilation (PSV), volume support ventilation (VSV), or no protocol.[131] There were no significant differences among the three treatment groups in extubation failure rates, and most children were weaned from the ventilator in 2 days or less.[131] In children who were successfully extubated, the median duration of ventilator weaning did not significantly differ according to mode of ventilation.[131]

Separating the infant or child with complex and/or chronic pulmonary disease from mechanical ventilation is challenging and requires an appreciation of the components of pulmonary dysfunction and timely recognition of acceptable mechanics and gas exchange in the spontaneously breathing patient. For example, the patient with a syndrome of alveolar hypoplasia is expected to be tachypneic at baseline, and this feature precludes the use of commonly applied criteria for extubation readiness. In these cases, weaning from mechanical ventilation can be guided by an ongoing assessment of tidal volume (measured at the endotracheal tube), work of breathing, serum pH, and evidence of appropriate daily weight gain as pressure support is decreased.

CONCLUSION

A fundamental understanding of age-specific diagnostic and treatment considerations is required when caring for the pediatric patient with pulmonary disease. Although the capacity for physiologic compensation in infants and children is remarkably efficient, these individuals are also prone to sudden and profound clinical deterioration, warranting the application of sophisticated supportive measures in the ICU. In recent years, work in the laboratory as well as the clinical arena has brought about an appreciation that in airways disease, alveolar disease, and complex conditions such as BPD and CDH, gentler strategies of mechanical ventilation may have a central role in improving functional outcomes. Thoughtful application of therapies proven to reverse pulmonary pathophysiology while promoting spontaneous ventilation as much as possible is likely to enhance already favorable survival statistics for even the most critically ill pediatric patients.

ANNOTATED REFERENCES

Arnold JH, Hanson JH, Toro-Figuero LO, et al: Prospective, randomized comparison of high-frequency oscillatory ventilation and conventional mechanical ventilation in pediatric respiratory failure. Crit Care Med 1994;22:1530-1539.

This prospective, multicenter, crossover trial showed that high-frequency oscillatory ventilation produced rapid and sustained improvements in oxygenation and decreased need for supplemental oxygen at 30 days when used to support pediatric patients with diffuse alveolar disease or air leak.

Courtney SE, Durand DJ, Asselin JM, et al: High-frequency oscillatory ventilation versus conventional mechanical ventilation for very-low-birth-weight infants. N Engl J Med 2002;347:643-652.

Large multicenter, well-controlled trial demonstrating significant benefit of high-frequency oscillatory ventilation compared to conventional ventilation in very low birth weight infants. Infants who received high-frequency oscillatory ventilation were successfully extubated earlier and were more likely to survive without need for supplemental oxygen at 36 weeks post menstrual age. No increase was observed in the occurrence of intracranial hemorrhage or other complications referable to prematurity.

Inhaled nitric oxide and hypoxic respiratory failure in infants with congenital diaphragmatic hernia. The Neonatal Inhaled Nitric Oxide Study Group (NINOS). Pediatrics 1997;99:838-845.

Multicenter trial in which infants with isolated congenital diaphragmatic hernia and hypoxic respiratory failure were randomized to receive inhaled nitric oxide or 100% oxygen. The study was unable to show a survival benefit or reduction in need for extracorporeal membrane oxygenation among those infants who received nitric oxide.

Randolph AG, Wypij D, Venkataraman ST, et al: Effect of mechanical ventilator weaning protocols on respiratory outcomes in infants and children: A randomized controlled trial. JAMA 2002;288:2561-2568.

Large multicenter trial that evaluated standardized ventilator weaning protocols versus no defined protocol in pediatric patients mechanically ventilated for acute illness. Most of the study population was successfully weaned from the ventilator in 48 hours or less. Use of protocols for the gradual weaning of mechanical ventilatory support had no impact on the duration of mechanical ventilation.

Ventilation with lower tidal volumes as compared with traditional tidal volumes for acute lung injury and the acute respiratory distress syndrome. The Acute Respiratory Distress Syndrome Network. N Engl J Med 2000;342:1301-1308.

Landmark multicenter trial showing that in adult patients with acute lung injury and ARDS ($PaO_2/FiO_2 = 300$), mechanical ventilation limiting tidal volumes to 6 mL/kg ideal body weight and plateau pressure = 30 cm H_2O results in decreased mortality and more ventilator-free days when compared with tidal volumes of 12 mL/kg ideal body weight and plateau pressure = 50 cm H_2O.

Chapter 90
PULMONARY EDEMA

Gad Cotter • Edo Kaluski • Zvi Vered

KEY POINTS

1. Under normal circumstances the **alveolar space is maintained free of fluids** mainly due to an active process of fluid clearances mediated by active Na$^+$ transport of the type II endothelial cells. Therefore, fluid can accumulate in the alveolar space when transudated at an increased rate, either due to physical pressure in-balance (significant increase in pulmonary capillary pressure or rapid shifts in thoracic pressure) or due to increased permeability of the capillary-alveolar barrier.

2. The **diagnosis of pulmonary edema** is based on presentation with acute respiratory distress accompanied by physical findings of diffuse "wet" rales over the lung fields that are most prominent on the bases and decreased peripheral perfusion associated with typical findings on chest radiography.

3. **Pulmonary edema can be divided into cardiovascular- and noncardiovascular-based types mostly on clinical grounds.** However, cardiovascular pulmonary edema is commonly associated with abnormal electrocardiographic findings, large cardiac silhouette on chest radiography, increased plasma levels of brain natriuretic peptide, abnormal echocardiographic findings, and high pulmonary capillary wedge pressure.

4. The **most common type of noncardiovascular pulmonary edema is ARDS,** the final common pathway for many injuries affecting the lung (e.g., infection, shock, and toxic damage).

5. Other causes of noncardiovascular pulmonary edema (postoperative, pregnancy related) are caused by **excessive administration of fluids and large fluid shifts** leading to abrupt increase in wedge pressure, although in other cases inflammatory damage to the alveolar capillary membrane (transfusion-associated pulmonary edema) as well as increased peripheral resistance (neurogenic pulmonary edema) play a pivotal role.

6. This syndrome is caused by a combination of **decreased myocardial contractility** (mostly caused by ischemic damage, valvular diseases, cardiomyopathy, or arrhythmias) combined with **increased systemic vascular resistance** caused by undetermined inflammatory-endothelial activation, leading

to a vicious cycle of decreased systemic oxygenation and perfusion, begetting respiratory failure, multi-organ failure, and death.

7. Although only examined in a few studies, reduced oxygen saturation, very high or very low blood pressure, high pulse rate and respiratory rate, and reduced myocardial contractility, evidenced by an increased wedge pressure on right-sided heart catheterization, seem to be **negative early prognostic signs** in patients admitted with pulmonary edema.

8. The **most important step in the treatment of pulmonary edema is the initial stabilization,** which can be achieved by improving systemic oxygenation (high-flow facemask and maybe noninvasive ventilation), administration of nitrovasodilators to patients with systolic blood pressure greater than 120 mm Hg, administration of small doses of furosemide and morphine, arrhythmia control, and mechanical ventilation to nonresponders.

9. Although no firm data exist on effective measures to prevent recurrence, early revascularization in patients with significant acute ischemia and surgical correction of severe valvular lesions are warranted. In the future, new drugs that increase left ventricular contractility without increasing oxygen demand and arrhythmias as well as neurohormonal inflammatory modulators may play a pivotal role in prevention of recurrence.

DEFINITION

Pulmonary edema is a life-threatening syndrome caused by accumulation of fluid within the alveoli leading to disruption of the normal gas exchange process, severe hypoxemia, failure of tissue oxygenation, acidosis, and widespread organ failure; if untreated, it rapidly progresses to death.

PHYSIOLOGIC BACKGROUND

Under normal circumstances the alveolar space is kept free of fluids by an active process of sodium (Na$^+$) and perhaps chloride (Cl$^-$) transport. Fluid is regularly transudated from the pulmonary capillaries through the thin gas exchange apparatus, composed of the capillary endothelial and type 1 alveolar cells, into the alveoli. This process is slowed considerably owing to the tight gap junctions existing between the cells that reduce potential fluid transudation. Some fluid, however, escapes these mechanisms and reaches the alveoli. In the past the common paradigm suggested that this fluid is removed from the alveoli by a simple oncotic pressure gradient. However, 20 years ago Matthay and coworkers[1] demonstrated that alveolar fluid clearance is not affected by the Starling forces but is rather an active process. Na^+ from the alveolar fluid enters the type II alveolar cells through amiloride-sensitive channels as well as cotransport with glucose, H^+, amino acids, phosphorus, and other yet undefined mechanisms and then is extruded at the basal side of the cells by an active process mostly (>90%) controlled by the Na^+,K^+-ATPase. The fluid follows the Na^+ by a simple osmotic mechanism, which is at least partially mediated by aquaporins.[2] Furthermore, some fluid reabsorption occurs also in the airways, although in these regions active Cl^- reabsorption probably plays a role in the overall fluid clearance.[3]

Therefore, fluid can accumulate in the alveolar space only when this protective mechanism fails. This can occur when fluid is transudated into the alveolar space at an increased rate, overwhelming the active reabsorption mechanism, or when active fluid clearance mechanisms become less effective (Fig. 90-1). Increased fluid transudation can be related either to physical pressures in-balance (significant increase in pulmonary capillary pressure or rapid shifts in thoracic pressure) or to increased permeability of the capillary-alveolar barrier.

DIAGNOSIS

Although the clinical syndrome of pulmonary edema might differ slightly because of its diverse etiologic factors, the diagnosis of pulmonary edema is, in most cases, rather easy to make if the clinician is experienced.[4] Patients usually present with acute severe respiratory distress. On inspection the patient is anxious, sometimes cyanotic, tachypneic, diaphoretic, and dyspneic and is sitting up and gasping for air and using accessory respiratory muscles to assist in the work of breathing. The patient often coughs up a pink frothy fluid. On examination the patient's extremities are cold, pale, and sweaty. On auscultation, symmetrical diffuse "wet" rales are heard over the lung fields that are most prominent in the bases.

The most useful ancillary test to establish the presence of pulmonary edema is the chest radiograph (Fig. 90-2).[5] In addition to the milder signs of pulmonary congestion such as "cephalization," that is, redistribution of the blood flow to the upper lung fields, and Kerley-B lines, one may observe predominant interstitial lines, reflecting pulmonary interstitial edema and diffuse small nodular opacities that progressively coalesce in the inner two thirds of the lung field producing the "butterfly" appearance. Differentiation between cardiovascular and noncardiovascular pulmonary edema based on the chest radiographic findings may be difficult. However, increased cardiac silhouette, widened pulmonary arteries, and central distribution of the pulmonary blood flow usually direct toward a cardiovascular etiology.

The differentiation between cardiovascular and noncardiovascular pulmonary edema is mostly based on the clinical circumstances. Patients presenting to the emergency department with acute pulmonary edema usually have cardiovascular pulmonary edema, especially when accompanied by a history of heart failure, valvular or ischemic heart disease in the presence of harsh cardiac murmurs, abnormal electrocardiogram, or a large cardiac silhouette on a chest radiograph. Recently, the measurement of brain natriuretic peptide (BNP) has become a useful immediate ancillary tool for the diagnosis of cardiovascular pulmonary edema. Noncardiovascular pulmonary edema occurs almost exclusively in typical clinical settings, commonly as a complication

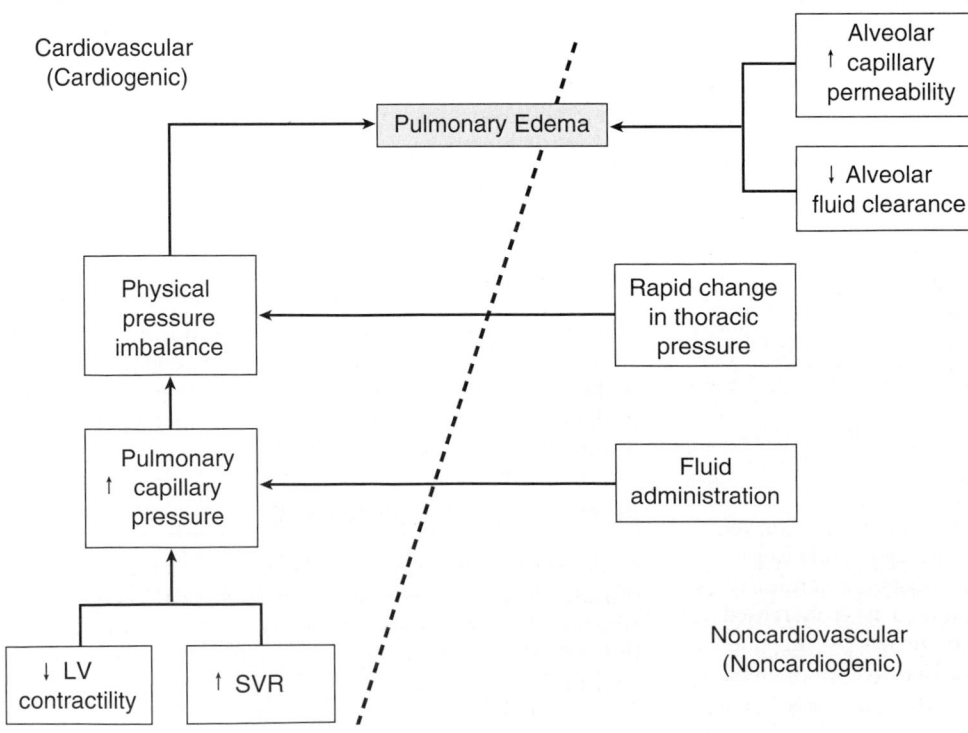

FIGURE 90–1. The pathophysiology of pulmonary edema.

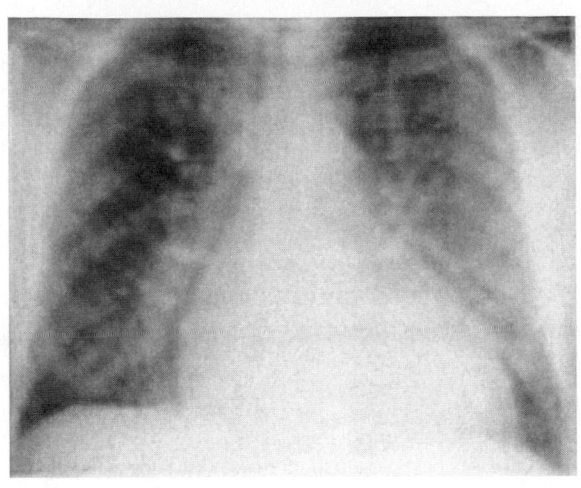

FIGURE 90–2. Chest radiograph of a patient with pulmonary edema.

of an obvious condition such as severe diseases related to acute respiratory distress syndrome (ARDS) or other clinical conditions such as climbing to high altitude, diving in cold water, transfusion-related acute lung injury (TRALI), a major operation, pregnancy, neurogenic events, opiate overdose, radiocontrast use, anticancer treatment, or inhalatory injury.

However, sometimes the differentiation between cardiovascular and noncardiovascular pulmonary edema is difficult based on clinical characteristics. In such cases the measurement of a low pulmonary capillary wedge pressure during right-sided heart catheterization is instrumental in the diagnosis of noncardiovascular edema. Reduced echocardiographic ejection fraction as well as reduced cardiac output during right-sided heart catheterization may occur in both syndromes and hence are not specific enough for differentiation between the two syndromes.

NONCARDIOVASCULAR (NONCARDIOGENIC) PULMONARY EDEMA

The most common cause of noncardiovascular pulmonary edema is ARDS. ARDS is the common final pathway of many injuries affecting the lung, including infections (both pneumonia and systemic infections), other primary systemic inflammatory reactions, various shock syndromes, inhaled toxins (both gaseous and gastric content and foreign materials), disseminated intravascular coagulation, and systemic toxic syndromes. Although damage to the alveolar-endothelial barrier combined with decreased alveolar fluid clearance leads to fluid accumulation within the alveoli, impairing the gas exchange mechanism, the clinical presentation, pathogenesis, and course of ARDS are significantly different from those of pulmonary edema and therefore this syndrome is reviewed in detail elsewhere (see Chapter 75).

In most other syndromes of noncardiovascular pulmonary edema a combination of factors including inflammation, direct damage to the capillary-alveolar membrane, and hypoxia causing leakage of the capillary-alveolar barrier and decreased alveolar fluid clearance are prominent pathogenetic mechanisms of pulmonary edema. However, increased vascular resistance and decreased left ventricular contractility, the main factors contributing to cardiovascular pulmonary

edema, may also be present in some of the syndromes that have traditionally been defined as noncardiovascular, whereas increased permeability of the alveolar-capillary membrane as well as decreased alveolar fluid clearance may be observed in cardiovascular pulmonary edema. Hence, it is possible that, in the future, the distinction between cardiovascular and noncardiovascular pulmonary edema will become less important.

The causes of noncardiovascular pulmonary edema are described in Table 90-1, and the most common causes are reviewed in the following sections.

POSTOPERATIVE PULMONARY EDEMA

Postoperative pulmonary edema is a relatively common finding, especially when the surgical procedures are extensive and the patient is elderly and suffers from significant cardiac comorbidities. Although previously reported to be a rare postoperative complication, with an incidence of less than 5%,[6] and in some minor procedures less than 1%,[7] in one study performed in a large hospital,[8] the rate of postoperative pulmonary edema was found to be 7.6%. In 5%, a comorbidity contributing to the pulmonary edema event was identified (e.g., acute myocardial infarction, acute renal failure, acute gastrointestinal bleeding, pneumonia, pulmonary embolism, or hyponatremia). However, pulmonary edema developed in 2.6% of patients without such risk factors. The mortality of postoperative pulmonary edema was 12% overall and 4% in patients with postoperative pulmonary edema without significant predisposing risk factors. The pathogenesis of postoperative pulmonary edema is diverse. Cardiovascular factors are major contributors to pulmonary edema in patients sustaining a postoperative myocardial

TABLE 90–1. ETIOLOGY OF NONCARDIOVASCULAR PULMONARY EDEMA
Increased Alveolar-Capillary Permeability and Reduced Alveolar Fluid Clearance
Acute respiratory distress syndrome
Neurogenic pulmonary edema
Preeclampsia
Drug Substance and Toxic Inhalation Pulmonary Edema
Opiate overdose
Anticancer therapy
Salicylate overdose
Thiazolidinedione-related pulmonary edema
Radiocontrast-related pulmonary edema
Environmental and toxic inhalation pulmonary edema
Other drugs[35]: tricyclic antidepressants, hydrochlorothiazide
Alveolar-Capillary Pressure Imbalance
Perioperative pulmonary edema
Elevated Capillary Pressure: Excessive Fluid Transfusion or Fluid Shifts
Peripartum pulmonary edema
Ovarian hyperstimulation syndrome[13]
Exertional pulmonary edema
Hypoxia-Related Pulmonary Edema
High-altitude pulmonary edema
Rapid Change in Thoracic Pressure
Post upper airways obstruction
Post pneumonectomy
Post evacuation of pleural effusion
Post evacuation of pericardial fluid (rare)

infarction, whereas alveolar capillary leakage and reduced alveolar fluid clearance play a major role in postoperative pulmonary edema related to major infections. In the absence of predisposing risk factors, fluid overload may be the main reason for pulmonary edema. In one study,[8] fatal pulmonary edema was associated with administration of an average of 9 L during 27 hours. Therefore, careful monitoring of perioperative net fluid retention as well as measures to prevent perioperative myocardial infarction, renal failure, bleeding, and infections are important in the prevention of this life-threatening complication.

PREGNANCY-RELATED PULMONARY EDEMA

Pulmonary edema is an uncommon complication of pregnancy. In one large prospective study[9] it was demonstrated that pulmonary edema complicates approximately 0.1% of all pregnancies. It usually occurs in the peripartum period from a combination of factors, including mobilization of fluids and fluid administration, use of tocolytic treatment, and preeclampsia. The diagnosis of pulmonary edema is made during the antepartum period in 47%, the intrapartum period in 14%, and the postpartum period in 39%. Tocolytic treatment use is the most common cause of pregnancy-related pulmonary edema (26%). In most cases, multiple tocolytics that include a beta-mimetic agent are administered, probably inducing a significant increase in systemic vascular resistance. In a further 26%, pulmonary edema is related to a preexisting cardiac disease that is exacerbated during the peripartum period and in combination with the large volume shifts during this period that induce pulmonary edema. Fluid overload per se is the main etiology of pulmonary edema in 22% of patients. In these cases pulmonary edema is related to a large volume transfusion of approximately 6 L over a short period of time. The administration of a large volume of fluids in the peripartum period has become common practice, aiming at reducing preterm delivery. However, such practice should be tempered to prevent this life-threatening complication. Finally, preeclampsia is the main cause of pulmonary edema in 18% of cases. Preeclampsia causes pulmonary edema through a combination of cardiovascular (reduced left ventricular contractility and increased systemic vascular resistance) as well as noncardiovascular factors (endothelial damage leading to increased fluid leak into the alveoli). Increased maternal age, parity, and history of hypertension increase the likelihood of pulmonary edema in patients with preeclampsia.

Although the differential diagnosis of peripartum pulmonary edema is extensive, it is imperative to rule out other possibilities, especially pulmonary emboli, before initiation of treatment. In most cases, interruption of fluid transfusion and tocolytics in combination with diuretics and measures to decrease blood pressure will promptly reverse the clinical symptoms.

Peripartum cardiomyopathy is an important entity causing pulmonary edema but should be listed among the causes of cardiovascular pulmonary edema.

POSTOBSTRUCTIVE PULMONARY EDEMA

This syndrome occurs after the relief of either acute or chronic obstructions of the upper airways.[10] The most common cause is relief of obstruction occurring during anesthesia, although other acute causes of upper airways obstruction such as epiglottitis, croup, foreign bodies, strangulation, tumors, goiter, vocal cord paralysis, and obstruction of endotracheal tubes have been reported. Furthermore, the relief of chronic upper airway obstruction after tonsillectomy or adenoidectomy may also lead to pulmonary edema. Pulmonary edema develops minutes to hours after the relief of obstructions, and its incidence may be up to 10% after relief of acute obstructions and up to 40% after relief of chronic obstruction.[11] The pathophysiology of postobstructive pulmonary edema is not known, but a combination of increased pulmonary capillary pressure owing to significant negative pressure during the obstructive period combined with hypoxia leading to decreased alveolar fluid clearance, increased systemic vascular resistance due to sympathetic overflow, and stress failure of the alveolar-capillary membrane have all been postulated as possible causative mechanisms.[12] The diagnosis is based on usual clinical and chest radiographic findings. Some authorities advocate the use of noninvasive positive-pressure ventilation as the main treatment modality.[10,12]

POSTPNEUMONECTOMY PULMONARY EDEMA

Pulmonary edema develops in 2.5% to 4.5% of patients after pneumonectomy.[13-15] The pathogenesis of this syndrome is unknown. However, a combination of large fluid transfusion, excessive negative pressure in the operated hemithorax due to underwater suction systems, major lymphatic interruption related to extensive surgery, and damage to the alveolar-capillary membrane have been implicated as possible causes. The fatality of this syndrome is significant, up to 85% in one series.[13] Hence, prevention by use of balanced pneumonectomy drainage and judicious fluid transfusions is of great importance. Once it is established, treatment should consist of positive-pressure ventilation and supportive measures.

RE-EXPANSION PULMONARY EDEMA

Pulmonary edema may occur after evacuation of a large pneumothorax or pleural effusion. In one series,[16] its incidence was reported to be 6%, mainly in relation to chronic cases. The pathogenesis is not known, but leaks in the alveolar capillary membrane after prolonged atelectasis and rapid re-expansion were suggested by some authors. The treatment is symptomatic. The prognosis is not known, although in some older series a mortality of up to 20% was described.

NEUROGENIC PULMONARY EDEMA

Neurogenic pulmonary edema is an uncommon complication of various neurologic insults such as head injury, intracranial and subarachnoid hemorrhage, as well as some acute neurologic diseases, including seizures, tumors, hydrocephalus, and neurosurgical procedures. The clinical course is highly variable. The syndrome is often acute and fulminant but may be subclinical and smoldering, manifesting as a mild progressive shortness of breath. The pathogenesis of neurogenic pulmonary edema[17,18] is probably related to a combination of increased sympathetic discharge leading to both increased systemic vascular resistance and decreased left ventricular contractility, as well as increased alveolar-capillary leakage. It is therefore possible that the large variability in clinical presentation is related to the specific contribution of each of the pathogenic mechanisms involved. The differential diagnosis of neurogenic pulmonary edema is extensive, and careful diagnosis is crucial before institution of treatment. In addition to the measures usually applied in pulmonary edema (see later), some authorities in the neurologic literature advocate the use of alpha-adrenergic blockers such as phentolamine and phenoxybenzamine owing to the possible role of sympathetic overflow in this syndrome. However, these treatment options have never been examined in a prospective, controlled study and hence should be used with caution.[17]

EXERTIONAL AND SWIMMING-INDUCED PULMONARY EDEMA

Pulmonary edema has been reported to occur during and especially after strenuous exercise and diverse sports activities[19,20] and is especially common (up to 60%) after prolonged swimming in cold water.[21] The pathogenesis of this syndrome is unknown. However, stress damage to the alveolar-capillary barrier owing to the dramatic increase in cardiac output as well as peripheral vasoconstriction, especially in cold water swimming, are possible mechanisms. The prognosis is usually benign, and some authorities advocate the use of inhaled beta-mimetics to expedite alveolar fluid reabsorption.[22]

HIGH-ALTITUDE PULMONARY EDEMA

High-altitude pulmonary edema is a syndrome related to climbing to high altitudes. Its exact pathophysiology is unknown, but in a few recent studies it was demonstrated that a combination of hypoxia-induced vasoconstriction leading to increased pulmonary capillary pressure and alveolar fluid transudation[23] together with decreased alveolar fluid clearance[24] leads to alveolar fluid accumulation and edema. The inflammatory changes previously described in these patients are probably secondary to pulmonary edema rather than a primary pathophysiologic event.[25] Important risk factors for high-altitude pulmonary edema include rapid ascent, significant excretion, cold ambience, and individual susceptibility. People who previously sustained an episode of high-altitude pulmonary edema are at an increased risk for repeated episodes when climbing to high altitudes, probably owing to a tendency for more hypoxia-related vasoconstriction or reduced alveolar fluid clearance. The clinical presentation is typical, ranging from cough to full-blown respiratory failure. The treatment includes oxygen administration, rapid descent to lower altitudes or simulated descent by a hyperbaric chamber, and possibly administration of calcium antagonists. Furosemide and dexamethasone are probably not efficacious. Recently, it has been suggested that the use of beta-mimetic drugs (e.g., salmeterol inhalation) by virtue of their effect to increase alveolar fluid clearance may become an effective measure in both the treatment and prevention of high-altitude pulmonary edema.[26]

DRUG-, SUBSTANCE- AND TOXIC INHALATION–INDUCED PULMONARY EDEMA

The most common cause of drug-induced pulmonary edema is the use of cardiodepressants such as beta-adrenergic blockers and some calcium blockers and antiarrhythmics. Even topical administration of beta-adrenergic blockers might provoke pulmonary edema[27]; hence, careful examination of all drug treatments and especially new drugs that have been administered is imperative when admitting a patient with pulmonary edema.

Pulmonary edema has been associated with the intake or toxicities of drugs that provoke edema through different mechanisms.

Opiate Overdose Pulmonary Edema

This type of pulmonary edema is observed with all opiate derivatives, including opium (as described in 1880 by William Osler),[28] heroin,[29] and methadone. Recently, opiate-related pulmonary edema is most commonly the result of heroin overdose. Its prevalence is unknown; however, in one retrospective study it has been reported to occur in approximately 10% of patients admitted with heroin overdose, related to a more severe respiratory depression but not co-intoxication with alcohol or cocaine ("speed ball"). In the past it had been suggested that opiate-related pulmonary edema is associated with the impurities of the intravenous preparation. However, more recent studies have suggested that opiates by themselves induce damage to the alveolar-capillary membrane, causing fluid transudation into the alveoli combined with depressed alveolar fluid clearance induced by the overdose-related hypoxia. Opiate-related pulmonary edema is rarely life threatening and is easily manageable by medical treatment. However, sometimes this complication occurs up to 36 hours after resolution of the heroin overdose; hence a period of observation is warranted in all patients admitted with such an overdose.

Anti-Cancer Therapy–Related Pulmonary Edema

Pulmonary edema has been described as a complication of anti-cancer therapies. Its incidence is unknown, and most reports in the literature are sporadic case reports. In one review,[30] Briasoulis and Pavlidis relate pulmonary edema to treatment with interleukin-2; granulocyte and granulocyte-macrophage colony-stimulating factors; cytotoxic drugs such as cytarabine, gemcitabine, docetaxel, vinblastine, methotrexate, and 5-fluorouracil; bone marrow transplantation; and the vitamin-A derivative ATRA. Although the pathogenesis of anti-cancer therapy–related pulmonary edema is unknown, and likely to be different for the different agents implicated, increased alveolar-capillary membrane permeability due to direct toxicity (by cytotoxic drugs) and inflammatory activation (by interleukin-2, bone marrow transplantation, and ATRA) are possible mechanisms. The prognosis is usually related to the underlying condition.

Salicylate Overdose

Although there are scattered reports of an association between pulmonary edema and nonsteroidal anti-inflammatory agents as a group, pulmonary edema has been mainly reported to complicate salicylate overdose.[31] It occurs in 10% to 60% of patients sustaining a salicylate overdose and exclusively in patients with blood levels greater than 30 mg/dL, but its incidence is not related to the exact blood levels. It is more common in older and sicker patients, especially when the intoxication is chronic. Treatment is symptomatic and includes all measures to treat salicylate toxicity per se. Importantly, pH should be maintained as close to normal as possible. In a few cases hemodialysis has been used, especially when blood levels were greater than 100 mg/dL; however, the reports on its efficacy are limited.

Thiazolidinedione-Related Pulmonary Edema

The thiazolidinediones currently include troglitazone, rosiglitazone, and pioglitazone. They are known to promote fluid retention and possibly diuretic resistance and have been reported to cause pulmonary edema.[32]

Radiocontrast-Related Pulmonary Edema

Pulmonary edema is a rare complication of radiocontrast administration with an unknown incidence. The pathophysiology is related to an increased leakage of the alveolar-capillary membrane owing to both direct toxic effects of the radiocontrast media and complement-mediated inflammatory activation.[33] The treatment is conventional (see later), and the prognosis is usually favorable.

Environmental and Toxic Inhalation Pulmonary Edema

Pulmonary edema is one of the more serious complications of inhalation of toxic gases and irritants.[34] The list of possible inhalatory causes of pulmonary edema is vast[34]; however, the most common causes include gases such as chlorine, hydrogen sulfite, fluorine, methyl isocyanate, paraquat, pesticides, insecticides, and fumigants. Other common causes include particulated fat emboli, low-dose irradiation particles, environmental air pollution ("metal fume fever" due to manganese), and, last, inhalation of recreational drugs such as cocaine and crack cocaine. The treatment is usually symptomatic. Both morbidity and mortality from this condition are high; hence, prevention of accidental exposure is of utmost importance.

TRANSFUSION-RELATED ACUTE LUNG INJURY (TRALI)

TRALI is a syndrome of sudden-onset noncardiovascular pulmonary edema occurring during or a few hours after transfusion of a blood product.[35,35a] The incidence is 1 to 5 in 10,000 transfusions, and it usually occurs after administration of products containing large amounts of plasma, although it has been reported to occur after administration of as little as 50 mL of whole blood or any plasma containing blood products including intravenous immunoglobulins. The pathogenesis is unknown; however, it has been suggested that leukocyte activation due to antibodies in donor plasma to antigens of recipient white blood cells or reactive lipids in aged cellular blood components are important contributing factors. Although host factors such as infection, cytokine administration, lung disease, and recent surgery may contribute to the incidence and severity of TRALI, the syndrome was also reported in healthy volunteers receiving blood products. Activated leukocytes are sequestered in the lungs and cause damage to the capillary-alveolar membrane leading to congestion, hypoxia, pulmonary edema, hypovolemia, hypotension, and fever. Laboratory findings include hemoconcentration, hypoalbuminemia, and neutropenia or neutrophilia. Differential diagnosis includes ARDS, other forms of pulmonary edema, and pneumonia. Early diagnosis is important to prevent administration of diuretics that may be detrimental in TRALI. Treatment includes oxygen administration and sometimes mechanical ventilation (required in approximately 68% of cases). Corticosteroids have been advocated by some authors, although their use has never been examined in a controlled prospective study. In contrast to ARDS the clinical course in TRALI is often benign, with improvement starting after 24 to 48 hours; if the patient survives, no sequela are observed. However, mortality remains high, at about 5%, and TRALI is the third cause of transfusion-related mortality. Prevention is the most important measure including avoiding unnecessary transfusions, increased use of red cells containing less plasma, and possibly avoiding the use of products containing large amounts of plasma derived from multiparous women, who often are autoimmunized against leukocyte antigens during pregnancy.

CARDIOVASCULAR (CARDIOGENIC) PULMONARY EDEMA

DEFINITION AND INCIDENCE

Cardiogenic pulmonary edema is the extreme form of acute heart failure. Although a standard definition of this syndrome does not exist we have previously defined cardiogenic pulmonary edema as an episode of acute heart failure accompanied by severe respiratory distress and oxygen saturation less than 90% on room air before treatment.[36] The incidence of cardiogenic pulmonary edema is not known. Although there are approximately 1 million annual hospital admissions due to heart failure in the United States,[37] the exact fraction of acute heart failure and pulmonary edema is not known.

PATHOGENESIS

Initiation Phase

Cardiogenic pulmonary edema is caused by a failure of the cardiovascular system, leading to an increase in left ventricular pressures transmitted backward to the pulmonary veins, inducing an increase in pulmonary capillary pressure and transudation of fluid from the capillaries to the pulmonary interstitium and alveoli, overwhelming the reabsorption ability of the alveolar cells.[3] The cardiovascular failure that causes pulmonary edema is the end product of a combination of reduced left ventricular contractility and increased systemic vascular resistance (Fig. 90-3), leading to a vicious cycle.[36] First, the decrease in left ventricular contractility induces a significant neurohormonal (sympathetic, renin-angiotensin, and endothelin) and inflammatory (interleukin-6–mediated) activation,[38] leading to peripheral vasoconstriction and increased systemic vascular resistance. Second, increased systemic vascular resistance imposes a significant afterload mismatch, further reducing left ventricular contractility. This vicious cycle causes a decrease in cardiac output and peripheral perfusion and also an increase in left ventricular pressure that leads to the pulmonary edema syndrome.

Amplification Phase

This vicious cycle is amplified by four distinct mechanisms (Fig. 90-4):

1. *Myocardial ischemia:* In many patients pulmonary edema coexists with significant coronary artery disease. In such patients the hypoxia, acidosis, and reduced cardiac output present during pulmonary edema may induce myocardial ischemia, thus further reducing left ventricular contractility, increasing left ventricular pressures, and further worsening the pulmonary edema syndrome.

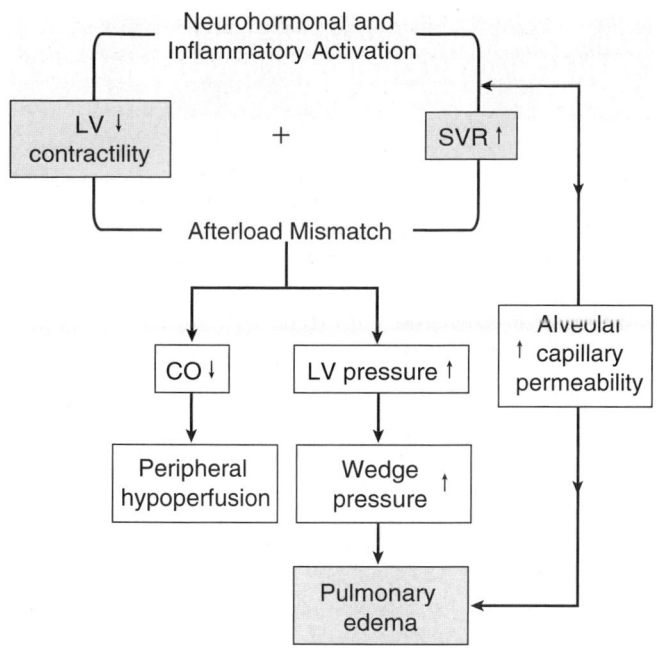

FIGURE 90–3. The initiation phase of pulmonary edema.

the acute inflammatory reaction leads to prolonged leakage of the alveolar-capillary membrane. This process may contribute to the initial event as well as to the known tendency of patients admitted with cardiovascular pulmonary edema to develop recurrent events during the days after the initial event.[40] Furthermore, the significant hypoxia present during the initiation of the acute heart failure event may depress the rate of alveolar fluid clearance, further enhancing pulmonary edema.[3]

Common Final Pathway

As the cycle leading to pulmonary edema progressively amplifies, the patient's condition deteriorates into a state of severe cardiovascular failure with low cardiac output, reduced oxygenation, significantly activated neurohormonal and inflammatory modulators, increased systemic vascular resistance, decreased peripheral perfusion, myocardial ischemia, respiratory failure, and, if untreated, death.

ETIOLOGY

As previously stated, in most cases cardiogenic pulmonary edema is caused by a combination of decreased left ventricular contractility and increased systemic vascular resistance. These two mechanisms exist to a certain degree in most forms of cardiogenic pulmonary edema. For example, in patients who sustain pulmonary edema due to severe acute ischemia, some increase in systemic vascular resistance is commonly observed owing to sympathetic activation, whereas in patients presenting with "flush" hypertensive pulmonary edema, left ventricular contractility by invasive hemodynamic measurements is at least to some extent decreased. Often, however, the etiologic factor is primarily related to either an acute decrease of left ventricular contractility or an increase in systemic vascular resistance (Table 90-2).

Although severe myocardial ischemia is a common etiology of cardiogenic pulmonary edema, minor ischemia, as evident

2. *Right ventricular failure:* The increased fluid content in the lungs and decreased oxygen saturation induce pulmonary vasoconstriction. This is translated into an increase in right ventricular pressure, again compromising left ventricular function through the ventricular interaction mechanism.[39]
3. *Respiratory failure:* The decreased oxygenation, acidemia, and reduced cardiac output may lead to depressed central respiratory drive and failure of the respiratory muscles, leading to respiratory failure superimposed on cardiovascular failure.
4. *Leakage of the alveolar-capillary membrane and decreased alveolar fluid clearance:* Although debated during recent years, it seems that in cardiovascular pulmonary edema

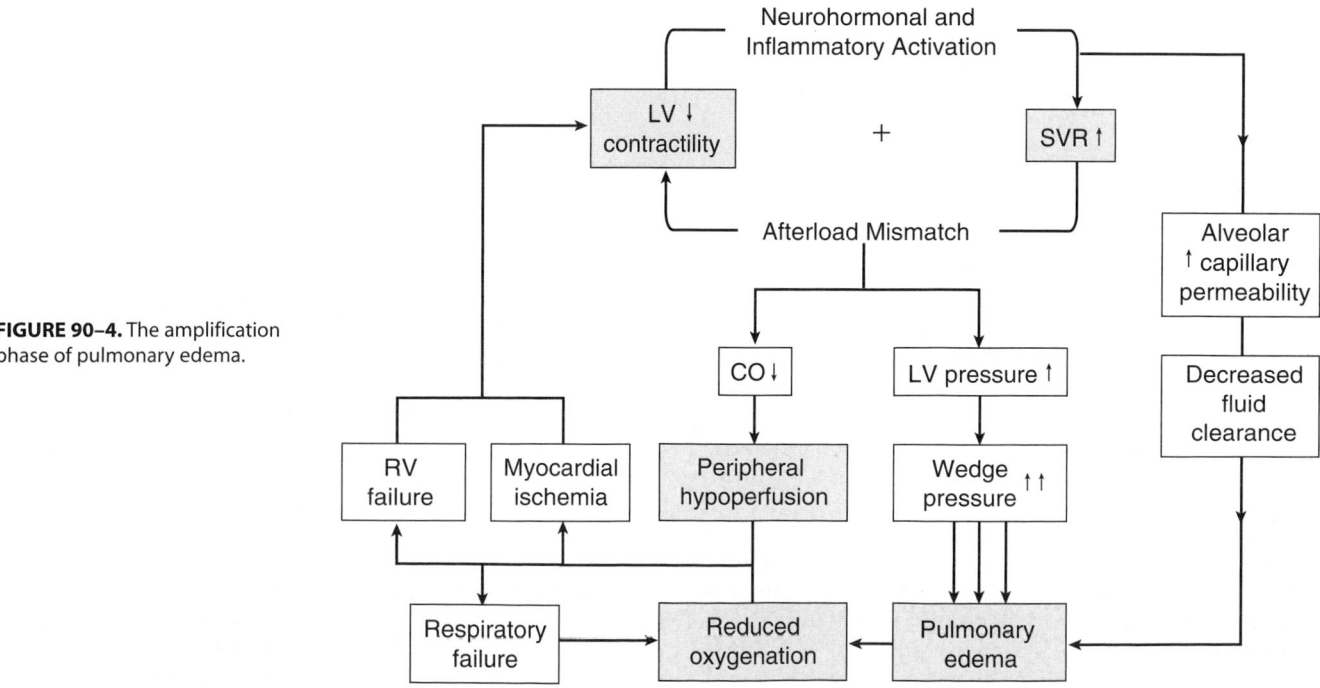

FIGURE 90–4. The amplification phase of pulmonary edema.

TABLE 90–2. ETIOLOGIC FACTORS OF CARDIOVASCULAR PULMONARY EDEMA

Reduced Left Ventricular Contractility

Severe acute myocardial ischemia
Valvular or mechanical factors (see Table 90-7)
Cardiomyopathies (dilated, hypertrophic, restrictive)
Myocarditis
Cardiodepressant drugs (beta-adrenergic blockers, calcium channel blockers, antiarrhythmics)
Severe arrhythmias

Increased Systemic Vascular Resistance

"Flush" hypertensive pulmonary edema
Renal artery stenosis
Pheochromocytoma, hypertensive crisis
Neurogenic pulmonary edema?
Cold immersion pulmonary edema?

TABLE 90–3. INITIAL EVALUATION OF PATIENTS WITH SUSPECTED CARDIOVASCULAR PULMONARY EDEMA

Immediate Work-Up

History of heart failure or regular intake of loop diuretics, previous myocardial infarction, or known significant valvular disease
Physical examination: check blood pressure, temperature, signs of peripheral edema, and cardiac and pulmonary physical findings
Arrhythmia monitoring
Pulse oximetry
12-Lead electrocardiogram
Chest radiograph

Advanced Work-Up

Complete blood gas analysis
Laboratory evaluation (complete blood cell count, electrolytes, urea/creatinine, creatine kinase, troponin)
Brain natriuretic peptide measurement (if available)
Echocardiographic evaluation
Right-sided heart catheterization

by minor electrocardiographic changes and mild increase in plasma markers (creatine kinase [CK], troponin), is part of the common final pathway of cardiogenic pulmonary edema. Hence, careful evaluation of these symptoms and signs should be implemented on an individual basis, because routine revascularization procedures in these patients are sometimes related to significant complications and restoring coronary flow to nonviable myocardial segments may not reduce recurrent heart failure events.[41] Furthermore, in recent years it has become apparent that the etiology of the cardiogenic pulmonary edema is often associated with a hypertensive event related to echocardiographic signs of diastolic dysfunction, increased endothelin levels, and sustained inflammatory activation at recovery.[38,42] This novel syndrome is related to older age, relatively preserved left ventricular ejection fraction, higher prevalence of female sex, and history of hypertension and is probably one of the more common causes of cardiovascular pulmonary edema.[42,43]

DIAGNOSIS AND INITIAL EVALUATION

Although immediate treatment is imperative to avert cardiovascular and respiratory failure and death, it is important in parallel to treatment administration that an initial evaluation is performed in patients admitted with pulmonary edema (Table 90-3). This evaluation has important goals:

1. *Establish the diagnosis of pulmonary edema.* Although the diagnosis can often be made with high certainty based on symptoms and clinical signs, further evaluation is essential to rule out other acute diseases leading to respiratory failure and/or hemodynamic insufficiency (Table 90-4). In patients with a known history of heart failure, significant ischemic heart disease, or valvular lesions, the classic symptoms and signs combined with typical chest radiographic findings (see earlier) are sufficient for diagnosis and initiation of treatment. Also, in patients without such history, typical symptoms and signs accompanied by chest radiographic findings in the presence of fever less than 38°C, reduced echocardiographic left ventricular ejection fraction, or elevated BNP or Pro NT-BNP are usually diagnostic of pulmonary edema. In some cases, however, the diagnosis remains uncertain and right-sided heart catheterization may be required to establish the

exact diagnosis. During right-sided heart catheterization findings of increased pulmonary capillary wedge pressure, reduced cardiac index, and cardiac power (the product of mean arterial blood pressure and cardiac output measured simultaneously) and increased systemic vascular resistance are usually indicative of pulmonary edema. Although no exact cutoff point exists regarding these hemodynamic variables for the diagnosis of cardiovascular pulmonary edema, if right-sided heart catheterization is performed while the patient is still in pulmonary edema, systemic vascular resistance of more than 3000 dynes is usually measured.[44]

2. *Determine whether pulmonary edema is the result of severe acute ischemia.* As previously stated, this distinction may be difficult to establish. However, patients with significant dynamic ST-segment elevation or depression or deep T-wave inversion on electrocardiography, especially if these changes are in the anterior wall (precordial leads) and not accompanied by pathologic Q waves or bundle branch block and accompanied by significant CK-MB or troponin elevation, should be regarded as suffering from pulmonary edema owing to severe acute ischemia and treated as such (see later).

3. *Determine the severity of pulmonary edema.* Although the data on the risk stratification of patients with cardiovascular pulmonary edema are limited, the following measures

TABLE 90–4. DIFFERENTIAL DIAGNOSIS OF CARDIOVASCULAR PULMONARY EDEMA

Conditions Leading to Respiratory Failure

Exacerbation of obstructive lung disease
Respiratory infections or pneumonia
Acute respiratory distress syndrome

Conditions Leading to Both Respiratory and Cardiovascular Failure

Pulmonary emboli
Sepsis
Cardiogenic shock

of disease severity have been established in patients with acute heart failure and cardiogenic pulmonary edema:

a. *Baseline characteristics:* Older age, male sex, lower weight, hyponatremia, and reduced hemoglobin and renal function have been correlated with worse outcome. No exact cutoff points have been determined for these measures, although age older than 65 years, weight less than 78 kg, sodium less than 135 mEq/L, hemoglobin less than 11 g/dL, and blood urea nitrogen greater than 45 mg/dL have been proposed as such.[45-47]

b. *Findings on admission:* As previously stated, oxygen saturation less than 90% is required for the diagnosis of pulmonary edema. However, as arterial oxygen saturation decreases, the chances of respiratory failure increase and the patient's prognosis becomes worse.[48] Admission blood pressure is also an important sign of disease severity; however, its correlation with outcome is "U"-shaped. Higher admission blood pressure is usually correlated with higher vascular resistance and, hence, worse outcome.[48] On the other hand, low blood pressure (<120 mm Hg systolic) on admission is correlated with decreased left ventricular contractility and is a negative prognostic sign.[44] Finally, higher pulse rate and respiratory rate at admission were correlated with increased rate of adverse events in patients admitted with pulmonary edema.[48]

c. *Cardiac contractility:* Cardiac power[49] is the product of simultaneously measured cardiac output (cardiovascular flow) and mean arterial blood pressure (MAP, cardiovascular pressure). Cardiac power output is calculated as $Cpo = CO \cdot MAP \cdot 0.022$, and its units are watts. In recent studies cardiac power output was demonstrated to be the strongest predictor of outcome in patients with chronic heart failure[36] and cardiogenic shock[50] as well as acute heart failure. Typically, cardiac power output of less than 0.5 to 0.6 watt on admission is associated with increased rate of recurrent heart failure events. However, the calculation of Cpo requires right-sided heart catheterization, which is currently performed less often. Reduced echocardiographic ejection fraction can be used as a measure of left ventricular contractility.[48]

d. *Measures of neurohormonal activation:* In patients with chronic heart failure, neurohormonal and inflammatory measures have been shown to be correlated with disease severity and outcome. The data on such measures in patients with acute heart failure and pulmonary edema are limited. However, it has been suggested that higher admission endothelin level is the mediator associated with worst outcome, whereas admission BNP is of limited value.[51-53] Currently, endothelin measurements are done only by specialized laboratories and hence cannot be used for immediate risk stratification.

4. *Determine whether the patient suffers from chronic heart failure that has deteriorated due to aggravating factors.* Cardiovascular pulmonary edema may occur owing to an acute aggravation of significant chronic heart failure (Table 90-5). The determination of existing chronic heart failure is important because in these patients acute pulmonary edema may occur as a result of an aggravating factor (Table 90-6) that may be easily manageable, hence improving our ability to treat the acute event and prevent early recurrence. On the other hand, in patients without

TABLE 90-5. CLINICAL SYMPTOMS AND SIGNS OF DETERIORATED CHRONIC HEART FAILURE VERSUS "TRANSIENT" PULMONARY EDEMA

	"Transient" Pulmonary Edema	Acute Decompensation of Chronic Heart Failure
Chronic heart failure symptoms (dyspnea/fatigue)	+	++++
Treatment with loop diuretics	+	+++
Peripheral edema	+	+++
Gain in body weight	I	III
Reduced ejection fraction (echo)	+	+++
Neurohormonal activation (endothelin)	+++	++
Aggravating factor	+	+++

a history of significant chronic heart failure symptoms, "flash" hypertensive pulmonary edema with relatively preserved left ventricular ejection fraction is a common cause of cardiogenic pulmonary edema, which may be associated with better prognosis.

5. *Determine whether pulmonary edema is related to preserved echocardiographic ejection fraction (HFnEF) or low ejection fraction (HF↓EF).* The distinction between HFnEF and HF↓EF was set by most investigators at EF equals 40%. Patients with HFnEF tend to be older, to be female, and to have a history of hypertension; their pulmonary edema is more often of the "flash" hypertensive type. On Doppler echocardiography they tend to demonstrate signs of diastolic dysfunction, in particular, shorter transmitral E-wave deceleration time and lower E/A-wave ratio; and their prognosis may be better. On the other hand, in patients with HF↓EF, acute ischemia is often a leading cause of pulmonary edema; and their prognosis is worse.[38]

6. *Rule out significant valvular and mechanical cardiac causes of pulmonary edema.* This evaluation underscores the role of early echocardiographic evaluation in patients with suspected cardiovascular pulmonary edema. The echocardiographic evaluation is especially indicated when a significant cardiac murmur is present and the patient's condition does not resolve immediately with conventional medical treatment. Table 90-7 depicts the main mechanical cardiac causes of pulmonary edema. If such a significant valvular or mechanical lesion is detected, the patient may require prompt surgical treatment.

TABLE 90-6. COMMON AGGRAVATING FACTORS LEADING TO DECOMPENSATION OF CHRONIC HEART FAILURE

Acute fluid and/or salt intake (diet noncompliance)
Medical treatment noncompliance
Acute ischemia or myocardial infarction
Sepsis or other infections (mostly upper respiratory tract)
Significant arrhythmias (atrial tachycardia, fibrillation or flutter, ventricular tachycardias, bradyarrhythmias)
Pulmonary embolism
Anemia
Hyperkalemia
Acute renal failure

TABLE 90–7. COMMON VALVULAR AND/OR MECHANICAL LESIONS THAT MAY LEAD TO PULMONARY EDEMA

Significant aortic stenosis or regurgitation
Significant mitral stenosis or regurgitation
Mechanical valve malfunction (thrombosis or pannus formation or leakage)
Acquired ventricular septal defect (associated with myocardial infarction)
Infective endocarditis
Aortic dissection

TREATMENT

Immediate Stabilization

Untreated pulmonary edema is a life-threatening situation. The progressive decrease in left ventricular contractility and increase in systemic vascular resistance culminate into a progressive decrease in organ perfusion and oxygenation, progressive acidemia, multi-organ failure, respiratory failure, and death. Accordingly, the immediate goals in the treatment of pulmonary edema are termination of the main aggravating vicious cycles leading to progressive heart failure, that is, improving systemic oxygenation and inducing rapid vasodilatation of both veins and arteries, thus decreasing vascular resistance, alleviating afterload mismatch, and reducing the preload of both the left and right ventricles.

Improving Systemic Oxygenation

This is usually achieved by positioning the patient in a sitting position and administering oxygen by a high-flow facemask. It has been suggested that noninvasive positive-pressure ventilation could further improve oxygenation.[54] However, this treatment might increase intrathoracic pressure, impairing cardiac function, and hence aggravate rather than improve congestion. Indeed, in a single study performed in patients with frank pulmonary edema, bilevel positive airway pressure (BiPAP) ventilation was found to be related to unfavorable outcome.[55] Therefore, the use of noninvasive ventilation in cardiovascular pulmonary edema should be regarded, at least for the time being, as optional and may be applied in patients with milder forms of acute heart failure or patients not responding to conventional oxygen supply and drug therapy.

Arrhythmia Control

In parallel to attempting to improve oxygenation, the patient should be connected to a rhythm monitor and malignant arrhythmias such as ventricular tachycardia, severe bradyarrhythmias, or significant atrial arrhythmias such as rapid atrial fibrillation should be immediately treated.

Intravenous Furosemide and Morphine

First-line treatment should be administered intravenously; hence, intravenous access should be established as soon as possible. Treatment should consist of intravenously administered furosemide at a dose of 40 to 80 mg given as a bolus and intravenously administered morphine up to 3 mg. This treatment combination induces mild diuresis and preload reduction and assists in reducing patient anxiety. Higher doses of furosemide are usually not recommended because such doses may lead to intravascular depletion and prerenal azotemia and are related to significant neurohormonal activation,[56] which can be deleterious in patients with cardiogenic pulmonary edema. Higher doses of morphine may induce respiratory depression and enhance respiratory failure[57] and thus should be avoided.

Intravenous Nitrates

Intravenous nitrates should be administered to all patients with cardiogenic pulmonary edema with a systolic blood pressure of greater than 120 mm Hg on admission. Intravenous nitrates are the only treatment modality that has been shown in a prospective randomized study to improve the outcome of patients admitted with pulmonary edema by averting respiratory failure and reducing the need for mechanical ventilation.[58] These agents can be administered as repeated boluses of 3 mg while monitoring blood pressure and oxygen saturation until either arterial oxygen saturation increases to greater than 90% or systolic blood pressure is reduced to less than 120 mm Hg. Nitrates can also be administered as a continuous drip, but the efficacy of such treatment has not been demonstrated in a prospective study.

Mechanical Ventilation

If the patient develops respiratory failure or pulmonary edema accompanied by significant hypotension, he or she should be classified as having cardiogenic shock and should be treated with mechanical ventilation. Patients not responding to medical treatment within 10 to 20 minutes, as evident by an increase in arterial oxygen saturation to more than 90%, accompanied by decreased tachypnea and blood pressure, are suffering from refractory pulmonary edema[48] and should be treated by mechanical ventilation. Tracheal intubation in patients with pulmonary edema may be difficult because the patient is hypoxic, anxious, and often uncooperative. Thus, tracheal intubation should be performed by the most skilled person available.

First 24 Hours

After the initial stabilization, as vascular resistance decreases toward normal values, cardiac index increases, and wedge pressure decreases, the main goals of treatment shift from rapid arterial and venous dilatation to preventing recurrence. Because decreased left ventricular contractility and increased systemic vascular resistance are important in the pathogenesis of pulmonary edema, traditional treatments employed during this time period are directed toward rapid increase in left ventricular contractility, prevention of recurrent vasoconstriction, and enhancement of diuresis. However, although some of the treatments are efficacious in accelerating symptom relief through their hemodynamic effects (increased left ventricular contractility or vasodilatation leading to reduced wedge pressure), their effect on outcome, as measured by prevention of recurrent events of pulmonary edema and death, when compared with placebo is limited.[59,60] Moreover, in some cases it has been suggested that some of these treatments might actually be associated with adverse outcomes. Therefore, all treatments should be administered with caution and only to patients with refractory symptoms of heart failure after the initial stabilization period.

Increasing Left Ventricular Contractility

Repair of Significant Valvular and Mechanical Lesions. Early echocardiography is warranted to evaluate global and regional cardiac function and detect any mechanical problem such as severe valvular lesion or septal rupture leading to pulmonary edema (see Table 90-7). If such a significant

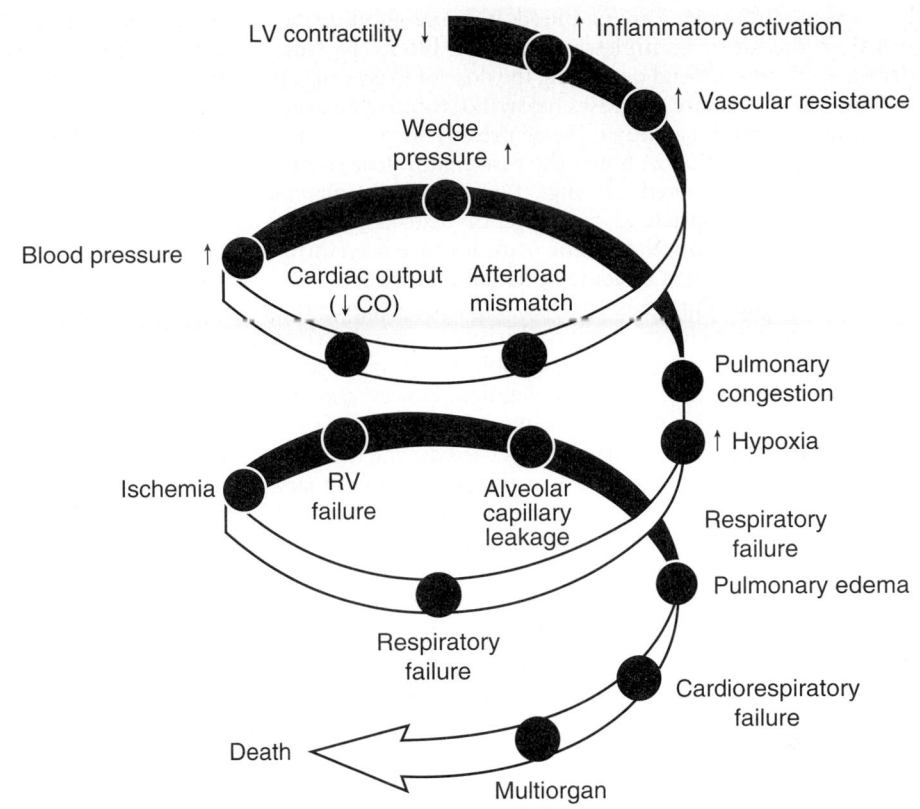

FIGURE 90–5. The common final pathway of cardiovascular pulmonary edema.

(Figure labels, clockwise from top:) LV contractility ↓ — ↑ Inflammatory activation — ↑ Vascular resistance — Wedge pressure ↑ — Blood pressure ↑ — Cardiac output (↓ CO) — Afterload mismatch — Pulmonary congestion — ↑ Hypoxia — Ischemia — RV failure — Alveolar capillary leakage — Respiratory failure — Pulmonary edema — Respiratory failure — Cardiorespiratory failure — Death — Multiorgan failure

mechanical problem is encountered and the patient's condition cannot be stabilized by medical treatment, all efforts should be directed to immediate surgical repair.

Treatment of Severe Acute Ischemia. If severe acute ischemia is considered to be the main etiologic factor leading to pulmonary edema, immediate efforts should be undertaken to relieve ischemia. In patients with acute ST segment elevation due to myocardial infarction, thrombolytic therapy or primary percutaneous coronary intervention should be executed promptly. In patients with a non–ST segment elevation ischemic event, maximal anti-ischemic treatment should be initiated followed by percutaneous coronary intervention if the ischemia or heart failure is refractory to medical treatment.[61] The intra-aortic balloon pump (IABP) as a tool of both immediate ischemia control and a way to improve effective cardiac power output may be efficacious in the treatment of acute heart failure complicating refractory ischemia or a mechanical complication.[62] Even if a patient sustaining pulmonary edema during an acute ischemic event is medically stabilized, the combination of these two syndromes has a grave prognosis. Therefore, after initial stabilization, these patients should be scheduled for immediate coronary angiography, followed by revascularization. Although in most cases, owing to significant stunning, this will not improve cardiac function immediately, it may improve left ventricular contractility over time, hence gradually decreasing the likelihood of recurrent episodes of acute heart failure.

Positive Inotropes. Positive inotropes aimed at improving cardiac systolic function, mostly sympathomimetic amines (i.e., dopamine, dobutamine, and phosphodiesterase inhibitors), are commonly used for the early treatment of pulmonary edema. These agents, although effective in the short term in relieving dyspnea and normalizing hemodynamic measurements,[63] may not be effective in the long-term

outcome of patients with acute heart failure or may even be harmful.[59,64] Thus, the administration of these agents should be reserved for refractory cases of primary pump failure (refractory heart failure accompanied by low ejection fraction or low cardiac power output) in which recurrent episodes of heart failure exacerbation cannot be prevented by conventional therapy. Lately, a new class of drugs has been developed that are aimed at improving cardiac systolic function in patients with heart failure. The first drug of this class to be reported, levosimendan, was examined in patients with acute heart failure.[65,66] When administered intravenously for 24 hours it improved subjective dyspnea and prevented recurrent episodes of heart failure exacerbation, as compared with dobutamine. No long-term follow-up data are available.

Preventing Recurrent Vasoconstriction. This goal has been traditionally achieved by the administration of vasodilators. This class of drugs currently includes nitrates and nitroprusside. The main obstacle in the use of such agents for a prolonged period of time is the rapid development of tolerance, limiting their effectiveness to 16 to 24 hours only. Moreover, these drugs have a "U"-shaped dose-response curve.[47] If given in suboptimal dose, vasodilators may have a limited effect in preventing pulmonary edema. However, administration of high doses may also reduce their effectiveness. In some cases vasodilators are given at doses aimed at achieving the maximal possible vasodilatation, leading to the largest increase in cardiac index and decrease in pulmonary wedge pressure achievable. However, in patients with heart failure with reduced left ventricular contractility, inappropriate vasodilatation may result in further decrease in blood pressure and cause hemodynamic instability, ischemia, renal failure, and even frank shock. Therefore, the administration of these drugs should be carried out under careful blood pressure monitoring, titrating the dose administered against blood pressure decrease. We recommend decreasing the dose of these drugs if systolic blood pressure decreases below 120 mm Hg and discontinue them permanently if blood pressure drops farther. Hence, during the first 24 hours the vasodilator dose should be progressively lowered, aiming at preventing recurrent episodes of inappropriate vasoconstriction instead of inducing true vasodilatation. Natriuretic peptides have been introduced for the treatment of acute heart failure owing to their vasodilatory and diuretic properties. The first drug of this class examined in a clinical study is nisiritide.[67] This drug was shown to be efficacious in improving subjective dyspnea score as well as inducing significant vasodilatation. However, in one analysis, concerns were raised regarding its safety.[60]

Diuretics. The third group of drugs used during the early period after initial stabilization of patients with pulmonary edema is diuretics, of which high-dose loop diuretics and especially furosemide are most commonly employed. However, studies examining the effect of high-dose furosemide administration have demonstrated that such treatment is associated with neurohormonal activation, increased renal failure, and other adverse events.[56,68-70] Therefore, the dose of furosemide administered to patients with acute heart failure should be restricted to the lowest possible dose achieving palliation of the congestive symptoms.

Treatment After the First 24 Hours

As a patient's condition stabilizes, long-term medical treatment should be established. First, as previously stated, in patients with obvious ischemia, coronary angiography and revascularization should be performed as soon as possible. Patients without clinical evidence of ischemia should be scheduled for a noninvasive test to assess the presence of ischemia and viability, either by radionuclide techniques or by dobutamine stress echo. In patients in whom significant ischemia and/or viability is demonstrated, in particular those demonstrating improved function of hypokinetic or akinetic segments during low-dose dobutamine and deterioration during high-dose dobutamine, coronary angiography should be considered. Concomitantly, oral medical treatment aimed at preventing repeated episodes of vasoconstriction should be administered. These drugs should be initiated at low doses and gradually titrated upward to achieve maximal effect while preventing excessive vasodilatation and hypotension. At present, only angiotensin-converting enzyme (ACE) inhibitors have been shown to be effective in this respect. However, even those drugs were examined only in patients with HF↓EF. ACE inhibitors can be substituted by angiotensin receptor I antagonists if side effects such as cough occur. Finally, beta-adrenergic blockers, which are extremely beneficial in the long-term treatment of heart failure, should not be administered to patients with acute heart failure until the patient's condition has stabilized.

It is important to emphasize that no study has examined the long-term treatment of patients with HFnEF; thus the administration of ACE inhibitors and beta-adrenergic blockers in these patients, although recommended by most authorities, remains unproven.

Outcome

As previously stated, the outcome of patients with cardiovascular pulmonary edema is strongly related to factors measured on admission, such as age, hemoglobin, creatinine, oxygen saturation, blood pressure, pulse, left ventricular contractility, and existence of significant ischemia as the main cause of the pulmonary edema. However, it has been demonstrated that a patient's response to treatment is also correlated with outcome.[47] Specifically, if oxygen saturation after 15 to 30 minutes of treatment remains below 95%, the patient is considered to have refractory pulmonary edema, which is correlated with a higher incidence of adverse outcome. Furthermore, significant blood pressure decrease at 15 to 30 minutes is also a predictor of outcome.

To date, the outcomes of patients with acute cardiovascular pulmonary edema have been described in only a few well-controlled prospective studies.[48,58] In these studies, the rate of early mechanical ventilation was approximately 20%, of which about half the patients required mechanical ventilation on admission and the rest required mechanical ventilation owing to early treatment failure (refractory pulmonary edema). Approximately 10% of patients sustained a myocardial infarction, and in 10% there was a further event of recurrent acute heart failure within 24 hours after admission. Cardiogenic shock was diagnosed in 2.5%. At 30 days, 38% of patients sustained a recurrent event of acute heart failure and the mortality was 5%.

DIFFERENCE BETWEEN PULMONARY EDEMA AND CARDIOGENIC SHOCK

Acute heart failure and cardiogenic shock are the two main syndromes of acute cardiovascular decompensation. In both, the main clinical manifestations are a combination of decreased peripheral perfusion and pulmonary congestion. Hemodynamically, the cardiac index is low and wedge pressure is high in both conditions. In one prospective study,[44] the cardiac index was similar in patients with cardiogenic shock and in patients with pulmonary edema.

Yet, the pathogenesis of these two syndromes is different, as is their treatment. In pulmonary edema the main hemodynamic finding is an increase in vascular resistance superimposed on impaired left ventricular contractility, whereas in cardiogenic shock the main findings include extreme pump failure expressed by a low cardiac power output and only a modest increase in vascular resistance. Therefore, vasodilators are very effective in the treatment of pulmonary edema while usually contraindicated for cardiogenic shock.

Accordingly, this distinction should be made early by clinical, echocardiographic, and hemodynamic evaluation. As a rule, vasodilator treatment should not be administered to patients with acute heart failure and systolic blood pressure less than 100 mm Hg. In these patients the initial treatment should be based on the SHOCK study[71] and include increasing doses of intravenous inotropes, intra-aortic balloon counterpulsation, mechanical ventilation, and elimination of precipitating factors. When signs of myocardial ischemia are detected, coronary angiography followed by coronary revascularization should be attempted. Preliminary data suggest that patients not responding to these measures may benefit from administration of L-NMMA (a nitric oxide synthase inhibitor).[72,73] A large, prospective, nonrandomized study is underway to investigate this novel treatment option.

ANNOTATED REFERENCES

Arieff AI: Fatal postoperative pulmonary edema: Pathogenesis and literature review. Chest 1999;115:1371-1377.

This review showed that postoperative pulmonary edema is common and related to excessive administration of perioperative fluids.

Cotter G, Moshkovitz Y, Milovanov O, et al: Acute congestive heart failure: A novel approach to its pathogenesis and treatment. Eur J Heart Fail 2002;4:227-234.
Potential pathogenetic mechanisms of cardiovascular acute heart failure are described.

Kaluski E, Kobrin I, Zimlichman R, et al: RITZ-5: Randomized intravenous tezosentan (an endothelin ET-A/B antagonist) for the treatment of pulmonary edema: A prospective randomized, multicenter, double-blind placebo controlled study. J Am Coll Cardiol 2003;41:204-210.
Different factors important in the risk stratification of patients with acute cardiovascular pulmonary edema are discussed.

Mathay MA, Landolt CC, Staub NC: Differential liquid and protein clearance from the alveoli of anesthetized sheep. J Appl Physiol 1982;53:96-104.
Alveolar fluid is not regulated by Starling forces but rather by active Na^+ transport by alveolar cells.

Pender ES, Pollack CV Jr: Neurogenic pulmonary edema: Case reports and review. N Engl J Med 1992;10:45-51.
The pathogenesis, course, and potential treatments of neurogenic pulmonary edema are examined.

Sciscione AC, Ivester T, Largoza M, et al: Acute pulmonary edema in pregnancy. Obstet Gynecol 2003;101:511-515.
The authors discuss the incidence and pathogenesis of pregnancy-related pulmonary edema.

Section V

CARDIOVASCULAR DISORDERS

Chapter 91

HEMODYNAMIC MONITORING

A. Rhodes • R. M. Grounds • E. D. Bennett

KEY POINTS

1. Hemodynamic monitoring now plays a major role in assessing and managing critically ill patients.

2. Arterial lines provide not only a continuous systemic pressure display but also provide easy access for blood gas analysis and other laboratory tests.

3. Central venous lines provide useful information from careful interpretation of waveforms. This information is usually used to guide fluid therapy. Unfortunately there is no threshold value of central venous pressure that can differentiate patients who will respond to a fluid challenge from those who will not.

4. The pulmonary artery flotation catheter is able to measure the cardiac output, pressures in the right atrium and pulmonary arteries, and the mixed venous oxygen saturation. Modern catheters perform all of these functions on a semicontinuous basis and can also provide information about right ventricular volumes and ejection fraction.

5. Transesophageal Doppler is a relatively noninvasive technique for the rapid beat-to-beat estimation of stroke volume and cardiac output. This can generally only be used in sedated and ventilated patients.

6. Pulse contour analysis of arterial waveforms provides beat-by-beat measurement and variability of stroke volume and cardiac output. There are a variety of proprietary monitors utilizing this technology. They all need calibration against an independent and accurate method of determining cardiac output.

7. The noninvasive methods of NICO and electrical bioimpedance are not widely used, and their accuracy is still unproven.

8. All of these techniques can be used to measure cardiac output and tissue oxygenation. Their therapeutic utility depends on correct training in their use and appropriate interpretation of the data they provide. Therapeutic decisions based on data obtained from hemodynamic monitors must also take into account information obtained from physical examination and laboratory results.

9. The use of a particular method of monitoring should be adapted to the type of patient and is largely dependent on available technical expertise, cost effectiveness, and individual preference in each unit.

10. Despite widespread use of these technologies there are limited data showing clinical benefit and thus their use should be weighed against their potential disadvantages and cost.

Hemodynamic monitoring is the intermittent or continuous observation of normal or altered physiologic parameters pertaining to the circulatory system with a view to early detection of need for therapeutic intervention. It also consists in observing how the cardiovascular system responds to illness, injury, and therapeutic intervention. Invasive hemodynamic monitoring has traditionally been within the realm of the ICU or operating theater, but attempts are now being made to improve noninvasive techniques and validate their use in other clinical settings.

The techniques of hemodynamic monitoring are evolving quickly, particularly over the past few years, and will undoubtedly continue to do so in the next decade. Consequently there are a number of different types of equipment utilizing a variety of different physical principles available for use in the ICU. The use of a particular method of monitoring should be adapted to the type of patient and is largely dependent on available technical expertise, cost effectiveness, and individual preference in each unit.

The primary objective of hemodynamic monitoring is to ensure that the patient is achieving an optimal tissue perfusion and oxygen delivery while maintaining adequate mean arterial pressures. Ideally targeting such goals should lead to significant reduction in morbidity and mortality. There is now evidence to show that such interventions can lead to reduced morbidity and mortality in some critically ill patients.[1-3]

ARTERIAL PRESSURE MONITORING

Noninvasive measurement of blood pressure is one of the most widely undertaken procedures in clinical medicine. Invasive techniques are more commonly employed in intensive care patients for several reasons. Most importantly, the accuracy provided by intra-arterial lines is vital in achieving optimal mean arterial pressure in critically ill patients when they are hemodynamically unstable. In addition, continuous surveillance of arterial pressure is of paramount importance when vasoactive agents are used. Furthermore, frequent noninvasive arterial pressure monitoring adds to the discomfort of the patient. Finally, an arterial line also permits frequent blood gas measurements.

Historically, it has been relatively easy to measure pressure in the major peripheral arteries. Reliance has therefore been put on the maintenance of systemic pressure under the assumption that adequate pressure will also provide adequate flow and thus adequate tissue perfusion.

Studies in intensive care patients where the focus has been the maintenance of blood pressure have not been particularly fruitful.[1,2,4] Hypotension is usually defined as a systolic pressure less than 90 mm Hg or a mean pressure less than 65 mm Hg.[5] Most intensivists accept that pressure needs to be kept at a level that allows adequate tissue perfusion particularly of the major organs and that the maintenance of flow is paramount.

Interpretation of the changes seen in the arterial waveform in relation to changes in intrathoracic pressure can now also give information about whether the patient is likely to respond to a fluid challenge.[6-9] A greater than 10% or 12% variability of systolic pressure and/or pulse pressure caused by the positive pressure associated with peak inspiration indicates that the patient is probably hypovolemic and is likely to respond to fluid resuscitation. This is an important technologic development because occult hypovolemia is probably not uncommon in critically ill patients and if unrecognized is likely to contribute to an increase in both morbidity and mortality.

CENTRAL VENOUS PRESSURE

Central venous pressure (CVP) is the intravascular pressure in the great thoracic veins, measured relative to atmospheric pressure. It is conventionally measured at the junction of the superior vena cava and the right atrium and provides an estimate of the right atrial pressure. The CVP is normally used as a marker of volemic status or preload.

The CVP is influenced by the volume of blood in the central venous compartment and also the compliance of that compartment (Table 91-1). Starling demonstrated the relationships between CVP and cardiac output and also between the venous return and CVP.[10] By plotting the two relationships on the same set of axes it can be seen that the "ventricular

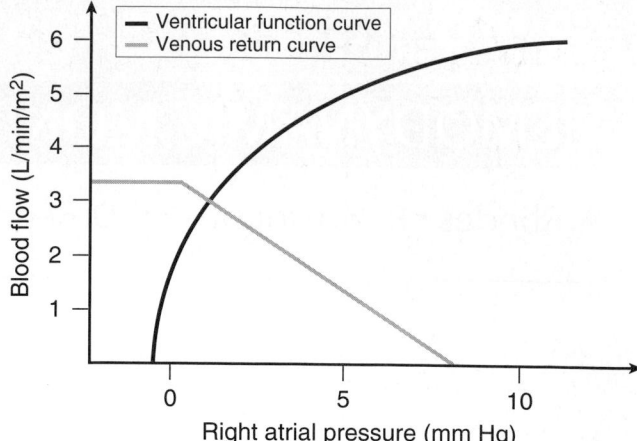

FIGURE 91–1. Ventricular function and venous return curves.

function curve" and the "venous return curve" intersect at only one point, demonstrating that if all other factors remain constant, that is, if nothing happens to alter the shape of either of the two curves, a given CVP can, at equilibrium, be associated with only one possible cardiac output and, similarly, a given cardiac output (or venous return) will, at equilibrium, be associated with a specific CVP (Fig. 91-1). Both curves can of course be affected by a number of factors: total blood volume and the distribution of that blood volume between the different vascular compartments (determined by vascular tone) will affect the venous return curve. The inotropic state of the right ventricle will affect the shape of the ventricular function curve. When any one of these factors is altered there will be an imbalance between cardiac output and venous return that will persist for a short time until a new equilibrium is reached at a new central venous blood volume and/or an altered central venous vascular tone.

The normal CVP exhibits a complex waveform as illustrated in Figure 91-2. The a wave corresponds to atrial contraction and the x descent to atrial relaxation. The c wave that punctuates the x descent is caused by the closure of the tricuspid valve at the start of ventricular systole and the bulging of its leaflets back into the atrium. The v wave is due to continued venous return in the presence of a closed tricuspid valve. The y descent occurs at the end of ventricular systole when the tricuspid valve opens and blood once again flows from the atrium into the ventricle. This normal CVP

TABLE 91–1. FACTORS AFFECTING THE MEASURED CENTRAL VENOUS PRESSURE

Central venous blood volume
- Venous return/cardiac output
- Total blood volume
- Regional vascular tone

Compliance of central compartment
- Vascular tone
- Right ventricular compliance
    Myocardial disease
    Pericardial disease
    Tamponade

Tricuspid valve disease
- Stenosis
- Regurgitation

Cardiac rhythm
- Junctional rhythm
- Atrial fibrillation
- Atrioventricular dissociation

Reference level of transducer
- Positioning of patient

Intrathoracic pressure
- Respiration
- Intermittent positive-pressure ventilation
- Positive end-expiratory pressure
- Tension pneumothorax

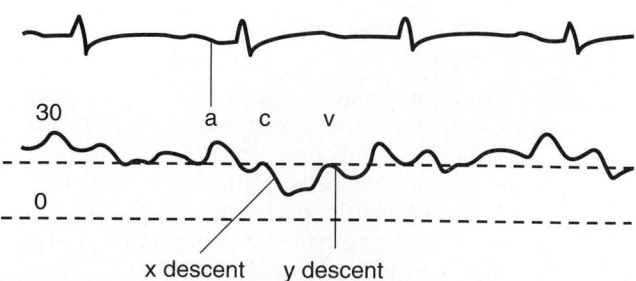

FIGURE 91–2. Central venous pressure waveform. Central venous pressure waveform from a ventilated patient *(bottom)* with time-synchronized electrocardiogram (ECG) trace *(top)*. The a wave represents atrial contraction and occurs immediately after atrial depolarization as represented by the p wave on the ECG. The c wave represents bulging of the tricuspid valve in early ventricular systole and is followed by the v wave, caused by atrial filling during ventricular systole.

TABLE 91–2. DISEASE STATES THAT MODIFY THE CENTRAL VENOUS PRESSURE WAVEFORM

- In atrial fibrillation the a wave is lost and the c wave may become more prominent.
- In the presence of atrioventricular dissociation or junctional rhythm when atrial contraction may occur during ventricular systole, extremely tall cannon a waves occur due to atrial contraction against a closed tricuspid valve.
- In tricuspid regurgitation blood is ejected backward during ventricular systole from the right ventricle into the right atrium. This produces a large fused c-v wave on the central venous pressure trace.
- In tricuspid stenosis, forward movement of blood from the right atrium into the ventricle occurs against a greater than normal resistance leading to an accentuated a wave and an attenuated y descent.
- Similarly, if right ventricular compliance is decreased by either myocardial or pericardial disease the a wave will be accentuated.
- With pericardial constriction a short steep y descent will also be seen that allows differentiation from cardiac tamponade where the central venous pressure will be monophasic with a single x descent.

TABLE 91–3. PARAMETERS MEASURED USING THE PULMONARY ARTERY CATHETER

- Pulmonary artery pressure
- Central venous pressure
- Cardiac output
- Pulmonary artery saturation
- Mixed venous oxygen saturation
- Core temperature

waveform may be modified by a number of pathologic processes (Table 91-2).

If the CVP is to be used as an index of cardiac preload, the end-diastolic pressure at end expiration must be identified. The c wave marks the closure of the tricuspid valve at the beginning of ventricular systole, and immediately before its onset the measured pressure should be equivalent to the right ventricular end-diastolic pressure (except in the case of tricuspid stenosis in which a pressure gradient will always exist between the two chambers). Where no c wave is clearly visible it is conventional to take the average pressure during the a wave. Where no a wave is visible (e.g., in atrial fibrillation) the pressure at the Z point (that point on the CVP waveform that corresponds with the end of the QRS complex on the electrocardiogram) should be used.

Taking all these factors into account, it is perhaps not surprising that the CVP will not provide a reliable estimate of preload in critically ill patients. The CVP correlates poorly with overall volemic status, right ventricular end-diastolic volume, stroke index, or an individual patient's response to a fluid challenge.[11] It is perhaps best used in non–critically ill patients when it can provide an estimate of the components to right ventricular filling and venous return and therefore can be used to guide fluid challenges by following the trend changes in the variable.

THE PULMONARY ARTERY CATHETER

Continuous, reliable, and accurate pressure and flow monitoring of cardiac performance helps in the early initiation of appropriate therapy toward precise hemodynamic goals. The pulmonary artery catheter with its measured and derived parameters (Tables 91-3 and 91-4) helps to direct therapy in the critically ill who balance their physiology precariously. The first double-lumen, balloon-tipped, flow-directed catheter was designed by Swan and Ganz in 1970.[12] Thereafter, there have been several modifications to the pulmonary artery catheter, which now enables the continuous monitoring of cardiac output from a thermodilution technique, of intravascular pressures, and of mixed venous oxygen saturation.

The pulmonary artery catheter is used to gain a comprehensive overview of the circulation. Information can be obtained about the preload, contractility, and afterload of the heart. Modern pulmonary artery catheters also measure the mixed venous oxygen saturation, enabling the clinician to make a judgment about the balance between the oxygen supply and demand. With this information, therapy can be tailored to the individual patient's requirements.

Once correctly positioned, the balloon tip is inflated temporarily occluding the pulmonary artery. Transducing the catheter port just distal to the balloon provides the pulmonary capillary occlusion pressure. The pressure in the left atrium becomes the main determinant of pressure distal to the inflated balloon because a static column of blood links the two points across the pulmonary capillary bed. This occlusion pressure therefore can provide an estimate of left ventricular preload. The accurate recognition of the waveform indicating the occlusion pressure is vital; however, the ability of clinicians to recognize this waveform is poor.[13-15] The catheter must be in the correct position and the point at the end of expiration must be identified to exclude interference from extravascular intrathoracic pressures.

For the pulmonary capillary occlusion pressure to give an accurate estimation of left ventricular preload, a number of criteria must be met:

- No impedance to flow across the pulmonary capillary beds
- No disease of the mitral valve
- A linear relationship between pressure and volume (compliance) in the left ventricle

Many of these criteria are not valid in the critically ill and thus much like with the CVP the pulmonary capillary occlusion pressure represents only a poor marker of systemic preload.

The appropriate use of the pulmonary artery catheter relies on the user achieving an adequate level of cardiac output for any given situation. The cardiac output can be increased by increasing the preload of the heart titrated from the pulmonary artery occlusion pressure (Table 91-5) and then by manipulation of either the right ventricular or left ventricular afterload. The adequacy of the cardiac output can be assessed in relationship to the body's overall energy balance by a coordinated assessment of cardiac output and mixed venous oxygen saturation.

TABLE 91–4. PARAMETERS CALCULATED USING THE PULMONARY ARTERY CATHETER

- Systemic vascular resistance
- Stroke volume
- Oxygen delivery
- Oxygen consumption
- Pulmonary vascular resistance
- Left ventricular stroke work index
- Right ventricular stroke work index

TABLE 91–5. NORMAL VALUES OF CARDIAC PRESSURES OBTAINED FROM A PULMONARY ARTERY CATHETER IN A SPONTANEOUSLY BREATHING PATIENT

	Mean (mm Hg)	Range (mm Hg)
Right atrium	4	3-6
Right ventricle		
Systolic	25	20-30
Diastolic	4	2-8
Pulmonary artery		
Systolic	25	20-30
Diastolic	10	5-15
Mean	15	10-20
Pulmonary artery occlusion pressure	10	5-14

The mixed venous oxygen saturation is the venous saturation of oxygen in the pulmonary artery. It enables a quantification to be made of the overall oxygen extraction of the blood. The normal value for this is in the region of 70% to 75%. Any decrease in this variable is due to either a decrease in oxygen delivery or an increase in oxygen utilization. A thorough understanding of the factors that derive these variables therefore enables a complete understanding of the circulatory dysfunction for any given patient.

In recent years use of the pulmonary artery catheter has been surrounded by controversy (Table 91-6) after the publication of a large observational study linking it with a poor outcome.[16] It is still unclear whether the catheter itself is responsible for the decreased survival rate seen in this study or whether the patients who were treated with the use of this tool were in fact sicker[17] or the measurements obtained by the clinicians were not accurate enough to appropriately guide therapy. The one fact that is now incontrovertible is that the appropriate use of the variables measured from the pulmonary artery catheter is the single most important fact. Unfortunately, there is often little consensus as to how to use these variables and, therefore, the controversy still exists.

PULSE CONTOUR ANALYSIS

Analysis of the arterial pulse wave contour obtained from an intra-arterial line can provide a great deal of information over and above just the value for arterial pressure. This has led to the development of technologies for the continuous monitoring of cardiac output obtained by analyzing the pulse

TABLE 91–6. COMPLICATIONS ASSOCIATED WITH THE PULMONARY ARTERY CATHETER

Complications Associated with Catheter Insertion	
Minor arrhythmias	48%
Sustained arrhythmias	Uncommon
Arterial puncture	1%
Pneumothorax	1%

Complications When Catheter Is in Place	
Infection of insertion site	0-22%
Catheter-related sepsis	2%
Mural thrombus	28-61%
Pulmonary infarction	0.1-7%
Rupture of pulmonary artery	<0.1%
Death	<0.1%

wave contour obtained from intra-arterial catheters placed in either the radial or femoral arteries.

Arterial pulse contour analysis is a technique of measuring and monitoring stroke volume on a beat-to-beat basis from the arterial pulse pressure waveform. This has several advantages over existing technologies, because the majority of critically ill patients already have arterial pressure lines transduced, allowing the technique to rapidly monitor changes in stroke volume and cardiac output on an almost continuous basis.

The fluctuations of blood pressure around a mean value are caused by the volume of blood (the stroke volume) forced into the arterial conduit by each systole.[18] The magnitude of this change in pressure—known as the pulse pressure—is a function of the magnitude of the stroke volume.

A number of factors exist that have made the transition of this concept into clinical reality technically challenging:

- The compliance of the aorta is not a linear relationship between pressure and volume. This nonlinearity prevents any simple approach for estimating volumes from the pressure change. There needs to be correction for this nonlinearity for any individual patient.[19]
- Wave reflection. The pulse pressure measured from an arterial trace is actually the combination of an incident pressure wave ejected from the heart and a reflected pressure wave from the periphery. To calculate the stroke volume, these two waves have to be recognized and separated. This is further complicated by the fact that the reflected waves change in size depending on the proximity of the sampling site to the heart and also the patient's age.
- Damping. As the change in pressure around a mean value describes the stroke volume, accurate pressure measurements are imperative. Unfortunately, pressure transducer systems used in routine clinical practice often suffer from being either underdamped or overdamped, leading to imperfect waveforms and measurements.
- Aortic flow during systole. Although the filling of the aorta is on an intermittent pulsatile basis, the outflow tends to be more continuous.

Despite these limitations a number of companies have developed systems to measure stroke volume from pulse contour techniques. Each of these companies has had to develop methods of calibrating the pulse contour changes for these factors on individual patients. This has been achieved with either transpulmonary thermodilution (PiCCO)[20] or lithium dilution (LiDCO)[21] methods. Whichever method is utilized, there is good clinical precision and accuracy demonstrated in a number of studies when compared with pulmonary artery catheterization.[22-24]

ESOPHAGEAL DOPPLER

The 19th century physicist Christian Doppler described the effect that bears his name, demonstrating that the frequency of signal transmitted toward or reflected from a moving object is altered proportionally to the velocity of the object. This observation has been widely used for measuring the speed of moving objects ranging from stars to cars to red blood cells.

Transcutaneous Doppler ultrasound is in general clinical use for measuring blood velocity in both peripheral and central veins and arteries. In the past 10 years or so the technology has been further developed to measure blood velocity in the descending aorta from which cardiac output can be calculated. The two most commonly used commercially systems both use a flexible probe, which is inserted down into the esophagus to a length of approximately 40 cm from the mouth.

One system (Deltex CardioQ[25]) has a piezoelectric crystal mounted at 45 degrees on the tip of the disposable probe, which produces ultrasound at a continuous frequency of 4 MHz. The probe tip is adjusted to lie in the esophagus at a point alongside the descending aorta. The ultrasonic beam is transmitted into the lumen of the aorta insonating the moving red cells. Some of the ultrasound is reflected back to the crystal at a frequency proportional to the velocity of the moving red cells.

This shifted frequency is converted to a velocity using the Doppler equation:

$$V = f \times C/(2 \times Fo \times cosQ)$$

where V = velocity of blood in cm/sec, f = Doppler shifted frequency, Fo = transmitted frequency, C = acoustic velocity in blood, and Q = angle of Doppler beam to blood vessel.

The velocity of the red blood cells thus obtained is converted to flow using a propriety algorithm, which assumes the cross-sectional diameter of the descending aorta based on a number of factors including age, gender, height, and weight. Because this measurement is made on the descending aorta it does not take into account flow to head and arms, which is assumed to be a constant 30% of the total cardiac output. Beat-by-beat values for cardiac output and stroke volume are calculated, and these values have been shown to correlate well with cardiac output measured by thermodilution.[25]

In contrast, the other commercially available product (Arrow Hemosonics[26]) uses a nondisposable probe over which is placed a disposable sheath; the whole device is then inserted into the esophagus. The pulsed Doppler transducer measures descending aortic red blood cell velocity. This is converted to flow by the continuous measurement of descending aortic diameter, which is obtained from an M mode echo signal provided by a separate transducer incorporated in the probe. Good correlation with independent measurements of cardiac output have also been obtained with this device. This technique allows cardiac output and stroke volume to be measured rapidly and relatively noninvasively and requires less training than required for use of the pulmonary artery catheter.

NICO HEMODYNAMIC MONITORING

The Novametrix noninvasive cardiac output monitor (NICO) measures cardiac output–based changes in respiratory CO_2 concentration caused by a brief period of rebreathing.[27] The measurement of cardiac output is accomplished by interpreting data collected by proprietary sensors that measure flow, airway pressure, and CO_2 concentration and then combining these signals to calculate CO_2 elimination. Using these variables, a technique known as Fick partial rebreathing is applied to calculate cardiac output. NICO can only be used effectively with mechanically ventilated patients in the operating room, ICU, or emergency department.

Potentially this device provides a completely noninvasive measurement of cardiac output. Its accuracy and reliability in critically ill patients is not yet proved, however, because clinical validation studies are not yet complete.[28]

ELECTRICAL IMPEDANCE CARDIOGRAPHY TECHNOLOGY

Electrical impedance cardiography technology measures the basal chest electrical impedance or resistance to flow in ohms.[29] The change of impedance across the chest wall is related to the change of flow of blood throughout the chest cavity. The impedance dz/dt (dz = change in impedance, dt = change in time) is produced by change in blood flow and volumes in the ascending aorta.

In devices using baseline impedance, large amounts of thoracic fluid such as in severe pulmonary edema may interfere with the impedance signal and dampen the waveform. The latest methods are baseline impedance independent. They provide continuous trend of heart rate and stroke volume and give derived cardiac output and index using stroke waveform morphology. Recent models of electrical impedance cardiography use advanced waveform morphology analysis to measure a filling index, the trend of which may be useful in monitoring response to therapy. Unfortunately, in view of its major limitations, its reliability in critically ill patients is very limited.

CONCLUSION

There are a number of different technologies for measuring cardiac performance. The simplest and most reliable of these are measurements of pressure. Measurements of flow and other variables of cardiac performance are more complex and less reliable. Individual clinicians must choose the appropriate parameters to measure and be aware of the various limitations of the measuring techniques. It is becoming clear that with the ability to measure the performance of individual parts of the cardiovascular system we are able to target therapy much more specifically, and there are a number of studies suggesting that selectively targeted therapy improves outcome.

ANNOTATED REFERENCES

Boyd O, Grounds RM, Bennett ED: A randomized clinical trial of the effect of deliberate perioperative increase of oxygen delivery on mortality in high-risk surgical patients. JAMA 1993;270:2699-2707.

Important trial that demonstrated that perioperative increase of oxygen delivery with dopexamine hydrochloride significantly reduces mortality and morbidity in high-risk surgical patients.

Connors AF Jr, Speroff T, Dawson NV, et al: The effectiveness of right heart catheterization in the initial care of critically ill patients. SUPPORT Investigators. JAMA 1996;276:889-897.

This prospective cohort study examined the association between the use of right heart catheterization (RHC) during the first 24 hours of care in the ICU and subsequent survival, length of stay, and intensity and cost of care in >5000 critically ill adult patients. The findings suggest that RHC was associated with increased mortality and increased utilization of resources.

Rhodes A, Cusack RJ, Newman PJ, et al: A randomised, controlled trial of the pulmonary artery catheter in critically ill patients. Intensive Care Med 2002;28:256-264.

This study compared the survival and clinical outcomes of critically ill adult patients treated with the use of a pulmonary artery catheter (PAC) to those treated without the use of a PAC. Their results suggest that the PAC is not associated with an increased mortality.

Chapter 92

ACUTE CORONARY SYNDROMES: PATHOPHYSIOLOGY AND DIAGNOSIS

William J. Brady • Chris A. Ghaemmaghami • Anna Baer • Andrew D. Perron

---

KEY POINTS

1. The electrocardiogram (ECG) is diagnostic for acute myocardial infarction (AMI) in only 50% of patients ultimately diagnosed with acute infarction. The remainder of these AMI patients demonstrate normal, nonspecifically abnormal, and confounding patterns.

2. Serum markers of myocardial injury are of value in ruling out myocardial infarction only when used in serial fashion. In most cases, isolated determinations are of little clinical value.

3. Echocardiography is a valuable tool in the AMI patient, enabling not only the determination of the diagnosis but also an assessment of current function and possible complication.

4. Atypical presentations of AMI are seen in up to 30% of infarct patients. The rate of atypical presentation is highest among the very elderly in whom mental status change, syncope, and other nonspecific symptom-sign complexes are seen.

5. The simultaneous presence of ST segment elevation and pathologic Q wave in the chest pain patient suspected of having AMI does not preclude the consideration for acute reperfusion therapies. Q waves can appear as early as 2 hours after the onset of AMI.

Angina pectoris was recognized in the 18th century; myocardial infarction (MI), however, was described approximately 200 years later. Simultaneous to the identification of MI was the initial introduction and subsequent application of the electrocardiogram (ECG)—the first objective method of assessing the coronary origin of the presentation. Over the next 50 years, angina pectoris and MI were further characterized and diagnosed; unfortunately, however, the management of ischemic heart disease did not progress as significantly. From this point in medical history until the 1960s, management consisted primarily of pain relief coupled with strict bed rest for prolonged periods and management of resultant congestive heart failure (CHF); acute complications such as cardiogenic shock and sudden cardiac death were invariably fatal events. Subsequently, the introduction and widespread use of cardiopulmonary resuscitation, external defibrillation, and antidysrhythmic agents gave the

clinician a powerful tool in the management of sudden cardiac death and other malignant dysrhythmias. Overall management, however, was still aimed at the complications of ischemic heart disease rather than the syndrome itself.

With the recognition of the thrombotic nature of the acute coronary syndrome within the last several decades, the stage was set for the next most significant advance in the management of the more acute forms of ischemic heart disease, namely acute myocardial infarction (AMI). Early coronary angiography coupled with intra-arterial administration of streptokinase ushered in the era of acute reperfusion therapies, certainly the most significant advancement in the recent past. Clinicians were now able not only to treat the acute complications of the illness but also to interrupt, if not halt, the primary process, thereby markedly reducing morbidity and mortality.

EPIDEMIOLOGY

In the last decade, approximately 3.5 million people were admitted to the hospital with heart disease. Approximately 20% of these patients had AMI. Myocardial infarction occurs most often in patients over age 40 years. Based on 1989 statistics, an estimated 6.2 million Americans have significant coronary artery disease. Many of these people are at increased risk for sudden death or AMI. Approximately two thirds of sudden deaths from coronary artery disease take place outside the hospital and usually occur within 2 hours after onset of symptoms.

Ischemic heart disease, particularly the acute forms of the illness, is the leading cause of death for adults in the United States today; approximately 50% of these deaths result from sudden cardiac death. Fifteen percent of the fatalities occur prior to age 65 years, with the majority in women. Interestingly, a marked drop in the rate of mortality from ischemic heart disease has been reported over the past 5 decades in the United States, likely resulting from an overall reduction in the incidence of AMI as well as a pronounced decline in the case-fatality rate of established MI.[1,2]

PATHOPHYSIOLOGY

Ischemic heart disease describes the entire spectrum of illness, ranging from acute to chronic entities, related to coronary artery disease, including angina pectoris, AMI, cardiomyopathy, and malignant dysrhythmia. Acute coronary syndromes, an important subset of ischemic heart disease, are defined as unstable angina and AMI. AMI is defined as myocardial necrosis. Consideration for the diagnosis of AMI requires two of the following three World Health Organization criteria: history of chest pain or equivalent, ECG change, or positive result on serum testing.[3] In the past, AMI was separated into Q wave (transmural) and non-Q wave (nontransmural) events. Recent opinion, however, has suggested that these descriptors fail to adequately describe the event, and the use of the terms ST segment elevation MI and non-ST segment elevation MI is urged.

In the ST segment elevation MI scenario, the patient's symptom presentation and diagnostic ECG provide the criteria for immediate diagnosis; a serum marker will ultimately become positive in the subsequent hours after onset. The non-ST segment elevation MI diagnosis is founded not only on the patient's clinical history and abnormal ECG but also on a positive serum marker. The actual pattern of serum marker abnormality has now become an important component of the definition of AMI. A sudden, marked increase in the serum troponin value that is not sustained over time (i.e., a clear peak in the serum concentration is found) is the first component of this pattern; this increase is then associated with a gradual decrease in the level over the next 7 to 10 days.[4] Importantly, no specific serum troponin value—either relative or absolute—is included in this description. Such elevations in the serum marker would, of course, require an association with a clinical event consistent with acute coronary syndrome, including evolutionary ECG changes. Furthermore, a minor elevation that is sustained over time, again not defined numerically, is not included in the definition as AMI; this scenario likely addresses the noncoronary elevation certain patients may exhibit. Non-ST segment elevation MI and ST segment elevation MI more appropriately describe the process with regard to the clinical presentation, underlying pathophysiology, urgent management considerations, and outcome.

The two primary intracoronary pathophysiologic events underlying the development of acute coronary syndrome include thrombus formation and vasospasm. The acute formation of thrombus within the coronary artery is considered a fundamental component in all forms of acute coronary syndrome. In the setting of either a structurally normal artery or preexisting coronary artery disease, initial endothelial damage produces platelet aggregation and resultant thrombus formation; in most cases, disruption of an atherosclerotic plaque provides the endothelial injury. Occlusion of the coronary artery then results, ranging from minimal, transient, asymptomatic obstruction to complete occlusion with prominent symptomatology—namely AMI. Coronary artery obstruction can lead to myocardial ischemia, hypoxia, acidosis, and ultimately MI.

In most instances of acute coronary syndrome, coronary vasospasm is also noted. The spasm results from both local and systemic events. Local vasoactive substances are released; autonomic nervous system stimulation increases with the proliferation of alpha-receptors; and endogenous sympathomimetic hormones such as epinephrine and serotonin are discharged into circulation—all culminating in coronary artery vasospasm and worsened myocardial perfusion. Coronary artery spasm with subsequent thrombus formation and without significant underlying coronary artery disease is involved in approximately 10% of cases of AMI.

Further myocardial injury at the cellular level occurs during the reperfusion phase, either by spontaneous or by therapeutically induced fibrinolysis. In particular, the introduction of calcium, oxygen, and cellular elements into ischemic myocardium can lead to irreversible myocardial damage that causes reperfusion injury, prolonged ventricular dysfunction (known as myocardial stunning), or reperfusion dysrhythmias. Neutrophils probably play an important role in reperfusion injury, occluding capillary lumens, decreasing blood flow, accelerating the inflammatory response, and resulting in the production of chemoattractants, proteolytic enzymes, and reactive oxygen species.

Additional issues to consider in the pathophysiology of AMI focus on initial, primary illness or concurrent medical events. Such considerations obviously have significant potential for impact on additional diagnostic and therapeutic issues; these presentations are reasonably likely in the undifferentiated, ill critical care patient. The patient with shock of varying cause may experience AMI due to the physiologic insult placed on the heart. For instance, the patient with distributive shock resulting from urosepsis or the patient with hypovolemic shock due to gastrointestinal hemorrhage may experience either non-ST segment elevation or ST segment elevation AMI. Furthermore, metabolic poisons such as cyanide, carbon monoxide, and hydrogen sulfide can disrupt myocardial cellular function, resulting in acute coronary syndrome.

CLINICAL FEATURES

THE HISTORY

The history—and the clinician's interpretation of the available history—is vital. In the critical care unit, however, the patient may be unable to offer a thorough history because of either active illness or instrumentation such as endotracheal intubation. If available, an appropriate history will enable the clinician to focus the evaluation, provide adequate therapies, secure a safe disposition, and minimize the need for additional investigations.

Angina pectoris, the chest pain associated with acute coronary syndrome, by definition includes a sense of choking, strangulation, or constriction. Common descriptions of the discomfort include not only pain but also pressure, squeezing, fullness, or heaviness. In some patients, the symptoms are perceived as gastrointestinal. The location for angina is substernal and left chest with radiation to the shoulders, arms, neck, or jaw. Patients with AMI, however, may also present with pain in the right chest. The duration of chest pain is valuable in determining its cause. Angina pectoris generally is short-lived, lasting less than 15 minutes. Patients with AMI usually experience more than 30 minutes of chest pain. Intermittent, sharp, localized chest discomfort lasting less than several seconds usually is not due to ACS. The symptoms of angina pectoris improve dramatically within 2 to 5 minutes after rest or nitroglycerin. If the pain persists for more than 10 minutes, the diagnosis of acute coronary syndrome or a noncardiac origin should be considered. Caution is also advised in the chest pain patient who appears to respond to antacid; over-reliance on this response as a major decision point in "ruling out" acute coronary syndrome is not encouraged. Many AMI patients experience associated symptoms such as dyspnea, diaphoresis, nausea, vomiting, dizziness, and anxiety; these various symptoms may be the primary complaint in patients presenting with AMI.

Risk factors that increase the likelihood for atherosclerosis and AMI—male gender, family history, cigarette smoking, hypertension, hypercholesterolemia, and diabetes mellitus—should be sought. Personal habits such as cigarette smoking and use of illicit drugs, particularly sympathomimetic substances such as cocaine, should be reviewed. Artificial or early menopause and the use of contraceptive pills may increase the likelihood of ischemic heart disease in women. If a patient has a history of coronary artery disease, a risk factor analysis is unwarranted because the risk of coronary artery disease is 100%.

There has been disagreement over whether these coronary risk factors should be considered in the clinician's medical decision-making. An early report[5] suggested that such factors, which were initially derived because of their ability to predict the development of coronary atherosclerosis and its complications over decades in association with other clinical variables such as ECG interpretation, have minimal predictive value acutely as to whether a patient is currently experiencing an AMI. More contemporary investigation in possible ACS patients suggests that the coronary risk factors, in fact, do have significant predictive value.[6]

Because angina is a visceral sensation that is often diffuse, some patients may have an anginal equivalent syndrome. Such anginal equivalent presentations describe patients who are experiencing acute coronary syndrome yet do not complain of typical chest pain; rather, these patients note atypical pain, dyspnea, weakness, diaphoresis, or emesis—these complaints, in fact, are the manifestation of the acute coronary syndrome event. Patients with altered cardiac pain perception (e.g., the elderly or patients with long-standing diabetes mellitus) are potentially at risk to present with anginal equivalent syndromes. A recent large survey of 434,877 confirmed AMI patients reported that a significant minority of these individuals—approximately 30%—lacked chest pain on presentation, noting only the anginal equivalent complaints.[7] The most frequently encountered anginal equivalent chief complaint is dyspnea, which is found in 10% to 30% of patients with AMI, often due to pulmonary edema.[7-9] Isolated emesis and diaphoresis are quite rare.[8,9]

The geriatric patient may also present atypically with acute weakness (3-8%) and syncope (3-5%).[10] Unexplained sinus tachycardia, bronchospasm resulting from cardiogenic asthma, and new-onset lower extremity edema have all been reported as anginal equivalent presentations for AMI in this age group. Among the very elderly, anginal equivalent syndromes typically involve neurologic presentations with acute mental status abnormalities and stroke. From the perspective of acute delirium, less than 1% of such patients in an emergency department population with altered mentation will be found to have AMI. AMI associated with acute stroke is noted in approximately 5% to 9% of patients.[10]

PHYSICAL EXAMINATION

The physical examination, although crucial to many life-threatening disease processes, is often not helpful in diagnosing AMI; AMI may be suggested, however, in the patient with obvious cardiac dysfunction, manifested by acute pulmonary edema or cardiogenic shock, or both. A change in mental status, poor peripheral perfusion, pronounced tachycardia, hypotension, diaphoresis, rales, jugular venous distension, and S3 and S4 heart sounds often provide evidence of significant myocardial dysfunction in patients with AMI. Patients with evidence of myocardial dysfunction, including S3 heart sound, S4 heart sound, or rales, on initial presentation are at much greater risk for adverse cardiovascular events, including nonfatal AMI, death, stroke, life-threatening dysrhythmia, and the requirement for cardiac surgery.

Caution should be exercised when attributing a chest wall source for pain based on palpation or movement. To safely relate the chest discomfort to a chest wall origin, the pain must be described as sharp or stabbing (i.e., pleuritic in nature) and be completely reproducible by palpation.[11] Up to 15% of patients with AMI may have some form of tenderness on chest wall palpation.[12]

DIAGNOSTIC STRATEGIES

ELECTROCARDIOGRAM

The ECG is used to establish the diagnosis of AMI or other noncoronary ailment, select appropriate therapy, determine the response to treatments, determine the correct in-patient disposition location, and predict risk of both cardiovascular complication and death. The ECG is an extremely powerful diagnostic study, which, if used in appropriate fashion, can guide the clinician in the evaluation of the chest pain patient suspected of AMI. An understanding of its shortcomings, however, in this application will only improve its use. From the perspective of the ECG diagnosis of AMI, the ECG has numerous shortcomings, including the "normal" and "nondiagnostic" interpretations, evolving AMI patterns, the non-ST segment elevation MI ECG presentation, confounding and mimicking patterns, and the isolated acute posterior wall AMI.

The ECG may manifest a range of ECG abnormalities (Fig. 92-1) in the patient with potential AMI, including the prominent T wave, T wave inversion, ST segment depression, ST segment elevation, and QA waves, among other findings. The earliest ECG finding resulting from ST segment elevation MI is the hyperacute T wave, which may appear minutes after the interruption of blood flow; the R wave also increases in amplitude at this stage. The hyperacute T wave, a short-lived structure that evolves rapidly on to ST segment elevation over a 5- to 30-minute period, is often asymmetric with a broad base; these T waves are also associated not infrequently with reciprocal ST segment depression in other ECG leads. Such a finding on the ECG is transient in the AMI patient; either apparent or progressive ST segment elevation is usually encountered at this stage. As the infarction progresses, the hyperacute T wave evolves into the giant R wave, particularly in the anterior wall AMI. The giant R wave is a transition structure from the hyperacute T wave to typical ST segment elevation; it essentially is a large monophasic R wave with pronounced ST segment elevation. Prominent T waves may be seen in patients with AMI as well as hyperkalemia, acute myopericarditis, benign early repolarization, left ventricular hypertrophy, and bundle branch block.

Within moments, the ST segment assumes a more easily recognized morphology. In approximately 85% of ST segment elevation MI patients, the initial upsloping portion of the ST segment is either convex or flat; if the ST segment is flat, it may be either horizontally or obliquely so. An analysis of the ST segment waveform can be particularly helpful in distinguishing

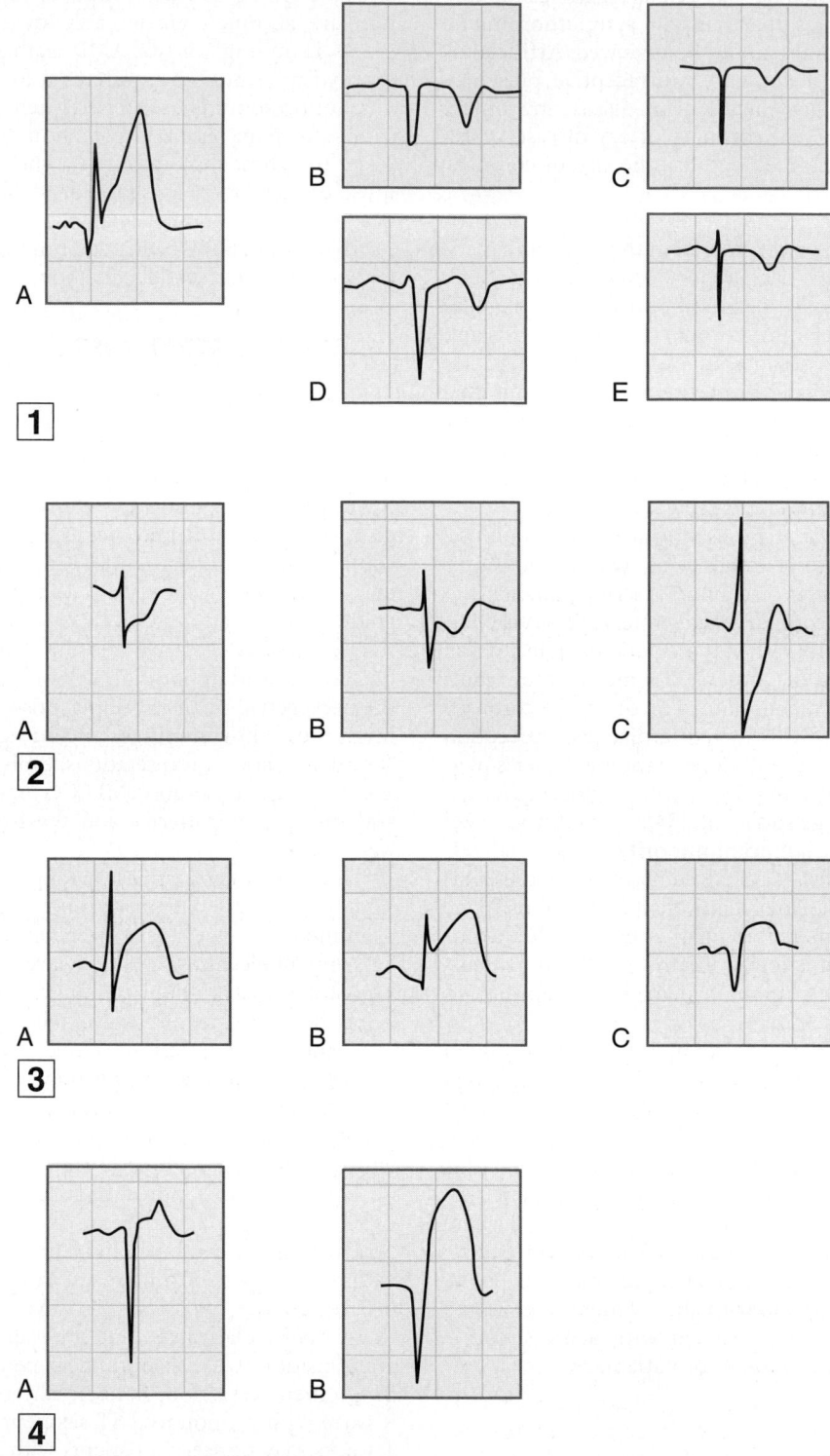

FIGURE 92–1. Electrocardiographic findings of acute myocardial infarction (AMI): **(1)** T wave abnormalities of AMI. **A.** Prominent, "hyperacute," T wave. **B-E.** T wave inversions of non-ST segment elevation MI. **(2)** ST segment depression. **A.** Flat. **B.** Downsloping. **C.** Upsloping. **(3)** ST segment elevation. **A.** Convex ST segment elevation. **B.** Obliquely straight ST segment elevation. **C.** Convex ST segment elevation. **(4)** Pathologic Q waves. **A.** Pathologic Q wave of completed myocardial infarction. **B.** Simultaneous ST segment elevation with pathologic Q wave 2 hours into the course of ST segment elevation MI.

among the various causes of ST segment elevation and identifying the AMI case. This technique uses the morphology of the initial portion of the ST segment/T wave—defined as beginning at the J point and ending at the apex of the T wave. Patients with noninfarctional ST segment elevation (i.e., early repolarization or left ventricular hypertrophy-related change) tend to have a concave morphology of the waveform. Conversely, patients with ST segment elevation due to AMI have either obliquely flat or convex waveforms. The use of this ST segment elevation waveform analysis in emergency room chest pain patients increases the specificity for the AMI diagnosis.[14] This morphologic observation should be used only as a guideline. As with most guidelines, it is not infallible.

Significant ST segment elevation occurring in at least two anatomically oriented leads is the primary ECG indication for fibrinolysis or urgent PCI. In that ST segment elevation represents a significant finding, a brief review of the various causes of ST segment elevation in the chest pain patient is warranted. Unfortunately, ST segment elevation in the chest pain patient less often results from AMI; in fact, only 20% to 30% of chest pain patients will have ST segment elevation MI—the remainder of these patients will have noninfarctional causes of the ST segment elevation.[14,15] Patients with chest pain may present electrocardiographically with ST segment elevation due to AMI, confounding patterns, or masquerading syndromes. In most instances, ST segment elevation resulting from AMI is easily noted. Confounding patterns such as left bundle branch block, ventricular paced rhythms, and left ventricular hypertrophy may obscure the typical ECG findings of AMI as well as produce noninfarctional ST segment elevation, which may lead the uninformed clinician astray. Other ST segment elevation patterns, including benign early repolarization and acute pericarditis, occur in the individual with chest discomfort and may suggest the incorrect diagnosis of AMI, exposing the patient to unnecessary and potentially dangerous therapies.

ST segment depression is generally considered to represent subendocardial, noninfarctional ischemia, although it may be the presenting ECG finding in the non-ST segment elevation MI patient. The morphology of subendocardial ischemic ST segment depression is classically horizontal or downsloping; upsloping ST segment depression is also seen, yet is less often associated with acute ischemia. With subendocardial ischemia, the ST segment depression is often diffuse and can be located in both the anterior and the inferior leads. ST segment depression also occurs as the primary ECG finding in non-ST segment elevation MI as well as a secondary, though important, manifestation in ST segment elevation MI, namely reciprocal ST segment depression; also, ST segment depression in the right precordial leads may represent posterior wall AMI. Nonischemic causes of ST segment depression include digoxin effect and repolarization changes seen in left ventricular hypertrophy, bundle branch block, and ventricular paced rhythm presentations.

Reciprocal ST segment depression, also known as reciprocal change, is defined as ST segment depression in leads separate and distinct from leads reflecting ST segment elevation. Importantly, this form of ST segment depression is not associated with situations in which altered intraventricular conduction produces deviation—such as bundle branch block, left ventricular hypertrophy, and ventricular paced rhythms. Reciprocal change in the setting of a ST segment elevation MI identifies a patient with an increased chance of poor outcome and, therefore, an individual who may benefit

from a more aggressive approach. Furthermore, its presence on the ECG supports the diagnosis of AMI with very high sensitivity and positive predictive values greater than 90%. The use of reciprocal change in both prehospital and emergency room chest pain patients increases the diagnostic accuracy in the ECG recognition of AMI.[16,17] Reciprocal change is seen in approximately 75% of cases of inferior wall AMI and much less often in cases of anterior wall MI (30%).

Inverted T waves produced by acute coronary syndrome are classically narrow and symmetric; they are morphologically characterized by an isoelectric ST segment that is usually bowed upward (i.e., concave) and followed by a sharp symmetric downstroke. The terms *coronary T wave* and *coved T wave* have been used to describe these T wave inversions. Prominent, deeply inverted, and widely splayed T waves are more characteristic of the noninfarctional, nonischemic conditions such as cerebrovascular accident. An important subgroup of patients with noninfarctional angina often have deep T wave inversions in the precordial leads (V1 through V4); the T wave may also be biphasic in this same distribution. The syndrome, termed the left anterior descending T wave or Wellen syndrome, is important to recognize because it is highly specific for stenosis of the left anterior descending coronary artery with anterior wall AMI as the natural history. T wave inversion can also be caused by non-ST segment elevation MI and evolving states of ST segment elevation MI.

In general, Q waves represent established myocardial necrosis and rarely are the primary finding in the AMI patient. Pathologic Q waves may be caused by a previously unrecognized prior infarction, or conversely, a prior MI may mask ischemic extension in the same anatomic location. Q waves usually develop within 8 to 12 hours after a transmural AMI, yet they can be noted as early as 1 to 2 hours after the onset of complete coronary occlusion. As such, the simultaneous presence of Q waves and ST segment elevation does not preclude consideration of fibrinolytic therapy.

The ECG changes discussed previously may all be encountered in the AMI patient. Two basic ECG presentations of AMI, the ST segment elevation MI and non-ST segment elevation MI, warrant further comment. The ST segment elevation MI presents with ST segment elevation in at least two anatomically contiguous leads—a reasonably straightforward principle. On the contrary, the non-ST segment elevation MI can manifest with a range of ECG abnormalities, representing a diagnostic challenge and a potential failing of the ECG. Patients with non-ST segment elevation MI may present with obvious abnormality, such as ST segment depression or T wave abnormalities; these findings can be transient. In these cases, symmetric convex downward ST segment depression or inverted or biphasic T waves are characteristically seen. Alternatively, the ECG may only reveal nonspecific findings or appear initially normal. Lastly, the non-ST segment elevation MI patient may demonstrate only a confounding pattern such as left bundle branch block. Regardless of the non-ST segment elevation presentation, the non-ST segment elevation MI patient is diagnosed with AMI only after the return of a positive serum marker.

Several ECG patterns confound the diagnosis of AMI, including left bundle branch block, ventricular paced rhythms, and left ventricular hypertrophy. In the patient with left bundle branch block, the anticipated or expected ST segment/T wave configurations are discordant, directed on the opposite side of the isoelectric baseline from the terminal

ECG Finding	Comment	Example
New LBBB	New onset and with appropriate clinical correlation	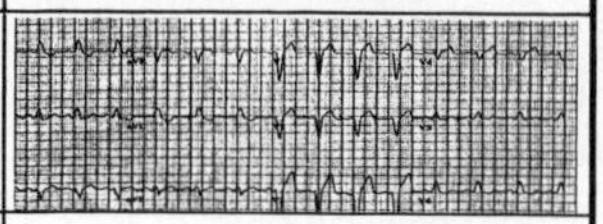
Concordant ST Segment Elevation	ST segment elevation >1 mm // concordant with QRS complex	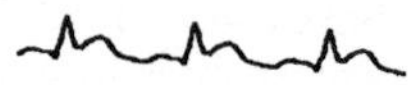
Concordant ST Segment Depression in leads V1, V2, and / or V3	ST segment depression >1 mm in leads V1, V2, or V3	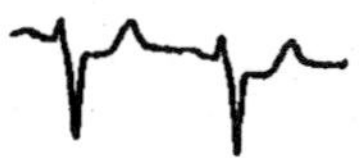
Discordant ST Segment Elevation	ST segment elevation >5 mm discordant with QRS complex	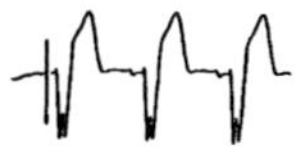

FIGURE 92–2. Electrocardiographic indications for reperfusion therapy in the left bundle branch block presentation.

portion of the QRS complex. This relationship is called QRS complex-T wave axes discordance (Fig. 92-2).[18,19] Loss of this discordance in patients with left bundle branch block may imply AMI. The clinician must realize, however, that the ECG is markedly compromised as a diagnostic tool in this setting. As with the left bundle branch block pattern, the right ventricular-paced rhythm and left ventricular hypertrophy patterns can both mimic and mask the manifestations of AMI. In ventricular paced rhythms, the principle of appropriate discordance should also be followed. An inspection of the ECG in patients with ventricular paced rhythms must be performed, looking for a loss of this QRS complex-T wave axes discordance. Loss of this normal discordance in patients with ventricular paced rhythms can suggest AMI.[20] Left ventricular hypertrophy is not uncommonly encountered on the ECG of chest pain patients. Its presence on the ECG, particularly the repolarization changes that alter the morphology of the ST segment and/or the T wave, can confound the early evaluation. These repolarization changes are seen in approximately 70% of cases and represent the new norm for the patient with electrocardiographic left ventricular hypertrophy.[21] Left ventricular hypertrophy is associated with poor R wave progression, producing a QS pattern in the right to mid-precordial leads. In most instances, the ST segment elevation is seen here along with prominent T waves. ST segment depression with inverted T wave is also seen in the lateral leads.

Several additional ECG tools can be employed by the clinician to further evaluate the chest pain patient suspected of AMI. These tools include additional ECG leads and ST segment surveillance. The additional-lead ECG improves the diagnostic power of the standard 12-lead ECG; with the addition of three leads, the 15-lead ECG is produced. In the 15-lead ECG, the posterior leads V8 and V9 image the posterior wall of the left ventricle (posterior AMI) and lead V4R evaluates the right ventricle (right ventricular infarction).

The use of the additional leads can not only confirm the presence of AMI but also alter treatment decisions in acute coronary syndrome patients. In a study of all emergency room chest pain patients initially evaluated with a 12-lead ECG, Brady el al[22] reported that the 15-lead ECG provided a more accurate description of myocardial injury in those patients with AMI yet failed to alter rates of diagnoses or the use of reperfusion therapies or change disposition locations. Looking at a more select population of chest pain patients, Zalenski and colleagues[23] investigated the use of the 15-lead ECG in chest pain patients with a moderate to high pretest probability of AMI who were already identified as candidates for critical care admission. In this study, the authors reported an approximate 12% increase in sensitivity for the diagnosis of AMI. Potential clinical indications for obtaining the 15-lead ECG in chest pain patients include: (1) ST segment depression in leads V1 through V3; (2) ST segment elevation MI of the lateral or inferior wall; (3) isolated ST segment elevation in lead V1 or ST segment elevation in leads V1 and V2; and (4) the inferior or lateral AMI complicated by hypotension on presentation or after preload reducing medication administration. Figure 92-3 is an example of a 15-lead ECG with inferoposterior AMI with right ventricular infarction. Note the ST segment elevation in leads II, III, and aVf (inferior AMI), RV4 (right ventricular infarction), and leads V8 and V9 (posterior AMI); the ST segment depression with prominent R wave is also seen in leads V1 to V3.

Serial monitoring of the ST segment can also aid the clinician in the diagnosis of AMI as well as monitor the response to therapy. This can be accomplished using two different approaches: serial 12-lead ECG acquisition or ST segment trend monitoring. Either technique can demonstrate the evolution of ST segment/T wave changes in a number of different clinical scenarios, including the initially nondiagnostic ECG, the continuous chest pain patient with an initially

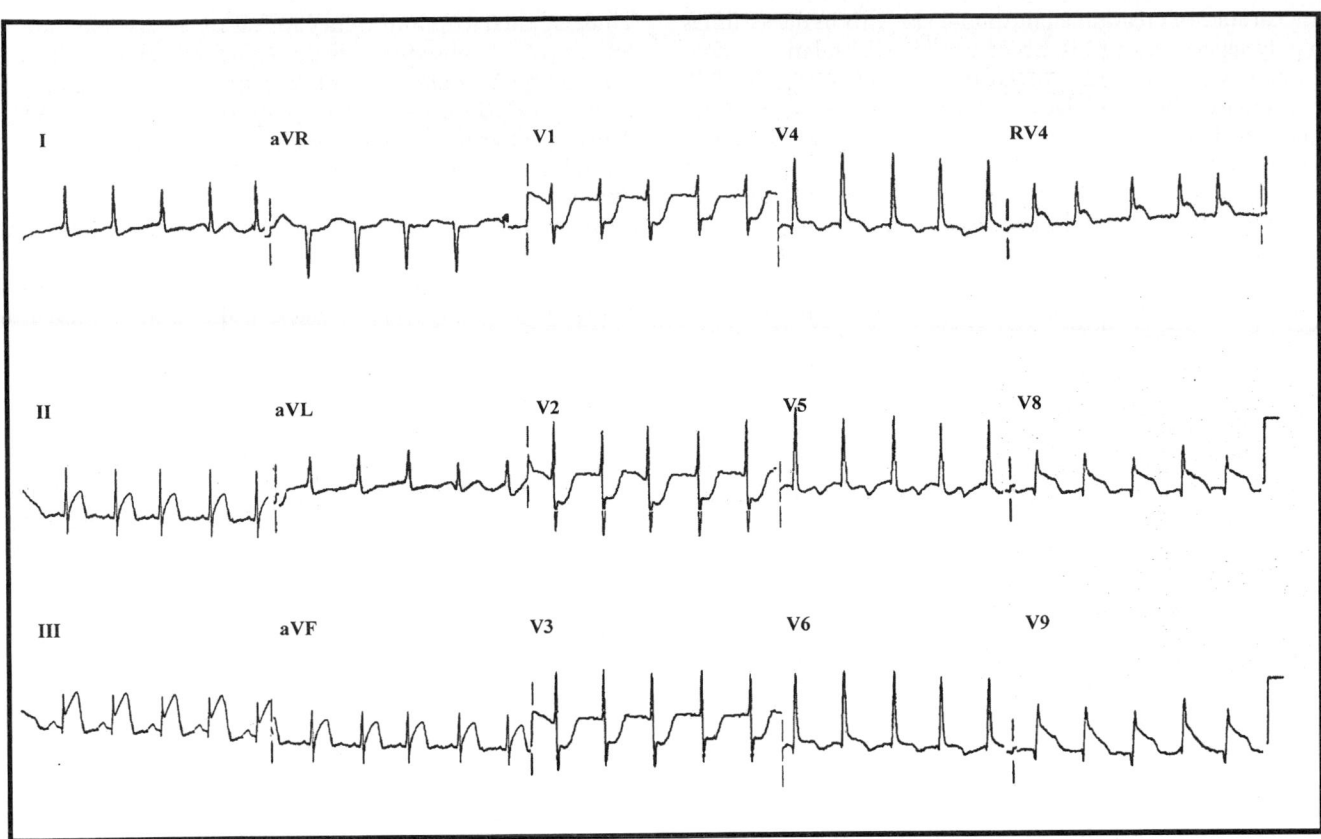

FIGURE 92–3. A 15-lead electrocardiogram showing inferoposterior acute myocardial infarction (AMI) with right ventricular (RV) infarction. Note the ST segment elevation in leads II, III, and aVf (inferior AMI), RV4 (RV infarction), and leads V8 and V9 (posterior AMI). The ST segment depression with prominent R wave is also seen in leads V1 to V3.

nondiagnostic ECG, and the individual with a confounding or masquerading ECG pattern. This increased level of monitoring may provide earlier evidence of coronary occlusion in patients with non-AMI acute coronary syndrome presentations. Potentially, serial ECGs can furnish an increased level of ECG monitoring in patients presenting with chest pain and a nondiagnostic ECG on presentation.[24-28] In the coronary care unit setting, serial ST segment surveillance initiated at admission offers additional clinical data with approximately 20% of patients revealing dynamic ECG change in the early stages of the hospital course.[29] ST segment monitoring has proved to be an effective method for non-invasive evaluation of reperfusion after delivery of fibrinolytic therapy in multiple investigations. In one series, Krucoff and colleagues[28] noted that angiographically proven reperfusion was detected with a sensitivity of 89% using serial ST segment trend monitoring, with a corresponding specificity of 82%.

SERUM MARKERS

The elevation of serum cardiac markers over several days of hospitalization has traditionally been the standard method for diagnosing AMI. Whereas creatinine phosphokinase-MB fraction once was the typical marker used by most clinical laboratories to indicate myocardial necrosis, now the troponins are the most commonly used serologic tests. Previously, detection of AMI by enzyme elevations over 48 to 72 hours was sufficient to establish the diagnosis of AMI. Because of the evolution of acute interventional modalities, however, significant time-sensitive pressure now exists to identify patients with AMI earlier after onset of the ailment. Particularly in patients with a nondiagnostic ECG, early serum markers of myocardial necrosis have the potential to alter the diagnostic course and treatment plans. Further, there are now clear data that indicate that elevations in serum markers, even in those not meeting traditional criteria for AMI, independently identify those patients at risk for poor outcome.[30-32]

Creatinine phosphokinase is an enzyme found in large quantities in cardiac and skeletal muscle. After AMI, increases in serum creatinine phosphokinase are detectable within 3 to 8 hours, with a peak at 12 to 24 hours after injury; assuming a single, one-time event, the levels will normalize within 3 to 4 days. The major problem that reduces the clinical utility of total creatinine phosphokinase as a diagnostic marker involves the widespread distribution of the enzyme in the body—not only in cardiac muscle but also in skeletal muscle, brain, kidney, lung, and gastrointestinal tract. The current major utility of the total creatinine phosphokinase determination in acute cardiac care is screening, to evaluate the need to perform the far more specific creatinine phosphokinase-MB assay.

Myocardial cells are by far the most abundant potential sources of creatinine phosphokinase-MB, and, as such, the appearance of creatinine phosphokinase-MB in the serum is highly suggestive of AMI. Unfortunately, skeletal muscle does contain small amounts of creatinine phosphokinase-MB, particularly the musculature about the pelvis. As a consequence, abnormal creatinine phosphokinase-MB elevations can be seen in patients after trauma, those with muscular dystrophies, myositis, or rhabdomyolysis, and in those who have undertaken vigorous exercise.

The kinetics of creatinine phosphokinase-MB parallel those of total creatinine phosphokinase. In the setting of AMI, the enzyme is released and is detectable in the serum as early as 3 hours after onset of the necrosis. Creatinine phosphokinase-MB characteristically peaks at 12 to 24 hours and normalizes within 2 to 4 days after injury. Elevated creatinine phosphokinase-MB values identify a patient at considerable risk for poor outcome. As with total creatinine phosphokinase measurement, however, the peak creatinine phosphokinase-MB value does not correlate well with infarct size; in fact, studies demonstrate that an elevated creatinine phosphokinase-MB level is associated with a poor prognosis, regardless of the magnitude of the elevation.

The sensitivity of a single creatinine phosphokinase-MB determination in diagnosing AMI is entirely dependent on the elapsed time from chest pain onset. Values obtained within 3 hours of onset are very poor diagnostic tools, with a sensitivity of only 25% to 50%. As the time from symptom onset further increases, however, so does the sensitivity for AMI detection, ultimately approaching 100% at 8 to 12 hours.[33,34] False-positive elevations can result from noncoronary disease states such as pericarditis, myocarditis, skeletal muscle disease, rhabdomyolysis, trauma, and exercise.

Two myocardial-specific proteins—myocardial troponin T and troponin I—have become extremely important in the evaluation of patients suspected of having AMI. The cardiac troponins I and T are genetically distinct from those forms found in skeletal muscle, making them highly cardiac-specific markers. The biokinetics of troponin release are related to the location of the protein within the cell. Normally, small quantities of troponins are free in the cytosol, whereas the majority is entwined in the muscle fiber. Following injury, a biphasic rise in serum troponins is seen. This two-component pattern corresponds to the early release of the free cytoplasmic proteins followed by a prolonged rise with disruption of the actual muscle fiber, resulting in a sustained release of the troponins for approximately 7 days. Serum troponin concentrations begin to rise measurably in the serum at about the same time as creatinine phosphokinase-MB elevations become detectable—as early as 3 hours after onset—and therefore offer no particular benefit over the creatinine phosphokinase-MB regarding early detection of the event; the troponins, however, remain elevated for prolonged periods of time, ranging from 7 to 10 days. The cardiac-specific troponins are highly sensitive for the early detection of myocardial injury in patients with AMI. A positive test result is associated with significant risk while negative study (i.e., serial troponins) findings predict low risk.[35]

The sensitivity of the troponins approaches 50% within 3 to 4 hours of the event. The test finding is positive for AMI in about 75% at 6 hours after onset of symptoms; at 12 hours, the test is almost 100% sensitive for AMI.[33] Moreover, the presence of a positive troponin, even in the face of a nondiagnostic ECG and negative creatinine phosphokinase-MB assay, independently confers a prognosis on the patient that is similar to those suffering ST segment elevation MIs.[36,37]

Thus, elevated troponin values appear to be excellent indicators of risk of subsequent death, AMI, and acute cardiovascular complications in all acute coronary syndrome patients, even those who do not meet traditional criteria for AMI. A negative test result, however, does not necessarily imply a favorable prognosis. One caveat for the troponins is that a number of systemic diseases can cause elevations in the serum levels of troponins without acute coronary syndrome (Table 92-1).

Myoglobin is attractive as an indicator for myocardial injury, because levels are elevated in the serum within 1 to 2 hours after symptom onset and peak 4 to 5 hours after AMI.[38] The sensitivity of myoglobin for AMI approaches 100% at 3 hours. Myocardial myoglobin is not currently distinguishable immunologically from skeletal muscle myoglobin, however, reducing its specificity to approximately 80% compared with 94% for immunochemical creatinine phosphokinase-MB determination 3 hours after emergency room presentation.[38] As with the troponins, myoglobin level is elevated in patients with renal failure because of reduced clearance, making this marker less useful in a patient population who tends to be at an elevated risk for acute coronary syndrome. Additionally, it also will be elevated in any clinical situation involving the skeletal muscle, such as trauma, exercise, and significant systemic illness.

Medical decision-making regarding serum marker use in the suspected AMI patient is complex. Serum markers are most often used in concert with each other and tested in a serial fashion. Relying solely on the result of a single negative assay can result in a missed diagnosis in up to 74% of patients.[39] Single testing strategies, however, may be of value when the clinician is evaluating a nonspecific presentation with illness course lasting greater than 72 to 96 hours. Trending results over time significantly reduces the chance of a missed diagnosis, particularly in acute presentations of short course. A number of studies support the assertion that the troponins approach 100% sensitivity and specificity for cardiac ischemia at 12 hours following an event.[33] These studies all caution, however, that such elevations will occur only with cell injury; hence, they are not appropriate markers for non-AMI acute coronary syndrome presentations. In the setting of an appropriate clinical history or diagnostic ECG changes, a strategy of serial cardiac marker testing is relatively

TABLE 92–1. DIFFERENTIAL DIAGNOSIS OF SERUM TROPONIN ELEVATIONS

Multiple trauma with shock
Cardiac trauma (contusion, cardioversion, myocardial biopsy, electrical injury)
Acute congestive heart failure
Hypertension
Renal failure
Hypothyroidism
Inflammatory states (myocarditis, Kawasaki disease, sarcoidosis)
Pulmonary embolism
Sepsis
Snake envenomation
Burns
Infiltrative diseases (amyloidosis, sarcoidosis, scleroderma)
Acute neurologic events (cerebrovascular accident, subarachnoid hemorrhage)

Data from Panteghini et al,[40] Wu et al,[41] and Armstrong et al.[42]

straightforward. Depending on the particular investigation employed, the clinician looks for the characteristic rise and fall of serial markers over a time-course for the diagnosis of AMI.[4] Most literature supports such serial testing in the acute setting for a period of 8 to 12 hours to adequately rule out myocardial infarction.[40,41]

The more challenging diagnostic situation is found in the critically ill patient with minimal rise in the serum marker and absence of a distinct cardiac event. It is clear, for instance, that troponin levels can be elevated in patients with renal failure or skeletal muscle diseases in the absence of ischemic coronary artery disease. In the renal failure patient, clinical suspicion of acute coronary syndrome must guide evaluation and management decisions; furthermore, the trending of values over time, seeking the characteristic rise and fall of serial markers as well as comparisons to "baseline" values will also improve the clinician's ability to use these diagnostic tests in appropriate fashion, thereby optimizing care. Patients with significant physiologic injury (e.g., sepsis, acute respiratory failure, multiple trauma, and shock) have also been found to have elevated troponin values. In these populations, the elevated levels correlate with left ventricular function and the presence of organ dysfunction, yet the data addressing hospital survival and length of stay are conflicting.

CHEST RADIOGRAPHY

In the setting of AMI, the chest radiograph does not assist in arriving at the diagnosis; other ancillary studies such as the ECG, serum markers, and echocardiography are the primary investigations. Rather, its use provides important information concerning the appropriate application of therapies (i.e., an evaluation of mediastinal width in the consideration of fibrinolytic agent use and the determination of pulmonary congestion in the consideration of acute parenteral beta-adrenergic blocking therapy). Further, the presence of CHF on the chest radiograph places the patient in a higher risk group of AMI patients who may benefit from an aggressive therapeutic approach.

The chest radiograph is obtained in the vast majority of patients who present with AMI. Evidence of pulmonary congestion is noted radiographically in approximately one third of such patients. Radiographic findings often parallel the clinical examination findings. AMI patients who develop CHF based on physical examination have an increased mortality risk, as reported by the Killip classification; the chest radiograph provides prognostic data. The chronicity of the CHF syndrome may also be suggested by the heart size. Patients who present with AMI complicated by pulmonary edema and who have a normal heart size most often have no past history of CHF. In fact, AMI is the most frequent cause of pulmonary edema with a normal cardiac size. In other instances, patients with AMI who manifest an enlarged cardiac silhouette on the chest radiograph frequently have a preexisting history of CHF, anterior wall infarct, and multiple-vessel coronary artery disease (Fig. 92-4).[42]

ECHOCARDIOGRAPHY

Echocardiography is a very useful diagnostic tool in the cardiac evaluation of the critically ill patient; an adequate echocardiogram is an excellent means of assessment of cardiac function at the bedside, including cardiac function

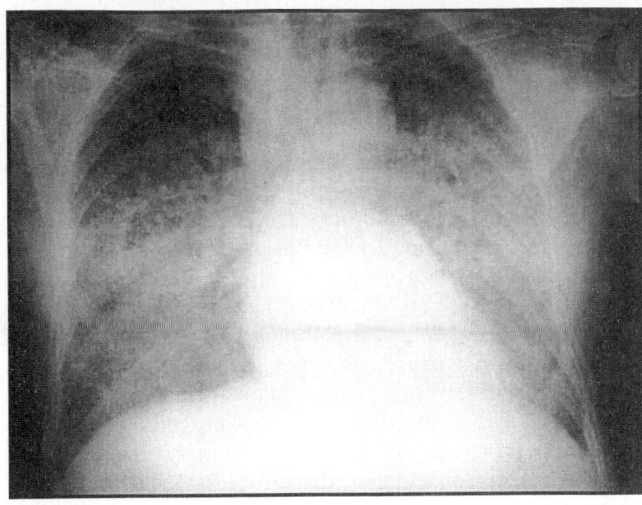

FIGURE 92–4. Chest radiograph showing cardiomegaly and pulmonary edema in an acute myocardial infarction patient with cardiogenic shock and multivessel coronary artery disease.

(ejection fraction) of the left ventricle, general cardiac anatomy, valvular anatomy and function, and the pericardial space. Perhaps most importantly in this application in the AMI patient, transthoracic echocardiography is used to evaluate left ventricular wall motion. The echocardiogram is able to detect regional wall motion abnormalities—an important data point in the clinical evaluation of the potential acute coronary syndrome patient. Chest pain patients with nondiagnostic, mimicking, or confounding ECGs represent a diagnostic problem; two-dimensional echocardiography may provide an answer to this clinical dilemma. The presence of a focal wall motion abnormality in a patient with an appropriate history suggestive of acute coronary ischemia provides strong clinical evidence of acute coronary syndrome, including AMI. In fact, the presence of a regional wall motion abnormality in these patients provides a sensitivity of 88% to 94% for the diagnosis of AMI in the coronary care unit.[43] The recent introduction of contrast echocardiography, the "bubble" echocardiogram, in this setting will only improve its diagnostic utility. In addition, a transthoracic echocardiogram not only allows for the diagnosis of the various mechanical and functional complications of AMI but also affords the opportunity to diagnose other pathology, including issues that may have contributed to the AMI (proximal aortic dissection with involvement of the coronary arteries) or alternative explanations of the chest discomfort.

Body habitus, patient cooperation, and ventilatory status can affect the quality of a transthoracic echocardiogram. Additional limitations include the experience of the operator as well as the expertise of the reader interpreting the study findings. Furthermore, the inability of the two-dimensional echocardiogram to distinguish between myocardial ischemia and myocardial infarction must be recognized by the clinician. Echocardiography is typically less expensive than radionuclide ventriculography and offers more anatomic detail while avoiding the use of radionuclides. Echocardiography can also be performed rapidly in the acute care setting. Transesophageal echocardiography can be performed in patients in whom more definitive information is required, particularly involving the cardiac valves and proximal aorta. The technique is similar, with the notable exception of probe placement, which is into the patient's esophagus. Compared with transthoracic echocardiography, transesophageal echocardiography offers a more precise image of valvular structure and function. Cardiac functional assessment is otherwise similar to transthoracic echocardiography. In unstable patients suspected of having aortic dissection, a transesophageal echocardiogram can be used at the bedside or in the surgical suite.

Candidates for transesophageal echocardiography must be NPO (nothing by mouth) for the procedure, be completely cooperative, and demonstrate the ability to swallow. Furthermore, these patients must have an adequate platelet count and lack esophageal pathologic conditions, including varices and other causes of upper gastrointestinal bleeding. Patients must receive adequate sedation and analgesia to lessen the discomfort associated with the procedure. As such, patients with potential respiratory compromise must be closely monitored during the procedure; "prophylactic" endotracheal intubation may be necessary in certain instances. Since transesophageal echocardiography is an invasive procedure, it is important to be certain that the information sought cannot be obtained from a transthoracic echocardiogram. Complications of transesophageal echocardiograms include injury to the teeth or mouth, bleeding, respiratory compromise, aspiration, and esophageal perforation.

INVASIVE HEMODYNAMIC MONITORING

Invasive hemodynamic monitoring in the AMI patient includes intra-arterial line placement and right heart catheterization. The need for an arterial line for continuous systemic blood pressure monitoring in the AMI patient is unusual. In most instances, noninvasive blood pressure monitoring coupled with serial, focused examinations of the patient suffice. Potential indications for intra-arterial line placement for continuous systemic blood pressure monitoring include the use of continuous infusion cardioactive medications (inotropic, vasopressor, vasodilator, and antihypertensive agents), cardiogenic shock, recurrent or persistent hypotension unresponsive to appropriate therapy, and severe pulmonary edema.

Right heart catheterization, the placement of a pulmonary artery catheter, allows for precise determination of the patient's hemodynamic status. Such information allows for determination of the cardiac output, vascular resistance, and pulmonary capillary wedge pressure. Although the array of clinical data provided by right heart catheterization is impressive, the vast majority of AMI patients do not require such extensive and invasive hemodynamic monitoring; in fact, many intensivists have questioned the utility of right heart catheterization.[44] More useful monitoring techniques include continuous ECG monitoring (for dysrhythmia), ST segment trend monitoring (for evolution of acute coronary syndrome), and noninvasive blood pressure determinations. Additionally, serial, focused physical examinations provide important clinical data: repeat assessments of the patient's general appearance, mental status, jugular venous pressure, lung fields, and peripheral perfusion provide, in most instances, appropriate and adequate information regarding the patient's hemodynamic status.

In general, a pulmonary artery catheter should be considered in patients with persistent or recurrent systemic hypotension unresponsive to adequate therapy; such patients with concurrent acute CHF can be more closely scrutinized

with adjustment of the various therapies. Such monitoring also allows for precise and immediate titration of cardioactive and vasoactive medications to the hemodynamic status. The diagnosis of the various functional and mechanical complications of AMI is best made using the examination and selected, noninvasive investigations (ECG, chest radiograph, and echocardiogram). Potential indications for placement of a pulmonary artery catheter in the AMI patient include cardiogenic shock, recurrent or persistent hypotension unresponsive to appropriate therapy, severe pulmonary edema, the combination of persistent hypotension with pulmonary congestion, concurrent use of intra-aortic balloon counterpulsation, and various complications of AMI (left ventricular rupture, pericardial tamponade, papillary muscle dysfunction, and profound right ventricular infarction).

CARDIAC CATHETERIZATION

Cardiac catheterization, also known as coronary angiography, is used to evaluate the anatomy of the coronary arteries; left ventricular function can also be assessed. Access is usually obtained through the right femoral artery; the left femoral artery and both brachial and radial arteries, however, can be used as well. Once the coronary anatomy has been evaluated, coronary lesions (Fig. 92-5) that are appropriate for intervention can be treated with balloon angioplasty or coronary stent placement, or both. Fractional flow reserve is a technique that can be used to evaluate the significance of a lesion by measuring the pressures proximally and distally to the lesion.

In the critically ill patient, many clinical issues and scenarios exist that can be evaluated and addressed via coronary angiography, including diagnostic and therapeutic considerations. The diagnosis of AMI can be established via coronary angiography, although such information is usually obtained via other, noninvasive means such as the ECG, serum markers, and echocardiogram. In situations in which the diagnosis is in question, however, coronary angiography provides information regarding the status of the coronary arteries and left ventricular function in the AMI setting. Furthermore, the patient who has suffered AMI and experiences recurrent ischemia or continued infarction despite

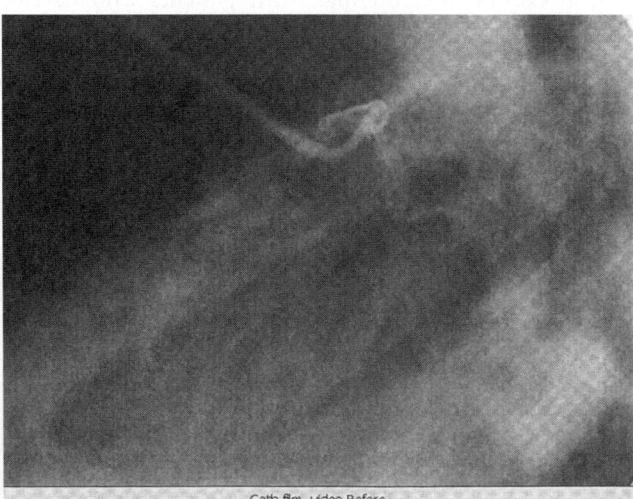

Cath film_video Before

FIGURE 92-5. Coronary angiography with obstructive coronary lesion and thrombus (arrow).

adequate revascularization therapy can be studied in the catheterization laboratory. Current information suggests that rescue angioplasty may be advantageous in patients whose infarct-related arteries fail to reperfuse after fibrinolytic therapy.[45] Some centers routinely catheterize patients after fibrinolytic therapy to determine whether successful reperfusion has occurred and to perform angioplasty if necessary and anatomically feasible. Other centers catheterize patients after fibrinolytic therapy only if there is clinical evidence that the infarct-related artery has failed to open, such as continued chest pain or persistent ST segment elevation. Routine performance of coronary angiography after fibrinolysis for risk stratification prior to discharge represents an additional, though controversial, indication for cardiac catheterization.

The structure and function of both native and prosthetic valves can be assessed at the time of coronary angiography. Additional information obtained in the catheterization laboratory includes right heart catheterization and myocardial biopsy findings. The diagnosis of aortic dissection or aortic aneurysm can also be made in the catheterization laboratory via aortography. If aortic dissection or aneurysm is suspected, however, it should be investigated via computed tomography-angiography or conventional aortography prior to cardiac catheterization.

When preparing a patient for the cardiac catheterization laboratory, several important issues must be considered and addressed, *assuming the clinical situation permits*, including contrast dye allergy, renal function, intravascular volume status, and platelet count and coagulation ability. The physician should obtain a detailed allergy history from the patient. Patients who are allergic to contrast dye or shellfish need to be premedicated with prednisone and diphenhydramine. Also, contrast dye is nephrotoxic; patients who have a history of renal insufficiency may be candidates for *N*-acetylcysteine therapy prior to the study. These patients should also be adequately hydrated prior to receiving dye. Patients should have adequate platelet counts and normal to minimally abnormal coagulation times. Careful consideration must be made prior to sending a patient with thrombocytopenia or coagulopathy for a catheterization procedure. Complications of cardiac catheterization include hemorrhage (both local at the puncture site and regional to the retroperitoneum), pseudoaneurysm, arteriovenous fistula, AMI, stroke, cholesterol embolism, cardiac dysrhythmia, cardiac valve damage, and death.

ANNOTATED REFERENCES

Brady WJ, Perron AD, Martin ML, et al: Electrocardiographic ST segment elevation in emergency department chest pain center patients: Etiology responsible for the ST segment abnormality. Am J Emerg Med 2001;19:25-28.

This study reports the cause of electrocardiographic ST segment elevation in adult chest pain patients presenting to the emergency department. Of note, AMI was an infrequent cause of the ST segment abnormality; the left bundle branch block and left ventricular hypertrophic patterns were the most frequent causes of ST segment elevation. Therapeutic considerations, such as fibrinolysis, must be made with this electrocardiographic differential diagnosis in mind.

The Joint European Society of Cardiology/American College of Cardiology Committee: Myocardial Infarction Redefined—A Consensus Document of the Joint European Society of Cardiology/American College of Cardiology Committee for the Redefinition of Myocardial Infarction. J Am Coll Cardiol 2000;36:959-969.

This consensus document redefines acute myocardial infarction with reference to patient complaint, electrocardiographic abnormality, and serum marker. Of importance is the description of the serum marker abnormality that continues to stress serial testing with the phrase "typical rise and fall" of the value relative to the clinical presentation. This issue is important with respect to the troponins, providing the clinician with information to distinguish noncoronary causes of elevated troponin values from ACS-related presentations.

Ornato JP, Peberdy MA, Jesse RL, et al: Value of coronary artery disease risk factors in judging whether chest pain accompanied by a normal or nondiagnostic ECG in the emergency department is due to acute cardiac ischemia. J Am Coll Cardiol 1996;27:31A.

This study explores the issue of classic CAD risk factors and their importance (i.e., impact) in the early medical decision-making of the possible ACS patient.

Zalenski RJ, Cook D, Rydman R: Assessing the diagnostic value of ECG containing leads V4R, V8, and V9: the 15-lead ECG. Ann Emerg Med 1993;22:786-793.

This study stresses the use of additional ECG leads in the chest pain patient. The right ventricular and posterior areas of the heart are poorly imaged with the ECG. These areas may harbor infarction not detected via standard ECG imaging. This study highlights the importance of the additional ECG leads and their impact on clinical care.

Hamm CW, Goldmann BU, Heeschen C, et al: Emergency room triage of patients with acute chest pain by means of rapid testing for cardiac troponin T or troponin I. N Engl J Med 1997;337:1648-1653.

This study stresses the importance of the serum troponin and its risk prognostication in the chest pain patient suspected of ACS—an elevated value is associated with high risk while a normal value is associated with very low risk.

Chapter 93

ACUTE CORONARY SYNDROMES: MANAGEMENT AND COMPLICATIONS

Steven M. Hollenberg

KEY POINTS

1. Myocardial infarction is diagnosed by a compatible clinical history, evolution of characteristic electrocardiographic changes, and an increase and decrease in cardiac enzyme levels.

2. All patients with suspected myocardial ischemia should be given aspirin upon presentation to the emergency department.

3. Patients with myocardial ischemia are divided by presentation with or without ST elevation, in accordance with treatment strategies. Patients with ST elevation benefit from immediate reperfusion with thrombolytic agents or direct angioplasty.

4. The promptness of reperfusion is more important than the mode by which it is accomplished. Reperfusion should be considered up to 12 hours after the onset of symptoms.

5. Risk stratification is the key to initial management of patients with non-ST elevation acute coronary syndromes.

6. In patients with high-risk non-ST elevation acute coronary syndromes, use of low-molecular-weight heparin, glycoprotein IIb/IIIa inhibition, and an early invasive approach should be considered.

7. Aspirin, beta-blockers, angiotensin converting enzyme inhibitors, and statins have been shown to decrease the rate of mortality after myocardial infarction.

8. Echocardiography is extremely useful for the diagnosis of complications after myocardial infarction. Invasive hemodynamic monitoring may be necessary in some cases as well.

9. Cardiogenic shock usually results from a myocardial infarction and is a medical emergency. The key to achieving a good outcome is an organized approach with rapid diagnosis and prompt initiation of therapy to maintain blood pressure and cardiac output.

10. Expeditious coronary revascularization is crucial in patients with cardiogenic shock. When available, emergency cardiac catheterization and revascularization with angioplasty or coronary surgery appears to improve survival and represents standard therapy at this time.

11. In hospitals without direct angioplasty capability, stabilization of patients with cardiogenic shock with intra-aortic balloon pump and thrombolysis followed by transfer to a tertiary care facility may be the best option.

DEFINITION AND CLINICAL MANIFESTATIONS

Acute coronary syndromes account for nearly 2 million hospitalizations annually in the United States, and, if patients who die before reaching the hospital are included, the mortality rate may be as high as 25%. Acute coronary syndromes are a family of disorders that share similar pathogenic mechanisms and represent different points along a common continuum. They include ST elevation myocardial infarction (MI), non-ST segment elevation MI, and unstable angina pectoris. The common link between the various types of acute coronary syndrome is the rupture of a vulnerable, but previously quiescent, coronary atherosclerotic plaque. Exposure of plaque contents to the circulating blood pool triggers the release of vasoactive amines and activation of platelets and the coagulation cascade. The extent of resultant platelet aggregation, thrombosis, vasoconstriction, and microembolization dictates the clinical manifestations of the syndrome.

The acute coronary syndromes have traditionally been classified into Q-wave MI, non-Q wave MI, and unstable angina. More recently, classification has shifted and has become based on the initial electrocardiogram (ECG): patients are divided into three groups: those with ST elevation (ST elevation MI), without ST elevation but with enzyme evidence of myocardial damage (non-ST elevation MI), and those with unstable angina. Classification according to presenting ECG coincides with current treatment strategies, since patients presenting with ST elevation benefit from immediate reperfusion and should be treated with thrombolytic therapy or urgent revascularization, whereas fibrinolytic agents are not effective in other patients with acute coronary syndrome.

ST ELEVATION MYOCARDIAL INFARCTION

Symptoms suggestive of MI may be similar to those of ordinary angina but are usually greater in intensity and duration.

Nausea, vomiting, and diaphoresis may be prominent features, and stupor and malaise attributable to low cardiac output can occur. Compromised left ventricular function may result in pulmonary edema with development of pulmonary bibasilar crackles and jugular venous distention; a fourth heart sound can be present with small infarcts or even mild ischemia, but a third heart sound is usually indicative of more extensive damage.

Patients presenting with suspected myocardial ischemia should undergo a rapid evaluation and should be treated with oxygen, sublingual nitroglycerin (unless systolic pressure is less than 90 mm Hg), and aspirin, 160 to 325 mg orally.[1] Narcotics should be used to relieve pain and also reduce anxiety, the salutary effects of which have been known for decades and should not be underestimated. A 12-lead ECG should be obtained and interpreted expeditiously.

ST-segment elevation of at least 1 mV in two or more contiguous leads provides strong evidence of thrombotic coronary occlusion, and the patient should be considered for immediate reperfusion therapy. The diagnosis of ST elevation MI can be limited in the presence of preexisting left bundle-branch block or permanent pacemaker. Nonetheless, new left bundle-branch block with a compatible clinical presentation should be considered acute MI and treated accordingly. Indeed, recent data suggest that patients with ST elevation MI and new left bundle-branch block may stand to gain greater benefit from reperfusion strategies than those with ST elevation and preserved ventricular conduction.[2]

THROMBOLYTIC THERAPY

Early reperfusion of an occluded coronary artery is indicated for all eligible candidates. Overwhelming evidence from multiple clinical trials demonstrates the ability of thrombolytic agents administered early in the course of an acute MI to reduce infarct size, preserve left ventricular function, and reduce short-term and long-term mortality.[3-5] Patients treated early derive the most benefit.[5] Indications and contraindications for thrombolytic therapy are listed in Table 93-1. Because of the small, but nonetheless significant, risk of a bleeding complication, most notably intracranial hemorrhage, selection of patients with acute MI for administration of a thrombolytic agent should be undertaken with prudence and caution. That is of special importance in intensive care unit (ICU) patients, who may have a predisposition to bleeding complications because of multiple factors. Contraindications can be regarded as absolute or relative. In the surgical patient, thrombolysis may pose a prohibitive risk and emergency coronary angiography (with percutaneous coronary intervention as clinically indicated) may be preferable.

In contrast to the treatment of ST elevation MI, thrombolytics have shown no benefit and an increased risk of adverse events when used for the treatment of unstable angina/non-ST elevation MI.[6] Based on these findings, there is currently no role for thrombolytic agents in these latter syndromes.

Thrombolytic Agents

Streptokinase is a single-chain protein produced by α-hemolytic streptococci. Streptokinase is given as a 1.5 million unit intravenous infusion over 1 hour, which produces a systemic lytic state for about 24 hours. Hypotension with infusion usually responds to fluids and a decreased infusion

---

TABLE 93–1. INDICATIONS FOR AND CONTRAINDICATIONS TO THROMBOLYTIC THERAPY IN ACUTE MYOCARDIAL INFARCTION

Indications

Symptoms consistent with acute myocardial infarction
Electrocardiogram showing 1 mm (0.1 mV) ST elevation in at least two contiguous leads, or new left bundle branch block
Presentation within 12 hours of symptom onset
Absence of contraindications

Contraindications

Absolute

Active internal bleeding
Intracranial neoplasm, aneurysm, or atrioventricular malformation
Stroke or neurosurgery within prior 6 weeks
Trauma or major surgery within prior 2 weeks that could be a potential source of serious rebleeding
Aortic dissection

Relative

Prolonged (>10 minutes) or clearly traumatic cardiopulmonary resuscitation*
Noncompressible vascular punctures
Severe uncontrolled hypertension (>200/110 mm Hg)*
Trauma or major surgery within prior 6 weeks (but more than 2 weeks ago)
Preexisting coagulopathy or current use of anticoagulants with INR >2-3
Active peptic ulcer
Infective endocarditis
Pregnancy
Chronic severe hypertension

*Could be an absolute contraindication in low-risk patients with myocardial infarction.

---

rate, but allergic reactions are possible. Hemorrhagic complications are the most feared side-effect, with a rate of intracranial hemorrhage of approximately 0.5%. Streptokinase produces coronary arterial patency approximately 50% to 60% of the time and has been shown to decrease mortality by 18% compared to placebo.[3]

Tissue plasminogen activator (t-PA) is a recombinant protein that is more fibrin-selective than streptokinase and produces a higher early coronary patency rate (70-80%). The Global Utilization of Streptokinase and Tissue Plasminogen Activator for Occluded Coronary Arteries (GUSTO) trial was a large (41,021 patient) clinical trial comparing streptokinase to t-PA in patients with ST elevation MI, and it demonstrated a significant survival benefit for t-PA (1.1% absolute, 15% relative reduction).[7] The GUSTO angiographic substudy showed that the difference in patency rates explains the difference in clinical efficacy between these two agents.[8] t-PA is usually given in an accelerated regimen consisting of a 15 mg bolus, 0.75 mg/kg (up to 50 mg) intravenously over the initial 30 minutes, and 0.5 mg/kg (up to 35 mg) over the next 60 minutes. Allergic reactions do not occur because t-PA is not antigenic, but the rate of intracranial hemorrhage may be slightly higher than with streptokinase, around 0.7%.

Reteplase is a deletion mutant of t-PA with an extended half-life and is given as two 10 U boluses 30 minutes apart. Reteplase was originally evaluated in angiographic trials that demonstrated improved coronary flow at 90 minutes compared to t-PA, but subsequent trials showed similar 30-day mortality rates.[9] Why enhanced patency with reteplase did not translate into lower mortality is uncertain.

Tenecteplase is a genetically engineered t-PA mutant with amino acid substitutions that result in prolonged half-life, resistance to plasminogen-activator inhibitor-1, and increased fibrin specificity. Tenecteplase is given as a single bolus, with the dose adjusted for weight. A single bolus of tenecteplase has been shown to produce coronary flow rates identical to those seen with accelerated t-PA, with equivalent 30-day mortality and bleeding rates.[10] Based on these results, single-bolus tenecteplase is an acceptable alternative to t-PA that can be given as a single bolus.

Because these newer agents in general have equivalent efficacy and side effect profiles, at no current additional cost compared to t-PA, and because they are simpler to administer, they have gained popularity. The ideal thrombolytic agent has not yet been developed. Newer recombinant agents with greater fibrin specificity, slower clearance from the circulation, and more resistance to plasma protease inhibitors are being studied.

PRIMARY PERCUTANEOUS CORONARY INTERVENTION IN ACUTE MYOCARDIAL INFARCTION

The major advantages of primary percutaneous coronary intervention over thrombolytic therapy include a higher rate of normal (TIMI grade 3-4) flow, lower risk of intracranial hemorrhage, and the ability to stratify risk based on the severity and distribution of coronary artery disease. Patients ineligible for thrombolytic therapy should obviously be considered for primary percutaneous coronary intervention. In addition, data from several randomized trials have suggested that percutaneous coronary intervention is preferable to thrombolytic therapy for several subsets of patients with acute MI who are at higher risk. The PAMI trial showed improved results with percutaneous coronary intervention in patients older than 75 years of age, those with anterior infarctions, and those with hemodynamic instability.[11] The largest of these trials is the GUSTO-IIb Angioplasty Substudy, which randomized 1138 patients. At 30 days, there was a clinical benefit in the combined primary endpoints of death, nonfatal reinfarction, and nonfatal disabling stroke in the patients treated with percutaneous transluminal coronary angioplasty compared to t-PA, but no difference in the "hard" endpoints of death and MI at 30 days.[12]

It should be noted that these trials were performed in institutions in which a team skilled in primary angioplasty for acute MI was immediately available, with standby surgical backup, allowing for prompt reperfusion of the infarct-related artery. More important than the method of revascularization is the time to revascularization, and that revascularization should be achieved in the most efficient and expeditious manner possible.[13] Procedural volume is important as well.[14]

Recent meta-analyses comparing direct percutaneous transluminal coronary angioplasty with thrombolytic therapy have suggested lower rates of mortality and reinfarction among those receiving direct percutaneous transluminal coronary angioplasty.[15,16] Thus, direct angioplasty, if performed in a timely manner (ideally within 60 minutes) by highly experienced personnel, may be the preferred method of revascularization, since it offers more complete revascularization with improved restoration of normal coronary blood flow and detailed information about coronary anatomy. There are certain subpopulations in which primary percutaneous coronary intervention is clearly preferred, and

TABLE 93–2. SITUATIONS IN WHICH PRIMARY ANGIOPLASTY IS PREFERRED IN ACUTE MYOCARDIAL INFARCTION

Clear Preference

Contraindications to thrombolytic therapy
Cardiogenic shock
Patients in whom uncertain diagnosis prompted cardiac catheterization, which revealed coronary occlusion

Possible Preference

Elderly patients (>75 years old)
Hemodynamic instability
Patients with prior coronary artery bypass grafting
Large anterior infarction
Patients with a prior myocardial infarction

other populations in which the data are suggestive of benefit. These subsets are listed in Table 93-2.

Coronary Stenting and Glycoprotein IIb/IIIa Antagonists

Primary angioplasty for acute MI results in a significant reduction in mortality but is limited by the possibility of abrupt vessel closure, recurrent in-hospital ischemia, reocclusion of the infarct-related artery, and restenosis. The use of coronary stents has been shown to reduce restenosis and adverse cardiac outcomes in both routine and high-risk percutaneous coronary intervention.[17] The PAMI Stent Trial was designed to test the hypothesis that routine implantation of an intracoronary stent in the setting of MI would reduce angiographic restenosis and improve clinical outcomes compared to primary balloon angioplasty alone. This large, randomized, multicenter trial involving 900 patients did not show a difference in mortality at 6 months but did show improvement in ischemia-driven target vessel revascularization and less angina in the stented patients compared to percutaneous transluminal coronary angioplasty alone.[18]

Glycoprotein IIb/IIIa receptor antagonists inhibit the final common pathway of platelet aggregation, blocking crosslinking of activated platelets, and their use in percutaneous intervention has become routine.[19] The benefits of glycoprotein IIb/IIIa inhibition and coronary stenting appear to be additive.[20,21] Thus, combining glycoprotein IIb/IIIa antagonism and stenting in acute MI makes theoretical sense and has now been tested in two large clinical trials. The ADMIRAL trial evaluated abciximab as an adjunct to primary percutaneous transluminal coronary angioplasty and stenting in 300 acute MI patients. Abciximab used in conjunction with stenting improved coronary patency before stenting and resulted in a nearly 50% relative risk reduction in the incidence of death, recurrent MI, and urgent revascularization at 30 days, although this was associated with an increased incidence of minor bleeding.[22] The CADILLAC trial randomized 2082 patients to either angioplasty alone, angioplasty plus abciximab stenting alone, or stenting plus abciximab. The composite endpoint of death, reinfarction, disabling stroke, and repeat revascularization was reduced with addition of abciximab to angioplasty, and outcomes were better with stenting (but abciximab added to stenting alone did not improve outcomes, although the event rate was low).[23] Based on the results of these trials, stenting has become routine for patients with percutaneous coronary intervention in the setting of acute MI, usually with the addition of glycoprotein IIb/IIIa inhibition.

In patients who fail thrombolytic therapy, salvage percutaneous transluminal coronary angioplasty is indicated, although the initial success rate is lower than that of primary angioplasty, reocclusion is more common, and the mortality rate is higher. The RESCUE trial focused on a subset of acute MI patients with anterior infarction and showed a reduction in the combined endpoint of death or congestive heart failure at 30 days in the group receiving salvage percutaneous transluminal coronary angioplasty.[24]

There is no convincing evidence to support empirical delayed percutaneous transluminal coronary angioplasty in patients without evidence of recurrent or provocable ischemia after thrombolytic therapy. The TIMI IIB trial and other studies suggest that a strategy of "watchful waiting" allows for identification of patients who will benefit from revascularization.[25]

ADJUNCTIVE THERAPIES IN ST ELEVATION MYOCARDIAL INFARCTION

Aspirin

Aspirin is the best known and the most widely used of all the antiplatelet agents because of low cost and relatively low toxicity. Aspirin inhibits the production of thromboxane A2 by irreversibly acetylating the serine residue of the enzyme prostaglandin H2 synthetase. Aspirin has been shown to reduce mortality among patient with acute infarction to the same degree as thrombolytic therapy, and its effects are additive to those of thrombolytics.[26] In addition, aspirin reduces the risk of reinfarction.[27,28] Unless contraindicated, all patients with a suspected acute coronary syndrome (ST elevation myocardial infarction, non-ST elevation MI, unstable angina) should be given aspirin as soon as possible.

Heparin

Administration of full-dose heparin after thrombolytic therapy with t-PA is essential to diminish reocclusion after successful reperfusion.[3,26] Dosing should be adjusted to weight, with a bolus of 60 U/kg up to a maximum of 4000 U and an initial infusion rate of 12 U/kg/hr up to a maximum of 1000 U/hr, with adjustment to keep the partial thromboplastin time between 50 and 70 seconds.[1] Heparin should be continued for 24 to 48 hours.

Nitrates

Nitrates have a number of beneficial effects in acute myocardial infarction. They reduce myocardial oxygen demand by decreasing preload and afterload and may also improve myocardial oxygen supply by increasing subendocardial perfusion and collateral blood flow to the ischemic region.[29] Occasional patients with ST elevation due to occlusive coronary artery spasm may have dramatic resolution of ischemia with nitrates. In addition to their hemodynamic effects, nitrates also reduce platelet aggregation. Despite these benefits, the GISSI-3 and ISIS-4 trials failed to show a significant reduction in mortality from routine acute and chronic nitrate therapy.[30,31] Nonetheless, nitrates are still first-line agents for the symptomatic relief of angina pectoris and when myocardial infarction is complicated by congestive heart failure.

Beta-Blockers

Beta-blockers are beneficial both in the early management of myocardial infarction and as long-term therapy. In the prethrombolytic era, early intravenous atenolol was shown to significantly reduce reinfarction, cardiac arrest, cardiac rupture, and death.[32] In conjunction with thrombolytic therapy with t-PA, immediate beta-blockade with metoprolol resulted in a significant reduction in recurrent ischemia and reinfarction, although the mortality rate was not decreased.[25]

Administration of intravenous beta-blockade should be considered for all patients presenting with acute myocardial infarction, especially those with continued ischemic discomfort and sympathetic hyperactivity manifested by hypertension or tachycardia. Therapy should be avoided in patients with moderate or severe heart failure, hypotension, severe bradycardia or heart block, and severe bronchospastic disease. Metoprolol can be given as a 5 mg intravenous bolus, repeated every 5 minutes for a total of three doses. Because of its brief half-life, esmolol may be advantageous in situations in which precise control of the heart rate is necessary or rapid drug withdrawal may be needed if adverse effects occur.

Oral beta-blockade has been clearly demonstrated to decrease mortality after acute myocardial infarction[33,34] and should be initiated in all patients who can tolerate it, even if they have not been treated with intravenous beta-blockers. Diabetes mellitus is not a contraindication.

Angiotensin-Converting Enzyme Inhibitors

Angiotensin-converting enzyme (ACE) generates angiotensin II from angiotensin I and also catalyzes the breakdown of bradykinin. Thus, ACE inhibitors can decrease circulating angiotensin II levels and increase levels of bradykinin, which in turn stimulates production of nitric oxide by endothelial nitric oxide synthase. In the vasculature, ACE inhibition promotes vasodilation and tends to inhibit smooth muscle proliferation, platelet aggregation, and thrombosis.

Angiotensin-converting enzyme inhibitors have been shown unequivocally to improve hemodynamics, functional capacity and symptoms, and survival in patients with chronic congestive heart failure.[35,36] Moreover, ACE inhibitors prevent the development of congestive heart failure in patients with asymptomatic left ventricular dysfunction.[37] This information was the spur for trials evaluating the benefit of prophylactic administration of ACE inhibitors in the post-myocardial infarction period. The SAVE trial showed that patients with left ventricular dysfunction (ejection fraction <40%) after myocardial infarction had a 21% improvement in survival after treatment with the ACE inhibitor captopril.[38] A smaller but still significant reduction in mortality was seen when all patients were treated with captopril in the ISIS-4 study.[31] The HOPE trial randomized 9297 patients with documented vascular disease or those at high-risk for atherosclerosis (diabetes plus at least one other risk factor) in the absence of heart failure to treatment with the tissue-selective ACE inhibitor ramipril (target dose 10 mg/day) or placebo.[39] An impressive 22% reduction in the combined endpoint of cardiovascular death, myocardial infarction, and stroke was observed, as well as improved survival that was additive to the benefits of aspirin and beta-blockers.[39] The mechanisms responsible for the benefits of ACE inhibitors probably include limitation in the progressive left ventricular dysfunction and enlargement (remodeling) that often occur after infarction, but a reduction in ischemic events was seen as well.

Immediate intravenous ACE inhibition with enalapril has not been shown to be beneficial,[40] but oral ACE inhibition should be started early in the hospital course. Patients should be started on low doses of oral agents (captopril 6.25 mg three times daily) and rapidly increased to the range demonstrated beneficial in clinical trials (captopril 50 mg three times daily, enalapril 10 to 20 mg twice daily, lisinopril 10 to 20 mg once daily, or ramipril 10 mg once daily).

Lipid-Lowering Agents

There is extensive epidemiologic, laboratory, and clinical evidence linking cholesterol and coronary artery disease. Total cholesterol level has been linked to the development of coronary artery disease events with a continuous and graded relation.[41] Most of this risk is due to low-density lipoprotein cholesterol. A number of large primary and secondary prevention trials have shown that low-density lipoprotein cholesterol lowering is associated with a reduced risk of coronary disease events. Earlier lipid-lowering trials used bile-acid sequestrants (cholestyramine), fibric acid derivatives (gemfibrozil and clofibrate), or niacin in addition to diet. The reduction in total cholesterol in these early trials was 6% to 15% and was accompanied by a consistent trend toward a reduction in fatal and nonfatal coronary events.[42]

More impressive results have been achieved using HMG-CoA reductase inhibitors (statins). Statins have been demonstrated to decrease the rate of adverse ischemic events in patients with documented coronary artery disease in the 4S trial[43] as well as in the CARE study[44] and the LIPID trial.[45]

The goal of treatment is a low-density lipoprotein cholesterol level less than 100 mg/dL.[46] Maximum benefit may require management of other lipid abnormalities (elevated triglycerides, low high-density lipoprotein [HDL] cholesterol level) and treatment of other atherogenic risk factors.

Calcium Channel Blockers

Randomized clinical trials have not demonstrated that routine use of calcium channel blockers improves survival after myocardial infarction.[47] In fact, meta-analyses suggest that high doses of the short-acting dihydropyridine nifedipine increase mortality in patients after myocardial infarction.[48] Adverse effects of calcium-channel blockers include bradycardia, atrioventricular block, and exacerbation of heart failure. The relative vasodilating, negative inotropic effects, and conduction system effects of the various agents must be considered when they are employed in this setting. Diltiazem is the only calcium channel blocker that has been proven to have tangible benefits, reducing reinfarction and recurrent ischemia in patients with non-Q-wave infarctions who do not have evidence of congestive heart failure.[49]

Calcium channel blockers may be useful for patients whose postinfarction course is complicated by recurrent angina, because these agents not only reduce myocardial oxygen demand but inhibit coronary vasoconstriction. For hemodynamically stable patients, diltiazem can be given, starting at 60 to 90 mg orally every 6 to 8 hours. In patients with severe left ventricular dysfunction, long-acting dihydropyridines without prominent negative inotropic effects such as amlodipine, nicardipine, or the long-acting preparation of nifedipine may be preferable; increased mortality with these agents has not been demonstrated.

NON-ST ELEVATION MYOCARDIAL INFARCTION

The key to initial management of patients with acute coronary syndromes who present without ST elevation is risk stratification. The overall risk of a patient is related to both the severity of preexisting heart disease and the degree of plaque instability. Risk stratification is an ongoing process that begins with hospital admission and continues through discharge.

Braunwald has proposed a classification for unstable angina based on severity of symptoms and clinical circumstances for risk stratification.[50] The risk of progression to acute myocardial infarction or death in acute coronary syndromes increases with age. ST segment depression on the ECG identifies patients at higher risk for clinical events.[50] Conversely, a normal ECG confers an excellent short-term prognosis. Biochemical markers of cardiac injury are also predictive of outcome. Elevated levels of troponin T are associated with an increased risk of cardiac events and a higher 30-day mortality rate and, in fact, were more strongly correlated with 30-day survival than ECG category or creatine kinase-MB level in an analysis of data from the GUSTO-II trial.[51] Conversely, low levels are associated with low event rates, although the absence of troponin elevation does not guarantee a good prognosis and is not a substitute for good clinical judgment.

ANTIPLATELET THERAPY

As previously noted, aspirin is a mainstay of therapy for acute coronary syndromes. Both the VA Cooperative Study Group[27] and the Canadian Multicenter Trial[52] showed that aspirin reduces the risk of death or myocardial infarction by approximately 50% in patients with unstable angina or non-Q-wave MI. Aspirin also reduces events after resolution of an acute coronary syndrome and should be continued indefinitely.

Clopidogrel or ticlopidine, thienopyridines that inhibit ADP-induced platelet activation and are more potent than aspirin, can be used in place of aspirin if necessary. Thienopyridines are used in combination with aspirin when intracoronary stents are placed. Clopidogrel is generally better tolerated than ticlopidine, since the risk of neutropenia is much lower.

In the CURE trial, 12,562 patients were randomized to receive clopidogrel or placebo in addition to standard therapy with aspirin, within 24 hours of unstable angina symptoms.[53] Clopidogrel significantly reduced the risk of myocardial infarction, stroke, or cardiovascular death from 11.4% to 9.3% ($P < .001$).[53] It should be noted that this benefit came with a 1% absolute increase in major, non-life-threatening bleeds ($P = .001$) as well as a 2.8% absolute increase in major or life-threatening bleeds associated with coronary artery bypass graft surgery (CABG) within 5 days ($P = .07$).[53] These data have raised concerns about giving clopidogrel prior to information about the coronary anatomy.

Clopidogrel has also been tested for secondary prevention of events. The CAPRIE trial, a multicenter trial of 19,185 patients with known vascular disease (prior stroke, myocardial infarction, or peripheral vascular disease), randomized patients to either 75 mg/day of clopidogrel or 325 mg aspirin.[54] After an average follow-up of 1.6 years, patients treated with clopidogrel had significantly fewer cardiovascular events than patients treated with aspirin (5.8% vs 5.3%, a relative risk reduction of 8.7%).[54]

ANTICOAGULANT THERAPY

Heparin is an important component of primary therapy for patients with unstable coronary syndromes without ST elevation. When added to aspirin, heparin has been shown to reduce refractory angina and the development of myocardial infarction,[28] and a meta-analysis of the available data indicates that addition of heparin reduces the composite endpoint of death or myocardial infarction.[55]

Unfractionated heparin, however, can be difficult to administer, because the anticoagulant effect is unpredictable in individual patients; this is due to binding of heparin to heparin-binding proteins and heparin inhibition by several factors released by activated platelets, most notably platelet factor 4. Therefore, the activated partial thromboplastin time must be monitored closely. The potential for heparin-associated thrombocytopenia is also a safety concern.

Low-molecular-weight heparins, which are obtained by depolymerization of standard heparin and selection of fractions with lower molecular weight, have several advantages. Because they bind less avidly to heparin binding proteins, there is less variability in the anticoagulant response and a more predictable dose-response curve, obviating the need to monitor APTT. The incidence of thrombocytopenia is lower but not absent, and patients with heparin-induced thrombocytopenia with anti-heparin antibodies cannot be switched to low-molecular-weight heparins. Low-molecular-weight heparin is less susceptible to inactivation by platelet factor 4. Finally, low-molecular-weight heparins have longer half-lives and can be given by subcutaneous injection. These properties make treatment with low-molecular-weight heparins at home after hospital discharge feasible. Since evidence suggests that patients with unstable coronary syndromes may remain in a hypercoagulable state for weeks or months, the longer duration of anticoagulation possible with low-molecular-weight heparins may be desirable.

Several trials have documented beneficial effects of low-molecular-weight heparin therapy in unstable coronary syndromes. The ESSENCE trial showed that the low-molecular-weight heparin enoxaparin reduced the combined endpoint of death, myocardial infarction, or recurrent ischemia at both 14 and 30 days when compared with heparin.[56] Similar results were found in the TIMI 11B trial comparing enoxaparin to heparin.[57] A meta-analysis of these two very similar trials demonstrated a 23% 7-day and an 18% 42-day reduction in the harder endpoint of death or myocardial infarction.[58] Dalteparin, another low-molecular-weight heparin, is also available, but the evidence for its efficacy is not nearly as compelling as that for enoxaparin.[59]

Although the low-molecular-weight heparins are substantially easier to administer than standard heparin, and long-term administration can be contemplated, they are also more expensive. Specific considerations with the use of low-molecular-weight heparins include decreased clearance in renal insufficiency and the lack of a commercially available test to measure the anticoagulant effect. Low-molecular-weight heparins should be given strong consideration in high-risk patients, but whether substitution of low-molecular-weight heparin for heparin in all patients is cost effective is uncertain.

GLYCOPROTEIN IIB/IIIA ANTAGONISTS

Given the central role of platelet activation and aggregation in the pathophysiology of unstable coronary syndromes, attention has focused on platelet glycoprotein IIb/IIIa antagonists, which inhibit the final common pathway of platelet aggregation. Three agents are currently available. Abciximab is a chimeric murine-human monoclonal antibody Fab fragment

that binds with relatively high affinity to platelet receptors, giving it a short plasma half-life (10 to 30 minutes) but a long duration of biologic action by virtue of the strength of the bond formed with the surface of the activated platelet. Tirofiban is a small-molecule, synthetic nonpeptide agent with a half-life of approximately 2.5 hours and a lower receptor affinity than abciximab. Eptifibatide is a small-molecule, cyclic heptapeptide with a 2-hour half-life.

The benefits of glycoprotein IIb/IIIa inhibitors as adjunctive treatment in patients undergoing percutaneous intervention have been substantial and consistently observed. Abciximab has been most extensively studied,[21,60,61] but a benefit for eptifibatide has also been demonstrated.[62] In acute coronary syndromes, the evidence supporting the efficacy of GP IIb/IIIa inhibitors is somewhat less impressive. Five major trials have been completed (the "4 P's" and GUSTO-IV). In the PRISM trial, tirofiban reduced the rate of death, myocardial infarction, or refractory ischemia when compared to heparin from 5.6% to 3.8% ($P < .01$) at 48 hours, but there was no difference at 30 days (7.1% vs 5.8%, $P = .11$).[63] In the subsequent PRISM-PLUS trial, tirofiban added to heparin reduced the rate of death, myocardial infarction, or refractory ischemia at 30 days from 11.9% to 8.7% ($P = .03$).[64] In the PURSUIT trial, eptifibatide reduced the rate of death or MI from 15.7% to 14.2% ($P = .04$) at 30 days.[65] The PARAGON trial with lamifiban did not show a significant benefit with glycoprotein IIb/IIIa inhibition.[66] In the GUSTO-IV acute coronary syndromes trial, however, abciximab did not produce an improvement; in fact, the rate of death or myocardial infarction was slightly higher with abciximab in the treatment group.[67] This trial included patients for whom percutaneous intervention was not planned; when patients with refractory angina and planned angioplasty were randomized to receive abciximab or placebo from 24 hours prior to the procedure through 1 hour following percutaneous transluminal coronary angioplasty in the CAPTURE trial, the primary endpoint, death, myocardial infarction, or urgent revascularization at 30 days, was reduced by glycoprotein IIb/IIIa inhibition, and the rate of myocardial infarction before percutaneous transluminal coronary angioplasty was reduced as well.[68] When patients were grouped into those with and without increased troponin, the benefit was confined to the positive troponin group.[68]

Recent meta-analyses have found a relative risk reduction of 40% for glycoprotein IIb/IIIa therapy adjunctive to percutaneous coronary intervention, and a reduction of 11% for glycoprotein IIb/IIIa inhibitors in non-ST elevation MI acute coronary syndromes.[19] Additional analysis suggests that glycoprotein IIb/IIIa inhibition is most effective in high-risk patients, those with either ECG changes or elevated troponin.[19] The benefits appear to be restricted to patients undergoing percutaneous intervention, which may not be entirely surprising.

INTERVENTIONAL MANAGEMENT

Cardiac catheterization can be undertaken in patients presenting with symptoms suggestive of unstable coronary syndromes for one of several reasons: to assist with risk stratification, as a prelude to revascularization, and to exclude significant epicardial coronary stenosis as a cause of symptoms when the diagnosis is uncertain.

An early invasive approach has now been compared to a conservative approach in several prospective studies.

Two earlier trials had negative findings. The TIMI IIIb study randomized 1473 patients to early angiography or conservative management with angiography and revascularization only for recurrent chest pain or provocable ischemia.[6] No significant difference was found in the combined endpoint of death, myocardial infarction, or positive treadmill test result at 6 weeks. There was, however, a high (64%) crossover rate from the conservative to the invasive arm, and hospital stays were lower with the early invasive approach.[8] The VAN-QWISH trial of 920 patients with non-Q wave myocardial infarction actually showed an increase in the primary endpoint of death or myocardial infarction with an invasive strategy, although overall mortality was not significantly different.[69] Difficulties with this trial included the fact that only 44% of patients randomized to the invasive arm underwent revascularization, compared with 33% in the conservative arm, and very high surgical mortality rate (11.6%).[69] It is important to realize that these trials were performed before widespread use of coronary stenting and platelet glycoprotein IIb/IIIa inhibitors, both of which have now been shown to improve outcomes after angioplasty.

More recently, a substudy of the FRISC II study, which used the low-molecular-weight heparin dalteparin, randomized 2457 patients to an early invasive or a noninvasive strategy and found a significantly lower mortality rate in the invasive group at 30 days, which was maintained at 1 year.[70] The TACTICS TIMI-18 trial used aspirin, heparin, and tirofiban in 2220 patients and found a significant reduction in the combined endpoint of death, myocardial infarction, or readmission for acute coronary syndrome with invasive management.[71] It is important to recognize that both of these trials selected high-risk patients (identified on the basis of either ECG changes or enzyme elevations) for inclusion. Addition of adjunctive antiplatelet therapy beyond the use of aspirin alone in conjunction with reperfusion may also have contributed to the improved outcomes with invasive strategies in these more recent trials.

Risk stratification is the key to managing patients with non-ST elevation MI acute coronary syndromes. One possible algorithm for managing patients with non-ST elevation MI is shown in Figure 93-1. An initial strategy of medical management with attempts at stabilization is warranted in patients with lower risk, but patients at higher risk should be considered for cardiac catheterization. Pharmacologic and mechanical strategies are intertwined in the sense that selection of patients for early revascularization will influence the choice of antiplatelet and anticoagulant medication. When good clinical judgment is employed, early coronary angiography in selected patients with acute coronary syndromes can lead to better management and lower morbidity and mortality.

COMPLICATIONS OF ACUTE MYOCARDIAL INFARCTION

POSTINFARCTION ISCHEMIA

Causes of ischemia after infarction include reduced myocardial oxygen supply due to coronary reocclusion or spasm, mechanical problems which increase myocardial oxygen demand, and extracardiac factors such as hypertension, anemia, hypotension, or hypermetabolic states. Nonischemic causes of chest pain, such as postinfarction pericarditis and acute pulmonary embolism, should also be considered.

Immediate management includes aspirin, beta-blockade, intravenous nitroglycerin, heparin, consideration of calcium-channel blockers, and diagnostic coronary angiography. Post-infarction angina is an indication for revascularization. Percutaneous transluminal coronary angioplasty can be performed if the culprit lesion is suitable. CABG should be considered for patients with left main disease, those with three-vessel disease, and those unsuitable for percutaneous transluminal coronary angioplasty. If the angina cannot be controlled medically or is accompanied by hemodynamic instability, an intra-aortic balloon pump should be inserted.

VENTRICULAR FREE WALL RUPTURE

Ventricular free wall rupture typically occurs during the first week after infarction. The classic patient is elderly, female, and hypertensive. Early use of thrombolytic therapy reduces

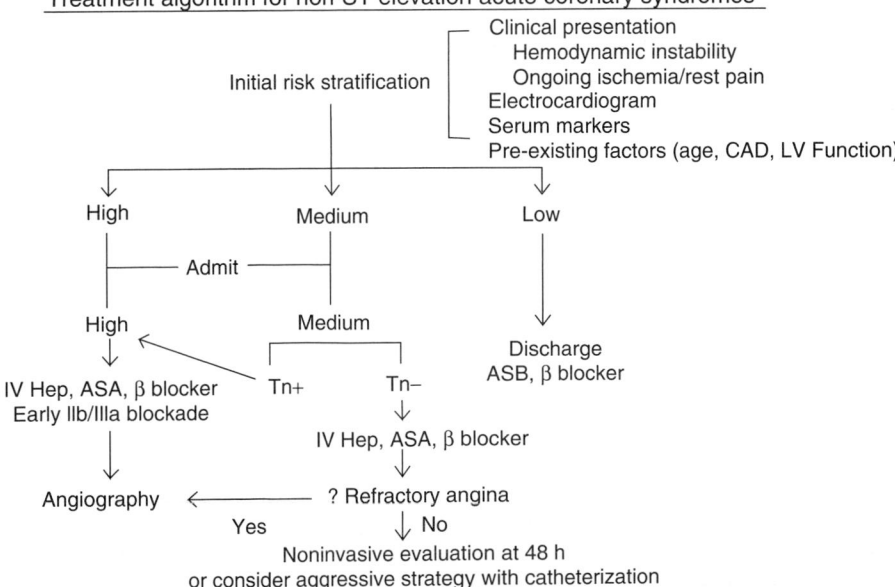

FIGURE 93–1. Possible treatment algorithm for patients with non-ST elevation acute coronary syndromes. ASA, aspirin; Hep, heparin; IV, intravenous; Tn, troponin.

the incidence of cardiac rupture, but late use may actually increase the risk. Free wall rupture presents as a catastrophic event with shock and electromechanical dissociation. Salvage is possible with prompt recognition, pericardiocentesis to relieve acute tamponade, and thoracotomy with repair.[72] Emergency echocardiography or pulmonary artery catheterization can help make the diagnosis.

VENTRICULAR SEPTAL RUPTURE

Septal rupture manifests as severe heart failure or cardiogenic shock, with a pansystolic murmur and parasternal thrill. The hallmark finding is a left-to-right intracardiac shunt ("step-up" in oxygen saturation from right atrium to right ventricle), but the diagnosis is most easily made with echocardiography.

Rapid institution of intra-aortic balloon pumping and supportive pharmacologic measures is necessary. Operative repair is the only viable option for long-term survival. The timing of surgery has been controversial, but most authorities now suggest that repair should be undertaken early, within 48 hours of the rupture.[73]

ACUTE MITRAL REGURGITATION

Ischemic mitral regurgitation is usually associated with inferior myocardial infarction and ischemia or infarction of the posterior papillary muscle, although anterior papillary muscle rupture can also occur. Papillary muscle rupture typically occurs 2 to 7 days after acute myocardial infarction and presents dramatically with pulmonary edema, hypotension, and cardiogenic shock. When a papillary muscle ruptures, the murmur of acute mitral regurgitation may be limited to early systole because of rapid equalization of pressures in the left atrium and left ventricle. More importantly, the murmur may be soft or inaudible, especially when cardiac output is low.[74]

Echocardiography is extremely useful in the differential diagnosis, which includes free wall rupture, ventricular septal rupture, and infarct extension with pump failure. Hemodynamic monitoring with pulmonary artery catheterization may also be helpful. Management includes afterload reduction with nitroprusside and intra-aortic balloon pumping as temporizing measures. Inotropic or vasopressor therapy may also be needed to support cardiac output and blood pressure. Definitive therapy, however, is surgical valve repair or replacement, which should be undertaken as soon as possible, since clinical deterioration can be sudden.[74,75]

RIGHT VENTRICULAR INFARCTION

Right ventricular infarction occurs in up to 30% of patients with inferior infarction and is clinically significant in 10%.[76] The combination of a clear chest x-ray with jugular venous distention in a patient with an inferior wall myocardial infarction should lead to the suspicion of a coexisting right ventricular infarct. The diagnosis is substantiated by demonstration of ST segment elevation in the right precordial leads (V_{3R} to V_{5R}) or by characteristic hemodynamic findings on right heart catheterization (elevated right atrial and right ventricular end-diastolic pressures with normal to low pulmonary artery occlusion pressure and low cardiac output). Echocardiography can demonstrate depressed right

ventricular contractility.[77] Patients with cardiogenic shock on the basis of right ventricular infarction have a better prognosis than those with left-sided pump failure.[76] This may be due in part to the fact that right ventricular function tends to return to normal over time with supportive therapy,[78] although such therapy may need to be prolonged.

In patients with right ventricular infarction, right ventricular preload should be maintained with fluid administration. In some cases, however, fluid resuscitation may increase pulmonary capillary occlusion pressure but may not increase cardiac output, and overdilation of the right ventricle can compromise left ventricular filling and cardiac output.[78] Inotropic therapy with dobutamine may be more effective in increasing cardiac output in some patients, and monitoring with serial echocardiograms may also be useful to detect right ventricular overdistention.[78] Maintenance of atrioventricular synchrony is also important in these patients to optimize right ventricular filling.[77] For patients with continued hemodynamic instability, intra-aortic balloon pumping may be useful, particularly because elevated right ventricular pressures and volumes increase wall stress and oxygen consumption and decrease right coronary perfusion pressure, exacerbating right ventricular ischemia.

Reperfusion of the occluded coronary artery is also crucial. A study using direct angioplasty demonstrated that restoration of normal flow resulted in dramatic recovery of right ventricular function and a mortality rate of only 2%, whereas unsuccessful reperfusion was associated with persistent hemodynamic compromise and a mortality rate of 58%.[79]

CARDIOGENIC SHOCK

Epidemiology and Pathophysiology

Cardiogenic shock, resulting either from left ventricular pump failure or from mechanical complications, represents the leading cause of in-hospital death after myocardial infarction.[80] Despite advances in the management of heart failure and acute myocardial infarction, until very recently, clinical outcomes in patients with cardiogenic shock have been poor, with reported mortality rates ranging from 50% to 80%.[81] Patients may have cardiogenic shock at initial presentation, but shock often evolves over several hours.[82,83]

Cardiac dysfunction in patients with cardiogenic shock is usually initiated by myocardial infarction or ischemia. The myocardial dysfunction resulting from ischemia worsens that ischemia, creating a downward spiral (Fig. 93-2). Compensatory mechanisms that retain fluid in an attempt to maintain cardiac output may add to the vicious cycle and further increase diastolic filling pressures. The interruption of this cycle of myocardial dysfunction and ischemia forms the basis for the therapeutic regimens for cardiogenic shock.

Initial Management

Maintenance of adequate oxygenation and ventilation are critical. Many patients require intubation and mechanical ventilation, if only to reduce the work of breathing and facilitate sedation and stabilization before cardiac catheterization. Electrolyte abnormalities should be corrected, and morphine (or fentanyl if systolic pressure is compromised) used to relieve pain and anxiety, thus reducing excessive sympathetic activity and decreasing oxygen demand, preload, and afterload. Arrhythmias and heart block can have major effects on cardiac output and should be corrected promptly with antiarrhythmic drugs, cardioversion, or pacing.

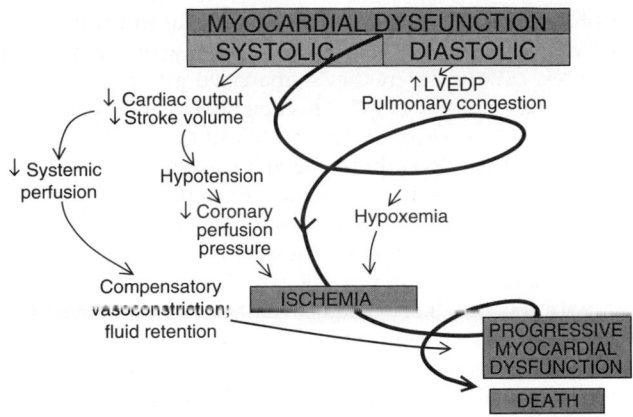

FIGURE 93–2. The "downward spiral" in cardiogenic shock. Stroke volume and cardiac output fall with left ventricular dysfunction, producing hypotension and tachycardia that reduce coronary blood flow. Increasing ventricular diastolic pressure reduces coronary blood flow, and increased wall stress elevates myocardial oxygen requirements. All of these factors combine to worsen ischemia. The falling cardiac output also compromises systemic perfusion. Compensatory mechanisms include sympathetic stimulation and fluid retention to increase preload. These mechanisms can actually worsen cardiogenic shock by increasing myocardial oxygen demand and afterload. Thus, a vicious circle can be established. LVEDP, left ventricular end-diastolic pressure. (Adapted with permission from Hollenberg SM, Kavinsky CJ, Parrillo JE: Cardiogenic shock. Ann Intern Med 1999; 131:47-59.)

The initial approach to the hypotensive patient should include fluid resuscitation unless frank pulmonary edema is present. Patients are commonly diaphoretic, and relative hypovolemia may be present in as many as 20% of patients with cardiogenic shock. Fluid infusion is best initiated with predetermined boluses titrated to clinical endpoints of heart rate, urine output, and blood pressure. Ischemia produces diastolic as well as systolic dysfunction, and thus elevated filling pressures may be necessary to maintain stroke volume in patients with cardiogenic shock. Patients who do not respond rapidly to initial fluid boluses or those with poor physiologic reserve should be considered for invasive hemodynamic monitoring. Optimal filling pressures vary from patient to patient; hemodynamic monitoring can be used to construct a Starling curve at the bedside, identifying the filling pressure at which cardiac output is maximized. Maintenance of adequate preload is particularly important in patients with right ventricular infarction.

When arterial pressure remains inadequate, therapy with vasopressor agents may be required to maintain coronary perfusion pressure. Maintenance of adequate blood pressure is essential to break the vicious circle of progressive hypotension with further myocardial ischemia. Dopamine increases both blood pressure and cardiac output and is usually the initial choice in patients with systolic pressures less than 80 mm Hg. When hypotension remains refractory, norepinephrine may be necessary to maintain organ perfusion pressure. Phenylephrine, a selective alpha$_1$-adrenergic agonist, may be useful when tachyarrhythmias limit therapy with other vasopressors. Vasopressor infusions need to be titrated carefully in patients with cardiogenic shock to maximize coronary perfusion pressure with the least possible increase in myocardial oxygen demand. Hemodynamic monitoring, with serial measurements of cardiac output, filling pressures, and other parameters, such as mixed venous oxygen saturation, allows

for titration of the dosage of vasoactive agents to the minimum dose required to achieve the chosen therapeutic goals.[84]

Following initial stabilization and restoration of adequate blood pressure, tissue perfusion should be assessed. If tissue perfusion remains inadequate, inotropic support or intra-aortic balloon pumping should be initiated. If tissue perfusion is adequate but significant pulmonary congestion remains, diuretics can be employed. Vasodilators can be considered as well, depending on the blood pressure.

In patients with inadequate tissue perfusion and adequate intravascular volume, cardiovascular support with inotropic agents should be initiated. Dobutamine, a selective beta$_1$-adrenergic receptor agonist, can improve myocardial contractility and increase cardiac output and is the initial agent of choice in patients with systolic pressures greater than 80 mm Hg. Dobutamine may exacerbate hypotension in some patients and can precipitate tachyarrhythmias. Use of dopamine may be preferable if systolic pressure is less than 80 mm Hg, although tachycardia and increased peripheral resistance may worsen myocardial ischemia. In some situations, a combination of dopamine and dobutamine can be more effective than either agent used alone. Phosphodiesterase inhibitors such as milrinone are less arrhythmogenic than catecholamines but have the potential to cause hypotension and should be used with caution in patients with tenuous clinical status.

Intra-aortic balloon counterpulsation reduces systolic afterload and augments diastolic perfusion pressure, increasing cardiac output and improving coronary blood flow.[85] These beneficial effects, in contrast to those of inotropic or vasopressor agents, occur without an increase in oxygen demand. Intra-aortic balloon counterpulsation does not, however, produce a significant improvement in blood flow distal to a critical coronary stenosis and has not been shown to improve mortality when used alone without reperfusion therapy or revascularization. In patients with cardiogenic shock and compromised tissue perfusion, intra-aortic balloon counterpulsation can be an essential support mechanism to stabilize patients and allow time for definitive therapeutic measures to be undertaken.[85,86] In appropriate settings, more intensive support with mechanical assist devices can also be implemented.

Reperfusion Therapy

Although thrombolytic therapy reduces the likelihood of subsequent development of shock after initial presentation,[83] its role in the management of patients who have already developed shock is less certain. The available randomized trials[3,7,26,87] have not demonstrated that fibrinolytic therapy reduces mortality in patients with established cardiogenic shock. On the other hand, in the SHOCK Registry,[88] patients treated with fibrinolytic therapy had a lower in-hospital mortality rate than those who were not (54% vs. 64%, $P = .005$), even after adjustment for age and revascularization status (OR 0.70, $P = .027$).

Fibrinolytic therapy is clearly less effective in patients with cardiogenic shock than in those without. The explanation for this lack of efficacy appears to be the low reperfusion rate achieved in this subset of patients. The reasons for decreased thrombolytic efficacy in patients with cardiogenic shock probably include hemodynamic, mechanical, and metabolic factors that prevent achievement and maintenance of infarct-related artery patency.[89] Attempts to increase reperfusion rates by increasing blood pressure with aggressive inotropic and pressor therapy and intra-aortic balloon counterpulsation make theoretical sense, and two small studies support the notion that vasopressor therapy to increase aortic pressure improves thrombolytic efficacy.[89,90] The use of intra-aortic balloon pumping to augment aortic diastolic pressure may increase the effectiveness of thrombolytics as well.

To date, emergency percutaneous revascularization is the only intervention that has been shown to consistently reduce mortality rates in patients with cardiogenic shock. An extensive body of observational and registry studies has shown consistent benefits from revascularization. Notable among these is the GUSTO-I trial, in which patients treated with an "aggressive" strategy (coronary angiography performed within 24 hours of shock onset with revascularization by percutaneous transluminal coronary angioplasty or bypass surgery) had significantly lower mortality (38% compared with 62%).[91] The National Registry of Myocardial Infarction-2 (NRMI-2) collected 26,280 shock patients with cardiogenic shock in the setting of myocardial infarction between 1994 and 1997, similarly supporting the association between revascularization and survival.[92] Improved short-term mortality was noted in patients who then underwent revascularization during the reference hospitalization, either via percutaneous transluminal coronary angioplasty (12.8% mortality vs 43.9%) or CABG (6.5% vs 23.9%).[93] These data complement the GUSTO-I substudy data and are important not only because of the sheer number of patients from whom these values are derived but also because NRMI-2 was a national cross-sectional study, which more closely represents general clinical practice than carefully selected trial populations. These studies cannot be regarded as definitive due to their retrospective design, but two randomized controlled trials have now evaluated revascularization for patients with myocardial infarction.

The SHOCK study was a randomized, multicenter international trial that assigned patients with cardiogenic shock to receive optimal medical management—including intra-aortic balloon counterpulsation and thrombolytic therapy—or cardiac catheterization with revascularization using percutaneous transluminal coronary angioplasty or CABG.[93,94] The trial enrolled 302 patients and was powered to detect a 20% absolute decrease in 30-day all-cause mortality rates. Mortality at 30 days was 46.7% in patients treated with early intervention and 56% in patients treated with initial medical stabilization, but this difference did not quite reach statistical significance ($P = .11$).[93] At 6 months, the absolute risk reduction with early invasive therapy in the SHOCK trial was 13% (50.3% compared with 63.1%, $P = .027$),[93] and this risk reduction was maintained at 12 months (mortality 53.3% vs 66.4%, $P < .03$).[94] Subgroup analysis showed a substantial improvement in mortality rates in patients younger than 75 years of age at both 30 days (41.4% versus 56.8%, $P = .01$) and 6 months (44.9% versus 65.0%, $P = 0.003$).[93]

The SMASH trial was independently conceived and had a very similar design, although a more rigid definition of cardiogenic shock resulted in enrollment of sicker patients and a higher mortality rate.[95] The trial was terminated early because of difficulties in patient recruitment, and enrolled only 55 patients. In the SMASH trial, a similar trend in 30-day

absolute mortality reduction similar to that in the SHOCK trial of 9% was observed (69% mortality in the invasive group vs. 78% in the medically managed group; RR = 0.88; 95% CI = 0.6-1.2; P = NS).[95] This benefit was also maintained at 1 year.

When the results of both the SHOCK and SMASH trials are put into perspective with results from other randomized, controlled trials of patients with acute myocardial infarction, an important point emerges: despite the moderate *relative* risk reduction (for the SHOCK trial 0.72, CI 0.54-0.95; for the SMASH trial, 0.88, CI 0.60-1.20) the *absolute* benefit is important, with 9 lives saved for 100 patients treated at 30 days in both trials, and 13.2 lives saved for 100 patients treated at 1 year in the SHOCK trial. This latter figure corresponds to a number needed to treat (NNT) of 7.6, one of the lowest figures ever observed in a randomized, controlled trial of cardiovascular disease.

On the basis of these randomized trials, the presence of cardiogenic shock in the setting of acute myocardial infarction is a class I indication for emergency revascularization, either by percutaneous intervention or CABG.[1]

ANNOTATED REFERENCES

Cannon CP, Weintraub WS, Demopoulos LA, et al: Comparison of early invasive and conservative strategies in patients with unstable coronary syndromes treated with the glycoprotein IIb/IIIa inhibitor tirofiban. N Engl J Med 2001;344:1879-1887.
TACTICS-TIMI 18 study, in which 2220 patients with unstable angina or non-ST elevation myocardial infarction were treated with aspirin, heparin, and tirofiban and randomized to an early invasive strategy of catheterization within 4 to 48 hours and revascularization as appropriate, or to a more conservative strategy, in which catheterization was performed only if the patient had objective evidence of recurrent ischemia or an abnormal stress test. The composite of death, myocardial infarction, and rehospitalization for an acute coronary syndrome at 6 months was decreased significantly, from 19.4% to 15.9%.

GUSTO Investigators: An international randomized trial comparing four thrombolytic strategies for acute myocardial infarction. N Engl J Med 1993;329:673-682.
A megatrial of 41,021 patients randomized to accelerated t-PA or streptokinase. Accelerated t-PA reduced mortality from 7.3% to 6.3% (reduction of 14%) compared to streptokinase, with a slight increase (0.2%) in the rate of disabling stroke.

Libby P, Ridker PM, Maseri A: Inflammation and atherosclerosis. Circulation 2002;105:1135-1143.
An excellent review of the concepts of the pathogenesis of acute ischemic syndromes.

Antman EM, Anbe DT, Armstrong PW, et al: American College of Cardiology/American Heart Association guidelines for the management of patients with ST elevation myocardial infarction. Executive summary. Am J Coll Cardiol 2004;44:671-719.
A comprehensive consensus statement regarding the indications for various invasive diagnostic and therapeutic maneuvers, when to consider temporary pacemakers, and the appropriate roles of assorted pharmacologic interventions, in ST elevation MI.

Yusuf S, Sleight P, Pogue J, et al: Effects of an angiotensin-converting-enzyme inhibitor, ramipril, on cardiovascular events in high-risk patients. N Engl J Med 2000;342:145-153.
This study involved 9297 high-risk patients (55 years or older, with vascular disease or diabetes plus one other cardiovascular risk factor) randomized to ramipril or placebo for a mean of 5 years. Ramipril significantly reduced the rates of death, myocardial infarction, and stroke.

Chapter 94

INVASIVE CARDIAC PROCEDURES: PERCUTANEOUS TRANSLUMINAL CORONARY ANGIOPLASTY, MITRAL AND AORTIC VALVULOPLASTY

Christian Spaulding • Olivier Varenne

KEY POINTS

1. **Percutaneous transluminal coronary angioplasty** (PTCA) is safe and effective. Stents are usually implanted during the procedure. A combination of clopidogrel and low-dose aspirin must be prescribed before and after the procedure. Platelet glycoprotein IIb/IIIa receptor inhibitors are effective primarily in patients with high-risk lesions or acute coronary syndromes.

2. **Restenosis** occurs in 30% to 50% of cases after balloon angioplasty, 3 to 6 months after the procedure. The incidence of restenosis is 25% to 50% less if stents are implanted. Drug-eluting stents further reduce this rate.

3. In patients with **unstable coronary artery disease and signs of ischemia** on electrocardiography or raised levels of biochemical markers of myocardial damage, an invasive approach with early (<24 hours) angiography is the preferred strategy. Preprocedure treatment includes aspirin, clopidogrel, heparin, and platelet glycoprotein IIb/IIIa receptor inhibitors.

4. **Primary PTCA is the most effective therapy for acute myocardial infarction**, especially in high-risk situations (cardiogenic shock, right ventricular infarction).

5. **Percutaneous mitral valvuloplasty is an accepted alternative to surgery in selected patients**. The mid- and long-term results of percutaneous aortic valvuloplasty are disappointing; it is therefore reserved for patients with severe comorbidities that preclude aortic valve replacement or as a "bridge" to definitive surgical correction.

PERCUTANEOUS TRANSLUMINAL CORONARY ANGIOPLASTY

Chronic ischemic heart disease is usually due to obstruction of the coronary arteries by atherosclerosis. It is the leading cause of mortality and morbidity in economically developed countries. Percutaneous transluminal coronary angioplasty (PTCA) has emerged as a major therapeutic option in patients with coronary artery atherosclerosis. The first PTCA in a patient was performed by Andreas Grüntzig in Zurich in September 1977.[1] PTCA was initially limited to the treatment of discrete stenoses in proximal segments of a coronary artery. Improvements in equipment and technique have increased the success rate and have led to its use in patients with complex stenoses or in high-risk clinical situations, such as acute coronary syndromes[2,3] or cardiac arrest.[4] PTCA is currently the most widely used coronary revascularization technique.

THE PROCEDURE

Vascular access is usually obtained through the femoral artery, where a sheath is introduced with the use of local anesthesia. A 5 to 8 Fr. guiding catheter is advanced through the sheath to the ostium of the coronary artery to be dilated. Once the guiding catheter is positioned in the coronary ostium, angiography of the diseased artery is performed to visualize the stenosis and the arterial segments proximal and distal to it (Fig. 94-1A). A flexible guidewire is advanced through the guiding catheter, navigated across the stenosis by rotating and advancing its angulated tip, and positioned in the distal arterial segment. The deflated balloon angioplasty catheter is advanced over the wire and positioned at the stenosis. The positions of the guidewire and balloon catheter are confirmed periodically by injecting contrast medium into the coronary artery through the guiding catheter. Once it is positioned, the balloon is usually inflated for 1 to 2 minutes at 3 to 12 atmospheres of pressure with a mixture of saline and contrast medium so that the inflation can be visualized (see Fig. 94-1B and C). Many patients have angina, electrocardiographic evidence of ischemia, or both during balloon inflation, because the coronary artery is temporarily occluded. Most often, a stent is implanted after balloon angioplasty (Fig. 94-2). Balloon-expandable stents are most commonly used. Before implantation, the stent is crimped on a balloon. The stent-balloon device is then positioned on the predilated site (see Fig. 94-1D), and the stent is implanted in the coronary artery wall by a short balloon inflation (see Fig. 94-1E). The balloon catheter is deflated

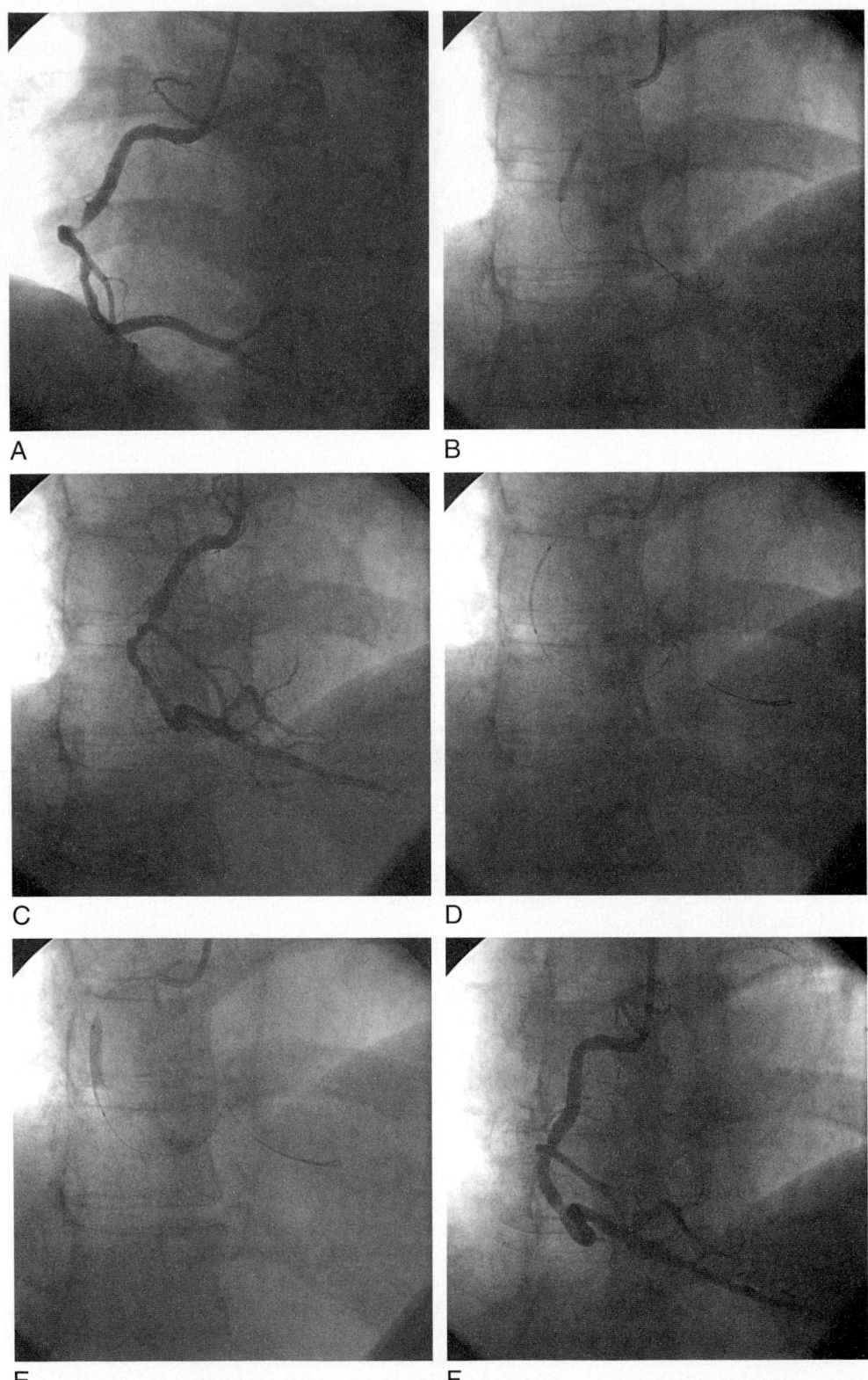

A

B

C

D

E

F

FIGURE 94–1. Coronary angioplasty procedure. *A,* Critical stenosis in the midsegment of a right coronary artery. *B,* Inflation of a 3.5-mm-diameter angioplasty balloon. *C,* Angiographic control after balloon inflation. *D,* Placement of a 3.5-mm-diameter, 18-mm-long metal stent. *E,* Inflation of the balloon. *F,* Final result.

and pulled out. The result is evaluated by injecting contrast medium (see Fig. 94-1*F*). If the result is satisfactory, the guidewire is removed. If the angiographic result is unsatisfactory, the guidewire remains in place. The balloon catheter can be replaced by a larger one, or another stent can be implanted. At the end of the procedure, a final angiogram is obtained to confirm that the result is satisfactory.

Recent improvements in stent profiles allow direct stent implantation without prior balloon dilatation. Direct stenting shortens the duration of the procedure and reduces

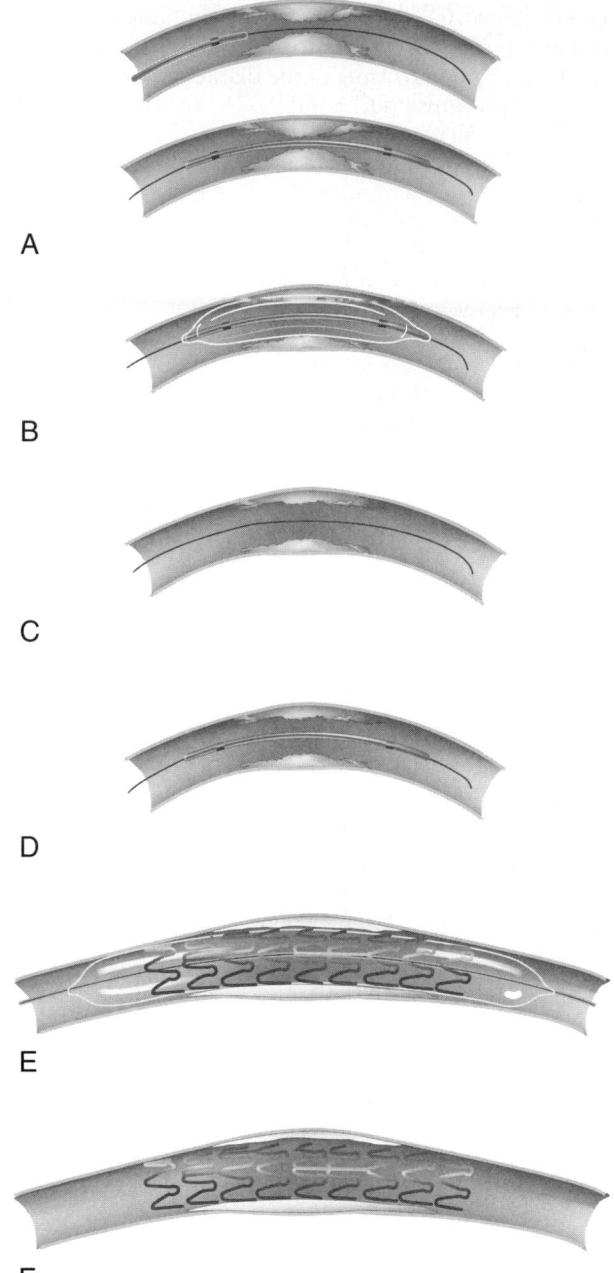

FIGURE 94–2. Implantation of a coronary stent. *A*, Placement of the balloon catheter. *B*, Predilatation with the balloon catheter. *C*, The balloon is withdrawn. *D*, Placement of the coronary stent, which has been crimped on a balloon catheter. *E*, Inflation of the balloon, and expansion of the stent. *F*, Withdrawal of the balloon catheter and the final result.

costs and can be applied in approximately 50% to 60% of cases.[5]

PRE- AND POSTPROCEDURE MANAGEMENT AND MEDICATIONS

The combination of low-dose aspirin (75 to 325 mg) and clopidogrel has been shown to reduce the incidence of acute stent occlusion after PTCA and is considered essential therapy before coronary interventions.[6,7] In the CREDO trial, patients were randomly assigned to receive a 300-mg clopidogrel loading dose (*n* = 1053) or placebo (*n* = 1063) 3 to 24 hours before PTCA. Thereafter, all patients received

clopidogrel, 75 mg/day, through day 28. From day 29 through 12 months, patients in the loading-dose group received clopidogrel, 75 mg/day, and those in the control group received placebo. Aspirin was administered in all patients. Long-term (1 year) clopidogrel therapy significantly reduced the risk of adverse events. A loading dose of clopidogrel administered at least 3 hours before the procedure did not reduce adverse events at 28 days, but subgroup analysis suggests that an interval of at least 15 hours between the loading dose and PTCA improves outcome.[8,9] Unfractionated heparin (typically 5000 to 10,000 units) is administered intravenously during PTCA to decrease the incidence of coronary artery thrombosis,[10] but it is usually not continued after the procedure. Intracoronary nitrates are given at the beginning of and during the procedure to prevent vasospasm.

Although the mainstay of antiplatelet and anticoagulation therapy for PTCA is the combination of clopidogrel and aspirin before and after the procedure and heparin during it, the use of platelet glycoprotein IIb/IIIa inhibitors has emerged as a powerful adjunctive therapy. The platelet glycoprotein IIb/IIIa receptor binds fibrinogen to crosslink platelets and can be blocked irreversibly by inhibitors such as abciximab, eptifibatide, and tirofiban. Several multicenter, randomized studies have compared heparin and aspirin to an additional treatment with platelet glycoprotein IIb/IIIa receptor inhibitors in patients undergoing PTCA and showed a significant reduction in major clinical events.[11-18] The greatest treatment benefit of platelet glycoprotein IIb/IIIa inhibitors appears to be in procedures on high-risk lesions or in patients with severe clinical patterns, such as acute coronary syndromes with ST segment changes or elevation of biologic markers of myocardial necrosis.[19] In this setting, platelet glycoprotein IIb/IIIa inhibitors should be administered before the procedure and continued at least 12 to 18 hours afterward.

The femoral arterial sheath is usually removed immediately after PTCA. Hemostasis is obtained by either manual compression or the use of closure devices. The patient remains in bed for 6 to 12 hours. Patients with stable angina and an uncomplicated procedure are usually discharged the day after removal of the sheath. Medications prescribed at the time of discharge depend on the underlying condition. Most often, the post-PTCA regimen includes low-dose aspirin (75 to 325 mg/day), clopidogrel (75 mg/day), a beta blocker or a calcium antagonist, and a statin.

Although the femoral artery remains the most widely used approach for diagnostic and therapeutic procedures, the radial artery is used increasingly to reduce the local complication rate and increase the patient's comfort. The sheath is pulled out immediately after the procedure, and hemostasis is obtained by applying a pressure dressing for several hours.[20] Immediate ambulation is feasible, and hospital discharge on the same day is possible in selected cases.[21]

EFFICACY OF THE PROCEDURE

PTCA of a nonoccluded coronary artery is successful in more than 95% of patients.[22] In the remaining patients, PTCA is unsuccessful because the stenosis cannot be crossed with either the guidewire or the balloon catheter, or because the stenosis is not adequately dilated despite the use of an appropriately sized balloon and stents. In 3% to 5% of cases, the vessel abruptly occludes (abrupt closure) during or immediately after the procedure. Reopening of the artery is attempted with repeat balloon inflations and multiple stent implantation. Stenting for abrupt closure (bailout stenting) has virtually eliminated the need for urgent coronary bypass surgery after failed PTCA. The most challenging lesions (long, angulated, calcified, or associated with intraluminal thrombus) carry a lower success rate.[23,24] PTCA also has a lower initial success rate (50% to 70%) in patients with chronically occluded arteries, because it may be difficult to manipulate the guidewire through a chronically occluded region.[25,26] In patients with recurrent angina after bypass surgery, the success rate of PTCA performed for properly selected stenoses of saphenous and arterial bypass grafts is close to that of native arteries, but the incidence of late events (myocardial infarction, repeat PTCA or other surgery) is higher.[27,28]

MECHANISMS OF CORONARY ARTERY DILATATION

The mechanisms by which PTCA increases the size of the arterial lumen have been studied in animals and cadavers.[29-32] Balloon-induced barotrauma causes endothelial denudation, cracking and disruption of the atherosclerotic plaque, and stretching or tearing of the media and adventitia (Fig. 94-3). These brutal and profound changes account for the post-PTCA angiographic features of intraluminal haziness, intimal flap, or dissection (Fig. 94-4). Intracoronary ultrasound imaging, which provides a cross-sectional view of the artery within the lumen, detects dissection of the arterial wall—sometimes extensive—in 50% to 80% of patients who have undergone successful PTCA.[33,34] These morphologic alterations open up new pathways for blood flow, leading to an increased luminal size. Balloon inflation may be deleterious, however, causing plaque hemorrhage, extensive dissection resulting in luminal compromise, platelet deposition, and thrombus formation.

In the weeks after successful PTCA, favorable remodeling of the disrupted plaque and endothelialization at the sites of intimal injury result in an increased luminal size. Angiographic studies indicate that intimal disruption usually resolves within 1 month after successful PTCA.[35]

RESTENOSIS

In patients who have undergone successful PTCA, recurrence of the stenosis, or restenosis, is the main limitation to long-term, event-free survival. Several definitions of restenosis have been suggested, but it is most commonly defined as more than a 50% narrowing of the diameter of the lumen at the site of a previously successful PTCA. Restenosis occurs in about 30% to 50% of patients in whom a coronary artery stenosis has been dilated by balloon alone.[36-38] Restenosis typically occurs 1 to 6 months after PTCA.[36]

The process of restenosis is multifactorial. Injury of the vessel initiates release of thrombogenic, vasoactive, and mitogenic factors.[39] Endothelial and deep-vessel injury leads to platelet aggregation, thrombus formation, inflammation, and activation of macrophages. These events induce the production and release of growth factors and cytokines, which in turn may promote their own synthesis and release from target cells.[40] A self-perpetuating process is initiated that results in the migration of smooth muscle cells from their usual location in the arterial media to the intima, where they change to a synthetic phenotype, produce extracellular matrix, and proliferate, thereby resulting in a stenosis within the vessel lumen. Intimal thickening accounts for about 30% of the loss in lumen diameter 6 months after coronary interventions. In addition, arterial remodeling occurs in the weeks after PTCA and can be evaluated using serial intravascular ultrasound imaging to measure the reduction in the cross-sectional area of the vessel.[41,42]

More than 70 trials enrolling more than 15,000 patients have evaluated various drugs to limit restenosis after PTCA.[43] Only one trial, using probucol, has shown beneficial results.[44] However, probucol must be administered 1 month before the procedure. In contrast, coronary stenting significantly reduces the incidence of restenosis because it produces large lumens and staves off pathologic remodeling.[45,46] Several multicenter, randomized trials showed that the incidence of restenosis is 25% to 50% lower after coronary stenting than after balloon angioplasty. Recently, drug-eluting stents have been developed to further reduce the restenosis rate. Stents are covered with a polymer that allows progressive delivery of antiproliferative drugs, such as sirolimus or paclitaxel, that inhibit smooth muscle cell proliferation. The restenosis rate is dramatically reduced with drug-eluting stents, with no increase in the acute complication rate. In the RAVEL trial, no restenosis was noted in patients receiving a drug-eluting stent, versus 26.6% in the bare metal stent group.[47] The SIRIUS trial included patients with more complex lesions, but a similar benefit was noted: restenosis occurred in 8.9% of patients receiving a drug-eluting stent, versus 36.3% of patients with bare metal stents.[48] Several large, ongoing randomized trials are testing

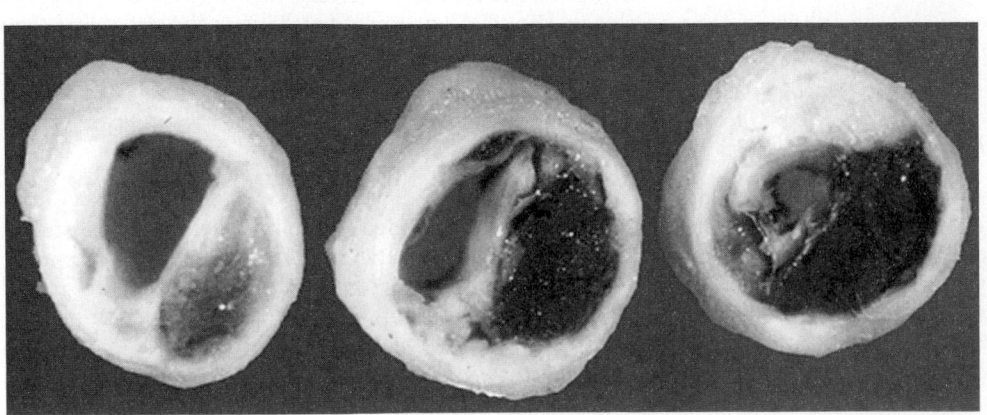

FIGURE 94–3. Pathologic specimen after coronary angioplasty. Balloon inflation has created plaque rupture with hemorrhage.

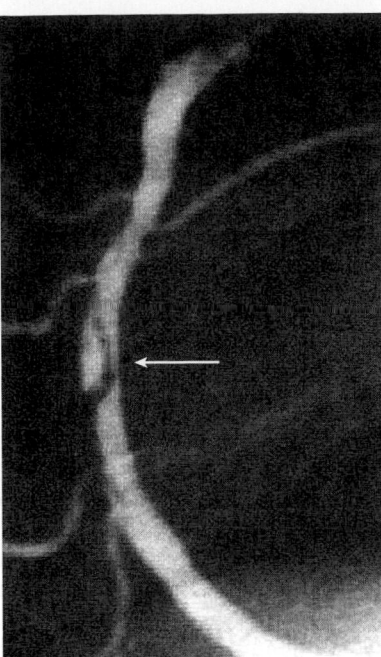

FIGURE 94–4. Arterial dissection (*arrow*) after balloon inflation in the midsegment of a right coronary artery.

the use of drug-eluting stents in various clinical situations, such as small vessels, acute myocardial infarction, and multivessel angioplasty. The widespread use of drug-eluting stents is currently limited by their availability and cost. Nevertheless, a sharp increase in the use of these devices is expected.[49]

OTHER CORONARY INTERVENTIONS

DIRECTIONAL ATHERECTOMY, LASER ANGIOPLASTY, AND ROTATIONAL ATHERECTOMY

Directional atherectomy extracts atherosclerotic tissue from the coronary artery with a cutting blade spinning at 5000 revolutions per minute in the tip of the atherectomy device.[50] During laser angioplasty, light emitted from optical fibers at the catheter tip vaporizes atheromatous tissue.[51] Rotational atherectomy uses a diamond-studded burr spinning at about 180,000 revolutions per minute to excavate calcified or fibrotic plaque.[52] In several randomized trials, these devices have not reduced the rates of late clinical events after coronary angioplasty,[53-55] and they are seldom used in current clinical practice.

CATHETER-BASED RADIOTHERAPY

Intracoronary gamma irradiation with iridium 192 has been proposed to prevent angiographic and clinical recurrence in patients undergoing treatment for in-stent restenosis.[56,57] Iridium 192 halves the need for repeat target lesion and vessel revascularization at 6 months and 5 years. However, this approach is time-consuming and technically difficult and is currently used only in selected cases of diffuse in-stent restenosis in highly specialized centers.

COMPARISON OF CLINICAL APPLICATIONS

Whether to recommend medical therapy, angioplasty, or surgical treatment remains a difficult decision in the care of individual patients with coronary artery disease. Nonetheless, the results of several clinical trials allow general guidelines to be developed.

PERCUTANEOUS TRANSLUMINAL CORONARY ANGIOPLASTY VERSUS MEDICAL THERAPY

PTCA has been compared with medical therapy for stable angina in several studies. In the Angioplasty Compared with Medicine study, patients with stable angina and single-vessel coronary disease were randomly assigned to treatment with PTCA or medical therapy.[58,59] In the Medicine, Angioplasty or Surgery study, patients with stable angina and a stenosis of the proximal left anterior descending artery were randomly assigned to medical therapy, PTCA, or bypass surgery of the left internal thoracic artery.[60] The Randomized Intervention Treatment of Angina (RITA-2) trial compared the long-term effects of PTCA and medical care in patients with coronary artery disease considered suitable for either treatment.[61] The Asymptomatic Cardiac Ischemia Pilot (ACIP) study randomized patients to three treatment strategies: angina-guided drug therapy, angina- plus ischemia-guided drug therapy, or revascularization by angioplasty or bypass surgery.[62] These studies suggest that PTCA provides more complete relief of angina than medical therapy does.

The TIMI IIIB study addressed the benefit of PTCA for patients with unstable angina or non–Q wave myocardial infarction.[63] This study enrolled 2220 patients with unstable angina and myocardial infarction without ST segment elevation who had electrocardiographic evidence of changes in the ST segment or T wave, elevated levels of cardiac markers, a history of coronary artery disease, or all three findings. Patients were randomly assigned to an early invasive strategy, which included routine catheterization within 4 to 48 hours and revascularization as appropriate, or to a more conservative (selectively invasive) strategy, in which catheterization was performed only if the patient had objective evidence of recurrent ischemia or an abnormal stress test. At 6 months, the rate of the primary endpoint (a composite of death, nonfatal myocardial infarction, and rehospitalization for acute coronary syndrome) was 15.9% with the early invasive strategy and 19.4% with the conservative strategy (odds ratio, 0.78; 95% confidence interval, 0.62 to 0.97; $P = 0.025$). In the FRISC II trial, 2457 patients were randomly assigned to invasive or noninvasive treatment and 3 months of dalteparin or placebo. After 1 year, in 100 patients, an invasive strategy saved 1.7 lives, prevented 2.0 nonfatal myocardial infarctions and 20 readmissions, and provided earlier and better symptom relief at the cost of 15 more patients with coronary artery bypass grafting and 21 more with percutaneous transluminal angioplasty.[64] An invasive approach with early (<24 hours) angiography is therefore the preferred strategy in patients with unstable coronary artery disease and signs of ischemia on electrocardiography or raised levels of biochemical markers of myocardial damage. Preprocedural treatment should include aspirin, clopidogrel, heparin, and platelet glycoprotein IIb/IIIa receptor inhibitors.

In patients with acute myocardial infarction, PTCA performed without prior thrombolytic therapy (primary PTCA) by an experienced team results in a lower risk of death or re-infarction than thrombolytic therapy does.[65-67] Stenting during primary angioplasty for acute myocardial infarction further reduces the occurrence of adverse events at 6 and 12 months.[68-70] Early administration of abciximab in patients with acute myocardial infarction improves coronary patency before stenting, the success rate of the stenting procedure, the rate of coronary patency at 6 months, left ventricular function, and clinical outcomes.[71] In patients with acute myocardial infarction complicated by cardiogenic shock, emergency revascularization improves survival at 6 months.[72] PTCA performed after failed thrombolytic therapy reduces adverse cardiac events and improves left ventricular function at 1 month.[73] In patients with right ventricular infarction, complete reperfusion of the right coronary artery by angioplasty results in dramatic recovery of right ventricular performance, as assessed by echocardiography, and an excellent clinical outcome.[74] In cardiac arrest, a strategy of immediate coronary angiography followed by angioplasty, if necessary, may increase survival.[4]

Thus, the results of clinical trials comparing PTCA with medical therapy suggest that the benefit of angioplasty depends on the severity and acuity of the clinical presentation. A gradient of risk extends across the spectrum of patients with coronary artery disease. At one end of the spectrum, patients with stable angina and one- or two-vessel disease treated medically are at low risk of nonfatal myocardial infarction. PTCA reduces angina more effectively, with a low risk of complications, but it does not lower the risk of death, myocardial infarction, or future revascularization procedures. In practice, initial revascularization by PTCA is proposed in this setting if the amount of myocardium at risk is high and if the lesions seem at low risk for procedure-related complications. At the other end of the spectrum, patients with acute coronary syndromes have a high risk of major complications and death that is significantly improved by PTCA and potent antithrombotic regimens.

PERCUTANEOUS TRANSLUMINAL CORONARY ANGIOPLASTY VERSUS BYPASS SURGERY

Several studies have compared PTCA with bypass surgery for patients with multivessel coronary artery disease. Despite the use of different protocols, the studies have yielded consistent results.[75-81] Major complications, such as death or myocardial infarction, occur with similar frequencies 1 to 5 years after angioplasty or bypass surgery. However, there is an increased need for repeat revascularization procedures in patients who are randomized to PTCA. In addition, in the BARI study, diabetic patients had higher rates of survival 5 years after treatment with bypass surgery.[75] New randomized trials comparing PTCA with bypass surgery are now being performed with the use of drug-eluting stents.

In practice, most patients with multivessel disease have diffuse lesions or chronic occlusions that are not amenable to PTCA. Bypass surgery therefore remains the preferred therapeutic option in this subset of patients, such as those with left main and triple-vessel coronary artery disease with critical obstruction of the proximal left anterior descending artery or left ventricular dysfunction. Nondiabetic patients with multivessel coronary disease who are good candidates for either PTCA or bypass surgery can be reassured that both revascularization approaches are followed by equivalent rates of major complications. However, the invasive nature of bypass surgery must be weighed against the likelihood of repeated procedures after PTCA. Whether the use of drug-eluting stents will reduce the rate of re-intervention after angioplasty in patients with multivessel disease and change these guidelines remains to be proved by ongoing trials

MITRAL VALVULOPLASTY

In patients with severe mitral stenosis, surgical mitral commissurotomy alleviates symptoms and improves mid- and long-term prognosis. Percutaneous mitral valvuloplasty was first applied in 1984 to young patients with rheumatic mitral stenosis using a transseptal approach.[82] The technique is widely accepted as an alternative to surgical repair or replacement in such cases, as well as in patients with more rigid calcific lesions. Selection of patients is based on the echocardiographic features of the mitral valve.[83]

The transseptal approach is the most commonly used technique. After puncture of the intra-arterial septum with a needle and a long sheath, a large (23- to 25-mm diameter) valvuloplasty balloon is advanced through the atrial opening and positioned across the mitral valve. Stepwise inflation of this balloon results in separation of the fused commissures, similar to the surgical technique of mitral commissurotomy.

Overall procedure mortality is 1% to 2%. Long-term follow-up studies demonstrate preservation of the improved mitral orifice.[84]

AORTIC VALVULOPLASTY

Calcific aortic stenosis in an adult is the most common indication for the more than 25,000 aortic valve replacements performed in the Unites States each year. With the evident success of balloon valvuloplasty for mitral stenosis, percutaneous aortic balloon valvuloplasty was proposed as an alternative to surgery. The balloon catheter is advanced retrogradely through the aortic stenosis using a femoral approach in most cases. Mid- and long-term results are disappointing; improvement in the orifice area is less than that obtained with a valve replacement, and echocardiographic follow-up shows recurrence of aortic stenosis in most cases.[85] Aortic valvuloplasty is therefore reserved for adult patients with severe calcific aortic stenosis who have severe comorbidities that preclude aortic valve replacement, or it is used in patients as a "bridge" to definitive surgical correction.[83,84] Preliminary results involving the percutaneous transcatheter implantation of a heart valve prosthesis for aortic stenosis are promising.[86]

CONCLUSION

The past 20 years have seen the explosive growth of interventional techniques. PTCA has become the most widely used method of coronary revascularization. Coronary stenting has revolutionized the practice of interventional cardiology by partially overcoming the limitations of coronary balloon angioplasty, such as abrupt vessel closure and restenosis. In patients with stable angina, PTCA reduces symptoms more effectively than medical therapy does, with a low risk of complications. Patients with acute coronary syndromes have a high risk of major complications and death that can be significantly reduced by PTCA. Drug-eluting stents further reduce the restenosis rate and will almost certainly enhance or expand clinical indications, especially in patients with multivessel disease. As with all new techniques, careful validation of their utility will be necessary to ensure their optimal use in patient care.

ANNOTATED REFERENCES

Andersen HR, Nielsen TT, Rasmussen K, et al: A comparison of coronary angioplasty with fibrinolytic therapy in acute myocardial infarction. N Engl J Med 2003;349:733-742.

In this study, 1572 patients with acute myocardial infarction were randomized to treatment with angioplasty or accelerated treatment with intravenous alteplase; 1129 patients were enrolled at 24 referral hospitals, and 443 patients were enrolled at 5 invasive treatment centers. The primary endpoint (a composite of death, re-infarction, or disabling stroke) was reached in 8.5% of the patients in the angioplasty group, compared with 14.2% of those in the fibrinolysis group (P = 0.002). A reperfusion strategy involving the transfer of patients to an invasive treatment center for primary angioplasty is superior to on-site fibrinolysis, provided the transfer takes 2 hours or less.

Bowers TR, O'Neill WW, Grines C: Effect of reperfusion on biventricular function and survival after right ventricular infarction. N Engl J Med 1998;338:933-940.

Echocardiographic studies were performed before and after angioplasty in 53 patients with acute right ventricular infarction. Complete reperfusion of the right coronary artery by angioplasty resulted in the dramatic recovery of right ventricular performance and an excellent clinical outcome. In contrast, unsuccessful reperfusion was associated with impaired recovery of right ventricular function, persistent hemodynamic compromise, and a high mortality rate.

Hochman JS, Sleeper LA, Webb JG: Early revascularization in acute myocardial infarction complicated by cardiogenic shock. SHOCK investigators: Should We Emergently Revascularize Occluded Coronaries for Cardiogenic Shock? N Engl J Med 1999;341:625-634.

Patients with shock due to left ventricular failure complicating myocardial infarction were randomly assigned to emergency revascularization (152 patients) or initial medical stabilization (150 patients). Revascularization was accomplished by either coronary artery bypass grafting or angioplasty. Intra-aortic balloon counterpulsation was performed in 86% of the patients in both groups. Six-month mortality was lower in the revascularization group than in the medical therapy group (50.3% versus 63.1%; P = 0.027). Early revascularization should be strongly considered for patients with acute myocardial infarction complicated by cardiogenic shock.

Moses JW, Leon MB, Popma JJ, et al: Sirolimus-eluting stents versus standard stents in patients with stenosis in a native coronary artery. N Engl J Med 2003;349:1315-1323.

Drug-eluting stents significantly reduce the occurrence of restenosis. It occurred in 8.9% of patients receiving drug-eluting stents, versus 36.3% of patients with bare metal stents.

Wallentin L, Lagerqvist B, Husted S, et al: Outcome at 1 year after an invasive compared with a non-invasive strategy in unstable coronary-artery disease: The FRISC II invasive randomised trial. Lancet 2000;356:9-16.

In this study, 2457 patients were randomly assigned to invasive or noninvasive treatment. After 1 year, in 100 patients, an invasive strategy saved 1.7 lives, prevented 2.0 nonfatal myocardial infarctions and 20 readmissions, and provided earlier and better symptom relief. An invasive approach with early (<24 hours) angiography is therefore the preferred strategy in patients with unstable coronary artery disease and signs of ischemia on electrocardiography or raised levels of biochemical markers of myocardial damage.

Chapter 95

SUPRAVENTRICULAR ARRHYTHMIAS

John Camm • Irina Savelieva

KEY POINTS

1. **Supraventricular tachycardia** (SVT) is characterized by narrow QRS complexes, but differentiating SVT from ventricular tachycardia may be necessary when bundle branch block, rate-dependent aberrancy, and antidromic atrioventricular (AV) reentry tachycardia are present.

2. **If the diagnosis of SVT cannot be proved**, the arrhythmia should be treated as ventricular tachycardia.

3. **Immediate direct-current (DC) cardioversion** is the treatment for any hemodynamically unstable tachycardia.

4. **In hemodynamically stable paroxysmal junctional tachycardias** (AV nodal reentry tachycardia and AV reentry tachycardia), vagotonic maneuvers should be tried first, because they may terminate tachycardia in about 50% patients without the need to resort to pharmacologic therapy.

5. Intravenous adenosine, verapamil, and esmolol are **first-line drug therapies for paroxysmal junctional tachycardias**, but adenosine and verapamil should not be used for wide complex tachycardias and atrial fibrillation with preexcitation.

6. **DC cardioversion or pharmacologic conversion** with intravenous ibutilide or flecainide is appropriate for the termination of atrial fibrillation associated with preexcitation syndrome.

7. **Intravenous verapamil, diltiazem, esmolol, metoprolol, and propranolol** can rapidly accomplish rate control in atrial fibrillation but may be less effective in atrial flutter.

8. **Beta blockers are preferable** in atrial fibrillation associated with thyrotoxicosis.

9. **Pharmacologic cardioversion of atrial fibrillation** in the absence of severe underlying heart disease can be attained using oral or intravenous flecainide or propafenone and intravenous ibutilide, but the last is more effective in atrial flutter.

10. **Propafenone and flecainide may result in atrial flutter** with slow atrial rates and 2:1 or 1:1 AV conduction, and verapamil, diltiazem, or beta blockers should be available to treat this complication; ibutilide can significantly prolong the QT interval and

cause polymorphic ventricular tachycardia that, if sustained, may require DC cardioversion.

11. **Intravenous amiodarone should be considered as first-line drug therapy** in patients with severely impaired left ventricular function.

12. Digoxin is not useful for **rate control** in the emergency setting.

13. **Accelerated AV rhythm and atrial tachycardia with AV block** commonly occur as a result of digitalis toxicity; digitalis withdrawal is the usual therapy.

14. **Anticoagulation is indicated if atrial fibrillation or flutter persists for more than 48 hours or if the duration is unknown**; anticoagulation and rate control should be the initial therapy in these patients.

15. **An alternative approach is transesophageal echocardiography**, to exclude the presence of atrial thrombi or dense spontaneous echo contrast, and short-term anticoagulation with low-molecular-weight heparin, followed by DC or pharmacologic cardioversion.

16. Patients with **paroxysmal junctional tachycardias, atrial tachycardia, atrial flutter, and first-onset or recurrent atrial fibrillation** should be referred to a cardiologist for long-term management; effective nonpharmacologic therapies are available for these arrhythmias.

CLASSIFICATION AND EPIDEMIOLOGY

Supraventricular arrhythmias include rhythms arising from the sinus node and the adjacent atrial tissue (inappropriate sinus tachycardia, sinoatrial reentry tachycardia), both the right and the left atria (atrial tachycardia, flutter, and fibrillation), the atrioventricular (AV) node (AV nodal reentry tachycardia, accelerated ectopic junctional rhythm), and the AV node with involvement of an accessory pathway or multiple pathways (AV reentry tachycardia) (Fig. 95-1).

ATRIOVENTRICULAR NODAL REENTRY TACHYCARDIA AND ATRIOVENTRICULAR REENTRY TACHYCARDIA

AV nodal reentry tachycardia and AV reentry tachycardia are usually referred to as paroxysmal supraventricular

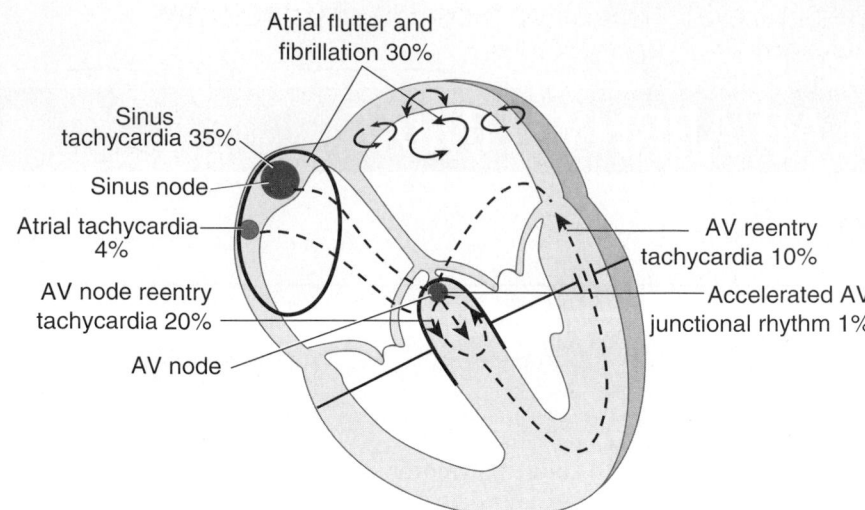

Sinus tachycardia 35%

Sinus node

Atrial tachycardia 4%

AV node reentry tachycardia 20%

AV node

Atrial flutter and fibrillation 30%

AV reentry tachycardia 10%

Accelerated AV junctional rhythm 1%

FIGURE 95–1. Supraventricular tachyarrhythmias encountered in the emergency setting. AV, atrioventricular.

tachycardias and are often seen in young patients with little or no structural heart disease, although a congenital heart abnormality giving rise to increased atrial pressure and dilatation (e.g., Ebstein's anomaly, atrial septal defect, Fallot's tetralogy) can coexist in a small percentage of patients with these arrhythmias.[1] The first presentation is common between age 12 and 30 years, and the prevalence is approximately 2.5 per 1000. Women are twice as likely as men to present with AV nodal reentry tachycardia.

ATRIAL FLUTTER AND FIBRILLATION

Atrial fibrillation is the most common supraventricular arrhythmia, affecting 1% to 2% of the general population, especially the elderly. It is usually associated with cardiovascular pathologies, among which hypertension and congestive heart failure prevail.[2] About one third of patients, however, present with no underlying heart disease and are considered to have "lone" atrial fibrillation. The epidemiology of isolated atrial flutter is largely unknown and is believed to be in the range of 0.037% to 0.88% per 1000 person-years, but nearly half these patients also have atrial fibrillation as a coexistent arrhythmia.

ATRIAL TACHYCARDIA

Atrial tachycardia affects 0.34% to 0.46% of patients with arrhythmias and is common in younger individuals following surgical correction of congenital heart disease and in the elderly, in whom it often occurs in association with atrial fibrillation.

OTHER SUPRAVENTRICULAR TACHYCARDIAS

Inappropriate sinus tachycardia and sinoatrial reentry tachycardia are less well defined clinical and electrocardiographic entities, and their prevalence and associated conditions are not well appreciated. Sinoatrial reentry tachycardia is found incidentally in 1.8% to 16.9% of patients undergoing electrophysiologic study for other supraventricular tachyarrhythmias.

CLINICAL PRESENTATION

The leading symptom of most supraventricular tachyarrhythmias, particularly AV nodal reentry tachycardia and AV reentry tachycardia, is rapid, regular palpitations, usually with an abrupt onset; they can occur spontaneously or be precipitated by simple movements. A common feature of tachycardias that involve circulation through the AV node is termination by Valsalva's maneuvers. In younger individuals with no structural heart disease, the rapid heart rate can be the main pathologic finding. Other symptoms may include anxiety, dizziness, dyspnea, neck pulsation, central chest pain, weakness, and occasionally polyuria due to the release of atrial natriuretic peptide in response to increased atrial pressures (more common in atrial tachycardia and AV nodal reentry tachycardia). Prominent jugular venous pulsations due to atrial contractions against closed AV valves may be observed during AV nodal reentry or AV reentry tachycardia.

True syncope is relatively uncommon unless uncontrolled tachycardia over 200 beats per minute is sustained for a long period, especially in patients who remain standing. Syncope has been reported in 10% to 15% of patients, usually just after onset of the arrhythmia or in association with a prolonged pause following its termination. However, in older patients with concomitant heart disease such as aortic stenosis, hypertrophic cardiomyopathy, and cerebrovascular disease, significant hypotension and syncope may result from profound hemodynamic collapse associated with only moderately fast ventricular rates.

It is essential to recognize that patients presenting with AV reentry tachycardia may also present with atrial fibrillation. If an accessory pathway has a short antegrade effective refractory period (<250 msec), it may conduct to the ventricles at an extremely high rate and cause ventricular fibrillation. The incidence of sudden death is 0.15% to 0.39% per patient-year, and it may be the first manifestation of the disease in younger individuals.

Irregular palpitations may be due to atrial premature beats, atrial flutter with varying AV conduction block, atrial fibrillation, or multifocal atrial tachycardia. Although highly symptomatic, these arrhythmias usually have a benign hemodynamic prognosis. However, in patients with depressed ventricular function, uncontrolled atrial fibrillation can reduce cardiac output and precipitate hypotension and congestive heart failure. Atrial fibrillation in association with slow AV conduction or complete block (Frederick's syndrome) may result in hemodynamic collapse. Inappropriate sinus tachycardia and nonparoxysmal accelerated junctional rhythm are characterized by relatively slow heart rates and gradual onset and termination.

ELECTROCARDIOGRAPHY

Whenever possible, a 12-lead electrocardiogram (ECG) should be taken during tachycardia. If a patient with an arrhythmia is hemodynamically unstable, a monitor strip should be obtained from the defibrillator before electrical discharge.

NARROW-COMPLEX TACHYCARDIAS

The typical ECG feature is narrow QRS complexes less than 120 msec. In this case, the tachycardia is almost always supraventricular, and the differential diagnosis relates to its mechanism (Fig. 95-2).

WIDE-COMPLEX TACHYCARDIAS

The differential diagnostic features of wide-complex tachycardias favoring a supraventricular origin of the arrhythmia include, but are not limited to, preexistent bundle branch block; rate-dependent aberrancy; antidromic AV reentry tachycardia, when an accessory pathway conducts and excites the ventricles retrogradely; and prominent electrolyte abnormalities (e.g., hypokalemia) resulting in QRS widening (Fig. 95-3). If the diagnosis of supraventricular tachycardia cannot be proved, the patient should be treated as if ventricular tachycardia is present. Immediate direct-current (DC) cardioversion is the treatment for any hemodynamically unstable tachycardia.

ATRIOVENTRICULAR NODAL REENTRY TACHYCARDIA

MECHANISM

In AV nodal reentry tachycardia, there are two functionally and anatomically different pathways within the AV node: one is characterized by a short effective refractory period and slow conduction, and the other has a longer effective refractory period and faster conduction. In sinus rhythm, the atrial impulse that depolarizes the ventricles usually conducts through the fast pathway. If the atrial impulse (e.g., an atrial premature beat) occurs early, when the fast pathway is still refractory, the slow pathway takes over in propagating the atrial impulse to the ventricles; it then travels back through the fast pathway, which by then has recovered its excitability, thus initiating the most common "slow-fast," or typical, AV nodal reentry tachycardia.

ELECTROCARDIOGRAPHIC PRESENTATION

In sinus rhythm, the ECG is usually normal, unless other unrelated abnormalities are present. During AV nodal reentry tachycardia, the rhythm is regular, with narrow QRS complexes and a rate of 140 to 250 beats per minute. The atria are activated retrogradely, producing the inverted P waves in leads II, III, and avF. Because atrial and ventricular depolarization occurs simultaneously, the P waves are often obscured by the QRS complexes and cannot be detected on the surface ECG (Fig. 95-4A). However, in about one third of cases of slow-fast AV nodal reentry tachycardia, a terminal positive deflection in lead avR or V_1 (or both), imitating right bundle branch block, or pseudo–S waves in the inferiorly oriented leads may be present, reflecting retrograde activation of the atria. Tachycardia using these pathways in reverse ("fast-slow," or long RP, tachycardia) is less common (5% to 10% of cases).

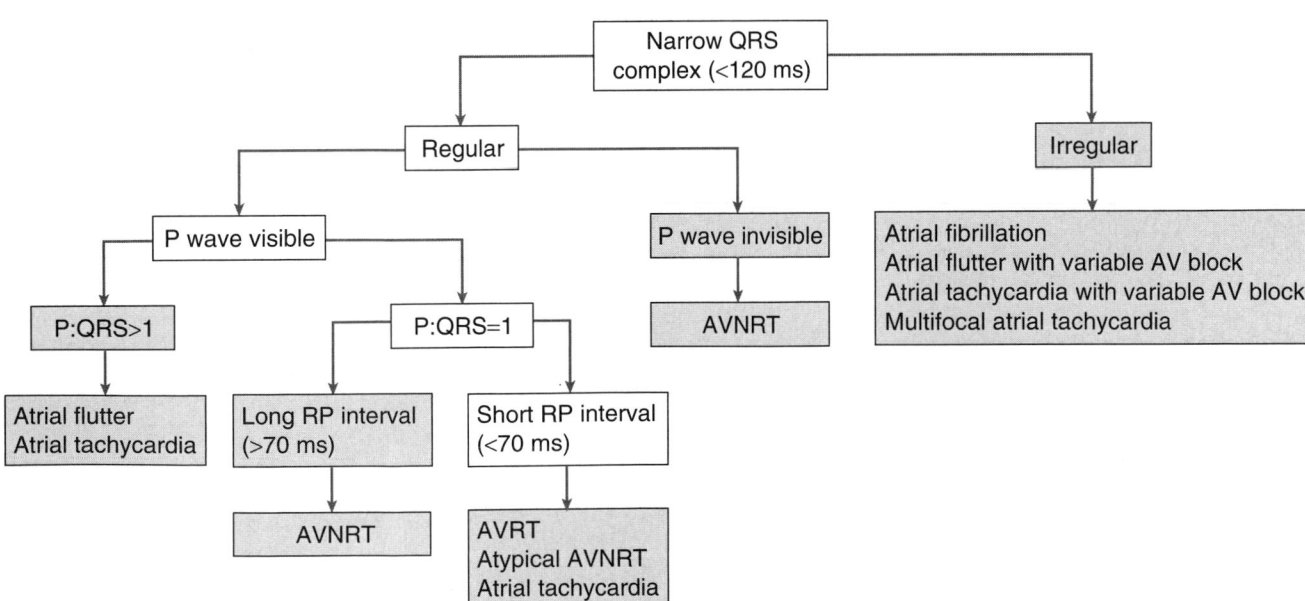

FIGURE 95–2. Differential diagnosis for narrow QRS complex (presumably supraventricular) tachycardias. Note that ventricular tachycardia may present with the narrow QRS complexes (e.g., fascicular tachycardia). AV, atrioventricular; AVNRT, atrioventricular nodal reentry tachycardia; AVRT, atrioventricular reentry tachycardia.

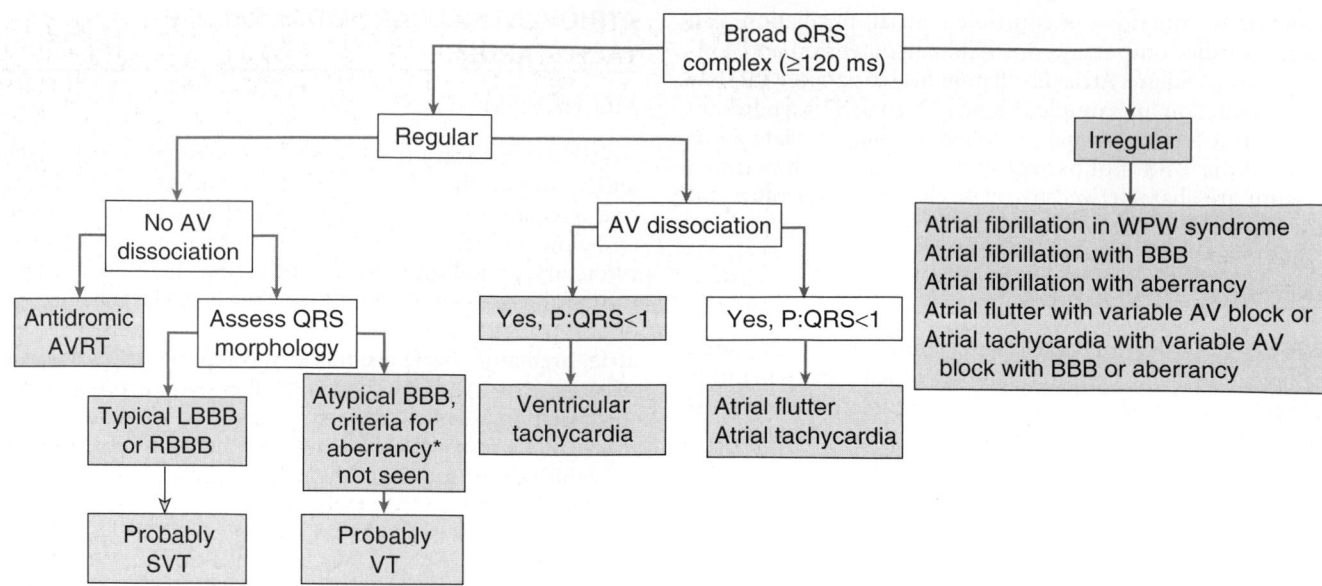

FIGURE 95-3. Differential diagnosis for wide QRS complex tachycardias. AV, atrioventricular; AVRT, atrioventricular reentry tachycardia; BBB, bundle branch block; LBBB, left bundle branch block; RBBB, right bundle branch block; SVT, supraventricular tachycardia; WPW, Wolff-Parkinson-White; VT, ventricular tachycardia.

*Criteria for aberrancy: rate dependency, triphasic QRS complexes, rSR in V$_1$, with R>, QRS width <140 msec, QRS deflections are discordant in precordial leads, absence of fusion and capture beats.

ATRIOVENTRICULAR REENTRY TACHYCARDIA

ACCESSORY PATHWAYS

AV reentry tachycardia occurs as a result of an anatomically distinct AV connection, termed an accessory pathway, produced by incomplete separation of the atria and ventricles during fetal development. The most common accessory pathways of the AV type (often called Kent's bundles) are located around the mitral or tricuspid annulus. In about 10% of cases, they are multiple.

Accessory pathways are capable of conduction in either or both directions. Accessory pathways that are capable of antegrade conduction are referred to as "manifest," demonstrating a delta wave during sinus rhythm when the atrial impulses conduct over the accessory pathway without encountering

AV delay. The PR interval is short (<120 msec), and the QRS complex is wide; this occurs because the atrial impulse enters a nonspecialized ventricular myocardium, and depolarization progresses slowly at first, giving rise to the delta wave before it is overtaken by a depolarization wavefront propagating via the normal conduction tissue. An accessory pathway that is capable of only retrograde conduction is termed "concealed" and does not produce a short PR interval or a delta wave during sinus rhythm.

MECHANISM AND ELECTROCARDIOGRAPHIC PRESENTATION

The reentry circuit of orthodromic AV reentry tachycardia involves the AV node and an accessory pathway, with the impulses conducting from the atria to the ventricles over

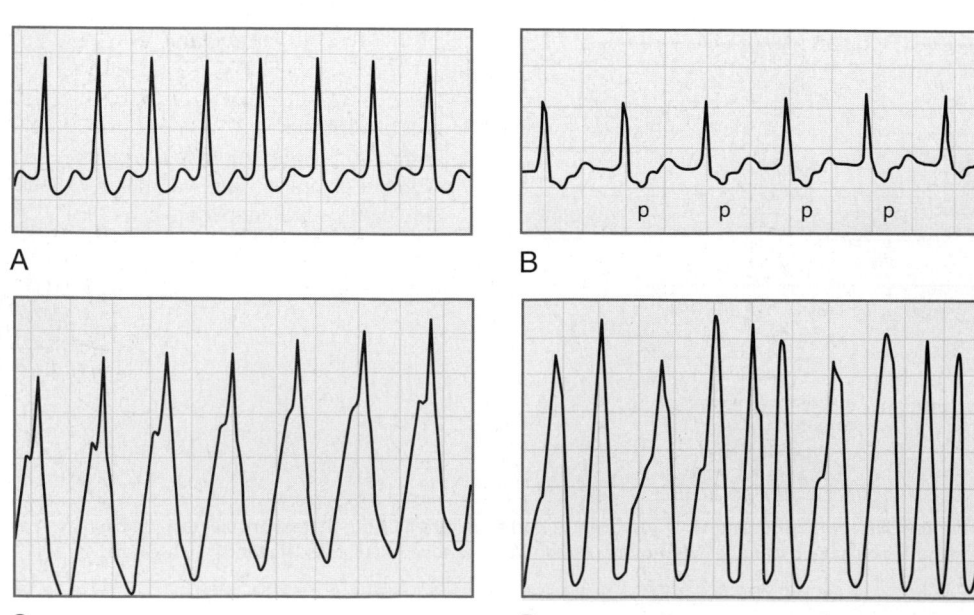

FIGURE 95-4. *A,* Atrioventricular nodal reentry tachycardia, slow-fast type. Note the narrow QRS complexes and the absence of P waves. *B,* Atrioventricular reentry orthodromic tachycardia. The retrograde inverted P waves follow the QRS complexes in leads II, III, and avF. *C,* Atrioventricular reentry antidromic tachycardia with wide QRS complexes. An electrocardiogram during sinus rhythm with a QRS complex morphology identical to that seen during tachycardia may be helpful in the diagnosis. *D,* Atrial fibrillation in preexcitation syndrome with a fast ventricular rate response.

TABLE 95–1. VAGAL MANEUVERS TO TERMINATE TACHYCARDIA

Carotid Sinus Massage

Ensure that there is no significant carotid artery disease (carotid bruits)
Monitor the electrocardiogram continuously
Place the patient in the supine position with the head slightly extended
Start with right carotid sinus massage
Apply firm rotatory or steady pressure to the carotid artery at the level of the third cervical vertebra for 5 sec
If no response, massage the left carotid sinus
Generally, right carotid sinus massage decreases sinus node discharge, and left carotid sinus massage slows atrioventricular conduction
Do not massage both carotids at the same time
A single application of carotid sinus pressure is effective in about 20% to 30% of patients with paroxysmal supraventricular tachycardias; multiple applications terminate tachycardia in about 50% of patients
Asystole is a potential but rare complication

Valsalva's Maneuver

Valsalva's maneuver involves an abrupt voluntary increase in intrathoracic and intra-abdominal pressures by straining
Monitor the electrocardiogram continuously
Place the patient in the supine position
The patient should not take a deep inspiration before straining
Ideally, the patient blows into a mouthpiece of a manometer against the pressure of 30-40 mm Hg for 15 sec
Alternatively, the patient strains for 15 sec while breath-holding
Transient acceleration of tachycardia usually occurs during the strain phase as a result of sympathetic excess
On release of strain, the rate of tachycardia slows because of the compensatory increase in vagal tone (baroreceptor reflex); it may terminate in about 50% of patients
Termination of tachycardia may be followed by pauses and ventricular ectopics

the AV node and traveling in the reverse direction through the accessory pathway (see Fig. 95-4*B*). In antidromic AV reentry tachycardia, the reentrant impulses conduct antegradely from the atria to the ventricles via an accessory pathway and retrogradely via the AV node or a second accessory pathway (see Fig. 95-4*C*). Antidromic AV reentry tachycardia is uncommon (<10% of cases). Atrial fibrillation is usually encountered in patients with antegradely conducting pathways (see Fig. 95-4*D*).

ACUTE MANAGEMENT

In an emergency, distinguishing between AV nodal reentry tachycardia and AV reentry tachycardia may be difficult, but it is usually not critical, because both tachycardias respond to the same treatment. If the patient is hemodynamically stable, vagal maneuvers, including carotid sinus massage, Valsalva's maneuver, and facial immersion in cold water, can terminate tachycardia in about 50% patients (Table 95-1).[3,4] Commercially available gel packs can be used as cold compresses instead of facial immersion, but the most important element is wet nostrils and breath-holding.

PHARMACOLOGIC TERMINATION

AV blocking agents, such as adenosine, verapamil, diltiazem, and beta blockers, are effective in terminating both AV nodal reentry and AV reentry tachycardia (Table 95-2).[1]

Adenosine

Intravenous (i.v.) adenosine is effective in diagnosing, rate slowing, and occasionally terminating the narrow-complex tachycardias.[5] Adenosine usually terminates AV nodal reentry tachycardia and AV reentry tachycardia but rarely interrupts the atrial flutter circuit and does not suppress automatic atrial tachycardia; it can, however, produce high-degree AV

TABLE 95–2. ACUTE PHARMACOLOGIC RATE CONTROL IN ATRIAL TACHYARRHYTHMIAS

Drug	Route of Administration	Dose	Onset	Potential Adverse Effects
Verapamil	Intravenous	5-10 mg (0.075-0.15 mg/kg) over 2 min; if no response, additional 5-10 mg after 15-30 min; 3-10 mg every 4-6 h for rate control	3-5 min	Hypotension, bradycardia, heart block, possible deterioration of ventricular function in the presence of organic heart disease
Diltiazem	Intravenous	0.25 mg/kg over 2 min; if no response, additional 0.35 mg/kg after 15-30 min; followed by 5-15 mg/h infusion for rate control	2-7 min	
Esmolol	Intravenous	0.5 mg/kg over 1 min, followed by 0.05-0.2 mg/kg/min for 4 min; if no response after 5 min, 0.5 mg/kg for 1 min, followed by 0.1 mg/kg for 4 min; infusion 0.05-0.2 mg/kg/min for rate control	2-3 min	Hypotension, bradycardia, heart block, possible deterioration of ventricular function in the presence of organic heart disease
Metoprolol	Intravenous	2.5-5 mg over 2 min followed by repeat doses if necessary (total 10-15 mg)	5 min	
Atenolol	Intravenous	2.5 mg over 2 min, followed by repeat doses if necessary (total 10 mg) or infusion 0.15 mg/kg for 20 min	5-10 min	
Propranolol	Intravenous	1 mg over 1 min (total 10-12 mg; 0.15 mg/kg)	5 min	
Digoxin	Intravenous	0.5-1 mg, followed by 0.25 mg every 2-4 h (maximum, 1.5 mg)	30-60 min	Bradycardia, atrioventricular block, atrial arrhythmias, ventricular tachycardia

Intravenous amiodarone can also be effective in rate control, especially in patients with poor left ventricular function, but there is insufficient evidence to support this recommendation. The rate-slowing effect of amiodarone is usually delayed by 1-2 hours.

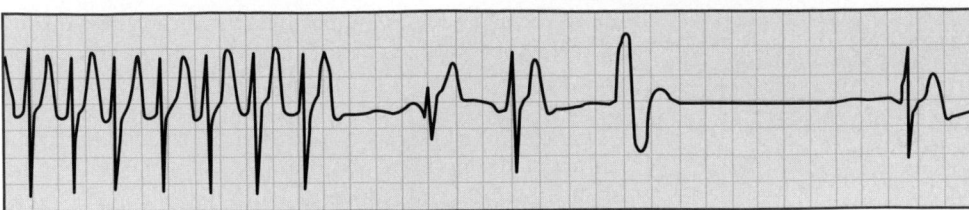

A

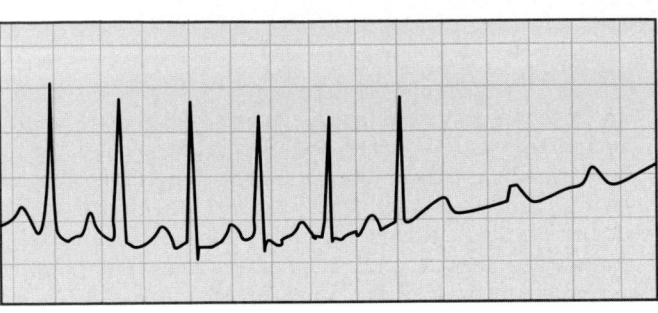

B

FIGURE 95–5. *A,* Adenosine usually terminates atrioventricular reentry tachycardias. *B* and *C,* It rarely interrupts the atrial flutter circuit or suppresses automatic focal atrial tachycardia but produces high-degree atrioventricular block during which the tachycardia persists.

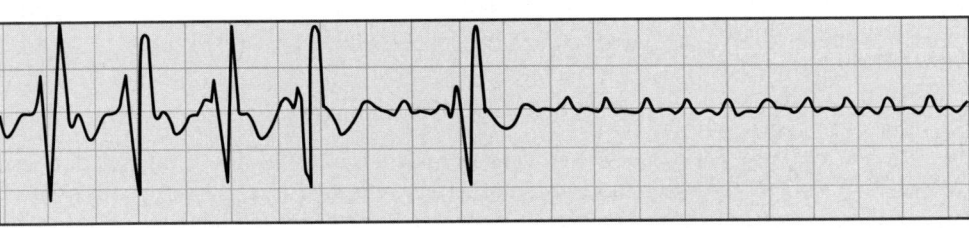

C

block during which the tachycardia persists (Fig. 95-5). It has no effect on most ventricular tachycardias. Adenosine is advantageous compared with verapamil because of its rapid onset and the absence of a negative inotropic effect in patients with poor left ventricular function and those with significant hypotension.

Adenosine is administered as a very rapid 3- to 6-mg i.v. bolus; if this is ineffective, another 6- to 12-mg bolus can be given 2 to 5 minutes later. Adenosine is metabolized very quickly, with an effective half-life of 10 seconds. Adverse effects, including dyspnea, facial flushing, and chest tightness, are therefore short-lived, but in about 12% of patients, adenosine may shorten the atrial effective refractory period and provoke atrial flutter or fibrillation or accelerate conduction over the accessory pathway and produce a rapid ventricular response. In a proportion of patients, ventricular premature beats and nonsustained ventricular tachycardia may occur after the successful termination of supraventricular tachycardia.[6] Some individuals, particularly heart transplant recipients, are unusually sensitive to adenosine and require a lower dose (1 mg).

Verapamil and Diltiazem

Verapamil is administered intravenously as a 5- to 10-mg bolus over 2 minutes, and the effect on tachycardia is expected in 5 to 10 minutes. If necessary, a second bolus of 10 mg can be given 30 minutes after the initial dose. Vagal maneuvers can be effective at this stage. Verapamil should not be used for wide-complex tachycardias. Intravenous verapamil is contraindicated in patients with poor left ventricular function or heart failure, and it should not be administered after pretreatment with oral and especially i.v. beta blockers. It should not be used for atrial fibrillation associated with preexcitation syndrome, because it may result in acceleration of conduction over antegradely conducting accessory pathway, especially with a short effective refractory period, a rapid ventricular response, and ventricular fibrillation. DC cardioversion or pharmacologic conversion with i.v. ibutilide or flecainide is appropriate for termination of atrial fibrillation with preexcitation. Diltiazem is an alternative to verapamil, but lower effective rates have been reported with this drug.[7]

Beta Blockers

Among beta blockers, esmolol, administered as an i.v. infusion at a rate of 50 to 200 µg/kg per minute, is the agent of choice because of its rapid onset. More readily available i.v. metoprolol, atenolol, and propranolol can also be considered (see Table 95-2). Excessive bradycardia caused by AV node blocking agents can be countered with i.v. injection of atropine 0.6 to 2.4 mg in divided doses of 0.6 mg.

Other Antiarrhythmic Agents

Because adenosine, verapamil, diltiazem, and beta blockers are so highly effective in terminating AV nodal reentry tachycardia and AV reentry tachycardia, specific antiarrhythmic drugs such as propafenone, flecainide, sotalol, ibutilide, and amiodarone are seldom needed in the acute setting. Digoxin is not useful because it is often ineffective and may facilitate conduction over the accessory pathway, shorten the atrial effective refractory period, and promote atrial fibrillation.

ATRIAL PACING

In patients with implantable devices, antitachycardia pacing facilities can be used to terminate the arrhythmia. However, there is also a risk of inducing atrial fibrillation with a rapid

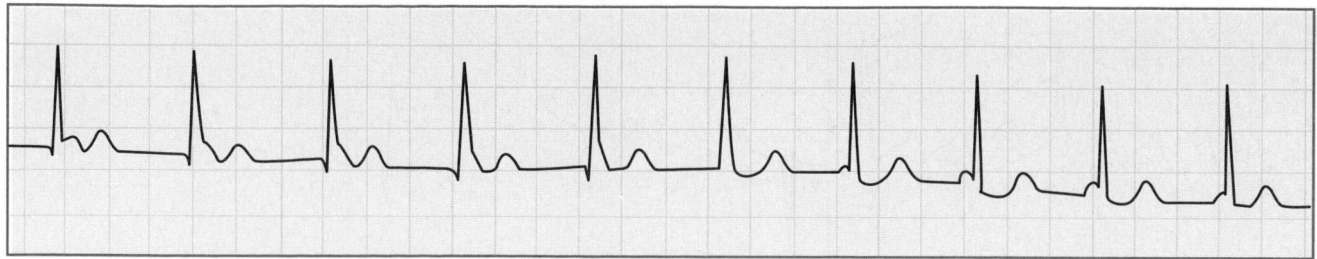

FIGURE 95–6. Accelerated junctional rhythm with independent sinus node activity.

ventricular response in a patient with an antegradely conducting accessory pathway.

LONG-TERM MANAGEMENT

Patients with AV nodal reentry tachycardia and AV reentry tachycardia should be referred to a cardiologist for electrophysiologic evaluation and long-term management. Both pharmacologic and nonpharmacologic alternatives, including ablation of an accessory pathway, are widely available.

ACCELERATED ATRIOVENTRICULAR RHYTHM

Accelerated AV rhythm is produced by abnormal automaticity in the AV node. It is a narrow QRS complex tachycardia (unless bundle branch block is present), with the ventricular rate ranging from 70 to 250 beats per minute. AV dissociation is also present, because the atria are activated normally by the sinus node impulse while the ventricles are depolarized from an accelerated junctional site (Fig. 95-6). This arrhythmia is commonly due to digitalis toxicity, and drug withdrawal is the usual therapy. If the rate of the AV node pacemaker is not fast, atropine can be given to increase the sinus node discharge until it resumes its dominance.

ATRIAL FIBRILLATION AND ATRIAL FLUTTER

Atrial fibrillation with a fast ventricular response is the most common supraventricular arrhythmia encountered in the emergency department in both younger adults with first-onset arrhythmia and older patients presenting with decompensation. Atrial flutter shares these clinical presentations and requires similar initial therapy. The acute management of both arrhythmias is therefore considered together.

ATRIAL FLUTTER

Mechanism
The classification of atrial flutter is based on the ECG presentation and electrophysiologic mechanisms. The most common type is typical isthmus-dependent atrial flutter. Incisional reentry atrial flutter occurs after surgical correction for congenital heart disease. There are also various forms of atypical flutters, such as atypical right atrial isthmus-dependent flutter (double-wave and lower loop reentry) and left atrial flutter, whose circuit contains the pulmonary vein or mitral valve annulus.[8]

Typical, or isthmus-dependent, atrial flutter involves a macro-reentrant right atrial circuit around the tricuspid annulus. The wavefront circulates down the lateral wall of the right atrium, through the eustachian ridge between the tricuspid annulus and the inferior vena cava, and up the interatrial septum, giving rise to the most frequent pattern, referred to as counterclockwise flutter. Reentry can also occur in the opposite direction (clockwise or reverse flutter).

Electrocardiographic Presentation
Atrial flutter is usually an organized atrial rhythm with an atrial rate typically between 250 and 350 beats per minute. In the more common counterclockwise flutter, F waves are negative in leads II, III, avF, and V_{5-6} and positive in leads V_{1-2} (Fig. 95-7A). Typical clockwise atrial flutter is characterized by positive F waves in leads II, III, and avF and negative waves in leads V_{1-2}.

Treatment with propafenone, flecainide, and amiodarone to prevent recurrent atrial fibrillation without adding an AV blocking agent (beta blocker or nondihydropyridine calcium antagonist) can organize the arrhythmia into typical atrial flutter with AV conduction of 1:1 or 2:1, producing a ventricular rate response of 150 beats per minute or higher (see Fig. 95-7B). The probability of 1:1 conduction is increased in the presence of an accessory pathway with a short effective refractory period.

Long-Term Management
The precise mechanism of atrial flutter is important for long-term management (e.g., catheter ablation) but has little influence on the initial approach. Patients with all types of atrial flutter should be referred for electrophysiologic evaluation with a view to ablation.

ATRIAL FIBRILLATION

Electrocardiographic Presentation
Atrial fibrillation is defined as rapid oscillations or fibrillatory f waves that vary in size, shape, and timing (see Fig. 95-7C). The ventricular response rate is variable and depends on the rate and regularity of atrial activity, the refractory properties of the AV node itself, and the balance between sympathetic and parasympathetic tone. The RR intervals are irregular unless the patient has complete AV block or a paced rhythm.

Classification
The clinical classification of atrial fibrillation includes first detected, paroxysmal, persistent, and permanent forms of the arrhythmia and is essential for deciding between rhythm restoration and rate control. First-onset atrial fibrillation, if the duration of the episode is less than 48 hours, is a clear

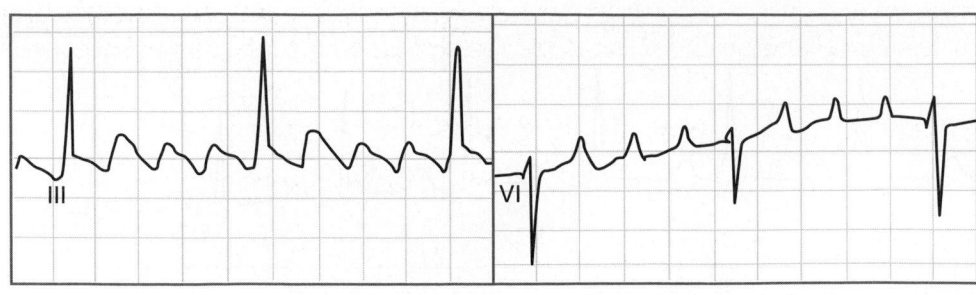

A

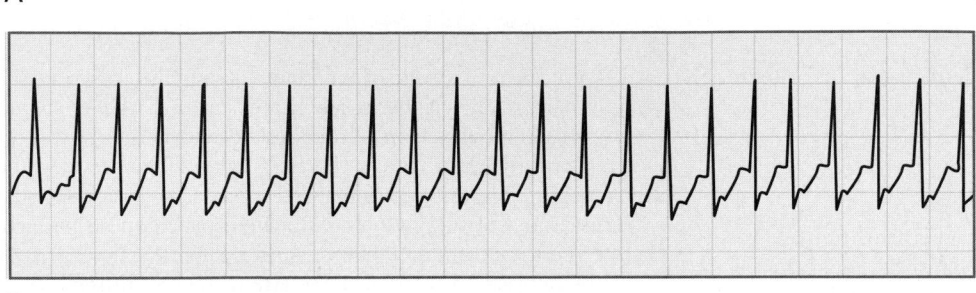

B

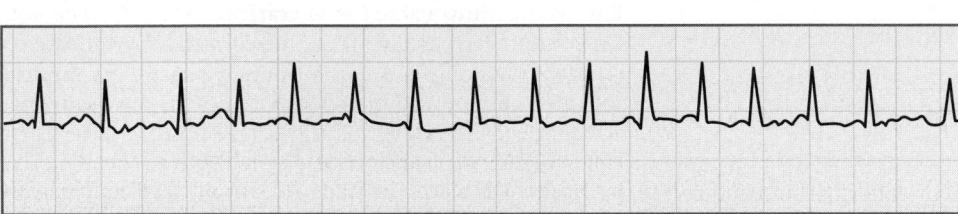

C

FIGURE 95–7. *A,* Typical counterclockwise atrial flutter. F waves are negative in leads II, III, avF, and V$_{5-6}$ and positive in leads V$_{1-2}$. *B,* Atrial flutter with 1:1 atrioventricular conduction and a ventricular rate of 270 beats per minute in a patient treated with flecainide. *C,* Atrial fibrillation with fast, uncontrolled ventricular rates.

indication to restore sinus rhythm by either electrical or pharmacologic means. Because atrial fibrillation may be asymptomatic, the "first detected episode" should not be regarded as necessarily the true onset of the arrhythmia, in which case formal anticoagulation (see later) and rate control may be preferential. Persistent or permanent atrial fibrillation should be treated initially by rate control and anticoagulation, when appropriate.

Long-Term Management

Recognition of the pulmonary veins as the source of atrial premature beats or rapid atrial tachycardia that triggers atrial fibrillation or drives the atria prompted the development of ablation techniques that may "cure" the arrhythmia. In symptomatic permanent or persistent atrial fibrillation, AV node ablation and permanent pacing are effective in rate and symptom control. Any patient with first-onset or recurrent atrial fibrillation should be referred to a cardiologist for long-term management.

ACUTE MANAGEMENT

Acute therapy for atrial flutter and atrial fibrillation depends on the clinical presentation. Emergency electrical cardioversion is indicated for patients with hemodynamic collapse and progressively deteriorating left ventricular systolic function.

Direct-Current Cardioversion

Atrial flutter can be converted with DC shock energy as low as 25 to 50 J, but because a 100-J shock is virtually always successful, it should be considered as the initial shock strength.

In recent-onset atrial fibrillation, sinus rhythm can be restored by a shock of 100 J, but it is recommended that cardioversion be started with an initial shock energy level of 200 J or greater. In patients with an arrhythmia of unknown duration, in heavier individuals, and in those with chronic obstructive lung disease and pulmonary emphysema, an initial setting of 300 to 360 J is appropriate. Success may occur on the third or subsequent attempt at an intensity that initially proved ineffective. For details, refer to Chapter 210.

Rate Control

Rate control is pertinent to all atrial tachyarrhythmias, particularly if restoration of sinus rhythm is deferred. Intravenous verapamil, diltiazem, and beta blockers can rapidly control the ventricular response rate in atrial fibrillation[2] (see Table 95-2), but the efficacy may be less in atrial flutter. The decrease in the ventricular rate (approximately 20% to 30%), time to maximal effect (20 to 30 minutes), conversion rate (12% to 25%), and adverse reactions (usually hypotension and bradycardia, although left ventricular dysfunction and high-degree heart block may occur) are reportedly similar with both classes of drugs. Beta blockers are preferable if thyrotoxicosis is suspected as a cause of the arrhythmia.

Intravenous digoxin is no longer the treatment of choice when rapid rate control is essential because of the delayed onset of its therapeutic effect (>60 minutes). However, because of its positive inotropic action, digoxin may be safer to use in patients with poor ventricular function and moderately fast ventricular rates. Digoxin may convert flutter to fibrillation, in which rate control is easier to accomplish.

TABLE 95–3. ANTIARRHYTHMIC DRUGS FOR PHARMACOLOGIC CONVERSION OF ATRIAL TACHYARRHYTHMIAS

Drug	Route of Administration	Dose	Potential Adverse Effects
Flecainide	Oral or intravenous	Loading oral dose 200-300 mg or slow injection 1.5-2 mg/kg over 10-20 min; if no response, infusion 1.5 mg/kg for 1 h, then 0.1-0.25 mg/kg over 24 h	Rapidly conducted atrial flutter, possible deterioration of ventricular function in the presence of organic heart disease, monomorphic ventricular tachycardia
Propafenone	Oral or intravenous	Loading oral dose 450-600 mg or 1.5-2 mg/kg over 10-20 min, followed by infusion 5-10 mg/kg if needed	
Ibutilide	Intravenous	1 mg over 10 min; if no response, additional 1 mg	QT prolongation, torsades de pointes, hypotension
Amiodarone	Intravenous (preferably central line)	5-7 mg/kg over 30-60 min, followed by infusion 20 mg/kg for 24 h (total 1200-1800 mg)	Hypotension, bradycardia, QT prolongation, torsades de pointes (?), gastrointestinal upset, constipation, phlebitis
Procainamide	Intravenous	1000 mg over 30 min, followed by 2 mg/min infusion	QRS widening, torsades de pointes, rapid atrial flutter

There is evidence that i.v. amiodarone may be effective in rate control when other AV node blocking agents have no effect on ventricular response or are contraindicated.

Pharmacologic Cardioversion

If the arrhythmia is hemodynamically stable and is of recent onset, pharmacologic cardioversion can be effective.

Flecainide and Propafenone

Pharmacologic cardioversion of atrial fibrillation can be accomplished with the IC class of antiarrhythmic drugs—flecainide and propafenone administered orally as a single dose of 300 and 600 mg, respectively (Table 95-3).[2] Placebo-controlled, randomized studies show an efficacy rate of 60% to 80% between the third and eighth hour after drug ingestion.[9,10] Both oral and i.v. routes of administration are equally effective, although with i.v. injection, restoration of sinus rhythm can be achieved more quickly.

Flecainide is given as a slow i.v. injection of 2 mg/kg over 10 to 30 minutes, up to the maximum dose of 150 mg. Propafenone is administered as a slow i.v. injection of 1.5 to 3 mg/kg, up to 300 to 600 mg. Because these drugs can significantly slow the atrial rate (from 300 to 350 beats/min to 200 beats/min), which may result in 1:1 AV conduction, beta blockers or calcium antagonists with negative dromotropic effects on AV node conduction (verapamil, diltiazem) should be used concomitantly. Other cardiovacular effects include reversible QRS widening and, rarely, left ventricular decompensation. Because of the negative inotropic effect, they are contraindicated in patients with severe structural heart disease and a poor ejection fraction.

Class IC drugs are usually ineffective for the conversion of atrial flutter, because they slow conduction within the reentrant circuit and prolong the flutter cycle length but rarely interrupt the circuit. These drugs pose the risk of increased (e.g., 2:1 or 1:1) AV conduction. Reported efficacy rates are as low as 13% to 40% with i.v. flecainide and propafenone.

Ibutilide

The class III agent ibutilide is administered intravenously as a 10-minute injection of 1 to 2 mg and is particularly effective in terminating atrial flutter, with a success rate of about 60%. Its administration may be associated with excessive QT interval prolongation, however, because of the rapid delayed rectifier potassium current (I_{Kr}) blockade and the risk of torsades de pointes.[11,12] It is less effective in atrial fibrillation. Higher doses of ibutilide administered as two successive infusions of 1 mg are usually required to terminate fibrillation. The advantage of ibutilide is that it may be effective in the conversion of arrhythmias of up to 30 days' duration, but the success rate drops significantly to 20% to 30%. The safety of ibutilide in patients with poor left ventricular function is unknown.

Amiodarone

Amiodarone administered intravenously at a dose of 5 mg/kg for 1 hour, followed by an infusion of 20 mg/kg over 24 hours, is effective in converting both atrial fibrillation and flutter, but the effect is significantly delayed.[13,14] However, because of its ability to control the ventricular rate, a low likelihood of torsades de pointes, and the absence of a negative inotropic effect, amiodarone can be used safely in patients with significant structural heart disease and those who are critically ill.

Procainamide and Sotalol

Procainamide administered as a slow i.v. injection of 1000 mg over 20 to 30 minutes, followed, if necessary, by an infusion of 2 mg/min over 1 hour, converts atrial flutter or fibrillation of less than 48 hours' duration, but its efficacy is limited in longer-lasting arrhythmias.[15] It is less effective than propafenone, flecainide, and ibutilide.

Sotalol is not indicated for the pharmacologic cardioversion of atrial flutter or fibrillation because its efficacy does not exceed 11% to 13%; however, it may satisfactorily control the ventricular rate.

Atrial Pacing

Burst overdrive atrial pacing can terminate atrial flutter in about 80% of cases and is feasible after cardiac surgery, when patients frequently have epicardial atrial pacing wires, or in patients with implantable dual-chamber pacemakers and defibrillators. High-frequency (50 Hz or 3000 beats/min) atrial pacing is available in some of the latest models for the termination of early-onset atrial fibrillation, but its efficacy has not yet been established. Atrial burst overdrive pacing may induce sustained atrial fibrillation, although short periods of fibrillation often precede conversion to sinus rhythm.

ANTICOAGULATION

Anticoagulation is imperative if the arrhythmia persists for more than 24 to 48 hours or if its duration is unknown.

TABLE 95–4. RISK STRATIFICATION AND INDICATIONS FOR ANTICOAGULATION IN ATRIAL FIBRILLATION AND FLUTTER

Risk of Stroke	Definition	Therapy
Low (1%/yr)	Age <65 yr; ejection fraction ≥0.50; no stroke or transient ischemic attack, hypertension, heart failure, or valvular heart disease	Aspirin 325 mg
Low to moderate (1.5%/yr)	Age 65-75 yr; no risk factors	Aspirin 325 mg
Moderate to high (2.5%/yr)	Age 65-75 yr and either diabetes or coronary heart disease	Warfarin (INR 2.0-3.0)
High (6%/yr)	Age <75 yr and hypertension, heart failure, or ejection fraction <0.50	Warfarin (INR 2.0-3.0)
	Age >75 yr, particularly women, even in the absence of risk factors	
Very high (10%/yr)	Age >75 yr and hypertension, heart failure, or ejection fraction <0.50	Warfarin (INR 2.0-3.0)
	Any age with a history of stroke or transient ischemic attack or valvular heart disease	

INR, International Normalized Ratio.
Modified from Straus SE, Majumdar SR, McAlister FA: New evidence for stroke prevention: Scientific review. JAMA 2002;288:1388-1395.

Atrial flutter and atrial fibrillation pose similar risks of thromboembolism, and the same criteria for anticoagulation should be applied in patients with either arrhythmia. In hemodynamically stable arrhythmias of more than 48 hours' or of unknown duration, rate control and 3 weeks' anticoagulation with warfarin (International Normalized Ratio 2.0 to 3.0) should be considered before any intervention (electrical or pharmacologic cardioversion, catheter ablation).[16]

TRANSESOPHAGEAL ECHOCARDIOGRAPHY–GUIDED CARDIOVERSION

If, for any reason, deferral of cardioversion is not indicated, the transesophageal echocardiography–guided approach, with short-term anticoagulation with low-molecular-weight heparin, is a safe and effective alternative.[17] It may be clinically beneficial in patients with recent-onset arrhythmias or in individuals at high risk of bleeding complications during prolonged anticoagulation therapy.[18] Compared with unfractionated heparin, low-molecular-weight heparin therapy does not involve prolonged i.v. administration or laboratory monitoring and therefore has the potential to greatly simplify cardioversion-related anticoagulation therapy in low-risk individuals. Post-cardioversion anticoagulation should be considered if thromboembolic risk factors are present (Table 95-4).[16,19]

ATRIAL TACHYCARDIA

MECHANISM

The mechanism of atrial tachycardia is attributed to enhanced automaticity, triggered activity, or intra-atrial reentry. Macro-reentrant atrial tachycardia often occurs after surgery for congenital heart disease. Focal atrial tachycardia typically originates along the crista terminalis in the right atrium, in the pulmonary veins in the left atrium, or around one of the atrial appendages.

ELECTROCARDIOGRAPHIC PRESENTATION

The heart rate varies from 120 to 250 beats per minute, P waves precede the QRS complex, and PP intervals are regular (see Fig. 95-5B). The PR interval is linked to the rate of tachycardia and is longer than in sinus rhythm at the same rate. P wave morphology is usually different from that during sinus rhythm and depends on the site of origin. Left atrial tachycardia presents with the negative P waves in leads I, avL, V_5, and V_6. Automatic atrial tachycardia may present as an incessant variety, leading to tachycardia-induced cardiomyopathy.

ATRIAL TACHYCARDIA WITH ATRIOVENTRICULAR BLOCK

Tachycardia with AV block occurs commonly in patients with organic heart disease, and in 50% to 75% of cases, it is due to digitalis toxicity (Fig. 95-8). Digoxin-specific antibody fragments (Digibind) are available for the reversal of life-threatening overdosage.

MULTIFOCAL ATRIAL TACHYCARDIA

This tachycardia presents as rapid, irregular atrial activity with discrete P waves of varying morphology and is considered a transitional rhythm between atrial tachycardia and fibrillation. However, it may occur in patients with chronic severe pulmonary disease as a result of theophylline or beta agonist overdose. Elimination of the causative factor may reduce the need for antiarrhythmic therapy. Intravenous verapamil can accomplish rate control.

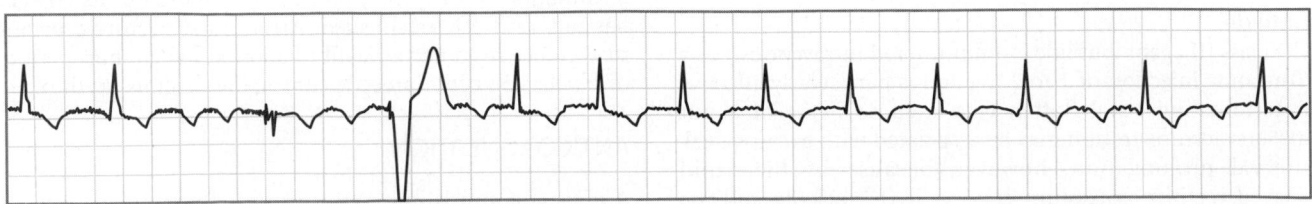

FIGURE 95–8. Atrial tachycardia with varying atrioventricular block as a result of digitalis toxicity.

ACUTE MANAGEMENT

DC cardioversion converts atrial tachycardia based on the reentry mechanism or triggered activity, but it may not terminate automatic tachycardia. Similarly, atrial overdrive pacing may slow the tachycardia rate but seldom suppresses the automatic focus.

It is generally accepted that beta blockers and calcium antagonists, particularly verapamil, can either terminate the tachycardia or produce rate control. Adenosine can terminate atrial tachycardia, but the most common response to adenosine is to create AV block and thereby reveal the unaffected tachycardia (see Fig. 95-5B, C).

Flecainide, propafenone, sotalol, and amiodarone are effective in converting the arrhythmia. If tachycardia occurs as a result of digitalis intoxication, therapy includes the cessation of digoxin and i.v. administration of potassium.

LONG-TERM MANAGEMENT

Patients with atrial tachycardia should be referred to a cardiologist, because the arrhythmogenic focus can be found and ablated in up to 86% cases.

INAPPROPRIATE SINUS TACHYCARDIA

Inappropriate sinus tachycardia is a persistent increase in resting heart rate unrelated to or out of proportion with the level of physical or emotional stress. It is found predominantly in women and is not uncommon in health professionals. Sinus tachycardia due to intrinsic sinus node abnormalities, such as enhanced automaticity, or abnormal autonomic regulation of the heart, with excess sympathetic and reduced parasympathetic input, is extremely rare. The usual therapy is beta blockers. In general, sinus tachycardia is a secondary phenomenon, and the underlying causes should be actively investigated. Depending on the clinical setting, acute causes include fever, hypotension, infection, anemia, thyrotoxicosis, hypovolemia, acute heart failure, acute pulmonary embolism, and shock. Sinus tachycardia may be associated with the abuse of drugs, such as amphetamines.

ANNOTATED REFERENCES

Albers GW, Dalen JE, Laupacis A, et al: Antithrombotic therapy in atrial fibrillation. Chest 2001;119(1 Suppl):194S-206S.
This paper focuses on the prevention of stroke in nonrheumatic atrial fibrillation and flutter and provides expert recommendations regarding risk stratification, anticoagulation strategies, cardioversion (including transesophageal echocardiography–guided cardioversion), and long-term management of patients at risk of thromboembolism. It contains a complete review of the evidence base for anticoagulation in atrial fibrillation.

Blomström-Lundvist C, Scheiman MM, Aliot EM, et al: ACC/AHA/ESC guidelines for the management of patients with supraventricular arrhythmias—executive summary. A report of the American College of Cardiology/American Heart Association Task Force on Practice Guidelines and the European Society of Cardiology Committee for Practice Guidelines (Writing Committee to develop guidelines for the management of patients with supraventricular arrhythmias). J Am Coll Cardiol 2003;42:1493-1531.
These practice guidelines describe a range of generally accepted approaches to the diagnosis and management of supraventricular tachyarrhythmias (excluding atrial fibrillation) and provide insight into the multiple mechanisms defined by electrophysiologic studies, with a focus on both acute and long-term therapies.

Camm AJ: Atrial fibrillation: Is there a role for low-molecular-weight heparin? Clin Cardiol 2001;24(3 Suppl):I15-I19.
This review paper summarizes evidence emerging from clinical studies that clearly supports both the use of transesophageal echocardiography–based cardioversion protocols and the introduction of low-molecular-weight heparin for anticoagulation in atrial fibrillation. Clinical settings in which low-molecular-weight heparin may offer advantages over unfractionated heparin and warfarin are discussed.

Fuster V, Rydén LE, Asinger RV, et al: Task force report: ACC/AHA/ESC guidelines for the management of patients with atrial fibrillation. Eur Heart J 2001;22:1852-1923.
These guidelines incorporate a comprehensive review of the latest information about the classification, epidemiology, mechanisms, and clinical presentations of atrial fibrillation. Practical approaches to acute and long-term management of this arrhythmia are discussed at length. An extensive list of references covers various aspects of atrial fibrillation.

Mehta D, Wafa S, Ward DE, Camm AJ: Relative efficacy of various physical manoeuvres in the termination of junctional tachycardia. Lancet 1988;1:1181-1185.
This paper compares the ability of four vagotonic physical maneuvers to terminate paroxysmal supraventricular tachycardias that involve the AV node as a part of their reentrant circuits. It shows that these tachycardias can be terminated without resorting to pharmacologic therapy in more than half of patients. The paper provides a detailed methodologic description and explains the physiologic effects of vagotonic maneuvers.

Chapter 96

VENTRICULAR ARRHYTHMIAS

Raúl J. Gazmuri • Prabhakaran Gopalakrishnan

KEY POINTS

1. **Hereditary and acquired abnormalities in cardiac ion channels** can alter the action potential and predispose to ventricular tachyarrhythmias, especially the torsades de pointes type.

2. Ventricular arrhythmias are the result of **abnormalities in impulse generation (automaticity and triggered activity) and impulse conduction (reentry)**.

3. Proper management of ventricular tachyarrhythmias requires the **assessment of precipitating and maintaining conditions**; often, the removal of these conditions is all that is needed.

4. **A long QT interval in the baseline electrocardiogram** should prompt a diligent search for possible drugs and metabolic conditions involved.

5. **Ventricular tachyarrhythmias in critically ill patients** are often precipitated by cardiac and respiratory processes.

6. **Atrioventricular dissociation is a reliable sign that a wide-complex tachycardia is ventricular**; this may be evident on the surface 12-lead electrocardiogram or after analyzing an esophageal lead.

7. **Direct-current synchronized cardioversion should be considered first-line treatment** in patients with ventricular tachycardia who are hemodynamically unstable or have heart failure.

Abnormalities in impulse generation and conduction leading to arrhythmic events are frequent in critically ill patients. They may result from primary cardiac events or may be secondary to a myriad of acute or acute-on-chronic conditions. The presence or anticipation of an arrhythmic event is frequently a reason for hospital admission to a unit with capability to continuously monitor the electrocardiogram (ECG) and with personnel proficient in the recognition and management of life-threatening arrhythmias (i.e., ICUs and telemetry units).

Abnormalities originating in atrial tissue and in pulmonary veins are considered supraventricular. They may compromise cardiac and hemodynamic function by means of an excessive heart rate or disruption of ventricular filling; yet, in the absence of accessory conduction pathways—bypassing the atrioventricular (AV) node—supraventricular arrhythmias are rarely life-threatening and can often be managed by non-emergent pharmacologic or mechanical means. In contrast, abnormalities originating in ventricular structures pose substantial risk of developing into life-threatening arrhythmias (e.g., ventricular tachycardia and ventricular fibrillation) that require immediate intervention to avert or reverse death.

In this chapter, ventricular arrhythmias that develop in critically ill patients are discussed, with primary focus on mechanisms, predisposing conditions, incidence, diagnosis, and acute clinical management. The technical aspects of electrical cardioversion and defibrillation are discussed in Chapter 210.

NORMAL ELECTROPHYSIOLOGY

ANATOMIC SYNOPSIS

The electrical impulse of the heart originates in the sinoatrial (SA) node, located high on the right atrium near its junction with the superior vena cava. The impulse then propagates through muscle fibers and specialized internodal pathways (composed of Purkinje-type fibers) to converge on the AV node, located in the interatrial septum near the tricuspid valve and the opening of the coronary sinus (Fig. 96-1). From the AV node, the impulse travels through the bundle of His, its left and right branches, and the Purkinje system to simultaneously activate the right and left ventricles. A ring of fibrous tissue interposed between the atria and the ventricles precludes spread of the electrical impulse through the muscle fibers. The AV node functions as a relay and filter, limiting the number of impulses that can be transmitted to the ventricles, thus preventing 1:1 conduction under conditions of very rapid atrial activation (i.e., atrial flutter, rate ≈300 cycles/sec; atrial fibrillation, rate ≈350 to 600 cycles/sec).

ACTION POTENTIAL AND PACEMAKER ACTIVITY

Action potential is the result of rapid depolarization and repolarization subsequent to changes in ion currents across the plasma cell membrane of polarized cells. The changes in ion currents result from a coordinated sequence of opening and closing of channels that regulate mainly the influx of sodium ions (Na^+) and calcium ions (Ca^{++}) (inward currents) and the efflux of potassium ions (K^+) (outward currents).[1-4] The action potential serves to propagate the electrical impulse throughout the conduction system and muscle fibers and to signal contractile activity.

The characteristics of the action potential vary, contingent on the type of cell. Cells from the Purkinje system and from atrial and ventricular muscle have a stable resting potential at approximately –90 mV (inside negative). This is largely

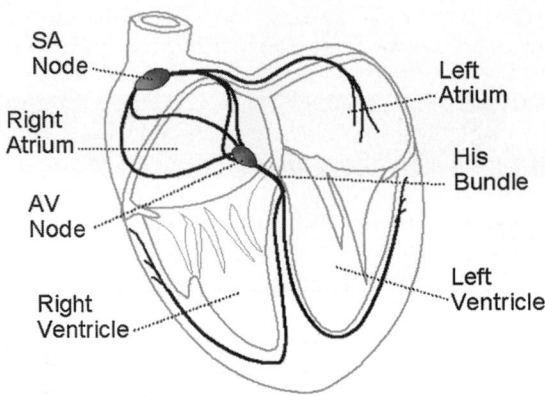

FIGURE 96–1. Conduction system of the heart. AV, atrioventricular; SA, sinoatrial.

the result of a K$^+$ current known as the inward rectifier (I_{K1}), which "anchors" the membrane potential to a voltage close to the equilibrium potential of K$^+$.[3] I_{K1} is turned off during depolarization (inward rectification) and then on during repolarization (see later). The arrival of an impulse that depolarizes the plasma membrane to between –70 and –80 mV (threshold potential) is needed for fast voltage-gated Na$^+$ channels to open and trigger an action potential.[4] The rapid Na$^+$ influx creates a current (I_{Na}) that drives the membrane potential toward the equilibrium potential of Na$^+$, causing further depolarization and reversal of the membrane potential to approximately +20 mV (overshoot). This phase is known as phase 0 of the action potential and ushers into a four-phase repolarization (Fig. 96-2). Phase 1 is the initial early repolarization (action potential notch) and results from rapid inactivation of Na$^+$ channels (inner gate) and the opening of K$^+$ channels carrying a transient outward

current (I_{to}). These channels turn on rapidly after depolarization and then quickly inactivate.[5-7] Because I_{to} is expressed in the subepicardial and midmyocardial regions but not in the subendocardial region, it contributes to the inhomogeneity of repolarization.[8] I_{to} has two components: one that is voltage-gated (I_{to1}) and one—less well characterized—that is presumably activated by changes in cytosolic Ca^{++} (I_{to2}).[6,7,9] Phase 2 is the plateau phase of the action potential and results mainly from a Ca^{++} current carried by the slow and prolonged opening of L-type voltage-gated Ca^{++} channels (I_{Ca-L}).[10,11] Opening of these channels begins during phase 0 at a membrane potential of –30 to –40 mV. These channels are inactivated in response to increases in cytosolic Ca^{++} and are strongly regulated by neurotransmitters. Phase 3 corresponds to late repolarization and follows the closing of Ca^{++} channels, along with the opening of K$^+$ channels, with slow activation kinetics carrying currents known as delayed rectifiers (I_K). These are the main repolarizing currents and have two components carried by distinct gene products: a rapid component (I_{Kr}) and a slow component (I_{Ks}).[12,13] Both are implicated in the heritable forms of long QT syndrome (see later).[14] In addition, opening of I_{K1} contributes to repolarization. Phase 4 represents the return to resting membrane potential and the interval during which ionic balance is restituted, largely through the action of the Na$^+$-K$^+$ pump.

Cells of the SA and AV nodes lack voltage-gated Na$^+$ channels, and phase 0 is carried by L-type Ca^{++} channels (I_{Ca-L}).[15] Because of their slower opening kinetics (relative to Na$^+$ channels), they give rise to a slanted phase 0 and in part determine the lower conduction velocity of the SA and AV nodes ($\approx$50 cm/sec) compared with the His-Purkinje system ($\approx$400 cm sec^{-1}) and muscle cells ($\approx$100 cm sec^{-1}). SA and AV node cells also have pacemaker activity and slowly depolarize during phase 4 to a threshold potential of approximately –40 mV. The slow depolarization is called prepotential or pacemaker potential and involves a background Na$^+$ current (I_{Na-B}), a decay of K$^+$ currents, the opening of T-type voltage-gated Ca^{++} channels (I_{Ca-T}) at a potential between the thresholds for I_{Na} and I_{Ca-L}, and the opening of L-type Ca^{++} channels, unleashing phase 0. Cells of the His-Purkinje system have latent prepotential activity and can become active when SA or AV node activity is depressed or their impulse is blocked. Atrial and ventricular muscle cells exhibit prepotential activity only under abnormal circumstances (see later).

The preceding description is succinct and oversimplified. Various other ion channels, antiporters, pumps, and receptors play important roles in specific physiologic states and disease processes. For example, there is a nonselective cationic channel that is gated at resting potential by intracellular Ca^{++} and produces an inward Na$^+$ current (I_{NS}).[16] This current may contribute to delayed afterdepolarizations following Ca^{++} release by the sarcoplasmic reticulum. $I_{K(ATP)}$ is a K$^+$ current carried through metabolically regulated channels that are inhibited by adenosine triphosphate (ATP) and opened under conditions of ischemia and hypoxia. $I_{K(ATP)}$ is the main contributor to the shortening of the action potential duration[17] and the characteristic ST segment elevation observed in the surface electrocardiogram[18] during ischemia.

The sarcolemmal Na$^+$-Ca^{++} exchanger is another important modulator of the action potential. Because it exchanges one Ca^{++} for three Na$^+$, it is electrogenic and generates a current ($I_{Na/Ca}$) whose direction is determined by the Na$^+$ and Ca^{++} gradients and the membrane potential.[19,20] In settings in which there is cytosolic Ca^{++} overload (e.g., ischemia and

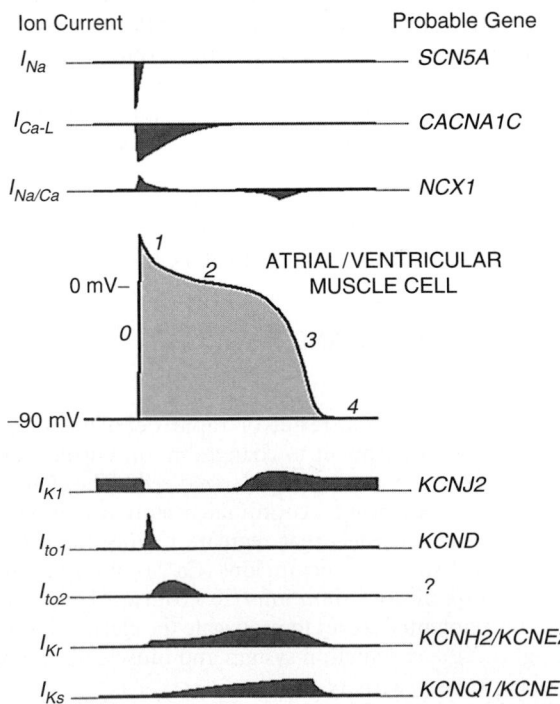

FIGURE 96–2. Action potential of a cardiac muscle cell depicting the main underlying inward and outward currents and their respective gene products. The distinctive phases of the action potential are numbered.

reperfusion, digitalis toxicity), Ca^{++} may trigger Ca^{++} release from the sarcoplasmic reticulum during phase 4, which in turn prompts reverse-mode operation of the Na^+-Ca^{++} exchanger, causing an inwardly directed $I_{Na/Ca}$ (Na^+ influx). This current contributes to the generation of delayed afterdepolarizations and triggered arrhythmias (see later).

Adrenergic receptors also play important roles in modulating the action potential by modifying channel activity.[21-23] For example, stimulation of beta-adrenergic receptors increases the activity of L-type Ca^{++} channels (leading to increases in $I_{Ca,L}$ and contractility). Beta-adrenergic receptor stimulation can also activate K^+ channels, shortening repolarization and the duration of the action potential.[24] $Alpha_1$-adrenergic receptors exert actions via G protein on the Na^+-K^+ pump, K^+ channels, and phospholipase C and can alter impulse initiation and repolarization. $Alpha_1$-adrenergic stimulation has been linked to triggered rhythms via early and delayed afterdepolarizations and the development of abnormal automatic rhythms in the setting of ischemia and reperfusion.[25,26]

Alteration in the proteins forming these various channels—mostly genetic, but also acquired—may distort the normal action potential, yielding distinctive electrocardiographic patterns (e.g., long QT syndrome, Brugada's syndrome) that are associated with increased risk of ventricular tachyarrhythmias.

MECHANISMS OF VENTRICULAR TACHYARRHYTHMIAS

The mechanisms by which ventricular tachyarrhythmias develop encompass abnormalities in impulse generation and abnormalities in impulse conduction. Both mechanisms often coexist and orchestrate the initiation and maintenance of ventricular tachyarrhythmias. Identification of the arrhythmogenic mechanism is important, because therapeutic strategies may be designed to target the so-called vulnerable parameter responsible for the genesis or maintenance of the arrhythmia.[27-29]

ABNORMALITIES IN IMPULSE GENERATION

Abnormalities in impulse generation are generally the result of automaticity (ectopic pacemaker activity) or triggered activity. Automaticity may result from enhanced normal automaticity in cells of the conduction system whose pacemaker potential is normally under overdrive suppression, or from the development of abnormal automaticity in muscle cells that normally do not exhibit pacemaker potential. Triggered activity refers to arrhythmias that arise from afterdepolarizations.

Enhanced normal automaticity occurs when cells from the AV node or His-Purkinje system fire at rates that escape the overdrive suppression of the SA node. This phenomenon may result from effects on phase 4 prepotentials that favor the earlier development of action potentials (i.e., less maximal polarization, faster depolarization, or lower threshold potential) or from shortening of the action potential duration, with an earlier return to phase 4. Enhanced normal automaticity is usually the result of adrenergic stimulation.

Abnormal automaticity refers to the generation of impulses in fibers that are partially depolarized as a result of a pathologic process, such as ischemia. Under these conditions, the reduction in the resting membrane potential

(less negative; to −70 or even −50 mV) shifts the balance during phase 4 toward depolarizing currents.[30] Through this mechanism, automaticity can developed in atrial and ventricular muscle cells, and the firing conditions of specialized tissues other than the SA node can be altered. Examples of abnormal automaticity include accelerated idioventricular rhythms and some ventricular tachycardias that develop 24 to 72 hours after acute myocardial infarction.[31,32]

Triggered activity refers to action potentials that result from afterdepolarizations, which are alterations in membrane potential that occur during repolarization without intervening external triggers or cell-to-cell interactions.[33] Afterdepolarizations that develop during phase 2, phase 3, or early phase 4 are called early afterdepolarizations and are characterized by transient retardations in repolarization, with or without upturn of the membrane potential (Fig. 96-3). When the upturn is of a magnitude sufficient to reach the threshold, an extra action potential is triggered before the cycle is over. Early afterdepolarizations are typically associated with conditions that prolong the action potential duration, such as decreased inactivation of fast I_{Na} (i.e., long QT3 syndrome) or decreased outward K^+ currents (i.e., I_{Ks} in long QT1 and I_{Kr} in long QT2 syndromes), prompting Ca^{++} entry through L-type Ca^{++} channels.[34] The development of early afterdepolarizations in this setting is thought to trigger torsades de pointes. Early afterdepolarizations are also associated with increased sympathetic tone, use of catecholamines, hypoxia, acidosis, and bradycardia. Afterdepolarizations that occur in late phase 4 are called delayed afterdepolarizations and are characterized by low-amplitude depolarizations that may reach threshold and trigger an action potential (see Fig. 96-3). The main underlying abnormality is intracellular Ca^{++} overload, promoting Ca^{++} release from the sarcoplasmic reticulum[34] and depolarizing currents (i.e., inward $I_{Na/Ca}$ currents). Delayed afterdepolarizations are classically associated with digitalis toxicity; however, many other conditions that favor cytosolic Ca^{++} overload can produce them, such as myocardial stretch, hypertrophy, catecholamines, ischemia, and reperfusion. Increased expression of Na^+-Ca^{++} exchanger, along with abnormalities in the ryanodine receptor, has been shown to predispose to delayed afterdepolarizations in the setting of heart failure.

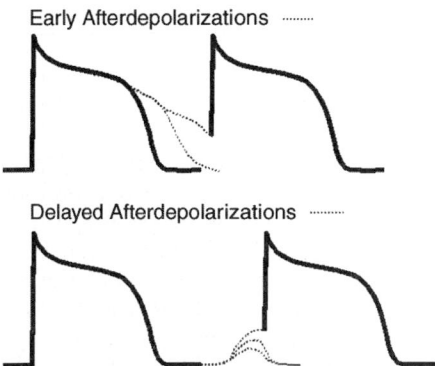

FIGURE 96–3. Afterdepolarizations (*dotted lines*). Early afterdepolarizations are retardations in repolarization, with prolongation in the action potential duration (*upper figure*). Delayed afterdepolarizations represent spontaneous depolarizations that occur after repolarization is over (*lower figure*). Afterdepolarizations that reach threshold trigger an action potential.

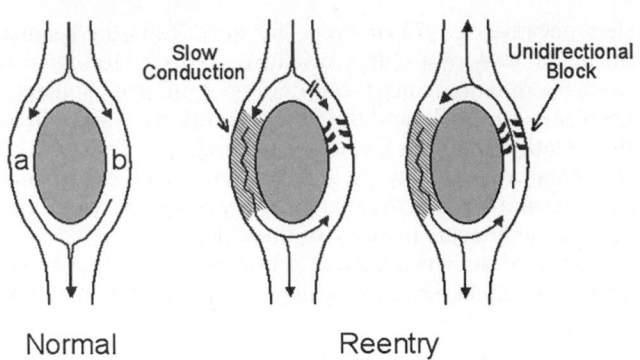

FIGURE 96–4. Ring model of reentry.

ABNORMALITIES IN IMPULSE CONDUCTION (REENTRY)

Abnormalities in impulse conduction leading to reentry account for the vast majority of sustained ventricular tachyarrhythmias. Reentry is a phenomenon in which a normally propagating impulse reenters previously excited tissue after its refractory period is over, and excites it again. Reentry can continue to repeat and establish a tachyarrhythmia. Several forms of reentry have been described, including circus movement reentry, phase 2 reentry, and reflection.[35]

Circus Movement

Circus movement is the most widely studied mechanism and encompasses four distinct models: ring, leading circle, figure of eight, and spiral wave.

The ring model is the simplest and illustrates the basic mechanism of reentry (Fig. 96-4).[36] This model requires two anatomically contiguous paths in specialized tissue or in muscle fibers separated by a central area of unexcitable tissue. One of these paths (*b* in Fig. 96-4) must exhibit a zone of unidirectional block, allowing the impulse to propagate in only one direction. The alternative path (*a* in Fig. 96-4) allows the impulse to circumvent the unidirectional block. Conduction through this alternative path should be slow, or refractoriness proximal to the path should be brief, to allow recovery of tissue excitability. Once the impulse reaches the distal end of the alternative path, it propagates in a retrograde manner through the path of unidirectional block to reenter the proximal end of the alternative path. For the cycle to repeat (and establish a reentry tachyarrhythmia), the wavelength of the circling impulse—defined as the product of conduction velocity and the duration of the refractory period—must be shorter than or at least equal to the length of the reentry circuit (path length), enabling its leading edge to find the tissue in an excitable state. Reentry is usually triggered by the arrival of a premature beat that finds the path of unidirectional block in a refractory period. Unidirectional block may result from increased refractoriness associated with either anatomic abnormalities (e.g., fibrosis, accessory pathway, bundle branch) or functional defects (e.g., ischemia, action of drugs). The ring model best applies to tachyarrhythmias that involve AV accessory pathways and the AV node.

The leading circle model is similar to the ring model but does not require anatomic obstacles and can develop in structurally uniform myocardium by a properly timed premature impulse.[37,38] The figure-of-eight model was first described in experimental myocardial infarction. It refers to two reentry circuits moving alongside a functional conduction block (ischemia or infarct) in opposite directions, forming a pretzel-like configuration.[39] The spiral wave model is considered a more complex version of the leading circle model. It involves a core and filaments and is usually described as reentry in two dimensions.[40,41] The spiral wave model has been used to explain the electrocardiographic patterns associated with monomorphic and polymorphic ventricular tachycardias and also ventricular fibrillation. In monomorphic ventricular tachycardias, the spiral wave is thought to be anchored and unable to drift within the myocardium, whereas in polymorphic ventricular tachycardias, such as torsades de pointes, the spiral is thought to drift. In the case of ventricular fibrillation, the spiral wave is believed to break up into multiple rotating spiral waves that are continuously extinguishing and re-creating. However, some authors have proposed a single rapidly shifting spiral, and others have postulated a stationary rotor whose frequency of excitation is exceedingly high, resulting in multiple areas of intermittent block.[42]

Phase 2

Phase 2 reentry refers to the generation of local re-excitation as a result of increased heterogeneity of repolarization. This phenomenon occurs when repolarization is markedly shortened in certain regions of the myocardium, essentially obliterating the action potential plateau (phase 2), but is maintained in others. This creates conditions conducive to local re-excitation, which may precipitate ventricular tachyarrhythmias during myocardial ischemia.[43] During ischemia, action potentials of normal duration alternate with ones of shorter duration, yielding beat-to-beat alternans (temporal dispersion) and site-to-site alternans (spatial dispersion) and promoting regions of conduction block and regions with injury current, leading to reentry and ventricular tachyarrhythmias. The degree of spatial and temporal dispersion progresses along with the duration of ischemia, suggesting that this mechanism may be an important trigger of ventricular tachycardia and ventricular fibrillation during acute myocardial ischemia.[44,45] In the surface electrocardiogram (ECG), dispersion of the action potential duration manifests as T-wave alternans, which is a powerful predictor of ventricular fibrillation.[46]

Reflection

Reflection refers to a back-and-forth propagation of the impulse over the same functionally unexcitable tissue, with recurrent activation of the proximal region as a result of electrotonic currents.[47,48] The area of unexcitable tissue could result from ischemia and lead to extrasystolic activity. Reflection differs from classic reentry, in that the impulse travels along the same pathway in both directions.

PREDISPOSING CONDITIONS

CHANNELOPATHIES

The term "channelopathies" has recently been coined to identify a group of diseases in which there are abnormalities in the proteins that form ion channels.[49,50] These abnormalities distort the normal action potential, primarily accentuating the inherent instability of repolarization and increasing the risk of polymorphic ventricular tachycardia of the torsades de pointes type. The intensivist should be able to promptly identify prolongation of the QT interval in the surface ECG. Channelopathies may be hereditary or acquired.

TABLE 96–1. CONGENITAL LONG QT SYNDROMES

Genetic Type	Gene	Chromosome	Protein
LQT1	KCNQ1	11	α subunit, I_{Ks}
LQT2	HERG	7	I_{Kr}
LQT3	SCN5A	3	α subunit, I_{Na}
LQT4	ANKB	4	Ankyrin-B
LQT5*	KCNE1	21	β subunit, I_{Ks}
LQT6†	KCNE2	21	Membrane protein, I_{Kr}

*KCNQ1 and KCNE1 gene products assemble to form a complete I_{Ks} channel.
†HERG and KCNE2 gene products assemble to form a complete I_{Kr} channel.

The hereditary channelopathies described so far result mainly from mutations in genes that encode for Na$^+$ and K$^+$ channels, with the most representative being long QT syndrome.[51-53] This syndrome was first described in 1957 by Jervell and Lange-Nielsen in a group of patients with long QT intervals, episodes of torsades de pointes, and deafness.[54] This syndrome is transmitted by autosomal recessive inheritance and is known as the Jervell and Lange-Nielsen syndrome. In 1963 and 1964, Romano and colleagues[55] and Ward[56] independently reported patients with an almost identical disorder but without deafness, in which the transmission was autosomal dominant (Romano-Ward syndrome). It is now recognized that long QT syndrome results from mutations in at least six genes, leading to distinct types designated LQT1 through LQT6 (Table 96-1). LQT1 is the principal genetic type responsible for both Jervell and Lange-Nielsen and Romano-Ward syndromes and accounts for nearly 50% of all genotyped families. LQT2 accounts for nearly 45%, and LQT3 for about 5%. The remaining types are much less frequent. With the exception of LQT3 and LQT4, these mutations affect K$^+$ channels, causing decreased activity of either I_{Kr} or I_{Ks} by mechanisms involving loss of function, dominant-negative transmission, or, more rarely, autosomal recessive transmission. LQT4 has recently been linked to a loss-of-function mutation in the ANKB gene.[57] This gene encodes ankyrin-B, which is a member of a family of versatile membrane adapters. Ankyrin-B—among other functions—coordinates the opening and closing of calcium, potassium, sodium, and chloride channels. The failure to properly coordinate the opening and closing of ion channels leading to long QT syndrome and arrhythmias illustrates a novel mechanism of arrhythmias. LQT3 stems from a mutation in SCN5A, the gene that encodes the α subunit of the fast cardiac Na$^+$ channel. SCN5A mutation leads to incomplete channel inactivation and persistence of I_{Na} during the plateau phase of the action potential.

The common mechanistic thread among long QT syndromes is perturbation of the balance between I_{Na} and I_K during the plateau phase of the action potential, yielding prolongation of repolarization, a reduced rate of I_{Ca-L} inactivation, late Ca^{++} influx, and early afterdepolarizations, predisposing to torsades de pointes.[58]

The diagnosis is suspected in young individuals who present with syncope or episodes of sudden death, typically during exercise, emotional distress, or exposure to factors that cause prolongation of the QT interval (see later). A family history of unexplained syncope or sudden cardiac death, especially in young kindred, should raise suspicion. Sudden cardiac death occurs in approximately 4% of affected individuals. The diagnosis should be suspected when the corrected QT interval (QTc = QT$_{(msec)}$/$\sqrt{R-R_{(sec)}}$) exceeds 470 msec in males (normal, <422 msec) and 480 msec in females (normal, <432 msec) in the absence of other conditions that may lengthen the corrected QT interval. In addition, there may be sinus bradycardia with sinus pauses in about one third of individuals (especially in LQT3), QT dispersion, and various T-wave abnormalities (e.g., notched, bifid, biphasic). Factors predisposing to sudden cardiac death include recurrent syncope, survival from cardiac arrest, congenital deafness, female sex, relative bradycardia, corrected QT interval greater than 600 msec, and kinship with a symptomatic patient.[51]

Another important hereditary channelopathy that also results from a mutation in the SCN5A gene is Brugada's syndrome.[59-62] In contrast to LQT3, this mutation leads to a loss of function, resulting in accelerated inactivation of I_{Na}; this unbalances the effects of I_{To} during phase 1, which prompts rapid repolarization and a very short action potential. Because I_{To} is expressed predominantly in the epicardium, the normally depolarized endocardium can re-excite the prematurely repolarized epicardium, leading to phase 2 reentry. Brugada's syndrome was described in 1992 by the Brugadas, who noticed an association between sudden cardiac death and ST segment elevation in V_1 to V_3, with a pattern resembling right bundle branch block in individuals with structurally normal hearts.[59] The ST segment can adopt various shapes, which have been related to the severity of the I_{Na}/I_{To} imbalance, including—in order of increasing severity—saddleback, coved, and triangular shapes.[58] Some authors have proposed that this SCN5A defect may be responsible for up to 50% of all sudden deaths in patients with apparently normal hearts, with an even higher incidence in younger individuals (idiopathic ventricular fibrillation).[63] The syndrome can present with the typical ECG pattern; however, patients may have concealed or intermittent forms, which can be unmasked by the administration of Na$^+$ channel blockers such as ajmaline, flecainide, or procainamide. This test is highly specific and should be considered in all patients who present with a history of syncope of unknown origin or idiopathic ventricular fibrillation. Patients with Brugada's syndrome must be treated with an internal cardioverter defibrillator. Antiarrhythmic agents have not been found to be effective.[62]

Acquired channelopathies may result from a broad spectrum of conditions. Advanced heart failure affects the expression of several ion channels.[64,65] There is down-regulation of I_{To1} and I_{K1}, which prolongs the QT interval; this allows more time for excitation-contraction coupling but predisposes to inhomogeneous repolarization and early afterdepolarizations. In addition, there is up-regulation of Na$^+$-Ca^{++} exchanger, yielding larger $I_{Na/Ca}$, which predisposes to delayed afterdepolarizations and triggered arrhythmias, especially in the face of cytosolic Ca^{++} overload.

Drugs represent an increasingly important cause of acquired channelopathies that manifest by a prolongation of the QT interval, mostly as a result of decreased activity in I_{Kr},[66] which is the same current responsible for congenital long QT2 syndrome. The list is long and includes antiarrhythmic agents, in which the primary target is ion channels, as well as many other drugs in which prolongation of the QT interval is an unintended effect (Table 96-2).[67] The intensivist should be familiar with this group of medications and capable of recognizing the clinical features of long QT syndrome. The University of Arizona, Health Sciences Center, maintains a complete and up-to-date list of drugs that prolong the QT interval; it is available at www.qtdrugs.org.

TABLE 96-2. DRUGS ASSOCIATED WITH QT PROLONGATION AND RISK OF TORSADES DE POINTES

Antiarrhythmic Agents

Amiodarone
Disopyramide
Ibutilide
Procainamide
Quinidine
Sotalol

Antibiotics

Clarithromycin
Erythromycin
Gatifloxacin
Halofantrine
Pentamidine
Sparfloxacin

Antipsychotic Agents

Chlorpromazine
Haloperidol
Mesoridazine
Pimozide
Thioridazine

Tricyclic Antidepressants

Amitriptyline
Clomipramine
Desipramine
Doxepin
Imipramine

Nonsedating Antihistamines

Astemizole
Terfenadine

Opiate Agonists

Levomethadyl
Methadone

Enterokinetic/Antinausea Agents

Cisapride
Domperidone
Droperidol

OTHER CONDITIONS

The QT interval may also be prolonged by electrolyte abnormalities, cocaine abuse, organophosphorus compound poisoning, subarachnoid hemorrhage, stroke, myocardial ischemia, fasting using liquid-protein-modified diets, autonomic neuropathy, and human immunodeficiency virus disease.[68-72] Some of these conditions are discussed below.

Electrolyte Abnormalities

Electrolyte abnormalities rarely precipitate but often contribute to the development of ventricular tachyarrhythmias, mostly in relation to abnormalities in serum K^+, Mg^{++}, and Ca^{2+}.[73]

Abnormalities in serum K^+ are among the most common electrolyte abnormalities in critically ill patients. Hypokalemia (serum $K^+ < 3.5$ mM) decreases the resting membrane potential (making it more negative), rendering cells less excitable and lowering the firing rate of pacemaker cells. Hypokalemia also prolongs the QT interval and flattens the T wave.[14] This effect is explained by the fact that conductivity of I_{Kr} is proportional to the square root of external K^+. Thus, at lower K^+, I_{Kr} is reduced, prolonging repolarization. This effect is more pronounced in cells from the midmyocardial region (which have a greater I_{Kr}/I_{Ks} ratio). Hypokalemia can develop in various settings, including the use of thiazide and loop diuretics, diabetic ketoacidosis, gastrointestinal fluid losses, alcohol abuse, hypomagnesemia, administration of insulin, and beta-receptor agonist stimulation. Hyperkalemia (serum $K^+ > 5.5$ mM) exerts opposite effects. It lowers the resting membrane potential (making it less negative), rendering cells more excitable; however, with severe hyperkalemia, the rate of rise of phase 0 is reduced, slowing conduction velocity and leading—at very high potassium levels—to widespread blocks (widening of the P wave and QRS interval). Rapidly rising serum K^+ can precipitate ventricular fibrillation, probably as a result of reentry that follows areas of conduction block. Hyperkalemia, by increasing I_{Kr}, accelerates repolarization and shortens the action potential duration, yielding the characteristic peaked and tall T waves.

Prompt treatment of these defects is important to avert life-threatening events.

Magnesium plays an important electrophysiologic role. Mg^{++} is a cofactor for the Na^+-K^+ pump and hence is important in maintaining the integrity of intracellular K^+ and the resting membrane potential. Mg^{++} also modulates the effects of various K^+ and Ca^{++} channels. Hypomagnesemia is associated with prolongation of the QT interval and increased risk of ventricular arrhythmias. This effect could be mediated in part through other electrolyte deficits, because hypomagnesemia is associated with hypokalemia and hypocalcemia.

Serum calcium is also important. Hypocalcemia increases the QT interval, predisposing to ventricular tachycardias. Hypercalcemia exerts the opposite effects, reducing the QT interval. Changes in intracellular calcium contribute to arrhythmias associated with acute ischemia and reperfusion and may be important in the genesis of ventricular tachycardia induced by exercise and by digitalis.

Hypothermia

Moderate (32°C to 35°C) and severe (<32°C) hypothermia can also predispose to ventricular tachyarrhythmias by causing prolongation of the QT interval, along with QT dispersion.[74] Typically, patients with hypothermia develop J waves (also known as Osborn waves) in the 12-lead ECG, which reflects accentuation of the inhomogeneity of repolarization caused by the predominant distribution of I_{To} in subepicardial and midmyocardial regions.[75] Accentuation of the action potential notch in the epicardium but not in the endocardium is responsible for the voltage gradient that manifests in the surface ECG as a J wave. Hypothermia may be complicated by the ingestion of drugs and the presence of electrolyte abnormalities that further increase the risk of ventricular tachyarrhythmias.

Arrhythmogenic Right Ventricular Cardiomyopathy

This disorder is characterized by progressive replacement of the normal right ventricular muscle cells by fibrous tissue and fat.[76] The condition may be familial, with autosomal

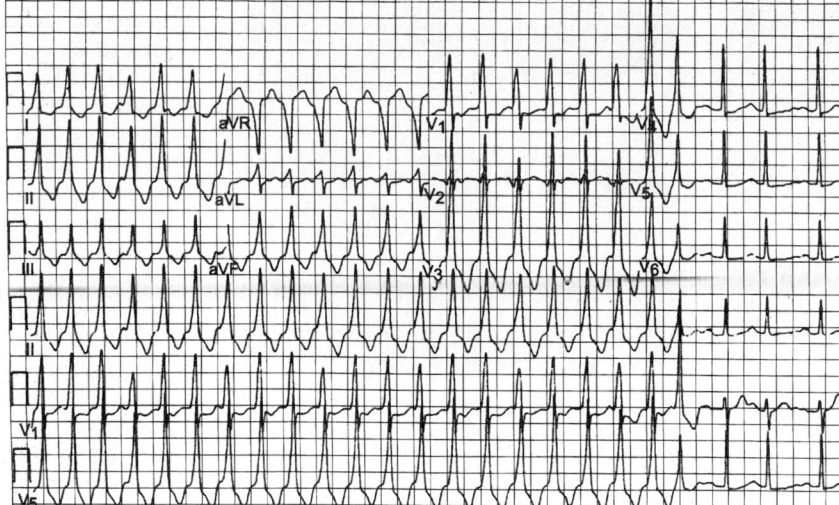

FIGURE 96–5. Representative monomorphic ventricular tachycardia with atrioventricular (AV) dissociation (P waves are best seen in V_1). The tachycardia ends into a sinus rhythm with first-degree AV block preceded by one fusion beat. (From Murphy JG [ed]: Mayo Clinic Cardiology Review, 2nd ed. Philadelphia, Lippincott Williams & Wilkins, 2000, p 657.)

dominant inheritance.[77] Patients present with palpitations, syncope, and sometimes sudden death. It is considered an important cause of sudden death in subjects younger than 35 years, especially when related to exercise.[78,79] The ECG is abnormal in 90% of cases, showing T-wave inversions beyond lead V_1 and epsilon waves in leads V_1 to V_3. The QRS complex may be widened (>110 msec), with complete or incomplete right bundle branch block morphology. There are ventricular premature beats with left bundle branch configuration.

CLINICAL DIAGNOSIS

Ventricular ectopic activity is suspected whenever wide QRS complexes dissociated from atrial activity appear in the ECG. Various types of ventricular arrhythmias can develop in critically ill patients, with different prognostic implications and management.

Premature ventricular contractions (PVCs) are isolated ventricular ectopic beats that may be found in normal, healthy individuals. However, they often accompany cardiac conditions (ischemia, cardiomyopathy, valvular heart disease), use of stimulants (caffeine, cocaine, alcohol, ephedrine, pseudoephedrine), electrolyte abnormalities (hypokalemia, hyperkalemia, hypomagnesemia), hypoxemia, catecholamine discharge, and medications (tricyclic antidepressants, antipsychotic medications, digoxin, flecainide, sotalol, quinidine). The ECG demonstrates a wide QRS complex with a bizarre axis, a T wave with polarity opposite to the QRS, and a full compensatory pause. PVCs usually do not produce symptoms.

Ventricular tachycardia is defined as three or more consecutive ectopic beats that originate below the AV node, with a rate that typically exceeds 100 beats per minute and often ranges between 130 and 170 beats per minute. Ventricular tachycardias usually have QRS complexes of 120 msec or longer and are therefore classified as wide-complex tachycardias. However, wide-complex tachycardias can also be supraventricular when the impulse originates above the bifurcation of the bundle of His but is conducted with aberrancy (see later).[80] Ventricular tachycardias are classified as monomorphic if all QRS complexes have similar morphology and polymorphic if they have variable morphology.

Monomorphic ventricular tachycardias are the most common form and are usually associated with structural heart disease, such as previous myocardial infarction and, less commonly, cardiomyopathy. The reentrant circuit can be small (microentry) or large (macroentry) and can be located in different regions of the myocardium, contingent on the infarcted sites. The mechanism is usually reentry operating within or around the damaged myocardium. A representative 12-lead ECG is shown in Figure 96-5.

Polymorphic ventricular tachycardias have irregular rhythms, usually compromise hemodynamic function, and may quickly degenerate into ventricular fibrillation. Variation in QRS morphology represents changes in the electrical axis. One special form of polymorphic ventricular tachycardia is torsades de pointes. This is a descriptive term denoting a rotating electrical axis in which the complexes rotate 180 degrees along an imaginary axis ("twisting points"); it is typically associated with long QT syndrome. Representative tracings are shown in Figure 96-6.

Ventricular tachycardias are considered sustained if they last 30 seconds or longer and nonsustained if they last less than 30 seconds. Most sustained ventricular tachycardias present with palpitations, chest discomfort, and weakness or with more severe symptoms such as dizziness, angina, syncope, seizures, and even sudden cardiac death.[81] On physical examination, the rhythm is usually regular. Hypotension may accompany the episode, especially in patients with underlying heart disease. Examination of the jugular veins may show cannon A waves, indicative of AV dissociation. Variability in S_1 occurrence and intensity and variations in blood pressure are also findings consistent with AV dissociation.

In nonemergency settings, a standard 12-lead ECG should be obtained to determine whether a wide-complex tachycardia is present and whether it is monomorphic or polymorphic. If monomorphic, the possibility of supraventricular tachycardia with aberrancy should be considered, although most wide-complex tachycardias are ventricular. The presence of shock, heart failure, or cardiac arrest favors ventricular tachycardia, and treatment should not be delayed.

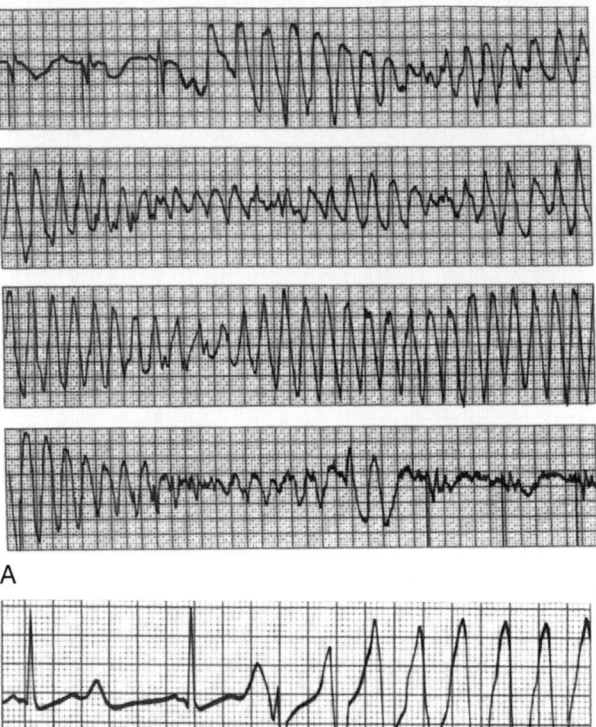

A

B

FIGURE 96-6. Torsades de pointes. *A*, A patient with a demand ventricular pacemaker developed QT prolongation (≈640 msec, seen during paced rhythm) after treatment with amiodarone for recurrent ventricular tachycardia. An episode of torsades de pointes developed that spontaneously terminated with resumption of a paced ventricular rhythm. *B*, Tracing from a young boy with congenital long QT syndrome and marked prolongation of the QTU interval (≈600 msec). TU alternans is noted before a late premature complex occurring on the downslope of the TU wave initiates an episode of ventricular tachycardia. (From Braunwald E, Zipes D, Libby P [eds]: Heart Disease: A Textbook of Cardiovascular Medicine, 6th ed. Philadelphia, WB Saunders, 2001, p 868.)

Supraventricular tachycardia with aberrancy (in a stable patient) should be suspected whenever there is a history of previous aberrant rhythms, accessory pathways, and baseline or rate-induced bundle branch block. The ECG should be carefully examined for evidence of AV dissociation, which is specific for ventricular tachycardia.[82] If P waves are not visualized in V_1 or in any of the other standard leads, a Lewis lead (arm electrode positioned on the parasternal area) or an esophageal lead can be used.[83] AV dissociation is indicated by P waves and QRS complexes that present at different and uncoupled rates. Other manifestations of dissociation include captured beats (narrow QRS conducted beats) and fusion beats (merge of ectopic with conducted beats).

Other ECG clues include regularity of the RR interval, which can be altered in supraventricular tachycardia but usually not in monomorphic ventricular tachycardia, and a QRS duration greater than 160 msec; however, the QRS duration can be shorter (110 to 114 msec) in instances of fascicular tachycardia. With respect to axis and morphology, the QRS in V_1 is usually predominantly positive (right bundle branch block morphology) or predominantly negative (left bundle branch block morphology). Occasionally, the QRS in V_1 has two peaks, leading to an RSr' pattern that is known as a "rabbit ear." In this instance, a taller "left ear" favors ventricular tachycardia, whereas a taller "right ear" is noncontributory.

The T waves are characteristically large and opposite for the main QRS deflection. Additional ECG criteria and algorithms are available to help differentiate ventricular from supraventricular tachycardia.[84-87] A widely accepted four-step algorithm developed by Brugada is shown in Figure 96-7.[85] A similar algorithm that incorporates pertinent clinical information can be found at http://www.anaesthetist.com/icu/organs/heart/ecg/wct.htm#step0.

Some special forms of ventricular tachycardia tend to be mistaken for supraventricular tachycardia with aberrancy.[88] These include bundle branch reentrant tachycardia, in which the impulse travels down the right bundle branch, across the interventricular septum, and up the left bundle branch.[89,90] The morphology resembles supraventricular tachycardia with left bundle branch block and is common among patients with nonischemic dilated cardiomyopathy.[91] Right ventricular outflow tract tachycardia is another condition caused by triggered activity from delayed afterdepolarizations that most commonly originate in the right ventricular outflow tract.[92] The tachycardia usually presents with left bundle branch block morphology and right axis deviation. Right ventricular outflow tract tachycardias occur in structurally normal hearts, typically in young individuals, and are responsive to verapamil or adenosine.[93] Finally, there are fascicular tachycardias that originate from either fascicle of the left bundle branch. They occur in structurally normal hearts, mimic supraventricular tachycardia with aberrancy, and are responsive to beta blockers and verapamil.[94]

Accelerated idioventricular rhythm is a form of automatic ventricular arrhythmia and is characterized by the presence of regularly wide QRS complexes with a rate between 50 and 120 beats per minute. It is often, but not always, slightly faster than the underlying sinus rhythm. Accelerated idioventricular rhythm is an electrocardiographic diagnosis and does not produce symptoms. Identifying this rhythm is important because it usually indicates underlying myocardial ischemia, and the treatments for ventricular tachycardia may not apply.

Ventricular fibrillation is defined as the abrupt onset of irregular waveforms of varying contour, duration, and amplitude without identifiable QRS and T waves. Ventricular tachycardia or supraventricular tachycardias that conduct through accessory pathways (e.g., Wolff-Parkinson-White syndrome) may be the initiating rhythm that degenerates into ventricular fibrillation. Ventricular fibrillation (and pulseless ventricular tachycardia) causes immediate cessation of blood flow, precipitating unconsciousness within seconds. Generalized seizures and agonal breathing may follow, which should not distract from the primary diagnosis and the emergency treatment of cardiac arrest.

INCIDENCE IN THE CRITICAL CARE SETTING

The incidence of ventricular arrhythmias in critically ill patients is difficult to ascertain with precision and varies in relation to the underlying condition, predisposing factors, structural abnormalities, and triggering events, as well as the method of detection.[95,96] Artucio and Pereira, using a chart review, reported in 1990 a 78% incidence for all types of brady- and tachyarrhythmias of atrial and ventricular origin in 2820 patients admitted to a general-purpose ICU over 12 years.[95] The incidence of ventricular tachyarrhythmias for the entire group was 22%, with the highest incidence in

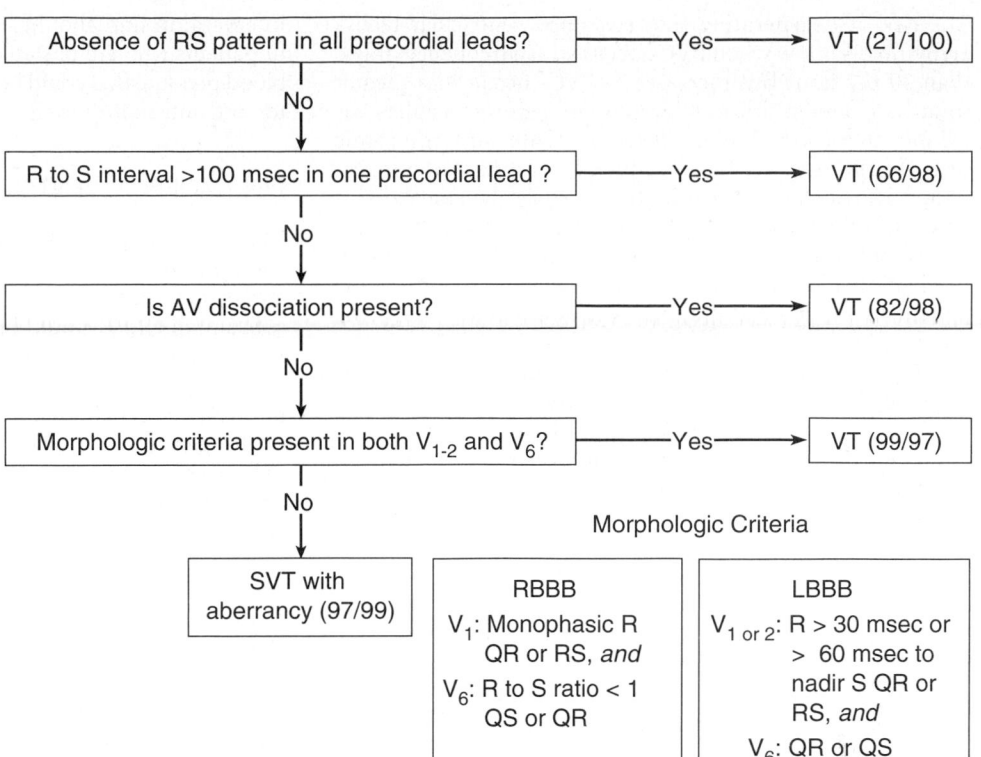

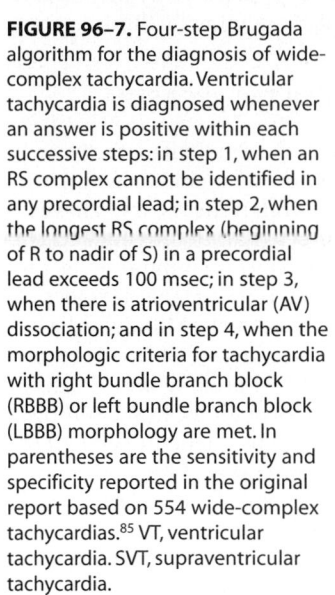

FIGURE 96–7. Four-step Brugada algorithm for the diagnosis of wide-complex tachycardia. Ventricular tachycardia is diagnosed whenever an answer is positive within each successive steps: in step 1, when an RS complex cannot be identified in any precordial lead; in step 2, when the longest RS complex (beginning of R to nadir of S) in a precordial lead exceeds 100 msec; in step 3, when there is atrioventricular (AV) dissociation; and in step 4, when the morphologic criteria for tachycardia with right bundle branch block (RBBB) or left bundle branch block (LBBB) morphology are met. In parentheses are the sensitivity and specificity reported in the original report based on 554 wide-complex tachycardias.[85] VT, ventricular tachycardia. SVT, supraventricular tachycardia.

patients with cardiovascular (460 of 1767; 26%) and respiratory (64 of 339; 19%) conditions and the lowest in patients with multiple trauma (7 of 107; 7%). Conditions such as sepsis, neurologic disorders, and intoxication had an intermediate incidence. Ventricular fibrillation occurred in 119 patients, representing 4% of the entire group and 19% of the subset with ventricular tachyarrhythmias. More recently, Reinelt and colleagues—using more restricted criteria (in which PVCs, couplets, and triplets were not included)—reported an overall incidence of cardiac arrhythmias of 18% (133 of 756 consecutive admissions) in a medical-coronary ICU.[96] The incidence of ventricular tachyarrhythmias for the entire group was 9% (65 of 756 patients); monomorphic ventricular tachycardia was the most common (54 of 65), followed by ventricular fibrillation (6 of 65) and polymorphic ventricular tachycardia (5 of 65). Factors present during the arrhythmic episodes included hypokalemia (10%), hypomagnesemia (12%), sedation (60%), mechanical ventilation (77%), and administration of catecholamines such as norepinephrine, epinephrine, and dobutamine (75%). In 23% of the episodes there was a history of previous myocardial infarction, and in 40%, a history of recent myocardial infarction. Fifty-two percent of the episodes occurred during a postoperative period, and 35% while a pulmonary artery catheter was in place. The presence of arrhythmias was associated with an increased length of stay and lower survival. However, fatal arrhythmic events occurred in only two patients, suggesting that arrhythmias were an indicator of severity rather than a cause of poor outcome.

Special consideration should be given to patients admitted for the evaluation of an acute coronary syndrome. Before the advent of thrombolysis in the 1980s, the incidence of ventricular tachycardia ranged between 3% and 39%.[97] With the widespread use of thrombolysis, the incidence has decreased.[98] This is thought to reflect less ventricular dysfunction and dilatation as a result of successful reperfusion.

For similar reasons, ventricular tachycardia is less frequent in patients with non–ST segment elevation (<1%) than in those with ST segment elevation (≈4%) myocardial infarction.[98]

Episodes of ventricular tachycardia have different implications, depending on whether they occur early or late in the course of myocardial infarction and whether they are sustained or nonsustained. Early is usually defined as the initial 48 hours after the onset of symptoms, although some authors use a 12-hour cutoff.[99] Early nonsustained ventricular tachycardias are relatively common, with an incidence between 9% and 12%.[100,101] They reflect electrical instability during the acute ischemic event but have little prognostic implication.[102] Early sustained ventricular tachycardias occur in less than 2% of patients,[103] but they identify a population with a poorer prognosis.[98]

Late ventricular tachycardias coincide with the phase of myocardial healing and may signal the presence of persistent ischemia, left ventricle dysfunction, or electrophysiologic instability.[99] Nonsustained ventricular tachycardias occur in approximately 6% of patients.[53,104] Sustained ventricular tachycardias occur in approximately 1% and convey a worse prognosis than do nonsustained episodes.[98,105]

One particularly arrhythmogenic period is during reperfusion after thrombolysis.[53,100] There are frequent PVCs and episodes of nonsustained ventricular tachycardia but rarely episodes of sustained ventricular tachycardia or ventricular fibrillation.[106] Accelerated idioventricular rhythm is also common, with an incidence as high as 50% to 75%. It occurs within 24 hours after the start of thrombolysis and then subsides.[106,107]

ACUTE MANAGEMENT

PVCs and episodes of nonsustained ventricular tachycardia have little immediate hemodynamic significance. Management should focus on identifying and removing contributing factors.

The risk of degenerating into sustained ventricular tachyarrhythmias is low when PVCs occur with a frequency of less than 30 per hour but increases as PVCs occur with greater frequency, are multifocal, present in pairs or triplets, or exhibit the R-on-T phenomenon. Acute antiarrhythmic drug therapy is typically not required. Treatment of nonsustained ventricular tachycardia that persists after the episode of critical illness should take into account the underlying cardiac substrate and may involve a thorough assessment of mechanical and electrical function. In general, asymptomatic patients without structural heart disease require no specific therapy.

The management of sustained ventricular tachyarrhythmias requires a dynamic approach in which therapeutic interventions often parallel and occasionally precede diagnostic evaluation. This is particularly true in instances of ventricular fibrillation and pulseless ventricular tachycardia, when delivery of unsynchronized electrical shocks and advanced life support cannot be delayed. In less urgent situations (or after reestablishment of cardiac activity), treatment should focus on identifying and removing precipitating and maintaining factors, paying close attention to (1) hemodynamic and respiratory abnormalities, (2) endogenous or exogenous adrenergic states, (3) acid-base and electrolyte imbalances, (4) presence of proarrhythmic agents, and (5) mechanical stimulation of cardiac structures. Not infrequently, treatment of these factors alone terminates the arrhythmic episode (e.g., repositioning of a pulmonary artery catheter, reversal of myocardial ischemia, discontinuation of drugs that prolong the QT interval, correction of electrolyte imbalances, discontinuation of sympathomimetic agents).

Specific antiarrhythmic interventions should take into consideration the type of rhythm and the degree of hemodynamic stability (discussed next).

MONOMORPHIC VENTRICULAR TACHYCARDIA

Antiarrhythmic agents and direct-current synchronized cardioversion are acceptable first-line options. Among the antiarrhythmic agents, lidocaine was previously recommended as the best diagnostic and therapeutic intervention. The initial diagnosis is often wide-complex tachycardia, and it was believed that lidocaine would be effective if the tachycardia was ventricular but not if it was supraventricular. However, more recent studies have demonstrated that lidocaine does not consistently terminate monomorphic ventricular tachycardia and is less effective than procainamide, sotalol, and probably amiodarone.[108-111] The 2000 international guidelines favor procainamide and sotalol (class IIa) over amiodarone and lidocaine (class IIb).[112,113] However, amiodarone is gaining popularity as a first-line drug for a wide variety of supraventricular and ventricular tachyarrhythmias.[114-117] In patients with impaired left ventricular function (ejection fraction <40%), amiodarone and lidocaine may be considered first-line antiarrhythmic agents because they have fewer antiinotropic effects. Lidocaine should also be considered when myocardial ischemia is the substrate for ventricular tachyarrhythmias.

Addition of a second antiarrhythmic agent is discouraged because their proarrhythmic effects are compounded. Thus, a single agent should be used and proceed to direct-current synchronized electrical cardioversion if optimal dosing fails. Electrical cardioversion is a highly effective and accepted intervention and should be considered first-line treatment in patients who are unstable or in those who have borderline blood pressure that could be further decreased by the vasodilator and anti-inotropic effects of most antiarrhythmic agents.

POLYMORPHIC VENTRICULAR TACHYCARDIA

The treatment of polymorphic ventricular tachycardia should aim at prompt restoration of a sinus rhythm with emergency electrical cardioversion if necessary. However, substantial effort should be directed at identifying and correcting associated precipitating and maintaining factors. Polymorphic ventricular tachycardia of the torsades de pointes type usually occurs in the setting of bradycardia and prolonged QT interval. The mainstay of management includes discontinuation of drugs that prolong the QT interval and correction of electrolyte abnormalities. In the setting of congenital long QT syndrome, beta blockers (or sympathetic interruption), pacing, and implantation of an internal cardioverter defibrillator device should be considered. In the acquired forms of long QT syndrome, intravenous magnesium, overdrive pacing (or isoproterenol, when pacing is not immediately available), and beta blockers after pacing are recommended interventions. Isoproterenol is contraindicated in congenital long QT syndrome because it can precipitate torsades de pointes.

Polymorphic ventricular tachycardia not of the torsades de pointes type is not responsive to magnesium. Ischemia should be suspected and treated accordingly. Use of beta blockers, including sotalol, and amiodarone is recommended. An algorithm for the treatment of stable monomorphic and polymorphic ventricular tachycardia is shown in Figure 96-8.[118]

VENTRICULAR FIBRILLATION AND PULSELESS VENTRICULAR TACHYCARDIA

The probability of survival after ventricular fibrillation and pulseless ventricular tachycardia is inversely related to the time elapsed between the onset of the arrhythmia and the delivery of electrical shocks.[119,120] Recent studies have shown that immediate defibrillation is highly effective and is associated with high survival rates when the duration of untreated ventricular fibrillation is short (<4 minutes).[121,122] With more protracted untreated ventricular fibrillation, mounting evidence from animal and human studies indicates that a period of closed-chest resuscitation before attempting defibrillation improves outcome.[121,123-125] For defibrillation, current evidence favors biphasic waveforms using nonescalating energy levels as low as 150 J (in contrast to the traditional 200-, 300-, 360-J sequence recommended when using monophasic waveforms).[126-128] For patients with shock-refractory ventricular fibrillation or pulseless ventricular tachycardia, use of amiodarone has been shown to facilitate the restoration of cardiac activity.[129,130]

Electrical storm is a rather uncommon but highly lethal phenomenon defined as recurrent episodes of ventricular fibrillation, occurring mainly in the course of an acute myocardial infarction. Conventional antiarrhythmic drug therapy—including lidocaine and procainamide—often fails to secure a stable sinus rhythm. The underlying mechanism seems to be excessive (and probably unbalanced) sympathetic activity. Recent studies have shown that outcome can be dramatically improved by sympathetic blockade

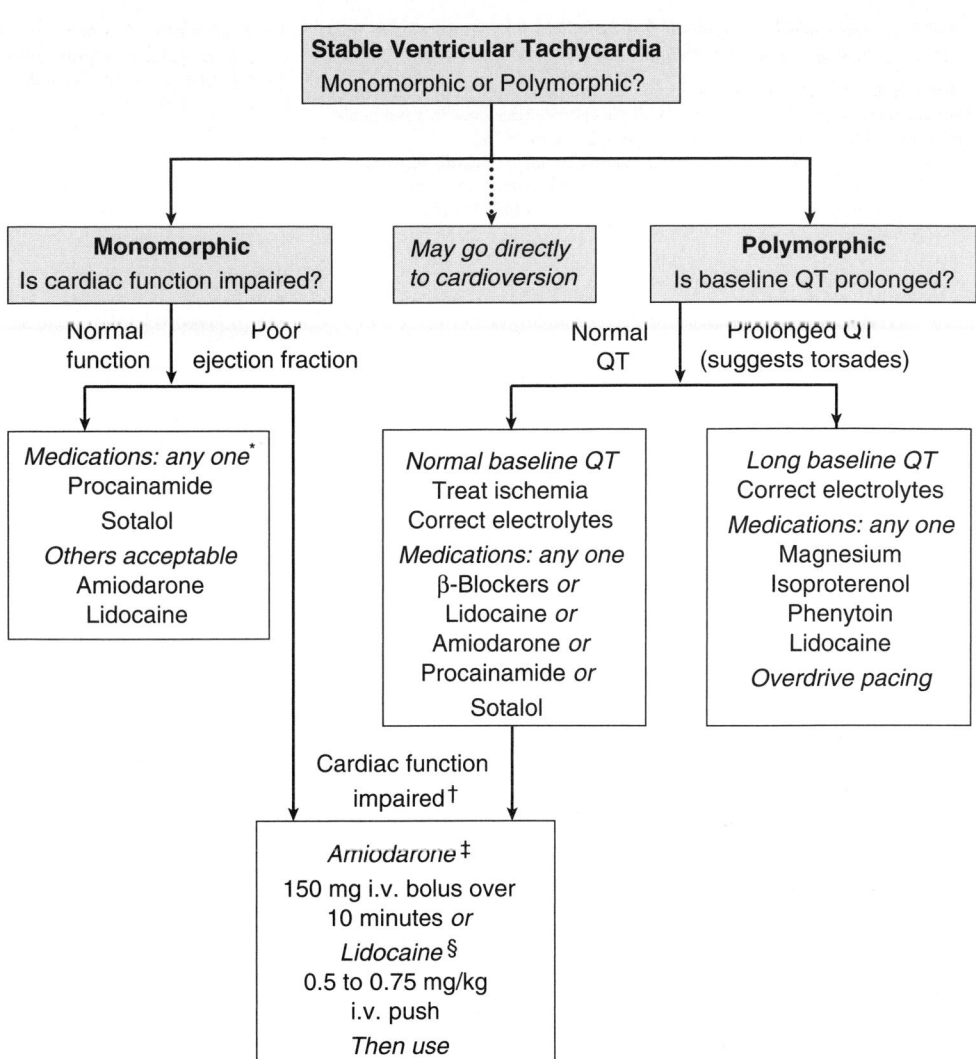

FIGURE 96–8. Algorithm for managing stable monomorphic or polymorphic ventricular tachycardia according to "Guidelines 2000 for Cardiopulmonary Resuscitation and Emergency Cardiovascular Care" (Circulation 2000;102:I158-I165). *Use only one agent to avoid proarrhythmic effects. †Ejection fraction <40% or clinical manifestations of congestive heart failure. ‡For amiodarone, give 150-mg bolus over 10 minutes and repeat dose if necessary every 10 to 15 minutes or infuse 360 mg over 6 hours (1 mg/min) followed by 540 mg over 18 hours (0.5 mg/min) to a maximal total cumulative dose of 2.2 g in 24 hours. §For lidocaine, give 0.5 to 0.75 mg/kg i.v. push and repeat dose if necessary every 5 to 10 minutes, followed by an infusion of 1 to 4 mg/min to a maximum of 3 mg/kg per hour.

using intravenous beta blockers or stellate ganglionic blockade.[131]

CONCLUSION

Ventricular tachyarrhythmias are important and prevalent manifestations of cardiac and extracardiac abnormalities in critically ill patients. In addition to the traditional assessment based on ECGs and hemodynamic manifestations, understanding and recognition of the processes that affect ion channels, pumps, exchangers, and signaling mechanisms are important for proper management. There is also increased awareness that mutations affecting cardiac channels are prevalent and clinically relevant. The intensivist should be alert and prepared to identify them and provide the necessary initial treatment and an appropriate referral. The initial enthusiasm for antiarrhythmic agents has diminished as the proarrhythmic effects of various compounds have become evident. Some drugs are no longer recommended as first-line agents, whereas others have become components of accepted algorithms. More emphasis is currently being place on understanding arrhythmogenic mechanisms and on correcting the precipitating and maintaining factors.

ACKNOWLEDGMENTS

The authors thank Maria E. Iliescu, MD, for reviewing part of the information presented. This work was supported in part by a VA Merit Review Grant and by NIH grant R01 HL71728-01.

ANNOTATED REFERENCES

Antzelevitch C: Basic mechanisms of reentrant arrhythmias. Curr Opin Cardiol 2001;16:1-7.
   Authoritative review of the mechanisms of reentrant arrhythmias.

Guidelines 2000 for cardiopulmonary resuscitation and emergency cardiac care. Part 6: Advanced cardiovascular life support. Section 5: Pharmacology I: Agents for arrhythmias, and Section 7D: The tachycardia algorithms. The American Heart Association in collaboration with the International Liaison Committee on Resuscitation. Circulation 2000;102:I112-I128, I158-I165.
   Current international recommendations for the acute pharmacologic management of cardiac arrhythmias.

Khan IA: Long QT syndrome: Diagnosis and management. Am Heart J 2002;143:7-14.
   Excellent and up-to-date review of long QT syndrome, addressing diagnosis and management.

New approaches to antiarrhythmic therapy. Parts I and II: Emerging therapeutic applications of the cell biology of cardiac arrhythmias. Circulation 2001;104:2865-2873, 2990-2994.

This two-part article provides a new paradigm for the assessment and management of cardiac arrhythmias.

Reinelt P, Karth GD, Geppert A, Heinz G: Incidence and type of cardiac arrhythmias in critically ill patients: A single center experience in a medical-cardiological ICU. Intensive Care Med 2001;27:1466-1473.

Report on the epidemiology of cardiac arrhythmias in critically ill patients. Although the authors found a high incidence of ventricular tachyarrhythmias accompanying critical illness, they are not causally related to adverse outcomes.

The Sicilian gambit: A new approach to the classification of antiarrhythmic drugs based on their actions on arrhythmogenic mechanisms. Task Force of the Working Group on Arrhythmias of the European Society of Cardiology. Circulation 1991;84:1831-1851.

This article provides an expanded classification of antiarrhythmic agents that takes into account their complexity and multiplicity of actions.

Chapter 97

CONDUCTION DISTURBANCES AND CARDIAC PACEMAKERS

Jason Knight • John Sarko

KEY POINTS

CONDUCTION DISTURBANCES

1. Atrioventricular (AV) node block is most often caused by medications, increased parasympathetic tone, or ischemia. Except when infarction permanently damages a portion of the conduction pathway, such blocks are usually reversible. Infranodal blocks, however, are rarely caused by physiologic abnormalities.

2. First-degree AV node block and Wenckebach block typically do not require treatment. Type II second-degree heart block and complete heart block usually do require treatment.

3. Therapy for AV block consists of atropine, adrenergic agents, Digibind (if appropriate), and pacing.

4. Bradyarrhythmias are common after cardiac surgery and may require temporary pacing, but a decision to place a permanent pacemaker should not be made until 5 to 7 days after surgery.

PACEMAKERS

1. A cardiologist or electrophysiologist should be consulted when a pacemaker or cardioverter-defibrillator malfunction is suspected.

2. Placing a magnet over the pacemaker disables the sensing mechanism, causing the pacemaker to fire at its preprogrammed rate, regardless of the underlying intrinsic rhythm.

3. Magnetic resonance imaging may be safe in a pacemaker patient if the unit is programmed to an asynchronous mode and the patient is watched carefully.

4. Failure to sense occurs when the pacemaker generates output regardless of the patient's underlying rhythm; this is rarely an urgent problem.

5. Failure to pace is noted when a pacemaker spike is not seen when expected (after the lower rate-limiting interval has been exceeded); this can be devastating for a pacemaker-dependent patient, and temporary pacing may be required.

6. Failure to capture occurs when a pacemaker fires as expected but fails to depolarize the myocardium. This complication may require temporary pacing.

CONDUCTION DISTURBANCES

Bradyarrhythmias and conduction blocks are common in the ICU. A broad range of clinical presentations and pathologic findings occurs in this group of arrhythmias. Some bradyarrhythmias are benign and asymptomatic and do not require treatment. Other atrioventricular (AV) blocks and arrhythmias are life threatening and warrant immediate intervention.

NORMAL CARDIAC CONDUCTION

Normal depolarization and impulse conduction are central to maintaining cardiac output. Two types of cells are found in the heart: (1) cells responsible for impulse generation and conduction, and (2) cells responsible for contraction. Depolarization of the myocardium begins in the sinoatrial (SA) node. The SA node is located in the posterior and superior portion of the right atrium and is innervated by the sympathetic and parasympathetic nervous systems.

The impulse is generated by a specialized group of cells with the ability to depolarize spontaneously. The initial depolarization of the SA node is not seen on the electrocardiogram (ECG). The P wave is generated when the impulse spreads throughout the atria. There is no specific conduction system in the atria to convey the SA node impulse to the AV node.[1] The impulse is transmitted by depolarization of adjacent atrial myofibrils. Approximately halfway through the P wave, the impulse reaches the AV node. The second half of the P wave is due to left atrial depolarization.

In a normal heart, the atria and the ventricles are electrically isolated from each other, except at the AV node. The AV node is located in the atrial septum near the apex of the triangle of Koch. The AV node is innervated by the sympathetic and parasympathetic nervous systems. Conduction through the AV node accounts for the majority of the PR interval. After emerging from the AV node, the impulse is conducted through the bundle of His. From there, the impulse travels down the right and left bundle branches and their fascicles to the Purkinje network, which causes ventricular contraction.

FAILURE OF IMPULSE CONDUCTION

Failure of conduction can occur anywhere along the conduction pathway. AV node block is most often caused by medications, increased parasympathetic tone, or ischemia. AV node blocks are usually reversible, except when infarction permanently damages a portion of the conduction pathway. Infranodal blocks are rarely caused by physiologic abnormalities. Structural heart disease and anatomic disruption of the conduction system are the main causes of infranodal heart block. Rare causes of infranodal block include disruption of the bundle of His from aortic valve calcification, Lenègre's disease (idiopathic degeneration of Purkinje fibers), and Chagas' disease.[2]

Once AV block is identified, it is helpful to determine the site of conduction pathology. The anatomic site can be identified in most cases by synthesizing the type of AV block, the width of the QRS complex, and the QRS morphology. When the QRS complex is narrow (<0.12 sec), the site of pathology is most likely supraventricular. When the QRS complex is wide, the most likely site of AV block is infranodal. Bundle branch and fascicular blocks produce various QRS morphologies that may aid in determining the specific anatomic location of pathology.

Clinical Presentation

Syncope and presyncope are the most dramatic symptoms of conduction disturbances; palpitations, dyspnea, angina, and fatigue are seen as well. Many patients are asymptomatic. A significant number of patients develop bradydysrhythmias after an acute myocardial infarction (MI) (Table 97-1).[3]

Diagnostic Evaluation

A high-quality ECG is paramount for the appropriate evaluation of P waves and various intervals. Routine monitoring in the ICU is usually accomplished with a single- or three-lead display at the bedside. The lead chosen should clearly delineate the P waves and QRS complexes. Complex arrhythmias may require Lewis leads, intra-atrial leads, or esophageal ECG monitoring. Calipers significantly aid in the diagnosis of AV blocks and are helpful to "march out" P waves and intervals. Holter or continuous loop monitoring can also be an important tool in the evaluation of AV block.[4] These monitors allow one to evaluate the cardiac conduction system during a patient's activities of daily living. A monitoring period of at least 24 hours is recommended so that both daytime and nighttime activities are included.

TABLE 97-1. INCIDENCE OF BRADYDYSRHYTHMIAS IN ACUTE MYOCARDIAL INFARCTION

Rhythm	Incidence (%)
Any bradydysrhythmia	25-30
Sinus bradycardia	25
Junctional escape rhythm	20
Idioventricular escape rhythm	15
First-degree atrioventricular (AV) node block	15
Second-degree AV block type I	12
Second-degree AV block type II	4
Third-degree block	15
Right bundle branch block	7
Left bundle branch block	5
Left anterior fascicular block	8
Left posterior fascicular block	0.5

SINUS NODE ABNORMALITIES

Sinus Bradycardia

Sinus bradycardia is defined as a sinus rhythm with a heart rate less than 60 beats per minute. Sinus bradycardia is divided into two categories: appropriate and inappropriate. Appropriate bradycardia is seen in young, healthy individuals and endurance athletes; the heart rate increases appropriately with exercise. Pathologic sinus bradycardia does not increase appropriately with exercise. Medications are the most common cause of inappropriate sinus bradycardia; autonomic influences, electrolyte abnormalities, and intrinsic structural disorders are others. In older individuals, sinus bradycardia can result from a decrease in the sinus node firing rate, which is a normal part of the aging process. Ischemia may also increase vagal tone and result in a slower heart rate.

Sinus Arrest

Sinus arrest occurs when the pacemaker cells in the SA node fail to depolarize. Pauses of less than 3 seconds may be seen in up to 11% of normal individuals and should not cause concern.[5] There is a higher incidence of sinus pause in athletes. Pauses longer than 3 seconds are usually considered pathologic and should be evaluated.

SA exit block and sinus arrest appear similar on ECGs, but they should be distinguished, if possible. The duration of the pause in exit block is a multiple of the PP interval. High-grade exit block cannot be distinguished from sinus arrest. The treatment is the same for both conditions.[6]

Noninvasive testing includes ECG, carotid sinus massage, and a tilt table test. Carotid sinus massage is useful to diagnose carotid sinus hypersensitivity. Risks of carotid sinus massage include transient ischemic attack and stroke, and the test should not be performed on patients with carotid bruits. The tilt table test is helpful to determine whether syncopal episodes are due to autonomic dysfunction. Invasive diagnostic testing of the SA node can also be performed, although this is rarely necessary.

The treatment of sinus node dysfunction can be temporary or permanent. Atropine or an isoproterenol drip can be used in the ICU as a bridge to permanent pacemaker placement. Temporary pacing is indicated for patients who fail to respond to medical therapy.

Carotid Sinus Hypersensitivity

Carotid sinus hypersensitivity is diagnosed when ventricular asystole greater than 3 seconds' duration (usually due to a sinus pause or arrest) or a drop in systolic blood pressure greater than 50 mm Hg occurs in response to carotid massage. If symptoms occur, a 30 mm Hg drop in systolic blood pressure defines a positive response. Treatment is permanent pacing in symptomatic patients only.[7]

Postsurgical Bradydysrhythmias

Bradyarrhythmias are common after cardiac surgery. Valve surgery and septal myectomy can cause significant damage to the conduction system. Prolonged ischemia during heart transplantation may also result in sinus node or conduction system damage. The decision to place a permanent pacer should not be made until 5 to 7 days postoperatively, however, because the bradyarrhythmia may be temporary. Medication administered during surgery or reversible ischemia is often implicated. Pacing is required in 2% to 3%

TABLE 97–2. CAUSES OF ATRIOVENTRICULAR NODE DYSFUNCTION

Drugs
  Digoxin
  Beta blockers
  Certain calcium channel blockers
  Membrane-active antidysrhythmic drugs
Primary cardiac disease
  Ischemic heart disease
  Idiopathic fibrosis of the conduction system
  Congenital heart disease
  Calcific valvular disease
  Cardiomyopathy
Metabolic
  Hyperkalemia
  Hypermagnesemia
Infiltrative disease
Infectious/inflammatory disease
Collagen vascular disease
Endocrine
  Addison's disease
Trauma
Radiation
Tumors
Neurally mediated
  Carotid sinus syndrome
  Vasovagal syndrome
  Neuromyopathic disorders

Adapted from Wolbrette DL, Naccarelli GV: Bradycardias: Sinus nodal dysfunction and atrioventricular conduction disturbances. In Topol EJ (ed): Textbook of Cardiovascular Medicine. Philadelphia, Lippincott-Raven, 1998, p 1655.

of patients with valve surgery and approximately 10% of patients with transplants.[8]

ATRIOVENTRICULAR NODE DYSFUNCTION

There are many causes and several manifestations of AV node dysfunction. Table 97-2 lists the causes of AV node abnormalities.

First-Degree Atrioventricular Block

First-degree AV block is characterized by a prolonged PR interval greater than 0.20 second in adults and 0.18 second in children who are not taking medications that can prolong the PR interval (Fig. 97-1). All the P waves are conducted to the ventricles, and the PR interval is typically fixed. Potential causes of first-degree AV block include delayed conduction through the atria from the SA node to the AV node, a delay in AV node conduction, or prolonged infranodal conduction.

Conduction delays from the SA node to the AV node are typically due to structural causes, such as right atrial enlargement or an ostium primum atrial septal defect. A delay in AV node impulse conduction is the most common

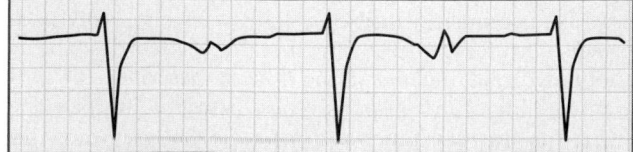

FIGURE 97–1. Electrocardiogram from a patient with first-degree atrioventricular block. The PR interval is approximately 0.34 second. All the P waves are being conducted to the ventricles. The PR interval is constant.

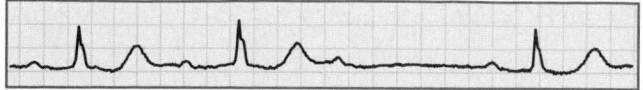

FIGURE 97–2. Electrocardiogram rhythm strip from a patient with second-degree atrioventricular block type I. Note the progressive prolongation of the PR interval until a failure of conduction occurs. Also note the reciprocal RP shortening. The pattern of conduction is 3:2.

cause of first-degree AV block. Patients with delayed conduction in the AV node often have a PR interval greater than 0.30 second. Infranodal causes of first-degree AV block are rare and are typically associated with a wide QRS complex due to disease in the fascicles or the bundle of His. First-degree AV block can also occur when each of these conduction times is at the upper limit of normal and summate to produce an overall prolongation of the PR interval.[7]

First-degree AV block is typically benign and asymptomatic. It can be seen in 0.5% of young adults without heart disease. In older people, first-degree block is most often the result of idiopathic degenerative disease. A prolonged PR interval is often an incidental finding when an ECG is ordered for other reasons. It rarely warrants further workup or treatment.

Second-Degree Atrioventricular Block Type I

Second-degree AV block type I, or a Wenckebach (or Mobitz type I) rhythm, is defined by a progressive prolongation of the PR interval with each successive beat, with eventual failure of a P wave to conduct to the ventricles (Fig. 97-2). This results in a dropped beat and failure of the ventricles to depolarize. The P waves occur at regular intervals. As the PR interval lengthens, the RR interval becomes shorter, which eventually results in decremental conduction. There is a reciprocal relationship between the RP interval and the PR interval.

The pathophysiology of second-degree AV block type I is similar to that of first-degree AV block, except that intra-atrial block is usually not a cause. For all practical purposes, second-degree AV block type I is caused by a block in AV node conduction. The QRS complex is generally narrow.

QRS complexes are typically grouped in twos, threes, fours, and so on. Group beating is characteristic of Wenckebach rhythms. The rhythm is described by recording the number of P waves and QRS complexes involved in the pattern of block (e.g., 4:3 or 3:2). During a dropped beat, a P wave is observed with no corresponding QRS complex. Second-degree AV block type I is a stable rhythm and has a much better prognosis than does a Mobitz type II rhythm. If the Wenckebach rhythm is due to medication, resolution of the block can be monitored with an ECG. Once the medication is discontinued, a shortening of the PR interval and a lengthening of the RP interval, with a corresponding improvement in AV node conduction, may be observed.

Second-Degree Atrioventricular Block Type II

Second-degree AV block type II (or Mobitz type II block) is characterized by a sudden nonconducted P wave without a change in the PR interval. A P wave with no corresponding QRS complex is observed on the ECG (Fig. 97-3). This is an inherently unstable rhythm, and serious pathology may be present. In contrast to the Mobitz type I rhythm, type II is described as a high degree of AV block, with P wave–to–QRS ratios of 3:1 and 4:1. A Mobitz type II rhythm is almost

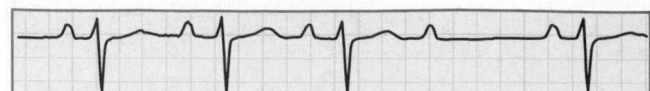

FIGURE 97–3. This electrocardiogram demonstrates second-degree atrioventricular block type II. The PR interval is constant before and after the blocked P waves. The QRS complex is widened.

always due to an infranodal conduction disturbance. The conducted QRS complexes are often wide, and a bundle branch block pattern is often observed. Second-degree AV block can result from anterior wall MI. Type II second-degree AV block can progress to complete heart block.

2:1 Atrioventricular Block

When conduction of every other P wave is blocked, 2:1 AV block is present. The PR interval of the conducted beat remains fixed. QRS complexes are regular and occur at half the atrial rate. 2:1 AV block can be caused by a Mobitz I (usually with a narrow QRS complex) or Mobitz II (with a wide QRS complex) rhythm, and the two entities are difficult to distinguish.

Third-Degree Atrioventricular Block

Third-degree AV block is characterized by complete AV dissociation. There is no conduction of the atrial signal through to the ventricle, so the atrial and ventricular systems operate independently. On ECGs, the P waves "march through" and are not associated with ventricular contraction. The PR intervals are irregular. The ventricular complexes may be junctional (narrow QRS complex; rate 40 to 60) or ventricular (wide QRS complex; rate <40). Depending on the escape heart rate, patients may present with tachypnea, dyspnea on exertion, fatigue, cyanosis, or syncope (Fig. 97-4).

Third-degree block can be divided into congenital and acquired causes. Sixty percent of patients with congenital heart block are female. Patients with congenital third-degree block often have an escape rhythm with an adequate rate.[9] Acquired third-degree block occurs most frequently in the seventh decade of life and usually requires permanent pacing; these patients are often male. Specific causes include medications, ischemia, progression from Mobitz type II rhythm, and infarction. Acute MI results in third-degree heart block in 14% of patients with inferior wall infarcts and 2% of patients with anterior infarcts. Third-degree block is usually observed within 24 hours after an MI. Third-degree block as a complication of inferior MI is usually temporary and may require only temporary pacing. Complete heart block as a result of anterior MI usually requires a permanent pacer.

Treatment involves correction of underlying disorders and immediate transcutaneous or transvenous pacing in unstable patients. If the primary cause cannot be medically managed, permanent pacing is required.

Diagnostic Pitfalls

Determining the degree of AV node block is usually straightforward if an adequate ECG has been obtained. There are

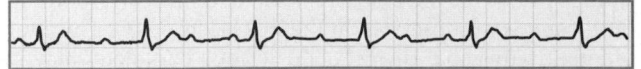

FIGURE 97–4. Complete heart block. The PR intervals are irregular, because the ventricles and atria represent two independent sources of depolarization.

circumstances, however, in which one may be misled to an incorrect diagnosis.

Third-degree block is occasionally misdiagnosed as second-degree block type II if there appears to be a constant PR interval. This may occur for short periods on an isolated rhythm strip. The clinician must therefore examine a strip for an appropriate length of time to make the correct diagnosis. Vagal maneuvers can also be attempted and may identify a second-degree AV block that is really a third-degree AV block.

With isorhythmic AV dissociation, the P waves and QRS complexes occur at a similar rate. The P waves may never "march out" long enough to determine whether they are all conducting. Interventions such as vagal maneuvers to change the P-QRS relationship may aid in diagnosis.

When second-degree AV block is fixed (2:1, 3:1, 4:1), some P waves may be concealed during the repolarization phase of the ECG. This may occur in acute MI or with ischemia. Vagal maneuvers and examination of multiple leads may be necessary to correctly identify the AV block.

When complete AV dissociation occurs with accelerated junctional or ventricular rhythms, it is possible that some of the atrial impulses would be conducted if the heart rate were slower. It is best to designate these rhythms as complex AV dissociation.

Therapy

Medical therapy for AV block consists of atropine, adrenergic agents, Digibind (if appropriate), and pacing. Atropine decreases vagal tone and is useful for hypervagotonia but not AV node ischemia. It is more useful in inferior wall MI than anterior wall MI. Atropine will not improve third-degree AV block or a Mobitz type II block if the pathology is below the AV node, and it is ineffective in heart transplant patients. Atropine should be used with caution in patients with Mobitz type II rhythms, because a paradoxical decrease in heart rate can occur.

Digibind should be used in symptomatic patients with digoxin-induced AV block. The number of vials of Digibind required is approximately equal to the patient's weight (in kilograms) times the digoxin serum level (in ng/mL) divided by 100.

PACEMAKERS

Although pacemakers are reliable, patients occasionally present with abnormalities in one or more pacemaker functions that may impact their current illnesses. Intensivists can expect to encounter patients with pacemakers routinely, and it is helpful to be familiar with the basics of their functions and malfunctions.

The North American Society of Pacing and Electrophysiology and the British Pacing and Electrophysiology Group created a code consisting of five letters to describe pacemaker functions, known as the NBG pacemaker code (Table 97-3).[10] The first three letters describe the antibradycardia functions, the fourth describes the programmability of rate responsiveness, and the fifth describes any antitachycardia functions. A pacemaker may carry one classification (e.g., DDD) but be capable of several modes of function, depending on how it is programmed. Indications for permanent pacing were updated by the American College of Cardiology in 2002.[11]

TABLE 97–3. NBG PACEMAKER CODE

Position Category	I Chamber paced	II Chamber sensed	III Response to sensing	IV Rate modulation or programmability	V Antitachycardia functions
Letters used	A = atria V = ventricular	A = atria V = ventricular	T = triggered I = inhibited	R = rate modulation P = simple programmable (rate or output)	P = pacing S = shock
	D = dual (A + V)	D = dual (A + V)	D = dual (T + I)	M = multiprogrammable O = none	D = dual (P + S)

From Bernstein AD, Camm AJ, Fletcher AD: The NASPE/BPEG generic pacemaker code for antibradyarrhythmia and adaptive rate pacing and antitachycardia devices. Pacing Clin Electrophysiol 1987;10:794-798.

The pacemaker itself consists of two components: a pulse generator, and wire leads connecting the generator to the heart. The pulse generator consists of a lithium-based battery and the circuitry to detect and analyze the cardiac rhythm and produce the output. The battery can last more than 10 years, depending on the type of programming, and at the end of its life it shows a gradual rate decrease, not an abrupt drop-off.[12]

Pacemakers also contain a reed switch that can be used to assess the pacemaker's pacing ability. When an external magnet is placed over the pulse generator, the reed switch closes, disabling the sensing mechanism. The unit then fires asynchronously, without regard for the patient's underlying rhythm. The pacing rate is unique to each model and manufacturer, and the magnet-programmed rate can vary, depending on whether the battery is at the beginning or end of its life or at a time of elective replacement.

Each patient is given a card when a pacemaker is implanted that describes the manufacturer, model, and pacing parameters. The pacemaker itself also contains a radiopaque code, visible on x-ray, that identifies the unit. Pacemakers can be interrogated with a manufacturer-specific program that retrieves ECG information about the unit that can help assess its functioning. An electrophysiologist should be consulted when a malfunction is suspected.

Two types of lead systems exist: unipolar and bipolar. Bipolar leads are considered standard, unless patient-specific factors warrant the use of a unipolar lead. Unipolar programming uses the lead in the endocardium as the cathode and the pacemaker unit itself as the anode. Because voltage in a unipolar lead is detected over a greater distance, the pacing spike is larger than with bipolar lead programming. Leads can be attached to the endocardium by active fixation (screwed into the myocardium) or passive fixation (held in place by fins). Passive fixation is associated with a greater incidence of dislodgment and perforation.[13]

Assessment of pacemaker function requires knowledge of its parameters. A pacing spike must be present on the ECG to properly evaluate the unit. If one is not present, a magnet can be placed over it and an ECG recorded. This can then be used with the clinical situation and prior ECG to determine its function.

Every pacer is programmed to fire after a maximum period in which no activity has been detected. This is called the lower rate-limiting interval, and it is the time between two consecutive paced beats. The escape interval is the time between a native complex and the following pacemaker spike. A slight delay beyond the lower rate-limiting interval can be programmed into the pacemaker when it senses a native QRS complex. This is an attempt to permit the heart to generate its own output and thus function in a more

physiologic manner; this is called rate hysteresis, and it is found most often in ventricular demand pacemakers.[14] Dual chamber pacers have an interval programmed between atrial and ventricular spikes, called the AV interval, which functions basically as the PR interval. The interval between a ventricular spike and the next atrial pacing spike is the ventriculoatrial interval. The AV and ventriculoatrial intervals sum to equal the lower rate-limiting interval.

COMPLICATIONS

Failure to Sense (Undersensing)

Undersensing occurs when the pacemaker generates output regardless of the patient's underlying rhythm (Fig. 97-5). A spike is seen at an interval earlier than the lower rate-limiting interval. Pacemaker output then competes with the patient's own intrinsic rhythm. Although ventricular pacing can present a problem when the threshold for ventricular capture has been altered (e.g., by ischemia), and atrial pacing can produce atrial fibrillation, these are rarely urgent problems.[15]

Specific causes of failure to sense are listed in Table 97-4. Blanking is not a true cause; rather, it is an instance of functional undersensing in dual chamber pacemakers. To prevent a pacemaker-induced tachycardia, a 12- to 125-msec period of inactivity is programmed into the ventricular component after an atrial complex. If an intrinsic QRS complex occurs during this period, it will not be sensed. Scar tissue does not conduct impulses as easily as normal myocardium does, so sensing may not occur. Most pulse generators begin asynchronous pacing at a critical point at the end of their life and will not sense intrinsic activity. Defibrillation can damage the unit; placing the defibrillator pad in an anteroposterior position may help. The unit should be observed closely after shocks are delivered.

Failure to Pace (Generate Output)

This complication is noted when a pacemaker spike is not seen after the lower rate-limiting interval has been exceeded

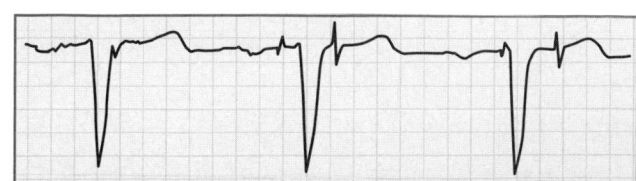

FIGURE 97–5. Failure to sense. Atrial and ventricular pacing spikes are seen around the intrinsic QRS complexes. Pacemaker activity does not lead to capture.

TABLE 97–4. CAUSES OF UNDERSENSING

Cause	Treatment
Lead fracture	Replace lead
Lead dislodgment	Reposition lead or increase sensitivity
Insulation defect in pacing lead	Replace lead
Magnet interrogation	Remove magnet
Blanking	Decrease ventricular refractory period
Amplitude of P wave or QRS complex too low to be sensed	Increase sensitivity
Myocardial fibrosis	Increase sensitivity or reposition lead
Myocardial perforation	Increase sensitivity or reposition lead
End of battery life	Replace battery
Acute myocardial infarction	Treat myocardial infarction
Electrolyte disturbance	Correct electrolytes
Antidysrhythmic drugs	Increase sensitivity, change drug
Magnetic resonance imaging	Reprogram to VOO, AOO, or DOO mode
Defibrillation	Place defibrillator pads as far from pacemaker unit as possible, place in anteroposterior position
Complexes occurring in pacemaker's refractory period	None, or use new generator with shorter refractory period

TABLE 97–5. CAUSES OF FAILURE TO PACE

Cause	Treatment
Lead fracture, loose connection, or insulation defect	Adjust or replace leads
Battery depletion	Replace battery
Pulse generator failure	Replace pulse generator
Cross-talk	Program a blanking period or safety pacing
Electromagnetic oversensing Sensing P or T or U waves	Decrease sensitivity, or advance tip deeper into right ventricle
Myopotential sensing	Decrease sensitivity, or use bipolar sensing
Electrocautery	Decrease sensitivity, or electrically isolate patient
Extracorporeal shock wave lithotripsy	Decrease sensitivity, or use minimal equipment necessary
Transcutaneous electrical nerve stimulator (TENS)	Decrease sensitivity, stop TENS unit
Magnetic resonance imaging	Program to DOO, VOO, or AOO mode

(except when hysteresis has been programmed; Fig. 97-6). Oversensing occurs when stimuli are erroneously sensed as pacemaker output. As a result, the expected, proper output is inhibited; this can be continuous or intermittent. Failure to pace can be a devastating complication for a pacemaker-dependent patient. It is important to determine whether output is truly occurring or not. A 12-lead ECG should be done, because spikes may be too small to be seen in a specific lead. Several causes are possible (Table 97-5).

Cross-talk is not a true malfunction of the pacemaker, but it can lead to an inhibition of activity. In a dual chamber system, the output of one chamber is sensed as the output of the other, and no pacemaker spike is generated; this occurs more often in unipolar leads. This problem is corrected by programming a blanking period. For a brief period after the atrial output (12 to 25 msec), the ventricular component is inhibited from firing. A second protection against cross-talk is to program the unit to fire depending on when in the AV interval the stimulus is detected. If it occurs immediately after the blanking period, a "safety" spike is generated, because it is assumed that it is impossible to differentiate cross-talk from a native QRS complex.

Failure to Capture

This complication occurs when a pacemaker fires as expected but fails to depolarize the myocardium. A pacer spike is seen on the ECG, but no QRS complex immediately follows it (Fig. 97-7). This can be dangerous for a pacemaker-dependent patient and may require temporary pacing until the problem is fixed. Most cases are due to problems with the lead-tissue interface, although isolated problems in the leads or the myocardium can also occur (Table 97-6).[13,16]

When a lead is placed into the myocardium, tissue fibrosis occurs over the first 4 to 6 weeks. Because scar tissue does not conduct as well as normal myocardium, the output voltage may need to be increased. Twiddler's syndrome is seen when a patient fidgets with the generator and ends up pulling the leads from their attachments to the myocardium. It is confirmed by chest x-ray. The pacemaker is replaced and fixed tightly to the underlying fascia. Perforation of the ventricle typically occurs shortly after the leads are placed and is confirmed by a chest x-ray showing the tip of the lead outside the heart. It is suggested by a change in pacing to a right bundle branch pattern, failure to capture, contraction of the diaphragm or intercostal muscles with pacing, or development of a pericardial friction rub. Provided the patient is not anticoagulated, the perforation is usually well tolerated.[14] Echocardiography can assess for the presence of pericardial effusion or tamponade. Repositioning of the lead is typically performed in the operating room after any coagulopathy has been reversed.

An increased threshold for capture can also be caused by myocardial ischemia, metabolic abnormalities, or certain drugs. Definitive treatment involves correcting the underlying disorder.

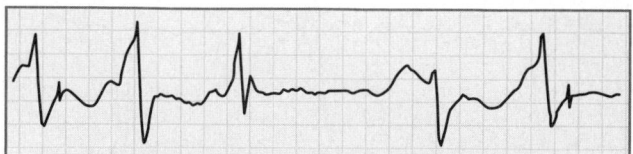

FIGURE 97–6. Failure to pace. An unduly long interval passes after the third QRS complex before another beat occurs. The pacemaker should have fired before this intrinsic beat.

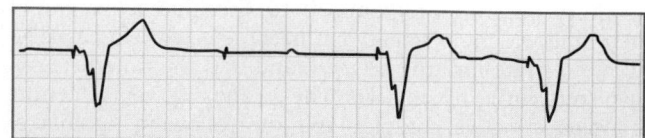

FIGURE 97–7. Failure to capture. After the first QRS complex, a small pacemaker spike occurs that does not result in depolarization of the ventricle. A nonconducted P wave follows, and then a pacemaker spike with capture occurs.

TABLE 97–6. CAUSES OF FAILURE TO CAPTURE

Cause	Treatment
Lead dislodgment from endocardial surface	Repair lead
Twiddler's syndrome	Fix unit to chest wall
Lead fracture or break in insulation	Replace lead
Improperly or inadequately programmed voltage	Reprogram voltage
Battery failure	Replace battery
Cardiac perforation	Reposition lead (in operating room) or increase voltage
Increased threshold for capture	
Fibrosis or scar tissue at contact site	Increase voltage or reposition lead
Myocardial ischemia	Treat ischemia
Metabolic	Treat abnormality
Hyperkalemia	
Hypercarbia	
Hypoxemia	
Hypothyroidism	
Drugs	Remove drug and replace with another
Beta blockers	
Class Ia antidysrhythmics	
Verapamil	
Flecainide	

When assessing for failure to capture, a distinction must be made between pseudofusion and fusion beats. A pseudofusion beat occurs when the pacemaker fires at the same time that an intrinsic beat occurs. The pacemaker output does not depolarize the myocardium, and instead, the pacemaker spike simply deforms the native QRS complex. It is an example of failure to capture. A fusion beat occurs when both the native complex and the pacemaker spike depolarize the myocardium, resulting in a QRS complex that is a hybrid of the two.

Other Problems

Pacemaker-mediated tachycardia, also called endless loop or pacemaker reentrant tachycardia, is a complication of dual chamber units. A premature atrial contraction or premature ventricular contraction that travels in a retrograde manner into the atria is sensed by the atrial component of the pacemaker, which induces the ventricular component to fire. The resulting ventricular depolarization reenters the atria, and the cycle continues. An upper rate limit is programmed into the pacemaker, so the tachycardia will not exceed this rate. A tachycardia paced by atrial and ventricular spikes is seen. Application of a magnet terminates the dysrhythmia; adenosine may not reliably block it.[17] A blanking period must be programmed.

Pacemaker syndrome is seen when only the ventricle is paced. Patients present with lethargy, syncope, dizziness, weakness, fatigue, palpitations, or congestive heart failure. It occurs because of an inability to raise the heart rate with exercise and because of the loss of AV synchrony. Dual chamber pacing is required to correct this.

The diagnosis of MI in a patient with a functioning pacemaker is difficult. Criteria similar to those in patients with left bundle branch block have been proposed, but sensitivity and specificity are lower.[15]

Advanced Cardiac Life Support protocols are not contraindicated by the presence of a pacemaker. Defibrillator pads should be kept as far away from the pulse generator as possible to minimize any damage to the unit.

Examination by magnetic resonance imaging has been considered contraindicated because of the interaction between the strong magnetic field and the pulse generator. Increased pacing rates, decreased rates, and pacing at the magnet rate have all been seen. However, programming the pacemaker to an asynchronous mode (AOO, VOO, or DOO) and close monitoring of the patient, along with the use of lower magnetic fields, may allow safe imaging.[18,19]

TEMPORARY PACING

Temporary cardiac pacing may be required for emergent or elective reasons. In general, any patient with bradycardia causing symptoms or hemodynamic instability that is unresponsive to atropine ought to be considered for temporary pacing (Table 97-7).[20] In most cases, this occurs after acute MI,[20,21] but certain drug poisonings may benefit from pacing,[22,23] and some interventions may, because of underlying disease, predispose a patient to significant bradycardia.

MODES OF PACING

Several modes of temporary pacing are available. Transcutaneous pacing involves placing the pacing pads on either the chest wall and back (the usual locations) or in an anterolateral position (especially if external defibrillation may be required). The negative electrode is placed over the apex of the heart. This is the easiest mode to use, but it is uncomfortable for a conscious patient and may require analgesia or sedation.

Transvenous pacing is usually well tolerated by patients but requires a high degree of skill to correctly place the pacing electrode in the right ventricle. Therefore, the American College of Physicians and the American College of Cardiology recommend that only physicians formally trained in their use place these electrodes.[24] The right internal jugular vein approach is best because of its more direct

TABLE 97–7. INDICATIONS FOR TEMPORARY CARDIAC PACING

Drug toxicity
  Beta blocker
  Calcium channel blocker
  Digitalis-induced dysrhythmia (when direct-current cardioversion is contraindicated)
Hyperkalemia with bradycardia or asystole
Hypothermia (transcutaneous pacing only)
Symptomatic bradycardia (including hemodynamic compromise, syncope, or ventricular ectopy in response to bradycardia) not responsive to atropine
Pacemaker malfunction with symptoms
Alternating BBB (after MI)
RBBB with alternating LAFB or LPFB (after MI not known to be old)
RBBB with LAFB or LPFB, or LBBB with first-degree heart block, not known to be old
Mobitz type II heart block
Asystole
LBBB not known to be old
Recurrent sinus pauses >3 sec not responsive to atropine
RBBB with first-degree heart block
Possibly helpful: bifascicular block or RBBB of unknown age

BBB, bundle branch block; LAFB, left anterior fascicular block; LBBB, left bundle branch block; LPFB, left posterior fascicular block; MI, myocardial infarction; RBBB, right bundle branch block.

route to the heart; the left subclavian vein approach can also be used but should be avoided, if possible, because it is a preferred site for placement of a permanent pacemaker.[20]

Transesophageal pacing allows pacing of either the atria or the ventricles, but it is not a commonly used modality. Transthoracic pacing, in which leads are placed percutaneously into the ventricular myocardium, is also possible but is fraught with complications, including pericardial tamponade, pneumothorax, visceral injury, and coronary artery laceration. Pacing leads placed during open heart surgery can also be used.

Pacing threshold should be determined, and the pacing energy should then be set at two to three times this minimum output. Thresholds should be checked daily.

ANNOTATED REFERENCES

American College of Cardiology: ACC/AHA/NASPE 2002 guideline update for implantation of cardiac pacemakers and antiarrhythmia devices: Summary article. Circulation 2002;106:2145-2161.

This guideline revises the indications for implantable pacemakers and cardioverter-defibrillators.

Bernstein AD, Camm AJ, Fletcher AD: The NASPE/BPEG generic pacemaker code for antibradyarrhythmia and adaptive rate pacing and antitachycardia devices. Pacing Clin Electrophysiol 1987;10:794-798.

The system for describing pacemakers is introduced and discussed in this article.

Sommer T, Valhous C, Lauch G, et al: MR imaging and cardiac pacemakers: In-vitro and in-vivo studies in 51 patients at 0.5 T. Radiology 2000;215: 869-879.

This study of several dozen pacemakers and patients with pacemakers suggests that magnetic resonance imaging is safe when performed under optimal conditions of asynchronous programming of the pacemaker, continuous patient monitoring, and low magnetic field strength.

Chapter 98

SUDDEN CARDIAC DEATH: IMPLANTABLE CARDIOVERTER-DEFIBRILLATORS

Michael McCready • Derek V. Exner

KEY POINTS

1. The implantable cardioverter-defibrillator (ICD) has a rapidly expanding role in the treatment of ventricular tachyarrhythmias. A general familiarity with its function, malfunction, and associated clinical problems is required of all acute care practitioners.

2. Current ICDs use nonthoracotomy leads and are often implanted subpectorally; all devices have pacemaker (ventricular, dual chamber, or biventricular) functions and advanced antitachyarrhythmia therapies, including low-energy cardioversion, antitachycardia pacing, and defibrillation.

3. Large clinical trials of ICDs demonstrate that device-based therapy is superior to medication-based approaches for preventing sudden death, particularly in patients with left ventricular systolic dysfunction and coronary artery disease.

4. Pacing malfunctions that may occur include oversensing, undersensing, failure to capture, and paced tachycardias. Chest radiographs to assess lead position and device interrogation can help define the cause of abnormal device behavior or lead failure.

5. ICD system infection is associated with high morbidity and mortality. Patients with unexplained fever, systemic inflammation, proven bacteremia, or pulmonary embolism should undergo careful examination of the pulse generator pocket and echocardiography to assess for lead vegetations.

6. Single ICD shocks are common, and multiple repetitive shocks can occur. It is important to distinguish appropriate from inappropriate shocks and identify possible precipitants of ventricular arrhythmias, such as exercise, myocardial ischemia, medication noncompliance, or electrolyte disturbance. If necessary, magnet application can suspend the tachyarrhythmia therapies to prevent repetitive shocks.

7. Important medical interventions that may affect ICD function in the ICU include surgical electrocautery, magnetic resonance imaging, external cardioversion-defibrillation, cardiopulmonary resuscitation, insertion of pulmonary artery catheters, and use of antiarrhythmic drugs.

8. Disabling ICD functions should be performed only after considering and thoroughly discussing the medical, ethical, and legal implications.

Since its initial development in the 1970s[1] and its introduction to clinical practice in the 1980s,[2] the implantable cardioverter-defibrillator (ICD) has revolutionized the management of patients with life-threatening ventricular arrhythmias. The effectiveness of these devices in preventing death due to ventricular tachycardia (VT) or ventricular fibrillation (VF) has been demonstrated in several large, well-conducted, randomized, controlled trials.[3-8] Far from being a "last resort," as previously conceived, device-based treatment of recurrent VT or VF is the initial treatment of choice for many patients who have experienced or are at high risk for experiencing these rhythm disturbances.[9] Device complexity makes a detailed understanding of ICD technology challenging for practitioners who are not electrophysiologists, but a general understanding of these devices and their associated clinical problems is increasingly important as device-based therapy becomes more widespread.

EPIDEMIOLOGY OF SUDDEN CARDIAC DEATH

Sudden cardiac death, arbitrarily defined as death from a cardiac cause occurring within 1 hour of symptom onset or without preceding symptoms,[10] is a major public health problem accounting for 450,000 deaths annually in the United States.[11] Out-of-hospital cardiac arrest carries a dismal prognosis, with reported rates of survival to hospital admission of 5% to 10% and minimal improvement in survival rates over the past several decades.[12] This poor outcome occurs in spite of public health efforts to improve public recognition of cardiac symptoms and shorten the time to therapy by means of bystander cardiopulmonary resuscitation (CPR) and better access to emergency medical services.[13] Among patients who survive to hospital admission, mortality and morbidity remain exceedingly high,[14,15] highlighting the need for preventive efforts.

A significant proportion of sudden cardiac deaths are due to a treatable arrhythmia such as VT or VF,[13,16] with the remainder being due to pulseless electrical activity or asystole. In autopsy studies, a majority of sudden cardiac death victims have pathologically apparent structural heart disease, particularly coronary atherosclerosis.[17] In many cases, recent unstable coronary disease can be demonstrated by pathologic evidence of recent plaque rupture, with or without thrombosis.[18] In cases in which cardiac monitoring was in place at the time of death, arrhythmia is commonly present.[19]

A significant proportion of sudden cardiac death occurs in patients without previously identified cardiac disease.[15,20] Currently, there is no feasible means of screening the population at large to identify all individuals who are at risk for this catastrophic event. Prediction and prevention strategies have therefore focused on identifying patients whose other clinical characteristics place them at particularly high risk for sudden cardiac death.[21,22] From the public health perspective, the most important conditions that predispose to a high risk of sudden cardiac death include cardiovascular risk factors, coronary artery disease, and left ventricular (LV) dysfunction of ischemic and nonischemic causes. Other conditions that predispose to sudden cardiac death in which the ICD has a role are listed in Table 98-1.

Sudden death is estimated to represent approximately 50% of all deaths due to chronic heart failure.[21,23] The majority of these are due to ventricular tachyarrhythmias,[19] but a significant proportion appear due to bradycardia.[24] Among the factors that predict sudden cardiac death, severity of LV systolic dysfunction and age are by far the strongest predictors.[25-27] For this reason, large clinical trials of ICD therapy have focused on patients with LV dysfunction, coronary disease, and spontaneous or inducible ventricular arrhythmias.[28]

PREVENTION OF TACHYARRHYTHMIC SUDDEN CARDIAC DEATH: NONDEVICE THERAPY

Before development of the ICD, antiarrhythmic drugs were the cornerstone of treatment and prevention of recurrent VT and VF. However, it is now recognized that these drugs are intrinsically hazardous owing to arrhythmogenicity and other adverse effects.[29-34] Currently, antiarrhythmic drugs retain a primary role in patients with a relatively low risk of sudden cardiac death. Among higher-risk patients, antiarrhythmic drugs are often used as adjuncts to ICD therapy.

An empirical approach to drug therapy has been extensively evaluated but remains controversial. Although class IC antiarrhythmic drugs, including encainide, flecainide, and moricizine, are effective for the suppression of ventricular ectopy, they were shown to significantly increase mortality in the landmark Cardiac Arrhythmia Suppression Trials.[30,31] D-Sotalol, which has class III antiarrhythmic properties, was evaluated in a randomized, controlled trial and, similar to class IC agents, was found to increase mortality.[35] The L-isomer that confers the beta-blocking effect may attenuate this hazard.[36] Another study demonstrated the relative safety of dofetilide, a class III agent, in patients with symptomatic heart failure and LV dysfunction, in that mortality was not increased when therapy was initiated in the hospital.[37]

Amiodarone remains the only reasonable empirical choice for arrhythmia prevention in patients with heart failure or LV dysfunction. Several trials have shown decreased risk of death among patients treated with amiodarone after myocardial infarction.[33,38] Among patients at risk for arrhythmic death, a meta-analysis of controlled trials showed a reduction in total, cardiac, and sudden cardiac deaths with amiodarone therapy.[39] In patients with heart failure, empiric amiodarone does not increase the risk of death (in contrast to class IC agents).[29,40]

Guided approaches to antiarrhythmic drug choice have also been evaluated.[41] The noninvasive approach uses serial ambulatory cardiac monitoring and assesses the arrhythmia's response to specific drug choices. An invasive approach is similar but uses serial programmed electrical stimulation to evaluate the effect of selected drugs on the inducibility of VT or VF. Both approaches have been evaluated and can predict response to medical treatment reasonably well.[42-44]

Both empirical and guided therapies are limited by high recurrence rates of VT and VF and medication-related adverse events.[34,45,46] For example, although amiodarone is the most effective antiarrhythmic drug for preventing the recurrence of VT and VF, a substantial proportion of patients (>20%) treated with amiodarone are unable to continue therapy in the long term owing to cumulative side effects, recurrent arrhythmia prompting a change in therapy, or death.[34,47]

Medications other than antiarrhythmic drugs have also been evaluated. Beta blockers clearly reduce the risk of death among patients with recent myocardial infarction[48,49] and LV dysfunction,[50-52] and it appears that approximately 50% of this decreased risk is due to reductions in sudden death.[49] Beta blockers have been shown to suppress ventricular arrhythmias among patients at elevated risk[53,54] and may reduce death when used as primary antiarrhythmic therapy.[55] Use of HMG-CoA reductase inhibitors ("statins") has been associated with a lower risk of sudden death compared with nonuse in several studies.[56,57] However, prospective randomized confirmation of this finding is lacking. Trials of angiotensin-converting enzyme inhibitors and angiotensin receptor blockers in patients with heart failure and coronary disease have shown reductions in the risk of sudden cardiac death in these populations.[58] Omega-3 fatty acids ("fish oils") appear to reduce the risk of sudden cardiac death in epidemiologic studies[36,59] and in prospective randomized trials.[60] Mechanisms, magnitude of benefit, and interactions with other potential therapies require further evaluation.

Catheter ablation and surgery are often effective in preventing recurrent VT in patients who are difficult to treat by other means. Both techniques attempt to damage or "ablate" involved myocardial tissue to interrupt reentrant VT circuits, thus preventing the development of sustained arrhythmias. In the past, VT surgery was considered a primary form of therapy in experienced centers, as it could offer a cure to patients with few other therapeutic options.[61-64] Currently, VT surgery has a limited role owing to very high operative morbidity and mortality and improved nonsurgical approaches. Catheter ablation is a developing technique whereby intracardiac catheters are used to induce VT, map the pathologic circuits, and, using radiofrequency energy or direct-current shock, ablate small areas of tissue to interrupt the circuit.[65,66] Although this technique may carry a lower procedural risk than open surgical approaches, a substantial number of patients have recurrent ventricular arrhythmias,[64,67]

TABLE 98–1. CAUSES OF VENTRICULAR ARRHYTHMIAS

Structural Disease

Left ventricular dysfunction
Coronary artery disease and acute myocardial infarction
Coronary artery anomalies
Hypertrophic cardiomyopathy
Arrhythmogenic right ventricular dysplasia

Primary Electrophysiologic Defects

Wolff-Parkinson-White syndrome
"Idiopathic" ventricular tachycardia or fibrillation
Catecholamine-sensitive polymorphic ventricular tachycardia
Long QT syndrome (congenital or acquired)
Brugada syndrome

and experience in most centers is limited. VT related to ischemic heart disease is especially difficult to manage with catheter ablative procedures,[67,68] owing to multiple pathologic intracardiac circuits.

Revascularization is of primary importance in patients with coronary artery disease and malignant ventricular arrhythmias. One study evaluated the role of ICD in patients undergoing coronary artery bypass grafting and showed no benefit in this population.[69] Until recently this was the only clearly negative trial evaluating the role of ICDs in the primary prevention of death in patients at risk for VT or VF. Other studies have demonstrated an association between coronary artery bypass grafting and decreased risk of sudden death.[70-72] A recent randomized trial of ICD therapy early following myocardial infarction (DINAMIT) also found no difference in mortality with usual medical care versus an ICD (see Table 98-4).

Several lifestyle factors have been associated with lower risks of sudden death. Tobacco avoidance, exercise, moderate alcohol consumption,[73] and a diet rich in fish[59] have all been shown to be protective, and lifestyle modification programs may prevent sudden cardiac death.[74,75]

IMPLANTABLE CARDIOVERTER-DEFIBRILLATORS

DEVICE BASICS

The ICD is composed of two parts: the pulse generator and the leads. The generator consists of batteries; a capacitor for charging and discharging ("shocking"); electronic circuits that monitor, analyze, and guide treatment of arrhythmias; and information storage capabilities. Additional capabilities are available in current devices.

The pulse generators of early devices were large (approximately 250 cm³) and required surgical implantation in the abdomen. Leads were large (150 to 180 cm²) epicardial pads placed via a thoracotomy. Separate epicardial screw-in sensing leads were also required. Implantation was associated with significant perioperative morbidity and mortality. Rhythm analysis was rudimentary and relatively insensitive. Only medium- or high-energy shock therapy was available. Data storage capacity was limited to information regarding the number of shocks. When intracardiac electrogram storage and analysis became available, it was apparent that inappropriate shocks, predominantly for atrial fibrillation, were common.[76,77]

The initial primary purpose of the ICD was to detect VT and VF and terminate these arrhythmias with effective defibrillation. Reports of early experiences suggested a substantially lower annual mortality among ICD recipients versus similar historical comparative groups.[78] More recent refinements in ICD technology have improved the safety and tolerability of the devices substantially, but effective defibrillation remains the crucial, lifesaving feature.

Current devices are much smaller, allowing subpectoral or subcutaneous implantation. Using nonthoracotomy lead systems, implantation methods are identical to permanent pacemaker implantation. Local anesthetic with mild sedation is used for implantation; heavy sedation or a brief general anesthetic is needed to test defibrillation thresholds. Operative mortality for nonthoracotomy systems is less than 0.5%.[79] The greatest intraoperative risk is related to the induction of VF and the resulting hemodynamic compromise.

Particularly in patients with severe LV dysfunction, the hemodynamic effects of even brief spells of VF can be persistent and detrimental.[80] Obesity or cachexia, limited vascular access, pulmonary hypertension, anticoagulation or bleeding disorders, and vascular or cardiac anomalies may increase the technical challenge of implantation. Tricuspid valve prosthesis or significant tricuspid valvular disease may preclude use of endocardial lead systems. Features of current devices are listed in Table 98-2. Common procedural risks are listed in Table 98-3.

THERAPEUTIC FUNCTIONS

Bradycardia and Pacing

Patients with significant heart failure commonly have symptomatic bradycardia due to conduction disturbances, inadequate chronotropic responses, and medications that induce bradycardia.[24] Further, postcardioversion and postshock bradycardia is common among ICD patients. To meet these

TABLE 98–2. FEATURES OF CURRENT IMPLANTABLE CARDIOVERTER-DEFIBRILLATORS

Size	30-80 cm³
Weight	70-150 g
Batteries	Low-resistance lithium or silver vanadium for charging defibrillation capacitor; separate battery for pacing functions
Leads	Steroid-eluting, silicone- or polyurethane-coated, 4-9 Fr. (1.3 to 3 mm) caliber, depending on type; ports for ventricular, atrial, left ventricular (coronary sinus), and superior vena cava leads
Output, charge	30-40 J, 750-800 V
Battery life	4-10 yr, depending on manufacturer, device, and use
Arrhythmia detection	Rate-based; enhanced ventricular tachycardia detection features vary by device and manufacturer
Arrhythmia management	Defibrillation with biphasic waveform, low-energy cardioversion, antitachycardia pacing features; atrial therapies, including antitachycardia pacing and cardioversion; bradycardic ventricular and dual chamber pacing; biventricular pacing
Storage capabilities	Device and lead identification, implantation date, physician contact; arrhythmia event data, including date and time, onset, heart rate, therapies delivered, shock counters, rate histograms, electrograms, marker channel; pacemaker functions, including pacing thresholds, lead impedances, R and P wave amplitude, percent pacing, heart failure diagnostic information
Programmable functions	Pacing parameters, tachyarrhythmic therapies, tiered therapy algorithms; many other refined programmed functions vary by manufacturer

TABLE 98–3. RISKS OF CARDIOVERTER-DEFIBRILLATOR IMPLANTATION

Anesthetic risk
Risk of fibrillation or defibrillation
Atrial and ventricular arrhythmias
Bleeding
Embolism (thrombus, air)
Vessel or organ injury
Cardiac injury or pericardial tamponade
Infection

needs, all current ICDs have pacing capabilities. Devices are available with ventricular, dual chamber, or biventricular pacing modalities.

Although ventricular and dual chamber pacemakers are frequently indicated for ICD patients, there are concerns about the potential adverse effects of right ventricular pacing. One major trial showed that atrioventricular sequential pacing at a rate of 70 beats per minute was associated with higher rates of heart failure, hospitalization, or death when compared with backup ventricular pacing at 40 beats per minute.[81] This effect was ascribed to the untoward hemodynamic effects of right ventricular pacing. Other studies have supported this finding.[82] Further, pacing can precipitate ventricular tachyarrhythmias in some patients.[83] Thus, the pacemaker backup rate should be turned down to the lowest acceptable rate in patients with LV dysfunction.

Biventricular pacing, or resynchronization therapy, is a new pacing modality incorporated into some devices. Biventricular pacing is not intended to treat bradycardia per se; instead, it coordinates synchronous left and right ventricular contraction.[84] In the presence of left bundle branch block or right ventricular pacing, the interventricular septum moves rightward during systole. This decreases the contribution of septal contraction to LV output, leading to less efficient LV systolic function. Biventricular pacing coordinates left and right ventricular contraction to minimize this effect. The left ventricle is approached through the venous system (coronary sinus) using specially designed catheters to allow epicardial LV pacing.

Several recent studies evaluated biventricular pacing in patients with advanced symptomatic heart failure and significant intraventricular conduction delay.[85-87] Results suggest improvements in symptoms, exercise tolerance, and quality of life[88] among a significant proportion of these selected patients. A survival benefit has also been recently demonstrated (see Table 98-4).[89]

Tachyarrhythmia Detection

The primary methods of detecting sustained VT are assessment of ventricular rate and duration of the tachycardia. Therapy is delivered for persistent heart rates exceeding a cutoff that is manually programmed. Different algorithms can be programmed for different rates (discussed later). The major limitation of an exclusively rate-based rhythm analysis is that tachycardias other than VT (e.g., supraventricular tachycardia) cannot be distinguished by rate alone.

Enhanced arrhythmia detection features in current dual chamber systems enable highly sensitive and specific detection of VT and VF, decreasing the occurrence of inappropriate therapies.[90-95] Onset criteria allow the distinction between sinus tachycardia, which generally has a gradual onset, and VT, which is abrupt. Rate stability criteria distinguish irregular

atrial fibrillation from VT. Devices also use the intracardiac electrogram to identify VT. Analysis of QRS width and slew rate (steepness of up- or downstroke of QRS) and comparison of QRS morphology during tachycardia with that during sinus rhythm aid further. Dual chamber devices use atrial lead sensing to evaluate the relationship between ventricular and atrial activity to distinguish supraventricular tachycardia from VT.[94]

Tachyarrhythmic Therapies: Tiered Therapy Algorithms

Using the methods outlined previously, the ICD detects arrhythmias and administers therapies as programmed. In contrast to early devices, current ICDs can deliver therapies other than defibrillation, including lower-energy cardioversion and antitachycardia pacing. Several devices also have atrial antitachycardia and cardioversion features, whose clinical benefit remains to be proved.[96,97] In a tiered therapy algorithm (Fig. 98-1), different "zones" of detection are programmed.

High-energy defibrillation is the primary and most important function of the ICD. It is the only effective therapy for VF or very rapid VT. The other available therapies are intended to abort hemodynamically tolerated VT to obviate a painful, high-energy shock.

If the ICD detects a ventricular rhythm in the VF zone, the battery charges the capacitor, which then discharges, or "shocks," if a second rhythm analysis confirms ongoing VF. Current is transmitted between the right ventricular lead and either the device itself ("active" or "hot" can) or other electrodes or coils.[98] The current passes through ventricular myocardium and depolarizes a proportion of myocytes with an energy of 27 to 35 J, depending on the manufacturer and configuration. This depolarized mass of myocardium interrupts the fibrillating electrical wave fronts and terminates VF. If defibrillation is ineffective, the device reinstates a diagnostic algorithm to detect ongoing VF. If VF is detected, the capacitor recharges, discharges, and continues this cycle of behavior until another rhythm is detected or the therapies are exhausted (4 to 6 consecutive high-energy shocks).

The major limitation of high-energy shocks is the associated discomfort experienced if the patient remains conscious during the arrhythmia. Most patients report that shocks are very painful, and fear, embarrassment, or other unpleasant emotions may be associated with the shock.[99] Quality of life is significantly impaired in patients who receive ICD shocks, although it is not known whether this impairment is due to the shock itself or the health condition necessitating the shock.[100,101]

Low-energy cardioversion is an established method of terminating hemodynamically tolerated VT, with a success rate greater than 80%.[102,103] When the device detects a rhythm in the slow VT zone, the capacitor is charged and a lower-energy shock is delivered, synchronized to the R wave. Energy outputs of 0.1 to 5 J can terminate some VTs. Patient discomfort increases substantially with increased output, particularly above 0.5 to 1 J. Above 5 to 10 J, no benefit is gained with low-energy cardioversion versus defibrillation in terms of patient comfort, although avoidance of high-energy output may prevent long-term device dysfunction[104,105] and prolong battery life. The other major risks of low-energy cardioversion are acceleration of the tachycardia rate, which occurs in up to 10% of cases, and delay of definitive therapy.[103] Less commonly, cardioversion can cause the rhythm to degenerate to polymorphic VT or VF, necessitating defibrillation.

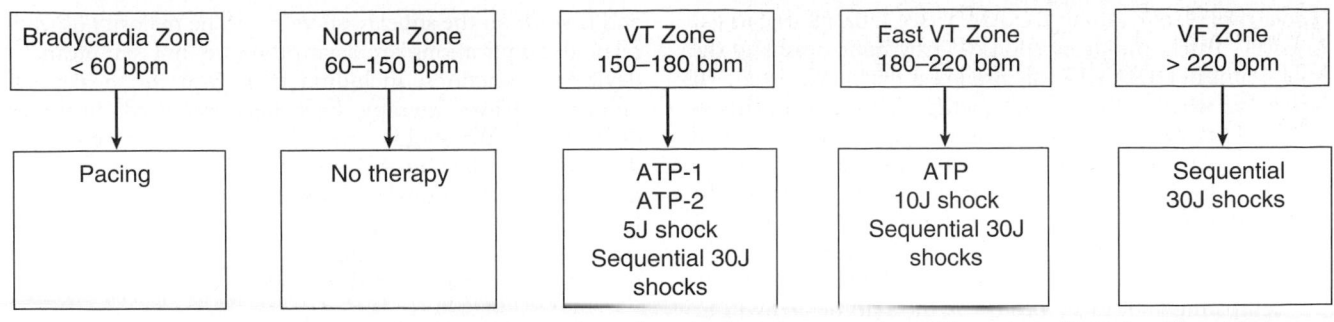

FIGURE 98-1. Example of a tiered therapy algorithm. ATP, antitachycardia pacing; bpm, beats per minute; VF, ventricular fibrillation; VT, ventricular tachycardia.

Antitachycardia pacing, when effective, is ideal therapy for terminating hemodynamically tolerated VT. Antitachycardia pacing is painless, although awareness of palpitations can occur. Antitachycardia pacing is usually the initial therapy attempted for episodes of VT, because success rates are similar to those obtained with low-energy cardioversion; up to 90% of VTs can be terminated with pacing.[106-108]

Antitachycardia pacing is more complex than defibrillation or cardioversion. The principle is to deliver pacing stimulation to the ventricle to gain control over the reentrant circuit that is perpetuating the tachycardia (overdrive suppression). If pacing is effective in entering the VT circuit, when pacing is terminated, the patient's native or paced control over ventricular depolarization is restored. In order to enter the circuit, pacing must occur in the excitatory gap when the ventricle is not refractory to stimulation, and the device must pace at a rate faster than the VT rate. Rates with a cycle length between 70% and 90% of the VT cycle length (i.e., approximately 10% to 40% faster) are most effective in terminating the tachycardia.[106,109] There are numerous pacing techniques intended to improve entry into the circuit and termination of the tachycardia. No standard nomenclature is shared by manufacturers to describe antitachycardia pacing algorithms, but each method employs several comparatively simple principles. Burst pacing delivers a series of several beats at a fixed cycle length. Ramp pacing progressively shortens cycle length (i.e., accelerates). Adaptive therapy modes allow pacing at differing rates, depending on the VT rate. Scanning allows the device to introduce pacing at varying points in the VT cycle. In the setting of slow VT, the device delivers several different antitachycardia pacing protocols in an attempt to terminate the tachycardia.

Atrial therapies incorporated in many newer devices include antitachycardia pacing and cardioversion. Their effectiveness in preventing and terminating atrial arrhythmias has been demonstrated,[97,110,111] but the clinical value of this approach remains controversial, except in selected patients in whom such therapies have proved individually beneficial and tolerable. Currently, it is rare to implant a device to treat atrial arrhythmias solely, but this is occasionally done in highly symptomatic patients who are intolerant of medical therapy.

CLINICAL TRIALS

As discussed earlier, prevention of sudden cardiac death has focused on a population of patients with LV dysfunction and heart failure, a large group that has been shown to be at high risk for arrhythmic death. In North America and western Europe, the majority of these patients have ischemic heart disease, although a substantial minority have nonischemic cardiomyopathy. Until recently, trials that enrolled only patients with nonischemic causes have shown neutral results related to mortality.[40,112,113] Three large recent trials indicate that ICD therapy reduces the risk of death versus amiodarone or best medical therapy (SCID-HEFT DEFINITE) (see Table 98-4).

Thirteen (n>100) randomized, controlled trials assessing the efficacy of ICD therapy have been completed (Table 98-4).[3,4,6,7,69,112-115] Three large trials assessed the role of ICD therapy as secondary prevention of sudden cardiac death among patients with ischemic LV dysfunction and sustained, hemodynamically significant ventricular arrhythmias.[3,4,114] The largest of these trials (Antiarrhythmics versus Implantable Defibrillators, or AVID) randomized 1016 patients with symptomatic VT or VF and LV dysfunction (LV ejection fraction < 0.40) to therapy with ICD versus antiarrhythmic drugs (82.4% amiodarone).[4] This study was stopped before completion of enrollment because of a statistically significant survival benefit (11.3% absolute risk reduction at 3 years) of the ICD. The Canadian Implantable Defibrillator Study (CIDS)[114] and the Cardiac Arrest Study Hamburg (CASH)[3] demonstrated trends toward decreased mortality, but these findings were not statistically significant. Meta-analysis of these three randomized trials supported data consistency, with a significant relative reduction in mortality risk of 28% (95% confidence interval 13% to 40%).[116]

The ten major primary prevention trials assessed the role of ICD therapy among patients at risk for but without clinically sustained VT or VF.[6-8,69] Although inclusion criteria varied somewhat, enrollment in these trials focused on patients with LV dysfunction. Similar to the secondary prevention trials, results of the primary prevention trials were consistent. Mortality reductions in the primary and secondary prevention trials have demonstrated similar results (Table 98-4). From these studies it is clear ICD therapy reduces annual mortality by 2% to 7% in most patient groups. These studies also indicate that patients with both ischemic and nonischemic etiologies of LV dysfunction benefit from ICD therapy and that amiodarone has a limited role in the prevention of sudden death in patients with heart failure.

All but two of the primary prevention trials demonstrated a mortality benefit from ICD therapy (Table 98-4). As previously discussed, routine aggressive coronary artery revascularization was likely responsible for the lack of benefit from routine ICD therapy in the CABG-Patch Trial.[69] This inference is supported by a lower than anticipated mortality rate in that trial and the fact that the ICD resulted in a significantly lower rate of arrhythmic death.[71] ICD therapy also did not reduce the risk of death in DINAMIT (see Table 98-4). Similar to CABG-Patch, the proportion of arrhythmic deaths to the total deaths in DINAMIT was also lower than anticipated.[72] It is not clear whether the lack of benefit from the ICD in DINAMIT reflects the influence of altered cardiac anatomic and electrical structure (remodeling) that occur in the initial three months following myocardial infarction or other factors. The lack of benefit from ICD therapy in these two trials illustrates that when considering a patient for an ICD, careful thought must be given to the long-term risk of arrhythmic death and the competing modes of death. As the rate of arrhythmic death is reduced, the impact of the ICD is significantly lessened.

A marked increase in the number of ICDs is anticipated to occur based on the results of recent trials (see Table 98-4). Issues of cost and identifying those patients most likely and least likely to benefit (risk stratification) from ICD therapy await the results on ongoing studies. It is worth emphasizing that ICD therapy is costly,[117,118] and the magnitude of benefit is sensitive to baseline risk.[119] Studies to date have assessed ICD therapy in relatively high-risk populations, but even within these populations, risk appears to vary substantially. For example, in AVID, no benefit was observed among the subgroup of patients with an LV ejection fraction greater than 0.35.[26] Whether ICD therapy is appropriate in lower-risk high-risk patients, particularly those with relatively preserved LV ejection fraction, remains to be determined. Further studies will aid in determining whether ICD therapy in such patients provides (1) no benefit, (2) a small but excessively costly benefit, (3) a small but clinically important benefit, or (4) excessive hazard.

DEVICE-RELATED ISSUES AMONG PATIENTS IN INTENSIVE CARE

DEVICE INTERROGATION

Device interrogation is performed by placing an analyzing header directly over the generator. Devices from different manufacturers require brand-specific programmers. ICD patients are provided with device information and contact telephone numbers so that device type can be determined in the event of an emergency. If this information is unavailable, an overpenetrated chest x-ray will reveal identifying markers on the pulse generator. Interrogation of the device determines the manufacturer, model, settings, recorded events, and battery and lead parameters. Implanting centers generally provide around-the-clock interrogation and reprogramming. In smaller facilities, if emergent device interrogation or reprogramming is required and a programming computer is available, the device manufacturer can provide guidance remotely and advise about the use of magnets for suspending therapies. It is worth reemphasizing that the application of a magnet will suspend detection of VT and VF by ICD. In contrast, a magnet results in reversion to a "safe pacing mode" when applied to a pacemaker.

LEAD FAILURE

Lead failure due to dislodgment, fracture, or insulation breach occurs in 5% to 10% of patients, and lead replacement is usually required.[120-122] Risk of lead failure is higher with a subclavian route compared with a cephalic vein approach, owing to the compressive effects of the clavicle

and first rib on the subclavian vein.[121] The majority of lead-related complications are asymptomatic, but symptomatic device malfunctions, including inappropriate shocks and failure to deliver therapy, have been reported. Increased defibrillation thresholds can occur in the absence of lead defects or dislodgment and are thought to be due to myocardial fibrosis at the point of contact of the defibrillation lead. Frequent shocks appear to exacerbate this response. Steroid-eluting leads attenuate the inflammatory-fibrotic myocardial response and the associated increase in thresholds.

PACING FUNCTION PROBLEMS

Oversensing occurs when the pacemaker detects electrical activity that is not due to chamber depolarization. It is suspected when the heart rate falls below the programmed lower pacing rate limit or when surface lead channels or intracardiac electrograms appear "noisy." This activity may be due to electrical activity in another cardiac chamber (far-field sensing), T-wave sensing, myopotentials from pectoral muscles, or electromagnetic interference. In this situation, the device fails to pace appropriately. Oversensing can be corrected by increasing sensing thresholds, switching from a unipolar to a bipolar pacing mode, avoiding electromagnetic interference, or either repositioning or replacing the lead.

Undersensing occurs when the device fails to detect chamber depolarizations. This is usually detected as extra pacing spikes, with or without associated capture. Undersensing may be due to poor lead contact with the myocardium, defects of the lead insulation or coil, myocardial infarction, or device malfunction. Chest x-ray to assess lead position and integrity as well as device interrogation to assess lead impedance are required.

Failure to capture occurs when pacemaker spikes do not effect ventricular depolarization. This may occur because the ventricle is refractory, insufficient energy is delivered, or the lead contact is inadequate. Chest x-ray and pacemaker interrogation are required to assess lead position and pacing thresholds.

Paced tachycardias can occur. This is due to either inappropriate tracking of atrial tachyarrhythmias or pacemaker-mediated (endless loop) tachycardia by a dual chamber device. Atrial tachycardias such as atrial fibrillation or atrial flutter may be sensed by a dual chamber pacemaker, and the ventricle may be paced at inappropriately rapid rates. This is treated by pharmacologic management of the atrial arrhythmia, decreasing the upper pacing rate of the ventricle, or turning on the mode-switching function, if available. Pacemaker-mediated tachycardia occurs with dual chamber devices but is less common than in the past because of automatic recognition and prevention algorithms. When ventricular pacing is associated with ventricle-to-atrium conduction, an endless loop of ventricular pacing, ventricle-to-atrium conduction, atrial sensing, and ventricular pacing can develop. Reprogramming to prevent immediate postventricular event detection of atrial events or prolonging the postventricular atrial refractory period ameliorates pacemaker-mediated tachycardia.

INFECTION

Infections involving ICDs have been reported to occur in up to 1% to 16% of patients.[123-125] This is a devastating complication carrying substantial morbidity; early mortality has been reported to be as high as 10%.[126,127] *Staphylococcus epidermidis*

TABLE 98–4. RANDOMIZED STUDIES OF IMPLANTABLE CARDIOVERTER-DEFIBRILLATORS (ICDs)

Trial and Year of Publication	Sample Size (n)	Treatment Arms	Patient Characteristics	Mortality Benefit (Annualized Absolute Risk Reduction)	Comments
Cardiac Arrest Survivors (Secondary Prevention)					
AVID[4] 1997	1016	ICD vs amiodarone	Mixed etiologies (81% CAD) LVEF ≤ 0.40	4%	Largest secondary prevention trial Quality-of-life assessment showed neutral effects of ICD
CIDS[114] 2000	659	ICD vs amiodarone	Mixed causes (80%-90% CAD)	2%	Result trends similar to AVID Quality-of-life assessment showed possible benefit of ICD
CASH[3] 2000	288	ICD vs amiodarone vs metoprolol	Mixed etiologies (75% CAD)	2%	Propafenone arm discontinued due to increased mortality Metoprolol and amiodarone performed similarly
Patients at High Risk of Sudden Death (Primary Prevention)					
MADIT[115] 1996	196	ICD vs no ICD	100% CAD LVEF ≤ 0.35 Inducible, nonsuppressible VT	5%	First study to demonstrate benefit of strategy of primary prevention
MADIT II[6] 2002	1232	ICD vs no ICD	100% CAD LVEF ≤ 0.30	3%	Largest primary prevention trial in patients wth CAD
CABG-Patch[69] 1997	900	ICD vs no ICD	100% CAD undergoing CABG LVEF ≤ 0.35 Abnormal signal-averaged ECG	None	Revascularization in both groups may have attenuated the benefits of ICD therapy
COMPANION[113] (2004)	1520	ICD + CRT vs Pacemaker + CRT vs no device	Mixed etiologies (54% to 59% CAD) LVEF ≤ 0.35 Highly symptomatic heart failure	7% ICD + CRT 4% Pacemaker + CRT	CRT lowers the risk of death The combination of an ICD + CRT resulted in the lowest risk of death CRT also improved quality of life
DEFINITE[112] (2004)	458	ICD vs no ICD	Heart failure not related to CAD LVEF ≤ 0.35 Symptomatic heart failure	3%	Largest primary prevention trial in non-CAD Extends the results of previous trials in patients with CAD
SCD-HeFT[40] (2004)	2521	ICD vs amiodarone vs placebo	Mixed etiologies (52% CAD) LVEF ≤ 0.35 Symptomatic heart failure	2%	Largest primary prevention trial ICD significantly reduced the risk of death Amiodarone had no impact on mortality
DINAMIT[72] (2004)	674	ICD vs no ICD	Early following myocardial infarction LVEF ≤ 0.35 Abnormal heart rate variability	None	A reduction in arrhythmic death (2%) but an unexplained increase in non-sudden death (2.5%) was observed with ICD therapy ICD therapy is not efficacious early after myocardial infarction, possibly due to changes in underlying substrate and risk of non-sudden death

AVID, Antiarrhythmics Versus Implantable Defibrillators; CABG-Patch, Coronary Artery Bypass Graft—Patch Trial; CAD, coronary artery disease; CASH, Cardiac Arrest Study Hamburg; CIDS, Canadian Implantable Defibrillator Study; COMPANION, Comparison of Medical Therapy, Pacing, and Defibrillation in Heart Failure; CRT, cardiac resynchronization therapy; DEFINITE, Defibrillators in Non-Ischemic Cardiomyopathy Treatment Evaluation; DINAMIT, Defibrillator in Acute Myocardial Infarction; LVEF, left ventricular ejection fraction; MADIT, Multicenter Automatic Defibrillator Trial; SCD-HeFT, Sudden Cardiac Death Heart Failure Trial.

and *Staphylococcus aureus* cause the majority of infections, although any pathogenic bacteria or fungus can theoretically seed the device. Infection in the first several months following implantation usually results from bacterial contamination with skin colonizers introduced during or immediately after the implantation procedure.[128] Late device infections (>1 year after implantation) are equally common,[129] and primary sources of bacteremia other than the ICD are usually implicated.[130-132]

Diagnosis of device infection is often challenging. Clinical suspicion must be high in patients with an implanted device who present with fever, weight loss, fatigue, systemic inflammation, or pulmonary embolism.[127,133] All ICD or pacemaker patients with fever of uncertain cause should undergo careful examination of the generator pocket site for signs of inflammation, and blood cultures should be performed. In all patients with proven bacteremia or fungemia, transthoracic and transesophageal echocardiography may be helpful.[134]

Treatment of confirmed ICD system infection requires extraction of all device components, a prolonged (e.g., 2 to 6 weeks) intensive antibiotic course, and reimplantation.[129] The optimal duration of antibiotic therapy is uncertain, and timing of reimplantation in patients at high risk for life-threatening arrhythmias or those who are pacemaker dependent must be individualized. When infection is suspected but unconfirmed, a trial of prolonged antibiotic therapy and close clinical vigilance for relapse may obviate system extraction. The risk of occult lead infection among patients with staphylococcal bacteremia is high,[134,135] and consideration should be given to extraction,[135] especially if relapse of infection occurs.

Current guidelines do not mandate antibiotic prophylaxis for pacemaker or ICD insertion,[136] but current evidence supports peri-implantation antistaphylococcal antibiotic prophylaxis.[137] Endocarditis prophylaxis for subsequent invasive procedures in patients with ICDs and pacemakers who have no other indications remains controversial and is not universally recommended.[136]

ARRHYTHMIAS AND ANTIARRHYTHMIC DRUGS

Patients with ICDs are at high risk for atrial and ventricular tachyarrhythmias. Management of these arrhythmias generally does not differ from the usual therapy for patients without ICDs. Indeed, more liberal use of rate-slowing and proarrhythmic medications is often permissible, owing to the protective effect of backup pacemaking and defibrillation. Observing device behavior during arrhythmias is important, because it may influence management decisions. For example, if rapid ventricular pacing is observed in a patient with rapidly conducted atrial fibrillation, it is likely that the device is undertaking an antitachycardia pacing algorithm for termination of VT. Urgent slowing of the ventricular rate may prevent escalation of therapy and inappropriate shocks. In patients with atrial or ventricular tachyarrhythmias, device-based termination with overdrive suppressive pacing should not be overlooked as a therapeutic option. Failure of the device to detect and treat ventricular and regular atrial arrhythmias may be solved by simply reprogramming the device by a practitioner familiar with its features.

ICD patients often receive additional antiarrhythmic therapy to prevent device-provided therapies[138] and to improve patient tolerance of these arrhythmias. Amiodarone[138] and sotalol[139,140] may decrease the frequency of VT and VF and thus decrease the need for defibrillation therapies, avoiding patient discomfort. Dofetilide does not appear to decrease the frequency of ventricular arrhythmias and may cause torsades de pointes.[141] Class I antiarrhythmic drugs, though avoided in general, are occasionally used in ICD patients to decrease occurrences of VT. Amiodarone often decreases the VT rate, which may limit the hemodynamic effects of the rhythm and facilitate pace termination. However, decreasing the VT rate can have several deleterious effects. The device may fail to detect the slower ventricular arrhythmia and may require reprogramming. Negative chronotropic and atrioventricular node blocking effects may lead to increased pacing, which can contribute to battery depletion and untoward hemodynamic effects in some patients.

Antiarrhythmic drug therapy has the potential to increase defibrillation thresholds. Class I drugs, except propafenone,[142] and chronic amiodarone use[143] have this effect, which may be clinically important in patients whose defibrillation threshold is close to the maximum output of the device. Acutely, in a monitored hospital setting, raising the defibrillation threshold may not be clinically important. However, if amiodarone therapy is initiated, consideration should be given to follow-up testing of device function.[47]

CARDIAC ARREST AND DIRECT-CURRENT CARDIOVERSION

Cardiopulmonary resuscitation and transthoracic direct-current cardioversion involve particular issues for patients with ICDs.[144,145] In principle, given the dire circumstances surrounding cardiac arrest, the presence of an ICD should not be a distraction; resuscitation should proceed as usual, but the potential for device-related problems should be recognized. Cardiac compressions theoretically increase the risk of lead dislodgment leading to asystole in pacemaker-dependent patients. Elective transthoracic cardioversion or emergent defibrillation exposes the device to potentially damaging high voltage.[146] Contemporary devices have incorporated elements that shunt energy away from the pulse generator. As a result, a circuit can develop, causing thermal damage at the lead-tissue interface and raise pacing and defibrillation thresholds.[147] Inadvertent reprogramming has been reported as well. Transient elevations in thresholds are common; however, failure to capture following cardiac arrest or cardioversion should prompt immediate assessment for lead dislodgment or potentially permanent lead failure. Direct-current cardioversion-defibrillation paddles should be placed as far from the pulse generator as possible in an anteroposterior position, and the lowest effective energy should be used.[144,145] The potential for electromagnetic interference due to transthoracic defibrillation should be recognized, and the device should be defunctioned by applying a magnet if inappropriate device defibrillations occur.

For elective cardioversion, there are several special considerations.[144] Thought should be given to attempting programmed cardioversion through the device rather than externally. If external cardioversion is necessary, a device programmer should be available in the room for immediate assessment of abnormal device function. Given the potential for a transient increase in capture threshold, the practitioner should be prepared to externally pace if necessary. Pacing and sensing thresholds should be checked immediately after a successful cardioversion and then again in 24 hours if feasible. The local device clinic should be contacted before attempting elective cardioversion, if possible, to ensure that immediate assistance is available and to identify any device peculiarities in advance.

EVALUATION AFTER A SHOCK

Most ICD patients experience a shock within 2 years of implantation,[148] and most isolated appropriate device therapies do not require a change in treatment, although addition or increase of a beta blocker, amiodarone, or sotalol may be considered. Symptoms and patient-perceived device behavior before the shock should be assessed. The presence of presyncope, syncope, or palpitations suggests that the shock was due to arrhythmia and was not spurious. It is important to identify precipitants of arrhythmia, such as exercise, angina, noncompliance with medications, or symptoms of worsening heart failure. Unstable myocardial ischemia and electrolyte disturbances should be excluded and treated. Diagnosis of ischemic events after a shock is challenging, because pacing, antitachycardia pacing, and shocks can cause nonspecific abnormalities of the ST segments,[149] and cardiac markers are often transiently elevated.[150]

In addition to baseline clinical parameters, the initial assessment of a patient after a shock includes device interrogation. Patients' memory of the sequence of events can be inaccurate, and interrogation provides information about the heart rate and rhythm before therapy initiation, therapy attempts, rhythm response to therapy, and definitive therapy, including number of shocks. Such information is crucial for evaluating the appropriateness of the shock and possible precipitating events, and it allows tailored programming of the device.

MULTIPLE SHOCKS AND ELECTRICAL STORM

Multiple, repetitive shocks can occur in 10% to 20% of ICD patients.[148,151,152] When these occur, it is crucial to rapidly determine whether such therapies are appropriate. Frequent shocks are often highly psychologically distressing[153] and can result in a syndrome similar to post-traumatic stress disorder.[154] Sedation with benzodiazepines improves patient comfort and may ameliorate catecholamine-dependent arrhythmias.[155] If the shocks are inappropriate, tachyarrhythmia detection should be disabled by magnet application. Urgent device reprogramming and therapy directed at the underlying condition (e.g., atrial tachyarrhythmias) are required. Frequent, repetitive appropriate therapies (electrical storm) are ominous and have been shown to predict an increased risk of nonsudden death in the next several months.[151] Recurrent VT or VF is most appropriately treated with beta blockade alone[156] or in combination with intravenous amiodarone,[148] and sedation with benzodiazepines may be beneficial. Additionally, deterioration in underlying conditions, including heart failure and myocardial ischemia, may precipitate electrical storm[148] and may require intensification of directed therapy.

ELECTROMAGNETIC INTERFERENCE

Several environmental and medical sources of electromagnetic interference can affect device functioning (Table 98-5).[144,157] Noise (electromagnetic interference) can be interpreted as rapid cardiac activity resulting in inhibition of pacing functions or spurious antitachycardia therapies. Noise reversion algorithms prevent prolonged inhibition of pacing by activating an asynchronous pacing mode when prolonged noise is detected; however, asynchronous pacing can have adverse hemodynamic effects and can initiate ventricular arrhythmias.

MAGNETIC RESONANCE IMAGING

The functioning of ICDs can be adversely affected by magnetic resonance imaging (MRI) techniques and can create artifacts that limit image quality. There are several major potential risks of exposure to clinically relevant magnetic field strengths (0.2 to 3 T).[144,158] Magnetic force induces significant device torque, which can cause motion of the pulse generator, resulting in local pain, tissue damage, or device dislodgment.[159,160] Electromagnetic interference can precipitate rapid pacing or inadvertent therapies or interfere with sensing functions, leading to therapy inhibition. ICDs are more sensitive to inhibition of pacing than pacemakers are. Lead heating is well described, but its clinical significance is not known. Theoretically, heating of the lead tip can cause local tissue damage, myocardial perforation, or scar and increase sensing and pacing thresholds.[158] In addition to the risk to the patient, the presence of any foreign body with ferromagnetic properties can create imaging artifacts, limiting the diagnostic value of MRI scanning in the area of the pulse generator or leads.

The absolute risk of adverse events in routine clinical situations is unknown, because there are no large-scale studies. With current technology, the presence of an ICD or implanted pacemaker is considered a contraindication to MRI. In the rare case in which a patient is foreseen to require an implantable device but also requires an MRI, implantation may be deferred if the potential diagnostic benefit of MRI in the near future outweighs the risk of delaying device implantation. In situations in which the diagnostic value of MRI is considered essential to the care of an ICD patient, scanning should be considered only after appropriately planning for the risks; a team prepared to address potentially life-threatening traumatic complications must be present to immediately attend to the patient.

SURGERY

With careful planning, most, if not all, surgical procedures can be safely performed in ICD patients. ICD patients have a high burden of cardiovascular morbidity, and perioperative cardiac events (ischemia, heart failure, arrhythmias) are relatively common. Adherence to established guidelines for perioperative assessment,[145] appropriate consultation, and anticipation of potential complications may reduce complications. The greatest risks related to the device itself are malfunction due to electromagnetic interference, arrhythmia precipitation due to catecholaminergic surge, and increased defibrillation thresholds due to anesthetic agents.[145] Strategies to prevent complications from electromagnetic interference are listed in Table 98-5.

DISEASE PROGRESSION AND END-OF-LIFE ISSUES

Many ICD patients inevitably develop end-stage heart failure due to underlying disease progression, possibly exacerbated by the presence of the ICD.[6] Upgrading of an existing ICD system to include resynchronization should be considered. When standard therapies are exhausted, heart transplantation may be an option. In patients who are not transplant candidates, a symptom-directed palliative approach is undertaken. When patients indicate a desire for permanent defunctioning of the ICD, possible reversible transient precipitants, such as depression or other mood disturbances, should be sensitively explored. In many cases, deterioration in health, such as an exacerbation of heart failure, causes frustration, and patients may feel that treatments are futile.

TABLE 98–5. SOURCES OF ELECTROMAGNETIC INTERFERENCE

Source	Potential Problems	Preventive Measures

Imaging techniques (MRI)[144]	Device motion
	Lead heating
	Oversensing
	Reprogramming
		MRI contraindicated
		If unavoidable, program to
		    asynchronous pacing mode and defunction
		    ATP therapies; resuscitation team must be available
		    during imaging

Surgical procedures involving electrosurgical (electrocautery) techniques[144,145,161]	Oversensing Spurious antitachyarrhythmia therapies	Use alternative cutting and hemostatic techniques Use bipolar electrocautery if working within 10 cm of the device and/or leads. Preoperative reprogramming (decrease sensitivity, asynchronous pacing, or noise reversion mode) Provide internal or external alternative pacing system for pacemaker-dependent patients Peripheral monitoring (e.g., pulse oximeter) Place ground pad on leg to direct current away from pulse generator Use brief bursts with pauses of at least 10 sec; use lowest power output possible and do not use near pulse generator Assess and reprogram device immediately after procedure
Muscle and nerve stimulators (including spinal, peripheral, and transcutaneous)	Oversensing	Test stimulator functioning and interrogate device's sensed activity and response before use
Radiotherapy	Cumulative dose-dependent pulse generator damage Prolonged charge time Battery depletion	Minimize dose Shield device Check device functioning after sessions
Temporary intracardiac foreign bodies (including pulmonary artery catheters, temporary pacemakers, and instruments used in percutaneous coronary interventions)	Lead dislodgment	Avoid these manipulations with recently implanted devices Use fluoroscopy or echocardiographic guidance if necessary
Environmental (including cellular telephones, security systems [retail and airport], electrical equipment [including household appliances])[162]	Usually not problematic in an inpatient setting Possible interference with device sensing functions	Proscribe cell phone use in monitored areas Observe for unusual device behavior (rapid pacing, pacing inhibition, shocks) during use of electrical equipment near patient Awareness of potential for interaction
Other medical procedures (e.g., radiofrequency ablation, percutaneous coronary interventions, extracorporeal shock wave lithotripsy)[144]	Several case reports of interaction with devices	Device interrogation following exposure

ATP, antitachycardia pacing; MRI, magnetic resonance imaging.

Psychosocial support and discussion of the goals of therapy often clarify patients' motivations and desires. In truly terminal patients or in those who are clear and firm about their desire to discontinue ICD therapy, device defunctioning (which remains reversible) should be undertaken after full discussion of the medical, ethical, and legal ramifications. Disabling pacing functions is more challenging, particularly in those who are pacemaker dependent. This should be undertaken only after extensive discussion with the patient and family and should be performed in accordance with local policies.

ANNOTATED REFERENCES

Exner DV, Klein GJ, Prystowsky EN: Primary prevention of sudden death with implantable defibrillator therapy in patients with cardiac disease: Can we afford to do it? (Can we afford not to?). Circulation 2001;104:1564-1570.
Review article of randomized trials of ICD therapy: Results of secondary prevention trials (cardiac arrest survivors) and initial primary prevention trials (patients at high risk for sudden death) comparing defibrillator therapy versus antiarrhythmic drugs or usual care are discussed along with issues of cost-effectiveness of ICD therapy.

Gregoratos G, Abrams J, Epstein AE, et al: ACC/AHA/NASPE 2002 guideline update for implantation of cardiac pacemakers and antiarrhythmia devices: A report of the American College of Cardiology/American Heart Association Task Force on Practice Guidelines. Circulation 2002;106:2145-2161. Available on-line:http://www.acc.org/clinical/guidelines/pacemaker/incorporated/index.htm
Consensus statement: Summarizes expert opinion and scientific evidence relevant to ICD utilization and provides guidelines for implantation and management of ICD therapy.

McAlister FA, Ezekowitz JA, Wiebe N, et al: Systematic review: Cardiac resynchronization in patients with symptomatic heart failure. Ann Intern Med 2004:141:381-390.
Review of cardiac resynchronization therapy: Systematic review of randomized trials, success rates, complications, as well as clinical outcomes (mortality/morbidity) and quality of life with cardiac resynchronization therapy.

Mirowski M, Reid PR, Mower MM, et al: Termination of malignant ventricular arrhythmias with an implanted automatic defibrillator in human beings. N Engl J Med 1980;303:322-324.
Historical interest: Original report of the effectiveness of the ICD to terminate recurrent life-threatening ventricular arrhythmias, heralding the era of "device-based" therapy.

Pinski SL, Trohman RG: Interference in implanted cardiac devices. Pacing Clin Electrophysiol 2002;25:1367-1381 (Part I) and 25:1496-1509 (Part II).
Two part review of electromagnetic interference and ICD function: Comprehensive summary of case reports and clinical studies. Recommendations for dealing wth electromagnetic interference related to device therapy.

Chapter 99

SEVERE HEART FAILURE

Michael D. Sosin • Gregory Y.H. Lip

KEY POINTS

1. Severe heart failure is a common emergency presentation associated with a high rate of mortality and a high rate of morbidity among survivors.

2. Ischemic heart disease is the most common underlying cause in the Western world, although the cause may differ between ethnic groups. Severe heart failure may be the first presentation of ischemic heart disease. Other common causes are hypertensive heart disease and dilated cardiomyopathy.

3. The diagnosis of heart failure is not always straightforward—it may be confused with asthma or chronic airway disease. Classic examination findings of heart failure are not sensitive or specific and require confirmation by the early use of investigations such as echocardiography.

4. Assessment for B type natriuretic peptide may be a useful method of ruling out heart failure in the acutely breathless patient but is not sufficiently sensitive to diagnose heart failure without additional investigations.

5. Initial therapy for an episode of severe heart failure should involve diuretic therapy, and a single dose of intravenous diamorphine can be considered. In patients with preserved systolic blood pressure, an infusion of vasodilator or recombinant brain natriuretic protein (nesiritide) may be considered. In patients with hypotension, inotropic agents can be considered, although studies suggest increased risk of mortality with such agents.

6. Patients who do not show evidence of improvement, or whose condition deteriorates, should be considered for additional support such as intra-aortic balloon counterpulsation or assisted ventilation early. Patients with cardiogenic shock due to ischemic heart disease should be considered for revascularization.

7. Once stabilized, patients must be established on appropriate secondary preventative therapy, including angiotensin-converting enzyme inhibitors and beta-blockers. Long-term follow-up is best provided by a specialist heart failure clinic.

Heart failure is a very common condition,[1] with high mortality and morbidity rates. Data from the Framingham heart study suggest that at 40 years of age, the lifetime risk for congestive heart failure is 21.0% (95% CI, 18.7-23.2%) for men and 20.3% (95% CI, 18.2-22.5%) for women.[2] Heart failure is increasing in prevalence,[3] partly due to improvements in treatment, so it is likely that severe heart failure will be seen more and more frequently in emergency departments throughout the world. Patients with severe heart failure often present in extremis, and their condition may deteriorate rapidly, so a sound knowledge of immediate treatment is vital for critical care and emergency physicians. Such patients often respond rapidly to appropriate treatment, making this a very satisfying condition to treat. However, it is important to note that outlook remains poor despite initial clinical improvement.

In this chapter, we will discuss causes, presentation, investigation, treatment, and prognosis of severe heart failure, including new developments in the investigation and management of this common, serious condition.

ETIOLOGY

Ischemic heart disease is the most common cause of heart failure, commonly related to previous myocardial infarction.[4] Although epidemiologic surveys such as the Framingham study suggest a high prevalence of hypertension as the "cause" of heart failure, it is likely that associated ischemic heart disease or arrhythmias also contribute. Other studies have demonstrated similar findings (Table 99-1).

It should be pointed out that epidemiologic studies such as the Framingham study have been carried out in almost exclusively white populations—etiologic factors may have different relative importance in other ethnic groups. For example, in Afro-Caribbeans, hypertension is the predominant etiologic factor, whereas in Indo-Asians, coronary artery disease and diabetes are common. It is important to note that different causes may coexist in the same patient.

ISCHEMIC HEART DISEASE

Ischemic heart disease is the most common cause of heart failure in the Western world. Many patients presenting with severe heart failure will give a history of previous myocardial infarction. However, an episode of severe heart failure may also be the first manifestation of ischemic heart disease, either due to massive myocardial infarction causing cardiogenic shock[5] or as a result of previous silent (or unreported) episodes of ischemia/infarction. It is therefore important to exclude myocardial infarction in all patients presenting with severe heart failure. Additionally, once the patient is stabilized, adequate secondary preventative strategies are vital to prevent

TABLE 99–1. EPIDEMIOLOGIC STUDIES OF ETIOLOGY OF HEART FAILURE

Etiology	Teerlink et al (31 Studies 1989-90) (%)	Framingham Heart Study* (%)		Hillingdon Study(%)
		Men	Women	
Ischemic	50	59	48	36
Nonischemic:	50	41	52	64
Hypertension	4	70	78	14
Idiopathic	18	0	0	0
Valvar	4	22	31	7
Other	10	7	7	10
Unknown	13	0	0	34

Because of rounding, totals may not equal 100%.
*Total exceeds 100% as coronary artery disease and hypertension were not considered as mutually exclusive causes.
Data from Lip GYH, Beevers DG: ABC of heart failure: Aetiology. BMJ 2000; 320:104-107.

TABLE 99–2. FINAL DIAGNOSES IN 1230 PATIENTS WITH INITIALLY UNEXPLAINED CARDIOMYOPATHY

Diagnosis	Number	Percentage
Idiopathic dilated cardiomyopathy	616	50
Myocarditis	111	9
Ischemic heart disease	91	7
Infiltrative cardiomyopathy	59	5
Peripartum cardiomyopathy	51	4
Hypertension	49	4
Human immunodeficiency virus infection	45	4
Connective tissue disease	39	3
Substance abuse	37	3
Familial	25	2
Valvular disease	19	1.5
Doxorubicin therapy	15	1
Endocrine disorder	11	1
Others	62	5.5

Data from Felker GM, et al: Underlying causes and long term survival in patients with initially unexplained cardiomyopathy. N Engl J Med 2000;342:1077-1084.

further ischemia or infarction. Some patients with ischemic cardiomyopathy may show evidence of "hibernation" of segments of myocardium,[6] and cardiac function in these patients may improve with revascularization (see later).

HYPERTENSIVE HEART DISEASE

Hypertension causes a significant proportion of cases of heart failure. An episode of severe heart failure may be the first presentation of hypertension—such patients have had unrecognized severe hypertension for many years. The onset of heart failure may result in a previously raised blood pressure becoming normal or even low, which can make the diagnosis difficult in a patient with previously undiagnosed hypertension. Electrocardiography and echocardiography may show evidence of left ventricular hypertrophy. Patients with hypertension also commonly have diastolic dysfunction as a cause for heart failure. In this situation, systolic contraction is normal or minimally impaired but the main abnormality is in diastolic relaxation and ventricular compliance.[7] The incidence of diastolic abnormalities increases with age, and while the mortality rate associated with diastolic heart failure appears to be lower than that of systolic heart failure, it is still significant. To date, the ideal method of defining abnormal diastolic function has not been clearly ascertained.

DILATED CARDIOMYOPATHY

Dilated cardiomyopathy is defined as left ventricular dysfunction of unknown cause. It is therefore a diagnosis of exclusion, and a firm diagnosis of dilated cardiomyopathy can only be made in the presence of a normal coronary angiogram. Intensive investigation of patients with a label of dilated cardiomyopathy may yield a definite cause in as many as 50% of cases (Table 99-2).

Dilated cardiomyopathy can manifest at any age, and, because heart failure may be perceived as a disease of the elderly, this can often result in misdiagnosis in younger patients.

VALVULAR HEART DISEASE

Structural Valve Disease

Valvular heart disease was, in previous years, a leading cause of heart failure in the Western world. Owing to the rise in ischemic heart disease, and the decrease in rheumatic fever, it is now less often the primary cause of an episode of severe heart failure. However, it is important not to discount significant valve disease in patients presenting with severe heart failure and to remember that signs may be difficult to elucidate in the acutely ill patient. Because all patients with severe heart failure should undergo echocardiography soon after admission, most if not all cases of significant valve disease should be detected. As noted earlier, after extensive myocardial infarction, acute mitral regurgitation can develop, causing sudden onset severe heart failure days after a patient's initial presentation with chest pain.

Functional Valve Disease

Patients with heart failure of any cause with dilatation of the left ventricle and mitral valve ring can develop functional mitral regurgitation. This further reduces left ventricular performance, and, in selected patients, mitral valve repair or replacement may be indicated.

DIABETES

In addition to the role of diabetes as a risk factor for the development of ischemic heart disease and resultant heart failure, there is evidence for a distinct diabetic cardiomyopathy.[8] Recognition of diabetes is important in the patient presenting with heart failure, as there is a growing body of evidence that rigorous control of blood glucose (using dextrose/insulin/potassium infusion, GIK) may improve outcome in cardiovascular disease,[9] although studies so far have not been directed specifically at patients with heart failure. All patients presenting with heart failure should be screened for diabetes, both for this reason and so that appropriate secondary prevention can be instituted.

OTHER POSSIBLE CAUSES OR EXACERBATING FACTORS

Patients with severe heart failure often have additional medical problems complicating management. Patients with a long history of stable heart failure may develop severe symptoms due to deliberate or accidental omission of medications, intercurrent infection, or the development of atrial fibrillation. Patients with heart failure tolerate anemia poorly. It is vital to consider and treat such exacerbating conditions where appropriate.

PRESENTATIONS OF SEVERE HEART FAILURE

Severe heart failure can manifest in several ways. The patient may or may not have a previous history of heart failure, or precipitating conditions such as angina or hypertension. It is important to note that gradual onset heart failure can easily be mistaken for asthma, and patients presenting to an emergency department may well have been given a diagnosis of asthma in the weeks or months preceding their admission.

ACUTE PRESENTATION: PULMONARY EDEMA

The classic presentation of heart failure is with acute pulmonary edema. Such patients present with extreme shortness of breath, often unable to speak due to their rapid respiratory rate. The symptoms may come on very suddenly. Even patients with ischemic heart failure may not report chest pain, either because the ischemia is silent or because the pain is being masked by the profound shortness of breath. Many patients will be unable to give a history due to their shortness of breath, and therefore examination findings and basic investigations are vital to make the diagnosis.

General Examination. Examination may often reveal pallor, sweating, and dyspnea. The patient will have a high respiratory rate and increased work of breathing, using accessory muscles of respiration. Peripheral edema is not always present, particularly in patients presenting with a first episode of heart failure. Equally, the jugular venous pulse may not be elevated.

Respiratory Examination. Percussion is unlikely to be of value, owing to difficulty in examining the patient. A pleural effusion large enough to cause such dyspnea as to simulate severe heart failure will usually be obvious on auscultation. Percussion can be performed afterward if needed to confirm such a diagnosis. Patients with heart failure may well have pleural effusions, but they are usually relatively small and unlikely to benefit from drainage. Auscultation usually reveals extensive fine crepitations, usually equal bilaterally and greatest at the lung bases. However, some patients have predominant wheeze, caused by edema of the bronchial walls, and this may cause diagnostic confusion. In such patients, the preferred option may be to treat both bronchospasm and pulmonary edema. Similarly, in the most severely affected and exhausted patients, the chest may be surprisingly silent, due to reduced tidal volumes. A single dose of an intravenous diuretic agent is unlikely to cause harm to patients with breathlessness of other causes, and in situations of diagnostic difficulty, a rapid response to diuretics may be helpful.

Cardiovascular Examination. Examination of the pulse may reveal atrial fibrillation. Patients in sinus rhythm are usually tachycardic, although patients with a history of ischemic heart disease may well be taking beta-blockers, which mask tachycardia. The blood pressure is preserved in approximately 80% of patients presenting with decompensated heart failure overall, but a significant number are hypotensive at presentation. This is the single most important factor affecting

treatment (see later) and is also likely to be altered by treatment, and so must be measured frequently. Palpation may or may not reveal a displaced apex beat, depending on the length of the history. There may be palpable heaves or thrills, but these are likely to be difficult to appreciate in the acutely breathless patient. Auscultation of the heart sounds may well be difficult. There may be a third or fourth heart sound, or there may be murmurs representing chronic stenotic or regurgitant valves, or an acute mitral valve prolapse or ventricular septal defect following myocardial infarction. (These latter two conditions can even occur several days after admission, in a patient with extensive myocardial infarction.) It is important to reexamine the patient regularly; once initial treatment has commenced, the patient may become less breathless, and previously inaudible signs may become clear.

Abdominal Examination. Examination of the abdomen can also be difficult in the acutely breathless patient. Where possible, such examination may reveal ascites, edema of the abdominal wall or genitalia, and enlargement of the liver. Pulsation of the liver can indicate tricuspid regurgitation.

SUBACUTE PRESENTATION: SHORTNESS OF BREATH/PERIPHERAL EDEMA

Many patients with severe heart failure present less acutely, with varying combinations of breathlessness and edema. This is often the case in patients with a previous diagnosis of heart failure and can be precipitated by intercurrent infection or withdrawal of diuretic or other medication (by the patient or a physician). In the early stages, edema may be more prominent unilaterally, and this may result in diagnostic difficulty. Such patients may be referred for exclusion of deep venous thrombosis (and it is important to be aware that the two conditions can coexist). Such patients often report gradually increasing breathlessness, with symptoms of orthopnea (shortness of breath occurring when lying supine) and paroxysmal nocturnal dyspnea (sudden shortness of breath waking the patient from sleep). Patients may resort to sleeping in a chair, leading to additional gravitational edema. Edema of the bowel can lead to reduced appetite, so called "cardiac cachexia," and further edema from hypoproteinemia. Peripheral edema is therefore often multifactorial in patients with heart failure. Differential diagnoses of peripheral edema are listed in Table 99-3.

Examination findings are similar to those for the acute presentation, although the patient is not in extremis and is able to speak sufficiently to give a full history. A full examination is possible more often in this situation, including auscultation of the heart sounds and abdominal examination. Peripheral edema may well be extensive, up to the abdominal wall and sacral areas. The jugular venous pulse may be elevated. Patients with extensive peripheral edema

TABLE 99-3. CAUSES OF PERIPHERAL EDEMA

Heart failure
Hypoproteinemia
Liver cirrhosis
Nephrotic syndrome
Lymphedema
Malnutrition
Gravitational edema

but a low jugular venous pulse may have hypoproteinemia rather then heart failure.

CHEST PAIN

As noted earlier, ischemic heart disease is an extremely common cause of heart failure. Patients presenting with chest pain thought to be ischemic in nature must be examined closely for subtle signs of heart failure. Patients presenting with extensive myocardial infarction may develop symptoms and signs of heart failure hours or days after admission. This may be precipitated by treatment (such as acute use of beta blockers or calcium channel blockers) or by a complication of the myocardial infarction, such as ventricular septal defect or mitral valve prolapse due to chordal rupture.

COLLAPSE/CARDIAC ARREST

Patients with severe heart failure of any cause are at high risk for malignant arrhythmias and thromboembolic disease such as pulmonary embolism. It is therefore not unusual for patients with severe heart failure to present with collapse or cardiac arrest. In such patients, the outlook is extremely poor. Even for patients presenting with ventricular tachycardia or ventricular fibrillation who are successfully cardioverted, the chance of surviving to discharge from hospital is low. Such patients can be considered for implantable cardioverter-defibrillators (see later). Pulmonary embolism and ventricular arrhythmias are covered in Chapters 79 and 96, and so will not be discussed in detail here.

INVESTIGATIONS

ELECTROCARDIOGRAPHY

All patients presenting with severe heart failure require at least one electrocardiogram (ECG). In cases of diagnostic difficulty, an entirely normal ECG virtually excludes systolic heart failure as the cause of symptoms.[10] In heart failure, an ECG is essential to diagnose arrhythmias such as atrial fibrillation, which may complicate management, as well as to look for evidence of myocardial ischemia or infarction, and conduction abnormalities such as left bundle branch block or bradycardia due to high degree atrioventricular block, which may respond to pacing. In patients in whom ischemia is suspected, serial ECGs are recommended, as changes may evolve during the course of the patient's treatment. Patients with acute severe heart failure should have continuous ECG monitoring during the acute phase, as they are at high risk for malignant ventricular arrhythmias.

CARDIAC ENZYMES

All patients presenting with severe heart failure, either as a first presentation or an exacerbation, should raise the question of myocardial infarction. As noted earlier, patients with ischemia often do not report chest pain in the setting of acute heart failure symptoms. Therefore, the use of biomarkers of cardiac muscle necrosis—ideally troponin I or T, assayed at presentation and repeated after 12 hours—is important for most patients presenting with heart failure, in conjunction with ECG findings, as noted earlier.

CHEST RADIOGRAPHY

Acutely, the chest radiograph is useful mainly in cases of diagnostic difficulty. In cases in which the diagnosis is reasonably clear from clinical information, treatment should not be delayed while waiting for a radiograph. However, most patients should have a chest radiograph early in the course of the admission.

The chest radiograph may show cardiomegaly, although this is poorly sensitive or specific for a diagnosis of heart failure (NB: portable films using anteroposterior projection may exaggerate the cardiac outline). A globular heart suggests the presence of pericardial fluid, which can be determined definitively by early echocardiography. Signs of pulmonary edema range from mild blunting of the costophrenic angles, perhaps with evidence of fluid in the horizontal fissure of the right lung, to upper lobe blood diversion (due to hypoxic vasoconstriction in the edematous dependent lung and opposite changes in the relatively edema-free upper lobes), to frank pulmonary edema. The chest radiograph may reveal signs of coexistent consolidation requiring antibiotic therapy.

ECHOCARDIOGRAPHY

Echocardiography should be carried out early in all cases of suspected heart failure. In recent years, bedside echocardiography devices have been developed that can be useful in the emergency department to assess the left ventricle and valves initially. In all cases, a full echocardiogram should be carried out when the patient is sufficiently stabilized.

Echocardiography is useful both to determine the extent of left ventricular dysfunction and to identify the cause. In cases of ischemic cardiomyopathy, regional wall motion abnormalities are commonly seen (although these can occasionally occur in cases of cardiomyopathy of other causes). Valve disease is readily identified by echocardiography. Echocardiography can be used to calculate the left ventricular ejection fraction, but in experienced hands, a qualitative assessment of left ventricular function can be equally useful. Some patients presenting with severe heart failure have preserved systolic function, and echocardiography can also be used to assess diastolic function. In the patient presenting with shortness of breath, in whom the cause is unclear, echocardiography can readily determine the presence or absence of heart failure.

BRAIN NATRIURETIC PEPTIDE

Natriuretic peptides are currently emerging as a novel test in cases of heart failure. The group includes three structurally related peptides, with variable activity at three distinct natriuretic peptide receptor subtypes, of which two are of potential use in patients with heart failure. Atrial natriuretic peptide is released from the atria in response to wall stretch. Brain natriuretic peptide, so called because it was first identified in brain tissue, is mainly released by the cardiac ventricles in response to wall stretch.[11] All the natriuretic peptides are elevated in acute coronary syndromes and myocardial infarction, due to release from myocytes. In addition, decompensated heart failure is associated with elevations of natriuretic peptide levels. Many possible applications for assays of these peptides have been proposed, but at present the most widely accepted indications for use of brain natriuretic protein (which appears to have the best sensitivity/specificity of all the natriuretic peptides) are as follows:

1. In the acutely dyspneic patient in whom there is diagnostic difficulty, a high brain natriuretic protein level is very suggestive of underlying cardiac failure.
2. In the dyspneic patient with no clinical signs of heart failure, a normal brain natriuretic protein level has a high negative predictive value, that is, it is useful in *excluding* heart failure as a cause.

The use of brain natriuretic protein for monitoring progress in heart failure is controversial: some studies have suggested that brain natriuretic protein may be useful to guide treatment. Indeed, many studies have found that brain natriuretic protein levels may have prognostic implications. It is also important to note that brain natriuretic protein levels must be used in conjunction with clinical assessment of the patient, as unexpected values may occur in some patients, such as a high brain natriuretic protein level in a stable patient. Of particular note is the fact that patients with severe heart failure due to cardiogenic shock may exhibit a paradoxically normal or even low brain natriuretic protein level. It has been suggested that myocytes in such a situation are unable to produce brain natriuretic protein. This theory is supported by studies of serial brain natriuretic protein levels in patients recovering from an episode of cardiogenic shock. An initially low brain natriuretic protein level is followed by a high level as recovery of myocardial function begins, and as recovery continues, the level returns to normal.

INVASIVE INVESTIGATIONS

Central Venous Pressure Catheter
Placement of a central venous catheter may be necessary for certain drugs, such as inotropic agents or amiodarone, which cannot be given into a peripheral vein. The central venous pressure measurement may give some idea as to right-sided filling pressure but does not give reliable information about the status of the left ventricle. In situations in which detailed information regarding filling pressures would affect management of a seriously ill patient, the Swan-Ganz catheter should be considered instead.

Swan-Ganz Catheter
Insertion of a Swan-Ganz catheter may provide additional hemodynamic information. The procedure has been associated with increased mortality and therefore should be used only in severely ill patients in whom the results are likely to influence management. It is important to note that echocardiography can provide much of the information obtainable by Swan-Ganz catheterization when adequate images can be obtained.

TREATMENT

ACUTE TREATMENT

Simple Measures
The patient should be in erect sitting position. High-flow oxygen therapy should be administered to hypoxic patients with pulmonary edema. A single small dose of opiate (such as diamorphine 2.5 mg) may alleviate distress and also temporarily reduce cardiac preload and is also clearly indicated for patients presenting with ischemic chest pain in addition to pulmonary edema.

Urinary catheterization is essential in the severely compromised patient to monitor urine output but may also be therapeutic to reduce the need for exertion, particularly if large doses of diuretics are to be used.

Diuretics
Although not supported by randomized trials, it is clear that intravenous diuretic therapy can cause rapid relief of pulmonary edema and symptoms of acute decompensated heart failure. Care is needed in patients with compromised renal function or hypotension, as diuretic therapy may exacerbate such problems. It is usual to give an initial bolus intravenous dose of diuretic, which should be tailored to the patient's previous use of diuretics. A diuretic naive patient will usually respond to a single 50 mg IV dose of furosemide, whereas patients already taking diuretics long term may need much larger doses. Subsequent therapy is often given as further boluses of intravenous diuretic at intervals, although there is some evidence that a continuous infusion of diuretic may be more efficacious and cause less renal dysfunction.

Some patients with significant fluid overload may require combination diuretic therapy, for example with the addition of a thiazide diuretic such as metolazone. Metolazone is a weak diuretic when used alone, but increased sodium delivery to, and reabsorption in, the distal renal tubule resulting from the use of a loop diuretic is blocked by metolazone, resulting in a profound diuresis. Care is needed to avoid dehydration and hyponatremia with this strategy. An alternative may be to combine furosemide with an aldosterone blocker in the acute phase.

Thromboprophylaxis
Patients with severe heart failure are often poorly mobile, due to breathlessness, peripheral edema, and the presence of monitoring and treatment equipment. They are at high risk for the development of deep venous thrombosis and pulmonary embolism.[12] The MEDENOX (prophylaxis in MEDical patients with ENOXaparin) trial, which included 1102 hospitalized patients, including 376 with NYHA class III/IV heart failure, found that 14.9% of placebo treated patients suffered venous thromboembolism. Importantly, in the group treated with enoxaparin, only 5.5% suffered venous thromboembolism.[13] This trial also included patients with other serious medical illnesses, including cancer, so this may be an overestimate of the risk of thromboembolism in heart failure. In cases of moderate to severe heart failure, particularly in hospitalized patients, some of this increased risk may be related to immobility, which is a well known risk factor for deep venous thrombosis.[14] Indeed, in previous years when bed rest was standard treatment for patients with heart failure, the rate of pulmonary embolism was very high. All patients with severe heart failure who are not anticoagulated and in whom there are no contraindications (such as active bleeding) should receive thromboprophylaxis with unfractionated or low-molecular-weight heparin, with the dose adjusted according to the patient's bodyweight.

Vasodilators: Glyceryl Trinitrate/Sodium Nitroprusside
Infusion of glyceryl trinitrate has been a standard part of therapy for pulmonary edema with preserved blood pressure

for many years. It is a direct acting vasodilator that reduces left ventricular preload and afterload, by release of the potent vasodilator nitric oxide. Glyceryl trinitrate has a very short half-life and is given by continuous intravenous infusion, with dose titrated according to response and the patient's blood pressure. The most frequent adverse effect is hypotension, which is readily reversible on stopping or reducing the rate of infusion. Glyceryl trinitrate is additionally anti-anginal and therefore of particular benefit in the patient with ischemic chest pain and pulmonary edema. Patients receiving glyceryl trinitrate rapidly develop tolerance to the drug, which can limit its effectiveness if given for long periods.

Sodium nitroprusside is an alternative vasodilator that is also effective in patients with heart failure and preserved blood pressure. The drug is given by continuous infusion and must be protected from sunlight. However, its use is limited by concerns over the toxic effects of the metabolites of sodium nitroprusside: cyanide and thiocyanide.

Nesiritide

The natriuretic peptides have a variety of beneficial effects on the heart and circulation, causing diuresis, increasing sodium excretion, and reducing pre- and afterload by causing venous and arterial dilatation. They may also reduce left ventricular remodeling and fibrosis.[15] These attributes have recently led to the therapeutic use of natriuretic peptides in heart failure, and short-term studies have shown that nesiritide infusion is at least as efficacious as standard therapy (dobutamine, milrinone, or glyceryl trinitrate) and is associated with reduced diuretic use in patients with acutely decompensated heart failure.[16] Nesiritide (recombinant human brain natriuretic peptide) has recently been approved by the American Food and Drug Administration for use in patients with acutely decompensated heart failure in whom systolic blood pressure is greater than 90 mm Hg. It is given by intravenous bolus (2 μg/kg) followed by continuous infusion (0.01 μg/kg/min), as an alternative to glyceryl trinitrate. Treatment is usually continued for 24 to 48 hours.

Inotropes

Approximately 80% of patients presenting with acute decompensated congestive heart failure have preserved blood pressure and can therefore receive cardiac load reducing therapy such as glyceryl trinitrate or nesiritide. However, these treatments are contraindicated in hypotensive patients with heart failure. If such patients do not respond to initial diuretic therapy favorably, or show evidence of deterioration, inotropic therapy may be considered. Long-term use of inotropic therapy is likely to be harmful in patients with heart failure,[17] but potentially appropriate uses of inotropes include use as temporary treatment of diuretic-refractory acute heart failure decompensations or as a bridge to definitive treatment such as revascularization or cardiac transplantation.

Intra-aortic Balloon Counterpulsation

Intra-aortic balloon counterpulsation is an invasive strategy to preserve coronary flow in the presence of very poor cardiac output. A percutaneous approach is used to position a balloon in the descending aorta. The balloon is inflated during systole, diverting blood into the coronary arteries. This technique may be used to maintain circulation to the heart and brain at the expense of other tissues as a bridge to transplantation or other surgical intervention. Use of intra-aortic balloon counterpulsation is associated with a significant adverse

event rate—up to 60% in one study of patients with cardiogenic shock.[18] There is no definite evidence that use of intra-aortic balloon counterpulsation improves the mortality rate among patients in heart failure; however, a comparison of patients from the Global Utilisation Of Streptokinase and Tissue Plasminogen Activator for Occluded Coronary Arteries (GUSTO-I) study showed a significantly lower rate of mortality in those undergoing intra-aortic balloon counterpulsation up to 1 day after admission as compared with all other patients (57% vs 67%).[19]

Assisted Ventilation
Noninvasive Ventilation

Noninvasive ventilation is a form of ventilatory support that does not require paralysis and intubation. Positive pressure is provided via a tight-fitting mask that may lie over the nose only or over the full face. Some patients are unable to tolerate the mask or the sensation of assisted ventilation.

Continuous positive airway pressure has an accepted role in the treatment of sleep apnea syndromes. Recently it has been recognized that sleep apnea is prevalent in patients with heart failure and may play a role in the development and progression of heart failure.[20] In addition, noninvasive ventilation has favorable effects on intrathoracic and left ventricular transmural pressures in patients with congestive heart failure.[21] Noninvasive ventilation has been used to treat acute heart failure. Several randomized trials have suggested that use of continuous positive airway pressure results in more rapid increase in PaO_2, decrease in PcO_2, and lower rates of intubation compared with standard treatment.[22] Noninvasive ventilation may be considered in patients with rising PcO_2 levels despite adequate medical therapy. Noninvasive ventilation results in decreased blood pressure, so may have a deleterious effect in patients who are already hypotensive. To be used successfully, noninvasive ventilation requires careful attention to mask fitting and close patient observation. Noninvasive ventilation should be used only in a high dependency setting, with appropriately trained staff.

Intermittent Positive Pressure Ventilation

Patients with evidence of exhaustion or worsening arterial blood gases despite adequate treatment may require invasive ventilation. The prognosis of patients with such refractory pulmonary edema is poor, but some patients show dramatic improvement after only a short period of intermittent positive pressure ventilation. Intermittent positive pressure ventilation results in decreased venous return due to increased intrathoracic pressure and therefore can have a deleterious effect on blood pressure. Blood pressure must be maintained (with inotropic agents if necessary) before intubation.

Surgery
Valve Replacement

Patients with severe heart failure due to valvular heart disease, or functional mitral regurgitation, may benefit from valve replacement or repair. Ideally, surgery should be delayed until the patient is stable, but selected patients not improving on initial therapy may benefit from emergency valve replacement, although such patients are inherently at high risk for such major surgery. A multidisciplinary team consisting of cardiologist, cardiovascular surgeon, and intensivist/anesthetist is needed to select suitable patients for intervention. A full discussion of indications for surgery is beyond the scope of this chapter.

Left Ventricular Assist Device

Left ventricular assist devices (LVADs) are surgically implanted devices developed to allow short- or long-term support to the failing left ventricle. Commonly, an inflow cannula receives blood from the left ventricle, which is then pumped out through a cannula in the ascending aorta. Although initially used as a bridge to transplantation, some studies have demonstrated recovery of function allowing explantation of the device after a period of left ventricular support in certain subgroups of patients together with appropriate pharmacologic therapy.[23] LVAD therapy for patients with terminal heart failure but who are not eligible for heart transplantation has been shown in the Randomized Evaluation of Mechanical Assistance for the Treatment of Congestive Heart Failure (REMATCH) trial[24] to be superior to medical therapy in ameliorating symptoms and to produce a 48% mortality reduction at 2 years' follow-up. However, the frequency of serious adverse events in the LVAD group was more than twice that in the medical-therapy group, mainly due to infection, bleeding, and malfunction of the device.

A number of devices are available. Choice depends on availability and local expertise.

The main complications of LVADs include thromboembolism, right ventricular failure, and device failure (equivalent to severe aortic regurgitation, as the devices do not have valves). Careful patient selection is necessary to gain most benefit from such devices.[25]

Revascularization

In recent years, the phenomena of "stunned" and "hibernating" myocardium have been recognized and widely investigated. Hibernating myocardium is defined as poorly functioning myocardium caused by reduced perfusion, which may recover function if perfusion is restored. Stunned myocardium results from an episode of ischemia. The segment of myocardium regains normal blood flow after the episode, but recovery of function is delayed (although recovery occurs spontaneously). In patients with chronic ischemic cardiomyopathy, revascularization may therefore result in improvement in left ventricular function. Patients with cardiogenic shock due to acute myocardial infarction have a very poor prognosis (see later), and in recent years several studies have addressed the possible benefits of acute revascularization in such patients. Retrospective analysis of the patients from the GUSTO-I study with cardiogenic shock (7.2%) showed that revascularization was associated with decreased mortality rate (overall 30-day mortality, 55%; patients undergoing coronary artery bypass grafting, 29%; patients undergoing percutaneous transluminal coronary angioplasty, 22%).[26]

The treatments were not allocated randomly, however. The two randomized controlled trials of medical therapy versus revascularization (Should We Emergently Revascularise Occluded Coronaries For Cardiogenic Shock [SHOCK][27] and Swiss Multicentre Angioplasty for SHOCK [SMASH][28]) had difficulties in recruitment, and both reported no significant difference in early mortality, although the SHOCK trial did show decreased mortality rate at 6 months in the intervention group. It is important to note that results from the SHOCK trial registry, which showed that patients selected to undergo angiography had better outcomes whether or not they went on to be revascularized, suggest that bias may be involved in the results of these studies.[29] Current evidence certainly does not support aggressive revascularization of all patients with cardiogenic shock, but revascularization may be appropriate in selected patients.

Stabilization and Chronic Treatment

A full discussion of long-term treatment for patients with heart failure is beyond the scope of this book. However, patients presenting with acute heart failure may need to be established on a variety of medications during their index admission, and so a brief summary of the main drugs used in heart failure maintenance is presented here.

Loop Diuretics

As noted earlier, loop diuretic therapy may provide rapid symptom relief in patients with fluid overload. However, loop diuretics may be associated with a number of adverse effects such as volume depletion, and no mortality benefit has been demonstrated in cases of heart failure. Although some patients with chronic heart failure may be able to have diuretic therapy withdrawn once they are appropriately stabilized, most require at least a small dose of maintenance diuretic, tailored to clinical evidence of fluid overload. Regular weighing is a simple method of monitoring the fluid status of heart failure patients. Care must be taken to monitor renal function in patients on high doses of diuretics. Diuretics may cause hypokalemia, although combining them with angiotensin-converting enzyme (ACE) inhibitors and potassium-sparing diuretics such as spironolactone (see later) may reduce this problem.

Angiotensin-Converting Enzyme Inhibitors/Angiotensin II Receptor Blockers

Multiple large randomized trials have shown that ACE inhibitors (e.g., ramipril, perindopril, lisinopril) are of unequivocal benefit in patients with heart failure and asymptomatic left ventricular dysfunction.[30] All patients should be started on an ACE inhibitor as soon as possible after a diagnosis of heart failure has been made—this is almost always during the index admission. Most patients will require gradual introduction of the drug, with monitoring of blood pressure and renal function. Effort should be made to achieve the highest tolerated dose of the chosen ACE inhibitor.

Some patients are unable to tolerate ACE inhibitors due to cough (caused by elevated levels of bradykinin, which is usually degraded by ACE). An alternative in such patients are angiotensin II receptor blockers, which directly block the angiotensin II receptor and do not cause bradykinin build-up. There is not yet sufficient evidence on angiotensin II receptor blockers to recommend them over ACE inhibitors as first-line therapy in heart failure patients. However, the recent Candesartan in Heart Failure—Assessment of Reduction in Mortality (CHARM) study demonstrated that in patients unable to tolerate ACE inhibitors, the angiotensin II receptor blocker candesartan provided similar mortality benefit.[31] Another arm of the CHARM study (CHARM-ADDED) showed additional benefit (reduction in the primary endpoint of cardiovascular death or hospital admission for congestive heart failure) when candesartan was added to ACE.[32]

Beta-Blockers

For many years, beta-blockers were thought to be harmful in patients with heart failure because of their negative inotropic effect. More recently, however, several large randomized trials have demonstrated consistent benefit of beta-blockers such as carvedilol,[33] bisoprolol,[34] and metoprolol.[35] Beta-blockers are indicated in patients with stabilized heart failure and are rarely started during the index admission. Their use involves careful dose titration, best supervised in a specialist heart failure clinic.

Aldosterone Inhibitors

The landmark Randomised Aldactone Evaluation Study (RALES) showed that, in patients with severe heart failure, spironolactone reduced mortality by 30%.[36] More recently, a more selective aldosterone inhibitor, eplerenone, has been developed, which (due to its lack of action at sex hormone and glucocorticoid receptor sites) lacks the unpleasant side effects of spironolactone such as painful gynecomastia. The recent EPHESUS study, which recruited 6642 post-myocardial infarction patients with left ventricular ejection fraction less than 40% and clinical heart failure and randomised them to receive eplerenone or placebo (in addition to otherwise optimized medical therapy), demonstrated a 15% reduction in all-cause mortality among the eplerenone group after a mean follow-up period of 16 months.[37] It is likely that aldosterone antagonists will be used increasingly in the management of patients with chronic heart failure.

Aldosterone blockers may cause hyperkalemia, particularly in combination with ACE inhibitors. Patients on this combination should have regular renal function testing.

Antithrombotic Therapy

Patients with heart failure and atrial fibrillation have clear indications for anticoagulation with adjusted-dose warfarin.[38] There is no clear evidence for the use of antithrombotic therapy in patients with heart failure in sinus rhythm, although such patients fulfill Virchow's triad (abnormal flow, abnormal vessel wall, abnormal blood constituents) for a prothrombotic state.[39] It is hoped that ongoing randomized trials comparing antiplatelet agents, warfarin, and placebo will provide more information on the optimal strategy for antithrombotic therapy in heart failure patients.

Direct-acting thrombin inhibitors, such as ximelagatran, may be an alternative to warfarin, and are currently being investigated for a number of indications.[40] Ximelagatran has advantages over warfarin in that dose adjustment and INR monitoring are not required.

Digoxin

Digoxin therapy in patients with heart failure in sinus rhythm (i.e., for inotropic effect) is common practice in North America but is less frequently used in Europe. Evidence of benefit is somewhat limited. Two trials showed withdrawal of digoxin from patients with symptomatic heart failure resulted in increased risk of heart failure decompensation.[41,42] The Digitalis Investigation Group (DIG) trial[43] demonstrated no difference in survival associated with the use of digoxin. A reduction in the risk of death from progressive heart failure in the DIG trial was balanced by an increase in the risk of sudden cardiac death. Digoxin may therefore be considered as additional therapy for patients on ACE inhibitors and beta-blockers but is not an alternative to these drugs.

Cardiac Resynchronization Therapy

Patients with heart failure may exhibit dyssynchronous contraction of the left ventricle, resulting from abnormal electrical conduction pathways. Typically this results in septal contraction occurring some time before contraction of the free wall of the left ventricle. Such dyssynchronous contraction results in significant circulation of blood in the left ventricular cavity, rather than forward flow of blood. The use of biventricular pacing to restore synchronous contraction of the left ventricle (cardiac resynchronization therapy) has increased in popularity in recent years. However, the optimal method for selecting patients for cardiac resynchronization therapy is unclear. Current guidelines use duration of the ECG QRS complex, but recent studies have shown that some patients with narrow QRS complexes may benefit from cardiac resynchronization therapy, and, equally, not all patients with wide QRS complexes benefit. Echocardiographic evidence of dyssynchronous contraction in combination with the ECG may prove to be a better method of selecting candidates for cardiac resynchronization therapy.[44]

Arrhythmia Therapy

Atrial Fibrillation

Atrial fibrillation can result in significant impairment of left ventricular function, due to loss of atrial contraction and abnormal left ventricular filling. Atrial fibrillation in the presence of reduced left ventricular function results in a very high risk of thromboembolic stroke, and so all patients with atrial fibrillation and reduced left ventricular function should be anticoagulated in the absence of contraindications. In the presence of poor left ventricular function or dilated left ventricle or left atrium on echocardiography, DC cardioversion is unlikely to cause sustained conversion to sinus rhythm but could be considered in situations in which palpitations due to atrial fibrillations cause significant distress to the patient. Pharmacologic rate control is likely to be more successful. Digoxin is commonly used for this purpose, although in the presence of renal impairment or diuretic-induced hypokalemia, toxicity is common. If tolerated, beta-blockers may achieve rate control, although the need to introduce such drugs gradually makes them less suitable for initial rate control. It may be possible to control the rate initially with careful digoxin therapy, then consider withdrawing digoxin once the patient is established on a sufficiently high dose of beta-blocker. Amiodarone is an alternative antiarrhythmic safe for use in heart failure patients, which can be used to control atrial fibrillation, although side-effects are problematic.

Ventricular Arrhythmias

Patients with heart failure frequently suffer from sudden death. Although it is now recognized that some episodes of sudden death are caused by thrombosis, such as pulmonary embolism, it is clear that malignant arrhythmias are a common cause of death in heart failure. Surprisingly, therefore, multiple trials of a variety of antiarrhythmic drugs in patients with heart failure have failed to show a mortality benefit (amiodarone),[45] or even shown a worsening of mortality (e.g., flecainide).[46] Routine use of antiarrhythmic drugs in patients with heart failure is therefore not recommended. In contrast, recent studies involving the use of implantable cardioverter-defibrillator devices in patients with reduced ejection fraction following myocardial infarction have shown reduced mortality. The recent COMPANION study,[47] which compared optimal medical treatment alone to optimal medical treatment plus cardiac resynchronization therapy plus or minus implantable cardioverter-defibrillator therapy, found

TABLE 99–4. INDICATIONS FOR IMPLANTABLE CARDIOVERTER-DEFIBRILLATOR THERAPY IN PATIENTS WITH HEART FAILURE

Cardiac arrest due to ventricular fibrillation or ventricular tachycardia
Spontaneous sustained ventricular tachycardia
Syncope of unknown origin with inducible ventricular tachycardia or ventricular fibrillation at electrophysiologic study
Nonsustained ventricular tachycardia with inducible ventricular fibrillation/ventricular tachycardia at electrophysiologic study
Left ventricular ejection fraction <30% at least 1 month after myocardial infarction or 3 months after coronary artery bypass grafting

that combined cardiac resynchronization therapy/implantable cardioverter-defibrillator reduced mortality but not hospitalization as compared with cardiac resynchronization therapy alone. At present, routine use of implantable cardioverter defibrillators (which in any case would be prohibitively expensive in most countries) in all heart failure patients cannot be recommended. Current indications for implantable cardioverter-defibrillator therapy in heart failure are listed in Table 99-4.

FURTHER MANAGEMENT: THE SPECIALIST HEART FAILURE CLINIC

Patients with heart failure are at high risk of further admissions and sudden death. Careful follow-up and adequate secondary prevention using the drugs and devices detailed here is essential to reduce the risk of readmission and other complications of heart failure. Ideally, such patients should be followed in a specialist heart failure clinic, with access to a cardiologist specializing in heart failure, specialist heart failure nursing, and access to investigations such as echocardiography, cardiac catheterization, and brain natriuretic protein. Nurse-led clinics are ideal for dose titration of beta-blockers and ACE inhibitors and also provide opportunities for monitoring of fluid status and symptoms.[48]

PROGNOSIS

Heart failure has a poor prognosis—diagnosis of chronic heart failure is associated with a mortality rate worse than that of many cancers.[49] As noted earlier, patients with severe heart failure often present in extremis but may respond rapidly to prompt effective management. However, their in-patient course is associated with a high risk of complications such as thromboembolism (particularly in the presence of atrial fibrillation) and sudden death, even in patients who show signs of recovery from their initial event. Close follow-up and secondary preventive measures are essential to improve prognosis in this high-risk group.

SUMMARY

Severe heart failure is a common disorder, with high rates of mortality and morbidity. Patients often present in extremis, so good knowledge of initial treatment is essential for all physicians and emergency department staff. Patients often respond rapidly to effective initial treatment, making this a satisfying condition to treat. However, patients may also deteriorate rapidly, and may require involvement of intensivists, cardiologists, and cardiac surgeons. Once stabilized, there are a number of evidence-based treatments that improve prognosis in these patients. Careful follow-up, ideally in a specialist heart failure clinic, is recommended after discharge.

SELECTED BIBLIOGRAPHY

Davies M, Hobbs F, Davis R, et al: Prevalence of left-ventricular systolic dysfunction and heart failure in the Echocardiographic Heart of England Screening study: A population based study. Lancet 2001;358:439-444.
  This recent general practice-based screening study provided a robust estimate of the prevalence of left ventricular systolic dysfunction.

Echt DS, Liebson PR, Mitchell LB, et al: Mortality and morbidity in patients receiving encainide, flecainide, or placebo. The Cardiac Arrhythmia Suppression Trial. N Engl J Med 1991;324:781-788.
  This important randomized placebo-controlled trial identified an increased mortality risk with type 1 antiarrhythmics in patients with cardiovascular disease.

Halperin JL, for the Executive Steering Committee, SPORTIF III and V Study Investigators: Ximelagatran compared with warfarin for prevention of thromboembolism in patients with nonvalvular atrial fibrillation: Rationale, objectives, and design of a pair of clinical studies and baseline patient characteristics (SPORTIF III and V). Am Heart J 2003;146:431-438.
  The ongoing SPORTIF III (open label, 23 countries) and V (double blind, 409 US centers) trials are comparing ximelagatran with adjusted-dose warfarin in patients with atrial fibrillation and at least one other risk factor (including heart failure).

MERIT-HF Investigators: Effect of metoprolol CR/XL in chronic heart failure: Metoprolol CR/XL Randomised Intervention Trial in Congestive Heart Failure (MERIT-HF). Lancet 1999;353:2001-2007.
  The benefit of beta-blockers in heart failure was proved in these randomized controlled studies (MERIT-HF, CIBIS-II, and US Carvedilol Heart Failure Study), bringing to an end the idea that beta-blockade could be harmful in patients with heart failure.

Rich MW, Beckham V, Wittenberg C, et al: A multidisciplinary intervention to prevent the readmission of elderly patients with congestive heart failure. N Engl J Med 1995; 333:1190-1195.
  This trial demonstrated that a multidisciplinary intervention involving nutritional advice, counselling, patient education, and exercise training could significantly reduce readmission rates and length of hospital stay in elderly patients with heart failure.

Chapter 100

MYOCARDITIS IN THE INTENSIVE CARE UNIT

Fredric Ginsberg • Joseph E. Parrillo

KEY POINTS

1. Myocarditis is most often caused by a viral infection. Myocardial damage is mediated through activation of cellular immune mechanisms.

2. The clinical course of myocarditis can be benign, with complete resolution, or the illness can be more severe, with the development of dilated cardiomyopathy and congestive heart failure.

3. The pharmacological therapy of heart failure associated with myocarditis is similar to therapy used in other forms of dilated cardiomyopathy. Severe cases may require the use of a ventricular assist device.

4. Fulminant myocarditis is an unusual complication with a rapidly progressive course resulting in cardiogenic shock. These cases should be aggressively managed with pharmacological therapy and ventricular assist devices, because significant improvement in left ventricular function will often occur.

5. Endomyocardial biopsy is frequently used to make the diagnosis of myocarditis and to direct therapy, although there are limitations in the interpretation of biopsy results.

6. Immunosuppressive therapy should not be used routinely in the treatment of myocarditis but should be strongly considered in patients who have severe heart failure early in the course of the illness or whose condition deteriorates despite the use of conventional heart failure treatment.

MYOCARDITIS IN THE INTENSIVE CARE UNIT

Myocarditis is defined as inflammation of heart muscle.[1] The study of myocarditis has been made difficult by a number of factors. The clinical picture of myocarditis varies widely, from asymptomatic patients who suffer no long-term sequelae, to critically ill patients with heart failure and cardiogenic shock. In addition, there are no standardized specific criteria for making the diagnosis of myocarditis or for determining a cause in individual patients.[2] Indeed, many different etiologic agents have been implicated in this disease. Lastly, there has been controversy regarding the most appropriate medical therapy for this condition.

On pathologic examination of myocardial biopsy specimens, or on autopsy series, myocarditis is usually apparent as infiltration of myocardium with lymphocytes and fibroblasts, accompanied by myocyte necrosis (myocytolysis).[2] It is this type of myocarditis, often termed *lymphocytic myocarditis*, that will be referred to in this chapter, unless otherwise specified. Other types of inflammatory reactions can be seen less frequently in cases of myocarditis, involving giant cells, eosinophils, or granulomas, which can be associated with specific clinical conditions.

In most patients with myocarditis, a specific cause is not found.[3] It is presumed, however, that in North America and Europe, the most common etiologic agent is viral.[1] Enteroviruses, specifically coxsackie B, are most commonly implicated. Other viruses have been associated with myocarditis, including adenoviruses, hepatitis C, and influenza virus.[4] Myocarditis is a common finding in patients infected with human immunodeficiency virus (HIV). However, the causative agent responsible in these cases is more likely to be a secondary viral or other infectious agent occurring in these immunocompromised hosts, rather than HIV itself.[1] Infectious illnesses such as Lyme disease, acute rheumatic fever, and diphtheria often have myocarditis as a prominent feature. In Central and South America, the most common cause of myocarditis is the protozoan *Trypanosoma cruzi*, the cause of Chagas' disease. Systemic diseases such as systemic lupus erythematosus, polymyositis, scleroderma, and sarcoidosis can be complicated by myocarditis, and myocarditis can be a feature of the infiltrative cardiomyopathies seen in hemochromatosis or amyloidosis. Lastly, myocarditis can be associated with doxorubicin cardiomyopathy or with peripartum cardiomyopathy, or can be a manifestation of a hypersensitivity reaction to medications (Table 100-1).[5,6]

Unfortunately, it is difficult to make a clinical diagnosis of a specific viral cause of myocarditis. This usually requires the measurement of antiviral antibody titers in acute and convalescent phase sera. Viral cultures of tissue specimens are unreliable.[3] The identification of viral genomes incorporated in myocyte DNA does not specifically indicate the virus as the etiologic agent (Table 100-2).

PATHOGENESIS

Based on observations of human myocarditis, as well as murine models of the disease caused by coxsackie B3, the pathogenesis of viral myocarditis can be described in three stages. The first stage is initiated by viral infection and replication within myocytes. Viral proteases and activation of cytokines may produce myocyte damage and apoptosis.[4] The presence of this viral replication phase is difficult to prove clinically, because patients may be asymptomatic during this phase or may only have nonspecific viremic symptoms.

TABLE 100–1. CAUSES OF MYOCARDITIS*

Infectious	Immune-Mediated	Toxic Myocarditis
Bacterial: brucella, *Corynebacterium diphtheriae*, gonococcus, *Haemophilus influenzae*, meningococcus, mycobacterium, *Mycoplasma pneumoniae*, pneumococcus, salmonella, *Serratia marcescens*, staphylococcus, *Streptococcus pneumoniae*, *S. pyogenes*, *Treponema pallidum*, *Tropheryma whippelii*, and *Vibrio cholerae* Spirochetal: borrelia and leptospira Fungal: actinomyces, aspergillus, blastomyces, candida, coccidioides, cryptococcus, histoplasma, mucormycoses, nocardia, and sporothrix Protozoal: *Toxoplasma gondii* and *Trypanosoma cruzi* Parasitic: ascaris, *Echinococcus granulosus*, *Paragonimus westermani*, schistosoma, *Taenia solium*, *Trichinella spiralis*, visceral larva migrans, and *Wuchereria bancrofti* Rickettsial: *Coxiella burnetii*, *Rickettsia rickettsii*, and *R. tsutsugamushi* Viral: **coxsackievirus**, cytomegalovirus, dengue virus, echovirus, encephalomyocarditis, Epstein-Barr virus, hepatitis A virus, hepatitis C virus, herpes simplex virus, herpes zoster, **human immunodeficiency virus**, influenza A virus, influenza B virus, Junin virus, lymphocytic choriomeningitis, measles virus, mumps virus, parvovirus, poliovirus, rabies virus, respiratory syncytial virus, rubella virus, rubeola, vaccinia virus, varicella-zoster virus, variola virus, and yellow fever virus	Allergens: acetazolamide, amitriptyline, cefaclor, colchicine, furosemide, isoniazid, lidocaine, methyldopa, penicillin, phenylbutazone, phenytoin, reserpine, streptomycin, tetanus toxoid, tetracycline, and thiazides Alloantigens: heart-transplant rejection Autoantigens: **Chagas' disease,** *Chlamydia pneumoniae*, Churg-Strauss syndrome, inflammatory bowel disease, giant-cell myocarditis, insulin-dependent diabetes mellitus, Kawasaki's disease, myasthenia gravis, polymyositis, **sarcoidosis, scleroderma, systemic lupus erythematosus**, thyrotoxicosis, and Wegener's granulomatosis	Drugs: amphetamines, **anthracyclines,** catecholamines, cocaine, cyclophosphamide, **ethanol,** fluorouracil, hemetine, interleukin-2, lithium, and trastuzumab Heavy metals: copper, iron, and lead Physical agents: electric shock, hyperpyrexia, and radiation Miscellaneous: arsenic, azides, bee and wasp stings, carbon monoxide, inhalants, phosphorus, scorpion bites, snake bites, and spider bites

*The most common causes are shown in **boldface** type.
From Feldman A, McNamara D: Myocarditis. N Engl J Med 2000;343:1388–1398.

In addition, there is no rapid screening test to confirm viral infection.

The second stage involves host immune activation. Stimulation of cellular immunity as well as humoral responses attenuates viral proliferation and can result in recovery from the illness. However, unabated immune activation can result in activated T cells targeting myocardial antigens, which cross-react with viral peptides. This leads to release of cytokines such as tumor necrosis factor, interleukin-1, and interleukin-6, resulting in further myocyte damage.[1,4] Activation of CD4 cells and antibody production seem to play a smaller pathogenetic role. It is believed that this secondary immune response to viral infection plays a greater role in disease pathogenesis than the primary infection.[4]

Evidence supporting these mechanisms includes the following: Myocardial biopsy with recombinant DNA techniques can detect viral genomes in 20% to 35% of patients. Tissue specific autoantibodies have been detected in 25% to 73% of patients with evidence of myocarditis on biopsy, and inappropriate expression of the major histocompatibility complex can frequently be demonstrated on biopsy specimens.[1] Enterovirus genome has been identified on biopsy specimens in less than 20% of myocarditis patients and 10% to 34% of idiopathic dilated cardiomyopathy patients. Elevated levels of inflammatory cytokines are detected in patients with active myocarditis.

TABLE 100–2. DISTINCT FORMS OF MYOCARDITIS

Active viral
Postviral (lymphocytic): common form of acute myocarditis
Hypersensitivity
Autoimmune
Infectious
Giant-cell myocarditis

From Haas G: Etiology, evaluation, and management of acute myocarditis. Cardiol Rev 2001; 9:88-95.

Either persistent overactivation of cellular immune activity or incomplete clearing and persistent or recurrent viral replication and host response can lead to the third stage, where significant myocardial damage occurs. This leads to left ventricular dilatation and remodeling, left ventricular systolic dysfunction, and manifestations of heart failure.[4] These processes can then abate, with reduction in left ventricular size and improvement of left ventricular function, or can continue to progress with development of chronic dilated cardiomyopathy and chronic heart failure.

CLINICAL PRESENTATION

The clinical presentation of myocarditis varies widely. Patients can be asymptomatic, as myocarditis is found in 1% to 10% of autopsy specimens of young adults who had no history of cardiac illness. Myocarditis can be found at autopsy in up to 20% of cases of young apparently healthy adults who die suddenly and unexpectedly.[1,3,6]

Patients ill with myocarditis most often present with chest pain, fatigue, dyspnea, and palpitations. Frequently they have recently experienced nonspecific symptoms of a viral infection including fever, malaise, and arthralgias. Physical examination can show fever, tachycardia, S3 and S4 gallop sounds, and a pericardial rub (if myopericarditis is present). Signs of heart failure can be present, including pulmonary rales and wheezes, hepatomegaly, ascites, elevated jugular venous pulse, and peripheral edema. Murmurs of mitral regurgitation and tricuspid regurgitation may be heard. Infrequently, patients can present with a fulminant course, with severe acute heart failure, pulmonary edema, and cardiogenic shock.[3]

The differential diagnosis includes acute myocardial infarction, pericarditis, or chest pain from pulmonary causes, including pulmonary embolism or pneumonia. Generalized sepsis is also a consideration.

Laboratory findings can include leukocytosis, eosinophilia, and an elevated erythrocyte sedimentation rate. Cardiac biomarkers such as CPK, troponin T, and troponin I are variably elevated depending in part on the chronicity of the process,[1] although recent data suggest that troponin may be useful in diagnosing myocarditis. Rheumatologic serologic markers and HIV status should be evaluated.

The 12-lead electrocardiogram shows sinus tachycardia and nonspecific ST segment and T wave changes most often. Patients may present with chest pain and ST segment elevation with a picture mimicking acute myocardial infarction. More severe cases can be associated with supraventricular or ventricular arrhythmias, conduction disturbances, and heart block.[1]

Echocardiography is essential to diagnose and quantitate regional or global left ventricular wall motion abnormalities, left ventricular and right ventricular size and function, and valvular regurgitation. Findings on myocardial nuclear scintigraphy are frequently abnormal, but this is an insensitive test for the diagnosis of myocarditis. Cardiac magnetic resonance imaging is currently being evaluated to assess the extent of cardiac involvement and to localize inflammation in cases of patchy nonhomogeneous myocarditis. This may aid in determining optimal sites for myocardial biopsy. Cardiac catheterization and coronary angiography are often necessary to exclude acute ischemia as the cause of chest pain or acute heart failure.

DIAGNOSIS

Myocarditis is a difficult diagnosis to make, as there are no specific clinical diagnostic criteria. Even though clinical and laboratory features of this illness, as described earlier, are insensitive and nonspecific,[2] myocarditis remains a diagnosis made on clinical grounds. Percutaneous endomyocardial right ventricular biopsy is currently used to aid in the diagnosis of myocarditis and is considered the most definitive diagnostic technique.

The Dallas criteria have been accepted as the standard for histopathologic diagnosis. These criteria define myocarditis as the presence of an active inflammatory myocardial infiltrate (more than 5 lymphocytes per high-power field) accompanied by myocyte necrosis. "Borderline myocarditis" is defined as active inflammation without myocyte necrosis. However, there is no difference in prognosis in patients with either of these biopsy results.[5] Thus, it appears that lymphocyte infiltration (with or without myocyte necrosis) is the most important diagnostic criterion.

Although endomyocardial biopsy is useful for diagnostic purposes, there are a number of significant limitations. A high frequency of interobserver variation has been noted among pathologists in applying the Dallas criteria. Biopsies are not sensitive in diagnosing myocarditis, as various series have reported positive biopsy results in only 10% to 67% of patients with myocarditis suspected on clinical grounds or recent-onset idiopathic dilated cardiomyopathy. This variability may relate to the timing of biopsies in respect to the stage or chronicity of the patient's illness. In addition, the myocardial inflammation may not be diffuse and may be patchy, or may predominantly involve the left ventricle, so random right ventricular biopsies may miss affected myocardium.[7] Thus, performing a biopsy earlier in a patient's clinical course and taking multiple biopsy specimens, possibly to include left ventricular sites, have been suggested as ways of improving the diagnostic yield. Biopsies should also be done in centers with a high-volume experience, with proven safety, and availability of appropriate pathologic techniques.[8]

However, it is important to emphasize that a negative biopsy finding does not preclude the diagnosis of myocarditis.

Although endomyocardial biopsy is an insensitive test with a number of problems, a positive biopsy finding has a high positive predictive value.[5] Some authors question the benefits of performing biopsy with standard staining techniques as a routine in suspected myocarditis cases, but this remains the best diagnostic test currently available. Other analyses such as examining specimens for viral genomes or using immunohistochemistry technology to identify up-regulated HLA proteins may offer improved diagnostic yield in the future.[7] Endomyocardial biopsy should be strongly considered in cases of suspected myocarditis when pathology results will affect management decisions, especially in patients with acute refractory heart failure or continued clinical deterioration despite appropriate aggressive heart failure therapy. Biopsy should also be considered in patients with worsening ventricular arrhythmias, with heart block, or with suspected causes such as sarcoidosis, collagen vascular disease, infiltrative cardiomyopathy, giant cell myocarditis, or eosinophilic myocarditis.[9] Endomyocardial biopsy should always be performed prior to initiating immunosuppressive therapy.

CLINICAL COURSE AND PROGNOSIS

The clinical course and prognosis of acute myocarditis is quite variable. Patients who are asymptomatic, with self-limited disease, or who present with a flu-like illness most often recover without complications. It is felt that some of these patients will progress to chronic dilated cardiomyopathy with manifestations of systolic heart failure,[2] although a precise incidence is not known. The majority of patients who present with manifestations of myocarditis will improve. Patients with heart failure and left ventricular dysfunction will experience spontaneous resolution of their illness in 6 to 12 months in up to 40% of cases, without long-term sequelae. However, a significant percentage of young, apparently healthy adults who die suddenly are found to have myocarditis at autopsy, suggesting that patients even with apparently mild illness can suffer fatal arrhythmias.

Patients with heart failure and myocarditis can recover normal left ventricular function or can progress to chronic dilated cardiomyopathy. Fifteen to 25% of patients who present with new-onset dilated cardiomyopathy have evidence for antecedent myocarditis.[2] There is a reported 1-year mortality rate of 20% in patients with lymphocytic myocarditis.[5] However, it is important to examine the patient population under study and the criteria used for diagnosing myocarditis in any series assessing prognosis and mortality.

A series of 21 patients with active myocarditis on biopsy was analyzed for predictors of disease course. Variables assessed included baseline hemodynamics, use of ventilatory and circulatory support, and serum cardiac biomarkers. Overall, there was a 37% mortality rate (8 of 21) with death occurring at 27.6 ± 6.9 days. Factors predicting a worse prognosis included hypotension (mean 84/49 mm Hg), higher pulmonary capillary wedge pressure (mean of 24 mm Hg), and use of mechanical ventilation. Factors that were not predictive of mortality included sex, age, heart rate, cardiac index, peak CPK or tumor necrosis factor levels, or the use of intra-aortic balloon counterpulsation for circulatory support.[10] However, no clinical markers reliably predict

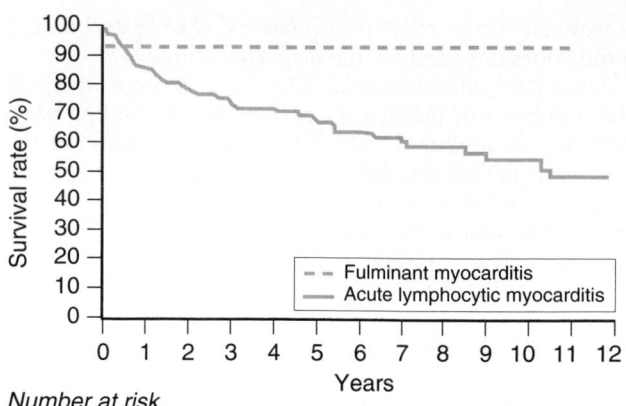

Number at risk

Acute myocarditis

    132 110 98 91 84 79 73 59 41 28 18 3 0

Fulminant myocarditis

    15 12 12 10 10 9 7 5 4 3 2 0 0

FIGURE 100–1. Unadjusted transplantation-free survival according to clinicopathological classification. Patients with fulminant myocarditis were significantly less likely to die or require heart transplantation during follow-up than were patients with acute myocarditis (*P* = 0.05 by the log-rank test). (From McCarthy R, Boehmer J, Hruban R, et al: Long-term outcome of fulminant myocarditis as compared with acute (nonfulminant) myocarditis. N Engl J Med 2000;342:690-695.)

which patients with myocarditis are more likely to recover or progress.[5]

FULMINANT MYOCARDITIS

A small percentage of patients with acute myocarditis present critically ill with acute severe heart failure and cardiogenic shock. This presentation is termed *fulminant myocarditis*. Most often these patients give a history of recent fever and symptoms of a viral illness, with a distinct time of onset of heart failure symptoms. This presentation can be contrasted with that of patients with myocarditis who have acute heart failure, but not cardiogenic shock, who demonstrate a less distinct time of onset of heart failure symptoms and less severe hypotension.

In a study of 147 patients presenting with heart failure due to biopsy-positive active myocarditis, with ejection fraction less than 40%, 10% of patients were believed to have fulminant myocarditis and 90% had acute lymphocytic myocarditis.[5] The patients with fulminant myocarditis needed hemodynamic support with high-dose vasopressors or left ventricular assist devices. The acute myocarditis patients had more stable hemodynamics and did not require vasopressors, or received them at low doses. Patients with fulminant myocarditis tended to be younger and have higher heart rates and lower systemic blood pressure. There was no difference between the groups in mean pulmonary capillary wedge pressure or cardiac index.

With aggressive treatment, patients with fulminant myocarditis actually had better survival rates, 93% at 1 year and 93% at 11 years. Patients with acute myocarditis had an 85% 1-year survival rate and a 45% survival rate at 11 years. Patients with lower pulmonary capillary wedge pressure or higher cardiac index at presentation also had better survival.

Thus, it is believed that fulminant myocarditis has a distinct clinical course, with critical illness at presentation but with excellent long-term survival once patients recover from the acute phase of their illness. Healing of myocardial injury and significant improvement of left ventricular systolic function can be expected. Therefore, an aggressive approach to therapy, including the use of ventricular assist devices or other mechanical assist devices, without resorting to early cardiac transplantation, is warranted (Fig. 100-1).[5]

GIANT CELL MYOCARDITIS

Giant cell myocarditis is a distinct form of myocarditis, generally with a rapidly progressive course, without significant likelihood of spontaneous resolution. On endomyocardial biopsy, infiltration with inflammatory giant cells is seen. Although the pathogenesis is not clear, it is believed to be an autoimmune disorder, and CD4 T-lymphocytes are thought to play an important role. A total of 63 patients with biopsy-confirmed giant cell myocarditis were studied retrospectively.[11] Heart failure was the presentation in 75% of cases; 14% presented with ventricular arrhythmias, and 11% presented with chest pain, an abnormal electrocardiogram, or heart block. There was an association with inflammatory bowel disease in 8% of cases. Survival was poor, with a median time of 5.5 months to death or cardiac transplantation (Fig. 100-2).

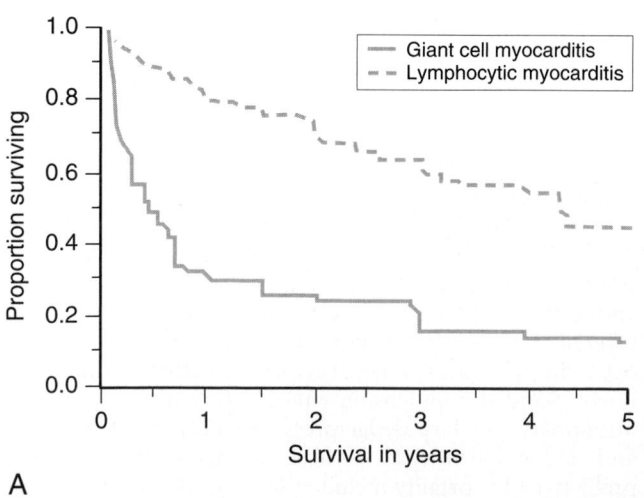

A

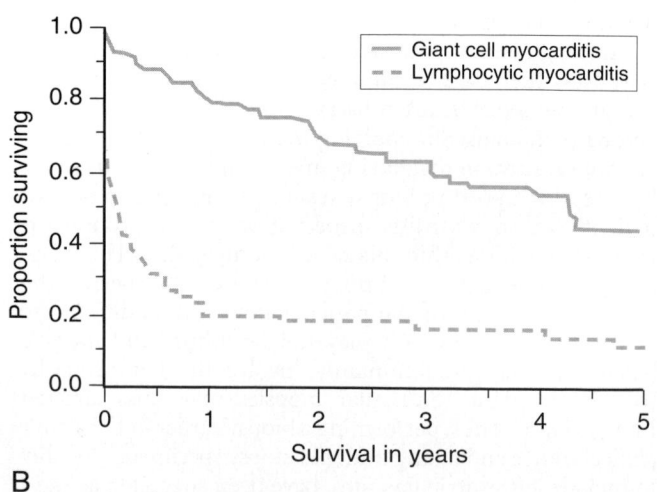

B

FIGURE 100–2. Line graphs showing the Kaplan-Meier survival curves for patients with giant cell myocarditis and lymphocytic myocarditis from the onset of symptoms (*A*) and from time of presentation to the referring center (*B*). In each case, survival was significantly shorter among those with giant-cell myocarditis. (From Cooper L, Berry G, Shabetai R, for The Multicenter Giant Cell Myocarditis Study Group Investigators: Idiopathic giant cell myocarditis—Natural history and treatment. N Engl J Med 1997;336:1862.)

In this uncontrolled series, immunosuppressive therapy was associated with prolonged survival from 3 months in 30 patients not given immunosuppressive drugs and 3.8 months in patients treated with prednisone, to 11.5 months in patients given prednisone plus azathioprine and 12.6 months in patients who were given cyclosporine as part of their regimen. Prognosis after cardiac transplantation was also worse when compared with other forms of heart disease, with a 30-day mortality rate of 15% and a 26% mortality rate during the 3.7-year post-transplant follow-up period. Twenty-six percent of patients had giant cell infiltrates seen in their transplanted heart at an average time of 3 years after transplant.

EOSINOPHILIC MYOCARDITIS

Eosinophilic myocarditis, sometimes termed *hypersensitivity myocarditis*, is a rare form of myocarditis characterized by eosinophilic infiltration and degranulation seen on endomyocardial biopsy. It is believed that pathogenesis involves a direct role of eosinophil-mediated myocyte damage. There can be associated arteritis. This entity is distinct from eosinophilic endocarditis (Loffler's endocarditis). The clinical manifestations are not specific, aside from a high incidence of eosinophilia in peripheral blood. Patients usually present with heart failure due to left ventricular systolic dysfunction. Fever and rash may be present. Untreated, the disease is often rapidly fatal.

The cause is believed to be a hypersensitivity reaction, usually to medication or, rarely, in association with parasitic infections. Drugs most often implicated are sulfonamides, diuretics, angiotensin-converting enzyme (ACE) inhibitors, cephalosporins, digoxin, or dobutamine. Eosinophilic myocarditis has been reported to occur weeks after smallpox vaccination, with an incidence of 1 in 16,000 vaccinated.[12] The clinical course is unfavorable, often with rapidly worsening heart failure and sudden death due to ventricular arrhythmia. Treatment involves the discontinuation of all potentially offending medication and the use of high-dose corticosteroids. Excellent responses to corticosteroids, as well as some spontaneously resolving illness, have been reported.[13,14]

Eosinophilic myocardial infiltration has been reported in 2% to 7% of myocardial biopsy specimens of patients awaiting cardiac transplantation, or in the explanted heart after transplant. The cause is unclear, but dobutamine therapy, sodium bisulfite used as a preservative in dobutamine solutions, and the use of left ventricular assist devices have been implicated. The presence of eosinophilic myocarditis in this setting did not have an adverse affect on post-transplant survival and did not recur in the transplanted heart.[15,16]

RELATIONSHIP BETWEEN MYOCARDITIS AND IDIOPATHIC DILATED CARDIOMYOPATHY

There are many data from animal models indicating that acute myocarditis often leads to chronic idiopathic dilated cardiomyopathy. An important question in humans is the incidence of unrecognized antecedent myocarditis in patients who present with heart failure and idiopathic dilated cardiomyopathy. The frequency of myocarditis as the cause of dilated cardiomyopathy is unknown, and the importance of immune-mediated mechanisms in the pathogenesis of dilated cardiomyopathy also needs to be defined. Analysis of endomyocardial biopsy specimens from patients with chronic dilated cardiomyopathy shows evidence of viral signals in 50% of cases and the presence of viral genome in 35%, although this does not prove causation.[17] Circulating autoantibodies to myocyte proteins and myocyte surface receptors have also been described in patients with dilated cardiomyopathy,[6,18] although these have also been described in a small number of patients (5%) with ischemic cardiomyopathy. These antibodies thus may be a secondary phenomenon and do not necessarily indicate a primary pathogenic role of immune-mediated injury.

THERAPY

GENERAL MANAGEMENT OF HEART FAILURE

The treatment of myocarditis is based on the clinical presentation. Patients with mild disease can be treated expectantly, with dietary sodium restriction, and avoidance of strenuous exercise for several weeks or months.[2] Animal models indicate that strenuous exercise can worsen myocarditis. Elimination of unnecessary medications is important in patients with eosinophilia.

Nonsteroidal anti-inflammatory drugs should be avoided because they may worsen myocarditis.[3] The routine use of anticoagulants for prophylaxis of systemic emboli is controversial. Patients who present with symptoms of arrhythmia or heart failure should be hospitalized, with continuous cardiac rhythm monitoring performed for evaluation of possible serious or life-threatening arrhythmias or conduction abnormalities. If these are diagnosed, they are treated in a similar matter as in patients with other causes of heart disease, utilizing antiarrhythmic drugs or pacemakers. However, patients should be observed over a period of time to see whether improvement or resolution of the disease takes place prior to implantation of the implantable cardiac defibrillator.

There are no controlled trials in humans that have evaluated standard heart failure medications in patients with myocarditis. However, there are data in murine models of myocarditis supporting the use of captopril,[2] and there are many data in humans supporting the use of ACE inhibitors, beta-blockers, and aldosterone antagonists in patients with dilated cardiomyopathy. Therefore, in patients with myocarditis and heart failure, the use of standard multidrug medical therapy for heart failure and left ventricular systolic dysfunction is indicated.[2,6] These medications have been shown to improve symptoms, prolong life, and regress the adverse left ventricular remodeling that occurs in patients with dilated cardiomyopathy of various causes.[19-21]

Administration of ACE inhibitors should be initiated in all patients with left ventricular systolic dysfunction. Treatment should begin at low doses, with upward titration to maximally tolerated doses. Patients should be closely monitored for potential side effects, including renal insufficiency, hyperkalemia, and angioedema. Relative contraindications to the use of ACE inhibitors include renal failure, hyperkalemia, bilateral renal artery stenosis, and hepatic failure. Patients with hypotension should be treated with parenteral vasopressors or circulatory assist devices prior to initiation of low-dose ACE inhibitor therapy.

Beta-adrenergic blockers have not been studied in humans with myocarditis, and their effects in the murine model have been mixed.[2] Nevertheless, beta-blocker therapy in large series of patients, which included patients with idiopathic dilated cardiomyopathy, have unequivocally shown benefit in patients with left ventricular systolic dysfunction,[22-26] and these agents should also be used in patients with heart failure due to myocarditis. Beta-blockers should be initiated after patients are on a stable dose of ACE inhibitors and when signs of fluid overload have resolved. Contraindications to beta-blocker therapy include bronchospastic disease or severe chronic obstructive lung disease, heart block, or significant underlying bradycardia. Hypotension should be corrected prior to initiating beta-blocker therapy.

Digoxin has been shown in animal models to decrease levels of cytokines, but digoxin was associated with adverse outcomes in one murine model of myocarditis. Digoxin can be useful in helping to control ventricular rates in patients with atrial fibrillation. The use of digoxin should be considered in patients with significant left ventricular systolic dysfunction, after ACE inhibitors and beta-blockers have been initiated. However, no survival benefit for digoxin has ever been shown in patients with heart failure due to dilated cardiomyopathy.[27] Contraindications to the use of digoxin include renal failure or heart block.

Lastly, the use of the aldosterone antagonist spironolactone has been shown to have symptomatic and survival benefit in patients with class III-IV systolic heart failure.[28] In experimental models, these agents can reverse the progressive myocardial fibrosis that occurs in the remodeling process of dilated cardiomyopathy. These agents have not been studied in patients with myocarditis, but their use should be strongly considered in patients with severe left ventricular dysfunction (ejection fraction less then 35%) and symptomatic heart failure.[2] Contraindications to the use of aldosterone antagonists include renal insufficiency, with serum creatinine levels above 2.0 mg%, or hyperkalemia. Serum potassium levels needs to be carefully monitored during initiation and dose titration.

In critically ill patients with severe heart failure and low cardiac index, parenteral vasodilators should be used. Intravenous nitroprusside is a powerful venous and arterial dilator, which significantly reduces systemic vascular resistance, mean systemic arterial pressure, and pulmonary capillary wedge pressure, raising cardiac index. It must be administered in the ICU with invasive hemodynamic monitoring with a pulmonary artery catheter, to best gauge the appropriate dose of medication and to accurately assess response to therapy. Prolonged use of nitroprusside is associated with accumulation of the toxic metabolites thiocyanate and cyanide, and serum levels of these compounds must be monitored. Intravenous nitroglycerin is also an effective venodilator and coronary vasodilator, with less arterial dilating property than nitroprusside. The use of nitroglycerin in cases of myocarditis has not been studied. Patients often develop tolerance to this drug.[29-31]

Nesiritide (B-natriuretic peptide) is a hormone produced by myocardial ventricular and atrial myocytes in response to stretch from chamber dilatation. It is a counter-regulatory peptide to the renin-angiotensin hormones, causing venous and arterial dilation, natriuresis, and diuresis.

These hemodynamic effects are favorable in patients with severe heart failure, and intravenous infusions of nesiritide are being used more widely in patients with severe heart failure due to left ventricular systolic dysfunction. Reduction in pulmonary capillary wedge pressure occurs more rapidly than with intravenous nitroglycerin. Nesiritide is not proarrhythmic, does not have toxic metabolites, and does not induce tolerance. Nesiritide use can cause significant hypotension in some patients.[32-35]

Patients with severe myocarditis may develop cardiogenic shock, with hypotension, respiratory failure, and signs of end organ hypoperfusion. In these instances, initial treatment with inotropic agents or vasopressors is indicated. Dobutamine is a potent beta$_1$-agonist with less beta$_2$- and alpha-agonist properties. Dobutamine has favorable short-term hemodynamic effects with increased myocardial contractility and reduced systemic vascular resistance and reduced pulmonary capillary wedge pressure. However, dobutamine can be proarrhythmic, and patients can develop tolerance to the drug. In studies utilizing routine use of dobutamine in patients with exacerbations of chronic systolic heart failure, the use of this drug was associated with increased mortality rates when compared with placebo.[36]

Milrinone is another parenteral inotropic agent, which works by inhibiting phosphodiesterase. This drug leads to increased inotropy and decreased systemic vascular resistance and pulmonary capillary wedge pressure, with resultant increased stroke volume and cardiac index. Milrinone may cause hypotension. It is less proarrhythmic than dobutamine and it does not induce tolerance.[37,38]

Arterial vasoconstrictors such as norepinephrine and dopamine can be used in patients with refractory hypotension for short-term urgent blood pressure support. However, these agents cause increased myocardial oxygen consumption and can have deleterious effects on myocardial function.

In patients with fulminant myocarditis or cardiogenic shock, the use of mechanical ventricular assist devices should be strongly considered. These devices offer hemodynamic support and left ventricular afterload reduction and may provide time for spontaneous improvement or recovery of normal left ventricular function. Ventricular assist devices (VADs) are mechanical pumps that take over the function of the failing ventricle, providing normal cardiac output. VADs are usually univentricular but can be biventricular, supporting both right and left ventricular function. They have been inserted via a midline sternotomy, with the inflow conduit to the pump inserted via the left ventricular apex. With improved technology, these devices are being made smaller and are being implanted through smaller incisions. A VAD is now available that can be inserted percutaneously. VADs are connected to an external power pack via a driveline through the skin. The power pack is now small enough so that it can be portable, and thus patients have freedom of movement and can participate in rehabilitation efforts during VAD use. Current devices have textured blood-contacting surfaces so routine anticoagulation therapy is not required. Complications of VADs include local site infection, sepsis, thromboemboli, right ventricular failure, and device failure.[39,40]

In patients with myocarditis, VADs can be used to provide circulatory needs and improve coronary flow during the time necessary for spontaneous resolution of myocarditis to occur. Beneficial reverse remodeling may occur while patients are on VAD support, resulting in improved myocyte structure and function. VADs can provide support for months or even years.

A retrospective study of 22 patients with nonischemic cardiomyopathy who were successfully weaned from left ventricular or biventricular assist devices was analyzed.[41] Patients had either myocarditis or acute onset of idiopathic dilated cardiomyopathy. The average age of patients was 32 years, and the average duration of VAD support was 57 days (range, 12-190 days). Twenty of 22 patients were discharged alive with their native heart, at an average of 22 days

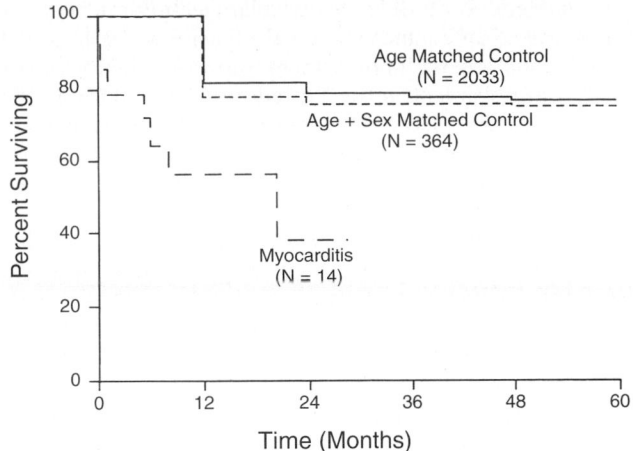

FIGURE 100–3. Graph showing the actuarial survival duration of heart transplant recipients with active lymphocytic myocarditis as compared with that of age-matched (—) and age- and sex-matched (- - -) control patients. (From Haas G: Etiology, evaluation, and management of acute myocarditis. Cardiol Rev 2001;9:88-95.)

after VAD removal. Two patients received cardiac transplants 1 year after VAD removal. Seventeen of the 22 patients remained alive and well with their native hearts at an average of 3.2 years after VAD removal. Sixteen patients were functional class I, and one was functional class II. Thus, the survival of native hearts in this series after being weaned successfully from VAD support was 86% at 1 year and was 77% at 5 years. This survival rate was indistinguishable from the survival rate of patients who received cardiac transplantation after a period of VAD support. These authors thus felt that patients with fulminant myocarditis should be given every opportunity to recover ventricular function, and that cardiac transplantation should be used only as a last resort, when severe heart damage is irreversible.[41]

There are several unresolved issues regarding VAD usage in patients with myocarditis. These include appropriate patient selection, timing of VAD placement, best medical therapy during VAD support, and optimal duration of VAD support. A 50-day course of VAD support in the above study allowed identification of 50% of those patients who ultimately recovered, and a 90-day course identified 80% of patients who recovered. The optimal means of serial assessment of native heart function while on VAD support needs to be delineated, and the best weaning protocol also needs definition.

Cardiac transplantation is the final option for treating critically ill patients with myocarditis. However, these patients have a higher rate of transplant rejection, and a lower survival rate when compared with patients transplanted for ischemic or other causes of cardiomyopathy. Myocarditis has been reported to recur in the transplanted heart (Fig. 100-3).[6]

IMMUNOSUPPRESSIVE THERAPY

Autoimmune mechanisms are believed to be responsible for the clinical manifestations of myocarditis and the development of myocardial necrosis and left ventricular dysfunction. Therefore, therapy with immunosuppressive drugs has been used. However, given the high rate of spontaneous recovery of left ventricular function (up to 40% of patients in some series), placebo-controlled trials are essential to properly evaluate the effects of therapy. In addition, heterogeneous patient populations, consisting of cases of both acute myocarditis and chronic dilated cardiomyopathy, have made it difficult to design effective immunosuppressive regimens.

High-dose daily prednisone therapy was used for a 3-month course in 102 patients with dilated cardiomyopathy, 59% of whom were classified as having "reactive" myocarditis on endomyocardial biopsy.[42] The authors found a significant improvement in left ventricular ejection fraction at 3 months in treated patients with reactive myocarditis (Fig. 100-4), but this improvement was not sustained at 9 months. Improvement did not occur in patients with nonreactive

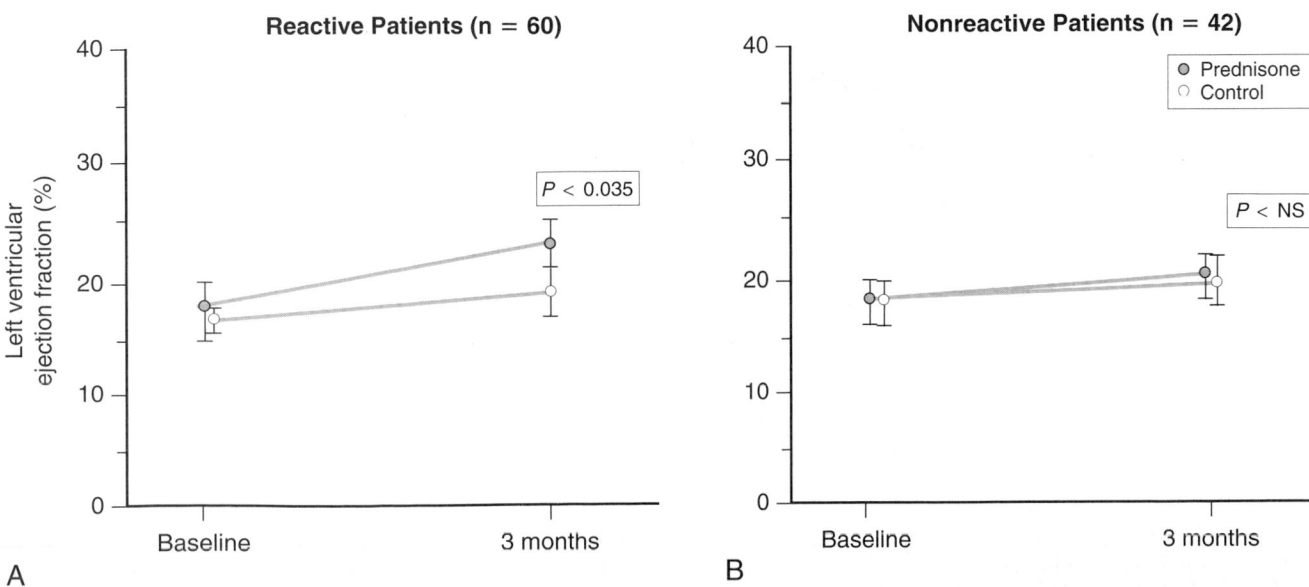

FIGURE 100–4. (A) Ejection fraction in reactive dilated cardiomyopathy patients at 3 months. (B) Prednisone does not change ejection fraction in nonreactive patients in 3 months. (From Parrillo J, Cunnion R, Epstein S, et al: A prospective, randomized, controlled trial of prednisone for dilated cardiomyopathy. N Engl J Med 1989;321:1061-1068.)

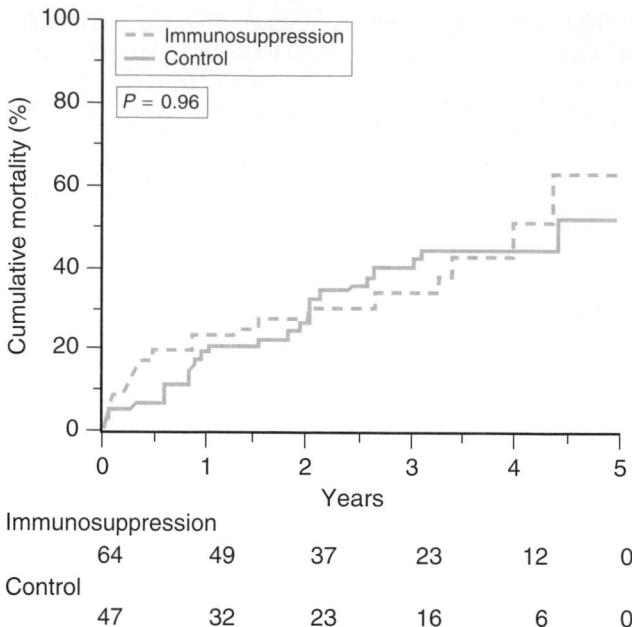

Immunosuppression

| 64 | 49 | 37 | 23 | 12 | 0 |

Control

| 47 | 32 | 23 | 16 | 6 | 0 |

FIGURE 100–5. Actuarial mortality (defined as deaths and cardiac transplantations) in the immunosuppression and control groups. The numbers of patients at risk are shown at the bottom. There was no significant difference in mortality between the two groups. (From Mason J, O'Connell J, Herskowitz A, et al, for The Myocarditis Treatment Trial Investigators: A clinical trial of immunosuppressive therapy for myocarditis. N Engl J Med 1995;333:269-275.)

biopsies treated with prednisone. No significant mortality benefit from immunosuppressive treatment was noted, although this was not a prespecified primary endpoint.

The Myocarditis Treatment Trial enrolled 111 patients with a positive endomyocardial biopsy finding and left ventricular ejection fraction less than 45%, with a duration of illness of less than 2 years.[43] Three treatment groups were compared: daily prednisone plus azathioprine, prednisone plus cyclosporine, and placebo. Overall, these patients had a 20% 1-year mortality rate and 56% 3-year mortality rate. These investigators found no difference in ejection fraction at week 28 or week 52, no change in left ventricular size at week 28, and no difference in 1-year mortality between treated and untreated groups. Their conclusion was that these immunosuppressive strategies were not beneficial. Significant limitations of this study include a 30% dropout rate and significant intraobserver variability among pathologists' diagnoses of biopsy specimens despite utilizing the Dallas criteria (Fig. 100-5).

In view of the limitations of histopathologic diagnosis using the Dallas criteria, another group of investigators utilized immunohistologic markers of inflammation, such as up-regulation of HLA, to diagnose active myocarditis as an indication for immunosuppressive therapy.[44] This criterion has the advantage of indicating that autoimmunity is playing a role in pathogenesis. Also, since HLA is distributed throughout the entire myocardium, biopsy sampling error is eliminated as a confounding variable in assessing response to therapy. In this study, 84 of 202 patients with chronic (>6 months) idiopathic dilated cardiomyopathy (ejection fraction <40%) were found to have strong expression of HLA in biopsy specimens and were randomized to receive placebo or prednisone plus azathioprine for 3 months. At 3 months' follow-up, a significant improvement in the prespecified

secondary endpoints of left ventricular ejection fraction, left ventricular volumes, and functional capacity was seen in the treated group, and this improvement was maintained at 2 years (71.8% improvement in the treated group vs. 30.8% in the untreated group). However, there was no improvement in the prespecified composite primary endpoint of death, cardiac transplant, or hospital readmission. This study was limited by a 31% dropout rate.

In another study, patients with positive endomyocardial biopsy specimens and progressive heart failure who responded to 6 months of therapy with prednisone and azathioprine were more likely to have circulating cardiac autoantibodies and no viral genome in their myocardium as compared with nonresponders.[45]

Studies have suggested that in patients with heart failure and low ejection fraction, intravenous immunoglobulin has a pronounced anti-inflammatory effect as measured by circulating levels of inflammatory markers.[46] Uncontrolled studies suggested benefit in patients with myocarditis from treatment with intravenous immunoglobulin.[47,48] However, a placebo-controlled double-blind trial of intravenous immunoglobulin in patients with myocarditis or idiopathic dilated cardiomyopathy of less than 6 months' duration showed no significant improvement with therapy as assessed by ejection fraction or functional capacity at 6 and 12 months.[49] In this study, average left ventricular ejection fraction improved from 25 ± 8% at baseline to 41 ± 17% at 6 months in both treated and untreated groups. One-year event-free survival rate was 91.9% in both groups. Another study suggested benefit with intravenous immunoglobulin as measured by improvement in ejection fraction in patients with chronic cardiomyopathy of greater than 6 months' duration.[46]

In summary, there is no evidence that patients with lymphocytic myocarditis or idiopathic dilated cardiomyopathy benefit from the routine use of immunosuppressive therapy. However, this treatment approach should be considered in patients with myocarditis and positive endomyocardial biopsy findings, those who develop early signs of severe heart failure, and those who are shown to experience progressive worsening of left ventricular function. In patients with idiopathic dilated cardiomyopathy who show worsening left ventricular function on weekly or monthly follow-up, immunosuppressive therapy should be strongly considered.[50] Lastly, immunosuppressive therapy should be used in patients with myocarditis associated with connective tissue diseases, eosinophilic or granulomatous forms of the disease, or giant cell myocarditis (Fig. 100-6).

Current investigations are evaluating antiviral therapies in the acute stage of myocarditis as well as the use of antiviral vaccine in the prevention of disease. Appropriately powered, controlled, prospective studies of homogeneous patient groups utilizing immunosuppressive therapy are still needed. Evaluating the mechanisms of myocardial recovery during VAD support may also help direct research toward other novel approaches to the treatment of myocarditis.

SUMMARY

Among many diverse causes, the most common cause of myocarditis is believed to be viral, with autoimmune mechanisms prominently involved in pathogenesis. Patients with myocarditis can present with acute chest pain, mimicking acute ischemic heart disease or other cardiopulmonary

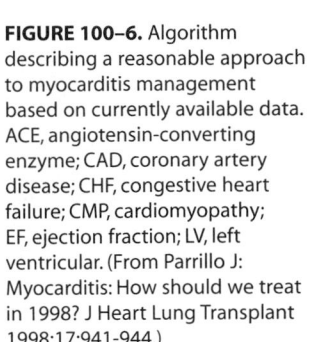

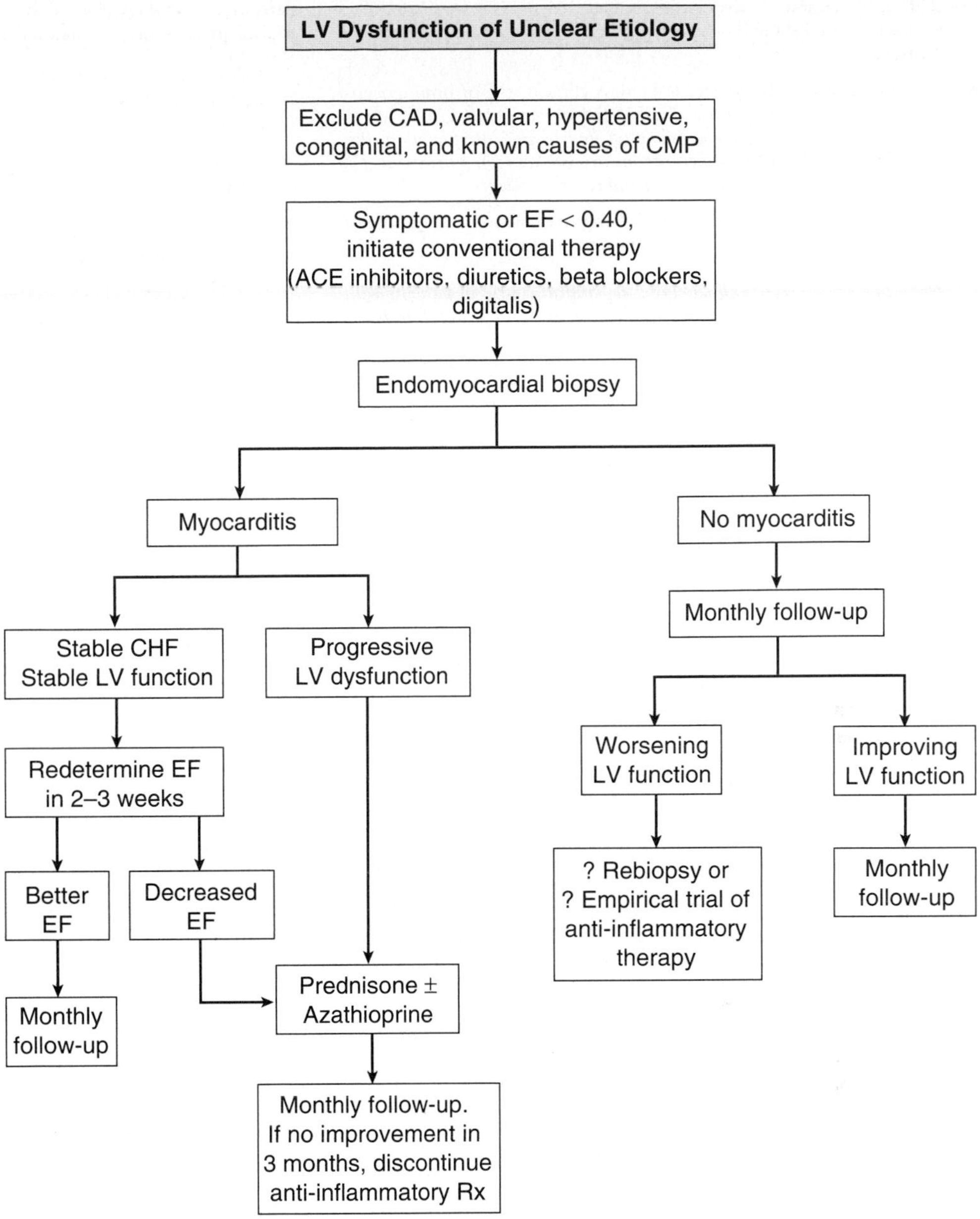

LV Dysfunction of Unclear Etiology

↓

Exclude CAD, valvular, hypertensive, congenital, and known causes of CMP

↓

Symptomatic or EF < 0.40, initiate conventional therapy (ACE inhibitors, diuretics, beta blockers, digitalis)

↓

Endomyocardial biopsy

Myocarditis | No myocarditis

Myocarditis:
- Stable CHF / Stable LV function → Redetermine EF in 2–3 weeks → Better EF → Monthly follow-up / Decreased EF → Prednisone ± Azathioprine
- Progressive LV dysfunction → Prednisone ± Azathioprine → Monthly follow-up. If no improvement in 3 months, discontinue anti-inflammatory Rx

No myocarditis:
- Monthly follow-up → Worsening LV function → ? Rebiopsy or ? Empirical trial of anti-inflammatory therapy / Improving LV function → Monthly follow-up

FIGURE 100–6. Algorithm describing a reasonable approach to myocarditis management based on currently available data. ACE, angiotensin-converting enzyme; CAD, coronary artery disease; CHF, congestive heart failure; CMP, cardiomyopathy; EF, ejection fraction; LV, left ventricular. (From Parrillo J: Myocarditis: How should we treat in 1998? J Heart Lung Transplant 1998;17:941-944.)

illnesses, or can present with heart failure due to dilated cardiomyopathy. A smaller percentage of patients present with acute heart failure due to severe left ventricular systolic dysfunction. Oral and parenteral pharmacological therapies that are used in patients with heart failure of the more common causes are also used in these patients. Patients can also present with fulminant myocarditis, characterized by severe heart failure and cardiogenic shock. These patients need intensive, aggressive pharmacological therapy as well as support with VADs, because they very often show significant improvement in left ventricular function so that pharmacological and VAD support can be weaned and discontinued, without having to resort to cardiac transplantation.

Endomyocardial biopsy is used in the diagnosis of myocarditis and for directing therapy, although it is limited by sampling error and by current histopathologic techniques for assessing disease activity. Newer immunohistologic methods may better define those patients who will respond to immunosuppressive therapy. Patients with myocarditis and progressive myocardial failure, despite conventional heart failure therapy, should be considered for immunosuppressive therapy on a case-by-case basis. Such patients should be followed with serial measures of left ventricular performance and endomyocardial biopsies.

ANNOTATED REFERENCES

Cooper L, Berry G, Shabetai R: Idiopathic giant cell myocarditis—natural history and treatment. N Engl J Med 1997;336:1860-1866.

The Multicenter Giant Cell Myocarditis Study Group investigators describe the clinical course, prognosis, and treatment of patients with this disease.

Farrar D, Holman W, McBride L, et al: Long-term follow-up of Thoratec ventricular assist device bridge-to-recovery patients successfully removed from support after recovery of ventricular function. J Heart Lung Transplant 2002;21:516-521.

This retrospective study describes the course of 22 patients with severe heart failure and myocarditis who were able to be successfully weaned from VAD therapy.

Feldman A, McNamara D: Myocarditis. N Engl J Med. 2000;343:1388-1398.

An excellent overview of the etiology, pathogenesis, diagnosis, and treatment of myocarditis.

Mason J, O'Connell J, Herskowitz A, et al: A clinical trial of immunosuppressive therapy for myocarditis. N Engl J Med 1995;333:269-275.

Despite limitations in patient follow-up and biopsy interpretation, this controlled trial showed no difference in survival between patients treated with an immunosuppressive regimen and control patients.

McCarthy R, Boehmer J, Hruban R, et al: Long term outcome of fulminant myocarditis as compared with acute (nonfulminant) myocarditis. N Engl J Med 2000;342:690-695.

These authors describe and compare the clinical course of patients with fulminant myocarditis with acute myocarditis, defining fulminant myocarditis as a distinct clinical illness.

Parrillo J, Cunnion R, Epstein S, et al: A prospective randomized controlled trial of prednisone for dilated cardiomyopathy. N Engl J Med 1989;321:1061-1068.

This placebo-controlled study showed a modest improvement in left ventricular ejection fraction in patients with inflammation on endomyocardial biopsy who were treated with prednisone.

Wu L, Lapeyre A, Cooper L: Current role of endomyocardial biopsy in the management of dilated cardiomyopathy and myocarditis. Mayo Clin Proc 2001;76:1030-1038.

This paper presents an overview of the use, complications, indications for, and yield of endomyocardial biopsy.

Chapter 101

ACQUIRED AND CONGENITAL HEART DISEASE IN CHILDREN

Duncan J. Macrae

KEY POINTS

1. The immature myocardium has little functional reserve, tolerating both increased preload and afterload poorly.

2. Cardiac output in the neonate is critically dependent on heart rate.

3. A hyperoxic test will usually differentiate cyanosis resulting from intracardiac shunting of deoxygenated blood and that from intrapulmonary ventilation-perfusion mismatch.

4. Manipulation of the pulmonary circulation, especially pulmonary vascular resistance, and the function of the subpulmonary ("right") ventricle are critical to understanding and managing many congenital heart lesions.

5. Mechanical circulatory support is effective in "bridging" many children with severe heart failure to recovery or cardiac transplantation.

6. In the era of mechanical circulatory support, acute fulminant myocarditis in children should be regarded as a condition from which a child can recover.

7. Appropriate intensive care management of the child with congenital heart disease must be based on a sound understanding of the anatomy and pathophysiology of the child's circulation.

8. Issues relating to the management of intracardiac shunts, cyanosis, and the pulmonary circulation and right ventricle are commonly of great importance in the child with congenital heart disease.

9. A specialist's advice should be sought early if children with known or suspected heart disease are admitted to nonspecialist pediatric or adult facilities.

PHYSIOLOGY

CIRCULATORY CHANGES AT BIRTH

During the transition from intrauterine to extrauterine life, major circulatory changes occur that have important implications for the clinical care of the newborn.[1,2] At birth in the normal newborn, the low-resistance placenta is eliminated from the circulation, resulting in an immediate increase in systemic vascular resistance (SVR), and the pulmonary vascular resistance (PVR) falls when the lungs become responsible for gas exchange. The fetal channels, the foramen ovale, and the arterial duct become redundant and close. In addition to the altered hemodynamics in infants born with congenital heart disease, some infants with structurally normal hearts have a persistent right-to-left shunt after birth owing to failure of the transition from fetal to postnatal circulation. Infants with this circulatory pattern, which is characterized by failure of the PVR to fall, have persistent pulmonary hypertension of the newborn (PPHN).[3] PPHN is one of the two principal causes of "nonpulmonary" cyanosis in the neonate, the other being cyanotic congenital heart disease.

The right ventricle (RV) and left ventricle (LV) contribute equally to fetal cardiac output. At birth, the LV becomes responsible for the systemic circulation, characterized by its high vascular resistance. The PVR falls suddenly at birth to approximately 50% of fetal levels to facilitate the required increase in pulmonary blood flow. It continues to fall to adult values during the first 6 to 8 weeks of life as the smooth muscle layer in the media of the pulmonary arterioles progressively thins out. The LV progressively adapts to its "high pressure" role by rapid myocardial growth, in contrast to the RV, which regresses to its "low pressure" subpulmonary role. The presence of congenital heart defects can profoundly alter these adaptive processes.

PHYSIOLOGY OF THE NEONATAL MYOCARDIUM

The neonatal myocardium is functionally immature. Age-dependent changes in intrinsic function and integration with a maturing circulation determine its response to insults such as hypoxia and ischemia.[4,5]

The myocardium matures in the postnatal period by increasing the number and the volume and conformation of its myocytes. The cell membrane (sarcolemma) develops the T tubular system, which facilitates rapid conduction of the action potential to the center of the cell, and the arrangement of myofibrils gradually becomes more uniform, improving its contractile function. In parallel with these structural changes, myocellular metabolism matures. Proper contractile function of the cardiac myocyte depends on an efficient excitation-contraction process, which is activated by the binding of calcium to troponin C. In the adult heart, calcium release from the sarcoplasmic reticulum (SR) is the predominant

TABLE 101–1. CHARACTERISTICS OF THE NEONATAL VENTRICLE

	Comparison to Mature Ventricle
Contractility	Contractility of the neonatal ventricle is reduced compared with the mature ventricle.
Compliance	Neonatal ventricle is inherently noncompliant compared with mature ventricle.
Augmentation Cardiac Output	There is little stoke volume reserve due to low compliance. Therefore, cardiac output is highly heart rate dependent in neonates.
Afterload	Neonatal ventricle tolerates increased afterload poorly.
Energy Substrate	Lactate is primary substrate of neonatal ventricle under aerobic conditions. Glucose is metabolized under anaerobic conditions. By 1 to 2 years there is changeover to primary "adult" substrate, free fatty acids.

source of calcium for troponin C activation whereas, in contrast, in the neonate, activation relies substantially on calcium influx through the "L"-type calcium channels. Optimal function of the neonatal myocardium is therefore exquisitely dependent on maintenance of normal extracellular calcium concentrations. Other elements of myocyte function are age dependent, such as the sarcoplasmic reticulum calcium/adenosine triphosphatase (SERCA), which is present in reduced quantities in the immature heart. This results in relatively inefficient calcium reuptake and therefore slower diastolic relaxation of the neonatal compared with the adult myocyte and is at least in part responsible for the prominence of diastolic dysfunction in the failing neonatal myocardium.

Healthy infants have higher plasma concentrations of catecholamines and higher density cardiac sympathetic innervation than older children and adults. This may partly explain the reduced ability of neonates to increase cardiac output in response to endogenous or exogenous catecholamines. Children in heart failure also have higher plasma catecholamine concentrations[6] but reduced densities of beta-adrenergic receptors compared with age-matched controls.[7] The effects of this are similar to those seen with exogenous agonist-induced desensitization. Children with severe heart failure show evidence of uncoupling of beta$_1$-adrenergic receptors from the enzyme adenyl cyclase[7] and other maladaptive responses, which result in reduced response to receptor agonists. In addition to heart failure, chronic hypoxia such as is seen in cyanotic congenital heart disease induces activation of the sympathetic nervous system with resultant adrenergic receptor desensitization.

Developmental aspects of myocardial support have been reviewed.[8] The clinical characteristics of the neonatal ventricle are presented in Table 101-1.

CONGESTIVE HEART FAILURE

Although the basic pathophysiologic mechanisms of heart failure have age-independent common mechanisms, the presentation and management of heart failure changes with age. The overwhelming cause of heart failure in the first year of life is congenital heart disease, usually with an intracardiac left-to-right shunt or a ventricular obstructive lesion (Table 101-2). By contrast, the primary abnormality in adult heart failure is usually LV dysfunction. Heart failure in adults is often gradual in onset; the neonate has little functional reserve, resulting in rapid decompensation and an emergent presentation.

The clinical findings[9] in an infant with heart failure are listed in Table 101-3. A prominent sign of cardiac failure in infancy is difficulty in feeding secondary to increased respiratory rate and effort. This equates to exertional dyspnea in the older child or adult. Failure to thrive results in the classic "wizened" appearance. Although hepatomegaly is a common sign of heart failure in infants (resulting from an increase in total circulating volume and hepatic venous congestion), peripheral edema, ascites, and pericardial or pleural effusions are much less commonly seen than in adults. One relatively common feature of severe heart failure in infancy is the occurrence of compression of the bronchial tree, particularly the left mainstem or lower lobe bronchus as a result of extrinsic compression by an enlarged left atrium or pulmonary artery. This can cause airway obstruction and associated lobar collapse or localized hyperinflation as a result of distal air trapping. Long-standing extrinsic compression may rarely cause tracheobronchomalacia, resulting in long-term respiratory difficulties even after resolution of heart failure.

CYANOSIS

Cyanosis is the visible manifestation of greater than 5 g/dL of reduced deoxygenated hemoglobin in cutaneous blood vessels and is a prominent feature in many types of congenital heart disease. *Peripheral cyanosis* results from high oxygen extraction ratios across the tissue vascular bed reflecting low tissue blood flow or high tissue oxygen demand. *Central cyanosis* results from desaturation of arterial blood, which may be

TABLE 101–2. COMMON CAUSES OF HEART FAILURE IN CHILDHOOD

Neonate < 2 Weeks of Age	Neonate > 2 Weeks of Age, Infant	Older Child
Congenital heart disease	Congenital heart disease	Congenital heart disease
Left-sided obstructive lesions	Left-to-right shunt lesions	Any lesion
Critical aortic stenosis	Ventriculoseptal defect	Following surgery
Aortic coarctation	Atrioventriculoseptal defect	Late deterioration of ventricle
Hypoplastic left heart syndrome	Truncus arteriosus	in palliated circulations
Arrhythmias	Total anomalous pulmonary	Acquired heart disease
Incessant supraventricular tachycardia	venous drainage	Cardiomyopathies (idiopathic or specific)
"Congenital" myocarditis		Myocarditis
Severe ventricular dysfunction due to birth		Rheumatic fever
asphyxia, sepsis, or severe metabolic disorders		Infective endocarditis
		Arrhythmias
		Severe anemia
		Nutritional deficiencies

TABLE 101–3. CLINICAL FEATURES OF HEART FAILURE IN INFANTS

Respiratory signs
  Initially tachypnea
  Dyspnea manifesting as poor feeding
  Later signs: retractions, intercostal recession, nasal flaring
  Pulmonary wheeze/rales
Tachycardia—little variability even at rest
Gallop rhythm
Hepatomegaly
Cardiomegaly
Poor peripheral perfusion—in severe failure "ashen" appearance

due to pulmonary disease or to right-to-left shunting of deoxygenated systemic venous blood in association with a congenital heart defect. The "pulmonary" and "cardiac" causes of central cyanosis can usually be differentiated by allowing the child to breathe 100% oxygen (a "hyperoxic test"). During administration of 100% oxygen, a PaO_2 above 160 mm Hg is highly suggestive of a noncardiac diagnosis and a PaO_2 of greater than 250 mm Hg excludes it. Occasionally, *differential cyanosis* is seen in which one or both of the upper limbs are normally saturated and the lower limbs cyanosed. This is caused by deoxygenated blood traversing the arterial duct to enter the aorta distal to the origin of one or both subclavian arteries and supplying the lower limbs while oxygenated blood from the LV predominantly supplies the upper limbs.

Chronic hypoxemia induces the twin physiologic responses of erythropoiesis, resulting in polycythemia and an increase in blood volume in a compensatory attempt to maintain oxygen-carrying capacity. However, as hemoglobin concentrations rise, blood viscosity increases and ultimately leads to sluggish flow in the peripheral circulation, cellular aggregation, and the occurrence of thrombotic lesions. Polycythemic patients are at high risk of thrombotic complications in situations of increased fluid loss (e.g., intercurrent diarrheal illness) or inadequate fluid intake (e.g., preoperative fasting). In addition to polycythemia, most children with chronic cyanosis develop finger clubbing, the result of an increased number of capillaries laid down in the vascular beds of the fingers and toes. Rare but important complications of severe cyanosis include cerebral and pulmonary thrombosis and cerebral abscess.

PULMONARY HYPERTENSION

The pulmonary vascular bed is of central importance to the manifestations of congenital heart disease from the first hours of life.[10] PVR usually falls dramatically in response to aeration of the lungs with first breaths. Thereafter, the smooth muscle of the pulmonary vascular bed thins gradually during the first months of life, with associated fall in PVR to "adult" values by approximately age 2 months. In infants with congenital heart lesions where an intracardiac communication between the systemic and pulmonary circulations is present, such as a ventricular septal defect (VSD), the fall in PVR encourages flow into the low-resistance pulmonary vascular bed and a left-to-right shunt develops. In response to the increased flow and subsequent shear stress this induces, progressive structural changes occur in the pulmonary arteries and arterioles. Initially, these changes consist of accelerated extension of muscle to the distal nonmuscular pulmonary arteries and medial muscular hypertrophy in the proximal muscular arteries. Later changes involve gradual hypertrophy of the arterial intima with deposition of collagen and elastin leading to gradual luminal obstruction and eventual occlusion. Associated with this is the development of plexiform lesions, the histologic hallmark of pulmonary vascular disease. Mild pulmonary vascular changes are of little significance to the cardiac intensivist, but children with more extensive medial muscular hypertrophy of the pulmonary arteries are at risk of labile pulmonary hypertension in the postoperative period. The extent of pulmonary hypertensive changes frequently determines the feasibility of surgical options. Children with established fixed high PVR are not suitable for corrective surgery, because surgical separation of the two circulations in the presence of fixed high PVR will result in immediate RV failure. Smaller elevation in PVR determines operability in the single-ventricle "Fontan" circulation (see later). Calculation of PVR and the response to varying vasodilators can be achieved following a pulmonary reversibility study in the cardiac catheter laboratory.[11]

CIRCULATORY SUPPORT IN CHILDREN

Children presenting with low cardiac output[12] must initially be assessed and managed according to standard resuscitation algorithms. These require that adequate oxygenation and circulating volume be achieved. If cardiac output remains low, cardiovascular drug therapy is usually indicated. The developmental differences noted earlier serve to emphasize the need to adopt age-appropriate pharmacologic strategies when supporting the failing myocardium of the neonate and infant. If cardiac output remains low despite application of such measures, mechanical circulatory support should be considered (Fig. 101-1).

PHARMACOLOGIC SUPPORT

Beta-adrenergic Agonists

Clinical and experimental studies have demonstrated marked age-related differences in the hemodynamic response to inotropic therapy. Although some of the observed differences may be accounted for by differences in drug pharmacokinetics, the variable maturation of the sympathetic nervous system, its receptors, and the cardiac myocytes militate against the recommendation of narrow, specific dose ranges for the use of catecholamines in neonates and children.[8]

In clinical practice, adrenergic agonists are used in a similar manner in children as in adults, that is, titrated to hemodynamic effect (Table 101-4). When systolic ventricular function is impaired, dopamine and dobutamine are commonly used as "first line" inotropes. Additional agents should be administered according to assessment of response judged clinically and from available hemodynamic monitoring. Epinephrine is occasionally useful when more potent inotropic stimulation is required. Norepinephrine or vasopressin can be used if refractory vasodilatation is present, such as occurs rarely after cardiopulmonary bypass (CPB) in children.[13] Isoproterenol is a nonspecific beta-adrenergic agonist whose principal cardiovascular effects are vasodilatation and increasing heart rate effects. The drug is rarely used in intensive care. Caution is needed when higher-dose catecholamine support is used in the neonate, because at high doses the agents induce a rise

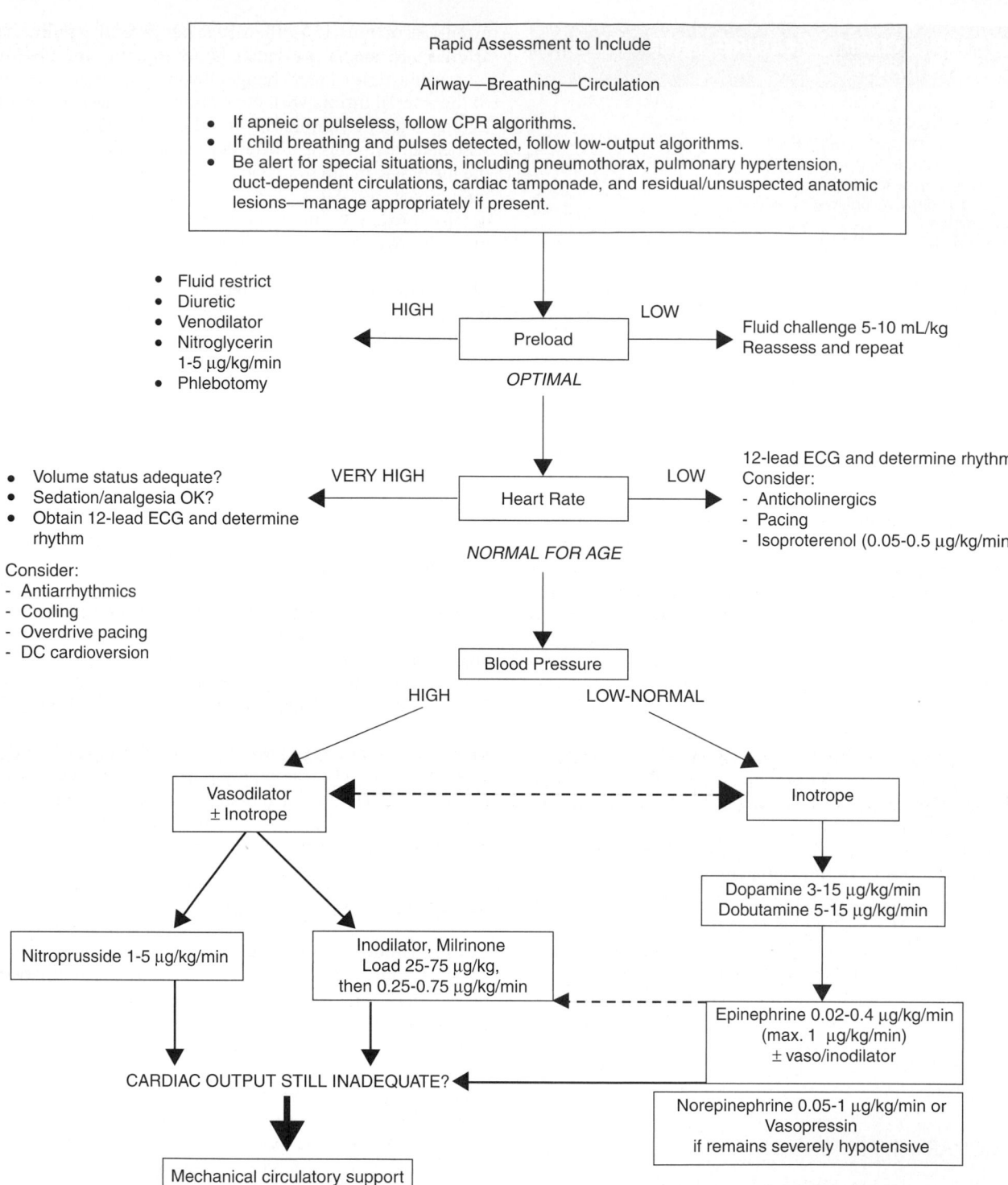

FIGURE 101–1. Guidelines for the management of low cardiac output in children.

in ventricular end-diastolic pressure in a ventricle that is already "developmentally" noncompliant. Catecholamine-induced myocardial necrosis has been identified in neonatal animal models.[14,15]

Phosphodiesterase (PDE) inhibitors have emerged as important agents in the management of neonates and children with cardiac failure. The cardiovascular actions of the clinically available PDE type III inhibitors amrinone,[16] milrinone,[17] and enoximone are similar (Table 101-5). By inhibiting

breakdown of cyclic adenosine monophosphate (AMP), intracellular calcium accumulation is promoted and augments the contractile state of the myocyte. In addition, the reuptake of calcium, which is a cyclic AMP–dependent process, is also augmented and these agents may therefore enhance diastolic relaxation, a particularly important aspect of neonatal cardiac function. In one multicenter randomized-controlled study of neonates and young children after cardiac surgery, the prophylactic administration of milrinone

TABLE 101–4. VASOACTIVE AGENTS IN CHILDREN: ADRENERGIC AGONISTS

Agent	Intravenous Dose Range	Alpha 1	Beta 1	Beta 2	Dopa	Comments
Dopamine	1-5 µg/kg/min	0	+/++		++	Beta-mediated inotropic effects at lower doses; alpha-mediated vasoconstriction at higher doses
	5-15 µg/kg/min	0/++	++		++	
Dobutamine	2-15 µg/kg/min	0	+/+++	0/++	0	
Epinephrine	0.02-0.1 µg/kg/min	0 /++	++/+++	++/+++	0	Beta$_2$ effect prominent at lower doses; alpha constrictor effects at higher doses
	0.2-0.4 µg/kg/min	++/+++	++++	+++	0	
Norepinephrine	0.2-0.5 µg/kg/min	++ /++++	+	0	0	Increases systemic vascular resistance. Reserved for treatment of severe hypotension associated with vasodilatation.
Isoproterenol	0.02-0.4 µg/kg/min	0	++++	++++	0	Prominent chronotropic activity. Beta 2 effects cause vasodilatation.

resulted in a lower incidence of low cardiac output.[18] Clinical studies in infants and children have demonstrated a synergistic effect when beta$_1$ agonists and PDE inhibitors such as amrinone, milrinone, or enoximone are co-administered, and this effect may be greater in neonates than in adults. In clinical use, the vasodilating action of the PDE III inhibitors is prominent, a useful property given the usual pattern low cardiac output associated with rising SVR and PVR that has been well documented in young patients after cardiac surgery.[19]

Systemic vasodilators are indicated in situations in which lowering SVR will reduce LV afterload and improve cardiac output. This is especially so in the neonatal setting, where elevation of the SVR is poorly tolerated by the myocardium. Vasodilators are also employed in the management of systemic hypertension as occurs in children after repair of aortic coarctation or other left-sided obstructive lesions. Vasodilators have variable effects on preload through concomitant venodilatation, the manifestations of which are dependent on the position the resultant end-diastolic pressure occupies on the

TABLE 101–5. VASOACTIVE AGENTS IN CHILDREN: CARDIOVASCULAR DRUGS OTHER THAN ADRENERGIC AGONISTS

	Dosage	Effects
PDE Type III Inhibitors		
Amrinone	*Neonates:* 4 mg/kg over 1 hour then 3-5 µg/kg/min i.v. *> 4 weeks of age:* 1-3 mg/kg over 1 hour then 5-15 µg/kg/min i.v.	Cardiac: Mild nonadrenergic inotropic and lusiotropic effects Vascular: Systemic and pulmonary vasodilator Amrinone may cause thrombocytopenia. Reduce amrinone dose in slow acetylators. Reduce milrinone dose in renal failure.
Milrinone	*All ages:* 50-75 µg/kg over 20 minutes *Maintenance:* 0.5-0.75 µg/kg/min i.v.	
Digoxin	Initial dose 15 µg/kg then 5 µg/kg after 6 hours. Thereafter, 5 µg/kg every 12 hr. Slow i.v. or p.o.	Delays atrioventricular conduction. Used in management of supraventricular tachycardia. Mild inotropic properties. May provide symptomatic relief in congestive heart failure. Bradycardia, supraventricular or ventricular dysrhythmias in overdose. Aim for plasma level 0.8-2.0 ng/mL Dose adjustment required in renal failure.
Esmolol	Short-term management of supraventricular tachycardia and perioperative hypertension 0.5 mg/kg, then 50-200 µg/kg/min i.v.	Bradycardia Hypotension Bronchospasm

Nitroprusside	0.5-5 µg/kg/min i.v.
	 Direct blood pressure monitoring required.
		Systemic and pulmonary vasodilatation
		 Systemic hypotension prominent
		 Cyanide toxicity
		     Metabolic acidosis earliest sign
		     Monitor thiocyanate levels when used > 48 hr or in renal failure

Captopril	Oral administration: 0.05 mg/kg as a test dose then incremental increase to 0.4 mg/kg (occasionally up to 1.0 mg/kg), titrated to effect (systemic blood pressure) every 8 hr.	Systemic vasodilatation/hypotension Small increase in plasma potassium levels
Nitroglycerin	0.5-8 µg/kg/min i.v. Direct blood pressure monitoring required.	Systemic and pulmonary vasodilatation
Propranolol	Relief of RV spasmodic RV outflow obstruction in the emergency management of hypercyanosis in tetralogy of Fallot 0.05-0.1 mg/kg i.v. stat Systemic hypertension 2-6 mg/kg in four to six divided doses	Bradycardia Hypotension Bronchospasm Lethargy

ventricular function curve. If preload reduction brings the end-diastolic pressure to the pre-plateau sloping portion of the ventricular function curve, stroke volume can only be maintained or augmented if preload is optimized by appropriate fluid administration. Directly placed left atrial pressure monitoring lines are commonly used to determine LV loading conditions in neonates and others too small for insertion of pulmonary arterial flotation catheters. Systemic vasodilators should be used with extreme caution in patients with systemic hypotension and those with LV outflow obstruction who are at risk of uncompensated severe systemic hypotension and myocardial ischemia.

In children, sodium nitroprusside is frequently the systemic vasodilator of choice because of its powerful arteriolar dilating properties and short half-life, which render it both effective and highly titratable (see Table 101-5). Nitroglycerin is an alternative short-acting drug that acts as an arteriolar dilator at higher doses but is an effective venodilator at lower doses. Phenoxybenzamine, a long-acting alpha-adrenergic blocker, is used in some centers in children undergoing surgery for congenital heart disease.[20]

For longer-term vasodilator therapy in children able to absorb enterally administered drugs, angiotensin-converting enzyme (ACE) inhibitors such as captopril and enalapril are used (see Table 101-5).[21] They have peripheral vascular and neurohormonal effects as well as direct effects on the myocardium through activation of intracellular signaling pathways involved in growth and apoptosis of cardiac myocytes and fibroblasts. Studies in adults have established that ACE inhibitors improve survival and symptoms in heart failure, owing in part to favorable effects on cardiac remodeling. Evidence for the use of ACE inhibitors in children is much less clear. Acute hemodynamic benefits have been demonstrated in children with heart failure caused by left-to-right shunts and systolic dysfunction of the systemic ventricle. Prolonged treatment with ACE inhibitors has been shown to be effective in reducing not only LV volume overload but also LV hypertrophy in the hearts of growing children with chronic LV volume overload.[22,23] The use of ACE inhibitors in the neonatal period has been questioned by the finding that they may influence the balance of apoptosis and cell growth, compromising necessary remodeling.[24]

Digoxin may have weak inotropic actions through its inhibitory effect on Na^+,K^+-ATPase and may also have peripheral effects that attenuate the actions of the neurohormonal system (see Table 101-5). Several adult studies have shown that digoxin improves symptoms in heart failure, but no studies have shown improvement in survival. Digoxin is widely used to treat heart failure in children, but there are few data to support or refute its use. Recommendations on its rational use in pediatric heart failure can only be implied by extrapolation of the 1997 U.S. Food and Drug Administration recommendations for adults, which state that digoxin can be used in symptomatic patients with heart failure in addition to diuretics, ACE inhibitors, and beta blockers.[21]

Diuretics

It is standard practice to use diuretics in virtually all children with heart failure. There are no pediatric studies showing that diuretic therapy reduces morbidity or mortality, but one adult study has shown that the diuretic spironolactone improves survival in adults with heart failure.[25]

Potent diuretics such as furosemide are widely used in heart failure treatment in childhood[26] and in the perioperative period when controlling fluid balance is crucial and renal function may be impaired. The intravenous route is preferred in these situations. Studies have shown that continuous infusion leads to smoother control of fluid and electrolyte shifts than intermittent intravenous bolus administration.[26]

Beta Blockers

Although there is increasing evidence of survival benefits accruing from beta-adrenergic blocker therapy in adults with moderate and severe heart failure,[27] evidence of similar benefits in children with heart failure is limited.[21,28,29] Although it might be reasonable to extrapolate adult survival advantages to older children with heart failure, extreme caution should be exercised in seeking to apply such therapy in the neonatal period.

Beta blockers have established roles in children in the management of hypertension and in the management of ventricular outflow tract obstruction, such as that which occurs in the tetralogy of Fallot.

Other Inotropic Agents

Triiodothyronine (T_3) has been shown in vitro and in animal studies to play an important role in up-regulating beta adrenoceptors and in increasing cardiac myocyte contractility.[30] Clinical studies have shown that T_3 supplementation can produce elevation in heart rate without concomitant decrease in systemic blood pressure[31] and may enhance cardiac functional reserve after CPB in infants. The calcium sensitizer levosimendan has both inotropic and peripheral vasodilating properties and has produced promising results in early adult studies.[32]

Pulmonary Vasodilators and Other Strategies to Prevent and Treat Pulmonary Hypertension

Oxygen alone is a potent dilator of the pulmonary vascular bed, with both high alveolar oxygen concentration and high systemic oxygen saturation having a favorable influence. PVR is also influenced by lung volume, being raised at both low and very high lung volumes. Most intravenously administered drugs used to treat pulmonary hypertension have nonselective effects, dilating both the pulmonary and systemic vascular beds. Tolazoline, prostaglandin E_1, and prostacyclin are among many agents that have been used as "pulmonary vasodilators." Prostacyclin is a short-acting vasodilator that acts via increasing levels of the intracellular messenger cyclic AMP, which has been widely used in the treatment of primary pulmonary hypertension in children.[33] In contrast, nitrates, nitroprusside, and, indeed, nitric oxide, act via the activation of guanylate cyclase and hence increase cellular levels of cyclic guanosine monophosphate, which is then inactivated by PDE type V. The pulmonary effects of intravenous vasodilators are frequently limited by their nonspecific action, leading to clinically important systemic hypotension.

Elevation of PVR is seen frequently in children after CPB,[19] which will exacerbate any underlying changes in pulmonary hemodynamics.[34] Reactive postoperative pulmonary hypertensive episodes typically occur in children after correction of left-to-right shunt lesions or in those with preoperative pulmonary venous hypertension. These "crises" are particularly associated with long CPB durations. In the current era, early corrective surgery has dramatically reduced the numbers of infants in whom pulmonary hypertension is a major perioperative issue. Postoperative pulmonary hypertension is still seen

TABLE 101–6. STRATEGIES TO PREVENT AND TREAT PULMONARY HYPERTENSION

Strategy	Comment
Perform anatomic investigation.	Rules out residual or undiagnosed anatomic abnormalities.
Permit right-to-left decompression.	Deliberate residual atrial septal defect acts as "pop off" in at-risk situations.
Provide analgesia/sedation.	Facilitates ventilation. Minimizes sympathetic influences.
Avoid acidosis.	Respiratory and metabolic acidosis raises pulmonary vascular resistance.
Maintain oxygenation.	Normal/high alveolar and mixed venous Po_2 lowers pulmonary vascular resistance.
Optimize hematocrit.	Ensures optimal oxygen delivery and higher mixed venous Po_2.
Optimize cardiac output.	Ensures optimal oxygen delivery and higher mixed venous Po_2.
Use pulmonary vasodilators.	Selectively reduces pulmonary vascular resistance.

in neonates and infants in association with lesions such as obstructed total anomalous pulmonary venous drainage, truncus arteriosus, and mitral valve replacement for congenital mitral stenosis. Children with lesser elevations in PVR may also benefit from pulmonary vasodilatation, including children with predominant RV dysfunction, for instance after cardiac transplantation[35] and in Fontan circulations and relatively high PVR.[36] General measures associated with the prevention and treatment of pulmonary hypertension should be considered before deploying specific pulmonary vasodilators (Table 101-6). In patients at high risk of pulmonary hypertension after cardiac surgery, LV filling can be maintained by right-to-left shunting through a small, surgically created atrial septal defect (ASD). Right-to-left shunt acts as a safety valve; and although some systemic desaturation occurs, LV filling and hence cardiac output are maintained.

Nitric oxide is an endogenous endothelial-derived vasodilator and a gas at room temperature. If added to inhaled gas mixtures in children with reactive pulmonary hypertension it induces selective pulmonary vasodilatation.[37] It is distributed to ventilated alveoli, from where it diffuses into the adjacent pulmonary arteriolar smooth muscle. Inhaled nitric oxide has been shown in randomized controlled trials to be effective and safe therapy in neonates with PPHN. Although the evidence for outcome benefit is limited to one randomized controlled study,[38] there is a substantial body of evidence to show that inhaled nitric oxide is effective in pediatric cardiac patients, including those with acute postoperative pulmonary hypertension after congenital heart surgery[39] and after pediatric heart transplantation. Inhaled nitric oxide can be used in the preoperative assessment of patients with pulmonary hypertension.[40]

Other candidate selective pulmonary vasodilators that are undergoing investigation in children include inhaled prostacyclin,[41] the PDE type V inhibitor sildenafil,[42] and bosentan, an endothelin-1 receptor blocker.[43]

MECHANICAL CIRCULATORY SUPPORT

Extracorporeal membrane oxygenation (ECMO) is a technically mature technique that has been used to support over 18,000 neonates with respiratory failure in whom survival rates of 70% to 80% are expected. Its use in this indication is supported by randomized controlled trials that demonstrate good short- and medium-term outcomes.[44] ECMO and ventricular-assist devices (VADs) have also been used to provide temporary circulatory support in children with intractable circulatory failure (see Chapter 70). Reported indications include severe ventricular failure, refractory arrhythmias, and cardiac arrest. The aim of mechanical circulatory support in such circumstances is to provide optimal cardiac output while resting the heart, awaiting its recovery, or to achieve survival by successful support of the child to cardiac transplantation. Single-center series[45] and collaborative registry figures[46] of ECMO or VAD for acute postoperative indications report similar figures for survival to hospital discharge (~40%) in children who it is assumed would not have survived without mechanical support. Rapid deployment ECMO has been reported as an effective intervention for the management of cardiac arrest in the pediatric cardiac ICU.[47] Hospital survival figures for CPR-ECMO seem encouraging,[47] but long-term neurodevelopmental follow-up studies are urgently needed before such strategies can be recommended unequivocally.

CARDIOMYOPATHIES

The two most common causes of heart failure in children are congenital heart disease and cardiomyopathy. Cardiomyopathies are primary myocardial diseases of either known or unknown cause characterized by left or biventricular dilatation and impaired contractility and occur in children and adults of all ages.

Nugent and colleagues reported the incidence of pediatric cardiomyopathy in a 10-year population-based study of Australian children as 1.24 cases per 100,000 children younger than 10 years of age,[48] a remarkably similar finding to a recently reported U.S. study.[49] Of 314 cases of cardiomyopathy reported by Nugent and colleagues, 184 of 314 (59%) were dilated cardiomyopathy, 80 (25%) were hypertrophic cardiomyopathy, 8 (2.5%) were restrictive cardiomyopathy, and 42 (13%) were unclassified, of which 29 (69%) exhibited LV noncompaction. Twenty percent of cardiomyopathy in this study was classified as familial, and in 8.9% specific mitochondrial or metabolic disease etiologically linked to cardiomyopathy was identified. Of the children in Nugent's study who underwent myocardial biopsy, 40.3% had histologic evidence of lymphocytic myocarditis according to the Dallas criteria,[50] which contrasts to an incidence of lymphocytic myocarditis in adult studies of only 10%.[51]

Presentation

Most children present with signs and symptoms of heart failure, including dyspnea, upper abdominal discomfort, nausea, and vomiting. Abdominal symptoms are often misdiagnosed as indicative of gastroenteritis, although the astute clinician will note the absence of diarrhea. It is presumed that these abdominal symptoms result from hepatic congestion and gut edema as a result of right-sided heart failure or ischemia (from splanchnic vasoconstriction). A history of an antecedent flu-like illness is strongly suggestive of a diagnosis of myocarditis. Some children with myocarditis follow a fulminant course typified by rapid onset of cardiogenic shock.[52,53]

The chest radiograph in the patient who presents acutely with a cardiomyopathy typically shows cardiomegaly and pulmonary venous congestion. An echocardiogram will reveal left atrial and ventricular dilatation and impaired systolic and diastolic function and often mitral or tricuspid regurgitation. ECG features are mostly nonspecific and include ST segment and T wave changes and arrhythmias. The presence of Q waves may indicate anomalous origin of the left coronary artery from pulmonary artery (ALCAPA). If ALCAPA cannot be unequivocally excluded by echocardiography, coronary angiography must be undertaken.

As cardiomyopathies result from a variety of acquired or inherited disorders, the differentiation of secondary (and possibly treatable causes of dilated cardiomyopathy) from the idiopathic form of the disease is of the greatest importance. Endomyocardial biopsies can be obtained to assist in the diagnosis of myocarditis and other specific myocardial diseases.

Prognosis

Recent studies have reported 5-year survival rates in childhood cardiomyopathy of 64% to 84%, although the impact of cardiac transplantation on survival rates is not clear in all studies. In contrast to myocarditis, sudden death is uncommon in children with other forms of dilated cardiomyopathy. Children with cardiomyopathies who fail to respond to conservative treatment and especially those with ongoing requirement for intravenous inotropic support, ventilatory support, or mechanical circulatory support and children with recurrent arrhythmias are candidates for early cardiac transplantation. Late recovery of ventricular function is however possible.[54] The prognosis for cardiomyopathy due to myocarditis in children appears to differ from that in adults, with survival of up to 80% among children who reach hospital alive.[55,56] Many children who survive the acute phase go on to recover normal cardiac function, in marked contrast to adults in whom mortality rates of 20% at 1 year increase to 56% at 5 years.[51]

ICU Management of Dilated Cardiomyopathy and Myocarditis

In children presenting with acute heart failure, hypotension, or cardiogenic shock, beta-adrenergic agonists may improve systolic ventricular function. PDE type III inhibitors such as milrinone are of hemodynamic benefit in acute heart failure, although large trials in adult heart failure have failed to show clear benefit from chronic administration.[57] Although metoprolol and carvedilol may be of benefit in chronic heart failure,[21,28,29] they should be avoided in hemodynamically unstable children. Nasal or mask continuous positive airway pressure (CPAP) has been shown to result in symptomatic improvement both by unloading of respiratory muscles and by lowering of LV afterload as a consequence of raising intrathoracic pressure.[58] Children in severe heart failure have high SVRs and no ventricular reserve. Great care is therefore needed if sedative agents are administered to facilitate tracheal intubation or ICU procedures. Agents with the least effects on the cardiovascular system should be chosen and allowance made for slow circulatory times when titrating sedative doses.

The use of mechanical circulatory support with ECMO or ventricular assist systems can be lifesaving in children with myocarditis or cardiomyopathy who develop cardiogenic shock.[59] A high proportion of children who receive mechanical support for fulminant myocarditis will recover ventricular function. Those who do not may be "bridged" to cardiac transplantation. Clearly, survival with a recovered native ventricle is a better outcome for a child than survival by means of cardiac transplantation. A multicenter series[56] documented a median time to return of ventricular function of 9 days in those who survived without transplantation. The absolute time limits for recovery of native ventricular function have not been established, although pragmatic decisions on whether to proceed to cardiac transplantation should probably be made if cardiac recovery has not occurred after 10 to 14 days of support.

Congenital Heart Disease

Congenital heart disease (CHD) classified as moderate or severe is detected in approximately 6 of 1000 live births, of whom between 2 and 3 will require expert cardiologic care soon after birth. The presence of extracardiac anomalies in children is associated with poorer outcomes.[54] Syndromes associated with cardiovascular involvement are of particular significance to the pediatric intensivist who must coordinate the cardiac and extracardiac aspects of care.[60] Trisomy 21 (Down syndrome) is associated with a high incidence of congenital heart disease, in particular, atrioventriculoseptal defects. Deletion of the q11 region of chromosome 22 is associated with a spectrum of cardiac (conotruncal defects, e.g., truncus arteriosus, hypoplastic left heart syndrome) and extracardiac abnormalities.[61] Of the latter, thymic aplasia places infants at risk for hypocalcemia secondary to hypoparathyroidism and impaired cellular immunity.

Many classifications of congenital heart lesions have been proposed. Although a sequential approach to the description of cardiac anatomy is most frequently employed by pediatric cardiologists, a broader physiologic approach is more useful to the nonspecialist. It is beyond the scope of this chapter to present a detailed overview of all aspects of congenital heart disease. A brief overview is presented, focusing on common lesions and information of particular importance to intensivists. Readers are directed elsewhere for more detailed coverage of pediatric cardiology,[62] pediatric cardiac surgery,[63] and pediatric cardiac intensive care.[64]

LESIONS WITH PREDOMINANT LEFT-TO-RIGHT SHUNT

VSD is the archetypal lesion associated with left-to-right shunting of blood. VSDs may occur in isolation or in association with other cardiac anomalies. Ventricular output will follow the path of least resistance, resulting in blood shunting across the defect and into the lungs as the PVR is lower than the SVR. The magnitude of the shunt, usually expressed as the ratio of pulmonary blood flow to systemic blood flow (Qp:Qs), depends on the size of the VSD and the level of the PVR. Small-diameter defects offer resistance at the level of the ventricular septum, limiting flow from the LV to RV and maintaining a pressure gradient between the two chambers. Larger-diameter defects are unrestrictive, with no pressure gradient between the two ventricles; and in this situation, flow is solely dependent on the ratio of PVR to SVR. Small restrictive VSDs rarely result in symptoms in infancy, typically presenting when a cardiac murmur is detected as an incidental finding. Infants with larger "unrestrictive" VSDs gradually develop congestive cardiac failure owing to the increase in pulmonary blood flow that occurs as the developmental fall in PVR occurs in the first weeks of life.[65] Thus, the consequences of a moderate or large "unrestrictive" VSD are increased pulmonary blood flow (high Qp:Qs) and extra volume work demanded of the LV. The volume overload of the LV results in LV enlargement and failure. If large left-to-right shunts are left untreated, PVR gradually rises. Although the initial rise is the result of pulmonary arteriolar muscular hypertrophy that is reversible, irreversible pulmonary vascular obstructive disease[66] eventually ensues and may result in the onset of right-to-left shunt (Eisenmenger's syndrome). For this reason, steps must be taken in all children with congenital heart lesions and raised pulmonary blood flow to correct the lesion or protect the lungs by either a corrective procedure or a palliative procedure such as pulmonary artery banding before severe pulmonary vascular changes develop. With the exception of isolated ASDs, most left-to-right shunt lesions that require surgical intervention present in the first year of life as heart failure and are associated with development of pulmonary hypertension. The principal lesions are described next.

VENTRICULAR SEPTAL DEFECT

Anatomy
VSDs occur in any part of the interventricular septum and are classified by location.[67,68]

Pathophysiology
Left-to-right shunting at ventricular level leads to left atrial dilatation, LV volume overload, and increased pulmonary blood flow. The degree of left-to-right shunt is determined by the size of the defect and the PVR. If a defect is "small," shunt flow is determined mainly by the size of the defect. Left-to-right flow across larger "unrestrictive" defects is determined principally by PVR—the lower the PVR, the greater will be the shunt and pulmonary blood flow.

Many small VSDs close spontaneously,[69] but if closure does not occur, infants with unrestrictive defects will fail to thrive and develop congestive heart failure as the PVR falls in early infancy. Untreated VSD leads to pulmonary hypertension and eventual progression to fixed pulmonary vascular obstructive disease. Eventually pulmonary artery pressure and vascular resistance exceeds that of the systemic circulation, leading to shunt reversal and cyanosis (Eisenmenger's syndrome). Patients with a fixed high PVR are not suitable for VSD closure because the RV will not tolerate the excessive afterload of the hypertensive pulmonary vascular bed.

Surgery
Most VSDs are repaired as a primary procedure.[70] Occasionally, pulmonary artery banding is undertaken to reduce pulmonary blood flow and protect the pulmonary vascular bed in neonates in whom primary repair is a high risk. This may be the case with complex conditions such as multiple defects and in very small premature infants. These conservative strategies are questioned by some surgeons.[71,72] VSDs are usually closed surgically on CPB using a sutured patch. Some defects can be closed at cardiac catheterization with an occlusion device.[68]

Postoperative Management
Most children undergoing elective VSD closure progress rapidly to extubation. Patients with severe cardiac failure or high pulmonary artery pressures preoperatively benefit from a more cautious approach in the early postoperative period

as do those with complex associated lesions. Low cardiac output or pulmonary edema may be noted in the early postoperative period as a consequence of generalized myocardial hypocontractility or due to the presence of a residual VSD. Pulmonary hypertension is relatively rare in the current era of "early" primary repair of VSD. Cases presenting late may have pulmonary hypertension, and life-threatening pulmonary hypertensive "crises" can occur in the postoperative period. Surgically placed pulmonary artery catheters greatly assist in the early detection and management of such episodes.[73] Junctional ectopic tachycardia (JET)[74,75] and complete heart block are generic risks of surgery in the vicinity of the ventricular septum. Compete heart block may be transient, but if atrioventricular synchrony has not returned by 7 to 10 days, a permanent pacing system is required.[76]

ATRIAL SEPTAL DEFECT

Anatomy
Anatomically, interatrial communications are of four types. Ostium secundum defects are the most common form of ASD and are centrally located in the atrial septum. Ostium primum type defects are part of the atrioventriculoseptal defect spectrum (see later). Sinus venosus defects occur close to the right atrium/superior vena cava or right atrium/inferior vena cava junction and are commonly associated with partial anomalous pulmonary venous drainage. Coronary sinus defects describe a type of ASD associated with absence of the wall between the left atrium and coronary sinus that allows left atrial blood to reach the right atrium via the coronary sinus.[67,77]

Pathophysiology
Left-to-right shunting of blood at atrial level leads to right atrial and ventricular dilatation with increased pulmonary blood flow. Congestive heart failure occurs in up to 5% of children with ASD in the first year of life. Pulmonary hypertension in association with ASD is relatively rare in childhood, with an incidence of 13% in unoperated children younger than age 10 years, although if defects are not closed, patients may progress to irreversible pulmonary hypertension.[78] Occasionally, infants or young children with primary pulmonary hypertension, pulmonary hypoplasia, or similar conditions present with apparently symptomatic ASD with right-to-left shunting. In these situations, the ASD is beneficial, decompressing the right side of the heart, with symptoms being a consequence of pulmonary hypertension rather than simply the presence of an ASD.

ASD CLOSURE

Centrally located secundum ASDs are frequently closed by placement of an ASD closure device at cardiac catheterization.[79] Large defects and non-secundum defects are closed surgically using CPB. Defects are typically closed if a child becomes symptomatic or electively between 3 and 5 years of age. There is essentially no mortality risk associated with closure of an isolated ASD, and good long-term morbidity-free survival is expected.[80]

Postprocedure Management
The vast majority of elective ASD closures progress rapidly to extubation post procedure (hours). Specific

postoperative problems seen after ASD closure include the following:

1. *Sinoatrial node dysfunction* manifests as an inappropriate chronotropic response or as atrial or junctional arrhythmias. The problem is caused either by direct trauma to the sinoatrial node or by interruption to its blood supply during surgery.
2. *Postpericardotomy syndrome* manifests as fever, malaise, lymphocytosis, nausea, vomiting, or abdominal pain in the weeks after surgery. The symptoms are caused by a sterile inflammatory process that can cause pericardial fluid to accumulate to the point at which pericardial tamponade is manifest. A history of recent cardiac surgery with symptoms as just mentioned should raise the suspicion of the syndrome and of potential tamponade, particularly if cardiomegaly is present on a chest radiograph.
3. *Pulmonary hypertension* is relatively rare in children after ASD repair. A previously undiagnosed ASD presenting in adulthood is more likely to be associated with pulmonary hypertension.
4. *Obstruction of pulmonary veins or vena cava* may occur in association with repair of sinus venosus defects.
5. *LV dysfunction* may occur. Transiently elevated left atrial pressure and pulmonary edema are occasionally seen after ASD closure in older patients owing to chronic RV overload and decreased LV compliance.

ATRIOVENTRICULOSEPTAL DEFECT (AVSD)

Anatomy

AVSDs result from failure of the lower part of the atrial septum to fuse with the upper part of the ventricular septum.[77] The hallmark of all AVSDs is the presence of a common atrioventricular (AV) junction and valve with two bridging and three smaller leaflets. The common AV valve has varying degrees of competence. There are three potential components of this defect, an ostium primum ASD, a VSD, and abnormal formation of the AV valves. The condition presents as partial AVSD (sometimes referred to as primum ASD), in which an ASD and cleft AV valve are present, and complete AVSD, which in addition has a VSD. AVSD-spectrum lesions commonly occur in children with Down syndrome.

Pathophysiology

Partial defects behave like a secundum ASD with left-to-right shunt at atrial level causing right atrial and RV volume overload. Associated incompetence of the left AV valve may lead to significant regurgitation and worsening symptoms. In complete defects, left-to-right shunting of blood at the ventricular level leads to congestive heart failure by about 2 months of age. Pulmonary hypertension and pulmonary vascular obliterative disease occur if repair is not undertaken by age 6 to 9 months.

Surgery

Partial or complete AVSDs are repaired under CPB. Partial defects are usually repaired electively at between 1 and 5 years,[81] whereas complete defects are usually repaired at 3 to 6 months to avoid severe pulmonary hypertensive complications.[82,83]

Postoperative Management

Afterload reduction with sodium nitroprusside or milrinone is useful if significant AV valve regurgitation is present post

repair. Problems seen after AVSD surgery include pulmonary hypertension,[84] which is however uncommon in the current era of early surgical repair. Residual lesions such as residual left AV valve regurgitation or residual VSD will slow postoperative recovery and require prompt diagnosis and aggressive management, including reoperation if necessary. Elevated left atrial pressure after AVSD repair can occur because of the presence of residual left AV valve regurgitation, left AV valve stenosis, LV outflow tract obstruction, residual VSD, and LV myocardial dysfunction. The precise cause of elevated left atrial pressure must be diagnosed and appropriate management instituted.

PATENT DUCTUS ARTERIOSUS (PDA)

Anatomy

A ductus arteriosus is a vascular communication, necessary in the fetal circulation, between the junction of the main and left pulmonary arteries and the lesser curvature of the aorta, which normally closes within 2 weeks of birth. Persistent patency occurs as an isolated defect, in premature neonates, and in association with other congenital heart lesions.

Pathophysiology

The key pathophysiologic abnormality in PDA, as in VSD, is left-to-right shunting leading to increased pulmonary blood flow, pulmonary hypertension, and LV volume overload. Neonates with this condition usually present with congestive heart failure, apneas, or respiratory problems. In term infants and older children, isolated PDA may present incidentally or with the onset of cardiac failure or problems with recurrent pulmonary infections. Pulmonary hypertension progressing to pulmonary vascular obstructive disease can occur within the first year of life, with the rate of onset of symptoms depending on the size of the duct.

Management

Indomethacin or ibuprofen is used to induce closure of patent ductus in premature neonates, acting through inhibition of the vasodilatory prostaglandin production, with success in approximately 70% of cases.[85] Transcutaneous catheter occlusion can be effective in suitable cases, with a low incidence of associated complications. Surgical ligation or division is required in very small subjects[86] and in older children with large ducts in whom occlusion devices cannot be safely deployed. Surgical closure is carried out via a lateral thoracotomy or as a video-assisted thoracoscopic procedure.[87]

Postprocedural Issues

The principal complications of conservative treatment of PDA with indomethacin or ibuprofen in preterm neonates are failure to induce closure and renal failure.[85] Surgical approaches may be complicated by occlusion failure and complications of thoracotomy, including infection and hemorrhage. Adjacent structures including the thoracic duct, phrenic nerve, and the recurrent laryngeal nerve may be damaged during surgery. Complications after transcatheter closure include residual shunt, embolization of closure device, and hemolysis.

TRUNCUS ARTERIOSUS

Truncus arteriosus is caused by the failure of the common arterial trunk to divide into the aorta and pulmonary artery.

Anatomy

A single arterial vessel originates from both ventricles, overriding the ventricular septum and supplying the coronary, pulmonary, and systemic circulations. Anatomic variations depend on the respective origins of the right and left branch pulmonary arteries from the common arterial trunk, main pulmonary artery, or aorta. A VSD lies immediately below a single ventriculoarterial truncal valve that is commonly dysplastic, leading to stenosis or regurgitation. Coronary artery abnormalities are common and may lead to difficulties when conducting surgical repair. Ten to 15 percent of patients have associated hypoplasia, coarctation, or interruption of the aortic arch, and a small proportion have stenosis or hypoplasia of the pulmonary arteries.

Aortopulmonary window is a rare lesion in which an abnormal vascular communication exists between the ascending aorta and the main pulmonary artery. Like truncus, this lesion is associated with 22q11 chromosomal deletion.[61,88]

Pathophysiology

The RV and LV are pressure and volume overloaded, particularly if truncal valve stenosis or regurgitation is present. Runoff into the pulmonary circulation due to low PVR and into the ventricles due to truncal valve regurgitation leads to a low diastolic pressure, which in the presence of high ventricular end-diastolic pressures may exacerbate myocardial ischemia. Pulmonary blood flow depends on the PVR and the presence or absence of stenoses in the proximal pulmonary arteries. Most commonly, therefore, pulmonary overcirculation and congestive heart failure result as PVR falls in the first weeks of life. The defect is commonly associated with 22q11 chromosomal deletion (DiGeorge syndrome, Shprintzen's syndrome). The important clinical manifestations associated with these include scanty or absent T cells[61,88] and the consequent risk of graft-versus-host reactions if transfused with viable leukocytes. Irradiation of all blood products is recommended unless normal T-cell status is confirmed.

Surgery

The pulmonary arteries are removed from the arterial trunk, leaving a vessel that becomes the neoaorta.[89,90] A valved conduit is then placed from the RV to the pulmonary arteries, and the VSD is closed. Mortality risk is less than 10% if the truncal valve is functionally normal, no other lesions are present, and the child is of an acceptable weight. Long-term results are encouraging, although the valved conduit will require upsizing during childhood.[91]

Postoperative Management

Specific postoperative problems associated with repair of truncus include pulmonary hypertension[84] and low cardiac output.[12] Inotropic support is required routinely, and delayed sternal closure may be employed to prevent tissue tamponade in the early postoperative period. Intensivists must be aware of the possibility of right-to-left shunting because surgeons may leave a smaller interatrial communication to decompress the RV. Failure to appreciate this mechanism may lead to an inappropriate focus on pulmonary causes of cyanosis. Right bundle branch block is common after truncus repair owing to the surgical right ventriculotomy. Heart block and atrial or junctional arrhythmias are also seen.

LEFT-SIDED HEART OBSTRUCTION

Obstruction to the exit of blood from the LV can occur at subvalvular, valvular, or supravalvular levels or more distally in the aortic arch. Infants with severe obstruction of the aortic valve or arch present in the neonatal period with either heart failure or cardiogenic shock. Aortic coarctation, aortic interruption, and critical aortic stenosis are associated with a duct-dependent systemic circulation and typically present in the first few days of life as the arterial duct closes. Less severe obstruction may be detected later as an incidental finding (murmur) or with the gradual onset of signs and symptoms, including those of LV failure. Chronic obstruction to LV outflow causes LV hypertrophy; and whereas systolic function may initially be well preserved, reduced diastolic compliance may occur early in the clinical course. If the obstruction is unrelieved, the subendocardial region becomes ischemic and endocardial fibrosis occurs. Papillary muscle ischemia may also occur and results in acquired mitral valve regurgitation.

VALVULAR AORTIC STENOSIS

Anatomy

Approximately 70% of aortic stenosis occurs only at the valvar level. Valvar aortic stenosis may be associated with other abnormalities, however, including supravalvar aortic stenosis, mitral valve anomalies, aortic insufficiency, and endocardial fibroelastosis. In neonatal aortic stenosis, the LV and other left-sided structures may be hypoplastic.

Pathophysiology

Neonates with clinically apparent valvular aortic stenosis present with acute LV failure or shock. Systemic perfusion may be maintained by right-to-left shunting of blood across a patent ductus with consequent systemic desaturation and the risk of reduced systemic perfusion if the ductus closes spontaneously. The LV exhibits poor performance in both diastole and systole, and as a consequence there are high left atrial pressures. Pulmonary edema is a prominent clinical feature. End organ ischemic damage including renal failure and necrotizing enterocolitis are frequently seen as a consequence of poor systemic perfusion. Less severe aortic stenosis typically presents later in infancy or childhood with exercise-induced syncope, chest pain, or sudden death. In these patients, concentric LV hypertrophy induced by chronic pressure overload is usually seen.

Surgery

A number of treatment options are available, with the choice of procedure dependent on age, clinical status of the child at presentation, associated anomalies, and anatomic complexity. The simplest procedure, percutaneous balloon valvotomy, is appropriate in patients with mild to moderate stenosis and favorable aortic valve anatomy.[92] Open aortic valve surgery is an alternative to balloon valvoplasty and may be favored if additional procedures (e.g., duct ligation) are required. If the native aortic valve cannot be salvaged or reconstructed, surgical choices include replacement of the aortic valve with a homograft or valved conduit or placement of the patient's own pulmonary valve into the aortic position with associated pulmonary homograft autograft (the Ross procedure).[93,94] A variant of the Ross procedure, the Ross-Konno procedure,[95] is indicated for complex LV outflow tract obstruction in which in addition to the Ross operation, annular enlargement or aortoventriculoplasty is undertaken.[94]

Postoperative Management

Most neonates presenting in heart failure or shock who undergo urgent procedures remain critically ill postoperatively and require ongoing multiorgan support.[96] If low cardiac output persists after repair, residual aortic stenosis or regurgitation must be excluded. Inotropic and vasodilator support of the failing myocardium should be guided by serial hemodynamic and echocardiographic evaluations. Relief of aortic stenosis in older children may be associated with systemic hypertension secondary to the unrestrained force of contraction of the hypertrophied LV. Children undergoing prosthetic valve replacement require long-term anticoagulation therapy.[97]

SUBVALVULAR AORTIC STENOSIS

Subaortic stenosis is seen in various forms including a fibrous diaphragm-like ring with a central orifice, a fibro-muscular tunnel (frequently associated with hypoplasia of ascending aorta and LV anomalies), or simply as dynamic obstruction due to hypertrophy of the LV outflow.[98]

Subaortic stenosis presents in neonates in association with other lesions including malalignment-type VSD, double-outlet RV, and aortic or aortic valvular lesions or as an isolated lesion in childhood.

Pathophysiology

Similar to valvular aortic stenosis, pressure overload in LV leads to hypertrophy with resultant raised pressure overload.

Surgery

The choice of surgical procedure depends on the anatomic substrate. Membranous subaortic stenosis requires simple resection. The tunnel form may be suitable for resection or require a more extensive Konno or Ross-Konno[94] type procedure. Finally, the hypertrophic form of subaortic stenosis requires a Ross-Konno operation with resection of LV myocardium.[99]

The perioperative course is usually uneventful after resection of membranous subaortic stenosis with mortality below 5%, although late recurrence is common. After surgery for tunnel and hypertrophic forms of subaortic stenosis the recovery pathway is determined by the age of the child, the nature and complexity of surgery performed, and, most critical of all, the presence of existing LV dysfunction. Specific postoperative problems include residual LV outflow tract stenosis, mitral regurgitation, VSD with left-to-right and left bundle branch block, or complete heart block secondary to resection of LV myocardium.

SUPRAVALVULAR AORTIC STENOSIS

Supravalvular aortic stenosis occurs in isolation and in association with Williams syndrome (supravalvular aortic stenosis, RV outflow tract obstruction (RVOTO), peripheral pulmonary stenoses, renal artery stenoses).[100-102] It may be a localized or diffuse narrowing above the sinotubular junction. The stenosis is occasionally associated with a hypoplastic ascending aorta, and there may be compromise to coronary filling.

Pathophysiology

Similar to valvular aortic stenosis, pressure overload in the LV leads to hypertrophy with resultant raised pressure overload. In addition, coronary arteries fill under high pressure and may become tortuous and dysplastic.

Surgery

Patch angioplasty is performed in most cases.[103]

Postoperative Management

Postoperative course is usually uneventful. Specific postoperative problems include residual aortic or LV outflow tract stenosis leading to cardiac failure and coronary ischemia that occurs if the repair has disturbed the coronary arteries or if LV hypertension and LV subendocardial ischemia persist.

AORTIC COARCTATION

Anatomy

A constriction of the thoracic aorta occurs in the region of the left subclavian artery where the ligamentum arteriosum originates. The complexity of the lesion varies from a discrete narrowing to more extensive aortic arch hypoplasia extending back to proximal aortic arch. Coarctation commonly coexists with VSD and can also be associated with other left-sided lesions, including aortic and mitral valve stenosis.[104]

Pathophysiology

In the neonatal presentation of aortic coarctation, a normal circulation is maintained until ductal tissue contracts, at which point distal aortic flow is severely reduced, leading to a clinical presentation of heart failure or shock and characteristic loss of lower limb pulses.[105] Prostaglandin E_1 or E_2 infusion should be started as soon as the diagnosis of a duct-dependent lesion is suspected, to reopen or maintain patency of the ductus arteriosus. After initial resuscitation, urinary output and resolution of metabolic acidosis are early indicators of successful reperfusion of the distal aorta. Early surgical repair is indicated.

Beyond the early neonatal period, aortic coarctation presents as progressive onset of cardiac failure or as an incidental finding (murmur, upper limb hypertension, absent weak femoral pulses) later in childhood. Thoracic aortic collaterals develop and may be noted as rib notching on a plain chest radiograph.

Surgery

Surgical resection of the narrowed aortic segment and associated ductal tissue and either end-to-end anastomosis or subclavian flap angioplasty are used to repair coarctation in the newborn, without CPB.[63] If aortic arch hypoplasia is more extensive, a homograft or prosthetic tube graft may be incorporated in the repair and CPB may be required.[106] Neonatal coarctation associated with VSD can be palliated by resection of the coarctation and banding of the pulmonary artery to restrict pulmonary blood flow, with delayed VSD repair. Alternatively, both lesions can be corrected in the neonatal period. The mortality rate for repair of neonatal coarctation is low. Kanter and colleagues reported 91% survival in a series that included both isolated and complex coarctation.[107] In older children it is less than 1%, although paraplegia secondary to interruption of spinal cord perfusion remains a concern.

Balloon angioplasty is frequently used to alleviate recurrent aortic coarctation and is increasingly being used with apparent success to address native coarctation particularly in older patients but is not favored in symptomatic neonates.[104,108]

Postoperative Management

Specific postoperative problems include systemic hypertension, which is thought to be due to multiple factors, including altered baroceptor and adrenal catecholamine and renin-angiotensin axes.[109,110] Persistent hypertension is less common after neonatal repair and when present it usually responds to short-term vasodilator therapy.[109,111] Additional beta-adrenergic blockade (esmolol,[112] propranolol, or labetalol) may be required, particularly with late-presenting coarctation. Some children have persistent hypertension after repair[113] and require long-term antihypertensive therapy. Postcoarctectomy syndrome[114] occurs in older patients and is thought to be the result of restoration of higher-pressure pulsatile flow to the mesenteric arterial tree and presents as abdominal distention, abdominal pain, ascites, or, occasionally, enteric infarction. The condition is best managed by avoiding enteral feeding for 24 hours after repair and aggressive treatment of systemic hypertension. The necessity of aortic clamping during surgical repair interrupts distal aortic flow and may result in spinal cord ischemia (rare in neonates, 0.4% incidence in older patients) or renal ischemia. The intensivist must seek positive confirmation of lower limb movement and adequate renal function in the early postoperative period. In neonates,[115] low cardiac output may persist owing to preexisting ventricular dysfunction, although residual coarctation should be excluded. Structures near the aortic arch prone to surgical injury include the thoracic duct, recurrent laryngeal nerve, and the phrenic nerve, leading to postoperative chylothorax, stridor, or hemidiaphragm paralysis.

INTERRUPTED AORTIC ARCH

Anatomy

In this condition the aortic arch is either atretic or interrupted, creating either complete disruption or luminal obstruction (without external interruption). A patent arterial duct is necessary to maintain perfusion of the distal aortic arch, closure of which leads to emergent presentation. A VSD and obstruction of the LV outflow tract commonly coexist. The more common form of interrupted aortic arch (type B) is associated with 22q11 chromosomal deletion (see earlier).[61,88]

Pathophysiology

Interrupted aortic arch should be regarded as a severe form of aortic coarctation, with duct-dependent distal aortic perfusion, and requires similar initial management.[105]

Surgery

Surgical reconstruction of the aortic arch and closure of the associated VSD are usually undertaken under CPB in the neonatal period.

Specific postoperative problems seen after repair of interrupted aortic arch include pulmonary hypertension, residual aortic arch obstruction, and residual VSD. There is a risk of transfusion-associated graft-versus-host disease and hypocalcemia in children with type B interrupted aortic arch with 22q11 deletion and DiGeorge phenotype.[116]

TOTAL ANOMALOUS PULMONARY VENOUS CONNECTION (TAPVC)

Anatomy

All of the pulmonary veins drain anomalously into a systemic venous structure and subsequently to the right atrium rather than directly into the left atrium. In supracardiac TAPVC (45% of cases) the pulmonary veins drain via a vertical vein to the innominate vein or connect directly into the SVC. In intracardiac TAPVC (25% of cases) the venous confluence drains via the coronary sinus into the RA, and in infracardiac TAPVC (25% of cases) the veins drain into the IVC or portal veins. Mixed forms also exist (5% of cases).[117] TAPVC is associated with an obligate ASD to allow mixing of systemic and pulmonary venous return to access the LV and systemic circulation.

Pathophysiology

Two patterns emerge depending on presence of obstruction to the pulmonary venous return. Obstruction of the pulmonary venous pathway is common and causes pulmonary venous hypertension, pulmonary venous edema, reflex pulmonary artery vasoconstriction, and subsequent right-sided heart failure. If obstruction is not present, the main pathophysiologic effects result from complete mixing of systemic and pulmonary venous blood in the right side of the heart with RV volume overload and failure.

Surgery

The pulmonary veins are anastomosed or baffled into the left atrium. In the current era the expected operative mortality is less than 5%,[118] although higher risks are reported in complex cases with associated lesions.[119]

Pulmonary hypertension, which may on occasion be severe or even life threatening, occurs frequently in infants after surgery for obstructed anomalous pulmonary veins.[84] If high pulmonary artery pressure occurs postoperatively it is essential to rule out residual pulmonary venous obstruction. Late re-stenosis is seen in up to 10% of cases and carries a poor prognosis, often related to a progressive fibrotic process occluding the lumen of the pulmonary veins.[120]

CYANOTIC LESIONS

TETRALOGY OF FALLOT

Anatomy

Tetralogy of Fallot (TOF) was initially described in the 19th century as an association of four anatomic findings: VSD, subpulmonary stenosis, aortic override of the ventricular septum, and RV hypertrophy.[63] The four lesions are actually the result of just one central problem, anterior and superior malalignment of the infundibular septum with respect to the muscular septum, which creates an obstruction in the RV outflow tract and leads to the four features seen.

Pathophysiology

Preoperative physiology depends mainly on the degree of RVOTO. Patients with minimal RVOTO have unrestricted pulmonary blood flow with left-to-right shunt through the VSD. Conversely, patients with severe obstruction will be cyanosed with saturations in the 70% to 80% range preoperatively as a result of right-to-left shunting across the VSD. RVOTO is often dynamic and may cause profound cyanosis (hypercyanotic spells), which requires treatment aimed at alleviating the dynamic RVOTO and maintaining right-sided heart output. Treatment of such episodes requires oxygen, sedation, and volume expansion. The knee-chest and over-shoulder positions compress the liver and increase RV filling. If such maneuvers fail, beta blockade (propranolol, 0.1 mg/kg) or vasoconstriction (e.g., phenylephrine, 5 to 20 μg/kg i.v.) may be required; and, as a last resort, preoperative ECMO support may be required.

Surgery

The timing and type of surgical intervention in TOF is controversial.[121] Complete repair is usually undertaken in the first year of life.[122,123] Some centers adopt a two-stage approach with initial placement of a modified Blalock-Taussig shunt in cyanotic infants. Complete repair is then undertaken when the child is bigger.

Residual VSD is poorly tolerated after TOF repair and requires early surgical closure. Moderate degrees of residual RVOTO may be well tolerated in the early postoperative period, but severe residual obstruction demands early re-investigation and reoperation with placement of a larger RV outflow tract patch or valved RV-PA conduit. All patients with a RV incision develop right bundle branch block. Junctional ectopic tachycardia is poorly tolerated after TOF repair.[74] Low cardiac output due to RV dysfunction is relatively common and should be suspected if the child is hypotensive, is tachycardic, and has a raised central venous pressure and hepatomegaly. The problem is predominantly one of poor RV compliance, often referred to as RV "restriction,"[124,125] and typically resolves in 3 to 5 days. Until recovery occurs, the heart should be supported by optimizing RV filling and ensuring AV synchrony. Negative-pressure ventilation has been shown to improve cardiac output where RV restriction exists.[12,126]

PULMONARY ATRESIA WITH INTACT VENTRICULAR SEPTUM (PA/IVS)

Anatomy

In this condition there is complete obstruction to the outflow of the RV, along with a variable degree of hypoplasia of the RV and tricuspid valve.[127] The tricuspid valve may also be incompetent. Pulmonary blood flow occurs via a PDA. Coronary artery sinusoids or fistulas are often found in "severe" PA/IVS with a small RV. Ten percent of cases will have an RV-dependent coronary circulation, in which coronary sinusoids/fistulas are associated with proximal stenosis and perfusion of areas of myocardium is dependent on flow via the RV. In some patients, the pulmonary arterial supply is abnormal with segments of the lungs being supplied solely or partially (dual supply) from systemic collateral vessels termed major aortopulmonary collateral arteries.[128,129]

Pathophysiology

Preoperatively there is complete mixing of systemic and pulmonary venous return in a duct-dependent circulation. The RV may be very hypertensive because there is no path for egress of blood. Some blood may pass via coronary sinusoids, if present, or back through a regurgitant tricuspid valve.

Surgery

The goal of surgery is to provide a secure source of pulmonary blood flow balanced to systemic flow and to permit the RV to develop to its maximal potential, always aiming for a two-ventricle repair where possible.[130] All infants need procedures in the neonatal period because of duct dependency. Subsequent strategies are chosen according to individual anatomic findings.

In severe forms of the condition (severe RV hypoplasia ± coronary fistulas), a two-ventricle repair will never be possible and a palliative approach is adopted. Initial palliation secures pulmonary blood flow with systemic-pulmonary artery shunts (30% to 40% PA/IVS) with the ultimate aim being a single-ventricle "Fontan" circulation (see later). In contrast, infants with a normal-sized RV may be suitable for RV outflow tract reconstruction in the neonatal period, therefore avoiding shunt and ending up with early anatomic correction (10% of cases). An intermediate group of patients, the majority of cases of PA/IVS, need initial palliation with decompression of the RV by radiofrequency perforation of the atretic pulmonary valve or outflow tract patch and often require a systemic-pulmonary artery shunt. They progress to either a single, one-and-a-half,[131] or biventricular repair, depending on subsequent development of the RV and pulmonary arteries.

Specific postoperative problems include low cardiac output due to excessive runoff through the shunt, myocardial ischemia due to decompressed coronary fistulas, or low systemic diastolic pressure due to excessive shunt runoff.

D-TRANSPOSITION OF THE GREAT ARTERIES (TGA)

Anatomy

In D-transposition, which accounts for 5% to 7% of all congenital heart lesions, the great vessels are transposed so that the aorta arises from the anatomic RV and the pulmonary artery from the LV.[63] The condition occurs with a VSD in approximately 40% of cases. Other commonly associated lesions include coarctation (10%), LV outflow tract obstruction (5%), and coronary abnormalities (33%).

Pathophysiology

The predominant finding in TGA is cyanosis due to parallel rather than serial function of the pulmonary and systemic circulations, with the greatest proportion of the output of a ventricle being recirculated to that ventricle. Survival is therefore dependent on the presence of mixing between the two circulations (Fig. 101-2). The presence of either a PDA or a VSD alone or in combination without an atrial communication does not ensure adequate mixing of the two circulations. If the diagnosis is suspected in a neonate, an infusion of prostaglandin E_1 or E_2 should be established to maintain ductal patency and, following echocardiographic confirmation of the diagnosis, a balloon atrial septostomy is performed to enlarge the foramen ovale and secure mixing at the atrial level. Saturations typically increase from very low levels (<50%) to 65% to 85% after these interventions, and it is then usually possible to discontinue the prostaglandin infusion.

Surgery

The preferred surgical option in the current era is the arterial switch (Jatene) operation,[63,132,133] although long-term results after Senning operations also appear to be acceptable.[134] The switch operation is usually performed within the first 2 weeks of life, beyond which the LV (functioning as a low-pressure subpulmonary or "right" ventricle since birth) is less able to

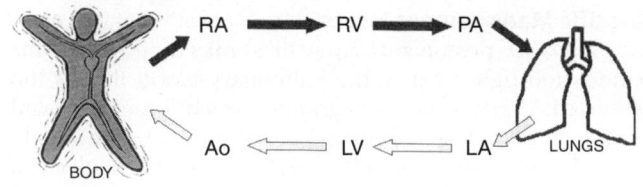

A

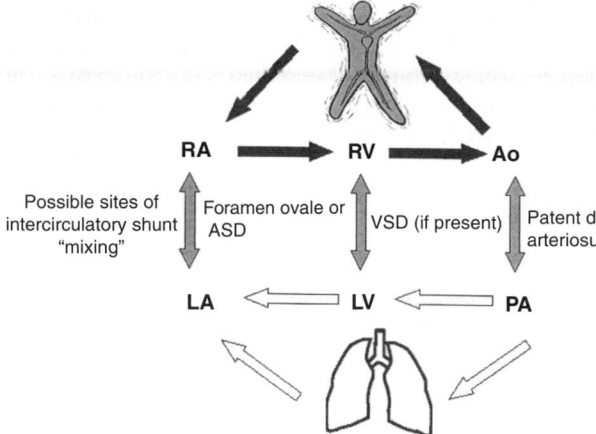

B

FIGURE 101–2. A, Normal series circulatory arrangement. **B,** Parallel circulation of transposition of the great vessels. RA, right atrium; RV, right ventricle; PA, pulmonary artery; LA, left atrium; LV, left ventricle; Ao, aorta.

cope with systemic pressures.[135] Infants with a large VSD have equal ventricular pressures, and repair can be delayed a little longer, although in practice most surgeons repair TGA with VSD within the first month of life. The operation consists of transection of the aorta and pulmonary artery with reconstruction of the vessels in their anatomic position, which necessitates transfer of the coronary arteries from the pulmonary artery to the neoaorta.

Specific Postoperative Problems after the Arterial Switch Operation

LV dysfunction is seen to some extent in all infants during the first 12 hours after the arterial switch operation.[19] It may be a sign of coronary insufficiency[136] or of acute dysfunction secondary to an "unprepared/involuted" LV or simply non-specific post-CPB "low cardiac output." In the absence of electrocardiographic or echocardiographic evidence of regional coronary ischemia, low cardiac output is managed conservatively. The postoperative LV of the neonate is poorly compliant. Rapid volume infusion should be avoided because LV distention and ischemia may result. Preload should be augmented gradually, titrating volume infused against measured left atrial pressure.

Alternative Surgical Techniques

Atrial switch operations (the Senning and Mustard procedures) are alternatives to the arterial switch operation and may be chosen in infants presenting beyond the early neonatal period in whom a one-stage arterial switch is not possible owing to deconditioning of the LV. In atrial switch operations, blood is diverted by an atrial baffle to establish a series circulation leaving the RV as the systemic ventricle. It is believed that the burden of late complications such as RV failure is greater after atrial switch procedures. An alternative

strategy for late-presenting transposition is a two-stage repair with initial banding of the pulmonary artery to condition the LV with "switch" once the ventricle is conditioned.[137]

Postoperative Care

Atrial switch procedures are usually performed outside the neonatal age group and, compared to "arterial" switch procedures, have a relatively uneventful postoperative course. Atrial volumes and compliance are reduced by the procedure such that postoperatively left and right atrial pressures must be maintained at higher than "normal" levels to maintain ventricular filling. Slow heart rates and arrhythmias are poorly tolerated.

COMPLEX "SINGLE VENTRICLE" CIRCULATIONS

Some defects are such that they can never be corrected to provide two functioning ventricles.[138] These complex arrangements include any heart in which one ventricle is hypoplastic such that it would be incapable of supporting either the pulmonary or systemic circulation independently. Examples of such situations include tricuspid atresia or double-inlet LV. In these examples, the RV has failed to develop adequately and is connected to a dominant LV via a VSD. Flow to the circulation supplied by the rudimentary ventricle originates from the dominant chamber and is dependent on an adequate VSD. Children with this type of anatomy will always have two ventricles, even if one is hypoplastic, but physiologically they behave as if the heart consists of only a "single" ventricle.

Complex "single ventricle" hearts can be palliated with a series of interventions leading to creation of a Fontan circulation when the systemic and pulmonary circulations are completely separated.[139] Initially, adequate intracardiac communications are established to ensure that both systemic and pulmonary venous return have unobstructed access to the dominant ventricle and supply both systemic and pulmonary blood flow. If necessary, pulmonary flow is augmented by the use of a systemic to pulmonary artery shunt (modified Blalock-Taussig shunt). Systemic and pulmonary blood flow is ensured at the expense of mixing of pulmonary and systemic venous returns, with consequent cyanosis and volume loading of the single ventricle.

Subsequently, if hemodynamic conditions are favorable, the Fontan circulation is established usually in a two-stage procedure. Initially, a bidirectional cavopulmonary anastomosis is created in which the superior vena cava is connected to the proximal right pulmonary artery. This has the benefit of reducing the volume load placed on the systemic ventricle by the previously placed systemic-pulmonary shunt. Finally, venous return from the inferior vena cava is also directed to the pulmonary circulation. This is achieved by forming a lateral tunnel[140] or the use of a synthetic extracardiac conduit[141] to channel blood from the inferior vena cava to the inferior aspect of the right pulmonary artery completing the total cavopulmonary connection or "Fontan" circulation.

In the Fontan circulation there is no "subpulmonary" ventricle, all ventricular tissue having been incorporated in the single ventricle, which receives pulmonary venous return and ejects into the systemic circulation. This establishes a form of series circulation and results in normal systemic oxygenation and equality of pulmonary and systemic blood flow. Pulmonary blood flow in the Fontan circulation is driven by the transpulmonary hydrostatic gradient and is only viable if the pulmonary vascular resistance and systemic ventricular end-diastolic pressures (pulmonary venous pressures) are low. The presence of good systemic ventricular function and low PVR are crucial determinants of operability. Patients with a Fontan circulation tolerate factors that impede systemic venous return such as dehydration, pneumothorax, pericardial effusion, positive-pressure ventilation,[58] raised pulmonary vascular resistance, or compromised ventricular or respiratory[142] function very poorly. Perioperative use of ACE inhibitors has been shown to reduce the severity and duration of pleural drainage,[143] a common problem caused by high postoperative systemic venous pressures.

Long-term follow-up studies have demonstrated that systemic ventricular function remains abnormal after Fontan procedures.[144] Ultimately, the Fontan circulation may fail and cardiac transplantation be considered.

Hypoplastic left heart syndrome (HLHS) encompasses a range of hypoplastic abnormalities of the left-sided cardiac structures and connections, including the ascending aorta. The condition is usually palliated in three stages, first described by Norwood. Some authorities prefer to offer cardiac transplantation without prior palliative surgery.[145] The stage 1 Norwood repair consists of reconstruction of the aortic arch with the establishment of pulmonary blood flow via a central systemic-pulmonary artery shunt. An alternative source of pulmonary blood flow, an RV-PA shunt, has been found to offer advantages (less diastolic runoff) over the central shunt of the classic Norwood 1 operation, which was a major clinical problem after the classic stage 1 operation.[146,147] In stage 2 of the Norwood procedure, undertaken at age 2 to 6 months, a bidirectional cavopulmonary (Glenn) shunt is fashioned with a completion to a Fontan circulation (stage 3) after 18 to 24 months of age. Fetal diagnosis facilitates early and appropriate management and may contribute to improved outcomes in HLHS.[146]

SURGICAL CONTROL OF PULMONARY BLOOD FLOW: PULMONARY ARTERY BANDING

Pulmonary artery banding is a surgical procedure in which a constriction is created in the main pulmonary artery with the aim of limiting pulmonary blood flow. It is performed without CPB through either a left thoracotomy or median sternotomy. The procedure is undertaken to restrict pulmonary blood flow, aiming to maintain a balance between the systemic and pulmonary circulations and to prevent the onset of pulmonary hypertension in some complex anomalies unsuitable for early anatomic repair.[148] Pulmonary artery banding is a palliative procedure and is usually a stepping stone to a more complex repair.

Physiology

A pulmonary artery band reduces pulmonary blood flow and therefore volume loading of the systemic or single ventricle. The intracardiac shunt is predominantly right to left after banding, and systemic arterial saturations are typically 75% to 85% after effective banding. The pressure gradient across an effective pulmonary artery band in a neonate is typically in the range of 40 to 60 mm Hg.

Specific Management Issues

Very low SaO_2 postoperatively (<70%) may indicate that the band is too tight, that is, the pulmonary blood flow is too restricted. Urgent echocardiographic evaluation of the band gradient and exclusion of other causes of hypoxemia should be undertaken. If hypoxemia persists, and particularly if significant metabolic acidosis develops, urgent removal of the band may be indicated. Pulmonary artery bands may occasionally be too loose to adequately reduce pulmonary blood flow, resulting in SaO_2 in excess of 90%. Signs of congestive cardiac failure may be noted and require medical treatment (diuretics) or further surgical intervention (rebanding or correction of lesion).

OTHER LESIONS

VASCULAR RINGS AND SLINGS

Vascular rings and slings[149] result from abnormal branching or positioning of the great vessels that results in encirclement or compression of the trachea and/or esophagus. They are seen in isolation or in association with intracardiac defects.

Anatomy

Three common types occur either in isolation or in association with other cardiac lesions, including right aortic arch, TOF, and AVSD.

Double Aortic Arch

This results from failure of the embryonic regression of one of the arches. The right arch, which is commonly dominant and usually larger, passes posterior to the esophagus and trachea to connect to the left-sided descending thoracic aorta forming a vascular ring. The left arch is commonly smaller and may exhibit varying degrees of hypoplasia, coarctation, or true atresia. The carotid and subclavian arteries originate from both arches. Sometimes a persistent ductus or ligamentum arteriosum forms a true ring around the trachea.

Right Aortic Arch with Aberrant Left Subclavian Artery

In this condition the left subclavian has its origin from the ascending aorta and courses to the left behind the esophagus with the vascular ring completed by the ligamentum arteriosum.

Pulmonary Artery Sling

The left pulmonary artery arises from the right pulmonary artery and crosses to the left by passing behind the trachea. The trachea is squeezed between the aorta and left pulmonary artery, and a true ring may be formed by a persistent ductus or ligamentum arteriosum.

Pathophysiology

Vascular rings have the potential to compress both trachea and esophagus. Pulmonary artery slings usually cause chronic tracheal compression, which eventually results in destruction of the tracheal skeleton with resultant tracheal stenosis in 50% of cases.

Surgery

Vascular rings are usually approached via a lateral thoracotomy (usually left). The left arch or ligamentum is divided to release the ring, and the descending aorta is dissected away from the esophagus. To correct pulmonary artery sling, the anomalous left pulmonary artery is transected and rerouted anteriorly and reanastomosed to the central pulmonary artery.[150,151]

Postoperative Care

This is usually uneventful. Extubation at the end of anesthesia or early in the ICU course is expected. Tracheomalacia may persist or present postoperatively, especially after pulmonary artery sling surgery, and may require long periods of respiratory support postoperatively via a tracheostomy.

ANOMALOUS LEFT CORONARY ARTERY FROM THE PULMONARY ARTERY (ALCAPA)

Anatomy

This usually occurs as an isolated lesion in which the left coronary artery arises from the pulmonary artery rather than the aorta.

Pathophysiology

Symptoms develop gradually as the PVR falls during early infancy. There is progressive onset of myocardial ischemia as left coronary flow falls in parallel with the fall in pulmonary artery pressure. The myocardium is initially well perfused by desaturated pulmonary artery blood, but as coronary flow falls, severe LV ischemia and dysfunction occur.

Surgery

Surgical intervention is necessary to reconnect the left coronary with the aorta, and this can be achieved either by creating a tunnel from the left coronary orifice to the aorta[152] (the Takeuchi operation) or by directly reimplanting the coronary artery.[153]

Postoperative Care

The principal perioperative problem in infants with symptomatic ALCAPA is management of low cardiac output. Beta-adrenergic agonists, PDE III inhibitors such as milrinone,[18] and occasionally mechanical circulatory support may be required.

SPECIFIC ISSUES FOR THE INTENSIVIST

DELAYED STERNAL CLOSURE

Complex cardiac surgery involving CPB results in edema of the myocardium and other mediastinal tissues. Under these circumstances, sternal closure may cause cardiac compression ("tissue tamponade"), which decreases ventricular compliance and leads to reduced cardiac output and elevated pulmonary venous pressures.[154,155]

INFECTIVE ENDOCARDITIS

Infective endocarditis is a condition characterized by microbial infection of the heart valves or other structures and is associated with substantial morbidity and mortality in both children and adults. The subject has been extensively reviewed.[156] Infective endocarditis can occur sporadically, but most patients have predisposing intracardiac structural abnormalities such as congenital heart disease, prosthetic heart valves, or acquired valvular regurgitation (e.g., post-rheumatic heart disease or mitral valve prolapse). Infection commonly occurs after a surgical procedure, including dental procedures, in which microorganisms are seeded into the bloodstream. In the pediatric cardiac ICU, infective endocarditis is often associated with the presence (and presumed colonization or infection) of indwelling central venous catheters. Intensivists should aim to minimize line-related infective complications by employing "best-practice" guidelines in the care and surveillance of central venous lines.[157] Consensus guidelines have been established that recommend the circumstances and type of antibiotic prophylaxis required to minimize the chances of at-risk patients acquiring infective endocarditis.[158]

ANNOTATED REFERENCES

Cullen S, Shore D, Redington A: Characterization of right ventricular diastolic performance after complete repair of tetralogy of Fallot: Restrictive physiology predicts slow postoperative recovery. Circulation 1995;91:1782-1789.
> *This paper characterized isolated diastolic dysfunction of the RV ("restrictive physiology") as a major cause of this low cardiac output state in children after surgical repair of tetralogy of Fallot. Knowledge of the presence of restrictive physiology allows the intensivist to adopt physiologically appropriate management strategies.*

Duncan BW, et al: Mechanical circulatory support for treatment of children with acute fulminant myocarditis. J Thorac Cardiovasc Surg 2001;122:440-448.
> *Viral myocarditis may follow a rapidly progressive and fatal course in children. This report demonstrates that mechanical circulatory support may be a lifesaving measure with a high proportion of survival attributed to recovery of native ventricular function.*

Hoffman TM, et al: Efficacy and safety of milrinone in preventing low cardiac output syndrome in infants and children after corrective surgery for congenital heart disease. Circulation 2003;107:996-1002.
> *Low cardiac output syndrome (LCOS), affecting up to 25% of neonates and young children after cardiac surgery, contributes to postoperative morbidity and mortality. This study evaluated the efficacy and safety of prophylactic milrinone in pediatric patients at high risk for developing LCOS. It is the largest randomized controlled trial in a pediatric cardiac surgical population, and one of the few double-blind randomized-controlled trials performed in this population.*

McElhinney DB, et al: Management and outcomes of delayed sternal closure after cardiac surgery in neonates and infants (comment). Crit Care Med 2000;28:1180-1184.
> *This study demonstrates that delayed sternal closure is an effective approach to the management of neonates and infants at risk for hemodynamic, respiratory, or hemostatic instability early after cardiac surgery.*

Nugent AW, et al: The epidemiology of childhood cardiomyopathy in Australia (comment). N Engl J Med 2003;348:1639-1646.
> *The incidence and age distribution of primary cardiomyopathy in children were previously not well defined. The centralization of pediatric cardiology services in Australia enabled these authors to undertake this retrospective, population-based cohort study of all Australian children who presented with cardiomyopathy over a 10-year period. The study succeeds in adding to our understanding of the distribution of cardiomyopathy types and the timing and severity of their presentation in children.*

Chapter 102

PERICARDIAL DISEASES

Bernhard Maisch • Arsen D. Ristic

KEY POINTS

1. **Diagnosis of acute pericarditis** is based on clinical presentation (chest pain, pericardial friction rub) and typical four-stage ECG changes. For etiologic diagnosis, pericardiocentesis, pericardioscopy, and pericardial/epicardial biopsy may be necessary.

2. **Echocardiography is essential** in all patients with pericarditis to detect pericardial effusion and determine its physiologic significance, as well as to check for signs of constriction, concomitant heart disease, or paracardial pathology.

3. A large proportion of patients usually classified as having **"idiopathic" pericarditis** actually have **viral and autoreactive pericarditis.** The diagnosis of viral pericarditis is not possible without the evaluation of pericardial effusion and/or pericardial/epicardial tissue, preferably by polymerase chain reaction (PCR) or in-situ hybridization.

4. PCR identification of *Mycobacterium tuberculosis*, high adenosine deaminase activity, and interferon gamma concentration in pericardial effusion are diagnostic with a high sensitivity and specificity for **tuberculous pericarditis.**

5. **Pericardiocentesis is indicated for** cardiac tamponade, for a high suspicion of purulent, tuberculous, or neoplastic pericarditis, or in patients with very large effusions without signs of tamponade (>20 mm in echocardiography in diastole). Electrical alternans and pulsus paradoxus are clinically important signs of advanced stage of cardiac tamponade and indicate the need for prompt pericardial drainage.

6. **Aortic dissection is a major contraindication** to pericardiocentesis. Relative contraindications include uncorrected coagulopathy, anticoagulant therapy, thrombocytopenia less than 50,000/mm[3], and small, posterior, and loculated effusions.

7. In cardiac wounds, postinfarction myocardial rupture, or dissecting aortic hematoma emergency **cardiac surgery** is lifesaving. Loculated effusions may require open surgery or thoracoscopic drainage.

8. **Postinfarction pericardial effusions** larger than 10 mm in diastole are frequently associated with cardiac rupture. Urgent surgical treatment is indicated.

9. **Intrapericardial instillation** of antineoplastic and/or sclerosing agents (e.g., cisplatin, thiotepa) can prevent recurrences of neoplastic pericardial effusions. Intrapericardial instillation of triamcinolone is highly efficient in preventing recurrences in patients with autoreactive pericardial effusion, mainly avoiding adverse effects of systemic corticosteroid therapy.

10. Pericardiectomy is the only treatment for permanent **constrictive pericarditis**. However, surgery should not be indicated too early (to avoid operating on patients with transient constriction). Even more important is not to perform surgery too late or in patients with myocardial fibrosis and/or atrophy. If the indication for surgery is established early, long-term survival after pericardiectomy corresponds to that of the general population.

ETIOLOGY AND CLASSIFICATION OF PERICARDIAL DISEASE

The spectrum of pericardial diseases consists of congenital defects, pericarditis (dry, effusive, effusive-constrictive, constrictive), neoplasm, and cysts. The etiologic classification comprises infectious pericarditis, pericarditis in systemic autoimmune diseases, type 2 (auto)immune process, post–myocardial infarction syndrome, and autoreactive (chronic) pericarditis.[1-3]

PERICARDIAL SYNDROMES

CONGENITAL DEFECTS OF THE PERICARDIUM

Congenital defects of the pericardium occur in 1 in 10,000 autopsies. Pericardial absence can be partial left (70%), right (17%), or total bilateral (rare). Additional congenital abnormalities occur in approximately 30% of patients.[4] Most patients with a total pericardial absence are asymptomatic. Homolateral cardiac displacement and augmented heart mobility impose an increased risk for traumatic aortic dissection.[5] Partial left-side defects can be complicated by herniation and strangulation of the heart through the defect (chest pain, shortness of breath, syncope, or sudden death).

TABLE 102–1. DIAGNOSTIC PATHWAY AND SEQUENCE OF PERFORMANCE IN ACUTE PERICARDITIS

Diagnostic Measure	Characteristic Findings
Obligatory	
Auscultation	Pericardial rub (monophasic, biphasic, or triphasic)
ECG*	*Stage I:* anterior and inferior concave ST segment elevation. PR segment deviations opposite to P wave polarity
	Early stage II: all ST junctions return to the baseline. PR segments deviated
	Late stage II: T waves progressively flatten and invert
	Stage III: generalized T wave inversions in most or all leads
	Stage IV: ECG returns to prepericarditis state
Echocardiography	Effusion types B to D (Horowitz)
	Signs of tamponade
Blood analyses	Erythrocyte sedimentation rate, C-reactive protein, lactate dehydrogenase, leukocytes (inflammation markers)
	Troponin I[†], CK-MB (markers of myocardial involvement)
Chest radiograph	Ranging from normal to "water bottle" shape of the heart shadow
	Performed primarily to reveal pulmonary or mediastinal pathology
Mandatory in Tamponade, Optional in Large/Recurrent Effusions or if Previous Tests Inconclusive in Small Effusions	
Pericardiocentesis/drainage	Polymerase chain reaction and histochemistry for etiopathogenetic classification of infection or neoplasia
Optional or if Previous Tests Inconclusive	
CT	Effusions, pericardium, and epicardium
MRI	Effusions, pericardium, and epicardium
Pericardioscopy, pericardial/epicardial biopsy	Establishing the specific etiology

*Typical lead involvement: I, II, aVL, aVF, and V3-V6. The ST segment is always depressed in aVR, frequently in V1, and occasionally in V2. Stage IV may not occur, and there are permanent T wave inversions and flattenings. If ECG is first recorded in stage III, pericarditis cannot be differentiated by ECG from diffuse myocardial injury, "biventricular strain," or myocarditis. ECG in early repolarization is very similar to stage I. Unlike stage I, this ECG does not acutely evolve and J-point elevations are usually accompanied by a slur, oscillation, or notch at the end of the QRS just before and including the J point (best seen with tall R and T waves—large in early repolarization pattern). Pericarditis is likely if in lead V6 the J point is greater than 25% of the height of the T wave apex (using the PR segment as a baseline).
†A cTnI rise was detectable in 38/118 patients (32.2%), more frequently in younger, male patients, with ST-segment elevation and pericardial effusion at presentation. An increase beyond 1.5 ng/mL was rare (7.6%), and associated with CK-MB elevation. cTnI increase was not a negative prognostic marker regarding the incidence of recurrences, constrictive pericarditis, cardiac tamponade, or residual left ventricular dysfunction (Imazio).
Data from references 2, 3, and 7 to 19.

Surgical pericardioplasty (Dacron, Gore-Tex, or bovine pericardium) is indicated for imminent strangulation.[6]

ACUTE PERICARDITIS

Acute pericarditis is dry, fibrinous, or effusive, independent of its etiology. Major symptoms are retrosternal or left precordial chest pain (which radiates to the trapezius ridge, can be pleuritic or simulate ischemia, and varies with posture) and shortness of breath. A prodrome of fever, malaise, and myalgia is common, but elderly patients may not be febrile. The pericardial friction rub can be transient and monophasic, biphasic, or triphasic. Pleural effusion may be present. Heart rate is usually rapid and regular. Echocardiography is essential to detect effusion and concomitant heart or paracardial disease (Table 102-1).[7-19]

Hospitalization and symptomatic treatment is warranted. Nonsteroidal anti-inflammatory drugs (NSAIDs) are the mainstay. Indomethacin should be avoided in elderly patients, owing to its effect on reducing flow in the coronaries. Ibuprofen (300 to 800 mg tid) is preferred for its rare side effects, favorable impact on coronary flow, and large dose range.[7] Colchicine (0.5 mg twice daily) added to an NSAID or as monotherapy also appears to be effective for the initial attack and for prevention of recurrences.[20] It is well tolerated with fewer side effects than NSAIDs. Systemic corticosteroids should be restricted to connective tissue diseases and autoreactive or uremic pericarditis. Intrapericardial application is effective and avoids systemic side effects.[2]

CHRONIC PERICARDITIS

Chronic (>3 months) pericarditis includes effusive (inflammatory or hydropericardium in heart failure), adhesive, and constrictive forms.[7] Symptoms are usually mild (chest pain, palpitations, fatigue), related to the degree of cardiac compression and pericardial inflammation. The detection of the curable causes (e.g., tuberculosis, toxoplasmosis, myxedema, autoimmune, and systemic diseases) allows successful specific therapy. Symptomatic treatment and pericardiocentesis should be applied if indicated. For recurrences, balloon pericardiotomy or pericardiectomy may be considered.[21,22]

RECURRENT PERICARDITIS

The term *recurrent pericarditis* encompasses (1) the intermittent type (symptom-free intervals without therapy) and (2) the incessant type (discontinuation of anti-inflammatory therapy ensures a relapse). Massive pericardial effusion, overt tamponade, or constriction is rare. Symptomatic management relies on exercise restriction and the regimen used in acute pericarditis. Colchicine may be effective when NSAIDs and corticosteroids fail to prevent relapses.[20,23,24] Corticosteroids should be used only in patients with poor general condition or in frequent crises.[7] A common mistake is to use a dose too low to be effective or to taper the dose too rapidly. The recommended regimen is prednisone, 1 to 1.5 mg/kg, for at least 1 month. If patients do not respond adequately, azathioprine (75 to 100 mg/day) or cyclophosphamide can be added.[25]

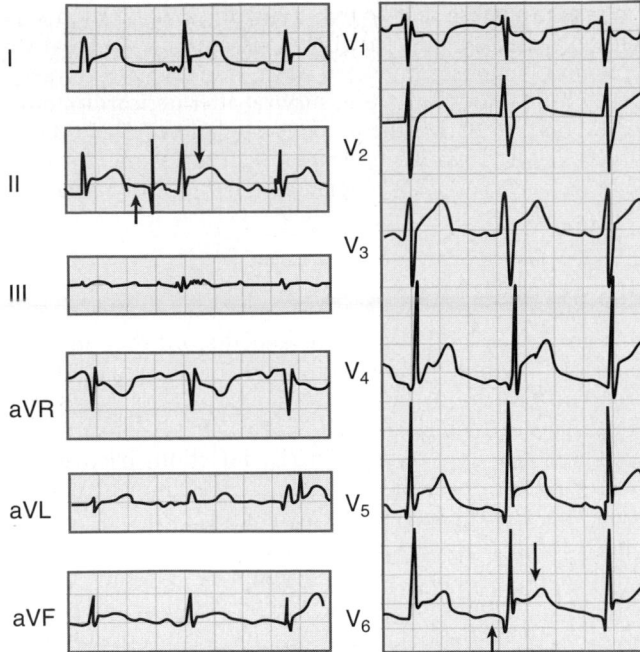

FIGURE 102–1. Typical electrocardiographic changes in acute pericarditis: PR depression *(small arrow)* and concave ST segment elevation *(large arrow)*.

Corticosteroids should be tapered over a 3-month period. Toward the end of the taper, introduce anti-inflammatory treatment with colchicine (0.5 mg bid or tid) or an NSAID. Renewed treatment should continue for 3 to 6 months. Pericardiectomy is indicated only in frequent and highly symptomatic recurrences resistant to medical treatment.[37] Before pericardiectomy, a corticosteroid-free regimen should be applied for several weeks.

PERICARDIAL EFFUSION AND CARDIAC TAMPONADE

Pericardial effusion may appear as transudate (hydropericardium), exudate, pyopericardium, or hemopericardium. Large effusions are common with neoplastic, tuberculous, cholesterol, uremic, myxedema, and parasitoses pericarditis.[27] Loculated effusions are more common when scarring has supervened (e.g., postsurgical, post trauma, purulent pericarditis). Effusions that develop slowly can be remarkably asymptomatic, whereas rapidly accumulating smaller effusions can present as tamponade. Cardiac tamponade is the decompensated phase of cardiac compression caused by effusion accumulation and the increased intrapericardial pressure. Heart sounds are distant. Orthopnea, cough, and dysphagia, occasionally with episodes of unconsciousness, can be observed. Insidiously developing tamponade may present as the signs of its complications (renal failure, abdominal plethora, shock liver, worsening of glaucoma,[28] and mesenteric ischemia). Tamponade without two or more inflammatory signs (typical pain, pericardial friction rub, fever, diffuse ST-segment elevation) is usually associated with a malignant effusion (likelihood ratio 2.9).[29]

Electrocardiography demonstrates low QRS and T-wave voltages, PR-segment depression (Fig. 102-1), ST-segment/T-wave changes, bundle branch block, and electrical alternans (rarely seen in the absence of tamponade).[7] Microvoltage and electrical alternans are reversible after effusion drainage.[19] In chest radiography large effusions are depicted as globular cardiomegaly with sharp margins ("water bottle" silhouette) (Fig. 102-2).[12] The size of effusions can be graded in echocardiography as (1) small (echo-free space in diastole < 10 mm), (2) moderate (10 to 20 mm) (Fig. 102-3), (3) large (≥20 mm), or (4) very large (≥20 mm and compression of the heart). In large pericardial effusions, the heart may move freely within the pericardial cavity ("swinging heart") inducing pseudoprolapse and pseudosystolic anterior motion of the mitral valve, paradoxical motion of the interventricular septum, and midsystolic aortic valve closure (Table 102-2).[30-40] Up to one third of patients with an asymptomatic large pericardial chronic effusion develop unexpected cardiac tamponade.[21] Triggers for tamponade include hypovolemia, paroxysmal tachyarrhythmia, and intercurrent acute pericarditis. Further details on cardiac tamponade and pericardiocentesis are available in Chapter 213.

CONSTRICTIVE PERICARDITIS

Constrictive pericarditis is a rare but severely disabling consequence of the chronic inflammation of the pericardium, leading to an impaired filling of the ventricles and reduced ventricular function. Until recently, increased pericardial thickness has been considered an essential diagnostic feature of constrictive pericarditis. However, in the large surgical series from the Mayo Clinic constriction was present in 18% of the patients with normal pericardial thickness.[41] Tuberculosis, mediastinal irradiation, and previous surgical

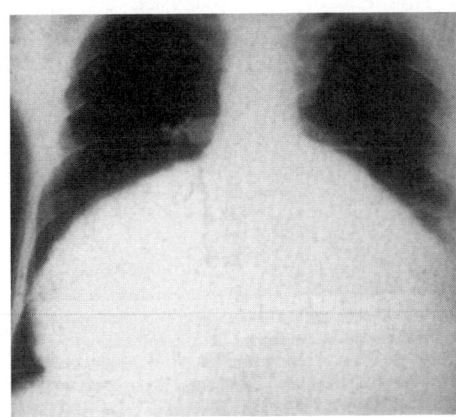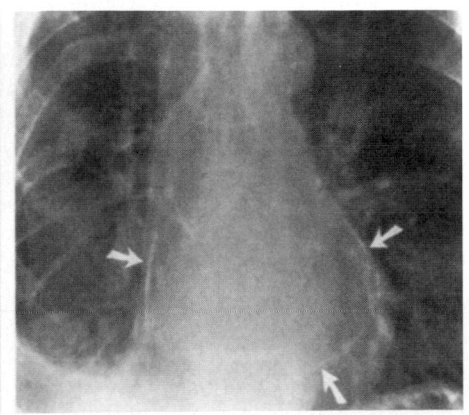

FIGURE 102–2. Chest radiographs in a patient with very large pericardial effusion—"water bottle" sign *(left)* and in a patient with constrictive pericarditis and pericardial calcifications *(white arrows)* *(right)*.

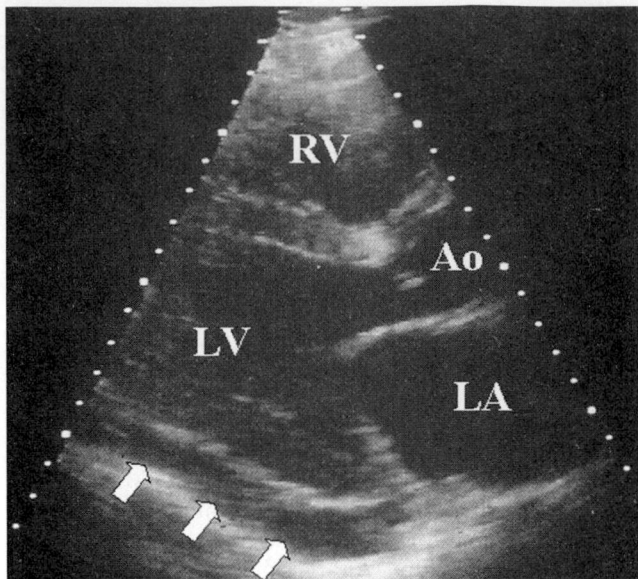

FIGURE 102–3. Echocardiographic findings in a small-moderate pericardial effusion *(white arrows)*. Long-axis parasternal view. LV, left ventricle; LA, left atrium; RV, right ventricle; Ao, aortic root.

procedures are frequent.[42] Constrictive pericarditis may rarely develop only in the epicardial layer in patients with previously removed parietal pericardium.[43] Transient constrictive pericarditis is an uncommon but important entity, because pericardiectomy is not indicated in these patients.[44]

Patients complain about fatigue, peripheral edema, breathlessness, and abdominal swelling, which may be aggravated by a protein-losing enteropathy. In decompensated patients venous congestion, hepatomegaly, pleural effusions, and ascites may occur. Hemodynamic impairment can be additionally aggravated by a systolic dysfunction due to myocardial fibrosis or atrophy. Differential diagnosis has to include acute dilatation of the heart, pulmonary embolism, right ventricular infarction, pleural effusion, chronic obstructive lung diseases,[45] and restrictive cardiomyopathy. The best way to distinguish constrictive pericarditis from restrictive cardiomyopathy is the analysis of respiratory changes with or without changes of preload by Doppler and/or tissue Doppler echocardiography,[46] but physical findings, electrocardiogram (ECG), chest radiography (see Fig. 102-2, right), computed tomography (CT) (Fig. 102-4, left), magnetic resonance imaging (MRI) (see Fig. 102-4, right), hemodynamics, and endomyocardial biopsy may be helpful as well.[7]

Pericardiectomy is the only treatment for permanent constriction. The indications are based on clinical symptoms, echocardiography findings, CT/MRI, and heart catheterization. A primary installation of cardiopulmonary bypass (CPB) is not recommended (diffuse bleeding following systemic heparinization). Pericardiectomy for constrictive pericarditis has a mortality rate of 6% to 12%.[47-50] The complete normalization of cardiac hemodynamics is reported in only 60% of patients.[47,49] Major complications include acute perioperative cardiac insufficiency and ventricular wall rupture.[51] Cardiac mortality and morbidity at pericardiectomy are mainly caused by the presurgically unrecognized presence of myocardial atrophy or myocardial fibrosis.[42] Exclusion of patients with extensive myocardial fibrosis and/or atrophy reduced the mortality rate for pericardiectomy to 5%. Postoperative low

cardiac output[51] should be treated by fluid substitution and catecholamines, high doses of digitalis, and intra-aortic balloon pump in most severe cases. If the indication for surgery is established early, long-term survival after pericardiectomy corresponds to that of the general population.[48,49] However, if severe clinical symptoms were present for a longer period before surgery, even a complete pericardiectomy may not achieve a total restitution.

PERICARDIAL CYSTS

Congenital pericardial cysts are uncommon; they may be unilocular or multilocular, with the diameter ranging from 1 to 5 cm.[52] Inflammatory cysts comprise pseudocysts as well as encapsulated and loculated pericardial effusions, caused by rheumatic pericarditis, bacterial infection, particularly tuberculosis, trauma, and cardiac surgery. Echinococcal *cysts* usually originate from ruptured hydatid cysts in the liver and lungs. Most patients are asymptomatic and cysts are detected incidentally on chest radiographs as an oval, homogeneous radiodense lesion, usually at the right cardiophrenic angle.[53] However, the patients can also present as chest discomfort, dyspnea, cough, or palpitations, owing to the compression of the heart. Echocardiography is useful, but additional imaging by CT (density readings) or MRI is often needed.[54] The treatment of congenital and inflammatory cysts is percutaneous aspiration and ethanol sclerosis.[55,56] If this is not feasible, video-assisted thoracotomy or surgical resection may be necessary. The surgical excision of echinococcal cysts is not recommended. Percutaneous aspiration and instillation of ethanol or silver nitrate after pretreatment with albendazole (800 mg/day 4 weeks) is safe and effective.[56]

SPECIFIC FORMS OF PERICARDITIS

VIRAL PERICARDITIS

Viral pericarditis is the most common infection of the pericardium. Inflammatory abnormalities are due to direct viral attack, the immune response (antiviral or anticardiac), or both.[3,57] Early viral replication in pericardial and epimyocardial tissue elicits cellular and humoral immune responses against the virus and/or cardiac tissue. Viral genomic fragments in pericardial tissue may not necessarily replicate, yet they serve as a source of antigen to stimulate immune responses. Deposits of IgM, IgG, and occasionally IgA can be found in the pericardium and myocardium for years.[57] Various viruses cause pericarditis (e.g., enteroviruses, echoviruses, adenoviruses, cytomegaloviruses, Ebstein-Barr virus, herpes simplex, influenzaviruses, parvovirus B19, hepatitis C, human immunodeficiency virus [HIV]). Attacks of enteroviral pericarditis follow the seasonal epidemics of coxsackievirus A+B and echovirus infections.[58] Cytomegalovirus (CMV) pericarditis has an increased incidence in immunocompromised and HIV-infected hosts.[59] Infectious mononucleosis may also present as pericarditis.

The diagnosis of viral pericarditis is not possible without the evaluation of pericardial effusion and/or pericardial/epicardial tissue, preferably by polymerase chain reaction (PCR) or in-situ hybridization. A fourfold rise in serum antibody levels is suggestive but not diagnostic for viral pericarditis.

Treatment of viral pericarditis is directed to resolve symptoms (see acute pericarditis), prevent complications,

TABLE 102–2. DIAGNOSIS OF CARDIAC TAMPONADE

Clinical Presentation	Elevated systemic venous pressure,* hypotension,† pulsus paradoxus,‡ tachycardia,§ dyspnea or tachypnea with clear lungs
Precipitating Factors	Drugs (cyclosporine, anticoagulants, thrombolytics), recent cardiac surgery, indwelling instrumentation, blunt chest trauma, malignancies, connective tissue disease, renal failure, septicemiaǁ
ECG	Can be normal or nonspecifically changed (ST-T wave), electrical alternans (QRS, rarely T), bradycardia (end stage), electromechanical dissociation (agonal phase)
Chest Radiograph	Enlarged cardiac silhouette with clear lungs
M mode/Two-Dimensional Echocardiogram	Diastolic collapse of the anterior RV free wall,¶ RA collapse, LA and rarely LV collapse, increased LV diastolic wall thickness "pseudohypertrophy," IVC dilatation (no collapse in inspiration), "swinging heart"
Doppler	Tricuspid flow increases and mitral flow decreases during inspiration (reverse in expiration)
	Systolic and diastolic flows are reduced in systemic veins in expiration and reverse flow with atrial contraction is increased.
M-mode Color Doppler	Large respiratory fluctuations in mitral/tricuspid flows
Cardiac Catheterization	Confirmation of the diagnosis and quantification of the hemodynamic compromise
	RA pressure is elevated (preserved systolic x descent and absent or diminished diastolic y descent).
	Intrapericardial pressure is also elevated and virtually identical to RA pressure (both pressures fall in inspiration).
	RV mid-diastolic pressure is elevated and equal to the RA and pericardial pressures (no dip-and-plateau configuration).
	Pulmonary artery diastolic pressure is slightly elevated and may correspond to the RV pressure.
	Pulmonary capillary wedge pressure is also elevated and nearly equal to intrapericardial and right atrial pressure.
	LV systolic and aortic pressures may be normal or reduced.
	Documenting that pericardial aspiration is followed by hemodynamic improvement**
	Detection of coexisting hemodynamic abnormalities (LV failure, constriction, pulmonary hypertension)
	Detection of associated cardiovascular diseases (cardiomyopathy, coronary artery disease)
RV/LV Angiography	Atrial collapse and small hyperactive ventricular chambers
Coronary Angiography	Coronary compression in diastole

LA, left atrium; LV, left ventricle; RA, right atrium; RV, right ventricle; IVC, inferior vena cava.

*Jugular venous distention is less notable in hypovolemic patients or in "surgical tamponade." An inspiratory increase or lack of fall of the pressure in the neck veins (Kussmaul sign), when verified with tamponade or after pericardial drainage, indicates effusive-constrictive disease.

†Heart rate is usually greater than 100 beats/min but may be lower in hypothyroidism and in uremic patients.

‡Pulsus paradoxus is defined as a drop in systolic blood pressure greater than 10 mm Hg during inspiration, whereas diastolic blood pressure remains unchanged. It is easily detected by simply feeling the pulse, which diminishes significantly during inspiration. Clinically significant pulsus paradoxus is apparent when the patient is breathing normally. When this sign is present only in deep inspiration it should be interpreted with caution. The magnitude of pulsus paradoxus is evaluated by sphygmomanometry. If the pulsus paradoxus is present, the first Korotkoff sound is not heard equally well throughout the respiratory cycle, but only during expiration at a given blood pressure. The blood pressure cuff is therefore inflated above the patient's systolic pressure. Then it is slowly deflated while the clinician observes the phase of respiration. During deflation, the first Korotkoff sound is intermittent. Correlation with the patient's respiratory cycle identifies a point at which the sound is audible during expiration but disappears when the patient breathes in. As the cuff pressure drops farther, another point is reached when the first blood pressure sound is audible throughout the respiratory cycle. The difference in systolic pressure between these two points is the clinical measure of pulsus paradoxus. Pulsus paradoxus is absent in tamponade, complicating atrial septal defect, and in patients with significant aortic regurgitation.

§Occasional patients are hypertensive, especially if they have preexisting hypertension.

ǁFebrile tamponade may be misdiagnosed as septic shock.

¶Right ventricular collapse can be absent in elevated right ventricular pressure and right ventricular hypertrophy or in right ventricular infarction.

**If after drainage of pericardial effusion intrapericardial pressure does not fall below atrial pressure, the effusive-constrictive disease should be considered.

Data from references 30 to 40.

and eradicate the virus. In patients with chronic or recurrent symptomatic pericardial effusion and confirmed viral infection the following specific treatment is under investigation[60]:

1. CMV pericarditis: hyperimmune globulin—once per day 4 mL/kg on days 0, 4, and 8; 2 mL/kg on days 12 and 16
2. Coxsackievirus B pericarditis: interferon alfa or beta 2.5 × 10⁶ IU/m² subcutaneously three times per week
3. Adenovirus and parvovirus B19 perimyocarditis: immunoglobulin treatment: 10 g intravenously on days 1 and 3 for 6 to 8 hours

Pericardial manifestation of HIV infection can be due to infective, noninfective, and neoplastic diseases (Kaposi's

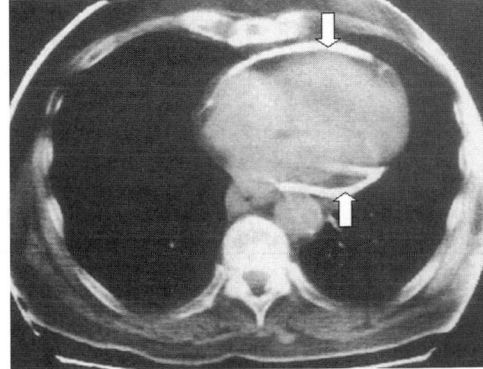
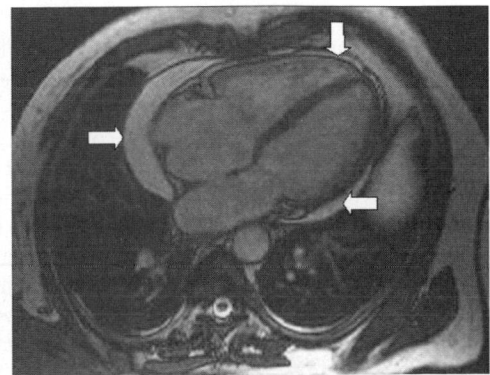

FIGURE 102–4. CT findings in constrictive pericarditis *(left). White vertical arrows* are depicting thickened pericardium and pericardial calcification. MR image of a patient with effusive-constrictive pericarditis is shown on the right-sided image. *Horizontal arrows* show loculated pericardial effusion, and the *vertical arrow* shows thickened pericardium.

sarcoma and/or lymphoma). Infective (myo)pericarditis results from the local HIV infection and/or from other viral (CMV, herpes simplex), bacterial *(Staphylococcus aureus, Klebsiella pneumoniae, Mycobacterium avium,* and *M. tuberculosis),* and fungal co-infections *(Cryptococcus neoformans).*[61] In progressive disease the incidence of echocardiographically detected pericardial effusion is up to 40%.[62] Cardiac tamponade is rare.[63] During treatment with retroviral compounds, lipodystrophy can develop (best demonstrated by MRI) with intense paracardial fat deposition leading to heart failure. Treatment is symptomatic, whereas in large effusions and cardiac tamponade pericardiocentesis is necessary. The use of corticosteroid therapy is contraindicated except in patients with secondary tuberculous pericarditis, as an adjunct to tuberculostatic treatment.[64]

BACTERIAL PERICARDITIS

Purulent pericarditis in adults is rare but always fatal if not treated.[65-68] The mortality rate in treated patients is 40%, mostly due to cardiac tamponade, toxicity, and constriction. It is usually a complication of an infection originating elsewhere in the body, arising by contiguous spread or hematogenous dissemination.[69] Predisposing conditions are pericardial effusion, immunosuppression, chronic diseases (e.g., alcohol abuse, rheumatoid arthritis), cardiac surgery, and chest trauma. The disease appears as an acute, fulminant infectious illness with short duration. Percutaneous pericardiocentesis must be promptly performed, and obtained pericardial fluid should undergo Gram, acid-fast, and fungal staining, followed by cultures of the pericardial and body fluids. Rinsing of the pericardial cavity, combined with effective systemic antibiotic therapy is mandatory (antistaphylococcal antibiotic plus aminoglycoside, followed by tailored antibiotic therapy according to pericardial fluid and blood cultures).[66] Intrapericardial instillation of antibiotics (e.g., gentamicin) is useful but not sufficient. Frequent irrigation of the pericardial cavity with urokinase or streptokinase, using large catheters, may liquefy the purulent exudate,[67,68] but open surgical drainage through subxiphoid pericardiotomy is preferable.[65] Pericardiectomy is required in patients with dense adhesions, loculated and thick purulent effusion, recurrence of tamponade, persistent infection, and progression to constriction.[66] Surgical mortality is up to 8%.

Tuberculous Pericarditis

In the past decade, tuberculous pericarditis in developed countries has been primarily seen in immunocompromised patients (acquired immunodeficiency syndrome [AIDS]).[70] The mortality rate in untreated effusive tuberculous pericarditis approaches 85%. Pericardial constriction occurs in 30% to 50%.[71,72]

The clinical presentation is variable: acute pericarditis with or without effusion; cardiac tamponade; silent, often large pericardial effusion with a relapsing course; toxic symptoms with persistent fever; acute constrictive pericarditis; subacute constriction; effusive-constrictive or chronic constrictive pericarditis; and pericardial calcifications.[3,73] The diagnosis is made by the identification of *M. tuberculosis* in the pericardial fluid or tissue and/or the presence of caseous granulomas in the pericardium.[70] Importantly, PCR can identify DNA of *M. tuberculosis* rapidly from only 1 µL of pericardial fluid.[74,75] Increased adenosine deaminase activity

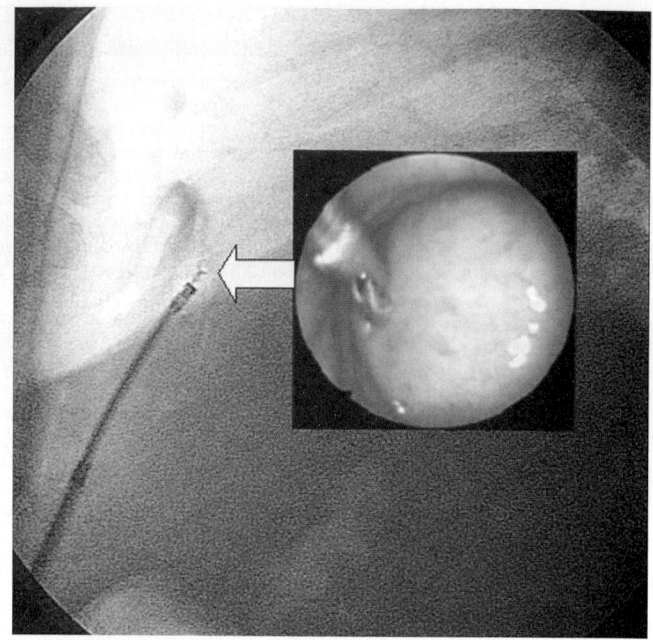

FIGURE 102–5. Flexible percutaneous pericardioscopy and epicardial biopsy *(arrow).*

and interferon gamma concentration in pericardial effusion are also diagnostic, with a high sensitivity and specificity. Both pericardioscopy and pericardial biopsy have also improved the diagnostic accuracy for tuberculous pericarditis (Fig. 102-5).[15] Pericardial biopsy enables rapid diagnosis with better sensitivity than pericardiocentesis (100% vs. 33%).

Pericarditis in a patient with proven extracardiac tuberculosis is strongly suggestive of tuberculous etiology (several sputum cultures should be taken).[76] The tuberculin skin test may be false negative in 25% to 33% of tests[71] and false positive in 30% to 40% of patients.[70] The more accurate enzyme-linked immunospot (ELISPOT) test detects T cells specific for *M. tuberculosis* antigen.[77] Perimyocardial tuberculous involvement is also associated with high serum titers of antimyolemmal and antimyosin antibodies.[78] The diagnostic yield of pericardiocentesis in tuberculous pericarditis ranges from 30% to 76% according to the methods applied for the analyses of pericardial effusion.[71,74] Pericardial fluid demonstrates high specific gravity, high protein levels, and high white blood cell count (from 0.7 to 54×10^9/L).[70]

Various antituberculous drug combinations of different durations (6, 9, 12 months) have been applied.[70,71,76,79-82] However, only patients with proven or very likely tuberculous pericarditis should be treated. Prevention of constriction in chronic pericardial effusion of undetermined etiology by "ex iuvantibus" antitubercular treatment was not successful.[79] The use of corticosteroids remains controversial.[76,80-83] A meta-analysis of patients with effusive and constrictive tuberculous pericarditis[81,82] suggested that tuberculostatic treatment combined with corticosteroids might be associated with fewer deaths and less frequent need for pericardiocentesis or pericardiectomy.[76,84] If given, prednisone should be administered in relatively high doses (1 to 2 mg/kg/day) because rifampicin induces its liver metabolism.[7] This dose is maintained for 5 to 7 days and progressively reduced in 6 to 8 weeks. If, in spite of combination therapy, constriction develops, pericardiectomy is indicated.

PERICARDITIS IN RENAL FAILURE

Renal failure is a common cause of pericardial disease, producing large pericardial effusions in up to 20% of patients.[85] Two forms have been described:

1. Uremic pericarditis—in 6% to 10% of patients with advanced renal failure (acute or chronic) before dialysis has been instituted or shortly thereafter.[86] It results from inflammation of the visceral and parietal pericardium and correlates with the degree of azotemia (blood urea nitrogen > 60 mg/dL).
2. Dialysis-associated pericarditis—in up to 13% of patients on maintenance hemodialysis[87] and occasionally with chronic peritoneal dialysis due to inadequate dialysis and/or fluid overload.[88] Pathologic examination of the pericardium shows adhesions between the thickened pericardial membranes ("bread and butter" appearance). The clinical features may include fever and pleuritic chest pain, but many patients are asymptomatic. Pericardial rubs may persist even in large effusions or may be transient. Because of autonomic impairment in uremic patients, heart rate may remain slow (60 to 80 beats/min) during tamponade, despite fever and hypotension. Anemia, due to induced resistance to erythropoietin, may worsen the clinical picture.[89] The ECG does not show the typical diffuse ST-segment/T-wave elevations observed with other causes of acute pericarditis, owing to the lack of the myocardial inflammation.[90] If the ECG is typical of acute pericarditis, intercurrent infection must be suspected.

Most patients with uremic pericarditis respond rapidly to hemodialysis or peritoneal dialysis with resolution of chest pain and pericardial effusion. To avoid hemopericardium heparin-free hemodialysis should be used. Hypokalemia and hypophosphatemia should be prevented by supplementing the dialysis solution when appropriate.[91] Intensified dialysis usually leads to resolution of the pericarditis within 1 to 2 weeks.[92] Peritoneal dialysis, which does not require heparinization, may be therapeutic in pericarditis resistant to hemodialysis or if heparin-free hemodialysis cannot be performed. NSAIDs and systemic corticosteroids have limited success when intensive dialysis is ineffective.[93] Cardiac tamponade and large chronic effusions resistant to dialysis must be treated with pericardiocentesis. Large, nonresolving symptomatic effusions should be treated with intrapericardial instillation of corticosteroids after pericardiocentesis or subxiphoid pericardiotomy (triamcinolone hexacetonide, 50 mg every 6 hours for 2 to 3 days).[87,93] Pericardiectomy is indicated only in refractory, severely symptomatic patients owing to its potential morbidity and mortality. After renal transplantation, pericarditis has also been reported in 2.4% of patients within 2 months.[94] Uremia or infection (CMV) may be the causes.

AUTOREACTIVE PERICARDITIS AND PERICARDITIS IN SYSTEMIC AUTOIMMUNE DISEASES

The diagnosis of autoreactive pericarditis is established using the following criteria[2]:

1. Increased number of lymphocytes and mononuclear cells greater than 5000/mm^3 (autoreactive lymphocytic) or the presence of antibodies against heart muscle tissue (anti-sarcolemmal) in the pericardial fluid (autoreactive antibody-mediated)
2. Inflammation in epicardial/endomyocardial biopsies by more than 14 cells/mm^2
3. Exclusion of active viral infection both in pericardial effusion and endomyocardial/epimyocardial biopsies (no virus isolation, no IgM-titer against cardiotropic viruses in pericardial effusion, and negative PCR for major cardiotropic viruses)
4. Tuberculosis, *Borrelia burgdorferi*, *Chlamydia pneumoniae*, and other bacterial infection excluded by PCR and/or cultures
5. Neoplastic infiltration absent in pericardial effusion and biopsy samples
6. Exclusion of systemic metabolic disorders and uremia. Intrapericardial treatment with triamcinolone is efficient with rare side effects.

Pericarditis occurs in systemic autoimmune diseases: rheumatoid arthritis, systemic lupus erythematosus, progressive systemic sclerosis, polymyositis/dermatomyositis, mixed connective tissue disease, seronegative spondyloarthropathies, systemic and hypersensitivity vasculitides, Behçet's syndrome, Wegener's granulomatosis, and sarcoidosis.[7] Intensified treatment of the underlying disease and symptomatic management is indicated.

THE POST–CARDIAC INJURY SYNDROME: POSTPERICARDIOTOMY SYNDROME

Post–cardiac injury syndrome develops within days to months after cardiac or pericardial injury or both.[7,95,96] It resembles the post–myocardial infarction syndrome, both appearing to be variants of a common immunopathologic process. Pericardial effusion also occurs after orthotopic heart transplantation (21%). It is more frequent in patients receiving aminocaproic acid during the operation.[97] Cardiac tamponade after open heart surgery is more common after valve surgery than coronary artery bypass grafting and may be related to the preoperative use of anticoagulants.[98]

Warfarin administration in patients with early postoperative pericardial effusion imposes the greatest risk, particularly in those who did not undergo pericardiocentesis and drainage of the effusion.[99] Symptomatic treatment is as in acute pericarditis (NSAIDs or colchicine for several weeks or months, even after disappearance of effusion).[100] Long-term (3 to 6 months) oral corticosteroids or preferably pericardiocentesis and intrapericardial instillation of triamcinolone (300 mg/m^2) are therapeutic options in refractory forms. Redo surgery is rarely needed. Primary prevention of postpericardiotomy syndrome using short-term perioperative corticosteroid treatment or colchicine is under investigation.[101]

POSTINFARCTION PERICARDITIS

Two forms of postinfarction pericarditis can be distinguished: an "early" form (pericarditis epistenocardica) and a "delayed" form (Dressler's syndrome).[102] Epistenocardiac pericarditis, caused by direct exudation, occurs in 5% to 20% of transmural myocardial infarctions but is clinically discovered rarely. Dressler's syndrome occurs from 1 week to several months after clinical onset of myocardial infarction with symptoms and manifestations similar to the post–cardiac injury syndrome. It does not require transmural infarction[103] and can also appear as an extension of epistenocardiac pericarditis. Its incidence is 0.5% to 5%[104] and is lower still in patients treated with thrombolytics (<0.5%)[105] but more frequent in cases of pericardial bleeding after antithrombotic treatment.[102,106] Of note, ECG changes are often overshadowed by myocardial infarction changes. Stage one ECG changes are uncommon and suggest "early" post–myocardial infarction syndrome, whereas failure to evolve or "resurrection" of previously inverted T waves strongly suggests myocardial infarction pericarditis.[107,108] Postinfarction pericardial effusion greater than 10 mm is most frequently associated with hemopericardium, and two thirds of these patients may develop tamponade/free wall rupture.[109] Urgent surgical treatment is lifesaving. If the immediate surgery is not available or contraindicated, pericardiocentesis and intrapericardial fibrin-glue instillation could be an alternative in subacute tamponade.[109,110] Ibuprofen, which increases coronary flow, is the agent of choice.[111] Aspirin, up to 650 mg every 4 hours for 2 to 5 days, has also been successfully applied. Corticosteroids can be used for refractory symptoms but may delay the healing after infarction.[7]

TRAUMATIC PERICARDIAL EFFUSION AND HEMOPERICARDIUM IN AORTIC DISSECTION

Direct pericardial injury can be induced by accidents or iatrogenic wounds.[112-115] Iatrogenic tamponade occurs most frequently in percutaneous mitral valvuloplasty, during or after transseptal puncture, particularly if no biplane catheterization laboratory is available and a small left atrium is present. Whereas the puncture of the interatrial septum is asymptomatic, the passage of the free wall induces chest pain immediately. If high-pressure–containing structures are punctured, rapid deterioration occurs. However, if only the atrial wall is passed, the tamponade may be delayed for 4 to 6 hours. Rescue pericardiocentesis is successful in 95% to 100%, with a less than 1% mortality.[116]

Transection of the coronary artery and acute or subacute cardiac tamponade occur very rarely during percutaneous coronary interventions.[117,118] A breakthrough in the treatment of coronary perforation has been the development of membrane-covered graft stents.[119,120]

During right ventricular endomyocardial biopsy the catheter may pass the myocardium, particularly when the bioptome has not been opened before reaching the endocardial border or it is directed to the right ventricular free wall instead of to the septum. Frank cardiac perforations are accompanied by sudden bradycardia and hypotension.[121] A perforation rate of 0.3% to 5% was reported, leading to tamponade and circulatory collapse in less than half of the cases.[121-123] The incidence of pericardial hemorrhage in left ventricular endomyocardial biopsy is lower (0.1% to 3.3%). Severe complications, leading to procedure-related mortality, were reported in only 0.05% in a worldwide survey of more than 6000 cases[122] and in none of the 2537 patients in our center.[123]

Pacemaker leads penetrating the right ventricle or epicardial electrodes may cause pericarditis with tamponade, adhesions, or constriction.[124-127] A right bundle branch block instead of a usually induced left bundle branch block is a clue.

Blunt chest trauma is the major risk of car accidents. The deceleration force can lead to myocardial contusion with intrapericardial hemorrhage, cardiac rupture, pericardial rupture, or herniation. Transesophageal echocardiography or immediate CT should be performed.[128] Pericardial laceration and partial extrusion of the heart into the mediastinum and pleural space may also occur after injury.[113]

In dissection of the ascending aorta, pericardial effusion can be found in 17% to 45% of the patients and in 48% of the autopsy cases.[128] In a clinical series of aortic dissection, pericardial tamponade was found by CT,[130] MRI,[131] or echocardiography[132] in 17% to 33% of patients with type I dissection, 18% to 45% in type II dissection, and 6% in type III dissection.[130] Pericardiocentesis is contraindicated, owing to the risk of intensified bleeding and extension of the dissection.[133,134] Surgery should be performed immediately.

NEOPLASTIC PERICARDITIS

Primary tumors of the pericardium are 40 times less common than metastatic ones.[7] Mesothelioma, the most common of the primary tumors, is almost always incurable. The most common secondary malignant tumors are lung cancer, breast cancer, malignant melanoma, lymphomas, and leukemia. Effusions may be small or large with an imminent tamponade (frequent recurrences) or constriction. Tamponade may even be the initial sign of malignant disease.[135] With small effusions most patients are asymptomatic. The onset of dyspnea, cough, chest pain, tachycardia, and jugular venous distention is observed when the volume of fluid exceeds 500 mL. Pulsus paradoxus, hypotension, cardiogenic shock, and paradoxical movement of the jugular venous pulse are important signs of cardiac tamponade. The diagnosis is based on the confirmation of the malignant infiltration within the pericardium by cytology or biopsy. Of note, in almost two thirds of the patients with documented malignancy pericardial effusion is caused by nonmalignant diseases (e.g., radiation pericarditis or opportunistic infections).[136,137] The chest radiograph, CT, and MRI may reveal mediastinal widening, hilar masses, and pleural effusion.[7] The analysis of pericardial fluid and pericardial or epicardial biopsy are essential for the confirmation of malignant pericardial disease.

Cardiac tamponade is an absolute indication for pericardiocentesis. In suspected neoplastic pericardial effusion without tamponade, systemic antineoplastic treatment as baseline therapy can prevent recurrences in up to 67% of cases.[135] However, pericardial drainage is recommended in all patients with large effusions because of the high recurrence rate (40% to 70%).[138-144] Prevention of recurrences may be achieved by intrapericardial instillation of sclerosing, cytotoxic agents, or immunomodulators. Intrapericardial treatment tailored to the type of the tumor indicates that administration of cisplatin is effective in secondary lung cancer, and intrapericardial instillation of thiotepa appears to be highly effective in breast cancer pericardial metastases.[145-150] No patient showed signs of constrictive pericarditis. Tetracyclines as sclerosing agents also control the malignant pericardial effusion in around 85% of cases, but side effects and complications are quite frequent: fever (19%), chest pain (20%), and atrial arrhythmias (10%).[135,143,144] Although intrapericardial administration of radionuclides has yielded very good results, it is not widely accepted because of the logistic problems connected with their radioactivity.[151] Radiation therapy is very effective (93%) in controlling malignant pericardial effusion in patients with radiosensitive tumors such as lymphoma and leukemia. However, radiotherapy of the heart can cause myocarditis and pericarditis by itself.[135]

RARE FORMS OF PERICARDIAL DISEASE

Fungal pericarditis occurs mainly in immunocompromised patients or in the course of endemic, acquired fungal infections.[152] It is mainly due to endemic (*Histoplasma, Coccidioides*) or opportunistic fungi (*Candida, Aspergillus, Blastomyces*) and semifungi (*Nocardia, Actinomyces*).[153-155] Diagnosis is obtained by staining and culturing pericardial fluid or tissue. Antifungal antibodies in serum are also helpful in establishing the diagnosis.[3] Treatment with fluconazole, ketoconazole, itraconazole, amphotericin B, liposomal amphotericin B, or amphotericin B lipid complex is indicated. NSAIDs can support the treatment with antifungal drugs. Patients with histoplasmosis pericarditis do not need antifungal therapy but respond to NSAIDs given for 2 to 12 weeks. Sulfonamides are the drugs of choice for nocardiosis. Combination of three antibiotics including penicillin should be given for actinomycosis. Pericardiocentesis or surgical treatment is indicated for hemodynamic impairment. Pericardiectomy is indicated in fungal constrictive pericarditis.

Radiation pericarditis may begin already during exposure (very rare) or months and years later—with latency of up to 15 to 20 years. Its occurrence is influenced by the applied source, dose, fractionation, duration, radiation exposed volume, form of mantel field therapy, and the age of the patient.[156] The effusion may be serous or hemorrhagic, later on with fibrinous adhesions or constriction, typically without tissue calcification. The symptoms may be masked by the underlying disease or the applied chemotherapy. Imaging should start with echocardiography, followed by cardiac CT or MRI if necessary. Pericarditis without tamponade may be treated conservatively. Pericardial constriction occurs in up to 20% of patients, requiring pericardiectomy. The operative mortality is high (21%) and the postoperative 5-year survival is poor (1%), mostly owing to myocardial fibrosis.[157]

Chylopericardium refers to a communication between the pericardium and the thoracic duct, as a result of trauma or congenital anomalies, or as a complication of open-heart surgery,[158] mediastinal lymphangiomas, lymphangiomatous hamartomas, lymphangiectasis, and obstruction or anomalies of the thoracic duct.[159] Infection, tamponade, or constriction may aggravate the prognosis.[160] The pericardial fluid is sterile, odorless, and opalescent with a milky white appearance and the microscopic finding of fat droplets. The chylous nature of the fluid is confirmed by its alkaline reaction, specific gravity between 1010 and 1021, Sudan III stain for fat, and the high concentrations of triglycerides (5 to 50 g/L) and protein (22 to 60 g/L).[161,162] Enhanced CT, alone or combined with lymphography, can identify not only the location of the thoracic duct but also its lymphatic connection to the pericardium.[163,164]

Treatment depends on the etiology and the amount of chylous accumulation.[165] Chylopericardium after thoracic or cardiac operation is preferably treated by pericardiocentesis and diet (medium-chain triglycerides).[166,167] If further production of chylous effusion continues, surgical treatment is mandatory. When conservative treatment and pericardiocentesis fail, a pericardioperitoneal window is a reasonable option.[168,169] Alternatively, when the course of the thoracic duct is precisely identified, its ligation and resection just above the diaphragm is the most effective treatment.[170]

Drug- and toxin-related pericarditis, tamponade, adhesions, fibrosis, or constriction may be induced by several drugs.[7,171] Mechanisms include drug-induced lupus reactions, idiosyncrasy, "serum sickness," foreign substance reactions, and immunopathy. Management is based on the discontinuation of the causative agent and symptomatic treatment.

Pericardial effusion in hypothyroidism occurs in 5% to 30% of patients.[7] Fluid accumulates slowly and tamponade occurs rarely. In some cases, cholesterol pericarditis may be observed. The diagnosis is based on serum levels of thyroxine and thyroid-stimulating hormone. Bradycardia, low voltage of the QRS and T wave inversion or flattening in the ECG, cardiomegaly on the radiograph, and pericardial effusion on echocardiography, as well as a history of radiation-induced thyroid dysfunction, myopathy, ascites, pleural effusion, and uveal edema may be observed.[172-176] Therapy with thyroid hormone decreases pericardial effusion.

Pericardial effusion and constriction in pregnancy may manifest as a minimal to moderate clinically silent hydropericardium by the third trimester. Cardiac compression is rare.[177] ECG changes of acute pericarditis in pregnancy should be distinguished from the slight ST-segment depressions and T-wave changes seen in normal pregnancy.[177,178] Occult constriction becomes manifest in pregnancy owing to the increased blood volume.[178] Most pericardial disorders are managed as in nonpregnant women.[179,180] Caution is necessary because high-dose aspirin may prematurely close the ductus arteriosus, and colchicine is contraindicated in pregnancy. Pericardiotomy and pericardiectomy can be safely performed if necessary and do not impose a risk for subsequent pregnancies.[180,181]

Fetal pericardial fluid can be detected by echocardiography after 20 weeks' gestation and is normally 2 mm or less in depth. More fluid should raise questions of hydrops fetalis, Rh disease, neoplasia, hypoalbuminemia, immunopathy, or maternally transmitted mycoplasmal or other infections.[182]

ANNOTATED REFERENCES

Maisch B, Seferovic PM, Ristic AD, et al: Guidelines on the diagnosis and management of pericardial diseases executive summary; The Task Force on the Diagnosis and Management of Pericardial Diseases of the European Society of Cardiology. Eur Heart J 2004;25:587-610.
 First ESC guidelines for the diagnosis and treatment of pericardial diseases.

Maisch B, Ristic AD, Pankuweit S: Intrapericardial treatment of autoreactive pericardial effusion with triamcinolone: The way to avoid side effects of systemic corticosteroid therapy. Eur Heart J 2002;23:1503-1508.
 First clinical study on autoreactive pericarditis and intrapericardial treatment with triamcinolone, showing high efficacy and low incidence of side effects during follow-up.

Maisch B, Ristic AD, Pankuweit S, et al: Neoplastic pericardial effusion: Efficacy and safety of intrapericardial treatment with cisplatin. Eur Heart J 2002;23:1625-1631.
 Study on intrapericardial treatment of neoplastic pericardial effusion revealing higher efficacy of cisplatin in lung cancer than in breast cancer patients.

Seferovic PM, Maisch B, Spodick DH (eds) and Maksimovic R, Ristic AD (assoc eds): Pericardiology: Contemporary Answers to Continuing Challenges. Belgrade, Science, 2000.

Most recent textbook on pericardial diseases covering advances in diagnosis and treatment, including original data on colchicine treatment, pericardioscopy, pericardial and epicardial biopsy as well as pericardiocentesis, percutaneous balloon pericardiotomy, and surgical procedures for pericardial diseases.

Seferovic PM, Ristic AD, Maksimovic R, et al: Diagnostic value of pericardial biopsy: Improvement with extensive sampling enabled by pericardioscopy. Circulation 2003;107:978-983.
Recent study on pericardial biopsy revealing contribution of endoscopic guidance to the diagnostic value of the procedure.

Chapter 103

EMERGENT VALVULAR DISORDERS

Catherine M. Otto

KEY POINTS

ACUTE MITRAL REGURGITATION

1. Causes include endocarditis, mitral prolapse, and acute myocardial infarction.
2. It presents as pulmonary edema.
3. Murmur may be soft or absent.
4. Prompt echocardiography is essential.
5. Pulmonary wedge v wave is not always seen.
6. Intra-aortic balloon pump improves hemodynamics.
7. Definitive treatment is mitral valve surgery.

ACUTE AORTIC REGURGITATION

1. Causes include endocarditis and aortic dissection.
2. Diastolic murmur may be soft.
3. Prompt echocardiography is essential.
4. Treatment is emergency surgery.

MITRAL STENOSIS

1. Rheumatic mitral stenosis typically occurs in young women.
2. It may present during pregnancy.
3. Echocardiography is diagnostic.
4. Acute decompensation can be treated conservatively.
5. Percutaneous balloon mitral valvuloplasty is the optimal intervention.

AORTIC STENOSIS

1. Aortic stenosis is common in the elderly.
2. Decompensation occurs with increased hemodynamic demand.
3. Physical examination shows a systolic murmur.
4. Echocardiography is diagnostic.
5. Conservative management for decompensation is appropriate.
6. Severe symptomatic disease requires aortic valve replacement.

PROSTHETIC VALVES

1. Mechanical valves are at risk of valve thrombosis.
2. Management of prosthetic valve thrombosis is controversial.
3. Tissue valves undergo degeneration 10 to 15 years after implantation.
4. Acute regurgitation is similar to native valve disease.

In the critical care setting there are two distinct presentations of valvular heart disease: (1) acute valve dysfunction resulting in acute heart failure and (2) chronic valve disease with decompensation due to increased metabolic demands (Table 103-1).[1] Valve regurgitation is the most common type of acute valve dysfunction. Valve stenosis, with rare exceptions, is a chronic, slowly progressive disease. However, in patients with asymptomatic chronic valve stenosis, acute deterioration can occur if there is a superimposed hemodynamic burden. For example, the patient with previously asymptomatic mitral stenosis may present with pulmonary edema in the setting of a systemic infection. Another example is the elderly adult with asymptomatic aortic stenosis who presents with cardiogenic shock in the setting of an acute gastrointestinal hemorrhage.

The key concepts in the management of the critically ill patient with valvular heart disease are the use of echocardiography to provide an accurate diagnosis of disease severity and the appropriate use of invasive hemodynamic monitoring to optimize loading conditions.

MITRAL REGURGITATION

ETIOLOGY

Mitral regurgitation may be caused by disease or distortion of any component of the mitral valve apparatus, including the mitral annulus, leaflets, chordae, and papillary muscles as well as by alterations in left ventricular (LV) geometry or systolic function (Fig. 103-1).[2] Primary causes of chronic mitral regurgitation include myxomatous valve leaflets (mitral valve prolapse) and rheumatic disease. Chronic secondary mitral regurgitation may be due to dilated cardiomyopathy or to coronary artery disease with regional or global left ventricular dysfunction.

Acute mitral regurgitation also may be due to involvement of the valve leaflets or the left ventricle. Patients with

TABLE 103–1. CAUSES OF ACUTE VALVE DYSFUNCTION

Mitral Regurgitation

Myxomatous disease with flail leaflet
Spontaneous chordal rupture
Endocarditis
Acute myocardial infarction
    Papillary muscle rupture
    Regional wall motion abnormality
    Left ventricular dilation and systolic dysfunction

Aortic Regurgitation

Endocarditis
Spontaneous rupture of a congenital fenestration
Aortic dissection

Tricuspid Regurgitation

Endocarditis
Penetrating chest trauma
Blunt chest wall trauma

Prosthetic Valves

Endocarditis
Valve thrombosis
Paravalvular dehiscence
Leaflet tear

myocardial wall underlying the posterolateral papillary muscle.[5-7]

CLINICAL PRESENTATION

Although patients with chronic mitral regurgitation may be asymptomatic for many years, the regurgitant lesion imposes a volume load on the left ventricle because an increased total stroke volume is needed to maintain a normal forward cardiac output. LV volume overload results in progressive LV dilation and may lead to an irreversible decline in ventricular contractility, even in the absence of clinical symptoms. Evaluation of ventricular contractility is problematic in patients with mitral regurgitation given that measures of ventricular performance are affected by preload and afterload.[8] However, based on outcomes after mitral valve surgery, the empirical parameters of ventricular end-systolic dimension and ejection fraction can be used to optimize the timing of surgical intervention. Thus, patients with moderate to severe chronic regurgitation undergo periodic echocardiography with valve repair or replacement recommended when the end-systolic dimension is 45 mm or more and the ejection fraction is 60% or less.[9]

Chronic mitral regurgitation usually is well tolerated even when there is a superimposed hemodynamic load such as systemic infection, pregnancy, or trauma. However, mitral regurgitant severity may acutely worsen by at least two mechanisms. First, an increase in afterload, for example with a hypertensive crisis, may increase regurgitant severity due to an increased driving pressure from the left ventricle to the left atrium. Second, alteration in LV geometry, for example with ventricular dilation due to decompensated heart failure, may change the orientation of the papillary muscles such that leaflet closure is impaired, resulting in a larger regurgitant orifice area.[10] In this situation, a vicious cycle may ensue in

myxomatous mitral valve disease may develop acute regurgitation due to spontaneous chordal rupture.[3,4] Bacterial endocarditis results in acute mitral regurgitation due to destruction of valve tissue, often with leaflet perforation. Mitral regurgitation complicates 3% to 16% of acute myocardial infarctions (AMIs) due to papillary muscle dysfunction or rupture as a result of impaired function of the

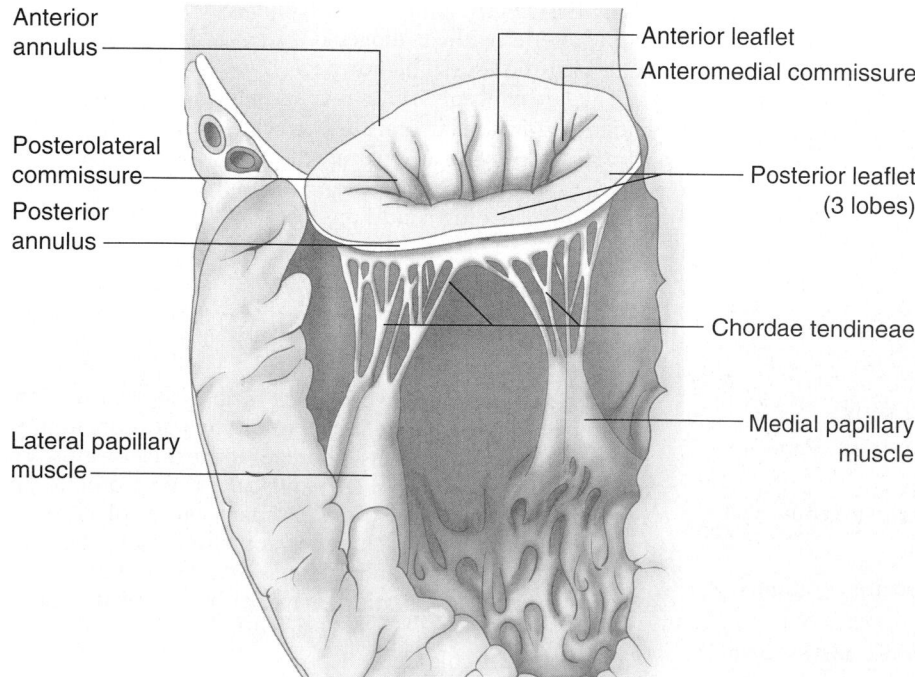

FIGURE 103–1. The mitral valve consists of the mitral annulus, anterior and posterior leaflets, chordae tendineae, and papillary muscles. Mitral regurgitation may be due to a disease that primarily affects the valve leaflets, such as mitral valve prolapse or rheumatic mitral valve disease, or may result from alterations in the function or structure of the left ventricle, such as those induced by ischemic disease or dilated cardiomyopathy. (From Otto CM: Clinical practice: Evaluation and management of chronic mitral regurgitation. N Engl J Med 2001;345:740-746.)

Anterior annulus
Posterolateral commissure
Posterior annulus
Lateral papillary muscle

Anterior leaflet
Anteromedial commissure
Posterior leaflet (3 lobes)
Chordae tendineae
Medial papillary muscle

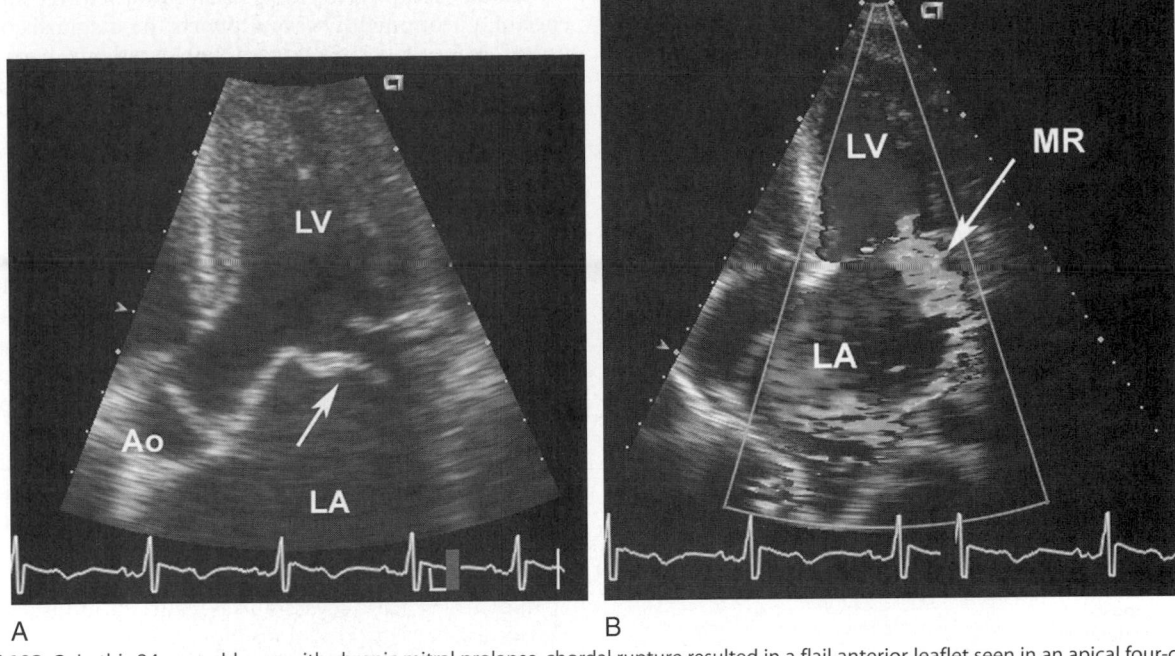

FIGURE 103–2. In this 24-year-old man with chronic mitral prolapse, chordal rupture resulted in a flail anterior leaflet seen in an apical four-chamber view (**A,** *arrow*). Severe mitral regurgitation (MR) was seen with a posterior and laterally directed jet on Doppler color flow imaging (**B,** *arrow*). Ao, aorta; LA, left atrium; LV, left ventricle. (See Color Section in this text.)

which LV dilation worsens mitral regurgitant severity, which increases LV dilation, and so forth.

Acute mitral regurgitation presents as acute pulmonary edema and is a surgical emergency (Figs. 103-2 and 103-3). Mitral chordal rupture results in the acute presentation of heart failure, often in patients who were unaware of a diagnosis of mitral valve prolapse. Patients with mitral valve perforation due to endocarditis present with pulmonary edema supcrimposed on signs and symptoms of endocarditis. Papillary muscle rupture or dysfunction after myocardial

infarction usually presents several days after AMI; in some cases, the initial presentation is acute pulmonary edema, with the myocardial infarction being clinically silent.[11]

DIAGNOSIS

A high level of clinical suspicion is needed to make the diagnosis of acute mitral regurgitation (Table 103-2). Acute pulmonary edema often obscures the signs and symptoms of the underlying disease process. The classical finding is a

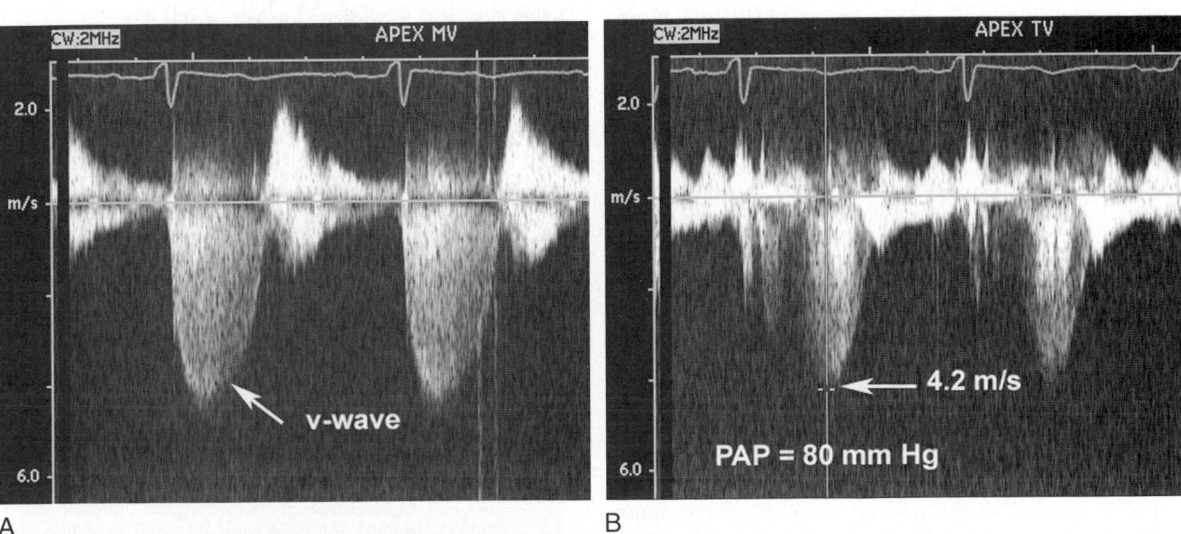

FIGURE 103–3. In the same patient as Figure 103-2 severe mitral regurgitation was recorded with continuous wave Doppler ultrasound (**A**). The rapid rise in left atrial pressure due to the regurgitant jet entering the left atrium results in a rapid decline in the Doppler velocity in late systole—the Doppler equivalent of the v wave seen on a pulmonary wedge pressure tracing. The continuous wave Doppler recording of the maximum tricuspid regurgitant jet velocity (**B**) of 4.2 m/s indicates a right ventricular to right atrial pressure difference of 70 mm Hg. The patient's right atrial pressure was estimated to be 10 mm Hg, based on the size and respiratory variation in the inferior vena cava, so that the estimated pulmonary systolic pressure is 80 mm Hg.

TABLE 103–2. DIAGNOSTIC APPROACH TO ACUTE VALVE DYSFUNCTION

Physical Examination	Unreliable
	Consider valve dysfunction in all patients with pulmonary edema
Echocardiography (transthoracic)	Accurate diagnosis of etiology of disease
	Quantitation of severity of stenosis or regurgitation
	Measurement of ventricular ejection fraction
	Estimation of pulmonary pressures
Transesophageal Echocardiography	Sensitive for detection of valvular vegetations
	Detection of paravalvular abscess
	Essential for prosthetic mitral valve dysfunction
	Useful for prosthetic aortic valve dysfunction
Right-Sided Heart Catheterization	Not reliable for diagnosis of valve disease
	May be helpful for optimizing loading conditions
Chest CT	Sensitive and specific for diagnosis of aortic dissection
Angiography	Used when coronary angiography is needed

holosystolic murmur at the apex radiating to the axilla.[12] However, although there is some correlation between the loudness of the murmur and regurgitant severity with chronic regurgitation, the murmur may be soft with acute severe mitral regurgitation. In patients with severe mitral regurgitation after myocardial infarction a murmur cannot be appreciated at all in up to 50% of patients.[13]

Thus, in patients presenting with acute pulmonary edema or cardiogenic shock, prompt echocardiography is essential. Transthoracic images often are diagnostic, allowing identification of the etiology of valve dysfunction, quantitation of regurgitant severity, estimation of pulmonary pressures, and measurement of ventricular size and systolic function. If transthoracic images are nondiagnostic, transesophageal echocardiography (TEE) can be performed at the bedside in the ICU. TEE provides excellent images of valve anatomy and Doppler evaluation of valve function.

Other diagnostic tests are based on the clinical presentation. Multiple blood cultures should be obtained in febrile patients with pulmonary edema to exclude the possibility of endocarditis. In patients with an abnormal electrocardiogram (ECG), chest pain, or a history of coronary artery disease, coronary angiography may be needed.

In the patient with acute pulmonary edema or cardiogenic shock after myocardial infarction, the differential diagnosis includes acute mitral regurgitation, a ventricular septal defect (VSD), or a contained rupture of the ventricular free wall. All these possibilities can be diagnosed by echocardiography, in an experienced center.

Invasive hemodynamic monitoring with a Swan-Ganz catheter for measurement of pulmonary pressures and cardiac output is needed in the patient with suspected acute mitral regurgitation. At the time of placement, oxygen saturations in the right atrium, right ventricle, and pulmonary artery should be measured; a VSD results in a "step-up" in oxygen saturation between the right atrium and ventricle due to oxygenated blood from the left ventricle entering the right ventricle. The pulmonary wedge pressure tracing should be examined for the presence of a v wave. The presence of a prominent v wave supports the diagnosis of acute mitral regurgitation, although some patients have severe regurgitation with no v wave and a v wave can be seen in the absence of severe mitral regurgitation in patients with a prosthetic mitral valve.[14,15]

MANAGEMENT

In patients with chronic mitral regurgitation and heart failure, management is directed at treating the process leading to decompensation and optimizing loading conditions (Table 103-3). For example, in a patient with a systemic infection, treatment of the infection, control of fever and tachycardia, and invasive monitoring to optimize preload and afterload are utilized. Medical therapy typically includes afterload reduction with nitroprusside or other vasodilators and preload reduction with diuretics.[16,17] The goal is to support the patient through the period of decompensation. Typically, hemodynamics return to the baseline compensated state after the acute illness.

In contrast, acute severe mitral regurgitation is a surgical emergency.[18] Medical stabilization should occur concurrently with consultation by a cardiac surgeon. Acutely, placement of an intra-aortic balloon pump (IABP) provides optimal afterload reduction while improving diastolic coronary blood flow.

The timing and risk of surgical intervention depend on the etiology of acute mitral regurgitation. Spontaneous chordal rupture usually can be treated early with mitral valve repair.[19] Compared with valve replacement, mitral valve repair is associated with a lower operative mortality, improved preservation of LV function, and better long-term survival. In addition, the risks of a prosthetic valve and anticoagulation are avoided.

The timing of surgery for endocarditis depends on the disease course in that individual, but most centers now advocate early surgical intervention in the patient with heart failure to prevent progressive valve damage and paravalvular abscess formation. Recent studies suggest that delaying surgery does not decrease the risk of recurrent infection. Valve repair is preferred but may not be possible depending on the extent of tissue destruction.

In patients with acute ischemic mitral regurgitation, treatment depends on the exact etiology of valve dysfunction.[20] In patients with acute mitral regurgitation due to a regional wall motion abnormality, myocardial function may improve after percutaneous revascularization.[6,21] In these patients, an

TABLE 103–3. THERAPEUTIC APPROACH TO ACUTE VALVE DYSFUNCTION

1. Accurate diagnosis with echocardiography—differentiate acute valve dysfunction from acute decompensation with chronic valve disease.
2. Treat the underlying disease process associated with decompensation (e.g., endocarditis, acute myocardial infarction, anemia).
3. Optimize loading conditions using diuretics, vasodilators, and other agents with invasive hemodynamic monitoring.
4. Consult the cardiac surgery team as soon as the diagnosis is made.
5. Use intra-aortic balloon pump for acute mitral regurgitation.
6. Consider surgical or percutaneous intervention for acute valve dysfunction.

IABP and medical therapy may be used during the acute episode with weaning of therapy as myocardial function improves.

Mitral regurgitation due to partial or complete papillary muscle rupture requires surgical intervention. Although the risk of surgery is high with an operative mortality rate of about 50%, outcome is even worse with medical therapy, with a mortality of 75% at 24 hours and 95% within 2 weeks after complete papillary muscle rupture.[5,22,23] With the use of echocardiography, partial papillary muscle rupture can be recognized; prognosis in these patients depends on the extent of myocardial damage and severity of mitral regurgitation.[24] With partial papillary muscle rupture, some surgeons prefer to stabilize the patient and delay surgery for 6 to 8 weeks after myocardial infarction to avoid operating on the necrotic myocardial tissue. However, many patients cannot be stabilized so acute intervention must be considered. Again, valve repair is preferred but myocardial necrosis may necessitate valve replacement. Risk factors for surgery include older age, female gender, and poor LV systolic function.[25] In some patients, the risk of surgical intervention may be so high as to be futile.

AORTIC REGURGITATION

ETIOLOGY

Chronic aortic regurgitation most often is due to a congenital bicuspid valve, rheumatic valve disease, or aortic root dilation. There are numerous causes of aortic root dilation, including hypertension, cystic medial necrosis, Marfan syndrome, and a bicuspid aortic valve.[26] The most common causes of acute aortic regurgitation are endocarditis, rupture of a congenital fenestration, and acute aortic dissection.[27] Endocarditis results in aortic regurgitation by destruction of the valve leaflet tissue, with a high percentage of cases also having paravalvular abscess formation. Aortic dissection results in acute aortic regurgitation either due to enlargement of the aortic annulus or to extension of the dissection into the valve region resulting in a flail aortic valve leaflet.

CLINICAL PRESENTATION

The acute backflow of blood from the aorta into the left ventricle in diastole results in an acute elevation in LV end-diastolic pressure with consequent pulmonary edema.[28] Because there has been no time for compensatory LV dilation, forward cardiac output falls abruptly due to the regurgitant flow across the valve in diastole so that patients with acute aortic regurgitation also may be in cardiogenic shock.[29] Decreased coronary perfusion pressure results in diffuse subendocardial ischemia, further impairing ventricular function.[30]

DIAGNOSIS

The clinical diagnosis of acute aortic regurgitation differs markedly from chronic aortic regurgitation (Fig. 103-4).[31] In contrast to the high-pitched diastolic decrescendo murmur of chronic aortic regurgitation, there is a "to-and-fro" murmur across the aortic valve that many clinicians fail to recognize as indicating aortic regurgitation. The pulse

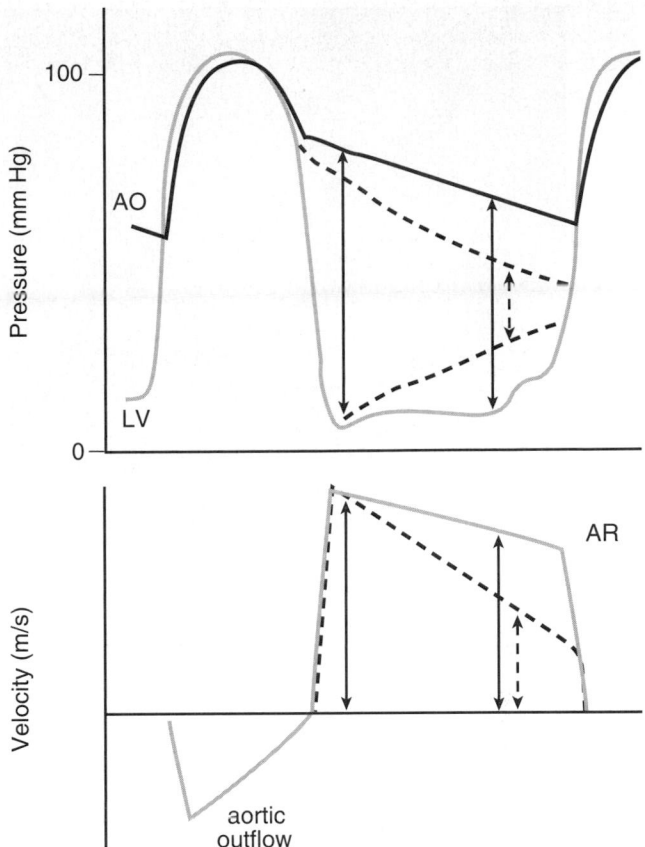

FIGURE 103–4. Left ventricular (LV) and central aortic (Ao) pressures and the corresponding Doppler velocity curves are shown for chronic *(solid lines)* and acute *(dashed lines)* aortic regurgitation. The shape of the velocity curve is related to the instantaneous pressure differences across the valve, as stated in the Bernoulli equation. With acute aortic regurgitation, aortic pressures fall more rapidly and ventricular diastolic pressure rises more rapidly, resulting in a steeper deceleration slope on the Doppler curve. (From Otto CM: The Textbook of Clinical Echocardiography, 3rd ed. Philadelphia, WB Saunders, 2004, p 326.)

pressure is narrow, owing to the low forward stroke volume, and peripheral signs of aortic regurgitation are not seen. As with acute mitral regurgitation, the physical examination findings often are subtle so a high index of suspicion and prompt echocardiography are needed to make this diagnosis.

Acute aortic regurgitation should be considered in the patient with signs or symptoms of endocarditis, in patients with a personal or family history of aortic root disease, and in those with a presentation consistent with acute aortic dissection.

Echocardiography allows imaging of the aortic valve and root and determination of the severity of aortic regurgitation based on a combination of two-dimensional imaging and pulsed, continuous wave, and color Doppler modalities (Figs. 103-5 to 103-7).[32] The continuous wave Doppler curve shows a steep diastolic slope corresponding to the rapid equalization of diastolic pressure in the aorta and left ventricle. With severe acute regurgitation, there is no pressure gradient at end diastole so that cuff diastolic blood pressure is equal to LV end-diastolic pressure. Echocardiography also allows accurate assessment of LV size and systolic function. When the differential diagnosis includes aortic dissection, transthoracic echocardiography is inadequate to exclude this

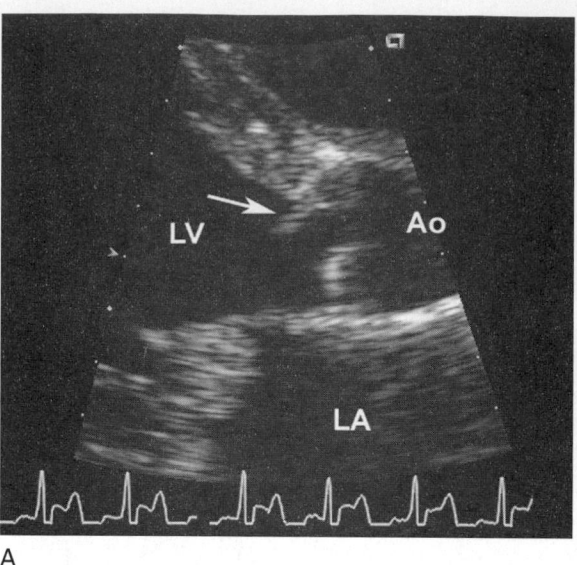

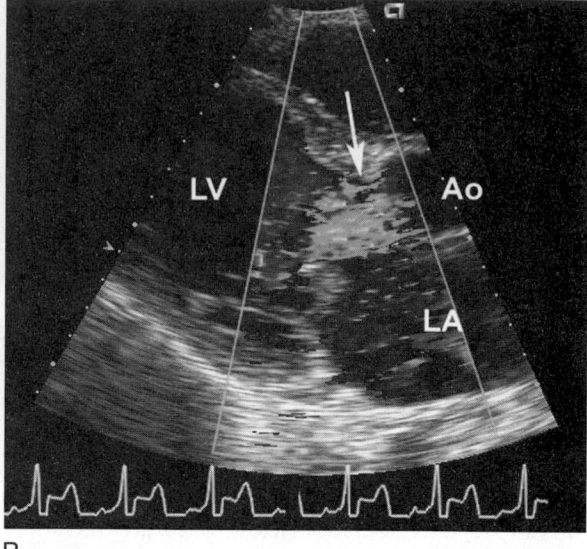

A

B

FIGURE 103–5. Endocarditis resulting in acute severe aortic regurgitation. In a long-axis view of the aortic valve (**A**) a flail aortic valve leaflet is seen *(arrow)* with the leaflet prolapsing into the left ventricular (LV) outflow tract in diastole. Color flow imaging (**B**) in the same view shows a broad jet of diastolic flow filling the outflow tract consistent with severe regurgitation. Ao, aorta; LA, left atrium; LV, left ventricle. (See Color Section in this text.)

possibility. Instead, TEE or computed tomography (CT) images should be obtained.

MANAGEMENT

Acute aortic regurgitation is a surgical emergency.[33] Preoperative management is supportive with ventilatory support and invasive hemodynamic monitoring. While the diagnosis is being made, therapy may include the use of diuretics, inotropic agents, and nitroprusside or other vasodilators in an attempt to stabilize hemodynamics.[17,34-36] However, an IABP is contraindicated because inflation of the balloon in the descending thoracic aorta in diastole will increase the amount of backflow across the aortic valve.

If acute aortic regurgitation is due to aortic dissection, acute surgical intervention is needed. The surgical approach may be replacement of the ascending aorta and valve with a Dacron or Gore-Tex valved conduit. When the valve leaflets are normal, some centers will preserve the native valve by re-suspension of the leaflets in a prosthetic conduit (called the David procedure).

When acute aortic regurgitation is due to endocarditis, surgical options include a mechanical valve, a heterograft tissue valve such as a porcine aortic valve or bovine pericardial valve, or a cryopreserved homograft aorta valve. Rarely, the patient may undergo valve repair if there is a simple perforation with adjacent normal leaflet tissue. Many surgeons prefer an aortic homograft in patients with endocarditis

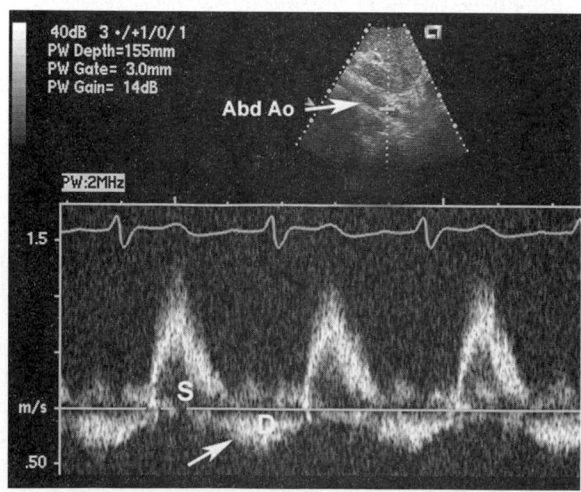

FIGURE 103–6. In the same patient as Figure 103-5, pulsed Doppler flow in the proximal abdominal aorta (Ao) shows normal forward flow in systole (S), with abnormal flow in diastole (D) that extends throughout diastole. This finding is highly specific for severe aortic regurgitation and can be helpful in the acute setting.

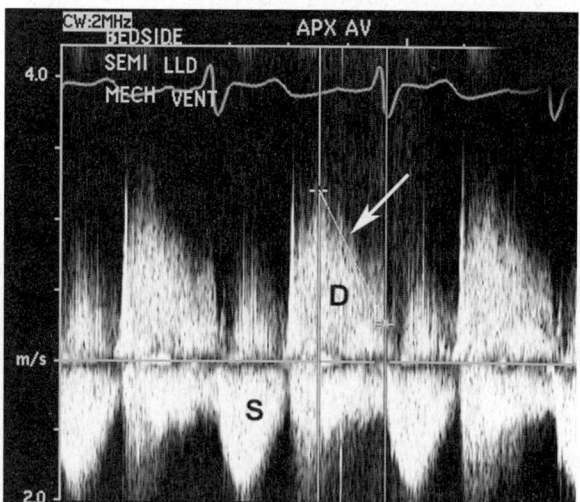

FIGURE 103–7. In the same patient as Figure 103-5, continuous wave Doppler flow of the flow across the aortic valve shows an increased antegrade velocity in systole (S) consistent with a high transaortic stroke volume. In diastole (D), a dense signal of retrograde flow is seen with a steep deceleration slope *(arrow)* consistent with equalization of pressures between the aorta and left ventricle in diastole.

because of relative resistance to reinfection and the frequent occurrence of paravalvular extension of the infection. A cryopreserved aortic homograft typically includes the valve, the ascending aorta, and the anterior mitral leaflet. The surgeon trims the homograft, retaining tissue to repair the aortic annulus, base of the ventricular septum, and anterior mitral leaflet as needed.

MITRAL STENOSIS

ETIOLOGY AND CLINICAL PRESENTATION

Mitral stenosis is nearly always due to rheumatic disease, with only rare cases of calcific mitral stenosis seen in the elderly. Rheumatic mitral stenosis is a slowly progressive disease with an insidious decline in exercise tolerance and symptom onset over many years.[37] However, in the asymptomatic patient with compensated moderate or severe mitral stenosis, acute decompensation can occur in the setting of increased systemic hemodynamic demands. Because mitral stenosis is more common in women (80% of cases) and occurs during the reproductive years, the most common emergency presentation of mitral stenosis is a pregnant woman with heart failure.[38,39] Many of these patients are unaware of underlying valve disease and are initially diagnosed during pregnancy. The clinical presentation may also be due to, or exacerbated by, the onset of atrial fibrillation.

A large atrial myxoma may mimic the clinical presentation of mitral stenosis, presenting as acute hemodynamic compromise due to obstruction of the mitral valve orifice by the tumor mass.

DIAGNOSIS

The apical diastolic rumble and opening snap of mitral stenosis is challenging to appreciate even in a quiet room with optimal patient positioning and frequently is inaudible in the ICU setting.[31] However, the diagnosis is easily made by transthoracic echocardiography with the mitral leaflet showing the characteristic findings of rheumatic disease: commissural fusion, chordal shortening and fusion, and restriction of the diastolic opening of the leaflets (Fig. 103-8).[40] Mitral stenosis severity can be quantitated by calculation of valve area by two-dimensional planimetry or by the Doppler pressure half-time method with moderate to severe stenosis defined as a valve area less than 1.5 cm² (Fig. 103-9). Transthoracic echocardiography also provides information on LV size and systolic function, left atrial size, pulmonary pressures, and any associated valve lesions. If evaluation for left atrial thrombus is needed, TEE has a sensitivity of only 60% compared with a sensitivity of nearly 100% from the transthoracic approach.

MANAGEMENT

Most patients with mitral stenosis and acute decompensation can be managed conservatively with treatment of the superimposed illness.[17] Efforts should be directed toward decreasing overall metabolic demand and increasing oxygen delivery by controlling fever, maintaining a normal hemoglobin level, and providing supplemental oxygen. If atrial fibrillation is present, rate control is essential, preferably with conversion back to sinus rhythm. Even when sinus rhythm is present, beta blockers may improve ventricular diastolic filling by prolonging the duration of diastole as heart rate is decreased.[41-44] Invasive hemodynamic monitoring and ventilatory support may be needed when severe heart failure is present.

In patients who do not respond to conservative therapy, emergency intervention should be considered. The optimal intervention is percutaneous balloon mitral valvotomy (PBMV), which typically results in an increase in mitral

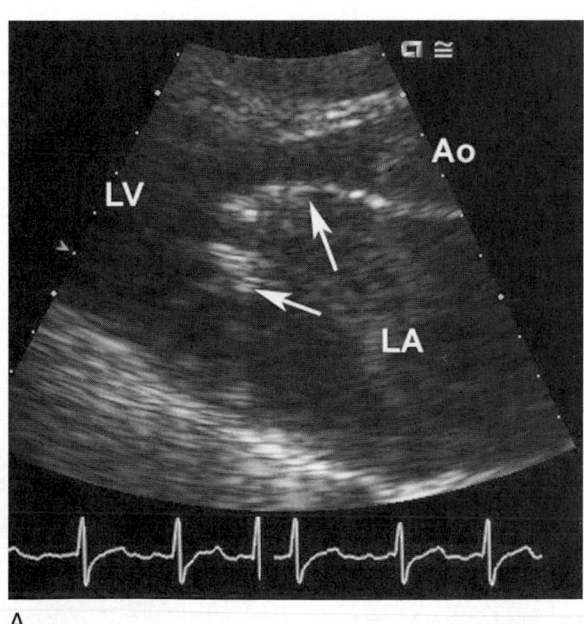
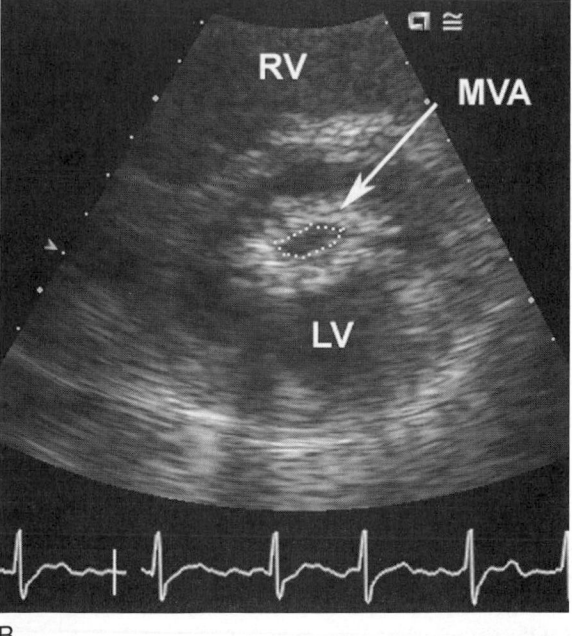

A B

FIGURE 103–8. In this patient with mitral stenosis, the long-axis view demonstrates the classic findings of diastolic doming of the leaflets (*arrows*) due to commissural fusion with thickening predominantly at the leaflet tips (**A**). In the short-axis view (**B**), the restricted mitral orifice with fusion of the commissures can be visualized, providing an accurate measurement of valve area (MVA) by direct planimetry. In this case, the valve area of 0.7 cm² indicates severe valve obstruction. Ao, aorta; LA, left atrium; LV, left ventricle; RV, right ventricle.

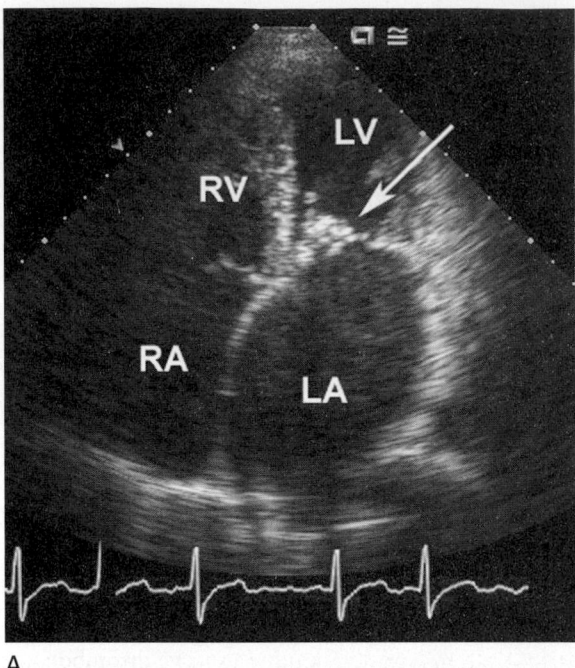

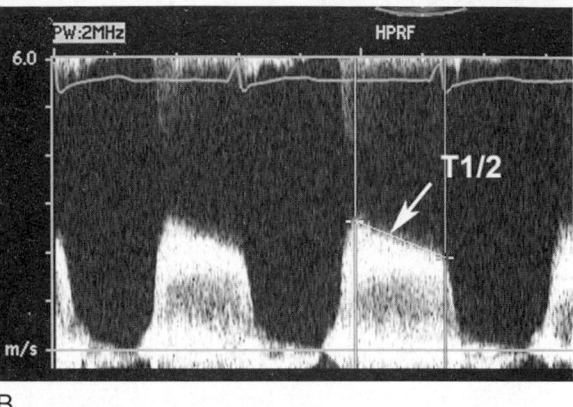

A
B

FIGURE 103–9. In the same patient as Figure 103-8, the apical four-chamber view (**A**) shows severe left atrial enlargement due to mitral obstruction with thickened valve leaflets *(arrow)*. The haziness in the left atrium is due to stasis of blood flow with spontaneous contrast medium enhancement on echocardiography. Continuous wave Doppler recording of flow across the mitral valve (**B**) shows an increased velocity corresponding to the transvalvular pressure gradient. The pressure half-time (T1/2) can be used to accurately calculate mitral valve area (0.7 cm²).

valve area to greater than 1.5 cm². PBMV can be safely performed even during pregnancy.[45-47] Patients with a left atrial thrombus, coexisting moderate to severe mitral regurgitation, or heavily calcified and deformed mitral valves are not candidates for PBMV; in these patients, surgical mitral valve replacement may be needed.

AORTIC STENOSIS

ETIOLOGY AND CLINICAL PRESENTATION

Valvular aortic stenosis in adults is most often due to calcification of a normal trileaflet or congenital bicuspid valve (Fig. 103-10). Rheumatic aortic stenosis is less common and is invariably accompanied by mitral valve involvement. In younger adults, congenital aortic stenosis may be encountered; some of these patients have restenosis after prior commissurotomy in childhood.

Like mitral stenosis, aortic valve stenosis is a chronic, slowly progressive disease that presents acutely only in patients who have not been receiving regular medical care.[48-50] As in mitral stenosis, acute decompensation may occur with a superimposed systemic condition. Young women with congenital aortic stenosis may present with angina or heart failure during pregnancy. In older adults, asymptomatic patients with moderate to severe valve obstruction may present with heart failure in the setting of pneumonia, anemia, or other conditions with increased metabolic demands.

DIAGNOSIS

The classic physical examination findings for aortic stenosis include a delayed and decreased carotid upstroke, a narrow pulse pressure, a single second heart sound (S_2), and a systolic

ejection murmur at the aortic region that radiates to the carotid. However, while a grade 4 murmur (palpable thrill) with a single S_2 and diminished carotids is specific for severe stenosis, these findings are very insensitive for the diagnosis.[51] Particularly when the patient is decompensated, the murmur may be soft and carotid upstrokes may be altered by coexisting vascular disease or loading conditions.

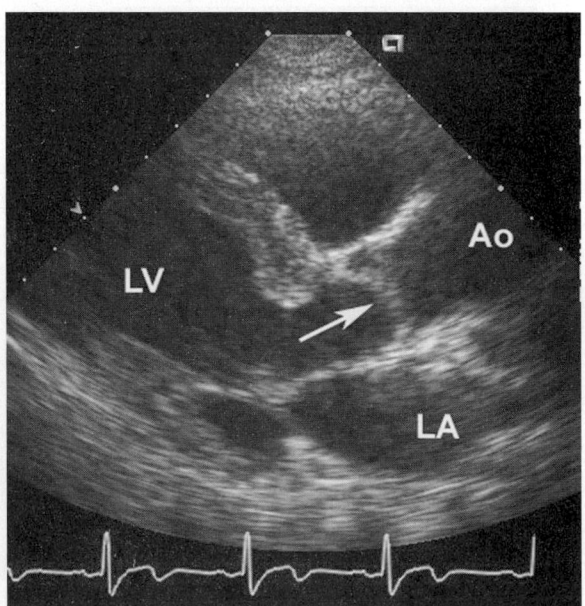

FIGURE 103–10. In this 26-year-old pregnant woman with a loud systolic murmur, the long-axis view shows doming of the aortic valve in systole *(arrow)*. Short-axis images confirmed a unicuspid aortic valve. Ao, aorta; LA, left atrium; LV, left ventricle.

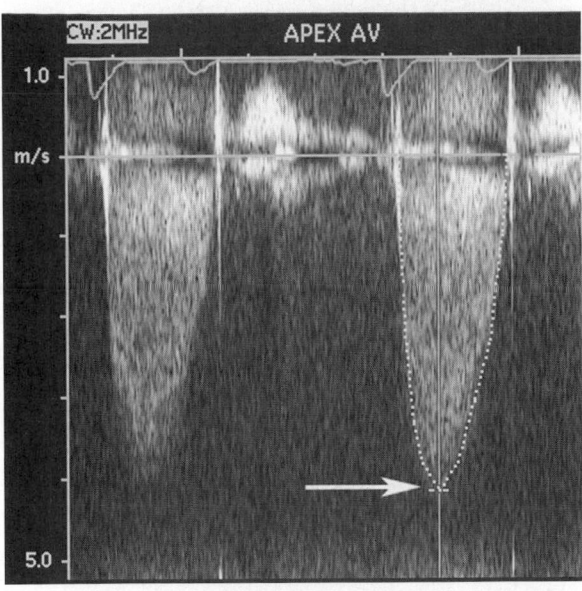

FIGURE 103–11. Continuous wave Doppler examination of the aortic valve in the patient shown in Figure 103–10 demonstrates a high-velocity signal consistent with severe aortic stenosis. The maximum velocity of 4.2 m/s corresponds to a maximum transaortic pressure gradient of 69 mm Hg and a mean gradient of 41 mm Hg. Valve area, calculated by the continuity equation, was 0.8 cm².

Echocardiography provides reliable evaluation of aortic stenosis severity based on the maximum velocity through the narrowed orifice and valve area, calculated with the continuity equation (Fig. 103-11). Disease severity is a continuum and velocities may be relatively low, despite severe stenosis, when cardiac output is reduced. In general, stenosis can be graded as severe (valve area < 1.0 cm² or jet velocity > 4 m/sec), moderate (valve area 1.0 to 1.5 cm² or jet velocity 3 to 4 m/sec), or mild (valve area > 1.5 cm² or jet velocity < 3 m/sec). Echocardiography also allows evaluation of ventricular systolic and diastolic function and any associated valve disease.[52]

MANAGEMENT

As with mitral stenosis, most patients with decompensated aortic stenosis can be managed conservatively by treating the underlying disease process that led to decompensation and restoring the patient's normal loading conditions. However, in the patient who has denied symptoms or has not been receiving medical care, the first presentation of aortic stenosis may be syncope or pulmonary edema. In these patients, aortic stenosis is the cause of decompensation, as evidenced by very severe valve obstruction, often with a low ejection fraction. Treatment is urgent aortic valve replacement. Some centers advocate the use of balloon aortic valvuloplasty in these patients, but this approach has no advantage over direct surgical intervention. A preliminary study suggests that cautious use of nitroprusside may improve hemodynamics before valve replacement in severe decompensated aortic stenosis if mean arterial pressure is greater than 60 mm Hg, but the utility and safety of this approach needs further evaluation.[53,54]

RIGHT-SIDED VALVE DISEASE

Pulmonic valve disease is nearly always congenital in origin with a chronic disease course. Tricuspid valve stenosis is rare and usually accompanies rheumatic mitral valve disease. However, tricuspid regurgitation can present acutely with severe regurgitation due to endocarditis or to blunt or penetrating chest wall trauma.[55-58] Rarely, acute tricuspid regurgitation is iatrogenic, related to a pacer wire or Swan-Ganz catheter.[59]

If due to penetrating chest wall trauma, valve dysfunction may be accompanied by pericardial effusion and tamponade physiology. Blunt chest wall trauma is accompanied by cardiac injury in 16% to 76% of cases in clinical series. The most common consequences are injury to the thoracic aorta or contusion of the right ventricle.[60] However, blunt chest wall trauma may result in valve rupture, with case reports of acute tricuspid and aortic regurgitation. Acute severe tricuspid regurgitation results in a low forward cardiac output and signs of an elevated right atrial pressure.

PROSTHETIC VALVES

MECHANICAL VALVES

Prosthetic mechanical heart valves are very durable, with complications most often due to valve thrombosis or paravalvular regurgitation.[61] Valve thrombosis occurs in the setting of inadequate anticoagulation and may result in functional valve stenosis if movement of the valve occluder is restricted or in valve regurgitation if clot prevents full closure of the valve. The clinical presentation of valve thrombosis is similar to that of native valve stenosis or regurgitation. Again, echocardiography provides key information on the presence and severity of valve dysfunction (Fig. 103-12).[62] TEE is especially important with mitral prosthetic valves because the valve itself blocks ultrasound penetration from a transthoracic approach.

Treatment of prosthetic valve thrombosis is controversial. When only a small thrombus and mild hemodynamic compromise is present, conservative therapy with full dose intravenous anticoagulation for several days may be adequate. With severe hemodynamic compromise, surgical intervention with repeat valve replacement may be necessary, although operative mortality is reported to be high, ranging from 17% to 40%.[9,63] Systemic thrombolytic therapy can restore valve function in some patients but is associated with death in 20%, systemic embolism due to fragmentation of the valve thrombosis in 16%, and the need for emergency surgery in 20%.[9] Thus, thrombolytic therapy typically is used only when surgical risk is high (see Fig. 103-12). The duration of thrombolytic therapy is based on Doppler echocardiographic evidence of resolution of thrombus and improvement in valve function. However, thrombolytic therapy should be stopped after 24 hours if there is no hemodynamic improvement and after 72 hours if only partial improvement. Guidelines for thrombolytic therapy for prosthetic valve thrombosis frequently are updated, so clinicians should check the latest guidelines and seek consultation from both cardiology and cardiac surgery before proceeding with therapy.[9,64]

Paravalvular regurgitation early after valve replacement may be related to suture dehiscence at a site of annular calcification. There may be associated hemolytic anemia, which can be treated conservatively if mild but may require reoperation if severe recurrent anemia is present. The new onset of paravalvular regurgitation should prompt careful evaluation for endocarditis (see Chapter 104).

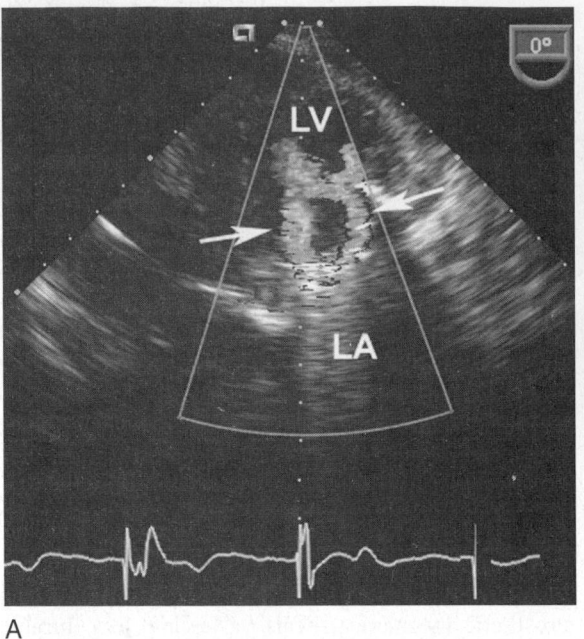

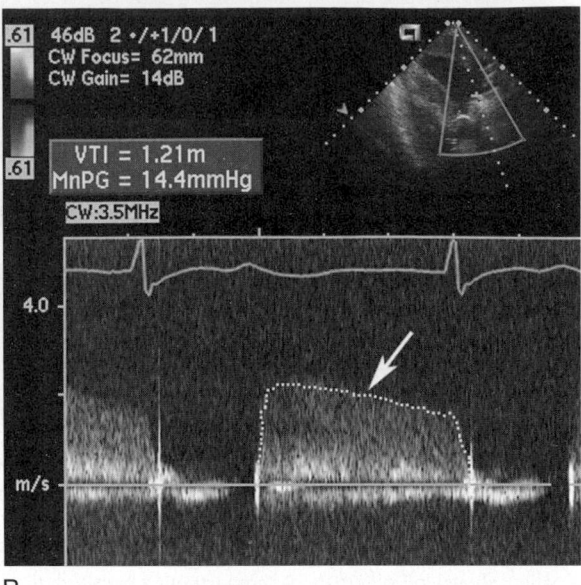

A   B

FIGURE 103–12. Acute prosthetic mitral valve thrombosis in an 82-year-old man 29 years after valve replacement. The patient presented acutely with pulmonary edema and a right upper extremity thrombotic occlusion after anticoagulation was temporarily discontinued owing to a gastrointestinal hemorrhage. Color Doppler imaging (**A**) shows only narrow jets *(arrows)* of flow antegrade across the mitral valve replacement and the continuous wave Doppler signal (**B**) shows a high gradient and very prolonged deceleration slope, consistent with severe obstruction to flow. After careful discussion given his high risk for surgery, he was treated with thrombolytic therapy, which resulted in normalization of his mitral valve Doppler flows and resolution of pulmonary edema. (See Color Section in this text.)

TISSUE VALVES

Tissue valves are subject to degeneration of the leaflets with superimposed calcification that may result in stenosis or regurgitation. Usually this is a slowly progressive process with presentation 10 to 15 years after valve implantation.[65,66] As with native valve disease, acute decompensation may occur in patients with chronic prosthetic valve dysfunction if there is a superimposed hemodynamic stress.

Acute regurgitation of a tissue valve can result from endocarditis or from a leaflet tear due to tissue degeneration. Tears in the valve leaflet typically occur adjacent to an area of calcification due to the increased stress on the normal leaflet tissue. As with mechanical valves, both transthoracic and transesophageal imaging are needed for full evaluation of suspected prosthetic tissue valve dysfunction. Treatment is similar to that for native valves with medical stabilization followed by surgery for repeat valve replacement.

ANNOTATED REFERENCES

Bonow RO, Carabello BA, deLeon AC, et al: ACC/AHA Guidelines for the Management of Patients with Valvular Heart Disease: A report of the American College of Cardiology/American Heart Association Task Force on Practice Guidelines (Committee on Management of Patients with Valvular Heart Disease). J Am Coll Cardiol 1998;32:1486-1588.
Consensus guidelines on the diagnosis, medical therapy, and timing of surgical intervention in valvular heart disease. Also provides a concise summary of our understanding of the natural history of valvular heart disease as the basis for an evidence-based approach to patient management.
Update in progress. Most recent version available on the website of the American College of Cardiology.

Carabello BA, Crawford FA Jr: Valvular heart disease. N Engl J Med 1997;337:32-41.
Concise review of the diagnosis and therapy of aortic and mitral stenosis and of aortic and mitral regurgitation with specific attention to the issues of acute valvular regurgitation. A readable and up-to-date summary with 99 references.

Iung B: Management of ischaemic mitral regurgitation. Heart 2003;89:459-464.
Ischemic mitral regurgitation is due to alterations in the alignment of the subvalvular apparatus, not to papillary muscle dysfunction. It often is associated with a soft murmur so that quantitative Doppler echocardiography is especially important in diagnosis. Treatment often includes concurrent mitral valve surgery at the time of coronary artery bypass grafting.

Pretre R, Chilcott M: Blunt trauma to the heart and great vessels. N Engl J Med 1997;339:626-632.
Mechanisms of injury due to blunt trauma include compression of the chest, direct injury, traction or torsion, and an acute elevation in blood pressure. Types of injury include tearing of the aorta (particularly at the aortic isthmus) or myocardium, valve rupture, and myocardial contusion. The importance of rapid diagnosis with bedside echocardiography and the indications for surgical intervention are discussed.

Vongpatanasin W, Hillis LD, Lange RA: Prosthetic heart valves. N Engl J Med 1996;335:407-416.
Prosthetic valve dysfunction may be suspected based on history or physical examination, but diagnosis usually requires echocardiography and other imaging techniques. Complications of prosthetic valves include valve thrombosis, embolization, structural failure, hemolysis, paravalvular regurgitation, and endocarditis. Careful antithrombotic therapy is needed to prevent mechanical valve complications. Therapy for prosthetic valve thrombosis is controversial.

Chapter 104

INFECTIOUS ENDOCARDITIS

Michel Wolff • Jean-François Timsit

KEY POINTS

1. Infectious endocarditis can be classified into **three types that differ markedly** in terms of incidence, clinical presentation, microbiologic features, and outcome: left-sided native valve, right-sided native valve, and prosthetic valve.

2. **Modifications of the Duke criteria** were recently proposed to take into account transesophageal echocardiography and to consider all *Staphylococcus aureus* bacteremia and positive Q fever serology as major criteria.

3. According to two recent large studies conducted in the United States and in France, streptococci remain the most common etiologic agents of infectious endocarditis, accounting for 58% of all pathogens. However, the microbiologic characteristics of the subset of patients who require ICU admission differ from those of the overall population. In ICU patients with infectious endocarditis, *S. aureus* is the leading pathogen.

4. Patients are generally referred to the ICU for cardiogenic or septic shock, pulmonary edema caused by valvular leak or prosthetic dysfunction, neurologic events, or renal failure. **Most complications occurred early during the course of infectious endocarditis.**

5. Mounting evidence shows that, for both complicated left-sided native valve endocarditis and *S. aureus* prosthetic valve endocarditis, **valve replacement combined with medical therapy** is associated with a better outcome than medical treatment alone. Improvement of outcome requires a multidisciplinary approach to optimize medical treatment and decision-making concerning indications and optimal timing of valve replacement.

Infectious endocarditis is associated with a myriad of complications, both cardiac and extracardiac, that may require transfer to the ICU. Local progression of the infection causes destruction of valve cusps or leaflets and chordae and may extend to peri- and paravalvular structures. Hemodynamic deterioration leads to secondary organ failure. Finally, embolization of infected tissues may damage vital organs and cause peripheral abscesses. Intensivists are often confronted with complex treatment decisions, such as the indication and timing of cardiac surgery and the management of hemodynamic and neurologic complications. Therefore, treatment of patients with complicated infectious endocarditis requires close cooperation among intensivists, infectious disease specialists, cardiologists, and cardiac surgeons. This chapter focuses on the changing epidemiology and progress made during the past 3 decades in the diagnosis and management of complicated infectious endocarditis.

PATHOPHYSIOLOGY

Infectious endocarditis is a microbial infection of the endocardial surface of the heart. The process is initiated by blood-borne microorganisms that adhere directly to the endothelium or by nonbacterial thrombotic endocarditis. The most important factors facilitating nonbacterial thrombotic endocarditis are organic valvular lesions, with associated perturbation of blood flow, and prosthetic valves. Circulating microorganisms can adhere to microscopic lesions, which explains why up to 50% of patients with infectious endocarditis have no previously known valvular abnormality.[1]

In simple infectious endocarditis, infection is limited to the valve cusps or leaflets and chordae and consists of vegetations, which are formed by pathogens, platelets, fibrin, and inflammatory cells. In advanced infectious endocarditis, deep tissue invasion results in the destruction or invasion of valvular and perivalvular structures. The infection may spread as cellulitis with the formation of an abscess or pseudoaneurysm, which can rupture to another heart chamber or even the pericardium. Infectious endocarditis can also occur at the site of a septal defect or on the mural endocardium.

In prosthetic valve endocarditis, lesions may differ according to the type of prosthesis. With biologic prostheses or homografts, the infection may be limited to cusps, whereas with mechanical prostheses, involvement of the sewing ring and the valve annulus is the rule.[2] Bacterial adherence to the prosthesis results from a complex relationship among the biomaterial, plasma proteins (e.g., fibronectin, laminin, thrombospondin, fibrinogen), and bacterial adhesion proteins. *Staphylococcus aureus* and coagulase-negative staphylococci express numerous surface factors: clumping factors A and B, which promote their adhesion to fibrinogen and fibrin, and fibronectin-binding proteins A and B, which permit adhesion to fibronectin.[3] In addition, once staphylococci have escaped the microbicidal effects of platelet peptides, they can bind to the platelet surface by a series of pathogenetic steps, including direct binding to the platelet surface, up-regulation of platelet surface receptors for fibrinogen, and interaction between specific bacterial proteins and platelet surface receptors.[4]

INCIDENCE AND CLASSIFICATION

The overall annual incidence of infectious endocarditis in Europe and the United States is between 15 and 60 cases per million. In a recent study conducted in France, the crude annual incidence of infectious endocarditis was 30 (95% confidence interval, 27 to 33) per million inhabitants. In the United States, the yearly incidence is estimated to be 15,000 to 20,000 cases.[5] Infectious endocarditis can be classified into three groups that differ markedly in terms of incidence, clinical presentation, microbiologic features, and outcome: left-sided native valve, right-sided native valve, and prosthetic valve endocarditis.

Left-sided native valve infectious endocarditis traditionally occurs in patients with underlying heart disease but may affect patients with no known valvular disease, especially when endocarditis is caused by highly virulent bacteria such as *S. aureus* or *Streptococcus pneumoniae*. Most infections are community acquired, but nosocomial cases are becoming more common.

Right-sided native valve infectious endocarditis is usually associated with intravenous drug use and has an estimated incidence of 1.5 to 20 per 1000 addicts.[6] Nosocomial cases are frequently a consequence of catheter-related infections. In most cases of pacemaker infectious endocarditis, vegetations are located only on leads, but tricuspid valve involvement occurs in at least 10% of patients.[7]

Prosthetic valve endocarditis accounts for 7% to 25% of infectious endocarditis episodes,[8] with a risk of approximately 1% at 12 months after valve implantation and 2% to 3% at 60 months.[9,10] The risk persists throughout follow-up, at a rate of approximately 0.4% yearly. The rates of endocarditis associated with mechanical versus biologic prostheses are controversial; some authors have found that bioprostheses present a greater risk of infection after the first postoperative year. Cases of prosthetic valve endocarditis occurring within 2 months of prosthesis implantation are called early and are usually of nosocomial origin; those developing more than 1 year after valve replacement are called late and are predominantly community acquired. Intermediate prosthetic valve endocarditis occurs between 60 days and 6 months after valve replacement and may be community or hospital acquired.[11] Proportional hazards functions based on 4189 consecutive patients indicated a significant decline in early prosthetic valve endocarditis and a slight increase in late prosthetic valve endocarditis.[12]

DEMOGRAPHICS AND ETIOLOGIC PROFILES

CLASSIC AND CHANGING PATIENT CHARACTERISTICS

The demographic characteristics of patients who develop infectious endocarditis have changed over the last few decades. Today, patients tend to be older, and their underlying diseases have changed.[13,14] In France, the infectious endocarditis incidence rises sharply for patients older than 50 years and peaks at 145 cases per million for men 70 to 80 years old.[1] In developing countries, rheumatic heart disease remains the most frequent underlying cardiac condition predisposing patients to infectious endocarditis. In contrast, in the United States and western Europe, nonrheumatic heart abnormalities, including mitral valve prolapse, aortic valve calcification, aortic bicuspid valve, and hypertrophic obstructive cardiomyopathy, are the main risk factors. For patients with mitral valve prolapse, risk factors include mitral regurgitation and thickened mitral leaflet. However, results of a recent 1-year survey of infectious endocarditis in France showed a significantly lower incidence of known underlying heart disease between 1991 and 1999.[1] This confirmed data from a Spanish study of native valve infectious endocarditis in nonaddicts, in which the percentage of patients with no prior heart disease increased from 22% in 1975-1985 to 46% in 1984-1992.[15] This trend can be explained, in part, by the markedly fewer postrheumatic valvular complications and improved antimicrobial prophylaxis. Nowadays, congenital heart diseases are rarely involved, except bicuspid aortic valve. Other conditions, including diabetes mellitus, long-term hemodialysis, and immunosuppression, are associated with a higher incidence of infectious endocarditis. At Duke University Medical Center, rates of hemodialysis dependence and immunosuppression among 329 patients with infectious endocarditis rose significantly between 1993 and 1999.[14] Moreover, several recent reports indicate that the incidence of nosocomial native valve infectious endocarditis is also rising.[16-18] Intravenous devices (catheters or fistulas for hemodialysis, vascular grafts) are the major sources of infection. Finally, patients with previous infectious endocarditis should be considered at risk for a new episode.

CLASSIC AND CHANGING CAUSES AND SOURCES OF INFECTION

Overall Distribution of Causative Microorganisms

Overall, streptococci remain the most common causative agent of infectious endocarditis, accounting for 58% of all pathogens in two recent large studies conducted in the United States and in France.[1,13] Changes in demographic characteristics probably explain the observed changes in organism frequency. Indeed, two major findings were lower rates of infectious endocarditis caused by oral streptococci[1,14] and higher frequencies of *S. aureus*. At Duke University, *S. aureus* was the single most common cause of infectious endocarditis in 1999, accounting for nearly 40% of episodes.[14]

Community-Acquired, Left-Sided Native Valve Infectious Endocarditis in Nonaddicts
Frequent Pathogens

Streptococci. *Streptococcus* species (mainly *Streptococcus mitis*, *Streptococcus sanguis*, *Streptococcus mutans*), which abound in the mouth and nasopharynx, are associated with dental procedures and diseases. Better application of appropriate prophylaxis for patients at risk probably explains the decreased frequency of *Streptococcus viridans*, but this organism is still responsible for 17%[1] to 36%[13] of episodes. Other factors, such as poor dental hygiene and minor or unrecognized periodontal disease, may be the source of *S. viridans* infectious endocarditis. *Streptococcus bovis*, isolated from up to 25% of patients with infectious endocarditis, may be involved in valve infection of dental or buccal origin. In addition, the association of *S. bovis* infectious endocarditis with carcinoma or other lesions of the colon (e.g., diverticulitis, polyps) is well known. Beta-hemolytic streptococci (groups A, B, C, and G) and *Streptococcus milleri* are isolated from 6% of patients with infectious endocarditis,[1] with the predominant species being group B. The majority of nonpregnant patients with group B streptococcal infectious endocarditis have an underlying condition such as diabetes mellitus, breast cancer, decubitus ulcer, or cirrhosis.[19]

Enterococci. Enterococci (mainly *Enterococcus faecalis* and *Enterococcus faecium*) account for only 8% to 11% of cases of infectious endocarditis.[1,13] These pathogens affect older patients, as demonstrated by a recent description of 93 episodes of enterococcal infectious endocarditis occurring in patients with a mean age of 74 years.[20] The portals of entry are the gastrointestinal and urogenital tracts through a lesion or a procedure (e.g., injection sclerosis of esophageal varices, transurethral prostate resection, urethral dilatation) resulting in transient bacteremia, in which case the infection is hospital acquired.

Staphylococcus aureus. *S. aureus* is implicated in approximately 30% of all cases of left-sided native valve infectious endocarditis[13] and is the causative agent in most acute infections, with about half of patients having no previously known heart disease. A clinically identifiable focus of infection (e.g., carbuncle, cellulitis, bursitis, ulcer, burn, osteomyelitis) may be present. However, in 50% to 60% of cases, no obvious portal of entry is detected, although the skin is probably the source in many of them. The relationship between *S. aureus* nasal carriage and infection has been established in specific subsets of patients, especially in intravenous drug users and patients with diabetes mellitus or on hemodialysis.[14]

Infrequent Pathogens

Enterobacteriaceae and HACEK Group. Despite the high frequency of Enterobacteriaceae bacteremia leading to severe sepsis or septic shock, infectious endocarditis caused by these pathogens is extremely uncommon, perhaps because Gram-negative bacilli adhere less avidly to the endothelium than Gram-positive cocci do. Most cases of infectious endocarditis develop in patients with severe comorbidities, including cirrhosis or immunosuppression. Bacteria of the HACEK group (fastidious organisms) originate from the oropharyngeal or urogenital flora and include *Haemophilus aphrophilus* or *paraphrophilus* (H), *Actinobacillus actinomycetemcomitans* (A), *Cardiobacterium hominis* (C), *Eikenella corrodens* (E), and *Kingella* species (K). These HACEK pathogens are implicated in less than 3% of cases of infectious endocarditis on either native or prosthesic valves.

Streptococcus pneumoniae. Pneumococcal infectious endocarditis occurs more commonly in alcoholics, but other patients, such as those with diabetes, malignancy, or chronic obstructive pulmonary disease, may be affected. Approximately 65% to 80% of patients have no known predisposing cardiopathy. The primary infection focus is the lungs, and meningitis is present in 40% to 60% of cases.[21]

Coagulase-Negative Staphylococci. Although they are the most common pathogens responsible for early prosthetic valve endocarditis, coagulase-negative staphylococci are also a well-documented cause of native valve infectious endocarditis. Most patients have documented valvular abnormalities, especially mitral valve prolapse. A substantial subset of coagulase-negative staphylococci infective endocarditis has been identified as being due to *Staphylococcus lugdunensis*, which causes destructive cardiac lesions, and its differentiation from other coagulase-negative staphylococci species in the laboratory may be difficult.[22]

Infectious Endocarditis in Intravenous Drug Users

It has been estimated that up to 76% of the infectious endocarditis cases in intravenous drug users are right sided, versus 9% in nonaddicts. The tricuspid valve is affected in 40% to 69% of episodes, a left-sided valve in 20% to 30%, and multiple valves in 5% to 10%. *S. aureus* is the most frequently isolated pathogen, especially for right-sided infectious endocarditis, where it is isolated in more than 80 % of cases.[23] Intravenous drug users are generally their own source of the infectious organism; many carry *S. aureus* in their noses or throats or on their skin. Most cases are caused by methicillin-susceptible strains. However, methicillin-resistant *S. aureus* infectious endocarditis has been reported in intravenous drug users in the United States and Europe. Other bacteria are involved much less frequently. Right-sided or left-sided infectious endocarditis caused by streptococci, enterococci, or coagulase-negative staphylococci has been reported, especially in those who inject drugs into the femoral vein. Enterobacteriaceae and *Pseudomonas aeruginosa* have also been observed to preferentially attack right-sided, previously undamaged heart valves in addicts, but these cases were attributed to preparation of the drug. Finally, although drug addiction is a classic predisposing factor for fungal endocarditis, a recent analysis of 270 cases of fungal endocarditis incriminated drug use in only 13%.[24]

Hospital-Acquired Native Valve Infectious Endocarditis

Several reports have indicated that hospital-acquired infectious endocarditis unrelated to cardiac surgery is a growing problem. Because intravascular devices are the main source of infection, the predominant role of *S. aureus* is not surprising. Other sources of nosocomial infectious endocarditis are gastrointestinal and urogenital procedures and surgical wounds. Other pathogens are Gram-negative bacilli, enterococci, coagulase-negative staphylococci, and fungi.[16,17] It should be emphasized that the diversification of care structures (long-term-care facilities, day-care centers) sometimes makes the distinction between community-acquired and nosocomial infection difficult, or even meaningless; this is particularly true for infections in hemodialysis patients. Infectious endocarditis developing in such circumstances is now included with the so-called health care–associated infections.

Prosthetic Valve Endocarditis

Although a broad spectrum of microorganisms may be involved in prosthetic valve endocarditis, staphylococci and streptococci predominate, with their frequency depending on the time interval after valve implantation. Coagulase-negative staphylococci and *S. aureus* are frequently responsible, regardless of interval. For late prosthetic valve endocarditis, microorganisms resemble those responsible for native valve infectious endocarditis, with a predominance of streptococci. Gram-negative bacilli are usually encountered in early and late prosthetic valve endocarditis; fungi, mainly *Candida* species, are responsible for approximately 8% and 3% of early and intermediate prosthetic valve endocarditis, respectively (Table 104-1).[8]

Specific Microbiologic Characteristics of Infectious Endocarditis in ICU Patients

The microbiologic characteristics of infectious endocarditis in patients who require ICU admission differ from those in the overall population. Analysis of a large series of infectious endocarditis patients hospitalized in two medical ICUs in a Parisian teaching hospital between 1994 and 2001 showed that *S. aureus* was the leading pathogen responsible for left-sided native valve and prosthetic valve endocarditis (see Tables 104-1 and 104-2). In a previous series of 122 ICU patients with prosthetic valve endocarditis, *S. aureus* was almost as frequent

TABLE 104–1. CAUSATIVE AGENTS OF PROSTHETIC VALVE ENDOCARDITIS (PVE)

Microorganism	Early and Intermediate PVE (%)		Late PVE (%)	
	International Studies[26, 44] (202 Patients)	Bichat Claude-Bernard ICUs (39 Patients)	International Studies[26, 44] (326 Patients)	Bichat Claude-Bernard ICUs (34 Patients)
Staphylococcus aureus	22	59	18	35
MSSA	NR	31	NR	32
MRSA	NR	28	NR	3
CoNS	33	5	16	6
Streptococci	3	5	25	26
Enterococci	9	8	14	3
HACEK	3	0	7	3
Gram-negative bacilli	10	1	NR	6
Fungi	8	8	3	3
Polymicrobial	2	0	1	0
Other	5	5*	9	9†
Culture negative	5	9	7	8

*Corynebacterium species in 2 patients.
†Corynebacterium species in 2 patients; Listeria monocytogenes in 1 patient.
CoNS, coagulase-negative staphylococci; HACEK, Haemophilus aphrophilus or paraphrophilus, Actinobacillus actinomycetemcomitans, Cardiobacterium hominis, Eikenella corrodens, and Kingella species; MRSA, methicillin-resistant S. aureus; MSSA, methicillin-susceptible S. aureus; NR, not related.

as streptococci in late-onset infections.[25] Those figures were confirmed by an Austrian study of 33 ICU patients with infectious endocarditis: S. aureus was isolated from 36% of them, versus 15% S. viridans and 12% enterococci.[26] Clearly, these findings are largely explained by S. aureus causing valve destruction, septic shock, and emboli to vital organs such as brain.

Patients with Negative Blood Cultures

Common causes of culture-negative infectious endocarditis have been reported in detail elsewhere.[5,8] Five main points should be emphasized: (1) Abiotrophia species (previously classified as nutritionally variant streptococci) are the main cause of culture-negative infectious endocarditis in patients who have recently received antibiotics. (2) Only 5% to 7% of patients who have not recently taken antibiotics have negative blood cultures. Polymerase chain reaction (in blood, excised vegetation, or systemic emboli) can be used to identify the causative organism, such as Bartonella species,[27] Tropheryma whiplei, or Coxiella burnetii. (3) Serologic tests are useful to diagnose infectious endocarditis caused by those organisms or by Brucella and Legionella species. (4) HACEK

organisms may require prolonged incubation and subculturing. (5) Candida (but not Aspergillus) species are usually isolated from routine blood cultures, but in some cases, fungi are recovered only from excised vegetations or peripheral emboli.

CLINICAL CHARACTERISTICS AND DIAGNOSIS

In 1994, a new set of diagnostic criteria for the diagnosis of infectious endocarditis, including two major and six minor criteria—known as the Duke criteria—was proposed.[28] Modifications of these criteria were recently proposed to take into account transesophageal echocardiography and to consider all S. aureus bacteremias and positive Q fever serology as major criteria.[29]

CLINICAL CHARACTERISTICS

In ICU patients, the clinical presentation of infectious endocarditis often includes extracardiac manifestations or findings associated with cardiac complications. Patients are generally referred to the ICU for cardiogenic or septic shock, pulmonary edema caused by valvular or prosthetic dysfunction, neurologic events, acute renal failure, or respiratory failure in the setting of pulmonary emboli complicating right-sided infectious endocarditis. Two salient features, usually associated with high-grade fever, strongly suggest the diagnosis of infectious endocarditis: a heart murmur (most commonly preexisting) or a prosthetic valve, and petechiae on the skin (especially the extremities; Fig. 104-1) and conjunctivae. A typical ICU candidate has an acute febrile and toxic illness with heart murmur, petechiae, and meningeal signs. Cerebrospinal fluid examination finds pleocytosis and Gram-positive cocci. Blood cultures yield S. aureus, and echocardiography confirms left-sided infectious endocarditis.

The onset of nosocomial infectious endocarditis is usually acute, and suggestive signs are often absent.[18] The diagnosis of infectious endocarditis is suggested by bacteremia persisting 3 to 5 days after the onset of antimicrobial treatment and removal of an infected catheter.

TABLE 104–2. CAUSATIVE AGENTS OF LEFT-SIDED NATIVE VALVE INFECTIOUS ENDOCARDITIS

Microorganisms	Connecticut Hospitals[13] (513 Patients): Number* (%)	Bichat-Claude Bernard ICUs (122 Patients): Number (%)
Streptococci	240 (47)	42 (34)
Staphylococcus aureus	143 (28)	52 (43)
Enterococci	58 (11)	3 (2)
CoNS	38 (7)	2 (2)
Gram-negative bacilli	NR	4 (3)
Streptococcus pneumoniae	NR	5 (4)
Other	21 (4)	7 (6)
Negative blood cultures	29 (6)	7 (6)

*The number of microorganisms exceeds the number of patients because some cases were polymicrobial.
CoNS, coagulase-negative staphylococci; NR, not reported.

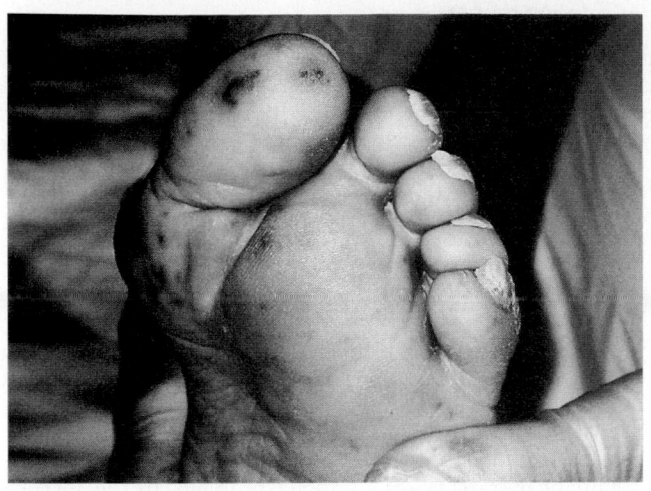

FIGURE 104–1. Typical purpuric lesions in a patient with *S. aureus* mitral valve endocarditis.

ECHOCARDIOGRAPHY

Echocardiography has the following objectives: (1) to detect vegetations and determine their size, (2) to diagnose paravalvular extension of the infection, (3) to evaluate myocardial function, (4) to detect pericardial effusion, and (5) if cardiac surgery is being considered, to measure the valve ring to choose the appropriate prosthetic valve for replacement. Transthoracic echocardiography is rapid and noninvasive, but its overall sensitivity is only about 65%. False-negative results are obtained when the examination is inadequate (in those with obesity or chronic obstructive pulmonary disease) or when vegetations are less than 5 mm. Transesophageal echocardiography associated with color Doppler techniques is more invasive, but its sensitivity for detecting vegetations is 90%.[18] Transesophageal echocardiography is particularly useful in patients with suspected valve perforation or extension of perivalvular infectious endocarditis and in those with prosthetic valve endocarditis. Its sensitivity and specificity for the detection of cardiac abscess are 80% and 95%, respectively. This technique is necessary for all patients undergoing valve surgery and may be repeated at close intervals to help the physician decide when to operate. However, transesophageal echocardiography should be used cautiously in nonintubated critically ill patients with respiratory failure.

COMPLICATIONS

Cardiac complications and hemodynamic failure, central nervous system (CNS) complications, and acute renal failure are the leading causes of ICU admission for patients with infectious endocarditis. Other complications are not addressed in detail.

CARDIAC COMPLICATIONS AND HEMODYNAMIC FAILURE

Congestive heart failure (CHF) is usually caused by infection-induced valvular damage or prosthesis dysfunction. In native valve infectious endocarditis, acute CHF is more frequently associated with aortic than mitral disease. CHF caused by aortic failure may require urgent valve replacement. Perivalvular extension of infectious endocarditis is frequently associated with CHF, and spread into the septum may lead to heart block. Erosion of a mycotic aneurysm of the sinus of Valsalva can cause hemopericardium and tamponade or can create fistulas to the right or left ventricle. Myocardial infarction due to coronary artery embolization is a rare event. Hemodynamic failure can also be caused by septic shock, especially during the bacteremic phase of *S. aureus* infectious endocarditis. All these complications may require the administration of positive inotropes or vasoconstrictors and the use of mechanical ventilation before valve replacement.

NEUROLOGIC COMPLICATIONS

CNS complications of infectious endocarditis occur frequently. They may be the first or predominant manifestation of the disease and can arise through several mechanisms. CNS complications are a leading cause of death due to infectious endocarditis, and their specific management may be complex.

Frequency, Microbiology, and Timing

In most series, CNS involvement during the course of infectious endocarditis occurs in 20% to 40% of cases, with an average of 30%; this figure has not changed much over time. Among 1329 episodes of infectious endocarditis from seven series described between 1985 and 1993, 437 (33%) were accompanied by CNS manifestations.[30] In a Finnish teaching hospital, 55 of 218 infectious endocarditis episodes (25%) were associated with neurologic complications.[31] Among 228 episodes of infectious endocarditis requiring ICU admission in our institution, 84 (37%) involved CNS complications. However, two other studies had lower rates: in France, strokes occurred in 17% of 264 infectious endocarditis cases caused by staphylococci or streptococci[1]; in the United States, among 513 episodes of complicated, left-sided native valve infectious endocarditis, focal neurologic signs or altered mental status were observed in 18% and 16% of cases, respectively.[13] Neurologic complications are a hallmark of left-sided abnormalities of either native or prosthetic valves. Despite some reported discrepancies, the infectious site does not influence the occurrence of neurologic complications. When neurologic complication rates were assessed as a function of the causative agent, the frequency of CNS involvement was two to three times higher with *S. aureus* than with other pathogens.[31,32]

Most neurologic complications are already evident at the time of hospitalization or develop within a few days. Indeed, neurologic manifestations were the first sign of infectious endocarditis in 47% of episodes and occurred in less than 1 week in another 29% of episodes.[31] The probability of developing these complications decreases rapidly once antimicrobial therapy has been started. Moreover, recurrent neurologic events, although possible even late, are uncommon.

Pathogenesis and Distribution

Neurologic complications of infectious endocarditis can arise through various mechanisms. Cerebral emboli result from dislodgment or fragmentation of cardiac vegetations, followed by vessel occlusion; this results in various degrees of ischemia and infarction, depending on the vessels and the collateral blood flow. Occlusion of cerebral arteries, with either stroke or transient ischemic attack, accounts for 40% to 50% of the CNS complications of infectious endocarditis.[30,31] Diffusion-weighted magnetic resonance imaging (Fig. 104-2)

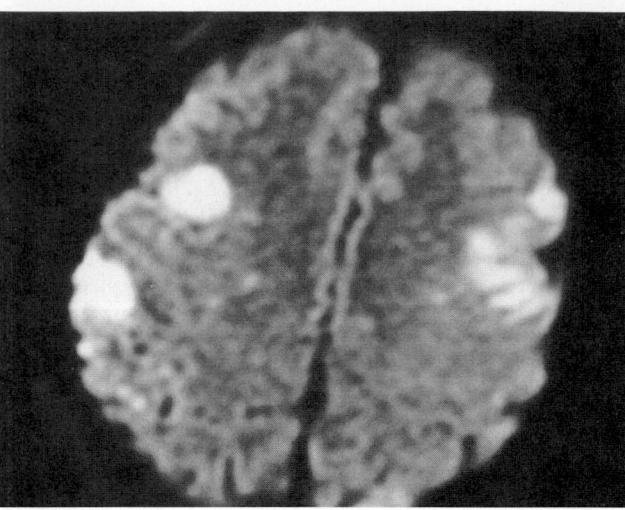

FIGURE 104–2. Diffusion-weighted magnetic resonance imaging showing multiple cerebral emboli in the same patient as in Figure 104-1.

has revealed a variety of patterns, including disseminated punctate lesions.[33] Cerebral hemorrhage may be the consequence of different mechanisms, each of which accounts for one third of bleeding complications: rupture of an intracranial aneurysm; septic erosion of the arterial wall, without a well-delineated aneurysm (acute necrotizing arteritis); or hemorrhagic transformation of ischemic brain infarcts, especially in anticoagulated patients. Overall, intracranial hemorrhage represents 10% of CNS complications (Fig. 104-3). Brain hemorrhage is more frequent during the bacteremic phase of *S. aureus* infectious endocarditis and is made more likely by severe thrombopenia and anticoagulant therapy.[34] Meningitis, occurring in 5% to 40% of patients with CNS manifestations of infectious endocarditis, can be the consequence of a wide variety of mechanisms; the cerebrospinal

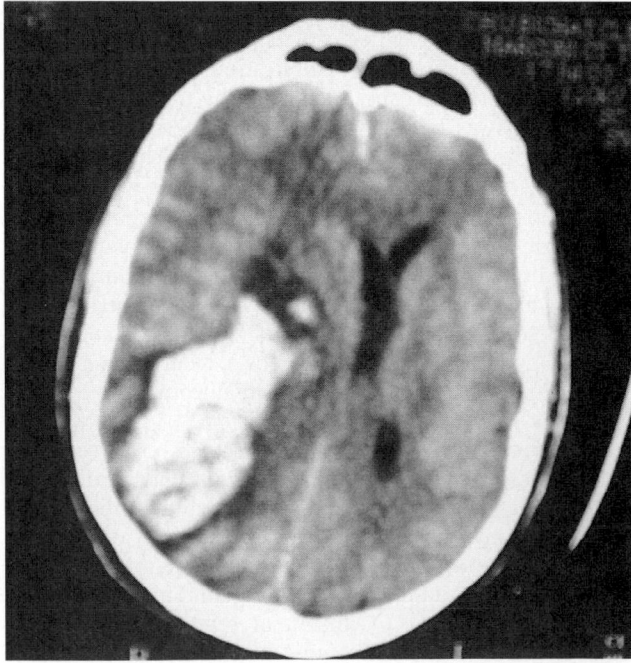

FIGURE 104–3. Cerebral hematoma in a patient with *S. aureus* prosthetic valve endocarditis.

fluid may be purulent with positive cultures, clear with moderate pleocytosis, or hemorrhagic. Brain abscesses associated with infectious endocarditis are uncommon; they account for less than 5% of CNS events, but the rate depends on the imaging technique used. In addition, many small abscesses or areas of cerebritis resolve with antibiotics alone. Finally, toxic encephalopathy, defined as mental changes or stupor without focal neurologic manifestations and without computed tomographic abnormalities, is often included among the CNS complications of infectious endocarditis. Obviously, this manifestation can have different causes, such as subtle cerebral lesions, or may be present in the setting of severe sepsis.

Specific Management

Infectious endocarditis occurring in patients receiving anticoagulant therapy poses a difficult problem. In the absence of CNS complications or in patients with nonhemorrhagic neurologic lesions, warfarin should be discontinued and replaced by heparin. However, in the presence of brain hemorrhage, anticoagulant therapy should be temporarily discontinued. Computed tomography scanning is essential for the diagnosis and management of CNS events associated with infectious endocarditis. In addition, it may be the only technique available for unstable ICU patients, especially those on mechanical ventilation. Computed tomography may show intracranial bleeding, ischemic lesions, or a pattern consistent with cerebral abscess. Magnetic resonance imaging is more sensitive for most lesions, except hemorrhage. Although conventional four-vessel angiography remains the gold standard for the evaluation of mycotic aneurysms, magnetic resonance angiography is a promising technique. In the absence of randomized trials, which are difficult (if not impossible) to organize, the respective roles of medical, endovascular, and neurosurgical treatment of intracranial aneurysms are not easily assessable. Endovascular treatment (coil embolization) seems to be a reliable and safe technique that should be considered when cerebral mycotic aneurysms are diagnosed.[35]

ACUTE RENAL FAILURE

Acute renal failure occurs in up to 40% of complicated infectious endocarditis cases necessitating ICU admission[26] and may result from several mechanisms. It is often the consequence of cardiogenic or septic shock (with or without multiorgan failure) leading to acute tubular necrosis. Drugs, such as the combination of a glycopeptide and an aminoglycoside, and the use of iodine contrast medium for radiologic investigations may further deteriorate renal function. In some patients with streptococcal or staphylococcal infectious endocarditis, acute renal failure is caused by severe glomerulonephritis. Acute renal failure may require the initiation of dialysis.

OTHER COMPLICATIONS

Systemic embolism can involve many organs, such as the spleen and kidneys; rarely, the liver or the iliac, mesenteric, or peripheral arteries are involved. Splenic abscesses are caused mainly by *S. aureus* or *S. viridans*. Abdominal computed tomography is the best procedure to detect splenic abscesses, which may require percutaneous drainage or splenectomy. Pulmonary emboli, the hallmark of right-sided

TABLE 104–3. ANTIBIOTIC TREATMENT OF COMPLICATED INFECTIOUS ENDOCARDITIS AS A FUNCTION OF VALVE TYPE, PATHOGEN, AND SUSCEPTIBILITY

Microorganism	Native Valve Infectious Endocarditis	Prosthetic Valve Endocarditis
Penicillin-susceptible streptococci (MIC ≤0.1 mg/L)	Penicillin G, amoxicillin, or ceftriaxone for 4 wk*	Penicillin G or amoxicillin for 4-6 wk + gentamicin for 2 wk*
Relatively penicillin-resistant streptococci (MIC >0.1-0.5 mg/L)	Penicillin G or amoxicillin for 4 wk + gentamicin for 2 wk*	Penicillin G or amoxicillin for 4-6 wk + gentamicin for 4 wk*
Streptococci with penicillin G MIC >0.5 mg/L, enterococci, and *Abiotrophia* spp	Penicillin G or amoxicillin for 4-6 wk + gentamicin for 4 wk*	Penicillin G or amoxicillin for 6 wk + gentamicin for 6 wk*
MSSA	Nafcillin or oxacillin for 4-6 wk + gentamicin for 3-5 days†	Nafcillin or oxacillin + rifampin for 6 wk + gentamicin for 2 wk†
MRSA	Vancomycin + rifampin for 4-6 wk + gentamicin for 3-5 days	Vancomycin + rifampin for 4-6 wk + gentamicin for 2 wk
HACEK organisms	Ceftriaxone or cefotaxime for 4 wk	Ceftriaxone or cefotaxime for 6 wk
Enterobacteriaceae	Ceftriaxone or cefotaxime for 4 wk + gentamicin or amikacin for 1 wk‡	Ceftriaxone or cefotaxime for 6 wk + gentamicin or amikacin for 2 wk‡
Bartonella spp	Amoxicillin or ceftriaxone for 4 wk + gentamicin for 1 wk	Amoxicillin or ceftriaxone for 4 wk + gentamicin for 1 wk
Coxiella burnettii	Doxycycline + rifampin + hydroxychloroquine for ≥ 18mo	Doxycycline + rifampin + hydroxychloroquine for ≥18 mo
Candida spp	Amphotericin B + flucytosine for 4-6wk + long-term suppressive treatment with fluconazole§	Amphotericin B + flucytosine for 6-8 wk + long-term suppressive treatment with fluconazole§

*Vancomycin or teicoplanin therapy is indicated for patients who are allergic to beta-lactam antibiotics. Optimal antimicrobial therapy is not available for high-level aminoglycoside-resistant and vancomycin-resistant enterococci. Eradicating these pathogens requires consultation with an infectious disease specialist or a microbiologist.
†A first-generation cephalosporin is indicated for patients who are allergic to penicillin, except for those with immediate-type hypersensitivity reactions to beta-lactam antibiotics, who should be treated with a glycopeptide.
‡The results of susceptibility tests might indicate the need to adapt the initial regimen.
§New molecules such as voriconazole and caspofungin should be evaluated.
HACEK, *Haemophilus aphrophilus* or *paraphrophilus, Actinobacillus actinomycetemcomitans, Cardiobacterium hominis, Eikenella corrodens,* and *Kingella* species; MIC, minimal inhibitory concentration; MRSA, methicillin-resistant *Staphylococcus aureus;* MSSA, methicillin-susceptible *S. aureus.*

endocarditis, may be responsible for respiratory failure or even acute respiratory distress syndrome, especially in intravenous drug users with *S. aureus* infectious endocarditis.[23]

MEDICAL AND SURGICAL TREATMENT

In the absence of large prospective, randomized studies, which present a considerable challenge, the overall strategy for infectious endocarditis treatment is derived mainly from retrospective series, clinical judgment, and expert recommendations.

ANTIBIOTIC TREATMENT

Certain general principles underlie the current guidelines for infectious endocarditis treatment.[36,37] In cases of streptococcal infectious endocarditis, determination of the minimal inhibitory concentration of penicillin is necessary to choose the best regimen. Parenteral antibiotics are recommended over oral drugs because of the importance of sustained antibacterial activity, which requires high dosages (e.g., 150 to 200 mg/kg of amoxicillin for streptococcal infectious endocarditis). However, oral antibiotics may be considered for right-sided infectious endocarditis after a few days of parenteral antibiotics when intravenous administration is not possible because of poor venous access. In that case, a combination of a fluoroquinolone and rifampin is an acceptable regimen. Many experts recommend using a combination of agents with activities against the cell wall (beta-lactams or glycopeptides) plus an aminoglycoside for most cases of infectious endocarditis, especially complicated cases such as those in ICU patients. The duration of aminoglycoside use depends on the pathogen and the presence of a prosthesis

(Table 104-3). Although a shorter course of aminoglycosides has been proposed for enterococcal infectious endocarditis,[20] no controlled study has confirmed the safety of this strategy. For staphylococcal infectious endocarditis, a triple regimen including rifampin is recommended,[38] especially for patients with prosthetic valve endocarditis. Short-term therapy (15 days) was shown to be effective in selected cases of noncomplicated *S. aureus* right-sided infectious endocarditis or left-sided native valve infectious endocarditis caused by highly susceptible streptococci. However, most current recommendations emphasize prolonged antibiotic administration (4 to 6 weeks, or even 8 weeks) for *S. aureus* prosthetic valve endocarditis. Valve cultures, but not positive Gram staining, should be taken into account to decide how long to continue antimicrobial therapy after valve replacement.[39]

SURGICAL MANAGEMENT

In recent series, 45% to 50% of patients (up to 75% in specialized medical-surgical centers) undergo valve replacement during the acute phase of infectious endocarditis before the completion of antibiotic treatment.

Indications for and Timing of Cardiac Surgery

Absolute indications are CHF caused by valvular insufficiency, prosthesis obstruction or dehiscence, periannular abscess, or *S. aureus* or fungal prosthetic valve endocarditis. These microorganisms cannot be eradicated without removal of the prosthesis. Development of CHF in the setting of infectious endocarditis generally requires cardiac valve replacement regardless of the number of days on antibiotics.

Relative indications, requiring case-by-case evaluation, are persistent bacteremia beyond 7 days, despite appropriate antibiotic therapy; non–*S. aureus* prosthetic valve endocarditis; and difficult-to-treat organisms such as *C. burnetii*, *Bartonella* species, multiresistant enterococci, or *P. aeruginosa*, especially in patients with prosthetic valve endocarditis.

With regard to other potential indications, contraindications, and timing of valve replacement, the following factors should be emphasized: (1) Although the risk of systemic embolization is higher in patients with large vegetations on the mitral valve, vegetation characteristics alone rarely justify valve surgery.[8] The decreasing risk of emboli with time, especially after the first week of effective antibiotic therapy, should be considered when deciding whether to operate. (2) In patients with neurologic complications, a conservative approach is to delay cardiac surgery for 2 or 3 weeks after an embolic event[40] and for at least a month after cerebral bleeding.[8] However, in the case of CHF, the valve can be replaced within 7 days or less after an embolic infarct, especially when it is of limited size and the patient's good mental status prevails. (3) True contraindications of valve surgery are rare and include uncontrolled septic shock, unhealed sternal wound infection, and severe coagulation disorders.

Surgical Technique

Surgery includes complete removal of all infected and necrotic tissue, followed by valve reconstruction. In selected cases, good results have been achieved with conservative mitral valve valvuloplasty. In most patients, valve replacement with a mechanical or biologic prosthesis or a homograft is necessary. An aortic homograft may be associated with a lower risk of relapse for patients operated on during the very early phase of infectious endocarditis.

OUTCOME AND PROGNOSTIC FACTORS

In a recent 1-year survey of infectious endocarditis in France, the overall in-hospital mortality rate was 16.6%.[1] This figure includes all types of infectious endocarditis and needs to be refined according to different categories of disease. Another recent cohort of 513 patients with complicated, left-sided native valve infectious endocarditis had a 6-month mortality rate of 26%.[13] Mortality rates for prosthetic valve endocarditis are much higher; rates of 33% and 44% have been reported,[41,42] and mortality may be higher than 50% for early prosthetic valve endocarditis.[25] Among 228 patients with infectious endocarditis referred to the two ICUs in our hospital, the in-hospital mortality rate was 45%. Nosocomial infectious endocarditis is associated with up to 68% mortality.[17] In contrast, the prognosis of right-sided infectious endocarditis in intravenous drug users is much better, with mortality being less than 10%.[23]

Prognostic factors of survival have been studied by several authors. In most cases, these reflect the site of infectious endocarditis (see earlier), comorbidities, causative agent, and type of complications. CHF, septic shock, neurologic events, and *S. aureus* are associated with a poor prognosis in most studies.[13,25,26] The hemodynamic status of the patient at the time of valve replacement is the main determinant of perioperative mortality, with a poorer prognosis for patients with

pulmonary edema or impaired left ventricular function.[43] Neurologic events markedly increase the risk of death, which can reach 50% in patients with altered mental status.[13] Among microorganisms, *S. aureus* is associated with higher mortality rates than streptococci for left-sided native valve and prosthetic valve endocarditis.[13,25] Finally, mounting evidence shows that, for both complicated left-sided native valve infectious endocarditis and *S. aureus* prosthetic valve endocarditis, valve replacement combined with medical therapy is associated with a better outcome than medical treatment alone.[13,25,42,45] The reoperation rate, mainly for prosthesis dehiscence or new infectious endocarditis, is 2% to 3% per year, and the 5-year survival rate is approximately 80% to 90% for native valve infectious endocarditis and 60% for prosthetic valve endocarditis. A scoring system taking into account mental status, comorbidity, CHF, microbiology, and the use of surgical treatment in left-sided native valve infectious endocarditis was recently published.[13]

CONCLUSION

Despite advances in both diagnosis and treatment, infectious endocarditis still carries high morbidity and mortality rates, especially for patients requiring ICU admission. Improvement of outcome requires a multidisciplinary approach to optimize medical treatment and decision-making concerning valve surgery.

ANNOTATED REFERENCES

Heiro M, Nikoskelainen J, Engblom E, et al: Neurologic manifestations of infective endocarditis: A 17-year experience in a teaching hospital in Finland. Arch Intern Med 2000;160:2781-2787.
> *Neurologic complications are evident before antimicrobial treatment is started in the vast majority of patients and are significantly associated with Staphylococcus aureus.*

Le T, Bayer AS: Combination antibiotic therapy for infective endocarditis. Clin Infect Dis 2003;36:615-621.
> *This is an excellent comprehensive review that focuses on in vitro and experimental basis of combination antibiotic therapy for infective endocarditis.*

Li JS, Sexton DJ, Mick N, et al: Proposed modifications to the Duke criteria for the diagnosis of infective endocarditis. Clin Infect Dis 2000;30:633-638.
> *The authors have reevaluated the Duke criteria. The main modifications are: redefinition of "possible endocarditis"; proposed clarifications and modifications of minor criteria; and redefinition of major criteria to take into account transesophageal echocardiography. Bacteremia due to S. aureus is a major criterion, regardless of whether the infection is nosocomially acquired or whether a removable source of infection is present. Positive Q fever serology is also changed to a major criteria.*

Mylonakis E, Calderwood SB: Infective endocarditis in adults. N Engl J Med 2001;345:1318-1330.
> *This review addresses epidemiologic, clinical, diagnostic and therapeutic aspects of infective endocarditis. Pertinent information is given on involved pathogens.*

Vickram HR, Buenconseyo Y, Uasbun R, et al: Impact of valve surgery on 6-month mortality in adults with complicated, left-sided native valve endocarditis: A propensity analysis. JAMA 2003;290:3207-3214.
> *This study suggests that valve surgery for patients with complicated, left-sided native valve endocarditis is independently associated with reduced 6-month mortality. The protective effect of surgery is more evident among patients with congestive heart failure.*

Chapter 105

HYPERTENSIVE CRISIS AND URGENCY

Catherine Lee Kelleher • Stuart L. Linas

KEY POINTS

1. Hypertensive crisis is defined as an elevated blood pressure associated with evidence of acute end-organ damage to vital organs, such as the kidney, heart, and brain. The absolute level of blood pressure and the rate of blood pressure elevation determine the development of hypertensive crisis.

2. Hypertensive encephalopathy is a distinct clinical syndrome that occurs when rapidly increasing central perfusion pressure exceeds the ability of the central nervous system to autoregulate.

3. Patients with hypertensive crisis are best treated parenterally with intensive care monitoring by arterial cannulation or automated blood pressure cuff measurement. The primary goal of blood pressure therapy is to lower the pressure at a rate that arrests or alleviates end-organ damage without causing ischemia of vital organs.

4. As a general rule, the choice of blood pressure medication and the rate at which the blood pressure is decreased are determined by the clinical setting.

Hypertension is a common problem in the United States affecting nearly 28.7% of adults in 1999 and 2000 (age-adjusted hypertension prevalence).[1] An analysis of self-reported rates of hypertension in the United States suggests that the incidence of hypertension may be increasing in adults.[1] Of hypertensive individuals, 30% are not aware of their diagnosis.[2] Of the 59% of hypertensive individuals being treated for hypertension, only 34% have a blood pressure less than 140/90 mm Hg.[2] The exact risk of hypertensive crisis is not clear; however, most authors estimate the risk to be less than 1%.[3,4] Data from the United States suggest that the hospital admissions for malignant or accelerated hypertension has doubled.[3]

Hypertensive crisis is defined as an elevated blood pressure associated with evidence of acute end-organ damage. With acute damage to vital organs, such as the kidney, heart, and brain, there is a significant risk of morbidity in hours without therapeutic intervention. The absolute level of blood pressure and the time course of blood pressure elevation determine the development of hypertensive crisis. In general, with hypertensive crisis, the diastolic blood pressure is greater than 130 mm Hg. In children, gravid women, and previously normotensive individuals, hypertensive crises

may occur with relatively minor increases in blood pressure. It is important to identify this syndrome early to prevent end-organ damage and to institute appropriate therapy as soon as the diagnosis is made. Malignant hypertension is a specific syndrome in which a markedly elevated blood pressure is associated with hypertensive neuroretinopathy.

Individuals with hypertensive urgency have an elevated blood pressure (diastolic pressure often >115 mm Hg) without evidence of acute end-organ damage. Hypertensive urgency may be associated with chronic stable complications, such as stable angina, previous myocardial infarction, chronic congestive heart failure, chronic renal failure, previous transient ischemic attacks, or previous cerebrovascular accident with no threat of an acute insult. Complications from hypertensive urgency are not immediate. In contrast to hypertensive crisis, a more gradual blood pressure reduction over hours is recommended.

An increased blood pressure can occur in the absence of acute or chronic target organ dysfunction. When the cause of hypertension is not identified, the blood pressure is lowered over days to weeks. Occasionally an elevated blood pressure may result from drug use, including over-the-counter medications such as pseudoephedrine and illicit substances such as cocaine. In these situations, the blood pressure is lowered rapidly. The focus of this chapter is hypertensive emergencies, including hypertensive crisis and hypertensive urgency.

PATHOPHYSIOLOGY OF HYPERTENSIVE CRISIS

The precise pathophysiology of hypertensive crisis is unknown. An abrupt increase in blood pressure is one of the initiating events in the transition from simple hypertension or normotension to hypertensive crisis. The product of cardiac output and peripheral vascular resistance determines blood pressure. The initial blood pressure increase is likely secondary to an increase in vascular resistance. Considerable evidence suggests that mechanical stress in the arteriolar wall leads to disruption of endothelial integrity.[5] With disruption of vascular integrity, diffuse microvascular lesions develop.[6,7] Fibrinoid necrosis of the arterioles is seen in vulnerable organs and is considered the histologic hallmark of hypertensive crisis.[6,7] It is unclear whether hypertension alone causes the development of hypertensive crisis or whether other factors are necessary. Increases in peripheral vascular resistance result in part from activation of the renin-angiotensin-aldosterone system. Evidence suggests angiotensin II may injure the vascular wall directly by activation of genes for proinflammatory cytokines (interleukin-6) and proinflammatory mediators regulated by nuclear factor-κB.[8,9] Other vascular-toxic influences may contribute to increased peripheral vascular resistance, including hyperviscosity, immunologic factors, and other hormones (e.g., catecholamines, vasopressin, and endothelin).[10-12] The end result of these changes is a significant increase in peripheral vascular resistance with ischemia of heart, brain, and kidneys.

In considering hypertensive crisis and treatment, the impact of blood pressure on cerebrovascular physiology is important. Hypertensive encephalopathy is a distinct clinical syndrome that occurs when rapidly rising central perfusion pressure exceeds the ability of the central nervous system to autoregulate. Autoregulation of cerebral blood flow refers to the ability of the brain to maintain a constant cerebral blood flow as the cerebral perfusion pressure varies from 60 to 150 mm Hg. In chronic hypertension, the range of autoregulation is increased from 60 to 150 mm Hg to 80 to 160 mm Hg. Autoregulation of cerebral blood flow is a function of cerebral perfusion pressure (mean arterial pressure – venous pressure) and cerebral vascular resistance:

$$\text{Cerebral blood flow} = \text{cerebral perfusion pressure (mean arterial pressure} - \text{venous pressure)} / \text{cerebrovascular resistance}$$

Under normal physiologic conditions the backflow in the cerebral venous system or venous pressure is near zero, and the arterial pressure determines the cerebral perfusion pressure. With acute brain injury, as seen with subarachnoid hemorrhage, stroke, and intracranial hemorrhage, the ability of the brain to autoregulate and maintain cerebral blood flow is impaired. Inability to autoregulate cerebral blood flow also is seen in hypertensive crisis when the mean arterial pressure is greater than 140 mm Hg.

DIAGNOSIS OF HYPERTENSIVE EMERGENCIES

Hypertension from any cause may enter a "crisis" phase. Although hypertensive crisis usually occurs in individuals with a history of essential hypertension, it also is seen in individuals with secondary hypertension and in individuals with no hypertensive history, as in preeclampsia, pheochromocytoma, drug withdrawal, and acute glomerulonephritis. A medication history, including over-the-counter medications and illegal drug use, should be obtained from every patient. Malignant hypertension is a unique clinical/pathologic syndrome that is associated with hypertensive crisis. Increases in blood pressure and target organ damage are caused by changes in the vasculature characterized by fibrinoid necrosis and a proliferative endarteritis. Risk factors associated with the development of malignant hypertension include age between 30 and 50 years,[13] male gender,[6] African-American background,[14] and smoking (increases risk by 2.5-fold to 5-fold).[15]

Patients with hypertensive crisis present with a variety of symptoms. The most common is headache. It is either sudden in onset or represents a change from a usual headache pattern and is often worst in the morning. The location is generally occipital or anterior with a steady quality. Other symptoms include visual complaints (scotoma, diplopia, hemianopsia, blindness), neurologic symptoms (focal deficits, stroke, transient ischemic attacks, confusion,

somnolence), ischemic chest pain, renal symptoms (nocturia, polyuria, hematuria), back pain (aortic aneurysm), and gastrointestinal complaints (nausea, vomiting). Weight loss occurs as high levels of circulating renin and angiotensin induce a diuresis.[16] These patients often present with intravascular volume depletion, which has strong implications for treatment.

The blood pressure is measured in both arms and with the patient lying and standing. In hypertensive crisis, diastolic blood pressures are usually greater than 120 to 130 mm Hg. Pathologic processes that cause stiffening of the vascular wall can prevent vessel compression by external compression with a blood pressure cuff; this results in an artificial increase (at times extreme) in the systolic and diastolic blood pressure, or "pseudohypertension." Pseudohypertension can occur in atherosclerosis, Mönckeberg's medial calcification, and metastatic calcification as experienced in end-stage renal disease. Clues to pseudohypertension include a markedly elevated blood pressure in an individual without evidence of end-organ damage. The diagnosis is suggested by a palpable radial artery after proximal compression (Osler's maneuver).[17]

A dilated funduscopic examination should be performed on all patients. Arteriolar thickening reflects chronic hypertension and is manifest by increased light reflex, vascular tortuosity, and arteriovenous nicking (grade I and II). Increased arteriole damage results in decreased blood flow manifest by a silver wire pattern to the vessels. These funduscopic findings reflect chronic hypertension and have no prognostic significance with regard to hypertensive crisis. During hypertensive crisis, there is loss of cerebral autoregulation. In malignant hypertension, additional findings are caused by the increased blood pressure and vasculitis in the retinal arteriolar and venous circulation, including flame-shaped hemorrhages, white cotton-wool spots, yellow-white exudates, and eventually, papilledema. The prognosis for these acute funduscopic findings is identical.[18,19]

With long-standing hypertension, there is often evidence of left ventricular hypertrophy. Examination of the abdomen should include evaluation for an aortic aneurysm. A careful neurologic examination should be done to rule out any evidence of a cerebrovascular accident. Alterations in mental status may indicate a stroke or hypertensive encephalopathy. Symptoms of hypertensive encephalopathy include headache, visual changes, and seizures. Focal neurologic symptoms are unusual without an associated cerebral bleed. Hypertensive neuroretinopathy is usually present but may be absent in patients in whom the pressure increase has been abrupt, such as in cases of acute glomerulonephritis or catecholamine excess states.

The initial laboratory evaluation should include serum sodium, chloride, potassium, bicarbonate, creatinine, and blood urea nitrogen levels; complete blood count (with a peripheral smear to identify schistocytes); electrocardiogram; and urinalysis. Evidence of intravascular hemolysis is common and may make it difficult to differentiate hypertensive crisis from primary vasculitis with secondary hypertension.[20,21] The renin-angiotensin-aldosterone axis is markedly activated, as evidenced by hypokalemia and metabolic alkalosis.[22,23] Blood urea nitrogen and creatinine are often elevated. Urinalysis may show small amounts of proteinuria and hematuria with occasional erythrocyte casts.[5] Marked increases in proteinuria suggest a primary glomerular process, such as glomerulonephritis, as the cause of the elevated blood pressure.

TABLE 105–1. DIFFERENTIAL DIAGNOSIS OF HYPERTENSIVE ENCEPHALOPATHY

Cerebral infarction
Subarachnoid hemorrhage
Intracerebral hemorrhage
Subdural or epidural hematoma
Brain tumor or other mass lesion
Seizure disorder
Central nervous system vasculitis
Encephalitis/meningitis
Drug ingestion
Drug withdrawal

If hypertensive encephalopathy is suspected, magnetic resonance imaging should be performed. With hypertensive encephalopathy, edema may occur in the posterior regions of the cerebral hemispheres, particularly in the parieto-occipital regions, a finding called *posterior leukoencephalopathy* on magnetic resonance imaging.[24] Brainstem involvement on magnetic resonance imaging also has been reported.[24] However, it is important to consider and eliminate other conditions with a similar clinical presentation (Table 105-1). Several important diagnostic considerations help exclude other causes of altered mental status: (1) Symptoms of generalized brain dysfunction tend to develop over time (12 to 24 hours) with hypertensive encephalopathy compared with acutely with ischemic stroke or cerebral hemorrhage; (2) focal neurologic findings are unusual with hypertensive encephalopathy, unless there is associated bleed; (3) papilledema almost always is noted with hypertensive encephalopathy and, if absent, should raise suspicion of another etiology; (4) compared with an acute central nervous system bleed, mental status with hypertensive encephalopathy improves within 24 to 48 hours of treatment.

TREATMENT OF HYPERTENSIVE CRISIS

Patients with hypertensive crisis are best treated parenterally with intensive care monitoring by arterial cannulation or automated blood pressure cuff measurement. The primary goal of blood pressure therapy is to lower the pressure at a rate that arrests or alleviates end-organ damage without causing ischemia of vital organs. Generally the rate of blood pressure control depends on conditions associated with the hypertensive crisis. In most settings, blood pressure can be reduced acutely by 20% to 25% within minutes to hours. After the patient is stabilized at this pressure, blood pressure is decreased to 160/100 to 160/110 mm Hg over the next 2 to 6 hours. If the patient is clinically stable, the blood pressure may be decreased toward a normal blood pressure over the next 24 to 48 hours. With these decreases in blood pressure, central nervous system blood flow autoregulation usually is maintained. In ischemic stroke, there are no large clinical trials to support rapid reduction of blood pressure. Rapid blood pressure reduction (e.g., 15 to 30 minutes) to the normal range is indicated with acute aortic dissection or in previously normotensive subjects with abrupt increases in blood pressure.

More rapid reduction in blood pressure also is recommended in patients with active unstable angina or congestive heart failure with pulmonary edema. In patients with malignant hypertension or hypertensive encephalopathy, a more controlled titration of blood pressure reduction over 1 to 3 hours is satisfactory. Exceptions to rapid blood pressure reduction include older patients with carotid stenosis. These individuals are particularly susceptible to central nervous system hypoperfusion. Blood pressure management in patients with stroke or intracranial bleeding is controversial because the loss of central nervous system blood flow autoregulation and the presence of brain edema require high systemic pressures to provide adequate cerebral perfusion.

Of hypertensive crises, 40% to 50% arise in patients with preexisting hypertension without identifiable secondary causes.[5,25,26] Essential hypertension is the underlying disorder in most African-American individuals.[27-29] In contrast, 50% to 60% of white patients with malignant hypertension have an identifiable cause (Table 105-2).

TABLE 105–2. SYNDROMES OF HYPERTENSIVE CRISIS

Malignant hypertension
Nonmalignant hypertension with target organ disorders
  Patient requiring emergency surgery with poorly controlled hypertension
  Hyperviscosity syndrome
  Postoperative patient
  Renal transplant patient: acute rejection, transplant renal artery stenosis
  Quadriplegic patient with autonomic hyperreflexia
  Severe burns
  Acute aortic dissection
  Intracranial hemorrhage, ischemic stroke, or subarachnoid hemorrhage
  Hypertensive encephalopathy
  Myocardial ischemia/acute left ventricular failure
  Preeclampsia/eclampsia
  Antiphospholipid antibody syndrome
  Acute renal failure
    Scleroderma renal crisis
    Chronic glomerulonephritis
    Reflux nephropathy
    Analgesic nephropathy
    Acute glomerulonephritis
    Radiation nephritis
    Ask-Upmark kidney
    Chronic lead intoxication
  Renovascular hypertension
    Fibromuscular dysplasia
    Atherosclerosis
  Endocrine hypertension
    Congenital adrenal hyperplasia
    Pheochromocytoma
    Oral contraceptives
    Aldosteronism
    Cushing's disease/syndrome
  Systemic vasculitis
  Atheroembolic renal crisis
  Drugs
    Oral contraceptives
    Nonsteroidal anti-inflammatory drugs
    Atropine
    Corticosteroids
    Sympathomimetics
    Erythropoietin
    Lead intoxication
    Cyclosporine
  Catecholamine excess states
    Pheochromocytoma
    Monoamine oxidase/tyramine interaction
    Antihypertensive withdrawal
    Cocaine intoxication, sympathomimetic overdose

Renovascular hypertension, secondary to either fibromuscular dysplasia or atherosclerosis, is common. Patients with underlying chronic glomerulonephritis account for 20% of cases of malignant hypertension.[30] Other renal causes include reflex nephropathy (particularly in children)[30] and analgesic nephropathy.[31]

SPECIFIC TREATMENT RECOMMENDATIONS FOR HYPERTENSIVE CRISIS BASED ON ETIOLOGY

GENERAL COMMENT ON MEDICATIONS USED TO TREAT HYPERTENSIVE CRISIS

The classes of parenteral antihypertensive agents available to treat hypertensive crisis include direct vasodilators (sodium nitroprusside, nitroglycerin), alpha/beta-adrenergic blockers (labetalol), alpha-adrenergic blockers (phentolamine), angiotensin-converting enzyme inhibitors (enalaprilat), calcium channel blockers, and dopamine agonists (fenoldopam). The advantages and disadvantages of these medications are summarized in Table 105-3. Their uses in specific clinical conditions are discussed in subsequent sections. In general, the vasodilator sodium nitroprusside is the most widely used agent because of it rapid onset of action (1 to 2 minutes) and short half-life (2 to 5 minutes). It is effective in most hypertensive emergencies, but should be used with caution in the setting of renal disease and liver dysfunction. There is no consensus on the most effective antihypertensive medications in the setting of a central nervous system insult, and

there are no randomized trials comparing different agents in hypertensive crisis and central nervous system insult. Most authors now caution, however, the use of nitroprusside in the setting of increased intracranial pressure. Vasodilators increase blood volume and have the potential to increase intracranial pressure. Animal and human studies in the setting of a normal intracranial pressure show no effect of nitroprusside on intracranial pressure.[32-34] In studies on animals and humans with preexisting increased intracranial pressure, however, nitroprusside increased the intracranial pressure, likely reflecting vasodilation on the background of decreased cranial compliance.[35-37] When sodium nitroprusside is contraindicated, other treatment options include labetalol and nicardipine. Fenoldopam, which is an agonist of the vasodilator dopamine-1 receptor, shares with nitroprusside a rapid onset and short duration of action. In addition, fenoldopam, in contrast to nitroprusside, increases renal blood flow, induces natriuresis, and produces no toxic metabolites.[38-42]

MALIGNANT HYPERTENSION

Malignant hypertension is specific syndrome characterized by markedly elevated blood pressures in conjunction with hypertensive neuroretinopathy. Funduscopic examination reveals flame-shaped hemorrhages, cotton-wool spots, or papilledema. Malignant hypertension also is associated with nephropathy, encephalopathy, microangiopathic hemolytic anemia, and cardiac ischemia. Untreated malignant hypertension is a rapidly fatal disorder, with a mortality of greater than 90% within 1 year, as reported in a classic series by

TABLE 105–3. TREATMENT OF HYPERTENSIVE CRISIS: INTRAVENOUS MEDICATIONS

Drug Name and Mechanism of Action	Indications/Advantages/Dose	Disadvantages/Adverse Effects/Metabolism/Cautions
Sodium nitroprusside: nitric oxide compound, vasodilator of arteriolar and venous smooth muscle, increases cardiac output by decreasing afterload	Useful in most hypertensive crises Onset of action immediate, duration of action 1-2 min Dose: Initial dose, 0.25 µg/kg/min, maximum dose 8-10 µg/kg/min Beware: 500 µg/kg over prolonged time, rate >2mEq/kg/min, cyanide is generated more rapidly than can be taken care of.	Contraindicated in high output cardiac failure, congenital optic atrophy. Anemia and liver disease at risk for cyanide toxicity—acidosis, tachycardia, change in mental status, almond smell on breath. Renal disease at risk for thiocyanate toxicity—psychosis, hyperreflexia, seizure, tinnitus. Cautious use with increased intracranial pressure. Do not use maximum dose for >10 min. Crosses the placenta
Nitroglycerin: directly interacts with nitrate receptors on vascular smooth muscle, primarily dilates venous bed, decreases preload	Use with symptoms of cardiac ischemia, perioperative hypertension in cardiac surgery Initial dose: 5 µg/min, maximum dose 200 µg/min	Contraindicated in angle-closure glaucoma, increased intracranial pressure. Blood pressure decreased secondary to decreased preload, cardiac output—avoid when cerebral or renal perfusion compromised. Caution with right ventricular infarct
Labetalol: beta-adrenergic blockade and alpha-adrenergic blockade, alpha/beta blocking ratio 1:7	Onset of action 2-5 min. Duration 3-6 h Dose: Bolus 20 mg, then 20-80 mg every 10 min for maximum dose 300 mg. Infuse at 0.5-2 mg/min	Avoid in bronchospasm, bradycardia, congestive heart failure, greater than first-degree heart block, second or third trimester pregnancy. Use caution with hepatic dysfunction, inhalational anesthetics (myocardial depression). Enters breast milk
Esmolol: cardioselective beta₁-adrenergic blocking agent	Used with aortic dissection, used during intubation, intraoperative and postoperative hypertension Onset 60 sec, duration 10-20 min Dose: 200-500 µg/kg over 1-4 min, then 50 µg/kg/min for 4 min, and titer, then infuse 50-300 µg/kg/min	See labetalol. Not dependent on renal or hepatic function for metabolism (metabolized by hydrolysis in red blood cells)
Fenoldopam: postsynaptic dopamine-1 agonist, decreases peripheral vascular resistance, 10 times more potent than dopamine as vasodilator	May be advantageous in kidney disease, increases renal blood flow, increases sodium excretion, no toxic metabolites Initial dose: 0.1 µg/kg/min with titration every 15 min, no bolus	Contraindicated in glaucoma (may increase intraocular pressure) or allergy to sulfites, hypotension especially with concurrent beta blocker. Check serum potassium every 6 h. Concurrent acetaminophen may significantly increase blood levels. Dose-related tachycardia

TABLE 105–3. TREATMENT OF HYPERTENSIVE CRISIS: INTRAVENOUS MEDICATIONS—CONT'D

Drug Name and Mechanism of Action	Indications/Advantages/Dose	Disadvantages/Adverse Effects/Metabolism/Cautions
Hydralazine: primarily dilates arteriolar vasculature	Primarily used in pregnancy/eclampsia Decrease blood pressure in 10-20 min, duration of action 2-4 h Dose: 10 mg every 20-130 min, maximum dose 20 mg	Reflex tachycardia, give beta blocker concurrently, may exacerbate angina. Half-life 3 h, may affect blood pressure for 100 h. Depends on hepatic acetylation for inactivation
Phentolamine: alpha-adrenergic blockade	Used primarily to treat hypertension from excessive catecholamine excess (i.e., pheochromocytoma) Onset of action 1-2 min, duration 3-10 min Dose: 5-15 mg	Beta blockade is generally added to control tachycardia or arrhythmias. As in all catecholamine excess states, beta blockers should never be given first because the loss of beta-adrenergically mediated vasodilation leaves alpha-adrenergically mediated vasoconstriction unopposed and results in increased pressure
Nicardipine: dihydropyridine calcium channel blocker inhibits transmembrane influx of calcium ions into cardiac and smooth muscle	Onset of action 10-20 min, duration 1-4 h Initial dose: 5 mg/h to maximum of 15 mg/h	Avoid with congestive heart failure, cardiac ischemia. Adverse effects include tachycardia, flushing, headache
Enalaprilat: angiotensin-converting enzyme inhibitor	Onset of action 15-20 min, duration 12-24 h Dose: 1.25-5 mg q6h	Response not predictable, with high renin states may see acute hypotension. Hyperkalemia with reduced glomerular filtration rate. Avoid in pregnancy
Trimethaphan: nondepolarizing ganglionic blocking agent, competes with acetylcholine for postsynaptic receptors	Used in aortic dissection Dose: 0.5-5 mg/min	Does not increase cardiac output. No inotropic cardiac effect. Disadvantages include parasympathetic blockade resulting in paralytic ileus and bladder atony, and development of tachyphylaxis after 24-96 h of use

Compiled from (1) Up to Date; (2) Varon J, Marik PE: The diagnosis and management of hypertensive crisis. Chest 2000;118:214-227; and (3) Abdelwahab W, Frishman W, Landau A: Management of hypertensive urgencies and emergencies. J Clin Pharm 1995;35:747-762.

Kincaid-Smith.[6] In this series, deaths were due to renal failure (19%), congestive heart failure (13%), renal failure plus congestive heart failure (48%), stroke (20%), and myocardial infarction (1%).

Aggressive therapy to prevent progressive ischemic injury in malignant hypertension is crucial. Although the autoregulatory range of central nervous system blood flow is reset upward in chronic hypertension, the lower limit of the autoregulation remains approximately 25% less than the resting mean arterial pressure in patients with normotension and chronic hypertension.[43] When the arterial blood pressure falls below this lower limit, cerebral blood flow decreases progressively, and symptoms of low central nervous system flow, including nausea, yawning, hyperventilation, clamminess, and syncope, develop. To protect cerebral function, after initial reduction of blood pressure by 20% within the first hour, blood pressure is reduced further over the next 2 to 6 hours to the 160/110 mm Hg range as long as the patient remains stable. Nitroprusside is one of the most useful intravenous agents for hypertensive crises. Some patients are highly sensitive to treatment owing to coexisting hypovolemia; low-dose nitroprusside is used to reach goal blood pressure. Many parenteral agents have been used as successful alternatives to nitroprusside, including labetalol, fenoldopam, and nicardipine. Premature discontinuation of parenteral therapy may cause rebound hypertension. Oral therapy is started after the pressure has been stabilized on parenteral therapy. Parenteral therapy then is slowly weaned.

Renal failure is common with malignant hypertension. For patients with worsening renal failure from malignant hypertension, renal failure exacerbates the hypertension. Aggressive treatment can arrest and reverse renal damage.

Because the arteriolopathy of malignant hypertension includes fixed anatomic lesions, initial lowering of blood pressure may worsen renal function. Dialysis may be required in patients with a presenting creatinine greater than 4.5 mg/dL.[44] In most patients, renal function begins to improve after 2 weeks of therapy. Of patients who require dialysis, 50% regain sufficient function to discontinue dialysis.[45] Recovery of renal function is predicted when the combined length of both kidneys is 20.2 cm or more, but is thought to be unlikely when the length is 14.2 cm or less.[46] The mean time to recovery is approximately 2 to 3 months, but recovery after 26 months has been reported.[47] In patients with malignant hypertension secondary to glomerulonephritis, eventual deterioration to end-stage renal disease may occur despite blood pressure control.[48] In contrast, renal function tends to remain well preserved in patients without underlying glomerulonephritis if blood pressure is well controlled. Nitroprusside is one of the preferred agents to treat hypertension and renal failure. The metabolism of nitroprusside results in the production of cyanide, which is taken up by red blood cells and conjugated to thiocyanate in the liver. Cyanide toxicity occurs in patients with anemia or liver disease, whereas thiocyanate toxicity is seen in renal disease (see Table 105-3). Thiocyanate levels should be monitored, and the duration of therapy should be kept to less than 72 hours whenever possible. Fenoldopam has no toxic metabolites and may protect renal function.[38-42]

Controversy exists regarding the management of relatively asymptomatic malignant hypertensive patients (i.e., with neuroretinopathy alone).[49-51] Although oral medication under close observation has been used successfully,[52] we prefer initial parenteral therapy. The progressive breakdown of central nervous system autoregulation in these patients enhances the sensitivity to ischemia with abrupt decreases in blood pressure. Of the oral agents, calcium antagonists and minoxidil are effective and safe. Angiotensin-converting enzyme inhibitors may cause hyperkalemia in undialyzed patients with significant renal insufficiency.

HYPERTENSIVE ENCEPHALOPATHY

In hypertensive encephalopathy, the mean arterial pressure exceeds the limits of autoregulation, and brain edema develops from extravasation of plasma proteins. If hypertensive encephalopathy is untreated, coma and death may follow.[53] The challenge of hypertensive encephalopathy is appropriate lowering of blood pressure in the setting of central nervous system ischemia and edema. The hallmark of hypertensive encephalopathy is improvement within 12 to 24 hours of adequate blood pressure reduction. The mean arterial pressure should be reduced cautiously by no more that 15% over 2 to 3 hours. Neurologic complications have been reported from reductions in mean arterial pressure of 40% or more.[54] In previously normotensive patients, including patients with eclampsia, blood pressure should be normalized. If the mental status worsens with treatment, the pressure should be allowed to increase until neurologic symptoms resolve, then be reduced to within the normal range over several days, to allow restoration of autoregulation.

ISCHEMIC CEREBRAL INFARCTION

When the cerebral perfusion pressure decreases below the level of autoregulation, ischemia develops. In response, there is a marked elevation in arterial blood pressure, which tends to return spontaneously to baseline 24 to 48 hours after the acute event. The role of blood pressure treatment in this setting is controversial. Data from animal studies show in the area surrounding the ischemic infarct that there are "neurons at risk" that rely on collateral circulation to maintain perfusion.[55] These neurons are nonfunctional, are not dead, and potentially can be "rescued" by reperfusion, a phenomenon referred to as *ischemic penumbra*.[55] The degree to which this phenomenon occurs in humans is unknown.[55] In addition, in acute stroke, autoregulation is impaired, and cerebral blood flow is not preserved in a predictable manner. As a result of these changes, acute reductions in blood pressure potentially could increase the area of infarct, resulting in severe clinical consequences. Recommendations from the American Stroke Association are as follows: In individuals with a recent ischemic infarct and a blood pressure greater than 220/120 to 220/140 mm Hg, the blood pressure may be decreased by 10% to 15%. During this reduction, the patient is monitored cautiously for any neurologic sequelae. If the diastolic blood pressure is greater than 140 mm Hg, the blood pressure is reduced with sodium nitroprusside by 10% to 15%.[56] Most clinicians do not treat hypertension in the setting of ischemic stroke, unless the blood pressure elevation is extreme (systolic blood pressure >220 mm Hg, diastolic pressures >120 mm Hg), or there is acute ischemic damage to vital organs (cardiac ischemia, aortic dissection). Hypotensive agents used in this setting include nitroprusside and labetalol. Intravenous labetalol may not elevate intracranial pressure as much as nitroprusside.[57,58]

SUBARACHNOID HEMORRHAGE

Approximately 10% of cerebrovascular accidents are due to subarachnoid hemorrhage.[59] Mortality rates are estimated at 40% to 50%.[60,61] Ruptured congenital berry aneurysms are the most common cause of subarachnoid hemorrhage. Subarachnoid hemorrhage increases intracranial pressure and decreases cerebral perfusion, causing global ischemia. Complications include an intracerebral hemorrhage or the development of hydrocephalus. The treatment of choice is surgical clipping. There is a significant risk of rebleed in the first 24 hours. Management of these patients is significantly different from patients with ischemic stroke. In contrast to ischemia, intracranial bleed induces intense vasospasm in neighboring vessels 4 to 12 days after the initial bleed, increasing the risk for significant cerebral ischemia. The mental status evaluation may be used to guide therapy. An intact mental status is evidence of adequate cerebral perfusion.

Markedly elevated pressures increase the risk of rebleeding. The goal is a 20% to 25% reduction in mean arterial pressure over 6 to 12 hours, but to not less than 160/100 to 180/100 mm Hg.[62] Labetalol is the preferred agent because there are no significant adverse effects on intracranial pressure or cerebral perfusion pressure.[58] Given the potential increase in cerebral blood volume and intracranial pressure associated with vasodilators, sodium nitroprusside and nitroglycerin are not usually first-line treatments. There are clinical data to show that treatment with oral nimodipine within 4 days of the acute event decreases vasospasm and cerebral ischemia.[63] Nimodipine also may directly protect nerve cells from ischemic damage by blocking calcium uptake into cells.

INTRACEREBRAL HEMORRHAGE

Intracerebral hemorrhage accounts for 10% to 20% of all strokes.[64] Hypertension is a major risk factor; 75% of affected individuals have preexisting hypertension.[65] Although patients with intracerebral hemorrhage may present with nausea, vomiting, change in mental status, hypertension, headache, and a focal neurologic examination, the definitive diagnosis must be made by neuroimaging. In contrast to ischemic stroke, in which blood pressure generally returns to normal in 24 to 48 hours, in intracerebral hemorrhage, although the most rapid decline in blood pressure occurs in the first 24 hours, the blood pressure may remain elevated for 7 to 10 days.[55,57] The hematoma compresses normal tissue, creating an area of ischemia, increasing intracranial pressure and further decreasing cerebral perfusion pressure. Autoregulation is altered, making cerebral perfusion critically dependent on systemic blood pressure.[57] There is no consensus on the treatment of hypertension in this setting, and no randomized studies have been done to look at the impact of blood pressure control on outcome. Some authors argue that decreasing blood pressure decreases risk of hemorrhage extension, edema, and associated systemic complications, particularly when systolic blood pressure exceeds 200 mm Hg, a level shown to be associated with hematoma growth.[57,64,65] Other authors argue that not treating hypertension allows continued perfusion of areas at risk from low blood flow.[57] It was thought previously that rebleeding was rare in the first 24 hours. More recent data suggest that rebleeding is more common than thought, occurring in one third of affected individuals.[65,66]

The greatest risk is in the first few hours after the initial insult.[66,67] An increased risk of bleed is associated with an initial large irregular bleed,[68] coagulopathy, liver disease,[69] and a low platelet count.[69] No studies have shown a clear relationship between acute hypertension after an intracerebral bleed and the risk of rebleed.[57] Extreme elevations of pressure (mean arterial pressure > 130 mm Hg) probably should be treated with reduction of blood pressure limited to 20%.[65] There is no consensus on the agent of choice.

Concern revolves around the impact of different antihypertensives on intracranial pressure. Common to all agents is a decrease in mean arterial pressure and a decrease in cerebral perfusion pressure. Vasodilating agents may increase cerebral blood flow and in the setting of decreased cranial compliance potentially may increase intracranial pressure, further decreasing cerebral perfusion pressure.[36,57] The combination of decreased cerebral compliance, decreased cerebral blood flow, and altered autoregulation as occurs in chronic hypertension makes the administration of any antihypertensive agent potentially dangerous. No large randomized studies are available to guide therapy. Combination alpha and beta blockers are recommended when antihypertensive treatment is indicated in intracerebral hemorrhage. Risks of this therapy include worsening of bradycardia associated with the Cushing response. In the setting of normal cranial compliance and an increased intracranial pressure, however, vasodilators are probably safe. Because of the high levels of circulating catecholamines with intracerebral bleed, beta blockade is added when vasodilator therapy alone is ineffective. In one study, barbiturates were found to reduce mean arterial pressure modestly, while markedly reducing the intracranial pressure, and should be considered in cases of severe hemorrhage.[70]

HEAD TRAUMA

Head trauma complications include skull fractures, epidural hematomas, subdural hematomas, intracerebral hematomas, and diffuse axonal damage. With trauma, there is often edema. Acute increases in intracranial pressure are prevented initially by flow of blood and cerebrospinal fluid from the cranial vault. With increasing edema, however, intracranial pressure eventually increases. In most trauma centers, intracranial pressure monitoring has become the standard of care.[71] Defective autoregulation may occur in 31% to 61% of patients with a closed-head injury.[71] If autoregulation is intact, increasing the mean arterial pressure causes vasoconstriction and produces no change in intracranial pressure. With altered autoregulation, increasing the mean arterial pressure may cause vasodilation, increasing blood volume, causing edema and increased intracranial pressure. The goal is to maintain a minimal cerebral perfusion pressure of 70 mm Hg and a mean arterial pressure greater than 90 mm Hg. If an antihypertensive agent is needed, a major consideration is its impact on intracranial pressure. A combination alpha and beta blocker may be preferred when there is decreased intracranial compliance and increased intracranial pressure. In the absence of increased intracranial compliance, vasodilators may be preferred.

AORTIC DISSECTION

Aortic dissection begins with a tear in the intima of the aorta that is propagated by the aortic pulse wave (dP/dt). Myocardial contractility, heart rate, and blood pressure contribute to the aortic pulse wave. There are two types of aortic dissection—type A and type B. Type A dissections often are associated with a tear in the intima of the proximal aorta next to a coronary artery and may extend to the aortic arch.[73] Type B dissections occur in the descending aortic arch and usually begin with an intimal tear next to the subclavian artery.[74] Risk factors for dissection include advanced atherosclerosis, Marfan syndrome, Ehlers-Danlos syndrome, and coarctation of the aorta.[75] Symptoms occur as the expanding hematoma causes pressure on the vasculature; this may cause myocardial infarction, stroke, spinal cord/bowel infarction, and acute renal failure. Ischemic kidney may develop leading to refractory hypertension.[76] Dissection to the aortic root can precipitate acute aortic insufficiency.[77] Rupture of the ascending aorta leads to hemopericardium and tamponade.[77]

Both types of dissection may present with severe, often tearing, pain in the chest, back, or abdomen, accompanied by diaphoresis, nausea, or vomiting. They are often, but not always, associated with hypertension.[78] Discrepancies in peripheral pulses may be observed. The chest x-ray may show widening of the mediastinum. An analysis showed a widened mediastinum was present in only half of individuals with type B dissection.[79] The diagnosis may be confirmed with computed tomography or magnetic resonance imaging.[78] Multiplane transesophageal echocardiography also is used.[78]

Type A dissections usually require surgery to prevent the catastrophic consequences of great vessel occlusion, aortic insufficiency, or tamponade. Type B dissections usually may be treated medically.

Treatment for type A and type B dissections is initiated based on clinical suspicion alone given the high mortality associated with this entity. The goal of treatment is first to decrease myocardial contractility and heart rate with beta blockade. Propranolol often is used. Labetalol also may be used, although its longer duration of action poses a disadvantage in patients going for emergency surgery. Next, the blood pressure is reduced to the lowest tolerable level until pain is relieved. Relief of pain suggests arrest of ongoing aortic dissection. The most widely used agent is nitroprusside. Nitroprusside is titrated to systolic pressure of 100 to 120 mm Hg or to diastolic pressure of 70 to 80 mm Hg. Prior treatment with beta blockade prevents reflex cardiac stimulation and a potential increase in the aortic pulse wave seen with nitroprusside.

An alternative regimen, preferred by some because of a more potent reduction in the steepness of the pulse wave contour, involves use of the ganglionic blocking agent trimethaphan.[79] This agent prevents increases in cardiac output and left ventricular ejection rate.[76,79] The rapid onset and short duration of action of this drug allow precise pressure control. Any mild reflex increase in heart rate may be treated with subsequent beta blockade. Hydralazine is avoided because it causes unwanted reflex cardiac stimulation. Even normotensive individuals should be treated with antihypertensive medications to keep the heart rate and shear forces low.

PULMONARY EDEMA

Many patients who present with pulmonary edema have long-standing antecedent hypertension with concentric left ventricular hypertrophy and well-preserved systolic contraction.[80,81] They develop acute diastolic dysfunction in response to abrupt increases in cardiac afterload secondary to increased systemic blood pressure.[82] With poor diastolic relaxation, the left ventricle requires markedly elevated filling pressures, leading to pulmonary venous hypertension and edema. The therapeutic goal is to decrease afterload, improve diastolic relaxation, and decrease pulmonary pressure. Vasodilators are the agent of choice because they improve diastolic relaxation and lower pulmonary venous pressure. A beta blocker also may be used. Nitroprusside often is used because it reduces preload and afterload, improving left ventricular function, and reduces myocardial oxygen demand. Modest decreases in pressure improve symptoms markedly. In less emergent settings, angiotensin-converting enzyme inhibitors or calcium channel antagonists have been shown to improve diastolic function and cause regression of concentric ventricular hypertrophy.[83]

In patients with left ventricular failure secondary to poor systolic function, vasodilators are the agents of choice. Nitroglycerin is preferred with cardiac ischemia. Nitroprusside may be used in patients refractory to nitrites. Although nitroglycerin dilates intercoronary collateral vessels more than small resistance arterioles and improves perfusion of ischemic myocardium, nitroprusside dilates resistance arterioles predominantly, resulting in a potential steal of blood flow away from ischemic areas. Diuretics are used to reduce left ventricular end-diastolic volume.

In acute myocardial infarction, acute catecholamine release and sympathetic outflow contribute to hypertension. The hypertension usually resolves in a few hours with sedation and pain control alone. Diastolic blood pressures greater than 100 mm Hg should be treated with nitroglycerin. The pressure is rapidly, but cautiously, reduced to near normotensive levels because overshoot hypotension can worsen coronary perfusion. Therapy usually can be stopped within 24 hours. There is considerable evidence that the early use of beta-blocking agents may reduce ultimate infarct size independent of blood pressure control.[84]

PERIOPERATIVE HYPERTENSION

Perioperative hypertension is a major risk factor for the development of postoperative hypertension.[85] It is recommended that elective surgery be deferred until the diastolic pressure is controlled at less than 110 mm Hg because patients with less severe hypertension do not seem to carry an increased risk.[86] The exception is in patients with end-organ damage secondary to hypertension, as with congestive heart failure, in which there seems to be an increased risk of adverse cardiac outcome.[87] In patients with chronic hypertension on adequate treatment, oral medications should be taken the morning of surgery.

Induction of anesthesia increases sympathetic activity, causing elevated blood pressure, a response that may be exaggerated in uncontrolled hypertension.[86] As anesthesia continues, there is generally a decrease in blood pressure. Rapid and wide fluctuations in blood pressure, leading to intraoperative hypotension, stroke, myocardial ischemia, or acute renal failure, are more common in individuals with a hypertensive history.

Patients taking hypertensive therapy before surgery should continue treatment after surgery, changing to an equivalent intravenous medication if they are unable to take oral medications. If patients have been on a beta blocker or clonidine, this medication should be continued postoperatively to prevent rebound hypertension. If intravenous medication is necessary, propranolol or methyldopa may be used. The high incidence of increased blood pressure results from the decreased use of "deep" anesthesia and absence of prolonged sedation after surgery. As a result, there is increased sympathetic response to surgical stimuli, such as pain, hypoxia, and the anesthetic agents themselves. Effective pain control and avoidance of hypoxia are sufficient to treat the hypertension. Adequate blood pressure control reduces the risk of bleeding from suture lines, premature graft closure, and ischemic damage to organs at risk. Nitroprusside is widely used. Nitroglycerin is preferred for post–coronary bypass patients. Fenoldopam, with its impact on increasing renal blood flow, also is recommended, especially in clinical settings where renal ischemia is a risk.

CATECHOLAMINE-ASSOCIATED HYPERTENSION

Hypertensive crisis related to excess catecholamine secretion can result from the ingestion of sympathomimetic agents, such as cocaine, amphetamines, phencyclidine, and phenylpropanolamine (diet pills); decongestants, such as ephedrine and pseudoephedrine; and other agents, including atropine, ergot alkaloids, and tricyclic antidepressants. It also may be caused by tyramine ingestion in conjunction with monoamine oxidase inhibitor therapy, autonomic dysfunction, withdrawal from certain antihypertensive medications, and pheochromocytoma. Critically elevated pressures can result and cause myocardial infarction, aortic dissection, and stroke.

Pheochromocytoma is a rare cause of hypertension.[88] Excess catecholamine secretion by the tumor results in a sustained elevation of blood pressure in most cases, whereas peripheral catecholamine uptake and storage lead to paroxysmal symptoms when the catecholamines are released in response to stimuli. Symptoms of pheochromocytoma include headache, palpitations, hypertension, anxiety, abdominal pain, and diaphoresis. Patients may present with orthostatic changes in blood pressure, a clue to the diagnosis.[89] For patients with hypertensive emergency, the treatment of choice is the short-acting parenteral alpha antagonist, phentolamine. After blood pressure reduction, beta blockade generally is added to control tachycardia or arrhythmias. As in all catecholamine excess states, beta blockers should not be used as initial therapy. Loss of beta-adrenergically mediated vasodilation leaves alpha-adrenergically mediated vasoconstriction unopposed and results in increased pressure. An oral regimen of the nonselective alpha antagonist, phenoxybenzamine, can be used in less critical situations. Labetalol has been effective in treating hypertension related to pheochromocytoma in selected patients. Because its beta-blocking effect exceeds its alpha-blocking effect, however, severe hypertension has been reported.[90]

Significant rebound hypertension may develop 12 to 72 hours after abrupt discontinuation of chronic beta-blocker therapy or a centrally acting alpha-agonist antihypertensive, such as clonidine or methyldopa, from increased sympathetic outflow. With severe hypertension, headache, diaphoresis, anxiety, nausea, tachycardia, and abdominal pain are reported. In cases of moderate hypertension, simply restarting the antihypertensive agent may control the blood pressure. With more severe blood pressure elevations, intravenous therapy should be started.

TABLE 105–4. TYRAMINE-CONTAINING FOODS
Chianti wine
Soy sauce
Avocados
Bananas
Coffee
Chocolate
Pickled herring
Chicken liver
Yeast
Fermented sausage
Canned figs
Certain beer
Unpasteurized cheese

In patients on monoamine oxidase inhibitor therapy, ingestion of foods containing tyramine or sympathomimetic amines can result in hypertension (Table 105-4). Tyramine is metabolized by an alternative pathway to octopamine, which releases catecholamines from peripheral sites by acting as a false neurotransmitter. Nitroprusside or phentolamine is used, with the addition of beta blockade as needed for tachycardia. The episodes are self-limited and last 6 hours or less.

GESTATIONAL HYPERTENSION, PREECLAMPSIA, AND ECLAMPSIA

Gestational hypertension is defined as a systolic blood pressure of at least 140 mm Hg and a diastolic blood pressure of at least 90 mm Hg on two separate blood pressure measurements done 6 hours apart. It occurs after 20 weeks of pregnancy in patients known to be previously normotensive.[91] Fifty percent of these women develop preeclampsia if gestational hypertension develops before 30 weeks of gestation.[94] *Preeclampsia* is defined as gestational hypertension with 300 mg of protein on a 24-hour urine (urine dipstick 1+).[91] A 24-hour urine is necessary because urine protein on dipstick correlates poorly with 24-hour urine protein in gestational hypertension.[92] Preeclampsia also should be suspected in patients with hypertension developing after 20 weeks of gestation and associated with nausea, vomiting, cerebral symptoms, abnormal liver function tests, and thrombocytopenia even in the absence of proteinuria. Preeclampsia develops in 7% of all pregnancies—70% in null gravidas and 30% in multigravidas. In the setting of molar pregnancy, it is seen in 70% of individuals.[93] During normal pregnancy, blood pressure initially is decreased, then slowly increases toward the normal range during the third trimester. In preeclampsia, intravascular volume is low despite peripheral edema, and the renin-angiotensin system is activated. Progression to seizures defines *eclampsia,* which may occur with diastolic pressures of 100 mm Hg. Clinical treatment includes bed rest and parenteral magnesium. With preeclampsia, to avoid compromise of placental blood flow, the goal is to keep the systolic blood pressure between 140 mm Hg and 150 mm Hg and diastolic blood pressure between 90 mm Hg and 105 mm Hg.[94] Hydralazine is the preferred agent. Labetalol also may be used. Nitroprusside should be avoided because of the risk of cyanide toxicity in the fetus. Angiotensin-converting enzyme inhibitors also should be avoided because of their potential impact on the fetus' kidney.

OTHER HYPERTENSIVE SITUATIONS

The renal crisis of scleroderma is an aggressive form of malignant hypertension in which proliferative endarteritis precedes hypertension. Ischemia-induced activation of the renin-angiotensin system causes hypertension. The incidence of this condition among patients with scleroderma ranges from 8% to 13%, and it is more common among blacks.[95] Progression to end-stage renal disease occurs in 1 to 2 months without treatment. Aggressive pressure control with angiotensin-converting enzyme inhibitors leads to a long-term survival of about 50% to 70%.[96]

Hypertension is a feature of primary and secondary antiphospholipid antibody syndromes, occurring in 93% of patients.[97] Malignant hypertension occurs in this syndrome secondary to microvasculopathy and emboli to the renal artery. Antihypertensive treatment is similar to malignant hypertension. Successful treatment outcomes have been reported with anticoagulation.[97]

One fourth of patients with extensive second-degree or third-degree burns develop severe hypertension in the first few days, likely owing to high levels of circulating catecholamines and renin. Nitroprusside and phentolamine are other treatments.

Patients with transverse spinal cord lesions at the T6 level or higher, including patients with Guillain-Barré syndrome, have dysreflexia, in which noxious stimuli in dermatomes below the level of the lesion trigger a massive sympathetic discharge. This discharge leads to severe hypertension, bradycardia, diaphoresis, and headache. In 90% of patients, distention of the bladder or bowel causes dysreflexia, and prompt decompression leads to resolution of hypertension.[98] Drugs that have been used successfully in treating this condition include nitroprusside, phentolamine, and labetalol.

Hypertension in the renal transplant recipient may be caused by acute rejection, vascular anastomotic stenosis, obstructive uropathy, corticosteroid use, cyclosporine, and native kidney renin release.[99] Oral calcium channel antagonists are effective and well tolerated in these patients. Other rare causes of hypertension include erythropoietin-associated hypertension. This condition is treated with phlebotomy and dose reduction in conjunction with antihypertensive drug.[100] Diabetics on beta blockers can experience severe hypertension with hypoglycemic episodes, presumably due to catecholamine release.

HYPERTENSIVE URGENCY

Hypertensive urgency refers to patients in whom blood pressure is severely elevated, but based on detailed history, physical examination, and laboratory evaluation, there is no evidence of acute end-organ damage. This clinical situation is different from that of patients with severe hypertension and chronic stable complications, such as patients with stable chronic renal failure or stable angina. The decision to treat the latter group in the inpatient or outpatient setting often depends on the associated end-organ involvement (Table 105-5) and reliability of patient follow-up.

The most common treatment category, termed *severe uncomplicated hypertension* (see Table 105-5), is used to describe patients with severe blood pressure elevation but no end-organ involvement. Despite markedly elevated pressures (e.g., diastolic pressures of 140 mm Hg at times), these patients are at low risk of immediate complications.

TABLE 105–5. SEVERE UNCOMPLICATED HYPERTENSION

Severe hypertension (diastolic >115 mm Hg) in association with one or more of the following:
Chronic renal failure
Chronic congestive heart failure
Stable angina
Previous myocardial infarction
Transient ischemic attacks
Previous cerebrovascular accident

Hypertension-related morbidity tends to occur over months to years. The treatment of choice is gradual pressure reduction over a few days in the outpatient setting. The major risk of therapy is rapid pressure reduction. The choice of antihypertensive agent is based on ease of administration and side-effect profile rather than on rapid blood pressure reductions. Frequently, restarting a previously effective regimen is all that is necessary. It is crucial to follow these patients over the next 24 to 48 hours to ensure the blood pressure is appropriately reduced. Although medicolegal issues may pressure physicians into loading these patients with medication to observe on-the-spot control of blood pressure, this practice has been questioned as having no clear rational scientific basis.

ANNOTATED REFERENCES

Hajjar I, Kotchen TA: Trends in prevalence, awareness, treatment, and control of hypertension in the United States, 1999-2000. JAMA 2003; 290:199-206.
Contrary to earlier reports, hypertension prevalence is increasing in the United States. Hypertension control rates, although improving, continue to be low. Programs targeting hypertension prevention and treatment are of utmost importance.

Chobanian AV, Bakris GL, Black HR, et al: The Seventh Report of the Joint National Committee on Prevention, Detection, Evaluation, and Treatment of High Blood Pressure. JAMA 2003.
Latest guidelines for hypertension prevention and management.

Blumenfeld JD, Laragh JH: Management of hypertensive crisis. Am J Hypertension 2001;14:1154-1167.
This article provides a detailed treatment algorithm to guide drug selection in patients presenting with a hypertensive crisis.

Adams HP Jr, Adams RJ, Brott T, et al: Guidelines for the early management of patients with ischemic stroke: A scientific statement for the Stroke Council for the American Stroke Association. Stroke 2000;34:1056-1083.
The management of patients with acute ischemic stroke is multifaceted, and indications for specific therapies vary among patients. There is strong evidence that outcomes after stroke can be improved and that death or disability from stroke can be reduced with appropriate treatment. This statement aims to provide guidance to physicians for the early treatment of patients.

Chapter 106

CARDIAC SURGERY: INDICATIONS AND COMPLICATIONS

Jacques P. Goldstein • Pierre Wauthy

KEY POINTS

1. Cardiac surgery includes mainly coronary and valve surgery. Indications for coronary artery bypass surgery are mainly based on symptoms and the presence of myocardial ischemia. Surgery is recommended in the presence of specific anatomical coronary lesions such as left main stenosis, triple vessel disease, or significant proximal left anterior descending stenosis.

2. Concerning aortic valve stenosis, aortic valve replacement is indicated when the effective valve area is ≤ 1cm². Aortic valve regurgitation requires surgery as left ventricular systolic dysfunction develops. Indications for mitral valve surgery have increased with the development of mitral valve repair.

3. Complications after cardiac surgery mainly include cardiac arrhythmias, bleeding, myocardial dysfunction, infectious problems such as mediastinitis, and pulmonary dysfunction. Neurologic complications and renal dysfunction also may develop. Acute complications such as aortic dissection after cardiac surgery or left ventricular rupture after mitral valve replacement are rarely observed but require early diagnosis and emergency reoperation.

Since the first clinical use of the heart-lung machine, developed by Gibbon in 1953, cardiac surgery has become a worldwide standard technique for the treatment of congenital and acquired cardiac diseases.[1] Over a period of more than 50 years with trials and errors, indications for surgical treatment of cardiac diseases have been well defined. The introduction of new surgical techniques, such as beating-heart surgery or new ministernotomy approaches, may improve some surgical results and may be applied to patients not suitable for the standard therapies. This chapter reviews the specific indications for cardiac surgery in patients with coronary and valvular diseases and discusses some of the most frequent complications encountered after cardiac surgery.

SURGICAL INDICATIONS FOR CORONARY ARTERY DISEASES

Chest pain is usually evaluated with a combination of noninvasive and invasive tests. Symptoms should be characterized in terms of duration, location, and severity using the Canadian Cardiovascular Society Classification System.[2]

Noninvasive tests, including resting and exercise electrocardiogram in combination with more complex isotope studies, confirm the presence of ischemic myocardial diseases. For the cardiac surgeon, coronary angiography remains the essential invasive test to describe the exact location and the extent of the coronary artery narrowing. Left ventricular function also should be evaluated using noninvasive or invasive tests. Because the aim of coronary artery bypass surgery is to eliminate symptoms and to prolong life, indications for surgery are based on symptoms (Canadian classification), left ventricular function, extension of regional ischemia, and anatomic localization of the coronary artery stenosis.

In the early 1990s, three large multicenter randomized trials were undertaken in Europe and in the United States: the Veterans Administration Cooperative Study, the European Coronary Surgery Study, and the Coronary Artery Surgery Study. Among all patients, patients who underwent coronary artery bypass grafting (CABG) always had extended survival compared with medically treated patients. Referring to the natural history of coronary artery disease and these three large multicenter randomized trials, Gibbons and colleagues[2] made some specific recommendations for myocardial revascularization, published by the American College of Cardiology/American Heart Association task force.[2] Anatomic criteria remain the key factors in favor of myocardial revascularization. The benefit of CABG is correlated with specific coronary lesions such as the following:

- Left main stenosis of more than 50% or a left main equivalent disease (>70% stenosis in the proximal left anterior descending and the proximal circumflex arteries)
- Triple-vessel diseases defined as significant lesions (>70%) in all three coronary territories (right, anterior, and lateral)
- Significant proximal left anterior descending stenosis with two-vessel disease

The improvement of long-term survival is even more striking when left ventricular function is depressed before surgery.[3] Since these three randomized trials were performed, however, several important factors have changed. The patient population is getting older, but patients older than age 65 were excluded from the early trials. Improvements in surgical techniques with systematic use of arterial grafts (intrathorax arteries, radial arteries) in combination with new medical therapies (platelet inhibitors or lipid-lowering agents) have been shown to improve the long-term survival rates after CABG.[2]

Besides specific coronary lesions, CABG should be evaluated taking into account some incremental risk factors that may increase morbidity or mortality, such as hemodynamic instability, older age, diabetes mellitus, and chronic obstructive pulmonary disease.[4] Nashef and coworkers[5,6] developed a simple and effective scoring system for the prediction of early mortality after cardiac surgery (Euroscore). Using the Euroscore online (www.euroscore.org), predictive mortality can be calculated according to several risk factors, including age, sex, chronic pulmonary disease, extracardiac arteriopathy, neurologic dysfunction, previous cardiac surgery, serum creatinine level, critical preoperative status, left ventricular function, pulmonary hypertension, and emergency operation.

New, less invasive CABG procedures may broaden the indications for surgery by reducing morbidity and mortality. Currently, evolving technology can be divided into three categories:

1. Off-pump CABG performed via sternotomy on a beating heart, avoiding cardiopulmonary bypass (CPB)
2. Minimally invasive CABG performed via a small left thoracotomy without CPB
3. Port-access CABG with femorofemoral CPB using thoracoscopic instruments

Early studies confirm the feasibility of these new techniques. Long-term benefits need to be evaluated, however.

SURGICAL INDICATIONS FOR AORTIC VALVE SURGERY

AORTIC STENOSIS

Echocardiography is the most efficient investigation to evaluate the degree of stenosis, degree of left ventricular hypertrophy, and evolution of left ventricular function in patients with aortic valve stenosis. The American College of Cardiology/American Heart Association Task Force on Practice Guidelines has graded the degree of aortic stenosis as mild (effective valve area >1.5 cm²), moderate (area >1 to 1.5 cm²), or severe (area ≤1 cm²).[7] When stenosis is severe and cardiac output is normal, the mean transvalvular pressure gradient is generally greater than 50 mm Hg. Most patients with aortic stenosis are symptomatic, mainly with angina pectoris and dyspnea.

Because aortic valve replacement is the only effective treatment for severe aortic stenosis, surgery is indicated in virtually all symptomatic patients except for patients with severe comorbid conditions. Cases involving patients undergoing CABG with mild-to-moderate aortic stenosis are controversial.[7-9] For asymptomatic patients with mild aortic stenosis (mean gradient ≤25 mm Hg) who require CABG, it may be reasonable to perform only revascularization given the slow evolution of aortic stenosis and the improvement in reoperation mortality and morbidity.[9]

AORTIC REGURGITATION

Patients with chronic aortic regurgitation are mainly asymptomatic for many years. During this period, increased volume and pressure are compensated by left ventricular hypertrophy. This balance between volume overload and hypertrophy may deteriorate, however, with a reduction in contractility. Patients develop dyspnea, orthopnea, and pulmonary edema, usually New York Heart Association functional class III or IV, which is a good indication for valve replacement.[7] Surgery also is indicated in patients with left ventricular systolic dysfunction (ejection fraction <0.25 or end-systolic dimension >60 mm or both).

Surgical treatment of asymptomatic patients with aortic regurgitation is controversial. Patients with aortic regurgitation and mild-to-moderate left ventricular dysfunction at rest (ejection fraction 0.25 to 0.49) also should be candidates for surgery knowing that most of them develop symptoms within 2 to 3 years. Aortic regurgitation also can be caused by aortic root dilation. Aortic root replacement with aortic valve replacement or aortic valve–sparing surgery should be performed when the aortic root dilation is 50 mm or greater.[10,11]

SURGICAL INDICATIONS FOR MITRAL VALVE SURGERY

Indications for mitral valve surgery have changed with the extension of mitral valve repair. With a better understanding of the specific anatomic lesions of the mitral valve associated with improvements in the surgical techniques, successful mitral repair can be achieved in specific ischemic and nonischemic mitral regurgitation.

MITRAL STENOSIS

Moderate or severe mitral stenosis (mitral valve area ≤1.5 cm²) in symptomatic patients (New York Heart Association class III or IV) represents a good indication for surgery.[7] Mortality may be 15% in older patients, however, with calcified valves and pulmonary hypertension.

MITRAL REGURGITATION

Mitral valve repair always should be attempted to avoid problems associated with prosthetic valves. Surgery is required in symptomatic patients with normal left ventricular function or mild or severe left ventricular dysfunction. In asymptomatic patients, surgery is advised only if the left ventricular function is mildly or moderately reduced. The acute onset of atrial fibrillation in patients with mitral regurgitation also is a good indication for surgery, even with normal left ventricular function.

Ischemic mitral regurgitation represents a specific entity related to left ventricular dysfunction, anulus dilation, or papillary muscle dysfunction. CABG alone sometimes may reduce left ventricular dysfunction and reduce mitral regurgitation. Echographic data were able to evaluate the regurgitated volume (proximal isovelocity surface area).[12] Mitral valve plasty should be undertaken when the regurgitated volume is greater than 35 mL. Usually, mitral ring annuloplasty is performed with a downsized ring enabling better mitral valve coaptation.[13,14]

COMPLICATIONS AFTER CARDIAC SURGERY

Most patients after cardiac surgery under CPB have a normal convalescence without complications. Convalescence may be abnormal, however, requiring intensive observation and prompt intervention if required. Numerous complications may occur after cardiac surgery; the most common are described here.

CARDIAC ARRHYTHMIAS

Postoperative cardiac arrhythmia is a major cause of morbidity and mortality in cardiac surgery. These arrhythmias may occur with normal cardiac function and in postoperative cardiac failure. Inotrope administration may increase the risk of such complications. Atrial and ventricular arrhythmias can occur in the postoperative period. Systemically, ventricular pacing wires are placed during the operation and left until patient discharge or a maximum of 10 postoperative days. Frequently, atrial and ventricular epicardial pacing wires are placed at the end of surgery. Pacing wires may help in the diagnosis and treatment of postoperative arrhythmias. To detect such arrhythmias, electrocardiogram monitoring is mandatory at least during the first 5 postoperative days.

Atrial Arrhythmias

Atrial fibrillation and flutter are common after cardiac surgery. After open cardiac procedures, 40% of patients may present with atrial fibrillation.[15] Flutter generally is recognized to be more difficult to treat than fibrillation. These complications rarely result in major morbidity or death, however. Age older than 65 years, history of intermittent atrial fibrillation, atrial pacing, male sex, and white race are risk factors of postoperative atrial fibrillation.[15] Intraoperative variables may influence the occurrence of atrial arrhythmias, such as Guiraudon atrial incision in mitral surgery. A postoperative increase in creatinine is also an independent risk factor for occurrence of atrial fibrillation.[16] Treatment of atrial fibrillation in the postoperative period is required. Beta blockers (sotalol) and amiodarone reduce the risk of postoperative atrial fibrillation with no marked difference between them.[17] Acquired long Q-T syndrome induced by class 3 antiarrhythmic agents may lead to spontaneous torsades de pointes, however, a fatal arrhythmia.[18] Acute administration of amiodarone is mandatory if the arrhythmia induces hemodynamic instability.[19] A bolus of 5 mg/kg is given initially over 20 minutes, followed by 15 mg/kg during the first 24 hours. This treatment is generally considered as the most appropriate after cardiac surgery.

Ventricular Arrhythmia

Ventricular electrical instability may occur after cardiac surgery. This instability may place the patient at high risk for sudden death from ventricular fibrillation. Electrocardiogram monitoring is mandatory during the first 48 hours after major cardiac procedures. The management of ventricular electrical instability is problematic; drugs generally used to treat these arrhythmias are often considered to induce these arrhythmias.[20,21] Electrophysiologic studies are essential in the immediate and long-term management of patients presenting with ventricular tachycardia in the postoperative period if the left ventricular ejection fraction is less than 40%.

BLEEDING AND CARDIAC TAMPONADE

Hemostasis is deeply altered after cardiac surgery under CPB. Altered platelet numbers and qualitative changes occur.

The fibrinolytic cascade and coagulation are activated, and the formation of fibrin clots is inhibited. All of these factors, associated with cytokine activation and kallikrein stimulation of neutrophils, lead to a propensity for patients to bleed after the procedure.[22] Continuous blood loss must be monitored as long as the drains are in place. Platelets and fresh frozen plasma administration may be considered if coagulation parameters are altered. Supplementary protamine administration must be considered if required. If bleeding persists despite correct coagulation tests, however, prompt reoperation must be considered if the bleeding rate exceeds 300 mL/h for 3 consecutive hours or 1000 mL/h during the first 4 to 5 hours after the procedure in adult patients. Early reexploration for bleeding is mandatory in 0.5% to 5% of cardiac surgery patients, essentially depending on institutional criteria. Using these parameters, early reoperation generally stops the bleeding, even if no bleeding origin is found. Reduction of homologous blood transfusion, cardiac tamponade, and easier patient subsystem management is the key point of early reoperation. Patience during the final steps of the primary procedure generally reduces the need for revision to nearly 0%.

Cardiac tamponade may occur if excessive bleeding persists. To prevent such a complication, chest drainage tubes must be placed properly in the operating room, and early suction is mandatory to avoid blood accumulation in the pericardium and the pleural space. Massive bleeding during the hours after the procedure and clot obstruction of the drains may lead to cardiac tamponade. Meticulous monitoring of drainage is required. If cardiac tamponade occurs, prompt reoperation is required. Delayed cardiac tamponade also may occur within the days after cardiac surgery. Clinical signs and symptoms must be tracked before patient discharge, including unexplained weakness; orthopnea and dyspnea; aggravation during exertion; and peripheral edema with hepatomegaly, ascites, and venous turgescence. Pulsus paradoxus must be checked, and a prompt chest radiograph must be done. A widened cardiac silhouette generally appears before clinical signs and symptoms. A large pericardial effusion develops postoperatively in 30% of patients after cardiac surgery and is more common if early postoperative bleeding is excessive.[23] Maximal effusion appears at approximately 10 days. Cardiac echocardiography generally is performed before patient discharge to exclude important pericardial effusion requiring drainage. If required, drainage is performed via a reopening of the incision below the xyphoid process. The pericardial fluid is evacuated using a surgical sucker. A chest tube may be placed if required to avoid early recurrence of the tamponade.

MYOCARDIAL DYSFUNCTION AFTER CARDIAC SURGERY

Low cardiac output after cardiac surgery when atrial pressures are elevated above usual postoperative values may be attributed to myocardial dysfunction in the absence of any other likely causes. Ventricular wall motion evaluation and end-diastolic and end-systolic ventricular volumes assessed by echocardiography are key in the diagnosis of myocardial dysfunction. Patients with normal preoperative left ventricular contractility and patients with depressed contractility are more likely to develop this complication. Chronic preoperative impairments of ventricular preload, afterload, or contractility by any mechanism are risk factors for postoperative myocardial dysfunction. Perioperative myocardial damage must be considered in the absence of preoperative risk factors in patients with postoperative contractility dysfunction. Incomplete operations, accuracy of myocardial protection management, and duration of global myocardial ischemia are intraoperative risk factors of further myocardial dysfunction. Poor postoperative function that reduces coronary blood flow explains the particular vulnerability of the heart in the early postoperative period. This coronary malperfusion may worsen myocardial function further. It generally is considered that heart vulnerability after cardiac surgery persists during the first 24 to 48 postoperative hours.

In the presence of postoperative myocardial dysfunction, the possibility of cardiac tamponade or cardiac compression (i.e., by pericardial restriction) must be excluded. If cardiac tamponade is diagnosed, prompt reoperation must be undertaken to relieve cardiac compression from blood accumulation in the pericardium. If cardiac dilation is observed at echocardiography, such as is observed during pulmonary hypertensive crisis, external heart compression by the sternum or the pericardium should be considered. The sternum and the pericardium must be opened rapidly if they were closed. This complication can be prevented in patients with increased risk factors for postoperative myocardial dysfunction by leaving the sternum open for the first 24 to 40 hours after the procedure. If cardiac restriction is believed not to be present, treatment is directed at increasing the cardiac output by manipulating preload and afterload, heart rate, and myocardial contractility. Preload may be manipulated by infusion of appropriate fluids. If the left ventricular wall thickness is unusually great or its compliance is restricted, as usually observed in aortic stenosis, the left atrial pressure may be elevated to 20 mm Hg. Left ventricular afterload should be reduced if required by vasodilator administration (e.g., nitroglycerin or nitroprusside). Nitroprusside is generally considered the drug of choice because of its short half-life and its potent arterial and lesser venous dilator effect. Heart rate must be optimally adapted by atrial pacing, sequential atrioventricular pacing, or ventricular pacing if the patient is in atrial fibrillation. If all these simple measures are not sufficient to restore cardiac performance, a catecholamine infusion must be started, although the disadvantages are recognized, particularly in the presence of a hypertrophic myocardium.

When all of these measures fail, the use of devices to support the circulation is indicated. All devices have advantages and risks. They generally are used as a last resort when the patient would not survive with standard approaches. The first device generally considered, if non contraindicated, is the intra-aortic balloon pump.[24] Contraindications include aortic insufficiency, severe aortic arteriosclerosis, and severe cardiac arrhythmias. Important complications do not exceed 3%.[24] Others devices must be considered if the intra-aortic balloon pump fails, including ventricular assist devices[25-27] and extracorporeal membrane oxygenation.[28] These supports generally require anticoagulation to avoid embolic complications and may induce severe hemorrhagic complications.

MEDIASTINITIS AND STERNAL DEHISCENCE

Wound complications and infections are uncommon in cardiac surgery and generally concern sternal dehiscence and mediastinitis. Deep sternal wound infection occurs in 1% to 4% of patients after cardiac surgery and has an overall mortality around 25%. Risk factors of mediastinitis are imperfect aseptic technique, prolonged operative time, harvesting both internal mammary arteries, undrained retrosternal hematoma, insecure sternal closure, obesity, diabetes mellitus, chronic obstructive pulmonary disease, prolonged mechanical ventilation, long-term corticosteroid treatment, and male gender. Early diagnosis is one of the cornerstones in the management of mediastinitis. Sternal puncture may facilitate the diagnosis of mediastinitis.[29] The gold standard treatment in early diagnosed mediastinitis includes early radical débridement to remove all the infected tissue and closed drainage techniques.[30] Severe mediastinitis necessitates complete sternal resection and associated techniques using omental[31,32] or bilateral pectoralis major flap transposition[33] to achieve chest stabilization and to restore pulmonary function.

PULMONARY DYSFUNCTION AFTER CARDIAC SURGERY

After the heart, the lungs are the organs that commonly have dysfunction after cardiac surgery. Nearly all patients after cardiac surgery with extracorporeal circulation have an increased alveolar-arterial oxygen gradient, resulting from right-to-left shunting in 3% to 15%.[34-36] Reasons for post–cardiac surgery lung dysfunction include the following:

1. During CPB, there is no blood flow in the pulmonary arteries.
2. The lungs are subject to an intense inflammatory reaction after CPB.
3. The alveolar-capillary barrier becomes more permeable after CPB.[37]
4. Atelectasis tends to develop, partially explained by the absence of pulmonary ventilation during CPB. Left lower lobe atelectasis is the most common.
5. Direct trauma to the lung or phrenic nerve paralysis by the surgeon may lead to pulmonary dysfunction.

Risk factors for acute pulmonary dysfunction after cardiac surgery include young age (particularly <2 years old),[38] which is associated with an increased tendency to develop whole-body edema; older age (>60 years old)[39]; pulmonary arterial hypertension; chronic obstructive pulmonary disease[40]; Down's syndrome[41]; amiodarone therapy[42-44]; elevated postoperative left atrial pressure; prolonged mechanical ventilation; and phrenic nerve paralysis.[45] In the presence of risk factors, pulmonary dysfunction may lead to acute respiratory distress syndrome. Mild pulmonary dysfunction generally resolves slowly after the patient is extubated and treated with ambulation and breathing exercises, but residual dysfunction may persist 10 days after operation.[46]

PHRENIC NERVE INJURY AND PARALYSIS

Phrenic nerve paralysis may enhance the tendency toward postoperative pulmonary dysfunction (Fig. 106-1).[47] Consequences of postoperative phrenic nerve palsy range from asymptomatic radiographic abnormality to severe pulmonary dysfunction requiring prolonged mechanical ventilation to other associated morbidities and even mortality.[48]

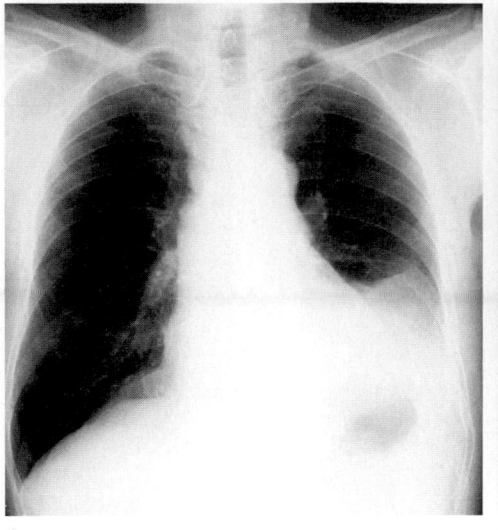

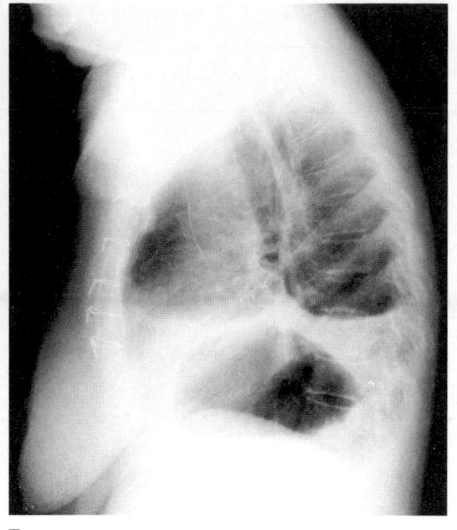

FIGURE 106–1. A, Posteroanterior chest x-ray of a left phrenic nerve injury after coronary bypass surgery. **B,** Lateral chest x-ray of a left phrenic nerve injury after coronary bypass surgery.

A

B

Several conditions in cardiac surgery may injure the phrenic nerve. The most common is a transient paralysis of the left phrenic nerve related to topical cooling application on the heart.[49] In the presence of topical cooling in contact with the pericardium containing the phrenic nerve, particularly on the pleural side of the pericardium, the phrenic nerve may be injured, and transient paralysis may result. The chest radiograph shows that when the patient was extubated, an elevation of the diaphragm related to this paralysis. At 1 week after surgery, radiologic evidence of diaphragm paralysis occurs in 30%[49] to 60%[50] if topical ice slush cooling is used. This paralysis may persist in 75% at 1 month and 30% at 1 year[49] after the procedure.

Transient or definitive phrenic nerve injury may be the result of internal mammary artery pedicle mobilization, ductus arteriosus closure, and aortic coarctation surgery. Reoperations in cardiac surgery enhance the risk of phrenic nerve injury, leading even to double phrenic nerve injury.[51]

NEUROLOGIC COMPLICATIONS

Neurologic complications after cardiac surgery under extracorporeal circulation may be attributed to hypoxia, metabolic abnormalities, emboli, or hemorrhage. Two types of complications, occurring in the same proportions, have been reported: A type 1 complication is major focal deficit, stupor, or coma, and a type 2 complication is intellectual dysfunction. After cardiac surgery with extracorporeal circulation, 6% of patients have been reported to develop an adverse cerebral outcome. Risk factors for developing neurologic impairment are advanced age and history of severe hypertension. Predictive factors for type 1 neurologic complications include severe proximal aortic atherosclerosis, history of prior neurologic disease, use of intra-aortic balloon pump, diabetes, hypertension, unstable angina, and increased age. Predictive factors for type 2 neurologic complications include history of excess alcohol consumption, arrhythmia (including atrial fibrillation), hypertension, prior CABG, peripheral vascular disease, and congestive heart failure.

RENAL DYSFUNCTION

Of patients who undergo cardiac surgery under extracorporeal circulation, 8% develop renal dysfunction in the postoperative period. Serum creatinine levels greater than 2 mg/dL are generally considered as the limit of appearance of renal dysfunction; 20% of these patients require dialysis. The overall mortality in patients who develop postoperative renal dysfunction is 20% and increases to 75% in patients who require dialysis. Predictive factors of renal dysfunction include advanced age, history of congestive heart failure, prior bypass surgery, type 1 diabetes, prior renal disease, and preoperative advanced renal dysfunction. The association between preoperative renal dysfunction and adverse events after cardiac surgery has been reported to be stronger if renal dysfunction is defined using creatinine clearance rather than the plasma creatinine level, particularly in patients with normal plasma creatinine levels.[52]

AORTIC DISSECTION AFTER CARDIAC SURGERY

Acute aortic dissection after cardiac surgery is a feared complication in which the blood leaves the normal aortic channel, the true lumen, and dissects the media to produce a false lumen (Fig. 106-2). An intimal tear generally is considered to be at the origin of this phenomenon.

Risk factors for spontaneous aortic dissection are systemic arterial hypertension, cystic medial necrosis of the aorta, Marfan syndrome, bicuspid aortic valve,[53] aortic coarctation (probably because it is associated with systemic arterial hypertension and aortic bicuspid valve), Turner's syndrome,[54] and Noonan's syndrome.[55] Cardiac surgery also may lead to aortic dissection. Aorta cannulation or partial clamping in the presence of excess aortic blood pressure may induce shear stress and subsequent intimal tears.

Diagnosis

Symptoms generally are induced by vessel occlusion. Cardiac ischemia and arrest may occur secondary to coronary arteries shearing off from their aortic origin after aortic dissection.

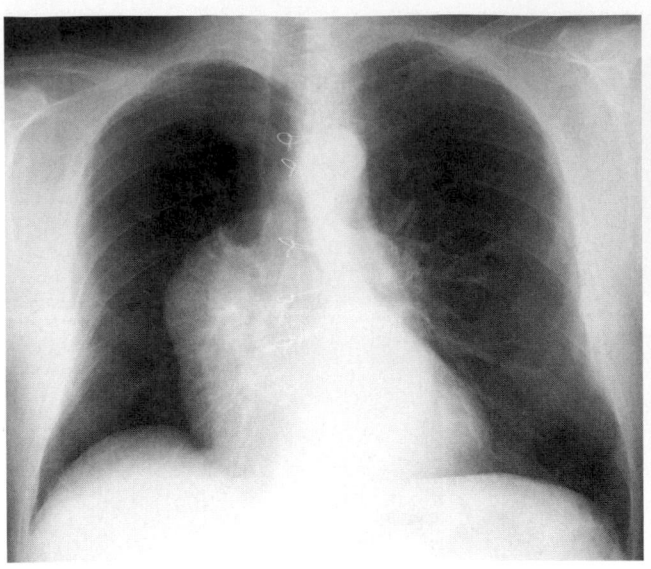
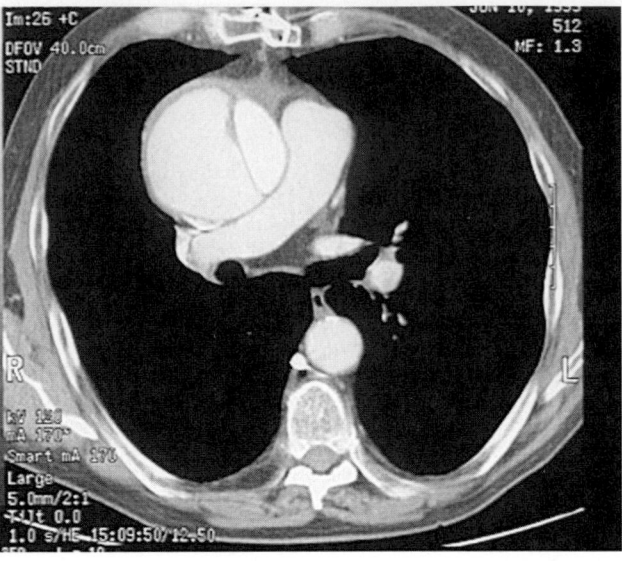

A   **B**

FIGURE 106–2. A, Chest x-ray of a patient with aortic dissection after aortic valve replacement. **B,** Computed tomography scan of a patient with aortic dissection after aortic valve replacement.

Massive hemorrhage after free rupture of the false lumen into the pericardium, the pleura, or the peritoneum also may occur. Aortic valvular incompetence may appear secondary to aortic valve involvement by the dissection. Oliguria or anuria also may appear. Neurologic complications, including stroke (secondary to aortic arch vessel occlusion) and paraplegia (secondary to intercostal arteries), may be observed. During or immediately after cardiac surgery, signs induced by aortic dissection and surgeon visualization of an important adventitial hematoma are important. The gold standard test to confirm aortic dissection is transesophageal echocardiography,[56] which is easily applicable in the operating room or in the ICU at the patient's bedside. The intimal flap is easily identified in the aortic lumen, and Doppler evaluation may help in identification and localization of the entry point of the dissection. This echocardiography may help to identify aortic valve regurgitation, left ventricular contractility, and eventually pericardial effusion. Computed tomography with contrast injection also has been used for the diagnosis of aortic dissection and evaluation of the extent of the dissection, including involvement of the abdominal aorta. Complications including stroke, renal hypoperfusion, and mesenteric ischemia also may be diagnosed using computed tomography.

Treatment

After diagnosis of an acute postoperative dissection, an aggressive surgical approach is mandatory. Surgery is performed to prevent death from hemorrhage and to reestablish blood flow in nonperfused organs. Limited ascending aortic replacement, associated with intimal tear resection, if any, is the standard procedure for a DeBakey type I and II dissection.[57]

LEFT VENTRICULAR RUPTURE AFTER MITRAL VALVE REPLACEMENT

Left ventricular rupture may occur immediately after discontinuing CPB in mitral valve replacement or within the first few hours in the ICU. Risk factors for this complication are the presence of a small left ventricle, female sex, and advanced age.[58] Excessive papillary muscle traction, decalcification of the mitral annulus, and ventricular mobilization (especially if the apex is tipped up) after valve replacement generally are involved in left ventricular rupture near the posterior atrioventricular groove. The midportion of the posterior wall also may be damaged by a pillar of a stented bioprosthesis. This complication, if it occurs in the ICU, is generally fatal. Some patients may be saved, however, if reoperation can be performed promptly. The patient must be placed rapidly on CPB and internal repair of the ruptured left ventricle done.[59]

ANNOTATED REFERENCES

Eagle KA, Guyton RA, Davidoff R, et al: ACC/AHA guidelines for coronary artery bypass graft surgery: Executive summary and recommendations: A report of the American College of Cardiology/American Heart Association Task Force on Practice Guidelines (Committee to revise the 1991 guidelines for coronary artery bypass graft surgery). Circulation 1999;100:1464-1480.

With the rapid evolution in diagnostic techniques and interventional cardiologic and surgical procedures, this publication presents significant guidelines in the diagnosis, evaluation, and treatment of coronary cardiac diseases. Written by more than 20 authors under the supervision of the American College of Cardiology and the American Heart Association, these guidelines represent an excellent summary of recent articles published in the English literature.

Funk M, Richards SB, Desjardins J, et al: Incidence, timing, symptoms, and risk factors for atrial fibrillation after cardiac surgery. Am J Crit Care 2003;12:424-433.

This article reports a prospective study concerning atrial incidence 2 weeks after patient discharge from the hospital. The authors emphasize that atrial fibrillation is frequent after cardiac surgery, with or without symptoms, and often occurs after discharge.

Gibbons RJ, Abrams J, Chatterjee K, et al: ACC/AHA 2002 guideline update for the management of patients with chronic stable angina—summary article: A report of the American College of Cardiology/American Heart Association Task Force on practice guidelines (Committee on the Management of Patients With Chronic Stable Angina). J Am Coll Cardiol 2003;41:159-168.

With the rapid evolution in diagnostic techniques and interventional cardiologic and surgical procedures, this publication presents significant guidelines in the diagnosis, evaluation, and treatment of coronary cardiac diseases. Written by more than 20 authors under the supervision of the American College of Cardiology and the American Heart Association, these guidelines represent an excellent summary of recent articles published in the English literature.

Wang F, Dupuis JY, Nathan H, Williams K: An analysis of the association between preoperative renal dysfunction and outcome in cardiac surgery: Estimated creatinine clearance or plasma creatinine level as measures of renal function. Chest 2003;124:1852-1862.

This was a prospective study comprising 6000 patients. The authors reported that routine preoperative estimation of creatinine clearance may improve the identification of high-risk patients, particularly patients with normal plasma creatinine levels preoperatively.

Chapter 107

PATHOPHYSIOLOGY AND CLASSIFICATION OF SHOCK STATES

Mark E. Astiz

KEY POINTS

1. The development of shock is related to alterations in one or more components of the circulatory system that regulate cardiovascular performance. These are intravascular volume, cardiac function, arteriolar resistance, the capillary circulation, the venules, the venous capacitance circuit, and mainstream patency.

2. Circulatory performance can be assessed from hemodynamic parameters, which include the underlying cardiac rhythm, arterial blood pressure, cardiac filling pressures, cardiac output, and systemic vascular resistance. Although shock is frequently defined by low pressure, the level of arterial pressure is not a reliable indicator of circulatory performance and tissue perfusion.

3. Circulatory shock can be divided into four subsets: hypovolemic, cardiogenic, distributive, and obstructive shock. This classification can be simplified into two broad categories with typical hemodynamic profiles. The first category is hypodynamic shock, which includes the hypovolemic, cardiogenic, and obstructive shock subsets. The second category, hyperdynamic shock, includes distributive shock. The common features of hypodynamic shock are a low cardiac output and vasoconstriction manifested by a high vascular resistance. Hyperdynamic circulatory shock is characterized by a high cardiac output and vasodilation manifested by a low vascular resistance.

4. Critical reductions in tissue perfusion elicit a complex set of reflexes that are directed at maintaining cardiac output and arterial pressure. Progression of the shock state is marked by declines in blood pressure that compromise coronary perfusion, cardiac performance, and microcirculatory integrity.

5. The primary metabolic defect in circulatory shock is impaired oxidative metabolism. This impairment is most commonly caused by decreases in tissue oxygen supply due to either global decreases in blood flow or maldistribution of blood flow. Cellular oxidative metabolism may also be impaired by mechanisms independent of tissue hypoperfusion. Accumulation of tissue carbon dioxide parallels the development of oxygen debt in circulatory shock.

6. Controversy exists over the optimal manner in which to monitor tissue perfusion in patients with circulatory shock. Commonly utilized parameters such as heart rate, arterial pressure, and cardiac output correlate poorly with survival in critically ill patients. These observations have led to the use of indices of tissue oxygen metabolism and carbon dioxide accumulation as markers of tissue perfusion and the adequacy of resuscitative efforts.

7. The primary causes of organ dysfunction in circulatory shock are ischemic injury related to tissue hypoperfusion, mediator-related organ dysfunction, and reperfusion injury. The relative importance of these mechanisms varies with the underlying cause of the shock state and the specific organ being examined.

8. The approach to patients with circulatory shock involves a rapid assessment of the underlying disease process and restoration of cardiopulmonary stability. The patient should be assessed by history and examination for clues as to the etiology of the patient's shock syndrome and for evidence of organ hypoperfusion. Efforts to achieve cardiopulmonary stability should occur simultaneously and should focus on ventilation, fluid infusion, and cardiac function. Definitive therapy depends on the etiology of the shock state.

9. There are several areas of active experimental interest. Therapies that modulate the activity of proinflammatory mediators and cellular apoptosis are being studied. The genetic underpinning of the immune response and its role in circulatory shock is another area of active interest.

PATHOPHYSIOLOGY OF SHOCK

Circulatory shock represents a final common pathway of cardiovascular failure. The mortality rate remains high, particularly for patients in cardiogenic and septic shock, among whom the overall mortality rates are 50% and 40%, respectively.[1,2] From a physiologic perspective, circulatory shock can be defined as a syndrome in which tissue perfusion is reduced such that blood flow is inadequate to meet cellular metabolic requirements. Clinical manifestations of shock are those of organ hypoperfusion: altered mental status; cool, clammy extremities; decreased blood pressure; decreased pulses; and oliguria.

MECHANISMS UNDERLYING IMPAIRED CARDIOVASCULAR PERFORMANCE

The development of shock is related to alterations in one or more components of the circulatory system that regulate cardiovascular performance. The first component is intravascular volume, which regulates mean circulatory pressures and venous return to the heart. Decreases in intravascular volume resulting from loss of plasma, water, or red blood cells limit venous return to the heart and cardiac output. The heart is the second component. Cardiac output is determined by heart rate, contractility, and loading conditions. Abnormalities in rhythm and heart rate may limit cardiac output. Impaired cardiac contractility decreases effective ventricular ejection and compromises stroke volume. Abnormalities in valvular function may also limit cardiac output. The third component is the resistance circuit and consists of the arteriolar bed, where the major decreases in vascular resistance occur. Arteriolar tone plays an important role in ventricular loading conditions, arterial pressure, and the distribution of systemic blood flow. Excessive decreases in arteriolar tone produce hypotension and limit effective organ perfusion, whereas excessive increases in arteriolar tone impede cardiac ejection by increasing ventricular afterload. Differences in arteriolar tone between organs can result in maldistribution of blood flow and mismatching of blood supply with tissue metabolic demands. The capillaries are the fourth component. They are the site of nutrient exchange and fluid flux between the intravascular and extravascular spaces. Increases in capillary permeability result in tissue edema and loss of intravascular volume. Decreases in capillary cross-sectional area, due to either obstruction or impairment in endothelial cell function, compromise tissue perfusion and nutrient blood flow. The opening of arteriovenous connections, which bypass the capillary network, may play a role in tissue hypoperfusion. The venules are the fifth component. They are the site of lowest shear stress in the circulatory system, and thus the site most prone to occlusion from alterations in cell rheology. Venular resistance contributes 10% to 15% of total vascular resistance. Increases in venular tone increase capillary hydrostatic pressures, thereby promoting the extravascular movement of fluid. The sixth component is the venous capacitance circuit. More than 80% of the total blood volume resides in the large capacitance vessels. Increases in venous tone decrease venous capacitance, redistributing blood volume centrally and thereby increasing venous return to the heart. Decreases in venous tone increase venous capacitance and decrease effective arterial blood volume and venous return. The seventh component is mainstream patency. Obstruction of the systemic or pulmonary circuit impedes ventricular ejection, while venous obstruction limits venous return to the ventricles.

HEMODYNAMIC ASSESSMENT

Circulatory performance can be assessed from hemodynamic parameters. A low heart rate may limit cardiac output, whereas increased heart rates can compromise stroke volumes

by limiting ventricular filling times. Bradyarrhythmias indicate structural abnormalities, the effects of drugs, hypoxia, or other metabolic stimuli. Severe bradyarrhythmias can also represent reflex-mediated responses, as occurs in cases of severe hemorrhagic shock, acute inferior wall myocardial infarction, and neurocardiogenic syncope. Tachyarrhythmias may be due to underlying cardiac disease or pharmacologic or environmental stimuli. Alternatively, increases in heart rate may reflect compensatory responses to maintain cardiac output and organ perfusion.

In patients with circulatory shock, blood pressure should be monitored using intravascular measurements. Vasoconstriction due to compensatory mechanisms to maintain arterial pressure or the use of pharmacologic agents limits the accuracy of noninvasive measurements. This is particularly true in hypodynamic forms of circulatory failure.[3]

For most vital organs, autoregulatory and neuronal mechanisms maintain blood flow independent of blood pressure at a mean arterial pressure of 60 mm Hg to 130 mm Hg.[4] At either higher or lower levels of pressure, blood flow becomes linearly dependent on blood pressure. Diseases such as hypertension can shift this relationship and increase the critical level of arterial pressure required for organ perfusion. Similarly, impaired autoregulatory mechanisms present in a variety of pathologic states expand the range of pressure-dependent blood flow.

The level of arterial pressure is not a reliable indicator of circulatory performance and tissue perfusion.[5,6] In states of hypodynamic circulatory shock, hypotension is a late marker of critical hypoperfusion. As cardiac output falls, blood pressure is initially maintained by increases in peripheral vascular resistance largely mediated by the sympathoadrenal system, and it is only after these mechanisms have been exhausted that hypotension develops. In this setting, tissue hypoperfusion may be present despite normal levels of blood pressure as blood flow is redirected toward more vital organs.[7,8] Conversely, hypotension may exist without evidence of organ hypoperfusion. In some vasodilated states, increases in cardiac output maintain vital organ blood flow despite decreased levels of arterial pressure.

Pulmonary artery wedge pressure and central venous pressure are indirect measures of ventricular preload. Filling pressures are determined by ventricular compliance, venous return, and systolic function. There is a poor correlation between filling pressures and blood volume measurements.[9] Factors such as ventricular interactions, positive airway pressure, and intrinsic cardiac disease may decrease ventricular compliance and lead to an overestimation of ventricular preload.[10] Measurements of ventricular volumes using echocardiographic techniques can provide more accurate assessment of ventricular loading conditions.

Cardiac contractility can be assessed by several techniques. End-systolic pressure-volume measurements are independent of loading conditions and are the most reliable measurement of cardiac contractility. Noninvasive methods, including radionuclide studies and echocardiographic measurements, can be used to assess ventricular ejection. The relationship between stroke volume and filling pressures can also be used to determine inotropic competence. In this regard, the response of stroke volume to changes in ventricular loading during fluid infusion is a measure of cardiac contractility. The adequacy of cardiac output in meeting tissue metabolic demands must be assessed independently

TABLE 107–1. CIRCULATORY SHOCK—HEMODYNAMIC PROFILES

	MAP	PAWP	CO	SVR	Svo$_2$	Lactate
Hypodynamic						
Hypovolemic hemorrhage, dehydration	↓	↓	↓	↑	↓	↑
Cardiogenic myocardial infarction	↓	↑	↓	↑	↓	↑
Obstructive pulmonary embolism, pericardial tamponade, tension pneumothorax	↓	↔↑	↓	↑	↓	↑
Hyperdynamic						
Distributive sepsis, adrenal insufficiency, anaphylaxis	↓	↔↓	↔↑	↓	↔↑	↑

CO, cardiac output; MAP, mean arterial pressure; PAWP, pulmonary arterial wedge pressure; Svo$_2$, venous oxygen saturation; SVR, systemic vascular resistance.

by monitoring indices of organ perfusion and systemic oxygen metabolism. A low cardiac output may be adequate in settings in which metabolic requirements are decreased, for example deep sedation or hypothermia. In contrast, an increased cardiac output may not be adequate when metabolic requirements are increased or maldistribution of blood flow exists, such as in septic shock.

Systemic vascular resistance is used as an indicator of arterial tone and is calculated from cardiac output and arterial pressure. Increases in systemic vascular resistance are most commonly due to vasoconstriction and represent compensatory mechanisms directed at maintaining blood pressure in the setting of a decreased cardiac output. Excessive increases in vascular resistance increase ventricular afterload and the impedance to ejection. Decreases in vascular resistance are due to vasodilation, decreases in blood viscosity, or the presence of arteriovenous connections. Vasodilation may be pathologic, as occurs in septic shock and liver disease, or it may be adaptive, as occurs in hyperdynamic stress following major surgery and traumatic injury. Venous tone is much harder to assess clinically. In most cases, changes in venous tone will parallel changes in arterial tone. Modest increases in central venous pressures in the setting of large-volume infusion and the absence of intravascular volume loss suggest decreased venous tone.

CLASSIFICATION OF SHOCK

Hinshaw and Cox proposed a classification of circulatory shock that was divided into four subsets: hypovolemic, cardiogenic, distributive, and obstructive shock.[11] This classification can be simplified into two broad categories with typical hemodynamic profiles (Table 107-1). The first category is hypodynamic shock, which includes the hypovolemic, cardiogenic, and obstructive shock subsets. The second category, hyperdynamic shock, includes distributive shock.

The common features of hypodynamic shock are a low cardiac index and a high-resistance vasoconstricted state. Increased oxygen extraction and lactic acidosis usually parallel the decrease in cardiac output. In cases of hypodynamic shock, the development of organ dysfunction is directly related to inadequate global blood flow. Common causes of hypovolemic shock are hemorrhage, dehydration due to gastrointestinal losses, and third spacing due to burns. Acute decreases in blood volume of 25% result in tachycardia and

orthostasis, whereas decreases of 40% are associated with hypotension. Decreased filling pressures are the hallmark of hypovolemic shock, in contrast to cardiogenic shock, in which situation they are elevated. Acute myocardial infarction involving 40% or more of the ventricular mass is the most common cause of cardiogenic shock.[12] Cardiomyopathies and severe valvular lesions are other important causes of cardiogenic shock. Finally, obstructive shock is related to a variety of causes, most commonly pericardial tamponade, acute pulmonary embolism, and tension pneumothorax. Since filling pressures are usually increased in these settings (due to outflow obstruction, impaired ventricular filling, and decreased ventricular compliance), distinguishing between obstructive shock and cardiogenic shock can be difficult.

Hyperdynamic circulatory shock is characterized by a high cardiac index and a low-resistance vasodilated state. Filling pressures can be increased or normal depending on the degree of volume repletion and the presence of myocardial incompetence. Common causes of hyperdynamic shock include sepsis, anaphylaxis, drug intoxications, spinal shock, and adrenal insufficiency. The underlying hemodynamic defect in each of these syndromes is maldistribution of blood flow and/or blood volume such that effective nutrient blood flow is compromised. In contrast to hypodynamic shock, oxygen extraction is normal or decreased despite evidence of hypoperfusion.[13] Direct mediator-related effects couple with tissue hypoperfusion to produce cellular injury and organ dysfunction in patients with septic shock.

Considerable overlap may exist between these different syndromes. Early in septic and anaphylactic shock, prior to fluid infusion, a significant hypovolemic component usually exists.[14] Hypovolemia may be present in a small group of patients presenting with shock due to acute myocardial infarction.[15] In the presence of severe sepsis-related myocardial depression, patients with septic shock can develop a hypodynamic profile. Similarly, patients in cardiogenic shock after cardiac surgery may demonstrate significant vasodilation due to the activation of mediator cascades while on cardiopulmonary bypass.[16]

PROGRESSION OF SHOCK

Critical reductions in tissue perfusion elicit a complex set of reflexes that are directed at maintaining cardiac output and

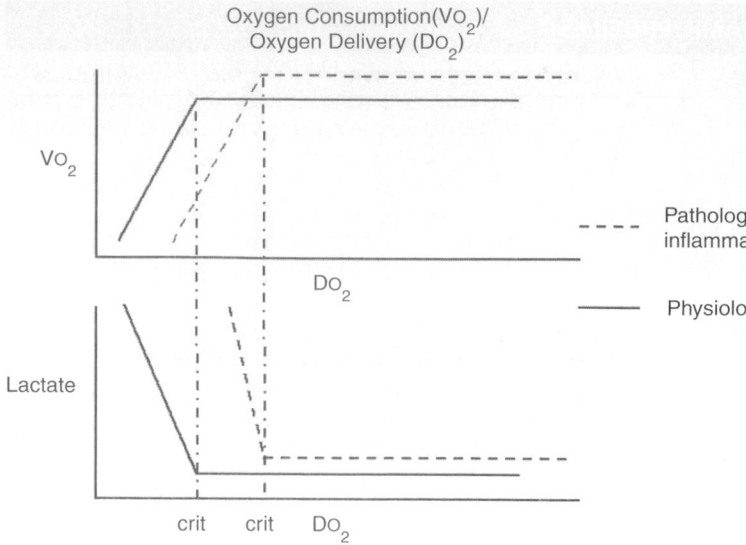

FIGURE 107–1. Oxygen consumption/oxygen delivery relationships. Oxygen consumption (Vo_2) is independent of oxygen delivery (Do_2) until a critical level of Do_2 is reached at which oxygen extraction has been maximized. At that level of oxygen delivery (Do_2crit), Vo_2 becomes linearly dependant on Do_2, and anaerobic metabolism manifested by lactic acidosis ensues. This relationship shifts upward and to the right when the ability of the tissues to extract oxygen is impaired due to alterations in the distribution of blood flow.

arterial pressure.[4] Activation of the sympathetic system increases heart rate and contractility. The release of catecholamines, angiotensin, vasopressin, and endothelins increases arteriolar and venous tone, thereby increasing arterial blood pressure and shifting blood volume from the capacitance vessels to the central circulation. In addition, blood flow is redirected from skeletal muscle, subcutaneous tissue, and the splanchnic circulation to the heart and brain. Vasopressin and activation of the renin-angiotensin system serve to enhance water and sodium retention, thereby protecting intravascular blood volume.

Progression of the shock state is marked by further declines in blood pressure that compromise coronary perfusion and cardiac performance. Increases in peripheral vascular resistance impede left ventricular ejection by increasing left ventricular afterload. Terminal phases of shock are marked by vasomotor dysfunction characterized by loss of arteriolar tone with paradoxical increased venular resistance. The resulting increase in capillary hydrostatic pressure leads to a loss of intravascular volume and worsening of the shock state. In animal models of hemorrhagic shock, a state of irreversible shock evolves from which the animals cannot be successfully resuscitated.[17]

This pathophysiology is altered in patients with hyperdynamic forms of circulatory failure such as septic shock. These patients are characterized by arterial and venous dilation, increased cardiac output, and misdistribution of blood flow. The influence of vasodilatory substances such as nitric oxide predominates over the effects of endogenous and exogenous vasopressor substances. In some forms of vasodilatory shock, inappropriately low levels of vasopressin and cortisol may contribute to vasodilation and refractoriness to catecholamines.[18,19] Progressive hypotension, which is refractory to fluid infusion and vasopressors, results in tissue hypoperfusion, acidosis, and organ failure. A hypodynamic circulation develops as a terminal event.

OXIDATIVE METABOLISM IN SHOCK

The primary metabolic defect in circulatory shock is impaired oxidative metabolism. This impairment is most commonly due to decreases in tissue oxygen supply caused by either global decreases in blood flow or maldistribution of blood flow. Systemic oxygen consumption may initially be

increased yet inadequate to meet tissue metabolic requirements; however, the terminal phases of all forms of shock are characterized by decreases in oxygen consumption. In experimental studies, the risk of mortality is directly related to the total amount of accumulated oxygen debt.[20]

Oxygen delivery is determined by cardiac output, hemoglobin concentration, and the arterial oxygen saturation. Under normal circumstances, oxygen consumption is independent of oxygen delivery and cardiac output (Fig. 107-1). Increases in cellular oxygen extraction, from a normal level of 25% to a maximum of level of 80%, maintain oxygen consumption as blood flow is reduced. When oxygen extraction is maximized, a critical level of oxygen delivery (Do_2crit) is reached, oxygen consumption falls, and anaerobic metabolism ensues. Alterations in vasomotor reflexes due to sepsis or drugs limit maximal oxygen extraction, resulting in critical tissue hypoxia and anaerobic metabolism at higher levels of oxygen delivery.[21,22]

Aerobic adenosine triphosphate (ATP) generation is dependent on glycolysis occurring in the cytoplasm and oxidative phosphorylation occurring in the mitochondria (Fig. 107-2). Under anaerobic conditions, ATP generation is limited to the two ATP generated in the cytoplasm, as compared to the 38 ATP generated aerobically. The decreased entry of pyruvate into the citric acid cycle results in the accumulation of lactic acid and the generation of additional hydrogen ions from the hydrolysis of ATP. Accordingly, the presence of lactic acidosis serves as an indicator of critical deficits in high-energy phosphate metabolism. The normal level of lactate is 0.4 mEq/L to 1.2 mEq/L levels greater than 2 mEq/L are associated with an increased rate of mortality.[23]

Oxidative metabolism may also be impaired by mechanisms independent of tissue hypoperfusion. A number of inflammatory mediators, including nitric oxide, endotoxin, oxygen radicals, calcium, and tumor necrosis factor impair mitochondrial function. Mitochondrial abnormalities have been observed in animal models of septic shock and in cases of reperfusion injury. Decreased mitochondrial activity has been reported in tissue taken from patients with septic shock.[24] Serum from patients with septic shock inhibits mitochondrial respiration and decreases cellular ATP concentration in vitro.[25] A potential pathway of direct mitochondrial impairment involves nitric oxide and its metabolite peroxynitrite.[25,26] Both of these substances can directly impair mitochondrial electron

Cellular Oxidative Metabolism

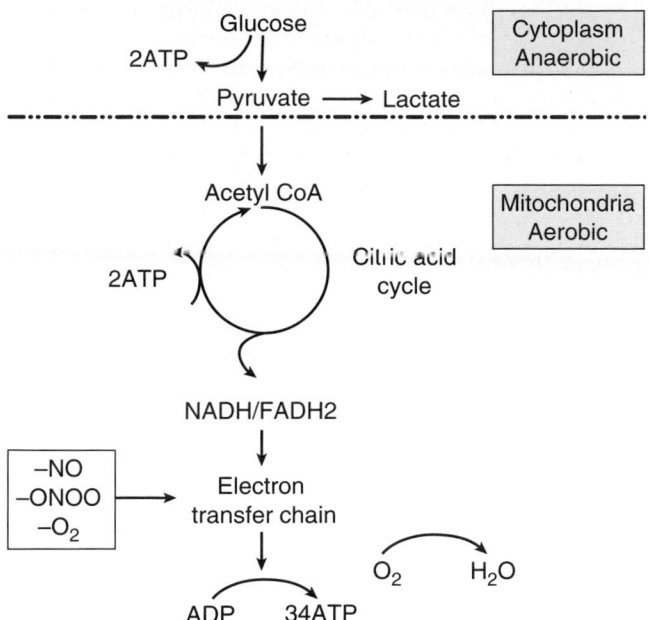

FIGURE 107–2. Cellular oxidative metabolism. Glucose is metabolized anaerobically in the cytoplasm and aerobically in the mitochondria under conditions of normal tissue perfusion. In conditions of shock, high-energy phosphate generation (ATP) is limited to anaerobic pathways. Nitric oxide (NO), peroxynitrite ($ONOO^-$), and superoxide (O_2^-) are potential inhibitors of the electron transfer chain.

chain complexes. In addition, peroxynitrite activates the mitochondrial enzyme polyadenosine-ribose-synthetase, leading to depletion of nicotine adenine dinucleotide and ATP.

Accumulation of tissue carbon dioxide parallels the development of oxygen debt in circulatory shock.[27] Clinically, increases in tissue carbon dioxide levels are manifested by venous hypercapnia and decreases in venous pH. The result is a widening of the arterial-venous carbon dioxide gradient proportional to the degree of circulatory failure. The normal gradient is less than 5 mm Hg, and it can increase to 40 mm Hg during cardiac arrest.[27] Decreased clearance of carbon dioxide generated by oxidative processes is responsible for the initial increase in tissue carbon dioxide levels. With the onset of anaerobic metabolism, tissue carbon dioxide excess is largely generated from titration of anaerobically derived acids by bicarbonate. The increase in tissue carbon dioxide levels may have physiologic significance and has been associated with impaired myocardial performance in vitro.[28]

MONITORING PERFUSION FAILURE

Controversy exists over the optimal manner in which to monitor tissue perfusion in patients with circulatory shock. Commonly utilized parameters, such as heart rate, arterial pressure, and cardiac output, correlate poorly with survival in critically ill patients.[5,6] This is particularly true in patients with septic shock and traumatic injury, in whom underlying deficits in tissue perfusion may exist despite initial resuscitative efforts.[5,29] These observations have led to the use of indices of tissue oxygen metabolism as markers of tissue perfusion and the adequacy of resuscitative efforts.

Mixed venous oxygen saturation (SvO_2), measured on blood taken from the pulmonary artery, is used as an index of tissue oxygenation. Venous blood is in equilibrium with the tissue and mixed venous blood, representing a weighted mean of all the venous effluents, and reflects overall tissue oxygenation. Mixed venous desaturation indicates the need for increased extraction to maintain oxygen consumption and the presence of tissue hypoxia. In cardiogenic shock, SvO_2 tracks cardiac function and systemic perfusion.[30] However, the same is not true in situations of septic shock and in other circumstances when the relationship between venous blood and tissue oxygenation is altered by maldistribution of blood flow.[13] In these circumstances, the ability of the tissues to extract oxygen is limited by decreases in effective nutrient flow such that SvO_2 may be increased or normal despite the presence of tissue hypoxia and anaerobic metabolism. Accordingly, although mixed venous desaturation is indicative of tissue hypoxia, normal levels do not preclude tissue hypoperfusion. Central venous oxygen saturation, measured on samples taken from the superior vena cava, may serve as an alternative measure of tissue perfusion.[31,32]

Arterial lactate concentration is a useful marker for the presence of anaerobic metabolism and therefore tissue energy deficits.[6,23] Although the initial level of arterial lactate has prognostic significance, the inability to clear lactate over time is more discriminating.[33,34] In patients with septic shock, factors other than hypoperfusion may contribute to lactate accumulation. These factors include increased hepatic flux of alanine from skeletal muscle, decreased pyruvate dehydrogenase activity, decreased hepatic clearance of lactate, and dysfunctional mitochondrial respiration. Despite these concerns, increases in lactate concentration are associated with decreases in the intracellular redox potential in patients with septic shock, suggesting that it is a useful marker of cellular energy metabolism in this setting.[35]

Oxygen consumption and oxygen delivery are global markers of systemic oxygen metabolism. Oxygen consumption, a measure of overall metabolic requirements, is calculated from cardiac index, hemoglobin, and arterial and venous oxygen saturation. It can also be measured directly from expired gases. Oxygen delivery is calculated from cardiac output, hemoglobin, and arterial saturation and is a measure of the total amount of oxygen being delivered to the tissues. Increased values of oxygen consumption and oxygen delivery have been observed in survivors and nonsurvivors, but considerable overlap exists between the two groups. Efforts to direct therapy at levels of these parameters associated with survival—"optimal goals"—have produced mixed results.[36,37] This, in part, reflects the varying metabolic requirements of individual patients.

The decrease in carbon dioxide (CO_2) clearance in circulatory shock is the basis for end-tidal carbon dioxide measurement and gastric tonometry. End-tidal CO_2 measurements are useful in monitoring perfusion during cardiopulmonary resuscitation.[38] Cardiac arrest results in marked decreases in pulmonary blood flow and accompanying decreases in carbon dioxide excretion. Consequently, end-tidal CO_2 values move toward zero during arrest and increase with successful resuscitation.

Gastric tonometry allows assessment of gastric mucosal perfusion. Because splanchnic blood flow is decreased early in patients in shock as blood flow is redirected to more vital organs, this measurement serves as an early marker of systemic hypoperfusion. Gastric tonometry measures intraluminal gastric carbon dioxide levels, which reflect mucosal carbon dioxide levels. In initial reports, intramucosal pH was calculated using arterial bicarbonate concentration.[39]

This calculation has been replaced with determination of the arterial-intramucosal P_{CO_2} gap. Widening of this gap or a decrease in the intramucosal pH is associated with an increased chance of mortality. Prospective randomized trials have not demonstrated that titration of therapy to tonometric values improves survival.[40] More recently, a technique for measuring sublingual CO_2 levels has been developed. Increases in sublingual P_{CO_2} and widening of the sublingual-arterial P_{CO_2} gradient are observed in nonsurvivors as compared with survivors.[41]

ORGAN FAILURE

The primary causes of organ dysfunction in circulatory shock are ischemic injury related to tissue hypoperfusion, mediator-related organ dysfunction, and reperfusion injury. Ischemic injury occurs when anaerobic metabolism ensues and high-energy phosphate production falls below the level required for cellular function and membrane integrity. It is the major factor contributing to organ failure in patients with cardiogenic and hypovolemic shock. The direct effect of inflammatory mediators, coupled with an ischemic injury, plays a major role in organ dysfunction in septic shock. Tumor necrosis factor, nitric oxide, and superoxide radicals are examples of mediators directly affecting cellular and organ function. Reperfusion injury occurs upon restoration of tissue perfusion following an absence of blood flow (Fig. 107-3). Activated neutrophils and oxygen radicals play important roles in this process.[42] Reperfusion injury may be important in hemorrhagic and traumatic shock; its role in cardiogenic shock and septic shock is less clear.

Cardiac dysfunction is frequently observed in patients in shock. In cases of acute myocardial infarction shock, cardiac dysfunction is related to ischemia and myocardial necrosis. Reperfusion injury may also play a role in patients who are acutely revascularized. Myocardial depressant substances cause myocardial depression in patients in septic shock and may also play a role in cases of hemorrhagic shock.[43] Down-regulation of beta-receptor density and affinity contribute to myocardial failure in sepsis and other syndromes.[44] Increases in pulmonary vascular resistance are the cause of acute right ventricular failure in patients with pulmonary embolism and may also be important in the situation of septic shock, particularly when it is complicated by the acute respiratory distress syndrome.

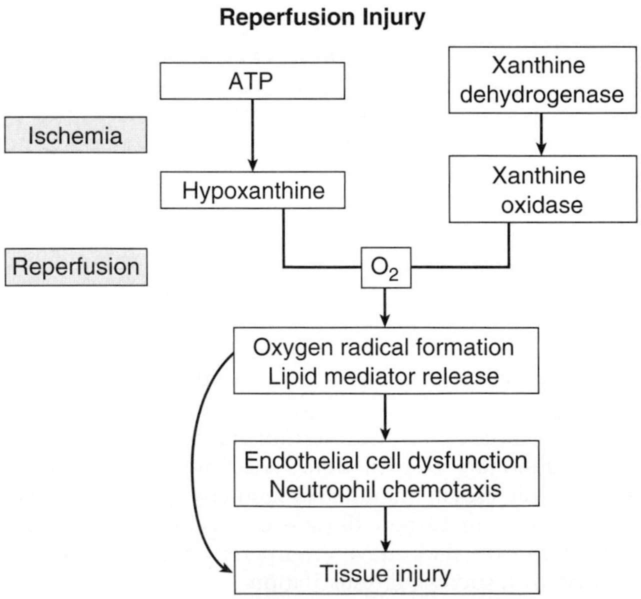

Minute ventilation and respiratory rate increase in patients with shock. Overt respiratory failure may result from pulmonary edema or acute lung injury and leads to additional increases in the work of breathing. Decreased respiratory muscle perfusion, coupled with hypoxia, contributes to respiratory muscle failure.[45] In patients with septic shock, inflammatory mediators may also directly impair respiratory muscle activity.

Renal dysfunction in shock is related to hypoperfusion. Initially, as cardiac output decreases, glomerular filtration is maintained by increases in efferent arteriolar tone. Release of atrial natriuretic peptide due to increased atrial pressures may help protect renal blood flow in patients with cardiogenic shock. However, as shock progresses, the increases in afferent arteriolar tone result in renal ischemia and acute tubular necrosis.[46] In septic shock, alterations in intrarenal blood flow may also impair effective glomerular filtration.

A characteristic pattern that involves centrilobar necrosis and marked transaminase elevation is observed in patients with ischemic hepatic injury associated with hypodynamic circulatory states.[47] Activation of Kupffer cells and the release of inflammatory mediators exacerbate ischemic injury in patients in septic shock and traumatic shock. In septic shock, canalicular cell function is impaired, resulting in intrahepatic cholestasis. Hepatic metabolic failure and impaired amino acid clearance are also a feature of septic shock.

Splanchnic mucosal blood flow is compromised early in shock. Intestinal injury may result from hypoperfusion or the release of oxygen radicals and activation of neutrophils during reperfusion.[48] Loss of the intestinal barrier can lead to translocation of bacteria and toxins, which in turn contributes to organ failure. Splanchnic hypoperfusion related either to shock or to the use of vasopressors also contributes to the development of stress ulceration, acalculous cholecystitis, intestinal necrosis, and pancreatitis. Pancreatic hypoperfusion may also predispose to the release of myocardial depressant factors.

Thrombocytopenia is observed in a majority of patients with septic shock. The coagulation cascade is activated in septic and traumatic shock by the cytokines, tissue factors, and bacterial toxins. Disseminated intravascular coagulation is marked by impaired fibrinolysis and increased consumption of clotting factors. Clinical manifestations are bleeding and vascular thrombosis. Large-volume asanguineous fluid resuscitation can also produce marked hemodilution of clotting factors and platelets.

Microvascular blood flow is impaired in all forms of circulatory failure.[49,50] Rheologic abnormalities of neutrophils and erythrocytes impede microvascular blood flow. Increased expression of the neutrophil integrins, platelet P-selectin, and the endothelial cell adhesion molecules result in cellular aggregation and microvascular obstruction.

Reperfusion Injury

FIGURE 107–3. Reperfusion injury. Under ischemic conditions, ATP is metabolized to hypoxanthine and xanthine dehydrogenase is converted to xanthine oxidase. During reperfusion, superoxide is produced from hypoxanthine and oxygen by xanthine oxidase. Superoxide and it metabolites produce cellular injury and membrane disruption, resulting in the release of prostanoids and leukotrienes. The lipid mediators and oxygen radicals act as chemoattractants for neutrophils, which injure tissues through the release of elastases, proteases, and additional oxygen radicals.

Platelet-fibrin interactions mediated through platelet expression of glycoprotein IIB/IIIA accentuate this process.[51] Decreased endothelial cell nitric oxide synthetase activity impairs normal vasodilatory reflexes and decreases the microvascular response to hypoxia. Increased microvascular permeability and tissue edema may also impede the diffusion of oxygen from the capillaries into the cells.

Disorientation and delirium are common in patients in shock. Hypotension, metabolic abnormalities, and hypoxia all contribute to neurologic dysfunction. Alterations in cerebral vascular reactivity and direct toxic effects of inflammatory mediators may also play a role in cerebral injury.[52] Severe hypotension, mean arterial pressure well below 60 mm Hg, can result in ischemic injury of the arterial border zones in the cortex and spinal cord.

The development of shock is associated with downregulation of immunologic function. Immunosuppressive substances, including interleukin-10, prostaglandin E_2, and adenosine, are released that decrease humoral immunity, monocyte, and neutrophil activity. An immunologic profile of decreased monocyte HLA-DR expression and impaired monocyte responsiveness to inflammatory stimuli has been associated with an increased risk of secondary infection and mortality.[53,54]

CLINICAL ASPECTS OF SHOCK

INITIAL APPROACH TO CIRCULATORY SHOCK

The approach to patients with circulatory shock involves a rapid assessment of the underlying disease process and restoration of cardiopulmonary stability. The patient should be assessed by history and physical examination for clues as to the cause of the patient's shock syndrome and for evidence of end-organ hypoperfusion. A complete blood cell count, coagulation studies, and blood gases and electrolytes measurement should be performed for all patients. Arterial lactate measurement is helpful to confirm the severity of the perfusion failure. An electrocardiogram and chest radiograph should also be obtained. The need for additional studies such as cultures, cardiac enzymes, and other tests depends on the suspected cause of the shock state. Efforts to achieve cardiopulmonary stability should occur simultaneously. The VIP approach can be used to prioritize these efforts by focusing on *v*entilation, *i*nfusion, and *p*ump activity.[55] The importance of early and vigorous resuscitation has recently been documented in patients in septic shock.[31]

Oxygenation and adequate ventilation must be ensured. High-flow oxygen systems can be employed initially; however, evidence of respiratory muscle fatigue, refractory hypoxia, or severe acidosis should prompt intubation and the initiation of mechanical ventilation. Reduction in the work of breathing may reduce physiologic stress and allow for redistribution of blood flow away from the respiratory muscles to other hypoperfused areas of the body.

Critical hypovolemia is present in the majority of patients presenting with circulatory shock in the medical-surgical setting and a significant portion of patients presenting with shock and acute myocardial infarction. Fluids should be infused in boluses and titrated to specific endpoints of heart rate, blood pressure, urine output, and clearance of arterial lactate. Attention should be given to the hemoglobin level, which will decrease with significant asanguineous fluid resuscitation. Although many patients tolerate a hemoglobin level

of 7 g/dL to 9 g/dL, increased levels may be required in patients with cardiac dysfunction. Placement of a pulmonary artery catheter should be considered in patients not responding to initial efforts and those with underlying cardiac or renal disease.

Disturbances of cardiac rhythm should be addressed rapidly. Bradycardia associated with hypotension may require a pacemaker or pharmacological therapy to increase the heart rate. Tachyarrhythmias that are not compensatory may require cardioversion. In the appropriate clinical setting, consideration should always be given to possible cardiac tamponade and tension pneumothorax, since these are potentially rapidly reversible causes of shock.

Continued evidence of hypoperfusion despite initial resuscitation efforts requires the initiation of vasoactive drugs. The choice of agents should be predicated on the goal of therapy. Persistent hypotension requires the use of a pressor agent such as norepinephrine to restore blood pressure to a mean arterial pressure of 65 to 70 mm Hg, which is associated with adequate organ perfusion. When hypotension is accompanied by impaired cardiac performance, an inotropic agent should be added.

The treatment of lactic acidosis with alkali solutions remains controversial. Sodium bicarbonate solutions increase serum osmolality and potentially worsen intracellular acidosis as bicarbonate is titrated to CO_2 and water. Prospective randomized trials have not demonstrated any benefit in either oxygen metabolism or circulatory function after alkali infusion for severe lactic acidosis.[56]

Definitive therapy depends on the cause of the shock state and may require additional diagnostic and therapeutic interventions. These efforts should be pursued in a timely manner. Endoscopic or surgical interventions may be required for patients in hemorrhagic and traumatic shock. Circulatory assist devices coupled with prompt efforts at revascularization enhance outcome in patients with cardiogenic shock.[1] Antibiotics and drainage procedures are required for septic shock. Activated protein C may also benefit patients with septic shock.[57] Acute pulmonary embolism and shock can be treated with thrombolysis, catheter embolectomy, or, in more extreme circumstances, surgical embolectomy.

NEWER THERAPIES

Newer fluids such as diaspirin-linked hemoglobin and ethyl pyruvate are being studied that, in addition to their volume-expanding capacity, may have anti-inflammatory activity.[58] Therapies that modulate the activity of proinflammatory mediators such as nitric oxide and polyadenosine-ribose synthase are being tested in situations of septic and hemorrhagic shock. Interventions that scavenge oxygen radicals, limit their production, and affect neutrophil activation are being studied to attenuate reperfusion injury in patients with hemorrhagic, septic, and cardiogenic shock. The role of apoptosis in the development of immune dysfunction and organ failure is being examined, with possible interventions directed at altering this process. Interferon-gamma and other agents that enhance immune function and reduce the incidence of secondary infections in patients surviving their initial shock episode are also being tested. Finally, the genetic underpinning of the immune response and its role in circulatory shock is another area of active interest.[59] This is particularly true in situations of septic shock in which tumor necrosis factor and interleukin-1 polymorphism have been associated with increased mortality. Progress in this important area will ultimately allow for the development of more focused interventions that have the greatest likelihood of benefiting individual patients.

ANNOTATED REFERENCES

Brealey D, Brand M, Hargreaves I, et al: Association between mitochondrial dysfunction and severity and outcome in septic shock. Lancet 2002; 360:219-223.

This study was one of the first studies to correlate evidence of mitochondrial dysfunction in patients with septic shock with nitric oxide-mediated pathways.

Hinshaw LB, Cox BG: The Fundamental Mechanisms of Shock. New York, Plenum Press, 1972.

The subsets of shock described in this text form the basis for all subsequent classifications of shock.

Rivers E, Nguyen B, Havstad S, et al: Early goal-directed therapy in the treatment of severe sepsis and septic shock. N Engl J Med 2001;345:1368-1377.

This study involves septic hypotensive patients. The study illustrates the importance of an integrated approach to resuscitating patients with shock, which includes hemodynamic and perfusion-related endpoints.

Weil MH, Afifi AA: Experimental and clinical studies in lactate and pyruvate as indicators of the severity of acute circulatory failure (shock). Circulation 1970;41:989-1000.

This is a classic study defining the importance of monitoring lactate in assessing perfusion failure in critically ill patients. A relationship between increased lactate levels and mortality was demonstrated. No added discrimination was observed when lactate levels were compared to lactate-pyruvate ratios.

Weil MH, Rackow EC, Trevino R, et al: Differences in acid-base state between venous and arterial blood during cardiopulmonary resuscitation. N Engl J Med 1986;315:153-156.

This study was one of the first to reexamine the significance of carbon dioxide accumulation in patients with circulatory failure. Marked increases in mixed venous PCO_2 in patients during cardiac arrest were reported.

Chapter 108

RESUSCITATION FROM CIRCULATORY SHOCK

Benoît Vallet • Eric Wiel • Gilles Lebuffe

KEY POINTS

1. Shock often, but not only, results from circulatory failure and decreased oxygen delivery (DO_2).

2. Shock occurs when a critical cellular partial pressure of oxygen (PO_2) is reached, a state at which inadequate tissue PO_2 produces cell dysoxia (cell oxygen consumption and ATP production are PO_2 limited) and injury.

3. Initial resuscitation from circulatory shock consists of (1) addressing the global adequacy of tissue oxygenation; (2) assessing the global flow; (3) diagnosing the shock type; and (4) deciding the best probabilistic treatment.

4. Treatment aims at (1) reducing preload dependency; (2) restoring cardiac contractility; (3) improving perfusion pressure; (4) reaching oxygen supply–to–oxygen needs independency; and (5) eliminating disease sources (e.g., anaphylaxis, infection, myocardial ischemia).

Circulatory failure results in a decrease in oxygen delivery (DO_2) associated with a decrease in cellular partial pressure of oxygen (PO_2). When a critical PO_2 value is reached, oxidative phosphorylation is limited and leads to a shift from aerobic to anaerobic metabolism. The result is a rise in cellular and blood lactate concentrations, associated with a decrease in adenosine triphosphate (ATP) synthesis. Adenosine diphosphate (ADP) and hydrogen ions accumulate and together with the raised serum lactate level lead to metabolic lactic acidosis. This state is called *dysoxia* and can be accepted as a definition for "shock," a state in which inadequate tissue oxygenation produces cellular injury. Shock often, but not only, results from circulatory failure and decreased DO_2.

Resuscitation from "circulatory shock" requires an emergency and global approach that is based on limited clinical features for establishing diagnosis and probabilistic therapy. The efficacy of this initial therapeutic strategy then becomes part of the diagnostic approach: if the chosen therapy is successful, it confirms the diagnosis retrospectively. This initial diagnostic approach is essentially based on physician knowledge of global hemodynamics and oxygen-derived parameters. It can be helped by rapidly available oxygen-derived biologic markers.

UNDERSTANDING THE UNDERLYING PATHOPHYSIOLOGY OF GLOBAL FLOW AND OXYGEN DELIVERY

ADDRESSING THE GLOBAL ADEQUACY OF TISSUE OXYGENATION

Adequacy of tissue oxygenation is defined as an adapted oxygen supply (or DO_2) to oxygen demand.[1] Oxygen demand varies according to tissue type and according to time. Although oxygen demand cannot be measured or calculated, oxygen uptake or consumption ($\dot{V}O_2$) and DO_2 both can be quantified; they are linked by a simple relationship:

$$\dot{V}O_2 = DO_2 \times ERO_2$$

where ERO_2 represents oxygen extraction ratio (ERO_2 in %; $\dot{V}O_2$ and DO_2 in mL O_2/kg/min). DO_2 represents the total flow of oxygen in the arterial blood and is given as the product of cardiac output ($\dot{Q}$) by arterial oxygen content (CaO_2): $DO_2 = \dot{Q} \times CaO_2$, with CaO_2 being the product of hemoglobin (Hb, g/100 mL) by arterial oxygen saturation (SaO_2, %) and Hb O_2 capacity (1.39 mL O_2/g Hb): $CaO_2 = Hb \times SaO_2 \times 1.39$.

Under physiologic control, oxygen demand equals $\dot{V}O_2$ (≈ 2.4 mL O_2/kg/min for a 12 mL O_2/kg/min DO_2, which corresponds to a 20% ERO_2). The rate of oxygen delivered by blood is physiologically larger than the rate of $\dot{V}O_2$: DO_2 is adapted to oxygen demand. When oxygen demand increases (e.g., during exercise), DO_2 has to adapt and increase.

During circulatory shock and/or severe hypoxemia, as DO_2 declines secondary to a decrease in $\dot{Q}$ and/or a decrease in CaO_2, $\dot{V}O_2$ can be maintained by a compensatory increase in ERO_2, $\dot{V}O_2$ and DO_2 remaining therefore independent. But as DO_2 falls further, a critical point (DO_2crit) is reached; ERO_2 can no longer compensate for this fall in DO_2 and, at this critical level, $\dot{V}O_2$ becomes DO_2-dependent (Fig. 108-1). At this DO_2crit (4 mL/kg/min), for a $\dot{V}O_2$ of about 2.4 mL/kg/min, ERO_2 reaches its critical point (ERO_2crit) of 60%. When $\dot{V}O_2$ is higher, DO_2crit is higher as well. Increase in oxygen extraction occurs via two fundamental adaptive mechanisms[2]: (1) redistribution of blood flow among organs via an increase in sympathetic adrenergic tone and central vascular contraction (this is responsible for a decreased perfusion in organs with low ERO_2, such as the skin and splanchnic area, and a maintained perfusion in organs with high ERO_2, such as heart and brain); and (2) capillary recruitment within organs responsible for peripheral vasodilation (opposite to central vasoconstriction).

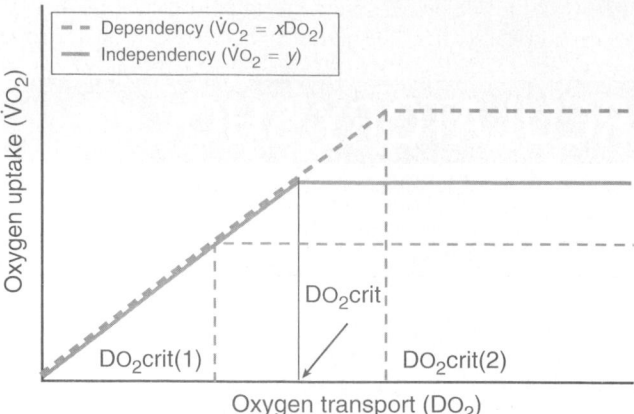

FIGURE 108–1. O_2 uptake ($\dot{V}O_2$)-to-O_2 supply (DO_2) relationship. When $\dot{V}O_2$ is supply independent ("independency") following the relation $\dot{V}O_2 = y$, whole body O_2 needs are met. When $\dot{V}O_2$ becomes DO_2 dependent ("dependency") according to the relation $\dot{V}O_2 = x \, Ta O_2$, $\dot{V}O_2$ starts to be linearly dependent on DO_2 at the critical DO_2 value (DO_2crit), which corresponds to dysoxia (insufficient ATP synthesis as related to needs) and shock state. DO_2crit is influenced by global organism O_2 needs: when $\dot{V}O_2$ is decreased (e.g., by rest, sedation, hypothermia), the DO_2crit is decreased as well [lower dotted line; DO_2crit(1)]; conversely, increased $\dot{V}O_2$ (e.g., by increased muscle activity, awakening, hyperthermia, sepsis) is associated with increased DO_2crit [upper dotted line; DO_2crit(2)].

USING MIXED VENOUS OXYGEN SATURATION AS A WAY TO ASSESS ADEQUACY OF GLOBAL TISSUE OXYGENATION

In the clinical setting, mixed venous oxygen saturation (SvO_2) can be used for assessing whole body $\dot{V}O_2$-to-DO_2 relationships. Indeed, according to the Fick equation, tissue $\dot{V}O_2$ is proportional to cardiac output: $\dot{V}O_2 = $ cardiac output $\times$ ($CaO_2 - CvO_2$), where CvO_2 is mixed venous blood oxygen content. To some extent, $\dot{V}O_2$ is approximately equal to cardiac output $\times$ ($SaO_2 - SvO_2$) $\times$ Hb $\times$ 1.39, and SvO_2 is approximately equal to $SaO_2 - \dot{V}O_2 /(\dot{Q} \times$ Hb $\times$ 1.39).

Four situations can be responsible for a decrease in SvO_2: hypoxemia (decrease in SaO_2), an increase in $\dot{V}O_2$, a fall in cardiac output, and a decrease in Hb. At DO_2crit, SvO_2 is

about 40% (SvO_2crit) with an ERO_2 of 60% and a SaO_2 of 100%. This SvO_2crit has been identified in humans.[3] It is important to emphasize that for the same decrease in CaO_2 (induced by a decrease of Hb or SaO_2), the decrease in SvO_2 will be more pronounced if cardiac output cannot adapt. Hence, SvO_2 represents adequacy of global flow to CaO_2 decrease. A 40% SvO_2 can be taken as an imbalance between arterial blood oxygen supply and tissue oxygen demand with evident risk of dysoxia. In the clinical setting, a decrease of SvO_2 of 5% from its normal value (77% to 65%) is representative of a significant fall in DO_2 and/or an increase in oxygen demand (Fig. 108-2). If initial probabilistic treatment (fluid resuscitation and/or low-dose inotropes and/or red blood cell transfusion) does not allow SvO_2 to be restored to a minimal 65%, Hb, SaO_2, and cardiac output should then be individually measured to introduce the appropriate treatment.

ASSESSING GLOBAL FLOW

Global flow is dependent on preload, myocardial contractility, afterload, and heart rate. Regional flow distribution is not homogeneous and is dependent on central and peripheral vascular tone, which ultimately results in the composite systemic vascular resistances (SVR). As an oversimplification, mean arterial pressure (MAP) can be estimated as the product of cardiac output by SVR. When flow decreases, MAP remains stable when SVR increases; this corresponds to increased sympathetic adrenergic tone and central vascular contraction in low ERO_2 organs, and preserved peripheral vasodilation in high ERO_2 organs. Overall, ERO_2 increases and SvO_2 decreases.

Minimal data exist to guide selection of the threshold for blood pressure maintenance. Arbitrary values of a systolic blood pressure of 90 mm Hg or a MAP of 60 to 65 mm Hg have traditionally been chosen. MAP is a better reflection of arterial pressure-head, but in the presence of an arterial line, systolic blood pressure is likely to be a more accurate pressure measurement and is typically used.[4]

Observation of an inappropriate tissue perfusion (e.g., raised blood lactate level, metabolic acidosis, SvO_2 <40%, decreased urinary flow) and its persistence despite probabilistic therapy (fluid, low-dose inotropes, red blood cells) should lead to optimizing flow according to the Frank-Starling curve. This can be assessed by invasive and noninvasive investigative procedure (see later).

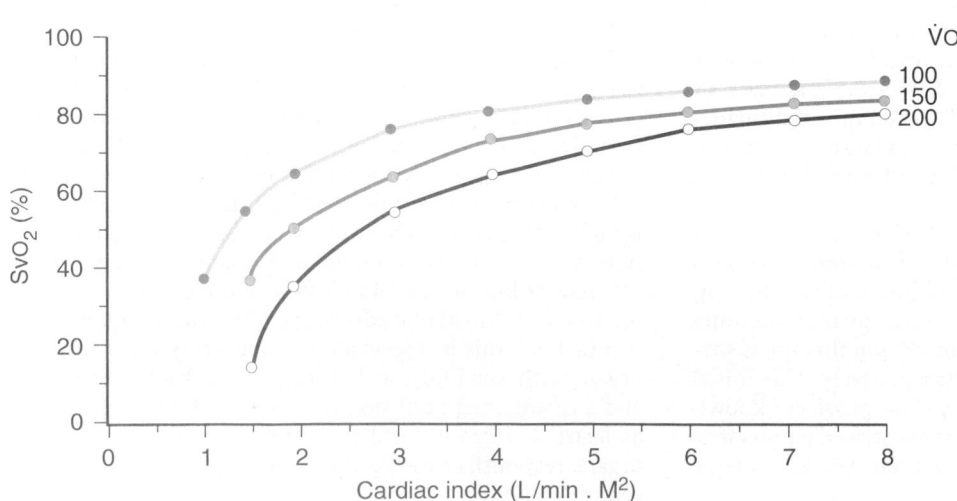

FIGURE 108–2. Venous O_2 saturation (SvO_2)-to-cardiac index (CI) relationship. According to the modified Fick equation, the relationship SvO_2/CI is curvilinear. Subsequently, when O_2 uptake ($\dot{V}O_2$) is constant, CI variations lead to large variations in SvO_2 when the initial CI value is low. In contrast, when initial CI values are already high, CI variations doe not influence SvO_2 very much. These relationships are modified when CI variations are associated with large modifications in $\dot{V}O_2$.

During circulatory shock, when ERO_2crit is reached, $\dot{V}O_2$-to-DO_2 dependency with a rise in blood lactate levels implies O_2 debt. Several authors have reported that oxygen debt is related to the likelihood of multiple organ failure and mortality in postoperative or polytrauma patients.[5,6] Patients who survive multiple organ failure have been shown to have higher cardiac index, lower SVR, higher $\dot{V}O_2$ and higher SvO_2 than nonsurvivors.[7,8] Rixen and Siegel[6] demonstrated that the degree of tissue oxygen debt is related to an enhanced inflammatory response, associated with an increased risk of acute respiratory distress syndrome, and higher mortality rates.

Recent research has emphasized the potential interest of central venous oxygen saturation ($ScvO_2$) for detecting global oxygenation impairment.[6] Experimental studies reported that changes in SvO_2 and $ScvO_2$ closely reflect circulatory disturbances during periods of hypoxia, hemorrhage, and subsequent resuscitation. Fluctuations in these two parameters correlated well, although absolute values differed.[9,10] Finally, observational data found $ScvO_2$ to be a useful parameter in detecting occult tissue hypoperfusion in both sepsis and cardiac failure.[11,12] An important feature with $ScvO_2$ monitoring is that $ScvO_2$ can be continuously provided by central venous catheters equipped with optic fibers (PreSep, Edwards Lifesciences). In initial resuscitation of circulatory shock, insertion of a central venous line is a standard, rapid, and easy approach, much easier than any other invasive or noninvasive hemodynamic monitoring, especially in patients who are not yet sedated, intubated, and ventilated.

In a recent study, patients admitted to the emergency department with severe sepsis and septic shock were randomized to standard therapy (n = 133) or to early goal-directed therapy (n = 130) targeted to achieve a central $ScvO_2$ of greater than 70%.[13] Standard therapy included antibiotics, fluid resuscitation, and vasoactive drugs to achieve a central venous pressure between 8 and 12 mm Hg, MAP greater than 65 mm Hg, and urine output greater than 0.5 mL/kg/h. The patients in the early goal-directed therapy group, in addition to the standard goals, had to reach an $ScvO_2$ of greater than 70% by optimizing fluid administration, hematocrit to greater than 30%, and/or prescription of inotrope (dobutamine to less than 20 µg/kg/min). Initial $ScvO_2$ in both groups was quite low (49 ± 12%), confirming that severe sepsis is hypodynamic before any fluid resuscitation has started. This study demonstrated a significant reduction in hospital mortality: 30.5% in the early goal-directed therapy group compared with 46.5% in the standard therapy group (P = .009). An important point in this study is that 99.2% of patients receiving early goal-directed therapy achieved their hemodynamic goals within the first 6 hours, compared with 86% of those receiving standard therapy. From the first to the 72nd hour, total fluid loading was not different between the two groups (approximately 13,400 mL); in contrast, from the first to the seventh hour, the amount of fluid received was significantly larger in the early goal-directed therapy patients (approximately 5000 mL vs 3500 mL). In the follow-up period between the seventh and the 72nd hour, in patients receiving early goal-directed therapy, mean $ScvO_2$ was higher (70.6 ± 10.7% vs. 65.3 ± 11.4%; P = .02), mean arterial pH was higher (7.40 ± 0.12 vs. 7.36 ± 0.12; P = .02), and lactate plasma levels were lower (3.0 ± 4.4 mmol/L vs. 3.9 ± 4.4 mmol/L; P = .02), as was base excess (2.0 ± 6.6 mmol/L vs. 5.1 ± 6.7 mmol/L; P = .02). The multiple organ failure score was significantly altered in patients receiving standard therapy when compared with early goal-directed therapy patients. This is the first study demonstrating that early identification of patients with sepsis, associated with early initiation of goal-directed therapy in order to achieve adequate tissue oxygenation by O_2 delivery ($ScvO_2$ monitoring) significantly improves mortality rates.[13]

DECIDING THE DIAGNOSTIC AND TREATMENT STRATEGY

Treatment strategy relies on shock definition (dysoxia) and starts with an early and rapid estimation of O_2 deficit, rapidly followed by an early probabilistic treatment (Fig. 108-3).

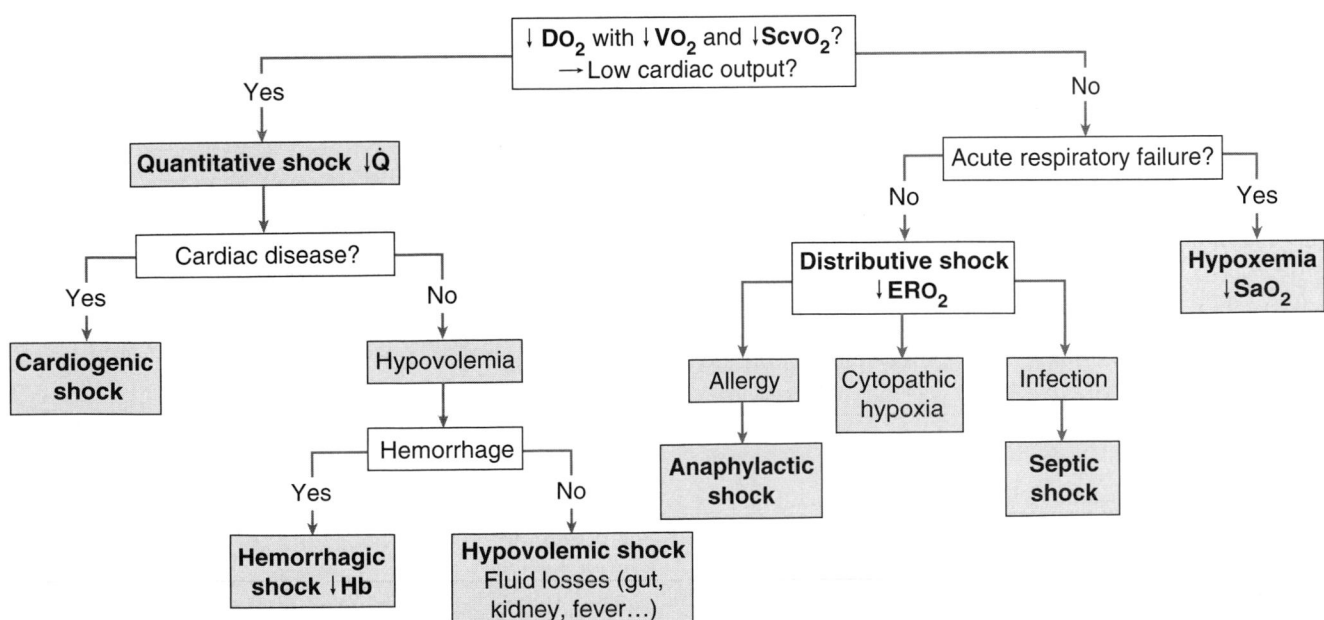

FIGURE 108–3. Initial interpretation of a shock state. DO_2, O_2 supply; $\dot{V}O_2$, O_2 uptake; Hb, hemoglobin; SaO_2, O_2 arterial saturation; $ScvO_2$, central venous O_2 saturation; $\dot{Q}$, cardiac output.

The response to this early probabilistic treatment (modification of lactate, arterial pH, $ScvO_2$ or SvO_2) then suggests which complementary investigation should be conducted (e.g., echocardiography, esophageal Doppler scan) and which type of monitoring should be installed (e.g., invasive systolic arterial blood pressure variations, Swan-Ganz catheter), which will help to refine the diagnosis and optimize treatment.

DIAGNOSING THE SHOCK TYPE

Quantitative Shock (Decreased Do_2)
Decreased Flow (Hypovolemic, Cardiogenic Shock)
Decrease in flow can be related to either a decrease in circulatory volume (absolute or relative hypovolemia) or to a failure of the cardiac pump.

Hypovolemia is "absolute" after severe hydration defects, plasma, or blood losses; it can be "relative" when fluid administration is insufficient to compensate a loss in vascular tone in the context of sepsis or anaphylaxis (or use of large doses of sedative drugs). In that context, there is an inadequacy between the content (volume) and the vascular capacity, and abnormal sympathetic tone is associated with an altered capillary recruitment. Relative hypovolemia is therefore often associated with altered redistribution of flow among and within organs. It is important to notice that shock can result from a mixture of quantitative and distributive features, and a mixture of absolute and relative hypovolemia.

Cardiac failure can result from either myogenic injury (infectious, viral, or ischemic disease), or "obstacle" to ventricular ejection (increased right ventricular afterload, increased vascular pulmonary resistance, increased left ventricular afterload, increased SVR), and/or a lack of ventricular filling (decreased right or left ventricular preload, valvulopathy, decrease in filling time by tachycardia).

Decreased Cao_2 (Hemorrhagic Shock, Acute Respiratory Failure, Poisoning)
A decrease in Hb is not necessarily associated with hypovolemia (hemodilution in which decreased Do_2 remains modest). When associated with an acute hemorrhage (hypovolemia), the decrease in Do_2 is higher inasmuch as the decrease in flow is larger.

Hemoglobin capacity to carry O_2 can also be limited. During carbon monoxide poisoning, a decrease in Do_2 results from a loading competition on Hb between carbon monoxide and O_2, and is "maximized" by abnormal O_2 utilization (carbon monoxide interacts with oxidative phosphorylation) and a decrease in ERo_2 capabilities. In this particular case, shock is both quantitative and distributive.

In an acute respiratory disorder (altered gas exchange or abnormal central or peripheral respiratory control), decreased Sao_2 leads to a decreased Cao_2 and Do_2 as soon as cardiac output can no longer compensate.

Distributive Shock (Decreased ERo_2)
This type of shock is linked to

- An altered flow redistribution among organs secondary to inflammation, anaphylaxis, or abusive use of sedation;
- A decrease in capillary recruitment secondary to altered vascular reactivity, increased intravascular coagulation, increased blood cell adhesion, and/or endothelial edema;

- An abnormal mitochondrial function (mitochondrial injury or dysfunction) such as described in "cytopathic hypoxia."[14]

Distributive shock often coexists with hypovolemic and/or cardiogenic shock.

DECIDING WHEN TO ADMIT THE PATIENT TO THE INTENSIVE CARE UNIT

Admission to the intensive care unit is requested when hemodynamic instability is present and requires use of inotropes (inoconstrictors or inodilators); this occurs when shock does not respond to initial therapy (fluid administration, low-dose inotropes, red blood cell infusion), requires ventilatory support (with a noninvasive interface or after intubation), or imposes hemofiltration (severe electrolyte disorder, fluid overflow, poisoning), and more generally when invasive procedures become necessary (invasive blood pressure monitoring). A patient becomes eligible for an intensive care unit bed at the time failure of one or more organs develops.

CHOOSING THE APPROPRIATE MONITORING

The discussion on monitoring type does not have any meaning until the cardiorespiratory emergency has been treated. The minimal monitoring device consists of an electrocardioscope, pulse oximeter, and rapid arterial pressure recordings (every 5 minutes and at the best continuous and invasive). A central venous catheter allows measurement of central venous pressure, which often cannot help much in deciding fluid administration (it is indicative at least when it remains lower than 5-8 mm Hg), but which facilitates infusion of drugs, crystalloids, or colloids. The central venous line also allows for monitoring and/or sampling of $ScvO_2$ (a surrogate for mixed SvO_2) if the catheter is not equipped with optic fibers. Central venous catheters are easier, should be cheaper, and carry less iatrogenic risk than Swan-Ganz catheters.

A Swan-Ganz catheter (at the best with continuous cardiac output and SvO_2 monitoring) and/or any noninvasive flow assessment (transesophageal echography, esophageal Doppler echography) is recommended when optimized cardiac output is doubtful according to the Frank-Starling curve. This requires that some preliminary cardiorespiratory stability has been obtained. In that context, fluid administration should be continued (the heart is preload-dependent) until cardiac output increases no further (becomes preload-independent); when cardiac output is not sufficient to maintain MAP or urine output, when SvO_2 remains low, or when lactate concentration remains elevated, an inotrope should be given. Cardiac echography must be done in the context of congestive heart failure and/or myocardial ischemia to diagnose ventricle or valve dysfunction. In the sedated, intubated, and ventilated patient, recordings of systolic pressure variation or pulse pressure variation can be helpful: the heart remains preload-dependent until systolic pressure variation is smaller than 10 mm Hg or pulse pressure variation is less than 10%, or both.[15] Arrhythmia limits this type of evaluation.

Iterative blood gas analysis (another approach justifying insertion of an arterial line), metabolic acidosis and lactate concentration evaluation, is a way to assess global tissue oxygenation and completes $ScvO_2$ or SvO_2 information.

THERAPEUTIC PRINCIPLES: SYMPTOMATIC AND ETIOLOGIC TREATMENTS

SYMPTOMATIC TREATMENT

Emergency therapeutic principles of care need to be decided at the time the initial diagnostic strategy is considered. It is necessary to give supplemental O_2 and ventilatory support in response to acute respiratory failure (acute lung injury, mechanical failure, respiratory distress) either through a face mask or by endotracheal intubation and ventilation. Acute circulatory failure is treated by initial fluid loading in the absence of left ventricular failure (see later). If decreased global contractility is present, inotropic support is considered with either dobutamine or dopamine. In case of anaphylactic shock, emergency treatment is to give intravenous epinephrine to treat allergy-induced vasodilation.

Fluid loading is the first step in treatment.[16] Its first goal is to optimize left ventricular preload to improve DO_2 by increasing cardiac output.[17] There is, however, an associated risk of interstitial edema, in particular pulmonary edema. Unless the patient has an acute lung injury, fluid loading aims at maximizing cardiac output[17] according to the Frank-Starling relationship, decreased lung gas exchange being detected by a decrease in SaO_2 (or by a decrease in its surrogate, pulse oximetry).

Swan-Ganz catheter derived pulmonary artery occlusion pressure has long been the most used static clinical variable for guiding fluid infusion. In septic shock, it was accepted that maximal cardiac output was obtained for values between 12 and 15 mm Hg.[17] To better estimate left ventricular preload, left ventricular end-diastolic surface has now been proposed. In fact, in the sedated, intubated, and ventilated patient, ventilatory-induced systolic pressure variation predicts increased systolic ejection volume to fluid loading much better than pulmonary artery occlusion pressure.[18]

Synthetic colloids are first-line agents. They may induce less pulmonary edema than crystalloids, especially in patients in septic shock. Crystalloids are recommended as first-line agents during anaphylactic shock. Normalization of hemoglobin concentration, [Hb], by red blood cell transfusion is not required. However, a [Hb] between 8 and 10 g/dL[117] might be preferred in patients with severe sepsis and/or coronary disease and/or decreased cardiac contractility. In those latter cases, decreased [Hb] is not compensated by increased cardiac output, and DO_2crit is reached more rapidly.

Catecholamines help in restoring perfusion pressure and maintaining cardiac output, thus allowing sufficient DO_2; this should allow regional flow distribution and improved ERO_2. All catecholamines are inotropes; they can be divided into (1) inodilators when they combine inotropic and vasodilatory properties (low-dose dopamine, any dose of dobutamine or dopexamine); or (2) inoconstrictors when they combine inotropic and vasoconstricting properties (high-dose dopamine, any dose of epinephrine or norepinephrine). Inodilators increase flow; inoconstrictors increase perfusion pressure. Because of variable individual sensitivity to catecholamines, dose titration is strongly recommended.[17] More potent vasopressors, such as vasopressin and derivatives, are now being tested.[19] It is important to emphasize that a rise in blood pressure may not be a surrogate of clinical benefit. Indeed, in a large placebo-controlled clinical trial, administration of the nonselective nitric oxide inhibitor N^G-methyl-L-arginine in septic shock produced both significant increases in blood pressure and significant increases in mortality.[20]

In septic shock, one study demonstrated that increasing MAP from 65 to 85 mm Hg was associated with no difference in organ perfusion variables.[21] Because increasing blood pressure through vasoconstriction may be associated with a decrease in flow, a trade-off may exist between raising blood pressure and decreasing cardiac index that will vary depending on the specific vasopressor or combined inotrope/vasopressor.[4]

OTHER THERAPEUTIC PRINCIPLES

The importance of correction of metabolic acidosis and the use of intravenous bicarbonate for shock-induced anion gap acidosis have been overemphasized in the past. Indeed, clinical studies, including one randomized, prospective trial, failed to show any hemodynamic benefit from bicarbonate therapy either to increase cardiac output or to decrease vasopressor requirements, regardless of the degree of acidemia. Cardiac function does not appear to be decreased for arterial pHs higher than 7.00. Bicarbonate infusion, apart from renal or digestive losses, is therefore not recommended, unless the patient requires hemodialysis or hemodiafiltration for hyperkalemia.[22]

In patients with septic shock, stress-dose (low-dose) steroid therapy (hydrocortisone 200 mg/day) needs to be considered, especially if the decrease in blood pressure requires high concentrations or an increasing concentration of vasopressors, once appropriate antibiotics are being given or the infectious site is controlled.[23] Intravenous hydrocortisone is administered after the serum cortisol level has been assessed (before and after corticotropin stimulation test). The duration of treatment is 5 days minimum when a positive clinical response is present. Beyond 72 hours, absence of any hemodynamic improvement suggests the hydrocortisone treatment is futile.

The place for high-volume hemofiltration in the treatment for septic shock remains to be defined. Although not oriented toward better circulatory efficacy, a number of treatments are essential in septic shock.[16] Control of the infectious source and eradication of it are essential. Empirical or probabilistic antibiotics need to be directed against gram-negative microorganisms but also against potentially resistant pathogens. This justifies double or triple antibiotherapy; it theoretically offers the following advantages: widening of the spectrum of activity, antibacterial synergy, increased bactericidal speed, and decreased risk for emergent resistant germs.

PROGNOSIS

The main prognostic factors for circulatory shock are the number of organ failures present on admission, the delay to start of treatment, and the response to symptomatic treatment; in cases of septic shock, control of the infectious source and its sensitivity to medical and surgical treatment is essential. The early timing of goal-directed therapy certainly influences the severity of multiple organ failure and the prognosis. This point has been clearly demonstrated by the recent trial from Rivers and colleagues.[13]

ANNOTATED REFERENCES

Dellinger RP, Carlet JM, Masur H, et al: Surviving Sepsis Campaign guidelines for management of severe sepsis and septic shock. Intens Care Med 2004; 30:536-555.

The objective of the Surviving Sepsis Campaign, an international effort to increase awareness and improve outcome in patients with severe sepsis, was to develop management guidelines for severe sepsis and septic shock that would be of practical use for the bedside clinician. The process included a modified Delphi method, a consensus conference, several subsequent smaller meetings of subgroups and key individuals, teleconferences, and electronic-based discussion among subgroups and among the entire committee. Evidence-based recommendations were made regarding many aspects of the acute management of sepsis and septic shock that will hopefully translate into improved outcomes for the critically ill patient. The impact of these guidelines will be formally tested and guidelines updated annually.

Dünser MW, Mayr AJ, Ulmer H, et al: Arginine vasopressin in advanced vasodilatory shock. A prospective, randomized, controlled study. Circulation 2003;107:2313-2319.

Arginine vasopressin was tested as a potent vasopressor agent to stabilize cardiocirculatory function even in patients with catecholamine-resistant vasodilatory shock. Forty-eight patients with catecholamine-resistant vasodilatory shock were prospectively randomized to receive a combined infusion of arginine vasopressin and norepinephrine or norepinephrine infusion alone. The combined infusion of arginine vasopressin and norepinephrine proved to be superior to infusion of norepinephrine alone in the treatment of cardiocirculatory failure in catecholamine-resistant vasodilatory shock.

Lopez A, Lorente JA, Steingrub J, et al: Multiple-center, randomized, placebo-controlled, double-blind study of the nitric oxide synthase inhibitor 546C88: Effect on survival in patients with septic shock. Crit Care Med 2004;32:21-30.

This multiple-center, randomized, double-blind, placebo-controlled study assessed the safety and efficacy of the nitric oxide synthase inhibitor N^G-methyl-L-arginine (546C88) in patients with septic shock. The trial was stopped early after review by the independent data safety monitoring board. Day-28 mortality rate was 59% (259/439) in the N^G-methyl-L-arginine group and 49% (174/358) in the placebo group (P < .001). The overall incidence of adverse events was similar in both groups, although a higher proportion of the events was considered possibly attributable to N^G-methyl-L-arginine. Most of the events accounting for the disparity between the groups were associated with the cardiovascular system (e.g., decreased cardiac output, pulmonary hypertension, systemic arterial hypertension, heart failure). There was a higher proportion of cardiovascular deaths and a lower incidence of deaths caused by multiple organ failure in the N^G-methyl-L-arginine group.

Michard F, Boussat S, Chemla D, et al: Relation between respiratory changes in arterial pulse pressure and fluid responsiveness in septic patients with acute circulatory failure. Am J Respir Crit Care Med 2000;162:134-138.

In mechanically ventilated patients with acute circulatory failure related to sepsis, the authors investigated whether the respiratory changes in arterial pulse pressure (ΔPP) could be related to the effects of volume expansion (VE) on cardiac index. It was concluded that in that particular population of patients, analysis of ΔPP is a simple method for predicting and assessing the hemodynamic effects of VE.

Rivers E, Nguyen B, Havstad S, et al: Early goal-directed therapy in the treatment of severe sepsis and septic shock. N Engl J Med 2001;345:1368-1377.

Goal-directed therapy involves adjustments of cardiac preload, afterload, and contractility to balance oxygen delivery with oxygen demand. The purpose of this study was to evaluate the efficacy of early goal-directed therapy before admission to the intensive care unit. Early goal-directed therapy provided significant benefits with respect to outcome in patients with severe sepsis and septic shock.

Ronco JJ, Fenwick JC, Tweeddale MG, et al: Identification of the critical oxygen delivery for anaerobic metabolism in critically ill septic and nonseptic humans. JAMA 1993;270:1724-1730.

The critical O_2 delivery for anaerobic metabolism was identified from the biphasic relationship between O_2 delivery and O_2 consumption in individual humans.

Chapter 109

INOTROPIC THERAPY IN THE CRITICALLY ILL

Jean-Louis Teboul • Xavier Monnet • Christian Richard

KEY POINTS

1. Inotropic therapy is often considered for patients with cardiogenic shock or for those with advanced heart failure whose condition is refractory to standard therapy. In these conditions, clinicians expect short-term positive effects of intravenous inotropic drugs, allowing cardiovascular stabilization.

2. Inotropic therapy can also be considered in high-risk surgical patients, even in the absence of a reduced myocardial contractility, to achieve supranormal levels of oxygen delivery during the perioperative period to prevent the onset of tissue hypoxia and organ dysfunction. Such a therapeutic attitude is not recommended for critically ill patients with established circulatory shock.

3. Most inotropic agents enhance myocardial contractility by increasing the Ca^{2+} concentration in the cytosol of cardiomyocytes after producing an increase in cytosolic cyclic adenosine monophosphate (cAMP) concentration. Synthetic and natural catecholamines enhance cAMP formation after fixing $beta_1$-adrenergic receptors at the cellular surface while phosphodiesterase inhibitors decrease cAMP degradation.

4. The $beta_1$-adrenergic agents, such as dobutamine, dopamine, and epinephrine, are the most potent inotropic agents.

5. Because of down-regulation of $beta_1$-adrenergic receptors, the myocardial effects of exogenous catecholamines are attenuated after a few days of administration.

6. Sepsis-induced decreased responsiveness of the myocardium to beta-adrenergic stimulation also results in attenuation of cardiac effects of exogenous catecholamine administration in patients suffering from septic shock.

7. The drugs given to increase cardiac contractility may also exert vasoactive effects that may interfere with vasoregulation of regional blood flow. The extent to which this interference is beneficial in increasing oxygen supply in hypoxic areas remains speculative. This emphasizes the need to monitor, as far as possible, perfusion and function of critical organs when such agents are given to patients in shock.

RATIONALE FOR USING INOTROPIC THERAPY IN CRITICALLY ILL PATIENTS

Two different objectives for using inotropes in critically ill patients have been considered: (1) the attempt to improve cardiac function in patients with low blood flow related to reduced myocardial contractility; and (2) the attempt to achieve supranormal values of cardiac output and oxygen delivery to prevent or reduce oxygen debt; in this situation, inotropes could be given after volume resuscitation, even in patients with normal myocardial contractility.

USE OF INOTROPES FOR REVERSING IMPAIRED MYOCARDIAL CONTRACTILITY

The first category of situations in which inotropic therapy is generally considered includes cardiogenic shock, acute heart failure, or acute exacerbation of chronic heart failure. However, although the use of such therapy in these clinical conditions seems logical on a classic pathophysiologic basis, no demonstration of a beneficial impact on morbidity and mortality can be found in the literature. Moreover, almost all the commercially available inotropes have been shown to be associated with an increased mortality rate when given on a long-term basis to patients with chronic heart failure. It has been postulated that the long-term use of inotropes may lead to deterioration of left ventricular function through acceleration of myocardial cell apoptosis.[1] Additionally, the beneficial effects on mortality of agents known to have negative inotropic effects, such as beta-blockers, is now well established in patients with chronic heart failure.[2,3] Therefore, inotropic therapy is generally reserved for patients with cardiogenic shock or for patients with advanced heart failure whose condition is refractory to standard therapy including diuretics, digoxin, beta-blockers, and angiotensin-converting enzyme inhibitors. Under these conditions, clinicians can expect short-term positive effects of intravenous inotropic therapy allowing cardiovascular stabilization. In patients with refractory heart failure who are candidates for cardiac transplantation, this therapy can be used as a bridge to transplantation. In those with potentially reversible causes of acute heart failure (such as myocardial infarction or acute myocarditis), short-term inotropic therapy must be considered as an appropriate bridge to coronary revascularization or recovery. The development of bedside echocardiography in the intensive care unit (ICU) should allow appropriate use of inotropic therapy, since this method provides a more accurate assessment of systolic cardiac function than traditional invasive methods such as pulmonary artery catheterization.

USE OF INOTROPES TO ACHIEVE SUPRANORMAL LEVELS OF OXYGEN DELIVERY

High-Risk Surgical Patients

The concept of attempting to achieve supranormal hemodynamic endpoints emerged from studies in high-risk surgical patients. In a preliminary study, Shoemaker and colleagues[4] examined the changes in hemodynamic patterns occurring during the perioperative period in survivors and nonsurvivors. Although during the first 12 postoperative hours there were minimal changes in the usual vital signs of both groups, the mean values of cardiac output, oxygen delivery, and oxygen consumption increased only in surviving patients.[4] The median postoperative values of cardiac index, oxygen delivery, and oxygen consumption observed in survivors were 4.5 L/min/m², 600 mL/min/m², and 170 mL/min/m², respectively.[4] The authors hypothesized that the higher hemodynamic values in survivors indicate a physiologic compensation for the increase in postoperative metabolic and oxygen requirements. In a prospective study in high-risk patients undergoing surgery, the same group showed that the use of these supranormal hemodynamic values as therapeutic endpoints was associated with a reduction in mortality from 33% to 4%.[5] In the protocol group, dobutamine and dopamine were given as inotropic drugs, even in the absence of evidence of reduced cardiac contractility, when volume resuscitation (and packed red blood cells, if necessary) failed to achieve supranormal values of oxygen delivery.[5] In another randomized study performed in high-risk patients undergoing surgery, the deliberate perioperative increase in oxygen delivery above supranormal values using dopexamine was associated with decreased rates of mortality and postoperative complications.[6] It is noteworthy that, in this study, oxygen consumption did not change significantly over the study period in any group, suggesting that the beneficial effects of dopexamine could have resulted from mechanisms other than prevention of global tissue hypoxia.[7] A reduction in the mortality rate was also reported in two other randomized studies performed in high-risk surgical patients.[8,9] In these studies, various inotropic agents, including dopexamine, epinephrine, and dobutamine, were given to achieve supranormal hemodynamic targets. However, in a multicenter randomized trial, dopexamine at doses that resulted in increased cardiac output after preoperative stabilization with fluids did not improve outcome after abdominal surgery as compared with fluids alone.[10] It is likely that in this study the patients had fewer risk factors than in the studies that demonstrated a beneficial effect of perioperative hemodynamic optimization. From all these findings, it is reasonable to consider the increase of cardiac output and oxygen delivery toward values higher than normal during the perioperative period in high-risk patients undergoing elective surgery.

CRITICALLY ILL PATIENTS

Whether this therapeutic approach could also be applied to patients admitted to the ICU for established acute illnesses has been a matter of debate. It was first postulated that critically ill patients could also benefit from aggressive hemodynamic treatment for at least two reasons: (1) the observation of higher median values of cardiac output and oxygen delivery in survivors in comparison with nonsurvivors in studies performed in patients with acute respiratory distress syndrome and sepsis[11-14]; and (2) the presence, in critically ill patients with sepsis,[15-17] acute respiratory distress syndrome,[18,19] and acute liver disease,[20,21] of an oxygen consumption/supply dependency occurring for supranormal values of oxygen delivery. Such a phenomenon was reported to correlate with the presence of increased blood lactate, a marker of global tissue hypoxia[15-17] and to be associated with a poor outcome.[22] This so-called pathologic oxygen consumption/supply dependency—ascribed to impaired oxygen extraction capacities associated with acute illnesses—would incite the clinician to increase oxygen delivery toward supranormal values to exceed its critical level. However, such an aggressive therapeutic approach has been seriously questioned for at least two major reasons. First, some authors using two independent methods to obtain oxygen consumption and oxygen delivery measurements no longer found any pathologic oxygen consumption/supply dependency in critically ill patients.[23-26] It has been suggested that a mathematical coupling of the shared variables (cardiac output and arterial oxygen content) could have explained the finding of oxygen consumption/supply dependency in the previous studies in which oxygen consumption and oxygen delivery were calculated using the same reverse Fick method.[27] Second, numerous randomized clinical trials performed in patients with acute illnesses did not demonstrate any benefit from deliberate manipulation of hemodynamic variables toward values higher than physiologic values.[14,26-31] In one of these studies, the mortality rate was even higher in the group of patients assigned to receive an aggressive treatment aimed at achieving supranormal values of oxygen delivery.[29] It was postulated that deleterious consequences of the use of high doses of dobutamine in patients of the protocol group were responsible for the increased mortality. It has to be noted that (1) the patients of the protocol group received high doses of the inotropic agent despite no evidence of any deficit of inotropic function, and (2) in most of these patients, the aggressive inotropic support failed to achieve the target value of oxygen consumption (170 mL/min/m²). The later analysis of the subgroup of septic patients of this study showed that the survivors were characterized by ability to increase both oxygen delivery and oxygen consumption regardless of their group of randomization.[13] The nonsurviving patients were characterized by inability to increase oxygen consumption despite the increase in oxygen delivery, suggesting a more marked impairment of peripheral oxygen extraction in nonsurvivors than in survivors.[13] In addition, the ability to increase cardiac output and oxygen delivery was also significantly reduced in nonsurvivors in comparison with survivors, suggesting a decrease in cardiac reserve in those patients who will die.[13] This is not a surprising finding, since the degree of myocardial dysfunction in septic shock correlates with increased risk of death. In this regard, it has been suggested that the response to a dobutamine challenge could have a prognostic value in septic patients, since, in two prospective studies, survivors were able to increase both oxygen consumption and oxygen delivery in response to dobutamine, whereas nonsurvivors were not able to increase either oxygen delivery or oxygen consumption.[32,33]

From all the results of randomized controlled studies, the deliberative attempt to achieve supranormal hemodynamic targets in the general population of critically ill patients is no longer recommended.[34-36] However, in the early phase of septic shock when blood flow and oxygen delivery are generally low, an aggressive hemodynamic therapy, including inotropes, aimed at rapidly normalizing oxygen delivery, was demonstrated to result in a better outcome in a randomized controlled trial.[37] Thus, in the early phase of septic shock and maybe in other acute illnesses, it is essential to rapidly restore normal global blood flow conditions to avoid further deleterious consequences of systemic hypoperfusion. In later stages of the disease, with inflammatory processes and organ dysfunction already developed, no evidence of benefit from a further increase in oxygen delivery has been shown in the literature. However, it seems to be likely that cardiac output should be kept in the normal range by using volume and/or inotropes to prevent worsening of the insult.

PHARMACOLOGIC PROPERTIES OF INOTROPIC AGENTS

Different inotropic drugs are available. Most of them act on adrenergic receptors located at the surface of the cardiomyocytes.

ADRENERGIC SIGNAL TRANSDUCTION IN CARDIOMYOCYTES

Natural as well as synthetic catecholamines enhance the Ca^{2+} cytosolic amount, which is directly related to the force of contraction (Fig. 109-1). Ca^{2+} fixes on the troponin C Ca^{2+}-specific binding site, inducing a conformational change that leads to the fixation of the myosin head to the actin filament.

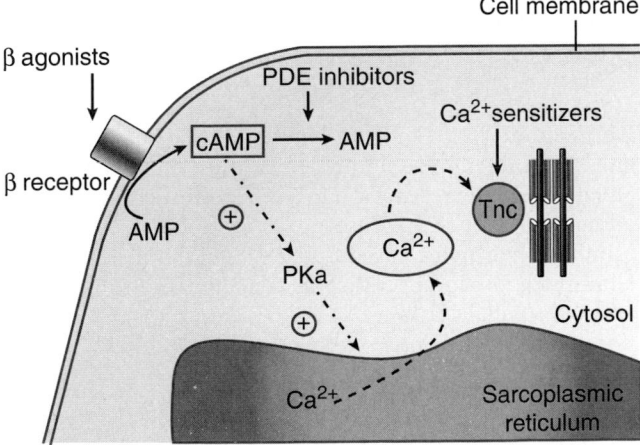

FIGURE 109–1. Mechanisms of action of inotropic agents at the cellular level. Schematic representation. Beta-agonist agents fix the beta receptor and stimulate the formation of cyclic adenosine monophosphate (cAMP) from AMP through adenylate cyclase. cAMP activates protein kinase A, which provokes the extrusion of Ca^{2+} from the sarcoplasmic reticulum into the cytosol through phosphorylated ryanodine receptors. Ca^{2+} fixes troponin C and finally activates the fixation of actin on myosin filaments. Phosphodiesterase (PDE) inhibitors also increase the cAMP concentration by inhibiting its degradation. The mechanism by which Ca^{2+} sensitizers increase inotropism is the enhancement of troponin C sensitivity for Ca^{2+}.

Hydrolysis of the adenosine triphosphate (ATP) molecule located on the myosin head to adenosine diphosphate (ADP) simultaneously induces the flexion of the myosin neck and the shortening of the contractile apparatus.

A rapid overview of the physiologic response to adrenergic receptor stimulation is essential to understand the pharmacologic properties of these drugs. Receptors of the adrenergic system are classed as α_1, α_2, β_1, β_2, and dopaminergic receptors.[38]

Beta₁-Adrenergic Receptors

Beta-adrenergic receptors are transmembrane proteins located in the sarcolemma. The beta₁-receptor subtype is mainly represented in the human heart. Its stimulation induces inotropic, lusitropic, chronotropic, and dromotropic effects, and all these effects result from the enhancement in Ca^{2+} cytosolic concentration. Binding of a beta₁-agonist agent to its receptor stimulates the G_s protein. The guanosine diphosphate, normally fixed to the stimulatory α_s subunit of G_s protein, is replaced by guanosine triphosphate and the α_s-guanosine triphosphate complex binds to adenyl cyclase, which then becomes activated. Cyclic adenosine monophosphate (cAMP) is formed from ATP and activates protein kinase A. Protein kinase A phosphorylates and activates several cellular structures, as follows:

- The ryanodine receptors of the sarcoplasmic reticulum, leading to enhanced extrusion of Ca^{2+} out of the sarcoplasmic reticulum. Indeed, the main part of the Ca^{2+} cytosolic content needed for contraction is provided by the sarcoplasmic Ca^{2+} store. The entry of Ca^{2+} through the membrane L-type channels modifies the molecular conformation of the ryanodine receptor of the sarcoplasmic reticulum. Parts of these ryanodine receptors are Ca^{2+} channels that enable massive release of Ca^{2+} out of the sarcoplasmic reticulum (see Fig. 109-1).
- The sarcolemmal L-type Ca^{2+} channels, increasing their opening time. This leads to an increased amount of cytosolic Ca^{2+} available for sarcoplasmic reticulum Ca^{2+} release and for contraction.

The increase in intracytosolic Ca^{2+} concentration also leads to the activation of calmodulin. This ubiquitous protein enables the phosphorylation of other proteins once it has fixed Ca^{2+}, as follows:

- The myosin light chain through the myosin light chain ATPase. This phosphorylation enhances the responsiveness of the cardiac contractile protein to Ca^{2+} and helps to increase the affinity of myosin for actin, thus participating in the inotropic effect.
- The phospholamban and the sarcolemmal Na^+/Ca^{2+} exchanger, leading to a faster decrease of Ca^{2+} cytosolic concentration after contraction and accounting for the lusitropic effect. Indeed, relaxation is dependent on Ca^{2+} reuptake by the sarcoplasmic reticulum through the sarcoendoplasmic reticulum calcium ATPase pump. The activity of the sarcoendoplasmic reticulum calcium ATPase pump is normally inhibited by the phospholamban located in the sarcoplasmic reticulum membrane near the Ca^{2+} pump. Phosphorylation of phospholamban relieves this inhibition and Ca^{2+} uptake by the sarcoplasmic reticulum is thus stimulated.

Beta$_2$-Adrenergic Receptors

The beta$_2$ receptor subtype is mainly represented in noncardiac structures. Beta$_2$-adrenergic stimulation induces arterial and venous relaxation. The effects of beta$_2$ stimulation in vascular smooth muscle result from a different activation pathway: once Ca^{2+} intracytosolic amount increases, it fixes the calmodulin regulatory protein, and the Ca^{2+}-calmodulin complex activates the myosin light chain kinase, leading to inhibiting phosphorylation of the myosin light chain, and finally smooth muscle relaxation.

Alpha-Adrenergic Receptors

When an agonist fixes the alpha$_1$ receptor, G$_h$, part of the G-protein family, stimulates phospholipase C, which splits phosphatidyl inositol into inositol triphosphate and 1,2-diacylglycerol. Inositol triphosphate stimulates the release of Ca^{2+} from the sarcoplasmic reticulum. Alpha$_2$-adrenoreceptor stimulation inhibits adenylate cyclase and reduces the cAMP intracellular content. Alpha-adrenoreceptors are not prominent in the cardiac tissue but are in the vascular wall. The cardiac alpha$_1$-stimulation induces a positive inotropic effect; alpha$_1$ and alpha$_2$ stimulation induces a potent arterial and venous constriction.

PHARMACOLOGIC PROPERTIES OF THE INOTROPIC AGENTS USED IN CLINICAL PRACTICE

Norepinephrine

Norepinephrine is the physiologic mediator released by the post-ganglionic adrenergic nerves.[38] It is a potent alpha$_1$ and beta$_1$-adrenergic agonist but has little activity on beta$_2$-receptors. Through its alpha-adrenergic effects, norepinephrine induces potent arterial and venous constriction. It increases systolic as well as diastolic blood pressure, left ventricular afterload, venous return, and cardiac filling pressures. The beta$_1$-stimulation results in a positive inotropic effect and an increase in stroke volume. However, the chronotropic effect is counteracted by baroreflex stimulation following vasoconstriction. Consequently, the heart rate is unchanged or reduced, and the cardiac output is generally unchanged. The coronary blood flow is enhanced by norepinephrine, because of coronary vasodilation secondary to enhanced cardiac metabolism and because of normalization of diastolic blood pressure when low.

Epinephrine

Epinephrine is the main physiologic adrenergic hormone of the adrenal medullary gland.[38] It is a potent stimulator of alpha, beta$_1$, and beta$_2$ receptors. The alpha-adrenergic effect is responsible for a marked arterial and venous vasoconstriction. Epinephrine increases systolic arterial pressure, but its effect on vasculature is partly counteracted by the beta$_2$-mediated vasodilation. The diastolic blood pressure is thus only slightly affected by epinephrine, and the increase in mean arterial pressure (MAP) is less than with norepinephrine. Through cardiac beta$_1$ stimulation, epinephrine increases heart rate and inotropism. The combination of the latter effects and the alpha-mediated venous constriction promoting venous return and cardiac preload results in an increase in cardiac output. Epinephrine also facilitates ventricular relaxation and enhances coronary blood flow through the increase in myocardial oxygen consumption.

Dopamine

Dopamine is the immediate physiologic precursor of norepinephrine and epinephrine. The cardiovascular effects of dopamine are mediated by several types of receptors that are activated at different levels of dopamine concentration and by norepinephrine produced by the transformation of dopamine.

At low rates of administration (<5 µg/kg/min), dopamine activates D1 receptors located in renal, mesenteric, cerebral, and coronary vessels and induces vasodilation without affecting arterial blood pressure. At higher and intermediate rates of administration (5-10 µg/kg/min), dopamine predominantly stimulates beta$_1$-adrenergic receptors and thus enhances inotropism and increases heart rate. At such rates of infusion, dopamine increases systolic blood pressure without altering diastolic blood pressure, because stroke volume is enhanced and arterial vascular tone only slightly altered.[38] Norepinephrine resulting from dopamine transformation contributes to these cardiovascular effects. At higher rates of administration (10-20 µg/kg/min), dopamine predominantly activates vascular alpha$_1$-adrenergic receptors and induces arterial and venous vasoconstriction, counteracting the D$_1$-receptor mediated vasodilation. This vasoconstriction increases arterial blood pressure, venous return, and cardiac filling pressures. At higher rates of administration, dopamine's hemodynamic effects are similar to those of norepinephrine.

Dobutamine

Dobutamine is a synthetic adrenergic agonist derived from dopamine. Its effects on adrenergic receptors are complex but do not result from endogenous transformation to norepinephrine.[38] Dobutamine simultaneously activates different adrenergic receptors with some opposite effects. In fact, the clinically used drug is a racemic mixture of a (−) enantiomer, activating alpha$_1$-adrenergic receptors, and of a (+) enantiomer activating beta$_1$ and beta$_2$ receptors.[39] The alpha$_1$- and beta$_1$-adrenergic stimulation results in inotropic and chronotropic effects. Dobutamine does not exert any intrinsic vascular effects, because the vasoconstriction induced by alpha$_1$ stimulation is counteracted by the beta$_2$ vasodilating effect.

Dopexamine

Dopexamine is a synthetic catecholamine inducing beta$_2$ and dopaminergic receptor activation, with no effect on alpha-adrenergic receptors and a weak direct effect on beta$_1$-adrenergic receptors. It also exerts indirect effects through inhibition of neuronal reuptake of norepinephrine. Its administration induces vasodilation and inotropic effects with substantially increased stroke volume.[38]

Isoproterenol

Isoproterenol is a potent synthetic beta-adrenergic agonist with a very low affinity for alpha-adrenergic receptors. Through its potent beta$_2$-vasodilating effects it induces a fall in diastolic and mean blood pressure, whereas systolic blood pressure is increased owing to the increase in stroke volume related to its beta$_1$-adrenergic activation.[38] The combination of the latter effect and the marked increase in heart rate leads to an enhanced cardiac output. The resulting increase in myocardial oxygen consumption is not compensated by coronary blood flow enhancement so that isoproterenol infusion may lead to myocardial ischemia, especially if there is preexisting coronary artery disease. Because of its proischemic and hypotensive effects, isoproterenol is no longer used as an inotropic agent in clinical practice.

Phosphodiesterase Inhibitors

Despite the major role of catecholamines in the management of critically ill patients with inadequate cardiac output, problems such as tachycardia, arrhythmias, increased myocardial oxygen consumption, excessive vasoconstriction, or loss of effectiveness may occur with prolonged exposure to beta-agonists. Thus, other inotropic drugs, such as phosphodiesterase inhibitors (amrinone, milrinone, and enoximone) have been proposed for the management of myocardial dysfunction. These synthetic drugs inhibit the peak III isoform of phosphodiesterase, which catalyzes cAMP (see Fig. 109-1). By increasing intracellular cAMP concentration, they induce a potent vasodilation of the arterial and venous systems through relaxation of vascular smooth muscle. The left ventricular preload is reduced to a greater extent than with dobutamine. At the cardiac level, phosphodiesterase inhibitors induce an inotropic effect similar to that induced by dobutamine. The heart rate is increased only at high rates of administration. The resulting effect is an increase in cardiac output. Because the enhancement of cAMP intracellular concentration also promotes the reuptake of Ca^{2+} by the sarcoplasmic reticulum, phosphodiesterase inhibitors facilitate ventricular relaxation. Finally, since beta-agonists exert their action by increasing the production of cAMP, phosphodiesterase inhibition could enhance their adrenergic effects. This is the pharmacologic basis for the synergic association of beta-agonists and phosphodiesterase inhibitors.

Calcium Sensitizers

Calcium sensitizers represent a new pharmacologic class of inotropic drug.[40] To date, levosimendan is the only calcium sensitizer approved for clinical use.[41] These drugs increase the sensitivity of troponin C for Ca^{2+} and hence the force of contraction (see Fig. 109-1). Their advantage over catecholamines would be to increase the force of contraction without enhancing the influx of Ca^{2+} into the cytosol and thus without increasing the risk of arrhythmias related to this ionic alteration. However, some degree of phosphodiesterase III inhibitory activity probably also contributes to their inotropic effect. These drugs also induce vasodilation by opening ATP-dependent K^+ channels.[40,41]

DECREASE IN BETA-ADRENERGIC RESPONSE

It is well recognized that response to beta-adrenergic stimulation is decreased in chronic cardiac failure. This may be a response to increased activity of the sympathetic nervous system, which may itself be a response to reduced cardiac output. Therefore, this negative retrocontrol of the beta-adrenergic response could act as a protection against excessive adrenergic stimulation. The cellular mechanisms involved are a down-regulation of $beta_1$-adrenergic receptors and a stimulation of the G_i protein of the adenyl cyclase system. The decrease in $beta_1$-adrenergic receptors could result from a decrease in beta-adrenergic receptor messenger RNA and to an increased internalization and degradation of these receptors. These latter mechanisms are mainly related to the phosphorylation of $beta_1$-adrenergic receptors by the beta-adrenoreceptor kinase, which is activated. The high level of nitric oxide (NO) production during heart failure

also contributes to attenuation of beta-adrenergic response. During exacerbations of chronic heart failure, the effects of exogenous catecholamines may thus be reduced.

Similarly, there is evidence for a decreased responsiveness of the myocardium to beta-adrenergic stimulation during septic shock.[42] This may be explained by the inhibition of adenyl cyclase activation due to an overexpression of G_i protein[43] at the gene level.[44]

HEMODYNAMIC EFFECTS OF INOTROPIC AGENTS IN CRITICALLY ILL PATIENTS

EFFECTS ON CARDIAC OUTPUT

Dobutamine and Dopamine

Dobutamine and dopamine are the beta-adrenergic agents most widely used in critically ill patients when an increase in cardiac output through an increase in myocardial contractility is desired. In patients with acute heart failure, the effects of these two agents were compared in a cross-over trial.[45] Whereas dobutamine (2.5-10 µg/kg/min) increased cardiac output through an increase in stroke volume in a dose-response fashion, dopamine increased stroke volume and cardiac output at 4 µg/kg/min but not at higher doses, presumably because of an increase in left ventricular afterload. It was also reported that pulmonary artery occlusion pressure decreased with dobutamine while it increased with dopamine. Similar findings were observed in patients with respiratory failure in whom dopamine also increased the left ventricular end-diastolic volume measured using isotopes while dobutamine did not.[46] This suggests an increase in left ventricular preload only with dopamine.

In cases of cardiogenic shock, dopamine is recommended as the inotropic agent of choice in the presence of severe hypotension whereas dobutamine is considered as a first-line therapy in the presence of predominant pump failure and volume overload but normal or moderately reduced blood pressure.[47,48] Accordingly, the SHOCK trial registry (1190 patients) reported that dopamine and dobutamine were used in 89% and 70%, respectively, of patients with cardiogenic shock due to massive acute myocardial infarction.[49] The combination of dopamine and dobutamine at low doses can be a therapy of interest when dobutamine alone fails to restore an adequate MAP.[50]

In patients with septic shock, in addition to hypovolemia, severe systemic vasodilation is associated with a variable degree of depressed myocardial contractility.[51] Accordingly, dopamine at median or high doses has been recommended as the catecholamine of choice when arterial pressure remains low despite adequate volume resuscitation, as it can exert both an alpha-mediated increase in arterial tone and a beta-mediated increase in myocardial contractility. In this regard, numerous studies in septic shock patients demonstrated that dopamine is able to increase both arterial pressure and cardiac output.[52-54] However, in these studies the restoration of an adequate MAP was mainly produced by the increase in cardiac output, through an increase in stroke volume and to a lesser extent an increase in heart rate, whereas minimal effects on systemic arterial resistance were observed despite relatively high doses of this agent. Dopamine was even demonstrated to increase cardiac output markedly while systemic resistance fell in septic patients without shock.[55] Conversely, in another study of patients with severe septic shock, cardiac output did not increase significantly with dopamine at doses up to 25 µg/kg/min while systemic vascular resistance (SVR) either did not change or significantly increased.[56] This emphasizes the great heterogeneity in the catecholamine response among septic patients and hence the difficulty in predicting clinical hemodynamic effects from pharmacologic properties because of interindividual differences in terms of severity of the insult, underlying diseases, comorbidities, integrity of the neurovegetative status, drugs concomitantly prescribed, and other factors.

Dobutamine is generally considered as the inotropic drug of choice when myocardial contractility is severely depressed in septic shock patients.[57] Comparison of dopamine and dobutamine has shown a similar increase in stroke volume (by 25%), heart rate (by less than 10%), and thus in cardiac output (by 33%) with the two agents but blood pressure increased only with dopamine, suggesting a vasodilatory (direct or indirect) effect of dobutamine.[52] Other authors reported decreased SVR with dobutamine in septic patients.[58,59] This emphasizes the absolute need to give a potent vasopressive agent to septic shock patients when dobutamine is chosen to support cardiac function in the presence of depressed myocardial contractility. One potential advantage of dobutamine is the decrease in cardiac filling pressures[60] that could allow an additional volume infusion to improve further cardiac output when necessary. A change from dopamine to dobutamine was shown to result in lower right and left ventricular filling pressures and an increase in right ventricular ejection fraction for the same pulmonary artery pressure and right ventricular end-diastolic volume, suggesting that dobutamine can exert a more favorable effect on cardiac contractility than dopamine.[61] This has justified the recommendation that dobutamine should be given rather than dopamine when the use of an inotropic drug is judged necessary in patients with severe sepsis or septic shock.[62] The detection of a marked decrease in left ventricular ejection fraction using bidimensional echocardiography[63] can help to diagnose a severe decrease in cardiac contractility and thus suggest the use of dobutamine when signs of peripheral hypoperfusion persist despite volume resuscitation and restoration of perfusion pressure with vasopressors. However, bedside bidimensional echocardiography is still not available in all general ICUs, so the recommendation of using an inotrope such as dobutamine is still based on the persistence of a low cardiac index (<2.5 L/min/m^2) after fluid resuscitation and an adequate MAP.[32] Because of the alteration of the beta-adrenergic pathway in the septic heart, the effect on stroke volume and cardiac output of a beta-agonist agent such as dobutamine may be attenuated in septic patients in comparison with nonseptic patients. In this regard, infusion of dobutamine at 5 µg/kg/min, a dose able to increase cardiac output substantially in healthy volunteers[64] or in patients with congestive heart failure,[65,66] has been reported to exert variable effects in the context of sepsis. For example, dobutamine at 5 µg/kg/min has been reported to induce a substantial increase in cardiac output in some studies in patients with severe sepsis[14,58,67] and to have no significant effect on cardiac output in studies investigating patients with a more severe septic shock.[68-70] It is likely that these differences in response to dobutamine were related to various individual factors, including differences in the vasopressive treatment coadministered, and in the degree of myocardial depression and/or beta receptor

down-regulation. In this regard, Silverman and associates[42] showed that incremental doses of dobutamine (0, 5, 10 µg/kg/min) produced a dose-related increase in cardiac output in septic patients without shock but no positive effect on cardiac output in patients with septic shock, even for the highest dose. Interestingly, they also showed that post-beta-adrenergic receptor signal transmission was impaired only in patients of the septic shock group and that impairment of beta-adrenergic receptor responsiveness found in both groups was significantly more marked in the septic shock group.[42] These findings, which allow the divergent results of numerous studies to be reconciled,[58,59,67-72] emphasize the unpredictability of the effects of beta-agonist agents in patients with sepsis. As a consequence, and because such agents have also potentially harmful effects (e.g., myocardial ischemia, cardiac arrhythmias), monitoring their effects on cardiac output to check their efficacy is the minimum required. However, no high-level recommendation on which method of cardiac output monitoring (e.g., pulmonary artery catheter, transesophageal Doppler, pulse contour method) is the more appropriate in this setting is currently available.

Epinephrine and Norepinephrine

Although these agents have beta$_1$-adrenergic properties and thus are able to increase myocardial contractility, they are used as vasoconstrictive agents in cases of severe hypotension, since they also have potent alpha-adrenergic properties. Yet significant increases in cardiac output with these drugs, consistent with potent inotropic effects, have been reported in septic patients.[54,73] In this regard, norepinephrine was shown to increase cardiac output to the same extent as dopamine for the same increase in MAP.[54] However, analysis of the existing literature indicates that the effects of norepinephrine on cardiac output are highly variable among septic patients.[74,75] By contrast, epinephrine appeared as a potent inotropic agent in most studies in septic patients.[70,76-78] However, epinephrine may impair splanchnic perfusion[79,80] and induce lactic acidosis,[81] despite its positive effects on cardiac output. Thus, epinephrine cannot be recommended as the first-choice drug when treatment of impaired cardiac contractility is considered. In the condition of depressed vascular tone and reduced myocardial function, epinephrine was even shown to be inferior to the combination of dobutamine and norepinephrine in terms of splanchnic perfusion, despite similar effects on systemic blood flow and pressure.[70,79,82]

Dopexamine

The pharmacologic properties of dopexamine should result in a combination of inotropic, afterload-reducing, and renal vasodilating effects, which could be useful for the management of acute exacerbation of congestive heart failure. In this regard, dopexamine was reported to substantially increase cardiac output in patients with heart failure without altering blood pressure: at doses up to 4 µg/kg/min, the majority of the effects resulted from an increase in stroke volume. At higher doses, the increase in heart rate made a greater contribution.[83] Similar results were found for the dose of 3 µg/kg/min in patients with acute respiratory failure and previous cardiomyopathy. In cases of human sepsis, dopexamine produced dose-dependent increases in stroke volume and heart rate but a dose-dependent decrease in SVR.[84] This underlines the marked vasodilating effect of this drug, which should not be administered in patients with severe sepsis in the absence of a potent vasopressor.

Under these conditions, dopexamine at doses ranging from 1 to 4 µg/kg/min could still enhance cardiac output without altering blood pressure.[85]

Phosphodiesterase Inhibitors

In patients with heart failure, phosphodiesterase inhibitors significantly increased cardiac output and stroke volume, while blood pressure slightly decreased due to a decrease in SVR, confirming the combined inotropic and vasodilating effects of these agents.[86] Because of the ability of beta-agonist agents to increase cAMP levels, thereby providing increased substrate for phosphodiesterase inhibitors, the combination of these two types of drugs would be attractive. Synergic effects on cardiac output of dobutamine and enoximone have been observed in patients with heart failure.[87] However, because of the disappointing results of trials of long-term oral phosphodiesterase inhibitor therapy in patients with chronic heart failure and of the OPTIME-CHF study in acute decompensation of congestive heart failure, the use of these agents is limited to a few categories of patients[88]: (1) patients with advanced heart failure awaiting transplantation, in whom intravenous milrinone may be better tolerated than dobutamine and its use may allow the continuation of beta-blocker therapy controlling arrhythmias or myocardial ischemia[89]; (2) patients with acute decompensation of chronic heart failure unable to achieve stabilization with standard treatment; and (3) patients with long-term beta-blocker use, in whom short-term intravenous milrinone may even be preferred to dobutamine. In septic patients, there is no recommendation to use these pharmacologic agents.

EFFECTS ON ARTERIAL OXYGEN CONTENT

The aim of inotropic therapy in critically ill patients with reduced cardiac contractility is not only to increase cardiac output but ultimately to improve oxygen delivery to the tissues. Thus, attention should be paid to the effects of these drugs on arterial oxygen content. Inotropes may affect arterial oxygen tension through several mechanisms. First, the reduction of lung filtration pressure resulting from improvement in cardiac function may decrease intrapulmonary shunt fraction and thus improve arterial oxygenation. Second, the increase in cardiac output may result in an increased venous admixture.[90] On the other hand, the increased mixed venous blood oxygen tension resulting from increased cardiac output may improve arterial oxygenation in the presence of ventilation/perfusion mismatching and thus may compensate for the increased venous admixture. Accordingly, when looking at the published data, it appears that even if venous admixture increased after dopamine[52,91,92] or dobutamine[52] administration, no significant change in arterial oxygen tension was observed with the use of any drug. Therefore, when an inotropic agent increases cardiac output in critically ill patients, it generally increases oxygen delivery to the same extent.[14,54,58,93]

EFFECTS ON TISSUE OXYGEN UTILIZATION

Even though an inotropic agent produces a large increase in oxygen delivery, its effectiveness in reducing oxygen deficit depends on its capacity to provide oxygen in the most hypoxic tissues. This concern is particularly crucial because, first, redistribution of blood flow is a characteristic pattern of shock states, and, second, inotropic drugs may also have vasoactive properties that interact with blood flow distribution.

Cardiogenic Shock

In this setting, redistribution of flow is recognized as a potent compensatory mechanism that, in response to reduced global oxygen delivery, attempts to deviate blood flow from nonvital organs with low oxygen extraction ratios toward vital organs with high oxygen extraction ratios, such as the heart or the brain. It must be kept in mind that administration of drugs with vasoactive properties may interfere with vasoregulation of regional blood flow. The extent to which this interference is beneficial in increasing oxygen supply and oxygen consumption in hypoxic areas remains speculative. This emphasizes the need to monitor, as far as possible, perfusion and function of critical organs.

Septic Shock

The maldistribution of flow at the macrocirculatory level as well as the microcirculatory level mainly contributes to defective tissue utilization and eventually to tissue oxygen debt in sepsis, even when systemic oxygen transport is greater than normal. Besides sepsis-induced microthrombosis, sepsis-induced alteration in vascular reactivity is a major cause of the altered distribution of blood flow between and within organs. In addition, severe sepsis can modify the impact of adrenergic drugs on regional blood flows, since a depressed vascular responsiveness to a vasoactive agent is likely to occur in this setting. This hypothesis may account for the absence of reduction of renal or splanchnic blood flow observed during vasoconstrictor therapy in endotoxic shock.[94] In cases of human sepsis, interference of sepsis-modified vasoactive drug properties by sepsis-induced macrocirculatory disturbances have been mostly investigated at the level of the splanchnic and the renal circulation.

Numerous clinical studies have examined the effects of adrenergic agents on splanchnic perfusion during sepsis. Their findings have sometimes varied, either because of differences in the methods used for assessing this regional circulation (e.g., gastric tonometry, laser-Doppler flowmetry, indocyanine green dilution) or because of the heterogeneity of the studied populations (e.g., differences in the severity of the septic insult, in the underlying diseases, in the therapy coadministered). However, from findings of the majority of these studies, some reasonable conclusions can be drawn. First, dobutamine is likely to exert a beneficial effect on the gut mucosal perfusion,[69,70,79,93] probably via a beta$_2$-adrenergic effect.[95] Second, dopamine may have deleterious effects on gut mucosal perfusion, despite its potential vasodilating action through mesenteric dopaminergic receptors. Third, epinephrine is probably the adrenergic agent with the least desirable effects on the splanchnic vasculature, as most studies showed a lower splanchnic blood flow with epinephrine than norepinephrine alone[80] or in combination with dobutamine,[69,70,79] even for global hemodynamic effects. Fourth, dopexamine can exert a favorable effect on splanchnic perfusion[19] comparable to that of dobutamine[69] and is likely to be related to a beta$_2$-adrenergic effect. Given all the available data, it is recommended that the combination of norepinephrine and dobutamine rather than epinephrine be used when an inotropic therapy is given to reverse cardiac dysfunction in severe sepsis.[32]

Regarding the effects of inotropic agents on the renal circulation in septic patients, two major points must be kept in mind. First, an alpha-adrenergic agent, such as norepinephrine, is able to increase renal blood flow and urine output,[56,87,96] despite its potential vasoconstricting effect on the afferent glomerular arteries. This is probably due to the beneficial effect of increasing MAP when the renal blood flow is dependent on arterial pressure, as occurs in cases of profound systemic hypotension. Otherwise, a sepsis-induced depressed responsiveness of afferent glomerular arteries to the action of norepinephrine cannot be excluded. Accordingly, there is no evidence in the available literature that norepinephrine is capable of decreasing renal blood flow and urine output when given to septic patients to increase MAP toward normal values. Moreover, it has been demonstrated in patients with septic shock that elevating arterial pressure up to 85 mm Hg with incremental doses of norepinephrine was not associated with a decrease in urine output.[97] Second, although dopamine at low doses (<5 μg/kg/min) is pharmacologically able to vasodilate renal arteries through its action on dopaminergic receptors, the systematic administration of low doses of dopamine in critically ill patients, including patients with sepsis, does not result in improved outcome[98] and must no longer be recommended.

Finally, inotropic drugs may also exert nonhemodynamic effects that could affect cellular metabolism and/or organ function.[7,99] For example, catecholamines may modulate cytokine response to sepsis, trauma, or major surgery through beta-adrenergic receptor activation.[7] Whether this effect (inhibition of proinflammatory cytokines and enhancement of proinflammatory cytokine production) plays a beneficial role in the reversal of tissue hypoxia and organ dysfunction remains to be evaluated.

ANNOTATED REFERENCES

Bellomo R, Chapman M, Finfer S, et al: Low-dose dopamine in patients with early renal dysfunction: A placebo-controlled randomised trial. Australian and New Zealand Intensive Care Society (ANZICS) Clinical Trials Group. Lancet 2000;356:2139-2143.

Despite the effect of dopamine at low doses on renal dopaminergic receptors, the administration of low-dose dopamine in critically ill patients at risk of renal failure does not result in any benefit in terms of renal dysfunction or outcome. This result underlines the difficulty of extrapolating pharmacologic properties of therapeutic agents to clinical effects, in particular in critically ill patients.

Boyd O, Grounds M, Bennett D: A randomized clinical trial of the effect of deliberate perioperative increase of oxygen delivery on mortality in high-risk surgical patients. JAMA 1993;270:2699-2707.

This monocentric randomized study demonstrated that deliberate increase in oxygen delivery toward supranormal values with dopexamine during the perioperative period was able to decrease mortality and complication rates dramatically in high-risk surgical patients.

Duranteau J, Sitbon P, Teboul JL, et al: Effects of epinephrine, norepinephrine or the combination of norepinephrine and dobutamine on gastric mucosa in septic shock. Crit Care Med 1999;27:893-900.

In this cross-over study in patients with septic shock, the addition of low-dose dobutamine to norepinephrine significantly increased gastric mucosal blood flow assessed with laser Doppler flowmetry while cardiac output and mean arterial pressure remained constant, suggesting a proper vasodilatory effect of dobutamine in this regional area. On the other hand, epinephrine at doses maintaining the same mean arterial pressure as norepinephrine did not produce any significant increase in gastric mucosal blood flow despite a large increase in cardiac output. This study confirms that catecholamines are not all equal in terms of regional blood flow.

Hayes MA, Timmins AC, Yau E, et al: Elevation of systemic oxygen delivery in the treatment of critically ill patients. N Engl J Med 1994;330:1717-1722.

This randomized study showed that attempting to achieve supranormal values of oxygen delivery in patients with an established critical illness may worsen rather than improve outcome.

Silverman HJ, Penaranda R, Orens JB, et al: Impaired beta-adrenergic receptor stimulation of cyclic adenosine monophosphate in human septic shock: Association with myocardial hyporesponsiveness to catecholamines. Crit Care Med 1993;21:31-39.

This clinical study demonstrated that patients with septic shock exhibit a decreased hemodynamic response to dobutamine when compared with septic patients without shock. Moreover, the stimulation of circulating lymphocytes of the studied population showed that in patients with septic shock, the degree of impairment of beta-adrenergic receptor responsiveness as well as that of post-beta-adrenergic receptor signal transmission was higher than in septic patients without shock. This study provides strong evidence of a septic shock-related myocardial hyporesponsiveness to catecholamines that may contribute to the reduced myocardial performance observed in this critical illness.

Chapter 110

MECHANICAL SUPPORT IN CARDIOGENIC SHOCK

Thomas G. Gleason • Mariell Jessup

KEY POINTS

1. The **leading cause of death among hospitalized patients** with acute myocardial infarction (AMI) continues to be cardiogenic shock.

2. **Intra-aortic counterpulsation for patients in shock after AMI** is used in only 22% of eligible patients.

3. Pioneering surgeons recognized by the 1960s that **left ventricular decompression and myocardial rest** could afford enhanced cardiac recovery after the insult of open-heart surgery.

4. The **physiologic rationale for the efficacy of the intra-aortic balloon pump (IABP)** includes (a) left ventricular systolic unloading directly reduces stroke work, which in turn reduces myocardial oxygen consumption during the cardiac cycle, and (b) diastolic augmentation raises arterial blood pressure and provides better coronary arterial perfusion during diastole, yielding increased oxygen delivery to the myocardium.

5. The **absolute indications for IABP placement** include cardiogenic shock, uncontrolled angina pectoris, acute postinfarction ventricular septal defect or mitral regurgitation, and postcardiotomy left-sided heart failure with low cardiac output.

6. In the aforementioned settings in the previous point, **IABP should be considered a primary therapy** that should not be delayed until noncardiac injury is clinically evident.

7. **Cardiogenic shock and high-risk angioplasty** are the most common indications for use of the IABP.

8. The SHOCK trial showed that **early revascularization of patients with coronary artery disease and shock after AMI**, often facilitated by IABP use (86%), yielded a lower 6-month mortality rate (50%) than with medical therapy alone (63%).

9. **Timing of IABP** can be synchronized in one of three ways: using an arterial (preferably aortic) pressure tracing in synchrony with the dicrotic notch, using the descent of the R wave on a rhythm tracing, or timed after a ventricular pacing spike when a pacemaker is in use.

10. The effectiveness of IABP is significantly improved by **proper timing of inflation and deflation.**

11. **Relative contraindications to IABP use** include severe atheromatous and atherosclerotic descending thoracic aorta, descending aortic aneurysm, recent descending thoracic aortic surgery, and mild to moderate aortic insufficiency.

12. The **incidence of major vascular complications** according to the STS National Database (1996-1997) and the Benchmark Registry (1997-1999) is 5.4% and 1.4%, respectively.

13. It is clear that the **mortality rate of cardiogenic shock after AMI remains high** at 39%.

14. **IABP support, combined with revascularization,** portends a better prognosis than adjunctive IABP use with medical therapy alone.

15. **Short-term cardiopulmonary support for cardiogenic shock has emerged as an important adjunctive therapy.** It is a relatively simple means of establishing immediate and complete circulatory support, requiring no additional equipment other than that needed for standard cardiopulmonary bypass support during cardiac surgery.

16. **VADs that utilize direct cardiac outflow cannulation** (VAD inflow) provide better ventricular decompression and rest than peripheral bypass support systems.

17. **Two advantages to the Thoratec system** are the ability of secure ventricular inflow (VAD) cannulation and the applicability of long-term utilization.

18. The **hallmarks of cardiogenic shock** are low cardiac output, hypotension, peripheral vasoconstriction, cold extremities, poor urine output, and altered mental status.

19. **Intrinsic causes of cardiogenic shock** can be divided into four pathophysiologic classifications: (a) acute valvular insufficiency, (b) acute myocardial infarction, (c) acute myocarditis, and (d) postcardiotomy cardiac failure.

20. **Insertion of a pulmonary arterial balloon catheter and echocardiography** should be done to help formulate a differential diagnosis.

21. **Cardiogenic shock after AMI requires immediate IABP placement,** often with additional pharmacologic support.

22. **Initial placement of implantable VADs** (e.g., HeartMate or Novacor) for mechanical support in patients with cardiogenic shock is generally not indicated.

An estimated 61.8 million people in the United States have heart disease, among whom 950,000 die annually.[1] Of these, 540,000 people suffer myocardial infarctions each year; 193,000 succumb to complications directly related to the infarction. The leading cause of death among hospitalized patients with acute myocardial infarction (AMI) continues to be cardiogenic shock.[2] The incidence of cardiogenic shock complicating AMI (approximately 7%) has remained constant over the past 25 years. Accurate statistics on the worldwide utilization of all mechanical support for cardiogenic shock are not known. However, estimates on the use of intra-aortic counterpulsation for patients in shock after AMI suggest a rate of use in only 22% of eligible patients.[3] The reasons for the apparent underutilization of this readily available modality are not clear. Accordingly, the indications, benefits, and limitations of mechanical cardiac support are outlined in this chapter.

HISTORICAL BACKGROUND

The evolution of mechanical cardiac support dates to the early 1950s when Gibbon developed the prototype cardiopulmonary bypass (CPB) apparatus.[4] In the years following, Lillehei, Kirklin, and others applied the heart-lung machine to facilitate open-heart surgery; their pioneering work and early observations led directly to the development of modern mechanical cardiac support systems.[5-7] These surgeons recognized that some patients had improved outcomes after surgery if they were weaned slowly rather than abruptly from CPB support. Their initial publications introduced the concept that left ventricular (LV) decompression and myocardial rest could afford enhanced cardiac recovery after the insult of open-heart surgery. Clinical use of extracorporeal CPB for heart surgery became widespread in the early 1960s. Simultaneously, several groups of investigators were testing means of mechanical cardiac assistance for use outside the operating room for support of patients in cardiogenic shock. The current modes of mechanical support are derivations of those originally developed and include aortic counterpulsation, continuous flow pumps with or without an oxygenator, and pulsatile pumps.

HISTORY OF AORTIC COUNTERPULSATION

The concept of arterial counterpulsation was introduced in 1961 by Clauss and coworkers and involved use of an external "ventricular" chamber that filled with blood from a catheter in the iliac artery[8] and was subsequently compressed by a piston. Compression of the "ventricle" was synchronized to either the QRS complex of an electrocardiogram (ECG) or the impulse of a pacemaker, so that a counter pulse of blood was delivered into the arterial system during diastole. It was

demonstrated in dogs that cardiac stroke work and LV end-systolic pressures could be substantially reduced with the use of a counterpulsation into the aorta. The following year Moulopoulus and associates adapted the model to create an intra-aortic balloon pump (IABP) that could provide a similar counterpulsation without the need for blood reservoirs.[9] The investigators used a balloon that was rapidly inflated and deflated with carbon dioxide during native diastole. The IABP was subsequently adapted and described for clinical use by Kantrowitz and colleagues in 1968.[10]

The original polyurethane balloon measured 1.8 cm in diameter by 14.8 cm in length when inflated (helium was used because its low density allows rapid delivery to and from the balloon) and displaced 32 mL of blood. There is little difference in the modern IABP and that originally described, other than the availability of different-sized balloons (30- to 50-mL balloons) and subtle differences in the materials used to make the catheters. The extracorporeal components of the IABP now include an electronically controlled pump with a solenoid valve in continuity with a pressurized helium source. The valve controls the flow of helium into and out of the balloon at intervals timed to either pressure changes on an arterial transducer, ECG signals (i.e., the QRS complex), or a ventricular pacer signal. This timing of balloon inflation and deflation is critical to attain optimal physiologic benefit of the cardiac support.

The physiologic rationale for the efficacy of the IABP is that balloon deflation provides a rapid, synchronized reduction in impedance (afterload) during isovolemic LV contraction. This is followed by a rapid, synchronized increase in aortic pressure during isovolemic LV relaxation (diastolic augmentation) caused by balloon inflation. In combination these events achieve two important goals. First, LV systolic unloading directly reduces stroke work, which in turn reduces myocardial oxygen consumption during the cardiac cycle. Second, diastolic augmentation raises arterial blood pressure and provides better coronary arterial perfusion during diastole, yielding increased oxygen delivery to the myocardium. The IABP does not directly move or redistribute blood flow; however, peak diastolic coronary flow velocity can be increased as much as 87% with IABP augmentation and peak diastolic flow velocity by as much as 117%.[11] Since introduction into clinical use in 1968, the IABP has remained an important adjunct to supporting patients in cardiogenic shock. Myocardial recovery is promoted by the reduction of cardiac work and the simultaneous increase in myocardial oxygen supply. However, therapeutic success is dependent on the patient having a minimum degree of left ventricular function that, in combination with IABP support, facilitates an adequate cardiac output to sustain end-organ function. When this minimal cardiac output is not met, alternative mechanical cardiac assistance must be considered.

HISTORY OF MECHANICAL ASSIST DEVICES

The need for effective mechanical cardiac assist devices became apparent in the 1950s during the development of CPB for open-heart surgery. Initial attempts with prolonged postoperative CPB demonstrated that the bypass circuit was damaging to both end-organ function and blood constituents after several hours of use.[12] The first attempt at isolated extracorporeal LV support was with a simple roller pump in 1962.[13] Subsequently, femoral venous-to-femoral arterial CPB was successfully used by Spencer and colleagues in four patients with postcardiotomy cardiac failure.[14]

Simultaneous to Spencer and colleagues' work with extracorporeal systems, DeBakey designed the first intracorporeal LV assist device (LVAD), the DeBakey blood pump.[15] This device consisted of a Dacron-reinforced silicone rubber tube with an inner chamber of blood from the left atrium that was connected to the descending thoracic aorta. Pressurized air was instilled into the outer chamber by an external pneumatic controller to compress the inner blood chamber, timed to the R wave of the QRS complex. Blood flow was directed from the left atrium to the descending aorta with the use of ball valves at both the inflow and outflow ends of the device. The DeBakey blood pump was first used in a patient who died 4 days postoperatively of neurologic complications. A remodeled extracorporeal version was subsequently used for postcardiotomy failure in a 37-year-old woman after aortic and mitral valve replacements. The device was needed for 10 days, but the patient survived.[16]

By 1972, investigators at the Texas Heart Institute had developed a pneumatically driven LVAD designed to be implanted in the abdomen.[17] This device had a blood chamber compressed by pulses of air delivered into the pump by a percutaneous driveline. Modern devices have chamber compression that is electrically powered via percutaneous drivelines. Paracorporeal, pneumatically driven devices were a parallel development. Paramount to the evolution of these devices was the sponsorship of the Artificial Heart Program of the National Heart, Lung, and Blood Institute, which was chartered in 1964.

By the 1960s, continuous flow, as compared to pulsatile, pumps were under development.[18,19] Over the subsequent 15 years, centrifugal pumps were perfected and introduced into clinical use. These pumps work on the principle of a forced, constrained vortex devised from three magnetic cones.[20-22] They have been shown to be useful in a variety of clinical settings where short-term mechanical support is needed and an IABP is inadequate. Several types of small, axial-flow or rotary pumps have also been developed.[23-36] These are generally constructed of a magnetically suspended impeller that rotates at extremely fast rates (25,000 to 35,000 rpm). The axial rotary pump technology has some potential advantages over pulsatile devices; they are quite small with few moving parts and do not require a compliance chamber.

CURRENT MECHANICAL SUPPORT DEVICES

COUNTERPULSATION/INTRA-AORTIC BALLOON PUMP

Indications

The absolute indications for IABP placement include cardiogenic shock, uncontrolled angina pectoris, acute postinfarction ventricular septal defect or mitral regurgitation, and postcardiotomy left-sided heart failure with low cardiac output. In these settings, IABP should be considered a primary therapy that should not be delayed until noncardiac injury is clinically evident. It is important to recognize that blood pressure alone is not an adequate indication of hemodynamic or cardiac stability. Limb perfusion, renal function, mental status, and even gastrointestinal function need to be considered in the assessment of adequate resuscitation and homeostasis. Additional measurable indices include arterial

(SaO_2) and mixed venous oxygen saturation ($S\bar{v}O_2$), acid-base status, urine output, and body temperature. A multivariate analysis of data accrued from 391 postcardiotomy patients requiring IABP demonstrated that epinephrine requirements greater than 0.5 µg/kg/min, a left atrial pressure greater than 15 mm Hg, urine output less than 100 mL/h, and $S\bar{v}O_2$ less than 60% correlated with mortality.[37] These criteria were used to help predict mortality and the need for subsequent mechanical support.

Other relative indications for IABP use include (1) high-risk, catheter-based interventional procedures such as left main coronary artery angioplasty, (2) after unsuccessful attempts at catheter-based intervention in patients with poorly controlled ventricular arrhythmias, and (3) concomitant poor LV function, and (4) in settings of persistent stunned, ischemic myocardium. These are all circumstances in which reduction of LV systolic wall tension and oxygen consumption by the IABP might enhance myocardial recovery after intervention. Conversely, the use of an IABP had no impact on mortality in a population of patients without hemodynamic instability undergoing high-risk angioplasty randomized in a prospective trial reported in 1997.[38] More recently, the Benchmark Counterpulsation Outcomes Registry of IABP use in 22,663 patients from 250 hospitals worldwide demonstrated that cardiogenic shock and high-risk angioplasty were the most common indications for utilization of the device.[39] Table 110-1 depicts a further characterization of the Benchmark report with respect to indications for use of the IABP and subsequent interventions.[40] Nevertheless, despite the widespread use of the IABP in over 150,000 patients worldwide each year,[41] no prospective, randomized trial has ever demonstrated a survival benefit with IABP use in the patient population undergoing high-risk catheter intervention. In contrast, the SHOCK trial showed that early revascularization of patients with coronary artery disease and shock after an AMI, often facilitated by IABP use (86%), yielded a lower 6-month mortality rate (50%) than with medical therapy alone (63%).[2] Additional studies have shown that in patients undergoing urgent or emergent revascularization after an AMI, those supported preoperatively with an IABP had a lower operative mortality than those in whom an IABP was not used (5.3% to 8.8% vs. 11.8% to 28.2%).[42,43] These data seem to justify a strategy of aggressive IABP use to facilitate early revascularization in the postinfarction patient.

Technical Considerations

The optimal site of insertion of an IABP is a common femoral artery that can be accessed either percutaneously with the use of a guidewire or by surgical cutdown. Modern intra-aortic balloon catheters are available for adults and children, according to the appropriate size and length for a given height and weight of the patient. Adult intra-aortic balloons have a range in volume filled between 25 and 50 mL, with a standard balloon size holding 40 mL of helium. IABP catheters placed through the femoral artery are positioned so that the tip is just distal to the takeoff of the left subclavian artery in the proximal descending thoracic aorta. Optimally, the tip of the catheter should be positioned with transesophageal echocardiographic (TEE) or fluoroscopic guidance.[44] To reduce the diameter of femoral cannulation, a sheathless IABP technique can be utilized and is our preferred method.[45]

Inflation of the balloon should be timed with closure of the aortic valve (at the dicrotic notch of the aortic pressure tracing) and should be inflated to nearly occlude the descending

TABLE 110–1. INDICATIONS FOR USE

	Total Population (n = 16,909)	Diagnostic Catheterization Only (n = 1,576)	Catheterization & PCI Only (n = 3,882)	Surgery CABG (n = 9,179)	Non-CABG (n = 1,086)	No Intervention (n = 1,186)
Support and stabilization (%)	20.6	21.4	54.4	9.7	5.0	7.8
Cardiogenic shock (%)	18.8	33.1	23.7	12.3	23.8	29.4
Weaning from cardiopulmonary bypass (%)	16.1	0.4	0.1	24.9	31.4	7.1
Preop: high risk CABG (%)	13.0	4.6	0.2	22.1	6.4	1.9
Refractory unstable angina (%)	12.3	15.3	8.3	15.8	2.2	3.0
Refractory ventricular failure (%)	6.5	9.1	2.5	5.9	15.7	12.7
Mechanical complication due to AMI (%)	5.5	9.8	7.0	4.2	5.2	5.1
Ischemia related to intractable VA (%)	1.7	1.6	1.5	1.9	1.7	1.6
Cardiac support for high-risk general surgery (%)	0.9	2.1	0.2	0.5	4.3	1.1
Other (%)	0.8	0.7	0.2	0.8	2.5	2.0
Intraoperative pulsatile flow (%)	0.4	0.1	0.1	0.7	0.5	0.2
Missing indication (%)	3.3	1.8	1.9	1.2	1.5	28.1

AMI, Acute myocardial infarction; CABG, coronary artery bypass graft; PCI, percutaneous coronary intervention; VA, ventricular arrhythmias.
Modified from Ferguson JJ 3rd, Cohen M, Freedman RJ Jr, et al: The current practice of intra-aortic balloon counterpulsation: Results from the Benchmark Registry. J Am Coll Cardiol 2001;38:1456-1462.

thoracic aorta. Timing can be synchronized in one of three ways: (1) using an arterial (preferably aortic) pressure tracing in synchrony with the dicrotic notch, (2) using the descent of the R wave on a rhythm tracing, or (3) timed after a ventricular pacing spike when a pacemaker is in use.[46-50] The effectiveness of IABP is significantly improved by proper timing of inflation and deflation, which can be difficult when there is an accelerated heart rate, cardiac rhythm disturbances, atrioventricular dyssynchrony, or low mean arterial pressure. IABP timing should be adjusted to maximize diastolic augmentation; hence, deflation should be as late as possible but just before opening of the aortic valve. If this cannot be gauged by the pressure tracing, it can be timed to the onset of the R wave on the ECG tracing or with the use of M-mode echocardiography.[51]

IABP catheters should not be left in place after weaning because of the risk of thrombus formation and embolization. An IABP should be weaned stepwise from a rate that is equivalent to heart rate (1:1) down to a ratio of 1:3 just before removal. Balloon catheters placed via an open surgical technique should also be removed surgically. Percutaneous removal of catheters placed in the iliac artery above the inguinal ligament (often done in obese individuals) can result in significant retroperitoneal bleeding. Consideration of operative removal is warranted.

When femoral arterial cannulation is not desirable due to aortoiliac occlusive disease or extensive peripheral vascular disease, the subclavian artery or the ascending aorta can be utilized.[52-56] With either technique, the IABP catheters are advanced antegrade down the descending thoracic aorta so that the balloon tip sits above the level of the diaphragmatic hiatus, and the most proximal end of the balloon is distal to the takeoff of the left subclavian. These antegrade balloons should always be placed with either fluoroscopic or echocardiographic guidance. They should be removed with open arterial repair in all cases.

Relative contraindications to IABP use include severe atheromatous and atherosclerotic descending thoracic aorta, descending aortic dissection or aneurysm, recent descending thoracic aortic surgery, and mild to moderate aortic insufficiency. Severe aortic insufficiency is an absolute contraindication to use because diastolic augmentation cannot be accomplished, and LV end-diastolic volume and pressure are actually increased rather than decreased.

Complications

The overall complication rate of IABP utilization is 6.5% to 8.1%. Major complications occur at a rate of 2.7% and include severe bleeding, major limb ischemia or amputation, infection, visceral or spinal cord ischemia, and attributable IABP mortality.[39,43] A summary of IABP complications as they occur in relation to subsequent percutaneous or operative coronary revascularization from the Benchmark Registry are listed in Table 110-2.[40] In this registry, rates of complications were quite low, the most common being access-site bleeding (4.3%) and limb ischemia (2.3%).[39] The rates of amputation, stroke, visceral or spinal cord ischemia and IABP-related mortality are all 0.1% or less.[39] Intra-aortic balloon entrapment is a rare complication.[57-59] The incidence of major vascular complications according to the STS National Database (1996-1997) and the Benchmark Registry (1997-1999) is 5.4% and 1.4%, respectively.[40,43] Ipsilateral limb ischemia should be immediately addressed after its recognition. This usually requires removal of the IABP with replacement at another location if it is still indicated. The ischemic limb may require thrombectomy with or without revascularization and fasciotomy.[60-66]

Outcomes

In the absence of prospective, randomized data it is difficult to ascribe outcome secondary to IABP placement. The Second Angioplasty in Myocardial Infarction (PAMI-II) Trial data examined high-risk patients with acute myocardial infarction revascularized by percutaneous intervention only and demonstrated a modest survival advantage at 6 months with the use of periprocedural IABP support.[38] When evaluating hospital mortality rates among patients undergoing coronary artery bypass graft (CABG) and/or valve surgery who received

TABLE 110–2. IABP OUTCOMES AND COMPLICATIONS

	Total Population (n = 16,909)	Diagnostic Catheterization Only (n = 1,576)	Catheterization & PCI Only (n = 3,882)	Surgery		No Intervention (n = 1,186)
				CABG (n = 9,179)	**Non-CABG** (n = 1,086)	
In-hospital mortality (%)	21.2	32.2	18.4	16.8	37.8	34.1
Mortality: balloon in place (%)	11.6	17.6	10.1	9.2	19.8	20.2
IABP-related mortality* (%)	0.05	0.1	0.1	0.0	0.0	0.1
Amputation[†]	0.1	0.0	0.1	0.1	0.1	0.0
Major limb ischemia[‡] (%)	0.9	0.6	0.5	1.2	1.0	0.5
Any limb ischemia (%)	2.9	3.2	1.9	3.5	2.5	1.7
Severe access site bleeding (%)	0.8	0.8	1.2	0.7	0.7	0.3
Any access site bleeding (%)	2.4	2.7	4.4	1.7	1.3	1.4
Balloon leak (%)	1.0	0.9	0.8	1.1	0.5	1.6
Composite Outcomes						
Major IABP complication[§] (%)	2.8	2.8	2.2	3.0	2.9	2.4
Any IABP complication[‖] (%)	7.0	7.6	7.5	7.1	6.0	5.2
Any unsuccessful IABP[¶] (%)	2.3	2.5	1.7	2.5	2.4	2.7

CABG, coronary artery bypass graft; IABP, intra-aortic balloon pump; PCI, percutaneous coronary intervention.
*Death as direct consequence of IABP therapy.
[†]All major limb ischemia.
[‡]Loss of pulse or sensation, abnormal limb temperature, or pallor, requiring surgical intervention.
[§]Balloon leak, severe bleeding, major limb ischemia, or death as a direct consequence of IABP therapy.
[‖]Any access site bleeding, any limb ischemia, balloon leak, poor inflation, poor augmentation, insertion difficulty, or death as direct result of IABP therapy.
[¶]Balloon leak, poor inflation, poor augmentation, or insertion difficulty.
From Ferguson JJ 3rd, Cohen M, Freedman RJ Jr, et al: The current practice of intra-aortic balloon counterpulsation: Results from the Benchmark Registry. J Am Coll Cardiol 2001;38:1456-1462.

preoperative IABP or required intraoperative/postoperative IABP support, it is evident that mortality was significantly lower among patients supported preoperatively, as depicted in Table 110-3.[40,43] Hence, there appears to be a survival advantage to earlier IABP support for patients with AMI and cardiogenic shock who need revascularization. In the setting of an acute ventricular septal defect (VSD) or acute mitral regurgitation after an AMI, IABP support can offer a dramatic improvement in the hemodynamic response of the patient.[67-71] Figures 110-1 and 110-2 stratify hospital mortality rates associated with IABP use in patients with AMI by principal usage indication or by performance of percutaneous or surgical coronary revascularization. It is clear that the mortality rate of cardiogenic shock after AMI remains high at 39%. However, IABP support, combined with revascularization, portends a better prognosis than adjunctive IABP use with medical therapy alone.[39]

CONTINUOUS FLOW PUMPS

Both roller pumps and centrifugal pumps deliver continuous flow, but have other, distinct limitations. Roller pumps remain in widespread use for cardiopulmonary support during cardiac surgery; applications outside the operating room have been virtually abandoned for several reasons. Roller pumps are insensitive to changes in arterial line resistance that may cause disruption of the apparatus. They require unobstructed venous flow. The rollers eventually cause spallation of tubing, leading to particle emboli and weakening of the tubing.[72] Roller compression causes hemolysis after prolonged use.[73]

Alternatively, centrifugal pumps are sensitive to both outflow resistance and filling pressure, offering a safer applicability outside the operating room. Centrifugal pumps like the Bio-Medicus Biopump (Medtronic, Corp., Minneapolis, MN) generate a constrained vortex within an acrylic shell

TABLE 110–3. HOSPITAL MORTALITY (OUTCOME PARAMETER) FOR PATIENTS UNDERGOING CARDIAC SURGERY WHO EITHER RECEIVED PREOPERATIVE IABP OR INTRA-/POSTOPERATIVE IABP SUPPORT

Type of Therapy	Benchmark Registry 1997-1999 Mortality/Total Operations with IABP, n (%)	STS National Database 1996-1997 Mortality/Total Operations with IABP, n (%)	STS National Database 1996-1997 Mortality/Total Operations without IABP, n (%)
Preoperative IABP	8.8 (329/3,721)	9.5 (2,487/26,077)	2.9 (10,919/378,810)
Intraoperative/ postoperative IABP	28.2 (954/3,380)	23.6 (3,528/14,933)	2.5 (9,878/389,954)

Based on data from the Benchmark Counterpulsation Registry 1997-1999 and the STS National Database 1996-97 compared with hospital mortality for patients who had neither preoperative nor intraoperative/postoperative IABP support.
From Christenson JT, Cohen M, Ferguson JJ 3rd, et al: Trends in intraaortic balloon counterpulsation: Complications and outcomes in cardiac surgery. Ann Thorac Surg 2002;74:1086-1090.

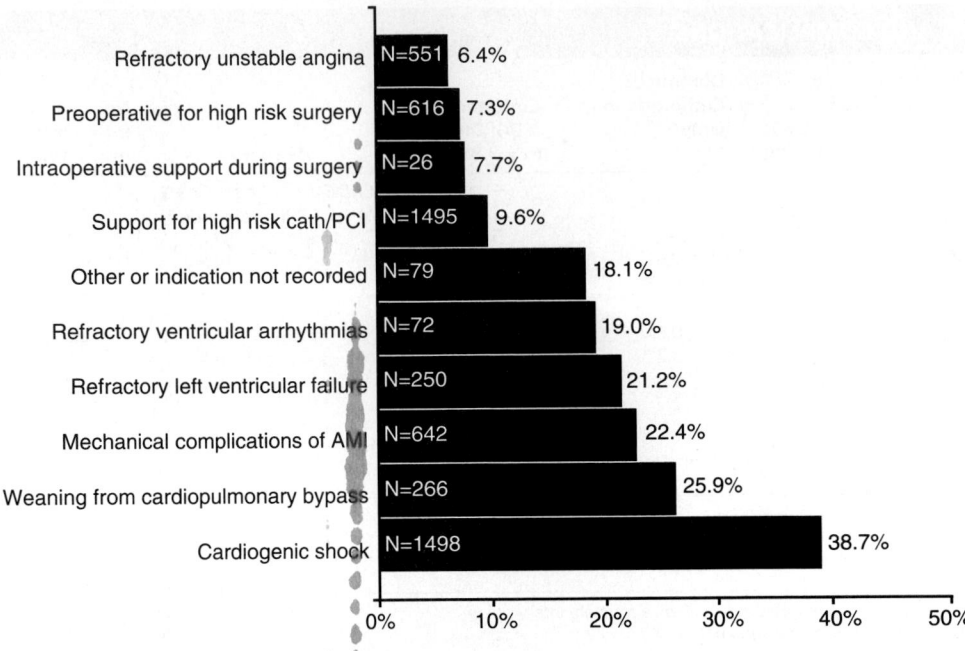

FIGURE 110–1. In-hospital mortality of 5,495 patients with acute myocardial infarction (AMI) requiring intra-aortic balloon pump counterpulsation, stratified by principal usage indication. PCI, percutaneous coronary intervention. (From Stone GW, Ohman EM, Miller MF, et al: Contemporary utilization and outcomes of intra-aortic balloon counterpulsation in acute myocardial infarction: The benchmark registry. J Am Coll Cardiol 2003;41:1940-1945.)

that houses concentric magnetic cones. The cones rotate as a magnetic rotary motor spins adjacent to the base of the cones[20-22] and can generate very high flows with less trauma to blood cells than roller pumps.[73-75]

The technology of centrifugal pumps, axial flow pumps, and membrane oxygenators has remarkably improved. Pump durability and reduced blood cell trauma have been demonstrated.[19,26,73-76] As a result, considerable experience has accumulated with the use of centrifugal pumps (cardiopulmonary support) for postcardiotomy LV failure, fulminant myocarditis, or cardiogenic shock after AMI.[32,77-93]

Indications

Short-term cardiopulmonary support for cardiogenic shock has emerged as an important adjunctive therapy. It is a relatively simple means of establishing immediate and complete circulatory support, requiring no additional equipment

other than that needed for standard CPB support during cardiac surgery. Cardiopulmonary support can be initiated percutaneously via the common femoral artery and vein. Alternatively, when faced with postcardiotomy LV failure, cardiopulmonary support can facilitate patient stabilization for subsequent transport to a tertiary medical center for VAD placement. Cardiopulmonary support circuits can be converted to longer-term support (beyond 6 to 8 hours) by upgrading the oxygenator.[94,95] A standard microporous hollow-fiber oxygenator (the type used in most CPB circuits) has a life span of 6 to 12 hours.[96] Changing to a solid-silicone membrane oxygenator (not microporous) will lengthen the life span of the cardiopulmonary support circuit up to 21 days; this conversion constitutes extracorporeal membrane oxygenation (ECMO) support. ECMO is generally used in the adult population for periods of 1 to 10 days when there is marked concomitant pulmonary insufficiency and cardiac failure.

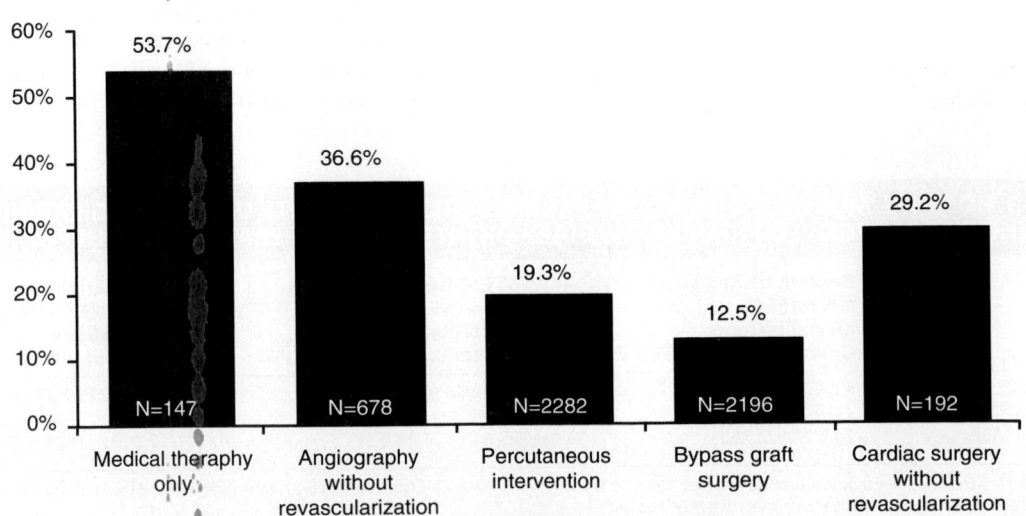

FIGURE 110–2. In-hospital mortality stratified by the performance of angiography and percutaneous or surgical coronary revascularization. (From Stone GW, Ohman EM, Miller MF, et al: Contemporary utilization and outcomes of intra-aortic balloon counterpulsation in acute myocardial infarction: The benchmark registry. J Am Coll Cardiol 2003;41:1940-1945.)

ECMO is also used for short-term (1 to 3 days) support when the neurologic status of a patient is unclear and longer-term support (i.e., VAD support) may not be appropriate until this status is clarified. Thus, ECMO can be used as a bridge to a longer-term, pulsatile flow assist device once the suitability of the patient is determined.

Technical Considerations and Complications

Disadvantages to the use of peripheral cardiopulmonary support or ECMO include the greater potential for ipsilateral limb complications, higher rates of hemolysis, the requirement for anticoagulation to prevent thrombosis of the oxygenator and circuit, and failure to adequately decompress the left ventricle.[97-103] Inadequate LV decompression with peripheral cardiopulmonary support/ECMO systems may be the mechanism responsible for some treatment failures. Regardless of the etiology of cardiogenic shock, a rested ventricle (i.e., decompressed) has a better chance of recovery than a distended ventricle.

Outcomes

The use of ECMO in the adult population for reasons other than primary cardiac failure with secondary pulmonary insufficiency has limited advantages over conventional therapies.[104,105] However, a substantial subset of patients who present with cardiogenic shock and are initially resuscitated with cardiopulmonary support/ECMO survive to revascularization, transplantation, or recovery, with survival rates as high as 75%.[77,78,81,82,106-112] ECMO used as a bridge to VAD placement for profound cardiogenic shock ("double bridge" mechanical assistance) can yield survival rates greater than 40%.[80] This strategy is pragmatic and offers immediate end-organ support while a subsequent definitive treatment plan can be designed.

VENTRICULAR ASSIST DEVICES

Pulsatile Pumps

There is a growing body of evidence suggesting that pulsatile assisted circulation, in the setting of acute cardiogenic shock, offers improved end-organ perfusion and lymphatic flow and is thus beneficial.[113-115] VADs that utilize direct cardiac outflow cannulation (VAD inflow) provide better ventricular decompression and rest than peripheral bypass support systems. There are now several mechanical assist devices that achieve these goals, including the extracorporeal ABIOMED BVS 5000 (ABIOMED, Inc., Danvers, MA) and the paracorporeal Thoratec VAD system (Thoratec Corp., Pleasanton, CA). Two other implantable, intracorporeal, pulsatile VADs that were designed for patients with chronic heart failure may have roles in certain subsets of patients with acute cardiogenic shock. These are the HeartMate LVAS XVE (Thoratec Corp., Pleasanton, CA) and the Novacor LVAS (World Heart Corp., Ottawa, Ontario).

Extracorporeal Short-term Support (ABIOMED)

The ABIOMED BVS 5000 was developed in the 1980s and was granted approval for use for postcardiotomy heart failure by the U.S. Food and Drug Administration in 1992.[116] Since that time, indications for the device have been broadened to include most patients with either postcardiotomy shock or precardiotomy shock who do not adequately respond to inotropes and an IABP. The ABIOMED system is a pneumatically driven, dual-chamber blood pump that delivers

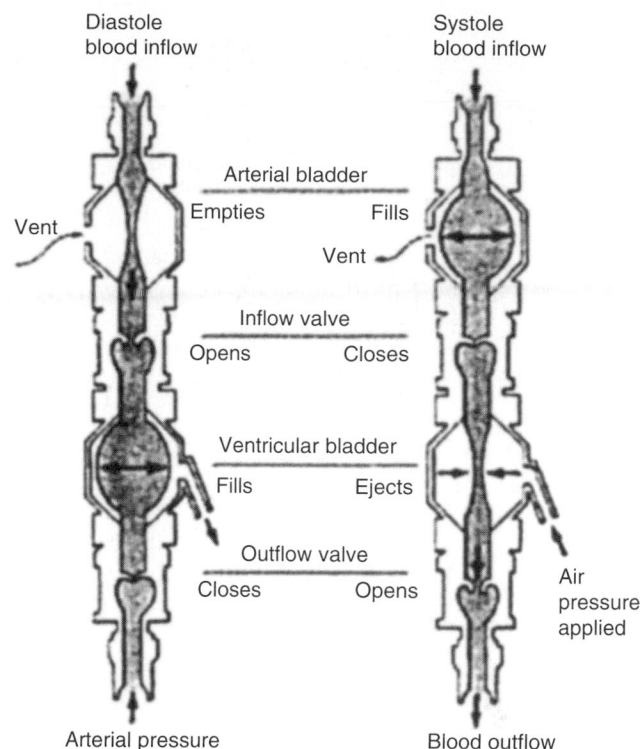

FIGURE 110–3. The ABIOMED BVS 5000. **Left,** The atrial chamber empties through a one-way valve into the ventricular chamber (diastole). **Right,** The pneumatically driven pump compresses the ventricular chamber and blood flows through a one-way valve into the patient (systole). The atrial chamber fills by gravity during pump systole. (From Moazami N, McCarthy PM: Temporary circulatory support. In Cohn LH, Edmunds LH Jr [eds]: Cardiac Surgery in the Adult. New York, McGraw-Hill, 2003.)

pulsatile flow. ABIOMED inflow cannulas are placed in the left and/or right atrium for univentricular or biventricular support. Outflow cannulas are housed with a Hemashield graft (Meadox Medicals Inc., Oakland CA) and are sewn to the aorta and/or pulmonary artery for left-sided and/or right-sided heart support. The pumps, as depicted in Figure 110-3, are extracorporeal. The upper (first) chamber fills passively by gravity, and the lower chamber serves as the pumping chamber. The two chambers are separated by a polyurethane trileaflet inflow valve; the lower chamber is separated from the arterial circulation by an outflow valve that prevents retrograde flow. As the pumping chamber is filled with blood, the surrounding air within the polycarbonate housing is displaced back into the drive console. This is sensed by the console; the console delivers compressed air back into the pumping chamber, which compresses the bladder and forces a pulse of blood into the arterial circulation.[116] The stroke volume that results is 70 to 80 mL with VAD output dependent on the rate of upper chamber filling. Flows of 5 L/min are typical for the ABIOMED system. This VAD requires anticoagulation, particularly for LV assistance. The device is generally useful for short-term (< 7 to 10 days) support because of the increased risk of thromboembolic complications or device malfunction beyond this period. If longer support is necessary, the ABIOMED pump can be exchanged with a new device or converted to a longer-term VAD system such as the Thoratec, HeartMate, or Novacor.

ABIOMED cannulation can be achieved either on or off CPB and with or without aortic cross-clamping. However, the condition of the patient is typically unstable, and cannulation,

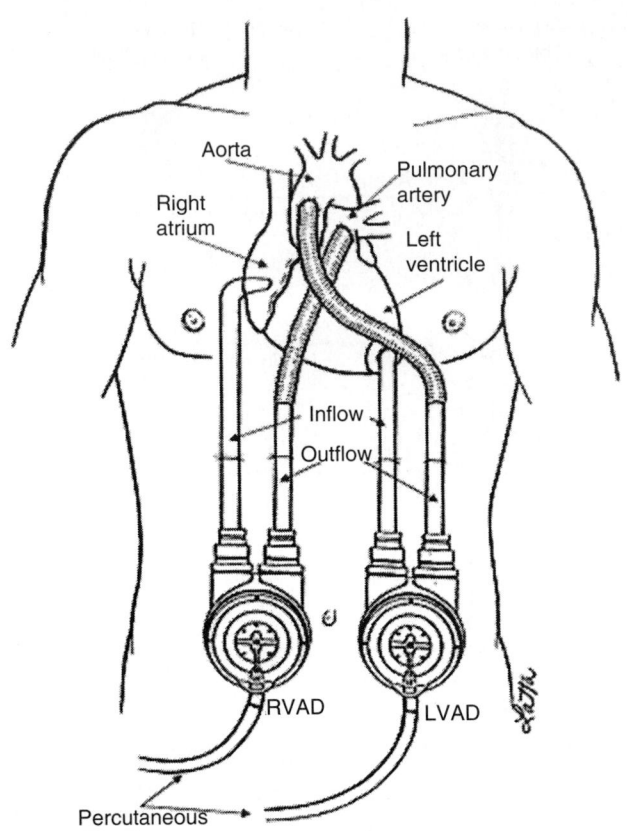

FIGURE 110–4. Thoratec ventricular assist system: a paracorporeal, pneumatically powered system configured for uni- or biventricular support. (From Hunt SA, Frazier OH: Mechanical circulatory support and cardiac transplantation. Circulation 1998;97:2079-2090. Copyright 1998, American Heart Association.)

and afterload. The pneumatically driven pulses (systole) can be controlled in three different modes: asynchronous, synchronous, and volume. The asynchronous mode maintains a fixed rate, but stroke volume may vary. The synchronous mode provides counterpulsation by timing ejection to the patient's R wave—this provides both a variable rate and variable stroke volume. The volume mode delivers a fixed stroke volume triggered by bladder filling, but the rate will vary. The volume mode is usually the most practical because the VAD output changes with the patient's physiologic condition.

The Thoratec system is paracorporeal, similar to the ABIOMED, but is more portable and has the potential for outpatient use in patients who are bridging to recovery or transplantation.[120-123] Two advantages to the Thoratec system are the ability of secure ventricular inflow (VAD) cannulation and the applicability of long-term utilization. LV cannulation provides better ventricular decompression than atrial cannulation.[124-128] This is important because LV distention or inadequate decompression will limit ventricular recovery in some patients. Ventricular cannulation also provides better VAD performance and reduces the risk of thrombotic complications, particularly in the setting of AMI.[108,124,126,128] Right ventricular cannulation provides similar advantages over right atrial cannulation. However, these advantages may not be manifest if the tricuspid valve is left intact, because the tricuspid leaflets are often in close proximity to the cannulation tip and can obstruct VAD inflow.[129] In this situation, the advantages and disadvantages of right atrial versus right ventricular cannulation must be weighed to direct the best approach.

Over 3700 Thoratec VADs have been placed worldwide in over 2400 patients[130]; more then half of these patients received biventricular support. Survival and hospital discharge rates vary widely between 20% and 80%, depending on the etiology of shock and the medical center.[77,80,120,127,131-133] Cases of acute

particularly of the pulmonary artery and aorta, may be safer on bypass with a decompressed, supported heart. Access is obtained via median sternotomy, with all cuffed cannulas brought out of the chest through separate subcostal incisions. The cuffs allow soft tissue in growth and adherence to reduce the incidence of infection of the cannulas and endocardium.

Approximately 6000 ABIOMED VADs have been placed worldwide for precardiotomy or postcardiotomy cardiac failure.[114,116-119] Survival and hospital discharge rates have ranged from 20% to 45%, depending on the indication for the ABIOMED and the hemodynamic condition of the patient before surgery.[114,116-118] The most common complications directly attributed to this VAD include bleeding, stroke, and infection, with rates of 20% to 40%.[114,116,118] Hemolysis is not a common problem.

Paracorporeal Longer-term Support (Thoratec)

The Thoratec VAD system is composed of a single chamber with a polyurethane, seamless bladder housed in a rigid casing (Fig. 110-4).[120] VAD inflow cannulas are either atrial or ventricular. Outflow cannulas have a polyester graft attached for direct connection to the aorta or pulmonary artery, similar to the ABIOMED cannulas. There are Bjork-Shiley tilting disc valves at both the inflow and outflow connections to the bladder to ensure unidirectional flow; they require anticoagulation. A pneumatic driveline is connected to the rigid casing and supplies alternating vacuum and pressure to facilitate bladder filling and emptying, respectively. The blood pump can be adjusted to accommodate changing preload

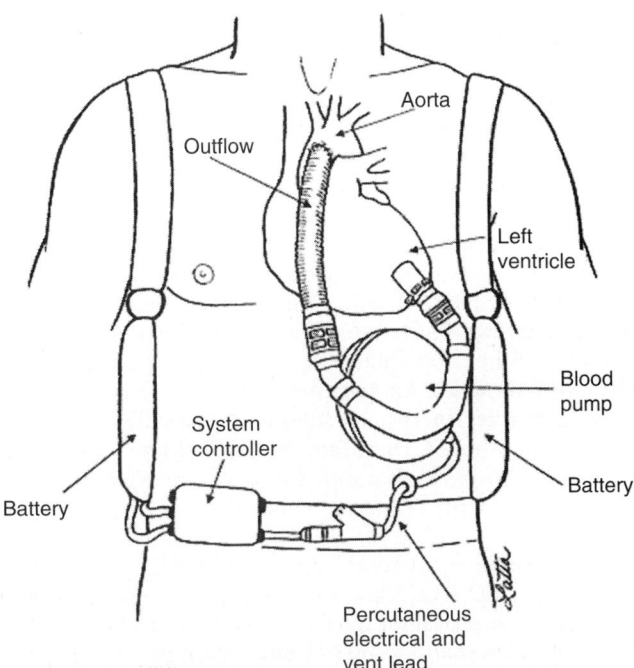

FIGURE 110–5. The HeartMate vented electric left ventricular assist device (HeartMate XVE): an intracorporeal, electrically powered system. (From Hunt SA, Frazier OH: Mechanical circulatory support and cardiac transplantation. Circulation 1998;97:2079-2090. Copyright 1998, American Heart Association.)

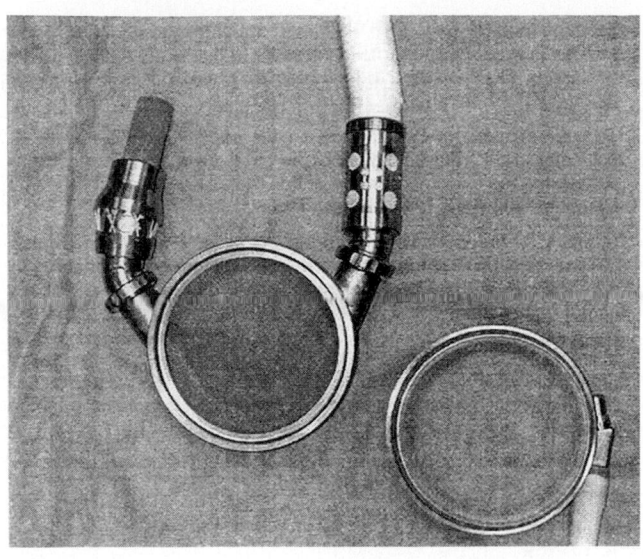

FIGURE 110–6. The HeartMate XVE left ventricular assist device in cross section depicting the pusher plate system responsible for displacement of blood within the chamber. (From Operating Manual for the HeartMate XVE LVAS, Thoratec Corporation, 2001.)

fulminant myocarditis with cardiogenic shock are among the best situations for VAD support with the Thoratec system, having an 88% recovery-with-discharge rate.[77] Complications of the Thoratec system are similar to other extracorporeal VAD systems when used for treatment of cardiogenic shock and include infection, stroke, bleeding, and acute renal failure. The rates of these complications vary among different series but range from 10% to 60%.[118,120,127,131,133-138]

Intracorporeal Long-term Support

The HeartMate LVAS XVE and Novacor LVAS have fully implanted pusher-plate blood pumps with externalized drivelines and are similar in their construction (Fig. 110-5). Each uses bioprosthetic valves to ensure unidirectional flow. The Novacor has bovine pericardial valves, and the HeartMate has porcine aortic valves. The Novacor has a seamless polyurethane pump sac between two pusher plates that generates a stroke volume of 70 mL. This surface requires anticoagulation. The HeartMate has a flexible polyurethane diaphragm that pushes against a titanium alloy housing generating a maximum stroke volume of 83 mL (Figs. 110-6 and 110-7). The blood contact surface is textured with polyurethane fibrils on one side and sintered titanium spheres on the housing. Fibrin and cellular components react and

bond to the surface creating a pseudointima, precluding the need for anticoagulation. Antiplatelet therapy is recommended for both systems.

Both systems have variable modes that can generate fixed rates or demand-sensitive rates. Both are approved for use for the treatment of end-stage heart failure, but they may have a selective role for cardiogenic shock. These devices are practical alternatives for use in a "double-bridge" setting with initial resuscitation using a temporary device (i.e., ECMO/cardiopulmonary support or ABIOMED) for stabilization and pulmonary recovery.[80,109,110,139,140] Results with the HeartMate and Novacor devices have been favorable and, in certain subsets of patients, better than longer-term support with other systems.[77,138,141-145] Complications have been similar to other VADs and include bleeding, infection, stroke, thrombotic complications, and renal insufficiency.

There are several miniaturized rotary axial flow pumps that have been designed for long-term (potentially permanent) mechanical assistance, including the MicroMed-DeBakey pump, the Jarvik 2000, and the HeartMate II.[146-155] These devices are being studied in clinical trials for use as a bridge to transplantation, recovery, or permanent replacement therapy.[147,156] They have not yet received widespread use for acute cardiogenic shock.

TREATMENT OF CARDIOGENIC SHOCK: AN ALGORITHM FOR MECHANICAL SUPPORT

The hallmarks of cardiogenic shock are low cardiac output, hypotension, peripheral vasoconstriction, cold extremities, poor urine output, and altered mental status. As the pathophysiologic state progresses, pulmonary insufficiency and pulmonary edema ensue. Extrinsic causes of cardiogenic shock most commonly manifest as circulatory collapse secondary to pericardial tamponade. Acute tamponade is easily diagnosed by echocardiography and requires surgical or percutaneous evacuation and subsequent treatment of that which caused the tamponade (e.g., traumatic injury, aortic dissection, ruptured aneurysm). Extrinsic causes of cardiogenic shock usually require immediate surgical intervention but rarely necessitate mechanical assistance. However, intrinsic causes of acute cardiogenic shock can be refractory to both medical and surgical therapies and may require mechanical assistance. Intrinsic causes of cardiogenic shock can be divided into four pathophysiologic classifications: (1) acute valvular insufficiency, (2) AMI, (3) acute myocarditis, and (4) postcardiotomy cardiac failure.

FIGURE 110–7. The HeartMate XVE blood pump compartment with the flexible polyurethane diaphragm within the housing pictured on the right. (From Operating Manual for the HeartMate XVE LVAS, Thoratec Corporation, 2001.)

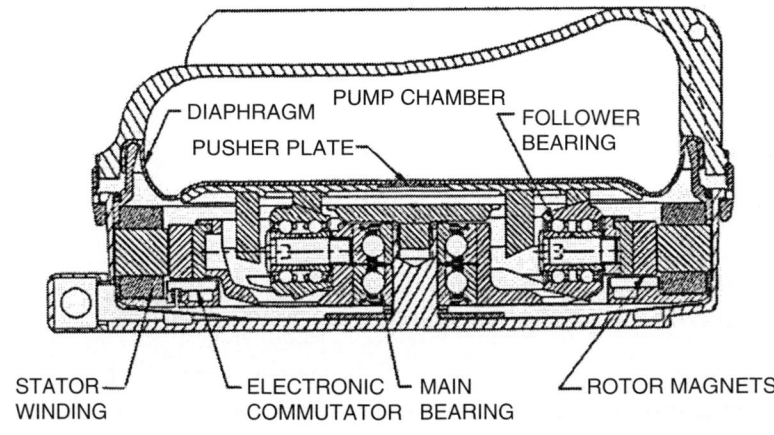

Irrespective of the etiology of cardiogenic shock, the approach toward the initial management of patients should be fairly uniform, and a suggested management algorithm is outlined in Figure 110-8.

First, insertion of a pulmonary arterial balloon catheter and echocardiography should be done to help formulate a differential diagnosis. Severe valvular insufficiency can usually be effectively excluded at this juncture. If severe aortic insufficiency is present, chronotropic control (heart rate 80 to 100 beats/min) and afterload reduction with inotropic support should be the initial maneuvers. An IABP is contraindicated because aortic regurgitation will worsen, and the patient should be prepared for immediate aortic valve replacement. Likewise, acute, severe mitral regurgitation can be readily identified with an echocardiogram and hemodynamic assessment. An IABP should be placed immediately in conjunction with inotropes and/or afterload reduction. Surgical intervention should proceed emergently and cardiac catheterization pursued preoperatively only if the patient can be adequately stabilized.

Acute fulminant myocarditis usually presents in a previously healthy individual with no history of cardiac disease. Patients with presumed myocarditis who do not stabilize after the insertion of an IABP and concomitant inotropic infusion should be diverted to VAD support expeditiously. A remarkable percentage of these patients will recover if adequately supported during the acute phase of this disease. Short-term to intermediate-term VADs are optimal in these patients because of the ease of their insertion and removal and the anticipation for relatively short-term recovery. Giant cell myocarditis is one exception to this rule, because most patients with this diagnosis will require transplantation.[157-160]

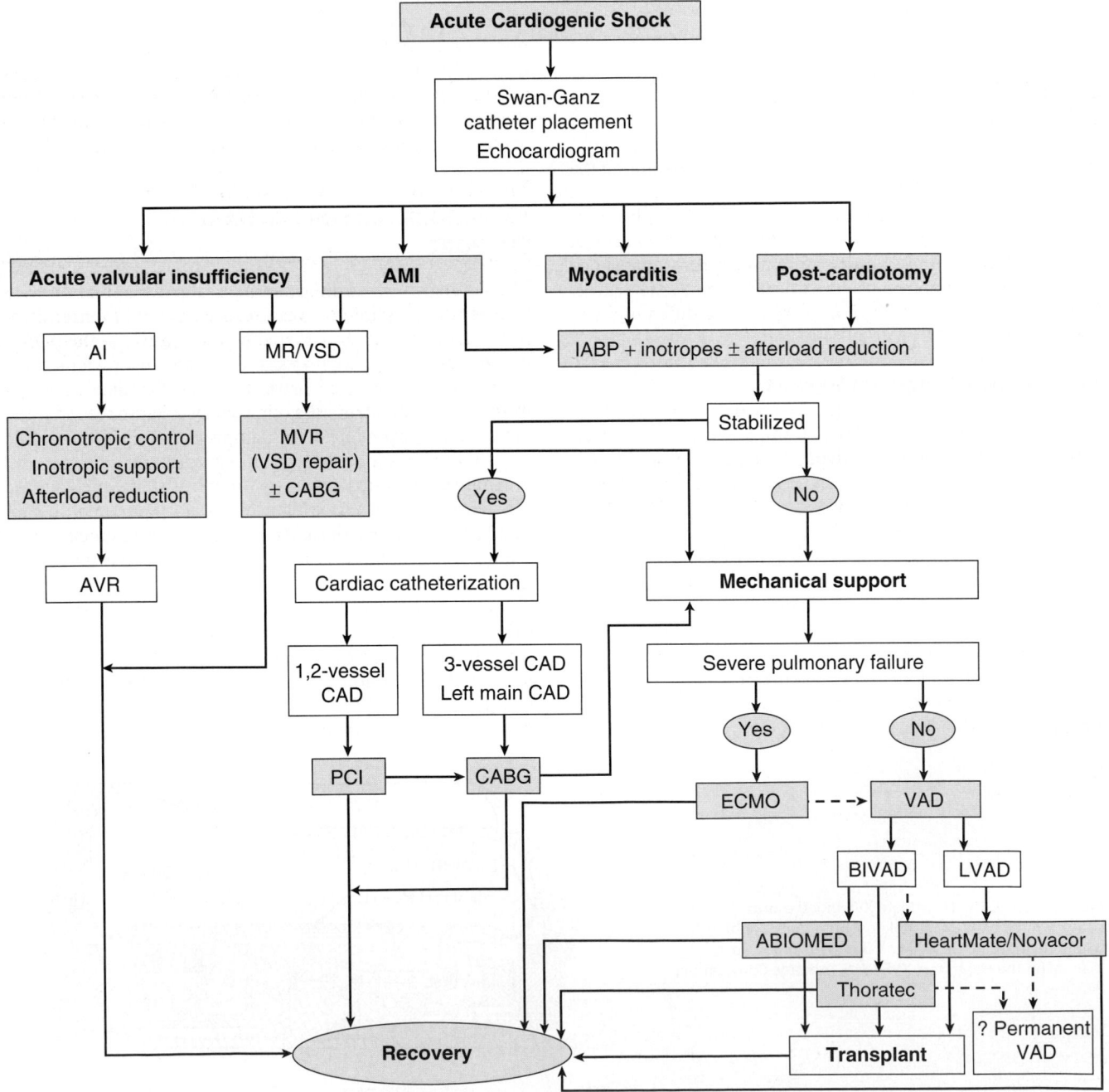

FIGURE 110–8. Algorithm for the management of acute cardiogenic shock.

Cardiogenic shock after AMI requires immediate IABP placement, often with additional pharmacologic support. If a mechanical complication (i.e., severe mitral regurgitation or VSD) has occurred, immediate surgical intervention is usually required. An expeditious cardiac catheterization is reasonable if the patient can be stabilized or placed on percutaneous bypass for the procedure. If no mechanical complication has occurred and the patient has been stabilized with IABP and medical therapy, cardiac catheterization may proceed. The number of diseased arteries usually determines subsequent allocation to percutaneous or surgical revascularization. Patients whose condition is unstable after an AMI, with continued cardiogenic shock despite IABP and inotropic support, should be considered for VAD support (see Fig. 110-6).

Postcardiotomy cardiogenic shock should be managed intraoperatively with an initial trial of IABP and inotropic support. If there is persistent shock or an inability to be weaned from CPB, VAD implantation is the next therapeutic step, provided a meaningful recovery is predictable or a plan for transplantation or permanent therapy can be clarified.

The mode of mechanical support used for cardiogenic shock is determined by a number of factors. The first is the degree of pulmonary insufficiency. If there is pulmonary failure with a very large alveolar-to-arterial oxygen gradient on maximal ventilatory support, ECMO support is indicated. A small percentage of ECMO patients in this setting will recover, some will require VAD placement as a bridge to transplantation, fewer still will bridge to VAD and then to recovery. If the degree of pulmonary insufficiency is limited to pulmonary edema that is likely to recover with adequate cardiac output, patients should undergo VAD placement directly. The choice of VAD in this situation is also dependent on several factors, including the predicted need for short- or longer-term support, the need for biventricular versus univentricular support, the chance of ventricular recovery, the institutional experience with different devices, and the relative risks of anticoagulation.

The ABIOMED system for postcardiotomy cardiac failure is preferred for those patients predicted to recover within days to a week of surgery, for cases when neurologic function is not known or is markedly compromised, and for patients who are not candidates for transplantation but may bridge to recovery or bridge to a longer-term and ambulatory device once stabilized with the ABIOMED. The ABIOMED system is the easiest to insert, so in cases of profound cardiogenic shock when operative brevity may be beneficial toward patient recovery, it may be the best choice. The system is also easy to convert to other longer-term VAD systems because the ABIOMED inflow cannulation is atrial and temporary.

The Thoratec system is the most versatile VAD and remains the support used most frequently at our institution for the treatment of refractory cardiogenic shock. The device is relatively easy to install, may be used for short-term or long-term univentricular or biventricular support, and allows the potential for ambulation. VAD inflow cannulation can be either via the atria or ventricles. Ventricular cannulation is preferable even in the case of AMI because of its hemodynamic efficiency, reliability, and better ventricular decompression. Despite the friability of freshly infarcted myocardium, the Thoratec ventricular cannulas are safe to insert through infarcted tissue. After review of our institutional data, we have observed no increase in VAD complications compared with those cannulas placed in uninfarcted

tissue (Gleason and Acker, unpublished data). Once a patient is stabilized with the Thoratec system, a management strategy can be mapped out as bridge to recovery, transplantation, or permanent therapy with an intracorporeal device.

Initial placement of implantable VADs (e.g., HeartMate or Novacor) for mechanical support in patients with cardiogenic shock is generally not indicated. These devices may be used as a second bridge ("bridge-to-bridge") toward recovery, transplantation, or permanency. There may be a select group of patients in whom these intracorporeal VADs have a primary role in cardiogenic shock: (1) patients who require a larger cardiac output than other devices can generate (large individuals needing a cardiac output greater than 6 L/min to reverse the shock state); (2) patients who are more stable, can sustain longer operative times, and are unlikely to achieve myocardial recovery; and (3) patients in whom anticoagulation is contraindicated, making the HeartMate device potentially safer.

CONCLUSION

Cardiogenic shock remains a lethal problem with a mortality rate as high as 75%.[2,161,162] Patients who cannot be stabilized with inotropic support and an IABP should be considered for mechanical assistance with a VAD. The ideal assist device that can be easily placed, is versatile and portable, has minimal risk of complication, offers a normal cardiac output with physiologically equivalent characteristics such as pulsatile flow, and is easily removed does not yet exist. Currently, there are three modes of mechanical cardiac assistance that have received widespread use in the patient population with cardiogenic shock, including ECMO/cardiopulmonary support, the ABIOMED BVS 5000, and the Thoratec VAD system. Implantable devices such as the HeartMate LVAS XVE and Novacor LVAS have occasionally been used in this moribund population but have a more defined role in the subacute and chronic heart failure population.

The use of mechanical assistance for acute cardiogenic shock has facilitated impressive improvements in survival for certain disease cohorts such as those with acute myocarditis, with survival rates over 70%.[77] VADs have had less remarkable an impact on patients with postcardiotomy shock or AMI-induced shock,[108] but results in these patient populations are improving annually. Inherent to achieving better results is our understanding that patients who present with cardiogenic shock typically have significant underlying comorbidities with multiple-system organ dysfunction and marked derangements in both coagulation and inflammatory mediators that complicate management. They need to be approached by an integrated multidisciplinary team, including cardiologists, cardiac surgeons, anesthesiologists, critical care specialists, and experienced nursing staff, to implement efficient and decisive treatment plans. These integrated systems offer the greatest chance for success. Technologies expand and improve exponentially every year, and it is clear that mechanical assistance will continue to play a pivotal role in the management of these difficult patients.

ANNOTATED REFERENCES

Farrar DJ: The Thoratec ventricular assist device: A paracorporeal pump for treating acute and chronic heart failure. Semin Thorac Cardiovasc Surg 2000;12:243-250.

The experience with use of the Thoratec system through May 2000 is reviewed. The results of over 1300 implants are discussed. Survival rates among patients transplanted and weaned from the Thoratec VAD support were 86% and 59%, respectively.

Hochman JS, Sleeper LA, Webb JG, et al: Early revascularization in acute myocardial infarction complicated by cardiogenic shock. SHOCK Investigators. Should We Emergently Revascularize Occluded Coronaries for Cardiogenic Shock. N Engl J Med 1999;341:625-634.

Results from the randomized SHOCK trial are reported. Emergency revascularization did not significantly reduce 30-day mortality, but it did reduce mortality at 6 months and IABP placement helped facilitate early revascularization.

Pagani FD, Lynch W, Swaniker F, et al: Extracorporeal life support to left ventricular assist device bridge to heart transplant: A strategy to optimize survival and resource utilization. Circulation 1999;100:II206-II210.

Experience using ECMO for the initial resuscitation and as a bridge to left ventricular assist device placement and subsequent heart transplantation in patients with severe hemodynamic instability is presented. ECMO can

be used to salvage some survivors from this very high-risk cohort before the utilization of LVAD resources.

Samuels LE, Holmes EC, Thomas MP, et al: Management of acute cardiac failure with mechanical assist: Experience with the ABIOMED BVS 5000. Ann Thorac Surg 2001;71:S67-S72; discussion S82-S85.

Results of use of the ABIOMED ventricular assist device in pre- and post-cardiotomy shock from one of the initial testing centers are outlined. An algorithm and standardized protocol for management of refractory cardiogenic shock with VAD insertion is presented.

Stone GW, Ohman EM, Miller MF, et al: Contemporary utilization and outcomes of intra-aortic balloon counterpulsation in acute myocardial infarction: The benchmark registry. J Am Coll Cardiol 2003;41:1940-1945.

This study reviews the indications and outcomes for the usage of the intra-aortic balloon pump (IABP) from 1996-2001. Data were collected prospectively in 250 medical centers with over 22,000 IABPs placed worldwide.

Chapter 111

PERIPHERAL ARTERIOPATHIES INCLUDING EMBOLISM

David Laithwaite • Krishna Lingam • Richard Donnelly

KEY POINTS

1. **Peripheral arterial disease** is common, often asymptomatic, and associated with atherosclerotic vascular disease in other arterial territories. A relationship exists between ankle-brachial pressure index (ABPI, a marker of severity of occlusive arterial disease in the lower limb) and patient survival: a lower ABPI is generally associated with a much higher 5-year mortality.

2. **Most patients with intermittent claudication are managed medically,** but critical limb-threatening ischemia requires urgent endovascular or surgical intervention to prevent limb loss. Acute limb ischemia is caused by either primary thrombotic occlusion (thrombus superimposed on a ruptured atherosclerotic plaque) or embolism arising from the heart or proximal vessels. The mode of presentation and symptoms and signs of acute limb ischemia depend on the site and cause of the arterial occlusion and the extent to which preexisting peripheral arterial disease has led to collateral vessel formation. **Acute limb ischemia still carries a 15% mortality rate at 30 days.**

3. **Endovascular approaches** (e.g., angioplasty and stenting) are especially useful for discrete, proximal, and isolated stenoses (e.g., in the iliac arteries), but patients with diffuse, distal, and/or bilateral disease are less suitable for endovascular treatment.

4. **Outcomes after revascularization for critical limb ischemia** depend on the patency of distal (run-off) vessels and the presence of coexistent risk factors (e.g., diabetes and smoking).

5. **New approaches to treatment** include therapeutic angiogenesis, that is, administration of naked DNA or recombinant protein for vascular growth factors to stimulate new collateral vessel formation from existing vascular structures.

CLASSIFICATION OF PERIPHERAL ARTERIAL DISEASE

Peripheral arterial disease generally refers to the various manifestations of atherosclerosis in the major vessels of the lower limb, including thromboembolic complications associated with acute limb ischemia. Peripheral arterial disease is common, is often asymptomatic, and shows a steep age-related incidence in older people.[1] The clinical and biochemical risk factors for atherosclerosis (e.g., cigarette smoking, diabetes, and hypercholesterolemia) are associated with more severe and progressive disease in the lower limb. Diabetes, in particular, distorts the clinical presentation by causing more diffuse and distal arterial involvement. This, in turn, often hampers clinical management, including revascularization, and results in poorer clinical outcomes, such as higher amputation and graft failure rates.

Fontaine classified the severity of chronic arterial insufficiency of the lower limb in 1954 (Table 111-1),[2] but intensive care specialists are mainly concerned with the management of critical limb ischemia and patients with acute limb-threatening arterial occlusion.

EPIDEMIOLOGY AND CLINICAL PRESENTATION OF LOWER LIMB ISCHEMIA

Based on an objective measure of arterial insufficiency (e.g., an ABPI < 0.95), the incidence of peripheral arterial disease has been reported as 7% in the 49- to 74-year age group, but only 22% of patients with peripheral arterial disease had symptoms.[3] The ABPI is obtained by dividing the ankle systolic BP at the level of the malleolus by the higher of two brachial systolic BPs. Under normal circumstances the ABPI is 1.0 and an ABPI less than 0.8 is invariably abnormal, reflecting significant arterial stenosis. The ABPI in an affected limb often falls after a short period of exercise (e.g., a walk test). Occasionally, the ABPI is falsely elevated, such as in patients with diabetes, when arteries are calcified and resistant to compression.

The most common symptom of peripheral arterial disease, intermittent claudication (Fontaine stage II), occurs in only 0.6% of people age 45 to 54 years but affects 9% of the over 70-year age group.[1] Although intermittent claudication is troublesome and disabling, most patients remain symptomatically stable in the medium to long term. Each year, however, 15 to 20 patients per 100,000 population progress to rest pain and critical limb ischemia (Fontaine stages III and IV).[4] In the United Kingdom, about 50,000 patients each year are admitted urgently to hospital for the management of severely disabling peripheral arterial disease (ABPI typically < 0.5).

Critical limb ischemia secondary to acute thromboembolic occlusion of a peripheral artery accounts for at least 10% to 16% of a vascular surgeon's caseload and still carries a 15% 30-day mortality despite recent developments in immediate

TABLE 111–1. FONTAINE CLASSIFICATION OF CHRONIC LEG ISCHEMIA

Stage I	Asymptomatic
Stage II	Intermittent claudication
Stage III	Ischemic rest pain
Stage IV	Ulceration, gangrene, or both

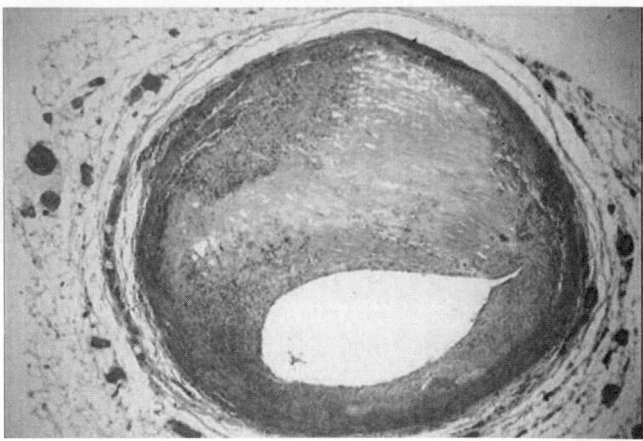

FIGURE 111–2. Histologic appearance of an atherosclerotic plaque illustrating infiltration with macrophages (which turn into foam cells) and acute inflammation, together with lipid accumulation and extracellular matrix expansion. A fibrous cap appears, which often ruptures, leading to platelet aggregation and acute thrombotic occlusion of the vessel.

management and revascularization techniques.[5] Patients with peripheral arterial disease have a considerably reduced survival (30% 5-year mortality) mainly due to atherosclerotic complications in other vascular territories.[6] Several studies have shown a clear relationship between ABPI and outcome (Fig. 111-1),[7] which highlights, not surprisingly, that more severe peripheral arterial disease tends to be associated with more severe coronary artery disease and shortened survival.

Cigarette smoking is the most powerful risk factor in the development of peripheral arterial disease. Smoking accounted for over 80% of cases of peripheral arterial disease in the Framingham study,[8,9] and most lower limb outcomes (e.g., amputation rates, patency of bypass grafts, and ischemic ulcer formation) are significantly worse in current or recent smokers. Similarly, diabetes and hypercholesterolemia are major risk factors associated with the development, progression, and complications of atherosclerosis in the legs. Amputation rates among diabetics are 15 to 70 times higher than in nondiabetics. Hypertension is also an important risk factor for peripheral arterial disease; high blood pressure increases the risk of intermittent claudication by a factor of three.

ATHEROSCLEROSIS OF LOWER LIMB ARTERIES

Atherogenesis is best described in three stages: initiation of the atherosclerotic lesion, progression, and plaque complications. During the initiation process, fatty streaks occur on the endothelial surface of the vessel and mononuclear leukocytes begin to invade the intima as part of a cytokine-mediated process of migration of inflammatory cells. These leukocytes (macrophages) steadily accumulate lipid and become foam cells. The fatty streak gradually progresses into an atherosclerotic plaque, which begins to encroach on the lumen of the vessel (Fig. 111-2). The iliac arteries and the superficial femoral artery in the lower limb are especially prone to

plaque formation. Smooth muscle cells also migrate and accumulate within the atherosclerotic plaque, and a fibrous extracellular matrix develops.

The complications that occur in atherosclerotic plaques include intraplaque hemorrhage and cap rupture or ulceration, which in turn lead to superimposed thrombus formation and complete vessel occlusion (Fig. 111-3). Such events are often limb or life threatening. Rupture or fissuring of a plaque exposes the lipid core, which in turn activates platelets and the clotting cascade. Clumps of platelets may remain firmly attached to the plaque, resulting in more severe stenosis or complete occlusion of the lumen, or they may detach to form emboli that will lodge in smaller vessels downstream from the culprit lesion.

ACUTE LIMB ISCHEMIA

CLINICAL PRESENTATION AND ETIOLOGY

Acute lower limb ischemia is common (14 cases annually per 100,000 population)[10] and can present with a range of different signs and symptoms. The Society for Vascular Surgery and the International Society for Cardiovascular

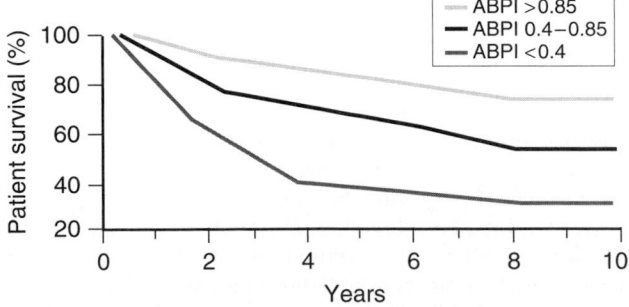

FIGURE 111–1. Relationship between ankle-brachial pressure index (ABPI) and survival in patients with symptomatic peripheral artery disease. This clearly illustrates how cardiovascular mortality increases in proportion to the severity of peripheral artery disease. (Modified with permission from McKenna M, Wolfson S, Kuller L: The ratio of ankle and arm arterial pressure as an independent predictor of mortality. Atherosclerosis 1991;87:119-128.)

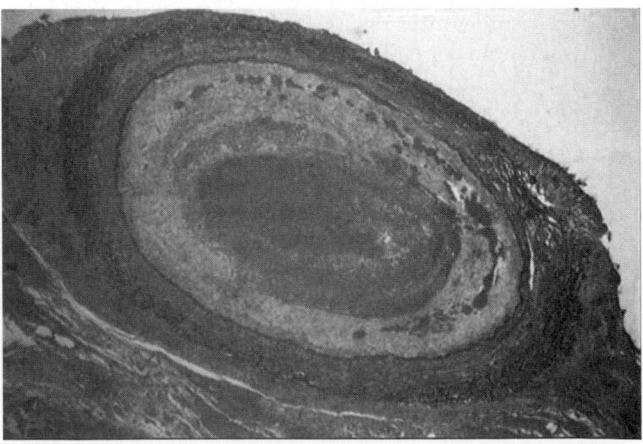

FIGURE 111–3. Acute thrombotic occlusion of a ruptured atherosclerotic plaque causing acute limb ischemia.

TABLE 111–2. CLINICAL CLASSIFICATION OF ACUTE LIMB ISCHEMIA

| Category | Description/Prognosis | Findings | | Doppler Signals | |
		Sensory Loss	Muscle Weakness	Arterial	Venous
I. Viable	Not immediately threatened	None	None	Audible	Audible
II. Threatened					
Marginally	Salvageable if promptly treated	Minimal (toes) or none	None	(Often) Inaudible	Audible
Immediately	Salvageable with immediate revascularization	More than toes, associated with rest pain	Mild, moderate	(Usually) Inaudible	Audible
III. Irreversible	Major tissue loss or permanent nerve damage inevitable	Profound, anesthetic	Profound, paralysis (rigor)	Inaudible	Inaudible

Surgery (SVS/ISCVS) have produced a classification system for acute limb ischemia that has been modified by Rutherford and colleagues[11] to improve its prognostic utility (Table 111-2).

The presentation of acute lower limb ischemia is strongly influenced by two factors: (1) the presence or absence of a preexisting collateral circulation and (2) the etiology of the occlusion (Table 111-3). In patients with previously normal arteries, the symptoms of acute lower limb ischemia are likely to be much more severe and abrupt in onset because there is unlikely to be any collateral circulation providing distal perfusion. Tissue ischemia downstream of the occlusion causes intense rest pain. In the absence of collateral flow, there is even greater urgency to restore perfusion to avoid irreversible tissue necrosis and/or permanent disability.

Inquiring in the history about the mode of onset of pain may allow some differentiation between primary thrombotic occlusion and those patients presenting with abrupt onset embolic occlusion. The presence or absence of any prior symptoms of peripheral arterial disease is important. Patients with moderate-to-severe intermittent claudication before the onset of acute lower limb ischemia are likely to have developed some degree of collateral circulation, and therefore the onset of acute lower limb ischemia may cause little more than a slight worsening of their usual lower limb symptoms.

Physical examination may reveal a classic acutely ischemic limb: it is pale, painful, cold, pulseless, paralyzed, and insensate. The presence of paralysis or paresthesia indicates a poor prognosis because of likely infarction of nerve and muscle tissue; at this stage primary amputation may be the most appropriate treatment option. Examination of the patient should also include the pulse rhythm and electrocardiogram to identify those patients in atrial fibrillation and a full assessment of the vascular supply to the contralateral limb.

The two most common causes of acute lower limb ischemia are primary thrombosis of a diseased native vessel or graft and embolic occlusion of an artery. Differentiation of these two causes is important because the approach to management is different. Embolectomy performed on a diseased artery may increase the risk of further thrombus formation and cause iatrogenic trauma to the vessel, in turn worsening limb ischemia. Primary thrombotic occlusion (e.g., following plaque rupture, see Fig. 111-3) is now the most common cause of acute lower limb ischemia because anticoagulants are used more widely in atrial fibrillation and the incidence of rheumatic heart disease is diminishing. Approximately 85% of acute peripheral arterial occlusions are now due to primary occlusion and 15% are secondary to embolism.[12,13]

UPPER LIMB ISCHEMIA

Acute limb ischemia is much more common in the leg compared with the upper limb. Upper limb ischemia accounts for 16.6% of all acute peripheral ischemic events.[14] Differentiation into acute and chronic ischemia in the upper limb is difficult owing to the rich collateral circulation present normally within the arm, allowing fairly severe disease to remain relatively asymptomatic. Embolic occlusion in the upper limb is much more common than primary thrombotic occlusion because the arm is seldom affected by atherosclerosis, but the principles of management are similar.

INVESTIGATIONS

Patients with a suspected embolic occlusion should ideally undergo radiologic investigation to confirm the level of occlusion, assuming time and expertise are available. Previously, this was routinely achieved by use of intra-arterial contrast angiography, but there have been concerns about delays to treatment and the risk of contrast nephrotoxicity. In addition, the technical limitations of angiography include poor resolution in low-flow states and the diagnosis of aneurysms is difficult (especially popliteal artery aneurysms). Thus, more recently, duplex ultrasound has been preferred for the diagnosis of acute arterial occlusion.

TABLE 111–3. ETIOLOGY OF ACUTE LIMB ISCHEMIA

Causes of Acute Occlusions of Peripheral Arteries in Patients With Preexisting Atherosclerotic Disease

- Thrombosis of native artery with atherosclerotic stenosis
- Thrombosis of arterial bypass graft
- Embolism from heart, aneurysm, atherosclerotic plaque, or critical stenosis upstream (including cholesterol or atherothrombotic emboli during endovascular procedures)
- Thrombosed aneurysm (especially popliteal)

Causes of Acute Critical Limb Ischemia in Patients Without Preexisting Atherosclerotic Disease

- Arterial trauma (especially iatrogenic)
- Arterial dissection
- Arteritis with thrombosis (e.g., giant cell arteritis)
- Spontaneous thrombosis with hypercoagulable state
- Popliteal cyst with thrombosis
- Popliteal entrapment with thrombosis
- Vasospasm with thrombosis (e.g., ergotism)

TABLE 111–4. CONTRAINDICATIONS TO USE OF THROMBOLYSIS IN ACUTE LIMB ISCHEMIA

Absolute Contraindications

- Active bleeding diathesis
- Acute gastroduodenal ulcers and/or recent gastrointestinal hemorrhage (within previous 10 days)
- History of stroke (excluding transient ischemic attack) in the previous 2 months
- Neurosurgery (intracranial, spinal) within the previous 3 months
- Intracranial trauma within the previous 3 months

Relative Contraindications

- Major nonvascular surgery or trauma within previous 10 days
- Cardiopulmonary resuscitation within previous 10 days
- Uncontrolled hypertension (systolic >180 mm Hg, diastolic >110 mm Hg)
- Puncture of uncompressible vessel
- Intracranial neoplasm
- Mitral valve disease
- Recent eye surgery
- Aneurysm, especially silent, intracerebral vascular malformations

Minor Contraindications

- Renal or hepatic insufficiency (especially if associated with coagulopathy)
- Bacterial endocarditis
- Pregnancy
- Diabetic hemorrhagic retinopathy
- Antiplatelet therapy

The use of duplex ultrasonography is well established in the diagnosis of chronic limb ischemia, but there is often difficulty in visualizing the aortoiliac segments owing to overlying bowel gas, obesity, and/or calcification and marked tortuosity of the iliac vessels. Nevertheless, a well-trained vascular technician acting in conjunction with a vascular surgeon can usually make an adequate assessment of the level of occlusion to plan management.

TREATMENT

Endovascular treatment of acute lower limb occlusion may involve suction embolectomy or local administration of thrombolytic therapy. A thrombolysis catheter is introduced into the thrombus, and a lytic agent such as urokinase or recombinant tissue plasminogen activator (rTPA) is delivered directly onto the occlusion.[27] Endovascular treatment of the underlying stenosis may also be attempted at this time (e.g., via balloon angioplasty or stent deployment).

Thrombolysis is indicated in patients who present early (<14 days' duration) with a primary thrombotic occlusion and those who are unsuitable or unfit for surgical embolectomy. The indications and contraindications for thrombolysis are shown in Table 111-4. Although direct thrombolysis avoids many of the risks of surgery, there are other potentially serious complications even though the thrombolytic is administered locally, such as stroke (1.2% to 2.3%), major hemorrhage (5.1%), distal embolization (5%), and compartment syndrome due to rapid reperfusion of the ischemic limb (2%).[10,15,16,28] In the case of an acute, severely ischemic limb, surgery is indicated to perform either embolectomy or primary amputation of an irreversibly infracted lower limb. Unless the history is clearly one of an embolic event, preoperative duplex or angiographic confirmation is required. Heparin (100 to 150 units/kg) is initiated immediately, and the patient is transferred to the operating room. For a femoral artery embolectomy, the procedure may be undertaken under local anesthesia, but close monitoring is mandatory given the high incidence of cardiovascular events in this population. In the case of primary thrombotic occlusion of a diseased vessel, arterial reconstruction is often required after angiography.

The outcome after peripheral artery embolism is often poor: mortality at 30 days is 15%, and amputation occurs in 10% to 30% of patients.[5] Identifying the source of the embolus is important by using echocardiography and ultrasound of the aorta.

CHRONIC CRITICAL LIMB ISCHEMIA

Critical limb ischemia is defined in nondiabetic patients as the presence of rest pain or tissue necrosis (ulceration or gangrene), with an ankle systolic pressure of less than 50 mm Hg or a toe pressure of less than 30 mm Hg[17] (ankle and toe pressures in diabetics may be artificially raised). These patients have a significant risk of limb loss, as well as a high cardiovascular and overall mortality rate. The management of chronic critical limb ischemia centers on restoring blood flow to the extremity by endovascular or surgical therapy.[29]

However, some patients present more urgently with an episode of "acute on chronic" limb ischemia. This requires prompt investigation and treatment to avoid long-term tissue loss and preserve the leg. These patients may, surprisingly, volunteer relatively few symptoms because their preexisting collateral vessels may be almost sufficient to nourish the limb. Patients without such well-developed collaterals will present more acutely with the classic findings of intense rest pain and signs of decreased perfusion. Some degree of tissue loss or necrosis may be present at diagnosis, and both lower limbs may be similarly affected.

TABLE 111–5. PATENCY RATES AFTER ENDOVASCULAR TREATMENT OF PERIPHERAL ARTERIAL DISEASE

| Study | Segment | Patency | | Time (yr) |
		Primary	Secondary	
Henry, et al.[19]	Superficial femoral	65%		4
	Popliteal	50%		4
Capek, et al.[26]	Femoropopliteal	81%		1
		61%		3
		58%		5
Jamsen, et al.[24]	Femoropopliteal	46%	63%	1
		31%	50%	3
		25%	41%	5

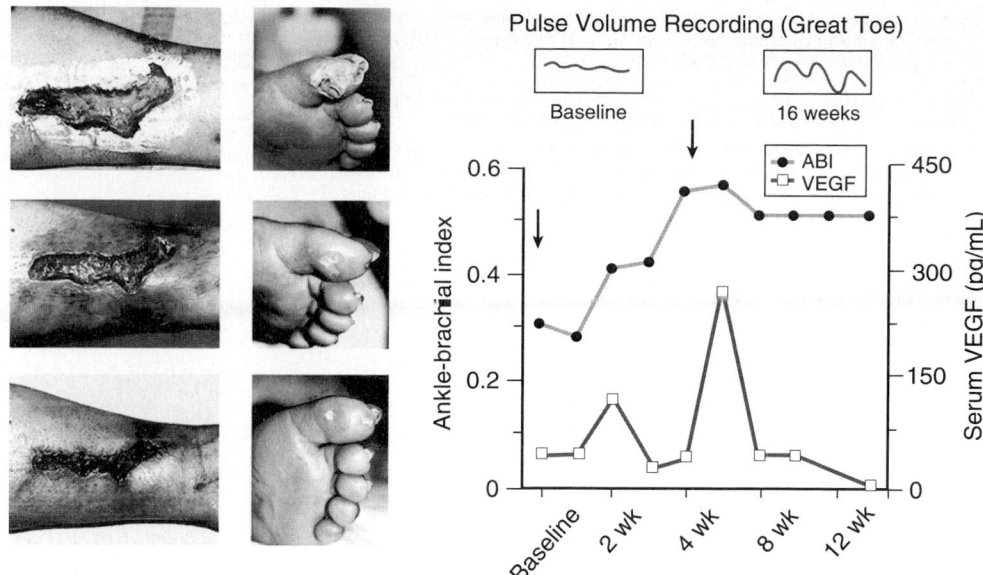

FIGURE 111–4. Therapeutic angiogenesis stimulates new vessel formation to develop collaterals. After intramuscular administration of naked DNA for VEGF in a patient with critical limb ischemia, there is evidence of VEGF formation and increased serum levels of VEGF associated with improved ABPI and resolution of ischemic tissue damage. (Reproduced with permission from Baumgartner I, Pieczek A, Manor O, et al: Constitutive expression of phVEGF165 after intramuscular gene transfer promotes collateral vessel development in patients with critical limb ischemia. Circulation 1998;97:1114-1123. Copyright 1998, American Heart Association.)

After angiographic assessment, the initial management should be endovascular. This is now accepted as first-line therapy and is usually successful (>85% restoration of perfusion). Patency rates for endovascular and surgical interventions depend on the site of intervention and the state of the distal vessels (degree of distal "run-off"). For example, iliac artery angioplasty has a 73% patency rate at 3 years if the run-off vessels are patent but only 30% patency if the distal vessels are also diseased.[18] Another study showed a 77% secondary patency rate at 6 years (secondary patency indicates that the vessel remains patent with the assistance of further interventions). Stenting in the iliac arteries is well established, increasing the patency of endovascular therapy to 86% at 4 years.[19] Results of angioplasty in the femoropopliteal vessels are less impressive, with a wide variety in the reported rates of primary and secondary patency. Some of these results are summarized in Table 111-5.

Analysis of pooled results from five separate studies[20-24] (n = 980) showed a 5-year patency rate after endovascular therapy of 41.9%, although the majority of these patients had intermittent claudication rather than critical limb ischemia. Surgery for similarly diseased segments, in those with critical ischemia, had a primary patency rate of 52% to 63% at 5 years, with corresponding limb salvage rates of 85% to 87%. Stenting in the infrainguinal arteries has not been shown to improve on the patency rates of bypass surgery and is therefore usually reserved for primary angioplasty failures.

NEW THERAPEUTIC APPROACHES

The management of peripheral arterial disease in general is steadily becoming more minimally invasive (e.g., with the wider application of endovascular approaches to abdominal aortic aneurysm repair and use of carotid artery angioplasty and stenting in place of endarterectomy). However, in the lower limbs, diffuse, distal, and/or bilateral disease is seldom amenable to a localized endovascular procedure. Angioplasty and stenting are mostly reserved for those patients with discrete, proximal, and unilateral stenoses (e.g., in the iliac vessels).

THERAPEUTIC ANGIOGENESIS

A novel development in this area includes therapeutic angiogenesis, which is the administration of naked DNA or recombinant proteins for vascular growth factors (e.g., vascular endothelial growth factor [VEGF] or basic fibroblast growth factor [bFGF]) to stimulate endothelial cell replication and migration to form new collateral vessels from existing vascular structures. Large placebo-controlled trials[25] have shown evidence that therapeutic angiogenesis may be effective in limb salvage in critical ischemia and in symptom relief for less acute forms of peripheral arterial disease, such as intermittent claudication (Fig. 111-4).

ANNOTATED REFERENCES

Bailey CM, Saha S, Magee TR, Galland RB: A 1 year prospective study of management and outcome of patients presenting with critical lower limb ischaemia. Eur J Vasc Endovasc Surg 2003;25:131-134.

A single-center prospective study of 134 patients with critical limb ischemia (Fontaine stages III and IV). Mortality and limb salvage rates of 27% and 61%, respectively, were achieved. This article includes data on both acute and chronic presentations of this disease.

Conrad MF, Shepard AD, Rubinfield IS, et al: Long-term results of catheter-directed thrombolysis to treat infrainguinal bypass graft occlusion: The urokinase era. J Vasc Surg 2003;37:1009-1016.

A prospective study assessing the efficacy and outcome of thrombolysis in 69 acute infrainguinal arterial bypass graft occlusions. Thrombolysis and endovascular therapy of any identified causative stenoses can achieve similar results to surgery in occluded vein bypass grafts.

Jamsen TS, Manninen HI, Jaakola PA, Matsi PJ: Long-term outcome of patients with claudication after balloon angioplasty of the femoropopliteal arteries. Radiology 2002;225:345-352.

A prospective single-center study indicating primary and secondary patency rates after percutaneous transluminal angioplasty (PTA) of the infrainguinal arteries in 218 limbs.

Ouriel K: Comparison of surgical and thrombolytic treatment of peripheral arterial disease. Rev Cardiovasc Med 2002;3(Suppl 2):S7-S16.

A review of the etiology of acute limb ischemia as well as of the efficacy of thrombolysis and surgery for the treatment of acute peripheral arterial occlusion. Included are data from the Rochester, STILE, and TOPAS trials.

Rutherford RB, Baker JD, Ernst C, et al: Recommended standards for reports dealing with lower extremity ischemia: Revised version. J Vasc Surg 1997;26:517-538.

A suggested revision of the standard used for analyzing and reporting lower extremity ischemia initially approved by the Joint Council of the Society for Vascular Surgery and the North American Chapter of the International Society for Cardiovascular Surgery.

Section VI

HEPATIC DISORDERS, GASTROINTESTINAL DISORDERS, AND NUTRITIONAL SUPPORT

Chapter 112

CRITICAL CARE NUTRITION

Stephen A. McClave • Daren K. Heyland

KEY POINTS

1. A paradigm shift in thinking has occurred, whereby nutritional therapy in the ICU is no longer considered adjunctive supportive care but rather a primary therapeutic strategy capable of favorably altering patient outcome.

2. Failure to use the gut following a major insult or injury leads to loss of functional and structural integrity, increased permeability, greater systemic bacterial challenge, increased oxidative stress, and a proinflammatory up-regulation of immune responses.

3. Providing enteral nutrition may set the tone for the systemic immune response by stimulating specific CD4 helper T-cell pathways and the release of associated cytokines involved with tolerance (Th3 and Tr1 cells) and down-regulation of inflammation (Th2 cells).

4. A number of management strategies help reduce the risk of enteral nutrition, such as feeding past the stomach directly into the small bowel, elevating the head of the bed 30 to 45 degrees, using promotility agents, and using nurse-directed feeding protocols.

5. The greater the severity of critical illness, the more important the issues of gut integrity and permeability become, and the more likely it is that enteral nutrition will improve clinical outcome compared with parenteral nutrition.

6. Small-volume "trophic" or "trickle" feeds may not be sufficient to maintain gut integrity and contain permeability; 50% to 60% of goal calories (i.e., caloric requirements) may be needed to achieve the therapeutic endpoints of enteral nutrition.

7. Arginine-supplemented immune formulas improve outcome (less infection and shorter hospital length of stay) in selected groups, such as patients undergoing major elective surgery, compared with standard enteral formulas; however, they may worsen outcome (excess mortality) in others, such as patients who are septic.

8. Glutamine supplementation (parenterally more so than enterally) may reduce mortality and infectious complications in certain critically ill populations.

9. Although the enteral route is always the first choice for nutritional support in critically ill patients, surprisingly, standard therapy (no artificial nutritional support) is associated with a better outcome than parenteral nutrition over the first 7 to 10 days when enteral nutrition is not feasible.

10. In the few specific circumstances in which parenteral nutrition is indicated, its efficacy may be maximized by strict control of blood glucose, permissive underfeeding, and withholding lipids for the first 7 to 10 days.

The overall efficacy of nutritional support, the need to start nutritional therapy in the first place, and its likelihood to impact patient outcome are all determined by a number of clinical factors. Not all patients need nutritional support. Individual patient selection and the specific disease processes involved are the most important issues. The appropriate route or specific design of therapy for one disease process cannot necessarily be extrapolated (or expected to be effective) for a different disease process. Severity of illness within the patient population, level of physiologic stress, and baseline nutritional status before injury often determine a patient's need for and response to nutritional therapy. Even in specific cases in which nutritional therapy is indicated, factors related to overall amount, content, route, and timing may determine whether nutritional support influences outcome or is rendered ineffective.

There has been a paradigm shift in the thinking about the true value of nutritional support in the intensive care setting. In the past, the goals of nutritional support were to provide adjunctive therapy to support the stress response, provide exogenous nutrients to reduce the drain on endogenous stores and the depletion of lean body mass, and prevent the consequences of protein calorie malnutrition. Today, the provision of early enteral feeding to critically ill patients is seen as a therapeutic tool or strategy to attenuate disease severity, modulate the immune response, reduce complications, and favorably impact patient outcome. Attaining access and initiating enteral feeding is considered part of the basic resuscitation of a critically ill patient. Although any artificial nutritional support involves some risk to the patient, providing early enteral feeding is clearly an integral component of what should be considered optimal care.

GUT USE AND THE DIFFERENTIAL RESPONSE TO FEEDING AND STARVATION

The functional and structural integrity of the gastrointestinal (GI) tract is affected by whether the gut is used and the patient receives enteral feeding. Animal and human studies suggest that enteral feeding maintains mucosal mass, stimulates cellular proliferation and production of brush border enzymes, and maintains villus height.[1-3] Enteral nutrients maintain the integrity of the tight junctions between the intestinal epithelial cells; stimulate blood flow to the gut; and promote the release of a variety of endogenous agents, such as cholecystokinin, gastrin, bombesin, and bile salts, that have trophic effects on the intestinal epithelium. Bombesin, for example, can reverse all the histologic and functional deficits caused by parenteral feeding,[4] and gastrin and cholecystokinin can encourage partial recovery of gut-associated lymphoid tissue after the use of parenteral nutrition (PN).[5] Secretory immunoglobulin A (sIgA) and the production of bile salts help coat bacteria within the GI tract, preventing adherence; along with the production of mucus and good GI contractility, this helps wash away bacteria in a caudad direction.[2] These mechanisms, together with antimicrobial secretions such as pancreatic enzymes, proteases, and lactoferrin, help keep the total number of bacteria in check. The normal, predominant, anaerobic flora of the gut is maintained, preventing overgrowth of more pathogenic organisms such as Enterobacteriaceae, a process referred to as colonization resistance.[6]

Gut disuse, with or without PN, can lead to deterioration of the functional and structural integrity of the gut. In animals, gut disuse is associated with a marked reduction in villus height, cellular proliferation, mucosal mass, and brush border enzymes. The intestinal changes caused by starvation in humans are less pronounced than in rodents. Whereas gut disuse may result in a 40% decrease of mucosal mass in rats, the decrease in humans is about 10% to 15%.[1] In humans, loss of villus height in response to pancreatitis is diminished by enteral feeding.[3] Villus atrophy is perpetuated in a time-dependent fashion with parenteral feeding.[3] Starvation alone may not be sufficient to increase gut permeability, but injury followed by starvation increases mucosal permeability.[2] The degree of increased gut permeability correlates directly with the severity of disease.[7] The degree of gut hyperpermeability correlates inversely with the percentage of goal calories provided by enteral feeding in burn patients.[8]

Lack of feeding in animals has been shown to result in bacterial overgrowth and loss of mucosal defenses against bacterial invasion.[6,9] Reduced peristalsis (ileus) can contribute to the bacterial overgrowth. Reduced secretions of bile salts and sIgA promote bacterial adherence to the mucosa. Bacterial translocation is associated with aerobic bacterial overgrowth and decreased intestinal sIgA levels.[2] Whether translocation involves live bacteria or simply their products (especially endotoxin) is not clear. Portal venous bacteremia has not been well documented in humans[10]; however, microbial DNA testing has shown that translocation of bacteria from the gut may be a major source of contamination in patients who appear to be septic but are culture negative and have no obvious site of infection.[11] Moreover, recent animal studies suggest that these gut-derived factors can reach the systemic circulation via the lymphatic system rather than via the portal bloodstream and thereby cause distant organ injury.[12] Infusion of even small doses of endotoxin in normal volunteers increases gut mucosal permeability.[6] Increases in gut permeability are associated with systemic endotoxemia in humans.[7,13] Among burn patients, infection is associated with increased gut

mucosal permeability.[8] Increases in gut permeability in critically ill patients correlate with the development of organ dysfunction.[14]

The intestinal secretion of sIgA is diminished within 5 days of gut disuse, with or without PN.[4,15] Respiratory secretion of IgA may be diminished even sooner. Reduction in the mucosal mass of gut-associated lymphoid tissue and decreased sIgA production increase susceptibility to infections normally controlled by IgA-mediated defenses in experimental animals.[16] In mice, as little as 5 days of gut disuse with PN results in loss of protection against respiratory viral infection and reduces clearance of the virus.[17] Refeeding with enteral nutrients restores antiviral defenses. Established antiviral mucosal immunity is lost when the GI tract is not stimulated by enteral feeding.[16]

The dendritic macrophages act as antigen-presenting cells, which release cytokines and activate naive CD4 T cells (Th$_O$).[18] Secretion of interleukin (IL)-12 stimulates the naive cells to differentiate into T helper 1 (Th1) lymphocytes, favoring a proinflammatory response and the release of other proinflammatory cytokines such as IL-2, interferon gamma (IFN-γ), and tumor necrosis factor (TNF). Th1 responses are associated with increased inflammation and are essential for host defenses against infection. Uncontrolled Th1 responses, however, can result in self-injury. Production of IL-4 also stimulates differentiation of Th$_O$ into T helper 2 (Th2) lymphocytes,[18] leading to secretion of (additional) IL-4, IL-6, and IL-10. The Th2 response tends to curb or check the Th1 inflammatory response. Th2 responses are essential to prevent self-injury caused by inflammation. However, excessive regulation of inflammatory responses by Th2 cytokines can lead to immune suppression.[18]

Normal enteral feeding stimulates the proliferation of Th2 CD4$^+$ helper T lymphocytes and the production and release of IgA-stimulating cytokines, including IL-4, IL-5, IL-6, IL-10, and IL-13.[19] This process is normally counterbalanced by the proliferation of Th1 CD4$^+$ helper T lymphocytes and IgA-inhibitory cytokines, including interferon-β (IFN-β), TNF, and IL-2. IL-4 stimulates naive CD4$^+$ helper T lymphocytes to convert to IgA-positive B cells in Peyer's patches. IL-10, IL-5, and IL-6 stimulate the differentiation of IgA-positive B cells into sIgA-secreting plasma cells in the lamina propria.[16]

Gut disuse, with or without PN, alters the balance of these lymphocyte populations and the profile of associated cytokines. In animals, gut disuse with PN for 5 days decreases IL-4 and IL-10 secretion and markedly reduces sIgA levels.[16] In human babies, use of PN reduces sIgA in intestinal immunocytes.[20] IFN-β, IL-5, and IL-6 production by Th1 lymphocytes is not affected by gut disuse and PN.[21] Thus, the absence of enteral nutrition (EN) can unbalance the ratio of pro- to anti-inflammatory responses.

Gut disuse affects the expression of adhesion molecules required for proper homing by naive B cells to the intestinal lamina propria and gut-associated lymphoid tissue. MADCAM-1 is the primary ligand required for the proper homing of B cells, and decreased expression of this molecule interferes with the normal migration of B cells from the vascular space into the lamina propria, leading to atrophy of Peyer's patches. In animals, there is a 60% decrease in MADCAM-1 expression within 4 days of initiating PN.[16] Within 3 days of starting PN, the number of T and B cells in the lamina propria and Peyer's patches decreases by about 50%.[2] In this model, secretion of the Th1 cytokine IFN-γ is unchanged, but secretion of the Th2 cytokines IL-4 and IL-10 decreases. Decreased production of IL-4 and IL-10 leads to increased expression of the adhesion molecules ICAM-1 and E-selectin in both the intestinal and pulmonary microvasculature. Increased E-selectin expression on endothelial cells in the pulmonary microvasculature promotes sequestration and extravasation of polymorphonuclear neutrophils.[22-24] As a result, any subsequent injury (e.g., ischemia-reperfusion) can promote the accumulation of polymorphonuclear neutrophils in the lungs, exacerbating organ injury and even increasing mortality.[25,26]

Approximately 1 ton of food passes through the intestinal tract of an adult human every year.[20] About 1/100,000 of this intake represents intact immunologic antigen.[20] Oral tolerance refers to the process whereby the immune response is down-regulated to prevent excessive responses to common antigens found in food and in the commensal bacterial flora of the GI tract. During the induction of oral tolerance, an alternative pathway for CD4+ helper T cell activation leads to proliferation of special regulatory T cells (Th3 and Tr1), which produce the counterregulatory cytokines IL-10 and transforming growth factor beta (TGF-β).[20] The stimulation and proliferation of Th3 cells induced by enteral feeding therefore promotes the expression of a balanced Th2-Th1 profile. The large dietary and indigenous microbial antigenic load is extremely important for maintaining normal mucosal immunity.[20] The antigenic constituents of food clearly exert a stimulatory effect on the intestinal B-cell system, helping to explain why enteral feeding supports a high density of IgA-secreting immunocytes within the intestinal lamina propria. Continued enteral feeding, as well as maintenance of the indigenous microbial flora in the gut, may help keep a balance between the Th1 and Th2 profile and prevent an exaggerated Th1 inflammatory response.

The importance of EN for modulating the inflammatory response was illustrated by a classic study of human volunteers challenged with a small dose of *Escherichia coli* lipopolysaccharide (endotoxin).[27] One group of subjects was maintained for 1 week without feeding and received PN, whereas another group was fed enterally during the same period. After 7 days of either PN or EN, both groups were challenged with lipopolysaccharide. The subjects in the PN group had an exaggerated response to the proinflammatory stimulus, manifested by higher circulating levels of cortisol and TNF, among other findings. Similarly, following injury or an inflammatory disease process, early enteral feeding can blunt the hypermetabolic response.[28,29] Among patients with acute pancreatitis, those fed enterally rather than parenterally had significantly lower circulating levels of C-reactive protein, less evidence of oxidative stress, faster resolution of systemic inflammatory response syndrome (SIRS), and a greater decreases in their acute physiology and chronic health evaluation (APACHE) II scores over a week of nutritional therapy.[13] In another study of patients with acute pancreatitis, there was faster resolution of the disease process among patients treated with enteral feeding compared with similar patients receiving PN.[30]

The traditional model of SIRS and the compensatory anti-inflammatory response syndrome (CARS) described in trauma and sepsis may be influenced by the differential immunologic response between enteral feeding and starvation or gut disuse.[31] In SIRS, there appears to be an up-regulated, nonspecific activation of the innate immune system, with an increase in the proinflammatory cytokines IL-1, TNF, IL-2, and IFN-γ. This profile is similar to that of the Th1 subset response (in which IFN-γ, TNF, and IL-2 are produced). Intracellular bacteria and viruses absorbed through the intestinal epithelium may activate dendritic cells, macrophages, and natural killer cells to produce IL-2 and IFN-γ, which causes naive CD4 cells to proliferate into Th1 cells. CARS, in contrast, appears to be a pattern of macrophage deactivation, reduced antigen presentation, and T-cell anergy, which results in a shift of the T helper cell pattern to a Th2 response.[31] Gut disuse following injury or illness may promote a SIRS response through stimulation of both the innate immune system (causing a hyperinflammatory response from macrophages and natural killer cells) and the acquired immune system (resulting in a shift from a Th2 to a Th1 profile).

Compared with the metabolic response to enteral feeding, this exaggerated stress response to gut disuse with or without PN has been shown to exacerbate disease severity, increase the rate of complications, and lead to prolongation of the disease process.[13,30]

THE IMPACT OF ENTERAL NUTRITION ON OUTCOME

Based on the theoretical rationale presented earlier, EN should be associated with improved clinical outcomes in critically ill patients. To evaluate the clinical evidence in support of using EN, we considered three groups of studies. The first are randomized trials that directly compared EN and PN. The second group includes studies that compared early EN (started within 24 to 48 hours of resuscitation) to more delayed forms of nutritional support (e.g., delayed EN, PN, or oral diet). The third group includes studies that evaluated various methods of delivering EN.

A recently published systematic analysis reviewed data from 13 randomized, controlled studies comparing EN and PN in heterogeneous populations of ICU patients, including those with head trauma, abdominal trauma, sepsis, and severe acute pancreatitis, among other conditions.[32] When a meta-analysis was carried out, there was no apparent difference in mortality rate between patients treated with EN and those treated with PN (relative risk [RR] 1.08; 95% confidence interval [CI] 0.70 to 1.65; Fig. 112-1). However, compared with PN, EN was associated with a significant reduction in infectious complications (RR 0.61; 95% CI 0.44 to 0.84; Fig. 112-2).

Eight randomized, controlled trials that compared early EN with more delayed forms of nutrition were recently reviewed and analyzed.[32] When these studies were aggregated, early EN was associated with treatment benefits that approached statistical significance. Early EN was associated with reduced mortality (RR 0.52; 95% CI 0.25 to 1.08; Fig. 112-3) and fewer infectious complications (RR 0.66; 95% CI 0.36 to 1.22; Fig. 112-4) compared with delayed nutrient intake. These differences approached but did not achieve statistical significance. No differences in length of hospital stay were observed between the groups. All seven studies that reported nutritional endpoints (e.g., nitrogen balance) showed a significant benefit for early EN. There were no differences in complications between the groups.

A number of strategies can be employed to maximize the delivery of EN while minimizing the risks of gastric colonization, gastroesophageal regurgitation, and pulmonary

Comparison: 01 EN vs PN
Outcome: 02 Mortality

Study	EN n/N	PN n/N	RR (95%CI Random)	Weight %	RR (95%CI Random)	Year
Adams	1/23	3/23		3.5	0.33(0.04,2.97)	1986
Borzotta	5/28	1/21		3.8	3.75(0.47,29.75)	1994
Cerra	7/31	8/35		14.1	0.99(0.40,2.41)	1998
Dunham	1/12	1/15		2.4	1.25(0.09,17.98)	1994
Hadfield	2/13	6/11		7.6	0.28(0.07,1.13)	1995
Hadley	3/21	2/24		5.5	1.71(0.32,9.30)	1986
Kalfarentzos	1/18	2/20		3.1	0.56(0.05,5.62)	1997
Kudsk	1/51	1/45		2.3	0.88(0.06,13.70)	1992
Moore 1992	8/118	11/112		14.5	0.69(0.29,1.65)	1992
Rapp	9/18	3/20		10.2	3.33(1.07,10.43)	1983
Woodcock	9/17	5/21		14.2	2.22(0.92,5.40)	2001
Young	10/28	10/23		18.9	0.82(0.42,1.62)	1987
Total (95% CI)	57/378	53/370		100.0	1.08(0.70,1.65)	

Test for heterogeneity chi-square = 14.70 df = 11 p = 0.2

Test for overall effect z = 0.34 p = 0.7

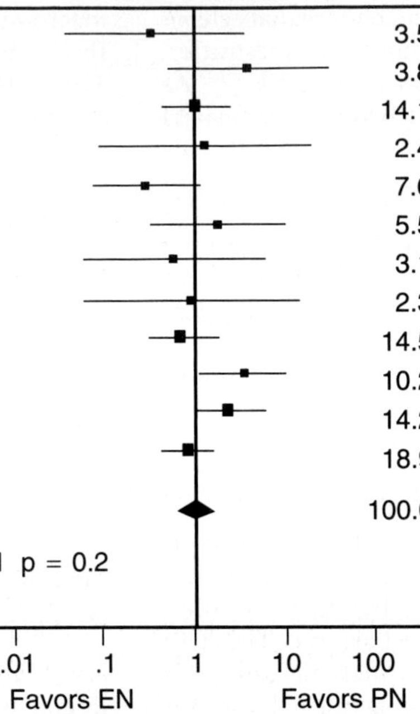

```
        .01    .1      1      10    100
           Favors EN         Favors PN
```

FIGURE 112–1. Studies comparing parenteral nutrition (PN) and enteral nutrition (EN) in terms of effect on mortality. CI, confidence interval; RR, relative risk.

aspiration (Table 112-1). By delivering enteral feeds into the small bowel beyond the pylorus, the frequency of regurgitation and aspiration is decreased.[33] In a recent meta-analysis, there were seven randomized trials that evaluated the effect of route of feeding on rates of ventilator-associated pneumonia.[34] When these results were aggregated, there was a significant reduction in ventilator-associated pneumonia with feeding distal to the pylorus (RR 0.76; 95% CI 0.59 to 0.99). These studies also demonstrated that small bowel feeding is associated with an increase in protein and calories delivered and a shorter time to attain the target dose of nutrition.

Unless logistic problems represent an unacceptable hurdle, we recommend the routine use of small bowel feedings. If routine use of this strategy is not feasible, small bowel feedings should be considered for patients at high risk for intolerance to EN (e.g., patients receiving inotropic or vasoactive drugs, continuous infusion of sedatives, or paralytic agents or those with large volumes of nasogastric drainage) or at high risk for regurgitation and aspiration (e.g., patients nursed in the supine position). Finally, if obtaining small bowel access is not feasible (e.g., because access to fluoroscopy or endoscopy is limited and blind techniques are not reliable), small bowel feedings should be considered for selected patients who repeatedly have large gastric residual volumes and are not tolerating adequate amounts of EN intragastrically.[32] Additional strategies to maximize the benefits of EN while minimizing the risks (see Table 112-1) include caring for the patient with the head of the bed elevated 30 to 45 degrees,[35] using GI promotility agents or reducing doses of opioids,[36] and using nurse-directed feeding

protocols that include frequent checking of gastric residual volumes.[37,38]

When data from all sources are considered, there is substantial clinical evidence, supported by a compelling theoretical rationale, that EN influences the clinical outcome of critically ill patients. EN is preferable to PN, and methods to maximize the delivery and minimize the risks should be considered in all critically ill patients receiving specialized nutritional support.

ASSESSMENT OF THE CRITICALLY ILL PATIENT

The clinician must first evaluate the level of stress in a critically ill patient to determine the likelihood of deterioration in nutritional status and to assess the overall need for aggressive nutritional support. If the patient is minimally stressed, nutritional support may not be required. Standardized scoring systems such as APACHE II or APACHE III, the injury severity score, and the abdominal trauma index (ATI) can be helpful for determining the level of stress and the likelihood of deterioration in nutritional status.[39,40] Scoring systems have also been used to assess the need for nutritional support in patients with acute pancreatitis.[41] Patients with an APACHE II score greater than 10 and having more than three Ranson criteria require additional nutritional support.[41]

It is difficult to discern the true incidence of protein calorie malnutrition (PCM) in the critical care setting. Identifying that a patient is significantly underweight, has sustained recent weight loss, or has remained NPO for some

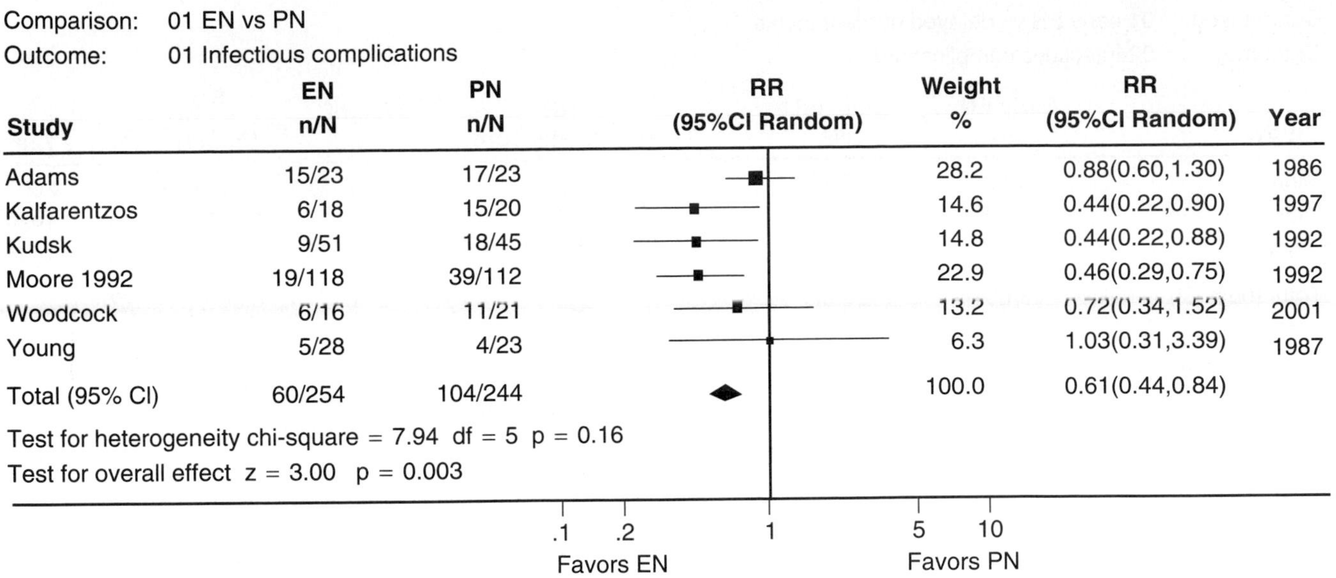

Comparison: 01 EN vs PN
Outcome: 01 Infectious complications

Study	EN n/N	PN n/N	RR (95%CI Random)	Weight %	RR (95%CI Random)	Year
Adams	15/23	17/23		28.2	0.88(0.60,1.30)	1986
Kalfarentzos	6/18	15/20		14.6	0.44(0.22,0.90)	1997
Kudsk	9/51	18/45		14.8	0.44(0.22,0.88)	1992
Moore 1992	19/118	39/112		22.9	0.46(0.29,0.75)	1992
Woodcock	6/16	11/21		13.2	0.72(0.34,1.52)	2001
Young	5/28	4/23		6.3	1.03(0.31,3.39)	1987
Total (95% CI)	60/254	104/244		100.0	0.61(0.44,0.84)	

Test for heterogeneity chi-square = 7.94 df = 5 p = 0.16
Test for overall effect z = 3.00 p = 0.003

```
.1   .2        1        5   10
    Favors EN        Favors PN
```

FIGURE 112–2. Studies comparing parenteral nutrition (PN) and enteral nutrition (EN) in terms of effect on infectious complications. CI, confidence interval; RR, relative risk.

period before the acute insult is the most reliable indicator that deterioration of nutritional status has occurred. Most clinical markers of PCM are confounded by the stress response. The critical care setting is certainly not the time or place to make up nutritional deficits and replete lean body mass. Poor nutrient intake and recent weight loss should alert the clinician that gut assimilation may be a problem, that more aggressive delivery of enteral or parenteral nutrients is appropriate, and that there is a greater need to meet calorie and protein requirements sooner in the hospital course (see Fig. 112-2).

If the overall level of stress and severity of illness indicate the need for nutritional support, the clinician must next evaluate the status of the GI tract. Intravascular volume status should be optimized before initiating enteral feeds.

It is not safe to infuse nutrients into the gut if there is ongoing ischemia or a high risk of mesenteric hypoperfusion. Feeding standard enteral formulas to patients with hypotension, hypovolemia, or septic shock, especially when vasopressors are being used to support blood pressure, may precipitate bowel ischemia.[42]

The concept of ileus and the clinical impression that the gut is "not working" can be misleading, because intestinal motility is segmental in nature. The adequacy of gastric emptying can be evaluated by determining the presence or absence of nausea and vomiting, high residual volumes, or high output from the nasogastric tube. Colonic motility is evaluated by determining whether the patient is passing stool or gas. Small bowel motility is evaluated by determining the presence or absence of abdominal distention and

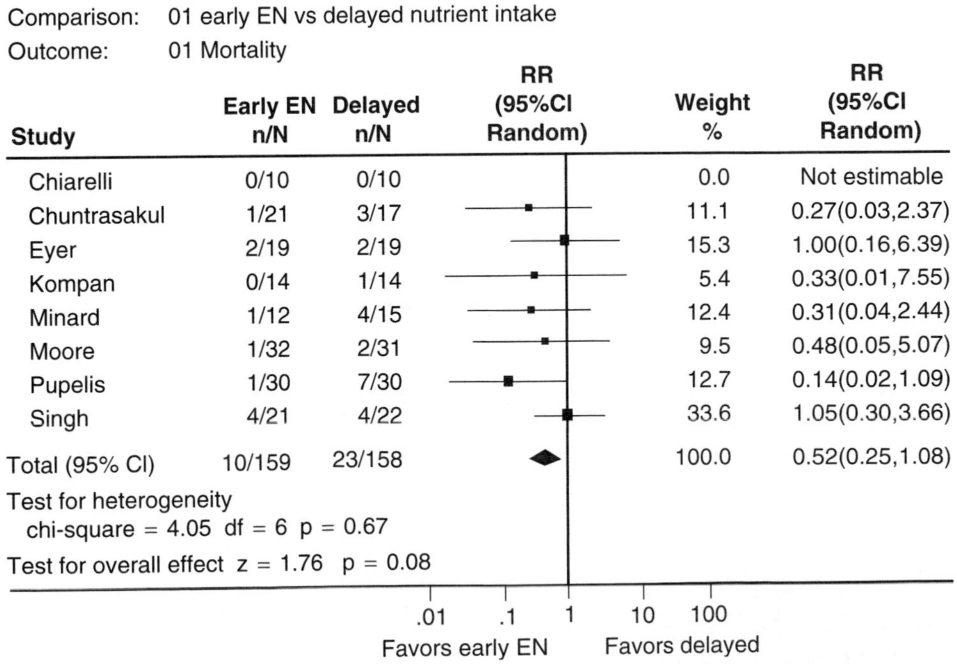

Comparison: 01 early EN vs delayed nutrient intake
Outcome: 01 Mortality

Study	Early EN n/N	Delayed n/N	RR (95%CI Random)	Weight %	RR (95%CI Random)
Chiarelli	0/10	0/10		0.0	Not estimable
Chuntrasakul	1/21	3/17		11.1	0.27(0.03,2.37)
Eyer	2/19	2/19		15.3	1.00(0.16,6.39)
Kompan	0/14	1/14		5.4	0.33(0.01,7.55)
Minard	1/12	4/15		12.4	0.31(0.04,2.44)
Moore	1/32	2/31		9.5	0.48(0.05,5.07)
Pupelis	1/30	7/30		12.7	0.14(0.02,1.09)
Singh	4/21	4/22		33.6	1.05(0.30,3.66)
Total (95% CI)	10/159	23/158		100.0	0.52(0.25,1.08)

Test for heterogeneity
chi-square = 4.05 df = 6 p = 0.67
Test for overall effect z = 1.76 p = 0.08

```
.01    .1        1        10   100
    Favors early EN    Favors delayed
```

FIGURE 112–3. Studies comparing early versus delayed nutrient intake in terms of effect on mortality. CI, confidence interval; EN, enteral nutrition; RR, relative risk.

Comparison: 01 early EN vs delayed nutrient intake
Outcome: 02 Infectious complications

Study	Early EN n/N	Delayed n/N	RR (95%CI Random)	Weight %	RR (95%CI Random)	Year
Minard	6/12	7/15		37.7	1.07(0.49,2.34)	2000
Moore	3/32	9/31		20.3	0.32(0.10,1.08)	1986
Singh	7/21	12/22		42.0	0.61(0.30,1.25)	1998
Total (95% CI)	16/65	28/68		100.0	0.66(0.36,1.22)	

Test for heterogeneity chi-square = 3.00 df = 2 p = 0.22
Test for overall effect z = 1.32 p = 0.19

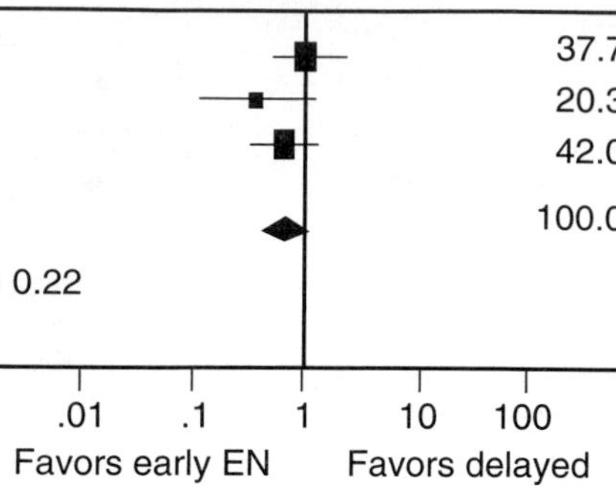

.01 .1 1 10 100
Favors early EN   Favors delayed

FIGURE 112–4. Studies comparing early versus delayed nutrient intake in terms of effect on infectious complications. CI, confidence interval; EN, enteral nutrition; RR, relative risk.

bowel sounds. However, absorption of nutrients from the small bowel does not require intestinal motility. Infusing nutrients into the lumen of the small intestine (with or without simultaneous gastric decompression) can actually stimulate intestinal motility via the release of gastrin, bombesin, motilin, and other promotility agents. Thus, ileus can actually resolve with aggressive attempts to provide nutrition enterally.

When EN is started soon after the onset of critical illness (i.e., enteral nutrients have been lacking only a short time), one can presume that the integrity of the intestinal mucosa is well maintained, and a standard enteral formula can be used. If the period of gut disuse has been more prolonged, the clinician must consider the possibility that mucosal integrity is not normal. If there is evidence of malassimilation and diarrhea, enteral formulas containing oligopeptides may enhance the absorption and assimilation of protein.[43] In a recent review of 19 prospective, randomized trials in humans, 11 studies showed evidence of clinical benefit when oligopeptide-containing formulas were used instead of standard enteral (intact protein) formulas. Although there was no impact on patient outcome, the benefits of oligopeptide-based diets included significantly improved nitrogen absorption, higher visceral protein levels, more weight gain, less frequent stooling, and reduced stool volume.[43]

Once EN is started, the clinician must monitor tolerance. Overall assimilation of nutrients by the enteral route is assessed clinically by checking for the presence or absence of diarrhea. Additionally, it is important to monitor circulating concentrations of glucose, triglycerides, urea nitrogen, and creatinine ratio. Risk factors for aspiration include age older than 60 years, decreased level of consciousness, bolus feeding, and supine position.[44-46] Gastric residual volumes, output from the gastric port of an aspiration or feeding tube, and passage of stool and gas are valuable indices of intestinal motility.

PRACTICAL CONSIDERATIONS

In some patients, nutritional support may not be necessary or the route of administration may not be an important consideration. However, in certain disease processes that are associated with high severity of illness, such as trauma, burns, acute pancreatitis, and acute respiratory failure requiring mechanical ventilation, the decision to use the parenteral rather than the enteral route for feeding can affect outcome.[47,48]

The greater importance of EN among sicker patients was first shown by evaluating septic complications in trauma patients, randomized at the time of surgery to receive either PN or EN.[49] Patients were ranked for severity of disease by their ATI scores. Among patients with ATI scores higher than 24, the incidence of septic complications was greater in the PN group than in the EN group (47.6% versus 11.1%; $P < 0.05$). Among patients with moderate illness and ATI scores lower than 24, there was no significant difference in the incidence of septic complications between the PN and EN groups (29.2% versus 20.8%; $P =$ NS).[49]

Further evidence of the importance of maintaining gut integrity in patients with more severe disease was provided by a series of prospective, randomized, controlled trials of EN versus PN in patients with acute pancreatitis.[13,50,51] In the first trial published, feeding by the enteral route was shown to be safe, but only 19% of the patients had severe pancreatitis, and there were no differences in the rates of nosocomial infection, organ failure, or overall complications.[51] In a second study, 38% of the patients had severe pancreatitis, and a significantly greater percentage of those fed enterally rather than parenterally had resolution of SIRS over the first week of therapy (81% versus 17%; $P < 0.05$); nevertheless, there were no differences between the groups with respect to rates of nosocomial infection or complications.[13] In a third study, 100% of the patients had severe pancreatitis, and septic complications were reduced from 50% in the PN group to 28% in the EN group ($P < 0.05$); the overall rate of

TABLE 112–1. STRATEGIES TO OPTIMIZE THE BENEFITS AND MINIMIZE THE RISKS OF ENTERAL NUTRITION

Initiate early, within 24-48 h of admission
Use small bowel feedings
Elevate head of the bed
Use motility agents
Reduce dose of narcotics prescribed
Use feeding protocol that enables consistent evaluation of gastric residual volume and specifies when feeds should be interrupted

complications was reduced from 75% in the PN group to 44% in the EN group ($P < 0.05$).[50]

For EN support, clinicians need to determine caloric requirements in order to set a goal or mandatory threshold for the volume, or "dose," of enteral feeding provided. Use of indirect calorimetry (see Chapter 225) or simplistic equations (e.g., 25 kcal/kg per day) to estimate caloric requirements can help identify this threshold amount. Focusing on such a goal volume allows clinicians to determine a dose-response effect of enteral tube feeding, that is, the percentage of this goal volume that is required to achieve the desired therapeutic endpoints (maintenance of gut integrity, containment of intestinal permeability, attenuation of the stress response, reduction of overall disease severity). In the early stages of critical illness, patients are in the throes of the hypermetabolic stress response and are more prone to ileus owing to higher doses of narcotics, electrolyte abnormalities, and shifts in fluid volume. In this situation, it is difficult to provide full caloric requirements. The minimum amount or volume of feeds (as a percentage of total caloric requirements) sufficient to achieve the desired therapeutic effect is not known. Recent evidence suggests that "trophic" or "trickle" rates of feeding (usually meaning 10 to 30 mL/h of a nutritional formula containing ≈1 kcal/mL) are probably inadequate to provide demonstrable benefits. Data from clinical studies indicate that 50% to 65% of goal calories are needed to prevent increases in intestinal permeability in burn victims[8,52] and bone marrow transplant patients (M. T. Demeo, personal communication), promote better and faster return of cognitive function in head injury victims,[53] and reduce the duration of mechanical ventilation and ICU and hospital length of stay in critically ill patients.[54] When higher feeding rates are not feasible, trickle feeds may have limited value and should be provided, but efforts to infuse greater volumes should be continued.

IMMUNONUTRITION

An additional strategy to maximize the benefits of EN is to use formulas supplemented with specific nutrients that are thought to modulate the immune system, facilitate wound healing, and reduce oxidative stress. Enteral formulas have been developed that contain certain compounds, such as L-glutamine, L-arginine, and omega-3 fatty acids, as well as selenium, vitamins E, C, and A, and beta carotene in supraphysiologic concentrations. The use of these products has been called "immunonutrition," and these products have been called "immune-enhancing diets." Although the overall effect of these individual nutrients in critically ill patients remains unknown, we have endeavored to review the efficacy and safety of products supplemented with arginine, glutamine, fish oils, and antioxidants.

L-ARGININE

The amino acid L-arginine plays fundamental roles in protein metabolism and polyamine synthesis and is a critical substrate for nitric oxide (NO) production.[55] It stimulates the release of growth hormone, insulin growth factor, and insulin, all of which may stimulate protein synthesis and promote wound healing. The enzyme L-arginase metabolizes L-arginine to L-ornithine, an amino acid implicated in wound healing. NO is produced by a family of enzymes

called nitric oxide synthases (NOSs), which exist in constitutive and inducible isoforms.[56] Under normal conditions and in some disease states, small quantities of NO are synthesized by the constitutive forms, which have a beneficial effect on tissue oxygenation and immune function.[57] Presumably mediated by constitutive NOS-dependent NO production, supplemental administration of L-arginine is associated with an increased lymphocyte and monocyte proliferation, enhanced T helper cell formation, activation of macrophages, reinforcement of natural killer cell function, and increased phagocytosis. These salutary effects of L-arginine on wound healing and antimicrobial defenses have prompted manufacturers to add supraphysiologic concentrations of the amino acid to immune-enhancing diets. However, excessive production of NO generated from inducible NOS (iNOS) can lead to excessive inflammation and vasodilatation, promote alterations in GI motility and mucosal integrity, and impair cellular respiration.[58] Induction of iNOS is mediated by Th1 cytokines (notably, IL-1, TNF, and IFN-γ), whereas L-arginase expression is induced by Th2 cytokines (notably, IL-4, IL-10, and TGF-ß).[59]

Data are lacking regarding the effects of L-arginine supplementation on clinically important outcomes in critically ill patients. In studies, L-arginine supplementation has been combined with the administration of other immune-modulating nutrients in critically ill patients, limiting the inferences that can be made about the role of L-arginine supplementation alone. In a recent updated meta-analysis, the results of 15 randomized trials were aggregated.[60] Overall, L-arginine-containing diets had no effect on mortality (RR 1.05; 95% CI 0.82 to 1.35) and no overall effect on the rate of infectious complications (RR 0.94; 95% CI 0.76 to 1.16). There was a trend toward reduction in hospital length of stay when L-arginine-containing diets were used, but the effect was statistically insignificant (weighted mean difference in days −3.5; 95% CI −8.8 to 1.9). The presence of significant statistical heterogeneity across studies weakened the estimate of the effect on length of stay.

Despite the absence of an overall effect on mortality, there may be some subgroups of critically ill patients that experience benefit (or harm) when treated with L-arginine-containing products. Based on the scientific rationale presented earlier, L-arginine-supplemented products might worsen the outcome for critically ill septic patients with increased iNOS expression,[61] but they might be beneficial in trauma patients with decreased circulating concentrations of L-arginine.[59] Accordingly, we performed a subgroup meta-analysis of the six studies that enrolled trauma patients and compared the results with those obtained in a meta-analysis of nine studies that enrolled nontrauma patients.[60] There was no difference in mortality when EN was carried out using an L-arginine-containing formula instead of a standard one in either trauma patients (RR 0.93; 95% CI 0.46 to 1.89) or nontrauma patients (RR 0.79; 95% CI 0.41 to 1.50). Nor was there a difference in the rate of infectious complications when EN was carried out using an L-arginine-containing formula instead of a standard one in either trauma patients (RR 1.09; 95% CI 0.80 to 1.49) or nontrauma patients (RR 0.97; 95% CI 0.78 to 1.19).

There are now three reports in the literature of excess mortality in critically ill septic patients treated with L-arginine-supplemented diets.[62-64] In a large multicenter, double-blind, randomized trial, Bower and colleagues compared Impact (an L-arginine-supplemented formula) with

Osmolite HN in critically ill patients.[62] More patients who received the L-arginine-supplemented formula died (24 of 153 [15.7%], versus 12 of 143 [8.4%] in the control group; $P = 0.055$), and all the excess mortality was observed in patients classified as septic at baseline (11 of 44 [25%], versus 4 of 45 [8.9%]; $P = 0.051$). In another study, 171 critically ill patients were randomized to receive either an experimental diet supplemented with L-arginine or an isonitrogenous control diet.[63] In the group that received the experimental formula, the mortality rate was significantly higher (20 of 87, or 23%) than it was in the control group (8 of 83, or 9.6%; $P = 0.03$). Despite similar baseline demographics and APACHE II scores in the two groups, more patients had pneumonia at baseline in the group that received the experimental formula. The excess mortality occurred in the subgroup of patients with pneumonia at baseline who received the experimental diet. Finally, Bertolini and colleagues published an interim analysis of data from a randomized multicenter trial that compared mortality in 39 severely septic patients treated with either an enteral immune-enhancing formula supplemented with L-arginine or PN.[64] In this small study, excess mortality was observed in the group treated with the L-arginine-supplemented diet (8 of 18 [44.4%], versus 3 of 21 [14.3%] who received PN; $P = 0.039$). Because PN is associated with worse outcomes in critically ill patients, these data support the view that administering large doses of L-arginine to septic patients increases mortality.

The only evidence to the contrary comes from a study by Galban and colleagues, who found that in critically ill patients with infection, treatment with an L-arginine-supplemented diet improved survival.[65] However, in this study, the majority of the treatment benefit occurred in the least sick patients (baseline APACHE II score <15). Thus, based on available evidence, L-arginine-supplemented diets should not be used in critically ill patients who are clearly septic. If a critically ill patient receiving an L-arginine-supplemented diet develops sepsis, that diet should be discontinued.

OMEGA-3 FATTY ACIDS

Dietary omega-3 and omega-6 fatty acids are incorporated into phospholipids and, thereby, influence the structure and function of cellular membranes. Omega-3 and omega-6 fatty acids also serve as substrates for the enzymes cyclooxygenase, lipoxygenase, and cytochrome P_{450} oxidase, leading to the formation of prostaglandins, thromboxanes, leukotrienes, and lipoxins. Metabolism of omega-6 fatty acids leads to the formation of arachidonic acid. Metabolism of arachidonate via the cyclooxygenase pathway results in the production of compounds containing two double bonds, which are called bisenoic prostanoids and are designated by a subscript 2 (e.g., prostaglandin [PG]E$_2$). Metabolism of omega-3 fatty acids leads to the formation of eicosapentaenoic acid (EPA). Trienoic prostanoids (e.g., PGE$_3$) are derived from EPA. Products derived from arachidonic acid via the 5-LO pathway are designated by a subscript 4 (e.g., leukotriene [LT]B$_4$), whereas products resulting from the action of 5-lipoxygenase (5-LO) on EPA are designated by a subscript 5 (e.g., LTB$_5$). The 2-series prostanoids and the 4-series leukotrienes are potent biologic mediators. In contrast, the 3-series prostanoids and the 5-series leukotrienes derived from EPA are much less active.

Experimentally, increasing the quantity of omega-3 fatty acids (found in fish oils) in the diet reduces platelet aggregation, slows blood clotting, and limits the production of proinflammatory cytokines.[66] Data from studies using animal models suggest that a diet enriched with fish and borage oils can ameliorate inflammation-induced acute lung injury.[67,68] The only clinical study of fish oil (omega-3 fatty acid) supplementation pertinent to the care of critically ill patients was carried out by Gadek and colleagues.[69] In a randomized, multicenter, double-blind clinical trial, these investigators studied the effects of a diet (Oxepa7, Ross Products, Columbus, Ohio) supplemented with fish oils (containing EPA and docosahexaenoic acid), borage oil (rich in γ-linolenic acid), and antioxidants on markers of lung inflammation and survival. One hundred forty-six patients with acute respiratory distress syndrome (ARDS) were randomized within 24 hours of meeting entrance criteria to either a high-fat, low-carbohydrate control diet or the experimental diet. Only 98 of the 146 patients were deemed "evaluable" and were included in the efficacy analysis. Among the evaluable patients, those who received the experimental diet had higher plasma phospholipid fatty acid levels (i.e., dihomo-γ-linolenic acid, EPA, and EPA/arachidonic acid ratio) and fewer total cells and neutrophils recovered from bronchoalveolar lavage fluid obtained on study days 4 and 7.

In addition, PaO$_2$/FiO$_2$ ratios on days 4 and 7 showed greater improvement in patients receiving the experimental diet compared with control patients. There was a nonsignificant improvement in survival in the experimental group compared with controls (16% versus 25%; $P = 0.17$). Patients fed the experimental diet required fewer days on supplemental oxygen (13.6 versus 17.1; $P = 0.078$), required significantly fewer days of ventilatory support (9.6 versus 13.2; $P = 0.027$), spent less time in the ICU (11.0 versus 14.8 days; $P = 0.016$), and had fewer new organ failures (10% versus 25%; $P = 0.018$). Thus, the findings from this study support the view that the administration of dietary lipids rich in omega-3 fatty acids can modify the lipid profile and favorably affect clinical outcome among critically ill patients with ARDS. However, a high-fat diet may be harmful, at least in critically ill burn victims.[70] Therefore, the results of the study by Gadek and colleagues may be confounded by the use of a high-fat control formula.[69] Further, because of the addition of supplements other than fish oils (e.g., antioxidants), it is not possible to definitively attribute the beneficial effects of the experimental diet to its higher content of omega-3 fatty acids.

L-GLUTAMINE

The amino acid L-glutamine plays a central role in nitrogen transport within the body. It is used as a fuel by rapidly dividing cells, particularly lymphocytes and gut epithelial cells,[71-73] and is also a substrate for the synthesis of the important endogenous antioxidant glutathione. Although L-glutamine is not an essential amino acid under normal conditions, plasma L-glutamine concentration decreases during critical illness, and low circulating levels of L-glutamine have been associated with immune dysfunction[74] and increased mortality.[75] Thus, L-glutamine may be regarded as a "conditionally essential" amino acid.

The effects of L-glutamine supplementation on clinically important outcomes have been assessed in several randomized trials of surgical and critically ill patients,[76] and the results from these studies have been subjected to meta-analysis.[60] In the aggregate, L-glutamine supplementation is associated with a significant reduction in mortality (RR 0.78; 95% CI 0.61 to 0.99; $P = 0.04$), a trend toward a reduction in infectious complications (RR 0.89; 95% CI 0.73 to 1.08; $P = 0.2$), and no overall effect on length of stay (weighted mean difference in days −1.30; 95% CI −4.77 to 2.17). When route of administration (parenteral versus enteral) was assessed in a subgroup analysis, the majority of the treatment effect with respect to mortality and infectious complications was associated with parenteral administration of L-glutamine in patients receiving PN. Because the majority of L-glutamine provided enterally is metabolized in the gut and liver, it may not have a systemic effect. Only one small study in burn patients demonstrated a reduction in mortality with enteral L-glutamine.[77] In a study of trauma patients, administration of an enteral formula supplemented with L-glutamine was associated with a nonsignificant decrease in the number of infections compared with the number of infections observed with administration of the control formula (20 of 35 [57%] versus 26 of 37 [70%]).[78]

Therefore, for critically ill patients requiring PN, we recommend L-glutamine supplementation as long as the patient remains on PN. Enteral diets supplemented with L-glutamine can be considered for patients with major burns or trauma. Recommendations regarding L-glutamine supplementation (enteral or parenteral) in other critically ill patient populations are premature and warrant further study.

ANTIOXIDANTS, VITAMINS, AND TRACE MINERALS

For a variety of inflammatory, infectious, and ischemic diseases, reactive oxygen species (ROS) represent a final common pathway. These toxic mediators (e.g., superoxide anion, hydroxyl radical, hydrogen peroxide, hypochlorous acid) can cause cellular injury by numerous mechanisms, including destruction of cell membranes through the peroxidation of fatty acids; disruption of organelle membranes, such as those bounding lysosomes and mitochondria; degradation of hyaluronic acid and collagen; and disruption of key proteins and enzymes, such as Na^+,K^+-ATPase or $alpha_1$-proteinase inhibitor. To protect tissues from ROS-induced injury, the body maintains a complex endogenous defense system, including enzymes such as superoxide dismutase, catalase, glutathione peroxidase, and glutathione reductase. These enzymes all have metals—notably, manganese, selenium, copper, or zinc—at their active sites. When these enzymatic antioxidants are overwhelmed, ROS are free to react with susceptible target molecules and cause cellular damage. Thus, cells have a secondary means of scavenging ROS using nonenzymatic antioxidants that are either water soluble, such as glutathione and vitamin C, or lipid soluble, such as vitamin E and beta carotene.[79]

In critical illness, oxidative stress arises due to an imbalance between protective antioxidant mechanisms and the generation of ROS. This imbalance may be caused by excess generation of ROS, low antioxidant capacity, or both. Plasma and intracellular concentrations of the various antioxidants are abnormally low in subpopulations of critically ill patients.[80-82] In critical illness, evidence of oxidative stress includes high circulating levels of byproducts of lipid peroxidation, markers of protein oxidation, nitration or nitrosylation, or increased activity of ROS-producing enzymatic systems.[83]

In a recent meta-analysis,[84] we aggregated results from 12 randomized trials that were designed to assess the value of administering exogenous antioxidants to critically ill patients.[83,85-95] Of the included studies, several examined the effects of a single nutrient with antioxidant properties.[86,88-90,92] In most cases, the nutrient evaluated was selenium,[86,88-90] but one study assessed the effect of zinc supplementation on outcome in ventilated patients with head trauma.[92] The effects of selenium combined with other antioxidants were assessed in four studies,[85-87,95] and four studies focused on the effects of vitamin A, vitamin C, vitamin E, N-acetylcysteine, and glutathione.[83,91,93,94] When the 12 trials were aggregated, antioxidants were associated with a significant reduction in mortality (RR 0.66; 95% CI 0.45 to 0.95; $P = 0.03$). Only five of these studies reported on infectious complications.[83,86,87,91,93] When these results were aggregated, antioxidants had no effect on infectious complications (RR 0.94; 95% CI 0.63 to 1.40; $P = 0.8$). In further subgroup analysis, the majority of the treatment effect seemed to be related to parenteral rather than enteral administration of antioxidants or antioxidant nutrients, especially selenium. Thus, for critically ill patients, selenium supplementation in combination with other antioxidants (vitamin E or alpha tocopherol, vitamin C, N-acetylcysteine, zinc) may be beneficial.

APPROPRIATE USE OF TOTAL PARENTERAL NUTRITION IN THE INTENSIVE CARE UNIT

The enteral route of feeding is always preferable to the parenteral route. However, EN is not always available, reliable, or safe. PN may be effective in specific circumstances when used correctly; in other circumstances, no nutritional therapy may be the most appropriate management. In the critical care setting, EN is clearly the first choice. In most cases, no nutritional support (other than glucose-containing intravenous fluids) is the second best alternative when EN is unavailable, impractical, or unsafe. PN is usually the choice of last resort.

PATIENT SELECTION

In almost all critical care patient populations, involving a wide range of disease processes (from surgery and pancreatitis to trauma, burns, and critically ill patients on mechanical ventilation), EN is first-line therapy and should be chosen before PN. The reduction of infections by the use of EN compared with PN is consistent, regardless of whether patients have cancer or protein energy malnutrition.[96] In the critical care of an average patient with an intact GI tract, PN should never be selected ahead of EN. When studies from diverse critical care patient populations are combined, "standard therapy" in which no artificial nutritional support is provided has a more favorable impact on patient outcome than PN does. In a recent meta-analysis, Braunschweig and colleagues showed a statistically significant reduction in infections with standard therapy compared with PN (RR 0.77; 95% CI 0.65 to 0.91).[96] If the patients were clearly well nourished, an even greater reduction in the incidence of infections was seen with standard therapy compared with PN (RR 0.61; 95% CI 0.50 to 0.76).[96] There was a trend toward reduced overall complications with standard therapy, which just missed statistical significance (RR 0.87; 95% CI 0.74 to 1.03).[96] Hospital length of stay was reduced significantly in 8 of the 14 studies reviewed by Heyland and coworkers in which standard therapy was compared with PN.[97]

The presence of PCM reverses the choice between standard therapy and PN. In general, PN has greater efficacy in patients with PCM, and the chance of a favorable impact on patient outcome is more likely with PN than with standard therapy. PCM is most commonly defined by a greater than 10% to 15% weight loss[97] or a low body mass index.[98] In patients with severe PCM, use of PN reduces infectious morbidity, overall major complications, and even mortality in comparison to standard therapy. In their meta-analysis, Heyland and coworkers showed a 48% reduction in risk of major complications with the use of total PN compared with standard therapy in malnourished surgery patients (RR 0.52; 95% CI 0.30 to 0.91).[97] In a diverse population of malnourished patients, giving no nutritional support and providing standard therapy are associated with a trend toward increased infection (RR 1.17; 95% CI 0.88 to 1.56) and a significant threefold increase in mortality (RR 3.0; 95% CI 1.09 to 8.56).[96] Those patients with severe PCM, the ones most likely to benefit from PN, usually represent a very small minority of patients. The prevalence of severe PCM in some studies of ICU patients ranged from 8.3% to 12.6%.[99-101]

Critically ill patients with sepsis and multiple organ dysfunction respond poorly to PN. Heyland and coworkers showed a trend toward a 2.5-fold increase in complications (RR 2.40; 95% CI 0.88 to 6.58) and a significant twofold increase in mortality (RR 0.178; 95% CI 1.11 to 2.85) from the use of PN compared with standard therapy with no nutritional support.[97]

Thus, for critical care nutrition in general, the clinician should rarely choose PN over EN. Aggressive EN appears to be the first-line therapy for nutritional support in critical care and is associated with lower infectious morbidity compared with the parenteral route. EN appears to be superior to both PN and standard therapy with no nutritional support across diverse patient populations. When EN is not feasible, aggressive nutritional support may need to be held for 7 to 10 days following an injury or an acute event. These patients, despite critical illness, sepsis, and multiple organ dysfunction, are better managed by standard therapy with no PN support over this initial period. Only if there is evidence of PCM (and EN is not feasible) should PN be given preferentially over standard therapy in the first week.

LIPID CONTENT

Use of emulsified lipids (Intralipid) with PN is controversial, because previous studies have shown that long-chain fats can cause immune suppression.[102] Intralipid can promote dysfunction of the reticuloendothelial system, enhance the formation of prostanoids and leukotrienes, increase the generation of ROS, and adversely affect the composition of cell membranes.[102]

Several reports demonstrate that intravenous lipids can adversely affect immune status and clinical outcome.[103,104] Results of a meta-analysis of PN suggest that the adverse effects of lipids may negate any beneficial effects of nonlipid PN supplementation.[97] Two studies compared the use of lipids to no lipids in PN.[102,105] Among trauma patients, the use of PN without lipids versus with lipids was associated with a significant reduction in pneumonia (48% versus 73%; $P = 0.05$), catheter-related sepsis (19% versus 43%; $P = 0.04$), length of ICU stay (18 versus 29 days; $P = 0.02$), and length of hospital stay (27 versus 39 days; $P = 0.03$).[102] In another study, the group that received no lipids (hypocaloric group)

showed a trend toward a reduction in infections compared with the group that received lipids (29% versus 53%; $P = 0.2$).[105] Combining these two studies, a meta-analysis showed a significant reduction in infections in the group that received no lipids (RR 0.63; 95% CI 0.42 to 0.93) and no difference in mortality (RR 1.29; 95% CI 0.16 to 10.7).[97]

The long-term effects of fat-free PN are unknown. However, some fat—at least 5% of total calories—needs to be provided as lipid emulsion to prevent essential fatty acid deficiency, although this issue is usually not important until after the first 10 days of hospitalization.[98] Therefore, lipid-free PN is probably best given to those patients requiring only short-term PN (<10 days). This recommendation cannot be extrapolated to those who have an absolute contraindication to EN and need PN for a longer duration.

EFFECT OF HYPERGLYCEMIA

Hyperglycemia might be a key factor in the reduced efficacy and increased rate of complications associated with PN. Hyperglycemia impairs neutrophil chemotaxis and phagocytosis,[96] leads to glycosylation of immunoglobulins,[106] impairs wound healing,[107] alters the function of the complement cascade,[108] and exacerbates inflammation.[109]

Compared with EN, PN more frequently leads to hyperglycemia. For a variety of reasons, patients receiving EN often receive fewer total calories than those receiving PN do.[96] Whereas PN formulas typically contain 60% to 75% carbohydrate, EN formulas usually contain 40% to 55% carbohydrate.[96] The parenteral route of feeding has been shown to lead to an increased stress response compared with enteral feeding. This effect, in turn, may increase endogenous glucose production and decrease glucose oxidation.[96]

The results from a number of early studies highlight the relationship between hyperglycemia and the incidence of nosocomial infection. In an early meta-analysis by Moore and associates comparing the parenteral and enteral routes of feeding in trauma patients, mean blood glucose concentration was greater than 200 mg/dL in the PN group on postoperative days 7 to 9, whereas it was only 132 mg/dL during the same period in patients receiving EN ($P < 0.05$).[109] The incidence of infection was 44% in the PN group and 17% in the EN group ($P < 0.05$).[109] In a different study, Kudsk and colleagues provided further evidence that hyperglycemia increases the risk of infection.[106] Among trauma patients randomized to EN or PN, those with a blood glucose concentration greater than 220 mg/dL had a 53% incidence of infection, whereas those with a blood glucose concentration less than 220 mg/dL had 23% incidence of infection ($P < 0.03$).

Van den Berghe and coworkers compared intensive insulin therapy (target range for blood glucose concentration, 4.4 to 6.1 mmol/L) and conventional treatment (target range for blood glucose concentration, 10.0 to 11.1 mmol/L) in critically ill patients receiving nutritional support.[110] This was a large study ($n = 1548$) of surgical ICU patients (predominantly elective cardiovascular surgery) with relatively low APACHE II scores (median, 9). Study patients were started on a glucose load (200 to 300 g/day) and then were advanced to PN, combined PN-EN, or EN after 24 hours of admission. Intensive insulin therapy was associated with a lower incidence of sepsis ($P = 0.003$), a trend toward a reduction in ventilator days, reduced ICU length of stay ($P < 0.04$), and decreased hospital mortality ($P = 0.01$) compared with conventional insulin therapy.[110]

From these studies, one can infer that intensive insulin therapy to achieve tight glycemic control may be associated with improved clinical outcomes in critically ill patients. The corollary is that high glucose loads in patients who are insulin resistant are associated with excess complications and increased mortality. Whether insulin has any therapeutic effect in patients who do not receive such high glucose loads or whether these results apply to other categories of ICU patients is unknown. Despite these limitations, in the absence of further studies, patients who are prescribed PN should receive intensive insulin therapy to obtain tight glycemic control. This can best be accomplished by using an insulin protocol or nomogram.[111]

CALORIC PROVISION—PERMISSIVE UNDERFEEDING

Several studies have shown a correlation between the provision of excessive amounts of calories and increased rates of insulin resistance, infectious morbidity, and mortality. Hyperglycemia (blood glucose concentration >220 mg/dL) has been shown to occur in greater than 50% of nondiabetic patients receiving PN in excess of 35 kcal/kg actual body weight per day.[112] In a retrospective study, patients who received a high dose of carbohydrates (77% of total calories and 42.4 kcal/kg per day, on average) were compared with patients who received a lower dose of carbohydrates (60.6% of total calories and 34.3 kcal/kg per day, on average).[113] The group that received more carbohydrates had significantly more episodes of sepsis (14 episodes in 26 patients versus 4 episodes in 17 patients; $P < 0.05$) and significantly higher mortality (28% versus 10%; $P < 0.05$).[113] Although the group on the higher-carbohydrate regimen received less protein than did the group on the lower-carbohydrate regimen (82.5 versus 98.7 g/day), this difference did not reach statistical significance.[113]

In another study, children with greater than 60% total body surface area burns were randomized to either a control group that received a high-carbohydrate, normal-protein regimen of PN or a study group that received a reduced-carbohydrate, high-protein regimen.[114] The control group received 87% of goal calories, whereas the study group received only 77.7% of goal calories ($P < 0.002$). The number of bacteremic days was 11% in the control group but only 8% in the experimental group ($P < 0.05$). Mortality was 44% in the control group and 0% in the experimental group ($P < 0.03$).[114]

Two additional studies evaluated the effect of hypocaloric feeding in critically ill patients. To achieve a hypocaloric dose of PN, Choban and colleagues[115] reduced both carbohydrates and lipids in morbidly obese critically ill patients, whereas McCowen and associates[105] withheld lipids in a heterogeneous group of patients, including critically ill patients. In the study by McCowen's group, hypocaloric feeding was associated with a trend toward a reduction in infectious complications ($P = 0.2$)[105]; infectious complications were not reported in the study by Choban's group.[115] There were no significant differences in mortality or length of stay between groups in either study.

Results of these studies suggest that insulin-resistant patients get hyperglycemic at lower rates of energy intake. Gain in body fat mass in response to excessive PN provision enhances the propensity to hyperglycemia and results in an increased incidence of sepsis. Isocaloric diets can have different effects, depending on insulin resistance. Malnutrition and loss of body fat may increase insulin sensitivity. Patients with

some degree of malnutrition seem to tolerate an infusion of carbohydrate and fat without hyperglycemia and hypertriglyceridemia and thus respond to nutritional support without added risk. Standard energy intake in patients with sepsis may actually exacerbate morbidity and mortality.

Thus, although increased protein intake is good, high nonprotein energy intake (from carbohydrates and fats) may reduce the benefits of nutritional support. "Permissive underfeeding," in which total caloric provision is set at 20 kcal/kg actual body weight (or even ideal body weight) per day may optimize the efficacy of PN in critically ill (especially septic) patients.

SUPPLEMENTAL TOTAL PARENTERAL NUTRITION

Few studies have looked at the impact of supplemental PN in patients receiving an insufficient volume of enteral feeding. In a study of 120 critically ill patients, Bauer and colleagues compared a control group receiving EN alone with a study group treated with EN supplemented with PN; both groups were fed for at least 4 to 7 days after starting nutritional support.[116] Overall, there was no difference in morbidity or mortality between the two groups. Duration of stay in the ICU, duration of mechanical ventilation, incidence of respiratory infection, and mortality were equal between the two groups. Hospital length of stay was shorter in the study group receiving supplemental PN than in the control group (31.2 versus 33.7 days; $P = 0.002$), but this effect was easily explained by a statistically significant earlier date of entry into the study (1.1 versus 1.5 days; $P = 0.002$). The cost of nutritional support was doubled by the addition of supplemental PN.

Of greater concern was a study by Herndon and colleagues of patients with greater than 50% total body surface area burns.[117] Mortality was significantly higher among the 16 study patients treated with EN and supplemental PN than it was in the 23 control patients treated with EN alone (63% versus 26%; $P < 0.05$). Supplemental PN added to the EN in the study group decreased the amount of enteral calories the patients tolerated. Although both groups exhibited depressed natural killer cell activity from days 0 to 14, the group receiving supplemental PN experienced greater depression of T cell helper–suppressor ratios from days 7 to 14.

A recent meta-analysis evaluated five randomized trials that addressed the clinical benefits of supplemental PN in critically ill patients.[118] The aggregated results demonstrated a trend toward increased mortality associated with the use of combination EN and PN (RR 1.27; 95% CI 0.82 to 1.94; $P = 0.3$). Supplemental PN was not associated with a difference in the incidence of infection (RR 1.14; 95% CI 0.66 to 1.96; $P = 0.6$). Supplemental PN had no effect on hospital stay (standardized mean difference –0.12 days; 95% CI –0.45 to 0.2 days; $P = 0.5$) or ventilator days. Thus, there appears to be no clinical evidence to support the practice of supplementing EN with PN when EN is initiated. Supplemental PN adds nothing and may actually worsen the outcome for patients already on EN.

DURATION AND TIMING OF PARENTERAL NUTRITION

When EN is not feasible, providing standard therapy with no artificial nutritional support may be better than PN in well-nourished patients, regardless of their disease process.

The timing of PN initiation is based on the underlying nutritional status of the patient. In a previously well-nourished but otherwise critically ill patient who has not resumed oral intake, it is reasonable to wait 7 to 10 days before initiating PN.[96,119] Some experts recommend a longer waiting period, 10 to 14 days, before initiating PN in a previously well-nourished patient who is not expected to resume oral intake soon.[98,100] However, after 14 days, increased mortality is seen in most patients who are not yet eating and remain on standard therapy with no nutritional support.[120] After 14 days, initiating PN is clearly associated with less mortality than is providing no nutritional support.[120] PN is indicated over standard therapy for the first 7 to 10 days when the enteral route is not available in malnourished patients (usually characterized by >10% to 15% weight loss). PN should not be initiated unless more than 7 to 10 days of therapy is anticipated. No studies of short-term PN (<7 days) have shown it to be efficacious or to impact favorably on patient outcome.

FUTURE CONSIDERATIONS

In the future, nutritional prescriptions will likely be complex recommendations that continue to consider protein and calorie requirements but, in addition, consider the key nutrients needed to modulate the stress response, maintain gut integrity, and ameliorate the pathophysiology of the underlying critical illness (Fig. 112-5). It may turn out that the prescription of key substrates will have a greater effect on outcome than the provision of calories or protein per se. For example, consider a critically ill patient with clinical or biochemical evidence of hypoperfusion. Early in the course of the illness, current thinking would say that EN is contraindicated. However, providing L-glutamine or antioxidants enterally may be exactly what this patient needs to recover from the oxidative stress associated with the critical illness. The need to meet protein and calorie requirements might occur much later in the course of the illness (see Fig. 112-5). Although this example represents an extreme case, nutritional prescriptions in the future will have to be more cognizant of the evolving pathophysiology and the ability of nutrients to modulate the integrity of the immune system, the systemic inflammatory response, and the underlying disease in the early phases of the clinical course.

As we move toward a more individualized nutritional prescription, we will need to give more consideration to the state of a patient's insulin resistance. The critical care community seems to have embraced the notion that "tight" glycemic control (keeping the serum glucose level at 4.4 to 6.1 mmol/L) is associated with a significant reduction in morbidity and mortality in critically ill patients.[110] However, providing high glucose loads to critically ill patients who are insulin resistant may result in harm, possibly even increasing mortality. In one study, the provision of glucose and insulin (maintaining glucose at the same level as in a control group that received saline) significantly amplified or prolonged key components of the systemic inflammatory and stress responses in human models of infection.[121] Although some may be saved with aggressive insulin therapy, withholding the carbohydrate loading in the first place makes more sense. Prescribing one product formulation for a given patient at a given rate for his or her entire stay may not be considered optimal care in the future.

Greater understanding of the pathophysiologic mechanisms that underlie critical illness and the systemic inflammatory response may help forge new strategies for nutritional support in the future. Early on, clinicians may separate pharmaconutrition from the provision of protein and calories, the latter of which may be limited by patient intolerance. Efforts to better delineate the dose-response effect of EN on gut integrity may help guide the "ramp-up" and degree of aggression with which feeding rates are advanced. Monitoring immune responses and alterations in the cytokine profile may help clinicians in the future decide whether to stimulate or up-regulate the immune response (through the provision of arginine or nucleotides) or to down-regulate responses (through the provision of omega-3 fatty acids and borage oil) as the patient proceeds through the hospital course.

ANNOTATED REFERENCES

Brandtzaeg PE: Current understanding of gastrointestinal immunoregulation and its relation to food allergy. Ann N Y Acad Sci 2002;964:13-45.
This paper provides an excellent review of gut immunology and provides the reader with an understanding of how events at the level of the gut serve to shape the stress response and modulate systemic immunity.

Taylor SJ, Fettes SB, Jewkes C, Nelson RJ: Prospective, randomized, controlled trial to determine the effect of early enhanced enteral nutrition on clinical outcome in mechanically ventilated patients suffering head injury. Crit Care Med 1999;27:2525-2531.
This study in trauma patients with head injury shows how modifying enteral feeding protocols to be more aggressive (faster ramp-ups in rate, higher gastric residual volumes) results in a greater percentage of goal calories being infused and better subsequent clinical outcome.

Van den Berghe G, Wouters P, Weekers F, et al: Intensive insulin therapy in critically ill patients. N Engl J Med 2001;345:1359-1367.
This landmark study clearly shows the tremendously favorable impact of tight glycemic control on patient outcome in critical illness.

Windsor AC, Kanwar S, Li AG, et al: Compared with parenteral nutrition, enteral feeding attenuates the acute phase response and improves disease severity in acute pancreatitis. Gut 1998;42:431-435.
This prospective, randomized trial of enteral versus parenteral feeding in patients with acute pancreatitis shows the degree to which enteral feeding can attenuate the stress response and thereby reduce overall disease severity (compared with parenteral feeding).

Young B, Ott L, Kasarskis E, et al: Zinc supplementation is associated with improved neurologic recovery rate and visceral protein levels of patients with severe closed head injury. J Neurotrauma 1996;13:25-34.
This meta-analysis beautifully outlines which patient populations benefit most from enteral feedings, describes situations in which standard therapy (no artificial nutritional support) is most appropriate, and delineates those few circumstances in critical illness when parenteral nutrition is indicated.

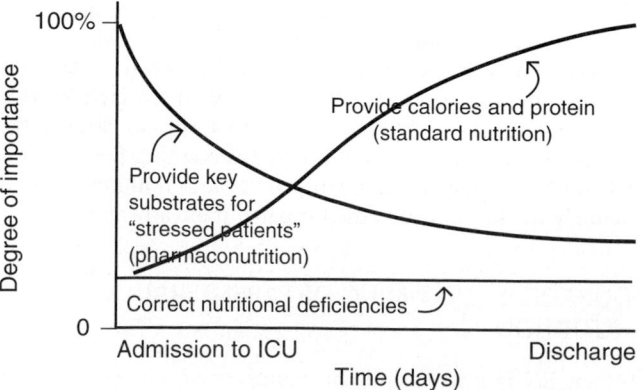

FIGURE 112-5. Pattern of prescriptions and goals of specialized nutritional support.

Chapter 113

NUTRITION ISSUES IN CRITICALLY ILL CHILDREN

David M. Steinhorn • Laura T. Russo

KEY POINTS

1. Assessment and monitoring of nutrition status is part of daily pediatric ICU care.

2. Nutrition support must be considered in all hospitalized children.

3. The goals are to minimize lean tissue loss and to optimize healing.

4. Growth is expected only during resolution of physiologic stress and convalescence.

5. Malnutrition may preexist or may develop progressively after hospitalization.

6. During acute illness, protein and calories should be provided in a controlled fashion: More is not always better.

7. During convalescence, protein and calories may be liberalized based on activity and tolerance.

Nutrition support of hospitalized children and infants has improved considerably in recent years. The improvements have come about largely through an increased understanding of nutritional biochemistry during physiologic stress and through the development of commercially available products that more closely meet the needs of ill children. As the knowledge base and resources for providing more appropriate nutrition to hospitalized children have increased, they have produced a staggering number of new products intended for specific subsets of pediatric patients. The optimal application of these products necessitates a fundamental understanding of the effects of injury and illness on children of different ages. In particular, the unique needs of young children and their responses to life-threatening disease need to be considered. Although contemporary resources for supporting the nutrition and metabolic needs of children have contributed to the care for patients with complex diseases, they also have provided new avenues for creating morbidities (e.g., total parenteral nutrition (TPN)–associated cholestasis, catheter-associated infections).

This chapter discusses many of the major issues affecting the nutrition support of hospitalized children. It is intended to be a practical resource for clinicians and to provide sufficient background information to allow the clinician to modify the nutrition approach as required by specific conditions. There can be no doubt that nutrition support of patients with prolonged or life-threatening disease has led to improved outcomes, which are achievable in most cases through the straightforward application of basic principles of nutrition.

NUTRITION ASSESSMENT

The nutrition assessment of hospitalized children is a central and crucial part of the initial examination and evaluation of all patients. The existence of chronic malnutrition and the development of acute malnutrition during critical illness have been recognized in pediatric critical care for many years.[1-3] Clinicians must assess newly admitted patients for the presence of malnutrition, which may complicate the response to therapies or impair recovery (Fig. 113-1). The presence of previous severe malnutrition may complicate critical care management through the presence of marasmic cardiomyopathy, severe intracellular energy deficiency, and the development of refeeding dysequilibrium when nutrients are provided in the ICU.

The initial nutrition evaluation consists of assessing the patient's weight, height, and historical evidence for recent weight loss and anthropometric measurements including midarm circumference and skin fold thickness (when edema is not present). Nutrition history must include the presence and duration of nausea, vomiting, diarrhea, fever, frequent infections, fatigue, food aversion, abdominal discomfort, or feeding intolerance. For growth standards, norms exist reflecting age and gender.[4] Ethnic background and considerations such as the presence of certain syndromes (e.g., Down's syndrome) or the child's birth status (e.g., premature, growth restricted) may affect the child's growth status. In particular, the determination of body mass index (previously known as *weight for height*) for children older than age 2 years provides important information regarding previous nutrition status. In children younger than age 2 years, weight for age in light of previous growth status is most useful. These straightforward measurements have withstood the test of time and were used by Pollack and coworkers[2] to estimate the risk of malnutrition in critically ill children admitted to a multidisciplinary ICU.[5] Their findings showed higher rates of preexisting malnutrition than had been previously thought. In addition, there was an unexpected deterioration in nutrition indices after admission, suggesting the powerful effects of life-threatening illness on nutritional stores and status even with excellent clinical care. Clinicians caring for children who will be in the hospital for more than a few days must be especially aware of the potential for acquired nutrition depletion.

Potential sources of error exist in interpreting anthropometric measurements which are primarily related to changes

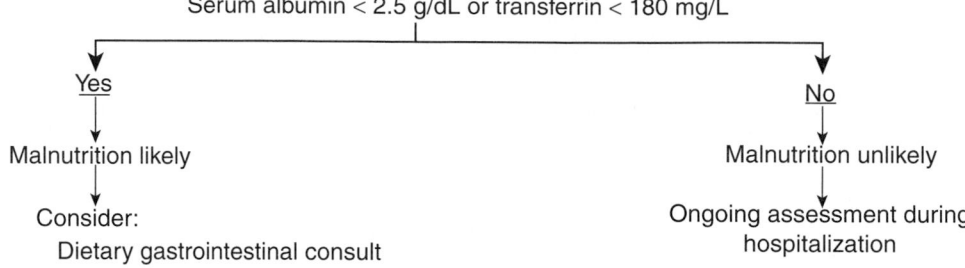

1. Physical examination: Obvious wasting? Skin and hair normal?

2. Plot on growth chart: Weight, height, head circumference (<24 months)

3. Determine: Percent height for age[4,†], and BMI[4,‡]

4. Measure: Serum albumin and transferrin

Height for age < 90 and BMI < 5 percentiles

Serum albumin < 2.5 g/dL or transferrin < 180 mg/L

FIGURE 113–1. Assessment of nutrition status on admission. BMI, body mass index. *Data from Waterlow.[5]

Yes

Malnutrition likely

Consider:
Dietary gastrointestinal consult
Nutrition support as soon as appropriate
Measure total protein, total lymphocyte count
Skin test for anergy (*Trichophyton, Candida*)
Anthropometrics: Measure triceps skin fold and midarm circumference

No

Malnutrition unlikely

Ongoing assessment during hospitalization

†Actual ht (cm) × 100/Expected ht at 50th percentile for age
‡Actual wt (kg)/[Actual wt (m)]^2

in body water associated with many acute critical illnesses in children (i.e., conditions producing capillary leak syndrome or defects in renal water clearance). These conditions may invalidate the measurement of skinfold or midarm circumference; however, their longitudinal use in patients can be helpful in estimating the accretion of fat and lean tissue stores. It is standard practice to measure these parameters in patients at risk for malnutrition, such as patients with cystic fibrosis, short bowel syndrome, and other conditions in which malabsorption or chronically elevated metabolic demands exist (e.g., congestive heart failure, bronchopulmonary dysplasia, and similar chronic conditions).

The triceps and scapular skinfolds measure the subcutaneous tissue compartment consisting primarily of adipose tissue, but also tissue edema in patients with anasarca from any cause. Triceps skinfold is measured by standardized skin caliper and is subject to considerable error if not performed in a consistent manner midway between the acromion and the olecranon. The midarm circumference should be measured at the same point with a nonstretchable tape measure. The two indices taken together permit a reliable estimate of the muscle mass. In general, good correlation exists between skinfold and arm circumference and weight-for-height percentile.[6] During critical illness, anasarca may obscure the loss of lean tissue, which may be apparent only after resolution of edema when successful diuresis has occurred. A reliable indicator of global loss of lean body mass can be seen in the wasting of the interosseous and thenar muscles of the hand, which becomes apparent 2 to 3 weeks after hospitalization with resolution of edema.[7,8]

In addition to anthropometric measurements, longitudinal determinations of specific plasma proteins, including albumin, transferrin, and prealbumin, have shown value in assessing the response of patients to nutrition support. Frequently, serum proteins are decreased during acute critical illness without reflecting preceding malnutrition. This phenomenon is seen frequently when endothelial permeability increases after sepsis, cardiopulmonary bypass, or ischemia-reperfusion injury. Through the loss of endothelial barrier function, large molecules such as albumin, which are normally three to four times more concentrated in the vascular compartment than in the interstitial fluid, move into the extravascular space, lowering their concentration without a concomitant decrease in the total body pool of albumin. This effect may be pronounced in patients who have received large volumes of crystalloid fluid during resuscitation. Clinicians must guard against the tendency to replace albumin during acute critical illness solely based on a low albumin level. Measures to correct the underlying pathophysiology should be considered before administering albumin. Otherwise, serum albumin in healthy children is generally greater than 3 g/dL, and edema is seen rarely in healthy children until the albumin decreases to less than 2 g/dL.

Shorter half-life serum proteins, such as prealbumin (half-life 2 days) and transferrin (half-life 7 days), also reflect nutrition status and respond more quickly to changes in anabolic state.[9] The pool of proteins in the plasma and interstitial space and some intracellular proteins represent a relatively labile pool of protein, referred to as the *visceral* protein pool. Visceral proteins are turned over rapidly relative to structural proteins, which comprise the *somatic* protein pool. In critical illness, the synthesis of specific proteins, such as C-reactive protein, ceruloplasmin, and alpha$_2$-macroglobulin, is increased, whereas the synthesis of other proteins, such as albumin (half-life approximately 20 days), is decreased.[10] These changes may be seen within 6 hours of the onset of severe physiologic stress. This response to physiologic stress is under the regulation of complex neurohumoral control and is referred to as the *acute phase response*. It is largely responsible for the increase in erythrocyte sedimentation rate associated with acute inflammatory conditions.[11] When followed longitudinally, the return of previously depressed levels of certain visceral proteins (e.g., albumin, transferrin, retinol binding protein, or prealbumin) represents the abatement of physiologic stress or improvement in nutrition when levels are low secondary to protein-calorie malnutrition. Such positive changes herald the impending return to a state of growth and tissue accretion—barring the re-entry into a new inflammatory state.

METABOLIC EFFECTS OF PHYSIOLOGIC STRESS IN CHILDREN

The events that lead to ICU admission are extremely varied, yet the body's response to acute physiologic stress tends to be similar whether the inciting event is sepsis, ischemia-reperfusion, trauma, burns, or other inflammatory conditions. Beyond low levels of stress, such as minor elective surgery, life-threatening illness, burns, organ transplantation, or major surgical procedures elicit dramatic systemic inflammatory responses as a result of activation of the immune system, clotting mechanisms, and the endothelium. The patient's ability to withstand the metabolic responses to such stresses and ultimately to reverse the process is central to recovery. A complete discussion of the metabolic response to stress is beyond the scope of this chapter, and the reader is referred to other sources.[12]

The initial response to injury is to activate endothelial cells and to prime inflammatory cells, such as neutrophils, macrophages, and lymphocytes, through proinflammatory mediators, including tumor necrosis factor, interleukin-2, histamine, eicosanoids, heat-shock proteins, free radicals, platelet-activating factor, and tryptases.[13] These same signals that produce activation of the endothelium lead to permeability changes and activation of clotting mechanisms and changes in hepatic and peripheral protein metabolism.[14] If recovery is to occur, this process must be extinguished by a decrease in the inflammatory state and an increase in tissue repair.[15] Although it may seem that simply shutting off the proinflammatory signals should lead to resolution, the process of resolving inflammation appears more complex.[16] Studies show the importance of many of the proinflammatory stimuli in regeneration and repair, and the timing of interventions is important.[16] In response to injury, a wide range of neurohumoral reactions occur, forming the classic "stress response," which includes elevation of growth hormone, endogenous catecholamines, glucagon, and cortisol. The recognition of the role of insulin-like growth factor-1 along with growth hormone in promoting protein synthesis and counterregulating the inflammatory states suggests important potential treatment options that have been best studied in burns.[17-19] Despite these studies showing benefit from growth hormone supplementation, evidence of increased mortality rate after growth hormone supplementation also has been reported.[20] Clinicians must balance the relative benefit of hormonal manipulation with potential risks.

In the inflammatory state, unremitting gluconeogenesis occurs through the release of glycerol and gluconeogenic amino acids from the periphery with their conversion to glucose in the liver and kidney. Hyperglycemia frequently is associated with this state and may induce glycosuria and an osmotic diuresis. Insulin activity becomes impaired at the tissue level, leading to so-called *insulin resistance* in the face of the powerful gluconeogenesis driven by the stress hormones. It seems that the impairment of insulin results from decreased phosphorylation of the insulin receptor and second messengers.[16] Evidence from adult ICU experience has suggested a benefit from the use of insulin infusions to maintain tight control over serum glucose level.[21] Although much of the preceding information derives from adult studies, it has found its way into contemporary pediatric practice in many centers in children of various ages. The use of insulin infusions to control hyperglycemia in premature infants continues to be standard practice.

The breakdown of protein is a central theme in the body's response to stress, which has wide-ranging significance beyond simple protein losses. The conversion of certain amino acids to glucose and the oxidation of others in peripheral tissues lead to the liberation of large quantities of amino-nitrogen, which would become toxic if not for the efficient conversion to urea. A dramatic increase in the rate of urea production is seen in critically ill patients. Concomitantly, other nonurea nitrogen is liberated in the form of uric acid and creatine and accounts for the dramatic increase in nitrogen wasting seen during stress states. Total urinary nitrogen losses in critically ill children may be 0.3 g/kg/d, which represents the loss of approximately 1.8 g/kg/d of protein.[22] In parallel with the increased turnover of proteins, the metabolic rate for the oxidation of energy substrates increases especially during the recovery phase of critical illness (see subsequent section on energy expenditure).

It has long been recognized that the body's response to withholding feeding (i.e., starvation) in healthy individuals is qualitatively and quantitatively different than that seen when nutrient intake is absent during periods of high physiologic stress. These differences are summarized in Table 113-1. In simple starvation, the body's regulatory mechanisms for sparing lean tissue and using triglycerides as the primary energy source are intact, whereas under the influence of the stress response, rapid depletion of lean tissues occurs with oxidation of amino acids, carbohydrate, and fat as energy substrates.

One of the major consequences of life-threatening physiologic stress is the net depletion of body protein representing structural (e.g., skeletal muscle mass) and functional (e.g., plasma proteins, enzyme systems, antibodies) tissues. With protein catabolism rates increased twofold,[23] synthesis does not keep pace, and a state of negative nitrogen balance ensues when patients are not given adequate calories and protein.[24,25] These changes produce depressed function of T and B lymphocytes, monocytes and neutrophils as cumulative protein loss increases. The synthesis of antibodies, chemotaxis, phagocytosis, and bacterial killing is impaired in the face of advanced protein-caloric malnutrition.[26]

TABLE 113–1. COMPARISON OF NUTRIENT METABOLISM IN STARVATION VERSUS SEPSIS/TRAUMA*

	Starvation	Sepsis/Trauma
Protein breakdown	+	+++
Hepatic protein synthesis	+	+++
Ureagenesis	+	+++
Gluconeogenesis	+	+++
Energy expenditure	Reduced	Increased
Mediator activity	Low	High
Hormone counterregulatory capacity	Preserved	Poor
Use of ketones	+++	+
Loss of body stores	Gradual	Rapid
Primary fuels	Fat	Amino acids, glucose, triglycerides

*Adapted from Barton R, Cerra FB: The hypermetabolism:multiple organ failure syndrome. Chest 1989;96:1153-1160.

A decrease in the total lymphocyte count may be seen in many patients, but a total lymphocyte count less than 1200/mm³ should raise concern for the presence of possible immune dysfunction. These alterations lead to impairment of host defense mechanisms. As noted earlier for the resolution of the inflammatory response, the patient's immune system plays a central role in recovery of wound healing and the recovery of immune competence.[27,28] It is likely that the syndrome of multiple organ dysfunction seen in critically ill patients is due in part to the inability of the immune system to down-regulate the inflammatory response to injury in specific organs. Nutrition support of a critically ill patient is thought to be essential to achieving recovery and minimizing the period of convalescence.

Considerable attention currently is focused on the use of modified nutrition support regimens in critically ill adults to modify the inflammatory response and to reduce secondary organ system dysfunction.[29] A wide range of substances have been shown to improve outcome or minimize nitrogen loss during critical illness in specific populations of patients.[30] Glutamine supplementation in critical illness continues to be a controversial subject with conflicting opinions regarding its value in either parenteral or enteral nutrition.[31] Reports have shown the beneficial effects of eicosapentaenoic acid, γ-linolenic acid, and antioxidants in critically ill adults. The preliminary results suggest that formulas supplemented with these products improve oxygenation[32] and reduce the alveolar inflammatory response during acute respiratory distress syndrome.[32,33] Trials of these agents are under way in critically ill children.

ENERGY EXPENDITURE

All cellular processes require energy generally in the form of adenosine triphosphate (ATP), which is produced through the oxidation of metabolic fuels with heat and water as byproducts. The production of ATP is closely coupled to cellular metabolism and must be maintained to prevent cell death. As ATP levels decline, ionic gradients cannot be maintained, excitatory cells cannot depolarize, the synthesis of new cells and repair of damaged cell constituents cannot occur, and mechanical work such as cardiac pump function and respiratory activity ceases. The body has numerous mechanisms for efficiently producing energy from a wide variety of substrates, including protein, fat, and carbohydrates. After the adaptation to decreased nutrient intake, an otherwise healthy individual relies on ketone bodies derived from the breakdown of fat stores to provide critical intracellular energy. Protein stores are relatively spared as the decrease in insulin output allows the metabolism to shift to a ketone-based state. As indicated in Table 113-1, critical illness impairs the normal conservational mechanisms of the body in response to decreased intake, leading to relatively rapid depletion of carbohydrate and available protein stores.

The close coupling between oxidative metabolism and substrate use is reflected in the amount of oxygen consumed (VO_2) and carbon dioxide produced (VCO_2) through the pathways of intermediary metabolism, which include the glycolytic pathway and the tricarboxylic acid cycle. Specific substrates, such as fat, protein, and various carbohydrates, have a characteristic relationship between VO_2 and VCO_2 based on the stoichiometry of their unique oxidation. This relationship is referred to as the *respiratory quotient* (RQ = VCO_2/VO_2) and may be measured through the quantification

of respiratory gas exchange through the patient's lung. The overall metabolic rate is determined most easily in the clinical setting through the process of *indirect calorimetry,* a process that estimates the resting energy expenditure based on VO_2 and VCO_2.[34] The respiratory quotient for fats is approximately 0.707 and for proteins approximately 0.809.[34] This concept is shown for the aerobic metabolism of glucose:

$$C_6H_{12}O_6 + 6O_2 \rightarrow 6CO_2 + 6H_2O \text{ (energy liberated = } 686 \text{ kcal/mol)}$$

$$RQ = 6CO_2/6O_2 = 1$$

The availability of equipment to perform indirect calorimetry reliably in children has been a major obstacle to its widespread application. Several factors limit the reliability with which indirect calorimetry can be performed in young children, including non–steady state due to patient movement and nursing interventions, the use of uncuffed endotracheal tubes producing loss of respiratory gases, high bias flows on infant ventilators, the use of elevated inspired oxygen concentration in nonintubated infants, and the small tidal volumes seen in the smallest patients. When indirect calorimetry is not feasible, VO_2 can be calculated in many patients via the Fick equation (A × VdO_2 × cardiac output) when a reliable measure of cardiac output is available. Based on a conversion factor of approximately 5 kcal of energy per liter of oxygen consumed, one can closely estimate metabolic rate[34] if the oxygen consumption is known.

Through indirect calorimetry, it has become clear that patients with similar clinical appearances may have widely differing metabolic rates when adjusted for age and weight.[35-40] These differences may be 300%, suggesting the potential for severe overnutrition[41] or undernutrition depending on the values assumed. Clinicians in the pediatric ICU generally must rely on information provided in controlled studies to guide the delivery of calories because most will not have a means of easily determining the resting energy expenditure. A wide range of predictive equations have been devised that attempt to predict energy requirements of critically ill children, but it is clear that no single method of estimating caloric expenditures would be successful for all critically ill children.[42]

In very young infants, the effects of environmental cold stress are recognized as a source of unnecessary morbidity. The thermal neutral zone in infants up to age 1 year tends to be several degrees higher than that for burned adults or older children. Heat lost to the environment produces rapid reductions in core temperature in young children with concomitant increase in metabolic demands. Maintaining the environment in a range of 30°C to 34°C through the use of servocontrolled heaters or other means can reduce energy requirements significantly in critically ill infants.

NUTRITION SUPPORT FOR A CRITICALLY ILL CHILD

The provision of nutrition support for critically ill children requires different considerations than conventional nutrition of healthy children.[43] During periods of critical illness, the use of nutrients for growth is markedly inhibited by the hormonal response to stress and the circulating inflammatory mediators. The use of calories for activity is much lower than under normal conditions. In addition, diet-induced thermogenesis is affected in hospitalized patients by the different routes and formulations of nutrients provided. Estimates of increased caloric and protein requirements during acute illness and recovery indicate that children have greater requirements for both on a body weight basis compared with critically ill adults. One of the most important points for clinicians prescribing nutrition support is to provide calories in a thoughtful manner based on the guidelines provided here and to *avoid excess caloric intake* during the acute phase of illness. During acute critical illness in children, many investigators have found resting energy expenditure to be increased less than previously expected[30,40,42] with significant risk for overfeeding.

MAINTENANCE FLUIDS

Maintenance fluids for most patients can be estimated based on body weight as indicated in Table 113-2. Children generally have increased requirements in relation to body weight for fluid, energy, protein, and many micronutrients. Water metabolism is closely coupled to metabolic activity because of the central place that water plays in intermediary metabolism. For a term newborn, these amounts should be reduced during the first few days of life because of their increased total body water. Premature infants have other considerations, and consultation with a pediatrician or neonatologist is crucial to provide appropriate and adequate fluid. The volumes must be increased for fever or persistent tachypnea because of increased insensible fluid losses. Additional fluids must be provided when abnormal losses are present, such as from diarrhea, nasogastric drainage, or wound loss in burns or from other sites. The composition of the replacement fluid is based on the content of sodium, potassium, bicarbonate, and chloride lost and conforms to conventional surgical and medical guidelines for fluid replacement. Typical maintenance fluids should provide sodium (3 to 5 mEq/kg/d) and potassium (2 to 3 mEq/kg/d) salts and a modest amount of glucose (5% or 10% if <1 year old). The provision of glucose in maintenance fluids is thought to spare lean tissue through the elicitation of insulin release, which exerts an anticatabolic effect in minimally stressed patients.

PRESCRIBING NUTRITION SUPPORT

The decision to provide nutrition via a parenteral or enteral route takes many factors into consideration, including the anticipated time to resumption of normal dietary intake, the available routes of nutrient administration, underlying metabolic or endocrine conditions, and the existence of organ dysfunction. When patients are not to receive conventional nutrition for a prolonged period, it is appropriate to consider support via the gut or intravenously. There is significant evidence that the enteral route is superior to TPN when it can be tolerated. Advantages of the enteral route include better maintenance of gut structure and function, reduced bacterial translocation, fewer metabolic complications, decreased intrahepatic cholestasis, greater ease and safety of administration, better outcomes, and reduced cost.[44,45]

Nutrition should be started as soon as the patient is metabolically stable. For a critically ill patient, sufficient metabolic stability has been achieved when aggressive correction of the electrolyte derangements has been achieved, and the acid-base status no longer requires aggressive correction.

When the decision has been made to start nutrition support, it is important to establish clear goals. During most acute critical illness, it is unreasonable to anticipate significant somatic growth, and the energy required for normal daily activities is markedly decreased. It is more realistic to employ nutrition support during this phase of illness to minimize the loss of lean body mass and to support the synthesis of critical visceral proteins required for organ function, antibody production, and the functioning immune system and to provide substrate for wound healing. The requirements for nutrients can be divided into macronutrients consisting of carbohydrate, protein, and fat and micronutrients consisting of minerals, vitamins, and trace elements. The vitamins and trace elements play key roles as essential cofactors in protein synthesis and intermediary metabolism.

CARBOHYDRATE

Carbohydrate serves predominantly as an energy source. The carbon backbone of the sugars also provides the basis for synthesis of many of the nonessential nutrients in the body. Carbohydrate is provided as sugars or starches in enteral formulas and as dextrose in parenteral nutrition. The caloric density of common dietary carbohydrate is generally 4 kcal/g except for dextrose solutions, which provide 3.4 kcal/g owing to energy lost through the process of hydration in solution. As the primary energy source, the rate of infusion should be adjusted to achieve the goals outlined in Table 113-3.

In general, the cellular energy requirements of most critically ill children and adults can be met through the infusion of 5 to 8 mg/kg/min of dextrose. This range represents approximately 25 to 40 kcal/kg/d of carbohydrate calories and is a close first approximation of basal energy expenditure seen in many hospitalized children. In healthy, nonstressed individuals, ketosis ensues when glucose entry into the circulation declines to less than 1.5 to 2 mg/kg/min. As an additional point of reference, infusion of greater than 10 to 12 mg/kg/min of glucose results in net lipogenesis and excess carbon dioxide production in most hospitalized patients. When hyperglycemia develops in the face of *appropriate* rates of glucose infusion, it has become routine to administer insulin as a continuous infusion. Reports in critically ill adults[21] and in an experimental animal model[46] strongly support the control of serum glucose in critically ill patients in a narrow euglycemic range. This practice has become commonplace

TABLE 113-2. APPROXIMATE MAINTENANCE FLUID REQUIREMENTS

Body Weight	Fluid Volume (mL/kg/d)
First 10 kg	100
Second 10 kg	50
Each additional kg	20

TABLE 113-3. TARGET GOALS FOR NONPROTEIN CALORIES (kcal/kg/d)

	Acute Phase (First 3-5 days)	Convalescent Phase (After 5 days)
Infants (<10 kg)	50-80	80-120
Children (1-7 years)	45-65	75-90
Children (>7 years)	30-50	30-75

in pediatric critical care, although rigorous evaluation of its benefit has not been established. The rate of insulin infusion required to control the serum glucose concentration may be two to three times higher than is routinely used in the treatment of diabetes as a result of the insulin resistance seen during critical illness.

FAT

A maximum of 20% to 30% of the caloric intake should be derived from fat. Intravenous fat should be infused as a 20% emulsion in infants to provide a concentrated calorie source (2 kcal/mL) and to supply essential fatty acids and lipid crucial to central nervous system development and cell membrane repair. Intravenous fat emulsions are administered continuously, unless rising plasma triglyceride levels suggest inadequate clearance. During periods of high physiologic stress, triglyceride levels frequently are elevated due to decreased peripheral clearance of triglycerides secondary to impaired lipoprotein lipase activity, increased generation of triglycerides from excess carbohydrate infusions, and elevation of lipolytic hormones in response to stress. To assess clearance, a minimal period of 4 hours without lipid infusion is needed to approximate the actual triglyceride level. A typical maximum for intravenous fat emulsion is 2.5 to 3.5 g/kg/d. Patients on enteral feedings may tolerate medium-chain triglycerides after bowel injury or with right-sided heart failure better than long-chain fats. Medium-chain triglycerides are absorbed directly into the portal circulation, avoiding the complex absorptive process needed to digest long-chain fats. Formulas developed for patients with biliary disease typically contain a greater content of medium-chain triglycerides, and many of the formulas developed for patients with absorption difficulties provide a significant portion of the triglyceride in the form of medium-chain triglycerides.

PROTEIN

Protein requirements are met through the provision of conventional enteral formulas or formulas containing hydrolysates of complex proteins that provide oligopeptides. Enteral formulas containing primary amino acids tend to be hypertonic with limited absorptive advantages due to the presence of mucosal transporter mechanisms that absorb dipeptides and tripeptides more efficiently. The high rate of protein turnover during critical illness is associated with an increase in ureagenesis and urinary nitrogen losses that may amount to 1 to 2 g/kg/d of protein equivalent. To minimize nitrogen loss and ensure that no amino acid concentration declines to a level that would limit protein synthesis, high-quality protein nutrition must be given through the acute and convalescent phase of illness. Conceptually, proteins must be administered in amounts sufficient to replace losses with additional protein to synthesize new tissue. Table 113-4 provides guidelines for the administration of protein to

children in the ICU. Nitrogen balance in response to nutrition support represents a continuum. In one study, the investigators found that nitrogen balance was obtained at an intake of 2.8 g/kg/d.[36] Positive nitrogen balance was achieved only with amino acid infusion rates at the upper end of the rates typically used by clinicians. Calories must be provided in sufficient quantity to ensure that protein can be used for synthesis rather than as an energy substrate.

The concept of calorie-to-nitrogen ratio derives from the concept that protein should be used for synthesis of functional and structural molecules rather than used as energy. Energy must be provided in adequate amounts. For a typical healthy individual, the ratio of enteral nonprotein calories to nitrogen ranges from 250:1 to 350:1. Because of the obligatory oxidation of amino acids during catabolic states, the nonprotein calories to nitrogen generally are much lower—in the range of 100:1 to 250:1. This ratio provides a convenient method for checking that the protein infusion is in line with the nonprotein calories. Low ratios suggest either excess protein delivery or inadequate calories.

SPECIAL CONSIDERATIONS

Patients with hepatic failure require a restriction of protein intake. Typically, patients with elevated plasma ammonia levels due to hepatic insufficiency should be restricted to approximately 1 g/kg/d of protein regardless of age. This protein may be provided as a conventional enteral formula or as parenteral nutrition. The blood products frequently administered in support of patients with liver failure contain significant amounts of protein that must be considered in the total nitrogen intake. Children with inborn errors of metabolism require care that is tailored to their specific metabolic lesion. Their nutrition needs are best determined by a clinician or dietitian experienced in the management of children with metabolic disorders.

Patients with renal insufficiency should receive nutrition that is optimized to achieve wound healing without excessive concern for the increase in blood urea seen. In general, the increase in nitrogen load is handled through dialysis so that optimal nutrition can be provided to promote recovery.

MICRONUTRIENTS

Multivitamin preparations are provided either as unit doses by the pharmacy in parenteral nutrition or as multivitamin infusion in the standard formulas. Occasionally, additional vitamins or trace elements are required for specific deficiency states or diseases, but fine-tuning of micronutrients other than minerals and electrolytes has been difficult to achieve clinically. Current recommendations are given in Table 113-5.

ROUTE OF ADMINISTRATION

Nutrition should be provided via the gastrointestinal tract whenever possible, supplementing with peripheral or central parenteral nutrition when adequate enteral intake cannot be achieved. In patients with significant burns, an enteral feeding tube should be placed within the first hours of hospitalization. Continuous drip feedings should begin within hours to minimize bowel dysmotility and feeding intolerance often seen if feeding is delayed in such patients. In other patients, initiating feedings on the second hospital day is feasible in

TABLE 113-4. PROTEIN REQUIREMENTS (g/kg/d)

	Acute Phase (First 3-5 days)	Convalescent Phase (After 5 days)
Infants/children (<7 years)	1.5-2.5	2-3
Children (>7 years)	1.5-2	1.5-2.5

TABLE 113–5. MICRONUTRIENTS

Weight (kg)	Copper	Zinc	Manganese	Chromium
<3	20 µg/kg/d	300 µg/kg/d	10 µg/kg/d	0.2 µg/kg/d
3-25	20 µg/kg/d	100 µg/kg/d	10 µg/kg/d	0.2 µg/kg/d
>25	1 mg/d	2.5-5 mg/d	0.25 mg/d	10 mg/d

Note. Multivitamins as per hospital standard per age.
From Joint FAO/WHO/UNU Expert Consultation: Energy and Protein Requirements. Geneva, WHO, 1985.

most cases and should be provided initially as a continuous infusion at a minimal rate of approximately 1 mL/kg/h and advanced as tolerated. The provision of *trophic* feedings is thought to provide many benefits, even though significant nutrition intake cannot be achieved. These benefits include maintenance of gut motility, improved mesenteric blood flow, and the release of trophic factors from the gut and pancreas that maintain enterocyte mass and hepatocyte function.[47] In addition, the enterocytes derive a significant portion of their nutrient and energetic requirements from the luminal contents during digestion, making enteral nutrition ideal when tolerated.

During acute critical illness, continuous drip feedings tend to be better tolerated than bolus feedings, especially in patients with respiratory distress. Transpyloric feeding when possible via weighted Silastic catheters should be used to minimize the risk of gastroesophageal reflux and aspiration. This approach has been used with excellent results in critically ill children.[44,45] Placement of transpyloric feeding tubes can be done blindly by some experienced clinicians or may be done by a radiologist under fluoroscopic guidance. Occasionally, metoclopramide or erythromycin may facilitate the passage of a transpyloric tube.[48] Even when a transpyloric feeding tube cannot be placed, continuous enteral feeding via a nasogastric tube may confer most of the benefits, although the risk of gastroesophageal reflux is increased. For young infants, breast milk is the optimal nutrient source and can be delivered easily by feeding tube when the infant cannot nurse. In older patients, the initial enteral nutrition formula for most critically ill children should be lactose-free, have some of the fat provided as medium-chain triglycerides, and contain easily absorbed proteins (i.e., dipeptides and tripeptides; see earlier). Most currently available formulas developed for children between ages 1 and 10 years conform to these recommendations. A wide variety of formulas exist, and the availability may vary from region to region. The hospital dietitian is best prepared to help in the selection of appropriate formulas and knows which products are available locally.

Although beyond the scope of the current discussion, a special consideration for premature infants and newborns includes the use of formulas supplemented with docosahexaenoic acid and arachidonic acid.[49] Docosahexaenoic acid and arachidonic acid are long-chain polyunsaturated fatty acids found in breast milk and added to infant formulas. Their importance in infant nutrition was recognized by the rapid accretion of these fatty acids in the brain during the first postnatal year. Subsequent reports of enhanced intellectual development in breast-fed children and recognition of the physiologic importance of docosahexaenoic acid in visual and neural systems from studies in animal models led to formulas being developed that contain them.[49] It is becoming routine in neonatal patients to supplement docosahexaenoic acid and arachidonic acid when providing enteral feedings.

Infants younger than 6 months old should receive isotonic or hypotonic feedings initially until tolerance has been shown. Young children between 1 and 5 years old should receive an age-appropriate formula or an adult formula with appropriate supplements of protein, vitamins, and trace elements. Critically ill children older than age 10 generally tolerate enteral formulas developed for adult patients with supplementation of vitamins and micronutrients as needed for age. Enteral formulas should be initially isotonic or hypotonic to minimize the possibility of diarrhea from excess osmotic load to the gut and to facilitate absorption. Infusion rates are begun conservatively at approximately 1 mL/kg/h with a stepwise increase every 4 to 6 hours as tolerated up to the desired final rate. When an acceptable rate is achieved, caloric density may be increased as tolerated. The clinician must maintain vigilance for evidence of feeding intolerance. In patients with poor tissue perfusion, enteral feedings are feasible; however, the risk of necrotizing enterocolitis is increased slightly when using the gut for nutrition. Any signs of pronounced abdominal distention, profuse diarrhea, severe gastroesophageal reflux, or the development of a new metabolic acidemia should lead to holding of feedings and assessing the abdomen before reinstituting feedings. Common manifestations of enteral feeding intolerance are outlined in Table 113-6.

PARENTERAL NUTRITION

One of the great achievements of nutrition science has been the development of effective and safe nutrients to provide TPN over prolonged periods intravenously. TPN has been invaluable in the survival of critically ill premature infants; children with congenital or acquired bowel defects; and children who do not tolerate enteral nutrition owing to malabsorption, surgery, or other causes of bowel dysfunction. TPN may come with a significant cost, however, in terms of iatrogenic electrolyte and acid-base disturbance, cholestasis, and hepatic fibrosis after prolonged TPN (especially in infants with short bowel syndrome), excess carbon dioxide production, and increased risk of bacterial and fungal infection.[50] The goals of TPN support during critical illness need to be clarified and kept realistic to avoid adding unnecessary metabolic stress to already compromised pulmonary, renal, and hepatic function. Excess TPN may contribute to organ dysfunction through the increased demands of the organs to regulate the nutrients that are infused directly into the circulation avoiding the first-pass counterregulation that occurs with enteral nutrition.

Amino acid solutions developed for neonates (e.g., TrophAmine) that contain taurine, tyrosine, cysteine, and histidine provide an advantage for select newborns and young

TABLE 113–6. ENTERAL FEEDING INTOLERANCE

Problem	Possible Reason	Possible Remedy
Diarrhea, malabsorption	Delivery too fast	Decrease delivery rate
	High osmotic load	Reduce volume
	Mucosal injury	TPN, continuous low-rate infusion to allow bowel recovery
	Substrate intolerance	Use elemental formula, especially disaccharide-free with MCT
Gastric retention/ gastroesophageal reflux	Hypertonic formula	Decrease osmolarity, dilute
	High long-chain fat content	Change to MCT-containing formula
	Hypodynamic gut	Positioning right-side down, consider prokinetic agent: metoclopramide (Reglan), opiate antagonist
Abdominal distention	Ileus, constipation	Rule out surgical abdomen, rule out constipation
		Add bulking agent or stool softener

MCT, medium-chain triglyceride; TPN, total parenteral nutrition.

infants with biliary disease, sepsis, or high physiologic stress. This effect derives from the increased content of branched-chain amino acids, the presence of amino acids that are conditionally "essential for age" in infants, and a reduction in nonessential amino acids. In premature infants or infants maintained on prolonged TPN, carnitine supplementation intravenously has been advocated to aid in triglyceride clearance through enhanced beta-oxidation of fatty acids.[51-53] In older children, conventional amino acid solutions (e.g., Aminosyn) provide adequate dietary nitrogen.

The provision of nutrients via TPN should be consistent with the guidelines set forth previously. Although an occasional patient may develop acute glucose intolerance or experience dramatic electrolyte changes after the initiation of TPN, it is generally well tolerated and can be advanced to full TPN within a few days. Pediatricians have had a habit of starting with dilute solutions of TPN and increasing protein and calorie intake slowly over many days as tolerance is shown. This approach has little scientific basis as long as nurses and physicians observe for signs of intolerance (e.g., hyperglycemia, glycosuria, acidemia, and hyperlipidemia).

A key point to the rapid achievement of the desired goal is to order the TPN solution at the intended final concentration and begin at half the intended ultimate infusion rate. If the goal for TPN is a 20% dextrose solution with 2 g/kg/d of protein to infuse at 44 mL/h, the pharmacy can prepare that goal solution, but it should be started at 22 mL/h until tolerance is evident by glucose monitoring. For comparison, this rate of infusion would be equivalent to a 10% solution with 1 g/kg/d of protein if it were running at the full 44 mL/h, a formulation that most clinicians would be comfortable starting. If the patient tolerates the infusion (e.g., no acidemia, hyperglycemia, or glycosuria) for 6 to 8 hours at the slower rate, the solution can be increased to 33 mL/h. After an additional period of demonstrated tolerance, the solution is increased to its intended final rate. This approach reduces the potential of waste of TPN and reduces a source of possible error in preparing the TPN for subsequent days. Daily changes in electrolyte content must be made as indicated by serum levels. The essential issue when taking this approach is to supplement with conventional maintenance intravenous fluids while TPN is being increased. Another useful approach to pediatric TPN is to plan for the entire day's nutrients to be placed in one half to two thirds of the total allowed daily fluid volume. The remaining maintenance volume of fluid is made up with proprietary crystalloid maintenance solutions

that can be increased or decreased as demanded by the fluid status of the patient without affecting the amount of nutrients delivered. Taking this approach also allows the clinician to reduce the total fluid intake without sacrificing the prescribed nutritional support. Using the two solutions allows one to titrate the intake as required by the changing clinical situation without abandoning the TPN for a given day.

ASSESSMENT OF RESPONSE TO NUTRITION SUPPORT

It is important to monitor the response to nutritional support. Intolerance of enteral support is frequently manifest through abdominal distention, vomiting, or other physical signs. With TPN, the intolerance is manifest in iatrogenic derangements of minerals, electrolytes, and acid-base status. Hyperglycemia was discussed previously, but may represent a complication of TPN administration. Standard nutrition assessment should be considered for each patient after the initial stress phase of critical illness. End-organ response to nutrition support is monitored by assessing whether serum transferrin or prealbumin is increasing or decreasing and whether genuine weight gain is occurring in convalescing patients.

In the event of inadequate response to nutrition support, a more detailed examination is necessary, including the measurement of albumin, total protein, and transferrin; a 24-hour urine collection to determine nitrogen balance; and, if possible, measurement of energy expenditure via indirect calorimetry. In extraordinary circumstances, consultation with a pediatric dietitian or gastroenterologist may be required to optimize the support. Total urinary nitrogen should be used to determine nitrogen balance in critically ill children due to the increased variability in the fraction of urinary nitrogen represented by urea in critical illness. As long as cardiopulmonary function is stable and lactic acidosis is not present, indirect calorimetry can provide practical information regarding overall energy expenditure and substrate use.

SUMMARY

Nutrition support of critically ill children is a central part of modern intensive care medicine. The complexity of pediatric disease and the wide range of nutrient options available necessitate close collaboration with dietary specialists who are familiar with children's nutrition requirements during critical illness. It has become almost axiomatic in critical care nutrition that giving ever more nutrition only produces undesired complications while not improving outcomes. Enteral nutrition will continue to be the preferred route of nutrition when it is tolerated, and it provides an efficient means of transitioning patients to conventional dietary intake when critical illness has resolved.

ANNOTATED REFERENCES

Bursztein S, Elwyn D, Askanazi J, et al: Energy Metabolism, Indirect Calorimetry, and Nutrition. Baltimore, Williams & Wilkins, 1989.

This book is a superb source of basic information regarding the measurement of energy expenditure. It includes theory and discussion of instrumentation and a clear explanation of the basis for fractionating energy expenditure into various substrates.

Chwals W, Lally K, Woolley M, et al: Measured energy expenditure in critically ill infants and young children. J Surg Res 1988;44:467-472.

This article contains a comprehensive discussion of energy use by young children after surgery and critical illness. The relatively limited caloric expenditure in such patients compared with healthy, age-matched children receiving normal nutrition is shown (see also references 36, 38, and 39).

Mizock B: Nutritional support in acute lung injury and acute respiratory distress syndrome. Nutr Clin Pract 2001;16:319-328.

The author gives an excellent overview of the cellular events in early acute respiratory distress syndrome. The author discusses the theory behind attempts at immune modulation of the pulmonary inflammatory response through manipulation of substrate delivery in enteral formulas (see also reference 32).

Shew S, Jaksic T: The metabolic needs of critically ill children and neonates. Semin Pediatr Surg 1999;8:131-139.

A comprehensive review is provided of metabolic responses in young children to physiologic stress. The senior author is experienced with in vivo stable isotope tracer studies in young children. This article is a good source for nutritional support versus underlying physiology.

Waterlow J: Classification and definition of protein-calorie malnutrition. BMJ 1972;3:566-569.

This is a classic article using weight for height as a measure of recent protein-calorie malnutrition and height for age as a measure of chronic protein-calorie deficits. These criteria were used in Pollack's observations of early nutritional depletion in critically ill children admitted to a tertiary care medical facility.

Chapter 114

PORTAL HYPERTENSION

Julia Wendon • E. Sizer

KEY POINTS

1. Portal hypertension is defined as the presence of a raised portacaval pressure gradient. The clinical implications and consequences of the presence of portal hypertension depend to some extent on the cause of the syndrome.

2. Those cases that have hepatic dysfunction as an integral component have a worse prognosis than those that do not.

3. Portal hypertension results from both increased resistance to portal flow and absolute increased portal flow, despite portosystemic collateral remodeling.

ANATOMY AND PHYSIOLOGY

The portal venous system drains blood from the gastrointestinal tract, pancreas, gallbladder, and spleen. The extrahepatic portal vein originates from the confluence of the splenic vein and the superior mesenteric vein and delivers blood to the liver. The inferior mesenteric vein and short gastric veins drain to the splenic vein. Flow in the portal vein is normally about 1 L/min (approximately 20% cardiac output) with a mean pressure of 7 mm Hg. Despite draining capillary beds and therefore having a relatively low oxygen content, 70% of hepatic oxygenation is derived from portal flow. The remainder of hepatic oxygen consumption is supplied by the blood flowing through the hepatic artery. Portal venous blood and hepatic arterial blood mix at the sinusoidal level and there exists a local hepatic arterial autoregulatory "buffer response" that increases arterial inflow in circumstances of low portal flow (adenosine mediated); nevertheless, total hepatic flow is not preserved where hepatic arterial flow is decreased.

Postsinusoidal blood drains through hepatic venules into hepatic veins and then into the inferior vena cava back to the systemic circulation. Hepatic venous pressure is normally 4 mm Hg.

A variety of pathologic processes can result in portal venous flow becoming "obstructed." Regardless of the cause (i.e., intra- or extrahepatic obstruction), this resistance to portal flow increases portal pressure and leads to the development of a collateral portosystemic circulation. Under these circumstances, only a small amount of the blood flow that originates within the portal system reaches the liver; the remainder is diverted and enters the systemic circulation directly.

The major sites of collateral remodeling are the gastroesophageal region, between the inferior mesenteric vein and the hemorrhoidal vein, the umbilical veins and cutaneous veins of the abdominal wall, and via retroperitoneal systems into the azygous system and the vena cava. Collateral vessels also may develop at the sites of previous surgery, trauma, or adhesions and may similarly be found at ileostomy or colostomy stoma (ectopic varices). In addition to the formation of discrete collateral vessels, there are also more generalized changes within the gastrointestinal tract, leading to vascular ectasia or so-called portal hypertensive enteropathy. Bleeding can occur from varices or there can be significant oozing from enteropathy.

Patients with portal hypertension exhibit characteristic splanchnic and systemic circulatory changes. Key to these manifestations is abnormal vasodilatation; this leads to splanchnic hyperemia and hypervolemia but effectively reduces central blood volume, leading to systemic hypotension. In turn, these circulatory changes prompt homeostatic systemic responses to hypovolemia, such as activation of the vasoconstrictor and sodium-retaining mechanisms. Overall, the changes comprise a hyperdynamic circulation, characterized by increased cardiac output, heart rate, and total plasma volume.

The origin of portal hypertension can be divided into cirrhotic and noncirrhotic and presinusoidal, sinusoidal, and postsinusoidal (Table 114-1).

DIAGNOSIS OF PORTAL HYPERTENSION

As mentioned earlier, portal hypertension is defined by pressure measurements: specifically, the gradient between portal and caval pressures (the portal pressure gradient). The normal value for the portal pressure gradient is 2 to 6 mm Hg. If this gradient is greater than 10 mm Hg, then clinically significant portal hypertension is present. Varices are rarely (maybe never) seen if the gradient is less than 10 mm Hg. Variceal bleeding is not observed if the pressure gradient is less than 12 mm Hg. Most importantly, protection from variceal bleeding is gained if the pressure gradient can be manipulated to less than 12 mm Hg.[1]

The direct measurement of this value is invasive. The most frequently adopted method involves transjugular catheterization. The advantage of this approach is that caval and hepatic venous pressures can be measured during the same procedure. Less frequently, a transhepatic approach is adopted and, rarely, direct surgical measurements are used. These less frequently used methods only measure absolute portal pressures, and a second measurement of caval pressure is still needed to calculate the gradient. Because of the

TABLE 114–1. ETIOLOGY OF PORTAL HYPERTENSION

Condition	Site of Increased Resistance	FHVP	WHVP	HVPG	SPP	Liver Disease
Cirrhosis	Intrahepatic sinusoidal	Normal	Increased	Increased	Increased	Yes
Alcoholic hepatitis	Intrahepatic sinusoidal	Normal	Increased	Increased	Increased	Yes
Extrahepatic portal, splenic, or mesenteric vein thrombosis	Extrahepatic presinusoidal	Normal	Normal	Normal	Increased	No
Early primary biliary cirrhosis, PSC, sarcoid, schistosomiasis, congestive heart failure, noncirrhotic portal fibrosis, NRH	Intrahepatic presinusoidal	Normal	Normal/ ?raised	Normal/ ?raised	Increased	No
Hemochromatosis, peliosis, infiltrative disease, acute fatty liver of pregnancy	Intrahepatic sinusoidal hypertension	Normal	Increased	Increased	Increased	Yes
Veno-occlusive disease, post-transplant rejection	Intrahepatic postsinusoidal hypertension	Normal	?Increased	?Decreased	Increased	Yes
Budd-Chiari syndrome (noncirrhotic)	Extrahepatic postsinusoidal hypertension	Increased	Increased	Normal	Increased	Depends on severity
Constrictive pericarditis, inferior vena cava obstruction, congenital inferior vena cava web, right heart failure	Extrahepatic postsinusoidal hypertension	Increased	Increased	Normal	Increased	Depends on severity

FHVP, free hepatic venous pressure; HVPG, hepatic venous pressure gradient; SPP, systolic pulse pressure; WHVP, wedged hepatic venous pressure.

invasiveness of this technique, it is usually only used intraoperatively during surgery for portal hypertension.

Indirect measurements also can be used to assess the portal pressure gradient. This procedure involves measurement of the free and wedged hepatic venous pressure using catheterization of the right hepatic vein. Wedged hepatic venous pressure (measured using a balloon-tipped catheter) reflects the pressure in a static column of blood from the hepatic vein to the sinusoid. It is an assessment of sinusoidal pressure rather than portal venous pressure, and, therefore, may underestimate the portal pressure gradient in disease states characterized by presinusoidal hypertension (see Table 114-1). The free hepatic venous pressure is obtained with the catheter in the hepatic vein and gives an assessment of caval pressure. Free hepatic venous pressure is not elevated in patients with diseases characterized by presinusoidal and sinusoidal portal hypertension, but it is characteristically raised in states of hepatic outflow block such as Budd-Chiari syndrome. The gradient between the two measurements is called the hepatic venous pressure gradient and is the most commonly quoted parameter in the medical literature regarding management of portal hypertension. Both the absolute value of hepatic venous pressure gradient and the change in hepatic venous pressure gradient with pharmacotherapy have prognostic significance related to the risk of variceal bleeding.[2] The splenic pulp pressure is a useful parameter in diseases with predominantly presinusoidal portal hypertension, when, as mentioned earlier, wedged hepatic venous pressure underestimates portal pressure.

It can be appreciated that even indirect methods of measuring portal pressure are not readily available in most settings. Instead, most clinicians rely on the clinical manifestations of portal hypertension: esophagogastric varices, splenomegaly, edema, and ascites.

COMPLICATIONS OF PORTAL HYPERTENSION

VARICES

Bleeding from varices is a major cause of morbidity and mortality in patients with significant portal hypertension. Life expectancy after variceal bleeding is considerably curtailed, both as an immediate consequence of hemorrhage (and its consequences, such as sepsis and renal failure) and in the longer term due to rebleeding.

Gastroesophageal varices are present in approximately 50% of cirrhotic patients and are large in 20%. Approximately one-third of patients with varices develop bleeding. The patients at greatest risk of bleeding are those with advanced liver disease and large varices. It is therefore important to identify the population at risk and modify their risk of bleeding. In patients with cirrhosis, the incidence of varices is 5% per year.[3] Patients with portal hypertension should undergo screening endoscopy to assess the severity of varices.[4] Once large varices are present, the risk of first bleeding is estimated at 15% per year.[5] At this point, it is generally accepted that patients have clinically significant portal hypertension, and primary prophylaxis (i.e., the prevention of a variceal bleed) may be appropriate.

ACUTE VARICEAL HEMORRHAGE

There is increasing evidence to suggest that an episode of infection is the precipitating event in most cases. Infection leads to a sudden rise in portal pressure and acute variceal hemorrhage. The vascular effect of infection in this setting is thought to relate to release of cytokines and inflammatory mediators, resulting in increased hepatic resistance and possibly increased portal venous flow with a sudden rise in portal pressure. A postprandial increase in splanchnic blood flow can also contribute to an acute rise in portal pressure.

Patients present acutely with hematemesis with or without melena. These patients can have significant hypovolemia and hypotension (especially if receiving beta-adrenergic antagonists) and an acute fall in hemoglobin concentration.

Resuscitation should follow standard guidelines, and steps should include securing the airway, ensuring adequate respiratory function, and obtaining intravenous access to enable circulatory resuscitation. In particular, early intubation should be considered in the face of the high risk of aspiration due to encephalopathy, the need for esophagogastroduodenoscopy, the presence of a full stomach, and a requirement for sedation.

TREATMENT

VOLUME REPLACEMENT

Resuscitation to normal arterial pressure results in acutely raised portal pressures with an attendant risk of rebleeding. Therefore, resuscitation to a systolic blood pressure of 90 mm Hg is adequate, although no class 1 evidence exists for this recommendation.[6] Large-volume blood loss will require support of coagulation with replacement of appropriate factors.

PHARMACOTHERAPY

At the same time as resuscitation, first-line treatment of suspected variceal hemorrhage in patients classified as high risk should include pharmacotherapy with a vasoactive drug prior to endoscopy. Treatment in this way will increase systemic pressure and possibly at the same time decrease portal flow, pressure, and variceal bleeding.

Terlipressin (Glypressin) is a prodrug of vasopressin that has some intrinsic activity. It acts on vasopressin 1 receptors within arteriolar smooth muscle and induces vasoconstriction via phospholipase C cascades. It causes splanchnic vasoconstriction and decreases splanchnic inflow, thus reducing portal pressure. Terlipressin also reduces collateral flow and variceal pressure. It is associated with decreased systemic ischemic events as compared with vasopressin and can be used without concomitant therapy with organic nitrates. Because of its structure, it requires cleavage of the glycol group before it becomes active. It has a longer half-life than vasopressin and can be administered intermittently. A dose of 2 mg IV given four times daily is as effective as endoscopic sclerotherapy in achieving initial control of variceal bleeding and preventing early rebleeding.[7] Terlipressin is well tolerated and has few side effects and may represent first-line treatment in acute hemorrhage until endoscopy can be performed in a controlled environment.

The duration of treatment should be governed by the clinical situation, but after 48 hours of therapy should be reviewed and the dose tapered (initially halved) with a total course being 6 to 7 days.

The role of some of the other vasoactive agents (somatostatin, octreotide, and the angiotensin 2 inhibitors) are less clearly defined. The somatostatin analogue octreotide may act by blocking the acute rise in portal pressure associated with fluid resuscitation in the face of gastrointestinal hemorrhage. Its use is associated with improved outcome after therapeutic endoscopy, but it is not associated with the salutary effect if used alone. Octreotide is a long-acting analogue of somatostatin; it acts by blocking the vasodilatory effects of glucagon and vasoactive intestinal peptide. The side-effect profile is more favorable than side-effect profiles for terlipressin or vasopressin.[8]

THERAPEUTIC ENDOSCOPY

As mentioned earlier, endoscopy should be undertaken after the patient is resuscitated. With the advent of pharmacotherapy, endoscopy does not need to be performed immediately, but should be carried out at the earliest opportunity by an experienced operator in the appropriate environment. None of the endoscopic methods of therapy reduce portal pressure; instead, they act by interrupting the abnormal collateral flow either by occlusion (band ligation, glue techniques) or by the induction of thrombosis (sclerotherapy).

Sclerosant Therapy Versus Banding Versus Glue

Endoscopic Sclerotherapy. In this approach, a sclerosant is injected directly into the varix. A variety of sclerosants are in use, but ethanolamine and sodium tetradecyl sulfate are the most common. No studies have shown any one to be superior to the others. The immediate effect of controlling bleeding is probably due to edema caused by the injection of sclerosant; thrombosis occurs later. Injection sclerotherapy can be accompanied by complications (Table 114-2). The rate of mortality related to severe complications is approximately 15%.[9] The most common long-term complication is esophageal stricture.

Endoscopic Band Ligation. In this method, a rubber band is placed on a variceal column that has been aspirated into a cylinder attached to the endoscope. The initial effect is caused by strangulation of the vessel that is the source of variceal hemorrhage; later, thrombosis and ischemia result, leaving a shallow mucosal ulcer. Endoscopic band ligation is associated with fewer complications than endoscopic sclerotherapy,[10] and systemic complications are rare. Although superficial ulceration is a side-effect of endoscopic band ligation, stricture formation is rare. The most hazardous complication is bleeding associated with early shedding of the band.

Glue. A recent report in small numbers of patients with decompensated liver disease and severe esophageal variceal hemorrhage suggests that injection of tissue glue rather than sclerosant may result in improved initial hemostasis, reduced rebleeding, and improved survival. However, this approach requires further study and comparison with endoscopic band ligation and other therapies before it is universally adopted.

TABLE 114–2. COMPLICATIONS OF ENDOSCOPIC SCLEROSANT THERAPY

Site	Complication
Local	Ulcers
	Bleeding
	Stricture
	Esophageal dysmotility
Regional	Perforation
	Mediastinitis
	Pleural effusion
Systemic	Sepsis
	Aspiration

Esophageal Varices Versus Gastric Varices

Gastric varices can be subclassified according to their anatomic position, relationship to esophageal varices, and whether they are primary in origin or whether they develop as a result of obliteration of esophageal varices. The Baveno III Consensus classifies gastric varices as gastroesophageal varices and isolated gastric varices. Endoscopic management of bleeding gastric varices can be technically demanding. Depending on local expertise, banding or glue injection may be attempted; however, some centers regard bleeding gastric varices as an indication for transjugular intrahepatic porto-systemic shunt (TIPS).

FAILURE OF THERAPY/SALVAGE

Therapy failure is defined as

- Inability to achieve initial control of bleeding
- Need for alternative therapy
- Early rebleeding
- Death within 5 days of first bleed

In 10% to 20% of patients, initial methods fail to control variceal bleeding. This group of patients are at high risk for having a poor outcome, as discussed later. Salvage management of failed therapy relies on other modalities for halting ongoing bleeding.

MECHANICAL SALVAGE METHODS

The use of balloon tamponade to control variceal hemorrhage has decreased dramatically with the widespread use of vasoactive agents and therapeutic endoscopy. Nonetheless, its role in the emergency management of uncontrollable bleeding varices cannot be doubted. Inflation of the gastric balloon results in tamponade of the varices, reduces blood flow into the plexus, and controls bleeding. The use of balloon tamponade effectively controls initial bleeding in 90% of patients. In the vast majority of cases, adequate control is achieved by inflation of the gastric balloon plus adequate traction without inflation of the esophageal balloon. It is rarely necessary to inflate the esophageal balloon, and it is important to appreciate that this maneuver contributes significantly to the incidence of potentially life-threatening complications. However, in approximately 50% patients, bleeding recurs upon deflation of the gastric balloon. Potential complications associated with the use of compression devices include pulmonary aspiration, esophageal mucosal ischemia and ulceration, and misplacement of the device with gastric balloon inflation in the esophagus, leading to esophageal perforation.

Ideally, the balloons should be filled with a mixture of water and radiocontrast material, allowing good delineation of position on chest radiograph. It is normally essential to intubate and ventilate patients who require balloon tamponade, to minimize the risk of aspiration and provide control of the airway. Balloon tamponade should be viewed as a short-term solution only, either until endoscopic therapy can be undertaken or until another definitive therapy can be undertaken if endoscopic management is not possible (e.g., TIPS). Regardless of other forms of salvage therapy, intermittent deflation of the gastric balloon is essential to avoid mucosal perfusion.

SHUNT SURGERY/INTERVENTIONAL RADIOLOGY

Traditionally, two types of surgical interventions have been used in the management of portal hypertension: operations aimed at decompressing the portal system and devascularization procedures. A third and more definitive alternative is liver transplantation.

Acute shunt surgery has been performed for more than 50 years. Although effective at lowering portal pressure (and thus decreasing the risk of further bleeding), shunting procedures can precipitate decompensation of liver function and encephalopathy by diverting portal blood flow away from the liver. The degree of these predictable events is somewhat dictated by whether the shunt is total, partial, or selective as well as the ability of the hepatic arterial autoregulation buffer response to increase hepatic arterial flow.

Side-to-side portacaval shunt is an example of a total shunt that is achieved either by direct anastomosis of the portal vein to the inferior vena cava or anastomosis using a short interpositional graft. Traditionally, the graft diameter is greater than 12 mm, producing total portal decompression. This procedure controls variceal bleeding in 95% to 98% of patients and ascites in more than 90% of patients. The encephalopathy rate is 30% to 40%. If the diameter of the graft is reduced to 8 mm, this type of shunt is known as a partial shunt. It does not provide total portal decompression, thus the risk of rebleeding is higher, but rates of both encephalopathy and ascites/liver failure are lower.

"Selective" shunts, such as the distal splenorenal shunt, aim to address the issue of portal flow diversion. The aim of this shunt is to decompress the gastroesophageal junction and the spleen through the splenic vein to the renal vein. Portal hypertension is thus maintained in the superior mesenteric and portal vein to maintain blood flow to the liver.

TIPS achieves the same effect in terms of decompression of the portal system without the operative risk. Depending on the diameter of the intrahepatic shunt, TIPS can be viewed as either a total or a partial shunt. It can be used in the setting of refractory acute hemorrhage when both endoscopic and pharmacologic strategies have failed. Use of TIPS, however, is not clearly associated with a survival benefit. TIPS carries a higher risk of precipitating encephalopathy and is significantly more expensive than either endoscopic or pharmacologic strategies. The exact subgroup of patients for whom salvage TIPS leads to a favorable outcome has not been characterized.

Devascularization procedures combine components of splenectomy and gastric and esophageal devascularization. The aim is to reduce inflow to variceal beds and therefore reduce the risk of bleeding. Because portal flow is maintained, the risk of encephalopathy is low (10-15%). In patients with extensive portomesenteric venous occlusion or previous splenectomy, devascularization may offer an alternative decompressive strategy in selected cases in which anatomic considerations make surgical or radiologic shunting impossible.

LIVER TRANSPLANTATION

Liver transplantation provides the ultimate in decompressive therapy, but its role in the salvage management of refractory variceal hemorrhage remains minor due to the scarcity of donor organs. In selected circumstances, however, orthotopic liver transplantation can successfully arrest both ongoing bleeding and, in the longer term, remodeling of the splanchnic circulation.

PROGNOSIS

The mortality rate following a variceal bleed is often quoted as in the range of 30% to 60%. Several reports of improved outcome since the introduction of therapeutic endoscopy may alter this estimate. The overall improvement in survival over the last 20 years is attributed to decreased early mortality, largely due to effective control of bleeding and prevention of rebleeding (due to treatment of the initial bleed, use of antibiotics, and secondary prophylaxis), rather than modification of the natural history of the disease. If survival analysis is commenced at 30 days after hemorrhage, there is no difference in survival rates in historical groups versus those treated contemporaneously.[12]

Poor prognostic indicators in the short term include the following:

- Failure to control bleeding (ongoing bleeding, early rebleeding)
- Sepsis
- Renal failure
- Severe liver disease (ascites, coagulopathy)
- Encephalopathy

Poor prognostic indicators in the long term include the following:

- Advanced age
- Presence of hepatocellular carcinoma
- Presence of complications
- Intolerance of secondary prophylaxis

COMPLICATIONS: SEPSIS, RENAL FAILURE, MULTIPLE ORGAN DYSFUNCTION SYNDROME

As mentioned earlier, failure to control initial bleeding is associated with high risk of death in the short term. The high risk of death is due to both the immediate consequences of massive blood loss and ongoing shock, as well as to the consequences of end-organ insults, leading to multiple organ dysfunction syndrome.

Significantly, bacterial infection is associated with both an increase in failure to control bleeding and early rebleeding. Bacterial infection is associated with poor short-term prognosis. The use of broad-spectrum antibiotics after variceal hemorrhage has been shown to reduce the infection rate, decrease the rebleeding rate, and, more importantly, improve early survival.[13]

A large proportion of the deaths attributed to variceal bleeding are not directly caused by hemorrhage but are a complication of variceal bleeding and decompensated liver disease. Importantly, renal failure in association with advanced liver disease (e.g., Child-Pugh score greater than 10) and variceal hemorrhage predicts a very poor short-term prognosis and correlates strongly with early death (<30 days). Development of renal failure is associated with severity of bleeding (reflected by hemodynamic parameters, transfusion requirement, and findings at endoscopic

examination), severity of liver disease (determined by Child-Pugh score), and presence or absence of bacterial infection. The prognosis of renal failure developing in association with variceal bleeding is similar to that for patients developing renal failure in association with spontaneous bacterial peritonitis and type 1 hepatorenal syndrome.

SECONDARY PROPHYLAXIS

After an initial variceal bleed, as many as 60% of untreated patients bleed again. Rebleeding is most frequent in the 6 weeks following an index variceal bleed and is seen in up to 40% of patients.[14] Risk factors for early rebleeding include age older than 60 years, severity of initial bleed, renal failure, ascites, active bleeding on endoscopy, red signs, clot on varix, hypoalbuminemia, and hepatic venous pressure gradient greater than 20 mm Hg. As mentioned earlier, aggressive volume resuscitation may cause a rebound increase in portal pressure and precipitate early rebleeding.[15] Survival during this period relates to the severity of liver disease (as determined by Child-Pugh score), the occurrence of rebleeding, and hepatic venous pressure gradient greater than 20 mm Hg. The risk of late rebleeding is related to the severity of liver disease, endoscopic findings indicative of high risk of rebleeding, and continued alcohol intake, along with the poor prognostic indicators mentioned earlier. Prognosis in this untreated group relates to the risk of rebleeding and of complications of variceal bleeding (e.g., liver failure, infection, exsanguination). At 1 year, 70% of patients have rebled or died.

Cirrhotic patients who survive an episode of variceal hemorrhage remain at high risk of rebleeding. Different modalities of treatment are all effective at reducing this risk. With the exception of therapeutic endoscopy, all act to reduce portal pressure. Adverse prognostic indicators include age, presence of renal failure or encephalopathy, and advanced Child-Pugh severity score.

All patients who survive an episode of variceal bleeding should receive some form of effective treatment to prevent rebleeding. The available options include pharmacotherapy, endoscopic therapy, radiologic TIPS, surgical shunt, and liver transplantation. Currently, first-line secondary prophylaxis of variceal hemorrhage consists of treatment using a nonselective beta-adrenergic antagonist. In patients who have contraindications, are intolerant, or are noncompliant, a variceal eradication program should be instituted. Endoscopic band ligation is better tolerated with fewer complications than sclerotherapy.

ANNOTATED REFERENCES

Escorsell A, Ruiz del Arbol L, Planas R, et al: Multicenter randomized controlled trial of terlipressin versus sclerotherapy in the treatment of acute variceal bleeding: The TEST study. Hepatology 2000;32:471-476.

This multicenter randomized controlled trial compared endoscopic sclerotherapy to terlipressin in 219 cirrhotic patients with endoscopy-proven acute variceal bleeding and found the two treatments equally effective in achieving the initial control of variceal bleeding and preventing early rebleeding. Both treatments are safe, but terlipressin is better tolerated and may represent a first-line treatment in acute variceal bleeding until the administration of elective therapy.

Ortega R, Gines P, Uriz J, et al: Terlipressin therapy with and without albumin for patients with hepatorenal syndrome: results of a prospective, nonrandomized study. Hepatology 2002;36:941-948.

Vasopressin analogues associated with albumin improve renal function in hepatorenal syndrome (HRS). This study concluded that terlipressin therapy reverses HRS in a high proportion of patients. Recurrence rate after treatment withdrawal is uncommon. Albumin appears to markedly improve the beneficial effects of terlipressin.

Moreau R, Durand F, Poynard T, et al: Terlipressin in patients with cirrhosis and type 1 hepatorenal syndrome: A retrospective multicenter study. Gastroenterology 2002;122:923-930.

This retrospective uncontrolled study shows that in patients with type 1 HRS, terlipressin-induced improved renal function is associated with an increase in survival.

Chapter 115

ASCITES

Lena M. Napolitano

KEY POINTS

1. The serum-ascites albumin gradient (serum albumin concentration–ascitic fluid albumin concentration) is the best diagnostic measure for the classification of ascites.

2. Diagnostic paracentesis must be performed in all patients with new-onset ascites.

3. Ascites is the most common complication related to liver disease and cirrhosis.

4. Ascites is characterized by three grades of severity, and treatment is based on grade.

5. The only definitive therapy for refractory ascites with cirrhosis is orthotopic liver transplantation. Other therapy includes large-volume paracentesis, peritoneovenous shunts, and transjugular intrahepatic portosystemic shunt.

DEFINITION AND DIAGNOSIS

Ascites is the abnormal accumulation of fluid in the peritoneal cavity.[1] Patients with ascites generally present on clinical examination with abdominal distention and a fluid wave or shifting dullness on abdominal percussion, but the abdominal examination findings may also be normal if the amount of ascites is not massive.

Diagnostic imaging can confirm the diagnosis of ascites. Ultrasonography is the easiest and most sensitive technique for the detection of ascitic fluid, being capable of visualizing very small volumes (5-10 mL). Computed tomography is also very sensitive for detecting ascites (Fig. 115-1). Small amounts of ascitic fluid localize in the perihepatic area and in Morrison's pouch (the hepatorenal space).

A diagnostic paracentesis (10-50 mL) is performed to evaluate the ascites as well as exclude or establish a diagnosis of spontaneous bacterial peritonitis. A diagnostic paracentesis should be performed in any person with new-onset ascites or in cirrhotic patients requiring hospitalization or experiencing clinical deterioration, such as worsening encephalopathy or unexplained fever. A missed or delayed diagnosis of spontaneous bacterial peritonitis could potentially lead to sepsis and significant morbidity and mortality.

Peritoneal fluid from patients with new onset of ascites of unknown origin should be assayed for cell count, albumin level, culture, total protein concentration, Gram stain, and cytology.[2] Serum albumin concentration should be measured as well.

The serum-ascites albumin gradient (serum albumin concentration–ascitic fluid albumin concentration) is the best diagnostic measure for the classification of ascites (Table 115-1).[3] The serum-ascites albumin gradient is very specific and sensitive in distinguishing ascites due to portal hypertension (serum-ascites albumin gradient >1.1 g/dL) from that occurring as a result of different pathogenetic mechanisms, such as inflammation or peritoneal malignancy (gradient ≤1.1 g/dL). Ideally, the specimens should be obtained simultaneously. In the past, ascites was classified as being an exudate (protein concentration ≥2.5 g/dL) or a transudate (protein concentration <2.5 g/dL), but this classification scheme is no longer used because of its poor sensitivity and specificity.[4] The total protein level may provide additional clues about diagnosis when used with the serum-ascites albumin gradient; that is, high serum-ascites albumin gradient and high protein is seen in most cases of ascites due to hepatic congestion, whereas low serum-ascites albumin gradient and high protein characterizes malignant ascites. The terms *high-albumin gradient* and *low-albumin gradient* should replace the terms *transudate* and *exudate* in the description of ascites.

The ascitic fluid cell count and differential cell count are important in evaluation of possible spontaneous bacterial peritonitis and other inflammatory peritoneal conditions. Normal ascitic fluid contains fewer than 500 leukocytes/μL and fewer than 250 polymorphonuclear leukocytes/μL. A neutrophil count of greater than 250 cells/μL is consistent with bacterial peritonitis. In tuberculous peritonitis and peritoneal carcinomatosis, a predominance of lymphocytes usually occurs. A sample of ascites should be inoculated into blood culture bottles for detection of spontaneous bacterial peritonitis. Gram stain is not sensitive for the detection of spontaneous bacterial peritonitis because of the low numbers of bacterial organisms present in the ascites.

The sensitivity of cytology for detecting malignancy is 58% to 75%, if a large volume of fluid is analyzed. Laparoscopy is an additional invasive diagnostic study that may also be indicated if a diagnosis of malignant ascites is considered. Peritoneal or tumor implant biopsy samples can be obtained at the same time for histologic diagnosis.

PATHOPHYSIOLOGY

Ascites is the most common complication related to liver disease and cirrhosis.[5] It is associated with profound changes in the splanchnic and systemic circulation and with renal

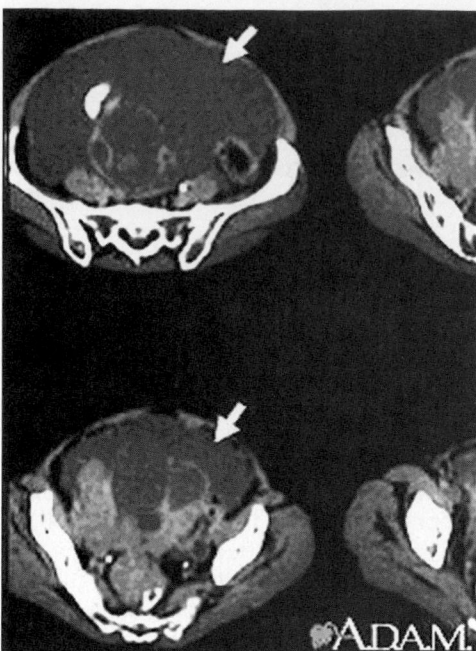

FIGURE 115–1. Ascites appearance on computed tomography scan of abdomen and pelvis. (From: http://www.nlm.nih.gov/medlineplus/ency/imagepages/1151.htm)

abnormalities. However, the pathogenesis of renal sodium retention and ascites formation in cirrhosis remains a subject of much controversy.

One accepted theory of ascites formation is the Forward Theory, which states that the development of ascites is related to the existence of severe sinusoidal portal hypertension that causes marked splanchnic arterial vasodilation and a forward increase in the splanchnic production of lymph.[6]

TABLE 115–1. CAUSES OF ASCITES BASED ON NORMAL OR DISEASED PERITONEUM AND SERUM TO ASCITES ALBUMIN GRADIENT (SAAG)

Normal Peritoneum

Portal Hypertension (SAAG > 1.1 g/dL)	***Hypoalbuminemia (SAAG < 1.1 g/dL)***
Hepatic congestion	Nephrotic syndrome
Congestive heart failure	Protein-losing enteropathy
Constrictive pericarditis	Severe malnutrition with
Tricuspid insufficiency	anasarca
Budd-Chiari syndrome	
Liver disease	***Miscellaneous Conditions***
Cirrhosis	***(SAAG < 1.1 g/dL)***
Alcoholic hepatitis	Chylous ascites
Fulminant hepatic failure	Pancreatic ascites
Massive hepatic metastases	Bile ascites
	Nephrogenic ascites
	Urine ascites
	Ovarian disease

Diseased Peritoneum (SAAG < 1.1 g/dL)

Infections	Pseudomyxoma peritonei
Bacterial peritonitis	Hepatocellular carcinoma
Tuberculous peritonitis	Other rare conditions
Fungal peritonitis	Familial Mediterranean fever
HIV-associated peritonitis	Vasculitis
Malignant conditions	Granulomatous peritonitis
Peritoneal carcinomatosis	Eosinophilic peritonitis
Primary mesothelioma	

Splanchnic arterial vasodilation also produces arterial vascular underfilling, a significant reduction of the effective blood volume, and arterial hypotension. These pathophysiologic changes lead to compensatory activation of sodium- and water-retaining mechanisms (the renin-angiotensin-aldosterone system, sympathetic nervous system, and nonosmotic release of vasopressin) and promote ascites formation. Therefore, according to this theory, derangements in the splanchnic arterial circulation, rather than the venous portal system, are primary in the pathogenesis of ascites formation.[7]

This theory is supported by the observation that interventions that markedly decrease portal pressure, such as surgical portacaval shunts or transjugular intrahepatic portosystemic shunts (TIPS), reduce ascites. In the advanced stages of cirrhosis, the extreme underfilling of the arterial circulation leads to maximal stimulation of vasoconstrictor mechanisms, which override the protective effects of renal vasodilator factors and cause renal vasoconstriction, further aggravating ascites formation and leading to functional renal insufficiency. Renal insufficiency is also one of the main causes of resistance to diuretic therapy.

Patients with advanced cirrhosis and portal hypertension often show an abnormal regulation of extracellular fluid volume, resulting in the accumulation of fluid as ascites, pleural effusion, or edema. The mechanisms responsible for ascites formation include alterations in the splanchnic circulation as well as renal functional abnormalities that favor sodium and water retention.[8] The renal functional abnormalities occur in the setting of a hyperdynamic circulatory state that is characterized by increased cardiac output, decreased systemic vascular resistance, and activation of neurohormonal vasoactive systems. This circulatory dysfunction, due mainly to intense arterial vasodilation in the splanchnic circulation, is considered to be a primary feature in the pathogenesis of ascites.

A major factor involved in the development of splanchnic arterial vasodilation is increased synthesis of nitric oxide (NO), a potent vasodilator that is elevated in the splanchnic circulation of patients with cirrhosis. This event decreases effective arterial blood volume and leads to fluid accumulation and renal function abnormalities, which are a consequence of the homeostatic activation of vasoconstrictor and antinatriuretic factors triggered to compensate for a relative arterial underfilling. The net effect is avid retention of sodium and water as well as renal vasoconstriction.

The Peripheral Arterial Vasodilation Hypothesis incriminates relative underfilling of the arterial vascular compartment as the primary problem. Relative arterial underfilling leads to the same neurohumoral responses that occur in states characterized by low cardiac output (e.g., chronic congestive heart failure).[9] Activation of the renin-angiotensin-aldosterone axis and the sympathetic system as well as nonosmotic release of vasopressin are well documented in cases of cirrhosis. This sequence of events results in renal water and sodium retention, failure to escape from the sodium-retaining effect of aldosterone, and renal resistance to atrial natriuretic peptide. Dilutional hyponatremia is the strongest predictor of the occurrence of hepatorenal syndrome.

The pathogenesis of the peripheral arterial vasodilation is not completely elucidated, but there is evidence for a major role of NO.[10] Increased vascular NO production has been demonstrated in cirrhosis. The hepatic artery in patients with ascites produces more NO than does the hepatic artery in patients without ascites. In a rat model of cirrhosis, normalization of vascular NO production with a NO synthase inhibitor corrects the hyperdynamic circulation, improves sodium and water excretion, and decreases neurohumoral activation. This insight into the mechanisms of the peripheral arterial vasodilation in cirrhosis should provide new tools in the treatment of edema and ascites, a major cause of morbidity and mortality in patients with cirrhosis.

The generally accepted peripheral arterial vasodilation hypothesis seems to best explain the mechanism of sodium retention and other clinical findings, such as hyperdynamic circulation in patients with cirrhosis. However, recent data in patients with pre-ascites or early ascites do not seem to conform to the peripheral arterial vasodilation hypothesis.[11] Renal sodium handling abnormalities can be demonstrated in patients with cirrhosis prior to the development of ascites when these individuals are challenged with a sodium load. These changes are apparent even in the absence of systemic vasodilation or arterial underfilling. Therefore, an alternative hypothesis with a direct hepatorenal interaction, acting via sinusoidal portal hypertension and/or hepatic dysfunction as the affector mechanism, is proposed to be the initiating event promoting renal sodium retention in patients with cirrhosis. The second and later process is the development of systemic arterial vasodilation, possibly due to the presence of excess systemic vasodilators and/or decreased responsiveness of the vasculature to endogenous vasoconstrictors. These changes, in turn, lead to a relatively underfilled circulation with consequent activation of neurohumoral systems, promoting further renal sodium retention as described by the peripheral arterial vasodilation hypothesis. When compensatory natriuretic mechanisms fail, refractory ascites develops and hepatorenal syndrome sets in. Thus, renal sodium retention in patients with cirrhosis is the result of interplay of many factors; direct hepatorenal interaction predominates in the earlier stages of the cirrhotic process, whereas systemic vasodilation becomes a more important pathogenetic mechanism as the disease progresses.

ETIOLOGY

Liver disease is a common cause of ascites. In patients with liver disease, ascites develops as a result of portal hypertension, which can be prehepatic (e.g., due to portal vein thrombosis), intrahepatic (e.g., due to cirrhosis), or posthepatic (e.g., due to Budd-Chiari syndrome). Patients with chronic liver disease develop portal hypertension and subsequent ascites from increased resistance of blood flow through the hepatic parenchyma. Circulatory changes, such as increased plasma volume and increased cardiac output, develop in conjunction with decreased systemic vascular resistance and blood pressure. Ascites is one of the most frequent complications of cirrhosis. Its appearance is considered a key marker of the transition from the compensated to the decompensated stage of the disease. The appearance of ascites also has prognostic significance, as it causes a sharp drop in the expected survival rate.

Most cases of ascites are due to liver disease. However, a number of disorders may be associated with ascites, and these include cirrhosis, hepatitis, portal vein thrombosis, cardiac disorders (constrictive pericarditis, congestive heart failure), liver cancer, nephrotic syndrome, protein-losing enteropathy, and pancreatitis (see Table 115-1). Nonhepatic causes include cardiac failure, malignancy, renal failure, and intra-abdominal inflammation. It is important to diagnose nonhepatic causes of ascites, such as malignancy, tuberculosis, and pancreatic ascites, since these occur with increased frequency in patients with liver disease.

MANAGEMENT

Ascites is the most common presentation of decompensated cirrhosis. It occurs in more than one half of all patients with cirrhosis, and its development heralds a poor prognosis (50% 2-year survival rate). Ascites is characterized by three grades of severity, and treatment is based on grade (Table 115-2). Effective first-line medical therapy for ascites includes dietary sodium restriction (2 g per day) and use of diuretics.[12] Diuretics are the mainstay of medical therapy in the treatment of ascites. Initially, an aldosterone antagonist (spironolactone) is used. Spironolactone competes with aldosterone for receptor sites in the distal renal tubules, increasing water excretion while retaining potassium and hydrogen ions. Spironolactone is usually initiated at a dose of 100 mg per day. The addition of a loop diuretic (e.g., furosemide) may be necessary in some cases to increase the natriuretic effect. The dosage of both the aldosterone antagonist and the loop diuretic should be increased sequentially until an adequate diuretic response is observed. Sodium restriction and diuretic therapy are initially effective in approximately 95% of patients. Water restriction is used only if persistent hyponatremia is present.

Paracentesis is reserved for patients refractory to medical management. As a therapeutic intervention, abdominal paracentesis is usually performed to drain a large volume of abdominal ascites.[13] When tense or refractory ascites is

TABLE 115–2. GRADES OF ASCITES AND RECOMMENDED TREATMENT

Grade	Definition	Treatment
Grade 1	Mild ascites only detectable by ultrasonographic examination	No specific treatment Dietary sodium restriction Careful follow-up
Grade 2	Moderate ascites, manifest by moderate symmetrical distention of the abdomen	Dietary sodium restriction Diuretics (spironolactone with or without furosemide, amiloride for patients with nonactivated renin-angiotensin-aldosterone system)
Grade 3	Large or gross ascites with marked abdominal distention	Paracentesis (total or large-volume, with colloid volume expansion) Dietary sodium restriction Diuretics

Adapted from Moore KP, Wong F, Gines P, et al: The management of ascites in cirrhosis: Report on the Consensus Conference of the International Ascites Club. Hepatology 2003;38:258-266.

present, large-volume paracentesis is safe and effective and has the advantage of producing immediate relief from ascites and its associated symptoms.[14] The removal of more than 5 L of fluid is considered large-volume paracentesis. Total paracentesis—removal of all ascites (even >20 L)—usually can be performed safely. Recent studies demonstrate that intravenous infusion of 5 g of albumin for each liter of ascites removed (>5 L) decreases complications of paracentesis, such as electrolyte imbalances and increased serum creatinine concentration, secondary to large shifts of intravascular volume. Large-volume paracentesis provides rapid resolution of symptoms with minimal complications and is well tolerated by most patients. Paracentesis-induced circulatory dysfunction may occur after large-volume paracentesis and is characterized by hyponatremia, azotemia, and increased plasma renin activity. Paracentesis-induced circulatory dysfunction is associated with increased mortality and may be prevented by administration of albumin intravenously (6-8 g/L of ascites removed).

The International Ascites Club, representing the spectrum of clinical practice from North America to Europe, has developed consensus guidelines for the management of cirrhotic ascites from the stage of early ascites to the stage of refractory ascites.[15] Mild to moderate ascites should be managed by modest salt restriction and diuretic therapy with spironolactone or an equivalent. Diuretics should be added in a stepwise fashion while maintaining sodium restriction. Gross ascites should be treated with therapeutic paracentesis followed by colloid volume expansion and diuretic therapy. Refractory ascites is managed by repeated large-volume paracentesis or insertion of a TIPS shunt. Successful placement of TIPS results in improved renal function, sodium excretion, and general well-being but has not been shown to improve survival. Clinicians caring for these patients should be aware of the potential complications of each treatment modality and be prepared to discontinue diuretics or not proceed with TIPS placement should complications or contraindications develop. Liver transplantation should be considered for all patients with ascites and cirrhosis. Ideally, liver transplantion should be performed prior to the development of renal dysfunction to minimize the risk of mortality.

REFRACTORY ASCITES

Refractory or recurrent ascites is a clinical challenge frequently encountered in patients with cirrhosis.[16-18] Ascites becomes refractory to medical treatment in nearly 10% of cirrhotic patients. The diagnosis of refractory ascites recently has been revised (Table 115-3). Refractory ascites is a poor prognostic sign; as many as 50% of patients with this condition die within 6 months of its development.

The only definitive therapy for refractory ascites with cirrhosis is orthotopic liver transplantation. The other options that are available include large-volume paracentesis, peritoneovenous shunts, and TIPS. The TIPS procedure has not been shown to have any influence on survival in patients with cirrhosis and refractory ascites, and TIPS is contraindicated in patients who have advanced liver failure because it can hasten death in such individuals. Peritoneovenous shunts are associated with a high incidence of complications and frequent occlusion. They are, therefore, rarely used for management of refractory ascites. Therefore, the initial treatment option for refractory ascites is repetitive large-volume or total paracentesis.[19,20]

TABLE 115–3. REVISED DIAGNOSTIC CRITERIA OF REFRACTORY ASCITES

Treatment duration: Patients must be on intensive diuretic therapy (spironolactone 400 mg/d and furosemide 160 mg/d) for at least 1 week and on a salt-restricted diet of less than 90 mmoles or 5.2 g of salt/day.

Lack of response: Mean weight loss of <0.8 kg over 4 days and urinary sodium output less than the sodium intake.

Early ascites recurrence: Reappearance of grade 2 or 3 ascites within 4 weeks of initial mobilization.

Diuretic-induced complications:

Diuretic-induced hepatic encephalopathy is the development of encephalopathy in the absence of any other precipitating factor.

Diuretic-induced renal impairment is an increase of serum creatinine by >100% to a value >2 mg/dL in patients with ascites responding to treatment.

Diuretic-induced hyponatremia is defined as a decrease of serum sodium by >10 mmol/L to a serum sodium concentration of <125 mmol/L.

Diuretic-induced hypo- or hyperkalemia is defined as a change in serum potassium to <3 mmol/L or >6 mmol/L despite appropriate measures.

Adapted from Moore KP, Wong F, Gines P, et al: The management of ascites in cirrhosis: Report on the Consensus Conference of the International Ascites Club. Hepatology 2003;38:258-266.

An early report describing the experience with TIPS for the management of refractory ascites documented that ascites was markedly reduced after this procedure.[21] In responders, plasma aldosterone and renin activity decreased, serum creatinine concentration decreased, and urinary sodium excretion increased. However, new-onset hepatic encephalopathy was seen in 14 of 30 patients studied. Severe disabling chronic encephalopathy occurred in five patients but was successfully reversed by balloon occlusion of the shunt in three patients. Cumulative survival in this study was 41% and 34% at 1 and 2 years, respectively.

Clinicians would find it useful to have a way to predict a favorable clinical response to TIPS for refractory ascites. A prospective cohort study of 53 cirrhotic patients without organic renal disease and with refractory ascites critically examined "responders" to TIPS, defined as those who survive for more than 6 months without severe chronic hepatic encephalopathy and with good control of ascites.[22] The following parameters were examined for prognostic value: age, creatinine clearance, plasma renin activity, plasma aldosterone concentration, and Pugh score. Good control of ascites was obtained in 90%, and 47% of patients were responders to TIPS. The cumulative survival rate was 54% at 6 months, 48% at 1 year, and 39% at 2 years. The majority of patients died of complications of hepatic insufficiency. Severe chronic hepatic encephalopathy developed in 26% of the patients. Creatinine clearance was the only factor that was a significant independent predictor of good clinical response to TIPS for refractory ascites. In patients with poor renal function, therefore, TIPS should not be considered.

A randomized prospective trial compared large-volume paracentesis and TIPS in 60 patients with cirrhosis and refractory ascites in Germany.[23] Multivariate analysis confirmed that TIPS was independently associated with survival without the need for transplantation ($P = .02$), with a mean follow-up of 45 months. At 3 months, 61% of the TIPS patients had no ascites, compared to 18% of the paracentesis group ($P = .006$).

A similar study, performed in Spain, randomized 70 patients with cirrhosis and refractory ascites to TIPS or repeated paracentesis plus intravenous albumin.[24] Recurrence of ascites and development of hepatorenal syndrome were lower in the TIPS group compared with the paracentesis group, whereas the frequency of severe hepatic encephalopathy was greater in the TIPS group. TIPS did not improve survival and was associated with higher costs.

The North American Study for the Treatment of Refractory Ascites, which was recently completed, enrolled a larger sample size than prior studies.[25] This was a multicenter, prospective, randomized clinical trial. One hundred nine patients with refractory ascites were randomized to medical therapy (sodium restriction, diuretics, and total paracentesis, n = 57) or medical therapy plus TIPS (n = 52). The principal endpoints were recurrence of tense symptomatic ascites and mortality. A technically adequate shunt was created in 49 of 52 subjects. TIPS plus medical therapy was significantly superior to medical therapy alone in preventing recurrence of ascites ($P < .001$), but no difference in mortality was identified (21 deaths occurred in each group). There was a higher incidence of moderate to severe encephalopathy in the TIPS group (20 of 52 versus 12 of 57, $P = .058$), but no difference in the incidence of liver failure, variceal hemorrhage, or acute renal failure. No differences in frequency of emergency department visits, medically indicated hospitalizations, or quality of life were identified. The authors concluded that although TIPS plus medical therapy was superior to medical therapy alone for the control of ascites, TIPS did not improve survival, affect hospitalization rates, or improve quality of life.

Historically, the peritoneovenous shunt was an alternative for patients with medically intractable ascites. There is no evidence that these shunts improved survival, and with the advent of the TIPS procedure, this form of therapy has been abandoned.

COMPLICATIONS

PARACENTESIS-INDUCED CIRCULATORY DYSFUNCTION

Paracentesis-induced circulatory dysfunction, or postparacentesis effective hypovolemia, is a recently described complication that may occur after large-volume or total paracentesis. This complication is characterized by hyponatremia, azotemia, and increased plasma renin activity. Paracentesis-induced circulatory dysfunction is associated with an increased mortality rate and can be prevented with the administration of plasma expanders. A recent study randomized 72 patients to receive albumin or saline after total paracentesis.[26] The incidence of paracentesis-induced circulatory dysfunction was significantly higher in the saline-treated group as compared with the albumin-treated group (33.3% versus 11.4%, $P = .03$). However, no significant differences were found when less than 6 L of ascitic fluid was evacuated (6.7% versus 5.6%, $P = .9$). Significant increases in plasma renin activity were found 24 hours and 6 days after paracentesis when saline was used, whereas no changes were observed when albumin was infused. Albumin was more effective than saline for the prevention of paracentesis-induced circulatory dysfunction but is not required when less than 6 L of ascitic fluid is evacuated. Therefore, the administration of intravenous albumin (6 to 8 g/L of ascites removed) is recommended with large-volume paracentesis.

Five randomized controlled trials have compared volume expansion with albumin to volume expansion with other agents, including dextran, collagen-based colloids, and hydroxyethyl starch.[27-31] All studies have documented that synthetic plasma expanders were as effective as albumin at preventing the clinical complications of paracentesis, namely hyponatremia or renal impairment. However, only one study examined prevention of paracentesis-induced circulatory dysfunction (defined by an increase in plasma renin activity or aldosterone concentration), and determined that albumin prevented this complication more effectively than synthetic plasma expanders.[25]

SPONTANEOUS BACTERIAL PERITONITIS

Spontaneous bacterial peritonitis is a common complication of cirrhotic ascites.[32] It can precipitate hepatorenal syndrome. The overall mortality rate from an episode of spontaneous bacterial peritonitis is approximately 20%. Following an episode of spontaneous bacterial peritonitis, the 1-year mortality rate approaches 70%.

The prevalence of spontaneous bacterial peritonitis in cirrhotic patients with ascites admitted to the hospital has been estimated at 10% to 30%. Any patient with ascites and fever or deterioration in renal or hepatic function should undergo diagnostic paracentesis. The fluid should be cultured and a cell count obtained. Antibiotic therapy should be initiated until the results of these tests are available.

To diagnose spontaneous bacterial peritonitis, ascitic fluid should be examined by microscopy and inoculated directly into blood culture bottles. An ascitic fluid neutrophil count of 250 polymorphonuclear cells/μL or greater is diagnostic of spontaneous bacterial peritonitis, but a Gram stain of the ascitic fluid is usually not informative.[33]

Gram-negative aerobic bacteria are the most common organisms isolated from ascites.[34] The three most common isolates are *Escherichia coli*, *Klebsiella pneumoniae*, and *Streptococcus pneumoniae*. Although the number of bacteria present in an episode of spontaneous bacterial peritonitis is very low, they excite an intensive inflammatory response. Hospitalized patients should be treated with appropriate intravenous antibiotics.

Patients who have survived an episode of spontaneous bacterial peritonitis have a 40% to 70% 1-year probability of a further episode. One randomized placebo-controlled trial examined the efficacy of antibiotic treatment purely for secondary prophylaxis of spontaneous bacterial peritonitis.[35] Long-term treatment with norfloxacin reduced the recurrence of spontaneous bacterial peritonitis at 1 year from 68% to 20%. The treatment effect was mostly due to a reduction in spontaneous bacterial peritonitis secondary to Gram-negative pathogens. On the basis of these results, long-term oral antibiotics are advised for patients recovering from an episode of spontaneous bacterial peritonitis until resolution of ascites, transplantation, or death (International Ascites Club recommendations). Furthermore, specific patients at high risk of a first episode of spontaneous bacterial peritonitis (patients with a protein level of less than 1 g/dL in ascitic fluid and those hospitalized with gastrointestinal hemorrhage) should also receive prophylaxis with orally administered antibiotics, usually quinolones.[30,31]

For a discussion of hepatorenal syndrome, see Chapter 117.

TABLE 115–4. CHILD-TURCOT-PUGH SCORING SYSTEM*

Clinical and biochemical measurements	Points Scored for Increasing Abnormality		
	1	2	3
Albumin (g/dL)	>3.5	2.8-3.5	<2.8
Bilirubin (mg/dL)	1-2	2-3	>3
For cholestatic disease: bilirubin (mg/dL)	<4	4-10	>10
Prothrombin time (seconds above normal)†	1-4	4-6	>6
or			
International normalized ratio†	<1.7	1.7-2.3	>2.3
Ascites	Absent	Slight	Moderate
Encephalopathy (grade)	None	1 and 2	3 and 4

*Scoring for Child class: A = 5-6 points; B = 7-9 points; C = 10-15 points.
†Prothrombin time or international normalized ratio can be used for scoring.
From Pugh RHW, Murray-Lyon IM, Dawson JL, et al: Transection of the esophagus for bleeding esophageal varices. Br J Surg 1983;60:646.

PROGNOSIS AND OUTCOMES

The short-term prognosis of acutely ill patients with cirrhosis is influenced by the degree of hepatic insufficiency and by dysfunction of extrahepatic organ systems. The Child-Turcot-Pugh classification (Table 115-4) was initially described for estimating outcome in cirrhotic patients undergoing surgery. One important component of the Child-Turcot-Pugh classification is the degree of ascites present, graded as absent, slight, or moderate.

A recent study[36] compared the Child-Pugh classification, the Acute Physiology and Chronic Health Evaluation (APACHE) II system, and the Sequential Organ Failure Assessment (SOFA) for predicting hospital mortality in patients (n = 143) with cirrhosis when used 24 hours after admission to a medical ICU. Cumulative mortality rates were 36% in the ICU, 46% in the hospital, and 56% at 6-month follow-up. By using the area under receiver operating characteristic (ROC) curves, the SOFA score showed an excellent discriminative power (0.94), which was clearly superior to the APACHE II (0.79) and the Child-Pugh system (0.74). Hospital mortality rates below and above a cutoff of 8 SOFA points were 4% and 88%, respectively ($P < .0005$). The SOFA score also reflected resource use during the ICU treatment as measured by daily workload and length of stay. The SOFA score is an easily applied tool with excellent prognostic abilities and can be used to enhance clinical judgment of prognosis as well as to provide patients and families with objective information. A similar study in 111 critically ill cirrhotic patients compared organ system failure scores obtained on the first day of ICU admission to the Child-Pugh classification in predicting hospital mortality.[37] The overall hospital mortality rate was 64.9%. Similarly, the organ system failure score (ROC 0.901) was superior to the Child-Pugh score (ROC 0.748) in prediction of hospital mortality in these ICU patients with cirrhosis.

In contrast, the prognostic accuracy of the Child-Pugh score was superior to either the APACHE II or III scores in prediction of short-term hospital mortality of patients with liver cirrhosis (n = 147) admitted to a medical ward and not the ICU.[38] Overall mortality in this study was 11.5%. Discrimination was excellent for Child-Pugh (ROC 0.859) and APACHE III (ROC 0.816) scores, and acceptable for APACHE II score (ROC 0.759). Although the Hosmer-Lemeshow statistic revealed adequate goodness-of-fit for Child-Pugh score ($P = .192$), this was not the case for APACHE II and III scores ($P = .004$ and .003, respectively). This study documented clearly that, of the three models, the Child-Pugh score had the least statistically significant discrepancy between predicted and observed mortality.

ANNOTATED REFERENCES

Rossle M, Ochs A, Gulberg V, et al: A comparison of paracentesis and transjugular intrahepatic portosystemic shunting in patients with ascites. N Engl J Med 2000;342:1701-1707.

This 2000 study suggested that the creation of a transjugular intrahepatic portosystemic shunt (TIPS) can improve the chance of survival without liver transplantation in patients with refractory or recurrent ascites.

Sanyal AJ, Genning C, Reddy KR, et al: The North American Study for the Treatment of Refractory Ascites. Gastroenterology 2003;124:634-641.

This multicenter, prospective, randomized clinical trial investigated the clinical utility of transjugular intrahepatic portosystemic shunt (TIPS) in the management of refractory ascites. Although TIPS plus medical therapy is superior to medical therapy alone for the control of ascites. it does not improve survival, affect hospitalization rates, or improve quality of life.

Sola-Vera J, Minana J, Ricart E, et al: Randomized trial comparing albumin and saline in the prevention of paracentesis-induced circulatory dysfunction in cirrhotic patients with ascites. Hepatology 2003;37:1147-1153.

This study compared the efficacy of saline versus albumin in the prevention of paracentesis-induced circulatory dysfunction (PICD), and found that albumin is more effective than saline in the prevention of PICD. Saline is a valid alternative to albumin when less than 6 L of ascitic fluid is evacuated.

Chapter 116

GASTROINTESTINAL HEMORRHAGE

Nathaniel L. Holzman • Clemens M. Schirmer • Stanley A. Nasraway, Jr.

KEY POINTS

1. When upper gastrointestinal hemorrhage is present, the clinician needs to preserve the patient's airway, resuscitate the host, and buy time for diagnosis and therapeutic intervention. Reliable large-bore venous catheterization is fundamentally necessary.

2. The most important sources of upper gastrointestinal bleeding are from peptic ulcer disease and variceal hemorrhage.

3. Use of a nasogastric tube and early endoscopy shows an upper gastrointestinal source.

4. Endoscopy is diagnostic and therapeutic.

5. Lower gastrointestinal bleeding usually takes a milder clinical course and is about 20% as common as upper gastrointestinal hemorrhage.

6. Colonoscopy offers diagnostic and therapeutic potential for colonic sources.

7. Diagnosis of acute small bowel bleeding can be made with tagged red blood cell scan or angiography.

8. Aggressive diagnostic approaches should be pursued in patients in whom surgery is being considered because of high morbidity and mortality associated with "blind" resections.

UPPER GASTROINTESTINAL HEMORRHAGE

Traditionally, patients with upper gastrointestinal bleeding present with hematemesis (bloody or coffee-ground appearance) and melena (black/tarry stools). Critically ill patients have accompanying orthostatic hypotension, shock, hematocrit less than 30% or decrease of greater than 6%, and requirement for packed red blood cell transfusion. All patients with acute bleeds require emergent assessment, aggressive resuscitation, accurate diagnosis, and appropriate hospital triage.[1]

Acute upper gastrointestinal bleeding is a common condition that accounts for greater than 300,000 hospital admissions in the United States each year. Despite advanced monitoring techniques and trends toward early endoscopic intervention, the mortality rate for acute upper gastrointestinal bleeding is 6% to 10%, unchanged in the last 50 years.[2] An aging population and presence of comorbidities, such as renal insufficiency, hepatic failure, or disseminated malignancy, contribute to the high mortality rate. Eighty percent of acute upper gastrointestinal bleeds remit spontaneously, and endoscopy results in greater than 90% hemostasis, but there still remains a 20% risk of rebleeding.[2]

APPROACH TO THE PATIENT

Management goals for acute upper gastrointestinal bleeding revolve around airway protection, preserving hemodynamic stability, and preventing unwanted complications, such as aspiration (Table 116-1). Immediately securing an airway and intubating early when necessary allows for more accurate airway monitoring and more aggressive resuscitation and gastric lavage. Nasogastric/orogastric lavage is used to remove fresh blood, clots, and other matter to prevent aspiration. Lavage is important for establishing a diagnosis (upper gastrointestinal bleed versus lower gastrointestinal bleed) or for determining recurrent bleeding.

It is crucial that resuscitation coincide with assessment. Venous access should be achieved with at least one or two large-bore intravenous catheters (≥16 gauge). Patients in critical condition require extensive blood pressure, electrocardiogram, and pulse oximetry monitoring. Important laboratory studies include complete blood count, serum electrolyte concentrations, prothrombin time or international normalized ratio or both, activated partial thromboplastin time, and type and crossmatch. Infusion of crystalloid or colloid solutions (or both) is crucial to maintain adequate arterial blood pressure. Packed red blood cells are infused to maintain hematocrit greater than 24%; in patients with comorbid disease, such as coronary artery disease, hematocrit is maintained greater than 30%. Coagulopathies and thrombocytopenia must be corrected.[2-4] Data from one uncontrolled study suggest that the administration of erythropoietin can increase red blood cell mass and stop chronic oozing from diffuse lesions.[5] Erythropoietin may improve platelet function and decrease the action of naturally occurring anticoagulants, improving hemostasis.[5]

Endoscopy

When the clinician has stabilized the patient, it is paramount to determine the bleeding source. Endoscopic stigmata are useful in predicting the risk of rebleeding.[6] An active bleeding ulcer has a 90% to 100% risk for rebleeding, a nonbleeding but visible vessel has a 40% to 50% risk of recurrent bleeding, and a visualized clot at an ulcer base has a 20% to 30% risk of rebleeding (Table 116-2). If there is no active bleeding and no vessels are visualized, the risk of rebleeding is much lower.[6]

Esophagogastroduodenoscopy is the modality of choice for visualizing the upper gastrointestinal tract and determining

TABLE 116–1. FIRST STEPS IN THE MANAGEMENT OF UPPER GASTROINTESTINAL BLEEDING

Airway protection
  Airway monitoring
  Endotracheal intubation
Hemodynamic stabilization
  Large-bore intravenous access
  Intravenous fluids, red blood cell transfusion
  Fresh frozen plasma, platelets
  Consider erythropoietin
Nasogastric and oral management
  Large-bore orogastric monitoring, with lavage
Clinical and laboratory monitoring
  Serial and frequent vital signs
  Serial hemograms, coagulation profiles, chemistries
  Electrocardiogram monitoring
  Hemodynamic monitoring (high-risk patients)
Endoscopic examination and therapy

From Conrad SA: Acute upper gastrointestinal bleeding in critically ill patients: Causes and treatment modalities. Crit Care Med 2002;30(Suppl 6):S365-S368.

the source of an upper gastrointestinal bleed. It is diagnostic and can play a therapeutic role. To improve visibility, before performing esophagogastroduodenoscopy, one should thoroughly lavage gastric contents to remove any remaining blood or clots and infuse one dose of 250 mg of erythromycin intravenously to promote gastric emptying. Complications from esophagogastroduodenoscopy are rare, occurring in approximately 1% of cases.[2,7] The most common complications include perforation, induced hemorrhage, and excessive sedation.

Aside from esophagogastroduodenoscopy, multiple radiologic tools can assist in localizing and treating the hemorrhage. Plain abdominal films, abdominal ultrasound, computed tomography, and magnetic resonance imaging are noninvasive entities that can be useful for identifying various underlying etiologies, such as bowel perforation, mechanical obstruction, or infarction. Another imaging modality is a nuclear bleeding scan. Although rarely used since endoscopy has proved to be more sensitive, this test is noninvasive, well tolerated, and safe. The most useful radiologic intervention is angiography. Similar to endoscopy, it has diagnostic and therapeutic capabilities and can diagnose bleeding rates of 0.5 mL/min. For patients with bleeding that is refractory to endoscopic therapy

or who are poor surgical candidates, intra-arterial vasopressin application and embolotherapy are valid therapeutic options.[8]

Triage

Because of the large volume of patients admitted to hospitals each year for gastrointestinal bleeding, it is important that patients be accurately triaged to the appropriate care setting to optimize care and use of hospital resources. Early physical and clinical assessment and endoscopy allow for accurate, swift risk stratification.[9] Criteria for ICU admission include presence of shock, presentation with hematemesis or hematochezia or both, presence of active bleeding and two comorbidities, and necessity for mechanical ventilation.[10] Other criteria that must be considered include transfusion requirements, setting in which bleeding occurred (e.g., during a hospital admission), age of the patient (age >60 years is associated with an increased risk for death), and need for more intensive monitoring.

Common Etiologies

A thorough, focused history and physical examination are essential for accurately establishing the cause of bleeding. Dyspepsia and midepigastric pain can be consistent with peptic ulcer disease. Heavy use of nonsteroidal anti-inflammatory drugs (NSAIDs) increases the risk for gastric ulcer. Tobacco use increases the risk for duodenal ulcer. Alcoholism increases the likelihood for esophageal varices. History of vomiting or retching may be associated with a Mallory-Weiss tear.[11] Past surgeries or recent illnesses also may prove to be important.

The most common reported cause of upper gastrointestinal bleeding is peptic ulcer disease. It accounts for more than 50% of acute bleeds each year. Two other common etiologies include esophageal and gastric varices and Mallory-Weiss tears. Other less common etiologies are listed in Table 116-3. A brief description of each etiology, course, and treatment regimen follows.

PEPTIC ULCER DISEASE

Accounting for greater than 50% of acute upper gastrointestinal bleeds, peptic ulcer disease costs exceed $20 billion per year in the United States.[12] Two major risk factors for developing peptic ulcer disease include *Helicobacter pylori* infection and NSAID use. Although the incidence of *H. pylori* infection has steadily decreased in recent years, the use of NSAIDs has increased.

TABLE 116–2. ENDOSCOPIC STIGMATA OF ULCER HEMORRHAGE

Endoscopic Appearance	Prevalence (%)	Rate of Rebleed, No Endoscopy (%)	Rate of Rebleed, with Endoscopy (%)
Active arterial bleeding	12	90	15-30
Visible vessel	22	50	15-30
Adherent clot	10	12-33	5
Oozing without stigmata	14	10-27	NA
Flat spot	10	7	NA
Clean ulcer base	32	3	NA

NA, not available.
From Zaharia-Czeizler: Erythropoietin stops chronic diffuse transfusion-dependent gastrointestinal bleeding. Ann Intern Med 2001;135:933.

TABLE 116–3. CAUSES OF SEVERE UPPER GASTROINTESTINAL BLEEDING IN 948 CONSECUTIVE PATIENTS

Diagnosis	%
Peptic ulcer	55
Gastric or esophageal varix	14
Angioma	6
Mallory-Weiss tear	5
Neoplasm	4
Gastric erosions	4
Esophagitis	4
Other	8

From Savides TJ, Jensen DM: Severe gastrointestinal hemorrhage. In Shoemaker WC, Ayres SM, Grenvik A, Holbrook PR (eds): Textbook of Critical Care, 4th ed. Philadelphia, WB Saunders, 2000, pp 1609-1616.

Colonization of *H. pylori* on the gastric mucosa induces an inflammatory reaction. This process results in mucosal damage, rendering the tissue more susceptible to further *H. pylori* colonization. Factors such as tobacco or NSAID use can increase the duodenal acid load, precipitating *H. pylori* colonization and further ulcer formation. Independent of *H. pylori* infection, NSAID use increases the risk for gastric ulcer formation and significantly increases the risk for gastrointestinal bleeding. Physiologic and psychological stress can activate ulcer formation, increasing the risk for acute bleeds.[13-15]

Management of Induced Peptic Ulcer Hemorrhage

Although *H. pylori* is a major contributing factor to peptic ulcer disease, there is no role for eradicating *H. pylori* infection when treating acute upper gastrointestinal bleeding. Acute treatment with H_2 receptor antagonists may reduce the risk of rebleeding from gastric but not duodenal ulcers.[16] Numerous studies directly show or support the notion that proton-pump inhibitors decrease the risk of rebleeding.[17-20] Compared with placebo in randomized controlled trials, treatment with the proton-pump inhibitor, omeprazole, decreases the rate of rebleeding episodes of all peptic ulcers.[16-20] Despite the short-term pharmacologic benefits on bleeding, no data have linked proton-pump inhibitor use with an overall decrease in mortality. To decrease the rebleeding rate, it is strongly recommended to continue antisecretory therapy and discontinue NSAID use after the acute bleeding episode.

Surgery is indicated for the treatment of bleeding ulcers refractory to two attempts of endoscopic hemostasis (using a thermal or laser device). Other indications for surgery include rapid deterioration secondary to exsanguination, large visible vessels not susceptible to endoscopic coagulation, and documented malignant ulcers.

VARICEAL HEMORRHAGE

The second most common cause of upper gastrointestinal bleeding is variceal hemorrhage. In the United States, portal hypertension, the predisposing factor for esophageal varices, most commonly results from cirrhosis. Around the world, presinusoidal causes of portal hypertension, notably schistosomiasis, also are important etiologic factors. The predicted risk for acute bleeding from a varix is based on many factors, including its size, location, endoscopic evidence of red stigmata, and presence of liver failure or ascites.[21] In a patient with cirrhosis, the Child-Turcotte-Pugh scoring system helps to assess the severity of disease and can act as an indirect determinant for risk of bleeding.[22] Although most acute upper gastrointestinal bleeds remit spontaneously, variceal hemorrhages stop bleeding spontaneously only about 50% of the time. The mortality rate for acute variceal hemorrhage has not changed dramatically over the past several years and remains approximately 40%, depending on the treatment regimen.[11]

Diagnosis usually is made with esophagogastroduodenoscopy. First-line therapy for variceal hemorrhage includes pharmacologic management consisting of infusion of vasopressin or octreotide and endoscopic sclerotherapy or ligation. Balloon tamponade initially was reported to achieve high rates of hemostasis (>60%).[9] The procedure has high risks for complications, however, such as pulmonary decompensation, and is associated with high rates of rebleeding after balloon removal and so is rarely used today. More invasive therapies used today include transjugular intrahepatic portosystemic shunt (TIPS) placement or open shunt surgery.

Medical Management

By activating the V_1 receptor found on vascular smooth muscle cells, vasopressin induces splanchnic and systemic vasoconstriction, reducing portal pressure. Although vasopressin infusion achieves hemostasis in greater than 50% of cases, use of this drug also can induce ischemic cardiac complications. The administration of nitroglycerin along with vasopressin decreases the likelihood of adverse vasoconstrictive events.[10,16] Although vasopressin can be dosed as a bolus, continuous infusion, or both, multiple controlled trials have shown that patients benefit most from the concomitant administration of nitroglycerin that allows for vasopressin to exert its full portal hypotensive effects.[23,24] Based on these data, it is recommended that intravenous vasopressin (0.4 U bolus followed by 0.4 to 1 U/min as an infusion) be combined with intravenous nitroglycerin (10 to 50 µg/min). Octreotide, a synthetic long-acting form of somatostatin, selectively vasoconstricts splanchnic vessels and is associated with far fewer cardiac complications than vasopressin.[23,25] Octreotide (50 µg bolus followed by 50 µg/h intravenous infusion for 5 days) has a rapid onset of action, selectively reducing portal and intravariceal pressures within seconds. A meta-analysis suggested that octreotide might be preferred over vasopressin, owing to a higher relative risk of achieving initial control of bleeding and a much lower adverse-effect profile.[26] Although vasopressin and octreotide have been shown to slow or arrest initial variceal hemorrhage, their efficacy is less striking in recurrences of bleeding. Neither vasopressin nor octreotide has been shown to decrease mortality.

Endoscopy

With the capability of being able to control greater than 80% of variceal bleeds, endoscopic sclerotherapy is an alternative to medical management. Endoscopy requires multiple sessions, does not reduce portal pressure, and cannot be used for control of bleeding from gastric varices due to technical considerations. Resulting in a lower rebleeding rate and fewer complications compared with sclerotherapy,[27] endoscopic variceal band ligation is proving to be more popular and successful. By encircling the varix with an elastic rubber band, this procedure ultimately leads to sloughing of thrombosed tissue.[27]

Invasive Intervention

If endoscopic intervention is unsuccessful or not feasible, a more invasive procedure—TIPS (percutaneous placement of an intrahepatic conduit between the portal and hepatic veins) or a surgically created portasystemic shunt—may be required. Although overall survival is not affected, the rate of rebleeding is decreased, and treatment of elevated portal pressures is achieved. Either procedure should be strongly considered in patients refractory to endoscopic treatment. Although the long-term management of bleeding may be improved over endoscopy, TIPS and surgical portosystemic shunts carry increased risks for worsening hepatic encephalopathy.[28,29] Based on published success rates, TIPS is considered the rescue therapy of choice compared with other emergent options, such as open shunt procedures. TIPS treats the acute hemorrhage and provides the bridge for the ultimate treatment, liver transplantation.[28,30,31]

OTHER CAUSES OF ACUTE UPPER GASTROINTESTINAL BLEEDING

Stress Ulceration

Critically ill patients are susceptible to stress-related mucosal damage in the esophagus, stomach, and duodenum. These lesions initially were thought to arise from excessive acid production, but are more likely due to insufficient mucosal perfusion. When first described in the 1960s, 10% of critically ill patients with multiple organ failure sustained extensive and even lethal hemorrhage, necessitating urgent gastrectomy.[32] In subsequent years, the combination of stress ulcer prophylaxis and improvements in resuscitation and other aspects of supportive care has been associated with a marked decrease in the incidence of hemorrhage from stress erosions. Antacids, H_2 receptor antagonists, gastric feedings, proton-pump inhibitors, and sucralfate are equally efficacious at limiting bleeding from stress ulcerations.[16] Cook and colleagues[33] showed that stress ulcer prophylaxis can be withheld safely for critically ill patients, unless either of two key risk factors, coagulopathy or severe respiratory failure, is present because the rate of clinically significant bleeding in low-risk patients is just 0.1%.

Esophagitis

Chemical, infectious, medication-induced, or reflux-induced esophagitis rarely results in acute severe bleeding. In rare cases of bleeding due to this cause, management consists of administering an H_2 receptor antagonist or proton-pump inhibitor, such as omeprazole. In addition, the offending agent should be removed immediately and other conditions treated. Generally a clinical diagnosis is made followed by pharmacologic management not requiring endoscopic or surgical intervention.

Mallory-Weiss Tear

A Mallory-Weiss tear develops at the distal esophagus and can extend across the gastroesophageal junction into the proximal stomach. Commonly associated with repetitive vomiting and retching, these longitudinal lacerations of the mucosa lead to submucosal arterial bleeds. Predisposing factors for the Mallory-Weiss syndrome include the presence of hiatal hernia, heavy alcohol use, and increasing age. Approximately 5% of acute upper gastrointestinal bleeds are caused by Mallory-Weiss tears.[34] The condition is primarily diagnosed by endoscopy. First-line treatment involves endoscopic injection or thermal coagulation therapy.[34-36]

Dieulafoy's Lesion

A Dieulafoy's lesion is a large, dilated, aberrant submucosal artery that precipitates the erosion of the overlying epithelium and ruptures into the gastrointestinal tract. Most commonly, the lesion arises on the lesser curvature of the stomach close to the gastroesophageal junction, but it has been discovered throughout the gastrointestinal tract.[37,38] Bleeding from Dieulafoy's lesion accounts for less than 1% of severe upper gastrointestinal bleeds.[36] The diagnostic modality of choice is endoscopy. Optimal management consists of endoscopic injection therapy, thermal coagulation, or possibly hemoclip placement.[39,40]

Other Arterial and Venous Malformations

Besides Dieulafoy's lesion, other vascular malformations lead to approximately 5% of acute upper gastrointestinal bleeds.[38] These malformations include idiopathic angiomas and the vascular lesions of Osler-Weber-Rendu syndrome, gastric antral vascular ectasia ("watermelon stomach"), and radiation-induced telangiectasia. These lesions more often present with occult bleeding but have the potential of causing more serious bleeding episodes. Endoscopy is used as a diagnostic and a treatment tool.

Upper Gastrointestinal Tumors

Upper gastrointestinal neoplasms account for approximately 1% to 3% of upper gastrointestinal bleeds.[41] Acute bleeding results from long-standing gastric or esophageal tumors that erode underlying vessels. Endoscopic injection therapy and thermal coagulation provide temporary stabilizing hemostasis until the patient can undergo palliative surgical resection. Upper gastrointestinal tumors that result in severe bleeding are associated with poor 1-year survival rates.[41]

Aortoenteric Fistulas

An aortoenteric fistula, a direct communication between the aorta and the gastrointestinal tract, forms in the presence of atherosclerotic aortic aneurysms or after abdominal aorta reconstruction. The incidence of such a fistula after aortic reconstructive surgery has been reported to be 0.6% to 1.5%; the interval between the operation and the onset of gastrointestinal bleeding ranges from a few days to many years.[42] Graft infection is usually a predisposing factor leading to fistula formation. Other less common causes include radiation, trauma, and tumor invasion. An aortoenteric fistula classically presents with a herald bleed (i.e., a self-limiting transient bleeding episode) before later presentation with exsanguinating hemorrhage. Aortoenteric fistula is a diagnosis of exclusion, requiring a keen clinical perspective and the modern advances of endoscopy, computed tomography, and arteriography. This condition is a surgical emergency, requiring removal of the aneurysm or infected graft and restoration of circulation to the lower extremities, usually by an extra-anatomic bypass procedure.[43,44]

LOWER GASTROINTESTINAL HEMORRHAGE

Acute lower gastrointestinal bleeding refers to blood loss from the intestinal tract emanating from a source distal to the ligament of Treitz and presentation with unstable vital signs, anemia, and the possible need for blood transfusions.[45] Lower intestinal bleeding,[46,47] rectal[48-51] or colonic bleeding,[52,53] and bloody diarrhea[54] are commonly used synonyms; more descriptive terms include bright red blood per rectum, maroon-colored or mahogany stools, and hematochezia.[46,47,55,56]

Making the distinction between upper and lower gastrointestinal hemorrhage is hard in many cases, considering that 80% of all patients with some form of gastrointestinal bleeding pass blood in some form per rectum,[57] and 11% of patients with an upper gastrointestinal bleed present exclusively with hematochezia.[55] Approximately 20% of all cases of apparent lower gastrointestinal bleeding have an upper gastrointestinal source; these patients characteristically are orthostatic because 500 to 1000 mL of blood must be lost rapidly from the upper gastrointestinal tract to pass through the distal gut and appear bright red as it exits the rectum.

EPIDEMIOLOGY

The reported incidence of lower gastrointestinal bleeding ranges from 20.5 to 27 cases per 100,000 adult population per year[46,53]; in contrast, the annual incidence of upper gastrointestinal bleeding ranges from 100 to 200 cases per 100,000.[58] The lower gastrointestinal tract is the source in 20% to 33% of cases of acute gastrointestinal bleeding.[46] Men are affected more often than women, and the incidence lower gastrointestinal bleeding increases with age such that the risk is 200-fold greater in persons in their 80s compared with persons in their 30s.[46,57]

PATHOGENESIS

The causes of lower gastrointestinal bleeding are summarized in Table 116-4.

Colonic Diverticula

Diverticulosis of the colon is more prevalent with older compared with younger individuals. The lesions consist of pseudodiverticula of the colonic wall, where the submucosa herniates through the submucosal layer of the gut. Bleeding occurs after asymmetric rupture of the intramural branch (vasa recta) of the marginal artery at the dome of the diverticulum, potentially secondary to erosions or ulcerations at the neck or the dome.[59] Diverticula are located predominantly in the descending and sigmoid colon and are asymptomatic in most patients. Prevalence is 50% in Western countries, but is only about 1% or less in African and Asian populations.

Bleeding occurs in 3% to 5% of all patients with diverticular disease,[60,61] and diverticulosis is thought to be responsible for 42% to 55% of cases of lower gastrointestinal bleeding.[46,47,52,53,56] The diagnosis of bleeding from diverticulosis as the cause of a lower gastrointestinal bleed should be made only after excluding other causes because using predetermined criteria lowers the rate to 10% to 20%,[51,56] and 87% of the diagnoses may be presumptive.[46]

In most patients, hematochezia is self-limited and accompanied by only mild left lower quadrant discomfort. Occasionally, severe bleeding occurs, however, resulting in anemia from acute blood loss. The differential diagnosis in the typical elderly patient includes internal hemorrhoids, ischemic colitis, angiodysplasia, polyps, and tumors.

Colonoscopy after urgent bowel cleansing is able to identify diverticula as the source of bleeding based on active bleeding or fresh blood in a segment of colon with no other lesions but diverticula. Mesenteric angiography and radionuclide bleeding scans also can show diverticular bleeding, if there is active bleeding, and contrast material extravasates into the colon lumen.

Endoscopic treatment using bipolar or heater probe coagulation or epinephrine injection is an efficacious treatment modality, leading to good acute control of hemorrhage and no recurrence of bleeding during 1 year of follow-up.[55,60,62,63] The bleeding diverticula can be shown on selective mesenteric angiography; embolization or infusion of vasopressin or

TABLE 116–4. FREQUENT CAUSES OF LOWER GASTROINTESTINAL BLEEDING

Lesion	Frequency (%)	Comments
Diverticular disease	17-42	In 80% of patients, spontaneous cessation of bleeding Surgery unlikely if < 4 U PRBCs/24 h required; surgery necessary in 60% of patients who required > 4 U PRBCs/24 h
Colonic vascular ectasia	2-30	Frequency of lesions varies in clinical series Acute bleeding more frequently associated with lesions in proximal colon
Colitis	9-21%	Abdominal pain and self-limited hematochezia is a common presentation of ischemic colitis, affecting the splenic flexure segment most often[106]
Ischemic		
Infectious		
Inflammatory bowel disease		
Radiation proctopathy		
Colonic neoplasia		
Postpolypectomy bleeding	11-14%	Usually self-limited, may occur 15 days after polypectomy
Anorectal causes	4-10%	Anoscopy and proctoscopy should be used in the initial evaluation
Hemorrhoids		Digital rectal examination
Rectal varices		
Upper gastrointestinal bleeding source	0-11%	Not excluded by negative nasogastric aspiration
Gastric ulcer		
Duodenal ulcer		
Varices		
Small bowel source	2-9%	Frequently diagnosed by radiologic or enteroscopic studies after cessation of initial bleeding episode
Crohn's ileitis		
Vascular ectasia		
Meckel's diverticulum		
Tumor		
Other	10%	
Unknown	11%	

PRBCs, packed red blood cells.
From Vernava AM 3rd, Moore BA, Longo WE, Johnson FE: Lower gastrointestinal bleeding. Dis Colon Rectum 1997;40:846-858; Longstreth GF: Epidemiology of hospitalization for acute upper gastrointestinal hemorrhage: A population-based study. Am J Gastroenterol 1995;90:206-210; and Jensen DM, Machicado GA: Colonoscopy for diagnosis and treatment of severe lower gastrointestinal bleeding: Routine outcomes and cost analysis. Gastrointest Endosc Clin N Am 1997;7:477-498.

both are used to achieve hemostasis, often followed by elective surgical resection of the affected area.[64,65] Some reports suggest that more serious bleeding arises from the right side of the colon.[66-69]

A segmental colectomy should be considered for uncontrollable bleeding in patients who fail medical resuscitation or when bleeding cannot be stopped with endoscopic or angiographic means. Surgery may be considered in cases of recurrent diverticular bleeding when the exact location of bleeding is certain. Bleeding from diverticular disease stops spontaneously in almost 80% of cases[70] and has a recurrence rate of 25%; 99% of cases require transfusion of less than 4 U of blood.[70]

Colonic Angiomas and Angiodysplasia

The presence of tortuous submucosal vessels is referred to as angiodysplasia; this condition is seen in 1% to 2% of cases in large autopsy and colonoscopy series.[59,71] Fewer than 1% of the general population has lower gastrointestinal angiodysplasia, and during a 3-year follow-up in one study, no bleeding episode was reported.[72] The incidence of angiodysplasia increases with age. Angiodysplasia accounts for 20% to 30% of all bleeding episodes[73,74] and may be the most prevalent cause of acute lower gastrointestinal bleeding in people older than age 65 years.[75]

Endoscopic coagulation (with bipolar probe or heater probes), injection sclerotherapy, and argon laser coagulation are effective for achieving hemostasis,[71] but these treatment modalities are associated with recurrence rates after local therapy of 30%.[71] Identification of upper gastrointestinal or small bowel angiodysplasia should prompt investigation to exclude additional lesions in the lower gastrointestinal tract.

Colon Cancer and Neoplasms

Acute and significant bleeding from a colon polyp or colon cancer is uncommon but can be a presenting symptom in 2% to 26% of cases.[47,53,76,77] Bleeding is thought to arise mainly from ulcerations of the luminal surface.[77]

Ischemic Colitis

Mesenteric ischemia is an important, life-threatening cause of lower gastrointestinal bleeding among critically ill patients.[78] Ischemia commonly is caused by mesenteric vasoconstriction in the setting of systemic hypoperfusion, resulting in watershed infarcts to segments of the bowel. Alternatively, ischemia may be secondary to arterial embolization of thrombi or atheromatous material secondary to atrial fibrillation or cardiac or aortic surgery. Other causes of colonic ischemia, including vasculitis,[80] polyarteritis nodosa,[80] Wegener's granulomatosis,[80] and rheumatoid vasculitis,[81] can present with lower gastrointestinal bleeding. Vasculitis causes an ulcerating, necrotizing process resulting in hemorrhage. Of patients with acute lower gastrointestinal bleeding, 3% to 9% bled from the colon secondary to ischemic colitis.[46,53,77] Diagnosis of mesenteric ischemia requires a high index of suspicion. Bleeding from ischemic colitis has a high mortality rate (approximately 50% to 60%), probably because the diagnosis is difficult to make and delays in interventions to improve mesenteric blood flow or resect infarcted bowel are common.[78]

Radiation Colitis

Ionizing radiation to the abdomen can cause acute and chronic damage to the colon and rectum. Approximately 75% of patients who receive a dose of 40 Gy develop acute, self-limited diarrhea, tenesmus, abdominal cramping, and rarely bleeding during the first few weeks.[82,83] Chronic effects occur later after approximately 6 to 18 months and are due to vascular damage, resulting in mucosal ischemia, thickening, and ulcerations. The median interval between the completion of radiation therapy and presentation with radiation colitis is 9 to 15 months.[82-84] Common findings are hematochezia and rectal pain, and patients often are anemic. Endoscopic findings include telangiectasias, strictures, ulcers, and signs of inflammation. Barium studies reveal flattened mucosa with loss of haustral markings.

Various endoscopic treatment modalities are used in the treatment of bleeding from radiation-induced mucosal changes,[85] including bipolar coagulation, heater probes, and argon plasma[86] or laser[87] coagulation. These approaches decrease the frequency of bleeding and reduce transfusion requirements. Corticosteroid and sucralfate enemas sometimes are helpful.[88] Iron supplements should be prescribed for chronically anemic patients. In refractory cases, hyperbaric oxygen, topical formalin, and antioxidant therapy with vitamins C and E also have been reported to be useful.[89-91] Surgery should be considered for significant and refractory bleeding.

Inflammatory Bowel Disease

Ulcerative colitis is the primary cause in 2% to 8% of cases of lower gastrointestinal bleeding, and 6% to 10% of emergency surgical resections for ulcerative colitis are due to acute lower gastrointestinal bleeding.[92,93] Lower gastrointestinal bleeding affects 0.6% to 1.3% of patients with Crohn's disease,[47,94] and Crohn's disease is responsible for about 1% of all lower gastrointestinal bleeds.[47,94]

Infectious Colitis

Infection with *Campylobacter jejuni, Salmonella* species, *Shigella* species, invasive *Escherichia coli, E. coli* O157,[95,96] or *Clostridium difficile* can result in acute onset of bloody diarrhea, leading to significant blood loss, fever, and abdominal pain. Diagnosis is made by stool cultures and flexible sigmoidoscopy. Except for cases of *C. difficile* infection causing pseudomembranous colitis with impending perforation, there is no role for surgical therapy, and antibiotic treatment may suffice.[97] Significant hemorrhage from the intestine also can be a problem in patients with graft-versus-host disease.[98]

Postpolypectomy Bleeding

Colonoscopic polypectomy harbors a 1% risk per case for developing a significant bleed 10 to 15 days after the procedure.[99,100] Colonoscopic polypectomy is responsible for 5% to 11% of cases of lower gastrointestinal bleeding.[47,53,76,77,95,101] Risk factors for this adverse outcome include polyp size greater than 2 cm; sessile polyp; elderly age; and use of aspirin, NSAIDs, or warfarin (Coumadin). Early bleeding may be due to separation of the polyp from the stalk, before adequate hemostasis of the blood vessels in the stalk has been achieved.[100] Late bleeding is thought to be due to sloughing of the coagulum.[100] In most of these cases, the bleeding stops spontaneously without requiring an intervention. Only 0.2% to 3% of cases have clinically significant hemorrhage, and there is a trend toward reduced incidence in later reports.[102-105] Hemostasis can be achieved by repeat colonoscopy with injection of epinephrine, application of hemoclips, or repeat snare coagulation.[99]

Vascular Causes

A history of aortic graft surgery predisposes patients to aortocolonic fistula formation 4 to 10 weeks to 14 years after the operation.[106] Although primary aortocolonic fistulas are rare and usually fatal,[107,108] fistulization between the aorta and the small bowel is less rare and clinically indistinguishable in presentation.[109]

Acquired Immunodeficiency Syndrome

Human immunodeficiency virus–associated thrombocytopenia can cause significant hemorrhage from hemorrhoids in this high-risk population.[111] Human immunodeficiency virus–associated colonic lesions have been implicated in 72% of cases of hematochezia in patients with acquired immunodeficiency syndrome; cytomegalovirus-induced colitis is the primary problem in 39% of the cases.[112,113] The attributable mortality from lower gastrointestinal bleeding in this patient population is low.[111,113]

INITIAL EVALUATION

The severity of the presentation may range from mild rectal bleeding without affecting normal vital signs to massive hemorrhage and shock, requiring urgent intervention and stabilization. Massive bleeding that warrants urgent surgery without waiting for results of diagnostic studies is uncommon, however.[69] About half of patients present with a decrease in hemoglobin and hemodynamic instability, 9% present with cardiovascular collapse,[53] 10% present with syncope,[53] and 30% have orthostatic changes.[47]

Compared with patients with lower gastrointestinal bleeding, patients with upper gastrointestinal bleeding are substantially less likely to present with shock (19% versus 35%) and are less likely to require blood transfusions (36% versus 64%).[96] The initial hemoglobin concentration of patients with upper gastrointestinal bleeding is significantly lower, and 85% to 90% of patients with lower gastrointestinal bleeding stop bleeding without intervention. Findings from angiographic studies indicate that the rate of bleeding changes frequently.[114] Table 116-5 summarizes criteria to define levels of certainty of the diagnosis of lower gastrointestinal bleeding on initial evaluation.

Bedside Diagnosis

A focused history and physical examination is an essential component of the evaluation of a patient with lower gastrointestinal bleeding. A minimal set of initial laboratory values includes complete blood count, serum electrolyte concentrations, blood urea nitrogen concentration, creatinine concentration, type and crossmatch, and coagulation profile. The initial hemoglobin or hematocrit value may reflect volume contraction and decrease substantially after volume resuscitation. In upper gastrointestinal bleeding, absorption of proteins from blood in the lower intestine can increase blood urea nitrogen concentration; however, measuring a normal blood urea nitrogen concentration does not rule out an upper gastrointestinal source.[115,116] In patients age 50 or older, an electrocardiogram always should be obtained; in younger patients, the decision to obtain an electrocardiogram should be made based on the patient's risk factors for coronary artery disease or complaints of chest pain or palpitations during the bleeding episode.

The history should elucidate the nature and duration of bleeding, including stool color and frequency. An effort

---

TABLE 116–5. HIERARCHY OF DIAGNOSTIC CERTAINTY FOR ACUTE COLONIC BLEEDING AFTER PRESURGICAL EVALUATION

Level I. Definitive Diagnosis

A. Actively bleeding lesion found at endoscopy (anoscopy, sigmoidoscopy, or colonoscopy) or angiography
B. Stigmata of recent bleeding (nonbleeding visible vessel, adherent clot) found at endoscopy
C. Positive TRBC scan if verified by IA or IB

Level II. Presumptive Diagnosis/Circumstantial Evidence

A. Fresh blood localized to colon segment inhabited by potential bleeding source
B. Positive TRBC scan localizing to the colon and colonoscopy that shows potential bleeding site in area of positive scan
C. Bright red blood per rectum confirmed by objective color testing and colonoscopy that shows single potential bleeding source in colon, complemented by negative upper endoscopy

Level III. Equivocal Diagnosis

A. Hematochezia or blood per rectum (without color specification) and colonoscopy that shows one or more potential bleeding sources

TRBC, tagged red blood cell.
From Zuckerman GR, Prakash C: Acute lower intestinal bleeding: Part II. Etiology, therapy, and outcomes. Gastrointest Endosc 1999;49:228-238; and Zuckerman GR, Prakash C: Acute lower intestinal bleeding: Part I. Clinical presentation and diagnosis. Gastrointest Endosc 1998;48:606-617.

---

should be made to elicit a history of associated symptoms, such as changes in bowel habits, fever, urgency, or weight loss. Potentially relevant findings in the past history include previous bleeding episodes, trauma, past abdominal surgeries, peptic ulcer disease, inflammatory bowel disease, radiation to the abdomen and pelvis, major organ dysfunction, and recent colonoscopy. Current medications, including aspirin, NSAIDs, and anticoagulants, should be recorded. The patient's allergies should be noted.

A physical examination should include at a minimum an immediate recording of vital signs, including changes with postural changes. If the blood pressure decreases by more than 10 mm Hg or the heart rate increases by more than 10 beats/min, the patient probably has had acute blood loss greater than 800 mL, representing approximately 15% of the circulating blood volume in an average adult. More marked hypotension and depressed mental status indicates acute blood loss greater than 1500 mL (30% of the circulating blood volume).[117] Cardiopulmonary, abdominal, and digital rectal examinations should be performed.

An important step in the initial workup is establishing prognosis so as to determine the most appropriate disposition for the patient.[118] Strate and colleagues[119] derived a set of independent prognostic factors to predict outcome in patients with acute lower gastrointestinal bleeding. Important factors include presence of tachycardia, hypotension, ongoing bleeding, or syncope. Also important are absence of tenderness on abdominal examination, history of aspirin use, and history of more than two active medical conditions (Table 116-6).[120] The Acute Physiology and Chronic Health Evaluation II (APACHE II) score correlates with poor outcome in patients with lower gastrointestinal bleeding.[121]

TABLE 116–6. INDEPENDENT RISK FACTORS FOR SEVERE LOWER GASTROINTESTINAL BLEEDING

Heart rate >100 beats/min
Systolic blood pressure <115 mm Hg
Syncope
Nontender abdominal examination
Bleeding in the first 4 h of evaluation
Aspirin use
More than two comorbid conditions

From Strate LL, Orav EJ, Syngal S: Early predictors of severity in acute lower intestinal tract bleeding. Arch Intern Med 2003;163(7):838-843.

DIAGNOSTIC PROCEDURES

Colonoscopy

Colonoscopy, previously considered of no value in the treatment of lower gastrointestinal bleeding,[122] is now an important method for diagnosis and treatment of lower gastrointestinal bleeding. The colonoscope can localize the bleeding site for the surgeon, if surgical therapy becomes necessary. Certain therapeutic interventions also can be performed using colonoscopy. One concern regarding the utility of colonoscopy has been poor visualization of the mucosa in an unprepared colon, leading to a relatively high risk of perforation or exacerbation of bleeding.[48,122] A variety of bowel preparation regimens are available, however, that can enahance visualization.[51,81] After initial stabilization, colonoscopy should be carried out within the first 24 hours.[69] For bowel preparation, 4 to 15 L of a balanced electrolyte solution should be administered enterally over 2 to 7 hours. With this preparation strategy, the diagnostic yield with colonoscopy is 74%.[55] Bowel preparation for colonoscopy has been reported to be safe and well tolerated in most instances.[47,51] Potential complications include fluid overload and heart failure.[55] In a large series of colonoscopic examinations for bleeding, only 2% were incomplete; the bowel preparation was inadequate in only 6% of cases.[55]

In two published series, a lesion could be demonstrable by colonoscopy in 48% and 90% of cases.[47,52] Table 116-7 lists criteria for diagnosing lesions detected at colonoscopy, including presence of active bleeding, a nonbleeding visible

TABLE 116–7. CRITERIA FOR COLONOSCOPIC DIAGNOSIS OF BLEEDING SITE

	Recurrence of Bleeding (%)
Active colonic bleeding site	50
Nonbleeding visible vessel	25
Adherent clot	29
Fresh blood localized to a colonic segment	
Ulceration of a diverticulum with fresh blood in immediate area	
Absence of fresh blood in terminal ileum with fresh blood in colon	

From Jensen DM, Machicado GA, Jutabha R, Kovacs TO: Urgent colonoscopy for the diagnosis and treatment of severe diverticular hemorrhage. N Engl J Med 2000;342:78-82; Zuckerman GR, Prakash C: Acute lower intestinal bleeding: Part II. Etiology, therapy, and outcomes. Gastrointest Endosc 1999;49:228-238; and Zuckerman GR, Prakash C: Acute lower intestinal bleeding: Part I. Clinical presentation and diagnosis. Gastrointest Endosc 1998;48:606-617.

vessel, or an adherent clot.[47,56,69] The likelihood of finding a lesion increases from 48% to 85% when colonoscopy is performed while the patient is still actively bleeding.[52] At colonoscopy, it is usually possible to visualize a small segment of the terminal ileum. The diagnosis of small bowel bleeding can be made by showing fresh blood in the terminal ileum or coming through the ileocecal valve in the absence of findings on upper endoscopy.[51,69]

Tagged Red Blood Cell Scan

In contrast to technetium 99m–sulfur colloid, which is taken up rapidly by the liver and spleen, technetium 99m–labeled red blood cells remain in the systemic circulation for 48 hours. In one study, technetium 99m–labeled red blood cells detected 93% of actively bleeding gastrointestinal lesions, and technetium 99m–sulfur colloid detected only 12%.[123] Technetium 99m–labeled red blood cells reportedly can detect bleeding at rates of 0.1 mL/min; however, in routine clinical practice, higher bleeding rates may be required. Approximately 45% of all scans are positive in patients with lower gastrointestinal bleeding.[125-128] The likelihood of a positive scan increases when the patient is actively bleeding when the radionuclide is injected.[125] The number of transfusions required and hemodynamic instability are not predictors of a positive scan.[128] Patients with a positive scan may require surgery more often and have higher rates of morbidity and mortality than patients with a negative scan.[126-128] A negative scan may be helpful in identifying a subgroup of patients who do not require therapeutic intervention.[126,127]

In one study, a radionuclide blush appeared on the scan immediately in 61% of the patients.[129] In these positive studies, a subsequently performed angiogram was always positive, and the location of the bleeding lesion on the arteriogram corresponded to the location of the lesion as determined by radionuclide scanning in all cases. Positive late scans matched the angiographic findings only 7% of the time.[129] The value of a positive scan depends on the interval between injection of the radionuclide and the positive scan; 57% to 67% accuracy is found after 2 hours compared with 95% to 100% within the first 2 hours. Scans that become positive after more than 6 hours may depict only blood that has migrated by peristalsis; the localizing value is less than 55%.[128,130] A history of NSAID or aspirin use lowers the yield of the technetium 99m–labeled red blood cell scan because bleeding in these cases is more likely to be diffuse.[131]

Recommendation for surgery should not be based on a technetium 99m–labeled red blood cell scan, given that localization is accurate in only 67% to 97% of studies.[125-127,129,131] Performing a confirmatory test before surgery lowers the rate of false localization.[125,126,129] Data are lacking to permit direct comparison of the diagnostic accuracy of colonoscopy and technetium 99m–labeled red blood cell scan.

Angiography

When used to identify the source of an acute lower gastrointestinal bleed, the sensitivity of angiography is 47%, and the specificity is 100%.[132] Angiography also can be therapeutic, but the procedure can be associated with complications. The overall risk of complications for noncerebral, noncoronary angiography is reported to be 9.3%; major complications include hematoma, dissection, femoral artery thrombosis, contrast reactions, contrast-induced nephropathy, and transient ischemic attacks.[133] To detect bleeding angiographically, the bleeding rate must be 0.5 mL/min or greater.[134]

The standard practice in many centers is to perform a technetium 99m–labeled red blood cell scan first. A negative scan implies a bleeding rate of less than 0.1 mL/min and makes a positive arteriogram unlikely.[126,136] An immediate blush on the technetium 99m–labeled red blood cell scan is a good predictor of a positive angiogram.[129] The arteriogram does not always show the actual bleeding site, however.[66] Identification of venous bleeding by arteriography is unlikely.[137]

Arteriograms are positive in 27% to 77% of cases.[52,66,73,126,129,138-143] If arteriography is performed only in the presence of active bleeding or hemodynamic instability, the study is positive in 67% to 72% of cases.[73] Using aggressive approaches, including administration of anticoagulants or vasodilators to prolong the bleeding, increases the detection rate to 32% to 65%.[66]

Esophagogastroduodenoscopy

Upper endoscopy has been variably used and should always be contemplated when evaluating a patient for lower gastrointestinal bleeding.[46,47,56,80] Although some studies reported that all examinations were negative,[46,47] in a study with a larger sample size, 11% of the patients presenting with severe hematochezia were found to have a lesion in the stomach or duodenum.[56] The role of upper endoscopy in the evaluation of lower gastrointestinal bleeding still needs to be defined.

Barium Enema

Barium enema has a low diagnostic yield and provides poor localization.[145,146] In one series, findings obtained by barium enema were misleading in 34% of cases.[147] Barium enema should be avoided because barium interferes with performing a subsequent colonoscopy or an angiogram.[47]

MANAGEMENT

Initial stabilization of the patient should be achieved before diagnostic measures are undertaken. Monitoring in an ICU is appropriate and recommended for patients with unstable vital signs. Patients with comorbid conditions and patients at risk for complications preferably should be treated in an ICU.

Several factors should be taken into consideration when deciding about the disposition of patients with lower gastrointestinal bleeding. The presence of comorbid condititons (e.g., cardiac, pulmonary, hepatic, renal, and neurologic dysfunction), low serum albumin concentration, prolonged prothrombin time, and elevated serum bilirubin level are common characteristics of patients with a higher risk for an adverse outcome.[57] Even if the vital signs are stable after initial resuscitation, admission to an ICU is warranted when patients fail to respond appropriately to initial resuscitation measures, display persistent hypotension and tachycardia, require blood transfusion, or have significant comorbid conditions.[147]

THERAPY

Resuscitation always should take precedence over any diagnostic measure or therapeutic procedure that might place the patient at risk. Resuscitation and diagnostic efforts overlap in most cases. In most cases, bleeding stops spontaneously. In the remaining cases, a combination of endoscopic, angiographic, and surgical techniques is required. The role of technetium 99m–labeled red blood cell scan is controversial.

Brackman and colleagues[120] prefer endoscopy or angiography over technetium 99m–labeled red blood cell scanning because the former two studies also offer the potential to be therapeutic.

Endoscopic Therapy

Endoscopic therapy includes the use of various heater, laser, and coagulation probes and injection of vasoconstricting or sclerosing agents. There are no good data comparing the efficacy of these methods.

Endovascular Therapy

After identifying a source for the lower gastrointestinal bleeding, endovascular therapy may be performed to achieve hemostasis. Approaches include intra-arterial injection of vasopressin or superselective embolization with thrombogenic coils, polyvinyl alcohol particles, or glue material.[148] Both methods have approximately a 70% success rate.[149,150]

Surgery

Many attempts have been made to establish stringent criteria to assess the need for surgery. Continued hemodynamic instability, transfusion requirements of more than 4 U in 24 hours or 10 U overall, and recurrent bleeding have been used to indicate a need for surgery.[70,151,152] Repeat bleeding from diverticular disease has been considered an indication for surgery[60,151]; however, some authors recommend waiting for a third bleeding episode.[153] Classically, total colectomy has been considered the last resort in the treatment of lower gastrointestinal bleeding. The impression of a higher morbidity and mortality involved with this procedure might be not supportable by current data. The authors argue that total resection of the colon may be an option, considering the time spent in repeat studies to obtain localization and determine the extent of the bleeding.[154]

OUTCOME

Historically, mortality rates for lower gastrointestinal bleeding are low (averaging <5%).[46] Patients with moderate-to-severe bleeding tend to have a better outcome, if triaged to a surgical service.[121]

SUMMARY

Diagnosis and management of lower gastrointestinal bleeding depends on the severity of the presentation, and although the initial differential diagnosis for hematochezia is complex, the initial triage process is crucial in determining the disposition of the patient. The prognosis can be made based on a variety of clinical scores, and use of the different diagnostic modalities usually leads to localization of the bleed.

ANNOTATED REFERENCES

Conrad SA: Acute upper gastrointestinal bleeding in critically ill patients: Causes and treatment modalities. Crit Care Med 2002;30(6 Suppl):S365-368.
This review illustrates the necessary principles for approaching and effectively treating a patient presenting with a gastrointestinal hemorrhage. It focuses on patient classification and highlights the criteria for identifying critically ill patients most at risk for rebleeding.

Jensen DM, Machicado GA, Jutabha R, Kovacs TO: Urgent colonoscopy for the diagnosis and treatment of severe diverticular hemorrhage. N Engl J Med 2000;342:78-82.

This article describes a prospective, nonrandomized study of 121 patients presenting with severe diverticular hemorrhage, the most common cause of lower gastrointestinal bleeding, who received hemicolectomy versus colonoscopic-guided local therapy. This study showed that timely colonoscopic intervention effectively prevents recurrent bleeding.

Savides TJ, Jensen DM: Therapeutic endoscopy for nonvariceal gastrointestinal bleeding. Gastroenterol Clin North Am 2000;29:465-487.

The use of endoscopy in the evaluation and treatment of upper gastrointestinal hemorrhage is steadily increasing in importance and timeliness.

This article thoroughly addresses patient assessment before endoscopy and effectively describes the role of endoscopy.

Zuccaro G Jr: Management of the adult patient with acute lower gastrointestinal bleeding. American College of Gastroenterology Practice Parameters Committee. Am J Gastroenterol 1998;93:1202-1208.

Practice guidelines for lower gastrointestinal bleeding issued by the American College of Gastroenterology are presented.

Chapter 117

HEPATORENAL SYNDROME

Àngels Escorsell • Vicente Arroyo

KEY POINTS

1. **Ascites is a common complication of liver cirrhosis preceding the development of severe complications** such as dilutional hyponatremia, refractory ascites, and hepatorenal syndrome (HRS) that carry an extremely poor prognosis.

2. **Renal functional abnormalities in cirrhosis start** with the reduced ability to excrete sodium, sodium retention, and accumulation of ascites. As the disease progresses, circulatory dysfunction increases as a consequence of the activation of endogenous vasoactive systems (sympathetic nervous system and the renin-angiotensin system).

3. The **final step leading to HRS is the decrease in renal perfusion** due to an imbalance between an extremely high vasoconstrictor tone and a decreased production of renal vasodilators.

4. **Patients with HRS respond poorly to diuretics.**

5. **Diagnosis of HRS follows the criteria of the International Ascites Club** (see Table 117-1) and mainly consists of the presence of a serum creatinine level greater than 1.5 mg/dL or a creatinine clearance lower than 40 mL/min in the absence of other potential causes of renal failure.

6. **HRS is classified into two types:**
   a. Type 1: severe and rapidly progressive renal failure, usually following a precipitating event and carrying an extremely poor prognosis (median survival: 2 weeks).
   b. Type 2: moderate and steady development of renal failure, clinically characterized by refractory ascites and with a slightly better prognosis (median survival: 6 months).

7. **Liver transplantation is the treatment of choice for HRS.** The recovery of renal function as well as the reversal of the hemodynamic and neurohumoral abnormalities associated with the syndrome may take 1 month after the operation.

8. **The 3-year probability of survival in transplanted patients with HRS is 60%,** slightly less than in recipients without HRS.

9. **Recent studies have shown that HRS type 1 is reversible** after treatment with intravenous albumin and vasoconstrictors, although the continuous infusion of vasoconstrictors is associated with ischemic complications.

10. **TIPS represents a promising approach to treat HRS type 1.**

11. **Successful prevention of HRS has been achieved in specific clinical settings,** such as spontaneous bacterial peritonitis (by administration of albumin + antibiotics) and acute alcoholic hepatitis (by giving pentoxifylline).

Ascites is a common complication of cirrhosis that develops late in the course of the disease, when there is severe portal hypertension and hepatic failure. Not surprisingly, it is associated with a poor survival (50% mortality at 3 years of follow-up).[1] In addition, it precedes the development of complications, such as dilutional hyponatremia, refractory ascites, and hepatorenal syndrome (HRS) that have an extremely poor prognosis. Consequently, liver transplantation should be performed before the development of these complications,[1,2] that is, when ascites develops. HRS has an annual incidence of approximately 8% in patients with ascites.[2] As previously mentioned, it develops at the latest phase of the disease and there is now evidence that it is an important determinant in survival.

MECHANISMS OF RENAL DYSFUNCTION IN CIRRHOSIS

Sodium retention, impaired free-water excretion, and decreased renal perfusion and glomerular filtration rate (GFR) are the main renal function abnormalities in cirrhosis. The onset of each of these abnormalities differs in time and, consequently, the course of cirrhosis can be divided in phases according to renal function. Renal dysfunction in cirrhosis usually follows a progressive course. Therefore, at the latest phase of the disease, when HRS develops, all three abnormalities are invariably present.

IMPAIRMENT IN RENAL SODIUM METABOLISM WITHOUT ACTIVATION OF VASOACTIVE SYSTEMS

Chronologically, the first renal functional abnormality in cirrhosis is reduced ability to excrete sodium. When cirrhosis is still compensated (i.e., ascites is absent), subtle abnormalities in renal sodium metabolism already can be detected.

Patients may not be capable of escaping from the effect of mineralocorticoids and develop continuous sodium retention.[3] Arterial vasodilatation is already present in compensated cirrhosis with portal hypertension.[4]

As the disease progresses, the impairment in sodium metabolism increases. At a critical point, patients are unable to excrete the amount of sodium normally ingested in the diet. Sodium is retained and accumulates as ascites. Renal perfusion, GFR, the renal ability to excrete a free water load, plasma renin activity, and the plasma concentrations of aldosterone and norepinephrine are normal.[5] Thus, sodium retention is unrelated to alterations in the renin-aldosterone system or the sympathetic nervous system, the two most important sodium-retaining systems so far identified.

STIMULATION OF THE RENIN-ANGIOTENSIN AND SYMPATHETIC NERVOUS SYSTEMS AND ANTIDIURETIC HORMONE WITH PRESERVED RENAL PERFUSION AND GLOMERULAR FILTRATION RATE

In cases of alcoholic cirrhosis, hepatic, circulatory, and renal function may improve if alcohol consumption is discontinued. In all other forms of cirrhosis and alcoholic cirrhosis with ongoing ethanol abuse, the degree of sodium retention increases progressively with progression of disease. When renal sodium avidity is extremely high, the plasma renin activity and the plasma concentrations of aldosterone and norepinephrine are elevated.[4,6-8] Circulatory dysfunction is greater at this stage of the disease because increased activity of the sympathetic nervous system and the renin-angiotensin system is needed fto maintain arterial pressure.

Renal perfusion and GFR are normal or moderately decreased, but renal perfusion is critically dependent on increased renal production of prostaglandins.[9] These lipid mediators are vasodilators that antagonize the vasoconstricting actions of angiotensin II and norepinephrine. A syndrome indistinguishable from HRS can be produced in patients with cirrhosis, ascites, and increased plasma renin activity if prostaglandin synthesis is inhibited with nonsteroidal anti-inflammatory drugs.[6,10] In addition, prostacyclin and nitric oxide cooperate to maintain renal perfusion in cirrhosis.[11,12]

PATHOGENESIS

Development of HRS represents the terminal phase of the disease. HRS is characterized by low arterial blood pressure; marked increased plasma levels of renin, norepinephrine, and antidiuretic hormone; and very low GFR (<40 mL/min).[13,19] Impairment in GFR in HRS occurs because of decreased renal perfusion secondary to renal vasoconstriction.[19] Renal histology is bland. Because renal vascular resistance correlates closely with activity of the renin-angiotensin and sympathetic nervous systems in cirrhosis,[20-25] HRS is thought to be related to extreme stimulation of these systems.

Urinary excretion of prostaglandin E_2, 6-keto-prostaglandin $F_{1\alpha}$ (a prostacyclin metabolite), and kallikrein is decreased in patients with HRS, indicating that renal production of these substances is reduced.[6,26] Renal failure in HRS, therefore, might be the consequence of an imbalance between the activity of vasoconstrictor systems and the renal production of vasodilators. The observation that HRS can be reproduced in nonazotemic, hyperreninemic cirrhotic patients with ascites with nonsteroidal anti-inflammatory drugs is compatible with this hypothesis.[9] Another possibility, however, is that renal vasoconstriction caused by the renin-angiotensin and sympathetic nervous systems is the primary cause of HRS. According to this hypothesis, reduced synthesis of prostaglandins and kallikrein is a secondary event that exacerbates renal insufficiency.

Because the pathogenesis of renal vasoconstriction in HRS is multifactorial, it is unlikely to be improved by pharmacologic treatment, which interferes with only one of the pathogenic mechanisms. Accordingly, it is not surprising that negative results have been obtained in studies using only inhibitors of the renin-angiotensin system, namely, alpha-adrenergic antagonists, endothelin receptor antagonists, adenosine antagonists, and prostaglandins.[27]

HRS is usually associated with an extremely low urinary sodium excretion. The renal ability to excrete free water is also markedly reduced, and most patients present with significant hyponatremia. Sodium retention in patients with HRS is caused by a decrease in filtered sodium and an increase in sodium reabsorption in the proximal tubule. Accordingly, the amount of sodium reaching the loop of Henle and distal nephron, the sites of action for furosemide and spironolactone, respectively, is very low. The delivery of furosemide and spironolactone to the renal tubules is also reduced because of renal hypoperfusion. Therefore, it is not surprising that patients with HRS respond poorly to diuretics.[28]

DIAGNOSIS

The first step in the diagnosis of HRS is demonstration of a reduced GFR, and this is not easy in advanced cirrhosis.[13,29] Muscle mass and, therefore, the release of creatinine is considerably reduced in these patients, and they can have a normal serum creatinine concentration despite having a very low GFR. Similarly, urea is synthesized by the liver, and urea synthesis may be reduced as a consequence of hepatic insufficiency. Therefore, failure to appropriately diagnose HRS is relatively common.[30,31]

The second step in the diagnosis of HRS is differentiation of this syndrome from other types of renal failure. In the setting of critical illness, differentiating HRS from other causes of renal insufficiency can be challenging.

In an effort to overcome both of these difficulties, the International Ascites Club proposed different diagnostic criteria of HRS.[32] Serum creatinine concentration should be greater than 1.5 mg/dL or creatinine clearance lower than 40 mL/min in the absence of other potential causes of renal failure (Table 117-1).

TABLE 117-1. MAJOR DIAGNOSTIC CRITERIA OF HEPATORENAL SYNDROME (INTERNATIONAL ASCITES CLUB)

Hepatic failure and portal hypertension
Creatinine >1.5 mg/dL or glomerular filtration rate < 40 mL/min
No shock, no ongoing bacterial infection, no nephrotoxic agents, no fluid losses
No improvement after diuretic withdrawal and IV saline infusion (1500 mL)
Proteinuria < 500 mg/day, normal renal echography

CLINICAL TYPES

HRS is classified into two types according to the severity and form of presentation of renal failure.[32] HRS type 1 is characterized by severe and rapidly progressive renal failure. It has been defined by doubling of the serum creatinine concentration to at least 2.5 mg/dL in less than 2 weeks. Although HRS type 1 may arise spontaneously, it frequently occurs in close relationship with a precipitating factor, such as severe bacterial infection, gastrointestinal hemorrhage, major surgical procedure, or acute hepatitis superimposed on cirrhosis. The association of HRS and spontaneous bacterial peritonitis has been carefully investigated.[33-35] HRS type 1 develops in approximately 30% of patients with spontaneous bacterial peritonitis despite rapid and successful treatment of the infection with non-nephrotoxic antibiotics. Patients with an intense systemic inflammatory response and high cytokine levels in plasma and ascitic fluid are especially prone to develop HRS type 1 after infection. Besides renal failure, patients with HRS type 1 after spontaneous bacterial peritonitis show signs and symptoms of severe liver failure (jaundice, coagulopathy, and hepatic encephalopathy) and circulatory dysfunction (arterial hypotension, very high plasma levels of renin, and norepinephrine) that worsen with the impairment in renal function. HRS type 1 is the complication of cirrhosis with the poorest prognosis. Median survival time after the onset of HRS is only 2 weeks.[2]

HRS type 2 is characterized by a moderate and steady decrease in renal function (serum creatinine less than 2.5 mg/dL). Patients with HRS type 2 show signs of liver failure and arterial hypotension but to a lesser degree than patients with HRS type 1. The dominant clinical feature is severe ascites with poor or no response to diuretics, a condition known as refractory ascites. Patients with HRS type 2 are especially predisposed to develop HRS type 1 after infections or other precipitating events.[33-35] The median survival of patients with HRS type 2 is 6 months, and it is worse than for patients with nonazotemic cirrhosis with ascites.[36]

TREATMENT

During the past decades, many vasoactive drugs (dopamine, fenoldopam, prostaglandins, misoprostol, saralasin, phentolamine, dazoxiben, norepinephrine, metaraminol, ocatpressin) have been evaluated as therapeutic agents to reverse HRS.[27] Unfortunately, none of these agents was shown to improve renal function. Therefore, HRS has been considered to be an intractable terminal complication of cirrhosis. However, in these studies, the drugs were given during only a few hours or days, and we now know that this is an insufficient duration of therapy to reverse HRS. Improvement of HRS after portosystemic shunt or liver transplantation does not occur until 1 week to 1 month after treatment. The same has been observed after the administration of volume expanders and vasoconstrictors.

The LeVeen shunt, introduced in 1974,[37] is another therapeutic modality that has yielded disappointing results in the treatment of HRS. For many years, the LeVeen shunt was considered to be an effective therapy for HRS. However, 15 years after its introduction, the LeVeen shunt was proved to be ineffective in HRS type 1.[38] In HRS type 2 with refractory ascites, it does not improve on the results obtained with therapeutic paracentesis.[39-40] The LeVeen shunt is associated with serious complications, such as superior vena cava thrombosis or intestinal obstruction, and a high rate of obstruction requiring reoperation. These features have led to the abandonment of this form of treatment.

Finally, the poor prognosis of patients with HRS has been traditionally considered to be caused by hepatic failure. Consequently, any improvement in renal function was expected to have little impact on survival. Treatment of renal failure in HRS, therefore, has not been taken as a real challenge to improve the natural history of the disease. The availability of liver transplantation has changed this perception. A small increase in survival may allow patients to obtain a transplant and to increase the 10-year probability of survival to 50%. The availability of hepatic transplantation, together with a better understanding of the pathogenesis of the syndrome, has stimulated clinical investigators to assess new treatment in HRS.

LIVER TRANSPLANTATION

Liver transplantation is the treatment of choice for HRS.[41-45] Immediately after transplantation, further impairment in GFR may be observed, and many patients require hemodialysis; 35% of patients with HRS compared with 5% of patients without HRS require renal replacement therapy.[41] Because cyclosporine or tacrolimus can contribute to impaired renal function, it has been suggested that administration of these drugs should be delayed until renal function begins to recover, usually 48 to 72 hours after transplantation. After the initial deterioration in renal function, GFR starts to improve and reaches an average of 30 to 40 mL/min by 1 to 2 months postoperatively. This level of moderate renal failure persists during follow-up and is more marked than is observed after hepatic transplantation in patients without HRS.[41] The hemodynamic and neurohormonal abnormalities associated with HRS disappear within the first month after the operation, and patients regain normal sodium and free water clearance.[46]

Patients with HRS who undergo transplantation have more complications, spend more days in the ICU, and have a higher in-hospital mortality rate than transplantation patients without HRS.[41-45] The long-term survival of patients with HRS after liver transplantation, however, is good. The 3-year probability of survival is 60%.[41-45] This survival rate is only slightly less than survival rate for liver transplant recipients without HRS (70% and 80%).[41,43]

Cirrhotic patients with HRS type 2 have a sufficiently prolonged predicted survival that they are not considered candidates for hepatic transplantation.

VOLUME EXPANSION AND VASOCONSTRICTORS

Treatment with arterial vasoconstrictors has only very recently been introduced as an approach for treating patients with HRS. This therapeutic strategy is based on clinical studies that showed that renal dysfunction in patients with cirrhosis is ameliorated when therapy is instituted with a combination of norepinephrine plus plasma volume expansion[47,48] or the short-term infusion of vasopressin.[49]

The first study showing that HRS can be reversed pharmacologically was performed by Guevara and coworkers.[50] These investigators assessed the hemodynamic, neurohormonal, and renal effects of combining intravenous albumin administration with a continuous infusion of ornipressin in 16 patients with HRS. Eight patients were treated for 3 days. Albumin was given at a dose of 1 g/kg on the first day and 20 to 60 g/day for the next 2 days. Ornipressin was given as an intravenous stepped dose infusion of 2 to 6 IU/h. Plasma levels of renin and norepinephrine normalized, indicating a marked improvement in circulatory function. However, only a slight increase in GFR (from 15 ± 4 mL/min to 24 ± 4 mL/min) was observed. The remaining 8 patients were treated for 15 days. Ornipressin was given at a dose of 2 IU/h. Albumin was given at a dose of 1 g/kg during the first day. The amount of albumin during the following days was adjusted according to plasma renin activity. In 4 patients, treatment was stopped after 4 and 9 days because of ischemic complications in three cases and bacteremia in one case. In these 4 patients, serum creatinine decreased substantially during therapy. Moreover, renal function deteriorated again after treatment was withdrawn. The course of treatment was completed in the remaining 4 patients. In these patients, mean arterial pressure increased significantly, plasma renin activity normalized, plasma norepinephrine concentration decreased, GFR increased, and serum creatinine concentration returned to normal. These 4 patients died 12, 60, 62, and 133 days after treatment; HRS did not recur in any of them during follow-up.

In a subsequent study, the same group treated 9 patients with HRS (6 with HRS type 1 and 3 with HRS type 2) with terlipressin (0.5 to 2 mg/4 h, i.v.) and intravenous albumin over 5 to 15 days.[51] Reversal of HRS (normalization of serum creatinine) was observed in 7 patients. No case developed ischemic complications. HRS did not recur in any patient. Five patients were transplant candidates, and 3 underwent transplant 5, 12, and 99 days after treatment. The 2 other patients died 30 and 121 days after the study. The remaining 4 patients died 13 to 102 days after treatment. In both studies, dilutional hyponatremia was corrected along with normalization of serum creatinine concentration. The results obtained in this group of 17 patients treated with ornipressin and terlipressin and intravenous albumin for more than 3 days are summarized in Table 117-2.

Other groups have confirmed these observations. Gülberg and colleagues[52] treated 7 patients with HRS type 1 with ornipressin (6 IU/h), dopamine (2 to 3 μg/kg/min), and intravenous albumin.[52] HRS was reversed in 4 patients after 5 to 27 days of treatment. In 1 patient, treatment had to be stopped because of intestinal ischemia. The remaining 2 patients did not respond. In 2 of the 4 patients responding to treatment, HRS recurred 2 and 8 months later, and they were re-treated. HRS was reversed in 1 patient. In the other patient, treatment had to be stopped because of ventricular tachyarrhythmia. In total, 2 patients reached liver transplantation and 1 patient was alive 1 year after inclusion after two successful treatments.

Mulkay and coworkers[53] treated 12 patients with HRS type 1 with terlipressin (2 mg q8-12h) and albumin infusion (0.5 to 1 g/kg day during 5 days) for 1 to 9 weeks. HRS was reverted in 7 patients. In the remaining five cases, serum creatinine concentration also decreased, but not to normal. Terlipressin was stopped in 6 patients without recurrence of HRS. No patient developed complications related to the treatment. Three patients underwent transplant 34, 36, and 111 days after being studied. The remaining patients died after a median survival time of 42 days.

Catecholamines are also effective for the treatment of HRS. Angeli and associates[54] used oral midodrine, an alpha-adrenergic agonist, intravenous albumin, and subcutaneous octreotride (to suppress glucagon) in 5 patients with HRS type 1. Midodrine dosage was adjusted to increase the mean arterial pressure by greater than 15 mm Hg. Patients received treatment for at least 20 days in hospital and subsequently continued treatment at home. In all cases, there was a dramatic improvement in renal perfusion, GFR, blood urea nitrogen concentration, serum creatinine concentration, and serum sodium concentration. Plasma levels of renin, aldosterone, and antidiuretic hormone decreased to normal or near-normal levels. Two patients were transplanted 20 and 64 days after enrollment while on therapy. One patient, who was not a candidate for liver transplantation, was alive without treatment 472 days after being discharged from the hospital. The remaining 2 patients died 29 and 75 days after enrollment. These results were compared with those obtained in 8 patients with HRS type 1 treated with intravenous albumin plus dopamine (2 to 4 μg/kg/min). In these 8 patients, a progressive worsening in renal function was observed. One patient underwent transplant but died 15 days later of a fungal infection. The remaining 7 patients died within 2 weeks after the initiation of treatment.

Duvoux and coworkers[55] treated 12 patients with HRS type 1 with intravenous albumin (to maintain central venous pressure over 7 mm Hg) and norepinephrine (0.5 to 3 mg/h) for a minimum of 5 days. A significant improvement in serum creatinine in association with a marked suppression of plasma renin activity was observed in 10 patients. Transient myocardial ischemia was observed in 1 patient. Three patients underwent transplantation, and 3 were still alive after 8 months of follow-up.

Finally, Ginès and colleagues[56] sought to determine whether albumin is necessary in the treatment of HRS

TABLE 117–2. EFFECT OF VASOCONSTRICTORS (ORNIPRESSIN AND TERLIPRESSIN) AND VOLUME EXPANSION IN HEPATORENAL SYNDROME

	Baseline (n = 15)	Day 3 (n = 12)	Day 7 (n = 9)	Day 14 (n = 7)
MAP (mm Hg)	70 ± 8	70 ± 8	77 ± 9	79 ± 12
PRA (ng/mL/h)	15 ± 15	4 ± 2	2 ± 3	1 ± 1
NE (pg/mL)	1257 ± 938	550 ± 382	550 ± 410	316 ± 161
Creatinine (mg/dL)	3 ± 1	3 ± 1	2 ± 1	1 ± 1

MAP, mean arterial pressure; NE, norepinephrine; PRA, plasma renin activity.
Normal values: PRA < 1.4 ng/mL/h, NE < 260 pg/mL; $P < .001$ for all values (analysis of variance).
Data from references 25 and 51.

with vasoconstrictors. Twenty-one patients with HRS were studied. The first 13 were treated with terlipressin (0.5 to 2 mg/4 h) and albumin (1 g/kg the first day; 20 to 40 g/day thereafter). The last 8 patients received terlipressin alone. Treatment was given until normalization of serum creatinine or for a maximum of 15 days. In patients treated with terlipressin plus albumin there was a significant increase in mean arterial pressure, a marked suppression of plasma renin activity, and a decrease in serum creatinine concentration. In contrast, no significant changes in these parameters were observed in patients treated with terlipressin alone. A complete response (normalization of serum creatinine concentration) was achieved in 10 patients treated with terlipressin plus albumin and in only 2 treated without albumin. HRS recurred in only 2 patients. One-month survival without transplantation was 87% in patients receiving terlipressin plus albumin and 13% in patients receiving terlipressin alone.

These studies show (1) HRS type 1 is reversible after treatment with intravenous albumin and vasoconstrictors; (2) both components of the treatment are important because HRS does not reverse when vasoconstrictors or plasma volume expanders are given alone; (3) the constant infusion of vasoconstrictors (ornipressin or norepinephrine) is associated with ischemic complications (a feature not observed when they are given intermittently); (4) there is a delay of several days between the improvement in circulatory function and the increase in GFR; and (5) reversal of HRS improves survival and a significant number of patients live long enough to obtain liver transplantation.

TRANSJUGULAR INTRAHEPATIC PORTOSYSTEMIC SHUNT

Because portal hypertension is the initial abnormality with regard to circulatory dysfunction in cirrhosis, decreasing of portal pressure by portosystemic anastomosis is a rational approach for the treatment of HRS. There are several case reports showing reversal of HRS after surgical portosystemic shunt.[57,58] However, major surgical procedures in patients with HRS are not likely to be tolerated. The development of transjugular intrahepatic portosystemic shunt (TIPS) has reintroduced the idea of treating HRS by reducing portal pressure.

Four studies assessing TIPS in the management of HRS type 1 have been reported[59-62] and reviewed by Brensing and coworkers.[63] In total, 30 patients were treated. In two series no liver transplantation was performed, whereas in the other two series 3 of 9 patients underwent transplant 7, 13, and 35 days after TIPS. TIPS insertion was technically successful in all patients. One patient died as a consequence of the procedure. GFR improved markedly within 1 to 4 weeks after TIPS and stabilized thereafter. In one study specifically investigating the neurohormonal systems, improvement in GFR and serum creatinine concentration was related to a marked suppression of the plasma levels of renin and antidiuretic hormone.[60] Follow-up data concerning hepatic function were obtained from 21 patients. De novo hepatic encephalopathy or deterioration of preexisting hepatic encephalopathy occurred in 9 patients, but in 5 encephalopathy could be controlled with lactulose. Survival rates based on the 27 patients without early liver transplantation at 1 month, 3 months, and 6 months were 81%, 59%, and 44%, respectively. These studies strongly suggest that TIPS is useful in the management of HRS type 1. Studies comparing TIPS with pharmacologic treatment in HRS type 1 are needed.

OTHER THERAPEUTIC METHODS

Hemodialysis and arteriovenous or venovenous hemofiltration are frequently used in patients with HRS, but the efficacy of these methods has not been adequately assessed.[64] Recently, extracorporeal albumin dialysis, a system that uses an albumin-containing dialysate that is recirculated and perfused through charcoal and anion-exchanger columns, has been shown to improve systemic hemodynamics and reduce plasma levels of renin in patients with HRS type 1.[65,66] In a small series of patients, improved survival was reported.[65] Further studies are needed to confirm these findings.

PREVENTION

Two randomized controlled studies enrolling large series of patients have shown that HRS can be prevented in specific clinical settings. In the first study,[67] the administration of albumin (1.5 g/kg IV at infection diagnosis and 1 g/kg IV 48 hours later) together with cefotaxime in patients with cirrhosis and spontaneous bacterial peritonitis markedly reduced the incidence of impaired circulatory function and the occurrence of HRS type 1 compared with a control group of patients receiving cefotaxime alone (10% incidence of HRS in patients receiving albumin vs. 33% in the control group). Moreover, the hospital mortality rate (10% vs. 29%) and the 3-month mortality rate (22% vs. 41%) were lower in patients receiving albumin plus antibiotics versus antibiotics alone. In a second study,[68] the administration of the tumor necrosis factor synthesis inhibitor pentoxifylline (400 mg tid), to patients with severe acute alcoholic hepatitis reduced the occurrence of HRS (8% in the pentoxifylline group vs. 35% in the placebo group) and hospital mortality (24% vs. 46%, respectively). Because bacterial infections and acute alcoholic hepatitis are two important precipitating factors of HRS type 1, these prophylactic measures may decrease the incidence of this complication.

CONCLUSION

HRS is a major clinical event during the course of decompensated cirrhosis. Although the most characteristic feature of the syndrome is functional renal failure caused by intense renal vasoconstriction, it is a more generalized process affecting the whole body. There are two types of HRS. Type 1 is characterized by rapid and progressive deterioration of circulatory and renal function. It usually develops in close chronologic relationship with a precipitating event, particularly severe bacterial infection; acute alcoholic, toxic, or viral hepatitis; or major surgical procedures. HRS type 1 carries a very poor prognosis (median survival rate < 2 weeks). HRS type 2 is characterized by steady deterioration of circulatory and renal function. Patients with HRS type 2 have a median survival of 6 months, and their main clinical problem is refractory ascites. The pathogenesis of HRS is decreased effective arterial blood volume because of splanchnic arterial vasodilatation and reduced venous return and cardiac output. The syndrome can be reversed by the simultaneous administration of intravenous albumin and arterial vasoconstrictors. Intrarenal mechanisms are also important and require a prolonged improvement in circulatory function to be deactivated. Systemic vasoconstriction, increased intrahepatic vascular resistance and portal pressure, and impaired hepatic function are other components of the syndrome. Long-term administration of intravenous albumin and vasoconstrictors and correction of portal hypertension with TIPS are effective treatments for HRS. These approaches improve survival and may serve as a bridge to liver transplantation, which is the ultimate treatment of choice in these patients.

ANNOTATED REFERENCES

Arroyo V, Ginés P, Gerbes A, et al: Definition and diagnostic criteria of refractory ascites and hepatorenal syndrome in cirrhosis. Hepatology 1996; 23:164-176.

This paper resulted from a large consensus conference that ended the confusion surrounding the definition of hepatorenal syndrome and providing a rationale basis for comparing different therapeutic approaches and performing meta-analysis.

Ginés P, Arroyo V, Vargas V, et al: Paracentesis with intravenous infusion of albumin as compared with peritoneovenous shunting in cirrhosis with refractory ascites. N Engl J Med 1991;325:829-835.

This prospective, randomized, controlled trial is the continuation of several investigations initiated by Quintero and Ginès in the 1980s showing that paracentesis is a rapid, effective and safe therapy for ascites, provided the plasma volume is expanded with albumin. In addition, the authors concluded that this therapeutic procedure is the treatment of choice in patients with tense ascites to replace peritoneovenous shunting treatment, nowadays abandoned.

Ginés A, Escorsell A, Ginés P, et al: Incidence, predictive factors, and prognosis of hepatorenal syndrome in cirrhosis. Gastroenterology 1993;105:229-236.

This retrospective study established the natural history of type 1 hepatorenal syndrome and provided epidemiologic and prognostic data to compare with and to design future prospective studies.

Guevara M, Gines P, Fernandez-Esparrach G, et al: Reversibility of hepatorenal syndrome by prolonged administration of ornipressin and plasma volume expansion. Hepatology 1998;27:35-41.

This paper followed the first investigation by the same authors introducing the pharmacologic treatment of hepatorenal syndrome by using systemic vasoconstrictors and plasma volume expansion, the most promising approach to the medical treatment of this syndrome.

Sort P, Navasa M, Arroyo V, et al: Effect of plasma volume expansion on renal impairment and mortality in patients with cirrhosis and spontaneous bacterial peritonitis. N Engl J Med 1999;341:403-409.

This important prospective, randomized, controlled trial showed that preventing renal impairment in spontaneous bacterial peritonitis resulted in an improvement in survival in those patients; and that this prevention was achieved by the administration of albumin to cause plasma volume expansion. The paper emphasizes the critical importance of improving renal perfusion in circumstances known to deteriorate it and to cause hepatorenal syndrome.

Chapter 118

HEPATOPULMONARY SYNDROME

Isabelle Michaud • David Kaufman

KEY POINTS

1. **Hepatopulmonary syndrome (HPS)** is defined as the association of liver dysfunction, intrapulmonary vascular dilatations, and gas exchange abnormalities. **Its clinical manifestations are nonspecific, and its natural history is unknown.**

2. The **exact mechanism leading to the pulmonary vasodilatation seen in HPS** is unclear, but inducible nitric oxide synthase (iNOS), endothelin-1, and heme oxygenase-1 have all been implicated in the pathophysiology.

3. The **differential diagnosis of HPS** includes other causes of hypoxia seen in end-stage liver disease, such as congestive heart failure, ascites, underlying lung disease, atelectasis, pleural effusions, and portopulmonary syndrome. This latter condition is characterized by elevated mean pulmonary artery pressures, as opposed to HPS in which the pulmonary artery pressure is normal to low.

4. **The diagnosis of HPS** is usually confirmed with the demonstration of an intrapulmonary shunt, either by lung perfusion scanning using technetium-Tc99 macroaggregated albumin or by contrast-enhanced echocardiography.

5. **Liver transplantation remains the only currently available treatment for HPS** and should be considered in symptomatic hypoxic patients. Promising results have been shown with the use of antimicrobial agents, but further studies are needed to confirm their possible benefit.

DEFINITION

Hepatopulmonary syndrome (HPS) is characterized by the presence of liver dysfunction, intrapulmonary vascular dilatation (IPVD), and gas exchange abnormalities, varying from increased alveolar-arterial oxygen gradient to severe hypoxia not explained by underlying cardiopulmonary disease.[1] This syndrome usually occurs with cirrhosis but also has been described with noncirrhotic portal hypertension. The clinical manifestations are nonspecific and include dyspnea, platypnea, orthodeoxia, clubbing, cyanosis, and spider nevi.[2]

INCIDENCE

Almost half of liver transplantation candidates have gas exchange abnormalities.[3] Hypoxemia secondary to HPS is present in 13% to 15% of patients with end-stage liver disease.[4] The natural history of HPS is unknown, but its association with increased morbidity and mortality seems to be due to worsening gas exchange over time.

PATHOPHYSIOLOGY

The exact mechanism leading to pulmonary vasodilation is still unclear. An imbalance in the expression of pulmonary vasodilating and vasoconstricting factors has been implicated in the pathogenesis of this phenomenon. Studies have reported that exhaled nitric oxide (NO) levels are increased in cirrhotic patients but return to normal after liver transplantation.[5] Nitric oxide is thought to be responsible for the vasodilatation and the blunted hypoxic pulmonary vasoconstriction seen in HPS.

In animal models of HPS there is increased expression of the enzyme inducible NO synthase (iNOS) in the pulmonary vasculature, possibly triggered by translocation of gut bacteria.[6] Increased activity of another enzyme that catalyzes the formation of NO, endothelial NO synthase (eNOS), is also implicated in the pathogenesis of HPS. Activation of eNOS might be mediated by increased circulating endothelin-1 levels seen in liver injury as well as increased expression of endothelin-B receptors in the lung vasculature noted in portal hypertension.[7] NO might not be the only factor implicated in pulmonary vasodilation. One study showed that expression of the enzyme heme oxygenase-1 (HO-1) is up-regulated in animals with HPS.[8] HO-1 catalyzes the oxidative degradation of heme to biliverdin, releasing carbon monoxide, a gaseous molecule that can cause pulmonary vasodilation.

It is important to differentiate HPS from portopulmonary syndrome (PPS). The latter is defined by a mean pulmonary artery pressure that is increased to greater than 25 mm Hg with increased pulmonary vascular resistance and normal or slightly elevated cardiac output.[9] HPS, in contrast, presents as normal to low pulmonary artery pressure, low pulmonary vascular resistance, and high cardiac output. These two entities are both part of the spectrum of vascular disorders seen in liver disease.

PATHOLOGY

The typical feature of HPS is the formation of IPVD manifested by dilation of precapillary and capillary vessels.

These lesions predominate at the bases of the lungs. Discrete arteriovenous communications can also be present, as well as peripheral pleural-based vascular spider angiomas.[2]

DIAGNOSTIC DILEMMAS

HPS must be differentiated from other causes of hypoxia in patients with end-stage liver disease. These include underlying lung diseases such as chronic obstructive pulmonary disease or pneumonia, congestive heart failure, massive ascites with associated atelectasis, or pleural effusion. Once these diagnoses are ruled out, HPS can be diagnosed by demonstrating abnormal oxygenation and the presence of an intrapulmonary shunt.

The arterial blood gas analysis typically shows decreased PaO_2 on room air in the standing position. PaO_2 may not improve when the inspired gas is switched to 100% oxygen. Pulmonary function tests reveal decreased diffusion capacity (DL_{CO}) in the majority of patients with HPS. However, this measure does not correlate with the severity of hepatic dysfunction.[3]

The demonstration of an intrapulmonary shunt can be made by a radionuclide lung perfusion scan using technetium-Tc99 macroaggregated albumin. In the presence of a cardiac or pulmonary shunt, the isotope is not trapped in the lung as it would normally be but is also taken up by the brain, liver, and kidneys. The disadvantage of this test is that it cannot distinguish between an intracardiac and an intrapulmonary shunt. This distinction can be made, however, using contrast-enhanced echocardiography. By using agitated normal saline injected into a peripheral vein, IPVD can be demonstrated when the microbubbles injected are visualized in the left atrium within three to six cardiac cycles after leaving the right heart chambers.

Pulmonary angiography may help differentiate between two patterns of IPVD: type I, the diffuse form, and type II, the focal form. This information may be useful because type II may improve after local embolization.[10]

MEDICAL MANAGEMENT

Many therapeutic agents have been tried in HPS, including methylene blue, indomethacin, octreotide, and garlic powder, but none has been clearly or consistently effective. Use of antimicrobial agents has shown interesting results[6] but needs validation by data from further studies. The rationale behind this therapy is that decreasing intestinal bacterial growth with antibiotics decreases the amount of endotoxin released in the bloodstream, leading to a reduction in iNOS-dependent NO production and vascular dilatation.[11] The use of a transjugular intrahepatic portosystemic shunt has

been described in a few case reports but is still considered experimental.[12]

TRANSPLANTATION

Symptomatic HPS is now recognized by the United Network for Organs Sharing as an indication for liver transplantation. Several reports have shown that liver transplantation can be performed safely in patients with significant hypoxia. Over 80% of patients have resolution or marked improvement in IPVD, although time to resolution of HPS is quite variable and may take more than a year.[13] The degree of preoperative hypoxia is not predictive of reversibility.[14]

Mortality after liver transplantation is higher in patients with HPS compared with patients without. Reported complications are pulmonary hypertension, cerebral embolic hemorrhages, and prolonged mechanical ventilation. In a recent prospective study, PaO_2 less than 50 mm Hg and an intrapulmonary shunt fraction equal to 20% were identified as predictors of post-transplantation mortality.[15] Despite these findings, liver transplantation remains the only currently available treatment for HPS and should be considered in patients with HPS having PaO_2 less than 60 mm Hg.

ANNOTATED REFERENCES

Arguedas MR, Abrams GA, Krowka MJ, Fallon MB: Prospective evaluation of outcomes and predictors of mortality in patients with hepatopulmonary syndrome undergoing liver transplantation. Hepatology 2003;37:192-197.
This study found that patients undergoing a liver transplantation for HPS had an increased mortality, particularly with more severe preoperative hypoxemia and significant intrapulmonary shunting.

Fallon MB, Abrams GA: Pulmonary dysfunction in chronic liver disease. Hepatology 2000;32:859-865.
This review article proposes a diagnostic algorithm aimed at facilitating the recognition of HPS in cirrhotic patients with pulmonary dysfunction.

Krowka MJ, Cortese DA: Hepatopulmonary syndrome: Current concepts in diagnosis and therapeutic considerations. Chest 1994;105:1528-1537.
This review article presents a detailed overview of HPS, from its clinical features to pathophysiology, diagnostic modalities, and therapeutic approaches.

Krowka MJ, Tajik AJ, Dickson ER, et al: Intrapulmonary vascular dilatations (IPVD) in liver transplant candidates: Screening by two-dimensional contrast-enhanced echocardiography. Chest 1990;97:1165-1170.
This prospective observational study screened 40 consecutive liver transplant candidates to determine the relationship between contrast-enhanced echocardiogram, arterial blood gases, and pulmonary function tests. Intrapulmonary vascular dilatations were found in 13.2% of patients, including some patients who were not hypoxemic.

Rabiller A, Nunes H, Lebrec D, et al: Prevention of gram-negative translocation reduces the severity of hepatopulmonary syndrome. Am J Respir Crit Care Med 2002;166:514-517.
This animal study showed that prophylactic norfloxacin given to cirrhotic rats reduced the severity of HPS by decreasing the incidence of gram-negative translocation and normalizing the activity and expression of lung-inducible nitric oxide synthase.

Chapter 119

HEPATIC ENCEPHALOPATHY

Gregory T. Everson

KEY POINTS

1. The spectrum of hepatic encephalopathy includes personality changes, impaired mental function, motor abnormalities (asterixis, tremor, hyperventilation, hyperactive reflexes), and altered consciousness.

2. Patients with chronic hepatic encephalopathy often have abnormal motor function, manifested as tremor, slowness of gait, ataxia, and even rigidity.

3. Several lines of investigation focus on ammonia as a key factor in the pathogenesis of hepatic encephalopathy. The ammonia (NH_3) hypothesis states that the major mechanism of hepatic encephalopathy is excessive accumulation of NH_3, which induces both neuronal metabolic derangements and also promotes astrocyte swelling.

4. Paradoxically, increased cerebral blood flow can aggravate cerebral edema and worsen neurological damage.

5. Of approximately 2000 cases of acute liver failure in the United States annually, the most common causes are acetaminophen toxicity, other forms of drug toxicity, hepatitis B, and hepatitis A. However, the second leading diagnostic category for fulminant hepatic failure is cryptogenic, cause unknown.

6. Infection is a leading comorbidity in patients with acute liver failure. Fever is not a feature in most cases of acute liver injury and, if present, usually signifies intercurrent infection.

7. One of the most common factors precipitating encephalopathy is noncompliance with prescribed out-patient medical treatment: low protein diet, lactulose, and neomycin.

Hepatic encephalopathy encompasses a spectrum of neuropsychiatric abnormalities that occur in patients with liver disease in the absence of other brain disease.[1,2] The spectrum includes personality changes, impaired mental function, motor abnormalities (asterixis, tremor, hyperventilation, hyperactive reflexes), and altered consciousness. A consensus panel of experts proposed classification of hepatic encephalopathy into type A, associated with acute liver failure; type B, associated with portal-systemic bypass without intrinsic liver disease; and type C, associated with chronic liver disease.[3]

The encephalopathy accompanying acute hepatic failure is commonly associated with cerebral edema and increased intracranial pressure, exhibits abrupt onset with a short prodrome and rapid progression, and often ends with the death of the patient.[4-6] Patients sequentially experience drowsiness, delirium, agitation or convulsions, decerebrate rigidity, unresponsiveness, and deep coma within a comparatively short period of time, usually hours to days. Irreversible neurologic damage may occur as a result of brain ischemia or herniation. Patients who develop coma in the setting of acute liver failure have a grave prognosis; less than 20% survive without hepatic transplantation.

In patients with chronic liver disease, encephalopathy develops insidiously and is often heralded by a change in mental or behavioral status. Encephalopathy may be episodic, persistent, or minimal and subclinical.[3] Episodes are sporadic, characterized by exacerbations and remissions, and are generally precipitated by inciting events.[1,2] Although the initial manifestation of portosystemic encephalopathy is usually a subtle change in mentation, the neurologic dysfunction may progress and be classified according to confusion, lethargy, and even coma (Table 119-1).[7] Neurologic signs vary and fluctuate but usually include asterixis, hyperreflexia, clonus, and extensor plantar response. Causes of chronic portosystemic encephalopathy may not always be apparent, but azotemia, sepsis, gastrointestinal bleeding, dehydration, electrolyte imbalance, and sedatives are frequent precipitants (Table 119-2). In some patients, chronic encephalopathy may not be clinically obvious but detectable only by psychometric testing. By these tests, about two thirds of cirrhotic patients with portal hypertension have unsuspected subclinical hepatic encephalopathy.[8-10]

PATHOGENESIS AND MECHANISMS OF ENCEPHALOPATHY

GENERAL PRINCIPLES

No single abnormality of hepatic or neurologic metabolism adequately explains all of the clinical, biochemical, physiologic or experimental findings of encephalopathy occurring in either patients or animal models.[1,2,6] Abnormalities of multiple neurotransmitters, including glutamate, gamma-aminobutyric acid (GABA), dopamine, serotonin, and opioids, have been described and plasma levels of a wide array of potential neurotoxins (ammonia, GABA, short-chain fatty acids, methanethiols) are increased (Table 119-3). Despite this seeming confusion, several lines of investigation focus on ammonia as a key factor in the pathogenesis of hepatic encephalopathy. Ammonia accumulation deranges glutamate and glutamine metabolism in the central nervous system (CNS) and alters the metabolism of GABA and its function

TABLE 119–1. STAGES OF ENCEPHALOPATHY IN CHRONIC LIVER DISEASE

Stage	Clinical Signs
Stage I	Mental slowness, euphoria or anxiety, shortened attention span, impaired calculating ability
Stage II	Lethargy or apathy, inappropriate behavior, personality change, more obvious problems with calculations
Stage III	Lethargic, somnolent, marked confusion and disorientation, but responds to verbal stimuli
Stage IV	Coma, patient may or may not respond to noxious stimuli

Patients with chronic liver disease rarely, if ever, demonstrate cerebral edema, regardless of the stage of encephalopathy.

TABLE 119–3. BRAIN NEUROTOXINS OR NEUROINHIBITORS THAT ACCUMULATE IN HEPATIC FAILURE

Ammonia
Manganese
Glutamine
GABA
Taurine
Benzodiazepine receptor ligands
Monoamines
Opioids
Methanethiols

as an inhibitory neurotransmitter. In addition, benzodiazepine receptors in the CNS are physically linked to GABA receptors. The latter finding provides an explanation for the increased sensitivity of patients with liver disease to the sedative and hypnotic effects of benzodiazepines and a rationale for use of benzodiazepine antagonists in the treatment of portosystemic encephalopathy. Hepatic encephalopathy, occurring in the setting of either acute liver failure or chronic liver disease, is also associated with marked changes in CNS glial cells on neuropathologic examination. Encephalopathy of acute liver failure is characterized by astrocytic swelling, but chronic encephalopathy is characterized by Alzheimer type II astrocytosis.

CEREBRAL BLOOD FLOW

In situations of acute liver failure, the brain is potentially subject to hypoxic injury due to complications, such as systemic arterial hypotension, respiratory failure, and reduction in cerebral blood flow, that commonly accompany cerebral edema and intracranial hypertension. Therapy is often directed at maintaining adequate arterial oxygenation (SaO_2 >90%), adequate cerebral perfusion pressure (>40 mm Hg), and optimal intracranial pressure (<20 mm Hg).[4,11] Paradoxically, increased cerebral blood flow can aggravate cerebral edema and worsen neurologic damage. In humans with acute liver failure, cerebral blood flow has been measured primarily using the 133-xenon wash-out technique.[12-15] These data suggest that cerebral blood flow is initially relatively low, but then increases with increasing blood concentration of ammonia, which decreases cerebral arteriolar tone.

TABLE 119–2. CLINICAL EVENTS PRECIPITATING HEPATIC ENCEPHALOPATHY IN CIRRHOTIC PATIENTS

Gastrointestinal hemorrhage
Infection
Spontaneous bacterial peritonitis
Pneumonia
Sepsis
Dehydration
Imbalance of electrolytes or acid-base
Renal failure
Drugs, toxins, medications
Illicit substances
Alcohol
Sedatives, hypnotics
Narcotics
Dietary indiscretion (excessive protein intake)

CEREBRAL GLUCOSE AND OXYGEN METABOLISM

Brain energy metabolism is unique in that glucose is the only substrate under normal physiologic conditions and its uptake and utilization by the brain is independent of insulin.[16-20] Under stress, the brain can utilize beta-hydroxybutyrate and acetoacetate. Ammonia accumulation during hepatic failure in humans or in experimental models of hyperammonemia is associated with altered cerebral glucose metabolism. In early acute liver failure, prior to the onset of intracranial hypertension, cerebral glucose metabolism and cerebral oxygen consumption are proportionately diminished.[16] There is no evidence of cerebral hypoxia, implying that the reduced glucose and oxygen utilization reflect diminished metabolic demand by the brain at this early stage. Cerebral lactate uptake is increased despite sufficient glucose delivery and preserved oxidative metabolism. Acute short-term mechanical ventilation, resulting in a moderate reduction in PCO_2 and cerebral blood flow, does not adversely affect oxidative brain metabolism. Thus, prior to development of intracranial hypertension, cerebral glucose and oxygen metabolism are reduced, but these changes are consistent with normal aerobic metabolism and physiologic regulation. After development of intracranial hypertension, oxygen metabolism remains reduced but measurements of cerebral glucose utilization vary from reduced to normal to increased, and glycolysis may be accelerated.[17,18,20] These findings suggest that progression of acute liver failure and development of intracranial hypertension is associated with relative cerebral hypoxia and switch to anaerobic metabolism.

AMMONIA HYPOTHESIS

The ammonia (NH_3) hypothesis states that the major mechanism of hepatic encephalopathy is excessive accumulation of NH_3, which induces neuronal metabolic derangements and also promotes astrocyte swelling.[21] In addition, NH_3 perturbs cerebral nitric oxide metabolism, which can mediate some of the pathophysiologic changes associated with hyperammonemia.[22] Studies using positron emission tomography and magnetic resonance spectroscopy have demonstrated that hepatic encephalopathy is associated with increased cerebral metabolic rate and increased permeability of the blood-brain barrier for NH_3.[23-29] Blood NH_3 originates mainly from four sources: intrahepatic deamination of amino acids, extrahepatic metabolism of nucleotides, gut metabolism of glutamine, and bacterial degradation of intestinal protein and urea.[30] More than 50% of blood ammonia is derived from bacterial degradation of protein.

NH_3 is normally metabolized by the liver to either urea or glutamine by the actions of carbamoyl-phosphate synthetase I (initiating enzyme of the urea cycle) and glutamine synthetase, respectively. Patients with hepatic failure have impaired NH_3 metabolism related to a reduction in liver metabolism and an increase in portal-systemic shunting. As a result, elevated blood NH_3 concentration is a characteristic feature of severely impaired hepatic function.

Certain clinical and experimental observations link the increase in blood NH_3 level to hepatic encephalopathy.[31-34] Hyperammonemia and elevated concentrations of NH_3 in the cerebrospinal fluid are features of acute and chronic hepatic encephalopathy, Reye's syndrome, deficiencies of urea cycle enzymes, and sodium valproate toxicity. In cirrhotic patients or patients with portacaval shunts, ingestion of NH_3-generating substances (i.e., proteins, amino acids, urea, ammonium salts) may precipitate encephalopathy. In animal models, chronic administration of ammonium salts results in Alzheimer type II astrocytosis, a change that is indistinguishable from that observed in patients with chronic hepatic encephalopathy.[31]

GLUTAMINE—GLUTAMATERGIC NEUROTRANSMITTER SYSTEM

The glutamatergic excitatory neurotransmitter system in the CNS is markedly altered in patients with both acute and chronic liver disease and in animal models of hepatic encephalopathy.[6,21,22] CNS astrocytes are a major regulatory cell in the glutamatergic system.[31] Normally, astrocytes avidly take up excess glutamate from the synaptic cleft (against a 3000- to 10,000-fold concentration gradient), an important function that terminates glutamate-induced neuroexcitation. Once glutamate is taken up by the astrocyte, it is metabolized to glutamine via the action of glutamine synthetase, which utilizes blood-derived NH_3 (Fig. 119-1). The hyperammonemia of liver failure favors the formation of glutamine but also impairs the release of glutamine from astrocytes. The accumulation of osmotically active glutamine in astrocytes is associated with cell swelling. Normally, glutamine is actively extruded from astrocytes and then taken up by presynaptic nerve terminals for conversion back to glutamate and subsequent utilization in neurotransmission. Under the conditions of liver failure and hyperammonemia, glutamate uptake into neurons and astrocytes is diminished and glutamate accumulates in the extracellular fluid. Clinically, levels of glutamine and glutamate increase in cerebrospinal fluid during hyperammonemic states, and cerebrospinal fluid concentrations of glutamine correlate loosely with the stage of encephalopathy. In animal models of acute encephalopathy, blockade of glutamine production by an inhibitor of glutamine synthetase, methionine sulfoximine, decreases cerebral edema and reduces astrocyte swelling. Production of NH_3 from the intestine is reduced by oral neomycin and nonabsorbable disaccharides, including lactulose, lactitol, or lactose (in lactase-deficient patients). These treatments lower plasma NH_3 concentration and improve subjective and objective measures of encephalopathy.

Other clinical and experimental observations refute the link between NH_3 and hepatic encephalopathy. Blood levels of NH_3 are elevated in cirrhotic patients, regardless of the presence or absence of encephalopathy. Furthermore, some patients with hepatic encephalopathy have normal blood levels of NH_3, and the grade of hepatic encephalopathy does

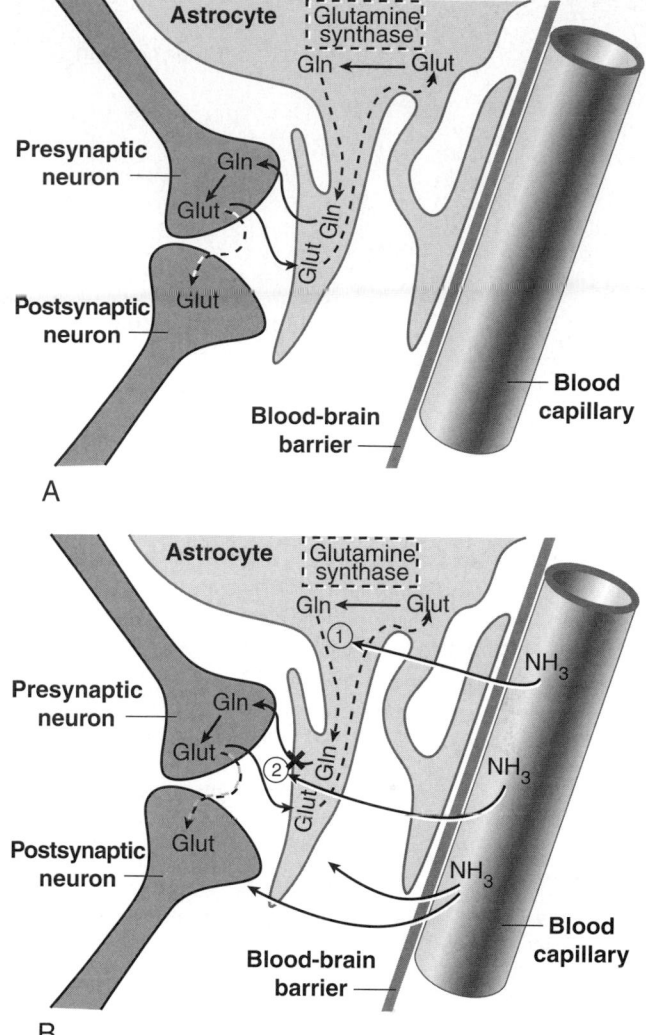

FIGURE 119–1. *A,* The formation of glutamine occurs predominantly in the astrocyte. Glutamine is pumped out of the astrocyte and taken up by presynaptic neurons, where it is converted to glutamate. Nerve stimulation releases glutamate from the presynaptic neuron to serve as an excitatory neurotransmitter. Astrocytes avidly take up glutamate from the synaptic cleft to abolish neuronal stimulation. *B,* Ammonia freely diffuses across the blood-brain barrier and stimulates formation of glutamine by the astrocyte via the action of glutamine synthase (1). Ammonia also blocks the export of glutamine from the astrocyte at the synaptic cleft (2). The net effect of these two actions is increased concentration of glutamine within astrocytes, which promotes astrocyte swelling.

not correlate with the blood concentration of NH_3. Seizures and hyperexcitability are commonly observed in animal models of NH_3 intoxication and in human congenital hyperammonemias but are rarely observed in patients with chronic hepatic encephalopathy. Administration of ammonium chloride to cirrhotic patients induces mild hyperkinesis but fails to exacerbate the typical symptoms of chronic encephalopathy.

GAMMA-AMINOBUTYRIC ACID-BENZODIAZEPINE RECEPTOR HYPOTHESIS

GABA is an inhibitory neurotransmitter that is found throughout the CNS.[35] The GABA hypothesis states that an excess of GABA or increased sensitivity to GABA is

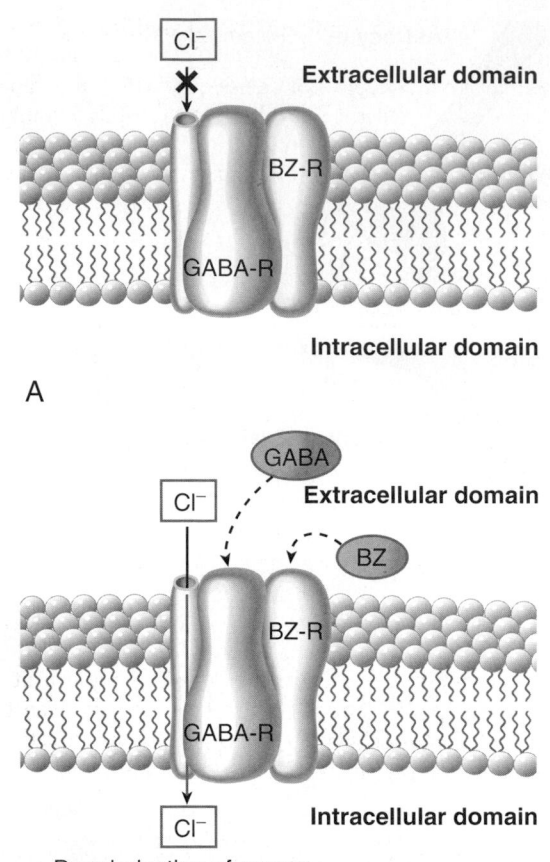

FIGURE 119–2. *A*, The GABA receptor complex is composed of the GABA receptor (GABA-R), central benzodiazepine receptor (BZ-R), and chloride channel (adjacent cylinder). *B*, Binding of GABA to GABA-R opens the chloride channel, hyperpolarizes the neuronal membrane, and inhibits neurotransmission. Activation of the BZ-R by BZ or BZ-like compounds potentiates the binding of GABA to GABA-R.

responsible for hepatic encephalopathy.[35-37] Observations in rabbits with galactosamine-induced hepatic failure provided the initial support for this hypothesis. GABA originates from the intestine and plasma levels increase with liver dysfunction due to inadequate hepatic extraction. During acute liver failure, the blood-brain barrier becomes more permeable and increased amounts of GABA enter the brain. Once in the brain, GABA binds to its receptor to produce neuronal inhibition and clinical encephalopathy. A key component to understanding the relationship of GABA and benzodiazepines was the recognition that the GABA receptor was tightly linked and modulated by the benzodiazepine receptor.[38-41] Binding of benzodiazepines to the benzodiazepine receptor induces a conformational change in the GABA receptor, enhancing the binding of GABA and neuronal inhibition. Activation of the GABA receptor opens a chloride channel, the third component of the GABA receptor complex (Fig. 119-2). In summary, GABA-induced inhibition of neurotransmission is enhanced by binding of benzodiazepines or related compounds to the benzodiazepine receptor, increasing the number of GABA receptors, increasing the activity of the GABA receptor, or opening the GABA-associated chloride channel.

The GABA hypothesis predicts that benzodiazepines would increase the severity of hepatic encephalopathy and that benzodiazepine antagonists, such as flumazenil, might ameliorate hepatic encephalopathy. Clinical experience

clearly suggests that cirrhotic patients, especially those with encephalopathy, are particularly sensitive to the amnesic and sedative effects of benzodiazepines. In our experience, use of benzodiazepines and other sedative/hypnotics is a common reason for worsening of hepatic encephalopathy. Recent studies have demonstrated that patients with hepatic encephalopathy have increased plasma levels of benzodiazepines or endogenous benzodiazepine-like compounds, which then can act as "false" neurotransmitters.[42-45] Some authors have suggested that patients with hepatic encephalopathy are particularly sensitive to GABA-mediated neuronal inhibition due to an increase in background stimulation of the GABA receptor by benzodiazepine-like compounds.

DOPAMINERGIC SYSTEM

Patients with chronic hepatic encephalopathy often have abnormal motor function, manifested as tremor, slowness of gait, ataxia, and even rigidity. Although these patients typically lack other features of parkinsonism (e.g., pill-rolling, resting tremor, mask-like facies, cogwheel rigidity), the motor abnormalities have prompted investigators to suggest that patients with hepatic encephalopathy may have impairment of the dopaminergic system. It is postulated that "false" neurotransmitters occupy dopaminergic binding sites within the CNS, thereby inhibiting dopaminergic activity. However, clinical trials in humans have failed to provide much support for this hypothesis. Both L-DOPA and bromocriptine, an L-DOPA agonist, are ineffective therapies for portosystemic encephalopathy (see later).

SEROTONERGIC SYSTEM

A number of alterations in CNS serotonin metabolism have been described in both humans and experimental animal models of hepatic encephalopathy. CNS levels of serotonin, serotonin receptors, and monoamine oxidases are increased. However, the exact role of serotonin in hepatic encephalopathy remains undefined.

TAURINE

Taurine is an inhibitory neurotransmitter, which is increased in brains of animal models of experimental hepatic encephalopathy and in the cerebrospinal fluid of primates with encephalopathy secondary to portacaval shunts. Plasma levels of taurine are greatest in patients with the greatest degrees of encephalopathy, suggesting that this inhibitory neurotransmitter may be involved in hepatic encephalopathy. Other neurotransmitters that may be altered in hepatic encephalopathy include (endogenous and exogenous) opioids and melatonin.

METHANETHIOL

Interest in methanethiol as a potential neurotoxin began with the finding of methanethiol in the urine of a patient with fetor hepaticus. Subsequently, levels of methanethiol, 4-methylthio-2-oxobutyrate, and methanethiol-mixed disulfides were found to be elevated in the plasma of cirrhotic patients.[46] It was suggested that these compounds may exacerbate the toxic effects of NH_3 and short-chain fatty acids. However, blood levels of methanethiol and related compounds are similar between deeply comatose patients and those with only mild cerebral dysfunction. Furthermore, there is little correlation between the grade of encephalopathy and the blood levels of these compounds.

FATTY ACIDS

The concentrations of short chain fatty acids are increased in the peripheral circulation of cirrhotic patients with hepatic encephalopathy. Normally, the liver metabolizes these fatty acids after absorption from the gut, but this function is impaired in cirrhotics; as a result, short chain fatty acid levels increase. The clinical severity of encephalopathy correlates poorly with plasma levels of acetic, propionic, butyric, valeric, and octanoic acids and short chain fatty acids have been administered to patients with cirrhosis without worsening of encephalopathy. Short chain fatty acids are not a likely cause of hepatic encephalopathy.

MANGANESE, ZINC

The liver is responsible for manganese excretion, and liver disease is associated with manganese accumulation. Magnetic resonance imaging (MRI) studies of the brain in patients with cirrhosis reveal pallidal hyperintensity on T1-weighted images (Fig. 119-3), a finding that correlates with the presence of extrapyramidal signs and symptoms and blood levels of manganese.[47] Markedly increased manganese concentrations have been detected in the globus pallidus when autopsy specimens from cirrhotic patients who died in hepatic coma were examined. Positron emission tomography reveals reduced cerebral glucose use in these areas. These findings suggest a relationship between manganese, brain hypometabolism, and some of the neuropsychiatric and motor abnormalities of hepatic encephalopathy.

Zinc deficiency is common in patients with long-standing cirrhosis. Its importance to the pathogenesis of hepatic encephalopathy is unknown, and three randomized, controlled trials of zinc supplementation have yielded conflicting results with respect to improvement in encephalopathy.

ENCEPHALOPATHY IN THE SETTING OF ACUTE HEPATIC FAILURE

DEFINITION

Acute liver failure is defined by the development of coagulopathy (prothrombin time >2 sec prolonged; international normalized ratio [INR] >1.5) in patients with acute hepatitis who do not have underlying chronic liver disease (an exception is Wilson's disease).[48-50] Patients with acute liver failure usually have extreme elevated circulating levels of aspartate aminotransferase and alanine aminotransferase with the initial injury; concentrations of both enzymes are typically 1000 to 5000 IU/L. These patients are often jaundiced and usually exhibit constitutional symptoms. They are at risk for encephalopathy, although most recover uneventfully. Progressive hepatic encephalopathy is a poor prognostic sign that signals the need for hepatic transplantation.

ETIOLOGY

There are approximately 2000 cases of acute liver failure in the United States each year.[51] The most common causes are acetaminophen toxicity, other forms of drug toxicity, hepatitis B, and hepatitis A. However, the second leading diagnostic category for fulminant hepatic failure is cryptogenic, cause unknown (Table 119-4). Recent data, collected since 1998, indicate that more than 50% of cases of fulminant hepatic failure in the United States are due to acetaminophen (38%) or other idiosyncratic drug reactions (approximately 14%).[52] Many cases of acetaminophen-induced liver failure are due to "therapeutic misadventure"; consumption of as little as 4 g/d of acetaminophen over several days can precipitate fulminant hepatic failure in the setting of fasting and alcohol use. Sporadic cases of fulminant hepatic failure due to drugs of abuse, notably cocaine and Ecstasy, have recently been described.[51,52] Fulminant hepatic failure from mushroom poisoning occasionally occurs among inexperienced amateur mushroom fanciers. Infiltration of the liver with rapid progression of tumor growth can lead to fulminant hepatic

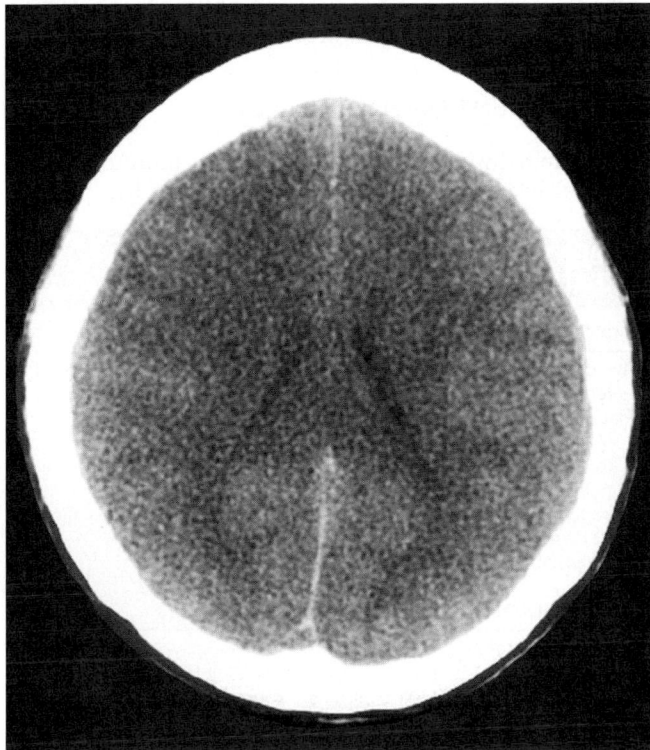

FIGURE 119–3. This magnetic resonance image (MRI) is a T1-weighted sagittal view of the brain demonstrating hyperintensity of the globus pallidus (whitish area), which may be related to manganese deposition.

TABLE 119–4. CAUSES OF ACUTE LIVER FAILURE

Acetaminophen	20%
Cryptogenic	15%
Non-acetaminophen drug toxicity	12%
Hepatitis B	10%
Hepatitis A	7%
Autoimmune hepatitis	6%
Wilson's disease	6%
Miscellaneous*	24%

*Budd-Chiari syndrome, herpes simplex, paramyxovirus, Epstein-Barr virus, *Amanita* poisoning, ischemia, malignant infiltration.
Adapted from Schiodt FV, Atillasoy E, Shakil O, et al: Etiologic factors and outcome for 295 patients with acute liver failure in the United States. Liver Transplant Surg 1999;5:29-34.

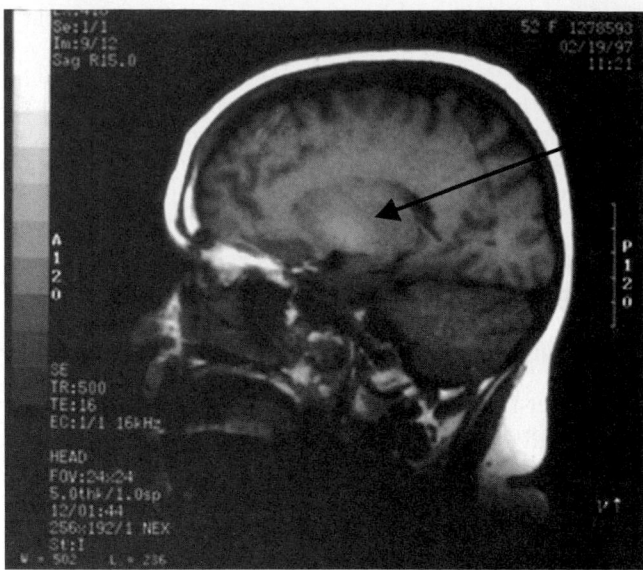

FIGURE 119–4. Computed tomographic scan of the brain of a patient with fulminant hepatic failure, stage IV hepatic coma, and cerebral edema. Note the diminished sulci and lack of distinction between white and grey matter. The cerebral edema resolved with medical management and the patient subsequently underwent transplantation. She achieved complete neurologic recovery after transplantation.

failure and has been described in patients with breast carcinoma, lymphoma, and melanoma. Biopsy of the liver is required to establish the latter diagnoses. Fulminant hepatic failure also may occur in the third trimester of pregnancy related to acute fatty liver of pregnancy, HELLP syndrome, or disseminated herpes infection.

PROGNOSIS

A major determinant of prognosis is the level of encephalopathy (see Table 119-1). Patients with acute liver failure who have progressed to higher stages of encephalopathy (stage III or IV) have the worst prognosis. The Glasgow Coma Scale is useful in assessing need for transplantation.[53] Cerebral edema on a computed tomography (CT) scan of the brain is a late feature of progressive encephalopathy (Fig. 119-4). Additional clinical features that indicate a poor prognosis include metabolic acidosis, renal failure, severe jaundice, or markedly prolonged prothrombin time.[50,53,54] The likelihood of survival varies with the cause of acute liver injury. Patients with acetaminophen overdose have a relatively favorable outcome: more than 50% survive. Patients with fulminant hepatitis A virus or hepatitis B virus infection have an intermediate prognosis; 30% to 50% of patients survive. In contrast, patients with a fulminant presentation of Wilson's disease or severe sporadic non-A, non-B, non-C hepatitis survive less than 10% of the time.

GENERAL CLINICAL MANAGEMENT

Once recognized, patients with acute liver failure with encephalopathy should be transferred to a center with expertise in managing hepatic failure that can offer liver transplantation.

All patients should be placed on needle (hepatitis B, non-A non-B hepatitis) and stool (hepatitis A) precautions, but not in isolation. Gloves should be worn when handling biologic specimens, and specimens should be clearly labeled ("Hepatitis patient"). All used instruments should be autoclaved or appropriately disposed of. No effective antiviral therapy exists for acute viral hepatitis or fulminant hepatic failure; corticosteroids are contraindicated because they may increase the risk of developing chronic hepatitis and are ineffective in the treatment of encephalopathy or cerebral edema in this setting. Removal of the offending drug, toxin, or alcohol is the mainstay of therapy of drug-induced and alcoholic hepatitis, respectively. *N*-acetyl cysteine is an effective primary intervention for hepatic injury related to acetaminophen[55] and is currently under investigation in the treatment of fulminant hepatic failure due to other causes (Table 119-5).

The coagulopathy of acute liver failure is due to depletion of clotting factors related to inadequate hepatic production. Some patients exhibit features of disseminated intravascular coagulation or primary fibrinolysis. Once the patient is diagnosed with severe acute liver failure or fulminant hepatic failure, we recommend administration of Mephyton (vitamin K) 10 mg/d SQ for 3 days. Prophylactic infusions of clotting factors are of unproven benefit. Use of clotting factors, such as fresh frozen plasma, cryoprecipitate, and platelets, should be restricted to patients with ongoing bleeding, such as gastrointestinal hemorrhage. Prophylaxis against peptic disease and gastrointestinal bleeding with proton-pump inhibitors is recommended.

Infection is a leading comorbidity in patients with acute liver failure.[50-54] Blood, urine, and sputum should be cultured frequently (even in the absence of fever or other signs of infection) and antibiotic therapy instituted only for positive cultures and directed against specific organisms. Fever is not a feature in most cases of acute liver injury and, if present, usually signifies intercurrent infection. Febrile patients should be cultured immediately and treated empirically with antibiotics. The most common sources of infection are the respiratory and urinary tracts and line sepsis. Currently we use vancomycin with a fluoroquinolone for initial treatment and then tailor the antibiotics once results of cultures are known.

MANAGEMENT OF ENCEPHALOPATHY

Encephalopathy is a hallmark of acute liver failure and is also observed in patients with underlying chronic liver disease

TABLE 119–5. USE OF *N*-ACETYL CYSTEINE IN TREATMENT OF ACETAMINOPHEN OVERDOSE
Oral Dosing Schedule
Avoid use of activated charcoal since it will bind *N*-acetyl cysteine, reducing its efficacy.
Place nasogastric tube for administration of *N*-acetyl cysteine. *N*-acetyl cysteine is highly unpalatable; most patients cannot tolerate its oral administration. The nasogastric tube is necessary to insure dosing of the medication.
Dosage: 140 mg/kg initially, followed by 70 mg/kg q4h, to a total of 17 doses of *N*-acetyl cysteine.
Toxicity: nausea, vomiting
Intravenous Dosing Schedule
Intravenous access for administration.
Dosage: Loading: 150 mg/kg in 200 ml D_5W; maintenance: 50 mg/kg in 500 ml D_5W over 4 hours, then 100 mg/kg in 1000 ml D_5W over 16 hours
Adverse reactions occur in approximately 15%: flushing and transient skin rash (usually responds to diphenhydramine), wheezing, nausea, vomiting. Patient should be monitored for anaphylaxis (treat with epinephrine, H1 and H2 blockers, supportive care).

TABLE 119–6. MEASURES USED TO MONITOR AND CONTROL CEREBRAL EDEMA DUE TO FULMINANT HEPATIC FAILURE

Correction of metabolic abnormalities.
Electrolytes (Na, K, Cl, HCO_3).
Acid-base (If patient is on mechanical ventilation, induce mild respiratory alkalosis).
Glucose (maintenance intravenous glucose infusion).
Avoid overtransfusion or overhydration.
Carefully match intake and output once patient is euvolemic.
Daily weights.
Avoid use of blood products unless indicated for ongoing bleeding and correction of coagulopathy or to maintain hemostasis when intracranial monitor has been placed. In the latter circumstance, diuresis of the patient may be necessary to avoid an excess intravascular volume, especially from plasma.
Institute dialysis in patients in renal failure.
Continuous arteriovenous or venovenous hemodialysis is preferred over standard hemodialysis.
Avoid severe volume shifts, stabilize blood pressure, maintain euvolemia, correct electrolyte and acid-base abnormalities.
Mechanical ventilation (worsening encephalopathy, $\geq$ grade II).
Main indication in liver failure is airway protection to prevent aspiration pneumonia.
Induce mild respiratory alkalosis (pH 7.45-7.50, Pco_2 20-30 mm Hg).
Elevate the head of the bed 15 to 30 degrees.
Use sedation to avoid having the patient "fight the ET tube".
Consider placement of intracranial pressure monitor in the epidural space.
Should be considered when patients evolve from stage II (agitated confusion) to stage III (stuporous) encephalopathy.
Maintain adequate platelet count (>60,000) with platelet transfusions and INR $\leq$1.5 with fresh frozen plasma, if necessary.
Mannitol is used to control intracranial pressure in patients with intact renal function or in those on dialysis. Mannitol is given in 0.5 to 1.0 g/kg doses. Serum electrolytes, glucose, and osmolarity should be checked every 4 to 6 hours. If intracranial pressure is elevated, osmolarity <310, and Na <145, then give mannitol. Mannitol should be held if the patient has excessive serum osmolarity or significant hypernatremia.

who sustain superimposed acute liver injury. The encephalopathy of acute hepatic failure is related to both metabolic factors, such as progressive elevation in blood NH_3 concentration, and cerebral edema. Progressively worsening encephalopathy is an ominous clinical feature; development of grade III or IV encephalopathy may herald the death of the patient due to cerebral edema, increased intracranial pressure, and central herniation of the brain. Efforts to control the encephalopathy of acute liver failure are directed at preventing or resolving cerebral edema (Table 119-6).[11,56-60] Because emerging evidence suggests that NH_3 may play a role in the development of cerebral edema, we recommend that dietary protein be limited to less than 40 g/d. We also recommend administration of lactulose to purge the bowel. However, one must exercise caution when using lactulose in the setting of fulminant hepatic failure; dosing should be monitored carefully and adjusted to avoid alterations in serum electrolyte concentrations or intravascular volume depletion. If oral lactulose (usual starting dose is 30 mL every 6 hours) is given simultaneously with intravenous mannitol, marked losses of free water may occur, inducing severe hypernatremia. Although one recent study suggested that infusion of hypertonic saline (30%) to maintain serum sodium concentration between 145 and 155 mmol/L is beneficial,[61] rapid shifts in sodium concentration have been associated with central pontine myelinolysis. Administration of terlipressin, a congener of vasopressin

used for treatment of hepatorenal syndrome, may worsen intracranial hypertension and should be avoided.[62]

Normalization of clotting parameters (INR <1.5; platelet count >60,000 cells/μL) prior to placement of intracranial pressure transducers is recommended. However, reversal of coagulopathy may be difficult and require infusing a large volume of fresh frozen plasma, potentially contributing to volume overload and worsening of cerebral edema. Some investigators have suggested that infusion of recombinant human factor VIIa is preferred in this setting, owing to the low fluid volume required and the ability of this agent to rapidly correct INR.

Hepatic glycogen, the main storage form of glucose, is depleted early in the course of acute liver failure. Depletion of hepatic glycogen predisposes to severe, potentially life-threatening hypoglycemia and worsening of cerebral energy metabolism. All patients with acute liver failure should be treated with glucose infusions, and blood glucose levels must be monitored frequently.

EXPERIMENTAL THERAPIES

Several methods have been used in patients with fulminant hepatic failure: exchange blood transfusion, plasmapheresis, cross-circulation with human and baboon donors, hemoperfusion through isolated human or animal liver, hemodialysis (conventional and polyacrylonitrate), and column hemoperfusion (microencapsulated charcoal, albumin-covered Amberlite XAD-7 resin). Only exchange transfusion and charcoal hemoperfusion have been evaluated in controlled trials, and in these studies, the mortality rate was either similar or greater in the treated group. Since none of these techniques has been demonstrated to improve survival, their use in patients with fulminant hepatic failure is not currently recommended (unless under IRB-approved protocols in major liver centers).

Albumin Dialysis. Stange and associates[63] recently reported use of an extracorporeal liver assist device based on albumin dialysis (MARS) in 26 patients with chronic liver disease who had either acute or chronic liver failure. The treatment lowered plasma levels of bilirubin and bile acids, but the effect on clinical outcome was unclear; nine patients with advanced liver disease (equivalent to UNOS 2A) died within an average of 15 days, but the remainder survived and were thought to have benefited. Further studies will be needed to define benefit and overall utility.

Bioartificial Liver. Bioartificial liver machines have recently emerged as potential therapeutic interventions in the treatment of fulminant hepatic failure. The major principal of the bioartificial liver is the use of a "bio-reactor," which contains liver cells external to the dialysis tubing in a dialysis cartridge through which blood or plasma flows. The liver cells used in these reactors vary from primary porcine hepatocytes to transformed human cells (HepG2-C3A). "Toxins" or metabolites diffuse across the capillary membrane, where the liver cells can remove, metabolize, or inactivate them. Experimental models suggest that removal of toxins and metabolites can reduce the neurotoxicity in case of fulminant hepatic failure by inhibiting the formation of cerebral edema. In clinical terms, the goal is stabilization of neurologic function to allow for hepatic regeneration or to bridge the patient to liver transplantation. To date, there has been only one large randomized multicenter trial of the use of the bioartificial liver in the setting of acute liver failure.

Demetriou and associates[64] reported the results of multi-center randomized controlled trial of porcine hepatocyte-based bioartificial liver in 171 patients with acute liver failure (n = 147) and primary nonfunction after liver transplantation (n = 24). In both the group as a whole and the subgroup of patients with acute liver failure, the 30-day patient survival rate was slightly, but insignificantly, higher in the bioartificial liver group (entire cohort: 71% vs 62%, P = NS; acute liver failure: 73% vs 59%, P = NS). A major confounding variable in this study was the overwhelmingly positive effect of hepatic transplantation. Transplanted patients (55% of cohort) experienced a 70% reduction in the relative risk (RR) of death (P < .0001). Additional analysis of survival in the subgroup of patients with acute liver failure, after controlling for the impact of transplantation, suggested survival benefit for bioartificial liver–treated patients (RR death = .56; P = .048). Although this initial report is encouraging, additional studies will be needed to determine the efficacy and role of bioartificial liver in the treatment of acute liver failure.

Hepatocyte Transplantation. The principles guiding use of hepatocyte transplantation are similar to those of the bioartificial liver: provide support during a period of critical need so that the patient can be bridged to recovery or transplantation.[65-67] One potential advantage of hepatocyte transplantation is the ability of liver stem cells to regenerate, raising the potential for repopulation of a dying or dead liver by allogeneic donor hepatocytes. The latter theoretical consideration has not been proven in humans with acute liver failure. Experience with hepatocyte transplantation in fulminant hepatic failure is limited. Our center reported outcomes for six patients, who were not candidates for liver transplantation due to active substance abuse or prohibitive underlying medical illness, and one patient, listed for transplantation, who had disseminated herpes infection.[67] Despite a suggestion of improvement in neurologic status after hepatocyte transplantation, all seven patients died. Currently hepatocyte transplantation for acute liver failure should be viewed as unproven and experimental.

LIVER TRANSPLANTATION

Liver transplantation is the only treatment that has been proven to improve survival in patients with acute liver failure and grade III or IV encephalopathy.[68] The rate of survival without transplantation is 10% to 20%. Survival rate increases to 60% to 80% with liver transplantation. In the study of bioartificial liver by Demetriou and associates,[64] the survival of patients with acute liver failure who underwent hepatic transplantation was 92%.

Resolution of Cerebral Edema
At some stage, cerebral edema is irreversible and patients, despite transplantation, go on to brain death or massive irreversible brain injury.[69,70] Risk of irreversible neurologic injury is greatest in those with cerebral perfusion pressure less than 40 mm Hg for more than 4 hours. Lesser increases in intracranial pressure may be associated with neurologic injury, but usually cerebral edema resolves in the post-transplant period and complete or partial neurologic recovery can be expected. In most cases of acute liver failure, all of the manifestations of the neurologic illness (cerebral edema, encephalopathy, coma) totally reverse without sequelae after successful hepatic transplantation. One complication, central pontine myelinolysis (CPM), may occur in the absence of cerebral edema and may be related to fluctuations in plasma sodium during resuscitative measures in the ICU, such as intravenous fluids, transfusions, antibiotics, sedatives, narcotics, invasive procedures, and ventilatory support. CPM can result in significant neurologic impairment requiring prolonged support and rehabilitation (e.g., physical therapy, speech therapy). Despite the serious nature of CPM, significant neurologic recovery can occur.[71]

Living Donor Liver Transplantation
Donor safety is a major concern in the performance of living donor liver transplantation. Current statistics suggest that the donor mortality rate is approximately 0.13% for adult-to-pediatric cases and 0.25% for adult-to-adult cases.[72] This procedure should be used with caution and performed only by centers with extensive experience and expertise in hepatic transplantation and liver resection.

Experience with living donor liver transplantation in cases of acute liver failure is limited. Outcome after living donor liver transplantation for fulminant hepatic failure was reviewed at a workshop sponsored by the National Institutes of Health in 2000.[73] Fourteen patients had undergone living donor liver transplantation for fulminant hepatic failure; all survived the surgical procedure and the survival rate at 1 year was 90%. These favorable results are encouraging and similar to results obtained using cadaveric liver transplantation.

ENCEPHALOPATHY IN THE SETTING OF CHRONIC LIVER DISEASE

Patients with cirrhosis of any cause and chronic portosystemic encephalopathy may present with a host of neuropsychiatric symptoms, ranging from subtle changes in mental status to coma.[1-3] Fetor hepaticus is common but not invariable. Asterixis, the "flapping tremor," is due to involuntary intermittent relaxation of sustained motor activity but is less specific than fetor hepaticus as a finding indicative of hepatic encephalopathy. Asterixis is usually only present during the late stages of encephalopathy. Asterixis is most easily elicited with the patient's arm outstretched, fingers separated, and wrists hyperextended. Although reported, cerebral edema rarely occurs in patients with encephalopathy in the setting of chronic liver disease. As the patient recovers from hepatic encephalopathy, asterixis and other manifestations of encephalopathy disappear.

RISK FACTORS AND PRECIPITATING EVENTS: IMPLICATIONS FOR DIAGNOSTIC TESTING AND TREATMENT

Flares of chronic encephalopathy may occur spontaneously and without an identifiable precipitating factor in patients with very severe hepatic impairment and extensive portosystemic shunting. However, in the majority of cases, acute worsening of chronic encephalopathy is precipitated by one or more of a number of common events.

Gastrointestinal Hemorrhage. Hemodynamically significant gastrointestinal hemorrhage is a major precipitating factor for hepatic encephalopathy. Delivery of a large protein load to the gastrointestinal tract (in the form of blood) stimulates bacterial metabolism and release of NH_3, GABA, and other compounds that may inhibit neurotransmission. Poor hepatic function or shunting of portal blood via portosystemic collateral vessels impairs hepatic clearance and enhances delivery of these molecules to the brain. Rapid diagnosis and treatment of gastrointestinal hemorrhage requires urgent esophagogastroduodenoscopy, initiation of endoscopic therapy, and administration of the somatostatin analog octreotide, or other vasoactive treatments. Transjugular intrahepatic portal-systemic shunt (TIPS) can be used to control recalcitrant hemorrhage, but encephalopathy may worsen after this procedure.

Infection. Infection, in particular sepsis, may precipitate hepatic encephalopathy in patients with chronic liver disease. Spontaneous bacterial peritonitis always should be considered when there is new-onset encephalopathy in a patient with ascites. Fever may be absent and clinical signs (i.e., abdominal pain, ileus) may be lacking. Spontaneous bacterial peritonitis is presumptively diagnosed if the absolute neutrophil count in ascites exceeds 250 cells/mL. Patients with cirrhosis and malnutrition are susceptible to infections because of reduced leukocyte migration, decreased serum bactericidal activity, depressed white blood cell mobilization, and impaired phagocytosis. Infection increases protein catabolism, releasing aromatic amino acids, which may contribute to the encephalopathy. Primary therapy is directed against the infection.

Medications (Sedatives). There are no safe sedatives for administration to cirrhotic patients with hepatic encephalopathy. Because liver metabolism is usually severely impaired in these patients, the clearance of benzodiazepines, barbiturates, chlorpromazine, morphine, and opioid derivatives such as methadone, meperidine, and codeine, is reduced. With repeated dosing, all of these compounds tend to accumulate in cirrhotic patients, increasing the degree and prolonging the duration of sedation.

Renal Failure. A common precipitating factor for hepatic encephalopathy is excessive diuresis, resulting in relative depletion of intravascular volume and prerenal azotemia. Factors contributing to the encephalopathy include electrolyte imbalance, disordered acid-base status, reduced intravascular fluid volume, and impaired renal clearance of metabolites, drugs, and toxins. Acute decompensation of intrinsic or chronic renal disease may be another cause of encephalopathy. Certain renal disorders have a predilection to occur in the setting of liver disease, including IgA nephropathy (Laennec's cirrhosis), membranoproliferative glomerulonephritis (viral hepatitis), nephrolithiasis (primary sclerosing cholangitis with inflammatory bowel disease), medullary sponge kidney (congenital hepatic fibrosis), and autosomal-dominant polycystic kidney (polycystic liver).

Fluid, Electrolyte, and Acid-Base Imbalance. Hepatic encephalopathy may be precipitated by dehydration, hypokalemia, and alkalosis. Metabolic alkalosis promotes an increase in nonionic NH_3 production, which diffuses very rapidly into the CNS. Diffusion of NH_3 into the brain and enhanced glutamine production may precipitate encephalopathy due to either astrocyte swelling and dysfunction or impairment of glutamatergic neurotransmission. With hepatic impairment, the kidneys produce glucose from branched-chain amino acids (gluconeogenesis) in an attempt to maintain peripheral energy supply. This process results in decreased circulating levels of branched-chain amino acids and a relative increase in the concentrations of the relatively more toxic aromatic amino acids, which may diffuse into the brain.

Hepatocellular Carcinoma. Hepatocellular carcinoma commonly occurs in cirrhotic patients; the estimated risk of developing this complication is 1% to 3% per year. Hepatocellular carcinoma can be heralded by the onset of spontaneous encephalopathy, usually in association with portal vein thrombosis. If all other precipitating factors for encephalopathy are excluded, the diagnosis of hepatocellular carcinoma should be entertained and serum alpha-fetoprotein concentration measured and imaging studies of liver (ultrasonography, computed tomography, magnetic resonance imaging) performed.

Surgical Shunt Procedure or TIPS. Hepatic encephalopathy is a common complication of portal diversion after surgical portal-systemic shunts or TIPS (Table 119-7).[74,75] Predictors of post-shunt encephalopathy include pre-shunt encephalopathy, severe liver disease (Child-Pugh score >10), poor clearance of indocyanine green and lidocaine, and elderly age. The mechanisms of hepatic encephalopathy after placement of a portal-systemic shunt include lack of compensatory dilation of the hepatic artery, lack of perfusion of the liver via the portal vein, and reduction in hepatocyte function. Clinically apparent encephalopathy after placement of a shunt usually responds to medical treatment (i.e., low protein diet, lactulose, neomycin). In rare circumstances, narrowing with a flow-reducing stent or occlusion of the shunt may be necessary to control the encephalopathy.[76]

Noncompliance with Therapy. One of the most common factors precipitating encephalopathy is noncompliance to prescribed outpatient medical treatment (i.e., low-protein diet, lactulose, and neomycin). A careful history, focusing on adherence to medical therapy, is necessary in the evaluation of the encephalopathic patient.

DIAGNOSIS

The diagnosis of portosystemic encephalopathy is based on clinical suspicion in the patient with chronic liver disease, and the impression is confirmed by resolution after medical therapy. Occasionally, it may be necessary to employ additional testing to confirm the diagnosis of portosystemic encephalopathy. Additional tests are particularly valuable when encephalopathy is the primary clinical manifestation of otherwise unsuspected liver disease or if the manifestations of encephalopathy are predominantly a change in behavior or an unusual neurologic syndrome (e.g., seizures, focal

TABLE 119–7. NEUROPSYCHIATRIC TESTS USED TO EVALUATE HEPATIC ENCEPHALOPATHY

Cerebral Function: Learning and Delayed Recall

Figure Memory Test	*Story Memory Test*
Concentration	Digit vigilance test
Fine motor coordination	Grooved pegboard
Sequential procedures	Trail making test
Problem solving	Wisconsin card sorting test
Attention	WAIS-R* digit symbol subtest
Vocabulary	WAIS-R vocabulary subtest
Verbal fluency skills	Controlled oral word association
Animal naming	Complex material
Auditory comprehension	WAIS-R block design subtest
Visual-spatial analysis	

Psychological Function
MMPI-2†

*WAIS-R, Wechsler Adult Intelligence Scale - Revised
†MMPI-2, Minnesota Multiphasic Personality Inventory

neurologic deficits). Rarely, cerebral edema complicates chronic liver disease.[77]

Plasma Ammonia Concentration. Elevated blood NH_3 levels are common in cirrhotic patients, especially those with encephalopathy. Some studies have demonstrated a correlation between blood NH_3 concentration and the presence and grade of encephalopathy, whereas others have not. In general, blood NH_3 levels might be useful as a marker of liver disease but are of little diagnostic or clinical value in managing the cirrhotic patient with hepatic encephalopathy.

Cerebrospinal Fluid Glutamine. Chronic elevation in NH_3 level leads to accumulation of glutamine in the CNS. Cerebrospinal fluid glutamine measurement may be useful in confusing cases in which the diagnosis of high-grade (III or IV) hepatic encephalopathy is uncertain or questionable. Measuring normal cerebrospinal fluid glutamine concentration virtually excludes the diagnosis of hepatic encephalopathy; increased cerebrospinal fluid glutamine provides evidence in favor of the diagnosis.

Electroencephalography. Electroencephalographic (EEG) abnormalities are relatively nonspecific in patients with hepatic encephalopathy and are similar to changes observed in patients with other causes of metabolic encephalopathy. Two findings have some specificity with respect to hepatic encephalopathy: reduced brainstem auditory-evoked potentials and diminished visual-evoked potentials. In various studies, the percentage of encephalopathic cirrhotic patients with EEG abnormalities is highly variable, ranging from 14% to 78% of patients.[4-11] Despite this variation in sensitivity, EEG findings are objective and can be used as an endpoint of response to therapy or medical interventions.

Radiologic Imaging. Standard computed tomography scans or radionuclide brain scans exhibit few distinguishing features, although loss of cortical volume may be common in patients with Laennec's cirrhosis and chronic encephalopathy (see Fig. 119-4). Computed tomography can be used to document cerebral edema or to exclude CNS complications, such as tumor, infection, or hemorrhage. Magnetic resonance imaging studies have revealed a few features relatively unique to hepatic encephalopathy. One feature, hyperintensity on T1-weighted images of globus pallidus (see Fig. 119-3), correlates with motor disorders (extrapyramidal symptoms), and excess accumulation of manganese.

Neuropsychiatric Testing. In general, neuropsychiatric testing is used primarily to monitor the efficacy of treatment. A battery of tests is employed to distinguish hepatic encephalopathy and organic brain syndrome from other causes of encephalopathy and underlying psychiatric disease. These tests are itemized in Table 119-7. Poor performance on number-connection tests correlates reasonably well with severity of encephalopathy and Child-Pugh classification.

THERAPEUTIC OPTIONS

The traditional treatment for hepatic encephalopathy is a restricted diet that provides 40 g or less per day of protein.[78-80] However, cirrhotic patients often develop severe muscle wasting, especially those with advanced disease, and unnecessary protein restriction might further worsen their poor nutritional state. Most hepatologists currently avoid the use of protein restriction in the management of chronic hepatic encephalopathy.

Branched-Chain Amino Acids. Early studies demonstrated that cirrhotic patients had increased levels of aromatic amino acids and decreased levels of branched-chain amino acids in blood samples. Subsequent clinical work suggested that patients with the greatest imbalances in plasma amino acids were more likely to be encephalopathic and to experience early death and higher rates of mortality. For this reason, there have been at least 14 controlled trials of the use of branched-chain amino acids in the treatment of cirrhotic patients with chronic encephalopathy. A recent well-controlled trial suggested efficacy.[81,82] However, results of these trials have been inconsistent, and separate meta-analyses yielded opposite conclusions regarding efficacy.[80,83] In addition, branched-chain amino acid preparations are much more expensive than standard amino acid supplements. A trial of branched-chain amino acids could be considered in patients who develop encephalopathy on standard protein diets and who manifest protein-calorie malnutrition. Branched-chain amino acid supplements may allow adequate protein intake in this select group of patients without increasing the frequency of attacks of encephalopathy.

Total Parenteral Nutrition. It is common for the wasted, cirrhotic patient to be considered for total parenteral nutrition (TPN). However, use of TPN is often inappropriate and expensive and leads to other complications (electrolyte imbalance, fluid overload, and infection). In most cases, TPN should be avoided and enteral feedings used in its place; care must be taken to avoid high enteral osmotic loads, which may precipitate diarrhea and fluid and electrolyte imbalances. In addition, many enteral preparations are relatively high in protein for the amount of calories delivered. Occasionally TPN is indicted because of the inability to deliver adequate calories by the enteral route or an intercurrent condition (e.g., infection, diarrhea, bowel obstruction, forced purgation) that makes it difficult or impossible to use the enteral route for nutritional support.

Lactulose. One of the most successful treatments for hepatic encephalopathy is lactulose, a nonabsorbable disaccharide that is fermented by bacteria in the intestine to yield acetic, butyric, propionic, and lactic acids.[84-88] The fermentation of lactulose produces an acidic milieu that alters the composition of the bacterial flora and produces an osmotic diarrhea. Each of these effects may be responsible for the ameliorative effects of lactulose on hepatic encephalopathy. Changing the composition of the bacterial flora may alter the metabolism of fecal contents and reduce the production of toxins, NH_3, and methanethiols that are responsible for the encephalopathy. The acidic luminal milieu creates an environment capable of trapping NH_3 as ammonium ion (NH_4^+):

$$NH_3 + H^+ =======>> NH_4^+$$

NH_3 is neutral and lipophilic and freely diffuses across the mucosal barrier of the colon, where it then can enter portal blood for delivery to the body. In contrast, NH_4^+ produced from the reaction of NH_3 with hydrogen ion, is ionized, is highly polar, and cannot readily diffuse across the lipid bilayer of mucosal cells. NH_4^+ is "trapped" in the fecal effluent and eliminated with passage of the bowel movement. In addition to these properties, the breakdown of each molecule of lactulose produces at least four osmotically active particles. Water diffuses into the lumen, down the osmotic gradient, increasing fecal water content, and, if enough lactulose is given, osmotic diarrhea. The purgative effect of lactulose may also be responsible for altering the composition of colonic bacteria and helps to eliminate toxins and wastes that might otherwise accumulate. The usual recommendation is to administer enough lactulose to produce two to three loose, semiformed stools each day. Excessive dosing with lactulose leads to severe diarrhea that can be associated with intravascular volume depletion and electrolyte imbalances; hence, excessive doses of lactulose should be avoided.

Neomycin. Neomycin is highly nephrotoxic and should never be given intravenously or parenterally. Orally administered neomycin is poorly absorbed and, therefore, is much less nephrotoxic. The goal of oral neomycin is to alter the bacterial composition of the colonic flora. The major advantage of neomycin over lactulose is that it does not cause diarrhea. The main disadvantage of this agent is that despite its poor absorption, some neomycin does gain entry to the circulation, which can contribute to nephrotoxicity. We recommend use of neomycin in patients who are intolerant of lactulose (usually due to diarrhea). Also, neomycin can be added to lactulose to improve the efficacy of the medical regimen in controlling the encephalopathy.[7,89-91] Some practitioners have recommended that neomycin (1 g bid) be given in short courses, lasting only 2 to 8 weeks.

Metronidazole. Studies have demonstrated that oral metronidazole 0.5 to 1.5 g/d given for 1 week was well tolerated, safe (no obvious neurotoxicity), and as effective as neomycin or lactulose in controlling encephalopathy. Others have not observed similar efficacy and have measured little effect of metronidazole on blood NH_3.[91] The advantages of metronidazole are that it does not cause diarrhea and it is not nephrotoxic. Disadvantages are that many patients complain of epigastric discomfort with its use and, hence, compliance with long-term treatment is often poor. In addition, maintenance therapy can be expected to cause peripheral neuropathy, which is already often a problem in patients with advanced liver disease. Finally, metronidazole has been reported to cause the "disulfiram reaction" when alcohol is consumed. The physician prescribing metronidazole to cirrhotic patients should also be aware that this drug undergoes extensive hepatic metabolism. One study of cirrhotic patients with encephalopathy revealed a threefold reduction in hepatic elimination and maintenance of therapeutic levels with as little as 500 mg given every 24 to 48 h.

Treatment of *Helicobacter pylori* Infection. Published reports had suggested that *Helicobacter pylori* infection might increase blood NH_3 levels and precipitate hepatic encephalopathy in patients with cirrhosis. Controlled treatment trials have failed to confirm this initial observation.[92-94]

Dopaminergic Agents. One of the theories regarding the pathogenesis of encephalopathy is that cirrhotic patients have a relative deficiency of dopaminergic activity within the CNS. There have been three trials of the use of L-DOPA and the dopaminergic compound bromocriptine in the treatment of hepatic encephalopathy. These studies were conducted in patients with chronic portosystemic encephalopathy and indicated the following: L-DOPA was ineffective in improving clinical encephalopathy, EEG, and encephalopathy scores. However, L-DOPA was also associated with impaired bowel motility and caused obstipation, an effect that counteracted the potentially beneficial CNS effects of the drug. For this reason, bromocriptine, an L-DOPA agonist that increases CNS L-DOPA concentrations without causing obstipation, was studied. However, it too failed to demonstrate a benefit. For these reasons, dopaminergic agents have not been used in the treatment of encephalopathy in clinical practice.

Benzodiazepine Antagonists. There have been several randomized controlled trials of short-term administration of flumazenil for the treatment of hepatic encephalopathy.[95-103] In some studies, flumazenil was superior to placebo in improving the grade of encephalopathy; 30% to 60% of encephalopathic patients improved after administration of flumazenil, and changes in the EEG paralleled the clinical improvement. In other studies, flumazenil was no better than placebo for ameliorating the symptoms of encephalopathy, and EEG abnormalities did not improve. A recent meta-analysis suggested benefit of flumazenil over placebo.[104] Flumazenil has a limited role in the treatment of hepatic encephalopathy, and additional trials enrolling larger numbers of subjects with varying grades of encephalopathy are needed.

These studies are provocative. The striking reversal of encephalopathy in some patients suggests that the GABA-benzodiazepine receptor system is one factor that may contribute to hepatic encephalopathy. These studies further emphasize the need to screen patients for use of benzodiazepines, which can be a cause of hepatic encephalopathy.

HEPATIC TRANSPLANTATION

The development of encephalopathy in a patient with chronic liver disease indicates severe portal-systemic shunting and hepatic dysfunction. The prognosis for patients developing this complication is grim; one recent study indicated 1-year survival of 42% and a 3-year survival rate of 23%.[105] In addition, there are numerous comorbidities in encephalopathic patients, including inability to continue gainful employment, poor function at home, nursing strains on spouse or family, inability to drive a vehicle, and inability to handle personal finances. Although medical therapies can ameliorate the major symptoms of encephalopathy, they rarely are effective enough to return the patient to full function. Often the patient with encephalopathy is at risk for other life-threatening complications of liver disease, such as variceal hemorrhage and spontaneous bacterial peritonitis. For all of these reasons, any patient with hepatic encephalopathy should be considered for hepatic transplantation (Fig. 119-5).

In contrast to acute liver failure, patients with chronic liver failure do not develop cerebral edema and virtually all manifestations of their encephalopathy resolve post-transplant.

POST-TRANSPLANT NEUROLOGIC COMPLICATIONS

Seizures. The complication of seizures, commonly observed in the past, is now a rare occurrence.[69,70] Risk factors for post-transplant seizures include intravenous cyclosporine or tacrolimus, rapid infusion of intravenous cyclosporine or tacrolimus, low plasma magnesium level, and low plasma cholesterol level. The type of underlying liver disease or pretransplant diagnosis of encephalopathy does not correlate with risk of post-transplant seizures. Early institution of oral

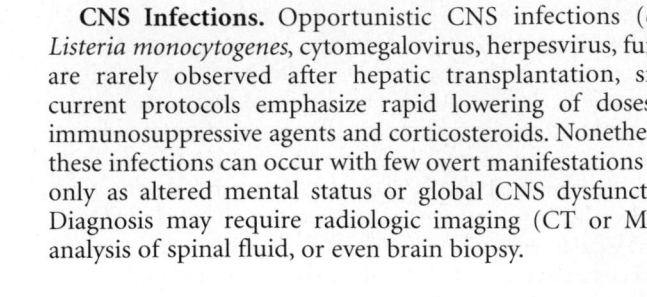

Survival in Patients with Encephalopathy

— Transplanted
- - Not transplanted

FIGURE 119–5. Survival for the first 10 years post-transplantation is shown for 785 adults who received transplants in our program at Colorado (solid line). The survival of patients after onset of encephalopathy who did not undergo hepatic transplantation[105] is also shown (dotted line) for comparison. A significant survival advantage is enjoyed by patients undergoing hepatic transplantation.

dosing of cyclosporine and tacrolimus, magnesium supplementation, and nutritional/vitamin support have markedly reduced the incidence of this complication.

Intracranial Hemorrhage. The incidence of post-transplant hemorrhagic stroke, subarachnoid bleed, or subdural hematoma is less than 1%. Most of these complications occur within days of the transplantation and manifest as either unexplained headache or rapidly evolving neurologic syndromes.

Ischemic Stroke. Ischemic stroke is usually a late complication, occurring years after successful liver transplantation. Reported rates of ischemic stroke after liver transplantation are low, at least for the first 5 post-transplant years, and are not increased above rates in the general population. Stroke rates may increase as patients survive longer, since they are at risk for accelerated atherosclerosis.

Central Pontine Myelinolysis. The patient at risk for central pontine myelinolysis usually experiences a prolonged ICU stay and requires numerous supportive measures. The patient presents with unresponsiveness to external stimuli even though sleep-wake patterns, spontaneous ventilation, and control of blood pressure and pulse are intact. In our experience, nearly all patients recover significant neurologic function, but prolonged rehabilitation is required.

Peripheral Neuropathy. Paresthesias and tremor are common after liver transplantation and are most often due to cyclosporine or tacrolimus. Usually symptoms are relieved simply by reducing the dose of these medications. Neuropathy is reportedly more common with tacrolimus, and switching to cyclosporine may alleviate symptoms. In rare cases, patients may require complete withdrawal of both cyclosporine and tacrolimus under coverage of alternate immunosuppression.

CNS Infections. Opportunistic CNS infections (e.g., *Listeria monocytogenes*, cytomegalovirus, herpesvirus, fungi) are rarely observed after hepatic transplantation, since current protocols emphasize rapid lowering of doses of immunosuppressive agents and corticosteroids. Nonetheless, these infections can occur with few overt manifestations and only as altered mental status or global CNS dysfunction. Diagnosis may require radiologic imaging (CT or MRI), analysis of spinal fluid, or even brain biopsy.

SUMMARY

This chapter discusses several key issues regarding hepatic encephalopathy, including definitions, clinical syndromes, diagnostic tests, precipitants, prognosis, and outcomes with therapy, including hepatic transplantation. The section on pathogenesis defines current knowledge regarding mechanisms of encephalopathy in both acute liver failure and chronic liver disease. The clinician faced with neuropsychiatric syndromes in patients with liver disease must differentiate the nature of the underlying liver disorder (acute liver failure vs. chronic liver disease), evaluate diagnostic test results, and institute appropriate therapy. Generally, the intensivist works in cooperation with a team composed of hepatologists, transplant surgeons, anesthesiologists, and nephrologists. Overall, outcomes of patients with encephalopathy depend on the general condition of the patient, severity of the underlying liver disease, comorbid conditions, and, in cases of acute liver failure, cerebral edema and intracranial hypertension. Liver transplantation, including the option of living donor liver transplantation, may yield favorable outcomes without neurologic sequelae if instituted prior to excessive and prolonged intracranial hypertension in the case of acute liver failure, or prior to multiorgan failure in the case of chronic liver disease.

ANNOTATED REFERENCES

Larsen FS: Optimal management of patients with fulminant hepatic failure: Targeting the brain. Hepatology 2004;39:299-301.
Good review article.

Clemmesen O, Ott P, Larsen FS: Splanchnic metabolism in acute liver failure and sepsis. Curr Opin Crit Care 2004;10:152-155.
The capability of the liver to extract oxygen, even under extreme conditions, renders the liver less prone to hypoxia. There is increasing evidence that both acute liver failure and sepsis are accompanied by a hypermetabolic state in the hepatosplanchnic area, characterized by enhanced glycolysis and hyperlactatemia. This should not be rigorously interpreted as an indication of hypoxia. In fact, clinically important splanchnic hypoxia may be a relatively uncommon phenomenon in such patients.

Als-Nielsen B, Gluud L, Gluud C: Dopaminergic agonists for hepatic encephalopathy. Cochrane Database Syst Rev 2004;4:CD003047.
Hepatic encephalopathy may be associated with an impairment of the dopaminergic neurotransmission, thus dopaminergic agonists may have a beneficial effect. This study did not find conclusive evidence that dopaminergic agonists are of benefit to patients with acute or chronic hepatic encephalopathy, or fulminant hepatic failure, but was limited by the small number of trials performed within this field and the low number of patients randomized in each trial.

Chapter 120

FULMINANT HEPATIC FAILURE, INCLUDING ACETAMINOPHEN TOXICITY

Murugan Raghavan • Peter K. Linden

KEY POINTS

1. **Fulminant hepatic failure (FHF) is distinguished from severe acute hepatitis** by the presence of hepatic encephalopathy and carries a transplant-free mortality of 50% to 80%.

2. Intentional and accidental **acetaminophen overdose remains the dominant cause of FHF** in the United States and is potentiated by concurrent alcohol ingestion, glycogen depletion, and anticonvulsant medication.

3. **The King's College Criteria** remain the most widely used prognostic scoring system for FHF; however, failure to fulfill the criteria does not reliably predict survival.

4. **Transjugular liver biopsy may be valuable for determining prognosis** based on the amount of hepatic necrosis and/or the presence of hepatic regeneration and may help to determine the etiology in enigmatic cases.

5. **The onset of grade III or IV hepatic encephalopathy** prognosticates a higher transplant-free mortality and is the most important clue to provide airway protection and perform both diagnostic and therapeutic modalities for intracranial hypertension.

6. **Intracranial hypertension is the major cause for early mortality** in FHF and is due to cerebral hyperemia, osmotic factors, and derangements of the blood-brain barrier.

7. **Cerebral hyperemia** can be detected by a decreased cerebral arteriovenous oxygen content difference or by transcranial Doppler showing elevated systolic blood flow velocity.

8. **Continuous monitoring of intracranial pressure** should begin with grade III encephalopathy and is most safely performed with an epidural pressure transducer.

9. **Elevated ICP** can be managed with hyperventilation, mannitol, mild hypothermia, therapeutic sedation, and other less proven interventions; however, the optimal management of this condition remains unknown.

10. **Prophylactic administration of fresh frozen plasma** does not improve survival and may aggravate volume overload and cerebral edema.

11. **Continuous venovenous hemofiltration is the optimal method for artificial renal replacement** to avoid hemodynamic fluctuations that may aggravate cerebral hyperperfusion or hypoperfusion.

12. **Liver transplantation is the only proven liver replacement therapy to reduce mortality**. Both biologic and nonbiologic artificial liver replacement therapies have shown promise but remain unproven to reduce transplant-free mortality.

Acute liver failure (ALF), also known as fulminant hepatic failure (FHF), embraces a spectrum of clinical entities characterized by acute liver injury, severe hepatocellular dysfunction, and hepatic encephalopathy. This condition is uncommon but not rare; it affects approximately 2000 people annually in the United States with a mortality ranging from 50% to 90% despite intensive care therapy.[1] Loss of hepatocyte function sets in motion a vicious multiorgan dysfunction syndrome, with ensuing death even when the liver has begun to recover. Complications of acute liver failure include encephalopathy, cerebral edema, sepsis, acute respiratory distress syndrome (ARDS), hypoglycemia, gastrointestinal bleeding, pancreatitis, and acute renal failure. Acetaminophen toxicity, idiosyncratic drug reactions, and hepatotropic viruses remain the most common cause of FHF in the United States. Orthotopic liver transplantation (OLT) is currently the only proven and definitive treatment option for these patients, who are unlikely to recover spontaneously. Unfortunately, many patients die before a suitable organ can be identified. Thus, the dominant medical interventions for acute liver failure in the critical care setting are supportive. Alternative "liver replacement" therapeutic strategies are under clinical investigation.

DEFINITIONS

Fulminant hepatic failure is defined as the appearance of hepatic encephalopathy in a patient with acute deterioration of liver function with no previous history of liver disease. Since the original definition of FHF proposed by Trey and

TABLE 120–1. CLASSIFICATIONS OF ACUTE LIVER FAILURE

Trey and Davidson[2]

Fulminant hepatic failure: development of HE within 8 weeks of onset of symptoms

British Classification[6]

Acute liver failure (includes only patients with encephalopathy)
Subclassification depending on the interval between jaundice and HE:
- Hyperacute liver failure: 0 to 7 days
- Acute liver failure: 8 to 28 days
- Subacute liver failure: 29 to 72 days
- Late-onset acute liver failure: 56 to 182 days

French Classification[3]

Acute hepatic failure: a rapidly developing impairment of liver function
Severe acute hepatic failure: prothrombin time or factor V concentration below 50% of normal with or without HE
Subclassification:
- Fulminant hepatic failure: HE within 2 weeks of onset of jaundice
- Subfulminant hepatic failure: HE between 3 and 12 weeks of onset of jaundice

International Association for the Study of Acute Liver Failure[5]

Acute liver failure (occurrence of HE within 4 weeks after onset of symptoms)
Subclassification:
- Acute liver failure—hyperacute: within 10 days
- Acute liver failure—fulminant: 10 to 30 days
- Acute liver failure—not otherwise specified
- Subacute liver failure (development of ascites and/or HE from 5 to 24 weeks after onset of symptoms)

HE, hepatic encephalopathy.

Davidson in 1970, several other classifications have emerged (Table 120-1).[2-6] In different classifications, the interval between the onset of symptoms or jaundice and the appearance of encephalopathy allows grouping of patients with similar causes, clinical characteristics, and prognosis.

ACUTE SEVERE HEPATITIS

Acute hepatitis with jaundice and coagulopathy without hepatic encephalopathy is referred to as severe acute hepatitis. Prognosis remains excellent. However, some people may progress to liver failure or develop chronic hepatitis, therefore mandating close observation.

FULMINANT HEPATIC FAILURE

Fulminant hepatic failure is defined as the development of encephalopathy within 2 weeks of onset of jaundice. The most common causes include acetaminophen toxicity, idiosyncratic drug reactions, and the viral hepatitides (A, B, D, and E). Although many with people with FHF die, recovery is possible without transplantation. Patients who survive FHF have no long-term sequelae with normal hepatic architecture and no chronic liver disease. Rarely, patients with viral hepatitis B or B with D coinfection develop chronic viral hepatitis.

SUBFULMINANT HEPATIC FAILURE

When jaundice develops more insidiously and the onset of encephalopathy is delayed for up to 8 to 12 weeks, the condition is classified as subfulminant hepatic failure (SFHF). Patients may develop liver failure several months after an initial insult. SFHF is most commonly caused by viral infections, idiosyncratic drug reactions, and autoimmune hepatitis. Prognosis is poor without transplantation, and those who survive may develop chronic liver disease.

ETIOLOGY

Whereas viral hepatitis remains the most common identifiable cause of FHF worldwide, acetaminophen toxicity and idiosyncratic drug reactions have replaced viral hepatitis as the most frequent apparent causes of acute liver failure in the United States in recent years.[7,8] Children have indeterminate causes, accounting for more than 50% of pediatric cases. Data from the National Institutes of Health Acute Liver Failure Study involving 308 patients (73% female with a median age of 38 years) from 17 centers in the United States were reported recently (Fig. 120-1).[7] Acetaminophen overdose was the most common apparent cause of acute liver failure, accounting for 39% of cases in the United States. Idiosyncratic drug reactions were the presumptive cause in 13% of cases, viral hepatitides A and B combined were implicated in 12% of cases, and 17% of cases were of indeterminate cause. Overall transplant-free patient survival at 3 weeks was 67%. Twenty-nine percent of patients had liver transplantation, and 43% survived without transplantation. Short-term transplant-free survival varied greatly, from 68% for patients with acetaminophen-related liver failure to 25% and 17% for those with other drug reactions and liver failure of indeterminate cause, respectively.

ACETAMINOPHEN TOXICITY

Acetaminophen overdose is now the leading cause of ALF in the United States and accounts for 39% of cases of FHF. This type of liver injury occurs both after attempted suicide by acetaminophen overdose and after unintentional "therapeutic misadventures" caused by use of the drug for pain relief in excess of the dose specified in the package labeling, typically over a period of several days.[9] A careful medical history clarifies the quantity ingested; blood levels can be confirmatory but may not be elevated in cases of unintentional overdose. Doses considered nontoxic (<4 g/day in adults, <8 mg/kg in infants) might cause hepatotoxicity if other concurrent factors exist, such as alcohol ingestion, fasting, or malnutrition. Hepatotoxicity usually develops 1 to 2 days after the overdose, and circulating alanine aminotransferase levels and prothrombin time reach their peak around day 3. A continued increase of prothrombin time after day 3 is associated with a 90% mortality rate. Acetaminophen is also nephrotoxic, and renal failure may occur in the absence of liver necrosis.

Acetaminophen undergoes phase 1 metabolism by hepatic cytochrome (CYP) P_{450} 2E1 enzymes to a toxic intermediate compound, N-acetyl-*para*-benzoquine-imide (NAPQI), which is rapidly detoxified by hepatic glutathione into a nontoxic metabolite. Under normal conditions, little NAPQI accumulates. However, in an overdose, owing to depletion of glutathione stores, unconjugated NAPQI accumulates and causes hepatocellular necrosis. The amount of liver injury is directly related to the amount of ingested acetaminophen and the amount of NAPQI that is produced. Enzyme inducers, such as alcohol, antiepileptic drugs, and cigarette smoke can

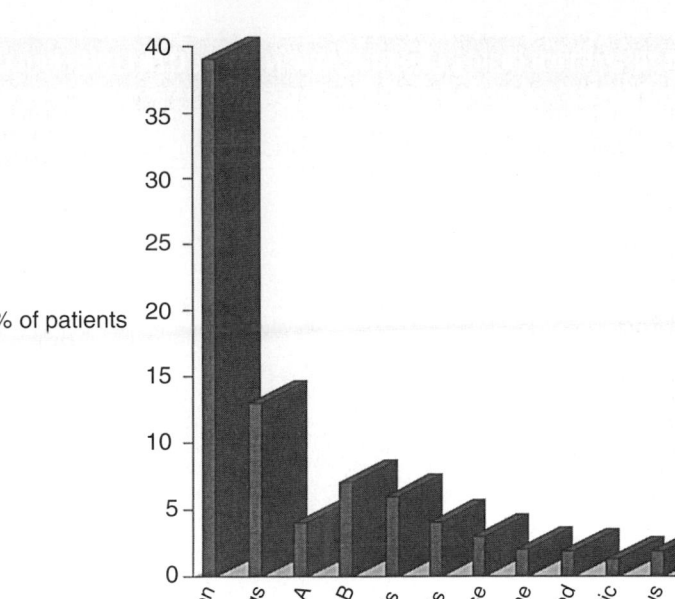

FIGURE 120–1. Etiology of acute liver failure in United States among patients referred for liver transplantation. (From Ostapowicz G, Fontana RJ, Schiodt FV, et al: Results of a prospective study of acute liver failure at 17 tertiary care centers in the United States. Ann Intern Med 2002;137:947-954.)

enhance acetaminophen-mediated hepatotoxicity. Chronic alcohol consumption induces synthesis of CYP2EI enzymes and, to a lesser extent, depletes glutathione stores. Substrate competition for cytochrome P_{450} 2E1 occurs between ethanol and acetaminophen when the two drugs are taken simultaneously. During the metabolism of acetaminophen, NAPQI formation is diminished when alcohol is present. The rate at which CYP2E1 degrades is also slowed, and the half-life of the enzyme increases, from 7 hours to 37 hours. As long as ethanol remains in the body there is competition between acetaminophen and ethanol for CYP2E1; however, once ethanol is removed, NAPQI formation is enhanced, resulting in enhanced hepatic injury in the 24 hours after cessation of alcohol consumption. Genetic variability within the population affecting expression of the cytokine, tumor necrosis factor-alpha (TNF-α) also has been implicated as a determining factor in the severity of drug reactions related to acetaminophen.[10]

IDIOSYNCRATIC DRUG REACTIONS

Drug-induced liver damage is a significant cause of death in patients with ALF in Western countries (Table 120-2). Idiosyncratic drug reactions constitute up 13% of cases of severe liver injury in United States. For reasons that are unclear, women generally predominate among patients with idiosyncratic drug-induced liver injury. Other risk factors for drug-induced hepatotoxicity include very young and very old age, abnormal renal function, obesity, preexisting liver disease, and concurrent use of other hepatotoxic drugs. Idiosyncratic drug toxicities are immunologically mediated by the drug itself or its metabolites. Most idiosyncratic reactions occur within 4 to 6 weeks after initiation of treatment, although rare cases have occurred months or years later. Idiosyncratic drug toxicities often culminate in SFHF and carry a poor prognosis without liver transplant.

Idiosyncratic hepatic injury is mediated by several mechanisms, including disruption of intracellular calcium homeostasis, injury to canalicular transport pumps, such as multidrug-resistance-associated protein 3 (MRP3), T cell–mediated immunologic injury, triggering of apoptotic pathways by TNF-α, and inhibition of mitochondrial beta oxidation.[11] Isoniazid, pyrazinamide, antimicrobials (amoxicillin-clavulanate, tetracyclines, and macrolides), anticonvulsants, antidepressants, nonsteroidal anti-inflammatory drugs, and halothane are most frequently implicated in FHF. Two histologic patterns are usually distinguished, one being characterized by confluent necrosis (isoniazid or halothane) and the other by hepatocyte microvesicular fatty change (valproic acid or tetracyclines). Reemergence of tuberculosis in the past decade has increased the frequency of FHF caused by isoniazid. Concurrent treatment with rifampicin and pyrazinamide may increase the risk of isoniazid toxicity.

Hepatotoxic herbal medicines (kava, St. John's wart) and certain dietary supplements are emerging as potential causes in a high proportion of patients with FHF.[12] Mushroom poisoning due to *Amanita phalloides* is relatively common in Europe, and more sporadic cases occur in the United States. Florid muscarinic effects such as sweating or watery diarrhea occur early, whereas FHF usually occurs 4 to 8 days after mushroom ingestion. Other toxins (e.g., carbon tetrachloride, yellow phosphorus, aflatoxins) are rare causes of FHF. Liver biopsy is seldom helpful for establishing the diagnosis.

VIRAL HEPATITIDES

Whereas viral hepatitides remain the most common identifiable cause of FHF worldwide, considerable geographic variation exists in the subtype of hepatitides. Thus, hepatitis B virus (HBV) is a common cause of FHF in the Far East and hepatitis E virus (HEV) is more prevalent in the Indian subcontinent.[13] In the United States, approximately 12% of FHF

TABLE 120–2. ETIOLOGIC CLASSIFICATION OF ACUTE LIVER FAILURE

Acetaminophen Toxicity

Idiosyncratic Drug Injury

Infrequent Agents
  Isoniazid
  Valproate
  Halothane
  Phenytoin
  Sulfonamides
  Propylthiouracil
  Amiodarone
  Disulfiram
  Dapsone
  Bromfenac
  Troglitazone
  Zidovudine
  Lamivudine
  Lamotrigine
  Gatifloxacin
  Methotrexate
Miscellaneous Agents
  Ecstasy
  Cocaine
  Phencyclidine
Rare Agents
  Carbamazepine
  Ofloxacin
  Ketoconazole
  Lisinopril
  Nicotinic acid
  Labetalol
  Etoposide
  Imipramine
  Interferon alfa
  Flutamide
  Tolcapone
  Nefazodone
  Oral contraceptives
Combination agents with enhanced hepatotoxicity
  Alcohol-acetaminophen

Trimethoprim-sulfamethoxazole
Rifampicin-isoniazid
Amoxicillin-clavulanic acid

Viral Hepatitides

Hepatitis A, B, C, D, E, G
Human herpesvirus
Cytomegalovirus
Epstein-Barr virus
Herpes simplex virus
Varicella-zoster virus
Paramyxovirus
Parvovirus B19
Adenovirus
Togavirus
Parvovirus
SEN virus
TT virus
Yellow fever virus

Toxins

CCL_4
Amanita phalloides
Yellow phosphorus
Herbal products

Vascular

Ischemic
Veno-occlusive disease
Budd-Chiari syndrome
Malignant infiltration
Non-Hodgkin's lymphomas

Miscellaneous

Wilson's disease
Autoimmune hepatitis
Acute fatty liver of pregnancy
Reye's syndrome

---

referred for liver transplants are due to hepatitis A and B. Occurrence of FHF within the larger number of patients with viral hepatitis, however, is rare (0.2% to 0.4% for hepatitis A, 1% to 4% for hepatitis B).

Hepatitis A virus (HAV) is associated with a higher risk of developing FHF if infection is acquired in older adulthood. Thus, vaccination is recommended for adults traveling from developed countries to endemic areas. The relevance of HAV as a cause of FHF in patients with preexisting chronic liver disease has been recognized recently. HAV vaccination in this high-risk group has been suggested. Postexposure prophylaxis with immune serum globulin may reduce the incidence of hepatitis A but only when administered within 14 days of exposure.

HBV can result in ALF through several mechanisms: acute primary HBV infections, reactivation of hepatitis B in patients with chronic HBV, superinfection with hepatitis D virus, and spontaneous seroconversion of individual from HBV e antigen to HBV e antibody. Acute HBV infection is diagnosed by the detection of IgM antibodies against hepatitis B core antigen (HbcAg) because a substantial number of patients have negative serum hepatitis B surface antigen (HBsAg) and serum HBV-DNA. Low or absent levels of HBsAg and HBV-DNA are associated with better prognosis and lower rate of recurrence after orthotopic liver transplantation.[14] FHF after reactivation of chronic hepatitis B has been

described mainly in immunosuppressed male patients; this form of the disease usually has a subfulminant course and a poor prognosis.

Most studies indicate that hepatitis C virus (HCV) infection alone does not result in FHF. However, isolated cases of HCV-RNA in serum or tissue of patients with FHF and negative markers for other viruses have been noted in Western countries.[15] Involvement of HCV in FHF is slightly more common in the Far East.[16] An increased risk of FHF in patients with chronic hepatitis B and superinfection by HCV has been suggested.

Acute liver failure is seen in 2.5% to 6% of hepatitis D virus cases. Coinfection with HBV and hepatitis D virus (HDV) or superinfection by HDV in patients with chronic hepatitis B can also cause FHF. The incidence of coinfection is higher when intravenous drug abuse is present. Diagnosis of acute infection by HDV is made by the presence of HDV antigen, anti-HDV IgM antibody, or HDV-RNA.

Infection by hepatitis E virus (HEV) is uncommon in Western countries but occurs in travelers to endemic areas. Pregnant women infected by HEV seem to have a special propensity for developing FHF. Diagnosis is made by detection of anti-HEV IgM antibodies.

Other viruses have been implicated in the pathogenesis of FHF of indeterminate etiology. These viruses include cytomegalovirus (CMV), human herpesvirus-6 (HHV-6),[17,18] Epstein-Barr virus (EBV), hepatitis G virus (HGV),[19] herpes simplex virus (HSV),[20,21] varicella-zoster virus (VZV), parvovirus B19 in children, and togavirus, adenovirus, paramyxovirus, yellow fever, Q fever, and, most recently, SEN virus and TT virus.[22] Although these causes are rare, they must be excluded because some patients may benefit from specific antiviral therapy.

Miscellaneous cardiovascular, metabolic, and other disorders account for 2% to 10% of cases of FHF. Acute liver ischemia secondary to shock states can result in hepatocellular necrosis; however, the prognosis remains good if the primary condition can be corrected. The prognosis is worse when FHF is due to other causes, such as Budd-Chiari syndrome, veno-occlusive disease, or malignancies associated with impaired hepatic blood flow. Rarely, the first manifestation of Wilson's disease is FHF, but underlying cirrhosis is always present. Death is universal without OLT. Acute fatty liver of pregnancy is rare, occurring in the third trimester of pregnancy, and usually responds well to fetal delivery. Other causes of FHF are autoimmune hepatitis, non-Hodgkin's lymphoma, or Reye's syndrome, the last being less common in the pediatric population since aspirin use has been curtailed.

PROGNOSTIC SCORING SYSTEMS

Survival in patients with ALF depends on many factors, including etiology, age, severity of liver dysfunction, degree of liver necrosis, nature of complications, and duration of illness. Patients with grade IV encephalopathy have greater than 80% mortality without liver transplantation. The successful use of OLT in FHF has created a need for early prognostic indicators to select patients most likely to benefit from OLT. Various prognostic scoring systems exist (Table 120-3).

For patients with acetaminophen overdose, HAV infection, shock liver, or pregnancy-related acute liver failure, the short-term survival without transplantation is 50% or greater. Patients whose liver disease was of indeterminate cause or was presumed to be related to drugs other than acetaminophen, HBV infection, autoimmune hepatitis, Wilson's disease, the Budd-Chiari syndrome, or cancer have lower rates of short-term transplant-free survival (<25%).

The King's College prognostic criteria are the most widely used. These criteria provide a reasonably accurate prediction of the likelihood of death and the need for transplantation in FHF patients.[23] The criteria are different for acetaminophen and non–acetaminophen-induced FHF (see Table 120-3). However, failure to fulfill King's College criteria does not predict survival. The APACHE II system has been found to be equal to King's College criteria for accuracy in predicting death in acetaminophen-induced FHF.[24] Other approaches include the Cliché criteria,[25] which uses factor V assay, factor VIII/V ratio, serial alpha-fetoprotein levels, and plasma group-specific component protein (Gc globulin) levels.[26,27] Liver volume decreases with progression of the disease, and its measurement with computed tomography (CT) may help to assess prognosis. Other proposed prognostic tools include the proportion of necrosis as assessed by histologic examination of specimens obtained by liver biopsy, the amount of fresh frozen plasma that is required to correct coagulopathy, or the determination of somatosensory evoked potentials. Recently, high serum levels of phosphate and lactate have

TABLE 120–3. VARIOUS PROGNOSTIC CRITERIA USED FOR LIVER TRANSPLANTATION IN PATIENTS WITH FULMINANT HEPATIC FAILURE

King's College Criteria[23]

Acetaminophen Overdose
- Arterial pH < 7.3 (irrespective of grade of encephalopathy)
  or
- PT >100 sec (INR > 6.5)
- Serum creatinine > 3.4 mg/dL (>300 µmol/L)
- Patients with grade III and IV hepatic encephalopathy

Non-acetaminophen Liver Injury
- PT > 100 sec (INR > 6.5) (irrespective of grade of encephalopathy) *or* any three of the following variables:
- Age < 10 or > 40 yr
- Non-A, non-B hepatitis, halothane hepatitis, idiosyncratic drug reactions
- Jaundice > 7 days before onset of encephalopathy
- Serum bilirubin 17.4 mg/dL (300 µmol/L)
- PT > 50 sec

Cliché Criteria[25]

- Factor V < 20% in person < 30 years
  or both of the following:
- Factor V < 30% in patients > 30 years
- Grade III or IV encephalopathy

Serum Gc Globulin Levels[26,27]

Decreasing Gc levels due to dying hepatocytes

Serum Alpha-Fetoprotein Level

Serial increase from day 1 to day 3 has shown correlation with survival

Liver Biopsy[31]

70% necrosis is discriminant of 90% mortality

PT, Prothrombin time; INR, International Normalized Ratio; Gc, plasma group-specific component protein.

been proposed as markers of poor prognosis in patients with acetaminophen-induced FHF.[28-30]

ROLE OF LIVER BIOPSY

Liver biopsy may confirm the suspected cause of FHF and determine the degree of hepatocyte necrosis. Greater than 70% necrosis in a liver biopsy specimen is associated with 90% mortality without transplantation.[31] Because severe coagulopathy precludes safe percutaneous liver biopsy, the transjugular approach is often preferred. Although a liver biopsy is not mandatory, it can be valuable both for determining prognosis and making the decision for early transplantation. Liver biopsy also can help to exclude occult malignancy in enigmatic cases. Liver biopsy also can be used to assess the liver for evidence of regeneration, as manifested by the presence of liver cell mitosis. In rare cases, the liver biopsy can provide etiologic information that enables specific therapy to be instituted, as in the cases of HSV, CMV, adenovirus, and paramyxovirus hepatitis infections. Because of the variable nature of liver biopsies in patients with FHF, a minimum of three, and ideally six, specimens of the hepatic parenchyma should be obtained for histologic evaluation. In addition, in patients in whom Wilson's disease or hepatic iron toxicity is possible, a separate core of liver tissue should be obtained for quantitative hepatic iron and copper determinations.

PATHOGENESIS AND CLINICAL FEATURES OF ACUTE LIVER FAILURE

Acute liver failure has a particular constellation of clinical features that are distinct from those seen with chronic hepatic insufficiency, regardless of the etiology. Typically, nonspecific symptoms, such as malaise or nausea, develop in a previously healthy person, followed by jaundice, rapid onset of altered mental status, and coma. Altered mentation and a prolonged prothrombin time are the hallmarks of the diagnosis. Supportive laboratory findings include high levels of serum aminotransferases, a variable elevation of serum total bilirubin concentration, low serum glucose levels, and arterial blood gas studies showing respiratory alkalosis and/or metabolic acidosis. Patients with SFHF have a more gradual onset of hepatic insufficiency, accompanied by ascites, renal failure, and a very poor prognosis. Cerebral edema is infrequent in such patients. The magnitude of elevation of aminotransferase levels and rate of decline does not affect the prognosis. When patients spontaneously recover, the serum bilirubin concentration and prothrombin time normalize, whereas when the disease progresses, bilirubin levels continue to increase (due to intrahepatic cholestasis) and prothrombin time remains prolonged, despite declining aminotransferase levels. The high mortality rates associated with ALF are caused by complications such as cerebral edema, renal failure, sepsis, pancreatitis, and cardiopulmonary collapse, which results in multisystem organ failure.

ENCEPHALOPATHY

The presence of encephalopathy is the essential clinical feature that differentiates FHF from acute severe hepatitis, and the time to onset after the appearance of jaundice distinguishes FHF from SFHF. The onset of encephalopathy is often abrupt and may occasionally precede the appearance of jaundice. Agitation, delusional ideas, and hyperkinesis are common but short-lived symptoms; coma rapidly ensues. The overall prognosis for those with stable grade I or II encephalopathy is good, whereas the prognosis for patients with grade III or IV encephalopathy is much poorer. In cases of acetaminophen overdose, encephalopathy usually occurs on the third or fourth day after ingestion and rapidly progresses to stage IV within 24 to 48 hours.

The pathophysiology of hepatic encephalopathy is poorly understood and is probably multifactorial. Ammonia and other putative markers have been identified and include endogenous substances, false neurotransmitters, short-chain fatty acids, benzodiazepines, and γ-aminobutyric acid. The electroencephalogram (EEG) typically shows diffuse slowing of cortical activity and high amplitude waveforms at 5 to 7 cycles per second. Subclinical seizure activity is often present in patients with grade III and IV encephalopathy, emphasizing the importance of EEG monitoring in these patients. Prophylactic therapy with phenytoin has been shown to reduce seizure activity and reduce cerebral edema.[32] Seizure activity in FHF has been linked to excessive central nervous system glutamine, the main excitatory neurotransmitter in the brain.

CEREBRAL EDEMA

Cerebral edema is estimated to occur in 75% to 80% of patients progressing to grade IV encephalopathy, and it is the leading cause of death in these patients. The mechanism(s) responsible for cerebral edema are only partially understood. Possible contributing factors include cerebral hyperemia, vasogenic edema due to disruption of the blood-brain barrier with rapid accumulation of low-molecular-weight substances, cytotoxicity due to the osmotic effects of ammonia, glutamine, and other amino acids, as well as the deleterious effects of proinflammatory cytokines and dysfunction of the sodium-potassium ATPase pump with loss of autoregulation of cerebral blood flow.[33,34] Intracranial blood flow is markedly reduced in patients with chronic hepatic encephalopathy; the decrease in perfusion appropriately matches the reduction in cerebral metabolic rate (CMR). However, patients with FHF often develop either relative or absolute cerebral hyperemia; thus, perfusion is not well matched to the reduced CMR present in evolving or established hepatic coma. An early indicator of this pathologic process is either a decrease in the transcranial oxygen content difference (arterial oxygen content – jugular bulb oxygen content) to less than 4 mL/dL blood or an increase in middle cerebral artery systolic blood flow velocity. Serial transcranial Doppler ultrasonographic monitoring of cerebral blood flow velocity helps to detect early cerebral hyperperfusion or hypoperfusion, suggesting impaired cerebral autoregulation.[35,36] Cerebral ischemia and permanent neurologic sequelae may occur (even after liver transplantation) if cerebral perfusion pressure (CPP), calculated as mean systemic arterial blood pressure minus intracranial pressure, is not maintained above 40 to 50 mm Hg. CT of the brain often fails to demonstrate cerebral edema in patients with elevated intracranial pressure. Late clinical stages of cerebral edema include systemic hypertension, decerebrate rigidity, hyperventilation, pupillary dilation, seizures, and brainstem herniation. An arterial ammonia level greater than 200 µg/dL in stage III and IV encephalopathy is a strong predictor of brain herniation.[37] Full recovery of cerebral function is the rule if normal liver function returns, but permanent brain damage has been observed in patients making an otherwise complete hepatic recovery.

COAGULOPATHY

Severe alterations in coagulation are typical of FHF and are due to impaired hepatic synthetic function, leading to inadequate production of coagulation factors. Decreased levels of factors II, V, VII, IX, and X account for the prolonged prothrombin time (PT) and activated partial thromboplastin time (aPTT) observed. Failure to observe an increase in circulating levels of the vitamin K–dependent factor VII by 25% after intravenous administration of vitamin K suggests that hepatic synthetic reserve is inadequate.[38] Many anticoagulation factors, such as proteins C and S, are synthesized by the liver, and activated coagulation factors are removed by the liver. Disruption of the balance between procoagulant and anticoagulant factors may result in excessive thrombosis and disseminated intravascular coagulation (DIC), and the laboratory distinction between the two is often difficult. Platelet counts are less than 100,000/mm³ in two thirds of patients at some point in their clinical course, and platelet function is altered. Hemorrhage from the gastrointestinal tract or elsewhere is common in FHF and most often correlates with a low platelet count; platelet transfusion may be necessary for patients with counts less than 50,000/mm³. Fresh frozen plasma has not been shown to be of value in the absence of bleeding.

METABOLIC DERANGEMENTS

FHF results in myriad metabolic abnormalities. Hypoglycemia is seen in up to 45% of patients with FHF. This abnormality is caused by depletion of hepatic glycogen stores and impaired gluconeogenesis and may be refractory to infusion of intravenous dextrose solution. Hepatic insulin resistance and impaired peripheral insulin sensitivity are often present.[39] Metabolic acidosis is common in acetaminophen-induced FHF and carries a poor prognosis. Hyponatremia, alkalosis, hypokalemia, hypophosphatemia, and lactic acidosis are common. Ionized hypocalcemia may indicate concomitant pancreatitis. Acute renal failure is seen in 30% to 70% of patients with acute liver failure and results from a combination of several factors, such as intravascular volume depletion, sepsis, DIC, or direct nephrotoxicity from drugs such as acetaminophen or nonsteroidal anti-inflammatory drugs (NSAIDs). Adrenal insufficiency has been described in up to 62% of patients with FHF when assessed by the change in plasma cortisol concentration after injection of synthetic ACTH (cosyntropin stimulation testing).[40] Hemodynamically unstable patients with adrenal dysfunction may benefit from replacement stress doses of hydrocortisone.

CARDIOVASCULAR, HEMODYNAMIC, AND RESPIRATORY COMPLICATIONS

Circulatory dysfunction accompanying FHF often mimics sepsis. Typically, patients are hyperdynamic and calculated systemic vascular resistance is low. Vasodilation is thought to be due to the proinflammatory effects of circulating endotoxin and cytokines. Relative hypovolemia secondary to reduced systemic vascular resistance can make it difficult to assess the adequacy of intravascular volume, prompting insertion of pulmonary artery catheters. Cardiac arrhythmias occur frequently owing to either electrolyte imbalances or increased circulating levels of catecholamines (from endogenous release or deliberate infusion). Severe peripheral shunting has been observed in acute liver failure and may result from the plugging of small vessels by platelets, interstitial edema, or abnormal vasomotor tone, although the exact mechanism is unclear. Severely diminished tissue oxygen extraction is more common in nonsurvivors. An abnormal pattern of oxygen supply dependency results in oxygen extraction over a wider-than-normal range of oxygen delivery, presumably as a compensatory mechanism. Prostacyclin, which has microcirculatory vasodilator effects, has been shown to increase peripheral oxygen uptake.[41]

Hyperventilation, hypercapnia, and respiratory alkalosis occur during acute liver failure and may worsen encephalopathy. Arterial hypoxemia is universal and is caused by a combination of intrapulmonary shunting, ventilation/perfusion mismatching, sepsis, aspiration, and ARDS.

SEPSIS

FHF results are associated with impaired host resistance to and enhanced risk for bacterial and fungal infections. Between 10% to 80% of FHF patients experience infections with an attributable mortality rate of 10% to 37%. Common infections are aspiration pneumonia and primary bloodstream infections, including candidemia. The most common microbial causes are gram-positive bacteria (*Staphylococcus aureus*,

enterococci), enteric gram-negative bacilli (*Escherichia coli*, *Klebsiella* species), and *Candida* species. Diminished hepatic reticuloendothelial function and opsonic activity, defective polymorphonuclear leukocyte function, and impaired cell-mediated and humoral immunity are the major predisposing mechanisms. In one prospective study of 50 patients, 80% had culture-proven infection, and in half of the remaining patients, infection was suspected but cultures were negative.[42] Regular microbial surveillance and aggressive treatment of presumed infection are essential, because prophylactic antibiotic regimens have shown little benefit.

MANAGEMENT

Optimal management of FHF begins with the recognition that any patient with acute liver disease may die suddenly and is best cared for in an intensive care unit. Because the transportation of patients with advanced levels of coma is hazardous and the disease often worsens rapidly, transfer to a liver transplantation center should be considered at the time of admission of any patient with altered mentation. Because the liver has a unique ability to regenerate after acute, self-limited injury, treatment is limited to general supportive measures until the liver recovers. Elucidation of the cause of hepatic failure allows some patients to benefit from specific therapies and may influence post-transplant management if a transplant is performed.

THERAPY DIRECTED AT THE SPECIFIC ETIOLOGY OF FHF

Depending on the suspected or confirmed FHF etiology, a number of therapies may exist that can ameliorate or reverse the degree of liver injury. *N*-Acetylcysteine (NAC) is used as a specific antidote for acetaminophen overdose. If given within the first 8 to 10 hours after an acute overdose, this drug replenishes glutathione stores and prevents the development of hepatotoxicity. The efficacy of NAC declines progressively thereafter, but it may be effective up to 72 hours after acetaminophen ingestion.[43] However, most authors recommend that NAC be given to all patients with acetaminophen-induced FHF, regardless of time of ingestion. It is used differently in Europe (intravenous formulation, total dose of 300 mg/kg over 20 hours) than in the United States (oral formulation, total dose of 1330 mg/kg over 72 hours). The poor oral bioavailability of NAC explains the high doses used in the United States. Although the intravenous formulation is not approved by the U.S. Food and Drug Administration, it has been utilized in patients with compromised gastrointestinal function due to gastroparesis, ileus, or pancreatitis. NAC is also used in Europe to treat established FHF of any cause, based on clinical reports from the King's College group. Benefits of NAC on survival, brain edema, hemodynamics, oxygen delivery, and oxygen consumption were found in patients with established FHF[43]; however, these effects were not confirmed by other groups.[44] A randomized, controlled trial of NAC by the U.S. Acute Liver Failure Study Group in patients with non–acetaminophen-induced FHF is underway and should clarify these issues.

In *Amanita* intoxication, beneficial effects have been reported with the use of penicillin G, cimetidine, silymarin, and forced diuresis. Activated charcoal and cathartic agents may be useful if they are given early after mushroom ingestion.

Hepatitis secondary to HSV may be missed because of its nonspecific presentation and the absence of typical mucocutaneous lesions. Most patients with HSV hepatitis are immunocompetent hosts. If HSV hepatitis is suspected, treatment with parenteral acyclovir or ganciclovir should be started.

In patients with Wilson's disease, plasma exchange with fresh frozen plasma replacement is preferred, because this intervention can remove relatively large amounts of copper in a short period of time.[45] Net copper removal is proportional to plasma concentration and can reach 12 mg per session. In the absence of renal failure, chelating therapy can also be employed. Hemofiltration and albumin dialysis have also been described as temporizing measures before OLT.[46]

Autoimmune hepatitis is usually treated with a course of methylprednisolone (40 to 60 mg every 6 hours). Acute fatty liver of pregnancy usually responds to fetal delivery. Urgent chemotherapy is indicated for FHF caused by massive infiltration of the liver by lymphoma. Acute Budd-Chiari syndrome may be amenable to thrombolytic therapy or to transjugular intrahepatic portosystemic shunt placement.

HEPATIC ENCEPHALOPATHY

The treatment of encephalopathy associated with FHF is directed at limiting gut ammonia production and the avoidance of aggravating factors such as infection, ileus, obstipation, gastrointestinal hemorrhage, and other central nervous system depressants. Lactulose may be useful in the treatment of patients with grade 1 or 2 encephalopathy; however, administration of lactulose does not improve survival in advanced encephalopathy. The efficacy of lactulose in FHF has not been tested in clinical trials. This agent should be used with caution because of the risk of hypernatremia, dehydration due to diarrhea, and ileus. Lactulose by enema remains an option in FHF patients who are unable to tolerate oral or nasogastric administration.

Oral metronidazole and neomycin directed against ammonia-producing gut flora have been employed; however, metronidazole may be neurotoxic in hepatic failure and neomycin, although minimally absorbed, can still cause nephrotoxicity and ototoxicity.

Endogenous benzodiazepine-like substances have been identified in the cerebrospinal fluid of patients with hepatic encephalopathy. Flumazenil, a benzodiazepine receptor antagonist, has been used (0.2 mg, up to 20 mg) with some success to provide short-term improvement in patients with hepatic encephalopathy.[47] Various experimental therapies such as exchange transfusion, charcoal hemoperfusion, and plasmapheresis have been used to lower ammonia levels; however, none of these has shown survival benefit.

CEREBRAL EDEMA

The optimal management of cerebral edema requires maintaining the delicate balance between mean arterial pressure and ICP to preserve adequate cerebral perfusion (Table 120-4). Combined cerebral edema and intracranial hypertension is the most common cause of death in patients with FHF when ICP exceeds 30 mm Hg. An arterial ammonia level higher than 200 μg/dL predicts brain herniation.[48] Therefore, ICP monitoring has been recommended for all patients with grade III and IV encephalopathy, especially candidates awaiting

TABLE 120–4. PREVENTATIVE AND THERAPEUTIC INTERVENTIONS FOR PATIENTS WITH CEREBRAL EDEMA AND INTRACRANIAL HYPERTENSION

General Measures

Head elevation at 30 degrees from bed
Minimize tactile and tracheal stimulation, including airway suctioning
Avoid hypovolemia and hypervolemia
Avoid hypertension
Avoid hypercapnia and hypoxemia
Monitor and maintain ICP < 15 mm Hg
Maintain CPP > 50 mm Hg
Monitor and maintain SvjO$_2$ between 55% to 85%
Use serial transcranial Doppler monitoring to titrate therapy

Management of Intracranial Hypertension

Mannitol boluses, 0.5 to 1.0 g/kg
Hyperventilation titrated to a PcO$_2$ of 28 to 30 mm Hg
Induced hypothermia to 32°C
Induced barbiturate coma with pentobarbital titrated to burst suppression of 5 to 10 cycles/sec
CVVH for oliguria and hyperosmolarity (>310 mOsm/L)

Other Unproven Therapies

Prophylactic phenytoin
Indomethacin
High-dose steroids
Plasmapheresis

ICP, Intracranial pressure; CPP, cerebral perfusion pressure; SvjO$_2$, jugular bulb oxygen saturation; CVVH, continuous venovenous hemofiltration.

transplantation; however, this form of monitoring has not been shown to increase survival.[49] ICP should be maintained at less than 15 mm Hg and CPP should be maintained at greater than 50 mm Hg, although transplant-free recovery has been reported in acetaminophen-induced FHF patients despite impaired cerebral perfusion for 2 to 72 hours.[50]

Most centers prefer epidural to subdural or intraparenchymal transducers, because of the lower rate of hemorrhagic and infectious complications.[51] Monitoring of jugular bulb oxygen saturation with a reversed jugular bulb venous catheter also can guide interventions to avoid or treat intracranial hypertension. Decreased venous oxygen saturations (<55%) indicate cerebral ischemia, and high venous oxygen saturations (>85%) indicate either decreased metabolic demands of the brain or cerebral hyperemia (more commonly the latter).

Current recommendations include maintaining the patient's head at a 30-degree upright angle to improve jugular venous outflow. In episodes of intracranial hypertension, a bolus of 0.5 to 1 g/kg of mannitol can be administered intravenously and repeated until plasma osmolarity reaches 310 mOsm/L. Patients with oliguria and renal failure may require hemodialysis to avoid hyperosmolarity. The role of high-dose corticosteroids has not been confirmed, and these agents are not effective in the treatment of cerebral edema associated with acute liver failure. Attempts should also be made to avoid prolonged coughing or tracheal stimulation during suctioning to prevent an acute rise in ICP.

Hyperventilation may reduce cerebral blood flow by 2% to 3% for every millimeter of mercury reduction in PcO$_2$. Moderate hyperventilation (PcO$_2$ = 28 to 30 mm Hg) can be employed to reduce cerebral hyperventilation; however, not all patients are PcO$_2$ responders, and this effect may wane after 48 hours owing to normal equilibration mechanisms.

Excessive cerebral vasoconstriction can be detected as widening of the cerebral arteriovenous oxygen content difference. Serial transcranial Doppler studies help to detect early changes in cerebral blood flow in response to therapy.[52] Induction of mild hypothermia induced with cooling blankets to 32°C has been shown to reduce ICP and cerebral blood flow and improve CPP in patients with FHF.[53] Care must be taken to avoid both cardiac depression and shivering during induced hypothermia. Induction of a barbiturate coma by administering parenteral sodium pentobarbital, sodium pentothal, or propofol titrated to the appearance of 5 to 10 cycles per second of EEG burst suppression can further reduce both cerebral metabolic rate and cerebral blood flow in refractory patients. However, adverse effects such as myocardial depression or arterial hypotension may create the need for inotropic or vasopressor support to preserve CPP in the minimally adequate range.

Indomethacin (25 mg i.v. bolus) has been shown to reduce cerebral blood flow and prevent brain edema in experimental models of FHF, and in isolated cases of FHF in humans, with encouraging results.[54] In a recent controlled clinical trial, prophylactic infusion of phenytoin (15 mg/kg, followed by 100 mg i.v. q 8 h) decreased the incidence of subclinical seizure activity and appeared to prevent brain edema.[32] However, clinical experience with these agents remains scarce, and therefore their efficacy and safety needs further studies.

COAGULOPATHY

Despite severe coagulopathy, patients with FHF seldom have spontaneous hemorrhage. A trial of vitamin K should be given to all patients with FHF, and serial measurements of factor V and VII can be used to help assess prognosis for spontaneous recovery. Routine use of fresh frozen plasma is not recommended unless spontaneous bleeding occurs or an invasive procedure is being contemplated. In those instances, 2 to 4 units of fresh frozen plasma should be administered every 6 to 12 hours, according to the severity of coagulopathy. Platelets should be transfused before invasive procedures if the platelet count is less than 50×10^9/L. Administration of fresh-frozen plasma does not increase survival and may cause volume overload and worsen cerebral edema. Recombinant activated factor VII offers advantages of shorter half-life and avoidance of volume overload, compared with fresh frozen plasma; however, more studies using this agent are needed.[55] When evaluation of mental state is not possible, monitoring of coagulation parameters helps to assess improvement or worsening of liver function.

ACUTE RENAL FAILURE

Patients with combined FHF and renal failure have a grave prognosis without renal support. Mechanisms leading to acute tubular necrosis (ATN) include renal hypoperfusion (due to intravascular volume depletion and reduced mean arterial pressure), deleterious effects of proinflammatory mediators, and direct toxic effects of the etiologic agent responsible for liver injury (e.g., acetaminophen). Optimal fluid balance is paramount in patients with acute liver failure to avoid prerenal azotemia and progression to ATN. Frequent monitoring of serum creatinine level, urinary output, and urinary sodium concentrations is required. Diuretics and "renal dose" dopamine (2 to 4 μg/kg/min) have no protective value in the therapy for acute renal failure

and are potentially harmful. Nephrotoxic drugs, such as aminoglycosides or radiographic contrast agents, should be avoided. Continuous venovenous hemofiltration (CVVH) is superior to intermittent hemodialysis, because this modality avoids the rapid fluid shifts and abrupt changes in ICP that are associated with intermittent dialysis.[56]

MISCELLANEOUS THERAPY

Glycemic control is vital in patients with deep encephalopathy. Constant infusion of 10% to 20% glucose is preferable to bolus administration for maintenance of euglycemia. FHF is a catabolic state, and protein-caloric malnutrition develops quickly. Thus, nutrition should be started soon and adjusted individually to maintain an adequate caloric intake. Enteral nutrition through a nasogastric or nasojejunal tube is preferred to parenteral nutrition. Although aromatic amino acid–free enteral formulas are commercially available, their clinical efficacy and cost-effectiveness are not established. Correction of hypomagnesemia, hypokalemia, or hypophosphatemia is accomplished by supplementation of these substances. H_2-receptor antagonists, proton-pump inhibitors, or sucralfate are used to reduce the incidence of gastrointestinal ulceration.

A high index of suspicion should be maintained for the presence of incubating infection, because fever and leukocytosis are absent in up to 30% of infected patients. Infection must be suspected in the presence of any sudden clinical deterioration, such as worsening encephalopathy or hemodynamic instability, especially if liver function has started to recover.[57] Microbiologic cultures should be obtained from appropriate sites, and empirical antibiotics covering both enteric gram-negative and gram-positive bacteria should be started. Antifungal coverage should be initiated, particularly in patients already on broad-spectrum antibacterial coverage, who have new onset of clinical deterioration. There are no generally accepted guidelines regarding use of prophylactic antibiotics. Their use is supported by recent studies that suggest that infection and progression to deep encephalopathy are highly correlated.[58,59] Two placebo-controlled, randomized studies demonstrated that selective enteral decontamination with a regimen directed at gram-negative bacilli and *Candida* species resulted in lower rates of infection in FHF patients but did not improve survival.[60,61] Selective enteral decontamination, however, does not add any benefit if the patient is already on intravenous antibiotics.

HEPATIC REPLACEMENT THERAPIES

Liver Transplantation
Orthotopic liver transplantation is the only measure that can radically influence the course of FHF. Ten to 15 percent of patients presenting each year with FHF undergo transplantation; 1-year survival is 65% to 89%.[62] However, transplantation is an expensive and high-risk procedure with considerable morbidity and represents a commitment to indefinite iatrogenic immunosuppression. Moreover, patients transplanted for FHF have a lower 1-year survival than those transplanted for other causes in most series, in part because of their poor clinical condition at the time of the procedure. Clinical liver transplantation continues to evolve, but availability of this therapy is hampered by continued shortages in donor organs. Contraindications to

transplantation include irreversible brain damage, uncontrolled infection, severe pancreatitis, and malignancy. Early identification of which patients would die if OLT were not performed is thus a very important objective. Both the King's College and the Cliché criteria are used most often to identify such patients (see Table 120-3). Liver biopsy, although not mandatory, may help to decide the need for early transplantation. In general, patients with 60% or less necrosis are likely to survive without the need for transplantation whereas those with 90% or more necrosis are unlikely to survive without transplantation.[25,63] Those patients who have hepatic necrosis greater than 60% but less than 90% have a less clear prognosis and require the most aggressive care and attention.

Decisions regarding transplantation do not have to be made at the time of admission but rather at the time a donor organ has been identified. This is because the typical waiting time for a donor organ for a United Network for Organ Sharing (UNOS) status 1 patient (those with FHF) is 2 to 3 days or more in the United States.[64] Currently, various surgical options exist for liver transplantation in patients with FHF (Table 120-5). The most frequently utilized procedure is cadaveric whole organ transplantation, with the donor organ being placed in the orthotopic position. However, continued efforts are being made to assess ways of expanding the donor pool by using marginal donors, living donor liver transplantation, cadaveric split liver transplantation, and various hepatic support systems to prolong survival long enough for the patient to undergo liver transplantation. Therapeutic hepatectomy with temporary portocaval anastomosis in FHF has been reported to stabilize FHF patients until a suitable liver donor organ was procured.[65-67] The anhepatic periods were 14 hours in two cases and 66 hours in a third report.

TABLE 120–5. HEPATIC REPLACEMENT THERAPEUTIC OPTIONS AVAILABLE TO PATIENTS WITH FULMINANT HEPATIC FAILURE

Liver Transplantation

Cadaveric transplantation
  Whole liver
  Reduced size liver
  Split liver
  Auxiliary partial liver
    Orthotopic position
    Heterotopic position
  Auxiliary whole liver
    Heterotopic position
Living-related transplantation
  Left lateral segment
  Left lobe
  Extended left lobe
  Right lobe

Artificial Liver Assist Devices

Non–cell-based systems
  Charcoal hemoperfusion
  High-volume plasmapheresis
  Continuous high-frequency hemodiafiltration
  Molecular adsorbent recirculating system (MARS)
Cell-based systems (bioartificial liver assist devices)
  Primary porcine hepatocytes
  Human hepatoblastoma cells
  (Extracorporeal Liver Assist Device [ELAD])

Hepatocyte Transplantation

Artificial Liver Assist Devices

Several novel modalities of artificial liver support have shown a benefit in FHF. A recent meta-analysis of 12 clinical trials of both biologic and nonbiologic hepatic support systems failed to demonstrate a survival benefit in acute liver failure but did show a 33% mortality reduction in acute-on-chronic liver failure.[68] The goals of artificial liver support systems are to (1) prevent irreversible neurologic damage, (2) provide time for possible regeneration of the liver to allow complete recovery, and (3) provide a bridge to liver transplantation. Charcoal hemoperfusion consists of the passage of plasma through columns of activated charcoal or resins with the goal of clearing lipophilic toxins. Clinical benefit was found in early reports, but randomized, controlled trials failed to confirm such results.[69] High-volume plasmapheresis improves mental status, corrects hyperdynamic circulation, and lowers ammonia levels.[70] In Japan, continuous high-flow hemodiafiltration (CHFHDF) employing a dialysate flow rate of 500 mL/min along with plasmapheresis has been used successfully in patients with advanced hepatic coma.[71] A few reports have also noted beneficial hemodynamic effects and lowering of ammonia levels with the molecular adsorbent recirculating system (MARS).[72,73] MARS is a modified dialysis method using an albumin-containing dialysate that is recirculated and perfused on-line through serial charcoal and anion-exchanger columns. MARS enables the selective removal of albumin-bound substances. However, currently no randomized clinical trials of the last two techniques in FHF are available.

Bioartificial Liver Assist Devices

Bioartificial liver assist devices use hollow-fiber cartridges housing hepatocytes in the extraluminal space. During extracorporeal perfusion of the system, hepatocytes provide metabolic function to the patient. The cells used in these devices are primary porcine hepatocytes (bioartificial liver device [BAL]) or human hepatoblastoma C3a line cells (extracorporeal liver assist device [ELAD]).

In the BAL system, plasma is separated from blood and is circulated through a charcoal column and then through the bioreactor. In several case reports, the BAL system was associated with significant improvements in blood glucose concentration, serum ammonia level, and bilirubin level; decreased ICP; increased CPP; and successful bridging to OLT.[74] In an interim analysis of the largest controlled clinical trial so far using a bioartificial liver assist device, 147 patients with FHF and 24 with primary graft nonfunction were randomly assigned to standard medical treatment alone or to standard medical treatment plus BAL. No significant differences were found in the endpoint (30-day survival) between standard medical treatment and BAL (59% vs. 70%; not significant), except in patients with acetaminophen overdose.[75] The final results of this study are currently awaited. An obvious safety concern of any porcine cell–based therapy is the transmission of porcine retroviruses to the human host. Although not described with this device, further investigation will need to closely monitor FHF patients for this complication.

In the ELAD, whole blood is perfused through the hollow fibers of the bioreactor. A controlled clinical trial of 24 patients showed improvement in galactose elimination time, encephalopathy, ICP, and hemodynamics in the group treated with the ELAD compared with standard medical therapy; no difference in survival was apparent.[76] In the absence of randomized controlled trials, the efficacy of liver-assist devices has been difficult to ascertain and remains unproved at this time.

Hepatocyte Transplantation

Hepatocyte transplantation has been attempted in patients with FHF to accomplish the same goals as with the hepatic liver assist systems. The rationale is to deliver a sufficient supply of hepatocytes to maintain liver function until regeneration of native liver occurs or a graft becomes available. Human hepatocytes from livers not used for transplantation can be cryopreserved, making them readily available if needed. Experimental studies in models of FHF showed engraftment and function of transplanted hepatocytes, with increased survival. In patients with stage III and IV encephalopathy and severe coagulopathy, intrasplenic or intrahepatic injection of human hepatocytes has been performed.[77,78] In two studies, improvements have been noted in several parameters, including encephalopathy score, hemodynamics, and serum ammonia and bilirubin levels. Pulmonary embolism of hepatocytes occurred in patients in whom the injection was intraportal but not in those with hepatocytes injected into the splenic artery.[77] Other concerns about this technique include transplantation and acquisition of an adequate number of hepatocytes (only 0.15 to 80 g have been injected compared with 300 g [20% of normal liver mass required] to replace liver function), use of immunosuppression in FHF, and the need for a 48-hour period for engraftment and function. Future trials using this concept are likely if results with hepatocyte liver assist systems prove disappointing.

CONCLUSION

Fulminant hepatic failure remains a rare but a devastating illness with high mortality. The treatment of FHF poses a great challenge to intensive care clinicians. A multidisciplinary approach to critical care management is clearly required to address the multitude of organ derangements that are sequelae of liver failure. Currently, only liver transplantation can radically alter the course of the disease process. Although transplant surgery including immunosuppressive therapy has considerably advanced over the past decade, this intervention is expensive and is associated with complications related both to the procedure and the need for life-long immunosuppression. Therefore, liver replacement strategies that are less invasive and permanent are urgently required. The current experience with nonbiologic and biologic artificial devices are encouraging but clearly require validation of their safety and efficacy by randomized, controlled trials.

ANNOTATED REFERENCES

Blei AT: Medical therapy of brain edema in fulminant hepatic failure. Hepatology 2000;32:666-669.
  A comprehensive and well-referenced review of the multiple pathologic mechanisms that culminate in FHF-related cerebral edema and of established or potential therapeutic measures for this problem.

Jalan R, Damink SW, Deutz NE, et al: Moderate hypothermia for uncontrolled intracranial hypertension in acute liver failure. Lancet 1999;354: 1164-1168.
  A small but very well performed case series demonstrating the efficacy and safety of hypothermia to reduce elevated intracranial pressures refractory to other modalities in patients with FHF.

Kjaergard LL, Liu J, Als-Nielsen B, Gluud C: Artificial and bioartificial support systems for acute and acute-on-chronic liver failure: A systematic review. JAMA 2003;289:217-222.
  A recent meta-analysis of published human clinical investigation of both biologic and nonbiologic extracorporeal liver replacement therapies and their impact on patient survival.

O'Grady JG, Alexander GJ, Hayllar KM, Williams R: Early indicators of prognosis in fulminant hepatic failure. Gastroenterology 1989;97:439-445.
  The classic paper that established the most widely used criteria (Kings College Criteria) for predicting liver transplant free mortality in a large cohort of patients with either acetaminophen- or non–acetaminophen-induced FHF.

Ostapowicz G, Fontana RJ, Schiodt FV, et al: Results of a prospective study of acute liver failure at 17 tertiary care centers in the United States. Ann Intern Med 2002;137:947-954.
  A relatively recent "snapshot" of the etiology of acute liver failure in the United States that documents the emergence of acetaminophen toxicity as the most common etiology, with clinical outcome and risk factors for nonsurvival.

Chapter 121

CALCULOUS AND ACALCULOUS CHOLECYSTITIS

Samuel A. Tisherman

KEY POINTS

1. Critically ill patients frequently do not present with the usual symptoms and signs of cholecystitis.
2. Laboratory tests for cholecystitis are not specific.
3. The best initial imaging study is ultrasonography, but scintigraphy or computed tomography also may be needed.
4. Management begins with antibiotics and bowel rest.
5. Although cholecystectomy is the most definitive procedure, image-guided percutaneous cholecystostomy is indicated for patients too unstable to undergo cholecystectomy.

Evaluating a patient with a possible acute abdomen in the ICU can be challenging. Patients frequently have multiple potential sources of sepsis and often are unable to describe symptoms or localize tenderness on physical examination. In addition, imaging studies, such as computed tomography (CT) and scintigraphy, may be difficult to obtain because of the risks associated with transport to the radiology suite or nuclear medicine facility. These confounding factors can be important in the evaluation of any intra-abdominal process, but may be especially troublesome in the case of acute cholecystitis.

The first reported case of acute, postoperative cholecystitis, described in 1844, was a lethal complication that occurred in a patient who had been treated for a strangulated femoral hernia.[1] Kocher and Matti[2] described a successful operation for gangrenous cholecystitis complicating a ventral herniorrhaphy in 1906. In 1962, Thompson and colleagues[3] reported a series of 98 patients who developed acute cholecystitis in the postoperative period. Of the patients, 76% were men, and 47% did not have gallstones; 12% of the patients developed perforation of the gallbladder. Glenn and Becker[4] showed that the incidence of acalculous cholecystitis and postoperative cholecystitis increased between 1955 and 1979.

The pathophysiology of cholecystitis in critically ill patients is different from that in the general population. At least half of the cases are acalculous.[5] Understanding this disease process can help increase the index of suspicion and lead to early diagnosis and treatment.

RISK FACTORS AND PATHOPHYSIOLOGY

In general, acute cholecystitis is associated with the presence of gallstones, which develop as a result of decreased solubility of cholesterol and bile salts in bile. Normally the concentrations of conjugated bile salts, cholesterol, and phospholipids in bile keep these components in solution. If the balance of these components is altered, stones may form. Risk factors include age, female sex, recent pregnancy, positive family history for gallstones, and hemolysis. Patients with gallstones may develop acute cholecystitis at any time. Occasionally, acute cholecystitis can occur during hospitalization for other reasons.

Acalculous cholecystitis also can occur spontaneously under certain circumstances. In outpatients, risk factors for acalculous cholecystitis include diabetes mellitus and vasculitis. Older age and male sex seem to be risk factors.[6] Acalculous cholecystitis also has been reported in cancer patients and patients with systemic infections and acquired immunodeficiency syndrome (AIDS). Acute cholecystitis is the most common indication for exploratory laparotomy or laparoscopy in AIDS patients.[7] Most AIDS patients have acalculous disease. The mortality rate is high. In children, most cases of acute cholecystitis are acalculous.[8] The cause seems to be dehydration or lymphadenopathy secondary to viral infections. Congenital biliary tract anomalies also need to be considered.

Acute cholecystitis has been described in multiple reports as a complication of a variety of surgical procedures,[9-14] trauma,[15-20] burns,[21] sepsis,[22] cardiovascular diseases, and malignancy.[23,24] There also has been an association with total parenteral nutrition and biliary stasis.[25-28] The pathophysiology remains unclear, however.

Theories regarding the pathogenesis of acalculous cholecystitis in critically ill and postoperative patients have evolved over the years. Sparkman[29] was the first to suggest that gastrointestinal hypomotility and biliary stasis were causative factors. Glenn and Wantz[30] added that the lack of enteral feeding in the postoperative period increased the concentration of bile salts and cholesterol in bile in the gallbladder. They further noted acute onset of cholecystitis with refeeding, suggesting impaction of stones or viscous bile in the cystic duct with gallbladder contractions. Thompson and colleagues,[3] having noted gallbladder mucosal necrosis, arterial thrombosis, gangrene, and perforation, suggested that hypoperfusion may be the crucial mechanism for acalculous cholecystitis. A more recent histopathologic study found that two thirds of surgical and trauma patients who developed acute cholecystitis had ischemic cholecystitis histologically.[31] Hakala and coworkers[32] performed ex vivo microangiography of gallbladders immediately after cholecystectomy. Patients with stones had normal vasculature, whereas patients with acalculous disease had poor and irregular capillary filling, suggesting that microvascular disturbances may play a role in the pathogenesis of this disease. Orlando and associates[33] suggested that, in addition to hypoperfusion, increased intraluminal pressure may be a crucial factor.

Hypoperfusion, particularly of the splanchnic circulation, is common in critically ill patients. Causative factors include hemorrhage, dehydration, heart failure, and sepsis. The use of vasopressors can exacerbate the situation. Mechanical ventilation with positive end-expiratory pressure can decrease portal perfusion and increase hepatic venous pressure.[34]

Biliary stasis secondary to fasting and narcotics may play a crucial role in increasing intraluminal pressure in the gallbladder. The combination of hypoperfusion and increased luminal pressure leads to a decrease in gallbladder perfusion pressure. Bacterial invasion subsequently can occur in the ischemic tissue.

The use of parenteral nutrition has been implicated in the pathogenesis of acalculous cholecystitis. In addition to the effects of fasting, parenteral nutrition can decrease bile production, worsening biliary stasis. Biliary sludge can be found in almost all patients on long-term parenteral nutrition.[25-28] Many patients subsequently form gallstones. Trauma patients also develop sludge over time, and this factor may play a role in the development of cholecystitis and pancreatitis.[35]

Eosinophilic infiltration of the inflamed gallbladder has been seen in patients developing acute acalculous cholecystitis after administration of antibiotics for other reasons, suggesting the possibility that a hypersensitivity reaction to the antibiotic played a causative role.[36] This theory has not been substantiated.

It has been suggested that the pigment load from massive transfusions can lead to changes in the relative concentrations of bile pigments compared with cholesterol and lecithin, increasing risk of acalculous cholecystitis. Long and coworkers[34] found no relationship, however, between transfusion requirements and risk of cholecystitis.

INCIDENCE

The incidence of acute cholecystitis in the ICU is difficult to determine given the great diversity of ICU patient populations and illness severity. Among cardiac surgical patients, acute cholecystitis is second only to upper gastrointestinal hemorrhage as an indication for abdominal operation.[37] About half of cases of acute cholecystitis in this patient population are due to acalculous disease. Visceral hypoperfusion related to left ventricular dysfunction has been implicated as a causative factor. Rady and associates[13] found that early predictors of acute cholecystitis included arterial occlusive disease, preoperative oxygen delivery less than 430 mL/min/m^2, longer cardiopulmonary bypass times, need for surgical re-exploration, cardiac arrhythmias, mechanical ventilation for 3 days or more, bacteremia, and nosocomial infections. The "common threads" of these factors are decreased tissue perfusion and oxygenation, significant surgical trauma (which would be expected to lead to production of inflammatory mediators), and perhaps bacterial translocation from the gut lumen. Rady and associates[13] suggested that patients who have had a complicated postoperative course should be followed by serial ultrasound studies of the gallbladder. Hagino and associates[14] found that 7 of 996 patients who had undergone aortic reconstruction developed postoperative cholecystitis. Six of the seven patients had had prolonged hypotension, all had multiple organ dysfunction, and five died.

Among postoperative patients in general, acute cholecystitis seems to occur with or without gallstones. Mortality is approximately 30%. Among trauma patients, about 90% of cases of acute cholecystitis are acalculous.[15-20] The percentage of cases of acute cholecystitis that are acalculous has increased significantly over time.[4] Because the incidence of the disease is low, but the many risk factors for the disease are common, it is difficult to identify specific groups of ICU patients who might benefit from selective screening for acute cholecystitis.

CLINICAL PRESENTATION

Given that the underlying pathophysiology of cholecystitis in the ICU often involves gallbladder wall ischemia, there is significant risk for rapid progression to gangrene and perforation. Consequently, although other causes of sepsis in the ICU are more common, one needs to have a low threshold for considering cholecystitis in the differential diagnosis of patients who may have intra-abdominal sepsis.

The signs and symptoms of acute cholecystitis generally do not differ between calculous and acalculous disease. Typically, patients with acute cholecystitis present with right upper quadrant or epigastric pain, often associated with a fatty meal. The pain may radiate to the back. Anorexia, nausea, and vomiting are common findings, as are fever and chills. If the patient is receiving enteral nutrition, the symptoms may be related to meals or tube feedings.

On examination, the most consistent finding is fever. Focal tenderness in the right upper quadrant or epigastrium is typically found, often with evidence of peritoneal irritation. Rarely the gallbladder is palpable. There may be abdominal distention and loss of bowel sounds. Jaundice may be present.

In critically ill patients, symptoms and physical findings are frequently difficult to assess because of alterations in the patient's mental status. Typical physical findings are frequently absent. Other concurrent disease processes often obscure the clinical picture.

The most consistent laboratory finding is a leukocytosis. Elevations of liver enzymes and bilirubin are common but not always present. Clinical findings and laboratory studies are not sensitive or specific for cholecystitis even in the general population[38,39] and are less so in critically ill patients. Consequently, radiologic studies are necessary.

IMAGING STUDIES

Ultrasonography has proved to be an accurate radiologic test for acute cholecystitis in the general population. In the ICU, the presence or absence of gallstones does not help with the diagnosis. The most useful ultrasound findings indicating acute cholecystitis are thickening of the gallbladder wall and pericholecystic fluid (Fig. 121-1). Ultrasound findings correlate well with operative findings. False-positive findings may occur with sludge, nonshadowing stones, cholesterolosis, ascites, hypoalbuminemia, and portal hypertension. Other ultrasound findings indicating acute cholecystitis include the "double wall" sign, representing edema of the gallbladder wall; the "halo" sign, representing sloughed gallbladder mucosa; intramural gas; distention of the gallbladder; and the sonographic Murphy's sign, showing point tenderness over the gallbladder. The sensitivity of ultrasound for

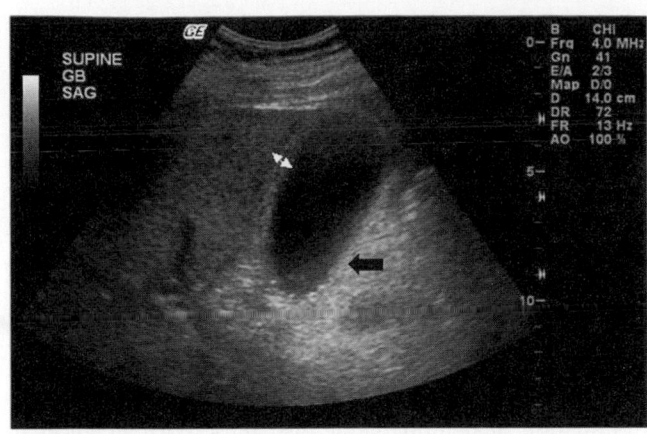

FIGURE 121–1. Ultrasound of the gallbladder shows wall thickening *(double arrow)* and sludge *(arrow)*.

findings characteristic of acute cholecystitis, suggesting that patients with several findings should undergo more aggressive diagnostic evaluation and, perhaps, therapeutic interventions.[40] In equivocal cases, serial ultrasound examinations may show increasing wall thickness, which should increase the suspicion for the diagnosis of cholecystitis.[42]

Scintigraphy of the gallbladder frequently has been used when acute cholecystitis is suspected, but when the findings from other tests, such as ultrasonography, are inconclusive or contradictory. Gallbladder scintigraphy is performed by administering technetium-labeled iminodiacetic acid. Cholecystitis is diagnosed if the radioactive tracer is visualized in the small bowel without visualization of the gallbladder within 4 hours, a pattern that suggests occlusion of the cystic duct (Fig. 121-2). Delayed visualization of the gallbladder may represent chronic cholecystitis. The rate of false-positive tests is significant in fasting patients, particularly patients receiving parenteral nutrition. The use of morphine to increase tone in the sphincter of Oddi and increase pressure within the biliary system can decrease the risk of a false-positive test.[44] The sensitivity of scintigraphy is 91% to 97%, and the specificity is 38% to 99%.[44-46] Scintigraphy is a useful complement to ultrasonography when ultrasonography alone does not provide enough information to permit a sufficiently early decision regarding intervention.[45]

CT of the abdomen can be used to make the diagnosis of acute cholecystitis.[47,48] The criteria for a positive study

detecting acalculous cholecystitis is 81% to 92%. The specificity is 60% to 96%.[38-44] One problem is that the typical ultrasound findings of cholecystitis can be seen in ICU patients without other evidence of cholecystitis. Boland and colleagues[40] performed ultrasound examinations of the gallbladder twice a week in a variety of ICU patients. Half of the patients without calculi developed at least one ultrasound finding of acute cholecystitis. Helbich and coworkers[41] attempted to apply a scoring system to the ultrasound

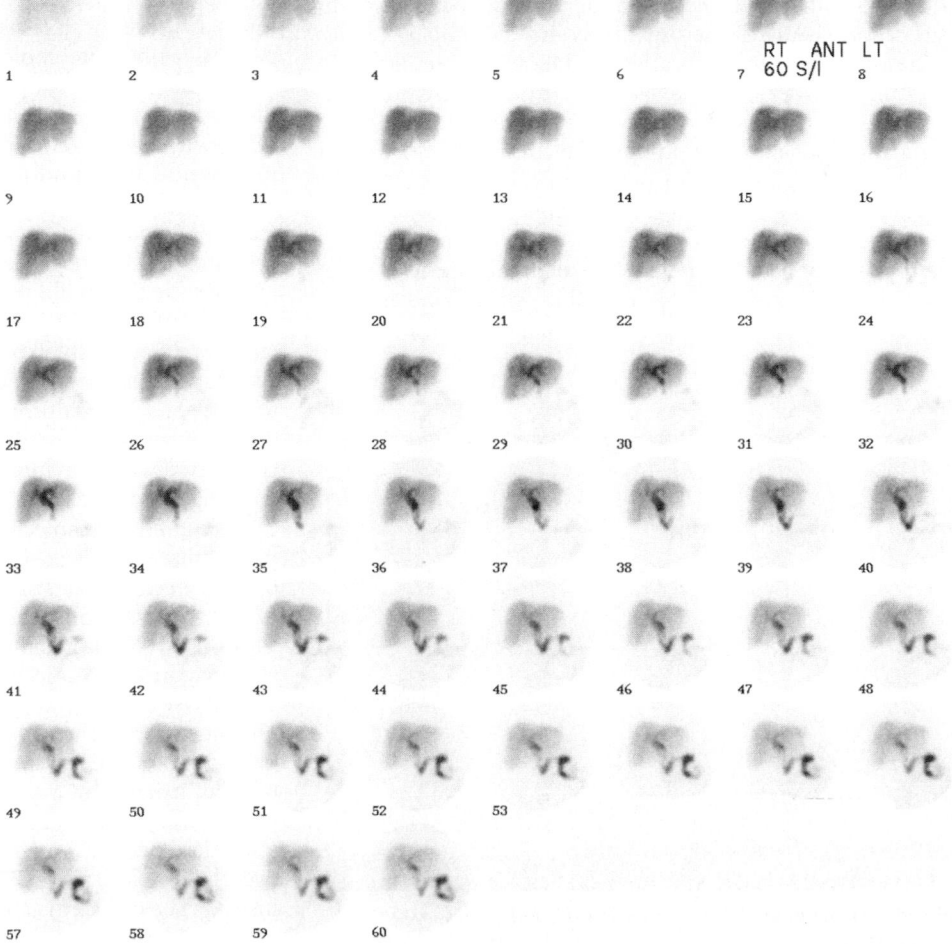

FIGURE 121–2. Scintigraphy of the biliary tree shows concentration of the tracer in the liver followed by flow into the biliary tree and small bowel. The gallbladder is not visualized, even after the administration of morphine.

include wall thickness greater than 4 mm, pericholecystic fluid or subserosal edema without ascites, intramural gas, or sloughed mucosa (Fig. 121-3). If intravenous contrast material is administered, enhancement of the gallbladder wall may be seen. Although CT may not be as sensitive as the other studies for determining the presence of gallstones or acute cholecystitis, it has the advantage of being able to detect or rule out other causes of an acute abdomen. A great disadvantage for critically ill patients is the need to transport the patient to the scanner.

In critically ill patients, ultrasound is usually the first test requested because it can be performed at the bedside in the ICU and carries no risk. It also can be repeated readily. The study is operator dependent; the reliability of the test, particularly its sensitivity, can be variable.[43] Specificity is good. Additional studies frequently are necessary, however. Ultrasonography and scintigraphy, in particular, complement each other well.[46] The results of any imaging studies need to be considered in the context of the patient's underlying disease, physical findings, and laboratory studies.

MANAGEMENT

The standard initial medical treatment for acute cholecystitis includes antibiotics, analgesia, and, at least during the early phase, bowel rest. Antibiotic coverage for uncomplicated cholecystitis should include enterococcal species and gram-negative rods, particularly *Escherichia coli* and *Klebsiella* species.[49] Among patients who have received antibiotics previously, more resistant and unusual organisms often are cultured from gallbladder bile in patients with acute cholecystitis. These organisms include *Staphylococcus* species, resistant gram-negative bacilli, anaerobic bacteria, and fungi. Older patients also are more likely to have infected bile. In patients with empyema of the gallbladder, Tseng and associates[50] found that bile cultures were positive in 83% of the cases. Gram-negative bacteria (e.g., *E. coli, Klebsiella pneumoniae, Morganella morganii, Pseudomonas aeruginosa,* and *Salmonella* species) were found in 75%, gram-positive bacteria (e.g., enterococcal species) were found in 30%, and obligate anaerobes were found in 7%. Broader coverage may be required for empirical coverage

until cultures are obtained and coverage can be more tailored.

The next question is whether to drain or remove the gallbladder acutely. Prospective, randomized trials to help clarify this issue are lacking. Early surgical consultation is crucial. The decision regarding radiographic or surgical intervention must be made with consideration of critical care and general surgical issues. If the patient can tolerate transport to the operating room and a general anesthetic, cholecystectomy is the most definitive therapy, particularly in light of the risk of gallbladder gangrene and perforation. Frequently, however, critically ill patients with acute cholecystitis are thought to be too ill for this approach. Of particular concern are patients who have significant respiratory dysfunction or hemodynamic instability. With advances in the ease of image-guided drainage, bedside cholecystostomy using ultrasound guidance has been used more commonly.

IMAGE-DIRECTED DRAINAGE

Image-directed cholecystostomy can readily be performed using either ultrasonography or CT. This procedure was first used for palliation of obstructive jaundice in 1979.[51] In 1980, successful drainage of empyema of the gallbladder was reported.[52] The first large series of percutaneous cholecystostomy for acute cholecystitis was reported in 1985.[53] Of 114 patients, 113 were treated successfully.

Percutaneous cholecystostomy and bile culture have been performed occasionally in patients with unexplained sepsis in the ICU. In patients who have cholecystitis, cultures are often positive if performed 72 hours after the onset of symptoms. Culture of bile is sterile in approximate 50% of patients with acute cholecystitis.[49] Boland and colleagues[54] tested the efficacy of percutaneous cholecystostomy as a diagnostic and therapeutic maneuver in 82 patients in the ICU with persistent unexplained sepsis; 48 patients improved. Ultrasound findings were not helpful in predicting response to percutaneous cholecystostomy. In a separate study of 24 such patients, 14 patients improved after cholecystostomy.[55] Of the remaining patients, three had pneumonia, and the others did not have a source of sepsis identified. Of the patients who improved, only four had positive bile cultures. In critically ill patients without a definitive diagnosis of acute cholecystitis, the role of percutaneous cholecystostomy and bile culture is unclear. Because the risk of this procedure is low, percutaneous cholecystostomy should be considered when the index of suspicion for acute cholecystitis is high enough.

Percutaneous cholecystostomy is contraindicated if the patient has evidence of diffuse peritonitis, suggesting gallbladder perforation. If imaging studies suggest a pericholecystic abscess, concomitant drainage of the abscess or surgical exploration is indicated.

Percutaneous cholecystostomy is most appropriate for patients with acute cholecystitis who are too unstable to tolerate a general anesthetic. The procedure is done under ultrasound or CT guidance. A needle is inserted into the gallbladder, usually via a transhepatic approach. A guidewire is passed through the needle and the needle tract is dilated using a standard Seldinger technique. A pigtail catheter is advanced over the wire into the gallbladder. Some use a trocar technique instead. The catheter is attached to a drainage bag.

Van Sonnenberg and coworkers[56] reported a series of percutaneous cholecystostomies in 127 patients.

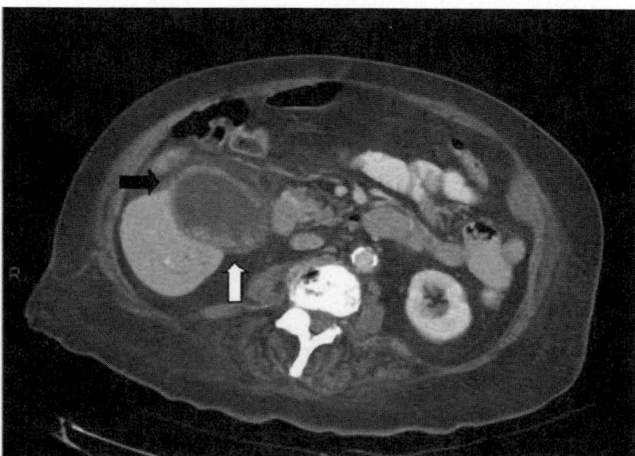

FIGURE 121–3. Computed tomography of the abdomen shows thickening of the gallbladder wall with infiltration of the pericholecystic fat *(black arrow)* and gallstones *(white arrow).*

Indications included acute cholecystitis, obstructive jaundice, gallbladder perforation, need for percutaneous removal or dissolution of gallstones, need for diagnostic cholecystocholangiography, and gallbladder biopsy. The procedure was successful in 125 cases. Eleven patients (8.7%) had major complications, whereas 5 (3.9%) had minor complications. Complications included bile peritonitis, bleeding, vagal reactions, hypotension, catheter dislodgment, and acute respiratory distress. No deaths were related to the procedure itself.

Overall mortality for percutaneous cholecystostomy is about 10%, being similar to open cholecystostomy.[56-59] The limiting factor for success of percutaneous drainage is the viability of the gallbladder. Focal ischemia or necrosis is unlikely to improve without cholecystectomy and predisposes the patient to perforation. Cholecystectomy should be considered in patients who do not improve with cholecystostomy. Lo and associates[57] found that all six patients in their series who failed to respond to cholecystostomy had transmural inflammation; five had a gangrenous gallbladder wall.

Cholecystostomy may obviate the need for cholecystectomy. The appropriate management after cholecystostomy is not completely clear, however. When the patient has recovered, one can readily obtain a cholangiogram through the catheter. If gallstones are present, elective cholecystectomy at a later date is recommended. If no stones are present, patients do well without cholecystectomy.[58,59]

Johlin and Neil[60] described a novel approach to achieve drainage of the gallbladder, using a transpapillary endoscopic approach. This approach may be helpful if other indications for endoscopic evaluation or intervention are present.

SURGICAL MANAGEMENT

Surgical options include cholecystostomy and cholecystectomy. Surgical cholecystostomy can be accomplished via a small right subcostal incision using local anesthesia or via laparoscopy. This procedure largely has been supplanted by image-guided, percutaneous cholecystostomy as described earlier.

Cholecystectomy may be advantageous compared with cholecystostomy because it allows one to examine the entire right upper quadrant for other pathology and to drain completely any fluid collections around the gallbladder. It also alleviates the risk of gallbladder perforation. When cholecystectomy is performed, a laparoscopic approach usually can be attempted, recognizing that one may need to abandon this approach and proceed with an open procedure because of difficulty with the dissection.

Bedside laparoscopy can be performed for evaluation of the acute abdomen in critically ill patients. If acute cholecystitis is identified, a cholecystostomy can be performed readily, or the patient can be taken to the operating room for a cholecystectomy.[61,62] If the diagnosis of cholecystitis is excluded, the patient may be spared an unnecessary trip to the operating room.

COMPLICATIONS AND OUTCOME

Complications of acute cholecystitis are much more common in critically ill patients than in the general population.

Among 27 patients with acalculous cholecystitis, Kalliafas and associates[38] found that 17 patients had gangrene, 4 patients had perforation, and 1 patient had an abscess. Mortality was 41%.

Gangrene may be present in 59% of cases.[9-22] Shapiro and coworkers[22] found gangrene or frank necrosis in 13 of 22 patients undergoing cholecystectomy for acute cholecystitis that developed in the ICU. Cornwell and colleagues[63] found necrosis or gangrene in 6 of 14 trauma patients who developed acute acalculous cholecystitis.

Compared with patients without gangrene, patients with gangrene are at greater risk of perforation or of failure of percutaneous drainage. Some of these patients have emphysematous cholecystitis (gas in the wall of the gallbladder), a diagnosis that carries an even greater risk of perforation. Emphysema can be identified by plain abdominal radiographs, CT, or ultrasound. Antibiotic coverage should include gasforming anaerobic organisms. Although percutaneous drainage may be effective,[64] early cholecystectomy is indicated if the patient does not improve promptly.

Perforation of the gallbladder occurs in approximately 10% of cases.[9-22] Usually the resulting fluid collection is localized and amenable to percutaneous drainage. Free perforation also can occur, and when it does, the risk of mortality is markedly increased.[65] The risk of perforation increases with delay in drainage or operation. Cholecystectomy is indicated for free perforation or for patients failing to respond rapidly to percutaneous drainage.

Empyema of the gallbladder also greatly increases mortality.[66] This complication may be amenable to percutaneous drainage,[50,67] but the risks of failure or perforation are substantial.

The risk of mortality from cholecystitis in the ICU mainly reflects the underlying disease processes and comorbidities. Overall mortality is approximately 30%.[9-22] Hadas-Halpern and colleagues[68] found that 10 of 80 patients undergoing percutaneous cholecystostomy for acute cholecystitis died of comorbid disease, whereas only 2 patients died of biliary peritonitis.

PREVENTION

No intervention has been shown conclusively to prevent development of cholecystitis in ICU patients. If the theories regarding the pathophysiologic mechanisms are correct, the incidence of the disease should be reduced by aggressively resuscitating patients with shock and avoiding biliary stasis by implementing early enteral feeding and minimizing the use of narcotics. Intermittent doses of cholecystokinin or deoxycholic acid have been shown to increase bile flow and may decrease the risk of acalculous cholecystitis in patients receiving parenteral nutrition.[69-71] Studies in ICU patients are needed.

SUMMARY

The diagnosis of acute cholecystitis in critically ill patients is difficult because patients frequently do not present with the usual symptoms and signs. Laboratory tests are nonspecific. The best initial radiographic study is ultrasound. Scintigraphy and CT also may be helpful. Management includes antibiotics and bowel rest. Percutaneous cholecystostomy may be used in unstable patients, although cholecystectomy remains the most definitive treatment, if this intervention can be accomplished safely.

ANNOTATED REFERENCES

Boland G, Lee MJ, Mueller PR: Acute cholecystitis in the intensive care unit. New Horiz 1993;1:246-260.

This article provides an extensive review of the pathophysiology, presentation, and management of acute cholecystitis in the ICU.

Flancbaum L, Alden SM, Trooskin SZ: Use of cholescintigraphy with morphine in critically ill patients with suspected cholecystitis. Surgery 1989;106:668-673.

The addition of morphine to cholescintigraphy can improve the diagnostic accuracy of this test for diagnosing cholecystitis in critically ill patients.

Helbich TH, Mallek R, Madl C, et al: Sonomorphology of the gallbladder in critically ill patients: Value of a scoring system and follow-up examinations. Acta Radiol 1997;38:129-134.

Ultrasound examinations of the gallbladder of patients in the ICU frequently reveal equivocal findings. This group tried to quantify these findings, coupled with serial examinations, to improve the diagnostic accuracy of ultrasonography in this setting.

Thompson JW III, Ferris DO, Beggenstoss AH: Acute cholecystitis complicating operation for other diseases. Ann Surg 1962;155:489.

This is one of the first articles to postulate that the crucial pathophysiologic mechanism for acalculous cholecystitis is hypoperfusion.

van Sonnenberg E, D'Agostino HB, Goodacre BW, et al: Percutaneous gallbladder puncture and cholecystostomy: Results, complications, and caveats for safety. Radiology 1992;183:167-170.

The authors describe a large series of patients who underwent percutaneous cholecystostomy with excellent results.

Chapter 122
ACUTE PANCREATITIS

Pamela A. Lipsett

KEY POINTS

1. Severe acute pancreatitis accounts for 10% to 15% of all patients presenting with pancreatitis and for virtually all the morbidity and mortality associated with the disease.

2. The early phase of severe acute pancreatitis is characterized by systemic inflammatory response syndrome and end-organ dysfunction, often requiring intensive support of the cardiopulmonary system. Respiratory dysfunction is a major component of multiple organ system dysfunction syndrome secondary to acute pancreatitis, and most patients with this syndrome require ventilatory support. In addition, initial management is intravascular volume resuscitation, regardless of the etiology and severity of acute pancreatitis. Sequestration of fluid can lead to loss of one third of plasma volume.

3. Pancreatic necrosis of more than 50% is associated with increased complications, especially pancreatic infection. Infected pancreatic necrosis is the most important risk factor for death secondary to necrotizing pancreatitis. Prevention, diagnosis, and treatment of infection in severe acute pancreatitis are crucial.

4. Understanding the cause of severe acute pancreatitis may dictate therapeutic options. A biliary origin should be suspected in female patients older than age 40 with a serum alanine aminotransferase level more than three times the upper reference limit.

5. Contrast-enhanced computed tomography (CT) is considered the gold standard for diagnosing pancreatic necrosis and peripancreatic collections and for grading acute pancreatitis. The Balthazar index ranges from 0 to 10 and is obtained by adding the points attributed to the extent of the inflammatory process to the volume of pancreatic necrosis. Although CT findings correlate with clinical course and severity of acute pancreatitis, it is not necessary to obtain this study in patients with mild pancreatitis.

6. Approximately 80% of deaths due to acute pancreatitis are related to infectious complications. It is reasonable to consider whether administration of prophylactic antibiotics can decrease the incidence of local or distant infections or the morbidity and mortality associated with pancreatic necrosis.

Although antibiotic prophylaxis is widely employed, the quality of evidence supporting this practice is relatively weak, and the increased microbial resistance seen in more recent trials suggests that this practice should not be widely employed without additional randomized controlled trials.

7. Patients with severe necrotizing acute pancreatitis require nutritional supplementation. Enteral nutrition is safe and efficacious but should be delivered distal to the pylorus. Some patients are so catabolic that enteral and parenteral nutrition may be required to support nutritional needs. Although triglyceride levels should be monitored, lipids can be used for supplementation in most patients.

8. Patients who fail to improve, patients who worsen, and patients with initial improvement who regress may have pancreatic infection. A contrast-enhanced CT scan and fine-needle aspiration should be considered to rule out infection.

9. Pancreatic débridement should be performed in patients with infected pancreatic necrosis. The specific surgical approach depends on local considerations, and no single method has been proven to be superior to another.

The term *acute pancreatitis* describes a wide spectrum of disease ranging from a mild edematous form of acute pancreatitis to severe acute necrotizing pancreatitis. The mild form of acute pancreatitis is a self-limited disease that is associated with little or no distant organ dysfunction. The mild form of acute pancreatitis has a mortality rate of less than 1% and usually resolves in 3 to 4 days. Patients with this form of acute pancreatitis rarely need ICU therapy or pancreatic surgery. Although most (80%) patients with acute pancreatitis have mild disease, 10% to 15% of patients develop the systemic inflammatory response syndrome (SIRS) and run a fulminant clinical course, leading to pancreatic necrosis and to multisystem organ injury.[1,2] The mortality rate for severe acute pancreatitis is 15% to 40%, whereas the overall mortality rate for all patients presenting with acute pancreatitis is less than 5%.[3-6] The natural course of severe acute pancreatitis occurs in two phases. The first 7 to 14 days of this disease process are characterized by SIRS and resulting end-organ dysfunction. Inflammatory mediators are released into the systemic circulation, and patients manifest signs and symptoms of cardiorespiratory and renal failure.[7] Pancreatic infection is uncommon during this early phase of acute pancreatitis and SIRS. Attempts to modify the course of the disease by instituting therapy with octreotide or platelet-activating factor receptor antagonists have been unsuccessful.[8,9]

Since the 1980s, the morbidity and mortality associated with acute pancreatitis have decreased substantially.[10-12] The reasons for the decrease in mortality in severe acute pancreatitis are uncertain, but may reflect improved critical care services and better strategies for surgical management. In general, mortality from severe acute pancreatitis is related to infection.[7] Infection of the necrotic pancreas (and associated tissues) typically develops in the second and third weeks of the disease and is reported to occur in 40% to 70% of patients with pancreatic necrosis.[13-16] Multiple organ system dysfunction syndrome is the main life-threatening complication, and mortality rates of 50% have been reported.[17] Infected necrosis is the most important risk factor for death secondary to necrotizing pancreatitis.[13-17] Prevention, diagnosis, and optimal treatment of infection in severe acute pancreatitis are crucial for improving outcome for patients with this disease.

This chapter discusses the etiology, pathophysiology, severity and staging, and management of patients with severe acute pancreatitis. Chronic pancreatitis is not discussed in this chapter. In 1998, the British Society of Gastroenterology published guidelines for the management of acute pancreatitis.[18] These guidelines proposed initial steps in the diagnosis, investigation, and treatment of this condition, but did not make recommendations regarding surgical management. Several additional authors have proposed guidelines and protocols for management of severe acute pancreatitis.[6,19-24]

ETIOLOGY AND EPIDEMIOLOGY

Acute pancreatitis has an annual incidence of 21 to 90 cases per 1 million, and the incidence of the disease is steadily increasing in some countries.[11,25] The increasing incidence of acute pancreatitis is believed to be related to increases in alcohol consumption and gallstone disease in some societies. Acute pancreatitis is slightly more common in men than in women. Biliary pancreatitis is more common in women, and alcohol-related acute pancreatitis is more common in men.

Understanding the etiology of pancreatitis may lead to important differences in evaluation and treatment. Familiarity with the causes of acute pancreatitis is important.[26,27] Gallstones are the leading cause of acute pancreatitis in developed countries and account for 45% of all cases. A biliary etiology should be suspected in female patients older than age 40 with a serum alanine aminotransferase level more than three times the upper reference limit.

Alcohol abuse typically accounts for about 35% of cases of acute pancreatitis; however, it is unclear whether acute alcoholic pancreatitis ever arises in the absence of chronic injury to the gland.[26] Infrequent, but not rare, causes of pancreatitis include drug reactions (usually idiosyncratic), pancreatic and ampullary tumors, hypertriglyceridemia, hypercalcemia (almost always secondary to hyperparathyroidism), hypothermia, congenital abnormalities of the biliary or pancreatic duct (e.g., choledochal cyst), trauma (including acute pancreatitis after endoscopic retrograde cholangiopancreatography), and infectious or parasitic organisms. Rare causes include bites of certain spiders, scorpions, and the Gila monster lizard. Unidentified causes are termed *idiopathic*. The roles of sphincter of Oddi dysfunction, pancreas divisum, and bile crystals or sludge in the development of acute pancreatitis are less clear.[26]

PATHOGENESIS

Regardless of the actual underlying cause, pancreatitis is an inflammatory process that can initiate SIRS.[7] Inappropriate activation of the proteolytic enzyme, trypsin, is thought to be the initial step in the development of acute pancreatitis. Trypsinogen is activated through hydrolysis of an N-terminal peptide called *trypsinogen-activating peptide*.[28] In rats, the site of localization and activation of this peptide is within small cytoplasmic vacuoles located within pancreatic acinar cells.[29] Trypsin also activates cells via the trypsin receptor, also known as *protease-activated receptor (PAR-2)*.[28] Pancreatic acinar and duct cells express abundant PAR-2. Trypsin activity in the pancreas is controlled mainly by the pancreatic secretory trypsin inhibitor (PSTI) also called *serine protease inhibitor Kazal type 1 (SPINK1)*.[30] PSTI is synthesized in pancreas acinar cells and acts as a potent natural inhibitor of trypsin. Normally, when trypsinogen is cleaved to release trypsin in the pancreas, PSTI immediately binds to the enzyme to prevent further activation of additional pancreatic enzymes (Fig. 122-1). PSTI also blocks further activation of pancreatic cells via the trypsin receptor, PAR-2.

Several additional protective systems prevent pancreatic autodigestion by trypsin, and the genetic expression of these systems may contribute to the risk of developing acute pancreatitis or modulate the severity of the disease when it occurs. Trypsin-activated, trypsin-like enzymes, such as mesotrypsin, degrade trypsinogen. Bicarbonate-rich pancreatic secretions are affected by abnormal expression of the cystic fibrosis transmembrane conductance receptor. A mutation in SPINK1, N34S, has been reported in people with familial pancreatitis,[30] in children with idiopathic chronic pancreatitis,[31,32] and in 2% of the control population.[31-33] Because these mutations in SPINK1 are much more common than pancreatitis, this

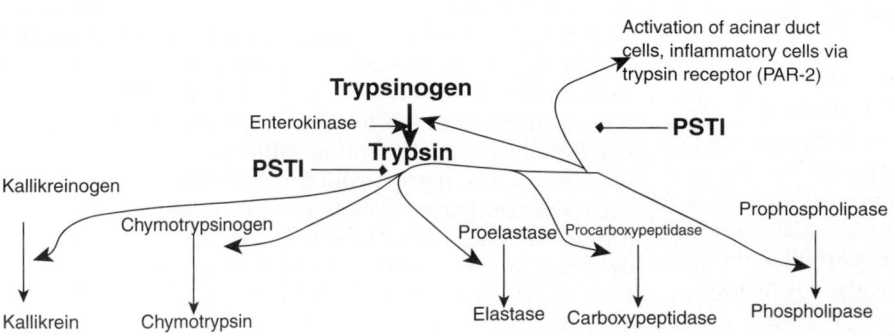

FIGURE 122–1. Activation pathways of proenzymes and protease activated receptor (PAR)-2 by trypsin. When trypsin is activated, it is capable of activating many digestive proenzymes. Trypsin also activates inflammatory cells via PAR-2. Trypsin activity in the pancreas is mainly controlled by pancreatic secretory trypsin inhibitor (PSTI). When trypsinogen is activated into trypsin in the pancreas, PSTI immediately binds to trypsin to prevent further activation of pancreatic enzymes.

mutation probably is a disease modifier rather than a causative factor underlying the development of acute pancreatitis.[26]

The causative genetic mutation of hereditary pancreatitis was identified in 1996 as the third exon of the cationic trypsinogen gene on chromosome 7q35.[34] This disorder occurs as an autosomal dominant, and 80% of individuals with at least one copy of this gene develop recurrent acute pancreatitis; all patients with penetrance (about 80%) develop chronic pancreatitis, and 40% of patients with hereditary pancreatitis subsequently develop pancreatic cancer.[35,36] Patients with this hereditary disorder and pancreatitis are clinically and pathologically similar to patients with sporadic causes of pancreatitis. Many genetic mutations affect the three-dimensional conformation of the trypsinogen-SPINK1 complex and might impair the activity of the SPINK1 defense system against activated trypsin.[34,37]

DIAGNOSIS

The diagnosis of acute pancreatitis is relatively straightforward when acute upper abdominal pain and tenderness, nausea, vomiting, and hyperamylasemia or hyperlipasemia are present.[26,38] These clinical and biochemical signs are nonspecific, however, and can be present in many other acute intra-abdominal conditions, such as acute perforation or mesenteric infarction. Many cases of acute pancreatitis still are diagnosed at autopsy. The diagnosis of acute pancreatitis can be particularly difficult in postoperative patients. Acute pancreatitis also can be hard to diagnose in patients receiving drugs for sedation and patients who are hypothermic or unable to complain of abdominal pain. The Cullen and Grey Turner signs (periumbilical and flank bruising) are rare and can be present with any disease associated with retroperitoneal hemorrhage. Although hyperamylasemia is common, normal circulating amylase levels are present in 10% to 20% of all cases of acute pancreatitis. Normal serum amylase concentrations are seen predominantly in acute pancreatitis secondary to hyperlipidemia, acute exacerbations of chronic pancreatitis, and late in the course of acute pancreatitis.[39] Advantages of serum amylase determination include its technical simplicity, wide availability, and sensitivity.[40] This diagnostic test is plagued by low specificity, however. Serum lipase concentration increases within 4 to 8 hours of the onset of acute pancreatitis, peaks at 24 hours, and returns to normal after 8 to 14 days.[41] The major advantage of serum lipase determination as a diagnostic test is its excellent sensitivity in acute alcoholic pancreatitis. Measurement of serum lipase activity also is valuable when patients present to an emergency department days after the onset of the disease because serum lipase levels remain elevated longer than do amylase levels.[40] Although serum lipase formerly was believed to be a specific marker for acute pancreatitis, increased circulating levels of serum lipase can occur in many other diseases. Simultaneous estimation of amylase and lipase levels does not improve accuracy.[40] Other pancreatic enzymes, such as P-isoamylase, macroamylases, immunoreactive trypsinogen, and elastase, generally are not considered useful for making the diagnosis of acute pancreatitis.

SEVERITY AND SCORING

Prediction of the severity of the disease at the time of admission can be difficult, and patients can appear clinically well at admission but clinically deteriorate within 48 hours. Several different prognostic scoring systems with clinical, laboratory, and radiologic criteria have been proposed. Ranson's criteria (Table 122-1),[42] the Imrie[43] (Glasgow) score, the Acute Physiologic and Chronic Health Evaluation (APACHE) II and III scores,[44] the simplified acute physiology score, and Balthazar's computed tomography (CT) index (Table 122-2)[45,46] are the most popular scoring systems and often are used to determine the need for admission to an ICU. Development of the Atlanta Classification system for severity of acute pancreatitis has allowed comparisons among clinical trials and different treatment strategies.[47] This classification system defined severe acute pancreatitis by its association with organ failure; local complications, such as necrosis, abscess, or pseudocyst; or both. By consensus, the Atlanta Classification also defined severe acute pancreatitis as the presence of three or more of Ranson's criteria or a score of 8 or more with APACHE II criteria. Most often, severe acute pancreatitis is a clinical expression of the development of pancreatic necrosis. Less commonly, patients with interstitial (edematous) pancreatitis may present with severe acute pancreatitis.[47] Serum concentration of C-reactive protein (CRP), neutrophil elastase, pancreatitis-associated

TABLE 122–1. RANSON'S CRITERIA FOR PATIENTS WITH NON–GALLSTONE-ASSOCIATED PANCREATITIS

At Presentation	During Initial 48 Hours
Age >55 years	Hematocrit fall >10%
White blood cell count >16,000/μL	Blood urea nitrogen >5 mg/dL
Blood glucose >200 mg/dL	Serum calcium <8 mg/dL
Serum alanine transferase >250 U/dL	Arterial PO$_2$ <60 mm Hg
Serum lactate dehydrogenase >350 IU	Base deficit >4 mEq/L
	Estimated fluid sequestration >6 L

Modified from Blamey SL, Imrie CW, O'Neill J, et al: Prognostic factors in acute pancreatitis. Gut 1984;25:1340-1346.

TABLE 122–2. CALCULATION OF BALTHAZAR'S COMPUTED TOMOGRAPHY SCORING SYSTEM FOR ACUTE PANCREATITIS

Inflammatory Process	Grade	Score	Subtotals
Normal	A	0	
Focal or diffuse enlargement Contour irregularity Inhomogeneous attenuation	B	1	
Grade B *plus* peripancreatic haziness/mottled densities	C	2	
Grades B, C *plus one* ill-defined peripancreatic fluid collection	D	3	
Grades B, C *plus two* ill-defined fluid collections or gas	E	4	
Necrosis			
None	0	0	
<30%		2	
50%		4	
>50%		6	
Total			

Modified from Balthazar EJ, Robinson DL, Megibow AJ, et al: Acute pancreatitis: Value of CT in establishing prognosis. Radiology 1990;174:331-336.

peptide, interleukin (IL)-6, IL-8, IL-1, IL-10, and soluble tumor necrosis factor receptors might be useful for the early prediction of severity of disease in acute pancreatitis. Circulating CRP concentration is an independent predictor of outcome in acute pancreatitis.[48] Wilson and colleagues[48] suggested that if the peak level of CRP is greater than 210 mg/L on day 2 to 4 or greater than 120 mg/L at the end of the first week, this simple test could be as predictive as multiple-factor scoring systems. Urinary trypsinogen activation peptide of 37 nmol/L after onset of acute pancreatitis predicts severity of the disease,[49] but this assay has not achieved wide use in clinical practice.

IMAGING

ULTRASONOGRAPHY AND ENDOSCOPIC ULTRASONOGRAPHY

Ultrasonography has little role in the grading of severity of acute pancreatitis or determination of extent of pancreatic necrosis.[50] The value of ultrasonography is compromised by overlying bowel gas in at least 25% to 30% of cases.[51] By aiding in the diagnosis of gallstones, common bile duct stones, common bile duct dilation, and free peritoneal fluid, ultrasonography can be useful for determining the cause of pancreatitis.[51] Ultrasonography should be considered as an initial test in all patients with pancreatitis, especially if gallstones are suspected.[52,53]

Endoscopic ultrasonography combines ultrasonography and endoscopic evaluation. It is less invasive than endoscopic retrograde cholangiopancreatography and has been shown to be clinically useful in diagnosing acute pancreatitis and choledocholithiasis.[54] Endoscopic ultrasonography may be useful when CT and ultrasonography fail to show common bile duct stones. Endoscopic ultrasonography also may be useful in selecting patients who would benefit from endoscopic retrograde cholangiopancreatography and early stone extraction. One advantage of endoscopic ultrasonography is that it can be performed in pregnant women, patients with metallic implants, and patients who are too unstable to be transported out of the ICU.[54]

COMPUTED TOMOGRAPHY

Contrast-enhanced CT is considered the gold standard for diagnosing pancreatic necrosis and peripancreatic collections and for grading acute pancreatitis (see Table 122-2).[45,46] Necrosis is detected by CT as focal or diffuse areas of diminished pancreatic parenchymal contrast enhancement (<50 Hounsfield units). The accuracy of this test is greater than 90%. CT findings of acute pancreatitis include diffuse or segmental enlargement of the pancreas (interstitial edema), irregularity of the contour of the pancreas with obliteration of the peripancreatic fat planes, heterogeneous appearance with areas of decreased density within the pancreas, and variable ill-defined fluid collections (see Table 122-2).[45,46] The Balthazar index ranges from 0 to 10 and is obtained by adding the points attributed to the extent of the inflammatory process to the volume of pancreatic necrosis. Although CT findings correlate with clinical course and severity of patients with acute pancreatitis,[53] it is not necessary to obtain this study in patients with mild pancreatitis.[18,21] CT can be helpful when the diagnosis is in doubt or when complications of pancreatitis may be developing. In general, contrast-enhanced CT scans should not be performed during the first 72 hours of the disease because necrosis may not be fully established until after 96 hours, and there have been isolated reports of intravenous contrast material causing derangements of the pancreatic microcirculation.[55,56] Contrast administration also can trigger or exacerbate renal insufficiency.

ENDOSCOPIC RETROGRADE CHOLANGIOPANCREATOGRAPHY

Endoscopic retrograde cholangiopancreatography is an effective means for treating common bile duct stones.[57] Endoscopic retrograde cholangiopancreatography is not indicated for the management of mild pancreatitis or nonbiliary pancreatitis.[57-59] This modality is indicated, however, in the management of patients with biliary pancreatitis and biliary obstruction or cholangitis.[60,61] There is controversy regarding the role of endoscopic retrograde cholangiopancreatography for the management of patients with biliary pancreatitis but without bile duct obstruction. Four clinical trials have sought to determine whether endoscopic retrograde cholangiopancreatography plus sphincterotomy or conservative management is more appropriate for patients with acute pancreatitis.[60,62,63] In a study of 121 patients randomized to endoscopic retrograde cholangiopancreatography or conservative treatment within 72 hours of onset, there was a significant reduction in morbidity (17% versus 34%; $P = .03$) but no significant difference in mortality (2% versus 8%; $P = .23$).[62] The differences in morbidity seen in this trial cannot be explained by differences in the severity of pancreatitis between the two groups.[62]

In another study that enrolled 195 patients, endoscopic retrograde cholangiopancreatography performed within 24 hours was compared with conservative therapy. Endoscopic retrograde cholangiopancreatography was associated with a significant reduction in morbidity (biliary sepsis; $P = .001$) without a significant reduction in mortality (five deaths with endoscopic retrograde cholangiopancreatography versus nine deaths with conservative treatment).[63] Included in this study were patients with nonbiliary pancreatitis, such as alcohol-related and parasite-related disease. A trial with similar design (endoscopic retrograde cholangiopancreatography within 24 hours versus conservative treatment) randomized 280 patients[64]; 75 of the 178 patients in the endoscopic retrograde cholangiopancreatography arm had impacted biliary stones. This study is the only one that showed a significant reduction in morbidity and mortality.

The study by Folsch and colleagues[60] was a multicenter trial of endoscopic retrograde cholangiopancreatography versus conservative management. Patients with biliary sepsis and obstruction were excluded from study entry because efficacy in this group has been established. In contrast to the previous studies, this study showed a significant increase in complications in the endoscopic retrograde cholangiopancreatography group compared with the conservatively managed group (respiratory failure, 12% versus 4% [$P = .03$]; renal failure, 7% versus 4% [$P = .10$]). In addition, the mortality rate was higher in the endoscopic retrograde cholangiopancreatography group compared with the control group (11% versus 6%), requiring premature termination of the study.[60] The results of this large clinical trial suggest that in the absence of biliary obstruction or sepsis, endoscopic retrograde cholangiopancreatography may be harmful, and a conservative approach is preferred.

The role of endoscopic retrograde cholangiopancreatography in idiopathic pancreatitis also is unclear.[65] Advances in ultrasonography and magnetic resonance cholangiopancreatography suggest that these modalities may have a preferred role when diagnostic considerations are the issue in acute pancreatitis, especially in view of the potential for complications with endoscopic retrograde cholangiopancreatography.[66-68]

MAGNETIC RESONANCE CHOLANGIOPANCREATOGRAPHY

Magnetic resonance cholangiopancreatography is a relatively recently developed tool for the noninvasive investigation of the hepatopancreatic biliary system.[69] Magnetic resonance cholangiopancreatography compares favorably with endoscopic retrograde cholangiopancreatography for assessing and diagnosing patients with extrahepatic bile duct abnormalities, such as choledocholithiasis and cholangiocarcinoma.[70] Magnetic resonance cholangiopancreatography can be performed when endoscopic retrograde cholangiopancreatography has failed or is not possible, although endoscopic retrograde cholangiopancreatography is not only a diagnostic modality, but also a therapeutic one because the endoscopic approach permits sphincterotomy and removal of common duct stones.[71]

Contrast-enhanced CT is the gold standard for documenting pancreatic necrosis and for assessing the severity of acute pancreatitis.[46,72,73] Nevertheless, results from a few studies suggest that magnetic resonance cholangiopancreatography compares favorably with contrast-enhanced CT for the diagnosis and grading of severe acute pancreatitis.[74,75] The major advantage of magnetic resonance cholangiopancreatography for severe acute pancreatitis is the ability to avoid infusing critically ill patients with iodinated contrast media.[69] Bowel peristalsis, vascular motion artifacts, gastrointestinal air, and the presence of metallic clips all can degrade the quality of the images obtained with magnetic resonance cholangiopancreatography.

MANAGEMENT

GENERAL SUPPORT

Monitoring and Resuscitation

Several publications suggest that patients with severe acute pancreatitis should be managed in an ICU, preferably by a specialist team.[21,76] Ongoing monitoring for signs of distant organ dysfunction is crucial. Initial management is intravascular volume resuscitation, regardless of the etiology and severity of acute pancreatitis. Sequestration of fluid into the so-called third space (i.e., the extravascular extracellular compartment) can lead to loss of one third of plasma volume.[76] Rapid restoration and maintenance of intravascular volume is essential because hypovolemia and shock probably are important factors contributing to the high incidence of acute renal failure among patients with severe acute pancreatitis.[77] It is common for patients with severe acute pancreatitis to require administration of crystalloid fluid at rates of 500 mL/h, at least for a while. When resuscitation has begun, ongoing monitoring of respiratory, cardiovascular, and renal function is essential. Ensuring adequate oxygen delivery to tissues and prevention of splanchnic ischemia are paramount.[78] Use of inotropes or vasoactive agents should be considered only after intravascular volume is optimized. Because ongoing

fluid sequestration may be pronounced in the abdomen, intra-abdominal pressure can increase, leading to the possibility of abdominal compartment syndrome.

Pulmonary Dysfunction

Respiratory dysfunction is a major component of multiple organ system dysfunction syndrome secondary to acute pancreatitis, and most patients with this syndrome require ventilatory support.[17,76,78] Acute respiratory distress syndrome is characterized by diffuse pulmonary infiltrates on the chest radiograph, arterial hypoxemia, pulmonary hypertension, and decreased pulmonary compliance.

Pulmonary Management

Patients with severe acute pancreatitis must be monitored closely for hypoxic and hypercarbic respiratory failure. Supplemental oxygen is almost uniformly required, and mechanical ventilation is often required.[21] Noninvasive positive-pressure ventilation may be used to avoid endotracheal intubation in carefully selected patients; severe acute pancreatitis often is associated with marked abdominal distention and diminished functional residual capacity, however, and noninvasive positive-pressure ventilation usually is not well tolerated. Management of acute lung injury and acute respiratory distress syndrome secondary to acute pancreatitis is similar to management of these conditions associated with other primary problems (e.g., sepsis).

Pain Relief

Provision of pain relief to patients with severe acute pancreatitis is not only humane, but also may improve pulmonary dysfunction. Although intravenous narcotics are useful and effective, epidural analgesia with local anesthetics may be advantageous.[84]

SPECIFIC SUPPORT

Nutrition

Traditionally, patients with acute pancreatitis have been managed by providing intravenous fluids and nutrition and avoiding enteral feeding to "rest" the inflamed pancreas and prevent stimulation of exocrine function and the release of proteolytic enzymes.[16] Nevertheless, most patients with mild acute pancreatitis can begin oral supplementation within a few days of their presentation with pain.[57,85] In the past, the primary approach for providing nutritional support for patients with severe acute pancreatitis was total parenteral nutrition (TPN).[86] TPN is expensive, however, and may increase the risk of sepsis or metabolic derangements.[86,87] TPN also has been associated with alterations in gut barrier function.[88] Accumulating data support the view that enteral nutrition is safe in patients with severe acute pancreatitis.[89-92] The Cochrane Database updated the topic of TPN versus enteral feeding in acute pancreatitis.[91] In two trials that enrolled a total of 70 patients, the relative risk of death with enteral nutrition versus TPN was 0.56 (95% confidence interval 0.05 to 5.62). The mean length of stay was reduced with enteral nutrition (median day −2.2; 95% confidence interval −3.62 to −0.078), and the relative risk for systemic infection with enteral nutrition versus TPN was 0.61 (95% confidence interval 0.29 to 1.28). In one trial, the relative risk for local septic complications and other local complications with enteral nutrition versus TPN was 0.56 (95% confidence interval 0.12 to 2.68) and 0.16 (95% confidence interval 0.01 to 2.86).[89-92] The Cochrane investigators concluded that although there is a trend in the reduction in adverse events after the administration of enteral nutrition, the available data are insufficient to support the conclusion that enteral nutrition is safer or more efficacious for improving outcome than TPN.[91] A study reported that the incidence of pancreatic sepsis and the number of surgical interventions are reduced among patients with severe acute pancreatitis treated with enteral nutrition supplemented with *Lactobacillus plantarum* 299.[93]

If a nasoduodenal or nasojejunal tube is placed, care should be taken if blind manipulation through the duodenum is attempted.[26] Although blind placement is possible, the duodenum is often distorted in patients with acute pancreatitis, and the risk of perforation is increased. Fluoroscopic or endoscopic guidance of the tube into a postpyloric, even jejunal, position is preferable.

Supplemental TPN may be valuable when nutritional requirements cannot be achieved using enteral nutrition alone, or enteral access cannot be established. Ileus is not an absolute contraindication to enteral feeding, and most patients tolerate continuous feeding at a slow rate. Although one article provided data to support the idea that gastric rather than jejunal feeding is safe in patients with acute pancreatitis,[94] consensus at this time is that enteral feeding should be initiated early and into the jejunum.[87-92,95]

Resting energy expenditure varies widely in acute pancreatitis patients, depending on the magnitude of the regional inflammatory process and the presence of additional complications, especially infection. Infection can increase energy expenditure by 5% to 20%, but overfeeding should be avoided, and tight glucose control should be employed.[90] Although triglyceride levels should be monitored and should not be allowed to escalate to levels above normal, administration of lipids is safe and appropriate.[90] Pancreatic secretion is not stimulated by intravenous lipids, whereas the anatomic site of nutrient administration determines the degree and extent of pancreatic stimulation after enteral nutrition. There is no proven causal relationship between infusion of exogenous fat and the development of pancreatitis.

The timing of oral refeeding must be based on clinical judgment. Consideration for feeding is based on resolution of ileus, improvement in signs of retroperitoneal inflammation, improvement in distant organ dysfunction, and absence of an enterocutaneous fistula.

PATHOGENESIS OF PANCREATIC INFECTION AND ANTIBIOTIC PROPHYLAXIS

Microorganisms can gain access to necrotic pancreatic and peripancreatic tissue via several routes, bacterial translocation from the colon being the most likely. Failure of the intestinal barrier permits bacteria and yeast to translocate from the lumen of the gut into ascites, mesenteric lymph, the bloodstream, and the pancreatic phlegmon.[96,97]

The notion that pancreatic infection in acute pancreatitis is due to infection by gut-derived organisms is supported by the observation that most pancreatic infections are monomicrobial and caused by gram-negative bacteria, at least when prophylactic antibiotics have not been administered.[5] Further support for the intestinal origin of pancreatic infection in acute pancreatitis derives from data obtained in a clinical trial of selective decontamination of the gut, wherein enteral administration of poorly absorbed antimicrobial agents was associated with a significant reduction in late mortality principally owing to decreased incidence of pancreatic gram-negative infection.[98] Microorganisms also can gain access to pancreatic necrosis through hematogenous dissemination from infected central venous catheters,[99] via the biliary tree, or via the pancreatic duct from the lumen of the duodenum (Figure 122-2).

The wisdom of using prophylactic antibiotics for the management of acute pancreatitis has been debated for more than 40 years. This question has been addressed by many small (relatively underpowered) randomized controlled clinical trials[98-108] and numerous observational or retrospective studies. Two meta-analyses have been published (Table 122-3).[98-108] When greater than 30% of the gland is necrotic, pancreatic infection occurs in more than 30% to 40% of patients with acute pancreatitis. Approximately 80% of deaths due to acute pancreatitis are related to infectious complications. It is reasonable to consider whether administration of prophylactic antibiotics can decrease the incidence of either local or distant infections or the morbidity and mortality associated with pancreatic necrosis. Initial work in this area focused on the specific characteristics of antibiotics and whether or not the drugs penetrate into pancreatic tissue.[109] Trials in the 1970s used antibiotics that either do not penetrate well into pancreatic tissue[107] or did not have an adequate spectrum of antimicrobial activity. Aminoglycosides penetrate tissues poorly, whereas cephalosporins (e.g., cefotaxime), ureidopenicillins (e.g., piperacillin), fluoroquinolones (e.g., ciprofloxacin, ofloxacin, perfloxacin), metronidazole, and imipenem all penetrate well into pancreatic tissue.[109]

The most widely quoted trials in support of antibiotic prophylaxis for acute pancreatitis include the trial by Pederlozi and colleagues[100] of 74 patients randomized to receive either imipenem (0.5 g every 8 hours for 14 days) or placebo, the trial by Sainio and associates[101] of 60 patients randomized to receive either cefuroxime (1.5 g intravenously every 8 hours) or placebo, and the trial by Luiten and coworkers[98] of 102 patients randomized to receive selective digestive decontamination versus standard therapy. In the trial by Pederlozi and colleagues,[100] the secondary rate of pancreatic infection decreased from 30% in the control group to 12% in the imipenem group ($P = .10$). There were three deaths in each group, and there were no beneficial effects on organ failure, mortality, or avoidance of surgery. The trial by Saino and associates[101] enrolled mostly young patients with alcoholic pancreatitis and found that infectious complications were more common in the group not treated with antibiotic prophylaxis compared with the group treated with cefuroxime (1.8 per patient versus 1 per patient; $P = .10$), as was mortality (7 versus 1; $P = .03$). Coagulase-negative *Staphylococcus* was a pathogen from an unspecified site in four of the eight patients who died. In the experimental arm of the selective digestive decontamination trial, colistin, amphotericin, and norfloxacin were administered via the oral and rectal routes. In addition, patients in this arm received a short course of therapy with cefotaxime in 50 patients versus 52 controls. There were 18 deaths among the 52 patients in the control group (35%) and 11 deaths among the 50 patients in the selective digestive decontamination group (22%) ($P = .048$).[98]

In a retrospective review of 180 patients with severe acute pancreatitis, Ho and Frey[105] found a mortality rate of 18%

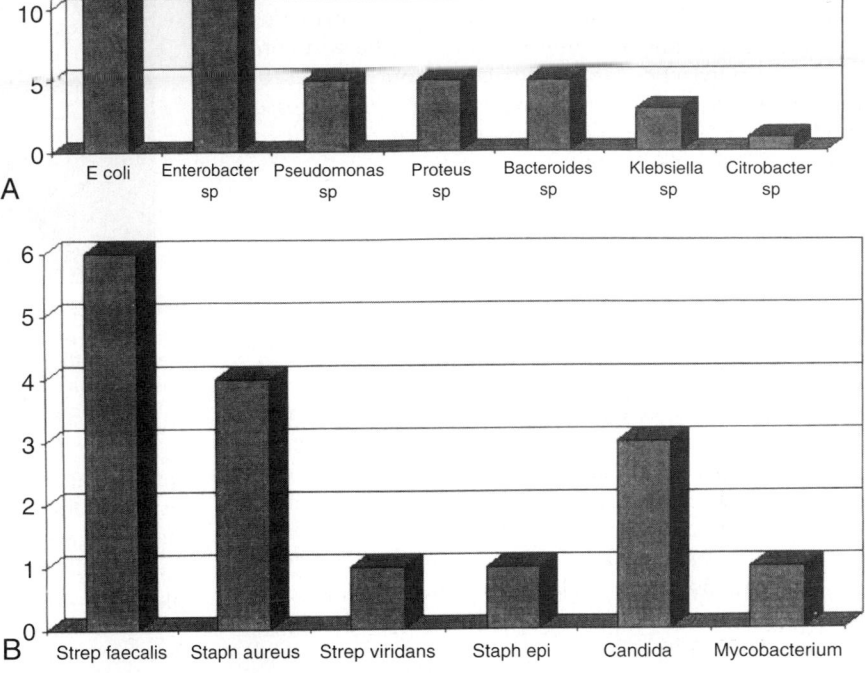

FIGURE 122–2. A, Gram-negative bacteria isolated from 45 patients with infected pancreatic necrosis in the preantibiotic era. **B,** Gram-positive organisms, yeasts, and mycobacteria isolated from 45 patients with infected pancreatic necrosis in the preantibiotic era. (From Hartwig W, Werner J, Uhl W, et al: Management of infection in acute pancreatitis. J Hepatobiliary Pancreat Surg 2002;9:423-428.)

and a pancreatic infection rate of 76% among patients who did not receive prophylactic antibiotics, whereas the mortality rate was only 5% and the infection rate 27% among patients who were treated with prophylactic imipenem. The two meta-analyses suggest a benefit in reduction of mortality when prophylactic antibiotics are used.[107,108]

Although antibiotic prophylaxis is widely employed, the quality of evidence supporting this practice is relatively weak and does not meet the criteria of two large randomized controlled trials showing the same clinical outcome. Improved outcome has not been shown adequately in a single well-done, convincing large trial with a diverse patient population and with endpoints of death or infection-related morbidity. Although the selective digestive decontamination trial does show a difference in mortality, because of the small number of patients enrolled in this trial, a change in outcome (death) of a single patient in this trial would have altered the fundamental finding of the trial. In addition, several reports of severe acute pancreatitis have documented changes in the microbial spectrum of pancreatic infections, characterized by

TABLE 122–3. RESULTS OF CLINICAL TRIALS OF ANTIBIOTIC PROPHYLAXIS IN PATIENTS WITH SEVERE ACUTE PANCREATITIS

Year	Antibiotic	No. Patients	Death	Pancreatic Infection	Sepsis
1993[100]	Imipenem (500 mg/8)	41	3	5	6
	Control	33	3	10	16
1995[101]	Cefuroxime (4-5 g/d)	30	1	9	11
	Control	30	7	12	13
1995[98]	SDD*	50	11		9
	Control	52	18		20
1996[103]	Ceftazidime/amikacin/metronidazole	11	1	0	4
	Control	12	3	4	7
1997[102]	Ofloxacin/metronidazole	13	0	8	6
	Control	13	2	7	0
1998[137]	Imipenem	30	3	10	
	Perfloxacin	30	7	3	
2001[106]	Imipenem	25	1		2
	Control	33	2		8

SDD, selective digestive decontamination.

an increased incidence of fungal species and more antibiotic-resistant bacterial species.[99,110,111] Fungal infection in severe acute pancreatitis is a risk factor for mortality.[110,111] These studies raise the possibility that prophylaxis with imipenem, a commonly employed antibiotic, may be associated with increased risk of infection with fungal species or imipenem-resistant bacteria. Prophylactic use of an antifungal agent may be warranted.[111] Although prophylactic antimicrobials administered intravenously or enterally are uniformly used in some institutions, I cannot recommend the widespread use of prophylactic antimicrobials without further data supporting the benefits of use over the apparent increase in antimicrobial resistance being reported in current series and seen in my own institution.

MANAGEMENT OF PANCREATIC NECROSIS AND ABSCESS

Pancreatic necrosis is defined by the presence of diffuse or focal areas of nonviable pancreatic parenchyma, often associated with peripancreatic fat necrosis.[47] Necrosis can be either sterile or infected; infection usually is confirmed by fine-needle aspiration.[112,113] Pancreatic infection occurs in about 10% of all cases of acute pancreatitis, but in 30% to 70% of cases with necrosis. Contrast-enhanced CT is currently the gold standard for documenting the presence of nonperfused pancreatic parenchyma. A pancreatic abscess is a circumscribed intra-abdominal collection of pus, usually in close proximity to pancreatic necrosis, which arises as a consequence of acute pancreatitis.[47]

Infected pancreatic necrosis should be suspected in patients with acute pancreatitis with clinical signs of sepsis. This diagnosis also should be suspected when patients fail to improve with supportive therapy or regress after an initial period of improvement (Figs. 122-3 and 122-4).[47] Patients suspected of having infected pancreatic necrosis should undergo contrast-enhanced CT scan or ultrasound-guided, fine-needle aspiration.[17,47,112,113] This approach is a safe and reliable way to differentiate between sterile and infected necrosis. Complication rates of this procedure are low. Rare serious complications include bleeding and aggravation of

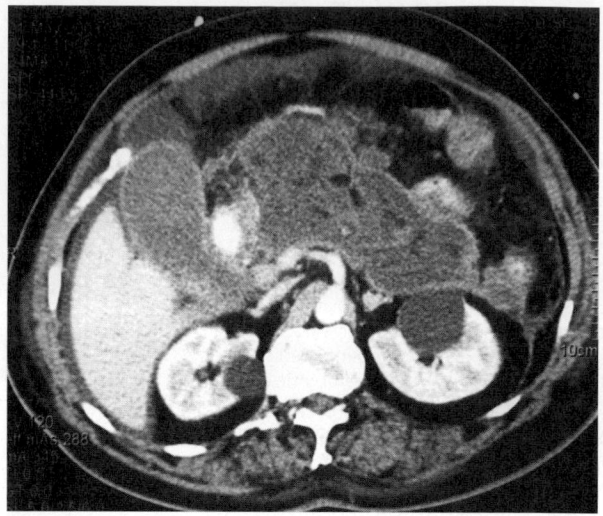

FIGURE 122–4. Computed tomography scan of a patient with severe necrotizing pancreatitis and Balthazar grade E scan; more than 50% necrosis of the gland was seen on previous scans of the gland, giving the patient a Balthazar index of 10. The patient developed pancreatic infection more than 4 weeks into his hospital course.

acute pancreatitis.[114,115] With Gram staining and culture of aspirated material, fine-needle aspiration by ultrasonography has a diagnostic sensitivity of 88% and specificity of 90%.[112] Fine-needle aspiration is indicated only in patients with signs and symptoms of sepsis, patients who fail to improve, and patients who worsen after initial clinical improvement because there is a possibility of contamination of sterile necrosis.[21] Outside of a clinical trial, fine-needle aspiration should not be performed as a matter of routine in a patient with severe acute pancreatitis who is clinically doing well. In one study, the proportion of patients with infection increased from 24% in the first week to 36% and 72% in the second and third weeks.[114] Several additional studies have confirmed infection rates of 2.8% to 22% in the first week and 28.8% to 55% in the second to fourth weeks.[15] The timing of fine-needle aspiration should be based on the probability of infection based on time of onset from the disease and the current clinical condition of the patient.

LABORATORY MARKERS OF INFECTED NECROSIS

No reliable blood test has been developed to establish the diagnosis of infected necrosis.[116-119] Measurement of serum CRP concentration is the best available blood test for identification of pancreatic necrosis; CRP concentration greater than 120 mg/L is associated with necrosis.[48] There is no correlation, however, between the serum CRP level and the presence of infected necrosis. Circulating levels of many other different mediators, including synovial phospholipase A_2, IL-8, procalcitonin, and tumor necrosis factor, have been tested for their ability to differentiate sterile pancreatic necrosis versus infected pancreatic necrosis. Procalcitonin is a 116-amino acid propeptide of calcitonin that has been shown to be a marker for severe bacterial and fungal infection. In a study of 32 patients with severe acute pancreatitis, serum levels of procalcitonin showed some predictive accuracy with regard to the presence or absence of pancreatic infection (using culture of material obtained by fine-needle aspiration as the gold standard).[117] Infected pancreatic necrosis was

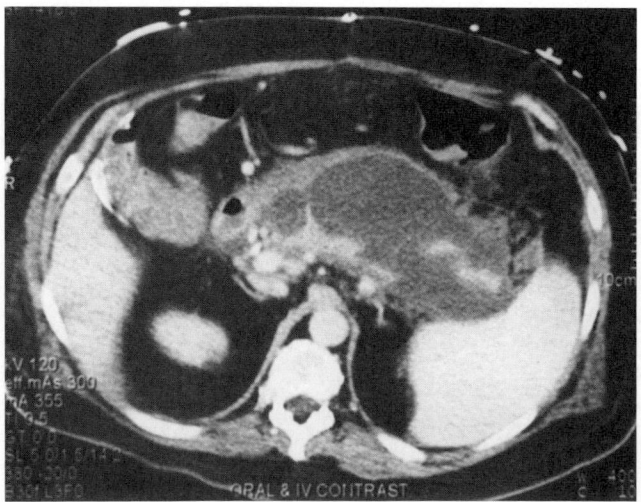

FIGURE 122–3. Computed tomography scan of a patient with severe acute pancreatitis, a large fluid collection, and significant (>50%) necrosis. Pancreatic infection occurred on hospital day 17.

predicted by a procalcitonin level greater than 1.8 mg/dL with a sensitivity of 94% and a specificity of 90%. These results could not be replicated in another study, however, or in a larger population of patients.[118] The true value of procalcitonin for identifying patients with infected pancreatic necrosis is unclear. An excellent review of serum markers in acute pancreatitis has been published.[119]

INDICATION AND TIMING OF OPERATIVE INTERVENTION

Although there is no consensus about the timing of operative intervention for pancreatic necrosis, most experts now recommend delaying operation until infection has been identified.[14,15,120] Theoretically, early surgery might aid in the diagnosis of infection and improve outcome by removing necrotic tissue and decreasing the stimulus for systemic inflammation. Early in the course of the disease, the pancreatic tissue is friable, however, and nonviable tissues are not well demarcated. In addition, viable tissue usually is present, even when the gland grossly appears to be completely necrotic. A randomized trial designed to answer the question of whether early versus late (beyond 14 days) necrosectomy offers a survival advantage was stopped before planned enrollment was completed because of a trend toward higher mortality (58%) in the early operation group compared with the late operation group (27%).[121] In another series of 121 patients with severe acute pancreatitis, few required early operation.[14] Early operation should be reserved for patients with proven infected necrosis or patients with other surgical complications, such as massive bleeding or bowel perforation.[120]

STERILE NECROSIS

Before 1990, the standard surgical practice was to débride necrotic pancreatic tissue operatively, even in the absence of infection (Table 122-4). Nonoperative management of sterile necrosis is now the standard of care, according to guidelines published by the American College of Gastroenterology,[19] Santorini Consensus Conference,[21] Bangkok World Congress of Gastroenterology,[122] and International Society of Pancreatology.[20] In selected cases, patients with extensive necrosis may not improve, and after a prolonged period of observation (6 to 8 weeks), operative débridement may be warranted.[123,124] Sterile pancreatic necrosis has a mortality rate of 0 to 10% when managed using a conservative nonoperative approach.[125,126] In a retrospective study, operative débridement of sterile necrosis caused conversion to infected necrosis.[126] Buchler and associates[127] reported a 3.5% mortality rate when sterile pancreatic necrosis was managed nonoperatively routinely. Only 1 of 57 patients

TABLE 122–4. RESULTS OF CONSERVATIVE TREATMENT OF PATIENTS WITH NECROTIZING PANCREATITIS AND STERILE NECROSIS

Year	Patients	Mortality—No. Patients (%)
1991[125]	11	0
1995[23]	65	4 (6)
2000[127]	56	1 (2)
2001[124]	62	7 (11)

TABLE 122–5. TREATMENT MODALITIES FOR NECROTIZING PANCREATITIS

Minimally Invasive[130]

Percutaneous drainage and peritoneal lavage[129]
Percutaneous necrosectomy, retroperitoneoscopy[130,131,138]
Endoscopic drainage[132]

Open

Conventional resection[106,133,134]
Necrosectomy and conventional tube drainage[125]
Necrosectomy and postoperative lavage[14,15,136]
Necrosectomy and re-laparotomy when needed[120,126]
Necrosectomy, drainage, and scheduled relaparotomy[12]
Necrosectomy, planned re-laparotomy, temporary abdominal wall closure[139]
Necrosectomy and laparotomy[136]

underwent surgical treatment; operation in the single case was performed because of rapid clinical deterioration.

OPERATIVE PROCEDURES

Although there is general agreement that infected necrosis requires operative débridement, there is no consensus about the best approach to achieve this goal.[14,15,122] All methods aim to remove infected tissue, while preserving most of the gland. There must be planning for continued evacuation of infected debris and exudates (Table 122-5).[6,127,128] At least three comparable techniques have been studied. All seem to offer equivalent outcomes but have never been compared in head-to-head comparison. These approaches are (1) necrosectomy combined with open packing technique,[128] (2) necrosectomy with planned staged re-explorations with repeated lavage,[12] and (3) necrosectomy followed by closed continuous suction lavage of the retroperitoneum.[6] In experienced hands, these techniques have lowered mortality rates for severe acute pancreatitis to less than 15%. Minimally invasive techniques also have been described, including percutaneous drainage, percutaneous necrosectomy, and endoscopic or laparoscopic approaches.[129-132] These limited drainage/débridement techniques have been successful, but are probably appropriate only for selected patients (Table 122-6).

Conventional Resection

Traditional formal pancreatic resections were performed for acute pancreatitis in the past. These procedures have been

TABLE 122–6. RESULTS OF CONSERVATIVE SURGICAL RETROPERITONEAL DRAINAGE

Series	Mortality (%)	Morbidity (%)	Repeated Surgery/Patient
N = 40	33	50	3.6
N = 18	22	38	2.6
N = 15	20	20	1.4
N = 14	0	42	5
N = 8	25	62	NA
N = 25	0	25	0
N = 15	27	40	0

Modified from Castellanos G, Pinero A, Serrano A, et al: Infected pancreatic necrosis: Translumbar approach and management with retroperitoneoscopy. Arch Surg 2002;137:1060-1063.

abandoned in the treatment of severe acute pancreatitis, however, because of excessively high rates for complications and mortality.[133-135] These procedures do not remove the surrounding necrotic tissue and needlessly remove healthy tissue.

Necrosectomy

Necrosectomy removes devitalized tissue from the pancreas and surrounding retroperitoneum.[12,13,17,124,127,136] The tissue generally is removed by gentle finger fracture technique. Necrosectomy is designed to remove most of the devitalized tissue without injuring major blood vessels.[12] Repeated operations are often necessary.

The open packing technique originally was popularized by Bradley[128] and was associated with a mortality of 15%, but morbidity was extensive and included external pancreatic fistulas in 46% of cases, hernias in 32% of cases, and massive venous hemorrhage in 7% of cases. Planned staged laparotomies and lavage were used by Sarr and coworkers[12] in 23 patients. In this series, the mortality rate was 17%, and the morbidity rate was 52%. Pancreatic and colonic fistulas occurred in 26% and 22% of cases. Fernandez-del Castillo and colleagues[123] reported a series of 64 consecutive patients with severe acute pancreatitis, including 36 with infected necrosis. Surgical management with drains was successful in 69%, and the overall mortality rate was only 6.2%. The authors noted a significantly better outcome when surgery was delayed beyond the fourth week.

In another large series of patients with severe acute pancreatitis, 42 patients (35%) required operative intervention.[126] The authors of this report preferred necrosectomy followed by closed suction lavage of the retroperitoneum using 35 to 40 L/d of peritoneal lavage solution for each of the first 7 postoperative days. In the series of 121 patients with necrotizing pancreatitis between 1993 to 2001, 35% (42 of 121) underwent necrosectomy with subsequent closed lavage.[15] Of the 121 patients, 12 (9.9%) died, including 9 patients who were treated surgically and 3 patients who were treated conservatively.[15] Morbidity included pancreatic fistulas in 8 of 42 (19%) surgically treated patients. Pancreatic fistulas after pancreatitis usually close spontaneously eventually, if pancreatic ductal obstruction is not present. In a few cases, enteric internal drainage or pancreatic resection may be required to achieve closure of pancreatic fistulas.

Aside from pancreatic infections, patients with severe acute pancreatitis are at risk for the usual gamut of nosocomial infections, including catheter-related bloodstream infections, urinary tract infections, and ventilator-associated pneumonia. Additional abdominal complications in patients with acute pancreatitis include concurrent biliary tract problems, stress gastritis and related bleeding, necrosis of the transverse colon, hemorrhage from gastric varices secondary to splenic vein thrombosis, and catastrophic bleeding from ruptured pseudoaneurysms involving the gastroduodenal artery or branches of the superior mesenteric artery. Should massive gastrointestinal bleeding occur and a gastric or proximal duodenal source is excluded, arteriography should be considered. Necrosis of the transverse colon should be considered in a patient with abdominal tenderness and distention and sepsis. Patients with colonic necrosis are usually dramatically ill. Enterocutaneous fistulas are seen commonly when the open packing technique is used and less commonly when other methods of management are employed.

OUTCOME

With an increasing number of patients surviving severe acute pancreatitis, attention has been focused on the quality of life and long-term outcome of surviving patients. This patient population is subject to a wide range of medical problems, including diabetes mellitus, symptoms of polyneuropathy, recurrent pancreatitis, and continual abdominal pain. Major social problems also can be an issue, especially among patients with alcohol-induced pancreatitis. Abdominal hernias may be present, especially in patients managed using open packing; future repair may be needed. Chronic pancreatitis and related problems, including pseudocysts, splenic vein thrombosis, and mesenteric pseudoaneurysms, can occur but are not discussed in further detail.

In one study, 145 patients after acute pancreatitis were compared with age-matched and gender-matched controls for results on the Short-Form 36 assessment of health-related quality of life.[136] Among this cohort of patients, 87% returned to work, 27% had recurrent attacks of pancreatitis, and 43% developed diabetes. Of the 113 patients with alcohol-induced pancreatitis, 30% were abstinent, and 28% remained problem drinkers, alcohol-dependent, or alcoholics.

SUMMARY

Acute pancreatitis is a widely variable disease that is usually mild in severity. Severe acute pancreatitis is a life-threatening disease, however, that can require intensive support, especially during the initial inflammatory period of SIRS, when massive fluid resuscitation and ventilatory, cardiovascular, renal, and nutritional support may be required. In patients with ongoing signs of SIRS beyond the second or third week of disease, progression from severe acute pancreatitis with sterile necrosis to infected necrosis should be considered. Fine-needle aspiration should be employed to diagnose pancreatic infection. Débridement of infected pancreatic necrosis is required, but the exact method of surgical débridement is controversial. Although severe acute pancreatitis is a life-threatening disease, in experienced hands the overall survival of patients with severe acute pancreatitis is about 90%.

ANNOTATED REFERENCES

Beger HG, Isenmann R: Acute pancreatitis: who needs an operation? J Hepatobiliary Pancreat Surg 2002;9:436-442.
This is a current review of surgical decision-making for patients with acute pancreatitis by two authorities in the field. The focus is on different approaches, timing, and controversy over the use of prophylactic antibiotics.

Frossard JL, Hadengue, Pastor CM: New serum markers for the detection of severe acute pancreatitis in humans. Am Respir Crit Care Med 2001;164: 162-170.
This article reviews the serum markers that might be useful for the diagnosis and management and staging of patients with acute pancreatitis. Specific limitations of current tests are discussed.

Hartwig W, Werner J, Muller CA, et al: Surgical management of severe pancreatitis including sterile necrosis. J Hepatobiliary Pancreat Surg 2002;9:429-435.
This article is a review of the surgical approach to patients with pancreatitis, including a discussion of the difficult problem of sterile necrosis. The focus is on the large local institutional experience.

Hartwig W, Werner J, Uhl W, et al: Management of infection in acute pancreatitis. J Hepatobiliary Pancreat Surg 2002;9:423-428.

This article discusses the pathogenesis of pancreatic infection and the microbiology. There is an extensive discussion of the data from previous small trials of prophylaxis.

Yousaf M, McCallion K, Diamond T: Management of severe acute pancreatitis. Br J Surg 2003;90:407-420.

This article is an excellent current review of the diagnosis, staging, and management of acute pancreatitis, with a special focus on changes in management since the 1970s.

Chapter 123
PERITONITIS AND INTRA-ABDOMINAL ABSCESS

Philip S. Barie • Addison K. May • Ajai K. Malhotra • Rao R. Ivatury

Patients who are critically ill and who have intra-abdominal infection represent a group that is at high risk of failure of management and other serious complications. Failure may occur because of inadequacy of surgical therapy (failure of primary source control) or the development of secondary complications, such as abdominal compartment syndrome or fistula formation. Ultimately, success or failure of management may be defined by the severity of the patient's illness. Optimal management of this diverse patient population is difficult to define and carry out; varies depending on the clinical situation; and is prone to wide variation in patterns of practice due, at least in part, to a lack of controlled studies in this patient population. Since there are few controlled studies of the management of critically ill patients with peritonitis, recommendations often are based on expert opinion and extrapolation from animal models and sometimes on clinical data.

Some basic principles can be applied broadly to this population. These principles include adequate and timely resuscitation to optimize tissue perfusion and oxygenation. Effective resuscitation may mitigate or avoid entirely certain manifestations of intra-abdominal infection in critical illness, such as ischemic colitis or acute acalculous cholecystitis. Source control also must be adequate and timely. Depending on the problem, source control may consist of débriding devitalized tissue, closing perforations, reducing the burden imposed by bacteria and their toxins, and providing appropriate and timely broad-spectrum antimicrobial therapy. However, to provide optimal management of these patients also requires a basic understanding of peritoneal defense mechanisms, the limitations of these defenses, relevant microbiology, and the factors that predict adverse outcomes in critically ill patients. Factors that predict failure of source control and management approaches to these challenging patients are presented in this chapter.

PATHOGENESIS

HOST DEFENSES

The healthy peritoneal cavity is a complex space lined with mesothelial cells that comprise the parietal and visceral peritoneum. The normal peritoneal cavity is quiescent immunologically but responds rapidly to bacterial contamination. Normally, about 50 to 100 mL of peritoneal fluid circulates freely among several potential and actual spaces within the peritoneal cavity.[1] Net fluid movement is upward toward the diaphragm, facilitated by normal peristalsis, normal diaphragmatic excursions, splanchnic blood flow, and factors that maintain normal membrane permeability of the microcirculation. Conversely, ileus, mechanical ventilation, splanchnic hypoperfusion, and intraperitoneal inflammation can disrupt normal fluid movement and result in fluid sequestration in the peritoneal cavity.

The three major intraperitoneal host defense mechanisms are clearance of bacteria by lymphatics, phagocytosis of bacteria by immune cells, and mechanical sequestration (abscess formation). A few phagocytic cells (peritoneal macrophages) circulate, and opsonic proteins that facilitate phagocytosis are present. Experimentally, if a small bacterial inoculum is placed in the peritoneal cavity, the bacteria are cleared within a few minutes from the peritoneal cavity when the peritoneal fluid is absorbed by specialized lacunae on the undersurface of the diaphragm.[1] The bacteria then pass into the central venous system via diaphragmatic and mediastinal lymphatics for disposition by systemic host defenses. When an infectious inoculum is introduced, there is a brisk inflammatory response that attempts to localize the infection, leading to abscess formation rather than generalized peritonitis. In this paradigm, formation of an intra-abdominal abscess can be considered "success"; indeed, mortality is higher for generalized peritonitis than for intra-abdominal abscess.[2,3]

Intra-abdominal infection is associated with both local and systemic inflammatory responses. Locally, the influx of phagocytes and activation of these cells (including neutrophils, monocytes, macrophages, and possibly, mast cells) promotes bacterial killing but also causes loss of microvascular integrity, interstitial edema, and exudative ascites. The surface area of the peritoneum is approximately the same as that of the skin; therefore, edema of the submesothelial interstitial space to a thickness of 1 mm sequesters about 1.7 L fluid in the prototypical 70-kg patient. Larger patients sequester relatively more fluid. Interstitial fluid can accumulate to a greater degree, and free peritoneal fluid can accumulate voluminously; thus, one can appreciate why large quantities of intravenous fluid must be infused to correct the intravascular hypovolemia that is characteristic of generalized peritonitis. Intraperitoneal fluid accumulation is detrimental to intra-abdominal host defenses, diluting opsonins and impairing neutrophil function, but there is no alternative to the administration of fluids to the hypovolemic patient.

When peritoneal injury occurs from inflammation, the mesangial cells that comprise the peritoneum are denuded, exposing the basement membrane. When platelets and fibrin come into contact with the basement membrane, fibrin polymerization occurs, evidenced by the exudative "rind" that forms on peritoneal surfaces. Fibrin contributes (along with apoptotic neutrophils) to the formation of adhesions and the walls of abscesses. Normally, the process is self-limited by up-regulation and/or activation of fibrinolytic factors (e.g., plasminogen) within the first week after mesothelial injury. If the insult is self-limited, peritoneal repair occurs within 3 to 5 days. Under local hypoxic conditions, the adhesions are invaded by fibroblasts and angiogenesis is up-regulated, and the adhesions become tenacious.[3a]

MICROBIOLOGY

Most of the bacteria normally resident in the gut are commensal flora that play little if any role in the pathogenesis of intra-abdominal infection. Most of the 500 to 800 bacterial species present in the healthy colon, where bacterial counts are highest and anaerobic species predominate, probably serve a role to support colonocyte metabolism and prevent overgrowth of the small numbers of potential pathogens (e.g., *Bacteroides fragilis*, *Escherichia coli*, *Klebsiella* spp, *Enterobacter* spp). Overgrowth of potential pathogens can occur after treatment with broad-spectrum antibiotics.

Perforation of a gastrointestinal tract hollow viscus releases bacteria into the peritoneal cavity, which vary in type and number with the site of perforation. In general, bacterial counts per gram of feces increase from proximal to distal, and likewise the numbers of anaerobes increase, both being highest in the colon. The bacteria must proliferate to cause infection, whereas local host defenses seek to prevent or contain the establishment of infection. In addition to the microbes present in peritoneal fluid, microbial colonization of peritoneal surfaces occurs rapidly after perforation or penetrating injury as a result of expression by the microorganisms of specific adherence factors. Enterobacteriaceae predominate early (within 4 hours) but are superseded within 8 hours by members of the *B. fragilis* group. Adherent bacteria are difficult to eradicate by operative peritoneal lavage; lavage with an antibiotic-containing fluid is also ineffective.[4]

Besides adherence factors, bacteria possess several other attributes that can enhance their virulence. Peptidoglycans and lipoteichoic acid in the cell walls of Gram-positive bacteria (especially streptococci and staphylococci) stimulate a proinflammatory response, and these organisms can elaborate exotoxins and proteases that cause tissue injury and promote their dissemination, whereas lipopolysaccharides that are constituents of the cell walls of Gram-negative bacteria can interact with many cell types to stimulate an inflammatory response. As bacteria proliferate and the size of the inoculum increases, acidic bacterial metabolites can impair neutrophil function.[3b] Larger inocula can render antibiotics (particularly beta-lactams) ineffective through what has been called the "inoculum effect."[3c] Additionally, bacteria can husband their substrates when inoculum size is sufficient through a "quorum-sensing" effect.[3d]

There are also mechanisms whereby bacteria, usually *B. fragilis* and either facultative Gram-negative bacilli or enterococci, act synergistically to suppress local host defenses and promote their survival and growth.[1] *B. fragilis* produces a capsular polysaccharide antigen that suppresses complement activation and inhibits leukocyte recruitment and function.[3e] Production of short-chain fatty acids by anaerobes can also interfere with neutrophil function (the pH within a typical intra-abdominal abscess is 5.0 to 5.5). Facultative bacteria consume the small amounts of oxygen in the microenvironment, favoring the survival and growth of anaerobes. Anaerobic bacteria lower the redox potential, thus also favoring their

TABLE 123-1. MICROBIOLOGY OF INTRA-ABDOMINAL INFECTION

Primary (Monomicrobial)	Secondary (Polymicrobial)	Tertiary (Polymicrobial)
Escherichia coli	Bacteroides fragilis group	Staphylococcus epidermidis
Klebsiella spp	Clostridium spp	Enterococcus spp
Streptococcus pneumoniae	Other anaerobes	Pseudomonas spp
Enterococcus spp	E. coli	Acinetobacter spp
	Klebsiella spp	Candida spp
		Enterobacter spp
		Enterococcus spp
		Streptococcus spp
		Staphylococcus spp
		Candida spp

growth. Either type of bacteria can enhance the growth of others by provision of crucial nutrients or the production of enzymes that destroy antibiotics.

In some respects, bacteria have evolved to take advantage of host defenses. For example, the adherence of bacteria to enterocytes (especially colonocytes) and their growth is enhanced by physiologic concentrations of norepinephrine,[5] which is secreted as part of the counter-regulatory response to stress, as well as being used therapeutically as a vasoconstrictor.

"Primary" peritonitis, infection that develops in the absence of gastrointestinal tract hollow viscus perforation, rarely causes critical illness. This type of peritonitis, which can afflict adults with hepatic cirrhosis or collagen vascular disease or children with certain glomerulopathies, is invariably monomicrobial. The typical pathogen is usually an enteric Gram-negative bacillus such as E. coli or Klebsiella spp, although infection with streptococci is also known to occur (Table 123-1). A high degree of suspicion is required, because definitive diagnosis is made by paracentesis and culture, and laparotomy or laparoscopy is not indicated. If polymicrobial flora (or an anaerobe) is isolated, the occult perforation must be found and treated.

A variant of primary peritonitis is device-associated peritonitis; although not "spontaneous" in the true sense of primary peritonitis, it shares with primary peritonitis the attribute of a single species of bacteria causing the infection, and the need to identify a site of perforation, if polymicrobial flora are recovered. The vast majority of cases are associated with catheters for chronic ambulatory peritoneal dialysis, which become infected as often as once per year of dialysis.[6] The most common infecting species are Staphylococcus aureus, Pseudomonas spp, and Candida spp. Removal of the catheter is usually necessary to eradicate these infections, especially those caused by the latter two organisms. Although rare, chronic ambulatory peritoneal dialysis-related recurrent methicillin-resistant S. aureus peritonitis has been associated with the emergence of vancomycin-resistant strains of S. aureus after treatment with multiple courses of vancomycin.[7]

Most patients with intra-abdominal infection sick enough to require critical care have "secondary" or "tertiary" peritonitis. Secondary peritonitis follows perforation of a hollow viscus of the gastrointestinal tract. The vast majority of cases are community-acquired; appendicitis is the most common cause. Accordingly, the polymicrobial bacterial flora responsible for the infection are highly susceptible to antibiotics (see Table 123-1). Thorough microbiologic analysis of

a carefully collected specimen of purulent peritoneal fluid from a patient with secondary peritonitis yields an average of five organisms (three anaerobes, with B. fragilis being the most common; two aerobes, with E. coli being the most common). Uncommon isolates include Enterococcus spp, Candida spp, Clostridium spp, and Pseudomonas spp. These uncommon isolates do not need to be "covered" by the antibiotic regimen, if the patient was previously healthy and does not have comorbid conditions that increase the risk for an adverse outcome (see later). Surgical "source control," or the "correct" operation, performed "correctly" and at the "correct" time,[8] combined with a short course of broad-spectrum antibiotic therapy, results in cure more than 85% of the time (more than 90% for appendicitis). Most community-acquired cases of peritonitis do not result in severe illness (severe sepsis, septic shock, multiple organ dysfunction syndrome) and are seldom encountered in the ICU.

"Tertiary" peritonitis describes recurrent or persistent intra-abdominal infection after failure of more than one source control procedure to control the infection.[9-11] The flora usually include one or more strains of staphylococci (often methicillin-resistant S. epidermidis or methicillin-resistant S. aureus)[12] and of Enterococcus spp, Candida spp, or Pseudomonas spp (see Table 123-1). It is controversial whether tertiary peritonitis represents invasive infection or colonization of the peritoneal cavity in the face of devastated host defenses. The notion that host defenses are compromised is supported by the observation that fluid collections are often poorly localized and serosanguineous rather than purulent. Also controversial is whether it is advantageous to leave the abdomen open (see later) or employ a temporary, resealable closure[13] to provide peritoneal toilet by frequent washouts. Cases of tertiary peritonitis are fortunately uncommon, but class I data regarding management are lacking owing to its rarity.

ADJUVANTS

The bacterial inoculum necessary to establish infection is decreased if adjuvant substances are present. Adjuvants may increase virulence or interfere with host defenses. Adjuvants are invariably present to some degree in every case of gastrointestinal tract perforation. In addition to ascites, adjuvants include blood, fibrin, bile, urine, chyle, pancreatic juice, and platelets.[14] The most important adjuvant is blood. Hemoglobin, fibrin, and platelets all impair host defenses. Iron is essential for bacterial growth and also depresses phagocyte function. Fibrin promotes trapping of bacteria and abscess formation and may sequester bacteria from neutrophils. Bile salts impair host defenses and are toxic to neutrophils, whereas pancreatic enzymes can be activated by bacterial infection, resulting in necrotic tissue that is an excellent culture medium.

Foreign materials can also act as adjuvants, serving as a prime locus for bacterial adherence, where the bacteria have an environment that is sequestered from phagocytes. The foreign material can also elicit an inflammatory reaction, thereby reducing the size of the inoculum necessary for infection. Drains, nonabsorbable suture material, fibers (e.g., from gauze sponges used during surgery), prostheses (e.g., vascular grafts, sheets of mesh), topical hemostatic agents, talc, barium sulfate (which produces a marked chemical peritonitis and can also activate coagulation via the intrinsic pathway), necrotic tissue, and feces can all act as

TABLE 123–2. RISK FACTORS FOR SEVERE SEPSIS IN PATIENTS WITH INTRA-ABDOMINAL INFECTIONS

Parameter	Relative Risk	95% Confidence Intervals
Age (years)		
<20		1.0
20-39	1.4	0.8-2.5
40-59	3.2	1.8-5.6
60-79	4.6	2.6-8.0
>79	6.5	4.7-11.8
Site		
Appendix		1.0
Gallbladder	2.7	1.9-3.8
Colon	3.9	2.6-5.8
Stomach/Duodenum	6.9	4.6-10.3
Small Bowel	9.0	6.1-13.4
Extent		
Localized		1.0
Abscess	1.2	0.8-1.8
Diffuse	1.5	1.1-1.9
Comorbidities		
Congestive heart failure	1.2	1.0-1.6
Stroke	1.8	1.2-2.7
Liver dysfunction	2.0	1.4-2.8
Renal dysfunction	2.0	1.4-2.9

Data from Anaya and Nathens.[2]

TABLE 123–3. RESULTS OF SURGICAL THERAPY OF PERITONITIS COMPLICATED BY SERIOUS ILLNESS*

	N	%
Total Cohort	239	100
Reoperations		
None	156	65
One		46
Two	15	6
Three or more	22	9
Mortality		
Overall	77	32
With reoperation	35/83	42
No reoperation	42/156	26
"Open" abdomen		31
"Closed" abdomen	42	

*APACHE II Score Greater than 10. This study was designed originally to include only patients with APACHE II scores ≥ 15, but was modified to scores > 10 owing to slow accrual. The mean APACHE II score of 18 reported in this series is thus lower than that reported in patients accrued entirely from ICUs, but the reoperation rate, morbidity, and mortality are high nonetheless. Data from Christou et al.[13]

adjuvants. The combination of barium and feces (introduced when colonic perforation is imprudently studied radiographically using barium sulfate as a contrast agent) elicits marked inflammation that can be lethal.

THE AT-RISK PATIENT

A recent population-based study of hospital discharges for peritonitis estimated that only 11% of patients develop severe sepsis (Table 123-2)[2] but that such patients have a 19-fold increased risk of death compared to those without severe sepsis. Only about 15% of patients enrolled in clinical trials of antibiotic therapy for secondary peritonitis have an APACHE II score greater than 15 points[15]; it is these patients who constitute most of the population who require critical care for intra-abdominal infection.

Some patients with community-acquired secondary peritonitis have critical illness as a result of delayed presentation, immunosuppression, or extremes of age. Splanchnic ischemia with perforation can complicate hypovolemia, distributive shock, atheroembolism, or thromboembolism in the setting of atrial fibrillation. However, most patients with critical illness have hospital-acquired peritonitis. The leading causes of hospital-acquired peritonitis are gastrointestinal anastomotic dehiscence and splanchnic ischemia in its protean manifestations. When peritonitis is hospital-acquired, peritoneal fluid cultures are more likely to grow *Enterococcus, Candida,* or *Pseudomonas,* and/or other antibiotic-resistant organisms, such as MRSA.[9-12]

The likelihood that intra-abdominal infection will be encountered in a particular ICU depends on local factors. Units that care for a high proportion of patients with multiple trauma or following emergency surgery are likely to have more cases of intra-abdominal infection than medical ICUs. However, low-prevalence units must be equally vigilant in their surveillance and assessment, because a missed intra-abdominal infection is almost always fatal.[16]

Mortality is high when patients are critically ill, ranging from 25% to 30% or more.[3-13] The risk of failure increases with increasing severity of illness,[15] inadequate empiric antibiotic therapy[17] (see later), delayed surgical therapy,[16,18] and failure of source control (need for reoperation) (Table 123-3).[13] Most clinical failures are not associated with multi-drug-resistant pathogens,[15] although some data suggest that clinical failure is associated with isolation of pathogens that are resistant to multiple antibiotics in cases of postoperative peritonitis.[17,19,20]

SPECTRUM OF DISEASE CAUSING CRITICAL ILLNESS

ABSCESS OF SOLID ORGANS

Abscesses of solid organs are unusual manifestations of intra-abdominal infection but must be recognized, as they can be lethal if untreated. Most cases arise as a complication of a community-acquired infection, but on occasion they may be a complication of medical care. The liver is affected most commonly; the spleen and kidney are affected less often. When of nosocomial origin, there is almost always an antecedent bacteremia (recognized or not) in cases of splenic abscess, whereas renal abscess/pyelonephritis is usually caused by an ascending infection of the urinary tract.

Liver abscess is associated most often with an ascending biliary infection (i.e., cholangitis) or portal bacteremia that complicates an enteric infection (e.g., diverticulitis). The most common causative organisms, including *E. coli, Klebsiella,* and *Enterococcus,* reflect these pathogenic mechanisms. Systemic sources for bacteremia, leading to liver abscess, are also possible and include dental abscess (viridans streptococci) or vascular catheters (*S. aureus, Candida albicans,* and others). Devitalized liver, as may occur after trauma, angioembolization, or ablation of neoplasms, is at particular risk for infection. The lesions may be solitary or multiple. In some rare instances, miliary liver abscesses develop. Treatment should be individualized. Antibiotics are mandatory, and a prolonged course (>2 weeks) may be necessary. Percutaneous drainage should be attempted for all lesions of amenable size and location. Overall mortality rate is approximately 25% but is higher for patients with multiple abscesses that are too small to drain.[21]

In general, the epidemiology of splenic abscess differs from that for liver abscess. The exceptions are cases due to bacteremia, rare fungal infections ("hepatosplenic candidiasis"), and cases associated with devitalized tissue. Patients at risk include those with a history of sickle cell disease, intravenous drug abuse, or traumatic injury (especially after splenic artery embolization).[22] *S. aureus* is the most common pathogen. Gram-negative organisms are relatively unusual as pathogens. Anaerobic infections (e.g., due to *Clostridium perfringens*) have been described. Empiric antibiotic therapy should address all likely pathogens. Percutaneous drainage may be attempted if conditions are favorable, but splenectomy and drainage are usually definitive as therapy. Overall mortality rate is approximately 20%.

Despite the high prevalence of "urosepsis," true abscesses of the kidney are uncommon as compared with either hepatic or splenic abscesses. Ascending infection of the lower urinary tract is the usual source; therefore, any common urinary tract pathogen (e.g., *E. coli, Klebsiella, Enterococcus, S. aureus*) can be causative, and broad-spectrum antibiotic therapy is necessary until microbiologic data become available. Surgical drainage may be required for nonresponders, or those with recurrent sepsis.

ACUTE ACALCULOUS CHOLECYSTITIS

Acute acalculous cholecystitis is an ischemic event and only secondarily an infection.[23] Although acute acalculous cholecystitis can complicate many illnesses, low flow to the splanchnic circulation is the common denominator. Medical patients at risk include those with congestive heart failure, diabetes mellitus, abdominal vasculitis, and malignant disease (including after bone marrow transplantation). The incidence of acute acalculous cholecystitis is even higher among surgical patients. Associations exist between acute acalculous cholecystitis and burns, trauma, cardiopulmonary bypass, biliary stents, and emergency aortic surgery.[23]

The diagnosis of acute acalculous cholecystitis can be challenging, and a high index of suspicion is required. Expedient diagnosis and therapy is necessary, as the disease can be fulminant; the incidence of gallbladder necrosis and perforation are approximately 50% and 20%, respectively. Commonplace findings are fever and hyperbilirubinemia.[23] These findings can occur in isolation or be associated with modest elevated circulating levels of transaminases or alkaline phosphatase. When signs and symptoms can be localized to the right upper quadrant, the differential diagnosis includes gastroduodenal perforation, acute pancreatitis, ischemia of the hepatic flexure of the colon, and acute hepatitis. Bedside ultrasonography is favored for the diagnosis of acute acalculous cholecystitis; the most accurate diagnostic features are gallbladder wall thickness greater than 3.5 mm and presence of pericholecystic fluid. Computed tomography (CT) is equally accurate and can be utilized when there are no localizing findings and the patient is a candidate for intrahospital transport. Hepatobiliary scintigraphy is not a good test to diagnose or exclude acute acalculous cholecystitis, owing to a high incidence of false-positive study findings that result, in part, from a lack of dietary stimulus for gallbladder contraction. Coadministration of morphine sulfate, which increases biliary hydrostatic pressure, can promote filling of the gallbladder and increase diagnostic accuracy of hepatobiliary scintigraphy.[24]

Increasingly, percutaneous cholecystostomy is the treatment of choice for acute acalculous cholecystitis. Success rates for patients so treated exceed 90% for control of acute acalculous cholecystitis; despite this, the overall mortality rate remains about 30%. When percutaneous cholecystectomy fails to provide adequate control of acute acalculous cholecystitis, the diagnostic possibilities include malposition of the drainage catheter, gallbladder perforation that has not been controlled, or a true diagnosis other than acute acalculous cholecystitis. If a cholecystostomy tube study confirms the absence of gallstones once the patient has recovered (gallstones are common in cases of postoperative cholecystitis but probably are irrelevant to the pathogenesis), the drain can be removed. Interval cholecystectomy is unnecessary if the drain is removable.

ISCHEMIC COLITIS AND ENTERITIS

Intestinal ischemia is a dangerous and relatively common complication of critical illness that can progress within hours to gangrene, perforation, and generalized peritonitis.[25] The splanchnic circulation is especially vulnerable to low cardiac output, particularly when the cardiac index is less than 2 L/min/M². Acquired protein C/protein S deficiency, which induces a hypercoagulable state, has been associated with either mesenteric arterial or venous thrombosis. Chronic atrial fibrillation or dilated cardiomyopathy can cause mesenteric arterial thromboembolism. Arteriography can cause "cholesterol" embolization, if an atherosclerotic plaque is dislodged from the thoracic aorta. Intestinal obstruction must also be considered, and this diagnosis may not be obvious if the point of obstruction is partial or proximal. However, most cases are caused by nonocclusive ischemia; the origin is often multifactorial, including hypovolemia, shock, and administration of vasopressors.

The pattern of injury is variable, depending on the mechanism, the presence of heart disease, and the status of the collateral circulation via the celiac artery and the inferior mesenteric artery. Large thrombi usually occlude the superior mesenteric artery where it narrows just distal to its first branch (the middle colic artery), which supplies the transverse colon, the distal duodenum, and the very proximal jejunum. The first 12 to 18 inches of small bowel and the left colon may be spared. Smaller emboli are more likely to infarct the small bowel and possibly the ascending colon (if the embolus is to the ileocolic artery) (Figs. 123-1 and 123-2); the distribution may be patchy. Nonocclusive ischemia occurs classically in "watershed" areas of the mesenteric circulation (e.g., splenic flexure of the colon), where collateral vessels bridge the two arterial distributions (i.e., between the superior and the inferior mesenteric artery). Although any segment of intestine can be affected by nonocclusive ischemia, the cecum (the point farthest from inferior mesenteric artery collaterals) (see Fig. 123-2) and the left colon are most likely to be affected. The left colon is particularly vulnerable after abdominal aortic surgery, especially if the inferior mesenteric artery has been ligated during the procedure.

Patients with intestinal ischemia are profoundly ill and will die without prompt intervention. The mucosal blood supply is more vulnerable than that of the seromuscular layers; therefore, transmural necrosis represents progressive disease. Patients may develop severe sepsis or septic shock

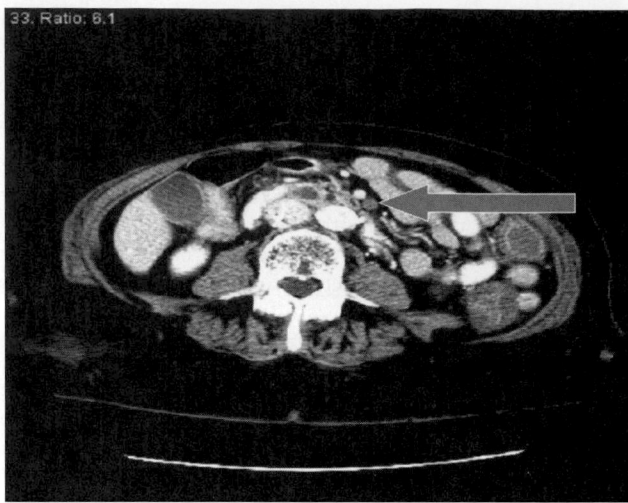

FIGURE 123–1. Computed tomographic scan after administration of oral and intravenous contrast in a patient with an embolism to the superior mesenteric artery and ischemia of the right colon. The arrow points to the embolus in the superior mesenteric artery.

before transmural gangrene or perforation. The protean manifestations of the syndrome, including the potential for ischemia anywhere from the ligament of Treitz to the peritoneal reflection over the distal rectum, make establishing the diagnosis difficult. Among communicative patients, pain that is disproportionately severe compared with tenderness and other objective findings is the diagnostic hallmark. Among intubated, sedated patients, the clinical features can be subtle. Abdominal distention, hypovolemia, hemoconcentration (due to sequestration of a large volume of fluid in the extracellular compartment), unexplained (and refractory) metabolic acidosis, or guaiac-positive stools may be the only signs. Hematochezia shortly following abdominal aortic surgery or resuscitation from shock is strongly suggestive of colon ischemia.

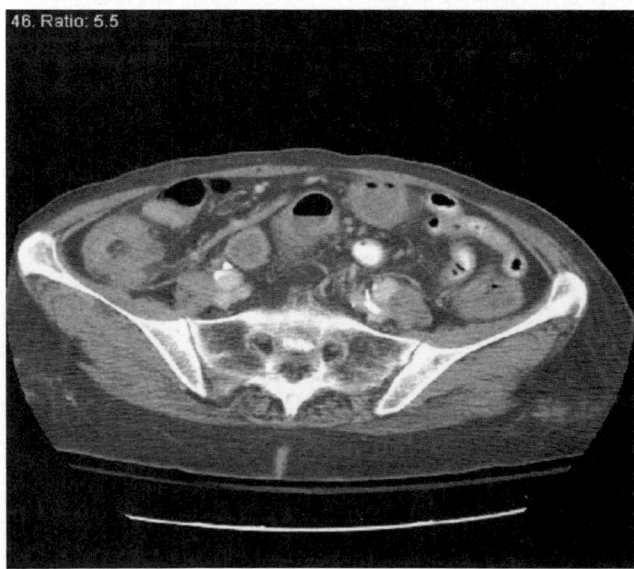

FIGURE 123–2. Computed tomographic scan after administration of oral and intravenous contrast material in a patient with an embolism to the superior mesenteric artery and ischemia of the right colon. Ischemia of the cecum is evident by the marked thickening of the wall of the cecum (left side of the image).

Given the propensity for left colon involvement, lower endoscopy at the bedside is usually the first diagnostic modality to be employed, but it is important to emphasize several caveats. Flexible sigmoidoscopy is easy and carries minimal morbidity but may miss ischemia at or proximal to the splenic flexure. Therefore, most experts prefer colonoscopy. Regardless of whether the procedure is performed using a sigmoidoscope or a colonoscope, endoscopy permits visualization of the mucosa only; hence, the assessment of severity of ischemia is only qualitative and may underestimate the extent of disease. CT is increasingly useful diagnostically and has largely supplanted arteriography (see Fig. 123-1). Diagnostic bedside laparoscopy is being evaluated for this indication (see later), but data are scant. Diagnostic testing should be foregone entirely in favor of celiotomy if signs of peritonitis are present.

Surgical therapy is individualized based on the location and extent of involvement and the physiologic state of the patient. Infarcted bowel is resected, but bowel of questionable viability may be left for reinspection by a "second-look" celiotomy in 12 to 24 hours. Anastomosis may be performed in the stable patient without peritonitis or deferred by leaving the occluded ends of bowel in temporary discontinuity in unstable patients. Creation of a temporary ostomy is a third option but is being performed with decreasing frequency. If there is confidence that a second-look procedure is unnecessary, the abdominal fascia can be closed. If reoperation is planned or if bowel edema and distention are such that definitive closure would risk the development of intra-abdominal hypertension and abdominal compartment syndrome (see later), a temporary abdominal wall closure can be performed (e.g., closure of skin only), or the abdomen can be left open with the viscera contained by packs, absorbable mesh, or plastic sheeting. Because of the wide spectrum of disease, it is difficult to generalize about the risk of mortality from ischemic enteritis. However, acute ischemic colitis in the aftermath of repair of a ruptured abdominal aortic aneurysm carries a risk of death as high as 80%.

ACUTE PANCREATITIS

Most cases of pancreatitis are neither iatrogenic nor severe. Choledocholithiasis and ethanol toxicity together account for about 80% of cases. Pancreatitis following trauma, upper abdominal surgery, or cardiopulmonary bypass accounts for only a small fraction of the remainder of cases. Approximately 85% of cases are self-limited and have a good outcome. The remaining 15% of cases account for most of the morbidity and all of the mortality. Infection is the most common complication and can lead to multiple organ dysfunction syndrome and death. Once established, the cause is less important than the severity of illness in determining outcome. The likelihood of mortality is associated with large intravenous fluid requirement, acidosis, and hypocalcemia.[26]

Infection can become manifest as an infected pseudocyst, a discrete pancreatic abscess, or infected pancreatic necrosis, which is a poorly localized process that affects the retroperitoneal fat as well as the pancreas itself. Infection can develop as early as 5 days after the onset of acute pancreatitis, and peak in incidence is at day 14. Almost any common organism can cause infection, including staphylococci, enteric Gram-negative bacilli, obligate anaerobes, *Pseudomonas aeruginosa*, and *Candida* spp. Assuming the choice is consistent with microbial susceptibility data, many authorities recommend treatment with imipenem or meropenem or a fluoro-quinolone plus metronidazole, based on kinetic studies of drug accumulation in normal pancreas or pancreatic juice. Fluconazole achieves adequate tissue concentrations, whereas aminoglycosides do not.[26a]

Almost everything else about the prevention and management of pancreatic infection is controversial, including the role of antibiotic prophylaxis, diagnostic methods, and techniques and timing of surgical drainage and débridement. Antibiotic prophylaxis of severe pancreatitis with imipenem is popular but unsubstantiated by Class I data and has been associated with an increased risk of fungal infection.[26b] Regardless of the severity of illness, all patients with pancreatitis should undergo ultrasonography of the biliary tree to detect the presence of gallstones. The optimal imaging study to quantify anatomic severity and assess for infection is CT. The study should be performed with thin "cuts" through the region of the pancreas, and imaging should be carried out during intravenous infusion of a contrast agent; devitalized pancreas can be discerned readily (Fig. 123-3). If the patient has systemic inflammatory response syndrome and infection (sepsis) is suspected, CT-guided fine-needle aspiration can be performed to obtain material for culture. If bacteria are identified, then surgery may be indicated. However, rare false-negative studies are problematic, because undrained pancreatic infection is invariably fatal.

Whether to operate for pancreatic necrosis and organ dysfunction without infection is a matter of debate; currently, opinion favors a conservative approach, such that operation is deferred as long as possible and is performed only for confirmed infections. This strategy allows the phlegmon to demarcate and minimizes the complications associated with what otherwise would be a difficult and potentially morbid dissection. These potential complications include hemorrhage, intestinal injury with fistula formation, multiple operations to gain source control, open abdomen, and abdominal wall hernia. Percutaneous drainage is of limited utility (approximately 30% success rate) owing to the tenacity of the necrotic tissue debris that must gain egress. Improvements in resuscitation and operative management of infectious complications have reduced the mortality rate by approximately one-half, to about 20%.

DIAGNOSIS

Patients may present critically ill from common causes of peritonitis (e.g., perforated duodenal ulcer or diverticulitis of the colon) and require resuscitation in the ICU, or they may develop intra-abdominal infection as a complication of critical illness (e.g., acute acalculous cholecystitis, ischemic colitis, missed traumatic injury). Anastomotic dehiscence and other postoperative complications are common in surgical ICUs, whereas ischemia from splanchnic hypoperfusion is more common in medical ICUs.[16]

Intra-abdominal infection is difficult to diagnose in critically ill patients. Historical information is often unobtainable, and altered mental status can mask the findings of physical examination. The clinical context is important. Bacteremia is uncommon with intra-abdominal infection but may be polymicrobial if present. At times, the only clue may be unexplained signs of sepsis or organ dysfunction. Radiologic corroboration must be obtained.

Radiologic studies, chosen with care, can often make the diagnosis before definitive intervention occurs. Although good-quality plain abdominal radiographs are difficult to obtain at the bedside, pneumoperitoneum (Fig. 123-4), intestinal obstruction, or signs of intestinal ischemia may be revealed. Of note, pneumoperitoneum may be a false-positive finding in mechanically ventilated patients, and for as long as 7 days after abdominal surgery.[26c,26d] Plain radiographs may be augmented by injection of water-soluble contrast into drains, fistulas, or sinuses to reveal the anatomy of complex infections or monitor the resolution after drainage.

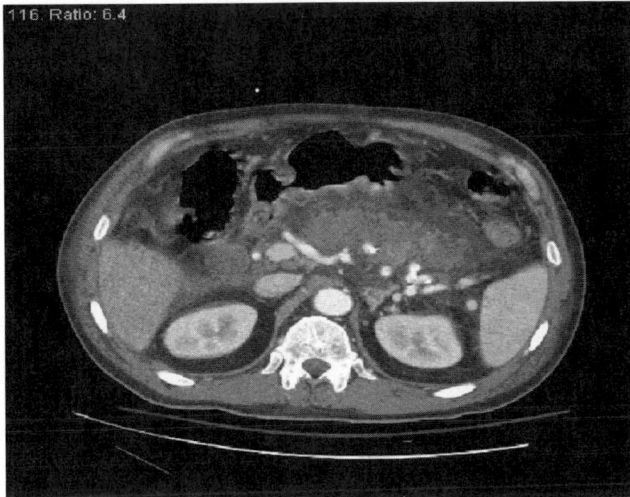

FIGURE 123–3. Computed tomographic scan after administration of oral and intravenous contrast material in a patient with severe acute pancreatitis. The borders of the pancreas are indistinct owing to marked surrounding inflammation. The hypodense area in the body of the pancreas is an area of pancreatic necrosis. Just posterior, note the extensive calcification of the celiac axis, splenic artery, and common hepatic artery.

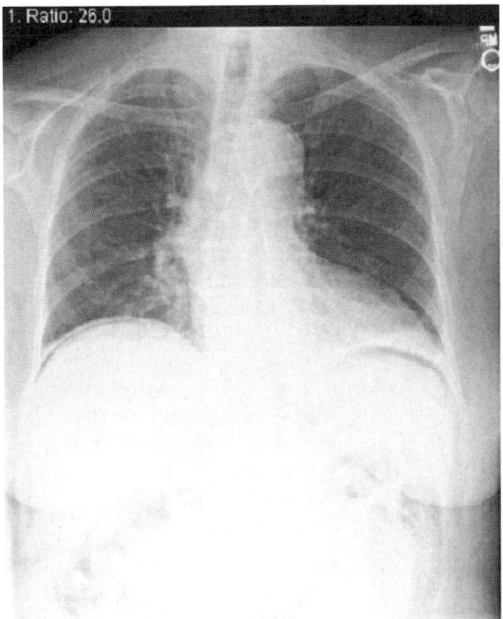

FIGURE 123–4. Pneumoperitoneum (crescent-shaped lucency) is evident under the right hemidiaphragm on this upright chest radiograph of a patient with perforated sigmoid diverticulitis. The crescent-shaped lucency under the left hemidiaphragm is the stomach bubble.

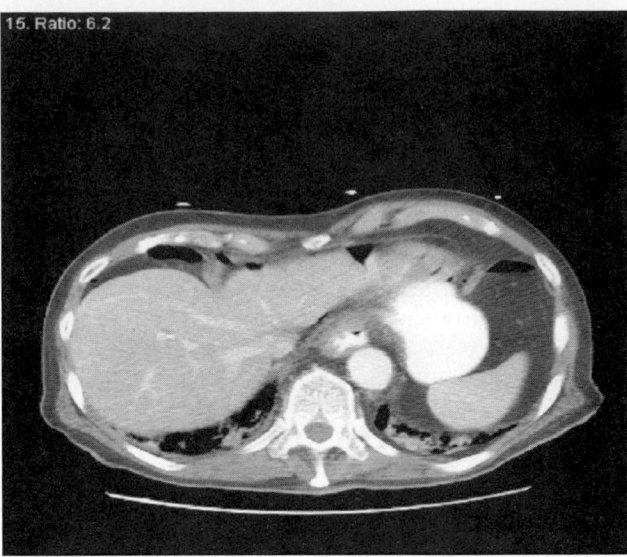

FIGURE 123–5. Computed tomographic scan after administration of oral and intravenous contrast in a patient with pneumoperitoneum from a perforated viscus. Multiple pockets of extraluminal gas are evident, particularly anterior to the liver.

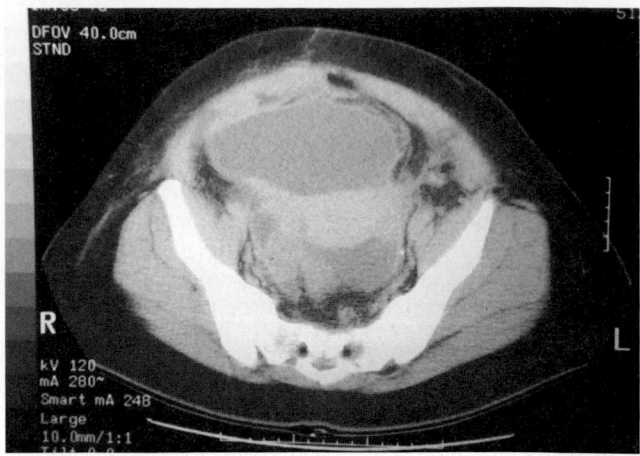

FIGURE 123–6. Computed tomographic scan after administration of oral and intravenous contrast material in a patient with a large pelvic abscess that is surrounding and compressing the urinary bladder. Note the compression and displacement of the rectum toward the right side of the pelvis (left side of the image).

Ultrasonography can be performed at the bedside and provides excellent visualization of the biliary tree. Ultrasonography can detect abscesses, particularly in the pelvis when transvaginal or transrectal probes are used. With the addition of color Doppler blood flow analysis, visceral blood flow can be assessed. However, ultrasonography is operator-dependent and provides limited visualization in the presence of increased bowel gas (e.g., ileus). Moreover, dressings can impede the positioning of the probe. Ultrasonography is effective when used to guide percutaneous drainage procedures.

When assessing critically ill patients, CT is the primary radiologic tool for imaging the abdomen and pelvis.[27,28] Most intra-abdominal infections can be diagnosed when contrast agents are administered by intravenous, oral, or rectal administration. Radiographic signs of intra-abdominal infection by CT include extraluminal gas (Fig. 123-5), free fluid, extravasation of contrast material, inhomogeneous radiographic density surrounding fat, and contrast-enhancing rim that is characteristic of abscess (Fig. 123-6). Intestinal obstruction can be diagnosed by intestinal distention proximal to a "transition point" of narrow-caliber bowel. Intramural gas may be identified when mesenteric ischemia is present; occasionally, a thrombus may be identified in a visceral vessel (see Fig. 123-5). The value of CT is mitigated by the need for transport to the radiology suite. When patients are hemodynamically unstable or dependent on a high level of mechanical ventilatory support, transport out of the ICU can be risky.[28a] Another mitigating factor is the need to administer iodinated contrast agents, which may precipitate or aggravate renal dysfunction. However, if the need for CT can be anticipated 24 hours in advance, pretreatment with *N*-acetylcysteine can limit the risk of contrast-induced nephropathy.[28b]

Radionuclide imaging is of limited utility in the setting of intra-abdominal infection and critical illness, owing to a lack of specificity and inability to support image-guided diagnostic or therapeutic aspiration. Magnetic resonance imaging is also

of limited usefulness, as the logistical obstacles inherent in not bringing ferrous metals (e.g., ventilators, pumps, pacemakers) near the magnet can be formidable.

Occasionally, an invasive diagnostic test is performed at the bedside. An existing surgical site can be probed judiciously with a gloved finger or sterile swab to identify a purulent collection adjacent to the site. Diagnostic peritoneal lavage may reveal bloody fluid (suggestive of acute ischemia), succus entericus, bile, or neutrophils. Bedside laparoscopy is an emerging technique; its utility is still being defined.[29] Although 2-mm instruments afford the opportunity to use local anesthesia, light transmission is decreased through smaller instruments, decreasing visibility. However, laparoscopy has been reported to avoid laparotomy in some cases, so its future value should not be discounted.

ILLUSTRATIVE PATIENT SCENARIO

The following patient narrative illustrates the use of multiple diagnostic and therapeutic methods for management of severe intra-abdominal sepsis. The key points of the case are highlighted in bold **type**.

A 50-year-old female patient on high doses of steroids for active Crohn's disease, with a past surgical history of multiple laparotomies and bowel resections, underwent laparoscopic cholecystectomy for symptomatic cholelithiasis. Apart from dense adhesions requiring extensive dissection, the surgery was uneventful and the patient was discharged the same evening. Seven days after discharge, the patient presented to the emergency department with severe abdominal pain. She was dehydrated, and the physical findings were suggestive of generalized peritonitis (**physical examination**) which may have been due to iatrogenic injury to bowel (**clinical setting**). Intravenous fluid resuscitation was started (**organ system support**) and a diagnostic work-up initiated. An erect chest radiograph (Fig. 123-7A) showed free intraperitoneal air, and erect and supine abdominal radiographs (Fig. 123-7B and C) showed evidence of ileus, with obliteration of renal and psoas shadows and also of the pre-peritoneal fat plane (**plane radiography**). An abdominal CT scan (Fig. 123-8)

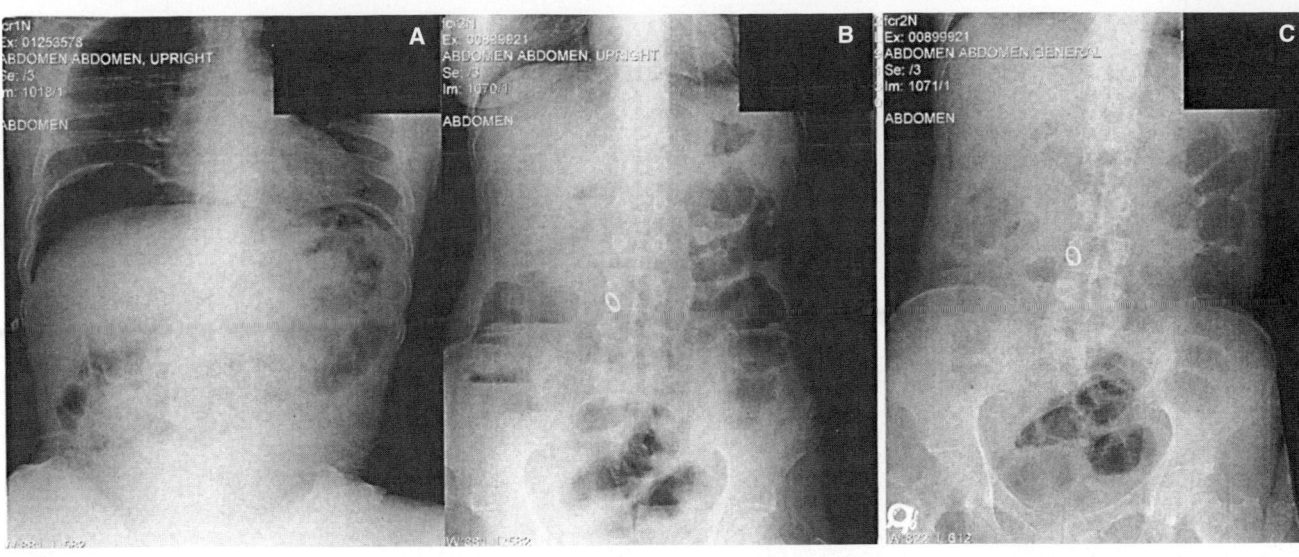

FIGURE 123–7. Acute series of a patient presenting with an acute abdomen 7 days after a laparoscopic cholecystectomy (see text). The erect chest radiograph (*A*) shows free intraperitoneal air. The erect (*B*) and supine (*C*) abdominal radiographs demonstrate evidence of ileus, with obliteration of the renal and psoas shadows and also of the preperitoneal fat plane.

demonstrated inflammatory changes in the right upper quadrant, with extraluminal air and contrast (**CT with intravenous and enteral contrast**). The patient was taken urgently to the operating room for exploratory laparotomy. There was moderate peritonitis caused by a 2-cm tear of the hepatic flexure. Purulent fluid and necrotic tissue were removed. A right hemicolectomy was performed, and the terminal ileum was anastomosed to the transverse colon (**source control**). The decision to perform an anastomosis, rather than create an ileostomy, was made because the patient had only 100 cm of small bowel, and it was believed that the management of a high-output ileostomy would be difficult. The patient was given cefoxitin started preoperatively and continued for 5 days (**second-generation cephalosporin for community-acquired bacterial peritonitis due to perforations >12 hours' duration**). The patient made an uneventful recovery and was discharged on the fifth postoperative day, tolerating a regular diet with regular bowel function and no fever.

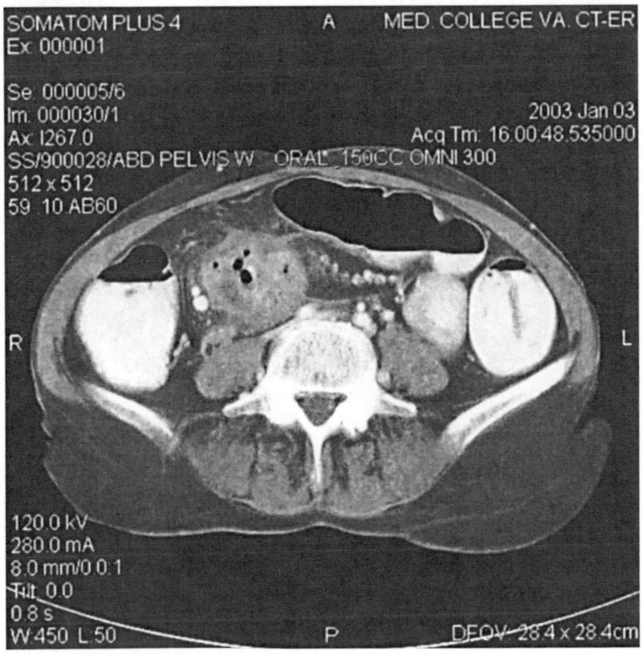

The patient returned to the emergency department 5 days after discharge in septic shock, with evidence of peritonitis on examination (**physical examination**), possibly due to anastomotic dehiscence (**clinical setting**). Resuscitation was initiated and the patient required intubation and ventilatory support (**organ system support**). A CT scan (Fig. 123-9) performed at this time showed extensive inflammatory changes in the right upper quadrant with extraluminal air and contrast (**CT with intravenous and enteral contrast**). The patient was taken again to the operating room, and the leaking anastomosis was resected with minimal extra bowel. The patient was unstable, hence the surgery was terminated after controlling ongoing soilage, and the abdomen was left "open" (**advanced operative technique: delayed definitive repair due to patient instability and also to guard against abdominal compartment syndrome**). The patient required pulmonary artery catheterization for ongoing management of resuscitation and advanced ventilatory support for acute respiratory distress syndrome. In addition, the patient was started on total parenteral nutrition (**nutritional support**) and administered activated protein C (**anticoagulant and anti-inflammatory antisepsis agent**). The patient returned to the operating room every 48 to 72 hours to control the advanced intra-abdominal infection (**peritoneal toilet**). She was given piperacillin-tazobactam that was continued for 7 days (**health care-acquired severe secondary bacterial peritonitis due to leaking ileocolic anastomosis**). At her third trip to the operating room, the bowel ends were anastomosed. With continued improvement and decrease in edema of the bowel, the patient's abdomen was closed on the fifth trip to the operating room. The patient continued to

FIGURE 123–8. Abdominal computed tomographic scan, obtained with intravenous and enteral contrast of the same patient as in Figure 123-7 (see text), demonstrates inflammatory changes (fat stranding), with extraluminal air and contrast, confirming suspicion of peritonitis secondary to a bowel perforation.

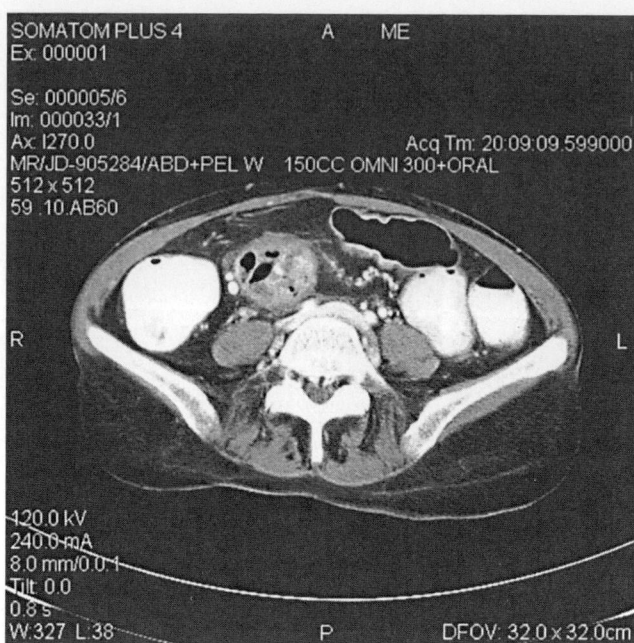

FIGURE 123–9. Abdominal computed tomographic scan, performed with intravenous and enteral contrast of the same patient as in Figures 123-7 and 123-8, performed a few days after an ileocolic anastomosis (see text). The scan demonstrates inflammatory changes (fat stranding), with extraluminal air and contrast, confirming suspicion of peritonitis possibly secondary to anastomotic dehiscence.

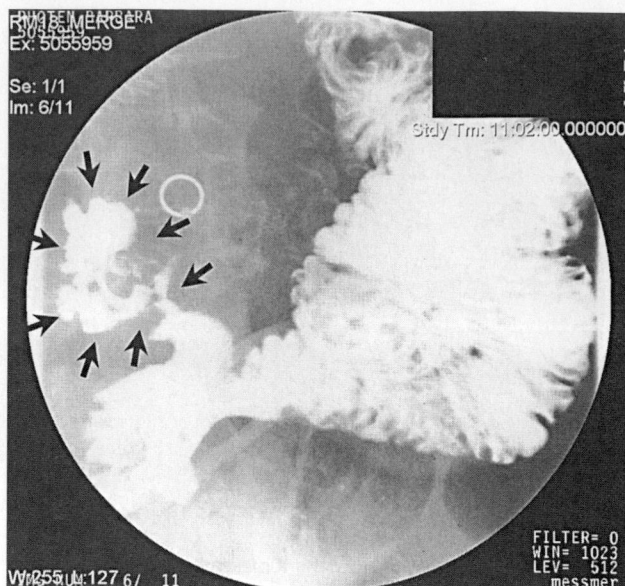

FIGURE 123–10. Contrast radiograph of the same patient as in Figures 123-7 to 123-9 performed for unexplained ileus and fever during recovery after advanced operation and intensive support for severe intra-abdominal sepsis (see text). The radiograph demonstrates a contained leak, probably from the anastomosis (*arrows*).

improve and had return of bowel function when oral intake was initiated. Ten days after closure of the abdomen, with the patient tolerating a regular diet and off antibiotics, she developed fever and new-onset ileus (**unexplained ileus**). A contrast radiologic examination (Fig. 123-10) was performed that showed a contained leak from the anastomosis (**contrast radiography**). This was confirmed by CT scan (Fig. 123-11; **CT with intravenous and enteral contrast**). Since the infection was contained, unilocular, with minimal solid debris, and the site of leak was small with no factors (apart from patient's inflammatory bowel disease) precluding spontaneous closure, a CT-guided drainage was performed (Fig. 123-12A-D; **percutaneous drainage**). The patient was started on imipenem/cilastatin (**hospital-acquired persistent intra-abdominal sepsis**). This was later changed to ampicillin, as the culture showed a highly sensitive *E. coli*, and continued for a total of 7 days. The patient was discharged 2 days after the drainage with the drainage catheter in place (Fig. 123-12E). The catheter was removed 4 weeks later when the collection had emptied itself and the anastomotic leak had healed (Fig. 123-12F).

PRINCIPLES OF MANAGEMENT

SOURCE CONTROL

Source control refers to the definitive control of amenable infections by appropriate and definitive surgical means. Stated succinctly, it is the right operation, performed correctly, at the proper time, leading to a good outcome. Definitive source control can be difficult to achieve, even when all technical considerations are met. Failure to obtain adequate source control reportedly occurs 10% to 25% of the time in cases of intra-abdominal infection, depending on the severity and

complexity of the infection.[30] The components of definitive source control include removal of infected or nonviable material and closure or control of perforations, restoration of hollow viscus continuity, and reduction of bacterial and toxin contamination of the peritoneal cavity. Achievement

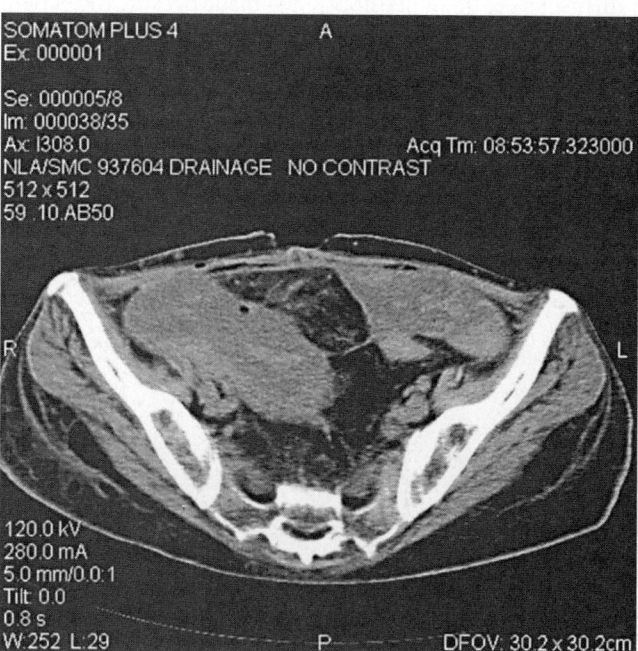

FIGURE 123–11. Abdominal computed tomographic scan of the same patient as in Figures 123-7 to 123-10, performed without any contrast after the contrast-enhanced radiograph suggested a contained leak from the ileocolic anastomosis (see text). The scan demonstrates a large collection in the same area, with visible extraluminal contrast (from the previous study, Fig. 123-10) and extraluminal air. In the absence of intravenous contrast, the inflammatory changes (ring enhancement and fat stranding) around the collection are not well visualized.

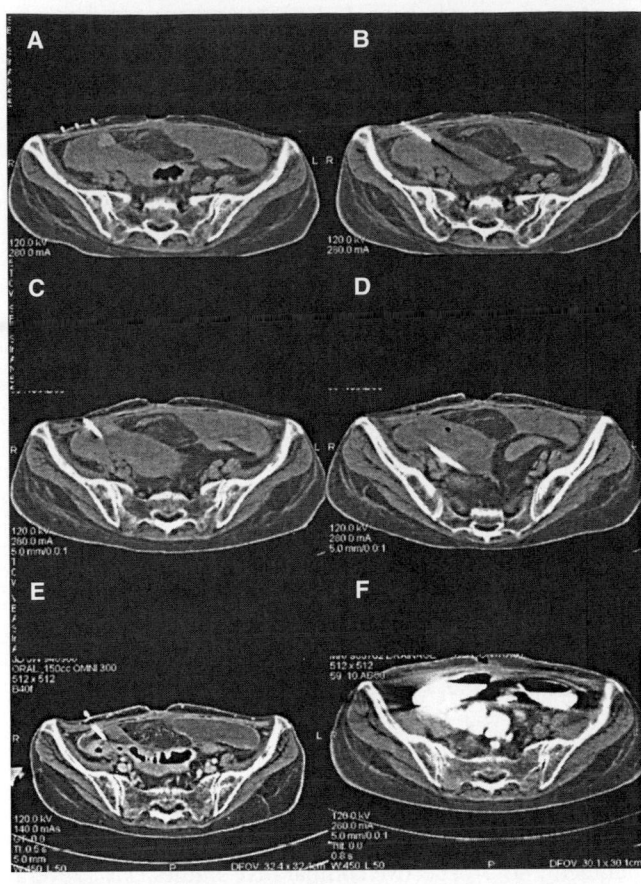

FIGURE 123–12. Computed tomography (CT)–guided percutaneous drainage of intra-abdominal abscess secondary to small anastomotic leak without generalized peritonitis (same patient as in Figs. 123-7 through 123-11; see text). A preliminary CT scan with radiopaque marker (*A*) identifies an accessible site. A needle is inserted at the chosen site (*B*) to access the abscess. Entry is confirmed by aspirating the abscess contents. A guidewire is inserted through the needle, and the tract is dilated over the guidewire. The drainage catheter is inserted into the tract (*C*) and placed in a dependent position (*D*). A follow-up CT scan (*E*) performed 2 days later confirms that the catheter remains in position and there is partial drainage of the collection. Another CT scan (*F*) performed 4 weeks later shows resolution of the abscess and no leakage of luminal contrast material, suggesting healing of the anastomotic leak.

of definitive source control in a single operation versus multiple, staged procedures is a function of the disease process itself, local and systemic factors including host-pathogen interactions, and surgical decision making.

To a large extent, the potential for infection is determined by the size of the bacterial inoculum and bacterial virulence relative to the host's resistance and ability to clear bacteria. Bacteria act synergistically to promote favorable conditions for the establishment and perpetuation of infection, through consumption of oxygen in the microenvironment, the inoculum effect (minimum inhibitory concentrations of antibiotics are increased by higher concentrations of bacteria), and the "quorum-sensing" effect, whereby bacteria sense when their numbers are optimal and regulate their growth accordingly. The ability of neutrophils to eliminate bacteria is altered by the presence of intraperitoneal fluid collections, low ambient oxygen tension (since oxygen is required for the oxidative burst used by phagocytes to kill ingested microbes), and the presence of adjuvants, such as bile or blood.[31,32]

Taken together, optimal surgical source control is management that ensures adequate perfusion and oxygen delivery, drains fluid collections and abscesses (which eliminates sanctuaries for bacterial growth while reducing the bacterial inoculum), debrides devitalized tissue, and removes (or does not implant) adjuvant substances. Combined with appropriate antimicrobial therapy, adequate source control restores conditions that permit recovery of intraperitoneal host defenses, increasing the host's ability to clear the infection.

ABSCESS

In a sense, abscess formation represents success of intraperitoneal host defense mechanisms, because the infection has been contained and generalized peritonitis has been prevented. However, success is incomplete, considering that an abscess is a milieu with characteristics that nurture and promote bacterial growth, including low pH, blood flow, and oxygen tension; altered redox potential; huge numbers of bacteria; and impediments to immune cell influx and penetration of antibiotics. An abscess may also be considered a "standoff" between the infection and host defenses, because neither progressive infection nor eradication occurs. However, an untreated intra-abdominal abscess should be considered only "meta-stable," because containment may fail suddenly with consequences that are catastrophic for the patient.

Small abscesses sometimes resolve with antibiotics alone. For example, adult males with appendicitis and a palpable mass have been treated in this way for decades, but prospective data are few. Numerous questions remain, including the maximum size of abscess that can be treated successfully with antibiotics in the absence of surgical or image-guided drainage. For hemodynamically stable patients with well-circumscribed, nonloculated abscesses, percutaneous drainage, and systemic antibiotics are indicated, if access to the abscess is safe and can be carried out without unduly risking damage to adjacent organs. Percutaneous decompression of abscesses is about 85% successful, resulting in rapid clinical improvement.[33] Percutaneous drainage may be definitive in some cases or may temporize to allow definitive management by a single operation under controlled circumstances rather than emergency surgery or multiple operations. If clinical improvement does not occur promptly following drainage, then formal operative intervention should be performed without further delay. If possible, a localized open drainage procedure (e.g., drainage of a right subphrenic abscess via a posterior approach through the bed of the 12th rib) can be as efficacious as laparotomy while minimizing bleeding and the risk of postoperative enterocutaneous fistula formation.[34]

GENERALIZED PERITONITIS

For unstable patients or those with generalized peritonitis, expeditious, formal operative intervention is generally required. Several factors must be considered at the time of operation: (1) Can the primary disease process be resected/repaired safely? (2) Can hollow viscus continuity be re-established? (3) If suture lines are created (e.g., as a result of carrying out an anastomosis or plication of a perforation), do they need to be protected by drains or fecal diversion? (4) What is the patient's risk of failure (e.g., recurrent/persistent peritonitis, abscess, suture line disruption, fistula formation)?

(5) What steps can be taken to reduce the risk of failure? (6) What clinical course will indicate that source control has failed and that reoperation is required?

The ability to resect/repair the disease process depends on the process itself and the clinical stability of the patient. However, with appropriate resuscitation and support, resection of diseased, necrotic, or infected tissue should be undertaken at the primary operation, in expectation of more rapid resolution of sepsis.[35]

Decisions regarding re-establishment of bowel continuity in patients with sepsis and peritonitis are complex. Three general approaches can be undertaken: (1) performance of a primary anastomosis at the first operation; (2) acceptance of temporary bowel discontinuity with planned reoperation (resection without immediate anastomosis); or (3) creation of a stoma for fecal diversion (with or without anastomosis). Factors weighed in the decision include the likelihood of suture line disruption or fistula formation, the ability to detect complications if they occur, and the likelihood of an adverse outcome if disruption occurs. Adequate blood flow must be present at the suture line for healing to occur. Thus, the risk of suture line failure is increased in patients with compensated or noncompensated shock, mesenteric ischemia, bowel wall distention, peritoneal inflammation, or bowel wall edema. In addition to inadequate blood supply, the extent of peritoneal inflammation also affects the likelihood of anastomotic failure. It is the inflammatory process in peritonitis that provides the disruptive influence, as prompt primary repair of intestinal traumatic wounds, in the presence of bacterial contamination but not established infection, is now standard.[36] Creation of a stoma should be considered when mesenteric blood flow is known or suspected to be inadequate or there is intense peritoneal inflammation. If suture lines must be created under adverse conditions, several maneuvers may minimize risk of dehiscence, including the placement of healthy, well-vascularized tissue over the suture line, tube decompression of the proximal bowel to prevent distention and the resulting increase in wall tension, and decreased perfusion pressure. Some authorities recommend placing drains to control leaks if they occur, although this approach is controversial.

PERITONEAL TOILET

As described previously, several local factors increase the likelihood of failed source control, including the size of the bacterial inoculum and the presence of adjuvant substances or collections of fluid.[32,37] However, adjunctive measures to cleanse the peritoneal cavity at surgery, including irrigation with a large volume of fluid (with or without added antibiotics) and débridement of fibrin from serosal surfaces, are unproved and may be deleterious. The value of irrigation is controversial. The practice is prevalent, despite a lack of evidence of benefit. Irrigation with antibiotic solutions is of no benefit if parenteral antibiotics are administered.[4] Moreover, experimental studies using animals suggest that irrigation fluids may increase the dissemination of infection by decreasing the viscosity of the purulent peritoneal fluid. On the other hand, studies of saline irrigation have generally examined small volumes instilled at low pressure.[4] Bacteria causing established infections adhere to serosal surfaces in peritonitis.[38-40] This adherence makes bacteria relatively resistant to removal by passive irrigation.[41] Pulse irrigation can dislodge adherent bacteria in other clinical settings and

may prove beneficial for management of intra-abdominal infection.[38,42] Neither continuous postoperative lavage nor radical peritoneal débridement have been demonstrated to be effective in randomized studies.[43,44] Radical débridement increases the risk of fistula formation.

Early recurrent fluid collections probably also enhance the risk of failure of source control by providing favorable growth conditions for residual bacteria. Loculated fluid collections are characterized by low oxygen tension, poor antibiotic penetration, and impaired leukocyte function. Despite widespread belief to the contrary, closed-suction drains do little to prevent recurrent fluid collections, because such systems are rapidly walled off from the general peritoneal cavity. In cases of diffuse peritonitis, prevention of recurrent fluid collections is much more difficult; it is impossible to drain the entire abdomen. In these situations, prospective consideration of scheduled repeat laparotomy is warranted.

THE OPEN ABDOMEN

Management using an "open abdomen" approach may be warranted in selected patients, including those with diffuse peritonitis, failed primary source control, increased intra-abdominal pressure that impairs vital organ (notably renal and pulmonary) function, or infections involving the anterior abdominal wall fascia (i.e., necrotizing fasciitis).[45,46] Whether laparotomy on demand, scheduled relaparotomy, or an open abdomen management technique is used for peritoneal toilet in diffuse peritonitis is a matter of clinical judgment; no prospective comparative studies exist. Several factors warrant consideration: (1) Recurrent fluid collections support substantial bacterial regrowth. (2) Exposed bowel is at risk of fistula formation and ileus; use of adherent dressings should be eschewed. (3) Abdominal domain is lost, as lack of fascial coaptation results in progressive contracture of the abdominal wall musculature. (4) If the abdomen cannot be closed primarily, then coverage of the abdominal contents with healthy tissue as soon as possible reduces the incidence of complications and metabolic stress.

Use of the open abdomen approach is considered because of on-going peritonitis or because the infection has extended to involve the tissue of the anterior abdominal wall.[47] The goal of open abdomen management is to substitute manual peritoneal toilet for intraperitoneal host defenses until they recover. Numerous variations in techniques have been reported. Most often, a negative-pressure system is utilized. A fenestrated nonadherent material is used to cover the bowel; drains are applied to aspirate fluid collecting above this layer; and an airtight adherent outer drape is applied to maintain a vacuum and prevent evisceration until adhesions form (Fig. 123-13). At re-exploration and washout, which may be performed daily at the bedside, the abdomen is lavaged and loculated fluid collections are broken up manually, with the operator remaining cognizant that the tolerance of inflamed bowel for manipulation is limited. If possible, all suture lines should be positioned beneath healthy tissue so as to avoid further injury. If drains are placed within the abdomen (their value is questionable in the absence of a fistula), these are brought laterally through the abdominal wall so that a fistula tract can form and heal spontaneously. Re-exploration and washout is repeated until no fluid collections persist and infection is controlled. Once the patient is resuscitated and infection is controlled, diuresis is undertaken to reduce anasarca and promote conditions for closure of the abdomen.

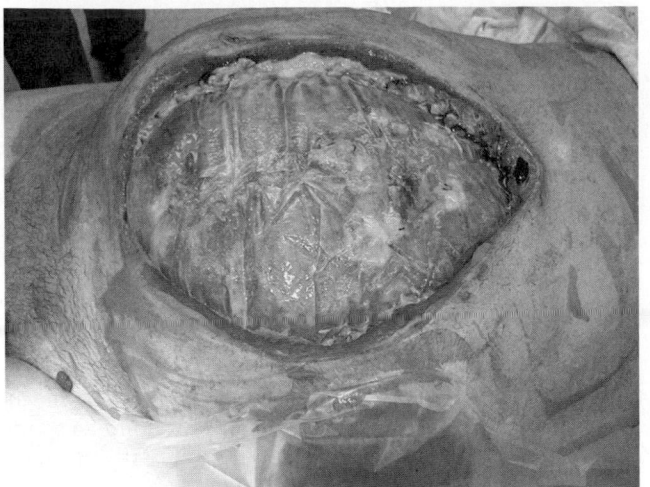

FIGURE 123–13. Open abdomen management of tertiary peritonitis. The vacuum dressing has been taken down to permit inspection. Absorbable mesh (woven polyglactin 910), sewn to fascial edges, covers the intestine. (Courtesy of Paul Kearney, M.D.)

TABLE 123–4. ANTIMICROBIAL AGENT REGIMENS FOR THERAPY OF SERIOUS INTRAABDOMINAL INFECTIONS

Single Agents

Imipenem
Meropenem
Piperacillin-tazobactam

Combination Agents

Aminoglycoside plus an anti anaerobic agent
- Amikacin, gentamicin, netilmicin, or tobramycin plus clindamycin or metronidazole

Aztreonam plus clindamycin
- Combination of aztreonam plus metronidazole is devoid of coverage against gram-positive cocci

Ciprofloxacin plus metronidazole
- Levofloxacin is likely comparable to ciprofloxacin

Third- or fourth-generation cephalosporin plus an anti-anaerobic agent
- Cefepime, cefotaxime, ceftazidime, ceftizoxime, or ceftriaxone plus clindamycin or metronidazole

Data from Mazuski et al.[48,49]

Nasogastric tube decompression is maintained and nutritional support is provided parenterally to prevent bowel distention. Once source control has been obtained, fascia that can be approximated without tension or increased abdominal pressure is closed. If primary closure of the fascia is feasible, then continued attempts to do so are undertaken. Some patients may tolerate skin closure without fascial closure as a short-term solution. However, in a substantial percentage of patients the fascia cannot be closed primarily, so mesh placement, enteral nutrition, and skin grafting prepare the patient for ventral hernia repair several months later.

ANTIBIOTIC THERAPY

It is firmly established that optimal antibiotic therapy for intra-abdominal infection (secondary peritonitis) requires an agent or combination of agents that are active against gut-derived facultative enteric Gram-negative bacilli as well as obligate anaerobes. However, because of limitations in trial design, no single regimen has been shown to be superior to all others, even though many class I studies have been carried out. The studies have been designed to prove equivalence, not superiority. The patients enrolled in clinical trials are not critically ill, for the most part, so new agents are not tested in the most challenging patients. Moreover, although antibiotics are an essential adjunct, it is surgery that is the crucial element of management for all but the most mild of cases.

Initial antibiotic therapy should be considered empiric, because the inciting cause of the infection is not always known at the time antibiotics must be started. Although anti-anaerobic therapy is not crucial for management of a fresh duodenal ulcer perforation (i.e., one that is less than 24 hours old), withholding such coverage for patients with complicated appendicitis or a colon perforation would be inappropriate. Considering that most regimens are equivalent (Table 123-4)[48,49] (except possibly for conventionally dosed aminoglycosides, which may be inferior),[50] the selection of a regimen should be based on considerations of cost and the risk of toxicity, including allergy to beta-lactam agents.

Local antimicrobial resistance patterns should be taken into account when infection develops after the patient has been hospitalized. Although mortality appears to be higher when an *Enterococcus* sp is isolated from polymicrobial intra-abdominal infections,[19] there is no evidence that specific antienterococcal therapy improves outcome.[19,51]

Making the decision of whether to treat fungal isolates is more difficult. Fungal species are common components of the normal intestinal flora; accordingly, isolation of fungi from peritoneal fluid is common at operation for a perforated viscus. Most fungal infections in surgical patients do not involve the blood stream but rather manifest as isolation of organisms from one or more sites that are normally sterile. Furthermore, fungal colonization usually precedes invasive infection in surgical patients. Therefore, some experts argue that it is wise to treat systemically when yeasts are recovered from peritoneal fluid.[52-54] However, there is no consensus regarding this issue, and antifungal therapy remains optional unless yeasts are cultured from the blood stream, yeasts are cultured (in the absence of other organisms) from an abscess, or the patient is profoundly immunosuppressed.[48,49]

The optimal duration of therapy is unknown, but the clinical trend is toward shorter courses of antibiotics. When source control is adequate, the role of antibiotics is a purely adjuvant one, and even generalized peritonitis can be treated with antibiotics for as little as 5 to 7 days.[55] When intestinal function returns, oral antibiotics with good bioavailability can be administered to complete the course of therapy.[48,49] For example, the bioavailability of fluoroquinolones is reduced from 100% to about 70% when the drug is administered by tube with enteral feedings, but dosage adjustments can be made to render the therapy effective.[56]

The role of antibiotics for tertiary peritonitis is even less well defined. There is little evidence that antibiotics make any difference whatsoever; moreover, most of the bacterial isolates tend to be resistant to commonly used empiric regimens. If used, antibiotics for tertiary peritonitis should probably be of narrow spectrum and administered briefly; anti-anaerobic therapy is probably unnecessary.

COMPLICATIONS

The complications of failed source control include abscess formation, anastomotic dehiscence, infection of the incision, recurrent or persistent (secondary or tertiary) peritonitis, fistula formation, sepsis, and multiple organ dysfunction syndrome, which is the leading cause of death. Whereas abscess, anastomotic dehiscence, and fistula formation are most commonly attributable to failure of the source control procedure itself, persistent peritonitis and sepsis are often attributable to failure of host defenses. There is undoubtedly overlap, and it can sometimes be impossible to attribute failure to anything other than a constellation of events. Regardless, if infection and sepsis persist, organ dysfunction, which can be fatal, is the expected result. Indeed, if organ dysfunction develops, achievement of source control thereafter may be unable to abrogate the response.

Management of these complications should be individualized, and it depends to some degree on the nature of the presentation. Discrete fluid collections may be amenable to percutaneous drainage, even if laparotomy was the initial mode of treatment. If there are more than two discrete fluid collections or there is diffuse peritonitis, drainage by laparotomy is generally required.

ENTEROCUTANEOUS FISTULA

Fistulas, abnormal epithelialized tracts between two hollow viscus structures or between a hollow viscus and the skin, usually manifest in a delayed fashion.[57-59] Fistulas result from prolonged inflammation, often in conjunction with an operative intestinal injury; 80% to 85% of fistulas occur in the postoperative period; fistulas that arise from infection alone (e.g., tuberculosis, abscess eroding directly into bowel) or in irradiated bowel are rare. A fistula may be an occult source of sepsis before drainage to the skin makes the diagnosis obvious. A fistula may occur with an abscess cavity (which requires drainage) along its tract. Alternatively, a fistula can be present without an intraperitoneal collection and not require surgical intervention.

Several basic requirements must be met for fistulas to heal spontaneously. Fistulas that drain more than 500 mL/day are more likely to have additional complications and to require surgical closure than are those that drain less than 200 mL/day.[59a]

Coexistent infection must be controlled. There must be neither distal obstruction nor foreign material present. Malignant disease must not involve the fistula tract, and there must be healthy tissue of sufficient depth in the abdominal wall to allow the tract to collapse and close. A fistula that develops within an open incision or during open-abdomen management is much less likely to heal.[59] Adequate blood flow and nutrition must be ensured.

When a fistula develops, initial care is supportive. Key elements include appropriate broad-spectrum antibiotic therapy, bowel rest, skin care (the drainage from a fistula can incite marked inflammation of surrounding skin), and parenteral nutritional support. Low-output, distal fistulas can sometimes be managed with enteral elemental feedings, if the amount of drainage does not increase when feedings are instituted. If the volume of drainage is high, fluid repletion with a balanced salt solution that resembles the electrolyte composition of the lost fluids (e.g., lactated Ringer's solution for small- or large-bowel fistulas) is indicated.

The next phase of management is delineation of the anatomy. Fistulas can occur at any point along the gastrointestinal tract, although the clinical context usually allows an estimate of the location to be made. Options are several, including barium studies of the gut, but the most expeditious manner may be to combine CT of the abdomen and pelvis with injection of a water-soluble contrast agent directly into the cutaneous opening of the tract. Once identified, a decision for surgery immediately versus medical management can be made. Thirty to 50% of all enterocutaneous fistulas close with nonoperative therapy, usually within 3 to 4 weeks.[59a]

The third phase of management is surgical correction if spontaneous closure does not occur. Infection must be controlled. If possible, resection of diseased bowel with primary anastomosis is preferred; bypass surgery is not recommended. In some cases, circumstances may dictate creation of a stoma and mucous fistula and restoration of continuity at a later date.

ABDOMINAL COMPARTMENT SYNDROME

Abdominal compartment syndrome may occur in critically ill patients with peritonitis and may be due to tissue edema, ascites, or packing materials placed temporarily at surgery. The diagnosis and management of abdominal compartment syndrome is discussed in Chapter 239.

MORTALITY

About 25% of critically ill patients with a perforated viscus die. The mortality rate is higher among older patients and those with greater severity of illness at the time of presentation. Severity of illness is so important as a determinant of outcome that, among critically ill patients, the site of infection within the abdomen is irrelevant.[3] Failure of the initial source control procedure is more likely to result in death than infection caused by a multi-drug-resistant pathogen. Although early, appropriate antibiotic therapy is important, changing antibiotics based on susceptibility data does not make a difference.[17,18]

Organ dysfunction is present to some degree in every patient dying with intra-abdominal infection. Implementation of strategies to prevent or reverse organ dysfunction have the potential to reduce the mortality risk of intra-abdominal infection. Early recognition of organ dysfunction can be a harbinger of persistent intra-abdominal infection and afford an opportunity to intervene while the process is still reversible.[60-63] The key elements in care to minimize mortality include early recognition of the problem, rapid resuscitation, timely and correct performance of the correct procedure for initial source control, and administration of appropriate broad-spectrum antibiotics. Important adjuncts may include tight control of serum glucose concentration,[64] administration of low doses of glucocorticoids,[65] and judicious transfusion of red blood cell concentrates,[66] but additional data are needed for confirmation. There is also some evidence that therapy with drotrecogin alfa (activated) may increase survival among these patients.[67]

ANNOTATED REFERENCES

Ayana DA, Nathens AB: Risk factors for severe sepsis in secondary peritonitis. Surg Infect 2003;4:355-362.

Most cases of peritonitis are caused by appendicitis; therefore, most patients with peritonitis are not sick enough to develop organ dysfunction or critical illness. The authors conducted a population-based study to determine risk factors for severe sepsis among patients with peritonitis.

Among several factors, increasing age, diffuse peritonitis as opposed to abscess formation, small bowel origin (likely owing to diagnostic difficulty/delay), and pre-existing hepatic or renal dysfunction increased the likelihood of the development of severe sepsis.

Gajic O, Urrurtia LA, Sewani H, et al: Acute abdomen in the medical intensive care unit. Crit Care Med 2002;30:1187-1190.

This is a large observational study of intra-abdominal infection in a medical intensive care unit, where the problem is rare in comparison to surgical ICUs. In addition to the differing epidemiology, two additional salient points should be noted. First, the index of suspicion must be high, because the diagnosis can be missed. Second, missed diagnoses and delayed therapy are both highly lethal.

Mazuski JE, Sawyer RG, Nathens AB, et al: The Surgical Infection Society guidelines on antimicrobial therapy for intra-abdominal infections: Evidence for the recommendations. Surg Infect 2002;3:175-233.

This document, from the Therapeutic Agents Committee of the Surgical Infection Society, is a comprehensive evidence-based review of the literature and recommendations for antibiotic therapy of intra-abdominal infections. Numerous regimens are equivalent for therapy of community-acquired infections among healthy, good-risk patients. There is a paucity of data regarding critically ill patients specifically, and data are also lacking regarding the optimal duration of therapy.

Sugerman HJ, Bloomfield GL, Saggi BW: Multisystem organ failure secondary to increased intraabdominal pressure. Infection. 1999;27:61-66.

The authors describe clearly the deleterious consequences of abdominal compartment syndrome, which results from increased intra-abdominal pressure from any of a number of causes, including bowel edema and distention, or packing within the abdomen. When pressure within the abdomen exceeds 20 to 30 mm Hg, there can be deleterious effects on either renal (decreased renal blood flow) or pulmonary function (decreased lung volumes from upward displacement of the diaphragm, decreased venous return), or both. Early recognition, and decompression of the intra-abdominal hypertension can prevent organ dysfunction or restore function.

Wittman DH, Schein M: Let us shorten antibiotic prophylaxis and therapy in surgery. Am J Surg 1996;172:26S-32S.

Surgeons overuse antibiotics for both prophylaxis and therapy. Surgical antibiotic prophylaxis is designed to protect the incision from surgical site infection while it is vulnerable (i.e., open). The surgical incision is ischemic for 24 to 48 hours after closure owing to the extensive efforts undertaken to ensure hemostasis. Postoperative doses of antibiotics after surgery of soft tissues increases the risk of superinfection and the emergence of resistant pathogens, without benefit to the patient. Likewise, surgical drainage of an intra-abdominal infection reduces the size of the bacterial inoculum and makes antibiotics more effective, while at the same time allowing host defenses to recover. Wittman and Schein outline the rationale for short courses of surgical antibiotic prophylaxis and therapy.

Chapter 124

ILEUS AND MECHANICAL SMALL BOWEL OBSTRUCTION

Vishal Bansal • Juan B. Ochoa

KEY POINTS

1. Ileus is **an often unrecognized condition** in the ICU. Its consequences can be disastrous, including abdominal compartment syndrome, respiratory embarrassment, severe electrolyte abnormalities, decreased renal blood flow, and intestinal necrosis.

2. There are **multiple causes of ileus**, including postoperative states; medications, particularly narcotics; and sepsis.

3. **Postoperative ileus is common in the ICU and can be avoided** by early feeding, limited use of nasogastric tubes, correction of electrolyte abnormalities, and optimal narcotic usage. Few medications have been shown to improve ileus; however, neostigmine can be used judiciously under careful observation.

4. New-onset ICU ileus may be a **marker of sepsis**, and possible sources should be carefully considered.

5. Mechanical small bowel obstruction presents with **early-onset vomiting and diffuse abdominal pain**. If unrecognized, it may quickly lead to intestinal ischemia and death.

6. **Surgical consultation is mandatory** if mechanical obstruction is suspected.

Often when managing critically ill patients, evaluation of the gastrointestinal (GI) tract consists of little more than perfunctory palpation of the abdomen, followed by brief auscultation with a stethoscope listening for bowel sounds. In contrast, other organ systems such as the heart and lungs are typically monitored using sophisticated technology that usually provides a quantitative measure of organ function. However, as with other organ systems, GI tract dysfunction can have profound consequences during critical illness, even when it is uninjured or not mechanically manipulated. Normal GI motility is essential for the adequate mixing of food with digestive fluids, maximal exposure of nutrients to absorptive mucosal surfaces, and prevention of bacterial overgrowth. Abnormal GI motility leading to gut stasis is called ileus and often occurs in critical illness. Mechanical intestinal obstruction is also observed frequently and is a result of physical extrinsic or intrinsic compression of the GI lumen. Mechanical obstruction and ileus can lead to severe GI dysfunction and possibly organ failure. Despite the fact that both ileus and mechanical intestinal obstruction result in lack of progression of a food bolus through the GI tract, there are major differences in their cause, diagnosis, and treatment; therefore, ileus and mechanical bowel obstruction are reviewed separately in this chapter.

ILEUS

The term *ileus* is derived from a Greek word meaning "obstruction." However, the etymology is misleading, because ileus actually denotes dysmotility in the absence of a mechanical obstruction. Ileus results from the loss of coordinated, propulsive muscle contractions from the smooth muscle coats of the bowel wall. Manifestations of ileus include failure to pass stool or flatus, coupled with abdominal distention and a decrease in bowel sounds. Clinical examination is the only practical tool to diagnose ileus.[1] Clinically, patients with ileus have abdominal distention, nausea, vomiting, and increased output of fluids through an existing nasogastric (NG) tube. There is no clear definition of what constitutes an abnormal degree of abdominal distention or an excessive amount of NG output. Most clinical and radiographic parameters used for the diagnosis of ileus are of questionable value, often revealing only diffuse intestinal air, bowel edema, or other nonspecific findings.[2] This means that the accuracy, sensitivity, and specificity with which we diagnose ileus are poor. Thus, the true incidence of ileus in critical illness is unknown.

The consequences of ileus can be disastrous (Table 124-1). In its most severe presentation, ileus can result in abdominal compartment syndromes, respiratory embarrassment, severe electrolyte abnormalities, decreased renal blood flow, and intestinal necrosis.[3] Prolonged ileus can result in decreased nutrient and medication absorption, bacterial overgrowth, and bacterial translocation. Paradoxically, an excessive fear of ileus may result in inadequate use of the GI tract and gut atrophy. This clinical attitude often results in the prescription of total parenteral nutrition in a naive effort to prevent the progression to malnutrition. Thus, new technology or mechanisms of diagnosing ileus are sorely needed.

NORMAL PHYSIOLOGY

Knowledge of normal GI physiology is useful in understanding some of the causes of and possible therapies for ileus. The GI tract consists of distinct tissue layers from inward to outward: mucosa, submucosa, circular muscle layer, longitudinal

TABLE 124–1. POTENTIAL CONSEQUENCES OF ILEUS IN A CRITICAL CARE SETTING

Nutrient malnutrition from "fear of feeding"
Bacterial overgrowth and translocation, worsening sepsis
Abdominal compartment syndrome
Vomiting and aspiration
Intestinal ischemia and necrosis
Longer hospitalization

muscle layer, and serosa. Within the GI tract are myenteric and submucosal nerve plexus, which communicate with the central nervous system via sympathetic and parasympathetic nerves.[4] The empty GI tract has a specific resting pattern of contractions that generates waves of pressure. These migratory motor complexes move in three distinct phases from the stomach to the distal ileum. Even though the gut maintains basal migratory motor complexes during fasting, these complexes are not noticeable in the colon under fasting conditions.

Introduction of a food bolus produces a radical and significant change in GI motor function. In the presence of a food bolus, the GI tract is distended, stimulating sympathetic and parasympathetic nerve endings. Food is thus "sensed" by the GI tract; as a result, migratory motor complex phases are abrogated, and the food bolus is propelled downstream by a series of pressure spikes initiated by electrical activity.[5] Colonic activity is also stimulated by the presence of a food bolus in its lumen, with the appearance of long, propulsive contractions. In healthy patients, the gut acts in a coordinated manner to establish motility, starting with the generation of membrane action potentials in the neuronal plexus, followed by contraction of smooth muscle cells in the muscular layers of the intestinal wall. This ring of serial concentric contractions is the basis for gut peristalsis, moving a food bolus from the mouth to eventual defecation. Various factors modulate gut motility in response to environmental and physiologic stimuli. Factors altering the gut membrane potential and stimulating gut contraction include an increased parasympathetic drive, releasing acetylcholine; cholecystokinin; gastrin; and direct stretching of the bowel.[6] Factors preventing gut depolarization and inhibiting contractility include an increased sympathetic drive, releasing norepinephrine and epinephrine; inflammation; and secretin.[6] Given this complex interplay between stimulation and inhibition of gut activity, it is clear that any deviation from homeostasis can induce ileus.

PATHOPHYSIOLOGY

The development of ileus in critically ill patients is almost always multifactorial. The most common cause of ileus, regardless of the setting, is manipulation of the intestine during laparotomy. Postoperative ileus has been recognized since the early 20th century and continues to be a major cause of prolonged ICU and hospital stays, adding almost a billion dollars a year to health care costs in the United States alone.[7] Postoperative ileus normally lasts for 3 to 5 days following major intra-abdominal surgery; small bowel function generally returns in the first 24 hours, followed by stomach and colon function in the next 24 to 48 hours.[6,8] In addition to causing discomfort and intolerance of oral feedings, ileus increases the risk of aspiration pneumonia, bowel ischemia, and sepsis.[9,10] Postoperative ileus may also cause clinicians to

eschew early enteral feedings in critically ill patients, even though there are abundant data supporting the benefits of such feedings (discussed later).[11,12]

The exact molecular pathophysiology of ileus is unresolved, but it involves a complex interplay among the central nervous system, inflammation, and medication regimens. It has long been taught that the dynamics of paralytic ileus are partly due to imbalance of splanchnic neural innervations.[13,14] Recent investigations, targeting the autonomic nervous system using animal models, suggest that splanchnic neurogenic dysfunction and mediators of inflammation are likely the two most important factors leading to the development of postoperative ileus.[15] As mentioned, gut motility is stimulated by the parasympathetic nervous system, whereas sympathetic stimulation is inhibitory. Postoperatively, the increased sympathetic drive and subsequent release of norepinephrine and epinephrine in neurons in the enteric nervous system play an important role in the pathogenesis of ileus.[16] In a study by Smith and coworkers, experimental laparotomies in dogs suppressed the movement of intraintestinal plastic balls.[16] This was measured in conjunction with increased blood concentrations of norepinephrine and epinephrine. Using this paradigm, several studies have achieved a significant reduction in postoperative ileus by blocking the sympathetic neural reflexes through the administration of epidural local analgesics.[17] Intra-abdominal release of phenylephrine, a potent sympathetic analog, directly on colonic tissue causes a dose-dependent decrease in the frequency of colon contractions.[18] Low-dose selective sympathetic antagonists, such as the alpha$_2$-antagonist atipamezole (0.06 mg/kg), have been shown to reverse postoperative ileus in rat models.[19,20] Further data, also obtained in postoperative rat models, suggest that central neuronal activity may inhibit gut motility via an efferent inhibitory, noncholinergic pathway that uses nitric oxide (NO) as a neurotransmitter.[21] NO causes smooth muscle relaxation and decreased contractility, as well as exerts a neurosuppressor effect on gut neuronal plexus. Reserpine, a drug that blocks sympathetic neurotransmission and possibly NO transmission, partially reverses ileus induced by laparotomy and small intestinal manipulation in rodents.[22] However, sympathetic and noncholinergic NO-dependent effects are insufficient to fully explain the pathogenesis of postoperative ileus, because combined treatment with a sympathetic antagonist and drugs to block NO synthesis fails to completely reverse ileus.[9]

A second important mechanism in the development of postoperative ileus is inflammation.[23] The role of inflammation in the pathogenesis of ileus can be explained by the large number of white blood cells residing within the muscular layers of the intestine.[24] Intestinal manipulation activates these white cells, inducing the production and release of proinflammatory cytokines and the up-regulation of neutrophil adhesion molecules (e.g., LFA-1). As a result, there is greater migration of neutrophils and an increase in the intestinal leukocyte population following surgery. Cytokines such as interleukin-1, interleukin-6, and tumor necrosis factor, and other substances such as NO and prostaglandins (via inducible NO synthase and cyclooxygenase-2, respectively), act to decrease intestinal motility through different mechanisms.[25,26] Specimens of whole human intestine, taken at different points during operations, show a clear, progressive increase in inducible NO synthase expression, develop leukocyte infiltrates, and display diminished in vitro muscle contractility.[27]

The exact mechanisms by which inflammation leads to the development of ileus are still unknown. It is clear, however, that neutrophils and macrophages play an essential role. For example, blocking leukocyte recruitment almost completely prevents the suppression of jejunal muscle contractility, as observed 24 hours after intestinal manipulation.[28] These findings strongly support the theory that inflammation and its mediators are important causative factors in the development of ileus.

Ileus is a common complication of sepsis and may be a single-organ example of the multiple organ failure that characterizes severe sepsis. The administration of lipopolysaccharide has already been shown to depress skeletal, cardiac, and smooth muscle contractility.[29,30] Further studies have shown that lipopolysaccharide impairs smooth muscle contraction in the small bowel and causes significant GI motility derangements, most likely linked through an NO-mediated mechanism.[31] This accords with an inflammatory pathophysiology of ileus, because a sublethal dose of endotoxin in rats suppresses gut motility and activates gut resident leukocytes.[32] This decrease in intestinal transit allows the overgrowth of bacteria within the lumen of the small intestine and eventual translocation of bacteria from the gut to the regional lymph nodes.[33,34] These observations indicate that ileus, in a critical care setting, may be not only a result of sepsis but also a cause of sepsis, particularly persistent and recurrent sepsis in a "vicious circle" paradigm. Hence, the presence of new-onset ileus in the critical care population may be a harbinger of sepsis and may also be a causative factor in persistent septicemia.

It is important to keep in mind that the neural and inflammatory mechanisms are not mutually exclusive, and the interplay between these complicated forces of biology are likely tightly related in abnormal GI motor function. The finding that activation of the sympathetic nervous system and the inflammatory response is responsible for the development of ileus has permitted the creation of an all-encompassing model. This has practical implications, as investigators are designing new strategies for the prevention and treatment of ileus.

CONTRIBUTING FACTORS

Narcotics. The constipating effects of morphine and other opiates have been recognized for centuries. Narcotics work primarily through the enteric nervous system by stimulating μ-receptors, an effect that decreases colonic propulsion and coordinated peristalsis and increases the resting tone of smooth muscle cells.[35] To provide adequate analgesia, the dose of morphine must be four times the amount needed to slow GI motility.[36] The opioid tolerance that occurs with long-term use to treat pain does not carry over to colonic dysmotility; therefore, progressively higher doses prescribed for analgesia have an even greater likelihood of promoting ileus.[36]

Electrolyte Abnormalities. Massive variations in systemic electrolytes can cause a significant imbalance in gut motility. In burn and VIPoma patients exhibiting ileus and pseudo-obstruction, severe hypokalemia has been linked as a causative factor.[37]

Catecholamines. Exogenous catecholamines, when infused systemically to support blood pressure or cardiac output, decrease GI motility not only by increasing sympathetic tone but also by promoting splanchnic vasoconstriction and mesenteric hypoperfusion. For example, more than

80% of hypotensive trauma patients treated with vasopressors exhibit signs of abnormal GI motor function.[38] This effect may be countered by early feeding (addressed later).

Anesthesia. General anesthetics, including enflurane, halothane, and nitrous oxide, may influence the duration of postoperative ileus, especially when the effects of these agents are added to those of systemic opioids.[39]

Medications. Anticholinergics, psychotropics, calcium channel blockers, benzodiazepines, and other medications have all been implicated as factors promoting ileus.[10]

CLINICAL MANAGEMENT

Diagnosis

As stated earlier, the diagnosis of ileus is made from clinical observation. A nonintubated, neurologically intact patient complains of bloating, which is described as an abnormal sensation of abdominal distention. In addition, the patient may complain of abdominal pain, although, at least early on, it is usually not severe. A frequent complaint is increased belching. In more advanced cases, nausea and vomiting eventually occur. Vomiting is an especially worrisome event, putting patients at risk for aspiration. Significant dehydration and electrolyte abnormalities may be observed and are especially frequent in a vomiting patient. Dehydration and electrolyte abnormalities also decrease blood flow and further contribute to abnormal GI motor function.

Postoperatively, surgeons often question patients about the passage of flatus or the presence of bowel movements and may limit oral intake until this occurs. To our knowledge, however, there has been no study that correlates flatus and normal GI motility.

It is often impossible to determine whether an intubated or heavily sedated critically ill patient has any of these complaints. Thus, clinicians rely on "signs" of ileus. High output of GI fluids, as well as the reflux of bile from the duodenum into the stomach through an NG tube, is often used to diagnose ileus; however, migration of the NG tube into the duodenum can be associated with high-volume, bile-tinged fluid in the absence of ileus. Gastric residuals refer to the volume of gastric aspirate obtained after feeding a patient a nasoenteral diet. Increased gastric residuals are also used in measuring ileus. There are no available data, however, to determine pathologic quantities of NG output or gastric residuals or how these volumes can be optimized.

Abdominal distention is common. On palpation, a patient with a distended abdomen feels abnormally tense and sometimes exhibits tachycardia during the abdominal examination. Generalized measures of abdominal distention are difficult to establish, because abdominal girth varies dramatically from patient to patient. Changes in the abdominal girth of a given patient during hospitalization are more reliable. We frequently use a tape measure to follow abdominal girth.

Plain abdominal films are often used to diagnose ileus. The classic radiographic picture of ileus is the presence of air in the small bowel. In addition, distended loops of small bowel are reported. Increasingly, abdominal computed tomography (CT) scans are being used to diagnose ileus. Again, patterns of air and distended loops of bowel may be observed. Perhaps more important than diagnosing ileus is the fact that CT has nearly 100% sensitivity and specificity for determining the presence of intestinal obstruction, which, in critically ill patients, can be confused with ileus.[40]

Treatment

The successful treatment of ileus involves adequately identifying and treating its cause, optimizing the dose of narcotics, correcting electrolyte imbalances, and eliminating contributing factors (see earlier).

Postoperative ileus is classically treated by NG decompression, nothing by mouth (NPO), opiate restriction, and correction of fluid and electrolyte disturbances. In addition, surgeons classically encourage ambulation in an effort to "resolve" postoperative ileus, although there is no proof that physical exercise induces or restores normal GI motility.[41]

Adequate hemodynamic resuscitation improves splanchnic blood flow and is essential in a patient with ileus. Adequate resuscitation also allows a decrease in the use of vasopressors (catecholamines), therefore eliminating an iatrogenic cause of ileus. However, intravenous fluids should be used sparingly; massive fluids can increase the incidence of bowel edema, which can contribute to abnormal GI motility.[42]

NG decompression is an essential aspect of treatment in patients with ileus. NG tubes decrease the incidence of vomiting and abdominal distention, and adequate GI decompression leads to better mucosal blood flow. Inadequate use of NG tubes does not benefit the patient and may increase morbidity significantly. However, Bauer and colleagues, in a randomized study of 200 patients, found no evidence that postsurgical patients without NG tubes had more wound infections, dehiscence, or anastomotic complications than did patients with NG tube decompression.[43] In other studies, there was an increased incidence (though not statistically significant) of pneumonia and atelectasis in patients treated traditionally with NG tubes until postoperative ileus resolved.[43,44] In addition, NG tubes may cause erosions of the GI tract and perforations and necrosis of the nose. Thus, we do not advocate the routine use of postoperative NG tubes.

A diagnosis of ileus is often used as an excuse to starve the patient and prevent the use of enteral nutrition. Nutrients, however, play a key role in maintaining normal GI motility, mucosal integrity, and mucosal trophism.[45] Several studies demonstrate that ileus resolves faster and patients recover more quickly when they are permitted a judiciously tailored oral intake.[46,47] In a meta-analysis of eight prospective, randomized trials of enteral versus parenteral nutrition that included 230 patients (118 receiving total enteral nutrition and 112 receiving total parenteral nutrition), 84% of patients tolerated early enteral feeding between 8 and 24 hours after a laparotomy. There was also a significant decrease in septic complications in enterally fed compared with parenterally fed patients (35% versus 18%).[11] Based on these findings, early enteral nutrition in critical illness has gained popularity and has become a standard of care. Lewis and associates performed a systematic review and meta-analysis of randomized, controlled trials comparing NPO management versus early feedings.[48] Early postoperative feedings were associated with a significant shortening of hospital stay and a reduction in the risk of infection ($P < 0.04$). A slight reduction in the incidence of anastomotic dehiscence, pneumonia, intra-abdominal abscess, and mortality was seen, but this failed to reach statistical significance.

Like all therapies, early enteral nutrition has to be used with care to avoid adverse effects, which may be especially severe in hemodynamically unstable ICU patients. In the ICU, it is routine to place feeding tubes past the pylorus, delivering nutrients directly into the small bowel. Delivery of nutrients through the enteral route increases oxygen consumption significantly and may lead to intestinal ischemia and bowel necrosis if oxygen demands are not met.[49,50] In addition, excessive volumes of nutrients may distend the bowel, further compromising mucosal blood flow. In severe hypovolemic or cardiogenic shock, the shunting of blood from the gut and kidney to the central circulation further decreases gut blood flow. This may be especially significant for a patient in shock, particularly one who is receiving aggressive medical hemodynamic support that causes additional splanchnic vasoconstriction. Intuitively, many clinicians do not feed patients at all during these dire circumstances; however, recent data suggest that a small amount of enteral nutrition increases splanchnic blood flow, even in a state of gut vasoconstriction in rats infused with vasopressin.[46] Despite some of the preliminary evidence suggesting that early enteral nutrition may restore splanchnic perfusion in a hemodynamically unstable patient, such feedings should be delayed until adequate resuscitation and perfusion have occurred. Overall, however, the goal of early enteral nutrition is to deliver a small amount of nutrients to maintain gut trophism and stimulate neural function and hormonal release, leading to quicker resolution of ileus.

A large amount of work has focused on identifying pharmacologic treatments of ileus (Table 124-2). Therapies include the use of nonsteroidal anti-inflammatory agents, NO synthase inhibitors, sympatholytic agents, parasympathomimetic agents, and opioid antagonists, in addition to more traditional agents such as metoclopramide and erythromycin. In recent years, there has been renewed interest in the use of sympatholytic agents. Early systemic sympatholytic drugs were successful in decreasing ileus, but side effects (e.g., severe bradycardia) prevented these agents from being used clinically.[51] Sympathetic blockade can also be achieved with epidural anesthesia and has been used as a strategy to resolve ileus.[3] In fact, it appears that bowel function returns more quickly and hospitalization is shorter when patients receive midthoracic (T8-T10) bupivacaine nerve blocks after surgery.[52] Epidural naloxone (to antagonize the effects of systemic opiates) also improves gut motility after operations.[53] Most critically ill patients do not have epidural catheters in place, however, and few would advocate inserting one for the sake of sympatholytic therapy to treat ileus.

TABLE 124–2. PHARMACOLOGIC STRATEGIES IN THE TREATMENT OF ILEUS

Treatment	Rationale
Epidural anesthesia (bupivacaine)	Blockade of splanchnic inhibitory sympathetic reflexes
Opioid antagonist (ADL 8-2698)	Selective antagonism of gut μ-receptors
NSAIDs (regimens under investigation)	Inhibition of COX-2 and subsequent decrease in inhibitory prostaglandins
Acetylcholinesterase inhibitor (neostigmine)	Increase in gut wall cholinergic activity
Beta-receptor antagonist (propranolol)	Sympathetic blockade (poor efficacy)
Motility agents (erythromycin, metoclopramide)	Motilin agonists (poor efficacy)
Cisapride	Acetylcholine agonist (taken off the market due to cardiac arrhythmias)

COX, cyclooxygenase; NSAID, nonsteroidal anti-inflammatory drug.

The opioid antagonist ADL 8-2698 (Adolor, Exton, Pa.) does not cross the blood-brain barrier and thus does not prevent the analgesic effects of opioids, making it a plausible therapeutic option. In 79 postlaparotomy patients randomized to receive placebo, 1 mg of ADL 8-2698, or 6 mg of the drug, the median time to the first passage of flatus decreased from 70 to 49 hours, and the median time to the first bowel movement decreased from 111 to 70 hours, in patients given the 6-mg dosage.[54] Further investigations using ADL 8-2698 are currently under way.

The cholinesterase inhibitor neostigmine is increasingly being used as a therapeutic agent to treat ileus. Neostigmine blocks the hydrolysis of acetylcholine and, therefore, increases the concentration of this neurotransmitter at neuromuscular junctions within the smooth muscle coats of the bowel. As a result, gut motility is enhanced. In 1999, Ponec and colleagues reported that a 2-mg bolus injection of neostigmine caused almost immediate defection in 10 of 11 patients with prolonged colonic ileus.[55] However, bolus administration of neostigmine can be associated with serious side effects, particularly profound bradycardia. One way to ameliorate the undesirable side effects is to administer neostigmine by continuous infusion. This approach was employed by van der Spoel and coworkers, who randomized critically ill patients to receive 0.4 to 0.8 mg/h of continuous neostigmine or placebo.[56] Among the patients treated with neostigmine, 79% defecated within 24 hours of starting therapy with the drug. Moreover, continuous infusion of neostigmine was associated with few cardiac or other major side effects. A 2-mg bolus of neostigmine is an effective therapy for patients with significant ileus, particularly in the ICU, where careful cardiac monitoring is already in place. However, after defecation, the ileus often returns.

Cisapride increases the release of acetylcholine within the mesenteric plexus, thereby increasing GI motility. Although cisapride was shown to ameliorate ileus in some studies, the drug was withdrawn from the market in the United States because it was associated with an increased incidence of cardiac arrhythmias, especially torsades de pointes.[57]

In a recent human study, the beta blocker propranolol (80 to 160 mg/day) failed to improve ileus in postoperative patients.[58] Similarly, other pro-propulsive agents such as erythromycin and metoclopramide, which are motilin agonists, yielded disappointing results in trials evaluating their effects on ileus resolution.[59,60] Therefore, a universally accepted medication regimen for the treatment of ileus has yet to be determined, and a multimodal approach optimizing the use of narcotics, electrolyte correction, and early enteral feeding is still the best treatment option.

MECHANICAL INTESTINAL OBSTRUCTION

Mechanical intestinal obstruction is the result of an identifiable anatomic barrier to the passage of luminal contents of the gut. The source of obstruction can occur within the bowel lumen or bowel wall, such as a tumor, or it can be extrinsic to the GI tract, as observed in patients with adhesions or incarcerated hernias. Intestinal obstruction, if untreated, will lead to stasis of intestinal contents, progressive dehydration, intestinal ischemia, shock, and ultimately death. This progression of disease is why surgical students often recite "never let the sun set or rise on a small bowel obstruction." Thus, it is essential to identify the presence of mechanical obstructions in critically ill patients.

CLINICAL PRESENTATION

Intestinal obstruction presents as a classic clinical picture of severe, cramping abdominal pain; nausea; protracted bilious vomiting; and, in patients with complete obstruction, the absence of flatus or bowel movements. This presentation is in stark contrast to that of an ileus, where nausea and vomiting are usually late signs and the progression of pain and discomfort is often much slower and more indolent. In mechanical obstruction, the cramping abdominal pain is eventually replaced by continuous pain as intestinal ischemia ensues. In more advanced cases, circulatory collapse is observed due to the loss of fluids and electrolytes and the development of sepsis.

On examination, patients with intestinal obstruction are in severe distress and pain. They may exhibit systemic symptoms such as tachycardia, diaphoresis, and shock. The abdomen is distended, sometimes causing respiratory embarrassment. Bowel sounds can be hyperactive and are often described as "metallic" in nature. Palpation can detect an extrinsic cause of obstruction, such as a hernia, or abdominal surgical scars, suggesting the presence of adhesions. Palpation of the abdomen may also reveal the presence of a mass. Patients normally do not exhibit signs of peritoneal irritation unless intestinal ischemia is present. A rectal examination generally reveals an empty rectal vault. Sarr and colleagues, in a famous study, prospectively evaluated the preoperative judgment of senior attending surgeons and preoperative physiologic parameters in 51 patients undergoing exploration for a mechanical small bowel obstruction.[61] No preoperative parameter, including abdominal pain, fever, peritoneal signs, leukocytosis, or acidosis, proved to be sensitive, specific, or predictive for intestinal ischemia. Moreover, the senior surgeons' clinical judgment detected strangulation in about 50% of patients. Ultimately, the need for surgery is based on the patient's clinical course, the surgeon's experience, and pure gestalt.

Patients with intestinal obstruction may become critically ill. Thus, intestinal obstruction is an important reason for admission to an ICU. It is not uncommon for patients to arrive in shock caused by intestinal obstruction or to be critically ill after surgical resection of infarcted bowel. The incidence of intestinal obstruction as a complication in critically ill patients admitted to the ICU for other reasons is unknown, however.

IMAGING AND LABORATORY SUPPORT

The radiographic picture of intestinal obstruction is classically described as the presence of air-fluid levels in the small bowel, dilatation of the small or large bowel, intestinal wall edema, and a "cutoff point" after which a paucity of air is observed. Plain abdominal films have to be taken in the upright position so that air-fluid levels can be observed. Plain abdominal films are often used to follow patients with intestinal obstruction.

CT has become a popular way of evaluating patients with intestinal obstruction, although the clinical picture should be sufficient to make the diagnosis in most patients. CT scans are quite useful, however, in identifying uncertain causes of intestinal obstruction and in alerting physicians to the presence of ischemia.[62,63] However, it must be emphasized that inappropriate performance of a CT scan may delay a much-needed surgical intervention.

Laboratory tests are often ordered for patients with intestinal obstruction. White blood cell counts are modestly elevated unless intestinal ischemia and sepsis are present. Patients with dehydration may present with hemoconcentration, acidosis, electrolyte abnormalities, and an abnormally elevated creatinine level.

The clinical picture of intestinal obstruction is quite different from that of ileus. However, differentiating the two conditions in critically ill, neurologically impaired, or heavily sedated patients may be difficult in the absence of a reliable clinical examination. Frequently, surgeons are asked to help determine whether "abdominal pathology" is preventing a critically ill patient from making progress. In addition, it may not be feasible to perform diagnostic tests, such as CT scans, because of the risks of transportation. Thus, if a surgeon is confronted with a patient who exhibits severe abdominal distention and high NG outputs, other tests such as diagnostic peritoneal lavage, diagnostic laparoscopy, or bedside laparotomy are sometimes used.

TREATMENT

As with ileus, successful treatment depends on the proper and prompt identification of a mechanical intestinal obstruction and the determination of its cause. Surgery is central to the appropriate management of patients with intestinal obstruction, and prompt collaboration with surgeons and critical care physicians is tantamount to adequate care. The need for eventual surgery is determined by the cause of the intestinal obstruction, whether the obstruction is partial or complete, and the presence of intestinal ischemia.

Decompression of the GI tract is achieved with an NG tube. An adequately placed NG tube controls vomiting, provides an estimate of GI fluid losses, and allows easier administration of contrast material for radiographic studies. NG decompression also controls abdominal pain, unless a closed-loop obstruction or intestinal ischemia is present. Antiemetics in the absence of an NG tube do not control vomiting and should not be used. Similarly, narcotics should be used with care or not at all if pain is adequately controlled with an NG tube. Once the episode of intestinal obstruction resolves (with or without surgical intervention), the NG tube should be removed as soon as possible, to minimize complications and side effects caused by the tube.

Fluid replacement, correction of electrolytes, and hemodynamic resuscitation are essential for the treatment of intestinal obstruction. An obstructed bowel exhibits enormous edema, leaching away large volumes. In addition, careful use of antibiotics should be considered in these patients.

CONCLUSION

Ileus and mechanical intestinal obstruction are two disease processes associated with dysfunction of the GI tract. Inadequate correction of either may result in GI failure, which is associated with increased morbidity and mortality. Ileus and mechanical intestinal obstruction present with distinct clinical pictures; however, differentiating these entities may be especially difficult in obtunded and heavily sedated ICU patients. In either case, early diagnosis, surgical consultation, and correction of the causes are essential aspects of caring for these patients.

ANNOTATED REFERENCES

Boeckxstaens GE: Understanding and controlling the enteric nervous system. Best Pract Res Clin Gastroenterol 2002;16:1013-1023.
This article provides a concise overview of normal GI physiology, specifically describing the physiology of the enteric nervous system.

Cheatham ML, Chapman WC, Key SP, Sawyers JL: A meta-analysis of selective versus routine nasogastric decompression after elective laparotomy. Ann Surg 1995;221:469-476.
This meta-analysis reviewed 26 trials (3964 patients) comparing selective versus routine NG decompression in an attempt to evaluate the need for it after elective laparotomy. This paper does not support the routine use of postoperative NG tubes to prevent ileus, given the higher incidence of complications.

Kalff JC, Carlos TM, Schraut WH, et al: Surgically induced leukocytic infiltrates within the rat intestinal muscularis mediate postoperative ileus. Gastroenterology 1999;117:378-387.
This study is one of the first showing that operative manipulation of the gut causes significant inflammation and infiltration by resident gut leukocytes, which has a significant role in the pathogenesis of postoperative ileus.

Ponec RJ, Saunders MD, Kimmey MB: Neostigmine for the treatment of acute colonic pseudo-obstruction. N Engl J Med 1999;341:137-141.
This prospective study evaluated the efficacy of a 2-mg bolus of neostigmine in 21 randomized patients with colonic pseudo-obstruction. Neostigmine had an immediate effect and can be considered in certain patients who fail conservative management.

Sarr MG, Bulkley GB, Zuidema GD: Preoperative recognition of intestinal strangulation obstruction: Prospective evaluation of diagnostic capability. Am J Surg 1983;145:176-182.
This prospective study evaluated preoperative diagnostic parameters and the preoperative judgment of senior attending surgeons for 51 patients who were about to undergo laparotomy for complete mechanical small bowel obstruction. No preoperative clinical parameter proved to be sensitive, specific, and predictive for strangulation.

Chapter 125

ACUTE MEGACOLON IN CRITICALLY ILL PATIENTS

H. M. Oudemans-van Straaten

KEY POINTS

1. Acute megacolon is a nonobstructive motility disorder of the colon associated with a large range of metabolic and pharmacologic conditions, such as sympathetic or dopaminergic stimulation, ischemia, inducible nitric oxide synthase activation, and use of opioids.

2. Clinical awareness and a strategy of care for the colon are needed to prevent the potentially lethal complications of acute megacolon.

3. In addition to the correction of conditions impairing colonic motility and withdrawal or replacing medications inhibiting gut motility, a continuous infusion of neostigmine is a safe and generally effective treatment for nonobstructive megacolon in critically ill patients.

4. Toxic megacolon is a complication of severe colitis in critically ill patients mostly due to infection with *Clostridium difficile*.

Acute megacolon refers to a syndrome presenting as marked colonic distention in the absence of mechanical obstruction that results from disturbed colonic motility. It may be a manifestation of Ogilvie's syndrome or of toxic megacolon. *Ogilvie's syndrome (acute colonic pseudo-obstruction)* is a disease of seriously ill hospitalized patients that is associated with a large range of metabolic, pharmacologic, and postoperative conditions that suppress colonic motility. In *toxic megacolon*, the distention is caused by severe colitis and is associated with systemic toxicity. Toxic megacolon classically is described as a complication of inflammatory bowel disease, usually ulcerative colitis, but in critically ill patients, toxic megacolon mostly occurs as a complication of severe infectious colitis, such as colitis caused by *Clostridium difficile*. In both manifestations of acute megacolon, progressive distention may lead to sepsis, ischemia, perforation, and multiple organ dysfunction, potentially life-threatening complications that must be prevented. This chapter focuses on acute megacolon in patients admitted to the ICU. A strategy to prevent megacolon is proposed.

CLINICAL FEATURES

OGILVIE'S SYNDROME (ACUTE COLONIC PSEUDO-OBSTRUCTION)

The hallmark of Ogilvie's syndrome is abdominal distention with or without tenderness in a patient with serious comorbid disease.[1-5] Patients may present with constipation, but flatus or stools may pass as well. Bowel sounds are normal, diminished, or high, and percussion is hypertympanic. Tenderness is most pronounced over the cecum. Nausea and vomiting may occur, but gastric retention is often minimal, and enteral feeding may be tolerated. If diagnosis and treatment are delayed, progressive distention may cause peritoneal signs, respiratory compromise, nutritional depletion, sepsis, multiple organ failure, ischemia, and perforation. Perforation most commonly occurs in the cecum. The risk of perforation is unlikely when cecal diameter is less than 12 cm, but increases sharply when the diameter of the cecum is greater than 12 cm.[2] Critical illness–related colonic ileus is characterized by the nonpassage of stools for many days without marked colonic distention. This syndrome has been described in ICU patients with multiple organ failure and may be an early presentation of acute megacolon.[6]

TOXIC MEGACOLON

Toxic megacolon is a serious complication of inflammatory bowel disease or infectious colitis. Patients present with fever, abdominal tenderness, and abdominal distention or with acute abdomen. Inflammatory bowel disease or infectious colitis commonly presents with diarrhea, but a decrease in stool frequency may herald the onset of megacolon and cause a delay in diagnosis.[7,8] Altered consciousness, dehydration, hypotension, tachycardia, leukocytosis, thrombocytopenia, hypoalbuminemia, and electrolyte disturbances are common. In severe cases, systemic toxicity may lead to septic shock and multiple organ failure.[9-11] Ascending pyelophlebitis and septic emboli in the superior mesenteric vein and liver are rare complications. Patients with ulcerative colitis are at the highest risk of developing toxic megacolon early in the course of disease, and some are affected at initial presentation.[12] Factors that may trigger toxic megacolon are early discontinuation or decrease in medications, use of antidiarrheals such as loperamide or opioids, severe hypokalemia, barium enema, and colonoscopy.

PATHOGENESIS AND PREDISPOSING FACTORS

OGILVIE'S SYNDROME

The pathophysiology of Ogilvie's syndrome is not fully understood. The syndrome may result from an imbalance between the *sympathetic* and *parasympathetic* regulation of motility, but neurotransmitters, inflammatory mediators, metabolic derangement, and pharmacologic interventions also play a role.[13] Intestinal motility is mainly under control of the local enteric nervous system, an independently functional network[14] connected to the central nervous system by parasympathetic nerves promoting motility and sympathetic nerves suppressing motility. The sympathetic innervation of the colon occurs via the celiac and mesenteric ganglia and the spinal cord. The parasympathetic nerves to the right and transverse colon originate from the *vagus* nerve, and the parasympathetic nerves to the distal colon result from the spinal cord (S2-4). Several types of motor activity are involved in intestinal propulsion; the migrating motor complexes during fasting and local-reflex peristalsis after feeding are the most important. Migrating motor complexes are initiated by the hormone motilin. The motilin receptor is expressed on enteric neurons of the human duodenum and colon.[15] A host of other mediators and conditions, such as opioids, dopamine, and nitric oxide, affect their activity. Local-reflex peristalsis is activated by intraluminal distention, stimulating the release of 5-hydroxytryptamine, which triggers activity of afferent neurons. Above the site of the stimulus, excitatory motor neurons are activated to release acetylcholine and substance P, resulting in contraction. Below the stimulus site, inhibitory neurons capable of releasing nitric oxide and vasoactive intestinal peptide are activated and cause relaxation.[16] This nonadrenergic, noncholinergic, intrinsic inhibitory innervation is more pronounced in organs with a reservoir function, explaining why the stomach and proximal colon are more susceptible to distention than is the small intestine.[17]

Clinical factors predisposing to Ogilvie's syndrome are summarized in Table 125-1.[1-5] The syndrome first was described by Ogilvie in two patients with malignant infiltration of the celiac plexus.[18] After surgery and trauma of spine, hip, and pelvis, dysfunction of the sacral parasympathetic nerves (S2-4) may impair motility of the distal colon, causing atony with functional obstruction.[19] In one series, 67% of the patients with Ogilvie's syndrome had cardiovascular disease.[4] Drugs and ischemia may play a role in the pathogenesis of Ogilvie's syndrome. In critically ill patients, increased sympathetic tone suppresses motility. Exogenous *catecholamines* have dose-dependent effects on intestinal motility; low doses promote motility, and high doses suppress motility.[20] Alpha-adrenergic agonists are stronger inhibitors of acetylcholine release than are beta-adrenergic agents.[21] The potential of dobutamine and dopexamine to block intestinal peristalsis is low. Dopamine inhibits not only upper gastrointestinal motility, but also distal colonic motility.[22,23] *Ischemia*, as a result of shock or its treatment

with vasopressors, initially suppresses motility but may progress to ischemic necrosis. An association between the development of late colonic ischemic complications and the use of dopamine has been reported.[6] Clonidine, a central alpha$_2$-adrenergic receptor agonist, decreases fasting colonic smooth muscle tone[24] and is associated with Ogilvie's syndrome.[25] *Opioids* suppress the phase III migrating motor contractions.[26] This inhibiting effect on gut motility is mediated by activation of mu opioid receptors in the gastrointestinal tract, whereas receptors in the central nervous system mediate the analgesic actions of opioids.[27] In patients with *sepsis*, proinflammatory cytokines and nitric oxide, generated by inducible nitric oxide synthase, suppress intestinal motility.[28-31]

TOXIC MEGACOLON

The incidence of toxic megacolon in inflammatory bowel disease has decreased substantially with better management of severe colitis. The most common cause of toxic megacolon in critically ill paitents is pseudomembraneous colitis with the overgrowth of *C. difficile*.[32] Sporadic cases of megacolon due to infections with *Salmonella*,[33] *Shigella, Amoeba*, herpes, or cytomegalovirus also have been described.[7] In patients with human immunodeficiency virus (HIV), toxic megacolon may be a primary manifestation of the HIV infection or be related to infection with *C. difficile* or cytomegalovirus.[34] The incidence of cytomegalovirus-related gastrointestinal disease in acquired immunodeficiency syndrome has decreased since highly active antiretroviral therapy has become available. Causes of toxic megacolon are summarized in Table 125-2.

The pathogenesis of toxic megacolon is not well understood.[7,8] Inflammation extends into the deeper layers of the colonic wall (i.e., the longitudinal muscle layer and the serosa) in toxic megacolon, whereas the inflammation is typically limited to the mucosa in ulcerative colitis. Deep infiltration, microabscesses, edema, and necrosis may paralyze colonic smooth muscle and lead to dilation. Bacterial toxins permeating through ulcerations activate the release of cytokines with subsequent systemic toxicity. There is increasing evidence that nitric oxide, locally generated in excessive amounts by an increased activity of inducible nitric oxide synthase in inflammatory and smooth muscle cells, is the key mediator of diminished smooth muscle function in toxic megacolon.[35] The amount and activity of inducible nitric oxide synthase are significantly increased in the muscular layers of resected colons of patients with toxic megacolon, but not of tumor and colitis controls.[36]

TABLE 125–1. CLINICAL FACTORS PREDISPOSING TO OGILVIE'S SYNDROME (ACUTE COLONIC PSEUDO-OBSTRUCTION)

Immobility and dehydration
Postoperative state, trauma, cesarean section and normal delivery
Drugs
    Alpha-adrenergic agonists, dopamine, clonidine, opioids, anticholinergics, calcium channel antagonists, theophylline
Gut ischemia
Sepsis and endotoxemia: nitric oxide
Metabolic factors
    Hypokalemia and hyperglycemia, hypothyroidism, diabetes mellitus, amyloidosis of chronic renal insufficiency
Miscellaneous
    Herpes zoster, β$_2$-microglobulin amyloidosis

TABLE 125–2. DISORDERS ASSOCIATED WITH TOXIC MEGACOLON

Inflammatory bowel disease
    Ulcerative colitis
    Crohn's disease
Infectious colitis
    Salmonella, Shigella, amebic colitis
    Clostridium difficile
    Cytomegalovirus colitis
Human immunodeficiency virus infection
Cancer chemotherapy
Ischemia

TABLE 125–3. FACTORS ASSOCIATED WITH COLONIZATION AND SUBSEQUENT INFECTION WITH *CLOSTRIDIUM DIFFICILE*

Disruption of indigenous microflora
    Antibiotics suppressing indigenous microflora
    Cancer chemotherapeutics with antimicrobial activity[41]
    Preoperative bowel preparation
Opportunity of infection
    Prolonged hospital stay
Microbial factors
    Toxigenicity and adhesion
Diminished gastrointestinal defense
    Reduced or suppressed gastric acid secretion
    Parenteral nutrition
    Postpyloric enteral nutrition
    Gastrointestinal surgery
Antibody response of the host
Poor underlying condition
    Advanced age
    Cancer
    Renal insufficiency
    Long-term use of corticosteroids
    Bedridden state

CLOSTRIDIUM DIFFICILE INFECTION

The most frequently identified clinical risk factor for *C. difficile*–associated diarrhea is the antecedent use of antibiotics that alter the indigenous colonic microflora.[37-39] The opportunity to acquire the organism increases with prolonged hospital stay. *C. difficile* may be detected in 10% to 25% of hospitalized patients, and the organism may spread by nosocomial transmission.[39-43] Whether a person remains an asymptomatic carrier or develops colitis depends on the size of the *Clostridium* population, the toxigenicity of the strain, the toxin-neutralizing effects of the indigenous gut flora, and other host factors (Table 125-3).[32,44,45] Susceptibility also is increased by poor gastrointestinal defense mechanisms as a result of a reduction in gastric acid secretion, total parenteral nutrition, enteral feeding (especially postpyloric), or recent gastrointestinal surgery.[40,46,47] A combination of factors increases the risk.

C. difficile is a gram-positive, spore-forming rod. Pathogenic strains produce two major exotoxins: A and B. Both toxins activate cell-signaling molecules, including the transcription factor nuclear factor-κB and mitogen-activated protein kinases in monocytes, leading to the production and release of proinflammatory cytokines. Both toxins induce colitis in humans. The colonic injury results from alterations of the enterocyte cytoskeleton with disruption of tight junction function with marked inflammation in the lamina propria. Severe pseudomembranous colitis occurs in 3% to 5% of carriers.[38] Severe recurrent sepsis[48] and toxic megacolon[49] are rare complications.

C. difficile cannot be detected in most adults. Colonization results from an alteration in the composition of the indigenous colonic microflora. After exposure, growth is under control of the indigenous flora suppressing its growth. Enemas containing normal human feces seem to be effective in the treatment of infected patients.[50] Mechanisms include the production of volatile acids, hydrogen sulfide, and secondary bile acids.[44]

DIAGNOSIS AND DIFFERENTIAL DIAGNOSIS OF ACUTE MEGACOLON

Besides history and clinical features, plain abdominal radiography is crucial for diagnosis and follow-up. Dilation is

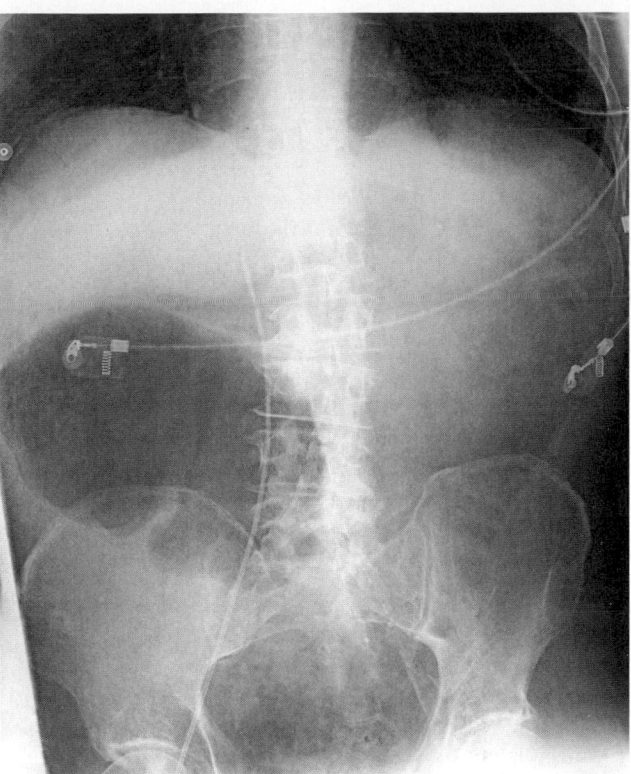

FIGURE 125–1. Plain abdominal radiograph of a patient with respiratory insufficiency resulting from severe emphysema and Ogilvie's syndrome 10 days after dynamic hip screw implantation for femoral fracture. Dilation is most pronounced in the cecum and ascending colon. Gas and fecal pattern in the distal colon are normal. The patient was treated successfully with intravenous neostigmine.

most pronounced in the cecum, ascending colon, and right transverse colon. The size of the cecum may range from 6 to 20 cm. In Ogilvie's syndrome, colonic diameter typically decreases gradually distally to a collapsed bowel and a normal gas and fecal pattern in the rectum (Fig. 125-1). Additional dilation of the left colon may occur, however, as well (Fig. 125-2). Mechanical obstruction is excluded if gas is visible in all colonic segments including the rectosigmoid. If not, an enema should be administered. The osmotic effect of a water-soluble medium is diagnostic and often therapeutic in decompressing the colon.[51] Barium enema is not advised because of the risk of peritoneal contamination in case of perforation. Air-fluid levels and dilation of the small bowel may be present. In Ogilvie's syndrome, the colonic haustral and mucosal pattern is maintained, whereas the pattern is disturbed or lost in toxic megacolon. Deep ulcerations may be visible between large pseudopolypoid projections into the lumen. Pneumatosis of the bowel wall is a sign of ischemic necrosis and free peritoneal air of perforation. Diagnosis of severe colitis can be made with computed tomography, but findings are nonspecific for the underlying cause.[52] Computed tomography shows a diffusely thickened or edematous colonic wall with pericolonic inflammation. Computed tomography may be helpful in patients presenting without diarrhea, with symptoms of acute abdomen, for differential diagnosis, or to show or exclude complications.

The underlying cause of toxic megacolon, inflammatory bowel disease or infectious colitis, must be identified (see Tables 125-1, 125-2, and 125-3). The history may reveal chronic abdominal complaints, diarrhea, bloody stools,

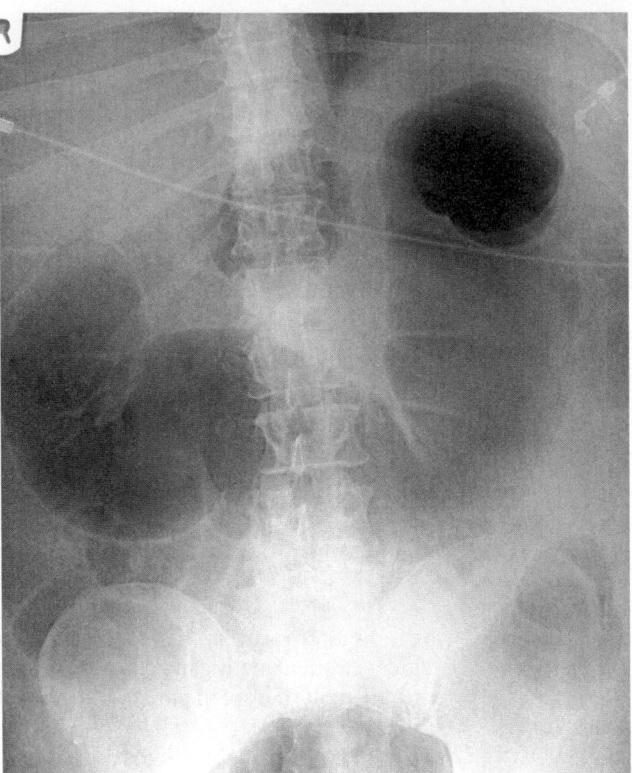

FIGURE 125–2. Plain abdominal radiograph of a patient with Ogilvie's syndrome 11 days after surgery for a ruptured aneurysm of the abdominal aorta. Dilation is present in the right and the left colon, probably owing to ischemia. The syndrome resolved with vasodilators and intravenous neostigmine.

familial occurrence of inflammatory bowel disease, recent travel, intake of contaminated food, hospitalization, use of antibiotics, risk factors for HIV infection, or immunosuppression. Infection with cytomegalovirus or *C. difficile* may precipitate toxic megacolon in ulcerative colitis. If unresponsive to therapy, Ogilvie's syndrome and ischemic colitis may be complicated by progressive distention with bacterial overgrowth and systemic toxicity mimicking toxic megacolon.

For microbiologic diagnosis of infectious colitis, a fresh fecal sample should be submitted immediately to the laboratory for culture on specific media.[38] For the diagnosis of a *C. difficile* infection, stool must be tested for the presence of toxicogenic *C. difficile*. The toxin can be detected using an enzyme-linked immunosorbent assay, which is inexpensive, quick, and highly specific; the sensitivity is low, however.[39] The gold standard diagnostic test to identify *C. difficile* toxin B in the stool is the tissue culture cytotoxicity assay. It is more sensitive than the enzyme-linked immunosorbent assay, but is costly and time-consuming; results take 24 to 48 hours. Although the test is positive in asymptomatic carriers, a positive test in a patient with antibiotic-associated megacolon makes infection with *C. difficile* highly probable. The stool culture for *C. difficile* is sensitive, but not specific for toxin-producing strains. In adults, cultures are useful in support of other diagnostic methods. Blood cultures are warranted in all cases of toxic megacolon. They are generally positive in severe cases of typhoid fever. If stool and blood cultures remain negative when antibiotics already have been initiated, a bone marrow culture still may yield *Salmonella* after 5 days.

Limited endoscopy with biopsy may provide useful information. Inflammatory bowel disease is characterized by diffusely abnormal crypt structure, whereas the architecture of the crypts is intact in bacillary colitis. In cytomegalovirus colitis, inclusion bodies are present. Mild cases of *C. difficile* are associated with nonspecific colitis. In severe cases, focal ulcerations covered by purulent material presenting as yellow or white plaques 2 to 4 cm in diameter are found with normal intervening mucosa. Pseudomembranous colitis may not be detected if only flexible sigmoidoscopy is performed.[53] A full colonoscopy in acute megacolon carries the risk of perforation, however. Some authors suggest that endoscopy is safe and valuable in timing surgical intervention.[38]

MANAGEMENT

OGILVIE'S SYNDROME

The classic treatment of Ogilvie's syndrome includes fasting, nasogastric suction, intravenous fluids, electrolyte replacement, and frequent positional changes. In some patients, colonic dilation improves over some days. A more proactive strategy in an earlier phase is now advocated, however. Awaiting resolution, the distended colon is at risk for complications that need prevention. First, if there is any doubt about diagnosis, the administration of a water-soluble contrast enema is advocated. Enemas are contraindicated if the patient displays peritoneal irritation. Concomitantly, conditions that can impair colon motility must be corrected. Specifically, it is important to withdraw all medications that can inhibit gut motility (see Table 125-1). Alternatives to these medications are generally available. Opioids might be replaced by epidural anesthesia, an intervention that can promote resolution of colonic ileus by inducing sympathetic blockade.[54,55] Efforts should be made to reduce infusion rates for vasoconstrictors. Lactulose may increase fecal gas formation. The knee-elbow position may relieve bowel distention.[56]

If these measures are not effective, neostigmine is the drug of choice. In a double-blind crossover trial in a non-ICU population, the use of a bolus of 2 mg of neostigmine intravenously led to rapid colonic decompression in most patients.[57] Because severe bradycardia is unwanted in critically ill patients, a continuous infusion with neostigmine is a safer option. In a double-blind, placebo-controlled, crossover study in critically ill, ventilated patients with ileus of the colon, continuous intravenous administration of neostigmine, 0.4 to 0.8 mg/h, resulted in defecation in 80% of the patients, whereas no defecation occurred during placebo infusion.[6] Treatment with neostigmine was tolerated well. By slowly increasing the dose, adverse events, such as bradycardia, present gradually, and the dose of neostigmine can be reduced or infusion of the drug stopped. Repeat radiographs are obtained for follow-up assessment of colonic diameter.

There are several case reports showing effective colonic decompression with cisapride in patients with Ogilvie's syndome.[58] Cisapride induces colonic contraction and shortens colonic transit time by enhancing acetylcholine release in the mesenteric plexus. Its use is limited by its ability to induce severe ventricular dysrhythmias as a result of prolongation of the Q-T interval, especially in combination with drugs metabolized by the cytochrome P (CYP3A4) system or other drugs prolonging the Q-T interval.[59] In the United States, the drug is not available anymore, but it still is available in Europe. Erythromycin, a motilin agonist, also may improve colonic motility.[60] The dose should be low (200 mg twice daily intravenously) because higher doses can inhibit motility.[61] Selective peripheral kappa opioid receptor agonists are a potential therapeutic intervention to improve motility.[27]

Colonoscopic decompression may be indicated if decompression with enema and neostigmine fails.[62] Colonoscopic decompression is seldom necessary. Colonoscopy in this setting is time-consuming, difficult to perform, and hazardous. The unprepared bowel contains copious amounts of stool. Inflation of air may increase colonic distention, impair ventilation, and lead to perforation. It is advocated to provide a watery enema before the procedure and avoid the liberal use of air.[63] Advancing the scope as far as the hepatic flexure may be sufficient to obtain adequate decompression.[64] Gas should be aspirated. Colonoscopy is successful in 70% to 80% of patients,[62,64] but the recurrence rate is 15% to 40 %.[3,62,64,65] Recurrence may be reduced if a decompressive tube is left in place,[66] but controlled trials with this intervention are not available. Mortality rates associated with colonoscopy are 1% to 5% in experienced hands.[64,67] If signs of ischemia are encountered, such as scattered areas of friable hemorrhagic or necrotic mucosa, the procedure should be discontinued and laparotomy performed.

Indications for surgery are failure of conservative treatment, clinical signs of impending or actual ischemia, and perforation. For surgical management, the reader is referred to the review by Dorudi and colleagues.[2] The type of surgery depends on the state of the colon. Tube cecostomy is the procedure of choice[2] and carries a lower mortality than resection.[1] A large Foley catheter is left in place for 2 to 3 weeks. The results of decompressive transverse colostomies and of diverting ileostomy are unsatisfactory and carry a higher mortality rate.[1] Median laparotomy should be performed if clinical signs suggest cecal ischemia or perforation. Percutaneous cecostomy might be an alternative in certain high-risk patients.[68]

TOXIC MEGACOLON

The main initial goal of treatment of toxic megacolon is to reduce the severity of colitis and restore motility.[7] Medical treatment is successful in about 50% of cases, but from the beginning the patient should be assessed daily by the intensivist and the surgeon. Apart from general support with intravenous fluids, electrolyte and vitamin replacement, early optimization of circulation, and, if necessary, mechanical ventilation, patients with toxic megacolon are treated with intravenous antibiotics, corticosteroids, and selective digestive decontamination. Conditions that can impair colon motility must be corrected (see Table 125-1). Antiperistaltic agents for diarrhea are absolutely contraindicated. These drugs worsen dysmotility and lead to retention of bacteria and toxins. Systemic antibiotics are necessary to reduce septic complications and peritonitis. In addition to intravenous metronidazole, systemic antibiotics should have a gram-negative spectrum guided by local susceptibility testing and adjusted to culture results. It is important to select antibiotics that give the least disturbance of the indigenous anaerobic flora, and in case of C. difficile, the culprit antibiotics have to be stopped. Selective digestive decontamination, using the correct antibiotics (polymyxin, tobramycin, and amphotericin B),[69] attacks overgrowth of aerobic gram-negative bacteria and yeasts, reduces the fecal endotoxin pool, and leaves the protective flora intact. Systemic toxicity and associated infections are limited.[70-72] In animal studies, decontamination of the bowel with oral, nonabsorbable, broad-spectrum antibiotics

reduced inducible nitric oxide synthase expression and prevented dilation.[35] Although there is no literature about the use of neostigmine in toxic megacolon, a trial with neostigmine may be useful to promote motility and defecation. By promoting defecation, neostigmine helps to clear bacterial overgrowth and associated systemic toxicity. Sulfasalazine and 5-aminosalicylic acid compounds should be given only after the acute attack starts to resolve.[7]

For antibiotic treatment of toxic megacolon due to C. difficile colitis, intravenous metronidazole, 500 mg every 8 hours, is recommended in addition to vancomycin, 500 mg every 6 hours, administered via the nasogastric tube.[38,39,73] Vancomycin retention enemas might be administered as well (500 mg of vancomycin in 100 mL of normal saline). Oral vancomycin is not absorbed, and high fecal concentrations are achieved. Intravenous vancomycin is not effective. Intravenous metronidazole may be secreted through an inflamed mucosa. In patients with active disease receiving oral or intravenous metronidazole, bactericidal fecal concentrations were achieved, concentrations decreased as the diarrhea improved, and neither oral nor intravenous metronidazole was detectable in the feces after recovery.[74] Cytomegalovirus colitis requires specific treatment with ganciclovir, 5 mg/kg intravenously, with adjustment of dose in patients with renal dysfunction.

Intravenous corticosteroids are recommended for patients with toxic megacolon. Hydrocortisone (100 mg every 6 hours) or an equivalent dose of another corticosteroid can be employed. Although there is consensus for the use of corticosteroids in inflammatory bowel disease, there are no randomized trials showing beneficial effects in patients with toxic megacolon due to infectious colitis. Corticosteroids have been shown, however, to improve mortality in patients with typhoid fever[75] and in patients with septic shock.[76] Corticosteroids are potent inhibitors of inflammation and specifically inhibit inducible nitric oxide synthase expression. By this mechanism, these drugs may prevent further colonic dilation.[35]

Probiotics are an attractive additional approach to the management of C. difficile colitis, especially in recurrent and severe cases, because the aim of this approach is to restore the colonization resistance provided by the colonic microflora.[39,77] Examples are (a mixture of) Lactobacillus, Bifidobacterium lactis, and Enterococcus faecium (10^{10} colony-forming units every 6 hours) or the yeast Saccharomyces boulardii (500 mg every 12 hours). Probiotics also may be beneficial in ulcerative colitis.[78] Probiotics seem to stimulate specific and nonspecific immune responses.[79] The preferred route of feeding is enteral.[80] Tolerance is monitored by gastric retention and abdominal signs. Total parenteral nutrition offers no proven benefit.[7] If probiotics are supplied, it seems logical to combine this treatment with fiber-enriched enteral feeding, but controlled trials are available only in other intensive care settings.[81,82]

Patients with toxic megacolon due to inflammatory bowel disease need surgery without delay if response to medical treatment is not rapidly apparent. Surgical intervention should be considered when the patient has progressive signs of organ failure despite medical treatment, a worsening computed tomography scan, or signs of peritonitis. Subtotal colectomy with end-ileostomy is the treatment of choice for urgent surgery.[7] Among patients with severe C. difficile infection, subtotal colectomy is the procedure of choice, even if the appearance of the colon at laparotomy is relatively normal. The outcome was worse when a more conservative surgical approach was applied.[32]

OUTCOME

With appropriate management, pseudo-obstruction usually resolves within a couple of days. Despite adequate treatment, mortality rate may be high, however, depending on comorbid diseases, cecal diameter, delay in decompression, the kind of the intervention, or the presence of an ischemic or perforated cecum.[1,2,7] After elective total joint arthroplasty, acute colonic pseudo-obstruction was not associated with mortality, but with prolonged hospitalization.[19] In patients with pseudo-obstruction needing surgery, mortality was 30% compared with 14% after early conservative treatment.[1] The patients treated with tube cecostomy alone had a similar mortality as patients treated conservatively. In one series, all patients who died had coronary artery disease.[4] In the presence of perforation, mortality rate may increase to 50%.[2] Even with early intervention before massive distention of the colon, hospital mortality in patients with multiple organ failure is high, mostly as a result of late death secondary to underlying diseases after resolution of ileus. These figures show that in the ICU, acute colonic pseudo-obstruction is a disease of patients with severe comorbidities. It is an organ failure, one that is not scored in the presently available organ failure scores.

In severe ulcerative colitis, the fatality of toxic megacolon is high, especially if surgery is delayed. The development of multiple organ failure predicts a fatal outcome.[11] Mortality of toxic megacolon secondary to *C. difficile* infection may be 80%.[40] In a cohort of 59 ICU patients with *C. difficile* colitis, one fifth of the patients required surgery for progressive toxicity or peritonitis. In the surgical patients, Acute Physiologic and Chronic Health Evaluation scores at diagnosis were higher, and mortality rate was 42% compared with 15% in medical patients.[32]

STRATEGY TO PREVENT ACUTE MEGACOLON IN CRITICALLY ILL PATIENTS

In contrast to the wide attention in the recent literature to gastric emptying, little notice is taken of defecation. Among critically ill patients, it is not unusual for the first stools to be passed after more than 1 week. Defecation removes bacteria from the gut and reduces overgrowth of pathogenic bacteria and yeasts. With respect to the potentially lethal complications of Ogilvie's syndrome and toxic megacolon, clinical awareness and a strategy of care for the colon are needed. This strategy includes providing early resuscitation of shock, avoiding prolonged infusion of high doses of alpha-adrenergic drugs, minimizing the use of dopamine and opioids, adjusting the standard antibiotic strategy of the unit, instituting early enteral feeding, and providing measures to promote defecation and early mobilization and ambulation. The use of antibiotics that affect the growth of indigenous protective colonic microflora should be avoided whenever possible. Selective digestive decontamination is advocated in patients with an expected stay of more than a few days. Proper selective digestive decontamination prevents overgrowth of aerobic gram-negative bacteria and yeasts and reduces fecal endotoxin pool, dilation and associated systemic toxicity, gram-negative infections, and possibly mortality.[35,69-72] With these measures, *C. difficile* colitis is virtually absent in the ICU. If and when prevention has failed and the resident flora is reduced due to the prolonged use of antibiotics and malnutrition, possible protective measures include the restoration of protective gut flora by the administration of probiotics in combination with fiber-enriched enteral feeding. Protective gut flora, such as *Lactobacillus*, breaks down fiber to short-chain fatty acids. These fatty acids are an essential fuel for the colon mucosa and stimulate immunocompetence.[79,82-84] If defecation does not occur spontaneously, an enema and oral polyethylene glycol 3350, preferentially supplemented with electrolytes (about 13 g every 6 to 8 hours), are advocated from day 3, and if stools do not pass and physical examination of the abdomen is without suspicion, neostigmine is started. By implementation of a protocol promoting defecation, deterioration of the patient's condition by dilation of the colon can be prevented.

ANNOTATED REFERENCES

Saunders MD, Kimmey MB: Colonic pseudo-obstruction: The dilated colon in the ICU. Semin Gastrointest Dis 2003;14:20-27.
   Prognosis in acute colonic pseudo-obstruction is determined by the severity of the underlying disease, the maximal cecal diameter, the delay in colonic decompression, and the status of the bowel.

Sheth SG, LaMont JT: Toxic megacolon. Lancet 1998;351:509-513.
   Nitric oxide may be involved in the pathogenesis of toxic megacolon.

Van der Spoel JI, Oudemans-van Straaten HM, Stoutenbeek CP, et al: Neostigmine resolves critical illness-related colonic ileus in intensive care patients with multiple organ failure—a prospective, double-blind, placebo-controlled trial. Intensive Care Med 2001;27:822-827.
   A continuous infusion of neostigmine is a safe and effective treatment for decompression of nonobstructive megacolon in critically ill patients.

Section VII

RENAL AND ELECTROLYTE DISORDERS

Chapter 126

CLINICAL ASSESSMENT OF RENAL FUNCTION

Todd W. B. Gehr • Anton C. Schoolwerth

KEY POINTS

1. **Acute deterioration of renal function is common in the ICU** and contributes significantly to overall morbidity and mortality.

2. The **serum creatinine concentration often underestimates the decrease in GFR** and may be abnormal only after marked reductions in GFR.

3. **Utilizing equations to estimate renal function should be routine in the ICU.**

Five to 15 percent of patients in ICUs experience acute deterioration in renal function.[1,2] Conversely, renal dysfunction adds substantially to the morbidity and mortality of these patients. Moreover, changes in renal function directly affect drug disposition. Thus, a means to assess renal function is essential for optimal management. The glomerular filtration rate (GFR) is the standard measure of renal function. It reflects overall renal functional capacity and, in renal failure, correlates with structural damage to the kidney. This chapter reviews selected aspects of renal physiology with an emphasis on measurement of renal function, consequences of altered function, and approaches to improving renal function. The focus is on measurement and optimization of GFR and renal blood flow (RBF).

RENAL BLOOD FLOW

Under physiologic conditions, blood flow to the kidneys is 20% of cardiac output. This high rate of blood flow (1 to 1.2 L/min) is particularly remarkable in that the kidneys make up only 0.5% of total body weight. The high blood flow rate is due, at least in part, to the unique anatomic arrangement of the renal vasculature, with the interlobar and arcuate vessels offering little resistance to flow. This, in turn, is because the interlobular arteries originate from the arcuates in a parallel arrangement and because the afferent arterioles also arise in a parallel arrangement from the interlobular vessels. It is this parallel arrangement that accounts for the low resistance because the total resistance of n equals parallel paths, each with a resistance R, is R/n^3. Major resistance vessels in the kidney are the afferent and efferent arterioles that bound the glomerular capillary network. Although total resistance is a function of resistance across each of these vessels, it is a unique feature of the kidney that variations in the individual resistances across the afferent and efferent arterioles, respectively, may lead to alterations in glomerular capillary pressure and, hence, in GFR.[3]

Despite a wide range of perfusion pressures, RBF and GFR are maintained relatively constant, a process described as autoregulation. The term *autoregulation* generally refers to the relative constancy of GFR over a range of perfusion pressures but also refers to the regulation of RBF. Emphasis has been placed on the preglomerular vasculature, mainly the afferent arterioles, as the major site at which renal perfusion is regulated. However, studies also suggest that the larger vessels, such as the interlobular vessels, may respond to a variety of vasoactive stimuli and participate in an autoregulatory phenomenon. A variety of hypotheses have been generated to explain the autoregulatory response of the kidney with respect to RBF. There is evidence to suggest mediation by neural, humoral, or intrarenal factors that regulate the renal circulation.[4]

The renin-angiotensin pathway has a significant effect on renal hemodynamics. Renin, elaborated in the juxtaglomerular cells, may be released in response to a decrease in renal perfusion pressure and to altered sodium chloride delivery to the ascending limb and macula densa cells. Increased renin secretion in turn leads to augmented angiotensin II (AII) formation at the local nephron level. AII, in turn, affects renal vascular resistance by an effect on both the afferent and efferent arterioles, with the effect predominating on the latter vessels.

Renal eicosanoids also affect renal hemodynamics. Eicosanoids are biologically active fatty acid products of arachidonic acid and are synthesized in the kidney in response to a variety of stimuli, with local release and effect on the renal vasculature. Stimulation of the cyclooxygenase pathway and prostaglandin synthetases leads to the formation of endoperoxides (PGG_2, PGH_2), prostaglandins (PGD_2, PGE_2, PGF_{2a}, PGI_2), and thromboxane A_2,(TXA_2). Leukotrienes are synthesized by another major pathway involving the enzyme lipoxygenase. In the kidney, the major products of arachidonic acid metabolism are PGE_2 and PGI_2 and, to a lesser extent, PGI_{2a}. These compounds have a predominant effect of relaxing renal vascular smooth muscle and lead to vasodilatation, whereas TXA2 is a vasoconstrictor prostanoid. It is believed that in disease states endogenous vasodilator prostaglandins serve a protective function to maintain renal perfusion and GFR in response to vasoconstrictor stimuli, including AII and enhanced sympathetic nervous system activity. In contrast, release is inhibited by nonsteroidal anti-inflammatory drugs.

Other vasoactive compounds that affect the renal circulation include the plasma and glandular kallikreins and kinins and endothelium-derived vasoactive factors, such as nitric oxide and endothelin.[4] Among the catecholamines, alpha- and beta-adrenergic agonists are known to affect renal vascular tone by causing vasoconstriction and vasodilatation, respectively.

In addition, dopamine in low doses leads to renal vasodilatation. Emphasis has more recently been placed on atrial natriuretic peptide and purinergic agents, such as adenosine. The effect is likely to be influenced by changes in salt intake and extracellular fluid volume as well as by hydration status. For example, the influence of AII on renal hemodynamics is greater in sodium depletion, which also activates the sympathetic nervous system. In response to mild nonhypotensive hemorrhage, renal hemodynamics are relatively well maintained. However, with further reductions in volume associated with a more severe hemorrhage, renal ischemia, mediated by activation of the renin-angiotensin system, renal efferent adrenergic nerves, and circulating catecholamines, may occur.[4]

Finally, modification of dietary protein and amino acid intake may affect renal hemodynamics. Dietary protein intake in excess of 1 g/kg/day has been associated with renal vasodilatation, as have infusions of casein hydrolysates and amino acids.[5,6] Conversely, chronic consumption of a low-protein diet may be associated with renal vasoconstriction.

MEASUREMENT OF RENAL BLOOD FLOW

Renal blood flow is measured conventionally by the clearance of infused para-aminohippurate (PAH), which is cleared almost totally from the arterial plasma by both filtration and secretion. Thus, its clearance approximates the rate of renal plasma flow (RPF):

$$RPF = U_{PAH} \cdot V/P_{PAH}$$

where U_{PAH} and P_{PAH} refer to urine and plasma PAH concentration, respectively, and V is urine flow rate in milliliters per minute.

RBF can be estimated by correction for the hematocrit (Hct):

$$RBF = RPF/[1 - Hct]$$

Although available, this test is rarely used in clinical practice. In fact, direct quantitation of RPF and RBF is rarely indicated outside research studies; however, sometimes it is necessary to document that the kidneys are being perfused. In this case, one of three additional methods may be utilized: (1) selective arteriography, (2) Doppler ultrasonography, and (3) external radionuclide scanning.

Because the latter two methods are noninvasive, they are preferred. With respect to the nuclide study, until recently, scanning was usually performed utilizing ^{125}I-iodohippurate sodium; however, the poor radiologic characteristics of ^{131}I limit its use in renal imaging.[7] More recently, other agents, such as [127]I-orthoiodohippurate and ^{99m}Tc-L,L-ethylenedicysteine may prove to be superior.[7,8]

CLINICAL CORRELATES

Although a significant body of data has been obtained to indicate a complex relationship between neurocirculatory factors and renal hemodynamics, several points can be made from a clinical perspective. Optimization of cardiac output and extracellular fluid (ECF) volume, including the intravascular space, is essential for the maintenance of renal perfusion. Particularly because the effects of vasoactive compounds such as AII and catecholamines are accentuated in the presence of renal hypoperfusion and volume contraction, attention should be directed to an assessment of ECF volume, with correction of any deficits, and to optimizing cardiac function. Frequently, pharmacologic agents have been employed to maintain renal perfusion in situations in which this may be compromised. Specifically, there has been widespread use of so-called low-dose or renal dose dopamine infusions. This is based on the observation that in low doses (<3 μg/kg/min) dopamine leads to renal vasodilatation.[9] At higher doses, renal vasoconstriction may occur.

The beneficial effects of dopamine infusion have not been documented in patients who are depleted of sodium chloride and volume, and the use of dopamine has not been shown to be effective beyond a short period of infusion.[9-11] That is, infusions of renal dose dopamine for 24 to 36 hours may be beneficial in the appropriate circumstance, but there is no evidence supporting the long-term use of this agent. Thus, justification for prolongation of its use beyond several days is not supported by available data. Furthermore, reports suggest that adverse outcomes may be associated with the use of dopamine.[11] Beyond anecdotal evidence, there are no compelling data to support the use of other potential vasodilator substances such as prostaglandins. Although high-protein feeding and amino acid infusions may increase RBF by an undefined mechanism, there is no justification for utilizing these therapies solely from a hemodynamic point of view.[5,6]

GLOMERULAR FILTRATION RATE

Of the 500 to 700 mL of plasma delivered per minute to the kidneys (corresponding to a renal blood flow of 1 to 1.2 L/min), 20% to 25% is filtered. Glomerular filtration is a major function of the kidney and averages approximately 130 mL/min/1.73 m² in normal males and 120 mL/min/1.73 m² in females. Estimation or direct assessment of GFR remains one of the most important measurements of renal function and is widely utilized in clinical practice.

MEASUREMENT OF GLOMERULAR FILTRATION RATE

GFR is classically measured as the clearance of inulin (C_{In}), a fructose polymer with a mean molecular weight of approximately 5 kDa. Because this substance is not present endogenously, it must be given by constant infusion after a loading dose. Inulin is available commercially but is expensive, often difficult to obtain, and cumbersome to utilize. As a result, C_{In} is rarely used in clinical practice except for research protocols. Although inulin is generally measured chemically, ^{3}H-labeled and ^{14}C-labeled inulin are also available but are expensive.

More recently, other radiolabeled nuclides have been found to be satisfactory substitutes for inulin and have advantages in the measurement of GFR.[7,8,12,13] Particularly ^{99m}Tc-labeled diethylenetriamine pentaacetic acid (DTPA) and [125]I- or ^{131}I-labeled iothalamate clearances closely approximate the C_{In}.[14,15] ^{99m}Tc-DTPA has been utilized and found to give measurements that correlate closely with C_{In} in ICU patients.[16,17] In addition, the clearance of gentamicin has been utilized in a limited fashion to measure GFR.[18,19] At the present time it is not common for GFR to be measured directly. Rather, GFR is estimated by the endogenous creatinine clearance or serum creatinine determination (see later).

The normal values for GFR given previously apply for individuals from the teenage years through approximately age 35. Thereafter, GFR declines in most individuals. Whereas this decline was formerly thought to occur at a relatively constant rate of approximately 10 mL/min per decade,[20-22] more recent data, obtained in a longitudinal fashion, indicate that this reduction is not so predictable.[23] In addition, a circadian rhythm for GFR has been described.[24,25] GFR is maximal in the daytime, whereas a minimal value during the night has been found in normal individuals. Whether this circadian pattern of GFR occurs in critically ill hospitalized patients is not known.

CREATININE CLEARANCE AND SERUM CREATININE

CREATININE CLEARANCE

The endogenous creatinine clearance (C_{Cr}) enjoys widespread use as a reasonable gauge of GFR when great precision is not demanded, which it rarely is in clinical practice. The use of creatinine as a marker of GFR has the advantage that creatinine is endogenously produced and is easily measured by inexpensive methods. Creatinine, like inulin, is freely filtered and absorbed minimally if at all by the tubules. However, creatinine is secreted and the contribution of secretion to total excretion is greater as the GFR decreases and serum creatinine rises. At GFRs below 40 mL/min, C_{Cr} exceeds C_{In} by 50% to 100%.[14,26] When GFR is significantly depressed and it is deemed important to get a more precise measurement of GFR, one of the previously mentioned methods to estimate GFR directly might be utilized. Additionally, because C_{Cr} overestimates GFR and the clearance of urea underestimates GFR, the mean value of simultaneously obtained creatinine and urea clearances has been shown to provide a close estimation of C_{In} when the latter is below 20 mL/min.[27]

Because cimetidine competes with creatinine for tubular secretion (see later), administration of cimetidine may increase the accuracy both of creatinine clearance in 24-hour collections (when given for several days beforehand) and of 4-hour, water-loaded clearances.[28-30] Taking advantage of this effect results in a more accurate estimate of GFR. Specifically, C_{Cr} obtained in the presence of cimetidine (400 mg as a priming dose followed by 200 mg every 3 hours) yielded values that closely approximated C_{In}.[28,29] Volume expansion in humans causes a small rise in GFR, whereas volume depletion, severe heart failure, hypotension, anesthesia, surgery, trauma, sepsis, and even mild intestinal bleeding without frank hypotension may depress GFR substantially.

Various methods are available to measure creatinine. Creatinine is frequently measured using the Jaffé alkaline picric acid reaction. Although this method is widely utilized, this reaction also measures other chromogens, which may lead to a false elevation in the estimated serum creatinine (S_{Cr}) measurement. Substances such as acetoacetate (in ketoacidosis), pyruvate, ascorbate, 5-flucytosine, certain (but not all) cephalosporin antibiotics, and very high urate artifactually raise S_{Cr} in normal subjects by 0.5 to 2 mg/dL.[31-37] These substances are excreted into the urine but contribute trivially compared with overall urine creatinine (U_{Cr}). Thus, noncreatinine chromogens affect the S_{Cr} but have little effect on the U_{Cr}.

In individuals with normal renal function, the contribution of serum noncreatinine chromogens to raising the S_{Cr} is approximately equal to the contribution of secretion to creatinine excretion such that the C_{Cr} closely approximates GFR. As GFR decreases, the contribution of noncreatinine chromogens to the total measured S_{Cr} becomes less than the

secreted moiety and the C_{Cr} overestimates GFR to a greater extent. Direct enzymatic creatinine measurements are not affected by noncreatinine chromogens. Very high levels of serum glucose (>1000 mg/dL) and 5-flucytosine may interfere with the enzymatic reaction, whereas high levels of bilirubin (>5 mg/dL) affect the autoanalyzer method[35] and lead to falsely low S_{Cr} values. It is therefore important to know the method by which a given laboratory measures S_{Cr}. Competing for the same proximal tubular organic base secretory site as creatinine, certain pharmacologic agents may suppress this process and lead to a rise in S_{Cr}. Trimethoprim, probenecid, and cimetidine, but not ranitidine, are organic bases that inhibit creatinine secretion competitively and can result in a mild elevation in S_{Cr}, usually 0.5 mg/dL or less.[38-41]

As with all clearance methods, the C_{Cr} is subject to errors that may amount to as much as 10% to 15% or more. In addition to potential problems in estimating S_{Cr} and U_{Cr}, errors in timing of urine collection, incomplete collection, and inaccurate measurement of urine volume are other factors that contribute to errors.[42] Although 24-hour U_{Cr} clearances have been widely utilized, no specified time period is required for the clearance to be obtained. In fact, shorter collection periods of several hours may be more accurate in patients passing adequate amounts of urine (not oliguric), particularly if the patient is not in a steady state (see later). To reduce errors in volume measurement, one can induce a water diuresis in stable subjects before beginning the test,[43] although this is rarely practical in the ICU setting. Nevertheless, because many ICU patients have indwelling Foley catheters, it should be possible for accurately timed urine collections to be obtained and for C_{Cr} to be measured with reasonable accuracy.

SERUM CREATININE

Because of the practical and technical problems in obtaining estimates of GFR by clearance methods, renal function is most commonly estimated by following the S_{Cr} in hospitalized patients. Creatinine is formed nonenzymatically from creatine and phosphocreatine in muscle cells and is normally present in the serum at a concentration of 0.8 to 1.4 mg/dL in adults and 0.3 to 0.6 mg/dL in children and pregnant subjects. The measured S_{Cr} depends on the method of measurement, as discussed previously, GFR, rate of creatinine production, volume of distribution (e.g., S_{Cr} is lower in anasarca), and extent of its tubular secretion and intestinal degradation.[3] Because creatinine production is closely related to muscle mass, S_{Cr} is generally less in females than in males and decreases as muscle mass is lost with aging or with debilitating illnesses.

The relationship between S_{Cr} and C_{Cr} (and hence GFR) can be described by a rectangular hyperbola[42]; however, this relationship applies in the steady state and assumes a constant rate of creatinine production (Fig. 126-1). Thus, a doubling of the S_{Cr}, reflects a 50% decrease in C_{Cr}, a fourfold increase in S_{Cr}, a 75% drop in GFR, and so on. Because creatinine production may not remain constant, S_{Cr} may underestimate the decrease in GFR in critically ill patients who have a decrease in muscle mass secondary to an ongoing catabolic state. Moreover, it should be appreciated that S_{Cr} is an insensitive marker of change early in the course of renal disease. Thus, a 33% fall in GFR may raise the S_{Cr} from 0.8 to 1.2 mg/dL, a value that is still within the normal range. If the prior value is not known, this fall in GFR may go unrecognized.

S_{Cr} provides a close estimate of GFR only in the steady state. With an abrupt decrease in GFR, as may occur in acute

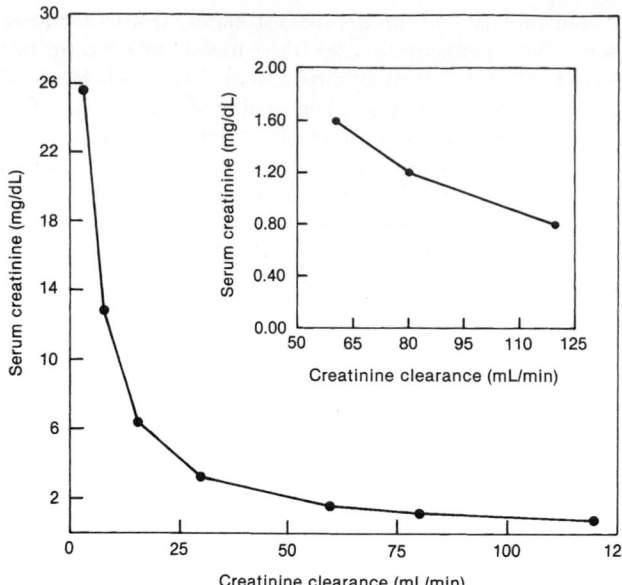

FIGURE 126–1. Relationship between creatinine clearance and serum creatinine. In the steady state, the serum creatinine should increase twofold for each 50% reduction in creatinine clearance. Inset represents an enlarged view of the changes in serum creatinine as creatinine clearance decreases from 120 to 60 mL/min. If serum creatinine is 0.8 mg/dL when the creatinine clearance is 120 mL/min, creatinine clearance can decrease by 33% such that the increased serum creatinine is still within the normal range.

renal failure, creatinine production would be expected to continue unchanged, but because of the decrease in GFR, creatinine excretion will be impaired. As a result, the S_{Cr} increases until a new steady state is obtained, at which time the amount of creatinine produced equals the amount filtered (GFR – S_{Cr}) and excreted (U_{Cr} – V). Depending on the extent of damage and decrease in GFR, it may take several days for a new steady state to be achieved (Fig. 126-2). Therefore, following an insult leading to an abrupt decrease in GFR, the S_{Cr} rises progressively over the next several days. This should not be interpreted as a new insult each day but, rather, that a steady state has not yet been obtained. While the S_{Cr} is changing, its absolute value cannot be used as an accurate measure of the decrease in GFR. If an accurate measurement of GFR is needed during this time, a short C_{Cr} can be obtained.

A variety of equations have been developed to estimate C_{Cr} based on the S_{Cr} without collection of urine. Table 126-1 is a compilation of the more commonly used equations.[44] These equations generally take into consideration muscle mass (estimated as body weight), sex (males having a higher GFR than females), and age. Aging, hepatic diseases, excessive muscle wasting, severe muscular atrophy or dystrophy, hyperthyroidism, paralysis, and chronic glucocorticoid therapy have been associated with reduced creatinine generation.[17] In addition, particularly at low levels of GFR, correction for nonrenal creatinine metabolism is also recommended.[45,46] One of the most commonly utilized equations is that developed by Cockcroft and Gault.[47]

$$C_{Cr} = \frac{(140 - age) \cdot lean\ wt\ in\ kg}{72 \cdot S_{Cr}}$$

where age is expressed in years. The preceding expression is used for men. The formula for women is the preceding formula multiplied by 0.85.

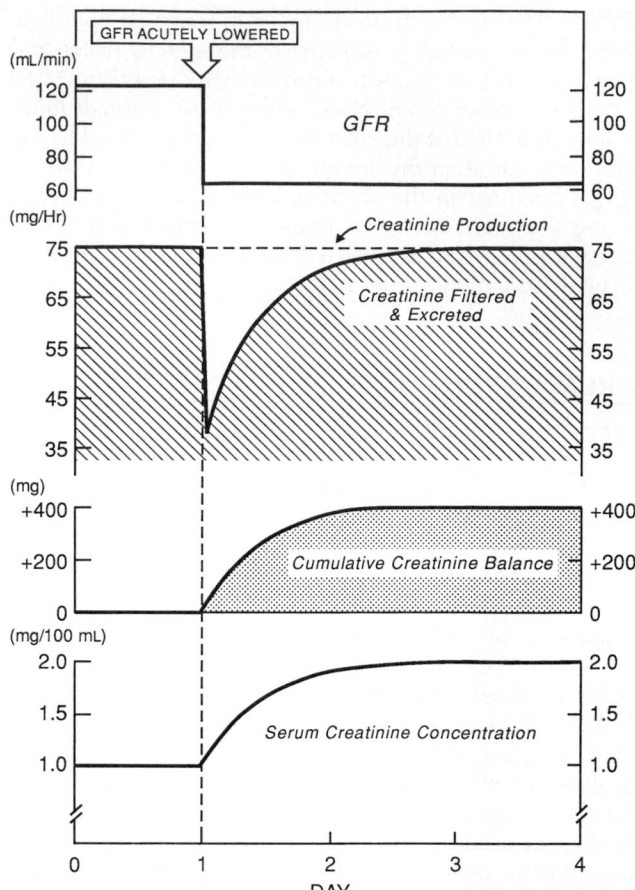

FIGURE 126–2. Expected changes in serum creatinine resulting from an acute fall in the glomerular filtration rate (GFR) and attainment of a new steady state. Between days 0 and 1, the patient is excreting all the creatinine that is produced and serum creatinine is stable at 1 mg/dL. A 50% reduction in GFR on day 1 results in an abrupt fall in filtered (and, therefore, excreted) creatinine. Release of creatinine from muscle remains constant; as a result, creatinine is retained and its serum concentration is increased. As the creatinine concentration rises progressively, filtered (and excreted) creatinine also increases until the excreted creatinine returns to control levels and matches creatinine production. This new steady state (days 3 to 4) is achieved by doubling of serum creatinine concentrations, which maintains the filtered creatinine load at control levels in the face of halving of the GFR. A larger decrease in GFR would lead to a greater increase in the steady state (e.g., a 90% reduction in GFR would lead to a 10-fold rise in serum creatinine) and would take a longer time to achieve. (From Kassirer JP: Clinical evaluation of kidney function-glomerular function. N Engl J Med 1971;285:385. Reprinted with permission from The New England Journal of Medicine.)

The reliability of this equation as a measure of GFR has been assessed in patients with diabetes, pregnant women with renal disease,[48] obese individuals,[49] elderly individuals,[50,51] and black Americans with hypertensive renal disease.[52] It has also been assessed in critically ill patients.[53] These studies have indicated that the accuracy of GFR estimates using the Cockcroft-Gault equation is similar to, or greater than, 24-hour C_{Cr} and the precision is better. This equation seems to be most accurate for estimating GFR when the latter is in the range of 10 to 100 mL/min.[43,49,52,53] An accurate prediction of GFR was derived by Walser and colleagues[54] in patients with advanced renal disease (S_{Cr} > 2 mg/dL) as follows:

For males,

$$GFR = 7.57\ [Cr]^{-1} - 0.103\ age + 0.096\ weight - 6.66$$

TABLE 126–1. COMMONLY USED EQUATIONS USED FOR THE ESTIMATION OF GLOMERULAR FILTRATION RATE OR CREATININE CLEARANCE

Cockcroft-Gault (C_{Cr} • BSA/1.73 m²)
   For men: $C_{Cr} = [(140 - age) • weight (kg)]/S_{Cr} • 72$
   For women: $C_{Cr} = ([(140 - age) • weight (kg)]/S_{Cr} • 72) • 0.85$
MDRD (1)
   GFR = $170 • [S_{Cr}]^{-0.999} • [age]^{-0.176} • [0.762$ if patient is female]
     • $[1.18$ if patient is black] • $[BUN]^{-0.170} • [Alb]^{0.318}$
MDRD (2)
   GFR = $186 • [S_{Cr}]^{-1.154} • [age]^{-0.203} • [0.742$ if patient is female]
     • $[1.212$ if patient is black]
Jellife (1) (C_{Cr} • BSA/1.73 m²)
   For men: $(98 - [0.8 • (age - 20)])/S_{Cr}$
   For women: $(98 - [0.8 • (age - 20)])S_{Cr} • 0.90$
Jellife (2)
   For men: $(100/S_{Cr}) - 12$
   For women: $(80/S_{Cr}) - 7$
Mawer
   For men: weight • $[29.3 - (0.203 • age)] • [1 - (0.03 • S_{Cr})]$
   For women: weight • $[25.3 - (0.175 • age)] • [1 - (0.03 • S_{Cr})]$
Bjornsson
   For men: $[27 - (0.173 • age)] • weight • 0/S_{Cr}$
   For women: $[25 - (0.175 • age)] • weight • 0.07/S_{Cr}$
Gates
   For men: $(89.4 • S_{Cr}^{-1.2}) + (55 - age) • (0.447 • S_{Cr}^{-1.1})$
   For women: $(89.4 • S_{Cr}^{-1.2}) + (55 - age) • (0.447 • S_{Cr}^{-1.1})$
Salazar-Corcoran
   For men: $[137 - age] • [(0.285 • weight) + (12.1 • height^2)]/(51 • S_{Cr})$
   For women: $[146 - age] • [(0.287 • weight) + (9.74 • height^2)]/(60 • S_{Cr})$

For females,

$$GFR = 6.05 [Cr]^{-1} - 0.08 \, age + 0.08 \, weight - 4.81$$

where creatinine (Cr) is expressed in millimoles, age in years, and weight in kilograms. More precision was obtained by including a value for 24-hour urinary urea nitrogen, as a measure of protein intake.[54]

SERUM UREA NITROGEN

Less accurate as a marker of GFR than the S_{Cr}, serum urea nitrogen (SUN) (or blood urea nitrogen [BUN]) is still used extensively in clinical practice to estimate renal function. Although this was the earliest available indicator of renal function, several other factors should be appreciated regarding the use of this substance. Urea, like creatinine, is freely filtered and is retained in the blood as GFR falls. However, in contrast to creatinine, urea may be reabsorbed to a significant extent, its excretion tending to be increased with increasing urine flow rates, whereas its excretion is reduced when tubular fluid reabsorption is enhanced. Of greater importance, urea production is more variable than creatinine. Produced in the liver, urea increases with high protein intake, amino acid infusions, and hypercatabolic states. In addition, endogenous sources of protein such as absorbed hemoglobin from gastrointestinal bleeding may contribute to increased urea synthesis. Even at a constant GFR, SUN may rise in subjects on high protein intake and fall with protein restriction or on refeeding of previously starved, nonhypercatabolic subjects.

Several pharmacologic agents also may affect urea nitrogen formation. Tetracyclines may lead to an increase in SUN by an antianabolic effect without any detectable change in GFR, whereas glucocorticoids and severe illnesses or trauma do the same by inducing endogenous protein hypercatabolism. Because of the widespread use of hyperalimentation in ICU patients, an impairment in renal function is often associated with a marked disproportion in the elevation of SUN compared with S_{Cr}. For this reason, the issue is raised as to whether SUN elevation itself poses an important threat to the patient if the GFR is in a range that should not lead to enhanced morbidity by itself. In those circumstances, it is useful to measure the rate of urea appearance (or generation) to estimate whether other factors, such as gastrointestinal bleeding, excessive amino acid infusions, and protein administration, are contributing to the increase in SUN above that expected by the decrease in GFR.[44,45] Urea nitrogen (UN) appearance can be determined from urine urea nitrogen (UUN), SUN, and body weight as follows:

$$UN = UUN • V + \Delta \, body \, pool \, UN$$

where UUN • V is 24-hour UN excretion and Δ body pool UN = 0.6 – nonedematous weight (kg) • ΔSUN/day.

If the weight is changing,[44,45]

$$\Delta \, body \, pool \, UN = (0.6 • nonedematous \, weight • \Delta SUN) + (\Delta \, weight • final \, SUN)$$

Nitrogen balance (BN) is equal to

$$BN = IN - UN - NUN$$

where IN is urea nitrogen intake and NUN is nonurea nitrogen excretions.[45]

NUN, which includes fecal nitrogen, urinary creatinine, uric acid, and unmeasured nitrogen, averages 0.031 g nitrogen/kg/day.[45] The data obtained from the just-described measurements may be quite useful in evaluating the cause of disproportionate elevations in SUN. If the patient is in a steady state (with a stable weight and SUN), BN = 0, and IN can be estimated from UN + NUN.[45] Because catabolism, except for *severe* trauma and burns, is usually 2 to 4 g nitrogen/day, additional conclusions can be drawn if the patient is not in the steady state. For example, if it is known that IN is less than UN + NUN, gastrointestinal bleeding with or without excess catabolism would be suggested. Similarly, one can evaluate if the increase in SUN is a reflection of excessive exogenous protein and amino acid administration (usually >1.5 g/kg/day; g UN 0.16 = g protein or amino acids). If IN is above UN, such as in severe liver disease, the clinician might more carefully evaluate changes in weight and SUN as well as clearances, because the latter may be more severely depressed than initially suspected.

SODIUM BALANCE AND EXTRACELLULAR FLUID VOLUME

Sodium is the primary cation of the ECF, present in a concentration of 140 to 142 mmol/L. The volume of the ECF is approximately 20% of total body weight and represents a third of total body water. Regulation of ECF volume is governed by factors regulating sodium balance and sodium excretion. The reader is referred to an excellent review on this topic.[55] For the purposes of this discussion, several factors are emphasized. Under physiologic conditions and in the steady state, sodium balance is maintained, because the amount of sodium excreted equals that which enters the body by oral and intravenous routes. Sodium excretion and the fraction of filtered sodium that is excreted (FE_{Na}) can be readily determined. Absolute sodium excretion is measured as the product of the urine sodium concentration and the urine volume,

$$Na^+ \text{ excretion} = (U_{Na} \cdot V)$$

FE_{Na} can be determined as follows:

$$FE_{Na} = U_{Na} \cdot V/GFR \cdot S_{Na}$$

For practical reasons, the C_{Cr} ($=U_{Cr} \cdot V/S_{Cr}$) is used to estimate GFR, such that

$$FE_{Na} = U_{Na} \cdot V/U_{Cr} \cdot V/S_{Cr} \cdot S_{Na}$$

Because the V term in the numerator and denominator cancels out,

$$FE_{Na} = U_{Na}/S_{Na} \cdot S_{Cr}/U_{Cr}$$

Thus, FE_{Na} can be calculated from the sodium and creatinine determined in a random urine sample and serum (or plasma) simultaneously. The resulting calculation is expressed as a percentage by multiplying by 100. This test is of value in the setting of acute renal failure to aid in distinguishing a prerenal from a renal parenchymal etiology.[56] It is not usually helpful in aiding in the diagnosis of urinary tract obstruction or in the presence of underlying chronic renal insufficiency. The reason for the difficulty in interpretation in chronic renal insufficiency can be illustrated by the following considerations. At a GFR of 130 mL/min and a dietary sodium intake of 3 g of sodium (130 mmol), an individual in sodium balance will excrete 0.5% of the filtered load ($FE_{Na} = 0.5\%$). For sodium balance to be maintained at lower levels of GFR with the same sodium intake, FE_{Na} must be increased progressively. Successive decreases in GFR by 2 from 130 would result in an FE_{Na} of 1%, 2%, 4%, and 8%, respectively. Thus, interpretation of the FE_{Na} in a patient with acute renal failure superimposed on chronic renal insufficiency is problematic unless the prior steady-state FE_{Na} is known. This is rarely the case.

The fractional excretion of chloride (FE_{Cl}) has been suggested to be more accurate than that of sodium in helping to distinguish prerenal from parenchymal causes of acute renal failure.[57] This is particularly so in the situation in which acute renal failure occurs with simultaneous metabolic alkalosis. If the urine contains substantial amounts of bicarbonate urinary pH ($U_{pH} > 7$), sodium excretion increases to maintain electroneutrality. Under these circumstances, the FE_{Na} may give misleading information but the FE_{Cl} can be used to obtain the same information.

Although urinary sodium excretion can be used to help make determinations with respect to ECF volume under certain circumstances, this may be fraught with potential errors. No laboratory test is available to provide this information. Rather, the astute clinician must rely on bedside evaluation complemented, where appropriate, with measurements of central venous pressure and pulmonary capillary wedge pressure to assist in making determinations with respect to ECF volume status. For example, a low FE_{Na} (<1%) in the setting of acute renal failure usually indicates a decrease in renal perfusion but does not provide information on the status of the patient's ECF volume. Because a low FE_{Na} can be seen with either ECF volume contraction or severe congestive heart failure, these conditions must be distinguished at the bedside. Moreover, sometimes a low FE_{Na} exists even in the presence of parenchymal renal disease, such as acute glomerulonephritis, severe burn, and radiocontrast nephropathy. Finally, administration of potent diuretic agents can alter the FE_{Na} and may result in misleading interpretations. For this reason, urine samples should be obtained before diuretics are administered.

A few additional points are worthy of note with respect to diuretic use. There is now ample evidence that in a patient in positive sodium balance, diuretic therapy should not be utilized without simultaneously restricting sodium intake, including intravenous saline, if negative sodium balance and reduction in edema fluid are desired.[58] In general, this requires restriction of dietary sodium intake, usually to less than 2 g of sodium per day (0.88 mmol) if the patient is in an edema-forming state. Although a diuresis can be effected even with liberal sodium intake, this requires higher doses of diuretics and more frequent administration of these agents. The coexistence of hyponatremia should not deter clinicians from restricting sodium intake but, rather, should cause them to address solute-free water intake as well. Of course, under certain circumstances, obligatory intakes make it difficult to achieve optimal restriction to assist diuresis. That is, with various pharmacologic drips, blood products, and feeding regimens necessary in acutely ill patients in the ICU, this may become a difficult problem. Under those circumstances, increasing doses of diuretics, including continuous infusions of loop diuretics, may be required.

ANNOTATED REFERENCES

Chertow GM, Sayegh MH, Allgren RL, Lazarus JM: Is the administration of dopamine associated with adverse or favorable outcome in acute renal failure? Am J Med 1996;101:49.

One of the first large, randomized trials exploring the use of low-dose dopamine (<3 μg/kg/min) and high-dose dopamine in ICU patients. The study revealed that there was no evidence that low-dose dopamine improved survival or obviated the need for dialysis, and its use should be discouraged.

Lin J, Knight EL, Hogan ML, Singh AK: Comparison of prediction equations for estimating glomerular filtration rate in adults without kidney disease. J Am Soc Nephrol 2003;14:2573.

Complete evaluation of most of the equations used to estimate GFR. Almost all of the equations have their limitations that are delineated in this article. The MDRD equation and Crockcroft-Gault equations are adequate for most situations.

Wharton WW, Sondeen JL, McBiles M, et al: Predictability of creatinine clearance estimates in critically ill patients. Crit Care Med 1993;21:1487.

Creatinine clearance, inulin clearance, and estimates of GFR based on the Cockcroft-Gault equation were compared in 20 ICU patients. This study emphasized the inaccuracies of obtaining creatinine clearances in the ICU setting. The Cockcroft-Gault equation accurately predicted GFR as determined by inulin clearances.

Wilcox CS, Mitch WE, Kelly RA, et al: Response of the kidney to furosemide: I. Effects of salt intake and renal compensation. J Lab Clin Med 1983;102:450.

Classic study on the pharmacodynamics of furosemide showing the importance of salt intake and homeostatic mechanisms activated by diuretic use.

Wharton WW 3rd, Sondeen JL, McBiles M, et al: Measurement of glomerular filtration rate in ICU patients using ^{99m}Tc-DTPA and inulin. Kidney Int 1992;42:174.

This study in 18 ICU patients compared clearances of inulin, creatinine, and ^{99m}Tc-DTPA to estimated Cockcroft-Gault clearance. The clearance of DTPA correlated best to inulin clearance throughout the entire range of clearances studied. DTPA clearance was also simple and inexpensive to perform in the ICU setting.

Chapter 127
METABOLIC ACIDOSIS AND ALKALOSIS

Thomas D. DuBose, Jr.

KEY POINTS

DIAGNOSIS OF TYPES OF DISTURBANCES

1. Simple and mixed disturbances can be differentiated through appreciation of the limits of compensation and calculation of the anion gap.
2. Mixed disorders are more common in critically ill patients.
3. A pathway to correct diagnosis involves a stepwise approach.

METABOLIC ACIDOSIS

1. Two broad types of acidosis can be defined by calculation of the anion gap.
2. Treatment of acidosis requires consideration of the concept of "potential" bicarbonate.

HIGH ANION GAP ACIDOSES

1. Four categories of high anion gap acidosis can be identified readily through simple clinical laboratory tests.
2. L-Lactic acid acidosis is the most common type of high anion gap acidosis in the ICU.

L-LACTIC ACIDOSIS

1. Lactic acid acidosis occurs with or without hemodynamic compromise in the ICU.
2. Bowel ischemia and therapy for HIV infection with nucleoside reverse-transcriptase inhibitors are now frequent causes.
3. Therapy should first be directed to correction of the abnormality responsible for lactate generation.
4. Alkali therapy has many disadvantages and should be administered with understanding of the pathophysiology of lactate generation.

KETOACIDOSIS

1. Diabetic ketoacidosis (DKA) is common, but alcoholic ketoacidosis is often missed. Distinguishing features include the degree of ketonemia and the relative level of β-hydroxybutyrate—the latter being a characteristic of alcoholic ketoacidosis, not DKA.

2. DKA responds to low doses of regular insulin (0.1 U/kg/h i.v.) and volume re-expansion with 0.9% NaCl.
3. Clearing of ketones in plasma is reflected by progressive correction of the anion gap.

DRUG- AND TOXIN-INDUCED ACIDOSIS

1. Toxins such as ethylene glycol and methyl alcohol increase the osmolar gap.
2. Treatment should not be delayed and should include intravenous ethyl alcohol or formepizole, intravenous fluids, $NaHCO_3$, thiamine, and hemodialysis.

NON-GAP OR HYPERCHLOREMIC METABOLIC ACIDOSES

1. Hyperchloremic acidosis is characterized by a normal anion gap (10 mEq/L), high chloride, and low bicarbonate.
2. Renal causes can be distinguished from gastrointestinal causes by calculation of the urine anion gap: $UAG = [Na^+ + K^+]_u - [Cl^-]_u$.

METABOLIC ALKALOSIS

1. Once generated by bicarbonate gain or acid loss, metabolic alkalosis is maintained by renal mechanisms that encourage bicarbonate retention rather than excretion.
2. Measurement of urine $[Cl^-]$ and clinical estimation of extracellular fluid volume (ECV) status is helpful in evaluation of the causes of chronic metabolic alkalosis.
3. Metabolic alkalosis in the ICU may occur in combination with other acid-base disorders (mixed acid-base disorders).
4. Combined metabolic and respiratory alkalosis can result in extreme elevation of the pH and is associated with high mortality.
5. Unique causes of alkalemia in the ICU include nasogastric suction, vomiting, diuretics, alkali administration, steroids, mechanical ventilation, hyperalimentation, magnesium deficiency, potassium deficiency, and third space sequestration of ECV.

The appropriate diagnosis and management of acid-base disorders in acutely ill patients necessitates accurate and timely interpretation of the specific acid-base disorder. Precise interpretation involves simultaneous measurement of plasma electrolytes and arterial blood gases as well as an appreciation by the clinician of the physiologic adaptations and compensatory responses that occur with specific acid-base disturbances. In most circumstances, these compensatory responses can be predicted through an analysis of the prevailing disorder. The severity of illness encountered in the ICU specifies that complicated acid-base disturbances are observed commonly and more regularly than on the typical internal medicine service. Hypotension, sepsis, multiorgan failure, drug overdose, diabetes, respiratory failure, renal failure, and hepatic dysfunction all result in disturbances of acid-base homeostasis. In addition, therapeutic interventions in the ICU may extend and complicate acid-base equilibrium. Because disturbances of pH affect a wide variety of physiologic functions and have clinically significant consequences, timely and accurate characterization of these disturbances becomes an essential component of critical care medicine. Identification of an acid-base disturbance should prompt a search for the cause of the disturbance itself. A thoughtful evaluation of all acid-base disturbances is of primary importance, and efforts to normalize pH should be cause specific and based on proven therapeutic efficacy.

LABORATORY ASSESSMENT OF ACID-BASE STATUS AND MONITORING

Evaluation of acid-base status requires analysis of both the arterial blood gas and an electrolyte panel. These collections should be obtained simultaneously or within a brief span. Collection into a low-friction syringe allows ease of arterial puncture and collection. Excess heparin should be avoided and air bubbles removed from the syringe promptly. Analysis should follow shortly. Mixed venous blood gas measurement is complicated by disassociation in arterial and venous $PaCO_2$, especially in the presence of poor tissue perfusion. On-line continuous monitoring of blood gas values may offer advantages in the future but is not yet generally available. The anion gap (AG) should be calculated from the electrolyte panel in every instance because it may reveal a high-AG metabolic acidosis, even in the setting of a mixed disorder where arterial pH may be in the normal range.

NORMAL ACID-BASE HOMEOSTASIS

Systemic arterial pH is maintained between 7.35 and 7.45 by extracellular and intracellular chemical buffering together with respiratory and renal regulatory mechanisms. The control of $PaCO_2$ by the central nervous system and respiratory systems and the control of the plasma bicarbonate by the kidneys stabilize the arterial pH by excretion or retention of acid or alkali. The metabolic and respiratory components that regulate systemic pH are described by the Henderson-Hasselbalch equation:

$$pH = pK_a + \log_{10} \frac{HCO_3}{P_{CO_2} \times 0.0301}$$

Under most circumstances, CO_2 production and excretion are matched, and the usual steady-state $PaCO_2$ is maintained

at 40 mm Hg. Underexcretion of CO_2 produces hypercapnia, and overexcretion causes hypocapnia. Nevertheless, production and excretion are again matched at a new steady-state $PaCO_2$. Therefore, the $PaCO_2$ is regulated primarily by neural respiratory factors and is not subject to regulation by the rate of CO_2 production. Hypercapnia is usually the result of hypoventilation rather than of increased CO_2 production. Increases or decreases in $PaCO_2$ represent derangements of neural respiratory control or are due to compensatory changes in response to a primary alteration in the plasma $[HCO_3^-]$.[1]

Primary changes in $PaCO_2$ can cause acidosis or alkalosis, depending on whether $PaCO_2$ is above or below the normal value of 40 mm Hg (respiratory acidosis or alkalosis, respectively). Primary alteration of $PaCO_2$ evokes cellular buffering and renal adaptation, a slow process that becomes more efficient with time. A primary change in the plasma $[HCO_3^-]$ as a result of metabolic or renal factors results in compensatory changes in ventilation that blunt the changes in blood pH that would occur otherwise. Such respiratory alterations are referred to as *secondary*, or compensatory, changes, because they occur in response to primary metabolic alterations.[1]

The kidneys regulate plasma $[HCO_3^-]$ through three main processes: (1) "reabsorption" of filtered HCO_3^-, (2) formation of titratable acid, and (3) excretion of NH_4^+ in the urine. The kidney filters approximately 4000 mmol of HCO_3^- per day. To reabsorb the filtered load of HCO_3^-, the renal tubules must therefore secrete 4000 mmol of hydrogen ions. Between 80% and 90% of HCO_3^- is reabsorbed in the proximal tubule. The distal nephron reabsorbs the remainder and secretes protons to defend systemic pH. Although this quantity of secreted protons, 40 to 60 mmol/day, is small, it must be secreted to prevent chronic positive H^+ balance and metabolic acidosis because metabolism of the average diet rich in protein produces fixed acids that consume bicarbonate on entry into the extracellular fluid. This quantity of secreted protons (net acid) is represented in the urine as titratable acid and NH_4^+. Metabolic acidosis in the presence of normal renal function increases NH_4^+ production and excretion. NH_4^+ production and excretion are impaired in chronic renal failure, hyperkalemia, and renal tubular acidosis.[1,2]

In sum, these regulatory responses, including chemical buffering, the regulation of $PaCO_2$ by the respiratory system, and of $[HCO_3^-]$ by the kidneys, act in concert to maintain a systemic arterial pH between 7.35 and 7.45.

DIAGNOSIS OF TYPES OF DISTURBANCES

The most common clinical disturbances are **simple** acid-base disorders, that is, one of the metabolic disturbances (metabolic acidosis or alkalosis) or one of the respiratory disturbances (respiratory acidosis or alkalosis) occurring alone rather than in combination. Because physiologic compensation is not complete and cannot achieve a normal pH, the pH is abnormal in simple disturbances. More complicated clinical situations can give rise to **mixed** acid-base disturbances through simultaneous expression of more than one simple disturbance.[1-3]

SIMPLE ACID-BASE DISORDERS

Primary respiratory disturbances (primary changes in $PaCO_2$) invoke compensatory metabolic responses (secondary changes in $[HCO_3^-]$), and primary metabolic disturbances elicit predictable compensatory respiratory responses.

TABLE 127–1. ACID-BASE ABNORMALITIES AND APPROPRIATE COMPENSATORY RESPONSES FOR SIMPLE DISORDERS

Primary Acid-Base Disorders	Primary Defect	Effect on pH	Compensatory Response	Expected Range of Compensation	Limits of Compensation
Respiratory acidosis	Alveolar hypoventilation ($\uparrow P_{CO_2}$)	$\downarrow$	$\uparrow$ Renal HCO_3^- reabsorption ($HCO_3^- \uparrow$)	Acute: $\Delta[HCO_3^-] = +1$ mEq/L for each $\uparrow \Delta P_{CO_2}$ of 10 mm Hg	$[HCO_3^-] = 38$ mEq/L
				Chronic: $\Delta[HCO_3^-] = +4$ mEq/L for each $\uparrow \Delta P_{CO_2}$ of 10 mm Hg	$[HCO_3^-] = 45$ mEq/L
Respiratory alkalosis	Alveolar hyperventilation ($\downarrow P_{CO_2}$)	$\uparrow$	$\downarrow$ Renal HCO_3^- reabsorption ($HCO_3^- \downarrow$)	Acute: $\Delta[HCO_3^-] = -2$ mEq/L for each $\downarrow \Delta P_{CO_2}$ of 10 mm Hg	$[HCO_3^-] = 18$ mEq/L
				Chronic: $\Delta[HCO_3^-] = -5$ mEq/L for each $\downarrow \Delta P_{CO_2}$ of 10 mm Hg	$[HCO_3^-] = 15$ mEq/L
Metabolic acidosis	Loss of HCO_3^- or gain of H^+ ($\downarrow HCO_3^-$)	$\downarrow$	Alveolar hyperventilation to $\uparrow$ pulmonary CO_2 excretion ($\downarrow P_{CO_2}$)	$P_{CO_2} = 1.5[HCO_3^-] + 8 \pm 2$ $P_{CO_2} =$ last 2 digits of pH $\times 100$ $P_{CO_2} = 15 + [HCO_3^-]$	$P_{CO_2} = 15$ mm Hg
Metabolic alkalosis	HCO_3^- or loss of H^+ ($\uparrow HCO_3^-$)	$\uparrow$	Alveolar hypoventilation to $\downarrow$ pulmonary CO_2 excretion ($\uparrow P_{CO_2}$)	$P_{CO_2} = +0.6$ mm Hg for $\Delta[HCO_3^-]$ of 1 mEq/L $P_{CO_2} = 15 + [HCO_3^-]$	$P_{CO_2} = 55$ mm Hg

Adapted from Bidani A, DuBose TD Jr: Cellular and whole body acid-base regulation. In Arieff AI, DeFronzo RA (eds): Fluid, Electrolyte, and Acid Base Disorders, 2nd ed. New York, Churchill Livingstone, 1995.

Primary changes in $PaCO_2$ or $[HCO_3^-]$ alter systemic pH and cause acidosis or alkalosis. To illustrate, metabolic acidosis due to an increase in endogenous acids (e.g., ketoacidosis) lowers extracellular fluid $[HCO_3^-]$ and decreases extracellular pH. This stimulates the medullary chemoreceptors to increase ventilation and to return the ratio of $[HCO_3^-]$ to $PaCO_2$, and thus pH, toward normal, although not to normal. The degree of respiratory compensation expected in a simple form of metabolic acidosis can be predicted from the relationship $PaCO_2 = (1.5 \times [HCO_3^-]) + 8$, that is, the $PaCO_2$ is expected to decrease 1.25 mm Hg for each mmol per liter decrease in $[HCO_3^-]$. Thus, a patient with metabolic acidosis and $[HCO_3^-]$ of 12 mmol/L would be expected to have a $PaCO_2$ between 24 and 28 mm Hg. Values for $PaCO_2$ below 24 or greater than 28 mm Hg define a mixed disturbance (metabolic acidosis plus respiratory alkalosis or metabolic acidosis plus respiratory acidosis, respectively). Nomograms are available, and may be helpful, but are not substitutes for an appreciation of the limits of compensation as displayed in Table 127-1.[1]

MIXED ACID-BASE DISORDERS

Mixed acid-base disorders, defined as independently coexisting disorders not merely compensatory responses, are more often seen in patients in ICUs and can lead to dangerous extremes of pH. A patient with DKA (high-AG metabolic acidosis) may develop an independent and superimposed respiratory problem leading to respiratory acidosis or alkalosis. Patients with underlying pulmonary disease may not respond to metabolic acidosis with an appropriate ventilatory response because of insufficient respiratory reserve. Such imposition of respiratory acidosis on metabolic acidosis can

lead to severe acidemia and a poor outcome. When metabolic acidosis and metabolic alkalosis coexist in the same patient, the pH may be normal or near normal. When the pH is normal, an elevated AG (see later) denotes the presence of a metabolic acidosis. A diabetic patient with ketoacidosis may have renal dysfunction resulting in simultaneous metabolic acidosis. Patients who have ingested an overdose of drug combinations such as sedatives and salicylates may have mixed disturbances as a result of the acid-base response to the individual drugs (metabolic acidosis mixed with respiratory acidosis or respiratory alkalosis, respectively). Even more complex are triple acid-base disturbances. For example, patients with metabolic acidosis due to alcoholic ketoacidosis may develop metabolic alkalosis due to vomiting and superimposed respiratory alkalosis due to the hyperventilation of hepatic dysfunction or alcohol withdrawal.[1]

PATHWAY TO DIAGNOSIS OF ACID-BASE DISORDERS

A stepwise approach to the diagnosis of acid-base disorders follows and is summarized in Table 127-2.[1-3] In the determination of arterial blood gases by the clinical laboratory, both pH and $PaCO_2$ are measured, and the $[HCO_3^-]$ is calculated from the Henderson-Hasselbalch equation. This calculated value should be compared with the measured $[HCO_3^-]$ (or total CO_2) on the electrolyte panel. These two values should agree within 2 mmol/L. If they do not, the values may not have been drawn simultaneously, a laboratory error may be present, or an error could have been made in calculating the $[HCO_3^-]$. After verifying the blood acid-base values, one can then identify the precise acid-base disorder.[1]

TABLE 127–2. STEPS IN ACID-BASE DIAGNOSIS

1. Obtain arterial blood gases (ABG) and electrolytes simultaneously.
2. Compare [HCO_3^-] on ABG and electrolytes to verify accuracy.
3. Calculate anion gap.
4. Know four causes of high–anion gap acidosis (ketoacidosis, lactic acid acidosis, renal failure, and toxins).
5. Know two causes of high Cl^- acidosis (bicarbonate loss from gastrointestinal tract, renal tubular defect).
6. Estimate compensatory response (see Table 127-1).
7. Compare Δanion gap and ΔHCO_3^-.
8. Compare change in [Cl^-] with change in [Na^+].

TABLE 127–3. ANION GAP IN THE DIAGNOSIS OF METABOLIC ACIDOSIS

Anion Gap = $Na^+ - (Cl^- + HCO_3^-)$ = 10 mEq/L

Decreased Anion Gap	*Increased Anion Gap*
Increased cations (not Na^+)	Increased anions (not Cl^- or HCO_3^-)
↑ Ca^{++}, Mg^{++}	↑ Albumin concentration
↑ Li^+	Alkalosis
↑ IgG	↑ Inorganic anions
Decreased anions	Phosphate
(not Cl^- or HCO_3^-)	Sulfate
↓ Albumin concentration	
(hypoalbuminemia)*	
Acidosis	↑ Organic anions
Laboratory error	Lactate
Hyperviscosity	Ketones
Bromism	Uremic
	↑ Exogenously supplied anions
	Toxins:
	Salicylate
	Paraldehyde
	Ethylene glycol
	Methanol
	↑ Unidentified anions
	Toxins
	Uremic
	Hyperosmolar, nonketotic states
	Myoglobinuric acute renal failure
	Decreased cations (not Na^+)
	↓ Ca^{++}, Mg^{++}

*Albumin is the major unmeasured anion. A decline in serum albumin of 1.0 g/dL from the normal value of 4.5 g/dL decreases the anion gap by 2.5 mEq/L. Correction is very important to diagnose anion gap acidosis in nephrotic syndrome or any cause of hypoalbuminemia.
Adapted from Emmett M, Narins RG: Clinical use of the anion gap. Medicine 1977;56:38-54, and from Oh MS, Carroll HJ: The anion gap. N Engl J Med 1977;297:814-817, 1977.

The most common causes of acid-base disorders should be kept in mind while probing the history for clues about the etiology. For example, established chronic renal failure is expected to cause a metabolic acidosis, and chronic vomiting frequently causes metabolic alkalosis. Patients with pneumonia, sepsis, or cardiac failure frequently have respiratory alkalosis, and patients with chronic obstructive pulmonary disease or a sedative drug overdose often display a respiratory acidosis. The drug history is important because loop or thiazide diuretics may cause metabolic alkalosis and the carbonic anhydrase inhibitor acetazolamide can result in metabolic acidosis.

Blood for electrolytes and arterial blood gases should be drawn simultaneously before therapy, because an increase in [HCO_3^-] occurs with metabolic alkalosis and respiratory acidosis. Conversely, a decrease in [HCO_3^-] occurs in metabolic acidosis and respiratory alkalosis.[1,3]

Metabolic acidosis often leads to hyperkalemia as a result of cellular shifts in which H^+ is exchanged for K^+ or Na^+. For each decrease in blood pH of 0.10, the plasma [K^+] should rise by 0.6 mmol/L. This relationship is not invariable, however. DKA, lactic acidosis, diarrhea, and renal tubular acidosis are regularly associated with potassium depletion because of urinary K^+ wasting.[1]

ANION GAP

All evaluations of acid-base disorders should include a simple calculation of the AG (Table 127-3); it represents those unmeasured anions in plasma (normally 10 mmol/L) and is calculated as follows:

$$AG = Na^+ - (Cl^- + HCO_3^-)$$

The unmeasured anions include predominately anionic proteins but, also, phosphate, sulfate, and organic anions. When endogenously produced acid anions, such as acetoacetate and lactate, accumulate in extracellular fluid, the AG increases, causing a high-AG acidosis. An increase in the AG is most often due to an increase in unmeasured anions and less commonly is caused by a decrease in unmeasured cations (calcium, magnesium, potassium) (see Table 127-3).[1] In addition, the AG may increase with an increase in anionic albumin, either because of increased albumin concentration or alkalosis, which alters albumin charge. A decrease in the AG can be due to (1) an increase in unmeasured cations; (2) the addition to the blood of abnormal cations, such as lithium (lithium intoxication) or cationic immunoglobulins (plasma cell dyscrasias); (3) a reduction in the major plasma anion, albumin, concentration (nephrotic syndrome); (4) a decrease in the effective anionic charge on albumin by acidosis; or (5) hyperviscosity and severe hyperlipidemia, which can lead to an underestimation of sodium and chloride concentrations.[1] A fall in serum albumin by 1 g/dL from the normal value (4.5 g/dL) decreases the AG by 2.5 mEq/L. This correction should be routinely applied when calculating the AG in hypoalbuminemic patients (see Table 127-3).[1]

In the face of a normal serum albumin, a high AG is usually due to non–chloride-containing acids that contain inorganic (phosphate, sulfate), organic (ketoacids, lactate, uremic organic anions), exogenous (salicylate or ingested toxins with organic acid production), or unidentified anions. By definition, therefore, a high-AG acidosis has two identifying features: a low [HCO_3^-] and an elevated AG. The latter is present even if an additional acid-base disorder is superimposed to modify the [HCO_3^-] independently. Metabolic acidosis of the high-AG variety concomitant with either chronic respiratory acidosis or metabolic alkalosis represents a situation for which [HCO_3^-] may be normal or high. Nevertheless, the AG is elevated and the [Cl^-] is depressed (Table 127-4).[1]

Similarly, normal values for [HCO_3^-], $PaCO_2$, and pH do not ensure the absence of an acid-base disturbance. For instance, an alcoholic who has been vomiting may develop a metabolic alkalosis with a pH of 7.55, $PaCO_2$ of 48 mm Hg, [HCO_3^-] of 40 mmol/L, [Na^+] of 135, [Cl^-] of 80, and [K^+] of 2.8. If such a patient were then to develop a superimposed alcoholic ketoacidosis with a β-hydroxybutyrate concentration of 15 mM, arterial pH would fall to 7.40, [HCO_3^-] to 25 mmol/L, and the $PaCO_2$ to 40 mm Hg. Although these blood gas findings are normal, the AG is elevated at

TABLE 127–4. CLINICAL CAUSES OF HIGH–ANION GAP AND NORMAL–ANION GAP ACIDOSIS

High Anion Gap

Ketoacidosis
  Diabetic ketoacidosis (acetoacetate)
  Alcoholic (β-hydroxybutyrate)
  Starvation
Lactic acid acidosis
  L-Lactic acid acidosis (types A and B)
  D-Lactic acid acidosis
Toxins
  Ethylene glycol
  Methyl alcohol
  Salicylate

Normal Anion Gap

Gastrointestinal loss of HCO_3^- (negative urine anion gap)
  Diarrhea
  Fistula, external
Renal loss of HCO_3^- or failure to excrete NH_4^+ (low net acid
  excretion = positive urine anion gap)
  Proximal renal tubular acidosis
  Acetazolamide
  Classic distal renal tubular acidosis (low serum K^+)
  Generalized distal renal tubular defect (high serum K^+)
Miscellaneous
  NH_4Cl ingestion
  Sulfur ingestion
  Dilutional acidosis

30 mmol/L, indicating a mixed metabolic alkalosis and metabolic acidosis.[1]

METABOLIC ACIDOSIS

Metabolic acidosis can occur because of an increase in endogenous acid production (such as lactate and ketoacids), loss of bicarbonate (as in diarrhea), or accumulation of endogenous acids (as in renal failure). Metabolic acidosis has profound effects on the respiratory, cardiac, and nervous systems.[1]

EFFECTS OF ACIDOSIS

The fall in blood pH is accompanied by a characteristic increase in ventilation, especially the tidal volume (Kussmaul respiration). Intrinsic cardiac contractility may be depressed, but inotropic function can be normal because of catecholamine release. Both peripheral arterial vasodilation and central venoconstriction can be present; the decrease in central and pulmonary vascular compliance predisposes to pulmonary edema with even minimal volume overload. Central nervous system function is depressed, with headache, lethargy, stupor, and, in some cases, even coma. Glucose intolerance may also occur.[1]

GENERAL MODEL FOR THE TREATMENT OF METABOLIC ACIDOSIS

The treatment of metabolic acidosis with alkali should be reserved for severe acidemia except when the patient has no "potential $[HCO_3^-]$" in plasma. Potential $[HCO_3^-]$ can be estimated from the increment (Δ) in the AG (ΔAG = patient's AG − 10).[1] It must be determined if the acid anion in plasma is metabolizable (i.e., β-hydroxybutyrate, acetoacetate, and lactate) or nonmetabolizable (anions that accumulate in chronic renal failure and after toxin ingestion). The latter requires return of renal function to replenish the $[HCO_3^-]$ deficit, a slow and often unpredictable process. Consequently, patients with a normal AG acidosis (hyperchloremic acidosis), a slightly elevated AG (mixed hyperchloremic and AG acidosis), or an AG attributable to a nonmetabolizable anion in the presence of renal failure should receive alkali therapy, either orally ($NaHCO_3$ or Shohl's solution) or intravenously ($NaHCO_3$), in an amount necessary to slowly increase the plasma $[HCO_3^-]$ into the 20 to 22 mmol/L range. Controversy exists, however, in regard to the use of alkali in patients with a pure AG acidosis from accumulation of a metabolizable organic acid anion (ketoacidosis or lactic acidosis).[1] In general, severe acidosis (pH < 7.15) warrants the intravenous administration of 50 to 100 mEq of $NaHCO_3$, over 30 to 45 min, during the initial 1 to 2 h of therapy. Provision of such modest quantities of alkali in this situation seems to provide an added measure of safety, but it is essential to monitor plasma electrolytes during the course of therapy, because the $[K^+]$ may decline as pH rises. The goal is to increase the $[HCO_3^-]$ to no more than 10 mEq/L and the pH to 7.25. The goal is never to increase these values to the normal values of 25 and 7.40, respectively.[1]

There are two major clinical categories of metabolic acidosis: high AG and normal AG (see Table 127-4).[1]

HIGH–ANION GAP ACIDOSES

High-AG acidosis is the most common form of metabolic acidosis encountered in the ICU. There are four principal causes of a high-AG acidosis: (1) lactic acid acidosis, (2) ketoacidosis, (3) toxin-induced, and (4) acute and chronic renal failure (Tables 127-4 and 127-5). Initial screening to differentiate the high-AG acidoses should include (1) a search in the history for evidence of drug or toxin ingestion (ethylene glycol, methyl alcohol, salicylates); (2) determination of whether diabetes mellitus is present (DKA); (3) a search for evidence of alcoholism or increased levels of β-hydroxybutyrate (alcoholic ketoacidosis); (4) observation for clinical signs of uremia and determination of the blood urea nitrogen and creatinine (uremic acidosis); (5) inspection of the urine for oxalate crystals (ethylene glycol); and (6) recognition of the numerous clinical settings in which lactate levels may be increased (hypotension, shock, cardiac failure, leukemia, cancer, and drug or toxin ingestion).[1]

L-Lactic Acidosis

An increase in plasma L-lactate may be secondary to the following (see Table 127-5)[4]:

- Poor tissue perfusion (type A)—circulatory insufficiency (septic, cardiogenic, or hypovolemic shock) or severe hypoxia (hypoxemia, carbon monoxide poisoning, cyanide, severe anemia)
- Aerobic disorders (type B1)—associated with systemic disorders (malignancies, diabetes mellitus, renal or hepatic failure, abnormal bowel flora, severe infections [e.g., cholera, malaria]), seizures, and AIDS
- Drugs/toxins (type B2)—metformin, ethanol, methanol, ethylene glycol, isoniazid, antiretroviral agents, and fructose
- Inborn errors of metabolism (type B3)—impaired mitochondrial oxidation of pyruvate, G6PD deficiency

TABLE 127–5. METABOLIC ACIDOSIS WITH HIGH ANION GAP

L-Lactic Acidosis

Type A
  Poor tissue perfusion
  Shock
    Cardiogenic
    Hemorrhagic
    Septic
  Acute hypoxemia
  Carbon monoxide poisoning
Type B
  Various common disorders
    Diabetes mellitus
    Renal failure
    Liver disease
    Infection (especially AIDS)
    Leukemia, lymphoma, large tumors
    ? Pancreatitis, anemia, poliomyelitis
  Ingestion or administration of drugs or other toxic substances
    Metformin
    Phenformin (historical)
    Ethanol
    Antiretroviral therapy for HIV infection with NRTIs
    Cancer chemotherapy
    Salicylates
    Sorbitol
    Xylitol
    Dithiazanine iodide
    Streptozotocin
    Isoniazid
    Cyanide
    Nitroprusside
    Jamaican vomiting sickness
  Hereditary forms
    Glucose 6-phosphate deficiency (type I glycogenosis)
    Fructose-1,6-diphosphatase deficiency
    Pyruvate carboxylase deficiency
    Pyruvate dehydrogenase deficiency
    Oxidative phosphorylation deficiencies
    Methylmalonicaciduria
  Miscellaneous
    Ingestion of lactic acid milk, Kombucha tea

D-Lactic Acidosis

  Short-bowel syndrome
  Ischemic bowel
  Small bowel obstruction

Ketoacidosis

  Diabetic
  Alcoholic
  Starvation
  Inborn errors of metabolism

Intoxication

  Ethylene glycol
  Methanol
  Salicylates
  Paraldehyde

Uremia (Late Renal Failure)

Adapted in part from Cohen RD, Woods HF: Clinical Biochemical Aspects of Lactic Acidosis. Oxford, Blackwell Scientific Publications, 1976; and Relman AS: Lactic acidosis. In Brenner BM, Stein JH (eds): Contemporary Issues in Nephrology. Acid-Base and Potassium Homeostasis, Vol 2. New York, Churchill Livingstone, 1978, p 65.

Among the most common causes of lactic acid acidosis in medical ICUs is unrecognized bowel ischemia or infarction in a patient with severe atherosclerosis or cardiac decompensation receiving vasopressors.[5] D-Lactic acid acidosis, which may be associated with jejunoileal bypass or intestinal obstruction and is due to formation of D-lactate by gut bacteria, may cause both an increased AG and hyperchloremia (see Table 129-5).[4,5] Lactic acidosis is among the most frequent and the critical of all AG acidoses observed in the acute care setting. Approximately 1% of all nonsurgical inpatients develop a lactic acidosis at some point during the course of the hospitalization.[6] Whether lactic acidosis represents a unique entity or is a consequence of a variety of other conditions common to the ICU has been debated. For purposes of definition, a serum L-lactate level greater than 5 mmol/L is thought to represent a clinically significant lactic acidosis. Nevertheless, some patients in the ICU maintain serum lactate levels between 2 to 5 mmol/L, and it is uncertain whether such patients progress to frank lactic acidosis.

L-Lactic acid is the product of the anaerobic metabolism of pyruvate. Pyruvate is derived from glucose by means of the Embden-Meyerhof pathway. Under aerobic conditions, pyruvate is oxidized to acetyl CoA. In the absence of oxygen, however, pyruvate is reduced, instead, to lactate. Lactate is converted back to pyruvate by both the liver and the kidney via the Cori cycle. Hepatic dysfunction, therefore, predisposes to the development of lacticacidemia in the presence of tissue hypoperfusion.

Whereas the lactic acid acidoses have been classified by Huckabee and Cohen into two types—type A (hypoxic) and B (nonhypoxic) subtypes as noted earlier[7]—it has been recognized that lactic acidosis is often the result of the simultaneous existence of both hypoxic and nonhypoxic factors, and in many cases the precise etiology is difficult to establish. Decreased oxygen delivery to peripheral tissues in shock, for example, results in L-lactic acid accumulation. Severe acidemia decreases portal blood flow and hepatic clearance of lactic acid.[8] Moreover, in sepsis there is both a decrease in tissue perfusion and a decrease in oxygen utilization. Technically, therefore, the classification of lactic acidosis is primarily of conceptual interest.

The numerous causes of lactic acidosis are outlined in Table 127-5. Numerous drugs have been implicated in the occurrence of lactic acidosis. Of particular note is the newer biguanide (metformin) and antiretroviral therapy, specifically with nucleoside reverse-transcriptase inhibitors (NRTIs). Risk factors for NRTI therapy–associated lactic acidosis include a creatinine clearance less than 70 mL/min and a low CD4+ T lymphocyte count.[4]

Critically ill patients with a significantly elevated AG or low serum bicarbonate should be suspected of having a lactic acidosis, particularly in the presence of hepatic insufficiency. A high index of suspicion must be maintained, however, because the AG is a relatively insensitive reflection of lactic acidosis. Iberti and coworkers reported a poor correlation between arterial pH, the AG, and serum lactate levels.[9] Fifty percent of patients with serum lactate levels above 5 and less than 9.9 mmol/L displayed a normal AG.

Several investigators have sought to characterize the prognostic value of serum lactic acid levels. Studies have found an inverse correlation between mortality and L-lactate levels above 2.0 to 2.5 mmol/L.[10-12] Prognosis is related to lactate concentration, as well as the ability to metabolize a lactic acid load after a resuscitative effort. Falk and associates observed that the ability to lower serum lactate levels by 50% within 18 hours after resuscitation correlated with a significantly greater rate of survival.[13] Other studies have reinforced these findings, revealing both significantly lower lactate levels and increased ability to clear lactate in survivors as opposed to nonsurvivors.[14] Presumably, the inability to clear lactate is an index of organ dysfunction.[15,16] Nevertheless, dichloroacetate, which decreases lactic acid levels, has not been shown to improve survival.[17]

Treatment of Lactic Acidosis

The first principle of therapy in lactic acid acidosis is that the underlying condition that disrupts lactate metabolism must first be corrected; tissue perfusion must be restored when it is inadequate. There has been controversy as to whether lactic acidosis contributes to mortality per se or is a marker of the severity of the underlying illness.[4,5] This debate has focused on recommendations for use of buffers in the management of lactic acidosis. Nevertheless, there is general agreement that the most judicious and initial management of lactic acidosis is the reversal of those processes that led to development. Optimizing cardiac output and tissue oxygenation through supportive therapies should be of primary consideration in management. Mechanical ventilation is instituted to reduce the metabolic work of breathing and optimize ventilation; fluids and inotropic agents are helpful in restoring adequate cardiac output. Vasoactive drugs should be used cautiously based on an understanding of the underlying hemodynamics and knowledge of the mechanisms of action of the drugs. Vasoconstrictors should be avoided, if possible, because they may worsen tissue perfusion. Alkali therapy is generally advocated for acute, severe acidemia (pH < 7.15) to improve cardiac function and lactate utilization. However, $NaHCO_3$ therapy may paradoxically depress cardiac performance and exacerbate acidosis by enhancing lactate production (higher pH stimulates phosphofructokinase). While the use of alkali in moderate lactic acidosis is controversial, it is generally agreed that attempts to return the pH or $[HCO_3^-]$ to normal by administration of exogenous $NaHCO_3$ are deleterious. Fluid overload occurs rapidly with $NaHCO_3$ administration because of the massive amounts required in some cases. In addition, central venoconstriction and decreased cardiac output are common. The accumulation of lactic acid may be relentless and may necessitate diuretics, ultrafiltration, or dialysis.[18,19] Hemodialysis can simultaneously deliver HCO_3^-, remove lactate, remove excess ECV, and correct electrolyte abnormalities. When conventional hemodialysis is necessary, sodium bicarbonate should be the dialysate base equivalent.[19,20] The use of continuous renal replacement therapy as a means of lactate removal and simultaneous alkali addition through dialysis is a promising adjunctive treatment in critically ill patients with L-lactic acidosis but requires additional study. The ultrafiltration accomplished with continuous renal replacement therapy offers additional benefits because volume administration is poorly tolerated in patients with severe lactic acid acidosis because of central venoconstriction and decreased cardiac output.

If the underlying cause of the L-lactic acidosis can be remedied, it is anticipated that the lactate will be reconverted to HCO_3^-. HCO_3^- derived from lactate conversion and any new HCO_3^- generated by renal mechanisms during acidosis and intravenously administered bicarbonate are all additive and may result in overshoot alkalosis.[21]

Sodium Bicarbonate

Traditionally, $NaHCO_3$ has been the buffer of choice in the treatment of metabolic acidosis. A reasonable approach is to infuse sufficient $NaHCO_3$ to raise the arterial pH to no more than 7.2 over 30 to 40 minutes. $NaHCO_3$ therapy can cause

fluid overload and hypertension because the amount required can be massive when accumulation of lactic acid is relentless. Fluid administration is poorly tolerated because of central venoconstriction, especially in the oliguric patient. If the underlying cause of the lactic acidosis can be remedied, blood lactate will be converted to HCO_3^- and may result in an overshoot alkalosis. Proponents of $NaHCO_3$ infusion argue that the acidosis is detrimental to normal physiologic function. Although severe acidosis *may* have a deleterious effect on cardiopulmonary performance, recent studies have actually shown an improvement in cardiac performance in the presence of a mild-to-moderate acidosis.[5] Accordingly, the pH below which most clinicians feel obligated to use $NaHCO_3$ has declined. Therefore, the recommendation for administration of $NaHCO_3$ in the treatment of severe acidoses when the pH is less than 7.15 seems reasonable. At this pH, as predicted by the Henderson-Hasselbach equation, minor changes in bicarbonate or PCO_2 will result in a large decrease in pH.[22] However, there are no data supporting a specific pH at which therapy must be instituted.

A prospective study evaluating $NaHCO_3$ in patients with lactic acidosis showed an increase in serum pH but no improvement in hemodynamics when compared with normal saline.[23] The use of $NaHCO_3$ also failed to increase hemodynamic responsiveness to circulating catecholamines, concomitant with a decrease in serum ionized calcium.[24-27] Sodium bicarbonate may also result in impaired utilization of oxygen and increase anaerobic metabolism through stimulation by alkalemia of phosphofructokinase. Finally, sodium bicarbonate administration intravenously generates CO_2 (HCO_3^- + $H^+ \rightarrow H_2O + CO_2$). With depressed cardiac output, CO_2 can accumulate, causing intracellular acidosis and a further reduction in cardiac output. While severe acidosis may require bolus therapy initially (1 mEq/kg; one ampule contains 50 mEq), chronic sodium bicarbonate therapy is most easily administered as a near isotonic infusion rather than bolus therapy. Subsequent administration should be guided by arterial blood gas analysis. Note that bicarbonate is distributed roughly in the total body water. Therefore, the typical desired bicarbonate of 8 to 10 mEq/L can be used to predict the bicarbonate deficit in mEq as follows:

$$\text{Bicarbonate deficit} = (\text{desired} - \text{actual } HCO_3^- [\text{mEq/L}]) \times 0.5 \text{ L/kg} \times \text{body weight (kg)}.$$

The possible adverse effects of bicarbonate infusion include volume overload, hypercapnia, alkalemia, hyperosmolality, hypocalcemia, and hypokalemia.

Dichloroacetate

Dichloroacetate stimulates the activity of pyruvate dehydrogenase, thereby increasing the rate of oxidation of pyruvate and limiting the generation of lactate. Initial animal studies showed improved aerobic glucose utilization and an increase in intracellular adenosine triphosphate. A large multicenter trial showed a significant reduction in serum lactate, an increase in arterial pH, and an increase in the number of patients able to resolve hyperlactatemia from 43% to 58%.[17] Nevertheless, although dichloroacetate was effective in improving lactic acidosis, there was no decrease in mortality. Chronic use of dichloroacetate has been associated with neurologic toxicity, including limb paralysis and neuropathies.[28] In summary, dichloroacetate is not recommended in the therapy for lactic acid acidosis.

Carbicarb

Carbicarb is an equimolar mixture of sodium bicarbonate and sodium carbonate designed to decrease the CO_2 burden that results from the administration of sodium bicarbonate.[29] It has been proposed that Carbicarb is superior to sodium bicarbonate because it has an equal buffering capacity but does not result in the generation of CO_2.[30] Animal studies examining the effects of Carbicarb have shown stabilization of serum lactate levels as well as improved acid-base profile. In contrast, sodium bicarbonate administration increased lactate, lowered intracellular pH, and increased P_{CO_2}.[31] Carbicarb administration also resulted in a significant increase in cardiac index when compared with normal saline and sodium bicarbonate. Controlled studies examining the effectiveness of Carbicarb in the clinical setting have not yet been reported. This buffer, however, is not presently available for use.

Tromethamine

Tromethamine (THAM) is rarely used for lactic acidosis. Theoretically, this biologically inert amino alcohol buffers both CO_2 and nonvolatile acids. THAM, which is available as the acetate salt (0.3 mol / L), acts as a proton acceptor and has a pK of 7.8, indicating that it should function as an effective buffer at a pH of 7.4. The maximum daily dose of THAM in a 70-kg patient is 3.5 L or 15 mmol/kg. THAM is excreted in the urine and should be avoided in renal insufficiency. Severe hyperkalemia, hypoglycemia, ventilatory depression, and hepatic necrosis in neonates have been reported.[32] Given the risks of serious side effects, THAM should be used only after careful consideration or not at all.

D-Lactic Acidosis

D-Lactic acidosis should be considered in patients with a history of intestinal disease who present with confusion and AG metabolic acidosis. Overproduction of D-lactate may occur when there is overgrowth of gut bacteria.[33] Patients present with an AG acidosis, normal L-lactate levels, and neurologic findings such as confusion, ataxia, and loss of memory (see Table 127-5). Symptoms are worsened after high carbohydrate meals or oral hyperalimentation or tube feedings. In patients with short bowel syndrome or who have undergone jejunal-ileal bypass there not only is an overgrowth of bacteria but also accumulation of carbohydrate in the colon. Sufficient D-lactate can be produced to overwhelm enzymatic clearance. Treatment is directed at decreasing the overgrowth of bacteria with antibiotics and the avoidance of high carbohydrate feeding.

Ketoacidosis

See Table 127-5.

Diabetic Ketoacidosis

This condition is caused by increased fatty acid metabolism and the accumulation of ketoacids (acetoacetate and β-hydroxybutyrate). DKA usually occurs in insulin-dependent diabetes mellitus in association with cessation of insulin or with an intercurrent illness, such as an infection, gastroenteritis, pancreatitis, or myocardial infarction. Each of these conditions increases insulin requirements temporarily and acutely. The accumulation of ketoacids accounts for the increment in the AG and is accompanied most often by hyperglycemia [glucose > 17 mmol/L (300 mg/dL)]. It should be noted that because insulin prevents production of ketones, bicarbonate

therapy is rarely needed except with extreme acidemia (pH < 7.1), and then in only limited amounts (see Treatment of Lactic Acidosis).

Treatment of Diabetic Ketoacidosis. The general principles of treatment of DKA include (1) use of a flow sheet with frequent monitoring and recording of electrolyte values, (2) fluid replacement to correct the consequences of the preceding osmotic diuresis, (3) identification of the precipitating cause of the ketoacidosis (infection), and (4) anticipation of the consequences of therapy, especially if alkali therapy is included in the regimen. Most patients with DKA require correction of the volume depletion that almost invariably accompanies the osmotic diuresis and ketoacidosis. The serum Na^+ concentration may be arithmetically corrected for the degree of hyperglycemia to determine the type of intravenous fluid needed (i.e., correct Na^+ by 1.6 to 1.8 mEq/L for each 100 mg/dL increment in plasma glucose). In general, it seems prudent to initiate therapy with isotonic saline at a rate of 1000 mL intravenously per hour. When the pulse and blood pressure have stabilized and the corrected serum Na^+ concentration is in the range 130 to 135 mEq/L, switch to 0.45% sodium chloride. Use of lactated Ringer's should be avoided. If the blood glucose level falls below 300 mg/dL, 0.45% sodium chloride with 5% dextrose should be administered.[34]

Low-dose intravenous insulin therapy (0.1 U/kg/h) smoothly corrects the biochemical abnormalities and minimizes hypoglycemia and hypokalemia.[34] Usually, in the first hour, a loading dose of the same amount is given initially as a bolus intravenously. Although regular insulin may also be administered intramuscularly (0.1 U/kg initially then 0.1 U/kg/hr), it should be noted that intramuscular insulin may not be effective in patients with volume depletion, which often occurs in ketoacidosis.

Total body K^+ depletion is usually present, although the K^+ level on admission may be elevated or normal. Because the plasma K^+ concentration should increase 0.6 mEq/L for each 0.1 unit decline in arterial blood pH, a normal or reduced K^+ value on admission indicates severe K^+ depletion and should be approached with caution. Administration of fluid, insulin, and alkali may cause the K^+ level to plummet. When the urine output has been established, 20 mEq of potassium chloride should be administered in each liter of fluid as long as the K^+ value is less than 4.0 mEq/L. Equal caution should be exercised in the presence of hyperkalemia, especially if the patient has renal insufficiency, because the usual therapy does not always correct hyperkalemia. Never administer potassium chloride empirically.

The arguments for and against alkali therapy have been summarized previously. The young patient with a pure AG acidosis ($\Delta AG = \Delta HCO_3^-$) usually does not require exogenous alkali because the metabolic acidosis should be entirely reversible. Elderly patients, patients with severe high-AG acidosis (pH < 7.15), or patients with a superimposed hyperchloremic component may receive small amounts of sodium bicarbonate by slow intravenous infusion (no more than 44 to 88 mEq in 60 minutes). Thirty minutes after this infusion is completed, arterial blood gas analysis should be repeated. Alkali administration can be repeated if the pH is 7.20 or less or if the patient exhibits a significant hyperchloremic component, but it is rarely necessary. The AG should be followed closely during therapy because it is expected to decline as ketones are cleared from plasma and herald an increase in plasma HCO_3^- as the acidosis is repaired. Therefore, it is not necessary to monitor blood ketone levels continuously. Hypokalemia and other complications of alkali therapy dramatically increase when amounts of sodium bicarbonate exceeding 400 mEq are administered. However, the effect of alkali therapy on arterial blood pH needs to be reassessed regularly and the total administered kept at a minimum, if necessary.[34]

Routine administration of PO_4^{-3} (usually as potassium phosphate) is not advised because of the potential for hyperphosphatemia and hypocalcemia.[34] A significant proportion of patients with DKA have significant hyperphosphatemia before initiation of therapy. In the volume-depleted, malnourished patient, however, a normal or elevated PO_4^{-3} concentration on admission may be followed by a rapid fall in plasma PO_4^{-3} levels within 2 to 6 hours after initiation of therapy.

Alcoholic Ketoacidosis

Chronic alcoholics can develop ketoacidosis when alcohol consumption is abruptly curtailed; it is usually associated with binge drinking, vomiting, abdominal pain, starvation, and volume depletion. The glucose concentration is low or normal, and acidosis may be severe because of elevated ketones, predominantly β-hydroxybutyrate. Mild lactic acidosis may coexist because of alteration in the redox state. The nitroprusside ketone reaction (Acetest) can detect acetoacetic acid but not β-hydroxybutyrate, so that the degree of ketosis and ketonuria can be underestimated. Typically, insulin levels are low and concentrations of triglyceride, cortisol, glucagon, and growth hormone are increased.

Treatment of Alcoholic Ketoacidosis. Extracellular fluid deficits should be repleted by intravenous administration of saline and glucose (5% dextrose in 0.9% NaCl). Hypophosphatemia, hypokalemia, and hypomagnesemia may coexist and should be corrected. Hypophosphatemia usually emerges 12 to 24 hours after admission, may be exacerbated by glucose infusion, and, if severe, may induce rhabdomyolysis, aspiration, and platelet dysfunction. Upper gastrointestinal hemorrhage, pancreatitis, and pneumonia may accompany this disorder.[35-38]

Drug- and Toxin-Induced Acidosis

(See Table 127-5)
Salicylates

Salicylate intoxication in adults usually causes respiratory alkalosis, mixed metabolic acidosis–respiratory alkalosis, or a pure high-AG metabolic acidosis. In the latter example, which is less common, only a portion of the AG is due to the salicylates. Lactic acid production is also often increased. Treatment should begin with vigorous gastric lavage with isotonic saline (not $NaHCO_3$) followed by administration of activated charcoal. In the acidotic patient, to facilitate removal of salicylate, intravenous $NaHCO_3$ is administered in amounts adequate to alkalinize the urine and to maintain urine output (urine pH > 7.5). While this form of therapy is straightforward in acidotic patients, a coexisting respiratory alkalosis may make this approach hazardous. Acetazolamide may be administered when an alkaline diuresis cannot be achieved, but this drug can cause systemic metabolic acidosis if HCO_3^- is not replaced. Hypokalemia may occur with an alkaline diuresis from $NaHCO_3$ and should be treated promptly and aggressively. Glucose-containing fluids should be administered because of the danger of hypoglycemia. Excessive insensible fluid losses may cause severe volume depletion and hypernatremia. If renal failure prevents rapid clearance of salicylate, hemodialysis can be performed against a bicarbonate dialysate.

Alcohols

Under most physiologic conditions, sodium, urea, and glucose generate the osmotic pressure of blood. Plasma osmolality is calculated according to the following expression:

$$P_{osm} = 2Na^+ + Glu + BUN \text{ (all in mmol/L)}$$

or, using conventional laboratory values in which glucose and BUN are expressed in milligrams per deciliter:

$$P_{osm} = 2Na^+ + Glu/18 + BUN/2.8$$

The calculated and determined osmolality should agree within 15 mmol/kg H_2O. When the measured osmolality exceeds the calculated osmolality by more than 15 to 20 mmol/kg H_2O, one of two circumstances prevails. Either the serum sodium is spuriously low, as with hyperlipidemia or hyperproteinemia (pseudohyponatremia), or osmolytes other than sodium salts, glucose, or urea have accumulated in plasma. Examples include mannitol, radiocontrast media, isopropyl alcohol, ethylene glycol, ethanol, methanol, and acetone. In this situation, the difference between the calculated osmolality and the measured osmolality (*osmolar gap*) is proportional to the concentration of the unmeasured solute. With an appropriate clinical history and index of suspicion, identification of an osmolar gap is helpful in identifying the presence of poison-associated AG acidosis.

Ethylene Glycol

Ingestion of ethylene glycol (commonly used in antifreeze) leads to a metabolic acidosis and severe damage to the central nervous system, heart, lungs, and kidneys. The increased AG and osmolar gap are attributable to ethylene glycol and its metabolites oxalic acid, glycolic acid, and other organic acids. Lactic acid production increases secondary to inhibition of the tricarboxylic acid cycle and altered intracellular redox state. Diagnosis is facilitated by recognizing oxalate crystals in the urine, the presence of an osmolar gap in serum, and a high-AG acidosis. Treatment should not be delayed while awaiting measurement of ethylene glycol levels in this setting. Treatment includes the prompt institution of a saline or osmotic diuresis, thiamine and pyridoxine supplements, fomepizole or ethanol, and hemodialysis. The intravenous administration of the alcohol dehydrogenase inhibitor fomepizole (4-methylpyrazole; 7 mg/kg as a loading dose) or ethanol intravenously to achieve a level of 22 mmol/L (100 mg/dL) serves to lessen toxicity because both compete with ethylene glycol for metabolism by alcohol dehydrogenase. Fomepizole, although expensive, offers the advantages of a predictable decline in ethylene glycol levels without the adverse effects, such as excessive obtundation, associated with ethyl alcohol infusion.

Methanol

The ingestion of methanol (wood alcohol) causes metabolic acidosis, and its metabolites formaldehyde and formic acid cause severe optic nerve and central nervous system damage. Lactic acid, ketoacids, and other unidentified organic acids may contribute to the acidosis. Due to its low molecular weight (32 Da), an osmolar gap is usually present. The treatment is similar to that for ethylene glycol intoxication, including general supportive measures, fomepizole or ethanol administration, and hemodialysis.

Ethanol

After absorption of ethanol from the gastrointestinal tract, it is oxidized to acetaldehyde, acetyl coenzyme A, and CO_2. A blood ethanol level greater than 500 mg/dL is associated with high mortality. Acetaldehyde levels do not increase appreciably unless the load is exceptionally high or the acetaldehyde dehydrogenase step is inhibited by compounds such as disulfiram, insecticides, and sulfonylurea hypoglycemia agents. Such agents in the presence of ethanol result in severe toxicity. Ethanol does not cause an increase in the AG or acidosis unless hypotension from profound intoxication ensues. The contribution of ethyl alcohol to osmolality can be estimated by dividing the blood alcohol level by 4.3.

Isopropyl Alcohol

Rubbing alcohol poisoning is usually the result of accidental oral ingestion or absorption through the skin. Although isopropyl alcohol is metabolized by the enzyme alcohol dehydrogenase, as is methanol and ethanol, isopropyl alcohol is not metabolized to a strong acid. Isopropyl alcohol is metabolized to acetone, and the osmolal gap increases as the result of accumulation of both acetone and isopropyl alcohol. Despite a positive nitroprusside reaction from acetone, the AG, as well as the blood glucose, is typically normal, not elevated, and the plasma HCO_3^- is not depressed. Thus, isopropyl alcohol intoxication does not typically cause metabolic acidosis. Treatment is supportive, with attention to removal of unabsorbed alcohol from the gastrointestinal tract, and intravenous fluids. Hemodialysis is effective but not usually necessary. Patients with severe isopropyl alcohol intoxication (blood levels greater than 100 mg/dL) may develop cardiovascular collapse and lactic acidosis. Such severe intoxication may benefit from more aggressive therapy, including hemodialysis.[39]

Paraldehyde

Intoxication with paraldehyde is now very rare but is due partly to acetic acid, the metabolic product of the drug from acetaldehyde[40] and other organic acids.[41-43]

Renal Failure

The hyperchloremic acidosis of moderate renal insufficiency is eventually converted to the high-AG acidosis of advanced renal failure. Poor filtration and reabsorption of organic anions contribute to the pathogenesis. As renal disease progresses, the number of functioning nephrons eventually becomes insufficient to keep pace with net acid production. Uremic acidosis is characterized, therefore, by a reduced rate of NH_4^+ production and excretion, primarily due to decreased renal mass. $[HCO_3^-]$ rarely falls below 15 mmol/L, and the AG rarely exceeds 20 mmol/L. The acid retained in chronic renal disease is buffered in part by alkaline salts from bone. Despite significant retention of acid (up to 20 mmol/day), the serum $[HCO_3^-]$ does not decrease further, indicating participation of buffers outside the extracellular compartment. Chronic metabolic acidosis results in significant loss of bone mass due to reduction in bone calcium carbonate. Chronic acidosis also increases urinary calcium excretion, proportional to cumulative acid retention.

Treatment of Renal Failure Acidosis

Both uremic acidosis and the hyperchloremic acidosis of renal failure require alkali replacement to maintain the $[HCO_3^-]$ between 20 and 24 mmol/L. This can be accomplished most

TABLE 127–6. DIFFERENTIAL DIAGNOSIS OF HYPERCHLOREMIC METABOLIC ACIDOSIS

Gastrointestinal Bicarbonate Loss

Diarrhea
External pancreatic or small bowel drainage
Ureterosigmoidostomy, jejunal loop
Drugs
    Calcium chloride (acidifying agent)
    Magnesium sulfate (diarrhea)
    Cholestyramine (bile acid diarrhea)

Renal Acidosis

Hypokalemia
    Proximal RTA (type 2)
    Distal (classic) RTA (type 1)
Hyperkalemia
    Generalized distal nephron dysfunction (type 4 RTA)
        Mineralocorticoid deficiency
        Mineralocorticoid resistance
        $\downarrow$ Na^+ delivery to distal nephron
        Tubulointerstitial disease
        Ammonium excretion defect
    Drug-induced hyperkalemia
Potassium-sparing diuretics (amiloride, triamterene, spironolactone)
Trimethoprim
Pentamidine
Angiotensin-converting enzyme inhibitors and angiotensin II
    receptor blockers
NSAIDs
Cyclosporine, tacrolimus
Normokalemia
Early renal insufficiency

Other

Acid loads (ammonium chloride, hyperalimentation)
Loss of potential bicarbonate: ketosis with ketone excretion
Dilution acidosis (rapid saline administration)
Hippurate
Cation-exchange resins

readily with relatively modest amounts of oral alkali (1.0 to 1.5 mmol/kg/day) on a chronic basis. It is assumed that alkali replacement prevents the harmful effects of H^+ balance on bone and prevents or retards muscle catabolism. For patients in the ICU oral bicarbonate therapy may not be possible and small amounts of daily intravenous bicarbonate supplement may be necessary. The development of acute renal failure with metabolic acidosis may necessitate the replacement of renal function by dialysis. Dialysis can provide sufficient replacement of bicarbonate through the use of bicarbonate in the dialysate. Bicarbonate is the preferred buffer for dialysate in the acute care setting whether dialysis is provided intermittently or continuously. Occasionally, citrate may be used in continuous renal replacement therapy as a regional anticoagulant. Citrate routinely results in both hypocalcemia and metabolic alkalosis requiring the administration of calcium chloride and 0.1N HCl intravenously, respectively.

NON-GAP OR HYPERCHLOREMIC METABOLIC ACIDOSES

Alkali can be lost from the gastrointestinal tract in diarrhea or from the kidneys (renal tubular acidosis [RTA]). In these disorders (Table 127-6) reciprocal changes in $[Cl^-]$ and $[HCO_3^-]$ result in a normal AG. In pure hyperchloremic acidosis, therefore, the increase in $[Cl^-]$ above the normal value approximates the decrease in $[HCO_3^-]$. The absence of such a relationship suggests a mixed disturbance.

Diarrhea

With diarrhea, stools contain a higher $[HCO_3^-]$ and decomposed HCO_3^- than plasma so that metabolic acidosis develops along with volume depletion. Instead of an acid urine pH (as anticipated with systemic acidosis), urine pH is usually around 6 because metabolic acidosis and hypokalemia increase renal synthesis and excretion of NH_4^+, thus providing a urinary buffer that increases urine pH. Metabolic acidosis due to gastrointestinal losses with a high urine pH can be differentiated from RTA because urinary NH_4^+ excretion is typically low in RTA and high with diarrhea. Urinary NH_4^+ levels can be estimated by calculating the urine AG (UAG):

$$UAG = [Na^+ + K^+]_u - [Cl^-]_u$$

When $[Cl^-]_u$ is greater than $[Na^+ + K^+]$, and the UAG is negative, the urine ammonium level is appropriately increased, suggesting an extrarenal cause of the acidosis. Conversely when the UAG is positive, the urine ammonium level is low, suggesting a renal cause of the acidosis.

Renal Tubular Disease

Loss of functioning renal parenchyma by progressive renal disease leads to hyperchloremic acidosis when the glomerular filtration rate (GFR) is between 20 and 50 mL/min and to uremic acidosis with a high AG when the GFR falls to less than 20 mL/min. Such a progression occurs commonly with tubulointerstitial forms of renal disease, but hyperchloremic metabolic acidosis can persist with advanced glomerular disease. In advanced renal failure, ammoniagenesis is reduced in proportion to the loss of functional renal mass, and ammonium accumulation and trapping in the outer medullary collecting tubule may also be impaired. Because of adaptive increases in K^+ secretion by the collecting duct and colon, the acidosis of chronic renal insufficiency is typically normokalemic (see Table 127-6).

Proximal RTA (type 2 RTA) is most often due to generalized proximal tubular dysfunction manifested by glycosuria, generalized aminoaciduria, and phosphaturia (Fanconi's syndrome). With a low plasma $[HCO_3^-]$, the urine pH is acid (pH < 5.5). The fractional excretion of $[HCO_3^-]$ may exceed 10% to 15% when the serum HCO_3^- is greater than 20 mmol/L. Because HCO_3^- is not reabsorbed normally in the proximal tubule, therapy with $NaHCO_3$ will enhance renal potassium wasting and hypokalemia (see Table 127-6).

The typical findings in classic distal RTA (type 1 RTA) include hypokalemia, hyperchloremic acidosis, low urinary NH_4^+ excretion (positive UAG, low urine $[NH_4^+]$), and inappropriately high urine pH (pH > 5.5). Such patients are unable to acidify the urine below a pH of 5.5. Most patients have hypocitraturia and hypercalciuria, so that nephrolithiasis, nephrocalcinosis, and bone disease are common. In type 4 RTA, hyperkalemia is disproportionate to the reduction in GFR because of coexisting dysfunction of potassium and acid secretion. Urinary ammonium excretion is invariably depressed, and renal function may be compromised, for example, owing to diabetic nephropathy, amyloidosis, or tubulointerstitial disease.

Hyporeninemic Hypoaldosteronism

This condition typically causes hyperchloremic metabolic acidosis, most commonly in older adults with diabetes mellitus or tubulointerstitial disease and renal insufficiency. This disorder is not uncommonly recognized in the ICU (Table 127-7). Patients usually have mild to moderate renal insufficiency and acidosis, with elevation in serum $[K^+]$ (5.2 to 6.0 mmol/L), concurrent hypertension, and congestive heart failure. Both the metabolic acidosis and the hyperkalemia are out of proportion to impairment in GFR. Nonsteroidal anti-inflammatory drugs, trimethoprim, pentamidine, and angiotensin-converting enzyme inhibitors can also cause hyperkalemia with hyperchloremic metabolic acidosis in patients with renal insufficiency (Table 127-8).

Hyperchloremic metabolic acidosis has been reported to occur in patients receiving total parenteral nutrition containing synthetic L-amino acid preparations (see Table 127-6). This effect is thought to be secondary to an excess of cationic amino acids as compared with anionic amino acids present in these formulas. The severity of the acidosis associated with the use of protein solutions is less than that encountered with the use of the older protein hydrosylate formulations.[5,44] To minimize the possibility of inducing acidosis, parenteral nutrition solutions should be buffered with acetate or other organic anion.

TABLE 127–7. ISOLATED HYPOALDOSTERONISM IN THE CRITICALLY ILL PATIENT

Elevated ACTH and cortisol levels in association with a decrease in aldosterone elaboration
  Inhibition of aldosterone synthase
    Heparin
    Hypoxia
    Cytokines
    Atrial natriuretic peptide (ANP)
Manifestations of hypoaldosteronism
  Hyperkalemia
  Metabolic acidosis
Potentiated by K^+-sparing diuretics, K^+ loads in parenteral nutrition, or heparin

---

TABLE 127–8. CAUSES OF DRUG-INDUCED HYPERKALEMIA

Impaired Renin-Aldosterone Elaboration/Function

Cyclooxygenase inhibitors (NSAIDs)
Beta-adrenergic antagonists
Spironolactone
Angiotensin-converting enzyme inhibitors and angiotensin II receptor blockers
Heparin

Inhibitors of Renal Potassium Secretion

Potassium-sparing diuretics (amiloride, triamterene)
Trimethoprim
Pentamidine
Cyclosporine
Digitalis overdose
Lithium

Altered Potassium Distribution

Insulin antagonists (somatostatin, diazoxide)
Beta-adrenergic antagonists
Alpha-adrenergic agonists
Hypertonic solutions
Digitalis
Succinylcholine
Arginine hydrochloride, lysine hydrochloride

Dilutional Acidosis

A rapid increase in ECV can result in the development of hyperchloremic metabolic acidosis (see Table 127-6).[5,45] This phenomenon is thought to occur as a result of a change in the volume of distribution of bicarbonate, which leads to a decrease in serum concentration. Nevertheless, Garella and associates have demonstrated that the serum bicarbonate is only diluted modestly by large increases in extracellular volume.[46] Thus, a clinically significant metabolic acidosis would occur only with massive fluid administration. Dilutional acidosis, however, is not uncommon in the ICU. Critically ill patients are frequently hypoproteinemic, and infusion of 0.9% NaCl (154 mmol chloride/L) increases chloride concentration [Cl^-]. The intensivist should recognize this phenomenon and consider using solutions with lower chloride concentrations if large amounts of intravenous fluids are administered.

METABOLIC ALKALOSIS

Metabolic alkalosis is revealed by an elevated arterial pH, an increase in the serum [HCO_3^-], and an increase in $PaCO_2$ as a result of compensatory alveolar hypoventilation. It is often accompanied by hypochloremia and hypokalemia. The patient with a high [HCO_3^-] and a low [Cl^-] has either metabolic alkalosis or chronic respiratory acidosis. As shown in Table 127-1, the $PaCO_2$ increases 6 mm Hg for each 10-mmol/L increase in the [HCO_3^-] above normal. Stated differently, in the range of [HCO_3^-] from 10 to 40 mmol/L, the predicted $PaCO_2$ is approximately equal to the patient's [HCO_3^-] + 15. The arterial pH establishes the diagnosis, because it is increased in metabolic alkalosis and decreased or normal in respiratory acidosis. Metabolic alkalosis frequently occurs in association with other disorders such as respiratory acidosis or alkalosis or metabolic acidosis.[1,47]

PATHOGENESIS

Metabolic alkalosis occurs as a result of net gain of [HCO_3^-] or loss of nonvolatile acid (usually HCl by vomiting) from the extracellular fluid. Because it is unusual for alkali to be added to the body, the disorder involves a generative stage, in which the loss of acid usually causes alkalosis, and a maintenance stage, in which the kidneys fail to compensate by excreting HCO_3^- because of volume contraction, a low GFR, or depletion of Cl^- or K^+.[1, 47,48]

Under normal circumstances, the kidneys have an impressive capacity to excrete HCO_3^-. Continuation of metabolic alkalosis represents a failure of the kidneys to eliminate HCO_3^- in the usual manner. For HCO_3^- to be added to the extracellular fluid, it must be administered exogenously or synthesized endogenously, in part or entirely by the kidneys. The kidneys will retain, rather than excrete, the excess alkali and maintain the alkalosis if (1) volume deficiency, chloride deficiency, and K^+ deficiency exist in combination with a reduced GFR, which augments distal tubule H^+ secretion or (2) hypokalemia exists because of autonomous hyperaldosteronism. In the first example, alkalosis is corrected by administration of NaCl and KCl, whereas in the latter it is necessary to repair the alkalosis by pharmacologic or surgical intervention, not with saline administration.[47,48]

DIFFERENTIAL DIAGNOSIS

To establish the cause of metabolic alkalosis (Table 127-9), it is necessary to assess the status of the ECV, the recumbent

TABLE 127–9. CAUSES OF METABOLIC ALKALOSIS

Exogenous HCO_3^- Loads

Acute alkali administration
Milk-alkali syndrome

Effective Extracellular Volume Contraction, Normotension, K^+ Deficiency, and Secondary Hyperreninemic Hyperaldosteronism

Gastrointestinal origin
  Vomiting
  Gastric aspiration
  Congenital chloridorrhea
  Villous adenoma
  Combined administration of sodium polystyrene sulfonate
    (Kayexalate and aluminum hydroxide)
Renal origin
  Diuretics (especially thiazides and loop diuretics)
    Acute
    Chronic
  Edematous states
  Posthypercapnic state
  Hypercalcemia-hypoparathyroidism
  Recovery from lactic acidosis or ketoacidosis
  Nonreabsorbable anions such as penicillin, carbenicillin
  Mg^{++} deficiency
  K^+ depletion
  Bartter's syndrome (loss-of-function mutation of Cl^- transport in
    thick ascending limb of Henle's loop)
  Gitelman's syndrome (loss-of-function mutation in Na^+-Cl^-
    cotransporter)
  Carbohydrate refeeding after starvation

Extracellular Volume Expansion, Hypertension, K^+ Deficiency, and Hypermineralocorticoidism

Associated with high renin
  Renal artery stenosis
  Accelerated hypertension
  Renin-secreting tumor
  Estrogen therapy
Associated with low renin
  Primary aldosteronism
    Adenoma
    Hyperplasia
    Carcinoma
    Glucocorticoid suppressible
Adrenal enzymatic defects
  11β-Hydroxylase deficiency
  17α-Hydroxylase deficiency
Cushing's syndrome or disease
  Ectopic corticotropin
  Adrenal carcinoma
  Adrenal adenoma
  Primary pituitary
Other
  Licorice
  Carbenoxolone
  Chewer's tobacco
  Lydia Pincham tablets

Gain-of-Function Mutation of ENaC with Extracellular Fluid Volume Expansion, Hypertension, K^+ Deficiency, and Hyporeninemic Hypoaldosteronism

Liddle's syndrome

and upright blood pressure, the serum [K^+], and the renin-aldosterone system.[1] For example, the presence of chronic hypertension and chronic hypokalemia in an alkalotic patient suggests either mineralocorticoid excess or that the hypertensive patient is receiving diuretics. Low plasma renin activity and normal urine [Na^+] and [Cl^-] in a patient who is not taking diuretics indicate a primary mineralocorticoid excess syndrome. The combination of hypokalemia and alkalosis in a normotensive, nonedematous patient can be due to Bartter's or Gitelman's syndrome, magnesium deficiency, vomiting, exogenous alkali, or diuretic ingestion. Determination of urine electrolytes (especially the urine [Cl⁻]) and screening of the urine for diuretics may be helpful. If the urine is alkaline, with an elevated [Na⁺] and [K⁺] but low [Cl⁻], the diagnosis is usually either vomiting (overt or surreptitious) or alkali ingestion. If the urine is relatively acid and has low concentrations of Na⁺, K⁺, and Cl⁻, the most likely possibilities are prior vomiting, the posthypercapnic state, or prior diuretic ingestion. If, on the other hand, neither the urine sodium, potassium, nor chloride concentrations are depressed, magnesium deficiency, Bartter's or Gitelman's syndrome, or current diuretic ingestion should be considered. Bartter's syndrome is distinguished from Gitelman's syndrome because of hypocalciuria and hypomagnesemia in the latter disorder. The genetic and molecular basis of these two disorders has been elucidated recently.[1,47]

ALKALI ADMINISTRATION

Chronic administration of alkali to individuals with normal renal function rarely causes alkalosis because the kidney has a high capacity for bicarbonate excretion. However, in patients with coexistent hemodynamic disturbances, alkalosis can develop because the normal capacity to excrete HCO_3^- may be exceeded or there may be enhanced reabsorption of HCO_3^-. Such patients include those who receive oral or intravenous HCO_3^-, acetate loads (parenteral hyperalimentation solutions), citrate loads (transfusions or continuous renal replacement therapy), or antacids plus cation-exchange resins (aluminum hydroxide and sodium polystyrene sulfonate).

METABOLIC ALKALOSIS ASSOCIATED WITH EXTRACELLULAR FLUID VOLUME CONTRACTION, K⁺ DEPLETION, AND SECONDARY HYPERRENINEMIC HYPERALDOSTERONISM (see Table 127-9)

Gastrointestinal Origin

Gastrointestinal loss of H⁺ from vomiting or gastric aspiration results in retention of HCO_3^-. The loss of fluid and NaCl in vomitus or nasogastric suction results in contraction of the ECV and an increase in the secretion of renin and aldosterone. Volume contraction causes a reduction in GFR and an enhanced capacity of the renal tubule to reabsorb HCO_3^-. During active vomiting, there is continued addition of HCO_3^- to plasma in exchange for Cl⁻, and the plasma $[HCO_3^-]$ exceeds the reabsorptive capacity of the proximal tubule. The excess $NaHCO_3$ reaches the distal tubule, where secretion is enhanced by aldosterone and the delivery of the poorly reabsorbed anion HCO_3^-.[47,48] Because of contraction of the ECV and hypochloremia, Cl⁻ is avidly conserved by the kidney as recognized by a low urinary chloride concentration (Table 127-10). Correction of the contracted ECV with NaCl and repair of K⁺ deficits corrects the acid-base disorder.

Renal Origin
Diuretics
Drugs that induce chloruresis, such as thiazides and loop diuretics (furosemide, bumetanide, torsemide, and ethacrynic

TABLE 127–10. DIAGNOSIS OF METABOLIC ALKALOSIS

Saline-Responsive Alkalosis	Saline-Unresponsive Alkalosis
Low Urinary [Cl⁻]	*High or Normal Urinary [Cl⁻]*
Normotensive	Hypertensive
Vomiting, nasogastric aspiration	Primary aldosteronism
Diuretics	Cushing's syndrome
Post hypercapnia	Renal artery stenosis
Bicarbonate therapy of organic acidosis	Renal failure plus alkali therapy
K⁺ deficiency	Normotensive
Hypertensive	Mg⁺⁺ deficiency
Liddle's syndrome	Severe K⁺ deficiency
	Bartter's syndrome
	Gitelman's syndrome
	Diuretics

acid), acutely diminish the ECV without altering the total-body bicarbonate content. The serum $[HCO_3^-]$ increases. The chronic administration of diuretics tends to generate an alkalosis by increasing distal salt delivery, so that K⁺ and H⁺ secretion are stimulated. The alkalosis is maintained by persistence of the contraction of the ECV, secondary hyperaldosteronism, K⁺ deficiency, and the direct effect of the diuretic (as long as diuretic administration continues). Repair of the alkalosis is achieved by providing isotonic saline to correct the ECV deficit.

Bartter's Syndrome
Three types of Bartter's syndrome have been described, and all are inherited as autosomal recessive disorders. Both classic Bartter's syndrome and the antenatal Bartter's involve impaired Cl⁻ absorption, which results in volume depletion and activation of the renin-angiotensin system. Excessive prostaglandin elaboration is in response to volume depletion, hypokalemia, and high angiotensin II levels.[49-54] These phenotypes are the result of loss-of-function mutations of one of the genes that encode three transporters involved in vectorial NaCl absorption in the thick ascending limb of Henle's loop.[55] The most prevalent disorder is a mutation of the gene that encodes the bumetanide-sensitive Na⁺ 2Cl⁻ K⁺ cotransporter (*NKCC2* or *BSC1*) on the apical membrane. A second mutation has been discovered in the gene that encodes the apical K⁺ conductance channel (*ROMK*),[55] which operates in parallel with the Na⁺ 2Cl⁻ K⁺ transporter to recycle K⁺.[56] A third defect, in the basolateral Cl⁻ channel, which transports Cl⁻ out of the cell, has been described. All three defects have the same net effect: loss of Cl⁻ transport in the thick ascending limb of Henle's loop.[57,58] Such defects would predictably lead to extracellular fluid contraction, hyperreninemic hyperaldosteronism, and increased delivery of Na⁺ to the distal nephron and thus alkalosis and renal K⁺ wasting and hypokalemia. Secondary overproduction of prostaglandins, juxtaglomerular apparatus hypertrophy, and vascular pressor unresponsiveness would then ensue.

Distinction from surreptitious vomiting, diuretic administration, and laxative abuse is necessary to make the diagnosis of Bartter's syndrome.[59-65] The finding of a low urinary Cl⁻ concentration is helpful in identifying the vomiting patient (see Table 127-10).[60,65] The urinary Cl⁻ concentration in Bartter's syndrome would be expected to be normal or increased rather than depressed.

Treatment of Bartter's syndrome is generally focused on the repair of hypokalemia by inhibition of the renin-angiotensin-aldosterone or the prostaglandin-kinin system. K⁺ supplementation,[66] Mg⁺⁺ repletion,[62,67] propranolol,[68,69] spironolactone,[68,69] prostaglandin inhibitors, and angiotensin-converting enzyme inhibitors[70,71] have all been advocated, but each has met with limited success.

Gitelman's Syndrome

Gitelman's syndrome resembles Bartter's syndrome in that an autosomal recessive Cl⁻-resistant metabolic alkalosis is associated with hypokalemia, a normal to low blood pressure, volume depletion with secondary hyperreninemic hyperaldosteronism, and juxtaglomerular hyperplasia. Gitelman's syndrome, which occurs more often in adults, is distinguished from Bartter's syndrome, which occurs more commonly in children, because of the presence of hypocalciuria, hypermagnesuria, and hypomagnesemia.[72-74] These unique features mimic the effect of chronic thiazide diuretic administration. Gitelman's syndrome is the result of missense mutations (several have been described) in the gene *SLC12A3*, which encodes the thiazide-sensitive distal convoluted tubule Na⁺-Cl⁻-cotransporter (NCCT).[74-77] Loss of activity of the NaCl cotransporter increases tubule Ca⁺⁺ absorption, leading to the classic finding of hypocalciuria. A recent study has demonstrated that peripheral blood mononuclear cells from patients with Gitelman's syndrome express mutated NCCT mRNA.[78] Treatment of Gitelman's syndrome, as with Bartter's syndrome, consists of liberal dietary sodium and potassium salts, but with the addition of magnesium supplementation in most patients. Angiotensin-converting enzyme inhibitors have been suggested to be helpful in selected patients but can cause frank hypotension.

Nonreabsorbable Anions and Magnesium Deficiency

Administration of large quantities of nonreabsorbable anions, such as penicillin or carbenicillin, can enhance distal acidification and K⁺ secretion by increasing the transepithelial potential difference (lumen negative). Mg⁺⁺ deficiency results in hypokalemic alkalosis by enhancing distal acidification through stimulation of renin and hence aldosterone secretion.

Potassium Depletion

Pure K⁺ depletion causes metabolic alkalosis, although generally of only modest severity.[79-83] One reason that the alkalosis is usually mild is that K⁺ depletion also causes positive sodium chloride balance with[84-87] or without mineralocorticoid administration. The salt retention, in turn, antagonizes the degree of alkalemia.[83] When access to salt as well as to K⁺ is restricted, more severe alkalosis develops.[83] Activation of the renal H⁺,K⁺-ATPase in the collecting duct by chronic hypokalemia likely plays a major role in maintenance of the alkalosis. Specifically, chronic hypokalemia has been shown to markedly increase the abundance of the colonic H⁺, K⁺-ATPase mRNA and protein in the outer medullary collecting duct. In animals, the alkalosis is maintained in part by reduction in GFR without a change in tubule HCO₃⁻ transport.[88] In humans the pathophysiologic basis of the alkalosis has not been well defined. Alkalosis associated with severe K⁺ depletion, however, is resistant to salt administration.[89] Repair of the K⁺ deficiency is necessary to correct the alkalosis.[79-83,89]

After Treatment of Lactic Acidosis or Ketoacidosis

When an underlying stimulus for the generation of lactic acid or ketoacid is removed rapidly, as with repair of circulatory insufficiency or with insulin therapy, the lactate or ketones are metabolized to yield an equivalent amount of HCO₃⁻. Other sources of new HCO₃⁻ are additive, with the original amount generated by organic anion metabolism to create a surfeit of HCO₃⁻. Such sources include (1) new HCO₃⁻ added to the blood by the kidneys as a result of enhanced acid excretion during the preexisting period of acidosis and (2) alkali therapy during the treatment phase of the acidosis. Acidosis-induced contraction of the ECV and K⁺ deficiency act to sustain the alkalosis.

Post Hypercapnia

Prolonged CO_2 retention with chronic respiratory acidosis enhances renal HCO₃⁻ absorption and the generation of new HCO₃⁻ (increased net acid excretion). If the $PaCO_2$ is returned to normal, metabolic alkalosis results from the persistently elevated [HCO₃⁻]. Alkalosis develops if the elevated $PaCO_2$ is abruptly returned toward normal by a change in mechanically controlled ventilation. Associated ECV contraction does not allow complete repair of the alkalosis by correction of the $PaCO_2$ alone, and alkalosis persists until Cl⁻ supplementation is provided.

METABOLIC ALKALOSIS ASSOCIATED WITH EXTRACELLULAR FLUID VOLUME EXPANSION, HYPERTENSION, AND HYPERALDOSTERONISM

Mineralocorticoid administration or excess production (primary aldosteronism of Cushing's syndrome and adrenal cortical enzyme defects) increases net acid excretion and may result in metabolic alkalosis, which may be worsened by associated K⁺ deficiency. ECV expansion from salt retention causes hypertension and antagonizes the reduction in GFR and/or increases tubule acidification induced by aldosterone and by K⁺ deficiency. The kaliuresis persists and causes continued K⁺ depletion with polydipsia, inability to concentrate the urine, and polyuria. Increased aldosterone levels may be the result of autonomous primary adrenal overproduction or of secondary aldosterone release due to renal overproduction of renin. In both situations, the normal feedback of ECV on net aldosterone production is disrupted and hypertension from volume retention can result (see Table 127-9).

Liddle's syndrome results from increased activity of the collecting duct Na⁺ channel (ENaC). Liddle's syndrome is a rare inherited disorder associated with hypertension due to volume expansion manifested as hypokalemic alkalosis and normal aldosterone levels.

SYMPTOMS OF METABOLIC ALKALOSIS

With metabolic alkalosis, changes in central and peripheral nervous system function are similar to those of hypocalcemia; symptoms include mental confusion, obtundation, and a predisposition to seizures, paresthesia, muscular cramping, tetany, aggravation of arrhythmias, and hypoxemia in chronic obstructive pulmonary disease. Related electrolyte abnormalities include hypokalemia and hypophosphatemia.

TREATMENT OF METABOLIC ALKALOSIS

The maintenance of metabolic alkalosis represents a failure of the kidney to excrete bicarbonate efficiently because of chloride or potassium deficiency, or continuous mineralocorticoid elaboration, or both. Treatment is primarily directed at correcting the underlying stimulus for HCO_3^- generation and restoring the ability of the kidney to excrete the excess bicarbonate.[1,47-48] Assistance is gained in the diagnosis and treatment of metabolic alkalosis by paying attention to the urinary chloride concentration, the arterial blood pressure, and the volume status of the patient (particularly the presence or absence of orthostasis) (see Table 127-10).[1] Particularly helpful in the history is the presence or absence of vomiting, diuretic use, or alkali therapy. A high urine chloride concentration and hypertension suggests that mineralocorticoid excess is present. If primary aldosteronism is present, correction of the underlying cause will reverse the alkalosis (adenoma, bilateral hyperplasia, Cushing's syndrome). Patients with bilateral adrenal hyperplasia may respond to spironolactone. Normotensive patients with a high urine chloride may have Bartter's or Gitelman's syndrome if diuretic use or vomiting can be excluded. A low urine chloride and relative hypotension suggests a chloride-responsive metabolic alkalosis such as vomiting or nasogastric suction. [H^+] loss by the stomach or kidneys can be mitigated by the use of proton-pump inhibitors or the discontinuation of diuretics. The second aspect of treatment is to remove the factors that sustain HCO_3^- reabsorption, such as ECV contraction or K^+ deficiency. Although K^+ deficits should be repaired, NaCl therapy is usually sufficient to reverse the alkalosis if ECV contraction is present, as indicated by a low urine [Cl^-].

Patients with congestive heart failure or unexplained volume overexpansion represent special challenges in the ICU. Patients with a low urine chloride concentration, which is usually indicative of a "chloride-responsive" form of metabolic alkalosis, may not tolerate normal saline infusion. Renal HCO_3^- loss can be accelerated by administration of acetazolamide (250 to 500 mg i.v.), a carbonic anhydrase inhibitor, if associated conditions preclude infusion of saline (elevated pulmonary capillary wedge pressure, or evidence of CHF). Acetazolamide is usually very effective in patients with adequate renal function, but can exacerbate urinary K^+ losses. Dilute hydrochloric acid (0.1 N HCl) is also effective but can cause hemolysis and may be difficult to titrate. If used, the goal should be to not restore the pH to normal but to a pH of approximately 7.50. Alternatively, acidification can also be achieved with oral NH_4Cl, which should be avoided in the presence of liver disease. Hemodialysis against a dialysate low in [HCO_3^-] and high in [Cl^-] can be effective when renal function is impaired. Patients receiving continuous renal replacement therapy in the ICU typically develop metabolic alkalosis with high bicarbonate dialysate or when citrate regional anticoagulation is employed. Therapy should include reduction of alkali loads via dialysis by reducing the bicarbonate concentration in the dialysate, or if citrate is being used, by infusion of 0.1 N HCl post filter.

ANNOTATED REFERENCES

Bonnet F, Bonarek M, Morlat P, et al: Risk factors for lactic acidosis in HIV-infected patients treated with nucleoside reverse-transcriptase inhibitors: A case-control study. Clin Infect Dis 2003;36:1324-1328.
The problem of NRTI-induced lactic acid acidosis in patients with HIV is evaluated by a case-controlled study to determine risk factors. Two factors were identified to be associated with an increased risk of lactic acidosis: (1) creatinine clearance less than 70 mL/min and (2) a low CD4+ T lymphocyte count before inception of therapy. Interestingly, the total cumulative exposure to NRTIs was not associated with an increased risk of lactic acid acidosis. Therefore, creatinine clearance and CD4+ T lymphocyte count should be monitored in patients infected with HIV and could lead to modifications in antiretroviral therapy to diminish the risk of occurrence of lactic acidosis.

Gudis SM, Mangi S, Feinroth M, et al: Rapid correction of severe lactic acidosis with massive isotonic bicarbonate infusion and simultaneous ultrafiltration. Nephron 1983;33:65.
Although this is an older study, the use of continuous forms of renal replacement therapy to control volume overload to allow infusion of massive amounts of isotonic bicarbonate solution deserves a more comprehensive evaluation as an approach to treatment in patients with severe lactic acid acidosis.

Halperin ML, Hammeke M, Jose RG, et al: Metabolic acidosis in the alcoholic: A pathophysiologic approach. Metabolism 1983;32:308.
Alcoholic ketoacidosis is underdiagnosed clinically. This disorder cannot only result in life-threatening acidemia but, as a result of malnutrition, causes life-threatening hypophosphatemia. This scholarly review explains the pathophysiology and provides a basis for appreciation of the clinical syndrome.

Ogedegbe AE, Thomas DL, Diehl AM: Hyperlactatemia syndromes associated with HIV therapy. Lancet Infect Dis 2003;3:329-337.
The incidence of hyperlactatemia, as revealed in this study, is now approaching 20% in HIV-infected patients receiving NRTIs. The reported incidence probably underestimates the actual occurrence of lactic acidosis in such patients, especially because recognition may be difficult because many patients remain asymptomatic. However, studies show that life-threatening metabolic acidosis with hepatic steatosis occurs with NRTI therapy. This important public health problem is summarized thoroughly in this paper.

Stacpoole PW, Nagaraja NJ, Hutson AD: Efficacy of dichloroacetate as a lactate-lowering drug. J Clin Pharmacol 2003;43:683-691.
This paper by the same senior author who performed the first controlled clinical trial of dichloroacetate for treatment of lactic acidosis in adults demonstrates that the maximum lactate-lowering effect of dichloroacetate is dose dependent but independent of time after administration. The study suggests that dichloroacetate could be effective in reducing lactate levels in patients with mild hyperlactatemia. This may be an important observation for ongoing investigation in low-level hyperlactatemia as it applies to a number of clinical circumstances.

Chapter 128

DISORDERS OF WATER BALANCE

Tomas Berl • Jeremy Taylor

KEY POINTS

1. **The concentration of sodium in extracellular fluid** is a reflection of the tonicity of body fluids, not of total body sodium content.

2. **The intake of water and the osmotic release of antidiuretic hormone** maintain the concentration of sodium in a very narrow range (138 to 142 mEq/L), despite great variation in water intake.

3. **Hyponatremia can occur with low, normal, or high total body sodium.** A measurement of urinary sodium is helpful in differentiating extrarenal and renal sodium losses in hypovolemic hyponatremia.

4. **Euvolemic hyponatremia** is the most commonly encountered form, and the syndrome of inappropriate antidiuretic hormone (SIADH) is most common in this setting.

5. **The duration of hyponatremia and the presence or absence of neurologic symptoms** determine the therapeutic approach.

6. **Acute hyponatremia should be treated rapidly, but chronic hyponatremia requires careful monitoring** to prevent an excessively rapid increase in serum sodium and demyelination.

7. **Vasoporessin antagonists** are now under investigation for the treatment of hyponatremia.

8. **Disorders in thirst** and vasopressin release or action lead to hypernatremia.

9. **Most patients admitted with hypernatremia are elderly**; most hospital-acquired hypernatremia is caused by inadequate water intake in patients with water losses due to either loop diuretics or high (parenteral or oral) protein loads leading to an osmotic urea diuresis.

10. **The treatment of hypernatremia** requires the administration (orally or parenterally) of electrolyte-free water; ongoing losses should not be ignored.

Water, the body's most abundant constituent, accounts for approximately 50% of lean body mass in females and 60% of lean body mass in males. As shown in Figure 128-1, total body water is distributed between the intracellular compartment (two thirds of total body water) and the extracellular compartment (one third of total body water). The extracellular compartment is subdivided into the interstitial compartment (three fourths of extracellular body water) and the plasma compartment (one fourth of extracellular body water).[1]

The concentration of solutes in body fluids, as reflected in extracellular fluid by the serum sodium ion concentration [Na$^+$], is tightly regulated between 138 and 142 mmol/L. This precise control is achieved by the maintenance of water balance; intake and losses are matched in a steady-state situation, despite marked fluctuations in daily solute and water intake. Water intake is determined primarily by thirst, as well as by learned social and cultural behaviors. Water excretion is controlled by the hypothalamic secretion of vasopressin (antidiuretic hormone [ADH]) and its target tissue, the renal collecting tubule. This allows for enormous flexibility, because the kidney is able to dilute or concentrate urine (osmolality as low as 50 mOsm/kg H_2O or as high as 1200 mOsm/kg H_2O), depending on the body's need to excrete or retain water, respectively. Thus under water loading conditions, the kidney can excrete up to 20 to 25 L of urine a day. Likewise, the kidney has the ability to excrete as little as 0.5 L of urine per day (under conditions of water deprivation).[1]

CONTROL OF SERUM SODIUM CONCENTRATION

Sodium is the most abundant cation in the extracellular compartment and is therefore the major determinant of plasma osmolality (Posm):

$$\text{Posm (mOsm/kg)} = 2[\text{Na (mEq/L)}] + [\text{Blood urea nitrogen (mg/dL)}/2.8] + [\text{Glucose (mg/dL)}/18]$$

Under normal physiologic conditions, plasma osmolality is maintained between 280 and 290 mOsm/kg. Fluctuations in plasma osmolality outside of this range are sensed by osmoreceptors in the hypothalamus, which is normally the primary determinant of the secretion of vasopressin (ADH), a cyclic octapeptide that is synthesized and secreted by supraoptic and paraventricular nuclei within the hypothalamus. The threshold for the osmotic release of vasopressin is 280 to 290 mOsm/kg, and the receptors are sensitive to changes in plasma osmolality of as little as 1% (Fig. 128-2). Alterations in this threshold occur in pregnancy, leading to an approximately 10 mOsm/kg decrease in this setting. The stimulus for vasopressin release is not limited to changes in osmolality; a number of nonosmotic stimuli can maintain vasopressin release, even in hypotonic conditions. The primary nonosmotic stimulus for vasopressin secretion is decreased

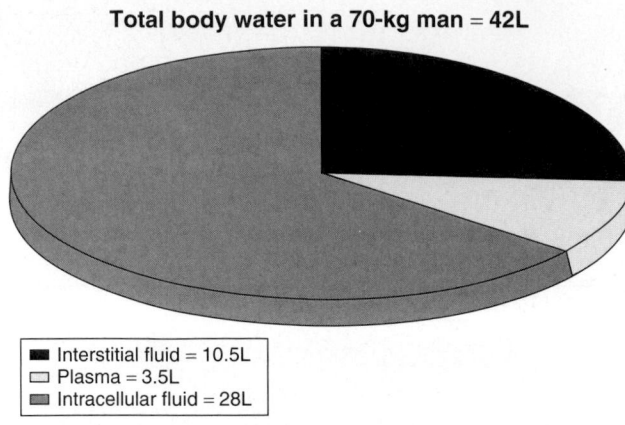

FIGURE 128–1. Body water distribution into different compartments. Extracellular fluid volume (14 L) is sum of interstitial fluid (10.5 L) and plasma fluid (3.5 L).

effective arterial blood volume, which can achieve a far greater rise in vasopressin levels than hyperosmolality can; however, a significant (>7%) fall in blood volume is required. Additional nonosmotic stimuli for vasopressin secretion include nausea, hypotension, and pain.

The primary site of action for vasopressin is within the principal cells of the renal collecting ducts. As illustrated in Figure 128-3, vasopressin binds to the V2 receptors on the basolateral membrane of these cells, which, through a G protein–activated cascade, results in the increased insertion of a specific water (aquaporin 2) in the luminal membrane.[2] This process renders the collecting tubule permeable to water.

Thirst also plays an important role in water balance. The most potent stimulus for thirst is hypertonicity; a change of 2% to 3% in plasma osmolality produces a strong desire to consume water. The threshold that triggers the sensation of thirst is higher than that for the release of vasopressin and usually occurs at a plasma osmolality of 290 to 295 mOsm/kg (see Fig. 128-2). A decrease in effective arterial blood volume also stimulates thirst, probably mediated by angiotensin II, a potent dipsogen.

Protection against states of water excess is provided by the normally functioning renal diluting system. The three essential components of the diluting mechanism are depicted in

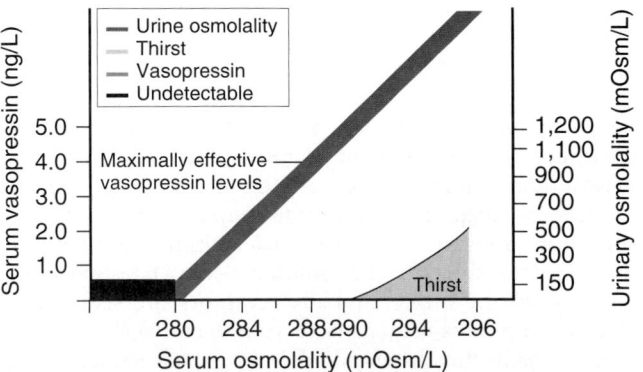

FIGURE 128–2. Mechanisms maintaining plasma osmolality. The response of thirst, vasopressin levels, and urinary osmolality to changes in serum osmolality. (From Johnson R, Feehally J [eds]: Comprehensive Clinical Nephrology. St. Louis, Mosby, 2003, p 83.)

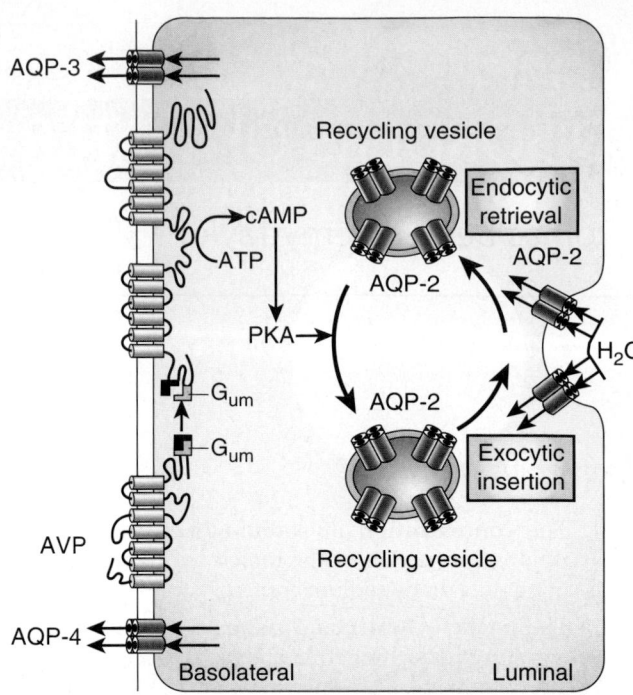

FIGURE 128–3. Intracellular action of vasopressin by its interaction with the V2 receptor on the basolateral membrane of the collecting duct. This interaction leads to increased adenylate cyclase activity via the stimulatory G protein (Gs), which in turn causes vesicles in the cytoplasm carrying the water channel protein aquaporin-2 (AQP-2) to move throughout the cell and fuse with the luminal membrane, thus increasing the water permeability of the collecting duct cells. These water channels are then recycled by endocytosis when the cell is no longer stimulated by vasopressin. ATP, adenosine triphosphate, AVP, arginine vasopressin; cAMP, cyclic adenosine monophosphate; PKA, protein kinase A. (From Kumar S, Berl T: Disorders of water metabolism. In Schrier RW [ed]: Atlas of Disease of the Kidney. Philadelphia, Current Medicine, 1999, pp 1.9-1.22.)

Figure 128-4. First, because the major site of urine dilution is the water-impermeable ascending limb of the loop of Henle and the distal convoluted tubule, it is necessary to have normal delivery of tubular fluid to the distal nephron. Therefore, either a decreased glomerular filtration rate or increased proximal tubule fluid reabsorption limits the volume of dilute urine available for excretion. Second, the diluting segment of the nephron (see Fig. 128-4) needs to be functioning normally. Thiazide diuretics, for example, impair the distal convoluted tubule's ability to maximally dilute tubular fluid by blocking the thiazide-sensitive Na^+/Cl^- channel. Third, in order to excrete a dilute urine, vasopressin must be absent so that the collecting duct remains impermeable to water. With this diluting system intact, the kidney can handle a large load of free water (up to 1 L/h) without changes in serum sodium and thus serum osmolality.

An individual's average daily solute load is approximately 600 mOsm. In states of low water intake, the kidney can concentrate the urine to 1200 mOsm/kg, therefore allowing for the excretion of as little as 0.5 L of urine per day. For this to occur, the renal concentrating mechanism must operate normally. The determinants of the renal concentrating mechanism are depicted in Figure 128-5. The water-impermeable thick ascending loop of Henle actively reabsorbs sodium chloride (NaCl) into the medullary interstitium while

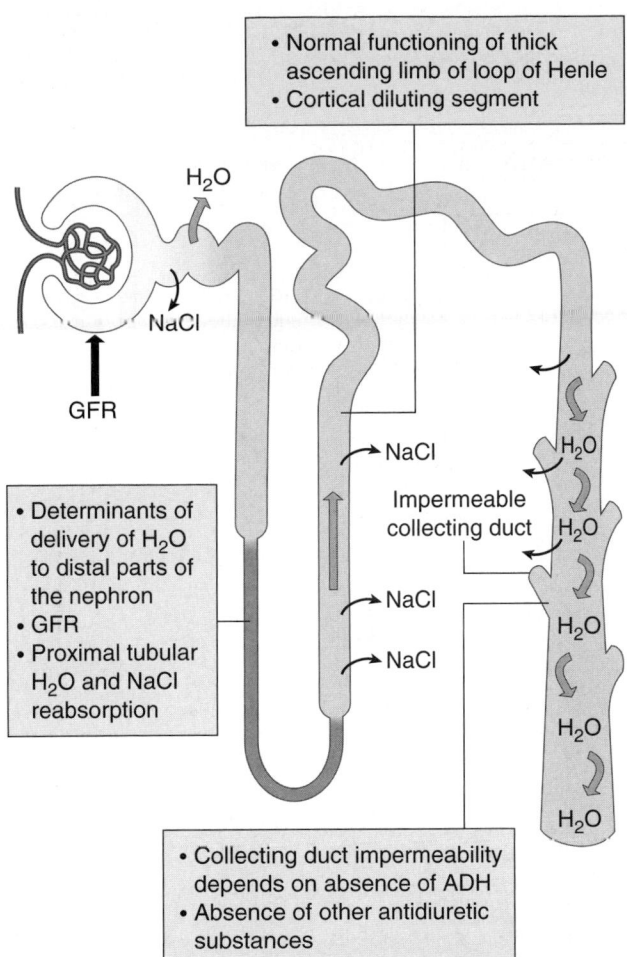

• Normal functioning of thick ascending limb of loop of Henle
• Cortical diluting segment

H_2O

NaCl

GFR

→ NaCl

Impermeable collecting duct

H_2O

H_2O

→ NaCl

→ NaCl

H_2O

• Determinants of delivery of H_2O to distal parts of the nephron
• GFR
• Proximal tubular H_2O and NaCl reabsorption

H_2O

H_2O

• Collecting duct impermeability depends on absence of ADH
• Absence of other antidiuretic substances

FIGURE 128–4. Determinants of the urinary dilution mechanism include (1) delivery of water to the thick ascending limb of the loop of Henle, distal convoluted tubule, and collecting system of the nephron; (2) generation of maximally hypotonic fluid in the diluting segments (i.e., normal thick ascending limb of the loop of Henle and cortical diluting segment); and (3) maintenance of water impermeability of the collecting system, as determined by the absence of antidiuretic hormone (ADH) or its action and other antidiuretic substances. GFR, glomerular filtration rate; H2O, water; NaCl, sodium chloride. (From Kumar S, Berl T: Disorders of water metabolism. In Schrier RW [ed]: Atlas of Disease of the Kidney. Philadelphia, Current Medicine, 1999 pp 1.9-1.22.)

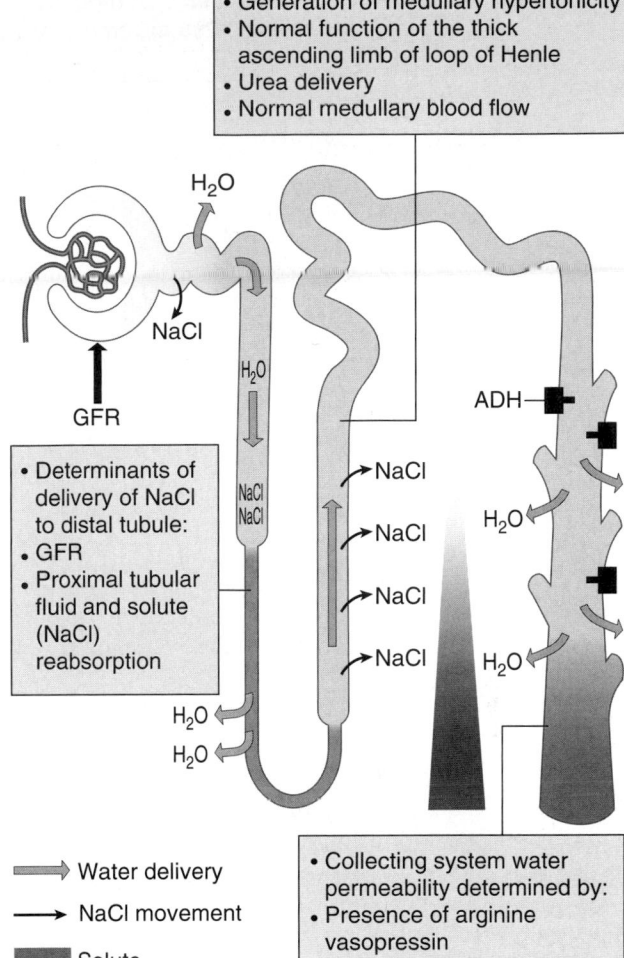

• Generation of medullary hypertonicity
• Normal function of the thick ascending limb of loop of Henle
• Urea delivery
• Normal medullary blood flow

H_2O

NaCl

GFR

H_2O

NaCl
NaCl

ADH

→ NaCl

H_2O

→ NaCl

→ NaCl

→ NaCl

H_2O

H_2O

H_2O

⟹ Water delivery
⟶ NaCl movement
▮ Solute concentration

• Collecting system water permeability determined by:
• Presence of arginine vasopressin
• Normal collecting system

FIGURE 128–5. Determinants of renal concentrating mechanisms: (1) Delivery of sodium chloride (NaCl) to the diluting segments of the nephron (thick ascending limb of the loop of Henle and distal convoluted tubule) is determined by glomerular filtration rate (GFR) and proximal tubule function. (2) Generation of medullary interstitial hypertonicity is determined by normal functioning of the thick ascending limb of the loop of Henle, urea delivery from the medullary collecting duct, and medullary blood flow. (3) Collecting duct permeability is determined by the presence of antidiuretic hormone (ADH) and normal anatomy of the collecting system, leading to the formation of a concentrated urine. (From Kumar S, Berl T: Disorders of water metabolism. In Schrier RW [ed]: Atlas of Disease of the Kidney. Philadelphia, Current Medicine, 1999 pp 1.9-1.22.)

leaving water behind in the tubular fluid. The reabsorbed sodium increases the osmolality of the interstitium, which reaches its maximum at the papillary tip of the medulla. In the presence of vasopressin, water in the collecting duct is able to travel down its osmotic gradient and is reabsorbed. Once vasopressin is secreted, the collecting duct must be able to respond to it. Any disorder or pharmacologic agent that impairs the ability of vasopressin to act on the collecting ducts will incapacitate the renal concentrating mechanism and lead to dilute urine excretion.

Figure 128-6 summarizes the mechanisms that maintain plasma tonicity and culminate in altered serum sodium values when impaired. These disorders arise whenever there is a disturbance in the body's regulation of the relative amount of water to sodium. Hyponatremia is caused by an increase in water relative to sodium (a water excess state), and hypernatremia results from a decrease in water relative to sodium (a water deficit state).

HYPONATREMIA

Hyponatremia is among the most common electrolyte disorders encountered in clinical practice.[3] It is defined as a serum sodium value less than 135 mEq/L.

Hyponatremia is usually associated with hypo-osmolality. There are, however, clinical settings in which this is not the case and plasma osmolality is normal or even high (Fig. 128-7). Translocational hyponatremia occurs when water moves from the intracellular space to the extracellular space in response to an osmotically active solute. The alteration in plasma sodium that occurs in this situation does not reflect a change in total body water. In clinical practice, translocational hyponatremia is most frequently seen in the setting of hyperglycemia,

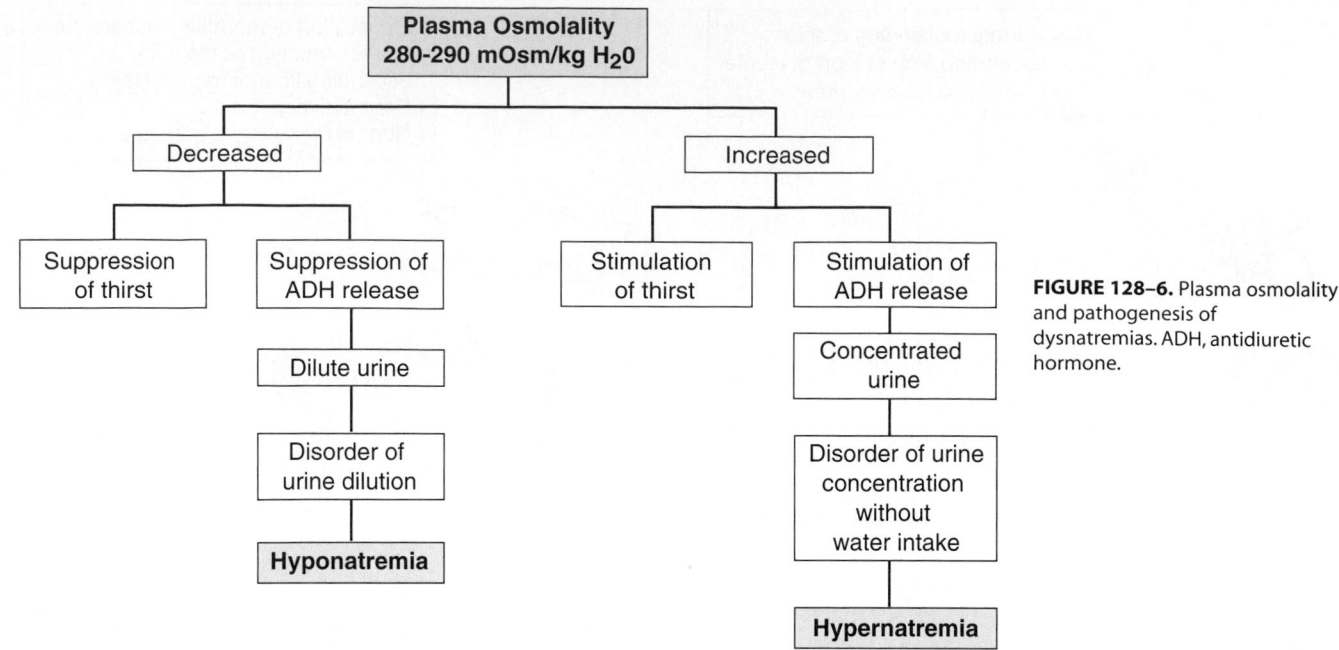

FIGURE 128–6. Plasma osmolality and pathogenesis of dysnatremias. ADH, antidiuretic hormone.

which accounts for 15% of hyponatremia in hospitalized patients.[4] The decrease in plasma sodium can be approximated as 1.6 mEq/L for every 100 mg/dL increase in plasma glucose concentration; it will return to normal with glycemia-lowering therapy. Recently, however, this correction factor has been challenged, in that it leads to a serious underestimation of serum sodium values in association with very high serum glucose concentrations (>500 mg/dL). It has been recommended that a correction factor of 2.4 be used in patients with severe hyperglycemia.[5]

Pseudohyponatremia occurs when the solid phase of plasma is increased by large quantities of lipids or proteins. A rise in plasma lipids of 4.6 g/L or plasma protein concentrations greater than 10 g/dL will decrease the sodium concentration by approximately 1 mEq/L. This occurs because the flame photometry method of measuring sodium uses whole plasma rather than just the liquid phase. This problem can be eliminated by employing methods that use only the liquid phase to measure sodium concentration, such as direct potentiometry in an undiluted sample.

Once it is established that a patient has true hypotonic hyponatremia, it is helpful to determine the patient's volume status. Placing the patient into one of three volume categories—hypovolemic, euvolemic, or hypervolemic—can narrow down the diagnostic possibilities. This method also helps define appropriate therapeutic approaches.[6] A thorough history and physical examination, supported by measurements of urinary sodium concentration, are essential in making this categorization (Fig. 128-8).

HYPOVOLEMIC HYPONATREMIA

Hypovolemic hyponatremia occurs when a patient has both a total body Na^+ deficit and a water deficit, with the former exceeding the latter. The underlying cause is the nonosmotic release of vasopressin in response to hypovolemia. Hypovolemia is the driving force, maintaining hormone secretion despite hypotonicity. Clinically, this occurs in patients with high gastrointestinal or renal losses of solute and water, in combination with an intake of hypotonic fluids.

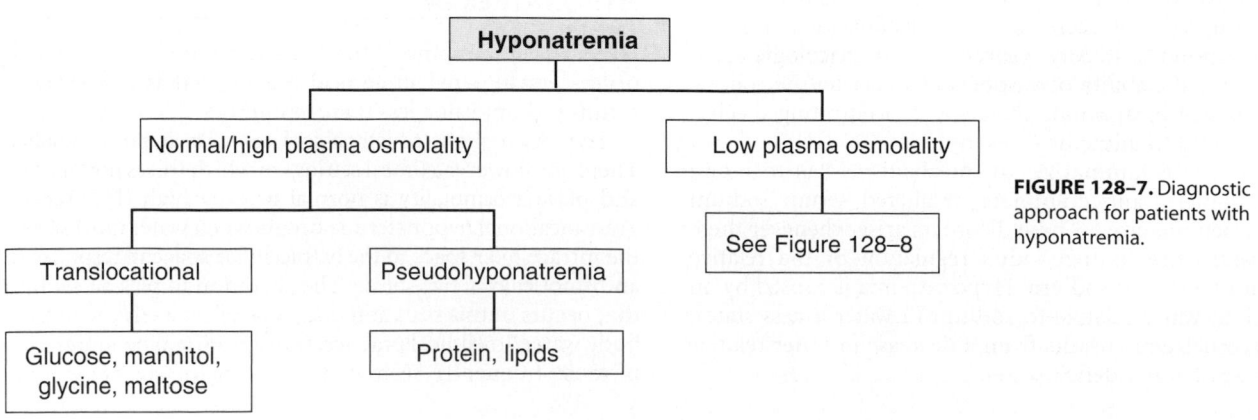

FIGURE 128–7. Diagnostic approach for patients with hyponatremia.

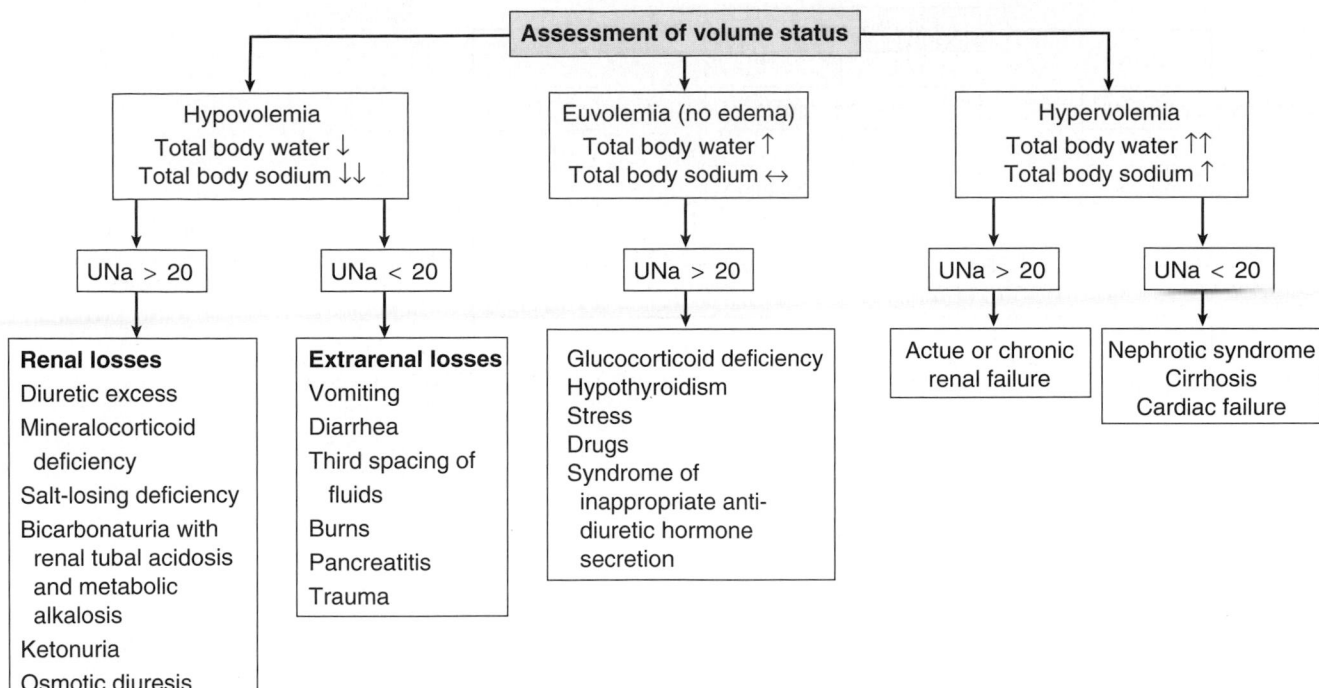

FIGURE 128–8. Diagnostic algorithm for hyponatremia. UNa, urinary sodium concentration. (Adapted from Parix G, Kumar S, Beil T: Disorders of water metabolism. In Johnson R, Feehally J (eds): Comprehensive Clinical Nephrology. St. Louis, Mosby, 2003, p 93.)

These patients exhibit signs of hypovolemia: tachycardia, orthostatic hypotension, flattened neck veins, dry mucous membranes, and decreased skin turgor. As illustrated in Figure 128-8, urinary sodium measurements can be instrumental in differentiating between extrarenal (urine $[Na^+] < 20$ mmol/L) and renal (urine $[Na^+] > 20$ mmol/L) losses.

Patients experiencing vomiting or diarrhea become volume contracted, and the kidney responds by avidly retaining Na^+ and chloride ions (Cl^-), thereby reducing the urinary $[Na^+]$ to very low levels (<10 mmol/L). A similar response is seen in disorders such as pancreatitis, peritonitis, or burns, in which third spacing of fluid leads to intravascular volume depletion and renal sodium conservation. An exception occurs in patients with vomiting and metabolic alkalosis. In this situation, bicarbonaturia results in higher urinary Na^+ excretion (>20 mmol/L), despite sometimes profound volume depletion. This results from the fact that bicarbonate (HCO_3^-) is a nonreabsorbable anion, and its excretion requires the excretion of cations as well, most notably sodium.

Diuretic use is one of the more common causes of hypovolemic hyponatremia, particularly thiazide diuretics. Diuretic-induced hyponatremia is associated with high urine $[Na^+]$. Loop diuretics inhibit the Na^+-K^+-$2Cl^-$ pump in the thick ascending loop of Henle (see Fig. 128-5) and therefore lead to renal salt loss (urine Na^+ >20 mmol/L). However, because this inhibition also interferes with generation of the hypertonic medullary interstitium, the responsiveness to vasopressin is decreased, and adequate urine dilution is still possible. In contrast, thiazide diuretics block the Na^+-Cl^- cotransporter in the distal tubule, directly impairing the urinary dilution capacity (see Fig. 128-4). Underweight women and elderly patients appear to be especially at risk for developing hyponatremia with thiazide use. Several proposed mechanisms for diuretic-induced hyponatremia,

which usually occurs within 2 weeks after starting the drug, have been put forth. One is that hypovolemia causes increased vasopressin secretion, decreased delivery of fluid to the diluting segment of the nephron, and potassium ion (K^+) depletion, resulting in increased thirst by alterations in osmoreceptor sensitivity.

Osmotically active, nonreabsorbable solutes also lead to renal sodium wasting (urine Na^+ > 20 mmol/L) and hypovolemia. As long as water intake persists, a diabetic patient with glucosuria, a patient with urea diuresis after recovery from postobstructive acute renal failure, and a patient with mannitol diuresis will all have urinary Na^+ losses in excess of water losses, leading to hyponatremia.

HYPERVOLEMIC HYPONATREMIA

Congestive heart failure, nephrotic syndrome, renal failure, and cirrhosis can all result in hypervolemic states with increased total body sodium and water. Hyponatremia occurs when the increase in total body water exceeds that of Na^+. All these conditions are associated with impaired water and salt excretion (Fig. 128-9).

In congestive heart failure, the decrease in effective arterial blood volume leads to vasopressin release through the activation of aortic and carotid baroreceptors. Water excretion is further limited by stimulation of the renin-aldosterone-angiotensin and sympathetic nervous system pathways. This results in a reduction in glomerular filtration rate. The low cardiac output and increased production of angiotensin II also potently stimulate thirst, leading to further hypotonicity. Patients with cirrhosis develop splanchnic arterial vasodilatation and arteriovenous fistulas, which also lead to a decreased effective arterial blood volume, increased vasopressin release, and, in the end, impaired water excretion and hyponatremia.

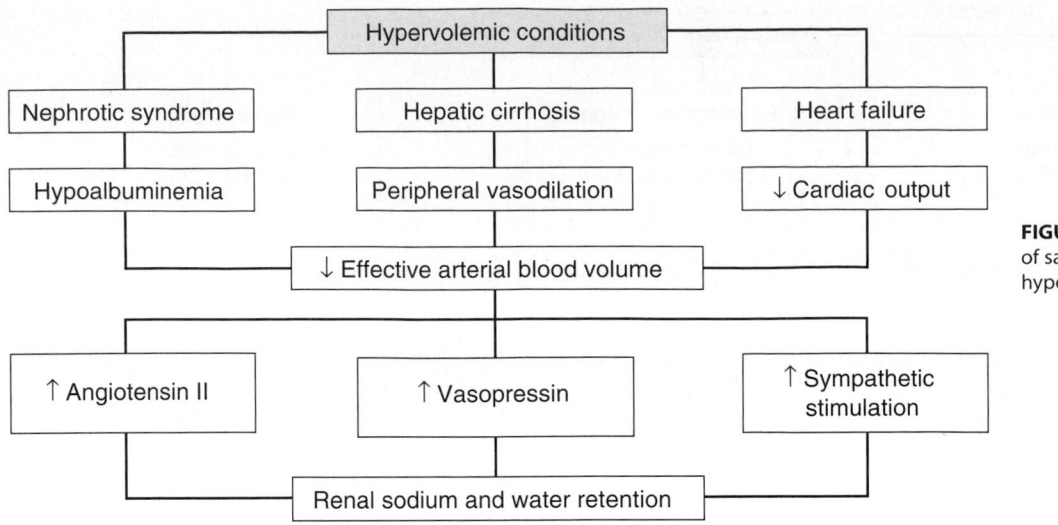

FIGURE 128–9. Pathophysiology of salt and water retention in hypervolemic disorders.

In contrast to those with congestive heart failure and cirrhosis, most patients with nephrotic syndrome have intravascular volume contraction resulting from an alteration in Starling forces from hypoalbuminemia and lowered plasma oncotic pressure. Volume contraction has been shown to stimulate vasopressin release in nephrotic subjects.[7] In advanced renal failure, the water-excreting capacity of the kidney is greatly reduced. Just as edema occurs when sodium intake exceeds the excretory capacity of the diseased kidney, hyponatremia occurs when the free water intake is greater than the ability to excrete solute-free water. Even with maximum suppression of vasopressin, a patient with a glomerular filtration rate of 5 mL/min may be able to excrete only a little more than 2 L of solute-free urine daily.[4]

EUVOLEMIC HYPONATREMIA

Euvolemic hyponatremia is the most commonly encountered dysnatremia in hospitalized patients. These patients have increased total body water but no clinical signs of increased total body Na^+. There are many causes of euvolemic hyponatremia (see Fig. 128-8), including many pharmacologic agents (Table 128-1), hypothyroidism, and glucocorticoid deficiencies. The most common cause, however, is the syndrome of inappropriate antidiuretic hormone (SIADH). This syndrome is characterized by an impaired suppression of vasopressin secretion relative to the degree of hypotonicity. Central nervous system disturbances, certain solid organ tumors (small cell cancer of the lung, pancreatic cancer, duodenal cancer), and human immunodeficiency virus (HIV) are some of the more notable causes, although many others exist. SIADH remains a diagnosis of exclusion, and certain criteria need to be met. The essential diagnostic criteria are a plasma osmolality less than 270 mOsm/kg H_2O; inappropriately concentrated urine osmolality greater than 100 mOsm/kg H_2O; clinical euvolemia; elevated urine Na^+ concentration under conditions of normal salt and water intake; and absence of adrenal, thyroid, pituitary, or renal insufficiency or diuretic use.[8]

SYMPTOMS

Patients with serum Na^+ concentrations above 125 mmol/L are usually asymptomatic, although some patients may have nausea and vomiting. Once serum Na^+ concentrations go below 125 mmol/L, neuropsychiatric symptoms predominate, mostly as a result of increasing cerebral edema. These include headaches, lethargy, ataxia, psychosis, seizures, coma, and death. Severe cerebral edema resulting in tentorial herniation can also occur, more commonly with the rapid development of hyponatremia. The mortality of severe hyponatremia approaches 50% if left untreated; therefore, the presence of any signs and symptoms warrants prompt intervention.[9,10]

TREATMENT

Certain patients have an increased risk of developing cerebral edema during hyponatremia (Table 128-2). Postoperative

TABLE 128–1. DRUGS ASSOCIATED WITH HYPONATREMIA

Vasopressin Analogs

Desmopressin (DDAVP)
Oxytocin

Drugs that Enhance Vasopressin Release

Chlorpropamide
Clofibrate
Carbamazepine, oxcarbazepine
Vincristine
Nicotine
Narcotics
Antipsychotics, antidepressants
Ifosfamide

Drugs that Potentiate Renal Action of Vasopressin

Chlorpropamide
Cyclophosphamide
Nonsteroidal anti-inflammatory drugs
Acetaminophen (paracetamol)

Drugs with Unknown Mechanism for Causing Hyponatremia

Haloperidol
Fluphenazine
Amitriptyline
Thioridazine
Fluoxetine
Sertraline

TABLE 128–2. HYPONATREMIC PATIENTS AT RISK FOR NEUROLOGIC COMPLICATIONS

Acute Cerebral Edema	Osmotic Demyelination Syndrome
Postoperative menstruant females	Alcoholics
Elderly women taking thiazides	Malnourished patients
Children	Hypokalemic patients
Psychiatric polydipsic patients	Burn patients
Hypoxemic patients	Elderly women taking thiazides

premenopausal women with hyponatremia are more likely to develop neurologic complications than are either postmenopausal women or men; thus, hypotonic fluids should not be used perioperatively in these patients. Patients on thiazide diuretics, particularly elderly women, are more susceptible to severe hyponatremia and its complications. Children, psychiatric polydipsic patients, and patients with hypoxia also seem to be at higher risk.

Certain subpopulations of patients are at greater risk of developing osmotic demyelination syndromes during treatment for hyponatremia (see Table 128-2). Susceptibility to osmotic demyelination is related to the severity and chronicity of the hyponatremia. Osmotic demyelination is rarely seen with serum Na^+ greater than 120 mmol/L or if the duration of hyponatremia is less than 24 to 48 hours. Severely hyponatremic patients with alcoholism, malnutrition, hypokalemia, or severe burns, as well as elderly women prescribed thiazide diuretics, appear to be at increased risk.[11] Osmotic demyelination initially presents as a generalized encephalopathy associated with the rapid correction of serum Na^+. The classic symptoms follow 2 to 3 days after the serum Na^+ is corrected; these include behavioral changes, cranial nerve palsies, and quadriplegia with a "locked-in" syndrome. Magnetic resonance imaging is diagnostic, but the typical lesions may not appear for up to 2 weeks after symptoms begin.[12]

An optimal treatment strategy for hyponatremia should focus on four factors: (1) presence or absence of symptoms; (2) duration of hyponatremia, if known; (3) patient's volume status; and (4) degree of hyponatremia (Fig. 128-10).

Rapid correction is indicated for patients with acute (<48 hours) symptomatic hyponatremia. In these circumstances, the risk of cerebral edema far exceeds the risk of treatment-related complications such as osmotic demyelination. The goal should be a rise in serum Na^+ of 2 mmol/L per hour until symptoms have resolved. Although it is not necessary to correct to normal serum Na^+ levels, doing so does not appear to be unsafe. Correction can usually be achieved using hypertonic saline solutions (3% NaCl) at a rate of 1 to

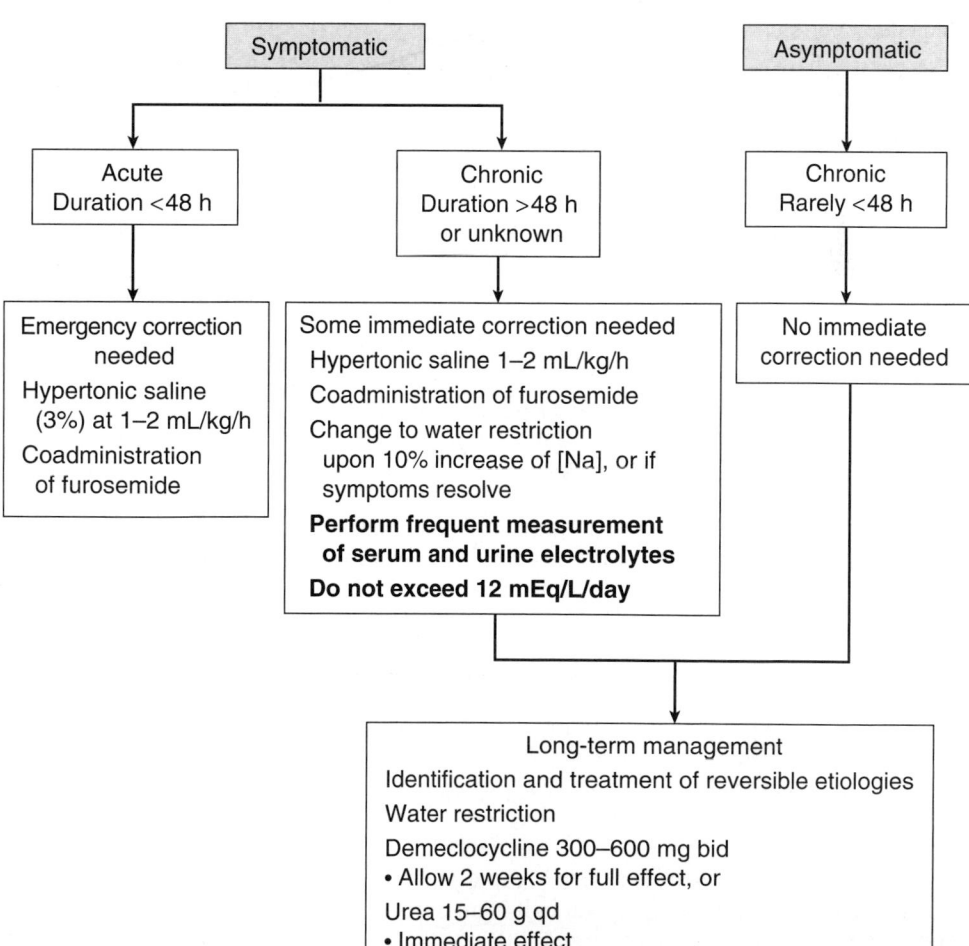

FIGURE 128–10. Treatment of severe (<125 mM/L) euvolemic hyponatremia. (Adapted from Thurman JM, Halterman RK, Berl T: Theory of dysnatremic disorders. In Brady H, Wilcox C (eds): Therapy in Nephrology and Hypertension, 2nd ed. Philadelphia, WB Saunders, 2003, pp 335-348.)

2 mL/kg per hour. If the patient is having severe symptoms (seizures, coma), higher rates of infusion can be used. The goal of this infusion is strictly to increase the serum tonicity rapidly, to prevent the development of life-threatening cerebral edema. Administration of a loop diuretic will help normalize the serum sodium concentration more readily by enhancing free water excretion and will prevent volume expansion from the administered NaCl. Patients receiving hypertonic saline solutions need to be monitored very closely, with frequent assessments of volume status, output, and electrolytes.

Symptomatic hyponatremia of longer than 48 hours' duration must be approached with extreme caution, because these patients have the greatest risk of complications. Partial correction of serum sodium in patients with chronic symptomatic hyponatremia should proceed without delay, because failure to correct is associated with poor outcome.[13] Cerebral water increases by about 10% during severe hyponatremia. With this in mind, it is safe to increase the serum sodium by 10% ($\approx$10 mmol/L), followed by water restriction. This aggressive treatment should continue until either the symptoms resolve or this 10% increase is reached. Thereafter, the correction rate should be less than 0.5 mmol/L per hour and should certainly not exceed 1 to 1.5 mmol/L per hour or 12 mmol/L per day. To prevent overcorrection, it is important to monitor the rate and electrolyte content of infused fluids and urine output. For example, if a patient is excreting large quantities of hypotonic urine and has already reached the desired magnitude or rate of correction, hypotonic fluids may need to be infused to prevent a too rapid rise in serum sodium concentration (for a detailed description of this approach, refer to reference 14).

The approach to patients with chronic asymptomatic hyponatremia is different. For those with euvolemic hyponatremia, a search for underlying, reversible causes should be undertaken. If SIADH is determined to be the diagnosis, and if the cause is either unknown or untreatable, a conservative approach is appropriate. The hallmark of this treatment strategy is fluid restriction. Calculating a patient's electrolyte-free water excretion can help guide the degree of water restriction necessary:

$$cH_2Oe = V[1 - (UNa + UK)/PNa],$$

where cH_2Oe is electrolyte-free water clearance, V is urine volume, UNa is urinary sodium concentration, UK is urinary potassium concentration, and PNa is serum sodium concentration.

To increase serum sodium, the amount of water intake needs to be less than the sum of the insensible losses and the free water excretion. This formula can be used to guide therapy, as follows:[15]

If (UNa + UK)/PNa is greater than 1, water intake should be less than 500 mL/day.
If (UNa + UK)/PNa is approximately 1, water intake should be 500 to 700 mL/day.
If (UNa + UK)/PNa is less than 1, water intake should be up to 1 L/day.

Free water restriction is usually successful as long as the patient is compliant. This becomes difficult in an outpatient setting if intake is restricted to less than 1 L/day. In these circumstances, alternative treatments, such as enhancing solute excretion or pharmacologic inhibition of vasopressin, may be necessary.

Demeclocylcine is the agent of choice to suppress vasopressin in patients with SIADH not responsive to free water restriction. The usual oral dose is 600 to 1200 mg/day, and this should be adjusted to the lowest dose that keeps the serum Na+ in the desired range with unrestricted water intake. Side effects of demeclocycline include skin photosensitivity and polyuria. Nephrotoxicity can also be seen, particularly in patients with liver disease who have impaired hepatic drug metabolism. However, the side-effect profile is far superior to that of lithium, which has been used in the past. Lithium, though effective in its antagonism of vasopressin, is limited by its neurotoxicity, nephrotoxicity, and narrow therapeutic window.

Specific vasopressin antagonists are under development and may soon supplement these other agents, as well as alleviate the need for strict water restriction. These oral, nonpeptide, V2-selective antagonists have had promising results in animal models of hyponatremia, as well as some success in treating SIADH patients.[16] In humans, these agents have demonstrated the ability to induce a water diuresis in healthy controls and in patients with SIADH.[16,17] One such antagonist, conivaptan, has been shown to be as effective as the more standard treatment of water restriction, furosemide, and urea. Conivaptan was well tolerated and appears to be safe for extended use.[18] Although some of these vasopressin antagonists also have V1 antagonistic properties, their overall effect appears to be aquaretic, without significant changes in blood pressure. In high doses, vasopressin antagonists might cause significant dehydration, so close monitoring is important.[19] Whether the oral V2 receptor antagonists will work in patients with high circulating levels of arginine vasopressin to produce an effective and sustained increase in serum sodium is not yet known. More clinical studies must be performed to determine appropriate dosing, particularly in the acute setting, where a too rapid correction could be deleterious. Nevertheless, these agents hold great promise, and from the patient's perspective, they would be a welcome alternative to water restriction.

Another option for patients who remain unresponsive to or noncompliant with fluid restriction is to enhance solute excretion. One approach is to increase Na+ intake (2 to 3 g of additional NaCl in the diet) in combination with a single dose of a loop diuretic (40 mg of furosemide is usually sufficient). The administration of urea (30 to 60 g/day) has a similar effect by promoting an osmotic diuresis. The major limitation to urea is the occurrence of gastrointestinal side effects.

Treatment of chronic hypovolemic hyponatremia requires repletion of volume. In this situation, neurologic symptoms are rare, because losses of both Na+ and water limit osmotic shifts within the brain. Restoring effective arterial volume will inhibit further vasopressin release and help normalize serum Na+ levels.

Hypervolemic hyponatremia can be very difficult to treat because it is often a sign of severe underlying cardiac, hepatic, or renal disease. Water restriction is important; however, these patients often experience extreme thirst, making compliance difficult. Loop diuretics increase free water excretion and can therefore be beneficial in raising serum Na+ values as well as treating edema. Thiazide diuretics should generally be avoided because they impair urinary dilution and may worsen the hyponatremia. Vasopressin receptor antagonists are also under investigation in these disorders but are not yet available for clinical use.[20] A study by Wong and colleagues investigated the efficacy of the vasopressin V2 antagonist VPA-985 in correcting hyponatremia in a group of patients, including 33 with cirrhosis and 6 with congestive heart failure.[19] VPA-985 produced a significant aquaresis, with significant increases in free water clearance and serum sodium levels. Unless the underlying disease process can somehow be improved, treating hyponatremia in these cases represents a significant clinical challenge.

HYPERNATREMIA

Hypernatremia is defined as a serum sodium concentration greater than 146 mEq/L. The incidence of hypernatremia in hospitalized patients ranges from 0.63% to 2.23%, with the elderly being more susceptible.[21] Hypernatremia results in significant morbidity and mortality, ranging from 42% to 70% in adult patients. Acute elevations of serum sodium above 160 mEq/L are associated with a mortality rate of 75%, whereas mortality in chronic hypernatremia is 10%.

Hypernatremia develops whenever intake is less than the sum of extrarenal and renal water losses or, less commonly, when too much salt is introduced without adequate water intake. The primary defense mechanism against water depletion and hyperosmolarity is the renal concentrating capacity. However, even maximally concentrated urine does not prevent all water losses. Thirst also plays an important role in preventing water depletion. As long as water losses can be replaced, normal serum sodium concentration can be maintained. Most hypernatremic patients therefore have either an inability to obtain free water or an impaired thirst sensation. Hypernatremic patients generally fall into one of three broad categories, based on overall volume status: hypovolemic, hypervolemic, or euvolemic. Categorizing patients in this way allows one to better identify the underlying cause and provides a guide for therapeutic intervention (Fig. 128-11).

HYPOVOLEMIC HYPERNATREMIA

Patients who sustain losses of both sodium and water, but with comparatively greater water losses, are at risk of developing hypovolemic hypernatremia. These patients present with signs of volume depletion, such as orthostatic hypotension, decreased skin turgor, dry mucous membranes, flattened neck veins, and tachycardia. The urinary sodium concentration can help determine whether the water losses are primarily renal or extrarenal in nature, with a urinary [Na+] greater than 20 mmol/L indicating renal losses and less than 20 mmol/L indicating extrarenal losses.

HYPERVOLEMIC HYPERNATREMIA

This is the least common form of hypernatremia and occurs when patients sustain an increase in total body sodium that exceeds any increase in total body water. It can be seen after the administration of hypertonic solutions such as 3% NaCl, intra-amniotic instillation for therapeutic abortions, administration of NaHCO$_3$, or inadvertent dialysis against a high Na+-containing dialysate. Congestive heart failure patients taking loop diuretics may also be prone to develop hypernatremia. Patients with primary sodium-retaining disorders such as Cushing's disease or hyperaldosteronism are also somewhat hypernatremic. These patients' basal serum [Na+] is approximately 143 to 144 mEq/L by virtue of an upward resetting of the osmotic threshold for vasopressin release in these hypervolemic states.

EUVOLEMIC HYPERNATREMIA

These patients have water losses without a change in total body sodium. Again, water losses alone do not always lead to hypernatremia; however, if water intake is also impaired, the serum sodium will increase. The water losses can be

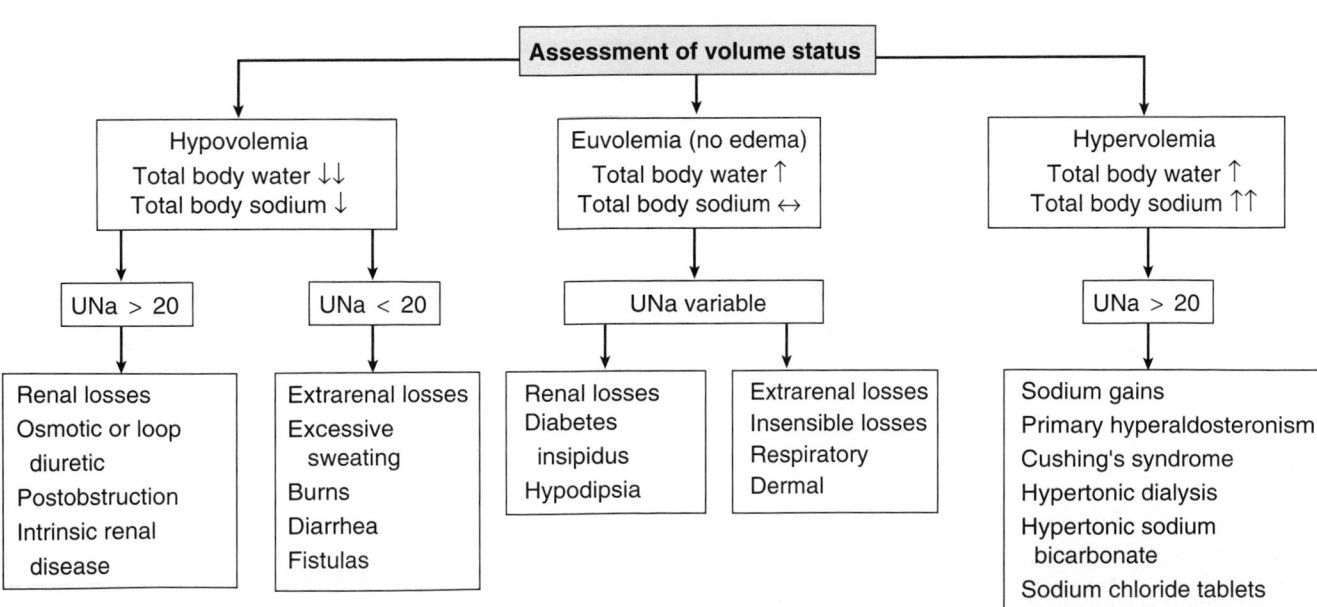

FIGURE 128-11. Diagnostic algorithm for hypernatremia. UNa, urinary sodium concentration. (Adapted from Parix G, Kumar S, Beil T: Disorders of water metabolism. In Johnson R, Feehally J (eds): Comprehensive Clinical Nephrology. St Louis, Mosby, 2003, p 93.)

TABLE 128–3. WATER DEPRIVATION TEST

Diagnosis	Urine Osmolality with Water Deprivation (mOsm/kg H₂O)	Plasma AVP after Dehydration	Increase in Urine Osmolality with Exogenous AVP
Normal	>800	>2 pg/mL	Little or none
Complete central diabetes insipidus	<300	Undetectable	Substantial
Partial central diabetes insipidus	300-800	<1.5 pg/mL	>10% of urine osmolality after water deprivation
Nephrogenic diabetes insipidus	<300-500	>5 pg/mL	Little or none
Primary polydipsia	>500	<5 pg/mL	Little or none

AVP, arginine vasopressin.

extrarenal (skin, respiratory tract), in which case urine osmolality will be elevated, or they can be renal, from impaired vasopressin production or collecting tubule response. The urine sodium in all cases varies, depending on the individual's water intake.

Specific Euvolemic Hypernatremic Disorders

Central Diabetes Insipidus

Central diabetes insipidus results from impaired secretion of vasopressin from the supraoptic and paraventricular nuclei of the hypothalamus. Differentiating central diabetes insipidus, nephrogenic diabetes insipidus, and primary polydipsia can be a clinical challenge, because all three present with polyuria and polydipsia. Distinguishing among them is best accomplished by measuring vasopressin levels and monitoring the response to a water deprivation test followed by vasopressin administration (Table 128-3). Pituitary magnetic resonance imaging can also be used to make the diagnosis of central diabetes insipidus. T1-weighted images of the healthy posterior pituitary gland demonstrate a hyperintense signal, whereas this signal is absent in most patients with central diabetes insipidus (although it may be present in the rare inherited forms of the condition).[22] Until either of these tests can be performed, some clinical features may help distinguish a patient with central diabetes insipidus from a compulsive water drinker. Central diabetes insipidus is often abrupt and memorable in onset, with

patients experiencing a constant need for water; a compulsive water drinker often provides a more vague history of onset. Nocturia is common in patients with central diabetes insipidus but is unusual in compulsive water drinkers. The plasma osmolality is also a helpful measurement, with values greater than 295 mOsm/kg suggestive of central diabetes insipidus and values below 270 mOsm/kg favoring a diagnosis of compulsive water drinking. One other finding that is often seen in patients with central diabetes insipidus is a strong preference for cold water.

There are many known causes of central diabetes insipidus (Table 128-4), including several inherited forms; however, about 50% of cases are idiopathic, with the remainder resulting mainly from infection, tumor, or trauma affecting the central nervous system. The treatment of central diabetes insipidus relies primarily on hormone replacement and pharmacologic agents (Table 128-5). In the acute setting, aqueous vasopressin (Pitressin) is advantageous; its short duration of action makes complications such as water intoxication less likely. For a patient with chronic central diabetes insipidus, desmopressin acetate (DDAVP) is the agent of choice; it has a long half-life and can be administered intranasally (10 to 20 µg) every 12 to 24 hours. DDAVP does

TABLE 128–4. CAUSES OF CENTRAL DIABETES INSIPIDUS

Congenital

Autosomal dominant
Autosomal recessive

Acquired

Post-traumatic
Iatrogenic (postsurgical)
Tumor (metastatic from breast, craniopharyngioma, pinealoma)
Histiocytosis
Granuloma (tuberculosis, sarcoid)
Aneurysm
Meningitis
Encephalitis
Guillain-Barré syndrome
Idiopathic

TABLE 128–5. TREATMENTS FOR DIABETES INSIPIDUS

Type of Diabetes Insipidus	Drug	Dose
Complete central	DDAVP	10-20 µg intranasally q12-24 h
Partial central	Aqueous vasopressin	5-10 U subcutaneously q4-6h
	Chlorpropamide	250-500 mg/day
	Clofibrate	500 mg tid-qid
	Carbamazepine	400-600 mg/day
Nephrogenic	Thiazide diuretics NSAIDs	
	Amiloride (for lithium-related disease)	5 mg/day
Gestational	DDAVP	As for complete central

DDAVP, desmopressin; NSAIDs, nonsteroidal anti-inflammatory drugs.
Adapted from Lanese D, Teitelbaum I: Nypernatremia. In Jacobson HR, Striker GE, Klahr S (eds): The Principles and Practice of Nephrology. Philadelphia, CV Mosby, 1998.

not have the strong vasoconstrictive properties of aqueous vasopressin, which must be used with caution in patients with coronary and peripheral vascular disease. In patients with partial diabetes insipidus, additional agents that increase the release of vasopressin, such as carbamazepine, chlorpropamide, and clofibrate, can be used.

Nephrogenic Diabetes Insipidus

The diagnosis of congenital nephrogenic diabetes insipidus is usually made early in infancy with a presentation of hypo-osmolar urine, severe dehydration, fever, vomiting, and hypernatremia. An intact thirst mechanism and access to free water are absolute necessities for survival, because neither hormonal nor pharmacologic treatments are effective. Rehydration therapy in patients with congenital nephrogenic diabetes insipidus should consist of hypotonic glucose solutions; isotonic solutions promote further water losses via the excretion of solutes. Solute intake should also be limited by using low-sodium and -protein diets.

One form of congenital nephrogenic diabetes insipidus follows an X-linked inheritance pattern, with only males exhibiting the complete disease phenotype. Females can have a subclinical form, which suggests the presence of variable penetrance. Affected males with X-linked congenital nephrogenic diabetes insipidus have an inability to concentrate urine in the presence of vasopressin. The defect has been located on the X chromosome where the V2 receptor protein is encoded. There appear to be multiple disease-causing mutations in this area of the X chromosome; 87 such mutations in the V2 receptor were found in 106 presumably unrelated affected families.[23] The autosomal recessive form of congenital nephrogenic diabetes insipidus is the result of mutations in the gene encoding for aquaporin-2 (*AQP-2*). This form is much less common than the X-linked variety, but multiple disease-causing mutations have been described.[24]

Acquired nephrogenic diabetes insipidus is more common but usually less severe, with partial preservation of urine-concentrating mechanisms. Urinary volumes are therefore much less (>3 to 4 L/day) compared with congenital nephrogenic diabetes insipidus, central diabetes insipidus, or compulsive water drinking. Common causes include hypercalcemia, hypokalemia, sickle cell anemia, demeclocycline therapy, lithium therapy, pregnancy, and chronic renal failure. Many of these entities have also been associated with decrements in aquaporin-2 expression in experimental models of these disorders.

SIGNS AND SYMPTOMS

Hypernatremia always represents a hyperosmolar state. Most of the signs and symptoms are reflections of central nervous system disturbances. These include altered mental status, lethargy, seizures, irritability, hyperreflexia, and spasticity. Patients can also exhibit nausea, vomiting, fever, respiratory distress, and intense thirst. Certain patients are at increased risk for developing severe, life-threatening hypernatremia. These include both elderly patients and infants, certain hospitalized patients (those receiving hypertonic infusions, tube feedings, osmotic diuretics, lactulose, or mechanical ventilation), patients with altered mental status, and those with uncontrolled diabetes or an underlying polyuric disorder.

TREATMENT

Much of hospital-acquired hypernatremia can be prevented by attention to hypotonic fluid losses and appropriate replacement. Once a diagnosis of hypernatremia has been made, it is important to initiate treatment promptly. This depends on first identifying the patient's volume status, with the end goal being restoration of serum tonicity (Fig. 128-12). The rate of correction of hypernatremia depends primarily on its rate of development and on the presence or absence of neurologic symptoms. If hypernatremia is corrected too rapidly, water can move into brain cells, resulting in cerebral edema. If symptoms are present and the hypernatremia is believed to be acute in onset, rapid correction over the first several hours is appropriate, with the maximum correction rate not exceeding 2 mEq/L per hour. An accepted goal is to correct half the water deficit over the first 24 hours, with the remaining deficit being corrected over the next 48 hours. Serum sodium should be closely monitored during the course of treatment, with careful assessment of ongoing fluid losses.

For patients with euvolemic hypernatremia, the primary therapy is 5% glucose solutions. It is important to replace not only the water deficit but also any ongoing water losses (urinary, respiratory, skin losses). The water deficit can be calculated from the serum sodium concentration, using the assumption that 60% of the body weight is water:

$$\text{Water deficit} = 0.6 \times \text{Body weight} \times (\text{PNa}/140 - 1)$$

To take into account any ongoing urinary water losses, it is necessary to calculate an electrolyte-free water clearance:

$$cH_2Oe = V[1 - (UNa + UK/PNa)]$$

The sum total of the water deficit combined with any ongoing losses can be used to guide the amount and duration of water replacement, with the understanding that these calculations are not static and may need frequent adjustments. In the case of acute, severe central diabetes insipidus, in addition to the preceding water replacement therapy, it may be necessary to use short-acting aqueous vasopressin (Pitressin) 5 U subcanteously every 6 hours, depending on the response to therapy. In the chronic setting, DDAVP can be used, as outlined previously. In patients with chronic nephrogenic diabetes insipidus, the primary intervention is treatment or removal of the underlying cause. A rare form of diabetes insipidus can occur with pregnancy when the placenta produces vasopressinase. These patients respond to treatment with DDAVP, which is not degraded by this enzyme.[25]

In the setting of hypovolemic hypernatremia, the initial management is fluid resuscitation using isotonic saline solutions or other plasma expanders. Once intravascular volume has been restored, administration of hypotonic solutions can further restore normal serum tonicity.

The final setting involves patients with hypervolemic hypernatremia, when the primary disorder is total body sodium excess. The goal, therefore, is to promote natriuresis with loop diuretics, along with the administration of 5% dextrose. Patients should be monitored closely to prevent too rapid sodium removal and volume depletion. If renal function is significantly impaired, volume overload and hypertonicity may require corrective dialysis therapy.

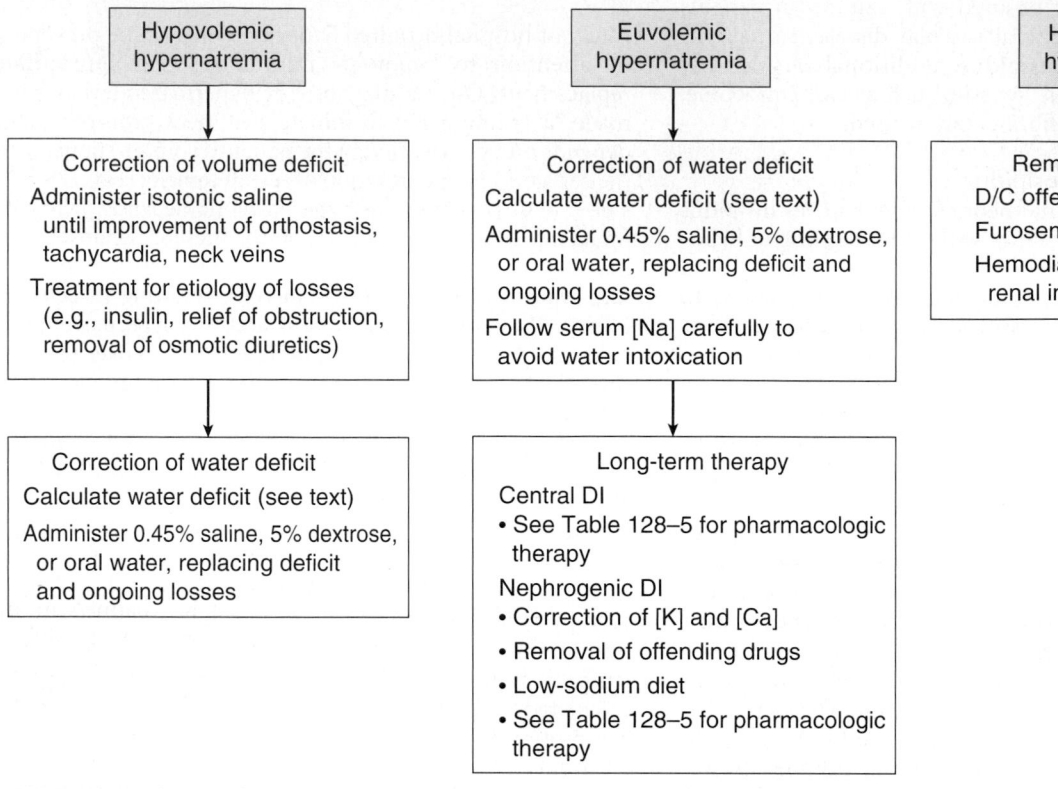

FIGURE 128–12. Therapeutic approach to hypernatremia. D/C, discontinue; DI, diabetes insipidus.

ANNOTATED REFERENCES

Ayus JC, Arieff AI: Chronic hyponatremic encephalopathy in post-menopausal women: Association of therapies with morbidity and mortality. JAMA 1999;281:2299-2304.

This retrospectively study in elderly women with hyponatremia analyzed neurologic outcome as a function of the magnitude of serum sodium correction.

Decaux G: Long-term treatment of patients with inappropriate secretion of antidiuretic hormone by the vasopressin receptor antagonist conivaptan, urea or furosemide. Am J Med 2002;110:582-584.

An excellent report on the use of a new V2 antagonist in the treatment of hyponatremia in SIADH. These drugs may soon be available for such purposes.

Furst H, Hallows KR, Post J, et al: The urine/plasma electrolyte ratio: A predictive guide to water restriction. Am J Med Sci 2000;319:240-244.

This physiologic analysis can serve as a guide to the degree of water restriction required to treat hyponatremia. An excellent review of the significance of urinary sodium and potassium concentrations.

Knepper MA: Molecular physiology of urinary concentrating mechanisms: Regulation of aquaporin water channels by vasopressin. Am J Physiol 1997;272:F3-F12.

This is an excellent review of the cellular biology of vasopressin action, with an emphasis on the regulation of AQP-2—the vasopressin-dependent water channel.

Palevsky PM, Bhagrath R, Greenberg A: Hypernatremia in hospitalized patients. Ann Intern Med 1996;124:197-203.

This study on the epidemiology of hypernatremia found that approximately 50% of patients admitted with this disorder are elderly.

Chapter 129

DISORDERS OF PLASMA POTASSIUM CONCENTRATION

Kamel S. Kamel • Mitchell L. Halperin

KEY POINTS

1. Movement of potassium ions (K^+) across cell membranes requires an open K^+ channel and a negative voltage in the cell. The electrogenic transport of sodium ions (Na^+) generates this negative voltage.

2. There are two major factors that cause K^+ to enter cells: hormones and acid-base influences.

3. Control of the renal excretion of K^+ maintains overall daily K^+ balance. Two factors influence the rate of excretion of K^+: flow rate in the terminal cortical collecting duct; and net secretion of K^+ by principal cells in the cortical collecting duct, which raises the luminal concentration of K^+.

4. The actual rate of K^+ excretion should be compared with the expected rate of K^+ excretion to assess whether the renal response is appropriate to the stimulus.

5. The rate of excretion of osmoles provides a minimum estimate of the flow rate in the terminal cortical collecting duct. A typical value is 0.5 mOsm/min; the major osmoles are urea and Na^+ plus chloride ions (Cl^-).

6. A reasonable approximation of the luminal concentration of K^+ in the cortical collecting duct can be obtained by adjusting the urinary K^+ concentration for the amount of water reabsorbed in the medullary collecting duct.

7. The basis for the change in the rate of electrogenic reabsorption of Na^+ can be deduced from an assessment of extracellular fluid volume, the ability to conserve Na^+ and Cl^- in response to a contracted effective extracellular fluid volume, and measurement of the activity of renin and the level of aldosterone in plasma.

8. It is imperative to recognize when a dyskalemia represents a medical emergency, because therapy must take precedence over diagnosis.

PATHOPHYSIOLOGY OF THE DYSKALEMIAS

Dyskalemias are common electrolyte disorders in the critical care setting that may have serious sequelae, notably cardiac arrhythmias.[1] The pathophysiology of these electrolyte disturbances is more easily understood if it is examined in the context of the transport of potassium ions (K^+) across membranes. This concept of K^+ transport has two components—an open membrane channel for K^+, and a force to cause K^+ to move.

K^+ Channels. There are insufficient K^+ channels in an open configuration in cell membranes to permit K^+ to diffuse to electrochemical equilibrium. When the number of open K^+ channels increases, K^+ moves out of cells, and the intracellular fluid (ICF) voltage becomes more negative (see Fig. 129-1 for an example to illustrate the importance of this physiology in the critical care setting).

Driving Force for the Movement of K^+. K^+ moves into a compartment that has a more negative voltage when K^+ channels are open. To create this negative voltage in cells, cations are exported at a faster rate than anions. The cation is usually sodium (Na^+), because of its abundance and the means to cause its transmembrane movement—activity of the electrogenic Na^+,K^+-ATPase.[2] This ion pump exports 3 Na^+ out of the cell but imports only 2 K^+ into the cell (Fig. 129-2). Because Na^+ movement is much greater than that of impermeable ICF anions (macromolecular phosphates such as RNA, DNA, and phospholipids), a negative intracellular voltage is generated.

REGULATION OF K^+ HOMEOSTASIS

Regulation of K^+ homeostasis has two important aspects. First, control of the transcellular distribution of K^+ is vital for survival, because it limits acute changes in the plasma K^+ concentration (P_K). Second, the regulation of K^+ excretion by the kidney maintains overall K^+ balance; this is a relatively slow process.

DISTRIBUTION OF K^+ BETWEEN THE EXTRACELLULAR AND INTRACELLULAR COMPARTMENTS

Na^+,K^+-ATPase Pump

The number of Na^+ ions pumped is greater when the concentration of Na^+ rises in cells or when the activity of the pump rises, but its impact on the net cell voltage depends on whether the Na^+ entry into cells is electroneutral or electrogenic.

Electroneutral Entry. This occurs when Na^+ enters cells in exchange for hydrogen ions (H^+) via the Na^+-H^+ exchanger (Fig. 129-2).[3] The Na^+-H^+ exchanger is normally

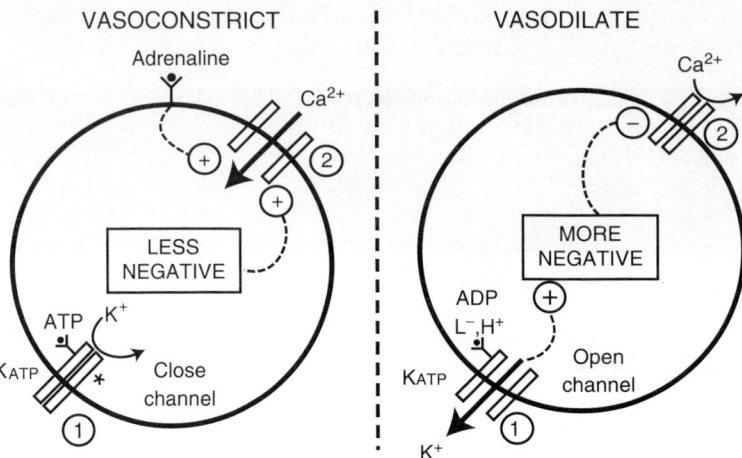

FIGURE 129–1. Vasoconstrictor tone in vascular smooth muscle cells (represented by circles). When the intracellular fluid (ICF) has a less negative voltage because its K_{ATP} ion channels are largely closed, the voltage-gated Ca^{++} channel (site 1) can be maintained in an open configuration, permitting a sustained rise in the ICF Ca^{++} concentration. Hence, vasoconstriction will be the dominant response (shown to the left of the dashed line). In contrast, when K_{ATP} channels are opened by adenosine diphosphate (ADP), L-lactate anions (L⁻), and H⁺ (site 2), this leads to a more negative ICF voltage and closure of the voltage-gated Ca^{++} channels. ATP, adenosine triphosphate. (From Halperin ML: The ACID truth and BASIC facts—with a Sweet Touch, an enLYTEnment, 5th ed. Toronto, RossMark Medical Publishers, 2004, p 4.)

inactive in cell membranes because it is an electroneutral exchanger and the concentrations of its substrates (Na⁺ in the extracellular fluid [ECF] compartment and H⁺ in the ICF compartment) are considerably higher than that of its products (Na⁺ in the ICF and H⁺ in the ECF) in steady state. The two major activators of the Na⁺-H⁺ exchanger are insulin[4] and a higher concentration of H⁺ in the ICF compartment (Fig. 129-3, *upper portion*).[3]

Electrogenic Entry. The Na⁺ channel in cell membranes is normally gated by voltage. When open, one cationic charge enters the cell per Na⁺ transported. Because only one third of a charge exits for each Na⁺ pumped via Na⁺,K⁺-ATPase (see Fig. 129-2), this diminishes the degree of intracellular net negative voltage, which leads to a net *exit* of K⁺ and hence a rise in the P_K.

Hormones that Affect the Distribution of K⁺

Catecholamines. An acute shift of K⁺ into cells and hypokalemia are seen in conditions associated with a surge of catecholamines (e.g., subarachnoid hemorrhage, myocardial ischemia, extreme anxiety).[5] Beta₂-adrenergic agonists cause a shift of K⁺ into cells via activation of the Na⁺,K⁺-ATPase pump (see Fig. 129-2).[6] This leads to the export of

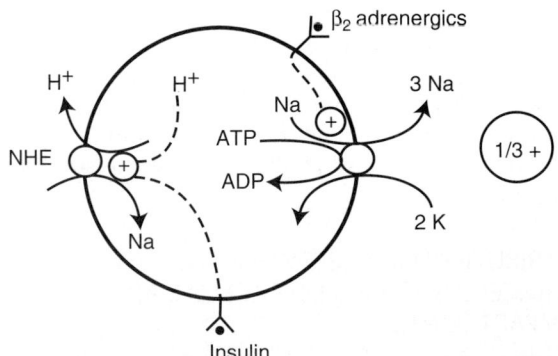

FIGURE 129–2. Na⁺,K⁺-ATPase activity and the export of positive voltage. The Na⁺,K⁺-ATPase pump generates the electrical driving force for K⁺ entry into cells, provided that the source of Na⁺ pumped is either Na⁺ that existed in cells (site 1) or the electroneutral entry of Na⁺ via the Na⁺-H⁺ exchanger (NHE) (site 2). If the source of Na⁺ pumped is the Na⁺ that entered cells via the Na⁺-specific ion channel (site 3), the voltage in cells will become less negative. ADP, adenosine diphosphate; ATP, adenosine triphosphate. (From Halperin ML: The ACID truth and BASIC facts—with a Sweet Touch, an enLYTEnment, 5th ed. Toronto, RossMark Medical Publishers, 2004, p 64.)

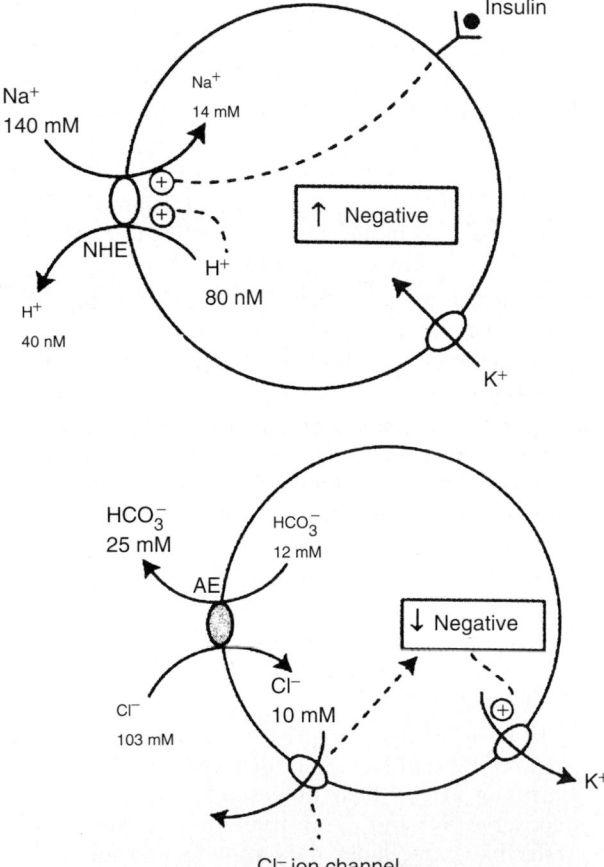

FIGURE 129–3. Role of the Na⁺-H⁺ exchanger (NHE) and the anion exchanger (AE) in the shift of K⁺ across cell membranes. The circle represents a cell membrane. The NHE and AE are normally *inactive* in cell membranes. Thus, concentrations of their substrates and products dictate the direction of ion flux when they become active. There are two major activators of the NHE: insulin and a higher concentration of H⁺ in the intracellular fluid (ICF) compartment. As Na⁺ exits via the Na⁺,K⁺-ATPase pump, the net effect is a more negative intracellular voltage and the entry of K⁺ into cells (see Fig. 129-2). When the AE is activated, HCO_3^- is exported, and Cl⁻ enters cells. The intracellular negative voltage drives the subsequent exit of Cl⁻ from cells, making the inside of cells less negative. As a result, K⁺ exits from cells in this setting. (From Halperin ML: The ACID truth and BASIC facts—with a Sweet Touch, an enLYTEnment, 5th ed. Toronto, RossMark Medical Publishers, 2004, p 109.)

intracellular Na^+. Beta$_2$ agonists are used to shift K^+ into cells in patients with hyperkalemia.[7] Beta blockers are used to treat the subtype of hypokalemic periodic paralysis associated with hyperthyroidism.[8,9]

Insulin. Insulin acts to shift K^+ into cells primarily because of augmentation of the electroneutral entry of Na^+ into cells via the Na^+-H^+ exchanger.[4,10,11] This, in conjunction with stimulation of the electrogenic Na^+,K^+-ATPase pump, causes the voltage in cells to become more negative (see Figs. 129-2 and 129-3). This effect of insulin has been used clinically in the emergency treatment of patients with hyperkalemia.[7]

Acid-Base Influences

When an acid is added to the body, most of the H^+ are buffered in the ICF compartment.[12] Monocarboxylic acids enter cells via a specific transporter, and this is an electroneutral event.[13] To shift K^+ out of cells, the mechanism of entry of H^+ into cells should be electrogenic—causing a less negative voltage in cells. For example, activation of the chloride ion (Cl^-)–bicarbonate (HCO_3^-) anion exchanger causes HCO_3^- to exit cells and Cl^- to enter cells (see Fig. 129-3, *bottom portion*).[14] Because cells have Cl^- channels in their membranes,[15] the rise in the concentration of Cl^- in the ICF, in conjunction with the usual negative voltage, forces Cl^- to exit cells. This exit of Cl^- is electrogenic and causes a less negative voltage in cells, resulting in the exit of K^+ from cells.[16]

Several clinical implications follow from this analysis. First, if hyperkalemia is present in a patient with metabolic acidosis due to a monocarboxylic organic acid, causes for hyperkalemia other than the acidosis should be sought (e.g., insulin lack in patients with diabetic ketoacidosis, tissue injury, lack of adenosine triphosphate to drive the Na^+,K^+-ATPase pump in patients with L-lactic acidosis due to hypoxia,[17] or a renal defect that causes reduced excretion of K^+). Second, although inorganic acidosis (addition of HCl) causes a shift of K^+ out of cells, patients with chronic hyperchloremic metabolic acidosis (e.g., those with chronic diarrhea or renal tubular acidosis) usually have a low P_K because of excessive loss of K^+ in the diarrhea fluid[18] or the urine.[19]

Although hypokalemia is a common finding in patients with metabolic alkalosis,[20] this reflects renal K^+ wasting largely due to the underlying disorder (e.g., vomiting, diuretic use, hyperaldosteronism) rather than small effect of alkalemia due to the shifting of K^+ into cells when H^+ exits. Respiratory acid-base disorders cause only small changes in the P_K, because there is little movement of Na^+ across cell membranes in these disorders.[21,22]

Tissue Anabolism and Catabolism

Hypokalemia may develop with rapid cell growth if inadequate K^+ is given. Examples include the use of total parenteral nutrition, the presence of rapidly growing malignancies, and during the treatment of diabetic ketoacidosis[23,24] or pernicious anemia. Hyperkalemia may be seen with crush injury and the tumor lysis syndrome.[25] In these patients, factors that compromise the kidney's ability to excrete K^+ are usually present as well. In patients with diabetic ketoacidosis, there is total body K^+ depletion[26] but hyperkalemia due to a shift of K^+ from cells, secondary to a lack of insulin.[11] The corollary is that during therapy, complete replacement of the K^+ deficit must await the provision of cellular constituents (e.g., phosphate, amino acids, Mg^{++}) and the presence of anabolic signals.

REGULATION OF K^+ EXCRETION BY THE KIDNEY

Control of the renal excretion of K^+ maintains overall daily K^+ balance. The usual intake of K^+ in adults eating a typical Western diet is close to 1 mmol/kg body weight, but K^+ excretion can decline to a nadir of 10 to 15 mmol/day when there is virtually no K^+ intake.[27] The rate of K^+ excretion can match an intake of more than 200 mmol/day with only a minor rise in P_K.

Control of K^+ secretion occurs primarily in the late distal convoluted tubule and the cortical collecting duct (CCD).[26] Two factors influence the rate of K^+ excretion: the flow rate in the terminal CCD (see equation 1), and the net secretion of K^+ by principal cells in the CCD, which raises the luminal concentration of K^+ ($[K^+]_{CCD}$).

$$K^+ \text{ excretion} = \text{Flow rate}_{CCD} \times [K^+]_{CCD} \qquad (1)$$

Flow Rate in the Cortical Collecting Duct

When vasopressin acts, the flow rate in the CCD is determined by the rate of delivery of osmoles, because the osmolality of fluid in the terminal CCD is equal to the plasma osmolality (P_{osm}). Because vasopressin acts throughout the 24-hour cycle,[28] a minimum estimate of the flow rate in the terminal CCD is obtained by dividing the rate of excretion of osmoles by the osmolality of luminal fluid (Fig. 129-4). During a water diuresis, although the rate of flow in the CCD is high, the rate of excretion of K^+ need not be, because vasopressin is required for K^+ secretion.

[K^+] in the Lumen of the Terminal Cortical Collecting Duct

The secretory process for K^+ in principal cells has two elements. First, a negative luminal voltage must be generated by electrogenic reabsorption of Na^+ via the epithelial sodium channel (ENaC). Aldosterone increases the activity of the

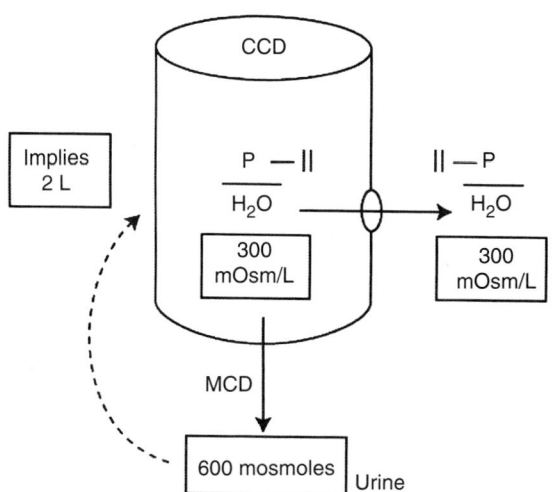

FIGURE 129–4. Noninvasive estimate of the flow rate in the terminal cortical collecting duct (CCD). The barrel-shaped structure represents the CCD. When vasopressin acts, the plasma osmolality (P_{osm}) and the osmolality of luminal fluid of the CCD are equal (represented as 300 mOsm/kg H_2O for easy math). For example, if 600 mOsm are excreted at a given time, the minimum flow rate to the CCD would be 2 L. MCD, medullary collecting duct. (From Halperin ML: The ACID truth and BASIC facts—with a Sweet Touch, an enLYTEnment, 5th ed. Toronto, RossMark Medical Publishers, 2004, p 65.)

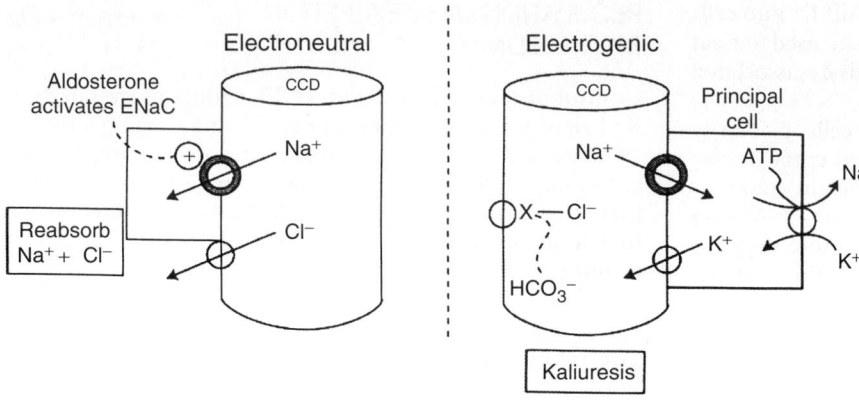

FIGURE 129–5. Electrogenic and electroneutral reabsorption of Na^+ in the cortical collecting duct (CCD). The barrel-shaped structure represents the CCD, and the rectangles represent principal cells. Na^+ is reabsorbed via the epithelial sodium channel (ENaC); this reabsorption is increased by aldosterone (shaded enlarged circle). Net secretion of K^+ occurs through its specific ion channel (ROM-K). Electroneutral reabsorption of Na^+ is shown on the left, and an example of electrogenic reabsorption of Na^+ (HCO_3^- or an alkaline luminal pH decreasing the apparent permeability of Cl^- in the CCD) is shown to the right of the dashed horizontal line. ATP, adenosine triphosphate. (From Halperin ML: The ACID truth and BASIC facts—with a Sweet Touch, an enLYTEnment, 5th ed. Toronto, RossMark Medical Publishers, 2004, p 66.)

ENaC (Fig. 129-5, left side).[29] The individual steps for aldosterone action include its binding to the cytoplasmic aldosterone receptor in principal cells, entry of this hormone-receptor complex into the nucleus, and the synthesis of new proteins, including serum and glucocorticoid-regulated kinase.[30] Second, open K^+ channels must be present in the luminal membranes. K^+ channels are abundant and have a high probability of being open; therefore, this does not seem to be a rate-limiting factor for the net secretion of K^+ in most instances.

Glucocorticoids do not usually stimulate the secretion of K^+ in the CCD, because principal cells have the enzyme 11 β-hydroxysteroid dehydrogenase (11 β-HSDH). This enzyme converts cortisol to a metabolite (cortisone) that does *not* bind the mineralocorticoid receptor (Fig.129-6). Cortisol, however, can exert a mineralocorticoid effect if the activity of 11 β-HSDH is decreased or if it is overwhelmed by an extreme abundance of cortisol.

Under most circumstances, variations in the luminal Na^+ concentration in the CCD do not regulate the secretion of K^+.[31] The reabsorption of Na^+ in the CCD can be electroneutral or electrogenic, depending on whether Cl^- is reabsorbed as fast as Na^+ (electroneutral) or slower than Na^+ (electrogenic) (see Fig. 129-5). The pathways for the reabsorption of Cl^- in the CCD are not well defined, but it is

likely that paracellular pathways play an important role.[32,33] A faster reabsorption of Na^+ than Cl^- in the CCD can occur for three reasons. First, Na^+ is delivered to the CCD with little Cl^-. A key finding in these patients is a Cl^--poor urine.[34] Second, reabsorption of Cl^- in the CCD may be inhibited; this mechanism is suspected when the urine is not Cl^- poor. It appears that HCO_3^- or an alkaline luminal pH in the CCD could inhibit Cl^- reabsorption.[35] Third, a more negative luminal voltage in the CCD could develop when the delivery of Na^+ and Cl^- is very high *and* the capacity for Cl^- reabsorption is less than that for Na^+. This requires a stimulated reabsorption of Na^+ via the ENaC in the CCD.

At times, Na^+ is *not* reabsorbed faster than Cl^- in the CCD, so an appreciably negative luminal voltage cannot develop.[32,36] The hyperkalemia in patients with type II pseudohypoaldosteronism (Gordon's syndrome) may be an example of this pathophysiology. Two factors are important to achieve this near-equal rate of ion transport in the CCD. First, low delivery of Na^+ and Cl^- to the CCD occurs because the reabsorption of Na^+ and Cl^- is augmented in the distal convoluted tubule because of increased activity of the Na^+-Cl^- cotransporter (NCC). Second, ECF volume expansion suppresses the release of aldosterone, leading to a less open ENaC; hence, the rate of reabsorption of Cl^- in the CCD may match that of Na^+.

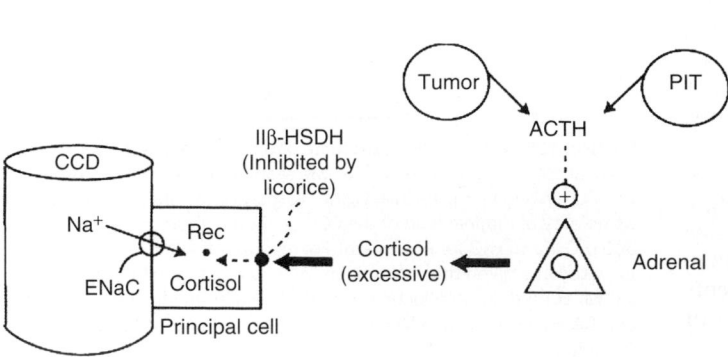

FIGURE 129–6. Conditions in which cortisol acts as a mineralocorticoid. Cortisol has a very high affinity to the aldosterone receptor. As cortisol enters principal cells of the CCD, 11 β-HSDH (larger solid dot in the membrane) inactivates it before it can bind to the aldosterone receptor (Rec; smaller dot in the cell). There are three circumstances in which cortisol will successfully bind to the aldosterone receptor: (1) when there is a deficiency of 11 β-HSDH (apparent mineralocorticoid excess syndrome), (2) when an inhibitor 11 β-HSDH is present (e.g., licorice), and (3) when the supply of cortisol exceeds the ability of 11 β-HSDH to inactivate it (e.g., ectopic production of adrenocorticotropic hormone [ACTH] by a tumor). ENaC, epithelial sodium channel; PIT, pituitary gland. (From Halperin ML: The ACID truth and BASIC facts—with a Sweet Touch, an enLYTEnment, 5th ed. Toronto, RossMark Medical Publishers, 2004, p 81.)

Tools to Assess Control of the Renal Excretion of K^+

Examine the Rate of K^+ Excretion. To assess the renal response in a patient with hypokalemia or hyperkalemia, we use the expected rate of K^+ excretion when these electrolyte abnormalities are due to nonrenal causes. With a K^+ deficit, the expected response is to excrete less than 15 mmol/day.[27] With a surfeit of K^+, the expected response is to excrete greater than 200 mmol/day, values observed in response to a K^+ load with a minor increase in P_K.[37]

To assess the rate of excretion of K^+, a 24-hour urine collection is not necessary. One can use the urinary potassium–urinary creatinine ($U_K/U_{creatinine}$) ratio (despite the diurnal variation in K^+ excretion),[38] because creatinine is excreted at a near-constant rate throughout the day.[39,40] Moreover, a $U_K/U_{creatinine}$ in a spot urine sample provides more relevant information because the stimulus to drive K^+ excretion (e.g., P_K) can be known at that time. The expected value in a patient with hypokalemia is less than 1 mmol K^+/mmol creatinine (<10 mmol K^+/g creatinine), whereas in a patient with hyperkalemia, the expected $U_K/U_{creatinine}$ ratio is greater than 15 mmol K^+/mmol creatinine (>50 mmol K^+/g creatinine).

Estimate the Flow Rate in the Terminal Cortical Collecting Duct. The critical factor is the rate of excretion of osmoles (equation 2), typically about 0.5 mOsm/min or 720 mOsm/day.

$$\text{Flow rate}_{CCD} = (U_{osm} \times \text{Urine flow rate})/P_{osm} \quad (2)$$

The major osmoles in the urine are urea and Na^+ plus Cl^-. A low flow rate in the terminal CCD could be due to a low rate of delivery of urea (low intake of protein) or of Na^+ and Cl^- (low effective circulating volume, low intake of salt). A high flow rate in the CCD could be due to inhibition of NaCl reabsorption in an upstream nephron segment due to high salt intake, diuretic use (osmotic or pharmacologic), or diseases that inhibit the reabsorption of Na^+ and Cl^- in an upstream nephron segment (e.g., Bartter's syndrome or Gitelman's syndrome).

Estimate the $[K^+]_{CCD}$. A reasonable approximation of the $[K^+]_{CCD}$ can be obtained by adjusting the U_K for the amount of water reabsorbed in the medullary collecting duct. This is done by dividing the U_K by the $(U/P)_{Osm}$ (the P_{Osm} equals the osmolality of the fluid in the terminal CCD when vasopressin acts; see Fig. 129-4 and equation 3). The assumption here (reasonable in most circumstances) is that little K^+ is secreted or reabsorbed in the medullary collecting duct.

$$[K^+]_{CCD} = [K^+]_{urine}/(U/P)_{Osm} \quad (3)$$

Calculate the Transtubular [K] Gradient (TTKG). To calculate the TTKG, divide the $[K^+]_{CCD}$ by the P_K (Fig. 129-7; equation 4). The TTKG provides a semiquantitative reflection of the driving force for K^+ secretion in the terminal CCD.[41] The expected value for the TTKG in a patient with hypokalemia due to a nonrenal cause is less than 2, whereas the appropriate renal response in a normal subject given a K^+ load is greater than 7.

$$\text{TTKG} = [K^+]_{CCD}/P_K \quad (4)$$

Establish the Basis for the Abnormal $[K^+]_{CCD}$. In a patient with hyperkalemia, a lower than expected $[K^+]_{CCD}$

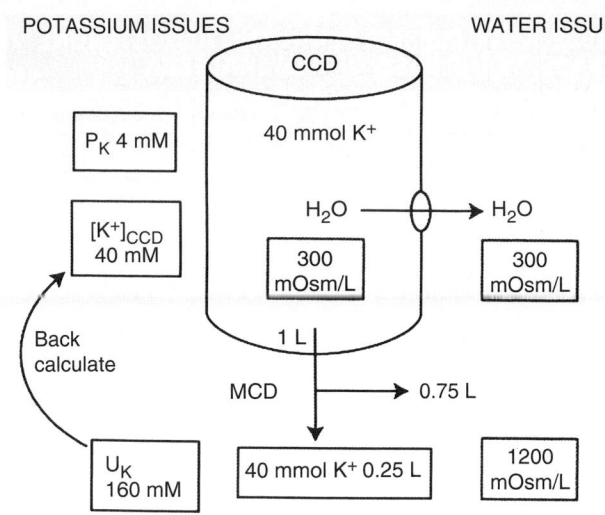

POTASSIUM ISSUES   WATER ISSUES

FIGURE 129–7. Transtubular K^+ concentration gradient. The barrel-shaped structure represents the cortical collecting duct (CCD), and the arrow below the CCD is the medullary collecting duct (MCD). In this example, the luminal K^+ concentration is 40 mM, or 10-fold larger than the peritubular K^+ concentration of 4 mM. Consider what happens when 1 L of fluid traverses the MCD, where 75% of the water is reabsorbed. In this example, no K^+ is reabsorbed or secreted in the MCD. Therefore, the U_K is fourfold higher (40 versus 160 mM), as is the U_{osm} (300 versus 1200 mOsm/kg H_2O). This should be taken into account in assessing the U_K. (From Halperin ML: The ACID truth and BASIC facts—with a Sweet Touch, an enLYTEnment, 5th ed. Toronto, RossMark Medical Publishers, 2004, p 69.)

implies that the negative luminal voltage is abnormally low due to less electrogenic reabsorption of Na^+. The converse is true in a patient with hypokalemia. The basis for the change in the rate of electrogenic reabsorption of Na^+ can be deduced from an assessment of the ECF volume, the ability to conserve Na^+ and Cl^- in response to a contracted effective ECF volume, and measurement of the activity of renin and the level of aldosterone in plasma (Table 129-1).[42] Alternatively, one can focus on changes in blood pressure (Table 129-2).

HYPERKALEMIA

CLINICAL APPROACH

It is imperative to recognize when hyperkalemia (or hypokalemia) represents a medical emergency, because therapy must take precedence over diagnosis. A step-by-step approach to the diagnosis of hyperkalemia is illustrated in Figures 129-8 and 129-9. Alternatively, one could use an approach that relies on changes in blood pressure (see Table 129-2).

1. *Are there any laboratory or technical explanations for hyperkalemia?* Hemolysis, megakaryocytosis, fragile tumor cells, a K^+ channel disorder in red blood cells,[40] and excessive fist-clenching during blood sampling[43] should be excluded. Pseudohyperkalemia may be present in cachectic patients because the normal T-tubule architecture in skeletal muscle may be disturbed. This permits more K^+ to be released into venous blood, even without excessive fist-clenching.

2. *Is hyperkalemia acute, or is K^+ intake very low?* If the answer is yes, proceed to an analysis of factors that could cause a shift of K^+ from cells.[44]

TABLE 129–1. PLASMA RENIN AND ALDOSTERONE TO ASSESS THE BASIS OF A DYSKALEMIA

	Renin	Aldosterone
Effective ECF volume		
Low	High	Should be high
High	Low	Should be low
Adrenal gland lesion		
Primary hyperaldosteronism or adrenal tumor	Low	High
ACTH causing aldosterone synthesis (GRA)	Low	High
Adrenal insufficiency	High	Low
Kidney lesions		
Renal artery stenosis	High	High
Malignant hypertension	High	High
Renin-secreting tumor	High	High
Liddle's syndrome	Low	Absent
Bartter's syndrome	High	Should be high
Gitelman's syndrome	High	Should be high
Gordon's syndrome	Low	Low
11β-HSDH fails to remove all cortisol		
Hereditary defect (AME)	Low	Low
Inhibition (e.g., licorice ingestion)	Low	Low
Saturation because of ectopic ACTH	Low	Low

ACTH, adrenocorticotropic hormone; AME, apparent mineralocorticoid excess; ECF, extracellular fluid; GRA, glucocorticoid-remediable aldosteronism; 11β-HSDH, 11β-hydroxysteroid dehydrogenase.

3. *What is the rate of K⁺ excretion?* If the rate is considerably less than 200 mmol/day (or <15 mmol K⁺/mmol creatinine), it is inappropriately low in the presence of hyperkalemia, and its basis should be determined by asking the following questions (see Fig. 129-9).

TABLE 129–2. DYSKALEMIAS AND BLOOD PRESSURE

Hyperkalemia

1. Associated with high blood pressure
   a. Enhanced Na⁺ and Cl⁻ reabsorption in the DCT (e.g., Gordon's syndrome, diabetes mellitus, calcineurin inhibitors)
   b. Advanced renal disease
2. Associated with low blood pressure
   a. Pseudohypoaldosteronism type I
   b. Adrenal insufficiency
   c. Use of drugs that block ENaC (e.g., trimethoprim)

Hypokalemia

1. Associated with high blood pressure
   a. Overactive renin-angiotensin system (e.g., renin-secreting tumor, renal artery stenosis, malignant hypertension)
   b. Adrenal hyperplasia or adenoma
   c. Liddle's syndrome
   d. Mineralocorticoid receptor mutation and pregnancy
   e. Apparent mineralocorticoid excess syndromes (e.g., mutations, licorice and related drugs)
   f. Use of diuretics to treat essential hypertension
2. Associated with low blood pressure
   a. Diuretics
   b. Vomiting, laxative abuse
   c. Bartter's and Gitelman's syndromes
   d. Stimulation of the calcium-sensing receptor

Because hyporeninemic hypoaldosteronism has multiple causes, it is not listed in this table.
DCT, distal convoluted tubule; ENaC, epithelial sodium channel.

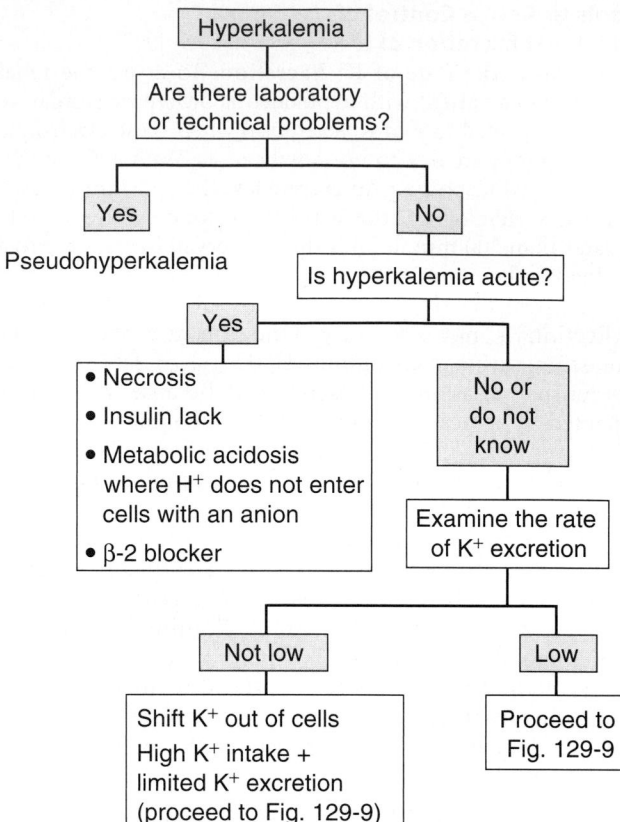

FIGURE 129–8. Initial steps in a patient with hyperkalemia. In the absence of an emergency that demands urgent therapy, proceed with this diagnostic algorithm. (From Halperin ML: The ACID truth and BASIC facts—with a Sweet Touch, an enLYTEnment, 5th ed. Toronto, RossMark Medical Publishers, 2004, p 90.)

a. *What is the reason for the low K⁺ excretion?* The two components of the K⁺ excretion formula need to be interpreted in terms of events in the terminal CCD (see equation 1). A low flow rate in the terminal CCD occurs if there is a low rate of excretion of NaCl, urea, or both.
b. *Why is the [K⁺]_CCD abnormally low?* Seek the basis for a diminished negative luminal voltage in the CCD—either slower Na⁺ reabsorption via the ENaC, or a very low delivery of Na⁺ and Cl⁻ to the CCD with diminished ENaC activity, such that Na⁺ cannot be reabsorbed faster than Cl⁻. An assessment of the ECF volume helps differentiate between these two settings.

If the effective ECF volume is low and the plasma renin activity is high, suspect a primary, slower Na⁺ reabsorption (see Table 129-1). If the urinary sodium (U_Na) and urinary chloride (U_Cl) levels are not very low in a patient with a low effective ECF volume, a renal defect in the reabsorption of Na⁺ is present (Table 129-3). Suspect a low level of aldosterone in plasma if there is a rise in the [K⁺]_CCD and a fall in the U_Na and U_Cl 2 hours after the administration of an exogenous mineralocorticoid (100 μg fludrocortisone). This diagnosis is confirmed by a very low concentration of aldosterone in plasma. In contrast, if the patient does not respond to exogenous mineralocorticoids, the presumptive diagnosis is that the slower Na⁺ lesion is due to an aldosterone receptor problem or a low ENaC activity in principal cells.

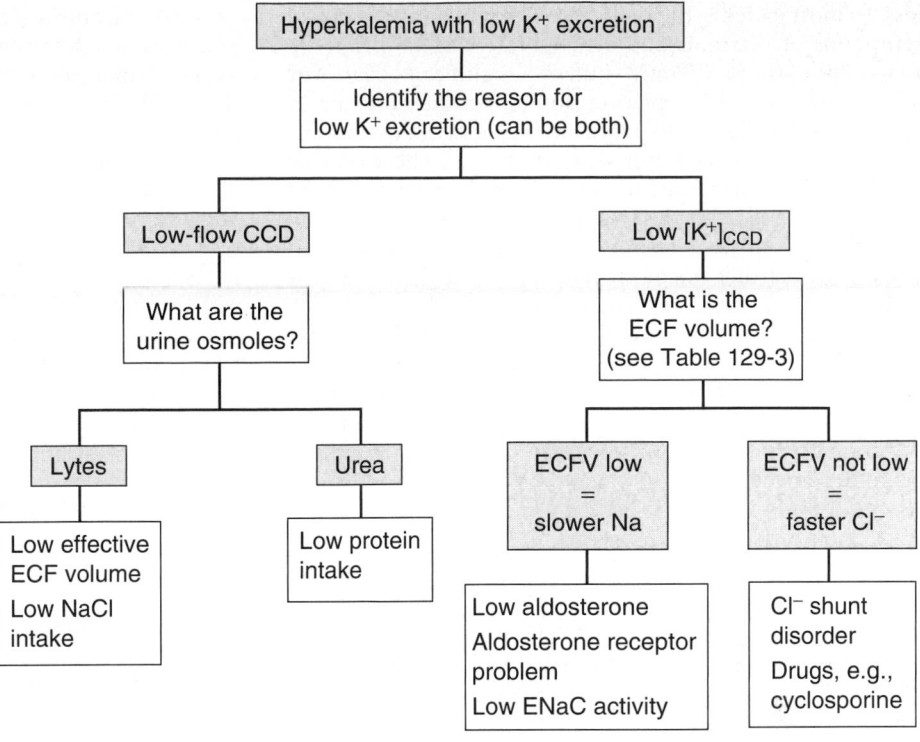

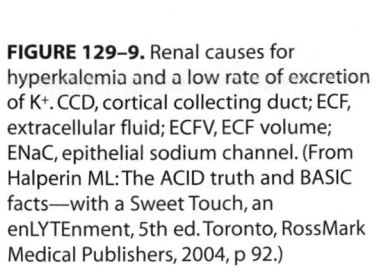

FIGURE 129–9. Renal causes for hyperkalemia and a low rate of excretion of K+. CCD, cortical collecting duct; ECF, extracellular fluid; ECFV, ECF volume; ENaC, epithelial sodium channel. (From Halperin ML: The ACID truth and BASIC facts—with a Sweet Touch, an enLYTEnment, 5th ed. Toronto, RossMark Medical Publishers, 2004, p 92.)

If there is a high effective circulating volume, low plasma renin activity, and low concentration of aldosterone in plasma in the face of hyperkalemia, suspect that excessive reabsorption of Na+ and Cl– is present in the distal convoluted tubule (see Table 129-1).[36] Hypertension may be present (see Table 129-2), and there is often an unusually large fall in blood pressure in response to thiazide diuretics.[45] A rise in the $[K^+]_{CCD}$ with bicarbonaturia (but not exogenous mineralocorticoids) supports the diagnosis of this lesion, which was previously called a Cl– shunt disorder.[46]

SPECIFIC CAUSES

A list of the causes of hyperkalemia based on the possible underlying pathophysiology is provided in Table 129-4.

Addison's Disease

In the past, the most common cause of this disorder was bilateral adrenal destruction with tuberculosis, but autoimmune adrenalitis now accounts for the majority of cases.[47] Additional causes include other infectious diseases (disseminated fungal infection), adrenal replacement by metastatic carcinoma or lymphoma, adrenal hemorrhage or infarction, and drugs that impair the synthesis of aldosterone (e.g., ketoconazole and possibly fluconazole).

Patients with chronic primary adrenal insufficiency may present with chronic malaise, fatigue, anorexia, and weight

---

TABLE 129–3. URINE ELECTROLYTES IN THE DIFFERENTIAL DIAGNOSIS OF HYPOKALEMIA

Condition	Urine Electrolyte*	
	Na+	*Cl–*
Vomiting		
Recent	High†	Low‡
Remote	Low	Low
Diuretics		
Recent	High	High
Remote	Low	Low
Diarrhea or laxative abuse	Low	High
Bartter's or Gitelman's syndrome	High	High

*Do not use urine electrolytes in this fashion during polyuric states.
†Urine concentration >15 mM.
‡Urine concentration <15 mM.

TABLE 129–4. CAUSES OF HYPERKALEMIA

High intake of K+
  Only if combined with low excretion of K+
Shift of K+ out of cells
  Cell necrosis
  Lack of insulin, beta-blockers
  Metabolic acidosis where the anion does not distribute in the ICF compartment
  Rare causes (e.g., hyperkalemic periodic paralysis, barium)
Lower K+ loss in the urine
  Low flow rate (low osmole excretion rate)
  Low $[K^+]_{CCD}$
    Na+ reabsorbed slower than Cl–
      Very low delivery of Na+ to the CCD
      Low levels of aldosterone (e.g., Addison's disease)
      Blockade of the aldosterone receptor (e.g., spironolactone)
      Low ENaC activity (hereditary disease)
      Block of ENaC (e.g., amiloride, triamterene, trimethoprim-like drugs)
    Na+ reabsorbed at a similar rate as Cl–
      Gordon's syndrome (e.g., WNK kinase-4 or -1 mutations)
      Drugs (e.g., cyclosporin)

CCD, cortical collecting duct; ENaC, epithelial sodium channel; ICF intracellular fluid.

loss. In most patients, the blood pressure is low, and postural symptoms of dizziness and syncope are common. The P_K is usually close to 5.5 mM unless a significant degree of intravascular volume depletion diminishes the flow rate in the CCD. Nevertheless, hyperkalemia is not seen on presentation in approximately one third of cases.[48] The diagnosis can be established by the findings of low plasma aldosterone and cortisol levels, high plasma renin activity (see Table 129-1), and blunted cortisol response to the administration of adrenocorticotropic hormone (ACTH). Both glucocorticoid and mineralocorticoid replacement is required.

Adrenal crisis is an emergency that requires immediate restoration of the intravascular volume (intravenous saline) and correction of the cortisol deficiency (dexamethasone or hydrocortisone). Beware of raising the plasma Na^+ too rapidly if hyponatremia is present, because of the higher risk of osmotic demyelination in a catabolic patient.[49]

Pseudohypoaldosteronism Type I

The underlying pathophysiology is a "closed" ENaC in the CCD. In the autosomal recessive form, most mutations are in the α subunit of the ENaC.[50] Patients usually present in the neonatal period with renal salt wasting, hyperkalemia, metabolic acidosis, failure to thrive, and weight loss. ENaC activity is also impaired in the lung, leading to excessive airway fluid and lower respiratory tract infections. The autosomal dominant disorder is due to mutations involving the mineralocorticoid receptor.[51] The clinical disorder is usually milder without lung involvement and may remit with time. Patients with this syndrome fail to respond to exogenous mineralocorticoids, and their plasma aldosterone levels and plasma renin activity are markedly elevated. Treatment includes supplementation with NaCl and inducing the loss of K^+ through the gastrointestinal tract.

Syndrome of Hyporeninemic Hypoaldosteronism

There are two causes of this syndrome. The less common cause is destruction of or a biosynthetic defect in the juxtaglomerular apparatus that leads to hyporeninemia and thereby to a low plasma aldosterone level. Hyperkalemia is due to a relatively slower reabsorption of Na^+ in the CCD. The ECF volume tends to be low, with clinical features that were described earlier. These patients should have a significant rise in the $[K^+]_{CCD}$ with the administration of mineralocorticoids. The second cause involves a low delivery of Na^+ and Cl^- to the CCD due to their enhanced reabsorption in the distal convoluted tubule. ECF volume expansion results in hyporeninemia and hypoaldosteronism.[52-54] Hyperkalemia is due to less electrogenic reabsorption of Na^+ in the CCD. This syndrome is most commonly seen in patients with diabetic nephropathy (see Table 129-2). The ECF volume in these patients is not low, and the clinical findings were described earlier. These patients do not have an appreciable rise in the $[K^+]_{CCD}$ with exogenous mineralocorticoids, but the $[K^+]_{CCD}$ may rise with thiazide diuretics (higher Na^+ and Cl^- delivery to the CCD) or the induction of bicarbonaturia (inhibition of Cl^- reabsorption in the CCD). Thiazide diuretics often lower the blood pressure.

Pseudohypoaldosteronism Type II (Gordon's Syndrome)

The activity of the thiazide-sensitive NCC is increased in this disorder.[36] Hypertension and hyperkalemia are common presenting features. The plasma renin activity is suppressed, and plasma aldosterone levels are inappropriately low with hyperkalemia (see Table 129-11). Thiazide diuretics are particularly helpful in these patients for treating both the hypertension and the hyperkalemia.[45]

Major deletions in the genes encoding for WNK kinase-1 and WNK kinase-4 (WNK stands for with no lysine [K is the abbreviation for lysine]) have been reported in these patients. WNK kinase-4 normally causes a decrease in luminal NCC activity.[36] Therefore, if WNK kinase-4 were deleted, reabsorption of Na^+ and Cl^- by the NCC in the distal convoluted tubule would be augmented. The molecular defect in WNK kinase-1 is the removal of intron bases, which leads to its activation (gain of function). WNK kinase-1 inactivates WNK kinase-4—the inhibitor of the NCC—hence a gain in WNK kinase-1 function leads to the activation of the NCC.

Cyclosporin-Induced Hyperkalemia

Hyperkalemia develops in some patients receiving cyclosporin following organ transplantation.[46] The pathophysiology of hyperkalemia and the clinical signs in these patients resemble those in Gordon's syndrome.[54]

Trimethoprim-Induced Hyperkalemia

The cationic form of trimethoprim causes hyperkalemia and salt wasting by blocking the ENaC in the CCD.[55] Although this was initially attributed to high doses of trimethoprim,[56-58] conventional doses may also cause a rise in P_K. Patients with human immunodeficiency virus (HIV) infection have other conditions that make them more prone to develop hyperkalemia (e.g., a shift of K^+ from cells due to alpha-adrenergic–mediated suppression of insulin release when the ECF volume is contracted).[59] K^+ excretion is also diminished because of low flow in the CCD due to a low rate of urea excretion.[60] Moreover, low flow in the CCD causes the trimethoprim concentration to be higher in the luminal fluid in the CCD and hence to become a more effective blocker of the ENaC. Loop diuretics may help by lowering the concentration of trimethoprim, but enough NaCl will be required to defend the ECF volume. Because only the protonated form of trimethoprim blocks the ENaC,[55] increasing the urine pH should cause less trimethoprim to be in its cationic form, and its antikaliuretic effect should be minimized. Inducing bicarbonaturia with acetazolamide is a rational therapeutic option when continuation of trimethoprim is necessary and blockade of the ENaC is likely. Enough alkali must be given to avoid the development of metabolic acidosis.

Hyperkalemic Periodic Paralysis

This syndrome has an autosomal dominant inheritance and is the result of a mutation in the α subunit of the skeletal muscle Na^+ channel gene.[61] This leads to failure to completely close these voltage-gated Na^+ channels when the concentration of K^+ in the ECF is raised—hence the decreased electrical excitability of the skeletal muscle. Symptoms of weakness and ultimately paralysis in association with hyperkalemia usually follow bouts of exercise. Acetazolamide seems to be effective in preventing these episodes, although its mechanism of action is not clear.

THERAPY

Medical Emergency

The major danger of a severe degree of hyperkalemia is a cardiac arrhythmia. Because mild electrocardiographic changes may progress rapidly to a dangerous arrhythmia, any such abnormality related to hyperkalemia should be considered a potential medical emergency. In certain circumstances, we would treat patients with a P_K greater than 7.0 mM aggressively, even in the absence of electrocardiographic changes; the exceptions include participants in extreme exercise (e.g., supramarathoners),[62] most patients on chronic hemodialysis, and infants.

Antagonize the Cardiac Effects of Hyperkalemia

Ca^{++} is the best agent, and its effects should be evident within minutes. It is usually given as 20 to 30 mL of a 10% calcium gluconate solution (2 to 3 ampules) or 10 mL of 10% $CaCl_2$ (1 ampule). This dose can be repeated in 5 minutes if electrocardiographic changes persist. The effect usually lasts 30 to 60 minutes. Extreme caution should be used in patients on digitalis, because hypercalcemia may aggravate digitalis toxicity.

Induce a Shift of K+ into the Intracellular Fluid

Insulin. A number of studies support the use of intravenous insulin to treat acute hyperkalemia.[63-67] Large doses of insulin (20 units of regular insulin) are needed to achieve the supraphysiologic plasma levels required for a maximal shift of K^+ into cells. Hypoglycemia must be avoided by monitoring the plasma glucose level and giving glucose as needed.

Beta₂-Adrenergic Agonists. Beta₂-adrenergic stimulation lowers the P_K in patients with renal failure.[64,66,68-73] Allon and colleagues used 10 and 20 mg of nebulized albuterol or placebo on three separate occasions and observed a decline in the P_K that was sustained for at least 2 hours.[71] The maximal decrease in P_K was 0.6 and 1.0 mM, respectively. There was a minimal increase in heart rate and a notable absence of cardiovascular side effects. However, 20% to 40% of patients are resistant to this therapy, and it is not possible to predict nonresponders. We do not recommend this treatment as the sole emergency therapy, and we are concerned about the safety of these drugs in the doses used to treat hyperkalemia—four to eight times the dose prescribed for the treatment of acute asthma. The combination of nebulized beta₂-agonists and insulin to lower the P_K was reported to produce a greater fall in P_K (1.2 mM) than either drug alone (~ 0.65 mM).[64] It should be noted that only 10 units of regular insulin were given in this study, and the magnitude of the fall in P_K was lower than that observed in other studies using higher doses of insulin.[63] Thus, it remains uncertain whether beta₂-agonists have a P_K-lowering effect additive to that of higher doses of insulin.

Sodium Bicarbonate (NaHCO₃). A number of recent studies found $NaHCO_3$ therapy to be ineffective as the sole treatment of hyperkalemia.[63,74,75] It is noteworthy that these studies were performed in stable hemodialysis patients who did not have significant acidosis (the Na^+-H^+ exchanger was presumably inactive). Thus the question remains: Would $NaHCO_3$ be effective in patients with a more significant degree of acidosis? There are no data in the literature to answer this question definitively (for a review, see reference 76). Studies that examined the combined use of $NaHCO_3$ and insulin had conflicting results.[65,67] Given this uncertainty, we use $NaHCO_3$ in addition to other therapies only to treat emergency acute hyperkalemia in patients with a significant degree of acidosis. Caution is warranted, because the excessive administration of $NaHCO_3$ risks inducing hypernatremia, ECF volume expansion, carbon dioxide retention, and hypocalcemia.

No Medical Emergency

Removal of K+ from the Body

It is important to appreciate that much less K^+ loss is needed to decrease the P_K from 7.0 to 6.0 mM than to decrease it from 6.0 to 5.0 mM.[77] Hence, creating a small K^+ loss can be very important when there is a severe degree of hyperkalemia.

Enhanced Excretion of K+ in the Urine

If K^+ excretion is low because of low urine volume, but there is high U_K, a loop diuretic may induce kaliuresis by increasing the flow rate in the CCD. One can avoid unwanted ECF volume contraction by replacing the NaCl lost in the urine. This NaCl should be given at the same tonicity as the urine to avoid creating a dysnatremia. If the U_K is unduly low, giving a mineralocorticoid (100 µg fludrocortisone) and possibly inducing bicarbonaturia with a carbonic anhydrase inhibitor may cause a substantial kaliuresis. HCO_3^- lost in the urine might need to be replaced.

Cation Exchange Resins

A cation exchange resin can exchange bound Na^+ or Ca^{++} for cations, including K^+. Sodium polystyrene sulfonate (Kayexalate) contains 4 mEq of Na^+ per gram, but only a small amount of Na^+ is exchanged for K^+ in the gastrointestinal tract.[78] The only favorable location for the exchange of Na^+ for K^+ is the lumen of the colon, but a number of factors limit the magnitude of this process. For example, other cations such as NH_4^+, Ca^{++}, and Mg^{++} may exchange for resin-bound Na^+ apart from K^+. Even if K^+ were secreted in the colon, the low stool volume would limit the total K^+ loss. For example, if the negative luminal transepithelial voltage were –90 mvolts and the P_K were 5 mM, the concentration of K^+ in stool water would be 100 mM. With a usual stool volume of 125 mL, of which 75% is water, only 10 mmol of K^+ would be lost by this route. Hence, we believe that there is virtually no benefit in using resins to treat acute hyperkalemia and little benefit in adding resins to cathartics in the setting of chronic hyperkalemia.[76]

Dialysis

Hemodialysis is more effective than peritoneal dialysis for removing K^+. Removal rates of K^+ can approximate 35 mmol/h with a dialysate bath K^+ concentration of 1 to 2 mM. A glucose-free dialysate is preferable to avoid the glucose-induced release of insulin and the subsequent shift of K^+ into cells, lessening the removal of K^+.

HYPOKALEMIA

CLINICAL APPROACH

As illustrated in Figures 129-10 and 129-11, a step-by-step approach using the following questions can determine the pathophysiology of hypokalemia.

1. *Might hypokalemia be acute?* Both the time frame and the clinical setting are important elements to consider. An acute shift of K^+ into cells may occur when there is a large surge of catecholamines (e.g., post myocardial infarction, head trauma)[79] or in patients with hypokalemic periodic paralysis.[80]
2. *What is the rate of K+ excretion?* To assess the renal response to hypokalemia, we use the expected rate of K^+

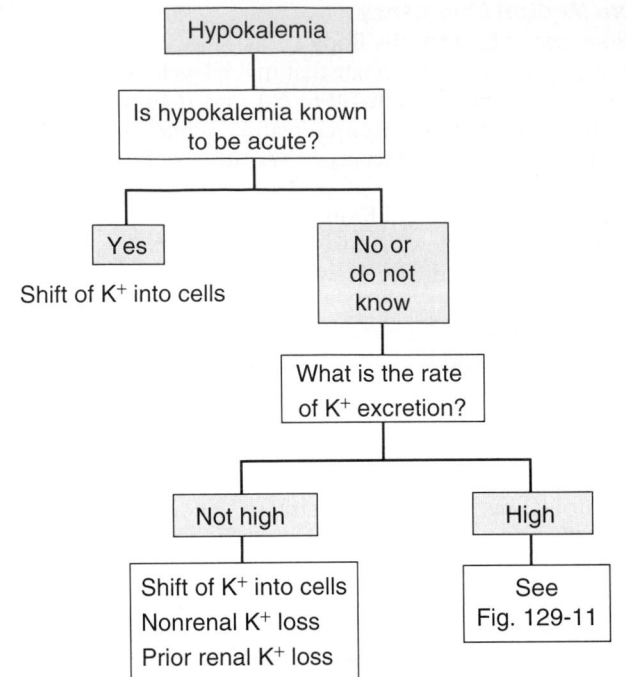

FIGURE 129–10. Approach to a patient with hypokalemia. (From Halperin ML: The ACID truth and BASIC facts—with a Sweet Touch, an enLYTEnment, 5th ed. Toronto, RossMark Medical Publishers, 2004, p 78.)

excretion when hypokalemia is due to nonrenal causes—less than 10 to 15 mmol/day, or close to 1 mmol K$^+$/mmol creatinine.[27] If the rate of K$^+$ excretion is higher than this minimum range, proceed to the questions outlined in Figure 129-13.

3. *What is the reason for the high rate of excretion of K$^+$?* The two components of the K$^+$ excretion formula need to be assessed and back-calculated to reflect events in the CCD.

4. *What osmoles account for the high flow rate in the CCD?* When the osmole excretion rate is much greater than 0.5 mOsm/min, one needs to determine which class of osmoles is responsible—organic compounds (glucose, urea, or mannitol, if it was administered) or electrolytes. A high rate of excretion of K$^+$ requires stimulation of the ENaC by aldosterone.[26]

5. *Why is the [K$^+$]$_{CCD}$ abnormally high?* A high [K$^+$]$_{CCD}$ in the presence of hypokalemia (TTKG >2) indicates a more negative luminal voltage in the CCD. Patients with an expanded effective ECF volume have a low plasma renin activity (see Table 129-1), and they may have hypertension (see Table 129-2). In contrast, patients with a low ECF volume have high plasma renin activity and Na$^+$ and Cl$^-$ poor urine (see Table 129-3).

6. *Why is the ECF volume low?* Possible diagnoses include the use (abuse) of diuretics or conditions that mimic the effect of diuretics (Bartter's or Gitelman's syndrome).[34] If the urine contains Cl$^-$ but not Na$^+$, the excretion of Cl$^-$ is obligated by a high rate of excretion of another cation, NH$_4^+$ (see Table 129-3). Conditions that cause metabolic acidosis due to diarrhea or laxative abuse should be suspected. In contrast, if the urine contains Na$^+$ but not Cl$^-$, the excretion of Na$^+$ is obligated by the excretion of another anion (e.g., bicarbonate in a patient with recent vomiting, hippurate in a glue sniffer, or a drug anion such as penicillin).

SPECIFIC CAUSES

A summary of the causes of hypokalemia is provided in Figure 129-12 and Table 129-5.

Hypokalemia with Low Extracellular Fluid Volume

Diuretic-Induced Hypokalemia

Two factors contribute to the development of hypokalemia in patients receiving diuretics: a high flow rate and increased secretion of K$^+$ in the CCD. The latter requires an enhanced electrogenic reabsorption of Na$^+$ via the ENaC (due to effects of aldosterone). Hypokalemia is usually modest in degree. A P$_K$ less than 3 mM is observed in less than 10% of patients and usually within the first 2 weeks of therapy.[81]

In the absence of diuretic use, Bartter's syndrome and Gitelman's syndrome should be suspected, because the urine consistently contains Na$^+$ and Cl$^-$ while the ECF volume is contracted. Diuretic abuse should be considered if one spot urine sample has little Na$^+$ and Cl$^-$, reflecting the normal renal response to a low ECF volume (see Table 129-2). The urine should be screened for diuretics.

Four issues about hypokalemia and diuretic use are worth highlighting. First, because the risk of developing hypokalemia is dose dependent, the lowest effective dose should be used. Second, restricting the intake of NaCl to less than 100 mmol/day may minimize the degree of renal K$^+$ wasting. Third, use of a K$^+$-sparing diuretic may reduce the renal loss of K$^+$. Fourth, whether a mild degree of hypokalemia due to diuretic use should be treated is debatable. Because patients with ischemic heart disease, with left ventricular hypertrophy, and patients treated with digitalis may be at increased risk for arrhythmias, they should be given KCl supplements.

Vomiting-Induced Hypokalemia

Because the K$^+$ concentration in gastric fluid is usually less than 15 mM,[18] hypokalemia in patients with vomiting or nasogastric suction results primarily from loss of K$^+$ in the urine due to the actions of aldosterone, along with distal delivery of HCO$_3^-$.[35] To a lesser extent, hypokalemia may be the result of a shift of K$^+$ into the ICF compartment due to alkalemia.[21] Key diagnostic elements are a history of vomiting or a strong concern about body weight, a significant degree of hypokalemia, metabolic alkalosis, and, especially, a very low U$_{Cl}$ (see Table 129-3). In a patient with recent vomiting, the urine may contain a considerable amount of Na$^+$ despite ECF volume contraction, because the excretion of HCO$_3^-$ obligates the excretion of Na$^+$. Other causes of hypokalemia with a low ECF volume must be considered (see Table 129-5). Therapy must also deal with the underlying cause of vomiting and should include the administration of KCl.[20,82] If the patient has a contracted ECF volume, NaCl should be administered as needed.

Hyperchloremic Metabolic Acidosis

Rare causes of excessive excretion of K$^+$ and metabolic acidosis include distal renal tubular acidosis due to a low rate of secretion of H$^+$ in the distal nephron[19] and inhibition of renal carbonic anhydrase. Hypokalemia is also seen in patients who sniff glue and overproduce hippuric acid.[83] If they also have a contracted ECF volume, there can be excessive excretion of K$^+$ due to an open ENaC in the CCD and the distal delivery of Na$^+$ with hippurate anions instead of Cl$^-$. In patients with

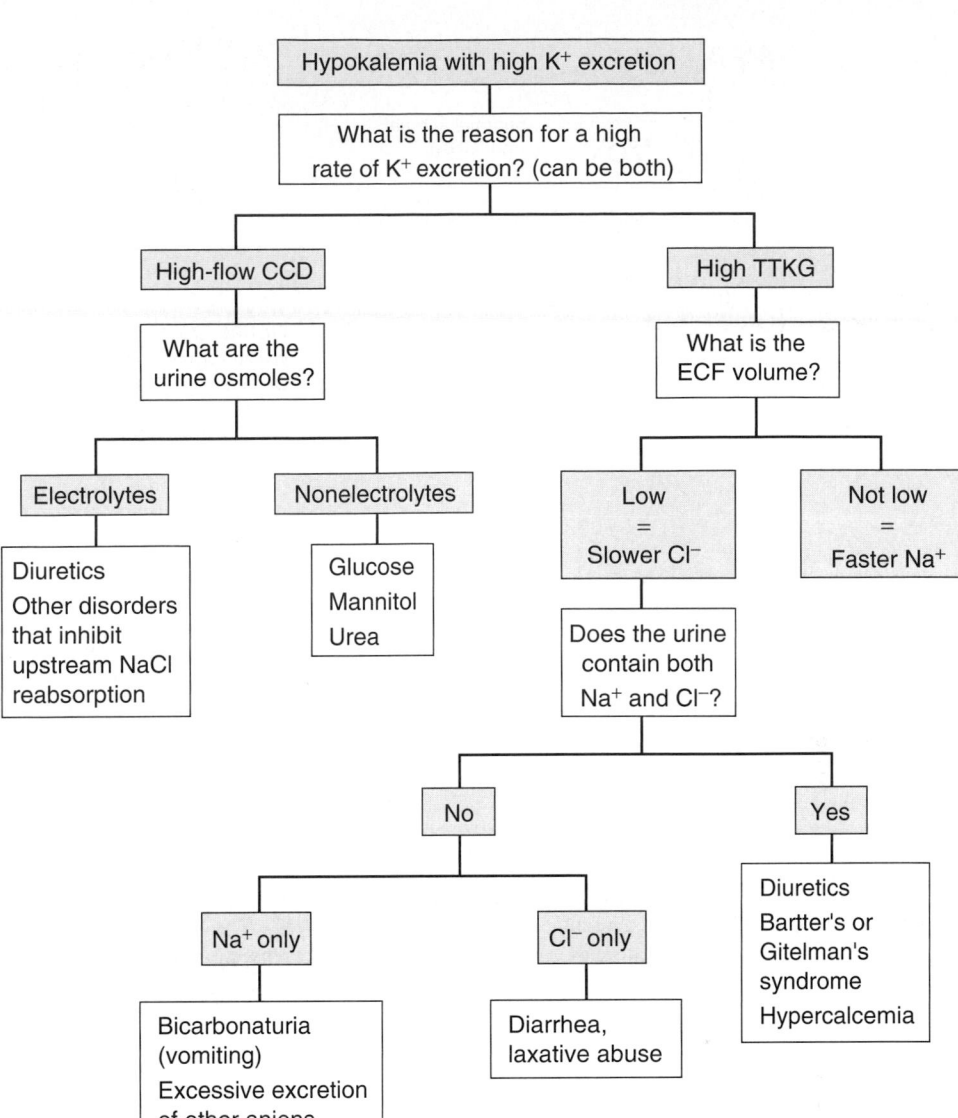

FIGURE 129–11. Renal causes of hypokalemia. CCD, cortical collecting duct; ECF, extracellular fluid; TTKG, transtubular [K] gradient. (From Halperin ML: The ACID truth and BASIC facts—with a Sweet Touch, an enLYTEnment, 5th ed. Toronto, RossMark Medical Publishers, 2004, p 79.)

gastrointestinal problems, much K$^+$ can be lost in colonic fluids.[18] A history of a diarrheal illness may be obtained, but abuse of laxatives may be denied. Measurement of the urine electrolytes can provide helpful clues (see Table 129-3). The U_{Na} will be low if the ECF volume is contracted, but the U_{Cl} is characteristically high, reflecting the high rate of excretion of NH$_4^+$ in response to metabolic acidosis or hypokalemia. One may have to rely on measurements of stool electrolytes and other evidence of laxatives in the stool to confirm the diagnosis.[80]

Bartter's Syndrome

Bartter's syndrome is a disease of children, for the most part. Mutations that cause Bartter's syndrome have been identified in five separate genes that affect NaCl transport in the thick ascending limb of the loop of Henle (see Fig. 129-13). There is often a positive family history or consanguinity. The clinical picture is dominated by ECF volume contraction, and the major laboratory features include hypokalemia; renal wasting of Na$^+$, Cl$^-$, and K$^+$; and metabolic alkalosis. The pathophysiology of Bartter's syndrome is similar to having a loop diuretic acting 24 hours a day, producing a higher than expected rate of excretion of Na$^+$ and Cl$^-$ in the face of a contracted ECF volume; an inability to maintain a sufficiently

high U_{osm} when vasopressin acts; and renal calcium wasting, as evidenced by a high urinary calcium–urinary creatinine ratio. Renal K$^+$ wasting is due to both a high flow rate in the CCD and a high [K$^+$]$_{CCD}$. The high [K$^+$]$_{CCD}$ occurs because of an enhanced distal delivery of Na$^+$ and Cl$^-$ to the CCD, together with a faster rate of reabsorption of Na$^+$ than Cl$^-$ in this nephron site. Although a considerable amount of magnesium is reabsorbed in the loop of Henle, hypomagnesemia is not a common finding in patients with Bartter's syndrome, because downstream sites can reabsorb virtually all of this higher distal delivery.

Gitelman's Syndrome

Gitelman's syndrome usually occurs in adolescent females. The main clinical symptoms are tetany and weakness.[84] The clinical picture is dominated by ECF volume contraction. Hypokalemia; renal wasting of Na$^+$, Cl$^-$, and K$^+$; and metabolic alkalosis are the major laboratory findings. Because the loop of Henle is not abnormal, patients can have a high U_{osm} when vasopressin acts. There is little calcium excretion in these patients (very low urinary calcium-creatinine ratio). Hypomagnesemia is a common finding in patients with long-standing Gitelman's syndrome.[85]

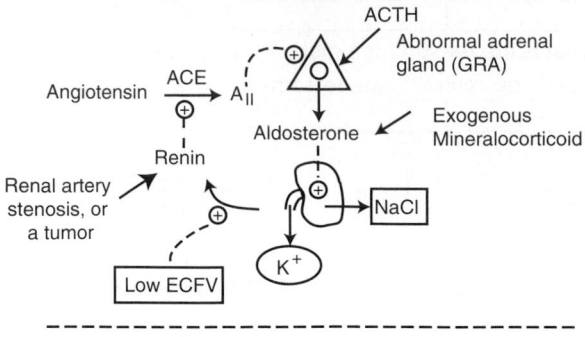

HIGH MINERALOCORTICOID ACTION

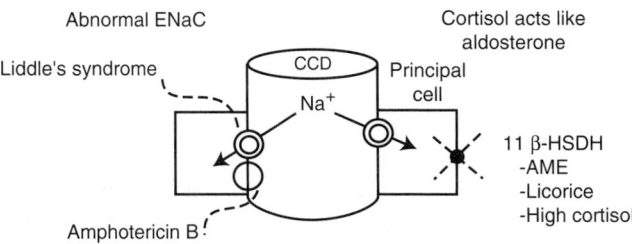

LOW ALDOSTERONE ACTION

FIGURE 129–12. Hypokalemia with augmented K⁺ secretion in the cortical collecting duct (CCD). ACE, angiotensin-converting enzyme; ACTH, adrenocorticotropic hormone; AME, apparent mineralocorticoid excess; ECFV, extracellular fluid volume; ENaC, epithelial sodium channel; GRA, glucocorticoid-remediable aldosteronism; HSDH, hydroxysteroid dehydrogenase. (From Halperin ML: The ACID truth and BASIC facts—with a Sweet Touch, an enLYTEnment, 5th ed. Toronto, RossMark Medical Publishers, 2004, p 73.)

TABLE 129–5. CAUSES OF HYPOKALEMIA

Decreased intake of K⁺
    Rarely a primary cause unless K⁺ intake is very low and duration is prolonged
    Can augment the degree of hypokalemia if there is ongoing K⁺ loss
Shift of K⁺ into cells
    Hormones (insulin and beta-adrenergics are most important)
    Metabolic alkalosis
    Anabolic state (e.g., recovery from diabetic ketoacidosis)
    Rare (e.g., hypokalemic periodic paralysis)
Excessive renal K⁺ loss
    Faster reabsorption of Na⁺ in the CCD
      High aldosterone levels
      Cortisol acts as mineralocorticoid
        Low 11 β-HSDH activity (AME)
        Inhibitors of 11 β-HSDH (e.g., licorice)
        Very high cortisol level (e.g., ACTH-producing tumor)
      Constitutively active ENaC (e.g., Liddle's syndrome)
      Artificial ENaC (e.g., amphotericin B)
    Slower reabsorption of Cl⁻ in the CCD
      Delivery of Na⁺ without Cl⁻ to the CCD and low ECF volume
      Inhibition of Cl⁻ reabsorption in the CCD (e.g., bicarbonaturia)
      High delivery of Na⁺ and Cl⁻ to the CCD and a V_{max} for Na⁺ reabsorption that exceeds that for Cl⁻ (inhibition of NaCl reabsorption in upstream nephron segment plus ECF volume contraction)
Loss of K⁺ via the gastrointestinal tract or skin

ACTH, adrenocorticotropic hormone; AME, apparent mineralocorticoid excess; CCD, cortical collecting duct; ECF, extracellular fluid; ENaC, epithelial sodium channel; 11β-HSDH, 11-β hydroxysteroid dehydrogenase; V_{max}, maximum velocity.

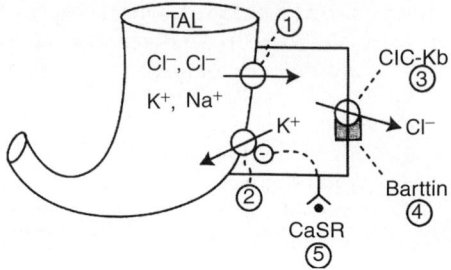

FIGURE 129–13. Possible molecular basis for Bartter's syndrome. The stylized structure is the thick ascending limb (TAL) of the loop of Henle. Defects that can lead to a diminished reabsorption of Na⁺ and Cl⁻ and thereby Bartter's syndrome involve the Na⁺-K⁺-Cl⁻ cotransporter (NKCC) (site 1),[97] the ROM-K channel (site 2),[98] lesions affecting the basolateral ClCN-Kb (site 3) or its β subunit protein barttin (site 4),[99,100] or, indirectly, the calcium-sensing receptor (CaSR) (site 5).[101,102] (From Halperin ML: The ACID truth and BASIC facts—with a Sweet Touch, an enLYTEnment, 5th ed. Toronto, RossMark Medical Publishers, 2004, p 221.)

Gitelman's syndrome is similar to having a thiazide diuretic acting 24 hours a day. Mutations that cause Gitelman's syndrome have been identified in three separate genes that affect NaCl transport in the distal convoluted tubule (see Fig. 129-14). One can anticipate other molecular causes that enhance WNK kinase-4 or lower WNK kinase-1 activity. The combination of enhanced distal delivery of Na⁺ and Cl⁻ to the CCD and a faster rate of reabsorption of Na⁺ than Cl⁻ in this nephron site leads to a more negative luminal voltage in the CCD and enhanced K⁺ secretion.

Correction of hypokalemia is extremely difficult in patients with Bartter's and Gitelman's syndromes, even with large supplements of K⁺. Correction of hypomagnesemia with oral magnesium is not successful because of gastrointestinal side effects. Angiotensin-converting enzyme (ACE) inhibitors have been used with variable success, but hypotension is a potential problem with this therapy. We are concerned about the prolonged use of nonsteroidal anti-inflammatory drugs because of the potential for chronic renal dysfunction. K⁺-sparing diuretics in large doses may help conserve K⁺ but may exacerbate renal salt wasting. A common clinical observation is that even high doses of

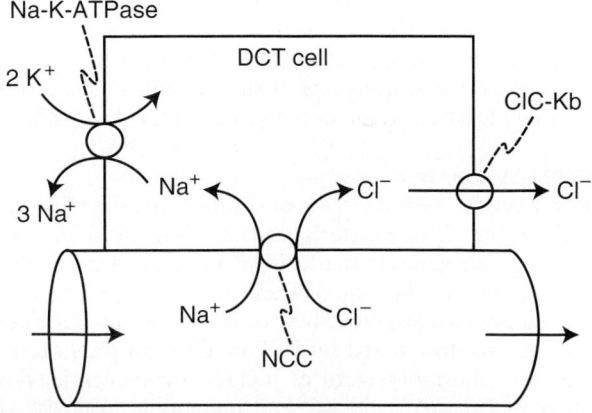

FIGURE 129–14. Possible molecular basis for Gitelman's syndrome. The most common defect causing Gitelman's syndrome is a mutation involving the Na⁺-Cl⁻ cotransporter (NCC),[94] but others include a lesion in the γ subunit of the Na⁺,K⁺-ATPase pump[95] or in Cl⁻ channels on basolateral membranes in this nephron segment (ClC-Kb).[96] DCT, distal convoluted tubule.

amiloride may fail to curtail the excessive kaliuresis in patients with Bartter's and Gitelman's syndromes. Part of the explanation for this diminished effect is the high-volume delivery to the CCD.

Cationic Drug–Induced Hypokalemia

Gentamicin and tobramicin are cationic antibiotics that bind to the calcium-sensing receptor on the basolateral aspect of cells of the loop of Henle (see Fig. 129-13).[86] This leads to inhibition of the luminal K^+ channel and to furosemide-like effects.

Hypokalemia with Normal or High Extracellular Fluid Volume

Primary Hyperaldosteronism

Hypersecretion of aldosterone may be due to an adrenal adenoma or bilateral adrenal hyperplasia. This diagnosis should be suspected in patients with hypertension and unexplained hypokalemia with renal K^+ wasting. Nevertheless, a significant proportion of these patients do not have hypokalemia or hypertension.[87] An elevated plasma aldosterone level and very low plasma renin activity are characteristic findings (see Table 129-1). A random plasma aldosterone (in ng/dL) to plasma renin activity (in ng/mL/h) ratio is an excellent screening test. This ratio is usually 4 to 10 in normal subjects or in patients with essential hypertension, but it can be as high as 30 to 50 in patients with primary hyperaldosteronism. To differentiate patients with adrenal adenoma from those with bilateral adrenal hyperplasia, imaging techniques are helpful (computed tomography or magnetic resonance imaging). If an adrenal adenoma is not detected, adrenal vein sampling or an iodocholesterol scan can help in the differential diagnosis.

The finding of very low plasma renin activity with high plasma aldosterone levels separates patients with primary hyperaldosteronism from those with other causes of hypertension and hypokalemia (see Table 129-1). The differential diagnosis includes glucocorticoid-remediable aldosteronism. Patients with this condition have elevated plasma aldosterone levels and suppressed plasma renin activity, but they are unique because aldosterone can be suppressed with the administration of dexamethasone.[88]

In patients with adrenal adenoma, unilateral adrenalectomy is usually the preferred treatment. In patients with bilateral adrenal hyperplasia and those with adrenal adenoma who are not candidates for surgery, medical therapy with K^+-sparing diuretics is recommended. Amiloride is generally better tolerated than spironolactone. The effects of amiloride are more evident in patients who are salt restricted (lower flow rate in the CCD and thereby a higher concentration of amiloride for any given amount of the drug).

ACTH-Producing Tumor or Severe Cushing's Syndrome

The clinical picture is similar to that of hyperaldosteronism, but the level of aldosterone in plasma is low. Because of an overabundance of cortisol, the activity of 11 β-HSDH is insufficient to inactivate all the cortisol that enters principal cells (see Fig. 129-6). As a result, cortisol binds to the mineralocorticoid receptor and exerts mineralocorticoid activity.

Plasma ACTH levels are markedly suppressed in patients with Cushing's syndrome and high if there is an ACTH-producing tumor (e.g., oat cell carcinoma of the lung). In patients with ACTH-producing tumors, overt signs of glucocorticoid excess may not be evident at the time of diagnosis. The P_K is often below 2 mM. Plasma aldosterone levels and renin activity are both suppressed. Therapy is directed at the primary disorder. Large supplements of KCl and drugs that inhibit the ENaC are often necessary to treat the hypokalemia.

Syndrome of Apparent Mineralocorticoid Excess

The clinical picture is of hyperaldosteronism, but the level of aldosterone in plasma is low. Because of decreased activity of the enzyme 11 β-HSDH, cortisol binds to the mineralocorticoid receptors and exerts mineralocorticoid activity.[89] Plasma aldosterone levels and renin activity are both suppressed (see Table 129-1). The diagnosis is confirmed by finding an elevated urinary cortisol to cortisone ratio. A similar clinical picture can be induced with chronic ingestion of licorice or licorice-like compounds.[90] The administration of dexamethasone, which does not bind the mineralocorticoid receptor, helps correct the hypertension and hypokalemia if it suppresses the endogenous production of cortisol.

Liddle's Syndrome

The clinical picture is of hyperaldosteronism, but the level of aldosterone is very low. The pathophysiology of this disorder is one of a constitutively active ENaC in the CCD.[91] Several mutations in the genes encoding for the β or γ subunits of the ENaC have been described in patients with Liddle's syndrome.[92,93] It is an autosomal dominant inherited disorder with early onset of severe hypertension and hypokalemia. Interestingly, however, a number of patients with this disorder do not have hypokalemia. A positive family history of early-onset hypertension and hypokalemia and very low plasma aldosterone levels and plasma renin activity are key elements in the diagnosis. There is no excess secretion of cortisol, and the urinary cortisol to cortisone ratio is not elevated. Control of hypertension and correction of hypokalemia are more likely to be achieved with the administration of ENaC blockers (amiloride, together with a low salt diet) than with mineralocorticoid antagonists (spironolacatone).

Drug-Induced Hypokalemia

Amphotericin B induces hypokalemia because there is an artificial and unregulated cation (Na^+ and K^+) channel that is permanently in an open configuration and permits K^+ secretion in the CCD. Treatment involves correcting the electrolyte abnormalities, discontinuing the drug if possible, and waiting for its side effects to wear off. Avoidance of large intravenous infusions of fluid when giving this drug will minimize the risk of a very high flow rate in the CCD when amphotericin B acts.

Hypokalemic Periodic Paralysis

This disorder is characterized by episodes of transient shifts of K^+ from the ECF to the ICF compartment of skeletal muscle. This shift of K^+ can be provoked by a high-carbohydrate meal (release of insulin) or strenuous exercise (adrenergic surge). The latter is particularly important in patients who have hyperthyroidism.[9] In the Asian population, the disorder is more frequent in males and is commonly associated with thyrotoxicosis.[80] The familial, nonthyrotoxic variety is inherited as an autosomal dominant disorder and usually manifests in the teenage years. Genetic analyses suggest that the abnormality in these patients is linked to the gene that encodes for the dihydropyridine-sensitive Ca^{++} channel in skeletal muscles; it is not clear how this leads to hypokalemia.

Laboratory findings are helpful to differentiate this acute hypokalemia from an acute shift of K^+ into cells in a patient with chronic hypokalemia.[80] First, there is an absence of acid-base disorders. Second, one should anticipate a low rate of excretion of K^+, as manifested by a low $U_K/U_{creatinine}$ ratio, low TTKG, or both. Patients with hypokalemic periodic paralysis usually need far less KCl to normalize the P_K than do patients who have a chronic K^+ wasting disease together with a reason to shift K^+ acutely into cells ($\sim$1 versus >3 mmol KCl/kg body weight).

Therapy is largely symptomatic or empirical. Hyperthyroidism, if present, is treated in the usual fashion. Patients are advised to avoid carbohydrate-rich meals and vigorous exercise. Nonselective beta blockers may reduce the number of the attacks of paralysis with little effect on the degree of fall in the P_K.[9] An acute attack is treated with the administration of KCl. There is, however, the risk of post-treatment hyperkalemia when K^+ moves back into the ECF compartment. Patients with the thyrotoxic variety of hypokalemic periodic paralysis can be treated with a nonselective beta blocker and a much smaller administration of KCl.[8] Acetazolamide 250 to 750 mg/day has been used successfully in patients with the familial form of hypokalemic periodic paralysis, although the basis of its beneficial effect is unclear.

THERAPY

Our approach is to first recognize when hypokalemia may be life-threatening.

Medical Emergency

These emergencies include cardiac arrhythmias, extreme weakness causing respiratory failure, and hepatic encephalopathy. When any of these conditions is present, enough K^+ must be given to raise the P_K quickly. The total body K^+ deficit should be replaced much more slowly. Because large doses and high concentrations of K^+ might be needed, K^+ must be administered via a central vein, and the patient should be on a cardiac monitor. In general, the infusion should not contain glucose or HCO_3^-, because this might aggravate the degree of hypokalemia.

No Medical Emergency

Hypokalemic Periodic Paralysis. In the absence of a cardiac or respiratory emergency, small doses of KCl should be given to patients with hypokalemic periodic paralysis to minimize the risk of severe rebound hyperkalemia, because they do not have large deficits of K^+. If associated with hyperthyroidism, a nonselective beta blocker (propranolol 3 mg/kg) can provide effective therapy.[8]

Magnitude of the K^+ Deficit. There is no useful quantitative relationship between the P_K and the total body K^+ deficit, because there may also be a shift of K^+ into cells.[77] Hence, careful monitoring of the P_K during replacement of the K^+ deficit is mandatory.

Route of K^+ Administration. The oral route is preferred if bowel sounds are present. When a peripheral intravenous route is used, the K^+ concentration should not be greater than 40 mM. The rate of K^+ administration should not be greater than 60 mmol/h in all but emergency settings.

K^+ Preparations. Increasing the intake of K^+-rich foods (e.g., bananas, fruit juice) has the danger of inducing a large

weight gain. Oral KCl (e.g., salt substitutes such as co-salt, which provide 14 mmol of K^+ per gram) are generally well tolerated and are inexpensive. Liquid K^+ supplements have an unpleasant taste and are often poorly tolerated. Most preparations used are "slow release," either microencapsulated or in a wax matrix. Although usually well tolerated, they may cause ulcerative or stenotic lesions in the gastrointestinal tract.

In patients with a deficit of KCl (e.g., chronic vomiting or diuretics), only KCl is needed, whereas in patients with a $KHCO_3$ deficit (e.g., diarrhea), $KHCO_3$ may be needed in addition to KCl. Because the administration of HCO_3^- may lead to a shift of K^+ into cells, KCl should be given initially, and alkali should be withheld until the P_K approaches a safe level ($\sim$3 mM), unless there are ongoing and large losses of HCO_3^-. K^+ phosphate may be needed when there is rapid anabolism and little oral intake. We give K^+ as KCl in the treatment of diabetic ketoacidosis and rely on the patient's diet to supply the phosphate needed to restore a normal ICF composition later. If phosphate is given, limit the infusion to less than 50 mmol every 8 hours to minimize the risk of hypocalcemia and metastatic calcification.

Adjuncts to Therapy

Renal loss of K^+ can be reduced by using K^+-sparing diuretics. This is feasible only on a chronic basis. Amiloride and triamterene are better tolerated than spironolactone, because they lack the latter's gastrointestinal and hormonal (amenorrhea, gynecomastia, decreased libido) complications. Hyperkalemia may develop when K^+ is given with K^+-sparing diuretics, especially if other conditions that compromise K^+ excretion are present; note that these drugs have a long half-life.

Risks of Therapy

With prolonged hypokalemia, the CCD may become temporarily hyporesponsive to the kaliuretic effect of aldosterone (reviewed in reference 41). Hence, it is important to monitor the P_K frequently during the treatment of hypokalemia. Hyperkalemia has been observed in approximately 4% of patients taking K^+ supplements. The risk is highest in patients with renal failure and diabetes mellitus. The simultaneous use of ACE inhibitors, beta blockers, or nonsteroidal anti-inflammatory drugs may also predispose to the development of hyperkalemia.

ANNOTATED REFERENCES

Halperin ML, Kamel KS: Potassium. Lancet 1998;352:135-142.
Concise overview of regulation of the rate of K^+ excretion by factors that affect both the voltage within the lumen of the CCD and the volume exiting from the CCD. Provides useful information concerning the pathophysiology of disorders of K^+ excretion, the accuracy of clinical diagnosis, and where leverage can be exerted in therapy.

Hebert SC: Extracellular calcium-sensing receptor: Implications for calcium and magnesium handling in the kidney. Kidney Int 1996;50:2129-2139.
Describes an important signaling pathway in the kidney—the calcium-sensing receptor—with broad clinical implications in areas other than disorders of K^+ excretion. For example, this explains the basis for the development of nonoliguric renal failure in patients who have aminoglycoside-induced acute tubular necrosis.

Kamel KS, Wei C: Controversial issues in treatment of hyperkalemia. Nephrol Dial Transplant 2003;18:2215-2218.
Broad overview of aspects of therapy for patients with hyperkalemia. The basis for selecting one therapy over another becomes clearer with a critical review of the literature.

Landry DW, Oliver JA: The pathogenesis of vasodilatory shock. N Engl J Med 2001;345:588-595.

Relevant for understanding the control of blood flow rate in an ICU setting. This provides a rationale for why drugs such as vasopressin and sulfonylureas can be useful in patients with multiorgan failure or septic shock.

Lin SH, Lin YF, Halperin ML: Hypokalemia and paralysis: Clues on admission to help in the differential diagnosis. Q J Med 2001;94:133-139.

Demonstrates a practical approach to the differential diagnosis of acute hypokalemia. Clues for recognizing hypokalemia due to an acute shift of K⁺ into cells are provided. and clinical implications for therapy are discussed.

Yang C-L, Angell J, Mitchell R, Ellison DH: WNK kinases regulate thiazide-sensitive Na-Cl cotransport. J Clin Invest 2003;111:1039-1045.

An example of how advances in molecular biology can be used at the bedside. The focus here is on patients with Gordon's syndrome who have an unanticipated molecular basis for the development of hyperkalemia and hypertension.

Chapter 130

DISORDERS OF CALCIUM AND MAGNESIUM METABOLISM

Mordecai M. Popovtzer

KEY POINTS

HYPOCALCEMIA

1. Serum levels of 25(OH) vitamin D serve as an estimate of body stores of vitamin D. Low serum concentrations of 25(OH) vitamin D indicate a state of vitamin D deficiency.

2. Hypoparathyroidism is a common cause of hypocalcemia. Magnesium depletion inhibits parathyroid hormone (PTH) secretion and peripheral responses to PTH and to vitamin D; it also blunts the calcemic effect of intravenous calcium. Thiazides enhance the calcemic effect of vitamin D, whereas furosemide aggravates the hypocalcemia.

3. Neuromuscular manifestations of hypocalcemia include focal and generalized seizures. The spasm of diaphragm and intercostal muscles may cause respiratory arrest. Cardiovascular complications of acute hypocalcemia are hypotension, bradycardia, and ventricular arrhythmias such as torsades de pointes.

4. Hypoparathyroidism, and particularly the variant autosomal dominant hypocalcemia, should be treated cautiously. Raising serum calcium levels may cause hypercalciuria with increased risk of nephrocalcinosis and renal failure.

HYPERCALCEMIA

1. Malignancy is the prevalent cause of hypercalcemia, accounting for 70% to 80% of all cases, and is most commonly seen in hospitalized patients. Primary hyperparathyroidism is common in the outpatient setting, accounting for 10% to 20% of all cases of hypercalcemia. Milk-alkali syndrome ranks third.

2. Hypercalcemia with undetectable PTH and high urinary cyclic adenosine monophosphate (AMP) is consistent with humoral hypercalcemia of malignancy (HHM). Detection of parathyroid hormone-related protein (PTHrP) does not rule out parathyroid adenoma; rather, the absence of PTH and the presence of PTHrP rule out adenoma and support HHM.

3. Familial hypocalciuric hypercalcemia is a form of parathyroid hyperplasia with autosomal dominant transmission. It is caused by an inactivating mutation of a calcium-sensing receptor. The clinical course is benign, without nephrolithiasis, but hypermagnesemia, pancreatitis, and chondrocalcinosis may occur.

4. Hypercalcemic crisis is a life-threatening emergency. It may be a complication of primary hyper parathyroidism, malignancy, and other hypercalcemic disorders. It warrants aggressive treatment to lower the serum calcium concentration.

5. The first goal in treating hypercalcemia is to restore the extracellular volume to normal by intravenous administration of normal saline. This usually requires 3 to 4 L of saline.

HYPOMAGNESEMIA

1. Hypomagnesemia is common in hospitalized patients (>10%) and even more so in the ICU setting (>50%). The concerns regarding hypomagnesemia are focused on its potential role in cardiac arrhythmias (e.g., torsades de pointes) and sudden death.

2. Hypomagnesemia leads to renal losses of potassium, and, vice versa, hypokalemia augments urinary losses of magnesium. In the former, hypokalemia may be refractory to potassium replacement unless magnesium repletion is accomplished first.

HYPERMAGNESEMIA

1. The most common cause of hypermagnesemia is concurrence of excessive magnesium loads in the presence of impaired renal function. Very often a large magnesium load comes from therapeutic use of magnesium salts as laxatives or enemas.

2. Neuromuscular manifestations of hypermagnesemia relate to its curare-like effect, leading to loss of reflexes, muscle paralysis, and apnea. Central nervous system abnormalities are lethargy, drowsiness, dilated and fixed pupils, and coma.

3. The cardiovascular effects of hypermagnesemia consist of bradycardia and hypotension. The electrocardiogram (ECG) shows increased PR interval and QRS complex. Complete heart block and cardiac arrest is the terminal event.

4. Severe hypermagnesemia is a medical emergency. Treatment includes intravenous administration of saline and loop diuretics. Calcium, an antagonist of magnesium, may be given intravenously at the dose of 100 to 200 mg elemental calcium over 5 minutes. Dialysis with magnesium-free dialysate quickly clears an excess of magnesium.

SERUM CALCIUM CONCENTRATION

The calcium concentration is essential to many physiologic phenomena, including preservation of the integrity of cellular membranes, neuromuscular activity, regulation of endocrine and exocrine secretory activities, blood coagulation, activation of the complement system, and bone metabolism.

TOTAL SERUM CALCIUM CONCENTRATION

The normal range for total serum calcium must be established for each laboratory and varies according to the method used. Total serum calcium concentration is divisible into protein-bound and ultrafiltrable (diffusible) calcium.[1,2]

Protein-Bound Calcium

Approximately 40% of total calcium is bound to serum proteins, and 80% to 90% of this calcium is bound to albumin. Variations in serum protein alter proportionately the concentration of the protein-bound and total serum calcium. An increase in serum albumin concentration of 1 g/dL increases protein-bound calcium by 0.8 mg/dL, whereas an increase of 1 g/dL of globulin increases protein-bound calcium by 0.16 mg/dL. Thus, it is obvious that changes in total serum calcium concentrations cannot be used for the assessment of the effect on bound calcium concentrations unless the changes in albumin and globulin concentrations also are determined. Marked changes in serum sodium concentration also affect the protein binding of calcium. Hyponatremia increases, whereas hypernatremia decreases, protein-bound calcium. Changes in pH also affect protein-bound calcium, and an increase or decrease of 0.1 pH, respectively, increases or decreases protein-bound calcium by 0.12 mg/dL. In vitro, freezing and thawing serum samples may decrease the binding of calcium as well.

Ultrafiltrable (Diffusible) Calcium

Serum ultrafiltrable calcium is obtained by applying pressure on serum against a semipermeable membrane. Thus, serum water is forced across the membrane, and the ultrafiltrate is analyzed for calcium concentration and then corrected for total serum solids. The samples must be handled anaerobically, because changes in pH may affect calcium binding.

Under normal conditions, ultrafiltrable calcium constitutes 55% to 60% of the total serum calcium concentration.

FREE (IONIZED) CALCIUM

The biologically active component of diffusible calcium is ionized calcium. Serum ionized calcium concentration in normal subjects ranges from 4.0 to 4.9 mg/dL or 47% of total serum calcium. The samples have to be handled anaerobically because changes in pH alter the concentration of ionized calcium. Storage of serum in oil does not prevent changes in pH, because carbon dioxide dissolves readily in oil. An increase in serum pH of 0.1 unit may cause a decrease in ionized calcium of 0.16 mg/dL. As with ultrafiltrable calcium, freezing and thawing of serum may alter the level of ionized calcium.

COMPLEXED CALCIUM

The nonionized portion of diffusible or ultrafiltrable calcium is called complexed calcium. The calcium complexes are formed with bicarbonate, phosphate, and acetate. The amount of complexed calcium is measured indirectly by subtracting the ionized calcium (47%) from the ultrafiltrable calcium (60%) and thus equals about 13% of total serum calcium. The complexed calcium has been found to be increased twofold in patients with uremia.

CYTOSOLIC FREE CALCIUM

Cytosolic free calcium can be measured by loading the tested cells with a fluorescent probe such as indo-1-acetoxymethyl ester and exciting the cells at 350 nM. The ratio of fluorescence emission at 410 nM to that at 490 nM is used as an index of free intracellular calcium.[3] The normal concentration of cytosolic calcium is 100 nM/L, that is, 10,000-fold lower than the concentration of extracellular calcium. This very steep gradient is maintained by an energy-driven calcium pump, known as the plasma membrane Ca^{++}-ATPase (PMCA). In certain types of cells a Na^+/Ca^{++} exchanger, energized by Na^+-gradient helps drive cytosolic calcium into the extracellular space. Part of cellular calcium is sequestered in intracellular organelles, including endoplasmic reticulum, sarcoplasmic reticulum in muscle cells, and mitochondria. These organelles are endowed with their own calcium pumps that help preserve the very low free cytosolic calcium. The calcium-dependent intracellular signaling generally requires a 10-fold increase in free cytosolic calcium. With each heartbeat the cytosolic calcium concentration in cardiac myocytes is elevated 10-fold, from a resting level of 100 nM to 1000 nM. Likewise, in other signaling events such as T-cell activation, which triggers the transcription of interleukin-2, a 10-fold increase in cytosolic calcium serves as the signal for the response. Elevation in cytosolic calcium is mediated by the activation of calcium channels, which allows passive calcium flux down its electrochemical gradient.[4]

HYPOCALCEMIA

Disorders associated with hypocalcemia can be classified into disorders related to vitamin D and disorders related to parathyroid hormone (PTH).

DISORDERS RELATED TO VITAMIN D DEFICIENCY

Vitamin D Deficiency

Hypocalcemia is a common feature of vitamin D deficiency. The common causes of vitamin D deficiency are listed in Table 130-1. Lack of sunlight exposure impairs endogenous vitamin D synthesis. Because vitamin D is a fat-soluble vitamin, nutritional osteomalacia usually is associated with a deficient intake of food products containing fatty substances. Gastrectomy may lead either to dietary deficiency due to avoiding fatty products and/or due to malabsorption of vitamin D, as noted with Billroth type II surgery, in which a vitamin D–absorbing bowel segment is bypassed. Bile salts deficiency impairs vitamin D absorption. Small bowel diseases, laxative abuse, and certain anticonvulsants (phenytoin) interfere with absorption. Urinary losses of vitamin D were linked to Fanconi's syndrome and nephrotic syndrome.[5] Because hepatic formation of 25(OH) vitamin D from vitamin D is not tightly controlled and depends primarily on the availability of vitamin D, the serum level of 25(OH) vitamin D_3 is utilized as a measurement of body stores of vitamin D; low levels of 25(OH) vitamin D indicate vitamin D deficiency.[2]

Impaired Metabolism of Vitamin D

Hypocalcemia in patients ingesting phenobarbital is associated with low levels of circulating 25(OH) vitamin D. Half-life of vitamin D and 25(OH) vitamin D are shortened by barbiturates, owing to induction of microsomal enzymes in the liver. The latter leads to rapid turnover of 25(OH) vitamin D and increased formation of inactive polar metabolites of vitamin D. Low circulating levels of 25(OH) vitamin D also have been observed in patients with hepatic failure due to reduced transformation of vitamin D to 25(OH) vitamin D in the liver.[6]

Dietary calcium deprivation, per se, in rats increases the clearance and inactivation of 25(OH) vitamin D and causes vitamin D deficiency. It has been suggested that this variety of vitamin D deficiency is caused by secondary hyperparathyroidism, which augments renal synthesis of 1,25(OH)$_2$ vitamin D, which, in turn, enhances the degradation of 25(OH) vitamin D to inactive metabolites.

TABLE 130–1. COMMON CAUSES OF VITAMIN D DEFICIENCY

Lack of exposure to sunshine
Nutritional
Malabsorption
  Following gastrectomy
  Tropical and nontropical sprue
  Chronic pancreatitis
  Biliary cirrhosis
  Ingestion of cathartics
  Intestinal bypass
  Anticonvulsant therapy
Abnormal metabolism of vitamin D
  Vitamin D–dependent rickets
  Ingestion of barbiturates and anticonvulsants
  Renal insufficiency
  Hepatic dysfunction
  Calcium deprivation
Renal losses of vitamin D
  Nephrotic syndrome
  Fanconi's syndrome

Hypothetically, this mechanism may account for vitamin D deficiency in clinical states of calcium malabsorption, including gastrointestinal diseases, anticonvulsant therapy (e.g., phenytoin), and certain drugs such as colchicine, fluoride, and theophylline. Likewise, increased intake of foods rich in phytate, oxalate, and citrate that chelate calcium in the gastrointestinal tract and render it nonabsorbable may cause vitamin D deficiency.[2,7]

Vitamin D–dependent rickets type I (VDDR-1), also designated as pseudo–vitamin D deficiency, is inherited as an autosomal recessive disorder in which 25(OH) vitamin D-1α-hydroxylase in the proximal tubules is deficient due to defects in the 1α-hydroxylase gene. It is manifested by early hypocalcemia, hypophosphatemia, severe secondary hyperparathyroidism, and severe rickets. The serum 1,25(OH)$_2$ vitamin D is undetectable or very low, whereas 25(OH) vitamin D levels are normal. The clinical abnormality can be reversed completely by the administration of pharmacologic doses of vitamin D or physiologic doses of 1,25(OH)$_2$ vitamin D. Linkage analysis in families with VDDR-1 mapped the disease locus to chromosome 12q13-14.[8,9]

End-Organ Resistance to 1,25(OH)$_2$ Vitamin D

Hypocalcemia refractory to 1,25(OH)$_2$ vitamin D_3 was described as type II vitamin D–dependent rickets, also known as hereditary 1,25(OH)$_2$ vitamin D_3–resistant rickets. This familial disorder is inherited by autosomal recessive transmission and is characterized by hypocalcemia, impaired intestinal absorption of calcium, rickets, and alopecia, which reflects a defect in the physiologic action of 1,25(OH) vitamin D in the skin. In contrast to vitamin D–dependent rickets type I, in type II the serum 1,25(OH)$_2$ vitamin D level is elevated and the patients either respond to pharmacologic doses of 1,25(OH)$_2$ vitamin D_3 or do not respond at all. In some patients with this disorder, an abnormal nuclear uptake, abnormal cytosol receptor binding of 1,25(OH) vitamin D, or both are present. These findings suggest that the mechanism of the end-organ resistance is a defect in the receptor. Mutations of vitamin D receptor genes have been identified.

DISORDERS RELATED TO PARATHYROID HORMONE

Reduced Production of PTH

Hypoparathyroidism

Hypoparathyroidism is a disorder characterized by hypocalcemia and hyperphosphatemia due to a deficient or absent secretion of PTH.

Hypoparathyroidism is a common cause of hypocalcemia. It commonly presents as paresthesias, muscle spasms (i.e., tetany), and seizures. However, very often, mild chronic hypoparathyroidism may cause hypocalcemia so gradually that the only symptoms may be visual impairment from cataracts after years of hypoparathyroidism.

Hypoparathyroidism may be either an acquired abnormality designated as secondary hypoparathyroidism, or primary hypoparathyroidism, also known as idiopathic hypoparathyroidism.

Secondary Hypoparathyroidism

Hypoparathyroidism may be caused by surgery. This variety of hypoparathyroidism may result from accidental removal of parathyroids or traumatic interruption of their blood supply.

Hypocalcemia that appears after excision of parathyroid adenoma results from functional suppression and hypofunction of the remaining normal glands. Very often the parathyroid deficiency is of short duration. More protracted hypocalcemia after parathyroidectomy has been reported in association with the "hungry bone" syndrome. In the latter, it is believed that the reduction in circulating PTH leads to reversal of the negative calcium balance at the bone level, and increased deposition with reduced release of calcium leads to hypocalcemia. Similarly, hypocalcemia has been reported to occur in 15% of patients after thyroidectomy.[10]

Hypoparathyroidism may be a component of multiple endocrine dysfunctions, including adrenal insufficiency owing to an autoimmune disorder. In hypoparathyroidism associated with pernicious anemia, an autoimmune mechanism has also been implicated. Hypoparathyroidism is a recognized complication of thalassemia and Wilson's disease. Deposition of iron and copper, respectively, in the parathyroid glands is the likely underlying mechanism.[6,11]

Hypocalcemia may occur in magnesium depletion.[12] It has been shown that the chronic state of low serum magnesium diminishes the release of PTH.[13] Hypomagnesemia has been reported to induce skeletal resistance to PTH.[14] It is interesting that some patients with hypoparathyroidism who also exhibit resistance to vitamin D may respond to it after administration of magnesium. Similarly, patients with symptomatic hypoparathyroidism who fail to respond to intravenous calcium become responsive after treatment with intravenous magnesium. The mechanisms that underlie the effects of hypomagnesemia on serum calcium are poorly understood. It may be speculated, however, that magnesium depletion may impair the activity of the calcium pump and thus alter the distribution of calcium between the extracellular and the intracellular spaces.

Hypocalcemia in association with hypomagnesemia has been reported in 60% of patients with severe acute respiratory syndrome (SARS).[15] Hypocalcemia may follow therapeutic use of magnesium sulfate (e.g., in preeclampsia) secondary to magnesium-induced suppression of PTH. Aminoglycosides and cytotoxic agents may exert a toxic effect on parathyroid glands, leading to hypocalcemia.[2,11]

Symptomatic hypoparathyroidism has been observed in association with HIV infection.[2]

Primary (Idiopathic) Hypoparathyroidism

Primary hypoparathyroidism may occur in association with other endocrine disorders or as an isolated entity. The latter is termed *isolated hypoparathyroidism,* and it may occur as a sporadic or familial disorder.[16]

Primary isolated hypoparathyroidism may be due to a mutation in the pre-pro-PTH gene. This variety of familial isolated hypoparathyroidism may be inherited both as an autosomal dominant and as autosomal recessive form. Patients may carry a mutation affecting the signal peptide–encoding region of the pre-pro-PTH gene or a donor splice site mutation of pre-pro-PTH gene. The former may be inherited both in an autosomal dominant and autosomal recessive form, whereas the latter is inherited as an autosomal recessive disorder. This form of primary isolated hypoparathyroidism that is caused by a defect in PTH synthesis is a very rare disorder.[17-19]

Autosomal dominant isolated hypoparathyroidism was described in families with activating mutations of the gene that encodes the extracellular calcium sensing receptor

(CASR) located in chromosome 3. It is associated with low or low-normal levels of PTH and relative hypercalciuria because of decreased absorption of calcium in Henle's loop and in the distal and the connecting tubules where CASR affects calcium absorption. This abnormality has been identified in many subjects with a mild variant of hypoparathyroidism, termed *autosomal dominant hypocalcemia.* Here the abnormality consists of relatively abnormal secretion of PTH due to hypersensitivity of the parathyroid glands to the inhibitory effect of calcium. In patients with familial autosomal dominant hypocalcemia, the hypocalcemia is mild and often asymptomatic. It should be treated cautiously, when mild, because raising the serum calcium concentration enhances the urinary excretion of calcium, increasing the risk of nephrocalcinosis and renal insufficiency.[20-22]

Autosomal recessive isolated hypoparathyroidism due to the absence of the *GCMB* gene (human orthologue of the *Drosophila* glial cell missing gene), which is located to 6p23-24, has been reported. The transcription factor GCMB is predominantly expressed in parathyroid cells and is critical for development of the parathyroid glands. This mutation causes agenesis of parathyroid glands with severe hypocalcemia and seizures at an early age.[23]

Aplasia or hypoplasia of the parathyroids is most commonly caused by the DiGeorge velocardiofacial syndrome, associated with deletions of chromosome 22q11.2. Most cases are sporadic, but familial cases with autosomal dominant inheritance have been reported. The affected patients present abnormalities in organs derived from the third and fourth branchial arches, including the parathyroid glands, thymus, and outflow tract of the heart. The affected patients typically present in the first week after birth with signs of hypocalcemia, such as tetany and seizures. They have characteristic facial features, an upturned nose, and a widened distance between the inner canthi (telecanthus) with short palpebral fissures. Cardiac defects include truncus arteriosus, tetralogy of Fallot, or interrupted aortic arch. Thymic hypoplasia leads to immune deficiencies. CATCH 22 syndrome is an acronym for *c*ardiac defects, *a*bnormal facies, *t*hymic hypoplasia, *c*left palate and *h*ypocalcemia caused by chromosome 22q11 deletions.[24]

A similar phenotype including hypoparathyroidism has also been associated with deletions of chromosome 10p. The HDR syndrome, consisting of *h*ypoparathyroidism, sensorineural *d*eafness, and *r*enal dysplasia, is due to defects in the *GATA3* gene at chromosome 10p15. GATA3 is a transcription factor that binds to the consensus motif A/TGATAA/G and regulates differentiation during embryonic development. The HDR syndrome is an autosomal dominant disorder that can present as hypocalcemia in early life, although the diagnosis of hypoparathyroidism may be delayed by many years.[25]

Autoimmune hypoparathyroidism is commonly a part of polyglandular autoimmune syndrome type I, which is a familial syndrome. It occurs during childhood and is inherited as an autosomal recessive trait, caused by mutations in the autoimmune regulator *(AIRE)* gene. It is associated with mucocutaneous candidiasis and adrenal insufficiency. Antibodies against the calcium sensing receptor were found in some patients. It can present as hypoparathyroidism in the absence of the two other disorders. Adrenal insufficiency is a late phenomenon in this syndrome. The acronym APECED stands for *a*utoimmune *p*olyglandular *e*ndocrinopathy with *c*andidiasis and *e*ctodermal *d*ystrophy, including vitiligo, alopecia, nail dystrophy, enamel hypoplasia of teeth, and corneal opacities.[26]

Very rare instances of hypoparathyroidism include an X-linked recessive disorder with mutations in Xq26-Xq27.[27] It has been described in only two families. Hypoparathyroidism was also reported in association with two mitochondrial cytopathies with mitochondrial DNA mutations: the Kearns-Sayre syndrome and the Kenny-Caffey syndrome.[28]

Impaired Action of PTH due to Peripheral Resistance
Pseudohypoparathyroidism

Pseudohypoparathyroidism is a rare inheritable disorder characterized by mental retardation, moderate obesity, short stature, brachydactyly, with short metacarpal and metatarsal bones, exostoses, radius curvus, and an expressionless face. The biochemical abnormalities are hypocalcemia and hyperphosphatemia. Some patients exhibit only the biochemical abnormalities. Thus, the disorder may be subdivided into pseudohypoparathyroidism type IA, which is also known as Albright's hereditary osteodystrophy, and type IB. Pseudohypoparathyroidism type IA is associated with both the somatic and biochemical abnormalities, and type IB presents as the biochemical defect without the somatic abnormalities. In patients with pseudohypoparathyroidism, the administration of PTH fails to increase urinary cyclic AMP and is not associated with phosphaturia. It has been shown also that the response to the administration of exogenous dibutyryl cyclic AMP is intact in pseudohypoparathyroidism and causes pronounced phosphaturia. It has been proposed that the skeletal refractoriness to PTH shows a certain degree of selectivity. Accordingly, the bone responds to the remodeling action of the hormone but is resistant to its calcemic-homeostatic effect.[29] Because of the hypocalcemic stimulus, secondary hyperparathyroidism may develop in some patients, leading to osteitis fibrosa cystica. Failure of the kidney to form $1,25(OH)_2$ vitamin D_3 in response to PTH results in a low circulating level of this metabolite. This deficiency may be responsible, at least partly, for the skeletal refractoriness to the calcemic action of PTH that requires the presence of $1,25(OH)_2$ vitamin D_3. It has been proposed that the hyperphosphatemia causes a reciprocal fall in serum calcium leading to hypocalcemia. The low $1,25(OH)_2$ vitamin D_3 may contribute to hypocalcemia as well.

Most patients with the type I form of pseudohypoparathyroidism manifest approximately 50% reduction in cellular activity of the α subunit of the G protein that stimulates adenylate cyclase (Gsα) encoded by the *GNAS1* gene. Patients with type IA show a generalized Gsα deficiency and often manifest resistance to other hormones whose effects are mediated by Gsα-coupled receptors (e.g., calcitonin, glucagon, and thyroid-stimulating hormone). Pseudohypoparathyroidism type IA is caused by an inactivating mutation of the α subunit of the G protein and is inherited as an autosomal dominant trait. At variance with type IA, patients with pseudohypoparathyroidism type IB manifest a selective end-organ resistance to PTH alone.[30]

An additional mechanism of target organ refractoriness to PTH has been identified. In one patient, the administration of PTH was associated with a normal increase in urinary cyclic AMP but failed to produce phosphaturia. The latter is designated as pseudohypoparathyroidism type 2. In this case the resistance to PTH resided more distal to the generation of cyclic AMP, possibly at the level of cyclic AMP/protein kinase A (PKA) interaction.[2]

Pseudo-pseudohypoparathyroidism occurs in families with pseudohypoparathyroidism type IA. It presents as inactivating mutations of *GNAS1* and features of Albright's osteodystrophy but without the resistance to PTH and other hormones.[2,31]

GNAS1 is imprinted in a tissue specific fashion, which accounts for the difference between the above subtypes. The renal expression of *GNAS1* is determined by the maternal allele. Thus, maternal or paternal transmission leads to different clinical disorders. With paternal transmission of a mutated *GNAS1*, Albright's osteodystrophy occurs without hypocalcemia, because the normal maternal allele preserves renal responsiveness to PTH, resulting in pseudo-pseudohypoparathyroidism. The mechanism of type IB is not readily understood.[31]

Calcitonin

Calcitonin binds to specific cell membrane receptors on bone-resorbing osteoclasts and depresses their activity. In this regard, it antagonizes the effect of PTH on bone.

Medullary carcinoma of the thyroid is derived from parafollicular cells of ultimobronchial organ, which secrete calcitonin. It may present as a familial and autosomal dominant or sporadic disorder. Patients with this tumor have high circulating levels of calcitonin. Hypocalcemia has been reported in some patients. However, it is absent in the escape phenomenon, probably owing to a secondary increase in PTH and/or an "escape" from the effect of calcitonin, which was observed in experimental studies.

Hypocalcemia has been described in critically ill patients admitted to ICUs. The incidence of hypocalcemia amounted to 88% in these patients. The degree of hypocalcemia correlated with the severity of the disease and was most commonly detected in patients who were septic. The mechanism of this abnormality is unknown. Circulating levels of calcitonin precursors (CTpr) increase up to several thousandfold in response to microbial infections, and this increase correlates with the severity of the infection and mortality. The relationship of elevated CTpr to the emergence of hypocalcemia needs to be investigated.[32]

Bisphosphonates

Hypocalcemia has been reported in patients with bone metastases of solid tumors who were treated with pamidronate[33] and in a patient treated with alendronate for osteoporosis. In both cases bisphosphonate induced skeletal resistance, and PTH was proposed as a possible mechanism. Hypomagnesemia may cause hypocalcemia by a similar mechanism.[34]

Rapid Removal of Calcium from the Circulation
Malignant Neoplasms

Hypocalcemia may develop in patients with malignant neoplasms in association with osteoblastic bone-forming metastases. These lesions may lead to rapid deposition of mineral in the newly formed matrix, thus causing hypocalcemia. Such hypocalcemia has been described in patients with carcinoma of the prostate or carcinoma of the breast with osteoblastic metastases. Although most of these patients have shown osteoblastic lesions on radiologic examinations, associated osteolytic lesions also have been present.

Hyperphosphatemia

The various causes of hyperphosphatemia that may lead to hypocalcemia are listed in Table 130-2.

The oral or intravenous administration of phosphate lowers serum calcium concentration in normal animals and hypercalcemic human subjects. This observation formed the basis for the clinical use of phosphate administration in states of hypercalcemia. The association of hyperphosphatemia and hypocalcemia has been reported to occur in a variety of circumstances. Hyperphosphatemia has been observed in persons ingesting large quantities of phosphate-containing laxatives or receiving enemas with phosphate. Hyperphosphatemia and hypocalcemia with tetany may develop in infants fed cow's milk, which contains 1220 mg of calcium and 940 mg of phosphorus per liter (human milk contains 340 mg of calcium and 150 mg of phosphorus per liter).[35,36]

The mechanism responsible for lowering the serum calcium concentration by the administration of phosphate is not entirely understood. One possibility is that the decrease in serum calcium concentration is caused by deposition of calcium phosphate in the bone, soft tissues, or both.

In chronic renal failure, a constant increase in serum phosphorus concentration is observed when the glomerular filtration rate is 30 mL/min or less; and hyperphosphatemia is a common accompaniment of acute renal failure.

In patients undergoing chemotherapy for neoplastic diseases, particularly of lymphatic origin, large quantities of phosphates may be released into the circulation as a result of the cytolysis. Spontaneous tumor lysis may cause hyperphosphatemia and, consequently, hypocalcemia.

Acute Pancreatitis

The hypocalcemia associated with acute pancreatitis is not well understood. The precipitation of calcium soaps in the abdominal cavity, which results from the release of lipolytic enzymes and fat necrosis, has been suggested as the mechanism of hypocalcemia. Recently, endotoxemia has been implicated.[37]

Citrate, Lactate, Bicarbonate, Na-EDTA, Foscarnet, and Poisoning with Ethylene Glycol

The citrate present in stored blood and blood products, such as fresh frozen plasma and Plasmanate and citrate used in the process of plasmapheresis, may not be immediately metabolized and can cause a reduction in the plasma concentrations of ionized calcium owing to complexing of calcium with citrate. The ionized hypocalcemia (with a normal total calcium concentration) can lead to tetany, myocardial dysfunction, or hypotension. The same applies to intravenous lactate and Na-EDTA, which causes ionized hypercalcemia. Bicarbonate may directly complex calcium or may increase protein binding of calcium from the resulting alkalosis. Low serum ionized calcium may be a complication of ethylene glycol (antifreeze) poisoning because of calcium binding by oxalic acid, which is the metabolite of the poison. An analogue of the pyrophosphate foscarnet used to treat cytomegalovirus infection in HIV-infected patients causes ionized hypocalcemia because of chelation of calcium by foscarnet.[2]

CLINICAL CONSEQUENCES OF HYPOCALCEMIA

The clinical presentation of hypocalcemia depends on its severity, the rapidity of the fall in serum calcium concentration, the age of the patient, the chronicity of hypocalcemia, and the comorbid conditions.

Most infants with hypocalcemia are asymptomatic. Among those who become symptomatic, the characteristic sign is increased neuromuscular irritability. Generalized or focal clonic seizures may be the first indication of hypocalcemia. Other manifestations may include stridor caused by laryngospasms and wheezing caused by bronchospasms. Vomiting may be caused by pylorospasm.

Neuromuscular manifestations in adults with hypocalcemia are variable. The characteristic symptom is tetany, which includes perioral numbness and tingling, paresthesias in the extremities, carpopedal spasm, laryngospasm, and focal and generalized seizures. The spasms of the diaphragm and of intercostal muscles may cause respiratory arrest and asphyxia.

The characteristic physical findings in patients with hypocalcemia that are indicative of latent tetany are Trousseau's sign (carpal spasm) and Chvostek's sign (facial muscle contraction).

Visual impairment may be caused acutely by papilledema whereas chronic hypocalcemia, usually, when due to hypoparathyroidism, causes cataracts.

Myocardial functional and anatomic abnormalities have been associated with hypocalcemia. Acute hypocalcemia may be associated with hypotension. Very often the absence of the compensatory reflex tachycardia aggravates the condition. The typical ECG change consists of prolongation of the QT interval (normal QT interval = 0.44 second). Hypocalcemia prolongs phase 2 of the action potential, and thus prolongs repolarization time, because inward calcium currents are one of the factors determining the plateau configuration of the action potential. QT prolongation is associated with a variety of ventricular arrhythmias, most characteristically torsades de pointes. These abnormalities can be reversed with calcium replacement. Calcium therapy significantly shortens the repolarization intervals and decreases the frequency of ventricular premature contractions.[38] Chronic hypocalcemia may cause infrequently hypocalcemic cardiomyopathy, which is a dilated cardiomyopathy. Partial recovery of cardiac function has been reported after restoration of normocalcemia.[39]

TREATMENT OF HYPOCALCEMIA

Symptomatic hypocalcemia generally responds promptly to the intravenous administration of calcium. The commonly

TABLE 130–2. HYPERPHOSPHATEMIA AS A CAUSE OF HYPOCALCEMIA

Administration of phosphate
    Oral phosphate
Cow's milk in infants
Laxatives containing phosphate
Potassium phosphate tablets
    Phosphate-containing enemas
    Intravenous phosphate
Renal diseases
    Acute renal failure
    Chronic renal failure
Neoplasms treated with cytotoxic agents
    Lymphomas
    Leukemia
    Tumor lysis
    Rhabdomyolysis

used preparations are 10% calcium gluconate (10-mL ampules containing 90 mg of elemental calcium) and 10% calcium chloride (10-mL ampules containing 360 mg of elemental calcium). The treatment should be instituted immediately, because delay may be associated with further aggravation of tetany and lead to generalized seizures and even cardiac arrest.

The intravenous administration of 100 to 200 mg elemental calcium (5 to 10 mEq) should be slow to avoid complications. Then the administration of calcium can be continued as a slow drip of 100 to 200 mg of elemental calcium, diluted in 250 to 500 mL of 0.45% NaCl or D5W, given over several hours, until oral calcium takes over. Calcium extravasation should be avoided because it causes local irritation and thrombophlebitis.

Chronic treatment with oral calcium should follow the intravenous therapy in patients with chronic hypocalcemia owing to irreversible causes such as hypoparathyroidism. Oral calcium administration constitutes the best initial therapy in mild cases. The commonly used preparations are in tablet form: calcium lactate, 300 mg (60 mg of elemental calcium); chewable calcium gluconate, 1 g (90 mg of elemental calcium); calcium carbonate (Os-Cal), 250 mg of elemental calcium; calcium carbonate, 650 mg (250 mg of elemental calcium); and calcium citrate, 950 mg (200 mg of elemental calcium).

Oral calcium also may be used for patients for whom the diagnosis of irreversible hypoparathyroidism has not been established with absolute certainty. In patients who fail to respond to oral calcium, vitamin D in large doses is the only available treatment. The commonly used preparations are capsules containing 1.25 mg (50,000 units) of vitamin D_2 (ergocalciferol). The average dose ranges between 1.25 and 3.75 mg/day. DHT3 is three times as potent as vitamin D_2 in raising serum calcium concentration. Each capsule contains 0.125 mg of DHT3. The average daily dose ranges between 0.25 and 1.00 mg of DHT3. Both vitamins are available in liquid oil solutions as well. Both hypoparathyroidism and pseudohypoparathyroidism respond to physiologic doses of $1,25(OH)_2$ vitamin D_3 and $1\alpha(OH)$ vitamin D_3 with restoration of serum calcium concentration to normal. Calcitriol is marketed as Rocaltrol and is dispensed in capsules containing 0.25 and 1.0 μg. Chlorothiazides may enhance the calcemic action of vitamin D and its analogs, whereas furosemide may aggravate the hypocalcemia through its hypercalciuric action.

Patients in whom hypocalcemia is associated with hypomagnesemia respond poorly to intravenous calcium, but the serum calcium concentration is restored to normal levels with correction of the hypomagnesemia.

Symptoms rarely develop in patients with chronic renal failure and hypocalcemia. However, very often reduction of elevated serum phosphorus with phosphate-binding antacids causes an increase in serum calcium concentrations.

Hypocalcemia associated with osteomalacia resulting from vitamin D deficiency is rarely symptomatic. It usually responds to physiologic doses of vitamin D and increased oral calcium intake.

HYPERCALCEMIA

Primary hyperparathyroidism and malignancy account for 80% to 90% of all cases of hypercalcemia.[40]

Primary hyperparathyroidism is the leading cause of hypercalcemia in the outpatient setting. Its incidence is 1% in the normal population.[41] Hypercalcemia is most often detected in routinely tested blood specimens. Malignancy is the prevalent cause of hypercalcemia in hospitalized patients.[42] The most common iatrogenic hypercalcemia is milk-alkali syndrome, which ranks third after malignancy and hyperparathyroidism and accounts for 10% to 15% of cases with hypercalcemia. The free over-the-counter access to the generic brands of calcium carbonate and their widespread use for heartburn, osteoporosis, and as an alleged prevention of colon cancer may be the underlying cause for the rise in the incidence of milk-alkali syndrome.[43]

Hypercalcemia presents a challenge to every clinician. In some instances, the cause of hypercalcemia is self-evident on the basis of the circumstantial clinical findings, whereas extensive efforts are required to establish the etiology in other situations. The important causes of hypercalcemia are listed in Table 130-3.

TABLE 130–3. DISORDERS ASSOCIATED WITH HYPERCALCEMIA

Primary hyperparathyroidism
Adenoma and carcinoma
  Hyperplasia
  Multiple endocrine adenomatosis
  Ectopic secretion of parathyroid hormone by neoplasms (rare)
Secondary hyperparathyroidism
  Malabsorption and vitamin D deficiency
  Chronic renal failure
  Following kidney transplantation
Familial hypocalciuric hypercalcemia
Hypercalcemia associated with malignancy
  Lytic bone metastases
Circulating tumor-secreted factors
  Parathyroid hormone-related protein
  1,25-Dihydroxyvitamin D3-induced hypercalcemia
Locally acting, noncirculating, tumor-secreted cytokines
  Interleukin–1 and IL–6
  Tumor necrosis factor-beta
  Granulocyte-macrophage colony-stimulating factor
  Transforming growth factor-alpha
  Prostaglandins
Hypercalcemia in patients with hyperabsorptive hypercalciuria
Hypervitaminosis D
Hypervitaminosis A
Granulomatous diseases
  Sarcoidosis
  Tuberculosis
  Histoplasmosis
  Coccidioidomycosis
  Leprosy
Foreign body granuloma
Hyperthyroidism
Adrenocortical insufficiency
Infantile hypercalcemia
Immobilization
Milk-alkali syndrome
Hypophosphatasia
Parenteral nutrition
Hypercalcemia associated with acute renal failure
Medications
  Thiazides
  Lithium
  Theophylline
  Calcium ion exchange resins
Near-drowning in Dead Sea

HYPERPARATHYROIDISM

Primary hyperparathyroidism is present in 10% to 20% of all patients with hypercalcemia.[2] Making the diagnosis of hyperparathyroidism is important because of its amenability of surgical cure. The disease is more common in females than in males; the incidence increases in women after menopause but is less frequent in older men. A single parathyroid adenoma is by far the most common cause of primary hyperparathyroidism. Carcinoma is very infrequent, occurring in less than 1% of all reported cases. Primary hyperplasia is found in less than 10% of all cases, but it is the most frequent cause in familial hyperparathyroidism.[2,42]

The morphologic differentiation between adenomas and hyperplasia sometimes is very difficult. The presence of a capsule and a rim of compressed normal gland tissue around the periphery of an adenoma may be helpful in making a definitive diagnosis. The persistence or recurrence of hypercalcemia after surgery for a purported adenoma warrants a more precise evaluation of the morphologic status of the parathyroid tissue to be removed—safe removal without allowing recurrence of the disease is a very difficult balance to achieve. If more than one gland shows histologic features of hyperplasia, then removal of more than one gland is recommended; generally, approximately 200 mg of parathyroid tissue should remain. Some patients with primary hyperparathyroidism have especially pronounced hypercalciuria despite a very mild degree of hypercalcemia and minimal or no bone disease. In patients with primary hyperparathyroidism, a very strong positive correlation was found between $1,25(OH)_2$ vitamin D_3 in the serum and the urinary calcium excretion. Patients with nephrolithiasis and hypercalcemia had circulating levels of $1,25(OH)_2$ vitamin D_3 higher than those present in hyperparathyroid patients without renal stones. The reason for this difference in the $1,25(OH)_2$ vitamin D_3 levels is unknown, but it stresses the importance of vitamin D metabolism in the clinical presentation of primary hyperparathyroidism.[2]

The high incidence of parathyroid adenomas in association with various malignant neoplasms is not well understood but warrants consideration in every case in which a malignant tumor is accompanied by hypercalcemia.

Molecular biology provides the means to study the role of genomic aberrations as the underlying mechanism of primary hyperparathyroidism. In parathyroid adenomas, changes were reported to occur in the gene that encodes PTH and is located on chromosome 11.[45] Likewise, alterations were identified in the X chromosome. The genomic abnormalities consist of loss of tumor-suppressor genes and/or overexpression of oncogenes on chromosome 11. Likewise, inactivation of tumor suppressor genes was found in the X chromosome. It is interesting that these genomic changes were found not only in patients with parathyroid adenoma but also in patients with parathyroid hyperplasia, including hyperplasia secondary to chronic renal failure.[46]

The familial occurrence of parathyroid adenomas with an autosomal dominant inheritance mandates biochemical screening of family members of patients with primary hyperparathyroidism. Establishing the diagnosis of familial hyperparathyroidism also may be important to the patient's surgeon, alerting him or her to the high incidence of hyperplasia and multiple adenomas in this group of patients. In some families, primary hyperparathyroidism is associated with other endocrine tumors as well. The syndrome of hyperparathyroidism, medullary carcinoma of the thyroid with amyloid stroma, pheochromocytoma, and multiple neuromas is known as multiple endocrine neoplasia type II (MEN II) or Sipple's syndrome. The syndrome described by Wermer consisted of hyperparathyroidism and tumors of the pituitary and pancreatic islet cells (MEN I).[47]

MEN I is an autosomal dominant familial neoplasia syndrome. Recently the gene of MEN I ("menin") has been cloned. The gene was mapped to the long arm of chromosome 11. *MEN1* is a tumor suppressor gene. Inactivating germline mutations of the *MEN1* gene lead to the growth of multiple endocrine neoplasia. Over 40 different germline mutations of *MEN1* have been identified in MEN I kindreds, suggesting the absence of a founder effect. By contrast, MEN II is caused by activating mutation of the *RET* proto-oncogene and is inherited as an autosomal dominant trait.[46-48]

The hyperparathyroidism/jaw tumor syndrome consists of hyperparathyroidism, cement-ossifying fibromas of the jaw, renal cysts, Wilms' tumor, and renal hamartomas. This syndrome is caused by a mutation of an unknown gene on chromosome 1q24 and is inherited as an autosomal dominant trait.[47,48]

A small minority of parathyroid adenomas have activating mutation of the cyclin D1 oncogene (*CCDN1*). These mutations result in overexpression of the protein cyclin D1. It is interesting in this regard that primary hyperparathyroidism was induced by parathyroid-targeted overexpression of cyclin D1 in transgenic mice.[47-50]

Primary hyperparathyroidism can best be diagnosed by demonstrating persistent hypercalcemia with elevated serum PTH. Patients presenting with bone, renal, gastrointestinal, or neuromuscular symptoms are considered symptomatic and usually require surgery. Conversely, in asymptomatic patients, objective manifestations of primary hyperparathyroidism that are indications for surgery include markedly elevated serum calcium concentration, a previous episode of life-threatening hypercalcemia, a reduced creatinine clearance, presence of kidney stones, hypercalciuria, and substantially reduced bone density.

The ^{99m}Tc-sestamibi scan is a new technique that helps detect and localize parathyroid adenomas with high precision and accuracy.[43] Furthermore, this technique makes it possible to identify the adenoma intraoperatively with use of a portable radioactivity detector probe (miniaturized handheld gamma probe) and to guide the surgeon directly to the tumor. This advanced technique allows the surgical procedure to be carried out under local anesthesia with reduced morbidity and with more successful outcome. Likewise, progress has been made with use of diagnostic ultrasonography. The close monitoring of PTH levels (PTH has a very short half-life during surgery) may assist in ascertaining the success of parathyroidectomy. A recent clinical study examined the clinical course and development of complications for up to 10 years in 121 patients with primary hyperparathyroidism; 101 (83%) of the patients were asymptomatic. During the study, 61 (50%) patients underwent parathyroidectomy and 60 were followed without surgery. Parathyroidectomy resulted in the normalization of biochemical values and increased bone mineral density. Most asymptomatic patients who did not undergo surgery did not have progression of disease; however, approximately one fourth of them did have some progression. The progression included recurrent kidney stones, decrease of more than 10% in bone density, rise to more than 12 mg/dL in serum calcium concentration, and the development of hypercalciuria. These findings raise serious questions regarding the choice of the optimal treatment for so-called asymptomatic patients with primary hyperparathyroidism.[51]

Familial hypocalciuric hypercalcemia is an unusual form of parathyroid hyperplasia with autosomal dominant transmission. There is a high incidence of neonatal primary hyperparathyroidism among the offspring of the affected families. The clinical course is relatively benign, with an absence of nephrolithiasis and an infrequent occurrence of pancreatitis and chondrocalcinosis. Mild parathyroid hyperplasia with modestly elevated levels of circulating PTH and increased urinary excretion of cyclic AMP have been reported in these patients. The unsatisfactory response to subtotal parathyroidectomy, however, suggests additional underlying abnormalities. The presence of hypocalciuria both before and after subtotal parathyroidectomy provides a strong argument that enhanced tubular reabsorption of calcium plays an important role in maintaining hypercalcemia. Hypermagnesemia, which appears to reflect increased tubular reabsorption of magnesium, is another unique feature of this hypercalcemic disorder. It has been proposed that a concurrence of defects in both the parathyroid glands and kidneys in their response to serum calcium concentration is an explanation for this disorder.[52]

Recent studies demonstrated that inactivating mutations in the human calcium-sensing receptor gene caused both familial hypocalciuric hypercalcemia (FHH) and neonatal severe hyperparathyroidism. The calcium-sensing receptor gene has been mapped to chromosome 3, the same chromosome to which the FHH disease locus was localized in the past. In most families with FHH, linkage to chromosome 3g predominates, although in one family linkage to chromosome 19f was demonstrated. Thus, the disease exhibits genetic heterogeneity. Inheritance of a single copy of mutated gene causes FHH, whereas homozygous patients who inherit two inactive genes develop neonatal severe hyperparathyroidism. The latter is associated with severe hypercalcemia owing to parathyroid hyperplasia that usually requires surgery. These mutations lead to a defective calcium-sensing receptor with a presumable impairment of signal transduction function, possibly resulting from abnormal coupling with G protein. This, in turn, appears to lead to abnormally reduced parathyroid and renal responsiveness to changes in extracellular calcium, resulting in increased PTH secretion and avid tubular reabsorption of calcium. Thus, the calcium-sensing receptor plays an important role in calcium-regulated secretion of PTH and tubular reabsorption of calcium. The FHH-associated excessive reabsorption of calcium, probably in the thick ascending limb of Henle and distal nephron, which persists even after parathyroidectomy, suggest that this abnormality is PTH independent.[52,53]

MALIGNANCY ASSOCIATED WITH HYPERCALCEMIA

A malignant neoplasm is the single most common cause of hypercalcemia. Hypercalcemia is most commonly produced by tumors of lung, breast, kidney, and ovary and by hematologic malignancies. Very often the hypercalcemia is uncontrollable and thus is a harbinger of the patient's demise. Indeed, survival after the appearance of hypercalcemia in association with malignancy is very poor, with a median of 3 months. Two main mechanisms are known to mediate the

hypercalcemia of malignancy: local and humoral. The local mechanism is manifested by the presence of osteolytic lesions in the skeleton. The malignant cells may act to destroy the bone directly; however, even local osteolysis is mediated by activated osteoclasts in most instances. Many tumors may produce hypercalcemia by a dual mechanism, that is, both local and humoral. It has become apparent that humoral hypercalcemia of malignancy (HHM) is caused by a circulating factor that is secreted by the neoplasm.[54] This circulating substance acts on the bone to induce osteoclastic resorption and on the kidney to reduce phosphate reabsorption, to increase calcium reabsorption, and to increase nephrogenous cyclic AMP excretion. All of these biochemical effects are characteristic of the actions of native PTH. However, only in two patients, one with small cell carcinoma of lung and the second with ovarian carcinoma, was the ectopic secretion of PTH demonstrated.[55,56] In the vast majority of patients with HHM, the circulating factor is PTH-related protein. PTHrP is a 141 amino acid protein that binds to the receptors common to the native PTH, but it is encoded by a distinct gene. Even though PTHrP shares structural homology of amino-terminal residues with PTH, immunoradiometric assay of PTH has been able to distinguish completely between patients with HHM and those with primary hypoparathyroidism. Thus, hypercalcemia with absence of detectable PTH by radioimmunoassay and presence of high urinary cyclic AMP supports the diagnosis of HHM. PTHrP was originally isolated from human malignant tumors associated with HHM. Subsequently, it was detected to be present in a variety of tissues, including parathyroid adenoma, skin, breast, placenta, testis, pancreas, and brain. With regard to the presence of PTHrP in parathyroid tissue, it has been suggested that PTH is produced by the chief cells (major component of parathyroid tissue), whereas PTHrP is produced by the oxyphil cells. Accordingly, the detection of PTHrP in circulation per se does not rule out parathyroid adenoma. Rather, the absence of PTH and the presence of PTHrP by radioimmunoassays in fact rule out parathyroid adenoma and support the diagnosis of HHM.[57]

In vitro PTHrP, similarly to native PTH, has been shown not only to stimulate renal adenylate cyclase and increase the formation of cyclic AMP but also to activate the 1α-hydroxylase and enhance the formation of 1,25(OH)$_2$ vitamin D$_3$. In vivo, however, contrary to patients with primary hyperparathyroidism who may have high levels of serum 1,25(OH)$_2$ vitamin D$_3$, patients with HHM have low serum levels of calcitriol. In this regard, it has been reported that certain solid neoplasms produce substances that may inhibit the activity of 1α-hydroxylase and suppress the formation of 1,25(OH)$_2$ vitamin D$_3$. This appears to be the most tenable explanation for the low calcitriol in patients with HHM.[58]

Another interesting feature that distinguished between patients with primary hyperparathyroidism and those with HHM are the findings of bone histomorphometry. Whereas in patients with primary hyperparathyroidism bone resorption is closely matched with bone formation, in patients with HHM bone resorption and formation are uncoupled; specifically in HHM, enhancement of bone resorption and suppression of bone formation occur. The cause of this discrepancy is not readily apparent. Additional studies are necessary to determine whether malignancies produce factors that suppress bone formation.[59]

High PTHrP levels are present in 80% of patients with bone metastases from breast cancer who present with hypercalcemia, whereas PTHrP was present only in 12% of patients with breast cancer and metastases at sites other than bone. These findings are consistent with the notion that PTHrP may promote the development and growth of metastases in the bones by its potent osteolytic activity, which provides the environment for the proliferation of malignant cells.[59]

Hypercalcemia is a recognized complication of lymphoma, including both Hodgkin and non-Hodgkin types. Serum levels of $1,25(OH)_2$ vitamin D_3 are either elevated or inadequately suppressed by the hypercalcemia in many patients with lymphoma-associated hypercalcemia. The elevated $1,25(OH)_2$ vitamin D_3 levels may play a role in the pathogenesis of hypercalcemia. In some cases, chemotherapy induced normalization of serum calcium and a concomitant fall in $1,25(OH)_2$ vitamin D_3. Conversely, reappearance of hypercalcemia was associated with a recurrent rise above normal of $1,25(OH)_2$ vitamin D_3 levels. Human T-lymphotrophic virus–transformed lymphocytes are able to produce $1,25(OH)_2$ vitamin D_3 from $25(OH)$ vitamin D_3. Thus, there is a possibility that in some cases of lymphoma the malignant cells may have a similar capacity to produce $1,25(OH)_2$ vitamin D_3, which may contribute to the development of hypercalcemia. However, it is noteworthy that the levels of PTHrP were elevated and considered to be responsible for the rise in serum calcium concentration in a number of patients with lymphoma-associated hypercalcemia. Obviously, both PTHrP and elevated $1,25(OH)_2$ vitamin D_3 may act synergistically to cause hypercalcemia.[60]

The Role of Osteoclast-Activating Cytokines in Hypercalcemia of Malignancy

Tumor cells in bone and tumor-associated macrophages release factors that are known as osteoclast-activating cytokines. These tumor-derived factors, implicated in the development of hypercalcemia of malignancy, are interleukin-1 (IL-1), interleukin-6 (IL-6), tumor necrosis factor-alpha (cachectin), tumor necrosis factor-beta (TGF-β, lymphotoxin), transforming growth factor-alpha (TGF-α), and arachidonic acid metabolites. In addition, tumor cells may produce mediators (e.g., granulocyte-macrophage colony-stimulating factor) that induce immune cells to produce tumor necrosis factor and IL-1. Cytokines are produced and act locally as osteolytic factors. In most instances, the osteoclast-stimulating activity of the cytokines requires the presence of osteoblastic cells. Intravenous infusion of cytokines causes hypercalcemia in animals; however, these factors are believed to act locally in a paracrine fashion in clinical circumstances.[59,61-63]

Tumor cells act indirectly by adapting to the physiologic mechanisms that promote bone resorption. Tumor cells release hormones (PTHrP), growth factors (TGF2), cytokines (IL-6), and eicosanoids (prostaglandins), which act on osteoblastic cells to enhance the production of osteoclast activating factors. Most important of these is the cell membrane–associated protein termed *receptor activator of NF-KB ligand* (RANKL), a member of the TNF family of cytokines. RANKL can then bind to its cognate receptor (RANK) residing on the cell surface membrane on osteoclast precursors and in the presence of macrophage colony-stimulating factor (M-CSF) can promote the differentiation and fusion of the preosteoclasts to form active multinucleated osteoclasts. Concomitantly, production of soluble decoy receptors for RANKL, termed *osteoprotegerin* (OPG), by osteoblastic cells inhibits osteoclastic osteolysis. Osteolytic bone matrix releases growth factors, including TGF-β, which accelerate tumor growth in the lysed area. Thus, a cycle is activated in which tumor cells and bone matrix interact to promote metastatic expansion. One study has demonstrated that prostatic tumor cells may produce a soluble RANKL (sRANKL) and thus directly, without the mediating role of osteoblastic cells, accelerate the osteoclastogenesis and osteolysis. In the same study, the administration of the decoy receptor for RANKL, OPG, prevented the establishment of osseous tumors. These observations bear on possible new therapeutic avenues in preventing spread of prostatic tumor.[64]

Hypercalcemia occurs in approximately one third of patients with myeloma. Osteolytic bone lesions are the most common skeletal radiographic findings. The bone destruction in myeloma is mediated by osteoclasts that accumulate adjacent to the collections of myeloma cells. This association of myeloma cells with osteoclasts is most likely related to the osteoclast-activating effect of cytokines that are locally secreted by the malignant cells. Myeloma cells produce in vitro several osteoclast-activating factors, including TGF-β, IL-1, and IL-6. The increase in bone resorption in most cases is associated with a suppressed osteoblastic bone-forming activity. This explains the depressed skeletal uptake of bone-seeking radiolabeled elements in myeloma, resulting in negative bone scans in the majority of the affected patients. Myeloma cells exhibit a unique capability to grow rapidly in the bone. Myeloma cells secrete osteoclast-mobilizing and osteoclast-stimulating cytokines, whereas osteoclasts secrete IL-6, which is a major growth factor of the myeloma cells. This relationship between myeloma cells and osteoclasts explains the rapid destruction of bone in this malignancy.[59,61-63]

VITAMIN D INTOXICATION AND HYPERCALCEMIA

All patients receiving vitamin D, other than in small doses, for the treatment of hypoparathyroidism may develop hypercalcemia, with the attendant risk of renal failure. The appearance of hypercalcemia in hypoparathyroid patients receiving pharmacologic doses of either ergocalciferol (vitamin D_2) or DHT3 is almost unpredictable, because the margin between normocalcemic and hypercalcemic doses of the vitamin is very narrow. Some episodes of hypercalcemia may pass unnoticed and yet may be the underlying cause of reduced renal function in these patients. The administration of thiazide diuretics also may be an aggravating factor in this situation, partly because they reduce the urinary excretion of calcium. Hypercalcemia associated with vitamin D intoxication may be present from 1 to 6 weeks after discontinuation of the treatment, and normocalcemia may persist for an additional 4 months without any treatment. The toxic effect of vitamin D excess is associated with a high circulating level of $25(OH)$ vitamin D_3, which is continuously produced by the liver from the adipose tissue stores of vitamin D. The serum level of $1,25(OH)_2$ vitamin D_3 generally is not elevated and even may be reduced; however, the free non–protein-bound $1,25(OH)_2$ vitamin D_3 levels may be elevated. The hypercalcemia associated with $1,25(OH)_2$ vitamin D_3 administration, however, is much more short lived (3 to 7 days).[65]

Various factors may alter the response to vitamin D. The inhibitory effect of estrogens on bone resorption may be absent after menopause, which allows more calcium to be released from the bone for any given dose of vitamin D. The administration of corticosteroids may reduce the effect of vitamin D; in fact, corticosteroids may be used to treat vitamin D intoxication. The most important precaution in preventing the complications of vitamin D intoxication is to measure serum calcium concentrations frequently in these patients. Likewise, the presence of excessive hypercalciuria, even in the absence of hypercalcemia, is a risk factor for nephrocalcinosis and renal failure. Thus, monitoring of urinary calcium excretion in these circumstances is recommended as well.

VITAMIN A INTOXICATION AND HYPERCALCEMIA

Hypercalcemia associated with vitamin A intoxication has been much discussed.[66] This condition has been associated with excessive intake of vitamin A, which is readily available for sale in various pharmaceutic preparations. Isotretinoin, a derivative of vitamin A that is effective in the treatment of severe nodulocystic acne, has been reported as a cause of hypercalcemia. The main symptom of vitamin A intoxication is painful swelling over the extremities. Prolonged hypercalcemia in this condition also has been associated with nephrocalcinosis and impairment of renal function. In experimental animals, excessive amounts of vitamin A cause fractures, increased number of osteoclasts, and calcification of soft tissues. In human subjects, periosteal bone deposition constitutes the typical radiographic feature.

SARCOIDOSIS AND HYPERCALCEMIA

Hypercalcemia in patients with sarcoidosis is associated with increased intestinal absorption of calcium and increased calcium release from the bone; it is found in about 17% of all patients with sarcoidosis. It is more frequent in males than females. In a small proportion of patients, very high serum calcium concentration leads to metastatic calcifications and eventual death from uremia. The hypercalcemia may disappear with the appearance of uremia.

Seasonal incidence of hypercalcemia in sarcoidosis is directly related to the amount of sunlight exposure. Plasma levels of $1,25(OH)_2$ vitamin D_3 have been found to be increased in patients with sarcoidosis and hypercalcemia, a finding that accounts for the abnormal calcium metabolism in this disease. In most of the patients, hypercalcemia may be corrected with the administration of glucocorticoids, which restores to normal both the elevated calcium and $1,25(OH)_2$ vitamin D_3 concentrations in the serum. Serum immunoreactive PTH has been found to be low in patients with sarcoidosis, regardless of the presence or absence of hypercalcemia.[67]

In vitro studies demonstrated production of $1,25(OH)_2$ vitamin D_3 by primary cultures of pulmonary alveolar macrophages harvested from patients with active sarcoidosis. Thus, the pathogenesis of hypercalcemia in sarcoidosis is extrarenal production of $1,25(OH)_2$ vitamin D_3 by the macrophage, which is a major constituent of the sarcoid granuloma. A similar mechanism appears to be responsible for the hypercalcemia associated with other granulomatous diseases. Hypercalcemia has been reported in tuberculosis, leprosy, foreign body–induced granulomas, silicone-induced granuloma, disseminated candidiasis and coccidioidomycosis, histoplasmosis, berylliosis, granulomatous lipid pneumonia, and eosinophilic granuloma. However, as opposed to the physiologic synthesis of $1,25(OH)_2$ vitamin D_3 by proximal tubular epithelial cells, which is regulated by PTH and serum levels of phosphate and calcium, the extrarenal formation of $1,25(OH)_2$ vitamin D_3 is not regulated physiologically. However, it may depend on the availability of its precursors cholecalciferol and $25(OH)$ vitamin D_3.[67-69]

HYPERTHYROIDISM, HYPOTHYROIDISM, AND HYPERCALCEMIA

The incidence of hypercalcemia in patients with hyperthyroidism varies from 10% to 22% in different reports. This hypercalcemia may be reversed by antithyroid therapy. Because the association of hyperthyroidism and hyperparathyroidism has been reported to be common, the therapeutic response of the hypercalcemia to the antithyroid therapy may be of some diagnostic significance. The effect of thyroid hormone on calcium metabolism primarily consists of increased bone turnover, increased urinary calcium excretion, and decreased intestinal absorption of calcium, with a resultant negative calcium balance. Thus, the action of thyroid hormone on bone is primarily responsible for the hypercalcemia. Thyroid hormone enhances the ability of PTH to increase bone resorption and directly enhances bone resorption in vivo in the absence of PTH. Serum phosphate may be elevated in hyperthyroidism, possibly because of suppression of parathyroid activity by the hypercalcemia and subsequent enhanced tubular reabsorption of phosphate.[70,71]

Serum calcium and phosphate levels are normal and alkaline phosphatase is low in the vast majority of patients with hypothyroidism; however, some patients may manifest hypercalcemia. Calcium balance in patients with hypothyroidism tends to be positive as a result of increased intestinal absorption and reduced urinary excretion. Both changes predispose to the development of hypercalcemia. The bone turnover in hypothyroid patients is reduced.

ADRENAL INSUFFICIENCY AND HYPERCALCEMIA

Hypercalcemia is a common abnormality in adrenal insufficiency. The mechanism of hypercalcemia in this clinical setting is not well understood. One study indicates that the increase in serum calcium concentration is due to an increase in the protein-bound fraction of serum calcium that results from accompanying volume depletion. The volume depletion also may cause an increase in the renal tubular reabsorption of calcium, and vitamin D's enhancement of calcium absorption from the intestine may be greater in the absence of glucocorticoid hormone.[72]

IDIOPATHIC INFANTILE HYPERCALCEMIA

Idiopathic infantile hypercalcemia encompasses a group of disorders characterized by hypercalcemia during infancy, mostly of a transient nature. It can be divided into benign and severe types according to the gravity of the clinical manifestation. The benign type is associated with minimal symptomatology and has an excellent prognosis. The severe form is associated with serious somatic sequelae, including mental deficiency, "elfin" facies with depressed nasal bridge, epicanthal folds, supravalvular aortic stenosis, bladder diverticula, degenerative renal disease, occasionally pulmonic stenosis, ventricular septal defects, and dental abnormalities. These somatic distortions, known as Williams' syndrome, are believed to reflect developmental defects resulting from hypercalcemia, probably already present in the fetal stage. The hypercalcemia is of limited duration; however, the somatic abnormalities are permanent. Thus, many patients suffering from Williams' syndrome who present with the clinical syndrome fail to show abnormalities in calcium metabolism. The primary genetic abnormality is deletion of one allele of elastin gene. Hemizygosity for this gene was detected in 75% of patients. This defect is probably responsible for the vascular, valvular, and developmental defects.[73]

Idiopathic infantile hypercalcemia has been attributed to hypersensitivity to vitamin D. In support of this possibility is the finding that hypercalcemia in this syndrome may occur with small doses of vitamin D, which are only two to three times larger that the physiologic dose. The high incidence of this syndrome in a group of infants in England who were drinking milk fortified with excessive amounts of vitamin D and its disappearance when vitamin D was eliminated from the diet supported the possibility that the syndrome was owing to hypersensitivity to vitamin D. However, there is no unifying pathogenesis underlying the abnormal calcium metabolism in idiopathic infantile hypercalcemia. Increased serum levels of $1,25(OH)_2$ vitamin D_3 have been considered to be the mechanism of hypercalcemia by some investigators. Others have failed to show that abnormality even in the presence of hypercalcemia. Abnormalities in the regulation of calcitonin secretion with reduced stimulation by hypercalcemia were advanced as the possible mechanism by others.

Hypercalcemia with fat necrosis is a peculiar variant of the disease. In this syndrome affecting infants, only hypercalcemia occurs, with areas of necrosis of subcutaneous fat tissue. In some cases, high levels of $1,25(OH)_2$ vitamin D_3 were reported. Some investigators maintain that hypercalcemia is not a primary but rather a secondary phenomenon. In the latter instance, it has been proposed that the rise in $1,25(OH)_2$ vitamin D_3 leading to hypercalcemia is secondary to the granulomatous inflammation of the fat necrosis. Irrespective of the mechanism, idiopathic infantile hypercalcemia is treated by dietary restriction of calcium and vitamin D.

JANSEN'S CHONDRODYSTROPHY

Jansen's chondrodystrophy is characterized by short limbs, mild hypercalcemia, and low serum PTH levels. It is caused by activating mutations of PTH/PTHrP receptor and is inherited as an autosomal dominant trait. It is associated with increased proliferation and delayed maturation of chondrocytes.

IMMOBILIZATION AND HYPERCALCEMIA

Immobilization may be associated with excessive loss of bone minerals, hypercalcemia, and rapidly developing osteoporosis. The lack of postural mechanical stimuli to the skeleton disturbs the balance between bone formation and resorption, thus leading to loss of bone mass and its minerals. Usually, the amount of calcium released from the bone is excreted in the urine and does not increase the serum calcium concentrations. However, in states of rapid bone turnover, which are present in normal children and adolescents and in patients with bone abnormalities such as Paget's disease, immobilization may result in overt hypercalcemia.[74]

HYPOPHOSPHATASIA

Hypophosphatasia is a syndrome characterized by low serum alkaline phosphatase, high serum levels of pyrophosphate, and skeletal abnormalities resembling osteomalacia. The disorder may be associated with hypercalcemia, especially in infants.

MILK-ALKALI SYNDROME

Milk-alkali syndrome may occur in patients who ingest large amounts of milk and alkali as a therapy to relieve the symptoms of peptic ulcers. The syndrome is characterized by hypercalcemia, hyperphosphatemia, alkalosis, metastatic calcifications, and progressive renal failure. It has been shown that these abnormalities may be reversed by discontinuation of the therapy. Large doses of calcium carbonate seem to be the major factor in the development of this syndrome, because the use of antacids other than calcium carbonate do not lead to hypercalcemia. Therefore, it appears that the hypercalcemia of milk-alkali syndrome results from high oral loads of calcium carbonate and causes renal retention of phosphate by suppressing PTH secretion.[75] The resulting serum calcium-phosphorus product leads to metastatic calcification and impairment of renal function. Increased oral intake of calcium carbonate also has been reported to induce hypercalcemia in uremic patients. Similarly, the use of calcium-containing exchange resins for the treatment of hyperkalemia may cause hypercalcemia because of the release of calcium from the resin in the intestinal lumen. Hypercalcemia has been described in patients recovering from acute renal failure. The etiology is not well understood, but in some patients it may result from the combination of secondary hyperparathyroidism and released calcium from traumatized, necrotic muscle and to high calcitriol levels produced by the traumatized muscles.

THIAZIDE DIURETICS AND HYPERCALCEMIA

Chronic administration of thiazide diuretics may lead to hypercalcemia in patients treated with large doses of vitamin D (hypoparathyroid patients and patients with osteoporosis) and in patients with hyperparathyroidism. The mechanism of action may involve: (1) reduced urinary excretion of calcium due to a direct tubular effect, or extracellular fluid depletion with secondary increase in tubular reabsorption of sodium and calcium, or both; and (2) increased bone responsiveness to the resorptive actions of vitamin D and PTH. It has been demonstrated that thiazides may acutely enhance the skeletal response to PTH in the absence of changes in extracellular fluid volume, but there is no evidence for such an effect in hypoparathyroid patients receiving large doses of vitamin D.[76]

LITHIUM AND THEOPHYLLINE TOXICITY

Patients treated chronically with lithium may develop hypercalcemia with elevated PTH levels. The incidence of primary hyperparathyroidism in patients with bipolar affective disorders treated with lithium is 47-fold higher than in the general population. To date, 50 cases of parathyroid adenomas and hyperplasia that were associated with chronic lithium therapy have been reported.[77,78] Theophylline toxicity may be associated with hypercalcemia probably due to stimulation of beta-adrenergic receptors in bone.

CLINICAL MANIFESTATIONS OF HYPERCALCEMIA

The symptoms of hypercalcemia depend on its rate of onset, its magnitude, its duration, the underlying disorder, and the comorbid conditions. Acute hypercalcemia may induce acute renal failure due to extracellular volume contraction and direct renal vasoconstriction. This abnormality is reversible, whereas chronic hypercalcemia may cause nephrolithiasis and nephrocalcinosis with tubulointerstitial scarring and chronic renal failure. Hypercalcemia may cause constipation, nausea and vomiting, and peptic ulcer disease. Polyuria is caused both by its natriuretic effect and impaired urinary concentration with features of nephrogenic diabetes insipidus.

Hypercalcemia leads to membrane hyperpolarization with shortened QT interval on an ECG. Cardiac arrhythmias are rare.

Neuromuscular effects include impaired concentration and memory, muscle weakness and fatigue, confusion, lethargy, stupor, and coma.

Bone pain can occur in patients with hyperparathyroidism or malignancy. Osteoporosis of the cortical bone is associated with hyperparathyroidism. Compression fractures of the vertebral bodies sometimes with sudden onset of paralysis may be the first manifestation of multiple myeloma.

Persons who nearly drowned in the Dead Sea presented with hyperosmolar coma and hypercalcemia, hypermagnesemia, and hypernatremia.

Familial hypocalciuric hypercalcemia is rarely associated with bone disease, but chondrocalcinosis and pseudogout have been reported to occur in high frequency.

Hypercalcemic crisis is a life-threatening emergency that warrants aggressive treatment. It may be a complication of primary hyperparathyroidism, malignancy, and other hypercalcemic disorders. It is characterized by very high serum calcium levels exceeding 15 mg/dL. The treatment is aimed at restoring extracellular volume to normal and lowering serum calcium levels. Acute hemodialysis with calcium-free dialysate may become a necessity.

TREATMENT OF HYPERCALCEMIA

Lowering of serum calcium concentration can be produced by (1) inhibiting calcium release from the bone, increasing its deposition in the bone and other tissues, or both; (2) increasing removal of calcium from the extracellular fluid or inhibiting its absorption in the bowel; and (3) decreasing the ionized fraction by complex formation with chelating substances.

Hypercalcemia augments urinary losses of sodium and water, resulting in the contraction of extracellular volume and reduced glomerular filtration rate. The latter leads to diminished urinary excretion of calcium and further aggravation of hypercalcemia. Therefore, the first therapeutic goal is to restore the extracellular volume to normal by intravenous administration of normal saline. This usually requires 3 to 4 L of saline. This therapeutic action per se lowers the serum calcium concentration, partly by the dilutional effect and partly by increased urinary excretion of calcium. There is a risk of extracellular volume overload during a rapid intravenous administration of saline, which is particularly hazardous in elderly patients. Therefore, monitoring of central venous pressure in this situation may be very helpful. Likewise, the addition of loop diuretics as an adjunct therapy not only may minimize the risk of fluid overload but also may substantially increase the urinary excretion of calcium. The effect of loop diuretics as calciuretic agents requires prompt replacement of urinary losses of sodium and water. The use of loop diuretics may be particularly beneficial in patients who develop hypercalcemia as a result of excessive secretion and high serum levels of PTH, PTHrP, or both. Hormone-induced, excessive tubular reabsorption of calcium plays a major role in the development and maintenance of hypercalcemia in these circumstances.

Bisphosphonates

Bisphosphonates (formerly diphosphonates) represent a group of drugs with a high therapeutic potential for the treatment of hypercalcemia in general and that associated with malignancy in particular. Bisphosphonates are related to an endogenous product of bone metabolism, pyrophosphate. The P–O–P bonds of pyrophosphates are cleaved by phosphatase in the process of bone mineralization and osteoclastic bone resorption. In the bisphosphonates, carbon replaces the oxygen moiety, generating a bond P–C–P, which is resistant to hydrolysis by phosphatase. Bisphosphonates have a great affinity for bone and bind tightly to calcified-bone matrix, impairing both the mineralization and resorption of bone. In addition, they interfere with the function of osteoclasts. They appear to have several direct effects on the osteoclast function, including prevention of osteoclast attachment to bone matrix and prevention of osteoclast differentiation and recruitment. Bisphosphonates also inhibit the motility of isolated osteoclasts. Thus, they are very potent inhibitors of bone resorption.

The first of the bisphosphonates, ethane hydroxybisphosphonate (etidronate [Didronel]), is available for clinical use, but its potency as an antihypercalcemic agent is limited, at least when given orally. Probably, this is because its effect to reduce bone resorption is offset by its effect to inhibit bone mineralization. Reduction of serum calcium concentration has been achieved more successfully with the second generation of bisphosphonates, including dichloromethylene bisphosphonate (clodronate) and amino-hydroxypropylidene bisphosphonate (pamidronate; ADP), which causes a reduction in bone resorption with a dose that has a negligible effect on bone mineralization. Pamidronate and etidronate are approved for treatment of hypercalcemia of malignancy in the United States. In clinical trials, pamidronate and clodronate have been demonstrated to inhibit hypercalcemia, bone pain, and pathologic fractures in patients with malignancy-associated hypercalcemia. Pamidronate is most effective when given intravenously; a single infusion of 30 mg achieved normocalcemia in 90% of patients in one study. When compared, the effect of 30 mg of pamidronate is equal to 600 mg of clodronate and 1500 mg of etidronate in controlling hypercalcemia. The third generation of bisphosphonates, including alendronate, risedronate, and tiludronate, in preliminary studies is 500 times more efficient in inhibiting bone resorption than clodronate. Zoledronic acid is one of a new generation of nitrogen-containing bisphosphonates that in clinical studies was superior to pamidronate. This agent has been approved for clinical use.

Glucocorticoids

Glucocorticoids are effective in lowering serum calcium in states of vitamin D intoxication; possible mechanisms are suppression of bone resorption and decreased intestinal absorption. It has been pointed out that glucocorticoids are more effective in hypercalcemia associated with lymphoma, leukemia, and multiple myeloma than with other neoplasms. This effect of glucocorticoids might be related to a tumor lytic effect, interference with the production of osteoclast-activating cytokines, or both. The average dose is 3 to 4 mg/kg/day of hydrocortisone given intravenously or orally. The fall in serum calcium concentration occurs 1 to 2 days after starting the therapy.

Calcitonin

Calcitonin lowers serum calcium concentration by inhibiting bone resorption and by increasing urinary calcium excretion. The administration of calcitonin is associated with negligible toxicity; however, its therapeutic action has a limited duration because of the osteoclast escape phenomenon, which is apparent several days after starting therapy. Addition of glucocorticoids may be helpful to maintain efficacy.

Mithramycin (Plicamycin)

Mithramycin is a cytotoxic substance derived from an actinomycete of the genus *Streptomyces* and is used mainly in the treatment of testicular tumors. Mithramycin lowers serum calcium concentration by suppressing bone resorption. The dose, which is lower than the antitumor dose and has fewer side effects, is 25 µg/kg, given intravenously. The drug is available commercially as Mithracin. The effect starts 24 to 48 hours after injection and lasts several days. Side effects are suppression of bone marrow activity and hepatocellular and renal toxicity, which usually occurs with repeated doses.

Phosphate

Oral and intravenous salts of phosphorus lower serum concentration and reduce urinary excretion of calcium. This effect has been variously attributed to (1) deposition of mineral in the bone; (2) increased deposition of calcium in soft tissues; and (3) suppression of bone resorption. The major untoward side effects of this therapy are extraskeletal calcifications, including nephrocalcinosis with resulting renal failure. Thus, the use of phosphates to treat hypercalcemia should be discouraged in patients with high serum phosphates and renal insufficiency. Phosphates may be given intravenously at a dose of 20 to 30 mg of elemental phosphorus per kilogram of body weight over 12 to 16 hours. Serum calcium concentration should be determined at close intervals. The commercially available preparation for intravenous use is InPhos; 40 mL of the solution contains 1000 mg of phosphorus, 65 mEq of sodium, and 8 mEq of potassium.

Other Therapies

Gallium nitrate has been approved by the Food and Drug Administration for treatment of hypercalcemia. It inhibits bone resorption by reducing the solubility of hydroxyapatite crystals. Nephrotoxicity is a major side effect of gallium nitrate. The use of a somatostatin congener (lanreotide) has been reported to successfully inhibit hypercalcemia in a patient with a PTHrP secreting pancreatic neoplasm. The calcium-lowering effect was associated with suppression of the serum levels of PTHrP.

The hypercalcemia associated with thyrotoxicosis and theophylline toxicity has been successfully treated with intravenous propranolol.

Intestinal absorption of calcium may be reduced by dietary restrictions and binding of calcium in the bowel with cellulose phosphate and sodium phytate to form nonabsorbable complexes.

Calcium also may be removed directly from the extracellular fluid with hemodialysis or peritoneal dialysis by employing calcium-free dialysate solution.

Reduction of serum-ionized calcium may be accomplished with intravenous Na-EDTA, which is a chelating agent. The complexed calcium then is excreted in the urine. The main disadvantage of this therapy is the nephrotoxicity of EDTA.

DISORDERS OF MAGNESIUM METABOLISM

Magnesium is the second most abundant intracellular cation. The intracellular concentration of magnesium ranges between 10 to 20 mEq/L; however, most of it is bound to organic compounds, including adenosine triphosphate (ATP). The free intracellular magnesium, as determined by magnesium-specific dyes, is lower than its concentration in the extracellular fluid. The latter favors a passive flux of magnesium into the cytosol down an electrochemical gradient and requires an active efflux from the cell. The exchange between the extracellular and intracellular compartments appears to be slow, and changes in intake and intestinal absorption are tightly balanced by parallel changes in urinary excretion.[79,80]

The renal tubular handling of magnesium displays a Tm (tubular maximum) with serum levels being close to the Tm threshold values. Thus, any rise in serum level and in the filtered load is counterbalanced by urinary spillover and, vice versa, a fall in filtered load leads to a sharp decline in urinary excretion almost down to zero. Therefore, in the presence of normal kidney function, serum levels are maintained at nearly constant values ranging form 1.4 to 1.7 mEq/L (1.7 to 2.1 mg/dL), most of which is ultrafiltrable with only 15% to 20% being protein bound. Hypermagnesemia can be encountered primarily with impaired kidney function and excessive oral or parenteral load. Hypomagnesemia results from decreased dietary intake, intestinal malabsorption, or renal losses.[79]

Intracellular magnesium plays an important role for protein synthesis, oxidative phosphorylation, nucleic acid stability, storing and utilization of energy, enzymatic reactions involving ATP, such as the activity of Mg^{++}, Na^+, K^+-ATPase, which are essential for maintenance of intracellular electrolyte composition. Extracellular magnesium has been regarded as essential to nerve conduction, neuromuscular transmission, cardiac conduction, and vascular tone.

HYPOMAGNESEMIA AND MAGNESIUM DEPLETION

Although hypomagnesemia is common in hospitalized patients (>10%) and ever more so in the ICU setting (>50%), its clinical significance is still a subject of investigation. The concerns regarding hypomagnesemia and magnesium depletion focused on its potential role in acute (cardiac arrhythmias and sudden death) and chronic (coronary artery disease) cardiovascular morbidity. Another pertinent issue is the common association of hypomagnesemia with other electrolyte abnormalities, including hypokalemia and hypocalcemia, which may confound the interpretation of the clinical correlations.[12,81]

The causes of hypomagnesemia can be divided into two major categories: (1) extrarenal magnesium losses, including deficient intake, and (2) renal losses. The best test to distinguish between these two entities is determination of urinary magnesium. In the former, the urinary magnesium is as low as or lower than 10 mg (0.8 mEq)/24 h, as compared with average normal excretion of 120 mg (10 mEq)/24 h. In the latter the excretion may exceed 40 mg (3.3 mEq)/24 h. Another way to discriminate between these two categories is the response to intravenous load of 40 mEq (480 mg) of magnesium as magnesium sulfate, infused over 4 hours. In magnesium-replete individuals, 80% of the intravenous load is excreted in the urine over 24 hours, whereas in magnesium-depleted patients most of the load is retained but not in the patients with renal leak.

EXTRARENAL LOSSES

Dietary deprivation, prolonged malnutrition, tube feedings, and parenteral nutrition deficient in magnesium may induce cumulative magnesium depletion and hypomagnesemia. Gastrointestinal losses may be caused by steatorrhea, possibly due to formation of magnesium soaps. Small bowel disease and chronic pancreatitis may be the underlying causes. Acute pancreatitis may precipitate magnesium in necrotic fat tissue similarly to calcium resulting in hypomagnesemia. Hypomagnesemia may follow surgery for morbid obesity with short bowel syndrome and diarrhea.[12,79]

Hyperthyroidism may cause hypomagnesemia due to severe diarrhea, possible shift of magnesium to intracellular space, and urinary losses due to hypercalcemia.

Chronic alcoholism is one of the leading causes of magnesium depletion. Poor nutrition, diarrhea, chronic pancreatitis, and possibly a renal tubular defect may contribute to hypomagnesemia.[82]

Severe burns may lead to sequestration of magnesium in the necrotic tissue, including necrotic fat, leading to magnesium depletion.

Hungry bone syndrome after parathyroidectomy may lead to both hypocalcemia and hypomagnesemia owing to increased deposition of both divalent ions in the newly deposited bone mineral. Acute dialysis for severe refractory hypercalcemia without addition of magnesium to the dialysate may cause hypomagnesemia.

Ionized hypomagnesemia may appear after transfusions with citrate-rich blood products and after foscarnet therapy for cytomegalovirus chorioretinitis due to chelation of magnesium by both agents.

PRIMARY INTESTINAL HYPOMAGNESEMIA OR HYPOMAGNESEMIA WITH SECONDARY HYPOCALCEMIA

Hypomagnesemia with secondary hypocalcemia (HSH) is an autosomal recessive disorder characterized by low serum magnesium and hypocalcemia. Hypocalcemia is secondary to parathyroid failure and peripheral resistance to PTH.

The defect is in intestinal magnesium transport and a mild renal defect. The patient presents within the first 3 months of life with muscle spasms, tetany, and seizures. If untreated, the disorder leads to permanent neurologic damage and may be fatal. The gene locus was mapped to chromosome 9q22. A mutation was identified in a novel gene *TRPM6*, which encodes an ion channel with magnesium conductance properties.[83] TRPM6 protein has been demonstrated along the entire small and large intestine and in distal renal tubules.

RENAL LOSSES

This category can be divided into noninherited and inherited disorders.

Osmotic diuresis induced by intravenous salt loads, diabetic ketoacidosis, and mannitol administration increases urinary excretion of many electrolytes, including magnesium. During recovery from ketoacidosis, especially after phosphate replacement, a precipitous fall in serum magnesium may require parenteral administration of magnesium.

Hypercalcemia as seen both with primary hyperparathyroidism, hyperthyroidism, and intravenous administration of calcium causes renal losses of magnesium as both divalent cations compete for the same reabsorption mechanism in Henle's loop. Similarly, loop diuretics cause renal magnesium and calcium wasting whereas thiazides enhance urinary excretion of magnesium but cause tubular retention of calcium. Primary hyperaldosteronism and SIADH are associated with modest increases in urinary magnesium excretion.

Renal magnesium wasting has been observed in patients treated with aminoglycosides, amphotericin B, and cisplatin.[83] These agents may lead to potassium wasting and renal tubular acidosis. Cyclosporine and tacrolimus cause magnesium wasting with potassium retention. Experimental data suggest that cyclosporine impairs paracellin-1–dependent absorption of magnesium at Henle's loop. Pentamidine was reported to be associated with hypomagnesemia due to renal wasting in a patient with AIDS treated for *Pneumocystis carinii* pneumonia.[85]

Inherited Disorders of Renal Magnesium Losses

Isolated Dominant Hypomagnesemia (IDH)
The patients present with generalized seizures in childhood, but the mothers may be asymptomatic with less pronounced hypomagnesemia. Many affected members of the family may be asymptomatic. Hypocalciuria but not hypocalcemia is present. The gene locus was mapped to 11a23 with a mutation Gly14Arg in the gene *FXYD2*, which encodes the alpha subunit of Na^+,K^+-ATPase in the distal tubule. Why a mutation in the alpha subunit would result in selective renal magnesium wasting is unknown.[86]

Isolated Recessive Hypomagnesemia (IRH)
The affected individual presents with symptoms of hypomagnesemia early during infancy. Hypomagnesemia due to increased urinary magnesium excretion is the only biochemical abnormality. Linkage analysis has excluded thus far all established gene loci.[83]

Familial Hypomagnesemia with Hypercalciuria and Nephrocalcinosis (FHHNC)
FHHNC is an autosomal recessive hypomagnesemia characterized by renal magnesium and calcium wasting, bilateral

nephrocalcinosis, and nephrolithiasis with progressive renal failure. FHHNC patients present during early childhood with recurrent urinary tract infection, polyuria and polydipsia, failure to thrive, abdominal pain, vomiting, tetanic episodes, and generalized seizures. PTH levels are increased before renal failure. Hypomagnesemia may disappear with decline in glomerular filtration rate. Renal transplantation corrects the abnormal renal handling of magnesium and calcium. Using positional cloning a model gene was mapped to chromosome 3q27-29. *CLDN16*, formerly *PCLN-1* gene (claudin 16, paracellin 1), mutations are the underlying cause of FHHNC. CLDN16 codes for paracellin-1 (claudin 16), a tight junction protein that is strongly expressed both in medullary and cortical segments of the loop of Henle. It is suggested that paracellin-1 contributes to the formation of calcium- and magnesium-selective paracellular pathways. Family analysis suggests that carriers of heterozygous *CLDN16* mutations may present with hypercalciuria, nephrolithiasis, and nephrocalcinosis.[83]

Autosomal Dominant Hypocalcemia

Activating mutations of the calcium sensing receptor (CASR) lead to hypocalcemia, hypocalciuria, and, in about 50% of patients, hypomagnesemia. The diminished PTH secretion and decreased reabsorption of divalent cations in the cortical thick ascending limb (CTAL) of Henle's loop and distal convoluted tubule lead to urinary loss of calcium and magnesium. The inhibition of calcium and magnesium reabsorption in the loop of Henle is thought to be secondary to selective reduction in paracellular permeability and/or the reduction in the lumen-positive transepithelial voltage. The disorder has been mapped to chromosome 3q13.3-21 with mutation of gene coding for CASR.[20-22]

Classic Bartter Syndrome

Classic Bartter syndrome is caused by mutations in the *CLC-NKB* gene encoding the basolaterally located renal chloride channel CIC-KB, which mediates chloride efflux from the tubular epithelial cells to the interstitium along the CTAL and distal convoluted tubule. Hypomagnesemia is detected in up to 50% of patients with mutations in *CLCNKB* in chromosome 1p36.[83]

Gitelman's Syndrome

Gitelman's syndrome (GS) is an autosomal recessive disorder. Major symptoms of GS include muscle weakness and tetanic episodes that are related to profound hypomagnesemia. Patients with GS always present with hypocalciuria. The presence of both hypomagnesemia and hypocalciuria is diagnostic for GS. Loss of function mutations in the gene coding for NaCl cotransporter (NCCT) of the distal convoluted tubule is the underlying abnormality. Hypocalciuria in GS is explained by reduced entry of NaCl into distal convoluted tubule cells leading to apical membrane hyperpolarization. This increases calcium absorption mediated by apical entry via the epithelial calcium channel and basolateral extrusion through the Na^+/Ca^{++} exchanger. The reason for the hypomagnesemia in GS is still unknown.[83]

CLINICAL CONSEQUENCES OF MAGNESIUM DEPLETION

The clinical manifestations of hypomagnesemia depend on its severity, duration, and coexistent electrolyte abnormalities.

Hypomagnesemia and depletion of intracellular stores especially in cardiac muscle have been considered to underlie cardiovascular and other functional abnormalities, including cardiac arrhythmias, such as atrial fibrillation and torsades de pointes, impairment of cardiac contractility, and vasoconstriction. ECG changes in magnesium depletion include widening of QRS complex and peaking of T waves, followed by prolongation of PR interval and diminution of T waves. The ventricular arrhythmias are more common during myocardial ischemia after cardiopulmonary bypass. Magnesium prevents the increase in action potential duration and the prolongation in membrane repolarization, which normally occurs in ischemic myocardium.[87]

One study in which 404 consecutive patients admitted with congestive heart failure were evaluated after being treated with furosemide showed that hypomagnesemia emerged as being associated with a shorter survival. This was shown after adjustment for comorbid conditions. The author recommended magnesium supplementation once hypomagnesemia is detected.[88]

Prolonged insufficiency of magnesium supply[89] results in anorexia, nausea, vomiting, and weakness within weeks and in paresthesias and muscle weakness, cerebral seizures, and cardiac manifestations within months. The neuromuscular abnormalities of magnesium depletion include positive Trousseau's and Chvostek's signs, which may occur in the absence of hypocalcemia, hypokalemia, and alkalosis.

Hypomagnesemia may lead to secondary renal losses of potassium, and, vice versa, hypokalemia may enhance urinary losses of magnesium. In the former, hypokalemia is refractory to potassium replacement unless magnesium repletion is accomplished first. The same applies to hypocalcemia secondary to magnesium depletion and/or associated with magnesium depletion. Correction of magnesium depletion must come first to achieve correction of hypocalcemia. Thus, in states of refractory hypokalemia and/or hypocalcemia, magnesium depletion may be the underlying mechanism.

TREATMENT OF HYPOMAGNESEMIA

The amount and the route of magnesium replacement depend on the degree of hypomagnesemia and the severity of the symptoms. In patients with asymptomatic hypomagnesemia, the treatment of the underlying disorder such as diarrhea and dietary adjustments may solve the problem. Unless the serum magnesium falls to and below 1 mg/dL (0.8 mEq/L, 0.4 mM/L), most of the patients remain asymptomatic. The goal of the replacement is to achieve levels above 1 mg/dL. In patients with minimal symptoms, oral replacement therapy may be beneficial. That route of administration is limited by the occurrence of diarrhea secondary to oral magnesium. Magnesium oxide tablets have high magnesium content: 550 mg of elemental magnesium per 1 g (46 mEq/g). Other oral preparations such as magnesium chloride, magnesium sulfate, and magnesium acetate contain approximately 100 mg of elemental magnesium per 1 g (8 to 10 mEq/g). Two to four tablets a day in divided doses may be sufficient in mild cases; the dose can be doubled if necessary. Slow-release preparations include Slow Mag containing magnesium chloride (60 mg, 5 mEq per tablet) and Mag-Tab SR with magnesium lactate (84 mg, 7 mEq per tablet). If hypomagnesemia is associated with the use of diuretics that need to be continued, addition of potassium-sparing diuretics such as amiloride may be helpful.

Amiloride may also be considered in other states of magnesium wasting such as Bartter's or Gitelman's syndrome and cisplatin nephrotoxicity.

Oral replacement also can be made with antacids that contain both magnesium and aluminum, such as Maalox, in patients who develop diarrhea from magnesium oxide.

In states of emergency, such as torsades de pointes tachyarrhythmia, 16 mEq (192 mg) of magnesium should be given intravenously over 5 to 15 minutes followed by 128 mEq (1536 mg) over the ensuing 24 hours. Magnesium has potentially a deleterious effect on arteriovenous conduction; therefore, it is relatively contraindicated in greater than first-degree arteriovenous block and sinus bradycardia. The same therapeutic regimen may be followed in patients with tetany and seizures due to hypomagnesemia. In severe preeclampsia, the intravenous loading dose of magnesium is 32 mEq (384 mg), followed by an infusion of 8 mEq/h, up to 24 hours ante partum.

HYPERMAGNESEMIA

The normal kidney can dispose of large filtered loads of magnesium by attenuating tubular reabsorption to minimum after the renal tubular Tm is exceeded. Thus, intact kidneys are the major regulating organ for maintaining magnesium balance. The most common cause of hypermagnesemia is concurrence of excessive magnesium load in the presence of impaired renal function. Very often a large magnesium load is the consequence of therapeutic employment of magnesium salts as laxatives or enemas. Attempts to release bowel obstruction with magnesium salts may be detrimental. The magnesium salt is retained in the bowel and by generating local hypertonicity it displaces large volumes of extracellular fluid into the distended bowel, leading to volume contraction with reduced renal function (prerenal azotemia). The trapped magnesium diffuses into the circulation in massive amounts, and in the presence of impaired renal function it is retained and raises the serum magnesium level (SMg). Endogenous magnesium loads may be released in rhabdomyolysis from necrotic muscles and in tumor lysis from malignant cells destroyed by chemotherapy.

Acute intravenous magnesium loads such as given in preeclampsia may cause transient hypermagnesemia occasionally accompanied by hypocalcemia as a result of acute suppression of PTH by high serum magnesium. The children born to mothers with preeclampsia may have hypermagnesemia as well.

Ingestion of massive quantities of magnesium has been reported to cause hypermagnesemia even in the absence of renal dysfunction. This observation needs further evaluation because increases in filtered magnesium sulfate may induce solute diuresis leading to hypovolemia and functional renal failure.

Hypermagnesemia may be more common in the elderly who often consume magnesium salts as antacids and laxatives and display aging-related reduction in renal function.

Hypermagnesemia was reported recently in 5% of patients with congestive heart failure treated with furosemide and was associated with a shorter survival. Hypermagnesemia was more frequent in the elderly and in those with impaired kidney function. However, the incidence of arrhythmias and sudden death was the lowest in patients with hypermagnesemia.

Patients with chronic renal failure may present with mild elevation of serum magnesium; however, ingestion of magnesium salts should be avoided because they may induce life-threatening hypermagnesemia.

Adrenal insufficiency, primary hyperparathyroidism, milk-alkali syndrome, and familial hypocalciuric hypercalcemia may be associated with hypermagnesemia. Lithium and theophylline have been reported to cause hypermagnesemia. Near-drowning in the Dead Sea is associated with hypernatremia, hypercalcemia, and hypermagnesemia.

CLINICAL MANIFESTATIONS

Mild hypermagnesemia with serum magnesium levels less than 3 mEq/L (3.6 mg/dL, 1.5 Mm/L) is usually asymptomatic. Above these values, the severity of symptoms parallels the magnitude of serum magnesium. The major manifestations are neuromuscular, central nervous system, and cardiovascular abnormalities.

Neuromuscular manifestations relate to the curare-like action of hypermagnesemia, hindering the neuromuscular impulse transmission. It is first manifested as reduced deep tendon reflexes (SMg ~ 5 mEq/L) progressing to areflexia (SMg ~ 8 mEq/L), muscle paralysis and apnea (SMg > 10 mEq/L). Central nervous system abnormalities consist of lethargy, drowsiness (SMg ~ 6 mEq/L), dilated and fixed pupils, and coma (SMg ~ 10 mEq/L).

The cardiovascular effects of hypermagnesemia may be related to its effects as ion channel blockers. These effects lead to bradycardia and hypotension (SMg ~ 8 mEq/L). ECG abnormalities consist of increased PR and QT intervals (SMg ~ 8 mEq/L) and QRS duration. With the rise in the serum magnesium above 10 mEq/L complete heart block and cardiac arrest are the terminal events.

TREATMENT OF HYPERMAGNESEMIA

Severe hypermagnesemia is a medical emergency that requires immediate attention because it can cause respiratory and cardiac arrest. Moderate elevations of serum magnesium in the range of 4 to 5 mEq (4.8 to 6.0 mg/dL) in the presence of normal kidney function may be managed with complete cessation of magnesium intake, restoration of extracellular volume with 0.9% or 0.45% NaCl solution, followed by intravenous loop diuretic. This may help increase urinary excretion of magnesium.

With higher serum magnesium levels and/or significant symptoms, calcium, an antagonist of magnesium, may be given intravenously over 5 minutes at the dose of 100 to 200 mg of elemental calcium (5 to 10 mEq i.v.). This may be repeated to alleviate the symptoms. If serum magnesium levels exceed 6 mEq/L and symptoms worsen, hemodialysis with magnesium-free dialysate may be effective to clear quickly the excess of magnesium.

ANNOTATED REFERENCES

Awad SS, Miskulin J, Thompson N: Hyperparathyroidism in patients with prolonged lithium therapy. World J Surg 2003;27:486-488.
   This report calls attention to the association of chronic lithium therapy for bipolar disorders with the development of hypercalcemia with elevated PTH levels. The incidence of primary hyperparathyroidism in patients treated with lithium is 47-fold higher than in the general population. The most common cause of primary hyperparathyroidism is parathyroid adenoma.

Konrad M, Weber S: Recent advances in molecular genetics of hereditary magnesium-losing disorders. J Am Soc Nephrol 2003;15:249-260.

> This is a comprehensive, in-depth review of recently unfolding information on abnormalities associated both with intestinal and renal causes of magnesium wasting. The paper focuses on the molecular aspects of hereditary genetically transmitted defects in tubular epithelial and in intestinal magnesium transport causing hypomagnesemia.

Moore EW: Ionized calcium in normal serum, ultrafiltrates and whole blood determined by ion-exchanged electrode. J Clin Invest 1970;49: 318-324.

> This is a seminal classic introducing the methodology to determine ionized calcium in different fractions of blood. This publication presents the first detailed protocol describing the techniques of the employment of calcium-sensitive ion exchange electrode for the assay of ionized calcium.

Nykjaer A, Dragun D, Walther D, et al: An endocytic pathway essential for renal uptake and activation of the steroid 25(OH) vitamin D_3. Cell 1999;96:507-515.

> This paper reports a novel finding that endocytosis mediated by apical megalin is the mechanism by which filtered 25(OH) vitamin D bound to a protein carrier gains access to tubular epithelial cytosol where it is converted to 1,25(OH)2 vitamin D. This contradicts the previously held view that free 25(OH) vitamin D diffuses passively from the circulation into cytosol through the basolateral membrane of tubular epithelial cells.

Zivin JR, Gooley T, Zager RA, et al: Hypocalcemia: A pervasive metabolic abnormality in the critically ill. Am J Kidney Dis 2001;37:689-698.

> This article presents an interesting finding that hypocalcemia was present in 88% of critically ill patients who were admitted to intensive care units. The level of hypocalcemia correlated with the severity of the disease. The mechanism of this abnormality is unknown.

Chapter 131

FLUIDS AND ELECTROLYTES IN PEDIATRICS

Desmond Bohn

KEY POINTS

1. **Total body water is higher in infants than in older children**, particularly in premature infants, who have a limited ability to excrete a concentrated urine.

2. **Hyponatremia (sodium <136 mmol/L) is the most common electrolyte abnormality** seen in hospitalized children and indicates the presence of antidiuretic hormone (ADH) and expansion of the intracellular fluid compartment. Acute hyponatremia is associated with the development of cerebral edema and can result in catastrophic neurologic injury and death.

3. Nonphysiologic secretion of ADH (i.e., not produced in response to increased osmolality or hypovolemia) leads to the **retention of electrolyte-free water in acutely ill children.**

4. The **widespread use of hypotonic fluids in children is not evidence based** and contributes to the problem of hyponatremia.

5. The **prescription of intravenous fluids** in children should be based on whether there is a need for extracellular free water and the measurement of serum sodium. Children with serum sodium levels <138 mmol/L should receive isotonic fluids.

6. Hypernatremia (sodium >150 mmol/L) is associated with contraction of the intracellular fluid compartment and a hyperosmolar state. The most common causes in children are diabetic ketoacidosis and gastroenteritis.

7. The **intracellular fluid deficit in hyperosmolar state needs to be corrected slowly** to prevent water shifts and the development of cerebral edema.

8. **The most significant morbidity and mortality risk in children presenting with severe diabetic ketoacidosis is cerebral edema.** These patients require close monitoring of level of consciousness and slow correction of the fluid and electrolyte deficit.

The fundamental principles that govern fluid and electrolyte physiology in children (particularly older children) are in many ways similar to those in adults. However, there are some important differences that apply mainly to infants and young children, and these must be taken into account when prescribing fluids in critical care. In addition, many of the principles used to estimate fluid losses and replacement requirements (maintenance fluids) are based on limited studies published 50 years ago, when the complexity of illness was not as well understood. Also, these formulas were based on principles established for normal physiology and did not take into account the hormonal influences that govern fluid and electrolyte balance, which may be seriously perturbed in critical illness. The challenge is to rethink some of these principles in the light of new knowledge of how acute illness may influence them.

BODY WATER DISTRIBUTION IN CHILDREN

Body water content changes significantly with age in children.[1,2] Total body water is high in the fetus and preterm infant. During early fetal life, total body water represents 90% of total body weight, with 65% being in the extracellular fluid compartment. By term, the extracellular and intracellular fluid volume has fallen to 45% and 30% of total body water, respectively (Fig. 131-1). The preterm infant has a relative expansion of both total body water and extracellular fluid volume, and a diuresis in the first few days of postnatal life is common. Fractional excretion of sodium is inversely correlated with age in the preterm infant, who is susceptible to both sodium loss and sodium and volume overload.[3] In addition, glomerular filtration rate is lower than in the term infant, and the large surface area–to–body weight ratio leads to considerable evaporative water losses.[4-7] Further discussion of fluid and electrolyte physiology in the preterm infant is beyond the scope of this chapter.

Significant changes occur in total body water over the first year of life—from 75% of body weight at birth to 65% at 6 months and 60% at 1 year (Table 131-1). Some of this is accounted for by an increase in body fat. By puberty, total body water is approximately 60% of body weight in males, with a slightly lower percentage in females. Extracellular fluid volume decreases over the first year of life to 30% of total body water; it decreases with age thereafter, reaching adult values early in childhood. The relatively high extracellular fluid volume in infancy is mainly due to the larger interstitial lymph space. In contrast, the intracellular fluid volume remains relatively constant during childhood.

FLUID HOMEOSTASIS IN CHILDREN

To achieve normal fluid homeostasis, fluid intake must balance losses. The latter consist of urine output and insensible losses (evaporative losses from the skin surface and respiratory tract), plus fluid loss in the stool, which, in the absence of

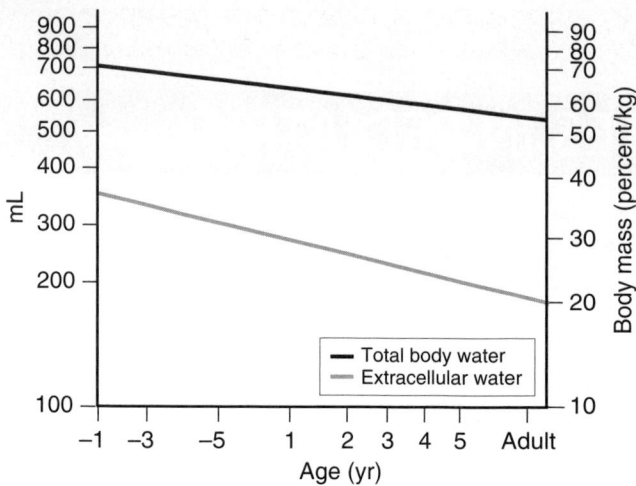

FIGURE 131–1. Changes in total body water (TBW) with age. The intracellular water is represented by the difference between the two diagonal lines. (Adapted from Kooh SW, Metcoff J: Physiologic considerations in fluid and electrolyte therapy with particular reference to diarrheal dehydration in children. J Pediatr 1963;62:107.)

diarrhea, is minimal. Insensible losses are mainly in the form of electrolyte-free water from the respiratory tract (15 mL/100 kcal/day). This loss is eliminated during positive-pressure ventilation. Sweat contains mostly water with a small amount of sodium, except in situations in which the sweat glands contain excessive amounts of sodium, such as in patients with cystic fibrosis. Evaporative losses also increase with elevation in body temperature, and during thermal stress, water losses may increase to as much as 25 mL/100 kcal per day (Table 131-2).

Obligate water excretion in the urine is dependent on solute load and the ability to concentrate and dilute the urine. The average osmolar excretion in newborn infants receiving infant formula is 16 to 20 mOsm/kg per day.[2] Infants are somewhat disadvantaged compared with older children and adults, in that they cannot maximally dilute (infants, 200 mOsm/L, versus adults, 80 mOsm/L) or concentrate (infants, 800 mOsm/L, versus adults, 1200 mOsm/L) the urine. In addition, infants' high metabolic rate and the solute load from enteral feeding formula mean that they require more water excretion per unit solute amount. The high solute load and the limited urine concentrating ability make them prone to significant extracellular fluid contraction (dehydration) when water loss is excessive. Typically, this occurs in gastroenteritis, when reduced oral intake is combined with excessive water and electrolyte loss in the stool.

TABLE 131–1. WATER CONTENT OF BODY COMPARTMENTS IN CHILDREN

Age	TBW (% Body Weight)	Extracellular Fluid (% Body Weight)	Intracellular Fluid (% Body Weight)
Premature	80	45	35
Full-term newborn	75	40	35
1 mo–1 yr	65	30	35
1–12 yr	60	20	40
Adolescent			
Male	60	20	40–45
Female	55	18	40

TBW, total body water

TABLE 131–2. WATER LOSSES IN NORMAL CHILDREN (mL/100 kcal/24 h)

Source	Newborn–6 Mo	6 Mo–5 Yr	5–10 Yr	Adolescent
Insensible	40	30	20	10
Urine	60	60	50	40
Fecal	20	10	—	—
Total	120	100	70	50

Urine is the major source of electrolyte loss in the body, except when there are fluid losses from the gastrointestinal tract. The commonly used values for sodium (Na) and potassium (K) requirements in parenteral fluids in children are 2 to 3 mmol/kg per day and 1 to 2 mmol/kg per day, respectively. These are the amounts of cations needed for normal homeostasis; however, in critically ill children, urinary Na and K concentrations may be much higher.

In normal, healthy individuals, water intake is regulated by thirst, which is stimulated by osmoreceptors in the hypothalamus. Infants and small children are unable to regulate their intake because they do not have access to water; this also applies to older children and adults in coma or with reduced levels of consciousness. When oral intake is replaced by parenteral fluids in children, the amount of fluid (i.e., water) given depends on body weight and energy expenditure. In 1957, Holliday and Segar published a formula that linked body weight to energy expenditure (Table 131-3).[8] An allowance of 50 mL/100 kcal per day was made for insensible water loss, with 66.7 mL/100 kcal per day to replace urine output. Factoring in a gain from water oxidation of 16.7 mL/100 kcal per day leaves a total of 100 mL/100 kcal per day for the replacement of normal losses. The estimates for sodium (3 mmol/100 kcal/day) and potassium (2 mmol/100 kcal/day) in maintenance fluids were calculated from the sodium and potassium concentration of cow's milk and breast milk.

This paper by Holliday and Segar has become the standard reference for parenteral fluid administration in pediatrics. Although the formula is convenient and simple to use, the assumptions made about daily requirements for sodium, potassium, and electrolyte-free water mandate the use of hypotonic intravenous solutions, which has been almost universal practice in pediatric medicine for almost 50 years (Table 131-4). However, nonphysiologic stimuli for antidiuretic hormone (ADH) secretion (e.g., pain, anxiety, narcotics, positive-pressure ventilation), which inhibits the excretion of electrolyte-free water, are common in critically ill patients. It is therefore not surprising that mild degrees of hyponatremia are common in pediatric patients receiving parenteral fluid therapy. In a study by Gerigk and colleagues of 103 children admitted to the hospital with acute medical illnesses, the median plasma Na value was 136 mmol/L, with

TABLE 131–3. REQUIREMENTS FOR MAINTENANCE PARENTERAL FLUIDS*

Body weight	0-10 kg	10-20 kg	>20 kg
Water requirements	100 mL/kg/day	1000 mL + 50 mL/kg/day for each kg >10	1500 mL + 20 mL/kg for each kg >20

*Based on the formula of Holliday MA, Segar WE: The maintenance need for water in parenteral fluid therapy. Pediatrics 1957;19:823-832.

TABLE 131–4. WATER AND ELECTROLYTE CONTENT OF COMMONLY USED INTRAVENOUS FLUIDS

Fluid Type	Na$^+$ (mmol/L)	Cl$^-$ (mmol/L)	Osmolality	Osmolality with 20 mmol KCl/L Added	pH	Electrolyte-Free Water/L
0.9 NaCl	154	154	308	348	5.5	0
0.45 NaCl	77	77	154	194	5.5	500
0.9 NaCl, 5% dextrose	154	154	560	600	4	0
5% dextrose, 0.45 NaCl	77	77	406	446	4	500
5% dextrose, 0.2 NaCl	34	34	321	361	4	780
4% dextrose, 0.18 NaCl	31	31	284	324	4	800
5% dextrose	0	0	252	292	4	1000
Ringer's lactate	130	109	272	312	6.5	114
Ringer's lactate 5%	130	109	525		6.5	114
3% NaCl	513	513	1027		5.5	0

plasma ADH levels that were higher than expected for that degree of hyponatremia.[9] In 31 control patients (elective surgical admissions), the median serum Na levels were 139 mmol/L, with lower ADH levels. A similar observation was made in patients with hospital-acquired hyponatremia who received twice as much electrolyte-free water compared with a control group.[10] The nonphysiologic secretion of ADH has been reported in association with many acute medical illnesses, including meningitis, bronchiolitis, encephalitis, traumatic brain injury, and gastroenteritis.[11-23] An increasing number of publications now recommend the use of isotonic or near-isotonic fluids for standard maintenance in pediatrics to avoid the administration of electrolyte-free water, which is potentially hazardous when ADH secretion is not inhibited.[10,24-27] Hypotonic fluids should be reserved for patients with a demonstrated need for electrolyte-free water (serum Na$^+$ >145 mmol/L).

PERIOPERATIVE FLUID MANAGEMENT

Standard practice in perioperative fluid management has been to replace intravascular volume loss with blood or colloid solutions and to use electrolyte solutions to provide for ongoing fluid requirements and to replace losses from exposed serosal surfaces in open body cavities in thoracic and abdominal surgery and losses from third space fluid sequestration (Table 131-5). Extra fluid is frequently administered to treat hypotension due to the vasodilating effects of anesthetic agents. The electrolyte solution preferred by most anesthesiologists for intraoperative fluid administration is Ringer's lactate or isotonic saline, because of concern about the development of postoperative fluid retention and hyponatremia associated with elevated ADH levels[28-31]; the potential for this is increased when hypotonic dextrose or saline solutions are used.[30,32-34] The inability to excrete a

sodium-free water load is amply illustrated in patients undergoing scoliosis surgery, who seem to be at particularly high risk for the development of hyponatremia.[35] Two nonrandomized studies have shown that the degree of hyponatremia is less when isotonic or near-isotonic solutions are used.[36,37] Burrows and coworkers, in a nonrandomized trial, compared Ringer's lactate with 0.2 sodium chloride (NaCl) in a group of children undergoing scoliosis surgery.[37] They found that the postoperative plasma Na level decreased in both groups, but the reduction was marked in those patients receiving the hypotonic fluid. Although, at first glance, the explanation seems to be electrolyte-free water retention due to nonphysiologic stimulation of ADH secretion, it does not explain the reduction in plasma Na seen with Ringer's lactate. Further insights came from the study by Steele and colleagues, in which plasma and urine Na levels were measured in adult patients undergoing elective surgery, all of whom received Ringer's lactate as the perioperative fluid.[38] They found that the urine Na concentration was consistently above 150 mmol/L and as high as 350 mmol/L in some instances. This was associated with a significant positive water balance and a fall in plasma Na, a process they termed postoperative "desalination." In a similar study of children undergoing elective surgery, all of whom received Ringer's lactate, we found similar levels of urinary Na loss (unpublished observations). We believe that this desalination process is consistent with the kidney's attempt to deal with volume overload after the vasodilating effects of anesthetic agents are no longer present but ADH is still being actively secreted. In this situation, it would be unwise to prescribe hypotonic fluids in the postoperative period and impose an extra burden of more electrolyte-free water to be excreted by the kidney.

SODIUM

Sodium is the principal cation of the extracellular fluid compartment. Movement of Na into the intracellular fluid compartment is reversed by activation of the Na$^+$,K$^+$-ATPase pump. Sodium is absorbed in the proximal tubule under the influence of aldosterone. The serum Na reflects the osmolality and the extracellular fluid water volume, which is tightly regulated by ADH secretion.

HYPONATREMIA

Hyponatremia (serum Na < 136 mmol/L) is the most common electrolyte disorder seen in a hospitalized population and implies an expansion of the intracellular fluid compartment.[39]

TABLE 131–5. ELECTROLYTE COMPOSITION OF BODY FLUIDS (mmol/L)

	Na$^+$	K$^+$	Cl$^-$	HCO$_3^-$
Sweat	50	5	55	
Saliva	30	20	35	15
Gastric juice	60	10	90	
Bile	145	5	110	40
Duodenum	140	5	80	50
Ileum	130	10	110	30
Colon	60	30	40	20

TABLE 131–6. CAUSES OF HYPONATREMIA

Water gain
  Excessive water ingestion
  Hypotonic fluid administration
  SIADH
  Congestive heart failure
  Chronic renal failure
Salt loss
  Gastroenteritis
  Cerebral salt wasting

SIADH, syndrome of inappropriate antidiuretic hormone.

It is caused by either water gain (e.g., use of hypotonic fluids) or salt loss (e.g., gastroenteritis) (Table 131-6).

Acute hyponatremia, defined as a decrease in plasma Na to less than 130 mmol/L within 48 hours, leads to rapid movement of water from the extracellular to the intracellular fluid compartment; this can cause cerebral edema, with catastrophic outcomes reported in children.[32,40,41] The clinical findings are those of raised intracranial pressure (nausea, vomiting, headache), but the condition is frequently undiagnosed until the onset of seizures. This is usually followed by apnea, suggesting that brainstem coning has occurred. Symptomatic hyponatremia rarely results from a serum Na level of 125 mmol/L. When it occurs, it constitutes a medical emergency. The primary objective is to raise the serum Na above this level to prevent seizures and cerebral herniation. This is most effectively achieved with the use of hypertonic saline.[42] Once this threshold has been reached, the serum Na can be allowed to correct by fluid restriction, with or without the use of furosemide. Intravenous mannitol has also been used successfully in the emergency treatment of acute symptomatic hyponatremia.[43]

Chronic hyponatremia is a common finding in patients with heart failure and renal failure and is associated with increased total body water and salt retention. It is not associated with cerebral edema, but correction of chronic hyponatremia with isotonic or hypertonic saline has been associated with central pontine demyelination.[44-46]

HYPERNATREMIA

Hypernatremia is defined as serum Na greater than 145 mmol/L and is caused by either water deficit or salt gain (Table 131-7). The former is seen in infants with severe gastroenteritis, with water loss in excess of sodium loss,

TABLE 131–7. CAUSES OF HYPERNATREMIA

Water loss
  Gastroenteritis
  Central diabetes insipidus
  Nephrogenic diabetes insipidus
  Use of loop diuretics
  Use of osmotic diuretics
  Use of radiology contrast medium
  Excessive insensible cutaneous loss (burns, sweating)
  Diabetic ketoacidosis or hyperosmolar nonketotic diabetes
Salt gain
  Use of high-Na solutions (hypertonic saline, i.v. bicarbonate)
  Use of hypertonic enteral feeding formulas
  Use of cathartic agents

sometimes compounded by increased solute intake from incorrect mixing of infant formula. The absence of ADH secretion, causing diabetes insipidus, is seen in patients with pituitary tumors, traumatic brain injuries, and central nervous system infections.[47-50] Water loss in critically ill children may also be associated with the use of loop diuretics or mannitol. Hypernatremia secondary to salt gain is seen with the excessive use of isotonic or hypertonic saline solutions or with the administration of intravenous bicarbonate.

An increase in serum Na is associated with movement of water from the intracellular to the extracellular fluid compartment and the development of a hyperosmolar state. Brain cells adapt with an increase in electrolytes and "ideogenic" osmoles (inositol, taurine), which tends to mitigate the fluid shift by partial restoration of intracellular osmolality and brain cell volume.[39,51,52] Na levels greater than 155 mmol/L are frequently associated with abnormal central nervous system findings, and there is an increased risk of subdural hemorrhage and infarction in infants with hypernatremic dehydration and serum Na levels greater than 160 mmol/L.[53-56] There is the added danger of the development of brain edema during the attempt to correct these hyperosmolar states rapidly by using solutions that are hypo-osmolar compared with the intracellular fluid compartment.[57-62] Published recommendations state that the rate of correction of serum Na should be less than 0.5 mmol/L per hour, using the following formula, which estimates the effect of 1 L of any infusate on serum Na:

$$\text{Change in serum Na} = (\text{Infusate Na} - \text{Serum Na})/(\text{Total body water} + 1)$$

In severe hypernatremia (serum Na >170 mmol/L), the level should not be corrected to below 150 mmol/L in the first 48 to 72 hours.[63]

The epidemiology of hypernatremia in children has changed. Whereas gastroenteritis with dehydration was once the principal cause, it is now a hospital-acquired problem associated with either excess salt administration or a free water deficit. In a recent study by Moritz and Ayus of children with serum Na levels greater than 150 mmol/L, the problem was hospital acquired in 60%, and the mortality rate was 11%.[64] In a similar series of adult patients, the ICU mortality rate for patients with plasma Na levels greater than 150 mmol/L was 30%.[65]

MANAGEMENT OF ACUTE WATER AND SODIUM DEFICITS IN CHILDREN

Two major problems of acute water and electrolyte deficits are worthy of specific mention because of the potential for serious adverse outcomes. These are gastroenteritis and diabetic ketoacidosis.

Gastroenteritis

Acute gastroenteritis is the most common cause of a disturbance in fluid and electrolyte homeostasis in childhood. Infants with diarrhea are particularly vulnerable to significant losses of fluid, sodium, chloride, and bicarbonate from the small intestine and present with what is frequently classified as hypotonic, isotonic, or hypertonic dehydration based on the serum Na level. This terminology is technically incorrect, because only in the hypertonic form is there loss of fluid from the intracellular fluid compartment; only these patients are truly dehydrated. Patients with diarrheal illnesses associated with fluid loss with normal or reduced serum Na levels have loss of total body water and extracellular fluid, with normal or increased intracellular fluid volume.[66] Infants with hypernatremic dehydration are at greatest risk for an adverse neurologic event, but seizures from severe hyponatremia have been reported in infants presenting with acute gastroenteritis due to oral salt-free fluids being given as replacement.[11,67,68] The assessment of the degree of extracellular fluid deficit is usually made on clinical grounds using the time-honored signs of delayed capillary refill, dry mucous membranes, decreased skin turgor, and the like.[69] However, these are open to subjective interpretation, and there may be a tendency to overestimate the degree of extracellular fluid contraction in less severely ill children. In a study by Mackenzie and associates, the fluid deficit in children with gastroenteritis and mild to moderate "dehydration" was overestimated, which resulted in the overuse of intravenous fluids.[70] Skin turgor, increased capillary refill time, high serum urea concentration, low arterial pH, and increased base deficit all correlated with the degree of extracellular fluid contraction but not the presence of thirst or oliguria. Other studies have shown that a reduced serum bicarbonate concentration is the most common electrolyte abnormality associated with significant extracellular fluid contraction in gastroenteritis.[71,72]

Patients with gastroenteritis whose serum is isotonic or hypotonic should be managed with isotonic saline; those who are hypertonic should receive solutions that contain electrolyte-free water. In infants with severe hypernatremia, the free water deficit should be corrected slowly because of the danger of rapid fluid shift to the intracellular fluid compartment (see earlier). There is an increasing trend to rapidly rehydrate these patients with intravenous solutions in the emergency department before discharging them home,[73,74] but a more simple and effective technique is to use oral rehydration therapy, which has a proven efficacy in clinical trials of patients with acute gastroenteritis. These solutions contain Na concentrations of between 45 and 90 mmol/L.[74-77]

CHLORIDE

Chloride (Cl) is the principal anion of the extracellular fluid compartment. It is filtered at the glomerulus, and 80% is reabsorbed in conjunction with sodium in the proximal tubule. It is also reabsorbed in the ascending limb of the loop of Henle, a process that is blocked by furosemide. Chloride is exchanged for bicarbonate (HCO_3) in the distal tubule. In extracellular fluid volume depletion, excess Cl along with Na is reabsorbed in the proximal tubule, resulting in reduced distal delivery and less HCO_3 secretion. With Cl depletion, less Na is reabsorbed in the proximal tubule. Increased distal delivery results in increased exchange with potassium and hydrogen ions. This contraction alkalosis is invariably associated with hypochloremia, most commonly due to overuse of loop diuretics. Hypochloremia is also caused by gastric suctioning and respiratory acidosis. In addition, many of the conditions that cause hyponatremia also result in hypochloremia.

Hyperchloremia is seen in association with respiratory alkalosis, hypernatremic dehydration, and the administration of isotonic saline. The use of large amounts of isotonic saline during fluid resuscitation can result in a hyperchloremic metabolic acidosis.[78] If the serum Cl is not measured, an increased base deficit could be misinterpreted as indicating inadequate volume resuscitation in shock.[79]

Plasma Cl measurements are an integral part of calculating the anion gap, which is important for the diagnosis of metabolic acidosis.[80] This is the difference between the measured cations (Na^+) and anions (Cl^- and HCO_3^-), which is normally in the range of 12 to 16. The anion gap is increased when unmeasured anions are present, such as lactate and the accumulation of β-hydroxybutyrate in diabetic ketoacidosis. A normal or reduced anion gap acidosis is seen in association with hyperchloremia from saline administration or other situations in which there is an increase in serum Cl.[78,81,82]

POTASSIUM

Potassium (K^+) is the major cation of the intracellular fluid compartment, with an intracellular concentration of 150 mmol/L. Measurement of serum K^+ reflects the extracellular fluid concentration, which is only 2% of the total body K^+. The gradient between the intracellular and extracellular fluid compartments is maintained by activation of the Na^+,K^+-ATPase pump in the cell membrane. The movement of K^+ from the extracellular to the intracellular fluid compartment is enhanced by insulin, hypothermia, alkalosis, catecholamines, and beta agonist therapy.

Potassium filtered at the glomerulus is reabsorbed in the proximal tubule and the thick ascending limb of the loop of Henle. It is secreted in the distal nephron under the influence of aldosterone, plasma K^+ concentration, and urine flow rate.

HYPOKALEMIA

Hypokalemia is commonly seen in children with gastroenteritis and diarrhea, when extracellular fluid contraction leads to stimulation of aldosterone secretion. There is also total body K^+ depletion in diabetic ketoacidosis, although the initial measured level is high due to the acidosis.[69] Adolescents with anorexia nervosa can present with profound degrees of hypokalemia, and it is a known cause of sudden death in this syndrome.[83] In the critical care setting, hypokalemia is most commonly associated with diuretic use, nasogastric suction, hypomagnesemia, and metabolic alkalosis. In acute metabolic alkalosis, each 0.1-unit rise in pH results in a reduction of 0.2 to 0.4 mmol/L in serum K^+.[84] In chronic metabolic alkalosis, K^+ is exchanged for hydrogen ion in the distal nephron. Increased K^+ output in the urine is also associated with renal tubular defects (Bartter's syndrome, renal tubular acidosis) and the use of drugs such as amphotericin, ticarcillin, carbenicillin, and steroids.[85]

Potassium supplementation therapy in the critical care setting is usually in the form of potassium chloride (KCl), as there is frequently an associated Cl deficiency. Acetate and phosphate can be used as alternative anions in the hyperchloremic state (e.g., diabetic ketoacidosis).

The clinical manifestations of hypokalemia include muscle weakness (which may prolong the effect of neuromuscular blockers), intestinal ileus, and cardiac arrhythmias. Arrhythmias are rarely a problem, except in children with congenital heart disease, particularly in the post–cardiopulmonary bypass setting. The potential for digoxin toxicity is enhanced with hypokalemia. In situations in which hypokalemia needs to be treated in the setting of fluid restriction, high-concentration K^+ infusions (up to 0.5 mmol/mL) can be infused through central lines, with frequent measurements of serum K+ levels. Hypokalemia may remain resistant to treatment when significant hypomagnesemia is present.

HYPERKALEMIA

Hyperkalemia is caused by either failure of potassium excretion (renal failure) or movement of K+ from the intracellular to extracellular fluid compartment. Common causes of the latter are cellular breakdown or injury, as occurs in tumor lysis syndrome, rhabdomyolysis, burns, and trauma. Use of the depolarizing neuromuscular blocker succinylcholine in this setting or in patients with muscle dystrophy or spinal cord injury can lead to an abrupt rise in serum K+ and cardiac arrest. Severe hyperkalemia is also seen in malignant hyperthermia, due to a combination of hemolysis and acidosis. Both captopril and propranolol can cause hyperkalemia by decreasing the amount of aldosterone synthesis. Propranolol also blocks beta-adrenergic-mediated movement of K+ across the cell membrane. Acute metabolic acidosis also results in a rapid movement of K+ from the intracellular to the extracellular fluid compartment, and severe hyperkalemia is frequently seen during cardiac arrest and cardiopulmonary resuscitation, without necessarily implying causality.

Acute hyperkalemia represents a medical emergency. Serum levels in excess of 6 mmol/L can result in cardiac arrest and sudden death, particularly in the post–cardiopulmonary bypass setting. Frequently, the only clinical manifestation is the finding of tall, peaked T waves and widening of the QRS complex on the electrocardiogram tracing, but the absence of these findings does not exclude the diagnosis. Patients with borderline high levels of serum K+ can develop life-threatening hyperkalemia with the development of an acidosis. Because it is the extracellular K+ level that is harmful, emergency measures should be directed at increasing the transmembrane flux from the extracellular to the intracellular fluid compartment. These include the use of bicarbonate to correct acidemia, beta agonist therapy, and glucose or insulin.[84,86] The use of intravenous calcium chloride helps protect the heart against the development of rhythm disturbances. These are temporizing measures while steps are taken to increase K+ removal from the body by the administration of Na-K exchange resins (rectally or via nasogastric tube) or acute dialysis.

CALCIUM

The calcium concentration is maintained under the control of vitamin D, parathyroid hormone, and calcitriol. The majority of calcium is in the bone; in the absence of parathyroid hormone, there is reduced calcium resorption from bone and increased urinary secretion because of the decreased renal production of calcitriol. Forty percent of calcium is protein bound, and the most common cause of a low total calcium level in critically ill children is hypoalbuminemia. In this situation, the ionized level is normal. Conversely, the ionized level is reduced when there is increased protein binding.

Hypocalcemia is seen in neonates with birth asphyxia, in preterm infants, in term newborns in the first week of life, and in infants of diabetic mothers. It is an invariable finding in newborn infants with DiGeorge syndrome, where it is seen in association with conotruncal congenital heart defects, typically truncus arteriosus and interrupted aortic arch. The majority of these infants have microdeletions of the long arm of chromosome 22 (22q– syndrome) and immunodeficiency. For this reason, all blood products transfused to these children need to be irradiated. Hypocalcemia is a common finding in critically ill older children, with a reported incidence of 49% in one study.[87] Causes include cardiopulmonary bypass, the use of citrated blood and blood products, albumin transfusions, burns, sepsis, and the use of loop diuretics and aminoglycosides. Hyperphosphatemia, seen in tumor lysis syndrome and renal failure, can also result in hypocalcemia.

Hypercalcemia in critically ill children is usually the result of excessive calcium administration, frequently in association with diuretic administration. The end result may be the development of nephrocalcinosis. Other less common causes include neonatal severe primary hyperthyroidism, caused by mutations of the *CaSR* gene, and Williams syndrome, where it is associated with supravalvular aortic stenosis and peripheral pulmonary artery stenosis.

CRYSTALLOID VERSUS COLLOID SOLUTIONS IN CRITICALLY ILL CHILDREN

The use of colloid solutions, particularly albumin, in preference to crystalloids is a widespread practice in pediatric critical care, especially in the setting of post–cardiopulmonary bypass, burns, and septic shock. Hypoalbuminemia is common in critically ill patients and has been shown to be associated with increased mortality rates in adults.[88] Although a study in critically ill children showed a similar high incidence of hypoalbuminemia, there was no evidence that it was an independent predictor of outcome.[89]

It is well established that early, aggressive fluid resuscitation improves outcome in both pediatric and adult septic shock,[90,91] but there is ongoing controversy over the type of fluid that should be used.[92-96] Two published meta-analyses by the Cochrane group reviewed randomized trials that compared crystalloids with colloids or crystalloids with albumin.[93,94] They concluded that the use of either colloid was associated with an increased mortality rate in critically ill patients. Most of the trials were small studies that were insufficiently powered to address mortality. There were only six pediatric studies analyzed, and five of these were in neonates. Despite the concerns raised by the publication of these papers, early, aggressive fluid resuscitation with albumin, specialist advice, and transfer to a pediatric ICU of patients with meningococcal sepsis in the United Kingdom reduced mortality from 50% in severely ill patients to less than 5%.[97]

Understanding the distribution of colloid and crystalloid in the different fluid compartments is fundamental to fluid resuscitation. Ernest and colleagues studied the distribution of normal saline and 5% albumin in septic patients.[98] Normal saline increased the extracellular fluid compartment by a 1:1 ratio, with only 20% remaining within the intravascular space, whereas 5% albumin more than doubled the extracellular fluid compartment and was distributed equally intravascularly and interstitially. Volume for volume, two to three times as much crystalloid as colloid is required to produce the same hemodynamic effect.

Meningococcal septicemia is frequently used as a clinical paradigm for fluid shifts in septic shock. Plasma proteins, including albumin, and water from the intravascular compartment leak out to the interstitium and result in hypovolemia and hypotension.[99] Fleck and coworkers showed that there is a 300% increase in the albumin escape rate from the vascular to the interstitial space associated with hypoalbuminemia in septic patients.[100]

The pathophysiology of increased capillary leak in dengue shock syndrome is similar to that in meningococcal sepsis. A recent randomized, controlled trial showed greater improvements in hematocrit and pulse pressure among children with dengue shock syndrome who received colloid compared with those who received crystalloid.[101] There is clearly a need for well-designed clinical trials to show whether the use of colloids rather than crystalloids improves outcome in critically ill pediatric patients.

ANNOTATED REFERENCES

Cardenas-Rivero N, Chernow B, Stoiko MA, et al: Hypocalcemia in critically ill children. J Pediatr 1989;114:946-951.

The definitive study showing that early and aggressive fluid resuscitation with a combination of crystalloid and colloid solutions decreases morbidity and mortality in children presenting with sepsis.

Gerigk M, Gnehm HE, Rascher W: Arginine vasopressin and renin in acutely ill children: Implication for fluid therapy. Acta Paediatr 1996; 85:550-553.

This study of acutely ill children admitted to the hospital found that nonphysiologic secretion of ADH is common in this patient population.

Moritz ML, Ayus JC: Prevention of hospital-acquired hyponatremia: A case for using isotonic saline. Pediatrics 2003;111:227-230.

A carefully argued opinion piece that draws attention to the problems of hyponatremia in children receiving intravenous fluids and advances the rationale for using isotonic solutions.

Steele A, Gowrishankar M, Abrahamson S, et al: Postoperative hyponatremia despite near-isotonic saline infusion: A phenomenon of desalination. Ann Intern Med 1997;126:20-25.

An adult study showing that serum Na falls in the perioperative period due to a combination of water retention and hypernatriuresis.

Chapter 132

ACUTE RENAL FAILURE

Brian D. Poole • Robert W. Schrier

KEY POINTS

PRERENAL CAUSES

1. Prerenal azotemia accounts for 70% of community-acquired acute renal failure (ARF) and 40% of hospital-acquired ARF.

2. Because there is no cellular injury in prerenal azotemia, it is reversible with correction of causative factors such as volume depletion, use of non-steroidal anti-inflammatory drugs, or congestive heart failure.

3. It is characterized by bland urine sediment and a fractional excretion of sodium (FE_{Na}) less than 1%.

POSTRENAL CAUSES

1. Postrenal azotemia occurs when there is bilateral obstruction to urine flow.

2. It is an uncommon cause of ARF in the ICU.

3. Evaluation includes renal ultrasonography and postvoid residual, which should be less than 50 mL.

INTRARENAL CAUSES

1. These causes are defined according to the anatomic location of injury—glomerulus, tubule, interstitium, or vasculature.

2. In the ICU, acute tubular necrosis is the most common form of ARF and includes both tubular and vascular injury.

3. Differentiation from prerenal azotemia is accomplished by examination of the urine sediment, which is characterized by muddy brown casts, as well as an FE_{Na} greater than 1%.

EPIDEMIOLOGY

1. ARF is a common complication, occurring in up to 25% of ICU patients.

2. In the majority of patients, it is multifactorial in nature, with components of hypotension, sepsis, and drugs.

3. Mortality is high—up to 80% of patients—and is generally part of multiorgan failure.

4. The risk of developing ARF increases with age and in the presence of baseline chronic kidney disease, oliguria, and sepsis.

DEFINITION

1. Qualitatively, ARF is an abrupt reduction in glomerular filtration rate, but clinically, it is defined in terms of small solute clearance.

2. Blood urea nitrogen (BUN) and creatinine are the most common parameters measured, but they are not sensitive indicators of renal dysfunction in the acute setting.

3. There is no standard definition of ARF in the literature, but it commonly includes a 50% increase in serum creatinine, or a level greater than 2 mg/dL.

4. Future directions include the measurement of injury markers.

TREATMENT

1. For the prevention of contrast-induced ARF in patients at risk, hydration with normal saline is most beneficial. The role of *N*-acetylcysteine is undetermined.

2. There is no role for dopamine in the treatment of ARF.

3. Diuretics can be used in the initial management of ARF, but if there is no response, they should be discontinued and initiation of renal replacement therapy considered.

HEMODYNAMIC MANAGEMENT

1. Early goal-directed management may reverse adverse hemodynamics before tissue injury occurs and result in a better outcome.

2. Recognition of the clinical entity pseudo–acute respiratory distress syndrome and management with ultrafiltration may improve patient outcome.

3. Controversy still exists over the optimal fluid resuscitation. In general, crystalloids should be used, but in capillary leak syndromes such as sepsis, colloids may be useful.

4. When vasopressors are indicated, the effect on systemic hemodynamics generally outweighs the direct renal vasoconstriction, but in cases of sepsis, vasopressin may be preferable because of its selective vasoconstriction in the splanchnic vasculature.

NUTRITIONAL SUPPORT

1. Patients with ARF have increased protein catabolism due to insulin resistance.

2. Enteral nutrition is recommended.

3. Caloric supplementation should be 25 to 30 kcal/kg per day.

4. Protein restriction has no role in the management of ARF.

INDICATIONS FOR NEPHROLOGY CONSULTATION

1. Early nephrology consultation may lead to improved outcome due to earlier recognition of ARF.

RENAL REPLACEMENT THERAPY

1. It is likely that early initiation of renal replacement therapy (BUN <60 mg/dL) is beneficial.

2. Further indications include volume overload, hyperkalemia, acidosis, and pericarditis.

3. In patients with moderately severe illness, it is likely that an increased dose of renal replacement therapy results in improved outcome.

4. With continuous venovenous hemofiltration, ultrafiltration rates approaching 35 mL/kg per hour should be attained.

5. With intermittent hemodialysis, daily dialysis should be initiated for catabolic patients in the ICU.

MODALITY

1. Patients with delayed recovery from acute tubular necrosis often have fresh areas of necrosis on renal biopsy. This is likely exacerbated by dialysis-associated hypotension.

2. Continuous renal replacement therapy (CRRT) provides better cardiovascular stability than intermittent modalities do.

3. CRRT also allows superior metabolic control in catabolic patients and improved fluid management in patients receiving parenteral nutrition or blood products.

4. Despite its theoretical benefits, CRRT has not been associated with improved patient outcome.

5. Drawbacks to the use of CRRT include an increase in nursing care and the need for continuous anticoagulation.

DIALYSIS MEMBRANE

1. The interaction between blood and the dialysis membrane can initiate an inflammatory response. This response has been shown to elicit vasoconstriction and may prolong the course of ARF.

2. Biocompatible membranes have been shown to result in improved outcome in some but not all studies.

3. The ability to bind inflammatory cytokines may contribute to the ability of synthetic membranes to improve outcome.

DIALYSIS BUFFER

1. Lactate buffer is associated with hyperlactatemia in patients with hypotension or liver dysfunction. Elevated serum lactate levels contribute to protein catabolism.

2. Lactate buffer is also associated with decreased hemodynamic stability.

3. Bicarbonate-based buffer is now the standard.

MEDICATION DOSING

1. In critical illness, both the volume of distribution and the extent of protein binding of drugs change.

2. Owing to potential toxicities, it is important to consider the degree of renal function when determining medication dosing.

Acute renal failure (ARF) is characterized by an abrupt decrease in the glomerular filtration rate (GFR) that results in the accumulation of nitrogenous waste products and an inability to maintain fluid and electrolyte homeostasis.[1] ARF can result from decreased renal perfusion that is not severe enough to cause cellular injury; an ischemic, toxic, or obstructive injury of the renal tubule; a tubulointerstitial process with inflammation and edema; or a primary reduction in the filtering capacity of the glomerulus. If renal tubular and glomerular function is intact but solute clearance is limited by factors compromising renal perfusion, the failure is termed prerenal azotemia. If renal dysfunction is related to obstruction of the urinary outflow tract, it is termed postrenal azotemia. Acute renal failure due to a primary intrarenal cause is called intrinsic renal failure or renal azotemia. Prerenal failure and intrinsic renal failure due to ischemia and nephrotoxins are responsible for most episodes of ARF.[2,3]

Renal blood flow is approximately 1200 mL/min and constitutes 20% of the cardiac output. Given this apparently generous perfusion, it may seem surprising that the kidneys are so susceptible to hemodynamic insults. The majority of this perfusion (80% to 90%), however, is to the renal cortex, where glomerular filtration occurs. The medulla is designed to concentrate and dilute the urine. During urine concentration, the high osmotic gradient required for reabsorption of water is associated with a low rate of blood flow. In fact, the oxygen tension in the outer medulla, in the region of the metabolically active thick ascending limb of Henle, is only around 10 mm Hg.[4] This combination of low blood flow and oxygen tension in a metabolically active environment makes the kidneys very susceptible to ischemic injury.

PRERENAL CAUSES

Prerenal azotemia is a consequence of reduction in renal perfusion without cellular injury. As such, this is a reversible process if the underlying cause is corrected. This may be secondary to decreased blood volume, as occurs with vomiting, dehydration, and hemorrhage, or it may be due to a reduction in the effective arterial blood volume, as in congestive heart failure and cirrhosis. Further, the administration of medications that interfere with the normal autoregulatory ability of the kidney can contribute to prerenal azotemia. In settings of diminished renal perfusion, the administration of nonsteroidal anti-inflammatory drugs or angiotensin-converting enzyme inhibitors can precipitate overt prerenal azotemia.[2]

During prerenal azotemia, the renin-angiotensin-aldosterone system becomes activated secondary to a decrease in renal blood flow, accompanied by increased activity of the adrenergic nervous system. The increased level of angiotensin II and the adrenergic activation serve to increase the proximal reabsorption of sodium, whereas aldosterone increases sodium reabsorption in the distal tubule. Together, these actions decrease the urine sodium concentration to less than 20 mmol/L and the fractional excretion of sodium (FE_{Na}) to less than 1%.[5]

Prerenal azotemia accounts for approximately 70% of community-acquired cases of ARF[6] and 40% of hospital-acquired cases.[3] Therefore, prerenal causes should be excluded in all cases of ARF. Therapy of prerenal ARF involves reversing the underlying cause, such as volume replacement or discontinuation of offending agents.

POSTRENAL CAUSES

Postrenal ARF occurs when there is bilateral obstruction of urine flow. Intratubular pressure increases and in turn decreases glomerular filtration pressure. Obstruction of urine flow is a relatively uncommon cause of ARF and is more common in the community than in the ICU. Several series have placed the incidence of postrenal ARF at 2% to 10% of all cases of ARF.[7-9] Postrenal ARF can be divided into renal and extrarenal causes. Extrarenal causes include prostatic disease, pelvic malignancy, and retroperitoneal disorders. Intrarenal causes include crystal deposition, as occurs in ethylene glycol ingestion, or uric acid nephropathy in tumor lysis syndrome. Cast formation and tubular obstruction also occur in light chain diseases such as multiple myeloma.

Postrenal causes of ARF should be evaluated with renal ultrasonography and measurement of postvoid residual urine in the bladder (>50 mL is abnormal). It is important to rule out these causes rapidly, because the potential for renal recovery is inversely related to the duration of obstruction.[10]

INTRARENAL CAUSES

Intrarenal causes of ARF can be classified according to the anatomic location of the injury, includilng the glomerulus, tubule, vasculature, and interstitium. Suspicion of glomerulonephritis or vasculitis should be raised in a patient with renal failure who has an active urine sediment with red cells and red cell casts. In contrast, acute interstitial nephritis classically presents with pyuria and white cell casts in the urine; on occasion, hematuria is also present. Most cases of ARF from interstitial nephritis are drug related, commonly due to antibiotics, nonsteroidal anti-inflammatory drugs, or diuretics. Recovery usually occurs with removal of the offending agent and may be hastened by a short course of steroids, such as 60 to 80 mg of prednisone for 10 days. Tubular injury is most often either ischemic or toxic in nature and presents as acute tubular necrosis (ATN). This is the most common form of ARF encountered in the hospital and the ICU[3,9,11-13] and is the focus of this chapter.

In ischemic ARF, there is both tubular and vascular injury. In the tubules, an increase in intracellular calcium after ischemic injury activates the cysteine proteases calpain and caspase. This leads to necrosis and apoptosis, as well as relocation of Na^+,K^+-ATPase from the basolateral membrane to the cytosol. Relocation interferes with the normal vectorial transport of sodium and increases the distal delivery of sodium chloride (NaCl). An increase in the delivery of NaCl to the macula densa in the distal tubule activates tubuloglomerular feedback and further decreases GFR. Further, ischemia increases production of nitric oxide, which also causes cellular damage and detachment of epithelial cells from the basement membrane. Much of the deleterious action of nitric oxide is mediated through the generation of peroxynitrite from the combination of reactive oxygen species and nitric oxide. The cellular detachment is responsible for cast formation and tubular obstruction. These mechanisms all independently contribute to the decrease in renal function seen in ATN.[14]

In ischemic injury, the vascular endothelium is damaged and displays an exaggerated response to vasoconstrictor stimuli such as angiotensin II and endothelin-1 and a decreased response to vasodilators such as acetylcholine and bradykinin. In addition, there is a loss of autoregulatory capability. This loss of autoregulation in the setting of otherwise minor hemodynamic changes is likely responsible for the fresh ischemic lesions often seen on biopsy when recovery from ARF is delayed.[15] In ARF secondary to sepsis, there is intrarenal vasoconstriction despite peripheral vasodilatation, causing a decrease in renal blood flow and GFR.[16,17]

The kidney's susceptibility to toxic injury can be attributed to its functional properties. The kidneys receive 20% to 25% of the cardiac output, and there is extensive reabsorptive capacity as well as concentrating ability. All these factors contribute to the delivery of large amounts of toxin to the tubular epithelial cells. In addition, there is extensive biotransformation, generating toxic metabolites, and the high energy consumption with marginal oxygen delivery renders the tubules susceptible to toxic injury.[18]

An increasingly common form of ARF in the hospital is secondary to the use of contrast media. Hou and colleagues found contrast nephropathy to be the third most common form of ARF in the hospital.[3] The pathogenesis involves both hemodynamic and toxic effects. Contrast media cause

TABLE 132–1. LABORATORY AND MICROSCOPIC FINDINGS IN PRERENAL AZOTEMIA AND ACUTE TUBULAR NECROSIS

Laboratory Test	Prerenal Azotemia	Acute Tubular Necrosis
Urine osmolality (mOsm/kg H_2O)	>500	<400
Urine sodium (mEq/L)	<20	>40
Urine-plasma creatinine ratio	>40	<20
Fractional excretion of sodium (%)	<1	>2
Urinary sediment	Normal, occasional hyaline cast	Renal tubular epithelial cells, granular and muddy brown casts

From Esson ML, Schrier RW: Diagnosis and treatment of acute tubular necrosis. Ann Intern Med 2002;137:744-752.

renal vasoconstriction and medullary ischemia, as well as direct tubular toxicity.[19] Patients with preexisting renal disease and diabetes are at high risk, as are patients who are volume depleted.

The differentiation of ATN from prerenal azotemia can be aided by the evaluation of urinary indices (Table 132-1).[20] In established ATN, tubular function is impaired, and tubular sodium reabsorption is hindered. This results in a urine sodium value greater than 40 mmol/L and an FE_{Na} greater than 2%. Urine concentrating ability is also abnormal, resulting in isosthenuria with urine osmolality less than 350 mOsm/kg H_2O.[21] However, a low FE_{Na} may be seen in entities causing ATN, such as rhabdomyolysis and myoglobinuria,[22] as well as contrast-mediated ARF[23] and sepsis.[24]

In patients with prerenal azotemia who are treated with diuretics that may obscure the FE_{Na}, the fractional excretion of urea or the urine-to-plasma ratio of creatinine may be more discriminatory. A fractional excretion of urea less than 35% or a urine-to-plasma ratio of creatinine greater than 15 is indicative of prerenal azotemia.[25]

EPIDEMIOLOGY

In the ICU, ARF is a common complication occurring in 1% to 25% of patients,[3,7,11,26,27] depending on the definition of ARF and the patient population. The most common cause of renal failure is ATN.[3,9,11,28] Specific causes of ATN can be classified as hemodynamically mediated ARF, such as in prolonged prerenal azotemia, hypotension, and sepsis; toxic ARF, secondary to antibiotics, chemotherapeutic agents, and contrast media; or postsurgical ARF. In a large prospective analysis by Liano and coworkers, sepsis was the most common cause (35%); postsurgical (25%) and toxic (31%) causes were also common.[9] However, many, if not most, patients have a multifactorial cause of ARF (Fig. 132-1).[9,29] Despite ever-improving supportive interventions in the ICU, the mortality rate for ARF has not changed in the last 3 decades, remaining at 40% to 80%, depending on the study.[11-13,26,30] It has been hypothesized that this continued poor prognosis is due to the changing patient population cared for in the ICU. Today, patients are older, with greater comorbidities, and their renal disease most often develops in the setting of multiorgan failure.[9,26,31] This high incidence of multiorgan failure has made it difficult to discern whether ARF itself causes increased mortality or whether it is a marker of severely ill patients. Several recent studies have found that ARF does in fact contribute to excess mortality in the setting of contrast nephropathy and cardiac surgery.[27,32,33]

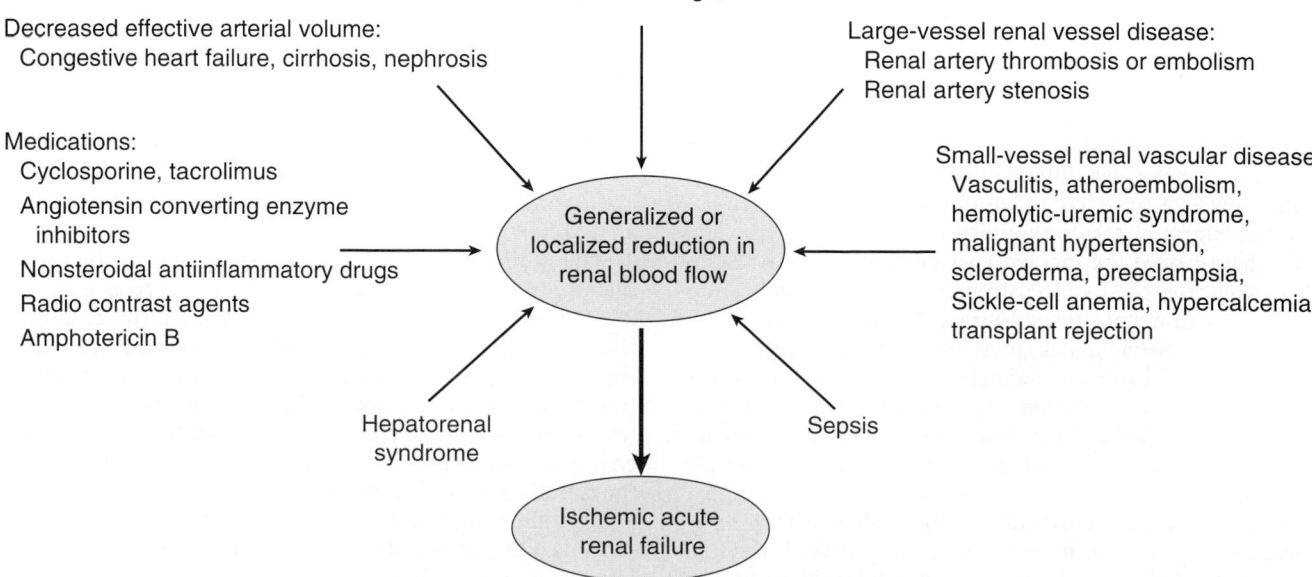

FIGURE 132–1. Conditions that lead to ischemic acute renal failure. (From Thadhani R, Pascual M, Bonventre JV: Acute renal failure. N Engl J Med 1996;334:1448-1460.)

TABLE 132–2. RISK FACTORS FOR DEVELOPING ACUTE RENAL FAILURE

Age >65 yr
Infection on admission
Cardiovascular failure
Cirrhosis
Respiratory failure
Chronic heart failure
Lymphoma or leukemia

Adapted from Vaz AJ. Low fractional excretion of urine sodium in acute renal failure due to sepsis. Arch Intern Med 1983;143:738-739.

In those patients who do survive, there is significant morbidity, with about 33% requiring long-term renal replacement therapy (RRT) and 28% requiring long-term institutionalization.[28]

The risk of developing ARF in the ICU was evaluated by de Mendonca and associates, who found that seven characteristics, if present on admission, were associated with a high risk of developing ARF (Table 132-2).[26] Several other studies addressed risk factors for mortality in the setting of ARF.[3,7,9,11,26,28,34] As indicated in Table 132-3, the risk of death in those with ARF is increased by the presence of nonrenal organ failure; more severe renal dysfunction, as indicated by oliguria; sepsis; advanced age; and male gender. Liano and colleagues found that as the number of organ failures increased, mortality increased.[9] With two organ failures, mortality was 53%; this increased to 80% with three organ failures and 100% with five organ failures.

To further stratify the probability of death in critically ill patients, several severity of illness scoring systems have been developed. These indices help in comparing patients enrolled in clinical trials, as well as in better utilizing finite resources to help those patients with the best chance of recovery. In large populations, these scoring indices have been successful in predicting outcome[35]; however, they do not discriminate well in patients with ARF.[36] The renal parameters used in these scores consist of blood urea nitrogen (BUN), serum creatinine, and total urine output per day. With the latest version of the Acute Physiology and Chronic Health Evaluation (APACHE III), oliguric ARF constitutes just 12.7% of the maximal score, thereby underestimating the effect of ARF on mortality.[37] Further, there is no correction for patients with ARF and a low serum creatinine, who also have a poor outcome, probably reflective of poor nutritional status.[37] An attempt has therefore been made to develop more disease-specific indices, such as Liano and colleagues' individual severity index, the Cleveland Clinic Foundation severity score, and the Project to Improve Care

TABLE 132–3. RISK FACTORS FOR MORTALITY IN ACUTE RENAL FAILURE

Higher severity index score
Age >65 yr
Male gender
Oliguric acute renal failure
Sepsis
Cardiovascular failure
Mechanical ventilation
Prior decreased health status

in Acute Renal Disease index. The majority of these indices were developed at single centers, and few have been validated outside the original institution. Also, the patient populations to which the indices were applied have differed, such as using all ARF patients or only dialyzed patients. Thus, there is no completely generalizable, validated bedside predictor for mortality in ARF patients.

DEFINITION

Defining ARF as an abrupt decrease in GFR is only a qualitative definition and is not very helpful clinically, where a quantitative definition is required. Unfortunately, there is no consensus definition of ARF, as highlighted by a review of 28 ARF studies in which each one used a different definition.[38] Some commonly used definitions include a decrease in GFR of 50%, a doubling of serum creatinine, or an absolute rise in creatinine of 0.5 mg/dL or above a certain cutoff, such as 2 to 3.5 mg/dL. With this lack of consensus, it is difficult to compare studies, and research in ARF is hindered.

Clinically, estimating renal function relies on measures of solute clearance, such as creatinine and BUN, as well as urine output. In the acute setting, this can be problematic, in that the solutes may not be at a steady-state level. The level of BUN depends on the exogenous urea load, which is categorized as intake, endogenous production from catabolism, and tubular reabsorption. In prerenal azotemia, there is enhanced reabsorption of urea from the medullary collecting duct, leading to a disproportionate increase in BUN compared to creatinine (ratio >10 to 15:1). Likewise, serum levels of creatinine in critically ill patients vary, depending on the level of catabolism and nutrition. Further, aggressive fluid resuscitation results in a diluted serum concentration of creatinine, and tubular secretion of creatinine occurs at low levels of GFR.[20] Moran and Myers modeled hemodynamically mediated ATN and found that there can be a significant delay in both the increase in creatinine with ATN and the decrease after recovery.[39] Therefore, reliance on blood levels of BUN and creatinine can be fraught with error. To develop a consensus definition of ARF, the Acute Dialysis Quality Initiative Task Force has been formed and is attempting to develop a definition that includes GFR criteria in the form of serum creatinine as well as urine output and the presence of acute on chronic disease.[40]

Given the difficulties of measuring function as an index of injury, there has been a search for identifying injury markers in the urine of critically ill patients. This approach would be optimal, because it could identify patients early in the course of ARF who would benefit from intervention. One such marker is kidney injury molecule-1 (KIM-1).[41] Other markers such as γ-glutamyl transpeptidase and alkaline phosphatase are also being investigated.[42] Currently, the urine sediment (i.e., epithelial cells) and urine indices (i.e., FE_{Na}) are the earliest and most sensitive harbingers of ATN.

TREATMENT

In light of its dismal outcome, it is imperative that therapies to prevent or ameliorate ARF be developed. To that end, several trials for both the prevention and the treatment of ARF have been conducted with multiple agents.

With the increasing use of contrast agents in diagnostic and therapeutic procedures, prevention of contrast-mediated nephropathy has been studied extensively. Intravenous fluids have long been used to prevent contrast nephropathy, but in patients with chronic renal insufficiency, the incidence is still greater than 10%.[43] Therefore, multiple other agents have been studied. Solomon and coworkers found that both furosemide and mannitol, when given with saline, produced a worse outcome than saline alone in patients with chronic renal insufficiency.[43] Dopamine[44] and atrial natriuretic peptide[45] have also failed to reduce contrast nephropathy. Two agents, acetylcysteine[46] and fenoldopam,[47] were found to decrease the incidence of contrast nephropathy in high-risk patients, but these findings were not verified in a study by Allaqaband and associates.[48] In that trial, acetylcysteine and fenoldopam offered no additional benefit in patients with chronic renal insufficiency undergoing cardiovascular procedures. Currently, our recommendation for the prevention of contrast nephropathy in high-risk patients (Table 132-4) is adequate hydration, preferably with normal saline,[49] and the use of low-osmolar[50] or iso-osmolar[51] contrast media.

Dopamine has long been used in the treatment of ARF. The renal effects of dopamine include an increase in GFR and an increase in sodium and water excretion. Clinically, the first response is an increase in diuresis.[52] These responses occur in patients with normal renal function; it is unknown whether these effects are also seen in those with ARF. In patients with early renal dysfunction (serum creatinine >1.8 mg/dL or urine output <0.5 mL/kg/h), dopamine did not alter the peak serum creatinine or the need for RRT.[53] This was confirmed in a meta-analysis to determine whether progression of ARF, need for RRT, or mortality was affected by dopamine.[54]

Aside from its lack of efficacy in ARF, dopamine has deleterious side effects. It hastened the onset of gut ischemia in an experimental model,[55] and clinically it worsened contrast nephropathy.[56] Higher doses may increase mortality,[57] perhaps by worsening myocardial ischemia.[58] Therefore, low-dose dopamine currently has no role in the treatment or prevention of ARF.

Diuretics are also frequently used in patients with ARF, especially in an attempt to convert oliguric into nonoliguric ARF, given the improved prognosis of the latter.[59-61] Loop diuretics, most commonly furosemide, inhibit Na+,K+-ATPase in the thick ascending loop of Henle and therefore decrease the active reabsorption of sodium. Theoretically, this has some potential benefits, such as decreasing energy expenditure and increasing flow rate to flush out tubular casts. In the experimental setting, loop diuretics can be protective if administered before the insult. However, even when patients are successfully converted to nonoliguria, there is no reduction in the need for RRT or mortality.[62,63] In patients with relatively severe ARF, Shilliday and colleagues found that loop diuretics resulted in a diuresis but did not change mortality or the need for RRT. In addition, patients with contrast nephropathy who were treated with furosemide had a worse outcome.[43] Recently, a study by Mehta and coworkers found an increased mortality in ARF patients treated with diuretics.[64] It is unclear why this occurred, but the authors speculated about a possible nephrotoxic effect of diuretics or a delay in the initiation of RRT because of increased urine output. However, the increased mortality occurred in patients who were not diuretic responsive, likely because of more severe ARF. These patients already had a worse prognosis, and whether diuretics may have worsened the outcome is unknown. Therefore, we recommend a diuretic challenge to determine responsiveness; if there is no response, discontinue the diuretic and consider RRT.

Atrial natriuretic peptide is a hormone secreted by the cardiac atria that increases GFR and glomerular filtration pressure by dilating the afferent arteriole and constricting the efferent arteriole.[65] It also decreases tubular reabsorption of sodium and chloride,[66] redistributes medullary blood flow,[67] disrupts tubuloglomerular feedback,[68] and reverses endothelin-induced vasoconstriction.[69] Given these characteristics, as well as animal studies showing improvement in GFR and renal histology,[70,71] a small clinical trial was undertaken that showed a decrease in the need for RRT with atrial natriuretic peptide infusion in patients with ARF.[72] This trial was followed up with a large, multicenter, placebo-controlled trial that did not show improved dialysis-free survival in patients with ATN, except for those with oliguria.[73] One potential reason for this lack of effect is that there were significant decreases in blood pressure in the treated group, potentially worsening ischemia. In a follow-up trial of patients with oliguric ATN, there was a nonstatistically significant trend toward improvement in dialysis-free survival in patients treated with atrial natriuretic peptide; again, however, there was a significant decrease in the systolic blood pressure among this group.[74] At this time, atrial natriuretic peptide cannot be recommended for therapy of ATN.

HEMODYNAMIC MANAGEMENT

Intravascular volume is critical in maintaining hemodynamic stability, tissue oxygenation, and organ function.[75] In critically ill patients, it is increasingly being recognized that accurate assessment of volume status and the appropriate use of fluid replacement may lead to better outcomes. In a study by Rivers and associates, it was shown that early goal-directed therapy based on optimizing the mixed venous oxygen saturation in the first 6 hours resulted in decreased mortality in septic patients.[76] However, supranormal levels of cardiac index or mixed venous oxygen saturation did not decrease mortality.[77] Further, studies have shown an increased mortality in patients with positive fluid balance and acute respiratory distress syndrome (ARDS).[78-81]

We have coined the term pseudo- or pre-ARDS to focus on a common and clinically important situation in ICUs. Just as prolonged prerenal azotemia may eventually lead to ischemic ATN, prolonged pseudo- or pre-ARDS may lead to ARDS in association with evidence of pulmonary capillary damage and stiff lungs, as diagnosed clinically by a decrease in pulmonary compliance. Thus, pseudo- or pre-ARDS describes a clinical syndrome of noncardiogenic pulmonary

---

TABLE 132–4. RISK FACTORS FOR CONTRAST NEPHROPATHY

Preexisting renal impairment
Diabetes mellitus
Decrease in effective arterial volume (congestive heart failure, volume depletion, cirrhosis)
High dose of contrast media
Concurrent use of nephrotoxic agents (nonsteroidal anti-inflammatory drugs, angiotensin-converting enzyme inhibitors)

edema in the absence of evidence of decreased pulmonary compliance. Although many clinicians group these clinical entities together as ARDS, independent of pulmonary compliance, we believe that, from a pathophysiologic, prognostic, and therapeutic viewpoint, these clinical entities may be substantially different.

Both pseudo-ARDS and ARDS are frequently associated with sepsis. Sepsis is a vasodilated state in which systemic vascular resistance decreases and cardiac output increases. Studies in renal experimental animals have shown that vasodilatation with an arterial vasodilator, such as minoxidil, is associated with an increased albumin distribution space and a failure of interstitial hydrostatic pressure to rise during saline administration.[75] These changes in interstitial Starling forces favor an increase in interstitial fluid volume during saline infusion. We frequently consult on ventilated ICU patients with ARF who have a 20-L positive fluid balance that has not been recognized in a quantitative sense because the pulmonary capillary wedge pressures are not considered elevated (<18 mm Hg). Excess saline fluid has been administered to resuscitate these vasodilated septic patients, leading to pulmonary edema, hypoxia, and ventilatory support. In the early stages, the majority of these patients do not have decreased pulmonary compliance (i.e., stiff lungs). However, these septic ICU patients with renal failure on prolonged respiratory support ultimately have a mortality as high as 80%. Patient mortality has been reported to begin increasing after 48 hours on a respirator. The potential barotrauma, oxygen toxicity, and pulmonary infections that may occur with prolonged ventilatory support frequently lead to stiff lungs and what virtually all authorities would term bona fide ARDS.

We believe that not distinguishing clinically between pseudo-ARDS and ARDS may be detrimental to ICU patients. Marked improvement in the pulmonary edema of pseudo-ARDS by diuresis or ultrafiltration may allow much earlier extubation and removal of ventilatory support before the development of pulmonary capillary damage and stiff lungs (i.e., ARDS). With ARDS and prolonged ventilatory support, a very high mortality occurs, particularly in the presence of renal failure and thus multiorgan failure.

Prospective, randomized studies need to be undertaken in septic patients to examine whether early resuscitation with limited volume expansion (e.g., 2 to 3 L of saline), albumin, and vasopressin (to constrict vasodilated areas associated with sepsis, including skin, muscle, and splanchnic circulation) rather than large volumes of saline (10 to 20 L is not uncommon) can decrease the need for ventilatory support and the development of ARDS and thereby improve survival.

To aid in appropriate hemodynamic support, invasive monitoring has been used to guide therapy. Techniques such as the pulmonary artery catheter rely on the measurement of filling pressures, such as central venous pressure and pulmonary artery occlusion pressure, to estimate preload responsiveness. In critically ill patients, the relation between filling pressures and ventricular end-diastolic volume (preload) is often obscured by changes in ventricular compliance or changes in the pericardium or thorax.[83] In addition, the pulmonary artery catheter has been linked to a worse outcome in patients.[84,85] A positive response to fluid challenge can be predicted in mechanically ventilated patients by analyzing the respiratory variations in pulse pressure. It has been shown that a change in pulse pressure greater than 15% during a single breath is more accurate in predicting an increase in cardiac output in response to volume loading than is either right atrial pressure or wedge pressure.[86,87]

Fluid management in critical illness is aimed at improving organ perfusion. However, in inflammatory states such as sepsis, there may be major fluid shifts resulting in tissue edema despite intravascular depletion. Aside from the inflammatory cascade, vasodilatation itself can result in an increase in interstitial fluid volume, likely secondary to albumin escape from the vasculature.[88] There are currently no clinical methods to detect the presence of capillary leak, apart from fluid administration having no effect on intravascular volume.[83] Therefore, if only transient improvements in hemodynamics occur with fluid administration or there is a continuing need for fluid, it is likely that the patient will best be served by a change to vasopressor agents.

When volume replacement is indicated, there is controversy over the optimal type of fluid. Crystalloids are the most common form of volume replacement, but their effect on plasma volume is limited. Each liter of fluid administered increases plasma volume 200 mL, but the intravascular half-life is only 20 to 30 minutes.[75] In models of hemorrhagic shock, crystalloids were unable to restore microcirculatory blood flow[89,90] and increased the risk of tissue edema in the gut and lungs.[91]

Colloidal substances such as albumin, dextran, and hydroxyethyl starches, because they are macromolecules, are retained within the intravascular space and have a greater effect on plasma volume. Albumin has been used for decades, but it is expensive and may cause an increase in mortality, according to the Cochrane Injuries Group.[92] In capillary leak, albumin shifts into the interstitium and can worsen interstitial edema.[91] Dextran cannot be recommended for plasma volume expansion because of serious side effects, such as coagulation abnormalities[93] and ARF.[94]

Hydroxyethyl starches (HESs) are polymers of amylopectin that vary in molecular weight and the number of substitutions of hydroxyethyl groups. As the molecular weight and number of substitutions increase, the side effects also increase. HES 200/0.5 is a compound with a middle molecular weight and low substitution number. It has been studied in a number of situations, such as perioperative volume replacement, cardiac surgery, trauma, and sepsis.[94-97] It has also been suggested that HES may be able to decrease capillary leakage.[98,99] In a clinical trial comparing 20% albumin to HES 200/0.5 for volume replacement in septic patients, the HES demonstrated improved regional microcirculation.[95] Aside from coagulation disorders, all hyperoncotic colloids can theoretically cause ARF. In patients with decreased renal blood flow, the addition of a hyperoncotic substance can cause a reduction or cessation of GFR[75] by altering the Starling forces governing ultrafiltration. This effect can be reduced by also giving crystalloid solutions.

Given the relative lack of efficacy but safety of crystalloids, it is prudent to begin with crystalloids in fluid resuscitation. However, in cases of microcirculatory disturbances and capillary permeability, such as sepsis, colloids may improve tissue perfusion and decrease tissue edema.

In sepsis and septic shock, there is hypotension despite normal or increased cardiac output.[100] The hypotension in sepsis is often not responsive to fluid and requires the administration of vasopressor agents. Because these agents cause vasoconstriction, there has been concern about their use in ARF. Norepinephrine causes a reduction in renal blood flow in healthy animals and humans.[101] The ultimate effect of norepinephrine on renal blood flow, however, depends on the resulting increase in blood pressure and vascular resistance. Norepinephrine increases blood pressure via an α_1-mediated increase in systemic vascular resistance and a β_1-mediated increase in cardiac output. The increase in resistance can potentially decrease cardiac output by increasing afterload. In the kidney, the effect on renal vascular resistance depends on the increase in systemic pressure, with a decreased renal sympathetic tone causing vasodilation as well as an autoregulatory vasoconstriction secondary to increased perfusion pressure and the α_1-mediated renal vasoconstriction.[102] In a study of septic patients, it was demonstrated that norepinephrine increased urine output and GFR.[101] In a randomized trial, norepinephrine resulted in higher blood pressure, systemic vascular resistance, and diuresis than did high-dose dopamine.[103]

Vasopressin is a hormone secreted by the posterior pituitary that increases systemic vascular resistance through the activation of V_{1a} receptors on vascular smooth muscle. During septic shock, there is a biphasic response, with early high levels of endogenous vasopressin, followed by a decrease.[104] The renal effects of vasopressin are complex and involve the interplay between V_1 and V_2 receptors that regulate the antidiuretic function of vasopressin.[104] A study of vasopressin in septic shock demonstrated that a 4-hour infusion improved the urine output and creatinine clearance.[105]

NUTRITIONAL SUPPORT

Nutritional support in patients with ARF does not differ significantly from that of critically ill patients in general. The goals of nutritional support are the preservation of lean body mass, stimulation of immune competence, repair, and wound healing. ARF affects water, electrolyte, and acid-base balance, but it also induces a change in protein, carbohydrate, and lipid metabolism.[106] In patients with uncomplicated renal failure, oxygen consumption is approximately that of normal subjects. In the presence of sepsis or multiorgan failure, however, oxygen consumption is increased 20% to 30%.[107] Therefore, energy expenditure is determined more by the underlying disease. Energy substrate should not exceed this requirement, and it is better to err on the side of slight underfeeding than overfeeding. Patients with ARF should be supplemented with 25 to 30 kcal/kg body weight per day. Even in hypermetabolic states such as sepsis, energy expenditure is rarely greater than 130% of calculated basic energy expenditure. Therefore, supplementation should not exceed 35 kcal/kg body weight per day.[106]

The hallmark of metabolic alterations in ARF is the activation of protein catabolism and the release of amino acids from skeletal muscle. This process is responsible for the negative nitrogen balance encountered in critically ill patients. An underlying mechanism of protein catabolism is insulin resistance.[108,109] Plasma insulin levels are elevated, but maximal insulin-stimulated glucose uptake is decreased by 50%. This insulin resistance leads to stimulated hepatic gluconeogenesis fueled by protein catabolism.[108] The elevated level of gluconeogenesis coupled with insulin resistance also frequently leads to hyperglycemia. Other factors such as inflammatory cytokines (namely, tumor necrosis factor) and catecholamines are also involved in the hypercatabolism.[110] To combat malnutrition in this setting, it is often necessary to use nutritional supplementation in the form of enteral or parenteral feeding.

Enteral nutrition has become the standard form of nutritional support in critically ill patients. Enteral feeding helps maintain gastrointestinal function, including acting as a barrier to microorganisms. Kudsk and coworkers found a decrease in infectious complications with enteral versus parenteral feeding.[111] In another study, infections, complications, and mortality were decreased in enterally fed patients.[112] A meta-analysis by Heyland and colleagues reviewed 26 randomized trials comparing total parenteral nutrition with standard care and found no survival benefit and possible harm in medical ICU patients fed parenterally.[113] Therefore, enteral support is recommended in critically ill patients with or without ARF.

Traditionally, nutrition has been delivered in the form of 50% to 80% carbohydrates. Recently, this has been the subject of study. Lipids, in addition to providing calories, also provide essential fatty acids. Essential fatty acids such as omega-3 polyunsaturated fatty acids and amino acids such as arginine have been found to stimulate the immune system. A prospective, randomized trial of "immune-enhancing" enteral nutrition found that in patients who received adequate nutrition, those who received the immune-enhancing diet had a decrease in mortality and hospital stay.[114] This study did not address ARF patients, but it is likely that they would also benefit.

In the past, protein restriction was employed in ARF patients to control uremia. However, this is likely to be detrimental to the patient and results in a profoundly negative nitrogen balance.[115] With the advent of continuous modalities of RRT, it is possible to adequately supplement protein and control uremia. Therefore, some authors recommend aggressive protein replacement at 2.5 g/kg per day, as opposed to the standard 1 to 1.5 g/kg per day.[115]

INDICATIONS FOR NEPHROLOGY CONSULTATION

Currently, there are wide variations in the timing of nephrology consultation in patients with ARF. Some physicians prefer to consult at the first rise in serum creatinine, whereas others wait until RRT is needed. In a study evaluating the effect of nephrology consultation on patient outcome, Mehta and associates found that a delay in nephrology consultation (>48 hours after ICU admission with ARF) led to higher mortality.[116] In this study, the patients with delayed consultation had a lower serum creatinine concentration and higher urine output but more organ failure and higher total body water. In the multivariate analysis, delayed consultation was no longer significant, but the trend was there. Why would early consultation affect mortality? It could result from delayed recognition of renal failure. Higher total body water likely leads to tissue edema and organ dysfunction (i.e., pulmonary edema). Therefore, in patients in the ICU, early recognition of ARF and its appropriate management may lead to better outcomes.

RENAL REPLACEMENT THERAPY

INDICATIONS

As mentioned previously, 1% to 25% of patients in the ICU develop ARF. Of those, 30% to 70% require RRT.[9,11,34,116] Many practitioners delay the initiation of RRT as long as possible because of concerns that dialysis may delay the recovery of renal function.[117,118] Indications for the initiation of RRT have traditionally been volume overload, hyperkalemia, acidosis, symptoms of uremia such as encephalopathy and pericarditis, and azotemia. The level of azotemia at which RRT should begin is unknown. Several early, retrospective studies suggested that early initiation of RRT resulted in survival improvements.[119,120] Kleinknecht, in 1972, evaluated the beneficial effects of "prophylactic" dialysis.[120] This retrospective study included 279 patients dialyzed before 1966 with a BUN greater than 164 mg/dL and 221 patients dialyzed between 1968 and 1970 with a BUN less than 93 mg/dL at the time of dialysis initiation. Prophylactic dialysis was associated with a decreased incidence of gastrointestinal bleeding, septicemia, and mortality. In 1975, a prospective trial by Conger on soldiers in Vietnam with traumatic ARF showed a decrease in complications such as bleeding and sepsis, as well as improvement in survival, in patients who underwent hemodialysis at a BUN less than 70 mg/dL compared with approximately 150 mg/dL.[121] This small study was followed by a larger, prospective trial of intensive hemodialysis by Gillum and colleagues in 1986.[122] In this trial, 34 patients with ATN were assigned to dialysis at a BUN less than 60 mg/dL or less than 100 mg/dL. The patients dialyzed earlier had less gastrointestinal bleeding, but there was no significant difference in mortality.

Even in the era of continuous renal replacement therapy (CRRT), there are still no evidence-based guidelines to determine when to initiate RRT. In a retrospective analysis of 100 patients with post-traumatic ARF treated with CRRT, dialysis was characterized as early (BUN <60 mg/dL) or late (BUN >60 mg/dL). The early patients, who started dialysis with a BUN of 40 mg/dL, had improved survival compared with the late patients, who had a BUN of 95 mg/dL at the time of dialysis initiation.[123] However, in Bouman and associates' randomized trial of both timing and dose of CRRT in critically ill patients who were ventilated and oliguric and had equivalent severity scores, early therapy had no survival advantage.[124] Nevertheless, based on the opinion of experts in the field, some guidelines have been proposed for the initiation of RRT (Table 132-5).[125]

ADEQUATE DOSING

In chronic hemodialysis patients, the adequacy of dialysis is currently determined by the level of small solute (urea) clearance. This is determined by the Kt/V formula, where K is the dialysis membrane clearance of urea, t is the time on dialysis, and V is the volume of distribution of urea, which is equal to total body water. In chronic hemodialysis, a Kt/V of 1.2 per session is considered adequate.[126] As can be seen from the formula, to increase urea clearance, one can increase the time on dialysis or increase the dialyzer clearance. Dialyzer clearance depends on blood flow and dialysate flow rates, as well as the inherent properties of the membrane.

In the United States, intermittent dialysis is still the most common practice in patients with ARF; 70% of patients are dialyzed three times a week, and 30% are dialyzed four times a week.[127,128] Currently, there is no standard Kt/V for adequate dialysis in ARF, but Paganini and coworkers showed that in patients with moderately severe disease, as indicated by the Cleveland Clinic Foundation severity score, there was a significant increase in survival among those with a higher Kt/V (Fig. 132-2).[125,129] This was followed by a study comparing daily to alternate-day hemodialysis. Schiffl and colleagues studied 160 patients with ARF who were divided into two groups: one received daily hemodialysis, and the other alternate-day hemodialysis. It was found that daily hemodialysis resulted in less hypotension, sepsis, gastrointestinal bleeding, and respiratory failure, as well as a significant decrease in mortality.[130] This study has been criticized because the Kt/V delivered to the alternate-day group was only 0.94, which is significantly less than the prescribed dose of 1.2. Therefore, it could be that the alternate-day group received inadequate dialysis.

The significant difference between prescribed and delivered dialysis dose was studied by Evanson and coworkers, who found that the prescribed dose was a Kt/V of 1.25, whereas the dose delivered was only 1.04.[127] These authors found that the most significant factor predicting actual delivered dose was the patient's predialysis weight. It follows that a higher weight in critically ill patients represents higher total body water and therefore a larger volume of distribution of urea. This would be expected to decrease the Kt/V if it were not accounted for in the prescription of dialysis.

TABLE 132–5. POTENTIAL INDICATIONS FOR RENAL REPLACEMENT THERAPY IN THE ICU

Nonobstructive oliguria (urine output <200 mL/12 h) or anuria
Severe acidemia
Azotemia (blood urea nitrogen >80 mg/dL)
Hyperkalemia (K+ >6.5 mmol/L)*
Uremia (encephalopathy, pericarditis, neuropathy, myopathy)
Severe dysnatremia (Na+ >160 or <115 mmol/L)
Hyperthermia (temperature >39.5°C)
Clinically significant organ edema (especially lung)
Drug overdose with dialyzable toxin
Coagulopathy requiring large amounts of blood products in a
    patient at risk for adult respiratory distress syndrome

Any one of these indications is sufficient to consider the initiation of renal replacement therapy. Two of these indications make renal replacement therapy desirable.
*Intermittent hemodialysis removes K+ more efficiently than do continuous modalities.
Adapted from Bellomo R, Ronco C: Continuous haemofiltration in the intensive care unit. Crit Care 2000;4:339-345.

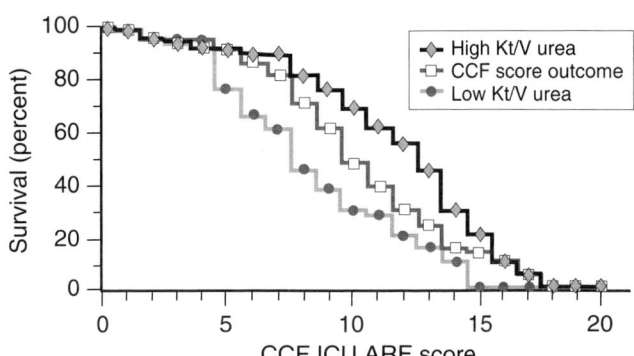

FIGURE 132–2. Dose of hemodialysis and survival. ARF, acute renal failure; CCF, Cleveland Clinic Foundation; Kt/V, formula in which K is the dialysis membrane clearance of urea, t is the time on dialysis, and V is the volume of distribution of urea. (From Paganini E, et al: Establishing a dialysis therapy/patient outcome link in intensive care unit acute dialysis for patients with acute renal failure. Am J Kidney Dis 1996;28[Suppl 3]:s81-s89.)

CRRT has been advocated in patients with ARF because of its ability to more efficiently remove solute,[131] as well as provide hemodynamic stability.[125] But the optimal dosing in CRRT is not known. Ronco and colleagues randomized 425 patients with ARF to increasing doses of continuous venovenous hemofiltration (CVVH).[132] This form of RRT depends on convection, not diffusion, for solute clearance. This means that there is no dialysate involved, and solute is removed with water during ultrafiltration. These investigators used three increasing doses of ultrafiltration—20, 35, and 45 mL/kg per hour—and found that mortality was 41%, 57%, and 58%, respectively. The mortality was significantly lower in the 20 mL/kg group than in the other two groups. If the patient was septic, using the highest dose was beneficial.[132,133] A more recent study by Bouman and coworkers in severely ill, ventilated patients with high severity scores was unable to detect a difference in mortality between high ultrafiltration volume (48 mL/kg/h) and low ultrafiltration volume (20 mL/kg/h).[124] It may be that because these patients were severely ill, their mortality was too high to detect any difference.[129]

MODALITY

When RRT is indicated in the ICU, physicians have to choose between intermittent techniques, such as traditional hemodialysis used in end-stage kidney disease, or continuous therapies such as CVVH. Intermittent hemodialysis (IHD) is complicated by hypotension in 20% to 30% of patients,[134] and in hemodynamically unstable patients, this can significantly limit therapy and delay the recovery of renal function. Renal biopsies from patients with ATN performed 3 to 4 weeks after the inciting incident showed areas of fresh injury. These patients had all undergone hemodialysis, and many of the sessions were complicated by transient decreases in blood pressure.[15] Solez and coworkers compared biopsies from patients with delayed recovery from ARF with biopsies from those who were recently recovered.[117] The biopsies were taken 3 to 4 weeks after injury, and those with delayed recovery had more areas of necrosis. To explain the continuing ischemic injury in response to blood pressure in the normal autoregulatory range, it was demonstrated that the hemorrhagic reduction of blood pressure in postischemic rats was associated with a paradoxical vasoconstriction, leading to a further decrease in renal blood flow.[135] This is likely due to increased sensitivity to vasoconstrictors and decreased sensitivity to vasodilators in the postischemic kidney secondary to endothelial damage.[136,137]

The response of renal function to dialysis mode has been evaluated. It was found that although creatinine clearance decreases in response to either mode, the decrease is much more substantial in IHD than in CRRT (−25% versus −7%).[138] In a clinical trial comparing CRRT and IHD, Mehta and associates found that in patients who survived ARF, the ones treated with CRRT had increased renal recovery compared with those receiving IHD.[139]

Control of both uremia and volume is the major goal of RRT in ARF. With IHD, the control of volume is episodic and is unable to respond to changing clinical scenarios. CRRT, in contrast, has the ability to change ultrafiltration based on changing needs, such as blood product or nutrition administration.[140] Further, it has been shown that solute removal is improved with CRRT,[131] and patients maintain lower BUN levels.[141] Other metabolic parameters include

control of the metabolic acidosis and hyperphosphatemia associated with renal failure. Comparative studies show a more rapid improvement and better control of both acidosis and phosphate with CRRT.[142]

Despite the improvements in hemodynamics and metabolic control, it has yet to be shown that these improvements translate into increased survival. Because the patient populations prescribed each modality are often quite different, it has been difficult to accurately compare the two modalities. In a retrospective analysis of 349 patients with ATN, the mortality rate was higher in patients treated with CRRT than in those treated with IHD (68% versus 41%). However, in a multivariate analysis adjusting for illness severity, there was no longer a difference in survival.[143] In a study at the Cleveland Clinic, where patients were equivalent in terms of severity scores and dose of dialysis delivered, there was no difference in mortality between CRRT and IHD.[144] In the largest randomized, prospective comparison of modalities, Mehta and colleagues randomized 166 patients with ARF to CRRT or IHD.[139] This trial found an increase in mortality with CRRT, but the patients were not well matched. Patients treated with CRRT had higher APACHE II and APACHE III scores, as well as higher rates of liver failure; when these factors were adjusted for, there was no longer a difference in mortality. Based on data by Paganini and associates, it could be that equivalent doses of dialysis confer no difference in mortality, but in hemodynamically unstable patients, it is often easier to deliver adequate dialysis with CRRT.[37,129]

In certain situations, CRRT is preferable to IHD, including in patients with or at risk for increased intracranial pressure. Studies have shown that CRRT prevents the increase in intracranial pressure that is associated with intermittent RRT.[145,146] Another group of patients better suited for CRRT are those with diuretic-resistant congestive heart failure. CRRT has been shown to restore dry body weight, improve urinary output, decrease neurohumoral activation, and prolong symptom-free time.[147] The hemodynamic instability of these patients makes them ideal candidates for CRRT.

The use of CRRT in patients with severe sepsis or septic shock has also received much attention. Sepsis is associated with hemodynamic instability, making CRRT an attractive option. It has been shown that CRRT has beneficial effects on hemodynamics in animal models of sepsis.[148] This is thought to be secondary to the removal of inflammatory cytokines by both convective and adsorptive measures. Hemofiltration membranes allow the ultrafiltration of mid-molecular-weight molecules such as cytokines. Further, the continuous blood-membrane contact allows the membrane to adsorb more mediators. The use of CRRT as an adjunctive measure in the treatment of sepsis in patients with or without ARF is being evaluated.[133]

Despite its advantages over IHD, CRRT has some disadvantages as well. With CRRT, there is generally a need for continuous anticoagulation to prevent clotting of the filter. Although this is usually done with low-dose heparin, there is the risk of bleeding or heparin-induced thrombocytopenia. When a patient is a bleeding risk, a trial of no anticoagulation can be tried, or regional anticoagulation with citrate is used in some centers.

CRRT also requires more nursing support and is thought to be more expensive than IHD. However, although CRRT may be somewhat more expensive,[149] if there is an increase in renal survival after ARF, it may be less expensive in the long run.

DIALYSIS MEMBRANE

When blood comes into contact with the hemodialysis membrane, the alternative complement and coagulation cascades are activated, resulting in inflammation as well as intense vascular smooth muscle constriction.[150] It has been postulated that this contributes to the prolongation of a course of ATN.[151] Early dialysis membranes were made of cellulose or its derivatives, and it has been shown that the hydroxyl radicals on the cellulose membranes were able to activate the complement system.[152] These older membranes were thus not biocompatible. Newer, synthetic polymers are less able to activate the complement cascade and also have the ability to bind the complement that is activated, thereby decreasing the systemic effects.[153] Because of this decrease in immune activation, these membranes are considered biocompatible. In CRRT, there is continuous contact between the blood and membrane, making this interaction quite important.

There is evidence of improved renal recovery after ARF when biocompatible membranes are used for dialysis.[138,154,155] The effect of biocompatible membrane use in patients with ATN has been evaluated, and early studies showed an improvement in survival.[134,154,156] More recently, however, several studies have been unable to show a survival advantage with biocompatible membranes.[157-159]

Membranes may also play a role in blood purification beyond that of solute clearance. There is interest in the ability of membranes to adsorb and bind cytokines from the blood. This is particularly attractive in sepsis, when there is dysregulation of the immune system with both pro- and anti-inflammatory effects. In an investigative technique called coupled plasma filtration adsorption, in which a resin cartridge that can bind mediators is placed in series with the filter, there is evidence that cytokine removal can restore monocyte responsiveness to lipopolysaccharide. In sepsis, there are increases in proinflammatory cytokines such as tumor necrosis factor and interleukin-1β, as well as increases in anti-inflammatory cytokines such as interleukin-10. By nonselectively removing both mediators, it may be possible to improve outcomes in sepsis.[160]

BUFFER

In determining the adequacy of dialysis, factors other than solute clearance must be considered. One goal of RRT is to maintain normal acid-base balance in patients with ARF to prevent the complications of acidemia with regard to cardiovascular performance, hepatic metabolism, and hormonal response.[161] To maintain normal pH, the dialysate must contain a buffer. Traditionally, bicarbonate buffer solution was unavailable because of its instability in the presence of calcium and magnesium.[162] Therefore, the anion lactate was most commonly used in RRT. This anion is converted in the liver to bicarbonate on an equimolar basis under physiologic conditions. However, in critically ill patients with organ dysfunction and disordered tissue perfusion, it is possible that not all the anion will be converted to bicarbonate, resulting in increased serum lactate levels. This is especially likely in patients with liver dysfunction. The increased lactate, without its redox partner pyruvate, can result in increased protein catabolism as well as myocardial depression.[163] Further, it can worsen acidosis in patients with preexisting lactic acidosis.[164,165]

Recently, bicarbonate-based solutions have become available in separated solutions that are mixed just before use. In a study by Barenbrock and colleagues, bicarbonate- versus lactate-based fluid replacement was studied in patients with ARF treated with CVVH.[166] They found that the serum lactate concentration was significantly higher and the bicarbonate was lower in patients treated with lactate-based solution. In addition, they showed an increase in cardiovascular events and hypotension in patients treated with lactate solution. In a study by McLean and coworkers comparing lactate and lactate-free dialysate, the mean arterial pressure rose during lactate-free dialysis with decreased inotrope use and fell during lactate-buffered dialysis with increased inotrope use.[167]

MEDICATION DOSING

During ARF, drugs normally eliminated by the kidney exhibit a markedly decreased clearance. The physiochemical characteristics of drugs affect their removal by dialysis. The molecular weight, volume of distribution, protein binding, intercompartmental rate constants, and fraction eliminated by the kidneys are important in determining drug clearance by RRT.[168] Drug clearance with CVVH is through convective transport, and it approximates the unbound drug concentration in plasma multiplied by the ultrafiltration rate.[169] Drugs with molecular weights of less than 500 Da are readily removed by either conventional hemodialysis or CVVH, but those with higher weights of 1000 to 5000 Da are eliminated more efficiently by CVVH because of the use of high-flux membranes that allow the passage of larger molecules.

The volume of distribution greatly impacts the clearance of a drug, in that those with large distributions are likely to be more bound in the tissues. Therefore, only a small amount has access to the vasculature at any time. For these drugs, clearance with CVVH is greater than with intermittent therapies because of the continuous nature of the clearance.[168]

The extent of protein binding of a drug is important because the protein-drug complex is generally greater than 50,000 Da. At this size, neither intermittent nor continuous therapies will efficiently remove the drug. However, the extent of protein binding is dependent on pH, uremia, concentration of free fatty acids, heparin therapy, and relative concentrations of drug and protein.[170-172] In critically ill patients, the serum albumin is often decreased, thereby making more drug available for clearance during RRT.

Because of the potential toxicities, as well as the need to maintain therapeutic levels of multiple medications, it is important to consider and adjust medication dose during ARF and its therapy with RRT. Dosages of medications must be adjusted for the type of RRT, as well as for the specific characteristics of the drug.

CONCLUSION

Despite extensive clinical experience and improvements in supportive care, the mortality rate of critically ill patients with ARF has not changed over the last 3 decades. However, new information is emerging about the diagnosis and treatment of ARF. Table 132-6 summarizes current recommendations for the care of patients with ARF.[20] These recommendations are based on evidence from clinical trials as well as clinical judgment.

TABLE 132–6. RECOMMENDATIONS FOR THE EVALUATION AND TREATMENT OF ACUTE RENAL FAILURE

Evaluate patient for ARF when serum creatinine increases by >0.5 mg/dL

Exclude prerenal causes (volume depletion, CHF, cirrhosis, NSAIDs, ACE inhibitors)

Exclude postrenal causes with renal ultrasonography and postvoid residual

Review urine sediment (muddy brown casts, ATN; RBC casts, glomerulonephritis or vasculitis; pyuria, acute interstitial nephritis; bland sediment, prerenal or postrenal azotemia)

Evaluate urine electrolytes in absence of diuretics

After exclusion of pre- and postrenal azotemia and confirmation of ATN by urine sediment and electrolytes, notify a nephrologist when serum creatinine >2 mg/dL

Note the projected need for dialysis: oliguric ATN (urine volume <400 mL/24 h), 85% of patients; nonoliguric ATN (urine volume >400 mL/24 h), 30%-40% of patients

Avoid excessive fluid resuscitation leading to pseudo-ARDS, ventilator support, and multiorgan complications

Avoid hypotension (generally there is no need to treat hypertension aggressively in the absence of hypertensive crisis)

Maintain fluid balance and treat hyperkalemia; do not use "renal-dose" dopamine

Review active medications for necessary dose adjustments

When indicated, use enteral rather than parenteral alimentation

Discuss timing for initiation and mode of renal replacement with nephrologist (intermittent vs continuous hemodialysis and use of biocompatible membrane)

ACE, angiotensin-converting enzyme; ARDS, acute respiratory distress syndrome; ARF, acute renal failure; ATN, acute tubular necrosis; CHF, congestive heart failure; NSAID, nonsteroidal anti-inflammatory drug; RBC, red blood cell. From Esson ML, Schrier RW: Diagnosis and treatment of acute tubular necrosis. Ann Intern Med 2002;137:744-752.

ANNOTATED REFERENCES

Brivet FG, et al: Acute renal failure in intensive care units—causes, outcome, and prognostic factors of hospital mortality: A prospective, multicenter study. French Study Group on Acute Renal Failure. Crit Care Med 1996;24:192-198.

This is an epidemiologic evaluation of the incidence, cause, and risk factors for death in patients with ARF in the ICU.

Gettings LG, Reynolds HN, Scalea T: Outcome in post-traumatic acute renal failure when continuous renal replacement therapy is applied early vs late. Intensive Care Med 1999;25:805-813.

This retrospective analysis evaluated the timing of RRT and found that initiating RRT early (BUN <60 mg/dL) results in superior outcomes.

Paganini E, et al: Establishing a dialysis therapy/patient outcome link in intensive care unit acute dialysis for patients with acute renal failure. Am J Kidney Dis 1996;28(Suppl 3):s81-s89.

This study established that patients with a moderate degree of disease severity have better outcomes when treated with an increased dose of RRT.

Ronco C, et al: Effects of different doses in continuous veno-venous haemofiltration on outcomes of acute renal failure: A prospective randomised trial. Lancet 2000;356:26-30.

This study using CRRT showed that higher doses of RRT, as assessed by ultrafiltration rates, resulted in improved mortality.

Schiffl H, Lang SM, Fischer R: Daily hemodialysis and the outcome of acute renal failure. N Engl J Med 2002;346:305-310.

In severely ill patients with ARF who were catabolic, daily dialysis, and hence a larger dose of dialysis as assessed by Kt/V, resulted in better outcomes than alternate-day dialysis.

Chapter 133

RENAL REPLACEMENT THERAPY IN THE ICU

Rinaldo Bellomo • Vincenzo D'Intini • Claudio Ronco

KEY POINTS

1. Uremia is the accumulation of uremic toxins of different molecular weights associated with pathogenicity secondary to kidney dysfunction.

2. Acute renal failure is a separate syndrome from chronic renal failure and should be approached in a distinct manner.

3. Specific indications exist for the initiation of renal replacement therapy in acute renal failure. Early initiation has been shown to be beneficial.

4. Multiple therapeutic modalities of renal replacement therapy exist to treat acute renal failure. No modality is clearly superior to another. Treatments should be tailored depending on the clinical scenario.

5. Knowledge of prescribed drug pharmacokinetics is important when dosing patients on renal replacement therapy.

Severe acute renal failure causes dysregulation in the homeostasis of fluid, potassium, metabolic acids, and waste products, which can lead to life-threatening complications. Extracorporeal blood purification techniques can be applied to prevent these complications and improve homeostasis. Various techniques of renal replacement therapy include continuous venovenous hemofiltration, intermittent hemodialysis, and peritoneal dialysis, each with its technical variations but with a common fundamental principle of removing unwanted solutes and water through a semipermeable membrane. The membranes used are either biologic (peritoneum) or artificial (hemodialysis or hemofiltration membranes) and have characteristics with advantages and disadvantages.

PRINCIPLES OF RENAL REPLACEMENT THERAPY

The principles of renal replacement therapy have been extensively studied and described.[1-3] The two fundamental principles of renal replacement therapy particularly relevant to critical care physicians are summarized here.

WATER REMOVAL

The removal of unwanted solvent (water) is therapeutically as important as the removal of unwanted solute (e.g., acid, uremic toxins, potassium). During renal replacement therapy, water is removed through a process called *ultrafiltration*. This process is essentially the same as that which occurs in the glomerulus. It requires a driving pressure, which is greater than the oncotic pressure, to drive fluid across a semipermeable membrane. This pressure is achieved by the following:

1. Generating a transmembrane pressure (as in hemofiltration or during intermittent hemodialysis) greater than the oncotic pressure
2. Increasing osmolality of the dialysate with osmotic agents (as in peritoneal dialysis)

SOLUTE REMOVAL

The removal of unwanted solutes can be achieved by creating an electrochemical gradient across the membrane by using a flow past system with toxin-free dialysate (diffusion) intermittent hemodialysis and peritoneal dialysis. This process is called *diffusion*. This term defines the movement of solute with a statistical tendency to reach the same concentration of solute in the available distribution space on each side of the membrane. Solute transport is governed by the following formula:

$$JD = DTA \, (dc/dx)$$

Where J is solute flux, D is diffusion coefficient, T is temperature of the solution, A is membrane surface area, dc is concentration gradient between the two compartments, and dx is diffusion distance (thickness of the membrane). In dialysis, blood and dialysate are separated by a membrane. Bidirectional diffusive transport of molecules occurs in response to a concentration gradient.

Solutes also can be removed by creating a "solvent drag"—solutes moving together with solvent across a porous membrane—convection. In this process, the ultrafiltrate is discarded and replaced with toxin-free replacement fluid—hemofiltration. Solvent drag occurs when water is driven by a hydrostatic or an osmotic force across a semipermeable membrane, carrying with it solutes that can pass through uninhibited. The solutes retain a similar concentration to the original solution, whereas larger molecules are retained. Filtration occurs in response to a transmembrane pressure gradient according to the formula:

$$Qf = Km \times TMP = Km \, (Pb - Puf - \pi)$$

Where Qf is filtration, Km is coefficient of permeability of the membrane, TMP is transmembrane pressure, Pb is hydrostatic pressure of blood, Puf is hydrostatic pressure in the ultrafiltrate compartment, and π is oncotic pressure of blood. In convective treatments, the transport (Jc) of solute x is governed by the formula:

$$Jc = UF\,[x]_{UF}$$

Where UF is volume of ultrafiltrate and $[x]_{UF}$ is concentration of solute x in ultrafiltrate. From this, we may derive that clearance in convective treatments is as follows:

$$K = Qf\,[x]_{UF}/[x]_{Pw}$$

Where Qf is ultrafiltration rate and $[x]_{UF}/[x]_{Pw}$ is the ratio of the solute concentrations in the ultrafiltrate and plasma water or the sieving coefficient S. From this formula, it may be observed that when the sieving coefficient is 1, clearance equals ultrafiltration rate.

Despite these distinctions, diffusion and convection often act simultaneously, and it is almost impossible to divide these transport mechanisms physically. The term *hemodialysis* may not describe aptly the mode of treatment in the case of highly permeable membranes. A more suitable term would be *hemodiafiltration* (if replacement solution is needed) or *high-flux dialysis* (if a filtration–back filtration mechanism is present and no replacement fluid is required). The various modalities are described in Figure 133-1.

The rate of diffusion of a given solute depends on its molecular weight, porosity of the membrane, blood flow rate, dialysate flow rate, protein binding, and concentration gradient across the membrane. If standard, low-flux, cellulose-based membranes are used, middle molecules of molecular weight of greater than 500 Da are insufficiently removed. Synthetic high-flux membranes (cutoff at 20 to 40 kDa) can remove larger molecules. When such membranes are used, convection is superior to diffusion in achieving the clearance of middle molecules. During peritoneal dialysis, larger molecules (albumin) also can be removed because of the porosity of the peritoneal membrane. Because blood flow rate across the peritoneal membrane is limited, however, clearances also are limited.

INDICATIONS FOR RENAL REPLACEMENT THERAPY

The treatment of acute renal failure requires a different style and philosophy from renal replacement therapy for chronic renal failure. In a critically ill patient, renal replacement therapy should be initiated early. It is physiologically irrational and clinically dangerous to wait for complications to appear before intervening. Fear of early dialysis stems from the well-known adverse effects of conventional intermittent hemodialysis with cuprophane membranes, especially hemodynamic instability, and from the risks and limitations of continuous or intermittent peritoneal dialysis.[4-6] If one uses continuous renal replacement therapy techniques,[7] however, these concerns are not justified. If extended dialysis techniques are used, they are minimized.[8] Accordingly the time-honored criteria for the initiation of renal replacement therapy in patients with chronic renal failure may be inappropriate in critically ill patients.[9] Modern criteria for the initiation of renal replacement therapy in the ICU are presented in Table 133-1.

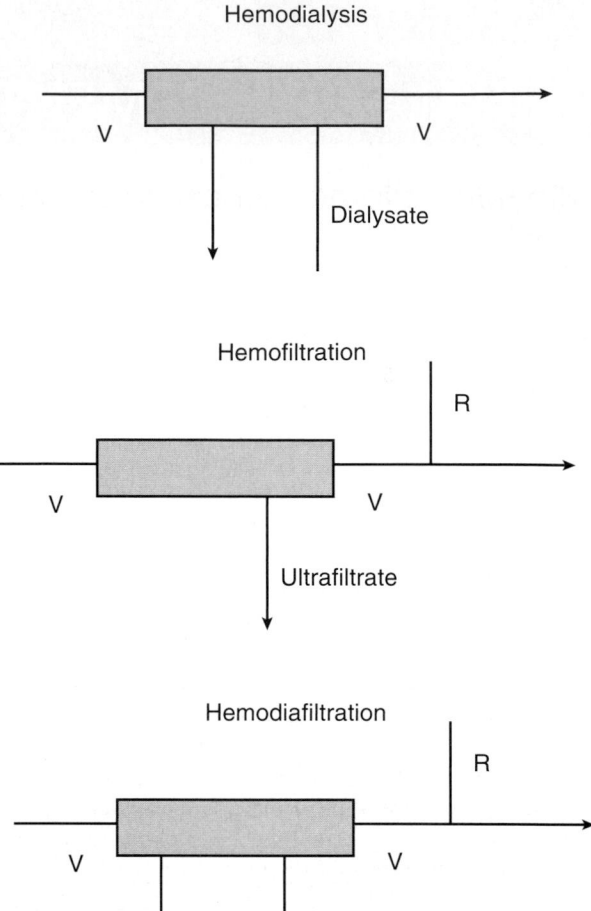

FIGURE 133–1. Solute removal methods: hemodialysis, hemofiltration, and hemodiafiltration. V, venous blood prefilter and postfilter; R, replacement fluid.

Once intermittent hemodialysis or continuous hemofiltration has been started, there are limited data on what is an "adequate" dose of dialysis. The concept of dialysis adequacy in acute renal failure remains controversial and ill defined,

TABLE 133–1. MODERN CRITERIA FOR THE INITIATION OF RENAL REPLACEMENT THERAPY IN THE ICU*
Oliguria (urine output <200 mL/12 h)
Anuria (urine output 0-50 mL/12 h)
[Urea] >35 mmol/L
[Creatinine] >400 µmol/L
[K+] >6.5 mmol/L or rapidly rising
Pulmonary edema unresponsive to diuretics
Uncompensated metabolic acidosis (pH <7.1)
[Na+] <110 mmol/L and >160 mmol/L
Temperature >40°C
Uremic complications (encephalopathy, myopathy, neuropathy, pericarditis)
Overdose with a dialyzable toxin (e.g., lithium)

*If one criterion is present, renal replacement therapy should be considered. If two criteria are simultaneously present, renal replacement therapy is strongly recommended.

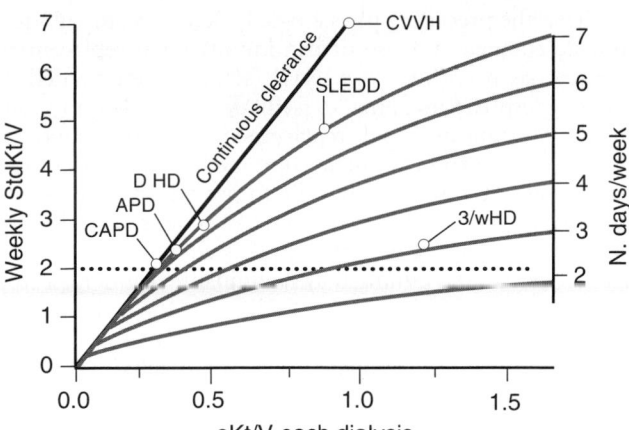

FIGURE 133–2. The various clearances affiliated with various dialysis techniques. Continuous and prolonged treatments, such as slow low-efficiency extended daily dialysis (SLEDD), can provide greater clearances. APD, automated peritoneal dialysis; CAPD, continuous ambulatory peritoneal dialysis; CVVH, continuous venovenous hemofiltration; HD, hemodialysis.

TABLE 133–2. QUANTITATIVE BLOOD PURIFICATION			
	Daily Short Hemodialysis	SLEDD	CVVH
Clearance (mL/min)	200	80	20
Urea [C]o (mg/dL)	110	110	70
Urea [C]t (mg/dL)	30	30	65
Treatment time (min)	180	480	1440
Kt/V	1.12	1.24	0.8
Total clearance (L)	36	30.4	20.0
Urea removed (g)	18	27	30.6

CVVH, continuous venovenous hemofiltration; SLEDD, slow low-efficiency extended daily dialysis; [C]o, concentration of urea at zero; [C]t, concentration of urea at end of treatment .

and the current goal is the maintenance of homeostasis at all levels.[10] Data are emerging that better uremic control may translate into better survival.[11-13] Patients at least should have urea levels maintained between 10 and 20 mmol/L throughout the treatment period. This level of uremic control should occur despite adequate nutrition support with a protein intake around 1.5 g/kg/d. This goal can be achieved easily using continuous renal replacement therapy at urea clearances of 36 to 48 L/d depending on patient size and catabolic rate. If intermittent hemodialysis is used, daily treatment and extended treatment are more desirable[8] with the goal of ensuring at least some adequacy for small solute removal. This means that intermittent hemodialysis must guarantee at least a daily urea clearance in liters greater than or equal to the patient's total body water. Total body water can be calculated from tables or simply as 60% of body weight. This relationship is expressed by the following equation:

Efficiency of renal replacement therapy = urea Kt/V

Where K is clearance in mL/min, t is time of treatment in minutes, and V is volume in liters of total body water. Kt/V is a fractional clearance, and its optimal value depends on the time of application of the technique and the intensity of clearance. For this reason, Kt/V is not an absolute parameter, and it must be adapted to the type and modality of therapy (Fig. 133-2). In this view, a more universal parameter used to compare different therapies is the standardized Kt/V, which requires higher single-session Kt/V for intermittent treatments to be similarly adequate as more frequent or continuous treatments (Table 133-2). These parameters guarantee a minimal acceptable level of blood purification for urea and other waste products in most patients.

MODE OF RENAL REPLACEMENT THERAPY

There is a great deal of controversy as to which mode of renal replacement therapy is "best" in the ICU. This controversy arises from the lack of randomized controlled trials comparing different techniques. Trials of sufficient statistical power are difficult to conduct and may never be performed. In the absence of direct comparisons of suitable statistical power and design, techniques of renal replacement therapy may be judged on the basis of the following criteria:

1. Hemodynamic side effects
2. Ability to control fluid status
3. Biocompatibility
4. Risk of infection
5. Uremic control
6. Avoidance of cerebral edema
7. Ability to allow full nutritional support
8. Ability to control acidosis
9. Absence of specific side effects
10. Cost

In our opinion, the evidence available supports the view that peritoneal dialysis and conventional intermittent hemodialysis (3 to 4 h/d, three to four times per week) are inferior to continuous renal replacement therapy and probably slow low-efficiency extended dialysis. Some salient aspects of continuous renal replacement therapy, intermittent hemodialysis, and peritoneal dialysis require discussion, however.

CONTINUOUS RENAL REPLACEMENT THERAPY

Continuous renal replacement therapy is now the most common form of renal replacement therapy in Australian and European ICUs. In the United States, however, continuous renal replacement therapy reportedly is used in only 10% to 20% of ICU patients.[14] Continuous renal replacement therapy has undergone several technical modifications since it was first described in 1977. Initially, it was performed as an arteriovenous therapy (continuous arteriovenous hemofiltration) in which blood flow through the hemofilter was driven by the patient's blood pressure. Clearances were low, however, and countercurrent dialysate flow soon was added to double or triple solute clearances (continuous arteriovenous hemodialysis/diafiltration) with or without spontaneous ultrafiltration. The need to cannulate an artery is associated with 15% to 20% morbidity, however. Double-lumen catheters and peristaltic blood pumps have come into use with or without control of ultrafiltration rate.

In a venovenous system, dialysate also can be delivered countercurrent to blood flow (continuous venovenous hemodialysis/hemodiafiltration) to achieve either almost pure diffusive clearance or a mixture of diffusive and convective clearance.

Whatever the technique of continuous renal replacement therapy, the clearances achieved can be adjusted by adjusting ultrafiltration rate or dialysate flow rate or both, typically aiming to achieve a daily clearance at least equal to the patient's total body water. A standardized nomenclature is now available for continuous renal replacement therapy techniques.[15] To make the reading easy and to make the reader familiar with the most accepted definitions and treatment schemes, we have summarized in Figure 133-3 the complete set of available techniques, including some hints on operational parameters. No matter what technique is used, the following outcomes are predictable:

1. Continuous control of fluid status
2. Hemodynamic stability
3. Control of acid-base status
4. Ability to provide protein-rich nutritional support, while achieving excellent uremic control
5. Control of electrolyte balance
6. Control of phosphate and calcium balance
7. Prevention of swings in intracerebral water
8. Minimal risk of infection
9. High level of biocompatibility

Given the preceding physiologic beneficence, the ubiquitous acceptance and use of continuous renal replacement therapy has been limited. Several factors have impeded its more widespread use. First, to facilitate a true 24-hour treatment, continuous renal replacement therapy mandates the presence of trained nursing and medical staff 24 hours a day. Small ICUs may not be able to provide such a level of support. Second, such personnel need to be trained. If continuous renal replacement therapy is used only 5 to 10 times a year, the cost of training may be unjustified, and expertise may be hard to maintain. Depending on the organization of patient care, continuous renal replacement therapy may be more expensive than intermittent hemodialysis. This cost difference is minimal or absent in some countries, such as Australia, but may be significant in the United States. Finally, the issues of continuous circuit anticoagulation and the potential risk of bleeding have been a major concern.

ANTICOAGULATION DURING CONTINUOUS RENAL REPLACEMENT THERAPY

The flow of blood through an extracorporeal circuit causes activation of the coagulation cascade and promotes clotting of the filter and circuit itself. To delay such clotting and achieve acceptable operational life (approximately 24 hours) for the circuit, anticoagulation frequently is used.[16]

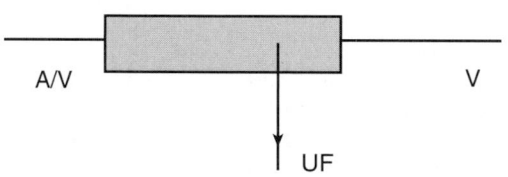

SCUF—Slow continuous ultrafiltration (AV or VV)

A/V   V

UF

Technique used for fluid control only
Convective mechanism
Ultrafiltrate isoosmotic to blood
Used in arteriovenous or venovenous mode
Qb = 50–100 mL/min
Ultrafiltration rate controlled

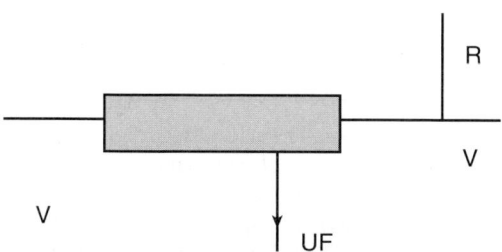

CVVH—Continuous venovenous hemofiltration

R

V

V

UF

Convective blood purification through high permeability membrane
Ultrafiltration rate controlled
Ultrafiltrate replaced by replacement solution
Qf = 50–200 mL/min   Qf = 8–25 mL/min
K = 12–36 L/24h
Can be used in arteriovenous mode

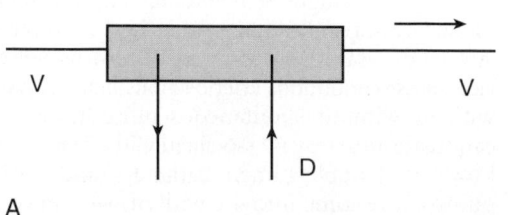

CVVHD—Continuous venovenous hemodialysis

V   V

D

A

Diffusive blood purification through low permeability dialyser
Dialysate solution in countercurrent flow
No replacement fluid used
Qb = 50–200 mL/min   Qf = 2–4 mL/min
Qd = 10–20 mL/min   K = 14–36 L/24h
Small molecule clearance only
Can be used in arteriovenous mode

FIGURE 133-3. Schematic representation and definitions of the different continuous renal replacement therapies according to standard nomenclature. Functional capabilities are described. A, artery; D, dialysate; K, clearance; Pf, plasma filtration rate; Qb, arterial flow; Qd, dialysate flow; Qf, ultrafiltration rate; UF, ultrafiltrate; UFc, ultrafiltrate control pump; V, vein.

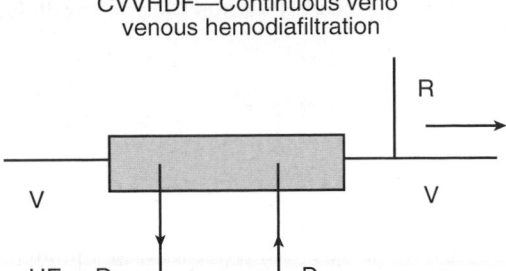

CVVHDF—Continuous veno venous hemodiafiltration

Diffusive and convective blood purification
Countercurrent dialysate flow
High permeability membrane utilized thus
    small and middle molecules removed
$Qb = 50–200$ mL/min $Qf = 8–12$ mL/min
$Qd = 10–20$ mL/min $K = 20–40$ L/24h

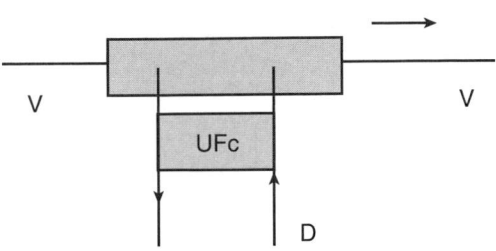

CVVHFD—Continuous high flux dialysis

Diffusive and convective blood purification
    through a highly permeable membrane
Back diffusion occurs in membrane
Dialysate in countercurrent flow
Accessory pumps to control ultrafiltration
Replacement not required since fine
    regulation of filtration and backfiltration
$Qb = 50–200$ mL/min $Qf = 2–8$ mL/min
$Qd = 50–200$ mL/min $K = 40–60$ L/24h

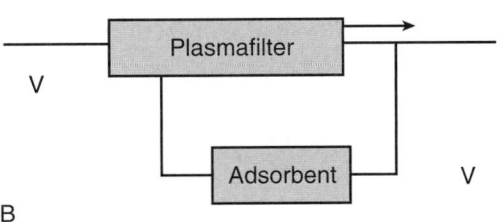

CPFA—Continuous plasmafiltration adsorption

A highly permeable plasmafilter filters Fluid
    plasma allowing it to pass through a bed
    of adsorbent material (carbon or resins)
Fluid balance maintained
Can be coupled with CVVH or CVVHD/F
$Qb = 50–200$ mL/min $Pf = 20–30$ mL/min

B

FIGURE 133–3.—CONT'D.

Circuit anticoagulation increases the statistical risk of bleeding for the patient, however. The clinician must weigh the risks and benefits of more or less intense anticoagulation. In this regard, the intensivist has several strategies available (Table 133-3).

In most patients, low-dose heparin (<10 IU/kg/h) is sufficient to achieve adequate filter life.[17] Heparin is easy and inexpensive to administer. It is easy to reverse and, at these doses, has almost no effect on the patient's coagulation tests. In some patients, a higher dose is necessary. In others (pulmonary embolism, myocardial ischemia), full heparinization may be indicated concomitantly and should be pursued. Regional citrate anticoagulation is effective but requires that the hospital pharmacy or ICU use a special dialysate or replacement fluid. Citrate anticoagulation is expensive and more complex to organize. Nonetheless, it provides excellent and effective anticoagulation at minimal risk to the patient.[16] Regional heparin/protamine anticoagulation also is complex, but may be useful if frequent filter clotting occurs and further anticoagulation of the patient is considered dangerous. Low-molecular-weight heparin also is efficacious but more expensive and hard to reverse because it accumulates in renal failure. It has not been shown to provide any advantages over unfractionated heparin. Heparinoids and prostacyclin may be useful if the patient has developed heparin-induced thrombocytopenia and thrombosis and citrate is not available. Serine proteinase inhibitors have been used but are not available outside Japan. Finally, in perhaps 10% to 20% of patients, anticoagulation is best avoided because of endogenous coagulopathy or recent surgery. In such patients, mean filter life of greater than 24 hours can be achieved, provided that blood flow is kept at 200 mL/min, and vascular access is reliable.[18]

Many circuits clot for mechanical reasons (inadequate access, unreliable blood flow from double-lumen catheter

---

TABLE 133–3. STRATEGIES FOR CIRCUIT ANTICOAGULATION DURING CONTINUOUS RENAL REPLACEMENT THERAPY

No anticoagulation
Low-dose prefilter heparin (<500 IU/h)
Medium-dose prefilter heparin (500-1000 IU/h)
Full heparinization
Regional anticoagulation (prefilter heparin and postfilter protamine usually at a 100 IU-to-1 mg ratio)
Regional citrate anticoagulation (prefilter citrate and postfilter calcium—special calcium-free dialysate needed)
Low-molecular-weight heparin
Prostacyclin
Heparinoids
Serine proteinase inhibitors (nafamostat mesilate)

depending on patient position, and kinking of catheter). Responding to frequent filter clotting by simply increasing anticoagulation without making the correct etiologic diagnosis (checking catheter flow and position, taking a history surrounding the episode of clotting, identifying the site of clotting) is often futile and exposes the patient to an unnecessary risk of bleeding.

CONTINUOUS RENAL REPLACEMENT THERAPY TECHNOLOGY

The increasing use of venovenous continuous renal replacement therapy has led to the development of a series of continuous renal replacement therapy technologies, which offer different kinds of machines to facilitate its performance.[19] Some understanding of these devices is important for the successful implementation of continuous renal replacement therapy in any ICU. The simplest technical approach is to allow ultrafiltration to occur spontaneously, measure it, and replace it as indicated. In such a system, hourly measurement of effluent is necessary, and the only requirement is that of a blood pump to deliver blood to the filter and of a volumetric pump to administer replacement fluid at the appropriate rate. This approach has been wryly called "chasing the bucket" to describe the nurse's need to monitor outflow and inflow continuously. Such a system is inherently unsafe and labor intensive. A volumetric pump can regulate effluent flow easily, however. One can have a simple blood pump with safety features (air bubble trap and pressure alarms) and use widely available volumetric pumps to control replacement or dialysate flow and effluent flow. Such adaptive technology is inexpensive (approximately $10,000 U.S. dollars) but is not user-friendly. Also, volumetric pumps have an inherent inaccuracy of about 5%, which in a system exchanging 50 L/d can cause problems.[19] Various manufacturers have produced custom-made machines for hemofiltration. For a detailed discussion of such machines, the reader is referred to specialist textbooks.[19] These machines are safer and have much more sophisticated pump control systems, alarms, and graphic displays. They are much more user-friendly especially with the setup procedure. Most, if not all, ICUs in developed countries now conduct continuous renal replacement therapy with new devices characterized by advanced built-in technology and a high degree of automation.

INTERMITTENT HEMODIALYSIS

Intermittent hemodialysis remains dominant in the United States. Vascular access is typically by double-lumen catheter as in continuous hemofiltration. Intermittent hemodialysis machines use high dialysate flows (300 to 400 mL/min), however, and generate dialysate by using purified water and concentrate. Conventionally, intermittent hemodialysis is applied for short periods (3 to 4 hours), usually every second day. These technical features have important implications. First, volume has to be removed over a short time. Critically ill patients tolerate such removal (1 to 2 L in 4 hours) poorly; this can lead to a high incidence of hypotension.[20] Repeated hypotensive episodes may delay renal recovery.[4] Second, solute removal is episodic; this translates into inferior uremic control.[20] These features are summarized in Figure 133-4. The same applies to acid-base control. Limited fluid and uremic control imposes unnecessary limitations on nutritional support. Rapid solute shifts increase brain water content and

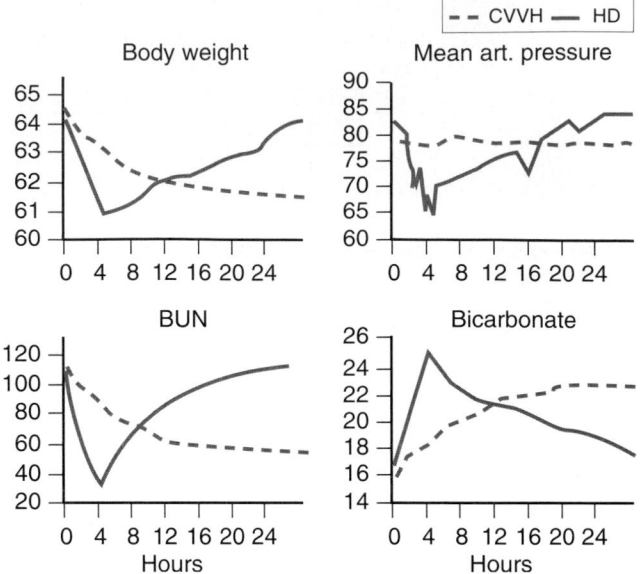

CVVH Versus Daily Hemodialysis

FIGURE 133–4. Comparisons of mean arterial pressure, body weight, blood urea nitrogen (BUN), and bicarbonate control with continuous and intermittent therapies, showing smoother and less varied control of all parameters with continuous treatment. CVVH, continuous venovenous hemofiltration; HD, hemodialysis.

increase intracranial pressure.[21] Finally, much controversy has surrounded the issue of membrane bioincompatibility. Standard low-flux dialyzing membranes made of cuprophane are known to trigger the activation of several inflammatory pathways, much more so than high-flux synthetic membranes (also used for continuous hemofiltration). It is possible that such a proinflammatory effect contributes to further renal damage and delays recovery or even affects mortality.[22,23]

The serious limitations of applying "conventional" intermittent hemodialysis (3 to 4 h/d every second day) to the treatment of acute renal failure have been highlighted,[8] and new approaches to intermittent therapies (so-called hybrid techniques), such as slow extended dialysis, slow low-efficiency daily dialysis, and intermittent extended hemofiltration, are emerging. These techniques seek to adapt intermittent hemodialysis to the clinical circumstance and increase its tolerance and its clearances. In our opinion, such hybrid approaches represent a welcome improvement in dialysis support and a clear recognition that acute renal failure patients should not receive the dialysis offered to patients with end-stage renal failure.

PERITONEAL DIALYSIS

Peritoneal dialysis is not commonly used in the treatment of adult acute renal failure either in the United States or elsewhere.[24] Typically, access is by the surgical insertion of an intraperitoneal catheter. Glucose-rich dialysate is inserted into the peritoneal cavity and acts as the "dialysate." After a given "dwell time," it is removed and discarded with the extra fluid and toxins that have moved from the blood vessels of the peritoneum to the dialysate fluid. Machines also are available that deliver and remove dialysate at higher flows through a double-lumen peritoneal catheter, providing intermittent treatment and higher solute clearances. Several major shortcomings make peritoneal dialysis relatively unsuited to the treatment of adult acute renal failure:

1. Limited, sometimes inadequate solute clearance
2. High risk of peritonitis
3. Unpredictable hyperglycemia
4. Fluid leaks
5. Protein loss
6. Interference with diaphragm function

There have been no reports since the 1980s of the sole use of peritoneal dialysis for the treatment of adult ICU patients with acute renal failure. Despite this, the new technique called *continuous flow peritoneal dialysis* might offer something new in this field. No studies have been conducted so far.

DRUG PRESCRIPTION DURING DIALYSIS THERAPY

Acute renal failure and the need for renal replacement therapy profoundly affect drug clearance. A comprehensive description of changes in drug dosage according to the technique of renal replacement therapy, residual creatinine clearance, and other determinants of pharmacodynamics is beyond the scope of this chapter and can be found in specialist textbooks.[25] Table 133-4 provides general guidelines for the prescription of drugs that are commonly used in the ICU.

CONTROVERSIES IN RENAL REPLACEMENT THERAPY

Several controversies currently surround the use, timing, dose, and choice of renal replacement therapy. The most pressing question is whether continuous renal replacement therapy offers an important survival advantage over intermittent hemodialysis in the management of acute renal failure. To address this question, a randomized controlled trial of large proportion with extremely strict criteria would be required. Such a task would be extremely difficult to undertake. Attempts to date have fallen short of decisive results.[26] A meta-analysis of all studies up to the end of 2000 showed a trend in favor of continuous renal replacement therapy.[12] One finding from the largest randomized controlled study to date showed that patients treated with continuous renal replacement therapy who survived were more likely to have renal recovery than patients treated with intermittent hemodialysis (92.3% versus 59.4%; $P < .01$).[26] These findings suggest that mortality may not be the only appropriate endpoint for future trials and that continuous renal replacement therapy may increase recovery of renal function after acute renal failure.

A single-center randomized controlled trial[27] compared daily with every-second-day hemodialysis and showed improved survival and greater renal recovery with daily therapy. Another single-center randomized controlled trial compared continuous venovenous hemofiltration with peritoneal dialysis in ICU patients with sepsis and found a dramatic reduction in mortality and in the cost of therapy per life saved when continuous hemofiltration was used.[24]

Finally, if continuous hemofiltration is used, the dose of treatment may be an important determinant of outcome. A single-center randomized controlled trial showed that increasing the ultrafiltration rate from 20 to 35 mL/kg/h significantly increased survival.[11]

TABLE 133–4. DRUG DOSAGE DURING DIALYTIC THERAPY*

Drug	CRRT	IHD
Aminoglycosides	Normal dose q36h	50% normal dose q48h—{2/3} redose after IHD
Cefotaxime or ceftazidime	1 g q8-12h	1 g q12-24h after IHD
Imipenem	500 mg q8h	250 mg q8h and after IHD
Meropenem	500 mg q8h	250 mg q8h and after IHD
Metronidazole	500 mg q8h	250 mg q8h and after IHD
Co-trimoxazole	Normal dose q18h	Normal dose q24h after IHD
Amoxicillin	500 mg q8h	500 mg daily and after IHD
Vancomycin	1 g q24h	1 g q96-120h
Piperacillin	3-4 g q6h	3-4 g q8h and after IHD
Ticarcillin	1-2 g q8h	1-2 g q12h and after IHD
Ciprofloxacin	200 mg q12h	200 mg q24h and after IHD
Fluconazole	200 mg q24h	200 mg q48h and after IHD
Acyclovir	3.5 mg/kg q24h	2.5 mg/kg/d and after IHD
Ganciclovir	5 mg/kg/d	5 mg/kg/48 h and after IHD
Amphotericin B	Normal dose	Normal dose
Liposomal amphotericin B	Normal dose	Normal dose
Ceftriaxone	Normal dose	Normal dose
Erythromycin	Normal dose	Normal dose
Milrinone	Titrate to effect	Titrate to effect
Amrinone	Titrate to effect	Titrate to effect
Catecholamines	Titrate to effect	Titrate to effect
Ampicillin	500 mg q8h	500 mg daily and after IHD

*These values represent approximations and should be used as a general guide only. Critically ill patients have markedly abnormal volumes of distribution for these agents, which affects dosage. CRRT is conducted at variable levels of intensity in different units, also requiring adjustment. The values reported here relate to continuous venovenous hemofiltration at 2 L/h of ultrafiltration. Vancomycin is poorly removed by continuous venovenous hemodialysis. IHD also may differ from unit to unit. The values reported here relate to standard IHD with low-flux membranes for 3 to 4 hours every second day.
CRRT, continuous renal replacement therapy; IHD, intermittent hemodialysis.

Cost comparisons have been analyzed by several authors, and the general consensus is that the difference in cost between continuous renal replacement therapy and intermittent hemodialysis is minimal and depends more on the structure of ICU and nephrologic care than on disposables.[28] If continuous renal replacement therapy is associated with a greater rate of renal recovery, it would be more cost effective than intermittent hemodialysis. Such evaluations require more information from large randomized controlled trials.

Finally, much evidence suggests that modifications of continuous renal replacement therapy techniques might provide substantial immunomodulatory effects in patients with combined acute renal failure and severe sepsis or multiorgan failure. Such effects may be mediated partly by the removal of soluble mediators[29-34] and are associated with significant beneficial physiologic effects in septic patients. Although no large randomized controlled trials of modified renal replacement therapy technology have been conducted yet in severe sepsis, these observations already suggest the notion that physicians always should consider carefully the broader aspects of extracorporeal organ support in their ICU patients.[34] The evidence basis surrounding most of the above-mentioned issues has been formally summarized and evaluated by the Acute Dialysis Quality Initiative consensus conference.[35]

SUMMARY

Renal replacement therapy has undergone remarkable changes and is continuing to evolve rapidly. Technology is being improved to facilitate clinical application, and new areas of research are developing. Continuous renal replacement therapy now is firmly established throughout the world as perhaps the most commonly used form of renal replacement therapy. Conventional dialysis, the usage of which was slowly decreasing, is reappearing, however, in the form of extended, slow-efficiency treatment, especially in the United States. Meanwhile, the use of novel membranes, of sorbents, and of different intensities of treatment is being explored in the area of sepsis management and liver support. Intensivists need to keep abreast of this rapid evolution if they are to offer their patients the best of care.

ANNOTATED REFERENCES

Bellomo R: Continuous hemofiltration as blood purification in sepsis. New Horiz 1995;3:732-737.

This article represents the beginning of the use of renal replacement therapy for the treatment of sepsis.

Bellomo R, Ronco C: Adequacy of dialysis in the acute renal failure of the critically ill: The case for continuous therapies. Int J Artif Organs 1996;19:129-142.

This is the first article to deal with adequacy of renal replacement therapy in critically ill patients.

Kellum JA, Mehta RL, Angus DC, et al: The first international consensus conference of CRRT. Kidney Int 2002;62:1855-1863.

This is the first consensus publication on renal replacement therapy in the ICU provided by the Acute Dialysis Quality Initiative.

Ronco C, Bellomo R: Acute renal failure and multiple organ dysfunction in the ICU: From renal replacement therapy (RRT) to multiple organ support therapy (MOST). Int J Artif Organs 2002;25:733-747.

This article describes the first approach to multiple organ dysfunction with a complex and articulated extracorporeal system as a platform for therapy.

Ronco C, Bellomo R, Homel P, et al: Effects of different doses in continuous veno-venous haemofiltration on outcomes of acute renal failure: A prospective randomized trial. Lancet 2000;355:26-30.

This article reports on the largest randomized prospective trial on dose of renal replacement therapy in the ICU. This article has set the standard for dialysis dose in the ICU.

COLOR FIGURES

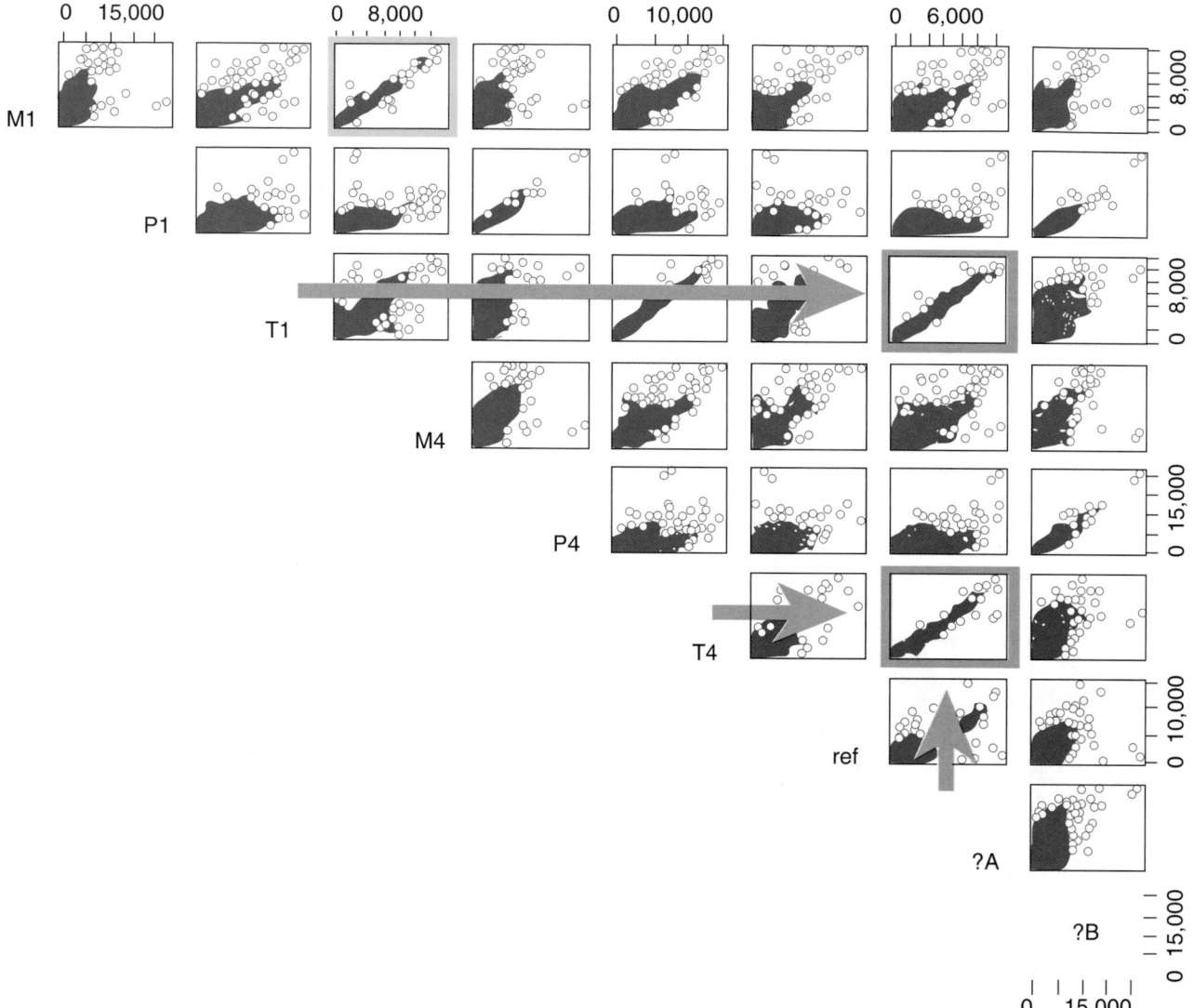

FIGURE 44–1. (A) Human transcriptome profiles of circulating T lymphocytes (T), monocytes (M), and mixed blood leukocytes (P) from normal volunteers (#1 and #4), compared with reference human RNA and two unknown samples (?A and ?B). At left, pair-wise comparisons of U95Av2 GeneChip expression signal for approximately 12,000 genes and expressed sequence tags show good pair-wise correlations between profiles of like cell types but not between different cell types in the same individual (e.g., compare good M1 to M4 correlation [yellow box] with poor M1 to T1 or P1 correlations). Moreover, assigning a cell type to the unknown samples A and B is easily accomplished, as shown by the orange arrows (?A to T cells, and ?B to mixed leukocytes). At right, the GenMAPP transforming growth factor-beta (TGF-β) pathway indicates differences in gene expression among T cell (red), monocyte (green), and PAXgene (blue). This program allows one to visually compare apparent levels of gene expression by color-coding genes that have increased expression in a given data set. In this example comparing blood leukocyte, isolated T cell, and isolated monocyte GeneChip signals, apparent gene expression for the type III TGF-β receptor (betaglycan) was greatest in T cells (red box); stress-induced protein 1 (SIP1) and c-FOS were greatest in monocytes (green boxes); and STAT3 was greatest in blood (mixed) leukocytes (blue box). The other genes shown (uncolored) were not changed. Thus, this figure indicates that apparent gene expression for the type III accessory receptor for TGF-β was greater in T cells, whereas apparent gene expression for SIP1 repressor and c-FOS cofactor was higher in monocytes. In contrast, there was higher apparent gene expression in blood (mixed) leukocytes only for the STAT3 cofactor.

Continued on next page

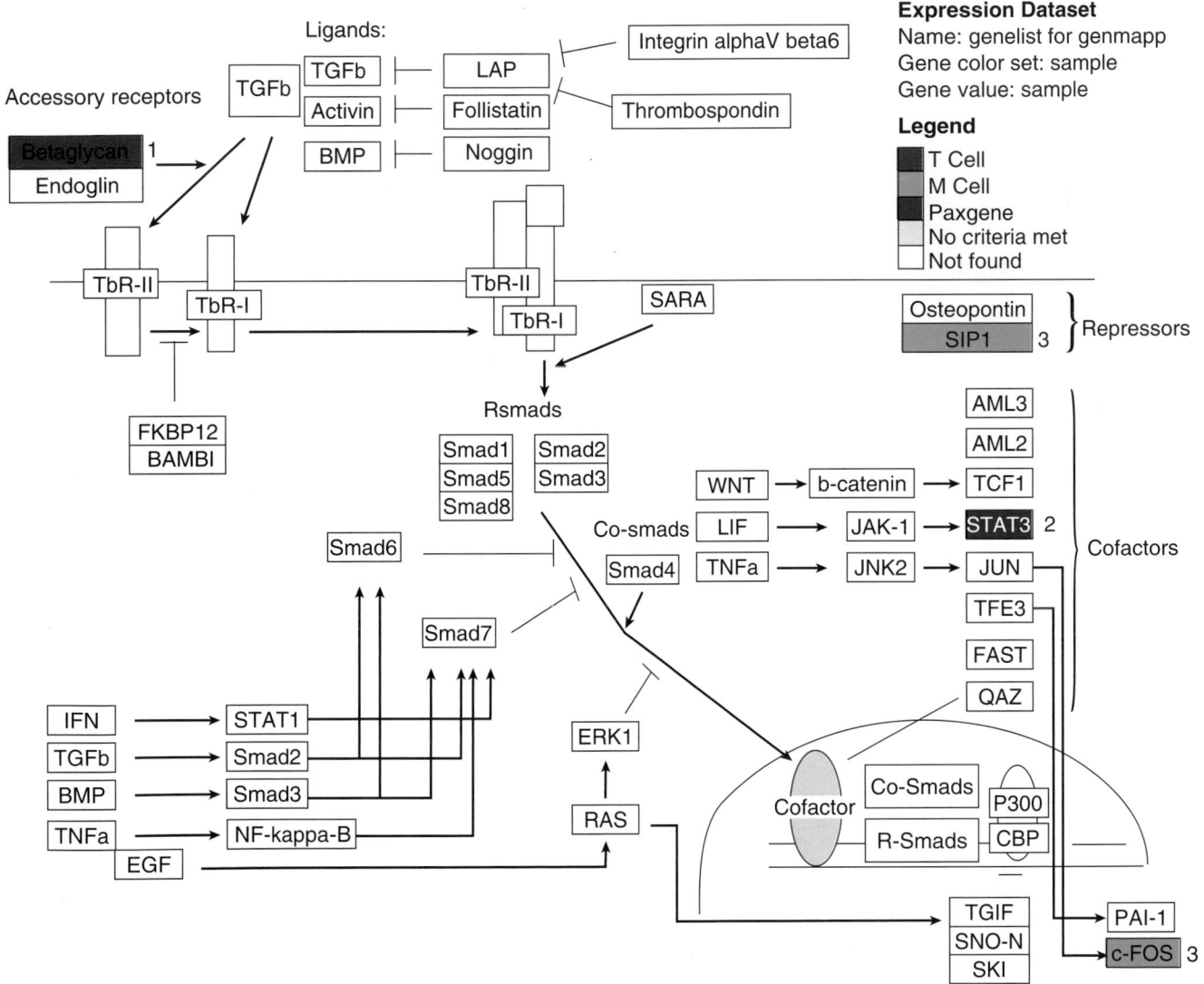

FIGURE 44–1. (B)

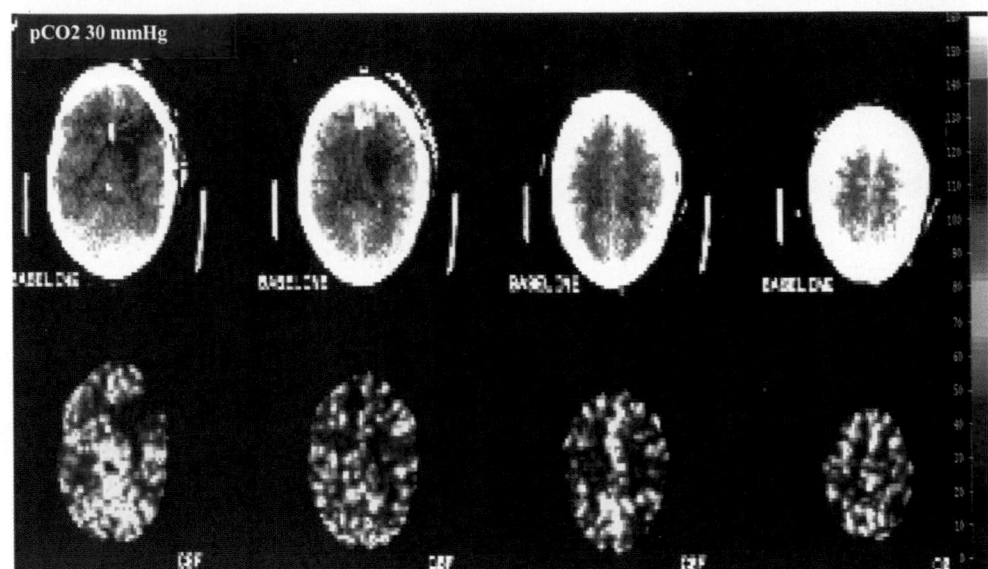

FIGURE 47–4. Computed tomography scans of a head-injury patient with an intracranial pressure (ICP) of 70 mm Hg and $Paco_2$ 30 mm Hg but diffusely normal to hyperemic cerebral blood flows. (Courtesy of Howard Yonas, University of Pittsburgh.)

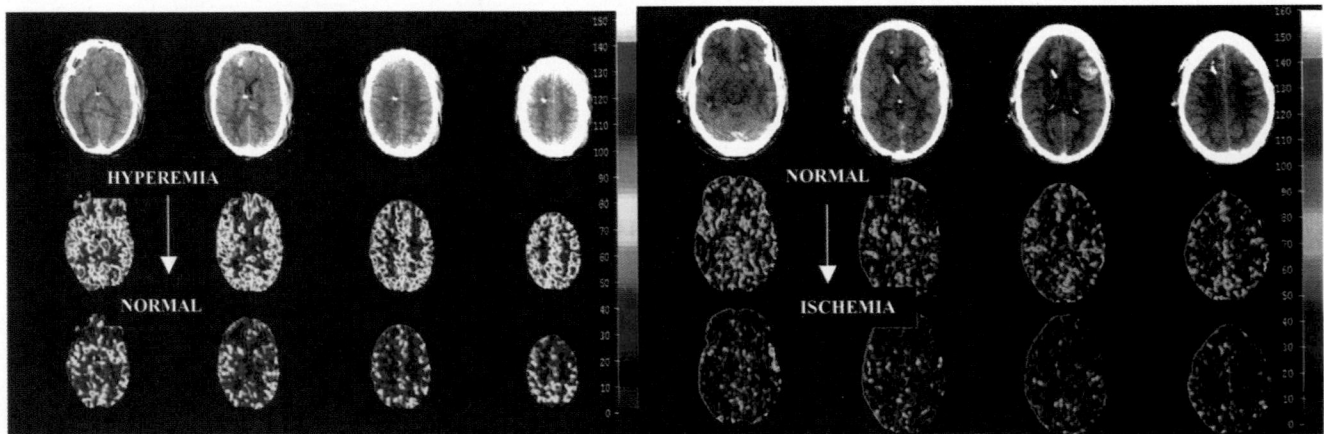

FIGURE 47–15. Effects of $Psco_2$ changes on cerebral blood flow (CBF). Two examples of disparate effects of hyperventilation on CBF. Both figures are stable xenon CBF scans in head trauma patients with and without hyperventilation. CBF scale is indicated on the right in mL/100 g/min and Pco_2 is indicated above each study. Computed tomography images are indicated in the upper figures and CBF maps in the lower figures. In the left figure, $Paco_2$ was decreased from 40 to 30 mm Hg. The baseline scan shows hyperemia and the hyperventilated scan shows CBFs of approximately 60 to 70 mL/100 g/min, probably acceptable flows. In the right figure, $Paco_2$ was decreased from 38 to 30 mm Hg. The baseline CBFs were acceptable. The effect of this modest extent of hyperventilation was to produce widespread areas of CBF less than 20 mL/100 g/min, probably unacceptable flows. (Courtesy of Howard Yonas, University of Pittsburgh.)

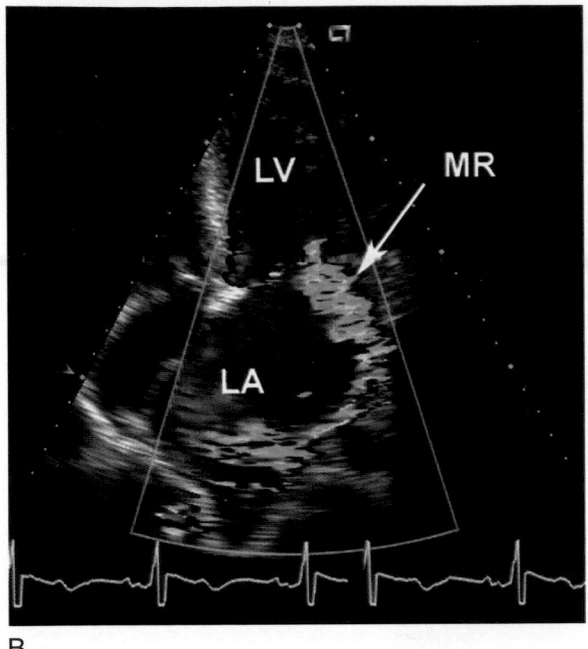

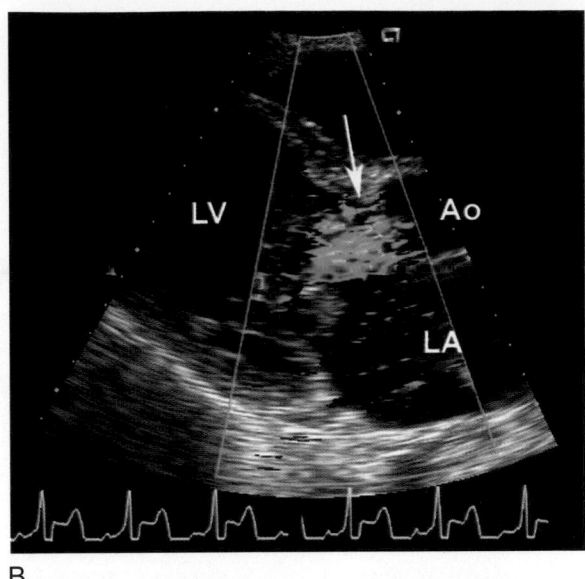

B

FIGURE 103–2. In this 24-year-old man with chronic mitral prolapse, chordal rupture resulted in a flail anterior leaflet. Severe mitral regurgitation (MR) was seen with a posterior and laterally directed jet on Doppler color flow imaging (**B,** *arrow*). LA, left atrium; LV, left ventricle.

FIGURE 103–5. Endocarditis resulting in acute severe aortic regurgitation. Color flow imaging (**B**) shows a broad jet of diastolic flow filling the outflow tract consistent with severe regurgitation. Ao, aorta; LA, left atrium; LV, left ventricle.

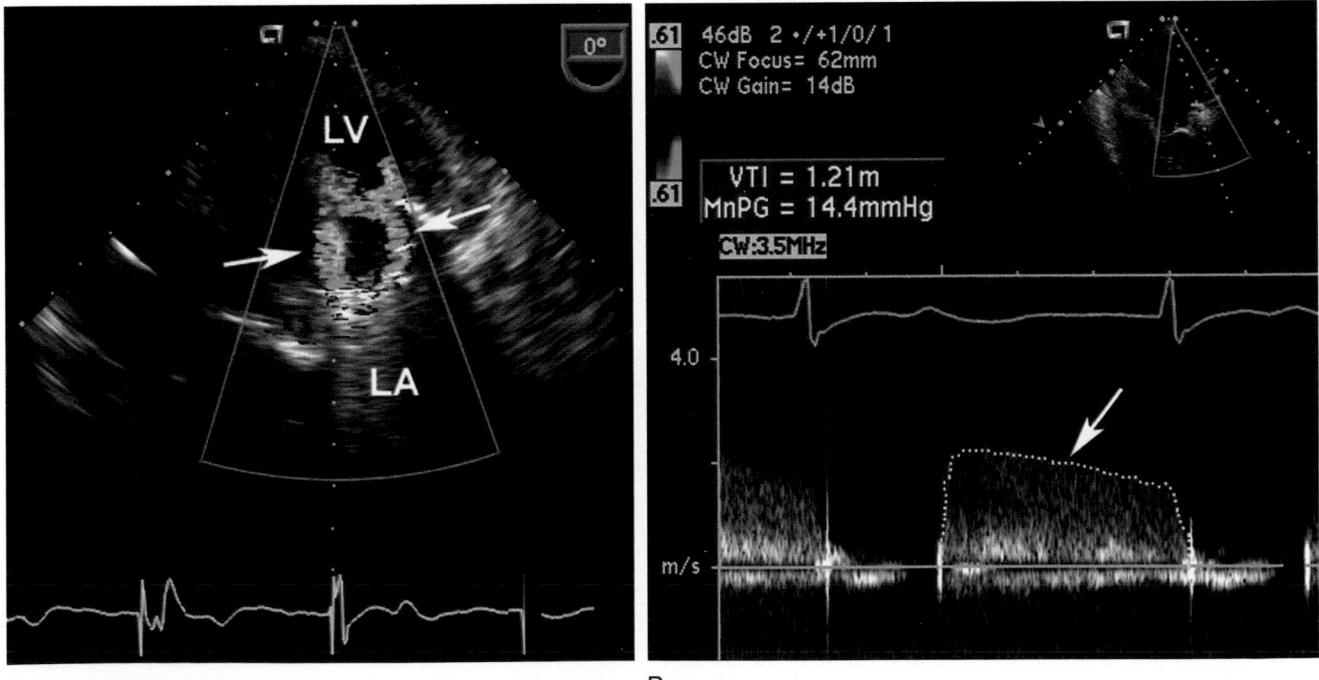

A **B**

FIGURE 103–12. Acute prosthetic mitral valve thrombosis in an 82-year-old man 29 years after valve replacement. The patient presented acutely with pulmonary edema and a right upper extremity thrombotic occlusion after anticoagulation was temporarily discontinued owing to a gastrointestinal hemorrhage. Color Doppler imaging (**A**) shows only narrow jets (*arrows*) of flow antegrade across the mitral valve replacement (MVR) and the continuous wave Doppler signal (**B**) shows a high gradient and very prolonged deceleration slope, consistent with severe obstruction to flow. After careful discussion given his high risk for surgery, he was treated with thrombolytic therapy, which resulted in normalization of his mitral valve Doppler flows and resolution of pulmonary edema.

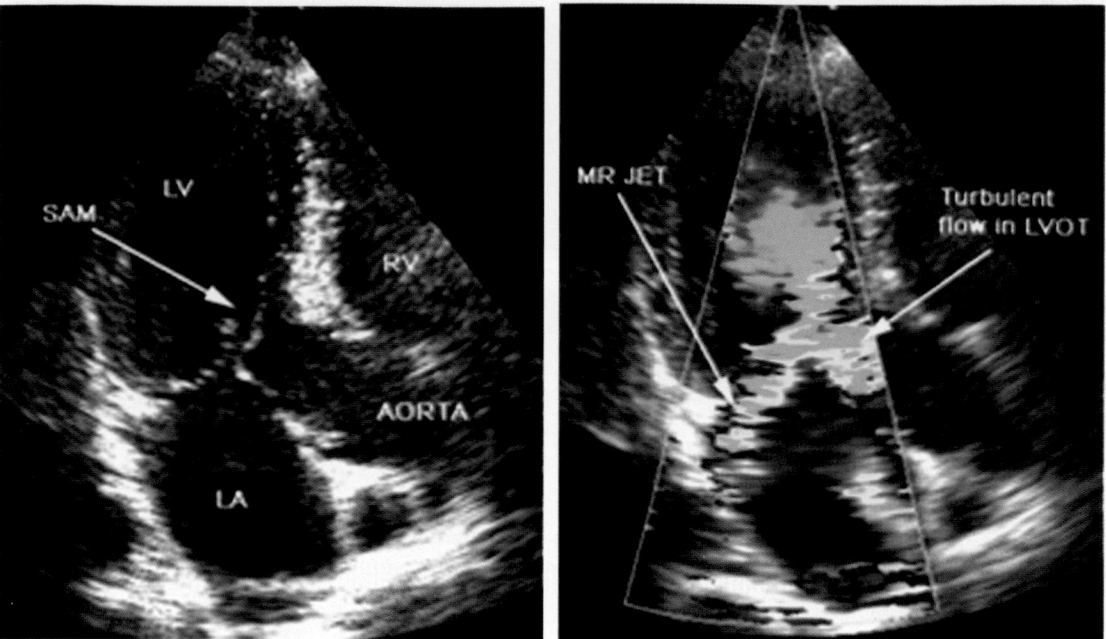

FIGURE 206–11. Systolic anterior motion (SAM) of the mitral valve in a patient with asymmetric left ventricular hypertrophy and dehydration. Two-dimensional transthoracic apical long-axis view shows movement of the anterior leaflet of the mitral valve *(arrow)* toward the interventricular septum during systole *(left)*. This creates a subaortic dynamic obstruction. The resulting high velocity and turbulence in the left ventricular outflow tract (LVOT) gives a "mosaic" pattern of flow on color Doppler *(right)*. A variable degree of asymmetric mitral regurgitation (MR) also may be present secondary to the systolic anterior motion as shown in this example *(right)*. LA, left atrium; LV, left ventricle; RV, right ventricle.

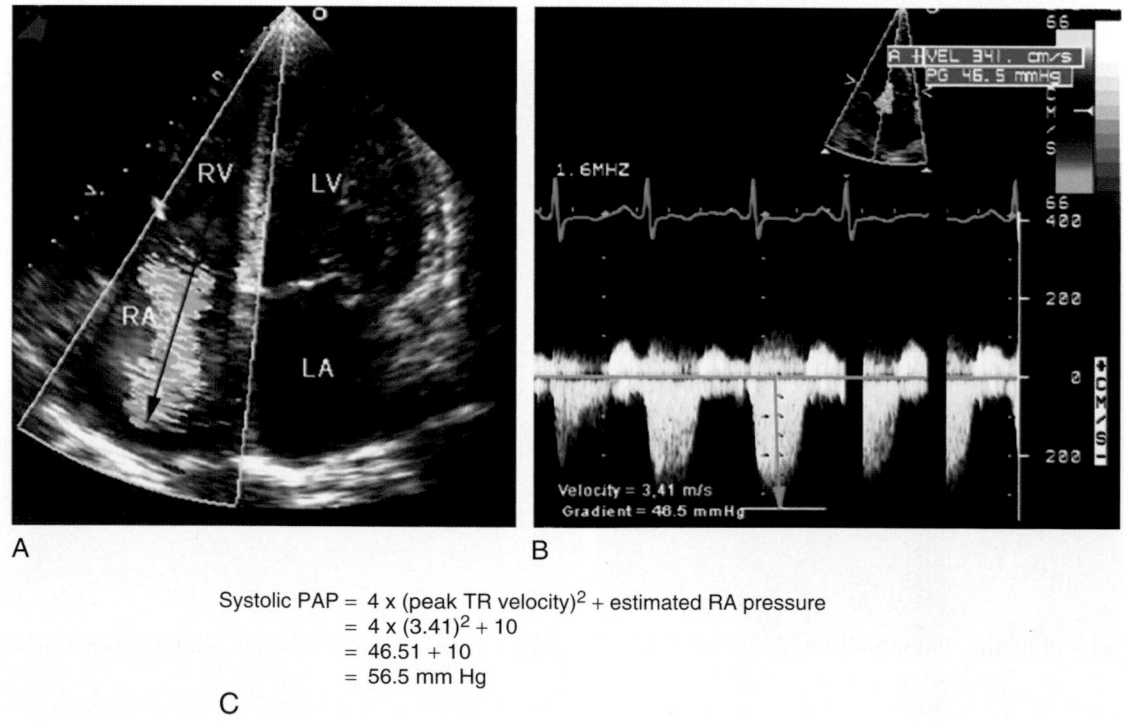

$$\text{Systolic PAP} = 4 \times (\text{peak TR velocity})^2 + \text{estimated RA pressure}$$
$$= 4 \times (3.41)^2 + 10$$
$$= 46.51 + 10$$
$$= 56.5 \text{ mm Hg}$$

C

FIGURE 206–12. Calculation of systolic pulmonary artery pressure (PAP). **A,** Color Doppler transthoracic apical four-chamber view shows a significant tricuspid regurgitation (TR) jet from right ventricle (RV) to right atrium (RA). The peak tricuspid regurgitation velocity is measured by placing the continuous wave Doppler in the center of the tricuspid regurgitation jet *(arrow)*. **B,** Spectral continuous wave Doppler profile of the tricuspid regurgitation jet. Peak tricuspid regurgitation velocity (3.41 m/s) and peak systolic pulmonary artery pressure gradient (46.5 mm Hg) can be obtained with this modality. **C,** Peak systolic pulmonary artery pressure also can be determined from the peak tricuspid regurgitation Doppler velocity using the modified Bernoulli equation: $\Delta P = 4 \times (\text{peak tricuspid regurgitation velocity})^2$. To this peak systolic pressure gradient between right ventricle and right atrium is added the estimated right atrial pressure (determined to be 10 in this example) to obtain the peak right ventricular systolic pressure. In the absence of pulmonic stenosis or right ventricular outflow obstruction, peak right ventricular systolic pressure is equal to systolic pulmonary artery pressure. LA, left atrium; LV, left ventricle.

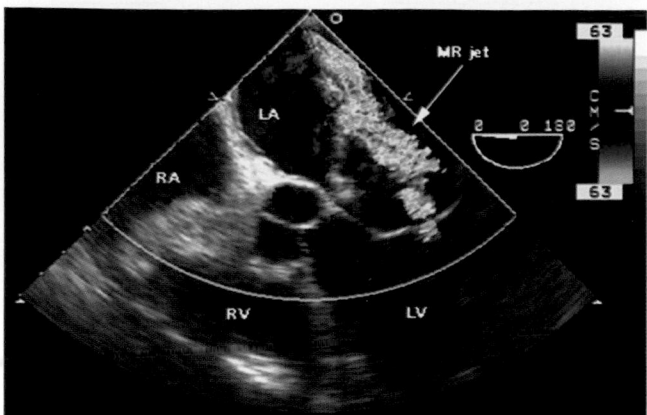

FIGURE 206–13. Severe mitral regurgitation (MR). Transesophageal five-chamber view shows severe mitral regurgitation with a large regurgitant jet *(arrow)* going far posteriorly in the left atrium (LA). In this case, systolic flow reversal in the pulmonary veins (another echocardiographic sign of severe mitral regurgitation) also was present (not shown on this picture). Because of its close anatomic proximity, transesophageal echocardiography is an excellent tool for the precise evaluation of the degree of mitral regurgitation. LV, left ventricle; RA, right atrium; RV, right ventricle.

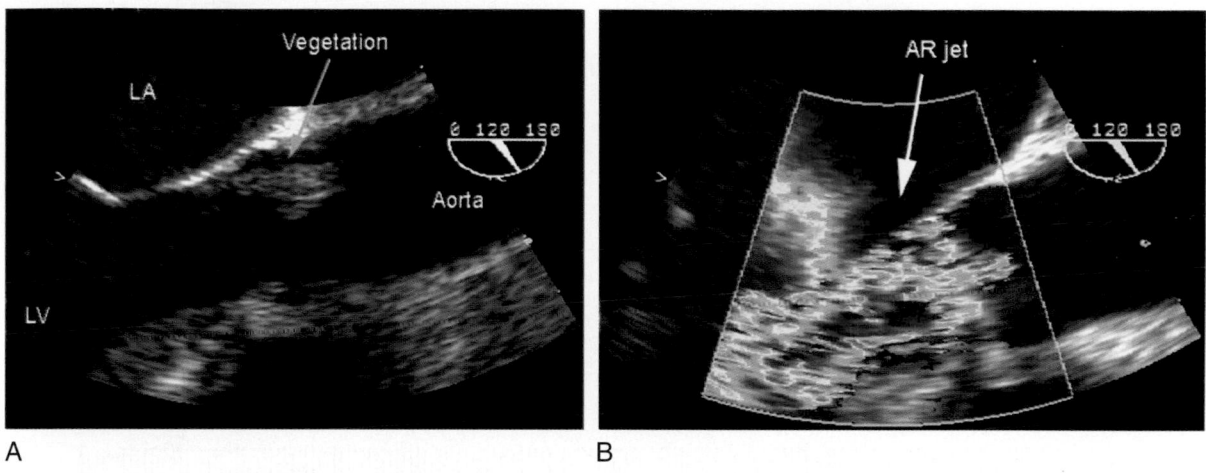

FIGURE 206–16. Infective endocarditis of the aortic valve. A 55-year-old patient was admitted to the ICU with fever, chills, hypotension, and respiratory distress for which he had to be intubated. He had 4/4 positive blood cultures for *Staphylococcus aureus*. Transthoracic echocardiography was performed initially, but the quality was suboptimal, and no definite conclusion could be reached. Subsequent transesophageal echocardiography revealed a large vegetation on the left aortic coronary cusp as seen in the midesophageal view at 120 degrees (**A**). Color Doppler examination (**B**) revealed the presence of associated severe aortic regurgitation (AR). The patient was treated with antibiotics and emergent aortic valvular surgery. LA, left atrium; LV, left ventricle.

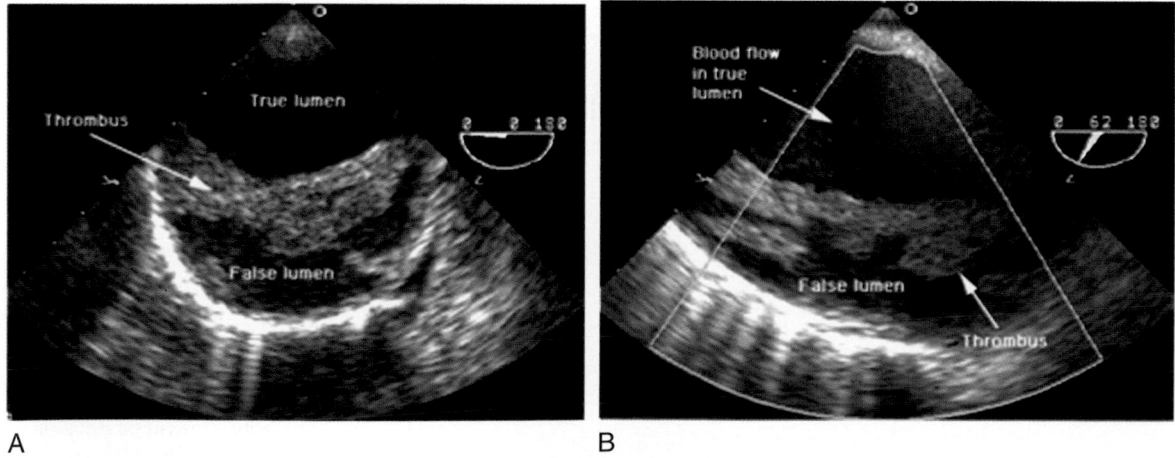

FIGURE 206–17. Dissecting thoracic aortic aneurysm. A 65-year-old patient presented to the emergency department with severe ripping chest pain radiating to the back. The initial electrocardiogram was unremarkable, and the chest x-ray showed a widened mediastinum. The patient underwent transesophageal echocardiography, which revealed the presence of a large dissecting aneurysm of the descending thoracic aorta. The short-axis view (**A**) revealed the presence of a large aneurysm with a true and a false lumen. The false lumen was filled with thrombus *(arrow)*. On the longitudinal view with color Doppler (**B**), blood flow in the true lumen is visualized. The patient was taken emergently to the operating room.

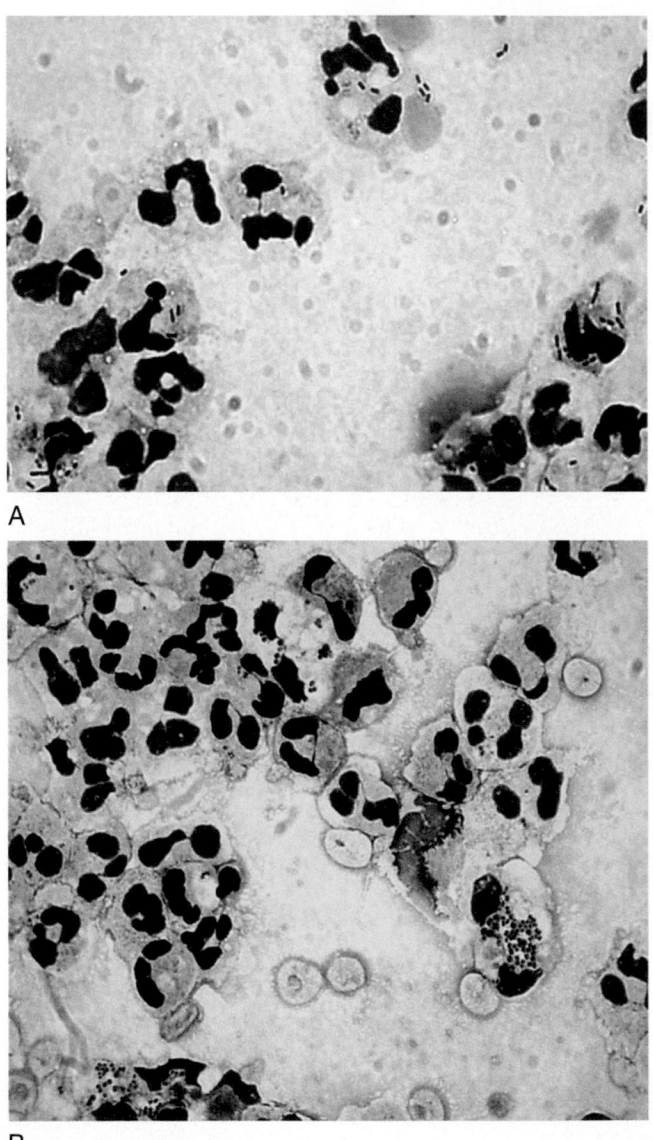

A

B

FIGURE 218–1. Light micrographs of neutrophils recovered by bronchoalveolar lavage (BAL) from a patient with pneumonia due to *Klebsiella pneumoniae* (**A**) and a patient with pneumonia due to *Staphylococcus aureus* (**B**). In each patient, the morphology and Gram staining of extra- and intracellular bacteria closely correlated with the results of BAL bacterial cultures.

Chapter 134

URINARY TRACT OBSTRUCTION

Scott Liebman • Isaac Teitelbaum

KEY POINTS

1. **Urinary tract obstruction is a fairly common disorder.** It should be considered in all cases of unexplained renal failure.

2. **The presence of urine output does not exclude the diagnosis of urinary tract obstruction.** Obstruction may present with any degree of urine output; the classic presentation of acute anuria is uncommon.

3. **Urinary tract obstruction may be a consequence of pathology anywhere between the renal tubules themselves and the tip of the urethra.** This may be divided into upper urinary tract obstruction (between the renal tubules and the ureterovesicular junction) and lower urinary tract obstruction (between the bladder and the urethra). The distinction is based on the fact that upper and lower urinary tract obstructions typically present as different constellations of symptoms and physical findings, and treatment of the two disorders is different.

4. **Urinary tract obstruction may be intrinsic** (due to pathology within the urinary tract itself) **or extrinsic** (compression of the urinary tract due to pathology in a different organ system). Intrinsic causes may be either intraluminal or intramural.

5. **The clinical presentation of urinary tract obstruction is quite varied.** It depends on many factors, including the anatomic location, the acuity with which the obstruction develops, and the severity of the obstruction (unilateral vs. bilateral, partial vs. complete). Patients may present with acute colicky pain, with nausea and vomiting mimicking an abdominal emergency, and with signs and symptoms of chronic renal failure, or they may be completely asymptomatic.

6. **There are no specific laboratory values that suggest obstruction.** Patterns that may be seen include renal insufficiency with associated hyperphosphatemia, hypocalcemia, and anemia or a hyperchloremic metabolic acidosis with or without hyperkalemia. Urine findings may mimic prerenal azotemia early on, with low urinary sodium and a fractional excretion of sodium less than 1%; typically this is not seen in a chronic obstruction. Alternatively, the laboratory values may be completely normal.

7. **Urinary tract obstruction leads to changes in all aspects of renal function.** Glomerular filtration rate and renal blood flow decrease. Tubular dysfunction is manifested by sodium wasting as well as defects in concentrating ability and urinary acidification.

8. **A postobstructive diuresis** may be seen after relief of complete bilateral obstruction or of obstruction of a solitary functioning kidney.

9. **Ultrasonography is very specific in detecting obstruction,** but false-positive findings may be seen in cases of increased urinary flow or with vesicoureteral reflux. Spiral computed tomography (CT) is often useful in determining the anatomic site of obstruction, especially in the case of urolithiasis or retroperitoneal causes. Isotope renography provides functional rather than anatomic information; it is especially helpful in diagnosing an obstruction when urinary flow rates are enhanced with diuretics. Excretory urography has been largely superseded by these modalities.

10. **Initial therapy of obstruction is directed at the management of potentially life-threatening complications such as gram-negative septicemia or hyperkalemia.** One must then decide whether it is necessary to intervene to establish or maintain patency or whether the obstruction may be managed conservatively. Finally, consideration should be given to disease-specific treatments.

11. **Data regarding recovery of renal function are inconclusive.** There is no imaging test that will predict whether renal function will return. Typically, recovery is dependent on the duration of obstruction; however, recovery has been observed even in patients who were dialysis dependent for months.

Urinary tract obstruction is a common disorder that affects all age groups. Autopsy studies show a rate of 3% to 4% in adults and 2% in children.[1] An obstructed urinary tract may lead to complications such as infection with ensuing sepsis, and renal dysfunction, which may be permanent if the obstruction is of long standing. The causes of obstruction are diverse, and often the clinical presentation is subtle. The clinician must maintain a high index of suspicion and be mindful of the fact that urinary tract obstruction only rarely presents classically with acute anuria. In fact, in partial obstruction, the urinary output may be high, low, or normal and often offers no clue to the underlying pathology. Obstruction must be considered in all cases of unexplained renal failure because prompt recognition and treatment can greatly impact the morbidity and mortality of this disorder.

Before beginning a discussion of urinary tract obstruction, it is useful to review the various terminologies used in referring to this entity.

Obstructive uropathy refers to disorders that interfere with drainage of the urine. It can occur at any level of the genitourinary tract. As is discussed later, obstructive uropathy can result from pathology within the urinary tract itself (intrinsic obstruction) or from pathology originating outside the urinary tract that eventually causes external compression of the system (extrinsic obstruction). It may be acute or chronic and partial or complete, and the resulting symptom complex typically depends on the acuity and severity.

Obstructive nephropathy refers to those cases in which obstructive uropathy causes a decline in renal function.

Hydronephrosis is a term that actually refers to dilatation of the urinary collecting system, with renal parenchymal changes due to back-pressure. Typically, however, the term is used to describe any dilatation of the urinary tract, regardless of renal parenchymal changes. Hydronephosis is usually, but not exclusively, seen in obstructive disorders. Nonobstructive pathogenesis of hydronephrosis may include vesicoureteral reflux or occur in conditions of excessive flow through the collection system, such as with habitual water drinking or diabetes insipidus.

ETIOLOGY

The disorders that lead to urinary tract obstruction may first be separated into congenital and acquired causes. This classification may be further refined by considering the anatomic level of obstruction, that is, from the renal pelvis to the ureterovesicular junction (upper urinary tract) or from the bladder to the urethra (lower urinary tract).

CONGENITAL CAUSES

There are many congenital malformations that may cause hydronephrosis, occurring at any level from the ureteropelvic junction (UPJ) to the urethral meatus. For purposes of this discussion, only congenital UPJ obstruction will be considered, because this is by far the most common congenital urologic disorder causing obstruction in adults.

Typically, congenital UPJ obstruction is due to the presence of an adynamic segment of the ureter, with resultant failure of peristalsis. Occasionally, but much less often, a patient may have a ureteral stricture at this site.[2]

UPJ obstruction may present in a variety of ways. Flank pain is quite common, often in the setting of increased urinary flow (i.e., with excess fluid or alcohol intake). Other, less common, presenting symptoms include nephrolithiasis, microscopic hematuria, pyelonephritis, gross hematuria, chronic renal insufficiency, or nonspecific abdominal pain. Alternatively, the disorder may be recognized when a patient undergoes a radiocontrast procedure for another reason.

The diagnosis is typically made by excretory urography (XU), which shows delayed excretion of tracer on the affected side accompanied by dilation of the renal pelvis and calyceal system. If the XU is equivocal, a diuretic enhanced study, which increases flow through the collecting system, may reveal the abnormality. Ultrasound and CT may be useful in ruling out other entities in the differential diagnosis of obstruction.

ACQUIRED CAUSES

In addition to categorization by anatomic level, acquired causes of urinary tract obstruction may be further divided into those causes that originate in the urinary tract (intrinsic causes) and those that are a result of external compression (extrinsic causes). Intrinsic causes may be further subdivided into intraluminal and intramural causes (Table 134-1).

Blockage of urinary flow at any site from the renal tubules themselves to the distal urethra may cause urinary tract obstruction. Processes above the bladder neck need to be bilateral, or occur in a solitary functioning kidney, to cause complete anuric obstruction.

Intrinsic Causes
Intraluminal Causes
Disorders that cause obstruction at the level of the renal tubules include crystal-induced disease, uric acid nephropathy, and cast nephropathy secondary to multiple myeloma.

TABLE 134-1. ACQUIRED INTRINSIC CAUSES OF URINARY TRACT OBSTRUCTION

Upper Urinary Tract		Lower Urinary Tract	
Intraluminal	**Intramural**	**Intraluminal**	**Intramural**
Renal tubules	Ureter (including UPJ and UVJ)	Bladder	Bladder
Casts (myeloma)	Strictures	Urolithiasis	Neuromuscular disease
Crystals (acyclovir, indinavir,	Neoplasms	Blood clots	Post CVA
sulfonamides)	Polyps	Neoplasms	Diabetes mellitus
Uric acid nephropathy	Schistosomiasis	Urethra	Multiple sclerosis
Ureter (including UPJ and UVJ)	Tuberculosis	Urolithiasis	Spinal cord injury
Urolithiasis		Blood clots	Medications
Blood clots		Neoplasms	Anticholinergics
Neoplasms			Narcotics
Sloughed papillae			Schistosomiasis
			Urethra
			Strictures

UPJ, ureteropelvic junction; UVJ, ureterovesical junction; CVA, cerebrovascular accident.

Crystal-induced renal failure is often a complication of acyclovir, indinavir, or trimethoprim therapy.

Nephrolithiasis is a common cause of an acquired, intraluminal obstruction at the level of the ureter. Typically the obstruction occurs at one of the three narrowest portions of the ureter: the UPJ, the UVJ, or the point at which the ureter crosses over the pelvic brim. Most renal stones cause acute, intermittent obstruction, but some of the rarer stone types, such as struvite and cysteine stones, may lead to chronic obstruction and permanent renal damage. Neoplasms, blood clots, sloughed renal papillae, and genitourinary tuberculosis are other, rarer causes of intrinsic obstruction at the level of the ureter.

Acquired intraluminal causes of obstruction at the level of the bladder and urethra are similar to those of the ureter, with urolithiasis, malignancies, and blood clots being the main offenders. Worldwide, infection with *Schistosoma hematobium* with resulting fibrosis is a common reason for bladder obstruction.[3] While rare in industrialized countries, it should be considered when confronted with patients from endemic areas such as Africa and the Middle East. In addition to the bladder, the ureters may be involved as well.

Intramural Causes

Intramural causes of upper urinary tract obstruction are uncommon; they include strictures, tumors, and polyps. Intramural obstruction is more common in the lower urinary tract, especially when one includes functional defects due to abnormal neuromuscular function. Common causes of functional obstruction include neurogenic bladder from diabetes, multiple sclerosis, spinal cord injury, or previous cerebrovascular accidents. Medications such as anticholinergic drugs or narcotic analgesics may cause functional urinary tract obstruction. The elderly are especially susceptible to the effects of medications.

Extrinsic Obstruction

There are many potential causes of extrinsic obstruction of the urinary tract; the more common of these are presented in Table 134-2.

Unilateral hydronephrosis of some degree, right side greater than left, is present in the majority of pregnancies by the third trimester. This is thought to be due to mechanical compression by the gravid uterus. Typically, the dilatation is asymptomatic, no treatment is needed, and it resolves after delivery. There are case reports, however, of bilateral ureteral obstruction by the gravid uterus with resultant renal failure.[4-6]

Malignancies with retroperitoneal lymphadenopathy may cause ureteral obstruction. The primary tumor varies but may include those of the colon, prostate, bladder, uterus, or cervix. Hematologic malignancies can also cause obstruction due to enlarged retroperitoneal lymph nodes.

Retroperitoneal fibrosis may also cause obstruction by encasement of the ureters. The etiology of retroperitoneal fibrosis is varied and may be either idiopathic or secondary to a variety of infectious (especially genitourinary tuberculosis), malignant, traumatic, autoimmune, or drug-related causes. The interested reader is referred to a general urology textbook for further details.

Often, retroperitoneal processes may cause obstruction without obvious evidence of hydroureter or hydronephrosis. Clinicians should always remain attuned to this possibility and consider using a functional study to establish the diagnosis.

TABLE 134–2. EXTRINSIC CAUSES OF URINARY TRACT OBSTRUCTION

Urinary System

Prostatic disease
  Benign prostatic hypertrophy
  Prostatic carcinoma
Other malignancies
  Bladder
  Renal cell carcinoma

Obstetric-Gynecologic

Pregnancy
Malignancies
  Cervical
  Ovarian
  Endometrial
Fibroids
Endometriosis
Ovarian abscess

Gastrointestinal System

Metastatic colon carcinoma
Crohn's disease
Diverticulitis

Hematologic System

Lymphoma
Leukemia (mainly in children)

Vascular Disease

Aortic aneurysm
Iliac aneurysm

Retroperitoneal Fibrosis

Other Retroperitoneal Diseases
Lymphadenopathy
Malignant
Infections
Hematomas
Granulomatous disease

Another cause of extrinsic obstruction at the level of the ureters is abdominal aortic aneurysms (AAA). Abdominal aortic aneurysms can cause obstruction via direct compression of the ureters, by fibrosis or, less commonly, inflammation. Iliac vessel aneurysms may also cause obstruction, although less frequently than AAA.

Extrinsic obstruction at the level of bladder and urethra is more common in men. It is typically due to prostatic pathology—either benign prostatic hypertrophy or prostate cancer.

CLINICAL PRESENTATION

The clinical presentation of urinary tract obstruction can be quite varied, depending on factors such as the acuity, severity (complete vs. partial, unilateral vs. bilateral), and the anatomic location.

PAIN

Patients with acute ureteral obstruction, as with nephrolithiasis, typically present with colicky pain, often severe, with nausea and vomiting, mimicking an abdominal emergency.

Partial ureteral obstruction may present as chronic dull flank pain. Acute lower urinary tract obstruction may present as abdominal pain due to a distended bladder or with back pain.

LOWER URINARY TRACT SYMPTOMS

Patients with lower urinary tract obstruction may be asymptomatic, or they may present with symptoms such as urgency, hesitancy, nocturia, weak stream, and frequency.

CHANGES IN URINE OUTPUT

Changes in urine output are common during obstruction. Complete bilateral obstruction (or unilateral in a patient with a solitary functioning kidney) is one of a small number of causes of complete anuria. However, it must be kept in mind that urinary tract obstruction may present with any degree of urine output: anuria, oliguria, normal urine output, or polyuria. As will be discussed later, urinary tract obstruction may interfere with tubular sodium reabsorption and the urinary concentrating mechanism. Therefore, a patient with partial obstruction and decreased glomerular filtration rate (GFR) may exhibit polyuria owing to defective tubular reabsorption of salt and water. These patients are at risk of volume depletion and dehydration.

RENAL FAILURE

Typically if the obstruction is unilateral, and the unaffected kidney is without disease, the plasma creatinine concentration will not change significantly. This type of obstruction may remain clinically quiescent for an extended period of time before coming to clinical attention. Slowly progressing, chronic causes of obstruction may not lead to any symptoms referable to the urinary tract. Patients with these disorders, such as prostatic disease or retroperitoneal fibrosis, may not come to medical attention until they present with complaints consistent with uremia, such as fatigue, anorexia, nausea, and vomiting.

INFECTION

An obstructed urinary tract is more susceptible to infection than an anatomically normal system, especially if the obstruction is at the level of the bladder. There is often residual urine in the bladder, which provides an excellent culture medium for bacteria. A renal stone causing the obstruction may also be a nidus for infection. Sometimes, the presence of recurrent infection may be the first clue to an anatomic abnormality. In fact, in men, a solitary urinary tract infection is cause for a workup to define urinary tract anatomy.

HYPERTENSION

Urinary tract obstruction may lead to hypertension by several mechanisms. The most common is that the ensuing renal insufficiency may lead to excess salt and water retention, culminating in volume-mediated hypertension. A situation in which the obstructed kidney produces excess renin, similar to renovascular disease, has also been described.[7-9]

LABORATORY VALUES

There are no specific findings in the laboratory examination to suggest that an obstruction is present. The urinalysis may be bland or may include red blood cells (in the setting of a stone or malignancy) or white blood cells (in the setting of infection). An experienced observer may also be able to discern crystals in a freshly voided urine. Calculation of the fractional excretion of sodium (FeNa) may reveal it to be less than 1% in acute obstruction, but greater than 1% when the obstruction is chronic, owing to tubule dysfunction. Blood tests may show no abnormalities or may show values consistent with renal failure, such as elevated blood urea nitrogen, creatinine, and phosphorus levels and decreased calcium, bicarbonate, and hemoglobin values. The blood tests may also be indicative of a renal tubular acidosis, with or without hyperkalemia.

PATHOPHYSIOLOGY

Over the past three decades various animal models have furthered our understanding of the renal response and adaptation to obstruction. There are changes in renal blood flow, GFR, and tubular function.

CHANGES IN RENAL BLOOD FLOW

Acute

There are no human data available, but animal models have suggested a transient increase in renal blood flow in the early stages of urinary tract obstruction.[10] Studies in anesthetized dogs have shown an acute increase in renal blood flow of about 30% within 15 minutes of complete ureteral obstruction.[11] Similar results have been seen in cat and rat models.[12] Local production of vasodilatory cytokines, such as prostaglandin E_2, seems to be at least partially responsible for this renal vasodilatation, because this response can be inhibited by pretreatment with prostaglandin inhibitors, such as indomethacin.[13] This phase of increased blood flow lasts approximately 2 hours.[12]

After this time period there is increased intrarenal resistance, with a decrease in renal blood flow. Canine studies reveal renal blood flow to be 40% to 50% of control after 24 hours of complete unilateral ureteral obstruction.[11,14]

Chronic

The decrease in renal blood flow seen at 24 hours persists in the chronic stage. Studies have demonstrated that blood flow in the affected kidney decreases to 12% to 50% of control values when the obstruction is of long standing.[14-16] This decrease in blood flow appears to be mediated by intrarenal vasoconstrictive agents, most notably angiotensin II and thromboxane A_2. Animal models have shown that angiotensin II levels are enhanced in obstructed kidneys,[10,12] and pretreatment with angiotensin-converting enzyme inhibitors can attenuate the vasoconstriction, and ultimately the decrease in GFR, after release of a 24-hour complete unilateral ureteric obstruction.[17,18] Thromboxane is thought to be produced both from intrinsic glomerular cells and leukocytes that have infiltrated the obstructed kidney.[12] Further studies have shown that treatment with thromboxane synthase inhibitors increases GFR after release of an obstruction.[19] Thus, it appears that angiotensin II and thromboxane

A_2 are important mediators of the postobstructive renal vaso-constriction and decrease in GFR.

Changes in Glomerular Filtration Rate

Ultrafiltration in the kidney, or the GFR, is determined by the interaction of Starling's forces between the glomerular capillary and the tubules.

In the immediate phase of obstruction, tubular hydrostatic pressure (P_t) rises and GFR may decrease on that basis. However, this cannot explain all of the ensuing decrease in GFR. With both bilateral obstruction and unilateral obstruction, P_t will decrease over time.[1] In unilateral obstruction, P_t may return to normal levels, whereas in bilateral obstruction the P_t will fall, albeit to a level that is still elevated compared with the baseline value.[1] Nonetheless, GFR does not improve as the P_t improves. On the contrary, GFR continues to decline. The main factor responsible for the decrease in GFR at this time is the decrease in glomerular hydrostatic pressure due to vasoconstriction as discussed in the preceding paragraphs.

Effects of Obstruction on Tubular Function

Urinary tract obstruction disrupts tubular function in several ways, resulting in impairments in sodium reabsorption, potassium secretion, urinary acidification, as well as urinary concentrating and diluting abilities.

Sodium Reabsorption

The effects of obstruction on sodium excretion are different depending on whether the obstruction is unilateral or bilateral. Animal data show that, after relief of a unilateral obstruction, there is little difference between the sodium excretion of the two kidneys.[20] Because the GFR of the affected kidney is low, this implies an increase in fractional excretion of sodium, and, therefore, a defect in tubular sodium reabsorption.

In contrast, relief of bilateral urinary tract obstruction may result in striking increases in salt and water excretion, up to five to nine times normal,[20] implying a considerable tubular defect. To a degree, this response is appropriate, ridding the body of excess salt and water accumulated during the obstruction. However, experimental evidence suggests that this does not account for all of the salt and water diuresis. Rats' after 1 day post relief of bilateral urinary obstruction show increased sodium and water excretion, even if food and water are withheld during this time.[1]

The tubular segments that may be affected have been evaluated using micropuncture techniques. Obstruction affects superficial (cortical) and deep (juxtamedullary) nephrons differently.

In unilateral obstruction, the superficial nephrons actually hyper-resorb sodium, with about 1.9% of the filtered sodium remaining at the junction between the distal convoluted tubule (DCT) and the cortical collecting duct (CCD) (compared with 5% in a nonobstructed kidney).[20] There is sodium wasting in the juxtramedullary nephrons, and when the superficial nephrons and the juxtamedullary nephrons combine their tubular fluid (i.e., at the tip of the renal papilla) the result is an increase in the fractional excretion of sodium (2.5% vs. ~ 1%).[20]

In bilateral obstruction, the situation is similar. The superficial nephrons have a slight defect, with 7% of the filtered sodium remaining at the DCT/CCD junction.[20] The juxtamedullary nephrons are more severely affected, with 62% of the filtered sodium remaining at the tip of the loop of Henle.[20] Furthermore, bilateral renal obstruction results in sodium addition, along the course of the medullary collecting duct, in stark contrast to its normal reabsorptive function. The combination of poor juxtamedullary nephron reabsorption and dysfunction of the medullary collecting duct leads to a sharp increase in both the fractional excretion of sodium and the absolute amount of sodium excreted. The defects in renal sodium handling are summarized in Figure 134-1. This tubular dysfunction is one of the mechanisms of postobstructive diuresis (see later).

Recent studies have elucidated a mechanism for the decrease in sodium reabsorption. Studies in rats have shown a down-regulation of the major sodium transporting proteins in the nephron. These include the sodium-hydrogen exchanger (Na^+-H^+) and the sodium phosphate (Na^+-Pi) cotransporter in the proximal tubule, the Na^+-K^+-2 chloride (Na^+-K^+-$2Cl^-$) transporter in the loop of Henle, and the thiazide-sensitive cotransporter (TSC) in the distal tubule.[21] Furthermore, activity of the Na^+, K^+-ATPase was also shown to be down-regulated, decreasing sodium efflux from the cell, thereby decreasing the transcellular concentration gradient that favors sodium reabsorption.[21]

Another factor when considering the defect in tubular sodium reabsorption is the role of circulating hormones. Studies have demonstrated that rats with bilateral, but not unilateral, obstruction have increased levels of circulating atrial natriuretic peptide.[22]

Urinary Concentration and Dilution Defects

Patients with urinary tract obstruction often have urine that is iso-osmotic to plasma, indicating the presence of concentration and dilution defects. The obstructed kidney is unable to establish the normal hypertonic medullary interstitium, owing at least in part to the decrease in Na^+-K^+-$2Cl^-$ transporter activity described earlier. This affects dilution capacity directly, as reabsorption of sodium without water in this nephron segment is the mechanism of urinary dilution. Urinary concentration is also affected, as the hypertonic medullary interstitium is necessary to promote water movement through aquaporin channels in the collecting ducts. In addition to the defect in generating a hypertonic interstitium, the obstructed kidney has a defect in response to antidiuretic hormone.[23,24] Normally, ADH causes the insertion of aquaporins into the luminal membrane of the collecting ducts. Obstructed kidneys do not respond normally to either endogenous or exogenous ADH. The defect appears to be reduced expression of aquaporin-2,[25,26] although there may be reduced trafficking into the membrane as well.[27]

Acidification and Potassium Secretion

Patients with obstructive uropathy may exhibit reduced ability to acidify their urine. There are several potential causes for the decreased hydrogen ion excretion. A hyperchloremic non–anion gap acidosis associated with hyperkalemia may be seen in some patients with obstructive uropathy.[28] This is thought to be due primarily to hyporeninemic hypoaldosteronism (a decrease in aldosterone secretion due to a decrease in renin release). Lack of aldosterone also directly decreases potassium secretion in the distal tubule. Hyperkalemia decreases proximal tubular ammoniagenesis; and because ammonia is needed to "trap" the secreted proton, the amount of acid that can be excreted is limited.

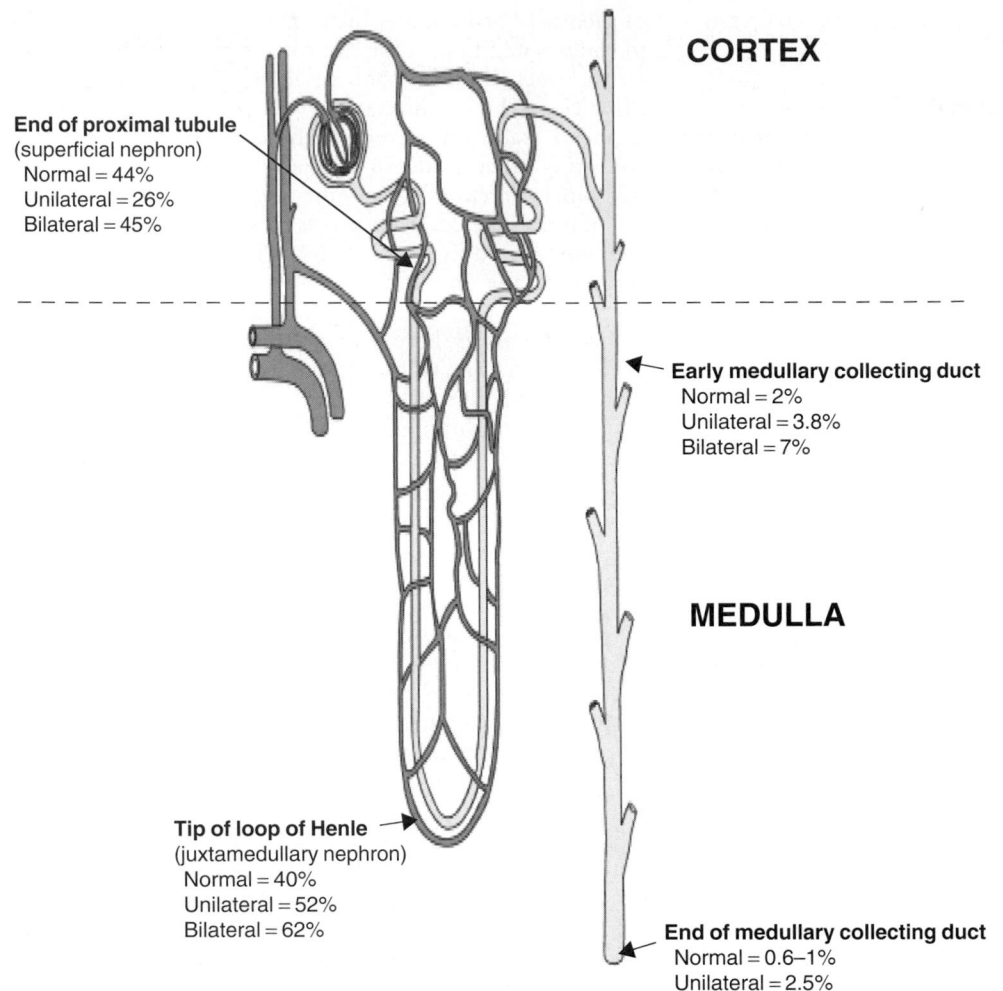

CORTEX

End of proximal tubule
(superficial nephron)
Normal = 44%
Unilateral = 26%
Bilateral = 45%

Early medullary collecting duct
Normal = 2%
Unilateral = 3.8%
Bilateral = 7%

MEDULLA

Tip of loop of Henle
(juxtamedullary nephron)
Normal = 40%
Unilateral = 52%
Bilateral = 62%

End of medullary collecting duct
Normal = 0.6–1%
Unilateral = 2.5%
Bilateral = 12%

FIGURE 134–1. Amount of sodium remaining at various points along the nephron in normal kidneys, after relief of unilateral obstruction and after relief of bilateral obstruction. Note the increase in sodium between the early medullary collecting duct and the end of the medullary collecting duct after relief of bilateral obstruction. (Data from Frøkiær J, Christensen BM, Marples D, et al: Down-regulation of aquaporin-2 parallels changes in renal water excretion in unilateral ureteral obstruction. Am J Physiol 1997;273: F213-F223.)

These patients, however, can acidify their urine in the setting of systemic acidosis (because titratable acidity is not affected), so the acidosis is typically mild and self limited. A minority of patients may present with a type I distal renal tubular acidosis, where hydrogen excretion itself (not ammoniagenesis) is affected.[12] These individuals cannot acidify their urine in the presence of an acidic serum pH and are therefore at risk for severe acidosis.

Postobstructive Diuresis

After relief of bilateral obstruction, or of obstruction of a solitary kidney, patients may experience copious urine output, referred to as a postobstructive diuresis. There are many factors that may lead to this large urine output. Poor renal function during obstruction leads to the retention of urea. When the obstruction is relieved, the urea acts as an osmotic diuretic, resulting in the excretion of water and salt.[29] Also, as previously discussed, bilateral obstruction leads to production of atrial natriuretic peptide.[22] When the obstruction is relieved, the atrial natriuretic peptide may lead to an appropriate diuresis to rid the body of excess sodium and free water.

At times, the diuresis may be inappropriate. As noted earlier, the tubules lose their ability to concentrate urine and to reabsorb sodium. The resulting water and sodium diuresis may be excessive and lead to hypernatremia and volume contraction. Finally, the postobstructive diuresis may be iatrogenic. When faced with a large, but appropriate, diuresis, physicians often reflexively administer intravenous fluids. The large diuresis after release of obstruction is often appropriate, and the physician may be driving further diuresis with the continued intravenous administration of fluid.

As illustrated earlier, patients need not receive intravenous fluid solely for a large urine output. Fluid administration should be reserved for those patients who appear clinically volume depleted. Of course, electrolytes need to be monitored and repleted regardless of the patient's volume status.

Other Tubular Functions

Magnesium excretion is increased after relief of both unilateral and bilateral obstruction.[20] The presumed mechanism is decreased absorption by the loop of Henle.[20] Data regarding calcium excretion are conflicting, and the exact fate of calcium is uncertain. Phosphate excretion is markedly increased after relief of bilateral obstruction, probably in part owing to decreased expression of Na⁺-Pi in the proximal tubule (the major site of phosphate reabsorption).[20] In contrast, phosphate excretion is decreased in unilateral obstruction.[20]

Figure 134-2 illustrates the tubular defects that may be encountered in the setting of urinary tract obstruction.

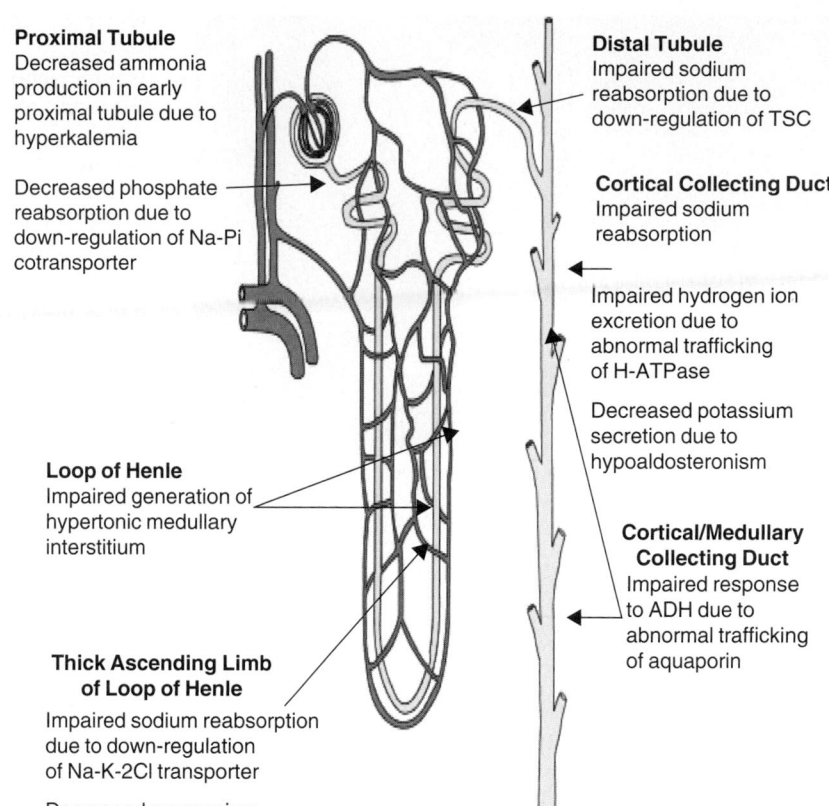

Proximal Tubule
Decreased ammonia production in early proximal tubule due to hyperkalemia

Decreased phosphate reabsorption due to down-regulation of Na-Pi cotransporter

Distal Tubule
Impaired sodium reabsorption due to down-regulation of TSC

Cortical Collecting Duct
Impaired sodium reabsorption

Impaired hydrogen ion excretion due to abnormal trafficking of H-ATPase

Decreased potassium secretion due to hypoaldosteronism

Loop of Henle
Impaired generation of hypertonic medullary interstitium

Cortical/Medullary Collecting Duct
Impaired response to ADH due to abnormal trafficking of aquaporin

Thick Ascending Limb of Loop of Henle
Impaired sodium reabsorption due to down-regulation of Na-K-2Cl transporter

Decreased magnesium reabsorption

FIGURE 134-2. Potential tubular defects after relief of bilateral obstruction. Not all defects will be present in every patient. Also note there is a difference in tubular function after relief of bilateral versus unilateral obstruction. See text for details. Na^+-K^+-$2Cl^-$, sodium-potassium-2 chloride transporter; TSC, thiazide sensitive cotransporter; ADH, antidiuretic hormone; H^+-ATPase, hydrogen ATPase.

RADIOLOGIC EVALUATION

PLAIN ABDOMINAL RADIOGRAPHY

Plain abdominal films may be useful in that they can detect radiopaque stones. There are severe limitations to this modality, however, because radiolucent stones or any other causes of obstruction will not be detected. Furthermore, it is not always easy to distinguish nephrolithiasis from vascular phleboliths.

EXCRETORY UROGRAPHY

Excretory urography was the modality of choice in the past, although ultrasound and CT have now largely superseded it. The benefit of XU is that it can provide both anatomic and functional information. Obstruction is suggested by the presence of a dense nephrogram, a nonexistent pyelogram, or dilatation of the collecting system.[30] There are several drawbacks to this modality. First, it requires a dose of intravenous contrast agent that one would rather avoid in a patient with renal insufficiency. Second, the uptake of the dye into the kidney is dependent on GFR, and thus the test is limited when GFR is impaired.

ULTRASOUND

Ultrasound has several advantages over XU, although it does have some drawbacks as well. Ultrasound is inexpensive, is usually readily available, and does not expose the patient to either contrast agent or radiation. It is very sensitive in detecting hydronephrosis, with documented sensitivities of 98% (Fig. 134-3).[30] The specificity is 78%.[30] The false-positive tests occur because there are nonobstructive causes of hydronephrosis, as previously mentioned. Furthermore, renal cysts may be mistaken for hydronephrosis, depending on anatomic location.[31] Another disadvantage is that ultrasound often does not provide anatomic information regarding the cause of the obstruction.

Several features of the ultrasound have been examined to better evaluate for obstruction. Ureteral jets are Doppler representations of urine flow from the ureters into the bladder.[30] The normal ureteral jet is pulsatile, corresponding to the pulsatile nature of ureteral peristalsis. The absence of ureteral jets suggests complete obstruction, although this may also be seen with other causes of anuria. Partial obstruction may present as an abnormal pattern of the ureteral jet, such as a slow continuous jet of weak intensity. In a study in patients with nephrolithiasis it was found that the ureteral jet patterns are usually abnormal (absent) in patients with high-grade obstruction but often not significantly different from controls in patients with low-grade obstruction.[32]

The resistive index (RI) has also been advocated as a means to detect obstructive processes. The RI is the difference between the peak systolic velocity and the peak diastolic velocity divided by the peak systolic velocity.[30] The theory behind using RIs is that during obstruction, increased tubular pressure will cause vascular compression and impede blood flow (both during systole and diastole) and the RI will rise. The major problem in using RIs to detect obstruction is the lack of specificity, because a large number of unrelated conditions, such as intrinsic kidney disease of any cause, will cause the RIs to rise. Furthermore, the RIs will not be elevated early in the course of obstruction, during the initial vasodilatory phase.

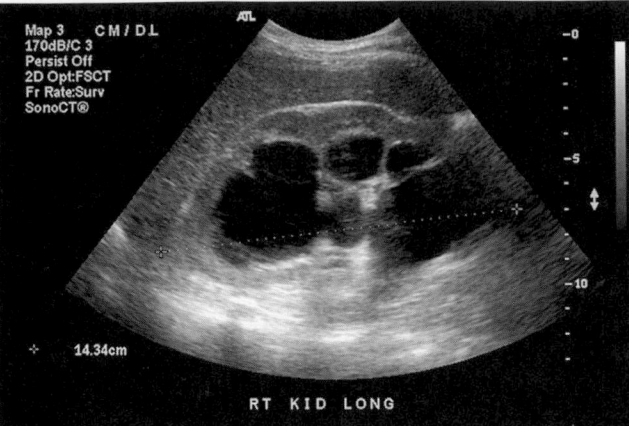

FIGURE 134–3. Typical appearance of a hydronephrotic kidney showing renal pelvis and calyceal dilatation. Note the increase in kidney length (14.34 cm) compared with normal (~10-11 cm).

COMPUTED TOMOGRAPHY

Computed tomography has become more popular since the advent of spiral scanning, which obviates the need for oral or intravenous contrast medium. Benefits of CT include visualization of renal stones that are radiolucent on plain film and excellent visualization of the retroperitoneal area. The latter benefit makes CT ideal to detect retroperitoneal fibrosis or obstruction due to retroperitoneal lymphadenopathy. Studies have shown that when compared with XU, CT is as accurate in detecting obstruction and more helpful in determining the anatomic site.[33] Spiral CT is now the imaging procedure of choice in most institutions for the evaluation of suspected nephrolithiasis. In addition to its excellent visualization of the collecting system, CT has the benefit of looking at other organ systems and ruling in or out other conditions in the differential diagnosis. The major drawback to CT is its cost and radiation exposure.

ISOTOPE RENOGRAPHY

Isotope renography is also employed in the evaluation of suspected obstruction (Fig. 134-4). Radiographic tracers are injected, and the patient is then imaged with a scintillation counter. Renal uptake and excretion can be measured. The utility of this test is more functional than anatomic. The sensitivity of renography can be improved by administering a loop diuretic such as furosemide before the scan. The increase in urine flow may unmask an obstruction and turn a previously negative scan positive. This test does not, however, provide the anatomic information that can be gained from an intravenous urogram or a CT scan.

TREATMENT

Urinary tract obstruction may be treated conservatively or with an intervention aimed at establishing patency of the urinary tract. Indications that mandate more aggressive intervention include the presence of infection, an unacceptable symptom complex (typically pain in an upper urinary tract obstruction or excessive lower urinary tract symptoms when this site is obstructed), or decrease in renal function.

Lower urinary tract obstruction may be relieved simply by inserting a urethral catheter. A suprapubic catheter may be needed for urethral trauma or strictures. Once patency is obtained further decisions regarding the timing and nature of definitive treatment should be made in conjunction with a urologist. If the patient's renal function is stable and there are no infectious complications, treatment need not be urgent.

Treatment of upper urinary tract obstruction may include specific therapies based on the cause (i.e., lithotripsy for urolithiasis or radiation therapy for obstructions due to malignancy) and nonspecific treatments designed to decompress the urinary system. For an upper urinary tract obstruction, the options include the placement of nephrostomy tubes and either antegrade or retrograde (i.e., cystoscopically inserted) ureteral stents. Concomitant with intervention

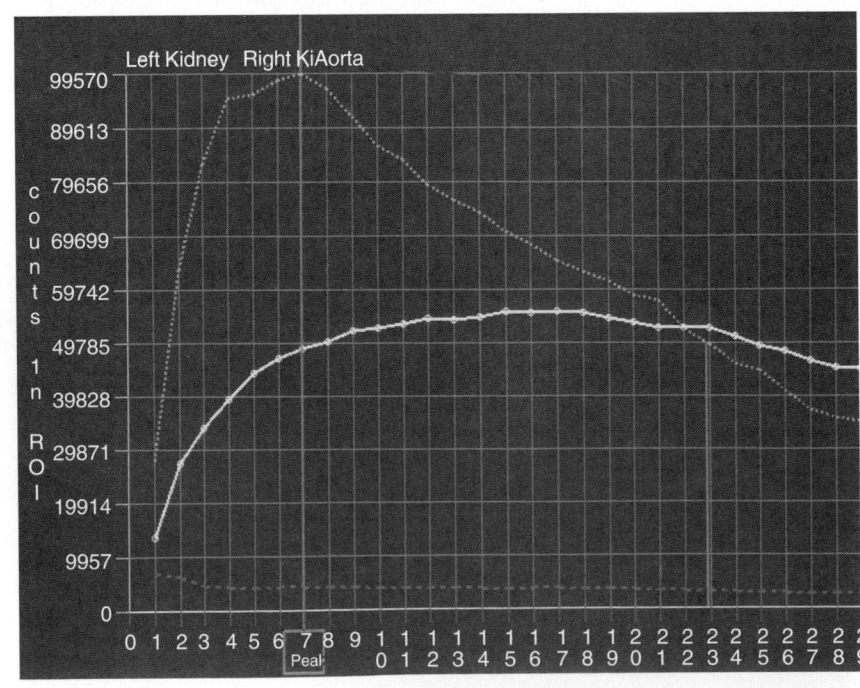

FIGURE 134–4. Renogram showing left-sided obstruction. Note that both kidneys take up the tracer. On the right side this is followed by an excretion of the tracer, whereas on the left the tracer remains at peak value.

efforts, medical therapy should include antibiotic support if infection is present. The metabolic derangements of acute renal failure, such as hyperkalemia, should be addressed, and dialysis should not be withheld while awaiting decompressive therapy. Once drainage is established one must then decide whether to proceed with definitive surgical correction or to consider nephrectomy. This decision requires an estimation of the potential of renal recovery.

RECOVERY OF RENAL FUNCTION

Unfortunately, the data regarding prediction as to whether and when an obstructed kidney will regain function are not conclusive. The degree of obstruction on ultrasound or XU does not correlate with the potential for renal recovery.[34] No imaging modality has proven reliable in estimating the potential for renal recovery, although cortical thinning on ultrasound and less than 10% value of GFR or renal blood flow on isotope scanning portend a poorer prognosis.[34]

In contrast, there is evidence that the likelihood of recovery of kidney function after an obstruction is related to the duration and severity of the obstruction. Animal studies indicate that the longer the duration of obstruction, the less the degree of recovery.[10] Further studies suggest that even if the GFR does return to normal, as many as 15% of nephrons may be lost and the normal GFR is due to hypertrophy and hyperfiltration of the remaining nephrons.[35] Human studies are lacking, but the data suggest that the majority of kidney function will be recovered within 14 days,[36] although some patients may take months for complete recovery. The maximum duration at which an obstructed kidney will regain function is unknown and is probably influenced by the severity of the obstruction (i.e., complete vs. partial).

Another avenue to estimate potential renal recovery is via a kidney biopsy. In obstruction, as in most other kidney diseases, the amount of tubulointerstitial fibrosis provides a guide as to the likelihood of recovery of function. Obviously, the more fibrosis present, the more significant the kidney injury, and the less chance of recovery; however, the exact relationship between the tubulointerstitial changes and the degree of recovery has not been established.

The fact that it cannot be concluded with confidence whether the kidney will recover mandates that patients with any degree of obstruction and renal insufficiency have the obstruction relieved and have serial determinations of renal function. Partial recovery has been seen even after months of hemodialysis.[37,38]

ANNOTATED REFERENCES

Li C, Wang W, Kwon T-H, et al: Altered expression of major renal Na+ transporters in rats with bilateral ureteral obstruction and release of obstruction. Am J Physiol 2003;285:F889-F901.
This article provides the molecular basis for the salt-wasting observed after relief of bilateral obstruction. The levels of expression of renal sodium transporters were examined in rats after 24 hours of bilateral ureteral obstruction and at days 3 and 14 after relief of the obstruction. This article demonstrates the down-regulation of essentially all transporters during obstruction and the rates at which transporter function begins to normalize.

Moody T, Vaughan ED Jr, Gillenwater J: The renal hemodynamic response to chronic unilateral complete ureteral occlusion. Invest Urol 1970;8:78-90.
The authors of this article were among the first to examine progressive hemodynamic changes in the ipsilateral and contralateral kidneys after total unilateral ureteral occlusion. This study showed that ipsilateral renal blood flow continued to decrease, despite the decrease in ureteral (i.e., tubular) pressure. This led future investigators to search for hemodynamic mediators of the changes in renal blood flow after obstruction and not simply ascribe the changes to changes in ureteral pressure.

Smith RC, Rosenfield AT, Choe KA, et al: Acute flank pain: Comparison of non–contrast-enhanced CT and intravenous urography. Radiology 1995;194:789-794.
This article directly compared nonenhanced CT with intravenous (or excretory) urography in the evaluation of obstruction in patients who present with acute flank pain. The major findings were that CT was as good as excretory urography in determining whether an obstruction was present, but CT was better at identifying stones as the cause of the obstruction. Subsequently, nonenhanced CT has become the modality of choice for suspected urolithiasis.

Wen J, Frokiaer J, Jorgensen T, et al: Obstructive nephropathy: An update of the experimental research. Urol Res 1999;27:29-39.
The authors review data obtained from animal models of ureteral obstruction. Both antenatal and adult models of complete and partial unilateral, as well as bilateral obstruction, are discussed. They also review the effects of obstruction on renal function, blood flow, and morphology, as well as data regarding the potential for renal recovery.

Yarger W, Schocken D, Harris R: Obstructive nephropathy in the rat: Possible roles for the renin-angiotensin system, prostaglandins, and thromboxanes in postobstructive renal function. J Clin Invest 1980;65:400-412.
This study examines the roles of the renin-angiotensin system, prostaglandins, and thromboxanes in the vasoconstriction of the postobstructed kidney. By using various inhibitors of these compounds the investigators concluded that angiotensin II, thromboxanes, and prostaglandins are important mediators of renal hemodynamic changes in the postobstructed kidney.

Chapter 135

CONTRAST DYE–INDUCED NEPHROPATHY

Brendan J. Barrett

KEY POINTS

1. **The likelihood of contrast nephropathy** is largely determined by the presence of risk factors, with preexisting renal impairment, with or without diabetes, reduced intravascular volume, and contrast dose being the major ones.

2. **The pathogenesis remains somewhat unclear** but seems to involve ischemic and direct toxic injury to renal tubules.

3. **Although contrast dye–induced renal dysfunction is often transient,** some cases require permanent renal replacement therapy and mortality is increased, particularly in those requiring dialysis.

4. **Management of established cases of contrast nephropathy remains supportive.**

5. **Prevention of contrast dye–induced renal injury** is important. The need for a contrast agent should be carefully considered and the dose used minimized in those at risk for nephropathy. Deliberate saline hydration may be indicated if volume excess is not a problem. Both *N*-acetylcysteine and theophylline are now recommended based on trials demonstrating efficacy, with the former being easier to use in very ill patients.

The nephrotoxicity of iodinated radiocontrast media was implicated as the third most common cause of acute renal failure in hospitalized patients in the early 1980s and again in the late 1990s.[1,2] The increasing use of procedures requiring radiographic contrast media, possibly combined with increasing age and comorbidity of the treated population, contributes to the continuing importance of contrast nephropathy. Contrast nephropathy is commonly defined as an acute decline in renal function after the administration of an intravascular iodinated contrast agent, in the absence of other causes. For research purposes, definitions such as a proportionate (e.g., 25% or 50%) or absolute (e.g., 0.5 mg/dL, 50 μmol/L) rise in serum creatinine concentration above the baseline value are commonly used. Awareness of the nephrotoxicity of contrast dye and the factors predisposing to it have improved over time to the point that clinicians may now overestimate the risk associated with some specific medical conditions.[3] Much of the recent research on contrast nephropathy has been directed at prevention, and this is discussed after a review of the epidemiology, pathogenesis, clinical features, diagnosis, and management.

EPIDEMIOLOGY AND RISK FACTORS

Very mild, transient changes in renal function occur in almost all patients given an intravascular radiocontrast agent.[4] The exact incidence of clinically significant contrast nephropathy is not clear, because prospective studies have produced a wide range of estimates. The inconsistencies are at least partly explained by differences in criteria used to define the condition, the level of risk in the population studied, and the degree to which other potential causes of acute renal failure have contributed. The risk of contrast nephropathy is strongly influenced by the presence of preexisting renal impairment, especially combined with diabetes mellitus, cardiac failure, and high doses of contrast media.[5,6] Most prospective studies have indicated that the risk begins to rise when the serum creatinine concentration before administration of the contrast agent exceeds 1.2 to 1.5 mg/dL (105 to 130 μmol/L). Diabetics with normal renal function do not have a significantly increased risk of contrast nephropathy.[7] Conditions that reduce effective arterial volume, including dehydration, cardiac failure, cirrhosis, and nephrosis, may also increase the risk. Other potential risk factors include advanced age and concurrent use of nonsteroidal anti-inflammatory agents.

One large observational study reported an incidence of 14.5% for contrast nephropathy among patients having cardiac angiography.[8] In the absence of risk factors, the risk of renal failure is lower than this, averaging about 3% in prospective studies.[9] The risk of contrast nephropathy rises dramatically with the number of risk factors present. In one study the incidence rose progressively from 1.2% to 100% as the number of risk factors went from zero to four.[10] Recently reported, prospectively collected registry data suggest that the general incidence of nephropathy requiring dialysis after percutaneous coronary intervention is 0.44%.[6]

PATHOGENESIS

In animals, pathologic findings of contrast nephropathy include vacuolization of proximal tubular cells and congestion of the subcortical medulla.[11] The pathogenesis is not entirely understood, but it is most likely to involve a combination of ischemic and direct tubulotoxic effects.[12] The mechanism of injury may vary by contrast type, partly as a result of differences in tubular secretion and pinocytosis of contrast medium.[13]

Injection of a contrast agent induces a biphasic renal hemodynamic change, with an initial transient increase and then a more prolonged decrease in global renal blood flow.[14] In the period of lower flow, there is cortical vasoconstriction and outer medullary vasodilation and congestion.[11] The cortical vasoconstriction may be due to compression of vessels by increased hydrostatic pressure in tubules and interstitium and by the effects of vasoactive substances, including endothelin, vasopressin, prostacyclin, nitric oxide, and adenosine.[14-18] Tubuloglomerular feedback may play a role with high-osmolality media.[19] Despite medullary vasodilation, medullary hypoxia occurs and may lead to injury due to an imbalance of oxygen demand and supply.[17] Demand is increased by the osmotic diuresis induced by contrast agent excretion.[17] This is reflected clinically by the lower incidence of contrast nephropathy associated with contrast media of low-osmolar or iso-osmolar type.[5,20-22] In addition, factors that impair medullary vasodilation, such as nonsteroidal anti-inflammatory drugs, may worsen contrast nephropathy. Many studies of preventive interventions affecting renal blood flow have been disappointing, but the drugs used may not specifically have moderated the impact of contrast agents on regional oxygen supply and demand. A potential role for direct tubular cell toxicity is suggested by in-vitro studies.[23,24] Oxidant-mediated injury may also play a role.[25-27] Although suggested, convincing data are lacking on the role of tubular obstruction by contrast dye–induced increases in Tamm-Horsfall proteins, uric acid, or oxalate crystals.

CLINICAL FEATURES AND DIAGNOSIS

Patients with contrast nephropathy are generally asymptomatic but have an acute rise in serum creatinine concentration 24 to 72 hours after administration of the contrast agent. The renal failure is usually nonoliguric, but it may be oliguric, especially if there is significant preexisting renal impairment.[28,29] Serum creatinine level typically peaks at 3 days and returns to baseline within 10 days.[14] Clinically significant deterioration is unlikely if the serum creatinine concentration does not increase by more than 0.5 mg/dL within 24 hours.[30] In a minority of cases, the renal failure is severe enough to require dialysis or renal function does not recover to precontrast values. To make an unequivocal diagnosis of contrast nephropathy, other potential causes of acute renal failure must be ruled out. Prerenal factors, atheroembolic disease, and other nephrotoxic insults are high on the list of differential diagnoses. As with acute renal failure in general, contrast nephrotoxicity may be only one of several factors leading to a decline in renal function in a given patient. The relatively rapid onset and typical course of events may help differentiate contrast nephropathy from other causes. Urinalysis may be unremarkable or may show granular casts, tubular cells, or proteinuria. Fractional excretion of sodium can be low.[14,28]

MANAGEMENT AND OUTCOME

In most instances contrast nephropathy never becomes clinically evident and renal function returns to baseline. In more severe cases the management is no different than that for acute renal failure of any other cause. Careful control of fluid and electrolyte balance, avoidance of further nephrotoxic insults, attention to nutrition, and surveillance for complications are generally all that is required, although dialysis may be necessary in the occasional patient.[6,20,31] Vasodilating agents have not been efficacious for the treatment of established contrast nephropathy.[32,33] Prophylactic hemodialysis

soon after administration of a contrast agent in patients with high serum creatinine concentrations has not been of benefit.[34,35] Dialysis does not need to be done for routine removal of contrast medium after imaging in previously dialysis-dependent cases.[36]

Although most patients recover fully, as many as 30% have some degree of permanent renal impairment, which may be partly due to other illnesses present or medications used at the time contrast nephropathy developed.[37] Contrast nephropathy can prolong a hospital stay[33] and may be associated with a twofold to threefold increase in mortality.[38,39] This is particularly true for those cases requiring dialysis.

PREVENTION

As outlined in Figure 135-1, the risk of contrast nephropathy can be reduced by general and specific measures. The first step is to assess the presence of risk factors and the indications for use of a contrast agent. Most risk factors can be detected with a routine history and physical examination. It is not practical or necessary to measure serum creatinine concentration on every patient before use of a contrast agent, but this should be done in those patients with other risk factors.[40] Some risk factors, such as dehydration or cardiac failure, can be at least partially corrected before administering contrast media. Advances in imaging modalities may permit avoidance of contrast agent use in some high-risk cases. If a contrast agent must be given to patients with uncorrected, or uncorrectable, risk factors, the lowest dose possible, preferably of an iso-osmolar agent, should be administered and serum creatinine concentration should be monitored after the procedure.[21,22] In addition, specific prophylactic measures are indicated for high-risk patients. Many specific pathogenetically based prophylactic measures have been tested. These include a "diuretic" approach with

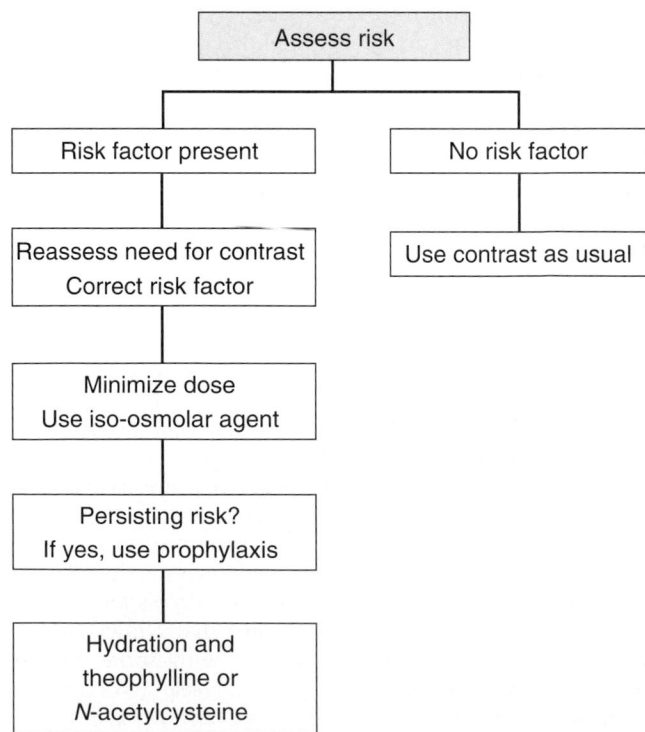

FIGURE 135–1. Recommended approach for minimizing the risk of contrast nephropathy.

deliberate hydration, furosemide, or mannitol, singly or in combination; a "vasodilator" approach with low doses of dopamine, fenoldopam, atrial natriuretic peptide (ANP), captopril, calcium channel blockers, prostaglandin E₁, or endothelin antagonist; and an "antioxidant" approach using theophylline or *N*-acetylcysteine (NAC). The evidence supporting the use of these measures varies.

Both furosemide and mannitol have been associated with increased risk of contrast nephropathy,[41,42] as has an endothelin antagonist.[43] Whereas intravenous infusion of low doses of dopamine has sometimes been associated with benefit in non-diabetics,[44-50] the therapy is cumbersome, costly, and not recommended for routine prophylaxis. Animal studies and initial data in humans suggest promise for a more selective dopamine receptor agonist, fenoldopam.[51,52] An initial clinical trial shows a trend to benefit, but more definitive data are required.[53] Infusion of ANP has also been disappointing.[32,54] Some promising data exist for prostaglandin E₁,[55] calcium blockers,[56-58] and captopril,[59] but further trials are warranted to better establish the efficacy of these approaches.

RECOMMENDED SPECIFIC PROPHYLACTIC REGIMENS

The value of deliberate hydration has been established in a randomized trial versus no therapy,[60] and this forms the basis of most prophylactic regimens. The mechanism of protective effect may include correction or prevention of volume depletion or prevention of protein precipitation in tubules. Although many institutions have used intravenous 0.45% saline at a rate of 1 mL/kg/h, beginning up to 12 hours before contrast agent administration and continuing for up to 24 hours, a recent trial found that 0.9% saline was more effective.[61] Intravenous hydration is not practical for many ambulatory cases, and a small trial suggests that oral prehydration, with intravenous fluid as just described for 6 hours post contrast agent use, may be adequate.[62] Whatever protocol is used, it should be adjusted based on patient tolerance and the degree of diuresis achieved.

In addition to deliberate hydration, either theophylline or NAC can be recommended based on benefit in several clinical trials. Theophylline has shown benefit in several small trials and toxicity has been minor.[4,63-67] No benefit was seen in one small early trial and in one nonrandomized comparative study.[33,68] The trials have included a reasonable proportion of diabetics and patients with renal impairment. Optimal dosing for theophylline is unclear, with single intravenous doses as low as 200 mg being effective. Oral dosing at about 200 mg every 12 hours for 2 days beginning before contrast agent administration also seems reasonable for now. NAC has been tested in many recently reported trials. The initial trial in patients having an intravenous contrast medium administered at a fixed dose of 75 mL was strongly positive.[69] Further trials have largely been done in patients having cardiac angiography.[70-75] All trials have been in patients with stable renal impairment of at least moderate degree, and most have included a high proportion of diabetics. Nonionic, low-osmolality contrast was used at varying doses for most studies. Some of the trials are hard to

interpret because of low power and a lack of blinding. Although the weight of evidence is in favor, a few of the trials failed to show a benefit with NAC.[72-74] There has been some evidence at the usual NAC dose of 600 mg every 12 hours for four doses beginning before contrast agent administration, but that benefit may be limited to those receiving lower doses of the contrast agent.[72] NAC has a short half-life and, because toxicity is very limited, higher or more frequent dosing could be considered in such cases.

CONCLUSION

Contrast nephropathy remains an important problem with significant consequences. The pathogenesis seems to relate to ischemic and possibly direct tubulotoxic injury, especially in the outer medulla. Contrast nephropathy is not common in the absence of other risk factors and these—existing renal impairment, especially with diabetes, and dehydration—are generally detectable with a history and physical examination plus or minus determination of a serum creatinine concentration. Risk factors should be corrected whenever possible, and when they cannot be, patients should receive the smallest dose of iso-osmolar contrast possible and have their creatinine value measured after the procedure. Deliberate hydration and either theophylline or NAC should be considered in high-risk cases. Supportive care is indicated if contrast nephropathy occurs.

ANNOTATED REFERENCES

Gruberg L, Mintz GS, Mehran R, et al: The prognostic implications of further renal function deterioration within 48 hours of interventional coronary procedures in patients with pre-existent chronic renal insufficiency. J Am Coll Cardiol 2000;36:1542-1548.
   This study, with others, establishes the overall negative prognostic impact associated with contrast nephropathy, particularly if renal replacement therapy is required.

Huber W, Ilgmann K, Page M, et al: Effect of theophylline on contrast material–induced nephropathy in patients with chronic renal insufficiency: Controlled, randomized, double-blinded study. Radiology 2002;223; 772-779.
   This trial, along with prior studies, supports the use of theophylline as a means to reduce the risk of contrast nephropathy.

Rich MW, Crecelius CA: Incidence, risk factors, and clinical course of acute renal insufficiency after cardiac catheterization in patients 70 years of age or older. Arch Intern Med 1995;150:1237-1242.
   The data in this trial clearly show the impact of increasing background risk on the likelihood of contrast medium–associated renal injury.

Tepel M, van der Giet M, Schwarzfeld C, et al: Prevention of radiographic contrast agent–induced reductions in renal function by acetylcysteine. N Engl J Med 2000;343:180-184.
   This trial is one of the first to demonstrate the efficacy of acetylcysteine in prevention of contrast nephropathy. The limited dose of contrast and the large treatment benefit have led some to question the applicability of the results and have led to many subsequent trials and more recent meta-analysis.

Trivedi HS, Moore H, Nasr S, et al: A randomized prospective trial to assess the role of saline hydration on the development of contrast nephrotoxicity. Nephron Clin Pract 2003;93:c29-c34.
   Although deliberate hydration has often been suggested as a way to reduce the risk of contrast nephropathy, this is the most definitive demonstration of its efficacy by a randomized trial comparing hydration to no therapy.

Chapter 136

GLOMERULONEPHRITIS AND INTERSTITIAL NEPHRITIS IN THE ICU

Debbie S. Gipson • David B. Thomas • Ronald J. Falk

KEY POINTS

1. **Serum complement** levels can be important tools in distinguishing causes of glomerulonephritis (GN): (a) normal serum complement (IgA nephropathy, Henoch-Schönlein purpura, pauci-immune necrotizing, and crescentic GN) and (b) depressed serum complement (postinfectious GN, lupus nephritis).

2. Many underlying causes for **renal-based acute renal failure are reversible.** However, transition of active glomerular lesions and acute tubulointerstitial disease to irreversible scar is rapid (measured in days) and necessitates early diagnosis and **early intervention.**

3. **Urinalysis** with **evaluation of urine sediment,** blood chemistry with **peripheral blood smear review,** and **serology** (for the patient's immunologic status, e.g., ASO, ANA, ANCA, viral serologies) complement the differential diagnosis and physical examination. Fundamental understanding of the urine sediment and peripheral blood review is key to accurate and rapid clinical diagnosis of acute renal failure.

4. Although clinical findings and laboratory studies may be highly suggestive of the etiology of renal dysfunction, **kidney biopsy** often is the only means to confirm the diagnosis of a specific GN or tubulo-interstitial nephritis.

5. Treatment of drug-induced tubulointerstitial nephritis begins with **discontinuation of the causative agent.** Subsequent use of a causative agent may result in prolonged renal failure.

Nearly 300,000 Americans are diagnosed with acute renal failure (ARF) each year. ARF may be a consequence of prerenal causes that result in hypoperfusion of the kidneys, renal causes, and postrenal or obstructive lesions. The focus in this chapter is on the renal causes of ARF, including GN and interstitial nephritis (Fig. 136-1). Interstitial nephritis should be distinguished from acute tubular necrosis (ATN) in that ATN is typically preceded by an acute ischemic event.

Although nearly 2 dozen forms of GN have been described, only some of these can lead to ARF (Fig. 136-2). The most aggressive form of GN is described clinically as rapidly progressive glomerulonephritis (RPGN). Rather than a single disease entity, RPGN is the severe form of many of the glomerular diseases that are divided into renal limited etiologies and systemic diseases that involve the kidneys (Table 136-1). RPGN is defined as rapidly declining renal function, progressive oliguria, hematuria, proteinuria, and hypertension.[1] The renal ultrasound documents a normal renal arterial and venous blood flow and normal to slightly enlarged kidneys. A renal biopsy reveals a high degree of glomerular injury with necrosis and crescent formation (see Fig. 136-2). The transition from an acute cellular crescent to a scarred fibrous crescent signifies a transition to a chronic lesion. In animal models, the transition from an active glomerular lesion to a chronic, nonreversible injury occurs in as little as 2 weeks. The presentation of a patient with RPGN constitutes a need for prompt diagnosis with early intervention and therapy to interrupt a natural progression to chronic renal failure.

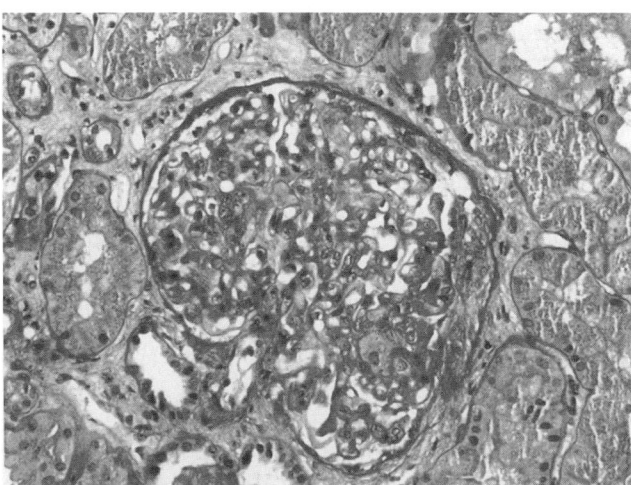

FIGURE 136–1. Glomerulonephritis. Focal endocapillary hypercellularity ("proliferative lesion") is present from the 2 to 6 o'clock positions of the glomerulus. The remaining portion of the glomerular capillary tuft has mesangial hypercellularity, and a fibrocellular crescent is present (2 to 4 o'clock positions) (original magnification × 200, periodic acid–Schiff).

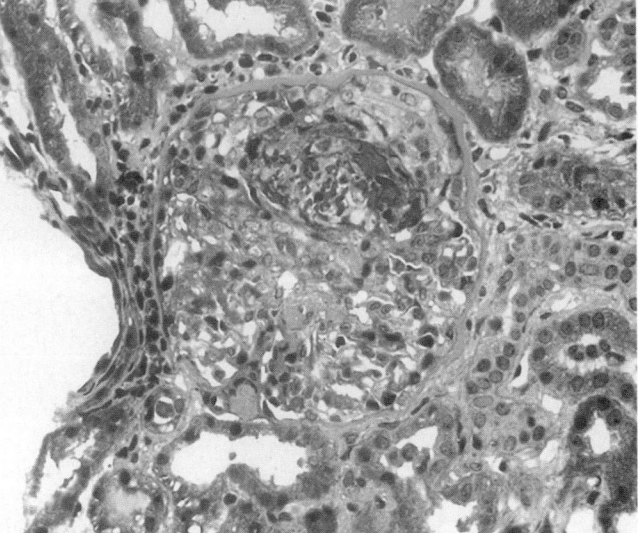

FIGURE 136–2. Rapidly progressive glomerulonephritis. A cellular crescent is present in the glomerulus (4 to 8 o'clock position) with fuchsinophilic ("bright red") fibrinoid necrosis of the glomerular capillary tuft (original magnification × 200, trichrome).

GLOMERULONEPHRITIS

The clinical manifestations of GN include hematuria, proteinuria, hypertension, and ARF. The hematuria may be microscopic or macroscopic with dysmorphic urinary red blood cells and, commonly, red blood cell casts. The abnormal red blood cell morphology includes blebs and budding with a clear variability in red cell shape and decrease in red cell size.[2] Dysmorphic hematuria is considered by some clinicians to be an indicator of glomerular bleeding rather than bleeding with a lower urinary tract origin. When grossly abnormal, the urine may be a rust or tea color. Urinary protein excretion typically exceeds 1 g per 24-hour period and in some instances ranges to 10 to 15 g/day. A large quantity of proteinuria (typically > 3.5 g/day and referred to as nephrotic range) is associated with edema, hypoalbuminemia, and hypercholesterolemia. Leukocyturia with or without white blood cell casts may be observed with GN of inflammatory origin.

Hypertension may be associated with acute or chronic GN. In an acute setting, hypertension is often associated with hypervolemia. Hypertension ranges from mild to severe and may be the indication for admission to the ICU. ARF is not universally present with GN but may portend a worse long-term prognosis. Renal failure may be manifest by elevation in serum creatinine and blood urea nitrogen values, hyperkalemia, oligoanuria, uremic symptoms of somnolence, anorexia, and nausea.

A comprehensive discussion of GN in children and adults is beyond the scope of this chapter. Consequently, the most common lesions are presented and a general approach to management follows.

POSTINFECTIOUS GLOMERULONEPHRITIS

Group A beta-hemolytic *Streptococcus* is the most common infectious antecedent of postinfectious GN. Patients present with a history of antecedent pharyngitis or pyoderma by 7 to 21 days.[3] Nephritogenic strains of streptococci include Lancefield group A type XII and M types 1 to 4, 18, 25, 31,

TABLE 136–1. DISEASES ASSOCIATED WITH THE DEVELOPMENT OF RAPIDLY PROGRESSIVE GLOMERULONEPHRITIS

Renal Limited

IgA nephropathy
Post infectious glomerulonephritis
Pauci-immune necrotizing and crescentic glomerulonephritis

Systemic Disorders

Henoch-Schönlein purpura
Wegener's granulomatosis
Microscopic polyangiitis
Goodpasture's syndrome
Systemic lupus erythematosus
Thrombotic microangiopathy

49, 52, 55 to 57, 59, and 61.[4-7] Streptococcal groups C and G and numerous other bacterial agents are also occasionally associated with postinfectious GN.[8-10] The peak age at onset of postinfectious GN is 2 to 6 years, although all ages may be affected. *Streptococcus*-associated disease may occur in sporadic or epidemic forms. In epidemics the attack rate may vary by streptococcal strain but averages 10% to 15% among the population at risk and approaches 38% among household contacts.[11-14]

Clinical features include microscopic hematuria in 70% and macroscopic hematuria in 30%. Proteinuria is common but may not reach nephrotic range (>3.5 g/day). Hypertension is found in approximately 75% of patients, the majority of whom will require short-term antihypertensive management. Edema is found in association with salt and water retention with or without nephrotic-range proteinuria in the majority of patients. The elderly are particularly susceptible to congestive heart failure with an S3 gallop rhythm, dyspnea, jugular venous distention, and confirmatory chest radiograph findings.[15,16] Encephalopathy is uncommon but may affect children with postinfectious GN. When present, the central nervous system manifestations may include confusion, lethargy, headache, and seizures.[15-18]

Laboratory findings are well characterized. In addition to the urinary findings just discussed, the acute phase of postinfectious GN is associated with activation of the alternate complement cascade with depressed levels of CH50 and C3. These values return to normal by 8 weeks from the onset of the nephritis.[15,19-25] Failure to do so suggests an alternative diagnosis such as membranoproliferative GN, a chronic infection such as endocarditis or abscess-associated GN, systemic lupus erythematosus (SLE), congenital complement deficiency, or atheromatous emboli. In some patients the classical complement pathway is activated with low levels of C4.[26] Serologic studies confirming a recent streptococcal infection may be found when postinfectious GN is associated with this organism. The Streptozyme test, including many streptococcal antibody assays, will often be positive.[27] The ASO titer is most likely to be elevated in streptococcal pharyngitis–associated postinfectious GN.[28] However, some strains of group A streptococci type XII and impetigo-associated streptococci do not produce streptolysin S or O, resulting in a normal ASO titer.[6] A positive skin or pharyngeal culture is found in as few as 25% of patients with postinfectious GN.

The prognosis of patients with postinfectious GN is generally excellent. The clinical symptoms of edema and hypertension are typically short term, lasting less than 2 weeks.[29] Hematuria and proteinuria may persist up to 1 year from the onset of the disorder. The most common long-term sequela is hypertension. Severe forms of postinfectious GN with glomerular crescent formation have been associated with hypertension, proteinuria, and renal insufficiency 10 or more years from the original diagnosis.[30-32]

IgA NEPHROPATHY

IgA nephropathy may be idiopathic, familial, or secondary to a variety of conditions such as chronic liver disease, chronic lung disease, or gastrointestinal disorders.[33-38] In the idiopathic form, IgA nephropathy is most commonly diagnosed in the second and third decades of life. It is uncommon in very young children and African Americans. IgA nephropathy may be familial in up to 10% of cases.

The clinical features of IgA nephropathy are those of macroscopic hematuria in up to 50% of patients and microscopic hematuria in the remaining patients. Hematuria may be episodic and, therefore, a history of previous episodes of tea-colored urine should be sought. Hematuria is often associated with a concurrent upper respiratory tract infection, including streptococcal pharyngitis. Proteinuria may be absent to severe. In the most severe forms, the nephrotic syndrome with hypoalbuminemia, edema, and hyperlipidemia may develop. Malignant hypertension is a presenting feature in approximately 5%,[39] and ARF may be present at the initial encounter in a minority.[40,41]

Laboratory features of IgA nephropathy are nonspecific. Serum IgA levels have not been shown to be either of diagnostic or prognostic value. Complement components C3 and C4 levels are normal to slightly elevated.[42] Urinary protein excretion is often less than 1 g/day. A high and sustained level of proteinuria (> 1 g/day) is considered an indicator of poor long-term renal survival. Renal biopsy is the definitive method of diagnosis for IgA nephropathy.

The long-term prognosis of patients with IgA nephropathy is highly variable. With long-term management, approximately 2% develop end-stage renal failure each year. Indicators of a higher risk of progression to kidney failure include sustained proteinuria over 1 g/day, nephrotic syndrome, sustained hypertension, and male gender.[43-46] An episode of ARF associated with macroscopic hematuria does not portend a worse long-term prognosis.[47-49] Secondary IgA nephropathy may resolve with treatment of the primary disorder, as has been documented after liver transplant in cases of liver failure–associated disease.

HENOCH-SCHÖNLEIN PURPURA

On renal histology, the kidney biopsies of Henoch-Schönlein purpura (HSP) and IgA nephropathy are identical. HSP is most common in males between the ages of 4 to 5 years.[50-55] The clinical features of HSP distinguish it from the renal-limited IgA nephropathy with the classic features of sudden onset of rash, progressing from nonblanching erythematous macules to urticarial papules to purpura.[56-57] The rash has a symmetrical distribution on the extensor surfaces of the distal extremities and buttocks. Localized edema on the dorsa of the hands and feet, face, and scalp is often seen. Joint pain without effusion occurs in up to 70%. Gastrointestinal involvement includes abdominal pain and vomiting in

50% to 70%. Melena is documented in approximately one half of those with abdominal pain.[51,58-60] Intussusception manifesting as severe abdominal pain and an abdominal mass is an uncommon manifestation in children, and protein-losing enteropathy has been reported in adults with HSP.[51,61-64] Nephritis occurs in 40% to 60%,[50,51,65-69] with severity ranging from mild to a severe rapidly progressive course. Central nervous system manifestations have been reported with confusion, somnolence, and seizures in a minority. Vasculitis effects on multiple other organ systems have been reported.

Laboratory findings of microscopic or macroscopic hematuria, proteinuria, and varying degrees of renal insufficiency are common. Coagulation studies are typically normal, including platelet count, prothrombin time, and partial thromboplastin time. Sedimentation rate is elevated. IgA and C3 complement studies are normal to elevated and are not helpful in the diagnosis or management.[55,70-72]

The long-term morbidity of HSP nephritis is observed as a 2% to 5% risk of end-stage renal failure.[66,69] Poor prognostic indicators include acute nephritic syndrome on presentation, persistent nephrotic syndrome, older age at presentation, and the presence of a greater percentage of glomerular crescents on renal biopsy.[51,66,69,73,74] A minority of affected patients will have long-term hematuria, proteinuria, and chronic glomerular disease documented as IgA nephropathy on subsequent renal biopsy.[75]

LUPUS NEPHRITIS

Approximately 80% of children and 40% of adults with SLE have renal involvement. Females are more likely affected by SLE but are no more likely to develop lupus nephritis than males with the systemic disorder.[76-81] Children and African Americans have more severe nephritis.[76-79,82,83] The diagnosis is made based on the systemic manifestations of SLE and laboratory confirmation with hypocomplementemia and elevated titers of antineutrophil antibody and anti–double-stranded DNA antibody in addition to the kidney biopsy.

Lupus nephritis has been categorized by the World Health Organization into six subtypes based on kidney histology.[84] The mildest forms—normal (class I) and mesangial (class II) lupus nephritis—have excellent prognosis and are managed within the care for the overall SLE disease process.[85-92] The focal segmental and diffuse proliferative lesions (classes III and IV), membranous lesion (class V), and sclerosing lesion (class VI) all have significant impact of the prognosis for long-term renal function.[93,94]

The proliferative lesions of lupus nephritis (classes III and IV) present as hematuria, proteinuria, and hypertension. The majority of patients with diffuse proliferative lesions tend to have acute renal insufficiency on presentation. Similarly, the diffuse proliferative lesion is the lupus lesion most likely considered in the differential diagnosis of RPGN with ARF. Therapy for the proliferative lesions is designed to control the inflammatory process in the kidney and prevent progression to renal failure.

Lupus membranous nephropathy is characterized clinically by nephrotic levels of urinary protein excretion. As a consequence, membranous nephropathy presents the challenge of management of nephrotic syndrome with peripheral and pulmonary edema, hypercoagulability with risk of venous thrombosis, pulmonary emboli, and risk of bacterial peritonitis. The risk of chronic kidney failure and complications associated with uncontrolled nephrotic syndrome makes the control of this lupus nephritis variant necessary. The 10-year renal survival of membranous lupus nephritis ranges between 75% and 93%, with an increased risk of renal failure in African Americans.[95-97]

Sclerosing lupus nephritis is a chronic lesion that has a poor prognosis; if it is an isolated lesion, it does not respond to immunosuppressive therapy. Patients with this lesion without additional active lesions tend to have normal anti–double-stranded DNA and complement levels.

Just as SLE is a remitting and relapsing disease, the nephritis that accompanies this vasculitis can remit, relapse, and change subtypes. The relapse or escalation of nephritis will often warrant a second renal biopsy to precisely classify the disease and guide therapy. Current estimates of overall renal survival are 70% to 90% at 5 years.[83,98-100]

PAUCI-IMMUNE NECROTIZING AND CRESCENTIC GLOMERULONEPHRITIS

Pauci-immune necrotizing and crescentic GN is defined by kidney biopsy features with glomerular crescents, necrosis, and an absence of immunoglobulin or complement within the glomeruli. This lesion may affect the kidney alone or may be a component of a systemic disorder. The small vessel vasculitides associated with antineutrophil cytoplasmic autoantibody, including renal-limited microscopic polyangiitis, Wegener's granulomatosis, Churg-Strauss syndrome, and other idiopathic renal-limited pauci-immune necrotizing and crescentic GNs, are included in this group of disorders.[101-103] These patients often present to the ICU setting with signs and symptoms of an RPGN and systemic vasculitis that may include pulmonary hemorrhage, cutaneous vasculitis, arthritis or arthralgias, and constitutional manifestations of fatigue, weight loss, and fever that may be life threatening if not treated promptly.

The pauci-immune necrotizing and crescentic GNs typically present with modest amounts of proteinuria (<3 g/day), hematuria, red blood cell casts, hypertension, and renal insufficiency. Approximately 85% of these patients will have abnormal levels of circulating antineutrophil cytoplasmic autoantibodies.[94,102,104-108] The renal biopsy is characterized by cellular or fibrous crescents, glomerular necrosis, and varying amounts of interstitial fibrosis. Immunofluorescence studies fail to show staining for immunoglobulin or complement, and electron microscopy of the kidney tissue shows a lack of immune complex deposition and basement membrane disease.

Although most patients improve with initial therapy, those patients who fail to respond are likely to progress to end-stage disease and possibly death.[109-111] The presence of pulmonary hemorrhage as a component of the systemic vasculitis with pauci-immune necrotizing and crescentic GN is a life-threatening condition with a 30% to 80% mortality rate.[105,112,113] The pauci-immune necrotizing and crescentic GNs tend to follow a remitting and relapsing course, making long-term monitoring a key component to patient and kidney survival.

ANTI–GLOMERULAR BASEMENT MEMBRANE GLOMERULONEPHRITIS

Nephritis caused by anti-glomerular basement membrane (anti-GBM) antibodies may occur in isolation or as a syndrome including pulmonary and renal manifestations of vasculitis. All affected patients have an elevated titer of anti-GBM antibodies. This type of nephritis most commonly affects adults: males in the second and third decades and females in the sixth and seventh decades. An affected patient may present with respiratory symptoms of cough, dyspnea, hypoxia, or pulmonary hemorrhage. The kidney biopsy shows clear linear deposition of antibodies, most commonly IgG and C3, along the GBM and glomerular crescent formation.[114-119]

Laboratory findings of nephritis with hematuria, red blood cell casts, and proteinuria are present. An elevated serum creatinine concentration, elevated erythrocyte sedimentation rate, anemia, and elevated anti-GBM antibodies are typical. Pulmonary infiltrates on chest radiography or computed tomography are evidence of lung involvement, as are hemosiderin-laden macrophages in pulmonary secretions.

Patient and kidney survival is dependent on prompt, aggressive therapy and typically includes corticosteroids, plasmapheresis, and cyclophosphamide or azathioprine. Overall patient survival is approximately 85%, and renal survival is 60% when treatment is initiated promptly.[120-125] Unlike the ANCA-associated crescentic GN, anti-GBM antibody disease does not tend to relapse after the initial control of the disorder.[126-129]

THROMBOTIC MICROANGIOPATHY

Thrombotic microangiopathy (TMA) includes thrombotic thrombocytopenic purpura (TTP) and hemolytic uremic syndrome (HUS). Thrombotic microangiopathy may be idiopathic, familial, or associated with autoimmune disorders such as SLE or scleroderma with pregnancy, or with an antecedent diarrheal illness typically observed in small children. The clinical presentation includes a microangiopathic hemolytic anemia, thrombocytopenia, neurologic symptoms and signs, and impaired renal function with or without fever. The neurologic symptoms of confusion, headache, seizures, and coma have been observed and may be the predominant findings.

Microangiopathic hemolytic anemia is defined as nonimmune hemolysis with schistocytes noted on peripheral blood smear. A decrease in serum haptoglobin and increase in lactate dehydrogenase level are consistent with hemolysis. Normalization of lactate dehydrogenase and platelet counts is a marker of therapeutic response. The urinary findings include hematuria, hemoglobinuria, and, rarely, red cell casts. Hypocomplementemia occurs in up to 50% of patients.[19,130] In children with diarrhea-associated HUS, stool cultures should be tested for *Escherichia coli* 0157:H7.

The prognosis for the thrombotic microangiopathies is dependent on the etiology of the disorder. Among patients with TTP the patient survival has improved dramatically from 6% to 87% with current management strategies, including plasma exchange.[131,132] Among children with diarrhea-associated HUS, plasma exchange has not proven to be effective in changing the clinical course. In this setting, supportive care is warranted, with expected patient survival of approximately 94%.

TREATMENT OF ACUTE GLOMERULONEPHRITIS

Hypertension

Patients with acute GN tend to be volume expanded and edematous owing to sodium and water retention. As a result, elevations in blood pressure are primarily caused by fluid overload. Renal ischemia may result in increased activity of the renin-angiotensin system, which may contribute to the hypertension observed in these patients. Consequently, the therapy for hypertension will often begin with control of the volume status with loop diuretics and fluid restriction. Care should be taken to avoid potassium-sparing diuretics owing to the risk of hyperkalemia. In the setting of anuria, dialysis may be required to control hypervolemia. The addition of antihypertensive agents is commonly indicated for severe hypertension or for hypertension in the setting of euvolemia.

Dialysis

The institution of dialysis for a patient with ARF adds the potential for dialysis-related morbidity, including hypotension, renal ischemia, dialysis membrane reactions, and fluid and electrolyte disorders. Consequently, dialysis is considered for patients with ARF with symptomatic uremia, severe fluid overload, or significant electrolyte abnormalities. Uremic symptoms may include somnolence or hemorrhagic pericarditis. In addition to refractory fluid overload, expected need for large fluid volumes in the management of an oligoanuric patient may be considered an indicator for acute dialysis.

Immunosuppression

The prognosis of some glomerulonephritides is substantially improved by the use of immunosuppressive agents. In the acute setting with a severe and rapidly progressive renal failure, intravenous corticosteroid therapy may be warranted in addition to supportive care. Intravenous boluses of corticosteroids are typically prescribed for patients with RPGN, proliferative lupus nephritis, and necrotizing and crescentic GN. Corticosteroid therapy alone is not sufficient for the management of proliferative lupus nephritis. In this disorder, therapeutic regimens with corticosteroids and additional immunosuppressive agents such as cyclophosphamide result in a substantial improvement in renal survival.[100,133,134] Six- to 12-month courses of glucocorticoid therapy have been studied in a limited number of high-risk patients with IgA nephropathy with variable results.[43,135-138]

The scleroderma renal crisis is a reminder that pulses of corticosteroids are not a universal component of the management of ARF. Indeed, pulse corticosteroids may contribute to the onset of a scleroderma renal crisis and are associated with a greater risk of patient demise.[139,140]

Cyclophosphamide is a mainstay of therapy for disorders such as proliferative lupus nephritis, pauci-immune necrotizing and crescentic GN, and Goodpasture's syndrome. In each of these instances, improved renal and patient survival has been documented with cyclophosphamide. Cyclophosphamide doses of 2 mg/kg/day orally or 500 to 1000 mg/m²/day by intermittent intravenous pulses are standard for GN.[111,141,142] Cyclophosphamide dose adjustment according to peripheral leukocyte counts may be necessary. The duration of cyclophosphamide induction and maintenance regimens are disease specific.

The inclusion of cyclophosphamide therapy for the management of an oligoanuric patient with pauci-immune necrotizing and crescentic GN is difficult, owing to the clearance of metabolites via the urinary tract and the risk of hemorrhagic cystitis and bladder cancer. Alternatives in this setting have not been rigorously studied but have included plasmapheresis, corticosteroids, and azathioprine.[143,144]

Recent studies have searched for alternatives to cyclophosphamide. Mycophenolate mofetil is an oral agent with early reports of success in the treatment of proliferative lupus nephritis in Asia.[145,146] Long-term follow up of these patients has suggested a higher relapse rate of lupus nephritis when compared with those treated with standard cyclophosphamide therapy. Cyclosporine has been used in combination with other immunosuppressive agents for those resistant to or intolerant of cyclophosphamide, or as a primary agent for disorders such as membranous lupus nephritis.[147-149] Although cyclosporine appears to be of benefit while on therapy, relapse risks with the discontinuation of therapy is a concern, especially for proliferative lupus nephritis.[150,151]

Plasmapheresis

Plasmapheresis effectively removes large-molecular-weight substances from the plasma, including autoantibodies and immune complexes. This technique may be considered in the management of RPGN, necrotizing and crescentic GN with renal failure, thrombotic microangiopathy, including TTP, and HUS occurring in the absence of diarrhea.[131,152] Plasmapheresis has been associated with improved patient survival among patients with vasculitis-induced pulmonary hemorrhage.[105,112,113]

Plasmapheresis has been a standard therapeutic option in the setting of acute GN associated with pulmonary hemorrhage. Before the initiation of plasmapheresis, the mortality rate approached 80% in affected individuals. The initial course of plasmapheresis is daily for 5 to 6 days, followed by alternate-day therapy. Factor VIIa has been used for the management of other bleeding disorders and may improve the control of pulmonary hemorrhage in vasculitis-associated pulmonary hemorrhage.[153-156]

INTERSTITIAL NEPHRITIS

CLINICAL PRESENTATION

Acute tubulointerstitial nephritis (TIN) accounts for approximately 7% of all cases of ARF.[157] The clinical presentation of acute TIN ranges from a mild renal insufficiency to oliguric renal failure. The urinary findings are typically bland, with mild proteinuria (<3 g/day). Granular, hyaline, or white blood cell casts may be noted. Microscopic hematuria is common. Eosinophiluria, based on Wright's or Hansel's stain, is suggestive of acute TIN but is neither sensitive nor specific for this disorder.[158,159] Serum studies may reflect tubular injury with impaired urinary absorption of glucose, bicarbonate, phosphorus, amino acids, and uric acid. Distal tubular injury may result in impaired potassium excretion, metabolic acidosis, and sodium wasting (Fig. 136-3).

Systemic manifestations of a hypersensitivity reaction may accompany a medication-associated acute TIN with fever, rash, and arthralgias.[160,161] A wide variety of medications have been associated with acute TIN, some of which have been listed in Table 136-2. The onset of drug-associated acute TIN ranges from days to weeks. With the removal of the offending agent, the duration of ARF is approximately 2 weeks in most individuals, although prolonged or chronic renal failure may occur.[162] Underlying causes of acute TIN have been documented in a large series of patients with 85% drug induced, 10% infection, and 5% idiopathic.[163] In general, no etiologic agent can be identified in approximately 20% of patients with biopsy-proven acute TIN with renal insufficiency.[164] A few cases of acute TIN associated with Chinese herbal remedies[165,166] and environmental allergens such as wasp stings[167] have been reported.

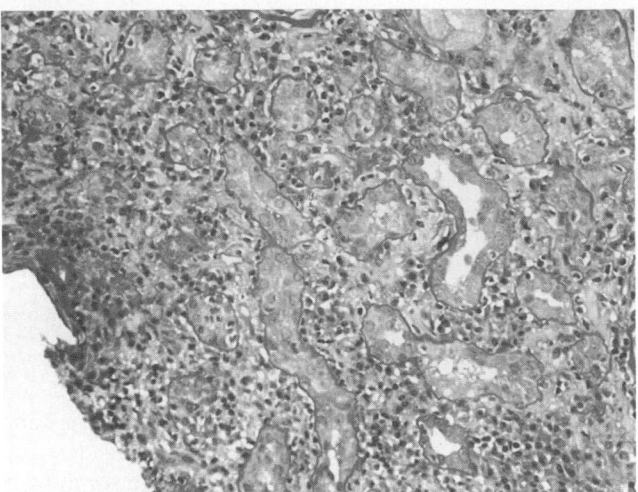

FIGURE 136–3. Acute tubulointerstitial nephritis. A diffuse, predominantly mononuclear cell infiltrate is present within an expanded and mildly edematous interstitium, and periodic acid–Schiff (PAS)-positive tubular basement membranes have wrinkling. Foci of tubulitis are also present. (Original magnification × 200, PAS.)

DIFFERENTIAL DIAGNOSIS

All causes of ARF are initially considered in the differential diagnosis of a suspected case of acute TIN. The differential diagnosis of acute TIN includes causes of renal dysfunction with accompanying bland urinary sediment. Acute tubular necrosis can present in a similar manor but does not have eosinophiluria. Because the absence of urinary eosinophils does not exclude the diagnosis of TIN, a definitive distinction between these disorders on clinical grounds may not be possible. The occurrence of pyelonephritis is associated with white blood cell casts, leukocyturia, hematuria, and mild proteinuria. The distinguishing feature is a confirmatory urine culture. Renal tubulopathy associated with direct nephrotoxins, medullary cystic kidney disease, and juvenile nephronophthisis will similarly present as a bland urinary sediment and renal insufficiency. When laboratory and radiographic studies do not allow a clear diagnosis, a kidney biopsy may be required to provide a precise diagnosis and guide medical therapy.

PROGNOSIS AND MANAGEMENT

The initial management of a patient with acute TIN is largely supportive, with dialysis as indicated. Identification of all candidate etiologic agents, elimination of potentially causative medications, and control of potential infectious causes are fundamental to the control of TIN.[168] When replacing medications, it is important to choose medications that are not likely to cross-react with the original agent.

The use of corticosteroid therapy remains controversial. Case series and uncontrolled studies have suggested a benefit from the use of daily or alternate-day prednisone tapered over 2 to 4 weeks or pulse methylprednisolone.[125,159,169] No prospective, controlled studies have been reported in the literature.

The prognosis for recovery of renal function in children with acute TIN is good, with a median recovery time of approximately 70 days and approximately 86% long-term

TABLE 136–2. ETIOLOGIC CLASSIFICATION OF ACUTE TUBULOINTERSTITIAL NEPHRITIS

Medications

Anticonvulsants
Nonsteroidal anti-inflammatory
Antibiotics
Diuretics
Miscellaneous

Diseases

Idiopathic (10%-20%)
Tubulointerstitial nephritis with uveitis
Systemic lupus erythematosus
Renal allograft rejection

Microorganisms

Bacteria	Virus
Leptospira species	Adenovirus
Rickettsia	HIV
Yersinia	Cytomegalovirus
(pseudotuberculosis)	Hantavirus
Mycoplasma	Polyoma
Streptococcus	Ebstein-Barr
Brucella	Hepatitis B
Corynebacterium diphtheriae	Rubella
Francisella tularensis	Paramyxovirus
Legionella pneumophila	Parasites
Salmonella typhi	*Ascaris*
Treponema pallidum	*Leishmania donovani*
	Toxoplasma gondii
	Fungi
	Histoplasma
	Candida

renal survival.[159,169] Adults with acute TIN may have a worse prognosis, with a 70% to 80% renal survival.[164,170] Prolonged renal failure has been reported when the causative pharmacologic agent has been reinstituted. Consequently, the avoidance of future use of agents known to have caused TIN in a patient may be warranted.

ANNOTATED REFERENCES

Dooley MA, Hogan S, Jennette C, et al: Cyclophosphamide therapy for lupus nephritis: Poor renal survival in black Americans. Glomerular Disease Collaborative Network. Kidney Int 1997;51:1188-1195.
The poor response of black Americans compared with white Americans to standard therapy for proliferative lupus nephritis is documented in this study.

Hedger N, Stevens J, Drey N, et al: Incidence and outcome of pauci-immune rapidly progressive glomerulonephritis in Wessex, UK: A 10-year retrospective study. Nephrol Dial Transplant 2000;15:1593-1599.
This study contributes to our understanding of the incidence of pauci-immune rapidly progressive glomerulonephritis.

Hu W, Liu Z, Chen H, et al: Mycophenolate mofetil vs cyclophosphamide therapy for patients with diffuse proliferative lupus nephritis. Chin Med J (Engl) 2002;115:705-709.
This randomized controlled trial compares the short-term response of lupus nephritis to mycophenolate mofetil and cyclophosphamide therapy.

Schwarz A, Krause PH, Kunzendorf U, et al: The outcome of acute interstitial nephritis: Risk factors for the transition from acute to chronic interstitial nephritis. Clin Nephrol 2000;54:179-190.
Bi- and multivariate analysis for risk factors in the development of chronic renal insufficiency following acute tubulointerstitial nephritis.

Tasic V, Polenakovic M: Occurrence of subclinical post-streptococcal glomerulonephritis in family contacts. J Paediatr Child Health 2003;39:177-179.
This observational study documents the significant frequency of post-streptococcal glomerulonephritis in household contacts.

Section VIII

INFECTIOUS DISEASES

Chapter 137

ANTIMICROBIALS IN CHEMOTHERAPY STRATEGY

Douglas N. Fish

KEY POINTS

1. The **continuing emergence of antimicrobial resistance in ICUs** is a major factor in the appropriate selection and use of antimicrobials in critically ill patients.

2. **Inadequate antimicrobial therapy,** defined as the use of drugs with poor in-vitro activity against infecting pathogens, has been demonstrated in numerous studies to be significantly associated with increased mortality and other measures of poor patient outcome.

3. **Hospital formulary–based antimicrobial restrictions may be effective in reducing drug costs and limiting specific outbreaks of resistant infections;** however, appropriate drug use must be based on basic principles of rational antimicrobial use rather than relying on such restrictions to prevent or overcome resistance problems.

4. **Antibiotic cycling,** in which a specific drug or an entire antibiotic class is periodically withdrawn from clinical use and replaced with a different drug or class, appears to be a promising means of decreasing antimicrobial resistance and improving patient outcomes.

5. Although **establishment of a definitive diagnosis of infection is paramount to the appropriate selection and use of antimicrobials,** the actual site of infection and specific pathogens are never identified in many critically ill patients.

6. **Patients who have a new fever, or who have previously been started on antimicrobial therapy and have persistent fever** despite the resolution of other signs and symptoms of infection, should also be evaluated for noninfectious sources of fever before continuing or instituting unnecessary antimicrobial therapy.

7. **The initial selection of adequate empirical drug therapy is of vital importance** in optimizing outcomes of antimicrobial use in critically ill patients.

8. **Empirical antimicrobial regimens for critically ill patients** should be sufficiently broad spectrum in pharmacologic activity to cover the most likely pathogens, initiated promptly, and given in relatively high doses to optimize the provision of adequate and aggressive therapy.

9. **Clinicians must utilize the results of culture and susceptibility tests,** when available, to reassess and make appropriate changes to empirical drug regimens.

10. **Antimicrobial regimens selected for either empirical or definitive therapy should provide suitable activity against suspected or known pathogens** while at the same time using the fewest required number of drugs, narrowing the spectrum of antimicrobial activity as much as possible, minimizing the risk of drug-related toxicities, and minimizing the cost of drug therapy.

11. **Combination antimicrobial regimens** are most appropriately used in the treatment of mixed infections and documented infections with difficult pathogens such as *Pseudomonas aeruginosa*, as well as to provide adequate empirical therapy in institutions with high rates of antimicrobial resistance.

12. **Basic knowledge and understanding of pharmacokinetic and pharmacodynamic properties of antimicrobials** are necessary to achieve the most effective and safe use of antimicrobials in critically ill patients.

13. Although **most antimicrobial use in critically ill patients should be administered by the intravenous route,** oral therapy may also be administered in selected patients and should be considered when appropriate.

14. Recent studies have shown that **shorter courses of antimicrobial therapy,** such as 8 days versus 15 days for ventilator-associated pneumonia, may be equal in efficacy to longer courses of therapy and may be associated with a decreased incidence of superinfections and decreased antimicrobial use, drug costs, adverse effects, and antimicrobial resistance.

15. **Careful monitoring of antimicrobial use is required in all critically ill patients** and should include evaluation of clinical response to therapy, changes in organ function that may necessitate changes in the dosing regimen, occurrence of drug-related adverse effects and toxicities, evaluation for adverse drug interactions, and monitoring of serum drug concentrations when appropriate.

Infections are frequently suspected or documented in critically ill patients. Patients are often admitted to the ICU for treatment of community-acquired or hospital-acquired infections, whereas many other patients require treatment for nosocomial infections acquired during their ICU stay. Although patients in ICUs represent only 8% to 15% of hospital admissions in the United States,[1] these patients suffer a disproportionately high rate of infectious complications and are exposed to very high rates of antimicrobial use.[2,3] The importance of antimicrobial drugs in the modern management of critically ill patients with a variety of bacterial, fungal, and viral infections can scarcely be understated. However, despite the availability of improved diagnostic techniques and a wide variety of potent, highly effective antimicrobials, the prevention and appropriate treatment of infections in ICU patients remain a formidable challenge to the clinician.

ANTIMICROBIAL RESISTANCE IN THE ICU

The continuing emergence of antimicrobial resistance in ICUs is a major factor in the appropriate selection and use of antimicrobials in the critical care setting. It has been estimated that 50% to 60% of all nosocomial infections occurring each year in the United States are caused by antimicrobial-resistant strains of bacteria.[3] The overall incidence of infections due to antibiotic-resistant pathogens, changes in the epidemiology of infections caused by specific pathogens, and increasing resistance to even the most potent, broad-spectrum agents make the selection of appropriate antimicrobial therapy extremely challenging in many institutions.[2-4] The difficulties in selecting antimicrobial therapy are particularly acute in ICUs because of the higher prevalence of antimicrobial resistance in these areas compared with other non-ICU settings.[5-8]

A number of factors are associated with high rates of antimicrobial resistance in the ICU. Chief among these is the heavy use of antimicrobial agents in critically ill patients. A number of studies have identified a close association between antimicrobial use and the subsequent development of antibiotic resistance.[9-18] While use of antibiotics is associated with the emergence of resistance during therapy, previous exposure to antibiotics is also a well-established risk factor for antimicrobial resistance.[2,3,8] The higher severity of illness found among ICU patients is related to several risk factors for antimicrobial resistance, including the presence of invasive devices such as endotracheal tubes and intravascular and urinary catheters,[3,19] prolonged length of hospital stay,[6,17,20] immune suppression,[2] and malnutrition.[2,3] The increasing prevalence of antimicrobial-resistant pathogens among residents in long-term care facilities is also an increasingly important source for resistant bacteria in ICUs.[2-4,8,21] Finally, antimicrobial-resistant pathogens are easily cross-transmitted among patients in ICUs owing to poor adherence of hospital personnel to infection control techniques, contamination of equipment, and frequent overcrowding of patients.[2,22,23] All of these various factors combine to make ICUs the epicenter of antimicrobial resistance in hospitalized patients.[5]

Increased antimicrobial resistance has been observed among both gram-positive and gram-negative bacteria as well as among certain fungi, particularly *Candida* species. Table 137-1 summarizes important trends in increasing resistance in the United States among selected pathogens and drug classes.[2,24,25] Much of the changing epidemiology of infection in the ICU has centered around the emergence of gram-positive organisms as predominant pathogens in the critically ill patient. Surveillance programs such as the National Nosocomial Infection Surveillance (NNIS) System sponsored by the Centers for Disease Control and Prevention have repeatedly documented impressive increases in antimicrobial resistance among pathogens such as methicillin-resistant *Staphylococcus aureus* (MRSA), vancomycin-resistant enterococci (VRE), and multidrug-resistant *Streptococcus pneumoniae*.[2,4,24] Rates of MRSA and methicillin-resistant coagulase-negative staphylococci have continued to steadily increase over the past decade and are most commonly associated with central catheter–associated bloodstream and wound infections,[2-4,7] whereas MRSA is also being increasingly documented as a frequent pathogen in ventilator-associated pneumonias.[4,26,27] Although MRSA has been traditionally regarded as a hospital-acquired pathogen, this pathogen has also emerged as a common cause of community-acquired infections[28-31]; approximately 30% of all MRSA isolates found in hospitals are now actually community acquired.[32] The increase in methicillin resistance among staphylococci has led to a heavy reliance on vancomycin as a drug of choice for infections due to these pathogens and is perhaps related to the dramatic increase in the number of infections caused by VRE among ICU patients. High-level penicillin resistance among *S. pneumoniae* has been increasing steadily over the past decade and is now approximately 20%.[33,34]

TABLE 137–1. TRENDS IN ANTIMICROBIAL RESISTANCE AMONG SELECTED NOSOCOMIAL PATHOGENS FROM ICU PATIENTS IN THE UNITED STATES, 1993-1997 AND 2002

Pathogen	Resistance Rate, 1993-1997	Resistance Rate, 1999	Percent change, 1993-1997 to 1999
Vancomycin-resistant enterococci	15.4	27.5	78%
Methicillin-resistant *Staphylococcus aureus*	35.6	57.1	60%
Methicillin-resistant coagulase-negative staphylococci	84.0	89.1	6%
3GC-resistant *Escherichia coli**	2.5	6.3	152%
3GC-resistant *Klebsiella pneumoniae**	10.0	14.0	40%
Imipenem-resistant *Pseudomonas aeruginosa*	12.9	22.3	73%
Fluoroquinolone-resistant *P. aeruginosa*	12.3	32.8	167%
3GC-resistant *P. aeruginosa*	20.8	30.2	45%
3GC-resistant *Enterobacter* species	32.4	32.2	−6%

3GC, Third-generation cephalosporin (cefotaxime, ceftriaxone, or ceftazidime).
*Rates reflect nonsusceptibility (resistant and intermediate susceptibility).

Additionally, penicillin-resistant pneumococci tend to be multidrug resistant; 25% to 30% of *S. pneumoniae* have decreased susceptibility to macrolide antibiotics, and rates of resistance to several other drug classes including sulfonamides, tetracyclines, and cephalosporins have also increased.[33,34] Although the prevalence of fluoroquinolone resistance among *S. pneumoniae* is still very low (1%),[33-35] there is significant concern regarding excessive use of fluoroquinolones and the potential for significant resistance in the future.[35,36]

Antimicrobial resistance also continues to be an increasingly important problem among gram-negative bacilli. Of particular concern is the rapid spread of resistance mediated by extended-spectrum beta-lactamases (ESBLs) among organisms such as *Klebsiella pneumoniae*. Organisms that produce ESBLs are usually resistant to multiple antimicrobials, including third- (e.g., ceftriaxone, ceftazidime) and fourth-generation (e.g., cefepime) cephalosporins and aztreonam,[37,38] and are also associated with high rates of resistance to aminoglycosides and fluoroquinolones.[38,39] The increase in ESBL-mediated resistance is reflected in rates of *K. pneumoniae* resistance to third-generation cephalosporins, as shown in Table 137-1. Antimicrobial resistance among *Pseudomonas aeruginosa* is also alarming in that agents currently being particularly affected include the fluoroquinolones and carbapenems such as imipenem.[4,24,25,40,41] Resistance of *P. aeruginosa* to fluoroquinolones and imipenem has increased rapidly and represents the most dramatic changes in antimicrobial susceptibilities detected by recent surveillance studies; nearly 10% of *P. aeruginosa* isolates are now resistant to multiple drug classes, including cephalosporins, carbapenems, aminoglycosides, and/or fluoroquinolones.[40] Multidrug resistance is also very common (approximately 25% of isolates) among strains of *Acinetobacter baumanii*. Fluoroquinolone resistance is also now being increasingly reported among organisms such as *Escherichia coli* that are usually considered to be extremely susceptible to this class of drugs.[41] Antimicrobial resistance among gram-negative organisms such as *P. aeruginosa* has been of great concern in the ICU setting for many years, but increasing resistance among previously susceptible organisms and the involvement of multiple drug classes clearly indicates that the problem continues to grow worse.

Candida albicans is the seventh most common pathogen associated with nosocomial infections in critically ill patients. While *C. albicans* is associated with approximately 7% of all nosocomial infections, it is the second most common cause of nosocomial urinary tract infections (15% of infections) and fourth most common cause of nosocomial bloodstream infections.[2] Resistance to antifungal agents among *Candida* species is usually considered to be quite infrequent. However, a recent multicenter study of 50 hospitals in the United States found that 10% of *C. albicans* isolates from bloodstream infections were resistant to fluconazole.[42] Because susceptibility testing for *Candida* species is not routinely performed in most hospitals, the true scope of resistance among *C. albicans* and other strains is not well characterized and may in fact be higher than currently assumed. It is well documented, however, that the relative frequency of fungal infections with *Candida krusei* and other strains with decreased susceptibility to azole antifungals is increasing among certain populations such as the critically ill and patients with hematologic malignancies.[43,44] While currently not considered to be a major problem, increasing antimicrobial resistance among fungal pathogens such as *C. albicans* is nevertheless of concern.

Infections caused by antimicrobial-resistant bacteria have been demonstrated to be associated with higher mortality rates and longer length of ICU and hospital stays.[45-48] Antimicrobial-resistant strains of bacteria have been demonstrated to express virulence factors that may be different from those expressed by antimicrobial-susceptible strains; this may explain some of the increased mortality associated with these infections.[12,48-51] However, increased mortality associated with infections caused by resistant bacteria may also be explained by the increased likelihood that patients will receive inadequate antimicrobial treatment. Inadequate antimicrobial therapy, defined as the use of drugs with poor in-vitro activity against the infecting pathogen, has been demonstrated in numerous studies to be significantly associated with increased mortality and other measures of poor patient outcomes.[52-61] Treatment with inadequate antimicrobial therapy is particularly problematic during the initial empirical treatment of infections when specific pathogens and antibiotic susceptibility information are not yet known.[54,57,59-61] It is logical to assume that selection of adequate empirical therapy becomes more difficult as the organisms become more resistant to antimicrobial therapy, and it has in fact been demonstrated in clinical studies that most inadequate treatment of nosocomial infections in the ICU is related to the presence of pathogens that are resistant to the selected antibiotics.[55-57] Furthermore, it has been shown in patients with nosocomial pneumonia that changing to more appropriate antibiotics when culture and susceptibility results became available (typically 48 to 72 hours after initiating therapy) did not significantly lower mortality rates compared with patients who received inadequate antibiotics for the entire duration of therapy.[53] The importance of antimicrobial resistance in terms of antimicrobial selection and patient outcomes is thus difficult to overstate.

STRATEGIES TO REDUCE ANTIMICROBIAL RESISTANCE

Various strategies have been recommended to decrease problems of resistance through improved use of antimicrobials. These strategies include the use of antimicrobial protocols and guidelines, hospital formulary–based antimicrobial restrictions, scheduled antimicrobial rotation or "cycling," improved techniques for detection and/or diagnosis of infections, use of combination antimicrobial therapy, decreased duration of antimicrobial therapy, and early involvement of infectious diseases specialists in the management of infected patients.[62] Among these various strategies, the roles of antimicrobial restrictions and antimicrobial cycling are two particularly controversial issues.

Hospital formulary–driven restriction of specific drugs or drug classes is a common method of controlling antimicrobial use within an institution. Formulary-based restrictions have historically been used to control drug costs; they may also reduce rates of adverse effects of high-risk agents.[63] More recently, antimicrobial restrictions have also been used in an attempt to either decrease overall emergence of antimicrobial resistance within an institution or to control acute outbreaks of resistance affecting specific drugs and pathogens.[16,64-66] The effectiveness of antimicrobial restrictions in reducing overall levels of resistance has not been consistently demonstrated. Indeed, it can be argued that antimicrobial restrictions cause intense selective pressure from a small number of agents and may actually promote the emergence of resistance rather than preventing it.[63] Antibiotic restrictions that are instituted in response to specific outbreaks of antibiotic-resistant infections, together with appropriate infection control measures, have been shown to successfully manage specific resistance problems.[64-66] However, it has also been shown that restriction of a drug in response to a resistance issue may in turn cause other resistance problems affecting other drugs.[16] This phenomenon is sometimes referred to as "squeezing the balloon" because the enforcement of antimicrobial restrictions leads to new selective pressures that may effectively solve the original problem but cause the development of new resistance issues.[67] A classic example involved restriction of ceftazidime and increased use of imipenem in response to an outbreak of ceftazidime-resistant *K. pneumoniae*; although ceftazidime resistance among *K. pneumoniae* isolates was effectively decreased by 44%, the rates of imipenem-resistant *P. aeruginosa* significantly increased by 69%.[16] Although antimicrobial restrictions may be effective in reducing drug costs and limiting specific outbreaks of resistant infections, the emphasis must clearly be on appropriate and rational drug use rather than relying on such restrictions to overcome resistance problems.

Antibiotic cycling, in which a specific drug or an entire antibiotic class is periodically withdrawn from clinical use and replaced with a different drug or class, has been investigated as a means of decreasing resistance by limiting narrow selective pressures and exposing organisms to a wide variety of different antimicrobials over time.[68-72] Although initial studies are promising and have demonstrated reduced antimicrobial resistance as well as decreased incidence of certain nosocomial infections and reduced patient mortality,[68,70-72] results of these studies have not been entirely consistent in the overall effectiveness of the antibiotic cycling strategy. In addition, a number of important questions concerning antibiotic cycling have not been adequately addressed by previous studies. These questions include which specific agents or classes are most appropriate to cycle; whether agents or classes of drugs should be cycled in a specific order; how often to change drugs within the scheduled cycle; and whether the potential effectiveness of antimicrobial cycling is maintained over long periods of time.[69] Further research is clearly needed to answer these and other relevant questions, but the cycling concept itself appears promising.

PRINCIPLES OF APPROPRIATE ANTIMICROBIAL USE

While many of the issues regarding antimicrobial use in critically ill patients are currently centered on issues related to antimicrobial resistance, adherence to basic principles of appropriate drug use is still crucial in overall optimization of drug therapy (Table 137-2).

DIAGNOSTIC ISSUES

Establishment of a definitive diagnosis of infection is paramount to the appropriate selection and use of antimicrobials. Once infection is suspected in the ICU patient, a comprehensive workup must be performed to identify the site of infection. The microbial causes of various ICU infections are reasonably predictable once the actual site of infection is known; appropriate drug selection thus properly begins with identification of a known or suspected site of infection. Unfortunately, the site of infection is often unable to be identified with any certainty; studies in septic patients have shown that no source of infection is identified in up to 30% to 40% of patients.[59,74] Modern ICU practitioners have access to a wide range of invasive and noninvasive diagnostic techniques, and these should be employed when appropriate. However, the institution of antimicrobial therapy should not be unnecessarily delayed for the sake of performing exhaustive diagnostic tests.[75]

Gram stain of appropriate specimens from potential sites of infection should also be utilized to help determine appropriate empirical or "definitive" (i.e., based on culture and susceptibility information) antimicrobial therapy. Although the yield of useful information from Gram stains is usually not high in critically ill patients, performing this test is nevertheless of value for those patients in whom causative pathogens are identified.[52,53,55] Gram stains from specimens obtained from certain sites such as the respiratory tract and wounds should be interpreted with caution, owing to high rates of colonization with nonpathogenic organisms, particularly in patients who have already been hospitalized for several days. Early studies clearly demonstrated the high frequency and rapid time course of microbial colonization of ICU patients. Classic studies demonstrated that rates of colonization of the oropharynx and bronchi of critically ill patients with gram-negative organisms reached 45% and 65% within 5 days after ICU admission, respectively, and over 90% at both sites by day 10.[76] These patients also become highly colonized with gram-positive cocci and particularly yeast soon after ICU admission. Great care must be taken to differentiate colonizing organisms from true pathogens when evaluating Gram stain and culture results from nonsterile areas of the body or areas that may become colonized after the placement of foreign devices such as catheters (e.g., urinary tract and respiratory tract). Colonization is often distinguished on the basis of Gram stain results showing multiple morphologic types of bacteria or the absence of clinically relevant signs and symptoms of infection despite the presence of microbial growth. However, in critically ill patients, colonization is often extremely difficult to distinguish from true infection and antimicrobials are initiated based on a presumptive diagnosis.

Clinicians must also keep in mind that there are numerous sources of fever in critically ill patients that are not associated with infection (Table 137-3). The occurrence of new fever in an ICU patient should prompt a thorough evaluation of noninfectious sources of the fever before initiation of antimicrobial therapy. Patients who have been started on antimicrobial therapy and have persistent fever despite the resolution of other signs and symptoms of infection should also be evaluated for noninfectious sources of fever.

SELECTION OF EMPIRICAL DRUG THERAPY

The initial selection of adequate drug therapy is of vital importance in optimizing outcomes of antimicrobial use in critically ill patients. Selection of inadequate therapy has been demonstrated in numerous clinical studies to be associated with increased patient mortality,[52-60] and the risk of inadequate therapy is often directly related to rates of antimicrobial

TABLE 137–2. BASIC PRINCIPLES OF APPROPRIATE ANTIMICROBIAL USE IN CRITICALLY ILL PATIENTS

1. Establish definitive diagnosis before initiating antimicrobials.
   a. Perform comprehensive clinical evaluation.
   b. Perform appropriate diagnostic tests.
   c. Obtain appropriate specimens for culture and susceptibility testing.
   d. Evaluate patient for noninfectious sources of fever.
2. Initiate appropriate empirical antimicrobial therapy.
   a. Consider known/probable site of infection and most likely pathogens.
   b. Consider colonization vs. infection when evaluating culture results.
   c. Consider rates of antimicrobial resistance among potential pathogens.
   d. Consider need for combination antimicrobial therapy vs. monotherapy.
   e. Initial therapy should be broad spectrum, parenteral, and at appropriately aggressive doses.
      (1) Consider pharmacokinetic properties of potentially used agents and potential alterations.
      (2) Consider pharmacodynamic properties of potentially used agents.
      (3) Consider age, organ dysfunction, and site of infection when determining proper dose.
      (4) Consider potential drug-related adverse effects and toxicities.
      (5) Consider potentially relevant drug/drug or drug/disease state interactions.
      (6) Consider use of less expensive agents when appropriate.
3. Change to appropriate definitive drug therapy when possible.
   a. Monitor culture and susceptibility test results.
   b. Spectrum of antimicrobial activity of selected agents should be as narrow as possible when pathogen(s) is/are known.
   c. Consider need for combination antimicrobial therapy vs. monotherapy.
   d. Therapy should be at appropriately aggressive doses.
      (1) Consider pharmacokinetic properties of potentially used agents and potential alterations.
      (2) Consider pharmacodynamic properties of potentially used agents.
      (3) Consider age, organ dysfunction, and site of infection when determining proper dose.
      (4) Consider potential drug-related adverse effects and toxicities.
      (5) Consider potentially relevant drug/drug or drug/disease state interactions.
      (6) Consider use of less expensive agents when appropriate.
4. Consider use of oral antimicrobials when appropriate.
   a. Patients clinically respond to parenteral therapy.
   b. Patients have functional gastrointestinal tracts.
   c. Suitable oral alternatives to parenteral therapy are available.
5. Perform careful patient monitoring for duration of antimicrobial therapy.
   a. Evaluate for clinical resolution of signs and symptoms and evidence of response to therapy.
   b. Evaluate for changes in organ function that may require change in drug-dosing regimen.
   c. Monitor serum drug concentrations when appropriate.
   d. Evaluate for drug-related adverse effects and toxicities.
   e. Evaluate for potential adverse drug interactions.
6. Carefully reassess patients who appear to be failing antimicrobial therapy.
   a. Evaluate patient for unidentified or new sources/sites of infection or superinfection.
   b. Obtain additional specimens for culture and susceptibility testing.
   c. Evaluate drug regimen for proper spectrum of activity against known or presumed pathogens.
   d. Consider emergence of antibiotic resistance among certain pathogens (e.g., *P. aeruginosa*).
   e. Evaluate drug regimen for proper dosing of individual antimicrobial agents.
   f. Consider pharmacokinetic and pharmacodynamic properties of agents and potential need for increased daily doses or alternative dosing methods.
7. Limit duration of therapy when possible.
   a. Short courses are desired over long courses in patients who have promptly responded to antimicrobial therapy.
   b. In patients with no documented infection/pathogens, discontinue antimicrobials after appropriate course of therapy and assess continued need for treatment.

resistance in certain pathogens.[55-57] A number of factors are therefore important to consider when choosing initial empirical therapy. These considerations should include suspected site(s) of infection and corresponding potential pathogens, rates of resistance of these pathogens to potentially used drugs, a patient's prior exposure to antimicrobial therapy that may potentially increase the likelihood of antimicrobial resistance, and the results of any pertinent prior diagnostic tests. A reasonable understanding of the pharmacology, pharmacokinetics, pharmacodynamics, potential toxicities, potential drug interactions, and appropriate dosing of individual antimicrobials is also important in the selection of a specific drug once the type of drug to be used has been decided on. These drug-specific considerations are discussed in more detail later in this chapter. In general, empirical antimicrobial regimens for critically ill patients should be aggressive, that is, sufficiently broad spectrum in pharmacologic activity to cover the most likely (rather than all possible) pathogens, initiated promptly, and given in relatively high doses when the presence of any significant renal or hepatic dysfunction is accounted for.

Clinicians should be familiar with patterns and rates of resistance of key pathogens involved in both community-acquired and nosocomial infections. Resistance rates for pathogens occurring in community-acquired infections may be very different from those same types of pathogens causing nosocomial infections. For example, *E. coli* causing community-acquired urinary tract infections may have a rate of resistance to ciprofloxacin of 1% to 2%, whereas *E. coli* associated with nosocomial urinary tract infections may display resistance to ciprofloxacin in greater than 10% of strains.[77,78] Likewise, *S. aureus* associated with community-acquired infections is predominantly susceptible to methicillin while the rate of methicillin-resistant *S. aureus* (MRSA) is now 60% to 70% in many hospitals in the United States.[2-5] Whereas information concerning rates of antimicrobial resistance in the outside community is often not as readily available as information concerning institutional susceptibilities, ICU practitioners should nevertheless be familiar with resistance rates in both settings to choose appropriate antibiotics. Although antibiograms summarizing drug susceptibilities of key pathogens are available in most institutions, clinicians should recognize that published susceptibilities often do not differentiate between ICU and non-ICU isolates. It is well recognized that resistance rates are often much higher among isolates obtained from patients in ICUs where antimicrobial use is heaviest and more risk factors for resistance (e.g., higher severity of illness, invasive devices, immune suppression) are present.[79-81] It is also known that

TABLE 137–3. NONINFECTIOUS SOURCES OF FEVER IN CRITICALLY ILL PATIENTS

Hemorrhage

Central nervous system
Gastrointestinal
Intra-articular
Pulmonary
Retroperitoneal

Inflammatory Conditions

Atelectasis
Blood product transfusion
Cholecystitis
Collagen vascular diseases
   Systemic lupus erythematosus
   Rheumatoid arthritis
Gout and pseudogout
Ischemic bowel
Pericarditis
Postoperative fever
Postpericardiotomy syndrome
Trauma
Vasculitis
   Cerebral angiitis
   Temporal arteritis
   Lymphomatoid granulomatosis
   Cholesterol embolism
   Drug-induced vasculitis
   Giant cell arteritis
   Henoch-Schönlein purpura
   Polyarteritis nodosa
   Radiation arteriopathy
   Wegener's granulomatosis

Medications

Allergic reactions
Idiopathic drug fever

Metabolic Conditions

Adrenal insufficiency
Alcohol withdrawal
Heat stroke/exhaustion
Hyperthyroidism
Malignant hyperthermia
Neuroleptic malignant syndrome
Seizures

Neoplasms

Colorectal carcinoma
Hepatoma
Hepatic metastases
Leukemia
Lymphoma
Renal cell carcinoma

Thromboembolism

Deep venous thrombosis
Dissecting aortic aneurysm
Graft/venous access thrombosis
Myocardial infarction
Pulmonary embolism
Thrombophlebitis
Thrombotic thrombocytopenia purpura

susceptibilities often differ markedly among different types of ICUs (e.g., medical, surgical, burn, trauma) owing to patients with varying risk factors and potential differences in the types and amounts of antimicrobials used in each of these areas.[79-81] When such information is available, ICU practitioners must be aware of any important differences between their unit-specific drug susceptibilities and resistance rates for the institution as a whole.

DEFINITIVE DRUG SELECTION

When the results of culture and susceptibility tests are available, clinicians must utilize this information to reassess and make appropriate changes to empirical drug regimens. Antimicrobial regimens should be selected that provide suitable activity against identified pathogens while at the same time using the fewest required number of drugs, narrowing the spectrum of antimicrobial activity as much as possible, minimizing the risk of drug-related toxicities, and minimizing the cost of drug therapy. It is common for patients to be treated empirically for the entire duration of therapy owing to the inability to identify the site(s) of infection, negative culture results, cultures suspected to be positive for colonizing organisms rather than pathogens, or other reasons. However, rational antimicrobial therapy dictates that culture and susceptibility information must be utilized in the selection of more definitive antimicrobial therapy when such information is available and felt to be reliable. It is inappropriate to continue empirically selected drug regimens simply because the patient is clinically responding to present therapy and the clinician is unwilling to make a change of any kind.

COMBINATION THERAPY

Combinations of drugs are often recommended and used in both empirical and definitive antimicrobial regimens as a means of increasing the spectrum of pharmacologic activity, providing potentially additive or synergistic activity against selected organisms such as *P. aeruginosa*, improving clinical efficacy, and minimizing the potential for emergence of resistance during therapy.[82-85] Combination regimens are also associated with the potential disadvantages of increased drug-related toxicities and increased drug costs. Although combination therapy is considered standard practice for certain specific infections such as some types of endocarditis,[86] the efficacy of combination therapy has not been well proven in respect to its presumed advantages. While combinations of drugs may increase the overall spectrum of activity compared with the same drugs used alone, single agents such as carbapenems (imipenem/cilastatin and meropenem) and piperacillin/tazobactam provide very broad ranges of pharmacologic activity that includes gram-negative (including *P. aeruginosa*), gram-positive, and anaerobic bacteria. A number of studies concerning the treatment of sepsis have shown that monotherapy with ceftazidime, cefepime, and carbapenems is similar in efficacy to combination regimens (77% to 93% and 76% to 94% clinical response rates, respectively) with no differences in the development of resistance during therapy.[87-93] However, these studies are now several years old and may not reflect the current spectrum of pathogens and antimicrobial resistance encountered in contemporary ICU practice. Although it is most appropriate to use antimicrobials with a narrow spectrum of activity whenever possible, monotherapy may not be feasible in many institutions in which high rates of antimicrobial resistance are present among common pathogens such *P. aeruginosa* and *S. aureus*. As previously discussed, the selection of adequate empirical antimicrobial regimens is becoming more difficult as bacteria become more resistant and the routine use of monotherapy regimens is very difficult in many institutions from this standpoint.

Aside from considerations regarding empirical antimicrobial regimens, combination regimens are appropriately used in the treatment of mixed infections caused by aerobic and anaerobic bacteria, gram-negative and gram-positive bacteria, and/or bacteria and fungi.[82,83] In these situations it is often more appropriate to select two or more agents with focused activity against known pathogens rather than treat with an excessively broad-spectrum single agent. Combination regimens are also recommended in the treatment of systemic infections caused by certain gram-negative organisms such as *P. aeruginosa*, *Acinetobacter* species, *Enterobacter* species, and *Serratia marcescens* as well as severe staphylococcal and enterococcal infections to achieve the potential benefits of antibiotic synergy, improved efficacy, and decreased resistance.[82,83,94-97] Although some studies indicate that combination regimens for gram-negative pathogens such as *P. aeruginosa* are no more efficacious than monotherapy with newer agents such as cefepime and the carbapenems,[61,98-100] use of combination regimens is recommended until better data supporting the efficacy of monotherapy are available. This is particularly true in critically ill patients with neutropenia or other conditions that cause them to be severely immunocompromised.[82,83]

DRUG DOSAGE AND ADMINISTRATION

Antimicrobials are selected based primarily on their pharmacologic activity against presumed or documented pathogens. However, because of the severity and high risk of morbidity and mortality associated with infections in critically ill patients, particular consideration must be given to other pharmacologic properties as well. Optimization of antimicrobial therapy requires that drugs be dosed in a manner that maximizes their pharmacologic activity while minimizing the risk of adverse effects and toxicities. Special consideration should be given to antimicrobial mechanisms of action, pharmacokinetics and pharmacodynamics, routes of administration, potential adverse effects, and potential drug interactions.

Mechanisms of Action

Because infections in critically ill patients are often severe and fulminant, it is theoretically most desirable to use antimicrobials that are "cidal" rather than "static" (i.e., merely inhibiting growth). The use of bactericidal agents has not specifically been shown to be superior to bacteriostatic agents in ICU patients. However, alterations in immune function that inherently accompany critical illness and the otherwise immunocompromised state of many ICU patients as the result of neutropenia, immunosuppressive diseases, or use of immunosuppressive drugs make it prudent to use antimicrobials that quickly reduce the antimicrobial burden at the site of infection and potentially result in eradication of pathogens through their bactericidal actions. Penicillins, cephalosporins, aminoglycosides, fluoroquinolones, vancomycin, metronidazole, and amphotericin B are examples of "cidal" antimicrobials commonly used for the treatment of ICU infections.

Pharmacokinetic Considerations

Pharmacokinetic properties that should be specifically considered in critically ill patients include distribution to various tissues and fluids and routes of metabolism and excretion. The ability of a drug to penetrate to the site of infection in sufficient quantities to have activity against a pathogen is crucial for achieving clinical and microbiologic efficacy. Although the distributional characteristics of antimicrobials are often only specifically considered in the treatment of central nervous system infections, good penetration to tissues and fluids present at the site of infection is a necessary consideration when selecting agents for any infection in ICU patients. Routes of drug metabolism and elimination are also important pharmacokinetic properties because of the prevalence of acute and chronic organ failures in most critically ill populations. Severe organ dysfunction, particularly of the liver or kidneys, should prompt clinicians to select agents that do not rely on that organ for metabolism or excretion from the body to avoid excessive drug accumulation and increased potential for unacceptable drug toxicities. Clinicians should also be mindful of the fact that some common antimicrobials (e.g., ceftriaxone, ciprofloxacin) are dependent on both the liver and the kidneys for metabolism and excretion, and their use may be particularly problematic in patients with dysfunction of both of these organ systems. Practitioners must be familiar with the pharmacokinetic properties of commonly used antimicrobials to use them in the most efficacious and safe manner.

Pharmacodynamic Considerations

Pharmacodynamics is the discipline that attempts to define and apply the relationships between concentrations of a drug and its pharmacologic effects (both desirable and undesirable).[101] Although both the pharmacologic activity of an agent and its pharmacokinetic disposition are important considerations in drug selection and dosing, it is the combination of these two properties that is critical to achieving optimal outcomes during treatment of infections. The pharmacologic activities of antibacterial drugs are commonly defined by their minimal inhibitory concentration (MIC) as determined by in-vitro testing. The MIC is the minimal concentration required to inhibit the growth of a target organism; highly active agents are associated with low MICs, that is, only low concentrations are required to inhibit bacterial growth, whereas agents with poor activity are associated with high MICs for the organism in question. It is logical that even extremely active agents with very low MICs will not be efficacious against a pathogen if the drug does not reach the site of infection in sufficient quantity; likewise, agents with relatively poor activity and higher MICs may be just as clinically efficacious if they are able to achieve high drug concentrations at the site of infection. Pharmacodynamic considerations combine MIC-defined activity and pharmacokinetic properties of a drug to make predictions regarding the drug's probable efficacy in the treatment of a given type of infection. Models of infection have allowed antibacterial drugs to be broadly classified into two major categories: concentration-dependent killing agents and time-dependent (concentration-independent) killing agents.[101]

Concentration-dependent agents, particularly aminoglycosides and fluoroquinolones, exert bactericidal activities when drug concentrations are well above the MIC of the organism; the higher the ratio of drug concentration at the site of infection to the MIC, the more rapid and/or complete the bacterial killing becomes. Previous studies have established that important pharmacodynamic predictors of clinical efficacy of concentration-dependent agents include the ratio of maximum serum concentration divided by the MIC (C_{max}/MIC) and the ratio of the 24-hour area under the serum concentration-versus-time curve divided by the MIC (AUC_{0-24}/MIC).[101-111] Although the ratios required to achieve maximal effects are not exactly known, in-vitro and in-vivo studies indicate that C_{max}/MIC ratios of at least 10 to 12 and, for the fluoroquinolones, AUC_{0-24}/MIC ratios of 30 to 50 for gram-positive and 125 to 250 for gram-negative organisms are required for optimal clinical and microbiologic outcomes as well as for the prevention of antimicrobial resistance.[101-111] Both C_{max}/MIC and AUC_{0-24}/MIC ratios appear to be important determinants of clinical and microbiologic outcomes, although it is less clear which of these parameters is most predictive of drug efficacy because they are closely linked by the pharmacokinetic properties of the drugs.

Time-dependent killing agents only exert antimicrobial effects when their concentrations at the site of infection are higher than the MIC of the pathogen; the so-called time above MIC (T > MIC) thus becomes the pharmacodynamic parameter of interest for these drugs.[101,112-114] Important time-dependent agents common in ICU practice include the penicillins, cephalosporins, carbapenems, clindamycin, and the macrolides. Studies indicate that T > MIC should be at least 40% to 50% of the dosing interval, although it has also been suggested that achieving T > MIC for 100% of the dosing interval may be desirable for optimal outcome.[101,112-114] These studies have also suggested that both the AUC_{0-24}/MIC as well as the T > MIC are important predictors of clinical efficacy and the risk of the development of microbial resistance.[101,112-114]

Because patients in the ICU are frequently infected with serious nosocomial pathogens that display decreased antimicrobial susceptibilities and are prone to developing resistance with inadequate therapy, failure to properly dose antimicrobial agents predisposes patients to clinical and microbiologic failure. The appropriate consideration of pharmacodynamic principles in the treatment of infection in critically ill patients enables clinicians to select dosing regimens that will maximize the potential effectiveness of the specific agent. Thus, aminoglycosides and fluoroquinolones, concentration-dependent killers, should be used in relatively high doses that facilitate their distribution into infected tissues and achieve concentrations manyfold higher than the MIC of pathogens. Direct application of these pharmacodynamic principles has resulted in the common use of extended-interval dosing (also referred to as once-daily or single-daily dosing) of aminoglycosides in which these drugs are administered in single doses of 6 to 9 mg/kg rather than smaller divided doses,[115] as well as the use of increased daily doses of fluoroquinolones (ciprofloxacin and levofloxacin) for severe infections such as nosocomial pneumonia and complicated skin and skin structure infections.[116] Likewise, beta-lactam antibiotics such as the penicillins and cephalosporins are best given as several smaller divided doses administered intermittently throughout the day, or even as a continuous infusion of drug, to maintain high concentrations of drug over long periods of time. Thus, beta-lactams are usually administered every 4 to 12 hours depending on achievable serum concentrations and the serum half-life of the specific agent.

The severity of infections encountered in the ICU population and the need for adequate C_{max}/MIC and AUC_{0-24}/MIC ratios are important considerations in these severely ill patients. However, the direct application of pharmacodynamic principles in routine patient care is still relatively new and there is still much to be learned in this area. Although it is assumed that serum concentrations of most drugs are related to their concentrations in various tissues, the use of serum C_{max}/MIC and AUC_{0-24}/MIC ratios does not always accurately predict tissue concentrations of drugs. A particularly important limitation of pharmacodynamic principles in the routine care of ICU patients is that they have not been thoroughly clinically validated in critically ill populations. Numerous studies have demonstrated that the pharmacokinetics of antimicrobials are often significantly altered in critical illness and that there is a high degree of interpatient (and even intrapatient) variability in this population.[115,117-124] Distribution of antimicrobials to infected tissues may also be affected by hemodynamic instability and regional or local changes in perfusion of various organs and tissues. The difficult combination of severe illness, pharmacokinetic variability, and life-threatening infections involving potentially drug-resistant pathogens makes the ICU population a difficult one in which to optimize drug therapy through appropriate application of pharmacodynamic principles. However, it is also only through the application of these principles that optimization of antimicrobial therapy is likely to be achieved in any consistent manner.

Dosing

Because of the severity of infections encountered in critically ill patients and because of the variability in pharmacokinetics, tissue penetration, and so on, the general recommendation for dosing of antimicrobials in ICU patients is to use high, aggressive doses. Use of high doses potentially compensates for pharmacokinetic variability that may be present and ensures that patients are receiving enough drug to achieve pharmacodynamic goals of antimicrobial use. However, use of high doses also puts patients at higher risk of drug-related adverse effects and toxicities, again partially owing to the pharmacokinetic variability in drug distribution and elimination. Although drug dosing should be aggressive, it must also be based on appropriate clinical considerations involving relevant issues such as drug toxicities, presence of renal or hepatic dysfunction that may lead to drug accumulation, the presumed site of infection and the ability of the drug to achieve adequate concentrations in that site, and susceptibilities of presumed or documented pathogens to the drugs in question.

Route of Administration

For initial therapy for serious infections, antimicrobials should generally be administered by the intravenous route to avoid any problems of drug absorption related to gut malperfusion and ensure rapid, adequate serum and tissue concentrations. However, although drugs are usually given intravenously at the initiation of therapy, drugs with good oral bioavailability may be effectively switched to oral formulations once patients are stable and responding to therapy. A number of drugs including levofloxacin, linezolid, fluconazole, and others have oral bioavailabilities approaching 100%; such agents may be administered orally without any apparent loss of therapeutic efficacy and with substantial cost savings.[122,125] Oral antibiotics are an option for many hospitalized patients, including those in the ICU, and should be considered when patients have responded favorably to parenteral regimens and are able to take oral medications.[122,125]

Adverse Effects and Toxicities

Critically ill patients are associated with higher rates of adverse effects from drugs compared to the general population of non-ICU patients. This is attributable to several factors, including the frequent presence of renal and/or hepatic dysfunction that may lead to excessive accumulation and high concentrations of drugs, administration of many concurrent medications that may have overlapping adverse effect profiles or additive toxicities, and underlying illness that makes them more predisposed to adverse effects such as central nervous system or renal toxicities. Clinicians must carefully evaluate patients for any predisposing conditions potentially associated with increased risk of drug toxicities, and either use high-risk antimicrobials with caution or avoid them altogether. A common example of this concept is the use of aminoglycosides. The overall incidence of aminoglycoside-induced nephrotoxicity is approximately 10% or less compared with rates of 16% to 36% in the critically ill.[115,126,127] Although they may be effectively used in such patients, aminoglycosides must be carefully dosed and monitored to decrease the risk of toxicities; alternatively, many clinicians would choose an agent such as a fluoroquinolone that may be used as part of combination regimens as alternatives to aminoglycosides and do not have the risk of nephrotoxicity. Clinicians must be familiar with the safety profiles of the various antimicrobials they commonly use and use appropriate benefit-versus-risk considerations when selecting agents for a specific patient. The use of multidisciplinary teams in the ICU has also been associated with a substantially decreased incidence of adverse effects in critically ill patients.[128-130]

Drug Interactions

Patients in ICUs are often managed with large numbers of drugs. With polypharmacy being the rule rather than the exception, clinicians must be alert to the potential for adverse drug interactions. Drug interactions involving delayed or decreased absorption of orally administered agents and metabolic interactions involving inhibition of hepatic enzyme systems (e.g., azole antifungals, macrolides) are among the most common types of interactions likely to be seen in this population and should be avoided whenever possible. Drug-disease state interactions involving antimicrobials and increased risk of adverse effects should also be considered and prospectively monitored.

DURATION OF ANTIMICROBIAL THERAPY

The appropriate duration of antimicrobial therapy for most infectious processes has been poorly studied. Beyond community-acquired urinary tract infections, endocarditis, and a handful of other infections, the appropriate duration of treatment for most infections remains incompletely defined. This is particularly true in critically ill patients. The general tendency has been to treat severe infections for long periods of time on the assumption that long courses of antimicrobials are required to provide good clinical efficacy, reduce the probability of treatment failure or relapse, and prevent the emergence of resistance due to the incomplete eradication of pathogens. However, long durations of therapy may

themselves contribute to the development of resistance by subjecting endogenous or colonizing bacterial flora to unnecessary antimicrobial exposure. Long durations of treatment may also increase the risk of drug-related toxicities and add unnecessary treatment costs. Recent studies have shown that shorter courses of antimicrobial therapy (e.g., 8 days versus 15 days for ventilator-associated pneumonia) are equal or superior in efficacy to longer courses and may be associated with a decreased incidence of superinfections and decreased antimicrobial use, drug costs, adverse effects, and antimicrobial resistance.[131-133] Despite the potential advantages of shorter treatment durations, the decision to discontinue antimicrobial use in seriously ill patients is often very difficult to make on clinical grounds. Clinical response to antimicrobial therapy may be masked by underlying illnesses or concurrent drugs, and critically ill patients may not always manifest an association between successful treatment of an infection and rapid improvement in clinical signs and symptoms.[134-136] Until additional research is able to better define optimal treatment durations for specific types of infections in ICU populations, the decision to discontinue therapy will largely rest on the clinical judgment of the ICU practitioner. Nevertheless, clinicians must remain cognizant of the desirability of limiting antimicrobial treatment durations and seek to discontinue drugs whenever appropriate.

MONITORING RESPONSE TO ANTIMICROBIALS

The appropriate use of antimicrobials in any population requires careful monitoring of patients for clinical response and adverse effects. This is particularly important in critically ill patients owing to the potential for a number of events that may indicate the need to modify drug selection or drug-dosing regimens to improve the probability of successful treatment, enhance patient safety, and decrease drug costs and antimicrobial resistance. Such events include inadequate initial drug selection, the availability of culture and susceptibility test results that may influence subsequent drug selection, emergence of bacterial resistance during therapy, rapidly changing organ function that would influence drug dosing, drug-related adverse effects and toxicities, and the occurrence of superinfection. Serum concentrations of drugs, particularly aminoglycosides, should be monitored to guide appropriate drug dosing.

Clinicians should be mindful that failure of patients to promptly respond to antimicrobial therapy does not necessarily imply that the patient is receiving inadequate therapy. Critically ill patients are often slow to respond to therapy due to the severity of the infection, concomitant disease states, advanced age, and a number of other patient-specific factors.[134-136] Thus, patients who are not clearly showing signs of clinical improvement within 24 to 48 hours after initiating antibiotics may merely require additional time to respond and do not necessarily require the modification of antimicrobial regimens. In addition, many noninfectious sources of fever are present in ICU patients and may confound assessment of a patient's response to therapy. The finding of a persistent fever while other clinical signs and symptoms are improving should thus prompt clinicians to carefully assess patients for other noninfectious sources of fever or failure to respond. Finally, it must be recognized that not every patient treated in the ICU will recover from their infection and failure to respond does not mean that the antimicrobial therapy is inadequate. Whether failure to respond to therapy is in fact related to inadequate drug therapy can only be discerned through careful patient monitoring and assessment. However, even with the most conscientious ongoing assessment, this is often a very difficult distinction to make. The appropriate management of patients who are initially unresponsive to antimicrobial therapy is one of the most challenging dilemmas in the treatment of infections in the ICU.

PROTOCOLS AND GUIDELINES FOR USE OF ANTIMICROBIALS

The use of prescribing guidelines and protocols has been shown to effectively improve overall antimicrobial appropriateness,[137-139] decrease the incidence of adverse drug effects,[140,141] avoid unnecessary antimicrobial use,[137,142] reduce or stabilize bacterial resistance rates,[67,142] and reduce drug costs.[139,142] The use of guidelines for the treatment of ventilator-associated pneumonia in ICU patients has also been associated with increased initial administration of adequate antimicrobial therapy and decreased durations of antibiotic therapy.[138] Although using clinical guidelines and protocols has been demonstrated to produce a number of favorable results, the implementation of such tools is often difficult because they are perceived as being too restrictive on clinical decision-making by individual practitioners. Properly prepared guidelines are multidisciplinary in their preparation and implementation, involve key physicians in their development to make them practical and promote support from other practitioners, and are tailored to the individual institution. Although numerous established guidelines are available in the literature and elsewhere, they must be adapted to each institution and based on specific needs and practice patterns. Guidelines and protocols must also involve intensive education of all affected parties, physicians and nonphysicians alike; this education must precede implementation and must also be ongoing to optimize guideline use. Finally, practitioners involved in use of the guidelines must be regularly updated regarding benefits already achieved and areas for continued improvement. Guidelines and protocols that are based on these principles are more likely to be successful and achieve the potential benefits associated with their use.

ANNOTATED REFERENCES

Chastre J, Wolff M, Fagon J-Y, et al: Comparison of 8 vs 15 days of antibiotic therapy for ventilator-associated pneumonia in adults: a randomized trial. JAMA 2003;290:2588-2598.

This prospective, randomized, double-blind, multicenter trial evaluated whether an 8-day course of antimicrobial therapy was as effective as a 15-day course in the treatment of ventilator-associated pneumonia. The shorter duration of treatment was associated with equal clinical efficacy as measured by mortality, recurrent infections, and ICU length of stay and was also associated with a statistically significant reduction in multidrug-resistant pathogens among those patients who experienced recurrence of pulmonary infection.

Kollef MH, Sherman G, Ward S, et al: Inadequate antimicrobial treatment of infections: A risk factor for hospital mortality among critically ill patients. Chest 1999;115:462-474.

This prospective cohort study evaluated the relationship between inadequate antimicrobial treatment of infection and hospital mortality in 2000 consecutive patients admitted to the medical or surgical intensive care units. Inadequate treatment of infection was demonstrated to be an important determinant of hospital mortality and other poor patient outcomes, and administration of inadequate therapy in both community-acquired and nosocomial infections was shown to be most commonly related to infection with pathogens associated with high rates of antimicrobial resistance.

Luna CM, Vujacich P, Niederman MS, et al: Impact of BAL data on the therapy and outcome of ventilator-associated pneumonia. Chest 1997;111:676-685.

This prospective observational study evaluated the impact of antibiotic selection on outcomes of patients with ventilator-associated pneumonia and determined the impact of bronchoalveolar lavage (BAL) on these outcomes. Although mortality rates were significantly reduced when adequate empirical therapy was administered before BAL, mortality was not reduced compared with patients receiving no therapy or who continued inadequate therapy if adequate therapy was not achieved until after BAL was performed or results were known.

Raymond DP, Pellitier SJ, Crabtree TD, et al: Impact of a rotating empiric antibiotic schedule on infectious mortality in an intensive care unit. Crit Care Med 2001;29:1101-1108.

This prospective cohort study evaluated the impact of implementation of a protocol-driven, rotating antibiotic schedule on infectious complications and mortality. Compared with the previous year of non–protocol-driven antibiotic use, rotation of empirical antimicrobial therapy was associated with significant reductions in infectious mortality and overall infections caused by antimicrobial-resistant bacteria.

U.S. Department of Public Health and Human Services, Public Health Service: National Nosocomial Infections Surveillance (NNIS) System Report, data summary from January 1992-June 2003, issued August 2003. Am J Infect Control 2003;31:481-498.

This latest report from the Centers for Disease Control and Prevention summarizes data related to antimicrobial use and resistance in intensive care units in the United States. Data regarding sites of infections and pathogen prevalence, infection rates, standardized measures of antibiotic utilization, and trends in antimicrobial resistance among key pathogens are presented.

Chapter 138

BETA-LACTAM DRUGS USED IN CRITICAL CARE

Steven J. Martin

KEY POINTS

1. **Beta-lactamase is largely responsible for bacterial resistance to the beta-lactam antibiotics.** Drugs that are stable to beta-lactamase enzymatic activity, such as the carbapenems and cefepime, are most reliable in institutions where significant beta-lactam resistance has occurred.

2. **Penicillin allergy is commonly reported, but true anaphylaxis is rare.** Cross reactivity among the other beta-lactam antibiotics is also low, and prudent consideration should be given to the type of reaction and response to skin testing before eliminating the beta-lactams from consideration.

3. In some institutions, extended-spectrum beta-lactamases have rendered most third-generation cephalosporins **unreliable for the treatment of** *Klebsiella* and *Enterobacter* infections. Alternatives include cefepime or carbapenems.

4. **Carbapenem toxicity is closely related to serum concentrations;** adjustment of dose for renal dysfunction is paramount to avoiding predictable side effects of these compounds.

The beta-lactam antibiotics are the most commonly prescribed antibiotics in the critical care setting. Their individual microbiologic spectra and relative safety have made them first-line therapy for prophylaxis and treatment of infection. From the oldest (penicillin) to the newest (ertapenem) agents discovered, beta-lactams continue to be useful for the myriad infectious complications of critical illness. Table 138-1 lists the parenteral beta-lactam antibiotics that are commonly used in the ICU. Several of these agents may be of more clinical value than others. The beta-lactam compounds share a similar mechanism of action, mechanisms of resistance, pharmacodynamic properties, and many common adverse effects. However, each individual class of beta-lactam has unique microbiologic spectrums and each of the agents has unique pharmacokinetic properties.

MECHANISM OF ACTION

Beta-lactam antibiotics are similar in that each contains a beta-lactam ring in addition to other pharmacologically active side chains stemming from this central structure. Side chain manipulation is largely responsible for both spectrum of activity as well as stability against enzymatic degradation, pharmacokinetics, and adverse effects. Beta-lactam antibiotics inhibit bacterial wall synthesis by binding to penicillin-binding proteins (PBPs). These PBPs are transpeptidases, carboxypeptidases, and endopeptidases involved in the structure and function of the cell wall structure.[1,2] The cell wall is made up of a peptidoglycan consisting of long polysaccharide chains of *N*-acetylglucosamine and *N*-acetylmuramic acid cross-linked by shorter peptide chains.[1-3] There are three stages to peptidoglycan formation, including accumulation of peptidoglycan precursors in the cytoplasm, linkage of precursor products in a long polymer, followed by cross-linking by transpeptidation. Beta-lactams inhibit this final transpeptidation step. Transpeptidation cross-links adjacent sugar chains via their pentapeptides. Peptidoglycan transglycosylase and D-alanyl-D-alanine transpeptidase activity is responsible for this activity. Beta-lactams inhibit D-alanyl-D-alanine transpeptidase activity by acetylation, forming stable esters with the open lactam ring attached to the enzyme's active site. The propensity of the D-alanyl-D-alanine trans- and carboxypeptidase to form stable bonds with beta-lactams provides these enzymes with their collective name of PBPs.[1-3] PBPs lie on the outer side of the cytoplasmic membrane in gram-positive bacteria and are shielded only by the peptidoglycan and outer capsule. In gram-negative bacteria most beta-lactams must cross the outer membrane via porin channels to reach PBPs. Entry through the porin channels is determined by size, charge, and hydrophobicity.

Bacterial killing and clinical efficacy for beta-lactam antibiotics is associated with the percent of time during the dosing interval that the drug concentration is above the minimal inhibitory concentration (MIC). In animal models, bacterial killing is maximized when the serum drug concentration exceeds the bacterial MIC for 60% to 70% of the dosing interval.[4] Carbapenems have faster killing rates than penicillins; cephalosporins have the slowest killing rates of the beta-lactam class.[5] Therefore, percentages for time above the MIC required for bacterial killing are highest for the cephalosporins and lowest for the carbapenems.[5] All intravenous beta-lactam antibiotics are recommended to be given in several daily intervals, but continuous infusion of these agents is an attractive administration method to maintain serum drug concentrations above the MIC. Several clinical trials have validated the use of this administration method in the critically ill, and institutions may institute continuous infusion protocols to reduce daily drug costs.[6-10]

Beta-lactams are commonly used in antibiotic combinations, which may include an aminoglycoside, a fluoroquinolone, a macrolide, or another beta-lactam. Combination therapy is used empirically to broaden the spectrum of activity

TABLE 138–1. BETA-LACTAM ANTIBIOTICS

Natural Penicillins

Penicillin GK

Penicillinase-Resistant Penicillins

Methicillin
Nafcillin
Oxacillin

Aminopenicillins

Ampicillin
Ampicillin/clavulanate

Anti-Pseudomonal Penicillins

Carboxypenicillins
  Carbenicillin
  Ticarcillin
  Ticarcillin/clavulanate
Ureidopenicillins and piperazine penicillins
  Azlocillin
  Mezlocillin
  Piperacillin
  Piperacillin/tazobactam

Cephalosporins

First Generation
  Cefazolin
Second Generation
  Cefoxitin
  Cefotetan
  Cefuroxime
Third Generation
  Cefoperazone
  Cefotaxime
  Ceftazidime
  Ceftriaxone
  Ceftizoxime
Fourth Generation
  Cefepime

Carbapenems

Imipenem/cilastatin
Meropenem
Ertapenem

Monobactams

Aztreonam

or minimize the likelihood of resistance. In documented infection with a known organism, combination therapy may be used to provide synergistic bacterial killing in an attempt to rapidly and thoroughly eradicate the pathogen. For combinations of aminoglycosides and beta-lactams there are ample in vitro data to substantiate the potential synergistic bactericidal activity of the drug in combination. These data are not clear for beta-lactam/fluoroquinolone combinations, and there are theoretical concerns about antagonistic interactions with this combination as well as combinations of two beta-lactam agents.

MECHANISMS OF RESISTANCE

Bacteria resist the cytotoxic activity of the beta-lactams by modifying the normal PBPs, bypassing the normal PBPs, reducing the permeability of drug through the outer membrane (gram-negative bacteria), actively removing drug from the cell through the efflux pump mechanism, and producing beta-lactamases. PBP modification and bypassing of normal PBPs are the most important mechanisms of resistance in gram-positive cocci, but beta-lactamases are important mechanisms of antibiotic resistance in gram-negative bacteria.[11]

Alteration of PBPs, including decreased expression of PBPs and structural modifications to the PBPs to decrease antibiotic binding affinity are seen in both gram-positive and gram-negative bacteria.[12] In gram-positive bacteria, altered PBPs occur commonly in *Streptococcus pneumoniae*, *Enterococcus faecium*, and *Staphylococcus aureus*. Genes encoding these PBP changes in *S. pneumoniae* contain segments from several different organisms, including the viridans streptococci.[13] In *S. aureus* and *E. faecium*, novel PBPs may be inducible through exposure to certain antibiotics.[14,15] These novel PBPs have a low affinity for beta-lactam antibiotics. PBP alterations are best illustrated in methicillin-resistant *S. aureus* (MRSA). Methicillin-resistance occurs through the actions of the *mec A* gene that encodes PBP2′ (PBP2a). MRSA produces PBP2′ as a fifth PBP in addition to the four PBPs found in all *S. aureus* strains.[16] Beta-lactam antibiotics have very low affinity for PBP2′, so the enzyme's function continues even in the presence of beta-lactams.

Gram-negative bacteria, including *Neisseria meningitides*, *Haemophilus influenzae*, and *Escherichia coli*, also produce altered PBPs.[17-20] Imipenem resistance due to altered PBPs has been reported in *Pseudomonas aeruginosa*, *Acinetobacter baumanii*, and *Proteus mirabilis*, although this PBP alteration is not the primary mechanism responsible for most imipenem resistance.[21-23]

Beta-lactamase production is largely responsible for beta-lactam antibiotic resistance among gram-negative bacteria in the critical care setting. Beta-lactamase hydrolyzes the beta-lactam ring structure within the antibiotic molecule, rendering the drug inactive. Most beta-lactamases function by a serine ester hydrolysis mechanism, but a few use a zinc ion to attack the beta-lactam ring.[11] Beta-lactamase can be chromosomal (inherent within the chromosome of the organism) or can be encoded by plasmids or transposons, which are mobile genetic elements that can carry genes for resistance mechanisms. Beta-lactamase production may be constitutive or inducible, and beta-lactam antibiotics vary in their ability to induce beta-lactamase production.[24,25] Penicillin G, ampicillin, cefoxitin, imipenem, clavulanate, and first-generation cephalosporins are strong beta-lactamase inducers.[25] Third-generation cephalosporins, ureidopenicillins, aztreonam, and semi-synthetic penicillinase-stable penicillins are weak beta-lactamase inducers.[25]

Some measure of beta-lactamase stability can be achieved through addition to the beta-lactam ring of a substituent that hinders hydrolysis.[26] For example, the semisynthetic penicillinase-stable drugs such as oxacillin and nafcillin remain active against methicillin-susceptible *S. aureus* owing to this ring structure manipulation. Beta-lactamase stability has been difficult to achieve in compounds with activity against gram-negative bacteria and may be due to the periplasmic location of beta-lactamase in the gram-negative cell structure.[11] Antibiotics, including the beta-lactams, have difficulty accessing the gram-negative cell wall owing to the presence of an outer membrane. Porins within the membrane permit limited access through to the peptidoglycan layer of the cell, but the periplasmic space between the membrane and peptidoglycan layer allows beta-lactamase to overwhelm the limited concentrations of drug that enter.

Third-generation cephalosporins have activity against beta-lactamase–producing Enterobacteriaceae because they do not induce enzyme synthesis. However, these drugs may select spontaneous "derepressed" mutants that constitutively produce beta-lactamase.[11] Emergence of derepressed mutants of Enterobacter species during third-generation cephalosporin therapy may be significant, particularly in pneumonia and bacteremia.[27] Through this selective pressure, organisms have developed that overproduce their chromosomal AmpC (class C) beta-lactamase.[28] This type of beta-lactamase is broad spectrum and inactivates most cephalosporins and aztreonam. AmpC resistance has been demonstrated in many clinically important gram-negative bacteria, including Acinetobacter species, Citrobacter freundii, Enterobacter species, E. coli, Morganella morganii, P. aeruginosa, and Serratia marcescens.[28] AmpC beta-lactamase is not inhibited by beta-lactamase inhibitors such as clavulanic acid, sulbactam, or tazobactam.[28] Unfortunately, these chromosomal AmpC beta-lactamases have been found on plasmids worldwide, suggesting that this broad-spectrum class of enzymes may be spread much more readily in clinical settings.[28]

Other plasmid-mediated beta-lactamases with more limited hydrolytic capacity have been found in Klebsiella pneumoniae, E. coli, Enterobacter species, and other common Enterobacteriaceae. These so-called extended-spectrum beta-lactamases (ESBL) are active against the oxyimino-cephalosporins and aztreonam, but not 7-α-methoxy-cephalosporins (cefoxitin, cetotetan), and are blocked by clavulanic acid, sulbactam, and tazobactam.[29] There are numerous reports of outbreaks of ESBL-producing Klebsiella and Enterobacter infections in ICUs.[27,30-37] Most organisms producing AmpC and ESBL enzymes remain susceptible to carbapenems, such as imipenem. However, beta-lactamase that uses zinc as an active site for beta-lactam hydrolysis is able to hydrolyze carbapenems, along with every other beta-lactam presently available.[38] These "metallo" beta-lactamases are produced by about 20 different bacterial strains. The genes that encode these enzymes tend to be chromosomal but have been identified on plasmids.[38] Beta-lactamase inhibitors are not active against "metallo" enzymes. Thus, there are several different types of beta-lactamases present for

the ICU clinician to consider. Understanding the resistance patterns that are likely to occur as a result of each type will help in making appropriate empirical antibiotic selection for nosocomial infection in the critically ill.

PENICILLINS

The microbiologic activity of the penicillins are shown in Tables 138-2 to 138-4. Natural penicillins are most active against non–beta-lactamase–producing gram-positive aerobic and anaerobic bacteria as well as selected gram-negative cocci, such as Neisseria species. Penicillin G is effectively the only natural penicillin used in the critical care setting. Gram-positive bacteria inhibited by natural penicillins in general are more susceptible to these penicillins than to semisynthetic penicillins. Penicillin and ampicillin remain the drugs of choice for enterococcal infections, although recent data suggest nearly 20% enterococcal resistance to ampicillin in North America.[39] Semisynthetic penicillins (oxacillin, nafcillin) are the agents of choice for penicillin-resistant S. aureus and Staphylococcus epidermidis, because penicillins exhibit faster bactericidal activity and improved clinical outcomes when compared with vancomycin.[40,41] Semisynthetic penicillins should be reserved for staphylococcal infections, even though they are active against streptococci. Methicillin is seldom used due to a higher incidence of interstitial nephritis than oxacillin or nafcillin. Nafcillin and oxacillin have similar antistaphylococcal activity and can be used interchangeably for this indication.

Ampicillin possesses the same spectrum as penicillin G and is active against gram-negative cocci and members of the family Enterobacteriaceae. Ampicillin alone is seldom used any longer in critical care settings, because beta-lactamase production is common for almost all Enterobacteriaceae and staphylococci. With the addition of sulbactam to ampicillin, activity is regained against most organisms within these categories. Use of the antipseudomonal penicillins is increasingly limited to ticarcillin/clavulanate and piperacillin/tazobactam, owing to the prevalence of beta-lactamase and the poor activity of these agents against this enzymatic activity. Carbenicillin and ticarcillin are less active than piperacillin against streptococci, enterococci, Haemophilus species, and P. aeruginosa. Ticarcillin and piperacillin have good clinical activity against

TABLE 138–2. MICROBIOLOGIC ACTIVITY OF BETA-LACTAM ANTIBIOTICS AGAINST AEROBIC GRAM-POSITIVE BACTERIA. PERCENT SUSCEPTIBLE BY NCCLS[58] INTERPRETATION (NO. OF ISOLATES TESTED)*

	Gram-Positive Bacteria					
Antibiotic	Staphylococcus aureus	Coagulase-negative Staphylococci	Streptococcus pneumoniae	Viridans Streptococci	Enterococcus faecalis	E. faecium
Penicillin G			53.2% (139)[61,64]	53.2% (139)[61,64]	94.3% (372)[61]	15.7% (127)[61]
Oxacillin	65.9% (4095)[59-63]	26.6% (1146)[61,62]				
Ampicillin/ sulbactam				87% (47)[65]	96% (372)[65]	18.1% (127)[61]
Cefuroxime			83.9% (341)[61]			
Cefotaxime			89.4% (341)[61]	87.8% (47)[65]		
Ceftazidime						
Ceftriaxone			94.8% (3550)[60,62]	86.6% (438)[66]		
Cefepime			95.5% (3891)[60-62]	87.7% (235)[66]		
Imipenem			87.8% (246)[60]	96% (47)[65]		

*When possible, data represent North American isolates from large, national susceptibility databases.

TABLE 138–3. MICROBIOLOGIC ACTIVITY OF BETA-LACTAM ANTIBIOTICS AGAINST AEROBIC GRAM-NEGATIVE BACTERIA. PERCENT SUSCEPTIBLE BY NCCLS[58] INTERPRETATION (NO. OF ISOLATES TESTED)*

Antibiotic	Gram-Negative Bacteria								
	Acinetobacter spp.	Citrobacter spp.	Enterobacter spp.	E. coli	H. influenzae	Klebsiella spp.	Proteus spp.	Pseudomonas aeruginosa	Serratia spp.
Ampicillin/sulbactam	79.2% (404)[63,67]	56% (66)[67]		77% (1076)[62,67]	100% (172)[67]	86% (246)[67]	91% (81)[67]		21% (47)[67]
Ticarcillin/clavulanate	72.9% (494)[68,69]	92.1% (89)[71]	88.6% (457)[59,71]	79.9% (1432)[59,71]		92.9% (986)[59,60,68]		63.1% (15,005)[59,60,67,71,72]	86.3% (226)[71]
Piperacillin/tazobactam	81.3% (494)[68,69]	97.8% (89)[71]	91.9% (2031)[59,69,71]	96.4% (1997)[59,62,71]	100% (199)[60]	94.9% (3754)[59,60,69,71]		89.6% (15,005)[59,60,67,71,72]	97.3% (226)[71]
Cefazolin			3.7% (81)[59]	88.8% (663)[59,62]		87.3% (71)[59]			
Cefotetan		83% (66)[67]	7.4% (81)[59]	99% (511)[67]	100% (172)[67]	93.2% (449)[60,67]	99% (81)[67]		96% (47)[67]
Cefoxitin			61.7% (81)[59]	94.4% (663)[59]		86.1% (274)[59,60]			
Cefuroxime				92.9% (98)[59]					
Ceftazidime	57.1% (404)[63,67]	79% (66)[67]	78.9% (1655)[59,69]	98.1% (1174)[59,62,67]	100% (371)[60,67]	95.6% (3288)[59,60,63,69]	99% (81)[67]	86.1% (15,340)[59,60,67,72]	98% (47)[67]
Ceftriaxone	53.4% (148)[63,68]	91.4% (155)[63,71]	90% (2031)[59,69,71]	99.6% (2410)[62,67,71]	100% (3742)[60,62,67]	97.4% (4000)[59,60,64,69,71]	88% (81)[67]		97% (273)[67,71]
Cefepime	71.6% (494)[68,69]	100% (89)[71]	99.6% (2031)[59,69,71]	99.7% (1997)[59,62,71]	100% (3570)[60,67]	100% (3542)[59,60,69]	88% (81)[67]	87.6% (15,005)[59,60,67,71]	100% (226)[71]
Imipenem	95.3% (404)[63,67]	100% (66)[47]	100% (1655)[59,69]	100% (1175)[59,62,67]	100% (3570)[60,67]	99.6% (2957)[60,70]	88% (81)[67]	88.1% (15,340)[59,60,67]	100% (47)[67]
Meropenem	99.2% (268)[70]	99.4% (878)[67]	99.6% (2480)[59,70]	99.7% (2262)[67,70]	99.7% (1453)[60,70]	99.6% (2163)[70]	100% (2163)[70]	87.5% (3965)[59,60]	99.1% (1048)[70]
Aztreonam	34.6% (404)[63,67]	83% (66)[67]	81% (1655)[59,69]	97.7% (1174)[59,62,67]	95.8% (371)[60,67]	95.3% (3288)[50,60,67,69]	96% (81)[67]	77.2% (15,340)[59,60,67,72]	94% (47)[67]

*When possible, data represent North American isolates from large, national susceptibility databases.

TABLE 138–4. MICROBIOLOGIC ACTIVITY OF BETA-LACTAM ANTIBIOTICS AGAINST ANAEROBIC GRAM-POSITIVE AND GRAM-NEGATIVE BACTERIA. PERCENT SUSCEPTIBLE BY NCCLS[73] INTERPRETATION (NO. OF ISOLATES TESTED)*

Antibiotic	Gram-Negative and Gram-Positive Bacteria		
	Peptostreptococcus	Fusobacterium	Bacteroides fragilis
Ampicillin/sulbactam	98.3% (116)[74,75]	100% (22)[75]	98.8% (961)[74]
Piperacillin/tazobactam	100% (61)[75,76]	100% (83)[75,76]	99.9% (961)[74]
Cefotetan	100% (12)[76]	100% (11)[76]	64.6% (961)[74]
Cefoxitin	100% (61)[75,76]	100% (33)[75,76]	93.35% (961)[74]
Imipenem	100% (21)[75,76]	100% (33)[75,76]	99.9% (961)[74]
Meropenem	100% (49)[75]	100% (22)[75]	99.1% (556)[75]
Ertapenem	100% (49)[75]	100% (22)[75]	99.1% (556)[75]

*When possible, data represent North American isolates from large, national susceptibility databases.

both gram-positive and gram-negative anaerobes, including *Bacteroides fragilis*, *Fusobacterium*, and *Prevotella* species. Mezlocillin and azlocillin have similar activity to piperacillin against *P. aeruginosa*, but the lack of a beta-lactamase inhibitor combination has dramatically reduced the use of either of these compounds in North America.

The pharmacokinetics of the penicillins and their dosing guidelines and administration are shown in Table 138-5. The pharmacokinetics of these agents has not been well investigated in critically ill patients, so extrapolation from healthy volunteers and less acutely ill patients is required. Although the pharmacodynamics of bacterial killing suggest that beta-lactams could be administered via continuous infusion, there are no data to demonstrate an improvement in efficacy for infusion compared with traditional bolus dosing. Oxacillin and nafcillin are inactivated largely by the liver, with some biliary secretion. The remainder of the drugs are eliminated unchanged through the kidneys.

TABLE 138–5. PHARMACOKINETICS OF BETA-LACTAM ANTIBIOTICS*

Antibiotic	Adult Dose†	Peak Serum Concentration	Renal Elimination	Half-life (h)	Dosing Alteration for Renal Dysfunction
Penicillin G	2-3 million units q 4-6h	20 μg/mL	90%	0.5	CrCl 10-50 mL/min: 50% of dose or full dose q 8-12h CrCl < 10 mL/min: 50% of dose or full dose at q 12-18h Post HD: 2 million units Post CV/VH: 2 million units
Oxacillin	1 g q 4-6h	52-63 μg/mL	50%	0.5-0.7	CrCl < 10 mL/min: 1 g q 12h Post HD, CVVH: none
Nafcillin	1 g q 4h	20 μg/mL	35%	0.5-1	Not necessary
Ampicillin/ sulbactam	1.5-3 g q 6h	40-71 μg/mL (after 1.5 g)	75-85%	1	CrCl 15-29 mL/min: q 12h CrCl: 5-14 mL/min q 24h Post HD: 1.5 g Post CVVH: 3 g
Ticarcillin/ clavulanate	3.1 g q 4-6h	330 μg/mL	60-70%	1.1	CrCl 30-60 mL/min: 2 g q 4h CrCl 10-30 mL/min: 2 g q 8h CrCl < 10 mL/min: 2 g q 12h Post HD: 3.1 g Post CVVH: 3.1 g
Piperacillin/ tazobactam	2.25-4.5 g q 6h	298 μg/mL (after 4.5 g)	68%	0.7-1.2	CrCl 40-60 mL/min: 3.75 g q 6h CrCl 10-39 mL/min: 2.25 g q 6h CrCl < 10 mL/min: 2.25 g q 8h Post HD: 2.25 g Post CVVH: 4.5 g
Cefazolin	1 g q 8h	185 μg/mL	80%	1.8	CrCl ≤ 35 mL/min: 500 mg q 12h CrCl < 10 mL/min: 500 μg q 18-24h Post HD: 500 mg Post CVVH: 1 g
Cefotetan	2-3 g q 12h	230 μg/mL	80%	3.5	CrCl 40-60 mL/min: 1 g q 12h CrCl 10-40 mL/min: 1 g q 24h CrCl < 10 mL/min: 1 g q 48h Post HD: 1 g Post CVVH: 2 g
Cefoxitin	2 g q 4-6h	150 μg/mL	80%	0.8	CrCl 40-60 mL/min: 1 g q 8h CrCl 10-40 mL/min: 1 g q 12h CrCl < 10 mL/min: 1 g q 24h Post HD: 1 g Post CVVH: 2 g
Cefuroxime	1.5 g q 8h	100 μg/mL	90%	1.3	CrCl 10-20 mL/min: 750 mg q 12h CrCl < 10 mL/min: 750 mg q 24h Post HD: 750 mg Post CVVH 1.5 g
Ceftazidime	1-2 g q 8h	160 μg/mL	90%	1.8	CrCl 30-50 mL/min: 1 g q 12h CrCl 15-30 mL/min: 1 g q 24h CrCl 5-15 mL/min: 500 mg q 24h CrCl < 5 mL/min: 500 mg q 48h Post HD: 1 g Post CVVH: 2 g
Ceftriaxone	1-2 g q 24h	123 μg/mL	40-50%	8	Not necessary Post CVVH: 1-2 g
Cefepime	1-2 g q 8-12h	130 μg/mL	85%	2.1	CrCl 10-30 mL/min: 1 g q 12h CrCl < 10 mL/min: 1 g q 24h Post HD: 1 g Post CVVH: 2 g
Imipenem	500 mg to 1 g q 6-8h	21-50 μg/mL (after 500 mg)	70%	1	CrCl 10-30: 500 mg q 12h CrCl < 10 mL/min: 250 mg q 12h Post HD: 250 mg Post CVVH: 500 mg

Continued

TABLE 138–5. PHARMACOKINETICS OF BETA-LACTAM ANTIBIOTICS*—cont'd

Antibiotic	Adult Dose†	Peak Serum Concentration	Renal Elimination	Half-life (h)	Dosing Alteration for Renal Dysfunction
Meropenem	1 g q 8h	49 µg/mL	70%	1	CrCl 25-50 mL/min:1 g q 12h CrCl 10-25 mL/min: 500 mg q 12h CrCl < 10 mL/min: 500 mg q 24h Post HD 500 mg Post CVVH: 1 g
Ertapenem	1 g q 24h	155 µg/mL	80%	4	CrCl <30 mL/min: 500 mg q 24h Post HD: 150 mg

*Data compiled from package insert information.
†All administration is intravenous; dosing is for serious, life-threatening infections.
CrCl, Creatinine clearance; HD, hemodialysis; CVVH, continuous veno-venous hemofiltration.

Ampicillin also undergoes some liver metabolism and biliary excretion, but about 75% of an intravenous dose is excreted unchanged in the urine. Intravenous ampicillin/sulbactam is administered in a 2:1 ratio. Sulbactam is principally excreted unchanged in the urine. Ticarcillin undergoes some metabolism in the liver, and small amounts of drug are secreted into the bile. Significantly more piperacillin is excreted into the bile, with some minor drug inactivation in the liver. The pharmacokinetics of piperacillin and mezlocillin are dose dependent, with nonproportional increases in serum concentration with increasing dosage. This occurs because of saturation of liver and biliary transformation pathways. Clavulanic acid undergoes approximately 50% elimination in the urine as unchanged drug, with 50% metabolism. Tazobactam is mainly eliminated unchanged in the urine, with some biliary secretion and liver metabolism.

The most common adverse event with the penicillins is hypersensitivity reactions. Recent data suggest that patients who report penicillin allergies are unlikely to experience hypersensitivity reactions if penicillin skin testing is negative.[42] Although some critically ill patients may be anergic, Arroliga and associates demonstrated that 106 of 117 ICU patients with a history of nonanaphylactic penicillin allergy responded to histamine control as part of a penicillin skin testing protocol and 105 (90%) tested negative for penicillin reaction.[43,44] Cross-reactivity between penicillins and cephalosporins has been reported at anywhere between 0.1% to 10%.[45] The true rate is probably closer to 1%.[45] In most allergic reactions to cephalosporin allergy, the side chain on the beta-lactam ring is responsible for the hypersensitivity response.[46] Because older cephalosporins have side chains similar to that of penicillin and may have contained penicillin contaminants, the rates of cross-reactivity reported with early use of the cephalosporins were high.[46] Cross-reactivity between penicillin and carbapenems is low, but this may reflect the low underlying rate of reaction with rechallenge of penicillin rather than a lack of cross-reactivity. Aztreonam is unlikely to elicit a reaction in penicillin-allergic individuals, owing to the unique side-chain structure on the monobactam chemical. Robinson and associates have published an approach to the treatment of patients with a possible or probable beta-lactam allergy.[46] For patients with a history suggestive of hypersensitivity to beta-lactams, such as urticarial rash, pruritus, angioedema, hyperperistalsis, bronchospasm, hypotension, or arrhythmia, a penicillin skin test should be performed before initiating therapy. If the test is negative, beta-lactam therapy can be started. Patients who react to the test should avoid beta-lactams or undergo desensitization.

Penicillin is rarely used in the ICU except for treatment of meningococcal meningitis, tertiary syphilis, streptococcal endocarditis, or streptococcal necrotizing fasciitis. The semisynthetic penicillins are indicated for nonurinary methicillin-susceptible staphylococcal infections. Ampicillin/sulbactam is useful for a variety of infections in the critically ill, including urinary tract infections, community-acquired respiratory tract infections, meningitis, endocarditis, biliary infections, skin and skin structure infections, and intra-abdominal infections. Piperacillin/tazobactam and ticarcillin/clavulanate are workhorse agents for many infections that arise in the critically ill, including pneumonia, bacteremia, urinary and biliary tract infections, intra-abdominal infections, and skin and skin structure infections. The agents can be used alone or in combination with aminoglycosides or fluoroquinolones. Piperacillin/tazobactam is reliably effective against *P. aeruginosa* and thus may be used empirically when this organism is suspected.

CEPHALOSPORINS

The microbiologic activity of the cephalosporins is shown in Tables 138-2 to 138-4. Only parenteral cephalosporins are useful in the critical care setting, because higher serum and tissue concentrations are required for serious infections, and these can be achieved only through parenteral administration. The cephalosporins can be divided into generations based on their microbiologic activity. Cefazolin is effectively the only parenteral first-generation cephalosporin in general use, although cephapirin and cephradine are also marketed in North America. Cefazolin has activity against methicillin-susceptible *S. aureus* and coagulase-negative staphylococci but may be susceptible to staphylococcal β-lactamase. Cefazolin is also active against most streptococci, but all cephalosporins lack clinically useful activity against the enterococci. Cefazolin activity against gram-negative bacteria is limited to *Moraxella catarrhalis, E. coli, P. mirabilis, K. pneumoniae, Salmonella* species, and *Shigella* species. The second-generation cephalosporins may be divided by their anaerobic activity, with cefoxitin and cefotetan (cephamycins) active against most gram-negative anaerobic organisms, including *Prevotella* species, *Fusobacterium* species, and *B. fragilis*. Cephamycins have less gram-positive potency than the first-generation cephalosporins but increased activity against Enterobacteriaceae such as *M. morganii*, *Proteus vulgaris*, *Providencia* species, and *S. marcescens*. Cefoxitin is a potent inducer of chromosomally mediated beta-lactamases.[47]

True parenteral second-generation cephalosporins include cefonicid and cefuroxime. Cefuroxime is stable to most beta-lactamases produced by gram-negative bacilli and is more active against methicillin-susceptible staphylococci and streptococci than is cefazolin. Cefuroxime has good potency against *H. influenzae* and is effective against most typical community-acquired respiratory tract pathogens. Third-generation parenteral agents include cefoperazone, cefotaxime, ceftazidime, ceftizoxime, and ceftriaxone. These agents have expanded potency against gram-negative bacilli and *S. pneumoniae*. Third-generation cephalosporins may be divided by their antipseudomonal activity, with cefoperazone and ceftazidime having clinically useful potency against *P. aeruginosa*. Cefoperazone possesses a methylthiotetrazole side chain that causes hypoprothrombinemia; this problem limits cefoperazone use in the critically ill who may be predisposed to bleeding due to underlying disease. Cefazidime has the greatest potency of the third-generation agents against *S. aureus*. Third-generation cephalosporins have excellent clinical activity against the Enterobacteriaceae but lack activity against enterococci, MRSA, *Listeria monocytogenes*, *Stenotrophomonas maltophilia*, and many *Acinetobacter* species. Third-generation cephalosporins may be hydrolyzed by ESBL-producing Enterobacteriaceae such as *Klebsiella*, *Enterobacter*, and *E. coli*. Cefepime, touted as a fourth-generation cephalosporin, has the same activity as the third-generation agents except it is stable to ESBLs.

The pharmacokinetics of the cephalosporins and their dosing guidelines and administration are shown in Table 138-5. Most cephalosporins have short half-lives and undergo extensive renal elimination. Cefoperazone and ceftriaxone, with significant biliary excretion, do not require dosing adjustments in renal dysfunction. The half-life of cefotaxime is not significantly increased in patients with renal failure; however, its active metabolite, desacetylcefotaxime, accumulates significantly, and thus dosing adjustments are required. Pharmacokinetics in the critically ill have been studied for ceftazidime, ceftriaxone, and cefepime. Ceftazidime volume of distribution (V_D) and terminal half-life were increased in critically ill patients without renal dysfunction.[9,48] Ceftazidime area under the concentration time curve (AUC) was increased 1.8-fold, clearance was increased 1.3-fold, V_D was increased 4.1-fold, and half-life was increased from 1.8 hours to 4.75 hours.[48] This expansion of the V_D may lead to inadequate serum concentrations throughout the dosing interval with intermittent bolus dosing.[49] Continuous infusion of ceftazidime, 60 mg/kg/day, in trauma patients was shown to maintain serum concentrations at well above the MIC_{90} for most ICU pathogens.[9] Continuous infusion of ceftazidime, 3 g/day, has been effective in treating nosocomial pneumonia, and the dose of drug administered is typically less than that required for intermittent bolus dosing.[6]

Ceftriaxone clearance in critically ill patients correlates to the degree of glomerular filtration function and is typically halved, even in patients with normal renal function.[50] V_D is also increased by up to 90% in the critically ill, possibly resulting in suboptimal serum concentrations with daily dosing of 2 g.[50] Cefepime V_D is also expanded in the critically ill, with a delay in renal clearance, resulting in serum trough concentrations below the MIC_{50} for many *P. aeruginosa* isolates with 2-g, every-12-hour dosing.[51] Pharmacokinetic

modeling suggests that shorter dosing intervals, such as 1 g every 4 hours, or continuous infusion could be used to improve serum trough concentrations.[51]

Continuous infusion of cefuroxime has also been studied in critically ill patients after coronary artery bypass grafting.[52] A continuous infusion of 3 g over 24 hours provided serum concentrations above the MIC for common ICU pathogens throughout the 24-hour dosing interval and prevented sternal wound infection in the 54 patients studied.[52]

Cephalosporins are generally well tolerated and cause minimal adverse effects. Agents with the methylthiotetrazole (MTT) side chain may cause hypoprothrombinemia via inhibition of synthesis and absorption of vitamin K and competitive inhibition of vitamin K–dependent clotting factors. Agents possessing the MTT side chain are cefamandole (no longer available), cefoperazone, cefotetan, and cefmetazole. Use of these agents may require vitamin K supplementation. The MTT side chain has also been associated with a disulfiram-like reaction.

Cephalosporins are perhaps the most commonly prescribed antibiotic class in the hospital and ICU setting. Because of their activity against gram-positive cocci and gram-negative bacilli, including *P. aeruginosa* and anaerobes, and their stability against beta-lactamase, these agents are used for prevention and treatment of nosocomial infection. Cephalosporins are commonly used in combination with aminoglycosides and fluoroquinolones for the treatment of serious infection.

CARBAPENEMS AND MONOBACTAMS

The carbapenems have a broad antibacterial spectrum of activity, including most aerobic and anaerobic gram-positive and gram-negative bacteria. They are useful for the treatment of infection due to gram-negative bacteria resistant to other antibiotics or to streamline complex polypharmacy. The microbiologic activity of the carbapenems is shown in Tables 138-2 to 138-4. Aztreonam, a monobactam, has broad aerobic gram-negative activity but lacks gram-positive activity or efficacy against anaerobes. Carbapenems are not active against MRSA. Imipenem has clinically useful potency against most enterococci, but meropenem and ertapenem have significantly less activity against these bacteria. Meropenem and ertapenem are less active against gram-positive aerobic bacteria than imipenem. Ertapenem and meropenem are more active than imipenem against Enterobacteriaceae. Imipenem and meropenem have similar activity against *P. aeruginosa* and *Acinetobacter* species, but ertapenem has no activity against important nonfermenting gram-negative rods, including *P. aeruginosa*, *S. maltophilia*, and *Acinetobacter* species. Aztreonam generally has activity against *P. aeruginosa*, but ceftazidime is usually twice as active.[53]

Carbapenems are generally stable against most beta-lactamases; however, metalloenzymes that can hydrolyze the carbapenems ring are increasing in the ICU setting.[54] Carbapenems are stable to ESBLs, but aztreonam is not. Carbapenems are also affected by multi-drug efflux pumps and porin channel changes, particularly in *P. aeruginosa*. Imipenem is not affected by the common efflux pump mediated by MexA-MexB-OprM.[55] However, imipenem readily selects resistant mutants of *P. aeruginosa* that lack a crucial porin channel (OprD) necessary for bacterial permeability to carbapenems but not other beta-lactamase drugs.[55] Loss of this porin channel produces imipenem MICs for *P. aeruginosa* of 8 to 32 mg/mL, conferring clinical resistance.[55] Meropenem is recognized and ejected by the Mex-B–mediated efflux pump, as well as being affected by the loss of the OprD porin channel.[55] Although either mechanism produces a threefold rise in meropenem MICs, neither mutation alone produces clinical resistance to meropenem. Rather, the combination of resistance mechanisms is required to preclude meropenem's clinical effectiveness.

Pharmacokinetics of the carbapenems and aztreonam is shown in Table 142-5. Ertapenem is highly protein bound and has a 4-hour half-life, compared with 1 hour for imipenem and meropenem. Consequently, it is administered once daily. In critically ill patients, both imipenem and meropenem have an expanded V_D and prolonged half-life.[10,56] Similar changes were observed for critically ill patients receiving aztreonam.[56] These data suggest that trough concentrations of carbapenems and aztreonam may be low in critically ill patients, and aggressive dosing may be warranted to minimize treatment failure and drug resistance. Continuous infusion of meropenem has been studied in the critically ill and produced steady-state serum concentrations well above the MIC_{90} for most common ICU pathogens, including *P. aeruginosa*. As with the cephalosporins, a lower dosage is required when administering the carbapenems by continuous infusion than by intermittent injection. Carbapenems and aztreonam are eliminated principally by the kidney, and dosage adjustment is necessary in renal dysfunction.

Imipenem is metabolized extensively by renal dehydropeptidase-1 (DHP-1), producing nephrotoxic metabolites that can produce proximal tubular necrosis. Cilastatin is a competitive inhibitor of DHP-1 that results in protection against the toxic metabolites of imipenem and increases the imipenem urine delivery to approximately 70%.[57] Neither meropenem nor ertapenem requires cilastatin coadministration. Imipenem has proconvulsive activity when administered in higher doses (4 g/day) or to patients with significant renal dysfunction in whom the drug may accumulate.

The carbapenems are used in the critical care setting for management of drug-resistant bacterial infections and in situations where broad-spectrum empirical therapy is necessary. There are not sufficient data to conclude that the carbapenems are interchangeable. Imipenem has the broadest spectrum of activity, but the potential for adverse effects in the ICU population may make meropenem an attractive option. Ertapenem will probably be reserved for use in non-critical care settings. Aztreonam is effective for gram-negative bacterial infections and has been used in place of aminoglycosides when renal toxicity is a concern. However, increasing gram-negative resistance to aztreonam and attractive alternatives, such as the third-generation cephalosporins and the fluoroquinolones, have relegated aztreonam to a second- or third-line choice for many infections.

Beta-lactam antibiotics have similar mechanisms of action, mechanisms of resistance, pharmacodynamic properties, and adverse effect issues. Their microbiologic activity varies with each category of drug, and individually within many categories, and the therapeutic use of each of these agents may be specific for certain agents (e.g., oxacillin or nafcillin) or broad (e.g., ceftriaxone). The beta-lactams are also used for prophylaxis of infection for many surgical and nonsurgical situations. The potential for resistance to develop appears to be significantly influenced by the degree of exposure that bacteria have to antibiotics. Given the extensive beta-lactam exposure to the microbiologic world over the past 50 years, newer changes to the beta-lactam ring structure, such as have been seen with carbapenems and cefepime, will be necessary to keep up with the challenging resistance problems that develop among pathogens common to the ICU setting.

ANNOTATED REFERENCES

Craig WA: Pharmacokinetic/pharmacodynamic parameters: Rationale for antibacterial dosing of mice and men. Clin Infect Dis 1998;26:1-10; quiz 11-12.
> This thorough review of pharmacodynamics serves as an essential primer for all clinicians. The paper describes pharmacodynamics of each antibiotic class and provides examples of the use of these principles in clinical practice.

Gonzalez C, Rubio M, Romero-Vivas J, et al: Bacteremic pneumonia due to *Staphylococcus aureus*: A comparison of disease caused by methicillin-resistant and methicillin-susceptible organisms. Clin Infect Dis 1999;29:1171-1177.
> This paper describes bacteremic episodes of both MRSA and MSSA treated with different antimicrobial therapy. The data support the notion that vancomycin is a poor choice for the treatment of MSSA infection compared with beta-lactam antibiotics.

Lipman J, Wallis SC, Rickard C: Low plasma cefepime levels in critically ill septic patients: Pharmacokinetic modeling indicates improved troughs with revised dosing. Antimicrob Agents Chemother 1999;43:2559-2561.
> This paper illustrates the pharmacokinetic variations that occur secondary to critical illness and objectively demonstrates the problems that occur with antibiotic therapy in this population.

Livermore DM: Of *Pseudomonas*, porins, pumps and carbapenems. J Antimicrob Chemother 2001;47:247-250.
> This is an excellent review of the mechanism of resistance for Pseudomonas aeruginosa against the carbapenems and compares resistance with imipenem to that of meropenem.

Robinson JL, Hameed T, Carr S: Practical aspects of choosing an antibiotic for patients with a reported allergy to an antibiotic. Clin Infect Dis 2002;35:26-31.
> Penicillin or other beta-lactam allergy is a common occurrence in clinical medicine. This paper provides a nuts-and-bolts approach to the use of antimicrobial therapy to which the patient may be allergic.

Chapter 139

AMINOGLYCOSIDES

Rose Jung

KEY POINTS

1. Most of the aminoglycoside use in ICUs consists of an **additive or synergistic role** with beta-lactam antibiotics against serious infections caused by aerobic gram-negative bacilli or aerobic gram-positive cocci.

2. Bactericidal activity is believed to be a result of **binding to and subsequent alteration of the cell envelope** in addition to ribosomal interaction causing inhibition of protein synthesis.

3. **Aminoglycosides have a broad spectrum of activity against aerobic gram-negative bacilli,** including Enterobacteriaceae (*Escherichia coli, Proteus mirabilis, Klebsiella* species, *Morganella* species, *Citrobacter* species, *Serratia* species, and *Enterobacter* species), *Pseudomonas* species, *Acinetobacter* species, and *Haemophilus influenzae.*

4. **The prevalence of bacterial resistance among Enterobacteriaceae has remained relatively low** and emergence of bacterial resistance during therapy rare; however, resistance in *Pseudomonas aeruginosa* isolates is increasing.

5. **Bacterial resistance to aminoglycosides** is achieved through enzymatic modification, alteration of the ribosomal target, decreased drug uptake, and efflux of antibiotics.

6. **Pharmacodynamic properties** consist of concentration-dependent bactericidal activity, postantibiotic effect, and synergism with beta-lactam compounds.

7. **Aminoglycosides are limited** by the potential for nephrotoxicity, ototoxicity, and, rarely, neuromuscular blockade.

8. **Serum concentration monitoring** is important for both efficacy and safety.

Aminoglycosides are important antibacterial agents in combating infections in critically ill patients. Commonly used antibacterials of this class include gentamicin, tobramycin, and amikacin. Although there are other members of this family with specific uses, most of the aminoglycoside use in ICUs consists of an additive or synergistic role with a penicillin or cephalosporin against serious infections caused by aerobic gram-negative bacilli or aerobic gram-positive cocci. Fortunately, the prevalence of bacterial resistance against these agents has remained relatively low and emergence of bacterial resistance during therapy rare.

Concentration-dependent bactericidal activity, postantibiotic effect, and synergism with beta-lactam compounds are clear advantages of aminoglycosides. However, their usefulness has been limited by the potential for nephrotoxicity, ototoxicity, and, rarely, neuromuscular blockade. As the mechanisms of activity and toxicities are better elucidated, the potential for adverse events may be reduced by modifying dosing strategies, avoiding risk factors, and using shorter duration of therapy. In addition, the cost of these agents is low in comparison to other antibacterials with similar spectrum of activity and efficacy. Consequently, in the era of increasing antibiotic resistance, the aminoglycosides will remain valuable weapons against infections in the ICU. The purpose of this chapter is to review the pharmacology, spectrum of activity, pharmacokinetics/pharmacodynamics, and safety of aminoglycosides in treatment of critically ill patients.

MECHANISM OF ACTION

The mechanisms of aminoglycoside activity are not completely understood, but binding to and subsequent alteration of the cell envelope in addition to ribosomal interaction causing inhibition of protein synthesis may contribute to their bactericidal activity. Aminoglycosides are cations that bind passively to negatively charged portions of outer membranes of gram-negative bacilli and competitively displace the cell wall Mg^{++} and Ca^{++} that link lipopolysaccharide molecules.[1,2] The result is a rearrangement of the cell envelope and subsequent formation of transient holes in the cell wall, which interrupts the normal permeability function of the bacteria.[3]

Once bound, aminoglycosides are transported slowly across the cytoplasmic membrane via an energy-dependent process and, thus, this is the rate-limiting step in the drug action.[4] The transmembrane electrical potential correlates with the uptake and antibacterial effect. This energy-dependent transport mechanism is impaired in an anaerobic environment, conditions of low pH, and high osmolality.[5] Thus, in certain clinical settings, such as in infections involving abscess, aminoglycoside transport is reduced and may not be as effective. In gram-positive bacteria, aminoglycoside uptake is decreased owing to the thicker outer cell wall membranes; thus, higher minimal inhibitory concentrations (MIC) are reported with these organisms.

Finally, aminoglycosides bind irreversibly to the 16S rRNA of the 30S subunit of ribosomes.[6] This aminoglycoside-ribosome interaction causes termination and miscoding of protein synthesis with subsequent bacterial cell death. Unlike most of the antibiotics that act to inhibit protein synthesis, aminoglycosides display bactericidal activity through multifactorial mechanisms, including ones yet to be determined.

SPECTRUM OF ACTIVITY

Aminoglycosides have a broad spectrum of activity against aerobic and facultative gram-negative bacilli. Most are active against Enterobacteriaceae (*Escherichia coli*, *Proteus mirabilis*, and species of *Klebsiella, Morganella, Citrobacter, Serratia*, and *Enterobacter*), *Pseudomonas* species, *Acinetobacter* species, and *Haemophilus influenzae*. Large surveillance studies involving both American and European ICUs reported that amikacin was the most active aminoglycoside against *P. aeruginosa* isolates, followed by tobramycin and gentamicin.[7,8] Although the differences were smaller, similar trends were reported for *E. coli* and *Klebsiella* species.[8,9] Against *Enterobacter* species, the susceptibility patterns were similar but gentamicin was more active than tobramycin.[8,9] Overall, the susceptibility rates approached approximately 90% or higher for Enterobacteriaceae.[8,9] However, against *P. aeruginosa* isolates, amikacin susceptibility rates ranged from 87% to 93%, depending on where the strains were isolated, and the susceptibility to gentamicin and tobramycin was much lower.[7,8]

Aminoglycosides are also sensitive to methicillin-susceptible *Staphylococcus aureus*.[8,10] For other gram-positive pathogens such as methicillin-resistant *S. aureus*, *Streptococcus* species, and *Enterococcus* species, aminoglycosides are limited only to provide synergistic activity with beta-lactam antibiotics. In *Enterococcus* species, the synergism is only observed in organisms that display low-level aminoglycoside resistance (4 to 250 μg/mL).[11] A poor active transport of drug due to the anaerobic metabolism and the thick cell wall is thought to be responsible for this type of resistance. Synergism is achieved in these organisms because aminoglycoside uptake is enhanced when combined with beta-lactam antibiotics. *Enterococci* may acquire one or more of the following resistance mechanisms to demonstrate high-level resistance: alteration of the target site, interference with drug permeability, or enzymatic inactivation of drug.[12] In these organisms, synergistic activity of aminoglycosides is not observed.

Whereas the rates of high-level aminoglycoside resistance in *Enterococcus* species vary markedly among institutions, the nationwide prevalence is estimated at 30% to 60%.[13] High-level resistance is low in *Enterococcus faecalis*, which is responsible for approximately 60% of nosocomial enterococcal bloodstream infections. However, this type of resistance is observed in greater than 50% of *E. faecium*, which causes approximately 20% of nosocomial enterococcal bloodstream infections.

Aminoglycosides also have activity against less common ICU pathogens. Streptomycin is the drug of choice for *Yersinia pestis* infection.[14] Both streptomycin and gentamicin have been reported to be effective for *Francisella tularensis* infection.[15] Amikacin has the best activity among aminoglycosides against *Mycobacterim avium-intracellulare*.[16] Streptomycin has activity against multidrug resistant *M. tuberculosis*.[17] Aminoglycosides also have in-vitro activity against *Legionella* species, but they are not clinically used owing to low intracellular penetration.[18]

MECHANISM OF RESISTANCE

Bacterial resistance to aminoglycosides is achieved through multiple mechanisms. These include enzymatic modification, alteration of the ribosomal target, decreased drug uptake, and efflux of antibiotics. The most common mechanism is inactivation by aminoglycoside-modifying enzymes. The exposed hydroxyl and amino groups of aminoglycosides are subject to potential inactivation by enzymes from both gram-positive and gram-negative bacteria.[19] There are three types of enzymes that transfer a functional group to the aminoglycoside structure resulting in inactivation: (1) aminoglycoside nucleotidyltransferases (ANTs) that transfer nucleotide triphosphates; (2) aminoglycoside acetyltransferases (AACs) that transfer the acetyl group from acetyl-CoA; and (3) aminoglycoside phosphotransferases (APHs) that transfer the phosphoryl group from ATP.[19,20] Aminoglycoside resistance genes that encode for these enzymes are usually found on extrachromosomal bacterial plasmids and transposons within the periplasmic space. Thus, they can be easily transferred from bacteria to bacteria.[21] Amikacin is the aminoglycoside most stable to these enzymatic effects because it has fewer sites for enzymatic attack.

Bacteria may protect themselves against aminoglycosides by changing ribosomal (16S rRNA) binding sites. Altering aminoglycoside attachment can be a result of either enzymatic activity or mutational modification. This phenomenon has been rare in most clinical isolates except for *Mycobacterium* species.[22]

Bacteria may also become resistant to aminoglycosides by preventing penetration of the drug through the outer bacterial cell membrane or by preventing active transport through the cytoplasmic membrane.[23] This may be a result of chromosomal mutations that result in alteration of transmembrane electrical potential and/or electron transport chain. Aerobic gram-negative bacilli and *Staphylococci* possessing this mode of resistance demonstrate cross-resistance to all aminoglycosides. Finally, as mentioned previously, uptake and subsequent activity may also be altered under anaerobic conditions.

PHARMACOKINETICS

All aminoglycosides have similar pharmacokinetic properties.[24-26] The distribution from the vascular to the extravascular space occurs rapidly within 15 to 30 minutes post infusion. The drug is primarily excreted by the glomerular filtration.[27] Thus, dosage adjustments are based on creatinine clearance. In patients with normal renal function, the half-lives of all aminoglycosides range from 1.5 to 3.5 hours. The half-life is shortened in febrile illnesses and prolonged in any conditions that decrease renal function. More than 90% of a parenterally administered dose is recovered in urine unchanged during the first 24 hours. The remainder is slowly recycled into the tubular lumen, where accumulation of the drug causes nephrotoxicity.[28]

Unfortunately, aminoglycoside concentrations are generally low in infected secretions and tissues, such as respiratory secretions, pleural fluid, cerebrospinal fluid, and aqueous humor. However, high drug concentrations are found in the proximal tubular cells of the renal cortex, which is thought to correlate with the nephrotoxic potential of aminoglycosides.[28]

PHARMACODYNAMICS

Pharmacodynamic principles associated with aminoglycosides include concentration-dependent bactericidal activity, postantibiotic effect (PAE), and synergism with other cell wall—active agents.[29] Aminoglycosides are rapidly bactericidal, and their rate of bacterial killing increases as the antibiotic concentration is increased.[30] Exposure of bacteria to the 24-hour aminoglycoside dose as a single bolus with the associated high peak drug concentration results in faster and a greater extent of bactericidal activity than those noted for the same total dose administered in divided doses.[31]

A PAE is a persistent suppression of bacterial growth after short antimicrobial exposure.[32] The higher the aminoglycoside concentration, the longer the PAE. In vitro, the aminoglycosides consistently demonstrate a PAE that varies from 1 to 3 hours in broth and serum for *P. aeruginosa* and from 0.9 to 2.0 hours for Enterobacteriaceae. A PAE can also be demonstrated after incubation with *S. aureus*.[33]

Synergy is frequently reported with a combination of an aminoglycoside and a cell wall–active antimicrobial (e.g., penicillin, cephalosporin, monobactam, carbapenem, glycopeptide).[34] Synergy is noted when significantly greater effect with two drugs is observed compared with those anticipated based on the effect of each individual drug. Enhanced aminoglycoside uptake in the presence of a cell wall–active drug has been demonstrated with *Streptococcus* species, *Enterococcus* species, *S. aureus*, and *P. aeruginosa*.[35-38]

ADVERSE EVENTS

The most common adverse event of aminoglycosides is nephrotoxicity.[39] The reported incidence ranges from 5% to 25%.[39-41] The variability results from differences in the definition of nephrotoxicity, the tests used to measure renal function, and the clinical setting in which the drugs were administered. In general, a decrease in the glomerular filtration rate is small, with most patients experiencing a nonoliguric decline in creatinine clearance. A progression to dialysis-dependent oliguric or anuric renal failure is rare. It takes several days of drug administration before nephrotoxicity of clinical consequence is apparent, and the resulting renal tubular necrosis is usually reversible.[39,40]

The risk factors for increased nephrotoxicity include older age, preexisting renal disease, hepatic dysfunction, frequent dosing interval, treatment lasting 3 or more days, previous aminoglycoside therapy, and concurrent nephrotoxic drugs (i.e., vancomycin, amphotericin B, furosemide, clindamycin, piperacillin, cephalosporins, methoxyflurane, foscarnet, and intravenous radiocontrast agents). In addition, ICU patients are at increased risk due to hypotension or contracted intravascular volume from volume depletion or diuretic therapy.

Nephrotoxicity is usually mild and reversible. Because aminoglycosides are useful in the treatment of serious infections, their use should not be avoided if the potential risk of nephrotoxicity is the only concern. Adjustment of dosage and close monitoring of serum drug concentrations will aid in minimizing this toxicity.[41] If deterioration in renal function does occur, it is advisable to discontinue therapy. Spontaneous recovery occurs within a few days in the absence of other nephrotoxins, hypotension, renal cortical necrosis of another etiology, or other clinical factors.

Aminoglycoside antibiotics may cause cochlear and vestibular damage.[39,40] Ototoxicity is of particular concern because it is usually irreversible and injury may appear after termination of drug administration. The incidence of cochlear toxicity is estimated to be 3% to 14%.[39,40] Toxicity may manifest unilaterally or bilaterally. The risk factors for ototoxicity include inherited susceptibility, patient's age,

dosage of therapy, renal function, and additive effects of other ototoxic agents (i.e., loop diuretics).[42] When aminoglycoside therapy is indicated, the risk of ototoxicity can be minimized by shortening the duration of therapy as clinically appropriate and by periodic assessments of renal function to avoid accumulation of drug. High-frequency audiometric testing may aid in early diagnosis and prevention of progressive damage in patients receiving more than 4 days of therapy.

The true incidence of vestibular toxicity in patients is very difficult to determine because symptoms are masked by compensatory mechanisms (i.e., visual and proprioceptive clues) over time. In addition, hair regeneration may be possible in the reversal of this toxicity.[43] Clinical manifestations include nausea, vomiting, and vertigo. These symptoms are exacerbated in the dark or in other situations that block compensatory pathways. Nystagmus may also be evident. Similar to cochlear toxicity, avoiding drug accumulation appears to be the most effective method of prevention.

The most life-threatening adverse reaction, although very rare, is neuromuscular blockade.[44] The resulting clinical manifestations include muscle weakness, respiratory depression with apnea, flaccid paralysis, and dilated pupils. A presence of deep tendon reflexes may be variable. The risk factors include a diagnosis of myasthenia gravis, hypomagnesemia, severe hypocalcemia, and concomitant administration of a neuromuscular blocking agent. A rapid rise in serum drug concentration due to short intravenous administration is also a risk factor. Blockade results from inhibition of the presynaptic release of acetylcholine and blockage of postsynaptic receptor sites of acetylcholine. Blockade is preventable by infusing aminoglycoside over a period of 30 minutes with traditional dosing. In patients receiving large doses once a day, the infusion time may be extended to 1 hour.

DRUG INTERACTION

Aminoglycosides interact chemically with beta-lactam antibiotics, such as the antipseudomonal penicillins (e.g., carbenicillin, ticarcillin, piperacillin, mezlocillin, and azlocillin).[45,46] The interaction results in a nucleophilic opening of the beta-lactam ring with acylation of an amino group of the aminoglycoside and mutual loss of antibacterial activity. When patients with renal failure were concomitantly administered an aminoglycoside and an antipseudomonal penicillin, the serum aminoglycoside concentration was reduced by 10% to 20%. Thus, the administration of these drugs should be separated by at least 1 hour.

EXTENDED INTERVAL DOSING VERSUS MULTIPLE DAILY DOSING

The aminoglycosides are licensed to be administered multiple times per day based on a patient's renal function.[47] In normal renal function (creatinine clearance ≥ 90 mL/min), empirical maintenance doses for gentamicin and tobramycin range from 1.5 to 2 mg/kg every 8 hours and for amikacin 5 to 7.5 mg/kg every 8 to 12 hours. Dose reduction and/or dosing interval prolongation may be necessary in those with renal dysfunction (Table 139-1). Dosing adjustments are usually required in patients with advanced age, decreased renal blood flow, intrinsic renal disease, and azotemia. Higher dosages or shorter intervals may be required in

TABLE 139–1. RECOMMENDED DOSING REGIMENS FOR SELECTED AMINOGLYCOSIDES BASED ON RENAL FUNCTION

			Recommended Regimen			
	Indication	Dose	CrCl ≥ 60 mL/min	CrCl = 40-60 mL/min	CrCl = 20-40 mL/min	CrCl < 20 mL/min or HD
Traditional Dosing						
Gentamicin	Pneumonia or other severe infections	1.5-2.0 mg/kg	q 8h	q 12h	q 24h	Re-dose based on trough levels < 1 µg/mL
	Synergy	1 mg/kg	q 8h	q 12h	q 24h	Re-dose based on trough levels < 1 µg/mL
Tobramycin	Pneumonia or other severe infections	1.5-2.0 mg/kg	q 8h	q 12h	q 24h	Re-dose based on trough levels < 1 µg/mL
Amikacin	Pneumonia or other severe infections	5-7.5 mg/kg	q 8h	q 12h	q 24h	Redose based on trough levels < 5 µg/ml
Extended-Interval Dosing						
Gentamicin	Pneumonia or other severe infections	5-7 mg/kg	q 24h	q 36h	q 48h	Re-dose based on trough levels < 1 µg/mL
Tobramycin	Pneumonia or other severe infections	5-7 mg/kg	q 24h	q 36h	q 48h	Re-dose based on trough levels < 1 µg/mL

CrCl, creatinine clearance; HD, hemodialysis.

neonates, in burn patients with serious pseudomonal infections, or in patients with cystic fibrosis.[48]

A dosing strategy that utilizes pharmacodynamic principles (concentration-dependent killing and PAE) of aminoglycosides has been used widely since its introduction in the 1980s. This strategy is frequently referred to as extended-interval aminoglycoside dosing (EIAD) or once-daily dosing. They both employ a large bolus dose over an extended period to achieve high serum concentrations to produce rapid bactericidal effect and undetectable trough concentrations at the end of the dosing interval to reduce accumulation of drugs, limiting toxicities.[49]

The bactericidal effects of the aminoglycosides are primarily a function of drug concentration relative to the MIC. The most rapid bacterial killing is typically observed when peak concentrations (Cmax) are approximately 10 times greater than the MIC of the organism. Enhanced patient outcome and decreased selection of resistant organism have also been demonstrated with higher peak concentrations (Cmax of ≥ 20 mg/L).[50,51] The EIAD also provides a drug-free period at the end of the dosing interval to reduce drug accumulation. Uptake of aminoglycosides into tissues of both the renal cortex and the inner ear has been shown to be most efficient at low-sustained concentrations resulting from continuous infusion or frequent intermittent drug administration. Reduced risk for nephrotoxicity and ototoxicity has been observed in patients receiving EIAD with at least 4 hours of drug-free period (serum concentration of < 0.5 mg/L). During this time, the regimen relies on PAE to provide therapeutic effect.

Numerous clinical studies of EIAD have been evaluated in patients with bacteremia, intra-abdominal infections, urinary tract infections, pelvic infections, cystic fibrosis, and febrile neutropenia.[52-54] Unfortunately, none of these studies specifically examined efficacy and safety in critically ill population, thus limiting its application in ICU patients. This is particularly troubling owing to the altered pharmacokinetics

of aminoglycosides in critically ill patients. The mean volume of distribution in critically ill patients ranges from 0.3 to 0.4 L/kg. However, in surgical and trauma ICU patients, volume of distribution of up to 0.8 L/kg has been reported.[55,56] Because the Cmax:MIC ratio is directly affected by large volume of distribution, the ratio in critically ill patients is expected to be less than optimal. In addition, several studies reported that critically ill patients had drug-free intervals ranging from 6 to 9 hours at the end of the dosing interval.[57] Because these drug-free intervals exceed the PAE observed for most organisms in vitro, this dosing strategy may not effectively inhibit regrowth of surviving organisms. Finally, a poor correlation between estimated creatinine clearance and aminoglycosides has been documented in ICU patients.[58] This variability in drug clearance may be secondary to unstable renal function, malnutrition, hemodynamic instability, and use of drugs such as vasopressors, diuretics, and other nephrotoxic drugs.

The lack of adequate efficacy and safety data in critically ill patients compounded with the alterations in pharmacokinetic parameters makes it difficult to advocate its routine use in ICU patients. On the other hand, aminoglycosides are most often used in combination with beta-lactam antibiotics in critically ill patients. Failure to achieve targeted concentrations or other potential disadvantages may be overcome by effective use of the other agent in the combination therapy. The theorized advantages of EIAD can be achieved in critically ill patients by individualizing the dosing based on serum levels rather than utilizing the Hartford nomogram.[59] Reasonable targets would be a peak concentration of 20 mg/L or a Cmax:MIC of 10 and concentration of less than 0.5 mg/L for 4 hours at the end of the dosing interval.

A recommended empirical dose in adults with serious gram-negative infections and normal renal function is 5 to 7 mg/kg/day for gentamicin or tobramycin. Once-daily or extended interval dosing of amikacin has not been adequately studied. The dosing interval may need to be prolonged if the patient's calculated creatinine clearance is below 60 mL/min. In those patients with normal renal function or in surgical or trauma patients, the dosing interval may need to be shortened to every 12 hours. Serum monitoring is necessary to recommend optimal dosing regimen.

SERUM CONCENTRATION MONITORING

Monitoring of serum concentrations is essential for both efficacy and toxicity. Monitoring schemes are different for two methods of administering aminoglycosides. For traditional multiple daily dosing regimens, peak concentrations should be checked 30 minutes after the end of an intravenous infusion.[47] Because the drug is often infused over a 30-minute period, it may be convenient to request the serum sample 1 hour after the start of the drug administration. The desired peak concentration may be different depending on the site of infection. For nosocomial infections involving tissues where aminoglycoside penetration is low (e.g., lower respiratory tract infections), the target peak concentration should range from 8 to 12 mg/L for gentamicin and tobramycin and 25 to 30 mg/L for amikacin. On the other hand, for infections where the drug concentrates heavily (e.g., urinary tract infections) the adequate peak concentration can range from 5 to 8 mg/L for gentamicin and tobramycin and 10 to 20 mg/L for amikacin.

Trough concentration is a good indication of accumulation and therefore a good predictor for nephrotoxicity and ototoxicity. A trough concentration should be less than 2 mg/L, although less than 1 mg/L is preferred in most critically ill patients. These serum concentrations should be measured during steady state, which is approximately after the third dose in most cases. The frequency of subsequent monitoring of serum drug concentrations will vary among patients (usually once weekly throughout therapy) but should be more frequent in patients with changing renal function or in those with a more resistant pathogen.

For the EIAD, there are two different methods of determining optimal regimen. The first and the more well-known method uses the Hartford nomogram.[59] According to this method, serum concentrations are drawn between 6 and 14 hours after the first dose and applied to a nomogram to determine the recommended fixed-dose and dosage interval. Although the use of a nomogram is simpler and less expensive owing to the reduced number of serum concentrations evaluated, available studies in critically ill patients indicate that the use of this nomogram did not reliably predict targeted Cmax:MIC ratio and allowed excessively long periods of drug-free period at the end of the dosing interval.[55,56]

Instead, in critically ill patients, monitoring of two serum drug concentrations to derive a dosing regimen is recommended. Obtaining a peak concentration at 1 hour post 1 hour infusion (2 hours after the start of infusion) and another serum concentration between 8 and 18 hours after the end of the infusion will allow adequate determination of a patient-specific regimen. This will allow assessment of peak serum concentration for the targeted Cmax:MIC ratio and the length of drug-free interval. Thereafter, in absence of worsening renal function, a periodic trough concentration should be monitored to ensure adequacy of renal clearance of drug. The targeted trough concentration with this dosing regimen should be undetectable (< 0.5 mg/L) for approximately 4 hours at the end of the dosing interval.

ANNOTATED REFERENCES

Buijk SE, Mouton JW, Gyssens IC, et al: Experience with a once-daily dosing program of aminoglycosides in critically ill patients. Intensive Care Med 2002;28:936-942.

This prospective, descriptive study evaluated a once-daily dosing program in 89 critically ill patients. An initial once-daily dosing regimen of 7 mg/kg produced Cmax:MIC ratios of greater than 10 in the majority of critically ill patients, but a dose adjustment or lengthening of interval was necessary in 49% of patients. Renal impairment occurred in 14% of patients. Individualized regimens based on serum concentrations are advocated in this study.

Karlowsky JA, Draghi DC, Jones ME, et al: Surveillance for antimicrobial susceptibility among clinical isolates of *Pseudomonas aeruginosa* and *Acinetobacter baumannii* from hospitalized patients in the United States, 1998 to 2001. Antimicrob Agents Chemother 2003;47:1681-1688.

In 2001, 92.5% and 75.9% of P. aeruginosa isolates from ICU patients were susceptible to amikacin and gentamicin, respectively. Among A. baumannii isolates, 84.5% and 52.9% were susceptible to amikacin and gentamicin, respectively.

Mingeot-Leclercq MP, Tulkens PM: Aminoglycosides: Nephrotoxicity. Antimicrob Agents Chemother 1999;43:1003-1012.

A review of the basic and the clinical research on aminoglycoside nephrotoxicity is presented.

Sader HS, Biedenbach, Jones RN: Global patterns of susceptibility for 21 commonly utilized antimicrobial agents tested against 48,440 Enterobacteriaceae in the SENTRY Antimicrobial Surveillance Program (1997-2001). Diagn Microbiol Infect Dis 2003;47:361-364.

In 1997-2001, Escherichia coli (46.1%), Klebsiella species (21.3%), and Enterobacter species (12.2%) were the frequently isolated pathogens. Among aminoglycosides, amikacin was the most active agent (97.3% susceptible), followed by gentamicin (90.6% susceptible) and tobramycin (89.8% susceptible) against Enterobacteriaceae from Asia-Pacific, Europe, Latin America, and North America.

Vakulenko SB, Mobashery S: Versatility of aminoglycosides and prospects for their future. Clin Microbiol Rev 2003;16:430-450.

A recent review of mechanism of activity and resistance as well as the epidemiology of the resistance is presented.

Chapter 140

FLUOROQUINOLONES

Douglas N. Fish

KEY POINTS

1. The fluoroquinolones have assumed an increasingly important role in the treatment of infections in critically ill patients owing to **their broad spectrum of antimicrobial activity, favorable safety profiles, and ease of administration.**

2. **The fluoroquinolones are rapidly bactericidal agents** that have a broad spectrum of activity against important gram-positive, gram-negative, and atypical pathogens.

3. Although ciprofloxacin has traditionally been considered the most active fluoroquinolone against *Pseudomonas aeruginosa* and other important gram-negative pathogens, **recent data suggest that there is little difference between ciprofloxacin and levofloxacin in terms of relative susceptibilities or clinical efficacy in the treatment of infections caused by these bacteria.**

4. **Newer fluoroquinolones, including levofloxacin, gatifloxacin, and moxifloxacin, are all more reliably active** than ciprofloxacin against penicillin-susceptible or penicillin-resistant strains of *Streptococcus pneumoniae*, methicillin-susceptible *Staphylococcus aureus*, and other gram-positive organisms against which these agents have clinically relevant activity.

5. **Resistance to the fluoroquinolones has tended to emerge rapidly in bacteria with lower intrinsic susceptibility** (e.g., *S. aureus*, *P. aeruginosa*, and *Acinetobacter* species); however, fluoroquinolone resistance among isolates from ICUs has also become an increasing problem among gram-negative bacilli such as *Enterobacter* species and *Klebsiella pneumoniae*.

6. **The fluoroquinolones as a whole have excellent pharmacokinetic properties** and are characterized by rapid oral absorption, extensive distribution into many fluids and tissues resulting in concentrations that are well above the minimal inhibitory concentration (MIC) for many gram-negative and gram-positive organisms, and serum half-lives that are sufficiently long to allow once- or twice-daily dosing.

7. **High doses of fluoroquinolones are often necessary** to minimize the pharmacokinetic variability and optimize the concentration-dependent pharmacodynamic properties of the drugs, particularly in the treatment of severe infections suspected or documented to be caused by pathogens with intrinsically higher MICs to the drugs (e.g., *P. aeruginosa* and *Acinetobacter* species).

8. **The fluoroquinolones have generally proven to be a safe and very well tolerated class of drugs,** and most drug-related adverse effects are mild and self-limiting.

9. Although **there are differences among the individual drugs in terms of clinically important drug interactions and the clinical relevance of these interactions,** fluoroquinolones are associated with drug interactions involving decreased drug absorption and inhibition of hepatic metabolism of drugs such as warfarin and theophylline.

10. **Consideration should always be given** to the susceptibility of presumed or documented pathogens, site of infection, severity of infection, presence of organ dysfunction, and pharmacodynamic characteristics of the fluoroquinolones when choosing an appropriate dosing regimen for a specific critically ill patient.

The fluoroquinolones are synthetically derived, broad-spectrum antibacterial agents designed for both intravenous and oral administration. Since the introduction of ciprofloxacin in the late 1980s, the fluoroquinolones have assumed an increasingly important role in the treatment of infections in critically ill patients. Their broad spectrum of antimicrobial activity, favorable safety profiles, and ease of administration have made the fluoroquinolones popular choices for both empirical and directed therapies of a wide variety of infectious diseases. However, widespread use of the fluoroquinolones has not come without some concern regarding appropriate uses and the development of resistance among certain nosocomial pathogens such as *Pseudomonas aeruginosa*. This chapter will briefly review fluoroquinolone pharmacology, antimicrobial activity, safety, and other clinically relevant issues regarding their use and will focus on the four agents most frequently used in the critical care setting: ciprofloxacin, levofloxacin, gatifloxacin, and moxifloxacin.

MECHANISM OF ACTION

DNA gyrase and topoisomerase IV are thought to be essential for the replication of DNA and partition of replicated chromosomal DNA.[1] DNA gyrase, a tetrameric enzyme consisting of two A and two B subunits, is known to be a primary target of fluoroquinolones in gram-negative bacteria and is the only known enzyme capable of introducing negative superhelical twists into bacterial DNA.[2,3] The two subunits of gyrase are encoded by *gyrA* and *gyrB*, which are also potential sites of mutation and subsequent quinolone resistance.[3-5] Topoisomerase IV, another topoisomerase, seems to be a primary target of many fluoroquinolones in gram-positive bacteria such as *Staphylococcus aureus* and *Streptococcus pneumoniae*. Bacterial topoisomerase IV appears to be the principal enzyme that resolves or "decatenates" interlocked daughter DNA circles occurring at the completion of a round of DNA replication, allowing segregation of daughter chromosomes into daughter cells.[2,4,5] Topoisomerase IV, like DNA gyrase, is composed of four subunits, two each of the *parC* and *parE* gene products.

As part of the topoisomerase reaction mechanism, DNA gyrase and topoisomerase IV transiently break the DNA backbone and pass a double strand of DNA through those breaks, thus introducing a negative supercoil into the DNA strand.[6] Fluoroquinolone antibiotics have been shown to target DNA gyrase and the topoisomerase IV while these enzymes are functionally attached to the DNA strand in the presence of adenosine triphosphate, resulting in a drug/enzyme/DNA complex in which the DNA probably remains broken.[6] Cell death apparently results from release of double-stranded DNA breaks from multiple drug/enzyme/DNA complexes throughout the chromosome.[1,6-9] This mechanism of action does not in itself explain why the fluoroquinolones kill bacteria so rapidly, and it has been suggested that additional protein synthesis mechanisms and/or interference with the "SOS" response involved in the repair of damaged DNA also play a role in the rapidly bactericidal effects of these drugs.

ANTIMICROBIAL SPECTRUM OF ACTIVITY

Fluoroquinolones have excellent in-vitro activity against a wide range of both gram-positive and gram-negative organisms. Representative activities of currently available fluoroquinolones are shown in Table 140-1. The entire fluoroquinolones class displays excellent activity against enteric gram-negative aerobic bacteria as well as *Haemophilus influenzae*, *Moraxella catarrhalis*, and *Neisseria* species. Gastrointestinal pathogens such as *Salmonella* species, *Shigella* species, and *Campylobacter* species are also highly susceptible to the fluoroquinolones. Although some differences in relative potency exist between individual drugs as determined by the MIC for these organisms, little difference in clinical efficacy should be expected in the treatment of infections due to susceptible strains. Activity against *P. aeruginosa* is more variable, however. Ciprofloxacin has traditionally been considered the most active fluoroquinolone against this organism, but recent data suggest that there is little difference between ciprofloxacin and levofloxacin in terms of relative susceptibility of *P. aeruginosa* strains.[10] Ciprofloxacin was active against greater than 95% of *P. aeruginosa* strains when first released to the market in 1987; by 2001 both ciprofloxacin and levofloxacin were active against only approximately 65% to 80% of strains.[10-12] Clinically relevant differences between ciprofloxacin and levofloxacin are further minimized when pharmacokinetic and pharmacodynamic properties are considered.[13] Gatifloxacin is usually somewhat less active against *P. aeruginosa* than either ciprofloxacin or levofloxacin, and moxifloxacin tends to be the least active agent.[10,14,15] Nearly all fluoroquinolones adequately inhibit *P. aeruginosa* at concentrations achieved in the urine.

Activity of the fluoroquinolones against other nosocomial pathogens is also highly variable. Levofloxacin and gatifloxacin tend to be slightly more active against *Acinetobacter* species, whereas moxifloxacin and gatifloxacin usually display the best activities and ciprofloxacin is consistently the least active agent against *Stenotrophomonas maltophilia*.[10,14,15] However, resistance to these latter organisms is quite common and even agents with the best relative in vitro activity are not reliably clinically effective against many isolates.[10,14,15]

Several studies have reported that fluoroquinolones produce synergistic activity against gram-negative bacilli when used in combination with beta-lactam antibiotics.[16-19] These studies primarily evaluated antibiotic synergy against *P. aeruginosa* due to the frequent use of fluoroquinolones in antipseudomonal treatment regimens; ciprofloxacin, levofloxacin, and gatifloxacin have all been shown to achieve synergy against 25% to 75% of tested strains. One previous study also demonstrated synergistic in-vitro activity against *P. aeruginosa* with the combination of moxifloxacin and either ceftazidime or cefepime[19]; however, additive or synergistic activity with moxifloxacin-containing combinations has not been extensively evaluated against other organisms. The ability of gatifloxacin and moxifloxacin to produce synergistic activity against *P. aeruginosa* may often be limited by clinically achievable drug concentrations; the use of ciprofloxacin and levofloxacin in combination regimens is most likely to result in synergistic activity owing to their more potent activity and higher serum concentrations relative to the bacterial MICs.[17]

Newer fluoroquinolones have improved activity against gram-positive bacteria relative to older agents such as ciprofloxacin. Moxifloxacin has the best overall activity against staphylococci and streptococci and is slightly more active than gatifloxacin, followed by levofloxacin and more distantly by ciprofloxacin.[14,15,20] Levofloxacin, gatifloxacin, and moxifloxacin are all reliably active against penicillin-susceptible strains of *Streptococcus pneumoniae*; this activity is also retained against strains of *S. pneumoniae* resistant to other drug classes, including penicillins, macrolides, and sulfonamides. Although ciprofloxacin has only moderate activity against methicillin-susceptible *Staphylococcus aureus* (MSSA), newer agents have excellent activity against this organism. None of the fluoroquinolones is reliably active against methicillin-resistant *S. aureus* (MRSA), and rates of fluoroquinolone resistance among MRSA are now quite high. The fluoroquinolones as a class also have only moderate activity against the enterococci, with great variability seen among the various agents and specific bacterial strains.[14,15,20] The fluoroquinolones have consistently excellent activity against *Listeria monocytogenes*.[15]

The activity of the various fluoroquinolones against anaerobic bacteria is highly variable. Trovafloxacin was the first commercially available fluoroquinolone with clinically relevant anaerobic activity in vitro as well as proven clinical efficacy for anaerobic infections including complicated intra-abdominal infection. Moxifloxacin has in-vitro activity against *Bacteroides fragilis*, *Bacteroides* group organisms, *Fusobacterium* species, *Clostridium* species, and other clinically important anaerobes that is generally comparable to trovafloxacin, and gatifloxacin is only slightly less active than moxifloxacin.[15,21] Although clinical data are lacking, both moxifloxacin and

TABLE 140–1. REPRESENTATIVE IN-VITRO ANTIBACTERIAL ACTIVITY (MIC$_{90}$) OF SELECTED FLUOROQUINOLONES

Organism	Ciprofloxacin ($\leq$ 1 mg/L)*	Levofloxacin ($\leq$ 2 mg/L)*	Trovafloxacin ($\leq$ 2 mg/L)*	Gatifloxacin ($\leq$ 2 mg/L)*	Moxifloxacin ($\leq$ 2 mg/L)*
Gram-Negative Aerobic Bacteria					
Escherichia coli	0.016	0.03	0.03	0.016	0.008
Klebsiella pneumoniae	0.06	0.13	0.13	0.13	0.13
Proteus mirabilis	0.06	0.25	0.5	0.25	0.25
Enterobacter cloacae	0.03	0.06	0.06	0.06	0.06
Serratia marcescens	4	8	8	4	8
Morganella morganii	0.03	0.06	0.03	0.25	0.13
Citrobacter freundii	0.25	0.5	1	1	1
Pseudomonas aeruginosa	8	32	16	32	32
Acinetobacter species	1	0.5	0.13	0.25	0.25
Stenotrophomonas maltophilia	16	8	4	4	4
Haemophilus influenzae	0.016	0.06	0.016	0.016	0.06
Moraxella catarrhalis	0.03	0.03	0.016	0.03	0.03
Gram-Positive Aerobic Bacteria					
Staphylococcus aureus (MS)	0.5	0.25	0.06	0.13	0.06
Staphylococcus aureus (MR)	32	16	4	16	4
Staphylococcus epidermidis (MS)	2	0.5	0.13	0.25	0.13
Staphylococcus epidermidis (MR)	4	1	1	0.25	0.13
Streptococcus pneumoniae (PS)	2†	1	0.25†	0.5†	0.25†
Streptococcus pneumoniae (PR)	2†	1	0.25†	0.5†	0.25†
Streptococcus pyogenes	1	1	0.25	0.5	0.25
Enterococcus faecalis	4	2	1	2	1
Enterococcus faecium (VS)	16	8	4	8	4
Listeria monocytogenes	1	2	0.5	0.5	0.5
Atypical Bacteria					
Chlamydia pneumoniae	1	0.25	0.12	0.25	0.03
Legionella pneumophila	0.12	0.03	0.06	0.03	0.016
Mycoplasma pneumoniae	1	2	0.06	0.06	0.06
Anaerobic Bacteria					
Bacteroides fragilis	8	2	0.5	1	1
Bacteroides species	32	4	1	2	1
Fusobacterium species	4	2	1	0.5	1
Clostridium perfringens	4	2	0.25	1	0.25
Clostridium difficile	16	8	1	2	2
Peptostreptococcus species	4	2	0.25	0.5	0.25

MIC$_{90}$, Minimal inhibitory concentration at which 90% of tested strains are inhibited; MS, methicillin-susceptible; MR, methicillin-resistant; PS, penicillin-susceptible; PR, penicillin-resistant; VS, vancomycin-susceptible.

*Recommended susceptibility breakpoints for staphylococci and Enterobacteriaceae.

†Recommended susceptibility breakpoints for testing of trovafloxacin, gatifloxacin, and moxifloxacin versus S. pneumoniae are $\leq$ 1 mg/L. No recommended breakpoint exists for ciprofloxacin.

gatifloxacin have appreciable anaerobic activity that should prove useful for the treatment of anaerobic infections.

The fluoroquinolones are highly active against atypical pathogens, including *Legionella pneumophila*, *Chlamydia pneumoniae*, and *Mycoplasma pneumoniae*. Many authorities now consider the fluoroquinolones to be the drugs of choice for treatment of severe pneumonias caused by atypical pathogens, particularly *Legionella*, because of their very potent in-vitro activity, bactericidal actions, and high serum and intracellular concentrations.

MECHANISMS OF FLUOROQUINOLONE RESISTANCE

Two basic mechanisms of fluoroquinolone resistance have been identified. One involves alteration of DNA gyrase and topoisomerase IV, whereas the other results in reduced drug accumulation within bacterial cells.[22] Although plasmid-mediated resistance has been reported,[23] this appears to be rare compared with the more typical chromosomally mediated mechanisms of resistance.

Quinolone-resistant mutations in topoisomerase enzymes prevent the formation of drug/enzyme/DNA complexes, allowing DNA synthesis to occur in the presence of the drugs. Mutations in the genes encoding DNA gyrase (*gyrA* and *gyrB*) have been most frequently identified. However, other quinolone-resistant mutations in *parC* and *parE*, the genes encoding topoisomerase IV, have also been identified.[9,22,24] Resistance to the fluoroquinolones appears to arise in a stepwise manner. In some species (e.g., gram-negative bacteria) first-step mutations occur in *gyrA* and occasionally in *gyrB*, whereas in other species (e.g., *S. aureus, S. pneumoniae*) first-step mutations occur in *parC* and less often in *parE*.[9,24] First-step mutations usually result in a low-level resistance (≤ fourfold increased MIC), whereas additional mutations in either primary or secondary enzyme targets (second-step mutations) result in high-level resistance to drugs at clinically relevant concentrations. Dual *gyrA* and *parC* mutations have been described in clinical isolates of *S. pneumoniae;* however, it is thought that these strains were selected by fluoroquinolones with less potent antipneumococcal activity (e.g., ciprofloxacin).[25-27]

The first efflux system for quinolones was identified in *E. coli,*[28] whereas the first evidence for efflux-mediated quinolone resistance came from the characterization of *S. aureus* with overexpression of the *norA* gene product, a protein that mediates efflux.[29] Such efflux may occur in both quinolone-resistant and quinolone-susceptible strains of *S. aureus*. In some species (e.g., *P. aeruginosa*), at least two different efflux systems may be present that mediate resistance to tetracycline and chloramphenicol as well as the fluoroquinolones.[30] Although most efflux proteins appear to be relatively nonspecific multidrug transporters whose substrates include hydrophilic fluoroquinolones as well as monocationic organic compounds, relatively substrate-specific efflux pumps have also been described.[31]

Many genetic mutations have been described that result in decreased intracellular accumulation of fluoroquinolones and low-level drug resistance. Nearly all of these mutations are associated with decreased expression of OmpF, a non-specific outer membrane porin channel that is a major route of passage of hydrophilic fluoroquinolones through bacterial cellular membranes into the periplasmic space.[22,32] Although decreased membrane permeability is relatively common and easily induced, this is an unusual mechanism for clinically significant resistance. Strains of *E. coli*, *S. aureus*, and *P. aeruginosa* have been identified that possess both altered outer membrane permeability as well as *gyrA* mutations, resulting in high-level resistance to all tested fluoroquinolones.[33,34] Strains of highly ciprofloxacin-resistant *Salmonella* with both outer membrane protein alterations and expression of efflux pumps have also been described.[35]

Fluoroquinolone resistance among pathogens such as *S. aureus* and *P. aeruginosa* has been particularly problematic since the introduction of these agents into clinical use. As fluoroquinolones have become more extensively used in the treatment of respiratory tract infections, reports of increasing resistance among *S. pneumoniae* have focused attention on newly recognized mechanisms of drug action and drug resistance.[25-27] Resistance to the fluoroquinolones has tended

to emerge rapidly in bacteria with lower intrinsic susceptibility (e.g., *S. aureus*, *P. aeruginosa*, and *Acinetobacter* species) because fewer mutational steps are required to confer clinically relevant MIC changes.[36] However, fluoroquinolone resistance has also been noted to be an increasing problem among gram-negative bacilli such as *Enterobacter* species and *Klebsiella pneumoniae*, species that are usually considered to be highly susceptible to the drugs; this problem is particularly an issue among isolates from ICUs.[12] Development of resistance is also accelerated by the use of drugs with lower in-vitro activity, use of inappropriately low doses to treat infections caused by less susceptible organisms, and treatment of infection at sites where quinolone penetration may be decreased.[36] Development of resistance to one fluoroquinolone usually causes decreased susceptibility to all other agents in the class, although clinically relevant resistance may not necessarily occur. Of note, fluoroquinolone use has also been associated with high rates of cross-resistance among drugs of unrelated antibiotic classes such as the carbapenems, cephalosporins, and aminoglycosides.[12,37,38] Although not well understood, such cross-resistance is probably mediated by up-regulation and/or reduction in multiple efflux pump systems involved in passage of antibiotics through cell membranes and intracellular drug accumulation.[39,40] Although the fluoroquinolones remain highly active and clinically effective against a wide variety of important pathogens found in critically ill patients, increasing resistance is clearly an important issue in the clinical use of these drugs.

PHARMACOKINETICS

Pharmacokinetic properties of the currently used fluoroquinolones are shown in Table 140-2. The individual agents in the class do exhibit differences in certain properties such as oral bioavailability, half-lives, and routes of elimination and excretion. However, the fluoroquinolones as a whole are characterized by rapid oral absorption, extensive distribution into many fluids and tissues resulting in concentrations that are well above the MIC for many gram-negative and gram-positive organisms, and serum half-lives that are sufficiently long to allow once- or twice-daily dosing. Ciprofloxacin and levofloxacin have both been studied specifically in critically ill patients; although large interpatient variability and some differences in mean parameters were observed compared with normal volunteers, pharmacokinetics of the

TABLE 140–2. SUMMARY OF MEAN PHARMACOKINETIC PARAMETERS OF THE FLUOROQUINOLONES

Parameter	Ciprofloxacin 400 mg i.v. q 12h	Ciprofloxacin 400 mg i.v. q 8h*	Levofloxacin 500 mg i.v. q 24h*	Levofloxacin 750 mg i.v. q 24h	Trovafloxacin 300 mg i.v. q 24h*	Gatifloxacin 400 mg i.v. q 24h	Moxifloxacin 400 mg i.v. q 24h
Peak (mg/L)	4.6	6.5	7.5	12.1	3.6	5.5	4.2
Volume of distribution (L/kg)	1.2	1.3	1.2	1.3	1.4	1.5	1.7
Half-life (h)†	4.0	3.3	8.0	7.9	11.6	7.4	14.8
AUC$_{0-24}$ (mg · hr/mL)	12.7	46.5	66.1	108	34.2	35.1	38.0
Renal excretion as unchanged drug (%)	50-70	NR	NR	>95	10	84	45

AUC$_{0-24}$, Area under the serum concentration-versus-time curve from time 0 to 24 hours; NR, not reported.
*Data from critically ill ICU patients.
†In patients with creatinine clearance > 40-50 mL/min.

drugs were generally similar enough to allow the use of normally recommended doses.[41,42]

Certain pharmacokinetic features are of particular importance during use of these drugs in critically ill patients. Limited data suggest that fluoroquinolones are well absorbed after oral administration to critically ill patients, although patients must be carefully selected for clinical stability and absence of gastrointestinal diseases or processes that may affect drug absorption.[42]

The fluoroquinolones have excellent distribution into many tissues and fluids and often reach concentrations manyfold higher than found in blood. For example, ciprofloxacin achieves tissue-to-serum concentration ratios of approximately 2 in bronchial and lung tissues, 2 in lung tissues, 13 in the kidneys, and up to 30 in the bile.[43] Levofloxacin has been shown to achieve pulmonary epithelial lining fluid:plasma and alveolar macrophage:plasma ratios of 2.1 to 2.3 and 8.9 to 12.0, respectively, 12 hours after multiple-dose administration of levofloxacin, 500 to 750 mg orally.[44] Such high tissue and fluid levels have important pharmacodynamic implications (see later) and increase the likelihood of successfully treating infections at these sites. In contrast, penetration of the fluoroquinolones into the cerebrospinal fluid is relatively poor and ranges from 20% to 40% of serum concentrations in the absence of inflamed meninges.

Ciprofloxacin, levofloxacin, and gatifloxacin are all excreted to a large degree through the kidneys as unmetabolized drug; doses should therefore be appropriately adjusted in the presence of moderate-to-severe renal dysfunction to avoid unnecessary drug accumulation. In contrast, elimination of moxifloxacin is relatively insensitive to changes in renal function; this drug is highly metabolized and even severe renal impairment does not influence dosing requirements. Mild to moderate hepatic impairment does not significantly affect the pharmacokinetics of most of these agents; however, most drugs have not been well studied in patients with severe or end-stage liver disease and consideration should be given to empirically decreasing the daily dosage of hepatically eliminated drugs. Ciprofloxacin has been shown to undergo compensatory increases in renal clearance in patients with severe liver disease and no dosage adjustments are required if renal function is normal[45]; however, caution is warranted when dosing ciprofloxacin in patients with both hepatic and renal dysfunction.[46]

PHARMACODYNAMIC CONSIDERATIONS

Studies have clearly demonstrated that the fluoroquinolones exhibit concentration-dependent bacterial killing.[47-55] A number of studies, including a prospectively developed model of the pharmacodynamic response to levofloxacin during treatment of respiratory tract, skin, and urinary tract infections, have provided evidence that achieving a ratio of fluoroquinolone peak serum concentrations to the bacterial MIC (peak/MIC ratio) of greater than 10 to 12 appears to be predictive of clinical drug efficacy and successful bacterial eradication.[47-49] The ratio of area under the 24-hour serum concentration-time curve to MIC (AUC/MIC_{24}) has also been shown in vitro and retrospectively in vivo to be predictive of favorable clinical response and reduced development of resistance.[50-52] Although the optimal AUC/MIC_{24} ratio breakpoints are still unclear, favorable AUC/MIC_{24} ratios appear to be 125 to 250 for gram-negative organisms and

30 to 50 for *S. pneumoniae*.[51-55] Whether either the peak/MIC ratio or AUC/MIC_{24} ratio is superior to the other parameter and which specific ratios are most predictive of drug efficacy remain somewhat controversial; however, the strong relationships between these pharmacodynamic parameters and clinical and microbiologic outcomes during fluoroquinolone therapy have been well established.

Certain principles of fluoroquinolone pharmacodynamics can be readily applied to the appropriate treatment of infections in critically ill patients. Fluoroquinolone pharmacokinetics are somewhat variable in the critically ill, and the drugs are often being used as empirical therapy for infections potentially caused by organisms with reduced fluoroquinolone susceptibility (i.e., higher MICs). High doses will thus often be necessary to minimize the variability in both pharmacokinetics and pathogen susceptibilities and optimize the concentration-dependent pharmacodynamic properties of the drugs in patients with severe infections. Use of higher doses is particularly recommended in the treatment of severe infections suspected or documented to be caused by pathogens with intrinsically higher MICs to the drugs (e.g., *P. aeruginosa* and *Acinetobacter* species). The fluoroquinolones readily penetrate into most tissues and fluids of the body, but the use of high doses in the treatment of serious infections should also maximize tissue penetration and more reliably achieve adequate drug concentrations at the site of infection. Based on the pharmacodynamic properties of the fluoroquinolones, the intensity of dosing and ability to achieve favorable peak/MIC or AUC/MIC_{24} ratios should also minimize the development of resistance. However, it should be noted that many pathogens found in critically ill patients (e.g., most of the enteric gram-negative bacilli, MSSA, streptococci) are highly susceptible to the fluoroquinolones and the use of high doses is not necessary to achieve concentrations adequate for the treatment of most infections.

ADVERSE EFFECTS

With some notable exceptions (e.g., most recently, trovafloxacin), the fluoroquinolones have generally proven to be a safe and very well tolerated class of drugs. The most common adverse effects associated with the fluoroquinolones are gastrointestinal effects such as nausea, vomiting, and diarrhea (~1% to 5% incidence); rash (< 2.5%); and central nervous system (CNS) effects, including headache, dizziness, and sleep disturbances (<1% to 2%). These adverse effects are generally mild and self-limiting and seldom result in discontinuation of fluoroquinolone therapy. With intravenous preparations, pain and inflammation at the injection site have also been reported.[56-58]

Adverse gastrointestinal effects of the fluoroquinolones are thought to be caused by a combination of direct gastrointestinal irritation and CNS-mediated effects; adverse gastrointestinal effects may be seen when these drugs are administered intravenously. *Clostridium difficile*–associated colitis has been only rarely associated with fluoroquinolone use, perhaps because of their minimal effect on gastrointestinal anaerobic flora. There is some concern that newer fluoroquinolones with enhanced anaerobic activity (e.g., trovafloxacin, moxifloxacin, gatifloxacin) may perhaps be associated with an increased risk of *C. difficile*–associated colitis, but this cannot be substantiated from data derived from clinical or surveillance studies.

CNS disturbances caused by fluoroquinolones can be broadly divided into two types: those resulting from direct effects of the drugs on the CNS caused by inhibition of gamma-aminobutyric acid (GABA) binding, and those resulting from adverse drug-drug interactions (either pharmacokinetic or pharmacodynamic). Of the fluoroquinolones, levofloxacin is associated with the lowest incidence of adverse CNS events and trovafloxacin with the highest. The occurrence of adverse CNS effects with ciprofloxacin, gatifloxacin, and moxifloxacin is similar and only slightly more frequent than with levofloxacin. Seizures have been only rarely reported during fluoroquinolone therapy and usually occurred in the presence of predisposing factors, such as seizure disorder, head trauma, anoxia, metabolic disturbances, or concomitant drug therapy with specific interacting agents (i.e., theophylline).[56-58]

Elevations in serum transaminase, alkaline phosphatase, and/or bilirubin levels have been noted to occur in 2% to 3% of patients receiving fluoroquinolone therapy.[56-58] These liver abnormalities are usually mild, are reversible, and do not necessitate discontinuation of therapy. Among the currently available agents, only trovafloxacin has been associated with clinically significant hepatotoxicity. Postmarketing surveillance of trovafloxacin in the United States detected nearly 150 cases of clinically symptomatic hepatic injury, including hepatitis and acute hepatic failure, among approximately 2.5 million patients who had been treated with the drug.[59] It is currently recommended in the United States that use of trovafloxacin be restricted to severe, life-threatening indications in hospitalized patients, that use of trovafloxacin be restricted to 14 days' duration, and that liver and pancreatic function tests be monitored or the drug be discontinued in patients who develop symptoms consistent with hepatitis and/or pancreatitis, as clinically indicated, during therapy with trovafloxacin.[59]

The fluoroquinolones, particularly gatifloxacin, have been implicated in causing abnormalities of glucose homeostasis. Both hypoglycemia and hyperglycemia have been reported, and patients with preexisting diabetes mellitus or other known glucose abnormalities are apparently at particularly high risk. Little specific information is currently available, and it is not entirely clear that these adverse effects are truly drug related.

Much recent attention has been focused on the potential of fluoroquinolones to cause cardiac toxicity manifested as electrocardiographic prolongation of the corrected QT (QTc) interval and arrhythmias including ventricular tachycardia, ventricular fibrillation, and torsades de pointes.[60-62] Considerable controversy exists as to the true risk of cardiac toxicity associated with the fluoroquinolones and whether specific agents might be associated with a greater degree of risk. It appears as though all of the currently available fluoroquinolones are capable of causing some degree of QTc prolongation. However, QTc interval prolongation is usually quite minor (mean of <5 to 10 ms), does not predictably occur in all patients exposed to fluoroquinolones, and is of no clinical significance in the vast majority of patients treated with these agents. Patients who may be at particular risk of drug-induced cardiac toxicity and who should be more closely monitored during fluoroquinolone use include those with the following characteristics: advanced age (>60 years), history of significant cardiac disease or previous arrhythmia, presence of electrolyte abnormalities (e.g., potassium, calcium, magnesium), and concomitant use of antiarrhythmic or other drugs known to cause prolongation of the QTc interval.[58,60,61]

Tendonitis and tendon rupture are rare complications of fluoroquinolone use. A total of only 33 cases have been reported in the medical literature with ciprofloxacin and levofloxacin; the number of cases related to other available agents is not known.[63] The median duration of drug use before the onset of symptoms was 6 to 7 days. Risk factors for the occurrence of tendinopathy are not well characterized but may include male sex, older age (median age of reported cases was 59 years), concurrent corticosteroid use, and presence of renal disease or history of renal transplantation.[63]

DRUG-DRUG INTERACTIONS

Concurrent administration of oral fluoroquinolones with multivalent cation-containing products such as aluminum- or magnesium-containing antacids and products containing calcium, iron, or zinc (including multivitamins with minerals) should be avoided. Concomitant use of these agents with a fluoroquinolone invariably results in a marked reduction of oral absorption of the antimicrobial; bioavailability of the fluoroquinolones may be reduced as much as 90% due to the formation of insoluble chelation complexes in the gastrointestinal tract that inhibit drug absorption.[58] Similar changes in oral antibiotic absorption have also been observed with concurrent administration of sucralfate or ferrous sulfate. Effects of enteral feeding formulas on the absorption of fluoroquinolones are variable, but concurrent administration should nevertheless be avoided. Concomitant administration of H_2 receptor antagonists and proton pump inhibitors have no clinically significant effects on the absorption of the fluoroquinolones.[58]

Ciprofloxacin has been shown to decrease theophylline clearance by a mean of approximately 25% to 30%, although increases in theophylline plasma concentrations of up to 308% have been reported.[64] Levofloxacin, trovafloxacin, gatifloxacin, and moxifloxacin have no significant effects on theophylline metabolism. Ciprofloxacin was also shown to reduce the clearance of the R-enantiomer of warfarin by 15% to 32%; however, the clearance of the S-enantiomer, which is more potent and is thought to cause the majority of warfarin's anticoagulant activity, was not affected. Therefore, this interaction was not believed to be clinically significant. No apparent effects on either the R- or S-warfarin concentrations or prothrombin times were noted during concomitant dosing of levofloxacin, trovafloxacin, moxifloxacin, or gatifloxacin.[58] Although significant pharmacokinetic or pharmacodynamic interactions between the fluoroquinolones and warfarin have not been documented through studies, several anecdotal case reports have described clinically significant interactions between warfarin and the fluoroquinolones. The anticoagulation of any patient receiving concomitant fluoroquinolone and warfarin therapy should be closely monitored.

DOSING

Recommendations for dosing of the currently available fluoroquinolones are given in Table 140-3. Recommended regimens in the presence of renal or hepatic dysfunction are also given when appropriate and where data are available. Consideration should always be given to the susceptibility of

TABLE 140–3. RECOMMENDED DOSING REGIMENS FOR SELECTED FLUOROQUINOLONES IN SEVERELY ILL PATIENTS

Drug and Indications	Recommended Regimen			
	CrCL ≥ 30 mL/min	CrCL < 30 mL/min	Hemodialysis	CVVH/CVVHDF
Ciprofloxacin				
Nosocomial pneumonia; severe/complicated LRTI, SSSI; febrile neutropenia	400 mg i.v. q 8h	200 mg i.v. q 8h or 400 mg i.v. q 12-18h	400 mg q 24h	400 mg i.v. q 24h
Complicated intra-abdominal; other systemic infections of mild-to-moderate severity	400 mg i.v. q 12h	400 mg i.v. q 24h	200-400 mg q 24h	200-400 mg i.v. q 24h
Levofloxacin	**CrCL ≥ 50 mL/min**	**CrCL < 50 mL/min**	**Hemodialysis**	**CVVH/CVVHDF**
Nosocomial pneumonia; complicated SSSI	750 mg i.v. q 24h	750 mg × 1, then 750 mg q 48h	500 mg q 48h	250-500 mg i.v. q 24h
Other systemic infections	500 mg q 24h	500 mg × 1, then 250 mg q 24-48 h	250 mg q 48h	250 mg IV q 24h
Trovafloxacin	**Normal/Impaired Renal Function**	**Mild-Moderate Cirrhosis**	**Hemodialysis**	**CVVH/CVVHDF**
Severe, life-threatening infections where benefits of use outweigh potential toxicities	300 mg i.v. IV q 24h	200 mg i.v. q 24h	300 mg i.v. q 24h	ND
Gatifloxacin	**CrCL ≥ 40 mL/min**	**CrCL < 40 mL/min**	**Hemodialysis**	**CVVH/CVVHDF**
All indications	400 mg i.v. q 24h	200 mg i.v. q 24h	200 mg i.v. q 24h	ND
Moxifloxacin	**Normal/Impaired Renal Function**	**Mild-Moderate Cirrhosis**	**Hemodialysis**	**CVVH/CVVHDF**
All indications	400 mg i.v. q 24h	400 mg i.v. q 24h	400 mg i.v. q 24h	ND

CrCL, creatinine clearance; CVVH, continuous venovenous hemofiltration; CVVHDF, continuous venovenous hemodiafiltration; LRTI, lower respiratory tract infection; ND, no data; SSSI, skin/skin structure infection.

presumed or documented pathogens, site of infection, severity of infection, presence of organ dysfunction, and pharmacodynamic characteristics of the fluoroquinolones when choosing an appropriate dosing regimen for a specific patient.

ANNOTATED REFERENCES

Fish DN: Fluoroquinolone adverse effects and drug interactions. Pharmacotherapy 2001;21(Suppl):253S-272S.

This review article provides a comprehensive evaluation of incidence and risk factors for fluoroquinolone-associated adverse effects and toxicities. The paper also discusses relevant drug-drug and drug-food interactions and highlights safety differences between individual fluoroquinolone agents.

Neuhauser MM, Weinstein RA, Rydman R, et al: Antibiotic resistance among gram-negative bacilli in US intensive care units: Implications for fluoroquinolone use. JAMA 2003;289:885-888.

This study evaluated susceptibilities to 16 commonly used antibiotics among clinical isolates gathered from intensive care units throughout the United States during the years 1994 to 2000. Whereas most antibiotics showed an absolute decreased susceptibility of 6% or less during the study period, overall susceptibility to ciprofloxacin decreased by 10% and was statistically associated with increased fluoroquinolone use.

Preston SL, Drusano GL, Berman AL, et al: Pharmacodynamics of levofloxacin: A new paradigm for early clinical trials. JAMA 1998;279:125-129.

This prospective study was one of the first clinical trials in humans to prospectively include a pharmacodynamic evaluation of clinical and microbiological success during fluoroquinolone therapy. As predicted from earlier in vitro and animal models, the ratios of both the maximum serum concentration divided by the pathogen minimum inhibitory concentration (MIC) and the pharmacokinetic area under the serum concentration-versus-time curve divided by the MIC were found to be the significant predictors of clinical and microbiological treatment success.

Rebuck JA, Fish DN, Abraham E: Pharmacokinetics of intravenous and oral levofloxacin in critically ill patients in a medical intensive care unit. Pharmacotherapy 2002;22:1216-1225.

This prospective study evaluated the pharmacokinetics of intravenous and oral levofloxacin in 30 severely ill patients in a medical intensive care unit. The pharmacokinetics of levofloxacin were found to be only slightly altered in comparison to those found in normal volunteers, and the bioavailability of oral levofloxacin was approximately 95%, highlighting the favorable pharmacokinetic and safety profile of this agent in severely ill patients.

Sahm DF, Critchley IA, Kelly LJ, et al: Evaluation of current activities of fluoroquinolones against gram-negative bacilli using centralized in vitro testing and electronic surveillance. Antimicrob Agents Chemother 2001; 45:267-274.

This large, prospective surveillance study evaluated activities of ciprofloxacin and levofloxacin versus clinical isolates of important gram-negative pathogens. Although ciprofloxacin is often considered to be more active than other fluoroquinolones, levofloxacin was comparable against most strains, including Pseudomonas aeruginosa, and was actually more active against certain problematic organisms such as Stenotrophomonas maltophilia.

Chapter 141
MACROLIDES

David T. Bearden

The macrolide class is based on the structure of erythromycin, the prototype natural macrolide isolated from *Streptomyces erythreus*.[1] Commonly, the term *macrolide* is expanded to include the azalide azithromycin. The newly developed ketolides, owing to their similar structural bases, are close members of the macrolide family. There are many macrolides available throughout the world. The most commonly used macrolides are erythromycin, clarithromycin, and azithromycin. Roxithromycin is available in Europe and Asia. Telithromycin is the only currently available ketolide.

MECHANISM OF ACTION

The macrolides inhibit bacterial protein synthesis by binding to the 50S ribosomal subunit.[2] The advanced macrolides have improved binding to the ribosomes compared with erythromycin. Telithromycin, the ketolide, has a similar target site, but its structure allows for enhanced binding, even in the presence of ribosomal mutations.

MECHANISMS OF RESISTANCE

There are three major mechanisms of bacterial resistance to macrolides: drug efflux, ribosomal mutations, and enzymatic inactivation. Active efflux, mediated by *mef* genes, and ribosomal methylation of the target site, mediated by *erm* genes, are the most clinically important resistance mechanisms. Organisms containing the *mef* gene commonly express low-level resistance that can often be overcome with larger doses of the antibiotic. In contrast, *erm*-containing organisms, expressing phenotypic macrolide-lincosamide-streptogramin B resistance, often express high-level resistance, rendering macrolides clinically ineffective.

ANTIMICROBIAL SPECTRUM OF ACTIVITY

The macrolides have activity against many classes of bacteria but have only sporadic activity within each of these groups. Their primary microbiologic activity is directed against respiratory and intracellular pathogens (Table 141-1).[3-23]

GRAM-POSITIVE AEROBES

Among the gram-positive aerobes, erythromycin activity is limited to the streptococci with reasonable activity against *S. pneumoniae*. The advanced macrolides (azithromycin, clarithromycin, dirithromycin, roxithromycin) have similar activity against *S. pneumoniae*. The utility of the macrolides against pneumococci is hampered by increasing resistance, commonly coupled with penicillin resistance. A 1999-2000 study from 25 countries reported 31% worldwide macrolide resistance.[24] The predominant worldwide resistance mechanism is *erm*(B) mediated high level resistance (56.2%), but there is considerable international variability. Resistant North American isolates most commonly contain low level *mef*(A) resistance, whereas most European and Far East countries report higher levels of *erm*(B)-containing pathogens. Resistance mechanisms are important, because low-level resistance may possibly be overcome with conventional dosing of the macrolides.[25] Pneumococcal resistance to one macrolide commonly confers resistance to all members of the class. The ketolides, however, maintain their activity against macrolide-resistant *S. pneumoniae* possessing both *erm*- and *mef*-mediated resistance.[24]

TABLE 141–1. ANTIBACTERIAL ACTIVITY OF THE MACROLIDES AND A KETOLIDE

Organism	MIC$_{90}$ Range (µg/mL)					
	Erythromycin	Clarithromycin	Azithromycin	Roxithromycin	Dirithromycin	Telithromycin
Gram-Positive Bacteria						
Staphylococcus aureus (MS)[3-5]	>128	>16->128	64	>128	>32->64	0.06-0.25
Staphylococcus aureus (MR)[3-5]	>128	>16->128	>64	>128	>32->128	0.5->128
Streptococcus pneumoniae (PS)[6,7]	0.5-1	0.06-0.25	0.5-1	2-4	0.5	0.03
Streptococcus pneumoniae (PR)[6-8]	>64-128	>64	>64-128	>64	>64	0.125-0.25
Viridans group streptococci[4,9-11]	8	>16	>64			0.12
Group A streptococci[3,12,13]	0.015-2	0.015-0.25	0.5	0.5-1	≤0.25	0.008-0.03
Group B streptococci[3,11,12]	0.03-0.12	0.015-0.06	1	0.06-0.25		0.008-0.06
Gram-Negative Bacteria						
Bordetella pertussis[14,15]	0.06-0.25	0.06	0.06	0.125-0.5		0.03
Haemophilus influenzae[3,13,16,17]	8	8-16	2	16	16	2
Moraxella catarrhalis[3,4,11-13,16,17]	0.06-0.5	0.03-0.25	≤0.06-≤0.25	0.12	1	0.03-0.12
Neisseria gonorrhoeae[3,11,17]	0.5-1	0.12-1	0.12	0.5		0.03-0.06
Neisseria meningitidis[3,11]	0.25	0.03-0.06		0.25		0.03
Listeria monocytogenes[17]	0.12	0.12	1			
Anaerobes						
Bacteroides fragilis group[18,19]	16->64	2->64	>64	>64		16->64
Clostridium difficile[3,18,19]	16->64	4->64	>64	16->64		1->64
Peptostreptococcus species[3,11,18-20]	4->128	2->32	>32->64	16-64		0.008-0.12
Prevotella species[18,21]	8	1	8	4		0.5-1
Porphyromonas species[18,20]	0.125-0.25	0.125	0.5	0.125		0.25
Atypical pathogens						
Legionella pneumophila[5,17]	1	0.015-0.78	2		4->16	
Mycoplasma pneumoniae[22,23]	≤0.004-0.06	≤0.001-0.03	≤0.001-0.03	0.25	0.25	0.008

MS, methicillin-sensitive; MR, methicillin resistant; PS, penicillin sensitive; PR, penicillin resistant.

GRAM-NEGATIVE AEROBES

The macrolides are largely ineffective against the Enterobacteriaceae and other nosocomial pathogens. With the exception of erythromycin, the macrolides and telithromycin have activity against *Haemophilus influenzae*. The activity of clarithromycin versus *H. influenzae* is enhanced in the presence of its active metabolite.[26] The macrolides and ketolide also display activity against *Moraxella catarrhalis, Bordetella pertussis, Neisseria gonorrhoeae,* and *N. meningitidis.* Clarithromycin has been the most commonly used macrolide against *Helicobacter pylori,* although resistance rates are currently 10% to 12% in the United States and have reached as high as 18% in Southern Europe.[27,28]

MISCELLANEOUS

The macrolides and the ketolide attain high intracellular concentrations and are active against *Legionella* species, *Chlamydia* species, and *Mycoplasma pneumoniae.* In vitro activity is also demonstrated against *Rickettsia, Bartonella,* and *Brucella* species,[29-31] as well as Lyme disease causing *Borrelia burgdorferi.*[32] In addition, azithromycin, clarithromycin, and telithromycin have activity against some strains of atypical nontuberculosis mycobacteria, including *Mycobacterium avium* complex.[33-35]

ANAEROBES

The macrolides and the ketolide have poor activity against obligate anaerobes but maintain moderate activity against a variety of oral anaerobes including *Prevotella* and *Porphyromonas* species.

PHARMACOKINETICS

Erythromycin base is acid labile but still adequately absorbed from the gastrointestinal tract. Food can decrease absorption (Table 141-2).[1,36-43] More stable oral formulations have complexed erythromycin with salts or esters to form erythromycin estolate, stearate, and ethylsuccinate. Erythromycin lactobionate has also been formulated to allow for intravenous delivery. Peak concentrations are 0.73 µg/mL after 250 mg base orally and 10 µg/mL after 500 mg intravenously.[1,36] The half-life is 1 to 1.5 hours.[37] Like all macrolides, erythromycin is widely distributed throughout the body, with higher tissue and intracellular concentrations compared with plasma. Erythromycin is not found in the cerebrospinal fluid in normal volunteers, but low levels have been reported in patients with meningitis.[37] Erythromycin is metabolized by cytochrome P450 (CYP) enzymes in the liver and excreted as inactive metabolites primarily in the feces.

Clarithromycin is well absorbed from the gastrointestinal tract (bioavailability 52% to 55%), with or without food. An intravenous lactobionate form is available in some countries. A peak concentration of 1.65 to 2.12 mg/mL is obtained after a 500-mg oral dose with a half-life of 3 to 5 hours.[38] Similar pharmacokinetics are observed after dosing with the oral suspension even in critically ill patients.[44] An extended-release formulation is available that delays the time to peak concentrations, provides similar total drug exposure, and allows for once-daily dosing.[45] Clarithromycin is well

TABLE 141–2. COMPARATIVE PHARMACOKINETICS OF MACROLIDES AND KETOLIDE

Drug	Normal Dosing	c_max	t_{1/2}	Absorption with Food
Erythromycin[1,36,37]	250-500 mg p.o. qid	0.7 µg/mL	1-1.5 h	Better fasting
	500 mg-1 g i.v. q 6h	10 µg/mL		
Clarithromycin[38]	250-500 mg p.o. bid	1.6-2.1 µg/mL	3-5 h	No effect
Azithromycin[39,40]	500 mg × 1, 250 mg p.o. qd	0.4 µg/mL	14-40 h	No effect
	500 mg i.v. qd	3.6 µg/mL		
Dirithromycin[41]	500 mg p.o. qd	0.1-0.5 µg/mL	30-44 h	Better after food
Roxithromycin[42]	150 mg p.o. bid	6.6-7.9 µg/mL	8.4-15.5 h	Better fasting
Telithromycin[43]	800 mg p.o. qd	1.9-2.3 µg/mL	7-10 h	No effect

distributed throughout the body, with respiratory tract tissue and fluid concentrations 3 to 30 times that of the plasma and alveolar macrophage concentrations 10^2 to 10^3 higher than plasma.[38] Cerebrospinal fluid concentrations are unknown. Hepatic metabolism is the major metabolic pathway and leads to the formation of 14-hydroxy-clarithromycin, an active metabolite with greater activity than the parent compound.[26,38] Clarithromycin is extensively metabolized, with 18.4% and 4.4% of unchanged drug excreted in the urine and feces, respectively, after a 250-mg dose.[38] Dosing changes are required in patients with moderate to severe renal dysfunction.

Azithromycin is 37% bioavailable when administered orally but is also available in an intravenous formulation.[39,46] Food has little effect on bioavailability. Peak concentrations in the plasma after a 500-mg dose range from 0.4 µg/mL for the oral formulation to 3.6 µg/mL for the intravenous formulation.[39,40] Azithromycin is unique in its extended half-life of 14 to 40 hours, thus providing low sustained plasma concentrations that persist after cessation of dosing.[39] While plasma concentrations are very low, azithromycin attains very high concentrations in tissues (100 times plasma) and phagocytes (3000 to 7000 times plasma).[40] Little to no azithromycin can be recovered from the cerebrospinal fluid, but brain tissue concentrations well exceed those in the serum.[47] Azithromycin is minimally metabolized and largely excreted via the biliary tract into the feces.

Dirithromycin is orally administered but has a poor bioavailability of 6% to 14% that is impaired further by administration with food.[41] Peak concentrations of 0.1 to 0.5 µg/mL are achieved after a 500-mg oral dose. Dirithromycin is largely hydrolyzed during absorption to erythromycyclamine, an active metabolite. The half-life of dirithromycin (and converted erythromycyclamine) is long, with a range of 30 to 44 hours. Dirithromycin attains high tissue concentrations that exceed those in plasma for the lung, bronchial secretions, phagocytes, and tonsils.[48] Fecal/hepatic elimination accounts for the majority (81% to 97%) of the excretion of orally administered dirithromycin and its major metabolite.

Roxithromycin is well absorbed orally, with peak plasma concentrations of 6.6 to 7.9 µg/mL after a 150-mg oral dose, and a half-life of 8.4 to 15.5 hours.[42] Fasting prior to dosing improves absorption. Tissue concentrations exceed those of the plasma. Roxithromycin is metabolized by multiple mechanisms, with the majority of the dose excreted in the feces.[42,49]

Telithromycin is 57% bioavailable, with peak plasma concentrations of 1.9 to 2.3 µg/mL after an 800-mg dose, regardless of food intake.[43] The half-life of telithromycin is 7 to 10 hours. Like the macrolides, telithromycin achieves high concentrations in respiratory tissues, alveolar macrophages,

and peripheral polymorphonuclear cells. Telithromycin is metabolized by CYP3A4 and non–CYP-related mechanisms. Fecal elimination of metabolites accounts for the majority of the excretion of telithromycin.

PHARMACODYNAMICS

The macrolides and ketolides appear to have time-dependent antibacterial activity that is a slowly bactericidal or bacteriostatic.[43,50,51] The relationships between drug concentration and bacterial effect that best explain the drug activity are the time above the MIC and the area under the inhibitory curve (AUC:MIC). Differences in the pharmacokinetics of the individual agents, and limited analyses, deter an absolute determination of the best dosing strategy. It should be noted that pharmacodynamic principles for antibacterials have generally been related to plasma concentrations.[52] As noted earlier, the plasma concentrations of the macrolides are usually lower than those of the tissues, where the majority of bacteria reside. It is difficult to relate tissue concentrations to the plasma concentration–derived pharmacodynamic parameters.

IMMUNE MODULATION

Increasing evidence suggests that antibacterial macrolides have anti-inflammatory effects.[53] An animal model of inflammation suggested that roxithromycin has greater anti-inflammatory activity than clarithromycin and azithromycin.[54] In addition to in vitro and animal models, clinical data suggest that macrolides may have activity in the treatment of inflammatory diseases including cystic fibrosis, diffuse panbronchiolitis, chronic sinusitis, and inflammatory skin diseases.[53,55] Early in vitro studies suggest that telithromycin may display little anti-inflammatory activity.[56]

ADVERSE EFFECTS

Gastrointestinal effects (nausea and diarrhea) predominate the common adverse events observed with macrolide therapy.[42,43,57] Erythromycin has the highest level of gastrointestinal effects.[1] Nausea with erythromycin may occur after intravenous dosing, as erythromycin is secreted into the gastrointestinal tract via the bile.[58] The advanced macrolides have a similar incidence of gastrointestinal adverse events. A review of azithromycin safety data from over 4000 patients reported gastrointestinal event rates of 4% for diarrhea and 3% for nausea.[57] In 3800 patients receiving clarithromycin, similar side effect rates were observed for nausea (3.8%) and diarrhea (3.0%). Roxithromycin was reported to have a 4% incidence of side effects in 32,405 patients, with 75% being mild to moderate gastrointestinal events.[42] In 4263 patients receiving dirithromycin, nausea and diarrhea each occurred in approximately 5% of patients.[59] From data in clinical trials, gastrointestinal side effects were reported frequently with telithromycin (7% to 20% diarrhea, 2% to 12% nausea), although considerable variability was observed across studies.[43]

More serious events include prolongation of the QT interval with torsades de pointes. In vitro estimations of *HERG* blockade suggest that clarithromycin ≈ roxithromycin > erythromycin.[60] In contrast, erythromycin was found to have a higher proarrhythmic potential than clarithromycin and azithromycin in an animal heart model.[61] Clinical torsades de pointes has been reported in patients receiving macrolides. Although the relative ability of the macrolides to cause arrhythmias is difficult to ascertain, clarithromycin was reported more frequently than erythromycin.[62]

PROKINETIC ACTIVITY

The intestinal prokinetic activity of the macrolides has been used to improve gastrointestinal mobility. Erythromycin has been shown to improve gastric emptying in a dose-dependent manner.[63] However, concerns have been raised over the potential to increase bacterial resistance with non-antibacterial macrolide use.[64] In a comparative trial in patients with enteral nutrition intolerability, erythromycin was inferior to metoclopramide and cisapride.[65]

DRUG-DRUG INTERACTIONS

Drug-drug interactions must be evaluated when considering macrolide therapy. The macrolides have variable degrees of inhibition of CYP3A4 and are also substrates of this enzyme. The use of macrolides with other drugs metabolized by CYP3A4 may result in increases in the second drug concentrations. Erythromycin is the most potent inhibitor of CYP3A4 followed by moderate inhibition with clarithromycin and roxithromycin and little to no inhibition by azithromycin or dirithromycin.[66] Erythromycin has been implicated in multiple drug interactions, including benzodiazepines, carbamazepine, cyclosporine, digoxin, HMG-CoA inhibitors, tacrolimus, and theophylline. Case reports of interactions with warfarin have been documented for many of the macrolides.[67] Clarithromycin, although in vitro a less potent

inhibitor of CYP3A4, has been associated with a similar scope of clinical interactions.[67] As expected by its limited CYP activity, few clinically important interactions have been reported with roxithromycin, dirithromycin, and azithromycin.[39,42,67]

The pharmacodynamic interaction between macrolides and other drugs known to increase the QT interval must not be overlooked (see Adverse Effects).

ANNOTATED REFERENCES

Farrell DJ, Morrissey I, Bakker S, et al: Molecular characterization of macrolide resistance mechanisms among *Streptococcus pneumoniae* and *Streptococcus pyogenes* isolated from the PROTEKT 1999-2000 study. J Antimicrob Chemother 2002;50(Suppl S1):39-47.

From S. pneumoniae isolates collected worldwide, erm-mediated (high level) resistance is seen in greater than half of all macrolide-resistant isolates. Large variations in resistance mechanism frequency are seen among countries, resulting in the need for local surveillance to guide empirical therapy.

Pankuch GA, Visalli MA, Jacobs MR, et al: Susceptibilities of penicillin- and erythromycin-susceptible and -resistant pneumococci to HMR 3647 (RU 66647), a new ketolide, compared with susceptibilities to 17 other agents. Antimicrob Agents Chemother 1998;42:624-630.

Telithromycin retains in vitro susceptibility against S. pneumoniae that are resistant to penicillin and other macrolides. Further in vitro testing via time-kill curve evaluation reveals uniform bactericidal activity against all tested strains.

Scaglione F, Rossoni G: Comparative anti-inflammatory effects of roxithromycin, azithromycin, and clarithromycin. J Antimicrob Chemother 1998;41(Suppl B):47-50.

In an animal model of inflammation, all tested macrolides decreased inflammation. Roxithromycin was the most potent anti-inflammatory macrolide, with activity close to the nonsteroidal anti-inflammatory nimesulide.

Shaffer D, Singer S, Korvick J, et al: Concomitant risk factors in reports of torsades de pointes associated with macrolide use: Review of the United States Food and Drug Administration Adverse Event Reporting System. Clin Infect Dis 2002;35:197-200.

A review of a spontaneous adverse event reports provided data on 156 cases of torsades de pointes in patients receiving macrolide antibiotics. Concomitant use of drugs known to increase the QT interval was found in half of the cases. Increased age, female sex, and comorbid diseases were other common risk factors.

Tessier PR, Kim MK, Zhou W, et al: Pharmacodynamic assessment of clarithromycin in a murine model of pneumococcal pneumonia. Antimicrob Agents Chemother 2002;46:1425-1434.

In a murine model of pneumonia, all three pharmacodynamic parameters (Cmax/MIC, AUC/MIC, and T > MIC) showed similar correlation with bacterial killing, animal survival, and time of survival. Based on these results, AUC/MIC ratio is suggested as the best composite to predict microbiologic and clinical efficacy of clarithromycin.

Chapter 142

AGENTS WITH PRIMARY ACTIVITY AGAINST GRAM-POSITIVE BACTERIA

Diane M. Cappelletty

KEY POINTS

VANCOMYCIN

1. Vancomycin is **slowly bactericidal** against dividing organisms except for *Enterococcus* and tolerant staphylococci, against which it is bacteriostatic. Vancomycin resistance of the VanA phenotype confers high-level resistance to both teicoplanin (minimal inhibitory concentration [MIC]: 16 to 512 µg/mL) and vancomycin (MIC: 64 to >1000 µg/mL). This was first identified in *Enterococcus* and relatively common within this genus. In 2002, this resistance gene was passed to two different *Staphylococcus aureus* isolates and for the first time conferred **high-level resistance to vancomycin within the *Staphylococcus* genus.**

2. The pharmacodynamic effect of vancomycin is time-dependent killing or time above the MIC. **The most important parameter or goal of therapy is to maintain a free serum trough concentration above the MIC** of the organism. Rate and extent of killing are maximized at four to five times the MIC. Vancomycin is approximately 55% protein bound; therefore, a total serum trough concentration of 8 to 9 µg/mL should be the target to provide the needed free concentration. **There is no documented correlation between serum peak concentrations and clinical outcomes.**

3. **Ototoxicity** rates range from 0% to 9%, and these numbers have not changed from initial studies conducted in the 1960s through studies conducted in the 2000s. There is no correlation between serum concentration and ototoxicity. The rate of **nephrotoxicity** when vancomycin is not administered with other nephrotoxic agents is 5% to 10%. Neither elevated peak nor trough concentrations correlated to nephrotoxicity.

DAPTOMYCIN

4. Approved by the FDA in September 2003 for skin and skin structure infections, this drug is active against vancomycin-resistant *Enterococcus*, methicillin-resistant *S. aureus*, vancomycin-intermediate *S. aureus*, and vancomycin-resistant *S. aureus*. Per the package insert it is **contraindicated for lung infections. Creatine phosphokinase concentrations increased** 2 to 3 days before clinical manifestation of symptoms and comprised 100% of the MM isoenzyme.

QUINUPRISTIN/DALFOPRISTIN

5. This drug is active against vancomycin-resistant *E. faecium*, methicillin-resistant *S. aureus*, vancomycin-intermediate *S. aureus*, and vancomycin-resistant *S. aureus*. It has **no activity against *E. faecalis*. Myalgias (6% to 7%) and arthralgias (9% to 9.5%)** are the most severe adverse effects and are the reasons for discontinuation of the drug.

LINEZOLID

6. The oral absorption is over 90%, making it **bioequivalent** to the intravenous formulation. Linezolid is **bacteriostatic** against staphylococci and enterococci.

7. **Reversible myelosuppression** is the most significant adverse effect associated with linezolid therapy. Anemia, neutropenia, and thrombocytopenia have all been reported, and the incidence **increases with durations of therapy exceeding 14 days.**

8. Linezolid is a **reversible nonselective inhibitor of monoamine oxidase;** therefore, the potential for interaction with adrenergic and serotonergic agents exists. Case reports of serotonin syndrome secondary to an interaction between linezolid and selective serotonin reuptake inhibitors have been reported.

Nosocomial infections in ICUs are associated with increased morbidity, mortality, and costs.[1] The causes of nosocomial infections have also changed in recent years. A 25-year study of nosocomial bacteremia demonstrated a change from *Staphylococcus aureus* and gram-negative bacilli as the predominant pathogens during the 1970s and 1980s to coagulase-negative staphylococci and *Enterococcus* along with *S. aureus* and *Pseudomonas aeruginosa* as the top pathogens.[2] There can also be differences in the predominance of pathogens in different ICUs and different types of nosocomial infections.

Nosocomial bacteremias were caused most often by coagulase-negative staphylococci and then by enterococci, followed by *S. aureus* in the medical ICU versus *S. aureus* and enterococci in the coronary care unit.[3,4] Nosocomial pneumonias were predominantly caused by gram-negative bacilli in the medical ICU versus *S. aureus* in the CCU.[3,4] Along with the increase in the prevalence of gram-positive cocci in the ICUs, these organisms are becoming multi-drug resistant. This chapter addresses these organisms and resistance issues within each of the antimicrobials with activity against these pathogens.

VANCOMYCIN

Vancomycin was discovered in 1956 and marketed in 1958. Early preparations of the drug contained pyrogens and impurities that produced a brownish, muddy appearance that provided vancomycin's nickname "Mississippi mud." In addition, these pyrogens and impurities caused high fevers, hypotension, severe phlebitis, and possibly nephrotoxicity.[5] However, by the time the preparation of vancomycin had been purified, methicillin and other agents active against gram-positive cocci were available and, because of their lower side-effect profile, became the preferred agents. In the past 15 to 20 years there has been resurgence in the use of vancomycin owing to the increase in infections caused by resistant gram-positive cocci.

MECHANISM OF ACTION AND MECHANISMS OF RESISTANCE

Vancomycin inhibits the synthesis of the cell wall by binding to the D-alanyl-D-alanine terminus of cell wall precursor units.[6,7] Vancomycin is slowly bactericidal against dividing organisms except for *Enterococcus* and tolerant staphylococci, against which it is bacteriostatic.[8]

Five types of resistance for vancomycin have been isolated from enterococci (VanA, VanB, VanC, VanD, VanE). The VanA phenotype confers high-level resistance to both teicoplanin (MICs: 16 to 512 µg/mL) and vancomycin (MICs: 64 to >1,000 µg/mL). Vancomycin can induce the expression of the VanA gene and has been identified in both *Enterococcus faecium* and *E. faecalis*. The VanB phenotype has also been identified in both *E. faecium* and *E. faecalis* and confers low-level resistance primarily to vancomycin. This resistance is inducible by vancomycin but not by teicoplanin; therefore, most strains remain susceptible to teicoplanin. There is very little information currently available about VanD or VanE types of resistance. VanA, B, D, and E are all transferable to other organisms. In contrast, the VanC phenotypes are endogenous (constitutively produced) and are components of *E. gallinarum* and *E. casseliflavus/E. flavescens* and confer resistance to vancomycin alone. The VanB gene has been identified in a strain of *Streptococcus bovis*. This gene showed 96% homology with the prototype VanB gene from *E. faecalis* V583, indicating the likelihood of the gene transfer from enterococcus to this strain of *S. bovis*.[9]

Vancomycin-intermediate *S. aureus* (MIC: 8 to 16 µg/mL) was first reported in 1996 from Japan, and as of June 2002 eight cases have been confirmed in the United States.[10] In June 2002, the first case of vancomycin-resistant *S. aureus* (MIC > 32 µg/mL) was identified in Michigan, followed in September 2002 by the second case in Pennsylvania.[10,11] No mechanism of resistance has yet been identified from the strains of vancomycin-intermediate *S. aureus*, but the two strains of vancomycin-resistant *S. aureus* both possessed the VanA gene.

Tolerance is another mechanism by which bactericidal activity is decreased. Tolerance can be measured or assessed by two methods: MBC:MIC ratio and time-kill curves. By definition, a MBC:MIC ratio of 32 or greater or less than 99.9% kill after 24 hours incubation in time-kill studies equates to tolerance. Handwerger and Tomasz suggested a change to the time-kill method and define tolerance as less than 90% kill after 6 hours of incubation.[12] Tolerance to vancomycin has been identified in *S. aureus*, *S. pneumoniae*, and group C and group G streptococci.[13-15]

SPECTRUM OF ACTIVITY

Vancomycin is active primarily against aerobic gram-positive cocci. The MIC_{90} against methicillin-susceptible *S. aureus* (MSSA) is 1 µg/mL, and against methicillin-resistant *S. aureus* (MRSA) it is 1 to 2 µg/mL.[16-18] The incidence of vancomycin-intermediate or -resistant *S. aureus* currently is very low and less than 1%. The activity of vancomycin against enterococci varies greatly with the species. *E. faecium* is the most resistant species of enterococci to vancomycin, with the resistant rates ranging from 30% to 90% depending on the institution. Overall, for all enterococci the vancomycin-resistance rates are 20% to 25%.[19] Vancomycin monotherapy is bacteriostatic against susceptible enterococci. Most streptococci are susceptible to vancomycin, although it is considered an agent of last resort against these organisms. Vancomycin has been the drug of choice for MRSA infections for the past 20 years; however, it is inferior to nafcillin or oxacillin for the treatment of MSSA infections. Treatment failures, prolonged treatment, and higher mortality rates have been demonstrated when vancomycin was used to treat MSSA infections compared with nafcillin or oxacillin.[20,21]

Vancomycin is active against anaerobic gram-positive organisms such as *Peptostreptococcus* species, *Propionibacterium* species, *Eubacterium* species, *Bifidobacterium* species, and most *Clostridium* species, including *C. difficile*.[22]

PHARMACOKINETICS/ PHARMACODYNAMICS

Vancomycin is administered orally and intravenously. The drug is poorly absorbed after oral administration, and the majority of the drug is excreted unchanged in the feces. Inflammation of the gastrointestinal tract may result in increased absorption of vancomycin, and concentrations of 5 µg/mL have been measured from the serum of patients with *C. difficile* colitis.[23] Intramuscular injections are extremely painful and should not be used. Distribution of the drug is complete 1 hour after a 1- to 2-hour intravenous infusion. Vancomycin is approximately 55% bound to plasma proteins. The volume of distribution corrected for weight is 0.4 to 0.9 L/kg.[24-30] Vancomycin does not penetrate well into noninflamed meninges or into aqueous humor.[31] Distribution into inflamed meninges is variable, with reported ranges of 1% to 37% of serum concentrations[32,33] and a mean concentration of 15% of serum or approximately 2.5 µg/mL.[34] Penetration into ascitic, pericardial, and synovial fluids is greater than 75% serum concentrations, 50% into pleural fluid, and 30% to 50% into bile.[28] Elimination is 80%

to 90% unchanged drug in the urine via glomerular filtration and the remaining via nonrenal elimination. The nonrenal elimination rate in healthy individuals is 40 mL/min, and in chronic renal failure patients it is 6 mL/min.[35] The half-life of the drug increases with decreased renal function; in patients with creatinine clearances greater than 80 mL/min the half-life is 4 to 6 hours. In patients with creatinine clearances less than 10 mL/min the half-life ranges 2 to 7 days, and in anuric patients it may be prolonged to 9 days.[24]

The pharmacodynamic effect of vancomycin is time-dependent killing or time above the MIC.[36] Therefore, the most important goal of therapy is to maintain a free serum trough concentration above the MIC of the organism. The vancomycin MIC of fully susceptible MRSA is 2 to 4 μg/mL; therefore, the free trough concentration should be at least 4 μg/mL. Vancomycin is approximately 55% protein bound; therefore, a total serum trough concentration of 8 to 9 μg/mL should be the target to provide the needed free concentration. With vancomycin-intermediate staphylococci MICs are 8 to 16 μg/mL, which would require total serum trough concentrations of 18 to 36 μg/mL to achieve a free concentration above these high MICs. If vancomycin were required to treat these vancomycin-intermediate pathogens, then continuous infusion would be the only reliable method to obtain concentrations above the MIC. There is no documented correlation between serum peak concentrations and clinical outcomes.

DOSAGE REGIMENS

Oral Administration

Oral administration of vancomycin is only for treating *C. difficile* colitis and is considered a second-line therapy. The dose is 125 mg orally every 6 hours and is not adjusted for renal dysfunction owing to the poor absorption. Two oral formulations (capsules or liquid) can be used, or the intravenous solution can be administered orally to treat *C. difficile*.

Average Adult

In nonobese adults with normal renal function, the usual dose is 1 g (~15 mg/kg) every 12 hours. This dose results in peak serum concentrations of 25 to 40 μg/mL 1 hour after completion of the infusion and trough serum concentration of 5 to 15 μg/mL. Dosing should be based on actual body weight. Several dosing guidelines have been developed to accurately and easily dose vancomycin. The most popular methods include the Moellering[26] and Matzke[27] nomograms. These methods use body weight and creatinine clearance to calculate a vancomycin dose. The weaknesses of these nomograms include the small number of patients used to develop and evaluate the nomogram and the fixed volume of distribution assumed for all patients (0.9 L/kg).[37,38] Matzke[27] found that for patients younger than 65 years old a volume of distribution of 0.7 L/kg may be more accurate and for those older than age 65 years it is 0.9 L/kg. Garaud evaluated critically ill patients and found an average volume of distribution of 0.6 L/kg in patients with creatinine clearances greater than 70 mL/min and 0.4 L/kg with creatinine clearances of 10 to 60 mL/min.[29] This variance in volume of distribution does affect the reproducibility of these nomograms when applied to different patient populations. The Cockcroft and Gault and modified Cockcroft and Gault methods of estimating creatinine clearance are reliable and accurate methods in patients of normal body mass.[39]

Morbidly Obese

Morbidly obese patients should receive approximately 30 mg/kg/day based on actual body weight; this should provide a peak serum concentration of 25 to 35 μg/mL. Because creatinine clearance is the best correlate to vancomycin clearance the most accurate method for estimating creatinine clearance should be used and varies with body mass. Creatinine clearance estimations in the obese patient are best predicted by the Salazar-Corcoran method.[40] Obese patients often require the dosing interval to be more frequent to achieve a trough serum concentration of 5 to 15 μg/mL. This is due to the faster rate of clearance of the drug (2.3 to 2.5 times higher) in obese compared with nonobese patients.[41,42]

Critically Ill Patients

Critically ill patients are often receiving medications to improve hemodynamics; these include dopamine, dobutamine, and furosemide. These medications result in increases in renal function and changes in volume status for the patient. In a study designed to assess the impact of these medications on vancomycin pharmacokinetics two observations were made.[43] First, some of the patients required larger total daily doses of vancomycin to achieve therapeutic concentrations than the Moellering nomogram predicted (26.78 + 3.01 mg/kg/day versus 18.95 + 3.41 mg/kg/day). Second, on discontinuation of these medications the serum trough concentrations increased despite no change in creatinine clearance or body weight. The theory is that these medications enhanced vancomycin clearance by improving renal blood flow and/or interacting with the renal anion transport system, thus increasing glomerular filtration and renal tubular secretion. Therefore, larger doses of vancomycin may be required while on these medications and smaller doses may be more appropriate on discontinuation of these medications.

Dialysis/Hemofiltration/Cardiopulmonary Bypass

The dialytic clearance of vancomycin by conventional membranes ranges from 0 to 15 mL/min.[44-47] The minimal clearance is due to the high molecular weight of the drug and the membrane's limited permeability.[47] The percentage of vancomycin removed by these low-permeability cellulose hemodialyzers is 4% to 6.9%.[44-46] Therefore, no supplemental vancomycin dosing is required after hemodialysis. The removal of vancomycin during intradialytic administration has been studied using three types of cellulose membranes: cellulose acetate (CA), cellulose triacetate (CT), and CA high performance-210 (CAHP-210). With the CA membranes 0% to 25% (mean of ~13%) of vancomycin is removed.[44,47] The CT membranes remove 16% to 44% (mean of ~26%) of vancomycin.[44,47] Vancomycin removal during intradialytic administration with the CAHP-210 membranes is 0% to 35% with a mean of 24%.[48] High-flux synthetic membranes such as polysulfone or polyacrylonitrile remove significantly more vancomycin than do the cellulose membranes. Each removes 30% to 55% and 25% to 40% of vancomycin, respectively.[44-46,49-51]

Continuous renal replacement therapy (CRRT) is a low-volume (1 to 2 L/h) therapy. The most frequently used methods of CRRT are continuous venovenous hemofiltration (CVVH), continuous venovenous hemodialysis (CVVHD), and continuous arteriovenous hemodialysis (CAVHD). Both CVVHD and CAVHD result in a greater total body clearance of vancomycin than do hemofiltration methods. The clearances achieved with each of these methods vary with blood flow rate, ultrafiltration rate, and membranes. The total clearance of vancomycin with CVVHD or CAVHD is 31 to 39 mL/min, and the half-life ranges from 14 to 25 hours.[35,52-55] Clearance of vancomycin in patients with normal renal function (CrCl > 70 mL/min) and with mild renal dysfunction (CrCl 40 to 70 mL/min) has been reported to be 88 and 48 mL/min, respectively.[56] High-volume hemofiltration (HVHF) with an ultrafiltration rate of 6 L/h increases vancomycin clearance to approximately 60 mL/min.[57] Therefore, patients receiving CAVHD or CVVHD should receive vancomycin every 36 to 48 hours and those undergoing HVHF should receive the drug every 12 to 24 hours.

Cardiopulmonary bypass (CPB) significantly impacts the pharmacokinetic parameters of vancomycin. Immediately after initiating CPB vancomycin serum concentration decreased by 7 μg/mL (5.7 to 8.4 μg/mL), which represented approximately a 38% decrease in concentration.[58] Over the next 30 minutes serum vancomycin concentration may increase 1 to 2 μg/mL but thereafter gradually and steadily decreases.[58] The half-life is not affected by CPB and does not change during the process.

Table 142-1 lists dosing regimens for the antimicrobials discussed in this chapter.

ADVERSE EFFECTS

Common toxicities that have been associated with vancomycin therapy include red man syndrome, thrombophlebitis, ototoxicity, and nephrotoxicity. Evidence establishing a clear relationship between these toxicities and vancomycin peak or trough concentrations or the incidence of these events is limited and contradictory.[5,38,59,60]

Red man syndrome comprises erythema, pruritus, and flushing of the upper torso and is often associated with too rapid an infusion of the drug. In general, the infusion rate should not exceed 1g/h. Less frequently, hypotension and angioedema can occur. It is believed that increased histamine release is the cause of this syndrome. The incidence of red man syndrome in healthy volunteers is significantly higher than is observed in patients (80% to 90% vs. 0% to 47%, respectively).[5,59-61] The higher rate of red man syndrome observed in healthy volunteers is thought to be attributed to differences in doses, rate of infusion, concomitant drugs, closeness of monitoring, and depletion of histamine stores by infection or trauma in patients.[62] A recent study in cancer patients demonstrated a 1% incidence of red man syndrome.[5] A comparative trial of once-daily versus twice-daily vancomycin found the incidence of this syndrome to be 13.7% and 9.6%, respectively.[59]

TABLE 142–1. DOSAGES FOR AGENTS WITH PRIMARY ACTIVITY AGAINST GRAM-POSITIVE BACTERIA

Drug	Dosage	Adverse Effects	Considerations
Vancomycin	Oral and intravenous administration Dose based on actual body weight (ABW) p.o.: 125 mg q 6h i.v.: 1 g (~15 mg/kg) q 12h for average-weight adult i.v.: For morbidly obese adult dose on ABW ~15 mg/kg/dose	Red man syndrome: Erythema, pruritus, flushing of upper torso Thrombophlebitis Ototoxicity: rare Nephrotoxicity: rare Maculopapular or erythematous rashes	Intramuscular injections painful Poorly absorbed orally Half-life of drug increases with decreased renal function Moellering and Matzke methods for dosing guidelines For obese patients and patients on dialysis, consider drug clearance
Teicoplanin	Intravenous administration Moderate infections: 400 mg (6 mg/kg) once followed by maintenance dose 200 mg (3 mg/kg) q 24h Severe infections: 400 to 800 mg (6 to 12 mg/kg) q 12h for two to three doses followed by 400 to 800 mg q 24h	Nephrotoxicity: rare Ototoxicity: rare Hypersensitivity	Special dosage considerations for patients with renal failure, patients on dialysis Compassionate use only in the United States (not FDA approved)
Daptomycin	i.v.: 4 mg/kg q 24h for average weight adult	Transient muscle weakness Myalgia	Contraindicated in pneumonia
Quinupristin/dalfopristin	i.v.: 7.5 mg/kg q 8-12h infused over 1 h	Arthralgia Myalgia Infusion-related Nausea, vomiting, diarrhea, rash	
Linezolid	Bioequivalence between oral and intravenous formulations Moderate infections: 600 mg twice daily Uncomplicated infections: 400 mg twice daily	Reversible myelosuppression Anemia Neutropenia Thrombocytopenia Diarrhea Headache Nausea and vomiting	

The effects of red man syndrome can be relieved by antihistamines.[63,64]

Thrombophlebitis is reported in 3% to 23% of patients and is more common in patients who receive vancomycin for more than 7 days or had peripheral catheter lines for prolonged durations.[5,59]

Ototoxicity rates range between 0% to 9%, and these numbers have not changed from initial studies conducted in the 1960s through studies conducted in the 2000s.[5,59,65-67] The definition of ototoxicity ranges from tinnitus to hearing loss. Ototoxicity is often believed to be associated with high peak serum concentrations of greater than 80 μg/mL. In one study in cancer patients only 4 of 19 patients with ototoxicity had elevated serum concentrations and only 1 had a concentration greater than 80 μg/mL.[5] Others have reported ototoxicity associated with peak serum concentrations of 37.5 to 152 μg/mL.[68,69] A trial comparing once-daily to twice-daily dosing of vancomycin demonstrated higher ototoxicity in the twice-daily dosed group (15.6% vs. 3.2%), which had a significantly lower peak concentration and similar trough concentration to the group receiving daily doses.[59] This lack of correlation between serum concentration and ototoxicity suggests that the observed toxicity was due to either another drug or to the combination of another drug with vancomycin. In the majority of cases the ototoxicity symptoms disappeared within a month of discontinuing vancomycin.

Nephrotoxicity associated with vancomycin is even more controversial than ototoxicity, and there are several confounding issues. The original formulation was very impure, and the impurities were associated with many toxicities, including nephrotoxicity. In addition, many definitions of nephrotoxicity have been used over the years, different patient populations studied, and different doses used, making it difficult to compare one study to another. In general, the rate of nephrotoxicity when vancomycin is not administered with other nephrotoxic agents is 5% to 10%.[59,70,71] Elting and colleagues identified older age, Acute Physiology and Chronic Health Evaluation (APACHE) III score greater than 40, and duration of therapy of greater than 14 days to be the best predictors for a patient to develop nephrotoxicity due solely to vancomycin therapy.[5] Neither elevated peak nor trough concentrations correlated to nephrotoxicity by multivariant analysis, but elevated trough concentrations did correlate by univariant analysis in this study. A number of other studies have found a relationship between vancomycin serum trough concentrations greater than 10 μg/mL and nephrotoxicity, but the percentage of patients developing nephrotoxicity is less than 50%.[70-72] As a result of the unreliability of vancomycin concentrations predicting toxicity, several authors and clinicians have suggested that routine monitoring of concentrations should be discontinued.[73-75] Studies have demonstrated higher rates of nephrotoxicity when vancomycin is used in combination with an aminoglycoside compared with either agent alone.[71,73,76] Goetz performed a meta-analysis of eight studies and found the incidence of nephrotoxicity associated with combination therapy was 13% greater than with vancomycin alone and 4% greater than with an aminoglycoside alone.[76] There are also studies that have not demonstrated an increase in toxicity with the combination of vancomycin and an aminoglycoside.[72,77,78] This lack of reproducibility further supports the theory that there is some other cause for the toxicity other than vancomycin.

Other toxicities associated with vancomycin include maculopapular or erythematous rashes (2% to 8%)[28,70,77] and anecdotal reports of neutropenia and thrombocytopenia.[79,80]

THERAPEUTIC DRUG MONITORING

Routine monitoring of vancomycin serum concentrations has become a highly debated issue over the past 10 years. Those who advocate routine monitoring cite the need to ensure therapeutic concentrations as well as minimize toxicities. To date there is only one trial that compared efficacy and toxicity with high dose once-daily versus twice-daily dosing of vancomycin in which peak serum concentrations were vastly different and trough serum concentrations were similar.[59] The mean peak serum concentrations in the once-daily and twice-daily dosed groups were 42.8 + 16.1 and 27.0 + 9.2 μg/mL, respectively. There were no differences in clinical efficacy, red man syndrome, thrombophlebitis, ototoxicity, and nephrotoxicity between the two groups. Studies over the past 20 years have proven that peak concentrations of vancomycin are not associated with toxicities. In addition, because vancomycin is a time-dependent killing agent and maximal killing is achieved at four to five times the MIC, peak concentrations are not associated with efficacy. Therefore, monitoring peak serum concentrations only adds to hospital and health care system costs and provides no beneficial clinical information. Some studies have demonstrated a correlation to serum trough concentrations greater than 10 μg/mL, whereas others have not. Given the lack of consensus it may be prudent to measure serum trough concentrations until studies that are more definitive are conducted to address this issue. In patients with end-stage renal disease the fluorescence polarization immunoassay (FPIA) overestimates vancomycin concentrations.[81] FPIA is the most common method for determining vancomycin concentrations, and when it was compared with the enzyme multiplied immunoassay technique it was found to produce higher peak serum concentrations by 7 to 11 μg/mL and higher trough concentrations by 4 to 6 μg/mL.

TEICOPLANIN

Teicoplanin is a glycopeptide antibiotic and is not approved for use in the United States. It is available for use in Europe, some Asian countries, Mexico, New Zealand, and Australia. It has a more favorable adverse effect profile than vancomycin; however, there is concern over teicoplanin's clinical efficacy in the treatment of severe gram-positive infections.

MECHANISM OF ACTION AND MECHANISMS OF RESISTANCE

Teicoplanin like other glycopeptide antibiotics inhibits the synthesis of the cell wall by binding to the D-alanyl-D-alanine terminus of cell wall precursor units.[82] Resistance has been reported in both staphylococci and enterococci. The VanA phenotype confers high-level resistance to both teicoplanin (MIC: 16 to 512 μg/mL) and vancomycin (MIC: 64 to greater than 1,000 μg/mL). The VanB phenotype has also been identified in both E. faecium and E. faecalis and usually confers low-level resistance to vancomycin but not to teicoplanin. There is a case report of a patient with E. faecium bacteremia developing resistance to teicoplanin, and the gene identified was the VanB gene.[83] This development may limit the utility of teicoplanin for some vancomycin-resistant enterococcal infections. Several reports of S. aureus resistance developing during therapy have been reported.[84-86]

The mechanism of the resistance was determined in one patient to be constitutive and non–plasmid mediated.[84]

SPECTRUM OF ACTIVITY

Teicoplanin is only active against gram-positive organisms. Activity against MSSA and MRSA is comparable to that of vancomycin. Coagulase-negative staphylococci have a varied pattern of susceptibility to teicoplanin. *S. haemolyticus* is the most resistant species to teicoplanin (30%).[87] These isolates are 25% more resistant to teicoplanin than to vancomycin. Against methicillin-resistant coagulase-negative staphylococci 39% of isolates have teicoplanin MICs greater than 8 µg/mL compared with 1% with vancomycin.[87,88] Teicoplanin is similar in activity to vancomycin against enterococci, although its reliability in treating infections with VanB resistance to vancomycin may be limited. Teicoplanin is active against other aerobic and anaerobic gram-positive organisms such as *Corynebacterium* species, *Clostridium* species, including *C. difficile* and *C. perfringens*, *Peptostreptococcus* species, and *Propionibacterium acnes*.

PHARMACOKINETICS/ PHARMACODYNAMICS

Teicoplanin is administered orally and intravenously. The drug is poorly absorbed after oral administration, and approximately 40% of the drug is excreted unchanged in the feces. The pharmacokinetic model that best describes the elimination of teicoplanin is the triexponential model. Intravenous and intramuscular administration of 6 mg/kg resulted in mean peak serum concentrations of 43 and 12 µg/mL attained at 0.5 and 4 hours after administration, respectively.[89] Despite the differences in peak concentrations the area under the concentration time curve for the intravenous and intramuscular administrations were similar; therefore, they are considered equivalent. Doses of 15, 20, and 25 mg/kg provide mean peak serum concentrations of 194, 197, and 253 µg/mL and trough concentrations (24 h) of 10.5, 13.6, and 19.8 µg/mL.[90] The volume of distribution is large at 0.8 to 1.6 L/kg, and teicoplanin is 90% protein bound.[89-91] Penetration into body fluids and tissues has not been extensively studied. Penetration into noninflamed meninges and fat is poor, but distribution into myocardium and pericardium is good.[92,93] Teicoplanin is primarily eliminated via glomerular filtration, and only 3% is metabolized.[94,95] The half-life is 155 to 168 hours in patients with normal renal function.[89] Because of the long half-life, it takes 14 days to reach steady state.[96,97] In patients with creatinine clearances of 13 to 25 the half-life was found to be 280 to 667 hours.[98,99]

DOSAGE REGIMENS/THERAPEUTIC DRUG MONITORING

AVERAGE ADULT

Despite the long half-life in patients with normal renal function teicoplanin should be administered daily and the dose is dependent on the severity of infection. For less serious infections involving the urinary tract, skin, soft tissue, and lower respiratory tract a loading dose of 400 mg (6 mg/kg) × 1 is administered followed by a maintenance dose of 200 mg (3 mg/kg) every 24 hours. For severe infections such as septicemia, endocarditis, and osteomyelitis 400 to 800 mg (6 to 12 mg/kg) is administered every 12 hours for two to three doses followed by 400 to 800 mg every 24 hours.[100-103] Although no therapeutic range has been established for teicoplanin, trough concentrations should be at least 10 µg/mL.[104]

Renal Failure/Dialysis

Teicoplanin is not removed by hemodialysis or continuous ambulatory peritoneal dialysis (CAPD).[105,106] The amount removed by CVVHD is dependent on the flow rate but is often minimal.[107] As renal function decreases, the clearance of teicoplanin decreases linearly with creatinine clearance.[98] Several dosing regimens exist for renal dysfunction, and the simplest method is administering the usual 6-mg/kg dose every 48 to 72 hours.

ADVERSE EFFECTS

Nephrotoxicity associated with teicoplanin is much lower than with vancomycin. The incidence from published and unpublished studies found the nephrotoxic rate to be 4%.[60] In addition, ototoxic rates with teicoplanin are similar to those with vancomycin.[60] Hypersensitivity reactions are the most common adverse reaction to teicoplanin (2% to 15%).[60]

DAPTOMYCIN

Daptomycin is a lipopeptide that was first discovered in the 1980s and was approved in September of 2003 by the U.S. Food and Drug Administration. In the 1980s it was also known as LY 146032. Currently, information concerning clinical efficacy is limited owing to the FDA review process.

MECHANISM OF ACTION AND MECHANISMS OF RESISTANCE

Daptomycin has a unique mechanism of action and has been found to inhibit lipoteichoic acid synthesis owing to binding to the membrane in the presence of calcium.[108-110] Minimal information is available on mechanism(s) of resistance to daptomycin. Limited in vitro studies have been performed attempting to create daptomycin resistance in the laboratory.[111] Mechanisms of resistance have not been elucidated, and the clinical relevance of in vitro resistance is unknown.

SPECTRUM OF ACTIVITY

Daptomycin's antibacterial activity is against most gram-positive bacteria, including vancomycin-resistant isolates and penicillin-resistant pneumococcus. The MICs of daptomycin are 8- to 16-fold lower in the presence of calcium. Therefore, all in-vitro testing must be supplemented with physiologic concentrations of calcium.[112] Breakpoints for susceptible and resistant interpretations have yet to be determined, but a tentative value of 2 µg/mL or less has been used.[112] The MIC$_{90}$ against MSSA, MRSA, *S. epidermidis*, and *S. saprophyticus* are all 0.5 µg/mL or less.[112,113] Against *E. faecalis* and *E. faecium*, including vancomycin-resistant strains the MIC$_{90}$ is 2 µg/mL or less, and for *S. pneumoniae* it is 0.25 µg/mL or less.[112,113] Daptomycin also appears active against vancomycin-intermediate and -resistant strains of *S. aureus*.[114,115]

PHARMACOKINETICS/PHARMACODYNAMICS

Healthy volunteers who received 1 mg/kg of daptomycin achieved a mean serum concentration of 1.1 μg/mL and demonstrated a drug half-life of 7 hours.[116] Daptomycin demonstrated linear pharmacokinetics from 0.5 to 6 mg/kg. The drug is 90% to 95% protein bound and is primarily eliminated by the renal route. After an intravenous 4 mg/kg dose the peak serum concentrations were 53 to 55 μg/mL and the half-life ranged from 10 to 15 hours in patients with creatinine clearances of more than 80 and down to 30 mL/min.[117] In patients with creatinine clearances less than 30 mL/min, end-stage renal disease/hemodialysis, and CAPD the peak serum concentrations range 40 to 50 μg/mL and the half-life is 30 to 33 hours.[117]

Daptomycin is rapidly bactericidal and exhibits concentration-dependent killing against gram-positive organisms including enterococci.[118]

DOSAGE REGIMENS AND THERAPEUTIC MONITORING

Average Adult

Routine dosing of daptomycin is 4 mg/kg every 24 hours. Phase III studies have been completed for complicated skin and skin structure infections and complicated urinary tract infections.[119] Phase II studies of its effectiveness against bacteremia have been completed, and there are ongoing phase III trials for its effectiveness against vancomycin-resistant enterococcal infections and endocarditis/bacteremia.[119]

Renal Failure/Dialysis

Dosing recommendations are not yet available, but adjustments do not need to be made until the creatinine clearance is less than 30 mL/min.

ADVERSE EFFECTS

At high doses, healthy volunteers reported transient muscle weakness and myalgia. Creatine phosphokinase concentrations increased 2 to 3 days before clinical manifestation of symptoms and were composed 100% of the MM isoenzyme. Weakness and moderate to severe myalgia was reported in the wrists, hands, and forearms. There was no change in mobility nor in electromyography.[120]

QUINUPRISTIN/DALFOPRISTIN

MECHANISM OF ACTION AND MECHANISMS OF RESISTANCE

Quinupristin/dalfopristin is a streptogramin antibiotic and is a mix of two different streptogramin components from groups A and B. The individual components are bacteriostatic, but the combination is often bactericidal. Each component binds to different sites on the 50S subunit of the ribosome, inhibiting translation of mRNA at the elongation step.[121] The resulting complex of drug and ribosome inhibits protein synthesis.

Streptogramins share similar sites of action with macrolide and lincomycin antibiotics. As a result, mechanisms of resistance are also shared. The most common type of resistance to streptogramins involves the erythromycin resistance methylase

(*erm*) genes, termed MLS$_B$.[122] These genes decrease the binding of antibiotics such as streptogramins group B, erythromycin, and clindamycin by dimethylating a residue on the 23S ribosome. Group A streptogramins are not affected, and the combination often retains its synergistic activity.[122] Enzymatic modification of both components is another mechanism of resistance that results in resistance to the drug.[123,124] The third mechanism involves efflux pumps: one that pumps out both macrolides and streptogramins and one specific for streptogramins.[123,125,126]

SPECTRUM OF ACTIVITY

Quinupristin/dalfopristin is active against a wide variety of gram-positive organisms as well as many anaerobes and oral flora organisms. An MIC of 2 μg/mL or less indicates susceptibility. The MIC$_{90}$ of most MSSA, MRSA, and coagulase-negative staphylococci is 1 to 2 μg/mL.[17,18,113] Against vancomycin-intermediate and -resistant *S. aureus* the drug is active with MICs of 0.25 to 1 μg/mL.[115,127] Both vancomycin-susceptible and -resistant *E. faecium* are susceptible to quinupristin/dalfopristin (MIC$_{90}$: 1 to 4 μg/mL); however, *E. faecalis* is resistant to quinupristin/dalfopristin (MIC$_{90}$:4 to 32 μg/mL).[128,129] Against a variety of streptococcal organisms, including penicillin-resistant pneumococci, the MIC$_{90}$ ranges from 0.5 to 2 μg/mL. Quinupristin/dalfopristin is also active against a variety of other organisms, including *Chlamydia* species, *Mycoplasma pneumoniae*, *Legionella* species, *Peptostreptococcus* species, *Fusobacterium* species, *Prevotella* species, *Actinomyces* species, and *Clostridium* species.

PHARMACOKINETICS/PHARMACODYNAMICS

Quinupristin/dalfopristin infusions should be administered over 1 hour, and the drug is incompatible with saline. In healthy volunteers and in patients undergoing CAPD the mean peak serum concentration of quinupristin was 2.6 and 2.9 μg/mL, respectively; and for dalfopristin it was 7.1 and 8.5 μg/mL, respectively, following a single 7.5-mg/kg dose.[130] Quinupristin/dalfopristin is hepatically metabolized to several active metabolites, and both the parent components and the metabolites are primarily eliminated via the bile into the feces.[131] Urinary excretion of quinupristin/dalfopristin and metabolites is 15% to 19%. The mean half-life ranges from 1.2 to 1.5 hours. The drug is 90% protein bound.[132]

Quinupristin/dalfopristin is bactericidal against staphylococci and streptococci, but it is bacteriostatic against *E. faecium*. The pharmacodynamic parameters that best predict efficacy have not been well characterized.

DOSAGE REGIMENS AND THERAPEUTIC MONITORING

Average Adult

The normal dose is 7.5 mg/kg every 8 to 12 hours and infused over 1 hour. Dosage reduction is likely required in patients with severe liver dysfunction, although specific recommendations are not available.

Renal Failure/Dialysis

Neither hemodialysis nor CAPD removes any appreciable amount of quinupristin/dalfopristin.[130,133] Penetration into the peritoneal cavity is negligible in CAPD patients. No dosage adjustment is needed in patients with renal insufficiency or on dialysis.

ADVERSE EFFECTS

Myalgias (6% to 7%) and arthralgias (9% to 9.5%) are the most severe adverse effect and are often the reason for discontinuation of the drug.[134,135] Elevations in direct and conjugated bilirubin and γ-glutamyl transferase are common. Infusion-related adverse effects occur in 30% to 45% of patients with peripheral lines used for the infusion.[134] The reactions include pain, burning, inflammation, and thrombophlebitis. Other toxicities include nausea, diarrhea, vomiting, and rash.

LINEZOLID

MECHANISM OF ACTION AND MECHANISMS OF RESISTANCE

Linezolid is an oxazolidinone antibiotic, which is a new class of synthetic agents. Linezolid binds to the 50S ribosome and inhibits the binding of mRNA, thereby preventing protein synthesis.[136] The binding site overlaps with that of chloramphenicol and lincomycin, but cross-resistance is not observed.[137] Clinical isolates of *S. aureus*, *E. faecium*, and *E. faecalis* resistant to linezolid have been identified. The mechanism of resistance is alteration of the 23S rRNA.[137] There are three case reports of vancomycin-resistant *E. faecium* infections in which the organisms were resistant to linezolid without the patient having any prior exposure to linezolid.[138,139] This may become a limiting factor in the widespread use of linezolid over vancomycin for infections caused by pathogens susceptible to both agents.

SPECTRUM OF ACTIVITY

Linezolid's breakpoint for susceptibility is 4 μg/mL. It is active against both methicillin-susceptible and -resistant staphylococci. The MIC_{90} against *S. aureus* and coagulase-negative staphylococci is 2 to 4 μg/mL.[140-142] Against vancomycin-intermediate and -resistant *S. aureus* the drug is active with MICs of 1 to 2 μg/mL.[115,127] Linezolid is equally active against both vancomycin-susceptible and -resistant enterococci with an MIC_{90} of 2 μg/mL.[115,143] Against both penicillin-susceptible and -resistant *S. pneumoniae* the MIC_{90} is 1 μg/mL.[144] Linezolid is also active against a variety of other organisms, including *Pasteurella multocida*, *Peptostreptococcus* species, *Fusobacterium* species, and *Prevotella* species.

PHARMACOKINETICS/ PHARMACODYNAMICS

Linezolid is available in both oral and intravenous formulations. The oral absorption is over 90%, making it bioequivalent to the intravenous formulation. The peak serum concentration and half-life at steady state after 600 mg twice daily were 14 to 18 μg/mL and 5 to 6 hours.[145-147] Linezolid is approximately 30% protein bound and penetrates quickly into bone, fat, and muscle, achieving 50% to 60% of serum concentrations in bone and 90% to 95% in muscle.[148] Elimination of linezolid is 30% renal and 70% metabolized with essentially no linezolid eliminated through the feces as

unchanged drug.[147] Linezolid is not an inducer of the cytochrome P_{450} enzyme system.

Linezolid is bacteriostatic against staphylococci and enterococci and is bactericidal against streptococci. It appears that the pharmacodynamic parameter best modeling the killing activity is the area under the concentration time curve to MIC ratio (AUC/MIC).[149] The AUC/MIC ratio required to produce a bacteriostatic effect varied from 22 to 97 (mean 48) for pneumococci and 39 to 167 (mean 83) for staphylococci. A dosage regimen of 600 mg twice daily achieves these values for organisms with MICs as high as 4 μg/mL.

DOSAGE REGIMENS AND THERAPEUTIC MONITORING

Average Adult
The usual dose of linezolid is 600 mg twice daily, and for uncomplicated skin and skin structure infections the dose is 400 mg twice daily.

Renal Failure/Dialysis
Hemodialysis removes approximately 30% of linezolid during a 3- to 4-hour session. However, no dosage adjustment is needed in patients with renal dysfunction or end-stage renal disease.

Adverse Effects
Reversible myelosuppression is the most significant adverse effect associated with linezolid therapy. Anemia, neutropenia, and thrombocytopenia have all been reported, and the incidence increases with durations of therapy exceeding 14 days.[150,151] The decrease in hemoglobin when linezolid therapy is greater than 2 weeks is 18% compared with 13% for comparator agents and linezolid therapy less than 2 weeks' duration.[150] The thrombocytopenia rate is 8% with the longer duration of therapy compared with 5% to 6% in all durations of therapy compared with 3% with comparator agents. Rates of neutropenia also increase to about 10% with extended durations of therapy. Complete blood cell counts should be monitored weekly, especially in patients in whom the duration of therapy is likely to exceed 2 weeks.

Linezolid is a reversible nonselective inhibitor of monoamine oxidase; therefore, the potential for interaction with adrenergic and serotonergic agents exists. Several case reports of serotonin syndrome (fever, agitation, tremors, and mental status changes) secondary to an interaction between linezolid and selective serotonin reuptake inhibitors (SSRIs) have been identified.[152-154]

Other adverse reactions to linezolid include diarrhea (8%), headache (7%), nausea and vomiting (6% and 4%), dizziness, rash, fever, constipation (2%), and abnormal liver function tests (1%).

ANNOTATED REFERENCES

Gerson SL, Kaplan SL, Bruss JB, et al: Hematologic effects of linezolid: Summary of clinical experience. Antimicrob Agents Chemother 2002;46:2723-2726.
  The clinical trial data are reviewed and the timeline for development of reversible myelosuppression is presented.

Gonzalez C, Rubio M, Romero-Vivas J, et al: Bacteremic pneumonia due to *Staphylococcus aureus*: A comparison of disease caused by methicillin-resistant and methicillin-susceptible organisms. Clin Infect Dis 1999; 29:1171.
  This is a 6-year prospective study that evaluated outcomes with staphylococcal bacteremic pneumonia. Mortality was just over 50% for each group;

however, mortality was greatest in patients with MSSA infection treated with vancomycin as compared with those treated with a beta-lactam.

Rodman DP, McKnight JT, Rogers T, et al: The appropriateness of initial vancomycin dosing. J Fam Pract 1994;38:473.

Forty-eight patients were evaluated for appropriateness of initial dosing and only 19 achieved what were determined to be appropriate peak and trough concentrations. In evaluating only for appropriate trough concentrations, 21 patients (43%) had values either too low or too high. Use of a dosing nomogram may improve the appropriateness of dosing vancomycin.

Rubinstein E, Prokocimer P, Talbot GH: Safety and tolerability of quinupristin/dalfopristin: Administration guidelines. J Antimicrob Chemother 1999;44:37-46.

Review of the most frequent adverse effects related to quinupristin/dalfopristin as well as drug-drug compatibility data.

Tally FP, Zeckel M, Wasilewski MM, et al: Daptomycin: A novel agent for gram-positive infections. Exp Opin Invest Drugs 1999;8:1223-1238.

Summary of daptomycin's new and novel mechanism of action, spectrum of activity and resistance. There is also a discussion of the phase II and III clinical trials.

Chapter 143

METRONIDAZOLE AND OTHER ANTIBIOTICS FOR ANAEROBIC INFECTIONS

Elizabeth D. Hermsen • John C. Rotschafer

KEY POINTS

1. **Metronidazole, a nitroimidazole antimicrobial, requires intracellular reduction** for pharmacologic activity and provides activity against both dividing and nondividing bacterial cells. Metronidazole's activity extends to many obligate anaerobes but not to aerobic bacteria.

2. **Anaerobes are often involved in mixed infections,** which present unique situations for antimicrobial use. The interactions between the different bacteria and the various antibiotics can be difficult to distinguish and/or predict.

3. **Standard dosing of metronidazole** (500 to 1000 mg q 6 to 8h) was established before the emergence of pharmacodynamics. Metronidazole is concentration dependent with a significant postantibiotic effect. Data from pharmacodynamic studies suggest that metronidazole can be dosed in larger doses (e.g., ≤1500 mg) every 12 hours or once daily for an effect similar to the standard regimens.

4. **Susceptibility patterns of anaerobes** have been changing over the years, and susceptibility to metronidazole cannot be assumed. Although susceptibility testing of anaerobes is difficult, clinicians must realize the importance of performing and analyzing the susceptibility tests.

5. **Several beta-lactam antibiotics, fluoroquinolones, and clindamycin possess antianaerobic activity.** However, resistance is a concern with all of these classes. A few investigational agents have the potential for use in anaerobic infections, but clinical data are needed.

METRONIDAZOLE

Metronidazole [1-(2-hydroxyethyl)-2-methyl-5-nitroimidazole], a nitroimidazole antimicrobial, was introduced in 1960 and quickly became the treatment of choice for *Trichomonas vaginalis*.[1] Initially, metronidazole was regarded as an antiprotozoal agent, proving to be an effective treatment for such infections as trichomoniasis, amebiasis, and giardiasis. The antibacterial activity of metronidazole versus obligate anaerobes was not widely recognized until the 1970s.[2-5] Since then, metronidazole has been used extensively for anaerobic infections such as *Clostridium difficile*–associated diarrhea (CDAD) and those involving *Bacteroides* species.

Because metronidazole has been in use for more than 40 years, a plethora of information exists regarding basic knowledge about this antimicrobial, including the mechanism of action, spectrum of activity, pharmacokinetics, adverse drug effects, and clinical uses. A brief discussion of these items follows. However, this chapter focuses on those topics of recent interest for metronidazole, namely, pharmacodynamics and resistance.

MECHANISM OF ACTION

Metronidazole possesses bactericidal activity against obligate anaerobes, although the mechanism of action has not yet been thoroughly elucidated. Metronidazole is a prodrug, requiring intracellular nitro-reduction to become active; thus, metronidazole, in the unchanged form, is not pharmacologically active.[1] During the process of reduction, cytotoxic intermediates are formed, and these intermediates are thought to be responsible for killing the cells. The reduction process depends on ongoing energy metabolism but not on ongoing cell multiplication, which translates into activity against both dividing and nondividing cells.[1]

SPECTRUM OF ACTIVITY

Anaerobic bacteria of the *Bacteroides fragilis* group are known to be the most clinically important anaerobic pathogens owing to their multidrug-resistant nature and the frequency with which they are involved in infectious diseases, including polymicrobial infections such as intra-abdominal infections, obstetric-gynecologic infections, and diabetic foot infections.[6,7] Nosocomial diarrhea and/or pseudomembranous colitis associated with antibiotic use are frequently caused by *Clostridium difficile*, another clinically important anaerobe.[8] Metronidazole is highly effective versus both of these medically relevant anaerobes (Table 143-1).

Metronidazole possesses significant antimicrobial activity against several obligate anaerobes but is not considered to be active versus aerobic bacteria. However, some investigators have previously contended that metronidazole exhibits activity against *Escherichia coli* when present with

TABLE 143–1. METRONIDAZOLE MINIMAL INHIBITORY CONCENTRATION (MIC) AND PERCENT SUSCEPTIBILITY FOR VARIOUS ANAEROBES

Anaerobe (No. of Isolates Tested)	MIC_{90} (mg/L)	% Susceptible
Clostridium difficile (186)	2	100
Peptostreptococcus (49)	2	94
Bacteroides fragilis group* (401)	1	100
Prevotella species (65)	2	100
Fusobacterium species (22)	2	100
Porphyromonas species (19)	2	100

*Includes *B. fragilis, B, distasonis, B. thetaiotamicron, B. ovatus, B. vulgatus, B. uniformis.*
Adapted and modified from Drummond LJ, McCoubrey J, Smith DG, et al: Changes in sensitivity patterns to selected antibiotics in *Clostridium difficile* in geriatric in-patients over an 18-month period. J Med Microbiol 2003;52:259-263; and Aldridge KE, Ashcraft D, Cambre K, et al: Multicenter survey of the changing in vitro antimicrobial susceptibilities of clinical isolates of *Bacteroides fragilis* group, *Prevotella, Fusobacterium, Porphyromonas,* and *Peptostreptococcus* species. Antimicrob Agents Chemother 2001;45:1238-1243.

Bacteroides fragilis,[9,10] although this effect could not be confirmed in a more recent mixed infection study.[11] Additionally, in 1980, Chrystal and coworkers found increased effectiveness of metronidazole against *B. fragilis* in the presence of *E. coli,* possibly owing to the ability of the cytotoxic intermediates to be formed in *E. coli* and then diffuse into the medium to kill the *Bacteroides* species.[12] Clearly, mixed infections are multifaceted and the interactions between the various microorganisms and the different antibiotics are difficult to distinguish.

PHARMACOKINETICS

Given orally, metronidazole is almost completely absorbed, with a bioavailability of greater than 90%.[13] Metronidazole is a relatively small molecular entity (molecular weight = 171.16) with low protein binding (<20%) and is widely distributed throughout the body.[14] The steady-state volume of distribution in adults is 0.51 to 1.1 L/kg.[13] The elimination half-life of metronidazole is 6 to 12 hours.[14,15] Metronidazole undergoes metabolism in the liver to form five known metabolites, two of which are 1-(2-hydroxyethyl)-2-hydroxymethyl-5-nitroimidazole (the hydroxy metabolite) and 2-methyl-nitroimidazole-1-acetic acid (the acid metabolite). The hydroxy metabolite exhibits 30% to 65% of the anaerobic activity of the parent compound.[13]

ADVERSE REACTIONS

The most common side effects of metronidazole treatment (at standard doses) are gastrointestinal disturbances, including mild nausea, a bad/metallic taste in the mouth, or furring of the tongue.[14] More rare adverse reactions to metronidazole include vaginal and/or urethral burning, dark/discolored urine, and central nervous system symptoms such as headache, ataxia, vertigo, somnolence, and depression.[16] Metronidazole is recognized for causing a disulfiram-like reaction with the concurrent ingestion of alcohol.[16] A study conducted by Visapää and coworkers found no evidence of disulfiram-like properties of metronidazole when it was given concomitantly with ethanol,[17] and this reaction has also been disputed by others.[18]

CLINICAL USES OF METRONIDAZOLE FOR ANAEROBIC INFECTIONS

Metronidazole is the drug of choice for *C. difficile*–associated diarrhea (CDAD) owing to its excellent oral bioavailability, low potential for selecting for vancomycin-resistant *Enterococcus* (VRE), and low cost.[8,19] However, recent data suggest that *empirical* use of metronidazole for CDAD should not be recommended owing to unnecessary antibiotic exposure and selection pressure for those patients in whom *C. difficile* is not the causative agent.[20] Metronidazole has been used successfully to treat anaerobic bacteremia, endocarditis, meningitis, brain abscesses, and mixed aerobic-anaerobic infections, although the addition of an antibiotic effective against aerobic bacteria is necessary for the latter.[2,3,5,14,21,22]

PHARMACODYNAMICS

The standard dosing regimen for metronidazole (500 to 1000 mg q 6 to 8h) was determined long before pharmacodynamics emerged as a science. Metronidazole exhibits concentration-dependent bactericidal activity along with a significant postantibiotic effect (>3 h).[13,23-25] These factors, in combination with a long half-life and a favorable safety profile, provide a wide corridor to manipulate metronidazole dose and dosage interval. Much more convenient regimens of larger doses (e.g., ≤1500 mg) given every 12 hours or once daily are plausible owing to the pharmacokinetic and pharmacodynamic characteristics.[23,24]

An in vitro pharmacodynamic model was used to compare the activity of four different metronidazole regimens, including a once-daily regimen and a standard thrice-daily regimen, against *Bacteroides* species.[24] All four regimens produced bactericidal activity (≥99.9% reduction in bacterial load) by 12 hours. No differences were found in the rate or the extent of bacterial killing for the different regimens, leading to the conclusion that the once-daily regimen was equally as effective as the standard thrice-daily regimen.

Knowledge of pharmacodynamic parameters and utilization of such parameters to more appropriately dose patients is of utmost importance in this era of antimicrobial resistance. Although resistance of anaerobes to metronidazole has remained low,[26] resistance should always be a concern. An understanding and application of pharmacodynamics to metronidazole should provide a more convenient dosing strategy for patients and may help stave off bacterial resistance.

MICROBIOLOGIC TESTING

A standard practice of identifying anaerobes is by placing a disc containing 5 µg of metronidazole on a streaked agar plate.[27] The infection is considered to have anaerobes if a zone of inhibition is present and is considered negative for anaerobes if no zone is identified. Even if a few colonies are seen within a zone of inhibition, they are assumed to be facultative anaerobes.[27] This method raises concern because the assumption is that the obligate anaerobes are always susceptible to metronidazole, which is not always the case. Elsaghier and colleagues exemplify this point with a case of *B. fragilis* that was completely resistant to the 5-µg disc but had a minimum inhibitory concentration (MIC) of only 6 mg/L, well below the resistance breakpoint of 32 mg/L.[28] Susceptibility testing of anaerobes is usually either not performed or not used to make clinical decisions because of several limiting factors, including the slow growth of anaerobes, the convolution of the testing method, the questions surrounding the appropriate testing media, the involvement of multiple organisms in anaerobic infections, and the generally held belief that susceptibility patterns of anaerobes have not changed over the years and remain forseeable.[29] Studies have proven the value and importance of susceptibility testing, showing that appropriate initial therapy is critical to a positive patient[30] and that in vitro susceptibility results reliably predict the clinical outcome of patients.[29] Therefore, clinicians must realize that susceptibility testing of anaerobes is necessary and that the susceptibility patterns have been changing over the years.

RESISTANCE

Worldwide resistance of anaerobes to metronidazole is estimated to be less than 5%.[26,31] A recent multicenter study conducted in the United States found no evidence of metronidazole resistance (all MICs < 8 mg/L) among 2673 isolates of B. fragilis group species.[31] Similarly, Aldridge and associates conducted an analysis of 542 blood isolates of the B. fragilis group, and only metronidazole was active against all of the tested isolates.[7] However, 6% of Peptostreptococcus isolates were not susceptible to metronidazole in another study published by Aldridge and associates.[32]

Reysett and colleagues have reported that four genes (chromosomally borne nimB and plasmid-borne nimA, nimC, and nimD) of Bacteroides species are commonly associated with metronidazole resistance.[33-35] The suggested mechanism of resistance mediated by these genes is the conversion of the nitro group of metronidazole to an amino group, foregoing the formation of the toxic nitro-radicals.[33,34] Evidence of transfer has been found within different Bacteroides species and between Bacteroides and Prevotella.[35]

Diniz and associates exposed B. fragilis group species to 4 mg/L of metronidazole and found that exposure to low levels of metronidazole increased both the virulence and the viability of the isolates.[6] Another factor to consider is the supposed protective effect of Enterococcus faecalis on B. fragilis when exposed to metronidazole.[36,37] The investigators found that E. faecalis was able to negate the bactericidal effect of metronidazole on B. fragilis. However, a more recent study conducted by Pendland and colleagues could not confirm these findings.[11]

Using a resistance breakpoint of 32 mg/L or higher for metronidazole, Peláez and coworkers, when studying 415 C. difficile isolates, found that 6.3% of the isolates were resistant.[19] Another more recent study conducted by Drummond and colleagues evaluated the susceptibility patterns of 186 C. difficile isolates from a geriatric population.[8] Contrary to the findings of Peláez and associates, no resistance to metronidazole was documented.

OTHER AGENTS EFFECTIVE AGAINST OBLIGATE ANAEROBES

Several classes of antimicrobials, including some broad-spectrum penicillins, clindamycin, carbapenems, beta-lactam/beta-lactamase inhibitor combinations, certain cephalosporins, and certain quinolones, exhibit activity versus certain anaerobic bacteria.[38] Metronidazole, imipenem, and piperacillintazobactam have proven to be the most reliable agents, whereas clindamycin, piperacillin alone, and cephalosporins such as cefotetan and cefoxitin have exhibited significantly decreased susceptibility rates.[7,31,38] Fifteen to 25 percent of B. fragilis group species are resistant to these compounds in the United States as well as in other parts of the world.[38]

BETA-LACTAM ANTIBIOTICS

Some beta-lactam antibiotics, including some broad-spectrum penicillins (piperacillin, ticarcillin), beta-lactam/beta-lactamase inhibitors (piperacillin-tazobactam, ticarcillin-clavulanate, ampicillin-sulbactam), certain cephalosporins (e.g., cefoxitin, cefotetan), and carbapenems (imipenem, meropenem, ertapenem) possess activity versus various anaerobic bacteria.[7,31,38] Because beta-lactams are generally regarded as concentration-independent or time-dependent antibiotics, the antibiotic concentration must remain above the MIC for a certain amount of time. Although several investigators have demonstrated antibacterial activity of beta-lactams with the time above MIC being as little as 40% of the dosing interval,[39] the pharmacodynamic characteristics of beta-lactam antibiotics against anaerobic bacteria have not been well characterized. However, owing to the existing knowledge of beta-lactam pharmacodynamics, once-daily regimens are unlikely. Although, when comparing the beta-lactams, some agents do have more convenient regimens than others owing to differences in their pharmacokinetics (e.g., ertapenem, 1000 mg q 24h, versus cefoxitin, 1000 mg q 6 to 8h).

Several beta-lactam antibiotics have circumvented much of the resistance among anaerobes, maintaining relatively high susceptibility rates. Of concern, Drummond and colleagues found that none of 186 tested C. difficile isolates was susceptible to cefoxitin, and only 1.1% of the isolates were susceptible to ceftriaxone.[8] Aldridge and associates showed that the susceptibility of Prevotella species, Fusobacterium species, Porphyromonas species, and Peptostreptococcus was the highest and the most consistent for piperacillin-tazobactam, imipenem, and meropenem (Table 143-2).[32] Resistance of B. fragilis group isolates to beta-lactams can be caused by beta-lactamase production, alteration in penicillin-binding proteins, changes in outer membrane permeability, and efflux.[38] Aldridge and associates found the order of activity of cephalosporins-cephamycins against B. fragilis group species to be cefoxitin > ceftizoxime > cefotetan = cefotaxime = cefmetazole > ceftriaxone, whereas no isolates were susceptible to penicillin G.[7] Piperacillin and ticarcillin alone exhibited 77% and 63% susceptibility, respectively, whereas piperacillin-tazobactam and ticarcillin-clavulanate showed 99.3% and 96% susceptibility, respectively. Ampicillin-sulbactam, another beta-lactam/beta-lactamase inhibitor combination, exhibited 93% susceptibility. All three carbapenems—imipenem, meropenem, and ertapenem—had favorable activity, with imipenem being the most active (Table 143-3).[7]

CLINDAMYCIN

Clindamycin has been used in clinical practice for many years now, but the pharmacodynamic properties had not been established against anaerobic bacteria until fairly recently. Klepser and colleagues examined the activity of clindamycin versus B. fragilis in an in vitro model.[40] The investigators

TABLE 143–2. ANTIBACTERIAL ACTIVITY OF VARIOUS ANTIBIOTIC AGENTS AGAINST SEVERAL ANAEROBES

Anaerobe and Antimicrobial Agent (No. of Isolates Tested)	MIC$_{90}$ (mg/L)	% Susceptible
Prevotella Species (65)		
Penicillin G	16	17
Piperacillin-tazobactam	≤ 0.06	100
Ampicillin-sulbactam	4	100
Cefoxitin	4	100
Imipenem	0.06	100
Meropenem	0.12	100
Ciprofloxacin	16	35
Clindamycin	4	89.2
Fusobacterium Species (22)		
Penicillin G	0.5	91
Piperacillin-tazobactam	0.12	100
Ampicillin-sulbactam	0.25	100
Cefoxitin	0.5	100
Imipenem	0.03	100
Meropenem	0.12	100
Ciprofloxacin	2	96
Clindamycin	0.12	91
Porphyromonas Species (19)		
Penicillin G	4	79
Piperacillin-tazobactam	1	100
Ampicillin-sulbactam	1	100
Cefoxitin	4	95
Imipenem	0.06	100
Meropenem	0.25	100
Ciprofloxacin	4	90
Clindamycin	8	90
Peptostreptococcus (49)		
Penicillin G	0.5	94
Piperacillin-tazobactam	0.25	100
Ampicillin-sulbactam	0.5	96
Cefoxitin	2	100
Imipenem	0.06	100
Meropenem	0.25	100
Ciprofloxacin	8	86
Clindamycin	2	92

Adapted and modified from Aldridge KE, Ashcraft D, Cambre K, et al: Multicenter survey of the changing in vitro antimicrobial susceptibilities of clinical isolates of *Bacteroides fragilis* group, *Prevotella, Fusobacterium, Porphyromonas,* and *Peptostreptococcus* species. Antimicrob Agents Chemother 2001;45:1238-1243.

TABLE 143–3. ANTIBACTERIAL ACTIVITY OF VARIOUS ANTIBIOTIC AGENTS AGAINST *B. FRAGILIS* GROUP ISOLATES

Antibiotic Agent (No. of Isolates Tested)	MIC$_{90}$ (mg/L)	% Susceptible*
Penicillin G (160)	128	0
Piperacillin (384)	128	77
Ticarcillin (137)	128	63
Piperacillin-tazobactam (142)	8	99.3
Ticarcillin-clavulanate (191)	8	96
Ampicillin-sulbactam (382)	8	93
Cefotaxime (384)	64	62
Ceftriaxone (138)	128	49
Cefoxitin (515)	32	84
Cefotetan (473)	64	64
Cefmetazole (84)	64	61
Ceftizoxime (358)	64	78
Imipenem (378)	1	99.5
Meropenem (127)	0.5	98
Ertapenem (92)	2	94
Clindamycin (542)	16	78

* Isolates categorized according to NCCLS breakpoints. Nonsusceptible isolates include both intermediate and resistant isolates.
Adapted and modified from Alridge KE, Ashcraft D, O'Brien M, et al: Bacteremia due to *Bacteroides fragilis* group: Distribution of species, β-lactamase production, and antimicrobial susceptibility patterns. Antimicrob Agents Chemother 2003;47:148-153.

susceptibility to other agents.[7] All of the antimicrobial agents listed in Table 143-3 exhibited further decreased susceptibilities when tested against isolates with decreased clindamycin susceptibility. Metronidazole was the only agent tested that did not show decreased susceptibility when exposed to these isolates.

FLUOROQUINOLONES

Both the peak/MIC ratio and the area under the curve (AUC)/MIC ratio have been identified as being predictive of fluoroquinolone activity versus gram-negative and gram-positive infections.[23] More specifically, AUC/MIC ratios of 125 and of 30 to 60 have been demonstrated to be predictive for fluoroquinolone activity in gram-negative and gram-positive infections, respectively.[42-44] However, limited data exist regarding the pharmacodynamics of fluoroquinolones against anaerobic bacteria. Peterson and colleagues conducted a study to explore whether the AUC/MIC ratio was predictive of quinolone activity versus *B. fragilis*.[45] Interestingly, the investigators found that the quinolones demonstrated concentration-independent activity versus *B. fragilis*, with an AUC/MIC ratio greater than or equal to 44 being predictive of activity. Of note, increased activity was not demonstrated when the AUC/MIC ratio was increased up to 200, and a paradoxical effect was noted with AUC/MIC ratios between 200 and 400 (antibiotic activity decreased). Furthermore, the authors suggest that the potential for the selection of resistant isolates may increase with an AUC/MIC ratio that is less than 44.

Resistance of *B. fragilis* group species to fluoroquinolones has become a concern, exemplified by Oteo-Iglesias and associates, who showed an increase from 0% to 12% fluoroquinolone resistance among *B. fragilis* isolates in just 3 years.[46] Moreover, Snydman and coworkers demonstrated significantly increased fluoroquinolone resistance among *B. fragilis* group species over a 4-year period.[31] The average resistance

found that clindamycin exhibited concentration-independent activity, which would suggest alternate-dosing regimens. Standard dosing for clindamycin ranges from 600 mg every 6 to 8 hours to 900 mg every 8 hours to 1200 mg every 12 hours, but the findings of Klepser and colleagues imply that doses of 300 mg every 8 to 12 hours may be more appropriate. Klepser and colleagues confirmed the effectiveness of this dosing regimen (300 mg q 8 to 12h) against *B. fragilis* by obtaining serum inhibitory and bactericidal titers (SIT, SBT) from the sera of 12 healthy volunteers.[41] The advantages of using a lower total dose include less drug exposure and decreased likelihood of adverse events.

The main concern with clindamycin is resistance. Drummond and coworkers examined the susceptibility of 186 *C. difficile* isolates to clindamycin and found that 66.7% of the isolates were resistant and 24.7% were intermediate.[8] Approximately 22% of *B. fragilis* group species are resistant to clindamycin.[7,31] Interestingly, Alridge and associates showed that clindamycin-intermediate or clindamycin-resistant isolates are more likely to have decreased rate for 1997 to 2000 was 17.5% for trovafloxacin and 13.6% for clinafloxacin (both now withdrawn from the market). Epitomizing the clinical relevance of these data, Oh and associates found fluoroquinolone-resistant isolates of *B. fragilis* in 9 of 12 healthy volunteers after a 7-day exposure to clinafloxacin (200 mg p.o. bid).[47] Decreased susceptibility to fluoroquinolones (ciprofloxacin) among other anaerobic bacteria is evident from Table 143-2.

INVESTIGATIONAL AGENTS

On a positive note, several investigational agents have shown potential for the treatment of anaerobic infections. Credito and coworkers evaluated the activity of garenoxacin, a novel des-quinolone, against various anaerobes, and garenoxacin compared favorably to the other agents tested, which included levofloxacin, moxifloxacin, piperacillin-tazobactam, imipenem, and metronidazole.[48] Likewise, Ednie and colleagues found ranbezolid, a new oxazolidinone, to possess significant anaerobic activity.[49] Furthermore, GAR-936, an investigational glycylcycline, and CS-834, an oral cephalosporin, have also demonstrated potential for use in anaerobic infections.[50]

ANNOTATED REFERENCES

Aldridge KE, Ashcraft D, O'Brien M, et al: Bacteremia due to *Bacteroides fragilis* group: Distribution of species, beta-lactamase production, and antimicrobial susceptibility patterns. Antimicrob Agents Chemother 2003;47:148-153.
This paper presents susceptibility data on 542 blood isolates of B. fragilis group tested over a 12-year period. Metronidazole, beta-lactam/beta-lactamase combinations, and carbapenems were consistently the most active agents. These data show the importance of susceptibility testing of the B. fragilis group and serve as a guide in the choice of empirical antimicrobial therapy.

Bryskier A: Anti-anaerobic activity of antibacterial agents. Expert Opin Investig Drugs 2001;10:239-267,
A comprehensive review of antibacterial agents with activity against anaerobic organisms.

Lamp KC, Freeman CD, Klutman NE, et al: Pharmacokinetics and pharmacodynamics of the nitroimidazole antimicrobials. Clin Pharmacokinet 1999;36:353-373.
This review presents a comprehensive overview of the pharmacokinetics, pharmacodynamics, and use of metronidazole and nitroimidazole antimicrobials.

Pelaez T, Alcala L, Alonso R, et al: Reassessment of *Clostridium difficile* susceptibility to metronidazole and vancomycin. Antimicrob Agents Chemother 2002;46:1647-1650.
C. difficile is generally assumed to be sensitive to metronidazole and vancomycin. However, this manuscript shows that some isolates are either resistant (6.3% for metronidazole) or have intermediate resistance (3.1% to vancomycin) to these agents.

VIII

Chapter 144

PREVENTION AND CONTROL OF NOSOCOMIAL PNEUMONIA

Richard G. Wunderink

KEY POINTS

1. The influence of endotracheal intubation is so dominant that **ICU-acquired pneumonia is almost synonymous with ventilator-associated pneumonia**.

2. A distinction should be made between the prevention of all nosocomial pneumonia and the prevention of **life-threatening nosocomial pneumonia, usually late-onset ventilator-associated pneumonia**.

3. **The pathogenesis of nosocomial pneumonia can be broken down into three basic steps:** colonization of the oropharynx with pathogenic microorganisms, aspiration, and overwhelming of the lower respiratory tract's host defense mechanisms.

4. The most important factor in colonization of the oropharynx with pathogenic microorganisms is the **use of systemic antibiotics, especially broad-spectrum antibiotics**.

5. Data from several sources (including a randomized, controlled trial) suggest that **prevention of pneumonia due to small-volume aspiration at the time of intubation** can be achieved by a short course of prophylactic antibiotics in selected patients.

6. The risk of ventilator-associated pneumonia is time dependent, so **any maneuver that decreases the duration of mechanical ventilation will decrease pneumonia rates**.

7. **Avoiding the supine position as much as possible in ventilated patients** is a simple and effective preventive measure that should be practiced in all ICUs.

8. Several lines of evidence suggest that **minimizing the number of manipulations of the ventilator tubing** will decrease the incidence of ventilator-associated pneumonia.

9. **Causes of the relative immunocompromise** that allows bacteria to overwhelm local host defenses in the lung are heterogeneous and patient dependent, unlike the stereotypical steps of colonization and aspiration.

Preventing pneumonia in the critically ill is a daunting task, and even controlling the incidence is difficult. Pneumonia is the most common nosocomial infection in the ICU.[1] The frequency of ventilator-associated pneumonia (VAP) varies from 8% to 28%.[2] A large 1-day point prevalence study of pneumonia demonstrated that nearly 10% of ICU patients were being treated for pneumonia.[1] The incidence of pneumonia also varies considerably, depending on the definition.[3] The risk of VAP is greatest early in the course of mechanical ventilation, dropping from a daily hazard rate of 3.3% at day 5 to a 1.3% rate at day 15.[4] The incidence also varies significantly among different types of ICU patients.[5] Postoperative patients, especially those undergoing cardiothoracic and trauma-related surgery, appear to have the highest rates. Coronary care unit patients appear to have the lowest rates; medical, respiratory, and other surgical patients demonstrate intermediate rates.

The influence of endotracheal intubation is so dominant that ICU-acquired pneumonia is almost synonymous with VAP. Endotracheal intubation increases the rate of nosocomial pneumonia between 3- and 21-fold.[2] Research on hospital-acquired pneumonia has been dominated by VAP, and very little is known about pneumonia in nonintubated ICU patients. Because the effect of nosocomial pneumonia on morbidity and mortality in nonintubated patients is so minor compared with that of VAP, concentration of VAP is appropriate.

A distinction should be made between prevention of all nosocomial pneumonia and prevention of life-threatening nosocomial pneumonia. The latter is almost exclusively VAP. The crude mortality rate for VAP ranges from 24% to 76%, with an estimated attributable mortality of 20% to 30%.[2,6] Early-onset VAP (within 5 to 7 days of intubation) has a minimal effect on mortality, if any. The greatest crude and attributable mortality rates are associated with typical late-onset microorganisms such as *Pseudomonas aeruginosa*, *Acinetobacter* species, and methicillin-resistant *Staphylococcus aureus*. Unfortunately, the most effective and well-documented strategies to prevent pneumonia work predominantly or exclusively in early-onset VAP and therefore do not result in a significant improvement in mortality. Conversely, one of the most consistent findings regarding VAP (including early onset) is a prolonged duration of mechanical ventilation. Because duration of ICU stay is the principal determinant of cost of care, prevention measures may be cost-effective even if they do not result in improved mortality.

PATHOGENESIS

The key to effective prevention and control strategies is a clear understanding of the underlying pathogenesis of nosocomial pneumonia. The essence of nosocomial pneumonia pathogenesis can be broken down into three basic steps—colonization of the oropharynx with pathogenic microorganisms, aspiration, and overwhelming of the lower respiratory tract's host defense mechanisms. Effective prevention and control measures can be analyzed by their effect on one or more of these steps.

Despite the convenience of this simple analysis, to assume that the pathogenesis of all types of nosocomial pneumonia and VAP is the same would be naive and incorrect. An example is the role of gastric colonization preceding oropharyngeal colonization, the basis for attention to enteral feedings and stress ulcer prophylaxis in VAP prevention. Although it may be an important factor for pneumonia due to Enterobacteriaceae, gastric and enteric colonization has no role in the pathogenesis of S. aureus or P. aeruginosa pneumonia, the two most common causes of VAP. Therefore, prevention strategies should be individualized to the pathogens and mechanisms prevalent in a specific ICU.

COLONIZATION WITH PATHOGENIC MICROORGANISMS

The antecedent event to most nosocomial pneumonias is colonization of the oropharynx with pathogenic bacteria. The oropharynx is not sterile normally, but the character of the normal flora is remarkably constant. A variety of factors alter the normal flora, allowing more pathogenic microorganisms to appear and to increase in number.

Time of exposure to these selective forces is a critical issue. Early-onset pneumonia, even early-onset VAP, tends to be caused by less pathogenic microorganisms such as streptococci, Haemophilus influenzae, or methicillin-sensitive S. aureus. Most of these selective forces are introduced in the hospital environment itself, rather than specifically in the ICU. Therefore, patients who develop pneumonia during the first few days of ICU admission or on mechanical ventilation should be considered to have late-onset pneumonia if the ICU admission was preceded by a 3- to 5-day hospital stay. Many of the same factors also operate in skilled-care nursing home facilities, blurring the distinction between hospital- and community-acquired pneumonia.

The major concern was once colonization of the oropharynx by Gram-negative enteric bacilli, generally from the Enterobacteriaceae family. These microorganisms are part of the normal bowel flora, but a variety of factors allow for their increased concentration and the selection of antibiotic-resistant strains. Oropharyngeal colonization is achieved by one of two main routes. The first is reflux of bacteria into the stomach from the duodenum, with subsequent gastroesophageal reflux into the esophagus and oropharynx. Colonization and proliferation in the stomach become critical intermediate steps in this pathway. Therefore, many prevention strategies logically target the stomach. The other route is self-inoculation by the fecal-oral route, through contamination of equipment or the hands of health care providers or the patient.

Recently, however, the focus has shifted away from the Enterobacteriaceae. S. aureus is now the most common microorganism causing ICU-acquired pneumonia, with P. aeruginosa the next most common. In addition, Acinetobacter species have become a common cause of VAP in many institutions. Of critical importance is the fact that none of these three microorganisms has a typical colonization pattern like that just described. S. aureus is a normal colonizer of the skin and the nasopharynx. Antegrade colonization of the oropharynx from the nose, especially with the use of nasogastric tubes in many critically ill patients, can occur quite easily. Similarly, Acinetobacter is found on moist body surfaces and in the gingival crevices of patients with poor oral hygiene. P. aeruginosa is usually not part of normal bowel flora but is ubiquitous in the environment. One of the unique aspects of Pseudomonas VAP is the appearance of tracheal colonization before oropharyngeal colonization.[7] The clinical implication is that because colonization of the stomach is not an important intermediary step, prevention measures directed at the stomach are not likely to affect pneumonia caused by these microorganisms.

A variety of strategies to prevent pneumonia are directed principally at preventing oropharyngeal colonization with pathogenic microorganisms.

AVOIDANCE OF ANTIBIOTICS

Clearly, the most important factor that leads to increased colonization of the oropharynx with pathogenic microorganisms is the use of systemic antibiotics, especially broad-spectrum antibiotics.[8] Most antibiotics kill the usual oropharyngeal flora, giving pathogens a selection advantage. The broader the spectrum of the antibiotic, the greater the likelihood that normal flora will be affected. In addition, some pathogens are eliminated. For this reason, antibiotics function more as amplifying agents rather than as true causes of colonization. The pathogenic microorganisms must still reside in the area normally, such as nasopharyngeal carriage of S. aureus, or be transferred from other sites, including the environment.

Thus, pneumonia can still occur despite the avoidance of antibiotics. However, the causative microorganisms are more likely to be less virulent pathogens or even normal flora, such as α-hemolytic streptococci. These microorganisms are less likely to lead to life-threatening pneumonia. Diagnostic strategies for fever in the ICU that result in the use of fewer antibiotics have been associated with lower mortality.[9] Shorter courses and fewer antibiotics for documented infections in critically ill patients have also been associated with a decreased risk of superinfection.[10,11] Although avoiding antibiotics may have only a small effect on the risk of developing the first episode of pneumonia, limiting their usage has a major effect on secondary pneumonia and infection-related death in the ICU.

USE OF TOPICAL ANTIBACTERIAL AGENTS

In contrast to the use of systemic antibiotics, the use of topical antibiotics for the prevention of colonization may be beneficial. This strategy remains controversial, however, and is an area of active research. In general, strategies rely on controlling pathogenic microorganisms at specific sites, despite the effect on normal flora. Topical agents generally do not have the toxicity of systemic agents, and although the use of topical antibiotics can lead to multi-drug-resistant isolates, the risk may not be as great as with systemic antibiotics.

Selective Digestive Tract Decontamination

By far the most extensively studied and most aggressive form of topical antibiotic strategy to prevent colonization is selective digestive tract decontamination. Although the specific agents used in different studies vary, the major focus is on controlling oropharyngeal colonization by almost sterilizing the bowel. Therefore, the antibiotics used are directed primarily at Gram-negative bacilli (usually polymyxin B and an aminoglycoside) and *Candida* (usually amphotericin B). Most regimens include two components—topical antibiotics in the oropharynx, and nonabsorbable antibiotics via a gastric tube. Some also include an initial short course of systemic antibiotics.

Despite more than 40 randomized, controlled trials, the benefit of selective digestive tract decontamination remains unclear.[12] Even meta-analyses performed to sort out the disparate results have been inconclusive regarding the overall benefit. However, several patterns have emerged. Selective digestive tract decontamination fairly consistently decreases the incidence of VAP when systemic antibiotics are used for the first 48 to 72 hours.[12,13] The rationale for the use of systemic antibiotics is to treat incipient endogenous infections and to prevent infection until sterilization of the bowel occurs. However, this really represents treatment of an episode of small-volume aspiration (discussed later), and an equivalent benefit has been found with a short course of prophylactic antibiotics alone.[14]

The efficacy of selective digestive tract decontamination in preventing life-threatening late onset VAP is less clear. Most studies do not demonstrate lower mortality in the treated group, despite lower rates of VAP. Treatment is directed primarily against the Enterobacteriaceae and yeast in the gastrointestinal tract, but because these microorganisms do not cause the majority of cases of VAP in the ICU, its benefit in preventing VAP due to these microorganisms may be diluted by the many cases of pneumonia caused by organisms that are not specifically addressed by the regimen.

The major drawback of selective digestive tract decontamination and the major criticism of its use is the potential for promoting antibiotic resistance. This theoretical risk has not been clearly demonstrated, even in ICUs that have used the regimen for prolonged periods.[13] The major determining factor is probably not the selective decontamination but rather the concomitant use of systemic antibiotics. If selective digestive tract decontamination truly decreases the incidence of VAP (and possibly other nosocomial infections), the resultant decrease in systemic antibiotic use may cancel out the risk of selecting for resistant isolates.

Selective digestive tract decontamination is practiced in only a few ICUs, mainly in Europe. Because the major benefit appears to be in preventing VAP due to Enterobacteriaceae, this strategy is probably best reserved for patient populations at increased risk for VAP due to these microorganisms. Postsurgical, trauma, and solid organ transplant patients are in this category, and not surprisingly, it has been suggested that selective digestive tract decontamination is more beneficial in surgical patients than in medical ICU patients. In addition, it appears to be very effective as part of the management of epidemics of antibiotic-resistant clones.

Topical Oropharyngeal Agents

Recently, controlling colonization of the oropharynx alone has generated interest. In a randomized, controlled trial of open heart surgery patients, use of a chlorhexidine oral rinse

lowered the risk of VAP from 9.4% to 2.9%, with the major effect being on Gram-negative bacteria.[15] This primary finding was accompanied by decreases in all nosocomial infections, fewer nonprophylactic antibiotic prescriptions, and a trend toward lower mortality. Other nonantibiotic agents are also being explored. This approach has the advantage of not disrupting the normal bowel flora by addressing only the primary area of concern. In addition, some of the newer agents under study have activity against pathogens other than Enterobacteriaceae.

Aerosolized Antibiotics

The earliest studied form of topical colonization prevention was the use of aerosolized antibiotics. Polymyxin B, a nephrotoxic antibiotic when used intravenously, is very active against most Gram-negative bacilli. In the early era of mechanical ventilation, daily aerosolized polymyxin B was used to prevent Gram-negative VAP. Routine use resulted in a dramatic decrease in the rate of VAP.[16] Not surprisingly, however, routine use was soon complicated by the emergence of antibiotic-resistant microorganisms, in this case, *Proteus* species (which have native resistance to polymyxin B). This feature, combined with a lack of mortality benefit, led to abandonment of this strategy.

AVOIDANCE OF INCREASED GASTRIC pH

Because the normally acidic environment of the gastric lumen is extremely effective in preventing colonization with either swallowed oropharyngeal flora or refluxed enteric flora, several prevention strategies have focused on this aspect. Once again, because bowel flora play only a secondary role in VAP, the overall effect of these manipulations on reducing the risk of VAP is blunted.

Stress Ulcer Prophylaxis

One of the most hotly debated issues in VAP prevention is the role of stress ulcer prophylaxis.[12,17] At one time, gastrointestinal bleeding from stress ulceration was a substantial problem in ventilated patients and was thought to be a major cause of death. Prophylaxis against stress ulceration was thus considered critical, and it still is by many. However, the incidence of gastrointestinal bleeding from stress ulceration has decreased markedly, and the risks do not appear to be as great as they were in the past. This change in risk may be a result of better hemodynamic resuscitation, improved ventilatory strategies, earlier use of enteral nutrition, or a combination of factors. The debate regarding the optimal gastrointestinal bleeding prophylaxis has therefore evolved over the last few decades.

Fairly early in the debate, antacids were found to be inferior to histamine type 2 blockers (H_2 blockers). In addition to increasing gastric pH, antacids have the disadvantage of increasing gastric volume, which is probably an independent risk factor for VAP.

The major controversy revolved around sucralfate versus H_2 blockers. Sucralfate had the advantage of providing adequate stress ulcer prophylaxis without affecting gastric pH. In addition, sucralfate was thought to have intrinsic antibacterial properties. Early studies tended to favor sucralfate over H_2 blockers. However, larger and more recent studies found no significant benefit of sucralfate in reducing the risk of VAP but a slightly greater risk of clinically significant gastrointestinal bleeding.[3] In addition, a multivariate analysis suggested that sucralfate use was associated with an increased risk of death in patients with acute respiratory distress syndrome (ARDS).[18]

After multiple randomized trials and several meta-analyses that reached contrasting conclusions, the difference between sucralfate and H_2 blockers appears to be minimal, and either class of agents is acceptable for gastrointestinal bleeding prophylaxis. Although not studied as extensively, proton pump inhibitors also appear to be a valid choice. The choice of agent should be individualized, based on the competing risks of stress ulceration and predisposition to VAP.

The major issue remaining is whether stress ulcer prophylaxis is needed at all in some mechanically ventilated patients.[3] Recent studies that included a placebo population suggested that both H_2 blockers and sucralfate may lead to an increased risk of VAP compared with controls. A subgroup of patients at increased risk for gastrointestinal hemorrhage can be identified, and mechanically ventilated patients without these high risk factors may not need prophylaxis.[19]

Enteral Nutrition Strategies

Malnutrition is clearly associated with an increased risk of pneumonia. Part of that increased risk may relate to increased binding of Gram-negative bacilli, including *Pseudomonas*, to epithelial cells.[7] Enteral administration of nutrition is the preferred route. Abdominal trauma patients randomized to early jejunostomy feedings versus total parenteral nutrition had significantly lower infection rates, including pneumonia.

However, continuous enteral nutrition infusions may increase both gastric pH and gastric volume. Therefore, enteral nutrition may theoretically increase the risk of VAP. Several multivariate studies have suggested that this potential risk is real.[4,20,21] A randomized trial found that the risk of VAP was increased with early aggressive feedings compared with low-level enteral nutrition (approximately 20% of goal feeding rate).[22] The latter was chosen to avoid atrophy of the microvilli of the enteric mucosa, a potential source of nosocomial infection. The increased risk of VAP was attributed to an increased risk of aspiration. A balance between the potential risks would be early initiation of enteral feeding but avoidance of aggressive prescriptions that might cause high gastric residuals and gastric distention.

Several strategies have been tried to provide enteral feeding yet prevent increased gastric colonization with pathogenic microorganisms. Theoretically, bolus feedings would allow intermittent lowering of the gastric pH, potentially sterilizing the stomach between doses. However, one randomized, controlled trial found that bolus feedings did not decrease the risk of VAP, and fewer patients achieved their goal feeding rates.[23] Acidification of enteral feedings has also been studied. Once again, VAP rates were not significantly improved, but the acid was clearly absorbed, causing some adverse consequences from the resultant metabolic acidosis.[24]

CROSS-INFECTION

The role of cross-contamination in the ICU should never be underestimated. Cross-contamination can cause colonization with specific pathogenic bacteria in a patient who has no other risk factors for that microorganism. In particular, *P. aeruginosa* and methicillin-resistant *S. aureus* appear to have the greatest potential to cause cross-contamination and subsequent infection.

By far the most important factor in cross-infection is hand washing among caregivers.[17] Multiple studies have documented the poor infection control practices of medical personnel, including physicians and bedside nurses.[25] The risk of poor hand washing increases with the intensity of care needed for an individual patient and with the number of patients per nurse. The use of an alcohol-based, self-drying hand wash appears to be effective and to increase compliance with hand washing.[26]

Avoiding cross-contamination via medical equipment is also important. Contaminated equipment is still a major cause of epidemic outbreaks of nosocomial pneumonia. Any clustering of VAP, especially when caused by an unusual agent, should raise this possibility. Respiratory therapy equipment is particularly suspect, and adherence to standards for the sterilization of ventilators, bronchoscopes, and other reusable equipment should be rigorous.

Probably the best strategy is a continuous, multifaceted, multidisciplinary program of infection control.[27] An important component of this program is monitoring VAP rates and providing feedback to individual units on infection rates. Although such a program is costly to develop, the substantial cost benefit of avoiding pneumonia usually justifies the expense.

ASPIRATION

The role of aspiration in nosocomial pneumonia is probably the least controversial. Evidence from a variety of sources documents the importance of aspiration, although the definition of aspiration may vary.

LARGE-VOLUME ASPIRATION

Large-volume aspiration is clearly a risk factor in nonintubated ICU patients. Although the aspirated material itself may not be infectious, such as enteral feedings, aspiration of a large bolus clearly predisposes to pneumonia. Probably a greater risk of large-volume aspiration is the development of ARDS, which is associated with a markedly increased risk of VAP. The greatest risk factors for this type of aspiration are gastrointestinal, such as protracted vomiting from bowel obstruction or gastrointestinal bleeding, and neurologic, including seizures, induction of anesthesia, and alcohol intoxication.

Appropriate use of endotracheal intubation is actually a protective factor for this type of aspiration. Once large-volume aspiration has occurred, selective use of bronchoscopy to extract solid material that might occlude a bronchus and cause a postobstructive pneumonia is one of the few preventive measures of benefit. Empirical antibiotics, especially prolonged courses, do not clearly prevent pneumonia but do select for more virulent microorganisms.

A form of large-volume aspiration unique to ventilated patients is the inadvertent instillation of ventilator tubing condensate. The condensate in tubing closest to the endotracheal tube frequently contains high levels ($>10^5$ organisms/mL) of pathogenic microorganisms. If this condensate is accidentally spilled back into the patient's tracheobronchial tree, VAP is very likely. This factor may be one explanation for the increased risk of VAP associated with patient transport out of the ICU.

SMALL-VOLUME ASPIRATION

Aspiration of a smaller volume of secretions is also associated with an increased risk of pneumonia in both intubated and nonintubated patients. Neurologic disease with inability to protect the upper airway is consistently documented as a risk factor for pneumonia. In this situation, aspiration occurs before or in conjunction with endotracheal intubation. The bolus can be either oropharyngeal secretions or gastric secretions. In the former situation, a large inoculum of oropharyngeal flora can reach the lower respiratory tract, and clinical pneumonia usually occurs within 48 to 72 hours.

Prevention of pneumonia from small-volume aspiration is probably best achieved by prophylactic antibiotics. Several prospective observational studies have suggested that antibiotics early in the course of mechanical ventilation are associated with a lower incidence of pneumonia.[4,20] However, the best evidence is a prospective, randomized trial of short-course cephalosporin prophylaxis (two doses) in patients intubated for nontraumatic coma.[14] The incidence of VAP was only 23% in the prophylaxis group, compared with 66% in the control group that did not receive any antibiotic. This randomized, controlled trial has been corroborated by the results of many studies of selective decontamination of the digestive tract. In most of these studies, the incidence of pneumonia was less only if a short course of systemic antibiotics was included with the topical antibiotics.

Prophylactic antibiotics have clearly been demonstrated to be of benefit only in the initial intubation of patients not previously hospitalized for a significant period. The efficacy of the short course is dependent on the fact that the aspirated bolus contains mainly normal oral flora rather than a high concentration of more pathogenic bacteria. These conditions may apply to patient groups other than those with nontraumatic coma, such as respiratory failure from nonbronchitic exacerbations of chronic obstructive lung disease, but the benefit must still be determined.

This prevention strategy seems to contradict the importance of avoiding unnecessary antibiotics discussed earlier. One very real risk is that preventing early-onset pneumonia, which does not have an attributable mortality, may increase the risk of more lethal late-onset VAP. Two aspects of this strategy outweigh the downside of increased risk of colonization of the oropharynx with more pathogenic bacteria. First, the antibiotics given are two doses of a single agent, and the antibiotic pressure is relatively low. Second, the 40% lower risk of pneumonia in patients given prophylaxis avoids a longer course of antibiotics, often with a wider spectrum.

MICROASPIRATION

Microaspiration is by far the most important form of aspiration in endotracheally intubated patients. Oropharyngeal secretions pool above the cuff of the endotracheal tube in most intubated patients. Extremely small volumes of secretions can pass below the cuff during small movements of the endotracheal tube associated with head repositioning, coughing, and other activities. Because oropharyngeal secretions contain 10^6 to 10^{10} colony-forming units per milliliter of secretions, even 0.1 mL of secretions can present a significant challenge to the host defenses of the lower respiratory tract. In addition, the endotracheal tube itself may become colonized with viable bacteria encrusted in the glycocalyx and deposited on the polyvinyl chloride surface of the tube.

Subsequent suctioning or other manipulations of the endotracheal tube can reintroduce bacteria into the lower respiratory tract. Several preventive therapies are directed at stopping or limiting this type of aspiration.

Shorter Duration of Endotracheal Intubation

Epidemiologic studies have demonstrated that the risk of VAP is not linear. The greatest risk occurs early, with a 3%/day risk in the first week, 2%/day in the second week, and 1%/day subsequently.[4] In addition, early-onset VAP (within the first 5 to 7 days of mechanical ventilation) has the lowest attributable mortality.[2,6] Therefore, the sooner the patient is extubated, the lower the cumulative risk of pneumonia and the lower the risk of lethal nosocomial pneumonia.

Probably the best strategy is avoiding intubation completely. Several studies have demonstrated a significantly lower incidence of nosocomial pneumonia in patients successfully managed with noninvasive ventilation.[28,29] The greatest documented benefit is for patients with exacerbations of chronic airflow obstruction. However, patients who fail noninvasive ventilation appear to have an increased duration of subsequent endotracheal intubation and thus an increased risk of VAP. Careful selection of candidates for noninvasive ventilation and early abandonment of this treatment in unsuccessful cases are critical to decreasing the pneumonia risk.

Even when patients are intubated, variations in the duration of mechanical ventilation for the same type and severity of critical illness suggest that efforts to shorten this duration are a viable approach to preventing VAP. Several strategies have demonstrated a significant benefit, including daily interruption of sedation[30] and daily assessment of ability to wean.[31] Although most of these studies did not specifically address the issue of VAP incidence, the overall benefit might be attributable in part to lower VAP rates.

The downside of these strategies is the association between re-intubation and increased risk of VAP. Several studies have demonstrated that re-intubation increases the risk of VAP threefold.[32,33] The need for re-intubation re-exposes the patient to the risk of small-volume aspiration discussed earlier. In addition, colonization of the oropharyngeal secretions by more pathogenic bacteria is more likely because of the prior episode of intubation. Therefore, although avoiding or shortening the duration of mechanical ventilation is clearly a laudable goal, an increase in the risk of VAP may occur with an overly aggressive approach.

Early Tracheostomy

The issue of early tracheostomy is still unsettled. Tracheostomy has some potential benefits in the prevention of VAP. The glottis is not held open by the endotracheal tube, and the vocal cords can be opposed. This may decrease the risk of aspiration significantly, and routine tracheostomy may be one explanation for the leveling off of the incidence of VAP after several weeks of mechanical ventilation. Probably just as important is that the security of a tracheostomy may allow greater mobilization of the patient and a greater amount of time spent in the upright position. Early reports of an increased risk of pneumonia with tracheostomy were compromised by lack of adjustment for prior duration of mechanical ventilation, inaccurate diagnosis (with some tracheostomy site infections classified as pneumonia), and variable surgical techniques. It has been suggested that early tracheostomy performed with the percutaneous dilatational technique is beneficial, but more data are needed.

Semirecumbent Positioning

For a variety of reasons, ventilated patients tend to be cared for in the supine position. Elegant clinical experiments have demonstrated that the degree of gastroesophageal reflux is significantly greater in supine patients than in semirecumbent patients.[34] Not only was reflux greater, but bowel flora colonized the oropharynx and bronchial tree in 68% of patients ventilated in the supine position, compared with only 32% in the semirecumbent position.

A prospective, randomized trial clearly demonstrated the benefit of semirecumbent positioning. Drakulovic and colleagues demonstrated that both clinically suspected and microbiologically confirmed cases of VAP were more common in patients ventilated in the supine position (8% of clinically suspected VAPs versus 34% for semirecumbent).[21] Supine body position (odds ratio 6.8) and enteral nutrition (odds ratio 5.7) were both independent risk factors for VAP, with the highest frequency in patients receiving enteral nutrition in the supine position (14 of 28; 50%). This finding suggests that gastric distention, whether caused by feedings or increased gastric secretions, may have an amplifying effect in the supine position.

Avoiding the supine position as much as possible is a simple and effective preventive measure that should be practiced in all ICUs. However, constant attention to patient positioning is required for efficacy.

Avoidance of Ventilator Tubing Manipulation

Several lines of evidence suggest that minimizing the number of manipulations of the ventilator tubing can decrease the incidence of VAP, possibly by decreasing the incidence of small-volume or microaspiration. Condensation of exhaled gas in the expiratory limb of the tubing or from humidifiers in the inspiratory limb can become heavily colonized with bacteria. Instillation of this liquid bolus into the patient's airway during manipulation of the tubing or movement of the patient can present a significant bacterial challenge to the lower respiratory tract defenses.

The use of heat and moisture exchangers rather than heater-humidifiers would theoretically alleviate some of this risk. However, randomized clinical trials have been inconclusive, although a trend toward decreased rates of VAP has been found.[35] This benefit is partially offset by increased rates of endotracheal tube occlusion secondary to inspissated secretions with the use of heat and moisture exchangers. Because the rate of VAP is clearly not increased with heat and moisture exchangers, other considerations determine the frequency of their use, especially cost.

The most consistent evidence that ventilator tube manipulation may increase the risk of VAP is that increasing the interval between changes of the ventilator tubing decreases the incidence of VAP. A series of studies progressively increased the duration of time between changes and found equivalent or less VAP with longer intervals.[17,35] These studies are so convincing that most institutions do not change ventilator tubing unless gross contamination is present.

Transporting patients outside the ICU, usually for diagnostic procedures, has also been associated with an increased risk of VAP.[32] In a prospective study, 24% of patients requiring transport outside of the ICU developed VAP, compared with only 4% of patients who did not. Unfortunately, more than half of ventilated patients required transport at least once. The need for bagging, changing ventilators, moving the patient out of bed, and other aspects of the process all increase the possibility of inadvertent introduction of condensate from the ventilator tubing into the patient. In addition, unintentional extubation is greater when transferring ventilated patients.

Continuous Aspiration of Subglottic Secretions

An innovative strategy to prevent microaspiration is the use of a specially modified endotracheal tube that allows continuous aspiration of subglottic secretions. This tube has an extra lumen on the dorsal surface, just above the level of the inflatable cuff. Oropharyngeal secretions that have pooled above the cuff can be continuously aspirated before being introduced into the distal trachea. One prospective, randomized trial demonstrated a decreased incidence of VAP (13% versus 29% with conventional endotracheal tubes).[36] All the studies of continuous aspiration of subglottic secretions have demonstrated a decrease only in early-onset VAP, usually due to *H. influenzae* and streptococci. No decrease in VAP due to multidrug-resistant microorganisms and no mortality differences have been demonstrated. In addition, the benefit is obviated if the patient receives antibiotics early in the course of mechanical ventilation,[37] probably because of the benefit of prophylactic antibiotics in early-onset VAP.[14] Pneumonia can also occur if the system malfunctions, usually due to plugging of the lumen or low cuff pressures allowing secretions to drain into the distal trachea rather than collecting above the cuff. These factors and the high cost have limited the use of this modality.

Avoidance of Gastric Overdistention

Unfortunately, even when in the semirecumbent position, many patients still have gastroesophageal reflux and microaspiration when given enteral feedings. The major issue is overdistention of the stomach, and two strategies have been studied to address this problem. The first is use of nasoenteric tubes rather than nasogastric tubes. Although this strategy is attractive theoretically, a small randomized, controlled trial did not show a benefit of postpyloric feeding compared with nasogastric feeding.[38] The major limitation is the difficulty in placing feeding tubes in the small bowel. Nevertheless, the theoretical benefit probably warrants placement of jejunostomy tubes whenever possible in critically ill patients undergoing abdominal surgery for other reasons.

The second strategy is the use of gastric prokinetic agents, such as metoclopramide. An additional benefit is that these agents increase the tone of the lower esophageal sphincter, potentially decreasing the risk of reflux while increasing gastric emptying. Once again, a randomized, controlled trial failed to confirm the benefit of using this agent to decrease the risk of VAP.[39] However, these agents' ability to increase the tolerance of enteral nutrition warrants their continued use, despite no demonstrated effect on VAP.

The adverse effect on gastric volume may cancel out the beneficial effect of bolus nasogastric feedings on gastric pH, contributing to this strategy's lack of benefit. Increased gastric volume may be an additional risk factor for VAP with antacid prophylaxis for gastrointestinal bleeding.

OVERWHELMING LOWER RESPIRATORY HOST DEFENSES

An underappreciated fact about nosocomial pneumonia is that despite aspiration of oropharyngeal secretions documented to contain pathogenic bacteria, only a minority of patients actually develop pneumonia. In the classic study of Johanson and associates, only 23% of patients with Gram-negative colonization of the oropharynx subsequently developed pneumonia.[40] Others have shown that quantitative culture levels of microorganisms equivalent to those found in pneumonia can transiently appear in routine non-bronchoscopic bronchoalveolar lavage samples without the subsequent development of clinical VAP.[41] Thus, the two steps described earlier—colonization by pathogens and aspiration—are necessary but not sufficient causes of nosocomial pneumonia.

The third step in the pathogenesis of nosocomial pneumonia, the overwhelming of lower respiratory tract defenses, is the least studied or understood. One major reason may be that the causes are heterogeneous and patient dependent, rather than the stereotypical steps of colonization and aspiration. Patients who develop VAP should generally be considered to have a form of acquired immunosuppression.[42] The more frequent occurrence of other nosocomial infections in patients with VAP supports this concept. In addition, a subgroup of VAP patients develops multiple separate episodes of VAP, suggesting even greater compromise of their lower respiratory tract defenses.

Many of the causes of compromised lower respiratory tract defenses are due to the underlying disease or critical illness precipitating ICU admission and the need for mechanical ventilation. However, several are common to most ICU patients and may be targets for prevention strategies.

MALNUTRITION

The overall rate of VAP appears to have decreased since early in the era of mechanical ventilation. Although a variety of factors may explain this finding, one important change is the aggressive use of nutritional support. In addition to increasing the risk of oropharyngeal colonization, malnutrition blunts many of the inflammatory responses to the bacterial challenge. The need for aggressive early nutrition may be somewhat debatable,[22] but provision of nutrition after 48 hours of mechanical ventilation is clearly the standard of care. Whether specialized immune-enhancing formulas are required to significantly impact the risk of infection is still unproved.

CORTICOSTEROIDS

Systemic corticosteroids have well documented anti-inflammatory effects that can clearly influence immune function. The difficulty in determining corticosteroids' effect on the risk of VAP is the competing effect of other risk factors for VAP. The most obvious example is that the use of corticosteroids may allow earlier extubation of a patient intubated for an exacerbation of asthma, thereby lowering the risk of VAP. This dual effect probably holds true for most cases in which corticosteroids are used acutely for critically ill patients. The potential benefits begin to be outweighed by clear adverse consequences after more prolonged courses.

TRANSFUSIONS

One common cause of immunosuppression is the use of red blood cell transfusions. This effect of transfusions has been known for several decades and was used therapeutically in pretransplantation management of patients with end-stage renal disease. Because the trigger for red blood cell transfusion varies widely among institutions and even among individual practitioners,[43] it is possible to avoid compromising host immunity with a more restrictive transfusion policy. Hebert and colleagues demonstrated that a conservative transfusion policy was associated with equivalent mortality in most ICU patients.[44] Adjunctive use of erythropoietin to maintain hematocrit without transfusion may also lower infection rates.[45] A complementary policy of routinely using leukoreduction filters with all blood transfusions decreased the incidence of post-transfusion fever as well as overall antibiotic use,[46] potentially decreasing the risk of pneumonia via several mechanisms.

ANNOTATED REFERENCES

Cook D, Guyatt G, Marshall J, et al: A comparison of sucralfate and ranitidine for the prevention of upper gastrointestinal bleeding in patients requiring mechanical ventilation. N Engl J Med 1998;338:791-797.

This large, multicenter, randomized trial did not demonstrate any difference in nosocomial pneumonia rates using various criteria for diagnosis, based on type of gastrointestinal bleeding prophylaxis. There was a slightly higher risk of gastrointestinal bleeding with sucralfate.

Drakulovic MB, Torres A, Bauer TT, et al: Supine body position as a risk factor for nosocomial pneumonia in mechanically ventilated patients: A randomised trial. Lancet 1999;354:1851-1858.

This randomized, controlled trial of body positioning clearly demonstrated a decreased risk with the semirecumbent position, providing strong evidence of the role of microaspiration in the pathogenesis of VAP.

Guerin C, Girard R, Chemorin C, et al: Facial mask noninvasive mechanical ventilation reduces the incidence of nosocomial pneumonia: A prospective epidemiological survey from a single ICU. Intensive Care Med 1997;23:1024-1032.

Prospective trial demonstrating that ventilator-associated pneumonia can more accurately be called endotracheal tube–associated pneumonia, providing further evidence of the role of microaspiration in VAP.

Sirvent JM, Torres A, El Ebiary M, et al: Protective effect of intravenously administered cefuroxime against nosocomial pneumonia in patients with structural coma. Am J Respir Crit Care Med 1997;155:1729-1734.

Randomized, controlled trial of true prophylactic antibiotic use to prevent VAP in a defined subgroup illustrated the two-edged sword of antibiotics—decreasing the risk of early pneumonia while selecting for more pathogenic microorganisms and possibly increasing the risk of late-onset VAP.

Valles J, Artigas A, Rello J, et al: Continuous aspiration of subglottic secretions in preventing ventilator-associated pneumonia. Ann Intern Med 1995;122:179-186.

Randomized trial demonstrating the decreased risk of early-onset VAP with a manipulation that decreases the amount of microaspiration. Even if the practical use of continuous aspiration of subglottic secretions is limited, the study illustrated the problem of secretions pooling above the cuff of the endotracheal tube and its role in VAP.

Chapter 145

VASCULAR CATHETER-RELATED INFECTIONS

Scott Norwood • Clyde E. McAuley

KEY POINTS

1. Primary bloodstream infection (BSI) is the fourth most common nosocomial infection; **intravascular devices are the source of most primary bloodstream infections.**

2. **A variety of factors,** including the patient "host," catheter composition, and microorganism-catheter surface interactions, **contribute to the ultimate development of a catheter-related bloodstream infection** (CR-BSI).

3. Although the risk of colonization and bacteremia increases with time, **the optimal time for catheter removal is not known** for peripheral arterial, central venous, and pulmonary artery catheters.

4. The **clinical diagnosis of a catheter infection** that requires treatment by catheter removal, antibiotics, or both, **is insensitive and nonspecific.**

5. Various **quantitative catheter culture techniques have been developed** to distinguish true infection from colonization; in general, **qualitative through-the-catheter (TTC) cultures should not be used** to diagnose CR-BSI.

6. **Skin preparation** before insertion and **appropriate site maintenance** are **crucial factors** in preventing CR-BSI.

7. Existing studies support the general guideline that central venous, pulmonary artery, and peripheral arterial **catheters should not be routinely changed at specific intervals to prevent infection.**

8. The **risk of infection for multiple-lumen catheters is not higher** than that noted for single-lumen catheters.

9. **Arterial catheters** are at **relatively low risk for colonization and CR-BSI.**

10. **Antiseptic and antibiotic impregnation of catheter surfaces** appears to be **a promising approach** for reducing catheter colonization and CR-BSI.

11. **Physicians in critical care units must study their own patient populations** to determine the incidence of significant catheter colonization and CR-BSI and to **develop appropriate guidelines** for catheter exchange and site maintenance.

Primary bloodstream infection (BSI) is the fourth most common nosocomial infection, preceded only by urinary tract infections, pneumonia, and surgical site infections.[1-3] Intravascular devices, particularly central venous catheters (CVCs), are the source of most primary BSIs.[2,4] It is estimated that approximately 80,000 CVC-associated BSIs occur yearly in ICUs in the United States,[2] with approximately 250,000 cases identified if entire hospital populations are considered.[2]

The cost of catheter-related bloodstream infection (CR-BSI) is substantial, both in terms of morbidity and financial resources expended.[2,5,6-8] Although multiple studies of risk factors and preventative strategies have been published, both the incidence and risk of death from all sources of nosocomial BSI and CR-BSI have increased progressively since the mid 1980s.[3] A 1995 survey of physicians' practices regarding the placement and subsequent maintenance of CVCs documented a high percentage of suboptimal catheter insertion and care practices.[9] This may explain the observed nationwide increase in the incidence of CR-BSI, and these suboptimal practices will more than likely continue to contribute to primary BSIs in patients with CVCs.[3]

In this chapter we clarify some of the commonly used terms associated with CR-BSI, discuss the various pathogenic theories, analyze patient- and hospital-related risk factors, discuss available diagnostic techniques, and review the existing data on infections associated with the most commonly employed types of vascular catheters.

DEFINITIONS

A consistent problem in the review of this subject is the absence of a consensus on precise definitions or terms for describing catheter bacterial or fungal colonization and CR-BSI.[10] Erroneous descriptions and definitions for contamination, colonization, and infection have resulted in confusion and misinterpretation of many clinical investigations.[11-13] Although it is clear that inanimate objects do not become "infected," there is strong evidence to suggest that bacteria may be able to live and multiply on catheter surfaces, deriving nutrients from catheter polymers, the deposited glycocalyx of certain bacterial species, and other nonviable bacteria.[14,15] Erroneous definitions of contamination, colonization, and true infection have led to confusion and incorrect interpretations by some investigators.[13] The following clinical definitions are derived from current guidelines from the Centers for Disease Control and Prevention (CDC)[2,16] and represent current standards for the accurate reporting of clinical and laboratory studies:

Catheter-related bloodstream infection (CR-BSI): a bacteremia or fungemia in a patient with an intravascular catheter with at least one positive blood culture obtained from a peripheral vein and clinical manifestations of infection (i.e., fever, chills, and/or hypotension) and no apparent source for the BSI except the catheter. One of the following should be present: a positive semiquantitative (>15 colony-forming units [CFUs]/catheter segment) or quantitative (>10^3 CFUs/catheter segment) culture whereby the same organism is isolated from the catheter segment and peripheral blood; simultaneous quantitative blood cultures with greater than 5:1 ratio CVC versus peripheral catheter; or a greater than 2-hour period between the initiation of growth of organisms on culture from a peripheral blood culture when compared with a simultaneously collected CVC culture.[17-19]

Localized catheter colonization: significant growth of a microorganism (>15 CFUs) from the catheter tip, subcutaneous segment of the catheter, or the catheter hub, by semiquantitive culture, without evidence of systemic infection. (This definition was commonly used in earlier studies as the definition for "catheter-related infection.")

Exit site infection: erythema or induration within 2 cm of the catheter exit site, in the absence of concomitant BSI and without concomitant purulence.

Clinical exit site infection (or tunnel infection): tenderness, erythema, or site induration greater than 2 cm from the catheter site along the subcutaneous tract of a tunneled (e.g., Hickman or Broviac) catheter, in the absence of concomitant BSI.

Pocket infection: purulent fluid in the subcutaneous pocket of a totally implanted intravascular catheter that might or might not be associated with spontaneous rupture and drainage or necrosis of the overlying skin, in the absence of concomitant BSI.

Infusate-related BSI: concordant growth of the same organism from the infusate and blood cultures (preferably percutaneously drawn) with no other identifiable source of infection.

Culture of drainage or of the skin around a catheter insertion site may, in some situations, be helpful in that a positive bacterial culture result assists in confirming the presence of an exit site infection. Cultures of the skin around the insertion site also have been shown to provide good negative predictive value.[20,21] It is important to also understand that values of 15 CFUs or less for semiquantitative and 10^3 CFUs or less for quantitative cultures can be regarded as a negative culture, a contaminant, or an insignificant infection that does not require treatment.

PATHOGENESIS

Investigators have shown that microbial colonization and biofilm formation on intravascular catheters are universal, occurring soon after catheter insertion.[14,15,22] The presence of bacteria or biofilm formation, in and of themselves, does not necessarily define a catheter infection. The final determinant of whether such colonization progresses to clinical infection is multifactorial. A variety of host factors, catheter composition, and the interaction between microorganisms and the catheter surface may all contribute to the ultimate development of a CR-BSI.[23]

There are four established pathogenic theories for the development of CR-BSI. Microorganisms found on patients' skin are the most common sources of CR-BSI.[24] The most

commonly accepted theory for the pathogenesis of CR-BSI is that bacterial colonization and subsequent CR-BSI begin at the interface between the catheter and the skin insertion site.[25] Host proteins such as fibronectin rapidly coat the catheter after insertion and provide a substrate for organisms such as *Staphylococcus aureus*. Multiple species of *Staphylococcus epidermidis* (also referred to as coagulase-negative staphylococci) are responsible for the majority of catheter colonizations causing CR-BSI.[2,24] These bacteria produce a glycocalyx or "slime" composed of a polysaccharide adhesive that mediates attachment of the bacteria to the catheter surfaces within 30 minutes after inoculation.[14,26] Microcolonies can develop within 1 hour, and heavy colonization occurs within 6 to 12 hours.[27] The glycocalyx coating may delay the penetration of some antibiotics and serve as a protective barrier against phagocytic neutrophils and macrophages.[14,28] In vitro studies also show that bacteria are able to grow on catheter surfaces even when externally supplied nutrients are lacking,[14,29,30] suggesting that bacteria are capable of using catheter components or other bacterial cells as nutrient sources. Catheter surface erosion does indeed occur, and it has been postulated that the catheter components, added antithrombogenic layers, or endogenous proteins that coat the catheter surface may serve as sustaining nutritional sources. Biofilm organisms have a slower growth rate, resulting in a delayed uptake of antimicrobial agents.[28]

A second theory of the pathogenesis of CR-BSI is that the catheter hub may be the primary source of infection.[31,32] This mode of infection is more commonly identified in patients with long-term catheterization.[31,33] Bacteria can be introduced via one or more hubs from frequent manipulations. As the biofilm grows, bacteria migrate down the inner luminal surface and gain access to the venous circulation. In low-flow regions, the biofilm attachment is weaker and breaks more easily, allowing entry of bacteria into the venous circulation.[28] A study by Segura and colleagues[31] identified a 10% rate of CR-BSI associated with hub contamination. The majority of patients in this study were not ICU patients. While 17% of catheter colonizations or CR-BSIs were due to hub contamination in one study evaluating pulmonary artery (PA) catheter infections, speciation antibiograms and plasmid profile analysis of bacterial isolates documented that 80% developed from skin entry sites.[34]

According to the third theory of CR-BSI pathogenesis, remote infections may produce bacteremia and subsequent seeding of the catheter. Although this scenario is plausible, hematogenous catheter seeding is considered an uncommon cause of CR-BSI.[22,35] It has been suggested that many catheter infections from fungal and enteric organisms, such as enterococci, *Escherichia coli*, and *Klebsiella*, may infect catheters by hematogenous spread.[36] In-vitro catheter experiments with gram-negative bacteria indicate that most gram-negative organisms show extensive bacterial adherence to catheter surfaces.[37] Antimicrobial-treated *Pseudomonas* species also develop a heavy mucoid film that is similar to that of *S. epidermidis* and is capable of coating catheter surfaces. In these in-vitro experiments, antibiotics did not eliminate gram-negative bacteria from the catheters, substantiating the clinical impression that it is very difficult (if not impossible) to eliminate gram-negative colonization of long-term vascular catheters by antibiotic therapy alone.[37]

Infusate contamination has been implicated as a fourth mechanism of CR-BSI.[38-40] Parenteral nutrition solutions[41] and lipid emulsions[42] can support bacterial and fungal growth,[35] but the risk from infusate contamination today is considered very low.

RISK FACTORS

Risk factors for catheter colonization and CR-BSI can be grouped as either *patient related* or *hospital related*. The following are patient-related risk factors for CR-BSI[35]:

- Age (i.e., <1 year or >60 years)
- Alteration of host defenses
- Severity of underlying disease
- Remote site of infection
- Heavy skin bacterial colonization
- Alterations in skin integrity from disease (e.g., psoriasis) or trauma (e.g., burns)

Whereas patient-related factors usually cannot be significantly modified during an acute illness, they must be considered when developing catheter maintenance protocols.

In contradistinction to patient-related risk factors for the development of CR-BSI, many hospital-related risk factors can be significantly modified and prevention protocols should focus on these risks.[43] A number of "performance indicators" have been proposed to assist in the prevention of CR-BSI[2,16]:

- Implementation of educational programs that include didactic and interactive components for those who insert and maintain catheters
- Use of maximal sterile barrier precautions during catheter placement
- Use of chlorhexidine for skin antisepsis
- Monitoring rates of catheter discontinuation when the catheter is no longer essential for medical management.[2,16]

Although the number of catheter manipulations and the experience of the individual performing the catheter insertion are considered risk factors, these typically cannot be changed or controlled for the individual patient at risk. Cutdowns should be avoided whenever possible because of the high incidence of catheter-related complications associated with the technique.[44] The most common risk factors for catheter colonization and CR-BSI that can be successfully altered or controlled are discussed separately.

ANATOMIC SITE OF INSERTION

A number of studies strongly suggest that the use of the internal jugular site is a significant risk factor,[34,45-47] possibly owing to the close proximity of oropharyngeal secretions, the greater catheter motion from adjacent neck movement, and the difficulty in maintaining sterile occlusive dressings.[34] However, the internal jugular site or the femoral vein site is recommended over the subclavian vein site for short-term hemodialysis catheters to reduce the risk of subsequent subclavian vein stenosis.[16]

The femoral site is also more likely to become heavily colonized and thus is also at a heightened risk for CR-BSI. A study by Kemp and associates[47] in patients receiving total parenteral nutrition found the overall incidences of catheter colonization to be 36% for femoral, 17% for internal jugular, and 5% for subclavian sites. "Catheter infection" was

defined as 15 or more CFUs in catheter-tip cultures by semiquantitative culture. The incidence of CR-BSI was not reported in the study.

Although several reports have noted the successful use of the femoral site for long-term parenteral therapy,[48,49] these studies incorporated a subcutaneous tunneling technique and the tip of the catheter was located in the inferior vena cava. Femoral vein cannulation is considered safe when the catheter site is used for 3 days or less and when dressing changes are frequent.[50] Data collected in our center suggest that colonization rates for femoral sites, even with the use of chlorhexidine and silver sulfadiazine-bonded catheters, is significantly higher than for subclavian or internal jugular catheter sites.[51]

DURATION OF CATHETER USE

The incidence of significant catheter colonization and CR-BSI is directly proportional to the length of time a catheter is used. Nonetheless, the optimal timing of catheter removal remains uncertain. The risk that an individual catheter will cause CR-BSI is low as long as the catheter is removed within 3 days. However, critically ill patients typically need venous access for prolonged periods and the timing of catheter removal must be weighed against ongoing clinical requirements. Several studies suggest that CVCs and Pulmonary artery (PA) catheters should not have predetermined life spans.[52-54] Another study in cancer patients provides evidence that peripheral arterial catheters should be removed within 4 to 6 days and PA catheters within 4 to 7 days of insertion.[55]

Recommendations and guidelines for catheter exchange may be used to minimize CR-BSI and to prolong access site use on the basis of existing published data. However, it is important to note that CR-BSI risk factors are multifactorial and that global recommendations for catheter removal may not be applicable to the individual patient. Generally, catheters should be removed (1) when they are no longer needed or (2) if CR-BSI is suspected on the basis of examination of the entry site and appropriate cultures confirm clinical suspicions (see section on diagnostic techniques). Individual hospitals, individual ICUs, and, in certain situations, individual practitioners should study their catheter infection rates to develop specific guidelines appropriate to their practice patterns and environment. Rates of CR-BSI per 1000 catheter-days can be calculated and compared with published standards.[2,16]

CRITICALLY ILL VERSUS NON–CRITICALLY ILL PATIENTS

A review of all prospective studies using quantitative culture techniques reported data varying from a low risk of 0.7% per day in catheters utilized for total parenteral nutrition to 3.3% per day for central venous monitoring catheters.[56] Many of these studies did not distinguish critically ill patients from other hospitalized patients and did not distinguish septic from nonseptic patients. One study examining multiple-lumen CVC infection rates in critically ill patients reported no infections or significant catheter colonization in critically ill nonseptic patients, compared with a 26.3% incidence of catheter colonization (previously termed *catheter-related infection*) and a 9.6% incidence of CR-BSI in critically ill septic patients.[57] This study also suggested that the number of days a patient is hospitalized before catheter insertion may contribute to a higher incidence of catheter colonization leading to CR-BSI.

CATHETER COMPOSITION

Older, stiffer catheters have been associated with a higher risk of thrombosis and infection.[58,59] Although newer, more flexible silicone and polyurethane catheters may be less thrombogenic and have diminished in-vitro adherence,[60] subsequent studies have questioned these assumptions. Gilsdorf and colleagues,[61] after studying four different intravenous catheter materials, concluded that the decreases seen with respect to in-vitro bacterial adherence and thrombogenicity did not translate into improved clinical resistance to catheter colonization and subsequent bacteremia. Their study demonstrated that *S. epidermidis* was adherent to polymeric silicone (Silastic), polytetrafluoroethylene (Teflon), and two types of polyurethane. These researchers speculated that bacterial adherence to these catheter materials in the absence of demonstrable nutrients reflects one of the following:[61]

- Organism resistance to nutritional deprivation
- Organism ability to utilize catheter materials as a nutrient base
- Organism expression of adherence factors independent of organism growth or nutrition

DIAGNOSTIC TECHNIQUES

The clinical diagnosis of a catheter infection that requires treatment by either catheter removal, antibiotics, or both is insensitive and nonspecific. Assuming that reasonable sterile technique during insertion and appropriate site care have been utilized, even the presence of erythema and purulent drainage is considered an unreliable indicator in certain situations.[17,62,63] Routine qualitative broth cultures are too sensitive for diagnosing CR-BSI,[56] yielding false-positive rates up to 50%.[64] Routine swab sampling and culture of the catheter exit site in the absence of local or systemic signs of infection may also be too sensitive, although some investigators suggest that periodic semiquantitative swab sampling and culture of CVC skin exit sites have a negative predictive value of at least 95%.[65]

The unreliability of clinical diagnosis has led to a variety of microbiologic diagnostic techniques. Because each method has advantages and disadvantages, some investigators have suggested that simply performing peripheral blood cultures and clinical evaluation may be all that is necessary and cost effective.[66] Both quantitative and semiquantitative catheter cultures require catheter removal to make the diagnosis of infection, prompting investigators to question the clinical utility of such techniques for the treatment of most hospitalized patients.[67]

The inappropriate removal of both long-term and short-term CVCs—with its attendant risks and added costs—has created a variety of catheter exit site and quantitative blood culture techniques.[68,69] Heavy colonization of the skin exit site is considered the most common precursor to CR-BSI. Conversely, catheter colonization and CR-BSI are associated with positive skin site culture results, especially quantitative cultures yielding 50 or more CFUs.[70] In a study of cancer patients with long-term nontunneled Silastic catheters,

surveillance cultures, quantitative skin cultures, and quantitative catheter cultures were nonspecific and insensitive in determining the presence of CR-BSI. However, when quantitative skin cultures were performed only in those patients with clinical findings suggestive of CR-BSI, this method was highly sensitive, specific, and predictive.[71] The technique of obtaining specimens for quantitative skin cultures has been thoroughly described by Bjornson and colleagues.[36]

QUANTITATIVE BLOOD CULTURES

The paired quantitative blood culture is a technique used for diagnosis of CR-BSI without the need for catheter removal. This technique, first described by Wing and associates,[72] involves obtaining blood culture specimens simultaneously through the catheter and peripherally and then performing quantitative comparisons of the bacterial concentrations in the two results. In the original report, a diagnosis of CR-BSI was confirmed if blood removed through the catheter had more CFUs per millimeter than blood obtained from a peripheral vein. Subsequent studies have shown that a 5- to 10-fold increase in the number of microorganisms grown from the catheter-drawn specimen is necessary to entertain the diagnosis of CR-BSI.[73-75] However, if the catheter blood quantitative culture value is positive at any level of colony count and the peripheral blood culture is negative, a diagnosis of CR-BSI cannot be made[3] and the catheter may merely be colonized. The technique of paired quantitative blood cultures has not gained widespread clinical application. Moonens and associates[76] showed that Gram's stains of blood removed through total parenteral nutrition catheters for paired quantitative blood cultures had a 100% positive predictive value and a 42% negative predictive value for diagnosing CR-BSI, enabling the rapid presumptive diagnosis of CR-BSI and earlier initiation of antimicrobial therapy.[76]

CATHETER CULTURE TECHNIQUES

Various quantitative catheter culture techniques have been developed to distinguish true infection from colonization.[56,68] The semiquantitative (roll-plate) technique developed by Maki and colleagues[64] is the best-studied and most commonly utilized method for surveillance cultures.[77] A 5-cm segment (either catheter tip or intracutaneous segment) is rolled across a blood-agar plate in a reproducible, defined manner. In the original study, a positive result was defined as 15 or more CFUs per plate, although most of the culture-positive catheters yielded confluent growth.[64] A positive catheter segment culture result (>15 CFUs, now defined as catheter colonization) resulted in a 16% risk of subsequent CR-BSI.

Many experts have recommended that both the catheter tip and the intracutaneous segment be cultured when CR-BSI is a diagnostic consideration. One study of infections in PA catheters showed that only 61% of semiquantitative tip cultures were positive in catheters known to be infected.[78] Intracutaneous segment cultures were positive in 83%, however, and culturing both the tip and the intracutaneous segment (of the PA catheter introducer) resulted in a 94% positive rate.[78]

Other, more complex techniques have been used to distinguish true infection from colonization, including

Gram's stain,[79] broth quantitative cultures,[80] and "sonicated" quantitative catheter cultures.[81] Moyer and associates[82] compared various culture techniques for diagnosis of catheter colonization and CR-BSI. They considered semiquantitative culture the best test for making the diagnosis of "catheter-related infection" but regarded paired quantitative blood culture of specimens simultaneously withdrawn through the catheter and peripherally as an acceptable approach in patients with very difficult venous access or long-term indwelling catheters.[72,82-84]

CULTURE RECOMMENDATIONS

It is generally recognized that the risk of infection is very low if catheters are placed under sterile conditions, receive appropriate care, and are removed within 5 days of insertion.[67] Therefore, routine culture of such catheters is not indicated except during surveillance periods for quality improvement purposes.

Sherertz[1] has provided the following recommendations for catheter cultures, which are both clinically useful and cost effective:

1. Unless conducting clinical research or investigating a problem, one should perform catheter cultures only when they are clinically indicated.
2. The roll-plate method for peripheral cultures should be used (semiquantitative culture method).
3. For removable CVCs, either the roll-plate technique (semiquantitative culture), vortex method, or sonication may be used.
4. Paired quantitative blood culture specimens obtained through the catheter and from a peripheral vein may be helpful in deciding whether to remove an implanted CVC.

Although Sherertz originally recommended that only the tip of the CVC be sampled for culture,[1] others have recommended simultaneously culturing both the tip and the intracutaneous segment of the catheter.[69,78] These latter recommendations also should be used for surveillance purposes if an institution identifies a CR-BSI rate greater than 2% to 3% (number of catheter infections per 100 catheters) or a catheter colonization rate greater than 15%.

A recurring question concerns the value of qualitative broth blood cultures of samples obtained through the central catheter (TTC) to diagnose CR-BSI or catheter colonization. Qualitative broth cultures have been advocated for confirming bacteremia from a variety of sources (e.g., pneumonia, abscess) but not specifically for CR-BSI.[83] This practice should be considered only when short-term catheters have been in place for relatively short periods of time (<4 days). Strict antiseptic preparation of the hub is mandatory to prevent false-positive culture results.[83] Catheter microbial colonization may contaminate TTC blood specimens. Thus, an important caveat to remember is that unless paired quantitative blood cultures are being performed, the TTC results should not be used to diagnose CR-BSI. Generally, qualitative TTC cultures should be avoided unless the physician knows precisely how the specimens are obtained and how long the short-term catheter has been in place. Thus, qualitative TTC cultures are indicated only if it is impossible to obtain blood culture specimens from peripheral venipuncture.

CATHETER AND SITE MAINTENANCE

Skin preparation before insertion and appropriate site maintenance are crucial factors in preventing CR-BSI. The long-term maintenance of catheters and insertion sites has been extensively studied, including the type and frequency of dressing changes, intravenous tubing changes, skin antiseptics, topical ointments, and guidewire exchange to diagnose or prevent infection. Great care should be taken in preparing the site for catheter insertion, including the use of careful antiseptic skin preparation and large, sterile drapes. Ideally, sterile gowns, gloves, surgical head covers, and masks are also employed during nonurgent situations.

ANTISEPTICS, OINTMENTS, AND DRESSING MATERIALS

A study assessing the efficacy of cutaneous antiseptics evaluated 668 catheterizations randomly assigned skin preparation with 10% povidone-iodine, 70% alcohol, or 2% aqueous chlorhexidine.[85] Chlorhexidine provided the best protection against catheter colonization, with an incidence of 2.3% versus 7.1% and 9.3% for alcohol and povidone-iodine, respectively ($P = .02$). The rate of CR-BSI was also lower: 0.5% versus 2.3% and 2.6%, respectively.[85] Another study evaluating epidural catheter colonization also strongly supported the use of chlorhexidine as the first-line skin antiseptic.[86]

Chlorhexidine, a cationic biguanide, is a potent germicide that is effective for nearly all nosocomial bacteria and yeasts.[85] Unlike povidone-iodine or alcohol, chlorhexidine provides residual cutaneous antibacterial activity that persists for several hours after application, and its germicidal activity is not neutralized by blood, serum, or other protein-rich biomaterials.[85] Another study compared a 4% alcohol-based solution of 0.25% chlorhexidine gluconate and 0.025% benzalkonium chloride with 10% povidone-iodine for care of CVC and arterial catheter insertion sites.[87] The rate of "catheter-related sepsis" in this study was 12 per 1000 catheter-days in the chlorhexidine-treated sites versus 21 per 1000 catheter-days for the povidone-iodine sites.[87]

Various ointments are also routinely used in an attempt to prevent catheter colonization and CR-BSI. In a large prospective study, Maki and Band[88] concluded that topical antimicrobial ointments conferred only a modest protective effect, primarily for peripheral venous catheters remaining in place for more than 4 days. If ointments are used at all, these researchers recommended topical polymyxin-neomycin-bacitracin ointment for peripheral catheters and iodophor ointment for CVC and arterial catheters.[89] However, the Healthcare Infection Control Practices Advisory Committee of the CDC recommends that topical antimicrobial ointments not be used on the insertion sites of peripheral venous catheters or short-term nontunneled CVCs.[2,16] Povidone-iodine ointment is recommended for short-term hemodialysis catheter insertion sites.[2,16]

The frequency and types of dressing changes have also been extensively studied. It is recommended that sterilely inserted peripheral intravenous catheters be removed at 72 to 96 hours to minimize the risk of phlebitis.[2,16] Peripheral catheters that were inserted under emergency conditions should be removed within 24 to 48 hours.[2,16] The dressing should be removed when the catheter is replaced (i.e., at 72 to 96 hours) or when the dressing becomes damp, loose, or soiled. It is important that the peripheral venous catheter site be inspected daily. Therefore, transparent dressings are almost universally employed for peripheral catheters.[90]

In a large study of dressing regimens for more than 2000 polytetrafluoroethylene peripheral venous catheters, Maki and Ringer[89] found no difference in skin site colonization, catheter colonization, or CR-BSI when comparing dry gauze, transparent polyurethane, and iodophor-transparent dressings. They recommended either sterile dry gauze or a transparent dressing for a peripheral catheter placed under sterile conditions, with subsequent dressing changes to coincide with catheter removal. Other studies suggest that transparent dressings enhance bacterial colonization of peripheral venous catheters, increasing both catheter colonization rates and hospital costs.[90]

Two studies have also implicated transparent dressings as contributing to CVC colonization and associated CR-BSI.[91,92] An analysis of previously published studies in the English literature documented (1) a statistically significant higher risk of catheter colonization for catheter sites with transparent dressings than for those with dressings of dry cotton gauze and tape and (2) a trend toward increased CR-BSI.[93] The study reported a 53% higher risk of catheter colonization (previously defined as catheter-related infection) for peripheral catheters and a 63% to 78% higher risk of significant colonization for CVCs. Conventional nonpermeable transparent dressings probably impede moisture evaporation from the insertion site and may, therefore, enhance bacterial colonization, especially in critically ill or diaphoretic patients.[90-92] Disadvantages of transparent dressings include poor adhesion in diaphoretic patients or with use of topical ointments and, depending on frequency of use, greater expense.[9]

However, it is important to understand that most of these earlier studies and the subsequent meta-analysis looked at conventional nonpermeable polyurethane dressings. A later study by Maki and associates[94] compared conventional (nonpermeable) polyurethane, highly permeable polyurethane, and sterile gauze and tape dressings for PA catheters. In this study, cutaneous bacterial colonization under the dressing at the time of catheter removal was lowest with gauze and tape ($10^{1.3}$ CFUs), intermediate with the highly permeable polyurethane dressings ($10^{1.8}$ CFUs; $P < .01$), and highest with the conventional (nonpermeable) polyurethane dressings ($10^{2.1}$ CFUs; $P < .001$). There were no significant differences in catheter segment colonization or CR-BSI among the three groups.[94] These researchers concluded that polyurethane dressings appear to be safe for use with PA catheters and may be left in place for up to 5 days between dressing changes.[94] If CVCs or PA catheters are used for prolonged periods, the authors believe that nonpermeable transparent dressings should be avoided.

REPLACEMENT SCHEDULES AND GUIDEWIRE EXCHANGE

Although it is well known that the risk of infection increases with time if catheters remain in place indefinitely, there are two schools of thought regarding catheter exchange for prevention of catheter colonization and CR-BSI. The first suggests that routine exchange of a catheter to a new site or by guidewire at a predetermined interval confers protection. The second advises that CVCs be left in place until the development of clinical suspicion or signs of catheter colonization or CR-BSI. Both practices have inherent risks.

With routine catheter exchange, the patient is exposed to the potential risk of pneumothorax or injury to major vessels.[13] Recontamination and subcutaneous tract infection may also occur during an improperly performed guidewire exchange.

Many studies evaluating guidewire exchange show that the technique is safe and effective for diagnosing CR-BSI and for prolonging catheter site utilization.[57,95-97] Guidewire exchange is effective in diagnosing catheter colonization and CR-BSI as long as every attempt is made to "sterilize" the entire external portion of the in situ catheter and the surrounding skin before the exchange. This practice not only prevents contamination of the new catheter during exchange but also yields more accurate semiquantitative culture results, because the catheters are removed through a "sterile field."[39] If bacteria are truly capable of growing and multiplying on catheter surfaces without external nutrient sources, as suggested by in vitro studies,[14,28,61,98] guidewire exchange may help prevent infection by removing significant numbers of externally and internally adherent bacteria before the development of a colony number sufficient to cause bacteremia or local infection.

One criticism of guidewire exchange is that intracutaneous tract colonization or contamination during the exchange may perpetuate local infection and allow for subsequent infection of the new catheter. One study reported this result as unlikely. Twelve culture-positive catheters were replaced with new catheters by guidewire exchange. Catheters removed from the same sites showed no growth in eight catheters (67%), probable contamination in one (8%), and the presence of microorganisms on cultures in only three (25%).[52] An observational cohort study of 2470 patients receiving CVCs showed that subsequent catheters exchanged over guidewires were at no higher risk for CR-BSI than a second catheter placed at a new anatomic site.[97] These studies suggest, as previously hypothesized by Bozzetti and colleagues,[99] that guidewire exchange may confer some protection against CR-BSI. However, when culture results for removed catheters are positive (semiquantitative culture >15 CFUs or quantitative culture >10^3 CFUs), it is recommended that the replacement catheter be removed from the colonized site.[64] Semiquantitative and quantitative cultures of removed catheters that are less than these values are not considered a precursor for CR-BSI. Therefore, the replacement catheter can remain in situ.

With the hope of clarifying this issue, two studies investigated the infection risk of different methods of managing long-term vascular catheters in critically ill patients.[52,53] Cobb and associates[53] studied four different methods of replacing CVCs and PA catheters. Patients were randomly grouped to receive (1) a new catheter at a new site every 3 days, (2) a guidewire exchange at the existing site every 3 days, (3) a new catheter and new site only when clinically indicated, or (4) a guidewire exchange only when infection was suspected. Of the 160 patients studied, 5% had CR-BSI, 16% had catheter colonization, and 9% had major mechanical complications. Not unexpectedly, insertions at new sites were associated with more mechanical complications when compared with the guidewire-exchanged catheters (5% vs. 1%; $P = .005$).[53] Although the results were not statistically significant, patients who were randomly assigned to guidewire exchanges were considered more likely to have bacteremia after the first 3 days of catheterization when compared with patients who received catheters at a new site

(6% vs. 0%; $P = .06$). The researchers concluded that routine replacement of central vascular catheters every 3 days does not prevent infection and that guidewire exchange may increase the risk of bacteremia.[53]

Eyer and colleagues[52] evaluated three different methods of site management for multiple-lumen, single-lumen, central venous, and PA catheters used for 7 days or more: (1) catheter exchange to a new site every 7 days; (2) no scheduled catheter change at any particular time but exchange to a new site when clinically indicated; and (3) guidewire exchange every 7 days. In all groups, a catheter change was mandatory for a positive blood culture, exit site infection (defined as purulent drainage, expanding erythema or cellulitis, or a positive qualitative swab culture result for the exit site specimen), or clinical signs of sepsis without a definite source. These workers found no difference in infection risk among the three methods of long-term catheter care, recommending that the method with the fewest complications and least expense be used.

These two studies support the following general guidelines[52]:

1. CVCs, PA catheters, and peripheral arterial catheters should not be routinely changed at specific intervals to prevent infection.
2. Guidewire exchange is appropriate when a damaged catheter needs to be replaced or when CR-BSI is suspected, because the technique is safer than placement of a new catheter.
3. If there is evidence of a skin exit site infection, removal of the existing catheter and placement of a new catheter at an alternate site is most appropriate.

Suggested Method for Guidewire Exchange

The following procedure of guidewire exchange is recommended:

1. Guidewire exchange begins with a complete sterilization of the external portion of the exiting catheter before the guidewire is placed: All intravenous tubing, including parenteral nutrition tubing, is carefully separated from the catheter hubs and replaced with sterile caps or plugs. The separated intravenous tubing tips are also sterilely protected until they are reconnected to the new catheter.
2. Sterile, disposable gowns and gloves are worn by personnel performing the procedure, along with surgical hats and masks, and a sterile field for the necessary equipment is prepared on a bedside table.
3. The distal ports of the catheter to be exchanged are placed on a sterile paper barrier (usually provided in the new catheter kit), and the insertion site, along with a 10-cm circumferential area of skin and the entire external portion of the catheter from insertion site to capped hubs, is scrubbed for 5 minutes with 10×10-cm gauze pads soaked in 4% chlorhexidine skin cleanser. The most important aspect of this preparation is that chlorhexidine be allowed to remain in contact with the skin and the entire external portion of the catheter for at least 5 minutes.
4. After this scrub, the excess soap is carefully removed from the area with dry 10×10-cm gauze pads and the skin sutures securing the catheter are removed with a No. 11 disposable scalpel.

5. The operator then exchanges sterile surgical gloves, and the entire area is widely draped with six sterile cloth surgical towels, or other large sterile barriers, with the distal catheter hubs being carefully removed from the now contaminated sterile paper barrier to the new sterile cloth barrier.
6. A sterile guidewire is carefully inserted through the distal port of the catheter after removal of the cap, with care taken that the wire does not touch the external portion of the hub.
7. The old catheter is carefully removed, with care taken to avoid contact with the surrounding skin.
8. Appropriate culture specimens are then obtained by amputating the 5-cm intracutaneous segment and the 5-cm distal tip of the catheter. This can be done with a sterile disposable suture removal kit (Johnson & Johnson Products, Inc., Stillman, NJ). The segments are placed into two separate culturettes (Baxter Healthcare Corporation, McGaw Park, IL) and transported immediately to the microbiology laboratory for semiquantitative cultures.
9. The portion of the guidewire protruding from the skin is then cleaned with 4% chlorhexidine. Before handling the new catheter, it is best to change to a third pair of sterile gloves. A new catheter is then placed over the guidewire into the proper anatomic position.
10. The catheter is sutured into place after the guidewire is removed.

A chest radiograph is generally not required after guidewire exchange.

For CVCs (16 to 30 cm in length), both the tip and the intracutaneous 5-cm segments from the removed catheter are sent for semiquantitative culture. For PA catheters and introducers, the 5-cm tip of the PA catheter and the 5-cm intracutaneous segment of the catheter introducer are sent in separate culturettes for semiquantitative culture.

INFECTION RISKS OF SPECIFIC CATHETER TYPES

PULMONARY ARTERY CATHETERS

Several studies have shown that the risk of infection from PA catheters has decreased substantially during the past decade.[34,94,100,101] Mermel and colleagues,[34] in an extensive study of the pathogenesis and epidemiology of PA catheter infections, found a 22% incidence of colonization and a 0.7% incidence of CR-BSI.

Another study of 69 PA catheters reported a 21.7% incidence of catheter colonization (>15 CFUs by semiquantitative culture).[78] Catheterization for longer than 5 days was associated with a higher risk of colonization and a 13.3% risk of CR-BSI if catheter colonization developed.[78] The risk of catheter colonization was 41.2% if the catheter remained in place longer than 5 days but only 15.4% if the catheter was used for 5 days or less. In a later study, all episodes of CR-BSI occurred with catheters that had been in place for 5 or more days.[94] These two studies and others[102-104] document that the risk of CR-BSI from PA catheters is relatively low when the catheters are used for 5 days or less and when reasonable insertion site care is provided.

MULTIPLE-LUMEN CENTRAL VENOUS CATHETERS

Multiple-lumen CVCs were first introduced into clinical practice in the early 1980s and have become ubiquitous, especially for use in critically ill patients.[10] These catheters have been implicated as a potential risk factor for CR-BSI. The risk of catheter colonization of multiple-lumen CVCs ranges from 6.9% to 11.5%, with an associated CR-BSI rate of 1.3% to 13.1%.[105-108] Kruse and Shah[10] reviewed all studies of CR-BSI in multiple-lumen CVCs from 1984 through 1992. They concluded that although a few trials suggest that the risk of infection is higher with multiple-lumen catheters, the majority of studies find no variance in infection rates when multiple-lumen catheters are compared with their single-lumen counterparts. Many of these studies used total parenteral nutrition as the entry criterion for patient selection; others combined PA catheter data. Such criteria and comparisons may bias the results of these studies because patients with multiple-lumen or PA catheters are usually more ill than are patients with single-lumen catheters. Therefore, the perceived higher infection rate may be related not to the type of catheter but rather to difficulty in maintaining sterility due to frequent catheter manipulations and the patients' compromised immunologic status.[6]

In a comparable study, Clark-Christoff and associates[107] examined the rate of CR-BSI in 78 patients with single-lumen catheters and 99 patients with triple-lumen catheters. All of the patients were considered to be at high risk for catheter colonization and associated CR-BSI. The researchers concluded that more frequent catheter manipulations with triple-lumen catheters caused a higher rate of infection and, therefore, these catheters should not be used routinely for total parenteral nutrition. Eyer and colleagues[52] reported a 3.4% incidence of catheter colonization with an associated 2.1% incidence of CR-BSI in triple-lumen catheters used for an average of 22.6 days. Several other studies also found no higher risk of CR-BSI associated with multiple-lumen catheters.[47,57,95,105,106,108]

Another study separated multiple-lumen catheter infections in critically ill surgical patients according to whether the patients were septic (with other sources of infection) or nonseptic (no source of infection identified).[57] There were no episodes of significant catheter colonization (defined as >15 CFUs by semiquantitative culture) or CR-BSI in the nonseptic critically ill patients. The incidence of catheter colonization in the septic group was 26.3%, and the incidence of CR-BSI was 9.6%.[57] The rate of catheter colonization (previously termed *catheter-related infection*) per 100 days was only 0.9 for both septic and nonseptic patients combined, which is very similar to rates previously published for single-lumen catheters.[57] This study concluded that the risk of infection for multiple-lumen catheters is no higher than for single-lumen catheters, but septic patients are probably at higher risk regardless of the type of catheter used.[57]

ARTERIAL CATHETERS

Band and Maki[109] have studied arterial catheter-related infections and have determined that the predominant variables for infection risk were percutaneous versus cutdown insertion (ninefold increase in CR-BSI with cutdowns) and extended arterial cannulation time (>4 days). The overall incidence of catheter-related infection (now considered significant catheter colonization) was 18%, with 70% of the infections occurring in catheters used longer than 96 hours. All five episodes of CR-BSI in this study occurred in patients with catheter sites used for more than 96 hours.

A later study also suggested that extended cannulation time is an important factor and reemphasized that the risk of infection for arterial catheters used less than 96 hours is virtually nonexistent.[110] In this later study, 27% of sites used for more than 96 hours became colonized, as evidenced by positive swab cultures of the entry sites. Significant catheter colonization (defined as >15 CFUs on semiquantitative culture) developed in 9.5% of radial and femoral artery sites used for up to 14 days (mean, 6.4 days), although there were no documented episodes of CR-BSI. Significant colonization (>15 CFUs by semiquantitative culture) developed in 44% of axillary sites after 96 hours of use.[110] The researchers concluded that (1) radial and femoral artery sites could be used for prolonged periods if skin site colonization were controlled with strict local site care and (2) guidewire exchange could also be used to confirm the presence of catheter colonization for arterial catheters. This relatively low risk of significant arterial catheter colonization and CR-BSI has been confirmed by others.[111]

LONG-TERM CENTRAL VENOUS CATHETERS

Although seldom used in the acute critical care setting, catheters for long-term central venous access in both the inpatient and outpatient setting are frequently employed for total parenteral nutrition and chemotherapy. In cancer patients, the catheters most frequently used have been long-dwelling tunneled devices (Hickman, Broviac, Groshong).[112] These catheters provide life-prolonging therapy over extended periods by allowing for nutritional support, antibiotics, and chemotherapy without the need for frequent intravenous line changes.[112]

The incidence of significant catheter colonization with tunneled CVCs is approximately 2 per 1000 catheter-days.[113] Early reports emphasized the importance of tunneling long-dwelling catheters to prevent infection, particularly when employed for chemotherapy.[112] However, several studies have shown no difference in infection rates between tunneled and nontunneled long-dwelling subclavian catheters.[114-116]

PERIPHERALLY INSERTED CENTRAL VENOUS CATHETERS

Although not very useful during acute critical illness, peripherally inserted central venous catheters (PICCs) have become a popular means for providing long-term venous access. These catheters are useful as "bridges" between short-term venous access (<2 to 3 weeks) and long-term access (>3 months). One review reported that the average duration of PICC use is in the range of 20 to 50 days.[117] These catheters are inserted through the basilic or cephalic vein and are used primarily to support patients outside the hospital setting. The majority of studies indicate a low rate of infection,[117,118] although one study reported a higher rate for PICCs than that for nontunneled silicone catheters placed directly into the subclavian vein.[114]

NOVEL TECHNOLOGY

ATTACHABLE SILVER-IMPREGNATED CUFFS

An attachable subcutaneous cuff made of an inner silicone sleeve and an outer layer of bovine collagen impregnated with silver ion (Vitacuff, Vitaphore Corporation, Plainsboro, NJ) was the first significant technologic advance specifically designed for preventing CR-BSI from short-term central venous catheterization. Two prospective randomized studies have suggested that the cuff may substantially reduce the risk of catheter colonization (defined as >15 CFUs on semiquantitative culture).[62,119] Although these studies reported reductions in rates of catheter colonization from 28.9% to 9.1% ($P = .002$)[62] and 34.5% to 7.7%,[119] no significant differences in the rates of CR-BSI were noted in either study.

Other studies have failed to demonstrate any benefit derived from the cuff in critically ill and septic patients.[13,95] One observational study documented a higher rate of catheter colonization (31%) and fungemia (20%) by *Candida* species.[95] Dahlberg and colleagues[120] also were unable to show any short-term or long-term benefits of the attachable silver-impregnated cuff in hemodialysis patients.

ANTISEPTIC-IMPREGNATED AND ANTIBIOTIC-IMPREGNATED CATHETERS

CVCs impregnated with various antiseptic and antibiotic agents have been developed in an attempt to reduce the frequency of CR-BSI.

A prospective, randomized study of 405 catheters compared a multiple-lumen catheter coated with silver sulfadiazine and chlorhexidine antiseptics with the standard polyurethane multiple-lumen CVC.[121] The antiseptic-coated catheters were only half as likely to become colonized as were their uncoated counterparts (1.0% vs. 2.5%, $P = .02$).

In another prospective randomized study, Collin[122] observed a ninefold reduction in catheter colonization (termed *catheter-related infection* and defined as >15 CFUs on semiquantitative culture) with the use of an antiseptic-bonded multiple-lumen catheter (2% vs. 18%, $P = .001$). These data translated to catheter-related infection rates (infections per 1000 catheter-days) of 2.27 for antiseptic-coated catheters and 24.68 for standard catheters ($P = .001$). The investigator concluded that the use of antiseptic-impregnated catheters significantly reduced the rate of "catheter-related infections" and ultimately led to fewer guidewire exchanges and catheter removals, thereby reducing patient risk and hospital costs.

Another study of 244 antiseptic-bonded catheters used for prolonged periods (mean, 11.7 + 8.74 days; range, 1 to 51 days) identified a rate of CR-BSI per 1000 days of 1.57,[51] which compared favorably with that for long-term tunneled central catheters.[113] The CR-BSI rate per 1000 days was even lower (0.98) when subclavian sites were analyzed separately.[51] Laboratory studies conducted in a variety of animal models have shown a significant reduction in skin and catheter bacterial colonization,[123] bacterial adherence,[124] and biofilm formation[124] with the use of catheters impregnated with silver sulfadiazine and chlorhexidine. Silver sulfadiazine and chlorhexidine are antiseptics possessing broad-spectrum antimicrobial properties, and the two agents exhibit a synergistic activity, reducing the risk of the emergence of resistant strains of bacteria.[124,125] Both chlorhexidine

and silver sulfadiazine are protective against the most virulent organisms associated with CR-BSI (*S. aureus* and *Candida* species).[121] Despite these favorable laboratory and clinical reports, other studies have failed to demonstrate a benefit from the use of antiseptic-impregnated catheters,[126,127] and reports of hypersensitivity to chlorhexidine have emerged as its use has become more commonplace.[128]

Trooskin and coworkers[129] first demonstrated the feasibility of antibiotic bonding to catheter surfaces.[124] Cefazolin,[129,130] rifampin and minocycline,[131-133] and teicoplanin[134] have all been used to impregnate CVCs to reduce infection. Concern remains that the widespread use of surface antibiotics for preventing CR-BSI may ultimately contribute to the emergence of antibiotic-resistant organisms. The strategy of impregnating catheter surfaces with either antiseptics or antibiotics appears to hold significant promise for future reduction in the rates of catheter colonization and CR-BSI.[125,132,135]

RECOMMENDATIONS

The following recommendations are based on the studies reviewed in this chapter and published CDC guidelines.[2,16]

Physicians in critical care units are encouraged to study their own patient populations to determine the incidence of significant catheter colonization and CR-BSI and to develop appropriate guidelines for catheter exchange and site maintenance. On the basis of currently available information, peripheral arterial catheters, CVCs, and PA catheters do not require "routine" exchange either to a different site or over a guidewire. Although the risk of colonization and bacteremia increases with time, the optimal time for catheter removal is not known for peripheral arterial catheters, CVCs, and PA catheters. Routine catheter exchange in critically ill patients does not alter infection risks.

Recommendations for short-term catheter placement are outlined in Table 145-1.

Any catheter (peripheral or central) that is placed under less than ideal conditions should be treated as a potential source of infection. Generally, such a catheter should be removed and a new catheter inserted at a different site if catheterization is needed for longer than 48 hours. Ideal conditions for catheter insertion include:

- Use of sterile, disposable surgical gowns, masks, hats, and gloves
- Careful preparation of the skin site with an appropriate antiseptic solution
- Wide draping of the area to create an adequate sterile field

The subclavian site is preferred over the internal jugular or femoral site for long-term (>72 hours) catheter use because of the higher colonization rates associated with neck and groin insertion sites. The only exception to this rule is for short-term hemodialysis catheters. In this situation, the internal jugular vein or femoral vein is preferred because of the risk for developing subclavian vein stenosis.

The absolute indication for removal of a catheter is the presence of an unexplained bacteremia. In the critical care setting fever is an unreliable indicator of CR-BSI. The authors believe that guidewire exchange *using the strict protocol described in this chapter* is an acceptable alternative to placing a catheter at a different site, particularly in patients

TABLE 145–1. RECOMMENDATIONS FOR SHORT-TERM CATHETER PLACEMENT

Catheter Type	Preferred Anatomic Site(s) (in Order of Preference)	Frequency of Catheter Exchange	Guidewire Exchange an Option?
Peripheral venous catheter	Upper extremity[†]	72-96 h[†]	No
Emergency peripheral venous catheter*	Upper extremity[†]	24-48 h[†]	No
CVC (single-lumen or multiple-lumen)	Subclavian[†,‡]	Routine replacement not recommended[†,‡]	Yes
	Internal jugular	Routine replacement not recommended[†,‡]	Yes
	Femoral	5 days[‡]	Yes
Peripherally inserted CVC	Upper extremity	Routine replacement not recommended	No
PA catheter and PA catheter introducer	Subclavian[†]	Routine replacement not recommended[†]	Yes
	Internal jugular		
Short-term hemodialysis	Internal jugular[†]	Routine replacement not recommended[†]	No recommendation[†]
	Femoral		
	Subclavian		
Peripheral arterial catheters	Radial[‡]	Routine replacement not recommended[†,‡]	Yes
	Femoral		
	Axillary		

CVC, central venous catheter; PA, pulmonary artery.
*Catheter inserted under emergency conditions, in which sterile preparation may have been less than optimal.
[†]Healthcare Infection Control Practices Advisory Committee guidelines. (Data from O'Grady NP, et al: Am J Infect Control 2002;30:477.[16])
[‡]Author's recommendation.

with difficult or compromised venous access. The most recent CDC guidelines discourage this practice[2,16] because 20% to 25% of catheters removed for suspected infection yield positive semiquantitative culture results. Despite these culture results, less than 10% of catheters removed are associated with CR-BSI.

In our experience, antiseptic-impregnated CVC and PA catheter introducers allow for prolonged catheter use without significantly increasing the risk of CR-BSI over time. Individual institutions and critical care units should review their infection rates and catheter insertion practices to determine whether this readily available technology is cost effective for their patients. We prefer daily site cleansing with 4% chlorhexidine and alcohol, followed by placement of a dry dressing consisting of sterile gauze and occlusive, porous tape. Antibiotic ointments do not seem to provide an added benefit, and there is insufficient evidence to strongly recommend the use of clear plastic dressings over tape and gauze, in terms of preventing infection and reducing costs. Adherence to strict protocols for both catheter insertion site preparation and subsequent catheter maintenance is crucial if catheters are to remain in place for prolonged periods without further increasing the risk for infection in the cohort of critically ill patients requiring vascular access.

ANNOTATED REFERENCES

Centers for Disease Control and Prevention: Guidelines for the Prevention of Intravascular Catheter-Related Infections. MMWR 2002; 51 (No. RR-10): 1-29.

An exhaustive and comprehensive review of catheter-related infections by a multidisciplinary panel of recognized experts. The guidelines are periodically reviewed and revised by the CDC to incorporate new scientific data and clinical recommendations.

Eggimann P, Harbath S, Constantin M, et al: Impact of a prevention strategy targeted at vascular-access care on incidence of infections acquired in intensive care. Lancet 2000;355:1864.
A multidisciplinary strategy to prevent infections from vascular-access devices was undertaken, including educational presentations, practical demonstrations, and the introduction of clinical pathways for inserting, using, and maintaining such devices. Exit site infections decreased dramatically, as did bloodstream infections.

Greenfield JI, Sampath L, Popilskis SJ, et al: Decreased bacterial adherence and biofilm formation on chlorhexidine and silver sulfadiazine-impregnated central venous catheters implanted in swine. Crit Care Med 1995;23(5):894.
An experimental laboratory study documented that antiseptic catheters had significantly fewer moderately and tightly adherent bacteria on outer and luminal catheter surfaces, and that antiseptic catheters prevented the development of a bacterial biofilm. Furthermore, antiseptic-impregnated catheters produced no local or systemic toxicity.

Mermel LA: Prevention of intravascular catheter-related infections. Ann Intern Med 2000;132:391.
Written by an acknowledged expert, this excellent and rigorous review article provides a survey of the recent medical literature.

Norwood S, Wilkins H, Vallina VL, et al: The safety of prolonging the use of central venous catheters: A prospective analysis of the effects of using antiseptic-bonded catheters with daily site care. Crit Care Med 2000;28:1376.
This large, prospective observational study of trauma patients documented that subclavian antiseptic-bonded CVCs may be used safely for more than 14 days when strict protocols for insertion technique and site maintenance are followed. Femoral and internal jugular antiseptic-bonded catheters are prone to earlier bacterial colonization and are not recommended for long-term venous access.

Chapter 146

PATHOPHYSIOLOGY OF SEPSIS AND MULTIPLE ORGAN DYSFUNCTION

K. Reinhart • F. Bloos • F. M. Brunkhorst

KEY POINTS

PATHOPHYSIOLOGY OF SEPSIS

1. Sepsis is an invasion of microorganisms or their toxins into the bloodstream, together with the host response to that invasion.
2. Any infection may be complicated by sepsis.
3. Microorganisms are recognized by their specific molecular patterns (cell wall products, exotoxins, bacterial DNA, viral RNA).
4. The host senses the presence of microbial molecules by specific receptors (i.e., Toll-like receptors).
5. Hyperinflammation is counteracted by an anti-inflammatory response, which may result in hypoinflammation.
6. Hemostatic balance is shifted to a procoagulant state due to activation of tissue factor and attenuation of natural anticoagulants.
7. Sepsis causes endothelial dysfunction, resulting in massive nitric oxide production.
8. Cardiac dysfunction in sepsis is mainly due to intramyocardial nitric oxide production and perhaps cardiac ischemia resulting in left ventricular diastolic dilatation and a rightward shift of the Frank-Starling curve.
9. Sepsis is accompanied by profound arterial hypotension due to massive endothelial nitric oxide production.
10. Microcirculatory dysfunction is a result of intravascular coagulation, endothelial cell swelling, activated leukocytes, and stiff red blood cells.

PATHOPHYSIOLOGY OF MULTIORGAN DYSFUNCTION

1. Multiorgan dysfunction refers to the parallel or sequential failure of at least two organs.
2. Tissue hypoxia is the most important factor in the development of multiorgan dysfunction.
3. Cytokine-induced apoptosis (programmed cell death) contributes to organ dysfunction.

4. Dysfunction of a single organ may affect the integrity of other organs.

PATHOPHYSIOLOGY OF SEPSIS

The term *sepsis* is derived from a Greek word meaning "putrid." It was believed that putrefaction of a wound was caused by contact with air and that death occurred when the process of putrefaction reached the blood (septicemia). In the 19th century, the concept of infection as a cause of sepsis was introduced by the Austrian obstetrician Semmelweis and the British surgeon Lister. From then on, the term *sepsis* was closely connected to bacterial infection. However, as the understanding of human immune physiology improved, the importance of the host response to infection in the pathophysiology of sepsis was recognized.

In this context, sepsis was defined as an invasion of microorganisms or their toxins into the bloodstream, together with the host response to this invasion.[1] Thus, the pathophysiology of sepsis combines the impact of infection with the host response of generalized inflammation, which finally leads to multiorgan dysfunction and death. This definition has been extended by the addition of several terms to more carefully describe the disease and its pathophysiology (Table 146-1). The ACCP/SCCM consensus conference defined sepsis as a systemic inflammatory response syndrome (SIRS) caused by infection.[2] More recently, it has been recognized that SIRS is counteracted by a hypoinflammatory state that also plays an important role in the further development of organ dysfunction.[3]

Sepsis is characterized by loss of hemostatic balance and endothelial dysfunction, which, in turn, severely compromises the cardiocirculatory system as well as intracellular homeostasis. Cellular hypoxia and apoptosis (programmed cell death) are then responsible for organ dysfunction and death. The network of organ systems affected by sepsis is depicted in Figure 146-1.

MICROBIOLOGIC STIMULUS

By definition, infection is a fundamental part of the pathophysiology of sepsis. Invasion by any microorganism able to induce infection in humans may be complicated by sepsis. Bacteria as well as fungi, parasites, and, to a lesser degree, viruses can trigger the mechanisms that lead to sepsis.

TABLE 146–1. DEFINITIONS

Term	Definition
Bacteremia	Presence of viable bacteria in the blood
Systemic inflammatory response syndrome (SIRS)	Generalized hyperinflammatory response to several impacts
Sepsis	SIRS caused by infection
Severe sepsis	Sepsis associated with organ dysfunction
Septic shock	Sepsis associated with arterial hypotension

From ACCP/SCCM Consensus Conference Committee: Definition for sepsis and organ failure and guidelines for the use of innovative therapies in sepsis. Crit Care Med 1992;20:864-874.

Although SIRS is the final common pathway of this process, the signal transduction pathway from infection to the complex host response differs among the microbiologic stimuli. Induction of an innate immune response is triggered by specific microbial molecules (e.g., bacterial wall components, exotoxins, bacterial DNA, viral RNA) called *pathogen-associated molecular patterns*. The presence of such patterns is sensed by recognition molecules called *pattern-recognition proteins*, which are able to initiate a host response. These proteins may be localized on the cell membrane or inside the cell. The Toll-like receptors (TLRs) represent the membrane-bound pattern-recognition proteins. Ten different TLRs have been discovered so far; however, for some TLRs, it is unclear which pathogen-associated molecular patterns they are activated by and what their specific functions are (Table 146-2).[4]

Gram-Negative Sepsis

In Gram-negative bacteremia, initiation of the immune response is mediated primarily by lipopolysaccharide (LPS), a bacterial cell wall product. In plasma, LPS is bound to the LPS binding protein. Bound LPS is transported to the opsonic receptor CD14, which is located on several cell membranes, especially on monocytes.[5] A soluble form of CD14 interacts with CD14-negative cells (i.e., dendritic cells). However, CD14 alone cannot explain the actions of LPS, because CD14 does not have an intracellular tail.

Another binding site of LPS is the transmembranous TLR4, which exists in combination with the accessory protein MD2.[6] The binding of LPS to CD14 and TLR4 induces, via other molecules, activation of nuclear factor kappa-B (NF-κB). Activated NF-κB migrates into the nucleus and activates gene promoter, which results in the transcription of cytokines and other proinflammatory mediators.[7] In monocytes, LPS also induces cytokine transcription via the triggering receptor expressed on myeloid cells-1 and the myeloid DAP12-associated lectin.[8] Intracellular pattern-recognition proteins in monocytes for LPS have recently been identified

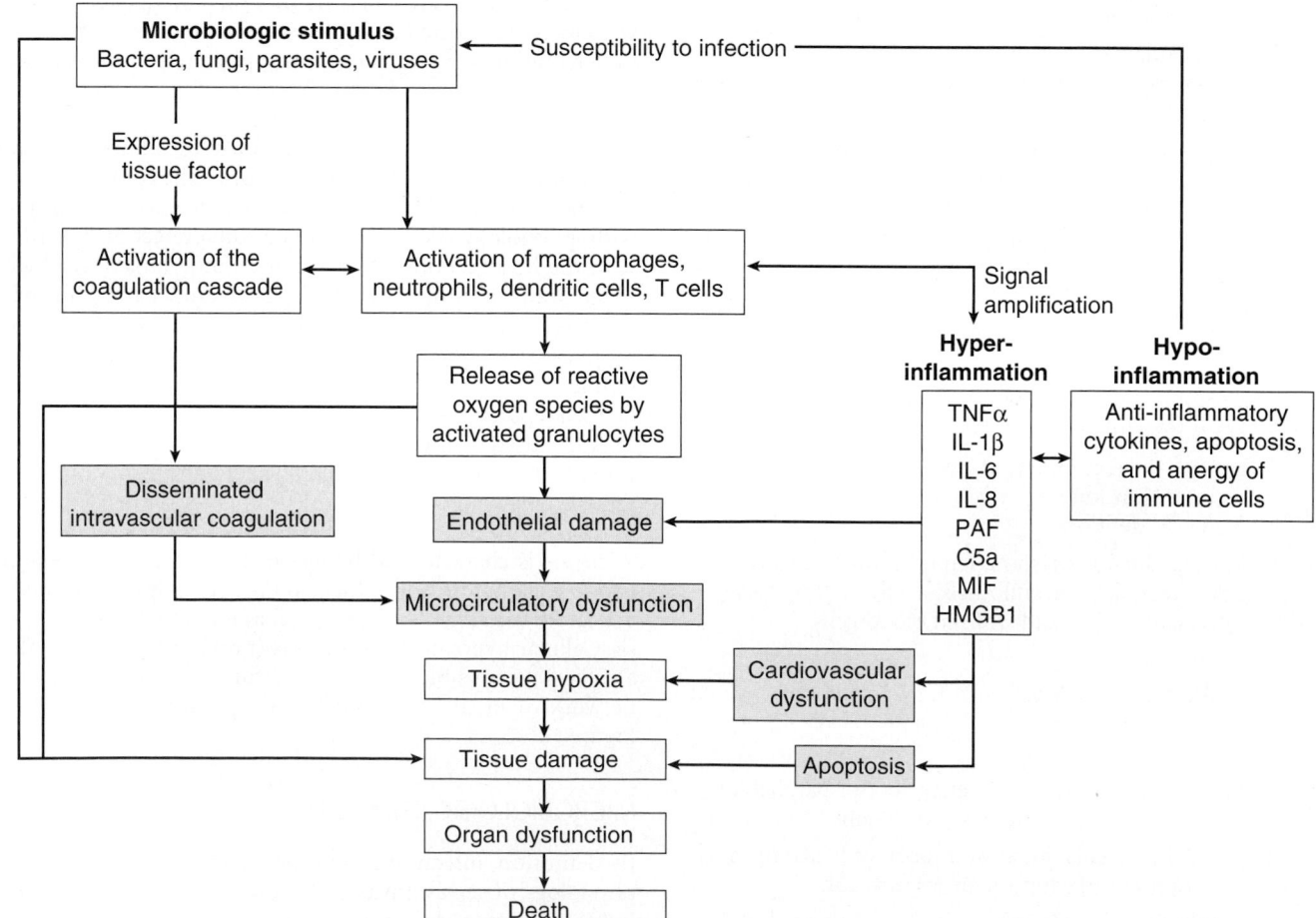

FIGURE 146–1. Pathophysiology of sepsis. HMGB, high-mobility group B protein; IL, interleukin; MIF, migration inhibitory factor; PAF, platelet-activating factor; TNF, tumor necrosis factor.

TABLE 146–2. TOLL-LIKE RECEPTORS (TLRs) AND THEIR NATURAL LIGANDS

TLR Type	Related Pathogen-Associated Molecular Pattern
TLR1 (via TLR2)	Bacterial products
TLR2	Gram-positive bacterial products, including peptidoglycans; some virus-related proteins
TLR3	Viral double-stranded RNA
TLR4	Endotoxin, other bacterial products, some fungal products
TLR5	Flagellin
TLR6 (via TLR2)	Some bacterial products
TLR7	Unknown
TLR8	Unknown
TLR9	Bacterial DNA
TLR10	Unknown

Modified from Heine H, Lien E: Toll-like receptors and their function in innate and adaptive immunity. Int Arch Allergy Immunol 2003;130:180-192.

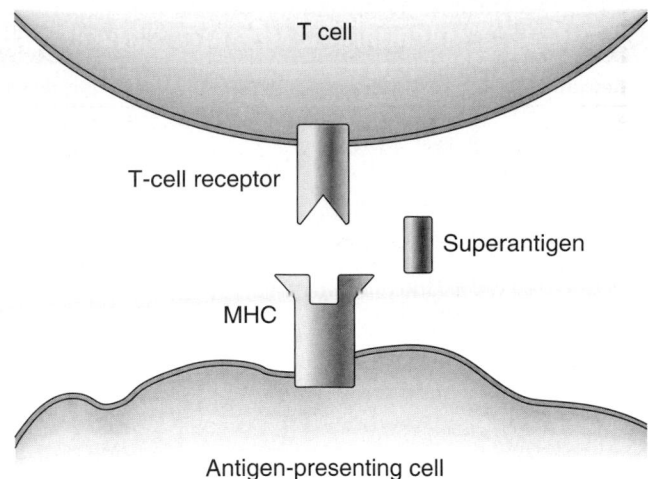

FIGURE 146–2. Pathophysiology of superantigen action. Superantigens work as a bridge between the T-cell receptor and the class 2 histocompatibility molecules (MHC).

as another pathway of cytokine expression, such as nucleotide-binding oligomerization domain 1 and 2 as LPS binding sites.[9]

Gram-Positive Sepsis

During the last decade, Gram-positive bacteria have gained greater importance as causative organisms for sepsis.[10] Gram-positive bacteria lack endotoxin and are recognized by cell wall components such as peptidoglycans and released bacterial toxins (exotoxins). Gram-positive and Gram-negative sepsis are not distinguishable clinically, suggesting a similar pathway of signal transduction. Indeed, the initial recognition of Gram-positive bacteria involves the CD14 receptor.[11] TLR2 has been identified as a pattern-recognition protein for Gram-positive bacteria.[12] The platelet-activating factor receptor also plays a role of signal transduction in some Gram-positive bacteria such as *Streptococcus pneumoniae*.[13] Both CD14 and the platelet-activating factor receptor are capable of initiating cytokine production via the NF-κB pathway.[14]

Some exotoxins cause a special type of septic shock called the toxic shock syndrome (TSS). TSS may be caused by the exotoxin TSS toxin-1, staphylococcal enterotoxins from *Staphylococcus aureus*, or streptococcal pyogenic exotoxins.[15] These toxins are capable of acting as so-called superantigens, which deploy their effects via the T-cell antigen receptor (TCR). The TCR consists of five variable elements: Vβ, Dβ, Jβ, Vα, and Jα. Conventionally, the T cell is activated if the major histocompatibility complex (MHC) of an antigen-presenting cell matches all five elements. Thus, T cells are activated by proper antigen contact only. This results in the stimulation of about 1 in 10,000 T cells. However, a superantigen such as TSS toxin-1 works as a bridge between the MHC and the Vβ-chain of the TCR only (Fig. 146-2). Because T-cell activation now occurs independently of a match between the MHC and TCR, about 20% of the entire T-cell pool may be activated at once. Besides further T-cell proliferation, T-cell activation causes the release of several cytokines, such as interferon-gamma, interleukin (IL)-2, and tumor necrosis factor (TNF) from T cells, as well as IL-1 and TNF from macrophages. Thus, the presence of superantigens ends in a release of cytokines, similar to Gram-negative sepsis. It is assumed that actions other than cytokine production may be responsible for superantigen actions in TSS; for example, superantigens may amplify the effects of LPS.[8]

Other Microbiologic Stimuli of Sepsis

Sepsis can also be induced by fungi, viruses, and parasites. Signal transduction by nonbacterial products, however, is not as well investigated as in bacterial sepsis. In part, this may be due to the fact that induction of cytokine release differs markedly not only among these microbiologic classes but also among species. Nevertheless, the release of proinflammatory mediators has been demonstrated during infections with *Candida albicans*,[16] coxsackie B virus,[17] and *Plasmodium falciparum*.[18] The signal transduction in viral infections is complicated by the fact that viruses can interfere with TNF-related cytokine release to avoid the host's antiviral activities.[19] Nevertheless, some pattern-recognition proteins were found to be responsible for virus recognition. Most importantly, TLR3 is able to sense viral double-stranded RNA.[4]

Cytokine response in *Candida* sepsis may be related to the binding of *C. albicans* to laminin. The protein laminin is a structural component in the basement membrane meshwork. It also has several biologic functions, such as cell differentiation, adhesion, migration, and proliferation. Hyphae express different sites that induce binding of *C. albicans* to laminin.[20] For *Aspergillus fumigatus* and *Cryptococcus*, TLR4 has been found to sense the presence of these fungi.[4]

THE IMMUNE RESPONSE IN SEPSIS

The cytokines TNF and IL-1 are released by activated macrophages and CD4 T cells within the first hour after infection. These primary mediators induce the release of several secondary mediators that amplify the signal of inflammation (Table 146-3). An important step in signal amplification is the activation of the complement system. Besides being activated by antigen-antibody complexes, the complement system may be stimulated by bacterial surface sugars and endotoxin. The complement fragment C5a, a cleavage product of the complement cascade, is a strong chemoattractant. C5a appears about 2 hours after the initiation of sepsis and stimulates macrophages to further produce proinflammatory mediators. Another mediator that amplifies the immune response is the macrophage migration inhibitory factor, which is produced by T cells, macrophages, monocytes, and pituitary cells in response to an infectious stimulus. Migration inhibitory

TABLE 146–3. MACROPHAGE MEDIATORS INVOLVED IN THE PATHOGENESIS OF SEPSIS

Mediator	Typical Effects
Cytokines IL-1, IL-6, IL-12, IL-15, IL-18, TNF, MIF, HMGB1, IL-10	Activate neutrophils, lymphocytes, and vascular endothelium; up-regulate cellular adhesion molecules; induce prostaglandins, nitric oxide synthase, and acute-phase proteins; induce fever IL-10 is predominantly a negative regulator of these effects
Chemokines IL-8, MIP-1α, MIP-1β, MCP-1, MCP-3	Mobilize and activate inflammatory cells, especially neutrophils; activate macrophages
Lipid mediators Platelet-activating factor, prostaglandins, leukotrienes, thromboxane, tissue factor	Activate vascular endothelium; regulate vascular tone; activate extrinsic coagulation cascade
Oxygen radicals Superoxide and hydroxyl radicals, nitric oxide	Antimicrobial properties; regulation of vascular tone

HMGB, high-mobility group B protein; IL, interleukin; MCP, monocyte chemoattractant protein; MIF, migration inhibitory factor; MIP, macrophage inflammatory protein; TNF, tumor necrosis factor.
From Cohen J: The immunopathogenesis of sepsis. Nature 2002;420:885-891.

factor appears about 8 hours after the onset of sepsis and activates T cells and macrophages to produce proinflammatory mediators. About 24 hours after the initiation of sepsis, levels of high-mobility group B1 protein increase and appear to play a role in endotoxin-related sepsis. High-mobility group B1 protein is a nuclear binding protein that, among other things, is capable of activating NF-κB. As a rather late mediator in sepsis, it is produced by macrophages and neutrophils and stimulates other phagocytic cells.[21]

Normally, the inflammatory process is well balanced and is necessary for the host to overcome the infectious impact. However, under certain conditions, the amplification process of inflammation is not limited to the site of infection and becomes generalized. This phenomenon has been called the systemic inflammatory response syndrome. SIRS is not restricted to infectious stimuli; it is present in a variety of other conditions, such as pancreatitis, burns, multiple trauma, and in patients undergoing heart surgery with cardiopulmonary bypass. Sepsis has been defined as SIRS due to an infectious stimulus.[2] The existence of genetic polymorphisms involving LPS binding sites or cytokines has an impact on the immunologic response in sepsis. Polymorphisms have been demonstrated for the TNF promoter IL-1Ra, CD14, TLR4, and LPS binding protein. Some of these polymorphisms seem to be associated with a higher mortality from sepsis or a greater susceptibility for sepsis.[8]

The immune response in sepsis does not involve only proinflammatory mediators. As in many other physiologic processes, the organism produces inhibitors to control certain reactions. Proinflammatory mediators are counteracted by anti-inflammatory molecules such as IL-4 and IL-10, because CD4 T cells can switch from the production of inflammatory cytokines (type 1 helper T cells) to the production of anti-inflammatory cytokines (type 2 helper T cells). Soluble TNF receptors and IL-1 receptor antagonists are released to inhibit the actions of the primary mediators of sepsis. T cells, neutrophils, and macrophages also may become unresponsive to infectious stimuli (anergy). Another mechanism of the anti-inflammatory response is the onset of apoptosis, a genetically programmed autodestructive release of proteases that induce cell death. In sepsis, apoptosis of immune cells such as CD4 T cells and follicular dendritic cells has been observed.[3] Absolute lymphocyte counts are significantly decreased in patients with sepsis.[22] Further, apoptotic cells impair the function of surviving immune cells.[23] The induction of apoptosis in sepsis is described in more detail in the section Pathophysiology of Multiorgan Dysfunction.

The anti-inflammatory response in sepsis has been termed the *compensatory anti-inflammatory response syndrome.*[24] It has been suggested that the first response to infection is hyperinflammation, which is followed by a hypoimmune state. From there, recovery would be possible, but the prolonged inability to eradicate microorganisms might result in the death of the patient.[3] However, serum levels of anti-inflammatory cytokines are increased in parallel with the increase of proinflammatory mediators.[25] Thus, anti-inflammation develops at the same time as the process of hyperinflammation. Although the persistence of high levels of anti-inflammatory mediators may contribute to mortality in these patients, the clinical role of a cyclic change between hyper- and hypoinflammation remains unclear.

LOSS OF HEMOSTATIC BALANCE

Sepsis is accompanied by activation of the coagulation cascade via the tissue factor– and factor VII–dependent generation of thrombin. Tissue factor is a 4.5-kDa protein that is bound to cell membranes, which are normally not in contact with blood. Tissue factor is capable of activating factor VII, which activates further steps in the extrinsic coagulation pathway. Activated factor VI of the extrinsic pathway activates factor XI of the intrinsic pathway (cross-talk), and thrombin is capable of activating factors VIII and XI of the intrinsic pathway (feedback). Thus, whereas the extrinsic pathway initiates coagulation, the intrinsic pathway serves as an amplifier of coagulation.[26]

Under normal conditions, the vascular luminal surface has anticoagulant properties. However, several cytokines as well as acute-phase proteins such as C-reactive protein, induce tissue factor expression on monocytes, neutrophils, and endothelial cells.[27-29] This induces intravascular thrombin formation initiated by the extrinsic pathway. Further thrombin generation is then maintained by the intrinsic pathway due to cross-talk and feedback. Because this process is not restricted to a local area, it is called disseminated intravascular coagulation. Disseminated intravascular coagulation causes a consumption of coagulation factors that may be followed by spontaneous bleeding. However, severe bleeding disorders are rare in septic patients (<3%).[30] The embolization of microvessels by the continuous and latent coagulation is believed to be more important, because it may be relevant in the development of microcirculatory dysfunction and organ failure. However, no direct evidence of this phenomenon is available.[31]

Physiologically, excessive coagulation is counteracted by several natural anticoagulants including antithrombin III, the thrombomodulin–protein C–protein S system, and tissue factor pathway inhibitor. In addition to the activation of tissue factor–dependent thrombin generation, anticoagulant function is attenuated in sepsis. Patients with sepsis demonstrate reduced levels of protein C and antithrombin III, due to consumption and reduced synthesis.[32,33] Thus, the physiologic balance between pro- and anticoagulant substances is altered in sepsis as there is a shift of the hemostatic balance toward a procoagulant state (Fig. 146-3).

Besides its anticoagulant actions, the protein C pathway is an important link between coagulation and inflammation, because activated protein C also seems to have anti-inflammatory properties. There is evidence that activated protein C reduces the production of cytokines such as TNF and IL-1, interferes with the LPS-CD14 interaction, and inhibits the response of macrophages to LPS.[34] The likely mode of action has been demonstrated in experimental sepsis, where activated protein C was able to block the migration of NF-κB into the nucleus.[35] Migration of NF-κB is an important step in the gene expression of cytokines (see Fig. 146-1). As mentioned earlier, protein C levels are significantly depressed in sepsis, supporting the hypothesis of loss of inflammatory control in this disease. However, the clinical importance of the anti-inflammatory actions of activated protein C in the pathophysiology of sepsis remains unclear.

ENDOTHELIAL DYSFUNCTION

Besides separating blood from tissue, endothelial cells have multiple physiologic functions involving the regulation of vascular tone, coagulation, and immune response.

The endothelium produces several vasoactive mediators, including nitric oxide (NO), prostacyclins, and endothelin. NO is a potent vasodilator that is produced by NO synthase (NOS) from the amino acid L-arginine. NO directly relaxes the vessel's smooth muscles. There are two different forms of endothelial NOS: the constitutional form (cNOS) and the inducible form (iNOS). Physiologically, cNOS—also referred to as endothelial NOS (eNOS)—produces only small amounts

of NO, and iNOS is expressed at low levels.[36] In sepsis, iNOS expression is stimulated by cytokines such as IL-1 and TNF.[37] This is followed by massive NO production and profound vasodilatation. Whether increased activity of cNOS also plays a role in sepsis is currently a matter of debate. During inflammation, endothelial cells express adhesion molecules on their surface, which causes the adherence of leukocytes. These adhesion molecules include endothelial leukocyte adhesion molecule-1, intracellular adhesion molecule-1, and vascular cell adhesion molecule-1. Endothelial leukocyte adhesion molecule-1 is a selectin that mediates the initial step of leukocyte adhesion, followed by leukocyte rolling along the endothelial surface. The leukocyte finally migrates through the endothelial layer into the tissue, mediated by intracellular adhesion molecule-1 and vascular cell adhesion molecule-1 expression on both endothelial cells and leukocytes.[38]

Migration of leukocytes into the tissue is a physiologic mechanism to move immune cells to the site of infection. However, in generalized inflammation, such as in sepsis, endothelial cells in several organs remote from the site of infection express adhesion molecules, inducing a generalized rolling and sticking of circulating leukocytes to the vascular surface. Adherence to endothelial cells activates leukocytes and induces a respiratory burst.[39] The respiratory burst involves the release of cytotoxic substances such as elastase, myeloperoxidase, and reactive oxygen species. These products are capable of damaging endothelial cells and the surrounding tissue. Endothelial cell damage causes capillary leakage whereby intravascular fluid penetrates the extracellular space, leading to tissue edema.

Endothelial cells have an anticoagulant surface produced by the expression of heparan sulfate on the cell membrane, release of plasminogen activator, and production of protein C. However, sepsis shifts the hemostatic balance toward a procoagulatory state. Endothelial cells share in this process by expressing tissue factor (see the previous section, Loss of Hemostatic Balance).

CARDIOCIRCULATORY DYSFUNCTION

Sepsis is frequently complicated by organ dysfunction and shock. Shock occurs when the cardiocirculatory system is

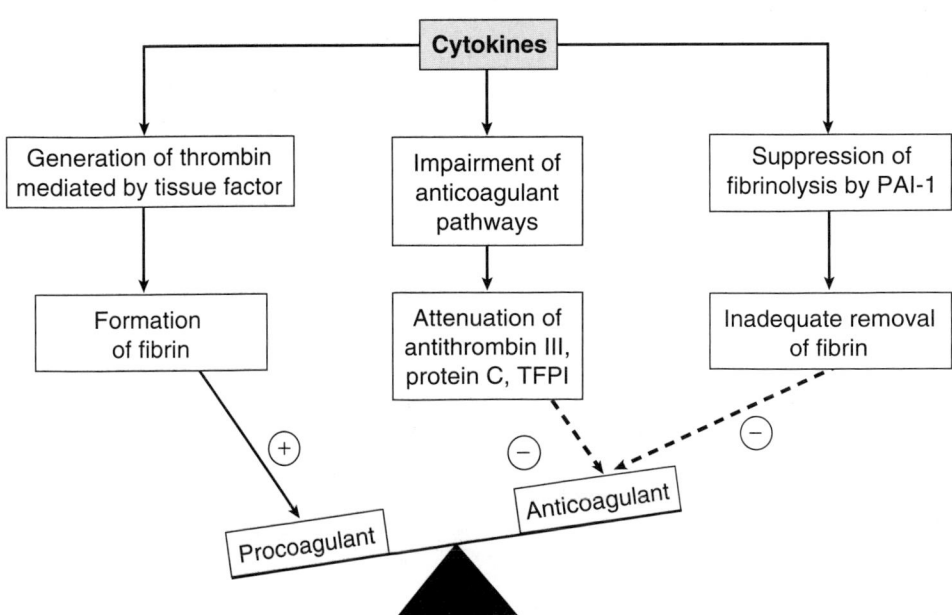

FIGURE 146–3. Shift of the hemostatic balance toward a procoagulant state in sepsis. PAI, plasminogen activator inhibitor; TFPI, tissue factor pathway inhibitor. (Modified from Levi M, Ten Cate H: Disseminated intravascular coagulation. N Engl J Med 1999;341:586-592.)

unable to transport sufficient amounts of oxygen to the tissues. In fact, sepsis compromises all levels of the cardiovascular system, resulting in cardiac dysfunction, vascular dysregulation, and microcirculatory damage. Impairment of the cardiovascular system causes a characteristic hemodynamic pattern that, in cases of adequate fluid loading and the absence of severe preexisting cardiac dysfunction, consists of a high cardiac output, arterial hypotension, and a low systemic oxygen (O_2) extraction. In sepsis, O_2 consumption is increased owing to higher metabolic needs (i.e., tachypnea, fever, increased cardiac work, increased rate of protein synthesis), further compromising the relationship between O_2 supply and demand (Fig. 146-4). The hepatic and splanchnic region is markedly affected by these changes associated with sepsis. Hepatosplanchnic O_2 uptake increases markedly during fever and bacteremia.[40]

Cardiac Dysfunction

In experimental septic shock, myocardial contractility is compromised shortly after the induction of sepsis.[41] This finding is confirmed in septic patients when a reduced ejection fraction is observed by echocardiography. The drop in myocardial contractility is accompanied by diastolic dilatation of the left ventricle, which causes the left ventricular end-diastolic volume to rise. This mechanism allows the heart to maintain a sufficient stroke volume despite impaired contractility. Clinically, a rightward shift of the Frank-Starling curve occurs. Thus, compared with healthy humans, patients with sepsis require greater cardiac filling pressures to maintain a similar stroke volume.[42] Septic patients without compensatory left ventricular dilatation have a significantly greater risk of death.[43] Cardiac dysfunction is reversible if the patient recovers from sepsis.

The presence of myocardial depressant substances was initially proposed in the 1980s, because the serum of septic patients was able to suppress the contractility of rat myocytes in vitro.[44] It was then discovered that cytokines such as TNF and IL-1 were responsible for these actions. As stated earlier, cytokines induce increased activation of iNOS, with subsequent enhanced NO production. NO affects myocytes in several ways: NO stimulates guanylate cyclase, and its product 3′,5′-cyclic guanosine monophosphate interferes with intracellular myocardial calcium metabolism. This includes a reduction in calcium's affinity to the contractile apparatus and an inhibition of the alpha-adrenergic–mediated increase in the slow inward calcium current. NO may directly damage myocardial cells by the formation of peroxynitrite via combination with superoxide ions. Peroxynitrite deploys toxic effects on many intracellular molecules by means of oxidation.[45,46] Another pathway of cytokine-mediated negative inotropy is the stimulation of intracellular sphingosine production by TNF.[47]

Sepsis is associated with alterations of regional and microregional blood flow, which results in a mismatch between regional O_2 supply and demand and, subsequently, multiple organ dysfunction (see later). It was therefore hypothesized that the heart shares in this type of injury. Although there were hints from experimental work that the coronary circulatory reserve is altered in sepsis,[48] clinical studies did not show a compromised coronary blood flow.[49,50] However, more recently it was demonstrated that patients with sepsis show elevated levels of troponin T.[51] This points to the fact that myocardial ischemia might exist despite normal coronary blood flow.

Vascular Dysfunction and Hypovolemia

In cardiogenic or hypovolemic shock, vasoconstriction is a common mechanism to avoid arterial hypotension. In sepsis, however, profound arterial vasodilatation occurs. Endothelial cells play an important role in the regulation of vascular tone because they release several vasoactive substances, such as NO and endothelin. Sepsis shifts the balance of these substances toward a vasodilatory state by uncontrolled NO production (discussed earlier). Severe arterial hypotension caused by profound systemic vasodilatation is one of the characteristic hemodynamic features of sepsis. The mechanism by which NO induces vasodilatation is complex. Important pathways include the activation of potassium channels and hyperpolarization of the plasma membrane of smooth muscle cells. These mechanisms, in turn, inhibit the actions of vasopressors

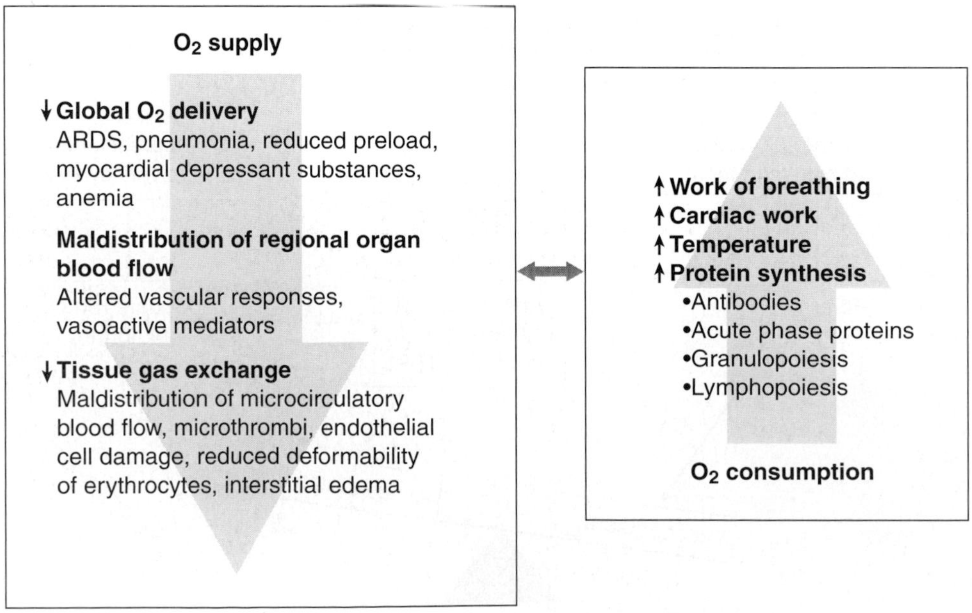

O₂ supply

↓ **Global O₂ delivery**
ARDS, pneumonia, reduced preload, myocardial depressant substances, anemia

Maldistribution of regional organ blood flow
Altered vascular responses, vasoactive mediators

↓ **Tissue gas exchange**
Maldistribution of microcirculatory blood flow, microthrombi, endothelial cell damage, reduced deformability of erythrocytes, interstitial edema

↑ **Work of breathing**
↑ **Cardiac work**
↑ **Temperature**
↑ **Protein synthesis**
•Antibodies
•Acute phase proteins
•Granulopoiesis
•Lymphopoiesis

O₂ consumption

FIGURE 146–4. The cardiocirculatory system of a septic patient is altered on the systemic, regional, and microregional levels. At the same time, sepsis increases O_2 consumption, further deteriorating the O_2 supply-demand relationship. ARDS, acute respiratory distress syndrome.

such as norepinephrine and angiotensin II, so that vasoconstriction does not occur despite high serum concentrations of these substances.[52]

Endothelial cells regulate vascular tone not only to maintain systemic blood pressure but also to control blood flow to single organs. Several mechanisms to preserve organ blood flow are impaired in sepsis. For example, there is a loss of coupling between the hepatic artery flow and the portal blood flow in endotoxic shock.[53] Similarly, the coronary circulatory reserve necessary to quickly adjust myocardial O_2 supply based on changes in myocardial O_2 requirements is reduced in sepsis.[48] The autoregulation of the intestinal perfusion of the mucosa is also depressed in experimental models of sepsis.[54]

Sepsis is accompanied by the development of significant tissue edema. The underlying mechanism is capillary leakage, which is another effect of endothelial damage.[55] This leakage also allows for the extravasation of albumin,[56] which reduces the intravascular oncotic pressure. Under conditions of capillary leakage, the Starling forces cannot counteract the development of tissue edema or reduce existing edema. Because endothelial damage affects all parts of the capillary network throughout the body, large amounts of intravascular fluid are shifted into the third space.

Microcirculatory Dysfunction

Severe sepsis and septic shock may be associated with high lactate levels and metabolic acidosis, despite a low systemic O_2 extraction. These signs of tissue hypoxia, which may be observed despite adequate fluid resuscitation, are interpreted as microcirculatory failure. Some parts of the microcirculation are extremely sensitive to physiologic stress, including hypoxia or ischemia. These areas are referred to as weak microcirculatory units.[57]

An increase in the number of weak microcirculatory units—and therefore increased microcirculatory shunting—is believed to play a major role in the O_2 extraction deficit in sepsis. This hypothesis has been confirmed in experimental sepsis. By using intravital microscopy, an increased number of capillaries with lack of flow was observed in septic animals.[58,59] More recently, capillary red blood cell oxygenation was measured in vivo by a spectrophotometric functional imaging system.[60] In the presence of sepsis, an increased proportion of perfused capillaries showed very high red blood cell velocities. These high-flow capillaries were interpreted as microcirculatory shunts. The remaining capillaries with normal flow showed a fivefold increase in O_2 extraction. However, this increase in O_2 extraction was insufficient to maintain O_2 supply to all regions, given the number of capillaries without flow.

Several factors may be responsible for microcirculatory shunting in sepsis. The underlying mechanism is the hindrance of blood flow by microvascular obstruction, which has several causes: (1) the onset of intravascular coagulation due to a shift to a procoagulant state causes the development of microthrombi[31]; (2) activation and damage of endothelial cells lead to endothelial cell swelling, narrowing the capillary lumen[61]; (3) activated leukocytes hinder red blood cell flow by rolling and sticking to endothelial cells[62]; and (4) red blood cells have reduced deformability in sepsis, which causes them to be captured in capillaries.[63]

Although there is good evidence from experimental work supporting the hypothesis of microcirculatory dysfunction in sepsis, there is considerable debate whether the O_2 extraction

TABLE 146–4. CHANGES IN HORMONE CONCENTRATIONS IN CRITICALLY ILL PATIENTS

Hormone	Acute Critical Illness	Prolonged Critical Illness
Catecholamines	++	+
Cortisol	++	+
Adrenocorticotropic hormone	Ø +	Ø –
Growth hormone	Ø –	–
Thyroid hormones	Ø –	–
Thyroid-stimulating hormone	Ø –	–
Androgen hormones	–	–
Prolactin	–	Unknown

From Ligtenberg JJ, Girbes AR, Beentjes JA, et al: Hormones in the critically ill patient: To intervene or not to intervene? Intensive Care Med 2001;27: 1567-1577.

deficit is due to a derangement of intracellular metabolic pathways rather than to microcirculatory dysfunction.[64,65] This hypothesis is contradicted by the fact that some capillaries are able to increase their O_2 extraction.[60] However, the assessment of tissue oxygenation on the cellular level is problematic, even in the experimental setting. Currently, it is believed that microcirculatory dysfunction has at least some part in the development of tissue hypoxia in sepsis. Clinically, this hypothesis is supported by the finding that early resuscitation guided by the central venous O_2 saturation improves survival in these patients.[66]

ENDOCRINE DYSFUNCTION

As depicted in Table 146-4, critical illness is associated with alterations in several endocrine functions. It is not clear whether these changes represent a physiologic response to critical illness or reflect a complex picture of endocrine dysfunction that needs diagnostic and treatment strategies. In sepsis, however, adrenal insufficiency and vasopressin deficiency contribute to the loss of vasomotor control.

Adrenal Insufficiency

Adrenal corticosteroids are involved in several physiologic pathways in the human body, including maintenance of vascular tone, vascular permeability, and distribution of total body water. In the clinical setting, corticosteroids also augment the effects of vasopressors.[67] Under normal conditions, they are secreted by the adrenal cortex in a diurnal pattern. Corticosteroid secretion is tightly controlled by a feedback mechanism called the hypothalamic-pituitary-adrenal axis (Fig. 146-5). However, several mechanisms may impair the physiologic stress response of the hypothalamic-pituitary-adrenal axis in critically ill patients (see Fig. 146-5), resulting in an inadequate increase of serum cortisol levels. This condition is referred to as relative adrenal insufficiency.[68]

Although the concept of relative adrenal insufficiency is a matter of debate, it has been demonstrated that an inadequate rise of cortisol after the corticotropin stimulation test is associated with an increased mortality in patients with septic shock.[69] Further, if these patients are treated with a stress dosage of hydrocortisone plus fludrocortisone, their survival rates increase.[70]

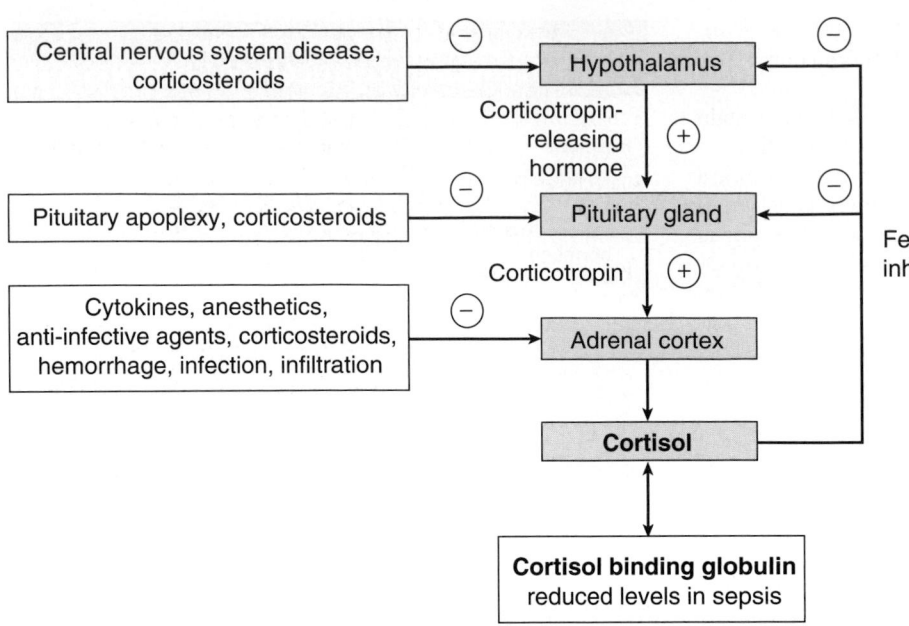

FIGURE 146–5. Hypothalamic-pituitary-adrenal axis. The physiologic control of cortisol release and its feedback mechanism are illustrated. This axis may be impaired on all levels in critically ill patients. +, stimulation; –, inhibition. (Modified from Cooper MS, Stewart PM: Corticosteroid insufficiency in acutely ill patients. N Engl J Med 2003;348:727-734.)

Vasopressin Deficiency

Vasopressin is excreted from the neurohypophysis in response to arterial hypotension or hypovolemia. Because septic shock is characterized by both arterial hypotension and hypovolemia, one would expect plasma vasopressin levels to be high; however, they are low in patients with septic shock.[71] Indeed, the administration of vasopressin or analogs can quickly restore blood pressure in these patients.[72] The pathophysiology of low vasopressin levels is not completely clear. Possible mechanisms include depression of the baroreflex, increased metabolism of vasopressin, and depletion of vasopressin stores in the pituitary gland.

Vasopressin is metabolized by plasma vasopressinase and by renal and hepatic clearance. Increased vasopressin metabolism seems unlikely in sepsis, because renal and hepatic functions are often compromised in this setting, and there is no evidence of increased vasopressinase activity in this disease. Depression of the baroreflex may play a role in vasopressin depletion. The baroreflex is mediated by sympathetic stimulation, and there is some evidence that sympathetic function might be impaired in sepsis.[73] This hypothesis is supported by the finding that in three septic shock patients with low plasma vasopressin levels, magnetic resonance imaging of the brain demonstrated low neurohypophysial concentrations.[74] In experimental septic shock, extremely high vasopressin levels are measured shortly after endotoxin infusion. This is followed by a marked drop in vasopressin levels, suggesting an exhaustion of vasopressin stores.[75,76] It is unknown whether such a process occurs in human sepsis.

Insulin Deficiency

Hyperglycemia is a common feature in critically ill patients, such as those with severe sepsis or septic shock. Although hyperglycemia may represent an adaptation to increased metabolism, there is evidence that pancreatic beta-cell function is impaired, causing inadequate serum insulin concentrations. Besides its effects on glucose utilization, insulin interferes with several pathways of the immune response, including inhibition of TNF and intracellular signal transduction by NF-κB.[77,78] Insulin also improves the function of macrophages. Thus, an insulin deficiency might be unfavorable in sepsis. In addition, the negative effects of hyperglycemia itself, such as reduced granulocyte function, delayed wound healing, and higher frequency of infections, can have an adverse effect on morbidity.

Treating critically ill patients with insulin to keep glucose levels in the physiologic range reduces the frequency of bloodstream infections and mortality rates, compared with patients whose glucose levels are elevated.[79] This may prove the hypothesis of the unfavorable effects of hypoinsulinemia. However, it is currently unclear whether the mortality reduction is an effect of normoglycemia or some immunologic action of insulin.

PATHOPHYSIOLOGY OF MULTIORGAN DYSFUNCTION

Multiorgan dysfunction is the parallel or sequential failure of at least two organs. It is a frequent complication of sepsis. Clinically, multiorgan dysfunction is termed the multiple organ dysfunction syndrome (MODS). MODS can involve any organ of a critically ill patient, even a remote organ that was not originally affected by the underlying disease. The development of MODS significantly contributes to ICU mortality. Scoring systems such as the Sequential Organ Failure Assessment or the Multiorgan Dysfunction Score, which assess the severity of MODS, correlate well with mortality.[80,81]

Some major components of the pathophysiology of MODS are depicted in Figure 146-6. The development of MODS includes a complicated network of inter- and intracellular actions. Because MODS can involve a variety of pathologic changes, different concepts of the pathophysiology of MODS have been generated (Table 146-5).[82]

Cellular dysfunction due to tissue hypoxia is likely an important factor in the onset of MODS. However, other factors also play a role, including the onset of programmed cell death (apoptosis) and the direct toxic effects of substances such as endotoxin and O_2 radicals. The development of SIRS does not require the presence of infection; severe trauma, burns, pancreatitis, and cardiac surgery with cardiopulmonary bypass are also associated with SIRS and increase the risk for MODS.[2,83]

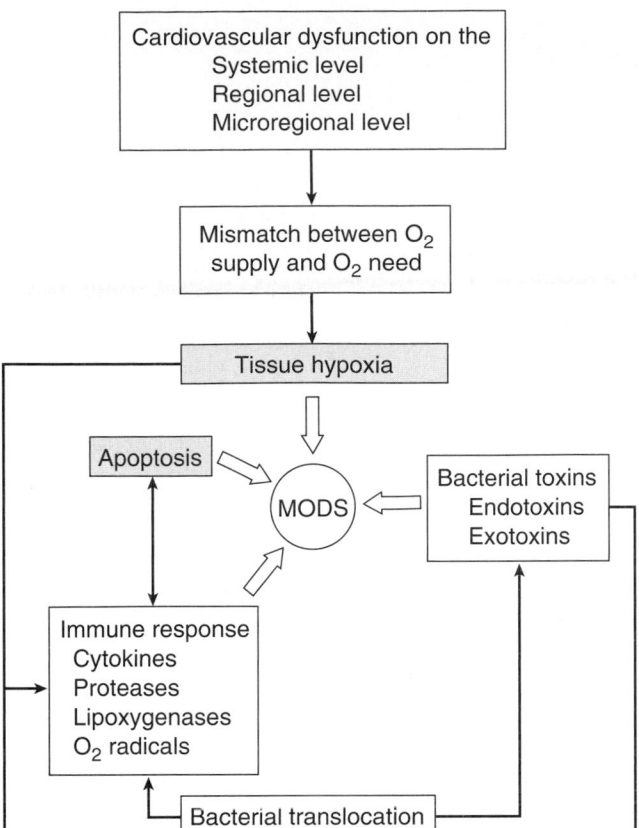

FIGURE 146–6. Pathophysiology of multiple organ dysfunction syndrome (MODS).

blood flow will persist or even progress if the underlying disease (e.g., sepsis) cannot be treated successfully. Tissue hypoxia may therefore be present even though treatment goals for adequate systemic hemodynamics have been achieved.

Tissue hypoxia is difficult to assess in a critically ill patient. It is therefore uncertain whether tissue hypoxia plays a leading role in organ dysfunction, because other mechanisms such as apoptosis have been identified as well.[84] In addition, it has been suggested that disturbance of mitochondrial O_2 utilization rather than tissue hypoxia is the motor of organ dysfunction. This hypothesis is supported by the observation that depletion of enzymes of the respiratory chain is associated with the development of MODS in septic patients.[85] Nevertheless, data are available that demonstrate the importance of tissue oxygenation in the development of MODS. For example, when central venous O_2 saturation was used to guide aggressive treatment to maintain O_2 delivery, there was a significant reduction in mortality,[66] supporting the concept of tissue hypoxia as an important mechanism in MODS. Further, critically ill patients who are unable to achieve an O_2 delivery of more than 600 mL/min/m² have an increased risk of death.[86] The onset of intestinal hypoperfusion, measured by a drop in gastric intramucosal pH, is also associated with higher mortality rates.[87]

APOPTOSIS

Apoptosis is a physiologic mechanism whereby activation of a specific DNA program induces cell death. Apoptosis is therefore a regulatory process for the proliferation and differentiation of cells. However, pathologic activation of apoptosis seems to be involved in the pathogenesis of MODS. Apoptosis is induced by a cascade system through either an extrinsic (receptor-dependent) or an intrinsic (receptor-independent) pathway. The extrinsic pathway is activated by the so-called death receptor superfamily, consisting of receptors such as the Fas-receptor (CD95) or the TNF-receptor. The intrinsic pathway may be induced by DNA damage. The process of apoptosis is mediated by an enzymatic cascade system in which active caspase-3 is the executioner protein that finally starts apoptosis. The receptors of the extrinsic pathway mediate the activation of procaspase-8 to active caspase-8 via several signaling proteins (Fig. 146-7). The intrinsic pathway works by altering the mitochondrial membrane potential through the signal protein p53, which mediates the activation of caspase-9. Both active caspase-8 and active caspase-9 activate the final common step in the apoptosis pathway (caspase-3).[88]

TISSUE HYPOXIA

As discussed previously, the host response to infection severely impairs the cardiovascular system through the development of cardiac dysfunction, systemic and regional vascular dysregulation, and microcirculatory damage. Systemic hemodynamics can be restored by measures such as fluid resuscitation or treatment with catecholamines. However, no clinically available measures allow for a differential diagnosis of regional or microregional disturbances of blood flow, nor are therapies available to specifically address such disturbances. Thus, microcirculatory dysfunction and maldistribution of regional

---

TABLE 146–5. CONCEPTUAL MODELS OF MULTIPLE ORGAN DYSFUNCTION

Pathologic Process	Manifestation
Uncontrolled infection	Persistent infection, nosocomial acquired infection, endotoxemia
Systemic inflammation	Cytokinemia (particularly IL-6, IL-8, TNF), leukocytosis, increased capillary permeability
Immune paralysis	Nosocomial infection, increased anti-inflammatory cytokine levels (IL-10), decreased HLA-DR expression; shift from type 1 to type 2 helper T cells
Tissue hypoxia	Increased lactate, low central venous O_2 saturation
Microvascular coagulopathy and endothelial dysfunction	Increased procoagulant activity, decreased anticoagulant activity (antithrombin III ↓, protein C ↓), high levels of fibrin derivatives, increased von Willebrand's factor, soluble thrombomodulin, increased capillary permeability
Dysregulated apoptosis	Increased epithelial and lymphoid apoptosis, decreased neutrophil apoptosis
Gut-liver axis	Increased infection with gut organisms, endotoxemia, Kupffer cell activation

IL, interleukin; TNF, tumor necrosis factor.
Modified from Marshall JC: Inflammation, coagulopathy, and the pathogenesis of multiple organ dysfunction syndrome. Crit Care Med 2001;29(7 Suppl):S99-S106.

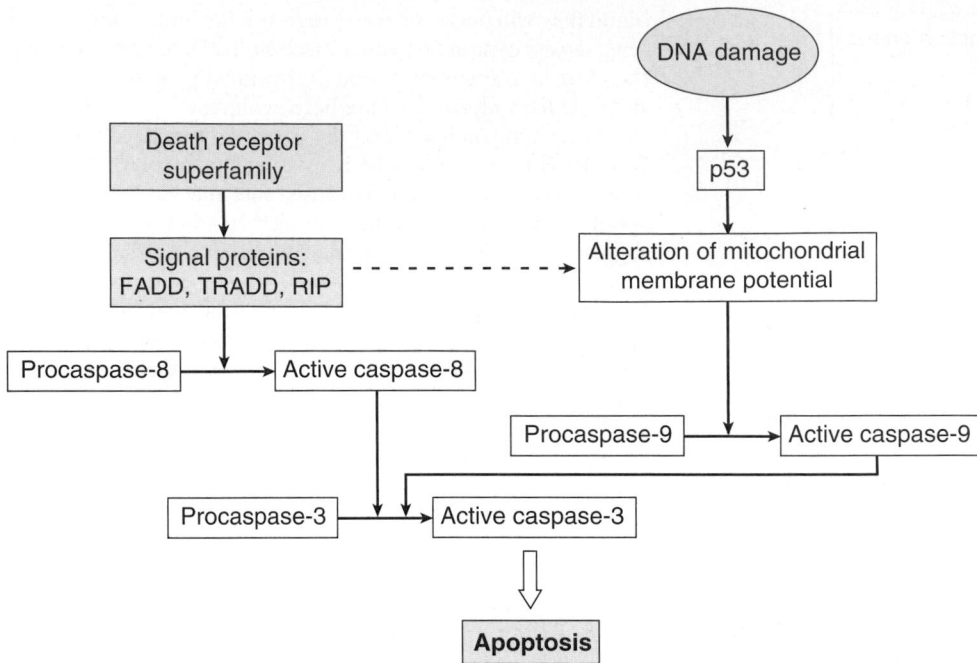

FIGURE 146–7. Extrinsic and intrinsic signaling process for apoptosis. FADD, Fas-associated death domain protein; RIP, receptor interacting protein; TRADD, TNF receptor 1–associated death protein. (Modified from Partrick DA, Moore FA, Moore EE, et al: Neutrophil priming and activation in the pathogenesis of postinjury multiple organ failure. New Horiz 1996;4:194-210.)

The extent to which apoptosis-related cell death contributes to the development of MODS is difficult to assess, because this pathomechanism has been investigated mainly in the experimental setting. However, there is some evidence that several substances present during SIRS can induce apoptosis in vitro. Hepatic cells in particular seem to be extremely vulnerable to endotoxin-related apoptosis.[89] Apoptosis of renal tubular cells has been observed after exposure to *Escherichia coli* toxins.[90]

THE "TWO-HIT" THEORY

Any severe impact to the human body, such as a traumatic or surgical injury or prolonged shock, can directly induce the development of organ dysfunction. Possible pathomechanisms include ischemia, reperfusion injury, or immediate tissue destruction due to trauma. Such an event is called a "first hit." This first hit may be severe enough to induce SIRS, with all the consequences to the cardiocirculatory system and cellular functions mentioned earlier.

Even if the first hit does not induce a primary MODS, a "second hit," such as an infectious insult (e.g., pneumonia, bacteremia due to catheter infection), could further activate an immune system that is already primed by the first hit. The "two-hit" theory hypothesizes that a second (or third) insult amplifies the inflammatory response to the first hit in such a way that SIRS occurs. If these events are followed by multiple organ dysfunction, the term secondary MODS is used.

The two-hit theory has been criticized for being somewhat arbitrary, because the differentiation between primary and secondary MODS is not always possible in the clinical setting.[91] However, our current understanding of the inflammatory response to injury supports the concept of priming.[92] Neutrophils are known to produce greater amounts of oxygen radicals and have increased adhesion properties after they have already been exposed to proinflammatory mediators. It has been demonstrated, at least in vitro, that priming followed by activation of neutrophils increases the extent of endothelial damage.

ANNOTATED REFERENCES

Cohen J: The immunopathogenesis of sepsis. Nature 2002;420:885-891.
  Cohen provides a general overview of the complicated pathways involved in the pathophysiology of sepsis.

Cunnion RE, Parrillo JE: Myocardial dysfunction in sepsis. Crit Care Clin 1989;5:99-117.
  Although written years ago, this article thoroughly describes the phenomenon of cardiomyopathy in patients with severe sepsis or septic shock.

Hotchkiss RS, Karl IE: The pathophysiology and treatment of sepsis. N Engl J Med 2003;348:138-150.
  This review article describes the immune response in sepsis, with a focus on the pathophysiology of immune suppression in sepsis and its influence on the development of multiple organ dysfunction.

Landry DW, Oliver JA: The pathogenesis of vasodilatory shock. N Engl J Med 2001;345:588-595.
  This review article describes the biochemical pathways that induce profound vasodilatation as it occurs in septic shock.

Marshall JC: Inflammation, coagulopathy, and the pathogenesis of multiple organ dysfunction syndrome. Crit Care Med 2001;29(7 Suppl):S99-S106.
  Marshall provides an overview of the proposed mechanism of multiple organ dysfunction. This supplement also contains several interesting articles about the interactions among inflammation, coagulation, and the endothelium.

Chapter 147

SEPTIC SHOCK

Jean-Louis Vincent

KEY POINTS

1. Septic shock affects 10% to 15% of ICU patients and has mortality rates of 50% to 60%.

2. Septic shock is most commonly caused by a bacterial infection, although fungi, viruses, and parasites can all be implicated. The most common source of the infection is the lung, followed by the abdomen.

3. Patients with sepsis can be classified according to their predisposing factors, the nature of the infection, the degree of immune response, and the associated organ dysfunction.

4. Septic shock is defined as severe sepsis (i.e., sepsis with organ dysfunction) with persistent arterial hypotension despite adequate fluid resuscitation, in the presence of perfusion abnormalities manifest by oliguria, reduced peripheral perfusion, altered mental status, and possibly altered skin perfusion.

5. Blood lactate levels are typically raised in septic shock, and persistently raised levels are a poor prognostic sign.

6. The management of septic shock must include infection control, hemodynamic stabilization, and immunomodulation.

INCIDENCE

Septic shock is the form of acute circulatory shock that occurs secondary to severe infection. The incidence of severe sepsis and septic shock is rising, partly related to medical progress, which allows patients to survive longer, resulting in increased numbers of older, debilitated, or immunocompromised patients passing through the ICU. Ten to 15 percent of ICU patients develop septic shock at one time or another, and the mortality rate is 50% to 60%.[1] Somewhat lower mortality rates have been reported in recent trials evaluating the effects of new therapeutic interventions,[2] but such studies include a number of exclusion criteria that are often associated with high mortality rates, such as cirrhosis, immunosuppression, or "do not resuscitate orders," so it is perhaps not surprising that mortality rates are lower in these therapeutic trials than in "real life."

ETIOLOGY

The organisms involved in severe sepsis and septic shock are most often bacterial. Although in the past gram-negative organisms were most commonly implicated, increasingly gram-positive organisms are isolated[1] such that roughly similar numbers of gram-positive and gram-negative organisms are now involved. Septic shock can also be caused by a fungal or parasitic infection, and in one third of patients no infectious agent is identified.[3] About one half of the infections are nosocomial. Although the infection can arise anywhere, the lung is the most common source of infection (40%), followed by the abdomen (20%), catheters and primary bacteremias (15%), and the urinary tract (10%).

PATHOPHYSIOLOGY

The pathophysiology of septic shock is complex and is covered in detail in Chapter 146. Essentially, the systemic sepsis response starts with the recognition of an invading organism or its toxins. Among the bacterial factors, one of the best-known toxins is lipopolysaccharide (LPS), which is part of the outer gram-negative bacterial membrane, but others include lipoteichoic acid and peptidoglycan. In certain cases, essentially infections involving *Staphylococcus aureus* or beta-hemolytic group A *Streptococcus,* the formation of superantigens results in the toxic shock syndrome.

The early humoral response involves notably the complement and contact (kinin-kallikrein) systems. The immune cells, principally monocytes/macrophages and polymorphonuclear neutrophils (PMNs), are able not only to recognize the pathogenic agents and their products so that they can phagocytose and destroy them but also to release a series of mediators that can themselves activate other cells. Among the cell membrane receptors implicated in the recognition of the pathogenic agents are the so-called Toll-like receptors (TLR), a family of 10 members. Of these, TLR4 is the receptor for gram-negative bacteria, TLR2 for gram-positive bacteria, mycobacteria, and yeasts,[4] and TLR9 for bacterial DNA.[5] In response to the cellular stimulation, intracellular signaling is activated, resulting largely in the activation of the transcriptional factor, nuclear factor-kappa B (NF-κB), which in turn is responsible for a series of proinflammatory reactions. A series of cytokines, two of the key players being tumor necrosis factor-alpha (TNF-α) and interleukin (IL)-1 that interact synergistically, is released by macrophages and other cells. TNF-α and IL-1 are particularly important proinflammatory cytokines whose administration in animals can reproduce all the features of septic shock, including hypotension and the development of multiple organ failure. A host of secondary mediators, including lipid mediators, oxygen free radicals, proteases, and arachidonic acid metabolites, are also released by macrophages, PMNs, and other cells. Vasodilator substances (e.g., nitric oxide [NO], prostaglandins) are released by endothelial cells and are responsible for the early hemodynamic changes of sepsis. NO, in particular, is a powerful vasodilator acting on vascular smooth muscle. Increased NO production is essentially caused by the induction of inducible NO synthase (iNOS) by proinflammatory cytokines. The formation of large quantities of NO can also have secondary toxic effects on cells. NO can block mitochondrial respiration, directly through inhibition of cytochrome aa3 and by reaction with superoxide radicals resulting in the production of peroxynitrite, which inhibits various phases of mitochondrial respiration.[6] These effects result in a depletion of cellular adenosine triphosphate and potentially severe detrimental effects on cell function. The inflammatory response also causes the release of vasoconstrictor substances (e.g., thromboxane, endothelins).

Other effects of the inflammatory reaction include the expression of adhesion molecules on the vascular endothelium and circulating cells (platelets, PMNs, and monocytes), allowing adhesion of activated leukocytes and their migration into subendothelial tissues. Alterations in the intercellular endothelial junctions result in increased capillary permeability and generalized edema. Alterations of coagulation and fibrinolysis complete the picture, with proinflammatory mediators creating a procoagulant state. Briefly, activation of tissue factor on the surface of various cells, particularly monocytes and endothelial cells, initiates the coagulation system.[7] In addition, sepsis causes a significant reduction in the plasma levels of natural anticoagulants, such as protein C, protein S, and antithrombin, by reducing their synthesis, increasing their consumption, and increasing their clearance. Thrombolysis is also stimulated with an increase in the levels of plasminogen activator inhibitor (PAI-1). The net result is a balance in favor of procoagulant processes, often leading to disseminated intravascular coagulation and participating in the microcirculatory disorder that leads to multiple organ failure and death in so many patients with severe sepsis.

During the sepsis response, anti-inflammatory mediators (IL-4, IL-10) are also released, which limit the effects of the proinflammatory mediators and can lead to a state of relative immunosuppression sometimes called immunoparalysis.[8] This reaction is responsible for a reduction in the expression of proteins of the major histocompatibility complex (HLA-DR) on the surface of monocytes.[9]

CLASSIFICATION

Following the recent recommendations from the Sepsis Conference,[10] patients with septic shock may be classified according to the letters: PIRO.

P = PREDISPOSING FACTORS

Each patient has specific characteristics.[11] For example, someone receiving long-term immunosuppressant therapy requires a different approach than someone who was previously healthy. Factors associated with lifestyle (e.g., alcoholism) may influence the course of septic shock.[12] Patient age and gender may also be important. Increasingly, genetics are being considered and studies are discovering which genetic factors can influence the development of, and survival from, severe sepsis. In particular, a polymorphism of the TNF-α promoter gene has been associated with an increased risk of

septic shock and a worse outcome from septic shock,[13] accompanied by the presence of increased blood levels of TNF-α.[14] Polymorphisms that may influence the response of the host to pathogenic organisms have also been described for IL-1 receptor antagonist (IL-1ra),[15] Toll-like receptor,[16] and mannose-binding lectin genes.[17] Improved understanding of these aspects should help better direct therapeutic strategies.

I = INFECTIOUS INSULT

This refers to the specific characteristics of the infection, that is, the agent or pathogen involved (e.g., gram-positive vs. gram-negative, bacteria vs. fungus), the source of the sepsis (e.g., urinary tract vs. respiratory tract), and the degree of extension of the infection (e.g., pneumonia confined to one lobe of one lung vs. generalized bilateral lung involvement, appendicitis vs. generalized peritonitis).[18] All these factors can influence the severity of the sepsis response and the patient's likely response to therapy.

R = HOST RESPONSE

This refers to the factors involved in the inflammatory response of the host to the infection, assessed largely by the presence or absence of the signs and symptoms of sepsis (e.g., degree of elevation of white blood cell count, C-reactive protein, procalcitonin).[19] Each patient mounts a different response dependent on various factors, including those discussed earlier, and the response will vary with time and treatment.

O = ORGAN DYSFUNCTION

This refers to the degree of organ dysfunction related to the sepsis[20] and can be evaluated using various scoring systems, including the MODS[21] (multiple organ dysfunction score) and the SOFA (sequential organ failure assessment) scores (Table 147-1),[22] which use objective, readily available measures to quantify the dysfunction of six organ systems. Dysfunction of each organ is rated according to a scale (0 [normal function] to 4 [organ failure] for the SOFA score) and individual scores can then be summed to provide a total. Individual organ function as well as a composite score can thus be followed during the course of disease and treatment.

CLINICAL PRESENTATION

It has been suggested that sepsis progresses in a continuum through severe sepsis to septic shock, but in the clinical situation such a progression is not always so clear cut or constant and it is difficult to predict which patients are going to develop septic shock and when. Septic shock can develop very abruptly without evidence of signs of sepsis in the preceding hours.

Septic shock is characterized by the persistence of severe arterial hypotension despite adequate fluid resuscitation in the presence of perfusion abnormalities manifest by oliguria, reduced peripheral perfusion, altered mental status, and possibly altered skin perfusion. Septic shock is typically associated with hyperlactatemia (blood lactate concentrations above 2 mEq/L).

One may anticipate that patients with septic shock will have fever, hyperleukocytosis, and all the other typical features

TABLE 147–1. THE SEQUENTIAL ORGAN FAILURE ASSESSMENT SCORE

	SOFA Score				
	0	1	2	3	4
Respiration					
PaO$_2$/FiO$_2$, mm Hg	> 400	≤ 400	≤ 300	≤ 200 with respiratory support	≤ 100
Coagulation					
Platelets × 10^3/mm^3	> 150	≤ 150	≤ 100	≤ 50	≤ 20
Liver					
Bilirubin, mg/dL (µmol/L)	< 1.2 (< 20)	1.2-1.9 (20-32)	2.0-5.9 (33-101)	6.0-11.9 (102-204)	> 12.0 (> 204)
Cardiovascular					
Hypotension	No hypotension	MAP < 70 mm Hg	Dopamine ≤ 5 or dobutamine (any dose)*	Dopamine > 5 or epinephrine ≤ 0.1or norepinephrine ≤ 0.1*	Dopamine > 15 or epinephrine > 0.1 or norepinephrine > 0.1*
CNS					
Glasgow Coma Scale score	15	13-14	10-12	6-9	< 6
Renal					
Creatinine, mg/dL (µmol/L) or urine output	< 1.2 (< 110)	1.2-1.9 (110-170)	2.0-3.4 (171-299)	3.5-4.9 (300-440) or < 500 mL/day	> 5.0 (> 440) or < 200 mL/day

*Adrenergic agents administered for at least 1 hour (doses given are in µg/kg/min).
From Vincomt JL, de Mendonça A, Cantralne F, et al: Use of the SOFA score to assess the incidence of organ dysfunction/failure in intensive care units: Results of a multicentric, prospective study. Crit Care Med 1998;26:1793-1800.

of sepsis, but unfortunately this is not always true. Fever may be an important clue, but moderate fever can be found in other types of shock. More importantly, fever is often absent in septic shock; in fact, hypothermia may be present in 15% to 20% of cases, and this symptom is associated with higher mortality rates.[23] Hyperleukocytosis is also very nonspecific and can be found in other types of circulatory failure. Likewise, lactic acidosis, a hallmark of all types of circulatory failure, is usually compensated by hyperventilation, so that tachypnea is not specific for septic shock. Similarly, tachycardia can be the result of the circulatory alterations associated with any type of shock.

A more typical characteristic of septic shock is the hyperkinetic pattern characterized by a high cardiac output (see later). Although such a hemodynamic pattern is not entirely specific—it can be found in other inflammatory states such as polytrauma or pancreatitis, or even anaphylactic shock—it should alert the attending physician to a likely diagnosis of septic shock.

HEMODYNAMIC CHANGES

The inflammatory reaction causes an intense vasodilation that increases vascular capacity and results in a fall in arterial blood pressure. Hypovolemia due to fluid loss (e.g., diarrhea, vomiting, sweating) and to alterations in capillary permeability contributes to the hypotension, and reduced myocardial contractility, largely owing to the release of mediators, can further aggravate the hemodynamic situation, although it is completely reversible when the septic shock resolves. The pathophysiology of the reduced myocardial contractility includes alterations in endothelial function, alterations in beta-adrenergic receptors, and alterations in myocardial calcium metabolism. These effects are caused largely by sepsis mediators such as TNF and IL-1, oxygen free radicals, platelet-activating factor (PAF), and NO, which all have negative inotropic effects.[24]

In less severe cases (i.e., severe sepsis without shock), arterial hypotension can be corrected by a fluid challenge. In more severe cases, even if there is a partial response to fluid repletion, the persistence of hypotension requires the use of vasopressor agents (see later). This differentiates severe sepsis from septic shock and indicates a very serious condition because acute circulatory failure (shock) systematically causes dysfunction of other organs.

After vascular filling, the hemodynamic status is characterized by a fall in vascular tone associated with reduced systemic vascular resistance (SVR) and a raised cardiac output. In addition, the reduced myocardial contractility causes a fall in the ventricular ejection fraction. The ejection volume, and particularly the cardiac output, may be maintained by an increase in the diastolic volumes. Hence, there is myocardial depression or dysfunction without any real cardiac failure (which would require a reduced cardiac output).

MONITORING

Any patient with septic shock requires monitoring with an arterial catheter to enable reliable and continuous assessment of arterial pressure. The catheter also facilitates blood sampling, notably for blood gas analysis.

THE PULMONARY ARTERY (SWAN-GANZ) CATHETER

The value of placing a pulmonary artery catheter (PAC) has been questioned.[25,26] However, although no study has conclusively demonstrated positive effects of this type of monitoring on outcome, it has been well demonstrated that information obtained from the PAC can help guide patient management.[27,28] Echocardiography can provide useful additional information, largely to visualize the degree of ventricular filling and the ejection volume. However, echocardiography requires an experienced operator, gives no information on the adequacy of the cardiac output for the patient's needs, and is difficult to perform continuously so that information is intermittent.

Importantly, the PAC is not necessary when there is a favorable response to fluid replacement but is likely to be of use in complex cases, particularly in patients with concomitant cardiopulmonary disease. In the absence of randomized controlled trials on the subject, one must rely on expert recommendations and guidelines.[29]

The PAC is useful not only for monitoring of the pulmonary artery occlusion pressure (PAOP) and the cardiac output but also the mixed venous oxygen saturation ($S\bar{v}O_2$), which is perhaps the most useful parameter because a fall in $S\bar{v}O_2$ is generally associated with inadequate oxygen transport.

BLOOD LACTATE LEVELS

The blood lactate level is an important biologic parameter in the determination of the adequacy of perfusion and oxygenation. The normal blood lactate level is around 1 mEq/L, and hyperlactatemia becomes pathologic above 2 mEq/L. Although in other forms of circulatory shock hyperlactatemia is due to cellular hypoxia, in septic shock additional mechanisms may play an important role in raising blood lactate levels. In sepsis, blood lactate levels may be raised by an increase in cellular metabolism, by inhibition of pyruvate dehydrogenase, and by reduced clearance. Repeated measurements enable one to assess the efficacy of treatment and have a predictive value superior to derived oxygenation parameters.[30] The evolution of blood lactate levels enables a global evaluation of the state of the shock, although in view of the relatively slow rate of change, blood lactate levels cannot be used to guide resuscitation.

PERIPHERAL PERFUSION PARAMETERS

Measurement of the gastric intramucosal pH (pHi) or its derivatives (mucosal P_{CO_2} or the difference between the mucosal and arterial P_{CO_2} [the P_{CO_2} gap]) is considered to reflect splanchnic perfusion and hence provide an idea of the adequacy of regional oxygenation. Such measures have a prognostic value in patients with severe sepsis[31] but have not been shown to be useful in guiding treatment in the individual patient.[32] Moreover, these techniques may be influenced by important technical considerations, including the influence of gastric acid and enteral nutrition.

Sublingual tonometry may provide a simpler way of directly visualizing the microcirculation. While the sublingual region is not one that would immediately seem to be of most interest, it is easily accessible; thus, by using techniques of orthogonal polarization spectral (OPS) imaging, changes in

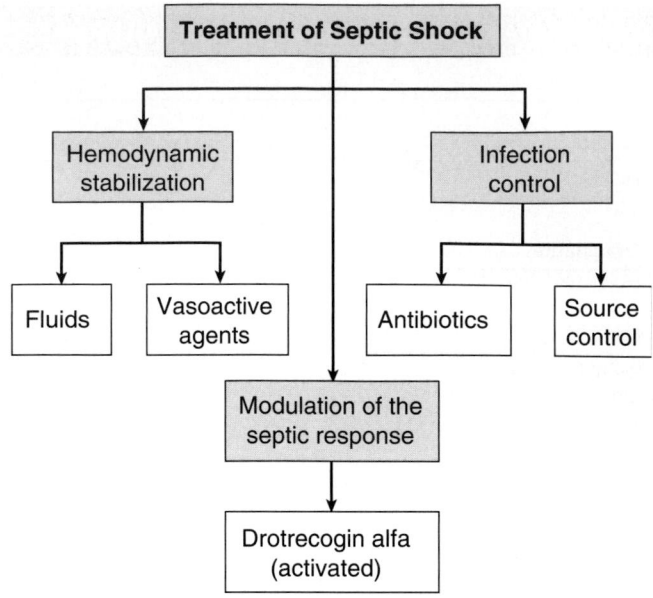

FIGURE 147–1. The three aspects of the treatment of septic shock

the microcirculation over time and after treatments can be monitored.[33,34]

MANAGEMENT

The management of the patient with septic shock involves three inseparable components[29]: the treatment of the infection, cardiovascular resuscitation,[35] and immunomodulation (Fig. 147-1).

CONTROL OF INFECTION

Infection must be treated effectively and rapidly. Antibiotic medication must be started quickly and must cover all likely organisms. This may depend on local microbiologic flora and resistance patterns. Most often, the microorganism(s) responsible for the sepsis is not known for sure and empirical broad-spectrum antibiotics must be given to ensure adequate coverage. This empirical therapy must then be adapted as soon as possible and within 24 to 48 hours at the latest, as microbiology culture results become available.

In addition to antibiotic treatment, any focus of infection must be removed or drained, by emergency surgery if necessary.

CARDIOVASCULAR RESUSCITATION

Here the VIP ruse proposed by Weil and Shubin[36] should be followed. Each patient is in fact a VIP, but the letters refer here to ventilation, infusion, and pump.

V = Ventilation

All patients with septic shock must be generously oxygenated with the aim of correcting any hypoxemia, regardless of whether it is due to an inadequate cardiac output, pulmonary edema, or pneumopathy. Severe cases require endotracheal intubation and mechanical ventilation. Noninvasive ventilation is not recommended in such hemodynamically unstable patients. Even though it may represent a temporary support rather than a treatment per se, mechanical ventilation allows not only an improvement in gaseous exchange but also has beneficial hemodynamic effects, notably by reducing the oxygen requirement of the respiratory muscles.

I = Infusion

Septic shock is accompanied by absolute and relative hypovolemia, the result of various mechanisms:

- External losses, which may be obvious such as vomiting and diarrhea, or less apparent such as sweating
- Internal losses via an increase in capillary permeability with development of edema and sometimes liquid effusions (peritoneal, pleural effusion)
- Increase in plasma volume associated with the arterial and venous dilatation

The hypovolemia needs to be corrected rapidly because it causes hemodynamic instability, both at the cardiac output level and in terms of peripheral perfusion.

Assessment of adequate volemia is essentially clinical: restoration of arterial pressure, improvement of cutaneous perfusion, improved diuresis, and improved mental state.[37] The central venous pressure (CVP) can be a useful guide, but it is not possible to define in advance the CVP level that should be reached in any individual patient. However, monitoring of the CVP or PAOP is essential to limit the risk of pulmonary edema. In fluid replacement, it is preferable to use a fluid challenge technique in which filling pressures are measured at regular intervals during the fluid administration (Table 147-2). If a PAC is in place, it is recommended that fluid replacement be given until the cardiac output reaches a plateau and further fluid causes no further increase in cardiac output.

There has been considerable debate as to which fluid should be used in sepsis, but it is the quantity of fluid rather than the type of fluid per se that is of greatest importance. Because of their propensity for leakage into the extravascular space, more crystalloid is needed to achieve the same effect as colloid,[38] thus potentially increasing the risk of edema, but colloids are more expensive and carry their own risks. In particular, there has been considerable controversy about the use of albumin in critically ill patients but a recent multicenter study performed in Australasia (the SAFE study) showed that albumin administration does not compromise outcome.

P = Pump (Vasoactive Agents)

If fluid administration alone is unable to restore an adequate perfusion pressure, vasoactive agents are required. Catecholamines are preferred for their rapid action and efficacy and their short half-lives. The adrenergic agents stimulate beta$_1$- (positive inotropes), beta$_2$- (essentially vasodilators and bronchodilatators), and alpha receptors (essentially vasoconstrictors) to varying degrees.

Dopamine is often recommended as the first-line drug for its mixed beta- and alpha-adrenergic effects.[37] Dopamine

also stimulates dopaminergic receptors, causing vasodilation primarily in the splanchnic and renal regions but the clinical relevance of this effect is uncertain. If hypotension persists despite doses of the order of 20 μg/kg/min, norepinephrine should be added. Some clinicians prefer norepinephrine as their first-line vasopressor and, indeed, there is little evidence to support the use of one over the other, with published guidelines now recommending either as the first-line drug.[35,37] Epinephrine should not be used as a first-line vasopressor in septic shock because it can have deleterious effects on the splanchnic circulation.[39] Dobutamine is often added to vasopressor therapy, particularly when using norepinephrine, to increase cardiac output by its positive inotropic effects.

IMMUNOMODULATION

Clinical trials assessing drugs that limit the effects of proinflammatory cytokines such as TNF (anti-TNF antibodies, TNF receptors) and IL-1 (IL-1 receptor antagonist inhibitors) have not given convincing results of a beneficial effects of these agents on outcome, probably largely because such cytokines have multiple effects, beneficial as well harmful.

The link between coagulation and inflammation led to the suggestion that some of the key coagulation proteins may have beneficial effects in sepsis. Although several clinical studies suggested a possible role for antithrombin in patients with severe sepsis, a large multicenter study failed to demonstrate any effect on outcome.[40] However, the administration of activated protein C (drotrecogin alfa [activated]) early in severe sepsis or septic shock reduced mortality[2] and morbidity.[41] In addition to its anticoagulation effects, activated protein C has important anti-inflammatory effects,[42-44] can influence cell signaling, and has antiapoptotic effects,[45] which may help explain why it has been shown to have beneficial effects in sepsis while other anticoagulants (antithrombin, tissue factor pathway inhibitor) have not. Drotrecogin alfa (activated) is infused at a dose of 24 μg/kg/hr via a continuous intravenous perfusion for 96 hours. Drotrecogin alfa (activated) administration is associated with an increased risk of hemorrhage,[46] such that it is contraindicated in patients with a high risk of bleeding. Infusions should be stopped 2 hours before any surgical intervention but may be restarted 12 hours after major interventions or sooner for more minor procedures if hemostasis is ensured. The high costs of the drug may also limit its use, although its cost-effective profile is similar to many other accepted ICU therapies.[47]

The administration of corticosteroids for patients with sepsis was proposed many years ago, but at the large doses studied (in the order of 30 mg/kg of methylprednisolone) was never shown to have a beneficial effect on survival.[48] More recently, the concept of relative adrenal insufficiency, based on the response to an ACTH test, has reawakened the interest in corticosteroids, and moderate doses of corticosteroids (hydrocortisone, 50 mg i.v. q6h) in patients with septic shock have been shown to restore the activity of vascular adrenergic receptors, without excessive immunosuppressive effects, thus improving hemodynamic status, and reducing mortality.[49] It is generally recommended that this treatment strategy be guided by an ACTH test, with treatment started immediately at the end of the test and stopped if the results show normal adrenal function.

The treatment of fever is controversial. Increased body temperature increases oxygen requirements, but the increased cellular metabolism may form part of the body's

TABLE 147-2. THE FLUID CHALLENGE TECHNIQUE

Define	Example
Type of fluid	Lactated Ringer's
Rate of infusion	500 mL in 20 minutes
Goal	Mean arterial pressure > 75 mm Hg
Limits	Central venous pressure 16 mm Hg

natural defense. Animal studies have suggested that control of fever may be detrimental[50] and that the release of heat shock proteins in fever may have important protective effects.[51] A multicenter study in patients with severe sepsis reported that ibuprofen, a cyclooxygenase inhibitor, was well-tolerated but did not reduce mortality.[52]

High-flow hemofiltration techniques can remove a range of bacterial products and mediators but are not without risk, notably because this process can remove beneficial products, including hormones and medications (antibiotics), as well as potentially harmful substances.[53] Experimentally, the most important effect of such techniques is improved cardiac function.[54]

METABOLIC SUPPORT

NUTRITIONAL SUPPORT

Malnutrition can prolong the course of sepsis and increase the risk of complications. In considering nutritional support in the patient with septic shock, several factors need to be remembered:

- Enteral route is preferable to the parenteral route.
- Enteral nutrition should probably not be started during the initial phase of resuscitation. Although studies are limited, increasing the oxygen requirements of the gut is probably not wise in the acute circulatory shock situation. However, as soon as the patient has achieved a degree of hemodynamic stability (after a maximum of 24 to 48 hours), enteral nutrition should be started.
- Careful control of blood glucose levels is recommended. A recent study[55] clearly showed reduced morbidity and mortality in surgical intensive care patients who followed a strict protocol to maintain blood glucose between 80 and 110 mg/dL (4.4 and 6.1 mmol/L).

ORGAN SUPPORT

Organ dysfunction can involve any organ and can be quantified using the SOFA score (see Table 147-1). Techniques for individual organ support are covered in separate chapters, but an overview is given here.

RESPIRATORY ALTERATIONS

Respiratory failure is a common complication of sepsis and is characterized by hypoxemia associated with the presence of bilateral infiltrates on the chest radiograph, with no evidence of left-sided heart failure (normal PAOP). The diagnosis of acute respiratory distress syndrome (ARDS) is made when the PaO_2/FIO_2 ratio is less than 200 mm Hg, and the less severe form, acute lung injury (ALI), is defined as a PaO_2/FIO_2 less than 300 mm Hg.[56]

When starting a patient on mechanical ventilation, several factors need particular attention:

- Worsening of arterial hypotension when starting mechanical ventilation suggests the presence of hypovolemia, responsible for a reduction in venous return (and hence in cardiac output) when intrathoracic pressures are increased.
- Tidal volume should be limited, not only for hemodynamic reasons but also to avoid a major inflammatory reaction.

In patients with ALI, mortality was reduced in patients given tidal volumes of 6 mL/kg predicted body weight as opposed to 12 mL/kg.[57]

- Excessive sedation must be avoided. Administration of sedative drugs and analgesics should be titrated in function with the needs of the individual patient. Excessive administration of these agents can compromise hemodynamic stability and prolong duration of mechanical ventilation and ICU stay.[58]

RENAL ALTERATIONS

Sepsis is the leading cause of acute renal failure in the ICU.[59] Renal function can worsen as a result of circulatory changes, associated with vasoconstriction of the afferent arteries and reduced glomerular filtration rate. In addition, management of the patient with sepsis often involves the administration of nephrotoxic agents, for example, certain medicines, notably aminoglycosides and amphotericin, and contrast agents for radiologic examinations.

Unfortunately, there is no prophylactic approach to renal failure other than to try and maintain adequate renal perfusion and overall volemia. The administration of low (renal)-dose dopamine is not effective at preventing renal failure,[60] and diuretics may be harmful.[61]

Renal epuration techniques are frequently necessary. In septic shock, continuous venovenous techniques, with or without dialysis, are generally preferred over intermittent techniques to facilitate control of fluid balance.

COAGULATION ALTERATIONS

Coagulation system alterations are generally systemic even when they do not meet all the criteria of disseminated intravascular coagulation. Treatment of these alterations revolves primarily around the cause, and there is no indication for heparin therapy. In severe cases associated with significant bleeding, fresh frozen plasma or platelet infusions may be indicated.

HEPATIC ALTERATIONS

Circulatory shock of any cause frequently results in the elevation of liver-associated enzymes, but the contribution of the various organs (e.g., muscles) is difficult to quantify. Often there is a rise in bilirubin after several days without evidence of hemolysis, major hematomas, or biliary pathology. Supplementary examinations (e.g., ultrasound) may be indicated to exclude any associated biliary pathology.

ALTERATION OF CEREBRAL FUNCTION

Circulatory shock is typically accompanied by an alteration of intellectual function, initially manifest as confusion without real coma and reversible with resolution of shock. Cerebral alterations can be prolonged, and the patient is then said to have septic encephalopathy. The exact cause of the encephalopathy is not clear, although various mediators of sepsis have been implicated.[62] Investigations are of little use except to exclude other causes. The electroencephalogram in general shows a slow diffuse slowing, whereas cerebral CT and cerebrospinal fluid examination are normal.

CONCLUSION

The optimal treatment of a patient with septic shock requires a rapid and effective management plan, with the assistance of the full ICU staff team. Infection control and hemodynamic stability must be approached simultaneously. The treatment of sepsis per se is currently limited to activated protein C and moderate doses of corticosteroids. Other interventions are undergoing clinical trials with the hope that they will improve microcirculatory changes of sepsis or beneficially modulate the host response. A better characterization of patients with septic shock, using for example the PIRO system, is necessary to better titrate therapeutic interventions to the individual patient.

ANNOTATED REFERENCES

Annane D, Sebille V, Charpentier C, et al: Effect of treatment with low doses of hydrocortisone and fludrocortisone on mortality in patients with septic shock. JAMA 2002;288:862-871.
Important study showing improve outcomes in patients with septic shock and relative adrenal insufficiency treated with moderate doses of steroids.

Bernard GR, Vincent JL, Laterre PF, et al: Efficacy and safety of recombinant human activated protein C for severe sepsis. N Engl J Med 2001;344:699-709.
Landmark study as it was the first phase III study to show beneficial effect of an immunomodulatory agent on survival from severe sepsis and septic shock.

De Backer D, Creteur J, Preiser JC, et al: Microvascular blood flow is altered in patients with sepsis. Am J Respir Crit Care Med 2002;166:98-104.
Study demonstrating the potential prognostic and monitoring uses of orthogonal polarization spectral imaging of the sublingual region in patients with sepsis.

International Sepsis Forum: Guidelines for the treatment of severe sepsis and septic shock. Intensive Care Med 2001;27(Suppl 1):S3-S134.
Supplement issue providing evidence-based guidelines on all aspects of the management of patients with severe sepsis and septic shock.

Levy MM, Fink MP, Marshall JC, et al: 2001 SCCM/ESICM/ACCP/ATS/SIS International Sepsis Definitions Conference. Crit Care Med 2003;31: 1250-1256.
Important report of the Sepsis Definitions Conference that introduces the PIRO concept.

Chapter 148

SEPSIS AND MULTIPLE ORGAN SYSTEM FAILURE IN CHILDREN

Joseph Carcillo • Jan A. Hazelzet

KEY POINTS

1. The mortality of severe sepsis in neonatal and pediatric patients has improved from 97% in 1963 to 9% in 1999. Previously healthy children have better outcomes than children with chronic illness.

2. Although outcomes are improving, the burden of newborn and pediatric sepsis is increasing in the United States. More children die with severe sepsis than die with cancer, with an estimated yearly health care cost of $4 billion in the United States for patients with this condition.

3. The physiologic differences in coagulation and fibrinolysis between adults and children might lead to an earlier exhaustion of coagulation factors and disseminated intravascular coagulation in infants and young children.

4. In contrast to adults, death from shock in children is most commonly associated with progressive cardiac failure, not vascular failure. Pediatric patients have low cardiac output/high systemic vascular resistance (60%), low cardiac output/low vascular resistance (20%), or high cardiac output/low vascular resistance (20%).

5. Genetic polymorphisms in components of the inflammatory pathways have been shown to be involved in the susceptibility, severity, and outcome of pediatric sepsis.

6. The American College of Critical Care Medicine published in 2002 evidence-based *Clinical Practice Parameters for Hemodynamic Support of Newborns and Children with Septic Shock*, based in part on the concept that early recognition and resuscitation improve outcome.

7. The moment of intubation should be estimated on the basis of clinical diagnosis of respiratory distress or hemodynamic instability, not on blood gas analysis.

8. Virtually all children with shock require aggressive volume resuscitation; this should be given as 20 mL/kg boluses of normal saline or colloid as intravenous push to a total of 60 mL/kg in the first 10 to 20 minutes.

9. Patients with multiple organ failure are at particular risk of toxicity with drugs that are metabolized by the cytochrome P-450 system.

DEFINITIONS OF SEPSIS, SEVERE SEPSIS, SEPTIC SHOCK, AND MULTIPLE ORGAN FAILURE

The 2001 International Sepsis Definitions Conference[1] centered discussion on whether *sepsis* should continue to be defined as systemic inflammatory response syndrome plus infection or infection plus systemic inflammatory response syndrome plus signs of organ dysfunction. It was agreed that the definitions of severe sepsis remain intact. Most pediatric literature defines inclusion criteria for *sepsis* as hyperthermia or hypothermia, tachycardia (may be absent in the hypothermic patient), evidence of infection, and at least one of the following signs of new-onset organ dysfunction: altered mental status, hypoxemia, bounding pulses, or increased lactate. S*evere sepsis* is uniformly defined as sepsis and organ failure determined by various organ failure scores.[2-5] *Septic shock* has been defined as infection with hypothermia or hyperthermia, tachycardia (may be absent with hypothermia), and altered mental status, in the presence of at least one, but usually more than one, of the following: decreased peripheral pulses compared with central pulses prolonged greater than 2 seconds (cold shock) or flash capillary refill (warm shock), mottled or cool extremities (cold shock), and decreased urine output (<1 mL/kg/h). Hypotension is observed in late decompensated shock.[6]

The American College of Critical Care Medicine[6] further defines shock according to response to therapy as fluid-refractory/dopamine-resistant, catecholamine-resistant, and refractory shock. *Multiple organ failure* is defined as more than one organ failure. The greater the number of concomitant organ failures, the greater the risk of mortality. Multiple organ failure generally is observed in septic shock patients who receive delayed resuscitation or inadequate source control therapies (inadequate nidus removal or ineffective antibiotic regimen). Multiple organ failure also is observed in patients with septic shock who have an underlying primary or acquired immunodeficiency that prevents timely eradication of infection.

CHANGING OUTCOMES AND EPIDEMIOLOGY

The mortality rate in neonatal and pediatric severe sepsis has improved from 97% in 1963 to 9% in 1999.[7-12] Previously healthy children have better outcomes than children with chronic illness. The randomized controlled trial of bactericidal permeability-increasing protein[13] for children with purpura fulminans/presumed meningococcal septic shock showed 10% mortality rates in the placebo groups. The reported outcomes in children with septic shock when using therapeutic approaches similar to those recommended in the 2002 American College of Critical Care Medicine *Clinical Practice Parameters for Hemodynamic Support of Pediatric and Neonatal Patients in Septic Shock*[6] show a decreasing tendency. In children with meningococcal septic shock in the United Kingdom, a 5% mortality rate was reported.[14] A single-center study in the United States reported a 10% mortality rate.[15] The investigators observed 0% mortality in previously healthy children but a 15% mortality rate in children with chronic illness (for the most part cancer patients). All of these children died with multiple organ failure. Ngo and colleagues[16] observed a 0% mortality rate in a randomized Dengue shock fluid resuscitation trial.

Although outcomes are improving, the burden of newborn and pediatric sepsis is increasing in the United States. More children die with severe sepsis than die with cancer, with an estimated yearly health care cost of $4 billion in the United States for patients with this condition.[12] Half are newborns with most of these having low birth weight.[9] Half of children with severe sepsis have underlying chronic illness. Neurologic and cardiovascular chronic illness is most common in infants with severe sepsis and cancer, whereas immune deficiency is most common in children with severe sepsis. Medical advances have affected etiology and epidemiology. In 1990, Jacobs and coworkers[17] reported that the most common causes of septic shock in children were, in descending order, *Haemophilus influenzae* b, *Neisseria meningitidis*, and *Streptococcus pneumoniae*. The 1995 and 1999 U.S. estimates suggest a change. *H. influenzae* type b is all but nonexistent, *N. meningitidis* is prevalent in only a few regions of the United States, and group B streptococcus is decreasing. The more recent use of *S. pneumoniae* vaccine is reducing the incidence of this infection. The Canadian government has implemented nationwide immunization in children younger than age 2 years for *N. meningitidis* serotype C.[18] The most prevalent causes of severe sepsis and septic shock in the United States now seem to be staphylococcal and fungal infections.[12]

PATHOPHYSIOLOGY AND DEVELOPMENTAL EFFECTS

MOLECULAR PATHOGENESIS

Controlled Inflammation with Eradication of Infection

Endotoxin, mannose and other glycoprotein moieties on the cell walls of yeast and fungi, superantigens, toxins associated with some gram-positive bacteria, mycobacteria, and viruses activate the innate immune system, comprising polymorphonuclear neutrophils, monocytes, and macrophages in part through Toll receptors, CD14 receptors (endotoxin), and other costimulatory molecules. These innate immune cells internalize microorganisms and kill them. Monocytes and macrophages present processed antigens from these killed microorganisms to circulating T lymphocytes and coordinate the adaptive immune response. This second wave of immune response includes B-cell activation and antibody production and generation of cytotoxic T cells and natural killer cells (particularly in viral and fungal infection). Opsonization with antibodies allows more efficient recognition, killing, and clearing of microorganisms by resident macrophages in the reticuloendothelial system.[19,20]

The activated inflammatory cells also initiate a series of biochemical cascades that result in phospholipase A_2, platelet-activating factor, cyclooxygenase, complement, and cytokine release that orchestrate an efficient and controlled inflammatory/immune response. The cytokines tumor necrosis factor (TNF) and interleukin (IL)-1β synergistically interact to promote positive feedback cascades that result in fever and vasodilation. These cytokines stimulate the production of many important effector molecules, including proinflammatory cytokines (e.g., IL-6, IL-8, and interferon-γ), which promote immune cell–mediated killing and anti-inflammatory cytokines (e.g., soluble TNF receptor, IL-1 receptor antagonist protein, IL-4, and IL-10), which turn the immune response off when the infection has been cleared. These cytokines also stimulate nitric oxide (NO) production, which leads to vasodilation. NO also combines with superoxide radicals to form peroxynitrite radicals ($ONOO^-$), which participate in intracellular killing of microorganisms. Cytokines also increase expression of endothelial-derived adhesion molecules, including E-selectin, which facilitates white blood cell rolling, and intercellular adhesion molecule and vascular adhesion molecule, which facilitate white blood cell adhesion and diapedesis. This activity guides activated inflammatory cells to the site of infection. The cytokines also induce a change in the endothelium to a prothrombotic and antifibrinolytic state. Expression of thrombomodulin is possibly decreased, and expression of the prothrombotic molecule tissue factor and the antifibrinolytic molecule plasminogen activator inhibitor-1 (PAI-1) is increased. The ensuing thrombus "walls off" the infection and allows vascular remodeling until anti-inflammatory cytokines turn off the proinflammatory cytokine response and restore the antithrombotic, profibrinolytic milieu after infection is cleared.

Uncontrolled Inflammation and Persistent Infection Lead to Septic Shock and Multiple Organ Failure

If the controlled activated immune cell response is ineffective in killing the infectious agent and clearing antigen, inflammation is uncontrolled, and systemic organ injury ensues. Increased TNF and NO production in cardiac cells and circulating myocardial depressant substances can lead to cardiac dysfunction and cardiovascular collapse. Peroxynitrite can cause DNA damage, and subsequent polyadenosyl ribose synthase (PARS) activation depletes cells of oxidized nicotinamide adenine dinucleotide and adenosine triphosphate (ATP), leading to secondary energy failure. Thrombosis and antifibrinolysis becomes systemic. Antithrombotic molecules, including protein C and antithrombin III, are consumed, and ongoing systemic release of tissue factor and PAI-1 results in unremitting thrombosis. At some point, consumption of procoagulant factors leads to a precarious state in which thrombosis is accompanied by bleeding because there are insufficient clotting factors. The anti-inflammatory response also becomes deleterious. IL-10 induces a T_H2 response and reduces the ability of immune cells to kill infection. Overactivated immune cells also release Fas and Fas ligand. Circulating Fas prevents activated immune cell apoptosis and ensures ongoing inflammation, and Fas ligand can induce apoptosis in liver cells. Ineffective and unresolving inflammation leads to systemic organ failure.

CLINICAL PATHOLOGIC CORRELATES

On the basis of in vivo biochemical analyses and autopsy histology, several forms of multiple organ failure could be characterized.[21-24] *Thrombocytopenia-associated multiple organ failure* (platelet count <100,000/µL or a 50% decrease in platelet count from baseline) was attributable to purpura fulminans and disseminated intravascular coagulation with increased tissue factor activity in vivo and fibrin thrombi at autopsy in only 20% of patients. Of these patients, 80% showed thrombotic thrombocytopenic purpura pathophysiology with increased ultralarge von Willebrand factor multimers, absent von Willebrand factor cleaving protease, increased PAI-1 activity in vivo, and platelet/fibrin thrombi at autopsy.

Sequential or liver dysfunction–associated multiple organ failure (shock/acute respiratory distress syndrome followed sequentially by liver and renal failure) was associated with viral sepsis and lymphoproliferative disease. These patients were found to have unremitting Epstein-Barr virus infection with lymphocyte Fas ligand–mediated destruction of liver and high circulating Fas and Fas ligand levels.

Unresolving multiple organ failure with prolonged monocyte deactivation (monocyte HLA-DR expression <30% or ex vivo TNF response to lipopolysaccharide <200 pg/mL for >5 days) was associated with secondary bacterial, fungal, or herpesvirus family infection. These patients had elevated IL-10 and IL-6 levels. Patients who died had infection at autopsy.

Lymphoid depletion syndrome (lymphocyte depletion of lymph nodes and spleen) was found at autopsy. All of these children had fungal, bacterial, or herpesvirus family infection at the time of death. Risk factors (odds ratio >10) for this process included lymphocytopenia (<1000/mm^3) or hypoprolactinemia or both for more than 7 days.

These *clinical pathologic correlates* support the following hypotheses: (1) Uncontrolled inflammation contributes to organ failure after septic shock; (2) uncontrolled inflammation contributes to systemic thrombosis; (3) uncontrolled inflammation leads to adrenal dysfunction not only through thrombosis, but also potentially through NO-mediated inhibition of cytochrome P-450 activity; and (4) uncontrolled inflammation is commonly associated with uneradicated infection. It is likely that genetic and environmental factors can increase an individual patient's risk for systemic thrombosis and uneradicated infection.

COAGULATION SYSTEM

As is generally accepted and explained in many reviews, coagulation and fibrinolysis are an integrative part of the immune system.[25] There are important physiologic differences in the hemostatic system in children compared with adults. The decreased levels of several crucial coagulants and increased levels of alpha$_2$-macroglobulin may contribute in part to the lower risk of thrombotic events in childhood during physiologic conditions.[26,27] In pathologic conditions, these physiologic differences might lead to an earlier exhaustion of coagulation factors and disseminated intravascular coagulation in infants and young children.[28] The coagulation system is a marker of organ dysfunction in sepsis. It is associated with subsequent endothelium activation and systemic clotting and finally antifibrinolysis.

CARDIOVASCULAR SYSTEM

Ceneviva and associates[29] found that in contrast to adults, who predominantly have high cardiac output/low vascular resistance shock, children with fluid-refractory/dopamine-resistant shock have varied hemodynamic states, including low cardiac output/high systemic vascular resistance (60%), low cardiac output/low vascular resistance (20%), and high cardiac output/low vascular resistance (20%), which can change with time and depend on age. In contrast to adults, death from shock is most commonly associated with progressive cardiac failure, not vascular failure. Infants and children frequently are insensitive to dopamine or dobutamine and respond to epinephrine (cold shock) or norepinephrine (warm shock).[29-31] Newborns are different as well. Adults can double their heart rate to improve cardiac output, but newborns cannot. Newborns, although tachycardic, depend on increased vascular tone to maintain blood pressure. Persistent pulmonary hypertension and right ventricular failure also complicate newborn septic shock.[32,33] Dopamine should be used only at low dosage, and norepinephrine should be discouraged to prevent worsening of pulmonary artery hypertension through alpha-adrenergic stimulation.

PREDISPOSING FACTORS AND PREVENTION STRATEGIES

Environmental and genetic factors associated with reduced immune function predispose children to the development of sepsis and septic shock. These factors include age (prematurity, neonate, and age <1 year), cancer and immunosuppressive chemotherapeutic agents, transplantation and immunosuppressive agents, primary immunodeficiency disorders (e.g., hypocomplementemia, hypogammaglobulinemia, chronic granulomatous disease), acquired immunodeficiency disorders (neutropenia, lymphocytopenia, monocyte deactivation), and malnutrition. Prolonged use of invasive catheters also predisposes to infection.

Among the community-acquired causes of sepsis, *N. meningitidis* has a diverse clinical picture, ranging from a self-limiting bacteremia to meningitis to a severe, rapidly fatal sepsis. After invasion of the bloodstream by the bacteria, three main cascade pathways are activated: the complement system, the inflammatory response, and the coagulation and fibrinolysis pathway. These pathways do not act independently, but are able to interact with each other. Genetic polymorphisms among components of these pathways have been shown to be involved in the susceptibility, severity, and outcome of meningococcal disease. Knowledge of genetic variations associated with susceptibility to and severity of meningococcal infection has been reviewed.[34]

Complement deficiencies and defects in sensing or opsonophagocytic pathways, such as the rare Toll-like receptor 4 single nucleotide polymorphisms and combinations of inefficient variants of Fcγ-receptors, seem to have the most important role in genetically established susceptibility. Effect on severity has repeatedly been reported for FcγRIIa and PAI-1 polymorphisms. Angiotensin-converting enzyme is associated with a proinflammatory response. The absence of a 284-base pair marker in the angiotensin-converting enzyme gene (D allele) is associated with higher circulating angiotensin-converting enzyme activity compared with the presence of this marker (I allele). The DD genotype is associated with increased disease severity, and although not significant, a twofold increase in mortality rate has been reported. Outcome effects have been confirmed for single nucleotide polymorphisms in properdin deficiencies, PAI-1 and combination of the −511C/T single nucleotide polymorphisms in IL-1β, and +2018C/T single nucleotide polymorphisms in IL RN. Conflicting results are reported for the effect of the −308G/A promoter polymorphism in TNF. These differences may reflect discrepancies in group definitions among studies or the influence of additional single nucleotide polymorphisms in the TNF promoter, which can form haplotypes representing different cytokine production capacity. For several single nucleotide polymorphisms, the potential effect on susceptibility, severity, or outcome has not yet been confirmed in an independent study.

The hallmark of pediatric medicine is prevention. Public health programs that reduce prematurity could be expected to have the greatest impact on the incidence of sepsis. The use of group B streptococcus prophylaxis in at-risk mothers has reduced the incidence of septic shock in premature and term infants. Immunization programs for diphtheria, pertussis, tetanus, measles, mumps, rubella, *H. influenzae* type b, *S. pneumoniae,* and *N. meningitidis* (type C for infants and type C, A, and Y for college students) all effectively reduce the incidence of sepsis in newborns and children. The primary immunodeficiency initiative is an important physician education program. Children with frequent pneumonia, sinus infections, or skin infections can benefit from early immunodeficiency workups, including quantitative immunoglobulins, complement levels, nitroblue toluene testing of polymorphonuclear neutrophil function, and antibody titer response to immunization. Early identification of these children can lead to use of therapies that reduce the incidence of sepsis.

DIAGNOSTIC APPROACH AND SCORING SYSTEMS

Several prognostic factors have been related to severity and nonsurvival, as follows:

- Increased levels of endotoxin, cytokines, lactate, PAI-1, adhesion molecules, procalcitonin, elastase, troponin, and adrenocorticotropic hormone
- Decreased levels of C-reactive protein, glucose, fibrinogen, coagulation factors, protein C, leukocytes, and platelets
- Many scoring systems in use: specific for pediatric patients, including pediatric risk of mortality[35] and pediatric organ failure,[5] and specific for certain categories of patients, including Rotterdam score,[36] Glasgow Meningococcal Septicaemia Prognostic Score,[37] disseminated intravascular coagulation,[38,39] and adapted adult scores (e.g., organ failure score).[40]

THERAPY

EARLY RECOGNITION AND GOAL-DIRECTED THERAPY TO IMPROVE OUTCOME

Early recognition, adequate resuscitation, appropriate therapeutic response, removal of the nidus of infection, and effective antibiotic therapy are crucial to optimal outcome.[41,42] In June 2002, the American College of Critical Care Medicine published its evidence-based *Clinical Practice Parameters for Hemodynamic Support of Newborns and Children with Septic Shock,* based in part on the concept that early recognition and resuscitation improve outcome (Fig. 148-1).[6]

IMMEDIATE RESUSCITATION (FIRST HOUR)

Airway and Breathing
Newborns and children usually have an adequate airway, but mechanical ventilation is required in 80% in shock. Intubation should be performed according to pediatric advanced life support and Neonatal Resuscitation Program guidelines on the basis of clinical diagnosis of respiratory distress or hemodynamic instability, not blood gas analysis. Volume resuscitation and the use of the non–cardiac depressant drug ketamine as an induction agent are recommended to prevent worsening positive-pressure ventilation–associated hypotension. It is clinical practice to intubate pediatric patients in an early stage of the disease, generally when they need more than 60 mL/kg of fluid resuscitation.[14]

Volume Resuscitation
Virtually all children with shock require aggressive volume resuscitation[10,43,44]; this should be given as 20 mL/kg boluses of normal saline or colloid as intravenous pushes to a total of 60 mL/kg in the first 10 to 20 minutes. If the liver edge becomes palpable, rales are heard, or the perfusion pressure (mean arterial pressure − central venous pressure) narrows, more fluid is not advised. Some children have required 200 mL/kg in the first hour. Many clinicians use crystalloid as the first fluid and follow with colloid if this is unsuccessful. Serum glucose should be checked because hypoglycemia can have devastating neurologic consequences. Glucose should be administered rapidly in this condition.

Cardiovascular Therapy
Children can present with low cardiac output and high systemic vascular resistance, high cardiac output and low systemic vascular resistance, or low cardiac output and low systemic vascular resistance shock.[29] Depending on which situation exists, inotropic support should be started in the case of fluid-refractory shock or a combination of an inotrope with a vasopressor or a vasodilator. Dopamine or dobutamine is probably the first choice of support for a pediatric patient with hypotension refractory to fluid resuscitation. The choice of vasoactive agent is determined by the clinical examination. Dobutamine-refractory or dopamine-refractory shock often can be reversed with epinephrine or norepinephrine infusion.[29] Pediatric patients requiring inotropic support are in a low cardiac output, not a high cardiac output, state. The use of vasodilators can reverse shock in pediatric patients who remain hypodynamic with a high systemic vascular resistance state, despite fluid resuscitation and implementation of inotropic support. Nitrosovasodilators (nitroprusside or nitroglycerin have a short half-life) are used as first-line therapy for children with epinephrine-resistant low cardiac output and elevated systemic vascular resistance shock.

Adrenal Insufficiency
Lack of response to epinephrine (cold shock) or norepinephrine (warm shock) can be caused by adrenal insufficiency or thyroid deficiency.[45-47] Children at risk for this condition (e.g., purpura fulminans, prior steroid exposure, central nervous system disease) should be treated with hydrocortisone. The proper dose has been poorly investigated and ranges from a

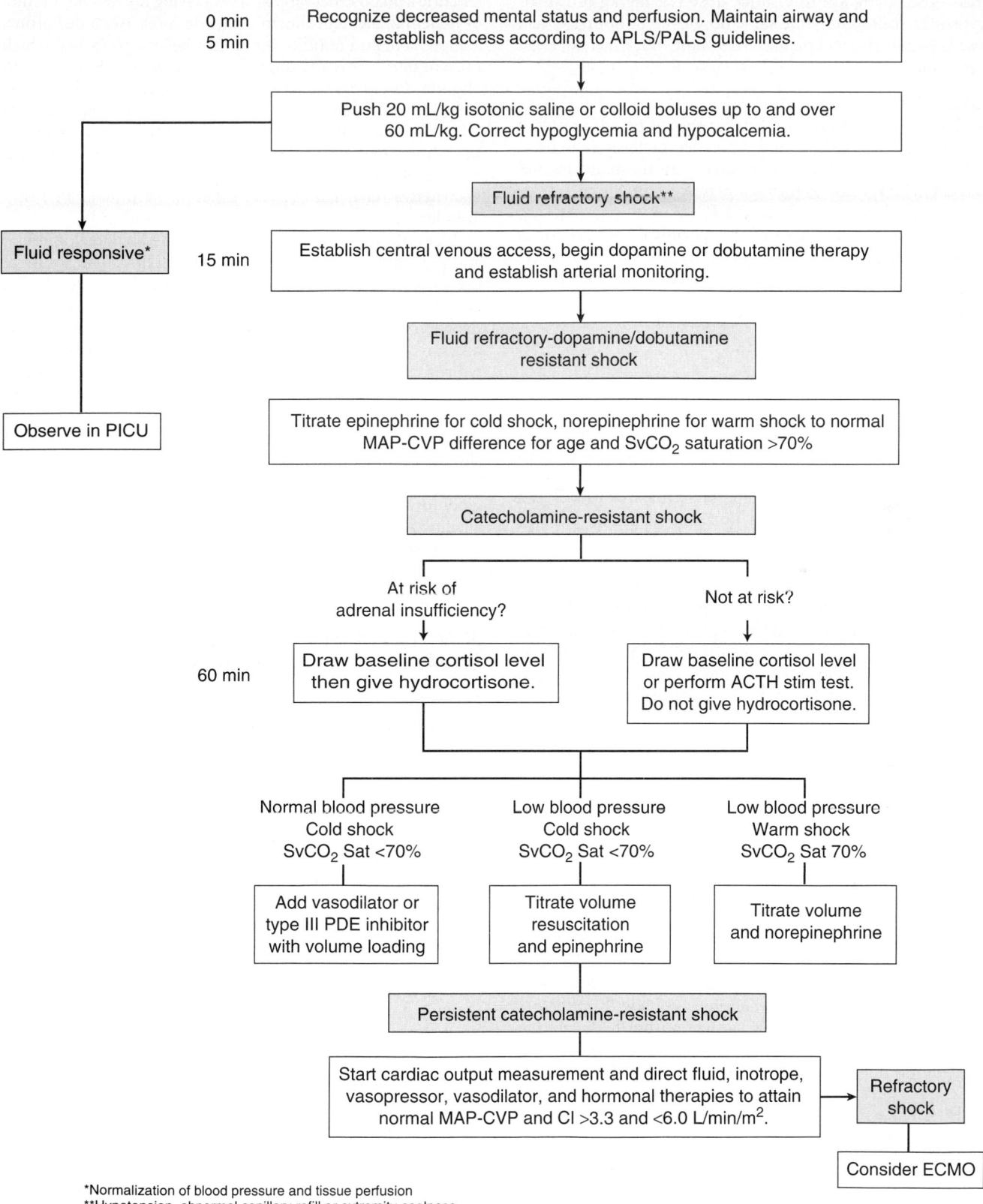

FIGURE 148–1. Clinical practice parameters for hemodynamic support of newborns and children with septic shock. This evidence-based treatment algorithm is based on early recognition and resuscitation to improve outcome. ACTH, adrenocorticotropic hormone; APLS/PALS, advanced pediatric life support/pediatric advanced life support; CI, cardiac index; CVP, central venous pressure; ECMO, extracorporeal membrane oxygenation; MAP, mean arterial pressure; PDE, phosphodiesterase; PICU, pediatric intensive care unit; SvCO₂, venous carbon dioxide saturation. (From Carcillo JA, Fields AI: Clinical practice parameters for hemodynamic support of pediatric and neonatal patients in septic shock. Crit Care Med 2002;30:1365-1378.)

stress dose (2 mg/kg) to a shock dose (50 mg/kg of hydrocortisone), followed by the same dose over 24 hours. Which dose is better in catecholamine-resistant shock has not been determined.

Antibiotics

Antibiotics and antifungal therapies should be administered according to age, setting, and resistance patterns (empirical therapy). The emergence of resistant organisms mandates that antibiotics be specific to regional practice. Some investigators advocate antibiotic cycling in the ICU.[48] Although survival from sepsis and septic shock can occur only if the infection is eradicated, administration of antibiotics should never supersede or postpone volume and cardiovascular resuscitation.

STABILIZATION OF SEPSIS AND SEPTIC SHOCK (AFTER FIRST HOUR OF RESUSCITATION)

Cardiovascular

The first hour of resuscitation is directed toward restoration of normal perfusion pressure; however, ensuing therapies should be directed toward obtaining normal central venous oxygen saturation. Children with persistent warm shock can respond to more volume and norepinephrine. In selected children with norepinephrine-resistant shock, vasopressin (at physiologic dose) or angiotensin can bypass alpha receptor desensitization and restore vascular tone; however, this can increase afterload and decrease cardiac output.[49-51] Children with cold shock and normal blood pressure respond to afterload reduction and volume loading.[29,52] When pediatric patients remain in a normotensive low cardiac output and high vascular resistance state, despite epinephrine and nitrosovasodilator therapy, the use of milrinone (if liver dysfunction is present) or amrinone (if renal dysfunction is present) should be strongly considered.[53] These type III phosphodiesterase inhibitors can bypass beta-adrenergic receptor desensitization.[53-55] Children with cold shock and hypotension are most worrisome. They can respond to more volume and epinephrine. Neonates and children with pulmonary hypertension and right ventricular failure can respond to inhaled NO.[56]

Extracorporeal membrane oxygenation is an effective therapy in refractory neonatal shock (80% survival) and should be considered as a possible therapy in refractory pediatric shock (50% survival).[57,58] This success is likely due to the fact that refractory shock in newborns and children is usually cardiac, not vascular, failure. Adults with refractory shock from Hantavirus (a low cardiac output/high vascular resistance state) have similar extracorporeal membrane oxygenation outcomes to newborns with refractory shock.[59]

Respiratory

Lung "protection" ventilation strategies reduced mortality rates in adults with acute respiratory distress syndrome (many who had sepsis).[60] Effective tidal volumes of 6 mL/kg are a reasonable compromise when ventilating septic children with acute respiratory distress syndrome. Positive end-expiratory pressure protects against volutrauma by maintaining functional residual capacity and optimal compliance. Optimal positive end-expiratory pressure can be determined using partial pressure of oxygen in arterial blood-to-inspired oxygen fraction ratio or compliance.

Renal Failure

Renal failure occurs if ischemia continues for greater than 60 minutes, thrombosis prevents perfusion, or myoglobin and uric acid obstruct tubular flow. During the first 60 minutes of ischemia, the neurohormonal system releases aldosterone, angiotensin, and antidiuretic hormone (vasopressin), which prevent natriuresis and diuresis; this manifests clinically with oliguria. Rapid resuscitation reverses ischemia and, because 20% of blood flow goes to renal perfusion, manifests as return of urine output greater than 1 mL/kg/h. If ischemia lasts more than 1 hour, ATP depletion causes epithelial cells to separate from and obstruct tubules, leading to tubulo-obstructive renal failure (also called *acute tubular necrosis*). Tubular regeneration requires 6 weeks to 3 months.

Blood flow to the kidney is autoregulated by preglomerular and postglomerular constriction and dilation. The ability of the preglomerular arterioles to dilate is impaired during endotoxemia and cirrhosis. Blood flow to the kidney depends on perfusion pressure (measured as mean arterial pressure – central venous pressure or, in the case of abdominal compartment syndrome, mean arterial pressure – intra-abdominal pressure) in children with sepsis.[61] Perfusion pressure should be maintained with volume, inotropes, and in some cases vasopressor therapies. Creatinine clearance should be measured daily to assess function. Diuretics are recommended to prevent fluid overload. Patients with myoglobinuria or uric aciduria should be treated with mannitol, alkalinization, and allopurinol (uric aciduria). Severe oliguria or anuria despite diuretics should be managed with daily or continuous hemofiltration/hemodialysis or peritoneal dialysis.

PURPURA FULMINANS AND DISSEMINATED INTRAVASCULAR COAGULATION

Disseminated intravascular coagulation is recognized clinically as a prolonged prothrombin time/partial thromboplastin time, reduced fibrinogen, increased fibrin degradation products, and thrombocytopenia.[38,39] When patients present with purpura fulminans/disseminated intravascular coagulation, with genetic proclivity (thrombophilias), or with rapidly growing organisms (meningococcus), the process is deadly unless reversed. Tissue factor is exposed by endothelial injury and released into the bloodstream. If tissue factor is unmatched by tissue factor pathway inhibitor, it activates factor VII–mediated coagulation. Ongoing coagulation consumes clotting factors (including fibrinogen), antithrombotic factors (antithrombin III and protein C), and platelets; this leads to a state of massive clotting and bleeding. Therapeutic strategies must restore a homeostatic milieu by removing or inhibiting tissue factor activity and replacing anticoagulant factors, procoagulant factors, and platelets. If systemic clotting is limb-threatening or life-threatening, fibrinolytic therapies may be required for reperfusion. Debate continues on whether specific therapies (e.g., antithrombin III, protein C, heparin, activated protein C, tissue plasminogen activator), nonspecific therapies (fresh frozen plasma and platelet replacement or plasma exchange), or a combination of both (plasma exchange plus antithrombin III, protein C, or activated protein C with tissue plasminogen activator added for limb-threatening or life-threatening thrombosis) is best. An activated protein C trial has been initiated in pediatric septic shock, but patients at risk of bleeding (low platelet counts) or receiving heparin-based continuous venovenous hemofiltration are being excluded. Some investigators believe that patients with meningococcemia cannot activate protein C,[62] whereas others believe that these children can activate protein C.[63] So far there is no evidence for benefit of either product.

NUTRITION, ELECTROLYTES, ENDOCRINE, AND METABOLISM

It is debated whether one should feed patients enterally when in shock; however, there is agreement the enteral route is best when shock resolves. Total parenteral nutrition should be considered in patients not tolerating enteral feeds and "calories given" directed to "calories expended" if a metabolic monitor is available. If a monitor is not available, calorie needs can be overestimated when using classic formulas in critically ill children. Hypoglycemia should be rigorously avoided and treated. Hypoglycemia is associated with devastating neurologic outcomes. Strict control of hyperglycemia with insulin infusion substantially reduced mortality in an adult surgical ICU by reducing deaths from multiple-organ dysfunction syndrome/multiple organ failure.[64] In general, infants are at risk for developing hypoglycemia when they depend on intravenous fluids; a glucose intake of 4 to 6 mg/kg/min or maintenance fluid intake with glucose 10% and sodium chloride 0.45% is advised. There are no studies in pediatric patients analyzing the effect of rigid glycemic control using insulin; this should only be done with frequent glucose monitoring in view of the risks for hypoglycemia.

IMMUNE MODULATION

Children who cannot kill invading organisms die from sepsis. Primary and acquired immunodeficiency states must be treated. Children with chronic granulomatous disease require white blood cell transfusions and interferon. Patients with hypogammaglobulinemia require treatment with intravenous immunoglobulin. Granulocyte-macrophage colony-stimulating factor was shown in a randomized controlled trial to improve survival in newborn neutropenic septic shock.[65] Transplant and nontransplant patients who develop septic shock while receiving immune suppression die unless the immune suppressants are rapidly tapered. Polyclonal intravenous immunoglobulin has been reported to reduce mortality rate and is a promising adjuvant in the treatment of sepsis and septic shock. All the trials have been small in children, however, and the totality of the evidence is insufficient to support a robust conclusion of benefit. Adjunctive therapy with monoclonal intravenous immunoglobulin is experimental.[67]

DRUG DOSING

Decreased cytochrome P-450 activity not only is manifest in impaired steroid synthesis, but also impaired drug metabolism is present in children with sepsis, septic shock, or multiple organ failure.[21] Patients with multiple organ failure are at particular risk of toxicity with drugs that are metabolized by the cytochrome P-450 system. Renal function also is impaired. Creatinine clearance–directed drug dosing of renally eliminated drugs is necessary in these patients. Drugs should be administered according to pharmacodynamic and pharmacokinetic goals.

MULTICENTER RANDOMIZED CONTROLLED TRIALS FOR PEDIATRIC SEPTIC SHOCK

Two studies were completed examining the role of endotoxin-neutralizing therapies in children with presumed meningococcal purpura fulminans/shock. Derkx and colleagues[68] reported a 25% reduction in mortality rate with the HA-1A antibody, and Giroir and others[13,69] reported a 25% reduction in mortality rate with rhBPI. Both studies were underpowered. Recombinant activated protein C resulted in a 20% reduction in mortality rate in a properly powered adult study and was approved for use in adults with severe sepsis and a 20% risk or greater of mortality. The drug was associated with increased intracranial hemorrhage in all patients. Further studies of activated protein C and protein C concentrate in pediatric patients are planned.

ANNOTATED REFERENCES

Carcillo JA, Fields AI: Clinical practice parameters for hemodynamic support of pediatric and neonatal patients in septic shock. Crit Care Med 2002;30:1365-1378.
  Evidence-based guidelines for the treatment of sepsis in neonates and pediatric patients are presented.

Emonts M, Hazelzet JA, de Groot R, et al: Host genetic determinants of *Neisseria meningitidis* infections. Lancet Infect Dis 2003;3:565-577.
  This is a review of the genetic polymorphisms and mutations known so far to be involved in the inflammatory process in meningococcal sepsis.

Leteurtre S, Martinot A, Duhamel A, et al: Development of a pediatric multiple organ dysfunction score: Use of two strategies. Med Decis Making 1999;19:399-410.
  This article describes an organ failure score useful in pediatric sepsis. The score is practical for use in daily practice.

Pollard AJ, Britto J, Nadel S, et al: Emergency management of meningococcal disease. Arch Dis Child 1999;80:290-296.
  An overview of the acute treatment of pediatric meningococcal sepsis is presented.

Watson RS, Carcillo JA, Linde-Zwirble WT, et al: The epidemiology of severe sepsis in children in the United States. Am J Respir Crit Care Med 2003;167:695-701.
  This is the first large overview of this size concerning epidemiology of pediatric sepsis in the United States.

Chapter 149

ACUTE BACTEREMIA

Philippe Eggimann • Didier Pittet

KEY POINTS

1. **A large proportion of all clinical forms of sepsis and a majority of cases associated with multiple organ failure are related to acute bacteremia.** These entities are responsible for significant mortality, morbidity, length of hospital stay, and resource utilization in almost all groups of patients studied.

2. **In most institutions, a shift in predominant organisms from Gram-negative bacilli to Gram-positive cocci has occurred** over the past 2 decades. This may be due in part to the fact that a large proportion of these infections are related to the presence of intravascular access devices, known to be largely colonized and infected by microorganisms from the skin flora.

3. **Blood cultures are negative in at least 40% to 60% of episodes of severe sepsis and septic shock,** but these conditions are associated with increased morbidity, mortality, and end-organ dysfunction even when blood cultures are negative.

4. **Delayed or inappropriate antibiotic treatment of acute bacteremia is associated with significantly higher mortality rates.** Accordingly, when bacteremia is suspected, empirical antimicrobial treatment should be prescribed in a majority of cases while awaiting the results of blood cultures.

5. As with other infections, the **prevention of acute bacteremia relies on strict adherence to the basic rules of hygiene,** particularly hand hygiene practices. Education-based measures targeted at controlling device-associated infections have also proved effective.

Acute bacteremia, which may be primary or secondary and community or hospital acquired, is one of the most severe forms of infection. Frequently observed among immunocompromised and critically ill patients, bacteremia is rarely asymptomatic. A large proportion of all clinical forms of sepsis and a majority of cases associated with multiple organ failure are related to acute bacteremia.[1-3]

DEFINITIONS

Bacteremia, which, strictly speaking, relates to the presence of viable bacteria in the blood, is not the appropriate term to describe the spectrum of diseases it includes. It may represent only the tip of the iceberg of a pathophysiologically comparable condition in which the presence of microorganisms in the blood is not identified; further, it does not describe episodes of fungemia or parasitemia. The term *bloodstream infection* has been proposed and progressively imposed in the literature and includes both primary and secondary forms (Table 149-1).[4-11] Bloodstream infection should be distinguished from *septicemia, clinical sepsis,* and *sepsis,* which refer to clinical syndromes discussed in other chapters of this book. Precise terminology is proposed in Table 149-1.

EPIDEMIOLOGY

Bloodstream infections represented 12% of all nosocomial infections reported in 10,038 patients from 1417 ICUs in the European Prevalence of Infection in Intensive Care (EPIC) study.[12] However, the epidemiology of bloodstream infection varies according to its source. Studies may include primary and secondary bloodstream infections and nosocomial or community-acquired infections, and they may report hospital-wide or only specific ward-related episodes (Table 149-2).[13-25] In series reporting mostly nosocomial episodes, primary bloodstream infection outnumbered infections originating from a distinct origin.

In addition, some surveillance systems may include clinical sepsis (see Table 149-1). This is the case for the largest existing surveillance network—the U.S. National Nosocomial Infection Surveillance System. This system, which took into account only data from ICUs, reported that most nosocomial bloodstream infections were related to intravascular access devices, with rates substantially higher among patients with central venous catheters than among those with peripheral lines.[26,27] There is limited information about the clinical importance of clinical sepsis, but recent data suggest that laboratory-based surveillance may grossly underestimate the real burden of primary bloodstream infection in intensive care.[28,29] Unsurprisingly, given that clinical sepsis and microbiologically documented bloodstream infection share the most important risk factor (i.e., exposure to intravascular access devices), underidentification of clinical sepsis may reduce the possibility of its prevention.[29,30]

The incidence of bloodstream infection in various patient populations is presented in Table 149-3.[13-15,17-19,22-24,31-48] However, an exact description of precisely what is reported is not systematically provided in the literature. Time trends should be considered when large study periods are reviewed.[20,21,24,27] In consideration of the large differences

TABLE 149–1. DEFINITIONS OF BLOODSTREAM INFECTION

Type of Bloodstream Infection	Criteria
Positive blood culture	Recognized pathogens* identified from one or more blood cultures and not related to an infection at another body site
Laboratory-confirmed	Positive blood culture with at least one of the following signs or symptoms: fever (>100.4°F [38°C]) or hypothermia (<98.6°F [37°C]); chills; low blood pressure (systolic blood pressure ≤90 mm Hg or a decrease >40 mm Hg from baseline)
Primary	Laboratory-confirmed bloodstream infection or clinical sepsis occurring without documented distal source of infection, including those resulting from catheter-related or catheter-associated infections
Secondary	Laboratory-confirmed bloodstream infection occurring in the presence of another documented site of infection
Catheter-associated	Primary bloodstream infection and presence of an intravascular access device
Catheter-related	Laboratory-confirmed bloodstream infection in a patient with an intravascular access device and at least one positive blood culture obtained from a peripheral vein, clinical manifestations of infection (fever, chills, hypotension), and no apparent source of bloodstream infection except the vascular access, plus one of the following: positive semiquantitative culture (>15 CFU/catheter segment) with the same organism;[5] positive quantitative culture (>10³ CFU/catheter segment) with the same organism,[7] simultaneous quantitative blood cultures with a ≥ 5:1 ratio CVC versus peripheral,[8] and differential period of CVC culture versus peripheral blood culture positivity of >2 h[9]

*One of the following: common skin contaminant (diphtheroids, *Bacillus* spp., *Propionibacterium* spp., coagulase-negative staphylococci, or micrococci) cultured from two or more blood cultures drawn on separate occasions; common skin contaminant cultured from one or more blood cultures from a patient with vascular access, and the physician institutes appropriate antimicrobial therapy; positive antigen test on blood *and* signs and symptoms with positive laboratory results not related to an infection at another site.

CFU, colony-forming unit; CVC, central venous catheter.

observed, extreme caution should be exercised when making rate comparisons and eventual benchmarking.[29,49-51]

MICROBIOLOGY

The distribution of microorganisms causing bloodstream infections varies according to the type of infection (Table 149-4).[13-15,17-19,22-25,37,40,45,52,53] In most institutions, a shift in predominant organisms from Gram-negative bacilli to Gram-positive cocci has been observed over the past 2 decades.[21,24,45,54] Several elements may explain this shift, which is more evident in series restricted to primary bloodstream infections. Many of these infections are related to the presence of intravascular access devices, known to be largely colonized and infected by microorganisms from the skin flora. Hospital-acquired bloodstream infections may be associated with the change in case-mix severity in many institutions, and the precise impact of a larger proportion of device-related infections is difficult to assess. A shift toward Gram-positive cocci has been reported in most series of empirical treatment of fever in neutropenic patients; these cases account for a significant proportion of bloodstream infections in some institutions, which explains the observed trends. The current high density of medical facilities and the unrestricted access to medical care for the majority of the population in most developed countries have played major roles in the prescription of antibiotics very early in the course of most infections. In addition, the widespread use of broad-spectrum antibiotics, either for therapy or for surgical prophylaxis, may be partially responsible for the increase in the relative proportions of coagulase-negative staphylococci and enterococci. The proportion of *Candida* species has considerably increased in many institutions as well. Prolonged treatment with multiple antibiotics, the use of indwelling intravascular devices, and prolonged neutropenia in patients with cancer have been demonstrated to be independent risk factors for the acquisition of nosocomial candidemia.

IMPACT ON MORBIDITY AND COSTS

Some studies have determined the impact of bloodstream infection on patient morbidity and hospital costs. In the ICU, a higher prevalence of nosocomially acquired infection is associated with a higher mortality rate. In the EPIC study, laboratory-proven bloodstream infection, pneumonia, and clinical sepsis were independently associated with increased mortality.[12]

The precise impact of infection can be determined by the attributable part of the confounding factors considered. Accordingly, the attributable mortality is defined as the difference in the death rate between infected and noninfected patients after adjustment for the presence of other confounding factors. Direct estimation is an easy method for determining the attributable fraction. An experienced clinician subjectively estimates whether death or any other parameter, such as excess length of stay or extra cost, is related to the infection. However, this technique underestimates the attributable part. Another method compares two groups of patients, one with and one without a specified infection; differences are expected to be attributable to the infection. However, this technique does not take into consideration potential confounding factors that may exist. These adjustments are generally insufficient, and the attributable part is often overestimated. So-called matched case-controlled studies (more appropriately, historical cohort studies with matching on potential confounders) are the method of choice to determine the true impact of an infection. Infected and noninfected patients are carefully matched for several confounding factors related to the investigated parameter. Among matching variables, age, severity of underlying disease, associated comorbidities, number of discharge diagnoses, and exposure time to risk factors are usually considered. Apart from when case and control patients are matched too closely, bias in the estimated impact is minimal with this approach.[55]

Nosocomial bloodstream infection is responsible for a significant increase in mortality, morbidity, length of hospital

TABLE 149–2. SOURCES OF BLOODSTREAM INFECTION

Author	No. of Cases	Primary (%)*	Secondary (%)	Urinary (%)	Abdominal (%)	Pulmonary (%)	Skin/Soft Tissue (%)	Bone/Joint (%)	Cardiovascular (%)	CNS (%)	Other (%)
Hospital-wide, community acquired											
Valles et al[13]	339	25	75	20	20	21	ND	ND	4	ND	10
Hospital-wide, nosocomial											
Lyytikainen et al[14]	1477	83	17	6	ND	ND	ND	ND	ND	ND	ND
Spengler et al[15]	935	51	49	16	9	11	12	ND	ND	ND	1
Pittet et al[16]	1745	62	38	7	2	11	10	ND	ND	ND	8
Hospital-wide, community acquired and nosocomial											
Brun-Buisson et al[17]	842	26	74	21	18	16	8	2	2	2	5
Petrosillo et al[18]	65	66	44	8	5	8	11	1	0	1	0
Endimiani et al[19]	521	79	31	14	0	11	3	0	0	0	3
ICU, community acquired and nosocomial											
Pittet et al[20]	176	21	79	6	31	28	ND	ND	ND	2	12
Hugonnet et al[21]	196	47	53	4	15	29	ND	ND	ND	1	4
ICU, nosocomial											
Valles et al[22]	590	65	35	6	6	18	2	ND	ND	ND	3
Renaud & Brun-Buisson[23]	111	55	45	ND	ND	ND	ND	ND	ND	ND	ND
Pittet & Wenzel[24]	3464	59	41	8	ND	12	10	ND	ND	ND	ND
Surgery, nosocomial											
Raymond et al[25]	363	53	47	ND	ND	ND	ND	ND	ND	ND	ND

*Catheter related or of unknown origin.
CNS, central nervous system; ND, not done.

TABLE 149–3. INCIDENCE OF BACTEREMIA IN DIFFERING POPULATIONS

Author	No. of Hospitals	Type of Hospital	Type of Infection	Per 1000 Admissions or Discharges	Per 1000 Patient-days
Hospital-wide series					
Elhanan et al[34]	1	Community	Any*	10.1	2.18
	1	University	Any*	12.0	2.64
Endimiani et al[19]	1	University	Any*	10.1	—
Brun-Buisson et al[17]	24	Any	Any*	9.8 (9.2-10.5)	—
Petrosillo et al[18]	17	Any	Any*,†	47.1	2.5
Lyytikainen et al[14]	4	Any	Nosocomial	2.7	0.8
NINSS[35]	61	Any	Nosocomial	—	0.6
Brun-Buisson et al[17]	24	Any	Nosocomial	4.4 (4.0-4.9)	—
Banerjee et al[36]	124	Community	Nosocomial	1.3	—
Spengler et al[15]	1	University	Nosocomial	4.1	—
Banerjee et al[36]	124	University	Nosocomial	6.5	—
Endimiani et al[19]	1	University	Nosocomial	7.4	—
Pittet & Wenzel[24]	1	University	Nosocomial	13.2	1.45
ICU series					
Valles et al[22]	30 mixed	Any	Community acquired	10.2	—
Luzzaro et al[52]	16 mixed	Any	Any*	6.8	—
Brun-Buisson et al[17]	24 mixed	Any	Any*	69 (59-80)	—
Richards et al[45]	205 mixed	Any	Nosocomial	7.5	2.4
Brun-Buisson et al[17]	24 mixed	Any	Nosocomial	41 (33-50)	—
Legras et al[46]	5 mixed	Any	Nosocomial	—	4.1
Renaud & Brun-Buisson[23]	15 mixed	Any	Nosocomial	50.4	4.5
Barsic et al[32]	1 mixed	University	Nosocomial	—	22.8
Kollef et al[33]	1 mixed	University	Nosocomial	—	9.6
Valles et al[22]	30 mixed	Any	Nosocomial	36.0	—
Richards et al[37]	112 medical	Any	Nosocomial	16.3	4.1
Eggimann et al[38]	1 medical	University	Nosocomial	15.2	3.8
Brooks et al[39]	1 medical	University	Nosocomial	—	3.0
Richards et al[40]	61 pediatric	Any	Nosocomial	14.6	3.7
Raymond & Aujard[41]	20 pediatric	Any	Nosocomial	—	3.4
Gastmeier et al[42]	72 pediatric	Any	Nosocomial	—	2.1
Simon et al[43]	1 pediatric	University	Nosocomial	—	4.8
Gilio et al[44]	1 pediatric	University	Nosocomial	—	1.5
Pittet & Wenzel[24]	1 surgical	University	Nosocomial	26.7	—
Richards et al[31]	93 coronary	Any	Nosocomial	—	1.8
Dettenkofer et al[48]	1 neurologic	University	Nosocomial	13.8	1.4

*Both community-acquired and nosocomial infections were reported together.
†HIV-positive patients.
NINSS, Nosocomial Infection National Surveillance Scheme.

stay, and resource utilization in almost all groups of patients studied (Table 149-5).[1,13-15,17-20,22,23,25,55-69] Importantly, microbiologic factors have been independently associated with increased mortality among patients with nosocomial bloodstream infection, even after adjustment for major confounders intrinsic to patients' underlying conditions.[16] These factors include pneumonia as a source of secondary bacteremia, polymicrobial infection, and infection caused by *Candida* species. Bloodstream pathogens such as *Staphylococcus aureus*, enterococci, *Pseudomonas aeruginosa*, *Enterobacter* species, and *Candida* species tend to be associated with higher mortality.

GENERAL PRINCIPLES OF MANAGEMENT

Blood cultures are usually performed in hospitalized patients if it is suspected that microorganisms are present in the blood. The clinical threshold for performing blood cultures is very low, and fever or systemic inflammatory response syndrome often justifies it. This may explain why only 10% to 15% of blood cultures performed are positive. It should be stressed that blood cultures are negative in at least 40% to 60% of severe sepsis and septic shock episodes.[1-3] Importantly, however, severe sepsis and septic shock are associated with increased morbidity, mortality, and end-organ dysfunction, even when blood cultures are negative.[70] Accordingly, when sepsis is suspected, it is generally not possible to wait until the results of blood cultures become available; empirical antimicrobial treatment is prescribed in a majority of cases (Fig. 149-1).

The management of bloodstream infection should combine early antimicrobial treatment and the active search for a source of infection that might require specific measures for eradication or therapy (Fig. 149-2). It has been shown repeatedly that either delayed or inappropriate antibiotic treatment is associated with significantly higher mortality rates.[21,33,71,72] In two studies, the appropriateness of antibiotic treatment was not found to be a risk factor for the development of septic shock in bacteremic patients,[13,58] but the mortality of those requiring vasopressors was significantly higher—85% versus 75% and 58% versus 24%, respectively—than that of patients who did not require them.

The choice of antibiotics should be based on susceptibility testing of the microorganisms identified from the bloodstream. In some conditions, pathogens identified from other body sites also need to be treated. However, in most cases, antibiotics are started empirically several days before any information becomes available from the laboratory. The choice

TABLE 149–4. MICROBIOLOGY OF BLOODSTREAM INFECTIONS

Author	Year of Publication	No. of Organisms	CoNS (%)	S. aureus (%)	S. pneumoniae (%)	Enterococci (%)	Other GPC (%)	E. coli (%)	Enterobacter (%)	P. aeruginosa (%)	Other GNB (%)	Yeasts (%)
Community acquired, hospital-wide												
Luzzaro et al[52]	2002	1031	5	19	10	6	12	42	3	4	7	2
Community acquired, ICU												
Valles et al[13]	2003	339	3	15	18	3	5	28	2	3	22	1
Nosocomial, hospital-wide												
Spengler et al[15]	1978	935	3	9	2	3	9	14	8	8	46	6
Edmond et al[2]	1999	10617	32	16	ND	11	1	6	7	4	16	8
Pittet & Wenzel[24]	1995	3464	26	16	ND	4	12	12	6	9	8	7
Raymond et al[25]	2000	245 primary	44	8	ND	13	11	4	10	3	4	5
Raymond et al[25]	2000	209 secondary	24	9	ND	17	6	8	11	10	10	5
Luzzaro et al[52]	2002	1478	13	23	1	9	12	15	8	9	11	9
Lyytikäinen et al[14]	2002	1477	31	11	ND	6	8	11	8	5	16	4
Nosocomial, ICU												
Valles et al[22]	1997	511	28	20	ND	6	3	6	10	9	15	5
Richards et al[37]	1999	2971	36	13	ND	16	ND	3	6	3	11	12
Richards et al[40]	1999	1887	40	9	6	ND	1	3	5	5	21	10
Renaud & Brun-Buisson[23]	2001	111	18	14	ND	7	5	ND	25	ND	15	7
Richards et al[45]	2000	4394	40	12	11	ND	7	2	7	4	5	12
Overall, any ward												
Brun-Buisson et al[17]	1996	812	11	22	9	6	10	30	5	4	11	2
Petrosillo et al[18,*]	2002	65	28	30	9	ND	1	6	5	7	1	15
Endimiani et al[19]	2003	521	16	24	ND	ND	10	ND	33	ND	7	10

*HIV-positive only.
CoNS, coagulase-negative staphylococci; GNB, Gram-negative bacilli; GPC, Gram-positive cocci; ND, not done.

TABLE 149–5. IMPACT OF NOSOCOMIAL BLOODSTREAM INFECTION IN CRITICALLY ILL PATIENTS

Author	Study Population	Year of Publication	Study Period	No. of Cases	Mortality (%) Crude	Mortality (%) Attributable	Attributable LOS (Days)	Attributable Costs (US$)**
Community acquired								
Ispahani et al[56]	Hospital-wide	1987	1983-86	875	NA	20	NA	NA
Valles et al[13]	ICU	2003	1998	339	43	32	NA	NA
Community acquired and nosocomial								
Pittet et al[20]	ICU	1996	1984-88	176	35	NA	NA	NA
Elhanan et al[34]	Hospital-wide	1995	1992-93	1048	27	NA	NA	NA
Brun-Buisson et al[17]	Hospital-wide	1996	1993	832	28	NA	NA	NA
Brun-Buisson et al[17]	ICU	1996	1993	832	55	NA	NA	NA
Leibovici et al[58]	Hospital-wide, appropriate antibiotics	1998	1988-94	2158	20	NA	9	NA
Leibovici et al[58]	Hospital-wide, inappropriate antibiotics	1998	1988-94	1255	34	NA	11	NA
Hugonnet et al[21]	ICU	2003	1994-97	521	17	NA	NA	NA
Endimiani et al[19]	Hospital-wide	2003	1999-00	521	17	11	34	NA
Zaragoza et al[59]	ICU, inappropriate antibiotics	2003	1995-99	39	56	30	NA	NA
Nosocomial								
Spengler et al[15]	Hospital-wide	1978	1968-74	935	37	NA	NA	NA
Forgacs et al[60]	ICU	1986	1971-85	468	61	NA	NA	NA
Wey et al[61]	Hospital-wide*	1988	1977-84	88	57	38	30.0	NA
Smith et al[62]	ICU[†]	1991	1986-89	34	82	30	NA	NA
Rello et al[63]	ICU[†]	1994	1990-92	111	65	35[‡]	NA	NA
Pittet et al[1]	ICU[†]	1994	1988-90	86	50	35	8.0	40,000
Pittet & Wenzel[64]	ICU, restricted to catheter-associated	1994	1988-90	20	45	25	6.5	29,000
Valles et al[22]	30 ICUs	1997	1993	590	42	19	NA	NA
Wisplinghoff et al[65]	Burn unit[§]	1999	1990-92	29	31	16	20.0	NA
Soufir et al[55]	ICU, restricted to catheter-associated	1999	1990-95	38	50	29	NA	NA
Di Giovine et al[66]	ICU[||]	1999	1994-96	68	35	4[¶]	10.0	35,000
Rello et al[68]	ICU, restricted to catheter-related	2000	1992-99	49	22	13[¶]	20.0	4000
Renaud & Brun-Buisson[23]	15 ICUs	2001	1998	96	52	35	5.5	NA
Renaud & Brun-Buisson[23]	15 ICUs[||]	2001	1998	28	50	2	8.0	NA
Renaud & Brun-Buisson[23]	15 ICUs, restricted to catheter-related	2001	1998	26	39	12[¶]	14.0[¶]	NA
Raymond et al[25]	Surgery	2000	1996-00	363	20	NA	NA	NA
Dimick et al[69]	ICU, restricted to catheter-related	2001	1998-99	17	56	35[‡]	20.0	71,443*
Petrosillo et al[18]	Hospital-wide[||]	2002	1998-99	65	25	17[‡]	16.0	NA
Lyytikainen et al[14]	Hospital-wide	2002	1999-00	1477	25	NA	NA	NA

*Candidemia only.
[†]Includes both primary and secondary bloodstream infections.
[‡]Attributable mortality was determined by a simple comparison with the crude mortality of all patients who did not develop a bloodstream infection.
[§]*Acinetobacter baumannii* nosocomial bloodstream infections only.
[||]Includes primary bloodstream infections after exclusion of catheter-related infections.
[¶]Differences are nonsignificant.
**Based on billing database.
LOS, length of stay; NA, not available.

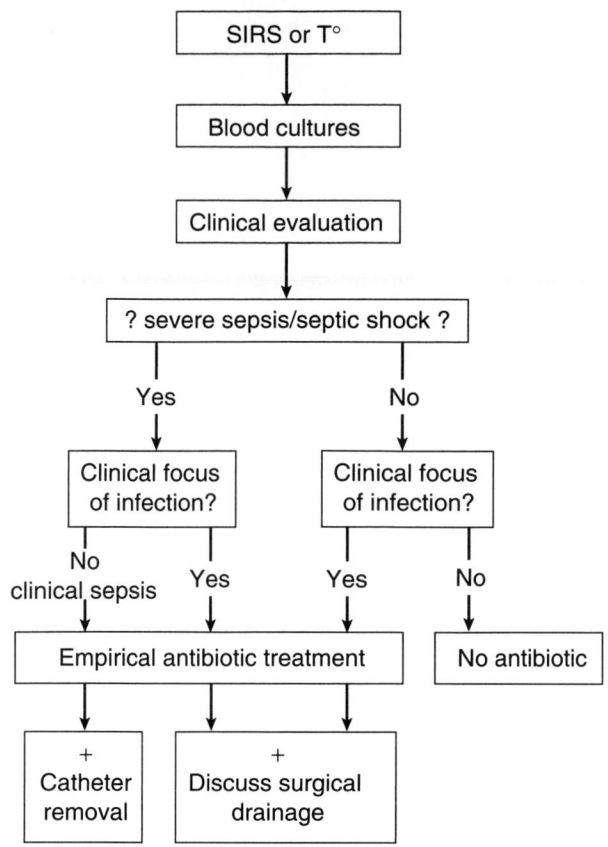

FIGURE 149–1. Management of a patient with suspected acute bloodstream infection. SIRS, systemic inflammatory response syndrome; T°, >100.4°F (38°C).

should be based on a precise knowledge of the epidemiology of all infections that could potentially be the source of bacteremia and any local patterns of resistance. Accordingly, a multidisciplinary approach, including close collaboration among the physician in charge of the patient, the infectious disease specialist, and the microbiology laboratory, is of paramount importance.

Specific measures should directly target all sources of infections. These include drainage of abscesses, adequate surgical management of peritonitis, and removal of infected prosthetic material.

The treatment of primary bacteremia and clinical sepsis should include the removal of catheters suspected of being infected. Catheter retention may result in a several-fold higher risk for recurrence of bloodstream infection. Removal is mandatory in severe or complicated infections in the presence of shock, persistent fever or bacteremia, or certain microorganisms (*S. aureus*, Gram-negative bacilli, *Candida* spp.).[10,26,73] Relapse, continuous fever, or bacteremia despite removal of the catheter requires an active search for complications, such as additional line-associated infection, metastatic abscess, septic thrombophlebitis, or endocarditis. After the completion of treatment, careful follow-up is mandatory owing to the frequent occurrence of late complications.[26,74]

PREVENTION

GENERAL MEASURES

As for any other infection, the prevention of bloodstream infection relies on strict respect for the basic rules of hygiene, particularly hand hygiene practices. This may be particularly

FIGURE 149–2. Workup following result of blood cultures. *A*, Evaluation at 48 to 72 hours of a patient treated for suspected acute bacteremia in the presence of a positive blood culture.

Continued

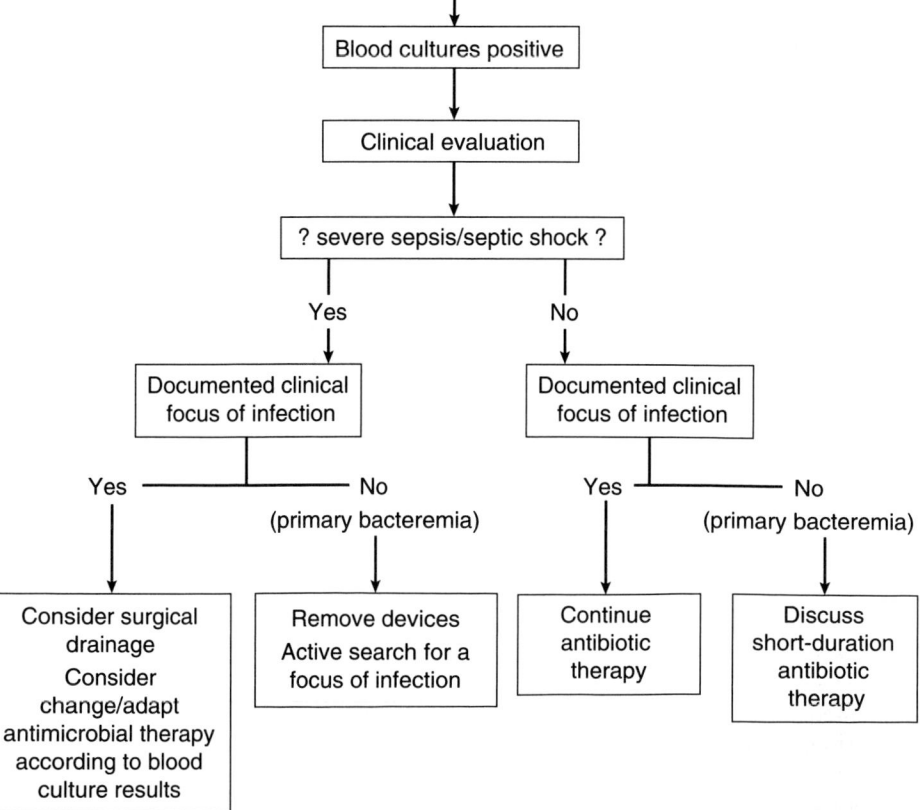

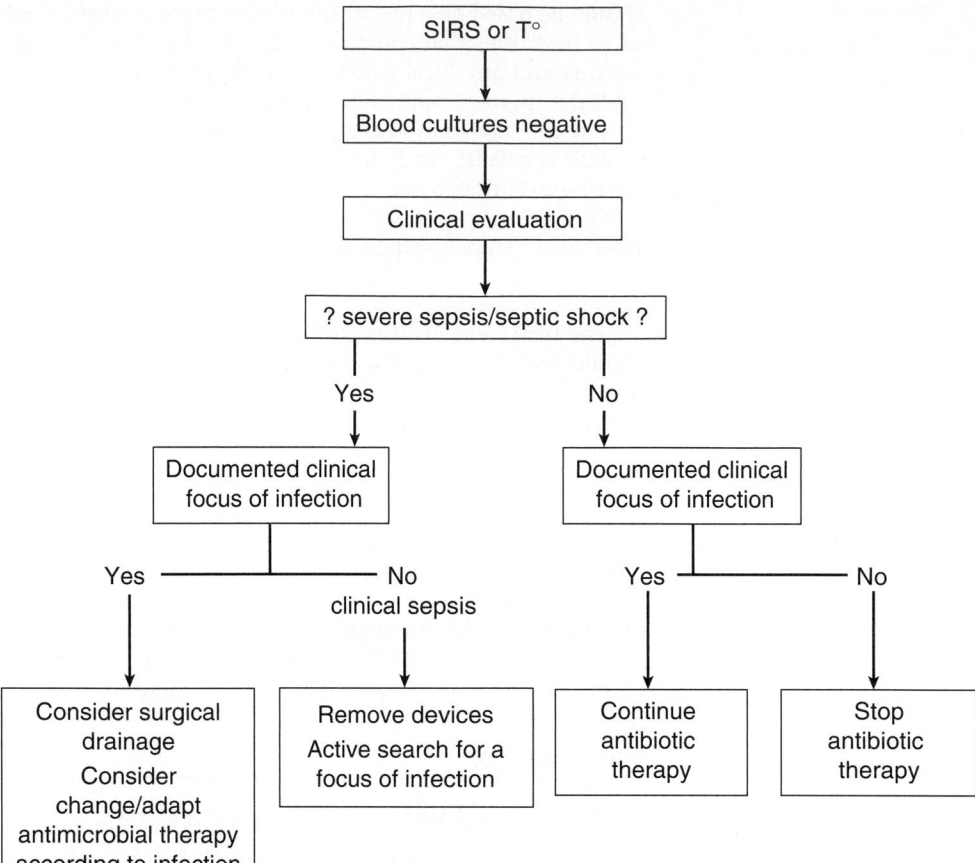

FIGURE 149–2—cont'd *B,* Evaluation at 48 to 72 hours of a patient treated for suspected acute bacteremia in the presence of a negative blood culture. SIRS, systemic inflammatory response syndrome.

important to prevent hospital-acquired bloodstream infections.

It is now clearly and firmly established that compared with traditional hand washing with soap and water, for which compliance rarely exceeds 40%, hand rubbing with alcohol-based solutions may result in significant and prolonged improvements in hand hygiene.[75,76] The latter combines the advantages of rapid-action, wide-spectrum antimicrobial efficacy; lower cost; and immediate availability at the bedside. Accordingly, guidelines for hand hygiene procedures have been completely reviewed and adapted to reflect these concepts.[77]

SPECIFIC MEASURES

The prevention of secondary bloodstream infections relies on specific measures that have been proved to prevent or cure particular types of infection, such as urinary tract, surgical site, and respiratory tract infections. Again, particular attention has to be paid to nosocomial infections; because most of these are device related, the majority must be considered preventable.[28] It was suggested that prevention could be achieved with the use of antibiotic- or antiseptic-coated devices, but their impact on the epidemiology of antibiotic resistance remains to be determined. Educational programs or global preventive strategies based on the strict application of specific preventive measures and careful control of all

factors associated with infection have proved to be even more effective in reducing infection rates.

ANNOTATED REFERENCES

Brun-Buisson C, Doyon F, Carlet J: Bacteremia and severe sepsis in adults: A multicenter prospective survey in ICUs and wards of 24 hospitals. French Bacteremia-Sepsis Study Group. Am J Respir Crit Care Med 1996;154:617-624.

This study examined the relationship between bacteremia and severe sepsis and assessed the influence of infection characteristics on the risk of severe sepsis and the outcome of bacteremia. Incidence rates of bacteremia and of bacteremic severe sepsis were 8 and 32 times higher in ICUs than in wards, respectively. Independent risk factors for severe sepsis during bacteremia included age and intra-abdominal, pulmonary, neuromeningeal, or multiple sources of bacteremia, but not the categories of organisms involved. The probability for death at 28 days was 25% and 54% in patients with bacteremia and bacteremic severe sepsis, respectively. The risk of death increased significantly with age, a rapidly or ultimately fatal underlying disease, the presence of severe sepsis, shock, and infection caused by Gram-positive organisms other than coagulase-negative staphylococci.

Harbarth S, Ferriere K, Hugonnet S, et al: Epidemiology and prognostic determinants of bloodstream infections in surgical intensive care. Arch Surg 2002;137:1353-1359.

This study explored the value of clinical variables available at the bedside to predict outcome in 224 critically ill patients with bloodstream infection. The 28-day fatality rate was 36%. By multivariate analysis, two independent predictors of mortality were the Acute Physiology and Chronic Health Evaluation (APACHE II) score at the onset of bloodstream infection and the number of evolving organ dysfunctions. Appropriate antimicrobial therapy was associated with improved outcome.

Hugonnet S, Harbarth S, Ferriere K, et al: Bacteremic sepsis in intensive care: Temporal trends in incidence, organ dysfunction, and prognosis. Crit Care Med 2003;31:390-394.

This study compared two cohorts of patients with bacteremic sepsis in the same surgical ICU during two separate periods (1984-1988 and 1994-1997). The incidence increased significantly from 3.2 to 4.3 per 100 admissions, with a comparable 28-day case fatality of 35% and 37%, respectively. The frequency of primary bacteremia increased from 21% to 47%, paralleled by an increase in the frequency of Gram-positive microorganisms. The proportion of patients with at least one organ dysfunction increased from 69% to 80%. For both cohorts, the two strongest predictors of mortality remained the APACHE II score at the onset of sepsis and the number of evolving organ dysfunctions.

O'Grady NP, Alexander M, Dellinger EP, et al: Guidelines for the prevention of intravascular catheter-related infections. Centers for Disease Control and Prevention. MMWR Morb Mortal Wkly Rep 2002;51:1-29.

This report of evidence-based recommendations to prevent catheter-related infections was prepared by a working group comprising members from at least 14 professional organizations. Major areas of emphasis include (1) educating and training health care providers, (2) using maximal sterile barrier precautions during central venous catheter insertion, (3) using a 2% chlorhexidine preparation as a skin antiseptic, (4) avoiding routine replacement of central venous catheters, and (5) using antiseptic- or antibiotic-impregnated short-term central venous catheters if the rate of infection is high despite adherence to other strategies.

Pittet D, Tarara D, Wenzel RP: Nosocomial bloodstream infection in critically ill patients: Excess length of stay, extra costs, and attributable mortality. JAMA 1994;271:1598-1601.

This study revealed the dramatic impact of nosocomial bloodstream infection in critically ill patients. A pairwise-matched (1:1) case-control study of critically ill surgical patients who developed nosocomial bloodstream infections showed that the crude mortality rates in cases and controls were 50% and 15%, respectively, corresponding to an attributable mortality of 35%. The extra hospital and ICU length of stay attributable to bloodstream infection was 24 and 8 days, respectively. Extra costs attributable to the infection averaged $40,000 per survivor.

Chapter 150

INFECTIONS OF THE UROGENITAL TRACT

F. M. E. Wagenlehner • K. G. Naber

KEY POINTS

1. **Complicated urinary tract infection** (UTI) is a very heterogeneous entity, with a common pattern of complicating factors.

2. **The bacterial spectrum of complicated UTI is much broader than in uncomplicated UTI,** comprising a variety of gram-negative and gram-positive pathogens and among these frequently multi-resistant pathogens.

3. **UTIs are frequent in ICUs. It would be pragmatic to stratify UTIs into those with nonurologic complicating causes,** in which the sole antimicrobial therapy is foremost, and those with urologic complicating causes, in which the complicating urologic anomaly needs to be effectively treated.

4. **Pathogens of nosocomial, complicated UTIs may be characterized by certain properties,** such as adaptation strategies to changing environments (i.e., hypermutator strains) or the propensity of biofilm formation.

5. **The diagnosis of UTI is based on medical history and thorough physical examination, including bedside ultrasound as well as investigations of urine (dipstick test, microscopy, and microbiology).** For clinical diagnosis, general accepted criteria should be employed. Symptomatic UTIs in ICU patients are especially difficult to evaluate.

6. **Not all bacteriuric patients in ICUs need to be treated.** Therapy should, however, be started in those with significant symptoms and morbidity; and in those even asymptomatic bacteriuria may be deleterious. Management of complicated UTI comprises adequate antibiotic therapy and successful treatment of complicating factors.

7. **Prophylaxis of UTI is important.** However, the percentage of infections that can be prevented is not known. Important points in prophylaxis encompass training of staff, hygiene measures, type of catheter and drainage, and patient care.

8. **Special clinical pictures of UTI and infections of contiguous organs are seen in the ICU.** UTIs of the upper urinary tract are distinguished from those of the lower urinary tract and infections of the male adnexal glands and fasciitis of the perineal and scrotal fascias. All these pictures can potentially merge into urosepsis if the UTI is not treated adequately. The urogenital tract is the source for sepsis in 20% to 30% of cases.

Infections in the ICU contribute significantly to patient morbidity. Depending on the type of ICU, nosocomial infections may account for 70% of infections.[1] Nosocomial infections of the urogenital tract are frequent[2] and sometimes underestimated in the ICU.

DEFINITION

Urinary tract infection can be the primary cause for admission to the ICU or can be acquired after intensive care procedures. Because patients are frequently sedated in the ICU, clinical diagnosis of UTI is often difficult. Nevertheless, UTI is an important cause of morbidity and antibiotic resistance in the ICU. Complicated UTI is a very heterogeneous entity, with a common pattern of the following factors:

- Anatomic, structural, or functional alterations of the urinary tract, which impede significantly urodynamic properties (e.g., stents, urine transport disturbances, instrumentation of the urinary tract, stones, tumors, neurologic disorders)
- Impaired renal function, caused by parenchymal diseases, or prerenal, intrarenal, or postrenal nephropathies (e.g., acute and chronic renal insufficiencies, cardiac insufficiency)
- Accompanying diseases impairing the patient's immune status (e.g., diabetes mellitus, liver insufficiency, immunosuppression, AIDS, hypothermia)

ETIOLOGY

Causative pathogens of UTI are almost exclusively bacteria and yeast. Viral pathogens are only found in patients with severe immunosuppression, such as after bone marrow transplantation. High antibiotic pressure and special circumstances in the ICU modulate the microbial spectrum. *Escherichia coli* is the most frequent pathogen, but it occurs less frequently than in uncomplicated, community-acquired UTI. Other Enterobacteriaceae may also be uropathogens (e.g., *Klebsiella, Proteus, Enterobacter, Serratia, Citrobacter,* or

TABLE 150–1. SPECTRUM OF PATHOGENS OF PATIENTS WITH URINARY TRACT INFECTION IN THE ICU, STRAUBING, GERMANY, 2001*

Pathogen	No. Patients	%
Escherichia coli	57	30.7
Klebsiella species	19	10.2
Proteus species	11	5.9
Enterobacter species	9	4.9
Serratia species	1	0.5
Citrobacter species	6	3.2
Morganella species	3	1.6
Enterobacteriaceae total	**106**	**57.0**
Pseudomonas species	13	7.0
Gram-negative bacteria total	**119**	**64.0**
Staphylococcus aureus	5	2.7
Coagulase-negative staphylococci	15	8.1
Streptococcus species	1	0.5
Enterococcus species	32	17.2
Gram-positive cocci total	**53**	**28.5**
***Candida* species**	**14**	**7.5**
Total	**186**	**100**

*For each patient only one isolate of each species (same antibiogramm) is included.

Morganella species). Nonfermenters, such as *Pseudomonas aeruginosa*, gram-positive cocci, such as staphylococci and also enterococci, and *Candida* species may also play an important role (Table 150-1). The microbial spectrum is likely to differ over time and from one institution to the other. To follow the spectrum and the development of antibiotic resistance, each ICU has to update its own analyses.

EPIDEMIOLOGY

The NIDEP (Nosocomial Infections in Germany: Surveillance and Prevention) study[3] showed that the highest prevalence rate of nosocomial infections in Germany was found in patients in ICUs (15.3%). The most frequent nosocomial infections in the hospital were UTI (42.1%), lower respiratory tract infections (20.6%), surgical site infections (15.8%), and primary sepsis (8.3%). The European Prevalence of Nosocomial Infection in Intensive Care (EPIC) study[1] revealed that 44.8% of patients were infected on the study day. Community-acquired infection was recorded in 13.7%, hospital-acquired infection in 9.7%, and ICU-acquired infection in 20.6%. The total occurrence of the most frequent types of ICU-acquired infection were pneumonia, 46.9%; lower respiratory tract infections, 17.8%; UTI, 17.6%; and bloodstream infections, 12.0%. The true incidence of UTI, however, may even be higher if meticulously looked for. About 80% of nosocomial UTIs are associated with indwelling urinary catheters; another 5% to 10% occur after other genitourinary manipulations.[4] At least 15% of complicated UTIs are febrile.[5]

Urinary tract infections in the ICU are divided into two groups:

1. UTIs with nonurologic complicating causes: diabetes mellitus, renal insufficiency, immunodeficiency, infectious foci contiguous to the urogenital tract, or trauma patients
2. UTIs with urologic complicating causes: renal transplantation, neurogenic bladder dysfunction, procedures in the urogenital tract, urinary stones or foreign bodies in the urogenital tract

In UTI with primary nonurologic causes, antimicrobial therapy is generally sufficient. However, in UTI with primary urologic causes, the complicating factors must be identified and treated. In this case antimicrobial therapy is only one component of the treatment

URINARY TRACT INFECTIONS WITH NONUROLOGIC COMPLICATING CAUSES

Poorly controlled diabetes mellitus is a risk factor for UTI because of impaired granulocyte function, a decreased excretion of Tamm-Horsfall protein, low interleukin-6 and interleukin-8 levels in the urine, leading to lower "cidality" of the urine, and altered microflora in the genital region. In addition, diabetic cystopathy and nephropathy may be complicating factors. The risk to develop UTI is 25 times higher in female diabetics and 20 times higher in male diabetics compared with nondiabetics.[6] Parenchymatous infections of the upper urinary tract are five times more frequent in diabetic patients than nondiabetics.[7-9] In diabetics, 75% of UTIs are caused by *E. coli*, *Serratia* species, *Klebsiella* species, *Enterobacter* species, and enterococci. Yeasts also frequently cause UTI in diabetics.[10,11] Treatment must address the metabolic situation. In pyelonephritis, usually a switch to insulin or to insulin-analogous therapy is necessary. Antimicrobial treatment may be prolonged.[6]

Immunosuppression is associated with increased risk of UTI. Patients with leukopenia (<1000/µL) show a higher rate of febrile UTIs and bacteremia due to UTI.[12] Symptoms and findings in these patients frequently are not diagnostic. Febrile episodes, however, are due to infections in approximately 60% of cases. Prompt empirical antibiotic therapy should therefore be instigated, encompassing gram-negative bacteria and *Pseudomonas* species.[13] Corticosteroids impair phagocytic and chemotactic activity of granulocytes as well as the production of cytokines and alter the function of lymphocytes, favoring UTI caused by *Pseudomonas* species and *Candida* species.[14] Twenty percent of patients with AIDS experience at least one episode of UTI, depending on their CD4 count. The spectrum of pathogens can be shifted to opportunistic pathogens.[15,16]

Pathogens may be translocated into the urinary tract from contiguous infectious foci (e.g., appendicitis, sigmoid diverticulitis, translocation by ileus). Symptoms and localization of pain can be misleading and may delay diagnosis. Operations or trauma may cause hypothermia, tissue hypoxia, and hemodynamic alterations that produce kidney dysfunction and impaired mucosal perfusion. The use of latex catheters in these critical situations (e.g., operations with heart-lung machine) can also lead to urethral strictures. Silicone catheters or suprapubic catheters are recommended in these patients.[17] Suprapubic catheters cannot prevent UTI. They can, however, lower the rate from 40% to 18%.[18]

URINARY TRACT INFECTIONS WITH UROLOGIC COMPLICATING CAUSES

Patients show a high risk to develop bacteriuria after renal transplantation, threatening patient and transplant. Early infections (up to 3 months after transplantation) are differentiated from late infections (more than 3 months after transplantation). Early infections may present with no symptoms. In this phase, occult bacteremia (60% of bacteremias after renal transplantation originate from the urinary tract), allograft dysfunction, and recurrent UTI after antibiotic therapy are frequently seen.[19] The newer immunosuppressive agents are associated with a lower incidence of rejection but a higher risk of late infection. In particular, mycophenolate mofetil is associated with an increasing incidence of UTI and with infections caused by cytomegalovirus.[20]

Early UTI after renal transplantation usually requires a longer antibacterial treatment (up to 6 weeks). The antibiotic must not possess renal toxicity or interfere with immunosuppressive agents. Possible agents can be trimethoprim, trimethoprim/sulfamethoxazole (TMP/SMX), or fluoroquinolones. Low-dose prophylaxis for 1 month with TMP/SMX starting after removal of the catheter is also a possible alternative.[21]

UTIs occurring more than 3 months post transplantation usually have a good prognosis, if there are no structural abnormalities, and need only be treated for 10 to 14 days.[22]

UTIs caused *by Candida* species are generally asymptomatic. There is, however, a risk of obstructive fungal balls leading to candidemia or invasion of the anastomosis in renal transplant recipients. Asymptomatic candiduria should therefore be treated in these patients.[21] Urine transport disturbances (e.g., from obstructive ureteral stone) require specific urologic therapy, such as percutaneous nephrostomy or stenting. In the case of bladder obstruction, an indwelling urinary catheter (suprapubic or transurethral) will be the primary therapy in the ICU. Long-term indwelling catheters (more than 30 days) are associated with a selected microbial spectrum of difficult-to-treat uropathogens (e.g., *Providencia* species, *Proteus* species, *Pseudomonas* species).[23,24] After initiation of antimicrobial therapy, the catheter should be exchanged to remove biofilm material. Treatment of UTI in these patients must be consistent to avoid emergence of resistance or cross-infection.[25]

PATHOPHYSIOLOGY

UTIs generally occur from organisms invading the urinary tract via the urethra. Pathogens originate from endogenous or exogenous nosocomial flora. Hematogenous spread to the urinary tract is rare.

In uncomplicated UTI, pathogens need to have very specific virulence factors enabling them to initiate an infection after invasion of the urinary tract. The medical conditions of an ICU patient may weaken physiologic barriers and defenses, thus facilitating entry of pathogens. In addition, the nosocomial environment in the ICU, including antibiotic pressure and decreased supply of oxygen or nutrients (e.g., iron) to tissues can select pathogens with specific resistance patterns. A general adaptation strategy is the formation of hypermutator strains, which show 100- to 1000-fold increased mutation frequencies, enabling the pathogens to rapidly adapt to new challenging environments and to thus invent effective mechanisms for infection and antibiotic resistance.[26,27]

A very important mechanism contributing to UTI is the formation of biofilms, associated with the increased number of biomaterials used in medical practice. Biofilm infections develop not only around foreign bodies, such as urinary catheters or stents, but also in urinary stones, scar or necrotic tissue, obstructive uropathies, or even chronic bacterial prostatitis. Biofilm has been defined as an accumulation of microorganisms and their extracellular products,

forming a structured community on a surface. The formation of biofilm generally consists of three steps:

1. Deposition of a host conditioning film
2. Attachment of microorganisms followed by microbial adhesion and anchorage to the surface by exopolymer production
3. Growth, multiplication, and dissemination of the organisms

The basic structural unit of a biofilm is a microcolony, that is, a discrete matrix-enclosed community consisting of bacteria of one or more species. The biofilm is usually built up of three layers[28-30]:

1. Linking film that attaches to the surface of a tissue or biomaterial
2. Base film of compact microorganisms
3. Surface film as an outer layer where planktonic organisms can be released to float freely and spread on the surface

Bacteria within the biofilms differ both in behavior and in phenotypic form from the planktonic, free-floating bacteria. The failure of antimicrobial agents to treat biofilms has been attributed to a variety of mechanisms:

- Organisms encapsulated in the biofilm grow more slowly than the planktonic ones, probably because the encapsulated bacteria have a decreased nutrient and oxygen supply leading to a decreased metabolic rate and antimicrobial susceptibility. This may select a less susceptible genotype, forming a resistant population. Furthermore, antimicrobial binding proteins are poorly expressed in these slow-growing bacteria.
- The biofilm matrix itself delays or impedes the diffusion of antibiotic molecules into the deeper layer of the film (extrinsic resistance).
- Bacteria within the biofilm are phenotypically so different from their planktonic counterparts that antimicrobial agents fail to eradicate them. Bacteria within a biofilm activate many genes that alter the cell envelope and molecular targets by altering the susceptibility to antimicrobial agents (intrinsic resistance). It is a current opinion that these phenotypic changes play a more important role in the development of antimicrobial resistance than the external resistance (biofilm matrix, glycocalyx).
- Bacteria within a biofilm can sense the external environment, communicate with each other, and transfer genetic information and plasmids within biofilms.
- Bacteria in biofilms can usually survive antibacterial concentrations 100 to 150 times higher than needed to kill planktonic bacteria of the same species.[31]

Antimicrobial treatment can be effective only in "young" biofilms (<24 hours). At present, combination therapy with fluoroquinolones and macrolides or fosfomycin seems to be the most effective against biofilm infections. During an acute febrile phase of a biofilm infection antimicrobial therapy is essential and can be effective because the planktonic bacteria are responsible for the febrile reactions and not the bacteria covered in the biofilm.[28] However, to eradicate pathogens from biofilm, the biofilm itself has to be removed (e.g., catheter change, extraction of infectious stones).

DIAGNOSIS

MEDICAL HISTORY AND PHYSICAL EXAMINATION

Sedated intubated patients often are difficult to evaluate regarding their signs and symptoms of UTI. The patient or a family member should be asked about previous episodes of UTI, as well as urologic diseases (e.g., stones, tumors) or operations.

The physical examination should include inspection and palpation of the costophrenic area, the lower abdomen, the pubic region, the inguinal lymph nodes, the genitals, and a digital transvaginal or transrectal examination. Ultrasound is an important diagnostic device, and its use should be frequently considered, because of the close proximity of the urogenital organs to the intestine, spleen, liver, pancreas, gallbladder, ovary, or uterus.

URINARY EXAMINATIONS

Urine specimens in the ICU patients are almost exclusively collected from catheters.

Because urine from catheters has to be collected into a closed system, the urine specimen should be taken from the puncture site at the catheter after disinfection, without opening the closed system. There are different complementary methods for laboratory examination of the urine specimen.

Dipstick Test

The dipstick test is done with undiluted urine and investigates the following infection-related parameters[32]:

- pH. An alkaline urine, pH > 8.0, points to urease producing organisms, such as *Proteus* or *Providencia*, and is associated with magnesium-ammonium-phosphate stones.
- nitrate. Most enterobacteria harbor a nitrate reductase that reduces nitrate to nitrite. Some common uropathogens, such as *Enterococcus* and *Staphylococcus*, lack nitrate reductase and will therefore not be detected using this parameter whatever their urinary concentration. Positive detection of nitrate requires its inclusion in the patient's diet.
- Leukocytes (positive leukocyte esterase). Granulocytes are the most frequently detected leukocytes in the urine of UTI patients. Macrophages appear fairly often in patients with UTI, but their significance remains unknown.
- Erythrocytes (positive hemoglobin). Hematuria remains a major sign of urinary tract and renal disease.
- Specific gravity/osmolality (degree of urine dilution).
- Protein. Total protein in urine is a mixture of high- and low-molecular-weight plasma proteins, from the kidney and the urinary tract, or bacteria.
- Glucose (metabolic condition of the patient).

Microscopy

Particles can be differentiated at basic or advanced levels. The basic level is for general laboratory service. Its target is a positive identification of the usually formed elements. The advanced level provides detailed evidence of renal damage or

TABLE 150–2. STANDARD VALUES FOR URINE IN COUNTING CHAMBER AND FIELD OF VISION

	Erythrocytes	Leukocytes
Uncentrifuged urine (chamber counting)	<10/mL	<10/mL

From European Urinalysis Guidelines, 2000.

specific details of microbes (e.g., Gram staining). There are two possibilities of microscopic evaluation[32]:

1. Chamber counting of uncentrifuged urine. (Standard values for urine are shown in Table 150-2.)
2. Urinary sediment findings. At least 10 fields of vision at 400× magnification are counted, and the mean value of particles is registered. However, centrifugation methods are never quantitative in counting erythrocytes and leukocytes because of variable loss during centrifugation.

Microbiology

To differentiate contamination in urine from significant bacteriuria, quantitative microbiology is needed. The microbial count has to be interpreted in relation to the urinary dilution.

CLINICAL DIAGNOSIS

To survey and compare infection rates in different institutions, UTIs should be classified according to widely accepted definitions, such as the definitions of the U.S. Centers for Disease Control and Prevention (CDC). The current CDC definitions[33] stratify nosocomial UTIs into symptomatic, asymptomatic, and other infections of the urinary tract. To be of value in determining a nosocomial infection, the urine specimens must be obtained aseptically using an appropriate technique, such as clean catch collection, bladder catheterization, or suprapubic aspiration.

Symptomatic UTI must meet one of the following criteria:

1. One of the following: fever (>38°C), urgency, frequency, dysuria, or suprapubic tenderness *and* a urine culture of greater than or equal to 10^5 colonies/mL urine with no more than two species of organisms
2. Two of the following: fever (>38°C), urgency, frequency, dysuria, or suprapubic tenderness *and* any of the following:
   a. Dipstick test positive for leukocyte esterase and/or nitrate
   b. Pyuria (≥10 white blood cells/μL or ≥3 WBC/high-power field of unspun urine)
   c. Organisms seen on Gram stain of unspun urine
   d. Two urine cultures with repeated isolation of the same uropathogen with greater than or equal to 10^2 colonies/mL urine in nonvoided specimens
   e. Urine culture with less than or equal to 10^5 colonies/mL urine of single uropathogen in a patient being treated with appropriate antimicrobial therapy
   f. Physician's diagnosis
   g. Physician institutes appropriate antimicrobial therapy
3. Patient 12 months of age or younger has one of the following: fever (>38°C), hypothermia (<37°C), apnea, bradycardia, dysuria, lethargy, or vomiting *and* urine

culture of greater than or equal to 10⁵ colonies/mL urine with no more than two species of organisms

4. Patient age 12 months or younger has one of the following: fever (>38°C), hypothermia (>37°C), apnea, bradycardia, dysuria, lethargy, or vomiting *and* any of the following:
   a. Dipstick test positive for leukocyte esterase and/or nitrate
   b. Pyuria
   c. Organisms seen on Gram stain of unspun urine
   d. Two urine cultures with repeated isolation of the same uropathogen with greater than or equal to 10^2 organisms/mL urine in nonvoided specimens
   e. Urine culture with less than or equal to 10^5 colonies/mL urine of a single uropathogen in a patient being treated with appropriate antimicrobial therapy
   f. Physician's diagnosis
   g. Physician institutes appropriate antimicrobial therapy

Asymptomatic bacteriuria must meet either of the following criteria:

1. An indwelling urinary catheter is present within 7 days before urine is cultured *and* patient has no fever (>38°C), urgency, frequency, dysuria, or suprapubic tenderness *and* has a urine culture of greater than or equal to 10^5 organisms/mL urine with no more than two species of organisms.
2. No indwelling urinary catheter is present within 7 days before the first of two urine cultures with more than or equal to 10^5 organisms/mL urine of the same organism with no more than two species of organisms, and patient has no fever (>38°C), urgency, frequency, dysuria, or suprapubic tenderness.

Other infections of the urinary tract (kidney, ureter, bladder, urethra, or tissues surrounding the retroperitoneal or perinephric spaces) must meet one of the following criteria:

1. Organism isolated from culture of fluid (other than urine) or tissue from affected site
2. An abscess or other evidence of infection seen on direct examination, during surgery, or by histopathologic examination
3. Two of the following: fever (>38°C), localized pain, or tenderness at involved site *and* any of the following:
   a. Purulent drainage from affected site
   b. Organism isolated from blood culture
   c. Radiographic evidence of infection. Radiographic evidence of infection includes abnormal results of ultrasound examination, computed tomography, magnetic resonance imaging, or nuclear medicine scan (e.g., gallium or technetium)
   d. Physician's diagnosis
   e. Physician institutes appropriate antimicrobial therapy
4. Patient age 12 months or younger has one of the following: fever (>38°C), hypothermia (<37°C), apnea, bradycardia, lethargy, or vomiting *and* any of the following:
   a. Purulent drainage from affected site
   b. Organism isolated from blood culture
   c. Radiographic evidence of infection
   d. Physician's diagnosis
   e. Physician-instituted appropriate therapy

By following these criteria, infection rates can then be calculated and compared with those of other institutions as they are published in the CDC web pages at http://www.cdc.gov/ncidod/hip/SURVEILL/NNIS.HTM/.

THERAPY

GENERAL PRINCIPLES

Not all bacteriuric patients in the ICU need to be treated. Therapy should only be started in patients with significant symptoms and morbidity and in whom asymptomatic bacteriuria may be deleterious (e.g., in case of renal transplant, pregnancy, severe diabetes mellitus, immunosuppression). In complicated UTI, antibiotic therapy can only be successful when the complicating factors can be eliminated or urodynamic functions restored. Treatment of complicated UTI therefore comprises adequate antibiotic treatment and successful urologic intervention.

ANTIBIOTIC THERAPY

For therapy for complicated nosocomial UTI, antibiotics must possess appropriate pharmacodynamic and pharmacokinetic prerequisites, that is, high renal, unmetabolized clearance, with good antibacterial activity, both in acidic and alkaline urine. Moreover, microbial resistance patterns must be considered in the choice of antibiotics. To diminish the selection pressure for resistant pathogens, antibiotics from different classes should be used.

Multiple antimicrobial agents are available for therapy for complicated UTI (Table 150-3): second- or third-generation cephalosporins, broad-spectrum penicillins with beta-lactamase inhibitors, monobactams, and carbapenems. For empirical therapy for severe UTI, broad-spectrum antibiotics should be used (e.g., broad-spectrum penicillins with beta-lactamase inhibitors, third- generation cephalosporins, fluoroquinolones, or carbapenems). Synergism with aminoglycosides, which block protein synthesis and thus block the forming of toxins or virulence factors, might be useful for initial therapy, but side effects have to be considered.

Candiduria is a common problem in ICUs. It may represent a harmless colonization, but it can also be an early sign of systemic candidosis.[34] A second urine culture after exchanging the catheter can rule out contamination. In the critically ill patient, systemic therapy for *Candida* species should be started according to susceptibility testing or species differentiation (see Table 150-3). Complicating factors, such as diabetes mellitus or urologic abnormalities, have to be treated concomitantly. Systemic antimycotic therapy is preferred to local instillation therapy because of the potentially systemic nature of candiduria in ICU patients.

UROLOGIC THERAPY

The urologic operative therapy of complicated UTI is divided into acute therapy and delayed drainage therapy. The primary aim of acute therapy is improved urinary flow with minimal patient contamination by infected urine. In primary therapy, catheters, stents, or drains are frequently used. Delayed drainage therapy of the urinary tract (e.g., lithotomy, prostatic resection, ureter reimplantation) is frequently performed with different urologic methods after days or weeks of stabilization.

TABLE 150–3. RECOMMENDATIONS FOR CALCULATED ANTIBIOTIC THERAPY FOR URINARY TRACT INFECTION

Diagnosis	Frequent Pathogens	Calculated Initial Therapy	Duration of Therapy
Cystitis uncomplicated	*Escherichia coli* *Klebsiella* species *Proteus* species Staphylococci	Trimethoprim/sulfamethoxazole Fluoroquinolone* Fosfomycin tromethamine Alternatively: aminoglycoside	1-3 days
Pyelonephritis acute, uncomplicated	*Escherichia coli* *Proteus* species *Klebsiella* species, other Enterobacteriaceae Staphylococci	Fluoroquinolone* Second-generation cephalosporin Alternatively: aminopenicillin/BLI, aminoglycoside	7-10 days

UTI, complicated
Nosocomial UTI
Pyelonephritis, acute, complicated
	Escherichia coli
	Enterococci
	Pseudomonas species
	Staphylococci
	Klebsiella species
	Proteus species
	Enterobacter species
	Other
	Enterobacteriaceae
	Candida species
		Fluoroquinolone*
		Aminopenicillin/BLI
		Second-generation cephalosporin
		Third-generation cephalosporin
		When initial therapy fails for 1-2 days:
		  Pseudomonas active
		  Acylaminopenicillin/BLI
		  Third-generation cephalosporin
		  Carbapenem
		In *Candida:*
		  Fluconazole
		  Flucytosine
		  Amphotericin B
			3-5 days until after defervescence and treatment of complicating factors

Prostatitis, acute, chronic
Epididymitis, acute
	Escherichia coli
	Other
	Enterobacteriaceae
	Pseudomonas species
	Enterococci
	Staphylococci
	Chlamydia
	Ureaplasma
		Fluoroquinolone*
		Alternatively in acute prostatitis:
		  second-generation cephalosporin,
		  third-generation cephalosporin
		If *Chlamydia* or *Ureaplasma* is
		  detected: doxycycline, macrolide
			Acute: 2 wk
			Chronic: 4-6 wk

Urosepsis	*Escherichia coli*
	Other Enterobacteriaceae
	After urologic procedures
	Multiresistant pathogens:
	  Pseudomonas species
	  Proteus species
	  Serratia species
	  Enterobacter species
		Third-generation cephalosporin
		  ± aminoglycoside
		Fluoroquinolone*
		Pseudomonas active
		Acylaminopenicillin/BLI
		Carbapenem
			3-5 days until after defervescence and treatment of complicating factors

BLI, Beta-lactamase inhibitor.
*Fluoroquinolone with sufficient urinary concentration.
From Naber KG, Bergman B, Bishop MC, et al: EAU guidelines for the management of urinary and male genital tract infections. Eur Urol 2001:40:576-588.

PROPHYLAXIS OF CATHETER-ASSOCIATED URINARY TRACT INFECTIONS

Eighty to 90 percent of nosocomial UTIs are associated with urinary catheters or instrumentation of the urinary tract. The best prophylaxis is to avoid a catheter or, if catheterization is necessary, to minimize catheter duration. Various techniques are applied to avoid catheter-related infections.

Silver coating of catheters may exert a bactericidal effect, but the concentration of free silver ions must be high whereas the exposure to albumin and chloride ions has to be low, because silver-chloride complexes can precipitate.[35] Heparin-coated catheters also demonstrate promising results. Suprapubic catheterization can decrease the rate of UTI from 40% to 18%, because the proximity to the anal region as well as the irritation of the urethral mucosa with the ensuing mucopurulent discharge are avoided.[18] Urinary drainage should be performed with a closed system that should not be opened either for emptying or for urinary sampling. The sites used for urinary sampling must be adequately sterilized. A rigid vertical, ventilated, drop chamber should be available to

prevent encrustation.[36] General hygienic procedures such as aseptic catheter insertion, wearing of disposable gloves, and hygienic hand disinfection to prevent cross-contamination or cross-infection are mandatory. Recommendations for the use of urinary catheters have been issued by the CDC to prevent health care–associated infections.[37]

RECOMMENDED EVIDENCE-BASED MEASUREMENTS FOR PREVENTING CATHETER-ASSOCIATED URINARY TRACT INFECTIONS (Table 150-4)[38]

Personnel

1. Only persons who know the correct technique of aseptic insertion and maintenance of the catheter (e.g., hospital personnel, family members, or patients themselves) should handle catheters. *Category I*
2. Hospital personnel and others who take care of catheters should be given periodic in-service training stressing the correct techniques and potential complications of urinary catheterization. *Category II*

TABLE 150–4. SUMMARY OF MAJOR RECOMMENDATIONS FOR PREVENTION OF CATHETER-ASSOCIATED URINARY TRACT INFECTIONS

Category I. Strongly Recommended for Adoption

- Educate personnel in correct techniques of catheter insertion and care.
- Catheterize only when necessary.
- Emphasize hand washing.
- Insert catheter using aseptic technique and sterile equipment.
- Secure catheter properly.
- Maintain closed sterile drainage.
- Obtain urine samples aseptically.
- Maintain unobstructed urine flow.

Category II. Moderately Recommended for Adoption

- Periodically reeducate personnel in catheter care.
- Use smallest suitable-bore catheter.
- Avoid irrigation unless needed to prevent or relieve obstruction.
- Refrain from daily meatal care with either of the regimens discussed in text.
- Do not change catheters at arbitrary fixed intervals.

Category III. Weakly Recommended for Adoption

- Consider alternative techniques of urinary drainage before using an indwelling urethral catheter.
- Replace the collecting system when sterile closed drainage has been violated.
- Spatially separate infected and uninfected patients with indwelling catheters.
- Avoid routine bacteriologic monitoring.

From Hooton TM, Carlet JM, Duse AG, et al: Definitions and epidemiology of nosocomial and health care associated infections in urology. In Naber KG, Pechere JC, Kumazawa J, et al (eds): Nosocomial and Health Care Associated Infections in Urology. Presented at the first international consultation on Nosocomial and Health Care Associated Infections in Urology, June 27-28, 2000, Paris. Plymouth, England, Health Publication Ltd, 2001.

Catheter Use

1. Urinary catheters should be inserted only when necessary and left in place only for as long as necessary. They should not be used for the convenience of the nursing staff. *Category I*
2. For selected patients, other methods of urinary drainage such as condom catheter drainage, suprapubic catheterization, and intermittent urethral catheterization can be useful alternatives to indwelling urethral catheterization. *Category III*

Hand Washing

1. Hand washing should be done immediately before and after any manipulation of the catheter site or apparatus. *Category I*

Catheter Insertion

1. Catheters should be inserted using aseptic technique and sterile equipment. *Category I*
2. Gloves, drape, sponges, an appropriate antiseptic solution for periurethral cleaning, and a single-use packet of lubricant jelly should be used for insertion. *Category II*
3. As small a catheter as possible, consistent with good drainage, should be used to minimize urethral trauma. *Category II*
4. Indwelling catheters should be properly secured after insertion to prevent movement and urethral traction. *Category I*

Closed Sterile Drainage

1. A sterile, continuously closed drainage system should be maintained. *Category I*
2. The catheter and drainage tube should not be disconnected unless the catheter must be irrigated (see Irrigation). *Category I*
3. If breaks in aseptic technique, disconnection, or leakage occur, the collecting system should be replaced using aseptic technique after disinfecting the catheter-tubing junction. *Category III*

Irrigation

1. Irrigation should be avoided unless obstruction is anticipated (e.g., during bleeding after prostatic or bladder surgery); closed continuous irrigation may be used to prevent obstruction. To relieve obstruction due to clots, mucus, or other causes, an intermittent method of irrigation may be used. Continuous irrigation of the bladder with antimicrobial agents has not proved to be useful and should not be performed as a routine infection prevention measure. *Category II*
2. The catheter-tubing junction should be disinfected before disconnection. *Category II*
3. A large volume sterile syringe and sterile irrigant should be used and then discarded. The person performing irrigation should use aseptic technique. *Category I*
4. If the catheter becomes obstructed and can be kept open only by frequent irrigation, the catheter should be changed if the catheter itself may contribute to the obstruction (e.g., formation of concretions). *Category II*

Specimen Collection

1. If small volumes of fresh urine are needed for examination, the distal end of the catheter, or preferably the sampling port if present, should be cleansed with a disinfectant, and urine then aspirated with a sterile needle and syringe. *Category I*
2. Larger volumes of urine for special analyses should be obtained aseptically from the drainage bag. *Category I*

Urinary Flow

1. Unobstructed flow should be maintained. *Category I* (It may be necessary to temporarily obstruct the catheter for specimen collection or other medical purposes.)
2. To achieve free flow of urine (a) the catheter and collecting tube should be kept from kinking; (b) the collecting bag should be emptied regularly using a separate collecting container for each patient (the draining spigot and nonsterile collecting container should never come into contact); (c) poorly functioning or obstructed catheters should be irrigated (see Irrigation) or, if necessary, replaced; and (d) collecting bags should always be kept below the level of the bladder. *Category I*

Meatal Care

1. Two studies have shown that cleansing with povidone-iodine solution twice daily and daily cleansing with soap and water do not reduce catheter-associated urinary tract infection. Daily meatal care with either of these two regimens is therefore not recommended. *Category II*

Catheter Change Interval

1. Indwelling catheters should not be changed at arbitrarily fixed intervals. *Category II*

Spatial Separation of Catheterized Patients

1. To minimize the chances of cross-infection, infected and uninfected patients with indwelling catheters should not share the same room or adjacent beds. *Category III*

Bacteriologic Monitoring

1. The value of regular bacteriologic monitoring of catheterized patients as an infection control measure has not been established and is not recommended. *Category III*

SPECIAL CLINICAL PICTURES

INFECTIONS OF THE UPPER URINARY TRACT AND CONTIGUOUS ORGANS

Pyelonephritis

The high osmolality of the renal medulla has a negative effect on leukocyte function. For that reason, the interstitium of the renal medulla is much more affected in pyelonephritis than the cortex. Clinical symptoms are unilateral or bilateral flank pain, painful micturition, dysuria, and fever (>38°C). Focal nephritis is limited to one or more renal lobules, comparable to lobular pneumonia. Ultrasonographic findings are of a circumscribed lesion with interrupted echoes, which break through the normal cortex-medulla-organization. The CT scan shows typical wedge-shaped, poorly limited areas of diminished sonographic density. As differential diagnoses, renal abscess, tumor, and renal infarction must be taken into account. Emphysematous pyelonephritis characteristically shows gas formation in the renal parenchyma and perirenal space. Diabetes mellitus or obstructive renal disease are predisposing factors. The most frequently isolated organisms are *E. coli*, *Klebsiella pneumoniae*, and *Enterobacter cloacae*. Fermentation of glucose in Enterobacteriaceae occurs via two different metabolic pathways: mixed acid fermentation and the butylene glycol pathway. Organisms of the *Klebsiella-Enterobacter-Hafnia-Serratia* group, and to a lesser extent *E. coli*, use the butylene glycol pathway and produce copious amounts of CO_2, which appears clinically as gas formation.[39] Aggravated by diminished tissue perfusion, the contralateral side is often affected as well.

Renal, Perirenal Abscess

Clinical symptoms are rigors, fever, back or abdominal pain, flank tenderness, mass lesion and redness of the flank, and protection of upper lumbar and paraspinal muscles. Respiratory insufficiency, hemodynamic instability, or reflectory paralytic ileus occurs frequently. Frequent signs of renal abscess formation are fever and leukocytosis for more than 72 hours, despite antibiotic therapy. Urinary culture may be negative in 14% to 20%.[40] Frequently isolated organisms are *E. coli*, *K. pneumoniae*, *Proteus* species, and *Staphylococcus aureus* from hematogenous spread. Caudad, the fascial limitations are open and the perirenal fat is in close contact with the pelvic fat tissue. A perinephritic abscess may therefore point to groin or perivesical tissue, or to the contralateral side, thus penetrating the peritoneum. Inflammation of flank, thigh, back, buttocks, and lower abdomen may occur. Because of late diagnosis the mortality can be as high as 57%. Blood cultures are positive in 10% to 40%, and urinary cultures are positive in 50% to 80%.[41]

INFECTIONS OF THE LOWER URINARY TRACT AND CONTIGUOUS ORGANS

Cystitis

Cystitis is frequently limited to the bladder mucosa and hence shows no systemic signs or symptoms. An ascending infection can, however, clinically result. Cystitis in the ICU is almost exclusively catheter associated and can cause hematuria. Spontaneous elimination is frequently found after removal of the indwelling catheter, but less frequently in elderly patients.[42] Patients with persistent bacteriuria after catheter removal may experience symptomatic UTI in the future and should therefore be treated with antibiotics.[43]

Epididymitis/Orchitis

Epididymitis in the ICU usually is an ascending infection and can also involve the testis as well. Possible causes are subvesical obstruction, transurethral resection of the prostate, or an indwelling, transurethral urinary catheter, in which case the pathogens are identical with the pathogens in the urine. Of note, epididymitis is frequently involved in urogenital tuberculosis. Orchitis with the formation of a sterile hydrocele can appear in the course of polyserositis or heart insufficiency and may point to a generalized systemic disease.

Cavernitis

Cavernitis of the penis is a rare phlegmonous infection of the cavernous bodies. Possible causes are indwelling, transurethral urinary catheters, penile operations, autoinjection for erectile dysfunction or trauma, pelvic operations, or trauma. Pathogens may represent skin flora or uropathogens. Treatment consists of suprapubic catheterization or, if needed, operative débridement and broad-spectrum antibiotic therapy.

Acute Prostatitis and Prostatic Abscess

Acute prostatitis and prostatic abscess are bacterial infections of the prostate gland. The bacterial spectrum consists of 53% to 80% *E. coli* and other enterobacteria, 19% gram-positive bacteria, and 17% anaerobic bacteria.[44] In regions with a high incidence of *Neisseria gonorrhoeae*, the prostate may be involved. Symptoms are high fever, rigors, dysuria, urinary retention, and perineal pain. Rectal palpation reveals an enlarged, tender prostate. Prostate massage is contraindicated. In acute prostatitis the pathogens are usually detected in urine. However, the urine may be sterile in prostatic abscess formation. Therapy consists of a combination of antibiotic therapy with broad-spectrum beta-lactam/lactamase inhibitors, antibiotics, and aminoglycosides as well as the insertion of a suprapubic catheter. In the case of a prostatic abscess urologic drainage is necessary.[45]

Fournier's Gangrene

Fournier's gangrene is a necrotizing fasciitis of dartos and Colles' fascias. It is mainly seen in men in the fourth to seventh decade but also occurs in women or the newborn. Causes are operations or trauma in the genital or perineal region, including microlesions, or infectious processes from the rectal or urethral areas. Important predisposing factors are diabetes mellitus, liver insufficiency, chronic alcoholism, hematologic diseases, or malnutrition. The infectious process follows anatomically preformed spaces. The superficial perineal fascia is fixed dorsally at the transverse deep perirenal muscle and laterally at the iliac bone and merges ventrally in the superficial abdominal fascia. Hence, a ventrally open and craniodorsally and laterally closed space is formed (Colles' space) that facilitates the spread of infection. In contrast to gas gangrene, the fascial borders are respected in Fournier's gangrene. A mixed bacterial flora is seen, consisting of gram-positive cocci, enterobacteria, and anaerobic bacteria. The released toxins facilitate platelet aggregation and entrapment of complement, which, in conjunction with the release of heparinase by anaerobic bacteria, leads to small vessel thrombosis and tissue necrosis.[46,47] The destruction of tissue enhances the potential of acute renal failure. Fournier's gangrene is a rapidly progressing infection leading to septic shock, if not treated in time.

Therapy consists of immediate, operative débridement followed by subsequent operations, until the infectious process has been controlled. A suprapubic catheter is advisable and a colostomy needs to be performed in cases in which fecal contamination of the wound is inevitable. A combination of antibiotic therapy with broad-spectrum beta-lactam/lactamase inhibitor antibiotics, fluoroquinolones, and clindamycin is necessary.

UROSEPSIS

In 20% to 30% of all septic patients the initial infectious focus is in the urogenital tract. The most frequent causes for urosepsis are obstructive diseases of the urinary tract, such as ureteral stones, anomalies, stenosis, or tumor. The bacterial spectrum in urosepsis consists of 50% *E. coli*, 15% *Proteus* species, 15% *Enterobacter* and *Klebsiella* species, 5% *P. aeruginosa,* and 15% gram-positive organisms.[48] If host defense is impaired, less virulent organisms such as enterococci, coagulase-negative staphylococci, or *P. aeruginosa* may cause urosepsis. Effective treatment eliminates the infectious focus and improves organ perfusion. Adequate antibiotic therapy ensures improved outcome in septic shock.[49] For broad-spectrum coverage, combination therapy should be used. If enterobacteria are expected, a third-generation cephalosporin, for example, ceftriaxone or cefotaxime in combination with an aminoglycoside or fluoroquinolone, can be used. In case of *Pseudomonas* species,

acylaminopenicillins (e.g., azlocillin, piperacillin) in combination with a beta-lactamase inhibitor, or a carbapenem should be chosen. In the case of methicillin-resistant *S. aureus,* glycopeptides have to be considered (see Table 150-3). In any case, microbiologic sampling (urine, blood, tissue culture) before the initiation of treatment is compulsory to tailor the initial empirical therapy according to laboratory results.

ANNOTATED REFERENCES

Garner JS, Jarvis WR, Emori TG, et al: CDC definitions for nosocomial infections. Am J Infect Control 1988;16:128-140.
> The Centers for Disease Control has developed a set of definitions for surveillance of nosocomial infections. This is a generally accepted, valuable tool for objective diagnosis of infections, although in critically ill patients it may be necessary to modify these criteria.

Goto T, Nakame Y, Nishida M, Ohi Y: Bacterial biofilms and catheters in experimental urinary tract infection. Int J Antimicrob Agents 1999;11:227-231.
> An experimental setup to study the antibiotic susceptibility of pathogens in biofilm. Fluoroquinolones, and perhaps macrolides, have advantageous effects in the treatment of biofilm infections.

Naber KG, Bergman B, Bishop MC, et al: EAU guidelines for the management of urinary and male genital tract infections. Eur Urol 2001;40:576-588.
> This is a short version of the UTI Guidelines elaborated by the Urinary Tract Infection Working Group of the Health Care Office of the European Association of Urology. The topics include classification, diagnosis, treatment, and follow-up of uncomplicated UTI, UTI in children, UTI in diabetes mellitus, renal insufficiency, renal transplant recipients and immunosuppression, complicated UTI due to urological disorders, sepsis syndrome, urosepsis, urethritis, prostatitis, epididymitis, orchitis, and principles of perioperative prophylaxis in urology.

Oliver A, Cantón R, Campo P, et al: High frequency of hypermutable *Pseudomonas aeruginosa* in cystic fibrosis lung infection. Science 2000;288:1251-1253.
> This study elucidates an excellent model for the special propensities of nosocomial pathogens. There were 36.7% of patients with cystic fibrosis who harbored P. aeruginosa isolates with 100- to 1000-fold increased mutation rates, thus enabling them to rapidly adapt to changing environmental needs.

Vincent J-L, Bihari DJ, Suter PM, et al: The prevalence of nosocomial infection in intensive care units in Europe. JAMA 1995;274:639-644.
> This multicenter, 1-day prevalence study on 1417 European ICUs investigated 10,038 patients, finding 44.8% of patients who were infected and 20.6% who had ICU-acquired infection; therefore, infection control in critically ill patients is important.

Chapter 151

CENTRAL NERVOUS SYSTEM INFECTIONS

Karen C. Bloch • Allen B. Kaiser

KEY POINTS

BACTERIAL MENINGITIS

1. **Fever, headache, and meningismus** are the classic presenting signs and symptoms of bacterial meningitis; however, absence of any one (or all) of these features, particularly in a patient with altered sensorium, may be seen.

2. **Neuroimaging studies** should precede lumbar puncture in the presence of **papilledema, focal findings on neurologic examination, immunocompromise** (human immunodeficiency virus [HIV] infection, malignancy, or transplant), **seizures** in the week prior to presentation, or **coma.**

3. **Empirical antibiotic therapy should begin as soon as possible after appropriate cultures have been obtained;** it can be modified later, based on results of cerebrospinal fluid Gram stain and culture.

4. Patients with negative cultures and **limited clinical response** after 48 hours of therapy should undergo **repeat lumbar puncture and head computed tomography (CT) or magnetic resonance imaging (MRI) scans.**

5. Corticosteroid treatment in adults is controversial, but **combination therapy with dexamethasone and antibiotics has been associated with improved outcomes** in patients with pneumococcal meningitis.

BRAIN ABSCESS

1. **MRI is superior to CT** for imaging brain abscesses, especially in the early stages of infection.

2. Microbiology of brain abscesses is dependent on the route of infection; abscesses spreading from a **contiguous focus are frequently polymicrobial.**

3. Treatment of brain abscesses typically requires **prolonged administration of antibiotics** tailored to culture results.

VIRAL ENCEPHALITIS

1. An **infectious cause** of encephalitis is found in **less than 50% of cases.**

2. **Herpes simplex virus** (HSV) must be included in the differential diagnosis of all cases of encephalitis, as this infection has a high morbidity and mortality unless treated with acyclovir. Herpes simplex encephalitis typically presents with **temporal lobe lesions on MRI, and HSV polymerase chain reaction is more than 95% sensitive for diagnosis.**

CENTRAL NERVOUS SYSTEM INFECTION IN HIV-INFECTED PATIENTS

1. HIV-infected patients are at risk for a number of opportunistic infections. Because many of these cause **mass lesions, CT or MRI should be performed before lumbar puncture.**

2. Ring-enhancing lesions seen on neuroimaging are most frequently due to either **toxoplasmosis or lymphoma.** In patients with positive *Toxoplasma* serology, empirical treatment for 2 weeks is indicated; brain biopsy should be performed in patients with lack of radiographic improvement.

3. Cryptococcal meningitis can be diagnosed by the detection of **cryptococcal antigen in either the serum or the cerebrospinal fluid.**

EPIDURAL ABSCESS

1. Epidural infections typically **present initially with back pain and fever,** with progressive neurologic impairment. Diagnosis is confirmed by MRI.

2. In the presence of **impaired neurologic function, surgical drainage is imperative;** there is little chance of recovery if symptoms have been present for more than 24 hours before decompression. Empirical antibiotics to cover **staphylococci and enteric Gram-negative rods** should be continued until culture results are available.

Physiologic and anatomic barriers make direct medical and surgical intervention difficult in critically ill patients with central nervous system (CNS) infections. Physiologically, the blood-brain barrier impairs delivery of many antimicrobials, and anatomic barriers are created by the bony calvaria and the central location of the ventricular system.

In addition, noninfectious conditions may mimic CNS infection. For example, a necrotic brain tumor may be clinically indistinguishable from a brain abscess. In general, it is prudent to address potentially reversible infectious possibilities immediately in such situations.

A final problem is that many pathogens produce identical clinical syndromes. Timely identification of the specific agent is crucial. Fortunately, most pathogens can be identified from laboratory tests, such as Gram stains of cerebrospinal fluid or pus aspirated from a brain abscess. Epidemiologic clues may also suggest specific microorganisms; pathogens associated with community-acquired infections differ from those acquired in a hospital. In short, proper therapy of infectious processes of the CNS demands an appreciation of the anatomy and physiology of the CNS, the pharmacokinetics of antimicrobial agents, and the epidemiology of infecting pathogens.

BACTERIAL MENINGITIS

ANATOMY

Bacterial meningitis is a pyogenic infection of the cerebral ventricles and the subarachnoid space, with bacteria usually confined to the nutrient-rich cerebrospinal fluid. Most cerebrospinal fluid is formed in the choroid plexus of the ventricles, flows into the subarachnoid space at the cisterna magna and around the cerebral hemispheres, and is reabsorbed by the arachnoid villi (Fig. 151-1). In adults, cerebrospinal fluid is produced at a rate of approximately 500 mL/day, yet the cerebrospinal fluid space averages only 140 mL in volume, consistent with rapid production and reabsorption. The cerebral and spinal subarachnoid spaces connect at the cisterna magna. Flow through the spinal subarachnoid space is of variable velocity and direction.

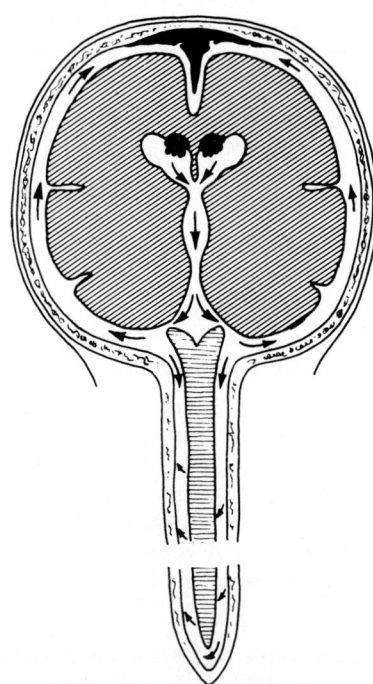

FIGURE 151–1. Cerebrospinal fluid flow within the central nervous system. Cerebrospinal fluid that forms at the choroid plexus of the cerebral ventricles rapidly enters the subarachnoid space at the foramina of Luschka and Magendie. From the cisterna magna, an organized flow of cerebrospinal fluid occurs around the convexities of the brain to the arachnoid villi. There are multiple pathways of bidirectional flow around the spinal cord.

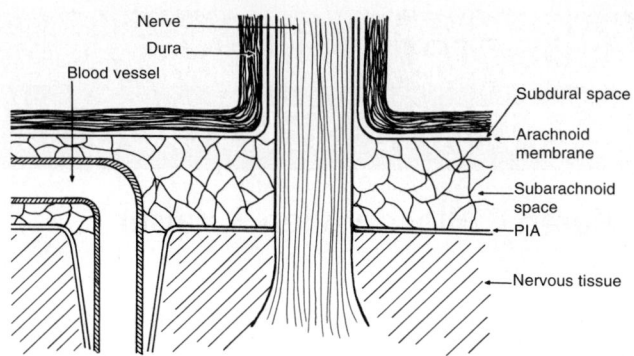

FIGURE 151–2. This diagram of the potential and actual spaces between the layers of the meninges shows the relationship of blood vessels and nerve roots to the subarachnoid space.

There are numerous potential and actual spaces among the layers of the meninges (Fig. 151-2). Meningitis involves the actual space (i.e., the subarachnoid space). The brain parenchyma is usually not infected in uncomplicated bacterial meningitis, even when the illness follows a fulminant course. Exceptions occur in neonates, in whom both *Citrobacter freundii* and *Haemophilus influenzae* may cause focal areas of cerebritis or microabscesses adjacent to the pia. In adults, acute meningitis due to *Listeria monocytogenes* may be complicated by rhomboencephalitis or brain abscess.

How does bacterial meningitis produce such profound CNS dysfunction when neural tissues are not directly infected? Neural damage likely occurs as a direct result of the host inflammatory response. Once in the cerebrospinal fluid, bacteria induce leukocyte migration into the subarachnoid space, resulting in occlusion of cortical blood vessels, damage to nerve roots that traverse the subarachnoid space (see Fig. 151-2), and impaired cerebrospinal fluid flow (see Fig. 151-1). Clinically, this manifests as cranial or spinal nerve dysfunction and hydrocephalus. Activation of these white cells leads to an inflammatory cascade, with the release of cytokines, oxidants, and proteolytic enzymes. At the cellular level, this chain of events results in disruption of the blood-brain barrier and impaired cerebrovascular autoregulation.[1] Increased intracranial pressure may result in transtentorial herniation or tissue hypoxia due to decreased tissue perfusion.

The cerebrospinal fluid–filled subarachnoid space consists of multiple interconnected compartments. The small size of the foramina of Luschka and Magendie probably ensures unidirectional caudal flow toward the cisterna magna, where the cerebrospinal fluid then moves either cephalad or into the spinal canal. This compartmentalization has implications for therapy, because the movement of medications and infectious agents depends on the rate and direction of cerebrospinal fluid flow. A blockage at any of these levels may restrict the entry of antibiotics into sites of ongoing infection.

Infectious agents can invade the cerebrospinal fluid by at least three routes (Table 151-1). First, the vascular structures of the choroid plexus and pia, and the vessels that traverse the subarachnoid space, may serve as conduits during systemic bacteremia. A second, less common route is direct invasion across the protective meninges. Physical disruption of the dura by trauma or surgery allows direct invasion of the subarachnoid space and should be considered in patients with a history of cerebrospinal fluid leakage, or rhinorrhea. Emissary veins provide another pathway for bacteria to spread from contiguous foci into the subarachnoid space.

TABLE 151–1. ROUTES BY WHICH BACTERIA MAY ENTER THE SUBARACHNOID SPACE

Vascular (Blood-Brain Barrier)

Mostly likely pathogens: pneumococci, meningococci, *Listeria*, *Escherichia coli* (neonates), group B streptococci (neonates), *Haemophilus influenzae*

Choroid plexus: may be common site of invasion for *H. influenzae*

Meningeal blood vessels: throughout the subarachnoid space; may be usual route for pneumococci

Arachnoid villi: possible route of invasion, located between the sagittal sinus and subarachnoid space

Transdural

Most likely pathogens: pneumococci, Gram-negative enteric bacilli, staphylococci (including coagulase-negative), *H. influenzae*

Surgery: including ventriculoatrial or ventriculoperitoneal shunts

Trauma: especially when cribriform plate or petrous bone is fractured

Parameningeal infective focus: including sinusitis, mastoiditis, otitis, or osteomyelitis; emissary veins may serve as conduit

Congenital defects: including myelomeningocele and spinal dermal sinus

Transparenchymal

Mostly likely pathogens: anaerobic bacteria, enteric Gram-negative bacilli.

Occurs when brain abscess ruptures directly into ventricles or subarachnoid space

These veins traverse the skull and dura, directly connecting the soft tissues of the head and neck with the venous system of the brain and meninges, including the arachnoid villi. Although blood in the emissary veins usually flows away from the brain, the CNS veins and dural sinuses do not contain valves, and retrograde flow of bacteria is possible. Congenital defects may occur at any point from the glabrata to the cauda equina, offering additional direct communication with the subarachnoid space.[2]

Rarely, organisms may reach the ventricles or subarachnoid space from within the neural tissue; for example, rupture of a brain abscess into the ventricles may cause a disastrous complication.

PATHOPHYSIOLOGY

The unique anatomy and composition of the cerebrospinal fluid–filled compartments, combined with a paucity of host immunologic defenses, create a microenvironment that allows the persistence and proliferation of microorganisms. Polymorphonuclear leukocytes are not normal inhabitants of the cerebrospinal fluid, and mobilization of these phagocytic cells is delayed during the early stages of infection. Similarly, the concentration of immunoglobulin in cerebrospinal fluid is 1/800 that in serum,[3] limiting the effectiveness of humoral immunity. Most important, complement, which plays a critical role in chemotaxis, phagocytosis, and intracellular killing, is virtually absent from normal cerebrospinal fluid. These features dictate that once the cerebrospinal fluid is inoculated with pathogens, resolution of infection without antibiotics is virtually impossible.[4]

Limited local defense mechanisms may explain the importance of using bactericidal rather than bacteriostatic antibiotics in bacterial meningitis. For instance, although tetracycline may be as effective as penicillin for many extra-CNS infections and produces acceptable cerebrospinal fluid

levels, treatment of pneumococcal meningitis with both penicillin and tetracycline is associated with a higher mortality than penicillin monotherapy.[5] Tetracycline neutralizes the bactericidal activity of penicillin, and its inferior performance suggests that host defenses cannot compensate for the lack of bacterial killing.

CLINICAL COURSE

Most patients with bacterial meningitis exhibit only modest impairment of cognition on presentation. Several days of malaise, fever, and headache are typical, and meningismus is usually present.[6] The cerebrospinal fluid indices are almost always abnormal, and Gram stain or culture of the fluid usually reveals the infecting pathogen, unless antibiotics were administered beforehand. Despite the availability of antibiotics that are active against all common causes of acute bacterial meningitis, in adults, the overall mortality remains approximately 25%.[7]

For unclear reasons, pyogenic meningitis follows a more fulminant course in some patients. These patients experience rapid (<48 hours) signs and symptoms of both systemic and CNS infections. In addition to having fever, headache, and meningismus, they exhibit early impairment of sensorium, ranging from lethargy to coma. Despite appropriate antimicrobial therapy, mortality rates of approximately 50% have been reported for such patients.[8] Predictors of an adverse outcome in adults include impaired level of consciousness, seizures, and hypotension,[9] with a threefold higher mortality among patients who are obtunded at presentation.[6]

SYNDROMES OF CENTRAL NERVOUS SYSTEM INFECTION

Definitive diagnosis of bacterial meningitis requires laboratory confirmation. Involvement of the CNS by other pathogens (e.g., viruses, fungi, mycobacteria) and noninfectious processes (e.g., subarachnoid hemorrhage) may produce identical syndromes. Subacute CNS infection syndrome is a slowly evolving syndrome characterized by fever, headache, and meningismus. These features plus an acute onset (<24 to 48 hours) and early impairment of higher integrative functions represent the acute meningitis syndrome (Table 151-2).

The following sections outline approaches to acute meningitis and subacute CNS infection syndromes. These approaches prioritize the competing needs of obtaining a precise etiologic diagnosis versus instituting early antimicrobial therapy.

Acute Meningitis Syndrome

Early recognition and therapy of acute meningitis syndrome are essential to minimize morbidity and mortality. The initial manifestation of the illness may be subtle, with a low-grade headache or fever. However, once meningeal symptoms (vomiting, severe headache, stiff neck) develop, the clinical course is dramatic. Patients appear "toxic," and higher integrative functions may deteriorate rapidly. In the elderly, the higher incidence of noninfectious conditions that may mimic acute meningitis syndrome (e.g., subarachnoid bleeding and malignancies involving the CNS) complicates the initial evaluation. In addition, the elderly have a higher morbidity and mortality associated with bacterial meningitis, and the

TABLE 151–2. CAUSES OF ACUTE AND SUBACUTE CENTRAL NERVOUS SYSTEM INFECTION SYNDROMES

Acute Meningitis Syndrome

Rapid onset (<24-48 h) of fever, headache, or meningismus, with early cognitive impairment

Common
Pyogenic meningitis (pneumococcal, meningococcal, *Listeria*, other)

Uncommon
Viral encephalitis (especially herpes simplex), subarachnoid bleed, brain abscess (with rupture)

Rare
Viral meningitis, granulomatous meningitis (cryptococcal, mycobacterial), carcinomatous meningitis, brain tumor

Subacute Central Nervous System Infection Syndrome

Subacute onset (>24-48 h) of fever, headache, or meningismus, with no or gradual cognitive impairment

Common
Viral meningitis, viral encephalitis, rickettsial infection

Uncommon
Brain abscess, brain tumor, granulomatous meningitis

Rare
Cerebrovascular accident, carcinomatous meningitis

percentage of unusual pathogens (i.e., other than *Neisseria meningitidis* or *Streptococcus pneumoniae*) is significantly higher than in younger patients (69% versus 34%).[10] Thus, particularly with the aging population, there is an increasing need to develop an approach to the diagnosis and therapy of bacterial meningitis that balances the competing agendas of obtaining cerebrospinal fluid for culture and rapidly administering antibiotics (Fig. 151-3).

Acute meningitis syndrome represents an infectious disease emergency. A delay in antibiotic therapy has been associated with adverse outcome, particularly when progressive neurologic impairment occurs before receiving therapy.[9] Coupled with the need for urgent treatment is the need for urgent diagnosis. Identification of a pathogen allows the clinician to tailor the antibiotic regimen based on susceptibility patterns, and it has prognostic and therapeutic implications. However, situations arise when lumbar puncture is unavoidably delayed. This may be due to anatomic factors that make lumbar puncture technically difficult or the need to perform neuroimaging studies to exclude a contraindication to lumbar puncture. If a significant delay in obtaining cerebrospinal fluid is anticipated, antibiotics should be given immediately after peripheral blood cultures are obtained. Depending on the pathogen, the yield of cerebrospinal fluid culture decreases sharply within 15 minutes to 4 hours after the administration of antibiotics.[11] Nevertheless, the risk of delaying treatment supersedes the need to make a microbiologic diagnosis. Despite the effect of prior antibiotics on culture and Gram stain, the absolute neutrophil count and differential are suggestive of bacterial meningitis,[12,13] and a full course of empirical therapy should be completed if cerebrospinal fluid parameters suggest this diagnosis.

Complicating the management of acute meningitis syndrome is the perceived risk (and legal consequences) of uncal herniation following lumbar puncture. Despite the failure of imaging to accurately predict the risk of herniation,[14-16]

empirical antibiotics followed by a head computed tomography (CT) scan before lumbar puncture has become the "standard of care" in many emergency rooms across the country. Recent studies challenge this practice, citing the potential deleterious effect of CT-related delays in the initiation of therapy or the compromising effect of premature sterilization of cerebrospinal fluid cultures.[9,11,17] Even among patients with an abnormal CT scan, only a minority of cases have radiographic findings precluding lumbar puncture. Papilledema, the presence of focal findings on neurologic examination, immunocompromise (human immunodeficiency virus [HIV] infection, malignancy, or transplant), seizures in the week before presentation, and coma are reasonable indications for obtaining a CT scan before lumbar puncture,[16] not only because of their correlation with space-occupying lesions but also because their presence suggests diagnoses unrelated to bacterial meningitis.

Subacute Central Nervous System Infection Syndrome

Febrile illness associated with a somewhat more gradual progression of signs and symptoms of CNS involvement represents the subacute CNS infection syndrome. Headache can be mild to severe, and neck stiffness can be minimum or marked. However, patients with this syndrome are typically oriented and clinically stable at the onset of illness, with a gradual progression of symptoms (>24 to 48 hours). Although bacteria may be causative, most cases are caused by other pathogens and noninfectious factors.

Herpes simplex encephalitis, brain abscess, and meningitis due to fungi, mycobacteria, fastidious bacteria (e.g., *Rickettsia*, *Treponema pallidum*), or viruses all produce fever, worsening headache, and progressive impairment of higher integrative functions. On occasion, carcinomatous meningitis, brain tumor, and subarachnoid bleeding cause similar findings (see Table 151-2). To avoid inappropriate therapy and unnecessary hospitalization, the decision to institute antimicrobial therapy should be carefully weighed. However, if pyogenic meningitis is still a possibility, empirical antimicrobial therapy should be begun, as outlined in the previous section.

The first priority when managing subacute CNS syndrome is rapid diagnosis (as opposed to the rapid-therapy approach to acute meningitis syndrome). With this syndrome, the physician has time to carefully evaluate the patient and relevant laboratory data (Fig. 151-4). Peripheral blood granulocytosis (>10,000/mm³), cerebrospinal fluid cell counts over 1000/mm³, cerebrospinal fluid protein concentration over 100 mg/dL, and cerebrospinal fluid glucose concentrations <40 mg/dL favor a bacterial cause, and these patients should be given empirical antibiotics for acute meninigits syndrome.

If history and examination findings suggest a space-occupying lesion, lumbar puncture and even antimicrobial therapy can be safely delayed, pending results of emergent CT or magnetic resonance imaging (MRI). However, if significant delays are likely, empirical therapy should be given. Other causes of subacute CNS infection syndrome are discussed later (see Brain Abscess and Viral Infections of the Central Nervous System).

Additional diagnostic studies may be indicated for subacute infections. Serologic testing for HIV should be performed, because the spectrum of infectious agents is much broader

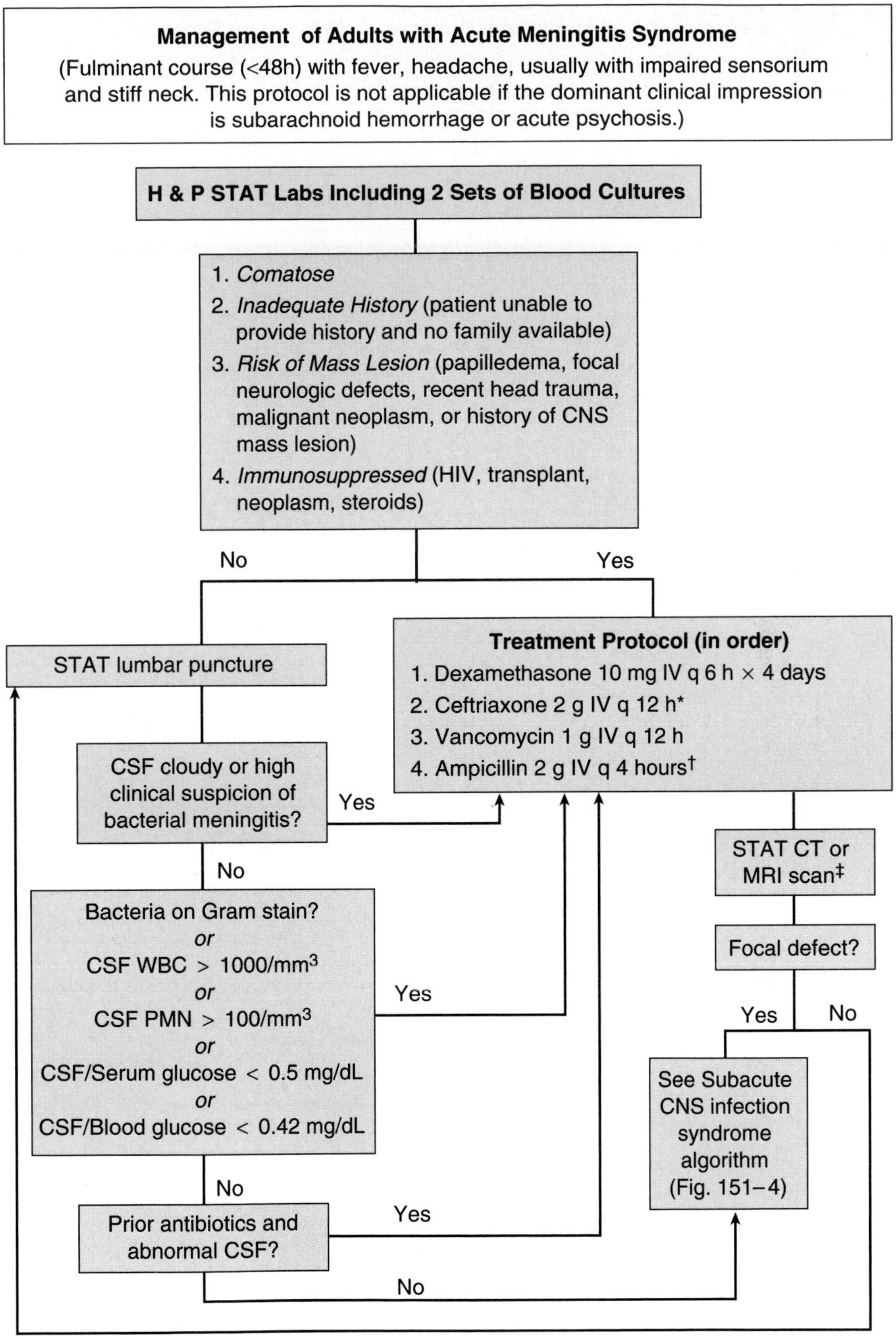

Management of Adults with Acute Meningitis Syndrome

(Fulminant course (<48h) with fever, headache, usually with impaired sensorium and stiff neck. This protocol is not applicable if the dominant clinical impression is subarachnoid hemorrhage or acute psychosis.)

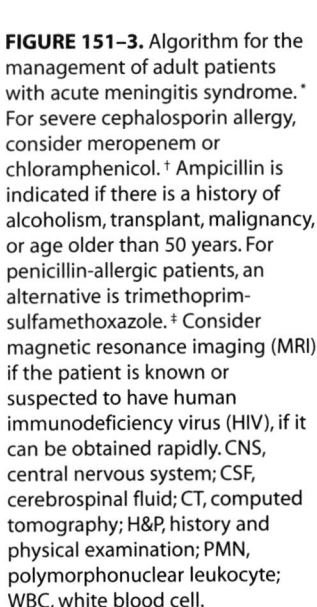

H & P STAT Labs Including 2 Sets of Blood Cultures

1. *Comatose*
2. *Inadequate History* (patient unable to provide history and no family available)
3. *Risk of Mass Lesion* (papilledema, focal neurologic defects, recent head trauma, malignant neoplasm, or history of CNS mass lesion)
4. *Immunosuppressed* (HIV, transplant, neoplasm, steroids)

No — Yes

STAT lumbar puncture

Treatment Protocol (in order)
1. Dexamethasone 10 mg IV q 6 h × 4 days
2. Ceftriaxone 2 g IV q 12 h*
3. Vancomycin 1 g IV q 12 h
4. Ampicillin 2 g IV q 4 hours†

CSF cloudy or high clinical suspicion of bacterial meningitis? — Yes

No

Bacteria on Gram stain?
or
CSF WBC > 1000/mm³
or
CSF PMN > 100/mm³
or
CSF/Serum glucose < 0.5 mg/dL
or
CSF/Blood glucose < 0.42 mg/dL

Yes

No

Prior antibiotics and abnormal CSF? — Yes

No

STAT CT or MRI scan‡

Focal defect?

Yes — No

See Subacute CNS infection syndrome algorithm (Fig. 151–4)

FIGURE 151–3. Algorithm for the management of adult patients with acute meningitis syndrome. * For severe cephalosporin allergy, consider meropenem or chloramphenicol. † Ampicillin is indicated if there is a history of alcoholism, transplant, malignancy, or age older than 50 years. For penicillin-allergic patients, an alternative is trimethoprim-sulfamethoxazole. ‡ Consider magnetic resonance imaging (MRI) if the patient is known or suspected to have human immunodeficiency virus (HIV), if it can be obtained rapidly. CNS, central nervous system; CSF, cerebrospinal fluid; CT, computed tomography; H&P, history and physical examination; PMN, polymorphonuclear leukocyte; WBC, white blood cell.

among HIV-infected individuals. Testing for enteroviruses (cerebrospinal fluid polymerase chain reaction [PCR] or viral culture), cryptococcal antigen, neurosyphilis, mycobacterial infection (culture or PCR of cerebrospinal fluid), herpes simplex virus (cerebrospinal fluid PCR), tick-borne infections (*Ehrlichia, Rickettsia,* Lyme disease), and arboviral encephalitides should be individualized, based on patient characteristics, severity of illness, knowledge of local pathogens, and season.

EPIDEMIOLOGY

The epidemiology of bacterial meningitis has evolved in the last decade, with a greater than 90% decrease in the incidence of *H. influenzae* meningitis following routine pediatric immunization.[18] In immunocompetent adults, *S. pneumoniae* remains the most frequent cause of bacterial meningitis, followed by *N. meningitidis. L. monocytogenes* is a significant cause of meningitis among the elderly,

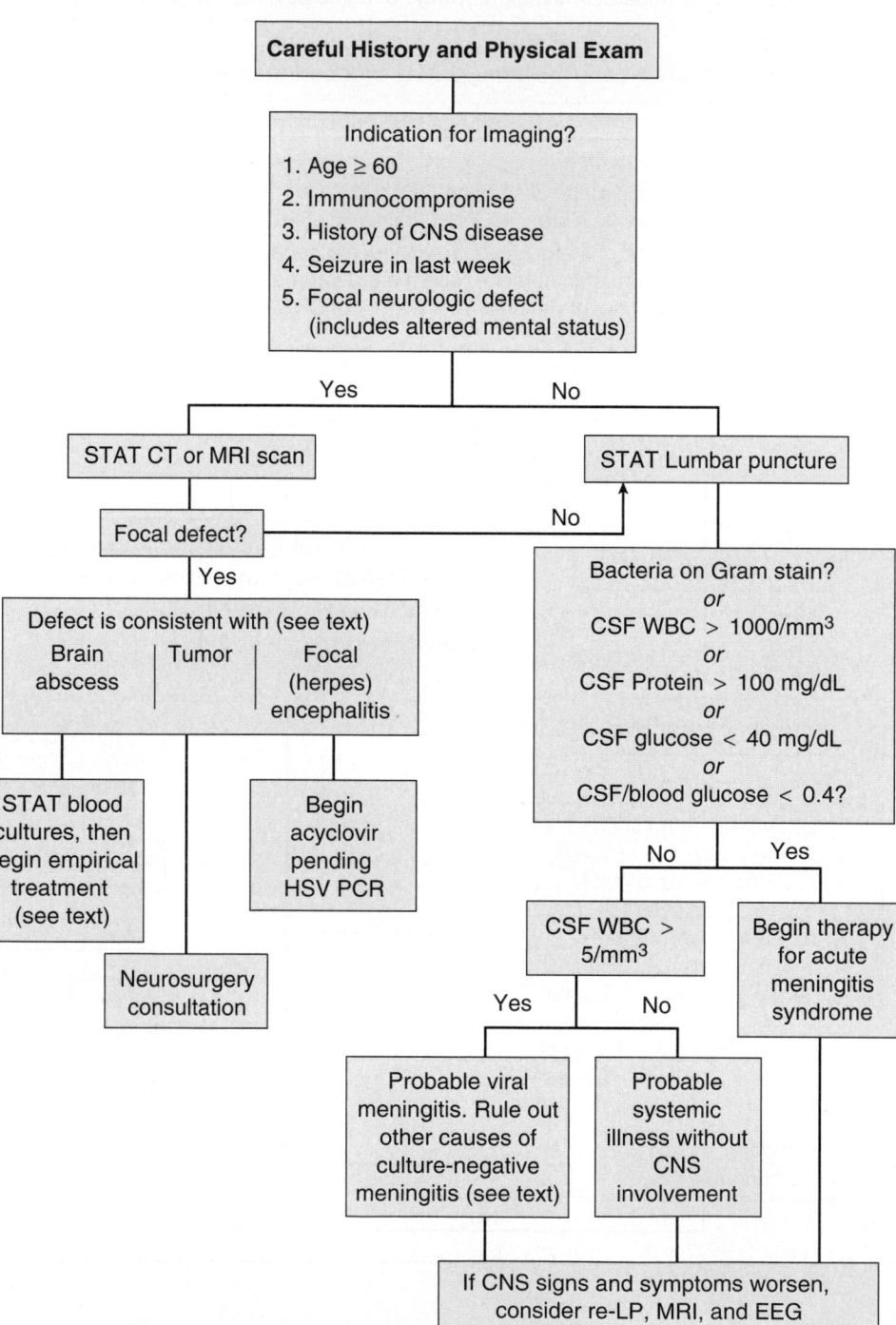

Management of Adults with Subacute CNS Infection Syndrome
(Subacute illness—3-7 days—with moderate fever and worsening headache; often with progressive impairment of higher integrative function and/or focal defects.)

Careful History and Physical Exam

Indication for Imaging?
1. Age ≥ 60
2. Immunocompromise
3. History of CNS disease
4. Seizure in last week
5. Focal neurologic defect (includes altered mental status)

Yes → STAT CT or MRI scan

No → STAT Lumbar puncture

Focal defect?

Yes

Defect is consistent with (see text) | Brain abscess | Tumor | Focal (herpes) encephalitis

STAT blood cultures, then begin empirical treatment (see text)

Begin acyclovir pending HSV PCR

Neurosurgery consultation

No → STAT Lumbar puncture

Bacteria on Gram stain?
or
CSF WBC > 1000/mm³
or
CSF Protein > 100 mg/dL
or
CSF glucose < 40 mg/dL
or
CSF/blood glucose < 0.4?

No → CSF WBC > 5/mm³

Yes → Begin therapy for acute meningitis syndrome

Yes → Probable viral meningitis. Rule out other causes of culture-negative meningitis (see text)

No → Probable systemic illness without CNS involvement

If CNS signs and symptoms worsen, consider re-LP, MRI, and EEG

FIGURE 151–4. Algorithm for the management of patients with subacute central nervous system (CNS) infection syndrome. CSF, cerebrospinal fluid; CT, computed tomography; EEG, electroencephalogram; HSV, herpes simplex virus; LP, lumbar puncture; MRI, magnetic resonance imaging; PCR, polymerase chain reaction; WBC, white blood cell.

immunocompromised individuals, alcoholics, and pregnant women. These groups are also at higher risk for infection with Enterobacteriaceae. *Pseudomonas aeruginosa* and *Staphylococcus aureus* are important pathogens in nosocomially acquired infections.

THERAPY

Antibiotics

The choice of empirical antibiotics is based on knowledge of the likely causative agents, which vary based on host characteristics (e.g., age, immunocompromise), site of acquisition (nosocomial versus community acquired), and local resistance patterns. Antimicrobial agents and doses commonly used for the treatment of CNS infections are listed in Table 151-3. Pneumococci and meningococci remain the most common causes of community-acquired meningitis in immunocompetent adults younger than 50 years.[17] In the last decade, pneumococci that are intermediately (minimum inhibitory concentration >0.12 to 1 µg/mL) or highly (minimum inhibitory concentration >2 µg/mL) resistant to penicillin have emerged as important pathogens.

TABLE 151-3. ANTIMICROBIAL DOSAGE FOR CENTRAL NERVOUS SYSTEM INFECTION

Drug	Dosage (by Total Body Weight)	Usual Dosage (for 70-kg Adult)
Acyclovir	10 mg/kg i.v. q8h	700 mg i.v. q8h
Ampicillin	30 mg/kg i.v. q4h	2 g i.v. q4h
Cefotaxime	30 mg/kg i.v. q6h	2 g i.v. q6h
Ceftazidime	30 mg/kg i.v. q8h	2 g i.v. q8h
Cefepime	30 mg/kg i.v. q8h	2 g i.v. q8h
Ceftriaxone	30 mg/kg i.v. q12h	2 g i.v. q12h
Meropenem	40 mg/kg i.v. q8h*	1 g i.v. q8h
Metronidazole	7.5 mg/kg i.v. q6h	500 mg i.v. q6h
Nafcillin	30 mg/kg i.v. q4h	2 g i.v. q4h
Penicillin G	60,000-70,000 U/kg i.v. q4h	4 million U i.v. q4h
Tobramycin or gentamicin†	2 mg/kg i.v. load, then 1.7 mg/kg q8h‡	140 mg i.v. load, then 120 mg i.v. q8h‡
Intrathecal	0.1 mg/kg/day	5-10 mg/day
Intraventricular	0.1 mg/kg/day	5-10 mg/day
Trimethoprim-sulfamethoxazole	5 mg/kg i.v. q6h	350 mg i.v. q6h§
Vancomycin	15 mg/kg i.v. q6h	500 mg i.v. q6h‡ or 1 g i.v. q12h

*Pediatric dose. Adults should receive usual dosage.
†Regardless of which aminoglycoside is used, only preservative-free preparations should be used.
‡Adjust dose based on serum levels.
§Dose indicates trimethoprim component.

Penicillin-resistant pneumococci are typically multidrug resistant; however, many isolates remain sensitive to third-generation cephalosporins, and all are susceptible to vancomycin. Initial therapy for most patients with meningitis should include a third-generation cephalosporin such as cefotaxime or ceftriaxone, as well as vancomycin. Vancomycin should never be used alone as initial therapy because of its marginal CNS penetration and lack of activity against Gram-negative organisms. Third-generation cephalosporins offer the advantage of excellent CNS penetration, and they are bactericidal; however, cephalosporin resistance among pneumococci is increasing. Initial antibiotic choices can be refined when sensitivity patterns become available, typically in 2 to 3 days. Patients infected with pneumococci with intermediate- or high-level cephalosporin resistance who do not respond clinically should have a repeat lumbar puncture within 72 hours to document decreasing inflammation.[19]

Gram-negative bacilli are significant causes of meningitis in the elderly. Fortunately, third-generation cephalosporins, which form the mainstay of empirical therapy, are highly active against enteric organisms (see Fig. 151-3). *Pseudomonas* is typically resistant to ceftriaxone and cefotaxime, and patients at risk for infection with this organism should receive an antipseudomonal cephalosporin (ceftazidime or cefepime). When Gram-negative bacilli are seen on the cerebrospinal fluid Gram stain, an antipseudomonal cephalosporin in combination with an aminoglycoside should be given. Imipenem is active against *Pseudomonas* and achieves therapeutic levels in the cerebrospinal fluid; however, because this agent lowers the seizure threshold, it is relatively contraindicated for meningitis. Meropenem, a related carbapenem, is less epileptogenic and may be used for this indication.[19]

Other CNS pathogens not reliably treated with the standard empiric therapy of a third-generation cephalosporin are listed in Table 151-4. Empiric ampicillin therapy for *L. monocytogenes* should be provided for elderly patients, particularly those with T-cell immunocompromise, and for those who are alcohol dependent or pregnant.[17] If the cerebrospinal fluid Gram stain shows Gram-positive rods, suggestive of *Listeria*, intravenous gentamicin should be added. For patients intolerant of penicillins, trimethoprim-sulfamethoxazole is an acceptable alternative.

The duration of therapy in bacterial meningitis varies with the pathogen and the clinical response. Although there have been few randomized studies evaluating the optimal duration of therapy, 7 days of treatment for *H. influenzae* and *N. meningitidis* meningitis is typically sufficient, whereas *S. pneumoniae* requires 10 to 14 days of therapy.[17,20] Adults with pneumococcal meningitis commonly have predisposing infections, including pneumonia, sinusitis, otitis, or, rarely, endocarditis.[6] Although therapy for meningitis usually treats the primary cause, endocarditis requires prolonged therapy with bactericidal antibiotics.

The response of patients with Gram-negative enteric meningitis is less consistent. Follow-up spinal taps every 2 to 4 days are required during therapy of enteric Gram-negative bacillary meningitis, including *P. aeruginosa*. Progressive improvement in cerebrospinal fluid parameters of infection or colony counts of organisms should be observed. Lack of clinical or microbiologic improvement should prompt consideration of intraventricular therapy. After the cerebrospinal fluid of patients with enteric Gram-negative meningitis has become sterile, an additional 7 days of antimicrobial therapy is warranted. Because antibiotic penetration into cerebrospinal fluid falls as meningeal inflammation subsides, parenteral antibiotics are recommended for the entire course.

TABLE 151-4. BACTERIAL MENINGITIS PATHOGENS NOT ADEQUATELY TREATED WITH CEFOTAXIME OR CEFTRIAXONE MONOTHERAPY

Organism	Effective Antimicrobial
Pseudomonas aeruginosa	Ceftazidime or cefepime plus tobramycin
Listeria monocytogenes	Ampicillin or trimethoprim-sulfamethoxazole
Staphylococcus aureus (methicillin susceptible)	Nafcillin
S. aureus (methicillin resistant)	Vancomycin
Pneumococci (high-level penicillin-resistant strains)	Vancomycin plus cephalosporin

For all causes of bacterial meningitis, abnormalities of the cerebrospinal fluid (high protein and cell counts) persist for days to weeks. Resolution of symptoms (e.g., fever, leukocytosis, meningismus) should serve as adequate evidence of successful therapy. In a patient who responds poorly to 48 hours of therapy, repeat lumbar puncture and head CT or MRI are indicated. Repeat lumbar puncture is particularly important for detecting clearance of bacteria from the cerebrospinal fluid in patients with cephalosporin-resistant pneumococcal meningitis who demonstrate a slow clinical response. Patients with culture-negative pyogenic meningitis and suboptimal clinical response should also have repeat lumbar puncture to ensure response to empirical antibiotics. Ongoing or worsening cerebrospinal fluid parameters suggest infection with either resistant bacteria or with a pathogen more typically associated with subacute meningitis syndrome (see Table 151-2).

Corticosteroids

Much of the morbidity of bacterial meningitis is caused by the vigorous host inflammatory response. Corticosteroids block inflammation, and animal studies have shown an improvement in outcome when corticosteroids are given as adjuvant therapy with antibiotics. Numerous pediatric studies support the use of immunomodulators; children receiving concomitant dexamethasone and antibiotics have decreased morbidity, particularly hearing loss.[21] However, the majority of pediatric cases were infected with *H. influenzae*, a rare cause of meningitis in developed countries since the introduction of vaccine, and questions remain regarding the utility of steroids for other pathogens.

Corticosteroid treatment in adults is also controversial. A randomized treatment trial found a significant reduction in both morbidity and mortality among adults receiving combination therapy with dexamethasone and antibiotics, particularly among the subgroup with pneumococcal meningitis.[22] In this study, most infections were due to penicillin-sensitive pneumococci, and patients were treated with aminopenicillins. Evaluation of steroid use for resistant pneumococci has not been done; however, data demonstrating reduced vancomycin levels in the cerebrospinal fluid when this antibiotic is administered with steroids have raised concern about adjuvant therapy when cephalosporin-resistant

pneumococci are prevalent. Further, in controlled studies in children and adults, the initial doses of steroids and antibiotics were given concomitantly, and it is unknown whether beneficial effects remain when steroid administration is delayed. At present, it is reasonable to give adjuvant dexamethasone (10 mg intravenously every 6 hours for 4 days) concomitantly with the first dose of antibiotics, with the caveat that patients found to be infected with cephalosporin-resistant pneumococci should be followed closely to ensure clearance of bacteria from the cerebrospinal fluid.

COMPLICATIONS

Systemic complications may dominate the clinical course of acute bacterial meningitis. Forty percent of patients with pneumococcal meningitis have concomitant sepsis. The sepsis is usually from an extra-CNS infection, such as pneumonia. Less commonly, sepsis represents seeding of the bloodstream from the infected meninges. Whether bacteremia precedes or follows meningeal infection, sepsis demands immediate attention. General supportive measures, including protection of the airway and hemodynamic support, are crucial. Although many of these patients may meet the criteria for the administration of activated protein C (drotrecogin alfa), limited data on its safety and efficacy in meningitis exist. Increased risk of intracranial hemorrhage, particularly in patients with thrombocytopenia, has been reported.[23]

Meningococcal meningitis presents unique public health and infection control challenges. This diagnosis is suggested by the presence of a petechial or purpuric rash; however, this finding is neither sensitive nor specific.[24] To prevent secondary cases of meningococcal meningitis among health care workers, all patients with presumed bacterial meningitis should initially be placed in respiratory isolation to prevent the spread of infection by droplet transmission.[25] Complications specific to meningococcal meningitis include purpura fulminans and necrotizing vasculitis, leading to skin necrosis and digital gangrene (Fig. 151-5). Nonspecific complications associated with meningococcal as well as other forms of meningitis include adrenal insufficiency due to infarction (Waterhouse-Friderichsen syndrome), renal failure (due to acute tubular necrosis in the setting of hypotension), deafness, hydrocephalus, and cognitive impairment.

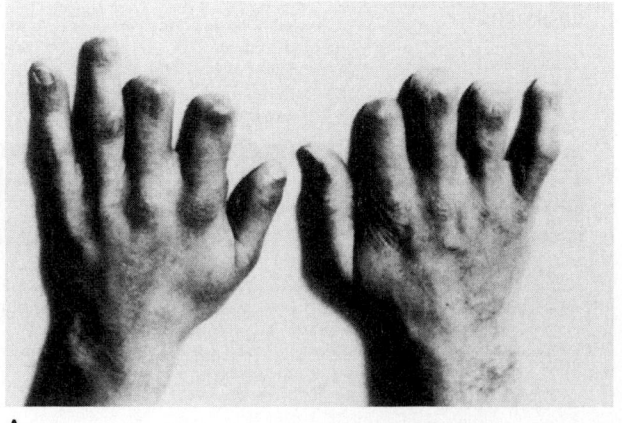
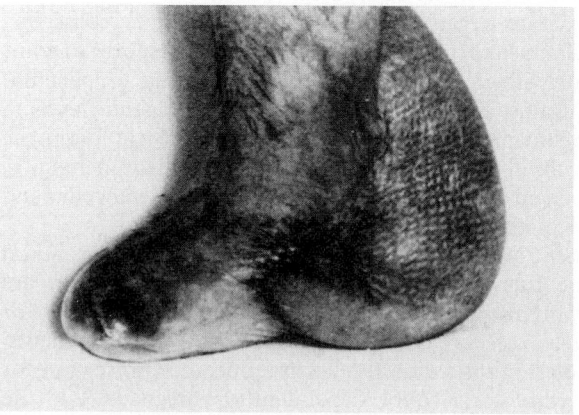

A   B

FIGURE 151–5. Extremities—hands *(A)* and foot *(B)*—of a 14-year-old boy observed by two physicians as his petechial rash progressed to "bruises" (purpura fulminans). Purpura were not recognized as the hallmarks of *Neisseria meningitidis*–induced sepsis. In addition to the loss of extremities from the necrotizing vasculitis of meningococcemia, the patient rapidly developed signs and symptoms characteristic of the acute meningitis syndrome.

BRAIN ABSCESS

Pyogenic brain abscess is a localized suppurative infection of parenchymal CNS tissue and may involve any region of the CNS from the cerebral cortex to the conus medullaris. Differentiating brain abscess from other CNS infections or brain tumors may be challenging, as there is significant overlap in the clinical and radiologic presentation (see Table 151-5). Even with modern antibiotic therapy and radiographic techniques, mortality remains as high as 20%. Rapid progression of symptoms and impaired mental status at presentation are predictors of an adverse outcome.[26] MRI is more sensitive than CT for detecting small or early lesions and allows better visualization of the cerebellum and brainstem.

PATHOPHYSIOLOGY

A brain abscess begins as a localized area of parenchymal inflammation (cerebritis), which evolves to necrosis and frank suppuration. The initial stage, characterized by vascular congestion, petechial hemorrhage, cerebral edema, and tissue softening, is demonstrable by MRI. As cerebritis progresses, CT findings become abnormal, revealing a capsule-like hyperemic zone surrounding the area of inflammation. In time, liquefaction results in frank abscess formation.

As the abscess matures, a dense capsule is formed. In relatively avascular areas of the brain, capsule formation is delayed. Once it forms, however, the capsule resolves slowly. When necrosis is rapid and capsule formation is delayed, as in the relatively avascular cerebral white matter, abscess rupture is more likely. In some cases, edema is the dominant process.

In the preantibiotic era, contiguous foci (middle ear, mastoids, sinuses) caused most brain abscesses. With the availability of antibiotics, however, such complications have become less common. An increasing number of cases are due to distant foci of infection or originate from unknown sites. With hematogenous seeding, abscesses tend to develop along the middle cerebral artery distribution. The etiologic pathogen differs according to the route of infection. Frequently, abscesses that arise from contiguous sites are polymicrobial. The bacteria most often isolated from brain abscess are aerobic and anaerobic streptococci, although other anaerobic organisms, enteric Gram-negative rods, staphylococci, pneumococci, and *Nocardia asteroides* may be present.[27] Fungi such as *Aspergillus* and even protozoa such as *Toxoplasma* can also be etiologic agents, particularly in immunosuppressed patients.

CLINICAL COURSE

The variable signs and symptoms of brain abscess relate to variations in location, size, and rapidity of development. At one extreme, the course may span weeks, with few constitutional symptoms. In this setting, signs and symptoms of a space-occupying lesion predominate, and neoplasm is the primary diagnostic concern. In contrast, a previously asymptomatic brain abscess may rupture into the subarachnoid space, causing death within hours. The differential diagnosis in this setting includes an acute cerebrovascular event and pyogenic meningitis. However, brain abscess usually progresses subacutely for 7 to 14 days. Classic symptoms include excruciating headache, low-grade fever, and focal neurologic signs. Occasionally, a patient has no symptoms referable to the CNS, and fever may be absent in as many as 50% of cases. Lumbar puncture may demonstrate increased cells and protein and normal or decreased glucose.

Organisms are identified in only 10% of cases. Because a lumbar puncture may be life threatening in the presence of an expanding brain abscess, this procedure should be deferred if neuroimaging studies reveal a mass lesion.

Parameningeal foci progress to brain abscess as the inflammatory process erodes through bone and meningeal tissues. Chronic otitis, sinusitis, or postsurgical and posttraumatic dural defects in a patient with progressive neurologic deterioration strongly suggest brain abscess.

Bacterial pathogens also invade neural tissues via hematogenous spread. The presence of chronic extrameningeal suppurative foci or illicit intravenous drug use predisposes to brain abscess. Filtration of bacteria by the pulmonary vasculature protects the brain from hematogenous seeding. However, when cardiac shunts or pulmonary arteriovenous fistulas are present, brain abscesses may occur. In as many as a third of patients, there is no obvious source of infection. Brain abscesses associated with endocarditis are rare but, when present, are often multiple and small. Bacterial meningitis is an infrequent cause of intracerebral abscess.

CNS complications of brain abscess relate to both tissue inflammation and increased intracranial pressure from a space-occupying lesion. Nonspecific complications common to all critically ill patients include aspiration and gastrointestinal bleeding. Specific complications include focal neurologic defects, altered mental status, or seizures. Although signs and symptoms related to the space-occupying effect help localize the infection to the brain, these findings do not differentiate infection from other intracerebral mass lesions. When surrounding edema is excessive, aggressive therapy with corticosteroids is warranted. If a brain abscess ruptures into the subarachnoid space or into a cerebral ventricle, rapid deterioration in mental status is the rule, and mortality in these cases is high.

IMAGING

CT and MRI techniques are particularly valuable in assessing brain abscesses. Changes in lesion size after the institution of therapy can be closely monitored from week to week. Neurosurgical intervention can be guided by assessing proximity to vital neural structures. An expanding abscess may be aggressively drained, or conversely, a stable or shrinking abscess can be assiduously observed.

CT scanning has some limitations, particularly if performed without contrast, and it may be insensitive for visualizing early cerebritis. In addition, the cerebellum, brainstem, and spinal cord may not be well visualized, and CT may not detect lesions 1.5 cm or smaller, as are typically seen with endocarditis. For such lesions, MRI enhanced with intravenous gadolinium is more sensitive.

Maturation of the brain abscess is associated with encapsulation, and this is suggested by ring enhancement on CT or MRI. Misinterpretation can occur, particularly when the abscess is in the white matter, where decreased vascularity may result in delayed encapsulation with minimal ring enhancement. Similarly, steroid therapy may decrease local inflammation, resulting in resolution of ring enhancement. Ring enhancement is not specific for bacterial abscesses and may be seen with other infections or brain tumors.

THERAPY

A combination approach of antimicrobials coupled with surgical drainage constitutes the accepted management of pyogenic brain abscesses. Choice of antimicrobials should be guided by culture results, given the diversity of potential pathogens and the need for prolonged therapy (e.g., 6 to 8 weeks). Because of the difficulty in getting therapeutic concentrations of antibiotics across the blood-brain barrier, additional pharmacologic considerations include CNS penetration and parenteral administration. Empirical therapy should be begun while awaiting culture results and should be guided by the likely microbiology based on the origin of the infection. In cases in which the source is unknown or metastatic spread from a distant focus is likely, empirical therapy with nafcillin, metronidazole, and a third-generation cephalosporin should be adequate.[27] Vancomycin may be substituted when resistant *S. aureus* is a concern, and an antipseudomonal cephalosporin should be used for postoperative infections or for an abscess arising from an otogenic site. Diagnostic aspiration is invaluable in identifying specific pathogens, and sensitivity testing is crucial for narrowing therapy. Fungal and mycobacterial cultures should be obtained on all aspirates. Positive cultures from blood or extra-CNS suppurative foci occasionally establish a presumptive etiologic agent. Ancillary testing for a culture-negative brain abscess includes HIV serology, serum cryptococcal antigen, and toxoplasmosis titers.

In selected cases, brain abscesses can be treated with antimicrobials alone, particularly when the causative agent is known and the lesion measures less than 2.5 cm.[28] Medical management without drainage may be necessary when the lesion is inaccessible or surgical intervention poses unacceptable risks. However, open or stereotactic drainage is indicated when (1) cultures of extra-CNS sites do not yield a pathogen, (2) deterioration from increased intracranial pressure occurs, and (3) there is no radiographic improvement on medical therapy. Patients treated without drainage may require a longer duration (e.g., 12 weeks) of parenteral antibiotics and should be followed closely for clinical and radiographic improvement. Steroids should not be routinely used unless significant edema is present.

VIRAL INFECTIONS OF THE CENTRAL NERVOUS SYSTEM

All components of the CNS are vulnerable to viral infection. The resultant clinical syndrome may be meningitis, encephalitis, or myelitis. Acute viral meningitis is characterized by meningeal irritation, cerebrospinal fluid pleocytosis, and a self-limited clinical course. Myelitis implies infection of the spinal cord and may be present in isolation (e.g., polio virus infection) or as part of an overlap syndrome of encephalomyelitis (e.g., acute flaccid paralysis associated with West Nile virus encephalitis). The hallmark of viral encephalitis is alteration in cognition lasting 24 hours or more. Personality changes may occur, with irritability and inability to concentrate. Patients may also develop fever, headache, nausea, and vomiting. As a result of parenchymal involvement, CNS function may deteriorate over several days; confusion, lethargy, somnolence, coma, and seizures are common. Meningismus may develop at any point during viral encephalitis or may remain absent.

PATHOPHYSIOLOGY

Most viral infections of the CNS occur through hematogenous spread. The virus may initially traverse mucous membranes (e.g., enteroviruses) or be inoculated into subcutaneous tissue (e.g., arboviruses). After local replication within extraneural tissues, sustained viremia occurs. Alternatively, the virus may gain access to the CNS by direct neuronal invasion, as occurs when rabies virus spreads retrograde along peripheral nerves into the CNS. The olfactory tracts may provide a route of entry for herpes simplex virus type 1.[29]

Individual viruses demonstrate affinities for different anatomic areas of the CNS. Enteroviruses and mumps viruses usually infect the ependyma and tissues of the subarachnoid space, producing meningeal irritation. In contrast, arboviruses and rabies viruses almost always involve the parenchyma and cause encephalitis. In older children and adults, herpes simplex virus type 1 characteristically causes temporal lobe encephalitis, whereas herpes simplex virus type 2 more typically causes meningitis. Such affinities are not absolute. For example, enteroviruses may on rare occasions cause encephalitis.

ACUTE VIRAL MENINGITIS

Although many viruses cause meningitis, in clinical practice, the specific pathogen is rarely identified. In most cases, extensive diagnostic evaluation is not indicated, as viral meningitis is typically a self-limited syndrome and does not require treatment. Epidemiologic studies suggest that enteroviruses are the most common cause of viral meningitis[30] and are particularly prevalent in children and young adults. Other viral causes of meningitis include arboviruses (see Viral Encephalitis), herpes simplex virus type 2, acute HIV infection, and lymphocytic choriomeningitis virus.

At the time of presentation, it may be difficult to differentiate viral meningitis from other forms of culture-negative meningitis that may be more aggressive or require directed therapy. The differential diagnosis for culture-negative or aseptic meningitis includes tick-borne infections such as *Ehrlichia* or *Rickettsia*, secondary syphilis, mycobacterial or fungal infections, irritation from a parameningeal focus, and partially treated bacterial infections (see Fig. 151-3). Signs and symptoms of viral and bacterial meningitis are indistinguishable. Cerebrospinal fluid findings suggestive of a viral cause include lymphocytic pleocytosis (typically with a total white blood cell count <1000), normal glucose, and normal to slightly elevated protein. Management is supportive, with fluid repletion for significant dehydration and pain control the mainstays of care. Meningeal symptoms usually resolve in the first 2 weeks, but malaise may be prolonged.

VIRAL ENCEPHALITIS

A host of viral agents infect the parenchyma of the brain or spinal cord to produce encephalitis or myelitis, respectively; however, despite intensive investigation, in the majority of cases, no organism is identified.[31,32] Viral encephalitis is typically an acute febrile illness associated with headache, an altered level of consciousness disproportionate to systemic illness, behavioral or speech disturbances, and focal neurologic signs such as seizures or hemiparesis. In contrast, viral myelitis causes hemiparesis or hemiplegia but spares higher integrative functions. Overlap syndromes of encephalomyelitis can occur.

Viral encephalitis is caused by acute invasion of brain parenchyma. Clinically, viral encephalitis must be differentiated from acute disseminated encephalomyelitis (ADEM), an autoimmune phenomenon that typically occurs 5 to 21 days after a viral respiratory or gastrointestinal illness. MRI in ADEM reveals enhancing, multifocal white matter lesions suggestive of demyelination.[33] Neuroimaging to distinguish these entities is important, because ADEM responds to high-dose steroids. With the exception of herpes simplex encephalitis (see later), management of viral encephalitides revolves around supportive care and control of seizures. Despite the lack of specific antiviral treatments, thorough evaluation is important to direct public health interventions (e.g., mosquito eradication for West Nile virus or other arboviruses) or provide prognostic information (e.g., rabies).

HERPES SIMPLEX ENCEPHALITIS

Herpes simplex encephalitis (HSE) is the most common cause of sporadic encephalitis in the United States. Although the mortality of untreated HSE exceeds 70%, timely administration of acyclovir has been shown to improve survival. Although clinical, laboratory, or radiographic findings may be suggestive of HSE, no combination of presenting features is sufficiently sensitive, and empirical acyclovir should be given to all patients with encephalitis until definitive diagnostic studies are completed.[34]

Common signs and symptoms of HSE include fever, personality change, and dysphasia. Hemiparesis and seizures occur in approximately 40% of cases.[34] Without treatment, progressive obtundation occurs. Cerebrospinal fluid typically exhibits a lymphocytic pleocytosis, but this is nonspecific. Suggestive findings include temporal lobe localization on neuroimaging studies, with MRI being superior to CT, and periodic lateralizing epileptiform discharges on the electroencephalogram. With the availability of noninvasive diagnostic methods such as PCR, it appears that up to 20% of cases manifest mild or atypical presentations.[35] Definitive diagnosis requires detection of herpes simplex in the brain or spinal fluid. PCR on cerebrospinal fluid, a noninvasive test with a sensitivity greater than 95%, is now considered the gold standard for diagnosis.[36] Empirical acyclovir can usually be discontinued if the PCR is negative, although there have been reports of false-negative results early in the course of the disease.[37] For PCR-confirmed cases, acyclovir therapy should be continued for a minimum of 14 days, with treatment extended if the cerebrospinal fluid remains PCR-positive at this point.[38]

CENTRAL NERVOUS SYSTEM INFECTION AND THE AIDS PATIENT

CNS dysfunction is common in patients with acquired immunodeficiency syndrome (AIDS). MRI, followed by lumbar puncture, is indicated for any patient with AIDS who has significant headache or altered mental status, even when CNS symptoms do not dominate the picture. This sequential approach to evaluation is recommended because mass lesions, including toxoplasmosis, lymphoma, and progressive multifocal leukoencephalopathy, are common. Ring-enhancing lesions on CT or MRI are suggestive of the first two entities, whereas focal white matter disease favors the last. Positive serologic testing for *Toxoplasma gondii* or the presence of multiple mass lesions increases the likelihood of

CNS toxoplasmosis, and if either of these is present, empirical therapy for toxoplasmosis should be begun.[39] Surgical intervention may be reserved for cases with signs of impending herniation or lack of radiographic response after 2 weeks of therapy.

Cryptococcal meningitis is also common in AIDS and typically presents as a slowly progressive syndrome marked by fever and headaches. Diagnosis of this infection can be made by either serum or cerebrospinal fluid cryptococcal antigen testing, both of which have a sensitivity greater than 90%. Cerebrospinal fluid testing provides important prognostic and therapeutic information. Treatment recommendations include induction therapy with amphotericin B and flucytosine for 2 weeks, followed by consolidation therapy with fluconazole.[40] Maintenance therapy with fluconazole must be continued for life.

PARADURAL ABSCESS

The epidural space is between the dura and the bony structures of the skull and vertebral column; the subdural space is between the subarachnoid membrane and the dura (see Fig. 151-2). Unlike the subarachnoid space, the paradural tissues are only potential spaces, with the arachnoid membrane and the dura resisting the spread of infection across their surfaces. Although subdural abscesses are more common within the cranium and epidural abscesses are more common within the vertebral column, the causes, pathophysiology, and therapies are similar. These abscesses usually develop from a contiguous infection, surgery, or trauma.

In the skull, the epidural tissues are dense, and abscess formation is unusual. The subarachnoid membrane is less adherent to the dura, making the subdural space the more likely site of infection. The reverse is true in the vertebral column, where a thin layer of fat and blood vessels separate the dura from the vertebral bony structures. Here, infection is more likely to involve the epidural space. Once established, infection may dissect within the epidural space for considerable distances.

Cranial subdural empyema may be clinically indistinguishable from a brain abscess. Subdural abscess is usually associated with infection of the paranasal sinuses and, less commonly, the ears or mastoids.[41] Trauma, surgical intervention, or hematogenous sources cause the remaining cases. Organisms common to sinusitis, including streptococci, pneumococci, *Haemophilus*, anaerobes, and staphylococci, cause most infections. Gram-negative enteric bacilli may be associated with middle ear and mastoid infections.

An epidural abscess of the vertebral column classically progresses rapidly from back pain to paraplegia to paralysis. *S. aureus* accounts for two thirds of cases of epidural abscess.[42] Although most cases are community acquired, approximately one fifth occur after spinal instrumentation (surgery or nerve block), and nosocomial flora such as methicillin-resistant *S. aureus* or *Pseudomonas* may be causative in this population. Other risk factors for spinal epidural abscess include intravenous drug use, diabetes mellitus, trauma, and comorbid conditions such as dialysis.

Paradural abscesses tend to evolve rapidly, often producing irreversible damage to underlying neural structures. Antibiotics alone are inadequate if there is evidence of nerve compression, and neurosurgical drainage remains the

TABLE 151–5. DIFFERENTIAL DIAGNOSIS OF CENTRAL NERVOUS SYSTEM INFECTION AND TUMOR

	Brain Abscess	Bacterial Meningitis	Herpetic Encephalitis	Brain Tumor
History				
Headache	Severe, often focal	Severe, generalized	Mild to severe	Absent to severe
Focal defect	Often	Occasional	Occasional	Usual
Progression	Days to weeks	Hours to days	Days	Days to months
Physical Examination				
Fever/degree	Usual/low grade	Always/high	Always/high	Rare
Early focal signs	Often	Occasional	Occasional	Usual
Pressure signs	Often	Rare	Occasional	Often
Distal infection	Often	Often	No	No
CT or MRI Scan				
Focal	Always*	No	Often	Always
Ring effect/onset	Often/late†	—	No	Often/early

*May be negative or nonspecific during first 48 hours of illness.
†Development of abscess wall may be delayed by steroid therapy.
CT, computed tomography; MRI, magnetic resonance imaging.

mainstay of therapy. MRI has greatly aided in the rapid localization and management of paradural abscesses.

SPINAL EPIDURAL ABSCESS SYNDROME

The spinal epidural abscess syndrome usually begins with localized spinal pain. Higher integrative functions generally remain intact; systemic manifestations are rarely severe enough to cause cortical dysfunction. Symptoms usually progress through four clinical phases: spinal ache, nerve root pain, radicular weakness, and paralysis. Back pain with fever, focal tenderness, and sensory or motor deficits strongly suggests this disease. A source of hematogenous seeding may be present in three fourths of patients.

Diagnosis hinges on visualization of a collection in the epidural space (Fig. 151-6). The diagnostic study of choice is MRI, which defines cord compression and the presence and extent of abscess, identifies drainable paraspinal fluid collections, and detects concomitant vertebral osteomyelitis. Other procedures such as myelography and CT scanning may be used if MRI cannot be performed. Emergency neurosurgical intervention is considered mandatory for this infection if there is clinical evidence of cord compression. In selected cases, patients may be successfully treated with antibiotics alone. Nonsurgical management might be considered if a pathogen is identified by peripheral blood cultures or by needle biopsy; if there is no progression of neurologic findings (e.g., weakness) on frequent examination; if pain improves with treatment; and if fever, peripheral white blood cell count, and sedimentation rate all decline on therapy.[43,44] Unfortunately, some patients develop sudden neurologic impairment even weeks into conservative therapy, presumably secondary to vascular compromise of the cord. Initially, neurologic deficits may be limited to a loss of pain sensation in the perianal region (second sacral dermatome). Progressive weakness indicates the need for immediate MRI and neurosurgical consultation, because decompression within 24 hours offers the best chance of neurologic recovery.[42]

Degenerative disease and metastatic tumor may mimic epidural abscess, especially if fever is present. A metastatic tumor of the spinal cord can produce rapidly progressive cord compression, and a history of malignancy may be suggestive. MRI usually distinguishes among degenerative spinal disease, metastatic tumor, hematoma, and epidural abscess.

Spinal epidural abscess demands empiric antimicrobial therapy pending the results of culture. Community-acquired abscess is usually due to *S. aureus* and should be treated with nafcillin. If methicillin-resistant staphylococci are a concern, vancomycin can be substituted. Recent urinary tract infection, decubitus ulcers, or vertebral surgery suggests the presence of Gram-negative bacilli, and a third-generation cephalosporin should be added. Treatment may be modified when culture results are available.

SEPSIS SYNDROME WITH CENTRAL NERVOUS SYSTEM INVOLVEMENT

In the sepsis syndrome, an acutely ill patient develops CNS dysfunction late in the course of the illness, typically in the setting of multiorgan system failure. Altered mental status, attributable to hypotension and hypoperfusion, ranges from confusion to obtundation. Seizures may occur due to metabolic abnormalities, ischemia, or hemorrhage. In treating such patients, general supportive measures take precedence over CNS concerns. After a brief assessment, general life-support measures should correct hypotension, hypoxia, and anuria. As soon as they are easily accessible, body fluid specimens are obtained for culture, and broad-spectrum antimicrobials should be administered. At this point, a careful history should be taken and a physical examination performed. The patient is treated as outlined for subacute CNS infection syndrome (see Fig. 151-4). Delays in directly assessing the CNS are justifiable only when the history is adequate to document that a clear-cut systemic illness preceded the onset of CNS symptoms and signs. Otherwise, a more aggressive use of lumbar puncture and CT or MRI is warranted (see Figs. 151-3 and 151-4).

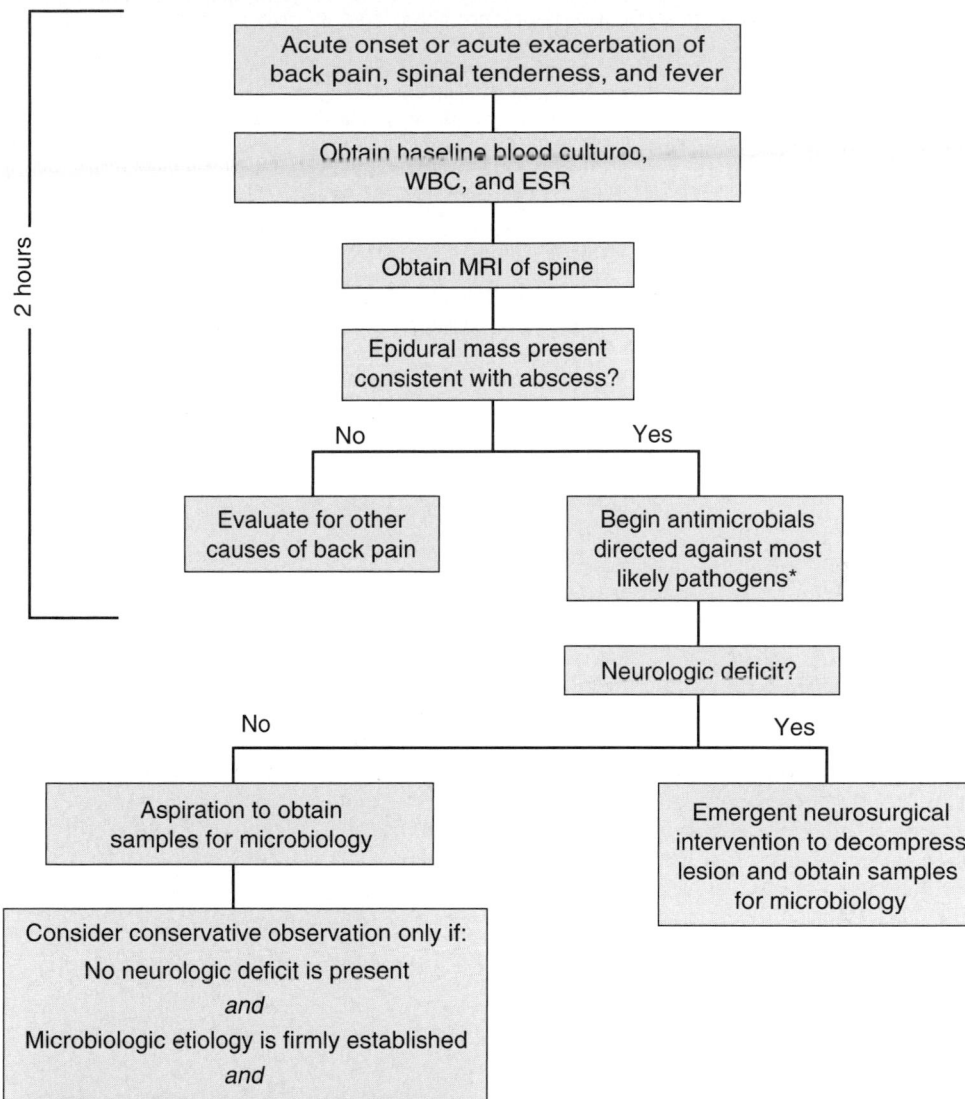

Management of Patients with Spinal Epidural Abscess Syndrome
(Acute onset of back pain and spinal tenderness plus fever.)
(Higher integrative functions are intact, but neck stiffness may be present.)

Acute onset or acute exacerbation of back pain, spinal tenderness, and fever

Obtain baseline blood cultures, WBC, and ESR

Obtain MRI of spine

Epidural mass present consistent with abscess?

No — Evaluate for other causes of back pain

Yes — Begin antimicrobials directed against most likely pathogens*

Neurologic deficit?

No — Aspiration to obtain samples for microbiology

Yes — Emergent neurosurgical intervention to decompress lesion and obtain samples for microbiology

Consider conservative observation only if:
No neurologic deficit is present
and
Microbiologic etiology is firmly established
and
WBC and ESR fall rapidly on antibiotics
and
Excruciating pain resolves
and
Paraspinous fluid collections have been drained percutaneously
(or if surgery is absolutely contraindicated for other reasons)

2 hours

FIGURE 151–6. Algorithm for the management of patients with the spinal epidural abscess syndrome. If magnetic resonance imaging (MRI) cannot be performed, myelography, high-contrast computed tomography (CT), or CT-myelography may be an acceptable alternative to localize an epidural abscess. * If abscess drainage can be performed promptly, antimicrobial drugs may be withheld until specimens for microbial analysis are obtained. WBC, white blood cell; ESR, erythrocyte sedimentation rate.

CONCLUSION

Acute infection of the CNS requires rapid therapeutic intervention. Because the four major syndromes of CNS infection (acute meningitis syndrome, subacute CNS infection syndrome, spinal epidural abscess syndrome, and sepsis syndrome) differ in their signs and symptoms, as well as in the approach to definitive diagnosis and therapy, it is important to distinguish among them. Moreover, diverse infectious and noninfectious causes may produce similar CNS syndromes. For therapy to be maximally effective, it must be instituted within minutes to hours of the initial evaluation. Thus, in the practice of critical care medicine involving CNS disease, the goal remains rapid institution of empirical therapy for treatable infectious syndromes while efficiently working to identify the specific disease process.

ANNOTATED REFERENCES

Aronin SI, Peduzzi P, Quagliarello VJ: Community-acquired bacterial meningitis: Risk stratification for adverse clinical outcome and effect of antibiotic timing. Ann Intern Med 1998;129:862.

This retrospective cohort study identified hypotension, altered mental status, and seizures as independent risk factors for death or sustained neurologic morbidity in patients with meningitis. A model incorporating these three variables into prognostic stages identified progression to a higher stage before the receipt of antibiotics as a predictor of poor outcome.

de Gans J, van de Beek D, Investigators EDiABMS: Dexamethasone in adults with bacterial meningitis. N Engl J Med 2002;347:1549-1556.

This prospective, randomized, double-blind, placebo-controlled study evaluated whether the addition of dexamethasone to standard antibiotic therapy improved the outcome for adults with meningitis. Mortality and morbidity were significantly reduced in the group that received dexamethasone 10 mg every 6 hours for 4 days starting at the time of presentation. This was particularly true in the subset of patients with pneumococcal meningitis.

Glaser CA, Gilliam S, Schnurr D, et al: In search of encephalitis etiologies: Diagnostic challenges in the California Encephalitis Project, 1998-2000. Clin Infect Dis 2003;36:731-742.

The California Encephalitis Project prospectively tested clinical specimens from 334 patients throughout the state with presumed encephalitis. In this cohort, 13% of cases had a probable or confirmed infectious agent identified, 12% had a possible infectious cause, 10% had a noninfectious diagnosis, and 62% remained undiagnosed despite extensive testing.

Hasbun R, Abrahams J, Jekel J, et al: Computed tomography of the head before lumbar puncture in adults with suspected meningitis. N Engl J Med 2001;345:1727-1733.

This prospective cohort study evaluated factors predictive of an abnormal head CT among patients presenting with presumed meningitis. The authors identified age older than 60 years, immunocompromise, history of CNS disease, seizure within 1 week before presentation, altered mental status, and abnormal focal neurologic examination as predictors of an abnormal study. Among patients with none of these features, the CT scan was normal in 93 of 96 patients, for a negative predictive value of 97%.

Redington JJ, Tyler KL: Viral infections of the central nervous system, 2002: Update on diagnosis and treatment. Arch Neurol 2002;59:712-718.

This paper provides a comprehensive review of the literature, with an emphasis on emerging pathogens, new diagnostic studies, and evolving treatment options for viral infections of the CNS.

Chapter 152

INFECTIONS OF SKIN, MUSCLE, AND SOFT TISSUE

Weidun Alan Guo • Steven M. Steinberg

KEY POINTS

1. Soft tissue infections include infections of the skin, subcutaneous tissue, and muscle. They are commonly encountered in ICUs and are **often severe and potentially life threatening.**

2. **Most serious soft tissue infections require some degree of tissue injury and break in the skin to establish the infection.** The break in the skin may be due to a surgical incision or trauma; it may be related to large wounds or very small ones. The tissue injury may be due to either blunt or penetrating trauma of any kind.

3. **The initial management of necrotizing soft tissue infections** (NSTIs) involves physiologic support, aggressive fluid resuscitation, appropriate broad-spectrum parenteral antibiotics, and, most importantly, expedient and radical surgical débridement. Other adjunctive therapies, such as hyperbaric oxygen and immunoglobulin, may be used, but their efficacy has not been as well established.

4. **Topical antimicrobial agents are commonly used in burn patients.** Their use has substantially decreased the incidence of conversion of partial-thickness to full-thickness wounds by local infection and thereby has reduced mortality associated with burn wound infection. Systemic antibiotics are not used prophylactically in burn patients.

5. **Pressure ulcers in ICU patients occur primarily in patients with impaired mobility** due to injury, weakness, sedation, or use of paralytic agents. **Pressure ulcers are almost entirely preventable,** and measures to prevent development of decubitus ulcers, including pressure relief and appropriate nutrition, should be taken in all patients who are thought to be at risk for decubitus ulcers.

Infections of skin, soft tissue, and muscle include a broad range of diseases from those originated from the skin (impetigo, ecthyma, erysipelas, pyoderma), superficial fascia (embolic ulcers, cellulitis), fascia cleft, and deep fascia (necrotizing fasciitis) to muscle (myonecrosis). Discussion of skin and soft tissue infections that are chronic and less life threatening, for which patients usually consult their primary care professionals, is out of the scope of discussion in this book.

In this chapter, we focus on infections of skin, soft tissue, and muscle that are commonly encountered in ICUs and are often severe and potentially life threatening. These infections include necrotizing soft tissue infections (NSTIs), soft tissue infections of the neck and head, and infectious complications of bites, burns, and pressure ulcers.

NECROTIZING SOFT TISSUE INFECTIONS

NSTIs represent a spectrum of infectious processes characterized by extensive, rapidly progressive infections. Based on the depth of skin and soft tissue involvement, NSTIs are divided into three categories: necrotizing cellulitis, necrotizing fasciitis, and myonecrosis. Table 152-1 shows the classification of NSTIs. The sine qua non of these infections is necrosis of subcutaneous tissue, fascia, and muscle with widespread undermining of the skin. The lack of anatomic boundaries and the fact that the infection is deep to the skin helps account for the severity of the infection as well as for the frequent delay in its recognition. Although the trunk and extremities are the most common sites of NSTIs, it is important to understand that any other anatomic site, including the perineum and head and neck, may be involved.[1] Retroperitoneal perforation of appendicitis or a cecal cancer can cause the infection to extend into the thigh along the psoas muscle and cause necrotizing infections of the thigh.[2,3] Cervical fasciitis due to dental abscess can extend to the mediastinum.[4]

Many different descriptive terms and eponyms have been used to describe NSTIs. The most common infections encountered in ICU patients are postoperative progressive bacterial synergistic gangrene, clostridial cellulitis, synergistic gangrene, necrotizing fasciitis, Fournier's gangrene, gas gangrene, and Meleney's synergistic gangrene. Although the terminology and depth of infection may be different, the severity of the infection and the emergent need for surgical intervention are common to all varieties of these infections.

PATHOGENESIS

Pathophysiologic factors that are involved in the development and progression of NSTIs are host resistance, the bacterial pathogens, and local barrier factors.

Host Resistance

As shown in Table 152-2, individuals who are immunocompromised or who have chronic diseases are more likely to develop necrotizing skin and soft tissue infections than those without such medical problems.

TABLE 152–1. CLASSIFICATION OF NECROTIZING SKIN, SOFT TISSUE, AND MUSCLE INFECTIONS

Disease	Bacteriology	Comments
Necrotizing Cellulitis		
Clostridial cellulitis	*Clostridium perfringens*	Local trauma, recent surgery; fascial/deep muscle spared
Nonclostridial cellulitis	Mixed: *Escherichia coli, Enterobacter, Peptostreptococcus* species, *Bacteroides fragilis*	Diabetes mellitus predisposes; produces foul odor
Meleney's synergistic gangrene	*Staphylococcus aureus*, microaerophilic streptococci	Rare infection; postoperative; slowly expanding, indolent, ulceration in superficial fascia
Synergistic necrotizing cellulitis	Mixed: aerobic and anaerobic, including *B. fragilis, Peptostreptococcus* species	Diabetes mellitus predisposes; variant of necrotizing fasciitis type I; involves skin, muscle, fat, and fascia
Necrotizing Fasciitis		
Type I	Mixed: aerobic and anaerobic. Staphylococci, *E. coli*, group A streptococci, *Peptostreptococcus* species, *Prevotella, Porphyromonas* species, *B. fragilis, Clostridium* species	Usually requires a breach in the mucous membrane layer either through surgery or penetrating injuries or from chronic medical conditions such as diabetes, peripheral vascular disease, malignancy, and anal fissures
Type II	Group A streptococci	Increasing in frequency and severity since 1985; very high mortality; often begins at site of nonpenetrating minor trauma such a bruise or muscle strain but often no identified precursor Predisposing factors: blunt/penetrating trauma, varicella (chickenpox), intravenous drug abuse, surgical procedures, child birth, NSAID use
Myonecrosis		
Clostridial myonecrosis	*Clostridium* species	Predisposing factors: deep/penetrating injury, bowel and biliary tract surgery, criminal abortion and retained placenta; prolonged rupture of the membranes; and intrauterine fetal demise or missed abortion in postpartum patients. Recurrent gas gangrene occurs at sites of previous gas gangrene.
Streptococcal myonecrosis	Streptococci	
Special Type of Necrotizing Soft Tissue Infection		
Fournier's gangrene	Polymicrobial with *E. coli* the predominant aerobe and *Bacteroides* the predominant anaerobe. Other microflora: *Proteus, Staphylococcus, Enterococcus*, aerobic and anaerobic *Streptococcus, Pseudomonas, Klebsiella*, and *Clostridium*	Necrosis of the scrotum or perineum that starts with scrotal pain and erythema and rapidly spreads onto anterior abdominal wall and gluteal muscle. It is more often seen in diabetics and can be associated with trauma.

Bacterial Pathogens

There are specific bacteria that are more likely than others to cause necrotizing soft tissue infections, as shown in Table 152-1.[5,6] Although necrotizing cellulitis and fasciitis may be caused by a single bacterial pathogen, such as group A *Streptococcus*, *Vibrio* species, or Zygomycetes, about 80% of necrotizing cellulitis or fasciitis results from polymicrobial infections with synergistic facultative aerobes and anaerobic gas-forming organisms. The former includes gram-positive and gram-negative aerobes, such as *Streptococcus pyogenes*, *Staphylococcus aureus*, *Enterococcus faecalis*, *Escherichia coli*, or *Pseudomonas aeruginosa*, and the latter includes *Clostridium perfringens*, *Bacteroides fragilis*, and *Peptostreptococcus*.[5,6] Certain predisposing conditions can be correlated with specific bacteria, for example, trauma with *Clostridium* species, diabetes mellitus with *Bacteroides* species, *S. aureus*, and Enterobacteriaceae, and immunosuppression with *Pseudomonas* species and Enterobacteriaceae.[7]

Traditionally, gas gangrene is synonymous with clostridial infection, and gas in the soft tissue is thought to be a grave finding. The majority of gas-producing infections do not involve *Clostridium* species but are instead necrotizing infections involving other bacterial pathogens. Many bacteria, especially facultative gram-negative bacilli (e.g., *E. coli*) produce insoluble gases, such as hydrogen, nitrogen, and methane, whenever they are forced to use anaerobic metabolism. Thus, the presence of crepitus in a soft tissue infection on physical examination or radiographs implies anaerobic metabolism and existence of a necrotizing soft tissue infection. However, it does not signify any specific microbiologic pathogen.

Local Barrier Failure

Most serious soft tissue infections require some degree of tissue injury and break in the skin to establish the infection. The break in the skin may be due to a surgical incision or trauma; it may be related to large wounds or very small ones. The tissue injury may be due to either blunt or penetrating trauma of any kind. However, in a significant percentage

TABLE 152–2. FACTORS PREDISPOSING TO NECROTIZING SOFT TISSUE INFECTIONS

Human, animal, or insect bites
Contaminated or dirty surgical procedures
Diabetes mellitus
Long-term corticosteroid use
Malignancy
Trauma/burns
Intravenous drug abuse
Chronic alcoholism
Malnutrition
HIV infection/AIDS
Cirrhosis
Peripheral vascular diseases
Chronic renal failure

of cases, it is difficult to find evidence of a break in the skin or soft tissue trauma.

CLINICAL MANIFESTATIONS AND DIAGNOSIS

The critical aspect of diagnosing NSTIs is maintaining a high index of suspicion, which allows for early recognition of the nonlocalized, necrotizing nature of the infection and the need for surgical intervention. Although necrotizing cellulitis and fasciitis may occur after significant tissue trauma or a relatively trivial injury, up to 40% of NSTIs have no identifiable cause. In necrotizing cellulitis, gas is invariably found in the skin, but the fascia and deep muscle are spared. Early clinical findings are similar to those of common wound infections, including local edema (89%), erythema (30%), fever (71%), and local cutaneous anesthesia (27%) due to cutaneous nerve necrosis.[8] These are followed by gangrenous skin changes with rapid extension beyond the borders of the original infection. Synergistic polymicrobial necrotizing fasciitis is characterized by "dishwater pus." Patients usually have high fever, but no obvious source of clinical infection can be detected. Pain in the area of infection is usually out of proportion to the physical findings. As the infection progresses, the patients develop shock and multiple organ failure.

Clostridial myonecrosis (gas gangrene) typically develops within 12 to 24 hours after a traumatic event or closure of a deep contaminated wound. Recurrent gas gangrene caused by *C. perfringens* has been described in individuals with non-penetrating injuries at sites of previous gas gangrene, where spores of *C. perfringens* remain quiescent in tissue and then germinate when minor trauma provides conditions suitable for growth.[5] Patients present with the triad of severe pain, tachycardia out of proportion to fever, and crepitus in the soft tissue. Once overt gangrene with edema and bronze, purplish, or brown discoloration with bullae and watery discharge occur, the disease is at an advanced stage. Gram stain of the exudate shows gram-positive rods occasionally accompanied by other flora.

In contrast, streptococcal myonecrosis usually develops over 2 to 4 days after trauma or closure of a wound. The onset is not as rapid, and patients do not appear as sick, the pain is not as severe, and the gas formation is not as obvious as those with clostridial myonecrosis.

MANAGEMENT

The initial management of necrotizing soft tissue infections involves physiologic support, aggressive fluid resuscitation, appropriate broad-spectrum parenteral antibiotics, and, most importantly, expedient and radical surgical débridement. Other adjunctive therapies, such as hyperbaric oxygen and immunoglobulin have been used, but their efficacy has not been as well established.

Antibiotics

For type I necrotizing fasciitis (mixed aerobic and anaerobic), antibiotic treatment should be based initially on results of the Gram stain. Early empirical treatment should be initiated with extended-spectrum penicillins (e.g., ampicillin-sulbactam, piperacillin-tazobactam, ticarcillin-clavulanic acid), or carbapenem antibiotics (e.g., imipenem/cilastatin). If there is a suspicion that resistant coliforms might be participating, such as in patients who have been hospitalized or who have been treated with antibiotics recently, a third-generation cephalosporin, aminoglycoside, or aztreonam combined with either clindamycin or metronidazole may be used. For those patients in whom clostridia are suspected, penicillin G plus clindamycin may be useful for inhibiting toxin production in patients with clostridial myonecrosis.

Although there are no data from clinical trials establishing the benefit of combined therapy in type II necrotizing fasciitis (group A streptococci), penicillin G combined with clindamycin is the antibiotic therapy of choice. Clindamycin, but not metronidazole, is recommended not for its anti-anaerobic properties but because of its additional activity against gram-positive organisms, including specific inhibition of toxin production.[9] Cefotaxime and ceftriaxone are acceptable alternatives. For patients allergic to penicillin, vancomycin is the recommended treatment.

Surgical Intervention

Surgical débridement is critical in the management of NSTIs. Aggressive surgical excision of all involved tissue with a margin of normal-appearing tissue is mandatory. All necrotic tissue should be excised back to healthy bleeding margins. Additional incisions parallel to cutaneous nerves and blood vessels may be used to assess fascial viability without elevating the skin. Aggressive fascial débridement of abdominal surgical wounds may necessitate the use of prosthetic material to replace an abdominal wall defect. In Fournier's gangrene, when infection involves the scrotum and testes, a colostomy for fecal diversion may be necessary to keep the wound clean. The testes generally survive because their blood supply is usually spared, but they may need to be temporarily implanted in the soft tissue of the medial thighs if the scrotum must be débrided. On rare occasion, NSTI of the extremities may require amputation.

Myonecrosis or gas gangrene requires radical débridement to viable muscle. When this process involves the extremities, control of the infection is more easily achieved, although, as mentioned previously, amputation may be necessary. In contrast, clostridial myonecrosis involving the trunk may present some very difficult therapeutic decisions because the removal of nonviable tissue may leave the peritoneal or thoracic cavities open and their contents exposed. Temporary coverage with prosthetic materials may be necessary. Trunk infections are therefore associated with a grim prognosis.

Adjunctive Therapy
Hyperbaric Oxygen

The use of hyperbaric oxygen (HBO) in NSTIs is controversial. Although there are no randomized, prospective studies of HBO in these infections, in-vitro data and reviews of clinical series seem to show beneficial effects of HBO when combined with antibiotics and surgical débridement in the management of clostridial infection.[10-15] Hyperbaric oxygen is toxic to clostridia and acts to inhibit bacterial growth, blocks the production of alpha toxin and preserves marginally perfused tissue.[10] Debate also exists about the use of HBO for nonclostridial necrotizing skin and soft tissue infection. In one report, the addition of HBO to the surgical and antimicrobial treatment of nonclostridial necrotizing fasciitis significantly reduced mortality and the need for débridement.[12]

Intravenous Immunoglobulin

Intravenous immunoglobulin (IVIG) has been administered to patients with streptococcal toxic shock syndrome and may be efficacious in the treatment of this toxin-medicated disorder.[16] Recent studies have demonstrated IVIG has some beneficial effect in the treatment of NSTIs, theoretically owing to its neutralization of circulating clostridial toxins and streptococcal superantigens.[17,18] However, in an animal study, addition of IVIG to penicillin and clindamycin did not significantly increase the clearance of bacteria compared with the control group.[16]

IMPORTANT SOFT TISSUE INFECTIONS OF THE HEAD AND NECK

LUDWIG'S ANGINA

In 1836, German physician Wilhelm Frederick von Ludwig described five patients with gangrenous induration of the connective tissues of the neck that progressed rapidly to involve the tissues covering the muscles between the larynx and the floor of the mouth.[19] Ludwig's angina is a potentially life-threatening, rapidly progressive, diffuse "woody" or brawny cellulitis of the submandibular and sublingual spaces that occurs most often in young adults with dental infections.

Pathogenesis

In adults, 52% of cases of Ludwig's angina are caused by dental caries and the disease has a mortality rate of 5% to 10%.[20-22] Submandibular and sublingual spaces freely communicate and, with involvement of the deep cervical fascia, infection may spread rapidly with grave consequences. Extension along the carotid sheath or the retropharyngeal space can cause mediastinitis.[23] Infection is commonly caused by oral cavity anaerobes such as *Fusobacterium*, anaerobic streptococci, *Bacteroides*, spirochetes, and hemolytic *Streptococcus* organisms, although the infection may be mixed with *Staphylococcus* and *Streptococcus* or a combination of aerobic or anaerobic organisms. The presence of anaerobes commonly accounts for the occurrence of gas in the tissues.

Clinical Manifestations

The patient is febrile and complains of severe neck pain and swelling, odynophagia, dysphagia, drooling, and leaning forward to maximize the airway diameter. Patients usually have a recent history of dental work or obviously poor dental hygiene.

Examination may reveal a tender, symmetrical, and indurated swelling, sometimes with palpable crepitus in the submandibular area. The tongue may be swollen or displaced upward and backward and the mouth is held open due to the lingual swelling. The presence of stridor, dyspnea, decreased air movement, or cyanosis suggests airway compromise. The appearance of significant asymmetry of the submandibular area is an ominous sign because it may represent an extension of the inflammation to the parapharyngeal space.

Radiographic views of the teeth may indicate the source of infection, and lateral views of the neck will demonstrate soft tissue swelling around the airway and, possibly, submandibular gas. Computed tomography of the neck may be recommended to determine the extent of inflammation.

The diagnosis of Ludwig's angina is usually made clinically according to four criteria: (1) cellulitis with little or no pus is present in both the submandibular and sublingual spaces; (2) the cellulitis is always bilateral; (3) gangrene is present with serosanguineous, putrid fluid; and (4) the cellulitis is rapidly spreading in the connective tissue, fascia, and muscles, without glandular tissue and lymphatic involvement.[20]

MANAGEMENT

Control of Airway

The progression from the first findings of symptoms to asphyxia may occur rapidly over several minutes to a few hours. Therefore, airway protection is a critical component of the initial management. Stridor, tachypnea, dyspnea, inability to handle secretions, and agitation are all indicative of impending airway loss. In the past, the standard of care for Ludwig's angina was early emergency intubation or tracheostomy to protect the airway. However, this practice has been gradually abandoned. Recent data show that most cases can be managed initially by close observation in a critical care unit and intravenous antibiotics.[21] If an artificial airway is required, then flexible fiberoptic-guided nasotracheal intubation is the preferred method of airway control. Tracheostomy, under local anesthesia and performed through the cellulitis, is still the most widely recommended means of obtaining a surgical airway. The violation of the tissue planes of the neck could hypothetically increase the risk of spreading the infection into the mediastinum.[22,24]

Antibiotics and Other Pharmacotherapy

Clindamycin is the antibiotic of choice for treating Ludwig's angina. Ampicillin-sulbactam, metronidazole and penicillin, imipenem/cilastatin, piperacillin/tazobactam, and cefoxitin are other reasonable choices for treating the obligate anaerobes that are most commonly encountered in this infection. In immunocompromised patients, a broader spectrum of antibiotic coverage against organisms such as facultative gram-negative rods and *S. aureus* (e.g., cefotaxime, ceftizoxime, ticarcillin-clavulanic acid, piperacillin-tazobactam, imipenem, or meropenem) may be required.[25-27]

Corticosteroids have been used empirically to treat airway edema. The value of corticosteroids in the setting of Ludwig's angina is unclear, and they probably are not indicated.[28]

Surgical Intervention

Surgical débridement may only moderately improve the airway. Surgical incision and drainage was the therapy of choice in the preantibiotic era. Unless antibiotic therapy is significantly delayed, it is unlikely that pus will be identified because pus collections develop relatively late. With the exception of dental extractions, surgery is reserved for those patients who do not respond to medical therapy and those with crepitus and purulent collections.[29-31] For the most part, the location of abscesses should be identified using computed tomography or magnetic resonance imaging. Any patient requiring surgical intervention should have an artificial airway in place before neck exploration.

ACUTE EPIGLOTTITIS

Acute epiglottitis is a potentially life-threatening bacterial infection causing inflammation and edema of the epiglottis, aryepiglottic folds, and surrounding tissues. Before the era of *Haemophilus influenzae* vaccine, epiglottitis used to be a primarily pediatric infection. However, in recent years, the incidence of adult epiglottitis has been on the rise. It is not clear so far if this increase in adult acute epiglottitis is due to increased recognition or to prevalence.[32-34] With the widespread use of the *H. influenzae* B (HIB) vaccine, the prevalence of HIB decreased from 23.8 cases per 100,000 in 1991 to 0.92 cases per 100,000 in 1996. However, in the past 4 years, its prevalence has started rising again nationwide to 1.88 cases per 100,000 in 2001 and 2.81 cases per 100,000 in 2002.[35]

Pathogenesis

Invading bacteria cause inflammation and edema of the epiglottis, aryepiglottic fold, and surrounding tissues. These structures then may protrude downward and over the glottic opening, causing airway obstruction. In the past, most of the cases (50% to 70%) were caused by HIB.[36] However, at the present time, other bacteria including group A beta-hemolytic *Streptococcus, Staphylococcus aureus,* and *Streptococcus pneumoniae* have become more common.

Clinical Manifestations and Management

Early signs of epiglottitis include hoarseness, dysphagia, odynophagia, and a sore throat. Some authors advocate direct or indirect laryngoscopy on adult patients without respiratory distress; it is safe to perform such procedures in the operating room or ICU where both the equipment and personnel required for emergency intubation are at hand. The most common misdiagnosis is streptococcal pharyngitis. Patients who can maintain their airway and adequate oxygenation should be closely observed in an ICU where definitive airway management can be achieved in a controlled fashion. Dyspnea and stridor indicate impending airway obstruction and emergency airway control should be established. Flexible fiberoptic laryngoscopy is usually used during intubation because it provides direct visualization of the airway while serving as a guide for intubation.

The third-generation cephalosporins cefotaxime and ceftriaxone are the antibiotics of choice for acute epiglottitis. These antibiotics are usually effective against *H. influenzae*, streptococci, and staphylococci. A number of other antibiotics, including cefuroxime, ampicillin-sulbactam, piperacillin-tazobactam, ticarcillin-clavulanic acid, levofloxacin, and chloramphenicol, are also effective in epiglottitis. Whereas they are at times used empirically, the role of corticosteroids and racemic epinephrine is unresolved and the doses used have been arbitrary.[32-34]

INFECTIONS OF BITE WOUNDS

It is estimated that 4.7 million dog bites, 400,000 cat bites, and 250,000 human bites occur in the United States annually. In addition to bites, exposure to mouth flora can also occur in what is described as clenched-fist injuries, finger or thumb sucking, and "love nips." The incidence of infection after cat bites can be more than 50%, and infection after dog or human bite wounds can be 15% to 20%. Wild animal bites also are a potential source of serious infection. Although the majority of patients with bite wounds do not seek medical attention, some bite wounds can become disasters, leading to severe infections and sepsis that result in loss of limb function or even require amputation.[37] There are four types of bite wounds: scratches, punctures, lacerations, and avulsions. Although many of these wounds may look innocuous initially, they may lead to serious infections

(i.e., NSTIs) and sepsis. Complications also include lymphangitis, septic arthritis, tenosynovitis, and osteomyelitis. In immunocompromised individuals, such systemic infections as endocarditis, meningitis, and brain abscess can occur.[38,39]

PATHOGENESIS

The microbiology of bite wounds generally is polymicrobial, reflecting the aerobic and anaerobic microbiology of the oral flora of the biter and the skin of the victim, as well as the environment.

Soft tissue infections caused by human mouth flora are usually due to a mixture of pathogens. It has been reported that the human mouth hosts 42 different species of bacterial flora, of which aerobes (*Eikenella corrodens, Staphylococcus, Streptococcus,* and *Corynebacterium* species) are the common isolates from infected bite wounds.[40] Commonly isolated anaerobes include *Bacteroides* and *Peptostreptococcus* species. *E. corrodens* is a slow-growing, gram-negative bacillus frequently associated with chronic infection and abscess formation in human bites.

As in human bites, polymicrobial infections are frequently encountered in animal bites. Whereas almost any oral flora isolate is a potential pathogen, *Pasteurella multocida* is the most prevalent organism found among isolates from dog bite wounds (20% to 50%) and is also a common pathogen in cat bite wound infections.[41,42] *Staphylococcus aureus*, alpha-, beta-, and delta-hemolytic streptococci, gram-negative organisms, and anaerobic microorganisms that are usually part of the normal mouth flora of animals also have all been isolated.[41]

MANAGEMENT

The goals of management of bite wounds are to prevent or appropriately treat infection and to minimize the soft tissue deformity. For domestic animal bites, unless the animal is suspected of having rabies, rabies prophylaxis is not necessary. Many wild animals, including skunks, raccoons, foxes, and bats, should be considered rabid unless proved otherwise, and a bite by such an animal should result in rabies prophylaxis. Tetanus immunization status must also be determined, and, if not up to date, tetanus toxoid should be administered. Tetanus immune globulin should also be considered for those victims whose last tetanus booster was more than 10 years before the bite injury. Radiography is indicated if there are any concerns that deep structures are at risk. These include hand wounds, deep punctures, and crushing bites, especially those over joints.

Meticulous wound care is the cornerstone of human or animal bite wound management. Copious irrigation of the wound decreases the incidence of wound infection. Careful débridement of devitalized tissue, particulate matter, and clot is also necessary to reduce the infection risk and to improve the cosmetic result. Puncture wounds and dog bite injuries of the hand should not be closely primarily. Other wounds with extensive crush injuries or those requiring extensive débridement can be approximated and be closed by delayed primary or secondary intention.

Cultures of clinically uninfected wounds are not indicated. However, it is recommended that cultures be performed in infected wounds that are not improving despite apparently adequate antibiotic treatment.[41,43] In human or animal bite victims, prophylactic broad-spectrum antibiotics are recommended for patients with high-risk bites. These high-risk factors for infection include wounds of the hand, foot, face, scalp, and perineum, puncture wounds, crush wounds that cannot be débrided, bites over vital structures (artery, nerve, or joint), patient age older than 50 years, or patients who are immunosuppressed.[43] In most patients, amoxicillin-clavulanic acid is the preferred antibiotic. Alternatives include moxifloxacin, gatifloxacin, amoxicillin, doxycycline, and cefuroxime.[43] In human bites, amoxicillin-clavulanic acid will cover *E. corrodens* and most other oral flora and is the recommended antibiotic. Other options include second- or third-generation cephalosporins, quinolones, or doxycycline. In patients who are allergic to penicillin, trimethoprim-sulfamethoxazole is an alternative for both dog and cat bites, whereas quinolones or erythromycin may be used for human bites.

Patients who require inpatient care for complex wounds, systemic toxicity, established infection, or suspicion of musculoskeletal, neurologic, or vascular involvement or patients who are at very high risk of invasive infection (e.g., immunosuppression) should be treated with parenteral antibiotics. In these patients, wound and drainage cultures should be obtained. Ampicillin-sulbactam and ticarcillin-clavulanic acid are the preferred antibiotics. Cefoxitin and quinolones are alternatives. However, antibiotic therapy is generally not sufficient, by itself, to produce the best results. In addition to antibiotic therapy, the wound must be cleansed with an antibacterial agent such as povidone-iodine, débrided of all necrotic tissue, and irrigated vigorously. Data have shown that wound irrigation, débridement, and antibiotics provided better results than débridement alone.[44,45] Management of cellulitis, fasciitis, or myonecrosis secondary to bite wound infections is the same as for those same disorders of other etiology. Consultation with a hand surgeon should be considered in those with hand wounds, because the risk of infection of bite wounds on a hand is higher than other sites.[46]

INFECTIONS OF BURN WOUNDS

Burn wound infection/sepsis is one of the most common causes of death in burn patients.[47] It is estimated that more than 100,000 of the 2.5 million burned patients in the United States require hospital admission and 12,000 patients die per year.[48] The highest risk of bacterial invasion from skin flora into the eschar occurs 5 to 7 days after burn. Mechanisms of burn wound infection include the breakdown of the natural cutaneous barrier, compromised host defenses, and exposure to pathogenic and opportunistic bacteria. The surface of a burn, which contains a large amount of necrotic tissue and protein-rich wound exudate, provides an excellent growth medium for surface bacteria leading to bacterial colonization and invasion. Burns are also associated with an immunocompromised status. The percentage of total body surface area (TBSA) burned and the duration of hospitalization correlate well with the incidence of wound infections.[49,50] The predisposing factors for the development of a burn wound infection are listed in Table 152-3.

PATHOGENESIS

After thermal injury, all burn wounds become contaminated with microorganisms, either from the patient's endogenous flora or from the resident microorganisms in the burn unit. This colonization is initially without clinical significance.

TABLE 152–3. PREDISPOSING FACTORS FOR BURN WOUND INFECTIONS

Burn wound greater than 30% total body surface area
Full-thickness burn
Extremes in patient age
Preexisting diseases: immunosuppression, diabetes mellitus, vascular insufficiency
Virulence and antibiotic resistance of colonizing pathogens
Failure of skin graft
Prolonged open burn wound
Improper initial burn wound care

However, surface-colonizing bacteria can penetrate the avascular eschar and proliferate beneath the eschar at the viable-nonviable tissue interface. When the host defense mechanisms are compromised, these bacteria can break this barrier and spread systemically, resulting in bacteremia and the sepsis syndrome.

The most common organisms found in burn wound infections are bacteria, and 70% to 90% are endogenous to the patient. The remainder is acquired by cross-infection, principally from the hands of health care professionals. Before the era of penicillin, streptococci and staphylococci were the predominant pathogens. Since the 1950s, *P. aeruginosa* has become the most important species.[51,52] Other important bacterial species include *S. aureus*, group A *Streptococcus*, *Enterobacter cloacae*, *Enterococcus faecalis*, and *Klebsiella* species.[51] Recently, *Acinetobacter* species are emerging as a significant pathogen in burn units.[53] Fungi, especially *Candida albicans* and *Aspergillus* species, and viruses (herpesvirus) are also pathogens that can be isolated from infected burn wounds.[54,55]

CLINICAL MANIFESTATIONS AND DIAGNOSIS

Successful treatment of burn wound infections and sepsis largely depends on early detection of infection. Burn wound infection is difficult to diagnose on the basis of clinical signs and symptoms, because burn-induced inflammatory responses (e.g., fever, leukocytosis) are indistinguishable from those of infection. The local signs of infection may be absent, minimal, or late. Diagnosis is generally based on a combination of clinical signs that indicate sepsis syndrome (e.g., fever, leukocytosis, organ dysfunction, hyperdynamic state) and the results of surveillance cultures. Any of the findings listed in Table 152-4 should raise a suspicion of burn wound infection.

The practice of culturing the burn wound surface does not accurately predict progressive bacterial colonization or incipient burn wound sepsis. Qualitative and quantitative correlations are poor between flora on the surface of the

TABLE 152–4. CLINICAL SIGNS SUGGESTIVE OF BURN WOUND INFECTION

Progression of second-degree to third-degree burn injury
Discoloration:
   Wound: red, brown or black
   Subcutaneous fat: green
   Wound margins: erythematous or violaceous
   Subeschar fat: hemorrhagic
Unexpected rapid eschar separation
Metastatic septic lesion in unburned tissue

burn wound and bacterial colonization and invasion of the deep layers of the eschar. It has been reported that biopsy of the wound with quantitative culture is an accurate indicator of invasive burn would infection.[56] On histologic examination, evidence of microvascular invasion connotes hematogenous dissemination of organisms. Studies showed that quantitative cultures of 10^5 CFU/gram of tissue, a 100-fold increase in concentration of organisms/gram of tissue within a 48-hour period, or histologic evidence of bacterial invasion of viable tissue correlate with a high (75%) mortality rate.[57,58] In recent years, real-time detection polymerase chain reaction (RTD-PCR) has been shown to be a good tool for rapid quantitative detection of pathogens in burn wound infection.[59] The application of these techniques provides early diagnosis as well as the identity of the organism and its sensitivity to antimicrobials.[59] It is important to differentiate bacterial colonization of dead tissue and invasion of viable tissue; the latter can be diagnosed by the histologic finding of organisms in viable subeschar tissue. When bacterial invasion to viable tissue is detected, excision of the infected wound is important and systemic antibiotics are mandated.

MANAGEMENT

Prevention of Burn Wound Infections

Although it was previously documented that manipulation of the burn wound leads to hematogenous spread and organ seeding of bacteria and, therefore, antibiotics were administered immediately before and during burn wound excision, more recent data suggest a lesser incidence of burn wound manipulation-induced bacteremia than reported in prior series.[60,61] Therefore, systemic antibiotic prophylaxis is not routinely administered to burn patients admitted to the hospital.

Frequent wound dressing changes with evaluation of the burn wound and surrounding tissue allows for early detection and therapy of cellulitis. In many burn units in the United States, early excision and grafting of burn wounds has become the standard of care. Early excision is defined as the staged excision of all deep partial- and full-thickness burns by the third to seventh post-burn day. The philosophy of early burn wound excision has resulted in improved survival in patients with TBSA burns greater than 30% to 40%, shorter hospital length of stay, lower costs of hospital care, and fewer painful dressing changes. If for some reason, such as hemodynamic instability or severe respiratory failure, the patient cannot undergo early excision and coverage, surveillance wound cultures should be performed several times per week to diagnose burn wound infection early. In addition, strict antiseptic measures, such as hand washing, barrier isolation, and equipment and room cleaning, decrease the incidence of wound infection.[62]

Topical antimicrobials are commonly used in burn patients. Their use has substantially decreased the incidence of conversion of partial-thickness to full-thickness wounds by local infection, and thereby has reduced mortality associated with burn wound infection. In addition, these agents may prolong the sterility of the full-thickness burn wound. However, they have not eliminated the need for aggressive removal of the necrotic tissue and closure of the wound with autografts. The commonly used topical agents are listed in Table 152-5. According to an international survey, silver sulfadiazine is the topical agent of choice for partial- to full-thickness burn wounds.[63]

TREATMENT OF BURN WOUND INFECTIONS

Antibiotics

As mentioned earlier, systemic antibiotics are not used prophylactically. Instead, they should be reserved for use in cases of known or suspected invasive infection. As long as bacterial culture results are available, antibiotics with the narrowest spectrum of activity should be used to minimize the development of resistant organisms. Currently there is no consensus on optimal antibiotic regimen for patients who require initiation of empirical antibiotic therapy before culture and sensitivity results have returned. Recommendations for empirical therapy are based on the length of time since the burn was sustained, previous administration of antibiotics to the patient, and the likely pathogens. Knowledge of the bacterial pathogens and antibiogram specific to the medical center is important. Combination of multiple antibiotics for a single infection is only used when bacteremia persists in the face of therapeutic doses of a single antibiotic.

TABLE 152–5. COMMONLY USED TOPICAL AGENTS IN BURN WOUNDS

Agent	Advantage	Dose	Precaution
Silver sulfadiazine	Useful in prevention of infections from second- or third-degree burns. Bactericidal activity against many gram-positive and negative bacteria; also effective against yeast.	Apply to open wounds twice or three times daily.	Does not penetrate eschar. Neutropenia. Caution in glucose-6-phosphate dehydrogenase deficiency.
Mafenide acetate cream	Topical. Diffuses freely into the eschar and is highly effective against gram-negative organisms, including *Pseudomonas* species.	Apply cream to open wounds twice or three times daily.	Pain/burning may occur. Metabolic acidosis due to inhibition of carbonic anhydrase.
Silver nitrate (0.5%)	Silver ion has broad-spectrum antibacterial activity but does not penetrate burn wound eschar; therefore, it is most effective when applied early.	Apply topically to wound to a thickness of approximately 1.5 mm daily or twice daily as moistened dressings.	Not for internal use. Stains wound and everything else. Does not penetrate eschar. Hyponatremia.
Mupirocin	Active against a wide variety of gram-positive bacteria, including methicillin-resistant *Staphylococcus aureus*. Also active against certain gram-negative bacteria. Exerts activity by binding to bacterial isoleucyl transfer RNA-synthetase.	Apply to affected areas three times a day and cover with gauze dressing.	Prolonged use may result in growth of resistant organisms; do not use on very large wounds where polyethylene glycol absorption is possible (especially in patients with moderate renal failure).

Inappropriate use of multiple antibiotics does not decrease mortality. Instead, it promotes overgrowth of resistant pathogens such as *Candida* species, enterococci, and multiple antibiotic-resistant species.

Surgical Intervention

Invasive bacterial or fungal burn wound infections are treated with surgical excision to the level of viable tissue. Recent data showed that early burn wound excision significantly reduces bacterial colonization and reduces the risk of invasive burn wound infection. Patients who undergo topical treatment and delayed burn wound excision exhibit greater bacterial colonization and increased rates of infection.[64] Wounds that can be excised completely should be covered with an allograft or autograft. If complete débridement is not possible, topical antimicrobials should be applied and the wound should be reexamined within 24 hours for possible repeat débridement.

INFECTIONS OF PRESSURE ULCERS

Pressure ulcers are caused by localized tissue necrosis and infection due to prolonged compression between a bony prominence and an external surface. Pressure ulcers in ICU patients occur primarily in patients with impaired mobility due to injury, weakness, sedation, or use of paralytic agents. Pressure ulcers result in significant morbidity in critically ill patients. Studies have shown that the incidence of pressure ulcers is increasing in critically ill patients.[65] Emergency ICU admission and ICU length of stay more than 7 days in elderly patients confer significant risk for the development of decubitus ulcers.[66,67] Although infection of decubitus ulcers is high in the nursing home setting or in spinal cord injury patients, it is an uncommon cause of infection or sepsis in ICU patients.[68-70] Pressure ulcers may pose a risk to other hospitalized patients by serving as a reservoir for resistant organisms such as methicillin-resistant *S. aureus*, vancomycin-resistant enterococci, and multiply-resistant gram-negative bacilli.[71]

PATHOGENESIS AND CLASSIFICATION

The risk factors for pressure ulcers in patients in ICUs are essentially the same as for those on a general hospital floor. They include limited physical activity, impaired sensory perception, poor nutritional status, chronic disorders (e.g., diabetes mellitus, cardiovascular disease, and cerebrovascular accident), fever, impaired circulation, low serum hemoglobin concentration, and increased blood urea nitrogen and serum creatinine concentrations.[65] Also, a number of infectious complications have been implicated in the development of pressure ulcers. In order of frequency, these are local infection, cellulitis of surrounding tissue, contiguous osteomyelitis, and bacteremia.[69]

Three different classification systems have been developed to describe the extent of pressure ulcers. Table 152-6 shows the most commonly used system promulgated by the National Pressure Ulcer Advisory Panel. Other systems, such as those proposed by Shea and Yarkony/Kirk, are similar.[72]

Infections of pressure ulcers are usually polymicrobial. Aerobes that are commonly recovered include staphylococci, enterococci, *Proteus mirabilis*, *E. coli*, and *Pseudomonas* species. Anaerobic *Peptostreptococcus*, *Bacteroides fragilis*, and *Clostridium* species are also found in these infections. Methicillin-resistant *S. aureus* has also become a prominent organism found in decubitus ulcers.[71,73] Pressure ulcers are a major reservoir of methicillin-resistant *S. aureus*. Making an accurate microbiologic diagnosis is usually impractical and difficult, because all pressure ulcers are colonized with microorganisms and a superficial culture will not distinguish between colonizing and infecting organisms. If it is necessary to determine the microbiology accurately, it is more appropriate to direct a needle through intact skin and aspirate a specimen for bacterial culture from the margin of the ulcer.[69]

MANAGEMENT

There are many different approaches to the treatment of these chronic wounds. However, none has been shown to be more effective than any other. Measures to prevent development of decubitus ulcers, including pressure relief and appropriate nutrition, are probably the best means of preventing infection in the ulcers. Once the ulcer has been established and infection is present, débridement of necrotic and marginally viable tissue is absolutely necessary to obtain healing. Topical agents, such as povidone-iodine, hydrogen peroxide, and others, have been widely used, but there is no difference in terms of outcome among these agents. Proper use of occlusive dressings increases patient comfort, enhances healing, decreases the possibility of infection, saves time, and reduces costs. Topical antimicrobial agents have not been shown to be effective. Systemic antibiotic therapy should be reserved for infected ulcers. Skin grafting of clean wounds, if the underlying cause of the pressure ulcer has been removed, is an accepted method of treating these chronic wounds, and it has been shown to be effective.

Staging	Description
TABLE 152–6. NATIONAL PRESSURE ULCER ADVISORY PANEL CLASSIFICATION OF PRESSURE ULCERS	
I	Observable pressure-related alteration of intact skin with one or more of the following changes: skin temperature (warmth or coolness); tissue consistency (firm or boggy feel); or sensation (pain, itching). Defined area of persistent redness (in lightly pigmented skin) or red, blue, or purple hues (in darker skin tones).
II	Partial-thickness skin loss involving epidermis and/or dermis. The ulcer is superficial and presents clinically as an abrasion, blister, or shallow crater.
III	Full-thickness skin loss involving damage or necrosis of subcutaneous tissue that may extend down to, but not through, underlying fascia. The ulcer presents clinically as a deep crater with or without undermining of adjacent tissue.
IV	Full-thickness skin loss with extensive destruction, tissue necrosis, or damage to muscle, bone, or supporting structures (e.g., tendon, joint capsule).

However, adequate treatment frequently requires much more complex therapies, including tissue flaps and, sometimes, even amputation to effect wound closure. The treatment of recalcitrant wounds can be difficult and costly. Currently, several new therapeutic strategies are under review, such as alginates, a variety of wound dressings, growth factor therapies (platelet-derived growth factor, fibroblast growth factor, transforming growth factor, recombinant human growth hormone, or insulin-like growth factor-1), tissue-engineered skin substitutes, and autologous outer root sheath cells that lead to wound closure.[74-76]

A variety of empirical antibiotic regimens have been suggested for patients with pressure ulcer-associated cellulitis, osteomyelitis, or bacteremia. In general, any regimen that is active against the majority of organisms that are usually causal is appropriate. Although advanced inanition is the most common cause of failure of these lesions to heal, osteomyelitis needs to be ruled out by physical examination and radiograph. If osteomyelitis is present, it requires a more extended course of therapy and, frequently, amputation.

Mechanical therapies aimed at healing decubitus ulcers must include removal of all necrotic tissue and some strategy to relieve the pressure that caused the ulcer. Once the dead tissue has been débrided, the ulcer may be covered with a moist dressing or with one of the new skin substitutes such as Apligraf or Granuflex hydrocolloid dressing or human skin equivalent (HSE).[75,76] Studies have shown that these dressings are more cost-effective in treating pressure ulcers.[75,76] However, before any such local therapy is chosen, it is very important that any infection be controlled and that the patient is in good nutritional balance.

ANNOTATED REFERENCES

Brook I: Microbiology and management of human and animal bite wound infections. Prim Care 2003;30:25-39.

> This article reviewed 79 publications on bite wound infections and described the microbiology, diagnosis, and management of human and animal bite wound infections. The authors pointed out that hand wounds present a special problem, because 30% or more become infected.

Cumming J, Purdue GF, Hunt JL, et al: Objective estimates of the incidence and consequences of multiple organ dysfunction and sepsis after burn trauma. J Trauma 2001;50:510-515.

> In this prospective study, a total of 85 patients with 20% total body surface area burns admitted to a single center were prospectively enrolled over 1 year. The study revealed that severe multiple organ dysfunction and severe sepsis/septic shock are both related to burn size, age, and male sex and to the length of ICU stay and duration of ventilatory support.

Eachempati SR, Hydo LJ, Barie PS: Factors influencing the development of decubitus ulcers in critically ill surgical patients. Crit Care Med 2001;29:1678-1682.

> This prospective study analyzed surgical ICU patients who developed decubitus ulcers and compared different factors in the development of decubitus ulcers in surgical ICU patients. The authors concluded that early nutrition, early mobilization, and possibly less noxious bedding surfaces may decrease the incidence of decubitus ulcers.

Elliot D, Kufera JA, Myers RA: The microbiology of necrotizing soft tissue infections. Am J Surg 2000;179:361-366.

> This retrospective study reviewed charts of 182 patients with NSTIs in a 100-bed level I trauma center. The authors reported that NSTIs are frequently polymicrobial, and the most common organisms are, in order, Bacteroides species, Escherichia coli, and other gram-negative rods.

Wang C, Schwaitzberg S, Berliner E, et al: Hyperbaric oxygen for treating wounds: A systematic review of the literature. Arch Surg 2003;138:272-279.

> This is a meta-analysis of the use of HBO for wound care and clinical outcomes on 57 studies, including randomized controlled trials, cohorts, and case series that reported original data. The studies suggest that HBO may be helpful as an adjunctive therapy for gas gangrene, chronic non-healing diabetic wounds, compromised skin grafts, osteoradionecrosis, and soft tissue radionecrosis, but there is insufficient evidence to determine the timing for HBO and whether patients will benefit.

Chapter 153

HEAD AND NECK INFECTIONS

Jeremy D. Gradon

KEY POINTS

SITES OF DEEP HEAD AND NECK INFECTION

1. **Normal oral flora** consists of mixed bacteria, primarily anaerobes.

2. **Oral fibronectin production** is decreased in the oral cavity of critically ill patients, allowing oral colonization with gram-negative organisms in this population.

3. **Deep neck infections** may occur in the submandibular, lateral pharyngeal, and retropharyngeal spaces.

4. **Internal jugular vein septic thrombophlebitis (Lemierre's syndrome)** is an anaerobe infection of the internal jugular vein caused by *Fusobacterium necrophorum*.

CLINICAL SYNDROMES

1. **Sinusitis** can be complicated by local invasion including brain abscess, meningitis, cavernous sinus thrombosis, and local osteomyelitis.

2. **Fungal sinusitis** may be caused by *Mucor*, which can complicate diabetic ketoacidosis, corticosteroid treatment, neutropenia, and desferrioxamine administration.

3. **Quinsy (peritonsillar abscess)** can be complicated by spread into the lateral pharyngeal space.

4. **Epiglottitis** is suspected when a patient is drooling saliva, sitting forward, and breathing "apprehensively."

5. **Diphtheria** can present as cranial nerve palsies, myocarditis, or respiratory obstruction.

6. **Retropharyngeal space infection** may be complicated by mediastinal infection via spread through potential tissue spaces (the "danger space").

7. **Ludwig's angina (submandibular space infection)** is "woody" induration of the submandibular space that may be complicated by airway obstruction due to posterior and upward displacement of the tongue.

8. **Lateral pharyngeal space infection** needs differentiation of whether the anterior or posterior spaces are involved (see text).

9. **Lemierre's syndrome** is classically complicated by the development of septic pulmonary emboli and septic arthritis.

Infections of the head and neck range in severity from minor to life threatening. The intensivist is called on to manage such patients either when they are critically ill or when airway compromise has occurred or is imminent. Besides airway management and control of sepsis, the intensivist must also be aware of the local anatomy and relevant microbiology. This knowledge will both help guide the choice of antimicrobial agents as well as allow the clinician to anticipate the potential for spread of infection to related anatomic spaces and subsequent complications thereof.

NORMAL HEAD AND NECK FLORA

Huge numbers of bacteria are resident in the oral cavity in health, with the bacterial load exceeding 10^{11}/mL in the gingival crevices of patients with teeth.[1] The main bacterial species are anaerobes, including *Bacteroides*, *Fusobacterium*, *Prevotella*, and *Peptostreptococcus*. Other common oral inhabitants include *Streptococcus mutans*, *Staphylococcus aureus*, *Actinomyces* species, and *Eikenella corrodens*. Pharyngeal colonization and subsequent infection with organisms such as *Streptococcus pneumoniae*, *Neisseria meningitidis*, and *Streptococcus pyogenes* may also occur.

In acute illness an additional modifying factor is the decreased production of oral mucosal fibronectin. This is of relevance to the clinician because fibronectin in normal physiologic amounts will preferentially bind gram-positive bacteria (such as *S. mutans*); however, when its production is decreased, there is rapid colonization of the oral cavity with gram-negative organisms, including species such as *Pseudomonas aeruginosa*.[2] These gram-negative organisms may then participate in head and neck infections of oral or odontogenic origin necessitating broad nosocomial type gram-negative antibiotic coverage when the patient has been recently hospitalized or acquired the infection in the ICU.[3]

TABLE 153–1. DIFFERENTIATING FEATURES OF DEEP NECK INFECTIONS

Space	Clinical Features*
Submandibular space (Ludwig's angina)	Woody submental induration, protruding swollen/necrotic tongue, no trismus, rotted lower molars commonly present
Lateral pharyngeal space	
Anterior	Fever, toxicity, trismus, neck swelling
Posterior	No trismus, no swelling (unless ipsilateral parotid is involved), cranial nerve IX-XII palsies, Horner's syndrome, carotid artery erosion
Retropharyngeal space	
Retropharynx	Neck stiffness, decreased neck range of motion, soft tissue bulging of posterior pharyngeal wall, sore throat, dysphagia, dyspnea
Danger space	Mediastinal or pleural involvement
Prevertebral	Neck stiffness, decreased neck range of motion, cervical instability, possible spread along length of vertebral column
Jugular vein septic thrombophlebitis (Lemierre's syndrome)	Sore throat, swollen, tender neck, dyspnea, chest pain, septic arthritis

*Fever and signs of systemic toxicity are common to all.

SITES OF DEEP HEAD AND NECK INFECTION

Serious infection of the head and neck can involve the following general anatomic areas[4]:

- Sinus
- Pharynx
- Epiglottis
- Retropharyngeal space and the "danger space"
- Submandibular space (Ludwig's angina)
- Lateral pharyngeal space (anterior and posterior)
- Internal jugular vein (Lemierre's syndrome)

Some of these spaces are connected via actual or potential spaces. Thus, infection beginning in one space may spread rapidly to involve others, with the potential resultant damage or destruction of vital structures. Such connections are discussed in this chapter, and differentiating features are highlighted in Table 153-1.

CLINICAL SYNDROMES

SINUSITIS

Acute bacterial sinusitis accounts for a high proportion of physician visits in the primary care setting.[5] In the ICU, patients who are critically ill with nasogastric tubes or endotracheal or nasotracheal tubes in place may develop acute sinusitis caused by resistant nosocomial organisms (e.g., methicillin-resistant *S. aureus*, *P. aeruginosa*) and anaerobes.[6] Treatment involves the use of broad-spectrum antimicrobial agents (Table 153-2) and close collaboration with an otolaryngologist to determine if drainage is needed. In addition, application of topical vasoconstrictors to the nasal mucosa is often recommended to help drain the sinuses.

Complications of nosocomial sinusitis are related to the local anatomy. Spread via the diploic veins can result in meningitis, brain abscess, contiguous osteomyelitis, or cavernous sinus thrombosis. Spread from the ethmoidal sinuses can result in frontal lobe brain abscesses, whereas sphenoidal

TABLE 153–2. THERAPEUTIC OPTIONS FOR SINUSITIS, PHARYNGITIS, AND EPIGLOTTITIS

Syndrome	Likely Flora	Antibiotic Options*
Sinusitis		
Community acquired	*Haemophilus influenzae*, *Streptococcus pneumoniae*, *Staphylococcus aureus*	Ampicillin-sulbactam (3 g i.v. q 6h) Levofloxacin (500 mg i.v. q 24h) Levofloxacin (500 mg i.v. q 24h) plus clindamycin (300 mg to 900 mg i.v. q 8h)
ICU acquired	*Pseudomonas aeruginosa* *Escherichia coli* and related coliforms Methicillin-resistant *S. aureus*	Ceftazidime (2 g i.v. q 8h) or piperacillin-tazobactam (3.375 g i.v. q 4h) plus an aminoglycoside, plus vancomycin (1 g i.v. q 12h)
Fungal	*Aspergillus* species *Mucorales* species	Amphotericin B (1 to 1.5 mg/kg/day i.v.) Liposomal amphotericin B (5 to 10 mg/kg/day i.v.) Caspofungin (70 mg i.v. day 1, then 50 mg/day i.v.) Voriconazole (6 mg/kg q 12h × 2 doses, then 4 mg/kg q 12h)† Itraconazole (200 mg i.v. q 12h × 4 doses, then 200 mg/day i.v.)
Pharyngitis	*Clostridium diphtheriae* Epstein-Barr virus (with airway compromise)	Intravenous penicillin or erythromycin *plus* diphtheria antitoxin No antiviral therapy effective Intravenous corticosteroids
Epiglottitis	*H. influenzae* type b *S. pyogenes* (group A *Streptococcus*)	Ceftriaxone (1 to 2 g i.v. q 24h) Ampicillin-sulbactam (3 g i.v. q 6h) Rifampin prophylaxis (600 mg p.o. q 24h) for close contacts for 4 days

*Antibiotic choices listed are examples, because for most infections multiple different antibiotics are effective and thus individual choice will be influenced by patient factors (e.g., allergies), local hospital bacterial resistance rates, and microbiologic culture results.
†*Note:* Voriconazole is *not* active against mucorales.

sinus infection can spread to involve the surrounding pituitary gland, optic chiasm, internal carotid artery, cavernous sinus, or temporal lobe of the brain.

Rhinocerebral mucormycosis or aspergillosis can develop in hosts with diabetic ketoacidosis, high-dose corticosteroid treatment, severe neutropenia, or history of desferrioxamine treatment. This infection can be rapidly fatal if the underlying problem cannot be corrected. The general teaching has been that high doses of antifungal therapy (see Table 153-2) plus extensive surgery is always required for any hope of survival.[7] However, the need for major surgery in all cases has come into question recently.[8] Close collaboration with appropriate surgeons and infectious diseases colleagues is required in such cases.

PHARYNGEAL INFECTIONS (see Table 153-2)

Life-threatening pharyngeal infections include acute anaerobic pharyngitis (Vincent's angina) caused by a combination of oral anaerobes and spirochetes. The clinical manifestations in the critically ill host include acute ulcerations and necrosis of the oral mucosa and gingiva. Secondary bacteremia with sepsis syndrome can complicate this entity.[9] Treatment involves adequate oral débridement and the administration of antibiotics with both aerobic and anaerobic activity.

Quinsy (peritonsillar abscess) can complicate prior tonsillitis and is most common among young adults.[10] Presenting symptoms include fever, pharyngeal pain, and unilateral pharyngeal swelling. If not adequately drained, the infection can spread into the lateral pharyngeal space, which was the most common cause of mortality due to quinsy in the preantibiotic era.

Diphtheria is rare owing to mass vaccination. It presents as a sharply demarcated adherent dark gray nasal or pharyngeal membrane. Clinical illness is due to release of a bacterial toxin that inhibits translocase (via inhibition of elongation factor 2). Myocardial dysfunction and central nervous system toxin–mediated injury may occur late, but fulminant infections can be complicated by death from acute respiratory obstruction or circulatory failure (bull-neck diphtheria). Culture of the organism (Corynebacterium diphtheriae) requires the use of specific Loeffler medium.

EPIGLOTTITIS

Acute epiglottitis is primarily a disease of children who have not received the Haemophilus influenzae type b vaccine and is thus rare at present.[11] It presents as an acute febrile illness usually of less than 12 hours' duration, with the child characteristically sitting forward, drooling saliva, and taking shallow and apprehensive breaths (because deeper breathing draws the epiglottis over the airway and produces obstruction). The diagnosis is made clinically although lateral neck radiography (if the child is stable enough to go for a radiograph), which shows enlargement of the epiglottis 30% to 57% of the time. Attempts to visualize the characteristic edematous cherry-red epiglottis directly may precipitate acute airway obstruction and should not be attempted unless the ability to secure an airway immediately is certain. Blood and epiglottis cultures usually grow H. influenzae type b.

Antibiotic options are outlined in Table 153-2. There is no clear consensus on the role of exogenous corticosteroids to decrease epiglottic edema. Rifampin prophylaxis should be administered for 4 days to close household and hospital contacts of persons (especially younger than the age of 4 years) with invasive H. influenzae type b disease.

RETROPHARYNGEAL INFECTIONS
(see Table 153-1)

The area situated between the pharynx anteriorly and the vertebrae posteriorly constitutes the retropharyngeal space that begins behind the pharynx and ends at the junction of the cervical and thoracic vertebrae. This anatomic region is subdivided into several distinct anatomic spaces (retropharyngeal, prevertebral, "danger"), some of which may provide the means of spread of infection from the initial retropharyngeal area to distant sites.

Located between the prevertebral space posteriorly and the retropharyngeal space anteriorly is a potential space called the "danger space" that connects the base of the skull with the posterior mediastinum and diaphragm. Infection may spread unimpeded within this space. In addition, infection occurring between the vertebrae and the prevertebral fascia may spread along the length of the vertebral column. For a detailed discussion of anatomic considerations see reference 1.

Infections of the retropharynx occur as:

- Primary infections
- Secondary to extension posteriorly from the pharynx or anteriorly from infected cervical vertebrae
- Via hematogenous spread

Clinically, retropharyngeal infections present as acute fever, systemic toxicity, sore throat, neck stiffness, dysphagia, and dyspnea. Airway obstruction may occur as a consequence of anterior bulging of the pharyngeal wall with supraglottic compression.[12]

Prevertebral infections usually involve the cervical vertebrae and present as neck pain, stiffness, and prevertebral soft tissue swelling.[13] Rarely, instability or destruction of the cervical vertebrae may develop with death due to acute spinal cord compression.[12]

"Danger space" infection is suspected when pleural or mediastinal infection or pain complicates a retropharyngeal infection.[14] Mediastinitis secondary to danger space infection is generally fulminant with pleural extension and a high mortality rate. Rarely, mediastinal infections, such as those that occur after coronary artery bypass graft surgery, may spread upward through the danger space and present in the retropharynx.

The microbiology of retropharyngeal infections is usually mixed aerobic/anaerobic oral bacteria. In the critically ill host with nosocomial infection, colonization of the oropharynx with resistant pathogens will necessitate modification of antimicrobial choice. The imaging techniques needed include plain lateral neck radiographs that will show loss of normal cervical lordosis and thickening of the retrotracheal area (usually < 22 mm) or the prevertebral fascia (usually < 7 mm). Bedside ultrasonography may provide information regarding the presence or absence of drainable collections, but if the patient is stable enough to go to the radiology suite, computed tomography (CT) or magnetic resonance imaging (MRI) provides the best definition studies. Close collaboration with appropriate surgical colleagues is necessary for

TABLE 153–3. THERAPEUTIC OPTIONS FOR DEEP NECK INFECTIONS

Syndrome	Likely Flora	Therapeutic Options*
Submandibular space infection		
Community acquired	Anaerobes, streptococci, *Staphylococcus aureus*	Ampicillin-sulbactam (3 g i.v. q 6h) Ceftriaxone (1 to 2 g i.v. q 24h) plus clindamycin (300 to 900 mg i.v. q 8h) or metronidazole (500 mg i.v. q 6h) Ertapenem (1 g i.v. qd)
Hospital/ICU acquired	*Pseudomonas aeruginosa* Methicillin-resistant *S. aureus* Anaerobes	Imipenem (500 mg i.v. q 6h) or piperacillin-tazobactam (3.375 g i.v. q 4h), plus vancomycin (1 g i.v. q 12h)
Retropharyngeal space infection	Anaerobes, streptococci, *S. aureus*	Ampicillin-sulbactam (3 g i.v. q 6h) Ceftriaxone (1 to 2 g i.v. q 24h) plus clindamycin (300 to 900 mg i.v. q 8h) or metronidazole (500 mg i.v. q 6h) Ertapenem (1 g i.v. qd)
Lateral pharyngeal space infection	Anaerobes, streptococci, *S. aureus*	Ampicillin-sulbactam (3 g i.v. q 6h) Ceftriaxone (1 to 2g i.v. q 24h) plus clindamycin (300 to 900 mg i.v. q 8h) or metronidazole (500 mg i.v. q 6h) Ertapenem (1 g i.v. qd)
Internal jugular vein Septic thrombophlebitis	*Fusobacterium necrophorum*	Metronidazole (500 mg i.v. q 6h) Clindamycin (300 to 900 mg i.v. q 8h) Ampicillin-sulbactam (3 g i.v. q 6h)

*Antibiotic choices listed are examples, because for most infections multiple different antibiotics are effective and thus individual choice will be influenced by patient factors (e.g., allergies), local hospital bacterial resistance rates, and microbiologic culture results.

successful management.[15] Therapy is outlined in Table 153-3. On occasion nonbacterial processes such as Kawasaki disease can mimic retropharyngeal abscesses.[16]

SUBMANDIBULAR SPACE INFECTION (LUDWIG'S ANGINA)

The submandibular space is contained between the mucous membranes of the floor of the mouth superiorly and the muscle and fascia attachments of the hyoid bone inferiorly. The most common route of infection into this space is via infected lower molar teeth, and infection is more frequent in persons with underlying diabetes, neutropenia, or systemic lupus erythematosus.

Clinical presentation is of an acutely ill patient with mouth pain, dysphagia, drooling of saliva, stiff neck, and fever. The submandibular tissues are woody but not fluctuant, and true "drainable" collections are uncommon. The tongue may be swollen and displaced upward against the palate and also protrude out of the mouth. Trismus is not present; however, if the infection spreads to the lateral pharyngeal space, then trismus may occur. Unrecognized lateral pharyngeal space involvement may be complicated by subsequent spread to the retropharyngeal space. Late complications of Ludwig's angina include death from airway obstruction, aspiration pneumonia, carotid artery erosion, and tongue necrosis.[17]

Lateral neck radiographs will demonstrate edema of the submandibular soft tissues. Pockets of gas may be seen if gas-forming organisms are involved. CT is most helpful diagnostically. However, attention must be paid to having qualified staff accompany the patient to the CT scanner in case acute airway obstruction develops. Should airway protection be needed, tracheotomy or cricothyroidotomy is advocated because of the risk of inducing acute airway obstruction with routine "blind" nasal or oral intubation. The infection is commonly polymicrobial, and appropriate antibiotic therapy options are described in Table 153-3.

In approximately 50% of cases, surgical drainage is required. In addition, causative rotted molar teeth (if present) should be removed.[18]

LATERAL PHARYNGEAL SPACE INFECTIONS

Infection of the lateral pharyngeal space is one of the most common deep neck infections encountered. In a review of 110 deep neck infections in adults seen at an academic medical center over a 10-year period, infections of the lateral pharyngeal space accounted for 55%.[19] In contrast, in children such infections are rare, with peritonsillar infection (quinsy) being the most common deep neck infection.

The lateral pharyngeal space is cone shaped, extending from the sphenoid bone down to the hyoid bone. Posteriorly it is bound by the prevertebral fascia (that separates it from the retropharyngeal space) and anteriorly by the buccinator and superior constrictor muscles. The parotid gland communicates with this space. The styloid process divides the space into an anterior compartment (containing fat, lymph nodes, and muscle) and a posterior compartment (containing the carotid artery, cranial nerves IX to XII, and the cervical sympathetic trunk).

Common precipitating causes of infection include dental disease (33%), injection drug use (inserting needles directly into the space) (20%), local trauma (9%), and tonsillitis (4%). Patients frequently have underlying diabetes or human immunodeficiency virus infection.

Clinically, anterior lateral pharyngeal space infections present as fever, pain, trismus, and systemic toxicity. Turning the head to the opposite side causes increased pain owing to stretching of the ipsilateral sternocleidomastoid muscle.

Infection of the posterior lateral pharyngeal space presents as fever, systemic toxicity, and parotid swelling. Trismus and external swelling do not occur. Involvement of local vital structures can occur, including carotid artery erosion or clot, septic thrombophlebitis of the internal jugular vein, cranial nerve IX to XII palsies, or Horner's syndrome.

Therapy involves urgent surgical intervention to drain infection and prevent spread of infection to the retropharyngeal space or erosion of the carotid artery. The choice of antibiotics for this frequently polymicrobial infection is shown in Table 153-3.

INTERNAL JUGULAR VEIN SEPTIC THROMBOPHLEBITIS (LEMIERRE'S SYNDROME)

Septic thrombophlebitis of the internal jugular vein is known as Lemierre's syndrome. It is a relatively rare entity usually caused by infection with the anaerobe *Fusobacterium necrophorum*, a normal inhabitant of the human gingival crevice.

Latest theories on the pathogenesis of this infection indicate that the first stage of infection is pharyngitis in approximately 87% of cases. This is then followed by invasion of the lateral pharyngeal space with the development of septic thrombophlebitis of the internal jugular vein. Subsequent to this, bloodborne infection develops with the classic findings of septic pulmonary emboli or cavitating pneumonia and septic arthritis.[20] Other precipitating factors include mastoiditis, lateral pharyngeal space infection, or trauma to the internal jugular vein.

Clinically, the syndrome begins with fever and sore throat. When internal jugular vein involvement develops, the patients complain of a swollen and/or tender neck, which is thus a warning sign of danger in a patient with recent pharyngitis. Dyspnea and pleuritic chest pain indicate pulmonary involvement.

Early diagnosis is critical to minimize the risk of infectious metastatic complications requiring surgical intervention or drainage. Blood cultures should be promptly obtained and empirical anti-anaerobic bacterial coverage begun. Radiologic diagnosis is made most reliably by CT, although bedside ultrasound examination of the internal jugular vein can be useful in the critically ill patient who cannot leave the ICU. If the infection occurred secondary to mastoiditis it is necessary to rule out intracerebral vein thrombosis by MRI.

Antibiotic choices are outlined in Table 153-3. There are no firm data to support or refute the use of anticoagulants in Lemierre's syndrome.[21] In addition, surgical ligation or excision of the internal jugular vein for uncontrollable sepsis was necessary in approximately 8% of cases in a recently published series.[20]

CONCLUSION

The intensivist will frequently be asked to assist in the care of patients with serious deep neck infections. The critical issues encountered include protection of the airway, sepsis management, and the potential for erosion of the infection into surrounding vital structures in the neck. Such infections are frequently polymicrobial, and thus broad-spectrum antibiotics with both aerobic and anaerobic coverage should be chosen.

Common critical issues to be decided for each patient individually include:

- Safety of performing an intraoral examination for fear of precipitating acute airway obstruction
- Safety of sending a patient out of the ICU for studies such as CT; although patients may appear stable initially, they are at risk for the sudden development of acute airway obstruction and thus should always be accompanied by a team capable of securing an airway when they travel out of the ICU for tests or procedures.
- Need for timing of possible surgical intervention: early close collaboration with otolaryngologists, head and neck surgeons, neurosurgeons, or vascular surgeons is critical for successful management of these complex and frequently critically ill patients

ANNOTATED REFERENCES

Chirinos JA, Lichstein DM, Gracia J, Tamariz LJ: The evolution of Lemierre syndrome. Medicine (Baltimore) 2002;81:458-465.

A detailed discussion of the latest thoughts on the pathophysiology of Lemierre syndrome indicating that it usually follows acute pharyngitis. The controversy regarding the need for anticoagulation is also discussed.

Chow AW: Infections of the oral cavity, neck and head. In Mandell GL, Bennet JE, Dolin R (eds): Principles and Practice of Infectious Diseases, 5th ed. New York, Churchill-Livingstone, 2000, pp 689-703.

A comprehensive review of the microbiology and anatomy of head and neck infections. Excellent diagrams of the relevant anatomy are included. In addition, a helpful explanation of how the deep neck spaces are interconnected is given explaining how infection of one space can spread to involve another.

Gradon JD: Space-occupying and life-threatening infections of the head, neck and thorax. Infect Dis Clin North Am 1996;10:857-878.

Extensive clinical descriptions of these infections. Numerous illustrative clinical photographs are included in the text.

Har-El G, Aroesty JH, Shaha A, et al: Changing trends in deep neck abscess: A retrospective study of 110 patients. Oral Surg Oral Med Oral Pathol Oral Radiol Endod 1994;77:446-451.

An article by authors with extensive experience in management of these infections describing the risk factors, microbiology and need for emergency surgical airway protection. The authors describe the need for emergency tracheotomy in 11 of 15 patients with Ludwig's angina. Of their total of 110 patients, the most common deep neck infection was lateral pharyngeal space infection (55%). The most common predisposing factors were dental infection, local injection drug use, mandibular fracture, and tonsillitis.

Chapter 154

HUMAN IMMUNODEFICIENCY VIRUS INFECTION

Alison Morris • John M. Luce

KEY POINTS

1. Intensive care survival of HIV-infected patients has improved over the course of the AIDS epidemic, and ICU care is now indicated for most patients.

2. Non–AIDS-related diagnoses have become more common since the introduction of highly active antiretroviral therapy (HAART), although many patients admitted to the ICU may not be receiving this therapy.

3. Mortality from *Pneumocystis carinii* pneumonia (PCP) can still be high, particularly if patients develop a pneumothorax while on mechanical ventilation.

4. Clinicians should have a high suspicion for PCP because many patients will not be aware that they are HIV-infected before ICU admission.

5. Early bronchoscopy with bronchoalveolar lavage should be performed in patients with pneumonia who do not have a definitive microbiologic diagnosis.

6. Trimethoprim-sulfamethoxazole is the treatment of choice for PCP, and corticosteroids should be given to those meeting the established criteria.

7. Fatal lactic acidosis can develop as a result of antiretroviral medications. Treatment consists of drug discontinuation and supportive care. Administration of riboflavin, thiamine, and L-carnitine may be beneficial.

8. Immune reconstitution syndrome after initiating HAART can occasionally lead to respiratory failure, particularly in patients with PCP.

9. Administration of HAART in the ICU is difficult, may lead to viral resistance, and is associated with many side effects and drug interactions; however, early HAART might improve ICU survival.

10. Adrenal insufficiency is more common in HIV-infected patients and should be suspected in patients with hypotension.

Many changes have occurred in the overall management and prognosis of patients with the human immunodeficiency virus (HIV). Management of HIV-infected patients early in the acquired immunodeficiency syndrome (AIDS) epidemic was based largely on the diagnosis and treatment of opportunistic infections and neoplasms. Because these disorders were diagnosed late in the course of HIV infection, treatment too often yielded poor results. In 1987, the first antiretroviral medication, zidovudine, became available and was followed by other nucleoside analogs.[1,2] In concert with chemoprophylaxis for opportunistic infections, these agents offered the first hope that HIV infection could be arrested, if not cured. As time has passed, other classes of medications have been developed to combat HIV. With the discovery of protease inhibitors and the use of combination therapies for HIV known as highly active antiretroviral therapy (HAART) there has been dramatic improvement in the morbidity and mortality of patients infected with HIV.[3] These combinations of medications can result in prolonged suppression of HIV viral RNA levels and sustained increases in CD4 cell counts.

Changes in the spectrum and survival of those patients with HIV admitted to an ICU have occurred since the widespread introduction of HAART in 1996. Unfortunately, not all patients have been able to benefit from HAART. Those not known to be HIV infected, those without access to HAART, and those not responding to HAART may still present with AIDS-associated opportunistic infections and neoplasms.[4] In this chapter, we discuss the recent trends in the epidemiology and survival of HIV-infected patients admitted to an ICU. Because PCP remains a leading cause of respiratory failure in HIV-infected patients and still carries a high mortality rate, we will also discuss diagnostic approaches and therapy for PCP. Finally, we will examine problems unique to the ICU care of HIV-infected patients, particularly those related to HAART.

INTENSIVE CARE TRENDS AMONG HIV-INFECTED PATIENTS

EPIDEMIOLOGY

Both the epidemiology of ICU admissions and views of the utility of ICU care for HIV-infected patients have undergone several shifts during the course of the AIDS epidemic. In the beginning of the epidemic, most patients with HIV infection admitted to the ICU had PCP and survival was poor.[5] ICU admission was often considered futile. Over the course of the epidemic, bacterial pneumonia, sepsis, and non–HIV-associated diagnoses have become increasingly common, although PCP remains an important cause of ICU admission with high mortality in certain groups of patients. With the widespread availability of HAART, there have been continued changes in ICU mortality and epidemiology and ICU care is again indicated for most patients. Unfortunately, with increasing reports of antiretroviral resistance and transmission of multidrug-resistant HIV,[6-8] ICU trends may shift again with an increase in opportunistic infections and poor outcomes.

The most extensive series documenting ICU epidemiology has come from San Francisco General Hospital where researchers have tracked the trends in ICU diagnoses, admissions, and survival throughout the different eras of the AIDS epidemic. During era I (1981-1985), overall hospital mortality for those admitted to an ICU was 69%, and median survival was only 7 months.[5] The number of ICU admissions peaked in 1984 and then decreased despite rising numbers of hospital admissions for AIDS patients. This decrease in ICU admissions was attributed to both physicians' and patients' views of ICU care as futile. In era II (1986-1988), mortality decreased, largely as a result of the use of adjunctive corticosteroids for PCP, which was still the leading cause of ICU admission.[9] Era III (1989-1991) actually saw an increase in mortality rates for PCP, likely from a bias away from withholding or withdrawing care.[10] In era IV (1992-1995), rates of ICU admission remained stable and overall mortality was 36.9%, a significant improvement from era I.[11]

Era V, or the HAART era (1996-1999), brought about significant changes in both mortality and admission rates.[12] The number of ICU admissions decreased significantly from an average of 111 per year in era IV to 88.5 per year in era V, and survival rate increased to 71.0%. Respiratory failure was still the most common cause of ICU admission (40.7% of diagnoses), but PCP only accounted for 10.7% of admissions compared with 17.6% in era IV. Admission demographics of patients reflected national trends in the HIV epidemic. During previous eras, the majority of patients were white, homosexual men.[11] During era V, African-Americans accounted for 44.6% of ICU admissions and women and intravenous drug users were also more commonly seen.

Because outcome and utilization of ICU care for HIV-infected patients vary according to hospital characteristics and geographic location, it is important to examine data from several centers.[13] In general, exact mortality and admission rates are different in different series but overall trends of decreasing mortality and changes in the spectrum of diagnoses remain similar. Afessa and green documented a mortality rate of 29.6% in a cohort of 169 ICU patients hospitalized between 1995 and 1999.[14] A series in Spain described a mortality rate of 40% in ICU patients between 1993 and 1998.[15] Nuesch and colleagues reported that ICU mortality remained stable at 28.5% and 25% in the time periods from 1994 to 1996 and 1997 to 1999, respectively.[16] Interestingly, the overall percentage of hospitalized HIV-infected patients admitted to the ICU in this study increased from 6.3% to 11.8% in the later years. The authors interpreted this increase as an indication of an improved prognosis for HIV resulting in more aggressive care.

In most series, respiratory failure remains the leading cause of ICU admission, although the percentage of respiratory admissions has declined. PCP accounted for as many as 62% of all ICU admissions in the early days of the epidemic and was by far the most common cause of respiratory failure.[5] Bacterial pneumonia is now becoming more common, although PCP still accounts for many cases of respiratory failure.[15,16] HIV-infected patients with bacterial pneumonia are more likely to become bacteremic, and mortality may be as high as 68% in this setting.[17] Non–AIDS-related diagnoses such as myocardial infarction and trauma may become more common during the current era of HAART, as may HAART-associated diagnoses (see later).

PROGNOSTIC FACTORS

Clinicians and patients making decisions regarding the utility of care should understand risk factors for ICU mortality. Studies have shown that there are several key factors that influence mortality, and these factors seem not to have changed over the years. Multivariate analysis of the cohort from era V at San Francisco General Hospital demonstrated that mechanical ventilation or a diagnosis of PCP predicted a higher mortality rate, whereas admission for a non–AIDS-associated diagnosis, an albumin level greater than 2.6 g/dL, and an Acute Physiology and Chronic Health Evaluation (APACHE) II score less than 13 all were associated with an increase in survival to hospital discharge.[12] These factors—particularly mechanical ventilation, serum albumin, and PCP—had been known to influence mortality before the HAART era as well.[9,11,14,15] Although use of HAART had a beneficial effect on survival in the San Francisco cohort, it was not an independent factor in outcome. Some studies have found that a higher CD4 cell count is associated with improved survival, but this finding is not universal.[11,12,14] Patients with a poor preadmission functional status and more advanced HIV may also not be expected to have a favorable prognosis.[18]

INTENSIVE CARE TRENDS IN PCP

Because PCP has historically been the most common cause of respiratory failure in AIDS patients and the most common reason for ICU admission, more is known about the outcome of intensive care for AIDS patients with PCP than for any HIV-infected group. Mortality for PCP in the ICU, particularly for patients requiring mechanical ventilation, has been high throughout the course of the AIDS epidemic, although there have been some improvements. In the 1980s, those who required intensive care had a mortality rate as high as 81% and mortality for patients requiring mechanical ventilation was 87%.[5] The introduction of adjunctive corticosteroids in the mid 1980s improved mortality for PCP-associated respiratory failure to approximately 60%.[9,19-22] Since that time little change has occurred in the outcome of severe PCP, with recent ICU mortality rates of 59% to 63%.[11,12] The main factors that influence mortality in PCP are the need for mechanical ventilation or the development of a pneumothorax. Both factors have been shown to increase mortality dramatically. Mortality among those requiring mechanical ventilation may still be as high as 76%; and if patients develop a pneumothorax while on mechanical ventilation, the outcome is almost uniformly fatal.[12,23]

DIAGNOSIS AND TREATMENT OF PCP

CLINICAL PRESENTATION

Although the number of cases of PCP has decreased, it remains a leading cause of respiratory failure among HIV-infected patients. PCP most commonly occurs in patients with CD4 cell counts below 200 cells/μL, and the risk of PCP increases exponentially as the CD4 cell count decreases below that level.[24,25] The clinical presentation of PCP ranges from the subtle to the fulminant. Most patients have most or all of the following symptoms and signs: fever, tachypnea, dyspnea with a nonproductive cough, and a chest examination that is normal or has a few dry rales.[26] In the HIV-infected patient, symptoms have generally been present for days to weeks before the diagnosis is made. Many patients may not be known to be HIV infected. Recent studies have shown that 28% to 57% of patients admitted to the ICU with PCP are not aware that they are infected with HIV.[23,27] Clinicians must remember to include PCP in their differential of respiratory failure, even in those not known to have HIV.

Severe PCP is often similar in presentation and pathogenesis to acute respiratory distress syndrome (ARDS). The organism appears to cause a widespread capillary leak,[28] and the chest radiograph usually resembles that in ARDS with diffuse, bilateral, interstitial infiltrates. Less commonly, PCP results in focal airspace consolidation. Infiltrates are occasionally unilateral or asymmetrical, and the pattern seen (reticular or granular) is more suggestive of the diagnosis than the distribution of the abnormalities. Cysts and pneumatoceles occur in 10% to 20% of cases, and patients with PCP are at risk for the development of a pneumothorax.[29,30] Finally, about 5% to 10% of patients who prove to have PCP initially have normal chest radiographs.[26]

DIAGNOSIS

Although PCP may have a typical clinical and radiographic presentation, definitive diagnosis is encouraged, particularly in those who are critically ill. Many respiratory diseases in HIV have overlapping presentations, and prompt initiation of appropriate therapy is important to prevent clinical deterioration and avoid unnecessary drug side effects. The diagnosis of PCP is made when the organism is identified in the pulmonary secretions of a patient with a compatible clinical presentation. PCP may be diagnosed by examination of induced sputum, which has a sensitivity of 79% and a negative predictive value of 61% in experienced hands.[26] The usefulness of sputum induction is often limited because many hospitals may not be experienced in performing the test and sputum induction is generally not tolerated in patients with respiratory distress.

When the sputum examination is negative or when it is not possible to obtain induced sputum, bronchoscopy with bronchoalveolar lavage (BAL) is the procedure of choice, with a sensitivity of over 90% for diagnosis of PCP in an HIV-infected individual.[31] Bronchoscopy with BAL should be performed as early as possible in undiagnosed patients. Although the addition of transbronchial biopsy generally adds little to the yield of lavage in the diagnosis of PCP, it is helpful in HIV-infected patients with other pulmonary infections.[32] Transbronchial biopsy is thus a reasonable initial invasive study when the probability of PCP is low and is a useful follow-up test when the BAL fails to demonstrate PCP.

TREATMENT

The mainstay of therapy for moderate to severe PCP is intravenous trimethoprim-sulfamethoxazole (TMP-SMX) (Table 154-1). The cure rate for TMP-SMX may be as high as 60% to 86%.[33,34] The drug should be administered at a total daily dose of 15 to 20 mg/kg of trimethoprim and 75 to 100 mg/kg of sulfamethoxazole divided into three or four doses per day. Approximately 25% of patients will have therapy-limiting toxicity from TMP-SMX, with most severe toxicities occurring between days 6 and 10 of treatment.[34-37] Side effects of TMP-SMX include nausea, rash, bone marrow suppression, hyponatremia, hyperkalemia, renal dysfunction, and transaminitis.

Intravenous pentamidine isethionate is an effective alternative for therapy in patients who cannot tolerate TMP-SMX or have failed treatment (see later). Although this agent has been reported to have success rates equivalent to TMP-SMX, some studies have found that it is somewhat less efficacious.[33,34,38] The recommended daily dose of pentamidine is 3 to 4 mg/kg administered over 1 hour. Pentamidine has a high rate of serious toxicity that includes nausea, hypotension, pancreatitis, hypoglycemia and hyperglycemia, bone marrow suppression, and nephrotoxicity. Because pentamidine is toxic to the pancreatic islet cells, initial hypoglycemia from a surge of insulin release followed by hyperglycemia from inadequate insulin may be seen, and the patient may progress to chronic diabetes mellitus. Adverse

TABLE 154-1. SUMMARY OF TREATMENT REGIMENS FOR SEVERE PCP IN DECREASING ORDER OF PREFERENCE

Agent	Dose	Side Effects
Trimethoprim-sulfamethoxazole	15-20 mg/kg/day trimethoprim with 75-100 mg/kg/day sulfamethoxazole, i.v., divided q 6 to 8h	Rash, nausea, bone marrow suppression, hyponatremia, hyperkalemia, nephrotoxicity, transaminitis
Pentamidine isethionate	3-4 mg/kg/day i.v.	Nausea, hypotension, hypo- or hyperglycemia, pancreatitis, bone marrow suppression, nephrotoxicity
Trimetrexate	45 mg/m^2 qd with leucovorin, 0.5-0.8 mg/kg q 6h	Nausea, bone marrow suppression, peripheral neuropathy, hepatotoxicity
Clindamycin-primaquine	900 mg i.v. q 8h (clindamycin) 30 mg p.o. qd (primaquine)	Nausea, diarrhea, rash, hemolytic anemia, methemoglobinemia, leukopenia
Adjunctive therapy: Prednisone if PaO$_2$ < 70 mm Hg or alveolar-arterial gradient > 35mm Hg	40 mg p.o. q 12h for 5 days, 40 mg p.o. qd for 5 days, 20 mg p.o. qd for 11 days	Hyperglycemia, psychosis

reactions may be seen in as many as 50% of patients treated with pentamidine.

When first-line therapies prove to be ineffective or toxic, trimetrexate may be used intravenously, but it is somewhat less effective than TMP-SMX and associated with a higher rate of relapse.[39] Because it is a very potent inhibitor of dihydrofolate reductase, it must be administered with leucovorin to rescue mammalian cells.[40] Intravenous trimetrexate should be given once daily at a dose of 45 mg/m². Leucovorin should be started before trimetrexate and continued for 3 days after completion of trimetrexate at a dose of 0.5 to 0.8 mg/kg every 6 hours. Clindamycin-primaquine can also be used as a salvage regimen. However, primaquine is administered orally and its use may therefore be limited in the ICU owing to impaired absorption.[41]

As discussed earlier, mortality due to severe PCP was extremely high at the beginning of the AIDS epidemic. The most profound improvement in mortality of PCP has occurred with the introduction of adjunctive corticosteroids.[19-22] It is recommended that patients with PCP and either a PaO$_2$ in room air of less than 70 mm Hg or an alveolar-arterial oxygen gradient greater than 35 mm Hg receive corticosteroids to reduce mortality.[42] Corticosteroid therapy should be administered at the onset of anti-*Pneumocystis* therapy because it acts to decrease the inflammation seen during the first few days of treatment. The usual recommended regimen is oral prednisone of 40 mg given twice daily for 5 days, followed by 40 mg once daily for 5 days, then 20 mg daily for 11 days. For those patients unable to take oral medications, intravenous methylprednisolone or dexamethasone may be substituted.

TREATMENT FAILURE

Clinical deterioration is commonly seen 3 to 5 days after initiation of treatment. Patients may experience worsening respiratory status with decreases in arterial oxygenation. These symptoms are likely due to an inflammatory response to dead or dying organisms that may increase capillary permeability and pulmonary edema formation. This edema formation may be inadvertently worsened by administration of excessive intravenous fluids.

Given that patients' conditions may deteriorate and that symptoms may be prolonged, it is difficult to determine when a treatment regimen is failing and should be abandoned for an alternative. Whether treatment failure is more likely in patients with previous prophylaxis use is unknown, but *Pneumocystis* has been shown to develop genetic mutations with exposure to sulfa- or sulfone-containing medications such as TMP-SMX and dapsone.[43,44] The relationship of these mutations to outcome is still controversial.[45-47] In general, treatment should be continued for 5 to 10 days before considering changing to a different agent.[38] It is also important to investigate alternative diagnoses that may be responsible for the patient's symptoms. Other causes of pneumonia including nosocomial organisms should be considered when treatment appears to be failing. Patients with PCP are also at increased risk of pulmonary edema that may explain worsening respiratory status with increasing radiographic infiltrates. Alternative diagnoses should be pursued with chest computed tomography, sputum cultures, or echocardiography as clinically indicated. Repeat bronchoscopy is helpful to diagnose agents other than PCP but is not useful in determining if PCP treatment is failing because *Pneumocystis* may persist in the bronchoalveolar lavage fluid for several weeks.[48]

VENTILATION OF THE PATIENT WITH PCP

The physiology of severe PCP resembles that of ARDS, and patients with PCP are at a high risk for developing barotrauma and pneumothoraces, often heralding a fatal outcome. Although no studies have examined ventilatory modes specifically in PCP, given the resemblance to ARDS and the high rate of barotrauma, low tidal volume ventilation should be employed. At San Francisco General Hospital, patients with severe PCP are ventilated with 6 mL/kg ideal body weight tidal volume according to the ARDSNet protocol.[49] Noninvasive positive-pressure ventilation (NPPV) has been studied in PCP and has been found to lower the rate of intubation, decrease the incidence of pneumothorax, and improve ICU survival.[50] Use of NPPV would be a reasonable first-line ventilation mode in patients with PCP and respiratory distress who can tolerate this form of ventilation and who can protect their airway.

HAART AND THE ICU

LACTIC ACIDOSIS

With the increasing use of HAART, ICU physicians need to be familiar with some of the life-threatening side effects that can occur with these medications. The syndrome of severe hepatic steatosis and lactic acidosis was first described in the 1990s.[51,52] The syndrome is most commonly associated with nucleoside reverse transcriptase inhibitors (NRTIs), particularly didanosine and stavudine, and results from mitochondrial toxicity of these agents.[53] The incidence of symptomatic lactic acidosis in HIV-infected patients taking NRTIs ranges from 1 to 25.2 cases per 1000 patient-years, and mortality rates may be as high as 77%.[54] A creatinine clearance less than 70 mL/min or a nadir CD4 cell count less than 250 cells/μL seems to predispose to development of the syndrome.[55] Patients often present with abdominal pain, nausea, and vomiting and may have myalgias or peripheral neuropathies. Serum lactate levels are elevated, and hepatic steatosis and elevation of transaminases occur frequently. Often, cessation of the antiretrovirals results in resolution of the syndrome; however, some patients can progress to life-threatening organ failure. An initial lactate level above 9 mmol/L seems to be associated with a higher risk of death,[56] and some authors believe that a level greater than 5 mmol/L should be considered life threatening.[57]

In patients presenting with lactic acidosis, the offending agent should be discontinued and usual supportive care administered. Although data regarding treatment outcomes are not extensive, treatment should be started in those patients with a lactate level above 5 mmol/L. Treatment with riboflavin, thiamine, and L-carnitine seems to reverse toxicity.[56-59] One recommended regimen is to administer 50 mg of riboflavin daily with 50 mg/kg of L-carnitine and 100 mg of thiamine until the lactic acidosis resolves. The exact length of treatment and the lactate level above which treatment is unlikely to succeed remain unclear.

IMMUNE RECONSTITUTION

The immune reconstitution syndrome leads to paradoxical worsening of an infection shortly after initiation of HAART.

This syndrome results from improvement in the immune system and a renewed inflammatory response directed against infectious agents.[60] While this syndrome has been reported to occur in diseases such as tuberculosis, cytomegalovirus (CMV), and *Mycobacterium avium* complex, it usually results only in a symptomatic worsening of these conditions.[60-62] There have been a few case reports of paradoxical worsening occurring during PCP.[63-65] Patients experienced increasing respiratory distress and hypoxemia, and some required mechanical ventilation.[63] All patients subsequently recovered, and there seemed to be some benefit from continuing or reintroducing corticosteroids. Patients admitted to the ICU with a presumed paradoxical worsening of PCP should receive corticosteroids, and appropriate testing should be performed to rule out other infections or respiratory disorders causing clinical worsening.

ADMINISTRATION OF HAART IN THE ICU

The question of whether to continue or initiate HAART while HIV-infected patients are in the ICU is an unresolved issue in critical care. Traditionally, antiretroviral regimens have been discontinued while patients are in intensive care, and clinicians have been reluctant to initiate HAART in this population. Many issues relating to the use of HAART exist in the ICU, including possible poor gastric absorption of antiretroviral medications, the potential for drug interactions and side effects, and concern about patient compliance in continuing HAART after discharge. There is also concern that initiating HAART in a patient with borderline respiratory status might lead to respiratory failure through paradoxical worsening and immune reconstitution.

HAART therapy is complicated in the ICU. Only zidovudine is available in an intravenous form. Other agents that are available as liquids and therefore could be administered via a feeding tube are listed in Table 154-2. If physicians choose to administer HAART to an ICU patient, they need to be particularly aware of possible side effects, including renal toxicity and hepatotoxicity, pancreatitis, and lactic acidosis. Many common ICU medications such as benzodiazepines, fluconazole, pentamidine, and amiodarone may have dangerous interactions or altered metabolism when given with antiretrovirals. Medications may also affect the serum levels of the antiretrovirals, resulting either in toxic or subtherapeutic concentrations. Consultation with a specialist familiar with the many antiretroviral regimens is advised.

Despite these potential difficulties, there is some reason to believe that critically ill patients may benefit from HAART. Morris and colleagues studied patients with PCP admitted to the ICU during the era of HAART. They found that mortality among those patients who did not receive HAART was 63%, whereas those patients either receiving HAART at time of admission or started on HAART in the ICU had a mortality rate of only 25%.[27] HAART might improve survival in patients with PCP through suppression of viral replication and improvement in immune function. It has also been postulated that protease inhibitors may have anti-*Pneumocystis* effects and aid in the treatment of PCP.[66] Until data from prospective, randomized trials are available, clinicians must make decisions about administering HAART on a case-by-case basis.

METABOLIC ABNORMALITIES IN THE ICU

METABOLIC COMPLICATIONS OF HAART

Many drugs included in HAART regimens have an adverse effect on lipids and glucose metabolism. Patients commonly develop metabolic abnormalities, including hyperlipidemia, hypercholesterolemia, glucose intolerance, and diabetes.[67-69] It has been postulated that these metabolic effects of HAART might lead to higher rates of cardiac and cerebrovascular disease among patients with HIV, potentially increasing the numbers admitted to intensive care with myocardial infarctions and strokes. Studies have had varying results, and the magnitude of the effect is not yet known. A recent study of over 36,000 HIV-infected patients from 1993 to 2001 demonstrated that there was no relationship between use of antiretroviral medications and cerebrovascular or cardiovascular events.[70] Follow-up may have been too short to detect an effect. In contrast, the HIV Outpatient Study (HOPS) found that risk of myocardial infarction increased among those using protease inhibitors (odds ratio for MI = 7.1).[71] Even if metabolic complications of HAART do not contribute to an increased rate of cardiovascular disease, clinicians can expect to see these problems more frequently as the HIV-infected population ages.

ADRENAL INSUFFICIENCY

Adrenal insufficiency is another important syndrome in the ICU that is more common among HIV-infected patients. The adrenal glands of patients with HIV may be damaged by infections such as CMV, by neoplasms such as lymphoma, and by drugs such as ketoconazole and rifampin.[72-74] At its most severe, adrenal insufficiency can present as refractory hypotension and may lead to death if not recognized. Marik and colleagues recently studied adrenal function in 28 critically ill HIV-infected patients. They found that depending on the criteria used, the rate of adrenal insufficiency varied from 7% to 75%.[75] Evidence of CMV infection was more common among the patients with adrenal insufficiency. Clinicians should have a high degree of suspicion for adrenal insufficiency in HIV-infected patients, particularly in those with CMV, and pursue testing with adrenocorticotropic hormone stimulation testing.

In summary, the outlook for ICU patients with HIV has improved dramatically since the beginning of the AIDS

TABLE 154–2. LIST OF ANTIRETROVIRAL AGENTS AVAILABLE IN LIQUID FORM

Protease Inhibitors

Amprenavir
Lopinavir
Nelfinavir
Ritonavir

Nucleoside Reverse Transcriptase Inhibitors

Abacavir
Lamivudine
Didanosine
Stavudine
Zidovudine (also intravenous)

Non-nucleoside Reverse Transcriptase Inhibitor

Nevirapine

epidemic. However, not all patients can benefit from HAART, and increasing viral resistance may lead to an increase in the incidence of opportunistic infections. Physicians caring for HIV-infected patients in the ICU need an understanding of both the HIV-associated and the non–HIV-associated conditions that can affect these patients. Knowledge of antiretroviral therapies and their side effects are also important because these therapies may lead directly to patients' ICU admissions and impact their morbidity and mortality. It is hoped that information will become available to guide clinicians in use of HAART in the ICU, and survival will continue to improve.

ANNOTATED REFERENCES

Bonnet F, Bonarek M, Morlat P, et al: Risk factors for lactic acidosis in HIV-infected patients treated with nucleoside reverse-transcriptase inhibitors: A case-control study. Clin Infect Dis 2003;36:1324-1328.

A case-control study assessing the risk factors for development of lactic acidosis in patients receiving nucleoside-reverse transcriptase inhibitors. The authors found that patients with a low creatinine clearance or a low nadir CD4 cell count were at increased risk for developing this complication.

Bozzette SA, Ake CF, Tam HK, et al: Cardiovascular and cerebrovascular events in patients treated for human immunodeficiency virus infection. N Engl J Med 2003;348:702-710.

This study of over 36,000 HIV-infected patients in Veterans Affairs facilities found that the rates of admission for cardiovascular and cerebrovascular disease decreased after the introduction of highly active antiretroviral therapy and that there was no relationship between use of any class of antiretrovirals and the development of cardiac or cerebrovascular disease.

Holmberg SD, Moorman AC, Williamson JM, et al: Protease inhibitors and cardiovascular outcomes in patients with HIV-1. Lancet 2002;360:1747-1748.

This large, multicenter cohort study followed 5,672 HIV-infected outpatients for development of myocardial infarction. The authors found that there was an increased incidence of myocardial infarction associated with the use of protease inhibitors.

Morris A, Creasman J, Turner J, et al: Intensive care of human immunodeficiency virus-infected patients during the era of highly active antiretroviral therapy. Am J Respir Crit Care Med 2002;166:262-267.

Fifth in a series of articles from San Francisco General Hospital documenting ICU epidemiology and mortality of HIV-infected patients throughout the course of the AIDS epidemic. In the most recent era of highly active retroviral therapy, intensive care admissions have decreased and survival has increased. Incidence of PCP has declined, although it is still a common cause of respiratory failure in this center.

Wislez M, Bergot E, Antoine M, et al: Acute respiratory failure following HAART introduction in patients treated for *Pneumocystis carinii* pneumonia. Am J Respir Crit Care Med 2001;164:847-851.

Report of 3 cases of respiratory failure in patients undergoing treatment for PCP who were started on highly active antiretroviral therapy. Respiratory worsening was secondary to immune reconstitution and occurred 7 to 17 days after initiating antiretroviral therapy. All patients recovered from the episode and corticosteroids appeared to be beneficial.

Chapter 155

INFECTIONS IN THE IMMUNOCOMPROMISED PATIENT

Andrew Githaiga • Magdaline Ndirangu • David L. Paterson

Many immunocompromised patients are managed in ICUs every year. The most common problem that these patients face is infection. Severe infection may be the cause of ICU admission. Common examples include community-acquired pneumonia, bacteremia, and CNS infections. The incidence of infections acquired by immunocompromised patients during ICU admissions also is significant.[1] Mortality exceeds 90% for certain infections in immunocompromised patients.[2] Early diagnosis and institution of appropriate antimicrobial and supportive therapy, especially when immunocompromise can be reduced, can improve outcome significantly, however. This chapter outlines some of the most common immunocompromising conditions and general principles regarding the epidemiology, diagnostic approach, and management of infections in immunocompromised patients.

COMMONLY ENCOUNTERED IMMUNOCOMPROMISING CONDITIONS

Immunocompromise can be broadly defined as a state in which the response of the host to a foreign antigen is subnormal. Immunocompromise could be congenital (primary) or acquired. Congenital immunodeficiencies are now much less common than acquired immunodeficiencies. In general, congenital immunodeficiency is observed more frequently in patients in pediatric ICUs than in adult ICUs. Patients with congenital immunodeficiencies usually have repeated infections, especially infections affecting the respiratory tree and sinuses. Congenital immunodeficiencies are usually "pure," in that the defects in response of the host to foreign antigens are usually specific and well defined. Bruton's X-linked agammaglobulinemia is associated with a defect in the normal maturation process of immunoglobulin-producing B cells. As a result, mature circulating B cells, plasma cells, and serum immunoglobulin are absent. The patient is susceptible to organisms that are normally dealt with by immunoglobulin, such as *Streptococcus pneumoniae* and *Haemophilus influenzae*. Other congenital immunodeficiency syndromes are listed in Table 155-1.

Most immunocompromised patients managed in ICUs for adults have acquired immunocompromise. Although the response of host defenses in the elderly, in diabetics, and in alcoholics is compromised, this chapter deals primarily with four categories of immunocompromised patients: (1) patients receiving chemotherapy for hematologic malignancies and solid tumors; (2) patients receiving immunosuppressive therapy in the context of solid-organ transplantation; (3) patients receiving corticosteroids, methotrexate, monoclonal antibodies to tumor necrosis factor, and other disease-modifying agents for rheumatoid arthritis, Crohn's disease, and autoimmune disorders; and (4) patients with HIV infection.

HEMATOLOGIC MALIGNANCIES AND SOLID TUMORS

The management of patients undergoing chemotherapy or transplantation for hematologic malignancies is discussed elsewhere in this textbook. In brief, prolonged neutropenia from chemotherapy has a significant risk of bacterial and

TABLE 155–1. CONGENITAL (PRIMARY) CAUSES OF IMMUNODEFICIENCY

Condition (Immunodeficiency)	Organisms with an Increased Tendency to Cause Infection in this Condition
T-lymphocyte Deficiencies	
DiGeorge's syndrome (thymic aplasia with reduced CD4 and CD3 cells)	Viruses (especially HSV and measles), sometimes *Pneumocystis carinii*, fungi, or gram-negative bacteria
Purine nucleoside phosphorylase deficiency (marked T-cell depletion)	*P. carinii* and viruses
B-lymphocyte Deficiencies	
Bruton's X-linked agammaglobulinemia (absence of B cells, plasma cells, and antibody)	*Haemophilus influenzae, Streptococcus pneumoniae, Staphylococcus aureus, Pseudomonas aeruginosa, P. carinii* (after first 4-6 mo of life when maternal antibody has been consumed)
Selective IgG subclass deficiencies	Variable
Selective IgA deficiency	*S. pneumoniae, H. influenzae*
Hyper-IgM immunodeficiency (elevated IgM but reduced IgG and IgA)	*S. pneumoniae, H. influenzae, P. carinii* (rarely)
Mixed T- and B-lymphocyte Deficiencies	
Common variable immunodeficiency (leads to various B-cell activation or differentiation defects and gradual deterioration of T-cell number and function)	*S. pneumoniae, H. influenzae,* cytomegalovirus, VZV, *P. carinii*
Severe combined immunodeficiency (severe reduction in IgG and absence of T cells)	*P. carinii,* viruses, *Legionella*
Wiskott-Aldrich syndrome (decreased T-cell number and function, low IgM, occasionally low IgG)	*S. pneumoniae, H. influenzae,* HSV, *P. carinii*
Ataxia-telangiectasia (decreased T-cell number and function; IgA, IgE, IgG$_2$, and IgG$_4$ deficiency)	*S. aureus, S. pneumoniae, H. influenzae*
Disorders of Complement	
C3 deficiency (congenital absence of C3 or consumption of C3 due to deficiency of C3b inactivator)	*S. pneumoniae, H. influenzae,* enteric gram-negative bacilli
Phagocyte Defects	
Chronic granulomatous disease (defect in NADPH oxidase in phagocytic cells)	*S. aureus, Escherichia coli, Klebsiella pneumoniae, Enterobacter cloacae, S. marcescens, P. aeruginosa, Aspergillus*
Chédiak-Higashi syndrome (impaired microbicidal activity of phagocytes)	*S. aureus, H. influenzae, Aspergillus*
Kostmann's syndrome, Shwachman-Diamond syndrome, cyclic neutropenia (low neutrophil count)	*S. aureus,* enteric gram-negative bacilli, *P. aeruginosa*

HSV, herpes simplex virus; NADPH, reduced nicotinamide adenine dinucleotide phosphate; VZV, varicella-zoster virus.

fungal infection. Classically, gram-negative organisms, such as *Pseudomonas aeruginosa,* and fungal organisms, such as *Aspergillus* species, have been associated with severe neutropenia. It has long been known that the severity and the duration of neutropenia influence the risk of infection.[3] It also has been well established that aggressive chemotherapy and radiotherapy for Hodgkin's disease, coupled with splenectomy, significantly impairs humoral defense against encapsulated organisms, such as *S. pneumoniae, H. influenzae,* and *Neisseria meningitidis.*[4] Transplantation is associated with a risk of graft-versus-host disease. Prophylaxis against and treatment of graft-versus-host disease may involve use of drugs such as cyclosporine or tacrolimus plus corticosteroids. Cyclosporine and tacrolimus inhibit calcineurin, an enzyme important in the lymphocyte activation cascade. Corticosteroids also affect lymphocyte function and depress functions of activated macrophages. As a result, patients receiving therapy for graft-versus-host disease may be prone to fungal, viral, and mycobacterial infections.

SOLID-ORGAN TRANSPLANTATION

Solid-organ transplantation also is covered in detail elsewhere in this book. Liver, kidney, pancreas, small intestine, heart, and lung transplantations are routinely performed in many medical centers. Solid-organ transplant recipients are uniquely susceptible to infection. They undergo significant surgery, breaching the defenses provided by the skin. They remain in ICUs for prolonged periods, requiring intravenous access and mechanical ventilation, and cutaneous and pulmonary barriers to infection are breached. Finally, solid-organ transplant recipients receive immunosuppressive therapy to prevent graft rejection. Commonly used immunosuppressive medications are listed in Table 155-2. Immunosuppressive regimens are in a constant state of flux—more recent trends have been toward aggressive "pretreatment" immediately before transplantation, coupled with decreased immunosuppression in the post-transplant period.[5]

In the early post-transplant period, transplant recipients are susceptible to nosocomially acquired bacterial infections, such as pneumonia and central line–associated bloodstream infection associated with general ICU care, and wound infections and intra-abdominal infections associated with the surgical procedure. Opportunistic infections may be acquired from the organ graft; cytomegalovirus is the most pertinent example, but a wide variety of infections, such as histoplasmosis and West Nile virus infection, have been acquired from the graft. Solid-organ transplant recipients,

TABLE 155–2. IMMUNOSUPPRESSIVE DRUGS USED IN SOLID-ORGAN TRANSPLANTATION AND THEIR MECHANISMS OF ACTIVITY

Immunosuppressive	Mode of Action
Corticosteroids	Negative regulation of cytokine gene expression
Azathioprine	Inhibits DNA and RNA synthesis; inhibits T- and B-cell function
Cyclosporine	Calcineurin inhibitor; inhibits cytokine expression
Tacrolimus	Calcineurin inhibitor; inhibits cytokine expression
Sirolimus (rapamycin)	Prevents translation of mRNAs encoding cell cycle regulators
Mycophenolate mofetil	Blocks purine biosynthesis; inhibits T- and B-cell proliferation
Polyclonal antilymphocyte	Lymphocyte depletion antibodies (e.g., Atgam, Thymoglobulin)
Muromonab-CD3 (OKT3)	Anti-CD3 monoclonal antibody
Alemtuzumab (Campath)	Anti-CD52 monoclonal antibody
Daclizumab, basiliximab	Anti-CD25 monoclonal antibody

TABLE 155–3. COMMONLY USED ANTICYTOKINES FOR MANAGEMENT OF RHEUMATOID ARTHRITIS

Drug	Mechanism of Action	FDA-Approved Indications
Adalimumab (Humira)	Recombinant, fully human anti-TNF monoclonal antibody	Rheumatoid arthritis
Anakinra (Kineret)	Recombinant human interleukin-1 receptor antagonist	Rheumatoid arthritis
Etanercept (Enbrel)	TNF receptor p75 Fc fusion protein	Rheumatoid arthritis, psoriatic arthritis, ankylosing spondylitis
Infliximab (Remicade)	Chimeric monoclonal antibody to TNF	Crohn's disease, methotrexate-refractory rheumatoid arthritis

FDA, Food and Drug Administration; TNF, tumor necrosis factor.

by virtue of their iatrogenic immunosuppression, also are susceptible to reactivation of latent infection (e.g., cytomegalovirus infection, tuberculosis, or histoplasmosis) or to infections acquired through the hospital environment (e.g., aspergillosis, legionellosis, or tuberculosis).

RHEUMATOID ARTHRITIS AND AUTOIMMUNE DISORDERS

Therapy for rheumatoid arthritis and other autoimmune disorders may be with simple analgesics or nonsteroidal anti-inflammatory drugs. Drugs with the potential to cause significant immunocompromise also are frequently used, however. Classically, therapy has been with corticosteroids or with disease-modifying antirheumatic drugs, such as azathioprine, cyclosporine, penicillamine, gold salts, hydroxychloroquine, leflunomide, methotrexate, or sulfasalazine. The effects of corticosteroids, azathioprine, and cyclosporine on host defenses have been noted previously (see Table 155-2). Methotrexate reversibly inhibits dihydrofolate reductase and interferes with DNA synthesis, repair, and cellular replication. In addition to its use in rheumatoid arthritis, it also can be used as an antineoplastic agent. Methotrexate can cause significant neutropenia.

A variety of anticytokine agents have become available for rheumatoid arthritis (Table 155-3). The use of these drugs also has been reported in treatment of Behçet's disease, Crohn's disease, graft-versus-host disease, hairy cell leukemia, psoriasis, pyoderma gangrenosum, sarcoidosis, and ulcerative colitis. Considerable attention has been paid to the possibility of pulmonary tuberculosis developing after treatment with such agents.[6] The risk is sufficiently high that it is recommended that tuberculin skin testing be performed for the presence of latent tuberculosis before the initiation of these anticytokine agents. Cases of invasive aspergillosis, coccidioidomycosis, cryptococcosis, histoplasmosis, and *Pneumocystis carinii* infection also have been reported associated with the use of these medications.[7-11] As is the case with transplant-associated immunocompromise, these infections may be reactivation of latent infection or new acquisitions of organisms acquired through the environment.

HUMAN IMMUNODEFICIENCY VIRUS INFECTION

HIV infection remains a relatively common infection, but acquired immunodeficiency syndrome (AIDS) has become less frequently encountered in ICUs since the advent of highly active antiretroviral therapy. As is discussed elsewhere in this book, HIV infection can be associated with substantial decline in CD4 lymphocyte counts. This decline creates a predisposition to *P. carinii* pneumonia, mycobacterial infection, fungal infection (e.g., cryptococcal meningitis), and viral infection (e.g., cytomegalovirus infection). Many patients with HIV infection are coinfected with hepatitis C virus, and as a result, liver failure is now a relatively common reason for ICU admission in HIV-infected patients. In some centers, liver transplantation is performed for HIV-infected patients with deteriorated liver function due to hepatitis viruses.[12]

GENERAL DIAGNOSTIC APPROACH TO IMMUNOCOMPROMISED PATIENTS WITH SEVERE INFECTIONS

Immunocompromised patients are a heterogeneous group. The infections commonly encountered by a patient with neutropenia as a consequence of chemotherapy may be different from infections observed in a patient with rheumatoid arthritis who is receiving infliximab. Even within a particular category of immunocompromise (e.g., kidney transplantation), patients may have a different degree of immunocompromise and a different susceptibility to infection. In solid-organ transplant recipients, the "net state of immunosuppression" (i.e., the cumulative burden of immunosuppression with a special weighting toward recent T-cell ablative therapy) influences the risk of infection. A renal transplant recipient who is receiving tacrolimus monotherapy twice per week would be less susceptible to opportunistic infection than a patient with recent acute cellular rejection treated with alemtuzumab. There have been more recent attempts to quantify immune function in solid-organ transplant recipients,[13] although it has not yet been definitively proved that such tests predict infection risk. In contrast, with HIV infection, CD4 lymphocyte count and HIV "viral load" predict risk of infection.[14] It is important to determine the recent CD4 lymphocyte count in patients with HIV infection. Patients with CD4 counts greater than 500 are unlikely to be infected with an opportunistic pathogen; patients with CD4 counts of 200 to 500 may be infected with organisms such as *Mycobacterium tuberculosis,* but are unlikely to be infected with opportunistic pathogens, such as cytomegalovirus or *Mycobacterium avium* complex; and patients with CD4 counts less than 200 have an increased risk of a wide variety of opportunistic infections.

Specific environmental exposures may be potentially important for immunocompromised patients. A travel history to the southwestern states of the United States may increase the likelihood that an immunocompromised patient has coccidioidomycosis (Fig. 155-1). Histoplasmosis is endemic in the Ohio River Valley. There may be environmental risks within the ICU. Outbreaks of invasive pulmonary aspergillosis have been linked to construction activity within the hospital. Outbreaks of legionellosis may be waterborne. (It is likely that many fungal and bacterial infections may be waterborne as well.[15,16]) Tuberculosis transmission has been well described in ICUs caring for transplant recipients or HIV-infected patients.[17] The net state of immunosuppression must be considered in the context of recent environmental exposures.

Although elements of history taking and physical examination may narrow the differential diagnosis of the causative agent of infection in immunocompromised patients, some of the "rules" applied to diagnosis in immunocompetent patients do not apply. Caution must be exercised in use of the diagnostic principle that follows "Ockham's razor" ("entities are not to be multiplied without necessity"). In an immunocompetent patient, given all the patient's symptoms, signs, and noninvasive laboratory test results, one unifying diagnosis usually explains all. Immunocompromised patients may have more than one infection simultaneously, however. A neutropenic patient may have bacterial pneumonia and invasive pulmonary aspergillosis simultaneously, whereas an

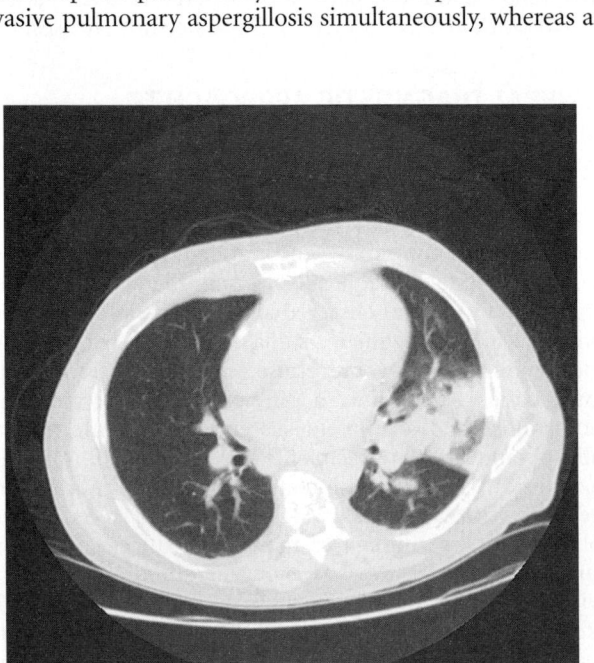

FIGURE 155–1. Computed tomography of the chest of a heart transplant recipient with recent travel to Arizona. *Coccidioides* IgG antibody was negative on admission, but *Coccidioides immitis* was grown from bronchoalveolar lavage.

TABLE 155–4. DIAGNOSTIC APPROACH FOR SEVERE INFECTIONS IN IMMUNOCOMPROMISED PATIENTS

History Taking and Review of Prior Records

Likely degree of immunocompromise
  Recent CD4 lymphocyte count and HIV viral load
  Time since transplantation
  Recent acute cellular rejection or graft-versus-host disease and
    treatment thereof
  Current or recent receipt of immunosuppressive medications
  Current or recent receipt of antiretroviral medications
Prophylaxis against opportunistic infections
  Receipt of antimicrobial prophylaxis against *Pneumocystic carinii,*
    herpes simplex virus, or cytomegalovirus
  Vaccination status (pneumococcus, influenza, *Neisseria meningitidis*)
Family history
  Personal or family history of tuberculosis or chickenpox
Potential environmental exposures
  Travel history to southwestern United States
  Exposure to hospital construction activity (aspergillosis)
  Exposure to hospital water supply (legionellosis, aspergillosis)
  Exposure to patients with tuberculosis or chickenpox
  Donor and recipient serostatus for cytomegalovirus or *Toxoplasma
    gondii*

Physical Examination

Skin
  Presence of cutaneous nodules consistent with cryptococcosis or
    nocardiosis
  Presence of cutaneous manifestations of graft-versus-host disease
  Kaposi's sarcoma
  Line insertion site erythema or pus
  Peripheral embolic phenomena
  Scars consistent with prior surgery
Mouth and other mucous membranes
  Presence of candidiasis
Respiratory system
  Presence of signs of focal versus multilobar pneumonia
Cardiovascular system
  Murmurs, prosthetic heart sounds
Abdominal examination
  Signs of peritonitis
  Hepatomegaly or splenomegaly
  Tenderness of renal allograft
Neurologic examination
  Nuchal rigidity
  Cranial nerve signs

Noninvasive Laboratory Tests

White blood cell count and differential
Blood and urine cultures
Serum cryptococcal antigen
Serum galactomannan antigen (aspergillosis)
Serum and urine *Histoplasma* antigen
Urinary *Legionella* antigen

Invasive Laboratory Tests

Bronchoalveolar lavage
Pleural fluid aspiration
Upper gastrointestinal endoscopy
Colonoscopy
Biopsy of liver, kidney, bone marrow

HIV, human immunodeficiency virus.

immunocompromised patient with HIV infection may have *P. carinii* pneumonia and pulmonary infiltrates due to human herpesvirus-8 infection (Kaposi's sarcoma).

The potential for multiple diagnoses underscores the need for early, invasive testing in immunocompromised patients with severe infection. Patients with unexplained severe community-acquired pneumonia may be best managed by early bronchoalveolar lavage before antimicrobial therapy aimed at numerous pathogens. Bronchoalveolar lavage could be sent for Gram stain, Ziehl-Neelsen stain, modified acid-fast stain, calcofluor stain, direct fluorescent antibody tests, and cytologic analysis to enable rapid diagnosis of infection with bacteria, mycobacteria, *Nocardia*, fungi, *Legionella*, viruses, and *P. carinii*. The bronchoalveolar lavage should be inoculated onto solid media and appropriate cell lines to enable culture of pathogens cultivable by such techniques. Molecular diagnostic testing may be appropriate in some instances. An outline of the diagnostic approach in immunocompromised patients is given in Table 155-4.

MAJOR MANIFESTATIONS OF INFECTION IN IMMUNOCOMPROMISED PATIENTS

Three major sites of infection in immunocompromised patients are discussed—pulmonary infection, CNS infection, and gastrointestinal tract infection. A large variety of organisms can cause infections at these sites. The organism causing infection in an individual immunocompromised patient sometimes can be inferred by the specific host defect in immunologic defense or the specific clinical manifestation. In most circumstances, the differential diagnosis is too broad, however, for definitive clinical diagnosis.

PULMONARY INFECTION

Pneumonia is a significant cause of morbidity and mortality in immunocompromised patients. In contrast to in the normal host, the impaired responsiveness of the immune system means that the disease presents in unusual ways, which may lead to challenges in establishing a diagnosis.

Infectious microorganisms usually gain access to the respiratory tract through inhalation, although hematogenous spread, direct inoculation, or pathogenic transformation of normal airway flora sometimes may occur. Mechanical defenses remove the bulk of potentially harmful agents from the lungs (Table 155-5). Inhaled particles greater than 10 μm in diameter usually become trapped in the upper airways or are removed by coughing or mucociliary clearance.

TABLE 155–6. OCCURRENCE OF PULMONARY INFECTION AFTER SOLID-ORGAN TRANSPLANTATION STRATIFIED BY TIME FROM TRANSPLANTATION

Time After Transplant (mo)	Organism
<1	Methicillin-resistant *Staphylococcus aureus*
	Gram-negative bacilli
	Legionella
	Aspergillus
1-6	Cytomegalovirus
	Aspergillus
	Legionella
	Gram-negative bacilli (if still mechanically ventilated)
>6	*Nocardia*
	Mycobacterium
	Cryptococcus
	Coccidioides immitis

Most bacteria range from 0.5 to 2 μm in size and are able to reach the terminal airways/alveoli and potentially cause infection. In the alveoli, the alveolar macrophages are the first line of defense. Subsequently an inflammatory response consisting of polymorphonuclear neutrophils is important. Finally, specific T-cell and B-cell immune responses are essential for successful defense against many pathogens.

As noted earlier in this chapter, although it may be possible to pinpoint a major immunologic deficiency, most immunocompromised individuals have an assortment of deficiencies in host defense working together. An organ transplant recipient who is on immunosuppressive medication also may be intubated, diabetic, and on corticosteroids and tacrolimus. All these factors contribute to the overall degree of immunity, each paving the way for its peculiar array of susceptibilities to pulmonary infection. In solid-organ transplant recipients, specific causes of pulmonary infection are most frequent at certain times post-transplantation (Table 155-6). In a similar manner, specific causes of pulmonary infection are more frequent at different CD4 lymphocyte counts for patients with HIV infection (Table 155-7).

A normal chest radiograph does not rule out pulmonary infection in immunocompromised patients. Additionally, although some diseases have suggestive radiologic findings (e.g., apical cavitations in tuberculosis), most radiographic findings need to be interpreted in the light of all other data available. Sometimes computed tomography may be required (e.g., in the evaluation of pulmonary nodules). Pulmonary nodules have a broad differential diagnosis in immunocompromised patients, including infections due to fungi (especially *Cryptococcus neoformans*, *Coccidioides immitis*, and *Aspergillus fumigatus*), *Nocardia*, mycobacteria, *Rhodococcus equi*, and *Bartonella*. Additionally, carcinomas and post-transplant lymphoproliferative disorders may present with pulmonary nodules. The differential diagnosis of cavitary lesions includes mycobacteria, invasive pulmonary aspergillosis (Fig. 155-2), legionellosis (especially that due to *Legionella micdadei*), and infection with *R. equi*. As noted earlier, the broad differential diagnosis of pulmonary infection in immunocompromised patients mandates early and aggressive diagnostic strategies, such as bronchoscopy with bronchoalveolar lavage sent for a comprehensive battery of microbiologic investigations.

TABLE 155–5. HOST DEFENSES AGAINST RESPIRATORY INFECTIONS AND HOW THEY ARE AFFECTED IN IMMUNOCOMPROMISED PATIENTS

Location	Host Defense	Defect
Upper airway	Filtration	Endotracheal intubation
	Mucociliary apparatus	Cystic fibrosis, cigarette smoking
	Cough	Impaired consciousness
Lower airway (nonspecific)	Alveolar macrophages	Immunosuppressive medication, corticosteroids
	Polymorpho-nuclear leukocytes	Corticosteroids, malnutrition, chemotherapy, malignancies
Lower airway (specific)	B lymphocytes	Hypogammaglobulinemia, CLL, multiple myeloma
	T lymphocytes	AIDS, malignancies, immunosuppressants

AIDS, acquired immunodeficiency syndrome; CLL, chronic lymphocytic leukemia.

TABLE 155–7. ETIOLOGY OF PULMONARY INFECTIONS IN PATIENTS INFECTED WITH HUMAN IMMUNODEFICIENCY VIRUS, STRATIFIED BY CD4 LYMPHOCYTE COUNT

	CD4 Count (cells/mm³)			
	>500	*200-500*	*50-200*	*<50*
Organism	*Streptococcus pneumoniae*	*S. pneumoniae*	*Pneumocystis carinii*	*P. carinii*
	Haemophilus influenzae	*H. influenzae*	*M. tuberculosis*	*Cryptococcus*
		Mycobacterium tuberculosis	*Cryptococcus*	*Cytomegalovirus*
				MAC
				Aspergillus

MAC, *Mycobacterium avium* complex.

CENTRAL NERVOUS SYSTEM INFECTIONS

Most infectious agents reach the CNS via hematogenous dissemination from an extraneural site. (Exceptions include retrograde propagation of infected thrombi within emissary veins, spread along olfactory nerves, and spread from a contiguous focus of infection.) The blood-brain barrier presents a natural and efficient barrier to hematogenous infection. The function of the blood-brain barrier in immunocompromised patients has not been well studied. It is well known, however, that when CNS infection is established, immune defenses (even in immunologically competent hosts) are inadequate to control the infection. Local opsonization is deficient within the brain. In animal models of bacterial brain abscess, corticosteroid administration led to a reduction in macrophage and glial response, with an increased number of viable bacteria in the brain abscess.[18]

Bacterial meningitis due to *N. meningitidis* is relatively uncommon in immunocompromised patients. In contrast, pneumococcal meningitis seems to occur with increased frequency in patients who have undergone bone marrow transplantation[19,20] and in patients with HIV infection.[21] Meningitis due to *Listeria monocytogenes* is classically associated with immunocompromise, reflecting the need for adequate T-cell function and interferon-gamma production to kill this intercellular pathogen.[22] In addition to meningitis, *Listeria* infection may be associated with brain abscess, particularly that occurring in the brainstem.[23,24] Enteric bacteria

(e.g., *Escherichia coli*) are rare causes of bacterial meningitis in immunocompromised patients. A classic association exists, however, between meningitis with such organisms and disseminated infection with *Strongyloides stercoralis*.[25,26] In the presence of immunosuppresssion (e.g., large doses of corticosteroids), *Strongyloides* can migrate from the gastrointestinal tract to the CNS, carrying enteric bacterial flora with it. Mortality is high without prompt recognition and treatment. *Nocardia* and mycobacteria also need to be considered in the differential diagnosis of CNS infections in immunocompromised patients, and diagnostic samples need to be sent for inoculation onto appropriate media for the isolation of these organisms.

Fungal infection of the CNS may cause meningitis or space-occupying lesions. Cryptococcal meningitis is associated with advanced HIV infection (CD4 lymphocyte count <100/mm³), but also can occur in transplanted patients.[27] The presentation is usually subacute, although dangerous elevations in intracranial pressure sometimes are observed. Space-occupying lesions in the brain may occur with disseminated mold infections (Fig. 155-3). These infections usually arise in the lung, but dissemination to the brain is part of multiorgan spread. Mortality is extremely high. Any of the pathogenic molds, such as *Aspergillus*,[2] Zygomycetes,[28]

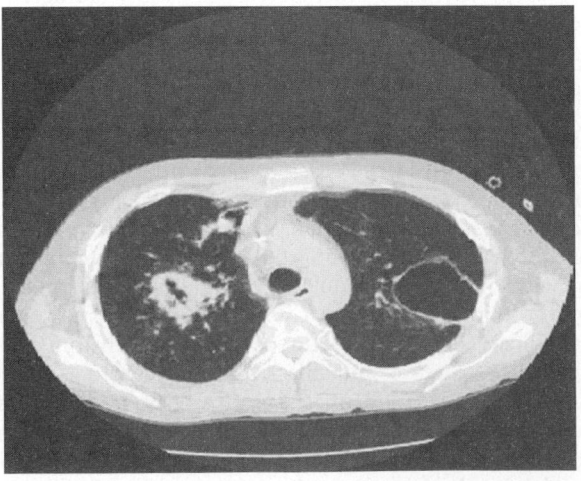

FIGURE 155–2. Computed tomography of the chest in a bone marrow transplant recipient with invasive pulmonary aspergillosis.

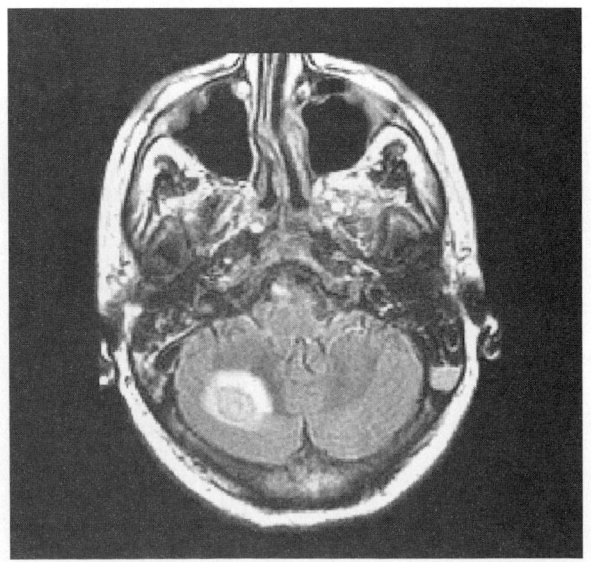

FIGURE 155–3. Magnetic resonance imaging of the brain in an intestinal transplant recipient with disseminated *Scedosporium apiospermum* infection.

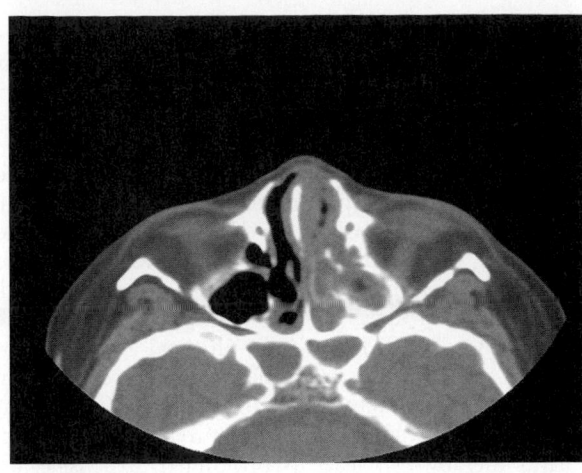

FIGURE 155–4. Invasive mucormycosis in a renal transplant recipient with a recent history of alemtuzumab administration for acute cellular rejection.

Scedosporium,[29] or *Fusarium*,[30,31] can undergo dissemination to the brain. The dimorphic fungi (e.g., *Histoplasma*, *Coccidioides*) also may disseminate from the lung, causing infection of the CNS. Zygomycetes also may be associated with frequently fatal infection arising within the nose or sinuses (rhinocerebral mucormycosis) (Fig. 155-4).[32]

The most common protozoal pathogen to affect the CNS is *Toxoplasma gondii*. The classic association is between *T. gondii* infection and advanced HIV infection, although cases have been reported associated with other forms of immunocompromise.[33] Amebic encephalitis has been reported occasionally in conjunction with advanced HIV infection.[34]

A variety of viruses can cause CNS infections in immunocompromised patients. Perhaps as a result of the widespread use of acyclovir prophylaxis in many immunocompromised populations, herpes simplex virus encephalitis is rare.[35] Some of the newer herpesviruses, such as human herpesvirus-6, have been associated with neurologic infection in transplant recipients.[36,37] Lack of diagnostic capabilities for these viruses may partially explain their apparent infrequency. Cytomegalovirus meningoencephalitis is well described in patients with advanced HIV infection[38] and occasionally has been reported in transplant recipients.[39] Disseminated infection with varicella-zoster virus in immunocompromised patients also may result in CNS infection. West Nile virus may be acquired from transplanted organs or blood transfusions and is associated with a significant meningoencephalitis in transplant recipients.[40,41]

As can be seen from the previous description of a wide variety of organisms causing CNS infection, there is a need for a broadly based diagnostic workup before empirical therapy is begun. If cerebrospinal fluid is collected, it should be sent for Gram stain and Ziehl-Neelsen stain for rapid diagnosis of bacterial and mycobacterial infections. Polymerase chain reaction can be applied to the diagnosis of some viral infections, such as herpes simplex virus, cytomegalovirus, and varicella-zoster virus. Cryptococcal antigens can be detected rapidly in cerebrospinal fluid, enabling a rapid diagnosis of this form of meningitis. Cerebrospinal fluid may not be able to be collected in patients with space-occupying lesions of the brain. Fine-needle aspiration may be performed in some circumstances. Before invasive diagnostic testing of the brain is performed, however, the patient's

skin is examined for lesions (such as may occur with cryptococcosis or nocardiosis), and the lungs are carefully reviewed by computed tomography. Because most CNS lesions have disseminated from other parts of the body, a diagnosis is often made more easily by microbiologic sampling of these body sites.

GASTROINTESTINAL INFECTIONS

Severe gastrointestinal infections in immunocompromised patients occasionally may warrant ICU admission because of dehydration or visceral perforation. As with respiratory and CNS infections, the differential diagnosis is usually broad, and a precise diagnosis rarely can be made based on clinical suspicion only. Immunocompromised patients have an increased predisposition to gastrointestinal infections depending on the type and degree of immunocompromise and exposure to certain pathogens.

The most commonly involved organisms in the etiology of infective esophagitis or gastritis are *Candida*, cytomegalovirus, and herpes simplex virus, although a variety of other organisms (e.g., mycobacteria, Zygomycetes) occasionally are implicated. Candidal esophagitis is the most common opportunistic infection in patients with AIDS. Rates of about 13.3 events of candidal esophagitis per 100 person-years occur in HIV-infected patients with CD4 counts less than $300/mm^3$.[42] A study of renal transplant patients in the United States showed that esophageal candidiasis is the most common fungal infection in these patients, making up 22% of all fungal infections.[43] Other predisposing factors for severe esophageal candidiasis include broad-spectrum antibiotic therapy, steroid therapy, cancer chemotherapy, diabetes mellitus, cutaneous burns, radiotherapy, and hematologic stem cell transplant. Although *Candida albicans* is the most frequently diagnosed organism, there is an increase

TABLE 155–8. CENTRAL NERVOUS SYSTEM INFECTIONS IN THE IMMUNOCOMPROMISED HOST

Etiologic Agent	Special Considerations
Meningitis	
Streptococcus pneumoniae	Especially in HIV-infected individuals
Listeria monocytogenes	Predilection for brainstem
Enteric bacteria	Associated with disseminated *Strongyloides* infection
Cryptococcus neoformans	Rapid diagnosis by cryptococcal antigen or India ink stain
Mycobacterium tuberculosis	Consider PCR for rapid diagnosis
Meningoencephalitis	
Herpes simplex virus	Rare in immunocompromised patients
Human herpesvirus-6	May be associated with lack of CSF pleocytosis
Varicella-zoster virus	Skin lesions yield diagnosis
West Nile virus	Transmitted via transplanted organ or blood
Space-occupying Lesions	
Nocardia	Pulmonary lesions usually also present
Toxoplasma gondii	Especially in HIV-infected individuals
Fungi	Pulmonary lesions usually also present

CSF, cerebrospinal fluid; HIV, human immunodeficiency virus, PCR, polymerase chain reaction.

of other species, including *Candida krusei* and *Candida glabrata*—this is notable because of the increase in resistance to fluconazole in these species. Finally, as noted previously in this chapter, patients with immunocompromise may have a combination of pathogens causing infection at any one time. Upper gastrointestinal endoscopy with biopsy is the gold standard for making the diagnosis.

Diarrhea is a common problem in immunocompromised patients with multifactorial etiologies. It may lead to diagnosis of immunosuppression in a previously undiagnosed patient when an opportunistic pathogen is found and appropriately investigated. Severe complications, such as malabsorption leading to malnutrition, dehydration, and wasting, can occur. Occasionally, intestinal perforation may result from gastrointestinal infection. In an immunosuppressed patient, it is important to differentiate diarrhea caused by opportunistic infections from diarrhea caused by neoplasms, graft-versus-host disease, drugs, and other therapeutic agents. Graft-versus-host disease accounts for more diarrhea in blood and bone marrow transplant patients than infective organisms.[44] In these patients, organisms that cause mild, self-limiting disease in the normal host may cause severe and life-threatening infections.[44]

Prolonged use of multiple antibiotics in high doses predisposes patients to colonization with *Clostridium difficile* and development of pseudomembranous colitis. Antibiotic prophylaxis to prevent *P. carinii* pneumonia or spontaneous bacterial peritonitis has been associated with *C. difficile*. In addition to the classic antibiotic risk factors of clindamycin or cephalosporin use, studies suggest that fluoroquinolones may increasingly predispose to *C. difficile*.[45]

Enteric bacterial pathogens, such as *Salmonella*, occur at increased frequency in immunocompromised patients, especially HIV-infected individuals. In some regions of Africa, nontyphoidal *Salmonella* infections are among the most common causes of bacteremia.[46] Severe *Salmonella* infections may be associated with intestinal perforation. *Shigella*, *Campylobacter jejuni*, *E. coli* (enterotoxigenic, enteroadherent, and enteroaggregative), and *Yersinia* species are other bacterial causes of diarrhea, although less commonly associated with bacteremia.

Protozoal infections are seen more commonly in HIV-infected patients than other immunocompromised groups. At CD4 counts less than 200 cells/mm³, patients with HIV infection may present with unusual protozoa (e.g., *Cryptosporidium* and *Microsporidium*). Occasionally, these pathogens also are seen in transplant recipients.[47-49] These pathogens are not detected on routine microscopic examination for ova, cysts, and parasites. Special stains and microbiologic techniques are needed. Routine examination usually detects *Giardia lamblia*, *Entamoeba histolytica*, and other more common pathogenic protozoa.

Cytomegalovirus can cause significant colitis in all immunocompromised populations. Cytomegalovirus colitis may occur in the absence of systemic evidence of infection (i.e., tests on peripheral blood, such as for the cytomegalovirus PP65 antigen, may be negative[50]). Intestinal biopsy may be required to make the diagnosis. Cytomegalovirus intestinal infection may present with diarrhea, but may have more profound presentations, such as with intestinal perforation.[51-53]

Finally, mycobacterial infections, such as tuberculosis, occasionally can be associated with colitis.[54] *M. avium* complex can be grown readily from the feces of patients with HIV infection and CD4 counts of less than 50/mm³, but it is frequently not the cause of diarrhea in such patients.

THERAPEUTIC DIFFICULTIES IN IMMUNOCOMPROMISED PATIENTS

EMPIRICAL THERAPY

The choice of empirical antimicrobial therapy is often difficult in immunocompromised patients because of the broad differential diagnosis involved. As emphasized earlier, management of infection in an immunocompromised patient can be simplified by narrowing the differential diagnosis by thorough history taking, review of prior medical records, and careful physical examination. Aggressive early diagnostic maneuvers, before beginning empirical antimicrobial therapy, can enable a definitive diagnosis to be made. Failure to collect cultures before beginning empirical therapy can lead to prolonged, expensive, and unnecessary therapy.

Empirical antibiotic therapy in suspected bacterial infections should be tailored to the individual patient to maximize the chance that empirical therapy is microbiologically adequate. There is a clear link between microbiologically adequate empirical therapy and successful outcome from infections in the ICU.[55] In settings such as severe pneumonia in the immuncompromised patient, empirical regimens comprising vancomycin, ciprofloxacin, meropenem, amphotericin, ganciclovir, and trimethoprim/sulfamethoxazole may be necessary to cover potentially lethal infection with methicillin-resistant *Staphylococcus aureus*, *P. aeruginosa*, *Legionella*, fungi, cytomegalovirus, and *P. carinii*. Amphotericin usually is preferred as empirical antifungal therapy for suspected fungal pneumonia because it has activity against Zygomycetes, which neither voriconazole nor the echinocandins possess. There is no established role for combination empirical therapy with antifungal agents. The decision to start empirical mycobacterial therapy is never an easy one. In general, we advise against it, unless there is a clear risk factor for tuberculosis. Empirical therapy for disseminated *Strongyloides* infection may have a place in immunocompromised patients coming from an endemic area and with the classic presentation of disseminated infection.

Immunocompromised patients presenting with acute meningitis should receive treatment that covers *S. pneumoniae* and *L. monocytogenes*. The combination of vancomycin, ampicillin, and ceftriaxone may be necessary (vancomycin and ceftriaxone for multidrug-resistant *S. pneumoniae* and ampicillin for *Listeria*). The combination of amphotericin and 5-flucytosine is recommended empirically for meningitis, in which India ink stain of cerebrospinal fluid reveals encapsulated fungi, consistent with *C. neoformans*. Immunocompromised patients with space-occupying lesions of the brain can be treated empirically with an antifungal drug (amphotericin or voriconazole) if suspicion of disseminated fungal infection is high, although nocardiosis, toxoplasmosis, or mycobacterial infection would not be covered without specific therapy.

For immunocompromised patients with severe diarrhea requiring ICU admission, empirical treatment with metronidazole (for *C. difficile*) and ganciclovir (for cytomegalovirus) may be given after fecal samples have been collected and colonic biopsy performed. For immunocompromised patients with intestinal perforation, antibiotic coverage against gut flora (i.e., treatment of peritonitis) plus treatment of the most likely causes of perforation (e.g., ganciclovir for cytomegalovirus) may be chosen.

PATHOGEN-DIRECTED THERAPY

The importance of appropriate specimen collection is that empirical therapy can be streamlined if cultures or other diagnostic tests are positive. With immunocompromised patients, antimicrobial therapy often is complicated by drug interactions or adverse drug reactions. Transplant recipients taking calcineurin inhibitors (e.g., cyclosporine or tacrolimus) or HIV-infected patients taking protease inhibitors are most at risk because these drugs may be metabolized by the cytochrome P-450 system. Significant interactions may occur between rifampin, macrolide antibiotics, azole antifungal drugs, and the calcineurin inhibitors.[56] Aggressive treatment of infections in immunocompromised hosts (e.g., with amphotericin, pentamidine, or foscarnet) may be associated with renal dysfunction, compounding the nephrotoxic effects of the calcineurin inhibitors. Antimicrobial agents, such as linezolid or ganciclovir, frequently may cause neutropenia, potentially adding further host defense defects.

CONCLUSION

Infection is likely to be the most significant problem an immunocompromised patient faces. Immunocompromised patients may present with severe infection or may acquire infection while critically ill for other reasons. Prevention of infection in the ICU is of primary importance. Pneumonia can be readily prevented by many strategies. Ventilator-associated pneumonia may be prevented by semirecumbent posturing and use of sucralfate (rather than H_2 blockers) for stress ulcer prophylaxis.[57] Aspiration of subglottic secretions and selective digestive tract decontamination are still controversial. Opportunistic pneumonia with *P. carinii* can be prevented by use of prophylaxis with trimethoprim/sulfamethoxazole, dapsone, or nebulized pentamidine. Environmental exposure to *Legionella, Aspergillus,* and *M. tuberculosis* can be prevented by ensuring water purification techniques (e.g., copper-silver ionization) and by preventing exposure of patients to construction activity or infected patients.

Many extrapulmonary infections can be prevented. Cytomegalovirus infection can be prevented by ganciclovir or valganciclovir prophylaxis, although some centers prefer a preemptive approach using serial monitoring of peripheral blood.[58] A similar preemptive approach may be useful in preventing aspergillosis by monitoring peripheral blood for the galactomannan antigen.[59,60] *C. difficile* infection is difficult to prevent because there is a clear need for antibiotic therapy for immunocompromised patients with infection. It remains to be seen whether experimental therapies, such as ramoplanin, play a role in this regard. Finally, attention to classic infection control practices, such as hand hygiene and contact isolation, is paramount in immunocompromised patients.

ANNOTATED REFERENCES

Anaissie EJ, Stratton SL, Dignani MC, et al: Pathogenic *Aspergillus* species recovered from a hospital water system: A 3-year prospective study. Clin Infect Dis 2002;34:780-789.

Although it is widely believed that inhalation of Aspergillus is the first step in development of invasive pulmonary aspergillosis, this study documented the occurrence of Aspergillus in hospital water systems. Protection against aspergillosis may be aided by prevention of exposure of immunocompromised patients to water that is not sterile.

DeSalvo D, Roy-Chaudhury P, Peddi R, et al: West Nile virus encephalitis in organ transplant recipients: Another high-risk group for meningoencephalitis and death. Transplantation 2004;77:466-469.

Emerging infectious diseases pose a considerable risk to immunocompromised patients. They may function as "the sentinel chickens" of societies. This study documented the effects of West Nile virus infection in an immunocompromised patient population.

Keane J, Gershon S, Wise RP, et al: Tuberculosis associated with infliximab, a tumor necrosis factor alpha-neutralizing agent. N Engl J Med 2001;345:1098-1104.

Although patients with rheumatoid arthritis may become immunocompromised by way of therapy with corticosteroids or methotrexate, the development of anticytokine agents for this condition has opened the way for a new range of opportunistic infections in this patient population. This study showed that tuberculosis occurs with increased frequency in patients receiving infliximab.

Kowalski R, Post D, Schneider MC, et al: Immune cell function testing: An adjunct to therapeutic drug monitoring in transplant patient management. Clin Transplant 2003;17:77-88.

The degree of immunocompromise and the subsequent risk of infection in transplant recipients have been difficult to quantify. This study examined the utility of an in vitro immune cell function assay as a means of quantifying global immune response in transplant recipients.

Neff GW, Bonham A, Tzakis AG, et al: Orthotopic liver transplantation in patients with human immunodeficiency virus and end-stage liver disease. Liver Transpl 2003;9:239-247.

Patients with HIV infection treated with highly active antiretroviral therapy are less likely to become immunocompromised than patients who do not receive this therapy. Many patients with HIV infection have coincident hepatitis C virus or hepatitis B virus infection, however. This study shows that liver transplantation, with all its attendant risks due to iatrogenic immunocompromise, can be performed safely in patients with HIV infection.

Chapter 156

INFECTIOUS ENDOCARDITIS

Helen Giamarellou • Anastasia Antoniadou

KEY POINTS

1. **ICU infectious endocarditis shares overlapping characteristics with nosocomial infectious endocarditis** (NIE) either acquired in the ICU or being an emergency necessitating critical care. NIE is defined as IE occurring 48 hours or more after admission or related to intervention performed 4 to 8 weeks before admission. It shares rather low incidence but high morbidity and mortality.

2. **NIE can involve either native valves (NVE) or prosthetic valves (PVE).** Mitral or aortic involvement is most often encountered, and medical/surgical interventions and instrumentations (e.g., intravascular devices, pacemakers) are the usual risk factors.

3. **Major pathogens in NIE** (90%) include staphylococci (*S. aureus* in device-associated endocarditis and coagulase-negative strains of *Staphylococcus* (–S. CNS) in PVE), *Enterococcus faecalis* as the second most common pathogen, and, among gram-negative organisms, *Pseudomonas aeruginosa* (mostly implicated in hemodialysis-associated NIE).

4. **Mortality of NIE** is higher in the elderly, in those with *S. aureus* and fungal endocarditis, and in those with early PVE. Early surgical intervention is mandatory.

5. **Fungal endocarditis** is rare, presenting as a complication of intravascular instrumentation or surgery or in the context of immunocompromise. *Candida* is the most common fungal causative agent. Delayed diagnosis, major embolic phenomena, and large vegetations are the rule. Combined surgical and medical treatment of long duration is needed to ameliorate the high (>50%) mortality rate.

6. **Nosocomial PVE** is classified as "early" (8 weeks to 1 year) or "late." *Methicillin-resistant S. epidermidis* is the pathogen predominating in early PVE, whereas *S. aureus* is the cause of the most lethal type of early PVE.

7. **Transesophageal echocardiography** (TEE) has enhanced our diagnostic approach in NIE (NVE or PVE) especially when the **DUKE diagnostic clinical criteria** are effectively used.

8. **ICU-acquired infectious endocarditis** shares a low but increasing incidence. It appears long after admission and is related to medical or surgical procedures and devices, and *S. aureus* is the predominating pathogen. Prolonged fever may be the only clinical feature, and TEE is a sensitive tool for effective diagnosis.

9. **NIE** requires early suspicion and pursuit of diagnosis and prompts initiation of antimicrobial therapy and cardiosurgical evaluation to perform early valve replacement as soon as this is indicated (by complication or pathogen type)

Nosocomial infectious endocarditis (NIE) is defined as the infective endocarditis (IE) that occurs 48 hours or more after admission to the hospital or as endocarditis that is related to an intervention performed in the hospital within 4 to 8 weeks before admission.[1-3] Early prosthetic valve endocarditis (PVE) is therefore NIE fulfilled by the latter definition. It has been estimated that NIE occurs in 0.8 of 10,000 hospital admissions and is diagnosed late during hospitalization (39 ± 25 days).[4] When compared with the 2.5 million cases (at least) of nosocomial infections occurring per year in the United States, the overall incidence of NIE seems to be low[5]; however, the associated morbidity and high mortality renders NIE of great importance for the clinician.

Because ICU-acquired endocarditis shares several overlapping characteristics with NIE in this review, NIE both on native and prosthetic valves is briefly described and IE "as an emergency" necessitating critical care is also discussed.

NOSOCOMIAL NATIVE VALVE ENDOCARDITIS

During the past decade 14% to 25% of all cases of IE have been considered as nosocomial.[6,7] It is, however, expected that the incidence will increase in the future because of (1) an increase in the incidence of nosocomial bacteremia; (2) improvement in survival of immunocompromised patients; (3) the steady increase in the number of ICU beds admitting seriously ill patients worldwide; and (4) the augmented survival rate of elderly patients in whom degenerative heart disease and/or prosthetic valves are more frequently encountered.[1,8]

Among episodes of NIE, 9.1% to 48% have been associated with central intravenous catheters and 6% to 22.7% with peripheral intravenous catheters, whereas 2% to 9% of Swan-Ganz catheterizations have been complicated with NIE.[3,4,9,10]

In 20% to 30% of patients with NIE, previous genitourinary tract surgery or instrumentation has been incriminated as the source of bacteremia.[3,4,9] The mitral and aortic valves are most often involved in NIE, with infected pacemaker leads or central intravascular catheters being the source of bacterial seeding to the tricuspid valve.[3,4,9] Excluding patients with early prosthetic valve endocarditis, 17% to 45% of cases with NIE have been reported to involve prosthetic valves.[3,4,11]

Staphylococci (both *S. aureus* and coagulase-negative strains) represent the major pathogens in NIE. *S. aureus* is responsible for 52% to 57% of NIE episodes, 91% of which have an intravascular device as the most probable source of bacteremia.[3,4,12,13] Coagulase-negative staphylococci, particularly *S. epidermidis,* has been isolated in approximately 40% of patients with NIE, 89% of whom have prosthetic valves in situ. When early prosthetic valve endocarditis is excluded, only 4% to 21% of NIE is attributed to coagulase-negative staphylococci.[6] *Enterococcus faecalis* represents the second most frequent pathogen in NIE, accounting for 5% to 30% of cases,[3,4,9] and the genitourinary tract is incriminated as the source of enterococcal bacteremia in 14% to 70% of NIE.[14] Gram-negative bacilli are rare causes of NIE, despite the fact that they cause lethal bacteremias in hospitals, probably as a result of their decreased ability to adhere to heart valves.[2] On the contrary, *P. aeruginosa* because of its adherence characteristics is often implicated in NIE, particularly in hemodialyzed patients.[15]

Fungal infectious endocarditis is a rare infection, comprising less than 10% of IE cases. However, in the past decade, an increased frequency of fungal endocarditis has been observed attributed to the increasing use of vascular lines, as well as to noncardiac surgery and increased numbers of immunocompromised patients.[2,16] The fungi most commonly described are *Candida albicans,* non-*albicans* species of *Candida* (28%), *Aspergillus* species (24%), and *Histoplasma capsulatum* (6%). In the past decade, the incidence of *C. parapsilosis* NIE has increased, with a mortality rate ranging from 36% to 50%.[17] The latter observation has been attributed to (1) the frequent colonization by this organism of the skin and subungual area[17]; (2) the ability of the pathogen to proliferate in glucose-containing solutions (hyperalimentation); (3) the ability to adhere to synthetic material because of slime production; and (4) contamination of intravascular pressure monitoring devices.

Contrary to *Candida* species, in which blood cultures in cases of IE are positive in 83% to 95%, blood cultures are positive in only 11% or less of patients with *Aspergillus* species. In cases of *Curvularia, Penicillium,* and *Phycomyces* infection, blood cultures are 100% negative.[18] In cases in which *Coccidioides immitis, Cryptococcus neoformans, Rhodotorula,* and *Saccharomyces cerevisiae* are involved, blood cultures are essentially positive, if properly collected.[18]

In cases of fungal endocarditis, prolonged symptoms before hospitalization and embolization of major arteries are classic findings. However, diagnosis is delayed or missed in 82% of patients.[16] For fungal endocarditis to be diagnosed early, it should be considered in the differential diagnosis and echocardiography performed, which then demonstrates large, bulky vegetations. Peripheral blood cultures should be obtained and accessible embolic specimens subjected to histologic examination.[16]

In NIE, the mortality rate has been found to be significantly higher in elderly patients (45.3%) than in the middle-aged (32.6%) and young (9.1%).[3] *S. aureus* and fungi are associated with the highest mortality. In the series of Fernandez-Guerrero and colleagues,[9] 75% of patients with *S. aureus* NIE died versus 20% suffering from community-acquired IE. Therefore, in addition to appropriate antimicrobial therapy, early surgical intervention is often mandatory. In fungal endocarditis, removal of the infected valve is indicated followed by postsurgical prophylaxis with oral azoles for 2 or more years and prolonged surveillance to detect relapses.[16,19]

NOSOCOMIAL PROSTHETIC VALVE ENDOCARDITIS

PVE accounts for 9.5% to 15% of all cases of IE, with mortality rates ranging between 25% and 60%.[20,21] It is a distinct and important form of IE because (1) more than 100,000 artificial heart valves are implanted annually in the United States[21] and (2) it is a major therapeutic challenge associated with the difficulty of eradicating infection on foreign material, which as a rule necessitates their surgical removal.

It has been reported that "early" PVE is found less often in porcine than mechanical valves, whereas it is almost absent from homografts.[22,23] However, studies with long-term follow-up have suggested that no significant differences exist in the incidence of PVE related to the valve type.[24]

PVE has been classified as "early" or "late," with the former occurring within 60 days of implantation.[20] Contamination of prosthetic valves at the "early period" occurs either directly at the time of implantation by a break in sterile surgical techniques or via transient episodes of bacteremia emanating mostly from infected intravascular catheters and wound or skin infections while the patient is still hospitalized, representing therefore a real nosocomial infection.[20] Based on the fact that *S. epidermidis,* which is the predominant isolate in "early" PVE, is often recovered up to 1 year after implantation, sharing with the strains isolated in the "early" period the common characteristic of resistance to methicillin, it has been recommended that antimicrobial therapy of "early" PVE should be extended to 1 year postoperatively.[21,24]

In the early postoperative period, the sewn ring and the valve annulus are not yet endothelialized and are therefore a site of thrombus formation and a target for adherence of bacteria.[21] Transient bacteremia can seed these thrombi and incite infection, leading to the formation of large vegetations that may cause functional obstruction or incompetence. As the infection advances, abscesses, fistulas, and progressive annular destruction may further complicate the underlying process, causing conduction blocks, mycotic aortic aneurysms, and even purulent pericarditis.

Microbiology of PVE is shown in Table 156-1. PVE may manifest as an indolent illness with low-grade fever and immune-mediated manifestations or as a fulminant acute febrile disease with hypotension. When early PVE is caused by *S. aureus,* the clinical picture is accompanied in more than 40% of cases by central nervous system (CNS) and intracardiac complications and a subsequent mortality ranging from 42% to 85%.[25]

Recent progress in transesophageal echocardiography (TEE), by applying a high-resolution biplane or multiplane transducer, has enhanced the diagnostic approach to PVE. Studies have demonstrated that the sensitivity of TEE in the diagnosis of PVE ranges from 82% to 96% versus 17% to 36% with transthoracic echocardiography (TTE).[26]

TABLE 156–1. ETIOLOGY OF PROSTHETIC VALVE ENDOCARDITIS VS. NOSOCOMIAL NATIVE VALVE ENDOCARDITIS

	Native Valve Endocarditis		Prosthetic Valve Endocarditis		
	Nosocomial	Community Acquired	≥2 mo	>2-12 mo	>12 mo
Streptococcus species	3%	32%	1.5%	10%	31%
Enterococcus species	10-30%	5-12%	9%	13%	11%
Staphylococcus aureus	37-57%	35-37%	23%	13%	18%
Coagulase-negative *Staphylococcus*	3-7%	5-6%	31%	35%	11%
Gram-negative bacilli	4-6%	4%	14%	3%	6%
Diphtheroids	3%	3%	7%		
HACEK		2%	0%	0%	6%
Fungi	≤10%	2%	9%	6%	1%
Miscellaneous	6-21%	5%	3%	6%	5%
Culture negative	4-7%	16%	3%	13%	8%

Modified from references 5-7, 12, 19, 23, and 26.

The Duke criteria have been used effectively to diagnose PVE, particularly when TEE is used to supplement non-diagnostic TTE.[27,28]

Mortality in PVE is still substantial, being higher in "early" PVE (77%) than in late-onset infection (42%). The leading causes of death in "early" PVE are septic shock (36%), congestive heart failure (29%), and renal failure (21%).[29] The survival rate with medical therapy alone in cases of moderate to severe chronic cardiac failure due to prosthesis dysfunction is almost nil. However, valve replacement in this group plus antimicrobial therapy will achieve a survival rate of 44% to 64%. Therefore, it has become a rule that *S. aureus* PVE should be treated with early surgical intervention. It is noteworthy that PVE recurs in only 6% to 15% of patients who are operated on with active bacterial invasive infection. After surgery for removal of the infected prosthetic valve, antibiotics should be continued for at least 6 weeks.[20,23]

INFECTIVE ENDOCARDITIS IN THE ICU (ICU-IE)

Although in large studies of patients with IE 9% to 14% of cases were considered as hospital acquired, few studies have focused on IE acquired or admitted in the ICU.[3,7,9] The most recent study to report on ICU-IE is that of Gouëllo and associates,[30] who among 4416 ICU hospitalized patients during a 6-year period (1992-1997) described 22 patients with ICU-IE defined by the Duke criteria. The prevalence was 5 cases per 1000 admissions, or 4 patients annually.

Although the incidence of ICU-IE seems to be low, the reported numbers are twofold higher than those previously published in 1988.[3] There are two possible explanations for the noted difference: (1) an increase in invasive procedures with subsequent augmentation of the infective risks and (2) a greater awareness of NIE that can be confirmed by echocardiographic detection. In the review of Gouëllo and associates,[30] for 6 patients NIE was the reason for the ICU admission, whereas for the remaining 17, the time elapsed between admission in the ICU and subsequent diagnosis was quite prolonged (range: 11 to 100 days; mean: 39 ± 25 days). According to the authors' analysis, 16 patients were predisposed to infection and 7 had underlying heart conditions that put them at risk for acute IE: 3 had prosthetic valves, 5 had valvular disease, and 2 had cardiac pacemakers.

In 21 cases NIE was the consequence of bacteremia related to a medical or surgical procedure: 11 intravenous devices, eight surgical wounds, a tracheal procedure, and a leg ulceration. It is also noteworthy that the mean time elapsed between ICU admission and the first positive blood culture was 30 (± 32) days with a range of 3 to 100 days. *S. aureus* predominated in 15 patients, whereas coagulase-negative *Staphylococcus*, *P. aeruginosa*, *Streptococcus* species, and *Candida* species were more rarely isolated. TTE and/or TEE showed vegetations in 9 patients, myocardial abscess in 5 patients, and valvular perforation in 1 patient. All patients were febrile, only in 9 a new murmur was found, whereas in 2 and 1, respectively, embolic events and cardiac failure were observed. The expected classic clinical features of IE should not be expected in ICU patients. For instance, central nervous system (CNS) signs because of sedation may be blunted and manifestations of renal failure are usually attributed to septic multiple organ dysfunction syndrome.

In the series by Gouëllo and associates,[30] the most common portals of entry were infected wounds and intravascular catheters, including peripheral ones. However, no case was directly related to a Swan-Ganz catheter, although the latter, by inducing endocardiac damage, may result in IE whenever patients become bacteremic. It is evident that bacterial seeding of foreign material, such as pacemakers, leads, defibrillators, and prosthetic valves, should be seriously considered in cases of fever of unknown origin in the ICU.[31-33] On the other hand, because the risk of NIE is proportionally increased with the duration of hospitalization, the diagnosis of NIE should always be suspected in the presence of fever of unknown origin with positive blood cultures after a prolonged stay in the ICU. The latter suspicion is strengthened in patients with prosthetic valves and those undergoing procedures that may damage the right side of the heart as well as whenever bacteremia lasts for more than 72 hours after catheter removal and/or positive blood cultures persist 3 days after starting appropriate antimicrobials.[31-33] Therefore, it can be assumed, as Gouëllo and associates[30] have stated, that "persistent fever in ICU patients is a sufficient symptom to promptly perform a cardiac echocardiography, especially a TEE, which is very sensitive for detecting vegetations and paravalvular abscesses."

Wolff and colleagues[25] tried to identify the prognostic survival factors among 122 patients with PVE admitted to the ICU. Despite the fact that their study was carried out between 1978 and 1992, the findings are still important. The predominant pathogens were *S. aureus* (33%), streptococci (20%), CNS (12%), enterococci (10%), and gram-negative bacilli (9%). At 4 months the overall survival was 66%, with *S. aureus* infection being the main predictor of death (75% vs. 15% with other pathogens). In *S. aureus* PVE, multivariate analysis identified prothrombin time less than 30%, concomitant mediastinitis, heart failure, and septic shock as death predictors, whereas in PVE due to other pathogens, prothrombin time less than 30%, renal failure, and heart failure were associated with death. As expected in *S. aureus* PVE, survival was higher in patients who received medical-surgical therapy than in those who received medical therapy alone (45% vs. 0%). In PVE due to other pathogens, no difference in survival between patients who underwent prosthetic valve replacement (89%) and those who received only medical treatment (81%) was observed. The authors concluded that non–*S. aureus* and uncomplicated PVE may be managed without valve replacement but prompt surgical intervention is required in all other situations. It should be also pointed out that the risk of infection of the new prosthesis in patients who undergo surgery before complete sterilization is considered low.

Zanutto and coworkers[34] described their 4-year (1997-2001) experience from 34 cases of acute IE requiring ICU hospitalization. Reasons for transfer to the ICU were severe sepsis in 11 patients, heart failure in 10, respiratory failure in 6, and neurologic or other disorders in 7. Comorbidities were present in 23 (diabetes, 11; intravenous drug abuse, 6). There was no previously known heart disease in 22 patients (65%), and 7 had early prosthetic valve endocarditis. TEE was performed in 31 patients, and vegetations were revealed in 30 (97%, mean diameter: 19 ± 9 mm), abscess in 2, and prosthetic dehiscence in 1. Responsible microorganisms were found in 32 patients (staphylococci: 18 (56%), streptococci: 13 (41%); group D streptococci: 8; and *Coxiella burnetii*: 1). Multiorgan failure developed in 13 patients (39%), 13 (39%) had acute renal failure, 14 patients (42%) were mechanically ventilated, and 12 (37%) required administration of inotropes. Valve surgery was performed in 29 patients (85%). In the remaining 4 patients, surgery was withheld, although it was clinically indicated, because of their poor clinical condition. The death rate was 44% (12 surgically and 3 medically treated patients).

IE in a neonatal ICU from 1983 to 1995 was examined retrospectively by Opie and coworkers using case-matched controls.[35] Of 12,246 infants admitted to this neonatal ICU, IE was identified in 8, an incidence of 0.07%. Presenting symptoms and signs were often vague and nonspecific. Gestation less than 32 weeks, birth weight less than 1500 g, thrombocytopenia, and neutropenia were common features. Infants with endocarditis had a significantly higher Clinical Risk Index for Babies score than those without endocarditis. The tricuspid valve was involved in seven infants, six of whom had a percutaneous central venous catheter in situ before diagnosis. Seven survived following prolonged antibiotic therapy. Because in the premature newborn, presenting signs and symptoms are often nonspecific, IE should be considered in the unwell very low birth weight infant.

In several studies the diagnostic value of echocardiography in the diagnosis of IE and particularly of the transesophageal view has been pointed out.[36-41] In case of a negative TEE, if clinical suspicion is high, a second examination has been advocated.[30] It should be noted that TEE provides an advantageous acoustic window on mechanically ventilated patients in comparison to TTE, where visualization may be poor.[40,42] Significant complications such as bronchospasm, hypoxemia, angina pectoris, pharyngeal bleeding, vomiting, and hematemesis have been reported in less than 4% of ventilated patients subjected to TEE.

NIE in the ICU requires prompt initiation of antimicrobial therapy and cardiosurgical evaluation, keeping in mind that mortality increases sharply with *S. aureus* as a pathogen, with age, and with the origin of the infection, that is, ICU versus community acquired. Of note, treatment duration of catheter-related staphylococcal (*S. aureus*) bacteremia aiming to treat successfully any seeded valve as occurs in 23% of the cases should never be shorter than 2 weeks, and echocardiography should be performed before treatment discontinuation.[43-45]

Prophylaxis of NIE, especially in ICU patients, mandates (1) intravenous access and intravascular procedures to be performed with the utmost aseptic care, (2) blood catheters to remain in place for as brief a duration as possible, and (3) tunnelization, although a controversial issue, to be considered either as an immediate approach for the temporary dialysis catheter or as a systemic procedure if the catheter has been or will be in place for more than 4 days. Antimicrobial prophylaxis is not justified before performing TEE.[46]

ANNOTATED REFERENCES

Durack GT, Lukes AS, Bright DK, and the Duke Endocarditis Service: New criteria for diagnosis of infective endocarditis: Utilization of specific echocardiographic findings. Am J Med 1994;96:200-209.
The initial proposal of Duke clinical diagnostic criteria as a tool to more accurate diagnosis of infectious endocarditis. These criteria have been validated during the past decade and are now widely accepted and used.

Giamarellou H: Nosocomial cardiac infections. J Hosp Inf 2002;50:91-105.
The latest comprehensive review on nosocomial infectious endocarditis includes risk factors, microbiology, types of infection, diagnosis, treatment, and prophylaxis.

Gouëllo JP, Asfar P, Brenet O, et al: Nosocomial endocarditis in the intensive care unit: An analysis of 22 cases. Crit Care Med 2000;28:377-381.
A prospective, cohort study of clinical features, microbiology, diagnosis, and outcome of infectious endocarditis in an ICU.

Heidenreich PA: Transoesophageal echocardiography(TEE) in the critical care patient. Cardiol Clin 2000;18:789-805.
A review of the validity of TEE imaging to the critical care patient, not only for the diagnosis of infectious endocarditis. It can be safely performed and effectively guide further management.

Wolff M, Witchitz S, Chastang C, et al: Prosthetic valve endocarditis in the ICU: Prognostic factors of overall survival in a series of 122 cases and consequences for treatment decision. Chest 1995;108:688-694.
Retrospective analysis of ICU patients with prosthetic valve endocarditis including prognostic factors and treatment outcome.

Chapter 157

FUNGAL INFECTIONS

Paul O. Gubbins

KEY POINTS

OVERVIEW

1. **Generally, fungal infections are more prevalent in ICUs than on the general medical wards.** Although *Candida* species are the most commonly isolated fungi in critically ill patients, infections caused by other opportunistic fungal pathogens (i.e., *Aspergillus, Fusarium, Cryptococcus neoformans,* and agents of zygomycosis) are also a concern in select critically ill populations.

2. The past decade has witnessed significant progress in the development of new antifungal agents. New antifungal agents differ in mode of activity, toxicity, and propensity to interact with other drugs. **Consequently, antifungal therapy can now be tailored to the specific needs of the patient.**

FUNGAL INFECTIONS IN THE CRITICALLY ILL

1. ***C. albicans* is the primary fungal pathogen in the ICU setting, but the prevalence of a given species may vary with age.** For example, candidemia among neonates is predominantly due to *C. albicans* and *C. parapsilosis* and rarely due to *C. glabrata* or other *Candida* species. In adults, *C. glabrata* and *C. albicans* predominate.

2. **Age differences in the isolation of specific species may have important repercussions for infection control, dosing, and selection of antifungal agents in older critically ill patients.**

3. **For the past decade, bloodstream infections (BSIs) due to *C. glabrata* have continually become more prevalent.**

4. **In the ICU *Candida* BSIs are common and difficult to detect, and consequently they carry a relatively poor prognosis.** Although isolation techniques have improved, blood cultures are shown to be positive in 50% of patients with hematogenous candidiasis. The attributable mortality rate associated with *Candida* BSIs is 38%, and *Candida* species are the only pathogens of BSIs that are an independent predictor of mortality. In surviving patients, candidemia adds approximately 1 month to the length of hospital stay.

5. Critically ill patients with hematologic malignancies are at high risk for infections due to *Candida* species and *Aspergillus* species. However, *Fusarium* species, *Pseudallescheria* species, and the Zygomycetes are increasing in frequency. Each of these emerging pathogens has particular clinical characteristics or tissue tropism, and they are often resistant to many antifungal agents. Not surprisingly, infections due to these pathogens are associated with high mortality.

SYSTEMIC ANTIFUNGAL AGENTS

1. Amphotericin B deoxycholate possesses a broad spectrum and a long history of use with little acquired resistance, but its toxicity is renowned and it is potentially costly. In low doses for short courses, this agent is tolerable.

2. Lipid amphotericin B formulations are safer than amphotericin B deoxycholate, but their cost drives their use. Future studies to assess earlier use and novel dosing strategies need to be developed.

3. Triazoles (azoles) possess a broad spectrum and are a relatively safe class of drugs, but they interact with vast array of drugs that are commonly used in ICU populations.

4. Echinocandins, the newest class, are seemingly safe and interact with few drugs, but their spectrum of activity is limited to primarily *Candida* and *Aspergillus* species.

TREATMENT OF FUNGAL INFECTIONS IN THE CRITICALLY ILL

1. **The three paradigms of preventive antimycotic therapy are prophylaxis, empirical therapy, and "preemptive therapy."** There are few data to support the prophylaxis paradigm in the ICU setting. "Empirical therapy," or the initiation of treatment with the first clinical suspicion of infection in the absence of any laboratory evidence of infection, and "preemptive therapy," the initiation of treatment in patients with nonspecific clinical risk factors and laboratory markers indicating high risk, differ little, and the two terms are often used interchangeably.

2. **Studies have demonstrated that in the ICU clinicians now have a choice of antifungal agents to treat candidiasis.** Most studies have focused on the prophylaxis paradigm. However, several prospective, randomized studies comparing empirical amphotericin B deoxycholate to fluconazole for the treatment of candidemia in non-neutropenic hosts have shown that fluconazole is effective and safer. Furthermore, in a prospective, randomized, double-blind study caspofungin has been shown to be at least as effective as amphotericin B deoxycholate for the treatment of invasive candidiasis. Although these studies included ICU patients, there are few comparative studies that assess the efficacy of amphotericin B deoxycholate in preventing or treating candidiasis specifically in the ICU setting.

3. The number of antifungal agents with activity against molds such as *Aspergillus* species is growing, yet options for empirical therapy of infections caused by these pathogens are still limited.

4. **The treatment of cryptococcosis, particularly that in the central nervous system, evolved from a series of classic clinical trials.** Elevations in intracranial pressure (ICP) occur in greater than 50% of patients and contribute significantly to the morbidity and mortality of this infection. **Therefore, in addition to antifungal therapy, elevations in ICP should be managed by sequential lumbar punctures.** Serum and cerebrospinal fluid antigen titers aid in the presumptive diagnosis and assessing the prognosis of infection. **A reduction in antigen titers during therapy is desired, but treatment decisions should be based on culture results.**

Medical advances during the past three decades have improved the prognosis of patients with cancer and other immunodeficiencies. Increasing sophistication in the field of transplantation and other significant medical advances during this time have greatly impacted the management of patients with renal, cardiac, and liver diseases. Moreover, in the past 30 years, advances in neonatology have also increased the survival of premature infants. While such advances have benefited society greatly, they have also fueled the emergence of systemic mycoses over this period. In the 1980s *Candida* species emerged as a significant nosocomial pathogen.[1] Increases in fungal infection rates were observed regardless of hospital type or size. The increases were attributed primarily to *Candida* species, which caused nearly 80% of all nosocomial fungal infections.[1] The rise in fungal infection rates occurred across all infection sites, especially in the bloodstream.[1] By 1990, *Candida* species caused nearly 8% of all nosocomial BSIs.[2,3] The rate of nosocomial candidemia had risen nearly 500% in large teaching hospitals and 200% or more in small teaching hospitals and large nonteaching hospitals.[2] *Candida* BSIs cause significant morbidity and mortality, and *Candida* species are now the fourth leading cause of nosocomial BSIs.[4]

Although *Candida* species are responsible for the vast majority of fungal infections among critically ill patients in general, infections caused by other opportunistic fungal pathogens such as species of *Aspergillus, Fusarium, Cryptococcus neoformans,* and agents of zygomycosis are also a concern in select critically ill populations (e.g., solid organ transplant, hematopoietic stem cell recipients, AIDS patients). Moreover, primary or endemic mycosis caused by *Blastomyces dermatitidis, Histoplasma capsulatum,* and *Coccidioides immitis* can cause severe disseminated infection in select populations as well.

In general, fungal infections are more prevalent in ICUs than on the general medical wards.[5-7] Therefore, the importance of preventing nosocomial fungal infections in the ICU setting is widely recognized. The importance of effective preventive measures against systemic mycosis is widely appreciated in critically ill oncology patients or hematopoietic stem cell transplant (HSCT) recipients. As our understanding of these infections improves, such measures are evolving in the general ICU setting. The past decade has witnessed significant progress in the development of new antifungal agents. These agents differ in mode of activity, toxicity, and propensity to interact with other drugs. Consequently, clinicians can now tailor antifungal therapy to specific patients. Moreover, our understanding of antifungal pharmacodynamics is developing and methods to measure antifungal susceptibility are improving. This chapter examines fungal infections in critically ill patients and reviews the growing selection of systemically acting antifungal agents available to treat these infections.

FUNGAL INFECTIONS IN THE CRITICALLY ILL

CANDIDA INFECTIONS IN THE ICU

Epidemiology

Fungal infections in the ICU setting most often occur in the bloodstream and urinary tract. In the ICU, during the 1980s, *Candida* species caused 10% of all BSIs and 25% of all urinary tract infections (UTIs) and were the fourth most commonly isolated pathogen.[4] Between 1986 and 1995 the proportion of UTIs in the ICU caused by fungi increased 33%, and between 1990 and 1995 *C. albicans* ranked second among all isolates from catheter-associated UTIs.[8]

C. albicans is also the fourth most common pathogen of BSIs in the ICU setting and is superseded by coagulase-negative staphylococci, *Staphylococcus aureus,* and enterococci.[8,9] An analysis of data from the ICU component of the National Nosocomial Infection Surveillance (NNIS) system reveals a significant decrease in the incidence of nosocomially acquired candidemia among ICU patients from 1989 to 1999.[10] A variety of surveillance reports show infection sites vary by ICU type. At a large teaching hospital during a 7-year period, 50% of all nosocomial fungal BSIs occurred in the surgical ICU and hematology unit. In addition, abdominal fungal infections occurred primarily in the bone marrow transplant and hematology unit. However, 33% of all nosocomial catheter-related fungal UTIs occurred in the surgical and medical ICUs.[5] In contrast, at another institution during a 2-year surgical ICU surveillance, surgical wounds and the urine were more common sites of fungal infection than the bloodstream.[11] Given the prevalence of UTIs in the nosocomial setting, NNIS data from 1986 to 1995 demonstrating that catheter-related UTIs were the most common nosocomial fungal infection in the ICU setting are somewhat intuitive.[4] However, in the National Epidemiology of Mycoses Survey

(NEMIS), a 2-year (1993-1995) study of fungal infections in the surgical and neonatal ICU settings of six different medical centers, BSIs were the most common nosocomial fungal infection.[12] In the NNIS data from 1989 to 1999, the highest rates of BSIs with *Candida* were observed in the medical and pediatric ICUs and the lowest rates were observed in the coronary and cardiothoracic ICUs.[10]

In general, *C. albicans* is the primary fungal pathogen in the ICU setting and is followed by *C. glabrata, C. parapsilosis, C. tropicalis, C. krusei, C. guilliermondii,* and *C. lusitaniae*.[9,10,12,13] This rank order varies little across infection site, but it may vary with age. Surveillance programs have noted that candidemia among neonates is predominantly due to *C. albicans* and *C. parapsilosis* and rarely due to *C. glabrata* or other *Candida* species.[14] In contrast, *C. glabrata* has become an increasingly common cause of candidemia in adult ICU patients. Data from NNIS demonstrate that from 1989 to 1999 there was a significant decline in the incidence of *C. albicans* BSIs and a significant increase in the incidence of *C. glabrata* BSIs among adult ICU patients.[10] *C. glabrata* was the only species that increased as a cause of BSIs during that decade.[14] Other surveillance programs have demonstrated similar age-based significant trends.[15,16] An international surveillance program noted significant declines in BSIs due to *C. albicans* with increasing age, and significantly higher rates of BSIs due to *C. glabrata* were observed in the younger adult groups. Moreover, isolates of *C. glabrata* from older patients had reduced susceptibilities to fluconazole.[15] Age differences in the isolation of specific species may have important repercussions for infection control, dosing, and selection of antifungal agents in older critically ill patients.

C. albicans is part of the normal flora of the gastrointestinal tract and other anatomic sites. BSIs caused by *C. albicans* arise endogenously from the gastrointestinal tract.[4] Patients become colonized with a unique strain over time at multiple body sites before infection finally develops.[4] In the ICU setting, depending on the body site, this colonization can occur for prolonged periods before the infection.[17] Generally, exogenous transmission of *C. albicans* is rare, but it has been reported in the neonatal ICU setting.[4] In contrast, exogenous transmission of non-*albicans Candida* species through indirect contact with the ICU environment is fairly common.[4] *C. parapsilosis* exemplifies this type of transmission. This species is not a human commensal, and colonization before infection is not necessary.[18-20] *C. parapsilosis* infections arise through indirect contact with the ICU environment or other patients.[19,20]

The increased prevalence of *C. albicans* and *C. parapsilosis* among neonatal ICU patients and the increasing prevalence of *C. glabrata* infections among adults has been widely appreciated.[4,10] Some speculate these trends may be a consequence of the preferential amphotericin B use in the pediatric and neonatal ICU settings and widespread use of fluconazole in adults.[5,15] Still, vertical transmission (i.e., mother to infant) of *C. albicans* and horizontal transmission of *C. parapsilosis* through indirect contact between the patient, the ICU environment, other patients, or personnel are well documented and may also contribute to these trends.[4,16] In fact, health care workers may be a primary reservoir for exogenous transmission of *C. parapsilosis* in the ICU. In one study 58% of ICU health care workers carried *Candida* species on their hands and *C. parapsilosis* was isolated from 52% of these health care workers' hands.[21]

Mortality

Candida BSIs are often difficult to detect. On the basis of symptoms, BSIs due to *Candida* species are often indistinguishable from BSIs of bacterial etiology. *Candida* species are cleared from the blood very efficiently by several organs, particularly the liver; and although isolation techniques have improved, not surprisingly, blood cultures are shown to be positive in only 50% of patients with hematogenously disseminated candidiasis.[22]

Candida BSIs carry a relatively poor prognosis, owing in part to the difficulty in establishing the diagnosis. Regardless of the cause, the overall attributable mortality of nosocomial BSIs, among critically ill patients, is 35%.[23] This mortality rate for BSIs in general is comparable to the mortality rate associated with BSIs due to *Candida* species. The crude mortality rate associated with *Candida* BSIs hospital-wide and in the ICU setting is 35% to 69%, and the attributable mortality is 38%.[24,25] Some centers report that mortality rates associated with *Candida* BSIs are among the highest of any BSI etiology.[24] Moreover, *Candida* species are the only BSI pathogens that have been identified as independent predictors of mortality.[24] In surviving patients, candidemia adds approximately 1 month to the length of hospital stay.[26]

Risk Factors

Among critically ill patients, risk factors for candidal infections are well described. Several, including broad-spectrum antimicrobial use, colonization, indwelling vascular catheters, and hemodialysis, have been identified as independent risk factors for *Candida* BSIs.[24] In most ICU settings many of these risk factors are unavoidable. For example, ICU patients account for less than 20% of hospital admissions yet broad-spectrum antibiotic use in this setting is significantly higher than in the non-ICU setting.[8,27] Studies have demonstrated that at a threshold inoculum *Candida* species can translocate from the intestinal tract to the bloodstream.[21,28] This threshold is often achieved as a consequence of antibiotic-induced changes in endogenous microflora. One study suggests that the number of antibiotics, and not the duration of antibiotic therapy, was a significant predictor of developing *Candida* BSIs.[24]

Although colonization with *Candida* species often precedes the development of infection, the inability to predict the likelihood a colonized site will progress to infection hinders the utility of this risk factor. Investigators have suggested colonization of the urinary tract (e.g., candiduria) is a harbinger of disseminated candidiasis in the ICU setting.[29] However, several studies have shown progression of infection from a urinary source to the bloodstream rarely occurs. Instead, candiduria may reflect a previously undetected BSI.[30]

OPPORTUNISTIC FUNGAL INFECTIONS IN IMMUNOCOMPROMISED CRITICALLY ILL PATIENTS

Invasive Aspergillosis in Critically Ill Patients with Hematologic Malignancies

Infections due to *Candida* species are common in the ICU setting. However, certain critically ill populations are also at risk for other opportunistic systemic mycoses as a consequence of their underlying disease. For example, *Aspergillus* species rarely cause infection in critically ill surgical patients but are important systemic pathogens in patients with significantly impaired immune function. Invasive aspergillosis is a frequent and deadly complication of cytotoxic chemotherapy, prolonged corticosteroid therapy, solid organ transplantation or HSCT, and other congenital or acquired immunodeficiencies. *Aspergillus* species are ubiquitous environmental molds, and most *Aspergillus* infections are acquired exogenously, via inhalation. In the absence of an effective immune response, airborne conidia invade sinus or lung vasculature. Although the lung is the most common site of invasive aspergillosis, *Aspergillus* species also demonstrate tropism for cutaneous, central nervous system, and cardiac vasculature.

In general, the incidence of invasive aspergillosis in patients with hematologic malignancies is approximately 10%, but it varies among specific populations.[31] Among patients with hematologic malignancies, patients with acute myelogenous leukemia have the highest incidence of invasive aspergillosis. The incidence of this disorder is higher among allogeneic HSCT recipients than among autologous HSCT recipients. In the HSCT population, data suggest the incidence of invasive aspergillosis is increasing.[32] The distribution is apparently bimodal, occurring early and late in the course of transplantation.[33] Prolonged neutropenia after cytotoxic chemotherapy or HSCT is the primary risk for early invasive aspergillosis in patients with acute leukemia or HSCT recipients. Excluding the spores from the patient's environment through the use of efficient air filtration is an effective way of preventing early invasive aspergillosis.[31] Late invasive aspergillosis primarily occurs in allogeneic HSCT recipients late in the post-engraftment period, typically in the absence of neutropenia.[33] The primary risk factor for late invasive aspergillosis is corticosteroid and immunosuppressant use in patients with moderate-to-severe acute and chronic graft-versus-host-disease.[31]

The clinical diagnosis of invasive aspergillosis has not improved over several decades, and new diagnostic methods are needed.[31] Lesions associated with invasive pulmonary aspergillosis evolve over a period of weeks. Radiographically, they appear as defined nodular densities. Classically, during a period of significant neutropenia the "halo sign" is detected, whereas in non-neutropenic hosts the "air crescent sign" is present. However, these findings may be nonspecific or absent in HSCT recipients.[34] The use of high resolution CT has increased the sensitivity of the radiographic diagnostic techniques for invasive aspergillosis. However, these improvements alone have not resulted in improved patient outcomes.[34] The serologic detection of fungal antigens such as galactomannan is a noninvasive technique that holds promise for improving the ability to diagnose invasive aspergillosis.

Miscellaneous Pathogens in Critically Ill Patients with Hematologic Malignancies

Candida species and *Aspergillus* species are the primary fungal pathogens in critically ill patients with hematologic malignancies. However, other pathogens such as *Fusarium* species, *Pseudallescheria* species, and the Zygomycetes are increasing in frequency. Each of these less common pathogens has characteristic clinical characteristics or tissue tropism. In addition, they are often resistant to many antifungal agents. Consequently, infections due to these pathogens are associated with high mortality.[34] Of these pathogens, the Zygomycetes (which cause mucormycosis) are the most common among critically ill patients, particularly in a surgical ICU. These angioinvasive pathogens are acquired through inhalation and produce a necrotic infection. Common risks are diabetic ketoacidosis, immunosuppression, organ transplantation, skin damage, and a prolonged ICU stay. Rhinocerebral and paranasal infections are common manifestations of these pathogens.

CRYPTOCOCCOSIS, HISTOPLASMOSIS, AND BLASTOMYCOSIS IN CRITICALLY ILL PATIENTS

Cryptococcus neoformans, H. capsulatum, and *B. dermatitidis* are not common pathogens in the ICU setting. These pathogens can cause infection in patients with intact immune function. However, with the exception of *B. dermatitidis,* severe infections due to these pathogens are more common among critically ill immunocompromised populations, particularly those with the acquired immunodeficiency syndrome (AIDS).

C. neoformans is a ubiquitous encapsulated yeast isolated from diverse environmental sources (i.e., soil, produce, and feces from a variety of birds). This pathogen is primarily acquired by inhalation. In the lung, the organism elicits a cell-mediated response involving neutrophils, monocytes, and macrophages. The cryptococcal polysaccharide capsule, an important virulence factor, facilitates laboratory identification and recognition by host cell-mediated immune response and possesses immunosuppressive properties.[35] For the past several decades the AIDS epidemic has significantly altered the incidence of cryptococcosis. Before the AIDS epidemic, cryptococcosis was an uncommon disease in the United States. However, in several U.S. cities during the mid 1990s, nearly 90% of cryptococcosis cases occurred in AIDS patients.[36] Recently, a decline in the annual incidence of AIDS-specific cryptococcosis was noted in several large cities in the United States and Australia. The decline corresponded to the advent of highly active antiretroviral therapy and other advances in the treatment of AIDS-associated opportunistic infections.[36]

Among critically ill immunosuppressed populations cryptococcal infections typically involve the central nervous system (CNS). The onset of this infection may be acute or gradual, and patients often present with nonspecific complaints. The disease frequently manifests as subacute meningitis or meningoencephalitis; thus, classic meningeal findings such as photophobia or nuchal rigidity may be absent. Although CNS infection likely results from dissemination of a primary infection, evidence of pulmonary disease or other extra-CNS infection is generally lacking in patients with CNS cryptococcosis.[37] The overall mortality associated with cryptococcosis is between 20% and 40%.[37] Mortality due to meningitis is nearly 25%.[37] There are few estimates of mortality associated with pulmonary cryptococcosis, but in AIDS patients this infection has a high mortality rate.

In cases of cryptococcal meningitis characteristic cerebrospinal fluid (CSF) findings may be present; however, CSF leukocyte count can be low and CSF protein and glucose values may be normal. Therefore, CSF analysis for cryptococcal antigen and culture of the organism are required to diagnose cryptococcal meningitis. Detection of organism by India ink stain is highly specific, but it is associated with a low sensitivity ($\approx$50%).[37] Determination of serum cryptococcal antigen using latex agglutination is a highly sensitive

(≈99%) and specific test, and therefore it is an important component of the diagnosis of cryptococcal disease. In patients with cryptococcal meningitis, particularly in those with AIDS, the serum cryptococcal antigen is almost always positive, and usually it is very high (i.e., >1:2048). Detection of antigen in the CSF strongly suggests infection, but in HIV-infected patients false-negative results can occur in up to 10%, even in the presence of positive cultures. The definitive diagnosis of cryptococcal infection requires a positive culture for *C. neoformans*.[37]

Histoplasmosis and blastomycosis are endemic mycoses found primarily in North America. *H. capsulatum* is endemically distributed primarily in the Mississippi and Ohio River Valleys, whereas *B. dermatitidis* is found primarily in the south central United States, in the Mississippi and Ohio River Valleys, and in certain regions of Illinois and Wisconsin. Both pathogens are acquired via inhalation of their spores.[38] The severity of histoplasmosis depends on host immune function and the extent of exposure, particularly in the immunocompetent host. Hematogenous dissemination from the lungs occurs in all infected patients; but in immunocompetent hosts, controlled and calcified granulomas develop in the reticular endothelial system.[38] However, among elderly hosts or those with cell-mediated immune disorders (e.g., HIV infection), progressive disseminated infection readily occurs.[38] After inhalation, *B. dermatitidis* can disseminate from the lungs to other organs as the yeast form. The initial inflammatory reaction involving monocyte-derived macrophages and polymorphonuclear cells results in the development of noncaseating granulomas.[38] The primary pneumonia is often undetected and resolves without sequelae. Endogenous reactivation in the lungs, skin, or bones is often the first sign of infection.

Among critically ill patients histoplasmosis manifests as either chronic pulmonary histoplasmosis or progressive disseminated (extrapulmonary) histoplasmosis. Chronic or cavitary pulmonary histoplasmosis occurs in middle-aged and elderly patients with underlying lung disease that compromises the ability of nonspecific host defenses to effectively clear the organism.[38]

Progressive disseminated histoplasmosis occurs in healthy or critically ill immunocompromised hosts, but it is more common and severe in the latter population (i.e., patients with malignancies or HIV infection). The infection can disseminate to a variety of organs including the reticuloendothelial system, oropharyngeal and gastrointestinal mucosa, skin, adrenal glands, and kidneys.

Blastomycosis occurs as an asymptomatic infection, acute or chronic pneumonia, or disseminated (extrapulmonary) disease.[38] Concurrent pulmonary blastomycosis is usually present with extrapulmonary disease. Extrapulmonary blastomycosis typically afflicts the skin, bones, and genitourinary system.[38] Cutaneous lesions are classically described as verrucous or ulcerative, and they are the most common skin manifestations of this disease.[38] Unless properly sampled and histologically analyzed, the verrucous lesions can be mistaken for a carcinoma. *B. dermatitidis* infects bone in up to 48% of cases.[38] The vertebrae, skull, ribs, and long bones are commonly involved, but any bone can be afflicted. Genitourinary system infection typically manifests as prostatitis only because there is a gender disparity in the incidence of blastomycosis.[38] The diagnosis of either histoplasmosis or blastomycosis is secured with the isolation and identification of the organism from tissue.[38]

SYSTEMIC ANTIFUNGAL AGENTS

AMPHOTERICIN B (AmB) FORMULATIONS

Amphotericin B Deoxycholate
AmB deoxycholate (AmB-d), a polyene antifungal agent, disrupts biologic membranes, thereby increasing their permeability. AmB-d also stimulates the release of cytokines, which causes arteriolar vasoconstriction in the renal vasculature.[39]

Pharmacology and Pharmacokinetics. Following a 0.6-mg/kg AmB-d dose, approximately 70% of the dose is recovered from the urine and feces over a 7-day period; the remaining 30% of the administered dose remains in the body a week after dosing.[40]

Overview of Toxicity. AmB-d causes "infusion-related" reactions, including hypotension, fever, rigors, and chills in approximately 70% of patients.[41] AmB-d also produces "dose-dependent" toxicities, including nephrotoxicity, azotemia, renal tubular acidosis, electrolyte imbalance, cardiac arrhythmias, and anemia.[39] Depending on the population, AmB-d–induced nephrotoxicity occurs in 15% to 80% of patients.[39] The "infusion-related" reactions occur early in therapy and often subside with time. Pretreatment regimens consisting of diphenhydramine (Benadryl), acetaminophen, meperidine, and hydrocortisone are used to prevent "infusion-related" reactions. The efficacy of these regimens is unclear, so their routine use is discouraged, until the "infusion-related" reactions occur, after which they should be employed with subsequent dosing.[41]

Although common and noxious, "infusion-related" reactions rarely cause early termination of AmB-d therapy or interfere with the use of other medicines. In contrast, AmB-d–induced nephrotoxicity, the primary "dose-related" toxicity, is somewhat unpredictable. In addition, in the ICU setting this toxicity often limits the use of AmB-d or interferes with the ability to use other medicines. Determining factors that predispose patients to AmB-d–induced nephrotoxicity has been difficult. Studies to date have used varying definitions of nephrotoxicity; and over the years, AmB-d has been used in a variety of patient populations.[42] Average daily dose, concomitant nephrotoxin use, particularly cyclosporine, and elevated baseline serum creatinine (Scr) have all been identified as risk factors for AmB-d–induced nephrotoxicity.[41,42] In some patient populations adequate saline hydration before dosing can reduce the incidence of AmB-d–induced nephrotoxicity. However, in the ICU setting the utility saline hydration may be limited by fluid restriction employed to manage the fluid status of critically ill patients. Most cases of AmB-d–induced nephrotoxicity in patients who are considered to be at low risk for the development of this complication are mild to moderate and reversible.[43] Severe nephrotoxicity is uncommon; and when it does occur, it, too, is often reversible.[43]

Lipid AmB Formulations
Amphotericin B lipid complex (ABLC), amphotericin B colloidal dispersion (ABCD), and liposomal amphotericin B (LAmB) are lipid formulations of AmB that have proven effectiveness in animal models of systemic mycoses and have demonstrated at least comparable efficacy to AmB-d in humans. They can be administered in higher daily doses for longer periods of time than AmB-d. Most importantly, all have significantly less associated nephrotoxicity than AmB-d.[44]

Pharmacokinetic Comparisons of Lipid AmB Formulations. The lipid AmB formulations differ in physicochemical properties and composition. These differences produce subtle differences in their pharmacokinetic behavior, which may ultimately prove to be clinically significant (Table 157-1). The disposition and activity of these formulations in human tissue is poorly characterized. However, animal data indicate high serum concentrations may influence the delivery of lipid AmB formulations to certain infection sites, such as the CNS and lungs.[45,46]

Toxicity Comparisons of Lipid AmB Formulations. The safety of the lipid AmB formulations is summarized in Table 157-1. Compared with AmB-d, the lipid formulations have significantly less associated nephrotoxicity.[44,47,48] These formulations differ in the incidence of "infusion-related" reactions and other adverse events associated with AmB-d infusion.[44] These reactions rarely result in early termination of therapy.[48,49] In general, compared with AmB-d, LAmB is better tolerated, ABLC is equally tolerated, and ABCD is less tolerated by most patients. Safety comparisons between ABLC and LAmB have produced conflicting results, but comparative data suggest LAmB may be somewhat safer than ABLC.[50] There are limited data comparing the safety of lipid AmB formulations to the triazole antifungal agents in critically ill patients. Given the safety of triazoles, it is unlikely the lipid AmB formulations will prove to be any safer.

In-vitro Susceptibility Testing. For many years clinically relevant antifungal susceptibility testing was nonexistent. Consequently, antifungal therapy in critically ill patients was largely empirical and not guided by susceptibility data. Clinically relevant antifungal susceptibility testing has developed over the past two decades. Currently, the National Committee for Clinical Laboratory Standards (NCCLS) has published an approved reference method for yeasts (M27-A). While this method is fairly established for interpreting susceptibility data for azole antifungal agents and flucytosine, use of this method and interpretation of its results with respect to the AmB formulations has been problematic.

Resistance to AmB formulations by *Candida* species, albeit rare, does exist. Fortunately, AmB resistance is uncommon among the four most commonly isolated species. Nonetheless, the ability of the M27-A method to identify AmB-resistant yeasts is limited and interpretive breakpoints have yet to be proposed for the AmB formulations.[51] Furthermore, although the method describes how to test *C. neoformans*, no interpretive breakpoints for any antifungal agent are specified.[51] The NCCLS has also published a proposed reference method for molds (M38-P). However, the development of this method is still in its infancy. Therefore, at this time caution should be exercised when using susceptibility data to help guide therapy with AmB formulations against yeast or molds. Susceptibility testing of *Candida* isolates from deep sites may be appropriate, but at present it is not widely recommended for other organisms or sites.[51]

AZOLE ANTIFUNGAL AGENTS

Fluconazole, Itraconazole, Voriconazole
In general, the systemic azoles exert a fungistatic effect by dose-dependent inhibition of cytochrome P450 (CYP)–dependent 14α-demethylase, the enzyme necessary for the conversion of lanosterol to ergosterol. This leads to the depletion of ergosterol, the essential sterol of the fungal cell wall, and ultimately compromises cell wall integrity. The degree of inhibition varies among the different azole agents, and this accounts for differences in spectrum of activity.

Pharmacology and Pharmacokinetics. The triazoles differ subtly in chemical properties, which form the basis of the pharmacokinetic differences between the agents and the propensity of this class to interact with other medications. These properties can limit the use of these agents, particularly itraconazole, in the ICU setting. For example, the lack of a liquid formulation often precludes the use of ketoconazole in critically ill patients.

Fluconazole pharmacokinetics have been studied in critically ill patients. Fluconazole clearance in surgical ICU patients correlates with creatinine clearance (CrCl).[52] In surgical ICU patients fluconazole volume of distribution correlates with body weight and is influenced by age.[52] Although fluconazole volume of distribution is higher than that of healthy volunteers, it likely diminishes with increasing age.[52] Consequently, the fluconazole half-life is markedly prolonged in surgical ICU patients.[52] Some authors have recommended dosage reductions of 50% in the patients with severe renal dysfunction (CrCl < 30 mL/min).[52] However, dosage reductions should be made cautiously in patients receiving fluconazole via enteral feeding tubes and with consideration to the infecting pathogen. Most data seem to indicate that the systemic availability of fluconazole is relatively unaffected by this mode of administration. However, one large study demonstrated that serum concentrations obtained with standard doses administered via an enteral feeding tube may not be adequate to treat *C. glabrata* infections.[53] Moreover, based on epidemiology and susceptibility data, higher fluconazole doses may be needed to treat *C. glabrata* BSI.[14]

Itraconazole is a highly lipophilic weak base and practically insoluble in water. It is available as a capsule and as an oral and intravenous solution formulated in hydroxy-propyl-β-cyclodextrin (HP-βCD).[54] Slow and erratic absorption of the capsule form precludes its use in critically ill ICU patients. HP-βCD enhances itraconazole solubility and improves its oral systemic availability. HP-βCD is poorly absorbed from the gastrointestinal tract, stimulates gastrointestinal secretion and propulsion, and causes diarrhea.

Under fasting conditions itraconazole is rapidly absorbed from the oral solution, and compared to the capsule there is less interpatient and intrapatient variability in serum concentrations.[55] Whereas HP-βCD improves itraconazole oral absorption, it hinders the intravenous form of this drug. After intravenous administration, renal elimination of itraconazole is negligible. However, HP-βCD is eliminated primarily by the kidneys (80% to 90%).[56,57] With severe renal impairment (CrCl ≤ 19 mL/min) renal elimination of HP-βCD decreases sixfold.[58] In patients with CrCl less than or equal to 30 mL/min intravenous itraconazole is contraindicated owing to concerns over the renal accumulation of HP-βCD.

Pharmacokinetics of itraconazole administered intravenously for 1 week followed by the oral solution administered either once or twice daily were assessed in 16 patients in the ICU setting. Mean itraconazole plasma concentrations in ICU patients were lower than in healthy volunteers or other patient populations.[59] This finding was attributed to larger volumes of distribution often observed in critically ill populations. The study demonstrated that with this regimen, adequate plasma itraconazole concentrations (= 250 ng/mL) may be achieved and maintained with the 1-week intravenous schedule followed by twice-daily oral administration, whereas

TABLE 157–1. COMPARISON OF PHYSICOCHEMICAL, PHARMACOKINETIC PROPERTIES, AND SAFETY OF THE LIPID-BASED AmB FORMULATIONS

Formulation	AmB Content (Mol%)	Phospholipid Composition	Phospholipid Molar Ratio	Size (µm)	Pharmacokinetic Comparison with AmB-d				Safety Compared with Am B-d			
					Mean C_{max}	Mean V_D	Mean CL	Mean AUC	Nephrotoxicity	IRAE	Electrolyte Disturbances	Cardiopulmonary AE
ABLC	33	DMPC DMPG	7 3	1.6–11.0	↓	↑	↑	↓	↓↓	↔	↓	↓
ABCD	50	Cholestryl sulfate	N/A	0.12–0.14	↓↑	↔↑	↔↑	↔↑	↓↓ ↓↓↓	↔↑	↕ ↕↓	↔↑
LAmB	10	HPC Cholesterol DSPG	2 1 0.8	0.08								

AmB-d, Amphotericin B deoxycholate; Cmax, maximum serum concentrations; VD, volume of distribution; AUC, area under the serum concentration curve; IRAE, infusion-related adverse event; AE, adverse event; ABLC, amphotericin B lipid complex; ABCD, amphotericin B colloidal dispersion; LAmB, liposomal amphotericin B; DMPC, dimyristoylphosphatidylcholine; DMPG, dimirystoylphosphatidylglycerol; HPC, hydogenated phosphatidylcholine; DSPG, distearoylphosphatidylglycerol; ↓, decreased; ↓↓, markedly reduced compared with AmB-d or other lipid AmB formulations; ↓↓↓, significantly reduced compared with AmB and other lipid AmB formulations; ↔, similar; ↑, increased.

the once-daily oral follow-up seems to be a suboptimal treatment.[59] During the oral dosing phase, diarrhea was the most common adverse event.

Voriconazole is a derivative of fluconazole with limited aqueous solubility and improved antifungal activity. It is available in intravenous and oral formulations. Intravenous voriconazole contains sulfobutyl ether β-cyclodextrin (SBECD) as a solubilizing agent. There are limited data on how critically ill patients handle voriconazole. In healthy volunteers, voriconazole exhibits good oral availability and wide tissue distribution, with hepatic metabolism and renal excretion of metabolites.[60] In patients with moderate to severe renal function, SBECD accumulates, and it is recommended that oral dosing be used in patients with a CrCl less than 50 mL/min.[60] Several case reports demonstrate that voriconazole achieves CSF concentrations that are approximately 30% to 70% of concurrent serum concentrations.[60]

Azole Drug Interactions. Drug interactions occur primarily in the intestine, liver, and kidneys by a variety of mechanisms. In the intestine they can occur as a result of changes in pH, complexation with ions, or interference with transport and enzymatic processes involved in gut wall (i.e., presystemic) drug metabolism. In the liver, drug interactions can occur as a result of interference with drug metabolizing enzymes. Drug interactions in the kidney can occur through interference with glomerular filtration, through active tubular excretion, or by other mechanisms. The azoles are one of the few drug classes that can cause or be involved in drug interactions at all of these sites by one or more of the above mechanisms. Drug interactions involving the azoles have been extensively reviewed.[61,62] Several of the drug-drug interactions involving the azoles occur classwide. Therefore, when using the azoles, the clinician must be aware of the many drug-drug interactions, both real and potential, associated with this class.

Interactions involving the azoles result as a consequence of their physicochemical properties. All azoles are somewhat lipophilic and thus undergo CYP-mediated metabolism. The azoles all inhibit one or more CYP enzymes. Of the three azoles reviewed here, only itraconazole appears to interact significantly with P-glycoprotein (P-gp), which is a transport protein involved in drug distribution.[61,62] Fluconazole is not affected by agents that increase gastric pH, but its potential to cause CYP-mediated interactions is more than that suggested by in-vitro studies. CYP-mediated interactions involving fluconazole are often dose dependent and can involve drugs metabolized by CYP3A4 (e.g., midazolam, rifampin, phenytoin) and CYP2C9 (e.g., warfarin).[61,62] Because of its linear and predictable pharmacokinetic properties, these interactions may sometimes be avoided or managed by using the lowest effective fluconazole dose.

Itraconazole is subject to pH-based and interactions involving CYP3A4 and P-gp. Drugs that will likely interact with itraconazole include agents that increase gastric pH (e.g., protonics) and lipophilic, CYP3A4 (e.g., HMG-CoA reductase inhibitors, benzodiazepines, immunosuppressives), and/or P-glycoprotein (P-gp) substrates (e.g., digoxin) with poor oral availability.[62] Voriconazole is not affected by agents that increase gastric pH. However, CYP-mediated interactions involving voriconazole can involve drugs metabolized by CYP3A4 (e.g., midazolam, rifampin, phenytoin), CYP2C9 (e.g., warfarin), or CYP2C19 (e.g., omeprazole).[60] Drug interactions involving the azoles that are relevant to the ICU setting are summarized in Table 157-2.

TABLE 157–2. DRUG INTERACTIONS INVOLVING THE AZOLES IN THE ICU SETTING

Drug	Effect
Drug Interactions that Decrease Itraconazole Plasma Concentrations	
Phenytoin, phenobarbital carbamazepine	Significantly decreases itraconazole concentration
Interactions with Itraconazole that Affect Other Drugs	
Midazolam, triazolam, diazepam	Increases effect of benzodiazepine
Haloperidol	Increases haloperidol concentration 30%
Cyclosporine, tacrolimus	Increases cyclosporine, tacrolimus trough concentration
Digoxin	Increases digoxin serum concentration
Fluconazole Drug-Drug Interactions	
Midazolam, triazolam	Increases effect of benzodiazepine
Cyclosporine	Increases cyclosporine trough concentration
Tacrolimus	No significant effect
Phenytoin	Increases phenytoin concentration
Voriconazole Drug-Drug Interaction	
Midazolam, triazolam	Increases effect of benzodiazepine
Cyclosporine, tacrolimus, sirolimus	Increases cyclosporine, tacrolimus, sirolimus trough concentrations

Adapted from Gubbins PO, McConnell SA, Penzak SR: Drug interactions associated with antifungal agents. In Piscitelli SC, Rodvold KA (eds): Drug Interactions in Infectious Diseases. Totowa, NJ, Humana, 2001, pp 185-217.

In-vitro Susceptibility Testing. Unlike AmB, interpretive breakpoints exist for *Candida* species tested against the azoles. For fluconazole these breakpoints were established based on data from mucosal and invasive disease. The breakpoints contain a unique category known as "susceptibility is dose dependent" (S-DD). This breakpoint considers the pharmacokinetics of fluconazole and emphasizes the importance of optimizing fluconazole blood and tissue concentrations for isolates with elevated minimal inhibitory concentrations.[54]

For itraconazole, breakpoints against *Candida* species exist only for mucosal infections.[54] Like fluconazole, there is an S-DD breakpoint that suggests the susceptibility depends on drug delivery to the infection site.[54] In contrast to the predictable and reliable bioavailability of fluconazole, itraconazole absorption is unpredictable and somewhat erratic. Therefore, lack of drug delivery to the infection site may be the true cause of the apparent reduced susceptibility. The correlation between itraconazole serum concentrations or minimal inhibitory concentrations and outcome are unclear.[54] The NCCLS has yet to establish breakpoints for voriconazole against clinically relevant fungal pathogens, and the relationship between clinical outcome and in-vitro susceptibility has yet to be determined.[60] Like AmB the interpretive breakpoints for *Cryptococcus* and other molds against the azoles have yet to be established.

Indications for Susceptibility Testing. Although the in-vitro susceptibility test for yeasts and molds will likely lead to more sensible use of antifungal agents, these methods are still evolving. Clinicians should not rely solely on the results of these methods to guide therapy. Moreover, antifungal susceptibility testing for yeasts should be done only when the results will impact therapy.

Emergence of Resistance and the Selective Pressure of the Azoles. Data indicate that BSI due to fluconazole-resistant Candida species, particularly *C. albicans,* continue to be rare occurrences.[4] Nonetheless, surveillances of BSI during the past decade consistently noted an increasing frequency of infections due *C. glabrata,* which is a species with reduced susceptibility to fluconazole.[4,10] The association between the selection of non-*albicans Candida* species and the use of fluconazole was first noted in the bone marrow transplant setting.[4] A possible association between azole use and the emergence of *C. glabrata* and *C. krusei* has also been noted in other hospital settings.[4,5] However, a definitive link between azole use and emergence of non-*albicans Candida* species is lacking. Nonetheless, growing evidence suggests the emergence of certain species, such as *C. glabrata,* particularly in the ICU setting, may be related to selective pressures exerted by the use of the azoles.[4,5,10]

ECHINOCANDIN ANTIFUNGAL AGENTS

Pharmacology and Pharmacokinetics. The echinocandin class of antifungal agents includes the first new antimycotics introduced in nearly 20 years. This class is fungicidal and disrupts cell wall synthesis by inhibiting a novel target, 1,3-β-D-glucan synthase. This enzyme is present in most fungal pathogens but is not present in mammalian cells.[63] The echinocandins are active against *Aspergillus* and *Candida* species. In addition, their spectrum of activity extends to *Pneumocystis carinii.* These agents have little or no activity against *H. capsulatum, B. dermatitidis,* or *C. neoformans.*[63] Currently, only caspofungin acetate is available in the United States, but within several years micafungin, and anidulafungin will likely be added to the list of available agents in this class.

The echinocandins are large lipopeptide compounds and thus cannot be formulated for oral dosing. Caspofungin acetate exhibits predictable linear pharmacokinetics, and with a half-life of 8 to 13 hours it can be dosed once daily.[63] The pharmacokinetics of caspofungin have not been evaluated in a critically ill population. In healthy male adults, following intravenous administration caspofungin undergoes minimal hydrolysis and/or *N*-acetylation and is slowly excreted unchanged primarily in the urine and to a lesser extent in the feces.[64] Caspofungin reaches high concentrations in the liver, kidney, and intestine.[63] No differences in pharmacokinetics were observed with age, gender, or race.[63] Dosage adjustment is not required in patients with impaired renal function, but the dose should be reduced by 50% in patients with significant hepatic impairment.[63]

Toxicity and Drug Interactions. In general, caspofungin is well tolerated, and in clinical trials the incidence of adverse events were significantly less than AmB. When adverse events were reported they were nonspecific (i.e., fever, headache, nausea, phlebitis, rash, elevated hepatic enzymes) and rarely were they severe enough to cause early discontinuation of therapy.[63] Similarly, caspofungin has a low potential to interact with other drugs. Clinically insignificant interactions with the cyclosporine tacrolimus have been reported, but the mechanism(s) of these interactions are unclear.[63]

Antifungal Susceptibility Testing. The NCCLS has not determined the optimal method to test the susceptibility of pathogenic fungi against the echinocandins. Therefore, interpretive breakpoints for caspofungin acetate have not been established.

PYRIMIDINE ANTIFUNGAL AGENTS (5-FLUOROCYTOSINE)

Pharmacokinetics and Toxicity. 5-Fluorocytosine (5-FC) is a fluorinated pyrimidine related to 5-fluorouracil, and it is the only agent in this therapeutic class. This antimycotic possesses a narrow spectrum of activity and is often associated with significant toxicity. Moreover, when used as monotherapy, resistance develops rapidly. Orally, 5-FC is nearly completely absorbed and distributes to total body water.[62] Hepatic metabolism and protein binding of 5-FC are negligible. Nearly 90% of a dose is renally excreted as unchanged drug and renal clearance is highly correlated with creatinine clearance (CrCl). Reductions in CrCl prolong the half-life of 5-FC.[62]

Myelosuppression is the primary toxicity associated with 5-FC. In addition, 5-FC can cause significant rash, nausea, vomiting, diarrhea, and liver dysfunction.[62] Flucytosine toxicity is associated with elevated drug concentrations and often occurs in the presence of renal dysfunction. Because 5-FC is primarily used in combination with AmB, the effects of renal dysfunction on 5-FC pharmacokinetics and the subsequent risk of toxicity cannot be ignored.

Dosing and Therapeutic Drug Monitoring. Therapeutic drug monitoring for 5-FC is beneficial. Ideally, 5-FC serum concentrations should be maintained between 25 to 100 µg/mL to minimize toxicity and avoid the emergence of resistance. There are several nomograms for dosing 5-FC based on CrCl in patients with renal dysfunction. However, the nomograms are based on serum creatinine measurements; thus, they should be used only with chronic renal dysfunction. In addition, they should be used cautiously in elderly patients. Furthermore, during therapy any necessary dosage adjustments should be made on the basis of plasma concentrations. Use of lower 5-FC doses (75 to 100 mg/kg/day) to minimize its toxicity has been advocated. In-vitro data suggest antifungal efficacy would not be compromised by such dosing.

TREATMENT OF FUNGAL INFECTIONS IN THE CRITICALLY ILL

CANDIDIASIS IN THE ICU

Options for empirical therapy of fungal infections in the ICU are expanding. Clinicians can now choose between the AmB formulations, fluconazole, itraconazole, voriconazole, and caspofungin. The poor prognosis associated with systemic candidiasis has fueled widespread use of antifungals, particularly fluconazole, in ICU patients with or without an established source of fungal infection. One center reported frequent use of fluconazole in ICU patients presumed to be at risk for yeast infections.[5] At that center AmB-d use declined slightly after fluconazole was introduced yet the proportion of patients treated with antifungals who received AmB-d declined markedly.[5] Over a 5-year period, fluconazole use in the surgical ICU at another institution increased nearly 16-fold, whereas surgical ICU admissions rose 26%

during that period but the number of surgical ICU beds remained constant.[65]

The three paradigms of preventive antimycotic therapy are prophylaxis, empirical therapy, and "preemptive therapy."[66,67] Prophylaxis is generally initiated in a population in anticipation of certain risk factors, regardless of whether they ever manifest. There are few data to justify the use of this paradigm in the ICU setting. Moreover, in view of growing concerns about selecting resistant fungal pathogens with indiscriminate antifungal use, this management strategy should be discouraged.[67] Empirical therapy is the initiation of treatment with the first clinical suspicion of infection, in the absence of any laboratory evidence of infection.[66,67] "Preemptive therapy" is treatment initiated in patients with nonspecific clinical risk factors (e.g., broad-spectrum antibiotic use, total parenteral nutrition, recent gastrointestinal surgery) and laboratory markers indicating high risk.[66,67] These paradigms differ little, and the two terms are often used interchangeably.

For many years, AmB-d had been the lone option for the prevention or treatment of candidiasis in the ICU setting. However, clinicians' reluctance to use this agent due to the risk of nephrotoxicity and the advent of safe and effective alternatives have limited its use in the ICU. There are few studies that demonstrate the efficacy of AmB-d in preventing or treating candidiasis specifically in the ICU setting. A retrospective study in general surgical patients with at least one blood culture positive for Candida species demonstrated that treatment with 210 mg or greater of AmB-d was associated with a significant protective effect.[68]

Lipid formulations of AmB have lowered the risk of nephrotoxicity associated with AmB, but there are no data regarding their use in the ICU setting. The results of studies assessing these formulations as empirical or salvage therapy in febrile neutropenic patients should not be extrapolated to the general ICU setting. The lipid formulations of AmB are suitable for critically ill, neutropenic, or otherwise immunocompromised patients who are at high risk for deadly non-Candida infections and will likely require high-dose AmB therapy for a prolonged period. Given the cost of these formulations, and the availability of other safe and less costly therapies, they are not likely a cost-effective means to prevent or treat candidiasis in the general ICU setting.

To date most studies of antifungal use in the ICU setting have evaluated the prophylactic paradigm using fluconazole. Prophylactic enteral fluconazole suspension has been evaluated in a double-blind, randomized, placebo-controlled trial as a means to prevent candidal infections in critically ill surgical patients who required ICU care for at least 3 days. A total of 117 patients with a median APACHE III score of 58 received an 800-mg loading dose followed by 400 mg daily for a median of 4 days.[53,69] Infections were approximately three times more prevalent in the control arm.[69] Based on these data, approximately 10 patients have to receive prophylactic therapy to prevent one fungal infection.[69]

Although the investigators concluded prophylactic fluconazole suspension is safe and effectively reduces the incidence of fungal infections in high-risk, critically ill surgical ICU patients the results should be interpreted cautiously.[69] This was a single center study; and true to the paradigm, patient selection was somewhat subjective and was based on an anticipated ICU stay of 3 or more days and the clinician's experience. Therefore, the results may not be widely generalized. Given the cost attributable to nosocomial fungal infections in the ICU, this mode of therapy may be attractive as a cost-effective approach to preventing systemic mycosis in critically ill patients. However, there is growing concern about the relationship between indiscriminate azole use and shifts in the isolation of more resistant Candida species, and the potential economic impact of these concerns needs to be assessed before this practice can be widely implemented.

Prophylaxis with fluconazole was evaluated in 220 mechanically ventilated ICU patients who were also receiving selective digestive decontamination (SDD) in a double-blind, randomized, placebo-controlled study. All patients received a standardized SDD regimen; and of those, 50% of patients also received fluconazole, 100 mg daily.[70] The incidence of candidal infections, particularly candidemia, was significantly less in the fluconazole-treated patients, and the risk of developing candidemia was reduced 90%.[70] In this study the intensity of colonization at the start of the study was similar, but colonization progressed more rapidly and intensified over the course of the study in the placebo group.[70] Patients in this study received intravenous fluconazole; and in addition to the concerns just mentioned, it is questionable whether this approach to preventing fungal infections in the ICU is cost effective.

Another prospective, randomized, double-blind placebo-controlled study evaluated the selective use of prophylactic fluconazole for the prevention of intra-abdominal candidal infections in abdominal surgery patients. This study included patients who had recurrent gastrointestinal perforations or anastomotic leakages; therefore, they were at very high risk of developing intra-abdominal candidiasis.[71] Although these patients were not critically ill (APACHE II score 13), prophylactic fluconazole prevented candidal colonization and dissemination of Candida species. Moreover, the occurrence of candidal peritonitis was significantly reduced by fluconazole.[71] This study suggests that perhaps when the prophylactic paradigm is selectively applied it can benefit specific patient populations. This has also been shown in the HSCT population.[72]

There have been several prospective, randomized studies comparing AmB-d to fluconazole for the treatment of candidemia in non-neutropenic hosts. These studies have shown that fluconazole is as effective and safer than AmB-d.[73-75] Furthermore, in a prospective, randomized, double-blind study caspofungin has been shown to be at least as effective as AmB-d for the treatment of invasive candidiasis.[76] Although these studies included ICU patients there are few comparative studies that assess the efficacy of AmB-d in preventing or treating candidiasis specifically in the ICU setting. Two small studies have evaluated AmB-d compared with fluconazole alone or in combination with 5-FC. In these studies there were little differences between the regimens.[77,78]

Itraconazole use in the ICU was limited by difficulty administering the capsule through feeding and nasogastric tubes. Although the oral solution solved this problem, there are few data assessing the effectiveness of this form of itraconazole in preventing or treating systemic candidiasis. Concerns about the accumulation of HP-βCD with the intravenous use of itraconazole in patients with compromised renal function limits the use of this formulation in the ICU setting. Furthermore, the use of itraconazole in the ICU is also limited by a significant drug-drug interaction profile with agents commonly used in the ICU. There are no comparative studies that assess the efficacy of voriconazole in preventing or treating candidiasis specifically in the ICU setting. The recommended antifungal therapy for candidiasis in the ICU setting is summarized in Table 157-3.[76,79]

TABLE 157–3. SUMMARY OF RECOMMENDED ANTIFUNGAL THERAPY FOR ASPERGILLOSIS AND CANDIDIASIS IN THE ICU SETTING

Infection	Recommended Treatment	Alternative Treatment
Aspergillosis		
Invasive pulmonary	AmB 1.0-1.5 mg/kg/day until desired response then consider ITZ ≥ 400 mg/day when disease progression slows	Lipid AmB formulations ≥ 5 mg/kg/day or ITZ ≥ 400 mg/day
Invasive Candidiasis (Candidemia)		
C. albicans	AmB ≥ 0.7 mg/kg/day for 2 wk	FCZ ≥ 6 mg/kg/day for 2 wk or caspofungin 70 mg × 1; then 50 mg/day for 2 wk
C. glabrata	AmB ≥ 0.7 mg/kg/day for 2 wk	FCZ 6-12 mg/kg/day for 2 wk or caspofungin 70 mg × 1; then 50 mg/day for 2 wk
C. krusei	AmB 1.0 mg/kg/day for 2 wk	Consider caspofungin*
C. parapsilosis	AmB 0.6-0.7 mg/kg/day for 2 wk	FCZ ≥ 6-12 mg/kg/day for 2 wk, caspofungin 70 mg × 1; then 50 mg/day for 2 wk†
Empirical Therapy		
Neutropenic fever	AmB 0.5-0.7 mg/kg/day, until neutropenia resolves	Liposomal AmB 3 mg/kg/day, until neutropenia resolves
Prophylaxis		
Neutropenic (HSCT)	FCZ 400 mg/day, while patients are at high risk	

AmB, amphotericin B; FCZ, fluconazole; ITZ, itraconazole; HSCT, hematopoietic stem cell transplant.
*Demonstrated similar results to AmB for primary treatment of invasive candidiasis; results with small numbers of C. krusei demonstrated clinical activity.
†Monitor for persistence; in-vitro susceptibilities reveal caspofungin MICs for C. parapsilosis higher than other Candida species and results of clinical trial demonstrated caspofungin to be effective in treatment of C. parapsilosis fungemia, but persistent cultures are common.
Adapted from references 76, 79, and 82.

INVASIVE ASPERGILLOSIS AND OTHER OPPORTUNISTIC MYCOSES IN BONE MARROW TRANSPLANTATION

Fever and neutropenia are common among critically ill immunocompromised individuals with hematologic malignancies. Although the fever can be due to many causes, these patients, particularly bone marrow transplant (BMT) or HSCT recipients, are at high risk of developing systemic mycosis due to Candida or Aspergillus species. Owing to the difficulty in diagnosing infections due to these pathogens, antifungal prophylaxis is standard in BMT patients. Fluconazole has been shown to decrease the incidence of invasive infections with Candida species and is widely used in the prophylactic paradigm.[72] As stated previously, invasive aspergillosis occurs early and late in the course of transplantation.[33] Therefore, persistently febrile BMT recipients should be treated empirically with antifungal agents with activity against molds, particularly Aspergillus species.

The number of antifungal agents with activity against molds such as Aspergillus species is growing, yet options for empirical therapy of infections caused by these pathogens are still limited. For many years "high-dose" AmB-d was employed as standard empirical therapy of invasive aspergillosis but its use was often curtailed over concerns about its toxicity profile. The lipid AmB formulations are costly; and although they are safer than AmB-d, they are not devoid of toxicity. Nonetheless, the use of these agents has been primarily limited by their cost. The azoles are safe, but their use may be limited by variable activity against Aspergillus species or for pharmacologic reasons.

Fluconazole lacks activity against molds. Itraconazole has activity against Aspergillus species, but, as discussed previously, the capsule dosage form is not suitable for many critically ill

patients, and it produces erratic blood levels. The oral solution is not well tolerated and is commonly associated with diarrhea, and concerns over administering the intravenous itraconazole solution in patients with diminished renal function have limited the use of this formulation in the critically ill. Voriconazole, a derivative of fluconazole with expanded activity against resistant Candida species and molds, has been evaluated in one of the few randomized comparative clinical trials for the empirical treatment of invasive aspergillosis. In that study in terms of the composite measurement of efficacy, LAmB slightly outperformed voriconazole, but in certain individual markers of efficacy (i.e., prevention of documented breakthrough infections, infusion reactions, and nephrotoxicity) voriconazole was safer and more effective than LAmB.[80]

With their lack of toxicity and low propensity for drug-drug interactions, the echinocandins are promising agents for empirical therapy of invasive aspergillosis in critically ill patients. Caspofungin was evaluated in an open-label, noncomparative study for the treatment of invasive aspergillosis. Favorable responses were observed in 41% of patients, which is similar to success rates (40% to 50%) observed with the azoles and lipid AmB formulations.[81] Given the limitations of existing choices, and the poor efficacy of monotherapy, new agents and/or therapeutic strategies are needed to improve the outcome of this devastating infection. The recommended antifungal therapy for the treatment of aspergillosis in the ICU setting is summarized in Table 157-3.[82]

CRYPTOCOCCOSIS, HISTOPLASMOSIS, AND BLASTOMYCOSIS

Although cryptococcosis, histoplasmosis, and blastomycosis are not considered nosocomial pathogens, patients with severe infections caused by these pathogens require intensive care. The treatment of cryptococcosis, particularly that in the CNS, evolved from a series of classic clinical trials. More recently, published guidelines by the Infectious Disease Society of America (IDSA) for the treatment of cryptococcal infections have recognized that with declining infection rates among HIV-infected individuals, waiting for randomized controlled trials to address unresolved questions surrounding the management of this infection may be impractical, and it made evidence-based recommendations on the best available data. The recommended antifungal therapy for the treatment of cryptococcosis in the ICU setting is summarized in Table 157-4.[83]

Management of Increased ICP in CNS Cryptococcosis. Elevations in ICP occur in more than half the patients with cryptococcal meningitis and contribute significantly to the morbidity and mortality associated with this infection.[83] The outcome and benefits of ICP management have been studied primarily in patients with HIV, and the influence of this treatment modality on the outcome of CNS cryptococcosis in non–HIV-infected patients is unknown. Therefore, ICP management may be an underutilized treatment modality in the management of non–HIV-infected patients with CNS cryptococcosis. In patients with or without HIV infection elevations in ICP should be managed by sequential lumbar punctures.[83] If necessary, more invasive procedures including insertion of a lumbar drain or placement of a ventriculoperitoneal shunt should be performed.[83] The frequency with which sequential lumbar punctures are performed depends on the initial opening pressure and symptoms. In patients with normal baseline opening pressure, the frequency of lumbar puncture is determined by the patient's response to therapy but the procedure should be repeated at a minimum of 2 weeks after the initiation of therapy.[83] For patients with elevated baseline opening pressure, lumbar puncture should be done to reduce the pressure 50% and performed daily to maintain the pressure in the normal range.[83]

Serum and CSF antigen titers are important in establishing the presumptive diagnosis and assessing the prognosis of infection. The test measures cryptococcal polysaccharide capsule antigens but does not differentiate viable from nonviable organism. Therefore, once therapy is started, treatment decisions should not be based on antigen test results.[83] A reduction in antigen titers during therapy is desired, but treatment decisions should be based on culture results.

Treatment of Histoplasmosis in Critically Ill Patients. Although there are no comparative studies, the efficacy of individual antimycotics for therapy of chronic and disseminated histoplasmosis has been well documented. AmB-d, ketoconazole, and itraconazole all have proven efficacy. The efficacy of 6 weeks to 4 months of AmB-d therapy for chronic infection is approximately 75%; however, relapse is common. The efficacy of itraconazole ranges from 75% to 85%, but, like for AmB-d, relapse may be common. In-vitro susceptibility of *H. capsulatum* to fluconazole is poor, and generally it is not used to treat this infection.[38]

The efficacy of AmB-d for therapy for disseminated histoplasmosis among immunocompetent patients is 70% to 90%. In a small study, all patients responded to itraconazole, 200 to 400 mg daily.[38] Therefore, AmB-d is recommended initially in severely ill patients. Once an adequate response is noted, therapy can be switched to itraconazole.[84] Few data exist concerning the efficacy of the lipid AmB formulations as therapy for disseminated histoplasmosis in immunocompetent patients. The recommended antifungal therapy for the treatment of histoplasmosis in the ICU setting is summarized in Table 157-4.[84]

TREATMENT OF DISSEMINATED (EXTRAPULMONARY) BLASTOMYCOSIS IN THE CRITICALLY ILL

Disseminated blastomycosis and diffuse pulmonary infection are both associated with notable mortality. Treatment of these infections produces cure rates ranging from 85% to 90%, and the effective agents cause little associated toxicity.[38]

TABLE 157–4. SUMMARY OF RECOMMENDED ANTIFUNGAL THERAPY FOR CRYPTOCOCCOSIS AND THE ENDEMIC MYCOSES IN THE ICU SETTING

Infection	Recommended Treatment	Alternative Treatment
Cryptococcosis		
CNS infection	Induction: AmB, 0.7-1 mg/kg, + 5-FC, 100 mg/kg/day, for 2 wk Consolidation: FCZ, 400 mg/day for minimum of 10 wk*	AmB, 0.7-1 mg/kg, + 5-FC, 100 mg/kg/day, × 6-10 wk
Histoplasmosis		
Acute pulmonary Extrapulmonary	AmB, 0.7 mg/kg/day, then ITZ, 200 mg, to finish 12 wk† AmB, 0.7-1.0 mg/kg/day, then ITZ, 200-400 mg/day for 6-18 mo	Lipid AmB formulation, 3 mg/kg/day
Blastomycosis		
Pulmonary	AmB, 0.7-1.0 mg/kg/day to 1.5-2.5 g total	AmB, 0.7-1.0 mg/kg/day to 0.5 g total then ITZ, 200-400 mg/day
Extrapulmonary CNS Non-CNS	 AmB, 0.7-1.0 mg/kg/day to 2 g total AmB, 0.7-1.0 mg/kg/day to 1.5-2.5 g total	 Lipid AmB formulation, FCZ 800 mg/day AmB, 0.7-1.0 mg/kg/day until patient is stable, then ITZ, 200-400 mg/day

CNS, Central nervous system; AmB, amphotericin B deoxycholate; 5-FC, 5-fluorocytosine; FCZ, fluconazole; ITZ, itraconazole.
*Has not been studied in non-HIV but has many aspects that lead to the successful treatment of this CNS infection.
†Consider corticosteroids 60 mg × 2 wk.
Adapted from references 83 to 85.

The optimal duration of therapy for the treatment of blasto-mycosis with existing antifungal agents is unknown and has been empirically derived from noncomparative studies and clinical experience. In cases of life-threatening infections or extrapulmonary disease and in patients who are severely immunocompromised or have already failed therapy with an azole, the risk of relapse is high.[38] Therefore, the duration of therapy is determined by the total AmB-d dose that will likely prevent relapse. Patients who receive a total AmB-d dose of less than 1.5 g often experience relapse.[38] For that reason, most experts recommend a total dose of 1.5 to 2.5 g of AmB-d in these cases.[38] Patients can be switched to safer azole therapy when significant improvement is observed.[85] The pharmacologic treatment of histoplasmosis in the ICU setting is summarized in Table 157-4.[85]

CONCLUSION

In the past several decades significant changes have occurred with regard to management of systemic mycoses in the ICU setting. First, systemic mycoses are now widespread in critically ill patients. Specifically, in the ICU setting *Candida* species are a common cause of nosocomial BSIs. There are many risks associated with the ICU environment or the patients' underlying disease state that predispose them to infections with these pathogens. In addition, historically, because of the high mortality associated with BSIs caused by *C. albicans*, this species has been the primary fungal pathogen of concern. In the past decade, growing evidence of a shift in the epidemiology of *Candida* isolates in the ICU has emerged. Whether the shift in epidemiology is a consequence of injudicious antifungal use is a matter of speculation and debate. Nonetheless, the steady increase in BSIs due to *C. glabrata*, a species with reduced susceptibility to antifungal therapy, is of concern. Furthermore, select populations of critically ill patients are at risk of developing life-threatening infections due to non-*Candida* species of fungi, such as *Aspergillus* species, *Fusarium*, and the Zygomycetes. These pathogens are angioinvasive and often respond poorly to antifungal therapy. The endemic mycoses (e.g., histoplasmosis, blasto-mycosis) are not typically a concern in the ICU setting, but patients with severe infections due to *B. dermatitidis*, *H. capsulatum*, or *C. immitis* will often require intensive care.

Second, methods to perform antifungal susceptibility tests on a variety of pathogens are still evolving, as is the clinicians' ability to interpret these tests. Along with this evolution has come an improved understanding of antifungal resistance and the pharmacodynamic actions of these drugs. This understanding may ultimately lead to more rational use of antifungals and perhaps improved outcomes in infected patients.

Last, in the past decade significant strides have been made in antifungal drug development. During this period there has been the development of safer, more bioavailable forms of existing agents and, for the first time in two decades, the marketing of a new class of agents, with a novel mechanism of action. Now the available drugs differ sufficiently in terms of toxicity and potential for drug-drug interactions that clinicians have the luxury of choice when tailoring antifungal therapy to a specific patient.

ANNOTATED REFERENCES

Mora-Duarte J, Betts R, Rotstein C, et al: Comparison of caspofungin and amphotericin B for invasive candidiasis. N Engl J Med 2002;347:2020-2029.
  A prospective, randomized, double-blind study that demonstrated caspofungin was at least as effective as amphotericin B deoxycholate for the treatment of invasive candidiasis. Although the study was not limited to ICU patients, the data suggest that caspofungin represents a reasonable alternative for the treatment of candidiasis when azoles cannot be used, or in the presence of azole-resistant strains. The potential value of this study to the ICU population is that caspofungin may be an effective nephro-sparing alternative to amphotericin B, in situations when an azole cannot be used.

Pelz RK, Hendix CW, Swoboda SM, et al: Double-blind placebo-controlled trial of fluconazole to prevent candidal infections in critically ill surgical patients. Ann Surg 2001;233:542-548.
  This study was perhaps the largest and most well-controlled trial to evaluate the prophylactic use of enteral fluconazole to prevent invasive candidal infections in critically ill surgical patients. After controlling for confounding variables this study demonstrated a 55% reduction in the risk of fungal infection among patients treated with fluconazole. Based on these data it was concluded that enteral fluconazole safely and effectively decreased the incidence of fungal infections in high-risk critically ill surgical patients.

Pittet D, Li Ning, Woolson RF, Wenzel RP: Microbiological factors influencing the outcome of nosocomial bloodstream infections: A 6-year validated, population-based model. Clin Infect Dis 1997;24:1068-1078.
  This article provides compelling data concerning the importance of Candida *species as bloodstream pathogens. The article provides data regarding the crude and attributable mortality rates of* Candida *bloodstream infections in the hospital. The study demonstrates that of all the microbial causes of bloodstream infections, only* Candida *species are an independent predictor of mortality due to bloodstream infection.*

Rex JH, Bennett JE, Sugar AM, et al: A randomized trial comparing fluconazole with amphotericin B for the treatment of candidemia in patients without neutropenia. N Engl J Med 1994;331:1325-1330.
  A landmark article that demonstrated that in patients without neutropenia, and without significant immunodeficiency, fluconazole and amphotericin B deoxycholate are not significantly different in their effectiveness in treating candidemia.

Wey SB, Mori M, Pfaller MA, et al: Risk factors for hospital-acquired candidemia: A matched case-control study. Arch Intern Med 1989;149:2349-2353.
  This study was one of the first rigorous epidemiologic assessments of the risk factors that predispose patients to candidemia. Established risk factors have been borne out on subsequent analyses.

Chapter 158

TUBERCULOSIS

Kathryn Lee Springer • Edward D. Chan

KEY POINTS

1. **Both primary and reactivation tuberculosis (TB) can cause bilateral alveolar infiltrates and hypoxic respiratory failure.** The presence of respiratory failure may cause physicians to inappropriately dismiss the diagnosis of TB.

2. **Disseminated or "miliary" TB may result from either primary or reactivation TB.** Disseminated TB typically presents subacutely but can manifest fulminantly with septic shock and multiorgan failure.

3. **Tuberculous meningitis** is typically a subacute disease. **Clinical syndromes include headache, altered mental status, stroke, hydrocephalus, and cranial neuropathies.** Classic features of bacterial meningitis, such as stiff neck and fever, may be absent.

4. **The diagnosis of tuberculous pericarditis can be difficult to prove.** Many individuals are treated empirically based on clinical suspicion, a positive purified protein derivative test, imaging studies, and exudative pericardial fluid with high protein and mononuclear white counts.

5. **Human immunodeficiency virus (HIV) is the most important host risk factor for TB, with a higher incidence of extrapulmonary TB.** With waning CD4+ counts, TB may be atypical in its presentation; for example, reactivation disease may mimic primary disease, with mediastinal adenopathy. In TB patients, treatment of HIV with highly active antiretroviral therapy may be associated with paradoxical reactions.

6. **Standard treatment of adults with TB consists of a three- or four-drug regimen for at least 6 months.** A 9- to 12-month regimen is suggested for tuberculous meningitis, for disease that is slow to respond to therapy, and when pyrazinamide is not used in the initial regimen. When multidrug-resistant TB is suspected or confirmed, an expanded regimen that includes amikacin, a fluoroquinolone, or other second-line oral agents is necessary.

The World Health Organization estimates that one third of the world's population is latently infected with *Mycobacterium tuberculosis*.[1] From this pool, approximately 9 million active tuberculosis (TB) cases emerge annually, resulting in 2 to 3 million deaths; this makes TB the most common cause of death by an infectious agent worldwide.[2] The acquired immunodeficiency syndrome (AIDS) epidemic is largely responsible for the rise in TB cases in much of the world (≈1.5 million patients with active TB are also infected with human immunodeficiency virus [HIV]), and coinfection with both agents contributes significantly to TB-related mortality. Ninety-five percent of cases of TB occur in the developing world. Incidence rates exceed 300 cases per 100,000 persons in much of sub-Saharan Africa, the Indonesian and Philippine archipelagos, Afghanistan, Bolivia, and Peru.[1,3] Areas with the most cases per year include India (1.9 million) and China (1.4 million). In North America, cases occur disproportionately among foreign-born individuals from TB-endemic countries, HIV-infected persons, institutionalized persons, and minorities. The United States saw a decline in TB cases up to the early 1980s, mostly due to public health programs, but HIV/AIDS, immigration, and waning TB programs led to a resurgence of TB in the late 1980s and early 1990s.[4] The annual number of cases is now declining again. As TB becomes rarer in the United States, decreased awareness of disease manifestations may lead to delays in diagnosis and treatment. In critically ill patients, early treatment is especially important to prevent TB-related mortality.

M. tuberculosis is classified as an acid-fast bacillus organism because it and other *Mycobacteria* species resist decolorization by acid alcohol during staining by Ziehl-Neelsen or Kinyoun methods. TB can be divided into two stages: infection and disease. Infection occurs by airborne transmission of tubercle bacilli that produce a localized (and usually lower lobe) pneumonia. Primary infection is usually asymptomatic but may present with mild nonspecific symptoms, symptoms of acute pneumonia, or severe disseminated disease. After primary infection, TB spreads from the lungs to the hilar lymph nodes and then throughout the bloodstream, resulting in latent infection (Fig. 158-1). Most cases of active TB are due to reactivation of latent infection. This occurs in about 10% of immunocompetent persons with TB infection and tends to occur within the first 2 years of infection. The result is usually a chronic destructive pneumonia involving the lung apices and superior segments of the lower lobes. Cavitation and fibrotic changes are common. There are many exceptions to this typical course; TB can involve any organ system and can present with severe and acute manifestations. In this chapter, selected critical care issues related to TB are discussed. Some disease forms, such as renal and peritoneal TB, are omitted because they are less likely to be seen in the ICU.

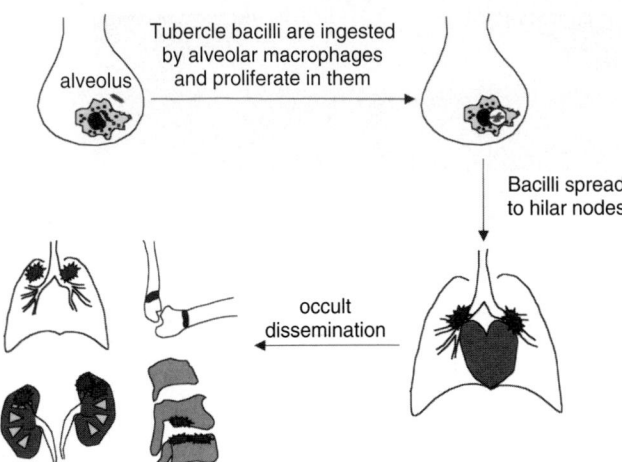

FIGURE 158–1. Drawing of primary tuberculosis infection and occult dissemination. *Mycobacterium tuberculosis* disseminates when infected mononuclear cells migrate throughout the body, particularly to the lung apices, kidneys, bone growth plates, and vertebrae, resulting in latent infection.

PULMONARY TUBERCULOSIS

Pulmonary disease is by far the most common manifestation of active TB and is the most common manifestation of TB requiring ICU admission. Severe disease is more likely to occur in patients with disseminated infection (see later) or with advanced immunodeficiency. Primary infection, though often asymptomatic in adults, can present with fever, hilar adenopathy, infiltrates, pleural effusions, and even severe pulmonary disease that may mimic viral or bacterial pneumonia. Reactivation and chronic TB can also present acutely with pulmonary destruction, respiratory failure, and death. Pulmonary gangrene, which carries a mortality of up to 75%, can ensue when rapid progression of infiltrate causes vascular damage and death of lung tissue.[5] Both primary and reactivation TB can cause bilateral alveolar infiltrates, hypoxic respiratory failure, and acute respiratory distress syndrome (ARDS).[6,7] In patients hospitalized with pulmonary TB, six factors are associated with respiratory failure or death: lymphopenia, advanced age, concomitant smear-positive extrapulmonary TB, alcoholism, a high percentage of neutrophils on the peripheral white blood cell count, and lack of radiographic cavitation.[8]

Studies have shown that the presence of respiratory failure may cause physicians to inappropriately dismiss the diagnosis of TB.[9-11] In older individuals (65 years and older) or patients with AIDS, the diagnosis of TB may also be delayed, in part due to atypical presentations.[12,13] The critical care physician should maintain a high index of suspicion and should consider primary or reactivation TB in any at-risk patient with respiratory failure or clinical ARDS. Respiratory failure due to TB is associated with a mortality of up to 50%; early recognition is important to reduce mortality and to prevent the nosocomial spread of TB.[11] Clinical presentation and chest radiograph findings vary greatly, depending on the stage of disease and host factors. Laboratory findings of anemia and hypoalbuminemia can be suggestive of a chronic process such as TB and have been shown to be predictors of death in patients with respiratory failure due to TB.[14] Pulmonary histology often reveals tuberculous bronchopneumonia, even when the presentation is consistent with ARDS. More details of diagnosis and treatment are discussed later.

Other life-threatening complications of pulmonary TB include hemoptysis, spontaneous pneumothoraces, bronchopleural fistulas, and pleural disease. Pleural TB can present as pleuritis or empyema. Pleural biopsy specimens are more likely to yield positive cultures than is pleural fluid.

DISSEMINATED TUBERCULOSIS

Disseminated or "miliary" TB is more likely to occur in the very young and very old and in patients with underlying diseases such as HIV. It may result from either primary or reactivation TB. Disseminated TB typically presents subacutely, with symptoms present for days to months, but it can manifest fulminantly with septic shock and multiorgan failure.[15] Typical signs and symptoms include fever, malaise, weight loss, dyspnea, and hypoxia. The characteristic chest radiograph (Fig. 158-2A) and computed tomography scan (see Fig. 158-2B) show a miliary pattern: a pattern of diffuse, small (<2 mm) nodules that resemble millet seeds (see Fig. 158-2C). In some cases of disseminated disease, the chest radiograph may appear normal. Other organs involved may include the adrenals, central nervous system (meningitis), gastrointestinal tract (hepatitis, cholestatic jaundice, pancreatitis), eyes, urinary tract (sterile pyuria), skin (abscesses), and bone marrow. Hematologic abnormalities such as anemia, leukemoid reaction, and thrombocytosis are nonspecific but characteristic features of miliary TB. Diagnosis can be difficult. If disseminated TB is suspected, sputum smears should be obtained, even when pulmonary disease is not apparent. Biopsy and culture of affected organs, such as the bone marrow, are often required. Culture of blood, urine, or stool may also yield results, especially in HIV-positive patients.[15]

NEUROLOGIC TUBERCULOSIS

TUBERCULOUS MENINGITIS

Tuberculous meningitis is rare in developed countries, with approximately 300 to 400 cases in the United States each year. It occurs via rupture of a subependymal tubercle that was seeded and formed during primary infection or disseminated disease. Individuals at high risk for tuberculous meningitis include very young children with primary TB and older patients with immunodeficiency disorders such as HIV. Most have no known history of TB, but evidence of extrameningeal disease (e.g., pulmonary, urinary) can be found in about half of patients.[16,17] The purified protein derivative (PPD) test is positive in only about 50%.

Tuberculous meningitis is typically a subacute disease. In one review of 58 cases, symptoms were present for 1 day to 9 months (median, 10 days) before diagnosis.[16] A prodromal phase of low-grade fever, malaise, headache, dizziness, vomiting, and personality changes may persist for 2 to 3 weeks before the patient presents for medical care. Typical findings at presentation include severe headache, altered mental status, stroke, hydrocephalus, and cranial neuropathies. These clinical features are the result of basilar meningeal fibrosis and vascular inflammation.[18] Classic features of bacterial meningitis, such as stiff neck and fever, may be absent. When allowed to progress, coma and seizures may ensue.

Diagnosis of tuberculous meningitis can be difficult and may be based on only clinical findings, without definitive

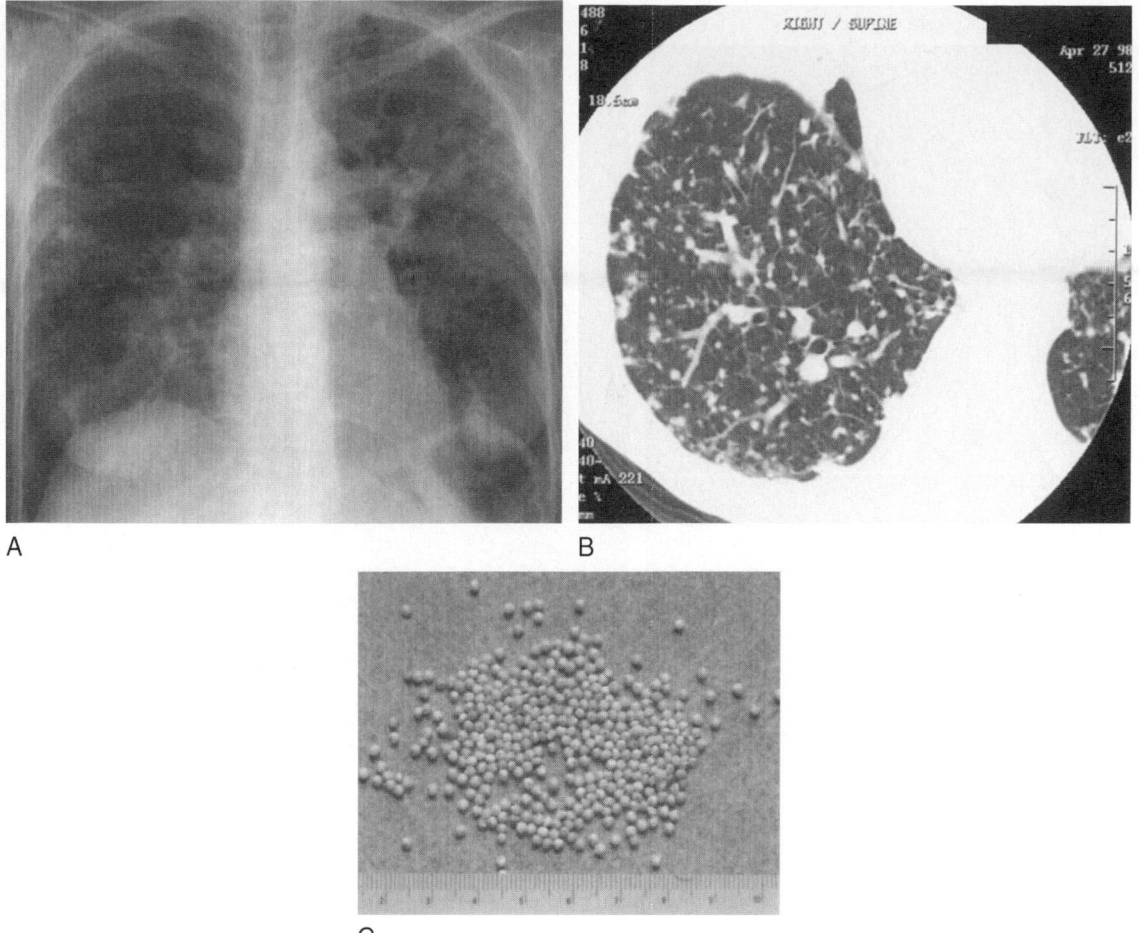

FIGURE 158–2. Miliary tuberculosis (TB). *A*, Chest radiograph of a patient with miliary TB. *B*, Chest computed tomography scan of the same patient. Both show the characteristically small, less than 2-mm nodules, which resemble millet seeds. *C*, Millet seeds are approximately 2 mm in diameter.

microbiologic proof. Certain clinical characteristics, such as longer duration of symptoms (>6 days), moderate cerebrospinal fluid leukocytosis and neutrophilia, and the presence of focal deficits, increase the probability of tuberculous meningitis.[19,20] Characteristic cerebrospinal fluid findings of tuberculous meningitis include:

- Leukocytosis with predominance of lymphocytes. White blood cell counts are usually between 100 and 500 cells/μL. Lower white blood cell counts and polymorphonuclear cell predominance may be seen very early in the course of disease.
- Elevated protein levels, usually between 100 and 500 mg/dL.
- Low glucose, typically less than 45 mg/dL.

Cerebrospinal fluid samples should be sent for acid-fast smears, but this has low sensitivity (<20%). Large volumes (10 to 15 mL) from several daily lumbar punctures are often needed. Sensitivity is increased if four spinal taps are performed. Culture can take weeks and is also associated with low sensitivity. Nucleic acid amplification-based tests (see later) are still considered investigational for use on nonrespiratory specimens. False-negative results may occur, but these tests are rapid and seem to have good specificity.[21] More study is needed to determine the appropriate use of polymerase chain reaction (PCR) and assays to detect mycobacterial antigens in the cerebrospinal fluid (ELISA,

radioimmunoassay). Stereotactic biopsy can be performed if tissue samples are needed.

Computed tomography or magnetic resonance imaging often reveals basilar meningeal enhancement (Fig. 158-3), hydrocephalus, or both.[17] Hypodensities due to cerebral infarcts and ring or nodular enhancing lesions can also be seen. Magnetic resonance imaging is superior for evaluating the brainstem and the extent of lesions.

Outcome is improved by timely treatment. Thus, empirical treatment is warranted when risk factors and clinical features suggest the presence of tuberculous meningitis. Recommended therapy is outlined in the treatment section later in this chapter. Therapy should be continued for 9 to 12 months. Corticosteroids may reduce long-term neurologic sequelae and improve long-term survival in patients with advanced disease.[18] One recommended corticosteroid regimen in patients with neurologic deficits is prednisone 1 mg/kg daily for 30 days, followed by gradual tapering over the next few weeks. Use of corticosteroids is better established in children.[22] Ventriculoperitoneal shunts or surgical decompression may be required for severe intracranial hypertension.

Prognosis depends largely on neurologic status at the time of presentation and the timing of treatment initiation. Most people die in 5 to 8 weeks if not treated. Various case series indicate a mortality rate between 7% and 65% in developed countries and up to 69% in underdeveloped areas.[16,17,23] Neurologic sequelae occur in up to 50% of survivors.[23] Mortality risk is highest in those with comorbidities, severe

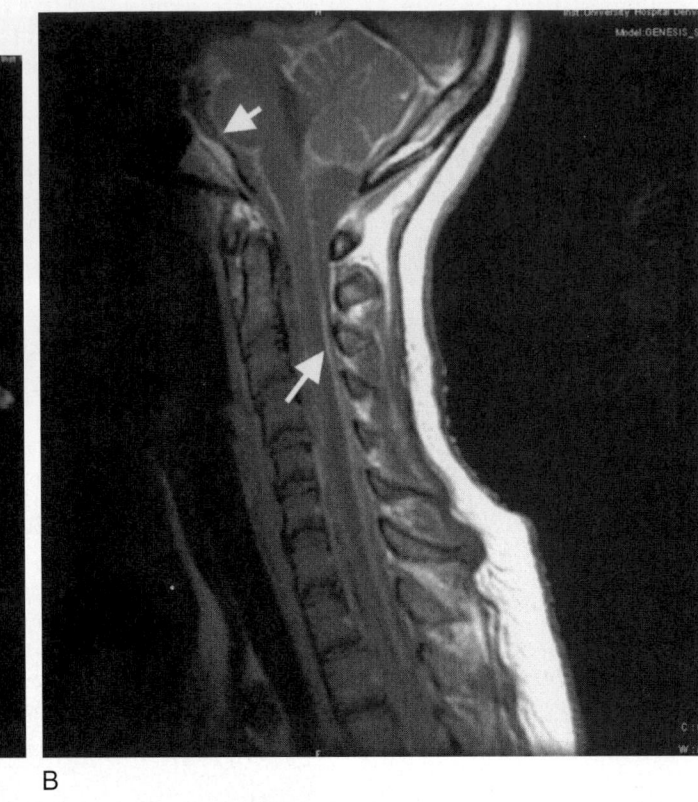

A   B

FIGURE 158–3. Tuberculous meningitis. T1-weighted transverse magnetic resonance imaging scan of the brain *(A)* and sagittal magnetic resonance imaging scan of the base of the brain and the spinal cord *(B)* in a patient with tuberculous meningitis. Note the enhanced meninges *(arrows)* in the basilar regions of the brain, brainstem, and spinal cord.

neurologic deficits on admission, and rapid progression of disease, and in advanced age.

OTHER CENTRAL NERVOUS SYSTEM MANIFESTATIONS

Other central nervous system manifestations of TB include brain abscess, intracranial tuberculoma, vasculitis, radiculomyelitis, and spinal arachnoiditis. These can occur in conjunction with tuberculous meningitis but are less likely to be seen in the ICU when isolated. Intracranial tuberculomas are more common among pediatric patients (especially infants) and can occur in any region of the brain. They result from hematogenous spread of TB. Tuberculous radiculomyelitis is a paradoxical reaction to the treatment of tuberculous meningitis and may respond to corticosteroids. Signs and symptoms include subacute paraparesis, radicular pain, bladder disturbance, and paralysis.[24]

CARDIOVASCULAR TUBERCULOSIS

TUBERCULOUS PERICARDITIS

Tuberculous pericarditis is an uncommon but important complication of TB. In countries with a low incidence of TB, it is primarily a disease of the elderly and those with HIV, but it should be included in the differential diagnosis of any patient with pericarditis or pericardial effusion. Tuberculous pericarditis can result from local spread from the lungs, tracheobronchial tree, lymph nodes, or adjacent bones or by disseminated infection. The onset is usually insidious. Presenting signs and symptoms include nonspecific

symptoms (fever, dyspnea, weight loss) and symptoms typical of pericarditis or cardiac tamponade. Large hemorrhagic effusions may develop, and pericardial inflammation and thickening may eventually cause a constrictive pericarditis. The presence of both pericardial effusion and constrictive pericarditis is physiologically characterized by continued elevation of diastolic pressure after pericardiocentesis. Such a finding should raise the suspicion of tuberculous pericarditis.

The diagnosis of tuberculous pericarditis can be difficult to prove. Culture of pericardial fluid is sensitive in only 30% of cases, and pericardial biopsy has a yield of approximately 60%. Biopsy tissue may reveal granulomatous changes consistent with TB or stain positive for acid-fast bacilli. The presence of elevated adenosine deaminase levels in the pericardial fluid has been touted as an indicator of tuberculous pericarditis, but confirmation is needed.[25] PCR holds promise as a more sensitive test in the diagnosis of tuberculous pericarditis.[26] Many individuals are treated empirically for tuberculous pericarditis based on clinical suspicion, positive PPD, imaging studies, and exudative pericardial fluid with high protein and mononuclear white counts. Treatment involves a standard four-drug regimen, as for other manifestations of TB. Corticosteroids (prednisone 60 mg/day, tapered over 11 weeks) are sometimes used in addition to antimycobacterial therapy and have been shown to reduce the need for operative intervention.[22] Pericardiectomy is sometimes necessary in the treatment of refractory or recurrent disease.

OTHER CARDIOVASCULAR MANIFESTATIONS

In addition to the pericardium, TB may affect the myocardium, endocardium, and epicardium (coronary arteries).

These conditions are all very rare. Tuberculous myocarditis occurs via direct spread from the pericardium or mediastinal lymph nodes or from disseminated disease.[27] Endocardial involvement may manifest as endocarditis or as mural thrombi with entrapped *M. tuberculosis*. TB that affects the coronary arteries results in coronary arteritis, with granulomatous inflammation of the arterial wall and obliterative intimal fibrosis.[28]

TB may also involve the aorta, resulting in aortitis, aortointestinal fistula formation, or rupture.[29,30] The pathogenesis of aortitis includes septic embolization from endocarditis, seeding of a preexisting aneurysm from bacteremia, or extension from a contiguous site of infection. Signs and symptoms include fever, abdominal or back pain, and a palpable abdominal mass. Blood cultures are positive for *M. tuberculosis* in about 15% of cases. Computed tomography findings include air in the aortic wall (pathognomonic), periaortic nodularity, saccular aneurysm in a noncalcified aorta, and rapidly increasing aortic diameter. Primary mycotic aneurysm of the aorta may be a sequela of chronic tuberculous aortitis.[31,32]

TUBERCULOSIS IN HIV-POSITIVE PATIENTS

HIV is the most important host risk factor for TB.[33] TB may be the initial manifestation of HIV infection; thus, all patients with TB should be tested for HIV. In many developing countries, TB is the most common opportunistic infection associated with HIV. In the United States, approximately 60,000 persons are coinfected with HIV and TB. The cell-mediated immune deficiency associated with HIV causes decreased interferon-γ production, contributing to poor immune control. This is likely responsible for the increased incidence of primary and reactivation disease in HIV-positive patients and the increased likelihood of atypical presentations such as miliary disease, TB sepsis, and central nervous system disease.[12] When the CD4+ count is above 200, TB is more likely to present with typical pulmonary disease. As the CD4+ count decreases, TB tends to become more severe and atypical. Reactivation disease may mimic primary disease, with mediastinal adenopathy and lack of cavitation on chest radiographs. Extrapulmonary TB is more common among HIV-positive patients, occurring in up to 70% of patients. Disease involving lymph nodes is especially common. The PPD is often negative in patients with low CD4+ counts, even in the setting of severe TB. Diagnosis can be further complicated by the fact that *M. tuberculosis* cannot be differentiated from *Mycobacterium avium* complex by acid-fast smear. Empirical treatment may be necessary before the diagnosis is confirmed. If rapid diagnosis is needed, nucleic acid amplification tests can be used. Although the risk for TB is highest among HIV-positive patients, other immunocompromised patients are also at increased risk. These include persons with cancer and those receiving high-dose and long-term corticosteroids or tumor necrosis factor inhibitors such as infliximab.[33]

In patients with TB, treatment of HIV with highly active antiretroviral therapy (HAART) may be associated with paradoxical reactions (apparent clinical worsening of disease).[34-36] This reaction is usually self-limited but may require corticosteroids and temporary discontinuation of HAART. Despite this potential complication, it is generally recommended that HIV therapy be continued during TB treatment when possible. In patients who are not already on HAART, it is usually advisable to delay HIV treatment for at least 4 to 8 weeks after TB therapy is begun. Another issue in HIV patients is that antituberculosis drugs may be improperly absorbed, which may increase the risk of treatment failure, relapse, and acquired drug resistance.[37] Treatment of TB in patients with HIV is similar to that in non-HIV-infected patients, but it may be complicated by drug interactions between TB medications and antiretrovirals.[38] The protease inhibitors and non-nucleoside reverse transcriptase inhibitors can either induce or inhibit the activity of the P450-3A (CYP3A) system. Rifampin can increase the activity of CYP3A, leading to decreased levels of several antiretrovirals. Rifabutin is a less potent inducer of the CYP3A system and is associated with fewer drug-drug interactions, but dose adjustments may be needed. Despite these potential drug interactions, a rifamycin-based regimen should be used whenever possible. Patients with liver disease (e.g., hepatitis C) may be at increased risk for drug-induced hepatotoxicity.

Because of the increased risk of rifamycin resistance, patients with HIV should *not* receive once-weekly isoniazid-rifapentine in the continuation phase of treatment, and twice-weekly isoniazid-rifampin or isoniazid-rifabutin should be avoided when the CD4+ count is less than 100/μL. Duration of therapy sometimes needs to be extended to 9 months. Recommendations regarding TB treatment in HIV patients are frequently revised as new drugs and information become available. The following resources can be used to assist with treatment decisions:

- Treatment guidelines published by the Centers for Disease Control and Prevention (CDC), American Thoracic Society, and Infectious Diseases Society of America.[39]
- CDC website: http://www.cdc.gov/nchstp/tb/.
- Medscape website (provides updated information on drug-drug interactions): http://www.medscape.com/updates/quickguide.

DIAGNOSIS

When TB is suspected, the first diagnostic test should be microscopic examination of an acid-fast smear and culture of relevant body fluids or tissues for mycobacteria. Several specimens are often required, especially for central nervous system disease. For suspected pulmonary TB, patients with respiratory symptoms should be placed in respiratory isolation until three serial sputum specimens are collected on different days for acid-fast smear and culture. Because patients with extrapulmonary disease may also have occult pulmonary disease, it is generally recommended that sputum smears be tested in these patients, regardless of chest radiograph findings.

Acid-fast smear does not differentiate between *M. tuberculosis* and atypical mycobacteria. Culture is used to confirm species and to determine drug susceptibility. This can be especially important in AIDS patients, who are at risk for atypical mycobacteria such as *M. avium* complex. Simultaneous culture on both liquid and solid media is suggested. Liquid media, such as the newer BACTEC systems, allow growth of the organism in about 14 days; growth takes 3 to 6 weeks on solid media (Löwenstein-Jensen or Middlebrook 7H11). Once sufficient growth is obtained, species identification can be performed via conventional biochemical tests or more rapid tests such as nucleic acid probes, high-performance

TABLE 158–1. CURRENT REGIMENS FOR TREATMENT OF DRUG-SUSCEPTIBLE TUBERCULOSIS

Regimen	Initial Phase	Continuation Phase
Daily* or 5 days/wk	8 wk of INH, RIF, PZA, ± EMB	18 wk of INH and RIF
Intermittent†	A. 2 wk of daily INH, RIF, PZA, and EMB (or SM)	A. 24 wk of twice-weekly INH and RIF
	B. 8 wk of thrice-weekly INH, RIF, PZA, and EMB (or SM)	B. 18 wk of thrice-weekly INH and RIF

*The daily regimen is used when patients self-administer their drugs. There is enough redundancy that, if patients miss some doses, the outcome will still be acceptable.
†The intermittent regimens are intended for directly observed therapy. Regimen A entails a total of 62 doses and has yielded over 95% success rates for the past 22 years in Denver, Colorado.[49] Regimen B involves 78 doses and has also resulted in success rates of approximately 95% in Hong Kong, where it is the standard regimen.[50]
EMB, ethambutol; INH, isoniazid; PZA, pyrazinamide; RIF, rifampin; SM, streptomycin.

liquid chromatography, the NAP test (p-nitro-α-acetylamino-β-hydroxypropiophenone), or molecular tests. Susceptibility testing on culture-positive specimens should be done only by experienced laboratories. Molecular fingerprinting by restriction fragment length polymorphism can be used to distinguish strain types when laboratory contamination is suspected.

The diagnosis of TB is sometimes based on classic histopathologic findings of caseating granulomas on tissue biopsy without smear or culture confirmation. If rapid diagnosis is needed, expensive nucleic acid amplification tests specific for *M. tuberculosis* complex can be used. Two such tests are available: Amplified *Mycobacterium tuberculosis* Direct Test (MTD, Gen-Probe) and AMPLICOR *Mycobacterium tuberculosis* Test (Roche). Both are currently approved by the Food and Drug Administration for use on smear-positive respiratory specimens, and an enhanced MTD is approved for respiratory specimens regardless of smear status. Sensitivity and specificity are both greater than 95% when used on smear-positive specimens. Use on nonrespiratory specimens is under investigation. The CDC has published guidelines on the use and interpretation of these tests.[40,41] Molecular tests such as PCR hold promise as rapid and sensitive diagnostic tests but have not been standardized across laboratories. ELISA or radioimmunoassays have detected mycobacterial antigens in the cerebrospinal fluid of patients with tuberculous meningitis.[42]

The PPD skin test is designed to diagnose TB infection, not disease. It should be used when TB is suspected, but a negative PPD never rules out any form of TB. Furthermore, a positive PPD suggests infection but does not confirm disease.

TREATMENT

Standard treatment of adults with TB consists of three- or four-drug regimens for at least 6 months.[43,44] The typical course of therapy for drug-susceptible disease includes 2 months of isoniazid, rifampin, pyrazinamide, and ethambutol, followed by 4 months of isoniazid and rifampin (continuation phase) (Tables 158-1 and 158-2). A 9- to 12-month regimen is suggested for tuberculous meningitis, for disease that is slow to respond to therapy, and when pyrazinamide is not used in the initial regimen. Ethambutol can be discontinued when drug susceptibility studies show sensitivity to isoniazid and rifampin. Streptomycin can be used instead of ethambutol if resistance is unlikely or susceptibility is shown. The continuation phase can be daily therapy, twice-weekly therapy, or thrice-weekly therapy (see Table 158-1). See the HIV section for details on the treatment of TB in HIV-positive patients. Specific guidelines, including information on first- and second-line agents, have been published by the CDC.[39]

When drug-resistant disease is suspected or confirmed, additional drugs that may be used include amikacin, a fluoroquinolone (levofloxacin, moxifloxacin, gatifloxacin, ofloxacin), capreomycin, ethionamide, cycloserine, and para-aminosalicylic acid. Local public health departments may provide assistance regarding resistance data. They should be contacted to meet reporting requirements and are usually responsible for treatment monitoring. Directly observed

TABLE 158–2. DOSAGES OF FIRST-LINE ANTITUBERCULOSIS DRUGS (IN ADULTS) AND MAJOR ADVERSE EFFECTS

Drug	Daily Dosage	Twice- or Thrice-Weekly Dosage	Adverse Effects
Isoniazid	5 mg/kg oral (max: 300 mg)	900 mg BIW 600 mg TIW	Hepatitis, peripheral neuritis, drug-induced lupus, seizures, hypersensitivity with rash and fever; drug interactions with phenytoin and disulfiram; pyridoxine can decrease neurotoxicity
Rifampin	10 mg/kg oral (max: 600 mg)	10 mg/kg 600 mg BIW 600 mg TIW	Orange body secretions, flulike syndrome, hepatitis, pruritus, thrombocytopenia, nausea, anorexia, diarrhea, renal failure, multiple drug interactions
Rifabutin*	10 mg/kg oral (max: 300 mg)	5 mg/kg	Neutropenia, uveitis, hepatotoxicity, orange discoloration of body fluids
Rifapentine*,†	10 mg/kg once weekly (max: 600 mg)		Similar to rifampin
Pyrazinamide	15-30 mg/kg oral (max: 2 g)	30-35 mg/kg	Hyperuricemia, hepatitis, rash, nausea, anorexia
Ethambutol	25 mg/kg initial 2 mo, then 15 mg/kg oral	50 mg/kg BIW 30 mg/kg TIW	Optic neuritis, gastrointestinal discomfort

*Rifabutin and rifapentine are considered first-line agents when intolerance to rifampin precludes its use or there is concern about drug interactions.
†Rifapentine is used in a once-weekly dose in HIV-negative patients with noncavitary and uncomplicated disease. It is not approved for use in children.
BIW, twice a week; TIW, three times a week.

TABLE 158–3. SELECTED PARENTERAL MEDICATIONS USED TO TREAT TUBERCULOSIS

Medication	Route	Initial Dosage in Adults* (Maximum Dosage)
Isoniazid	p.o., i.v., i.m.	5 mg/kg/day (300 mg)
Rifampin	p.o., i.v.	10 mg/kg/day (600 mg)
Streptomycin	i.v., i.m.	10-15 mg/kg/day or 750-1000 mg/day
Amikacin	i.v., i.m.	Same as streptomycin
Kanamycin	i.v., i.m.	Same as streptomycin
Capreomycin	i.v., i.m.	Same as streptomycin
Aminosalicylic acid	p.o., i.v.	8-12 g/day in 2 or 3 doses
Levofloxacin	p.o., i.v.	500-1000 mg/day
Moxifloxacin	p.o., i.v.	400 mg/day
Gatifloxacin	p.o., i.v.	400 mg/day

*Routine daily doses are given. Dosages may differ in children and in patients undergoing intermittent therapy. Persons older than 59 years should receive the lower dose for aminoglycosides (750 mg).
From Centers for Disease Control and Prevention: Treatment of tuberculosis. MMWR 2003;52:1-80.

therapy should be used whenever possible. Patients with multidrug-resistant TB require longer therapy and directly observed therapy. Surgical resection after 2 to 3 months of treatment may improve outcome.[39]

Parenteral therapy may be required in ICU patients and is recommended for patients with fulminant disease (Table 158-3). Isoniazid and rifampin are available in parenteral forms; ethambutol and pyrazinamide are not. Other active medications available for intravenous use include the aminoglycosides, fluoroquinolones, and capreomycin. In patients with renal failure, dose adjustments are required for drugs such as ethambutol, pyrazinamide, cycloserine, aminoglycosides, and fluoroquinolones. Isoniazid and pyrazinamide should probably be withheld in the setting of severe liver failure. An expert in the treatment of TB should be consulted when treating complicated ICU patients or those with multidrug resistance.

Corticosteroids are generally recommended in the treatment of several conditions, including tuberculous meningitis and pericarditis (see earlier sections).[45] Their role in patients with respiratory failure due to TB and in patients with severe AIDS-associated TB has not been proven, but many have used corticosteroids for these conditions. Typical therapy includes prednisone 40 to 80 mg/day tapered over many weeks.

Paradoxical reactions (clinical or radiographic worsening after treatment initiation) may occur in certain patients, especially those with HIV and alcoholics.[46,47] They are more common in patients with extrapulmonary disease (especially lymphadenitis) and may improve with nonsteroidal anti-inflammatory agents and corticosteroids.

RISK TO HEALTH CARE WORKERS

Pulmonologists are at higher risk for occupational exposure to TB compared with other specialists. Atypical presentations of TB can put providers at increased risk when TB is not suspected and proper precautions are not taken.[48] Bronchoscopy, which requires close contact with patients and provokes coughing, is likely associated with the 11% tuberculin skin test conversion rate among pulmonary fellows.[48] DMF-HEPA respirators should be used when performing bronchoscopy on patients with known or suspected TB.[48]

ANNOTATED REFERENCES

Barnes PF, Lakey DL, Burman WJ: Tuberculosis in patients with HIV infection. Infect Dis Clin North Am 2002;16:107-126.
This is a thorough review of the clinical manifestations of TB in HIV-infected patients. The authors discuss that nucleic acid amplification tests may be helpful in patients with acid-fast bacilli smear–positive sputum when the clinical suspicion of TB is intermediate or low.

Centers for Disease Control and Prevention: Treatment of tuberculosis. MMWR 2003;52:1-80.
This is the official statement of the American Thoracic Society, the CDC, and the Infectious Diseases Society of America regarding the treatment of TB. It includes recommendations for the treatment of special populations and lists common reactions and drug interactions associated with TB therapy.

Dooley DP, Carpenter JL, Rademacher S: Adjunctive corticosteroid therapy for tuberculosis: A critical reappraisal of the literature. Clin Infect Dis 1997;25:872-887.
The role of corticosteroids in the treatment of TB is controversial. This article reviews all major studies that compared corticosteroid therapy versus no corticosteroid therapy for many manifestations of TB.

Verdon R, Chevret S, Laissy JP, et al: Tuberculous meningitis in adults: Review of 48 cases. Clin Infect Dis 1996;22:982-998.
This retrospective review of 48 cases of tuberculous meningitis seen over 10 years confirms that outcome depends largely on clinical stage at admission and timing of treatment initiation. Clinical characteristics of tuberculous meningitis are also discussed.

Woods GL: The mycobacteriology laboratory and new diagnostic techniques. Infect Dis Clin North Am 2002;16:127-144.
This article summarizes the results of studies evaluating new screening and diagnostic tools (nucleic acid amplification, culture techniques, nucleic acid probes, restriction fragment length polymorphism, and susceptibility testing). The proper use of such tests is reviewed.

Chapter 159

MALARIA AND OTHER TROPICAL INFECTIONS IN THE INTENSIVE CARE UNIT

Daniel G. Bausch

KEY POINTS

1. A detailed history of the patient's travel itinerary, activities, exposures, and any pretravel prophylaxis and general knowledge of the prevalent diseases and their incubation periods and drug resistance patterns in the region of travel are imperative when evaluating patients with exposures overseas.

2. Most "nontropical" infections also are common in developing countries and need to be considered.

3. Infection with multiple tropical pathogens is common in individuals living in endemic areas.

4. Assessment of the patient's immune status, based on the history of exposure to tropical pathogens, is essential to diagnostic workup and to management.

UNCOMPLICATED MALARIA

1. Malaria is the most common serious infection in most tropical countries and in returning travelers and should be considered in any patient reporting travel in malaria-endemic areas or with exposure to unscreened blood products ("transfusion malaria") or blood-contaminated needles.

2. The risk of acquiring severe falciparum malaria is highest for individuals traveling to sub-Saharan Africa and New Guinea, moderate in India, and comparatively low in South East Asia and Latin America.

3. Malaria classically produces a three-stage "paroxysm" progressing over 8 to 12 hours and consisting of rigors and chills ("cold stage"), followed by fever ("hot stage"), and sweating with resolution of all symptoms ("defervescent stage"). The paroxysms classically occur with periodicity specific to each malaria parasite. In practice, neither the classic paroxysm nor the periodicity is invariably seen. Their absence should not be used to exclude the diagnosis.

SEVERE AND COMPLICATED MALARIA

1. Most severe and complicated malaria cases warranting attention in an ICU are due to *Plasmodium falciparum* in nonimmune children and adults and in pregnant women.

2. The most frequent severe complication is cerebral malaria, mostly seen in children and manifesting

as unrousable coma, convulsions, changes in sensorium, or focal neurologic signs. Other severe complications include severe anemia, hypoglycemia, lactic acidosis, acute renal failure, pulmonary edema, acute respiratory distress syndrome, shock, and bacterial superinfection.

3. Potentially severe complications due to nonfalciparum malaria include splenic rupture (*Plasmodium vivax*) and chronic nephrotic syndrome (*Plasmodium malariae*).

DIAGNOSIS

1. Most patients with *P. falciparum* present within 6 months of exposure.

2. Laboratory diagnosis traditionally is made through microscopy of thick and thin Giemsa-stained smears. Low or fluctuating parasitemias or altered parasite morphology may complicate diagnosis, especially with an inexperienced microscopist. Asymptomatic parasitemia is common in children from endemic areas.

3. Radiographic imaging of the abdomen is indicated when splenic rupture is suspected.

CLINICAL MANAGEMENT

1. Patients with evidence of severe or complicated malaria should be admitted to the ICU for aggressive supportive care and urgent intravenous (i.v.) drug therapy. In critically ill patients, chloroquine-resistant *P. falciparum* should be assumed until proved otherwise.

2. The quinolines, quinine and quinidine, are the drugs of choice in severe malaria. Artemisinin and its derivatives and various combination regimens may be equally efficacious, but generally should be reserved for cases of quinoline resistance or severe toxicity.

3. Side effects in response to quinoline therapy are frequent, but usually are mild, dose related, and reversible. Prolongation of the Q-T interval with i.v. quinoline therapy is common but rarely clinically significant. Cardiac monitoring should be performed. Most nonquinoline and newer quinoline drugs are well tolerated.

4. Ancillary therapies proposed for severe malaria include exchange transfusion, erythrocytapheresis,

iron chelation, antioxidants, monoclonal antibodies, and dichloroacetate. In most cases, insufficient controlled data are available on which to judge their efficacy. Steroids are detrimental in severe malaria and should not be used.

5. Hemoglobin and hematocrit, electrolytes, platelet count, glucose, lactate, arterial blood gas, blood urea nitrogen and creatinine, liver function and coagulation enzymes, and level of parasitemia in response to therapy should be monitored closely.

6. Case-fatality rates in severe malaria range from 2% to 50%. Factors that correlate with a poor prognosis include the infecting species and resistance profile, central nervous system involvement, pulmonary edema, hypoglycemia, lactic acidosis, renal failure, severe anemia, younger age, level of parasitemias, and treatment in a rural health facility as opposed to an ICU. Persistent neurologic sequelae are common in children with cerebral malaria, but children who survive without obvious neurologic defects subsequently seem to develop normally neuropsychologically.

7. Many patients with splenic rupture can be managed conservatively with supportive therapy, although splenectomy may be necessary.

Although the spectrum of possible "tropical" infections in a patient with exposures overseas initially may seem daunting, a detailed history of the travel itinerary, activities, and exposures often can narrow the differential diagnosis significantly (Table 159-1). This history must include more than simply recording the countries to which the patient traveled. Exposures of a business traveler staying at hotels and dining in fine restaurants in a major city may differ drastically from exposures of a student backpacking through rural areas of the same country. General knowledge of the diseases endemic in a given area and their incubation periods and drug resistance patterns is vital (Fig. 159-1 and Table 159-2; see Table 159-1). In addition, most "nontropical" infections also are common in developing countries. Although the differential diagnosis must be expanded to include tropical pathogens, common illnesses seen in developing and industrialized countries must be considered.

Patients prone to tropical infections can be divided into three groups: (1) nonimmune persons who have no history of exposure to tropical pathogens, primarily tourists and young children, regardless of geographic origin, after the waning of maternal antibody (around age 6 months); (2) immune or semi-immune persons residing in tropical countries who are repeatedly exposed; and (3) persons originally from tropical countries but now residing elsewhere who, in the absence of continued exposure, have waning immunity. The degree of immunity may exert profound effects on the presentation and severity of illness. A returning traveler may develop severe malaria at a relatively low parasitemic load, whereas a resident of sub-Saharan Africa with an equal degree of parasitemia may be asymptomatic. Genetic differences in susceptibility also may exist, such as resistance to *Plasmodium vivax* in blacks due to the absence of Duffy factor, which serves as the receptor, or the relative protection from severe malaria of *P. falciparum* afforded to persons carrying the sickle cell trait.[1-3]

In returning travelers, knowledge of pretravel vaccinations and prescribed and administered chemoprophylaxis (which often turn out not to be the same) is imperative, although these preventive measures do not confer 100% protection and should not be used to discard completely a given entity from the differential diagnosis. Physicians and patients frequently err in the prescribing of and adherence to appropriate prophylactic regimens.[4,5] Complete or partial chemotherapy may prolong the incubation period or alter the presentation of the illness. Individuals initially from tropical countries are often less likely to seek pretravel medical advice before making a visit home and often have considerably more exposures to tropical pathogens during their visit than do short-term travelers from industrialized countries.[6] People living in resource-poor tropical countries may be more likely to have complicating health problems, but less likely to have them previously diagnosed or controlled. Underlying diabetes, hypertension, malnutrition, chronic anemia, intestinal parasites, tuberculosis, human immunodeficiency virus (HIV), or hepatitis B infection may be discovered at the time of the acute illness.[7] Infection with multiple tropical pathogens is common in persons living in endemic areas. The finding of a given pathogen cannot automatically be assumed to be the cause of the patient's current illness.

UNCOMPLICATED MALARIA

Four species of *Plasmodium* cause malaria in humans: *P. falciparum*, *P. vivax*, *P. ovale*, and *P. malariae* (see Table 159-2). Malaria is the most common serious infection in most tropical countries and in returning travelers and should be considered in any patient reporting travel in malaria-endemic areas or with exposure to unscreened blood products ("transfusion malaria") or blood-contaminated needles. Growing travel and immigration over the past few decades have resulted in increases in imported malaria in most industrialized countries.[8,9] The risk of acquiring severe falciparum malaria is highest for individuals traveling to sub-Saharan Africa and New Guinea, moderate in India, and comparatively low in South East Asia and Latin America.[10,11] Malaria occasionally is reported in individuals without reported travel.[12] This exposure may result from the carriage of malaria-infected passengers (who may be asymptomatic) or anopheline mosquitoes on aircraft arriving from endemic areas. The parasite may be secondarily transmitted by anopheline mosquitoes endemic in some industrialized countries.

Malaria classically produces three stages of symptoms, which progress over 8 to 12 hours, constituting a "paroxysm." These stages correspond with and are attributable to the period of schizont rupture and the appearance of ring forms (merozoites) in the blood, which are accompanied by the release of many host inflammatory mediators. The paroxysm classically begins suddenly with a "cold stage," in which the patient experiences rigors and chills, often accompanied by headache, nausea, and vomiting. Intense peripheral vasoconstriction may result in pale, goose-pimpled skin and cyanosis of the lips and nail beds. Within a few hours, the "hot stage" ensues, with high fever, flushed skin, throbbing headache, and palpitations. The paroxysm concludes with the "defervescent stage," consisting of a drenching sweat and resolution of the fever. The exhausted patient often then sleeps. Although a

TABLE 159–1. TROPICAL DISEASES THAT MAY MERIT MANAGEMENT IN AN INTENSIVE CARE UNIT*

Disease and Organism	Distinguishing Clinical Features	Incubation Period	Geographic Distribution	Mode of Transmission and Typical Risk Factors
Nonspecific Febrile Syndromes				
African trypanosomiasis, hemolymphatic stage (*Trypanosoma brucei gambiense* and *T.b. rhodesiense*)	Lymphadenopathy, HSM, edema, rash, 30% have history of chancre, rarely DIC and thrombocytopenia	3-21 d	Sub-Saharan Africa	Tsetse fly bite; camping, safari
Babesiosis (*Babesia* spp.)	Hemolytic anemia, HSM	3-28 d	North America, Europe, sporadic cases worldwide	Tick bite, blood transfusion (rare); especially severe in asplenic persons
Brucellosis (*Brucella* spp.)	Subacute presentation over weeks-months, HSM, weight loss, may involve large bones, joints, spine	2-8 wk	Worldwide, especially Mediterranean, Middle East, and Latin America	Ingestion of contaminated dairy products; respiratory, skin, or conjunctival inoculation from contact with farm animals; abattoir workers, butchers, farmers
Candidiasis, disseminated (*Candida* spp.)	May involve any organ, skin or mucosal lesions not always present	1-4 wk	Worldwide	Usually in IH or after administration of long-term antibiotics or maintenance of indwelling catheters
Cat-scratch disease (*Bartonella henselae*)	Papule or eschar at site of inoculation, regional lymphadenopathy, fever may be mild, may progress to CNS involvement or endocarditis	1-2 wk	Worldwide	Cat scratch or bite, severe disease most often seen in IH
Coccidioidomycosis (*Coccidioides immitis*)	May see pneumonia with cavities, meningeal, skin, and bone involvement, eosinophilia	1-4 wk, often RD† in IH	Desert areas of the Americas	Inhalation of spores from soil; disseminated disease more common in Filipinos, blacks, Hispanics, IH, and pregnant women
Echinococcal cyst, leak, or rupture (*Echinococcus* spp.)	Allergic symptoms: urticaria, pruritus, anaphylaxis	Years	Worldwide	Ingestion of eggs in feces of infected carnivores, such as dogs and wolves; raising of domestic livestock
Erlichiosis (*Ehrlichia* spp.)	Rash (<50%), leukopenia, thrombocytopenia, HSM; may progress to GI, renal, pulmonary, or CNS involvement	7-21 d	Sporadic foci worldwide	Tick bite; camping, safari
Histoplasmosis, disseminated (*Histoplasma capsulatum*)	Mucocutaneous lesions, lymphadenopathy, HSM, DIC, any organ may be involved	1-4 wk, usually RD	Tropics worldwide	Inhalation of spores from soil, severe disease usually IH
Leptospirosis (*Leptospira* spp.)	Icterus, jaundice, conjunctival suffusion, rash, HSM, may be biphasic, may develop hepatorenal syndrome, CNS involvement, or pulmonary disease with hemorrhage	2-20 d	Worldwide	Contaminated urine of many types of small mammals, either directly or through soil or standing water; hunting, military exercises
Malaria (*Plasmodium falciparum, P. vivax, P. ovale, and P. malariae*)	See text	See Table 159-2	See Figure 159-1 and Table 159-2	Mosquito bite, transfusion
Measles	Conjunctivitis, coryza, cough, rash, Koplik's spots	5-14 d	Worldwide	Person-to-person via aerosol
Melioidosis (*Burkholderia pseudomallei*)	May develop pneumonia or local suppurative infection, shock (especially if IH)	2-21 d	South East Asia (especially Thailand), Australia, sporadic foci in tropics worldwide	Exposure to contaminated soil or infected animals, person-to-person (rare), often IH
Monkeypox (monkeypox virus)	Diffuse vesicular rash resembling chickenpox but involving palms and soles, lymphadenopathy	3-21 d	Central and West Africa	Person-to-person and from exposure to infected small mammals and monkeys; exotic pets; rule out smallpox/bioterrorism
Mycobacterium avium-intracellulare, disseminated	Usually subacute, HSM, weight loss	Months-years	Worldwide	Environmental organism causing opportunistic infection in IH
Oroya fever (*Bartonella bacilliformis*)	Acute anemia, jaundice, HSM, lymphadenopathy	2-3 wk	Peru, Ecuador, and Colombia	Sandfly bite; hiking, camping

Continued

TABLE 159–1. TROPICAL DISEASES THAT MAY MERIT MANAGEMENT IN AN INTENSIVE CARE UNIT*—cont'd

Disease and Organism	Distinguishing Clinical Features	Incubation Period	Geographic Distribution	Mode of Transmission and Typical Risk Factors
Paracoccidioidomycosis (*Paracoccidioides brasiliensis*)	May involve lungs, bones, skin, lymph nodes, adrenal glands, or mucous membranes	1-4 wk, often RD	Tropical America	Inhalation of spores from soil; more severe in IH
Penicilliosis (*Penicillium marneffei*)	Mucocutaneous lesions, HSM, lymphadenopathy, may have skeletal or pulmonary involvement	Unknown, probably ≥1 wk	South East Asia	Reservoir unknown, most often IH
Plague (*Yersinia pestis*)	Localized tender lymphadenitis (bubo), pneumonia, shock	2-8 d	Worldwide	Flea bite or person-to-person; areas of heavy rat infestations, rule out bioterrorism
Q fever (*Coxiella burnetii*)	HSM; may develop pneumonia, endocarditis, hepatitis, osteomyelitis, or neurologic abnormalities	2-29 d	Worldwide	Inhalation of organism from products of infected livestock or pets, especially birth products, but also milk, urine, and feces; farmers, ranchers
Rat-bite fever (*Spirillum minus* or *Streptobacillus moniliformis*)	Peripheral rash, sometimes with desquamation, polyarthritis in *S. moniliformis*, eschar or ulcer at site of bite in *S. minus*	2-28 d	Worldwide, especially Asia and North America	Bite of rat or other animal that preys on rats; ingestion of food contaminated by rat
Relapsing fever (*Borrelia* spp.)	Recrudescent fever pattern, HSM, petechiae, epistaxis, neurologic abnormalities	4-18 d	Worldwide (especially East Africa)	Body louse (*B. recurrentis*) or tick bite (various *Borrelia* spp.); conditions of poor hygiene, outdoor exposures, refugee camps, camping, safari
Rickettsiosis, spotted fever group (*Rickettsia rickettsii, R. conorii, R. africae, R. australis, R. sibirica, R. japonica, R. honei*, and *R. akari*)	Peripheral skin rash, eschar at site of tick bite may be seen (tache noire), may progress to GI, renal, pulmonary, or CNS involvement	7-14 d	Worldwide (with circumscribed distributions of each specific organism)	Tick bite (mite for *R. akari*); camping, safari
Rickettsiosis, typhus group (*Rickettsia prowazekii, R. typhi,* and *R. felis*)	Centripetal rash (~50%), no eschar	7-14 d	Worldwide, especially cold climates	Feces from infected louse (*R. prowazekii*) or flea (*R. typhi* and *R. felis*) rubbed into broken skin; crowding, poor hygiene, abundant rodents, refugee camps, flea-infested cats
Scarlet fever (group A *Streptococcus pyogenes*)	Pharyngitis, "sandpaper" rash, cervical adenopathy	1-4 d	Worldwide	Person-to-person via aerosolization/droplets
Schistosomiasis, Katayama fever (*Schistosoma* spp., especially *S. japonicum*)	Lymphadenopathy, HSM, eosinophilia	1-2 mo	Africa, Asia, Middle East, South America, Caribbean	Skin penetration of cercaria; swimming or bathing in contaminated water
Scrub typhus (*Orientia tsutsugamushi*)	Centripetal rash, conjunctival suffusion, lymphadenopathy, eschar at site of chigger bite (~50%), hearing loss in one third of cases	6-18 d	Asia, Australia, Pacific Islands	Chigger bite; outdoor rural or suburban exposures
Strongyloidiasis, disseminated (*Strongyloides stercoralis*)	Abdominal pain and distention, shock, pulmonary and CNS involvement common	2-3 wk, may be maintained via autoinfection for decades	Tropics worldwide	Skin contact with contaminated soil; military exercises, dissemination may occur in IH (AIDS, steroid treatment)
Toxic shock syndrome (*Staphylococcus aureus*, group A *S. pyogenes*)	Rash, extremity or abdominal pain, skin desquamation, soft tissue infection (70%)	2-10 d	Worldwide	Wound or vaginal colonization with toxin-producing bacteria; history of minor trauma (often without break in skin), previous surgery or varicella infection, staphylococcal syndrome often associated with menses
Trench fever (*Bartonella quintana*)	Rash, HSM, shin pain, may develop endocarditis and angioma-like lesions	1-2 wk	Worldwide	Body louse bite; areas of crowding or poor sanitation, more severe in IH
Trichinellosis (*Trichinella* spp.)	Diarrhea followed by myalgias, periorbital edema, eosinophilia, may involve heart or CNS	7-30 d	Worldwide	Ingestion of contaminated meat, including pork (*T. spiralis*), wild boar, horse, bear, and walrus

TABLE 159–1. TROPICAL DISEASES THAT MAY MERIT MANAGEMENT IN AN INTENSIVE CARE UNIT*—cont'd

Disease and Organism	Distinguishing Clinical Features	Incubation Period	Geographic Distribution	Mode of Transmission and Typical Risk Factors
Tularemia, typhoidal form (*Francisella tularensis*)	Pulse-temperature dissociation, diarrhea (~40%), may develop pneumonia	1-21 d	Sporadic foci worldwide, mostly Northern Hemisphere	Tick or fly bite, direct exposure to small mammals; hunting, camping, military exercises, rule out bioterrorism
Typhoid fever (*Salmonella typhi*)	Pulse-temperature dissociation, abdominal pain, rash, intestinal perforation and bleeding, HSM, 10% with extraintestinal manifestations	8-28 d	Worldwide	Fecal-oral
Vibrio infection, nonepidemic type (*Vibrio vulnificus*)	Bullous skin lesions, DIC, thrombocytopenia, GI bleeding, shock	1-2 d	Worldwide	Contaminated saltwater or seafood; severe disease mostly in IH, history of alcoholism, liver disease
Viral hemorrhagic fever (dengue, yellow fever, Ebola, Marburg, Lassa, Junin, Machupo, and Rift Valley fever viruses, many others)	Capillary leak syndrome, may or may not exhibit frank hemorrhage, GI hemorrhage, shock	3-21 d, depending on specific virus	Select areas worldwide	Depending on specific virus: exposure to rodent excreta, infected nonhuman primates, person-to-person, tick or mosquito bite, some unknown; rule out bioterrorism
Viral hepatitis (hepatitis viruses A, B, C, D, E; Epstein-Barr and cytomegalovirus; others)	HSM, light-colored stools, dark urine, jaundice	2 wk-5 mo, depending on specific organism	Worldwide	Fecal-oral or ingestion of seafood from contaminated sea beds (hepatitis A, E); percutaneous (blood exposure), sexual, or mother-to-child transmission (hepatitis B, C, D); hepatitis D requires coinfection with hepatitis B virus
Visceral leishmaniasis (*Leishmania* spp.)	Weight loss, HSM, neutropenia	Months-years	Tropics worldwide, especially Indian subcontinent, Middle East, and North Africa	Sandfly bite; military exercises, outdoor exposures

Gastrointestinal Syndromes

Disease and Organism	Distinguishing Clinical Features	Incubation Period	Geographic Distribution	Mode of Transmission and Typical Risk Factors
Amebic dysentery (*Entamoeba histolytica*, rarely other amebae)	Abdominal pain and diarrhea, sometimes bloody, minority may develop ameboma, toxic megacolon, peritonitis, or abscesses in solid organs (usually liver)	2-4 wk (usually longer for solid-organ involvement)	Worldwide	Fecal-oral; may be transmitted through anal sex
Anthrax, GI or oropharyngeal (*Bacillus anthracis*)	Abdominal pain and bloody diarrhea, neck swelling, pharyngitis, mucosal lesions, shock	2-10 d	Worldwide	Ingestion of spores; exposure to domestic animals or animal by-products; rule out bioterrorism
Ascending cholangitis (*Clonorchis sinensis* and *Opisthorchis* spp.)	May be recurrent and accompanied by pancreatitis	Months-years	Asia, former USSR	Ingestion of raw infected freshwater fish; sushi consumption
Bacterial dysentery (*Shigella* spp., *Campylobacter* spp., invasive and hemorrhagic *Escherichia coli*, nontyphi *Salmonella* spp., *Vibrio parahaemolyticus*, others)	Abdominal pain and diarrhea, sometimes bloody	10 h-7 d, depending on specific organism	Worldwide	Fecal-oral
Cholera (*Vibrio cholerae*)	Copious "rice water" diarrhea, abdominal pain, severe hypovolemia, fever minimal or absent	1-3 d	Tropics worldwide	Contaminated water or food, especially seafood; ceviche consumption
Clostridial gastroenteritis (*Clostridium difficile*)	Abdominal pain and diarrhea, sometimes with mucus or blood, toxic megacolon	~1 wk to months	Worldwide	Alteration of GI flora through previous antibiotic administration or GI manipulation
Eosinophilic gastroenteritis (*Angiostrongylus costaricensis*)	Mimics appendicitis or inflamed Meckel's diverticulum, right lower quadrant abdominal pain and mass, eosinophilia	Estimated 3-4 wk	Latin America	Ingestion of larvae in undercooked mollusks, crustaceans, or frogs
Hemolytic uremic syndrome (*Escherichia coli* O157:H7)	Bloody diarrhea followed by hemolysis and renal failure	2-5 d	Worldwide	Ingestion of poorly cooked meat, fecal-oral

Continued

TABLE 159–1. TROPICAL DISEASES THAT MAY MERIT MANAGEMENT IN AN INTENSIVE CARE UNIT*—cont'd

Disease and Organism	Distinguishing Clinical Features	Incubation Period	Geographic Distribution	Mode of Transmission and Typical Risk Factors
Neurologic Syndromes				
African trypanosomiasis, meningoencephalitic stage (*T. b. gambiense* and *T. b. rhodesiense*)	Headache, HSM, cervical lymphadenopathy, somnolence, change in mental status, extrapyramidal and cerebellar signs	Months-years	Sub-Saharan Africa	Tsetse fly bite; camping, safari
Antiretroviral syndrome (HIV-1)	Usually asymptomatic or mild flulike illness, meningoencephalitis occurs rarely	2-4 wk	Worldwide	Sexual transmission or percutaneous blood exposure; unprotected sex, intravenous drug use
Arboviral encephalitides (eastern equine, Japanese encephalitis, West Nile, Murray Valley encephalitis, St. Louis encephalitis, and Venezuelan equine encephalitis viruses, many others)	Encephalitis, focal neurologic deficits, seizures, change in mental status	3-21 d	Sporadic foci worldwide	Mosquito bite, seasonal
Bacterial meningitis (*Neisseria meningitidis*, *Streptococcus pneumoniae*, *Haemophilus influenzae* type B, *Listeria monocytogenes*, others)	Petechiae, ecchymoses, and bleeding suggest *N. meningitidis*	2-10 d, depending on specific organism	Worldwide, *N. meningitidis* more frequent in African "meningitis belt"	Person-to-person, asymptomatic carrier states, seasonal fluctuations
Botulism (*Clostridium botulinum*)	Bilateral cranial nerve deficits with symmetric descending weakness, fever absent	1-3 d	Worldwide	Toxin ingestion or wound contamination; home-canned foods, soil contamination
Brain abscess (various bacteria, fungi, and parasites)	Focal neurologic signs	Days-months, depending on specific organism	Worldwide	Varies with infecting organism
Cryptococcosis (*Cryptococcus neoformans*)	Mild meningitis with low-grade fever, nonfocal neurologic examination, sometimes seizures or pulmonary involvement	1-4 wk	Worldwide	Inhalation of spores from soil and bird and bat excreta; usually IH
Eosinophilic meningitis (*Angiostrongylus cantonensis*)	Headache, meningitis, sometimes cranial nerve involvement, fever minimal	1-7 d	South East Asia, South Pacific, sporadic foci worldwide	Ingestion of larvae in undercooked mollusks, crustaceans, or frogs
Gnathostomiasis (*Gnathostoma* spp.)	Migratory skin and subcutaneous swellings, epigastric pain and vomiting, eosinophilia, may invade any organ, especially CNS	Weeks-years	South East Asia, with sporadic cases from Central and South America	Consumption of raw freshwater fish, frogs, snakes, crustaceans, or poultry; sushi consumption
Herpes encephalitis (various herpesviruses)	Encephalitis, focal neurologic deficits, seizures, change in mental status, may show vesicular eruption	2-20 d, depending on specific virus	Worldwide; herpes B virus via monkey exposure in Asia and North Africa (wild monkeys) or captive monkeys worldwide	Person-to-person, often more severe in IH; herpes B virus via bite or other exposure to monkeys of the genus *Macaca*, person-to-person transmission reported; researchers, animal handlers
Mucormycosis (various fungi from the order *Mucorales*)	CNS infiltration with loss of consciousness, black exudate around mucous membranes of face, pulmonary infiltrates	1-7 d	Worldwide	Inhalation of spores from soil, traumatic inoculation of wound; usually IH (diabetes mellitus or steroid use)
Neurocysticercosis (*Taenia solium*)	Seizures, headache, change in mental status, muscle pain	Years	Worldwide, especially Latin America and India	Ingestion of cysticerci in contaminated pork; areas where pigs roam freely
Paragonimiasis, cerebral (*Paragonimus* spp.)	Meningoencephalitis, often accompanied by pulmonary disease	Years	Sporadic foci worldwide, especially East Asia, Peru, Ecuador, West Africa	Ingestion of raw infected crustaceans; sushi consumption
Poliomyelitis (poliovirus)	Acute flaccid paralysis, meningeal signs, muscle pain	9-12 d	Sporadic foci in Africa, Asia, and eastern Mediterranean	Fecal-oral
Primary amebic meningoencephalitis (*Naegleria fowleri*)	Fulminant meningoencephalitis	3-7 d	Sporadic foci worldwide	Entry of trophozoite through the nose; swimming in contaminated fresh warm water; hot springs

Disease and Organism	Distinguishing Clinical Features	Incubation Period	Geographic Distribution	Mode of Transmission and Typical Risk Factors
Rabies (rabies virus)	Change in mental status, autonomic instability, photophobia, aerophobia, paralysis	20-90 d	Worldwide	Animal bite or bat exposure; spelunking, caring for injured animals
Schistosomiasis, CNS (*Schistosoma* spp.)	Encephalopathy, meningoencephalitis, transverse myelitis, seizures	Weeks-months	Africa, Asia, Caribbean, Middle East, South America, Caribbean	Skin penetration of cercaria; swimming or bathing in contaminated water
Tetanus (*Clostridium tetani*)	Diffuse muscle spasms, opisthotonos, trismus, autonomic dysfunction	3-21 d	Worldwide	Soil contamination of wound, commonly involves umbilical stump in neonates
Tick-borne encephalitis (tick-borne encephalitis virus)	Encephalitis, focal neurologic deficits, seizures	7-14 d	Central and East Asia, Europe, North Africa, North America	Tick bite
Toxoplasmosis, cerebral (*Toxoplasma gondii*)	Meningoencephalitis, HSM, focal neurologic deficits, seizures, change in mental status	Usually RD	Worldwide	Ingestion of cysts in undercooked meat or oocysts from exposure to cat feces; usually IH
Variant Creutzfeldt-Jakob disease (prion)	Change in mental status, myoclonus, spasticity, rigidity, extrapyramidal and cerebellar signs and symptoms, occasionally seizures	Months-years	United Kingdom, with sporadic cases elsewhere in Europe, Canada, and United States	Recipients of cadaver transplants or injections of biomedical products derived from infected patients, contaminated surgical apparatus, person-to-person (?), ingestion of contaminated beef or lamb (?)
Visceral larva migrans (*Toxocara canis*)	Cough, wheezing, HSM, eosinophilia, may develop CNS or other solid-organ involvement	Weeks-years	Worldwide	Ingestion of eggs in puppy feces

Pulmonary Syndromes

Disease and Organism	Distinguishing Clinical Features	Incubation Period	Geographic Distribution	Mode of Transmission and Typical Risk Factors
Anthrax, inhalation (*B. anthracis*)	Pulmonary infiltrates with widened mediastinum, shock, CNS involvement	2-60 d	Worldwide	Inhalation of spores, exposure to domestic animals or animal by-products; rule out bioterrorism
Aspergillosis (*Aspergillus* spp.)	Pulmonary "fungus ball" (aspergilloma), transient infiltrates and allergic symptoms in allergic bronchopulmonary aspergillosis	1-4 wk	Worldwide	Inhalation of spores from soil
Bacterial pneumonia (*S. pneumoniae, Legionella pneumophila, Mycoplasma pneumoniae, Haemophilus influenzae, Chlamydia* spp., others)	Extrapulmonary findings frequent in legionnaires' disease and psittacosis	2-21 d, depending on specific organism	Worldwide	Person-to-person spread, legionnaires' disease associated with colonized air/water systems, psittacosis associated with bird exposure
Blastomycosis (*Blastomyces dermatitidis*)	Subacute pneumonia; bone, skin, and genitourinary tract involvement	1-4 wk, usually RD	Sporadic foci worldwide	Inhalation of spores from soil
Diphtheria (*Corynebacterium diphtheriae*)	Low-grade fever, cough, pharyngitis, oropharyngeal membrane, neck swelling, mucosal bleeding, myocarditis, polyneuritis	3-7 d	Worldwide, especially temperate areas	Person-to-person through respiratory route and breaks in the skin
Eosinophilic pneumonia (various parasites, helminthes, and filaria)	Eosinophilia, asthma-like condition, elevated IgE	Days-weeks, depending on specific organism	Worldwide, depending on specific organism	Lung passage of larvae or adult helminthes, mosquito bite (filaria), filarial disease occurs primarily in people living in endemic areas with continued exposure
Hantavirus pulmonary syndrome (various hantaviruses)	ARDS, thrombocytopenia, leukocytosis, hemoconcentration, circulating immunoblasts	1-5 wk	Americas	Contaminated rodent urine or feces; outdoor exposures
Pertussis (*Bordetella pertussis*)	Low-grade fever, coryza, rhinorrhea, paroxysmal dry cough	5-21 d	Worldwide	Person-to-person, adults vaccinated as children again susceptible to milder disease
Pneumocystosis (*Pneumocystis jiroveci*)	Dyspnea, dry cough, hypoxemia, often only mild findings on pulmonary auscultation and chest x-ray	Usually RD	Worldwide	Inhalation; usually IH

Continued

TABLE 159–1. TROPICAL DISEASES THAT MAY MERIT MANAGEMENT IN AN INTENSIVE CARE UNIT*—cont'd

Disease and Organism	Distinguishing Clinical Features	Incubation Period	Geographic Distribution	Mode of Transmission and Typical Risk Factors
Tuberculosis (*Mycobacterium tuberculosis*)	Upper lobe infiltrates and cavities; miliary tuberculosis, meningitis, and genitourinary involvement all common	Usually RD	Worldwide	Person-to-person via aerosol/droplet, increased frequency and likelihood of extrapulmonary involvement in IH
Tularemia, pneumonic form (*Francisella tularensis*)	Pulse-temperature dissociation, diarrhea (~40%)	1-21 d	Sporadic foci worldwide, mostly Northern Hemisphere	Tick or fly bite, or direct exposure to small mammals; hunting, camping, military exercises, rule out bioterrorism
Viral pneumonia (influenza, parainfluenza, respiratory syncytial, and SARS coronavirus; many others)	May be complicated by bacterial suprainfection	Days-weeks, depending on specific organism	Worldwide, depending on specific organism	Person-to-person spread and zoonotic, depending on specific virus; contact with farms or live-animal markets, birds, or pigs (zoonotic influenzas), civet cats suspected to be a reservoir of SARS coronavirus
Localized Infections				
Mycetoma (various fungi and bacteria)	Chronic swollen limb with nodules, sinus tracts, drainage of pus and "grains"	Weeks-months	Tropics worldwide	Traumatic implantation of organism into skin; soil exposure
Necrotizing fasciitis (group A *S. pyogenes*, *Clostridium* spp., *S. aureus*)	Rapid progression of edema, erythema, tenderness, bullae, necrosis, and gangrene	~24 h	Worldwide	Posttraumatic or surgical

*Only diseases that typically have acute or subacute presentations and may cause severe disease are included. Diseases are classified by the most typical associated severe syndrome. In practice, significant variation may exist.
†Initial infection is usually asymptomatic or mild. Reactivation with severe disease may occur years later, usually in immunocompromised hosts.
AIDS, acquired immunodeficiency syndrome; ARDS, acute respiratory distress syndrome; CNS, central nervous system; DIC, disseminated intravascular coagulopathy; GI, gastrointestinal; HIV-I, human immunodeficiency virus type I; HSM, hepatosplenomegaly; IH, immunocompromised host; RD, reactivation disease; SARS, severe acute respiratory syndrome.

classic periodicity is described for the different malaria species (see Table 159-2), this occurs only when the infection has persisted untreated long enough to allow for synchronization of schizont rupture. Schizont rupture tends to be asynchronous in *P. falciparum* and in most primary infections of any *Plasmodium* species. Malaria often may result in persistently spiking fevers difficult to distinguish from fever produced by many other infections. The absence of a classic paroxysm and periodicity should not be used to exclude the diagnosis. Paroxysms may be accompanied by

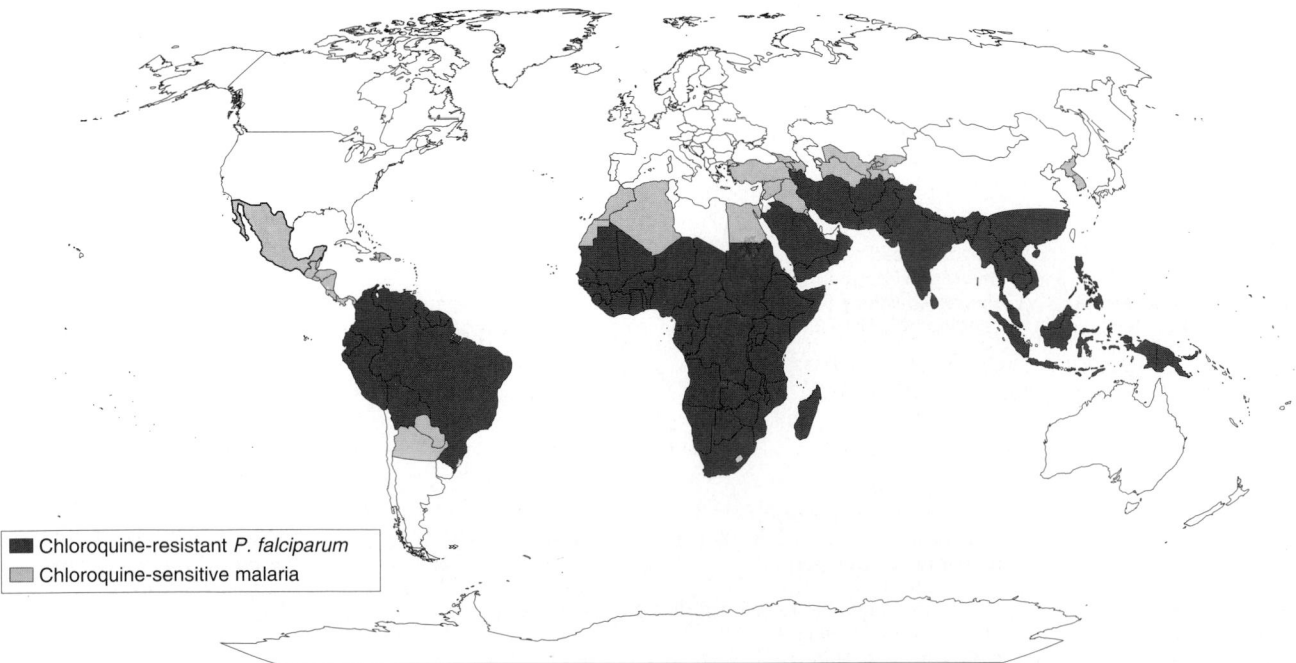

- ■ Chloroquine-resistant *P. falciparum*
- ▨ Chloroquine-sensitive malaria

FIGURE 159–1. Global distribution of malaria. The risk of malaria may vary within specific regions of each country. (Modified from Health Information for International Travel 2003-2004. Atlanta, Centers for Disease Control and Prevention, 2004.)

TABLE 159–2. FEATURES OF THE FOUR SPECIES OF MALARIA

	P. falciparum	P. vivax	P. ovale	P. malariae
Incubation period (d)	6-25	8-27	8-27	16-40
Asexual cycle (h)	48 (tertian)	48 (tertian)	48 (tertian)	72 (quartan)
Relapse	No	Yes*	Yes*	No[†]
Chloroquine resistance	Yes[‡]	Rare[§]	No	No[‖]
Characteristic on thin blood film	Rings predominate, multiply infected RBCs, high parasitemia, rings with threadlike cytoplasm, double nuclei, banana-shaped gametocytes	Enlarged RBCs, Schüffner's dots, trophozoite cytoplasm ameboid, 12-24 merozoites in mature schizont	Oval RBCs with fringed edges, Schüffner's dots, trophozoites cytoplasm compact, 6-16 merozoites in mature schizont	Trophozoite cytoplasm compact (band forms), 6-12 merozoites in mature schizont, RBCs unchanged

*Relapses may appear months to years after initial infection due to dormant hypnozoites in the liver.
[†]Although relapse does not occur, P. malariae can produce persistent infections that remain below detectable limits in the blood for 20 to 30 years or more.[108]
[‡]P. falciparum resistance to sulfadoxine/pyrimethamine (Fansidar), mefloquine, halofantrine, and artemisin also has been reported in some areas, along with partial resistance to quinine and quinidine.[109-114]
[§]P. vivax resistance to chloroquine now reported in some areas of South East Asia, Oceania, and South America.[115-126]
[‖]Chloroquine-resistant P. malariae also has been reported in south Sumatra, Indonesia.[127]
RBCs, red blood cells.
Modified from Miller LH, Warrell DA: Malaria. In Warren KS, Mahmoud AA (eds): Tropical and Geographical Medicine, 2nd ed. New York, McGraw-Hill, 1990, p 246.

cough, sore throat, myalgias, back pain, postural hypotension, abdominal pain, nausea, vomiting, diarrhea, and weakness. These symptoms are more common in children and may falsely suggest a diagnosis other than malaria. Rash and lymphadenopathy are not typical of malaria and suggest another diagnosis.

SEVERE AND COMPLICATED MALARIA

Although all species of malaria may produce severe consequences in a debilitated patient, potentially fatal malaria that warrants attention in an ICU can be grouped into three categories: (1) severe complications of P. falciparum in nonimmune children and adults; (2) splenic rupture, which occurs most frequently with P. vivax; (3) chronic nephrotic syndrome due to immune complex nephritis associated with P. malariae, usually seen in children and often complicated by overwhelming bacterial infection.

P. falciparum accounts for most severe malaria as a result of (1) its ability to infect red blood cells (RBCs) of all ages, resulting in overwhelming parasitemias (70% of RBCs); (2) its adherence to and obstruction of the microvasculature; (3) its induction of severe metabolic derangements directly through glucose consumption and lactate production and indirectly through the induction of cytokines; and (4) the high prevalence of chloroquine resistance to P. falciparum in many parts of the world (see Tables 159-2 and 159-3, Fig 159-1). Nonimmune persons and pregnant women are at greatest risk.

In contrast to the other species of malaria parasite, P. falciparum causes decreased RBC deformability and produces small protrusions or "knobs" on parasitized RBC membranes, which mediate their adhesion to the venular endothelium (Fig. 159-2). The rupture of schizont stage parasites exposes glycosyl phosphatidylinositol anchors on the parasite and RBC surface that induce macrophages and other inflammatory cells to release a host of inflammatory mediators, including tumor necrosis factor, interleukin-1, and various kinins and reactive nitrogen intermediates.[13-15] These cytokines play a role in up-regulation and activation of endothelial adhesion molecules, such as intercellular adhesion molecule type 1 and E-selectin, enhancing cytoadherence of parasitized cells and mediating such pathologic processes as hypoglycemia, lactic acidemia, shock, gut mucosal

damage, and increased permeability and neutrophil aggregation in the lung. The sum total of this cascade is sequestration of parasitized RBCs in the microvasculature, where they not only are sheltered from removal, but also cause sluggish flow and obstruction resulting in impaired oxygen delivery and organ dysfunction.[13,16] The most profound effects are usually on the cerebral capillaries, although a host of tissues may be affected, including the kidney, liver, spleen, placenta, intestine, lung, bone marrow, heart, and retina. Histopathologic changes are usually minimal, but ring hemorrhages and perivascular infiltrates sometimes develop at the sites of obstructed vessels, perhaps facilitated by thrombocytopenia due to splenic sequestration of platelets. Clinical deterioration usually appears 3 to 7 days after onset of fever. Genetic differences in the host and differences in parasite strains probably play roles in the ultimate course of the disease.

CEREBRAL MALARIA

Cerebral malaria is the most frequent severe complication of plasmodium infection, accounting for most fatalities and chronic sequelae. It is most frequent in children age 3 to 5 years. Strictly defined, cerebral malaria implies unrousable coma due to P. falciparum.[17] Hyperpyrexia and febrile convulsions in young children may produce transiently altered mental status without true involvement of the cerebral microvasculature and technically do not constitute cerebral malaria. In clinical practice, seizures or persistent changes in sensorium that cannot be attributed to other disease processes should be considered cerebral malaria, however, until proved otherwise. Although cerebral malaria is classically attributed to cytoadhesion and microvascular obstruction in the brain, other ongoing processes, including hypoglycemia, metabolic acidosis, and impaired oxygenation due to anemia and pulmonary edema, likely contribute.

The altered sensorium of cerebral malaria may develop gradually within a few days of onset of illness or manifest as persistent coma after a generalized convulsion. Compared with adults, children with cerebral malaria have a shorter history of fever before progressing to coma (average about 2 days). The most common neurologic picture is of a symmetric upper motor neuron lesion with hypertonia, hyperreflexia, clonus, absent abdominal reflexes, and extensor Babinski responses.

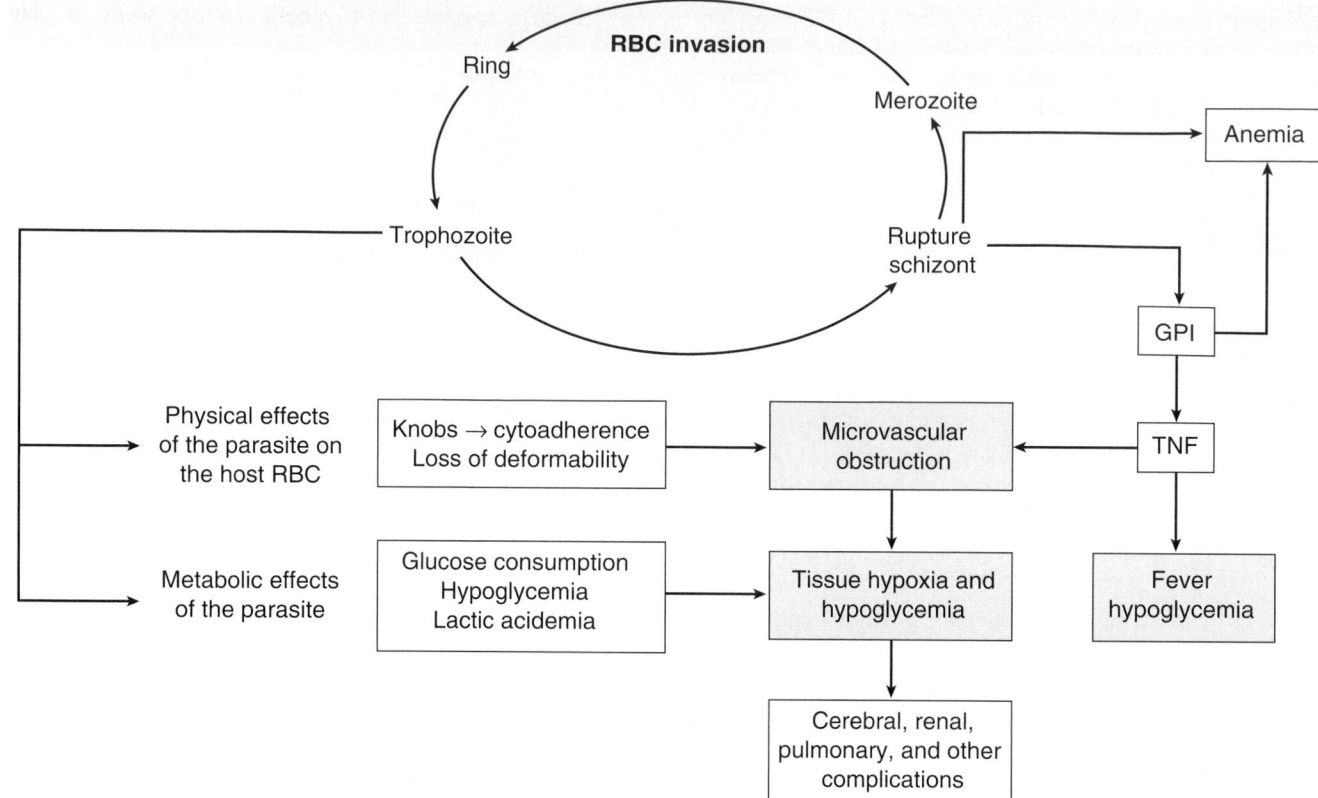

FIGURE 159–2. Pathogenesis of severe and complicated *Plasmodium falciparum* malaria. GPI, glycosyl phosphatidylinositol; RBC, red blood cell; TNF, tumor necrosis factor. (Modified from Krogstad D: *Plasmodium* species (malaria). In Mandell GL, Bennett JE, Dolin R [eds]: Principles and Practice of Infectious Diseases, 5th ed. Philadelphia, Churchill Livingstone, 2000.)

Hypotonia and acute cerebellar ataxia have been observed, especially in India and Sri Lanka. There is usually a diffuse, symmetric encephalopathy, sometimes with signs of frontal lobe release, such as a pout reflex and bruxism, although there is usually no grasp reflex, and the gag reflex is normally maintained. Decorticate and decerebrate posturing may occur. Meningismus, opisthotonos, and a dysconjugate gaze are seen frequently. Nystagmus and a sixth nerve palsy are more rare. Pupils are usually symmetric with intact pupillary, corneal, oculocephalic, and oculovestibular reflexes. Photophobia, severe neck rigidity, and papilledema are almost never seen.

Convulsions may occur in 50% of cases of cerebral malaria. In children older than 3 to 4 years, seizures become more likely to represent cerebral malaria, rather than febrile convulsions.[18] Generalized seizures classically are reported, but partial motor seizures, with or without secondary generalization, may occur. Although often showing only diffuse cortical dysfunction, electroencephalogram studies sometimes may reveal underlying status epilepticus even when it is not clinically noted.[19]

ANEMIA

Although some degree of anemia is often seen in all types of malaria, severe anemia (hemoglobin <5 g/100 mL) occurs almost exclusively with *P. falciparum* infections due to high parasitemias. Anemia is most common and often severe in pregnant women and young children (<1 year), in whom it may be the presenting sign.[20] In addition to the acute hemolytic destruction of parasitized RBCs, the more chronic processes of removal of parasitized cells from circulation by the spleen and cytokine inhibition of erythropoiesis may contribute.[21] Nonimmune subjects may develop anemia within days after infection, whereas anemia usually develops more slowly in patients who are semi-immune. The degree of anemia generally correlates with the bilirubin level and level of parasitemia. It may be exacerbated by underlying glucose-6-phosphate dehydrogenase deficiency in the setting of administration of oxidant antimalarial drugs, such as quinine and sulfadoxine, and iron deficiency anemia due to malnutrition. Significant jaundice and hemoglobinuria may result.

HYPOGLYCEMIA AND LACTIC ACIDOSIS

Hypoglycemia and lactic acidosis are frequently seen and sometimes major complications, especially in pregnant women and young children. Although sometimes asymptomatic in pregnant women, hypoglycemia often causes convulsions, impaired consciousness, and extensor posturing and may be confused with cerebral malaria. In addition to direct glucose consumption by the malaria parasite, decreased oral intake, depletion of liver glycogen, cytokine inhibition of gluconeogenesis, and insulin release stimulated by quinine or quinidine may contribute to hypoglycemia (see later). Serum insulin, lactate, alanine, and counterregulatory hormones are appropriately elevated.[56]

ACUTE RENAL FAILURE

Acute renal failure is seen in about 30% of adult patients with cerebral malaria but is uncommon in children. Because of the lessened magnitude of hemolysis, acute renal failure is rare among semi-immune patients. Acute renal failure is usually due to acute tubular necrosis, is oliguric in nature (<400 mL urine per 24 hours for adults), and is most often reversible. Renal ischemia due to hypovolemia, renal vasoconstriction, microvascular obstruction, and pigment nephropathy due to hemolysis all may contribute. Electrolyte abnormalities, such as hyponatremia, hypocalcemia (usually related to albumin loss), hypophosphatemia, and metabolic acidemia, and fluid overload with pulmonary edema may result. "Blackwater fever" refers to a severe syndrome characterized by low or absent parasitemia, intravascular hemolysis, hemoglobin-uria, and acute renal failure classically seen in people of northern European descent chronically exposed to *P. falciparum* and irregularly taking the antimalarial drugs quinine or quinidine. The syndrome virtually disappeared after 1950 when chloroquine superseded quinine. It is now said to be resurgent, however, albeit with lower mortality, in relation to mounting chloroquine resistance and consequent increased use of other quinines and the newer quinolines (mefloquine and halofantrine).[22]

PULMONARY EDEMA AND ACUTE RESPIRATORY DISTRESS SYNDROME

Pulmonary edema, which may progress to acute respiratory distress syndrome, occurs frequently and typically is the most lethal complication of malaria. It usually occurs late in the course of the illness in adult patients with other complications.[17] The pathology is one of a capillary leak syndrome with normal intracardiac pressures.[23,24] Interstitial edema and inflammatory cell infiltrates are seen at autopsy.[25] Tumor necrosis factor and other cytokine effects seem to be the causative factors because sequestration of parasitized RBCs in the lung is uncommon, even in patients with significant pulmonary involvement.

SHOCK AND BACTERIAL SUPERINFECTION

So-called algid malaria, referring to hypotension and shock, may resemble and sometimes be due to gram-negative sepsis secondary to impaired flow in intestinal capillaries with resultant mucosal erosion. This condition is often seen in hyperparasitemia with concomitant hypoglycemia and lactic acidemia and may progress to multiorgan system failure and death. Similar to most malaria complications, severe hemo-dynamic derangements are seen most often in nonimmune persons.[26] Whether bacteria are isolated or not, a classic septic shock picture is typical, with elevated cardiac index and decreased systemic vascular resistance.[27] Hemodynamic decompensation due to splenic rupture may mimic algid malaria.

TROPICAL SPLENOMEGALY AND SPLENIC RUPTURE

Splenomegaly is common in infection with all four malaria parasites. Tropical splenomegaly syndrome, also sometimes termed *hyperreactive malarial syndrome,* refers to a condition of massive splenomegaly, high titers of total serum IgM and malarial antibodies, scanty or absent parasitemia, and response to antimalarial agents. It is seen in individuals with a history of residence in an endemic area and can be associated with

any malaria species. Host genetic factors seem to play a role.[28]

In contrast to virtually all the other complications of malaria, which most often are associated with *P. falciparum,* acute splenic complications occur most commonly in *P. vivax,* especially with the first infection. Although the term *spontaneous splenic rupture,* with catastrophic implications, traditionally has been used, in reality a range of hematomas or tears of varying severity may occur. The rupture or tear usually occurs 2 to 3 months after infection, typically associated with trauma of varying degrees. Overeager examiners have been suggested to play a role in the pathogenesis, although no cases of clear palpation-induced rupture are reported. Fever, tachycardia, vomiting, prostration, abdominal pain or guarding, tender splenomegaly, hypovolemia, and rapidly worsening anemia are common presenting features. Abdominal pain may be localized or diffuse, mild or severe. Shock may ensue. Diaphragmatic irritation after rupture may cause referred pain to the left shoulder, supraclavicular, or scapular regions (Kehr's sign). This pain is present in about half of cases and is said to have good specificity for rupture.

OTHER COMPLICATIONS

Although rarely clinically significant, mild hepatocellular damage may occur and be manifested by elevated hepatic transaminases and jaundice. At least theoretically, metabolic clearance of antimalarial medications and lactate could be impaired, and deficits in the production of coagulation factors and albumin could be present. Disseminated intravascular coagulation is seen in less than 10% of severe cases. Thrombocytopenia, although frequent, is not usually associated with bleeding or correlated with disease severity. Although subendocardial and epicardial hemorrhages have been noted at autopsy, myocarditis does not occur, and primary cardiac events are relatively rare in malaria.

A host of secondary complications, including aspiration pneumonia, gram-negative septicemia (especially with nontyphoid salmonella), parvovirus infection, and endemic Burkitt's lymphoma, may be related to falciparum malaria. Although initially unrecognized, more recent studies have shown that malaria occurs with increasing frequency and severity in HIV-infected patients, especially during pregnancy.[29-32] Acute malaria can up-regulate HIV replication, leading to higher plasma viral loads. An association between severe malaria infection and hepatitis B surface antigen carriage has been noted.[33]

MALARIA IN PREGNANT WOMEN AND CHILDREN

In addition to pregnant women and their fetuses being more susceptible to infection, malaria is particularly dangerous in pregnant women and their fetuses, with increased risk of pulmonary edema, hypoglycemia, severe anemia, premature delivery, low birth weight, and maternal and fetal death. Malaria parasites often can be found in the placenta and may impair oxygen and nutrient transport to the fetus. Disease is most severe in primiparae, especially if nonimmune. In contrast, women from endemic areas are usually asymptomatic, with the exception of the effects of anemia, which is more severe in primiparae. Congenital malaria is rare except in infants born to nonimmune mothers.[34]

DIAGNOSIS

CLINICAL DIAGNOSIS

Because malaria often presents with nonspecific signs and symptoms, making a clinical diagnosis may be difficult. Although almost all patients have a history of fever, they frequently may be afebrile at the time of examination.[35] Physicians in industrialized countries who are unfamiliar with the disease may not include malaria initially in the differential diagnosis. Delayed diagnosis is frequent and is associated with a poor outcome.[6,36] Although patients with other species of malaria parasite may not present for months or years after infection, most patients with *P. falciparum* present within 6 months of exposure.[4] Incomplete chemoprophylaxis is often implicated in the delay. The differential diagnosis includes most febrile illnesses found in the tropics, including typhoid fever, bacterial pneumonia, leptospirosis, relapsing fever, enteropathogenic *E. coli* and other enteric pathogens, influenza, hepatitis, meningococcal infection, rickettsial infections, viral hemorrhagic fevers, and arboviral infections (see Table 159-1). Babesiosis may present clinically and microscopically similar to malaria in patients without travel to malaria-endemic areas. Cerebral malaria must be distinguished from bacterial meningitis, the viral meningoencephalitides, metabolic coma, and intoxications by lumbar puncture.[37] In cerebral malaria, the cerebrospinal fluid opening pressure is usually normal. A few lymphocytes and moderate elevation of protein may be seen. High cerebrospinal fluid lactate and low glucose indicate a poor prognosis.

CONVENTIONAL MICROSCOPY

Specific laboratory diagnosis traditionally has been made via the examination of thick and thin Giemsa-stained smears. Thick smears are more sensitive in generally diagnosing malaria, whereas thin smears allow identification of the specific parasite. Either smear can be used to quantify the level of parasitemia, but thick smears are theoretically more sensitive for this purpose.[38] Simultaneous infections with multiple strains of *P. falciparum* are common in some areas of sub-Saharan Africa and may occur with *P. vivax* in South East Asia and Latin America.[39,40] Blood obtained by pricking a fingertip or earlobe is preferred because parasite densities are higher in these capillary-rich areas, although blood obtained by venipuncture collected in heparin or ethylenediamine tetraacetic acid anticoagulant–coated tubes is acceptable if used shortly after being drawn to prevent alteration in the morphology of white blood cells and malaria parasites.[41]

TABLE 159–3. COMPLICATIONS OF *P. FALCIPARUM* MALARIA

Cerebral malaria
Anemia
Hypoglycemia
Lactic acidosis
Acute renal failure
Pulmonary edema and ARDS
Shock and bacterial suprainfection
Tropical splenomegaly and splenic rupture
Premature labor, abortion, and low birth weight

ARDS, acute respiratory distress syndrome.

Smears should be taken as soon as the diagnosis of malaria is considered, without waiting for manifestation of a classic paroxysm. Parasitemia may be undetectable in patients in the early stages of the illness, in patients with partial immunity, and in patients who have previously self-administered antimalarials, a common practice in malaria-endemic areas.[42] Levels of parasitemia may fluctuate over time, necessitating repeated smears for diagnosis. *P. falciparum*–parasitized RBCs may be sequestered in the deep capillaries of the spleen, liver, and bone marrow. Although a blood film is unlikely to be falsely negative in a patient with severe disease, negative smears should not prevent the prompt administration of antimalarial therapy if the diagnosis is strongly suspected.[11] Conversely, asymptomatic parasitemia is common in children from endemic areas, and a positive smear does not signify a clinical case under these circumstances.

Considerable expertise at reading malaria smears may be necessary to detect and distinguish the parasites (see Table 159-2). The most important point is to distinguish *P. falciparum*, with its concomitant risk of severe complications, from the other plasmodia. Superimposed platelets, particles of stain, pits in the slide, RBC inclusions such as Howell-Jolly bodies and inclusions seen in siderocytes, and other intracellular pathogens such as *Bartonella* and *Babesia* must be distinguished from malaria parasites. Alterations in parasite morphology may occur related to strain variation, drug pressure, and blood collection method.

NEWER LABORATORY METHODS

Various new diagnostic techniques for malaria have been developed, including microscopy with fluorescent stains (QBC), dipstick antigen detection of HRP2 and pLDH (Parasight-F, ICT Malaria Pf, OptiMAL), DNA probes, polymerase chain reaction assays, and automated blood cell analysis.[43-49] Each technique has unique advantages and disadvantages, but the sensitivity and specificity for *P. falciparum* are generally similar or better than conventional microscopy. Use of one of these new modalities should be considered when a high suspicion of malaria remains despite repeatedly negative blood smears, especially if the microscopist has limited experience with reading malaria smears; this is often the case in hospitals in industrialized countries where malaria is seen infrequently. Because of its greater sensitivity (down to approximately 5 parasites/μL), polymerase chain reaction may be a particularly valuable tool in nonimmune persons and may help determine whether multiple parasites of the same species but differing resistance profiles are present.

IMAGING

Computed tomography or magnetic resonance imaging of the abdomen is the usual diagnostic modality when splenic rupture is considered, although ultrasonography, arteriography, bleeding scans, or exploratory laparotomy sometimes may be needed. Although findings such as increased brain volume and occasionally brain swelling have been noted in computed tomography and magnetic resonance imaging studies in cerebral malaria, these tests are generally not helpful clinically and are indicated only to rule out suspected mass lesions when the diagnosis of cerebral malaria is uncertain.[50]

CLINICAL MANAGEMENT

INDICATIONS FOR ADMISSION TO THE INTENSIVE CARE UNIT

Features that indicate severe disease warranting admission to an ICU and urgent i.v. therapy include change in mental status, seizures, or other neurologic findings suggesting cerebral malaria; acute renal failure; pulmonary edema; shock; hypoglycemia; spontaneous bleeding or disseminated intravascular coagulation; acidemia; hyperparasitemia (>250,000 parasitized RBCs/μL or >5% of RBCs); jaundice; hyperpyrexia; and severe anemia. The threshold for ICU admission should be especially low for nonimmune patients, as they are more susceptible to severe disease. In these critically ill patients, chloroquine-resistant *P. falciparum* should be assumed until proved otherwise.

GENERAL MANAGEMENT

Careful attention to fluid balance is imperative, especially considering the poor prognosis when pulmonary edema or acute respiratory distress syndrome develops. Measurements of urine output and daily weights should be performed routinely. Monitoring of central venous pressure should be considered in delicate cases, such as cases with respiratory distress or compromised renal function. Considering that the prognosis associated with pulmonary failure is considerably poorer than that of acute renal failure, some authors recommend the early use of inotropes rather than excessive fluids in the setting of hypotension, although a beneficial effect on the overall hemodynamic profile has yet to be shown conclusively.[35,51] Dialysis is indicated for acute renal failure and may aid not only through improved fluid balance and control of acidemia, but also through the removal of circulating cytokine mediators of inflammation. Although observations are limited, the quinolines appear not to be dialyzed.[52] Cautious transfusion of packed cells is usually indicated when the hematocrit declines to less than 20%. In addition to improved oxygen transport, blood transfusion may reduce the parasite load and the cytokine mediators of inflammation.[35,53]

Concurrent administration of diuretics or low-dose dopamine may be warranted to avoid fluid overload. Metabolic acidosis should be treated by improving pulmonary gas exchange, correcting hypovolemia and hypoglycemia, and treating associated septicemia. Supplemental oxygen and mechanical ventilation may be required. Extracorporeal oxygenation also has been employed.[54] In patients with profound shock, blood cultures should be drawn and broad-spectrum antibiotics begun due to the risk of concomitant bacterial septicemia. Blood glucose should be checked frequently, especially in pregnant patients, and 50% dextrose should be administered when needed. Results of studies on the efficacy of continuous i.v. infusion of 5% dextrose have been mixed.[55,56] Quinoline-induced hypoglycemia may be prevented by the administration of somatostatin analogs followed by glucagons.[57] Seizures can be prevented with a single intramuscular injection of phenobarbital (3.5 mg/kg).[58] Although the risk of bleeding is low, aspirin should be avoided in the presence of thrombocytopenia. Many patients with splenic rupture can be managed conservatively with supportive therapy, although splenectomy may be necessary.[28]

In late pregnancy, fetal monitoring should be started before the initiation of quinoline therapy so that the effects of the disease can be distinguished from the effects of drug toxicity. Although fetal distress is usually the result of placental insufficiency, it sometimes may be related to high maternal temperature and hypoglycemia. These should be monitored carefully and treated accordingly. Fluid balance is particularly crucial in pregnant patients because the sudden increase in peripheral vascular resistance postpartum may precipitate pulmonary edema. Early obstetric intervention should be considered for the benefit of mother and fetus. In young children prone to febrile convulsions, extra efforts should be made to control fever by the use of acetaminophen, cooling blankets, and baths.

ANTIMALARIAL CHEMOTHERAPY

Because delay of therapy is associated with increased mortality, empirical treatment should be implemented immediately in all suspected cases after obtaining appropriate blood specimens. The cinchona alkaloids, quinine and quinidine, remain the drugs of choice in severe malaria (Table 159-4 and Table 159-5). Initial therapy should be i.v., unless intravascular access cannot be obtained. In the United States, where i.v. quinine is no longer available, quinidine gluconate is used.[59] Artemisinin and its derivatives (not available in the United States) and various combination regimens may be equally efficacious, but generally should be reserved for cases of quinoline resistance or severe toxicity.[60-62]

ADVERSE EFFECTS OF THERAPY

Side effects of quinine and quinidine, known as *cinchonism,* are common and typically include nausea, vomiting, headache, dysphoria, vasodilation, tinnitus, and changes in auditory and visual acuity. These alterations are dose-related and reversible. Less common side effects include rash, urticaria, angioedema of the face, pruritus, agranulocytosis, hepatitis, blackwater fever, and psychiatric disorders. Overdoses are associated with depressed respiration, circulatory collapse, and central nervous system alterations, including seizures and coma, which may be difficult to distinguish from cerebral malaria.[63] The simultaneous use of two quinolines or retreatment with the same quinoline within a short time may predispose to severe side effects.[64] The cinchona alkaloids are metabolized in the liver and excreted in the urine. Monitoring of blood levels is recommended for patients with impaired renal or hepatic function, and dose reduction is necessary in patients with severe renal impairment. Quinine metabolism seems to be decreased in children with kwashiorkor but increased in children with marasmus.[65]

Although rarely clinically significant, prolongation of the electrocardiogram Q-T interval with i.v. quinoline therapy is common.[66] Severe conduction abnormalities may occur along with hypotension, blindness, deafness, and coma when serum quinoline levels exceed 20 mg/L.[66,67] Dysrhythmias and hypotension also may result from too-rapid infusion. Cardiac monitoring should be performed with i.v. quinoline use, especially with quinidine, which, although more potent against the malaria parasite, also is generally more toxic.[66] Infusion rates of quinidine should be decreased if the Q-T interval increases by more than 25% of its baseline level.

Quinoline-induced stimulation of insulin may elicit significant hypoglycemia, especially in pregnancy.[56,68] Hypophosphatemia also may be precipitated by quinoline and

TABLE 159–4. DRUG REGIMENS FOR TREATMENT OF SEVERE MALARIA IN ADULTS

Drug	Route of Administration	Loading Dose	Maintenance Dose	Duration of Treatment
Quinidine gluconate*	i.v. in normal saline	10 mg salt/kg (maximum 600 mg) over 1–2 h[†]	0.02 mg salt/kg/min (constant infusion)	7 d[‡]
Quinine dihydrochloride*	i.v. in 5% dextrose	20 mg/kg over 4 h[†]	10 mg/kg q8h over 1–2 h	7 d[‡]
Quinine dihydrochloride*	i.m.	10 mg/kg q8h (maximum 1800 mg/d)	Same as loading dose	7 d[‡]
Artemether	i.m.	3.2 mg/kg	1.6 mg/kg q24h for ≥3 days	4 d
Artesunate	Rectal suppository *or*	200 mg/kg at 0, 4, 8, 12, 16, 24, 36, 48, and 60 h		60 h
	Oral	100 mg	50 mg q12h × 5 d	5 d
Plus Mefloquine[§]	Oral	750 mg at 72 h and 500 mg at 84 h		84 h
Or Mefloquine[§]	Oral	750 mg	500 mg 12 h after loading dose	12 h
Or Halofantrine[∥]	Oral	500 mg q6h × 3 doses	Repeat in loading dose 1 wk	2 treatment regimens 1 wk apart
Or Atovaquone/proguanil[¶]	Oral	2 tablets q12h	Same as loading dose	3 d
Or Quinine sulfate	Oral	650 mg q8h	Same as loading dose	3–7 d
Plus Doxycycline**	i.v.	100 mg q12h	Same as loading dose	7 d
Or Sulfadoxine/pyrimethamine[††]	Oral	3 tablets taken at once on last day of quinine	None	Single dose
Or Clindamycin	i.v.	600–900 mg q8h	Same as loading dose	7 d

*Although few prospective studies exist, it seems that the quinolines can be given in standard doses in pregnant patients. Despite theoretical concerns of their abortifacient properties, this has not been shown to be a practical problem even with extensive use.[128,129]

[†]If quinine or mefloquine has been taken within the previous 12 hours, the loading dose is omitted.

[‡]Intravenous therapy should be maintained until the patient can swallow quinine sulfate capsules (650 mg q8h for adults and 25 mg/kg/d [maximum 2 g] divided q8h for children). The dose should be reduced by 30% to 40% in patients requiring more than 72 hours of intravenous treatment due to decreased renal clearance and volume of distribution. Doses also must be diminished in patients with renal insufficiency.

[§]Mefloquine is teratogenic in animals but has not been observed to cause birth defects in humans.[130] It is contraindicated in the first trimester of pregnancy and should be avoided in the last two trimesters if possible.

[∥]Halofantrine is contraindicated in pregnancy.

[¶]Atovaquone/proguanil is packaged in the United States in fixed-dose combination tablets of 250 mg of atovaquone and 100 mg of proguanil (Malarone). Safety in pregnancy is not established.

**Doxycycline is contraindicated in pregnant women and children younger than age 8 years. Substitute clindamycin. Therapy can be converted to oral as the patient improves.

[††]Sulfadoxine/pyrimethamine is packaged in fixed-dose combination tablets of 25 mg of sulfadoxine and 500 mg of pyrimethamine (Fansidar). *P. falciparum* resistance to sulfadoxine/pyrimethamine is common. Efficacy of sulfadoxine/pyrimethamine against nonfalciparum plasmodia has not been shown. Sulfadoxine/pyrimethamine is contraindicated in near-term pregnancy and in patients with glucose-6-phosphate dehydrogenase deficiency.

i.v. dextrose, causing central nervous system dysfunction.[35] Levels of digoxin, mefloquine, neuromuscular blocking agents, and oral anticoagulants all may be increased with quinoline administration. Quinine can cause hemolysis in patients with glucose-6-phosphate dehydrogenase deficiency. Quinolines are contraindicated in patients with myasthenia gravis because of their curare-like effect on skeletal muscle.

In contrast to the cinchona alkaloids, the newer quinoline compounds, mefloquine and halofantrine, are generally better tolerated. Mild side effects include gastrointestinal symptoms, dizziness, vivid dreams, paresthesias, pruritus, and rash.[69] More severe neuropsychiatric reactions, such as seizures, acute psychosis, anxiety neurosis, and disturbances of the sleep-wake cycle, have been estimated to occur in 0.5% of users after treatment doses of mefloquine.[70] Mefloquine is contraindicated in persons with a history of epilepsy or psychiatric disorders. Although less so than with the cinchona alkaloids, cardiac conduction abnormalities may occur, especially with halofantrine, making these drugs contraindicated in patients with a history of dysrhythmias.[71] Other isolated adverse effects include exfoliative dermatitis and Stevens-Johnson syndrome, agranulocytosis, cutaneous vasculitis, and paresthesias.[72-75]

Side effects associated with artemisinin and its derivatives are infrequent and generally mild. Side effects include abdominal pain, diarrhea, contact dermatitis, decreases in reticulocyte and neutrophil counts, and elevated hepatic transaminases.[76] Cerebellar dysfunction in persons treated with artesunate has been reported.[77]

Rare but severe cutaneous reactions, including toxic epidermal necrolysis, erythema multiforme, and Stevens-Johnson syndrome, have been reported with sulfadoxine/pyrimethamine (Fansidar) use and have been attributed to the sulfadoxine component.[78] Other serious but unusual side effects with sulfadoxine include serum sickness, bone marrow suppression, hepatitis, hepatic granuloma, and pneumonitis.

Atovaquone/proguanil (Malarone) is usually well tolerated. Gastrointestinal symptoms, skin rash, headache, insomnia, and, rarely, hematologic and renal effects have been reported, especially at high levels.[79,80] The side effects of the commonly used drugs doxycycline and clindamycin are reported elsewhere.

ANCILLARY THERAPIES

Various ancillary therapies have been proposed for severe malaria. In most cases, insufficient controlled data are available on which to judge their efficacy. Exchange transfusion and erythrocytapheresis have been employed with apparent benefit in cases of severe disease with high parasitemia (>15%) and should be considered in such situations, especially if the patient's condition is worsening despite adequate chemotherapy.[81-86] The rationale for this form of therapy is

TABLE 159–5. DRUG REGIMENS FOR TREATMENT OF SEVERE MALARIA IN CHILDREN

Drug	Route of Administration	Loading Dose	Maintenance Dose	Duration of Treatment
Quinidine gluconate, quinine dihydrochloride, and artemether		Same as adult dosages (see Table 163-4)		
Artesunate	Oral	4 mg/kg	2 mg/kg/d divided in doses of 1 or 2 mg/kg q12h or q24h (total 10 mg/kg)	3 d
Plus Mefloquine	Oral	25 mg/kg on either day 1 or 2	None	Single dose on day 1 or 2
Or Mefloquine	Oral	15 mg/kg	10 mg/kg 8-12 h after loading dose	2 doses
Or Halofantrine	Oral	8 mg/kg q6h × 3 doses	Repeat loading dose in 1 wk	2 treatment regimens 1 wk apart
Or Atovaquone/proguanil*	Oral	Daily dose based on weight: 11-20 kg: 1 tablet; 21-30 kg: 2 tablets; 31-40 kg: 3 tablets; >40 kg: 4 tablets	Same as loading dose	3 d
Or Quinine sulfate	Oral	25 mg/kg/d divided q8h	Same as loading dose	3-7 d
Plus Doxycycline‡	i.v.	2 mg/kg/d	Same as loading dose	7 d
Or Sulfadoxine/pyrimethamine‡	Oral	<1 yr: {1/4} tablet; 1-3 yr: {1/2} tablet; 4-8 yr: 1 tablet; 9-14 yr: 2 tablets	None	Single dose
Or Clindamycin	i.v.	20-40 mg/kg/d divided q8h	Same as loading dose	7 d

*Atovaquone/proguanil is packaged in the United States in fixed-dose combination tablets of 250 mg of atovaquone and 100 mg of proguanil (Malarone).
†Doxycycline is contraindicated in children younger than age 8 years. Substitute clindamycin. Therapy can be converted to oral as patient improves.
‡Sulfadoxine/pyrimethamine is packaged in fixed-dose combination tablets of 25 mg of sulfadoxine and 500 mg of pyrimethamine (Fansidar). *P. falciparum* resistance to sulfadoxine/pyrimethamine is common. Efficacy of sulfadoxine/pyrimethamine against nonfalciparum plasmodia has not been shown. Sulfadoxine/pyrimethamine is contraindicated in patients with glucose-6-phosphate dehydrogenase deficiency.

based on (1) rapid reduction of parasite load, (2) removal of toxic substances, and (3) reduction of microcirculatory sludging. In some studies, iron chelators, such as desferrioxamine, have been shown to hasten malaria parasite clearance and shorten the duration of cerebral malaria coma.[87,88] Proposed mechanisms include depriving the parasite of necessary iron, enhancing the T helper immune response, and protecting against iron-mediated peroxidant cerebral tissue damage.[54] Antioxidants, such as pentoxifylline and inhaled nitric oxide, have been used, but attempts to attenuate the immune response in malaria generally have met with mixed results.[89-91] Monoclonal antibodies directed against tumor necrosis factor had no impact on mortality and may increase morbidity (neurologic sequelae), probably reflecting the participation of multiple cytokines in the pathogenesis of severe and complicated malaria.[92,93] Dichloroacetate to counter lactic acidosis also is under investigation.[94] Steroids are detrimental in severe malaria and should not be used.[95]

LABORATORY MONITORING

Uncomplicated cases may manifest mild hemolytic anemia, thrombocytopenia, leukopenia (of neutrophils and lymphocytes), and albuminuria. Findings in severe malaria may include profound anemia and thrombocytopenia; leukocytosis with a left shift; prolonged coagulation factors with increased fibrin split products and diminished fibrinogen reflecting disseminated intravascular coagulation; hyponatremia; hypoalbuminemia; hypophosphatemia; hypoglycemia; lactic acidemia; and elevated hepatic enzymes, lactate dehydrogenase, bilirubin, blood urea nitrogen, and creatinine.

Urinalysis may reveal proteinuria, RBCs and RBC casts, and hemoglobinuria. Coagulation defects and thrombocytopenia often correlate with the degree of parasitemia.

The level of parasitemia should be monitored via blood smear every 12 hours after the initiation of therapy. A decrease of 75% should be noted within 48 hours. If parasitemia does not decrease, partial quinine/quinidine resistance should be suspected, and the regimen should be changed accordingly (see Tables 159-4 and 159-5). Except in pregnant women and young children, doxycycline is usually added.[96] Clindamycin can be substituted for doxycycline in pregnant women.[34]

PROGNOSIS

Case-fatality rates in severe malaria range from 2% to 50%.[97-101] Factors that correlate with a poor prognosis in most studies include the infecting species and resistance profile, central nervous system involvement, pulmonary edema, hypoglycemia, lactic acidosis, renal failure, severe anemia, younger age, and treatment in a rural health care facility as opposed to an ICU.[35,101-106] There is a semiquantitative relationship between level of parasitemia and risk of death, especially in nonimmune patients. Although less than 10% of adults with cerebral malaria have persistent neurologic sequelae, this number may be 40% in children, especially if associated with hypoglycemia.[55,97] Commonly seen sequelae include hemiparesis, cerebellar ataxia, and extrapyramidal rigidity.[99] Children who survive without obvious neurologic sequelae subsequently seem to develop normally neuropsychologically.[107]

ACKNOWLEDGMENTS

The author thanks Emily Jentes, Corina Monagin, Nikki Maxwell, Torrey Theall, Christina Styron, Kent Wagoner, Laura Morgan, Don Krogstad, and Frederique Jacquerioz for their advice and assistance preparing the manuscript.

ANNOTATED REFERENCES

Bruneel F, Hocqueloux L, Alberti C, et al: The clinical spectrum of severe imported falciparum malaria in the intensive care unit: Report of 188 cases in adults. Am J Respir Crit Care Med 2003;167:684-689.

The clinical spectrum of imported malaria and the factors associated with a poor prognosis are reviewed in this retrospective study of 188 adult patients admitted to an ICU. Of the patients, 94% were infected with P. falciparum acquired in sub-Saharan Africa, and 96% had taken inadequate antimalarial chemoprophylaxis. Mortality was 11% in patients with severe disease. The main factors associated with death were the Simplified Acute Physiology Score, shock, acidosis, coma, pulmonary edema, and coagulation disorders. Bacterial coinfection also may have been a factor in some fatal outcomes.

Marsh K, Forster D, Waruiru C, et al: Indicators of life-threatening malaria in African children. N Engl J Med 1995;332:1399-1404.

In this prospective study of 1844 children admitted to the pediatric ward with malaria, the mortality rate was 3.5%. Of the deaths, 84% occurred within 24 hours of admission. Key prognostic indicators were impaired consciousness, respiratory distress, hypoglycemia, and jaundice. The authors propose a simple bedside index that identified 84.4% of the fatal cases compared with 79.7% identified by the current World Health Organization criteria.

Moody A: Rapid diagnostic tests for malaria parasites. Clin Microbiol Rev 2002;15:66-78.

Malaria presents a diagnostic challenge to laboratories in most countries. Accuracy, sensitivity, cost, efficacy, rapidity, capability of detecting all malaria parasite species, semiquantitative measurement, and ease of performance and training all are important considerations. This article reviews newer technologies and compares them with the gold standard of conventional microscopy.

Svenson JE, MacLean JD, Gyorkos TW, Keystone J: Imported malaria: Clinical presentation and examination of symptomatic travelers. Arch Intern Med 1995;155:861-868.

This chart review of 482 returning travelers with malaria illustrates the challenges in diagnosis. Presenting signs and symptoms were nonspecific. Almost all patients had a history of fever, but only half were febrile at presentation. Thrombocytopenia occurred in 50%. Only 46% of patients were prescribed or used chemoprophylaxis. Of patients with falciparum malaria, 87% presented within 6 weeks of return from travel. Diagnosis often was delayed in patients who sought care outside referral centers. Given the nonspecific and varied clinical presentation, malaria should be considered in any febrile patient with a history of travel to a malaria-endemic area.

Turner G: Cerebral malaria. Brain Pathol 1997;7:569-582.

Understanding the pathogenesis of cerebral malaria, the most common severe complication associated with the disease, is fundamental to good clinical management. This review details the central neuropathologic feature: parasite-induced activation of cytokines and cerebral endothelial cells resulting in the preferential sequestration of parasitized red blood cells in the cerebral microvasculature, ultimately impairing blood flow and producing the varied manifestations of cerebral malaria.

Chapter 160

RICKETTSIAL DISEASES

Florence Fenollar • Didier Raoult

KEY POINTS

1. **Three families of diseases are grouped under the name rickettsial diseases:** diseases caused by bacteria belonging to the *Rickettsia* genus, ehrlichioses, and Q fever. The *Rickettsia* genus is divided into the spotted fever group, which comprises about 15 different species of human pathogens, and the typhus group.

2. The spotted fever group causes arthropod-borne diseases. The four main symptoms that may be observed during spotted rickettsial diseases include **fever, a rash, an inoculation black eschar at the site of the arthropod bite, and lymphadenopathies.** The evolution of spotted fevers is usually mild.

3. The **typhus group** comprises *Rickettsia prowazekii*, causing louse-borne epidemic typhus, and *Rickettsia typhi*, the agent of the flea-borne, murine typhus. The scrub typhus group includes *Orientia tsutsugamushi*, a mite-borne disease.

4. The **prognosis of murine typhus is usually favorable,** with a fatality rate of 1%. The spontaneous fatality rate of epidemic typhus is 20% to 30%. Brill-Zinsser disease is a late relapsing form of exanthematic typhus.

5. Rickettsial diseases, mainly Rocky Mountain spotted fever, Mediterranean spotted fever, and typhus can be responsible for **multiple organ dysfunction syndrome.** In very severe cases, skin necrosis or even gangrene involving the digits or the limbs may be present.

6. American **human monocytic ehrlichiosis** (HME) has only been described in the United States. The prognosis of HME depends on early antibiotic treatment; it has a fatality rate of 2.5%. **Human granulocytic ehrlichiosis** (HGE) is observed in the United States and in Europe. The evolution is mild, with a fatality rate of 0.7%.

7. *Coxiella burnetii,* the agent of Q fever, causes a zoonosis, infecting many mammalian species. Humans are usually contaminated by aerosols. Q fever is divided into acute and chronic diseases. An acute primary infection may eventually be followed by a chronic disease in the presence of predisposing factors, such as cardiac valve damage.

8. The **diagnosis of rickettsial diseases is based on serology.** Culture is restricted to a specialized laboratory with biohazard and cell culture facilities.

Polymerase chain reaction (PCR) could also be performed on various samples.

9. **Doxycycline is the treatment of choice for rickettsial diseases.** It could be prescribed in adults and in children but not in pregnant women and allergic patients. A single-day treatment of 200 mg of doxycycline is sufficient for most of the rickettsioses.

Rickettsial diseases are due to strictly intracellular bacteria. Three families of diseases are grouped under this name: diseases caused by bacteria belonging to the *Rickettsia* genus, ehrlichioses, and Q fever.[1] The *Rickettsia* genus, which belongs to the α1 subgroup of proteobacteria, is divided into the spotted fever group (SFG), which comprises about 15 different species of human pathogens, the typhus group, and the scrub typhus group.[1] The spotted fever group causes arthropod-borne diseases and comprises mainly *Rickettsia rickettsii*, the agent of Rocky Mountain spotted fever, and *Rickettsia conorii*, the agent of Mediterranean spotted fever.[1] The four main symptoms that may be observed during spotted rickettsial diseases include fever; rash, which is usually maculopapular; inoculation black eschar, named "tache noire" at the site of the arthropod bite; and lymphadenopathies, draining this lesion or generalized. The typhus group comprises *Rickettsia prowazekii*, causing louse-borne epidemic typhus, and *Rickettsia typhi*, the agent of the flea-borne, murine typhus. The scrub typhus group includes *Orientia tsutsugamushi*, a mite-borne disease.[1] Ehrlichioses are zoonoses caused by bacteria constituting another branch of the α1 subgroup of proteobacteria.[2] This large group of bacteria is increasingly recognized as potential human pathogens. *Coxiella burnetii*, the agent of Q fever, belongs to the gamma proteobacteria group and causes a zoonosis, infecting many mammal species, including pets. The bacterium is excreted in birth products and milk. Humans are usually contaminated by aerosols. An acute primary infection may eventually be followed by a chronic disease in the presence of predisposing factors. The features of the main rickettsial diseases are summarized in Table 160-1.

RICKETTSIAL DISEASES

SPOTTED FEVER GROUP

Rocky Mountain spotted fever (RMSF) is caused by *R. rickettsii*, which is transmitted by *Dermacentor* ticks.[1,3,4] The disease mainly occurs during late spring and summer.

TABLE 160–1. FEATURES OF THE MAIN RICKETTSIAL DISEASES

Disease	Organism	Geographic Distribution	Vector	Eschar	Rash Distribution	Complications	Treatment	Fatality Rate in Absence of Treatment (%)
Spotted Fever Group								
Rocky Mountain spotted fever	*Rickettsia rickettsii*	United States	Ticks	No	Extremities to trunk	MODS	Doxycycline, 200 mg/day for 7 days	High
Mediterranean spotted fever	*R. conorii*	Mediterranean area	Ticks	Yes	Trunk, extremities, face	MODS	Doxycycline, 200 mg/day for 1 day	Moderate
Typhus Group								
Murine typhus	*R. typhi*	Worldwide	Flea	No	Trunk to extremities	Respiratory distress, seizure, coma	Doxycycline, 200 mg/day for 1 day	Low
Epidemic typhus	*R. prowazekii*	Worldwide	Body louse	No	Trunk to extremities	MODS	Doxycycline, 200 mg/day for 1 day	High
Brill-Zinsser disease	*R. prowazekii*	Worldwide	None	No	Trunk to extremities	No	Doxycycline, 200 mg/day for 1 day	Low
Scrub typhus	*Orientia tsutsugamushi*	Australia, Asia, South Pacific	Mite	Yes	Trunk to extremities	MODS	Doxycycline, 200 mg/day for 7 days	High
Ehrlichioses								
Human monocytic ehrlichioses	*Ehrlichia chaffeensis*	United States	Ticks	No	None	MODS	Doxycycline, 200 mg/day for 1 day	Moderate
Human granulocytic ehrlichioses	*Anaplasma phagocytophila*	United States, Europe	Ticks	No	None	Opportunistic infections	Doxycycline, 200 mg/day for 1 day	Low
Q fever	*Coxiella burnetii*	Worldwide	Ticks	No	None	ARDS	Doxycycline, 200 mg/day for 2 wk	Moderate

MODS, Multiple organ dysfunction syndrome; ARDS, Acute respiratory distress syndrome.

Patients develop high fever and headaches from 2 to 14 days after a tick bite. The association of fever, headache, and rash is observed in 44% of confirmed cases. The inoculation eschar is very rarely found. A macular rash is described for 66% of the patients. The disease is sometimes associated with general manifestations linked to increased vascular permeability and may lead to multiple organ dysfunction syndrome (MODS). This form is mainly observed in old people, in patients with glucose-6-phosphate dehydrogenase (G6PD) deficiency, and in alcoholics. The untreated patient worsens progressively, and there is a high level of mortality (20% to 25%). *R. conorii* belongs to a different but related serogroup: The strain Malish is the most common (Europe and Africa), and the other serotypes are Israel (Israel and Southern Europe), Astrakhan (on the Caspian sea), and Indian (India).

Mediterranean spotted fever is caused by *R. conorii sensu stricto.* The disease is transmitted by the dog tick *Rhipicephalus sanguineus,* which seldom bites humans.[1] Most cases are observed in the Mediterranean area during the summer. The classic presentation is that of a patient with fever, rash, and a single eschar. The rash, mainly papular, is observed in 97% to 99% of patients. The eschar is observed in 50% to 80% of cases. The spontaneous evolution is milder than that of RMSF. A fatality rate of 1% of diagnosed patients is still observed. The malignant form of the disease, such as shock and MODS, is found in approximately 5% of patients, mainly the elderly, in G6PD deficiency, and in alcoholics.

Israeli spotted fever, caused by *R. conorii* serotype Israel, transmitted by *R. sanguineus,* is found in Israel, Portugal, and Sicily. The disease is clinically similar to Mediterranean spotted fever. However, the eschar is more rarely observed and the spontaneous evolution is mild.[1] Astrakhan fever, caused by *R. conorii* serotype Astrakhan, is transmitted by *Rhipicephalus pumilio.* The disease, mainly observed in Astrakhan, is very similar to Mediterranean spotted fever, but the eschar is rarely observed and the severity is mild.[1] Indian tick typhus, caused by *R. conorii* serotype Indian, is transmitted by *R. sanguineus.* The disease has been observed in India and is close to Mediterranean spotted fever.[5] The rash is often purpuric, and the eschar is rarely found. The disease is mild to moderately severe.

African tick bite fever, caused by *R. africae,* is transmitted in sub-Saharan Africa and West Indies by *Amblyomma* ticks.[6] These ticks typically attack human in groups, thus explaining why grouped cases and multiple eschars are described. One week after the tick bite, 46% of the patients develop a rash, which is vesicular in half of them. Nearly all the patients present with an inoculation eschar, and 54% of them present with multiple eschars. The evolution is much milder than Mediterranean spotted fever.

Spotted fever caused by *R. slovaca,* also known as TIBOLA (tick-borne lymph adenopathy), is a disease common in Europe transmitted by *Dermacentor* ticks.[1,3,7-9] These ticks bite preferentially in cold months and in the scalp, because they prefer hairy areas. This disease is more prevalent in children and women. One week after the tick bite an eschar appears composed of a lesion ranging 2 to 8 cm in diameter associated with cervical adenopathy. Fever and rash are rarely observed. A postinfectious asthenia and residual alopecia at the site of the tick bite have been reported.

Queensland tick typhus, caused by *R. australis,* is transmitted by *Ixodes holocyclus* in Australia.[1,10] The patients present with a rash, which can be vesicular. An inoculation eschar is also frequently observed. The evolution is mild. **Japanese or Oriental spotted fever,** caused by *R. japonica,* is transmitted by *Haemaphylasis longicornis* and *Dermacentor taiwanensis* in Japan but also probably in Eastern China. The patients present with fever, headache, inoculation eschar, and a maculopapular rash.[1,3] Severe cases, such as meningoencephalitis and fulminant cases, have been reported.[11-13] **Flinders Island spotted fever,** caused by *R. honei,* presents as a febrile illness associated with an erythematous rash. It is also found in continental eastern Australia and probably in Thailand. An eschar is described in 25% of the patients, and regional adenopathy occurs in 55% of the patients.[1,3]

Siberian tick typhus, caused by *R. sibirica,* is transmitted by *Dermacentor marginatus* and *Haemaphysalis concinna.* The disease is found in Siberia and China. After 1 week of incubation, an ulcerated necrotic lesion appears at the inoculation site, often accompanied by regional lymphadenopathy. *R. mongolotimonae,* related to *R. sibirica,* is transmitted by the *Hyalomma asiaticum* tick in Mongolia and sub-Saharan Africa. Patients show a discrete rash, an inoculation eschar, and satellite lymphadenopathy.[3,14,15]

R. aeschlimannii has been isolated from *Hyalomma marginatum* in Africa, Corsica, and Spain and is responsible for a disease similar to Mediterranean spotted fever.[16] **Rickettsialpox or smallpox rickettsia** is due to *R. akari,* which is transmitted by *Allodermanyssus sanguineus.*[1] One week after a mite bite, a vesiculous rash appears. Even untreated, the patients recover spontaneously. **The infection due to *R. helvetica*** is not yet well characterized.[8,17,18] This bacterium has been isolated from *Ixodes ricinus*[17] and has been mainly associated with sudden death due to myocarditis.[8] Cases of fever without rash or eschar have also been reported.[17] **Flea-borne spotted fever** is worldwide. It is due to *R. felis,* which is transmitted by cat fleas.[19] The disease is characterized by fever, rash, headache, and central nervous involvement.[20,21]

TYPHUS GROUP

Murine typhus or endemic typhus, caused by *R. typhi,* is transmitted by rat fleas through scratching contaminated pruritic lesions after flea bites.[1,22] The disease begins with fever, nausea, myalgias, arthralgias, and headache. Six days on average after the onset, a maculopapular rash is observed in 40% of patients. Nonspecific digestive symptoms are sometimes present. One third of the patients have a cough. An interstitial pneumonia is less frequently observed. In severe forms, respiratory distress can be observed. Neurologic symptoms can be present, ranging from confusion and stupor to seizures and coma in severe forms. One third of patients present with a cough, and one fourth present with an unspecific interstitial pneumonia sometimes associated with pleural effusion. Prognosis is usually favorable, with a fatality rate of 1%.

Epidemic typhus or exanthematic typhus, caused by *R. prowazekii,* is transmitted by the human body louse.[1,22,23] The human body louse lives in clothes and multiplies rapidly when cold weather and lack of hygiene allow, such as during war, in poor countries, and in the homeless population in developed countries. The disease begins abruptly with fever, headaches, and myalgias. Neurologic involvement, such as stupor and confusion, are common. The fatality rate in untreated cases is 20% to 30%. Brill-Zinsser disease is a late relapsing form of typhus. It is frequently underdiagnosed, because the rash as well as recent exposure can be lacking. The disease is mild, and the prognosis is good.

Scrub typhus is transmitted by the bite of mite larvae infected by *O. tsutsumagushi*.[22] The disease is present in Japan, eastern Australia, eastern Russia, China, and the Indian subcontinent mainly in autumn and spring. One week after the bite, patients present with fever, headaches, and myalgias. An eschar may be observed for 50% of the patients that is often associated with draining lymph nodes. Generalized lymphadenitis and rash may be observed. Meningeal symptoms are relatively common. Severe forms can present as septic shock with MODS. The fatality rate ranges from 0% to 30%.

SEVERE FORMS OF SPOTTED FEVER AND TYPHUS

Rickettsial diseases, mainly RMSF, Mediterranean spotted fever, and typhus can be associated with increased vascular permeability and multiple organ involvement leading to MODS. In these severe forms, the patients may suffer from edema, hypovolemia, hypoalbuminemia, and hypotension leading to shock. In very severe cases, skin necrosis or even gangrene involving the digits or the limbs may be present. In some instances, noncardiogenic pulmonary edema develops. Renal failure is also frequently observed in severe cases. This renal failure may be related to acute tubular necrosis and require hemodialysis. In severe cases, delirium, coma, and seizures are described. Heart involvement can cause dysrhythmias. In severe cases, upper gastrointestinal hemorrhage can cause death. Cerebral hemorrhages may also occur.

DIAGNOSIS

The leukocyte count is classically within normal limits, but a leukopenia can be observed.[24] Thrombocytopenia can occur and may be marked in severe cases, as well as anemia, specifically when hemolysis is observed (frequently in patients with G6PD deficiency).[24] Coagulopathy with decrease in clotting factors (including fibrinogen) and prolonged coagulation times may contribute to bleeding. C-reactive protein and hepatic enzyme levels can be increased.[24] Hyponatremia and hypocalcemia can be observed and correlate with increased severity. Lactate dehydrogenase and creatine phosphokinase levels usually reflect the severity of organ involvement, including the lung, heart, and liver, and multifocal rhabdomyolysis.

Currently, the biologic diagnosis of rickettsioses is based on serology.[25] Two sera samples should be tested. The indirect immunofluorescence assay (IFA) is the reference test.[26] The early serum is often negative. A cutoff value of 1/64 for total immunoglobulins and 1/32 for specific IgM is usually required for the diagnosis. Cross-reactive antibodies have been observed with infections caused by other rickettsioses, *Ehrlichia*, *Bartonella*, *Legionella*, and *Proteus*. Other techniques, such as latex agglutination, enzyme-linked immunosorbent assay (ELISA), and immunoperoxidase assays are also available.[26] Western immunoblot assay is the most specific and sensitive serologic assay.[26] Cross adsorption is used to discriminate cross-reacting antibodies between two or more antigens, but the technique is limited by the large amount of antigen needed.[26] In skin biopsies, the bacteria could be detected

before the seroconversion but also retrospectively.[1,26] Biopsy specimens of the skin, preferably petechial lesions and eschar, may be tested. Both immunofluorescence and immunoperoxidase techniques are available.[26] Detection can be performed on frozen or fixed samples, as well as on paraffin-embedded material. Skin biopsies specimens, peripheral white blood cells, or suspected arthropods may be used for polymerase chain reaction (PCR) diagnosis. The blood should be collected in tubes containing EDTA or sodium citrate. Sera can also be tested. In parallel to regular PCR, a new technique called suicide PCR has been introduced. This technique corresponds to a nested PCR using a single-time PCR. Testing is done in a blinded fashion with one negative control used every seven samples. All positive PCR products must be sequenced for the identification of the pathogenic rickettsiae. The isolation of rickettsiae can be performed from human samples (decanted plasma or skin biopsies, ideally from the eschar) and from arthropods.[26] Culture is restricted to specialized laboratories with biohazard and cell culture facilities. Usually, culture of rickettsiae takes 3 to 7 days. This technique is fundamental for the identification of new rickettsial pathogens.

TREATMENT

Doxycycline is the treatment of choice for rickettsioses.[27] It can be prescribed in adults and children[28] but not in pregnant women and patients with specific allergies to it, tetracycline, or related antibiotics. A single day treatment of 200 mg of doxycycline is sufficient for most of the rickettsioses. The treatment should be given orally except in patients with gastric intolerance or coma, for whom it should be given intravenously. For RMSF, scrub typhus or the severe form of spotted fever, the treatment duration is usually longer than 1day. For RMSF and a severe form of spotted fever, it can be stopped 3 days after apyrexia. For scrub typhus, the currently recommended regimen is doxycycline, 200 mg daily for 7 days. In RMSF and in typhus, chloramphenicol is the only available alternative to doxycycline in pregnant women and in allergic patients and is prescribed at a dose of 2 g daily for 10 days. In other spotted fever, except for *R. felis*, josamycin at a dosage of 3 g daily for 7 days is sufficient. Severely ill patients must be treated in ICUs. Fluid administration should be carefully monitored. Anemia and coagulation abnormalities should also be corrected. Mechanical ventilation must be used in case of respiratory distress. Hemodialysis may be required in patients with renal insufficiency. Antiepileptics should be given in case of seizure. In cases of gangrene, amputation is sometimes necessary. Glucocorticoids have not proved useful. There is no current vaccination, and prevention is based on the avoidance of tick, flea, and body lice bites. Lice are fragile, so changing and boiling clothes is effective. Repellents and/or protective garments could also be used. After a possible exposure, ticks can be removed by forceps followed by skin disinfection.

EHRLICHIOSES

American human monocytic ehrlichiosis (HME) is due to *Ehrlichia chaffeensis,* which is transmitted by *Amblyomma* ticks.[29] This disease has only been described in the United States, mainly from April to September.[22,30] After an incubation period of 1 week, patients present with fever, headache, myalgia, and malaise. Cough, dyspnea, and vomiting are present less commonly. In one third of the cases, a rash, mainly maculopapular and rarely petechial, is observed. Central nervous system infection manifests in many forms, from confusion to coma. If not treated, patients may develop severe signs and require intensive care. In severe cases, shock and MODS may be observed with hypotension, tachycardia, respiratory distress, seizures, renal insufficiency, myocardial failure, and coma. The prognosis of HME depends on early antibiotic treatment, with a fatality rate of 2.5%.

Human granulocytic ehrlichiosis (HGE) is due to *Anaplasma phagocytophila*, which is transmitted by *Ixodes* ticks.[22,24,30] The disease is observed in the United States and in Europe, mainly in spring and autumn. Many infections are asymptomatic. When symptoms are observed, they are similar to those described for HME. However, a rash is rarely observed in HGE in comparison to HME, and the evolution of the disease is more favorable with a fatality rate of 0.7%. Neurologic symptoms may include confusion. Most deaths are the consequence of induced immunodepression. Patients may develop septic shock, herpes esophagitis, cryptococcosis, candidiasis, and aspergillosis, which can be fatal.

Canine granulocytic ehrlichiosis (CGE) is due to *E. ewingii*, an uncultured bacterium, which is transmitted by *Amblyomma americanum*. The disease is prevalent on immunosuppressed hosts in the United States, those infected with human immunodeficiency virus, or those receiving immunosuppressive drugs. Patients present with fever, thrombocytopenia, leukopenia, and various nonspecific symptoms, including meningitis.[24,30]

Canine monocytic ehrlichiosis is caused by *E. canis*, which is transmitted by *Rhipicephaleus sanguineus*. In 1996, a single case of infection was reported in an asymptomatic man from Venezuela who owned an infected dog.[31] In 1991, a immunohistology examination identified an organism antigenically related to *E. canis* in tissues from a patient who died of ehrlichiosis.[32] **Sennetsu ehrlichiosis** is due to *Neorickettsia sennetsu*. In 1953, one case was described in Japan. The bacterium was isolated from the blood, bone marrow, and lymph node of a 25-year-old man who had fever, headaches, myalgia, and anorexia.[33]

DIAGNOSIS

Leukopenia, thrombocytopenia, and elevated hepatic enzymes may be observed in ehrlichioses.[30] The diagnosis is based on acute and convalescent serologic examination with IFA, which shows a fourfold rise in specific antibody titers.[30] Cross reactivity among Ehrlichieae prevents definitive identification of the etiologic agent by serology alone. Inclusions, called morulae, may be seen rarely in monocytes and macrophages of patients with HME and occasionally in neutrophils of patients with HGE and CGE. PCR amplification may also be performed on blood samples.

TREATMENT

A single dose of 200 mg of doxycycline is the recommended treatment.[30] Rifamycins are effective in vitro against these bacteria. Chloramphenicol may not be effective for ehrlichioses. Prevention relies on avoidance of tick bites as described for rickettsioses. Severely ill patients must be treated in ICUs with reanimation measures.

Q FEVER

Q fever is a worldwide zoonosis caused by *C. burnetii*.[34] The reservoir of this bacterium is extensive, including mammals, ticks, and birds, but it is only partially known. The most commonly identified sources of human infection are cattle, goats, and sheep.[34] *C. burnetii* is currently considered as a potential warfare agent and classified in category B of the biological agents of the Centers for Disease Control and Prevention. Humans are usually infected by aerosol from amniotic fluid, placenta, or contaminated wool or, less frequently, by milk products.[34] Q fever is polymorphic and nonspecific. After contamination by *C. burnetii*, 60% of patients seroconvert without apparent disease, 38% present a self-limited disease, and only 2% necessitate an exhaustive diagnostic procedure.[34,35] After the primary infection, approximately 0.5% of patients develop chronic Q fever.

Patients with acute infection may present with a variety of symptoms, including pneumonia or hepatitis. Complications associated with acute Q fever are rare and may include encephalitis, renal failure, congestive heart failure, respiratory failure with acute respiratory distress syndrome, myocarditis, or pericarditis. The fatality rate is lower than 3%. Death can occur in patients with previous pulmonary or cardiac defects. Less common manifestations of acute Q fever include hemolytic anemia, mediastinal lymphadenopathy, optic neuritis, Guillain-Barré syndrome, and extrapyramidal neurologic disease. Post Q fever chronic fatigue has also been described.[36] The clinical course is usually favorable even without treatment, except in special hosts. In pregnant women with or without symptoms, Q fever compromises the pregnancy and can be responsible of abortion, fetal death, or prematurity.[37] Patients with cardiovascular abnormalities are at risk of chronic infection, such as endocarditis or vascular infection. Patients with Q fever endocarditis have a very chronic low-grade fever, progressive deterioration of valve function, and progressive heart failure. Vegetations are not frequently observed on echocardiography. If not diagnosed, the disease progressively worsens and emboli, most often cerebral, may be observed. Renal insufficiency, splenomegaly, or hepatomegaly may develop. Digital clubbing may also be present.[34] Cases of chronic osteomyelitis, hepatitis, and infection of aneurysm and vascular prosthesis have been also reported.

DIAGNOSIS

Leukopenia may be observed. Thrombocytopenia is frequent, as are increases in hepatic enzymes.[34] Circulating anticoagulants associated with antiphospholipid may be observed as well as anti–smooth muscle antibodies. Diagnosis is mainly based on serology, the most commonly used method being the IFA with the test of phase I and phase II antigens.[34] Acute Q fever is diagnosed when a seroconversion or a fourfold increase is obtained using phase II antigen. A single serum sample exhibiting IgG antibodies greater than or equal to 200 and greater than or equal to an IgM titer of 50 against phase II antigen is also diagnostic.[34] During chronic Q fever, antibodies are at higher titers and directed against both phase I and phase II antigens. IgG to phase I antigens at a titer at least of 800 is diagnostic of chronic infection as is an IgA titer greater than or equal to 100. Serology is useful for follow-up of patients with acute Q fever and underlying disease and in those with treated chronic Q fever. The other diagnostic tools are direct detection by cell culture performed in a specialized laboratory with biohazard facilities, PCR, or immunochemistry of cardiac valve, liver, or blood samples, but serology by IFA is the best test.[34] Liver biopsy, when performed, shows granulomas that may be characterized by a lipid vacuole and surrounded by a fibrinoid ring in the form of a doughnut.[34]

TREATMENT

In acute Q fever, doxycycline (200 mg/day) should be prescribed for 3 weeks in most cases.[34] In patients with a valvular abnormality, the recommended treatment of acute Q fever is based on the association of doxycycline (200 mg/day) and hydroxychloroquine (600 mg/day).[38] Clinical benefit has been described with the combination of prednisone and antibiotic therapy in cases in which slow regression of symptoms is found in patients with Q fever hepatitis.[34] Prednisone should be administered at a dose of 40 mg for 48 hours, then 20 mg for 48 hours, and then 10 mg for an additional 48 hours in such patients when apyrexia is not obtained after 3 days of antibiotic therapy.[34] In pregnant women, cotrimoxazole (sulfamethoxazole 1600 mg/day and trimethoprim 320 mg/day) continued throughout the pregnancy was associated with favorable outcome.[37] In patients with endocarditis, the recommended treatment is doxycycline (200 mg/day) and hydroxychloroquine (600 mg/day) for at least 18 months.[34] Prevention is based on veterinary controls in animals. A vaccine is available in Australia.

ANNOTATED REFERENCES

Dumler J, Walker D: Tick-borne ehrlichioses. Lancet Infect Dis 2001; 21-28.
Description and phylogeny of Ehrlichieae are detailed. The epidemiology and transmission, the clinical and laboratory presentation, the diagnosis, and the treatment of human granulocytic ehrlichiosis, human monocytic ehrlichiosis, and other human ehrlichioses are precisely described.

La Scola B, Raoult D: Laboratory diagnosis of rickettsioses: Current approaches to diagnosis of old and new rickettsial diseases. J Clin Microbiol 1997;35:2715-2727.
All the techniques available for the diagnosis of rickettsioses are specified and described. The advantages and the inconveniences of each assay are reviewed.

Maurin M, Raoult D: Q fever. Clin Microbiol Rev 1999;12:518-553.
All the knowledge on Q fever and Coxiella burnetii are reviewed in this article. Historical background, bacteriology, epidemiology, pathogenesis, clinical findings, laboratory diagnosis, treatment, and vaccine prophylaxis are carefully detailed.

Raoult D, Olson J: Emerging rickettsioses. In Scheld W, Craig W, Hughes J (eds): Emerging Infections. Washington, DC, ASM Press, 1999, pp 17-31.
This book chapter reviews most of the newly described rickettsioses such as African tick bite fever, tick-borne lymphadenopathy, Japanese spotted fever, Astrakhan fever, Flinders Island spotted fever, spotted fever due to Rickettsia mongolotimonae, and flea-transmitted rickettsioses.

Raoult D, Roux V: Rickettsioses as paradigms of new or emerging infectious diseases. Clin Microbiol Rev 1997;10:694-719.
This article reviews the previously and the newly described rickettsioses. The Rickettsiae not linked to human diseases and the diseases possibly due to Rickettsiae are also detailed around the world.

Chapter 161

ACUTE VIRAL SYNDROMES

Fernanda Silveira • Mesut Yilmaz • David L. Paterson

KEY POINTS

1. For a generalized vesicular rash, scraping the base of the lesion and using direct fluorescent antibody testing can assist in the rapid diagnosis of chickenpox or disseminated herpesvirus infections.

2. Cytomegalovirus infection should be rapidly excluded as a cause of fever in an immunocompromised patient by way of detection of antigen or DNA in peripheral blood.

3. Travelers from Africa, Asia, or South America who present with thrombocytopenia and fever should be assessed for the viruses that cause hemorrhagic fevers. Strict contact isolation should be used.

4. Herpes simplex virus, varicella-zoster virus, and enteroviruses can be detected by polymerase chain reaction of cerebrospinal fluid, enabling a rapid diagnosis.

5. Dosage adjustment is necessary for most commonly used antiviral agents in patients with renal dysfunction. Failure to adjust dosage may lead to adverse effects, such as neurotoxicity.

Acute infections with viruses produce a variety of clinical manifestations with a wide spectrum of clinical severity. Viral upper respiratory tract infections in immunocompetent hosts are usually trivial, although they may be life-threatening and associated with subsequent lower respiratory tract infection and disseminated disease in immunocompromised hosts. Viral infections can affect virtually every organ system of the body.

VESICULAR RASH

POXVIRUSES, INCLUDING SMALLPOX AND MONKEYPOX

Poxviruses are double-stranded DNA viruses that have reentered the spotlight because of concerns regarding bioterrorism with smallpox.[1] Additionally an outbreak of monkeypox infection in humans was detected in the United States for the first time,[2] which has triggered alarm about these infections. The poxviruses and their major clinical manifestations are listed in Table 161-1. In general, a common feature of poxviruses is that they cause vesicular skin eruptions.

Smallpox

The last case of endemic smallpox occurred in Somalia in 1977, and eradication of the disease was declared in 1980.[3] The virus (variola) has been maintained, however, in some laboratories—the last known case of laboratory-acquired smallpox occurred in the United Kingdom in 1978. In part as a result of this accident, the number of laboratories that retained the virus was reduced from 76 to just 2. These laboratories are at the Centers for Disease Control and Prevention in Atlanta in the United States and the Vektor Institute in Novosibirsk, Russia. It is unknown if all other laboratories destroyed their virus—the potential exists for a deliberate release of variola as an act of bioterrorism.

The incubation period for smallpox is 7 to 17 days (mean 10 to 12).[3] A prodromal phase occurs, which consists of abrupt onset of severe headache, backache, and fever. The fever is often 40°C, but then subsides. Then the rash begins; initial lesions are small, red macules, which over 2 to 3 days become macular then vesicular. The lesions start on the face and extremities, then cover the entire body. The palms and soles are affected. The lesions subsequently may umbilicate and crust.

The rash of smallpox could be confused with monkeypox, generalized vaccinia and eczema vaccinatum, chickenpox, coxsackievirus infection, herpes simplex virus infection (especially eczema herpeticum), rickettsialpox, insect bites, drug eruptions, and acne. A classic feature of smallpox is that the lesions are all at the same stage of development. In contrast, with chickenpox, individual lesions are present at different stages. With chickenpox, the fever occurs with the onset of the rash.

It is well known that smallpox is associated with significant mortality, although it is not clear what the likelihood of mortality would be in patients who receive good supportive care, such as exists in modern ICUs. There are many reasons for the mortality associated with smallpox. Substantial amounts of fluid and protein can be lost by febrile persons with numerous, weeping lesions. Some patients have a fulminant course with smallpox infection. In some patients, death may occur before the appearance of any rash. (The prodromal period is associated with significant viremia.) A hemorrhagic form of smallpox also is associated with high mortality.[3] Encephalitis occurs in fewer than 1% of patients infected. Secondary bacterial infections of the skin lesions may occur and are heralded by a second temperature spike.[3] Although cough is not usually a prominent symptom of smallpox, secondary bacterial pneumonia may occur, particularly in patients with severe disease.

TABLE 161–1. COMMON CLINICAL MANIFESTATIONS OF POXVIRUSES

Virus	Clinical Manifestations
Variola (smallpox)	Diffuse vesicular rash; systemic disease
Monkeypox	Vesicular rash
Vaccinia (cowpox)	Vesicular rash; postinfectious encephalitis
Parapoxvirus	Orf (localized vesicular lesion)
Molluscipoxvirus	Molluscum contagiosum
Tanapox virus	Vesicular rash

The Centers for Disease Control and Prevention recommends an algorithmic approach to the diagnosis of smallpox (this is described in detail at http://www.bt.cdc.gov/agent/smallpox). Patients can be subdivided into low-risk, moderate-risk, and high-risk groups depending on a variety of variables (Tables 161-2 and 161-3). Patients at low or moderate risk for smallpox should undergo direct fluorescent antibody testing of the skin lesion for varicella-zoster virus infection and herpes simplex virus plus polymerase chain reaction for varicella-zoster virus, herpes simplex virus, and enterovirus (where these tests are available). Patients at moderate risk should undergo consultation by infectious diseases or dermatology specialists. Electron microscopy should be performed if it is readily available, and viral culture or biopsy for erythema multiforme may be performed as indicated. If rapid testing for varicella-zoster virus and herpes simplex virus is negative for a moderate-risk patient, the adequacy of specimen collection needs to be confirmed. If there is ongoing clinical suspicion for smallpox, local and state health departments should be consulted. For patients at high risk for smallpox, all testing should be performed at the Centers for Disease Control and Prevention. This testing should include variola real-time polymerase chain reaction, *Orthopoxvirus* real-time polymerase chain reaction, and nonvariola *Orthopoxvirus* real-time polymerase chain reaction, in addition to tests for varicella-zoster virus, herpes simplex virus, and enteroviruses.

There is no approved treatment for smallpox. The patient should be vaccinated, especially if the illness is in an early stage.[3] Prevention of secondary cases is crucial. A suspected case of smallpox should be managed in a negative-pressure room. Additionally, strict respiratory and contact isolation is essential (detailed instructions are available at http://www.bt.cdc.gov/agent/smallpox).[3]

Vaccinia

Vaccinia is another poxvirus that is used in the immunization of people against smallpox. Primary vaccination results in a

TABLE 161–2. CRITERIA FOR THE SUSPICION OF SMALLPOX IN PATIENTS WITH ACUTE, GENERALIZED VESICULAR OR PUSTULAR RASH

Major Smallpox Criteria

Febrile prodrome
  >101°F, 1-4 days before rash onset
  With headache, backache, or abdominal pain
Firm, deep-seated, well-circumscribed vesicles/pustules
Lesions in the same stage of development in any one area of the body

Minor Smallpox Criteria

Centrifugal distribution
First lesions in the pharynx, oral mucosa
Patient appears "toxic"
Slow evolution of the rash
  1-2 days each stage: macule, papule, vesicle
Lesions on the palms and soles

TABLE 161–3. CATEGORIZATION OF RISK OF SMALLPOX FROM CLINICAL CRITERIA*

High Risk of Smallpox

Febrile prodrome *and*
Classic smallpox lesion *and*
Lesions in the same stage of development

Moderate Risk of Smallpox

Febrile prodrome *and* one other *major* smallpox criterion *or*
Febrile prodrome *and* four or more minor smallpox criteria

Low Risk of Smallpox

No febrile prodrome *or*
Febrile prodrome *and* fewer than four minor smallpox criteria

*The major and minor criteria are listed in Table 161-2.

vesicle at the site of vaccination, usually within 3 to 5 days. This vesicle becomes pustular or is surrounded by induration or congestion 6 to 8 days after vaccination. Rarely a generalized rash characterized by multiple, small vesicular lesions occurs. Occasionally, severe complications result from smallpox vaccination. If vaccinia is administered to a person with an immunologic deficiency, progressive necrosis at the site of vaccination may occur (vaccinia necrosum). Secondarily, metastatic lesions may spread to other parts of the body. Such cases may be fatal. Patients with eczema may develop dissemination of vaccinia virus in the abnormal skin, leading to a generalized rash (eczema vaccinatum or Kaposi's varicelliform eruption). Vaccinia immunoglobulin (0.6 mL/kg every 24 hours) is often prescribed for disseminated infection.

A generalized encephalitis may occur 1 to 2 weeks after vaccination and is associated with a mortality of 10% to 30%. Myocardial infarction, pericarditis, myocarditis, and dilated cardiomyopathy have been observed after smallpox vaccination, although the relationship between these findings and the vaccination has not yet been elucidated.[4,5]

From December 2002 to January 2004, the U.S. Department of Defense vaccinated 578,286 military personnel with vaccinia.[6] Thirty cases of suspected contact transfer of vaccinia were reported.[6] *Contact transfer* is the spread of vaccinia from a recipient of the smallpox vaccine to another person. This spread occurs because the live virus used in the vaccine is present on the skin at the site of the vaccination. Spread of the virus to other parts of the body (autoinoculation) also can occur via the same mechanism. No cases of vaccinia necrosum or eczema vaccinatum were observed in the people with contact transfer of the virus.

Monkeypox

Monkeypox was first recognized in 1958 as a disease of primates. The disease subsequently was recognized in rodents. Beginning in 1970, cases in humans were reported in central Africa.[7] In 2003, cases occurred in the United States in residents of the Midwest who had contact with imported prairie dogs.[2] Patients developed vesicular skin lesions and fever/sweats. Although case-fatality rates of 4% to 22% have been observed in outbreaks of the infection in Africa, none of 11 patients in the American outbreak died.[2]

HERPESVIRUSES

Herpes simplex virus, varicella-zoster virus, and herpes B virus all are capable of causing vesicular skin rash and other systemic manifestations of disease. The herpesviruses are large, DNA-containing, enveloped viruses that exhibit lifelong latent infection in people infected with them.[8,9] There are eight known herpesviruses: herpes simplex virus types 1 and 2; varicella-zoster virus; cytomegalovirus; human herpesvirus types 6, 7, and 8; and Epstein-Barr virus.

Herpes Simplex Virus

Herpes simplex viruses are found worldwide. Characteristically, herpes simplex virus 1 is associated with orolabial disease, and herpes simplex virus 2 is associated with genital infection, although this is not a rigid distinction. Primary infection (first infections with herpes simplex virus 1 or herpes simplex virus 2) usually is associated with mucosal lesions and systemic signs and symptoms. Mucosal and cutaneous lesions are vesicular and usually localized, although disseminated infection rarely may occur. Patients with atopic eczema or severe burns may develop severe extensive infections.

Primary herpes simplex virus infection may have severe complications. Aseptic meningitis may occur and is more common with herpes simplex virus 2. Meningeal symptoms usually start 3 to 12 days after the onset of genital lesions. Transverse myelitis and autonomic nervous system dysfunction also may occur in conjunction with primary genital herpes simplex virus infection. Herpes simplex virus encephalitis in adults usually is not associated with primary infection. Potentially, reactivation of latent herpes simplex virus 1 infection in trigeminal or autonomic nerve roots may be associated with extension of virus into the central nervous system via the innervation of the middle cranial fossa. Occasionally, patients with primary herpes simplex virus infection develop hepatitis, pneumonia, or thrombocytopenia.

By virtue of the establishment of latency, herpes simplex virus 1 or herpes simplex virus 2 may reactivate. Herpes simplex virus reactivations may be less severe than primary infections. In immunocompromised hosts, however, reactivation of herpes simplex virus 1 or herpes simplex virus 2 may be associated with disseminated infection or severe local esophagitis, hepatitis, or pneumonia. Neonatal herpes, occurring in an infant of a mother with primary or reactivation infection at the time of delivery, carries a high risk of disseminated, fatal infection.

Diagnosis of herpes simplex virus 1 or herpes simplex virus 2 infection causing a vesicular skin lesion can be suspected clinically by the presence of multiple vesicular lesions on an erythematous base, occurring in the orolabial or anogenital areas. A precise diagnosis can be established easily by use of antigen detection methods (e.g., direct fluorescent antibody testing) on scrapings from lesions. Results can be available within hours of specimen collection. If scrapings from lesions are collected, they also can be cultured for the presence of virus. Polymerase chain reaction is an alternative method. Staining of scrapings from the base of lesions with Giemsa stain (Tzanck smear), revealing giant cells or intranuclear lesions of herpes simplex virus infection, is rarely performed now, and few clinicians have experience in correctly identifying giant cells.

Varicella-Zoster Virus

Primary varicella-zoster virus infection causes chickenpox, whereas reactivation infection causes shingles (zoster). Chickenpox is characterized by multiple vesicular lesions all over the body, whereas shingles is characterized by a unilateral vesicular eruption with a dermatomal distribution. Immunocompromised patients with shingles may develop disseminated cutaneous infection, however, resembling chickenpox.

Chickenpox usually is associated with fever, constitutional symptoms, and a vesicular skin rash. Most skin lesions are small vesicular lesions, with an erythematous base. Successive crops of lesions occur over 2 to 4 days so that lesions appear at all stages from fresh vesicles to crusted lesions. Many life-threatening complications may occur.

Secondary bacterial infection of vesicular lesions is relatively common. The typical superinfecting organisms are *Staphylococcus aureus* and *Streptococcus pyogenes*. One manifestation of secondary bacterial infection is the occurrence of fever after the fever associated with onset of chickenpox has subsided. Frequently, severe infection with toxic shock syndrome may result.[10,11]

Chickenpox infection is associated with pneumonia in 1 in 400 cases of infection.[12] A larger proportion of people probably have some pulmonary involvement, but it is typically asymptomatic. Pregnant women and immunocompromised patients with chickenpox seem to have a high risk of life-threatening pneumonia. Chickenpox pneumonia is generally manifested by cough and shortness of breath 3 to 5 days after the onset of the rash. Chest radiography typically shows a reticulonodular infiltrate. Respiratory failure may occur.

Neurologic complications of chickenpox infections include encephalitis, acute cerebellar ataxia, and cerebral angiitis. Encephalitis due to varicella-zoster virus is less common than pneumonia but nevertheless may be life-threatening. The typical manifestation is onset of headaches followed by depression in level of consciousness occurring in an adult within 2 weeks of chickenpox. Acute cerebellar ataxia is more common in children 1 to 3 weeks after the onset of chickenpox. Ataxia and slurred speech may occur, but there is usually complete resolution of these abnormalities.

As with herpes simplex virus infections, the rash of chickenpox or shingles usually can be diagnosed confidently on clinical grounds or confirmed by direct fluorescent antibody testing or culture of scrapings of a skin lesion. Polymerase chain reaction can be performed on cerebrospinal fluid to diagnose varicella-zoster virus encephalitis.

Herpes B Virus

Herpes B virus infection is a relatively benign disease of monkeys. Herpes B virus infection of humans, usually occurring from monkey bites or scratches, is a severe and potentially fatal disease, however. Monkeys of the *Macaca* genus (rhesus and cynomolgus monkeys) are considered highest risk. An incubation period of 2 to 14 days usually is observed after the bite or scratch. Initial symptoms are nonspecific but include fever, malaise, and headache. A cluster of small vesicles may occur at the bite site. A severe encephalomyelitis may ensue, with death occurring in days. In the United States, only one reference laboratory is equipped to identify the virus. Prompt and exhaustive cleaning of wounds, followed by early initiation of acyclovir or valacyclovir, may prevent the occurrence of severe disease.[13]

FEVER IN IMMUNOCOMPROMISED PATIENTS

Numerous viruses can cause fever as a presenting symptom. The manifestations of viral infections in immunocompetent hosts are too numerous to discuss. In the absence of specific manifestations, such as pneumonia or encephalitis, viral infections are rarely life-threatening. The onset of fever in immunocompromised individuals may be the harbinger of severe, overwhelming viral infection, however. This section describes some of the potentially life-threatening clinical manifestations of viral infections in immunocompromised hosts.

CYTOMEGALOVIRUS

Cytomegalovirus infection is a classic cause of severe infection in immunocompromised hosts, especially solid-organ transplant recipients and patients with human immunodeficiency virus (HIV) infection. The infection can be primary or a reactivation infection. The risk of end-organ cytomegalovirus infection depends on the degree of immunosuppression and probably whether infection is primary or reactivation. For solid-organ transplant recipients, there is a significant risk of primary infection in patients who were seronegative for cytomegalovirus before transplantation, who received an organ from a person seropositive for cytomegalovirus infection.

The organs commonly affected by cytomegalovirus infection include the esophagus, colon, retina, and lungs. Virtually any organ can be infected, however, including the central nervous system. Some patients present with a syndrome of fever, malaise, and hematologic abnormalities, without any specific end-organ abnormalities.

Given the high risk of cytomegalovirus infection in solid-organ transplant recipients, strategies should be employed to prevent cytomegalovirus infection. Two options are prophylaxis or preemptive therapy. *Prophylaxis* implies the administration of preventive therapy to all persons at risk.[14-19] In contrast, *preemptive* therapy is the administration of antiviral therapy only to persons at highest risk, as determined by a positive result on a regularly monitored blood test for cytomegalovirus infection.[20-22] Such therapy is given even if the patient is asymptomatic. Detection of the cytomegalovirus PP65 antigen and polymerase chain reaction are used most often for early detection of cytomegalovirus infection.

EPSTEIN-BARR VIRUS

Primary Epstein-Barr virus infection may be associated with fever, malaise, and hematologic abnormalities in immunocompromised patients (as it is in some immunocompetent individuals). Epstein-Barr virus infection can be associated with development of malignancies, such as post-transplant lymphoproliferative disorder.[23-28] In some transplant populations, regular quantitative monitoring of Epstein-Barr virus in peripheral blood by polymerase chain reaction is performed to determine the risk of significant Epstein-Barr virus infection.

HUMAN HERPESVIRUS 6

Human herpesvirus 6 is a ubiquitous viral infection that usually occurs in infancy. Primary human herpesvirus 6 infection and possibly reactivation human herpesvirus 6 infection in immunocompromised patients can be associated with serious disease. Human herpesvirus 6 seems to have neurotropism—in addition to substantial fever, human herpesvirus 6 infection may be associated with confusion, coma, and seizures.[29,30] Occasionally, cerebrospinal fluid examination is normal apart from increased protein and the finding of human herpesvirus 6 by polymerase chain reaction.

HUMAN HERPESVIRUS 8

Human herpesvirus 8 is the virus associated with Kaposi's sarcoma, primary effusion lymphoma, and Castleman's syndrome.[31-34] It may be transmitted via the organ allograft in solid-organ transplantation. Primary infection in immunosuppressed patients may be associated with high fever, thrombocytopenia and other severe cytopenias, and mental state abnormalities.[35] Detection of human herpesvirus 8 by polymerase chain reaction in whole blood may establish the diagnosis.

WEST NILE VIRUS

In the 1990s, West Nile virus infection was detected in North America for the first time.[36-40] Although many cases of infection were directly from the vector of infection (mosquitoes), other cases were via blood transfusion or organ allograft. West Nile virus exhibits neurotropism; infected patients may have confusion and headache in addition to fever and other, more general symptoms.

ADENOVIRUS

Adenoviruses have a myriad of presentations in immunocompetent and immunocompromised hosts. Adenovirus infection in immunocompetent individuals rarely is associated with severe disease. Although adenovirus infection in immunocompromised hosts also may have trivial manifestations, in some patients disseminated disease may occur with catastrophic consequences.

POLYOMAVIRUSES

The most commonly encountered polyomaviruses are JC virus and BK virus. JC virus may be associated with progressive multifocal leukoencephalopathy, a progressive and ultimately fatal neurologic disease occurring in profoundly immunosuppressed individuals, such as patients with advanced HIV infection. BK virus is associated more commonly with renal infection in renal transplant recipients. This infection is usually not accompanied by systemic manifestations, such as fever. Infected patients have steadily rising serum creatinine, however. This presentation may be mistaken for acute rejection. Treatment with augmented immunosuppression is contraindicated, however, in patients with BK virus–associated nephropathy. Instead, immunosuppression should be minimized.

HEMORRHAGIC FEVER

Hemorrhagic fevers may be due to Filoviridae, Bunyaviridae, Arenaviridae, or Flaviviridae. Dengue hemorrhagic fever is not discussed in this chapter because it is reviewed in detail elsewhere in this book (see Chapter 165).

MARBURG AND EBOLA VIRUS HEMORRHAGIC FEVERS

Marburg virus and Ebola virus are members of the *Filovirus* genus. Marburg virus appears to have originated in Uganda and western Kenya, where it has infected monkeys and subsequently humans. *Marburg* refers to a town in Germany, where monkeys from Uganda infected medical researchers, who infected hospital staff. The major subtypes of Ebola virus have occurred in central Africa. An additional subtype (Reston) was discovered in Reston, Virginia, among infected monkeys imported from the Philippines.[41] The source of infection has never been definitively determined.

Marburg and Ebola virus infections have an incubation period of 5 to 10 days and begin with the abrupt onset of fever, myalgia, and headache. Somnolence and delirium usually follow. Most patients have abdominal pain and diarrhea. Many have a maculopapular rash on the trunk. Hemorrhagic manifestations, such as bleeding around needle puncture sites and bleeding from the mucous membranes, become prominent. Most patients have significant thrombocytopenia, leukopenia, and elevated transaminase levels. Viral culture, serology, and polymerase chain reaction methods all have been used to establish the diagnosis. At present, management is purely supportive. Additionally, strict contact isolation precautions are necessary.

HANTAVIRUSES AND CRIMEAN-CONGO HEMORRHAGIC FEVER

Hantavirus and the *Nairovirus* that causes Crimean-Congo hemorrhagic fever are from the Bunyaviridae family of viruses. Hantaviruses cause severe hemorrhagic fever with renal syndrome in China, Korea, and eastern Russia, whereas they cause a pulmonary syndrome in North America. *Hantavirus* usually is transmitted via aerosols of virus-contaminated rodent urine or feces. The incubation period is typically 2 weeks. Initially, patients develop fever, headache, dizziness, blurred vision, abdominal pain, and back pain. Petechiae may be evident on the palate and the trunk; most patients have significant thrombocytopenia. After 4 to 7 days, significant hypotension occurs. In patients who survive, oliguria and mucosal hemorrhage occur. Finally, polyuria occurs.

Crimean-Congo hemorrhagic fever is a severe hemorrhagic fever occurring in Russia, the Balkans, the Middle East, and Africa. The virus is transmitted by ticks. Patients have severe thrombocytopenia, disseminated intravascular coagulation, and extensive bleeding. Most patients are diagnosed via serologic tests.

LASSA FEVER AND SOUTH AMERICAN HEMORRHAGIC FEVERS

Lassa fever and South American hemorrhagic fevers are due to the Arenaviridae. Lassa fever occurs in West Africa. South American hemorrhagic fevers occur in Argentina, Bolivia, and Venezuela. Lassa fever is transmitted via rodents, but subsequent nosocomial transmission has been extensive. Many cases of Lassa fever are only mildly symptomatic. Some patients develop high fever, pharyngitis, and retrosternal chest pain, however, accompanied by significant mucosal bleeding. Hypotension, renal failure, and pulmonary edema may follow. Serology can be used to establish the diagnosis, but the virus also is isolated easily from the blood during the first week of illness, when viremia is often striking. Ribavirin use has been associated with a decrease in mortality.[42]

South American hemorrhagic fevers (Argentine, Bolivian, and Venezuelan) usually present with unremitting fever accompanied by a variety of nonspecific symptoms.

TABLE 161–4. VIRUSES THAT CAUSE ASEPTIC MENINGITIS OR ENCEPHALITIS

Virus	Important Clinical Features
Enteroviruses	Common cause of aseptic meningitis; rapid diagnosis available via PCR of CSF
Herpes simplex virus	In adults usually due to reactivation; rapid diagnosis available via PCR of CSF
Varicella-zoster virus	Uncommonly may cause encephalitis after chickenpox
Human herpesvirus 6	Causes encephalitis in transplant recipients
JK virus	Causes progressive multifocal leukoencephalopathy
Japanese encephalitis	Endemic in parts of Asia
St. Louis encephalitis	Outbreaks have occurred in all U.S. states
West Nile virus	Now common in U.S. and Canada
Tick-borne encephalitis	Several foci of infection
Nipah virus	Zoonosis occurring in Malaysia and Singapore
Hendra virus	Zoonosis occurring in Australia
Rabies virus	Well-known zoonosis
California encephalitis	La Crosse virus is responsible for most cases
Human immuno-deficiency virus	May cause acute encephalitis

CSF, cerebrospinal fluid; PCR, polymerase chain reaction.

Petechiae are often present on the palate and the skin, especially the axilla; mucosal bleeding may result. Pulmonary edema may occur; management is extremely difficult due to the combination of hypotension and refractory pulmonary edema. The diagnosis can be established by serologic tests. No specific therapy is widely available.

OTHER ACUTE VIRAL SYNDROMES

Many viruses can cause aseptic meningitis, encephalitis, pneumonia, or hepatitis. These viruses are summarized in Tables 161-4, 161-5, and 161-6 and are described in detail in other chapters.

ANTIVIRAL DRUGS

Since the advent of HIV infection, there has been an increase in development of drugs active against viruses. This section describes the currently available antiviral drugs, with the exception of drugs for HIV and viral hepatitis.

TABLE 161–5. VIRUSES THAT CAUSE PNEUMONIA

Virus	Important Clinical Features
Respiratory syncytial virus	Common cause of infection in infants
Influenza	Well-known cause of respiratory infection
Parainfluenza virus	Croup and pneumonia
Measles virus	Leading cause of pneumonia in children in underdeveloped nations
Coronaviruses	Severe acute respiratory syndrome
Cytomegalovirus	Important cause of pneumonia in immunosuppressed hosts
Varicella-zoster virus	Pneumonia can complicate chickenpox
Adenovirus	Ubiquitous virus; severe pneumonia in immunosuppressed hosts
Hantavirus	Severe pneumonia in immunocompetent hosts
Hendra virus	Zoonosis in Australia

TABLE 161–6. VIRUSES THAT CAUSE HEPATITIS

Virus	Important Clinical Features
Hepatitis A virus	Fecal-oral transmission
Hepatitis B virus	Parenteral, sexual, vertical transmission
Hepatitis C virus	Parenteral transmission
Hepatitis D virus	Requires coinfection with hepatitis B
Hepatitis E virus	Fecal-oral transmission

ACYCLOVIR

Acyclovir is a deoxyguanosine analog that inhibits viral DNA polymerase. When incorporated into viral DNA, it additionally acts as a chain terminator. Acyclovir has greatest clinical utility for herpes simplex virus 1, herpes simplex virus 2, and varicella-zoster virus. It has some activity against cytomegalovirus, but it is far inferior to ganciclovir for infections with this virus. Acyclovir-resistant herpes simplex virus has been well described, whereas acyclovir-resistant varicella-zoster virus is rare. Acyclovir is available in oral and intravenous forms. It penetrates the cerebrospinal fluid reasonably well, and cerebrospinal fluid levels are about 50% plasma levels.[43] Dosing for acute mucosal herpes simplex virus infections is 200 mg five times a day administered orally and for varicella-zoster virus infections is 800 mg five times a day administered orally. In herpes simplex virus encephalitis, a typical dose is 10 mg/kg given intravenously every 8 hours. Dose reduction is required in the presence of renal dysfunction. In the absence of appropriate reduction in dosage for renal dysfunction, neurotoxicity is observed, usually manifesting as confusion, hallucinations, and occurrence of tremor. Acyclovir can cause crystalline nephropathy; patients receiving the drug should be well hydrated.

VALACYCLOVIR

Because the bioavailability of orally administered acyclovir is low, valacyclovir (the L-valyl ester prodrug of acyclovir) was developed. It is usually administered twice per day for herpes simplex virus infections and three times per day for varicella-zoster virus infections.

FAMCICLOVIR

Famciclovir lacks antiviral activity but is the prodrug of penciclovir, which is active against herpes simplex virus and varicella-zoster virus. Similar to acyclovir, penciclovir is an inhibitor of viral DNA synthesis. In general, acyclovir-resistant strains also are resistant to penciclovir. Dose adjustment of famciclovir is needed in renal insufficiency.

GANCICLOVIR

Similar to acyclovir, ganciclovir is a deoxyguanosine analog. It has activity against herpes simplex virus and varicella-zoster virus. Its primary use has been in the treatment or prevention of cytomegalovirus infections. Ganciclovir acts by inhibiting viral DNA polymerases. Patients with end-organ disease due to cytomegalovirus usually are treated initially with ganciclovir, 5 mg/kg intravenously every 12 hours. Alterations in dose and frequency are required in patients with renal dysfunction. Typically, maintenance therapy is given at a reduced frequency (e.g., once per day) in patients who have received 2 to 3 weeks of induction therapy. Myelosuppression is the major toxicity of ganciclovir. Neutropenia typically begins to occur week 2 of ganciclovir therapy. Regular monitoring of hematologic parameters is mandatory for patients receiving ganciclovir. Central nervous system abnormalities, such as headache but including confusion, have been well described in patients receiving ganciclovir. In addition to an intravenous preparation, ganciclovir is available in an orally administered form. This form may be useful in prophylaxis against cytomegalovirus infection.[44] Ganciclovir also can be administered into the eye via an ocular implant.[45] Ganciclovir is less active against acyclovir-resistant herpes simplex virus strains than against acyclovir-susceptible strains. Resistance of cytomegalovirus to ganciclovir has been well described,[46] but usually occurs only in patients who have received prolonged courses of ganciclovir therapy.

VALGANCICLOVIR

The oral bioavailability of ganciclovir is poor. Valganciclovir, a prodrug of ganciclovir, can be used to enhance bioavailability. Valganciclovir is widely used as prophylaxis against cytomegalovirus infection.[47]

FOSCARNET

Foscarnet is used most frequently in patients with cytomegalovirus infection refractory to or who are intolerant of ganciclovir. Foscarnet also has activity against herpes simplex virus and varicella-zoster virus, including acyclovir-resistant and ganciclovir-resistant strains. Although foscarnet and ganciclovir may have synergistic activity against cytomegalovirus, there is no proven usefulness of combination therapy.[48] Use of the combination of ganciclovir and foscarnet is associated with greater toxicity than use of ganciclovir alone.[48] Foscarnet is available in an intravenous, but not an oral, formulation. Toxicity is common with foscarnet. Nephrotoxicity is a major dose-limiting side effect. Electrolyte abnormalities also are common, especially hypocalcemia, hypophosphatemia, hypomagnesemia, and hypokalemia. Hypocalcemia may be symptomatic. Foscarnet may produce painful genital ulcerations; saline loading may diminish the likelihood of nephrotoxicity or genital ulceration.

CIDOFOVIR

Cidofovir is a nucleotide analog that is active against many herpesviruses and other DNA viruses, including polyomaviruses, poxviruses, and adenovirus. It is active against acyclovir-resistant and ganciclovir-resistant herpes simplex virus and cytomegalovirus. Cidofovir is administered intravenously once a week or once every 2 weeks. Its use is accompanied by high rates of nephrotoxicity. Neutropenia also occurs in 20% of patients receiving this drug.

RIBAVIRIN

Ribavirin has found wide use as part of combination therapy for hepatitis C virus infection, but is discussed here in the context of its use against other viruses. In vitro, ribavirin has activity against a wide range of DNA and RNA viruses. Ribavirin (aerosolized) is approved by the U.S. Food and

Drug Administration for the treatment of bronchiolitis and pneumonia due to respiratory syncytial virus. It has been used systemically in the treatment of some hemorrhagic fevers. Systemic ribavirin administration is associated with hemolytic anemia. Use of aerosolized ribavirin is frequently controversial because the drug is teratogenic. Health care worker exposure to the drug potentially may occur when the drug is used in conjunction with mechanical ventilation, and use of aerosol containment systems is recommended.

ANTI-INFLUENZA DRUGS

Amantadine, rimantadine, zanamivir, and oseltamivir are potentially useful against the influenza viruses. They have found use as treatment of influenza and as postexposure prophylaxis against influenza. Amantadine and rimantadine are active only against influenza A virus, whereas zanamivir and oseltamivir are active against influenza A and B viruses. In patients who have not had reduced doses of amantadine or rimantadine given in the setting of renal dysfunction, serious neurotoxic reactions (including confusion and seizures) have been observed.

ANNOTATED REFERENCES

Breman JG, Henderson DA: Diagnosis and management of smallpox. N Engl J Med 2002;346:1300-1308.
Many textbooks have progressively diminished their coverage of smallpox since the 1970s. This review article fills in the gaps in a timely fashion.

Luppi M, Barozzi P, Schulz TF, et al: Bone marrow failure associated with human herpesvirus 8 infection after transplantation. N Engl J Med 2000;343:1378-1385.
Occurrence of significant viral syndromes after organ transplantation may be associated with primary infection transmitted via the graft or reactivation of prior infection. In this study, human herpesvirus 8 infection occurred after renal transplantation and was associated with severe pancytopenia.

Paya C, Humar A, Dominguez E, et al: Efficacy and safety of valganciclovir vs. oral ganciclovir for prevention of cytomegalovirus disease in solid organ transplant recipients. Am J Transplant 2004;4:611-620.
The availability of antiviral medications has opened the way for prevention of viral infections in high-risk groups. One such example is the prevention of cytomegalovirus by valganciclovir therapy.

Pealer LN, Marfin AA, Petersen LR, et al: Transmission of West Nile virus through blood transfusion in the United States in 2002. N Engl J Med 2003;349:1236-1245.
Just as viruses may be transmitted via solid organs, similarly they may be transmitted via blood transfusion. West Nile virus is one example.

Reed KD, Melski JW, Graham MB, et al: The detection of monkeypox in humans in the Western Hemisphere. N Engl J Med 2004;350:342-350.
There are numerous more recent examples of viral syndromes moving out of their traditional geographic locations. One is the occurrence of monkeypox in the United States.

Chapter 162

CLOSTRIDIUM DIFFICILE COLITIS

John G. Bartlett

KEY POINTS

1. Most cases of antibiotic-associated diarrhea are caused by *C. difficile* or are enigmatic.

2. Major complications of *C. difficile*–associated colitis are toxic megacolon, devastating diarrhea, and sepsis.

3. Clinical and laboratory clues to this diagnosis are exposure to antibiotics, watery diarrhea and cramps, evidence of colitis, leukocytosis, and hypoalbuminemia.

4. The diagnosis is made with tests for *C. difficile* toxin in stool, usually enzyme immunoassay.

5. The usual treatment is (a) discontinue the implicated antibiotic; (b) treat with oral metronidazole; (c) avoid antiperistaltics, and (d) maintain contact precautions to avoid nosocomial spread.

6. The intensivist is likely to see this as a common complication of antibiotic use in vulnerable patients when treatment is straightforward if the diagnosis is considered.

7. The intensivist may also see the complicated case with ileus, which poses treatment problems because the only treatment with established merit is oral antibiotics that may never reach the colon.

Antibiotic-associated colitis was recognized soon after antibiotics were introduced in the 1940s, but the cause was not known until 1978 with the original reports of the role of *Clostridium difficile* as the putative agent in nearly all cases of antibiotic-associated pseudomembranous colitis and 10% to 15% of those with uncomplicated antibiotic-associated diarrhea.[1] Subsequent work has identified pathophysiology, epidemiology, diagnostic methods, and treatment. The major challenges continue to be prevention and the management of patients with advanced disease, particularly those with ileus.

ETIOLOGY

C. difficile causes a spectrum of enteric complications of antibiotic use ranging from nuisance diarrhea to severe and sometimes life-threatening pseudomembranous colitis. There are occasional cases of antibiotic-associated colitis due to other pathogens (*Staphylococcus aureus,* enterotoxin-producing strains of *Clostridium perfringens* or *Salmonella*), but most cases are either due to *C. difficile* or are enigmatic.[2]

PATHOPHYSIOLOGY

There are six relevant issues:

1. **Colonization with *C. difficile:*** This organism is found in the colonic flora of 2% to 3% of healthy adults and 20% to 30% of hospitalized patients.[3,4]

2. **Toxin production:** *C. difficile* produces two toxins, designated toxin A and toxin B.[5] Most studies have implicated toxin A as the major cause of enteric disease based on animal studies that show florid colitis with injection into a bowel loop; more recent studies suggest that toxin B may also be a pathogen in humans. Most strains of *C. difficile* produce both toxins, but there are exceptions.[6]

3. **Antibiotic exposure:** This appears to be the most important identifiable risk and presumably reflects inhibition of the colonic flora with the opportunity for *C. difficile* to convert from the spore form to the vegetative form. It is the vegetative forms that replicate and produce toxin. Virtually every antibiotic with an antibacterial spectrum has been implicated, but the most frequent are clindamycin, cephalosporins, and broad-spectrum penicillins (e.g., ampicillin, piperacillin).[2] In general, the antibiotic most likely to cause this complication is clindamycin, so much so that at one time the terms *pseudomembranous colitis* and *clindamycin colitis* were used synonymously.[7] However, in current practice, cephalosporins account for the majority of cases, presumably reflecting their enormous usage rates.

4. **Epidemiology:** As noted, *C. difficile* is relatively infrequent in ambulatory persons but rates of colonization and disease are much higher as a result of exposure to the hospital environment.[4] *C. difficile* now represents an important nosocomial pathogen, so many laboratories initially test patients with nosocomial diarrhea only for this enteric pathogen because the others are almost never responsible. Nursing homes are another setting in which there are clustering of vulnerable patients with high rates of antibiotic use where *C. difficile* may be endemic or epidemic.[8]

5. **Age:** There is increasing susceptibility to this complication and especially severe disease in the elderly.[9]

6. **Immunologic susceptibility:** Many patients harbor *C. difficile* with no clinical expression even with extensive antibiotic exposure and sometimes have toxin in the absence of diarrhea.[10] The best explanation for this paradox is the presence of neutralizing antibody. Nevertheless, patients may have multiple cases of *C. difficile* enteric disease, and relapses after treatment are common.

CLINICAL SIGNS AND SYMPTOMS

The typical presentation is a patient who is receiving an antibiotic who develops diarrhea that is watery and associated with cramps.[2] It is not possible to distinguish this from antibiotic-associated diarrhea due to "nonspecific causes," but factors that support the probability of *C. difficile* include the following: (1) evidence of colitis by fecal leukocytes by endoscopy or characteristic changes on computed tomography (thickened bowel restricted to the colon often associated with ascites); (2) clinical features of severe disease including fever and profuse diarrhea with dehydration; and (3) laboratory tests, especially leukocytosis sometimes with a leukemoid reaction and hypoalbuminemia. Nearly all cases are associated with diarrhea, but occasional postoperative patients will not have this history or there will be no good record of it. Laboratory clues that are underappreciated are hypoalbuminemia reflecting this as a protein-losing enteropathy and leukocytosis with a white blood cell count greater than 20,000/mm³, which may be another one of the most important clues.[11]

MANAGEMENT (Table 162-1)

DIAGNOSIS

The diagnosis is based primarily on detection of the *C. difficile* toxin using a standard assay. The classic test is the cytotoxin assay with tissue cultures showing neutralization with the antitoxin.[2] More recently, most laboratories use an enzyme immunoassay test, which is easier and faster but somewhat less sensitive. The recommendation is to obtain a single test; if this is negative despite a probable diagnosis, the test should be repeated. The preferred test is an enzyme immunoassay that detects both toxin A and toxin B.[2]

TABLE 162–1. MANAGEMENT OF *CLOSTRIDIUM DIFFICILE* COLITIS

Diagnosis

1. Stool for *C. difficile* toxin × 1.
2. Repeat if negative and clinical features strongly suggestive.

Treatment

1. Stop implicated antibiotic.
   Note: If need antibiotic, use agent from a different class that is unlikely to cause this complication.
2. Avoid antiperistaltics.
3. Use standard antimicrobial treatment.
   a. Metronidazole, 250 mg p.o. three times a day for 7 to 10 days
   b. Vancomycin (alternative treatment for metronidazole intolerance or failure, or contraindication such as pregnancy), 125 mg p.o. four times a day for 7 to 10 days
4. If seriously ill with ileus:
   a. Vancomycin: high dose (500 mg four times a day) by enema or by long enteric tube
   b. Metronidazole: 500 mg i.v. every 6 hours
   c. Colectomy
5. *Infection control*
   a. Single room with bathroom if possible, especially if incontinent
   b. Hand washing with soap; use vinyl gloves; perform terminal room cleaning with sporicidal agent; avoid rectal thermometers.

TREATMENT

The most important immediate step is to discontinue the implicated antibiotic. If there is a need for antibiotic treatment, pick a drug that is unlikely to cause *C. difficile* colitis. *C. difficile* is retained totally within the colonic lumen so that treatment is based on antibiotic active against this organism that can be delivered intact to the colonic lumen. The two favored drugs are metronidazole and vancomycin, both given by mouth.[2,12,13] Metronidazole is often preferred because it is less expensive, avoids the promotion of vancomycin-resistant *Enterococcus* (VRE), and seems to work as well as vancomycin.[2] Nevertheless, many authorities prefer vancomycin for patients who are seriously ill based on the observations that resistance has never been found with this drug and the colonic levels are about 1000 times the minimal inhibitory concentration. The expected response with either drug is for rapid decrease in fever and a gradual elimination of diarrhea, which usually resolves in 4 to 6 days.[2,13] It is generally not advised to obtain a post-treatment stool toxin assay because many patients continue to shed the toxin despite a good clinical response.[8]

PREVENTION

C. difficile is an important nosocomial pathogen, and the current recommendations to prevent cases are hand washing with soap, cleaning of environmental surfaces with sporicidal agents in case-associated areas, isolation of symptomatic patients especially those who are incontinent, avoidance of rectal thermometers,[8] and, in some cases, institution of antibiotic control mechanisms. For antibiotic control, the best results during epidemics have been to control the use of clindamycin.[14]

COMPLICATIONS

The major complication of *C. difficile* for the intensivist are toxic megacolon and sepsis.[2,15] Toxic megacolon poses two problems: first is the severity of this complication per se, but more important is the inability to deliver vancomycin to the site of infection. Methods to deal with toxic megacolon include the use of high doses of vancomycin by mouth (500 mg four times daily), the use of long tubes from above or below (but these may not reach the site of infection), and the use of intravenous metronidazole (but the record here is checkered, in part owing to the relatively low colonic levels achieved). Some patients will be severely ill with the sepsis syndrome, but bacteremia is rare, colonic perforation virtually never occurs, and *C. difficile* bacteremia virtually never happens.[2,15] These patients require standard management of sepsis with particular attention to rehydration while attempting to control disease with oral vancomycin or metronidazole. It is critical to discontinue the implicated antibiotic.

CONCLUSION

C. difficile has emerged as a major nosocomial pathogen that is associated with antibiotic use, may cause a devastating colitis, is easily detected with the standard stool toxin assay, and usually responds rapidly to the combination of discontinuing the implicated antibiotic with or without the addition of oral vancomycin or metronidazole. An issue that is important for the intensivist is that this is a nosocomial pathogen that requires implementation of careful infection control procedures. Some patients present with toxic mega-colon, which may be difficult to manage, and the sepsis syndrome, in which *C. difficile*–induced enteric disease may be overlooked.

ANNOTATED REFERENCES

Bartlett JG: Clinical practice: Antibiotic-associated diarrhea. N Engl J Med 2002;346:334.
  Recent review of practical approach to antibiotic-associated diarrhea. Most cases are caused by C. difficile (10% to 30%) or are enigmatic (70% to 90%). The toxin assay usually distinguishes.

Gerding DN, Johnson S, Peterson LR, et al: *Clostridium difficile*–associated diarrhea and colitis. Infect Control Hosp Epidemiol 1995;16:459.
  SHEA infectious control guidelines for a patient with C. difficile diarrhea, which include (1) single room with bathroom, especially with incontinence; (2) contact precautions; (3) restrict use of rectal thermometers; and (4) restrict use of antibiotics (especially clindamycin) if necessary.

Lipsett PA, Samantaray DK, Tam ML, et al: Pseudomembranous colitis: A surgical disease? Surgery 1994;116:491.
  The Hopkins experience with 17 patients who had C. difficile colitis unresponsive to antibiotics due to ileus. These patients required colectomies and represented 1% of all C. difficile cases.

McFarlan LV, Mulligan ME, Kwok RYY, et al: Nosocomial acquisition of *Clostridium difficile* infection. N Engl J Med 1989;320:204.
  The authors emphasize the role of the hospital as a source of large numbers of cases presumably due to clustering of vulnerable patients and high rates of antibiotics. About 30% of hospitalized patients acquire C. difficile colonization of the colonic flora.

Wenisch C, Parschalk B, Hasenhundl M, et al: Comparison of vancomycin, teicoplanin, metronidazole, and fusidic acid for the treatment of *Clostridium difficile*–associated diarrhea. Clin Infect Dis 1996;22:813.
  The authors show that metronidazole and vancomycin are equally effective even with documented pseudomembranous colitis.

Chapter 163

TETANUS

C. Louise Thwaites • Lam M. Yen

Tetanus is caused by toxin from the bacterium *Clostridium tetani* and is characterized by muscle rigidity, spasms, and disturbance of the autonomic nervous system.

EPIDEMIOLOGY

Tetanus is now rare in the Western world, with only 35 cases in the United States in 2000,[1] but it is still a common problem in developing countries, where 80% of cases occur in Africa and Southeast Asia. Immunization programs targeting infants and pregnant women have coincided with a decline in the incidence of tetanus over recent years, but the estimated global incidence remains between 700,000 to 1 million cases/year.[2] In developing countries neonatal deaths account for a large proportion of cases, and neonatal tetanus is the second leading cause of death from vaccine-preventable diseases worldwide, responsible for an estimated 248,000 deaths/year (Fig. 163-1).[3] In developed countries the elderly are particularly at risk owing to missed boosters and reduced antibody levels. A recent study showed that only 31% of Americans older than age 70 years have adequate antibody concentrations.[4]

PATHOPHYSIOLOGY

Tetanus is caused by a potent neurotoxin from the gram-positive bacterium *C. tetani* (Fig. 163-2). *C. tetani* is a ubiquitous organism, capable of surviving in the environment as highly resistant spores, and has been isolated from soil, street dust, and human and animal feces.[5] Once in a suitable anaerobic environment these spores germinate, the bacteria multiply, and toxin is released. The most common sources of infection are minor lacerations to the limbs or the umbilical stump in neonates (Fig. 163-3).[6] In 20% of cases no source of infection can be found.[7] More unusual entry sites include dental infection, ear piercing, unsterile surgery, or injections.[8]

Toxin is preferentially taken up by motor nerves, either locally or after circulation in the bloodstream, and then transported retrogradely into the central nervous system.[9] Tetanus toxin is a zinc-dependent endopeptidase that cleaves vesical-associated membrane protein II (VAMP II or synaptobrevin) at a single peptide bond.[10] This molecule is essential for synaptic release of neurotransmitters, and cleavage disrupts synaptic transmission. The toxin preferentially affects the gamma-aminobutyric acid (GABA) inhibitory interneurons afferent to motor nerves in the spinal cord and the brainstem. By preventing inhibitory discharge, unrestricted motor nerve activity occurs, resulting in the increased muscle tone and spasms characteristic of tetanus. In severe forms of tetanus the autonomic nervous system is also affected, perhaps as a result of toxin action within the brainstem,[5,11] giving rise to marked cardiovascular instability.[12]

CLINICAL FEATURES

Two main forms of tetanus exist. The majority of tetanus cases are generalized, affecting all muscle groups. However, a milder form, localized tetanus, also exists, affecting muscle

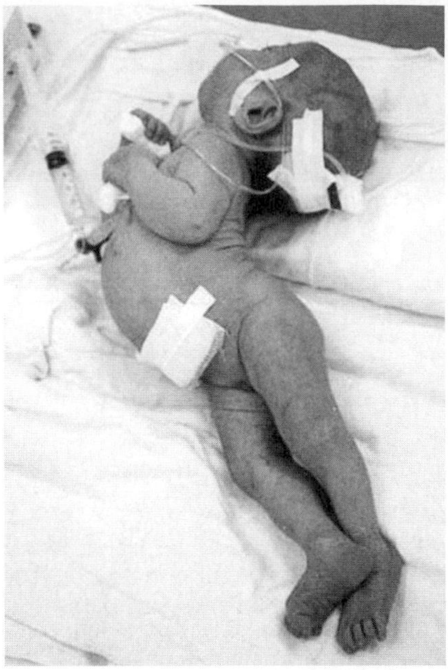

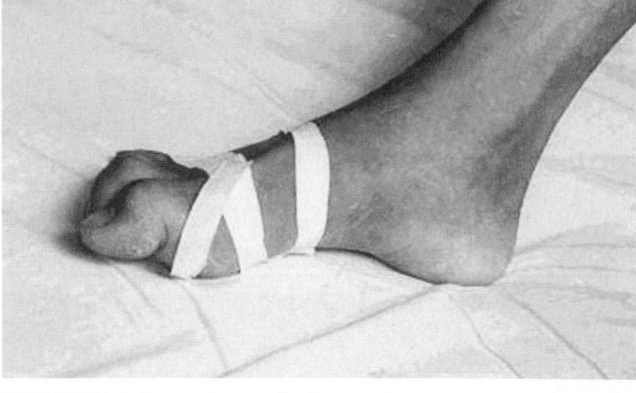

FIGURE 163–3. Lacerations to the feet are the most common focus of *C. tetani* infection. Note clawing of toes secondary to increased tone in surrounding muscles.

FIGURE 163–1. Neonatal tetanus.

groups in the immediate vicinity of a wound. A subgroup of localized tetanus, cephalic tetanus, is also recognized and is associated with a higher mortality,[13] perhaps owing to early laryngospasm or autonomic disturbance resulting from brainstem involvement. Cephalic tetanus is often associated with lower motor neuron palsies affecting the third or seventh cranial nerves (Fig. 163-4). Localized tetanus of any variety may progress to the generalized form.

After infection, a period of time (the incubation period) elapses before symptoms arise. This is usually between 4 and 14 days, with 90% of cases presenting within 15 days.[14]

Initial symptoms include muscle stiffness, with muscle groups with short neuronal pathways affected first; hence, trismus and back pain are present in more than 90% of cases on admission.[7] Involvement of the facial and pharyngeal muscles produce the characteristic "risus sardonicus" and dysphagia (Fig. 163-5). Increased tone in the muscles of the trunk results in opisthotonus. Muscle groups adjacent to the initial site of infection are often particularly severely affected, producing an asymmetrical picture.

The time from the first symptom to the first spasm is termed the period of onset. Both the period of onset and incubation period have prognostic significance, with shorter times being associated with more severe disease (< 48 hours for period of onset and < 7 days for incubation period).[15] Spasms may be spontaneous but can also be provoked by physical or emotional stimuli. Laryngospasm can occur early in the disease process, often in isolation, resulting in acute upper airway obstruction. Respiration may also be affected by spasms involving the chest muscles. Without facilities

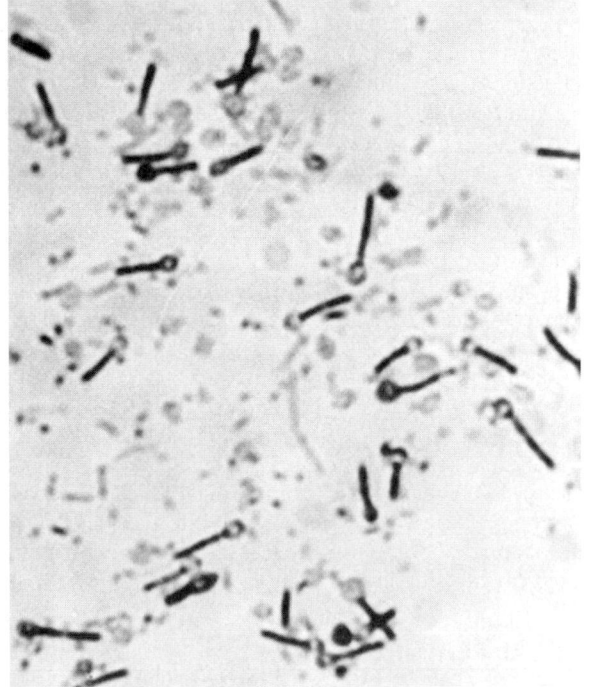

FIGURE 163–2. *Clostridium tetani:* a gram-positive bacillus with terminal spores. (Courtesy of J. Campbell, Oxford University Clinical Research Unit, Hospital for Tropical Diseases, Ho Chi Minh City, Vietnam.)

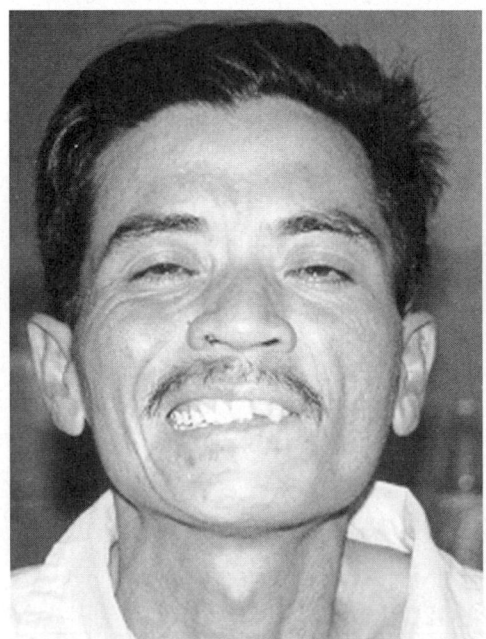

FIGURE 163–4. Cephalic tetanus associated with lower motor neuron palsy of seventh cranial nerve on the left side of the face.

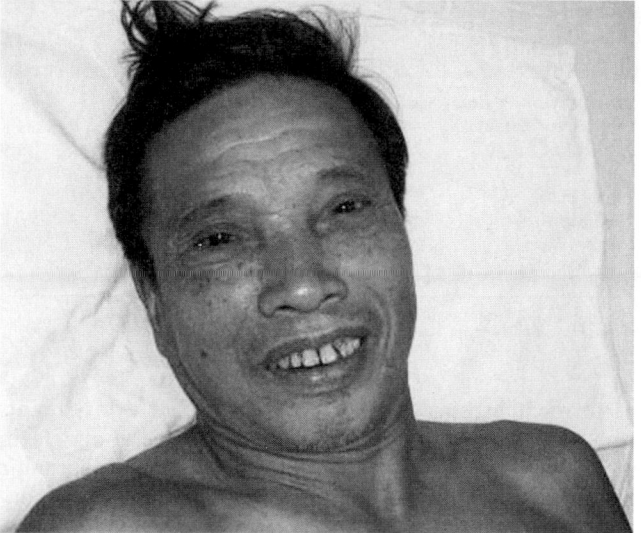

FIGURE 163–5. Facial muscle involvement in tetanus producing the characteristic "risus sardonicus."

for mechanical ventilation, respiratory failure due to muscle spasm is the most common cause of death.[5] Hypoxia is common in tetanus[16] either due to spasms or difficulties clearing the copious bronchial secretions and aspiration.

Muscle spasms are usually most severe during the first and second weeks of illness but may persist for 3 to 4 weeks, after which rigidity may remain for several more weeks. In severe tetanus, autonomic disturbance usually appears during the second week. Signs of sympathetic overactivity usually predominate, evident as periods of tachycardia and hypertension. Severe tetanus is associated with a hyperkinetic circulation, particularly if muscle spasms are poorly controlled.[17] Changes in blood pressure are mainly due to changes in systemic vascular resistance, with little change in the cardiac index.[18] Circulating catecholamines are raised[19] and may have a direct toxic effect on the myocardium.[20]

Acute renal failure is a recognized complication of tetanus, with dehydration, rhabdomyolysis due to spasms, and autonomic disturbance all contributing.[21,22] Other complications include tendon avulsions,[5] vertebral fractures secondary to muscle spasm,[23] gastrointestinal bleeding, venous thrombosis, and thromboembolism (Table 163-1).[24]

TABLE 163–1. COMPLICATIONS OF TETANUS

System	Complication
Cardiovascular	Hyper/hypotension
	Tachy/bradycardia
	Arrhythmias
	Ischemia
	Venous thrombosis/thromboembolism
Respiratory	Type I and type II respiratory failure
	Acute respiratory distress syndrome (ARDS)
	Aspiration pneumonia
	Ventilator-associated pneumonia
Other	Acute renal failure
	Gastrointestinal bleeding
	Sepsis
	Vertebral fractures
	Bed sores

DIAGNOSIS

Diagnosis is clinical, based on history and examination findings. Strychnine, a glycine agonist, may give rise to a similar clinical picture, but muscle tone is usually normal between spasms. Urinary or plasma measurement of strychnine will exclude this as a cause. Because abdominal muscle rigidity is often an early sign, the disease may mimic an acute abdomen. Other differential diagnoses include orofacial infections causing trismus, dystonic drug reactions, or hysteria. Culture of *C. tetani* from a wound is difficult, and a positive culture is supportive of the diagnosis but not confirmatory.

MANAGEMENT

Tetanus patients should be nursed in a quiet environment and all stimuli minimized. To prevent further toxin release, wounds should be cleaned and débrided of any necrotic material and antibiotics given. Metronidazole (400 mg rectally or 500 mg i.v. every 6 hours for 7 days) is the antibiotic of choice,[7] although penicillin (100 to 200,000 IU/kg/day) remains the standard therapy throughout most of the world. In one open study, metronidazole was associated with a lower mortality than penicillin (7% compared with 24%),[25] although no significant difference was found by a much larger study by Yen and associates.[7] There was, however, a reduction in sedative requirements in the metronidazole group, perhaps as a result of the proconvulsant activity of penicillin.

Antitoxin should be administered to neutralize any unbound toxin. Ideally, human immune globulin (100 to 300 IU/kg intramuscularly as a single dose) should be given. If this is unavailable, equine antitoxin (500 U/kg i.m.) can be used, but it is associated with a higher incidence of anaphylaxis.[7]

Tetanus infection does not result in immunity; therefore, all patients should be actively immunized with a full primary immunization course.

Further management consists of supportive care until the effects of the bound toxin wear off. The evidence base for most of the treatments listed below is limited. Many older therapies have never been subjected to trials, although their use is now routine. Small case series and case reports exist describing the use of newer agents, but few randomized controlled trials have been published.

Airway management is a priority in tetanus. Generalized muscle spasm, laryngospasm, aspiration, or large doses of sedatives may all impair respiration, and airway compromise should be anticipated. Tracheostomy is the preferred means of securing the airway, although endotracheal intubation is acceptable as an initial measure. Copious bronchial secretions are produced in tetanus, and patients need frequent suctioning to remove secretions.

Sedation with benzodiazepines is the standard therapy for tetanus. They inhibit endogenous antagonists of GABA$_A$ receptors and may counteract the effects of tetanus toxin. Intravenous diazepam or midazolam is usually used, and doses up to 200 mg/day are frequently required. Phenobarbitone and chlorpromazine have historically been used to provide adjunct sedation, and their use may be beneficial in patients with autonomic disturbance. Alternatively, if spasms are not sufficiently controlled using benzodiazepines, then nondepolarizing muscle relaxants and intermittent positive-pressure ventilation (IPPV) are indicated. Cardiovascularly, inert drugs, such as vecuronium, should be used if possible, and pancuronium should be avoided owing to its sympathomimetic side effects.[26,27]

Autonomic instability is difficult to treat. Rapid fluctuations in blood pressure mean drugs with short half-lives are desirable. The use of beta blockers is controversial because their use has been associated with episodes of profound hypotension.[28] Esmolol may confer some advantage in this setting, but little data have been published to support its use. Conventional therapy consists of heavy sedation, using high-dose benzodiazepines, morphine, and/or chlorpromazine.[29] Other treatments reported include clonidine and epidural bupivacaine, but data supporting their use are limited.[8,17] Bhagwanjee reports the use of epidural bupivacaine in 11 patients with severe tetanus. Fluctuations in blood pressure and heart rate were reduced after blockade, although two patients still required additional agents to control sympathetic overactivity.[30] In addition to hypertension, hypotensive episodes may also occur; and if they are unresponsive to volume expansion, inotropes are required.

Recently, interest has focused on the use of intravenous magnesium sulfate to control spasms and treat autonomic dysfunction, either as an adjunct to sedation or as a first-line agent.[31,32] Doses of 1 to 3 g/h have been used to achieve serum concentrations of 2 to 4 mmol/L. The first trial studied the effect of magnesium on cardiovascular instability on 10 patients already receiving heavy sedation for autonomic dysfunction. Results showed favorable changes in systemic vascular resistance, heart rate, and systolic blood pressure fluctuations when patients were receiving magnesium. The most recent study used magnesium as a first-line therapy in place of benzodiazepines,[32] and reported adequate spasm control in 38 of 40 patients, with 17 of the 24 patients aged younger than 60 years avoiding IPPV. Unfortunately, respiratory support was required for 10 of the 16 patients older than age 60 years. Concerns still exist regarding the safety of magnesium in sites without facilities for IPPV, and on the basis of the published data its routine use in this setting cannot yet be endorsed.

Patients with severe tetanus often require 2 or 3 weeks of IPPV until spasms subside, and nosocomial infection, particularly pneumonia, is an important problem. In one series the incidence of ventilator-associated pneumonia in tetanus patients was reported to be 52.6%, with autonomic disturbance an independent risk factor (RR, 31.65; 95% CI 2.68 to 373.74).[33]

OUTCOME

Outcome in tetanus depends on the severity of the disease and the facilities available for treatment. Adverse prognostic factors are given in Table 163-2. If the disease is not treated, the mortality from tetanus is greater than 60% and higher in neonates.[5,34,35] In units with good facilities mortality rates of 13% to 25% have been reported.[35,36] Few studies have been

TABLE 163–2. ADVERSE PROGNOSTIC FEATURES IN TETANUS*	
Incubation Period	<7 days
Period of Onset	<48 hours
Portal of Entry	Umbilicus, uterus, burns, open fractures, postoperative, intramuscular injections
Spasms	Present
Temperature	>38.4°C
Heart Rate	>120 beats/min (adult)
	>150 beats/min (neonate)

*Presented at 4th International Conference on Tetanus, Dakar, 1975.[39]

performed investigating the long-term effects on patients who survive, but it appears that recovery is complete in most, although some persistent electroencephalographic abnormalities and difficulties in balance, speech, and memory have been reported.[37,38]

ANNOTATED REFERENCES

Attygalle D, Rodrigo N: Magnesium as first line therapy in the management of tetanus: A prospective study of 40 patients. Anaesthesia 2002;57:811-817.

A prospective observational study of magnesium sulfate for control of spasms and autonomic dysfunction in 40 patients. Only two patients achieving target serum magnesium concentrations needed additional neuromuscular blocking drugs. Sympathetic overactivity was controlled without supplementary sedation. However, 17 patients, particularly the elderly, required additional ventilatory support.

Cavalcante NJ, Sandeville ML, Medeiros EA: Incidence of and risk factors for nosocomial pneumonia in patients with tetanus. Clin Infect Dis 2001;33:1842-1846.

Study of tetanus patients in ICU to identify risk factors associated with nosocomial pneumonia. Results from univariate analysis showed the degree of severity of tetanus, dysautonomy, use of neuromuscular blockers, use of higher doses of diazepam, and lower arterial oxygen and oxygen fractions as risk factors. However, results of multiple logistical regression found only dysautonomy to be significant.

Kerr JH, Corbett JL, Prys-Roberts C, et al: Involvement of the sympathetic nervous system in tetanus: Studies on 82 cases. Lancet 1968;2:236-241.

Description of syndrome of autonomic dysfunction, describing features of labile hypertension, tachycardia, peripheral vasoconstriction, profuse sweating, pyrexia, and increased urinary catecholamine excretion.

Patel JC, Mehta BC, Modi KN: Prognosis in tetanus. In Patel JC (ed): 1st International Conference on Tetanus. Bombay, Study Group of Tetanus, King Edward Memorial Hospital, 1963, vol 1, pp 181-201.

Patel and colleagues examined records of 4013 patients with tetanus. From the results, they concluded that "only 4 factors need to be considered when assessing prognosis: period of onset < 48 hours; presence of spasms on admission; incubation period of less than 7 days and rectal temperature of ≥ 100° F within 24 hours of admission." Furthermore, he suggested that if the first and second factors are present, the last two are unimportant.

Trujillo MH, Castillo A, Espana J, et al: Impact of intensive care management on the prognosis of tetanus: Analysis of 641 cases. Chest 1987;92:63-65.

Historical study of 671 patients, comparing the results of intensive care management of tetanus patients before and after institution of an ICU. Results showed a decrease in mortality, from 43.58% to 15%, with the main cause of mortality changing from early acute respiratory failure to unexplained cardiac arrest, probably related to autonomic dysfunction.

Chapter 164

BOTULISM

Vern C. Juel • Thomas P. Bleck

KEY POINTS

1. Botulinum toxins are zinc endopeptidases that cleave specific sites of proteins mediating the release of acetylcholine at the neuromuscular junction, in autonomic ganglia, and in parasympathetic nerve terminals.

2. Food-borne botulism is caused by the ingestion of preformed toxin from contaminated food sources. Food-borne disease may present in outbreaks involving several individuals.

3. Intestinal botulism is caused by ingestion of clostridial spores in susceptible individuals with colonization of the intestinal tract and in vivo toxin production.

4. Wound botulism is caused by clostridial colonization of individuals with devitalized tissues due to in vivo toxin production. Subcutaneous injection of illicit drugs, particularly black tar heroin, is responsible for a recent increase in cases.

5. Inhalational botulism from aerosolized toxin causes a neuroparalytic syndrome indistinguishable from the other forms of human botulism.

6. Outbreaks due to deliberate release of toxin may be characterized by numerous cases, rare toxin types, a common geographic factor without a common dietary exposure, and multiple simultaneous outbreaks.

7. The cardinal clinical features of botulism include a symmetrical, descending paralysis with multiple cranial neuropathies evolving rapidly in the absence of fever or altered sensorium. In food-borne disease, initial symptoms may include nausea, vomiting, diarrhea, and abdominal cramping. In infant intestinal botulism, the initial symptom is often constipation.

8. Differential diagnosis of botulism includes Guillain-Barré syndrome and its variants, myasthenia gravis, Lambert-Eaton myasthenic syndrome, tick paralysis, and acute brainstem lesions. For infant intestinal botulism, the differential diagnosis includes sepsis, meningoencephalitis, Werdnig-Hoffmann disease, congenital myasthenia gravis, and metabolic disorders.

9. Electrodiagnostic studies may help to support the diagnosis, although the findings may not be specific. The mouse bioassay is the confirmatory test for botulism.

10. Airway protection and ventilatory support are the main issues for supportive care.

11. Antitoxin may shorten the course of the disease when administered early to bind circulating toxin.

Botulism is the neuroparalytic disorder resulting from intoxication with the exotoxins produced by *Clostridium botulinum* and several other strains of clostridia. *C. botulinum* are spore-forming obligate anaerobic bacilli[1] whose heat-resistant spores are widely distributed in soil and marine sediment throughout the world.[2] The term *botulism* is derived from the Latin word for "sausage," *botulus*. Botulism initially was recognized as sausage poisoning in Europe in the early 19th century. Kerner, a German health official, recognized the relationship between sausage ingestion and paralysis in 230 people in 1820.[3] The toxin and the bacterium were initially demonstrated by Van Ermengem[4] in his study of an epidemic of food-borne botulism following raw ham consumption at a Belgian funeral music festival in 1895. In addition to food-borne botulism after ingestion of preformed toxin, forms of botulism owing to in vivo toxin production subsequently were recognized, including wound botulism in 1943,[5] infant botulism in 1976,[6,7] and adult intestinal botulism in 1986.[8] Inhalational botulism has been identified only in a single outbreak in humans[9] but has received more recent attention related to the potential for aerosolized toxin used as a biologic weapon.[10]

TOXIN CHARACTERISTICS

Seven distinct serotypes of botulinum toxin, A through G, are defined by the absence of cross-neutralization with antitoxin.[11] Human disease is produced by types A, B, E, and rarely F toxin, whereas types C and D produce disease in birds and mammals.[12] Type G has been implicated in human disease only rarely.[12,13] Neurotoxigenic strains of *Clostridium baratii* may produce type F toxin,[14,15] and some strains of *Clostridium butyricum* may produce type E toxin.[16]

Botulinum toxins are 150-kDa polypeptides that are converted during bacterial lysis by proteases into an active form consisting of a 50-kDa light chain and a 100-kDa heavy chain joined by a disulfide bond.[17] After absorption into systemic circulation, the carboxy-terminal domain of the heavy chain facilitates binding of the toxin to polysialoganglioside receptors on neuronal membranes, whereas the amino-terminal domain of the heavy chain mediates translocation of the toxin into motor or autonomic neurons.[18,19] The light chain is a zinc endopeptidase that cleaves a toxin-specific location of one or more of the *SNARE* (*s*oluble *N*-ethylmaleimide-sensitive *f*usion *a*ssociated protein *r*eceptor) proteins mediating the docking and fusion of acetylcholine vesicles with the presynaptic membrane at the neuromuscular junction, in autonomic ganglia, and in parasympathetic nerve terminals.[20] SNARE proteins SNAP-25 (synaptosomal-associated protein of 25 kDa) and syntaxin are associated with the presynaptic membrane, whereas synaptobrevin or vesicle-associated membrane protein (VAMP) is located on the synaptic vesicle membrane. SNAP-25 is cleaved by types A, C, and E toxin, and syntaxin is cleaved by type C toxin.[21-23] Synaptobrevin is cleaved by types B, D, F, and G and tetanus toxin.[24-26] After cleavage of SNARE proteins by botulinum toxin, the release of acetylcholine is permanently halted at affected synapses. Recovery from botulism occurs when the presynaptic neuron sprouts another nerve terminal to reform the cholinergic synapse.[27-29]

Botulinum toxin is the most toxic substance by weight known,[30] with a lethal dose in humans estimated to be approximately 1 ng/kg of type A toxin.[31] By extrapolation from primate studies,[32] the lethal dose of type A toxin for a 70-kg man is estimated to be 70 μg by mouth, 0.70 to 0.90 μg by inhalation, and 0.09 to 0.15 μg by intramuscular or intravenous routes.[33] In contrast to the heat-resistant spores of *C. botulinum,* the toxins are heat-labile and are inactivated by heating to 85°C for at least 5 minutes.[34]

FORMS OF HUMAN BOTULISM

FOOD-BORNE BOTULISM

Ingestion of contaminated food with absorption of toxin from the duodenum and jejunum causes food-borne botulism. Because several individuals may be exposed to a single contaminated food source, food-borne botulism often presents in outbreaks. The average annual number of food-borne botulism cases in the United States between 1973 and 1998 was 24 (range 14-94),[35] with an average of 9.4 outbreaks/year between 1950 and 1996.[12] The most frequently implicated foods include home-canned vegetables, fruits, and fish.[12] Failure to use a proper combination of heat, pressure, and time to kill spores during home canning, particularly with low-acid (pH >5) foods, may permit survival and germination of spores.[36] Although restaurant and commercially prepared foods are responsible for fewer outbreaks (7% from 1950-1996),[12] nearly half of food-borne cases may arise from these relatively larger outbreaks.[37] Fish preparation using fermentation among Alaskan natives is responsible for a large fraction of the total cases (29% from 1973-1998).[12]

Food-borne botulism due to type A toxin is most common in the United States, constituting 45% of outbreaks compared with 36% of outbreaks due to type E and 13% due to type B toxin during the period 1990 to 1996. Type F food-borne outbreaks are rare in the United States.[12] The geographic distribution of food-borne botulism outbreaks mirrors the type of spores residing in soil. Type A spores predominate in the western United States, and type B spores predominate in the northeastern and central United States.[38,39] Type E spores are found in marine life and sediments.[40,41] In a corresponding fashion, during the period 1950 to 1996, 86% of the type A outbreaks occurred west of the Mississippi River, whereas 61% of the type B outbreaks were from eastern states. Marine products have been implicated in 91% of type E outbreaks.[12]

Signs and symptoms of food-borne botulism generally develop within 12 to 36 hours of ingestion of contaminated food, with the acuity and severity of illness related to the amount of toxin absorbed. In general, a symmetrical, descending paralysis with multiple cranial neuropathies evolves rapidly in the absence of fever or altered sensorium. In food-borne botulism, the initial symptoms are often gastrointestinal and include nausea, vomiting, diarrhea, and abdominal cramping, which may be due to ingestion of other bacterial metabolites along with botulinum toxin in contaminated food.[42] Parasympathetic dysfunction may present early with dry mouth and blurred vision associated with dilated, poorly reactive pupils. Diplopia often develops secondary to extraocular muscle weakness with paretic, dysconjugate eye movements. With paralysis of bulbar muscles, patients may exhibit flaccid dysarthria, chewing difficulty, and dysphagia. The upper extremities, trunk, and lower extremities may become paretic in a descending fashion. Autonomic dysfunction may manifest as gastrointestinal dysmotility, orthostatic hypotension, altered resting pulse, urinary retention, or hypothermia.[43]

Respiratory compromise may occur due to a combination of upper airway obstruction from weak oropharyngeal muscles and diaphragmatic weakness. Requirements for mechanical ventilation are more prolonged for patients with type A disease (mean 58 days) compared with patients with type B disease (mean 26 days).[44] The clinical findings related to intoxication with various types of botulinum toxin are varied (Table 164-1), with type A disease causing more frequent extraocular and bulbar muscle weakness and with type B and E disease causing relatively more pupillary and autonomic dysfunction.[45-47]

With improvements in respiratory care, the case-fatality rate has improved from 60% during 1899 to 1949 to 12.5% during 1950 to 1996.[12] The fatality risk for the index case in an outbreak is 25%, with a 4% fatality risk for subsequent cases after recognition of an outbreak.[48] Because of the potential for exposure of other individuals to a contaminated food source and for additional cases accumulating from previous exposure, every case of suspected food-borne botulism should be reported to local and state public health authorities.

WOUND BOTULISM

Wound botulism results from in vivo toxin production in abscessed and devitalized wounds.[49] In the event of contamination by spores, these wounds provide an ideal anaerobic environment for spore germination and local colonization by *C. botulinum* with absorption of toxin into systemic circulation. In contrast to the rapid onset of botulism in food-borne disease with ingestion of preformed toxin, the incubation period for wound botulism is 7 days (range 4 to 14 days).[50] Single cases occur in isolation with a case-fatality rate of approximately 15%.[51] Before 1980, wound botulism was a rare disorder generally associated with deep wounds containing avascular areas. Between 1943 and 1985, 33 cases

TABLE 164–1. SYMPTOMS AND SIGNS IN HUMAN BOTULISM TYPES A, B, AND E

	Type A (%)	Type B (%)	Type E (%)
Neurologic Symptoms			
Dysphagia	96	97	82
Dry mouth	83	100	93
Diplopia	90	92	39
Dysarthria	100	69	50
Upper extremity weakness	86	64	NA
Lower extremity weakness	76	64	NA
Blurred vision	100	42	91
Dyspnea	91	34	88
Paresthesias	20	12	NA
Gastrointestinal Symptoms			
Constipation	73	73	52
Nausea	73	57	84
Vomiting	70	50	96
Abdominal cramping	33	46	NA
Diarrhea	35	8	39
Other Symptoms			
Fatigue	92	69	84
Sore throat	75	39	38
Dizziness	86	30	63
Neurologic Findings			
Ptosis	96	55	46
Reduced gag reflex	81	54	NA
External ophthalmoparesis	87	46	NA
Facial weakness	84	48	NA
Tongue weakness	91	31	66
Pupils fixed or dilated	33	56	75
Nystagmus	44	4	NA
Upper extremity weakness	91	62	NA
Lower extremity weakness	82	59	NA
Ataxia	24	13	NA
DTRs reduced or absent	54	29	NA
DTRs hyperactive	12	0	NA
Initial mental status			
Alert	88	93	27
Lethargic	4	4	73
Obtunded	8	4	0

DTRs, deep tendon reflexes; NA, not available.
Adapted from Bleck TP: *Clostridium botulinum* (botulism). In Mandell GL, Bennett JE, Dolin R (eds): Principles and Practice of Infectious Diseases, 5th ed. Philadelphia, Churchill Livingstone, 2000, pp 2543-2548. Data from references 45, 46, and 47.

were reported in the United States.[12] During the period 1986 through 1996, 78 cases of wound botulism were reported in the United States, most related to subcutaneous injection or "skin popping" of black tar heroin.[12,52] Wound botulism due to sinusitis after repeated cocaine inhalation also has been observed.[53] The neurologic signs and symptoms are virtually identical to food-borne disease except for the absence of prodromal gastrointestinal symptoms.[12] When present, fever is related to the wound infection.[54] The diagnosis should be suspected in patients with a drug injection history and without known exposure to a contaminated food source.[55]

INTESTINAL BOTULISM

Infant Intestinal Botulism

Infant and adult intestinal botulism result from the ingestion of *C. botulinum* spores that germinate, colonize the large intestine, and produce botulinum toxin in vivo.[6] Infant intestinal botulism is now recognized as the most common form of botulism in the United States with approximately 100 cases reported annually. About half of the cases relate to type A toxin, and the other half to type B intoxication.[12] Most individual cases occur sporadically, although rare, unexplained clusters are reported.[56-58] Since the recognition of infant intestinal botulism in 1976, nearly half of the reported cases have occurred in California. The geographic distribution of infant botulism is unexplained, with the highest incidence rates observed in Delaware, Hawaii, Utah, and California.[12] The average age of onset is 13 weeks, and most cases occur before 6 months, although some cases have occurred at 15 months of age.[12]

Ingestion of ambient *C. botulinum* spores, distributed widely in soils and dust, is thought to represent the primary route of exposure.[56] Honey is also a source of spores and has been implicated as a significant risk for infant intestinal botulism.[59-61] In an animal model of infant intestinal botulism, mice between 7 and 13 days old proved susceptible to intestinal colonization with *C. botulinum* after intragastric injection of spores.[62] Epidemiologic studies suggest a parallel peak human susceptibility to intestinal colonization by *C. botulinum* between 2 and 4 months of age.[63] This susceptibility appears related to the intestinal flora in the immature infant gastrointestinal tract. The resident flora are influenced by an infant's food sources,[64] although the potential significance of breast-feeding versus formula feeding as a risk for infant intestinal botulism is unresolved.[65]

A clinical spectrum of disease exists, with some infants exhibiting relatively mild and limited disease involving several days of constipation, poor feeding, and lethargy and other infants developing acute tetraparesis and respiratory failure.[65] In classic cases, constipation is often the initial symptom followed by lethargy, poor feeding, and weak cry. Examination reveals hypotonia with head lag; ptosis; reduced facial expression; and reduced gag, suck, and swallow reflexes. Deep tendon reflexes are reduced or absent. Extraocular movements are often paretic, and pupils may be large and poorly reactive. In one series, more than half of the patients were intubated and mechanically ventilated, usually following loss of protective upper airway reflexes.[66] Although the course is variable, most hospitalized infants reach maximal paralysis at approximately 1 to 2 weeks after hospitalization and begin to improve after 1 to 3 weeks.[65] In California between 1976 and 1991, the average length of hospitalization was 4.9 weeks. A longer length of stay was documented for type A cases (5.7 weeks) compared with type B cases (3.6 weeks), suggesting that type A intoxication causes more severe disease.[65] The case-fatality rate is less than 1% in hospitalized patients in the United States.[56]

Adult Intestinal Botulism

Children and adults also may be susceptible to intestinal colonization and in vivo toxin production by *C. botulinum*, *C. baratii*, or *C. butyricum* when the gastric barrier is compromised and the intestinal flora are altered.[8,15,67,68] Previously classified by the Centers for Disease Control and Prevention (CDC) as "botulism of undetermined origin," adult intestinal botulism has occurred in the setting of intestinal surgery, gastric achlorhydria, broad-spectrum antibiotic treatment, and inflammatory bowel disease.[69-71] Although adult intestinal botulism is uncommon (10 cases reported between 1986 and 1996),[71] it is probably underdiagnosed.

INHALATIONAL BOTULISM

Inhalational botulism does not occur in nature but is the result of an attempt to use the toxin in aerosolized form as a bioweapon.[10] The three documented human cases were reported from Germany in 1962, when botulinum toxin type A became accidentally reaerosolized during disposal of laboratory animals.[9] These patients initially developed dysphagia on day 3 after exposure and exhibited tonic pupils, paretic eye movements, dysarthria, and diffuse weakness by day 4. In animal experiments, monkeys became symptomatic 12 to 18 hours after exposure to aerosolized toxin with descending paralysis and death in some animals.[72] Aerosolized botulinum toxin was released by the Japanese religious cult Aum Shinrikyo on several occasions in the 1990s in Japan, although the attacks were not known to have produced human illness.[10] By the time of the 1991 Persian Gulf War, the state of Iraq had produced large quantities of concentrated botulinum toxin, which were loaded onto weapons for military use but never deployed.[73]

Release of aerosolized toxin has the potential to produce a botulism outbreak. The features of such an outbreak that might suggest a deliberate release of toxin[10] include numerous cases within an outbreak (the mean number of cases in food-borne outbreaks has averaged 2.5 for many years),[12] toxin types within an outbreak that rarely cause natural disease (type C, D, F, G, or E not related to marine sources), outbreaks with a common geographic factor without a common dietary exposure, and multiple simultaneous outbreaks.

IATROGENIC OR INADVERTENT BOTULISM

The therapeutic use of botulinum toxin for dystonia, spasticity, hyperhidrosis, sialorrhea, and other conditions occasionally has resulted in inadvertent paresis of nearby noninjected muscles, such as dysphagia in neck muscle injections for cervical dystonia[74] and jaw dislocation after parotid injections for sialorrhea in amyotrophic lateral sclerosis.[75] Although there are rare reports of paretic muscles distant to the site of injection,[76,77] it has been estimated that healthy patients would require a 10-fold toxin overdosing to develop systemic symptoms.[78] Nevertheless, single-fiber electromyography studies showed abnormal neuromuscular transmission in muscles distant to botulinum toxin injections.[79-81] Patients with underlying neuromuscular disorders seem to be predisposed to develop generalized weakness after therapeutic intramuscular botulinum toxin injections.[82-84] Systemic autonomic dysfunction also has been noted after therapeutic injections of type B toxin.[85]

DIAGNOSIS

DIFFERENTIAL DIAGNOSIS

The differential diagnosis for botulism includes Guillain-Barré syndrome and its variants, particularly Miller-Fisher syndrome and polyneuritis cranialis. Classic Guillain-Barré syndrome generally occurs with limb weakness and sensory disturbances and is readily distinguished from botulism. Patients with polyneuritis cranialis who exhibit extraocular and bulbar muscle weakness may be difficult to distinguish clinically from botulism in the early phases of illness. Despite prominent extraocular muscle weakness and areflexia in Miller-Fisher syndrome, the presence of limb ataxia helps to distinguish it from botulism. Myasthenia gravis also commonly produces weakness of extraocular and bulbar muscles, but the temporal course of the weakness is often fluctuating, with diurnal variation and improvement with rest or acetylcholinesterase medications. In contrast to botulism, myasthenia gravis does not affect autonomic function in general or pupillary function in particular. The presence of acetylcholine receptor antibodies is extremely specific for myasthenia gravis. Lambert-Eaton myasthenic syndrome often is associated with a neuroendocrine carcinoma of the lung and the presence of voltage-gated calcium channel antibodies. Although the symptoms and findings may be similar to botulism, the degree of bulbar paralysis is not as marked, and the clinical course is rarely acute or rapidly progressive. Tick paralysis produces an acute flaccid paralysis due to neurotoxins of ixodid ticks. A meticulous physical examination of the scalp and intertriginous regions should be performed for an attached tick. Acute brainstem lesions, including strokes, may also be diagnostic considerations, particularly if consciousness is impaired. In suspected infant botulism, the differential diagnosis includes sepsis, meningoencephalitis, Werdnig-Hoffmann disease, congenital myasthenia gravis, and metabolic disorders.

ELECTRODIAGNOSTIC STUDIES

Electrodiagnostic studies may confirm the presence of a presynaptic neuromuscular junctional disorder and strongly suggest the diagnosis of botulism or may support an alternative diagnosis. In botulism, sensory nerve conduction studies should be normal, and no evidence for segmental demyelination on motor nerve conduction studies (e.g., prolonged F latencies, conduction block, temporal dispersion) should be observed to suggest Guillain-Barré syndrome. Compound muscle action potential amplitudes commonly are reduced in clinically affected muscles.[86] The more affected muscles are often proximal ones, however, and routine motor nerve conduction studies recorded in intrinsic hand or foot muscles may fail to detect this nonspecific abnormality. In distinction to myasthenia gravis[87] and Lambert-Eaton myasthenic syndrome,[88] low-frequency (2 to 3 Hz) repetitive nerve stimulation studies rarely show a decremental response in terms of reduced amplitude and area of the compound muscle action potential elicited by stimulating a motor nerve.[86]

The characteristic finding in a presynaptic neuromuscular junctional disorder such as botulism is postexercise facilitation or post-tetanic facilitation with high-frequency (20 to 50 Hz) repetitive nerve stimulation. Although Lambert-Eaton myasthenic syndrome and botulism share this finding, post-tetanic facilitation may be less prominent[89] and more sustained[90] in botulism. Proximal muscles also may exhibit a comparatively greater degree of facilitation in botulism.[89] Post-tetanic facilitation may be more common in type B botulism compared with type A disease.[91]

Needle electromyography may reveal low-amplitude, short-duration motor unit potentials with an unstable firing pattern, although this nonspecific finding may be observed in many motor unit disorders.[89] Positive sharp waves and fibrillation potentials also are observed in about half of the cases.[92]

Single-fiber electromyography uses statistical analysis of muscle fiber action potentials generated by the same motor neuron to evaluate neuromuscular transmission. It is the most sensitive diagnostic test for detecting abnormal neuromuscular transmission, although it cannot distinguish reliably between presynaptic neuromuscular disorders. In botulism, it is more sensitive than repetitive nerve stimulation studies for showing neuromuscular junctional pathology.[93-95]

MOUSE BIOASSAY

Confirmatory testing for botulism currently involves a mouse bioassay, which is available only through the CDC and several state laboratories. In the mouse bioassay, mice are inoculated with type-specific antisera and patient serum or extracts from samples of body fluids or suspicious foodstuffs. In a positive mouse bioassay, all the mice die except those receiving the antisera matching the botulinum toxin type present in the patient or food specimens. Test results are generally available within 1 or 2 days after inoculation.[10] Details regarding specimen preparation and handling are available on-line.[12] Specimen samples in suspected cases of food-borne botulism should include serum, feces, gastric aspirates, vomitus, and foods suspected to be contaminated. In wound botulism, serum, feces, exudate, débrided tissue, and wound swab samples should be examined. In intestinal botulism, serum and feces should be sampled.[12] To obtain an adequate fecal sample, particularly in infant botulism, in which constipation is common, an enema using sterile, non-bacteriostatic water may be necessary. In addition to administering extracts to mice, the samples are anaerobically cultured, and the culture isolates are evaluated using the mouse bioassay.

MANAGEMENT

All cases of suspected botulism should be reported to the hospital epidemiologist or infection control officer and to local or state health departments or the CDC. This reporting is essential to coordinate laboratory testing and shipment of antitoxin and to initiate investigation of the toxin source.[10] Patients with suspected or confirmed botulism should be monitored carefully in an ICU with particular attention to their ability to protect the upper airway. Many patients require intubation and mechanical ventilation. Purgatives or activated charcoal may be useful if there is suspicion of residual contaminated food in the gastrointestinal tract.[54] The use of antibiotics that impair neuromuscular transmission should be avoided, particularly aminoglycosides and macrolides.[96,97]

Botulinum antitoxins may reduce the duration and severity of neurologic dysfunction associated with botulism if administered early in the course of disease. The effect of antitoxin is limited to circulating toxin, and the paralytic effects of previously bound and internalized toxin are not reversed by antitoxin.[48,65] Four types of antitoxin currently are available in the United States: (1) a licensed bivalent (A, B) human antiserum for infant botulism, (2) a licensed bivalent (A, B) equine antiserum, (3) an investigational monovalent (E) equine antiserum, and (4) an investigational heptavalent (A, B, C, D, E, F, G) antiserum.[98]

BOTULISM IMMUNE GLOBULIN INTRAVENOUS (HUMAN)

Botulism immune globulin intravenous (BIG-IV) is a licensed, bivalent human antiserum (type A, B) available for treatment of infant botulism. A 5-year randomized, double-blinded, placebo-controlled treatment trial demonstrated the safety and efficacy of botulism immune globulin intravenous in infant botulism. The mean length of hospital stay was significantly reduced in patients receiving botulism immune globulin intravenous (from 5.5 weeks to 2.5 weeks).[65] BIG-IV was officially licensed by the FDA in October, 2003, for the treatment of infant botulism types A and B under the proprietary name of BabyBIG. BIG-IV is available through the California Department of Health Services (24-hour telephone: 510-231-7600).

EQUINE ANTITOXIN

A licensed, bivalent equine antiserum (type A, B) is available through the CDC via state health departments for cases of suspected botulism. Investigational monovalent equine antiserum (type E) is also available through the CDC if type E intoxication is suspected. When state health departments are unavailable, the CDC 24-hour telephone number is 770-448-7100. Although controlled trials are lacking, use of the equine antitoxin is supported by inferential studies.[48,99] The equine origin of the antiserum resulted in hypersensitivity reactions in 9% to 20% and anaphylaxis in nearly 2% of patients between 1967 and 1977 when a larger dosage of antitoxin was used.[100] Skin testing for horse serum hypersensitivity is recommended before the use of the equine antitoxin; procedural details appear in the *U.S. Army Medical Research Institute of Infectious Diseases (USAMRIID) Medical Management of Biological Casualties Handbook*.[98] A "despeciated" investigational heptavalent equine antiserum against all known types of botulinum toxin (type A, B, C, D, E, F, and G) was developed by the USAMRIID. The antitoxin is prepared by cleaving the Fc fragments from equine IgG molecules, leaving $F(ab')_2$ fragments and approximately 4% equine antigens.[98,101] The product is available from USAMRIID and would be potentially useful in an outbreak of an atypical type of botulism (type C, D, F, G).

PENTAVALENT TOXOID

An investigational pentavalent toxoid (type A, B, C, D, E) for pre-exposure prophylaxis is available for military personnel and laboratory workers. A primary series of immunizations is given at 0, 2, and 12 weeks, followed by a 1-year booster.[98,102] Because it induces immunity over several months, the toxoid is not appropriate for postexposure prophylaxis.[10]

ANNOTATED REFERENCES

Arnon SS: Infant botulism. In Feigin RD, Cherry JD (eds): Textbook of Pediatric Infectious Diseases, 5th ed. Philadelphia, WB Saunders, 2004, pp 1758-1766.

This chapter summarizes the known pathophysiology of infant intestinal botulism and contemporary treatment guidelines.

Arnon SS, Schechter R, Inglesby TV, et al: Botulinum toxin as a biological weapon: Medical and public health management. JAMA 2001;285: 1059-1070.

This consensus report by the Working Group on Civilian Biodefense reviews the clinical and laboratory findings, differential diagnosis, and treatment recommendations for the various forms of human botulism. The features of a botulism outbreak suggesting a deliberate release of toxin are highlighted.

Centers for Disease Control and Prevention: Botulism in the United States, 1899-1996: Handbook for Epidemiologists, Clinicians, and Laboratory Workers. Atlanta, Centers for Disease Control and Prevention, 1998. Available at: http://www.cdc.gov/ncidod/dbmd/diseaseinfo/botulism.pdf.

This comprehensive work provides contemporary epidemiologic information relating to all forms of human botulism and detailed information relating to laboratory confirmation and specimen preparation and handling.

Hughes JM, Blumenthal JR, Merson MH, et al: Clinical features of types A and B foodborne botulism. Ann Intern Med 1981;95:442-445.

This classic series delineates the clinical symptoms and findings in a large series of patients with the most common toxin types in human food-borne botulism.

Chapter 165

DENGUE HEMORRHAGIC FEVER

Jeremy Farrar

KEY POINTS

1. Dengue is the most widely distributed mosquito-borne viral infection of humans, affecting an estimated 100 million people worldwide each year, with 40% (2.5 billion) of the world's population estimated to be at risk for infection. Dengue should be considered in any patient with fever, particularly if there is a recent travel history to endemic regions.

2. Of the many clinical features associated with dengue infections, from the standpoint of threat to life and clinical intervention, the most important is increased vascular permeability leading to the dengue shock syndrome.

3. During the critical phase of illness, regular review (every 15 to 30 minutes) of the dengue vital signs—pulse rate, blood pressure, peripheral temperature, and hematocrit—is necessary.

4. The mainstay of treatment is prompt, vigorous, but careful fluid resuscitation. If appropriate volume resuscitation is instituted at an early stage, shock is usually reversible. Careful clinical judgment is required throughout the patient's stay in the hospital to maintain an effective circulation while assiduously avoiding fluid overload.

Millions of individuals across the tropical and subtropical world become infected with dengue viruses every year. A small percentage of individuals infected with dengue develops overt clinical illness, and an even smaller percentage develops the severe forms of the disease, dengue hemorrhagic fever and dengue shock syndrome. With the enormous increase in tourism, business-related travel, and global deployment of military and international nongovernmental organizations in recent decades, dengue cases have been seen more frequently outside endemic areas. The daytime biting habits of the *Aedes* mosquito and the urban habitat visited by most international travelers make it all but impossible to avoid exposure (bed nets offer only limited protection). There is no vaccine or prophylaxis available. Dengue infections in travelers are monitored by TropNetEurop (www.tropneteurope/dengue) and in the United States by the Centers for Disease Control and Prevention (www.cdc.gov/dengue). Most infections in travelers (78%) manifest after short holidays or business-related travel to South and South East Asia and the Americas.[1]

Of the many clinical features associated with dengue infections, from the standpoint of threat to life and clinical

intervention, the most important is increased vascular permeability leading to dengue shock syndrome. Children are particularly prone to the development of shock, probably because of age-related differences in capillary fragility that may make them more susceptible than adults to the capillary leak syndrome.[2]

EPIDEMIOLOGY

Dengue is the most widely distributed mosquito-borne viral infection of humans, affecting an estimated 100 million people worldwide each year, with 40% (2.5 billion) of the world's population estimated to be at risk of infection.[3] It is endemic in parts of Asia and the Americas and has been reported increasingly from many tropical countries in recent years.[4] It has been classified by the World Health Organization into *dengue fever, dengue hemorrhagic fever,* and *dengue shock syndrome* (Table 165-1).[5] It is among the leading causes of hospitalization in Asia during the rainy season, with 500,000 cases reported annually to the World Health Organization. When shock becomes established, mortality rates of 12% to 40% have been reported.

The dengue virus is a single-stranded, positive sense RNA virus of approximately 11 kb in length and encodes three structural and seven nonstructural genes.[6] It is a member of the *Flavivirus* genus, which also includes yellow fever, Japanese encephalitis, West Nile virus, and hepatitis C virus.[7] There is considerable genetic diversity in the dengue virus family with four serotypes (Den-I, Den-II, Den-III, and Den-IV), all of which may produce a nonspecific febrile illness, dengue fever, or may result in the more severe manifestation of dengue hemorrhagic fever and dengue shock syndrome.

The dengue viruses are transmitted from viremic individuals to susceptible hosts by mosquitoes of the subgenus *Stegomyia*; the major global vector is *Aedes aegypti*, although other species may be more important in restricted geographic areas. The *A. aegypti* lays individual eggs in the damp walls of artificial and natural water containers, and these eggs can remain viable for months. The adult mosquito is strongly anthropophilic; prefers resting in sheltered dark areas inside houses; and has a diurnal feeding pattern, usually peaking in the midmorning and late afternoon. The female usually feeds twice during a single gonotrophic cycle, and the average life span is 8 to 14 days.

PATHOPHYSIOLOGY

Dengue hemorrhagic fever is characterized by increased vascular permeability and plasma leakage, thrombocytopenia,

TABLE 165–1. CASE DEFINITION

Dengue Fever

Probable
  Acute febrile illness with two or more of the following:
    Headache
    Retro-orbital pain
    Myalgia
    Arthralgia
    Rash
    Hemorrhagic manifestations
    Leukopenia
  And
  Supportive serology

Dengue Hemorrhagic Fever

The following must all be present:
  Fever or history of fever lasting 2-7 d
  Hemorrhagic tendencies evidenced by at least one of the following
    A positive tourniquet test
    Bleeding from the mucosa, gastrointestinal tract, injection sites, or other
    Hematemisis or melena
  Thrombocytopenia (<100,000/mm)
  Evidence of plasma leakage due to increased vascular permeability, manifest by at least one of the following
    Rise in hematocrit ≥20% above the average for sex, age, and population
    Drop in hematocrit after volume replacement ≥20% of baseline
    Signs of plasma leakage (i.e., pleural effusions, ascites, and hypoproteinemia)

Dengue Shock Syndrome

All of the above four criteria for dengue hemorrhagic fever must be present, plus evidence of circulatory failure manifested by
  Rapid and weak pulse
  Narrow pulse pressure (<20 mm Hg)
  Hypotension for age
  Cold clammy restless

grades III and IV) through circulatory failure (reduced pulse pressure and hypotension).[5] The capillary leak predisposes to pulmonary edema, pleural effusion, ascites, intravascular compromise, and hemoconcentration.

The most widely cited hypothesis to explain the vascular leak and hemorrhage is increased viral replication due to enhanced infection of monocytes in the presence of preexisting antidengue antibodies at subneutralizing levels—antibody-dependent immune enhancement.[8] This observation, which has strong epidemiologic and in vitro experimental evidence to support it, argues that in the primary asymptomatic dengue infection the moderate viremia is well controlled. The host immune system develops long-lasting immunity to the serotype of the infecting strain and short-lived cross-protection against heterologous serotypes. After a few months, the levels of cross-protective antibody directed against the heterologous serotypes fall below neutralizing levels, however, and from this stage onward infection with a second heterologous strain may result in increased viral uptake via Fcγ receptors into monocytes and enhanced viral replication. Severe disease has been reported during apparently primary infections, however, and not all secondary infections lead to severe disease, so other theories (viral and host genetic factors) have been suggested to try to explain the complex epidemiologic and immunopathogenetic features.[9-12]

CLINICAL FEATURES

Dengue fever is a mild, self-limited febrile episode that is associated with a rash. It usually begins with fever, respiratory symptoms (sore throat, coryza, and cough), anorexia, nausea, vomiting, and headache. Back pain, myalgias, arthralgias, and conjunctivitis also may occur. The initial fever usually resolves within 1 week, and a few days later a generalized morbilliform or maculopapular rash may develop. Fever may return with the rash. Dengue hemorrhagic fever has been classified into four grades of severity by the World Health Organization (Table 165-2; see Table 165-1). Grades I and II have only mild capillary leak, insufficient to result in the development of shock, and are differentiated by the absence (grade I) or presence (grade II) of spontaneous bleeding. In grade III, circulatory failure occurs, manifested by a rapid and weak pulse with narrowing of the pulse pressure to 20 mm Hg or less. In grade IV, shock is severe with no detectable pulse or blood pressure. Dengue hemorrhagic fever grades III and IV are collectively referred to as *dengue shock syndrome.*

Dengue fever begins with fever, respiratory symptoms (sore throat, coryza, and cough), anorexia, nausea, vomiting,

and hemorrhage, and the degree of each of these parameters usually correlates with clinically graded disease severity. Mild dengue hemorrhagic fever (dengue hemorrhagic fever grades I and II) is normally characterized by only mild hemorrhage, as indicated by spontaneous petechiae and a positive tourniquet test, whereas bruising often at injection sites, purpura, and other hemorrhage manifestations are usually present in the more severe grades III and IV of dengue hemorrhagic fever.

Vascular permeability is the most important parameter determining dengue hemorrhagic fever severity and precipitates dengue shock syndrome (dengue hemorrhagic fever

TABLE 165–2. WORLD HEALTH ORGANIZATION CLASSIFICATION OF DENGUE

Grade of Severity	Platelets	Plasma Leakage	Circulatory	Other Collapse
Dengue fever	Variable	Absent	Absent	TT variable ± hemorrhage
Dengue hemorrhagic fever				
Grade I	<100,000	Present	Absent	+TT No hemorrhage
Grade II	<100,000	Present	Absent	+TT hemorrhage
Dengue shock syndrome				
Grade III	<100,000	Present	PP <20 mm Hg	±TT ± hemorrhage
Grade IV	<100,000	Present	Absent BP	+TT ± hemorrhage

BP, blood pressure; PP, pulse pressure; TT, thrombin time.

and headache. Back pain, myalgias, arthralgias, and conjunctivitis also are common. The initial fever usually resolves within 1 week, and a few days later a generalized morbilliform or maculopapular rash develops (Fig. 165-1). Fever often returns with the rash.

Dengue hemorrhagic fever (grades I and II) is the more severe form of the disease and is characterized by hemoconcentration, thrombocytopenia, and coagulation abnormalities. Dengue shock syndrome (dengue hemorrhagic fever grades III and IV) is the most severe form of the disease (approximately 25% of cases), characterized by severe hypovolemia and shock. Petechiae and bleeding at injection sites is characteristic (see Fig. 165-1). Severe bleeding, including intracerebral hemorrhage usually associated with multiorgan dysfunction, is rare but is often fatal. Mortality rates vary from 1% to 5%, although much higher rates have been reported. Complications include severe bleeding, pleural effusions, shock, pneumonia, liver dysfunction or failure, encephalopathy, and pulmonary hemorrhage. The differential diagnosis is extensive and varies depending on where the patient is seen, but would include in Africa malaria, typhoid, leptospirosis, septicemia, other viral hemorrhagic fevers (e.g., Ebola, Lassa fever), chikungunya, West Nile fever, o'nyong-nyong fever, and Rift Valley fever (usually without a rash).

A pulse pressure of less than 20 mm Hg is one of the earliest manifestations of shock, before the development of systolic hypotension. The mainstay of treatment is prompt, vigorous, but careful fluid resuscitation. If appropriate volume resuscitation is instituted at an early stage, shock is usually reversible; in certain severe cases and in patients who are inadequately resuscitated, patients may progress to irreversible shock and death. Careful clinical judgment is required throughout the patient's stay in the hospital to maintain an effective circulation while assiduously avoiding fluid overload. Close attention and regular review (every 15 to 30 minutes during episodes of shock) of the hematocrit, pulse pressure, and peripheral perfusion are essential.[13,14] For patients with dengue shock syndrome, the World Health Organization recommends immediate volume replacement with isotonic crystalloid solutions, followed by the use of plasma or colloid solutions, specifically dextrans, for profound or continuing shock.[5]

Thrombocytopenia is universal in dengue hemorrhagic fever, and platelet function is abnormal. Mild prolongation of the prothrombin and partial thromboplastin times with reduced fibrinogen levels is common, but fibrin degradation products have not been found to be elevated to a degree consistent with classic disseminated intravascular coagulation. Patients with dengue shock syndrome have significant abnormalities in all the major pathways of the coagulation cascade.[15]

DIAGNOSIS

Classic dengue illness can be an easy diagnosis to make in endemic regions with experienced clinical staff and a high prior probability that a febrile illness with rash and thrombocytopenia is caused by dengue. Most of the symptoms and signs accompanying dengue infection are common to many febrile illnesses with few features that reliably discriminate dengue especially early.[16,17] The differential diagnosis invariably is large; it is region, country, and season specific. The differential diagnosis includes measles, rubella, enterovirus, influenza, typhoid, chikungunya, scarlet fever, malaria, leptospirosis, hepatitis A, rickettsiosis, bacterial sepsis, Hantaan infection, viral hemorrhagic fevers (including Ebola, Lassa fever), West Nile virus, o'nyong-nyong fever, and Rift Valley fever (usually without a rash). Because of the variation in clinical findings and the multiplicity of possible causative agents, the descriptive term *dengue-like disease* should be used until the laboratory provides a specific etiologic diagnosis.

The diagnosis is a clinical one with supportive laboratory tests. Proof of a dengue infection depends on confirmatory dengue serology and viral isolation if available. Serologic confirmation of acute dengue infection relies on the demonstration of specific IgM and IgG antibodies against dengue in the serum of patients. Ideally, acute and convalescent sera should be tested.

Viral isolation is performed by culturing the patient's serum with *Aedes albopictus* C6/36 cell monolayers. Virus infection of C6/36 cells is confirmed by immunofluorescent assay using a flavivirus-specific monoclonal antibody. Dengue virus RNA

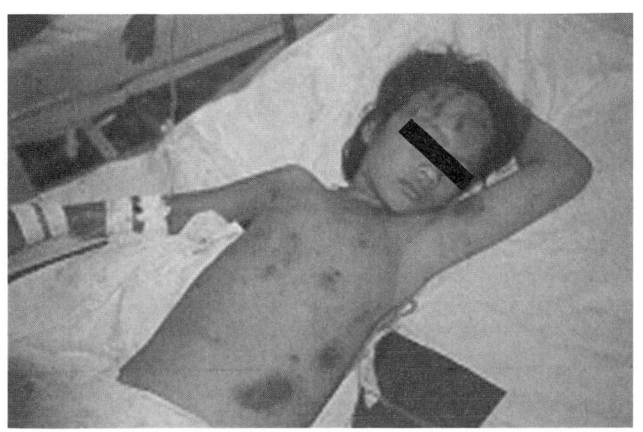

A

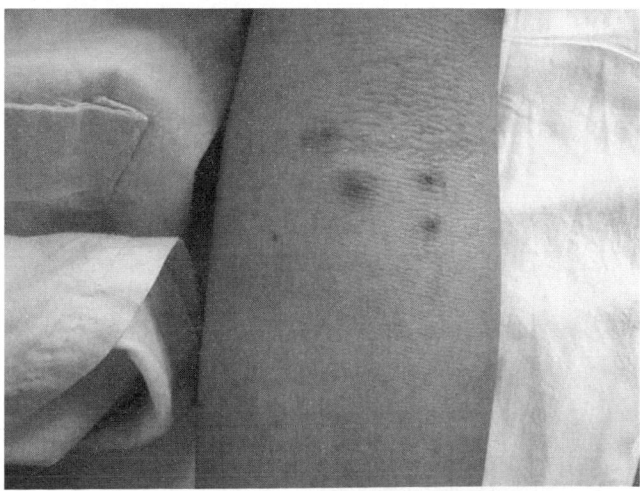

B

FIGURE 165–1. Characteristic acute skin manifestations of dengue. **A,** Bleeding at injection sites. **B,** Rash in established dengue shock syndrome.

also can be amplified by reverse transcriptase nested polymerase chain reaction from serum (Fig. 165-2).[18]

MANAGEMENT

There is no specific therapy for dengue, and the only effective treatment currently available for symptomatic dengue infections is supportive, focusing primarily on judicious fluid management (Fig. 165-3). Prompt restoration of circulating plasma volume is the cornerstone of therapy for patients with dengue shock syndrome. For the less severe syndromes of dengue fever and dengue hemorrhagic fever without shock, less aggressive parenteral fluid therapy frequently is indicated. This section focuses on the management of dengue shock syndrome; the management of unusual manifestations, such as dengue encephalopathy or fulminant hepatitis, is not addressed, being in general similar to the standard management of these disorders.

Patients admitted with established dengue shock syndrome should be cared for in an ICU, staffed by experienced medical and nursing personnel. Immediate restoration of a stable and effective circulation with parenteral fluid therapy is the primary aim of treatment. Extreme care is needed to balance the requirement for intravenous fluid to maintain plasma volume against the inherent risk of leakage of the administered fluid into the interstitial space. The leaked fluid may contribute to the development of pleural effusions, ascites, and respiratory compromise and the potential downward spiral toward multiorgan failure, disseminated intravascular coagulation, and death. As is often the case in looking after the critically ill, patients with the most severe capillary leak syndrome and most at risk of these complications also are the patients most in need of the most aggressive circulatory support. Getting this balance of fluid resuscitation and ongoing capillary leak right is the most difficult issue in looking after patients with dengue shock syndrome.

Rapid clinical assessment of cardiovascular status (pulse, blood pressure, peripheral perfusion, urine output, and mental state) determines initial management. The results of basic laboratory investigations, including hematocrit and platelet count, are useful, but initiation of treatment must not be delayed pending their availability. Detailed examination should be carried out when resuscitation is in progress. The following features are commonly associated with severe disease and a complicated clinical course:

- Unrecordable pulse and blood pressure with poor peripheral perfusion (grade IV dengue hemorrhagic fever).
- Narrow pulse pressure (≤10 mm Hg) with poor peripheral perfusion (severe grade III dengue hemorrhagic fever).
- Any evidence of compromised cerebral perfusion (lethargy, irritability, drowsiness, or restlessness).
- Presentation with shock early in the course of the disease (before day 4 of fever).

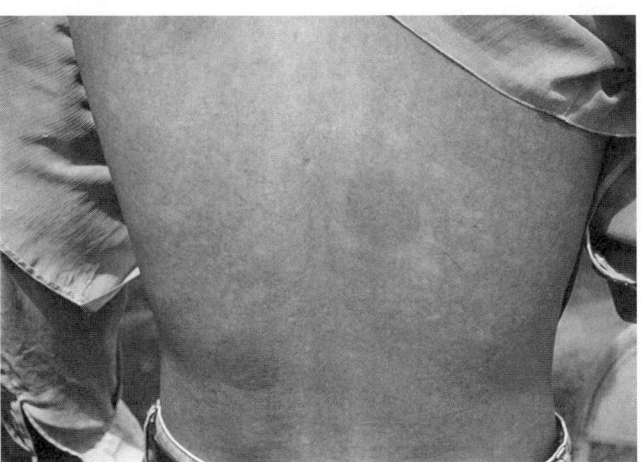

A

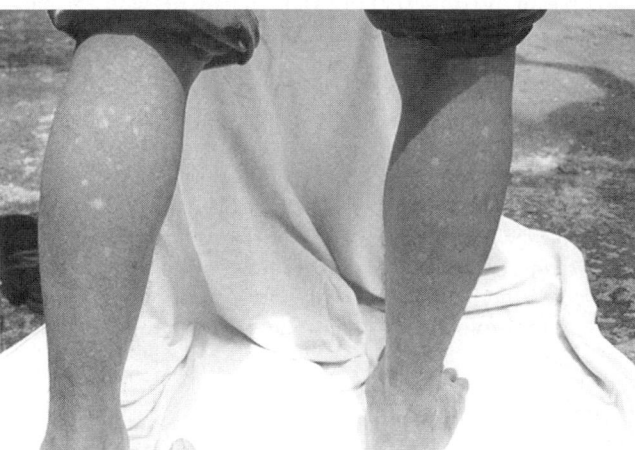

B

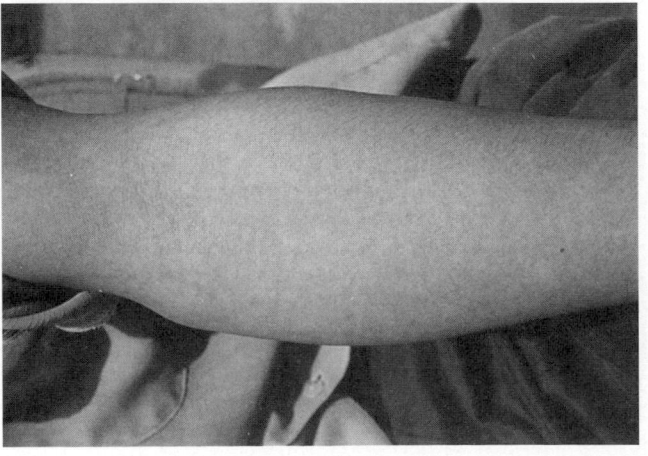

C

FIGURE 165–2. A-C, Characteristic skin manifestations in convalescent dengue.

- Age younger than 1 year. Dengue hemorrhagic fever/dengue shock syndrome occurs infrequently in infants younger than 1 year, but special care must be taken regarding fluid management in this age group. In infants, fluid accounts for a greater proportion of body weight, and minimal daily requirements are correspondingly greater; cardiovascular and renal function still are developing, and there is less reserve to cope with disturbance; finally, capillary beds are intrinsically more permeable than the capillary beds of older children or adults. All infants must be treated as high-risk patients and warrant early intervention with careful colloid-based resuscitation similar to older children with grade IV disease (see later).
- Marked elevation of hematocrit.
- Clinically apparent pleural effusions or ascites at the time of presentation with shock. Large volumes of fluid must be present to be clinically detectable, implying either recent onset of catastrophic leak or a steady loss of fluid over a longer time before the development of hemodynamic compromise.

After the initial rapid assessment, resuscitation with parenteral fluids should be started immediately. Reliable intravenous access must be secured as soon as possible, and rarely, in patients with profound shock, a venous cutdown or insertion of an intraosseous line may be necessary. All patients with shock or respiratory compromise should receive oxygen by facemask or nasal cannulae. A regular schedule of clinical observation every 0.5 to 1 hour should be instituted with a detailed record of all fluid intake and output. The hematocrit should be measured every 2 hours for the first 6 hours and thereafter every 4 to 6 hours until the patient is stable.

GRADE III DENGUE HEMORRHAGIC FEVER

For most patients with grade III dengue hemorrhagic fever, resuscitation should be started with an isotonic crystalloid solution (physiologic saline, Ringer's lactate, or Ringer's acetate) at a rate of 10 to 15 mL/kg over 1 hour. If the patient's clinical condition has stabilized after this time (wider pulse pressure, warm peripheries, and a reduction in heart rate), the rate of fluid administration may be reduced to 10 mL/kg/h for 2 hours, then gradually reduced to maintenance levels over the next 6 to 8 hours. A suitable schedule might be as follows: 10 mL/kg/h for 2 hours, 7.5 mL/kg/h for 2 hours, 5 mL/kg/h for 4 hours, then 2 to 3 mL/kg/h for 24 to 36 hours. For most patients, intravenous therapy can be stopped at this time, provided that the clinical condition has been stable for 24 hours.

If there is evidence of ongoing cardiovascular compromise after the first hour of treatment (no improvement in pulse pressure or pulse rate, persisting peripheral shutdown, a rising hematocrit) a colloid solution (6% dextran 70 or 6% starch solution) should be substituted for the crystalloid solution, at an initial rate of 10 to 15 mL/kg over 1 hour. Hyperoncotic preparations, such as 10% dextran, have been implicated in the development of renal failure when used in hypovolemic patients and should be avoided. If large volumes of colloid are infused, regular assessment of the coagulation profile is required.

Frequent observation of vital signs, mental state, and urine output and serial hematocrit measurements are used to assess the response to treatment. After initial resuscitation, most patients can be managed successfully with the reducing schedule of isotonic crystalloid fluid until the reabsorptive phase of the illness begins around day 6 to 7. If there are further episodes of cardiovascular decompensation after the initial episode, supplementary treatment with small infusions of 5 to 10 mL/kg of colloid may be required.

GRADE IV DENGUE HEMORRHAGIC FEVER

Patients with no recordable pulse or blood pressure (dengue hemorrhagic fever grade IV) should be managed more vigorously. Profoundly shocked patients require colloid therapy (6% dextran 70 or 6% starch solution) immediately. Despite initial severity, most patients improve with aggressive volume replacement and can be managed subsequently as suggested earlier for patients with grade III dengue hemorrhagic fever. Central venous pressure monitoring provides useful information to direct fluid therapy, but insertion of lines should be carried out only by experienced personnel and with careful attention to the coagulation state. Inotropic support may be required in addition to volume support. Significant pleural effusions and respiratory compromise are likely to develop, and pleural and ascitic drainage and artificial ventilation all may prove to be necessary. Metabolic and electrolyte derangements are common in these critically ill patients and should be actively sought and treated.

BLOOD TRANSFUSION

Blood transfusion is indicated only for patients with major bleeding and should be undertaken with extreme care because of the problem of fluid overload. In patients with dengue shock syndrome, major bleeding almost always is associated with severe or prolonged shock and is usually from the gastrointestinal tract. Underlying causes include profound thrombocytopenia and disseminated intravascular coagulation in combination with gastritis or stress ulceration. Internal bleeding may not become apparent for many hours until the first melena stool is passed. Blood transfusion should be considered in all patients who fail to improve clinically after appropriate fluid resuscitation, particularly if the hematocrit is stable or falling. Platelet concentrates and fresh frozen plasma also can be helpful but are effective only for a few hours.

Significant bleeding is more common in adults. Capillary leak syndrome occurs but is generally less severe than in children; in adults with shock, hemorrhage is often the major factor. More aggressive transfusion may be necessary although care still is required to avoid the pitfalls of fluid overload.

Steroids are not recommended in the management of dengue shock syndrome; the evidence for this comes from a series of small trials performed in the 1970s and 1980s. The total number of patients with dengue shock syndrome randomized to steroids (each study used a different form of steroid in varying doses, and not all studies were controlled) in the international literature is 150 in five published studies.[19-23] Most of these reported no benefit in the small number of patients investigated, although one trial reported a remarkable reduction in mortality.[19] The evidence from these five studies would not now be considered sufficient to base a global recommendation. There is an argument for revisiting this recommendation via a large double-blind, randomized clinical trial.

VIII

1416

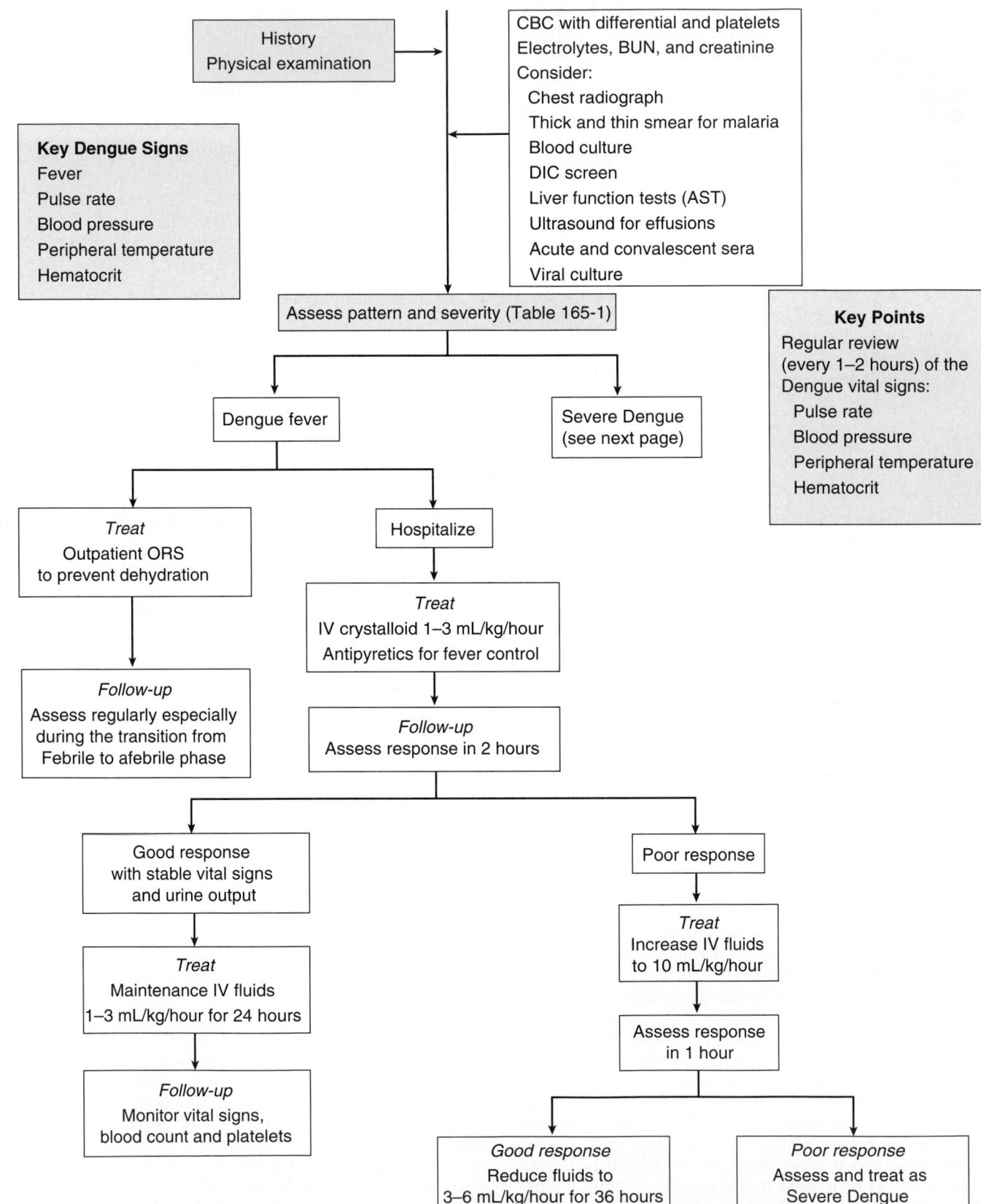

FIGURE 165–3. Clinical algorithm for a child with dengue infection. AST, aspartate aminotransferase; BP, blood pressure; BUN, blood urea nitrogen; CR, cardiac rhythm; DIC, disseminated intravascular coagulation; HR, heart rate; ORS, oral rehydration solution; PEEP, positive end-expiratory pressure; PR, pulse rate; RR, respiratory rate.

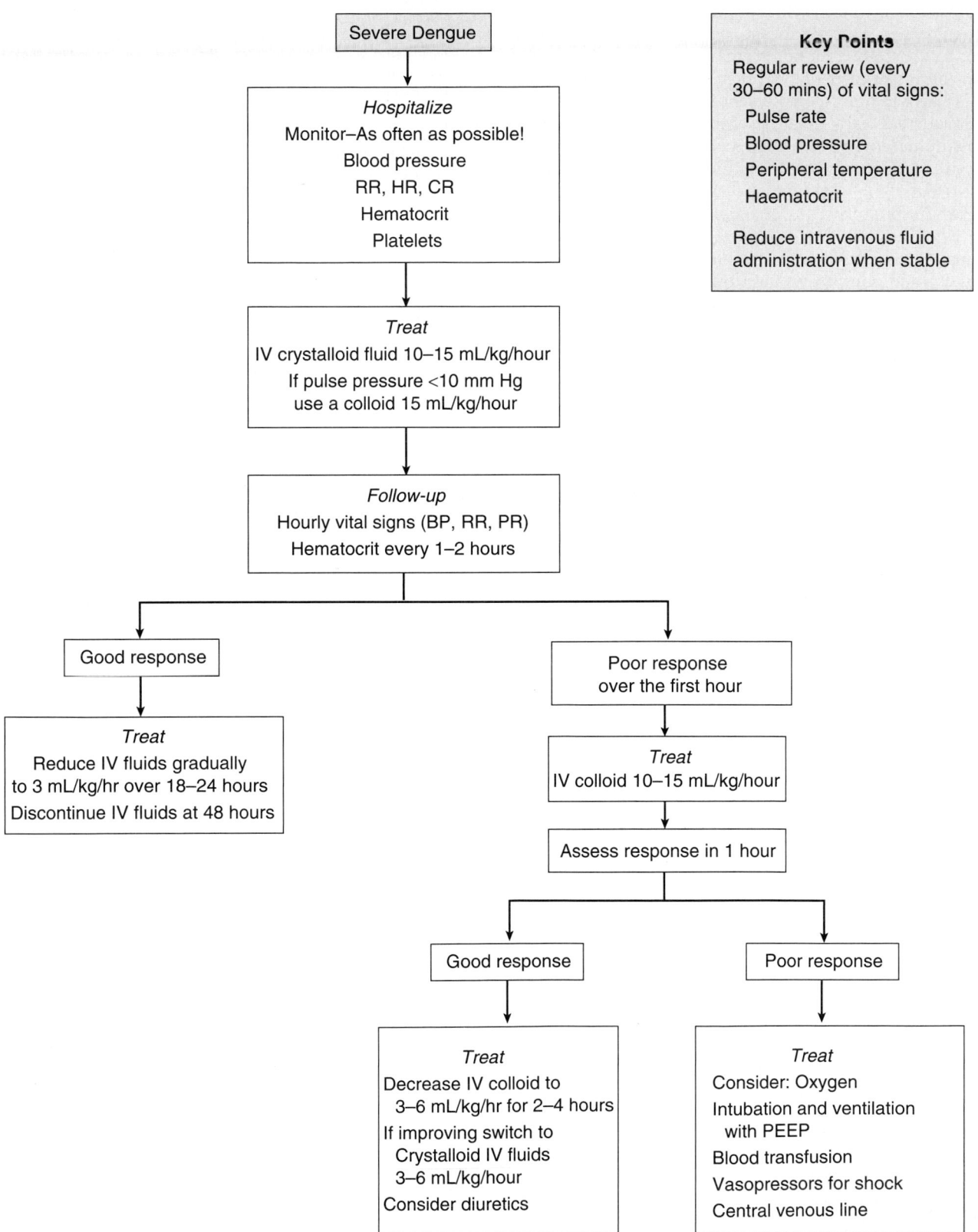

FIGURE 165–3.—cont'd.

Clinically significant fluid overload develops in several situations. Most commonly, it follows either administration of intravenous fluid in excessive amounts or too rapidly to patients with moderate capillary leak or continued parenteral fluid therapy when leak has resolved and the reabsorptive phase of the disease has begun. Rarely, it may be seen in patients with catastrophic leak for whom support of the circulation is not possible without administration of large volumes of fluid. Finally, fluid overload may occur in patients with underlying chronic diseases, particularly cardiac or renal disorders. Careful attention to management guidelines and frequent reassessment of the patient by experienced personnel should help to limit the occurrence of iatrogenic fluid overload, whereas early identification of rare patients with catastrophic leak or severe underlying disease may allow pre-emptive intervention before significant respiratory compromise occurs.

Early respiratory signs include tachypnea and recession and evidence of ascites and pleural effusions; pulmonary edema, cyanosis, and respiratory failure are late manifestations. In addition, severe fluid overload may compromise cardiac function, resulting in hypotension and circulatory failure. Measurement of central venous pressure is helpful in differentiating between hemodynamic instability resulting from severe overload and instability caused by inadequate treatment of the underlying hypovolemia.

CONCLUSION

Over the past 40 years, the incidence of dengue infections, particularly the more severe manifestations of dengue hemorrhagic fever and dengue shock syndrome, has increased dramatically, and dengue is now one of the most common reasons for hospital admission in Asia and the Americas during the rainy seasons. The mortality rate for patients admitted with established dengue shock syndrome is 1% to 5%, even with the best available care. The most important clinical feature of dengue is increased vascular permeability leading to dengue shock syndrome. Children are particularly prone to the development of shock. The judicious management of fluid balance in dengue shock syndrome is the most important therapeutic intervention. Overzealous resuscitation in the presence of ongoing capillary leak should be avoided.

ANNOTATED REFERENCES

Hales S, de Wet N, Maindonald J, Woodward A: Potential effect of population and climate changes on global distribution of dengue fever: An empirical model. Lancet 2002;360:830-834.
> *There is clear evidence that the world's climate is changing and that global warming (whatever the cause) is a real phenomenon. There has been much interest in the impact this change will have on the distribution of diseases, particularly vector-borne diseases. Projections for the future spread of dengue using conservative predictions of changes in humidity and population suggest that 4.1 billion people (44% of the world's population) will be at risk for dengue by 2055.*

Halstead SB: Pathogenesis of dengue: challenges to molecular biology. Science 1988;239:476-481.
> *Dengue viruses replicate in cells of mononuclear phagocyte lineage, and subneutralizing concentrations of dengue antibody enhance dengue virus infection in these cells. This antibody-dependent enhancement of infection regulates dengue disease in humans, although disease severity also may be controlled genetically, possibly by permitting and restricting the growth of virus in monocytes.*

Mongkolsapaya J, Dejnirattisai W, Xu XN, et al: Original antigenic sin and apoptosis in the pathogenesis of dengue hemorrhagic fever. Nat Med 2003;9:921-927.
> *Many dengue-specific T cells are of low affinity for the infecting virus and show higher affinity for other, probably previously encountered strains. Profound T-cell activation and death may contribute to the systemic disturbances leading to dengue hemorrhagic fever, and original antigenic sin in the T-cell responses may suppress or delay viral elimination, leading to higher viral loads and increased immunopathology.*

Ngo NT, Cao XT, Kneen R, et al: Fluid replacement in dengue shock syndrome: A randomized double blind comparison of four intravenous fluid regimens. Clin Infect Dis 2001;32:204-213.
> *The largest clinical trial of fluid resuscitation in dengue shock syndrome is reported. There were indications in patients presenting with more severe shock and an admission pulse pressure of 10 mm Hg or less that there are benefits of primary resuscitation with colloid fluids in this group.*

Wills BA, Oragui EE, Stephens AC, et al: Coagulation abnormalities in dengue hemorrhagic fever: Serial investigations in 167 Vietnamese children with Dengue shock syndrome. Clin Infect Dis 2002;35:277-285.
> *The bleeding in dengue hemorrhagic fever may result from a combination of thrombocytopenia, impaired platelet function, and increased fibrinolysis rather than classic disseminated intravascular coagulation. Despite the name dengue hemorrhagic fever, the main clinical problem in dengue is increased vascular permeability rather than bleeding.*

Section IX

HEMATOLOGIC AND ONCOLOGIC DISORDERS

Chapter 166

ANEMIA AND RED BLOOD CELL TRANSFUSION IN CRITICALLY ILL PATIENTS

Paul C. Hébert • Alan Tinmouth

KEY POINTS

1. Anemia is very common among critically ill patients, ranging in **incidence from 29% to 37%.**

2. **Patients with ischemic heart disease may appear to be at increased risk for adverse consequences from anemia.**

3. Randomized trials clearly indicate that **restrictive transfusion strategies decrease the need for red blood cell transfusions** and do not result in adverse clinical consequences.

4. **Further studies are required in high-risk populations** (acute coronary syndromes and early septic shock) as well as children.

Anemia is a common problem in critically ill patients admitted to ICUs.[1] Indeed, in a recent cross-sectional study, 29% of patients had a hemoglobin concentration below normal values and 37% of patients required a red blood cell (RBC) transfusion.[2] Allogeneic RBC transfusions are complex biologic products prepared from donated blood and may be considered unique in many respects when compared with other health interventions. Decisions concerning the use of RBC transfusion in the treatment of anemia and hemorrhage require a clear understanding of the risks and the benefits of both the condition and its treatment. Although we have developed a much clearer appreciation of the infectious and immunomodulatory risks of RBC transfusion over the past two decades, the risks of anemia in many clinical settings and the benefits of RBC transfusion are still inadequately characterized. We presume that the most significant risk associated with anemia is the harm resulting from the decrease in oxygen-carrying capacity and plasma volume. The development of adverse health consequences from anemia will, in part, depend on the capacity of the individual patient to compensate for these changes. The benefit of transfusion refers to the capacity of RBCs to correct these risks and possibly provide additional benefits such as increasing oxygen delivery to supranormal ranges. Such a framework highlights the concept of tradeoffs of risks and benefits. With the exception of patients who refuse blood for religious reasons, it is impossible, outside a randomized clinical trial, to distinguish clearly between these competing risks and benefits to patients.

NATURAL HISTORY OF UNCORRECTED ANEMIA

Numerous laboratory experiments indicate that extreme hemodilution is well tolerated in healthy animals. Animals subjected to acute hemodilution tolerate decreasing hemoglobin concentrations down to 50 to 30 g/L, with ischemic electrocardiographic changes and depressed ventricular function, occurring, respectively, at these levels of hemoglobin concentration.[3] However, acute hemodilution is less well tolerated in experimental animal models of coronary stenosis, with ischemic electrocardiographic changes and depressed cardiac function occurring at hemoglobin concentrations between 70 and 100 g/L. Human data regarding the limits of anemia tolerance are inadequate and often conflicting. Leung and associates[4] found electrocardiographic changes that may have been indicative of myocardial ischemia in 3 of 55 conscious resting volunteers subjected to acute isovolemic hemodilution to a hemoglobin concentration of 50 g/L.

While providing insight into the human physiologic response to acute anemia, the above-mentioned experimental data are of limited applicability to the perioperative setting, where many of the factors that influence oxygen consumption, including muscle activity, body temperature, heart rate, sympathetic activity, and metabolic state, are altered. Instead, we need to determine the risk of withholding RBC transfusions in the perioperative setting. From a systematic review completed for the Canadian Guidelines on Red cells, Hébert and associates[5] identified numerous reports of severe anemia being well tolerated in surgical patients.[6-18] Additional reports or case series[16,19-21] describe successful outcomes in patients with chronic anemia as a result of renal failure. Finally, descriptive studies in patients refusing red blood cell transfusion[7-9,15] and from regions experiencing limited blood supplies[10,22] have demonstrated that patients can survive surgical interventions with hemoglobin levels as low as 45 g/L.

In examining some of these studies in more detail, there appears to be an association between preoperative hemoglobin concentrations, intraoperative estimated blood loss, and postoperative mortality.[8,9] Indeed, there were no reported deaths in more than 100 patients undergoing major elective surgery when preoperative hemoglobins were greater than 80 g/L and the estimated blood loss was less than 500 mL. In a single center series of 542 Jehovah's Witness patients undergoing a cardiac surgical procedure, the overall mortality rate was 10.7%; only 2.2% of the deaths observed were considered to be a direct consequence of anemia. More recently, Viele and Weiskopf[18] identified 134 Jehovah's Witness patients with a hemoglobin concentration less than 80 g/L or hematocrit below 24% who were treated for various medical and surgical conditions without the use of blood or blood components. There were 50 reported deaths, 23 of which were attributed primarily or exclusively to anemia (defined as deaths with hemoglobin concentration below 50 g/L). For those patients who died of their anemia, 60% were older than 50 years. However, in 27 survivors with hemoglobin concentration below 50 g/L, 65% were younger than 50 years. Although publication bias must be kept in mind in examining these data, young healthy patients may survive without transfusion at hemoglobin concentrations in the range of 50 g/L. From these data, it is clear that extreme anemia is often tolerated in the perioperative setting but also appears to increase the risk of death. However, these observations should not be interpreted as support for a restrictive or conservative transfusion strategy, especially because most of the literature related to tolerance of anemia has not explored patient characteristics that predispose patients to adverse outcomes from moderate to severe anemia.

ANEMIA IN HIGH-RISK GROUPS

A number of risk factors for adverse outcomes associated with anemia have been identified in clinical practice guidelines[23-25] and reviews.[26-28] Anemia is believed to be less tolerated in older patients, in the severely ill, and in patients with clinical conditions such as coronary, cerebrovascular, or respiratory disease. However, the clinical evidence confirming that these factors are independently associated with an increased risk of adverse outcome is lacking. One small case-control study following high-risk vascular surgery suggests an increase in postoperative cardiac events with increasing severity of anemia.[12] In perioperative[29] and critically ill patients,[30] two large cohort studies have documented that increasing degrees of anemia were associated with a disproportionate increase in mortality rate in the subgroup of patients with cardiac disease. In 1958 Jehovah's Witness patients,[29] the adjusted odds of death increased from 2.3 (95% confidence interval, 1.4-4.0) to 12.3 (95% CI, 2.5-62.1) as preoperative hemoglobin concentrations declined from the range of 100 to 109 g/L to the range of 60 to 69 g/L in patients with cardiac disease (Fig. 166-1). There was no significant increase in mortality in noncardiac patients with comparable levels of

anemia. In a separate study of critically ill patients,[30] those with cardiac disease and hemoglobin concentrations less than 95 g/L also had a trend toward an increased mortality rate (55% versus 42%; P = .09) as compared with anemic patients with other diagnoses. Although both cohort studies were retrospective in nature and may not have controlled for a number of important confounders, the evidence suggests that anemia increases the risk of death in patients with significant cardiac disease.

Severity of illness also appears to be a risk factor in critically ill patients.[8,30] Two retrospective studies document that the degree of blood loss contributes to perioperative mortality.[8,30] However, there are no studies examining the independent contribution of age, cerebrovascular disease, and respiratory disease to an increased mortality risk in anemic patients. This relationship may well be complex, given that age and cerebrovascular disease are risk factors associated with coronary artery disease. Smoking-related respiratory diseases may have similar associations to cardiac disease. Therefore, the association between anemia and increased rates of adverse outcomes in these patients can best be described as speculative at this time.

RISKS AND BENEFITS OF TRANSFUSION

Four large observational studies that were specifically designed to compare clinical outcomes at varying hemoglobin concentrations in transfused and nontransfused patients have been conducted in various clinical settings. In the first of these, Hébert and colleagues[30] used a combined retrospective and prospective cohort design to examine 4470 critically ill patients admitted to six Canadian tertiary-level ICUs during 1993. In patients with cardiac diagnoses (ischemic heart disease, arrhythmia, cardiac arrest, or cardiac and vascular surgical procedures), there was a trend toward increased mortality when hemoglobin concentrations were less than 95 g/L. Furthermore, analysis of a subgroup of 202 patients with anemia, an Acute Physiology and Chronic Health Evaluation (APACHE) II score greater than 20, and a cardiac diagnosis revealed that transfusion of 1 to 3 units or 4 to 6 units of RBCs was associated with a significantly lower mortality rate as compared with those patients who did not receive a transfusion (55% [no transfusions] versus 35% [1 to 3 units] or 32% [4 to 6 units]; P = .01). Although the design of the analysis attempted to control for the confounding influence of disease severity, it is quite possible that the complex interrelationship between disease severity, the number of transfusions, and the degree of anemia may have resulted in a spurious association between a cardiovascular diagnosis and the reported mortality risk with anemia.

Wu and associates[31] retrospectively studied Medicare records of 78,974 patients older than 65 years who were hospitalized with a primary diagnosis of acute myocardial infarction. The authors then categorized patients according to their admitting hematocrit. Although anemia, defined in the study as a hematocrit less than 39%, was present in nearly half the patients, only 3680 patients received an RBC transfusion. Lower admission hematocrit values were associated with increased 30-day mortality rate with a mortality rate approaching 50% among patients with a hematocrit of 27% or lower who did not receive an RBC transfusion. Unfortunately, this study did not have any data on nadir hemoglobins and their relationship to mortality. Interestingly, RBC transfusion was associated with a reduction in 30-day

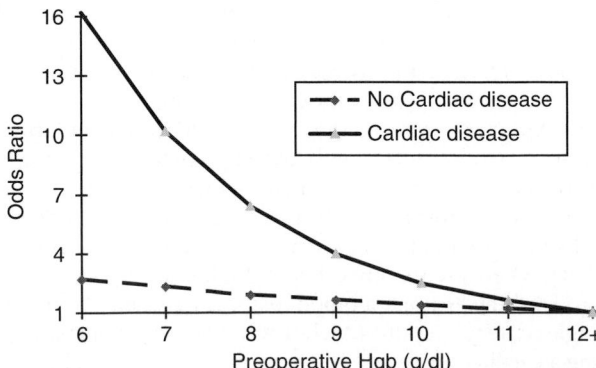

FIGURE 166–1. Adjusted odds ratio for mortality by cardiovascular disease and preoperative hemoglobin (Hgb). (Adapted from Carson JL, Spence RK, Poses RM, Bonavita G: Severity of anemia and operative mortality and morbidity. Lancet 1988;1:727-729.)

mortality for patients who received at least one RBC transfusion if their admitting hematocrit was less than 33%, whereas RBC transfusion was associated with increased 30-day mortality for patients whose admitting hematocrit values were 36.1% or higher. In the analysis, these associations were present even when adjustments were made for clinical patient factors, including APACHE II scores, location of myocardial infarction, and presence of congestive heart failure, and treatment factors, including use of reperfusion therapies, aspirin, and beta-adrenergic blockade.

In the only study exclusively focusing on the perioperative period, Carson and associates[32] attempted to determine the effect of perioperative transfusion on 30- and 90-day postoperative mortality with a retrospective cohort study involving 8787 patients with hip fractures undergoing repair between 1983 and 1993 in 20 different U.S. hospitals. This was a large, high-risk, elderly (median age, 80.3 years) population with extensive coexisting disease and with an overall 30-day mortality rate of 4.6%. A total of 3699 patients (42%) received a perioperative transfusion within 7 days of the surgical repair. After controlling for trigger hemoglobin concentrations, cardiovascular disease, and other risk factors for death, the results suggested that patients who had hemoglobin concentrations as low as 80 g/L and did not receive transfusion were no more likely to die than those with similar hemoglobin concentration levels who received a transfusion. (With hemoglobin concentrations less than 80 g/L, nearly all patients received a transfusion, so investigators were unable to draw conclusions about the effect of transfusion at these lower hemoglobin concentrations levels.) However, as the authors point out, despite the large sample size, inadequate power may still explain the inability to detect a reduction in mortality related to transfusion and they estimated that the study would need to be 10 times larger to detect a 10% difference in 30-day mortality with 80% power.

More recently, Vincent and coworkers[33] completed a prospective observational cross-sectional study involving 3534 patients admitted to 146 western European ICUs during a 2-week period in November 1999. Thirty-seven percent of these patients received an RBC transfusion during their ICU admission, with the overall transfusion rate increasing to 41.6% over a 28-day period. For those patients who received a transfusion, the mean pretransfusion hemoglobin concentration was 84 ±13 g/L. In an effort to control for confounding factors created by illness severity and the need for transfusion, these investigators used a strategy of matching transfused and nontransfused patients based on their propensity to receive a transfusion, thereby defining two well-balanced groups (516 patients in each group) to determine the influence of RBC transfusions on mortality. Using this approach, the associated risk of death was increased instead of decreased by 33% for patients who received a transfusion as compared with similar patients who did not receive blood. However, as pointed out in the accompanying editorial,[34] the results may have differed if the propensity scores were derived separately for categories of pretransfusion hemoglobin concentrations (e.g., <80, 80-100, and >100 g/L) instead of hemoglobin concentrations at ICU admission. For example, if one were to consider groups of patients with a pretransfusion hemoglobin concentration of less than 60 g/L, it is unlikely that the observed 33% increase in mortality would hold true or blood transfusion would never be recommended.

Unfortunately, as evidenced by a recent systematic review, there is a paucity of clinical trials comparing restrictive to liberal transfusion studies to examine the efficacy of RBC transfusion. Carson and coworkers[35] (Fig. 166-2) were able to identify only 10 randomized clinical trials of adequate methodologic quality in which different RBC transfusion triggers were evaluated. Included were a total of 1780 surgery, trauma, and ICU patients enrolled in trials conducted over the past 40 years. The transfusion triggers evaluated in these trials varied between 70 and 100 g/L. Data on mortality or hospital length of stay were available in only six of these trials. Conservative (low hemoglobin) transfusion triggers were not associated with an increase in mortality rate; on average, the rate of mortality was one-fifth lower (relative risk, 0.80; 95% CI, 0.63–1.02) with conservative as compared with liberal transfusion triggers. Likewise, cardiac morbidity and length of hospital stay did not appear to be adversely affected by the lower rate of RBC transfusions. There were insufficient data on potentially relevant clinical outcomes such as stroke, thromboembolism, multiorgan failure, delirium, infection, and delayed wound healing to perform any pooled analysis. Carson and colleagues[32] stated there were insufficient data to address the full range of risks and benefits associated with different transfusion thresholds, particularly in patients with coexisting disease. They also noted that their meta-analysis was dominated by a single trial: the Transfusion Requirements in Critical Care (TRICC) trial,[36] which enrolled 838 patients and was the only individual trial identified that was adequately powered to evaluate the impact of different transfusion strategies on mortality and morbidity.

The TRICC Study[36] documented an overall nonsignificant trend toward decreased 30-day mortality (18.7 versus 23.3%; $P = .11$) and significant decreases in mortality among patients who were less acutely ill (8.7 versus 16.1%; $P = .03$) in the group treated using a hemoglobin transfusion trigger of 70 g/L compared with a more liberally transfused group that received 54% more RBC transfusions. The investigators also noted that the 30-day mortality rates were significantly lower with the restrictive transfusion strategy among patients who were less acutely ill (APACHE II scores less than 20) and among patients who were younger than 55 years of age (Fig. 166-3).

A number of additional questions arose from the TRICC trial. The investigators were particularly interested in the risks and benefits of anemia and transfusion in patients with cardiovascular disease and in patients attempting to wean from mechanical ventilation. In the first of these subgroup analyses,[37] 357 patients (43%) were identified with cardiovascular disease. Of these, 160 had been in the restrictive RBC transfusion group and 197 in the liberal transfusion group. The two groups were fairly equally balanced with regard to baseline characteristics and concurrent therapies, with a few exceptions: there was less frequent diuretic use in the restrictive group (43% vs 58%; $P < .01$) and the use of epidural anesthetics was greater in the restrictive group (8% vs 2%; $P < .01$). Overall, in this subgroup analysis, there was no significant difference in the mortality rate between the two treatment groups. However, there was a nonsignificant ($P = .3$) decrease in overall survival rate in the restrictive group for patients with confirmed ischemic heart disease, severe peripheral vascular disease, or severe comorbid cardiac disease.

The subgroup analysis of patients receiving mechanical ventilation was limited to 713 (85% of the 838 patients in the TRICC trial who required invasive mechanical ventilatory support).[38] Of these, 357 had been in the restrictive RBC

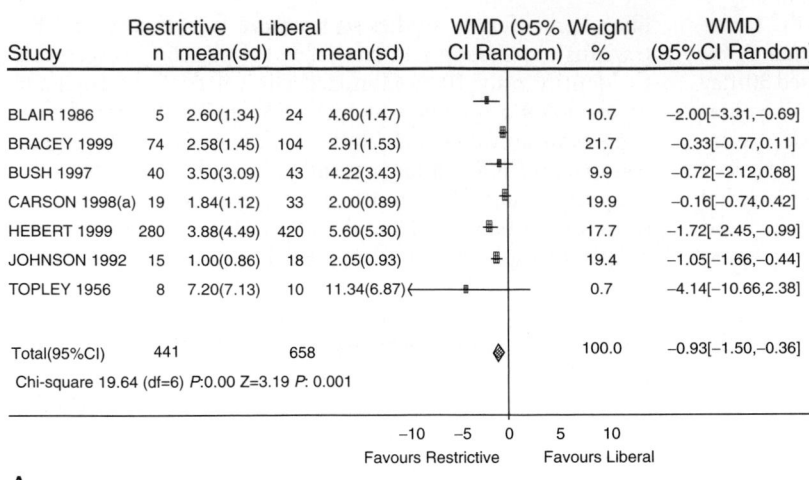

A

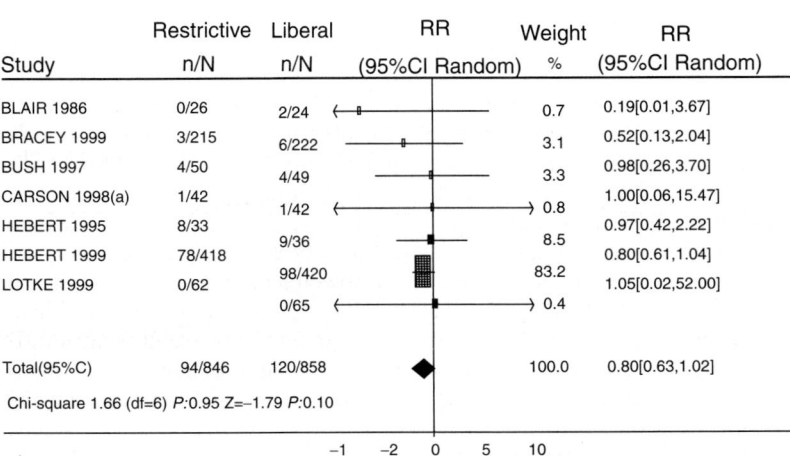

B

FIGURE 166–2. Effect of restrictive transfusion triggers on the use of allogeneic blood transfusion. (Adapted from Carson JL, Hill S, Carless P, et al: Transfusion triggers a systematic review of the literature. Trans Med Rev 2002;16(3):187-199.)

transfusion group and 356 in the liberal group. The mean duration of mechanical ventilation was 8.3 ± 8.1 days in the restrictive group and 8.8 ± 8.7 days in the liberal group ($P = .48$). Ventilator-free days were 17.5 ± 10.9 and 16.1 ± 11.4 in the restrictive and liberal RBC transfusion groups, respectively ($P = .09$). Eighty-two percent of the patients in the restrictive transfusion group were considered successfully weaned and extubated for at least 24 hours, compared with 78% in the liberal group ($P = .19$). Among the 219 patients who required mechanical ventilation for more than 7 days, there were no differences in the time to successful weaning (Fig. 166-4). The independent effects of RBC transfusions and hemoglobin concentration were also examined. Each additional transfusion was associated with an increased duration of mechanical ventilation (RR = 1.10; 95% CI, 1.14-1.06; $P < .01$) after adjusting for the effect of age, APACHE II score, and comorbid illnesses. Hemoglobin concentrations did not influence the duration of mechanical ventilation (RR = 0.99; 95% CI, 1.01-0.98; $P = .45$). Complications, including pulmonary edema and acute respiratory distress syndrome, were increased in patients in the liberal strategy group.

Even though a large randomized controlled trial has been completed, a number of questions remain to be answered. One of the most important questions is why the liberal RBC transfusion strategy failed to improve 30-day mortality rate and rates of organ failure in critically ill patients. It is conceivable that the greater number of allogeneic RBC units in the liberal group significantly depressed host immune responses[38,39] or resulted in altered microcirculatory flow as a consequence of prolonged storage times.

Subsequent to the publication of the TRICC trial, a study published by Rivers and colleagues[40] documented that the use of early goal-directed care based on a mixed central venous saturation decreased mortality from 46.5% in the control group to 30.5% in the goal-directed therapy group ($P = .009$). As one of the many interventions in patients with early septic shock, hematocrit concentrations were increased to greater than 30% if the central venous saturations fell to less than 70%. As a consequence of goal-directed therapy, 64% of patients as compared with 18.5% of the control group received RBC transfusions ($P < .0001$). The significant differences in patient populations studied by Rivers and colleagues and the TRICC trial may account for the apparently conflicting results between the studies. The new finding from the early goal-directed therapy study does highlight the need to perform additional studies in subpopulations of critically ill patients.

ALTERNATIVES TO TRANSFUSION

Numerous strategies have been explored and are recommended to decrease or to eliminate the need for blood transfusions during major surgery and critical illness. Some are

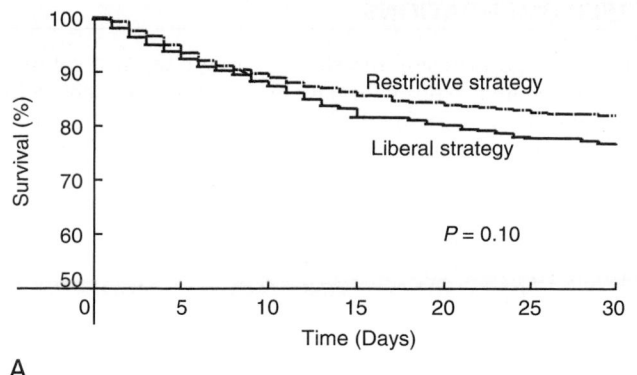

A

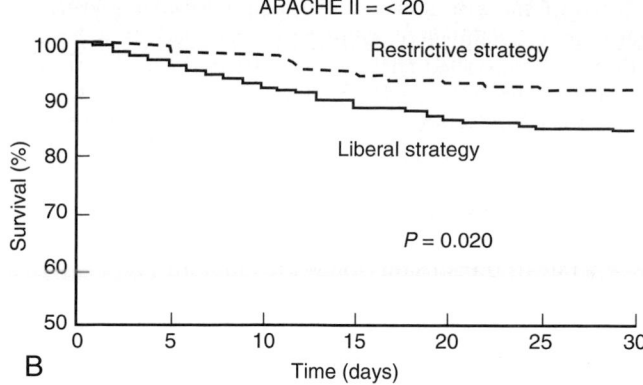

B

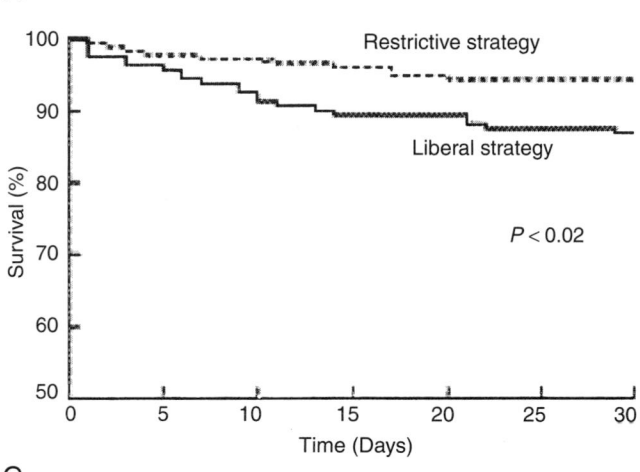

C

FIGURE 166–3. ICU survival over 30 days in study patients in the restrictive and liberal allogeneic RBC transfusion strategy groups. (*A*) Kaplan-Meier survival curves for all patients in both study groups. There is a trend toward lower mortality in patients in the restrictive group (dotted line) as compared to the liberal group (solid line) (*P* = .10). (*B*) In the subgroup with an APACHE II score less than 20, fewer patients died in the restrictive group than in the liberal group (*P* = .02). (*C*) There were also significant differences in survival among groups in the subgroup with ages less than 55 years (*P* = .02). (Adapted from Hébert PC, Wells G, Blajchmann MA, et al: A multicentre, randomized, controlled trial of transfusion requirements in critical care. N Engl J Med 1999;340:409-417.)

relatively benign, but others carry their own risks that must be weighed against the administration of RBCs. Alternatives include decreasing the use of medications that result in perioperative bleeding (such as nonsteroidal anti-inflammatory drugs and acetylsalicylic acid), avoidance of unnecessary phlebotomy and the use of blood conservation strategies (such as pediatric test tubes and arterial catheter reinfusion set-ups), medications to decrease blood loss (such as antifibrinolytic agents), and medications to increase hemoglobin production. In addition to a restrictive transfusion strategy, the two most useful approaches to decreasing RBC transfusions in critically ill patients appear to be blood conservation techniques such as decreased phlebotomies and erythropoietin therapy. Other therapeutic strategies are better suited to patients undergoing high-risk surgical procedures.

Decreased RBC production is one of the causes of anemia observed in the critically ill. Indeed, critical illness is characterized by blunted erythropoietin production and response.[41] This blunted erythropoietin response observed in critically ill patients appears to result from inhibition of the erythropoietin gene by inflammatory mediators.[42,43] It has also been shown that these same inflammatory cytokines directly inhibit RBC production by the bone marrow and may produce the distinct abnormalities of iron metabolism.[44,45] In patients with multiple organ failure, recombinant human erythropoietin therapy (600 IU/kg) has been shown to stimulate erythropoiesis.[46] Similarly, in a small randomized placebo-controlled trial (160 patients), therapy with recombinant human erythropoietin resulted in an almost 50% reduction in RBC transfusions as compared to patients treated with a placebo.[47] Erythropoietin was given at a dose of 300 U/kg daily for 5 days followed by every-other-day dosing until

ICU discharge. Despite receiving fewer RBC transfusions, patients in the recombinant human erythropoietin group had a significantly greater increase in hematocrit.

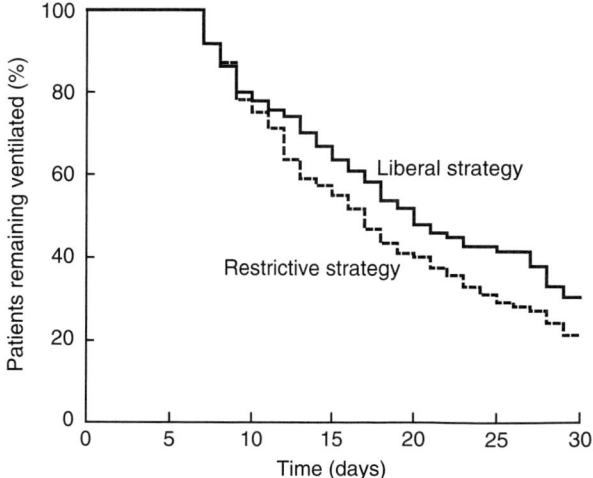

FIGURE 166–4. Time remaining on mechanical ventilation in the 283 patients requiring mechanical ventilation for more than 1 week. The time to successful weaning from mechanical ventilation is illustrated using Kaplan-Meier survival curves in patients who required mechanical ventilation for more than 1 week. Weaning success is defined as remaining off mechanical ventilation, once extubated, during the 30 days of observation. The hatched line refers to the restrictive group and the solid line refers to the liberal group. Survival curves were not statistically different when compared using a log rank test (*P* = .08). (Adapted from Hébert PC, Blajchmann MA, Cook DJ, et al: Do blood transfusions improve outcomes related to mechanical ventilation? Chest 2001;119:1850-1857.)

Recently, the efficacy of recombinant human erythropoietin in critically ill patients was evaluated in a large randomized controlled trial of 1302 patients.[48] In this trial, recombinant human erythropoietin was given weekly at a dose of 40,000 units. All patients received three weekly doses, and patients who remained in the ICU on study day 21 received a fourth dose. Treatment with recombinant human erythropoietin resulted in a 10% reduction in the number of patients receiving any RBC transfusions. The authors reported a 60.4% rate of transfusions following randomization in the placebo group as compared with 50.5% in the recombinant human erythropoietin group (OR, 0.67; 95% CI, 0.54–0.83; $P < .0004$) and a 20% reduction in the total number of RBC units transfused in patients receiving recombinant human erythropoietin ($P < .001$). All clinical outcomes including mortality rates, rates of organ failure, and lengths of stay in the ICU and the hospital were comparable between groups (all P values $> .05$). Taken together, these studies[47-49] demonstrate that recombinant human erythropoietin therapy in critically ill patients will result in a decrease in RBC transfusion and a rise in hemoglobin level. This is consistent with the hypothesis that the anemia in critically ill patients is similar to the anemia of patients with chronic disease and is characterized, at least in part, by a relative erythropoietin deficiency.[50] Given the high costs of erythropoietin and the lack of clinical benefit demonstrated in the randomized controlled trial, we do not yet recommend this blood conservation strategy in routine practice.

CONCLUSIONS

Despite the frequent use of RBC transfusions, there is only one large randomized trial that has examined RBC administration perioperatively and in the critical care setting. However, the TRICC trial does not provide sufficient evidence to determine optimal transfusion practice in postoperative care, in critically ill children, in situations of early septic shock, or in patients with a myocardial infarction or acute coronary syndromes. In addition, most transfusion practice guidelines published prior to the completion of the TRICC trial[35-37] are now dated and need to have expert opinion by solid evidence in diverse clinical settings. In the next several years, several randomized trials will provide additional evidence in support of bedside decision-making. For example, two transfusion studies will be evaluating transfusion triggers, one in premature infants and the other in critically ill children. At this juncture, high-quality clinical evidence is not yet available for many decisions related to RBC transfusions and alternatives such as human recombinant erythropoietin. We anticipate that risks and benefits of RBCs and alternatives will be elucidated in the coming years.

RECOMMENDATIONS

1. Adopt a transfusion threshold of 70 g/L in most volume-resuscitated critically ill patients, including patients with a history of coronary artery disease.
2. Aim to maintain patients' transfusion volume between 70 and 90 g/L.
3. Transfuse 1 RBC unit at a time and measure after every transfusion if anemia or bleeding remains a concern.
4. Exceptions to the previous recommendations include cases of patients with acute coronary syndromes (acute myocardial infarction and unstable angina) and patients with early septic shock.
5. There is insufficient evidence to recommend the routine use of erythropoietin in critically ill patients.

ANNOTATED REFERENCES

Corwin HL, Krantz SB: Anemia of the critically ill: "Acute" anemia of chronic disease. Crit Care Med 2000;28:3098-3099.
    Good review article.

Corwin HL, Gettinger A, Pearl RG, et al: Efficacy of recombinant human erythropoietin in critically ill patients: a randomized controlled trial. JAMA 2002;288:2827-2835.
    This study found that in critically ill patients, weekly administration of 40,000 units of recombinant human erythropoietin (rHuEPO) reduces allogeneic RBC transfusion and increases hemoglobin. Further study is needed to determine whether this reduction in RBC transfusion results in improved clinical outcomes.

Napolitano LM, Corwin HL: Efficacy of red blood cell transfusion in the critically ill. Crit Care Clin 2004;20:255-268.
    This article evaluates the literature on the efficacy of RBC transfusions in the critically ill. It concludes the RBC transfusion does not improve tissue oxygen consumption consistently in critically ill patients; it is not associated with improvements in clinical outcome and may result in worse outcomes in some patients; specific factors that identify patients who will improve from RBC transfusion are difficult to identify; and lack of efficacy of RBC transfusion likely is related to storage time, increased endothelial adherence of stored RBCs, nitric oxide binding by free hemoglobin in stored blood, donor leukocytes, host inflammatory response, and reduced red cell deformability. Taken together, these studies generally support conservative RBC transfusion strategies in critical care to reduce the risk of transfusion-related adverse effects.

Corwin HL: Erythropoietin in the critically ill—is it more than just blood? Crit Care 2004;8:325-326.
    Erythropoietin (EPO) has been in clinical use for the treatment of anemia for over 15 years. Recently it has been demonstrated that EPO has actions other than stimulating the bone marrow. It has been suggested that due to its tissue protecting effect, EPO may be effective in improving outcome in the critically ill.

Chapter 167

BLOOD COMPONENT THERAPY

James P. Isbister

KEY POINTS

1. An evidence-based approach to blood component transfusion has resulted in many long-standing transfusion dogmas being challenged and better guidelines for their use being developed.

2. The decision to transfuse should be supported by the need to relieve clinical signs and symptoms of impaired oxygen transport and to prevent morbidity and mortality.

3. It is not possible or necessary for fresh blood components to be immediately available for all acutely hemorrhaging patients, but use of blood less than 1 week from the collection date is desirable to minimize problems associated with the storage lesion.

4. The classic symptoms and signs of an acute hemolytic transfusion reaction include apprehension, flushing, pain (e.g., infusion site, headache, chest, lumbosacral, abdominal), nausea, vomiting, rigors, hypotension, and circulatory collapse.

5. A clinician needs a basic working knowledge of red blood cell (RBC) serology to ensure patient safety.

Blood component therapy has had a central role in the development and practice of numerous medical advances, especially in modern surgery. It is only in more recent years that blood transfusion is no longer regarded as essential for a wide range of medical and surgical conditions. Most major surgery now can be conducted without homologous blood component therapy.[1] Blood component transfusion is generally supportive therapy for the correction of one or more hematologic deficiencies until the basic disease process can be controlled or corrected. Appropriate attention to accurate diagnosis of the hematopoietic deficiency and consideration of the range of therapeutic options available and their potential hazards are essential before accepting blood component therapy as indicated.[2]

Blood component therapy and its immediate endpoints are part of a medical management process. Although appropriate endpoints may be achieved in terms of measurable parameters or clinical response, the clinician needs evidence that these traditional "outcomes" are relevant in relation to the final outcome for the patient. The human immunodeficiency virus (HIV) crisis shocked clinical medicine into a realization that there were many transfusion practices exposing patients to potential hazards without evidence for identifiable short-term or long-term benefits.

Evidence-based medicine is increasingly influencing the practice of transfusion medicine. In many areas of transfusion medicine, evidence from trials is not available, and the clinician must base therapy on a good understanding of the problem in terms of pathophysiology and indicators of severity. Transfusion medicine decision-making can be difficult, and there is ongoing debate regarding the indications for various homologous blood components. Unnecessary homologous transfusion can be avoided or minimized by giving attention to the clinical time frame, hematologic defect, alternatives, and knowledge about blood components and the potential hazards. There have been considerable advances in minimizing homologous transfusion and the development of transfusion alternatives.[3,4] Identifying patients at high bleeding risk and giving attention to surgical and anesthetic techniques (e.g., controlled hypotension, hypothermia prevention, reduction of venous pressure at operative site) and the application of pharmacologic agents substantially reduce blood loss. Autologous methodologies, including perioperative hemodilution, blood salvage, fibrin glue, and platelet fibrin gel, all may have a part to play.

GUIDELINES FOR BLOOD COMPONENT THERAPY

The following is a brief summary of the guidelines for use of commonly available blood components. An evidence-based approach to blood component transfusion has resulted in many long-standing transfusion dogmas being challenged and better guidelines for their use being developed. Figure 167-1 illustrates the general approach to the decision to transfuse blood components. The emphasis is on blood management and where blood component therapy fits into the bigger picture.

RED BLOOD CELL CONCENTRATES

The appropriate and inappropriate use of red blood cell (RBC) transfusions in acute medicine has received considerable attention in recent years; however, identifying the benefits of RBC transfusion in many circumstances has been difficult.[5] The question of the lowest safe hematocrit continues to receive considerable attention. Pushing any aspect of a system to its limits risks "sailing close to the wind" and may be appropriate in some situations, but potentially hazardous in others. In an otherwise stable patient, the transfusion of RBC concentrates is likely to be inappropriate when the hemoglobin level is greater than 100 g/L. Their use may be appropriate when hemoglobin is in the range 70 to 100 g/L if there are other defects in the oxygen transport system. The decision to transfuse

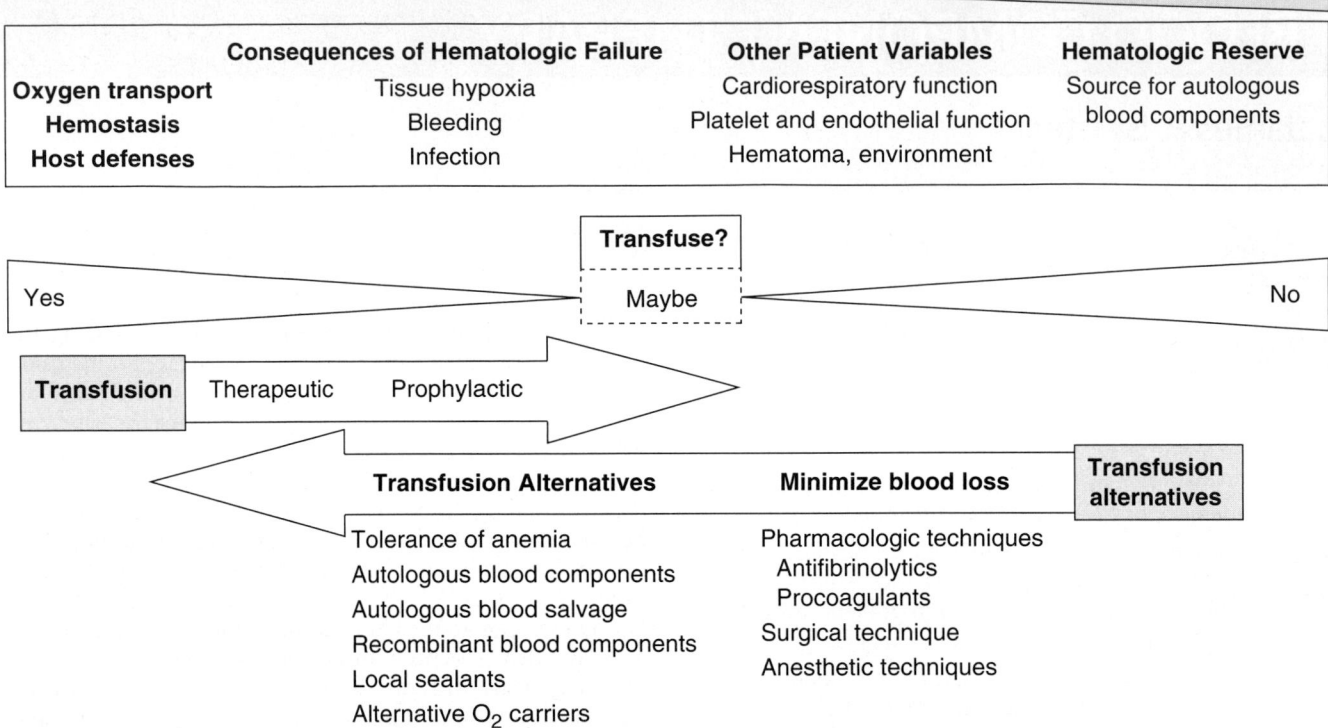

FIGURE 167–1. Overview of blood management and where blood component therapy may be appropriate.

should be supported by the need to relieve clinical signs and symptoms of impaired oxygen transport and to prevent morbidity and mortality. The transfusion of RBC concentrates is likely to be appropriate when hemoglobin is less than 70 g/L and the anemia is not reversible with specific therapy in the short-term, but lower levels may be acceptable in patients who are asymptomatic.

PLATELET CONCENTRATES

Platelet transfusions may benefit patients with platelet deficiency or dysfunction, and the general recommendations for their use are as follows.[6,7] Prophylactic transfusion of platelet concentrates is indicated in patients with bone marrow failure when the platelet count is less than $10 \times 10^9/L$, and there are no associated risk factors for bleeding or less than $20 \times 10^9/L$ in the presence of additional risk factors.

In patients undergoing surgery or invasive procedures, the platelet count should be maintained at greater than $50 \times 10^9/L$. In patients with qualitative defects in platelet function, platelet count is not a reliable indicator for transfusion, and transfusion decisions and monitoring of efficacy must be based on the setting and clinical features.

Platelet transfusions are indicated in hemorrhaging patients in whom thrombocytopenia is secondary to marrow failure and is considered a contributory factor to the bleeding. In massively hemorrhaging patients, platelet transfusions, in conjunction with correcting plasma coagulation factor deficits, are indicated when the platelet count is less than $50 \times 10^9/L$ or less than $100 \times 10^9/L$ in the presence of diffuse microvascular bleeding. The transfusion of platelet concentrates is not generally considered appropriate when thrombocytopenia is due to immune-mediated destruction, in patients with thrombotic thrombocytopenic purpura and hemolytic uraemic syndrome, or in uncomplicated cardiac bypass surgery.

FRESH FROZEN PLASMA AND CRYOPRECIPITATE

Fresh frozen plasma is widely used, but there are limited specific indications for its use, and evidence for efficacy in many clinical settings is minimal.[8] The use of fresh frozen plasma may be appropriate in patients with a coagulopathy who are bleeding or at risk for bleeding when a specific therapy or factor concentrates are not appropriate or unavailable. Fresh frozen plasma generally is indicated in hemorrhaging patients for replacement of labile plasma coagulation factors (e.g., massive transfusion, cardiac bypass, liver disease, or acute disseminated intravascular coagulation). Fresh frozen plasma may be indicated, in conjunction with vitamin K, in cases of excessive warfarinization, in which there is potentially life-threatening bleeding. The use of fresh frozen plasma generally is not considered appropriate in cases of hypovolemia; in plasma exchange procedures, unless postexchange invasive procedures are planned; or in treatment of immunodeficiency states.

Compatibility tests before transfusion are not necessary, but plasma should be ABO group compatible with the patient's RBCs, and volume transfused depends on the clinical situation and patient size. As a guide, initial dosing of 10 to 15 mL/kg is recommended, and efficacy should be monitored by laboratory tests of coagulation function.

Cryoprecipitate is prepared by thawing fresh frozen plasma between 1°C and 6°C and recovering the precipitate, which is refrozen. The component contains factor VIII, fibrinogen, factor XIII, von Willebrand's factor, and fibronectin and is principally indicated for fibrinogen deficiency or dysfibrinogenemia when there is clinical bleeding, invasive procedures, trauma, or acute disseminated intravascular coagulation. Cryoprecipitate should not be used for the treatment of hemophilia or von Willebrand's disease, unless factor concentrates are unavailable.

PLASMA-DERIVED PRODUCTS

A wide range of highly purified plasma-derived blood products is available for use in a plethora of clinical conditions. It is beyond the scope to this chapter to discuss their use in detail; Table 167-1 summarizes commonly used fresh and plasma-derived blood products.

RECOMBINANT BLOOD PRODUCTS

The development and introduction of recombinant blood components continues to be one of the most exciting advances in transfusion medicine. Recombinant growth factors (cytokines), such as erythropoietin and granulocyte stimulating factors, have had a major impact in the management of anemia and neutropenia. There are further promising recombinant cytokines in development that could have a role in a plethora of clinical conditions, especially as anti-inflammatory and tissue-protecting agents. Recombinant hemostatic factors have improved the management of hemophilia, and more recently the expansion of the clinical indications for the use of recombinant activated factor VII (factor VIIa) beyond the management of hemophiliac patients with coagulation factor inhibitors is having an impact on the management of a range of hemostatic disorders.[9,10] Because factor VIIa is dependent on tissue factor, which is usually available in limited quantities within the circulation, its clinical use is safe from a thrombosis-inducing point of view, and its use is now being recommended as a "panhemostatic agent." Factor VIIa initiates the extrinsic coagulation pathway only when complexed to tissue factor at sites of injury. It may have a role in a wide range of hemostatic disorders (e.g., massive blood transfusion, liver disease, uremia, severe thrombocytopenia, and platelet disorders). Recombinant activated protein C has antithrombotic, anti-inflammatory, and profibrinolytic properties and is finding a role in the treatment of patients with severe sepsis.[11]

BLOOD SUBSTITUTES

Efforts have been ongoing for many years to develop substitutes for RBCs and platelets. We have not seen the success, however, with development of substitutes for cellular blood components that there has been with recombinant plasma components. As their introduction into clinical medicine remains in the research phase, the reader is referred to reviews for further information. Promising progress is now being made, however, and clinical use of these agents may not be too far away.[12,13]

TABLE 167–1. BLOOD PRODUCTS

Blood product	Main indications
Whole blood*	Rarely indicated in acute hemorrhage if other blood products are unavailable
Red blood cell concentrates*	Hemorrhage and anemia
Leukocyte-depleted blood*	In patients having febrile reactions, to avoid leukocyte immunization in selected patients (especially patients with hematologic malignancy). Universal prestorage leukodepletion is more widely used and has the added benefit of minimizing storage lesions
Platelet concentrates*	Thrombocytopenia due to marrow hypoplasia or platelet functional defect
Granulocyte concentrates*	Occasionally in patients with sepsis associated with profound and prolonged neutropenia secondary to marrow suppression
Fresh frozen plasma*	Specific or multiple plasma protein deficiencies (especially coagulation)
Cryoprecipitate*	Hypofibrinogenemia and rarely in factor VIII and von Willebrand's disease, when concentrates are unavailable
4% or 5% albumin solutions†	Plasma volume expansion. Use is controversial, and the role of albumin solutions in critically ill patients remains under deliberation
Concentrated albumin†	Severe hypoalbuminemic states with complicating hypovolemia
Concentrate of coagulation Factors II, IX, and X†	Vitamin K–dependent factor II, IX, and X deficiency
Specific factor concentrates†	Factor VIII and IX concentrates have an established role in management of hemophilia, but others are in the process of establishing their clinical efficacy and indications. Antithrombin concentrates are available for thrombophilia due to antithrombin deficiency and are increasingly recommended in other disorders in which antithrombin may be depleted (e.g., DIC, MODS)
Gamma globulin†	Generally used intravenously for replacement in hypogammaglobulinemia or in high dosage in autoimmune disorders (e.g., idiopathic thrombocytopenic purpura, autoimmune polyneuropathy)
Specific immune gamma globulins†	Rhesus prophylaxis, specific infection prophylaxis (e.g., tetanus, zoster, hepatitis B)

*Fresh products.
†Fractionated plasma products.
DIC, disseminated intravascular coagulation; MODS, multiorgan dysfunction syndrome.

TRANSFUSION MANAGEMENT OF MASSIVE ACUTE HEMORRHAGE

Homologous blood may be required for the restitution of blood volume and oxygen-carrying capacity in the bleeding patient.[14] Massive or continuing blood loss of greater than one blood volume in 24 hours may result in depletion of hemostatic factors and the requirement for specific component therapy.[15] Previously healthy patients sustaining a loss less than 25% of their blood volume require only volume restoration.

Minimization of homologous blood transfusion can be achieved by close monitoring of the hematocrit, and hemodilution to low levels is now accepted practice. Ongoing and massive blood loss requires a coordinated, priority-oriented clinical and laboratory approach. The rapid infusion of large volumes of aged blood has potential problems that can compound with others in critically ill patients. It is not possible or necessary for fresh blood components to be immediately available for all acutely hemorrhaging patients. Whenever possible, however, blood less than 1 week from the collection date is desirable in a patient continuing to bleed to minimize the problems associated with the storage lesion. Potential complications of massive transfusion are discussed subsequently.

A protocol approach to blood component therapy generally is not recommended because each patient should be assessed and treated individually. In an elective situation in which there is severe or ongoing blood loss when defects can be predicted and identified, a preemptive protocol approach may be justified. Improvements in point of care testing of hemostasis (especially activated partial thromboplastin time, prothombin time, fibrinogen, and thromboelastography) allows better real-time management of hemostatic failure and rapid initiation of appropriate pharmacologic or blood component therapy.[16] Close interaction with the hematology and transfusion service is essential.

HAZARDS OF HOMOLOGOUS TRANSFUSION

The pathophysiology of transfusion reactions can be divided broadly into three categories:

1. Reactions may occur due to *immunologic differences* between the donor and recipient resulting in varying degrees of blood component incompatibility. In general, for a reaction to occur, the recipient needs to have been previously immunized to a cellular or plasma antigen.[17]
2. A wide range of *infectious agents* may be transmitted by homologous blood component therapy.
3. *Alterations in blood products due to preservation and storage* may result in quantitative or qualitative deficiencies in the blood components that reduce transfusion efficacy and expose the patient to potentially adverse consequence from storage accumulants in the component (Table 167-2).

In terms of causation of an adverse clinical event, the possible role of transfusion can be classified broadly into three categories on the basis of probability (Fig. 167-2):

1. *Definite—unifactorial.* The well-understood and well-reported hazards of transfusion (i.e., immunologic, technical, infectious) are generally unifactorial with a 1:1 causal relationship between the blood component transfused (usually a specific individual unit) and the adverse consequence for the patient. ABO blood group incompatibility, transfusion-related infection transmission, transfusion-associated graft-versus-host disease, and transfusion-related lung injury due to donor leukoagglutinins are examples in this category.
2. *Probable—oligofactorial.* Some adverse consequences of transfusion result from interaction with other insults, pathophysiology, or host factors, but the contribution of the transfusion usually can be specifically identified. Fever, allergic reactions, hypotensive reactions, pulmonary edema, some cases of transfusion-related lung injury, hyperbilirubinemia, and cytomegalovirus transmission are examples of this category.

TABLE 167–2. RED BLOOD CELL STORAGE LESION AND POSSIBLE CLINICAL CONSEQUENCES

Storage lesion	Potential clinical consequences
Alterations in red blood cell structure and function	
ATP depletion	Echinospherocyte formation, increased osmotic fragility, impaired RBC deformability with adverse effects on oxygen transport and delivery
Microvesiculation and loss of membrane lipid, lipid peroxidation and hemolysis, and irreversible damaged RBCs	Reduced RBC viability and cell death
	Hyperbilirubinemia, LDH, increased serum iron, free radical generation (?), hyperkalemia
Reduced 2,3-DPG	Increased hemoglobin affinity for oxygen and impaired unloading
Decreased CD47 antigen (integrin-associated protein) expression	Reduced post-transfusion survival due to premature clearance post-transfusion
RBC adhesion to endothelial cells	Adverse effects on microcirculatory hemodynamics
Storage temperature	Hypothermia unless pretransfusion warming
Additives	
Citrate	Hypocalcemia, acid-base imbalance, initial acidosis alkalosis
Glucose	Hyperglycemia
Sodium	Hypernatremia
Cytokines: IL-1, IL-6, IL-8, TNF	Fever, hypotension, flushing
Enzymes: Myeloperoxidase, elastase, arginase, secretory phospholipase A$_2$	Transfusion-related immunomodulation, neutrophilia
Reactive proteins: Defensins, annexin, soluble HLA, Fas ligand, soluble endothelial cell growth factor, and others	Proinflammatory, potential "priming" for ARDS, TRALI, and MODS
Histamine and kinin accumulation	Hypotension, anxiety, flushing, pain syndromes, proinflammatory
Microaggregates and procoagulants	Blockade of reticuloendothelial system
	Risk factor for development of ARDS, MODS, TRALI
	Activation of hemostasis > DIC (?), VTE (?), arterial thrombotic events (?)

ARDS, acute respiratory distress syndrome; ATP, adenosine triphosphate; DIC, disseminated intravascular coagulation; 2,3-DPG, 2,3-diphosphoglycerate; HLA, human leukocyte antigen; IL, interleukin; LDH, lactate dehydrogenase; MODS, multiorgan dysfunction syndrome; RBC, red blood cell; TNF, tumor necrosis factor; TRALI, transfusion-related acute lung injury; VTE, venous thromboembolism.

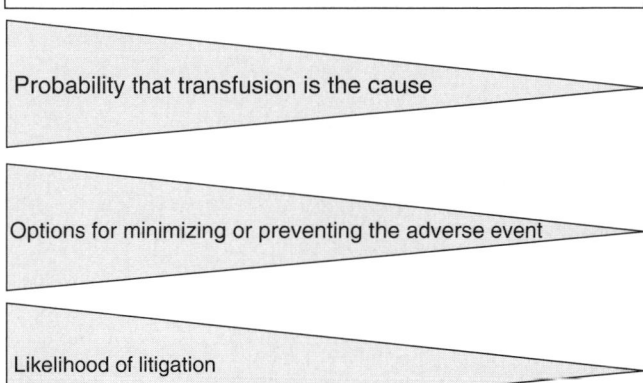

Unifactorial	Oligofactorial	Multifactorial
Definite	*Probable*	*Possible*
1:1 Causation	1:1 Causation + other factors	Transfusion as risk factor

Compatibility	Anaphylactoid reactions	ARDS
HIV	CMV	MODS
Hepatitis	Allergic reactions	TRIM
Endotoxemia	Fever	Thrombosis
GVHD	TRALI	
Technical error		

Probability that transfusion is the cause

Options for minimizing or preventing the adverse event

Likelihood of litigation

FIGURE 167–2. Hazards of homologous blood transfusion. ARDS, acute respiratory distress syndrome; CMV, cytomegalovirus; GVHD, graft-versus-host disease; HIV, human immunodeficiency virus; MODS, multiorgan dysfunction syndrome; TRALI, transfusion-related acute lung injury; TRIM, transfusion-related immunomodulation.

3. *Possible—multifactorial.* Transfusion may contribute to a complication or poor clinical outcome. In these circumstances, it is usually difficult to implicate transfusion directly in an individual case, and it is not necessarily the major factor. Transfusion-induced immunomodulation and the clinical consequences of storage lesions fall into this category. The role of transfusion contributing to such adverse consequences can be identified only by large well-conducted, controlled trials using powerful multifactorial statistical analysis. If transfusion can be identified as a significant contributory factor to a specific complication, its role is considered more as a risk factor rather than a direct 1:1 causal factor. Potential adverse clinical consequences of the storage lesions fall into this group, with product preparation method, dosage, and age of blood component being relevant. Often the specific details of component preparation (e.g., method of leukoreduction) are not stated, making it difficult to compare studies. Prevention of complications from the storage lesion focuses on the quality of preservation and minimizing transfusion rather than elimination of the risk, as is the case with ABO incompatibility or HIV.

HEMOLYTIC TRANSFUSION REACTIONS

Most severe acute hemolytic transfusion reactions usually have an identifiable and avoidable cause and result from an error at some point along the compatibility chain, most commonly incorrect patient identification. ABO incompatibility is the most common potentially fatal complication of blood transfusion, and meticulous attention to patient and sample identification is crucial. Various strategies are advocated to eliminate the possibility of ABO incompatibility, including bar coding vein-to-vein patient identification, bedside compatibility testing, and double patient sample collection. All of these strategies have problems, however, and the human factor remains important.

Most delayed hemolytic reactions are also immune in nature and usually cannot be prevented because the blood is serologically compatible at the time of transfusion. The clinician should always be on the outlook for the possibility of hemolytic episodes in critically ill patients, however, because these are commonly due to reactions to blood transfusion or medications.

Clinical features of hemolytic transfusion reactions are as follows:

- *Initial symptoms and signs.* The classic symptoms and signs of an acute hemolytic transfusion reaction include apprehension, flushing, pain (e.g., infusion site, headache, chest, lumbosacral, and abdominal), nausea, vomiting, rigors, hypotension, and circulatory collapse. In unconscious or anesthetized patients, these symptoms are unlikely to be noted.
- *Hemostatic failure.* Coagulopathy due to disseminated intravascular coagulation may be a feature, resulting in generalized hemostatic failure, with hemorrhage and oozing from multiple sites. Because the responsible transfusion is likely to have been administered for hemorrhage, increasing severity of local bleeding may be the first clue to an incompatible transfusion, especially if the patient is under anesthesia.
- *Oliguria and renal impairment.* Renal failure may complicate a hemolytic transfusion reaction, and early recognition and prevention are crucial. If circulating volume and urinary output are rapidly restored, established renal failure is unlikely to develop. Death from acute renal failure directly caused by an incompatible blood transfusion is preventable and is likely to occur only if expeditious action is not taken, or there are complicating clinical problems.
- *Anemia and jaundice.* A severe hemolytic transfusion reaction may be suspected from the development of jaundice or anemia.

ALLERGIC AND ANAPHYLACTOID REACTIONS

Noncellular blood (plasma and plasma derivatives) components rarely are considered to be a major cause for adverse reactions to transfusion therapy, but considering the complexity of plasma and component preparation processes, a broad range of potential adverse effects is possible.[18] Plasma reactions may be related to immunologic differences between the donor and the recipient; either the component is antigenic to the recipient or the plasma contains an antibody reacting with a recipient antigen. There may be physico-chemical characteristics of the plasma component, such as temperature, additives, alterations due to preparative processes, and accumulation of metabolites or cellular release products on storage. Clinical severity may range from minor urticarial reactions or flushing to fulminant cardiorespiratory collapse and death. Many such reactions are probably true anaphylaxis, but in others, mechanisms have been less clear, and the term *anaphylactoid* has been used.

Immunologic reactions to normal components of plasma may occur in two ways. First, plasma proteins may contain epitopes different from those on the recipient's functionally identical plasma proteins (e.g., anti–immunoglobin A [IgA] antibodies). Second, there may be antibodies in the donor plasma that react with cellular components of the recipient's blood cells or plasma proteins (e.g., transfusion-related lung injury).

Various contaminants in donor plasma or plasma components, related to the fractionation process, may be implicated in some reactions. Processing of plasma and its freezing may lead to activation of some of the proteolytic systems. Of particular importance in this respect are the complement and the kinin/kininogen systems. If these systems are activated, there may be generation of vasoactive substances and anaphylotoxins. Subjective sensations that may be missed in an unconscious patient and hypotension occurring during rapid infusion of a hypovolemic patient may be misinterpreted as further volume loss. Histamine levels may be increased in stored blood components, and histamine levels may correlate with nonfebrile, nonhemolytic transfusion reactions.

TRANSFUSION-RELATED ACUTE LUNG INJURY

Transfusion-related acute lung injury is a potentially fulminant complication of blood transfusion, characterized by acute respiratory distress arising within hours of a transfusion.[19,20] Most patients who are well resuscitated improve within 48 hours and usually make a full recovery. The pathophysiology of transfusion-related lung injury is classically due to the presence of leukoagglutinating or human leukocyte antigen (HLA)-specific antibodies in the plasma of the donor of the implicated components. When complement is activated, C5a promotes neutrophil aggregation and sequestration in the lung microvasculature causing endothelial damage. The concept of transfusion-related lung injury has been expanded to embrace a broader spectrum of acute lung injury after transfusion to include cases of post-transfusion lung injury in which other mechanisms may be responsible (e.g., anaphylactic reactions, cytokine reactions, platelet reactions, granulocyte transfusions, poorly stored blood). The patient's lungs may be "primed" by other pathologic factors, and transfusion becomes an additional risk factor.

POST-TRANSFUSION PURPURA

Post-transfusion purpura is a potentially life-threatening complication of transfusion in which platelet-specific alloantibodies develop at 5 to 10 days with the patient developing severe thrombocytopenia.[21] Paradoxically, in contrast to other immunologically mediated transfusion reactions, the patient's own platelets are destroyed during the immunologic reaction. Early recognition of this rare complication, which typically occurs in women, is essential to minimize morbidity and mortality. Platelet transfusions are usually ineffective even if crossmatch compatible, and high-dose intravenous immunoglobulin (2 g/kg given over 2 to 5 days) is the recommended treatment.

TRANSFUSION-ASSOCIATED GRAFT-VERSUS-HOST DISEASE

Transfusion-associated graft-versus-host disease is due to the infusion of immunocompetent lymphocytes precipitating an immunologic reaction against the host tissues.[22,23] It is most commonly observed in immunocompromised patients, but also may be seen in recipients of directed blood donation from first-degree relatives and occasionally when donor and recipient are not related due to homozygosity for HLA haplotypes for which the recipient is heterozygous. Transfusion-associated graft-versus-host disease is generally a devastating and fatal condition, with onset of the syndrome 2 to 4 weeks after homologous transfusion with fever, liver function test abnormalities, profuse watery diarrhea, erythematous skin rash, and progressive marrow failure.

TRANSFUSION-RELATED IMMUNOMODULATION

Transfusion-related immunomodulation is an evolving and complex area of research and new knowledge.[24] Leukocytes seem to be the main blood component responsible for the immunomodulatory effects of transfusion. Space does not permit detailed analysis; however, it is likely that prestorage leukodepletion would minimize the effects. Homologous transfusion has been shown to be an independent risk factor for postoperative infection. Many infections are distant from the wound site, suggesting a systemic reduction in host resistance. Immunomodulation also may be responsible for increased cancer recurrence rates after surgery, but this remains under investigation.

FEVER

The term *nonhemolytic febrile transfusion reaction* defines an acute complication of blood transfusion characterized by fever with or without chills and rigors. These reactions are generally not life-threatening, but they cause discomfort; involve the use of medications; and employ resources of medical, nursing, and laboratory personnel. The effects of rigors and pyrexia in critically ill patients are concerning, and temperatures greater than 38°C should not be ignored. Most febrile reactions are due to immunologic reactions against one or more of the transfused cellular or plasma components, usually leukocytes. The use of leukocyte-depleted blood products minimizes the likelihood of nonhemolytic febrile transfusion reaction.

TRANSFUSION-RELATED INFECTIONS

Transfusion-related infections have received much attention ars and have been the drivers for many changed blood donation and processing policies.[25] The reader is referred to detailed references on the infectious complications.[26] Table 167-3 summarizes current risk estimates for important transfusion-transmitted viral infections on the basis of full donor screening.[27]

BACTERIAL CONTAMINATION

Bacterial contamination of stored blood can cause fulminant endotoxic shock.[28] In recent years, the storage of platelets at

TABLE 167–3. RISK OF TRANSFUSION-RELATED INFECTIONS

Hazard	Minimization/prevention	Risk*
Bacterial contamination	Donor selection and collection technique	up to 1 in 80,000
HIV	Donor selection and viral testing	~1:4 × 10⁶
HCV	Donor selection and viral testing	~1:3 × 10⁶
HBV	Donor selection and viral testing	~1:1 × 10⁶
HTLV I and II	Viral testing	~1:1 × 10⁶

*Calman Chart assessment of risk:
High: >1:100 (e.g., transmission of chickenpox to household contacts)
Moderate: 1:100-1:1000 (e.g., smoking 10 cigarettes per day)
Low: 1:1000-1:10,000 (e.g., road accident)
Very low: 1:10,000-1:100,000 (e.g., accident at work)
Minimal: 1:100,000-1:1 million
Negligible: <1 million (e.g., hit by lightning)
HBV, hepatitis B virus; HCV, hepatitis C virus; HIV, human immunodeficiency virus; HTLV, human T-cell lymphotropic virus.

room temperature has made this blood component particularly susceptible to bacterial contamination. The clinical features of transfusion-related endotoxic shock in a nonanesthetized patient include violent chills, fever, tachycardia, and vascular collapse with prominent nausea, vomiting, and diarrhea. Anesthetized patients may have delayed onset of symptoms.

BLOOD STORAGE LESIONS AND POTENTIAL CLINICAL CONSEQUENCES

Blood is altered from the moment of its initial collection and subsequent storage. Physical and biochemical characteristics may be of particular importance when large volumes are infused rapidly. Warming of all rapid blood transfusions should minimize the possibility of hypothermia. Patients receiving massive blood component therapy are likely to be seriously ill and to have multiple problems. Potential adverse effects must be considered in conjunction with the injuries and multiorgan dysfunction. It is not always possible to define complications caused or aggravated by massive blood transfusion.

The storage lesions progressively increase until the time of expiry, and the extent of these changes is determined by the specific blood component, preservative medium, container, storage time, and storage conditions. Storage results in quantitative or qualitative deficiencies (or both) in blood components, which may reduce the efficacy of a transfusion. Quantitative deficiencies may result in reduced RBC survival, failure to achieve anticipated endpoints, and excessive donor exposure, increasing immunization and infection risks. Qualitative deficiency includes decreased membrane flexibility and increased adhesion to endothelium, which may impair microcirculatory hemodynamics. Reduced 2,3-diphosphoglycerate decreases hemoglobin oxygen affinity, impairing oxygen unloading.

In parallel with these storage changes is an accumulation of degenerate material (e.g., microaggregates and procoagulant material), release of vasoactive agents, cytokine generation, and hemolysis (Fig. 167-3). Many of the changes occurring during storage are related to the presence of leukocytes (especially granulocytes) and can be minimized by prestorage leukoreduction. The clinical significance of storage lesions continues to be debated; in some cases, the effects are widely accepted, in others, further studies are needed.[29] There is evidence that the storage lesion is clinically significant in several respects. Transfusion may result in significant increases in unconjugated bilirubin and lactic dehydrogenase, neutrophilia, and saturation of serum iron. The transfusion of biologically active lipids in stored blood may be associated with the development of acute lung injury in patients with predisposing conditions. Blood transfusion has been shown to be an independent risk factor for the development of postinjury multiorgan failure and acute respiratory distress syndrome and this relationship is stronger with the age of the transfused blood. There is an increased rate of infection associated with the transfusion of old blood after severe injury, suggesting that transfusion-related immunomodulation may not be related only to allogeneic transfusion, but contributed to by the storage lesion. Transfusion of stored blood older than 15 days in trauma patients is a predictor of a greater likelihood of admission to the ICU and predicted doubling of the length of stay in the ICU. Further information about the storage lesion and the possible clinical implications is summarized in Table 167-2. The commonly recognized potential hazards of rapid blood transfusion are as follows:

- *Citrate toxicity.* A patient responds to citrate infusion by the removal of citrate and mobilization of ionized calcium. Citrate is metabolized by the Krebs cycle in nucleated cells, especially the liver. A marked elevation in the citrate concentration is seen with transfusions of greater than 500 mL in 5 minutes; the citrate level rapidly falls when infusion is slowed. Citrate metabolism is impaired by hypotension, hypovolemia, hypothermia, and liver disease, and toxicity may be potentiated by alkalosis, hyperkalemia, hypothermia, and cardiac disease. There are many potential consequences of citrate-induced depression of ionized calcium, but a warm, well-perfused adult patient with normal liver function can tolerate a unit of blood every 5 minutes without requiring calcium replacement.

- *Acid-base and electrolyte changes.* Transfusion of stored blood presents a patient with an appreciable acid load, which may be of particular importance if there is a pre-existing metabolic acidosis. The acidity of stored blood is mainly due to the citric acid of the anticoagulant and the lactic acid generated during storage. Their intermediary metabolites are metabolized rapidly with adequate tissue perfusion, ultimately resulting in metabolic alkalosis. The routine use of sodium bicarbonate is unnecessary, and acid-base abnormalities should be corrected only in the context of the clinical situation. Although controversial, it is unlikely that the high serum potassium levels in stored blood have pathologic effects in adults except in the presence of acute renal failure. In contrast, hypokalemia may be a problem 24 hours after massive transfusion as the transfused cells correct their electrolyte composition and potassium returns into the cells. The sodium content of whole blood and fresh frozen plasma is higher than the normal blood levels due to the sodium citrate. This fact should be taken into account when large volumes of plasma are being infused into patients who have disordered salt and water handling (e.g., renal, liver, or cardiac disease).

ACCUMULANTS

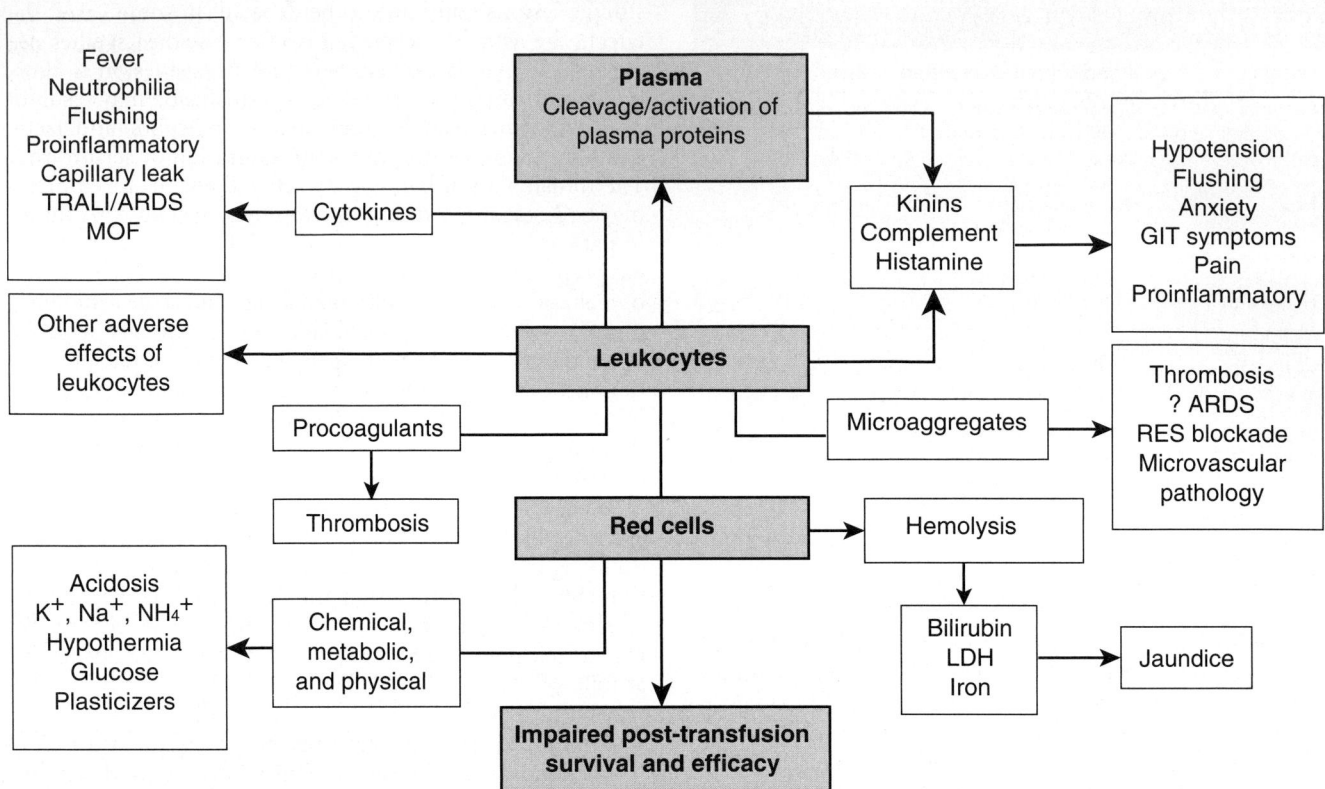

FIGURE 167–3. Red blood cell storage lesions. ARDS, acute respiratory distress syndrome; GIT, gastrointestinal tract; LDH, lactate dehydrogenase; MOF, multiple organ failure; RES, reticuloendothelial system; TRALI, transfusion-related acute lung injury.

HYPERBILIRUBINEMIA

Hyperbilirubinemia is common after massive blood transfusion because a significant proportion of RBCs transfused (30% if aged blood is used) may not survive, and the resulting bilirubin load causes varying degrees of hyperbilirubinemia. If the patient has been hypovolemic and shocked, biliary transport functions may be impaired, particularly in the presence of sepsis or multiorgan dysfunction. An important rate-limiting step in bilirubin transport is the energy-requiring process of transporting conjugated bilirubin from the hepatocyte to the biliary canaliculus. Bilirubin from destroyed transfused RBCs may be conjugated, but delayed excretion may lead to conjugated hyperbilirubinemia. A hemolytic transfusion reaction and resorbing hematoma also need to be considered as possible causes of hyperbilirubinemia.

BASIC IMMUNOHEMATOLOGY

RBC serology is a highly specialized area of knowledge, and it is not possible to expect clinicians to have more than a basic working knowledge essential for patient safety. This section summarizes core knowledge for the clinician.

SALINE AGGLUTINATION

Safe RBC transfusion has revolved around the traditional serologic technique of saline agglutination. A saline suspension of RBCs is mixed with serum and observed for agglutination. Saline agglutination is used for ABO blood grouping and is one of the techniques for compatibility testing of donor blood.

DIRECT AND INDIRECT ANTIGLOBULIN TEST

In RBC serology, the antiglobulin test (Coombs' test) is used to detect IgG immunoglobulins or complement components. The direct antiglobulin test detects immunoglobulin or complement components present on the surface of the RBCs circulating in the patient. The result is positive in autoimmune hemolytic anemia and hemolytic disease of the newborn and during a hemolytic transfusion reaction. The indirect antiglobulin test detects the presence of nonagglutinating antibodies in the patient's plasma, usually IgG type. Antibody screening for atypical antibodies and pretransfusion compatibility testing are the main applications of the indirect antiglobulin test.

REGULAR AND IRREGULAR (ATYPICAL) ANTIBODIES

The regular alloantibodies (isoagglutinins) of the ABO system are naturally occurring agglutinins present in all ABO types (except AB), depending on the ABO group. Group O people have anti-A and anti-B isoagglutinins, group A people have anti-B, and group B people have anti-A. Group A cells cause the most common and most dangerous ABO-incompatible hemolytic reactions. Atypical antibodies are not normally present in the plasma, but may be found in some people as naturally occurring antibodies or as immune antibodies. Immune antibodies result from previous exposure due to blood transfusion or pregnancy. Naturally occurring antibodies more frequently react by saline agglutination, and although they may be stimulated by transfusion, they usually are of minimal clinical significance. In contrast, many of the immune atypical antibodies are of major clinical significance, and their recognition is the raison d'être for pretransfusion compatibility testing and antenatal antibody screening. Most clinically significant immune atypical antibodies are detected by the indirect antiglobulin test. Blood group antigens vary widely in frequency and immunogenicity. The D antigen of the Rhesus (Rh) blood group system is common and highly immunogenic. When an Rh-negative (i.e., D-negative) patient is exposed to D-positive blood, there is a high likelihood of forming an anti-D antibody. For this reason, the D antigen is taken into account when providing blood for transfusion, in contrast to the numerous other RBC antigens that are less common or less immunogenic. Beyond the Rh (D), and sometimes the Kell (K) blood group antigens, it is not practical, or necessary, to take notice of other blood group antigens, unless an atypical antibody is detected during antibody screening procedures.

ANTIBODY SCREEN

On receipt of a blood sample by the transfusion service, the RBCs are ABO and Rh D typed, and the serum is screened for atypical antibodies. This screen consists of testing the patient's serum with group O screening cells. The screening panel consists of RBCs obtained usually from two group O donors containing all common RBC antigens occurring with a frequency of greater than approximately 2% in the community. If an atypical antibody is detected on the antibody screen, further serologic investigations are done to identify the specificity of the antibody. These investigations are time-consuming and when possible should be carried out electively.

CROSSMATCH (COMPATIBILITY TEST)

The crossmatch is the final compatibility test between the donor cells and the patient's serum. The crossmatch test tends to be overemphasized to the detriment of the antibody screen. With sophisticated knowledge of serology, the emphasis in the supply of compatible blood is now concentrated on the steps before the final compatibility crossmatch.

TYPE AND SCREEN SYSTEM

As precompatibility testing has assumed the major role in the selection of blood for transfusion, there has been a rethinking of policies relating to the supply of blood for elective transfusions. Whenever elective surgery is planned for a patient who is likely to require blood transfusion, the transfusion service must receive a clotted blood sample well before the anticipated time of surgery. The precompatibility testing should be carried out during routine working hours when facilities are geared for large workloads and enough staff are available to handle all contingencies.

PROVISION OF BLOOD IN EMERGENCIES

When quick clinical and laboratory decisions are made under conditions of stress, it is frequently difficult for all involved personnel to appreciate the difficulties of others. The decision to give uncrossmatched or partially crossmatched blood or to wait for crossmatch-compatible blood is not easy, and certain basic serologic considerations may clarify for the clinician some of the problems faced by the serologist. Depending on the degree of urgency and the extent of previous knowledge about the patient's RBC serology, blood can be provided with varying degrees of safety. When a patient is exsanguinating and likely to die, however, the giving of ABO-compatible, uncrossmatched blood, especially if the antibody screen is negative, is safe and appropriate therapy.

UNIVERSAL DONOR GROUP O BLOOD

Group O blood under normal circumstances is ABO compatible with all recipients. The transfusions should be given as RBC concentrates screened for high-titer A or B hemolysins and used only in extreme emergencies. If the recipient is of childbearing age, every attempt should be made to give Rh D-negative blood until the patient's blood group is known.

ABO GROUP–SPECIFIC BLOOD

Transfusion of blood of the correct ABO type circumvents the isoagglutinin problems alluded to earlier. Simple as this approach may seem, its safety depends on meticulous attention to grouping. Previous blood group information, such as a "bracelet" group or "unofficial" group written in the patient's records, may be incorrect, and there may be considerable risk if blood is administered on the basis of this information alone.

SALINE-COMPATIBLE BLOOD

The administration of saline-compatible blood is, for practical purposes, the administration of ABO group–specific blood.

ANNOTATED REFERENCES

Isbister JP: Decision making in perioperative transfusion. Transfus Apheresis Sci 2002;27:19-28.
> This papers reviews in detail the transfusion decision making process, overviewing all the interacting factors needing consideration when assessing the need for transfusion of blood components

Isbister JP: Is the clinical significance of blood storage lesions underestimated? Transfus Altern Transfus Med 2003;5:356-362.
> The importance of the blood storage lesion and its clinical consequences are increasingly recognized. Studies are establishing clinical significance in relation to morbidity, mortality and increased length of hospital stay. This paper reviews the current laboratory and clinical evidence for the storage lesion.

Kovesi T, Royston D: Pharmacological approaches to reducing allogeneic blood exposure. Vox Sang 2003;84:2-10.
> There are many pharmacologic approaches to minimizing blood loss and reducing the need for transfusion. This paper is a comprehensive review of the methods available.

Martyn V, Farmer SL, Wren MN, et al: The theory and practice of bloodless surgery. Transfus Apheresis Sci 2002;27:29-43.
> This review from an experienced blood conservation team summarizes comprehensively and systematically an approach to minimizing homologous blood transfusion.

Silliman CC, Boshkov LK, Mehdizadehkashi Z, et al: Transfusion-related acute lung injury: Epidemiology and a prospective analysis of etiologic factors. Blood 2003;101:454-462.
> The important complication of transfusion related lung injury (TRALI) is receiving increasing attention. This group has been making major contributions in this area that are presented in this important paper, which is recommended as a starting point for studying TRALI.

Chapter 168

MANAGEMENT OF NEUTROPENIC CANCER PATIENTS

Michaël Darmon • Élie Azoulay

KEY POINTS

1. Patient selection for ICU admission is based on the clinical status of the patient and on available treatment options for the malignancy. By working together, oncologists and intensivists can arrange for early ICU admission, before multiple organ failure develops.

2. The number of organ failures at ICU admission is the cornerstone of the prognostic evaluation in neutropenic patients. Together with shock, acute respiratory failure is the most common organ failure leading to ICU admission of neutropenic patients.

3. Neutropenia diminishes the ability to ward off infectious agents. Low neutrophil counts are associated with risk: the lower the count, the greater the risk. Infections are far more likely to occur when the count declines to less than 500/mm³. Duration of neutropenia also influences the rate and severity of infections.

4. High risk of serious infection in neutropenic patients has led to a consensus that probabilistic antibiotic therapy should be given routinely if a fever develops. The antibiotics should be active against gram-positive cocci and gram-negative rods. When the organism is recovered and identified, antimicrobial therapy should be adjusted accordingly.

It is now widely recognized that patients with neutropenia can benefit from admission to the ICU. Among patients with chemotherapy-induced neutropenia, 1% to 5% experience toxic side effects or infections that require ICU management.[1] Three factors have contributed to improved survival in ICU patients with neutropenia: (1) Oncologists and intensivists have made progress in selecting patients likely to benefit from ICU admission,[2,3] (2) the overall survival of cancer patients has improved in recent years,[4] and (3) survival has improved among cancer patients admitted to ICUs.[2,3,5-8] This chapter discusses factors that influence survival in neutropenic patients admitted to the ICU and describes more recent developments in management.

NEUTROPENIC PATIENTS IN THE INTENSIVE CARE UNIT

The outlook for cancer patients requiring ICU admission has long been considered dismal. The concept of *futility* was used to support either denial of ICU admission or treatment limitation decisions after ICU admission of cancer patients with neutropenia or bone marrow transplantation.[9-12] Several more recent studies have shown improved outcomes after ICU admission, however, in the overall population of patients with hematologic malignancies[2,3,6,8] and in patients with neutropenia or after autologous bone marrow transplantation.[5,13,14]

Several factors have contributed to improve the survival of neutropenic cancer patients admitted to the ICU:

- Better selection of patients likely to benefit from ICU admission has been achieved via close cooperation between oncologists and intensivists.[2] Selection is based on the clinical status of the patient and on available treatment options for the malignancy. By working together, oncologists and intensivists can arrange for early ICU admission, before multiple organ failure develops.

- Overall survival has improved in recent years in patients with hematologic or solid malignancies. The reasons include the introduction of new treatments,[15-17] advances in the management of treatment side effects,[18,19] and development of new ways to use existing treatments.

- Advances have been made in the life-supporting treatments used to manage cancer patients in the ICU. Two studies have established the benefits of noninvasive mechanical ventilation, which was independently associated with better survival in patients requiring respiratory support.[3,20] Survival rates in patients with septic shock have climbed steadily over the years.[7] The diagnostic benefits provided by widespread use of bronchoscopy and bronchoalveolar lavage in ICU patients with acute respiratory failure[21] have improved the survival of cancer patients in this setting.[22-24]

The number of organ failures at ICU admission is the cornerstone of the prognostic evaluation in neutropenic patients. The proliferative potential and other characteristics of the underlying malignancy seem to have a far smaller impact on survival.[25-27] Widely used physiologic scores (Simplified Acute Physiology Score II and Acute Physiology and Chronic Health Evaluation II)[28] are of limited assistance for several reasons: (1) They are intended for evaluating patient groups and do not perform well in the individual patient. (2) Although they have been validated in cancer patients, their calibration and discrimination for predicting survival are poor in this subset of patients. (3) The prognosis in cancer patients admitted to the ICU is not related to physiologic variables, but rather to organ failures and organ support therapies. The number of organ failures at ICU admission and, to an even greater extent, the time course of organ failures during the first few ICU days govern the chances for survival.[7,29] Finally, although bone marrow transplantation has been recorded to be of adverse prognostic significance in many studies,[10,30,31] these studies failed to separate autologous from allogeneic bone marrow transplant recipients or bone marrow transplant recipients from patients given "peripheral" hematopoietic stem cells (i.e., cells collected after mobilization out of the marrow). Allogeneic bone marrow transplant recipients who require ICU management have extremely high mortality rates in our experience[32] and in studies by other groups,[33] and mortality is highest when the need for life-supporting treatment arises late after the transplantation procedure.[31] Allogeneic bone marrow transplantation differs from autologous bone marrow transplantation in important ways, including the risk of graft-versus-host disease and the intensity of the immunosuppressive treatment required for this complication.

MANAGEMENT OF NEUTROPENIC CANCER PATIENTS IN THE INTENSIVE CARE UNIT

IMMUNODEFICIENCY

Vulnerability to infections occurs in cancer patients for several reasons. Neutropenia diminishes the ability to ward off infectious agents. Neutrophil counts less than 1000/mm³

are associated with a significant risk, and the lower the count, the greater the risk[34]; infections are far more likely to occur when counts fall to less than 500/mm³, and a further risk increase is noted at counts less than 100/mm³. The duration of neutropenia also influences the rate and severity of infections.[35]

Qualitative abnormalities in the functions of neutrophils, phagocytes, and lymphocytes contribute to the susceptibility of cancer patients to infection. An increased risk of infection by intracellular agents occurs in patients with hairy cell leukemia or T-cell acute lymphoblastic leukemia and in association with specific treatment agents.

FEVER

The high risk of serious infection in neutropenic patients has led to a consensus that probabilistic antibiotic therapy should be given routinely if a fever develops. The antibiotics should be active against gram-positive cocci (e.g., streptococci infecting mucositis lesions or staphylococci in intravascular catheters) and gram-negative rods (enterobacteria or *Pseudomonas aeruginosa*) (Table 168–1). The Infectious Diseases Society of America has updated its recommendations.[36] A good first-line regimen in an ICU patient with prolonged neutropenia (as often occurs in hematologic malignancies) is a penicillin that is active against *P. aeruginosa* and gram-positive cocci given in combination with either an aminoglycoside or a fluoroquinolone active against *P. aeruginosa*. Although not given routinely, vancomycin usually is added because many neutropenic ICU patients meet Infectious Diseases Society of America criteria for introducing a glycopeptide. These criteria include suspected catheter-associated infection, methicillin-resistant *Staphylococcus aureus* colonization, gram-positive cocci in blood cultures before identification of the organism, shock, and two situations associated with infection by gram-positive cocci—grade III or IV mucositis and abrupt body

TABLE 168–1. CLINICAL SEPSIS WITH BACTERIAL IDENTIFICATION IN THE SAINT-LOUIS HOSPITAL COHORT*

	All (59), n (%)	Pulmonary Infection, n (%)	Bacteremia, n (%)	Gastrointestinal Infection, n (%)	CNS Infection, n (%)	Urinary Tract Infection, n (%)
Gram-negative	**27 (45.8%)**	**11/27 (40.7%)**	**10/27 (37%)**	**3/27 (11.1%)**	**1/27 (3.7%)**	**1/27 (3.7%)**
Klebsiella spp.	2 (3.4%)	0	0	0	1	1
Escherichia coli	11 (18.7%)	4	5	2	0	0
Proteus spp.	1 (1.7%)	1	0	0	0	0
Pseudomonas aeruginosa	10 (16.9%)	5	5	0	0	0
Enterobacter spp.	1 (1.7%)	1	0	0	0	0
Acinetobacter spp.	1 (1.7%)	0	0	1	0	0
Stenotrophomonas maltophilia	1 (1.7%)	0	0	0	0	0
Gram-positive	**21 (35.6%)**	**12/21 (57.1%)**	**8/21 (38.1%)**	**1/21 (4.8%)**	**1/21 (4.8%)**	**0**
Staphylococcus spp.	10 (16.9%)	4	6	0	0	0
Corynebacterium spp.	1 (1.7%)	1	0	0	0	0
Streptococcus spp.	4 (6.8%)	2	1	0	0	0
Streptococcus pneumoniae	3 (5.1%)	2	0	0	1	0
Enterococcus spp.	2 (3.4%)	1	1	0	0	0
Clostridium difficile	1 (1.7%)	0	0	1	0	0
Miscellaneous	**11 (18.6%)**	**10/11 (90.1%)**	**0**	**0**	**1/11 (8.9%)**	**0**
Aspergillus	7 (11.8%)	7	0	0	0	0
Histoplasma capsulatum	1 (1.7%)	1	0	0	0	0
Epstein-Barr virus	1 (1.7%)	0	0	0	1	0
Cytomegalovirus	1 (1.7%)	1	0	0	0	0
Respiratory syncytial virus	1 (1.7%)	1	0	0	0	0
		33/59 (55.9%)	18/59 (30.5%)	4/59 (6.8%)	3/59 (5.1%)	1/59 (1.7%)

*Among 82 neutropenic patients with sepsis, 59 bacterial identifications were documented in 55 patients.
CNS, central nervous system.

temperature elevation to greater than 40°C.[36] Fluconazole, 400 mg/d, as prophylactic treatment of fungal infections, has been found to be beneficial only in allogeneic bone marrow transplant recipients.[18] After 5 to 7 days with febrile neutropenia, the risk of fungal infection (not only *Candida,* but also *Aspergillus*) is sufficiently high to warrant routine antifungal therapy in combination with antibacterial agents. In our ICU, we use amphotericin B as the first-line drug. Finally, the need for antiviral agents or trimethoprim-sulfamethoxazole should be evaluated on a case-by-case basis according to patient-related factors and to the clinical picture.[36] Initiation of treatment for herpesvirus infection should be considered in all patients with grade III or IV mucositis.

When the organism is recovered and identified, antimicrobial therapy should be adjusted accordingly. ICU patients whose body temperature returns to normal on the third treatment day but who have negative tests for causative organisms should continue to receive antibiotics until their blood cell counts return to normal.[36]

The cause of the fever should be looked for on chest radiographs, blood cultures, urine sediment and cultures, and stool cultures with tests for *Clostridium difficile* in patients with diarrhea or a high risk of infection with this agent (including patients with hematologic disease). The herpes consensus polymerase chain reaction test and a serum *Aspergillus* antigen assay should be done once or twice a week in patients who have been neutropenic for longer than 1 week.

HEMATOPOIETIC GROWTH FACTORS

Among available hematopoietic growth factors, granulocyte colony-stimulating factor (G-CSF) is the most widely used in patients with hematologic or solid malignancies. G-CSF increases neutrophil counts and enhances neutrophil functions. In non-ICU patients, G-CSF has been shown to decrease the duration of neutropenia, reducing the rate of serious infections.[37,38] G-CSF also decreased mortality related to bone marrow transplantation complications[39] or dose-intensive chemotherapy.[40]

Intensivists and hematologists place considerable emphasis on correcting neutropenia. Nevertheless, neutropenia recovery during the ICU stay was not associated with better survival in a study conducted at our institution.[13] G-CSF therapy was associated with more prompt recovery from neutropenia. This important finding from a statistical model

appropriate for the time dependency of neutropenia recovery contradicted two earlier studies in which G-CSF provided no benefits in ICU patients (Table 168-2).[41,42] G-CSF should be given to all neutropenic ICU patients in whom neutropenia recovery can be expected to occur within 7 days.[43] Examination of a bone marrow smear has been suggested as a more accurate tool for predicting the time to neutropenia recovery but is not performed routinely in patients given standard chemotherapy regimens. A bone marrow smear may be useful, however, after dose-intensive chemotherapy with bone marrow transplantation or after the first induction course for leukemia. G-CSF can stimulate the leukemic clone in patients receiving induction chemotherapy for acute leukemia and is contraindicated in this setting.

In contrast, G-CSF is given to nearly every patient with malignant Hodgkin's or non-Hodgkin's lymphoma. Close monitoring is needed in patients with respiratory symptoms or lung infiltrates before neutropenia recovery. It is imperative that G-CSF be discontinued as soon as bone marrow function improves (neutrophils >500/mm^3).[44] G-CSF can be given intravenously or subcutaneously; in the ICU, the simplest method is to use the venous line. Dosages recommended for adults are 10 μg/kg/d for filgrastim and 150 μg/m^2/d for lenograstim; however, the optimal dosages in ICU patients have not been determined. The daily dose is given as a single injection. No dosage adjustment is required in patients with kidney dysfunction. Blood cell counts should be obtained daily, and the G-CSF should be stopped as soon as the leukocyte count increases to greater than 1000/mm^3, or the neutrophil count increases to greater than 500/mm^3.

ISOLATION MODALITIES

Protective isolation involves reducing the patient's exposure to potentially infective microorganisms via geographic measures and technical measures (routine use of nonsterile gloves, gown, head covering, mask, and, in some cases, overshoes). Because the gut lumen is a reservoir for bacteria that can cause bacteremia, selective digestive decontamination was added to isolation measures in many studies. In our ICU, we use oral colimycin capsules and oral amphotericin B. Efficacy data on these regimens come from old and methodologically flawed studies that often produced conflicting results. No data are available on neutropenic ICU patients.

TABLE 168–2. COMPARISON OF STUDIES EVALUATING THE IMPACT OF COLONY-STIMULATING FACTORS ON OUTCOME OF NEUTROPENIC PATIENTS IN THE ICU

	Bouchama et al[41]		Gruson et al[42]		Darmon et al[13]	
Year	1999		2000		2001	
Method	Case-control		Cohort		Cohort	
Multivariate analysis	No		No		Yes*	
	With CSF	*Without CSF*	*With CSF*	*Without CSF*	*With CSF*	*Without CSF*
No. patients	30	30	28/33	33	53	49
Day of fever	Unknown	Unknown	103	72†	Unknown	Unknown
NR (%)	36.6	33.37	25	33.3	71.2	57.2†
Time before NR (days)	7.8 (±1.4)	5.7 (±1.3)	14 (±2.5)	13 (±3.5)	11 (6.7-16.5)	8 (2-16)
ICU survival (%)	23	10	18	18	55	61.5†

*Two models of multivariate analyses were compared, logistic regression and Cox model, in which neutropenia recovery was introduced as a time-dependent variable. In both models, 30-day mortality was the outcome variable of interest.
†P < .05.
CSF, cerebrospinal fluid; NR, neutropenia recovery.

Finally, there is a paucity of studies comparing isolation measures. A combination of geographic isolation with air filtering (laminar flow or high-efficiency particulate-arresting filters), technical isolation (usually involving use of a mask, head covering, and gown, although variations occurred across studies), and selective digestive decontamination has been found to decrease the mortality rate or the infection rate in many prospective and retrospective studies.[45] Although the optimal modalities for protective isolation and their usefulness in the ICU have not been determined, a reasonable approach to the management of neutropenic ICU patients is maximal protective isolation, including geographic isolation with air filtration, technical isolation with at least a mask and gown, and selective digestive decontamination.

SPECIFIC ORGAN FAILURES

ACUTE RESPIRATORY FAILURE

Together with shock, acute respiratory failure is the most common organ failure leading to ICU admission of neutropenic patients.[20] In neutropenic patients, acute respiratory failure often stems from a combination of factors that may be closely intertwined, such as infection and cardiogenic edema or alveolar hemorrhage. The causes of acute respiratory distress in cancer patients can be divided into infectious and noninfectious categories. At least three distinctive features characterize acute respiratory failure in cancer patients: (1) In contradistinction to patients with human immunodeficiency virus–related conditions, only 50% of cancer patients derive diagnostic benefit from bronchoscopy with bronchoalveolar lavage, and the proportion is smaller still in the subsets with neutropenia, bone marrow transplant, or mechanical ventilation. (2) Chances for survival are better when the cause is identified (allowing adjustments in management), a finding that has prompted bronchoalveolar lavage in patients managed with noninvasive mechanical ventilation or a laryngeal mask.[24] (3) Noninvasive diagnostic tools are being developed (e.g., antigen assays in serum and urine and polymerase chain reaction testing for viruses) and, when incorporated into current diagnostic strategies, should enable the noninvasive diagnosis of opportunistic pneumonia,[21] obviating the need for bronchoscopy and protecting the patient from the morbidity associated with this procedure.

SEPTIC SHOCK

Survival rates in cancer patients with septic shock have increased over the years.[7] Earlier treatment is one contributor to this improvement. There is a need for studies evaluating the impact of new management strategies in these patients, who were excluded from large multicenter randomized studies.[46-48]

MACROPHAGE ACTIVATION SYNDROME

Lymphohistiocytic activation syndrome is another name for macrophage activation syndrome, which may develop in a neutropenic patient or cause neutropenia. Multiple organ failure with vasoplegic shock may occur.[49] Fever, thrombocytopenia, and hepatosplenomegaly are almost universally present. Other manifestations include low counts of other cell lines, cholestasis with jaundice, high serum levels of ferritin and triglycerides, and low serum albumin and fibrinogen. Bone marrow smear findings are typical, with activated macrophages phagocytizing platelets, erythrocytes, and leukocytes, although false-positive results are encountered occasionally. Corticosteroids and etoposide are the mainstays of treatment and should be considered on an emergency basis.[50]

TYPHLITIS OR NEUTROPENIA-ASSOCIATED ENTEROCOLITIS

Typhlitis occurs chiefly after dose-intensive chemotherapy and manifests as any combination of abdominal pain, fever, and diarrhea.[34,51] The protean nature of the manifestations raises diagnostic challenges. Typhlitis is probably a multifactorial condition related to chemotherapy-induced colonic mucosal damage, thrombopenia-related bleeding within the colonic wall, and bowel colonization by pathogenic microorganisms.[51] Complications include bacteremia (28% to 82% of typhlitis episodes), gastrointestinal bleeding (65% of patients), and gastrointestinal perforation (5% to 10% of patients).[52] Ultrasonography or computed tomography of the gastrointestinal tract confirms the diagnosis and evaluates the severity of the disease. Computed tomography may show pneumoperitoneum or colonic pneumatosis indicating severe parietal damage with imminent perforation. Bowel wall thickening on ultrasound scan confirms the diagnosis.[53] In a retrospective study, bowel wall thickening was significantly associated with death (29% versus 0%), and mortality was highest when the bowel wall was thicker than 10 mm.[54] Conservative treatment should be used if possible, but surgery remains necessary in patients with life-threatening gastrointestinal bleeding, perforation, or uncontrolled sepsis.[52] A diagnosis of typhlitis requires prior elimination of other abdominal conditions, most notably classic surgical conditions and pseudomembranous colitis.[52]

ACUTE TUMOR LYSIS SYNDROME

Although the onset usually antedates the development of neutropenia by several days, the two problems of acute tumor lysis syndrome and neutropenia frequently are interlinked. The risk of tumor lysis syndrome varies with the tumor burden and with the nature and intensity of induction chemotherapy. Neutropenia develops soon afterward. Although a detailed description of tumor lysis syndrome is beyond the scope of this chapter, five key words come to mind: *Hyperuricemia* stems from the metabolism and lysis of tumor cells and can cause precipitates to form within the renal tubules if the urine is acidic. Recombinant *urate oxidases* (rasburicase) completely prevent this problem, obviating the need for alkalinization.[55] *Hyperphosphatemia* is an absolute contraindication to alkalinization (the risk being nephrocalcinosis related to precipitation) but can be controlled by hyperhydration and *renal support therapy*. *Dehydration* is almost always present and requires volume repletion with nonalkaline isotonic solutions.

CONCLUSION

The last few years have seen improvements in the survival of cancer patients managed in the ICU. Neutropenia no longer indicates a poor prognosis. The type and number of organ failures at ICU admission and their course during the first few days are the main determinants of survival. The potential benefits of early ICU admission need to be evaluated. Similarly, rather than routine denial of ICU admission, neutropenic patients should be allowed as a *therapeutic trial,* in which high-intensity ICU management (with no treatment limitations) is provided for a few days, and the prognosis is then reappraised based on the course of the organ failures to determine whether further aggressive treatment is in order.

ANNOTATED REFERENCES

Brenner H: Long-term survival rates of cancer patients achieved by the end of the 20th century: A period analysis. Lancet 2002;360:1131-1135.

Analysis of the Surveillance, Epidemiology, and End Results Database, of the United States National Cancer Institute, over a 25-year period. This study confirms the improvement in long-term survival rates of cancer patients and gives an estimation of 5-year, 10-year, 15-year, and 20-year relative survival rates for many types of cancer.

Darmon M, Azoulay E, Alberti C, et al: Impact of neutropenia duration on short-term mortality in neutropenic critically ill cancer patients. Intensive Care Med 2002;28:1775-1780.

This study confirms that organ failure, not disease progression or neutropenia duration, affects 30-day mortality of neutropenic, critically ill cancer patients.

Hughes WT, Armstrong D, Bodey GP, et al: 2002 guidelines for the use of antimicrobial agents in neutropenic patients with cancer. Clin Infect Dis 2002;34:730-751.

This article, prepared by the Infectious Diseases Society of America (IDSA) Fever and Neutropenia Guidelines Panel, updates the guidelines published in 1997 by the IDSA.

Larche J, Azoulay E, Fieux F, et al: Improved survival of critically ill cancer patients with septic shock. Intensive Care Med 2003;29:1688-1695.

Study demonstrating an improvement of the 30-day survival of critically ill cancer patients with septic shock over time.

Massion PB, Dive AM, Doyen C, et al: Prognosis of hematologic malignancies does not predict intensive care unit mortality. Crit Care Med 2002;30:2260-2270.

Observational study over a 10-year period concluding that severity of the underlying hematologic malignancies does not influence intensive care unit or hospital mortality of critically ill cancer patients but may affect 6-month mortality.

Chapter 169

VENOUS THROMBOEMBOLISM IN MEDICAL-SURGICAL CRITICALLY ILL PATIENTS

Deborah J. Cook • Mark A. Crowther

KEY POINTS

1. Venous thromboembolism is a multicausal disease, and critically ill medical-surgical patients have many baseline and time-dependent venous thromboembolism risk factors.

2. The true frequency of deep vein thrombosis and pulmonary embolism in critically ill patients is unclear, but likely to be substantial.

3. Unrecognized venous thromboembolism is likely to be associated with significant complications, including death, prolonged need for ventilation, and prolonged hospital and ICU stay.

4. The test of choice for the diagnosis of deep vein thrombosis in the ICU is compression ultrasonography because it is easy to perform at the patient's bedside, and it has been shown in symptomatic outpatients to be sensitive and specific for acute deep vein thrombosis.

5. Large randomized clinical trials are required to determine which types of thromboprophylaxis are most effective and cost-effective in medical-surgical ICU patients. Results of these trials would need active implementation strategies to ensure that they are used appropriately and safely in practice, individualized according to each patient's thrombosis and bleeding risks.

Venous thromboembolism is a common complication of serious illness, conferring considerable morbidity and mortality in hospitalized patients. Patients with deep vein thrombosis are at risk of subsequently developing pulmonary embolism, which may be fatal if untreated. Approximately 90% of cases of pulmonary embolism are believed to arise in the lower limbs[1] so that deep vein thrombosis can be viewed as an important precursor to more serious disease. Most clinical research on venous thromboembolism in the ICU is focused on deep vein thrombosis, and deep vein thrombosis is a major focus of this chapter.

In the ICU, patients with deep vein thrombosis are significantly more likely to have pulmonary embolism,[2] and patients with deep vein thrombosis have a longer duration of mechanical ventilation ($P = .02$), ICU stay ($P = .005$), and hospitalization ($P < .001$) than patients without deep vein thrombosis.[3] Clinically unsuspected deep vein thrombosis and pulmonary embolism are found frequently at autopsy in critically ill patients.[4-6]

Increased attention has focused on the risk factors, prevalence, incidence, clinical importance, and prevention of venous thromboembolism in critically ill patients in the ICU. Concerns have arisen for several reasons: (1) ICU patients have multiple predispositions to venous thromboembolism, including acute severe inflammatory conditions that affect the coagulation cascade and major and minor surgical procedures.[7-9] (2) Critically ill patients rarely can communicate their symptoms, sharply curtailing any possibility that patient self-reported symptoms would prompt intensivists to pursue the diagnosis of venous thromboembolism. (3) The physical examination is devalued in the high-technology critical care environment, and patients with acute venous thromboembolism may not manifest cardinal signs seen in non–critically ill patients, making detection of venous thromboembolism using clinical skills infrequent. (4) The clinical consequences of venous thromboembolism may be more serious in the ICU because of the decreased cardiorespiratory reserve of critically ill patients, which makes it less likely that they would tolerate pulmonary embolism, which in healthy patients would not lead to clinical sequelae.[10] (5) When screening ultrasound studies are conducted in heterogeneous ICU patients, deep vein thrombosis is diagnosed frequently, despite the infrequent clinical detection.[11]

Prophylaxis against venous thromboembolism was rated the number one patient safety initiative for hospitalized patients in the US Agency for Health Care Policy Research Evidence Report and Technology Assessment document.[12] Juxtaposed against the foregoing is the invisibility of medical-surgical critically ill patients in publications such as the National Institutes of Health Consensus Conference on Prevention of Venous Thrombosis and Pulmonary Embolism,[13] the European Consensus Statement on Prevention of Venous Thromboembolism,[14] the Thromboembolic Risk Factors Consensus Conference,[15] the Fifth American College of Chest Physicians Antithrombotic Consensus Conference,[16] and the American Thoracic Society Clinical Practice Guideline on Diagnosis of Venous Thromboembolism.[17] An editorial in 1998 stated that the medical-surgical ICU was "the last frontier for prophylaxis."[18]

RISK FACTORS FOR VENOUS THROMBOEMBOLISM IN MEDICAL-SURGICAL INTENSIVE CARE UNIT PATIENTS

Established risk factors for venous thromboembolism can be classified broadly under the framework of stasis, vascular injury, and congenital and acquired hypercoagulable states. This section presents evidence categorizing risk factors as (1) conventional clinical risk factors, (2) congenital hypercoagulable states, and (3) acquired hypercoagulable states based on thrombophilic markers.

CLINICAL RISK FACTORS

One conceptualization of risk factors for venous thromboembolism in the ICU is to consider ICU admitting diagnosis as a risk factor. Medical-surgical ICU patients are at higher risk of venous thromboembolism than general medical or surgical patients cared for on the ward, but at lower risk than other subgroups of critically ill patients, such as trauma victims or neurosurgical patients (Fig. 169-1). In the largest prospective cohort study using venographic diagnosis, of 716 trauma patients who did not receive prophylaxis, 201 (58%) had deep vein thrombosis between days 14 and 21, one third of which were in the proximal venous circulation (and likely of clinical significance).[19] Of these 201 patients, only 3 patients had symptoms of deep vein thrombosis. Among neurosurgical patients, in three cohort studies using radioactive iodine leg scanning, the deep vein thrombosis rate was 35% without prophylaxis; in seven randomized clinical trials that included a nonprophylaxis arm, the pooled incidence of deep vein thrombosis was 22%.[7] Patients with acute spinal cord injury have been evaluated in four randomized trials and six cohort studies, five of which did not use prophylaxis.[7] Four studies using either radioactive iodine fibrinogen or impedance plethysmography identified deep vein thrombosis

in 39% to 90% of patients. In the single study using the reference standard for the diagnosis of deep vein thrombosis, which is ascending venography, 81% of the subgroup of trauma patients with spinal cord injury had deep vein thrombosis.[19]

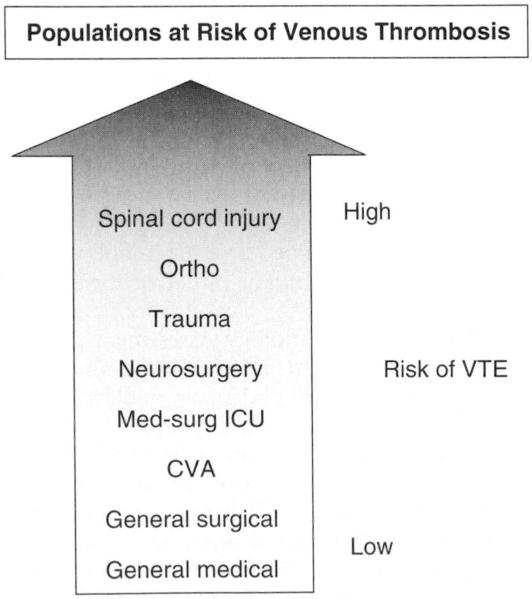

Another conceptualization of risk factors for venous thromboembolism in the ICU is to consider patient characteristics, events, and exposures that increase the risk of venous thromboembolism. Critically ill patients have an increased risk of venous thromboembolism due acute and chronic illnesses, immobility propagated by sedatives and paralytic drugs, and thrombin-generating invasive procedures. Observational studies in medical-surgical ICU patients have identified venous thromboembolism risk factors,[11,20] including patient demographics (e.g., female sex), prior venous thromboembolism events (i.e., personal history of venous thromboembolism), morbidity (e.g., malignancy), ICU procedures (e.g., central venous catheters), treatments (e.g., mechanical ventilation), and venous thromboembolism prophylaxis (i.e., decreasing risk). Inferences about many of these risk factors are limited due to small sample sizes and infrequent use of multiple logistic regression to evaluate rigorously baseline and time-dependent risk factors.

Studies large enough to perform multivariate analysis are most helpful.[2,3,21,22] In a prospective cohort study of patients ventilated for at least 1 week, the only independent risk factor for venous thromboembolism was central venous catheterization; each day that the catheter was in place was associated with a relative risk increase of 1.04.[2] In another prospective cohort study,[3] we enrolled consecutive medical-surgical patients 18 years old or older expected to be in the ICU for 72 hours or more. Exclusion criteria were an admitting diagnosis of trauma, orthopedic surgery, pregnancy, and life-support withdrawal. We performed bilateral lower extremity compression ultrasound within 48 hours of ICU admission, twice weekly, and if venous thromboembolism was clinically suspected. Thromboprophylaxis was protocol-directed and universal using ultrafractionated heparin. We recorded deep vein thrombosis risk factors at baseline and daily, using multivariate regression analysis to determine independent predictors. Patients were followed to hospital discharge. Among 261 patients with a mean Acute Physiology, Age, and Chronic Health Evaluation (APACHE) II score of 26, we identified four independent risk factors for ICU-acquired deep vein thrombosis: personal or family history of venous thromboembolism (hazard ratio 3.9; 95% confidence interval [CI] 1.5 to 10), end-stage renal failure (hazard ratio 3.7; 95% CI 1.3 to 11.2), platelet transfusion (hazard ratio 3.2; 95% CI 1.2 to 8.5), and vasopressor use (hazard ratio 2.8; 95% CI 1.1 to 7.2).

CONGENITAL HYPERCOAGULABLE STATES

A growing number of epidemiologic studies have highlighted how inherited and acquired abnormalities in the coagulation system predispose to venous thromboembolism. Activated protein C resistance due to factor V Leiden is the most common hereditary biochemical defect that predisposes to venous thrombosis, found in 5% of the population, followed by the prothrombin 20210A regulatory sequence mutation, found in 2%.[23-25] Although the impact of these prothrombotic states on the risk of venous thromboembolism is confounded by the use of prophylactic anticoagulants, there is some evidence that these states increase the risk of first deep vein thrombosis in patients in high-risk clinical situations. Lowe and colleagues,[26] in a large prospective cohort study of patients undergoing elective hip replacement, found

Populations at Risk of Venous Thrombosis

Spinal cord injury	High
Ortho	
Trauma	
Neurosurgery	Risk of VTE
Med-surg ICU	
CVA	
General surgical	Low
General medical	

FIGURE 169–1. The underlying population risk of venous thromboembolism (VTE) in hospitalized patients. Medical-surgical ICU patients have a midrange risk of venous thromboembolism, higher than ward patients with medical or surgical problems and lower than patients with spinal cord injury or trauma. (CVA, cerebrovascular accident.)

in a univariate analysis that patients with the factor V Leiden mutation had an increased risk of postoperative venous thrombosis. No large-scale studies have yet reported on the incremental risk of deep vein thrombosis in high-risk situations for patients with factor V Leiden; however, it is known that the prothrombin gene mutation predicts deep vein thrombosis in otherwise healthy outpatients (odds ratio [OR] 2.8).[27] Additional, but less common, inherited hypercoagulable states include deficiencies of antithrombin, protein C, and protein S, each of which is a naturally occurring anticoagulant protein. The ORs for venous thrombosis are 8.1 to 13.7 for antithrombin deficiency, 7.3 to 11.9 for protein C deficiency, and 8.5 to 10 for protein S deficiency.[28-30] Antiphospholipid antibodies, including the lupus anticoagulant and anticardiolipin antibody, are strong predictors of first and recurrent venous thrombosis. Elevations in the levels of homocysteine and coagulation factors VIII, IX, and XI also predispose to venous thromboembolism in other settings.[31-35]

In the observational study described earlier, we evaluated the frequency and clinical importance of thrombophilia markers at the time of ICU admission and during the ICU stay.[36] To examine whether baseline markers of activation of the coagulation system and known thrombophilic risk factors predicted the development of deep vein thrombosis, a comprehensive battery of tests was done at the time of enrollment, including activated protein C ratio (with confirmation of factor V Leiden where appropriate), protein C level, protein S level, antithrombin level, anticardiolipin antibody titer, and screening and confirmatory assays for the lupus anticoagulant. The receiver operating curves for four baseline coagulation tests at the time of ICU admission showed areas under the curve for each of the activated protein C ratio, antithrombin, protein C, and protein S tests that were not significantly different than 50%; that is, the presence of these abnormalities did predict the presence of deep vein thrombosis at the time of ICU admission. Tests with areas under the curve of 0.75 to 0.80 represent moderate diagnostic power. Baseline coagulation tests also were not useful predictors of deep vein thrombosis developing during the ICU stay.

ACQUIRED HYPERCOAGULABLE STATES

Coagulation abnormalities acquired in the ICU have received considerable attention. Acquired thrombophilic markers associated with thrombosis include lupus anticoagulant, anticardiolipin antibody, and increased levels of homocysteine. In critically ill patients, acquired reductions in the levels of antithrombin, protein C, and protein S due to consumption may be common, and it is possible that these deficiencies are associated with a high risk of venous thromboembolism and other complications of ICU stay, including death. The relationship between the inflammatory and coagulation cascades has been the focus of intense discussion in the sepsis literature.[37] Longitudinal studies have shown that protein C levels in sepsis are inversely correlated with mortality.[38] A randomized trial of recombinant activated protein C in 1690 patients with systematic inflammation and organ dysfunction showed a decrease in 28-day mortality from 30.8% to 24.7% (number needed to treat 16).[39] Approximately 80% of patients had protein C deficiency on entry into the trial, highlighting the prevalence of this acquired thrombophilic marker. The efficacy of recombinant activated protein C was the same, however, in patients with and without protein C deficiency. In another large

randomized trial of antithrombin administration in patients with sepsis, antithrombin levels were less than 60% of normal functional levels in more than 50% of patients, but antithrombin administration did not decrease mortality.[40]

In the study of deep vein thrombosis incidence described earlier,[3] we also evaluated whether quantitative D-dimer tests at the time of ICU admission and during the ICU stay[41] were associated with deep vein thrombosis. At the time of enrollment, twice weekly during the ICU stay, and at the time of any suspected venous thromboembolic events, patients had a battery of D-dimer tests, including whole-blood SimpliRed D-dimer tests and five D-dimer assays performed including D-dimer Plus, IL test DD, MDA-DD, Sigma DD, and Biopool. For the five quantitative baseline D-dimer tests in relation to deep vein thrombosis detected at the time of ICU admission, the areas under the curve for each of D-dimer Plus ($P = .01$), MDA-DD ($P = .002$), and Sigma DD ($P = .054$) were significantly different from .50. The receiver operating curves for time-dependent quantitative D-dimer tests and deep vein thrombosis developing during the ICU stay did not differ from 50%, indicating that D-dimer tests are not useful for predicting the development of venous thromboembolism in the ICU.

SUMMARY

Venous thromboembolism is a multicausal disease.[42] In considering clinical risk factors for venous thromboembolism, it is useful to classify them into risk factors that are fixed, such as admitting diagnoses, and risk factors that are modifiable, such as invasive procedures. Modifiable risk factors can form the basis of venous thromboembolism prevention strategies. Studies to analyze the relative contributions of congenital and acquired thrombophilia markers suggest that these markers are not useful for screening or diagnostic purposes in the ICU.

Awareness of risk factors for venous thromboembolism has at least four consequences. First, these risk factors may increase attention to the problem of venous thromboembolism in the ICU. Second, these risk factors could be used to risk stratify patients to identify patients who should have limited exposure to other venous thromboembolism risk factors (e.g., minimal sedation and short periods of central venous cathetherization). Third, high-risk patients may be considered for intensified venous thromboembolism prevention (e.g., low-molecular-weight heparin prophylaxis). Fourth, high-risk patients may warrant surveillance screening with lower limb ultrasounds.

PREVALENCE AND INCIDENCE OF DEEP VEIN THROMBOSIS IN MEDICAL-SURGICAL INTENSIVE CARE UNIT PATIENTS

The incidence of venous thromboembolism in the ICU depends on whether the events are clinically diagnosed or detected by screening methods. Venous thromboembolism rates observed in usual clinical practice are much lower than the rates observed during systematic screening because the former represent primarily diagnoses prompted by signs or symptoms. For example, 10%[43] to 100%[11,44] of proximal deep vein thromboses found by ultrasound screening were clinically unsuspected. In this section, we report the incidence of venous thromboembolism in critically ill patients based on studies using systematic screening methods for case identification.

Understanding deep vein thrombosis rates requires distinguishing events diagnosed at the time of ICU admission (prevalence at a point in time) from the events that develop over the course of critical illness (incidence over the ICU stay). Cross-sectional studies at the time of admission to a medical ICU[45] and surgical ICU[44] suggest a 10% prevalence of deep vein thrombosis diagnosed by screening compression ultrasonography. As mentioned earlier in the section on risk factors, however, the prevalence of deep vein thrombosis on admission to any ICU is influenced heavily by the case mix of patients.

The risk of deep vein thrombosis developing over the ICU stay was established in three longitudinal studies using systematic screening.[11,43,46] Among ICU patients not receiving prophylaxis, 76% of whom were mechanically ventilated, radioactive iodine fibrinogen scanning for 3 to 6 days identified deep vein thrombosis in 3 of 34 (9%) patients.[46] Using Doppler ultrasound twice weekly then at 1 week after ICU discharge in 100 medical patients expected to stay more than 48 hours, 70% of whom were ventilated, deep vein thrombosis was diagnosed in 32% of 100 patients receiving no prophylaxis, in 40% of patients receiving ultrafractionated heparin, and in 33% of patients who received mechanical prophylaxis.[11] In a third study of 102 medical-surgical ICU patients undergoing duplex ultrasound during days 4 to 7 and as clinically indicated,[43] deep vein thrombosis rates were 25%, 19%, and 7% in patients receiving no prophylaxis, mechanical prevention, and ultrafractionated heparin.

Earlier studies suggest that the prevalence of proximal deep vein thrombosis on admission to a medical-surgical ICU is estimated to be 10%, and the incidence of deep vein thrombosis developing over the ICU stay based on systematic screening ranges from 9% to 40%. Two of these studies performed surveillance for approximately 1 week,[43,46] however, and one study used radioactive iodine fibrinogen scanning for detection,[46] which likely underestimated the risk of ICU-acquired deep vein thrombosis. No studies used systematic screening for pulmonary embolism, and the true incidence of pulmonary embolism is not known.

More recent studies suggest a lower rate of venous thromboembolism in medical-surgical ICU studies, partly due to the administration of thromboprophylaxis. In a single-center cohort of 239 medical ICU patients who did not undergo systematic screening ultrasound, 44 (18.4%) patients had lower extremity deep vein thrombosis.[47] Ibrahim and colleagues,[2] in a cohort study involving twice-weekly upper and lower extremity ultrasound screening, found a 26.6% incidence of deep vein thrombosis. Among 261 patients with a mean APACHE II score of 25.5 (±8.4), the prevalence of deep vein thrombosis was 2.7% (95% CI 1.1 to 5.5) on ICU admission, and the incidence was 9.8% (95% CI 6.5 to 14.2) over the ICU stay.[3]

SUMMARY

The risk of deep vein thrombosis is highest for acute spinal cord injury patients, followed by trauma, neurosurgery, and medical-surgical ICU patients. From observational studies and randomized trials, it can be concluded that critically ill patients have an incidence of deep vein thrombosis that is dependent on (1) whether the event is detected by screening, (2) the diagnostic test method used, and (3) the type of prophylaxis. Specifically, deep vein thrombosis rates are higher among patients undergoing screening compared with patients

who have clinically detected events, among patients undergoing venography compared with patients undergoing compression ultrasound or leg scanning, and among patients not receiving prophylaxis compared with patients who receive it.

DIAGNOSIS OF DEEP VEIN THROMBOSIS IN MEDICAL-SURGICAL INTENSIVE CARE UNIT PATIENTS

A helpful constellation of signs and symptoms in a mathematically derived and validated clinical model has been developed and validated for its prediction of deep vein thrombosis in outpatients.[48] Diagnosing deep vein thrombosis in the ICU is more challenging, however. Symptoms rarely are elicited from mechanically ventilated patients, most of whom receive sedation and analgesia, rendering the notion of symptomatic deep vein thrombosis unhelpful in this setting. Compounding the problem is the fact that physical examination of the lower extremities may be devalued in the high-technology ICU environment compared with cardiopulmonary monitoring. In a survey of Canadian ICU directors, respondents stated that physical examination did not yield information that was helpful in the diagnosis of deep vein thrombosis.[49]

The reference standard for deep vein thrombosis remains ascending contrast lower limb venography, despite its widespread replacement by ultrasonography. Venography is able to detect all clinically important forms of deep vein thrombosis. Venography can reliably detect calf thrombosis, thrombosis in the pelvis, and thrombosis of the muscular veins of the thigh, all of which are not reliably detected by ultrasonography. Despite its utility, venography rarely is performed in practice in the ICU. In a Canadian ICU directors' survey, the use of venography to detect thrombosis was reported rarely (56%) or never (9%).[49] Concern about transporting potentially unstable patients to the radiology department,[50] the invasive nature of the test, and the risk of contrast dye–induced nephropathy[51] may contribute to the aversion to venography in this setting; however, it is also possible that many intensivists are unaware of the limitations of ultrasonography for the diagnosis of deep vein thrombosis. Studies conducted in the 1980s cited contrast nephropathy as the third leading cause of new-onset renal failure in hospitalized patients.[52] Although currently employed nonionic contrast media are associated with a lower rate of nephrotoxicity than ionic contrast media,[53] the volume of contrast administered remains an independent predictor of nephrotoxicity.[54] Additional risk factors for acquired renal insufficiency in medical ICU patients include common problems, such as sepsis, volume depletion, mechanical ventilation, and surgery.[55] The high rate of renal dysfunction in critically ill patients with normal serum creatinine is concerning, and even mild renal insufficiency in these patients is associated with an increased attributable mortality. For patients undergoing venography, intravenous fluid loading before and after the contrast dye and acetylcysteine, 600 mg twice daily by nasogastric tube, the day before and the day after the procedure reduce the rate of contrast-induced nephropathy as shown in a randomized trial.[56]

The test properties of lower extremity bilateral Doppler ultrasound in medical-surgical ICU patients have not been determined. A meta-analysis reported a pooled sensitivity of Doppler ultrasound for proximal deep vein thrombosis in symptomatic patients of 97% (95% CI 96% to 98%) and in asymptomatic patients of 62% (95% CI 53% to 71%).[57] Ultrasound is more insensitive for distal deep vein thrombosis (pooled sensitivity for symptomatic patients, 73% [95% CI 54% to 93%] and asymptomatic patients, 53% [95% CI 32% to 74%]). Symptomatic outpatients with suspected deep vein thrombosis and serially negative screening ultrasound studies have a 1% likelihood of subsequently developing a deep vein thrombosis or pulmonary embolism, suggesting that serially negative ultrasound studies safely and effectively rule out clinically important deep vein thrombosis.[58-60] It is unclear, however, to what extent serially negative ultrasound studies in medical-surgical ICU patients indicate the absence of deep vein thrombosis. Finally, ultrasound also inaccurately diagnoses some patients with deep vein thrombosis who do not have deep vein thrombosis by venogram, highlighting the false-positive rate of ultrasonography. Robinson and colleagues[61] performed ultrasonography and contrast venography in a large group of asymptomatic patients at the time of hospital discharge after joint replacement surgery; in this study, 6 of 19 positive compression ultrasound studies were not confirmed by venography.

Despite the advantages of using ultrasonography to diagnose deep vein thrombosis in the ICU, it is associated with a false-positive and false-negative rate that is not yet clearly established in the critical care setting. Nevertheless, bilateral lower extremity ultrasound is the most widely used diagnostic test for deep vein thrombosis according to venous thromboembolism researchers in the medical-surgical ICU[11,43-46] and according to a survey of radiologists from the United Kingdom.[62] A recent review referred to ultrasonography as the imaging procedure of choice for the diagnosis of deep vein thrombosis.[63] The American College of Radiology cited bilateral lower extremity ultrasound as the most appropriate test for deep vein thrombosis.[64] Finally, bilateral lower limb ultrasound is also the most feasible diagnostic test in the ICU. An ultrasound diagnosis of deep vein thrombosis requires noncompressibility of one or more lower limb venous segments, including (1) the trifurcation of the deep calves, (2) distal popliteal, (3) proximal popliteal, (4) distal femoral, (5) mid femoral, and (6) common femoral veins.

There is no diagnostic test for deep vein thrombosis that is highly accurate and feasible in the ICU population for daily practice. Nevertheless, Doppler ultrasound is the most widely accepted deep vein thrombosis diagnostic test. Because the likelihood of embolization from undiagnosed, untreated proximal deep vein thrombosis is high, strategies that screen for proximal deep vein thrombosis in these critically ill patients have the potential to reduce the risk of pulmonary embolism and its cardiopulmonary consequences through early treatment. Universal screening for deep vein thrombosis with ultrasonography cannot be recommended currently, however.[44,65] Development of a reliable screening test for venous thromboembolism in critically ill patients should be a high clinical priority because it is possible that the most widely used screening test today (ultrasonography) has an unacceptably high rate of false-positive tests. A false-positive ultrasound study is likely to lead to unneeded anticoagulant therapy (with its attendant risks).

THROMBOPROPHYLAXIS IN MEDICAL-SURGICAL INTENSIVE CARE UNIT PATIENTS

Only two published randomized trials have tested deep vein thrombosis prophylaxis in medical-surgical ICU patients.[66,67]

One double-blind, single-center trial allocated 119 medical-surgical ICU patients at least 40 years old to ultrafractionated heparin, 5000 U twice daily, or placebo subcutaneous injections.[66] Using serial fibrinogen leg scanning for 5 days, the rate of deep vein thrombosis was 13% in the ultrafractionated heparin group and 29% in the placebo group (relative risk 0.45, $P < .05$). Rates of bleeding and pulmonary embolism were not reported. In a more recent multicenter trial by Fraisse and colleagues,[67] 223 patients with an acute exacerbation of chronic obstructive pulmonary disease requiring mechanical ventilation for at least 2 days were allocated to the low-molecular-weight heparin nadroparin, 3800 or 5700 IU once daily, or placebo. Patients were screened with weekly duplex ultrasound studies and on clinical suspicion of deep vein thrombosis; venography was attempted in all patients. The rate of deep vein thrombosis was 16% in the nadroparin group and 28% in the placebo group (relative risk 0.67, $P < .05$). A similar number of patients bled in each group (25 versus 18 patients, $P = .18$). Although patients were not screened for pulmonary embolism, no patients developed pulmonary embolism during the trial.

A third trial of some relevance to the ICU enrolled acutely ill medical patients hospitalized with heart failure, respiratory failure not requiring mechanical ventilation, or one of the following if associated with an additional venous thromboembolism risk factor: infection without septic shock, musculoskeletal disorder, or inflammatory bowel disease.[68] Patients were excluded if they required intubation, had a coagulopathy, or had serum creatinine greater than 150 μmol/L. Patients were randomized to receive daily subcutaneous low-molecular-weight heparin enoxaparin, 40 mg or 20 mg, or placebo for 6 to 14 days. Patients had venography between days 6 and 14 or as clinically indicated. Ultrasonography was performed if venography was not feasible. Of 1102 randomized patients, 236 were not included in the main analysis (because the venogram could not be evaluated [n = 72], was technically unfeasible [n = 12], was not performed [n = 4], was not performed at the investigators' discretion [n = 58]; the patient refused [n = 62]; or the patient died [n = 28]). Among the remaining 866 patients, the deep vein thrombosis rate was 6% in patients receiving enoxaparin, 40 mg, compared with 15% among patients receiving either enoxaparin, 20 mg, or placebo (relative risk 0.37). Major hemorrhage developed in 12, 4, and 7 patients ($P =$ not significant). Clinically suspected and objectively confirmed pulmonary embolism developed in one patient in the low-dose enoxaparin group and three patients in the placebo group, although pulmonary embolism events were not evaluated per protocol. The fact that these patients, although requiring medical admission to the hospital, were not critically ill limits the generalizability of these findings to the critical care setting. Nonpharmacologic approaches, such as pneumatic compression devices and antiembolic stockings, although widely used, have not been evaluated in medical-surgical ICU patients, and their effectiveness must be extrapolated from other settings.

SUMMARY

Only two randomized trials evaluating venous thromboembolism prophylaxis in the ICU have been published. One trial of medical-surgical patients showed that ultrafractionated heparin is better than no prevention (the number of patients who needed to receive prophylaxis with 5000 U twice daily of subcutaneous ultrafractionated heparin to prevent one deep vein thrombosis was four).[66] The second trial of exclusively ventilated chronic obstructive pulmonary disease patients showed that nadroparin is better than no prevention (the number of patients who needed to receive prophylaxis with weight-adjusted, low-molecular-weight heparin to prevent one deep vein thrombosis was eight).[68] There are no trials comparing ultrafractionated heparin with low-molecular-weight heparin for venous thromboembolism prophylaxis in medical-surgical ICU patients. In contrast, in trauma patients, low-molecular-weight heparin is clearly superior to ultrafractionated heparin based on randomized trials.[69]

THROMBOPROPHYLAXIS COMPLIANCE IN MEDICAL-SURGICAL INTENSIVE CARE UNIT PATIENTS

Several prospective single-center usage reviews of venous thromboembolism prophylaxis provide evidence about the use of venous thromboembolism prophylaxis in practice. Prophylaxis was prescribed in 33% of 152 medical ICU patients in one study[70] and 61% of 100 medical ICU patients in another.[11] In contrast, in a medical-surgical ICU in which a clinical practice guideline was in place, venous thromboembolism prophylaxis was prescribed for 86% of 209 patients.[71] In another study of medical-surgical ICU patients, after excluding patients receiving therapeutic anticoagulation and for whom heparin was contraindicated, 63% of 96 patients received ultrafractionated heparin thromboprophylaxis.[20]

In a 1-day cross-sectional multicenter usage review of Canadian surgical ICU patients whose procedure was no more than 1 week earlier, ultrafractionated heparin was used predominantly.[72] We considered a range of patients including those with an admission diagnosis of hemorrhage and the potential for immediate postoperative bleeding to highlight the dual risks of thrombosis and bleeding. Two methods of venous thromboembolism prophylaxis were prescribed for 20 of 89 (22.5%) patients. Prophylaxis with ultrafractionated heparin or low-molecular-weight heparin was significantly less likely for postoperative ICU patients requiring mechanical ventilation compared with patients weaned from mechanical ventilation later in their ICU course (OR 0.36, $P = .03$). Use of intermittent pneumatic compression devices was significantly associated with current hemorrhage (OR 13.5, $P = .021$) and risk of future hemorrhage (OR 19.3, $P = .001$).

In a 1-day binational cross-sectional usage review of medical ICU patients in France and Canada,[73] we found that among 1222 patients (65% of whom were mechanically ventilated), heparin venous thromboembolism prophylaxis was administered to 63.9% of patients, similarly between the two countries. Excluding patients with contraindications to heparin and patients receiving therapeutic anticoagulation, 91.7% of medical ICU patients appropriately received either ultrafractionated heparin or low-molecular-weight heparin prophylaxis. Independent predictors of any type of heparin prophylaxis were invasive mechanical ventilation (OR 2.4; 95% CI [1.4 to 4.3]) and obesity (OR 3.1; 95% CI 1.1 to 8.8). Low-molecular-weight heparin was less likely to be prescribed for patients with renal failure (OR 0.1; 95% CI 0.0009 to 0.9) or receiving antiembolic stockings (OR 0.4; 95% CI 0.1 to 0.9) and much more likely to be prescribed in French ICUs (OR 9.2; 95% CI 5 to 16.9); however, among patients receiving low-molecular-weight heparin, high doses were more likely to be prescribed in Canadian ICUs (OR 8.7; 95% CI 2 to 37.6). Patients who were pregnant or postpartum (OR 7.7; 95% CI 1.3 to 44.3), had neurologic failure (OR 2.1; 95% CI 1.3 to 3.4), or were Canadian (OR 3; 95% CI 2.1 to 4.4) were most likely to receive mechanical venous thromboembolism prophylaxis (with antiembolic stockings or pneumatic compression devices), whereas patients who already were receiving heparin were less likely to receive mechanical prophylaxis (OR 0.5; 95% CI 0.3 to 0.7).

SUMMARY

Use of effective venous thromboembolism prophylaxis ranges widely, according to usage reviews. One inference from this health services research is that insufficient attention is paid to venous thromboembolism prevention in the critical care setting. When deciding on the type and intensity of prophylaxis, clinicians seem to risk stratify, in that patients with a greater number of venous thromboembolism risk factors are more likely to receive more intensive prophylaxis than patients with fewer risk factors. The variety of prophylactic approaches used highlights the diverse and dynamic competing risks of bleeding and thrombosis in heterogeneous ICU patients, underscoring population-based and individual risk-to-benefit ratios and delineating the need for large definitive studies to guide prophylaxis. Venous thromboembolism prevention methods should be individualized based on current and potential risks of bleeding and thrombosis. More randomized trials of venous thromboembolism prophylaxis in medical-surgical critically ill medical patients would better inform practice. These trials should be followed up with effective implementation strategies designed to change clinician behavior and improve patient outcomes.[74]

ANNOTATED REFERENCES

AHCRQ Evidence Report/Technology Assessment: Prevention of Venous Thromboembolism After Injury. Rockville, MD, Agency for Health Care Research and Quality, 2002.
> *This is a comprehensive review of thromboprophylaxis and clinical recommendations relevant to the ICU.*

Attia J, Ray JG, Cook DJ, et al: Deep vein thrombosis and its prevention in critically ill patients. Arch Intern Med 2001;161:1268-1279.
> *This is a comprehensive systematic review of the incidence of venous thromboembolism and thromboprophylaxis randomized trials in several types of ICU patients (medical-surgical, trauma, neurosurgical, and spinal cord injury patients).*

Ibrahim EH, Iregui M, Prentice D, et al: Deep vein thrombosis during prolonged mechanical ventilation despite prophylaxis. Crit Care Med 2002;30:771-774.
> *This is a well-conducted cohort study involving ultrasound screening for deep vein thrombosis in ICU patients; incidence and risk factor data are established.*

Kearon CJ, Julian JA, Newman TE, et al: Noninvasive diagnosis of deep vein thrombosis. McMaster Diagnostic Imaging Practice Guidelines Initiative. Ann Intern Med 1998;128:663-677.
> *This is a systematic review of the properties of ultrasonography for the diagnosis of deep vein thrombosis.*

Lacherade JC, Cook DJ, Heyland DK, et al, for the French and Canadian ICU Directors Groups: Prevention of Venous Thromboembolism (VTE) in Critically Ill Medical Patients: A Franco-Canadian cross-sectional study. J Crit Care 2003;18:228-237.
> *This is a Franco-Canadian survey of thromboprophylaxis patterns in medical ICU patients.*

Chapter 170

HEMATOLOGIC MALIGNANCIES IN THE INTENSIVE CARE UNIT

Delphine Moreau • Élie Azoulay • Benoit Schlemmer

KEY POINTS

1. The care of patients diagnosed with acute leukemias or aggressive lymphomas should always be left to highly trained hematologists, but **for some patients admitted with inaugural life-threatening complications, emergency cytotoxic treatment must be initiated by intensivists.**

2. In case of emergency chemotherapy, **appropriate samples of blood, marrow, or lymph nodes should be obtained before chemotherapy is initiated** and stored at room temperature to increase the chances of ultimately reaching a precise diagnosis.

3. Clinical situations requiring urgent treatment are cerebral or pulmonary leukostasis, leukemic infiltration of the lungs, central nervous system involvement, bulky mediastinal involvement with vascular or tracheobronchial compression, threatening disseminated intravascular coagulation (DIC), and severe hemophagocytic syndrome.

4. **All patients with high tumor burden should receive adequate preventive therapy for an acute tumor lysis syndrome** before initiation of the cytotoxic treatment.

5. In hematologic malignancy–related DIC, initiation of the **cytotoxic treatment is often followed by a temporary exacerbation of the coagulation disorder that requires intensive transfusion support.**

6. The use of low-dose heparin in hematologic malignancy–related DIC is not supported by the current literature and therefore cannot be recommended for patients in intensive care.

7. **The clinical presentation of severe lymphoma-related hemophagocytic syndromes can be misleading, mimicking that of septic shock,** but their early recognition is necessary, because a fulminant course is the rule without specific treatment.

With the rapid improvement in chemotherapy and supportive care of hematology patients, almost all hematologic malignancies are potentially curable in children and adults with chemotherapy, either alone or in combination with immunotherapy or radiotherapy and bone marrow transplantation if indicated. If the malignancy is not curable, prolonged remission with excellent quality of life is achievable for most patients. Nevertheless, delay in treatment of some aggressive malignancies can greatly jeopardize the chances of recovery for some acutely ill patients. In addition, intensivists may be confronted with hematologic emergencies, which they must learn to manage adequately.

EMERGENCY MANAGEMENT OF HEMATOLOGIC MALIGNANCIES IN THE INTENSIVE CARE UNIT

EMERGENCY DIAGNOSIS

Emergency diagnosis of a hematologic malignancy is rarely necessary, and most patients with suspected or confirmed hematologic malignancies can be admitted directly to the hematology unit with simple supportive care (e.g., management of febrile neutropenia, transfusion if appropriate). Indeed, the specific care of patients diagnosed with acute leukemias or aggressive lymphomas should always be left to highly trained hematologists. For most of these patients, emergency initiation of induction chemotherapy is not required; chemotherapy can easily be delayed for 1 day or longer, until an attending hematologist and cytologist can be reached and the necessary samples can be drawn and adequately processed.

In rare cases, patients present with life-threatening complications when no attending hematologist is available. Especially for leukemias, one should always try to obtain the following blood and marrow samples to allow for a precise diagnosis (i.e., cytologic characterization of the myeloid or lymphoid lineage, precise subtyping, and immunocytometric studies):

- 15 to 30 mL of peripheral blood (depending on leukocytosis) in heparinized tubes for molecular biology and flow cytometry studies (stored at room temperature)
- Bone marrow smears obtained by sternal or iliac aspiration, air-dried, and stored at room temperature (four to six slides) for cytology and immunohistochemistry studies
- Whenever possible, 1 mL of bone marrow aspirate (heparinized tube) for molecular biology and flow cytometry studies and another 1 mL for karyotyping (growth can be obtained even for some samples stored overnight at room temperature)

- If pleural or peritoneal effusions are accessible or emergency pericardial drainage is performed, a few milliliters of the fluid, stored at room temperature in heparinized tubes
- If superficial lymph nodes are present, a fine-needle aspiration for cytologic examination of smears whenever possible

CLINICAL SITUATIONS REQUIRING URGENT CHEMOTHERAPY

A small number of patients are admitted directly to ICUs with life-threatening complications[1] and require emergency cytotoxic treatment before a specialized attendant can be reached. In these cases, chemotherapy must be initiated by intensivists, then completed and "tailored" according to local protocols by a trained hematologist as soon as possible.

From the intensivist's point of view, emergency chemotherapy may be indicated in seven main clinical situations, independent of the absolute circulating blast counts:

1. Cerebral leukostasis, which should be suspected in the presence of any alteration of consciousness, even a simple slowing down of cognitive functions, once an emergency computed tomography (CT) scan has ruled out an intracranial hemorrhage.
2. Pulmonary leukostasis, which is generally observed in hyperleukocytotic leukemias, with circulating blast counts greater than 30,000 to 50,000/mm³ for acute myeloid leukemia (AML) or greater than 100,000/mm³ by definition for acute lymphoid leukemia (ALL). However, symptomatic leukostasis is very rare in ALL, even for greatly elevated blasts counts, because of the smaller size and higher plasticity of these blasts.
3. Leukemic infiltration of the lungs, which is different from leukostasis, can occur with low blast counts, and is often associated with AML5. These patients should be admitted to the ICU early in the course of their induction, because rapid deterioration of hematosis is frequent, both spontaneously and after initiation of the chemotherapy.[2]
4. Central nervous system (CNS) involvement suspected on the basis of clinical signs, such as focal deficits, seizures, or any degree of alteration of consciousness.[3] Here again, intracranial hemorrhage must first be ruled out by a CT scan.
5. Bulky mediastinal involvement with vascular compression (superior vena cava syndrome) or tracheobronchial repercussion, especially as seen in T-cell ALL.
6. Threatening disseminated intravascular coagulation (DIC) with low fibrinogen levels and a prolonged prothrombin time.
7. Severe hemophagocytic syndrome, with failure of one or more than one organ.

The choice of cytoreductive regimen depends on the type of malignancy, which is not always precisely known on arrival of the patient in the ICU. For acute leukemias, efforts should be made to characterize the lineage (ALL or AML) before treatment is initiated, but if lineage cannot be determined, a non–lineage-specific cytotoxic regimen should be chosen. Intensivists can, therefore, be confronted with five main situations, depending on whether the lineage diagnosis has been established: ALL, AML, promyelocytic leukemia (AML3), acute leukemia of unknown lineage, non-Hodgkin's lymphoma (NHL), and, very rarely, Hodgkin's disease (HD).

EMERGENCY CHEMOTHERAPY IN LEUKEMIAS

ACUTE LYMPHOBLASTIC LEUKEMIA

Classic induction therapy is based on a combination of prednisone, vincristine, and an anthracycline (daunorubicin in most studies), with or without the addition of cyclophosphamide.[4-6] In cases of compressive emergency or high tumor burden, progressive steroid therapy should be prescribed first (beginning with 0.5 mg/kg prednisone for the first dose); patients with high tumor burden should be carefully monitored, because they can rapidly develop a severe acute tumor lysis syndrome (ATLS).[7-10]

The steroid dose should be increased to 1 mg/kg/day prednisolone (or equivalent) 8 to 12 hours after the first dose, in the absence of an uncontrolled ATLS. If ATLS is present, half-dose steroids should be used until metabolic control is regained, and in severe ATLS the second steroid dose could even be postponed. In most cases of ALL, steroids alone will be able to halt the rising white blood cell (WBC) count or to initiate the reduction of bulky mediastinal tumors. On day 2 or 3, full-dose vincristine (1 mg/m² of body surface, with a maximum dose of 2 mg/day) and daunorubicin (30 to 60 mg/m², or equivalent anthracycline) should be added; combination with other drugs will be decided by a hematologist according to local protocols.

For patients with increasing or stagnating WBC counts or without biologic indicators of tumor response for lymphomas (especially increasing lactate dehydrogenase [LDH] levels) after two full doses of steroids, emergency adjunction of vincristine with or without daunorubicin as early as day 2 is required.

ACUTE PROMYELOCYTIC LEUKEMIA

The main complication of acute promyelocytic leukemia (APL) is DIC, with early mortality essentially related to hemorrhages located in the CNS.[11] Nevertheless, although leukostasis in APL is almost never a problem, because these patients are usually pancytopenic, their leukemia should be considered (and treated) as hyperleukocytic APL as soon as the WBC count is higher than 5000/mm³. "Variant" type AML3 can be misleading, because patients are not always cytopenic, but they can display true hyperleukocytosis, sometimes greater than 100,000 cells/mm³.

Although APL is remarkably sensitive to anthracyclines, the emergency treatment of APL with severe coagulation disorder now relies on early administration of all-trans-retinoic acid (ATRA).[12,13] There is no indication for progressive dosing of this drug, which should be prescribed immediately at 45 mg/m²/day in two oral doses taken at 12-hour intervals. Initial worsening of the DIC is the rule, and patients should receive abundant transfusion support to ensure a platelet count greater than 50,000/mm³, and at least 1.5 g/L of fibrinogen at all times. ATRA is available only in sealed, thick-walled, hardly soluble capsules that contain an oil-based solution. No parenteral form is available. Therefore, administration of ATRA is problematic through nasogastric tubes in mechanically ventilated patients; there is currently no other way than piercing the capsule, emptying its content, and carefully resuspending it in oil to allow injection into a gastric tube.

In hyperleukocytic APL, immediate coadministration of ATRA with daunorubicin is required, starting with half the usual dose (20 to 25 mg/m²/day) for at least 4 days, because transient exacerbation of DIC is almost universal.

ACUTE MYELOID LEUKEMIA OTHER THAN PROMYELOCYTIC LEUKEMIA

Urgent induction is derived from the classic reference treatment, a combination of 3 days of an anthracycline (classically daunorubicin, but idarubicin is one of the many possible alternatives), with 7 days of cytarabine.[4,14] The difference is that the scheme of administration is progressive: daunorubicin should be administered alone and at half the usual dose (20 to 25 mg/m²/day for a total of 6 days, equivalent to the 3 days of the standard full-dose regimen) before the continuous infusion of cytarabine (200 mg/m²/day for 7 days) is started on day 3 or 4.

ACUTE LEUKEMIA OF UNDETERMINED LINEAGE

In cases in which the lineage cannot be determined (e.g., no specialized cytologist on duty, poorly differentiated leukemia requiring complementary immunohistochemical study) and the patient requires urgent chemotherapy, then daunorubicin should be chosen, because of its activity on all types of blasts (AML or ALL). In contrast, empirical steroid therapy could be efficient in ALL but not in AML. The scheme of administration would again be half doses of daunorubicin (20 to 25 mg/m²/day), and the priority should be to have blood or marrow smears reviewed as soon as possible by a trained cytologist, so as to get at least the lineage determination within 24 hours. Chemotherapy can then be adjusted accordingly.

SPECIFIC PRECAUTIONS FOR LEUKEMIC PULMONARY INFILTRATION

Acute respiratory failure revealing a leukemia is rare, but intensivists should be aware that respiratory failure with bilateral consolidation can reveal nonhyperleukocytic monocytic leukemias (AML5).[2] This condition should be recognized promptly, because it appears to be associated with a high risk of rapid respiratory deterioration after initiation of chemotherapy. However, this should not be viewed as a hopeless complication of a rapidly fatal disease. On the contrary, these patients should receive early invasive or noninvasive ventilatory support and immediate chemotherapy, even if they are not hyperleukocytic and their respiratory impairment is still moderate. The induction treatment is based on low-dose daunorubicin alone (20 to 25 mg/m²/day) for 2 to 3 days, followed by the introduction of cytarabine. Aggressive supportive care should be initiated in case of respiratory deterioration, because, in our experience, 50% of these patients can survive these difficult inductions.

THE ROLE OF LEUKAPHERESIS

Therapeutic leukapheresis has been reported to be of benefit for patients with AML who have high WBC counts, and it is routinely used in some centers for acute hyperleukocytic leukemia.[15] However, controversial data have been published, and the results suggest that, despite a potential reduction in early mortality, there is no overall improvement on long-term survival.[16-18] Optimal supportive care based on hyperhydration, hypouricemic drugs, and prompt induction yields similar results, whether preceded or not preceded by a single oral dose of 2 to 4 g of hydroxyurea, without the complications inherent to the leukapheresis procedure. Based on the currently available literature and the fact that this technique is not available 24 hours a day or during weekends in most centers, we cannot recommend its use for unstable ICU patients, and chemotherapy-based cytoreduction protocols should be the first choice.

EMERGENCY TREATMENT OF NON-HODGKIN'S LYMPHOMAS

Emergency initiation of chemotherapy in non-Hodgkin's lymphomas (NHLs) can be necessary in the following clinical situations[1]:

1. Massive pleural or pulmonary involvement compromising hematosis
2. Bulky mediastinal tumor with compression of trachea or main bronchi
3. Poorly tolerated superior vena cava syndrome
4. CNS localization with alteration of consciousness
5. Spinal cord compression
6. Airway compromise in case of pharyngeal localization
7. Pericardial or cardiac involvement
8. Occlusive syndrome in massive abdominal tumors
9. NHL-related severe hemophagocytic syndrome

In these cases, initiation of chemotherapy may be required before exhaustive assessment of the disease has been completed, or even before definitive typing of the lymphoma has been established, thus complicating the therapeutic choices. Nevertheless, most of these life-threatening complications occur in the setting of aggressive, large cell lymphomas, and the important point is not to choose the optimal protocol for a specific NHL but to be efficient in ensuring survival with limited toxicity in these patients with compromised respiratory, cardiac, renal, or hepatic functions.

All of these patients should receive adequate preventive treatment for ATLS, and they should be closely monitored for the occurrence of this syndrome during the first 3 days.[7-9]

Rituximab (Rituxan, MabThera), an anti-CD20 monoclonal antibody, should never be prescribed as an empirical emergency treatment without both formal documentation of the CD20 positivity of the tumor cells and the approval of an experienced hematologist.[19]

BURKITT'S LYMPHOMAS

The risk of an overwhelming ATLS is so high in patients with Burkitt's lymphomas that steroids alone should be administered first and in increasing doses. Most protocols recommend that known or suspected Burkitt's lymphomas with high tumor burden be treated with a cytoreductive course of chemotherapy, before full-dose chemotherapy is administered.[20-23] The consensual choice is to deliver a first initial dose of 0.25 to 0.5 mg/kg of methylprednisolone, with the following dose administered 8 to 12 hours later if no uncontrolled metabolic disorder related to an ATLS is observed. In "steroid responders," lysis will be obvious on biologic criteria, especially the elevation of LDH, even in the absence of an obvious ATLS; dosing should then be increased to 1 mg/kg/day on day 2, before infusion of one dose of vincristine and one dose of cyclophosphamide (dosing specified below) on day 2 or 3, depending on the response to steroids. If no sign of lysis occurs after two doses of steroids (as revealed by stable LDH levels), the addition of one dose of vincristine is usually sufficient to initiate a spectacular response. The cyclophosphamide dose is delivered on the following day if the ATLS is controlled.

THREATENING NON-BURKITT'S, NON-HODGKIN'S LYMPHOMAS

With the exception of confirmed or suspected Burkitt's lymphomas (which require smaller doses of steroids on day 1), treatment of bulky NHLs should be started with steroids at 1 mg/kg/day of methylprednisolone or equivalent on day 1 and completed as early as day 2 with vincristine (1 mg/m² once, maximum total dose 2 mg, in the absence of severe preexisting peripheral neuropathy) and cyclophosphamide (500 to 700 mg/m²) on day 2 in the absence of uncontrolled ATLS.[20-22]

Whether bulky or not, NHLs with immediate life-threatening localization can require that all three drugs be infused on day 1, but intensivists should then be aware of the increased risk of uncontrolled ATLS, which may require extrarenal replacement.

CENTRAL NERVOUS SYSTEM INVOLVEMENT

Patients with NHL of the CNS who display focal deficits, alterations of the level of consciousness, or seizures should receive emergency steroid therapy with at least 2 mg/kg/day of methylprednisolone or equivalent. The optimal dosing is controversial in the literature, and doses ranging from 2 to 4 mg/kg/day can be considered as appropriate. Administration of high-dose methotrexate, a key drug in the treatment of CNS NHL, is not necessary in an emergency situation and should be prescribed only by a hematologist.[3,24]

EMERGENCY TREATMENT OF HODGKIN'S DISEASE

Emergency chemotherapy is a rare necessity in HD, but life-threatening mediastinal or cardiac involvement is possible, compromising oxygenation or hemodynamic stability. Nevertheless, one should remember that HD is a slow-responding tumor, so no spectacular reduction of tumor burden should be expected within 24 or 48 hours after the initiation of chemotherapy, and decisions regarding supportive care should take into account this parameter.

HD is not a steroid-sensitive disease; no single drug is rapidly efficient, and no recommendation is available in the literature regarding urgent cytoreduction in HD. Therefore, if a decision for emergency chemotherapy is made, a standard combination may be recommended: bleomycin, 10 units/m²; vinblastine, 6 mg/m²; doxorubicin, 25 mg/m²; and dacarbazine, 375 mg/m²—all administered

on day 1, in the absence of cardiac or pulmonary contraindications.[25-27]

BLASTIC MENINGITIS

Although prophylactic intrathecal chemotherapy is required in all patients with ALL or hyperleukocytic AML, very few patients require urgent intrathecal chemotherapy (coma, seizures, cauda equina syndromes).[3] Therefore, specialized consultation should always be obtained before administering any intrathecal chemotherapy, even in the presence of highly suggestive symptoms such as peripheral radicular pains or deficits, or hyposensitivity or dysesthesia of the chin (infiltration of the dental nerve). In addition, lumbar puncture, even for exploratory purposes, is contraindicated in patients with hyperleukocytosis, to prevent any seeding of the cerebrospinal fluid with blasts during the procedure, and in those patients with marked DIC. Moreover, intensivists should be aware that some cases of ATLS have been described after therapeutic lumbar punctures.

Nevertheless, if the indication of an emergency intrathecal treatment is confirmed, samples of cerebrospinal fluid should always be drawn for biochemical, cytologic, and bacteriologic examination before the chemotherapeutic agents are injected (usually a combination of 15 mg cytarabine, 15 mg methotrexate, and 40 mg conservative free methylprednisolone or equivalent).

ORGAN FAILURES RELATED TO HEMOPHAGOCYTIC SYNDROME

Severe hemophagocytic syndrome is now well recognized as a common presenting feature in NHL and HD.[28-30] In many cases, the organ failures are related to the intensity of the histiocytic activation and not to the aggressivity of the lymphoma itself, which can have a very low tumor burden, making the etiologic diagnosis all the more difficult. The clinical course of these patients is generally fulminant, especially once ICU admission is required.[31,32] The clinical presentation is confounding—it precisely mimics a septic shock, with fever, chills, vasoplegic shock, acute respiratory distress syndrome, and oliguric renal failure—but severe pancytopenia, high blood transfusion requirements, organomegaly, lymph node enlargement, and hepatic dysfunction several days or weeks before the occurrence of this pseudo-septic shock should suggest the diagnosis of severe hemophagocytic syndrome.[33] Biologic features such as elevated serum ferritin and hypertriglyceridemia are precious but inconstant markers of the disease, and the identification of hemophagocytosis on marrow smears or in lymph node or hepatic biopsy samples sometimes requires an experienced cytologist.

If sufficient clinical and biologic elements are highly suggestive of the diagnosis, treatment should be promptly administered, to allow emergency control of the cytokine-induced organ failures. The treatment of the underlying lymphoma itself can be postponed for 2 or 3 days if the diagnosis is not yet confirmed, until urgent processing and reading of smears or biopsies have been conducted. No randomized trial of chemotherapy has been conducted in lymphoma-related hemophagocytic syndrome, so no consensus is available in the literature regarding the optimal strategy. However, etoposide-based regimens seem to be the most appropriate choice for these high-risk patients,[33,34] frequently in combination with steroids. Based on case reports and our experience, the administration of 150 to 200 mg of etoposide, depending on the severity of the renal and hepatic failures, combined with 1 to 2 mg/kg/day of methylprednisolone, is rapidly effective in most cases (within 12 to 48 hours). The effect is only transient, and recurrence of the initial symptoms is the rule within 6 to 10 days in the absence of a specific treatment of the lymphoma, which should be started by a hematologist as soon as the lymphoma has been identified. If an aggressive NHL is highly suspected on preliminary results of smears (lymph node, marrow, or pleural effusion), a nonspecific cytoreductive combination of steroid, vincristine, and cyclophosphamide can be administered while awaiting the definitive results of the cytologic, histologic, and immunochemistry techniques.

MANAGEMENT OF DISSEMINATED INTRAVASCULAR COAGULATION

DIC is a common and serious complication of hematologic malignancies, but most of the time the bleeding is only moderately threatening, with mainly mucosal and cutaneous hemorrhagic manifestations.[35] In fact, DIC is often triggered by the initiation of chemotherapy in several types of ALLs and AMLs (AML4, AML5, and to a lesser extent AML1). However, severe forms of coagulation disorders are typically observed as a presenting symptom in untreated acute promyelocytic leukemias (APL or AML3), frequently combining DIC and a severe hyperfibrinolytic state.[13,36] Optimal treatment includes both symptomatic measures to reduce the risk of life-threatening hemorrhage (in the CNS, but also in lungs and gastrointestinal tract) and specific treatment of the leukemia.

Supportive care is essential in DIC and should include repeated platelet transfusions to reach a minimum platelet count greater than 50,000/mm³ permanently; correction of the prothrombin time and of hypofibrinogenemia with fresh-frozen plasma (2 to 4 units to start with) to ensure a prothrombin time less than 2.5 times normal; and a fibrinogen level greater than 1 g/L before the start of the treatment.[37] The use of low-dose unfractionated heparin (100 IU/kg/day) is controversial, requires platelet counts permanently superior to 50,000/mm³, and cannot be recommended for patients with active bleeding.[12,36,38,39] Its prescription in DIC with thrombotic tendencies should be discussed according to local protocols. As soon as appropriate transfusion support is initiated, chemotherapy should be started, always with progressive dosing, to reduce the leukemic load as quickly as possible. Transient worsening of the DIC is common and justifies the intensification of transfusions as required by biologic and clinical manifestations.

In DIC caused by hematologic malignances, the use of antithrombin III cannot be recommended based on currently available data, with the exception of severe DICs occurring after infusion of L-asparaginase.[40-42] In uncontrolled and life-threatening bleeding in nonhematology patients, the adjunctive use of recombinant factor VIIa has yielded some response, but this treatment has never been evaluated in the peculiar case of hematologic malignancies, and further well-designed evaluation of this molecule in severe malignancy-related DIC is needed to recommend its use in hematology patients.[43-47]

MULTIPLE MYELOMA AND OTHER CAUSES OF HYPERVISCOSITY SYNDROMES

Severe infectious complications and metabolic emergencies (e.g., hypercalcemia, acute renal failure) can lead myeloma patients to the ICU, and these conditions are detailed elsewhere in this text. Myeloma patients can also present with severe organ failures early in the course of their disease. Intensivists should not be discouraged from admitting these patients to the ICU if the disease is not refractory and the patient is in poor condition, because prognosis in the ICU has improved over the years and can justify their admission.[48] Hyperviscosity syndrome is one specific complication that can initially require ICU admission.

Hyperviscosity syndromes may be encountered in multiple myeloma and Waldenström's macroglobulinemia, symptomatic forms being more common in the latter.[49,50] Clinical manifestations are mainly neurologic (headaches, alteration or slowdown of cognitive function, stupor, even coma, and rarely seizures), ocular (visual impairment, papillary edema with dilated retinal veins, retinal hemorrhages), and excessive bleeding (mainly mucosal, cutaneous, and retinal). Emergency management is directed at rapidly decreasing blood viscosity through plasmapheresis, which leads to rapid alleviation of the initial symptoms. Long-term management, whether based on high-dose steroids or chemotherapy, is aimed at reducing the production of the monoclonal immunoglobulin and can be postponed until a hematologist consultant has been reached. Plasmapheresis is the only therapeutic option with immediate efficacy[51,52]; it consists of the exchange of 1 to 1.5 plasma volumes (5 L maximum), with 100% replacement by 4% human albumin solution. Plasmapheresis should preferably be conducted by a trained hemapheresis team, using specifically designed machines. If no such team is available, plasmapheresis can be performed by intensivists on several machines designed for ICU continuous renal replacement (e.g., Spectra-Cobe, Prisma-Hospal), equipped with plasma exchange kits. The rate of plasma exchange is then lower, but these devices allow easy exchange of 1 plasma volume, with standard anticoagulation of the filter (whereas "classic" plasmapheresis is generally performed with citrate anticoagulation). The hemodynamic tolerance is usually correct, even if most patients require volume expansion because of a moderate hypotension after 60% or 70% of the plasma exchange (due to rapid removal of the osmotically active paraprotein).

ANNOTATED REFERENCES

Azoulay E, Fieux F, Moreau D, et al: Acute monocytic leukemia presenting as acute respiratory failure. Am J Respir Crit Care Med 2003;167:1-5.
   This is a recent report of pulmonary leukemic infiltration with acute respiratory failure as a presenting feature in 20 patients with acute monocytic leukemia. Intensivists should be aware of both its rapid progression after initiation of chemotherapy and its potential reversibility with adequate ICU management.

Barbui T, Finazzi G, Falanga A: The impact of all-*trans*-retinoic acid on the coagulopathy of acute promyelocytic leukemia. Blood 1998;91:3093-3102.
   A comprehensive review of DIC in APL, the interactions between ATRA and the hemostatic system, and the impact of ATRA on the early hemorrhagic events in the treatment of APL.

Giles FJ, Shen Y, Kantarjian HM, et al: Leukapheresis reduces early mortality in patients with acute myeloid leukemia with high white blood cell counts but does not improve long term survival. Leuk Lymphoma 2001;45:67-73.

One of the only randomized trials testing early leukapheresis in hyper-leukocytic patients with acute leukemia, it demonstrated the absence of benefit on long-term survival. These patients should, therefore, be treated urgently with chemotherapy, without wasting time organizing leukapheresis or transfer to a medical center performing leukapheresis.

Lister A, Abrey LE, Sandlund JT: Central nervous system lymphoma. Hematology 2002:283-296.

This is a complete and meticulous review of up-to-date management of all type of CNS involvement in lymphoma (primary CNS lymphoma, blastic meningitis, secondary CNS lymphoma).

Patte C, Sakiroglu O, Sommelet D: European experience in the treatment of hyperuricemia. Semin Hematol 2001;38(Suppl 10):9-12.

This study, comparing the rate of dialysis required for ATLS-related renal failure, demonstrated the superiority of urate oxidase over allopurinol in the prevention of acute tumor lysis during the induction chemotherapy of diseases with high tumor burden.

Chapter 171

THE HEMATOPOIETIC STEM CELL TRANSPLANTATION PATIENT

Vinay Maheshwari • Alexander C. White

KEY POINTS

1. **Effective prophylaxis and screening** have reduced the incidence of opportunistic infections among patients undergoing hematopoietic stem cell transplantation (HSCT). Invasive fungal disease remains an important problem and is difficult to both prevent and treat.

2. **The engraftment syndrome, diffuse alveolar hemorrhage, and the idiopathic pneumonia syndrome** are all characterized by diffuse multilobar infiltrates, a widened alveolar-arterial gradient, and the absence of any identifiable infection. These syndromes may be related, but they need to be distinguished clinically, because they have different outcomes.

3. The **safety and diagnostic utility of fiberoptic bronchoscopy in stable HSCT patients** has been established. Bronchoscopy findings can result in a change in management in about 30% of cases. In HSCT patients with worsening respiratory failure, bronchoscopy needs to be undertaken with caution, because the procedure can precipitate the need for mechanical ventilation.

4. HSCT patients who require prolonged mechanical ventilation and vasopressor support and have evidence of other organ failure **tend to have a very high mortality rate.**

5. **End-of-life care in the HSCT patient population is complicated** and remains a difficult problem in the intensive care unit.

6. **The use of nonmyeloablative HSCT is increasing.** Use of these low-intensity transplantation regimens in older patients is likely to change the range of complications seen in the HSCT population in the future.

Bone marrow transplantation was developed as a treatment for hematologic malignancies in the early 1970s. It is now possible to use either peripheral blood stem cells or umbilical cord blood as additional sources of donor stem cells, so the term *bone marrow transplantation* has been replaced by the more inclusive *hematopoietic stem cell transplantation* (HSCT). The most common indications for HSCT at present are acute and chronic leukemia, aplastic anemia, hemoglobinopathies, Hodgkin's and non-Hodgkin's lymphomas, and multiple myeloma. HSCT has also been used as a treatment for solid tumors of the breast, ovaries, and testicles.

Critical illness, often involving the lung, develops in up to 40% of patients undergoing HSCT.[1,2] Respiratory failure accounts for up to 50% of admissions to the intensive care unit (ICU), and almost half of those admitted to the ICU require mechanical ventilation. Certain pulmonary complications are unique to the HSCT patient. These relate to cumulative lung damage from repeated courses of chemotherapy and radiation, pulmonary infections from immunosuppression, and lung manifestations of the underlying hematologic disease.[3] In addition, the HSCT patient remains at risk for common pulmonary diseases such as pulmonary embolus and community-acquired pneumonia. A number of risk factors for mechanical ventilation per se have been identified, including older age at transplantation, hematologic disease in relapse at the time of transplantation, and receipt of a nonidentical HSCT graft.[4] Other reasons for ICU admission include septic shock, hypotension, mucositis, cardiac dysfunction, neurologic complications, bleeding, and hepatic veno-occlusive disease.[1,5]

The field of HSCT continues to evolve. Less toxic, "nonmyeloablative" transplantation regimens are being developed in an attempt to limit regimen-related organ toxicity. The increased use of peripheral blood stem cells instead of bone marrow results in more rapid engraftment and hematopoietic reconstitution, which may reduce some of the infectious and bleeding complications that arise from cytopenias.[6]

Some of the complications of HSCT follow a temporal pattern. This pattern relates to changes that occur in the immune system in response to the conditioning treatment and subsequent transplantation and engraftment. There is an initial 2- to 3-week period of pancytopenia, followed by engraftment with a gradual reconstitution of the immune system over the next year. The complications that may result in critical illness are shown in Tables 171-1 and 171-2. Space does not permit an in-depth discussion of all of these issues. Therefore, this chapter focuses on the pulmonary complications of HSCT, with discussion also of mechanical ventilation, bronchoscopy, and outcomes of critical illness.

PULMONARY INFECTIONS

Pulmonary complications can occur in up to 50% of patients undergoing HSCT[7]; they are more frequent in recipients of allogeneic or matched unrelated transplants than in those receiving autologous transplants. The intensive pretransplantation conditioning therapy used to ablate the native bone marrow, post-transplantation immunosuppression, and graft-versus-host disease (GVHD) appear to be the major risk factors for pulmonary complications in this population.[8] Pneumonia that develops during the first 100 days after HSCT is usually caused by gram-negative enteric bacilli (see Table 171-1). As the immune system recovers and the patient spends less time in the hospital, this pattern changes, and gram-positive organisms become more common. Cytomegalovirus (CMV) infection used to be a major cause of pulmonary morbidity and mortality in the HSCT population. The introduction of CMV antigen surveillance and the use of preemptive treatment with ganciclovir have reduced the incidence of CMV pneumonitis to less than 10%.[9] The incidence of *Pneumocystis carinii* pneumonia in the HSCT population has also been reduced, to about 2%, with the effective use of antibiotic prophylaxis.[10]

These advances have helped to prevent some of the most serious pulmonary infectious complications that may result in critical illness in the HSCT population. However, the prevention and treatment of invasive fungal infection remains a serious problem in the HSCT population. Invasive pulmonary aspergillosis remains the leading causes of infectious death in recipients of allogeneic or matched unrelated transplants,[11] despite the development of newer antifungal agents such as caspofungin and voriconazole.[12-14] The immunocompromised HSCT population is also vulnerable to outbreaks of pneumonia from *Legionella pneumophila*[15] and respiratory syncytial virus.

NONINFECTIOUS PULMONARY DISEASE

Noninfectious pulmonary complications are an important cause of critical illness in the HSCT population. It is important to keep in mind when caring for HSCT patients that infectious and noninfectious pulmonary complications may occur contemporaneously in the same patient.

Respiratory failure that develops within days after transplantation may be caused by cardiogenic pulmonary edema. There is usually a brisk response to aggressive treatment, and intubation and mechanical ventilation can sometimes be avoided. Pulmonary edema causing respiratory failure in the HSCT patient is a positive predictor of survival in those requiring mechanical ventilation.[16] The large volumes of intravenous fluids and blood products used during HSCT can increase the circulating blood volume. Cyclophosphamide is commonly used in the preparative regimen and may cause acute cardiac toxicity.[17] This combination of increased circulating volume and myocardial damage increases the risk of cardiogenic pulmonary edema in some patients. Findings that suggest cardiogenic pulmonary edema in this population include diffuse pulmonary infiltrates, a rapid response to diuretics, and a reduced left ventricular ejection fraction on echocardiogram. The risk-benefit ratio of hemodynamic monitoring with a pulmonary artery catheter in this setting is not clear. These subjects often have a significant bleeding diathesis in addition to leukopenia, increasing the risk of hemorrhage and infection with catheter use.

TABLE 171-1. COMPLICATIONS OF HEMATOPOIETIC STEM CELL TRANSPLANTATION THAT MAY LEAD TO INTENSIVE CARE

Infection

Bacteria
  Escherichia coli, Pseudomonas, Klebsiella, Acinetobacter
  Staphylococcus species, *Enterococcus, Streptococcus*
  Clostridium species
Viral
  Herpesvirus
  Varicella-zoster virus
  Influenza, parainfluenza, adenovirus, respiratory syncytial virus
  Cytomegalovirus
Fungal
  Candida species
  Aspergillus species
Protozoal
  Toxoplasma
  Pneumocystis carinii

Cardiac Complications

Cardiogenic pulmonary edema
Arrhythmias
Pericardial effusion
Myocarditis

Neurologic Complications

Seizures
Encephalopathy
Polyneuropathy
Intracranial hemorrhage
Subarachnoid hemorrhage

Pulmonary Complications

Noncardiogenic pulmonary edema
Acute respiratory distress syndrome
Idiopathic pneumonia syndrome
Diffuse alveolar hemorrhage syndrome
Infectious pneumonia
Aspiration pneumonia
Bronchiolitis obliterans/airflow obstruction
Engraftment syndrome
Delayed pulmonary toxicity syndrome
Pleural effusions
Interstitial fibrosis

Gastrointestinal Complications

Mucositis
Diarrhea
Drug-induced hepatotoxicity
Hepatic veno-occlusive disease
Pancreatitis

Renal Complications

Drug toxicity
Hepatorenal syndrome

Graft-versus-Host Disease

Acute
Chronic

A syndrome characterized by noncardiogenic pulmonary edema can occur at about the time of neutrophil engraftment. This syndrome is known as the capillary leak syndrome or the engraftment syndrome.[18] The engraftment syndrome, as the name implies, occurs within 96 hours after the neutrophil count increases to greater than 500/μL for two consecutive days.[18] Three major diagnostic criteria have been proposed: fever greater than 38.3°C without evidence of infection, erythrodermatous rash, and noncardiogenic pulmonary edema. Minor criteria that may be part of the syndrome include hepatic dysfunction, renal insufficiency, weight gain, and transient encephalopathy. Progressive or symptomatic engraftment syndrome should be aggressively treated with high-dose corticosteroids. Hemodynamic collapse with multisystem organ failure is reported in up to 50% of patients with the engraftment syndrome.[2] The syndrome can be self-limited, so aggressive support in the ICU is warranted.[18]

Diffuse alveolar hemorrhage (DAH) is a clinical syndrome characterized by cough, fever, hypoxemia, and diffuse infiltrates on chest radiograph[19,20]; it may be a variant of the engraftment syndrome. The incidence of DAH in the HSCT population in the past was reported to be between 10% and 20%.[19,21,22] More recent data indicate that the incidence may be closer to 2%, with an increased frequency of DAH in recipients of allogeneic transplants.[23] Despite the name of the syndrome, hemoptysis is unusual and occurs in fewer than 15% of patients.[20] DAH is a recognized complication of both autologous and allogeneic HSCT.[19,24] A number of risk factors for DAH have been identified, including severe oral mucositis, intensive pretransplantation chemotherapy, total-body or thoracic irradiation, and evidence of airway inflammation on screening bronchoscopy before HSCT.[19,25,26] The pulmonary infiltrates seen in DAH develop approximately 11 days after transplantation and often predate the clinical diagnosis of DAH by up to 3 days.[27] The typical pattern is bilateral interstitial or alveolar infiltrates that are primarily central and involve the middle and lower lung zones.[28] Unilateral infiltrates may also occur, but they progress to bilateral involvement.[28] Computed tomography of the chest reveals bilateral lung consolidation or ground-glass opacification.[29] Diagnostic criteria have been developed to help diagnose DAH. These criteria include diffuse multilobar infiltrates, a widened alveolar-arterial gradient, the absence of any identifiable infection, and progressively bloodier return on bronchoalveolar lavage (BAL).[20,30] However, a postmortem study found BAL to be neither sensitive nor specific for DAH.[24] High-dose corticosteroids have been shown to provide a survival benefit in DAH, compared with low-dose corticosteroids and supportive therapy alone.[21] However, the efficacy of high-dose steroids has not been studied in a randomized controlled trial. Recombinant factor VIIa is a potential new therapeutic modality that may improve the clinical and radiographic abnormalities in DAH.[31] It is difficult to obtain accurate outcome data for a clinically defined syndrome such as DAH. Earlier data suggested that DAH had a poor prognosis and was associated with high mortality rates, ranging from 64% to 100%.[21,25,28,32] A more recent study showed a 48% overall mortality for HSCT patients with DAH, with recipients of autologous transplants having a lower mortality rate than those receiving allogeneic transplants.[20] The most common causes of death in patients with DAH are sepsis, multiorgan failure, and respiratory failure.[21,23]

The term *idiopathic pneumonia syndrome* (IPS) refers to a diffuse interstitial pneumonia without any specific infectious cause that occurs in HSCT patients. A National Heart Lung and Blood Institute workshop defined IPS as "evidence of widespread alveolar injury in the absence of active lower respiratory tract infection" in HSCT patients.[33] Additional features of the syndrome include abnormal pulmonary physiology and multilobar infiltrates on chest radiography

or chest computed tomography. The incidence of IPS is about 7%, and it occurs at a median time of 21 days after HSCT.[34] Although there is no difference in incidence of IPS between autologous and allogeneic HSCT recipients, significant risk factors have been identified only in allogeneic transplantation patients. These risk factors include an underlying diagnosis other than leukemia, grade 4 acute GVHD, and CMV-seropositive donor status.[34] Other potential risk factors identified for IPS include exposure to pretransplantation radiation, busulfan, and cyclophosphamide.[35 37] These data suggest that IPS may be caused by cumulative damage to the lung from chemotherapy, radiation, and GVHD. Almost 70% of patients who develop IPS require mechanical ventilation for respiratory failure. The hospital mortality rate for IPS is greater than 70%, and respiratory failure leading to death occurs in 62% of patients with IPS.[34] It is important to differentiate IPS from the other syndromes outlined in this section that may also manifest with bilateral pulmonary infiltrates.[34] The treatment of IPS is mainly supportive, and, even with aggressive care, the prognosis remains poor.[34,38]

Patients who develop transfusion-related acute lung injury (TRALI) may also present with bilateral pulmonary infiltrates. The pulmonary infiltrates are caused by granulocyte antibodies present in donor blood, which bind granulocytes within the pulmonary microvasculature of the transfused patient.[39] The clinical presentation of TRALI may be difficult to distinguish from that of cardiogenic pulmonary edema, engraftment syndrome, or acute respiratory distress syndrome (ARDS). TRALI usually develops about 4 hours after the transfusion of blood products and resolves within 4 days.[39] The treatment of TRALI is supportive, with some patients requiring a period of mechanical ventilation. There have been case reports of improvement with corticosteroids, but randomized controlled trials of their use in TRALI are lacking.

BRONCHOSCOPY

It is important to identify the cause of respiratory failure in the HSCT patient if the information can be obtained without increasing morbidity and mortality. A correct pulmonary diagnosis allows for focused treatment and avoids the use of unnecessary drugs. In this vulnerable population, spiral chest computed tomography has become invaluable in helping define subtle infiltrates seen on plain chest radiography and in targeting procedures. Several observational and prospective studies have established the safety and diagnostic utility of flexible fiberoptic bronchoscopy in the evaluation of the immunocompromised host with focal or diffuse pulmonary infiltrates.[27,34,40-42]

The yield of BAL, with or without a protected specimen brush, in the HSCT patient has been gradually falling over the past 20 years.[27,40,42-45] For example, in a 2000 study pulmonary complications were diagnosed accurately in only 42% of all fiberoptic bronchoscopies performed in a HSCT cohort.[43] The lower yields in recent studies appear to reflect improvements in prophylaxis and a consequent reduction in infections after HSCT.

Fiberoptic bronchoscopy is three times more likely to be performed in recipients of allogeneic or matched unrelated transplants, compared with autologous transplant recipients,[41] because of the higher incidence of pulmonary complications in the former group as a result of GVHD and increased need for immunosuppressive medication. Most bronchoscopies performed in the HSCT population result in a diagnosis of infection,[22,41,43] with the yield from fiberoptic bronchoscopy being higher in patients with diffuse compared with more focal infiltrates.[27,41] Pneumonia caused by CMV or *P. carinii* is now less common because of the availability of effective antibiotic prophylaxis and screening.[22,41,43] Pulmonary complications that are not caused by infection can also be diagnosed with fiberoptic bronchoscopy. These complications include DAH, IPS, bronchiolitis obliterans with or without organizing pneumonia, and radiation-induced lung injury.[22,43]

The results obtained from fiberoptic bronchoscopy have been reported to change management in 24% to 63% of HSCT patients undergoing the procedure.[27,44,45] A significant proportion of the changes in management include withdrawal of unnecessary antibiotics. Therefore, it is not surprising that, despite the change in management, diagnostic fiberoptic bronchoscopy had little effect on 30-day hospital mortality or overall mortality compared with nondiagnostic fiberoptic bronchoscopy.[27,44,45]

There is a significant complication rate associated with performing fiberoptic bronchoscopy in the HSCT patient population. The serious complications that have been reported include respiratory failure, hypotension, epistaxis, pulmonary hemorrhage, pneumothorax, and death.[27,41] The complication rate was significantly higher in those undergoing protected specimen brush and transbronchial biopsies, as opposed to BAL alone.[27,41,46]

The decision to perform fiberoptic bronchoscopy in the HSCT patient with pulmonary disease can be difficult. The risk-benefit ratio of the procedure must be carefully considered in this vulnerable population. BAL appears to be safe in most patients, but transbronchial biopsy appears to add significant risk to the procedure. Severe hypoxemia can be a contraindication to fiberoptic bronchoscopy in the nonintubated HSCT patient with worsening respiratory failure. The risk of an elective intubation for fiberoptic bronchoscopy must be balanced against the benefits of empiric treatment. An important factor in this decision is the high mortality rate among HSCT patients undergoing invasive mechanical ventilation. Although there have been some advances in technology that allow fiberoptic bronchoscopy to be performed safely in patients while they are receiving noninvasive mechanical ventilation, bronchoscopy in the unstable HSCT patient remains a challenge.[47-49]

SEPSIS

HSCT recipients have a number of risk factors for infection and septic shock, including immunosuppression, mucositis from preparative regimens, and the use of long-term indwelling catheters for vascular access. There is a temporal pattern to some of the infections, as shown in Table 171-2. Some of the more common organisms isolated are grampositive cocci, gram-negative enteric bacilli, *Candida* species, and *Aspergillus* species. Infection with CMV and herpes viruses also occurs. The impaired host defenses in the HSCT patient may prevent the localization of infection, and, as a result, septic shock may develop. Septic shock is the admitting diagnosis in about 18% of HSCT patients transferred to the ICU, and the diagnosis of septic shock is made in about 60% of all HSCT patients receiving ICU care.[50,51] HSCT patients

TABLE 171–2. TIMELINE OF COMPLICATIONS AFTER HEMATOPOIETIC STEM CELL TRANSPLANTATION

Pre-engraftment Complications (Days 0-30)

Regimen-related toxicity
  Mucositis
  Hemorrhagic cystitis
  Hypervolemia
Cardiogenic pulmonary edema
Engraftment syndrome
Diffuse alveolar hemorrhage
Idiopathic pneumonia syndrome
Veno-occlusive disease
Drug toxicity
Graft failure
Infections
  Coagulase-negative *Staphylococcus* species, methicillin-resistant *Staphylococcus aureus*
  Gram-negative bacilli
  Candida and *Aspergillus*
  Herpes simplex virus, adenovirus, influenza virus, respiratory syncytial virus

Immediate Post-engraftment Complications (Days 30-100)

Acute graft-versus-host disease (GVHD)
Idiopathic pneumonia syndrome
Diffuse alveolar hemorrhage
Infections
  Bacterial infections that occur during early phase
  Encapsulated bacteria
  Fungi, including *Aspergillus*
  Viruses, including cytomegalovirus, respiratory viruses
  Pneumocystis carinii

Late Post-engraftment Complications (Beyond Day 100)

Chronic GVHD
Bronchiolitis obliterans
Airflow obstruction
Disease relapse
Infections
  Encapsulated bacteria
  Gram-negative bacilli
  Nocardia
  Aspergillus
  Cytomegalovirus, varicella-zoster virus, Epstein-Barr virus
  P. carinii

with septic shock require vasopressor support in most cases and may progress to multisystem organ failure. The prognosis of septic shock in the HSCT patient is poor, and the 30-day mortality rate after ICU admission exceeded 80% in one recent study.[50] The need for more than 4 hours of vasopressor support has been shown to increase mortality among mechanically ventilated HSCT patients.[5] Empiric antibiotics and antifungal agents, along with blood products, form an important part of the management of critical illness in the HSCT patient. To date there has been no randomized controlled trial evaluating the efficacy and safety of recombinant human activated protein C in the treatment of sepsis in the HSCT population.[52]

A severe form of the engraftment syndrome with hemodynamic collapse and multisystem failure has been described; it closely mimics septic shock.[18] Because infection does not appear to play any role, the term *aseptic shock* has been used to describe this syndrome. Aseptic shock may be associated with widespread organ dysfunction. Increased levels of proinflammatory cytokines such as interleukin-6 (IL-6)[53,54] and C-reactive protein[55] may be useful in identifying patients at risk for major transplantation-related complications such as aseptic shock and organ dysfunction.[53]

HEPATIC VENO-OCCLUSIVE DISEASE

Veno-occlusive disease is the most common cause of liver failure in HSCT patients; it is reported in about 5% of the HSCT population.[56,57] The diagnosis should be suspected if jaundice, painful hepatomegaly, and ascites develop within the first 4 weeks after HSCT. As the liver fails, encephalopathy, coagulopathy, bleeding, fluid retention, and renal failure may develop and result in critical illness. A number of risk factors for veno-occlusive disease have been identified, including receipt of an allogeneic transplant, abnormal liver function tests before transplantation, high-dose chemotherapy, and previous abdominal radiation.[57]

Right upper quadrant ultrasonography with color Doppler typically shows hepatomegaly, ascites, and reversal of blood flow through the hepatic vein. Liver biopsy carries significant risk in the HSCT population and is rarely performed. Severe veno-occlusive disease with progressive liver failure occurs in 25% of cases and has a mortality rate of almost 100%.[56,57] The treatment of veno-occlusive disease is mainly supportive, with careful fluid balance, preservation of renal function, and judicious diuresis for management of ascites. Thrombolytics and heparin have been used but have a success rate of less than 30%. These treatments carry a high risk of bleeding complications in the HSCT population.[58] Promising results with defibrotide, a thrombolytic agent with minimal systemic effects, have been reported in patients with severe veno-occlusive disease.[59]

OUTCOMES OF CRITICAL ILLNESS

Forty percent of HSCT patients may require admission to the ICU at some point in their course. Published data on the survival of HSCT patients admitted to the ICU have a number of limitations. The studies are usually observational, retrospective, and performed in a single institution with no comparison group. In addition, transplantation centers may focus on different hematologic diseases and may have varied expertise, all of which may make it difficult to extrapolate from one study to the transplantation population as a whole. Critical care may also be delivered outside the ICU in some transplantation centers. These sources of bias need to be kept in mind when comparing outcome studies performed in the HSCT population.

There has been evidence of a gradual reduction in ICU mortality for HSCT patients over the past 15 years.[50] In two recent studies, based on different populations, ICU survival varied between 26% and 48%.[50,60] ICU survival is closely associated with the amount of organ damage that occurs during critical illness. For example, patients who require more than 4 hours of vasopressor support and have failure of two other organs (e.g., serum bilirubin greater than 4 mg/dL and serum creatinine greater than 2 mg/dL), have a mortality rate of almost 100%.[5,50,51,60] There are conflicting data on any association between ICU outcome and the timing of ICU admission after transplantation.[5,16,50] Earlier data demonstrating a survival benefit to early post-transplantation admission have not been reproducible. ICU survival is more likely if the critical illness is the result of infection.[61] The need for endotracheal intubation to manage

respiratory failure and the need for more than 15 days of mechanical ventilation have been associated with a survival rate of less than 5%.[1,5,16,62,63]

Noninvasive positive-pressure ventilation (NPPV) has been shown to be effective in immunocompromised patients with hypoxemic respiratory failure. In a small, prospective, randomized study of 52 neutropenic patients with hypoxemia and pulmonary infiltrates, the use of intermittent NPPV was associated with a lower intubation rate, fewer serious complications, and improved ICU and hospital survival, compared with spontaneous breathing and supplemental oxygen alone.[64] Only 17 (33%) of the subjects enrolled in this study had undergone HSCT. Sources of bias included patient selection and the inability to blind the study. In another study with a similar design, NPPV was also shown to be beneficial in subjects undergoing solid-organ transplantation.[65] These data suggest that NPPV may be useful in the HSCT population. Mucositis and severe GVHD of the oropharynx are complications unique to the HSCT population that may interfere with NPPV. In general, it is important not to delay intubation if the patient does not improve with NPPV.

The utility of the Acute Physiology and Chronic Health Evaluation II (APACHE II) scoring system in predicting ICU mortality in the HSCT population is unclear, but there is evidence that a score higher than 45 is associated with poor survival.[1,51] A recent study suggested that APACHE III scores better predict ICU mortality.[50] However, the APACHE scoring system does not take into account important features unique to the HSCT population. For example, the presence of GVHD[66] or the total amount of chemotherapy administered before transplantation may have an important impact on ICU survival rates in the HSCT population. Survival doe not appear to be affected by either age or the source of the donor graft.[1,62]

END-OF-LIFE ISSUES

This chapter has discussed some of the complications associated with HSCT that can lead to critical illness. Patients consent to undergo HSCT hoping to be cured of a potentially life-threatening hematologic disorder. The expectations from medical care in this patient population are high, and these same expectations are brought to the ICU if the patient develops critical illness. Personnel who work primarily in the ICU setting may have a different perspective on the outcome of critical illness in the HSCT patient. As a result, there may be disagreement between transplantation caregivers and ICU staff regarding the benefit of aggressive care in the HSCT patient. Efforts to educate physicians regarding the poor prognosis of HSCT patients who require aggressive intensive care support have not changed the use of ICU resources in this population.[67]

The overall high mortality rate associated with critical illness in the HSCT population has resulted in attempts to develop either guidelines for the withdrawal of care or parameters that may indicate futile care. For example, it has been shown that patients with acute lung injury requiring mechanical ventilation who had a prolonged need for vasopressors or sustained hepatic and renal failure had a mortality rate of almost 100%.[5] In this nested case-control study, the investigators demonstrated that death could be predicted within 4 days after initiation of mechanical ventilation in more than 50% of the patients who did not survive. The study was limited by population bias and retrospective design, as has been noted in other HSCT-related publications. In addition, only the first episode of mechanical ventilation after the first HSCT was studied. Referral bias makes it difficult to generalize the findings to other HSCT populations. The indications for intubation, NPPV, and vasopressor use may vary among transplantation centers and are another possible source of bias. The authors developed guidelines to help medical decision-making in the critically ill HSCT population.[5] The recommendations included the presentation of outcomes of mechanical ventilation in HSCT patients at the particular institution to the patient and family; in addition, the very poor survival of HSCT patients who have suffered massive intracranial hemorrhage,[68] tumor relapse despite transplantation, and fungal infection with progressive GVHD should be discussed. Guidelines to help medical decision-making could ease some of the burden on HSCT patients, their families' members, and the caregivers charged with their care.

The issue of withdrawal of care in the ICU continues to be an area of intense interest. One recent study explored the reasons for withdrawal of mechanical ventilation in anticipation of death in the ICU.[69] This was a prospective cohort study performed in 15 ICUs in four different countries. Four factors were identified that significantly determined the withdrawal of mechanical ventilation in this general ICU population: the physicians' perception that the patient preferred not to use life support, the physicians' prediction of ICU survival, poor cognitive function, and the use of inotropes or vasopressors. The critically ill HSCT patient differs from the general ICU patient, but these types of observation may have relevance for the HSCT patient.

THE FUTURE

The HSCT patient brings unique and difficult questions to the critical care arena. The field of HSCT continues to evolve, and over the past 3 years nonmyeloablative stem cell transplantation regimens have been developed.[70] These less toxic regimens have expanded the use of HSCT to older patients with more comorbid illnesses.[71] The subsequent development of donor-host mixed chimerism[72-74] may affect

pulmonary complications after transplantation and subsequent lung repair. Studies comparing critical care outcomes in nonmyeloablative versus conventional ablative transplantation are needed.

ANNOTATED REFERENCES

Afessa B, Tefferi A, Hoagland HC, et al: Intensive care unit support and Acute Physiology and Chronic Health Evaluation III performance in hematopoietic stem cell transplant recipients. Crit Care Med 2003;31: 1715-1721.

This was a retrospective cohort study of the APACHE III scoring system as a way to predict mortality in HSCT patients admitted to the ICU. The results suggest improved outcomes for critically ill HSCT patients over the past decade.

Feinstein MB, Mokhtari M, Ferreiro R, et al: Fiberoptic bronchoscopy in allogeneic bone marrow transplantation: Findings in the era of serum cytomegalovirus antigen surveillance. Chest 2001;120:1094-1100.

This retrospective review studied the diagnostic yield and management impact of fiberoptic bronchoscopy in the bone marrow transplantation population. The study showed that infection was the most common diagnosis, followed by DAH. Current prophylaxis and screening strategies have reduced the need for bronchoscopy to diagnose CMV disease or P. carinii pneumonia.

Hilbert G, Gruson D, Vargas F, et al: Noninvasive ventilation in immunosuppressed patients with pulmonary infiltrates, fever, and acute respiratory failure. N Engl J Med 2001;344:481-487.

This was a prospective, randomized trial of intermittent noninvasive ventilation compared with standard treatment (supplemental oxygen without ventilatory support) the immunosuppressed population. Fifty-two subjects with pulmonary infiltrates, fever, and hypoxemic acute respiratory failure were studied. Early initiation of noninvasive ventilation was associated with significant reductions in the rates of endotracheal intubation and serious complications and an improved likelihood of survival to hospital discharge. The study included only 17 HSCT subjects, limiting its generalizability.

Rubenfeld GD, Crawford SW: Withdrawing life support from mechanically ventilated recipients of bone marrow transplants: A case for evidence-based guidelines. Ann Intern Med 1996;125:625-633.

This nested case-control study evaluated the prognostic factors associated with increased mortality in mechanically ventilated HSCT patients. The authors developed guidelines to help medical decision-making in the critically ill HSCT patient.

Spitzer TR: Mini-review: Engraftment syndrome following hematopoietic stem cell transplantation. Bone Marrow Transplant 2001;27:893-989.

This is a review article that covers the clinical features and pathophysiology of the engraftment syndrome. Criteria for a uniform definition of the syndrome are proposed.

Chapter 172

ORGAN TOXICITY OF CANCER CHEMOTHERAPY

Lionel Karlin • Sophie Rigaudeau • Élie Azoulay

KEY POINTS

1. Hospital mortality among cancer patients admitted to the ICU is approximately 50%, which is not higher than in other patient groups for whom ICU admission is standard practice.

2. When seeking to establish a diagnosis of cancer drug toxicity, intrinsic evidence should continuously be confronted with extrinsic evidence to ensure optimal selection of diagnostic investigations.

Pulmonary toxicity:

- **Bleomycin** toxicity occurs in 3% to 40% of patients, the lung being the main target.

- **Methotrexate** causes acute or subacute pneumonitis simulating an infection, usually with interstitial involvement, in 1% to 7% of patients.

- With **fludarabine**, lung toxicity occurs in 8% of patients.

- **Gemcitabine** use causes pulmonary toxicity in 5% of patients.

- Within 8 days after **cytarabine** initiation, respiratory distress of variable severity develops in 13% to 28% of patients.

- **Cyclophosphamide** leads to clinical lung toxicity in almost 1% of patients.

Cardiac toxicity:

- **Anthracyclines** (doxorubicin, daunorubicin, epirubicin, idarubicin, and mitoxantrone) are the main culprit of cardiac toxicity.

- Drugs of the **taxane** class, most notably **paclitaxel, given in combination with anthracyclines,** lead to cardiotoxicity occurs in more than 20% of patients treated with this combination.

Hematologic toxicity:

- Severity of myelosuppression varies with mechanism of action of the anticancer agent and patient-dependent factors.

- **L-Asparaginase**

Neurologic toxicity:

- Peripheral nervous system toxicity: vinca alkaloids and platin derivatives

- Central nervous system toxicity: high doses of methotrexate and cytarabine, or intrathecal infection

Urologic and renal toxicity:

- Acute renal failure occurs chiefly with high doses of methotrexate.

- Tubulopathy occurs most often with platin derivatives.

- Hemorrhagic cystitis is a common adverse effect with cyclophosphamide and isosfamide.

Metabolic toxicity:

- Spindle poisons can cause SIADH, often with concomitant peripheral neuropathy and intestinal ileus.

Substantial improvements in survival rates among cancer patients admitted to the ICU have been achieved over the last decade.[1-6] Three factors have contributed to this advance: (1) patient selection, following reports in the 1980s of dismal outcomes[7-10] and ensuing recommendations that ICU admission be denied in many situations involving cancer patients[11-13]; (2) improved overall survival of cancer patients[14] as a result of therapeutic innovations and measures to prevent infections and drug toxicity; and (3) recent advances in ICU management of acute respiratory failure[2,15] and septic shock.[4]

Today, hospital mortality among cancer patients admitted to the ICU is approximately 50%, which is not higher than in other patient groups for whom ICU admission is standard practice (e.g., pancreatitis, extensive burns). In addition, parameters such as neutropenia, autologous bone marrow transplantation, or progression of malignancy no longer predict mortality.[16-18] New treatments, such as granulocyte colony-stimulating factor (G-CSF), shorten the duration of bone marrow failure,[19,20] thereby diminishing the risk of treatment-related infection, and medications that have limited toxicity can achieve remissions in patients initially considered as having relentlessly progressive disease.[21-23] As a result of these major therapeutic advances, the number of cancer patients referred for ICU admission is increasing steadily, with infection and treatment-related toxicity being the most common reasons for ICU admission.[5]

Intensivists are aware that further progress in diagnostic, prophylactic, and therapeutic strategies used in the ICU should provide additional survival gains in these patients. Better knowledge of the adverse effects of cancer chemotherapy would help intensivists to recognize drug toxicity earlier in patients admitted with suggestive symptoms, to administer specific treatments if available, and to anticipate and prevent toxic effects of medications started in the ICU.

This chapter focuses on the main toxic effects of cancer chemotherapy. Although not exhaustive, it supplies a long list of readily accessible references. It is written for intensivists who are called on to care for cancer patients with chemotherapy-related toxicity affecting the lungs, heart, metabolism, kidneys, nervous system, and bone marrow.

PULMONARY TOXICITY

Many anticancer agents can cause lung disease, usually with infiltrates. Lung toxicity may be life-threatening. Extrinsic evidence of causality varies widely. Abundant documentation of lung toxicity is available in the literature for some drugs, such as bleomycin, whereas only anecdotal case reports have been published for others. Consequently, the diagnostic strategy should follow the rules that apply to all drug-induced lung disorders:

1. Rule out pulmonary edema due to congestive heart failure.
2. Rule out lung infection due to an opportunistic or nonopportunistic organism (this is a diagnosis of exclusion).
3. Rule out lung infiltration by the cancer cells.
4. Check that the time from chemotherapy administration to respiratory symptom onset matches cases reported in the literature and determine whether the respiratory symptoms recur with each chemotherapy course (rechallenge).
5. Check that the clinical manifestations and laboratory test abnormalities are consistent with lung toxicity induced by the suspected drug (intrinsic evidence of causality).
6. Determine whether the symptoms resolve after the drug is stopped and glucocorticoids are given if needed.

When seeking to establish the diagnosis, intrinsic evidence should continuously be confronted with extrinsic evidence to ensure optimal selection of diagnostic investigations.

BLEOMYCIN-INDUCED LUNG TOXICITY

Bleomycin is a glycopeptide antibiotic that has been used since the 1970s in a wide range of solid tumors (lung cancer, esophageal cancer, head and neck cancer, germ-cell tumors of the ovary and testis, Kaposi's sarcoma), as well as Hodgkin's disease and non-Hodgkin's lymphoma. Bleomycin toxicity occurs in 3% to 40% of patients, the lung being the main target. Pneumonitis with diffuse infiltrates and fibrosis is the most typical manifestation, and it has a fatal outcome in 1% to 15% of cases.[24,25] Mean time to onset is 4 months after bleomycin administration.[26] Earlier lung toxicity responsible for clinical and radiographic manifestations reminiscent of bronchiolitis obliterans or hypersensitivity pneumonitis is less common.[24]

Available knowledge of the pathophysiology of bleomycin-induced lung toxicity stems mainly from animal models. Injury to the lung endothelium seems to be the initial event. Subsequently, there is an influx of inflammatory cells (macrophages, lymphocytes, and neutrophils) and of fibroblasts, and progression to lung fibrosis can occur.[24]

Established risk factors include the cumulative bleomycin dose, although the toxic amount varies across patients, most notably according to renal function. There is no threshold for toxicity but rather a linear relation between the bleomycin dose and the incidence of lung toxicity.[24] Simpson and colleagues[27] reported that lung toxicity rates were 5% with a cumulative bleomycin dose smaller than 450 mg, 13% with 450 to 550 mg, and 17% with more than 550 mg. However, because bleomycin is excreted through the kidneys, cumulative doses smaller than 100 mg have caused lung toxicity in patients with renal failure.[24] Other risk factors for bleomycin-induced lung fibrosis include age older than 70 years, tobacco use, concomitant radiation therapy to the chest, use of high fractional concentrations of inspired oxygen (often during surgery), and concomitant use of G-CSF or of other cancer chemotherapy agents exhibiting lung toxicity.[24,25,28,29]

A dry cough, dyspnea on exertion and then at rest, a fast breathing rate, and fever are the earliest symptoms.[24] Cyanosis may be visible. Fine crackling rales are heard over both lung bases, and, later in the course, rhonchi or a friction rub may be found. Infiltrates in both lung bases are typically seen on the chest radiograph, and progression to diffuse interstitial fibrosis may occur.[24] Computed tomography shows earlier changes consisting of subpleural linear and nodular opacities in the lung bases that may suggest lung metastases.[30] Asymmetric or more focal images can pose diagnostic challenges.[30] Blood gas measurements show hypoxia and hypocapnia, and lung function testing discloses a restrictive defect with decreases in vital capacity and in the diffusing capacity of the lung for carbon monoxide (DLCO).[24]

To decrease the risk of bleomycin-induced lung toxicity, the total dose should be determined according to the patient's risk factor profile, the objective being to find the best compromise between minimizing toxicity and optimizing the anticancer effect. Other drugs may be preferable in patients who are at high risk for bleomycin-induced lung toxicity. Suggested prophylactic agents include anti–tumor necrosis factor-α (TNF-α) and anti–transforming growth factor-β (TGF-β) antibodies, interleukin-1 (IL-1)–receptor antagonists, and antioxidants such as dexrazoxane, pentoxifylline, and amifostine.[24] Curative treatment starts with discontinuation of all chemotherapy agents known to cause lung toxicity and with respiratory function support, often in the ICU. Glucocorticoid therapy in a dosage of 60 to 100 mg/day is usually given, although compelling proof of efficacy is lacking. This practice is warranted given the possibility of bronchiolitis obliterans–organizing pneumonia or hypersensitivity pneumonitis, both of which respond to glucocorticoid therapy.[24] In survivors, the symptoms resolve completely and respiratory function returns to normal.[24]

METHOTREXATE PNEUMONITIS

Methotrexate is a cytotoxic agent belonging to the antimetabolite class. It antagonizes folic acid, thereby inhibiting the enzyme dihydrofolate reductase. Methotrexate is used not only in various solid tumors and hematologic malignancies, but also in nonmalignant diseases such as rheumatoid arthritis and severe psoriasis. Acute or subacute pneumonitis simulating an infection,[31] usually with interstitial involvement, occurs in 1% to 7% of patients receiving methotrexate.[32] The symptoms may also develop gradually over several weeks or months. Dyspnea, a dry cough, and, less often, a fever and headaches are the main clinical symptoms. Extrapulmonary manifestations may include erosive mucositis, a rash, and hepatic cytolysis.[32] Crackling rales are heard on lung auscultation. Peripheral blood eosinophil counts are moderately and transiently elevated. Hypoxemia (mean oxygen tension, 50 mm Hg), a restrictive defect, and a decrease in DLCO are typically found. Bronchoscopy with bronchoalveolar lavage (B-BAL) is mandatory.[33] The BAL fluid contains an abundance of cells with a predominance of lymphocytes; the CD4/CD8 ratio varies, most notably with the time from methotrexate administration to respiratory symptom onset.[34] Lung biopsy, whose use is declining, shows lymphocytic infiltration of the interstitial tissue and, rarely but distinctively, granulomas in areas of type II pneumocyte hyperplasia[32] with a variable degree of lung fibrosis.[35]

Again, the diagnosis rests on a set of converging arguments and on the principles reviewed earlier. Special attention should be directed to the toxicity of other anticancer agents (most notably bleomycin and cyclophosphamide) and to opportunistic lung infections (e.g., *Pneumocystis carinii* pneumonia, tuberculosis). Surgical or transbronchial biopsy is rarely appropriate but may deserve consideration if there is no response to treatment (methotrexate discontinuation and glucocorticoid therapy) or if there is a strong suspicion of lung infection despite negative B-BAL findings.

OTHER ANTICANCER AGENTS WITH LUNG TOXICITY

The purine analog fludarabine is an antimetabolite used mainly to treat advanced chronic lymphocytic leukemia and selected cases of low-grade lymphoma. Lung toxicity occurs in 8% of patients. Few cases have been published, the largest series to date being that of Helman and associates.[36] Fludarabine lung toxicity is a distinctive entity inasmuch as the specific immune function disorders induced by the drug promote the development of *P. carinii* pneumonia. Consequently, the diagnosis of fludarabine toxicity can be accepted only if two BAL examinations find no evidence of *P. carinii* infection. A favorable outcome is the rule after discontinuation off ludarabine and administration of systemic glucocorticoid therapy.

Gemcitabine is an antimetabolite used to treat solid tumors and hematologic malignancies. Although the bone marrow is the main target of gemcitabine toxicity (with at times profound myelosuppression), pulmonary toxicity occurs in 5% of patients.[37] Uncertainty continues to surround possible risk factors, although most patients seem to be older than 65 years of age; also, recent or concomitant mediastinal radiation therapy (e.g., for lung cancer) may increase the likelihood of lung toxicity.[37,38] The symptoms may set in within a few hours after the injection (usually at about the sixth injection) and include respiratory distress, a dry cough, a fever, crackling rales, and bilateral interstitial involvement on the chest radiograph.

Cytarabine, an agent similar to gemcitabine, has a longer history of use in acute myelogenous leukemia, in combination

with anthracyclines. Respiratory distress of variable severity develops in 13% to 28% of patients within 8 days of cytarabine initiation.[39]

BiCNU (carmustine) is an alkylating agent used to treat breast cancer and Hodgkin's disease. Interstitial pneumonitis with a potential for fibrosis is a rare adverse effect of BiCNU. The clinical presentation is similar to that of bleomycin-induced pneumonitis, and systemic glucocorticoid therapy has been found to be effective.[40]

Cyclophosphamide is widely used, not only to treat solid tumors and hematologic malignancies, but also as an immunosuppressant in patients with vasculitis or connective tissue disease. Clinical lung toxicity occurs in almost 1% of patients. There are two clinical variants: (1) acute lung toxicity with onset within 1 to 6 months after cyclophosphamide initiation and usually a favorable outcome after discontinuation of the drug and administration of glucocorticoid therapy, and (2) chronic lung fibrosis that worsens relentlessly and fails to respond to glucocorticoid therapy.[41]

Finally, a few cases of interstitial pneumonitis have been reported with melphalan, procarbazine, chlorambucil, mitomycin, vinblastine, etoposide, hydroxyurea, taxanes, and platin derivatives. An exhaustive list of drugs potentially responsible for lung toxicity and the corresponding clinical presentations can be found on the World Wide Web at http://www.pneumotox.com.

CARDIAC TOXICITY

Anthracyclines are the main culprits of cardiac toxicity. Evidence of cardiac toxicity for other agents (taxanes, antimetabolites, alkylating agents, and spindle poisons) is limited to anecdotal case reports.[42]

ANTHRACYCLINE-INDUCED CARDIAC TOXICITY

The anthracycline class—which includes doxorubicin, daunorubicin, epirubicin, idarubicin, and mitoxantrone—plays a major role in the treatment of many solid tumors (breast cancer, esophageal cancer, osteosarcomas) and hematologic malignancies (Hodgkin's disease, non-Hodgkin's lymphoma, acute leukemia). Anthracycline-induced myocardial toxicity can be life-threatening or dose-limiting, thereby affecting the prognosis of the disease by precluding optimal anticancer treatment.[43]

Anthracyclines induce cell death of dividing cells via inhibition of topoisomerase-2, intercalation to nucleus DNA, and production of free radicals.[44] The myocardium is vulnerable to free radicals because antioxidant enzyme activity is weaker in myocytes than in other tissues (e.g., liver, kidney). The cumulative anthracycline dose is the main risk factor for cardiac toxicity. Other risk factors include female gender, age at either end of the life span, black race, and Down syndrome.[43] Opinions are divided regarding the roles of prior radiation therapy to the chest, lymphoma, preexisting heart disease, and a preexisting decrease in the left ventricular ejection fraction.[43,45]

Two clinical presentations can be distinguished based on the timing of symptoms relative to anthracycline therapy—acute cardiotoxicity and chronic cardiotoxicity, which may be early (subacute) or delayed.[46] Acute cardiotoxicity manifests as a rapid deterioration in cardiac function during or within

1 week after the administration of anthracycline therapy, usually with reversal of the abnormalities after discontinuation of the drug.[43] Congestive heart failure with or without cardiogenic shock is the most common clinical presentation, although myocarditis or pericarditis may occur.[45] Adjustments in chemotherapy regimens have noticeably reduced the rate of acute cardiac toxicity, which now occurs in fewer than 1% of patients.[45] Chronic cardiotoxicity is far more common. The subacute form is characterized by irreversible dilated cardiomyopathy within 1 year after anthracycline discontinuation.[47-49] The delayed form develops insidiously after more than 1 year and runs a slowly progressive course.[47-49]

Electrocardiographic (ECG) changes are nonspecific and include sinus tachycardia, flat T waves, QT prolongation, and low amplitudes. Ventricular tachycardia and supraventricular rhythm disorders have been reported in patients with acute cardiac toxicity.[45] Troponin T elevation indicates myocardial damage with myocyte injury. Troponin I may be a good marker for cardiac dysfunction after high-dose chemotherapy and seems closely correlated to reduction in the left ventricular ejection fraction.[50] Echocardiography is a noninvasive and sensitive investigation.[43,45] Myocardial scintigraphy with technetium 99m is also used to document reductions in left ventricular ejection fraction and may be more informative than transthoracic echocardiography, most notably in obese patients. Dobutamine stress echocardiography has also been suggested as a diagnostic tool.[51] Finally, myocardial biopsy is an invasive diagnostic method whose sensitivity and specificity are controversial. Histologic analysis shows myofibril loss, dilation of the sarcoplasmic reticulum, and intracytoplasmic vacuoles in myocytes.[45]

Shock in a patient with a history of anthracycline therapy should prompt investigations for septic shock, even if there is evidence of cardiac dysfunction. Neutropenia strengthens the need to rule out sepsis. A diagnosis of congestive heart failure can be accepted only if fluid depletion induces full normalization of respiratory function and defervescence. B-BAL is mandatory in doubtful cases. Finally, the possible effects of other anticancer agents should be evaluated.

Curative Treatment

Standard treatment for congestive heart failure should be given, and anthracycline and other potentially cardiotoxic agents should be stopped, bearing in mind the negative consequences of this action on the chances of recovery from the malignant disease. Administration of an inotropic agent may be required in cases of acute cardiotoxicity. In chronic cardiotoxicity, angiotensin-converting enzyme inhibitors, diuretics, digitalis, and β-blockers are valuable. Heart transplantation has been used in patients with delayed cardiotoxicity and no evidence of active cancer.

Preventive Treatment

The mainstay of prevention is routine evaluation of cardiac function (measurement of left ventricular fraction ejection by echocardiography or cardiac scintigraphy) before starting anthracycline therapy. The anthracycline doses should be selected according to the patient's risk factor profile and the results of cardiac function evaluation. Close monitoring and in some cases cardioprotective therapy should be considered. Cardiac function should be tested at regular intervals throughout anthracycline therapy.

Epirubicin and idarubicin may be less likely to induce cardiotoxicity than the other anthracyclines. Continuous administration over several hours also seems to reduce the cardiotoxicity of anthracyclines. Available cardioprotective agents include dexrazoxane, an antioxidant that chelates iron.[52] Finally, liposomal encapsulation of anthracyclines reduces their cardiotoxicity without altering their anticancer effects.[53]

CARDIAC TOXICITY OF OTHER ANTICANCER AGENTS

Drugs of the taxane class, most notably paclitaxel, given in combination with anthracyclines, are effective in the treatment of breast cancer. However, cardiotoxicity occurs in more than 20% of patients treated with this combination.[54]

Furthermore, cardiotoxicity has been reported with high-dose 5-fluorouracil (5-FU) and with cyclophosphamide, cisplatin, and vincristine. The clinical presentation may be congestive heart failure, pericarditis or pancarditis, or supraventricular or ventricular rhythm disorders. These severe manifestations are fairly uncommon, and the cardiac abnormalities are usually reversible.

HEMATOLOGIC TOXICITY

In addition to the myelosuppressive effects expected with all anticancer agents, alterations in hemostasis are common after L-Asparaginase injection, and leukemia can occur in patients with a history of chemotherapy for cancer (Table 172-1). Furthermore, a number of anticancer agents induce impairments in cell-mediated immunity, thereby promoting the development of opportunistic infections. Infection and bleeding are the main complications of myelosuppression.

Whereas febrile neutropenia has been associated with 90% mortality in the absence of antimicrobial therapy,[55] mortality among neutropenic inpatients is now less than 10% in hematology wards[56] and 50% in ICUs.[17] This improved survival can be ascribed to the development of recommendations for the prophylaxis and treatment of infections in neutropenic patients,[57] use of autologous or allogeneic peripheral stem cell injections, improved knowledge of the pharmacokinetics and toxicity of anticancer agents, use of hematopoietic growth factors,[19,20] and introduction of medications with greater efficacy in fungal infections.

MYELOSUPPRESSION

Myelosuppression is virtually inevitable and usually reversible. The mechanism of action of the anticancer agent (i.e., the cell cycle phase affected by the drug) determines which cell lines are affected and governs the severity of marrow toxicity. For instance, nitrosoureas and mitomycin selectively destroy stem cells, causing severe and in some cases irreversible myelosuppression. In contrast, myelotoxicity is less marked with drugs that act more selectively on a specific cell cycle phase, such as vincristine, bleomycin, and cisplatin. Table 172-2 recapitulates the severity of myelosuppression seen with various agents.

The severity of myelosuppression varies also with patient-dependent factors such as age, extent of bone marrow invasion by tumor, prior treatments (radiation therapy and/or chemotherapy associated with myelofibrosis), and nutritional status. The World Health Organization has suggested a scheme for classifying the severity of myelosuppression based on peripheral blood cell counts, as shown in Table 172-3.

TABLE 172–1. HEMATOLOGIC TOXICITY OF CANCER CHEMOTHERAPY AGENTS

Toxic Effect	Anticancer Agents	Diagnostic Findings	Treatments
Anemia	Methotrexate, 5-FU, cytarabine, 6-mercaptopurine	Macrocytic anemia with normal levels of vitamin B_{12} and folate	Erythropoietin, blood transfusion
Thrombocytopenia	Nitrosoureas	Onset 4 to 6 weeks after chemotherapy	Transfusions
Marrow hypoplasia	Nitrosoureas, anthracyclines, busulfan	Anemia, thrombocytopenia, leukoneutropenia; nadir between 6 and 15 days after chemotherapy	Transfusions, erythropoietin, growth factors (G-CSF), stem cell reinjection
Thrombotic microangiopathy	Gemcitabine, mitomycin	Mechanical hemolysis (anemia, profound haptoglobin decrease, negative Coombs' test, schizocytes), high levels of LDH and free bilirubin, thrombocytopenia, renal failure	VIP transfusion, plasmapheresis, glucocorticoids, aspirin, dialysis
Hemostasis disorders	L-Asparaginase	Decreased PT, increased APTT; decreased fibrinogen, AT III, and plasminogen	Symptomatic: VIP transfusion, injection of AT III
Induced leukemia	Alkylating agents, nitrosoureas, etoposide, methotrexate, anthracyclines	AML 2 to 10 years after initial chemotherapy; complex karyotype abnormalities	—
Impaired cell-mediated immunity	2-CdA (cladribine, Leustatin), fludarabine (Fludara), pentostatin (Nipent), anti-CD52 (alemtuzumab, Campath)	Lymphopenia, opportunistic infections	Prophylaxis for *Pneumocystis carinii* infection

AML, acute myeloid leukemia; APTT, activated partial thromboplastin time; AT III, antithrombin III; 5-FU, 5-fluorouracil; G-CSF, granulocyte colony-stimulating factor; LDH, lactate dehydrogenase; PT, prothrombin time; VIP: virus-inactivated plasma.

Transfusion of packed red blood cells and platelets is the cornerstone of the treatment of myelosuppression. If there is time for planning in advance, mobilized peripheral stem cells (autologous or allogeneic) can be injected, a measure that shortens the duration of neutropenia to about 10 days. Bone marrow transplantation is followed by approximately 3 weeks of marrow failure.[19,20] Injections of G-CSF also reduce the severity of neutropenia.[19,20] Anemia induced by chemotherapy can be minimized by regular injections of erythropoietin.[58] Finally, careful attention should be given at all times to correcting nutritional deficiencies, particularly deficiencies of folic acid, iron, and vitamin B_{12}.

HEMOSTASIS DISORDERS INDUCED BY L-ASPARAGINASE

L-Asparaginase is widely used to treat acute lymphoblastic leukemia. Produced from strains of *Escherichia coli*, L-asparaginase hydrolyzes asparagine, an amino acid required by cells for protein synthesis. However, the effect of L-asparaginase is not confined to blast cells, and it causes a global decrease in protein synthesis. In particular, the decrease in clotting factor production by the liver manifests as a reduction in serum fibrin levels in 70% of patients, usually with no symptoms. If the alterations in hemostasis are severe, they manifest a both bleeding and thromboembolism (stroke and cerebral vein thrombosis). Clotting tests show low levels of prothrombin, antithrombin, and plasminogen, as well as an increase in the activated partial thromboplastin time.[59]

The treatment rests on symptomatic measures, most notably administration of virus-inactivated plasma or antithrombin. Neurologic complications, if present, should be treated appropriately.

SECOND LEUKEMIA AND MYELODYSPLASIA

Myelodysplasia and acute leukemia can occur within 10 years after treatment for breast cancer, ovarian cancer, or Hodgkin's disease with alkylating agents, nitrosoureas, mitoxantrone, VP-16, or methotrexate. Cytogenetic (karyotypic) abnormalities are common.[60] The prognosis is dismal, because resistance to chemotherapy is the rule.

TABLE 172–2. SEVERITY OF MYELOSUPPRESSION SEEN WITH VARIOUS CHEMOTHERAPY AGENTS

Mild	Moderate	Severe
Cisplatin	Antipurine	Anthracycline
Bleomycin	Podophyllin	Nitrogen mustard
Vinca alkaloids	Alkylating agents	Antifolates
	Hydroxyurea	Antipyrimidines
	Mitomycin	Nitrosoureas
	Procarbazine	(carmustine, lomustine)
		Busulfan
		Dacarbazine

TABLE 172–3. WORLD HEALTH ORGANIZATION SCHEME FOR CLASSIFYING THE SEVERITY OF MYELOSUPPRESSION

Toxicity Grade	Hemoglobin (g/dL)	Leukocytes (×1000)	Neutrophils (×1000)	Platelets (×1000)
0	Normal	Normal	Normal	Normal
1	9.5-10.9	3-4.5	1.5-1.9	75-100
2	8-9.4	2-2.9	1-1.4	50-74
3	6-7.9	1-1.9	0.5-0.9	25-49
4	4-5.9	0.5-0.9	0.1-0.4	<25
5	Death	Death	Death	Death

TABLE 172–4. NEUROLOGIC TOXICITY OF CANCER CHEMOTHERAPY AGENTS

Toxic Effect	Drugs	Diagnostic Findings	Treatments
Encephalopathies (headache, confusion, seizures)	BiCNU, cisplatin, cytarabine, 5-FU, ifosfamide, asparaginase, methotrexate, procarbazine	—	—
Cerebellar syndrome	Cytarabine, 5-FU	Clinical, imaging studies	—
Myelopathy (paraplegia, cauda equina syndrome)	Intrathecal methotrexate, cytarabine, thiotepa	—	—
Peripheral neuropathy	Vincristine, cisplatin, and taxanes	Clinical, electrophysiologic testing	Prevention: glutathione, amifostine for cisplatin; pain control
Stroke and cerebral vein thrombosis	Asparaginase, high-dose methotrexate, BiCNU or cisplatin by intracarotid injection	Clinical, imaging (CT, MRI)	—
Ototoxicity	Cisplatin	Audiogram	Amifostine, glutathione
SIADH	Vincristine	Low serum sodium	—
Cranial nerve involvement	Vincristine (nerves IV, V, and VI), ifosfamide	—	—
Aseptic meningitis	Intrathecal methotrexate and cytarabine	Spinal tap	—
Leukoencephalitis	Methotrexate	MRI	Hydration, folinic acid rescue therapy
Ophthalmologic involvement	Cisplatin, vincristine	Transient cortical blindness, retrobulbar optic neuropathy, retinal involvement, extraocular nerve palsy	Glutathione IV, amifostine

BiCNU, carmustine; CT, computed tomography; 5-FU, 5-fluorouracil; MRI, magnetic resonance imaging; SIADH, syndrome of inappropriate secretion of antidiuretic hormone.

IMPAIRED CELL-MEDIATED IMMUNITY

Lymphocyte depletion occurs with 2-CdA, fludarabine, pentostatin, and the recently introduced monoclonal antibody to CD52, alemtuzumab (Campath). Lymphodepletion can be profound and promotes the development of opportunistic infections. Prophylactic treatment is mandatory, most notably to prevent *P. carinii* infection.

NEUROLOGIC TOXICITY

Neurologic adverse effects of anticancer agents are both common and severe (Table 172-4). They may preclude the administration of optimal chemotherapy, thereby compromising the chances for recovery. The peripheral and central components of the nervous system may be affected. The diagnosis is one of exclusion; infections, trauma, and infiltration by malignant cells should be ruled out first.[61]

CONSEQUENCES OF INTRATHECAL INJECTIONS

Transient aseptic meningitis occurs within a few hours after direct intrathecal or intracerebral injection of anticancer agents in about 30% of cases. Introduction of a pathogen during the injection should be ruled out. Typically, meningeal symptoms and a fever develop (60% of cases). Concomitant radiation therapy may attenuate the symptoms by blunting the inflammatory response. A number of less common complications have been reported, such as myelopathy with paraplegia or cauda equina syndrome after cytarabine injection,[62] apparently ascribable to axonal damage due to a direct toxic effect on myelin. Repeated methotrexate injections can be

followed by progressive leukoencephalopathy.[63] The risk increases with the cumulative methotrexate dose; other risk factors include persistently high methotrexate levels in the cerebrospinal fluid, concomitant radiation therapy, and concomitant systemic methotrexate therapy.[63] Cerebral imaging studies may show multiple foci of atrophy and demyelination selectively affecting the periventricular white matter and the centrum semiovale, ventricular dilation, and calcifications. Optimal hydration, together with injectable folate supplements in patients receiving concomitant systemic methotrexate therapy, may decrease the risk of leukoencephalopathy.[64]

PERIPHERAL NERVOUS SYSTEM TOXICITY

Peripheral neuropathy may affect the sensory, motor, or autonomic nerve fibers (Table 172-5). One or more nerves may be affected, and multifocal forms may be symmetric or asymmetric. Demyelination or direct axonal damage is the

TABLE 172–5. CLASSIFICATION OF TOXIC NEUROPATHY

Toxicity Grade	Deep Tendon Reflexes	Paresthesia	Transit
0	Normal	Absent	Normal
1	Decreased	Present	Irregular
2	Absent	Severe	Constipation
3	Absent	Painful	Subobstruction
4	Paralysis	Autonomic disorders	Obstruction
5	Death	Death	Death

underlying abnormality. Vinca alkaloids and platin derivatives are the main causes of chemotherapy-related peripheral neuropathy.[61] Bilateral symmetric paresthesia in the hands and feet develops gradually. Physical findings may include absence of deep tendon reflexes, distal symmetric hypesthesia predominantly affecting thermal and pain sensations, and a variable degree of motor loss ranging from mild muscle weakness to paresis. Autonomic nervous system involvement results in transit time prolongation ranging from constipation to paralytic ileus, postural hypotension, and erectile and ejaculatory dysfunction. Electrophysiologic testing shows distal axonal dysfunction with blunting of action potentials.[65] The sensory fibers are predominantly affected.

Risk factors for peripheral neuropathy include alcohol abuse, diabetes mellitus, liver dysfunction, and a history of treatment with neurotoxic anticancer agents (platin derivatives).[61] Acute reversible peripheral neuropathy has been described in patients receiving vincristine for Hodgkin's disease; G-CSF may potentiate the toxicity of vincristine. In addition, the neurotoxicity of vincristine is dose-dependent: neurotoxicity can occur with cumulative doses of 5 to 6 mg and is seen consistently with doses greater than 15 to 20 mg. The abnormalities resolve slowly, over a few weeks to a few months. Vitamin supplementation does not seem to reduce the risk of neurotoxicity.

A number of other anticancer agents can induce peripheral neuropathy. Although the kidney is the main target of cisplatin toxicity, peripheral neuropathy similar to that seen with vincristine has been reported in more than 50% of patients.[65] Cisplatin may selectively affect proprioceptive and vibratory sensations. Motor loss is moderate. Autonomic system dysfunction may occur. Cisplatin neurotoxicity seems to be more common in female than in male patients, and it may be preventable by intravenous glutathione administration and by amifostine. Gradual recovery is the rule after cisplatin discontinuation, although a slowly progressive course occurs in a few patients.

Peripheral neuropathy has been reported with ifosfamide, procarbazine, taxanes (paclitaxel and docetaxel), and spindle poisons. Amitriptyline is effective in relieving the pain.

CENTRAL NERVOUS SYSTEM TOXICITY

Most anticancer agents are high-molecular-weight or water-soluble compounds that do not cross the blood-brain barrier. Central nervous system toxicity therefore is uncommon but may occur with high doses (methotrexate, cytarabine) or with routes of administration that bypass the blood-brain barrier (intrathecal injection, intracarotid injection, osmotherapy, direct intracranial chemotherapy). Cerebellar syndrome has been reported with cytarabine (cytosine arabinoside) and 5-FU (particularly in patients with dihydropyrimidine dehydrogenase deficiency). High-dose cisplatin can cause encephalopathy (headache, behavioral or personality disorders, confusion, drowsiness, seizures, and coma); concomitant optic nerve involvement may occur (Table 172-6). Ifosfamide is responsible for reversible, non–dose-dependent neuropsychiatric disorders including visual or auditory hallucinations, a dreamlike state, confusion, personality disorders, and anxiety. Seizures or a coma may occur. Extrapyramidal manifestations with myoclonus and spasticity are classic manifestations of ifosfamide neurotoxicity. Among patients treated with methotrexate in doses greater than 1 g/m², 15% experience spontaneously reversible

TABLE 172–6. CLASSIFICATION OF ENCEPHALOPATHY ACCORDING TO SEVERITY

Severity Grade	Description
0	No symptoms
1	Agitation, drowsiness
2	Bedridden
3	Requires treatment
4	Coma, manic episode, suicidal behavior
5	Death

encephalopathy, which must be differentiated from leukoencephalopathy with irreversible chronic pseudodementia. L-Asparaginase treatment causes encephalopathy in 15% to 60% of patients. Fludarabine is associated with a high rate of neurotoxicity (15% of patients), which is dose dependent and can be prevented by using low doses (25 mg/m³, 5 days per month). Encephalopathy is less common with 5-FU, BiCNU, and procarbazine.

CRANIAL NERVE INVOLVEMENT

Vincristine is responsible for involvement of the fourth, fifth, and sixth cranial nerves, facial palsy, laryngeal nerve palsy, and transient cortical blindness. Hearing loss is common with cisplatin; this effect is dose dependent and can be irreversible, with loss of ciliated cochlear cells.

UROLOGIC AND RENAL TOXICITY

Many factors can cause renal dysfunction in patients receiving anticancer chemotherapy,[66] including radiation-induced nephritis, tumor lysis syndrome, hyperuricemia, hyperphosphatemia, hypercalcemia, lysozymuria, thrombotic microangiopathy, disseminated intravascular coagulation, infiltration by the cancer cells, amyloidosis, and renal consequences of obstructive uropathy. Exacerbation of renal dysfunction occurs if nephrotoxic agents are used (e.g., aminoglycosides, antifungal agents, antiviral agents, iodine).

A number of anticancer agents can cause renal failure (Table 172-7). This effect is dose-limiting and therefore compromises the chances of recovery from the malignancy.[67] However, except for a few drugs such as carboplatin, pharmacokinetic data for guiding dosage adjustment are scarce.[68-71] In addition to renal failure, tubular disease or, more rarely, glomerular disease or thrombotic microangiopathy may occur with some agents.[66,72] The distal urinary tract may be affected by ifosfamide or cyclophosphamide.

The World Health Organization has developed a grading system for chemotherapy-related renal failure, based on urine output and serum creatinine levels, as shown in Table 172-8.

RENAL FAILURE

Methotrexate nephrotoxicity occurs chiefly with high doses (greater than 1 g/m²)[73] and is fatal in 20% of cases. The underlying mechanism involves precipitation of methotrexate and its even less soluble metabolite, 7-hydroxymethotrexate, within the renal tubules.[66] Precipitation is more likely to occur at acidic pH values, so urine alkalinization is mandatory, in combination with administration of folinic acid to antagonize the effects of methotrexate.[74]

TABLE 172–7. RENAL AND UROLOGIC TOXICITY OF CANCER CHEMOTHERAPY AGENTS

Toxic Effect	Drugs	Diagnostic Findings	Treatments
Chronic renal failure (cumulative dose)	Carmustine, semustine, streptozocin, platin derivatives, ifosfamide, pentostatin	Renal biopsy	Discontinuation of the anticancer agent
Acute renal failure	Methotrexate	—	Prevention: appropriate hydration, urine alkalinization
Glomerular disease	Carmustine, semustine, streptozocin	—	—
Tubular disease	Streptozocin, cisplatin, carboplatin, ifosfamide, cytarabine	Hypophosphatemia, hypokalemia, hypomagnesemia, hypouricemia, metabolic acidosis, glucosuria, aminoaciduria	Hyperhydration and forced diuresis for platin derivatives; amifostine; thiosulfate sodium
Hemorrhagic cystitis	Ifosfamide, cyclophosphamide		Hyperhydration, mesna
Dysuria, hematuria	Methotrexate, pentostatin	—	Appropriate hydration

Prolonged ifosfamide therapy can result in progressive renal failure; mesna protects against the bladder toxicity but not the renal toxicity of ifosfamide.[70,71]

With platin derivatives, nephrotoxicity is common, dose dependent, tubular, and potentially irreversible. Nephrotoxicity is the main dose-limiting adverse effect of these agents. Cisplatin therapy is consistently associated with a 20% to 40% decrease in the glomerular filtration rate.[68,70,75-77] Fluid and sodium repletion together with dose fractionation diminish the nephrotoxic effects of platin agents. Antidotes have been tested, but the results have been inconclusive.[78]

TUBULOPATHY

Platin derivatives can induce acute alterations in electrolyte levels. Severe hypomagnesemia is the earliest sign of tubular toxicity and may persist several years after the last chemotherapy course. Hypocalcemia and, less often, hypokalemia can occur as a result of the hypomagnesemia. Urinary concentrations of alanine aminopeptidase, N-acetyl-β-glucosaminidase, and β_2-microglobulin are elevated, indicating preferential involvement of the proximal tubules. If a renal biopsy is performed, histologic analysis shows tubular dilation, epithelial cell necrosis, interstitial edema and fibrosis, and thinning of the tubular basement membrane.

Ifosfamide also damages the proximal tubules. The suspected mechanism is inhibition of the Na^+/H^+ pumps and impairment of the sodium-dependent transporters of glucose, phosphate, and L-alanine by two ifosfamide metabolites, chloroacetaldehyde and 4-OH-ifosfamide. Laboratory tests show renal failure with urinary wastage of electrolytes (most notably phosphate), glucose, and amino acids. Urinary levels of alanine aminopeptidase, N-acetyl–β-glucosaminidase,

and β_2-microglobulin are high, indicating damage to the proximal tubules. Risk factors for ifosfamide-induced tubulopathy include a cumulative dose greater than 45 g/m[2], age younger than 5 years, a history of cisplatin therapy, and preexisting renal dysfunction from any cause.[66,70,71]

GLOMERULOPATHY

The glomerules are susceptible to damage from a number of alkylating agents. Prolonged administration of carmustine or semustine, for instance, can cause renal dysfunction with proteinuria. Histologic study shows glomerulosclerosis, thinning of the glomerular basement membranes, and foci of interstitial necrosis or tubular atrophy. In most patients, renal function fails to improve after treatment discontinuation.

THROMBOTIC MICROANGIOPATHY

Thrombotic microangiopathy manifests as acute renal failure. Although most cases occur as paraneoplastic syndromes, most notably in patients with metastatic mucus-secreting tumors, chemotherapy can induce hemolytic-uremic syndrome (10% of patients receiving mitomycin C). A few cases have been reported in patients treated with gemcitabine, CCNU (lomustine), and platin derivatives, and combinations such as daunorubicin/cytarabine or bleomycin/cisplatin have also been reported to cause thrombotic microangiopathy.

Mitomycin-induced thrombotic microangiopathy occurs after 5 to 12 months of treatment and within 1 to 2 months after the last dose.[66] The risk is higher with cumulative doses greater than 60 mg. Pulmonary edema, arterial hypertension, and oliguria or anuria are the typical manifestations; 17% to 25% of patients have central nervous system manifestations such as confusion, seizures, or coma.[72] Laboratory tests show acute renal failure, proteinuria, mechanical hemolytic anemia (with schizocytes), and peripheral thrombocytopenia. The reticulocyte count is high. Levels of free bilirubin and lactate dehydrogenase are high, whereas haptoglobin levels are dramatically decreased. The Coombs test is negative. The treatment is the same as for idiopathic thrombotic microangiopathy: virus-inactivated plasma transfusions, plasmapheresis, glucocorticoid therapy, blood pressure control, antiplatelet agents, and renal replacement therapy. The disorder continues to progress after discontinuation of mitomycin, and the outcome is usually fatal.[72]

TABLE 172–8. WORLD HEALTH ORGANIZATION GRADING SYSTEM FOR CHEMOTHERAPY-RELATED RENAL FAILURE

Grade	Urine Output	Serum Creatinine (μmol/L)
0	Normal	Normal
1	Transient decrease	115-180
2	Diuretic agents	181-354
3	High-dose diuretic agents	355-530
4	Dialysis	531-800
5	Death	Death

HEMORRHAGIC CYSTITIS

Hemorrhagic cystitis is a common adverse effect with the alkylating agents cyclophosphamide and ifosfamide.[79,80] Degradation of oxazaphosphorine in the kidneys produces acrolein, which has direct toxic effects on the bladder mucosa.[79,80] Prevention relies on appropriate saline hydration and administration of mesna,[78,81,82] which binds to acrolein, producing a stable, water-soluble thioester that is promptly eliminated. Mesna has no curative effects.[82] If cystitis occurs despite preventive measures, a double-lumen urinary catheter should be inserted for continuous bladder irrigation until the bleeding stops completely.[79]

METABOLIC TOXICITY

Metabolic disorders in patients receiving cancer chemotherapy fall into two groups: disorders related directly to the tumor (e.g., urinary tract compression, spontaneous lysis, syndrome of inappropriate secretion of antidiuretic hormone [SIADH]: Schwartz-Bartter syndrome) and disorders related to anticancer agents (e.g., drug-induced tumor lysis, electrolyte disturbances).[83] Hyponatremia (related chiefly to SIADH) is the main source of clinical symptoms.[84] Spindle poisons (vincristine, vinblastine, and, more rarely, vinorelbine [Navelbine]) can cause SIADH, often with concomitant peripheral neuropathy and intestinal ileus.[85,86]

Alkylating agents such as cyclophosphamide (lymphomas and solid tumors) or melphalan (myelomas) and, more rarely, chlorambucil and thiotepa can induce SIADH.[83,84] Cisplatin (used to treat cancer of the lung, ovary, or testis and relapsing lymphoma) is associated with hyponatremia related to SIADH or tubular wasting in 4% to 10% of patients.

Six criteria are used for the diagnosis of SIADH: (1) hyponatremia lower than 130 mmol/L; (2) plasma osmolality lower than 275 mOsm/kg; (3) urinary osmolality greater than plasma osmolality and greater than 500 mOsm/kg; (4) no clinical evidence of fluid and sodium depletion; (5) normal renal and adrenal gland function; and (6) normal thyroid function.[87] However, a diagnosis of chemotherapy-induced SIADH requires prior elimination of other causes, including paraneoplastic syndromes, central nervous system disorders, lung infections, and SIADH induced by other drugs.[87] The treatment is the same as for other causes of SIADH.[88,89]: fluid and sodium restriction to slowly correct the hydroelectrolytic disorders and to minimize the risk of central pontine myelinolysis. Blocking the effects of ADH on the renal collecting tubes by administration of diphenylhydantoin, lithium, or demeclocycline has been suggested.[88,89] In patients receiving cisplatin, failure of the renal tubule to reabsorb sodium results in excessive urination with hypovolemia and should be treated by sodium repletion. Finally, the decision whether to continue the causal chemotherapy agent must be made after careful consideration and close monitoring of electrolyte levels.

ANNOTATED REFERENCES

Kintzel PE: Anticancer drug-induced kidney disorders. Drug Saf 2001;24:19-38.
  Renal toxicity of chemotherapy, physiopathological explanations.

Lewis C: A review of the use of chemoprotectants in cancer chemotherapy. Drug Saf 1994;11:153-162.
  The interest of chemoprotectants in onco-hematology.

Singal PK, Iliskovic N: Doxorubicin-induced cardiomyopathy. N Engl J Med 1998;339:900-905.
  Diagnostic procedures of doxorubicin-induced cardiomyopathy.

Sleijfer S: Bleomycin-induced pneumonitis. Chest 2001;120:617-624.
  Clinical features, pathogenesis, risk factors, and treatment of bleomycin-induced pneumonitis.

Verstappen CC, Heimans JJ, Hoekman K, Postma TJ: Neurotoxic complications of chemotherapy in patients with cancer: Clinical signs and optimal management. Drugs 2003;63:1549-1563.
  Recent review of neurologic toxicity of chemotherapy.

Chapter 173

HEMATOLOGY AND ONCOLOGY IN CHILDREN

Guillaume Emeriaud • Jacques Lacroix

KEY POINTS

1. Anemia occurs in 37% of critically ill children.

2. Five types of events can be life-threatening in sickle cell disease: vaso-occlusive crisis, acute splenic sequestration, aplastic crisis, hyperhemolytic crisis, and infection.

3. A red blood cell (RBC) transfusion must be given to critically ill children who present with a hemoglobin (Hb) concentration lower than 5 g/dL. Above this value, the Hb concentration that should prompt a pediatric intensivist to prescribe RBC transfusion is unknown.

4. To limit exposure to multiple donors, packed RBCs should be administered on a unit-by-unit basis; packed RBCs are also available in half-units and in small units of 75 mL.

5. Disseminated intravascular coagulation is the most frequent hemorrhagic disorder observed in the pediatric intensive care unit (PICU).

6. Catheter-related thrombosis is common in PICU.

7. An acute oncologic emergency can be the initial presentation of an undiagnosed cancer, or it can be the consequence of a complication of the malignancy or its treatment.

8. Many system dysfunctions observed in critically ill children with malignancy are attributable to side effects of chemotherapy and radiation therapy.

9. Infections observed in oncologic patients are frequently caused by unusual germs.

10. In children with recurrent or refractory malignancies and those who have undergone bone marrow transplantation with prolonged mechanical ventilation and sustained multiple organ failure, outcomes are often poor and aggressive support may be unwarranted or futile.

This chapter is an overview of the main hematologic and oncologic problems that can be observed in pediatric intensive care units (PICUs). Differences between critically ill children and adults are emphasized.

HEMATOLOGY

ANEMIA

A normal decrease in the hemoglobin (Hb) level is observed during the first weeks of life, because of a limited release of erythropoietin. For this reason, the normal range of Hb concentration changes with age: 18.5 ± 2.0 g/dL (mean ± 2 standard deviations) during the first week of life, 11.5 ± 1.2 g/dL at 2 months, 12.0 ± 0.7 g/dL at 12 months, 13.5 ± 1.0 g/dL at 9 years, and 14.0 ± 1.0 g/dL after 12 years of age.[1] Based on these ranges, anemia occurs in 37% of critically ill children.[2]

Causes of anemia are multiple in critically ill children. Hemorrhage, phlebotomy, hemolysis (immunologic, infectious, microangiopathic, or toxic), and decreased production (invasion of the bone marrow, side effect of therapy, nutritional deficiency, blunted production of erythropoietin in response to hypoxia)[3] are frequently involved. Causes relatively specific to pediatric practice include congenital anemias (e.g., sickle cell disease, thalassemia, Blackfan-Diamond disease), glucose-6-phosphate dehydrogenase deficiency, and metabolic disorders. Sickle cell disease merits specific comment.

Sickle Cell Disease

Many types of abnormal Hb are observed in sickle cell disease. However, only Hb SS (homozygous sickle cell Hb), Hb SC, and Hb S–β-thalassemia can cause severe clinical problems. Five types of events can be life-threatening: vaso-occlusive crisis, acute splenic sequestration, aplastic crisis, hyperhemolytic crisis, and infection.

Vaso-occlusive crisis can affect any vascular bed, but the most dangerous manifestations are the acute chest syndrome, which can progress rapidly to severe acute respiratory distress syndrome (ARDS), and stroke. Stroke must be considered in patients who present with monoplegia, hemiplegia, or focal seizures. Painful crises involving joints or extremities are frequent during the second and third year of life. Infarction of abdominal structures (e.g., liver, gut) may also be observed. Hypoxemia, acidosis, polycythemia, and a high proportion of abnormal Hb are the main risk factors for vaso-occlusive crises. Transfusion of packed red blood cells (RBCs) is the main treatment. The goal of therapy is to decrease abnormal Hb to less than 30%, while maintaining the hematocrit at less than 35%. An exchange transfusion should be considered in severe cases, especially in acute chest syndrome or stroke. Oxygen, hyperhydration, pain-killing drugs, and sedation are also part of treatment.[4] Treatment of the precipitating cause is very important (e.g., antibiotics are urgently needed if an infection is possible). Noninvasive or invasive mechanical ventilation may be required. Some experts would also give bicarbonate if there is a severe metabolic acidosis. Nitric oxide destruction by free Hb is probably increased in sickle cell anemia[5]; one small trial suggested that inhaled nitric oxide (80 ppm) may be useful,[6] although this finding remains to be validated. Surgical treatment is rarely needed, most abdominal crises being caused by vaso-occlusion. Cholecystitis is not rare, but surgery may be postponed in most instances until after the vaso-occlusive crisis.

During a sequestration crisis, the amount of blood retained in the spleen may lead to hypovolemic shock and even death. An acute reduction of Hb concentration of 2 g/dL or more, with no other cause of blood loss, is considered diagnostic.

Aplastic crises can also cause an acute and severe anemia. The half-life of RBCs is severely shortened (15 to 20 days) in patients with major sickle cell diseases, and their production is increased. During aplastic crises, the reticulocyte count is low and the Hb level can decrease rapidly. An infection with parvovirus B19 is sometimes identified. Mortality rates associated with both sequestration crises and aplastic crises are significant, and these conditions must be treated aggressively, with volume administration and RBC transfusion (the Hb level must be increased by at least 5 g/dL).

Most hyperhemolytic crises are caused by an infection. The hematocrit decreases within a few days, and the reticulocyte count can increase by more than 35%. Treatment involves volume administration, RBC transfusion, and treatment of the infection.

Sickle cell disease can cause a functional asplenia with increased susceptibility to bacterial infections; these children are at high risk of contracting severe infections with *Streptococcus pneumoniae*, osteomyelitis, and septicemia.

Preventive measures must be used if possible. Patients with sickle cell disease should be monitored in the PICU after significant surgery to prevent dehydration, hypoxemia, and pain and to maintain the hematocrit between 30% and 35%. Long-term prevention can include chronic transfusion therapy and hydroxyurea[7]; other treatments that are under investigation include clotrimazole[8] and bone marrow or umbilical cord stem cell transplantation.[9] Genetic correction of sickle cell disease has been carried out with success in transgenic mice.[10]

Red Blood Cell Transfusion

The management of anemia in critically ill patients is discussed in Chapters 19 and 166; management includes prevention of blood loss, transfusion of blood products, and administration of folic acid and iron. The usefulness of erythropoietin is under investigation.[11]

The risks and benefits of RBC transfusion are not similar in adults and children. Some adverse events, such as necrotizing enterocolitis in neonates[12] or erythrocyte alloimmunization in young girls (up to 8% of patients),[13] are significant problems in the PICU. RBC transfusion to neonates increases the ratio of adult to fetal Hb, which decreases the affinity of blood for oxygen.[14] Nevertheless, RBC transfusion improves oxygen transport in critically ill children,[15-18] although the improvement in clinically significant outcomes resulting from transfusion, and specifically the definition of the optimal transfusion threshold, remain to be determined. Two studies completed in Africa suggested

that maintaining the Hb concentration of hospitalized children higher than 5.0 g/dL decreased the risk of death.[19,20] The critical Hb concentration may be higher in ICU patients because disease and stress increase oxygen consumption. In fact, the threshold Hb concentration with the best risk-benefit ratio in critically ill children is unknown,[21] and there is large variation among intensivists in transfusion practice patterns.[22,23]

Some points unique to pediatric practice must be considered when transfusing RBCs to a critically ill child. Packed RBCs should be administered on a unit-by-unit basis to limit exposure to multiple donors. Packed RBCs are available in half-units (standard division) or in small units of 75 mL (Pedipak) for young children. Packed RBC units must be warmed to 37°C if the patient is small (weight less than 10 kg) or if the amount given is substantial (greater than 20% to 30% of the blood volume).

Transfusion-associated graft-versus-host disease is a significant problem in immunodeficient patients. It can even occur in immunocompetent patients who receive dedicated blood donations from their parents, because the recipient may be unable to recognize white blood cells of a closely related donor as foreign.[24] Children with immunodeficiency and recipients of dedicated (directed donor) packed RBC units should receive irradiated RBCs.

HEMORRHAGIC DISORDERS

Disseminated intravascular coagulation (DIC) is the most frequent hemorrhagic disorder observed in the PICU. Its causes, pathophysiology, and treatment are similar to those in adults (see Chapters 21 and 34), even though purpura fulminans is more frequent in the PICU.

Congenital deficiencies of coagulation factors, as in hemophilia A (factor VIII), hemophilia B (factor IX), or factor VII deficiency, can cause severe hemorrhage. Congenital or acquired (dietary, antibiotics) vitamin K deficiency can also cause severe bleeding. Massive transfusion of packed RBCs is another cause of coagulation factor deficiency frequently seen in the ICU.

Thrombocytopenia in critically ill patients is related most often to sepsis, DIC, or multiple organ dysfunction syndrome or is drug-induced (see Chapter 20). Heparin-induced thrombocytopenia must also be considered. Immune-mediated thrombocytopenia in newborns can be secondary to maternal disease (e.g., maternal lupus erythematosus). Idiopathic thrombocytopenic purpura is frequent in children, but it rarely causes severe bleeding. Hemolytic uremic syndrome (HUS) and thrombotic thrombocytopenic purpura (TTP) can be associated with bleeding, but it is usually the renal failure or central nervous system involvement that leads the patient to the PICU. Platelet transfusion should be avoided in HUS and TTP, because it can accelerate the microangiopathy. However, platelet transfusion may be required in such cases if a critically ill child is bleeding and has significant thrombocytopenia. A platelet colony-stimulating factor is under investigation.

THROMBOSIS AND EMBOLI

Elsewhere in this book, there are chapters on pulmonary emboli (Chapter 79), thromboembolic diseases (Chapter 169), and their prophylaxis. Most thromboses observed in pediatric critically ill patients are acquired during the stay in the ICU. The causes and the sites of thrombosis in children are different than in adults. Children rarely are admitted to the PICU with a thrombosis of the limb, but catheter-related thrombosis is common, appearing rapidly after insertion of a catheter.[25] Heparin-coated catheters may prevent catheter-related thrombosis,[26] but their costs and benefits remains to be determined. DIC, allergy to heparin, prothrombic states (e.g., G20210A prothrombin-gene mutation, factor V Leiden, anticardiolipin antibody, antithrombin III, or protein C deficiency), and blood flow stasis are common risk factors for thrombosis in children.

Cerebral venous sinus thrombosis and renal vein thrombosis are more frequent in children than in adults. Symptoms of cerebral venous sinus thrombosis include seizures, coma, paresis, cranial nerve palsies, signs of increased intracranial pressure, and venous infarcts. Head and neck infections, chronic diseases such as connective tissue disorders, and prothrombic states are frequently associated.[27] Symptoms of neonatal renal vein thrombosis are acute renal insufficiency, hematuria, and hypernephrosis.

IMMUNODEFICIENCY

A significant proportion of critically ill children are immunodeficient. Most cases of acquired immunodeficiency are caused by chemotherapy and immunosuppressive drugs, but any severe condition, such as severe head trauma, sepsis, or burns, can induce immunodeficiency. Congenital immunodeficiencies are not rare in the PICU. For example, DiGeorge syndrome is frequent among patients with congenital heart disease. These patients have an increased risk of contracting infections, with unusual pathogens, in unusual sites, and with increased severity.

ONCOLOGY

The initial presentation of an undiagnosed cancer can occasionally represent an acute emergency requiring critical care. Consequences of a complication of a malignancy or its treatment commonly result in the need for PICU admission. Any organ or system can be involved. This section gives a brief overview of the most frequent cancers that are seen in critically ill children, describes the most frequent causes of system dysfunction that are encountered in such patients, and discusses the special case of pediatric bone marrow transplant recipients. Finally, some ethical considerations that are specific to these patients are presented.

CANCER IN CHILDREN

The most frequent cancers in children are leukemias, lymphomas, neuroblastoma, Wilms' tumor, central nervous system solid tumors, bone tumors, and soft tissue cancers. Cancer patients may need a stay in a PICU for any of the following reasons: (1) need for close monitoring during or after a high-risk procedure; (2) life-threatening complications of a cancer (e.g., compression of airways); or (3) malignancy or therapy-related complications. The prognosis of the patients in the first group is usually good, and their length of stay in the PICU is short. Most of the discussion in the subsequent sections involves the two other presentations.

Respiratory System

Causes of respiratory dysfunction in cancer patients include those observed in patients without cancer (see Chapter 89 on acute parenchymal disease in children and Chapter 75 on ARDS). However, many more specific diseases merit comment.

Respiratory infections are frequently caused by unusual pathogens. Primary lung malignancy is rare in children (histiocytosis), but leukemia, lymphoma, and metastases (neuroblastoma, bone cancer, Wilms' tumor) can invade the lungs. Airways can be obstructed by an intraluminal malignant mass, by an extrinsic bronchial or tracheal compression, or by vocal cord paralysis (e.g., after surgery for a thyroid cancer). Severe pulmonary hemorrhage can contribute to respiratory complications. Graft-versus-host disease and idiopathic pneumonia syndrome can be seen after bone marrow transplantation.[28] Respiratory dysfunction can also be related to cancer therapy (see Chapter 172 on adverse effects of cancer therapies).

Invasive investigation is sometimes required, such as bronchoalveolar lavage (see Chapter 218) or lung biopsy. Unusual organisms, such as *Mycobacterium, Pneumocystis,* and fungi, should be considered, as should invasion by malignant cells. Lung biopsy may be useful in some instances. However, the risk of severe complications (death, barotrauma, hemorrhage) is high in patients requiring mechanical ventilation,[29,30] and lung biopsy is generally contraindicated in cases of ongoing hemorrhage, significant coagulopathy, or arterial blood oxygen saturation less than 90%.[31]

Noninvasive mechanical ventilation is an effective means of preventing endotracheal intubation in immunocompromised patients with acute respiratory failure.[32] Nevertheless, invasive ventilation is frequently required.

Cardiovascular System

All types of shock can be observed in patients with malignancy. However, some cardiovascular diseases are more commonly seen in such patients.

The incidence of septic shock is high in pediatric patients with malignancies. Tumor can also cause heart failure by obstruction (e.g., mass in the auricula), compression, hemorrhagic or septic pericardial effusion, infection or inflammation of cardiac structures (endocarditis, myocarditis, pericarditis), fibrosis (i.e., restrictive myocarditis), or irritation of the cardiac electrical system. Congestive heart failure may also be caused by chemotherapy (especially with anthracycline or cyclophosphamide).

Arterial hypertension is frequently present, usually as a result of treatment side effects, particularly with corticosteroids. Severe hypertensive crisis can also result from malignant synthesis of sympathic mediators (neuroblastoma, Wilms' tumor, and, rarely, pheochromocytoma).

Neurologic System

Causes of seizures include mass effect, metastasis, infection, vasculitis, thrombosis, hemorrhage, adverse reaction to drugs or radiation therapy, hyponatremia, hypocalcemia, and hypertensive crisis.

Intracranial hypertension can be caused by infection, hemorrhage, a volume-expanding tumor, or hydrocephalus caused by an infratentorial brain tumor blocking spinal fluid flux.

Meningitis can be caused by the cancer itself or by an infectious process. Unusual organisms may be involved, such as *Cryptococcus neoformans, Toxoplasma gondii, Listeria monocytogenes,* and gram-negative rods.

Coma or paralysis can be caused by cerebral or spinal cord insults from compression, ischemia, or hemorrhage. Opsoclonus, raccoon eyes, and Horner's syndrome are suggestive of a neuroblastoma. Side effects of radiation therapy include Guillain-Barré–like syndrome, transverse myelitis, paraplegia, and brain necrosis. Myasthenia gravis may be the mode of presentation of thymoma.

Digestive System

Stress gastritis, peptic ulcer, and upper gastrointestinal bleeding are frequent in the PICU in children with malignancies. Bleeding from the gut or from a digestive cancer is rare in children, but it can be severe. Epstein-Barr virus, herpes simplex virus, or cytomegalovirus can cause hemorrhagic necrosis of the gastrointestinal tract with severe bleeding. *Candida* esophagitis is another cause of bleeding. Upper and/or lower gastrointestinal endoscopy must be done in case of severe bleeding.

Typhlitis is an inflammation of the cecum and surrounding tissue. It has been reported in 10% of leukemic patients at postmortem examination.[33] Usual signs of abdominal inflammation can be absent in neutropenic patients; therefore, typhlitis must be feared in all patients with suspicion of infection. Abdominal computed tomography is a good diagnostic test for this condition. Secondary sepsis or bleeding (or both) is the usual cause of death. Diarrhea is also quite frequent. *Clostridium difficile* colitis must be suspected in patients who have recently received antibiotics (see Chapter 162). Gastroenteritis may be caused by unusual organisms such as *Cryptosporidium.*

Hepatic dysfunction can be caused by viral infection, drug toxicity (methotrexate), or veno-occlusive disease resulting from chemotherapy or radiation therapy. Lymphoma can mimic veno-occlusive disease.[34] Most cases of pancreatitis result from cytotoxic reactions to chemotherapy.

Renal System

Cancer-related causes of acute renal failure include chemotherapy (e.g., cyclosporine, methotrexate), obstruction of the urinary tract by a tumor or by breakdown byproducts (uric acid, calcium-phosphate precipitate), radiation nephritis, invasion of the kidneys (leukemia, lymphoma), or multiple organ dysfunction syndrome. Acute tumor lysis syndrome can cause an acute renal insufficiency, but prevention is usually effective.

Metabolic Problems

Electrolyte disorders are frequently observed. These disorders are discussed in Sections I and VII. Malignant hypercalcemia is rare in childhood malignancies (incidence, less than 0.4%).[35] On the other hand, hypoparathyroidism and hypocalcemia can occur after thyroid surgery in adolescents. Moreover, hypocalcemia is frequent after massive transfusion. Hypercalcemia and hypocalcemia are discussed in Chapters 17 and 130.

Lactic acidosis in critically ill patients is usually a consequence of respiratory or cardiovascular dysfunction, sepsis, or multiple organ dysfunction. However, cancer with rapid and large turnover of malignant cells (e.g., leukemia, lymphoma) can be associated with lactic acidosis.[36,37]

Craniopharyngioma, some types of histiocytosis, and intracranial metastases can cause panhypopituitarism.

Fasting hypoglycemia is not rare in children with malignancy. Anorexia is a frequent symptom of cancer, as are nausea and vomiting, which are common side effects of cytotoxic chemotherapy. Enteral feeding should be attempted, but it is frequently limited by intolerance or abdominal complications. Therefore, parenteral nutrition is frequently required. Insulinoma is another cause of hypoglycemia in this population; it is associated with multiple endocrine neoplasia type I (MEN I) syndrome and Beckwith's syndrome. Hyperglycemia is also frequent, and insulin therapy may be indicated, to avoid limitation of caloric intake.

Steroids are part of many therapeutic protocols. Secondary adrenal insufficiency may appear if steroid treatment is inadvertently suspended.

Hematologic Problems

The proportion of cancer patients receiving chemotherapy who present with a significant hemorrhage is about 10%.[38]

Thrombosis is also a concern. Many types of cancer are associated with a hypercoagulable state because they release procoagulant mediators. DIC, heparin-induced thrombocytopenia, and catheter-related thrombosis are also frequent.

Bone marrow failure is extremely frequent in patients with cancer. It is an expected side effect of cytotoxic and radiation therapies, but it can also result from the cancer itself, infection, and many other causes. A reactive hemophagocytic syndrome can also occur in patients with severe multiple organ dysfunction syndrome.[39]

Causes of anemia and thrombocytopenia were discussed earlier. Causes of neutropenia include increased destruction (sepsis, hypersplenism) and decreased production (e.g., infections, malignant invasion of the bone marrow, radiation, drug toxicity). The risk of infections increases if the neutrophil count is lower than 1000/mm³. The use of various colony-stimulating factors (CSFs), such as granulocyte-macrophage (GM)-CSF, granulocyte (G)-CSF, and macrophage-granulocyte inducer, is advocated by some clinicians to shorten neutropenia. However, the number of transfusions required, the incidence of infection, and the survival rate are not ameliorated, even in neutropenic patients.[40,41] Even though CSFs are frequently used in patients with cancer and in recipients of bone marrow transplants, their usefulness remains to be determined.

Infectious Problems

Children with cancer must always be considered immunodeficient. Community-acquired pneumonia (Chapter 83), nosocomial pneumonia (Chapter 84), infections in the immunocompromised patient (Chapters 85 and 155), catheter-related infections (Chapter 145), and prevention as well as control of nosocomial infection (Chapter 144) are of considerable importance in these patients and are discussed in other chapters of this textbook.

Many symptoms anticipated in normal patients are attenuated in immunocompromised patients. For example, abdominal palpation can be normal in cases of peritonitis in neutropenic children, but some signs are suggestive of infection. For example, tender purpuric pustules or nodules suggest septic bacterial or fungal emboli.

Aggressive empirical antibiotic treatment must be initiated as soon as an infection is suspected, and sometimes antifungal or antiviral agents are included. A wide array of pathogens can be involved, including saprophytes, parasites, and fungi. G-CSF may be considered in neutropenic patients.

TABLE 173–1. OUTCOMES OF PATIENTS WITH MALIGNANCY OR BONE MARROW TRANSPLANTATION ADMITTED TO A PEDIATRIC INTENSIVE CARE UNIT

Patient Category	First Author (ref. no.)	Year of Admissions	Number of Days in PICU	Survival Rate (%)
Patients with cancer	Butt* (52)	1988	133	52
	Meert* (53)	1991	63	73
	Sivan* (54)	1991	72	49
	Heney* (55)	1992	70	51
	van Veen* (49)	1996	57	68
	Hallahan (56)	2000	172	84
	Heying* (57)	2001	48	73
Bone marrow transplant recipients	Rossi (58)	1999	39	44[†]
	Keenan (51)	2000	121	16[†‡]
	Hallahan (56)	2000	34	38
	Schneider (59)	2000	28	50
	Hagen (60)	2003	86	41[†]
	Jacobe (61)	2003	40	56[†]

PICU, pediatric intensive care unit.
*Study did not include bone marrow transplant recipients.
[†]Study included only patients who required mechanical ventilation.
[‡]Survival after 30 days.

BONE MARROW TRANSPLANTATION

Chapter 171 is devoted to bone marrow transplantation in adults. The adverse events that are observed after transplantation are quite similar in children and adults.

ETHICAL CONSIDERATIONS

The concept of "lethal condition futility" has been introduced to emphasize that curative care is futile if it only lengthens the agony of a patient, without promising a reasonable quality of life.[42] The current consensus among PICU caregivers is that intensive care is inappropriate if the chance of even short-term survival is poor because the patient is in the late stage of a chronic disease.[43-46] However, conflict about end-of-life decisions may arise with family members. Such problems must be overcome to provide the best and most appropriate palliative care and to open the way to what has been called "good death."[47]

End-of-life decisions about patients with cancer and bone marrow transplant recipients must be addressed by a multidisciplinary team, including the patient if he or she can express his or her will, family members, nurses, oncologists, and intensivists. It must be based on the chance of recovery from the acute disease, the chance of survival from the underlying disease, the quality of life before the acute problem, and the wishes of the patient and the parents.[48] The Pediatric Risk of Mortality (PRISM) score is not accurate in critically ill children with cancer and those who have received a bone marrow transplant.[49] A new score has been created for that purpose, but it remains to be validated.[50] Therefore, these scores cannot be relied upon to direct end-of-life decisions in these children. Survival rates of critically ill children with a newly diagnosed malignancy are good enough to merit a stay in the PICU in most instances. The outcomes for children with long cancer histories was so poor in the 1980s that these children were sometimes managed in palliative care outside the PICU. However, outcomes in these patients have improved in recent years (Table 173-1), and increasingly more intensivists would now admit such patients to the PICU.

The outcomes for bone marrow transplant recipients who require a stay in a PICU is worse than for patients with other malignancies, but the survival rate is significant. However, most recipients will die if they require mechanical ventilation for longer than 7 days, if they contract a multiple organ dysfunction syndrome with respiratory failure,[50] or if organ dysfunction syndrome includes more than one organ failure 7 days after intubation.[51]

ANNOTATED REFERENCES

English M, Ahmed M, Ngando C, et al: Blood transfusion for severe anaemia in children in a Kenyan hospital. Lancet 2002;359:494-495.
  The data in this paper suggest that the risk of mortality increased significantly in African children who required hospitalization if their Hb level was less than 5 g/dL.

Experts Working Group: Guidelines for red blood cell and plasma transfusions for adults and children. Can Med Assoc J 1997;156(Suppl 11):S1-S24.
  This is a very good summary of the available evidence on RBC and plasma transfusions. Comments specific to children are provided.

Heying R, Schneider DT, Korholz D, et al: Efficacy and outcome of intensive care in pediatric oncologic patients. Crit Care Med 2001;29:2276-2280.
  The outcome of children with cancer who require a stay in a PICU has improved so much in recent years that many of these patients would profit from critical care medicine.

Hilbert G, Gruson D, Vargas F, et al: Noninvasive ventilation in immunosuppressed patients with pulmonary infiltrates, fever, and acute respiratory failure. N Engl J Med 2001;344:481-487.
  This paper suggests that noninvasive mechanical ventilation may improve the prognosis and may prevent invasive mechanical ventilation if applied soon in the progression of acute respiratory diseases in immunosuppressed patients.

Jacobe SJ, Hassan A, Veys P, et al: Outcome of children requiring admission to an intensive care unit after bone marrow transplantation. Crit Care Med 2003;31:1299-1305.
  The outcome of children requiring admission to an ICU after bone marrow transplantation also has improved in recent years; however, it is inappropriate to maintain mechanical ventilation for more than 1 week in most instances, because almost all of these patients will die.

Section X

ENDOCRINE DISORDERS

Chapter 174

HYPERGLYCEMIC COMAS

P. Vernon van Heerden

KEY POINTS

1. Diabetic ketoacidosis (DKA) and hyperosmolar nonketotic hyperglycemia syndrome (HNHS) are life-threatening syndromes with a 6.2% overall mortality rate. The mortality rate for DKA is 1.2% to 4.9%, and for HNHS it is 2% to 41%.

2. DKA is a syndrome of hyperglycemia, metabolic acidosis, ketosis, and severe volume depletion. Severe insulin deficiency is the hallmark of this syndrome. Fluid and electrolyte depletion is a major component of the pathophysiology, as is unfettered lipolysis, which leads to the formation of ketoacids.

3. Precipitating factors for DKA include lack of insulin (either relative or absolute), physical stressors, postsurgical management, and substance abuse. Presenting clinical features of DKA include dehydration, ketosis, and metabolic acidosis. Laboratory tests usually show hyperglycemia, spurious hyponatremia, hyperosmolality, metabolic acidosis, elevated serum urea and creatinine levels, and elevated serum ketone levels.

4. Defining features of HNHS include hyperglycemia, dehydration, and hyperosmolality, but without ketoacidosis, indicating the presence of at least some insulin. HNHS is associated with a degree of renal dysfunction and impaired water intake.

5. Clinical features of HNHS that differentiate it from DKA are that it is less common than DKA, occurs in an older age group, and has a higher mortality rate; that hyperosmolality may be severe but metabolic acidosis is not as severe; and that normal anion gap and serum ketone levels are present. Precipitating factors for HNHS include mental obtundation, severe dehydration, renal dysfunction, and inappropriate diuretic use. Main metabolic derangements of HNHS are severe dehydration, relative insulin deficit, electrolyte depletion, and metabolic acidosis.

6. Neurologic sequelae of the hyperglycemic syndromes include altered mental state, cerebral edema, focal neurologic deficits, cognitive impairment, posthyperglycemic syndrome, seizures, and pain associated with hyperglycemic syndromes.

7. Diagnosis of hyperglycemic syndrome includes metabolic derangement on laboratory testing, hyperglycemia, and, usually, identification of a precipitating cause. Neuroradiologic testing may be required to exclude focal neurologic pathology (e.g., subdural hemorrhage), and specific diagnostic tests may be required to determine the exact type of metabolic acidosis (e.g., lactic acidosis versus ketoacidosis), to identify the precipitating cause of the hyperglycemic syndrome, or to exclude differential diagnoses.

8. The principles of management of hyperglycemic syndrome are as follows:
   - Treat the patient in a safe environment.
   - Institute treatment promptly, even if it means delaying precise diagnosis.
   - Airway protection is a priority.
   - Sedation of the delirious patient may be required to allow treatment to proceed safely.
   - Monitoring is important and is tailored to the severity of illness of the patient.
   - Serial laboratory testing is essential to guide therapy.
   - Treatment of the precipitating cause is important.
   - Serial clinical examinations and investigations allow more accurate therapy.
   - Treatment of comorbidities (e.g., severe ischemic heart disease) must not be forgotten in the critically ill patient.

9. Complications of treatment must be anticipated and dealt with expeditiously and may include hypokalemia, hypoglycemia, hyperchloremic metabolic acidosis, fluid overload, and cerebral edema.

Diabetic ketoacidosis (DKA) and hyperosmolar nonketotic hyperglycemia syndrome (HNHS) are life-threatening syndromes caused by metabolic derangement associated with diabetes mellitus. Although a distinction is made in the definitions of the two syndromes, there is much commonality between them, with up to 30% of presentations having features of both syndromes. DKA is approximately three times as common as HNHS in patients presenting with hyperglycemic syndromes.[1]

Although the metabolic derangement seen in DKA and HNHS is extreme, the death rate associated with these syndromes is low with appropriate and meticulous therapy. Surveys of patients presenting with hyperglycemic syndromes have found a 6.2% overall mortality rate, with 1.2% to 4.9% of deaths associated with DKA and 2% to 41% of deaths associated with HNHS.[1,2] Most deaths are not caused by the metabolic derangement but occur as a result of coexisting disease (e.g., myocardial infarction), sepsis (particularly pneumonia), or, less frequently, the management methods employed.[2,3]

HYPERGLYCEMIC SYNDROMES

DIABETIC KETOACIDOSIS

DKA is a syndrome of hyperglycemia, metabolic acidosis, ketosis, and severe volume depletion. DKA occurs in insulin-dependent diabetics, and severe insulin deficiency is the hallmark of this syndrome. Raised levels of stress hormones (glucagon, catecholamines, cortisol, and growth hormone) are also a feature. The hyperglycemia results in a glucose load in the glomerular filtrate that overwhelms the reabsorptive capacity of the renal tubules, resulting in an osmotic diuresis, with fluid and electrolyte depletion. Ketone bodies contribute to this osmotic diuretic effect. The lack of insulin causes unfettered lipolysis and the formation of ketoacids.

DKA accounts for approximately 6% of all diabetic admissions to hospital[3] and occurs in a younger age group (mean age, 33 years) compared with DKA-HNHS (44 years) or HNHS (69 years).[1]

Precipitating factors associated with the development of DKA include the following[3-5]:

- Lack of insulin, either relative or absolute
  Newly diagnosed or undiagnosed insulin-dependent diabetes
  Noncompliance with treatment or inadequate treatment in diagnosed diabetes
  Dietary mismanagement
- Physical stressors
  Acute infective illness (e.g., pneumonia, cholecystitis, urinary tract infection)
  Myocardial infarction
  Systemic inflammatory syndromes (e.g., pancreatitis)
  Medication interactions or mismanagement
  Glucocorticoid, phenytoin, or diuretic therapy
- Postsurgical management
- Substance abuse

Although there are many "stressors" in the ICU environment that could potentially cause or predispose to DKA (e.g., sepsis, altered caloric intake, use of total parenteral nutrition, catecholamine use), new development of DKA in the ICU is not common, presumably because of the high level of vigilance in this environment.

Presenting clinical features of DKA reflect the underlying metabolic derangements of dehydration, ketosis, and metabolic acidosis and include the following:

- Thirst and polyuria
- Tachycardia and hypotension
- Reduced skin turgor
- Dry mucous membranes
- Kussmaul respiration and ketotic fetor
- Evidence of infection/inflammation (e.g., fever)
- Altered mental state (discussed in detail later)

Laboratory tests supporting the diagnosis of DKA commonly reveal the following:

- Hyperglycemia
- Usually spurious hyponatremia

- Preserved or high levels of serum potassium (reflecting the acid-base status and not the severe total body depletion of potassium that is present)
- Variable levels of serum magnesium, calcium, and phosphate (although these are usually low or are revealed to be low on commencement of therapy)
- Hyperosmolality
- Metabolic acidosis, with low pH, low serum bicarbonate, raised anion gap, and raised serum ketone levels and a compensatory hypocapnia
- Elevated serum urea and creatinine levels
- Elevated serum ketone levels, as measured by the concentrations of β-hydroxybutyrate and acetoacetone

HYPEROSMOLAR NONKETOTIC HYPERGLYCEMIA SYNDROME

The defining features of HNHS include hyperglycemia, dehydration, and hyperosmolality, without ketoacidosis. The main differentiation from DKA appears to be the presence of at least some insulin (i.e., relative, rather than absolute, lack of insulin), more variable levels of stress hormones or counter-regulatory hormones, and the fact that renal dysfunction is commonly present. Renal dysfunction and impaired tubular function result in less capacity to deal with high solute and osmotic loads. This, together with impaired water intake, results in severe dehydration.

As mentioned earlier, HNHS is less common than DKA, occurs in an older age group, and has a higher mortality rate. Mortality may be associated with missed diagnosis (especially if the patient's mental state is impaired), comorbidity, or delayed or inappropriate therapy.

For HNHS, particularly in elderly patients, the precipitating factors (in addition to those listed for DKA above) commonly feature the following:

- Mental obtundation, dementia, or physical impairment limiting access to water (e.g., previous cerebrovascular accident)
- Severe dehydration
- Renal dysfunction
- Inappropriate diuretic use

Laboratory test results are similar to those listed for DKA but differ somewhat in degree, in that

- Serum glucose levels are usually higher
- Serum sodium levels may be normal (inappropriately so for the degree of hyperglycemia)
- Markers of renal dysfunction are worse
- Hyperosmolality is more marked
- Metabolic acidosis is not as severe
- Normal anion gap and serum ketone levels are present

METABOLIC DERANGEMENTS IN HYPERGLYCEMIC SYNDROMES

The main metabolic derangements that result in morbidity and must be urgently addressed in the management of both DKA and HNHS are severe dehydration, insulin deficit, electrolyte depletion, and metabolic acidosis. These are discussed in detail in Chapters 12 and 18.

Severe dehydration is estimated to be a water deficit in the range of 100 to 200 mL/kg.[4] Although there is no consensus on the ideal approach to fluid management in these patients, prompt restoration of the circulation with isotonic fluid (e.g., normal saline solution), followed by more moderate replacement of the water deficit using hypotonic fluid, are the underlying principles.

The insulin deficit should be treated initially with intravenous soluble insulin to produce normal blood glucose levels within 12 to 24 hours.

Electrolyte depletion is treated by appropriate replacement of sodium, potassium, magnesium, calcium, and chloride, as indicated by frequent testing during the early phase after presentation.

Metabolic acidosis rarely requires specific therapy and corrects with volume expansion and insulin therapy. Bicarbonate therapy is controversial but currently is not advocated, regardless of the presenting pH, because of the possibilities of exacerbation of hypokalemia, intracellular acidosis, reduced myocardial contractility, and reduced tissue oxygenation.

Figure 174-1 shows serial measurements taken from a typical patient with DKA on presentation and during his treatment in the ICU.

Therapy may be complicated if there is severe comorbidity, such as acute or acute on chronic renal failure or severe congestive heart failure, and in the patient who requires complex postsurgical care. In all cases, treatment of hyperglycemic syndromes should occur in an appropriate ICU environment with adequate monitoring and meticulous attention to detail to avoid the neurologic sequelae associated with these syndromes.

NEUROLOGIC SEQUELAE OF THE HYPERGLYCEMIC SYNDROMES

Neurologic sequelae of the hyperglycemic syndromes are not uncommon. They may occur before presentation (and may in fact be the precipitating cause), during the period of severe metabolic derangement, or after apparently uneventful correction of the hyperglycemic syndrome. The following sections describe recognized neurologic sequelae associated with the hyperglycemic syndromes.

ALTERED MENTAL STATE

Patients who present with DKA or HNHS commonly have an altered mental state, which may range from delirium to coma. Often the patient is very unwell and as a consequence is stuporous and uncommunicative, requiring continual prompting to elicit responses to questioning. This condition

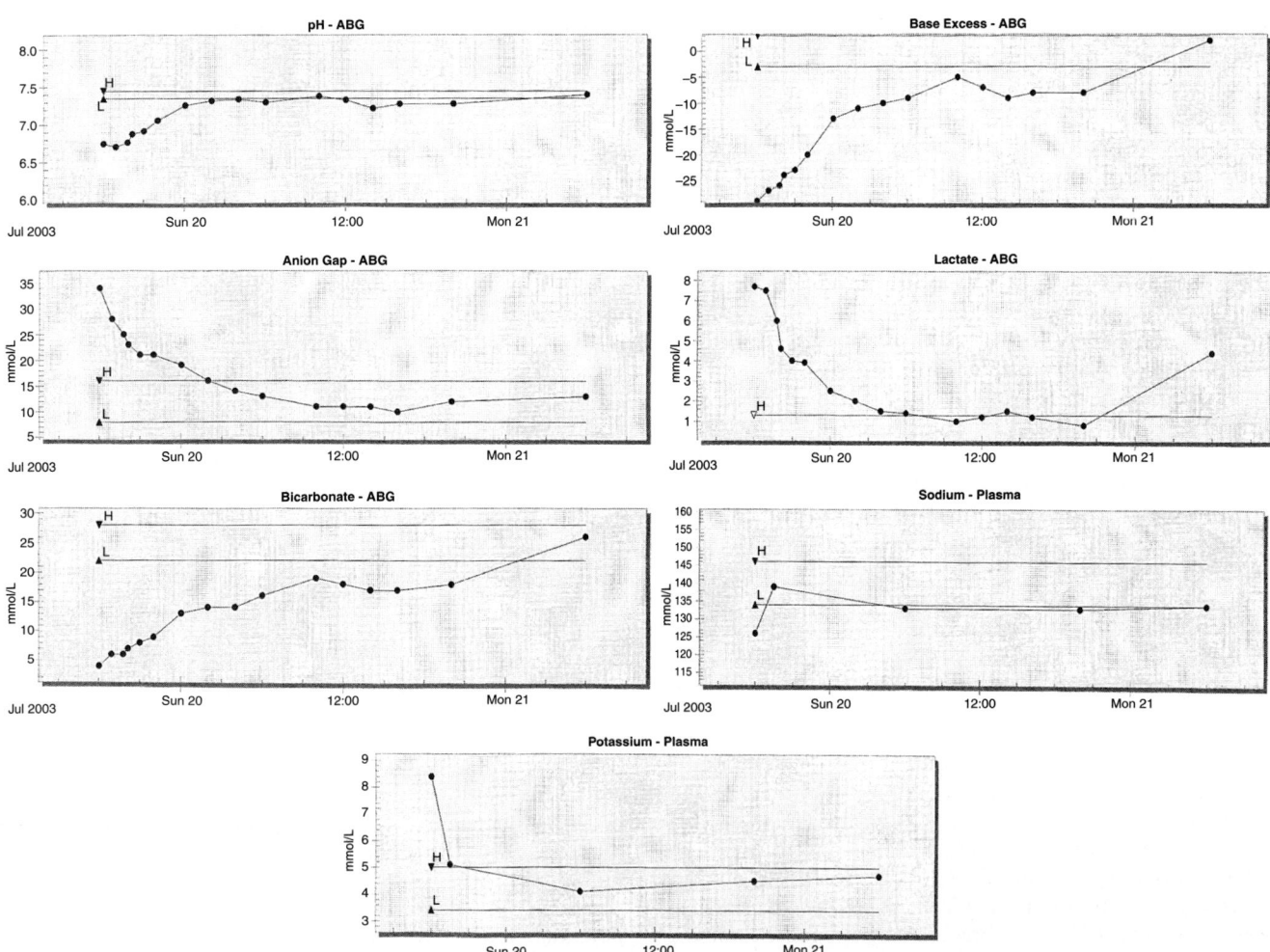

FIGURE 174–1. Trends in metabolic parameters monitored during treatment of diabetic ketoacidosis. ABG, arterial blood gases.

rapidly improves after rehydration, correction of the hyperglycemia, and correction of acidemia, if present, provided there is no underlying neurologic disease. Occasionally, a patient is completely unresponsive, even to painful stimuli, and requires management appropriate to the unconscious patient during treatment of the hyperglycemic syndrome (see later discussion). Clinically, there is no good correlation between blood glucose level, osmolality or pH, and the presenting mental state, which appears to be more a function of the patient's general health, comorbidities, the precipitating cause, and the duration of the hyperglycemic syndrome before presentation.

Clinical features of the comatose patient include all of the features of the hyperglycemic syndrome and, in addition, reduced level of consciousness as determined by the Glasgow Coma Scale (GCS), reactive pupils, variable reflex responses (due to the possibility of diabetic peripheral nerve disease), and occasional lateralizing motor signs. Lateralizing signs and lack of improvement in level of consciousness with correction of the metabolic derangement mandate further investigations, such as urgent computed tomographic (CT) scanning of the cranium or toxicology screening for sedative or illicit drugs.

Less commonly, the main feature of altered mental state is delirium. Delirium is marked by features of disorientation and psychomotor agitation. Delusions and hallucinations may also be manifested, particularly if drug intoxication has been a precipitant of the hyperglycemic episode. These patients can be very difficult to manage, presenting a danger to themselves and to their caregivers (e.g., pulling out venous or monitoring lines, refusing to cooperate with treatment regimens). Adequate sedation with either minor or major tranquilizers may be necessary to allow treatment to proceed smoothly.

CEREBRAL EDEMA

Rapid correction of hyperglycemia and hyperosmolality is associated with the development of cerebral edema in patients with hyperglycemic syndromes. Animal experiments suggest that this effect is not caused by sodium movement into the brain but by the rapid correction of glucose and osmolality.[6] Acidosis does not appear to play a role. This work negates somewhat previous theories[6-9] on the development of cerebral edema in hyperglycemic states, which suggested that the edema might be due to an effect of pH on the Na^+/K^+ exchange pump, causing entry of sodium and water into brain cells; osmotic disruption of the blood-brain barrier; or accumulation of osmotically active solutes ("pseudo-osmoles") such as amino acids, polyols, and trimethylamines, as an adaptation to the hyperosmolar environment. Other theories of the mechanism of cerebral edema include paradoxical central nervous system acidosis and a left shift in the oxygen-hemoglobin dissociation curve that reduces tissue oxygenation.[10]

The use of isotonic, rather than hypotonic, solutions for rehydration and the avoidance of a too-rapid correction of hyperglycemia appear to offer some protection against the development of cerebral edema. Cerebral edema is more common after treatment of DKA than after treatment of HNHS.[6] In patients with DKA, it is more common in the young, in whom the incidence is as high as 6.8 per 1000 episodes of DKA.[11] Cerebral edema is also more common in newly diagnosed diabetics.

Cerebral edema after treatment for a hyperglycemic syndrome usually manifests as prolongation of the altered mental state seen on presentation or new development of an altered mental state, with features as described previously. In adults, the signs and symptoms may be very subtle and abate over the course of a few days. Usually no specific therapy is required, besides good supportive care. Rarely, cerebral edema can produce focal and permanent neurologic damage.[12] Cerebral edema associated with DKA in children is a much more serious condition with a considerable mortality.[11,13-15] Urgent treatment of severe cerebral edema relies on intravenous mannitol in the first instance, followed by steroids and loop diuretics as second-line therapy.[10]

FOCAL NEUROLOGIC DEFICITS ASSOCIATED WITH HYPERGLYCEMIC SYNDROMES

There are isolated reports in the literature describing focal neurologic damage in patients with hyperglycemic syndromes. Most commonly, cerebrovascular accidents (CVA), particularly hemorrhagic and thrombotic types, have been associated with HNHS. This is not surprising, because CVA may be the precipitating factor for the development of HNHS in diabetic patients, and the hyperosmolar state in both DKA and HNHS may predispose to thrombotic CVA. Intracerebral venous thrombosis has also been reported[16] and has a poor outlook.

CVA may result in neurologic deficit evident on presentation, but often the final clinical picture is obscured by the altered mental state and only becomes clear after treatment of the hyperglycemic syndrome. The high incidence of neurologic signs and symptoms in diabetics may make the detection of new neurodeficits difficult. Many of the focal neurologic signs seen in these patients, particularly those with HNHS, disappear after treatment of the hyperglycemic syndrome. This may represent unmasking of focal areas of cerebrovascular insufficiency by the dehydration.[5]

Focal neurologic damage may also occur as a result of fluid and electrolyte shifts produced during treatment of the hyperglycemic syndromes (e.g., putaminal hemorrhage,[12] lateral pontine and extrapontine myelinolysis[17]). In patients who are treated for prolonged periods in the ICU for complications related to their episode of hyperglycemic syndrome critical illness polyneuropathy is also a possibility. This presents as profound, but reversible, tetraplegia.[18]

Adequate investigation of a residual or new focal neurologic deficit is mandated. This may include CT scanning, magnetic resonance imaging (MRI), and nerve conduction studies.

COGNITIVE IMPAIRMENT AFTER HYPERGLYCEMIC SYNDROMES

Cognitive impairment may occur after hyperglycemic syndrome. This impairment may be gross and clinically apparent (more common in elderly patients) or very subtle (e.g., poor concentration, loss of memory). It may be associated with focal or global neurologic deficit, as described previously, or it may be apparent in the presence of a structurally normal brain. Most cognitive impairment that is not caused by structural brain damage improves with time. Sensory-evoked potentials have shown promise as a sensitive test to detect subclinical brain dysfunction in patients with severe DKA.[19]

SEIZURES ASSOCIATED WITH HYPERGLYCEMIC SYNDROMES

Focal and generalized seizures are common in patients with hyperglycemic syndromes and may be resistant to treatment with the usual anticonvulsant agents.[5] Epilepsia partialis continua, an unusual form of seizure typified by abnormal MRI signal intensity in the precentral gyrus, can occur in DKA or HNHS.[20]

PAIN ASSOCIATED WITH HYPERGLYCEMIC SYNDROMES

Pain may be a prominent clinical feature of patients with hyperglycemic syndromes. Pain, often neuropathic in origin, may be so severe as to mimic the acute surgical abdomen. Pleuritic chest pain and headache are also common. Proper evaluation of pain is very difficult in the patient with emergent hyperglycemic syndrome. Frequent clinical evaluation, while addressing the main pillars of therapy (fluid and electrolyte replacement and insulin therapy) is important to detect early the true surgical cause of pain. Pain caused by the hyperglycemic syndrome itself usually diminishes with time and appropriate treatment, whereas other pathologic causes of pain may not. To complicate matters, chronic pain syndromes are also common in diabetics. A careful history is essential to differentiate the known ("old") pain from the new pain.

HYPERGLYCEMIA AND POOR NEUROLOGIC OUTCOME AFTER HEAD INJURIES AND CEREBROVASCULAR ACCIDENTS

Hyperglycemic syndromes are possible in diabetics who have suffered head injury or CVA. In these patients, it is vital to regain control of metabolic function and to provide adequate resuscitation to prevent secondary neurologic damage. Both hypovolemia and hyperglycemia have been shown to contribute to poorer neurologic outcomes.

CLINICAL APPROACH TO THE OBTUNDED HYPERGLYCEMIC PATIENT IN THE INTENSIVE CARE UNIT

The clinical approach to the obtunded hyperglycemic patient presenting to the ICU requires strict attention to the principles of management of the patient with a depressed level of consciousness, together with management of the underlying hyperglycemic syndrome.

DIAGNOSIS

Metabolic derangement is a differential diagnosis for all obtunded patients, even those who present with a much more graphic confounding diagnosis such as traumatic brain injury, because such injuries may be the result of an altered mental state associated with a hyperglycemic syndrome, or they may be the precipitating cause of a hyperglycemic syndrome. The usual clinical pathway of careful history, clinical examination, and appropriate laboratory testing will reveal the underlying hyperglycemic syndrome. Once the hyperglycemic syndrome is detected, the precipitating cause for DKA or HNHS should also be carefully sought. In particular, blood sputum and urine cultures should be taken early, and a chest radiograph may reveal pneumonia. If the initial tests do not reveal a source of sepsis, a more extensive series of tests for sepsis (e.g., cerebrospinal fluid examination) may be deferred until the metabolic state has been improved. Similarly, extensive neuroradiologic testing (CT or MRI) usually can wait until the patient has been appropriately resuscitated and treated. Because many of the neurologic signs resolve with the acute treatment, unnecessary testing is thereby avoided.

Specific diagnostic tests that are useful in the diagnosis and management of DKA or HNHS in the obtunded patient include the following:

- Blood glucose level and hemoglobin (HbA1C) concentration
- Arterial blood gas analysis, including bicarbonate level and anion gap
- Serum urea and electrolytes
- Serum osmolality (calculated and measured)
- Serum magnesium, calcium, and phosphate levels
- Full blood count
- Serum ketone levels, if available

MANAGEMENT PRINCIPLES

Sound management principles must be followed in the obtunded patient with DKA or HNHS.

Treatment must be provided in a safe environment, preferably in an ICU, with adequate monitoring of the cardiovascular system (blood pressure, heart rate, electrocardiographic parameters) and the respiratory system (pulse oximetry and serial blood gas measurements). More invasive monitoring techniques, such as central venous or pulmonary arterial catheterization, should be reserved for patient with severe comorbidities (e.g., renal or cardiac failure). Catheterization of the urinary bladder provides a sample for culture as well as a monitor of urine flow.

Treatment for the DKA or HNHS (as described above and in detail elsewhere) must be promptly initiated.

Fluid resuscitation is vital.

Insulin therapy is mandatory.

Electrolyte replacement (particularly potassium, and to a lesser extent magnesium and calcium) is important. Phosphate replacement is controversial but currently is not advocated.[3,21]

Airway protection is a priority, including proper posturing, placement of a nasogastric tube to avoid gastric distention and aspiration of gastric contents, and intubation of the trachea, if necessary.

Sedation of the delirious patient, with either minor or major tranquilizers, may be necessary to allow treatment to proceed. The major tranquilizers are probably safer, because they have a lower risk of respiratory depression.

Monitoring of response to these therapeutic measures should be charted either manually or electronically on a suitable bedside chart so that trends may be viewed as treatment proceeds.

Serial laboratory testing is necessary, at a frequency that allows timely adjustment in fluid, electrolyte, and insulin therapy (e.g., hourly or more often to begin with, with a decreasing frequency as the patient improves). Arterial cannulation is helpful in providing access for serial blood sampling. Access to a "stat" laboratory or good laboratory service is essential.

Treatment of the precipitating cause of the hyperglycemic syndrome, if one has been identified, should be initiated. This may involve, for example, antibiotic therapy or withholding of precipitating drugs.

Serial clinical examinations should be performed, as well as investigation and treatment of new problems that arise or neurologic problems that are not resolving. This may include imaging of the brain by CT or MRI to delineate cerebral edema or focal neurologic pathology or treatment of complications seen with variable frequency in patients with hyperglycemic syndromes, such as acute respiratory distress syndrome (ARDS), gastric distention, rhabdomyolysis, and thrombotic episodes.[10]

Treatment of comorbidities (e.g., renal replacement therapy for acute or acute on chronic renal failure, treatment of acute myocardial ischemia) is also important.[22] This may prove challenging, and the requirements may be diametrically opposed to those necessary for treatment of the hyperglycemic syndrome. For example, high-dose catecholamine therapy for cardiogenic shock after myocardial infarction may worsen insulin resistance.

COMPLICATIONS OF TREATMENT

The complications of the treatment itself must also be dealt with and may include the following:

- Hypokalemia—monitoring and necessary potassium supplementation should be provided long before there is a risk of cardiac arrhythmia
- Hypoglycemia due to overenthusiastic insulin therapy—avoid by adequate blood glucose level monitoring
- Hyperchloremic metabolic acidosis due to loss of bicarbonate precursors (ketones) in the urine and use of chloride-containing solutions such as normal saline for resuscitation—reduce by using of lactated Ringer's solution for resuscitation and 0.45% saline for subsequent rehydration
- Fluid overload
- Cerebral edema—described previously

ONGOING CARE

Once the patient is stable and has been adequately resuscitated and metabolic control has been reestablished, arrangements should be made for the smooth transition of care to an endocrinologist familiar with the chronic care of diabetic patients. This may be facilitated by the institution of enteral feeding and conversion from short-acting intravenous insulin to longer-acting subcutaneous insulin before handover. Ongoing care of the patient must address preventable precipitating factors (e.g., prompt treatment of septic foci, compliance with diabetic treatment regimens).[3,21]

ANNOTATED REFERENCES

Chiasson J, Aris-Jilwan N, Belanger R, et al: Diagnosis and treatment of diabetic ketoacidosis and the hyperglycemic hyperosmolar state. CMAJ 2003;168:859-866.
This paper provides an excellent review of DKA and the hyperglycemic hyperosmolar states. Insulin deficiency and raised counterregulatory hormone levels are the major underlying abnormalities. Clinical observations (dehydration and raised blood sugar levels) and simple confirmatory laboratory tests (pH, serum bicarbonate, and serum osmolality) are all that are required to make the diagnosis.

Kitabachi AE, Umpierrez GE, Murphy MB, et al: Management of hyperglycemic crisis in patients with diabetes. Diabetes Care 2001;24:131-153.
This review article discusses in depth the precipitating causes, pathogenesis, and management of diabetic comas and provides clear treatment algorithms.

MacIsaac RJ, Lee LY, McNeil KJ, et al: Influence of age on the presentation and outcome of acidotic and hyperosmolar diabetic emergencies. Intern Med J 2002;32:379-385.
This review of diabetic presentations to an Australian tertiary hospital showed that a combination of ketoacidosis and hyperosmolality was present in 30% of admissions for diabetic hyperglycemic emergencies.

Magee MF, Bhatt BA: Management of decompensated diabetes. Crit Care Clin 2001;17:75-106.
This review of the management of decompensated diabetes includes a section on the pathogenesis of cerebral edema seen during the treatment of diabetic comas as well as other potential complications of the treatment process.

Silver SM, Clark EC, Schroeder BM, et al: Pathogenesis of cerebral oedema after treatment of diabetic ketoacidosis. Kidney Int 1997;51:1237-1244.
This animal study into the causes of cerebral edema after treatment of DKA suggests that the rapid reduction in plasma glucose and osmolality, and not sodium movement into the brain, is to blame.

Chapter 175

HYPERGLYCEMIA AND BLOOD GLUCOSE CONTROL IN THE INTENSIVE CARE UNIT

Dieter Mesotten • Greet Van den Berghe

KEY POINTS

1. Unlike the diagnostic criteria for diabetes mellitus, there were, until recently, no clear guidelines for defining **stress-induced hyperglycemia** or for its treatment.

2. The Diabetes and Insulin-Glucose Infusion in Acute Myocardial Infarction Study (**DIGAMI Study**) was the first to show that maintenance of blood glucose at less than 12 mmol/L (220 mg/dL) with subcutaneous insulin for at least 3 months improved survival of diabetic patients with acute myocardial infarction.

3. A large prospective, randomized, controlled trial **recently challenged the classic dogma** that stress hyperglycemia, up to 12 mmol/L (220 mg/dL), is a beneficial response in nondiabetic patients. Indeed, glycemic control at less than 6.1 mmol/L (110 mg/dL) with exogenous insulin reduced mortality and morbidity among critically ill patients in a surgical intensive care unit.

4. **Blood glucose control and the concomitant improvement in dyslipidemia achieved by intensive insulin therapy,** rather than the insulin dose per se, explains a large part of its clinical benefits.

5. **Immune-enhancing as well as anti-inflammatory effects of intensive insulin therapy** jointly play a role in protecting the host during critical illness.

With the discovery of insulin by Banting and Best in 1922, it became possible to treat patients with type 1 diabetes mellitus, a disorder that was previously lethal due to the development of ketoacidosis. At the end of the 19th century, Claude Bernard described the link between acute trauma and the development of hyperglycemia irrespective of underlying diabetes, which was considered to be an adaptive stress response. Hyperglycemia also is commonly present during other types of critical illness. Until recently, treatment of hyperglycemia during critical illness was considered necessary only if blood glucose levels became excessively elevated, a strategy primarily based on anecdotal grounds. It was only recently that evidence became available in favor of treating even moderate hyperglycemia in critically ill patients.[1]

ALTERED GLUCOSE REGULATION IN STRESS

The concept of "stress diabetes" or "diabetes of injury" has been in the literature for almost 150 years. Stress-induced hyperglycemia is evoked by integrated hormonal, cytokine, and nervous "counterregulatory" signals on glucose metabolic pathways. In the acute phase of critical illness, it is assumed that increased levels of glucagon,[2] cortisol,[3] and growth hormone jointly increase hepatic gluconeogenesis. In addition, the catecholamines epinephrine and norepinephrine, released in response to acute injury, promote hepatic glycogenolysis.[4] The cytokines interleukin-1 (IL-1),[5,6] IL-6, and tumor necrosis factor (TNF)[7] may directly or indirectly enhance both of these hyperglycemic responses.

With the development of intensive care medicine over the last three to four decades, patients are able to survive conditions such as severe sepsis, multiple trauma, and extensive burns. Hence, such patients now frequently enter the chronic phase of critical illness.[8] The regulatory mechanisms for hyperglycemia during protracted critical illness remain less clear. Although in this more chronic phase the changes in glucagon levels are not well documented, growth hormone, cortisol, catecholamine, and cytokine levels[9] are usually decreased compared with the levels observed during the acute phase of critical illness.[10]

On the other side of the balance, glucose uptake is also changed during critical illness. Foremost, the important exercise-stimulated glucose uptake in skeletal muscle totally disappears because of the immobilization of the critically ill patient. But insulin-stimulated glucose uptake is hampered also, through a combined inhibition of glucose transporter-4 (GLUT-4)–dependent insulin-stimulated glucose uptake and glycogen synthase activity.[11,12] Although some studies have shown decreased glucose oxidation[13] through pyruvate produced by the glycolysis, others have demonstrated an opposite effect during critical illness.[14] However, the decrease in insulin-stimulated glucose uptake in skeletal muscle and adipose tissue is completely offset by a massive increase in total body glucose uptake, of which the mononuclear phagocyte system in liver, spleen, and ileum is the main receiver.[15]

The overall increased peripheral glucose uptake[16] in light of hyperglycemia underscores the pivotal role of increased hepatic glucose production during critical illness, which cannot be suppressed by exogenous glucose.[17] Normally, gluconeogenesis and glycogenolysis, the components of hepatic glucose production, are inhibited by insulin.

Increased serum insulin levels in combination with impaired peripheral glucose uptake and elevated hepatic glucose production indicate insulin resistance during critical illness.[18]

HYPERGLYCEMIA IN THE CRITICALLY ILL

In a normal individual, blood glucose levels are tightly regulated within the narrow range of 3.3 to 7.7 mmol/L (60 to 140 mg/dL), both in fed and fasted states. Diabetic hyperglycemia is defined by the World Health Organization as a fasting blood glucose concentration of 6.1 mmol/L or higher and fed blood glucose levels higher than 8.1 mmol/L. Unlike the diagnostic criteria for diabetes mellitus, no clear guidelines have been set for defining hyperglycemia in a critically ill patient. This explains the wide variations in the reported prevalence of hyperglycemia in critically ill patients, which ranges from 3% to 71%.[19] Until recently, it was considered state of the art to tolerate blood glucose levels up to 12 mmol/L (220 mg/dL) in fed critically ill patients.[20] Motivation for treatment of blood glucose levels higher than 12 mmol/L was primarily the occurrence of hyperglycemia-induced osmotic diuresis and fluid shifts once glycemia exceeds that threshold. Also, from the diabetes literature it was known that uncontrolled and pronounced hyperglycemia predisposes to infectious complications.[21,22] And finally, it was commonly accepted that this moderate hyperglycemia in critically ill patients was beneficial for organs, such as the brain and the blood cells, which rely solely on glucose for their energy supply and do not require insulin for glucose uptake.

MAINTENANCE OF NORMOGLYCEMIA IN THE CRITICALLY ILL

In 2001, our large prospective, randomized, controlled trial[1] was the first to challenge the classic dogma of beneficial stress hyperglycemia and to examine the effect of strict glycemic control (at less than 6.1 mmol/L) with exogenous insulin on mortality and morbidity of critically ill patients. Over a 1-year period, 1548 mechanically ventilated patients admitted to the ICU, predominantly after extensive or complicated surgery or trauma, were randomly allocated to either intensive insulin therapy with blood glucose levels kept tightly between 4.5 and 6.1 mmol/L (80 to 110 mg/dL) or the conventional approach, which recommended insulin therapy only if blood glucose levels exceeded 12 mmol/L. Strict blood glucose control at less than 6.1 mmol/L reduced ICU mortality of critically ill patients by more than 40% (Fig. 175-1). The effect occurred particularly in the population with prolonged critical illness, among whom mortality was reduced from 20.2% to 10.6% ($P = .005$). Even patients in the conventional insulin treatment schedule with only moderate hyperglycemia (6.1 to 11.1 mmol/L) showed higher mortality compared with the patients in the strict glycemic control schedule.[23] This is the first intervention since the introduction of mechanical ventilation to have such a pronounced beneficial effect on intensive care mortality. Intensive insulin therapy also had a major effect on morbidity. It decreased the duration of ventilatory support and ICU stay, reduced the need for blood transfusions, and lowered the incidence of bloodstream infections and excessive inflammation. Even more striking, intensive insulin therapy caused a highly significant decrease in the development of critical illness polyneuropathy and of acute renal failure.

COMPLICATIONS OF DERANGED GLUCOSE REGULATION

MILESTONE STUDIES ON GLYCEMIC CONTROL IN DIABETES MELLITUS

The publication of the Diabetes Control and Complications trial (DCCT) in 1993 settled the previously vigorous debate about whether tight glycemic control was beneficial for subjects with type 1 diabetes. The study was powered to detect a significant difference in the rates of progression of diabetic retinopathy, which is the most prevalent complication in type 1 diabetes, but showed a highly significant decrease in retinopathy, nephropathy, and peripheral and autonomic neuropathy.[24] Similarly, evidence for the importance of tight glycemic control in patients with type 2 diabetes became available with the publication of the United Kingdom Prospective Diabetes Study (UKPDS) in the late 1990s.[25] This trial showed that a 0.7% decrease in hemoglobin A1C lowered the incidence of retinopathy by 21%, microalbuminuria by 33%, cataracts by 24%, and myocardial infarction by 16% and resulted in a nonsignificant 5% decrease in the incidence of cerebrovascular accident. Although the UKPDS showed a trend to decreased mortality, neither study was appropriately powered to detect a significant decrease in diabetes-related mortality.

Patients with diabetes have a 1.5 to 2 times greater risk of death after an acute myocardial infarction (AMI), compared with nondiabetic AMI patients.[26] Furthermore, in AMI patients without previously diagnosed diabetes, hyperglycemia on admission has been associated with larger infarct size, a higher incidence of cardiac failure, and decreased survival at 1 year.[27] A number of studies have examined the outcome benefits of tightening glycemic control in diabetic patients with myocardial infarction. The largest study, with the longest follow-up period, was the Diabetes and Insulin-Glucose Infusion in Acute Myocardial Infarction (DIGAMI) study.[28] In that study, diabetic patients admitted to the hospital with an AMI were randomly assigned to standard treatment (at the physician's discretion), or to "intensive insulin therapy," which comprised an infusion of glucose and insulin, started as soon as possible and continued for 48 hours, after which the patients were submitted to a "stricter" blood glucose control regimen (less than 12 mmol/L) with subcutaneous insulin continued for at least 3 months after discharge. Patients in the intensive treatment arm had improved 30-day and long-term survival (29% relative risk reduction at 1 year).[29,30] Also, there was a significant decrease in reinfarction and new cardiac failure.[31]

For other disease states such as cerebrovascular ischemic insults, adverse outcome was shown to be significantly related to hyperglycemia on admission. Indeed, high blood glucose levels were associated with increased mortality and poorer neurologic recovery.[32] Also, in patients with traumatic head injuries, postoperative hyperglycemia was found to be an independent predictor of mortality.[33] The Glucose-Insulin in Stroke Trial (GIST) examined the effect of glucose-insulin-potassium (GIK) infusion. This trial, in which patients with acute stroke were allocated to standard therapy or a 24-hour infusion of GIK, did not significantly lower glycemia or mortality.[34]

It should be noted that studies on the benefits of GIK infusions in either cardiac or neurologic ischemic insults never targeted normoglycemia (in contrast to the insulin in

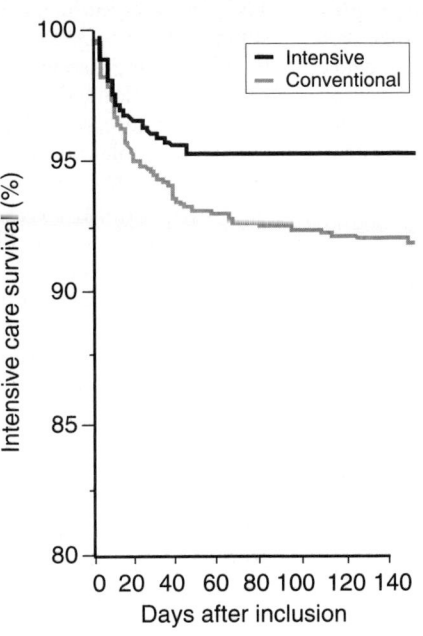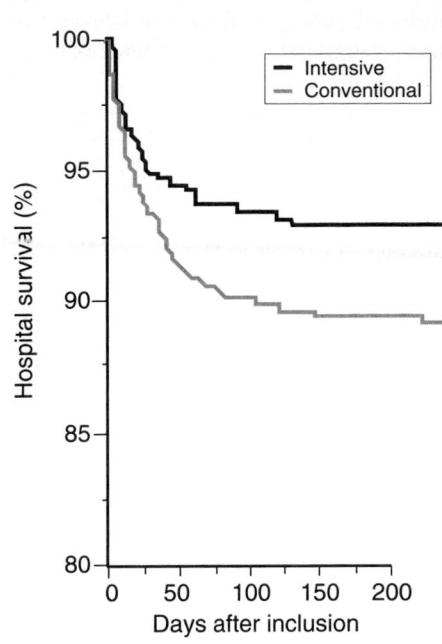

FIGURE 175–1. Kaplan-Meier cumulative survival plots for intensive care and in-hospital survival, showing the effect of intensive insulin treatment in a study of 1548 critically ill patients. Patients discharged alive from intensive care (*left panel*) and from hospital (*right panel*) were considered survivors. *P* values were obtained by log-rank (Mantel-Cox) significance testing. The difference between the intensive insulin group and the conventional group was significant for intensive care survival (unadjusted *P* = .005; adjusted *P* < .04) and for hospital survival (unadjusted *P* = .01). (From Van den Berghe G, Wouters P, Weekers F, et al: Intensive insulin therapy in critically ill patients. N Engl J Med 2001;345:1359-1367, with permission.)

the ICU trial). As such, they cannot provide conclusive evidence as to whether the degree of hyperglycemia simply reflects the severity of illness or is actually contributing to the adverse outcome of those insults.

NEPHROPATHY AND NEUROPATHY

The pathophysiology of diabetic nephropathy is different from that associated with critical illness. Diabetic nephropathy is mainly a glomerular disease, whereas renal failure in the critically ill is mostly caused by acute tubular necrosis. Currently, the only therapeutic option for the latter remains bridging time to spontaneous recovery through extracorporeal hemofiltration or dialysis, with the continuous venovenous mode being the preferred method for unstable critically ill patients.[35] Hence, preventive strategies are crucial, and these include maintaining or optimizing renal perfusion, diligence with monitoring of nephrotoxic therapies such as aminoglycosides, and limiting the use of nonionic radiocontrast materials. Evidence for specific preventive measures for acute renal failure in the critically ill patient was not available until the recently published study of intensive insulin therapy.[1] This study indeed revealed a 42% reduction in the occurrence of acute renal failure requiring extracorporeal replacement therapy.

In the diabetic patient, distal sensory neuropathy with the classic "stocking" distribution is the most frequent presentation of neuropathy.[36] Long-term critically ill patients often suffer from a diffuse axonal polyneuropathy.[37] It presents as a tetraparesis with muscle atrophy, but the diagnosis should be confirmed by electromyography. In most cases, the course is self-limited, and good recovery should be expected if the underlying critical illness resolves. However, this critical illness polyneuropathy severely impairs weaning from the ventilator and early mobilization.[38] Factors that are known to contribute to the development of critical illness–related polyneuropathy include sepsis, use of high-dose corticosteroids, and use of

neuromuscular blocking agents. However, the exact pathogenesis is not understood, and, until recently, specific prevention of or treatment for critical illness–associated polyneuropathy was unavailable.[39] Bolton[40] described a strong link between the risk of critical illness polyneuropathy on the one hand and on the other hand increased blood glucose levels and decreased serum albumin levels, both of which are metabolic manifestations of multiple organ failure and sepsis. Sepsis, with its accompanying release of cytokines, was considered to be the causal factor. Cytokines may indeed induce microangiopathy, which may play a role, as in diabetic polyneuropathy. The Leuven insulin in ICU study showed an important preventive effect of strict glycemic control with insulin on the occurrence of critical illness polyneuropathy, which was associated with a decrease in the duration of mechanical ventilation in patients with protracted critical illness.[1]

METABOLIC CONTROL AND INFECTIONS

It has long been known that the hyperglycemia of diabetes predisposes to infection.[21] Possible mechanisms include the hyperglycemia-induced inhibition of release of IL-1 from macrophages and oxygen radicals from neutrophils.[41] Hyperglycemia also impairs phagocytosis by macrophages.[42,43] Importantly, the impairment of the leukocyte oxidative burst and phagocytotic activity can be reduced by tight glycemic control.[44,45] In diabetic critically ill patients, such as those who have undergone open-heart surgery, an association between a higher risk of infectious complications[46] and blood glucose levels higher than 11 mmol/L (200 mg/dL) has been documented. In a follow-up study, it was also shown that continuous intravenous insulin infusion reduced the incidence of postcardiac surgery deep sternal wounds (0.8% versus 2% for subcutaneous insulin injections).[47] Uncontrolled hyperglycemia in burn patients also has been associated with failure of skin graft take and outcome.[48] Again, the causal link between hyperglycemia and a higher risk of serious infections, regardless of a previous history of diabetes, was provided only recently by the Leuven insulin in ICU study.[1] Indeed, strict maintenance of normoglycemia using exogenous insulin during critical illness was found to reduce the incidence of bacteremia to almost half and to a large extent prevented sepsis-associated mortality. This suggests an immune-enhancing effect of insulin-titrated blood glucose control. An improved capacity to clear bacterial invaders was recently shown to mediate this benefit in a novel rabbit model of prolonged critical illness.[49,50]

METABOLIC CONTROL AND DYSLIPIDEMIA

As in diabetes mellitus,[51] deranged metabolism during critical illness is reflected not only by hyperglycemia but also by an abnormal serum lipid profile.[52-54] Elevated triglyceride levels, caused by an increase in very-low-density lipoprotein (VLDL) cholesterol and low circulating high-density lipoprotein (HDL) cholesterol, are the most characteristic during critical illness.[55] Low-density lipoprotein (LDL) cholesterol levels are also decreased.[55] The latter change is offset by an increase in circulating small dense LDL particles,[56] which are supposedly more proatherogenic than the medium and large LDL particles.[57] It has now been shown, for the first time, that intensive insulin therapy can partially restore the deranged serum lipid profile during critical illness.[58] The strongest effect of this therapy was on the hypertriglyceridemia, which was totally obliterated. Serum levels of HDL and LDL also increased significantly, but they remained lower than those of healthy subjects.

The role of triglycerides in energy provision and the coordinating position of the lipoproteins in transportation of lipid components (cholesterol, triglycerides, phospholipids, lipid-soluble vitamins) are well established.[59] Lipoproteins have also been shown to act as endotoxin scavengers and hence to prevent deaths in animal models.[60,61] For that reason, intensive insulin therapy may improve the overall endotoxin-scavenging function. Contrary to the proposed infusions of lipoproteins,[55,62] intensive insulin therapy would be a more integrated approach to correct the deranged serum lipid profile. This was demonstrated by the multivariate logistic regression analysis, in which the improvement of the deranged lipidemia explained a significant part of the beneficial effect on mortality and organ failure, surprisingly surpassing the effect of glycemic control and insulin dose. Likewise, the effect of intensive insulin therapy on inflammation, reflected by a lowering of the concentration of serum C-reactive protein (CRP),[63] was no longer independently related to the outcome benefit when the changes in lipid metabolism were taken into account. This may suggest a link between the anti-inflammatory effect of intensive insulin therapy and its amelioration of the lipid profile. However, a mechanistic explanation for the dominant effect of serum lipid correction still needs to be delineated.

METABOLIC CONTROL, INFLAMMATION, AND COAGULATION

In diabetes mellitus and critical illness, the inflammatory cascade is activated. It has been clearly shown that intensive insulin treatment in critically ill patients prevents excessive inflammation.[1,63] The exact underlying mechanisms of insulin-induced anti-inflammatory effects have not yet been unraveled,[64] but it has been suggested that insulin may suppress the secretion and antagonize the harmful effects of TNF,[65,66] macrophage migration-inhibitory factor,[67] and superoxide anion.[68] The anti-inflammatory effect of intensive insulin therapy also was confirmed in an experimental rabbit model of prolonged critical illness.[50]

Furthermore, both diabetes mellitus and critical illness are hypercoagulable states.[69,70] Putative causes in diabetes include vascular endothelium dysfunction,[71] increased blood levels of several clotting factors,[72,73] elevated platelet activation,[74,75] and inhibition of the fibrinolytic system.[73] Levels of the anticoagulant protein C are also decreased.[76] In view of the similarities with critical illness[77,78] and the powerful preventive effect of intensive insulin therapy on septicemia, multiple organ failure, and mortality,[1] the effect of this simple and cheap metabolic intervention on the balance between coagulation and fibrinolysis in critically ill patients should be investigated.

SHOULD HYPERCALORIC, NORMOCALORIC, OR HYPOCALORIC NUTRITION BE PRESCRIBED?

It has been well documented that providing hypercaloric nutrition (hyperalimentation, 35 to 40 kcal/kg) to critically ill patients[79] can lead to infections and severe metabolic complications. These range from hyperglycemia, hypertriglyceridemia, and azotemia to hepatic steatosis, fat-overload syndrome, and hypertonic dehydration.[80] Since the introduction of more accurate means to estimate energy expenditure and a cautious approach toward obese or highly edematous patients, serious complications of feeding have been dramatically reduced.

On the other hand, in an attempt to decrease hyperglycemia and hence infectious complications, McCowen and colleagues[81] evaluated the efficacy of hypocaloric total parenteral nutrition (TPN) feeding (14 kcal/kg) compared with a standard weight-based regimen (18 kcal/kg). Contrary to expectation, the hypocaloric TPN did not lower the incidence of hyperglycemia or infections. Caloric restriction only seems to be effective in conjunction with a hyperproteinic approach—about 1.8 g protein per kilogram ideal body weight (IBW), compared with the standard 1.2 g/kg IBW.[82] This was also shown in a hypocaloric parenteral regimen using 2 g protein per kilogram IBW in patients with morbid obesity.[83] Overall, however, there does not appear to be a clearcut benefit of hypocaloric over normocaloric nutrition. This might be attributed to the ineffectiveness of hypocaloric nutrition in lowering blood glucose levels.

The potential benefit of hypercaloric feeding combined with insulin infusions to enhance the anabolic effects of insulin still needs to be assessed. This strategy would be quite similar to GIK infusions, in which high doses of insulin (0.1 to 1 IU/kg/hour) and glucose (30 to 80 g/hour) are combined. A meta-analysis of all published randomized trials investigating the effects of GIK infusion in previously nondiabetic subjects with AMI supported the concept that this intervention indeed may be life-saving.[84] So far, however, GIK infusions should be seen as a distinct intervention, because infusion of GIK is not targeted to maintain normoglycemia. The primary aim of GIK is to enhance myocardial metabolism of glucose instead of fatty acids when oxygen supply is compromised. Recently, interest in preoperative carbohydrate loading has been rekindled through the studies of Ljungqvist and colleagues,[85] which revealed that carbohydrate treatment, instead of overnight fasting, before surgery reduced both postoperative insulin resistance and hospital stay.

DOES A HISTORY OF DIABETES MANDATE A SPECIFIC METABOLIC MANAGEMENT DURING CRITICAL ILLNESS?

The beneficial effect of intensive insulin therapy on morbidity and mortality in critically ill patients was present equally among those patients with and without previously diagnosed diabetes.[1] Therefore, we believe that strict normoglycemia (less than 6.1 mmol/L) should be the therapeutic goal regardless of whether a history of diabetes is present. In both diabetic and nondiabetic patients, blood glucose control during intensive care is best achieved with a continuous insulin infusion, and oral agents should be discontinued during critical illness. Because the nutritional intake of critically ill patients is continuous in nature, either with TPN or with a combination of parenteral and enteral feeding, it is also logical to administer insulin in a continuous fashion. In addition, intravenous administration is more reliable and consistent than subcutaneous injections. Titration of a continuous insulin infusion is preferred to the use of a sliding scale, because the former not only provides a baseline insulin level but is also more easily and precisely adapted in response to the actual blood glucose levels. Insulin has a short half-life, which allows rapid cessation of effect if the patient develops hypoglycemia.

This risk of hypoglycemia is a major concern of intensive insulin therapy during critical illness. Clinical symptoms of the autonomic response (sweating, tachycardia, tremor) and central nervous symptoms such as dizziness, blurred vision, altered mental acuity, confusion, and eventually convulsions are often masked by concomitant diseases and by inherent intensive care treatments such as sedation and mechanical ventilation. Brain damage could be an irreversible complication of severe (less than 1.67 mmol/L) or prolonged hypoglycemia. Another insidious complication of hypoglycemia is the induction of cardiac arrhythmias, ranging from dispersed QT segments[86] and sinus bradycardias[87] to ventricular tachycardias.[88] To prevent hypoglycemia in the critically ill, insulin should be administered together with carbohydrates, either dextrose or feedings, and blood glucose levels should be measured frequently and regularly. In the Leuven insulin in ICU study,[1] blood glucose levels were measured every 1 to 2 hours during the first 12 to 24 hours of the patient's admission to the ICU. Once the targeted blood glucose level was reached on a stable insulin dose, measurements were scaled down to every 4 hours. If hypoglycemia occurred, it usually took place after the first week of ICU stay, at a time when blood glucose levels were stable. Inadequate insulin dose reduction during interruption of enteral feeding was often the precipitating factor for the hypoglycemia. Evidently, the hazard of hypoglycemia warrants a strict and detailed insulin titration protocol, combined with sufficient training of the nursing and medical staff.

SHOULD THE FOCUS BE ON INSULIN OR GLYCEMIC CONTROL?

Whether the effects of intensive insulin therapy during critical illness[1] were caused by maintenance of normoglycemia or by a direct insulin effect remains speculative. It is conceivable that insulin had a direct role in the functional improvement of the insulin-sensitive organs. In a normal individual, the bulk of the insulin-stimulated glucose uptake is situated in the heart and skeletal muscles. Also, muscle catabolism is aggravated in hyperglycemic conditions. This could partially explain the beneficial effects of intensive insulin therapy on the duration of mechanical ventilation in critically ill patients in the intensive insulin therapy trial. At the molecular level, steady-state messenger RNA levels of GLUT-4 and hexokinase II (HXK-II) in skeletal muscle were increased by intensive insulin therapy, which suggests a stimulation of peripheral glucose uptake.[58]

The liver, the major site for gluconeogenesis, is another important insulin-sensitive organ that could be involved in the improved outcome of the patients intensively treated with insulin. However, a recent study showed that serum and gene expression levels of insulin-like growth factor binding protein-1 (IGFBP-1) and those of phosphoenolpyruvate carboxykinase (PEPCK), the rate-limiting enzyme in gluconeogenesis, are not regulated by insulin in critically ill patients. This may indicate that control of gluconeogenesis was not the major factor in bringing about normoglycemia with exogenous insulin in the critically ill.[89] However, only glucose turnover studies would be able to give a reflection of true glucose kinetics. Nevertheless, such a study, using a well-designed canine model of critical illness, recently endorsed our findings to a great extent.[90] It revealed that the presence of an infection decreased hepatic glucose uptake, which was unresponsive to insulinization. In contrast, peripheral glucose uptake did respond to insulin infusion. Contrary to our findings, Donmoyer and colleagues[90] reported that there was a suppression of hepatic glucose production and that inhibition of glycogenolysis, rather than diminished hepatic uptake of gluconeogenic amino acids and gluconeogenesis by insulin therapy, appeared to be the determining factor.

Another major insulin-responsive organ is adipose tissue. The increased serum free fatty acid and triglyceride levels present during critical illness and the relative accruement of adipose tissue compared with lean body mass (muscle and bone tissue) with feeding in the patient with protracted critical illness jointly point to a deranged lipid metabolism. Although intensive insulin therapy partially restored the imbalance in serum lipids, with a significant contribution to the reduced ICU mortality, its direct effects on adipocytes remain to be investigated.[58]

The positive effects of intensive insulin therapy on kidney function and the decreased incidence of critical illness–related polyneuropathy may in part be explained by maintenance of normoglycemia, because both organs are supposedly, at least in part, insulin insensitive. Here, although on a totally different time scale, a parallel with type 2 diabetes emerges. Long-term studies have shown that meticulous blood glucose control decreases the incidence and severity of diabetic nephropathy, and the onset of diabetic neuropathy and "glucose toxicity" may be the underlying mechanism. However, the rapid onset of critical illness–related polyneuropathy and acute renal failure suggest that other factors, which predispose the critically ill to the toxic effects of hyperglycemia on neurons and kidneys, must play a role. Similarly, avoidance of hyperglycemia may be important for prevention of bloodstream infections. The suppression of the immune system conceivably results in an increased risk of postoperative infections, as discussed earlier. However, the exact underlying mechanisms of the clinical benefits of intensive insulin therapy in critically ill patients remain unknown. Future clinical and experimental studies should provide the answer to this fascinating pathophysiologic question.

ANNOTATED REFERENCES

Capes SE, Hunt D, Malmberg K, et al: Stress hyperglycemia and increased risk of death after myocardial infarction in patients with and without diabetes: A systematic overview. Lancet 2000;355:773-778.

This paper reviewed the literature, available in 2000, on the relationship between hyperglycemia and risk of death after acute myocardial infarction.

Malmberg K, Ryden L, Efendic S, et al: Randomized trial of insulin-glucose infusion followed by subcutaneous insulin treatment in diabetic patients with acute myocardial infarction (DIGAMI study): Effects on mortality at 1 year. J Am Coll Cardiol 1995;26:57-65.

This paper reported the results of the DIGAMI study, showing for the first time that reduction of blood glucose levels to less than 215 mg/dL after AMI improves outcome.

McCowen KC, Malhotra A, Bistrian BR: Stress-induced hyperglycemia. Crit Care Clin 2001;17:107-124.

This paper reviewed the literature, available early 2001, on the relationship between hyperglycemia and outcome of severe illness.

Van den Berghe G, Wouters PJ, Bouillon R, et al: Outcome benefit of intensive insulin therapy in the critically ill: Insulin dose versus glycemic control. Crit Care Med 2003;31:359-366.

This study investigated the relative impact of insulin and blood glucose control in bringing about the clinical benefits of intensive insulin therapy in the surgical ICU.

Van den Berghe G, Wouters P, Weekers F, et al: Intensive insulin therapy in critically ill patients. N Engl J Med 2001;345:1359-1367.

This paper reported on the first, large (N = 1548), prospective, randomized, controlled study showing that insulin-titrated maintenance of normoglycemia (less than 110 mg/dL) during intensive care improves outcome of (surgical) ICU patients.

Chapter 176

ADRENAL INSUFFICIENCY

Herwig Gerlach

KEY POINTS

1. The **definition of adrenal insufficiency** is based on the inability of the adrenal gland to produce adrenocortical steroid hormones.

2. The three major regulatory influences that affect the **hypothalamic-pituitary-adrenal (HPA) axis** and lead to the secretion of corticotropin (ACTH) as the main stimulatory factor for the adrenal cortex to release its hormonal products are circadian diurnal rhythms, stress, and feedback from free cortisol levels in blood and body fluids.

3. Each case of **physical or emotional stress** leads to an immediate, significant, and possibly continual increase in ACTH and cortisol excretion. This is typically paralleled by a loss of the circadian rhythm. The response to stress is proportional to the intensity of the stimulus.

4. The main cause of **primary adrenal insufficiency** (70% to 80% of cases) is autoimmune disorders, inducing morphologic destruction of greater than 90% of the adrenal cortex. The result is a critically decreased synthesis of steroids with typical clinical manifestations.

5. In contrast, **secondary adrenal insufficiency** is characterized by reduced stimulation of the intact adrenal gland due to low ACTH levels (hypothalamic-pituitary insufficiency), which also result in reduced cortisol levels.

6. **Tertiary adrenal insufficiency** is caused by long-term treatment with steroid hormones, which induces a feedback inhibition of the HPA axis.

7. The definition of **relative adrenal insufficiency** in critically ill patients is based on plasma cortisol levels. The critical threshold is a basal cortisol level of 18 to 25 μg/dL without preceding stimulation. Whereas absolute adrenal insufficiency is rare in critical care medicine, relative adrenal insufficiency has received considerable attention.

8. The **clinical manifestations of adrenal insufficiency** are usually nonspecific and include weakness, anorexia, orthostatic hypotension, and general gastrointestinal symptoms. Typical signs of primary adrenal insufficiency are hyperpigmentation due to increased ACTH levels, vitiligo in cases of autoimmune disorders, and hyperkalemia. Secondary forms cause milder symptoms because of maintained mineralocorticoid effects.

9. The **evaluation of adrenal insufficiency** includes measurement of the basal serum cortisol concentration as well as the incremental increase after stimulation with ACTH. In general, a high-dose test (250 μg ACTH) is preferred, with cortisol levels measured at 30 and 60 minutes after stimulation. Long-term tests or low-dose tests (1 μg ACTH) are used only for special indications. Basal values of less than 3 μg/dL serum cortisol indicate severe, absolute hypocortisolism requiring immediate intervention. In critically ill patients with septic shock, basal cortisol levels of less than 18 to 25 μg/dL may also indicate the need for low-dose replacement therapy.

10. **Acute adrenal insufficiency** (addisonian crisis) requires immediate intervention. Establishing intravenous access, infusing saline, monitoring the serum glucose concentration, and administering dexamethasone after drawing a blood sample may be lifesaving. ACTH stimulation tests should be used for diagnosis. Once the results are known, the use of hydrocortisone is preferred because of its mineralocorticoid effects.

11. **Chronic adrenal insufficiency** may require long-term replacement therapy with glucocorticoids and mineralocorticoids (for primary forms). Any physical or emotional stress must be considered as possibly harmful, with the need for 3 to 10 times increased doses of glucocorticoids.

12. In patients with **septic shock,** replacement with low-dose hydrocortisone (200 to 300 mg/day) seems to provide benefit, although further investigations are necessary to evaluate the optimal dosing. A cutoff level for random basal serum cortisol of less than 18 to 25 μg/dL is recommended to indicate which patients may benefit from low-dose therapy.

The adrenal gland is an important endocrine organ that supports the human organism's reaction to factors threatening the integrity of the body, either acutely or in a more chronic/adaptive manner. During the stress response, the central nervous system induces an activation of both the sympathoadrenergic system, by release of catecholamines, and the hypothalamic-pituitary-adrenal (HPA) axis, by release of steroid hormones (glucocorticoids and mineralocorticoids), with the aim of maintaining homeostasis by influencing metabolic, cardiovascular, immunologic, and endocrine functions. In this context, the adrenal gland plays the key role, combining the location for synthesis and expression of catecholamines and glucocorticoids, as well as androgenic hormones and factors of the renin-angiotensin-aldosterone (RAA) system. In acute and chronic inflammatory diseases, the HPA axis is stimulated by the immune system, which leads to morphologic and functional changes, especially of the adrenal cortex. This phenomenon has been described for acute infectious diseases and for other forms of severe sepsis and septic shock.

More than 50 years ago, the seminal observation was made that administration of an adrenocortical steroid extract to a patient with progressive, active rheumatoid arthritis stopped the disease. This led to the development of synthetic adrenocortical steroids, which gained a remarkable reputation in the treatment of a wide range of inflammatory and autoimmune disorders. However, it soon became apparent that this efficacy did not come without a cost in terms of potentially serious adverse effects. In patients with severe sepsis and septic shock, negative results of trials with high doses of glucocorticoids evoked skepticism for many years. Now, with encouraging results from studies of low-dose corticosteroid administration in patients with septic shock, the trend oscillates in the opposite direction. However, there is still controversy concerning which patients profit most from this therapy, as well as how to define and evaluate adrenal gland disorders. This chapter reviews recent data and focuses on the clinical relevance of adrenal insufficiency in critical care.

HISTORICAL REVIEW

"The unknown function of the adrenal gland safeguards this organ against annoying questions in medical science."

—Hyrtl, *Textbook of Anatomy,* 19th century

In 1564, the roman anatomist Bartholomeus Eustachius (1520-1570) discovered the adrenal gland and called them "glandulae quae renibus incumbent"—glands with an unknown function. Multiple hypotheses concerning their possible role were formed over the centuries, for example by the anatomist Adrianus Spigelius (1570-1625), who described the adrenal gland as an "upholstering space holder" between the kidney and the diaphragm. In 1855, Thomas Addison (1793-1860) first described the phenomenon that, in some deceased patients, the only pathologic finding was a morphologic destruction of the adrenal gland. He concluded that this organ must have a crucial function, and he called the described syndrome "Morbus Addison" (Addisons's disease). One year later, Brown-Séquard confirmed this hypothesis after performing a series of bilateral adrenalectomies in cats, demonstrating that these endocrine glands were necessary for life. However, Addison's conclusions were not accepted, and even 2 years after Addison's death, the famous pathologist Rudolf Virchow declared that he had never heard such an illogical statement.

In the 19th and early 20th centuries, several key findings were made. In 1856, von Koelliker described the anatomic division of the adrenal gland into cortex and medulla, and in 1903, Biedl confirmed that the adrenal cortex is the essential portion. In 1894, epinephrine (adrenaline) was isolated from the adrenal medulla as the first hormone; its chemical structure was described 3 years later, and, in 1901, epinephrine was synthesized. In patients with Addison's disease, however, the administration of epinephrine had no success, whereas the use of an animal extract of the adrenal cortex was lifesaving. The purification techniques were rapidly improved, and the resulting "cortin" was the first-choice drug for treatment of Addison's disease until the middle of the 20th century. Three independent groups of biochemists (Kendall, Winterstein, and Reichstein) successfully isolated 17-hydroxy-11-dehydrocorticosterone (later called "cortisone") from the adrenal cortex; the physiologic compound cortisol was first described by Reichstein in 1937. The extraction of cortisone, however, was arduous and uneconomical. Bovine adrenal glands of more than 20,000 animals were necessary to produce 1 kg of cortisone. The first synthesis and pharmaceutical preparation of cortisone was described in 1947 by an industrial company. Until this time, cortisone was only used in patients with Addison's disease.

In the same decade, Hench and Kendall, two rheumatologists at the Mayo Clinic, found that patients with various forms of rheumatism showed temporary remissions of their symptoms during pregnancy and during inflammatory diseases such as hepatitis. They speculated that this phenomenon might be the result of a general stimulation of the endocrine system and concluded that the use of cortisone might be beneficial in patients with acute rheumatoid arthritis. In September, 1948, a bedridden female patient with severe and painful rheumatism, which was resistant to all standard therapies at the time, provided the first documented case of cortisone treatment in inflammatory diseases. After 3 days, the patient was able to stand up; 1 week later, she left the clinic without pain and on her own feet. Retrospectively, the speculations regarding pregnancy and hepatitis were obviously wrong, but the anti-inflammatory character of cortisone was a key finding in pharmaceutical research. In contrast to Selye, who described cortisone as a crucial promoter of the physiologic stress response, the aforementioned findings (that the adrenal gland cortex as the location for endogenous production of cortisone is an important inhibitor of stress and inflammation) have been confirmed. In 1950, Kendall, Hench, and Reichstein received the Nobel Prize in Medicine for their historical findings on the physiologic role of the adrenal gland.[1-4]

ANATOMY OF THE ADRENAL GLAND

The two, paired adrenal glands are located in the retroperitoneal soft tissue near the top of each kidney. In neonates, the adrenal glands are relatively large (approximately one third of the kidney's size) compared with other organs. In the postnatal period, the partition of the cortex shrinks, which leads to a smaller organ in both relative and absolute terms. In adults, each adrenal gland weighs 4 to 5 g, and each has a flat form, with a sagittal diameter of less than 1 cm, a transverse diameter of 3 cm, and a craniocaudal diameter of 4 to 5 cm. The right gland has a triangle or pyramid-like shape, whereas the left organ has the form of a half-moon. The adrenal gland is composed of two embryologically distinct tissues. The adrenal cortex develops during the fifth week of gestation from a clump of mesodermal cells within the urogenital ridge, known as the adrenal primordium. Later, during the 12th gestational week, the adrenal medulla grows from neuroectodermal cells of the embryonic neural tube. In the fetal period, the cortex surrounds the medullar cells, resulting in the typical "sandwich" structure consisting of a flat, grey medulla with a yellow cortex.

The circulatory supply, with a flow rate of about 5 mL/minute, is maintained by up to 50 arterial branches from the aorta, the renal arteries, and the inferior phrenic arteries for each adrenal gland. The blood flow is directed from the capsule into the subcapsular arteriolar plexus, through the cortex and toward the medulla, where a single vein drains the blood entering the vena cava (right side) or the renal vein (left side), respectively. A direct blood supply to the medulla is maintained by medullary arteries. The adrenal cortex receives afferent and efferent innervation. Direct contact of nerve terminals with adrenocortical cells has been suggested, and chemoreceptors and baroreceptors present in the adrenal cortex infer efferent innervation. Diurnal variation in cortisol secretion and compensatory adrenal hypertrophy are influenced by adrenal innervation. Splanchnic nerve innervation has an effect on the regulation of adrenal steroid release. The adrenal medulla secretes the catecholamines epinephrine and norepinephrine, which affect blood pressure, heart rate, sweating, and other activities that are also regulated by the sympathetic nervous system. The adrenal cortex is divided into three layers: the zona glomerulosa, just under the capsule; the zona fasciculata or middle layer; and the zona reticularis, the innermost, net-like patterned area, with reticular veins draining into medullary capillaries. The zona glomerulosa exclusively makes the mineralocorticoid, aldosterone; the zona fasciculata and zona reticularis produce glucocorticoids and androgens.[5]

PHYSIOLOGY OF THE HYPOTHALAMIC-PITUITARY-ADRENAL AXIS

The adrenal glands are part of a complex system that produces interacting hormones to maintain physiologic integrity, especially during stress response.[6,7] This system, the HPA axis, includes the hypothalamic region, which produces corticotropin-releasing hormone (CRH). The pituitary gland, which is triggered by CPH, comprises two major structures—the adenohypophysis (anterior pituitary) and the neurohypophysis (posterior pituitary). The anterior pituitary is responsible for the secretion of corticotropin (adrenocorticotropic hormone [ACTH]), thyroid-stimulating hormone (TSH), growth hormone (GH), β-lipotropin, endorphins, prolactin, luteinizing hormone (LH), and follicle-stimulating hormone (FSH). The posterior pituitary secretes vasopressin (antidiuretic hormone, ADH) and oxytocin. ACTH regulates the production of corticosteroids by the adrenal glands. Hypothalamic neurons receive input from many areas within the central nervous system; they integrate these inputs and initiate an output to the anterior pituitary via the median eminence. The median eminence secretes releasing hormones into a hypophyseal portal network of capillaries that connect the median eminence with the pituitary hormones.

The anterior pituitary gland secretes ACTH under stimulation from hypothalamic CRH. ACTH, in turn, stimulates the synthesis and release of glucocorticoids, mineralocorticoids, and androgenic steroids from the adrenal gland. In terms of a feedback loop, ACTH release is inhibited by glucocorticoids,

which act on both the pituitary corticotropic cells and hypothalamic neurons. ACTH is also released during stress, independent of the circulating serum cortisol level. CRH, vasopressin, and norepinephrine act synergistically to increase ACTH release during stress. Endorphinergic pathways also play a role in ACTH regulation. Acute administration of morphine stimulates release of ACTH, but chronic administration blocks ACTH secretion.

ACTH and cortisol are secreted normally in a diurnal pattern, with lowest concentrations between 10 PM and 2 AM, and highest levels at about 8 AM. From a practical point of view, these rhythms are important because adequate assessment of endocrine function must take into account the variability of hormone levels in the blood; samples obtained at different times can provide useful, dynamic information regarding HPA function. Loss of diurnal rhythm may indicate hypothalamic dysfunction.

The HPA axis is stimulated not only by physical or psychic stress, but also by peptides such as ADH and cytokines. Therefore, the HPA axis plays an important role during infections and immunologic disorders.[8,9] Because of its interaction with the RAA system, regulating fluid and salt balance, synthesis of androgens (e.g., dehydroepiandrosterone) with possible impact on immunomodulation, and the sympathoadrenergic system, the HPA axis is probably the most important organ of stress response.

Stimulation of the immune system by infections induces the release of proinflammatory cytokines such as tumor necrosis factor-α (TNF-α), interleukin-1β (IL-1β), or IL-6. Following a cascade, these cytokines stimulate both the hypothalamus and the anterior pituitary gland, which finally leads to the release of glucocorticoids. IL-6 is also able to induce steroid release directly from the adrenal gland. The adequate increase of glucocorticoids during inflammation is a crucial factor for appropriate stress response. During acute infections, this release maintains metabolic and energetic integrity. If the process is chronic, the HPA axis adapts, with resultant typical clinical manifestations, such as hypercatabolic states, hyperglycemia, and suppression of androgens, GH, and thyroid hormones. These changes, however, may increase the risk of secondary infections.

The increased cortisol levels suppress higher regulatory levels of the HPA axis (negative feedback loop). After major surgery, or during sepsis and septic shock, high cortisol and low ACTH levels are detectable.[10,11] Even the infusion of dexamethasone or CRH is not able to suppress increased cortisol levels in these patients.[12,13] This phenomenon leads to the question of how the cortisol release is induced. Several investigations have demonstrated that adrenal cortisol synthesis in critically ill patients is not regulated by ACTH but by paracrine pathways via endothelin, atrial natriuretic peptide (ANP), or cytokines such as IL-6.[14-16] IL-6 directly induces the adrenal cortex to release cortisol, which, in chronic cases, can worsen the prognosis.[17]

CELLULAR RESPONSE TO ADRENOCORTICAL HORMONES AND RELATED DRUGS

Cortisol, the major free circulating adrenocortical hormone, is a hydrophobic hormone (being a steroid) and therefore circulates bound to protein. The complex with cortisol-binding globulin (CBG, or transcortin) accounts for about

95% of circulating cortisol, but only the free form is biologically active. Its plasma half-life is 60 to 120 minutes; cortisol is metabolized by hydroxylation in the liver, and metabolites are excreted with the urine. Steroid hormones enter the cytoplasm of cells, where they combine with a receptor protein. Metabolic, immunologic, and hemodynamic responses to adrenocortical steroid hormones are regulated in a very complex manner that includes transactivation, transrepression, post-transcriptional/translational regulation, and nongenomic effects. The immediate, nongenomic effects of steroid hormones were primarily attributed to mineralocorticoids (aldosterone). A rapid activation of the sodium-proton exchanger, increase of intracellular Ca^{2+}, and activation of second messenger pathways have been described.[18,19] A randomized trial in patients during cardiac catheterization revealed that, within minutes after aldosterone injection, cardiac index and arterial pressure increased significantly for 10 minutes and returned to baseline afterwards.[20] Interestingly, genomic effects of aldosterone seem to be mediated by binding to glucocorticoid receptors and not to mineralocorticoid receptors.[21] There is evidence that glucocorticoids, like cortisol, also modulate immune functions by rapid, nongenomic effects via nonspecific interactions with cellular membranes and specific binding to membrane-bound glucocorticoid receptors.[22] Nonspecific membrane effects have been demonstrated for inhibition of sodium and calcium cycling across plasma membranes (i.e., impairment of Na^+, K^+-ATPase and Ca^{2+}-ATPase). Moreover, the rapid activation of lipocortin-1 and inhibition of arachidonic acid release after glucocorticoid administration was independent of glucocorticoid receptor translocation. Finally, high-sensitivity immunofluorescence staining revealed membrane-bound glucocorticoid receptors on circulating B lymphocytes and monocytes.[22]

The multiple mechanisms by which glucocorticoids modulate cellular responses mainly involve genomic pathways.[23-25] Nongenomic effects are thought to account primarily for the immediate immune effects of high doses of glucocorticoids, whereas membrane-bound receptors probably mediate low-dose glucocorticoid effects. The classic model is that glucocorticoids bind to the cytoplasmic ligand-regulated glucocorticoid receptor-α (GRα), which is an inactive multiprotein complex consisting of two heat shock proteins (HSP70 and HSP90), which act as molecular chaperones, and other proteins (Fig. 176-1).

On glucocorticoid binding to GRα, conformational changes cause dissociation of HSP70 and HSP90, with subsequent nuclear translocation of GRα homodimers, binding of GRα to glucocorticoid response elements (GREs) of DNA, and transcription of responsive genes (transactivation), such as lipocortin-1 and β_2-adrenoreceptors. Alternatively, GRα may bind to negative GRE (nGRE) and repress transcription of genes (transrepression), such as pro-opiomelanocortin (POMC). More important, transrepression without direct binding of GRα to GRE by protein-protein interactions of GRα with transcription factors such as nuclear factor-κB (NF-κB) (as well as activator protein-1 [AP-1]) has been recognized as a key step by which glucocorticoids suppress inflammation,[26] inhibiting the synthesis of TNF-α, IL-1β, IL-2, IL-6, IL-8, inducible nitric oxide synthase (iNOS), cyclooxygenase-2 (COX-2), cell adhesion molecules, and growth factors and promoting apoptosis.[27] In addition, NF-κB repression may be mediated by glucocorticoid-induced up-regulation of the cytoplasmic NF-κB inhibitor, IκBα (see Fig. 176-1), which

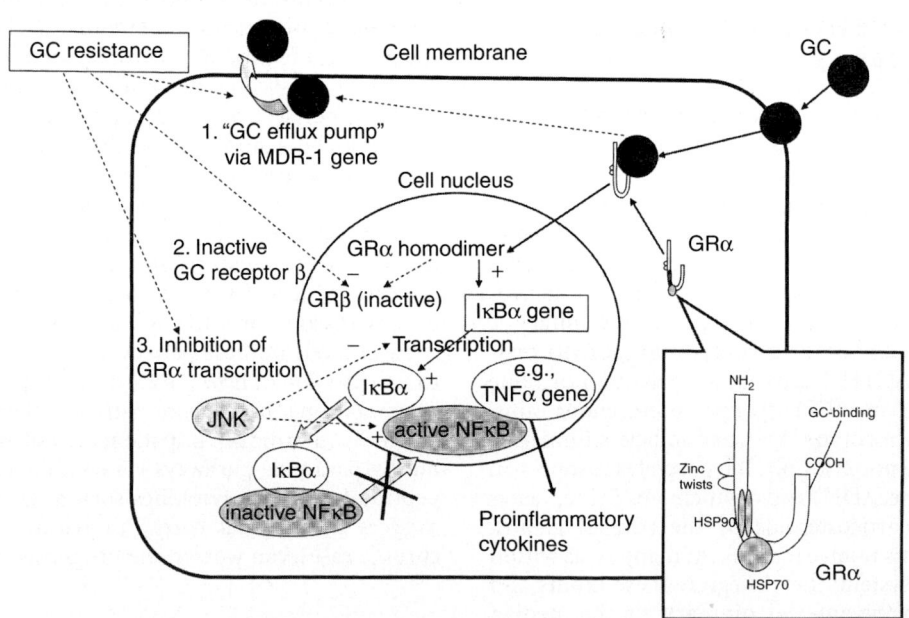

FIGURE 176–1. Cellular mechanisms of glucocorticoid effects *(right)* and glucocorticoid resistance *(left)*. After passive transport through the cell membrane, glucocorticoids (GCs) bind to the intracellular GC receptor-α (GRα), which is sequestered in the cytoplasm, bound to the heat-shock protein (HSP) complex that comprises chaperone molecules HSP70 and HSP90. Binding of GC to GRα allows formation of a homodimer, which is transported into the nucleus. GR-mediated transcription induces the inhibitor IκBα, which binds to and inhibits nuclear factor κB (NFκB). Thus, GC inhibit the NFκB-mediated synthesis of proinflammatory cytokines such as tumor necrosis factor-α (TNFα). Impaired GC sensitivity (GC resistance) includes three major pathways *(dotted arrows)*: (1) decreased cytoplasmic GC concentrations secondary to increased P-glycoprotein–mediated efflux of GC due to overexpression of the multidrug resistance gene, MDR-1; (2) increased expression of a truncated splice variant of the GR that is unable to transactivate GC-sensitive genes (GRβ); and (3) activation of proinflammatory mediators via upstream kinases (JNK) that can directly inhibit GR transcription activity. GR, glucocorticoid receptor; JNK, c-Jun NH₂-terminal kinase.

prevents translocation of NF-κB.[28] Clinical investigations provide support for the presence of endogenous glucocorticoid inadequacy in the control of inflammation and peripheral glucocorticoid resistance.[29] With glucocorticoid treatment, the intracellular relations between the NF-κB and GRα signaling pathways change from an initial NF-κB-driven and GRα-resistant state to a GRα-sensitive one. However, the data are conflicting and probably do not explain the early (less than 2 hours) suppressive effects of glucocorticoids; rather, they may account for the longer-term dampening effects of glucocorticoids on inflammatory processes.[23]

Besides transcriptional regulation, post-transcriptional, translational, and post-translational processes have been described for glucocorticoid-induced modulation of COX-2, TNF-α, granulocyte-macrophage colony-stimulating factor (GM-CSF), IL-1β, IL-6, IL-8, and interferon-γ (IFN-γ).[23] Furthermore, glucocorticoids act at multiple levels to regulate iNOS expression through decreased iNOS gene transcription and messenger RNA stability, reduced translation and increased degradation of the iNOS protein by the cysteine protease calpain,[30] limitation of the availability of the NOS cofactor tetrahydrobiopterin, reduced transmembranous transport and de novo synthesis of the NOS substrate L-arginine, and lipocortin-1–induced inhibition of iNOS.[31,32] Altogether, these complex mechanisms result in the considerable ability of glucocorticoids to inhibit inflammation and to stabilize hemodynamics. Finally, glucocorticoid receptors have been found in almost every nucleated cell in the body, and, because each cell type has its own expression of glucocorticoid effect, it follows that glucocorticoids (whether endogenously produced or exogenously administered) have many effects in the body. Both increase hepatic production of glucose and glycogen and decrease peripheral use of glucose. Steroids also affect fat and protein metabolism. They increase lipolysis, both directly and indirectly, by elevating free fatty acid levels in the plasma and enhancing any tendency to ketosis. Glucocorticoids further stimulate peripheral protein metabolism, using the amino acid products as gluconeogenic precursors.

DEFINITIONS OF ADRENAL INSUFFICIENCY

Adrenal glands may stop functioning if the HPA axis fails to produce sufficient amounts of the appropriate hormones. Primary adrenal insufficiency is defined by the inability of the adrenal gland to produce steroid hormones even if the stimulus by the pituitary gland via ACTH is adequate or increased. Primary adrenal insufficiency affects between 4 and 6 of every 100,000 people. The disease can strike at any age, with a peak between 30 and 50 years, and it affects males and females about equally. In 70% of cases, the cause is a primary destruction of the adrenal glands by an autoimmune reaction ("classic" Addison's disease or autoimmune adrenalitis), with about 40% of patients having a history of associated endocrinopathies. Most adult patients have antibodies against the steroidogenic enzyme 21-hydroxylase,[33] but their role in the pathogenesis of autoimmune adrenalitis is uncertain. In the other 30% of patients, the adrenal glands are destroyed by a cancer, amyloidosis, antiphospholipid syndrome, adrenomyeloneuropathy, acquired immunodeficiency syndrome (AIDS), infections (e.g., tuberculosis, cytomegaly, fungi), or other identifiable diseases (Table 176-1). In these cases, the typical morphologic changes of the adrenal cortex

TABLE 176–1. CAUSES OF ADRENAL INSUFFICIENCY

Primary Adrenal Insufficiency

Autoimmune adrenalitis (Morbus Addison), often with concomitant endocrinopathies
Hemorrhage (trauma, anticoagulants)
Infarction, thrombosis
Tumors
Infections (tuberculosis, cytomegaly, fungi, acquired immunodeficiency syndrome)
Amyloidosis, hemochromatosis, sarcoidosis
Congenital hyperplasias or hypoplasias
Congenital corticotropin (ACTH) resistance
Adrenomyeloneuropathy

Secondary Adrenal Insufficiency (Lesions of Pituitary and/or Hypothalamic Regions)

Tumors
Hemorrhages, apoplexy
Infections, inflammations
Autoimmune lesions
Trauma, surgery
Radiation
Congenital syndromes (e.g., familial deficiency of cortisol-binding globulin [CBG])

are atrophy, inflammation, and/or necrosis. In primary adrenal insufficiency, the whole adrenal cortex is involved, resulting in a deficiency of glucocorticoids, mineralocorticoids, and adrenal androgens.[34,35]

Secondary adrenal insufficiency is characterized by adrenal hypofunction due to the lack of pituitary ACTH or hypothalamic CRH. Diseases of the anterior pituitary that can cause secondary adrenal insufficiency include neoplasms (e.g., craniopharyngiomas, adenomas), infarction (e.g., Sheehan's syndrome, trauma), granulomatous disease (e.g., tuberculosis, sarcoidosis), hypophysectomy, and infection.[36] Causes also include hypothalamic dysfunction, such as after irradiation or surgical interventions (see Table 176-1). Because aldosterone secretion is more dependent on angiotensin II than on ACTH, aldosterone deficiency is not a problem in secondary adrenal insufficiency. Selective aldosterone deficiency can occur as a result of depressed renin secretion and angiotensin II formation.[34] Rare patients have an isolated deficiency of CRH,[37] and lymphocytic hypophysitis with subsequent adrenal insufficiency has been described in women.[38] These disorders may lead to an isolated ACTH deficiency.[34]

So-called tertiary adrenal insufficiency, which is often grouped together with secondary forms, commonly occurs after withdrawal of exogenous glucocorticoids. Many of these patients do well during normal activities but are unable to mount an appropriate glucocorticoid response to stress. This effect depends on the dose and duration of treatment and varies greatly from person to person. It should be anticipated in any patient who has been receiving more than 30 mg of hydrocortisone per day (or 7.5 mg of prednisolone or 0.75 mg of dexamethasone per day) for longer than 3 weeks.[35] If supraphysiologic doses of glucocorticoids have been administered to a patient for longer than 1 to 2 weeks, the drug should be tapered to allow for adrenal gland recovery. It may take 6 to 12 months for the adrenal glands to recover fully after prolonged use of exogenous glucocorticoids.[39] Because ACTH is not a major determinant of mineralocorticoid production, the basic deficit in adrenal insufficiency is that of deficient

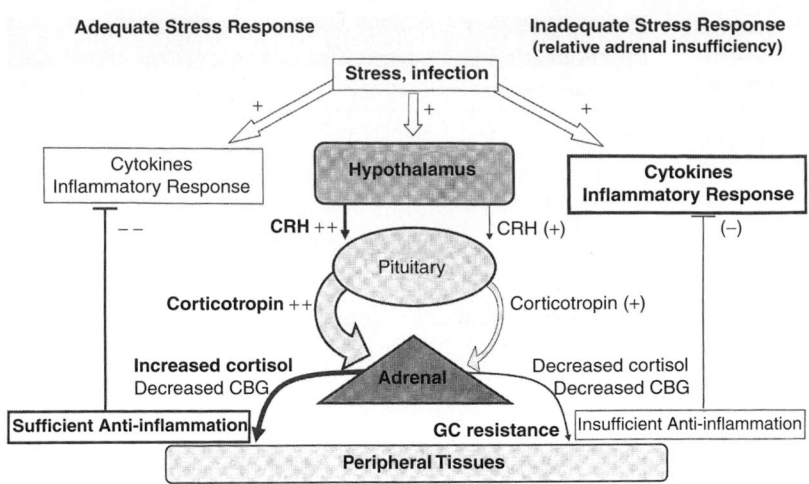

FIGURE 176–2. Concept of relative adrenal insufficiency. In contrast to the adequate stress response *(left)*, relative adrenal insufficiency *(right)* may occur when causal or additional factors impair the function of the hypothalamic-pituitary-adrenal (HPA) axis. This impairment may be caused by microcirculatory failure, additional drugs such as antibiotics, anesthetic drugs, infections, long-term use of steroids, or hemorrhages. The impaired HPA axis function results in insufficient anti-inflammatory effect, with an increased inflammatory response. +, activation; −, inhibition; CBG, cortisol-binding globulin; CRH, corticotropin-releasing hormone; GC, glucocorticoid.

glucocorticoid production. It is important that neither the dose of applied glucocorticoids, nor the time of treatment, nor the basal plasma level of cortisol allows adequate assessment of the function of the HPA axis. Some drugs have been described that induce adrenal insufficiency, either by directly affecting adrenocortical steroid release (e.g., fluconazole, etomidate)[40,41] or by enhancing the hepatic metabolism of cortisol (e.g., rifampicin, phenytoin).[35]

Isolated hypoaldosteronism is very rare and should be suspected in cases of hyperkalemia in the absence of renal insufficiency. The main causes for isolated deficiency of aldosterone secretion are congenital deficiency of aldosterone synthetase, hyporeninemia due to defects in the juxtaglomerular apparatus, and treatment with angiotensin-converting enzyme inhibitors that leads to loss of angiotensin stimulation. Other forms of hypoaldosteronism usually occur in patients with chronic renal disease or diabetes mellitus or both.

RELATIVE ADRENAL INSUFFICIENCY

The aforementioned forms of adrenal insufficiency, which lead to an absolute deficiency of steroids, are rare in critically ill patients (0% to 3%).[42] They are mostly characterized by morphologic changes in the HPA axis. To reflect the notion that subnormal adrenal corticosteroid production during acute severe illness can also occur without obvious structural defects in the HPA axis, deficiency syndromes resulting from a dysregulation have been termed "functional adrenal insufficiency."[43] Functional adrenal insufficiency can develop during the course of an illness and is usually transient.[35] In addition, decreased levels of glucocorticoids, which might be sufficient in normal subjects but are too low for stress situations because of the higher need, are encountered much more often and are associated with a worse prognosis for outcome.[44] This led to the concept of "relative adrenal insufficiency."

The major cause of relative adrenal insufficiency is an inadequate synthesis of cortisol by cellular dysfunction. In contrast to absolute adrenal insufficiency, the morphologic changes in relative adrenal insufficiency may be minor, sometimes being characterized by cellular hyperplasia within the adrenal cortex. This is often combined with a peripheral resistance of the target cells to glucocorticoid, which is caused by inflammatory events and aggravates the clinical course, even though the absolute cortisol serum levels may be normal.[45]

In septic shock, relative adrenal insufficiency may be caused by impaired pituitary ACTH release, attenuated adrenal response to ACTH, and reduced cortisol synthesis (Fig. 176-2).[35,46,47] In addition, cortisol transport capacity to affected sites may be reduced and response to cortisol may be impaired at the tissue level by cytokines modulating glucocorticoid receptor affinity to cortisol and/or GRE.[48,49]

In clinical trials, it was demonstrated that prolonged treatment of systemic inflammation with methylprednisolone in patients with severe acute respiratory distress syndrome (ARDS) improves the decreased glucocorticoid response by increasing glucocorticoid GC receptor affinity and reducing NF-κB–mediated DNA binding and transcription of proinflammatory cytokines.[29] Therefore, if relative adrenal insufficiency can be identified, treatment with supplemental corticosteroids may be of benefit.[35] The prevalence of relative adrenal insufficiency in the critically ill varies from 0% to 77% with various definitions, cutoff points, study populations, and adrenal function tests,[34,35,46,50,51] and it may be as high as 50% to 75% in severe septic shock.[52]

EVALUATION OF ADRENAL INSUFFICIENCY

In clinical practice, assessment of adrenal function is difficult, especially in critically ill patients, because the diurnal rhythm is lost. Values indicating normal adrenocortical function are listed in Table 176-2. Normally, morning (8 AM) serum cortisol concentrations less than 3 μg/dL (80 nmol/L) are strongly suggestive of absolute adrenal insufficiency,[53] whereas values lower than 10 μg/dL (275 nmol/L) make the diagnosis likely. Basal urinary cortisol and 17-hydroxycorticosteroid excretion is low in patients with severe adrenal

TABLE 176–2. VALUES INDICATING NORMAL ADRENOCORTICAL FUNCTION	
Parameter	**Normal Values**
Plasma cortisol (7-8 AM)	5-25 μg/dL (135-700 nmol/L)
Plasma corticotropin (ACTH, 7-8 AM)	<70 pg/mL
Urine excretion rate of free cortisol	20-90 μg/day
Urine excretion rate of 17-hydroxycorticosteroid (17-OHCS)	4-10 mg/day

insufficiency but may be low-normal in patients with partial adrenal insufficiency. Generally, baseline urinary measurements are not recommended for the diagnosis of adrenal insufficiency. To differentiate among primary, secondary, and tertiary adrenal insufficiency in cases of low cortisol, it is recommended that plasma ACTH concentrations be measured simultaneously. Inappropriately low serum cortisol concentrations (see earlier discussion) in association with increased ACTH concentrations are suggestive of primary adrenal insufficiency, whereas the combination of low cortisol and ACTH concentrations indicates secondary or tertiary disease. However, this conclusion should be confirmed by stimulation of the adrenal gland with exogenous ACTH. In secondary or tertiary adrenal insufficiency, the adrenal glands release cortisol, but in primary adrenal insufficiency the adrenal glands are partially or completely destroyed and do not respond to ACTH.

The so-called high-dose ACTH stimulation test usually consists of administering 250 µg (40 IU) of ACTH. For long-term stimulation tests, which are considered to be favorable for differentiating between secondary and tertiary adrenal insufficiency, 250 µg of ACTH is infused over 8 hours, or over 2 days.[54] Serum cortisol, 24-hour urinary cortisol, and 24-hour 17-hydroxycorticosteroid (17-OHCS) concentrations are determined before and after the infusion. This test may be helpful in distinguishing primary from secondary or tertiary adrenal insufficiency. In primary adrenal insufficiency, there is no response, or only a minimal response, of plasma or urinary cortisol and urinary 17-OHCS. Increases in these values in the 2 to 3 days of the test are indicative of a secondary or tertiary cause of adrenal insufficiency. In normal subjects, the 24-hour urinary 17-OHCS excretion increases 3- to 5-fold above baseline. Serum cortisol concentrations reach 20 µg/dL (550 nmol/L) at 30 to 60 minutes and exceed 25 µg/dL (690 nmol/L) at 6 to 8 hours after initiation of the infusion. Today, this test is not used very often, because clinical manifestations of the adrenal insufficiency combined with basal cortisol levels, short-term ACTH stimulation test results, and CRH tests (discussed later) usually provide sufficient information.

A short-term stimulation test with 250 µg ACTH, which is used mostly in non–critically ill patients, determines the basal serum cortisol level and the induced response concentration 30 and 60 minutes after intravenous administration of ACTH. The advantage of the high-dose test is that pharmacologic plasma ACTH concentrations can be achieved by either intravenous or intramuscular injection.[55] However, this test dose may be too high to identify mild cases of secondary adrenal insufficiency or chronic deficiencies.[56] Furthermore, it should not be used when acute secondary adrenal insufficiency (e.g., Sheehan's syndrome) is presumed, because it takes several days for the adrenal cortex to atrophy, and it will still be capable of responding to ACTH stimulation normally. In these cases, a low-dose ACTH test (discussed later) or an insulin-induced hypoglycemia may be required to confirm the diagnosis.[57,58] A rise in serum cortisol concentration after 30 or 60 minutes to a peak of 18 to 20 µg/dL (500 to 550 nmol/L) or greater is considered a normal response to a high-dose ACTH stimulation test and excludes the diagnosis of primary adrenal insufficiency and almost all cases of secondary adrenal insufficiency except those of recent onset.[59-61]

To further differentiate between secondary and tertiary adrenal insufficiency, the laboratory investigations may be completed by a CRH stimulation test. In both conditions, cortisol levels are low at baseline and remain low after CRH. In patients with secondary adrenal insufficiency, there is little or no ACTH response, whereas in patients with tertiary disease there is an exaggerated and prolonged response of ACTH to CRH stimulation, which is not followed by an appropriate cortisol response.[62,63] Formerly, the HPA axis was also tested by a stimulated hypoglycemia test. After administration of 0.1 IU insulin per kilogram body weight, which induces a hypoglycemic state of less than 40 mg/dL serum glucose, an intact HPA axis induces a serum cortisol concentration of greater than 20 µg/dL. Nowadays, this procedure is considered obsolete because of the high risk of hypoglycemia.

In critically ill patients, primary causes of absolute or relative adrenal insufficiency are multiple and often not detectable, if no specific hypothesis exists. Volume-resistant septic shock or any other form of life-threatening hypotension with increasing need for catecholamines and no reasonable explanation should give reason to evaluate adrenal function. Formerly, a serum cortisol value lower than 20 µg/dL suggested the diagnosis. Now, it is acknowledged that several factors complicate investigations of the HPA axis in patients with critical illness.

If possible, a short-term ACTH stimulation test should be performed for all critically ill patients with suspected adrenal insufficiency. In most patients, relative adrenal insufficiency is present, especially in patients with severe sepsis and septic shock. However, a clear definition of relative adrenal insufficiency is lacking, and the pathophysiology is rather complex, which makes it difficult to define clear cutoffs for both basal serum cortisol concentrations and incremental increases after short-term ACTH stimulation tests. Proposed cutoff points may depend on the method used to measure cortisol, with variations when compared with high-performance liquid chromatography (HPLC) as the reference method.[64] In addition, consideration of free cortisol or the increase in free cortisol in response to ACTH could increase the accuracy of adrenocortical function tests.[48] Furthermore, extrapolation of the diagnosis from reference values obtained from healthy people or from patients with HPA disorders may be misleading, because normal or high-normal cortisol concentrations in septic shock may indicate inadequate adrenal response to stress.

In a large series of patients, receiver operating characteristic curve (ROC) analysis reached highest sensitivity (68%) and specificity (65%) to detect nonresponders for the reference value less than 9 µg/dL (incremental increase).[52] A basal cortisol of 34 µg/dL and an incremental increase of 9 µg/dL after stimulation were the best cutoff points to discriminate between survivors and nonsurvivors. The higher the basal plasma cortisol and the weaker the cortisol response to ACTH, the higher was the risk of death. Some investigators have questioned the discriminative power of the incremental increase in cortisol after stimulation in patients with high basal cortisol values, because increases may reflect adrenal reserve more than adrenal function. Therefore, relative adrenal insufficiency was defined based on the hemodynamic response when a randomly measured cortisol concentration was less than 25 µg/dL.[46]

The routine use of the low-dose ACTH stimulation test in critically ill patients cannot be recommended at present, although it is preferred in patients with secondary or tertiary adrenal insufficiency.[65] After stimulation with 250 µg ACTH, circulating ACTH concentrations are typically 40 to 200 pg/mL during stress but may be as high as 60,000 pg/mL.[35] Stimulation of the adrenal gland with low doses of ACTH (1 µg) was shown to increase the sensitivity and specificity to detect adrenal insufficiency in patients with HPA disorders, who respond normally to traditional high-dose stimulation.[35,66-69] The test is performed by measuring serum cortisol concentrations immediately before and 30 minutes after intravenous injection of ACTH at a dose of 1.0 µg (160 mIU) per 1.73 m[2] body surface.[34] This dose stimulates maximal adrenocortical secretion up to 30 minutes after injection and in normal subjects results in a peak plasma ACTH concentration about twice that of insulin-induced hypoglycemia.[70] A value of 18 µg/dL (500 nmol/L) or more at any time during the test is indicative of normal adrenal function. The advantage of this test is that it can detect partial adrenal insufficiency that may be missed by the standard high-dose test.[57,58]

Based on these findings, it was suggested that the 1 µg ACTH stimulation test be used to uncover patients with relative adrenal insufficiency in septic shock more precisely. However, the 1-µg stimulation test has not been well validated in critically ill patients or in patients with septic shock.[34,35] In addition, studies evaluating low-dose and high-dose ACTH stimulation tests in septic shock may have been flawed by methodologic problems. At present, the 1-µg ACTH stimulation test cannot be recommended for routine use until further data from well-designed, randomized studies in patients with septic shock are available. Today, a three-level therapeutic guide for evaluation of relative adrenal insufficiency in critically ill patients, especially those with septic shock, is recommended. Patients with a random basal cortisol value lower than 15 µg/dL are designated as to likely profit from low-dose corticosteroid therapy, whereas corticosteroid replacement is unlikely to be helpful if the basal cortisol concentration is greater than 34 µg/dL. If a random basal cortisol value is between 15 and 34 µg/dL, adrenocortical stimulation with 250 µg ACTH should discriminate responders (incremental increase, 9 µg/dL or greater) from nonresponders (less than 9 µg/dL increase). However, no cutoff values are entirely reliable.[35]

CLINICAL SYMPTOMS

Approximately 25% of patients with adrenal insufficiency present with adrenocortical crisis.[34] The symptoms are not specific and include a sudden dizziness, weakness, dehydration, hypotension, and shock (Table 176-3). In many cases, the clinical picture is indistinguishable from that of shock, owing to loss of intravascular fluid volume. Other features, such as anorexia, nausea, vomiting, diarrhea, abdominal pain, and delirium, may be present, but they are also common in patients with other acute illnesses. Therefore, these symptoms may not be helpful and are often misleading. Hypoglycemia is rare in acute adrenal insufficiency but more common in secondary adrenal insufficiency. Hypoglycemia is a common manifestation in children and in thin women with the disorder. It remains extremely difficult to recognize an acute, absolute adrenal insufficiency based on clinical symptoms, especially in patients in the ICU. However, if the diagnosis is missed, the patient will probably die. Therefore, the threshold for laboratory investigations in cases of unexplained catecholamine-resistant hypotension should be low. It is important to note that the onset of an acute adrenocortical crisis does not necessarily mean an acute

onset of the causative disease itself. The preceding disease is often gradual and may go undetected until an acute illness, stress, trauma, pregnancy, or other condition precipitates an adrenal crisis.[34,71]

In most cases, primary adrenal insufficiency is the underlying disorder. Therefore, typical symptoms such as hyperpigmentation, scanty axillary and pubic hair, hyponatremia, or hyperkalemia may be diagnosed in the acutely ill patient. Adrenal crisis can occur in patients receiving appropriate doses of glucocorticoid if their mineralocorticoid requirements are not met.[72] After spontaneous events (e.g., hemorrhage, infarction, adrenal-vein thrombosis), these signs are absent. If an acute adrenal crisis is suspected, a blood sample should be obtained to confirm the diagnosis. The main clinical problem is hypotension and shock, which is caused by an acute mineralocorticoid deficiency. This is one reason for the fact that an acute adrenal crisis after secondary adrenal insufficiency is not so typical. However, glucocorticoid deficiency may also contribute to hypotension by decreasing vascular responsiveness to angiotensin II, norepinephrine, and other vasoconstrictive hormones, reducing the synthesis of renin substrate, and increasing production and effects of prostacyclin and other vasodilatory hormones.[73,74] Finally, panhypopituitarism may be associated with symptoms caused only by the lack of ACTH but also by the lack of TSH, gonadotropin, and GHs.

In chronic adrenal insufficiency, the major clinical features (see Table 176-3) may be detected; they may also be absent, if adrenal gland insufficiency develops over a prolonged period. There is a period characterized by normal basal steroid secretion but inability to respond to stress, in which case the patient may be asymptomatic. In other cases, there may also be signs and symptoms suggestive of other hormone deficiencies, such as decreased thyroid and gonadal function. Independent of the underlying cause, the most common clinical manifestations are general malaise,

TABLE 176–3. CLINICAL MANIFESTATIONS OF ADRENAL INSUFFICIENCY

Acute Adrenal Insufficiency

Acute apathy
Nausea, vomiting
Fever
Acute dehydration, tachycardia
Craving for salt
Hypotension, shock

Chronic Adrenal Insufficiency

Weakness, fatigue
Lack of appetite
Orthostatic hypotension
Weight loss, anorexia
Hyperpigmentation (only in primary Addison's disease due to increased corticotropin [ACTH])
Vitiligo
Nonspecific gastrointestinal symptoms (diarrhea, nausea, abdominal pain)
Nonspecific pain (myalgia, arthralgia, headaches)
Nonspecific psychic symptoms (depression, lack of concentration, confusion, psychosis)
Hypoglycemia
Hyponatremia
Hyperkalemia
Acidosis, prerenal azotemia
Lymphocytosis, eosinophilia

fatigue, weakness, anorexia, weight loss, nausea, vomiting, abdominal pain, arthralgia, postural syncope, diarrhea that may alternate with constipation, hypotension, electrolyte abnormalities (hyponatremia, hyperkalemia, metabolic acidosis), decreased axillary and pubic hair, and loss of libido and amenorrhea in women.[34,71]

In primary adrenal insufficiency, hyperpigmentation, and autoimmune manifestations (vitiligo) are typical because of the increased ACTH concentrations; these conditions are not seen in secondary or tertiary adrenal insufficiency. Soon after the disease develops, the skin becomes dark, which may appear similar to tanning but occurs on both sun-exposed and nonexposed areas. Black freckles develop on the forehead, face, and shoulders, and a bluish-black discoloration may develop around the lips, mouth, rectum, scrotum, or vagina. Another specific symptom of primary adrenal insufficiency is a craving for salt.[35] Typical laboratory abnormalities are hyponatremia, hyperkalemia, acidosis, slightly elevated creatinine concentration, mild normocytic anemia, and, rarely, hypercalcemia.[35]

In secondary adrenal insufficiency, because the production of mineralocorticoids by the zona glomerulosa is mostly preserved, dehydration and hyperkalemia are not present, and hypotension is less prominent than in primary disease. Especially in the early stages of the disease, chronic adrenal insufficiency is often insidious and the diagnosis can be difficult. Some patients initially present with gastrointestinal symptoms such as nausea, vomiting, diarrhea, and abdominal cramps.[35,75] In other patients, the disease may be misdiagnosed as depression or anorexia nervosa.[76,77] Hyponatremia and increased intravascular volume may be the result of "inappropriate" increase in vasopressin secretion. Decreased libido and potency as well as amenorrhea may occur. Hypoglycemia is more common in secondary adrenal insufficiency, possibly because of concomitant GH insufficiency, and in isolated ACTH deficiency. Clinical manifestations of a pituitary or hypothalamic tumor, such as symptoms and signs of deficiency of other anterior pituitary hormones, headache, or visual field defects, may also be present.[34,71] Finally, in young patients with suspected adrenal insufficiency, delayed growth and puberty point to the presence of hypothalamic-pituitary disease, as do headaches, visual disturbances, or diabetes insipidus in patients of any age.[35,36] Laboratory screening in patients with chronic adrenal insufficiency usually reveals hyponatremia, hypoglycemia, lymphocytosis, and eosinophilia.[35]

THERAPEUTIC STRATEGIES

Treatment of adrenal insufficiency involves eradication of the precipitating cause (e.g., tumor, infection) and hormone replacement. In acutely ill patients, if the diagnosis of adrenal crisis is suspected but not known, blood should be taken for measurement of cortisol concentrations, followed by administration of 250 μg ACTH in patients with an unknown history. Independent of a diagnosis, therapy for absolute adrenal insufficiency should be started immediately while awaiting results of testing.[78] Dexamethasone (1 mg every 6 hours) may be given as the initial glucocorticoid replacement, because it does not cross-react with cortisol in the plasma while adrenal testing is being performed. Patients usually are given intravenous fluids in the form of isotonic saline to restore intravascular volume and to replace urinary salt losses. Dextrose infusion may be added prevent hypoglycemia.

Hydrocortisone (100 mg intravenous bolus or over 30 minutes, followed by a continuous infusion of 10 mg/hour, or 50 mg every 4 hours, or 75 to 100 mg every 6 hours, resulting in a total daily dose of 240 to 300 mg hydrocortisone) is frequently given for hormonal replacement.[34,78] However, equivalent glucocorticoid doses of methylprednisolone or dexamethasone may also be used. Typically, mineralocorticoid replacement therapy is not required in adrenal crisis as long as the patient is receiving isotonic saline. Prophylactic use of antibiotics is not beneficial, but specific infections should be treated aggressively with appropriate antibiotic therapy.

Once the patient is stable, or in cases of chronic adrenal insufficiency, glucocorticoids can be tapered to maintenance doses. Long-term replacement doses consist of hydrocortisone 30 mg/day, with two thirds (20 mg) given in the morning and one third (10 mg) at night, or prednisone 7.5 mg in a similar regimen (5 and 2.5 mg, respectively). The daily dose may be decreased to 20 or 15 mg of hydrocortisone as long as the patient is well and physical strength is not reduced.[34] The goal should be to use the smallest dose that relieves the patient's symptoms, in order to prevent the side effects of weight gain and osteoporosis.[34,78,79]

If the patient continues to experience weakness or other symptoms of glucocorticoid deficiency, the dose can be increased. Excessive glucocorticoid therapy should be avoided to minimize complications of this therapy. In addition, a mineralocorticoid effect is provided with fludrocortisone (50 to 100 μg/day orally) to prevent sodium loss, intravascular volume depletion, and hyperkalemia, especially when the dose of hydrocortisone decreases to less than 100 mg/day. The therapy can be guided by measurements of blood pressure, serum potassium, and plasma renin activity, which should be in the upper-normal range.[34,61] However, clinical response is the best indicator of adequacy of replacement.

The optimal dosage of mineralocorticoids remains stable over long periods. Excessive mineralocorticoid replacement can cause congestive heart failure, alkalosis, hypokalemia, or hypertension. Patients receiving prednisone or dexamethasone may require higher doses of fludrocortisone to lower their plasma renin activity to the upper-normal range, whereas patients receiving hydrocortisone, which has some mineralocorticoid activity, may require lower doses. The mineralocorticoid dose may need to be increased in the summer, particularly if patients are exposed to temperatures greater than 29°C (85°F). In cases of isolated hypoaldosteronism, treatment includes liberal sodium intake and daily administration of fludrocortisone. In patients with secondary adrenal insufficiency due to panhypopituitarism, replacement with other hormones may also be necessary. In women, the adrenal cortex is the primary source of androgens in the form of dehydroepiandrosterone and dehydroepiandrosterone sulfate. Although the physiologic role of these androgens in women has not been fully elucidated, their replacement is being increasingly considered in the treatment of adrenal insufficiency.[80,81]

Once the patient is stable and is receiving maintenance doses of steroids, ACTH testing can be repeated to document adrenal recovery. Patients with primary adrenal insufficiency require lifelong glucocorticoid and mineralocorticoid replacement therapy and should carry a card containing information on current therapy, as well as some type of bracelet or necklace with recommendations for treatment in emergency situations. One of the important aspects of the management of chronic primary adrenal insufficiency is patient and family education. Patients should understand the reason for lifelong replacement therapy, the need to increase the dose of glucocorticoids during minor or major stress, and the need to inject hydrocortisone, methylprednisolone, or dexamethasone in emergencies. Patients should also have supplies of dexamethasone sodium phosphate and should be educated about how and when to administer them. The survival rate for patients with chronic primary adrenal insufficiency has gone from 2 years or less before the availability of steroid replacement to that of a normal population now that glucocorticoids are readily available. In acute adrenal insufficiency, prompt recognition and treatment usually result in a favorable outcome, provided the underlying disease process can be treated.

GLUCOCORTICOID REPLACEMENT FOR PATIENTS WITH SEPTIC SHOCK

In patients with severe sepsis and septic shock, the individual clinical course is extremely varied. The impact of the primary disease, as well as immunologic factors (cytokines), affect the HPA axis, and functional testing is aggravated. In contrast to the early phase of septic shock, adrenal cortisol release may recover, leading to relative adrenal insufficiency with absolute steroid levels near or even higher than the normal range.[82] In refractory septic shock, the prevalence of relative adrenal insufficiency may be as high as 50% to 75%.[52] Furthermore, dynamic testing is not always available in ICUs, which makes it difficult for the physician considering hormone replacement therapy, because decisions must be made within hours in severe forms of septic shock to improve prognosis. The rationale for the use of high-dose glucocorticoids in infection, sepsis, and shock can be attributed to well defined anti-inflammatory and hemodynamic effects recognized for decades. Proposed mechanism of protection includes improvement in hemodynamic, metabolic, endocrinologic, and phagocytic functions, resulting in the maintenance of normal morphologic-functional status of tissues, including brain, liver, heart, kidneys, and adrenals.[83] In addition, glucocorticoids inhibit key features of inflammation: endothelial cell activation and damage, capillary leakage, granulocyte activation, adhesion and aggregation, complement activation, and formation and release of eicosanoid metabolites, oxygen radicals, and lysosomal enzymes.[84-89]

However, experimental results have been confirmed in only one long-term prospective study in humans, in which high doses of methylprednisolone (30 to 60 mg/kg) or dexamethasone (2 to 4 mg/kg) given to 179 bacteremic septic shock patients over a period of 8 years reduced mortality from 38% to 10%.[90] Another study provided evidence that prolongation of treatment might have been beneficial, because shock reversal and improved survival occurred after bolus glucocorticoid application in an early time window but vanished after several days.[91] Two meta-analyses included 9 and 10 randomized trials, respectively, involving patients with severe sepsis and septic shock who received up to 42 g hydrocortisone equivalent or more, and concluded that high doses of corticosteroids were ineffective[92] or harmful.[93] This conclusion was confirmed by a large randomized trial in 1987.[94] Patients with proven gram-negative infections probably had profited more from glucocorticoids.[92] In one analysis, studies with the highest quality had the worst outcome for corticosteroids.[93] High-dose glucocorticoids were associated with

increased risk of secondary infections, increased mortality,[93] and increased incidence of renal and hepatic dysfunction.[95] Taken together, these studies indicate that high-dose glucocorticoids are not effective in septic shock in the long term, most probably because of breakdown of the immune system.

As with high-dose glucocorticoid treatment, numerous randomized controlled trials with low-dose corticosteroids in patients with septic shock also confirmed shock reversal and reduction of vasopressor support within a few days after initiation of therapy in most patients.[96-101] In a crossover study, mean arterial pressure and systemic vascular resistance increased during low-dose hydrocortisone treatment, and heart rate, cardiac index, and norepinephrine requirement decreased significantly.[102] All of these effects were reversible with cessation of hydrocortisone. Some studies indicated that corticosteroid-induced increase of sensitivity to norepinephrine is more pronounced in patients with relative adrenal insufficiency, compared with patients without relative adrenal insufficiency.[46,101,103] There are many potential mechanisms by which corticosteroids may modulate vascular tone.[104] There is considerable evidence that cytokine-induced formation of nitric oxide (NO) plays a central role in vasodilation, catecholamine resistance, maldistribution of blood flow, and mitochondrial and organ dysfunction and that the amount of NO production correlates with shock severity and outcome.[105,106] In a crossover trial, norepinephrine requirements could be reduced by low-dose hydrocortisone in almost all patients within 1 to 2 days. Hydrocortisone treatment also induced a significant and prolonged decline in nitrite/nitrate levels, which significantly correlated with the reduction in norepinephrine requirements during hydrocortisone infusion.[102] Considering the complex genomic and nongenomic actions of corticosteroids described earlier, it is probable that NO is not the only target. However, inhibition of NO synthesis by hydrocortisone at least contributes to shock reversal.

It is recognized that glucocorticoids modulate the stress response in a very complex manner, which includes not only anti-inflammatory and immunosuppressive actions to protect the host from overwhelming inflammation but also immune-enhancing effects.[27] The final effect of corticosteroids may depend on multiple factors such as the dose, the type of cell or tissue, the time point of action, and the balance of proinflammatory and anti-inflammatory cofactors. Markers of the inflammatory response; anti-inflammatory response; granulocyte, monocyte, and endothelial activation; antigen-presenting capacity; and innate immune response were investigated in septic shock patients.[102] In summary, hydrocortisone significantly attenuated the inflammatory and anti-inflammatory response, as well as granulocyte, monocyte, and endothelial activation. Monocyte human leukocyte antigen HLA-DR expression was depressed, but receptor downregulation was limited and was followed by a rebound increase after drug withdrawal.[102] In conclusion, immune effects of low-dose hydrocortisone treatment in septic shock may be characterized as immunomodulatory rather than immunosuppressive. Attenuation of a broad spectrum of the inflammatory response without causing severe immunosuppression might be a promising therapeutic approach, one that goes far beyond hemodynamic stabilization.

Although data on outcome in septic shock patients after low-dose corticosteroid treatment are limited, up to 300 mg/day of hydrocortisone appears to improve survival. In most trials with low-dose corticosteroids,[96-100] 28-day all-cause mortality was reduced, whereas in high-dose trials there was no significant effect. In a multicenter trial involving 300 patients with severe volume- and catecholamine-refractory septic shock, survival time was significantly increased in patients with relative adrenal insufficiency but not in responders to an ACTH stimulation test.[97] Similar results were obtained for ICU and hospital mortality, but not for 1-year follow-up. Significant increases in the incidence of serious adverse events during treatment with low-dose hydrocortisone have not been reported. The incidence of gastrointestinal bleeding, superinfection, or hyperglycemia has not been different in patients treated with corticosteroids or placebo, and wound infections were even less frequent in patients treated with low-dose hydrocortisone.[97] Treatment with low-dose hydrocortisone may induce an increase in sodium levels within a few days, and hypernatremia with values greater than 155 mmol/L has been reported during prolonged treatment.[100] Nevertheless, the indication for low-dose corticosteroids should be weighed against the possible risks, and treatment should be limited to the shortest possible duration.

Dosing of hydrocortisone in septic shock is similar to that used in adrenal crisis (100 mg initial bolus, followed by 200 to 300 mg/day), and the dose should be tapered after the patient stabilizes. Hydrocortisone is preferred, although a comparative study of various corticosteroids has not been performed in septic shock, because most experience of low-dose corticosteroid treatment in septic shock was derived from studies using hydrocortisone (see earlier discussion). Furthermore, hydrocortisone is the synthetic equivalent to the physiologic final active compound, cortisol, so treatment with hydrocortisone directly replaces cortisol, independent of metabolic transformation. Finally, hydrocortisone, in contrast to dexamethasone, has intrinsic mineralocorticoid activity. Fludrocortisone supplementation might be indicated if glucocorticoids without mineralocorticoid activity are used. It has not been established whether a weight-adjusted regimen (e.g., 0.18 mg/kg/hour)[56] is superior to a fixed regimen; moreover, a comparative study of bolus versus infusion regimens has not been performed so far.

Patients should be weaned from low-dose hydrocortisone over several days to avoid hemodynamic and immunologic rebound effects. In patients with septic shock, abrupt cessation of low-dose hydrocortisone was followed by significant reversal of many hemodynamic and immunologic effects observed during corticosteroid therapy, even after a short treatment period of 3 days.[102] Adrenal function tests with 250 μg ACTH can be performed in patients with septic shock; however, at present, exclusion of responders or patients with high random cortisol values from low-dose corticosteroid therapy cannot be recommended.[35] If basal serum cortisol concentrations are less than 15 μg/dL in a patient with septic shock, low-dose hydrocortisone replacement is recommended; levels greater than 34 μg/dL are considered to be sufficient. Between 15 and 34 μg/dL, an incremental increase of less than 9 μg/dL serum cortisol makes relative adrenal insufficiency likely, and therapy may be considered according to the clinical state.[35] Others recommend a randomly assigned cutoff level of 25 μg/dL serum cortisol.[46] Routine use of the low ACTH stimulation test (1 μg ACTH) cannot be recommended until further data from well-designed, randomized studies in septic shock patients are available.

Most importantly, it must be realized that all the aforementioned studies were performed in patients with catecholamine-resistant septic shock. So far there are no data justifying the use of low-dose steroids in patients with sepsis or severe sepsis! Significant effects on outcome have been observed only in patients with systolic blood pressure less than 90 mm Hg despite vasopressor therapy.[97] It is not known yet whether low-dose corticosteroids are also effective in patients with less severe shock. Finally, sufficient data on the dose-response characteristics of glucocorticoids in septic patients are still lacking, and the current recommended strategy of using 200 to 300 mg hydrocortisone per day is based on empiric recommendations, and further investigations are needed.

FURTHER IMPLICATIONS FOR ANESTHESIA AND CRITICAL CARE

Surgical stress increases serum cortisol levels fivefold to sixfold postoperatively, with return to normal at 24 hours unless stress continues. Patients who have received glucocorticoids equivalent to 30 mg/day cortisol for longer than 3 weeks may have impairment in this stress response, and steroid supplementation should be considered. However, short-term treatment of heterogeneous groups of patients with critical illness is controversial, and supraphysiologic doses of glucocorticoids are not beneficial and may even be harmful.[107] Therefore, outside situations in which benefit has been proven, supraphysiologic doses of glucocorticoids (e.g., 30 mg methylprednisolone per kilogram of body weight per day) in patients with critical illness are not indicated. Nevertheless, some successful indications have been described; in patients with unresolving ARDS, pharmacologic doses of methylprednisolone (2 mg/kg/day) reduced mortality and improved organ function.[29] Furthermore, early treatment with dexamethasone may improve the outcome in bacterial meningitis.[108,109] The positive effects of steroid treatment on tissue-specific resistance to glucocorticoids have already been described. However, despite the frequent suggestion that unexplained intraoperative hypotension and even death reflect unrecognized hypocortisolism, there is no evidence that primary adrenal insufficiency is a likely explanation for this response.

Patients with known chronic adrenal insufficiency must be advised to double or triple their dose of hydrocortisone temporarily whenever they have any febrile illness or injury.[34] In stressful situations or during major surgery, trauma, burns, or medical illness, high doses of glucocorticoids, up to 10 times the daily production, are required to avoid an adrenal crisis, although no data from randomized trials are available. A continuous infusion of 10 mg of hydrocortisone per hour, or the equivalent amount of dexamethasone or prednisolone, eliminates the possibility of glucocorticoid deficiency. This dose can be halved on the second postoperative day, and the maintenance dosage can be resumed on day 3. However, it is important, with regard to possible detrimental effects and the possibility of decreased resistance to infections, that this treatment should not be used for prolonged periods in the absence of evidence of corticosteroid insufficiency. General perioperative management should include avoidance of etomidate as an anesthetic drug (selection of other drugs and muscle relaxants is not influenced by the presence of treated hypocortisolism); infusion of sodium-containing fluids; minimal doses of any anesthetic drugs to avoid increased sensitivity to drug-induced myocardial depression; invasive monitoring of hemodynamics, glucose, and electrolytes; and decreased initial doses of muscle relaxant with monitoring of the effect using a peripheral nerve stimulator. Especially if acute adrenal insufficiency has been detected in a critically ill patient with a previously unknown disorder, thorough diagnostics are demanded even after improvement.

Observations suggest that control of cortisol secretion in response to stress is more complex than originally thought. Interactions among corticotropin-releasing factor (CRF), vasoactive intestinal polypeptide, arginine vasopressin, catecholamines, and other hormones in the control of cortisol secretion have been described.[110] α_2-Adrenergic receptor antagonists (e.g., clonidine), which are widely used in ICUs, may suppress the cortisol response to surgical stress. On the other hand, increases in intracranial pressure stimulate cortisol release without increasing ACTH levels, and adrenalectomy (but not adrenal demedullation) increases the permeability of brain tissue to macromolecules.[111] Further evidence also suggests that white blood cells may release ACTH-like peptides that can stimulate adrenal gland secretion of cortisol, and that primary adrenal insufficiency is associated with increases in serum levels of angiotensin-converting enzyme.[112]

There are many interactions between drugs and the HPA axis that must be considered if absolute or relative adrenal insufficiency is suspected. In patients with hepatic dysfunction, glucocorticoid doses should be tapered, especially prednisone, because hydroxylation to the active component requires considerable metabolic capacity. Special attention is required in the concomitant use of glucocorticoids with other drugs because of potential interactions, and because some drugs may affect the metabolism of the steroids, leading to a decreased or increased glucocorticoid effect on their target tissues.[113,114] Briefly, glucocorticoids decrease the drug blood levels of aspirin, coumarin anticoagulants, insulin, isoniazid, and oral hypoglycemic agents but increase the levels of cyclophosphamide and cyclosporine. Conversely, antacids, carbamazepine, cholestyramine, colestipol, ephedrine, mitotane, phenobarbitone, phenytoin, and rifampicin decrease glucocorticoid blood concentrations, but cyclosporine, erythromycin, oral contraceptives, and troleandomycin increase them. Furthermore, the combination of exogenous glucocorticoid administration and amphotericin B, digitalis glycosides, or potassium-depleting diuretics may induce or worsen hypokalemia; frequent monitoring of potassium levels is required. Finally, the general risk of immunosuppression by glucocorticoids forbids any use of vaccines from live-attenuated viruses, so as to avoid severe generalized infections.[113,114]

CONCLUSIONS

Underproduction of adrenal hormones can lead to serious illness. Glucocorticoids play a critical permissive role in intermediary metabolism, are counterregulatory in relation to insulin, modulate inflammatory and immune responses, and optimize cardiovascular and central nervous system function. Therefore, diseases involving primary adrenocortical dysfunction and those leading to secondary adrenal insufficiency may have severe sequelae, which are often life-threatening. The concept of relative adrenal insufficiency in critically ill patients with functional disorders of the HPA axis has attracted attention in recent years. Especially in patients with severe sepsis and septic shock, this phenomenon

is suspected to have a major impact on the severity of illness and the prognosis. Both absolute and relative adrenal insufficiency should be diagnosed by the use of adequate laboratory investigations. In most cases, the basal level of cortisol, combined with the results of a short-term stimulation test using 250 µg ACTH, can identify the disease. In patients with critical illness, however, it continues to be difficult to diagnose relative adrenal insufficiency.

In cases of severe, volume- and catecholamine-resistant shock with suspicion of adrenal crisis, immediate replacement therapy is indicated. If the diagnosis is not certain, dexamethasone should be administered to allow functional diagnostics. Once the diagnosis is made, hydrocortisone is the preferred drug, because it provides both glucocorticoid and mineralocorticoid effects. After stabilization, the patient's dose of glucocorticoids should be tapered down to a total of 20 to 35 mg hydrocortisone per day or equivalent analogs.

The fundamental role of glucocorticoids in the stress response to infection, together with increasing knowledge of the anti-inflammatory and immunosuppressive pharmacodynamic profiles, has been the rationale for their use in sepsis trials for decades. Timing, dosage, and duration of glucocorticoid administration were adapted to different disease pathophysiologic models and had a major impact on outcome. Randomized, controlled trials of high-dose glucocorticoid therapy failed to improve outcome, leading to skepticism and avoidance of any glucocorticoids in septic patients by most ICU physicians for years, with the exception of some special indications. However, recent randomized, controlled trials with low doses of hydrocortisone in patients with septic shock have evoked a corticosteroid renaissance. Based on current data, an incremental increase of less than 9 µg/dL after a 250-µg ACTH stimulation test may be used in patients with severe septic shock to determine relative adrenal insufficiency. Meanwhile, prolonged treatment of septic shock with low doses of corticosteroids is a therapeutic option to promote shock reversal and to increase vascular sensitivity to vasopressors.

ANNOTATED REFERENCES

Annane D, Sebille V, Charpentier C, et al: Effect of treatment with low doses of hydrocortisone and fludrocortisone on mortality in patients with septic shock. JAMA 2002;288:862-871.

This was the first multicenter clinical trial able to demonstrate that low-dose hydrocortisone combined with fludrocortisone reduces mortality in patients with severe, volume-restrictive septic shock.

Annane D, Sebille V, Troche G, et al: A 3-level prognostic classification in septic shock based on cortisol levels and cortisol response to corticotropin. JAMA 2000;283:1038-1045.

With a combination of testing both basic cortisol levels and incremental increases after ACTH stimulation in acutely ill patients, this study proved that the phenomenon of relative adrenal insufficiency has a crucial impact on outcome.

Auphan N, Didonato JA, Rosette C, et al: Immunosuppression by glucocorticoids: Inhibition of NF-kappa B activity through induction of I kappa B synthesis. Science 1995;270:286-290.

This paper is probably one of the most important publications on the cellular pathways of glucocorticoid response. It demonstrates how steroids inhibit NF-κB, which represents a key pathway of inflammatory diseases.

Cooper MS, Stewart PM: Corticosteroid insufficiency in acutely ill patients. N Engl J Med 2003;348:727-734.

This review presents the current concepts of pathophysiology, diagnosis, and treatment of corticosteroid insufficiency in acutely ill patients.

Keh D, Boehnke T, Weber-Carstens S, et al: Immunologic and hemodynamic effects of "low-dose" hydrocortisone in septic shock: A double-blind, randomized, placebo-controlled, crossover study. Am J Respir Crit Care Med 2003;167:512-520.

The authors performed a randomized trial in patients with septic shock, using a crossover design, which demonstrated that (1) hemodynamic stabilization by low-dose steroids is paralleled by reduced synthesis of endogenous nitric oxide, (2) low-dose hydrocortisone modulates rather than suppresses immunologic functions, and (3) rapid withdrawal of steroids induces rebound phenomena with impairment of the clinical course.

Chapter 177

THYROID GLAND DISORDERS

Alan P. Farwell

KEY POINTS

1. Synthesis and secretion of the thyroid hormones are under the control of the anterior pituitary gland in a classic negative feedback system. The major pathway of metabolism of the thyroid hormones is by sequential monodeiodination in peripheral tissues. Although greater than 99% of the thyroid hormones circulate bound to plasma proteins, only the free hormone has any metabolic activity (free hormone concept).

2. Nonthyroidal illness affects all aspects of thyroid hormone economy. In all critically ill patients, conversion of thyroxine (T_4) to 3,5,3′-triiodothyronine (T_3) is markedly impaired, resulting in serum T_3 concentrations often in the low range. Thyroid-stimulating hormone secretion by the anterior pituitary is blunted by a variety of endogenous and exogenous factors. Similarly, drugs and endogenous factors inhibit the binding of thyroid hormones to thyroid-binding globulin.

3. The routine screening of ICU patients for the presence of thyroid dysfunction is not recommended because of the high prevalence of abnormal thyroid function tests and low prevalence of thyroid dysfunction. No single laboratory test can diagnos the presence or absence of thyroid dysfunction. Determination of thyroid-stimulating hormone and free T_4 concentrations in patients with a high index of suspicion for thyroid dysfunction is an appropriate initial evaluation.

4. Critical illness causes multiple alterations in thyroid hormone concentrations that are nonspecific and relate to the severity of the illness (sick euthyroid syndrome). These alterations represent a continuum of changes that can be characterized into several distinct stages. Whether these changes represent a physiologic or pathologic response to illness is unclear; however, there is no evidence that thyroid hormone treatment provides any beneficial effect.

5. Thyroid storm is an acute, life-threatening complication of hyperthyroidism, representing the extreme manifestation of the disease, and usually is precipitated by a concurrent illness. The diagnosis remains a clinical one, with the cardinal features including fever, tachycardia, and mental status changes.

Thyroid hormone levels serve only as confirmatory tests in the appropriate setting. Combined therapy directed at blocking thyroid hormone production and treating the precipitating cause is essential.

6. Myxedema coma represents the extreme expression of severe, long-standing hypothyroidism, and even with early diagnosis and treatment, mortality has been reported to be 60%. Similar to thyroid storm, myxedema coma usually is precipitated by a concurrent illness, and the diagnosis remains a clinical one. Cardinal features include hypothermia, which can be profound, altered mental status, and cardiovascular depression. The mainstays of therapy include ventilatory and hemodynamic support, rewarming, correction of electrolyte disturbances, treatment of the precipitating incident, and administration of thyroid hormone.

Thyroid storm and myxedema coma are life-threatening emergencies that represent the extreme ends of the spectrum of thyroid dysfunction in a decompensated patient. Their presentation usually is dramatic and often is precipitated by a nonthyroid illness or event. Recognition of these disorders requires a high degree of clinical suspicion because the thyroid hormone abnormalities and other biochemical parameters do not differ significantly from uncomplicated thyrotoxicosis and hypothyroidism. Because thyroid storm and myxedema coma are clinical diagnoses, measurement of serum thyroid hormones serves as confirmation in the appropriate setting.

In contrast to these dramatic clinical presentations, critical illness also causes multiple alterations in thyroid hormone concentrations in patients without intrinsic thyroid dysfunction, which are nonspecific and relate to the severity of the illness. Because a wide variety of illnesses tend to result in the same changes in serum thyroid hormones, such alterations in thyroid hormone indices have been termed the *sick euthyroid syndrome*. The differentiation between patients with the sick euthyroid syndrome and patients with intrinsic thyroid disease is a frequent diagnostic problem in the ICU.

This chapter first reviews normal thyroid physiology and discusses the changes in thyroid hormone metabolism seen with critical illness. Evaluation of these patients and the identification of patients with intrinsic thyroid disease are discussed. Finally, diagnosis and management of the sick euthyroid syndrome, thyroid storm, and myxedema coma are reviewed.

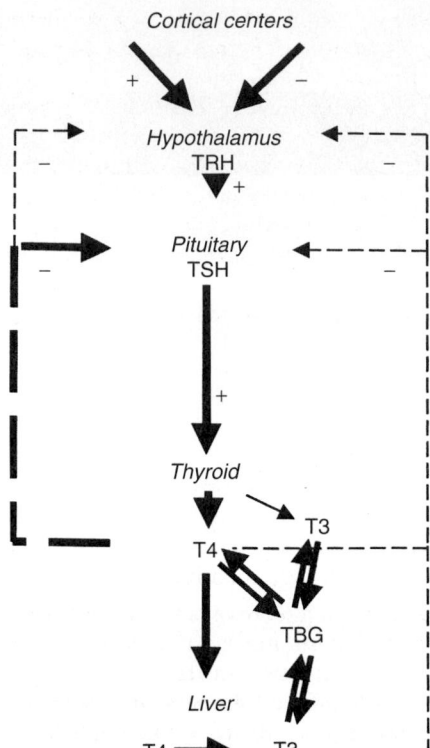

FIGURE 177–1. Diagram of the hypothalamic-pituitary-thyroid axis. The inhibitory effect of thyroxine (T_4) and 3,5,3'-triiodothyronine (T_3) on thyroid-stimulating hormone (TSH) secretion is shown by the dashed line and minus sign, and the stimulatory effects of thyrotropin-releasing hormone (TRH) on TSH secretion and TSH on thyroid secretion are shown by the solid lines and plus signs. T_4 and T_3 also may have an inhibitory effect on TRH secretion. TBG, thyroid-binding globulin.

NORMAL THYROID HORMONE ECONOMY

REGULATION

Synthesis and secretion of thyroid hormone is under the control of the anterior pituitary hormone, thyrotropin, or thyroid-stimulating hormone. Thyroid-stimulating hormone secretion increases when serum thyroid hormone levels decrease and decreases when levels increase, in a classic negative feedback system (Fig. 177-1). Thyroid-stimulating hormone also is under the regulation of the hypothalamic hormone, thyrotropin-releasing hormone. The negative feedback of thyroid hormone is targeted mainly at the pituitary level, but probably affects thyroid-releasing hormone release from the hypothalamus as well. In addition, input from higher cortical centers affects thyroid-releasing hormone secretion. Under the influence of thyroid-stimulating hormone, the thyroid gland synthesizes and releases thyroid hormone. Thyroxine (T_4) is the principal secretory product of the thyroid gland, comprising approximately 90% of the secreted hormone under normal conditions.[1] Although T_4 may have direct actions in some tissues, for the most part T_4 functions as a hormone precursor that is metabolized in peripheral tissues to the transcriptionally active T_3.

METABOLIC PATHWAYS

The major pathway of metabolism of T_4 is by sequential monodeiodination.[2] Removal of the 5'-, or outer ring, iodine by type I iodothyronine 5'-deiodinase is the "activating" metabolic pathway, leading to the formation of T_3. Removal of the inner ring, or 5-, iodine by type III iodothyronine deiodinase is an "inactivating" pathway, producing the metabolically inactive hormone, 3,3',5'-triiodothyronine (reverse T_3). Type I deiodinase is found predominantly in the liver and kidney, whereas type 3 deiodinase has a more widespread distribution. Under normal conditions, approximately 41% of T_4 is converted to T_3; approximately 38% is converted to reverse T_3; and approximately 21% is metabolized via other pathways, such as conjugation in the liver and excretion in the bile.[3,4]

T_3 is the metabolically active thyroid hormone and exerts its actions via binding to chromatin-bound nuclear receptors and regulating gene transcription in responsive tissues.[5] Important in the understanding of the alterations in circulating thyroid hormone levels seen in critical illness is the fact that only approximately 10% of circulating T_3 is secreted directly by the thyroid gland, whereas greater than 80% of T_3 is derived from conversion of T_4 in peripheral tissues.[1,2] Factors that affect peripheral T_4 to T_3 conversion have significant effects on circulating T_3 levels. Serum levels of T_3 are approximately 100-fold less than levels of T_4, and similar to T_4, T_3 is metabolized by deiodination to form diiodothyronine and by conjugation in the liver.

SERUM BINDING PROTEINS

T_4 and T_3 circulate in the serum bound to several proteins that are synthesized in the liver.[6] Thyroxine-binding globulin is the major serum binding protein and binds approximately 80% of the serum thyroid hormones. The affinity of T_4 for thyroxine-binding globulin is approximately 10-fold greater than that of T_3 and is part of the reason that circulating T_4 levels are higher than T_3 levels. Other serum binding proteins include transthyretin, which binds approximately 15% of T_4 but little, if any, T_3, and albumin, which has a low affinity but a large capacity for binding T_4 and T_3. Overall, 99.97% of circulating T_4 and 99.7% of circulating T_3 are bound to plasma proteins.

FREE HORMONE CONCEPT

Essential to the understanding of the regulation of thyroid function and the alterations of circulating thyroid hormones seen in critical illness is the "free hormone" concept: Only the unbound hormone has any metabolic activity. Because of the high degree of binding of T_4 and T_3 to the serum binding proteins, changes in either the concentrations of these proteins or the binding affinity of thyroid hormone to the serum binding proteins would have major effects on the total serum hormone levels. Because the pituitary responds to and regulates the circulating free hormone levels, however, minimal changes in the free hormone concentrations and overall thyroid function would be seen.

THYROID HORMONE ECONOMY IN CRITICAL ILLNESS

The widespread changes in thyroid hormone economy in a critically ill patient occur as a result of (1) alterations in the peripheral metabolism of the thyroid hormones, (2) alterations in thyroid-stimulating hormone regulation, and (3) alterations in the binding of thyroid hormone to thyroid-binding globulin.

TABLE 177–1. FACTORS THAT INHIBIT TYPE I 5′-DEIODINASE ACTIVITY

Acute and chronic illness
Caloric deprivation
Malnutrition
Glucocorticoids
Beta-adrenergic blocking drugs (e.g., propranolol)
Oral cholecystography agents (e.g., iopanoic acid, sodium iopodate)
Amiodarone
Propylthiouracil
Fatty acids
Fetal/neonatal period
Selenium deficiency

PERIPHERAL METABOLIC PATHWAYS

One of the initial alterations in thyroid hormone metabolism in acute illness is the acute inhibition of type I deiodinase, resulting in impairment in T_4 to T_3 conversion in peripheral tissues. Type I deiodinase is inhibited by a wide variety of factors (Table 177-1),[2] resulting in a marked decrease in T_3 production. T_3 levels decrease quickly after the onset of acute illness. In contrast, inner ring deiodination of T_4 to produce reverse T_3 is unaffected by acute illness. Because reverse T_3 subsequently is deiodinated by type I deiodinase, however, degradation of reverse T_3 decreases, and levels of this inactive hormone increase in proportion to the decrease in T_3 levels.

THYROID-STIMULATING HORMONE REGULATION

Serum thyroid-stimulating hormone levels are usually normal early in acute illness.[7,8] Thyroid-stimulating hormone levels often decrease, however, as the illness progresses as a result of the effects of a variety of inhibitory factors that are common in the treatment of critically ill patients (Table 177-2). Most common is the use of dopamine[9] and the increased levels of glucocorticoids, either endogenous or exogenous, which have a direct inhibitory effect on thyroid-stimulating hormone secretion. Pressor doses of dopamine may decrease thyroid-stimulating hormone levels to normal in patients with preexisting primary hypothyroidism.[10] Pulsatile thyroid-stimulating hormone secretion may be altered,[11] and the nocturnal thyroid-stimulating hormone surge often is decreased and may be absent in patients with nonthyroidal illness.[11,12] Decreased thyroid-releasing hormone secretion due to inhibitory signals from higher cortical centers and impaired thyroid-releasing hormone metabolism also may play a role in decreasing thyroid-stimulating hormone secretion.[13] Finally, certain thyroid hormone metabolites that are increased in nonthyroidal illness may play a role in the inhibition of thyroid-stimulating hormone and thyroid-releasing hormone secretion.[14]

SERUM BINDING PROTEINS

The binding of thyroid hormones to serum proteins also is altered with acute illness (Table 177-3). Serum levels of transthyretin decrease rapidly after the onset of acute illness.[15] Serum albumin levels decrease, especially during prolonged illness, in malnutrition, and in high catabolic states. Thyroxine-binding globulin levels may be increased, as seen with liver dysfunction[6] and human immunodeficiency virus infection,[16] or decreased, as seen with severe or prolonged illness.[17] Thyroxine-binding globulin also may be degraded rapidly by protease cleavage during cardiac bypass, providing some insight into the rapid decrease in serum T_3 levels in patients undergoing cardiac surgery.[18] An acquired binding defect of T_4 to thyroxine-binding globulin is seen commonly in patients with critical illness[17] and is believed to result from the release of some as yet unidentified factor from injured tissues that has the characteristics of unsaturated nonesterified fatty acids[19] and inhibits T_4 to T_3 conversion.[20] In systemically ill patients, nonesterified fatty acid levels increase in parallel with the severity of the illness,[21] and drugs such as heparin stimulate the generation of nonesterified fatty acids.[22] Many drugs, including high-dose furosemide,[23] antiseizure medications,[24] and salicylates,[24] also alter binding of T_4 to thyroid-binding globulin. These alterations in serum binding proteins in critical illness make the estimation of free hormone concentrations difficult (see later).

TABLE 177–2. FACTORS THAT DECREASE THYROID-STIMULATING HORMONE SECRETION

Acute and chronic illness
Adrenergic agonists
Bexerotene
Caloric restriction
Carbamazepine
Clofibrate
Cyproheptadine
Dopamine and dopamine agonists
Endogenous depression
Glucocorticoids
Insulin growth factor type 1
Metergoline
Methysergide
Opiates
Phenytoin
Phentolamine
Pimozide
Somatostatin
Serotonin
Surgical stress
Thyroid hormone metabolites

TABLE 177–3. FACTORS THAT ALTER BINDING OF THYROXINE TO THYROXINE-BINDING GLOBULIN

Increase binding	Decrease binding
Drugs	
Estrogens	Glucocorticoids
Methadone	Androgens
Clofibrate	Asparaginase
5-Fluorouracil	Salicylates
Heroin	Mefenamic acid
Tamoxifen	Antiseizure medications (phenytoin, carbamazepine)
Raloxifene	Furosemide
Capecitabine	Heparin
Systemic factors	
Liver disease	Inherited
Porphyria	Acute illness
HIV infection	Nonesterified free fatty acids
Inherited	

HIV, human immunodeficiency virus.

EVALUATION OF THYROID FUNCTION IN A CRITICALLY ILL PATIENT

DIAGNOSTIC TESTS

Thyroid-Stimulating Hormone Assays

Abnormal thyroid-stimulating hormone values have been reported in 20% of acutely ill patients, with greater than 80% of these patients having no intrinsic thyroid dysfunction on follow-up testing when healthy.[4,25,26] In a study of 1580 hospitalized patients, only 24% of patients with suppressed thyroid-stimulating hormone values (thyroid-stimulating hormone less than assay limit of detection) and 50% of patients with thyroid-stimulating hormone values greater than 20 mU/L were found to have thyroid disease.[4,25] None of the patients with subnormal but detectable thyroid-stimulating hormone values and only 14% of patients with elevated thyroid-stimulating hormone values less than 20 mU/L subsequently were diagnosed with intrinsic thyroid dysfunction. Although a normal thyroid-stimulating hormone level has a high predictive value of normal thyroid function, an abnormal thyroid-stimulating hormone value alone is not helpful in the evaluation of thyroid function in a critically ill patient.

Serum Thyroxine and Triiodothyronine Concentrations

Measurement of free thyroid hormone concentrations in a patient with nonthyroidal illness is fraught with difficulty.[27] The gold standard is determination of free hormone levels by equilibrium dialysis. This technique is labor intensive and time-consuming, however, and is rarely used. The most commonly available laboratory tests of thyroid hormone concentrations, the free T_4 index and free T_4 and free T_3 measured by analog methods, represent estimates of the free hormone concentration and are subject to inaccuracies.[28,29]

The free T_4 index is determined by multiplying the total T_4 concentration by the T_3-resin uptake or T_4-resin uptake, which is an inverse estimate of serum thyroid-binding globulin concentrations.[29] Measurement of free T_4 levels by the analog method, which seems to be supplanting the free T_4 index owing to a lower cost, is likely no more accurate than the free T_4 index.[30] In a healthy population, there is a close correlation between the free T_4 index and free T_4 levels. In a critically ill patient, this correlation breaks down, mainly because of difficulties in estimating thyroid-binding globulin binding with the resin uptake tests. Despite this breakdown, the sensitivity of the free T_4 index in a large study of hospitalized patients was 92.3% compared with 90.7% for the sensitive thyroid-stimulating hormone test.[25]

Serum T_3 concentrations are affected to the greatest degree by the alterations in thyroid hormone economy resulting from acute illness. There is no indication for the routine measurement of serum T_3 levels in the initial evaluation of thyroid function in a critically ill patient. This test should be obtained only if thyrotoxicosis is suspected clinically in the presence of a suppressed sensitive thyroid-stimulating hormone value and an elevated or high normal free T_4 index or free T_4 determination. At this time, the total T_3 assay is preferable to the free T_3 (analog) assay, owing to the variability between laboratories with the latter test.[29]

Autoantibodies

Autoantibodies to thyroglobulin and thyroid peroxidase, two intrinsic thyroid proteins, are commonly available.[29] Although significant titers of either or both of these antibodies indicate the presence of autoimmune thyroid disease, the presence of thyroid autoantibodies alone does not indicate thyroid dysfunction. Thyroid autoantibodies add to the sensitivity of abnormal thyroid-stimulating hormone and free T_4 index values in diagnosing intrinsic thyroid disease.[4,25]

Imaging Studies

Imaging studies are rarely essential to the diagnosis of thyroid disorders in a critically ill patient. Occasionally, functional analysis of the thyroid gland using the radioisotope iodine-123 may be useful in a patient with suspected thyrotoxicosis and equivocal laboratory tests. These studies are labor intensive, however, and management of the underlying acute illness often overshadows the benefits of obtaining these studies. Although anatomic studies, such as ultrasound, isotopic imaging, computed tomography, and magnetic resonance imaging, are useful in the evaluation of thyroid nodules and goiter, these conditions rarely are the cause of acute illness; as such, these studies usually are not helpful in a critically ill patient.

DIAGNOSIS

The routine screening of ICU patients for the presence of thyroid dysfunction is not recommended because of the high prevalence of abnormal thyroid function tests and low prevalence of true thyroid dysfunction. When thyroid function tests are ordered in a hospitalized patient, it should be with a high clinical index of suspicion for the presence of thyroid dysfunction. Whenever possible, it is best to defer evaluation of the thyroid-pituitary axis until the patient has recovered from his or her acute illness. Because every test of thyroid hormone function can be altered in a critically ill patient, no single test definitively can rule in or rule out the presence of intrinsic thyroid dysfunction.

A reasonable approach to the initial evaluation of thyroid function in a critically ill patient is to obtain either free T_4 index or free T_4 and thyroid-stimulating hormone measurements in patients with a high clinical suspicion for intrinsic thyroid dysfunction. Assessment of these values in the context of the duration, severity, and stage of illness of the patient allows the correct diagnosis in most patients. A mildly elevated thyroid-stimulating hormone coupled with a low free T_4 index or free T_4 is more likely to indicate primary hypothyroidism early in an acute illness as opposed to the same values obtained during the recovery phase of the illness. Similarly the combination of an elevated thyroid-stimulating hormone and low normal free T_4 index or free T_4 is more likely to indicate thyroid dysfunction in a hypothermic, bradycardic patient than in a tachycardic, normothermic patient. If the free T_4 index or free T_4 and thyroid-stimulating hormone are normal, thyroid dysfunction is effectively eliminated as a significant contributing factor to the clinical picture. If the diagnosis is still unclear, measurement of thyroid antibodies is helpful as a marker of intrinsic thyroid disease and increases the sensitivity of the free T_4 index or free T_4 and the thyroid-stimulating hormone. Measurement of serum T_3 levels is indicated only in the case of a suppressed thyroid-stimulating hormone and a mid to high normal free T_4 index or free T_4.

SICK EUTHYROID SYNDROME

As discussed earlier, critical illness causes multiple alterations in thyroid hormone concentrations in patients without

FIGURE 177–2. Alterations in thyroid hormone concentrations with critical illness. Schematic representation of the continuum of changes in serum thyroid hormone concentrations in patients with nonthyroidal illness. These alterations become more pronounced with increasing severity of the illness and return to the normal range as the illness subsides and the patient recovers. A rapidly increasing mortality accompanies the decrease in total and free thyroxine (T$_4$) concentrations. rT$_3$, reverse triiodothyronine (3,3′,5′-triiodothyronine; T$_3$, 3,5,3′-triiodothyronine; TSH, thyroid-stimulating hormone. (From Farwell AF: Sick euthyroid syndrome in the intensive care unit. In Irwin RS, Rippe JM [eds]: Intensive Care Medicine, 5th ed. Philadelphia, Lippincott Williams & Wilkins, 2003.)

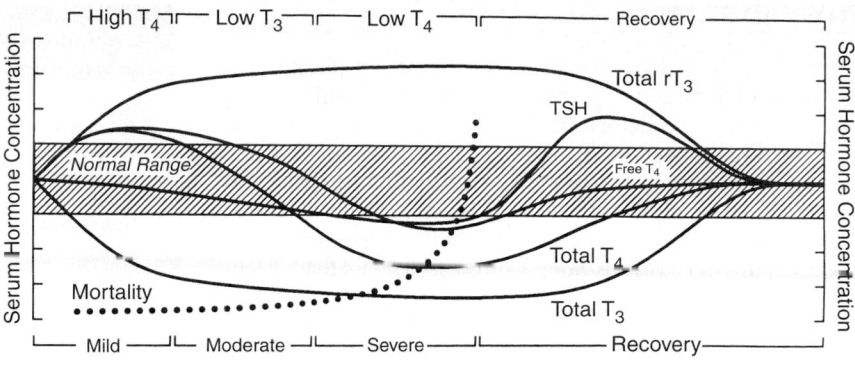

intrinsic thyroid dysfunction that are nonspecific and relate to the severity of the illness.[31-34] These alterations in thyroid hormone parameters represent a continuum of changes that depends on the severity of the illness and that can be categorized into several distinct stages (Fig. 177-2).[31,32] The wide spectrum of changes observed often results from the differing points at which the thyroid function tests were obtained during the course of the illness. These changes are rarely isolated and often are associated with alterations in other endocrine systems, such as reductions in serum gonadotropin and sex hormone concentrations[35] and increases in serum adrenocorticotropic hormone and cortisol levels.[36] The sick euthyroid syndrome should not be viewed as an isolated pathologic event, but as part of a coordinated systemic reaction to illness that involves the immune and the endocrine systems.

LOW TRIIODOTHYRONINE STATE

Common to all of the abnormalities in thyroid hormone concentrations seen in critically ill patients is a substantial depression of serum T$_3$ levels, which can occur 24 hours after the onset of illness.[8] More than half of patients admitted to the medical service show depressed serum T$_3$ concentrations.[4,25] The development of the low T$_3$ state can be explained solely by the impairment of peripheral T$_4$ to T$_3$ conversion through the inhibition of type I deiodinase (discussed earlier), which results in a marked reduction in T$_3$ production and reverse T$_3$ degradation and leads to reciprocal changes in serum T$_3$ and serum reverse T$_3$ concentrations.

HIGH THYROXINE STATE

Serum T$_4$ levels may be elevated early in acute illness due to either the acute inhibition of type I deiodinase or increased thyroid-binding globulin levels. This elevation is seen most often in elderly patients and in patients with psychiatric disorders. As the duration of illness increases, nondeiodinative pathways of T$_4$ degradation increase and return serum T$_4$ levels to the normal range.[4]

LOW THYROXINE STATE

As the severity and duration of the illness increase, serum total T$_4$ levels decrease into the subnormal range. Contributing to this decrease in serum T$_4$ levels are (1) a decrease in the binding of T$_4$ to serum carrier proteins, (2) a decrease in

serum thyroid-stimulating hormone levels leading to decreased thyroidal production of T$_4$, and (3) an increase in nondeiodinative pathways of T$_4$ metabolism. The decline in serum T$_4$ levels correlates with prognosis in the ICU, with mortality increasing as serum T$_4$ levels decline to less than 4 µg/dL and approaching 80% in patients with serum T$_4$ levels less than 2 µg/dL.[8,37,38] Despite marked decreases in serum total T$_4$ and T$_3$ levels in a critically ill patient, free hormone levels have been reported to be normal or even elevated,[27,28] providing a possible explanation for why most patients appear eumetabolic despite thyroid hormone levels in the hypothyroid range. The low T$_4$ state is unlikely to be a result of a hormone-deficient state and is probably more of a marker of multisystem failure in these critically ill patients.

RECOVERY STATE

As acute illness resolves, so do the alterations in thyroid hormone concentrations. This stage may be prolonged and is characterized by modest increases in serum thyroid-stimulating hormone levels.[39] Full recovery, with restoration of thyroid hormone levels to the normal range, may take several months after the patient is discharged from the hospital.[25]

TREATMENT OF SICK EUTHYROID SYNDROME

The question of whether the sick euthyroid syndrome in critically ill patients represents an adaptive or a pathologic response to illness is unclear. If therapy is considered, T$_3$ would be the logical choice, given the impairment of T$_4$ to T$_3$ conversion in an acutely ill patient (see earlier). Support for liothyronine therapy has come from animal studies related to cardiac surgery. The administration of T$_3$ to dogs undergoing cardiac bypass improved the postoperative clinical course.[40] Several prospective randomized clinical trials failed to show a similar benefit in humans undergoing cardiac surgery.[41-43] Liothyronine also has been used in organ donors to improve cardiac graft function in the recipients, and a minor benefit is suggested in this limited situation.[44,45] The available prospective randomized clinical studies to date in the general medical patient with the sick euthyroid syndrome fail to show, however, that supplemental thyroid hormone therapy, in the form of levothyroxine or liothyronine, provides any beneficial effect on outcome, and it is not indicated in a routine patient.[46-48]

THYROID STORM

Thyroid storm is an acute, life-threatening complication of hyperthyroidism and represents the extreme manifestation of the disease.[49-52] Historically, thyroid storm frequently was associated with surgery for hyperthyroidism and approached an incidence of 10% in some series, depending on the diagnostic criteria employed.[53,54] Currently, because of better recognition of the disease and improved perioperative management, thyroid storm is rare, accounting for less than 2% of all hospital admissions related to thyrotoxicosis.[50,52] Most often, thyroid storm is precipitated by an intercurrent medical problem in untreated or partially treated hyperthyroid patients.[49-52] The diagnosis of thyroid storm is a clinical one because there are no distinctive laboratory features, and thyroid hormone concentrations are similar to what is observed in uncomplicated thyrotoxicosis. Although the cause of the rapid clinical decompensation is unknown, a sudden inhibition of thyroid hormone binding to plasma proteins by the precipitating factor, causing an increase in free hormone concentrations in the already elevated free hormone pool, may play a role in the pathogenesis of thyroid storm.[55]

CLINICAL MANIFESTATIONS

Thyroid storm is primarily a clinical diagnosis; as such, the varying incidence of this disorder in patient series likely results from how strictly the diagnostic criteria are employed. Clinical features are similar to features of thyrotoxicosis, but more exaggerated (Table 177-4). Cardinal features of thyroid storm include fever (temperature usually >38.5°C), tachycardia out of proportion to the fever, and mental status changes. Tachyarrhythmias, especially atrial fibrillation in the elderly, are common. Nausea, vomiting, diarrhea, agitation, and delirium are frequent presentations. Vascular collapse and shock, owing to dehydration and cardiac decompensation, are poor prognostic signs, as is the presence of jaundice. Coma and death may ensue in 20% of patients, frequently secondary to cardiac arrhythmias, congestive heart failure, hyperthermia, or the precipitating illness.

Most patients display the classic signs of Graves' disease, the most common cause of thyrotoxicosis, including ophthalmopathy and a diffusely enlarged goiter.[56] Thyroid storm also has been associated with toxic nodular goiters. In the elderly, severe myopathy, profound weight loss, apathy, and a minimally enlarged goiter may be observed.[57]

TABLE 177-4. CLINICAL FEATURES OF THYROID STORM

Fever (>38.5°C [>105.8°F])
Tachycardia/tachyarrhythmias
Mental status changes
Delirium/agitation
Congestive heart failure
Tremor
Nausea and vomiting
Diarrhea
Sweating
Vasodilation
Dehydration
Hepatomegaly
Splenomegaly
Jaundice

TABLE 177-5. PRECIPITATING FACTORS FOR THYROID STORM

Surgery
  Thyroidal
  Nonthyroidal
Infections
  Pneumonia
  Upper respiratory
  Enteric
  Other
Stress
Trauma
Diabetic ketoacidosis
Labor
Cardiac disease
Iodinated intravenous contrast agents
Radioactive iodine therapy

PRECIPITATING FACTORS

In the past, thyroid storm frequently was associated with surgery for hyperthyroidism (Table 177-5), with symptoms beginning a few hours after thyroidectomy in patients prepared for surgery with potassium iodide alone. Most of these cases occurred in patients who were not appropriately prepared for surgery by current standards. Because of better recognition of the disease, preoperative treatment with thionamides to deplete the gland of thyroid hormone before surgery, and improved perioperative management with beta blockade, thyroid storm now is rarely a postoperative complication of thyroid surgery.

Currently, thyroid storm appears most commonly after infection, causing the thyrotoxic state to decompensate.[50,51] Pneumonia, upper respiratory tract infections, and enteric infections are common precipitating infections. Other precipitating factors include stress, trauma, nonthyroidal surgery, diabetic ketoacidosis, labor, heart disease, and iodinated contrast studies in an unrecognized or partially treated hyperthyroid patient.[58-62] Iatrogenic thyroid storm has been reported secondary to thyroid hormone overdose.[63] Thyroid storm occurring after iodine-131 therapy is extremely rare,[64,65] especially considering the frequency of the use of radioactive iodine in the definitive treatment of hyperthyroidism. When reported, radioactive iodine–induced thyroid storm usually occurred if there was no pretreatment with antithyroid drugs.[64]

DIAGNOSIS

As mentioned earlier, the diagnosis of thyroid storm is a clinical one. Burch and Wartofsky[49] developed a modified APACHE (Acute Physiology, Age, and Chronic Health Evaluation) score, with criteria including temperature, central nervous system effects, gastrointestinal effects, cardiovascular effects, and precipitant history, to assist in the diagnosis. There are no distinct laboratory abnormalities outside of elevated thyroid hormone concentrations, which are similar to abnormalities found in uncomplicated thyrotoxicosis. Serum T_3 concentrations often are elevated to a greater degree than serum T_4 concentrations owing to the preferential secretion of T_3 in the hyperthyroid gland.[52] There is little correlation between the degree of elevation of thyroid hormones and the presentation of thyroid storm. Serum thyroid-stimulating hormone concentrations are typically undetectable; however, because of the influence of nonthyroidal illness on thyroid-stimulating hormone secretion (see earlier), a low thyroid-stimulating hormone concentration by itself is insufficient to make a diagnosis of thyroid storm. Serum T_4 and T_3 concentrations in the normal range, regardless of the thyroid-stimulating hormone concentration, effectively eliminate thyroid storm as a tenable diagnosis.

Abnormal liver function tests are common. Hypocalcemia may be observed due to increased osteoclast-mediated bone resorption in a hyperthyroid patient. Hematocrit concentrations may be elevated due to volume contraction, and leukocytosis is common, even in the absence of infection.

The differential diagnosis of thyroid storm includes sepsis, neuroleptic malignant syndrome, malignant hyperthermia, and acute mania with lethal catatonia, all of which can precipitate thyroid storm in the appropriate setting. Clues to the diagnosis of thyroid storm are a history of thyroid disease, history of iodine ingestion, and presence of a goiter or stigmata of Graves' disease. The physician must have a high clinical index of suspicion for thyroid storm because therapy must be instituted before the return of thyroid function tests in most cases.

TREATMENT

Thyroid storm is a major medical emergency that must be treated in an ICU.[49-52] Therapy can divided into two major categories (Table 177-6):

1. *Thyroid-directed*—treatment aimed at decreasing thyroid hormone production, conversion, and secretion and at blocking the peripheral manifestations of thyroid hormone
2. *Supportive*—treatment aimed at controlling the fever, stabilizing the cardiovascular system, and managing the precipitating cause

Thyroid-Directed Treatment

Prompt inhibition of thyroid hormone synthesis and secretion is essential. Antithyroid drugs are given in large doses to inhibit synthesis of the thyroid hormones and to block the uptake of iodine. Propylthiouracil is preferred over methimazole because of its additional advantage of inhibiting type I deiodinase and impairing peripheral conversion of T_4 to T_3.[2] Because other, more powerful inhibitors of type I deiodinase are usually part of the therapeutic regimen in thyroid storm, however, the main beneficial effects of propylthiouracil are on inhibition of iodide uptake and hormone synthesis. Propylthiouracil and methimazole can be administered by nasogastric tube or rectally if necessary.[66,67] These preparations are not available for parenteral administration.

Iodides, the most effective drugs to block release of thyroid hormone from the thyroid gland, should be used only after antithyroid drugs have been administered. Monotherapy with iodides increases the synthesis of new thyroid hormones and markedly worsens the hyperthyroidism when the gland escapes from the initial iodide-induced blockade of hormone secretion (Wolf-Chaikoff effect).[68] The iodide preparation of choice is the radiographic contrast dye iopanoic acid (Telepaque) owing to its high iodine content (0.6 mg/g of iodine per dose) and the ability for the drug to inhibit type I deiodinase directly and block T_4 to T_3 conversion.[2] If iopanoic

acid is unavailable, Lugol solution or saturated solution of potassium iodide (SSKI) is an alternative source of therapeutic iodides. Use of iodides precludes the use of radioactive iodine as a definitive therapy for hyperthyroidism for several months. Lithium also has been reported to be effective in inhibiting thyroid hormone release to a similar degree as iodides.[69]

High-dose dexamethasone is recommended as supportive therapy as an inhibitor of T_4 to T_3 conversion and as management of possible coexistent adrenal insufficiency. Beta-adrenergic blockers, specifically propranolol, also are weak inhibitors of T_4 to T_3 conversion, although their main beneficial effect is on heart rate control.[70] Orally administered ion-exchange resin (colestipol or cholestyramine) can trap hormone in the intestine and prevent recirculation.[71,72] Plasmapheresis, peritoneal dialysis, and charcoal hemoperfusion also have been used in severe cases.[73]

TABLE 177–6. TREATMENT OF THYROID STORM

Thyroid-directed Therapy

Direct
Inhibition of thyroid hormone synthesis
  Propylthiouracil—800 mg orally/per rectum first dose, then 200-300 mg orally/per rectum q8h, *or*
  Methimazole—80 mg orally/per rectum first dose, then 40-80 mg orally/per rectum q12h
Block release of thyroid hormones from the gland
  Telapaque (iopanoic acid)—1 g orally qd, *or*
  SSKI—5 drops orally q8h, *or*
  Lugol solution—10 drops orally q8h, *or*
  Lithium—800-1200 mg orally qd; achieve serum lithium levels 0.5-1.5 mEq/L

Adjunctive
Block T_4 to T_3 conversion
  Iopanoic acid
  Corticosteroids (e.g., dexamethasone)—1-2 mg orally/i.v. q6h
  Propylthiouracil
  Most beta blockers (e.g., propranolol)—40-80 mg orally q6h
Remove thyroid hormones from the circulation
  Cholestyramine—4 g orally q6h, *or*
  Colestipol—20-30 mg orally qd, *or*
  Plasmapheresis, *or*
  Peritoneal dialysis

Supportive Therapy

Hyperthermia
Intravenous fluids
Antipyretics
Cooling blanket

Hemodynamic
Beta-adrenergic blocking drugs
  Propranolol—1 mg/min i.v. to a total dose of 10 mg, then 40-80 mg orally q6h, *or*
  Esmolol—500 mg/kg/min i.v., then 50-100 mg/kg/min, *or*
  Metoprolol—100-400 mg orally q12h, *or*
  Atenolol—50-100 mg orally daily
Other
  Vasopressors
  Digoxin

Etiology
Treatment of underlying illness(es)

Other
Anxiolytics (when mental status clears)

T_3, 3,5,3'-triiodothyronine; T_4, thyroxine.

Supportive Treatment

Simultaneously with antithyroid-directed therapy, treatment aimed at cooling the patient to a reasonable temperature and providing hemodynamic support should be instituted. Intravenous fluids, antipyretics, and cooling blankets all are effective. Beta-adrenergic blockers, such as propranolol (orally or intravenously) and esmolol (intravenously), are given for heart rate control. Calcium channel blockers also may be used to control tachyarrhythmias. Anxiolytics frequently are helpful when the patient's mental status improves. Finally, treatment of the underlying precipitating illness is essential to survival in thyroid storm.

LONG-TERM THERAPY

When the acute phase of thyroid storm is controlled, antithyroid drug therapy should be continued until euthyroidism is achieved, and the adjunctive therapy can be discontinued. Definitive therapeutic options for hyperthyroidism include radioactive iodine (after a few months to allow excretion of the excess iodides used during the acute management of thyroid storm) and surgery.[74,75] Long-term (1 to 2 years) treatment with antithyroid drugs in the hopes of achieving a remission is an option for patients with Graves' disease.[76]

MYXEDEMA COMA

Myxedema coma is a rare syndrome that represents the extreme expression of severe, long-standing hypothyroidism.[43,51,52,77-79] It is a medical emergency, and even with early diagnosis and treatment, mortality can be 60%.[79,80] The name *myxedema coma* is a misnomer because actual coma is rare.[77] The syndrome includes decompensated hypothyroidism, central nervous system impairment, and cardiovascular compromise. Myxedema coma occurs most often in the elderly and during the winter months; in one series, 9 of 11 patients with myxedema coma were admitted in late fall or winter.[79] As with thyroid storm, myxedema coma usually is caused by a precipitating event in an untreated, or partially treated, hypothyroid patient.

CLINICAL MANIFESTATIONS

The cardinal features of myxedema coma are (1) hypothermia, which can be profound; (2) altered mental status; (3) cardiovascular depression; and (4) a precipitating cause (Table 177-7). A severely hypothyroid patient becomes essentially poikilothermic because of disordered thermoregulation. This is the reason many cases occur in the winter

months. Body temperatures of 23.3°C have been reported; rectal temperatures are essential in making the diagnosis. Excessive lethargy and sleepiness may have been present for weeks to months, often interfering with meals. Rarely, psychosis and delirium have been reported. Bradycardia and hypotension may be profound, and the respiratory rate often is depressed. Because hypothyroidism by itself is insufficient to produce the clinical syndrome of myxedema coma, a precipitating cause must be assumed to be present.[77]

In addition to the aforementioned features, most patients have the physical features of severe hypothyroidism,[81,82] including macroglossia; delayed reflexes; dry, rough skin; and myxedematous facies, which results from periorbital edema, pallor, hypercarotenemia, periorbital edema, and patchy hair loss. Hypotonia of the gastrointestinal tract is common and often so severe as to suggest an obstructive lesion. Urinary retention due to a hypotonic bladder is related but less frequent. Pleural, pericardial, and peritoneal effusions may be present.

PRECIPITATING FACTORS

As mentioned earlier, cold stress is a common precipitant to myxedema coma (Table 177-8). Other common precipitating factors include pulmonary and urinary tract infections, cerebrovascular accidents, trauma, surgery, congestive heart failure, and intravascular volume loss from acute or chronic gastrointestinal bleeding or the overuse of diuretics.[51,52,77] The clinical course of lethargy proceeding to stupor and coma often is hastened by drugs, especially sedatives, narcotics, antidepressants, and tranquilizers. Many cases of myxedema coma have occurred in an undiagnosed hypothyroid patient who has been hospitalized for other medical problems.

DIAGNOSIS

Similar to the diagnosis of thyroid storm, myxedema coma is a clinical diagnosis. Although rare, the diagnosis of myxedema coma should be considered in any hypothermic, obtunded patient. Because the patient is obtunded, a prior history of hypothyroidism often must be obtained from other sources.

TABLE 177-7. CLINICAL FEATURES OF MYXEDEMA COMA

Mental obtundation
Hypothermia
Bradycardia
Hypotension
Coarse, dry skin
Myxedema facies
Hypoglycemia
Atonic gastrointestinal tract
Atonic bladder
Pleural, pericardial, and peritoneal effusions

TABLE 177-8. PRECIPITATING FACTORS FOR MYXEDEMA COMA

Cold stress
Infection
   Pneumonia
   Urinary tract
   Other
Stroke
Congestive heart failure
Trauma
Burns
Surgery
Intravascular volume contraction
   Gastrointestinal blood loss
   Diuretic use
CNS drugs
   Analgesics/narcotics
   Sedatives/hypnotics
   Tranquilizers
   Anesthetic agents

CNS, central nervous system.

Friends, relatives, and acquaintances might have noted increasing lethargy, complaints of cold intolerance, and changes in the voice. Clues to the diagnosis include an outdated container of levothyroxine discovered with the patient's belongings, which suggests that the patient has been remiss in taking medication. The medical record also may indicate that the patient was supposed to be taking thyroid hormone or refer to previous treatment with radioactive iodine, or there may be a thyroidectomy scar present.

Because greater than 95% of cases of myxedema coma are due to primary hypothyroidism,[51,52,77-79] the laboratory findings include an elevated serum thyroid-stimulating hormone and low or undetectable total and free serum T_4 concentrations. These thyroid hormone abnormalities are similar to the abnormalities in uncomplicated overt hypothyroidism. In a patient with central hypothyroidism, the diagnosis of myxedema coma may be difficult because serum thyroid-stimulating hormone concentrations are normal or low. Other symptoms of pituitary dysfunction usually are present in these rare patients, however.

Dilutional hyponatremia is common and may be severe. Elevated creatine kinase concentrations, sometimes markedly so, are encountered frequently and may misdirect the clinical picture toward cardiac ischemia.[83,84] In most cases, the MB fraction is normal, however, and an electrocardiogram often shows the low voltage and loss of T waves that is characteristic of severe hypothyroidism. Elevated lactate dehydrogenase concentrations, acidosis, and anemia are common findings. Lumbar puncture reveals increased opening pressure and high protein content.

Few of the signs and symptoms discussed previously are unique to myxedema coma. Protein-calorie malnutrition, sepsis, hypoglycemia, exposure to certain drugs and toxins, and cold exposure can cause severe hypothermia. Hypotension and hypoventilation, other cardinal features of myxedema coma, occur in other disease states. Low thyroid hormone concentrations may be seen in a critically ill patient with nonthyroidal illness (see earlier). As with thyroid storm, the physician must have a high clinical index of suspicion for myxedema coma because therapy must be instituted before the return of thyroid function tests in most cases.

TREATMENT

Treatment of myxedema coma is a medical emergency and should be managed in an ICU. The mainstays of therapy are (1) supportive care, with ventilatory and hemodynamic support, rewarming, correction of hyponatremia and hypoglycemia, and treatment of the precipitating incident, and (2) administration of thyroid hormone (Table 177-9).[51,52,77] Sedatives, hypnotics, narcotics, and anesthetics must be minimized or avoided altogether because of their extended duration of action and exacerbation of obtundation in a hypothyroid patient. Hypothermia is one of the hallmarks of myxedema coma, and its severity may be underestimated if the thermometer does not register less than 30°C. At core temperatures less than 28°C, ventricular fibrillation is a major threat to life. Despite its gravity, the management of the hypothermia of myxedema coma differs from the treatment of exposure-induced hypothermia in euthyroid subjects. In myxedema coma, the patient should be kept in a warm room and covered with blankets. Active heating should be avoided because it increases oxygen consumption and promotes peripheral vasodilation and circulatory collapse.

TABLE 177–9. TREATMENT OF MYXEDEMA COMA
Supportive
Assisted ventilation
Hemodynamic support
Passive rewarming for hypothermia
Intravenous glucose for hypoglycemia
Water restriction or hypertonic saline for severe hyponatremia
Intravenous hydrocortisone (100 mg q8h)*
Treatment of precipitating factor(s)
Avoidance of all CNS-acting medications
Thyroid Hormone Replacement
Levothyroxine—200-300 μg loading dose i.v., up to 500 μg i.v. in the first 24 h* *and/or*
Liothyronine—12.5 μg i.v. q6h

Active heating is recommended only for situations of severe hypothermia in which ventricular fibrillation is an immediate threat. In these cases, the rate of rewarming should not exceed 0.5°C per hour, and the core temperature should be raised to approximately 31°C.[51,52,77]

Because of a 5% to 10% incidence of coexisting adrenal insufficiency in patients with myxedema coma, intravenous steroids (i.e., hydrocortisone, 100 mg intravenously every 8 hours) are indicated before initiating T_4 therapy. Parenteral administration of thyroid hormone is necessary because of uncertain absorption through the gut.[85,86] A reasonable approach is an initial intravenous loading dose of 200 to 300 μg of levothyroxine. If there is inadequate improvement in the state of consciousness, blood pressure, or core temperature during the first 6 to 12 hours after administration, another dose of levothyroxine should be given to bring the total dose during the first 24 hours to 0.5 mg. This dose should be followed by 50 to 100 μg intravenously every 24 hours until the patient is stabilized. Alternatively, in the most severe cases, some clinicians recommend using liothyronine, 12.5 to 25 μg intravenously every 6 hours, until the patient is stable and conscious. Caution must be used to avoid overstimulation of the cardiovascular system. When the patient is stable, the patient should be switched to levothyroxine. The dose of thyroid hormone should be adjusted on the basis of hemodynamic stability, the presence of coexisting cardiac disease, and the degree of electrolyte imbalance.

Although myxedema coma is associated with a high mortality,[79,87] survival can be maximized by correcting the secondary metabolic disturbances and reversing the hypothyroid state in a sustained but gradual fashion. An effort to correct hypothyroidism too rapidly may completely negate the beneficial effects of the initial treatment.

LONG-TERM THERAPY

When the patient with myxedema coma is clinically stable, thyroid hormone replacement can be switched to oral levothyroxine. The dose of levothyroxine should be adjusted over the ensuing weeks and months to achieve serum T_4 and thyroid-stimulating hormone concentrations in the normal range.

SUMMARY

Thyroid storm and myxedema coma are medical emergencies, diagnosed by their clinical presentation, with serum thyroid hormone concentrations serving as confirmatory tests. The interpretation of thyroid function tests in the ICU patient outside of these dramatic presentations often is fraught with difficulty. The identification of patients with intrinsic thyroid dysfunction must take into consideration the clinical assessment of the patient and the duration and severity of the illness. Whenever possible, it is best to defer the evaluation of thyroid function until the patient has recovered from the critical illness.

ANNOTATED REFERENCES

Burman KD, Wartofsky L: Thyroid function in the intensive care setting. Crit Care Clin 2001;17:43-57.

This article is a more recent in-depth review on the changes in thyroid hormone parameters that occur in critically ill patients.

Chopra IJ: Simultaneous measurement of free thyroxine and free 3,5,3'-triiodothyronine in undiluted serum by direct equilibrium dialysis/ radioimmunoassay: Evidence that free triiodothyronine and free thyroxine are normal in many patients with the low triiodothyronine syndrome. Thyroid 1998;8:249-257.

The current clinically available tests that report free T_4 and T_3 levels actually only estimate the free fraction and as such may not reflect hormone levels accurately in critically ill patients. This important article shows that free T_4 and free T_3 levels in sick patients are normal and suggest that the changes in thyroid hormone levels during illness are not reflective of thyroid dysfunction.

Ringel MD: Management of hypothyroidism and hyperthyroidism in the intensive care unit. Crit Care Clin 2001;17:59-74.

This is an in-depth review of thyroid storm and myxedema coma that provides another perspective on the treatment of these thyroid emergencies.

Yamamoto T, Fukuyama J, Fujiyoshi A: Factors associated with mortality of myxedema coma: Report of eight cases and literature survey. Thyroid 1999;12:1167-1174.

The authors compared their experience with the literature and suggested that high-dose levothyroxine replacement in patients older than 55 years old or with cardiac complications may be associated with a higher mortality. Aggressive levothyroxine replacement seems to be tolerated by younger patients without cardiac complications.

Yeung SC, Go R, Balasubramanyam A: Rectal administration of iodide and propylthiouracil in the treatment of thyroid storm. Thyroid 1995;5: 403-405.

Treatment of thyroid storm in a patient unable to take pills or with gastrointestinal abnormalities is a challenge because of the lack of intravenous preparations of antithyroid drugs. This article offers an effective alternative in these patients.

Chapter 178

DIABETES INSIPIDUS

Serge Brimioulle

Diabetes insipidus is a disorder of water metabolism associated with polyuria, urine hypotonicity, and hypernatremia. The quantitative criteria include urine output greater than 200 mL/h or 3 mL/kg/h, urine osmolality less than 150 mOsm/kg, and serum sodium greater than 145 mEq/L. If urine osmolality measurement is not available, hypotonicity can be assessed from a urine specific gravity less than 1.005.

CENTRAL DIABETES INSIPIDUS

Neurogenic or central diabetes insipidus is characterized by a lack of antidiuretic hormone (ADH) that may result from any injury to the anterior hypothalamus, pituitary stalk, or posterior hypophysis.[1-3] In acute critically ill patients, the most common causes of diabetes insipidus are surgery for pituitary tumors, cerebral trauma, intracranial hypertension, and brain death (Table 178-1). Diabetes insipidus also may occur as a complication of bacterial meningitis or encephalitis, vascular aneurysm or thrombosis, drug administration, or alcohol intoxication. Injuries to the hypothalamus most often yield permanent diabetes insipidus because ADH is synthesized in the hypothalamus itself. Injuries to the pituitary stalk and neurohypophysis more commonly cause transient

diabetes insipidus because hypothalamic ADH secretion can be effective even in the absence of anatomic pathways to the normal site of release. Chronic diabetes insipidus in critically ill patients generally results from tumors of the pituitary region and from the sequelae of cerebral trauma.

CLINICAL PICTURE

In complete hypothalamic or pituitary injuries, diabetes insipidus generally develops 6 to 24 hours after the injury because previously released ADH remains circulating this long. Patients with untreated diabetes insipidus usually develop urine outputs of 10 to 15 L/day. When the thirst mechanism is preserved, it is activated as soon as osmolality or volemia decreases. If the patient remains conscious and is given free access to water, he or she may be able to drink large amounts and compensate for the urine losses. In other cases, the large amounts of dilute urine rapidly result in dehydration with hypovolemia and hypotension and in hypernatremia with neurologic deterioration. It is important that diabetes insipidus is recognized and treated rapidly, especially in comatose or noncommunicative patients. In patients with partial diabetes insipidus, the onset of polyuria may be delayed, and the volume of urine may be lower. Nevertheless, if urine is hypo-osmolar and the diabetes insipidus is not treated, dehydration and hypernatremia finally occur and cause symptoms.

Clinical signs of hypernatremia usually appear only when the serum sodium concentration increases to greater than 155 to 160 mEq/L or serum osmolality increases to greater than 330 mOsm/kg. Signs may appear sooner if hypernatremia is associated with other metabolic disorders, particularly with disorders that also increase serum osmolality. Symptoms mainly include confusion and lethargy. Severe hypernatremia results in coma and sometimes seizures. Acute and severe dehydration and hypernatremia may lead to cerebral shrinkage, sometimes associated with subdural or intraparenchymal hemorrhages.

Clinical signs of dehydration include blood volume depletion and hypotension in the most severe cases. Biologic markers of dehydration usually are absent in ICU patients with central diabetes insipidus because the urine loss begins abruptly and commonly reaches more than 1 L/h. The free water deficit can be estimated by the following formula:

$$\text{Deficit (L)} = \text{body weight (kg)} \times 0.6 \times (\text{Na}^+ - 140)/\text{Na}^+$$

The formula assumes that only free water has been lost and that sodium stores are normal. Most often, some sodium has been lost together with additional water, and the total water

TABLE 178–1. CAUSES OF DIABETES INSIPIDUS

Central
   Congenital anomalies: corpus callosum agenesis, cleft palate
   Granulomatous disease: sarcoidosis, tuberculosis, Wegener's disease
   Histiocytosis
   Sickle cell disease
   Idiopathic
   Tumors: suprasellar, infrasellar, aneurysms
   Infection: meningitis, encephalitis
   Head trauma, neurosurgery
Nephrogenic
   Congenital disease
   Renal disease: obstructive uropathy, reflux nephropathy, cystic
     disease
   Renal involvement in systemic disease: sarcoidosis, amyloidosis,
     sickle cell disease
   Drugs: phenytoin, aminoglycosides, amphotericin,
     demeclocycline, lithium

TABLE 178–2. MANAGEMENT OF DIABETES INSIPIDUS

Control polyuria with DDAVP or vasopressin
Calculate and replace free water loss
Monitor and replace urine losses hourly
Monitor serum electrolytes and adapt therapy every 4 h

DDAVP, 1-deamino-8-D-arginine vasopressin.

deficit is even higher than that estimated from the formula. A moderate level of hypernatremia (e.g., 155 mEq) already is associated with a free water deficit of more than 4 L, and a total water deficit that may be much higher if sodium has been lost.

DIFFERENTIAL DIAGNOSIS

The differential diagnosis of polyuria includes the intake of diuretic drugs, hyperglycemia, fluid overload, and fluid mobilization. The search for diuretic administration should include not only conventional diuretics, but also mannitol and iodinated contrast agents. The administration of diuretics may not be evident when these substances have been given before admission to the ICU (e.g., in another hospital before patient transfer; in an ambulance during transfer; or in the operating room during neurosurgery, trauma surgery, or vascular surgery). Preventive administration of furosemide and mannitol is given routinely in some neurosurgical procedures and may result in marked polyuria during and after the operation. Hyperglycemia-induced osmotic diuresis is common, can be suspected from polyuria or from hyperglycemia, and is confirmed or ruled out by the presence or absence of glucosuria. Hypervolemia, resulting from fluid overload or unmasked by discontinuation of sustained positive-pressure ventilation, may increase urine output to greater than 5 L/day for several days in patients with normal renal function. Mobilization of edema, at the time of recovery from disease or from surgery, also can result in sustained polyuria. In all these conditions, however, urine remains close to isotonic (osmolality about 300 mOsm/kg). Abundant intake of hypotonic fluid can cause polyuria and urine hypotonicity, but does not result in hypernatremia if renal function is normal. The observation of decreased urine output after ADH administration is not diagnostic of diabetes insipidus because ADH is able to reduce urine output and to increase urine osmolality in all conditions except nephrogenic diabetes insipidus.

TREATMENT

The management of diabetes insipidus includes two components (Table 178-2): (1) reduction of excessive urine output and (2) correction of water deficit. The polyuria of central diabetes insipidus is treated effectively by vasopressin (ADH) or by its synthetic analog desmopressin acetate (DDAVP

[1-deamino-8-D-arginine vasopressin]).[4] As indicated by its multiple names, vasopressin not only has antidiuretic, but also vasoconstrictive and oxytocic, effects, whereas desmopressin essentially retains the antidiuretic action. The effects of aqueous vasopressin (4 to 10 U subcutaneously or intramuscularly) on diuresis begin rapidly but last for only a few hours. Vasopressin must be repeated every 4 to 6 hours, and it has been recommended only for diagnostic purposes or in acute conditions (e.g., trauma) in which the diabetes insipidus might be transient. The effects of vasopressin tannate in oil emulsion (2 to 5 U intramuscularly) last 48 to 96 hours, but the preparation requires close attention to warming and mixing the suspension before injection. Vasopressin tannate previously used to be the standard therapy in patients with central diabetes insipidus, but now it has been abandoned in favor of desmopressin. Vasopressin tannate, where available, still may be used in patients who are refractory to desmopressin or who experience significant side effects. Desmopressin has prolonged effects (8 to 20 hours) and is appropriate for intravenous, subcutaneous, and intranasal routes. Lypressin is another ADH analog that is appropriate for intranasal use, but its effectiveness is limited by its duration of action of only 4 to 6 hours. Desmopressin is well known to increase factor VIII and von Willebrand's factor levels and is used for this purpose in patients with coagulation disorders and in surgical procedures associated with potential significant bleeding. In the ICU and acute central diabetes insipidus, desmopressin is initially given as 10 to 20 μg intranasally and repeated every 30 to 60 minutes until urine output is reduced to less than 100 mL/h. The initial dose required to maintain a normal urine volume ranges from 10 to 60 μg in most patients. The total appropriate dose is given again when the urine output increases again to greater than 200 mL/h (i.e., after 8 to 24 hours). The dosage must be reduced if urine output is excessively decreased. Systematic administration is not recommended because most cases of diabetes insipidus seen in ICUs are associated with acute events and may be incomplete or intermittent or both. The subcutaneous route is seldom used because absorption may be erratic in vasoconstricted patients and because an intravenous line is virtually always available in ICU patients. Desmopressin is injected intravenously when the intranasal route is not available (i.e., in cases of rhinorrhea and facial trauma). The required initial dose ranges from 2 to 20 μg and is given as repeated 2- to 4-μg boluses.

Vasopressin therapy can be associated with arterial hypertension, myocardial infarction, mesenteric infarction, peripheric ischemia, and uterine cramps. Vasopressin tannate may cause allergic reactions, ranging from urticaria to anaphylaxis, and sterile abscesses at sites of injection. Desmopressin may interfere with anticoagulant drugs and cause hypercoagulability. When given in excess, all these antidiuretic agents can result in oliguria, hyponatremia, and water intoxication. The severity of diabetes insipidus may vary over time, even in patients with chronic diabetes insipidus, and some patients with chronic diabetes insipidus who are used to drinking large amounts of water may continue to do so even if urine output is limited by a diuretic drug.

Patients with acute diabetes insipidus should receive a sufficient amount of water to match their urine output until the polyuria is controlled and to correct the deficit of free water that already exists at the time of diagnosis. If the gastrointestinal system is functional, water can be infused at rates of 1 to 2 L/h through a gastric tube. Otherwise, isotonic dextrose should be infused intravenously in appropriate amounts (hypotonic dextrose administration can be obtained by infusing equal amounts of water and isotonic dextrose in a central vein, but this procedure has been associated with vascular injuries). Practically the dedicated gastric or intravenous infusion rate is adjusted at least hourly to match the urine output of the last equivalent period. Additional water is provided to correct the initial water deficit over a few hours. Serum electrolytes should be monitored every 4 hours until a normal natremia is restored and stabilized. Blood glucose must be monitored closely and hyperglycemia treated aggressively using intravenous insulin. Failure to control hyperglycemia may be associated with osmotic diuresis due to glucosuria and superimpose an equivalent of diabetes mellitus on the already present diabetes insipidus.

NEPHROGENIC DIABETES INSIPIDUS

Nephrogenic diabetes insipidus is characterized by the inability of the renal parenchyma to concentrate urine in response to ADH.[5] The disorder usually is more severe when it is congenital. It is seldom diagnosed in the ICU. Nephrogenic diabetes insipidus generally is best treated with thiazide diuretics, sometimes combined with amiloride, that are helpful to limit urine volume to acceptable values. Prostaglandin inhibitors, such as indomethacin, also may be useful.

ANNOTATED REFERENCES

Fukuda I, Hizuka N, Takano K: Oral DDAVP is a good alternative therapy for patients with central diabetes insipidus: Experience of five-year treatment. Endocr J 2003;50:437-443.
   This study summarizes experience on the effectiveness of DDAVP therapy in central diabetes insipidus.

Maghnie M: Diabetes insipidus. Horm Res 2003;59(Suppl 1):42-54.
   This general review focuses on etiology and on clinical and radiologic features.

Maghnie M, Cosi G, Genovese E, et al: Central diabetes insipidus in children and young adults. N Engl J Med 2000;343:998-1007.
   This is a study on the etiology of central diabetes insipidus.

Morello JP, Bichet DG: Nephrogenic diabetes insipidus. Annu Rev Physiol 2001;63:607-630.
   This physiologic review on genetic aspects discusses the role of aquaporins in nephrogenic diabetes insipidus.

Verbalis JG: Diabetes insipidus. Rev Endocr Metab Disord 2003;4:177-185.
   This is a general review on diabetes insipidus.

Chapter 179

METABOLIC AND ENDOCRINE CRISES IN THE PEDIATRIC INTENSIVE CARE UNIT

Andrew C. Argent

Increasing numbers of metabolic and endocrine conditions are being recognized, and the number of children being treated for these conditions is increasing. Although improved screening programs and therapy may decrease the number of children requiring critical care for these conditions, it is likely that these conditions will be recognized in increasing numbers of critically ill children for the foreseeable future. General principles of ICU management apply to patients with endocrine and metabolic crises (Table 179-1).[1,2] Crises may cause damage with long-term sequelae for the child and family; however, they also present unique diagnostic opportunities. The intensivist has a particular responsibility to:

- Be aware of metabolic and endocrine problems
- Consider them in the differential diagnosis of particular clinical syndromes

- Perform appropriate clinical and biochemical investigations
- Seek advice from specialists in the clinical and laboratory diagnosis and management of the conditions

With the possible exception of diabetes mellitus, endocrine and metabolic crises are uncommon, and most intensivists do not see sufficient case numbers to become expert at managing these disorders. It is crucial to manage children with suspected or proven endocrine or metabolic crises in conjunction with specialist teams. The laboratory investigation of inborn errors of metabolism may be complex, and there are relatively few laboratories worldwide that have the capacity to elucidate fully most of the inborn errors of metabolism. Close cooperation with specialist laboratory centers is essential for accurate diagnosis and management.

A specific problem of endocrine and metabolic crises is that laboratory investigation of specific conditions may take time, and patients require urgent therapeutic intervention. Because it is often not possible to follow algorithms of investigation, the only reasonable response is to collect all appropriate specimens immediately,[3] store them appropriately, and liaise with the laboratory services to use the specimens in a logical and cost-effective manner to confirm the diagnosis.

ENDOCRINE CRISES

Endocrine crises present in a limited number of ways that include abnormalities of glucose control, fluid and electrolyte balance, and blood pressure control. Management of these crises consists of identifying the problem, investigating the cause, and correcting the abnormality directly or managing the underlying problem. This chapter provides a clinical overview of pediatric endocrine crises; detailed pathophysiology is discussed in other chapters.

ABNORMALITIES OF GLUCOSE CONTROL

Abnormalities of glucose control, including diabetic ketoacidosis, are the most common endocrine crises encountered in the PICU. Hypoglycemia and hyperglycemia are associated with increased mortality[4,5] in sick children and may be part of a wide variety of disease processes. Measurement of blood glucose is part of the initial biochemical evaluation of any sick child, particularly if a depressed level of consciousness or shock is present. When an abnormal glucose level has

TABLE 179–1. PRINCIPLES OF MANAGEMENT OF METABOLIC AND ENDOCRINE CRISES

Principle	Specifics of Conditions
Airway management	Many patients have depressed level of consciousness, and airway management is essential to prevent complications
Breathing support	Acidotic patients may make huge respiratory effort; ventilatory support may help to decrease the metabolic demands on these patients. Although administration of sodium bicarbonate may help to settle some of the acidosis-related symptoms, such as hyperventilation, bicarbonate may aggravate some problems seen in conjunction with urea cycle defects. Give bicarbonate only if the plasma bicarbonate <10 mmol/L and then only half correct deficits
Circulatory support	Ensure that there is adequate circulating volume; this may be a particular issue if there has been excessive fluid loss from vomiting or diarrhea
Disability	Control seizures using anticonvulsant agents Administer pyridoxine if possibility of pyridoxine dependency
Dialysis to remove toxins where necessary	Hemodialysis is the most efficient means of removing toxins such as ammonia and leucine. Hemofiltration is less efficient, but may be more applicable in critically ill children. Peritoneal dialysis is slower, but has the advantage of ease of initiation.[1] In some conditions, it may be possible to remove toxins by stimulating alternative pathways of metabolism
Ensure that glucose is normal	A normal glucose level should be maintained at all times. Excessive administration of glucose in the mitochondrial energy chain problem may exacerbate lactic acidosis. Also, attempt to provide an adequate energy supply (may use medium-chain fatty acids where appropriate). Minimize energy demands on patient
Fluids	In general, provide 1.5× normal fluid maintenance requirements to accelerate excretion of water-soluble toxins. In the context of encephalopathy (maple syrup urine disease or urea cycle defects), be careful to avoid overhydration, which may contribute to development of cerebral edema.
Feeds	If there is accumulation of a product, this needs to be eliminated from the diet (e.g., fructose, galactose). Start with protein-free diet, but do not continue that beyond 2 days because the catabolic state also creates problems. If diagnosis not identified, need gradual reintroduction of feeds and nutrition. If there is deficiency of any nutrient (e.g., carnitine, which may have a primary or a secondary deficiency), supplement that nutrient. Ensure that there is an adequate energy source along a metabolic route that is functional. Provide specific vitamin therapy where indicated
Family support and information	The diagnosis of an inborn error of metabolism has major implications for families, and considerable support is required[2]
Treat infection	Infections are an important component of pediatric ICU presentation of inborn errors of metabolism. Some conditions, such as galactosemia, are related to specific infections, such as Escherichia coli. Other conditions are related to pyogenic infections because of neutropenia. Children who are in a poor nutritional or metabolic state are more susceptible to infection. Intercurrent infections may be the precipitating factor for metabolic decompensation
Investigations	A wide variety of investigations are relevant to inborn errors of metabolism. Biochemical testing on a range of body fluids and on tissues is fundamental to the accurate diagnosis of the problem. Biochemical tests may range from simple screening tests to more complex tests on tissue culture. Imaging techniques, such as CT, MRI, magnetic resonance spectroscopy, and echocardiography, may be relevant. Functional tests, such as EEG, ECG, and EMG, may be useful in diagnosis. Increasingly, genetic diagnosis is available, if children have recognized genetic mutations
Monitor response to therapy	Clinical monitoring is essential. Biochemical monitoring of the appropriate metabolites is essential to ensure that metabolic control is established

CT, computed tomography; ECG, electrocardiogram; EEG, electroencephalogram; EMG, electromyogram; ICU, intensive care unit; MRI, magnetic resonance imaging.

been identified, levels must be remeasured at appropriate intervals until the problem has been resolved.

Hypoglycemia

Hypoglycemia is associated with potentially devastating damage to the brain and requires immediate correction. Although the exact definition of hypoglycemia in children is controversial, a minimal level of 2.6 mmol/L or greater should be maintained to ensure normal neural function.[6,7] It probably is safer to maintain a level of greater than 3.5 mmol/L. Because there are multiple causes for hypoglycemia, and symptoms may not be due to the hypoglycemia alone, it is essential to identify the cause of hypoglycemia.

Hypoglycemia is associated with severe illness. A wide range of illnesses, including infections, cyanotic and acyanotic congenital heart disease, and cardiomyopathy/myocarditis, has been associated with hypoglycemia. Hepatic failure from infection, toxin ingestion, or drug reactions may be associated with severe hypoglycemia, and Reye's syndrome classically presents with hypoglycemia. Toxins, such as salicylates and ethanol, also may cause hypoglycemia. Hypoglycemia has been linked with increased mortality from malaria,[8-10] gastroenteritis,[11] and acute bacterial meningitis,[12] among

other conditions. Hypoglycemia also has been described as a complication of therapy for leukemia with mercaptopurine and methotrexate[13,14] and malaria, although there is controversy about the role of quinine in hypoglycemia.[15] Although severe illness or sepsis may be an adequate explanation for hypoglycemia, a diagnosis of sepsis should not exclude the possibility of an endocrine or metabolic crisis.

The clinical signs of hypoglycemia may be nonspecific, ranging from lethargy, poor feeding, hypotonia, and "jitteriness" to convulsions, apneic episodes, cardiovascular collapse, and sudden infant death syndrome (SIDS). Because the signs are poor predictors of hypoglycemia,[16] regular monitoring of blood glucose is an important component of the management of any critically ill child.

Symptomatic hypoglycemia occurs more frequently during the neonatal period than in any other period of childhood. Infants at particular risk include infants with poor hepatic glycogen stores (e.g., preterm or small-for-gestational-age infants); poor glucose intake (e.g., preterm or ill infants); and hyperinsulinism, either primary or secondary to high intrauterine glucose levels (e.g., infants of diabetic mothers).[17] Hypoglycemia also may be a feature of perinatal illness, including asphyxia, polycythemia, hypothermia, septicemia, and respiratory distress syndrome. Much less common causes include growth hormone or adrenal insufficiency, inborn errors of metabolism, and glucagon insufficiency. Drugs administered to the mother during pregnancy, including oral hypoglycemic agents, also must be considered.

In childhood, hypoglycemia may result from inadequate glucose intake (prolonged starvation, malabsorption), defects in gluconeogenesis (glycogen storage disorders or deficiency of gluconeogenic hormones, such as adrenaline, corticosteroids, glucagons, growth hormone, and thyroid hormone), excessive insulin secretion (hyperinsulinism), and excessive use of glucose (fatty acid oxidation defects). Hypoglycemia also may be associated with abnormalities of amino acid metabolism.

The amount of glucose required to achieve normoglycemia and the duration of fast that can be endured without the development of hypoglycemia may assist in identifying a likely cause. Transient hypoglycemia that can be reversed with normal infusion rates of glucose (4 to 6 mg/kg/min) and does not recur is unlikely to be associated with an endocrine problem. Hyperinsulinemia is associated with rapid development of hypoglycemia and high glucose requirements (>6 to 8 mg/kg/min to >15 to 20 mg/kg/min). Hypoglycemia associated with adrenal insufficiency, growth hormone deficiency, and hypothyroidism tends to occur after several hours of fasting, is associated with ketosis, and can be reversed with normal infusion rates of glucose. Fatty acid oxidation defects are associated with hypoglycemia after a fast of some hours.

As soon as hypoglycemia is noted, specimens should be collected immediately for appropriate tests (Table 179-2). Treatment of hypoglycemia with intravenous glucose should be initiated promptly. An initial bolus dose of 0.5 g/kg of glucose (may need 0.5 to 2 g/kg in neonates) should be given as a 10% or 25% (in older children) dextrose solution, followed by an ongoing infusion of glucose at a rate of 4 to 8 mg/kg/min. The concentration of the ongoing infusion depends on the fluid requirements of the child and the availability of central venous access (for higher concentrations). Glucagon may be given at a dose of 0.1 to 0.3 mg/kg (intravenously or intramuscularly), but is unlikely to be effective in patients with low glycogen stores, glycogen storage disorders, or hepatic dysfunction. Hydrocortisone at a dose of 5 mg/kg every 12 hours may be useful in some patients. Diazoxide and intravenous octreotide decrease insulin release and may be useful in the management of hyperinsulinemia.

If non–glucose-reducing substances are present in the urine, galactosemia, hereditary fructose intolerance, or tyrosinemia should be considered. In the absence of reducing substances, low urinary ketones with hypoglycemia suggest hyperinsulinism or defects of fatty acid oxidation. The latter can be distinguished from hyperinsulinemia by the presence of high serum free fatty acids. Assays of insulin levels can confirm the diagnosis of hyperinsulinism.

Abnormalities of growth hormone, cortisol, or thyroid hormone typically are associated with high urinary ketones, the absence of hepatomegaly, and increased lactate. Hypoglycemia also may occur as a complication of insulin therapy for diabetes mellitus. Patients with diabetes mellitus may have inadequate responses to hypoglycemia.[18,19]

Hyperinsulinemic Hypoglycemia

Hyperinsulinism is the most common cause of persistent or recurrent hypoglycemia in infancy.[20] Hyperinsulinemia occurs in association with the Beckwith-Weidemann syndrome, maternal diabetes,[17] rhesus incompatibility, and perinatal asphyxia.[21] Hyperinsulinemia also occurs after maternal glucose treatment during delivery.[22]

Although most patients with hyperinsulinemic hypoglycemia present in the neonatal period, first presentation may be during infancy and occasionally during childhood.[23] The characteristic features of hyperinsulinism include hypoglycemia with glucose requirements of greater than 6 to 8 mg/kg/min to maintain normoglycemia, absence of ketonemia and ketonuria, low plasma free fatty acids, detectable insulin at the time of hypoglycemia, and response to glucagon administration.[20] Neonates with hypoglycemia may have the macrosomia typical of infants of diabetic mothers, but hyperinsulinemic hypoglycemia may occur in apparently normal infants of normal or low birth weight.

Hyperinsulinemic hypoglycemia is caused by abnormalities in the beta cells of the pancreas, which may be focal (associated with loss of the maternal allele from chromosome 11p15) or diffuse (associated with many genetic disorders).[24] Pancreatectomy often is necessary to prevent recurrent hypoglycemia in patients who do not respond to medical therapy. de Lonlay-Debeney and colleagues[24,25] used transhepatic portal vein catheterization and selective catheterization of the pancreatic vein combined with intraoperative histology to identify patients with focal or diffuse beta cell abnormalities. Patients with diffuse abnormalities had near-total pancrea-tectomy, whereas patients with focal lesions had partial pancreatectomy. Patients who had focal lesions removed did not have ongoing hypoglycemia postoperatively and did not develop glucose intolerance. By contrast, 13 of 30 patients with diffuse lesions had persistent hypoglycemia, 8 developed type 1 diabetes, and a further 7 had developed abnormal glucose tolerance within a mean follow-up time of 4.6 years. These investigations can be performed only in specialist centers. Even in specialist centers, pancreatic resection may be associated with significant postoperative morbidity.[26] Poor neurologic outcome remains a problem due to previous hypoglycemia, despite modern surgical approaches.[27]

Initial stabilization therapy consists of glucose infusions to achieve normoglycemia. Because there may be extremely high glucose requirements, and any cessation of infusion may be associated with severe hypoglycemia, it is essential to ensure that secure vascular access is *always* available, and central venous access may be required for concentrated glucose infusions. Glucagon always must be available and can be used as short-term, emergency therapy to maintain normoglycemia if there are problems with vascular access. Administration of glucagon may be associated with rebound hypoglycemia, and frequent glucose monitoring must be continued. Glucose polymers can be added to the diet to provide an enteral source of glucose, but care must be taken to limit the osmolar load on the gut, particularly in premature infants. When normoglycemia has been achieved, the child should be transported to a center with specific expertise in the management of hyperinsulinemia. Great care must be taken to ensure that hypoglycemia does not occur during transport.

The aim of further management is to confirm the diagnosis and ensure normoglycemia without the ongoing use of glucose infusions. Glucose intake can be supplemented using glucose polymers, but care must be taken in infants at risk of necrotizing enterocolitis. Pharmacologic therapy[28,29] should be tried in all patients, but is less likely to be successful in infants presenting in the neonatal period and in infants from certain genetic backgrounds. Medical therapy may be particularly

TABLE 179–2. INVESTIGATION OF HYPOGLYCEMIA

Blood glucose	Measurement of glucose using blood from capillary specimens and using test strips may be unreliable (particularly in poorly perfused patients or patients with high hematocrit); where possible, low glucose levels should be confirmed using laboratory assays on venous or arterial blood
Actual glucose intake	Hypoglycemia in the presence of normal glucose intake or after brief fast suggests hyperinsulinism. Hypoglycemia after hours of fasting is associated with fatty acid oxidation defects and endocrine insufficiency
Non–glucose-reducing substances in the urine	Particularly in neonates and probably not relevant in older children. If present in the urine, consider galactosemia, hereditary fructose intolerance, or tyrosinemia
Serum and urinary ketones	Low ketones suggest hyperinsulinism or fatty acid oxidation problem
Serum free fatty acids	Free fatty acids are low in hyperinsulinism but high in fatty acid oxidation defect
Serum insulin (and C peptide), cortisol, glucagon, growth hormone, and thyroid levels	Normal serum insulin in the presence of hypoglycemia is evidence of hyperinsulinism. C peptide may be necessary to ascertain whether exogenous insulin was administered. Release of C peptide may not be as pulsatile as that of insulin
Serum ammonia	To recognize hyperinsulinism/hyperammonemia syndrome
Urinary organic acids and serum amino acids	To diagnose fatty acid oxidation defects (urinary organic acids). Aminoacidopathies such as maple syrup urine disease, propionic acidemia, isovaleric acidemia, methylmalonic acidemia, and tyrosinemia may also present with hypoglycemia
Total and free carnitine with acylcarnitine profile	To recognize primary and secondary deficiency of carnitine and fatty acid oxidation defects

effective in patients with hyperinsulinemia/hyperammonemia syndrome.

Diazoxide (10 to 20 mg/kg/day in two to three divided doses) and chlorothiazide (7 to 10 mg/kg/day in two divided doses) are recommended as first-choice therapy because they can be given orally. Many patients respond to this therapy. Alternatives include nifedipine (0.25 to 2.5 mg/kg/d) and glucagon (infusion rates of 5 to 10 μg/kg/h or 1 μg/kg/h together with 10 μg/kg/day of octreotide) to decrease requirements for glucose infusion. If the therapy is successful, it may need to be continued for many years. If the response to therapy does not allow safe discontinuation of intravenous therapy, surgical resection of the pancreas with histologic support is required.[29-34] Close long-term follow up is essential.[35]

Hyperinsulinemic Hypoglycemia with Hyperammonemia

Hyperinsulinemic hypoglycemia with hyperammonemia (previously called *leucine-sensitive hypoglycemia*) is well described[36-38] and is attributed to mutations in the gene for glutamate dehydrogenase.[38] Patients generally respond well to therapy with diazoxide, and consumption of extra carbohydrate before protein meals may help to ameliorate symptoms.[40] Special low-leucine milks are available.

Ketotic Hypoglycemia

Although ketotic hypoglycemia ("accelerated starvation") is probably the most common cause of hypoglycemia in previously healthy children,[41] it is unlikely to present in the pediatric intensive care unit (PICU). This condition usually affects children age 6 months to 8 years, and the clinical features include ketosis, severe nausea, and hypoglycemia, usually occurring in the morning after a moderate fast. Treatment consists of ensuring that there is an adequate and regular intake of glucose, particularly during intercurrent infections. Urinary ketones may act as a warning signal because the ketosis usually precedes the onset of hypoglycemia by several hours.

Adrenal Insufficiency

Adrenal insufficiency after high-dose inhaled corticosteroid therapy has presented with hypoglycemia[42-46] and should be considered if there is a past history of inhaled steroid use (particularly fluticasone). Adrenal insufficiency also may occur after adrenal bleeds (e.g., after meningococcal septicemia or difficult delivery), as part of adrenal disease (e.g., congenital adrenal hyperplasia or hypoplasia) in which ambiguous genitalia may (or may not) be a pointer in females, or as part of hypopituitarism (e.g., congenital, after craniopharyngioma, or after cranial irradiation[47]). One study reported that 18% of patients with primary adrenal insufficiency presented with hypoglycemia.[48] Adrenoleukodystrophy should be considered as part of the etiologic diagnosis in any male patient with Addison's disease (pigmentation may be a clue) and should be tested for by measurement of very-long-chain fatty acids.[49] Not all patients with adrenal insufficiency present with hypoglycemia.

There is increasing evidence that adrenocorticoid deficiency may be a significant component in shocked children with sepsis.[50,51] The criteria for the diagnosis of adrenal insufficiency in critical illness are controversial,[52] but some adult data suggest that shock may be improved by the use of stress doses of glucocorticoids.[53-56]

Adrenocorticoid deficiency also has been shown in preterm infants. One study showed that five preterm infants with hypotension resistant to volume and inotropic therapy responded to administration of corticosteroids despite normal circulating levels of adrenocorticotropic hormone.[57] Another study showed that hydrocortisone had equivalent effect to dopamine in treatment of hypotensive, very-low-birth-weight infants.[58]

Congenital adrenal hyperplasia is associated rarely with hypoglycemia. Female patients are usually diagnosed early in life as a result of virilization, whereas male patients tend to present later. Patients with the salt-losing form of congenital adrenal hyperplasia present with hyponatremic dehydration and shock, usually associated with hyperkalemia. Because patients with salt-wasting 21-hydroxylase deficiency also may have catecholamine deficiency, shock may be a significant feature. Diagnosis is based on the clinical picture, typical electrolyte pattern, hypoaldosteronism, and hyperreninemia.[59] Long-term treatment consists of hydrocortisone (to suppress excess secretion of corticotropin-releasing hormone and corticotropin), 10 to 20 mg/m² of body surface area per day in three divided doses, although larger doses may be required during adrenal crises, together with mineralocorticoid replacement (0.1 to 0.2 mg of fludrocortisone daily) and sodium chloride supplementation. Little is known about the dose of hydrocortisone required during critical illness, although Charmandari and associates[60] showed that when 6-hourly bolus doses of 15 mg/m[2] of hydrocortisone are given, high immediate serum levels are achieved, followed by rapid decline to undetectable levels by 4 hours after administration. These authors postulated that continuous infusion of hydrocortisone may be more appropriate in critical illness.

Growth Hormone Deficiency

In the neonatal period, growth hormone deficiency presents with hypoglycemia (possibly with seizures), prolonged jaundice, and micropenis and undescended testes (in boys). Growth failure becomes apparent only toward the end of the first year of life. In later childhood, growth failure is a more common presentation, and hypoglycemia rarely occurs[47] unless associated with adrenocorticotropic hormone deficiency.

Hyperglycemia Other than Diabetes Mellitus

Hyperglycemia is relatively common in the PICU, with 51.9% of admissions having hyperglycemia in one study.[61] Hyperglycemia is common in patients with head injuries, after cardiac bypass surgery, after cardiac transplantation, with hemolytic uremic syndrome,[62] with tetanus,[63] and with toxin ingestion (e.g., theophylline poisoning[64]). Hyperglycemia was present in 55% of infants admitted to the hospital with severe gastroenteritis in one study,[65] and intravenous rehydration corrected hyperglycemia within 36 to 48 hours. The hyperglycemia was associated with increased cortisol, glucagon, and growth hormone levels. Another study of severe infantile gastroenteritis showed that hyperglycemia was associated with increased mortality.[5] Increased glucose on admission is associated with poor patient outcomes after head injury, although it is still unclear whether the high glucose level directly leads to exacerbation of brain injury or whether it reflects the severity of the insult.[66]

Iatrogenic causes of hyperglycemia in the PICU include resuscitation using glucose-containing fluids, parenteral nutrition, and high-dose corticosteroid therapy. Continuing hyperglycemia may be an indication of ongoing stress or undiagnosed type 1 diabetes and should prompt the clinician to investigate further.

Evidence from adult studies has shown that close control of glucose levels in the ICU using insulin infusions is associated with a significant improvement in patient outcome.[67] The study was conducted in an adult surgical ICU and showed a dramatic effect of insulin therapy with a 40% overall reduction in mortality in the group treated with insulin to achieve normoglycemia. This effect seems to be related to the glucose control achieved and not to the dose of insulin that was administered.[68] No data are available as yet on the effect of tight glucose control in the ICU for children. There is some evidence that hyperglycemic children may be extremely sensitive to insulin administration. Management consists of ensuring that ongoing stress has been resolved, limiting the intake of glucose, and administering low-dose insulin (0.05 U/kg/h) as an infusion if the preceding measures are inadequate to decrease levels of hyperglycemia.

Diabetes Mellitus

Children with diabetes mellitus have a higher mortality than healthy children, with standardized mortality ratios of 2.09 to 3.39, depending on age group.[69,70] The highest mortality is in children age 1 to 4 years, in whom the standardized mortality ratios may be 9.2[70] to 13.7.[71] Most deaths attributable to diabetes mellitus occur as a consequence of diabetic ketoacidosis or hyperglycemia, with the remainder attributable to hypoglycemia.[70] Although the incidence of type 1 diabetes mellitus has been increasing in many parts of the world, the hospitalization rate for diabetic ketoacidosis in established and new cases of type 1 diabetes mellitus has not increased in Canada and Europe since the 1990s[72,73] because of earlier diagnosis and safer ambulatory management with the help of a multidisciplinary team.

The mortality rate in the developed world for diabetic ketoacidosis ranges from 0.15% to 0.31%.[74] The most common cause of death among patients with diabetic ketoacidosis is cerebral edema.[70,75-77] Other causes of death in diabetic ketoacidosis include electrolyte disturbances, hypoglycemia, pulmonary edema, rhabdomyolysis, infections (including mucormycosis), and thrombosis. The management of diabetic ketoacidosis in childhood has been extensively reviewed elsewhere[74] with current recommendations.

Cerebral Edema in Diabetic Ketoacidosis

The incidence of cerebral edema in diabetic ketoacidosis in more recent reports ranges from 0.7%[75] to 0.9%.[78] The mortality rate is 21%, with 27% of survivors having neurologic sequelae[78] or a mortality or survival in vegetative state of 28% with 13% mild-to-moderate neurologic handicap.[79]

The exact mechanisms of cerebral edema in diabetic ketoacidosis and the risk factors that are involved are not clear. The clinical signs of cerebral edema in diabetic ketoacidosis are variable and include headache, deterioration in level of consciousness, inappropriate slowing of pulse rate, and increased blood pressure.

The risks of cerebral edema are higher in younger children and children with newly diagnosed diabetes. Cerebral edema may be present before therapy for diabetic ketoacidosis in 5% of cases,[78,80] although most cases develop 4 to 12 hours after initiation of therapy. Factors that have been associated with the development of cerebral edema include the administration of bicarbonate, a higher plasma urea, lower arterial partial pressure of carbon dioxide (PCO_2),[78] and a smaller increase in plasma sodium concentration during therapy.[78,81] Adverse outcomes have been associated with greater neurologic depression at the time of diagnosis, high initial serum urea nitrogen,[78,79] and intubation with hyperventilation to a PCO_2 less than 22 mm Hg.[79]

Although the biochemical derangements of hyperglycemia, metabolic acidosis with ketosis, and electrolyte abnormalities are the most obvious problems in diabetic ketoacidosis, significant derangements in other systems have been documented, including plasma tryptophan levels,[82] cytokine[83] and lymphocyte responses,[84] and coagulation abnormalities. There is little doubt that diabetic ketoacidosis is associated with a thrombotic state[85] (which may explain an increased incidence of cerebrovascular accidents), and care should be taken about the use of femoral central venous access because this may have a higher than usual complication rate in these patients.[86] A reported case of myocardial infarction related to diabetic ketoacidosis[87] may be a complication of the thrombotic state. Although myocardial function is generally normal in diabetic ketoacidosis,[88] myocarditis[89] has been noted in occasional case reports, whereas pulmonary edema may be more common than previously recognized.[90]

Principles of Management. Management of diabetic ketoacidosis should be coordinated by an experienced diabetes team. Children with severe diabetic ketoacidosis should be managed in a specialized diabetic unit or in the PICU.

Fluid Management. Protocols for fluid therapy in the management of diabetic ketoacidosis often provide specific volume guidelines. As pointed out by Inward and Chambers,[91] however, there is a wide range in the amount and rate of fluid and electrolyte loss in patients presenting with diabetic ketoacidosis (depending on the rate of onset and duration of symptoms, the severity of vomiting or diarrhea or both, and the fluid ingested by the patient). There is a wide range of intravascular status ranging from normovolemia to severe hypovolemia (uncommon). Clinical assessment of dehydration is notoriously inaccurate, and there is an unpredictable rate of ongoing fluid loss related to the osmotic diuresis.

Rapid replacement of intravascular volume has been shown to be a significant risk factor for the development of cerebral edema.[92] In the presence of hypovolemic shock, it is reasonable to infuse 0.9% saline using aliquots of 5 to 10 mL/kg until an acceptable blood pressure is obtained.[93] Typically, 10 to 20 mL/kg needs to be infused over 1 to 2 hours.[74] Ringer's lactate may be a reasonable alternative because administration of large volumes of 0.9% saline has been associated with the development of hyperchloremic acidosis.[94,95] There is no evidence to support the use of colloid solutions.

Thereafter the acceptable principles are that hypovolemia, rapid changes in plasma osmolality, and large volumes of sodium uptake should be avoided. Fluid therapy should be calculated to achieve rehydration over 48 hours.[96,97] Careful monitoring of fluid balance is essential to ensure that patients are neither losing excessive fluid (via osmotic diuresis) nor gaining excessive fluid. Fluid with a tonicity less than that of 0.45% saline should not be used, and a positive balance of approximately 6 mmol of sodium chloride per kilogram over 24 hours should be regarded as the upper limit.[93] The rate of fluid infusion rarely exceeds 1.5 to 2 times the usual daily requirement.

Despite the fact that almost all patients with diabetic ketoacidosis are potassium depleted, serum potassium levels frequently are increased at presentation. With initiation of insulin therapy and correction of acidosis, there is rapid intracellular movement of potassium, and careful monitoring of potassium levels is essential. As soon as potassium levels are less than 5.5 mEq/L, 30 to 40 mEq/L of potassium should be added to the fluid infusions, and 0.5 to 1 mEq/kg/h of potassium may be required to correct potassium deficits. Potassium may be given as chloride or phosphate. Although severe hypophosphatemia is relatively common,[98] and extreme hypophosphatemia has been reported,[99] there is no evidence that phosphate administration is routinely necessary in the management of diabetic ketoacidosis, and the clinical effects of severe hypophosphatemia rarely are seen in diabetic ketoacidosis. Theoretically, phosphate administration may reduce insulin resistance and depletion of adenosine triphosphate and have positive effects on 2,3-diphosphoglycerate.[100,101] Administration of potassium phosphate helps to decrease the chloride load given to patients with diabetic ketoacidosis. Potassium phosphate may be used safely,[102] provided that calcium levels are monitored carefully.[103,104] Glucose must be added to the infusion of fluids when the glucose levels are 14 to 17 mmol/L to avoid hypoglycemia.

Bicarbonate. The use of bicarbonate in diabetic ketoacidosis is extremely limited. Many studies have shown no clinical benefit from bicarbonate administration.[105-107] More recently, bicarbonate administration has been associated with the development of cerebral edema. Bicarbonate should not be given routinely, not in bolus form, and possibly only in patients who have a pH of less than 7.0 despite appropriate correction of intravascular volume and despite ongoing adequate insulin therapy.

Insulin Therapy. Intravenous insulin should be provided as a continuous low-dose infusion starting at 0.1 U/kg/h. If there is no response to insulin therapy, the infusion should be reviewed for technical problems (incorrect preparation, adhesion of insulin to infusion tubing), and the patient should be reviewed for ongoing hypovolemia or uncontrolled sepsis. There is no place for a bolus of intravenous insulin or an initial loading dose, other than in the management of life-threatening hyperkalemia. The insulin infusion should be continued until ketoacidosis is resolved, and the patient is fully conscious and retaining solid food.

Treat Underlying Cause. In previously undiagnosed patients, the cause of diabetic ketoacidosis is insulin deficiency. Even in previously diagnosed patients, most episodes of diabetic ketoacidosis probably are related to insulin omission or treatment error,[108] although children 3 years old or younger are more likely to have a bacterial infection.[109]

If infection is suspected as the precipitating cause of diabetic ketoacidosis, aggressive therapy with antibiotics and drainage of any pus should be instituted. Routine prophylactic antibiotic therapy is not indicated in diabetic ketoacidosis.

Monitoring. Although some patients are hypovolemic on presentation, there is little evidence that invasive hemodynamic monitoring is necessary. Careful monitoring of sodium levels is essential because smaller changes in serum sodium with therapy have been associated with development of cerebral edema.[78] Hyperlipidemia may decrease the aqueous phase of serum and artificially reduce sodium levels; this can be corrected using the following formula[110]:

$$[\text{True sodium}]\ (\text{mEq/L}) = [\text{reported sodium (mEq/L)}] \times [0.021 \times [\text{triglycerides (mg/dL)}] + 0.994])$$

The osmotic load of glucose also decreases serum sodium levels, with a decrease in sodium concentration of approximately 1.6 mEq/L per 100 mg/dL increase in glucose. The expectation is that with decreasing levels of hyperglycemia and hyperlipidemia, sodium levels should increase. This increase may be offset, however, by urinary losses of sodium secondary to osmotic diuresis.

Careful and frequent monitoring of potassium and glucose levels is essential. If phosphate is being administered, calcium levels should be monitored. Regular acid-base monitoring is required.

A more recent study has suggested that monitoring of end-tidal P_{CO_2} could be used as a noninvasive method for continuous monitoring of response to therapy for diabetic ketoacidosis.[111] The only proviso (as pointed out by the authors and in an accompanying editorial[112]) is that any changes in respiratory drive or efficiency of the respiratory system may mask changes in acid-base that otherwise might be reflected by capnometry.

Investigations for Possible Cerebral Edema in Diabetic Ketoacidosis. Although cerebral edema is the most common cause of depressed level of consciousness in diabetic ketoacidosis, there are other causes that are amenable to alternative therapy, including cerebral venous thrombosis[113] and acute hydrocephalus.[114] Other abnormalities, such as brain infarction[115] and extrapontine myelinolysis,[116] have been shown. Computed tomography of patients with a depressed level of consciousness may be recommended to exclude other treatable pathology. Because the risks are relatively low, however, excluding other pathology must be balanced against the risks associated with moving ill patients to the radiology suite.

Mannitol has been used for the management of cerebral edema[117] (0.25 to 1 g/kg over 20 minutes), although there are no controlled studies. Hypertonic saline (5 to 10 mL/kg of 3% saline) may be an alternative to mannitol.[118] Hyperventilation after intubation for cerebral edema may be associated with worse outcomes.[79]

Summary. Despite improvements in the management of diabetic ketoacidosis, it remains a serious illness with significant morbidity and mortality. In addition to improving management of the condition, strong focus must be brought to ensure that the condition is avoided where possible and diagnosed and treated promptly when it occurs.

Thyroid Insufficiency

Neonates exposed to large amounts of iodine in iodine-containing antiseptics may develop transient hypothyroidism[119-122] (also called the *Wolff-Chaikoff effect*) as a result of transcutaneous absorption of iodine. This condition also has been shown in infants undergoing cardiac catheterization and cardiac surgery.[123] Care should be taken to limit the exposure of infants to iodine-containing agents. Triiodothyronine supplementation may be considered in children who have been exposed to significant amounts of iodine before or during a critical illness.

The sick euthyroid syndrome has been well documented in the PICU, particularly in patients undergoing cardiac surgery. The subject has been reviewed elsewhere.[124] Although there may be benefit to some children from triiodothyronine supplementation after cardiac surgery,[125-128] there is no established role for triiodothyronine supplementation after cardiac surgery.

Children with Down syndrome have a high incidence of hypothyroidism.[129-131] Attention should be paid to the possible need for triiodothyronine supplementation in critically ill children with Down syndrome.

METABOLIC CRISES

EPIDEMIOLOGY

Population data on inborn errors of metabolism suggest that there is a minimal incidence of 35 to 40 per 100,000 live births[132,133] in predominantly white populations. In addition, some conditions have a particularly high incidence in particular population groups (e.g., maple syrup urine disease has an incidence of 568 per 100,000 births in the Mennonite community in Pennsylvania). Inborn errors of metabolism have a diverse presentation and are part of the differential diagnosis of many children admitted to the PICU with acute illness. Until more recently, only conditions such as phenylketonuria and galactosemia had been identified at birth using screening programs. With increasing availability of technology such as tandem mass spectrometry, screening of other inborn errors of metabolism (including fatty acid oxidation abnormalities and aminoacidopathies) has been introduced in some parts of the world,[134] and this potentially may decrease the number of children presenting with acute metabolic decompensation.

There is evidence that SIDS may be related to inborn errors of metabolism in at least 1% to 5% of cases,[135,136] and inborn errors of metabolism must be considered as part of the differential diagnosis of any infant who presents to the PICU or neonatal ICU after a near-SIDS episode. A family history of SIDS also should raise the possibility of inborn errors of metabolism in siblings presenting to the PICU with acute illness.

Inheritance is generally autosomal recessive, but there are conditions that are sex-linked recessive (e.g., ornithine transcarbamoylase deficiency). Many conditions inherited via maternal mitochondrial DNA are being recognized, and there may be a considerable range in these conditions (in terms of organ systems involved and the severity of involvement).[137]

Although there are a bewildering number of inborn errors of metabolism (the number of recognized conditions is expanding rapidly), many are amenable to therapy, and screening may be performed using relatively simple tests. Patients with incurable conditions may derive considerable relief of suffering from diagnosis and appropriate therapy. Even when a condition is not amenable to therapy, it is important to make a diagnosis to facilitate counseling for the family involved and prevent unnecessary suffering in future children. Long-term management of most inborn errors of metabolism requires a team approach, including metabolic experts, dietitians, geneticists, biochemists, and social workers, to elucidate the exact nature of the problem, provide appropriate therapy and therapeutic plans, and give genetic and family counseling. Although many screening tests for inborn errors of metabolism can be done in most diagnostic laboratories, the specialized tests required to identify the exact nature of an inborn error of metabolism can be done at relatively few laboratories. Despite the complexity of inborn errors of metabolism, there are principles that apply to the management of all children who are admitted to a PICU, and these should apply in inborn errors of metabolism (see Table 179-1).

WHEN TO CONSIDER AN INBORN ERROR OF METABOLISM IN THE PEDIATRIC INTENSIVE CARE UNIT

Inborn errors of metabolism may be classified into three diagnostically useful groups[138]: (1) disorders involving complex molecules in which symptoms are permanent, progressive, and independent of intercurrent events (e.g., peroxisomal disorders, lysosomal disorders, and congenital defects of glycosylation); (2) disorders that give rise to intoxication (e.g., organic acidemias and urea cycle defects); and (3) disorders involving energy metabolism (e.g., fatty acid oxidation defects and respiratory chain defects). The conditions most likely to present acutely in the PICU are conditions involving intoxication and energy metabolism. There is overlap, however, between all of these groups in terms of clinical presentation. There also may be considerable variation in the clinical presentation of conditions that have the same underlying genetic abnormality; this may apply even within families.

Although the clinical features of an inborn error of metabolism may be related primarily to the accumulation of a toxic metabolite, the condition may be complicated by the relative deficiency of another compound or increased stress put on other metabolic pathways by the primary problem.[139] Management may involve limiting the intake of potentially toxic substances, increasing the removal of toxic substances, supplementation of deficient substances, and supplementation of other metabolic pathways that are being stressed.

Inborn errors of metabolism should be considered as part of the differential diagnosis of any child or infant who presents with a severe illness, particularly during the neonatal period.[140] Acute symptoms that are particularly associated with inborn errors of metabolism include encephalopathy (acute or acute on chronic), intractable seizures, hepatic failure, cardiomyopathy, metabolic acidosis, and hypoglycemia (Table 179-3). Family history of SIDS or of previous childhood deaths may suggest an inborn error of metabolism. Particular attention should be paid to the identification of particular risk factors for the differential diagnoses, including drug exposure, prolonged rupture of membranes, and perinatal asphyxial episodes.

SPECIFIC CLINICAL PRESENTATIONS

Intractable Seizures

Seizures generally are an uncommon presentation of inborn errors of metabolism and, with the exception of the pyridoxine-dependent seizures, tend to be associated with other clinical and metabolic abnormalities. In a neonate presenting with intractable seizures, pyridoxine-dependent seizures[141] must be considered. These seizures have characteristic electroencephalogram patterns and respond to treatment with pyridoxine, although the dose required may vary considerably.[142] The diagnosis can be confirmed by correction of the electroencephalogram abnormalities and termination of seizure on administration of intravenous pyridoxine (initially 100 mg with increased doses to 500 mg if there is no initial response[142]). There is a considerable range in clinical presentation, and pyridoxine-dependent seizures probably

should be considered in any infant up to age 18 months presenting with seizures.[143] Data suggest that pyridoxine supplementation may improve seizure control in children with long-term convulsive disorders.[144]

Patients with defects in transport of glucose across the blood-brain barrier associated with mutations in the *GLUT1* gene may present with seizures. The only clue is the presence of low cerebrospinal fluid glucose in the presence of normal blood glucose. Patients may improve on a ketogenic diet.

Inborn errors of metabolism that may present with seizures associated with lactic acidosis include biotinidase deficiency, disorders of mitochondrial energy metabolism (including pyruvate dehydrogenase deficiency and mitochondrial electron transport chain defects), and peroxisomal and storage disorders. Biotinidase deficiency may present with myoclonic seizures,[145] although other forms of seizure also may occur.[146] The seizures occur in association with failure to thrive, a skin rash, and a severe metabolic acidosis, although the seizures may precede the occurrence of other clinical signs. Deafness is also a common feature.[147] Onset of symptoms is usually during infancy, but there are reports of onset of symptoms during childhood and adolescence.[148] Diagnosis can be made from analysis of organic acids in urine, whereas an enzyme assay can be done on blood. Administration of 20 mg of biotin causes resolution of symptoms.

Intractable tonic-clonic seizures also may be a feature of molybdenum cofactor deficiency.[149,150] This condition presents in early infancy with seizures, encephalopathy in the absence of metabolic acidosis, hypoglycemia or hyperammonemia, and failure to thrive. Imaging of the brain initially shows cerebral edema, which may progress to cerebral atrophy. There are typical computed tomography and magnetic resonance imaging findings.[151,152] Clinical features, computed tomography findings, and neuropathology may be similar to that seen in severe hypoxic-ischemic brain injury.[153,154] Lens dislocation may be a clinical feature.[155] Uric acid levels are low, whereas urinary amino acid analysis shows increased

TABLE 179–3. FACTORS THAT SHOULD ALERT THE INTENSIVIST TO THE POSSIBILITY OF AN INBORN ERROR OF METABOLISM

History

General	Population group with high incidence of inborn errors of metabolism
	Consanguinity of parents
	Previous history of apparent SIDS or childhood deaths in the family
	Presence of dysmorphic features associated with inborn error of metabolism
In neonatal period	Deterioration after apparently being normal at birth, particularly if Apgar scores and early neonatal period were normal
	Earliest signs of inborn error of metabolism in the neonatal period may include lethargy and poor feeding, which may progress rapidly to obvious depressed level of consciousness
	Depressed level of consciousness without obvious explanation
	Vomiting is an unusual clinical feature of illness in neonates and is strongly associated with inborn errors of metabolism
	Strange odors
In childhood	Previous history of being "sickly" with episodes of intermittent vomiting

Examination

General In neonatal period	Dysmorphic features that may be associated with inborn errors of metabolism
	Strange odors
	Neurologic signs in inborn errors of metabolism tend to include increased tone and abnormal movements, in contrast to the features of sepsis, which usually is associated with decreased tone
In childhood	Acute or intermittent ataxia is a common feature of inborn errors of metabolism in children

SIDS, sudden infant death syndrome.

S-sulfocysteine. Sulfite may be demonstrated on fresh urine specimens. Electrospray tandem mass spectrometry of urine or urine-soaked filter paper may facilitate rapid diagnosis.[156]

Seizures may be part of the clinical presentation of many other disorders, including seizures with lactic acidosis (Leigh disease; mitochondrial encephalopathy, lactic acidosis, and strokelike episodes [MELAS]; mitochondrial encephalopathy with ragged red fibers [MERRF]), GM$_2$ gangliosidosis, and peroxisomal disorders. Other clinical features predominate in these conditions and should direct investigation.

Investigation and Management

In infants presenting primarily with intractable seizures, investigations should include measurement of blood glucose, blood acid-base status, blood lactic acid (in association with pyruvate levels), cerebrospinal fluid glucose, lactic acid and pyruvic acid levels, urinary organic acids, and sulfite. Computed tomography and magnetic resonance imaging help to diagnose disorders of abnormal accumulation of metabolites and exclude structural brain problems that are responsible for symptoms.

Treatment focuses on control of the airway and respiration together with control of seizures. Pyridoxine or biotin should be administered early in appropriate doses if indicated.

Encephalopathy

The onset of acute encephalopathy always constitutes a medical emergency, and the cause must be elucidated as rapidly as possible. The differential diagnosis includes trauma, infection, intracranial space-occupying lesions, toxin ingestion, acute hepatic failure or Reye's syndrome, intracranial vascular problems (including thrombosis, hemorrhage, and embolic phenomena), and seizure disorders. There is often a strong tendency to attribute neurologic symptoms to hypoglycemia or hypocalcemia, but because these may be associated with inborn errors of metabolism it is vital to consider the inborn error of metabolism as part of the cause of the hypoglycemia.

The inborn errors of metabolism that present with acute encephalopathy vary with age. In the neonatal period, the common inborn errors of metabolism include urea cycle defects (with hyperammonemia), maple syrup urine disease, nonketotic hyperglycinemia, and organic acidopathies.[131] All of these conditions, with the exception of nonketotic hyperglycinemia, also may present during childhood. During childhood, the common inborn errors of metabolism presenting with acute encephalopathy include fatty acid oxidation defects and maple syrup urine disease.

Investigation

The specimens that normally would be collected for diagnosis of sepsis should be collected, including blood culture, hemoglobin, white blood cell count (including differential), and platelets. Serum electrolytes should be checked, including sodium, potassium, calcium, phosphate, and magnesium. Liver function tests are essential because acute hepatic failure may cause acute encephalopathy, and the liver may be affected by inborn errors of metabolism. Specimens for testing for inborn errors of metabolism must be collected at the time of presentation because this may provide the best opportunity for diagnosis (Table 179-4).

Blood Glucose Levels. The reader is referred to the earlier discussion of the approach to hypoglycemia. Hypoglycemia may be a particular feature of fatty acid oxidation defects and organic acidurias. Immediate correction of hypoglycemia is an essential element of treatment.

Plasma Ammonia Levels. Plasma ammonia levels should be checked in all children, particularly neonates, with unexplained depressed level of consciousness, particularly if there is hypotonia and apnea (see section on hyperammonemia for management and investigation). Treatment of severe hyperammonemia is an emergency.

Liver Function Tests. Reye's syndrome is part of the differential diagnosis of acute encephalopathy, but fatty acid oxidation defects, such as medium-chain acyl-CoA dehydrogenase deficiency, carnitine deficiency (usually with associated myopathy), and, far less frequently, long-chain acyl-CoA dehydrogenase deficiency and short-chain acyl-CoA dehydrogenase deficiency, may present with encephalopathy (usually in the neonatal period).

Blood Gas Analysis. Arterial blood gas analysis should be performed with particular attention to the presence of metabolic acidosis and calculation of the anion gap (this should be corrected for the presence of hypoalbuminemia).[157-159]

Blood Lactate Levels. Blood lactate levels may be increased in many situations, but typically are very elevated in mitochondrial electron transport chain defects.

Plasma Carnitine. Levels of carnitine may be substantially decreased in organic acidurias and fatty acid oxidation defects. Analysis of acyl carnitine and amino acid profile may help to make the diagnosis of isovaleric aciduria, methylmalonic aciduria, and propionic acidemia.

Quantitative Amino Acid Analysis. Quantitative amino acid analysis is necessary to identify the aminoacidopathies. This test is not always available, and results may take some time. Screening tests on the urine may point in the direction of certain conditions.

Urinary and Blood Ketones. Ketones are unusual in the neonatal period but tend to be a feature of maple syrup urine disease and propionic, isovaleric, and methylmalonic acidemia. Quantitative determination of blood ketones (acetoacetate using urine ketone strips or β-hydroxybutyrate by specific blood strip) may be a useful bedside screen.

Urinary Organic Acids. Urinary organic acids are abnormal in maple syrup urine disease, organic aciduria, and fatty acid oxidation defects.

Management

The principles of therapy are as follows:

1. Maintain airway control and breathing.
2. Maintain circulation.
3. Treat underlying or associated sepsis.
4. Remove toxic compounds.
5. Ensure an appropriate energy source for the body.
6. Provide any specific therapy that is available.

The toxic compounds that potentially can be removed include ammonia and leucine (see details subsequently).

Specific Conditions

Maple Syrup Urine Disease. If there is no acidosis and the ammonia is not increased, maple syrup urine disease should be considered. Patients typically are not dehydrated, are not acidotic, have no hyperammonemia, and have no hematologic abnormalities. Cerebral edema is a feature of maple syrup urine disease within the neonatal period and during later presentations.

TABLE 179–4. SPECIMEN COLLECTION FOR INBORN ERRORS OF METABOLISM

Substance	Tests	Comments on Technique	Conditions Identified
Urine	Detecting odors	Urine odors are best identified from urine drying on filter papers or from urine that has been kept in a closed container at room temperature for a while	MSUD (smell of maple syrup; some describe this as burnt sugar[133]) Isovaleric acidemia (sweaty feet odor) 3-methylcrotonyl glycinuria (catlike)
Urine Screening tests	Ketones		Urinary ketones are rare in neonates and are almost diagnostic of an inborn error of metabolism in a neonate
	Dinitrophenylhydrazine		Strongly positive with MSUD, PKU, or in ketoacidosis
	Ferric chloride		Green color with PKU; other colors may occur with other conditions
	Merckoquant 10013 Sulfit test	Urine specimen must be fresh because sulfite oxidizes rapidly at room temperature	Molybdenum cofactor deficiency
	Reducing substances		Galactosemia
Urine	Measurement of organic acids and amino acids	Specimen collected and frozen at −20°C	All aminoacidemias and organic acidurias
	Measurement of acyl carnitines and acyl glycines	Can increase the sensitivity of these tests by the use of loading dose of levocarnitine, 100 mg/kg orally	Many fatty acid oxidation defects
Blood	Anion gap	Correct for hypoalbuminemia	Screen to identify generally unmeasured anions
	Tandem mass spectrometry	Collected as blood on filter paper	All fatty acid oxidation defects, many of the aminoacidemias Abnormalities of the carnitine pathways
	Galactose-1-phosphate uridyltransferase	Collected as blood on filter paper	Galactosemia
	Estimation of ammonia, lactate, pyruvate, and ketoacids	All of these substances may be unstable; must collect on ice and transport immediately to laboratory	Aminoacidopathies, urea cycle defects
	Genetic studies	Before blood transfusion	All problems with identified genetic abnormalities Enzyme defects, organelle defects
Skin, liver, muscle, and endocardial biopsy	Fibroblast culture, enzyme identification, identification of abnormal collections and organelles		

MSUD, maple syrup urine disease; PKU, phenylketonuria.

The urine may smell like maple syrup, but the smell is also similar to that of burned sugar.[137] The urine smell may be difficult to detect in the first few days of life, then may be detected on diapers that have been allowed to dry.[160] Urine tests for ketones are usually strongly positive, and dinitrophenylhydrazine is usually positive, although both tests may be negative before 3 days of age.[160] Tandem mass spectrometry is the quickest and most efficient screening test in neonates. Leucine levels can be checked rapidly on whole-blood filter paper specimens, or quantitative amino acid analysis should be done on plasma or serum. Principles of management have been to remove leucine using dialysis and to reduce the production of leucine by dietary manipulation. Hemodialysis has been shown to decrease leucine levels rapidly,[161] particularly if used in conjunction with dietary therapy. Previously, exchange transfusion, peritoneal dialysis, and hemofiltration were reported to decrease leucine levels. Morton and colleagues[160] have used a protocol consisting of total caloric intake of 120 to 140 kcal/kg/day with lipid forming 40% to 50% of calories; 3 to 4 g/kg/day of protein as essential and nonessential amino acids with 80 to 120 mg/kg/day each of isoleucine and valine and 250 mg/kg/day each of glutamine and alanine, with tyrosine, histidine, and threonine supplemented to normalize plasma amino acid ratios; careful attention to sodium balance to ensure that serum sodium is kept at greater than 140 mEq/L; and hyperosmolar therapy if cerebral edema develops. This protocol produces decreases in leucine equal to that seen after dialysis.

Isovaleric Aciduria, Methylmalonic Aciduria, and Propionic Acidemia. Isovaleric aciduria, methylmalonic aciduria, and propionic acidemia may present in the neonatal period with encephalopathy, hyperammonemia, ketoacidosis (occasionally hyperammonemia may induce a respiratory alkalosis), moderate lactic acidosis, and hypocalcemia. The smell associated with isovaleric aciduria may be distinctive ("sweaty feet"). Blood glucose levels may be extremely variable from hypoglycemia to hyperglycemia. Dehydration is a feature of the clinical presentation, partly related to vomiting and poor intake and partly related to poor renal concentrating ability. One third of patients may present later during infancy, childhood, adolescence, or adulthood.

Strokelike episodes are a feature of isovaleric aciduria, methylmalonic aciduria, and propionic acidemia in later life, although there may be a wide range of neurologic presentations, including hypotonia and developmental delay. Extrapyramidal signs related to infarction of the basal ganglia may be a feature of methylmalonic aciduria and propionic acidemia. Neutropenia, thrombocytopenia, and anemia are common in the neonatal presentation, whereas neutropenia also may be a feature of a later presentation. Sepsis may be a significant component of clinical exacerbations, particularly in propionic acidemia.[162] Pancreatitis has been reported to be associated with these disorders.[163] Cardiomyopathy also may develop, particularly during metabolic decompensation.[164] Isovaleric aciduria, propionic acidemia, and methylmalonic aciduria are diagnosed by the organic acid profiles, and tandem mass spectroscopy may be useful by looking at the acyl carnitine profiles.

Patients presenting in the neonatal period with encephalopathy require treatment with limitation of protein intake (this rapidly requires adjustment to a diet with appropriate amino acid profile), removal of toxin (exchange transfusion may be useful; methylmalonic aciduria can be cleared renally if adequate fluid volumes are given), ensuring normal glucose levels, promoting anabolism, fluid management to avoid overhydration and dehydration, and management of sepsis. Some patients with methylmalonic aciduria may respond to therapy with hydroxycobalamine, and this should be given for several days to assess response. Supplemental glycine should be given to patients with isovaleric aciduria, and carnitine supplementation is useful for all. Some patients with propionic acidemia may benefit from metronidazole to decrease propionate metabolites from the bowel.

Nonketotic Hyperglycinemia. Nonketotic hyperglycinemia (nonketotic hyperglycinemia) presents in early infancy with severe encephalopathy in the absence of acidosis, ketosis, hypoglycemia, hyperammonemia, or any other clinical abnormalities. Although the outcome is almost invariably poor, there have been more recent descriptions of transient neonatal hyperglycinemia.[165] There also is an association of abnormality of the corpus callosum with nonketotic hyperglycinemia.[166] Diagnosis is confirmed by the presence of high cerebrospinal fluid glycine, although this may be difficult to interpret in some patients. The enzyme defect can be confirmed on a liver biopsy specimen.[167] Sodium benzoate may be helpful in therapy,[168] possibly in combination with imipramine.[169]

Hypoglycemia

The reader is referred to the section on endocrine crises for an endocrine approach to hypoglycemia. In hyperinsulinemia, the hypoglycemia typically develops soon after the intake of a feed, whereas patients with defects in fatty acid oxidation tend to be able to tolerate fasts of 4 to 8 hours. In hyperinsulinemia, it often is difficult to provide adequate amounts of glucose to correct the hypoglycemia (may require >12 mg/kg/min together with glucagon to control the hypoglycemia). In defects of gluconeogenesis, the hypoglycemia is relatively easy to control, but usually does not respond to glucagon administration. In hereditary fructose intolerance, the onset of hypoglycemia is concurrent with the introduction of sucrose (source of fructose) into the diet. In patients with defects in fatty acid oxidation, hypoglycemia does not usually develop after a short period of fasting. Although hypoglycemia may occur in association with sepsis, many inborn errors of metabolism are associated with sepsis (e.g., direct association with *Escherichia coli* and galactosemia, sepsis as precipitant of crisis, or ill health from inborn error of metabolism causing increased risk of sepsis) and should be considered diagnostically even if sepsis is proven.

Investigation and Management

If the glucose level is low, a venous specimen of blood should be collected immediately for laboratory glucose estimation (because bedside measuring techniques may be inaccurate at low levels of glucose). The clinician should give 0.5 g/kg of 10% to 25% dextrose in water (diluted with water for injection) promptly as a bolus intravenously followed by administration of 4 to 8 mg/kg/min of glucose. The glucose level should be reviewed within 30 minutes. The rate of glucose infusion may need to be increased, and high requirements suggest hyperinsulinemia.

Urine for Reducing Substances. Glucose should be excluded, but in the setting of hypoglycemia this is unlikely unless there have been substantial doses of glucose given. If reducing substances are positive, this suggests galactosemia, hereditary fructosemia, or tyrosinemia.

Urinary Ketones. If urinary ketones are positive, the clinician should look for abnormalities of the amino acids or organic acids (urinary and plasma organic acids and quantitative amino acids). High urinary ketones in the presence of hepatomegaly suggest of glycogen storage disease type 1, fructose-1,6-diphosphatase (FDPase) deficiency, or β-ketothiolase deficiency.[170] In the last-mentioned condition, lactate levels are normal, whereas they are increased in glycogen storage disease type 1 and FDPase deficiency. In the absence of hepatomegaly, high ketones suggest ketotic hypoglycemia or deficiencies of growth hormone or glucocorticoids.

Plasma Free Fatty Acids. If plasma free fatty acids are elevated, the patient is likely to have a fatty acid oxidation defect, but if they are low, hyperinsulinemia is more likely.

Lactate Levels. Lactic acidosis in association with hypoglycemia is characteristic of defects of gluconeogenesis, such as glycogen storage diseases.

Urinary Organic Acids, Plasma Amino Acids, and Ammonia Levels. Urinary organic acids, plasma amino acids, and ammonia levels should be measured as part of the diagnostic approach to hypoglycemia because hypoglycemia may be a feature of abnormalities of all these systems.

Specific Conditions

Galactosemia. The reader is referred to the subsequent section on hepatitis. Hypoglycemia may be a prominent feature of galactosemia, whereas hepatitis may be a more common presentation.

Hereditary Fructose Intolerance. Hereditary fructose intolerance is characterized by the onset of severe vomiting and hypoglycemia after the ingestion of fructose or sucrose.

Glycogen Storage Disease Type 1. Glycogen storage disease type 1 may present in the neonatal period with hypoglycemia. The hypoglycemia may be mild or easily controlled, however, with the result that the patients present later with hepatomegaly and lactic acidosis. Characteristically, hypoglycemia related to glycogen storage disease type 1 does not respond to therapy with glucagon.

Fatty Acid Oxidation Defects. Fatty acids are metabolized primarily via the β-oxidation cycle in the mitochondria and to a lesser extent in the peroxisomes (β-oxidation) and the microsomes (ω-oxidation). Defects in the mitochondrial oxidation of free fatty acid result in the accumulation of fatty acid oxidation products, which may be responsible for encephalopathy; hepatocellular dysfunction; and cardiac arrhythmias, which are a potentially fatal complication of fatty acid oxidation defects. Defects in fatty acid oxidation also may result in failure to meet the energy requirements of tissues such as skeletal muscles or cardiac muscles, resulting in myopathy or cardiomyopathy. Because tissues have to rely on glucose for energy, hypoglycemia may result. Finally, secondary carnitine deficiency may arise resulting in hypoglycemia, hyperammonemia, myopathy, and cardiomyopathy.

Many studies have suggested that fatty acid oxidation defects may be an important cause of sudden infant death.[136] Fatty acid oxidation defects are an important cause of cardiomyopathy[171] (see discussion of cardiomyopathy). Disorders such as medium-chain acyl-CoA dehydrogenase deficiency typically present with acute or recurrent Reye-like episodes with vomiting, encephalopathy, hypoglycemia, and hyperammonemia.

Medium-chain acyl CoA deficiency is the most common of the fatty acid oxidation defects and most frequently presents with a Reye-like episode. Cardiomyopathy never occurs in medium-chain acyl CoA deficiency. Cardiomyopathy is a more common presentation of carnitine deficiency and long-chain acyl-CoA dehydrogenase deficiency.

Diagnosis is based on the clinical features described earlier: tolerance of 8 to 24 hours of fasting, high plasma free fatty acid levels, normal to low ketone levels, increased urinary organic acids (C-6 to C-10 dicarboxylic acids), and low plasma carnitine levels. The abnormal findings may not be present between acute exacerbations, and it is crucial to collect specimens during the acute illness. Urine specimens must be collected; blood can be collected on filter paper for tandem mass spectrometry (these assays may be abnormal while the child is well). Specific mutation analysis is available for the most common medium-chain acyl-CoA deficiency. Treatment consists of supplying adequate glucose, supplementing carnitine, and providing symptomatic support.

Hyperammonemia

Transient hyperammonemia may occur in preterm infants in so-called transient hyperammonemia of the newborn, which is not associated with an inborn error of metabolism. Aggressive therapy may be associated with completely normal outcome. Hyperammonemia results in a marked encephalopathy, although patients typically are more hypotonic than in other metabolic encephalopathies and may develop a respiratory alkalosis, which is uncommon in other encephalopathies.

Primary hyperammonemia occurs in the urea cycle defects, but a secondary hyperammonemia may occur in defects of fatty acid oxidation (including carnitine-acyl-carnitine acyltranslocase), organic acidemia (including propionic acidemia, methylmalonic acidemia, isovaleric acidemia, holocarboxylase synthetase deficiency, and 3-hydroxy-3-methylglutaryl-CoA lyase deficiency). Hyperammonemia also may be a consequence of acute hepatic failure (e.g., with acute viral infection; toxin ingestion; and drug reactions, particularly antituberculosis drugs).

Investigation

Ammonia is potentially toxic, and therapy must be instituted urgently to remove ammonia. It is crucial to collect appropriate diagnostic specimens at the time of presentation because it may be difficult to establish a diagnosis when dialysis and other therapy have been instituted. The following tests enable an approach to diagnosis.[172]

Plasma Ammonium Levels. Hyperammonemia with levels of greater than 250 μmol/L typically are associated with urea cycle defects or transient hyperammonemia of the newborn.

Arterial Blood Gas Analysis. Hyperammonemia with urea cycle defects and transient hyperammonemia of the newborn are not associated with acidosis. Patients often may have a respiratory alkalosis. A metabolic acidosis is more likely to be associated with organic acidopathies.

Tests of the Urea Cycle. Tests of the urea cycle include plasma citrulline, urinary argininosuccinic acid synthetase, and urinary orotic acid.

Amino Acids (Quantitative). Quantitative amino acids may be difficult to interpret, but help with diagnosis of conditions such as methylmalonic aciduria, isovaleric aciduria and propionic acidemia.

Carnitine Levels and Acyl Carnitine Analysis. Carnitine and the acyl carnitines may be affected as part of the aminoacidemias.

Management

Principles of management for hyperammonemia consist of the following:

1. Provide intravenous glucose and lipid to decrease ammonia production from endogenous protein breakdown.
2. Administer intravenous arginine (L-arginine hydrochloride, 600 mg/kg intravenously over 1 hour, followed by 2 to 4 mmol/kg/24 h in four divided doses).
3. Administer intravenous sodium benzoate (250 mg/kg intravenously followed by 250 mg/kg/day in four divided doses) and sodium phenylacetate (250 mg/kg intravenously immediately followed by 250 mg/kg/24 h in four divided doses).
4. Dialyze to remove excessive ammonia. Hemodialysis is the most efficient means to remove ammonia, hemofiltration is the next option (and may be particularly useful in neonates who are too unstable to tolerate hemodialysis), and finally peritoneal dialysis may be used. Exchange transfusion has been performed, but is relatively inefficient at removal of ammonia.

Metabolic Acidosis

Metabolic acidosis can occur in many ways. It may be related to inadequate excretion of acid via the kidneys (e.g., proximal and distal renal tubular acidosis) or excessive production of acid in the body. In the case of inadequate excretion of acid from the kidneys, the pH of the urine almost always is inappropriately high. In addition, there is no anion gap. In the context of excessive acid production, there is an excessive anion gap.

The most common acids related to an increased anion gap are lactic acid and ketoacids, such as acetoacetate and 3-butyrobutyrate. All the organic acidopathies and aminoacidopathies may be associated with an increased anion gap, however. A variety of inborn errors of metabolism may be associated with proximal renal tubular acidosis, particularly cystinosis and Lowe syndrome.

Acid also may be produced by bacterial overgrowth in the bowel and absorbed as occurs in D-lactic acidosis.[173] D-Lactic acid is not detected by routine blood tests for lactic acid, which employ a lactic dehydrogenase, but is detected by urinary assays for organic acids. These patients present with acidosis with increased anion gap.

Patients with organic acidemias rarely present with metabolic acidosis as a primary feature of the illness, and the rest of the clinical presentation frequently provides clues as to the appropriate line of investigation. Investigation of organic acids remains an important component of the investigation of any patient, however, with unexplained metabolic acidosis.

Lactic Acidosis

Lactic acidosis is associated with inadequate oxygenation of tissues, as occurs in hypoxemia or in shock. In this situation, treatment consists of ensuring adequate oxygen content of blood and appropriate cardiac output.

So-called primary lactic acidosis occurs in the absence of hypoxemia and shock. Lactate accumulates either as a consequence of increased production of lactate or because of inadequate clearance and metabolism of lactate (primarily in the liver). Accumulation of lactate may occur without the development of acidosis, depending on the compensatory mechanisms. Many patients with congenital lactic acidosis have increased lactate levels with no acidosis between episodes of exacerbation, although episodes of exacerbation usually are associated with severe lactic acidosis.

Congenital lactic acidoses are variable in presentation, ranging from severe neonatal lactic acidosis with generally poor prognosis to children with milder defects and other children with syndromes such as the MELAS and MERRF syndromes and Leigh disease. In many of these conditions, the lactic acidosis is completely or partially overshadowed by the other clinical features of the conditions. Not all children with defects of mitochondrial energy metabolism have elevated levels.

Lactate production may be caused by increased glycolysis (e.g., glycogen storage disease type 1, hereditary fructose intolerance) or by decreased oxidation of pyruvate. Oxidation of pyruvate can be limited by many conditions, including the following:

1. Pyruvate dehydrogenase complex deficiency
2. Primary pyruvate carboxylase or holocarboxylase deficiency (this is related to biotin/biotinidase deficiency)
3. Electron transport chain defects (associated with increased lactate pyruvate ratios in blood and cerebrospinal fluid)

The clinical course of pyruvate dehydrogenase deficiency may be extremely variable, and diagnosis is confirmed by studies of enzyme activity in cultured fibroblasts. The lactic acidosis in pyruvate dehydrogenase deficiency can be ameliorated by a ketogenic diet,[174] although many factors must be considered before embarking on a ketogenic diet, including the protein content of the diet, particularly if there is associated renal failure, and the long-term problems of ketogenic diets.[175] Dichloroacetic acid may be helpful in some cases.[176] Many cases have been reported in which thiamine was associated with clinical improvement, although high levels may be required.[177]

Lactic acidosis occurs in all of the conditions affecting the metabolism of pyruvate through the tricarboxylic acid cycle. Abnormalities include pyruvate dehydrogenase deficiency and mitochondrial energy cycle defects. The mitochondrial energy cycle problems frequently are associated with persistent lactic acidosis, myopathy, failure to thrive, psychomotor retardation, and seizures. Other symptoms that may be present in mitochondrial energy conditions in children include antenatal problems,[178] cardiomyopathy[179,180] and cardiac arrhythmias,[181] sensorineural hearing loss,[182]

stroke and abnormalities of central respiratory drive,[183] and diabetes mellitus.[184]

Acquired defects in mitochondrial function have been associated with severe lactic acidosis in adults and children on antiretroviral therapy.[185] Lactic acidosis also may be a secondary phenomenon of defects of organic acid metabolism, including 3-hydroxy-3-methylglutaryl-CoA lyase deficiency, propionic acidemia, and methylmalonic acidemia.

Ketoacidosis

Primary defects in ketone use are rare but include β-ketothiolase deficiency, which may respond rapidly to administration of intravenous glucose. Ketoacidosis is a common feature of many of the organic acidemias, including maple syrup urine disease, methylmalonic acidemia, propionic acidemia, and isovaleric aciduria. Investigation of patients with ketoacidosis should include measurement of urinary organic acids.

Cardiomyopathy

A wide variety of inborn errors of metabolism may present with cardiomyopathy or cardiac arrhythmias. In most of these conditions, other clinical problems and symptoms predominate (e.g., in glycogen storage disease, organic acidopathies), and the cardiomyopathy is just part of an overall picture. In these situations, the diagnosis is assisted by the associations.

A few conditions may present with cardiac problems apparently in isolation. In the differential diagnosis of myocarditis/cardiomyopathy, many conditions need to be excluded, including carnitine deficiency, trifunctional protein defects or isolated long-chain 3-hydroxyacyl-CoA dehydrogenase deficiency. In the latter two conditions, urinary organic acid analysis *at the time of the acute illness* shows the presence of medium-chain and long-chain dicarboxylic acids. At least one form of very-long-chain acyl-CoA dehydrogenase deficiency can present as an acute cardiomyopathy. For all these conditions, measurement of acyl carnitines using tandem mass spectrometry allows diagnosis. Diagnosis is confirmed using enzyme activity in cultured fibroblasts. At least one case report[186] shows that substantial clinical improvement can be achieved by elimination of long-chain fatty acids from the diet (replacing with medium-chain fatty acids). Many of the disorders of the mitochondrial energy chain have poor myocardial function as a component of their multiple symptoms, but echocardiography may be needed to show more subtle features of poor contractility.

Hepatopathology

Inborn errors of metabolism can affect the liver in a variety of ways. Patients may present with symptoms ranging from acute hepatic failure to hepatomegaly to chronic hepatitis to cirrhosis. The hepatic dysfunction may present in apparent isolation or in association with cardiac, cerebral, muscle, and renal disease. The presentations of "hepatitis" may be virtually indistinguishable from the presentation of acute viral hepatitis or toxin ingestion.

In one study of infants presenting to a transplant service in acute hepatic failure, inborn errors of metabolism were responsible for the hepatic failure in 42.5% of the patients. Of these patients, 35% had hepatorenal tyrosinemia, whereas 50% had mitochondrial abnormalities. Hereditary fructose intolerance and galactosemia together were present in less than 9% of patients.[187]

Hepatorenal tyrosinemia may present in the neonatal period as acute hepatic failure. It is difficult to distinguish from acute viral hepatitis because plasma amino acid levels may be similar in both situations. Alpha-fetoprotein levels may be substantially elevated in hepatorenal tyrosinemia and may be a distinguishing feature. The coagulopathy tends to be relatively severe in hepatorenal tyrosinemia, and coagulopathy may be the only presenting feature of hepatorenal tyrosinemia.[188] Patients tend to have moderate-to-severe anemia. The response to treatment with 2-(2-nitro-4-trifluoromethylbenzoyl)-1,3-cyclohexandion (NTBC) may be dramatic,[189,190] although some patients do not respond. Hepatocellular carcinoma has occurred in some patients after response to NTBC.[191]

Galactosemia is characterized by the development of hypoglycemia in the neonatal period in association with jaundice (initially unconjugated, but subsequently conjugated), marked increase in transaminase levels, some abnormality of coagulation, and moderate hypoalbuminemia. Severe cerebral edema occasionally may be a dominant feature. Management has been reviewed elsewhere.[192] There is a close association with *Escherichia coli* septicemia, and any infant presenting with *E. coli* septicemia should be investigated for galactosemia. Galactosuria clears rapidly if feeds are stopped.

A screening test is available on blood collected on filter paper (semiquantitative measure of galactose-1-phosphate uridyltransferase). The diagnosis can be confirmed on a quantitative measurement of galactose-1-phosphate uridyltransferase. Wilson's disease may present as acute hepatitis, but rarely before age 5 years.

ANNOTATED REFERENCES

Boles RG, Buck EA, Blitzer MG, et al: Retrospective biochemical screening of fatty acid oxidation disorders in post-mortem livers of 418 cases of sudden death in the first year of life. J Pediatr 1998;132:924-933.

The authors devised a biochemical protocol for evaluation of frozen post-mortem liver specimens for defects of fatty acid oxidation. On review of specimens from 418 cases of sudden death in the first year of life, *the authors were able to identify 14 cases that closely matched the biochemical profiles seen in fatty acid oxidation defects. No cases of death due to abuse or accidents tested positive. Of deaths that had been classified as infectious, 20% showed multiple abnormalities in the liver specimens, suggesting that fatty acid oxidation defects should be considered as part of the differential diagnosis of sudden or unexpected death, even when an infectious agent has been identified.*

Dunger DB, Sperling MA, Acerini CL, et al: ESPE/LWPES consensus statement on diabetic ketoacidosis in children and adolescents. Arch Dis Child 2004;89:188-194.

This is an extensive evidence-based review of acute diabetic ketoacidosis in children and adolescents. Consensus guidelines are presented with appropriate references for the management of acute diabetic ketoacidosis in children and adolescents.

Durand P, Debray D, Mandel R, et al: Acute liver failure in infancy: A 14-year experience of a pediatric liver transplantation center. J Pediatr 2001;139:871-876.

This article presents a 14-year review of 80 infants (children <1 year old) admitted to the pediatric hepatology unit or ICU of a French hospital with acute liver failure (defined as prothrombin time >17 seconds and factor V plasma levels <50% of normal). Acute liver failure was a result of inherited metabolic disorders in 42.5% of cases, including mitochondrial respiratory chain disorders, type 1 hereditary tyrosinemia, and urea cycle defects.

Marcin JP, Glaser N, Barnett P, et al: Factors associated with adverse outcomes in children with diabetic ketoacidosis-related cerebral edema. J Pediatr 2002;141:793-797.

This is a retrospective study of 61 children (≤18 years old) from 10 U.S. pediatric centers admitted between 1982 and 1997 with diabetic ketoacidosis and cerebral edema. Only 59% survived without neurologic sequelae, and 28% died or survived in a vegetative state. Intubation with hyperventilation was associated with adverse outcome after adjustment for confounding variables. Poor outcome also was associated with greater neurologic depression at the time of diagnosis and a higher initial serum urea nitrogen concentration.

Morton DH, Strauss KA, Robinson DL, et al: Diagnosis and treatment of maple syrup disease: A study of 36 patients. Pediatrics 2002;109:999-1008.

This article evaluates an approach to the diagnosis and treatment of maple syrup urine disease. Eighteen neonates were diagnosed as having maple syrup urine disease between 12 and 24 hours of age using amino acid analysis of plasma or whole blood collected on filter paper. No infant identified before 3 days of age and treated with the protocol became ill during the neonatal period. A further 18 neonates who were intoxicated at the time of diagnosis responded rapidly to the management protocol without the need for dialysis or hemoperfusion. Follow-up of the 36 infants over more than 219 patient-years showed generally good metabolic control, with good developmental outcome. A management protocol is presented.

Section XI

THE OBSTETRIC PATIENT

Chapter 180

CARDIOVASCULAR AND ENDOCRINOLOGIC CHANGES ASSOCIATED WITH PREGNANCY

Marie R. Baldisseri

KEY POINTS

1. Normal pregnancy is associated with numerous physiologic changes that affect almost all maternal organ systems.

2. **Hemodynamic, metabolic, hormonal, and structural changes that occur during pregnancy are adaptive mechanisms for** maintaining a healthy homeostasis between the mother and the fetus.

3. **Maternal hemodynamic alterations and poor fetal outcome can occur if the physiologic adaptive mechanisms are insufficient to** maintain the normal homeostasis between the mother and the fetus.

4. The physiologic changes occur at different stages throughout the pregnancy.

5. The normal physiologic changes of pregnancy may alter the presentation of a maternal disease process, confound the diagnosis, or alter the endpoints of treatment.

6. **Cardiac output is increased significantly, up to 50%** above prepartum values, by the 24th week of gestation. The value then plateaus until term. **During labor and delivery, cardiac output is further increased** with uterine contractions and the "autotransfusion" effect of increased preload after delivery of the fetus and placenta.

7. **The increase in cardiac output** early in pregnancy is primarily **caused by an increase in blood volume.** Later in pregnancy, **an increase in the heart rate** by 15 to 20 beats/min is mainly responsible for the increase in cardiac output. Improved myocardial contractility may account in part for an improvement in cardiac output in pregnancy.

8. Maternal body position directly affects cardiac output and stroke volume. **In the supine position, the gravid uterus causes aortocaval compression and decreased preload.** An extreme manifestation of this effect is the "supine hypotensive syndrome" of pregnancy.

9. **After the 20th week of gestation,** pregnant women should not be placed supine but rather in the **left lateral recumbent position,** which maximizes

maternal hemodynamics. During cardiac resuscitation, the pregnant patient should be placed in this position, or **manual displacement of the uterus to the left is acceptable.**

10. Left ventricular end-diastolic volume is increased during pregnancy, but **filling pressures are relatively unchanged;** this may reflect the decrease in afterload caused by a decrease in systemic and pulmonary vascular resistance.

11. **Blood volume increases by 30% to 50%** by the end of gestation. However, red blood cell mass increases by only 15% to 20%, creating the **"physiologic anemia"** of pregnancy.

12. **A pregnant woman can lose up to 35% of her blood volume before tachycardia and hypotension occur as** a result of acute hemorrhage or severe hypovolemia.

13. Blood flow is increased to many organs during pregnancy, especially to the breasts, uterus, and kidneys. Renal blood flow increases by 25% to 50%, and the **glomerular filtration rate increases by up to 50%,** with a decrease in the plasma creatinine and blood urea nitrogen concentrations.

14. **A decrease in the diastolic blood pressure by 10% is seen in the second trimester,** secondary to the decrease in systemic vascular resistance. By the end of pregnancy, blood pressure levels should increase to prepartum values.

15. Blood vessel remodeling and changes in the coagulation system during pregnancy, including an increase in most clotting factors, makes the **pregnant woman hypercoagulable and more susceptible to venous thromboembolism** throughout pregnancy and in the postpartum period.

16. Remodeling of the heart causes enlargement of all four chambers. The pregnant woman may be more **susceptible to supraventricular and atrial arrhythmias** because of left atrial enlargement.

17. Systolic ejection murmurs and a third heart sound can commonly be heard during pregnancy. **Diastolic, pansystolic, and late systolic murmurs should prompt the clinician to look for an underlying cardiac problem.**

18. Pregnant patients with mild to moderate cardiac disease usually tolerate the hemodynamic changes of pregnancy. Those patients with **pulmonary hypertension and right-to-left shunts have mortality rates as high as 50%.**

19. There are numerous endocrine and metabolic alterations during pregnancy that primarily affect the hypothalamus, pituitary, and adrenal glands. As with cardiac disease, the presentation of a patient with endocrine and metabolic disorders may be difficult to differentiate from the normal hypermetabolic state of pregnancy.

20. Both corticotropin (ACTH) and cortisol levels are elevated in pregnancy. Cushing's syndrome can be exacerbated by pregnancy. **Acute adrenal crisis may be precipitated by the stress of labor and delivery.** The treatment is immediate glucocorticoid administration.

21. In preparation for lactation, prolactin levels are increased 10-fold throughout the pregnancy, as a result of estrogen and progesterone stimulation. This increase in prolactin may increase the size of pituitary adenomas and precipitate symptoms during the pregnancy.

22. Thyroid hormones are increased during pregnancy as a result of increased synthesis of thyroxine-binding globulin. Free levels are unchanged. Despite the complex thyroidal changes that occur during pregnancy, **pregnant women have no untoward complications if their daily iodine intake is sufficient.**

23. Transient diabetes insipidus can develop during pregnancy, secondary to a state of vasopressin resistance.

24. Large fluctuations in glucose and insulin levels are seen in pregnancy, depending on the nutritional state of the mother. Fasting glucose levels can decrease by 10% to 20%.

25. During pregnancy, there is **increased insulin secretion, with a relative state of insulin resistance.**

26. **Obese women with insulin resistance** and women with marginal pancreatic reserve **can develop gestational diabetes mellitus.**

27. **Fetal and neonatal mortality rates are low if strict metabolic glucose control with insulin therapy** is maintained.

28. Maternal lipid metabolism is increased during pregnancy, allowing for increased glucose utilization by the fetus.

Fundamental to the management of a critically ill pregnant woman is a thorough knowledge of the physiologic changes that occur during gestation and immediately after delivery. Clinicians must have a clear understanding of the extent of these changes, which occur in all pregnant women, to appropriately treat the critically ill patient whose additional pathology complicates the altered metabolic homeostasis and hemodynamics of the normal pregnant state. It is important to recognize that these physiologic changes add a level of complexity to diagnosis and management in the critically ill pregnant woman. The normal physiologic changes of pregnancy may alter the presentation of a disease process or illness during pregnancy. These physiologic changes may alter the interpretation of clinical and diagnostic examination findings in the pregnant woman. Subsequently, the endpoints of treatment can be significantly different than those for nonpregnant patients. Some of the physiologic changes associated with pregnancy occur early in the normal course of gestation, whereas others occur during the middle or later stages. The clinician must be aware of the timing of the physiologic changes in order to render the most effective care of critically ill pregnant patients. The physiologic changes of pregnancy affect almost all organ systems to varying degrees, depending, in part, on the gestational age of the fetus. Hemodynamic, metabolic, hormonal, and structural changes all occur during pregnancy. These changes allow for the natural growth and development of the fetus. The pregnant woman adapts remarkably well to these changes, as does the fetus, allowing the two to coexist without harm to the other. However, if the pregnant woman is ill, either from a preexisting, underlying disease process or from a new process that occurs during the pregnancy, the normal physiologic adaptive mechanisms of pregnancy can be insufficient to maintain the normal healthy union between mother and fetus. Depending on the severity of the underlying process or the new illness, the hemodynamic ramifications to the pregnant woman and the fetus can be devastating and life-threatening.

CARDIOVASCULAR CHANGES IN PREGNANCY

Cardiovascular and blood volume changes are among some of the more dramatic changes that occur in pregnancy (Table 180-1). These changes are primarily adaptive mechanisms, allowing the pregnant woman to accommodate her additional metabolic needs as well as those of the fetus during gestation and immediately after delivery. Cardiac output is significantly increased during pregnancy, by as much as 50% compared with nonpregnant values. Cardiac output is further increased in twin pregnancies and multiple gestations.[1] The dramatic rise in cardiac output is seen as early as the first 6 to 8 weeks of pregnancy.[2-4] After the 10th week of pregnancy, the cardiac output is increased by 1 to 1.5 L/min. Cardiac output reaches a maximum value by approximately the 20th to 24th week of gestation. The early increase in cardiac output is primarily caused by a significant increase in stroke volume. However, stroke volume decreases as the pregnancy advances because of aortocaval compression by the uterus and the pressure of the fetal presenting part on the common iliac vein. Caval compression occurs because the large gravid uterus rests on the vena cava, effectively decreasing venous return to the heart and therefore decreasing ventricular preload. In the latter half of pregnancy, a progressive increase in the maternal heart rate by 15 to 20 beats/min is primarily responsible for maintaining the elevated cardiac output. The additional increase in cardiac output before labor and delivery is caused by a further increase in heart rate. Resting cardiac output either is maintained or decreases slightly as term approaches.[2]

THE INFLUENCE OF BODY POSITION

Venous return is further compromised with changes in body position, particularly if the pregnant patient is supine. As a

TABLE 180–1. NORMAL HEMODYNAMIC CHANGES DURING PREGNANCY

Physiologic Parameter	Term Pregnancy	Labor and Delivery	Postpartum
Cardiac output	Increases 30-50%	Increases 50%	Increases 60-80% within 15-20 min
Blood volume	Increases 30-50%	Additional 300-500 mL with each contraction	Decreases to baseline
Heart rate	Increases by 15-20 beats/min	Increase depends on stress and pain relief	Decreases to baseline
Blood pressure	Decreases by 5-10 mm Hg in midpregnancy	Increase depends on stress and pain relief	Decreases to baseline
Systemic vascular resistance	Decreases	Increases	Decreases to baseline
Oxygen consumption	Increases by 20%	Increases with stress of labor and delivery	Decreases to baseline
Red blood cell mass	Increases by 15-20%	—	—

result, cardiac output can be diminished by as much as 25% to 30%. The effects of changes in body position are most obvious in the latter half of pregnancy, when the fetal size and gravid uterus can effectively tamponade the vena cava.[5] This phenomenon is exaggerated in women with poorly developed venous collaterals. With compression of the vena cava in the supine position, these women exhibit signs of severe hypoperfusion (hypotension and bradycardia), a phenomenon that is described as the "supine hypotensive syndrome" of pregnancy. The symptoms quickly resolve after the patient is repositioned to the left lateral recumbent position.[6] Cardiac output can decrease by 30% to 40% in patients with this syndrome. This vasovagal phenomenon underscores the influence of maternal body position on the hemodynamic alterations occurring in pregnancy.

Hemodynamic changes associated with a decrease in preload and, subsequently, a reduced cardiac output are less pronounced when the gravid uterus is minimally compressing the vena cava. This is optimally achieved by maintaining the pregnant woman with more than 20 weeks gestation in the full left lateral position whenever she is recumbent. Alternatives to this position, less optimal than the left lateral position but preferable to the supine position, are a left lateral tilt to 15 degrees or manual displacement of the gravid uterus. The latter maneuver of left uterine displacement can be performed by manually moving the uterus away from the midline to the left side when the patient is supine. This maneuver is particularly useful when performing cardiac compressions in a pregnant patient. In the supine position, the gravid uterus, which accounts for as much as 10% of the cardiac output, hinders successful resuscitation because of its adverse effects on intrathoracic pressure and venous return. Although hemodynamics are optimized in the left lateral position, it is difficult to achieve optimal chest compressions with the patient tilted all the way into the left lateral decubitus position. Acceptable alternatives are to perform cardiac compressions with the patient supine but with concurrent manual displacement of the uterus to the other side; it is also satisfactory to place a wedge under the right hip of the patient.[7,8]

OXYGEN CONSUMPTION AND VENTRICULAR PERFORMANCE

As cardiac output progressively increases, maternal oxygen consumption also increases. However, the increase in cardiac output is seen earlier than the rise in maternal oxygen consumption. Accordingly, the arteriovenous oxygen difference actually narrows early in pregnancy. The arteriovenous oxygen difference widens at the end of gestation. By term, there is a 20% increase in maternal oxygen consumption, mostly as a result of the increase in metabolic needs of the fetus. The increase in oxygen consumption is also a result of the increased work of ventilation during pregnancy, the increase in myocardial oxygen demand, and the increase in renal oxygen consumption. Oxygen extraction also gradually increases throughout gestation. The increase in cardiac output is probably the result of a combination of factors, including increased uterine blood flow, increased maternal circulating blood volume (and, hence, ventricular preload), and possibly estrogen- and prolactin-induced augmentation of myocardial contractility. Walters and Lim[9] suggested that ventricular dynamics may be improved during pregnancy as a direct result of the action of steroid hormones on the pregnant myocardium. In animal models, estrogens have been shown to increase cardiac output and decrease peripheral vascular resistance.[10] Echocardiographic studies performed in healthy pregnant women have demonstrated a decrease in the pre-ejection period of left ventricular systole but an increase in the left ventricular end-diastolic dimension.[11-13] It may be that a combination of improved myocardial contractility and increased ventricular diastolic area may be responsible for increases in cardiac output during normal pregnancy.[14,15]

HEMODYNAMIC CHANGES DURING LABOR AND DELIVERY

Although cardiac output remains relatively constant in the latter half of pregnancy, there is a significant increase during active labor and immediately after delivery. With each uterine contraction, cardiac output dramatically increases as an additional 300 to 500 mL of maternal blood volume from the uterus is returned to the heart. Cardiac output can rise to 50% greater than normal when the pregnant woman is pushing in the second stage of labor. The amount of blood returned to the heart is accentuated in the supine position. When the pregnant patient is supine, uterine contractions can cause a 25% increase in cardiac output, a 15% decrease in maternal heart rate, and a 30% to 35% increase in stroke volume. In the lateral recumbent position, the hemodynamic changes associated with uterine contractions are less pronounced; cardiac output and stroke volume may rise by only 6% to 7%, and there may be only a small change in the maternal heart rate. Cardiac output may be preferentially diverted to the heart if there is partial obstruction of the abdominal aorta by the uterus during contraction.

The hemodynamic changes seen during labor and delivery are influenced by anesthetic and analgesic techniques. The increase in cardiac output is less if caudal anesthesia is used. Within the first 20 to 30 minutes after delivery of the fetus and the placenta, there is an even greater increase in cardiac output because blood is no longer diverted to the uteroplacental vascular bed. Approximately 500 mL is redirected to the maternal circulation in the so-called "autotransfusion" effect of pregnancy. This effect can cause cardiac output to increase by 60% to 80% after aortocaval compression is removed and blood volume is increased. Most of the physiologic changes of pregnancy resolve and revert to normal within several days after delivery. Cardiac output returns to normal within 2 weeks to 3 months after delivery as sodium and water balances normalize.[16]

BLOOD VOLUME CHANGES

The changes in maternal blood volume during pregnancy are dramatic. Plasma volume increases by 30% to 50% by the end of gestation. This value is increased in the multigravida patient compared with primigravidas, but the exact mechanism responsible for this effect is unclear. The increase in blood volume can be as high as 70% with twin pregnancies. An increase of 10% to 15% in blood volume is seen as early as the seventh week of gestation. Blood volume is maximal at 30 to 34 weeks, after which the value plateaus until term.[17] Ventricular filling pressures do not increase despite the large increases in plasma volume.[18] This is most likely the result of concurrent decreases in systemic and pulmonary vascular resistance.

The increase in blood volume is a striking adaptive mechanism that permits additional blood flow to the uterus and other maternal organs, in particular the kidneys. Uterine blood flow increases to 100 mL/min by the end of the first trimester and reaches 1200 mL/min at term. Both sodium and water retention contribute to the increase in plasma volume. Total body water increases by approximately 6.5 to 8 L. Most of this increase is seen in the extracellular space and is preferentially distributed in the lower extremities. The total increase in body water includes approximately 3.5 L of amniotic fluid, placental fluid, and water in the fetus. The maternal blood volume increases by 1 to 2 L. Red blood cell (RBC) mass accounts for only 300 to 400 mL of the increase in total blood volume.

Plasma renin and aldosterone levels are elevated during pregnancy despite expansion of the maternal blood volume. Activation of the renin-angiotensin-aldosterone system may result from the concomitant decrease in peripheral vascular resistance and the increase in vascular capacitance seen as early as the first 6 weeks of pregnancy.[2] Both estrogens and progesterone increase aldosterone levels, increasing sodium and water retention.[19] At 12 weeks of gestation, atrial natriuretic peptide levels also increase, most likely in response to the increase in plasma volume.

The increase in blood volume is an adaptive mechanism that provides some level of protection for the inevitable blood loss that accompanies delivery of the fetus and placenta. The average blood loss during vaginal delivery is 500 mL; the average blood loss during cesarean delivery is approximately 1000 mL. Although providing some degree of protection from peripartum blood loss, the increased plasma volume associated with pregnancy also can lull the clinician into a false sense of security. A pregnant woman can lose up to 35% of her blood volume before the usual signs of hypovolemia and acute hemorrhage are obvious. Although the pregnant woman may appear to have stable vital signs up to this point, the fetus may be severely compromised and deprived of adequate maternal blood flow. Tachycardia, hypotension, and other signs of hemodynamic instability are late manifestations of a significant deficit in maternal blood volume.

THE PHYSIOLOGIC ANEMIA OF PREGNANCY

Accompanying the increase in blood volume is an increase in RBC mass stimulated by increased circulating levels of erythropoietin. The RBC mass increases during the second trimester and continues to increase progressively throughout the pregnancy. However, the increase of 15% to 20% in RBC mass is disproportionate to the 30% to 50% increase in blood volume. As a result, the hematocrit decreases, resulting in the "physiologic hemodilutional anemia" of pregnancy. Hemodilution is most notable during the 30th to 34th gestational weeks. The hemoglobin concentration can decrease by as much as 9%. In the second trimester, the hemoglobin level can decrease to 11 to 12 g/100 mL, compared with the normal nonpregnant value of 13 to 14 g/100 mL. The decrease in blood viscosity associated with the anemia of pregnancy allows for decreased resistance to blood flow and facilitates placental perfusion. The hematocrit decreases until the end of the second trimester but increases later in the pregnancy, when the increase in RBC mass is proportionate to the increase in plasma volume. The hematocrit stabilizes at that point or even increases slightly as term approaches.

The degree of change in RBC mass during pregnancy depends, in part, on whether iron is supplemented. With the increase in RBC mass, there is a need for additional iron to prevent the development of iron deficiency anemia. Maternal requirements for iron can increase to 5 to 6 mg/day. The fetus uses iron from maternal stores to prevent fetal anemia, but the presence of significant maternal iron deficiency anemia has been shown to result in a higher incidence of fetal complications, including preterm labor and late spontaneous abortions.[20-22]

RENAL BLOOD FLOW DURING PREGNANCY

Under the influence of circulating hormones, there is a preferential redistribution of blood flow to the uterus, breast, and kidneys during pregnancy. Each kidney increases in length and weight, and the renal pelvis and ureters dilate. The glomerular filtration rate (GFR) increases by 50%, and renal blood flow increases by 25% to 50%. Changes in GFR and renal blood flow occur by the sixth week of gestation. The increase in renal blood flow plateaus early in pregnancy and remains unchanged or decreases slightly as term is approached. Urine flow and sodium excretion are increased and are influenced by position, especially in late pregnancy. Flow rates and the sodium excretion rate are significantly higher in the lateral recumbent position compared with the supine position. The concentrations of serum creatinine and blood urea nitrogen are reduced proportionately to the increase in the GFR. Glycosuria may also occur during pregnancy as a result of the increase in the GFR and impaired tubular reabsorption of glucose.

CHANGES IN BLOOD PRESSURE AND IN THE VASCULAR SYSTEM

Arterial blood pressure decreases as early as the sixth week of pregnancy; the lowest diastolic pressures are recorded during the second trimester. By the eighth week of gestation, diastolic blood pressure decreases by approximately by 10%. Diastolic pressure reaches a nadir at 16 to 24 weeks and is typically 5 to 10 mm Hg less than normal. After the 16th gestational week, blood pressure progressively increases and is back to baseline by term. With the increase in venous return associated with uterine contractions and the additional factors of pain, anxiety, and stress during labor and delivery, an increase in blood pressure usually occurs during this time. The decrease in blood pressure during pregnancy is associated with a significant decrease in peripheral vascular resistance. The decrease in arteriolar tone is influenced by several factors, including hormonal changes that induce vasodilatation and lack of responsiveness to the pressor effect of angiotensin II.[23,24] There is evidence for blood vessel remodeling in pregnancy, leading to increased venous compliance.[25,26] During pregnancy, circulating levels of numerous endogenous procoagulant and anticoagulant proteins change, leading to a hypercoagulable state. As a consequence, the risk of venous thrombosis increases during pregnancy. The reported incidence is 0.7 cases per 1000 women, and this rate increases threefold to fourfold in the postpartum period.[27]

The treatment of choice for severe hypotension resulting from acute hemorrhage, sepsis, or other critical illness during pregnancy is, ideally, aggressive fluid resuscitation. However, in cases of fluid-unresponsive hypotension, vasopressors must be used to prevent detrimental consequences to both the mother and the fetus as a result of inadequate uterine blood flow secondary to hypotension. Most vasopressors increase maternal blood pressure at the expense of fetal blood flow, inducing vasoconstriction of the uterine vessels. There are few human studies of these agents in pregnant women. However, animal studies animals indicate that ephedrine and dopamine increase uterine blood flow while at the same time increasing maternal blood pressure.[28,29]

STRUCTURAL REMODELING OF THE HEART

The heart is dramatically remodeled during the first few weeks of pregnancy. There is enlargement of all four chambers. The valvular annular diameters increase, as does the thickness of the left ventricular wall. End-diastolic volume increases, although end-diastolic pressure remains unchanged.[26,30] Chamber enlargement, particularly of the left atrium, may be a predisposing factor for supraventricular and atrial arrhythmias. Nonspecific ST-T wave changes may also be found in asymptomatic pregnant woman.

As the uterus enlarges and the diaphragm elevates, the heart is rotated upward and to the left. The apical impulse on physical examination is heard best over the fourth intercostal space, lateral to the midclavicular line. Left axis deviation is seen on the electrocardiogram as a result of the rotation of the heart. Because of the displacement of the heart, pregnant women may appear to have cardiomegaly on the chest radiograph. In addition, lung markings may be more prominent, suggesting vascular congestion. These changes can be similar to those seen in patients with heart disease. Even in women with no underlying cardiac pathology, the normal physiologic changes of pregnancy can result in signs and symptoms that are difficult to differentiate from those associated with cardiac disease. Symptoms such as fatigue, decreased exercise tolerance, peripheral edema, palpitations, chest pain, dyspnea, and orthopnea are common complaints as pregnancy advances.

New murmurs often appear during pregnancy. Systolic flow murmurs and a third heart sound are common but are soft. Mild pulmonic and tricuspid regurgitation occurs in more than 90% of healthy pregnant woman.[31] One third of pregnant women have evidence of clinically insignificant mitral regurgitation. Diastolic, pansystolic, and late systolic murmurs are rare in normal pregnancy and may indicate underlying heart disease. Bruits originating from the internal mammary artery and venous hums with diastolic components are common during pregnancy. These findings can initially confuse the diagnosis of a more serious underlying cardiac illness.

CARDIAC DISEASE AND PREGNANCY

In women with significant cardiac pathology, the hemodynamic aberrations associated with pregnancy can be life-threatening. The incidence of significant cardiac disease in pregnancy is less than 2% but is increasing.[32,33] Advances in medical therapy and in cardiac surgery have allowed female cardiac patients to survive to childbearing age and to have successful term pregnancies.[34] For women with severe cardiac problems, such as pulmonary hypertension, Eisenmenger's syndrome, severe mitral stenosis, or Marfan's syndrome (in which the risk of aortic dissection is high during pregnancy), the physiologic changes of pregnancy can increase both maternal and fetal morbidity and mortality by transiently or permanently worsening the underlying heart disease.[35] Increases in blood volume, stroke volume, cardiac output, and heart rate and the decrease in systemic vascular resistance are poorly tolerated by pregnant women with severe underlying cardiac disease. Maternal mortality is less than 1% for patients with less severe cardiac problems, but it increases to 50% if pregnancy is associated with the presence of underlying primary pulmonary hypertension or cyanotic disorders such as Eisenmenger's syndrome.[33,36]

Approximately 90% of pregnant women with cardiac disease are rated as New York Heart Association (NHYA) functional class I or class II. These patients tolerate the hemodynamic changes of pregnancy and can be managed well with medical therapy, although the incidence of heart failure and arrhythmias tends to be higher in this group of patients.[37,38] The 10% of pregnant patients with NYHA functional class III or IV heart disease account for 85% of cardiac deaths.[39] Fetal morbidity and mortality are increased in these patients, and there is a higher incidence of prematurity, miscarriage, and intrauterine growth retardation.[40,41] Cardiac telemetry, fetal monitoring, and hemodynamic monitoring are usually necessary for these high-risk patients during labor and delivery and, because of the large changes in intravascular volume after delivery, during the first few postpartum days.

ENDOCRINOLOGIC AND METABOLIC CHANGES IN PREGNANCY

There are numerous endocrine and metabolic alterations during pregnancy, many of which are directly attributable to hormonal signals originating from the fetoplacental unit. Maternal adaptations to hormonal changes that occur during pregnancy directly influence the growth and development of the fetus and placenta. In pregnancy, there is also a change in the normal hormonal feedback mechanisms that control the synthesis and release of hormones. As with cardiac disease, the presentation of endocrine and metabolic disorders may be difficult to differentiate from the normal hypermetabolic state of pregnancy.

HYPOTHALAMIC AND PITUITARY ALTERATIONS

As in the nonpregnant state, the hypothalamic-pituitary axis is responsible for regulating many aspects of metabolism. Circulating levels of most of the releasing hormones of the hypothalamus increase during pregnancy because of increased production by the placenta rather than increased production and release by the hypothalamus. The target organ of the hypothalamus, the pituitary gland, undergoes remarkable structural and metabolic changes in pregnancy. Its size increases almost threefold secondary to estrogen stimulation.[42,43] Gonadotropin and growth hormone production decrease during pregnancy. However, synthesis of ACTH, prolactin, and thyroid-stimulating hormone (TSH) increases.

Free and bound cortisol levels are increased in pregnancy, even though circulating ACTH concentrations are elevated. These changes suggest that the normal negative feedback loop between ACTH and cortisol concentrations is altered in the pregnant state.[44] Free plasma cortisol concentrations may be two to three times higher than normal at term. Diurnal variation of cortisol is blunted but maintained throughout pregnancy. The clinical signs of weakness, peripheral edema, glucose intolerance, and weight gain associated with Cushing's disease are sometimes difficult to differentiate from the clinical features of normal gestation. The symptoms of Cushing's disease are exacerbated by pregnancy but often resolve after delivery. Improved outcomes are seen with surgical therapy intrapartum, if pituitary or adrenal tumors are discovered during the course of the pregnancy.[45,46] In normal pregnancy, cortisol release may not be suppressed with a low intravenous dose (1 mg) of dexamethasone.[47] An 8-mg dose of dexamethasone is usually needed to suppress cortisol secretion if a tumor is present. In patients with occult adrenal insufficiency, a life-threatening adrenal crisis may be precipitated by the stress of labor and delivery. During pregnancy, the signs and symptoms may be vague and nonspecific but with the stress of labor, these symptoms are exaggerated. The clinical diagnosis is made in conjunction with laboratory evidence of a low cortisol level or even a low-normal level and no increase in the plasma cortisol concentration with an ACTH stimulation test. Immediate treatment with stress doses of hydrocortisone is indicated in these patients.

In preparation for lactation, circulating prolactin levels progressively increase to about 10 times normal during the course of pregnancy, secondary to stimulation of the anterior pituitary by placental estrogens and progesterone.[42,43,48] The dramatic increase in plasma prolactin concentration may lead to an increase in size of preexisting pituitary adenomas larger than 1 cm.[49] Symptoms resulting from an increase in prolactin secretion usually subside within 6 weeks after delivery, if the patient is not breastfeeding.

TSH secretion is transiently decreased in the first trimester, but circulating TSH concentrations are usually increased by term.[50,51] Circulating levels of thyroxine (T_4) and triiodothyronine (T_3) increase as a result of a twofold estrogen-stimulated increase in the synthesis of thyroxine-binding globulin. Levels of free (dialyzable) T_4 and free T_3 are unchanged. The thyroid gland does not increase in size, despite the increase in production of thyroid hormones. Pregnant women who obtain sufficient dietary iodine (more than 200 µg daily) have no untoward complications from the changes in thyroid function.[50]

Posterior pituitary hormones are altered in pregnancy. Circulating oxytocin levels increase, but the vasopressin concentration remains essentially unchanged. Plasma osmolality decreases by 5 to 10 mOsm/kg, suggesting that the threshold for secretion of vasopressin decreases during gestation. Although vasopressin levels remain unchanged, some women develop transient diabetes insipidus during pregnancy.[52,53]

CHANGES IN GLUCOSE METABOLISM

Early in pregnancy, glucose metabolism is influenced primarily by increased levels of estrogens and progesterone, which induce pancreatic beta-cell hyperplasia and increased insulin secretion.[54] Glucose metabolism is primarily controlled by placental hormones later in the pregnancy, in response to the increased nutritional and metabolic demands of the fetus. Circulating glucose and insulin levels fluctuate widely, depending on the nutritional state of the mother. Morning fasting levels of glucose can decrease to less than 55 mg/dL. Fasting blood glucose levels decrease by 10% to 20% because of increased peripheral glucose utilization, decreased hepatic glucose production, and increased consumption of glucose by the fetus.

Pregnant women with diabetes mellitus experience more hypoglycemic episodes in the first trimester, because hepatic gluconeogenesis is decreased during this period. Insulin secretion increases during pregnancy. There is a relative state of insulin resistance, as evidenced by postprandial maternal hyperglycemia.[53-56] Normally, women adapt to the state of relative insulin resistance during pregnancy. However, those women with marginal pancreatic reserve or preexisting insulin resistance due to obesity may not produce sufficient insulin, leading to the development of gestational diabetes mellitus. Pregnant women with preexisting diabetes mellitus require as much as 30% more insulin than before pregnancy. There is a close correlation between maternal blood glucose levels and glucose uptake and utilization by the fetus, because glucose crosses the placental barrier. Poor maternal glucose control worsens fetal morbidity. For patients with preexisting insulin-dependent diabetes mellitus, fetal and neonatal mortality rates have decreased significantly, from 65% to between 2% and 5%, as a result of implementing strict metabolic glucose control with insulin.[57]

Lipid metabolism is accelerated in pregnancy, and the circulating concentrations of triglycerides and cholesterol increase. Increased production of triglycerides allows for maternal consumption while sparing glucose for use by the fetus.[58] Lipolysis is stimulated in adipose tissue, and there is a release of glycerol and fatty acids that decreases maternal glucose utilization, additionally sparing glucose for the fetus.

ANNOTATED REFERENCES

Capeless EL, Clapp JF: When do cardiovascular parameters return to their normal preconception values? Am J Obstet Gynecol 1991;165:883.

The objective of this study was to determine whether the normal physiologic hemodynamic parameters observed during pregnancy persisted after delivery, and for how long. The authors performed serial echocardiographic studies of 13 women before pregnancy and at 6 and 12 weeks after delivery. None of the pregnant women had known cardiac or hypertensive disorders before delivery. Cardiac output, stroke volume, and end-diastolic volume were calculated with M-mode echocardiography from the left ventricular dimensions. Measurements were performed with the patients in the left lateral recumbent position. Systemic vascular resistance was calculated from cardiac output and simultaneous measurements of blood pressure. Stroke volume and end-diastolic volume remained consistently elevated over preconception values at 6 and 12 weeks. Systemic vascular resistance remained decreased, compared with baseline, at 12 weeks. In this small study, the authors showed that cardiovascular parameters had not returned to prepregnancy values by 6 to 12 weeks postpartum. Previous authors have suggested that, with delivery of the fetus and placenta and the rapid mobilization of fluids, most hemodynamic changes resolve within several days after delivery. These authors suggest that prior studies have underestimated the contribution of stroke volume to the total change in cardiac output during pregnancy.

Clark SL, Cotton DB, Lee W, et al: Central hemodynamic assessment of normal term pregnancy 1989;161:1439.

This paper presents central hemodynamic data obtained with the use of a pulmonary artery catheter during pregnancy and after delivery. Ten primigravidas patients in late pregnancy (between the 36th and 38th weeks of gestation) underwent pulmonary artery catheter and arterial catheter placement. These same patients were restudied with a pulmonary artery catheter at 11 to 13 weeks after delivery. All measurements were performed with the patient in the left lateral recumbent position. The authors found significant decreases in systemic vascular resistance, pulmonary vascular resistance, colloid oncotic pressure, and colloid oncotic pressure-pulmonary capillary wedge pressure gradient in the third-trimester measurements (P < .05). A significant rise in cardiac output and heart rate was seen in all patients before delivery (P < .05). No significant changes in pulmonary capillary wedge pressure, central venous pressure, left ventricular stroke work index, or mean arterial pressure were found. Although blood volume and preload are elevated in pregnancy and end-diastolic volume increases, there were no substantial increases in the filling pressures of the heart as measured by the pulmonary artery catheter, suggesting a decrease in afterload with the decrease in the systemic and pulmonary vascular resistance.

Elkayam U, Gleicher N: Cardiac Problems in Pregnancy: Diagnosis and Management of Maternal and Fetal Heart Disease, 3rd ed. New York, Wiley-Liss, 1998.

This is an excellent expanded textbook that reviews the clinically relevant cardiac diseases associated with pregnancy. The normal physiologic changes during pregnancy, including hemodynamics and cardiac function, are discussed in detail. The editors include consideration of management of preexisting cardiac diseases as well as cardiac disorders occurring de novo during pregnancy (e.g., peripartum cardiomyopathy). Newer medical treatments and surgical options for the specific cardiac disorders are discussed. Chapters on cardiovascular imaging, drugs, and cardiac transplantation offer current and relevant information for the practicing clinician.

James DK, Steer PJ, Weiner CP, et al. (eds): High Risk Pregnancy: Management Options. London, WB Saunders, 1994.

This textbook offers an in-depth and comprehensive review of all organ system disorders that can occur during pregnancy and in the postpartum period. In each chapter, the authors discuss the expected hemodynamic, hormonal, structural, or metabolic changes seen during normal pregnancy in reference to a specific organ system. They give ample evidence from the literature, citing both animal and human pregnancy studies. Critical care, anesthetic, and surgical management of the pregnant patient are also presented in depth. Fetal and neonatal physiology, anomalies, and outcomes are presented as well. For the critical care specialist, obstetrician, or high-risk neonatologist, this textbook covers all aspects of prenatal, intranatal, and postnatal care and management of both healthy and ill pregnant patients.

Whitty JE: Maternal cardiac arrest during pregnancy. Clin Obstet Gynecol 2002;45:377.

This excellent review paper describes maternal deaths during pregnancy in the context of basic life support (BLS) and advanced cardiac life support (ACLS) resuscitation. The obstetric and nonobstetric causes of cardiac arrest in pregnancy are discussed. The article describes the physiologic cardiopulmonary changes of pregnancy that impede and affect normal cardiopulmonary resuscitative efforts. Specific maneuvers for resuscitation of the pregnant woman are described, including mask ventilation and the use of a wedge while performing cardiopulmonary resuscitation. As a critical adjunct to maternal resuscitation, the need for performing a perimortem cesarean section is discussed in relation to available data on fetal and maternal outcomes.

Chapter 181

HYPERTENSIVE DISORDERS IN PREGNANCY

Marie R. Baldisseri

KEY POINTS

1. **Hypertensive disorders** associated with pregnancy are not uncommon and **can either predate the pregnancy or be precipitated or unmasked by the pregnancy.**

2. Women with a prenatal history of diabetes mellitus, renal disease, vascular disease, or a family history of hypertension are predisposed to developing hypertension during pregnancy.

3. **Treatment is recommended if the systolic blood pressures (BPs) are 160 mm Hg or higher, or the diastolic BPs are 110 mm Hg or higher,** or with lower BPs if the patient is symptomatic.

4. **BP measurements should be consistently taken in** either the sitting position or in the inferior arm in the lateral recumbent position with each evaluation.

5. Cardiac output and blood volume are dramatically increased during pregnancy, and there is a decrease in systemic vascular resistance, particularly during the second trimester. **Diastolic BP is lowest during the second trimester.**

6. Elevated BPs caused by essential hypertension may transiently improve during the second trimester of pregnancy.

7. **Consistently elevated systolic BPs greater than 200 mm Hg** should prompt the practitioner to consider undiagnosed essential hypertension or some of the less common causes of hypertension, such as **primary aldosteronism, renal artery stenosis, or pheochromocytoma.**

8. **Pregnancy-induced hypertension presents early** in the pregnancy and **resolves after delivery.**

9. **Preeclampsia most often appears after the 32nd week of gestation** and resolves with delivery of the fetus.

10. **Preeclampsia may initially present after delivery as the HELLP syndrome** (hemolysis, elevated liver enzymes, and low platelets).

11. The classic **triad of peripheral edema, hypertension, and proteinuria is seen in preeclampsia.**

12. Preeclampsia is a multisystem disease. **Severe preeclampsia manifests** with signs and symptoms of **end-organ involvement.**

13. The antihypertensive drugs most frequently used in pregnancy have not been associated with significant fetal abnormalities.

14. **First-line antihypertensive drugs** for moderate hypertension are **oral α-methyldopa and oral labetalol.**

15. **Parenteral antihypertensive agents** are used for more severe elevations of BP. The agents most commonly employed are **labetalol, hydralazine, and sodium nitroprusside.**

16. Caution should be exercised with the administration of hydralazine, particularly in patients with decreased plasma volume.

17. Most forms of hypertension that are precipitated by pregnancy resolve in the postpartum period.

Hypertensive disorders associated with pregnancy are relatively common, occurring in approximately 10% of pregnancies. These disorders are most commonly divided into two groups: those that predated the pregnancy, such as preexisting essential hypertension superimposed on pregnancy, and those that were precipitated or unmasked by the pregnant state. Significant predisposing factors for development of hypertension during pregnancy are a family history of hypertension, preexisting diabetes mellitus, vascular or renal disorders, primigravid state, and multiple gestational pregnancies.

BLOOD PRESSURE MEASUREMENTS IN PREGNANCY

The definition of hypertension during pregnancy has been controversial. Earlier case series of normotensive pregnant women suggested that the normal systolic blood pressure (SBP) is less than 125 mm Hg and the normal diastolic blood pressure (DBP) is less than 85 mm Hg.[1,2] In a study of 15,000 pregnant women, Page and Christianson[2] reported that the perinatal mortality rate increased if there was a sustained increase in BP during the pregnancy.[2] However, more recently, there has been a general consensus that the amount of increase in systolic and diastolic BPs is more important than the baseline values. Many authors now agree that significant hypertension in pregnancy is defined by an increase of at least 30 mm Hg in the SBP and an increase in the DBP of at least 15 mm Hg. Some investigators have advocated treatment if a DBP is greater than 110 mm Hg or a SBP is greater than 160 mm Hg because of the increase in maternal complications with this degree of hypertension.[3-5]

Sustained (rather than transient) increases in BP are the key risk factor; accordingly, BP should be measured on at least two separate occasions. BP measurements need to be made in a standardized fashion (e.g., with the patient sitting in the same position) at each evaluation. Measurements in the upper arm in the lateral recumbent position may give falsely low values. BP is best recorded with the patient in the sitting position or in the inferior arm in the lateral recumbent position. Gant and associates[6] first proposed the "supine pressor" or "rollover" test as a specific and sensitive marker of risk for preeclampsia later during pregnancy. They suggested that the risk of preeclampsia is increased if the BP increases by more than 20 mm Hg when position is changed from the lateral recumbent to the supine position. Subsequent studies have not confirmed the validity or usefulness of this test in predicting the development of preeclampsia.[7,8]

Previously, some experts were concerned that aggressive management of hypertension in pregnancy might be detrimental, perhaps because hypertension improved uterine blood flow. These concerns appear to be unfounded, because later studies showed that uterine blood flow either increases or shows no change after hypertension is controlled. Nevertheless, caution must be exercised to ensure that treatment of hypertension during pregnancy does not induce hypotension, which adversely affects maternal hemodynamics and compromises fetal well-being. There is significant correlation between maternal BP control and fetal morbidity, and evidence now suggests that antihypertensive treatment for severe hypertension results in improved perinatal outcome.[9-11] However the benefits of strictly controlling BP in cases of mild hypertension in pregnancy are less clear.[12,13]

PHYSIOLOGIC CHANGES IN PREGNANCY

Essential to the management of hypertension in pregnancy is an understanding of the normal physiologic changes in cardiac output, vasomotor tone, and systemic BP that occur. During pregnancy, cardiac output increases by 30% to 40% in the second trimester, peaking at about the 24th week of gestation. The increase in cardiac output during the first two trimesters of pregnancy is primarily caused by increased maternal blood volume. Cardiac output plateaus for the remainder of the pregnancy until labor. An increase in cardiac output is seen with each uterine contraction. Cardiac output increases again during the immediate postpartum period, after delivery of the fetus and the placenta. It is during this period that cardiac output is highest as a result of the so-called "autotransfusion" effect (see Chapter 184).

Systemic vascular resistance and, consequently, BP decrease during the second trimester. Increased synthesis of vasodilating prostaglandins may play a role in the regulation of BP and uterine blood flow in pregnancy. In normal pregnancy, vascular resistance is determined by a proper balance of the effects of vasoconstricting factors and vasodilating factors, including prostaglandins. This balance may be disturbed in hypertensive states, due to inadequate prostaglandin synthesis.

In pregnancy-related hypertensive states, there is a paradoxical increase in the systemic vascular resistance, compared with pregnancy without hypertension. It is noteworthy that all patients with newly acquired or preexisting hypertension in pregnancy have a relative decrease in DBP during the second trimester, reflecting a relative decrease in systemic vascular resistance. Indeed, BP normalizes during the second trimester in some patients with preexisting hypertension.

CAUSES OF HYPERTENSION IN PREGNANCY

There are multiple causes of hypertension during pregnancy (Table 181-1). The most common hypertensive states are pregnancy-induced hypertension (gestational hypertension without the presence of proteinuria), essential hypertension, and preeclampsia (gestational hypertension with significant proteinuria). This classification is clinically useful to the practitioner, but the risk from systemic hypertension is significant for all three conditions, regardless of the specific cause of high BP. Hypertension during pregnancy may precipitate intrauterine growth retardation and is associated with an increased risk of death for both mother and fetus.

Pregnancy-induced hypertension is defined as primarily diastolic hypertension that occurs transiently during the pregnancy, usually manifesting after the 20th gestational week, and resolves within 1 to 2 months after delivery. Women who develop pregnancy-induced hypertension have a high rate of recurrence of hypertension with subsequent pregnancies and often develop chronic hypertension at a later time.

Essential hypertension (i.e., hypertension that was present prepartum, whether diagnosed or undiagnosed) persists in the postpartum period and accounts for approximately one third of all cases of hypertension during pregnancy. Essential hypertension may manifest during the first 20 weeks of pregnancy. Women who develop hypertension without proteinuria in the last trimester of pregnancy may have essential hypertension, either unmasked or precipitated by the pregnancy. In these cases of de novo presentation of hypertension, care must be exercised to rule out other non–pregnancy-related causes of hypertension, such as renal artery stenosis, pheochromocytoma, coarctation of the aorta, primary aldosteronism, and Cushing's syndrome. Essential hypertension, previously undiagnosed, is a consideration, particularly in older, multiparous women. As the age of parturients has increased, the incidence of essential hypertension in pregnant women has also increased. For some patients, the initial diagnosis of hypertension may be made during a routine prenatal visit with an obstetrician.

TABLE 181–1. CAUSES OF HYPERTENSION IN PREGNANCY
Pregnancy-induced hypertension (gestational hypertension without proteinuria)
Essential hypertension
Preeclampsia (gestational hypertension with proteinuria)
Primary aldosteronism (Conn's syndrome)
Renal artery stenosis
Coarctation of the aorta
Pheochromocytoma
Cushing's syndrome

For some patients, this prenatal visit is their first encounter with a physician as an adult. Essential hypertension should be suspected if there is a family history of hypertension, diabetes, or obesity. If there is a suspicion of preexisting essential hypertension, then cardiac echocardiography should be performed to evaluate for left ventricular hypertrophy, which would suggest that hypertension has been a problem for an extended period. There is no significant worsening of maternal and perinatal outcomes for pregnant patients with essential hypertension, particularly if extremes of BP are avoided with treatment. Complications related to intrapartum hypertension, such as placenta previa, placental abruption, and preeclampsia, are less likely with judicious treatment of elevated BP. Patients with essential hypertension have not been shown to have a higher incidence of preeclampsia, particularly if BP is well controlled.[14]

PATHOLOGY OF PREECLAMPSIA

Preeclampsia is a pregnancy-related multisystem disease process that usually occurs after the 32nd week of gestation. It is typically described as a triad of symptoms: peripheral edema, systemic hypertension, and significant proteinuria (0.3 g or greater in a 24-hour urine collection). Clinical onset is usually characterized by rapid weight gain associated with generalized edema, followed by onset of hypertension or proteinuria or both. The incidence of preeclampsia in the United States is 7%. The highest frequency occurs in young primigravidas, and the second highest incidence is in older multiparous women, a group that has a higher maternal mortality rate than the young primigravidas. The incidence is higher in patients with preexisting hypertension or renal vascular disease, and the symptoms may present earlier than the 32nd gestational week in these patients. Diastolic hypertension is most often seen in association with preeclampsia. It is less common to record SBP values greater than 160 mm Hg. If the SBP is greater than 200 mm Hg, the clinician should consider the possibility of underlying essential hypertension, which may be superimposed on the preeclamptic state. Because preeclampsia is a multisystem disease process, it may imitate or mask other pathologic conditions, and a thorough investigation to rule out other coexisting pathologies should be carried out.[15] Familial prevalence of preeclampsia has been reported.[16] In some cases, preeclampsia manifests 1 to 7 days after delivery. Most commonly, if preeclampsia is present in the postpartum period, it manifests as the HELLP syndrome, a severe variant of the preeclamptic spectrum of diseases.[17,18] This syndrome always includes some, if not all, of the following features: microangiopathic hemolytic anemia (H), elevated liver enzymes (EL), and low platelets (LP). The syndrome can develop without substantial BP changes or with no significant changes compared with BP readings taken during the pregnancy.

Olney and Kaulhausen[19] showed that a significant elevation of the BP in the second trimester is associated with an increased risk of preeclampsia later in the pregnancy. One third of pregnant women with mean arterial pressures greater than 90 mm Hg in the second trimester developed preeclampsia later during pregnancy. Only 2% of women with mean arterial pressures less than 90 mm Hg developed preeclampsia. Relatively mild hypertension early in pregnancy, which might be ignored in nonpregnant patients, should not be overlooked or dismissed in the parturient.

As many as 25% of all pregnant women have slightly elevated BPs in the last month of pregnancy, but the incidence of preeclampsia is also highest during this period. Accordingly, clinicians must remain vigilant when faced with new-onset hypertension and look for other signs and symptoms that might suggest the presence of the preeclamptic syndrome.

The exact pathogenesis of preeclampsia is still unknown, although it is believed to be related to endothelial cell injury and dysfunction that occurs in most maternal organs as a result of toxic substances released from a poorly perfused placenta. Genetic and immunologic factors also have been implicated in the pathogenesis of preeclampsia.[16,20] The generalized vasospasm that occurs in preeclampsia is responsible for many of the organ-specific signs and symptoms seen in this multisystem disease. The widespread vasospasm is associated with increased circulating levels of vasoconstrictors, increased sensitivity to angiotensin II, and decreased levels of vasodilators. Walsh and others have suggested that an imbalance in the ratio of prostacyclin to thromboxane production contributes to the pathogenesis of preeclampsia.[21,22] This idea has prompted studies of low-dose aspirin to prevent development of preeclampsia.[23] The maternal organs that are most affected in preeclampsia are the kidneys, brain, liver, and hematologic system. Despite a lack of understanding of the exact pathogenesis of preeclampsia, significant improvements in identification of the disease, monitoring, and management of these complex cases has improved perinatal and maternal morbidity and mortality. If vasospasm affects the uteroplacental bed, the incidence of intrauterine growth retardation, stillbirths, and neonatal deaths increases dramatically.[24]

Peripheral edema is a common symptom and complaint of pregnant women that cannot be ignored, because it may herald the onset of preeclampsia. Eighty-five percent of women with preeclampsia present with generalized edema, and significant weight gain is the first symptom.[9] Preeclampsia, first manifested by peripheral edema, is usually accompanied by a gradual increase in BP. Sodium retention is partly responsible for edema formation and hypertension. In normal pregnancy, the glomerular filtration rate increases by as much as 50%. There is a concomitant increase in sodium reabsorption by the renal tubules and a 60% to 80% increase in renal blood flow.[25] Renal blood flow increases because of the increase in cardiac output and a decrease in renal vascular resistance. In preeclampsia, sodium retention is caused by a decrease in the glomerular filtration rate, possibly resulting from vasospasm of the renal vasculature, commonly seen in preeclampsia. Renin and aldosterone secretion decrease in patients with preeclampsia, probably as a result of extracellular volume expansion and associated edema. The exact cause of the decreased activity of these factors is unknown, but it may be related to decreased renal prostaglandin synthesis, increased systemic BP, or expansion of extracellular volume.[26] In spite of the decreased levels of renin and aldosterone, sensitivity to angiotensin II is increased, a factor that may play a role in the pathogenesis of hypertension in preeclampsia.[27] Although sodium retention occurs in preeclampsia, blood volume actually can be diminished, compared with that in normotensive pregnant patients.[28] Plasma volume contracts as extracellular fluid is preferentially shifted from the vascular space to the interstitium. However, the decrease in plasma volume does not indicate volume depletion in patients with preeclampsia. In contrast to hypovolemic patients, cardiac output is increased and central venous and pulmonary capillary wedge pressures are normal to high in patients with preeclampsia.[29,30] These data guide the management of preeclampsia, because efforts should be directed to BP control rather than injudicious volume resuscitation.

Hyperuricemia in preeclampsia occurs, at least in part, because of decreased renal excretion of uric acid. However, the development of hyperuricemia frequently predates increases in serum blood urea nitrogen and creatinine, suggesting that other mechanisms are involved as well. Hyperuricemia has been used as a marker of severity of preeclampsia, and it is a risk factor for fetal mortality.[31]

CLINICAL PRESENTATION OF PREECLAMPSIA

Severity of illness is defined as mild, moderate, or severe, depending on the presenting signs and symptoms and associated comorbidities. Because of the multisystem nature of the process, preeclampsia may manifest with a wide spectrum of organ-specific abnormalities in addition to the general findings of edema, hypertension, and proteinuria. Because the pathologic abnormalities associated with preeclampsia are not necessarily secondary to hypertension, the severity of preeclampsia does not always correlate with the degree of BP elevation.[32] BP elevations are classified as mild, moderate, or severe. Hypertension in preeclampsia may result from increases in systemic vascular resistance and cardiac output.[33,34]

In mild preeclampsia, SBP is 130 to 140 mm Hg and DBP is 80 to 95 mm Hg. Peripheral edema is minimal, and there are no associated visual or cerebral symptoms. In moderately severe preeclampsia, the SBP may increase to as high as 150 to 160 mm Hg, and the DBP can be as high as 110 mm Hg. An increase in SBP of 25 mm Hg or more and an increase in DBP of 15 mm Hg or more suggests the presence of moderate to severe preeclampsia. Peripheral edema, hyperreflexia, and visual symptoms are present with moderately severe preeclampsia. In severe forms of preeclampsia, the SBP is greater than 160 mm Hg and the DBP is 110 mm Hg or greater. In severe preeclampsia, there are signs of multiple organ system involvement. Pulmonary, cardiac, renal, and neurologic disturbances may be present. Severe renal involvement in preeclampsia leads to glomeruloendotheliosis, which manifests as marked proteinuria (excretion of greater than 5 g protein daily). Oliguria (urine output less than 500 mL/day) is also common, and the serum creatinine concentration is usually greater than 1.6 mg/dL. Acute renal failure is relatively rare, although clinical evidence of renal involvement in preeclampsia significantly increases perinatal mortality.[35] Hepatic involvement is manifested by epigastric or right upper quadrant pain with elevated circulating levels of bilirubin and transaminases. Severe hepatic pathology can result in subcapsular hematomas and lacerations that may require surgical intervention.[36,37] Neurologic changes may include persistent headaches, visual disturbances, focal neurologic deficits, and severe hyperreflexia with or without clonus. Computed tomography of the brain may show cerebral edema, especially in the occipital region.

Severe preeclampsia associated with central nervous system irritability, manifesting as generalized tonic-clonic seizures not caused by other cerebral pathology, is defined as eclampsia. Eclampsia can occur without significant hypertension or proteinuria.[38,39] Cardiovascular and respiratory changes can manifest as pulmonary edema, resulting from iatrogenic fluid overload, acute systolic left ventricular failure, or diastolic left ventricular dysfunction secondary to chronic essential hypertension. Pulmonary edema may also result from increased capillary permeability or from a decrease in colloid osmotic pressure that occurs to some extent during normal pregnancy but can be accentuated by preeclampsia.[29,40] Hematologic disturbances consist of thrombocytopenia, disseminated intravascular coagulation, and hemolysis.[41,42]

It is unknown whether preeclampsia leads to persistent ("essential") hypertension after delivery, although it seems that this is unlikely. Nevertheless, an episode of preeclampsia may identify a subgroup of women with increased risk for eventual development of essential hypertension at a later time.[43] Some data suggest that the incidence of permanent hypertension after delivery is higher in multiparous women with preeclampsia.[44,45] Debate continues as to whether the presence of preeclampsia or the duration of the disease process may be responsible for influencing factors that later lead to the development of essential hypertension. Women who develop preeclampsia, superimposed on previously undiagnosed essential hypertension or underlying renal disease, are predisposed to the later development of essential hypertension.

OTHER CAUSES OF HYPERTENSION IN PREGNANCY

Some of the less common causes of hypertension are listed in Table 181-1.

Primary aldosteronism in a pregnant women has been reported but is uncommon. The treatment of hypertension in these patients is directed toward medical management during the pregnancy and postpartum operative intervention if an adenoma is present.

Renal artery stenosis can be associated with preeclampsia. Medical therapy with antihypertensive agents is recommended. Although ideal therapy for these patients would include angiotensin-converting enzyme (ACE) inhibitors, these agents are contraindicated during pregnancy, and other alternatives must be employed.[46-49]

Coarctation of the aorta is a rare cause of hypertension. It may be previously undiagnosed and then initially diagnosed during a patient's first pregnancy. It can be associated with preeclampsia. The greatest risk to these patients is aortic rupture caused by cystic medial necrosis of the aortic wall. This risk is amplified because the normal physiologic changes of pregnancy place further stresses on the abnormal aorta. Increases in BP, cardiac output, and the strain of labor with contractions can increase this risk. Aggressive medical management with antihypertensive medications, including β-adrenergic blockers, improves outcome in these high-risk patients.

Pheochromocytoma is a rare cause of hypertension, but patients have a poor outcome if the tumor is not diagnosed and treated. These patients can present with nausea, vomiting, profuse diaphoresis, severe headache, generalized weakness, palpitations, and seizures. The immediate causes of sudden death are secondary to pulmonary edema, cerebral hemorrhage, and cardiovascular collapse. Because of the risk of significant morbidity and mortality to both mother and fetus, it was previously recommended that immediate surgical intervention be carried out during pregnancy. Currently, most experts advocate medical therapy with α- and β-adrenergic blockade during pregnancy and tumor removal after delivery.

GENERAL TREATMENT PRINCIPLES

General recommendations for management and monitoring of hypertension in pregnant patients include stabilization and treatment of acute changes in BP. Specific goal-directed therapy is indicated for various organ-system abnormalities that may be present, particularly in those patients with moderate to severe preeclampsia. If proteinuria is not present and there is no suspicion of preeclampsia conservative management on an outpatient basis is usually adequate. Immediate hospitalization with bed rest is recommended for patients presenting with proteinuria if there is a high index of suspicion for the diagnosis of preeclampsia.

ANTIHYPERTENSIVE DRUG THERAPY

There is now an extensive pharmaceutical armamentarium available for the treatment of hypertension in pregnancy. In 1979, the U. S. Food and Drug Administration (FDA) established categories for all drugs with potential and real adverse effects on the fetus.[50] Although helpful to the clinician, these categories most often do not reflect current scientific knowledge regarding specific teratogenic effects of the drugs.[51]

The FDA categories are listed in Table 181-2. Most antihypertensive drugs used during pregnancy are classified as category C. Thiazide diuretics, prazosin, and α-methyldopa are designated as category A; metoprolol is a category B agent. Because most antihypertensive drugs are used later in

TABLE 181–2. FDA CATEGORIES OF FETAL DRUG TOXICITIES

Category	Description
A	Controlled studies in pregnant women have not demonstrated any risk to the fetus in the first trimester. These drugs are considered to be relatively safe for use during pregnancy.
B	No known specific risks are associated with use of the drug in pregnancy, but controlled human studies are lacking. If adverse effects were shown in animal reproduction studies, these were not confirmed in controlled human trials.
C	Studies in women and animals are not available or studies in animals have revealed adverse effects on the fetus. Most new drugs fall into this category. These drugs should be given only if the potential benefit justifies the potential risk to the fetus.
D	These drugs have shown a definite fetal risk in controlled human trials. However, their use may be necessary during pregnancy, and a risk-benefit assessment needs to be considered for the use of these agents.
X	These drugs have shown a definite risk to the fetus and their use is contraindicated because the potential risks to the fetus outweigh the potential benefits.

FDA, U. S. Food and Drug Administration.

pregnancy, the potential teratogenic effects of these drugs is usually not of concern. However, if treatment is initiated for patients with preexisting essential hypertension or early-onset gestational hypertension, teratogenic effects must be considered when choosing antihypertensive drugs. It may be necessary to change antihypertensive therapy early in pregnancy, if the patient is taking drugs that could increase the risks of fetal abnormalities.

The goal of hypertensive therapy in pregnancy is prevention of maternal complications such as intracerebral hemorrhage, stroke, and decompensated heart failure. There are no convincing data to determine the optimal BP goal with drug therapy.[52] There is disagreement concerning the proper normal values for BP during pregnancy, but most agree that acute treatment is mandated (1) if the SBP is greater than 160 mm Hg or the DBP is 110 mm Hg or greater or (2) if the SBP is more than 30 mm Hg greater than the baseline value or the DBP is more than 15 mm Hg greater than baseline. If acute and urgent drug therapy management is required, some patients may need to be hospitalized, depending on their compliance with drug therapy and the urgency of lowering the BP based on concomitant organ system involvement. For patients presenting with SBP 140 mm Hg or higher and DBP 90 mm Hg or higher, urgent drug therapy should be implemented if there is concurrent evidence of symptoms, underlying essential hypertension, or end-organ involvement. If the patient presents after the 24th gestational week and fetal viability is ascertained, both cardiac and fetal telemetry may be required. For patients presenting with SBP less than 140 mm Hg and DBP less than 90 mm Hg and no evidence of significant proteinuria, management and treatment can be provided on an outpatient basis, with frequent office visits and close maternal and fetal assessments. If the hypertension is refractory to standard therapy, hypertension worsens despite adequate drug therapy, or the suspicion of preeclampsia arises, then immediate hospitalization is recommended.

Conservative drug therapy is advocated for moderately severe preeclampsia, but the treatment of choice for severe preeclampsia and associated end-organ involvement is immediate delivery of the fetus. Delay in delivery for patients with severe preeclampsia and end-organ involvement can result in serious maternal and fetal complications.[53] If the fetus is of mature gestational age, factors influencing the decision to deliver are dependent on progression of the disease process, assessment of fetal lung maturity, and status of the cervix. Conservative management of preeclamptic patients at a gestational age less than 24 weeks is associated with serious maternal complications, and termination of the pregnancy should be considered. For patients at 28 to 32 weeks of gestation, conservative management with vigilant monitoring and assessment needs to be performed in a hospital setting.

A first-line drug still used today in the pregnant patient, although less commonly in the general populace, is oral α-methyldopa, a central α$_2$-adrenergic agonist. Historically, this has been a first-line drug of choice for many obstetricians over the years, and there has been little evidence to convince them otherwise. The starting dose is 250 mg orally two to three times a day for the first 48 hours of treatment. Dosing can be increased every two days until the desired BP level is achieved.[54] The maximum daily dose is 4 g. β-Adrenergic blocker therapy with oral labetalol, a combined α- and β-adrenergic antagonist, has become popular as a single-agent antihypertensive. The recommended initial dose is 100 mg orally twice daily. The dose can be increased as indicated, either semiweekly or weekly. The maintenance dose is usually 200 to 400 mg administered twice daily. The benefits of β-adrenergic blockade make this an attractive drug for parturients with underlying chronic essential hypertension and possible cardiac and vascular involvement. Diuretics also may be used, although care must be exercised to prevent excessive fluid losses, which can exacerbate the decrease in blood volume associated with preeclampsia. As mentioned previously, ACE inhibitors and angiotensin II receptor antagonists should be avoided intrapartum, because these agents can increase perinatal morbidity and mortality.

For acute and emergent drug therapy for severe hypertension, intravenous antihypertensive drugs should be used. Intravenous infusions are particularly attractive because they provide rapid control of BP and can be titrated easily. Intravenous hydralazine, a direct arteriolar vasodilator, remains the standard for many obstetricians, although other drugs may be preferable, because hydralazine decreases BP precipitously. Excessive lowering of BP is a particular problem when hydralazine is administered to preeclamptic patients with contracted blood volume.[55] If hydralazine is used, it should be given as 5- to 10-mg intravenous boluses every 15 to 30 minutes until BP is controlled. Onset of the hypotensive effect is 10 to 20 minutes, and duration of action about 8 hours. A meta-analysis of 11 trials in 570 women found that parenteral hydralazine was associated with an increase in the incidence of maternal hypotension, compared with other antihypertensives.[56,57] Infusions of hydralazine are difficult to titrate and are associated with increased incidence of fetal distress.[58]

Intravenous labetalol, a nonselective β- and α-adrenergic receptor blocker, is also commonly used for the acute management of hypertension. Labetalol rapidly decreases BP, but not at the expense of uteroplacental blood flow.[59] Labetalol crosses the placenta but rarely causes significant neonatal bradycardia.[60] An initial intravenous bolus of 10 or 20 mg should be given, followed by boluses of 40 to 80 mg at 10- to 15-minute intervals as needed to control hypertension. Labetalol also can be given by continuous intravenous infusion; the usual dose is 1 to 4 mg/min. Contraindications to the use of labetalol are the same as those for other β-adrenergic antagonists, notably heart block and acute asthma.

Sodium nitroprusside is a potent arterial and venous vasodilator that quickly decreases the BP. Rapid titration with a continuous intravenous infusion can be instituted starting at a dose of 0.25 to 0.5 μg/kg/min and adjusted every few minutes and titrated to effect. Invasive arterial monitoring is often recommended in conjunction with its use. As with all potent vasodilators, care must be taken when using sodium nitroprusside, because patients with volume depletion may be particularly sensitive to its effects. Despite a paucity of data, concern regarding the risks of fetal cyanide toxicity prompts some practitioners to avoid using this drug in pregnant patients. Careful attention to dosing and duration of use should minimize the risk of toxicity.

Other, less frequently used agents include intravenous nitroglycerin, oral clonidine, and β-adrenergic blockers other than labetalol. Intravenous nitroglycerin is easily titrated and is especially attractive for the management of patients with pulmonary edema. However, its antihypertensive potency is somewhat limited. Oral clonidine, a centrally

TABLE 181–3. ANTIHYPERTENSIVE DRUGS COMMONLY USED IN PREGNANCY

Type	Agents
Oral	α-Methyldopa
	Labetalol
	Clonidine
	Diuretics
Parenteral	Labetalol
	Hydralazine
	Sodium nitroprusside
	Nitroglycerin

acting α₂-adrenergic agonist, is an effective antihypertensive drug, but concerns about the risk of rebound hypertension after cessation limit its use.

There remains considerable debate concerning the use of β-adrenergic blockers in pregnancy, because of the potential risks of fetal bradycardia and a decrease in perfusion to the uteroplacental bed.[61] Esmolol has been used widely for heart rate control in pregnancy, but its efficacy is limited as an antihypertensive agent.

Hypertensive drugs commonly used during pregnancy are listed in Table 181-3.

MANAGEMENT OF HYPERTENSION DURING LABOR AND DELIVERY

Management of hypertension during labor and delivery is directed toward avoiding acute and maternal complications. Antihypertensive drug therapy with judicious use of intravenous fluids is of paramount importance to avoid unnecessary complications.[62] Postpartum monitoring is advocated for high-risk, chronically hypertensive patients. Hypertension associated with preeclampsia usually resolves spontaneously within a few weeks after delivery. These patients are at risk for development of acute complications such as hypertensive encephalopathy, pulmonary edema, and acute renal failure. The choice of antihypertensive medications or the doses used may need to be adjusted after delivery. Minute amounts of all antihypertensive agents are found in breast milk. Although limited data are available, adverse perinatal effects have not been observed with the more commonly used drugs, such as α-methyldopa, hydralazine, and the various α-adrenergic blockers.[4,63]

ANNOTATED REFERENCES

Buchbinder A, Sibai BM, Caritis S, et al: Adverse perinatal outcomes are significantly higher in severe gestational hypertension than in mild preeclampsia. Am J Obstet Gynecol 2002;186:66.

> The objective of this study was to compare the frequency of adverse fetal outcomes in women who developed hypertensive disorders with or without proteinuria during pregnancy. The study design was a secondary analysis of data from 598 women who had had preeclampsia in a previous pregnancy and were enrolled in a multicenter trial of aspirin for the prevention of preeclampsia. There were no statistically significant differences in perinatal outcomes between subjects with normotension or mild gestational hypertension and those with mild preeclampsia. Women with severe gestational hypertension had increased rates of preterm delivery and delivery of small-for-gestational-age infants. This information underscores the need for BP management in the high-risk, severely hypertensive patient but questions the benefits of treating less severe hypertension.

Magee L, Cham C, Waterman EJ, et al: Hydralazine for treatment of severe hypertension in pregnancy: Metanalysis. BMJ 2003;327:955.

A meta-analysis was performed to review outcomes in randomized controlled trials, published between 1966 and 2002, comparing hydralazine with other antihypertensive agents for severe hypertension in pregnancy. In 13 trials comparing hydralazine with either nifedipine or labetalol, hydralazine was an effective antihypertensive drug for severe hypertension but was associated with an increased incidence of maternal hypotension, cesarean section, placental abruption, oliguria, adverse effects on fetal heart rate, and lower Apgar scores. These data do not support the use of hydralazine as first-line therapy for severe hypertension in pregnancy.

Sibai BM: Chronic hypertension in pregnancy [High-risk pregnancy series: An expert's view]. Obstet Gynecol 2002;100:369.

In this excellent review article, Sibai describes the maternal outcomes of pregnant women with chronic essential hypertension. He makes a distinction between those women with "high-risk" versus "low-risk" chronic hypertension. He presents the lack of evidence of the benefits of treatment of low-risk essential uncomplicated chronic hypertension. The data strongly suggest treatment of severe hypertension in pregnancy to avoid poor maternal and fetal outcomes. However, the recommendations to treat less severe hypertension are based on dogma rather than scientific evidence, and he cautions against following them.

Sibai BM: Diagnosis and management of gestational hypertension and preeclampsia [High-risk pregnancy series: An expert's view]. Obstet Gynecol 2003;102:181.

This is an extensive review of gestational hypertension and preeclampsia. Sibai discusses the differences in maternal and perinatal complications and outcomes of women with mild hypertensive disease compared with severe hypertension. He recommends that women with diagnosed gestational hypertension require close evaluation of maternal and fetal conditions for the duration of the pregnancy. Those with severe disease should be managed as inpatients. He advocates the need for randomized trials to determine the efficacy and safety of antihypertensive drugs in pregnant women with mild-to-moderate hypertension.

Von Dadelszen P, Ornstein MP, Bull SB, et al: Fall in mean arterial pressure and fetal growth restriction in pregnancy hypertension: A meta-analysis. Lancet 2000;355:87.

These authors investigated the relation between fetoplacental growth and the use of oral antihypertensive drugs to treat mild-to-moderate hypertension. The study design was a metaregression analysis of published data from randomized trials. A greater mean difference in mean arterial pressure with antihypertensive therapy was associated with a higher incidence of small-for-gestational-age infants and lower mean birth weights. These data suggest that decreases in maternal BP of women with only mild-to-moderate pregnancy hypertension may adversely affect fetal growth and offer no benefits to maternal outcome.

Chapter 182

ACUTE PULMONARY COMPLICATIONS IN PREGNANCY

Cornelia R. Graves

KEY POINTS

PREGNANCY

1. Tidal volume (Vt) is increased during pregnancy; however, functional residual capacity (FRC) is decreased.

2. A normal arterial blood gas determination in pregnancy reflects a compensated respiratory alkalosis.

3. Respiratory distress occurs more rapidly in the gravid patient owing to changes in pulmonary physiology.

ASTHMA IN PREGNANCY

1. The treatment of asthma in pregnancy does not differ significantly from treatment in the nongravid state.

2. Because FEV_1 does not change during pregnancy, a peak flowmeter is a useful tool in monitoring patients with asthma.

3. A $PaCO_2$ of greater than 35 mm Hg in the setting of severe asthma represents respiratory distress in the gravid patient.

ARDS IN PREGNANCY

1. Caution should be used when considering treatment for preterm labor in patients requiring respiratory support. Correction of oxygenation is usually more effective than pharmacologic therapy.

2. The need for mechanical ventilatory support **does not mandate** delivery of the fetus. Most studies do not report significant maternal improvement after delivery.

3. Sedatives, hypnotic drugs, anxiolytic agents, and nondepolarizing neuromuscular blockade agents are not contraindicated in pregnancy.

EMBOLISM IN PREGNANCY

1. Pregnancy is a hypercoagulable state that increases the risk of thromboembolic phenomenon.

2. Radiographic studies should not be avoided in the gravid patient with respiratory compromise.

3. Anticoagulation therapy is not contraindicated in pregnancy; however, warfarin is contraindicated for use in the first trimester.

4. Amniotic fluid embolism occurs in about 1 in 80,000 pregnancies. It is associated with significant maternal morbidity and mortality.

During pregnancy, the respiratory system undergoes a number of changes and is subject to functional and anatomic stresses. The critical care provider must remember these changes to appropriately care for the maternal-fetal unit. Although the need for ventilatory support is rare in pregnancy, respiratory insufficiency is still the most common indication in pregnancy for admission to a critical care unit. In this chapter, the unique physiologic changes that occur during pregnancy are addressed and guidance is provided to the critical care specialist who may encounter pregnancies that are complicated by acute pulmonary complications.

PULMONARY PHYSIOLOGY IN PREGNANCY

A number of physiologic changes affect respiration during pregnancy. Normal pregnancy is associated with a 20% increase in oxygen consumption and a 15% increase in metabolic rate. During the first trimester, minute ventilation is increased while respiratory rate remains the same. Although one might assume that lung volume during pregnancy would decrease owing to the rise in the maternal diaphragm, tidal volume (VT) is actually increased by 40% over baseline values. The increase in VT is thought to be due to the increase in circulating progesterone that affects the respiratory center.[1] Arterial blood gas measurements reflect a respiratory alkalosis that is compensated by a metabolic acidosis that results in a relatively normal pH. $PaCO_2$ usually ranges from 28 to 32 mm Hg. Functional residual capacity (FRC), residual volume, and total lung volume are decreased near term. Because of this decrease, respiratory distress occurs more rapidly in the gravida than in the nonpregnant state. The function of the large airways as measured by forced expiratory volume at 1 second (FEV_1), and peak expiratory flow rate (PEFR) is essentially unchanged throughout pregnancy.[2]

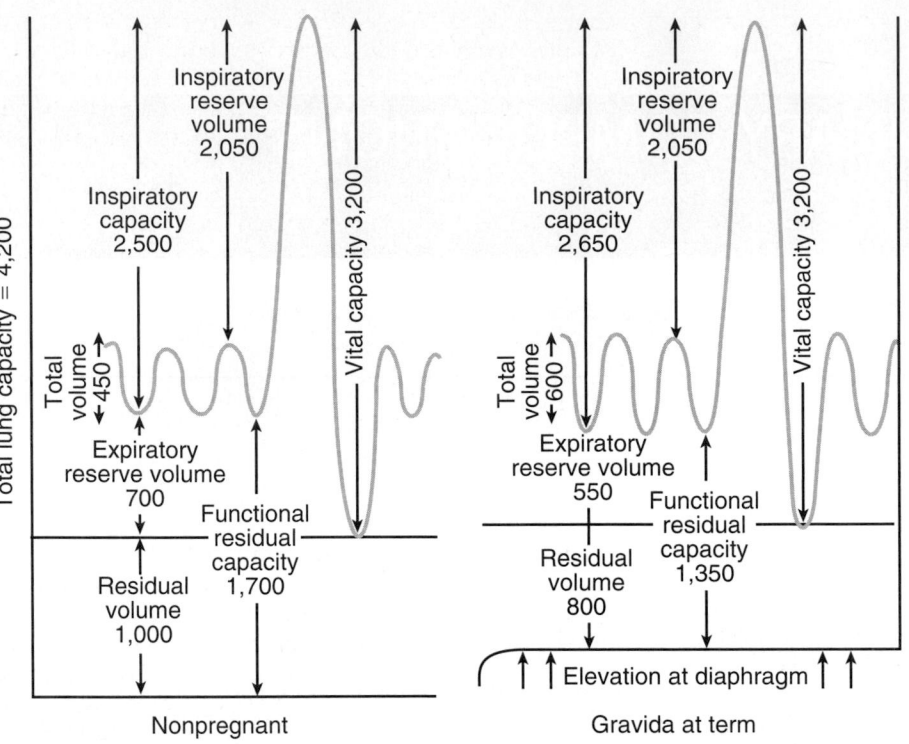

FIGURE 182–1. Respiratory changes in pregnancy.

Colloid osmotic pressure is decreased by 20%. This change in hydrostatic pressure results in a propensity for the pregnant patient to develop cardiogenic and noncardiogenic pulmonary edema.

Dyspnea on exertion is common, especially in the third trimester of pregnancy, making diagnosis of respiratory problems more difficult than in the nongravid state.

Figure 182-1 illustrates the graphic relationship of pulmonary changes.

ASTHMA

EPIDEMIOLOGY

Asthma is one of the most common pulmonary problems in pregnant women. Retrospective studies have estimated its prevalence from 1% to 4% in the gravid population.[3] The disease is characterized by hyperactive airways, leading to episodic bronchoconstriction. The role of inflammatory mediators in the pathogenesis of asthma has become apparent in recent years, leading to earlier use of inflammatory medications in the treatment of exacerbations.

The cause of asthma is unknown; however, it has been observed that its prevalence in the general population is increasing.

EFFECTS OF ASTHMA ON PREGNANCY

Asthma may be triggered by environmental allergens, medications, especially aspirin or nonsteroidal anti-inflammatory medications, or stress.[4] Most exacerbations are marked by cough, wheezing, and dyspnea. Rapid therapeutic intervention at the time of an exacerbation is imperative to prevent impaired maternal and fetal oxygenation because uncontrolled asthma can increase maternal morbidity. Affected women

are three times more likely to have hyperemesis gravidarum and twice as likely to undergo uterine hemorrhage.[5] Demissie and coworkers noted in a retrospective study of 2289 pregnant women that there was a twofold increase in pregnancy-induced hypertension, especially in women who were corticosteroid dependent. Preterm labor also was more common in patients who were corticosteroid dependent.[6]

Whereas historical data have shown an increase in perinatal death and low birth weight,[7] Fitzsimmons and colleagues observed low birth weight in only those patients treated for status asthmaticus.[8] In addition, Schatz and colleagues noted that intrauterine growth restriction was directly related to lung function as measured by FEV_1.[9]

EFFECT OF PREGNANCY ON ASTHMA

Numerous studies have observed that the course of asthma may be affected by pregnancy. Gluck and associates reviewed nine studies performed between 1930 and 1967 and found that on average, asthma improved in 36% of women during pregnancy, remained unchanged in 41%, and worsened in 23%.[10] Schatz and coworkers, in an analysis of 366 pregnancies in which patient status was followed by objective criteria, found that asthma improved in 28%, remained unchanged in 33%, and worsened in 35%. Fifty-nine percent of the patients had similar asthma control in successive pregnancies.[11]

Fetal sex may influence asthma in pregnancy. In one study, mothers who gave birth to boys were more likely to report improved asthma symptoms.[12] Dodds and colleagues also found that the use of medications to treat asthma was less common in mothers of boys.[13] While a number of hypotheses have been proposed, including alterations in progesterone and the role of leukotrienes, changes in not one of these mediators can explain the varied course of the pregnant asthmatic.[14]

MANAGEMENT

The National Asthma Education and Prevention Program (NAEP) issued specific guidelines regarding asthma treatment. In 1993, the Working Group on Asthma and Pregnancy established criteria for diagnosis and treatment in the gravid population.[15]

The goals of treatment during pregnancy are to control exacerbation and to prevent status asthmaticus, thereby reducing maternal and fetal hypoxemia.

The initial step in treatment involves monitoring of pulmonary function. FEV_1 is the single best measure of pulmonary function. Physical examination and chest radiography are poor measures of disease severity. A portable, hand-held peak flowmeter gives a quick, accurate assessment by measuring the PEFR. Most authorities believe that airways remain essentially unchanged throughout pregnancy; therefore, every patient with asthma should be given a peak flowmeter and be educated in its use. The patient should obtain a baseline PEFR during a quiescent period. The severity of disease is determined by the occurrences of exacerbations and the changes in FEV_1 and PEFR. The PEFR can be used as a guide to refer the patient for emergency care.

Pharmacologic therapy is the mainstay of asthma treatment. Most drugs used in the treatment of asthma are thought to be safe in pregnancy. Inhaled beta agonists are the most frequently used in asthma treatment. A prospective study of inhaled beta agonists in 259 pregnancies showed no change in the rate of congenital malformation, perinatal mortality, low birth weight, or complications of pregnancy.[16] There is little role for the use of oral beta agonists, which may have more adverse systemic symptoms and are no more effective than inhaled drugs.

Inhaled corticosteroid therapy remains the mainstay of the anti-inflammatory treatment of asthma. They have also been advocated as first-line therapy in patients with mild asthma.[17] In a prospective, observational study of 504 pregnant women with asthma, those taking an inhaled corticosteroid were four times less likely than their nontreated counterparts to suffer an exacerbation.[18] Another randomized study noted that there was a 55% reduction in readmission rates for acute asthma in patients using inhaled beclomethasone.[19] Inhaled corticosteroids can increase the effectiveness of beta-adrenergic agents by inducing the formation of new beta receptors. Because beclomethasone is the most studied of the inhaled corticosteroids in pregnancy, it is recommended as the first line of therapy.[15] However, if patients are well controlled on other corticosteroid preparations, it is suggested that they be continued on their current medication because all inhaled corticosteroids are labeled by the Food and Drug Administration (FDA) as pregnancy class C. Other nonsteroidal anti-inflammatory medications used in the treatment of asthma (e.g., cromolyn sodium and nedocromil sodium) appear to be less effective than inhaled corticosteroids in reducing asthma symptoms.

Systemic corticosteroids should be reserved for the periodic treatment of acute asthma exacerbations. Chronic oral corticosteroid therapy may increase the risks of gestational diabetes mellitus, preterm labor, low-birth-weight infants, and preeclampsia; however, it is evident that the benefits of controlled severe asthma outweigh the potential risks to the mother and the fetus.

Intravenous corticosteroids have no increased benefits over oral corticosteroids in the treatment of acute exacerbations.[20] Methylprednisolone, hydrocortisone, and prednisone are safe for use in pregnancy, unlike betamethasone or dexamethasone, because very little active drug crosses the placenta.

Leukotriene pathway moderators have been shown to improve pulmonary function, as measured by FEV_1.[21] Zafirlukast and montelukast are rated FDA category B; however, there is little experience with these drugs in pregnancy, and their role is undetermined.

The treatment of asthma requires patient education to provide optimization in the preconceptional period and during the pregnancy to provide optimum outcome. Table 182-1 offers a suggested schematic for the treatment of asthma in pregnancy.

STATUS ASTHMATICUS

Status asthmaticus is a rare complication in pregnancy. Diagnosis is established by a $PaCO_2$ of less than 70 mm Hg, a $PaCO_2$ of greater than or equal to 35 mm Hg, or a measured expiratory flow of less than 25% of expected. Because of impending respiratory failure, these patients should be managed in a critical care unit. Aggressive treatment of status asthmaticus is mandatory to protect the mother and the fetus. Maternal mortality may be as high as 7% and fetal mortality as high as 11% despite adequate treatment. Epinephrine is not contraindicated in pregnancy during a respiratory emergency. Criteria for intubation in the gravida with status asthmaticus include (1) inability to maintain PaO_2 of greater than 60 mm Hg despite supplemental oxygen; (2) inability to maintain a PCO_2 of less than 40 mm Hg; (3) evidence of maternal exhaustion with worsening acidosis despite intensive bronchodilator therapy (pH < 7.2); and (4) altered maternal consciousness.[15]

When traditional treatment proves to be ineffective, a number of therapies have been reported beneficial. The use of a helium-oxygen mixture that has been reported to be effective in nonpregnant studies has been used safely in pregnancy.[22]

TABLE 182–1. TREATMENT OF ASTHMA IN PREGNANCY

Mild Asthma

Characterized by FEV_1 or PEFR $\geq$ 80%
Brief (<1 hour) exacerbations
Treatment: inhaled beta$_2$ agonist

Moderate Asthma

Characterized by FEV_1 or PEFR range from 60% to 80%
Exacerbations more than twice per week; exacerbations may last for several days and occasional emergency care needed
Treatment: inhaled corticosteroids and inhaled beta$_2$ agonist

Severe Asthma

Characterized by a FEV_1 or PEFR < 60% of baseline
Continuous symptoms, limited activity, frequent exacerbations and nocturnal symptoms, occasional hospitalization and emergency treatment needed
Treatment: inhaled corticosteroids, inhaled beta$_2$ agonist, sustained release theophylline; oral corticosteroid taper for active symptoms

PULMONARY EDEMA

Pulmonary edema can be divided into two categories during pregnancy. Cardiogenic pulmonary edema is the result of high intravascular pressures creating a hydrostatic pressure gradient that results in the extravasation of fluid into the lung tissues despite the integrity of the normal lung microcirculation. Noncardiogenic edema is the result of a leaky pulmonary capillary bed despite normal intravascular pressures.

During pregnancy, the distinction between these two types of edema may be blurred owing to disease states that exacerbate the hypo-oncotic state of pregnancy.

ETIOLOGY

There are a number of causes of pulmonary edema in pregnancy. Some are pathologic in their process, others are due to idiopathic causes. One of the most common associations with pulmonary edema during pregnancy is hypertensive disease. In patients with hypertensive disease, pulmonary edema may be cardiogenic owing to fluid overload or left ventricular dysfunction or noncardiogenic owing to decreased oncotic pressure.

Another common cause of pulmonary edema in pregnancy is tocolytic therapy. Most cases described have resulted from the intravenous use of beta sympathomimetics. The use of magnesium sulfate therapy as well as the use of corticosteroids in association with tocolysis for preterm labor has been shown to exacerbate the condition. The incidence of edema is increased in multiple gestations and in patients with subclinical infection.

Other causes of acute pulmonary edema in pregnancy include amniotic fluid embolism, aspiration, and the need for massive transfusion after hemorrhage.[23]

TREATMENT

The treatment of pulmonary edema during pregnancy depends on its etiology. Determination of the cause is best obtained by the use of pulmonary artery catheterization and the measurement of pulmonary capillary wedge pressure. Although all patients may not require this intervention, it is recommended in patients in whom the clinical picture may be unclear (e.g., those with hypertensive disease) and in those who do not respond to standard diuretic therapy.

For patients who not improve rapidly with diuretic therapy, intubation and ventilation with positive pressure is recommended. In addition to the use of diuretic therapy, reduction of preload and afterload may be achieved by the use of vasodilators such as nitrates, hydralazine, or calcium channel blockers. All are safe for use in pregnancy.

Table 182-2 offers a guide for treatment of patients with pulmonary edema.

ACUTE RESPIRATORY DISTRESS SYNDROME

ETIOLOGY

The causes of ARDS[24-27] in pregnancy include preeclampsia, sepsis, aspiration pyelonephritis, intrauterine infections, acute fatty liver of pregnancy, and amniotic fluid embolism.[28]

TABLE 182–2. TREATMENT IN PATIENTS WITH PULMONARY EDEMA

1. Determine the etiology, stop fluids, tocolysis, etc
2. Treat with a diuretic (the author prefers furosemide in increments of 10 to 20 mg i.v. push)
3. Consider the use of morphine sulfate for patient comfort, 1 to 2 mg i.v. push q2-3h
4. Proceed with hemodynamic monitoring if the patient does not rapidly respond to the above measures
5. Consider intubation and mechanical ventilation with positive pressure for those patients with noncardiogenic pulmonary edema and those patients with cardiogenic pulmonary edema who need further support

---

In a review of 83 cases of ARDS associated with pregnancy, it was noted that among the causes of ARDS, 35 cases were attributed to uniquely obstetric conditions.[29] In addition, it was noted that varicella pneumonia and pyelonephritis were associated with ARDS. These conditions rarely trigger ARDS in immunocompetent adults. De Vaciana and colleagues pointed out that the development of lung injury in pregnancy correlates with known physiologic changes, including increased blood volume, decreased colloid osmotic pressure, and an unchanged critical lung closing volume despite a diminished FRC.[30]

MANAGEMENT

The management of ARDS includes diagnosis, maternal stabilization, fetal monitoring, investigation and treatment of underlying causes, and, in many cases, evaluation for delivery.[29]

Maternal stabilization includes intubation for mechanical ventilation, if necessary. The clinician should consider intubation sooner rather than later in the presence of respiratory deterioration, keeping in mind that the decreased FRC exacerbates respiratory distress.

Contemporary thinking regarding the treatment of ARDS has found that a lung protective ventilator strategy is the first therapy that has been found to improve outcomes in ARDS.

It has been noted in numerous studies that decreasing the V_T from the standard of 12 mL/kg to 6 mL/kg or less and peak inspiratory pressures to less than 30 cm H_2O from 50 cm H_2O have resulted in decreased morbidity and mortality in patients with ARDS.[31] There has been much discussion in the literature concerning permissive hypercapnia and its use in preventing lung injury. However, there have been no controlled studies in pregnancy, and I believe that increasing $PaCO_2$ in the pregnant patient should not be undertaken.

The judicious use of fluids is important in the management of ARDS. Although some authors have advocated the use of fluid restriction, the clinician must consider the volume-dependent status of pregnancy. It is recommended that fluid management be carefully guided by the use of hemodynamic monitoring.

Whereas oxygenation is important, it should be noted that oxygen should be used at the lowest concentration possible, because it is toxic to lung tissue in high doses. The goal of therapy is to keep the SaO_2 greater than or equal to 95%.

A number of other methods have been discussed in the treatment of ARDS, including inhaled nitric oxide, prostacyclin, surfactant, and inverse ratio ventilation. Currently, these modalities cannot be recommended because they have

TABLE 182–3. MANAGEMENT OF PATIENT WITH ARDS

1. Evaluate the patient in respiratory distress; calculate PaO_2/FiO_2 ratio; consider intubation if ≤ 200 mm Hg. The PEEP or CPAP mask is not recommended in pregnancy owing to the high risk of aspiration.
2. Set tidal volume at 8 to 9 mL/kg to prevent increased peak pressures. Given recent evidence, aim to keep peak pressures less than 40 cm H_2O.
3. Use PEEP starting at 5 to 8 cm H_2O to assist in recruiting alveoli.
4. Aim to keep FiO_2 less than 60%; keep SaO_2 greater than or equal to 95%.
5. Use a pulmonary artery catheter to assist in fluid management and to guide hemodynamic parameters.
6. Consider the use of tocolysis only after the patient has been adequately hydrated and oxygenated.
7. Consider delivery if indicated for obstetric conditions or if continuing the pregnancy has no clear benefit.

TABLE 182–4. TREATMENT OF PULMONARY EMBOLISM IN PREGNANCY

1. Begin therapy immediately, based on strong clinical suspicion while awaiting complete diagnostic work-up.
2. Establish the diagnosis with appropriate diagnostic imaging test.
3. Maintain maternal and fetal oxygenation.
4. Administer intravenous heparin and maintain full anticoagulation for 7 to 10 days prior to changing to subcutaneous injections (antepartum) or warfarin (postpartum). Oral anticoagulation should be continued 6 to 8 weeks after delivery.
5. Keep International Normalized Ratio, activated partial thromboplastin time, or factor Xa level in therapeutic range.

not been shown to decrease morbidity and mortality. Other trials considering prone ventilation and corticosteroids in late ARDS appear promising but have not been proven in large, prospective randomized trials.[32]

Fetal surveillance during ARDS may be more difficult owing to the drugs that are used to sedate the mother affecting fetal heart rate and variability. Sedatives, anxiolytics, hypnotics, and nondepolarizing agents are not contraindicated in pregnancy. In addition, preterm contractions and labor may present a problem due to maternal hypoxemia. The clinician is cautioned against starting tocolytic therapy before achieving adequate maternal oxygenation. If tocolysis in needed, beta agonists, such as terbutaline, should be avoided, owing to the risk of increased pulmonary capillary permeability and the increased demands on cardiac load. Magnesium sulfate is not strictly contraindicated but also may increase pulmonary capillary permeability. The use of NSAIDs may be the best choice for tocolysis because they have been proven to improve ARDS in animal models.[29] Consultation with a maternal-fetal specialist is recommended to assist the intensivist in caring for these complex patients.

The timing of delivery is a question that comes to the mind of the clinician taking care of the patient with ARDS. Some authors advocate delivery after maternal stabilization, citing the possible "therapeutic effect" of delivery. Whitty and colleagues failed to demonstrate any significant benefit to delivery. It is my opinion that delivery should be considered on a case-by-case basis, carefully weighing the risk:benefit ratio to the mother and the fetus.

Table 182-3 represents a reasonable management scheme for the patient with ARDS.

EMBOLISM

Because of the hypercoagulable changes in the coagulation cascade associated with pregnancy, there is an increased risk of venous thromboembolism. It has been estimated that clinically symptomatic pregnancy-related venous thromboembolism occurs in 1 to 2 per 1000 pregnancies. Maternal age (>40 years) and ethnic and genetic factors may increase this risk. Postpartum thromboembolism is three to five times more common than antepartum thrombotic events. Cesarean section confers a risk of 3 to 16 times that of a vaginal delivery.

Clinical signs of a pulmonary embolism include unexplained tachycardia, dyspnea, diaphoresis, and a nonproductive cough. The workup for a suspected pulmonary embolism should include normal laboratory studies (arterial blood gases) and an electrocardiogram in conjunction with radiographic testing. Pregnancy should not prevent obtaining appropriate radiographic studies. In patients with a high clinical index of suspicion for thromboembolic phenomena, definitive diagnosis is imperative. Ventilation-perfusion scans are recommended as the first diagnostic test. Spiral computed tomography has replaced ventilation-perfusion scanning in many centers as an initial test. Pulmonary angiography is still the "gold standard" for offering definitive diagnosis. All of the aforementioned tests use less than the 5 rads of radiation exposure that has been associated with fetal teratogenesis. The use of an abdominal shield further decreases fetal exposure.

D-Dimer may not be useful for the diagnosis of thromboembolism during pregnancy because it may be elevated in the absence of a thrombus. Heparin is the anticoagulant of choice in the antepartum patient. Unfractionated or low-molecular-weight heparin can be used. Neither of these drugs cross the placenta, owing to the size of the drug molecule. Patients on low-molecular-weight heparin should be monitored with factor Xa levels to ensure a therapeutic level.

Warfarin may be used in the second and third trimesters in patients in whom heparin therapy may be contraindicated. It is the anticoagulant of choice in the postpartum period and is compatible with breastfeeding.

The goals of therapy during the antepartum and postpartum period (6 to 8 weeks post delivery) should be an activated partial thromboplastin time of 2.0 to 2.5; a factor Xa level of 0.6 to 1.1, or an International Normalized Ratio of 2.5 to 3.0.

Amniotic fluid embolism is a rare phenomenon that may initially present as severe respiratory distress. Risk factors include rapid labor, multiple gestation, polyhydramnios, and uterine rupture. Patients with amniotic fluid embolism usually have symptoms of acute respiratory distress, cardiovascular collapse, and profound disseminated intravascular coagulation. Treatment is supportive; however, maternal mortality may be as high as 80%.

CONCLUSION

Because of the rare need for mechanical ventilation, there are no randomized controlled trials to determine the treatment modalities that are most effective in pregnancy. A recent retrospective study noted a maternal mortality rate of 14% and a fetal mortality of 11% in patients who required mechanical ventilation during pregnancy.[35] The critical care specialist, perinatologist, anesthesiologist, and other members of the health care team should work closely to provide coordinated care. Understanding of the physiologic changes during pregnancy combined with aggressive treatment of early pathologic changes will assist in providing improved management in gravid patients with potentially lethal pulmonary complications.[36]

ANNOTATED REFERENCES

Catanzarite VA, Wilms D: Adult respiratory distress syndrome in pregnancy: Report of 3 cases and review of the literature. Obstet Gynecol Surv 1997;52:381-392.

This is one of only a few reviews in the obstetrical literature evaluating ARDS and its effect on pregnancy.

Jenkins TM, Troiano NH, Graves CR, et al: Mechanical ventilation in obstetric population: Characteristic and delivery rates. Am J Obstet Gynecol 2003;188:549-552.

This retrospective review evaluates 51 women admitted during pregnancy for mechanical ventilation. Fetal and maternal morbidity and mortality are discussed.

Tan KS, Thompson NC: Asthma in pregnancy Am J Med 2000;109:727-733.

An excellent review article that evaluates asthma, pregnancy, and considerations for treatment.

Tomlinson MW, Caruthers TJ, Whitty JE, Gonik B: Does delivery improve maternal condition in the respiratory-compromised gravida? Obstet Gynecol 1998;91:108-111.

A retrospective review is presented of 10 pregnant patients requiring mechanical ventilation. Outcome variables are reviewed, including respiratory improvement after delivery.

Townson-Dizon D. Pregnancy-related venous thromboembolism. Clin Obstet Gynecol 2002;45:363-368.

Provides a summary regarding the treatment of venous thromboembolism during pregnancy.

Chapter 183

POSTPARTUM HEMORRHAGE

Marie R. Baldisseri

KEY POINTS

1. Postpartum hemorrhage (PPH) is defined as excessive bleeding after a vaginal or cesarean delivery which can be associated with hemodynamic instability if the bleeding is severe.

2. The usual signs of **tachycardia and hypotension** associated with severe bleeding **may not manifest early because of the relative hypervolemic state** of pregnancy or in cases of concealed hematomas with ongoing blood losses.

3. **PPH is the leading cause of maternal death** worldwide and one of the three leading causes of death in the United States, along with embolism and hypertensive disorders of pregnancy.

4. **Massive blood loss can occur from the uterus** because of the significant physiologic increase in blood flow to the uterus at term.

5. **Occult bleeding occurs most frequently with retained placental fragments, uterine atony, and concealed hematomas** in the pelvis, perineum, or retroperitoneal space.

6. Women with a prior history of PPH have a 10% risk of recurrence with a subsequent pregnancy.

7. **Many women have predisposing factors leading to the development of PPH.** Antenatal identification of potential predisposing factors allows for close monitoring of the high-risk patient.

8. **The most frequent cause of PPH is uterine atony,** which occurs in 1 of every 20 deliveries. Risk factors for uterine atony include overdistention of the uterus, retained placenta, uterine muscle fatigue, and use of halogenated anesthetic agents.

9. The **diagnosis of uterine atony is made clinically** by palpation of a boggy and enlarged uterus.

10. The **second most frequent cause of PPH is lacerations of the lower genital tract** that occur as a result of traumatic labor or spontaneously.

11. Manual exploration of the uterus confirms the diagnosis of retained placental fragments. Placental retention is most commonly associated with several types of placental anomalies.

12. **Disseminated intravascular coagulation (DIC) is associated with placental abruption,** the HELLP syndrome (hemolysis, elevated liver enzymes, and low platelets), acute fatty liver of pregnancy, intrauterine fetal death, sepsis, and amniotic fluid embolism.

13. **Amniotic fluid embolism syndrome usually manifests as sudden and acute respiratory failure,** cardiogenic shock, and DIC.

14. In the United States, most obstetricians practice expectant management of the third stage of labor, allowing for spontaneous delivery of the placenta. Active management of the third stage of labor involves the use of an oxytocic drug and gentle traction on the umbilical cord with countertraction of the uterus to facilitate delivery of the placenta.

15. **General treatment measures include aggressive and early fluid resuscitation** while investigating the potential source of the bleeding. Higher maternal mortality rates are seen when blood losses are underestimated and treatment is delayed.

16. Patients with **ongoing severe bleeding, blood losses greater than 2 L, or hemodynamic compromise require blood transfusions** in addition to volume resuscitation.

17. **Specific treatment** modalities include the administration of **oxytocic drugs, uterine packing, tamponade procedures** with arterial balloon occlusion, and selective arterial embolization.

18. **Surgical therapy** is reserved for cases of uterine atony and after all other modalities have failed. **Uterine, ovarian, and iliac artery ligations** have been successful in controlling bleeding.

19. **Total or partial hysterectomy is the definitive surgical procedure.** Uterine rupture necessitates a hysterectomy.

20. **Complications from PPH are the same as those of hemorrhagic shock,** with risk of multiple organ failure, acute respiratory distress syndrome, dilutional coagulopathy, and Sheehan's syndrome.

21. **Sheehan's syndrome results from severe PPH** and **manifests as severe hypopituitarism.**

22. The prognosis of PPH depends on the cause of the bleeding, its extent and duration, and the speed of diagnosis and treatment.

DEFINITION

The commonly accepted definition of postpartum hemorrhage (PPH) is excessive and life-threatening bleeding, after 20 weeks of gestation, that occurs at the time of delivery of the fetus or the placenta. Primary PPH is excessive blood loss within 24 hours of delivery. Secondary PPH is any abnormal or excessive bleeding that occurs between 24 hours and 12 weeks after delivery. Most commonly, bleeding occurs in the third stage of labor, which refers to the time between delivery of the fetus and delivery of the placenta after its separation and expulsion from the uterus. Defining excessive bleeding is somewhat problematic, because it can be difficult to determine the exact amount of blood loss, and clinicians tend to underestimate blood loss. With a normal vaginal delivery, blood loss is typically 500 mL or less; after a normal cesarean section, it is usually 800 to 1000 mL. Blood loss greater than these amounts has been used to define PPH. However, uncomplicated vaginal and cesarean deliveries can occasionally occur with greater amounts of blood loss but without hemodynamic compromise. Therefore, a more comprehensive definition of PPH is bleeding (regardless of the volume of shed blood) that is severe enough to cause hemodynamic compromise.

Some authors also have used a decrease in hematocrit greater than 10% as a diagnostic criterion, although the change in hematocrit depends on when the blood test is performed after the onset of bleeding.[1] The hematocrit level initially may be in the low-normal to normal range despite excessive bleeding, because hematocrit does not change quickly in response to rapid hemorrhage. The hematocrit is also determined, in part, by the volume of infused resuscitation fluid. Because the parturient's blood volume is increased by 30% to 50%, she may not manifest signs of tachycardia and hypotension until blood loss exceeds 1500 mL.[2] If the patient is hemodynamically unstable but the amount of blood visualized externally is relatively insignificant, then occult sites of internal bleeding should be suspected immediately.

INCIDENCE AND MORTALITY

Maternal mortality has significantly decreased over the past 50 years in developed countries, in part because of improvements in obstetric care. The pregnancy-related mortality rate is approximately 7 to 10 maternal deaths per 100,000 live births in the United States.[3,4] The mortality rates are significantly higher for African-American and for Asian or Pacific Island women compared with Caucasian women.[3,4] The three leading causes of death for all women are hemorrhage, embolism, and hypertensive disorders of pregnancy.

In developing countries, PPH remains the leading cause of maternal mortality, and it complicates approximately 1 of every 1000 deliveries.[5] Data from the World Health Organization indicate that 25% of maternal deaths are secondary to postpartum bleeding, accounting for more than 100,000 deaths annually worldwide.[6,7] It is estimated that 2% to 5% of deliveries are complicated by PPH.

PATHOPHYSIOLOGY

At term, blood flow to the uterus and placenta increases to 600 to 1200 mL/min, accounting for 10% of the maternal cardiac output.[8] In order to stem the flow of blood and to provide immediate hemostasis after delivery of the fetus, the uterus begins to contract. Myometrial contraction is the primary mechanism for both placental separation and hemostasis. The myometrial muscle fibers of the uterus contract and simultaneously retract, causing compression and occlusion of the blood vessels. Uterine atony results when this adaptive mechanism fails and the myometrial fibers are unable to contract and retract normally. Excessive bleeding from the uterus and lower genital tract from many causes, including lacerations, placental anomalies, and trauma, is directly related to the increase in blood flow to the uterus and placenta. At term, there is a physiologic increase in the circulating concentrations of various clotting factors. This adaptive response also helps to control the bleeding that is a normal consequence of delivery. However, these factors are overwhelmed by the excessive bleeding of PPH.

PRESENTATION

PPH often manifests as brisk and excessive flow of blood from the vagina. This finding is easily observed on physical examination. If the placenta has been delivered, blood can be seen at the vaginal entrance. Maternal hemodynamics may be unaltered initially. If the bleeding is left untreated, the typical presenting signs of hypovolemic shock (i.e., tachycardia, tachypnea, and hypotension) become apparent. Bonnar[9] described the symptoms related to PPH in relation to the amount of blood loss (Table 183-1).[9] However, the signs and symptoms of hemorrhagic shock may not occur immediately and may extend over a longer period of time if shed blood is sequestered in the uterus. Occult bleeding occurs most frequently with retained placental fragments, uterine atony, and concealed hematomas in the pelvis, perineum, or retroperitoneal space. Occult hemorrhage in the uterus or hematomas should be suspected in patients who are in the third stage of labor with hemodynamic instability but little or no evidence of external bleeding. Signs and symptoms of excessive bleeding also may be delayed because of the relative hypervolemic state of the patient and by the position of the patient after delivery with the legs elevated in stirrups.[10]

CAUSES OF POSTPARTUM HEMORRHAGE

Obtaining a detailed antenatal history is important in helping to determine a possible cause of PPH. A history of prior bleeding episodes associated with heavy menses or with dental or surgical procedures should raise the possibility of an underlying coagulation or bleeding disorder. Significant predisposing risk factors for the development of PPH include previous episodes of PPH, multiparity, and

TABLE 183–1. PRESENTATION OF SYMPTOMS IN POSTPARTUM HEMORRHAGE

% Blood Loss (mL)	Systolic Blood Pressure (mm Hg)	Signs and Symptoms
10-15 (500-1000)	Normal	Tachycardia, palpitations, dizziness
15-25 (1000-1500)	Low-normal	Tachycardia, weakness, diaphoresis
25-35 (1500-2000)	70-80	Restlessness, pallor, oliguria
35-45 (2000-3000)	50-70	Collapse, air hunger, anuria

TABLE 183–2. PREDISPOSING RISK FACTORS FOR POSTPARTUM HEMORRHAGE (PPH)

Previous PPH
Prolonged third stage of labor
Augmented or stimulated labor
Multiple gestation
Multiparity
Coagulation abnormalities
Cervical, vaginal, or perineal lacerations
Preeclampsia
Arrest of descent of the fetus
Mediolateral episiotomy
Nulliparity
Polyhydramnios
Maternal hypotension
Asian or Hispanic ethnicity

multiple fetuses. Women with a prior history of PPH have a 10% risk of recurrence with subsequent pregnancies.[11] Risk factors associated with the development of PPH are listed in Table 183-2. Early recognition of these risk factors may aid in the diagnosis and subsequently in the management of PPH. A randomized controlled trial (RCT) comparing oxytocin administration before and after delivery of the placenta found that birth weight, labor induction with augmentation, chorioamnionitis, the use of magnesium sulfate infusions, and previous episodes of PPH increased the risk of developing PPH.[12] However, a significant number of patients with PPH have no obvious predisposing factors.

Potential causes of PPH are listed in Table 183-3. The most frequent cause of PPH is uterine atony after delivery of either the fetus or the placenta. Bleeding is from the uterine vessels or from the placental site of implantation, if the placenta has been delivered. The incidence of uterine atony is approximately 1 in 20 deliveries. Uterine atony can lead to rapid and severe PPH. Overdistention of the uterus secondary to multiple gestation, fetal macrosomia, or polyhydramnios is a major predisposing risk factor for the development of uterine atony. Other predisposing factors are retained placenta, chorioamnionitis, uterine structural abnormalities, and muscle fatigue after prolonged or stimulated labor. General anesthesia, particularly with halogenated anesthetics, and magnesium sulfate infusions can inhibit effective uterine contractions and lead to uterine atony. The diagnosis of uterine atony is a clinical diagnosis that is made by assessing the tone of the uterus and its size by manually palpating the uterus externally. Bimanual examination of the uterus also can be performed to diagnose uterine atony. A boggy uterus associated with heavy vaginal bleeding or with an appreciable increase in the size of the uterus is diagnostic of uterine atony. The size of the uterus may be larger than normal as a result of accumulated blood within.

TABLE 183–3. CAUSES OF POSTPARTUM HEMORRHAGE

Uterine atony
Cervical or vaginal lacerations
Retention of placental fragments
Placental anomalies
Traumatic hematomas of the perineum or pelvis
Coagulation disorders
Uterine rupture
Uterine inversion

Lacerations of the lower genital tract are the second most frequent cause of PPH. Lacerations of the vagina and cervix can result from a number of causes. These lesions occur most commonly as a result of prolonged or tumultuous labor, particularly with uterine hyperstimulation with oxytocic agents. Nevertheless, lacerations can occur spontaneously as well. They are seen in deliveries associated with instrumentation, such as forceps deliveries, or with extrauterine or intrauterine manipulations of the fetus. Attempts to remove the placenta or placental fragments manually or with instrumentation can lead to traumatic lesions or hematomas. Excessive vaginal bleeding or traumatic hematomas can result from these lacerations. Careful examination with palpation of the vagina and cervix may reveal the presence of lacerations.

Retention of placental fragments or the entire placenta can lead to severe and life-threatening hemorrhage, which may be immediate or delayed depending on the extent of accumulated blood in the uterus. The World Health Organization uses retention of the placenta for 60 minutes or longer after delivery of the fetus as the criterion for placental retention.[13] Retained placenta is more likely to occur with a preterm gestation of less than 24 weeks. Placental abnormalities (i.e., placenta accreta, placenta increta, and placenta percreta) have been associated with retained placenta and failure of complete separation of the placenta from the uterus. Placenta accreta occurs when a portion or the entire surface of the placenta is abnormally attached to the uterus. Placenta increta involves actual invasion of the uterus by the placenta. If the placenta has been delivered, it is imperative to closely examine the placenta to look for missing fragments, a finding that suggests retained placental tissue.

Another less frequent cause of PPH is uterine rupture. Rupture is more common in patients with prior cesarean incisions and in those with any prior operative procedures of the uterus (e.g., intrauterine device placement, laparoscopy, hysteroscopy). Uterine rupture may manifest with severe and acute abdominal pain and hemodynamic instability, but there may not be significant bleeding initially. Uterine inversion is relatively uncommon but may be associated with blood losses of up to 2 L.

A defect in hemostasis resulting from an underlying coagulopathy should be considered if the uterus is contracting normally and manual exploration has excluded either placental retention or uterine rupture. Disseminated intravascular coagulation (DIC) associated with placental abruption (premature separation of a normally implanted placenta), the HELLP syndrome (hemolysis, elevated liver enzymes, and low platelets), intrauterine fetal death, acute fatty liver of pregnancy, sepsis, or amniotic fluid embolism may precipitate PPH. The incidence of severe DIC associated with PPH is estimated at 0.1% of pregnancies.[14,15]

Amniotic fluid embolism syndrome (AFES) is a catastrophic condition that can occur either during the pregnancy or after the delivery. AFES manifests with acute respiratory failure, cardiogenic shock, and/or DIC.[16] As many as 80% of these patients develop DIC, and in some DIC is the major clinical abnormality.[17,18] Oozing from intravenous or skin puncture sites, mucosal surfaces, or surgical sites should raise the suspicion of DIC; confirmation of the diagnosis is made by laboratory coagulation studies. Although the coagulation profile is unlikely to be abnormal with acute postpartum bleeding in the absence of DIC, coagulation parameters are clearly abnormal in the presence of DIC regardless of the cause. In late pregnancy, the circulating fibrinogen level usually is two to three times the normal prenatal value, but fibrinogen concentration is dramatically decreased if DIC is present. Preexisting or pregnancy-acquired disorders of coagulation are relatively infrequent causes of significant PPH.

DIAGNOSTIC STUDIES

Although the diagnosis is obvious with significant and excessive bleeding after delivery, not all patients present with immediate bleeding, because of hematoma formation or accumulations in the interior of the uterus. Bedside ultrasonography can be used for the detection of clots, hematomas, and retained placental products. For patients who are at high for risk for development of PPH, periodic ultrasound examinations during pregnancy can offer invaluable information concerning the extent and progression of placental disease. Angiography with selective arterial embolization can be used both diagnostically and therapeutically. Bleeding sites can be visualized and embolized simultaneously. For evaluation of a proven or suspected case of PPH, the following laboratory studies are almost always indicated: complete blood count with platelet count, coagulation studies with prothrombin and activated partial thromboplastin times, fibrinogen, and D-dimer level. With acute hemorrhage, the measurements of hemoglobin concentration and hematocrit may be of limited use.

PREVENTION

There has been much controversy concerning the preferred methods of managing the third stage of labor in terms of decreasing bleeding complications. The debate concerns active versus expectant management. Expectant management consists of waiting for separation and expulsion of the placenta, with minimal intervention except for gentle fundal massage. Active management of the third stage of labor involves three components. The first consists of administering a uterotonic drug, usually oxytocin, immediately after delivery of the fetus to promote contraction of the uterus and subsequent expulsion of the placenta. The second component involves early clamping and cutting of the umbilical cord. The third maneuver consists of gentle traction on the umbilical cord after the uterus is well contracted, using countertraction against the uterine fundus. Opponents of active management have cited a higher incidence of retained placental fragments due to the vigorous uterine contractions. The two modalities were compared in five randomized, controlled trials in a Cochrane meta-analysis of studies enrolling more than 6000 women. A 60% decrease in PPH was associated with active management of the third stage of labor.[19-21]

TABLE 183–4. GENERAL TREATMENT MEASURES FOR POSTPARTUM HEMORRHAGE

Oxygen administration
Gentle massage of the uterine fundus
Placement of large-caliber intravenous catheters for rapid and aggressive fluid resuscitation with isotonic solutions using the "3:1" rule
Blood product administration depending on the extent of bleeding and coagulation abnormalities

GENERAL TREATMENT MEASURES

Many deaths associated with PPH may have resulted because clinicians underestimated the extent of blood loss and failed to provide rapid and aggressive resuscitation with fluids and blood products. Several authors have suggested the use of specific management protocols for the care of patients with PPH.[9,22] These guidelines can expedite rapid diagnosis and management of obstetric hemorrhage. The general treatment measures for PPH are the same as those for any patient with acute hemorrhage (Table 183-4). Oxygen should be administered routinely. At least one to two large-caliber intravenous lines should be placed immediately. Central venous access is usually unnecessary, unless peripheral access cannot be obtained quickly. Aggressive volume resuscitation should be instituted immediately, because this intervention can be life-saving in patients with ongoing bleeding and hemodynamic instability. Isotonic saline or lactated Ringer's solution is the preferred fluid for aggressive resuscitation. Isotonic electrolyte solutions provide transient intravascular volume expansion. Monitoring of changes in blood pressure, heart rate, and pulse pressure can help the clinician to determine the amount of blood loss, particularly in cases in which bleeding is internal (Table 183-5).

General guidelines for fluid resuscitation of patients with hemorrhagic shock are based on the "3:1" rule. This recommendation derives from the empirical observation that patients require about 300 mL of crystalloid fluid replacement for every 100 mL of blood loss. This rule must be applied in the context of the clinical scenario. Applied blindly, this guideline can result in either excessive or inadequate volume resuscitation. Patients with expanding hematomas or areas of concealed active bleeding have hypotension out of proportion to the obvious blood loss and require resuscitation in excess of the 3:1 recommendation. In contrast, patients with ongoing blood losses that are being replaced with blood transfusions typically require less electrolyte fluid replacement.

Blood transfusions usually are necessary for patients with severe ongoing PPH. Healthy pregnant patients usually do not require transfusion if blood loss is 2000 mL or less. However, if blood loss is greater than 2 L or there is ongoing hemorrhage and hemodynamic instability, transfusion can

TABLE 183–5. THERAPEUTIC RESPONSE TO INITIAL FLUID RESUSCITATION

Response	Description	Follow-up Treatment
Rapid response	<20% of blood volume lost	No additional fluids or blood are needed
Transient response	20-40% of blood volume lost; responds to initial fluid bolus but later has worsening vital signs	Continue fluids and consider blood transfusions
Minimal or no response	Ongoing severe hemorrhage with >40% blood volume lost	Continue aggressive fluid and blood product replacements

TABLE 183–6. BLOOD PRODUCT REPLACEMENT

Crossmatched blood
Type-specific or "saline crossmatched" blood
Compatible ABO and Rh blood types
Rh-negative blood is preferable
Warm the blood, if possible, especially if the rate of infusion is >100 mL/min or if the total volume transfused is high; cold blood is associated with an increased incidence of arrhythmias and paradoxical hypotension
Administer calcium if blood is transfused rapidly at >100 mL/min because of binding of calcium by anticoagulants in banked blood
Give 6-10 units fresh-frozen plasma (FFP) for every 10 units of packed red blood cell (PRBC) transfusions, or give 1 unit FFP for every 5 units PRBC for patients requiring continued transfusions
Give 10 to 12 units of platelets, if the platelet count decreases to $<50 \times 10^9$/L
Cryoprecipitate can be given to replace fibrinogen in addition to the FFP

be lifesaving. Crossmatched packed red blood cells or type-specific blood can be infused rapidly using a blood warming device in cases of severe ongoing hemorrhage (Table 183-6). Manual external uterine massage should be performed immediately to stimulate uterine contractions and to express clots if uterine atony is suspected or confirmed. If the uterus does not respond to vigorous manual external massage and the rapid administration of oxytocin, then bimanual massage with one hand on the uterus and the other hand placed anterior to the cervix in the vagina should be performed. Aggressive uterine manipulation can result in uterine inversion. Direct pressure should be maintained over visible perineal, vaginal, or cervical lacerations. These general treatment measures can control excessive bleeding and even stop the hemorrhage in a significant proportion of patients.

SPECIFIC TREATMENT MEASURES

Oxytocic (uterotonic) drugs administered intravenously, intramuscularly, or intramyometrially are used to stimulate the uterus by producing rhythmic contractions and to control the degree of hemorrhage. Dosing regimens for oxytocic drugs are listed in Table 183-7.

Oxytocin (Pitocin) remains first-line therapy for most obstetricians. Prophylactic oxytocin, given either before or after placental delivery, decreases the incidence of PPH up to 40%.[23,24] Some authors advocate its use prophylactically

TABLE 183–7. DOSING REGIMENS FOR OXYTOCIC DRUGS

Drugs	Regimens
Oxytocin (Pitocin)	5-unit IV bolus
	Add 20-40 units oxytocin to 1 L of fluids
	10 units intramyometrially
Methylergonovine (Methergine)	0.2 mg IM every 2-4 h
Ergonovine (Ergotrate Maleate)	100-125 µg IM or intramyometrially every 2-4 h
	200-250 µg IM
	Total dose 1.25 mg
Carboprost (Hemabate)	250 µg IM or intramyometrially every 15-90 min
	Total dose 2 mg
Misoprostol	800 µg PR

IM, intramuscular; IV, intravenous; PR, per rectum.

after delivery of the fetus but before delivery of the placenta, to decrease the duration of the third stage of labor and the amount of blood loss.[25] In an RCT, the incidence of PPH was similar regardless of whether oxytocin was given before or after placental delivery.[12] Additionally, the incidence of retained placenta was similar for patients treated with oxytocin before or after delivery of the placenta.[12] Oxytocin should be used with caution in patients with hyperactive uterine contractions or hypertension, because the pressor effect of sympathomimetic drugs can increase if they are used with oxytocin.

Methylergonovine (Methergine) is now considered to be second-line therapy. It is a direct uterotonic agent that reduces uterine bleeding and shortens the third stage of labor. Hypertension is a relative contraindication for the use of methergine. Carboprost tromethamine (Hemabate), a synthetic prostaglandin, is now used in some centers as a second-line uterotonic agent. Asthma is a relative contraindication to the use of carboprost. Carboprost has been shown to be 80% to 90% effective in decreasing PPH refractory to oxytocin and ergonovine. Hayashi[26] reported that prostaglandins are superior to oxytocin and ergonovine for controlling PPH.[26] Misoprostol, prostaglandin E_1, causes uterine contractions, and rectal administration of this drug has been shown to be useful in refractory PPH.[27-29]

The practice of uterine packing to control bleeding remains somewhat controversial. Although this practice had been abandoned for many years, it has recently resurged as an effective method for tamponade of bleeding from the uterus.[30] Opponents of this practice argue that significant amounts of blood may be sequestered behind the uterine packing and that infection risks are increased. The packing can conceal the actual amount of bleeding, leading to gross underestimation of the extent of hemorrhage. The packing usually is removed in 24 to 36 hours. Uterine packing has been proposed as a temporizing maneuver to stop or decrease PPH before surgery or selective arteriography. Balloon occlusion catheters also have been used in the treatment of PPH.[31] Placement of a Sengstaken-Blakemore tube also has been used for control of bleeding.[32]

If there is a suspicion of retained placenta, examination of the uterus is both diagnostic and therapeutic. The uterus must be explored digitally and retained placental fragments removed either manually or with instruments. Because this procedure can be difficult and quite painful, it may be necessary to use regional or general anesthesia to obtain optimal visualization and manipulation of the uterus. Administration of oxytocic drugs should continue during manual extraction of placental fragments. Administration of broad-spectrum antibiotics has been recommended whenever there is manipulation or instrumentation of the uterus.[33]

Compression of the abdominal aorta against the vertebral column, which can be achieved by pressing a fist on the abdomen cephalad to the umbilicus, can be a lifesaving temporizing maneuver to control hemorrhage before surgery in the presence of fulminant bleeding with severe hemodynamic compromise. Military antishock trousers (MAST) also have been used as a temporizing measure before surgery.

If there is persistent and significant bleeding despite the therapeutic measures described, then consideration should be given to arteriography with selective arterial embolization. This procedure requires the expertise of an interventional radiologist and may not be readily available in many hospitals. Successful embolization of the bleeding sites can be accomplished, obviating the need for surgical intervention.[34-36] Fertility can be preserved with this procedure.[37] Some authors have advocated prophylactic placement of embolectomy catheters in patients at high risk for PPH, to minimize the procedural delay in the presence of active bleeding.[38,39] If embolization is unsuccessful, balloon catheter occlusion of the hypogastric arteries has been successfully performed as a temporizing measure before surgery.[40] Complications are minimal, and postprocedural fever appears to be the most common complication of the procedure.[41]

SURGICAL THERAPY

Surgical therapy is reserved for cases not amenable to medical therapy. Patients with ongoing hemorrhage despite aggressive medical therapy are candidates for operation. Surgery is the treatment of choice for uterine rupture. Lacerations, if visible, are directly repaired and oversewn. Lacerations high in the vaginal vault or in the cervix may require operative repair, primarily for improved visualization of the lesions. Hematomas of the lower genital tract are incised and drained. Arterial embolization of vaginal and vulvar lesions has been used. Hematomas of the broad ligament and in the retroperitoneal space are often managed conservatively if there is only minimal further expansion of the hematoma, but surgical exploration or embolization is mandated if additional significant bleeding occurs. Radiographic imaging with computed tomography, magnetic resonance imaging, and/or ultrasonography is a useful adjunct to monitor the expansion of these hematomas.

Ligation of the uterine, ovarian, or internal iliac (hypogastric) arteries can be performed. Most commonly, ligation of the uterine arteries controls bleeding, but in some cases additional surgical tamponade is required. These arteries provide 90% of uterine blood flow, and ligation is an effective means of controlling PPH.[42,43] If hemostasis is not achieved with uterine artery ligation, the ovarian arteries can be ligated as well. Ligation of the internal iliac arteries is a surgical option, but it is technically more difficult and usually is done only if ligation of the uterine and ovarian arteries has proved unsuccessful in halting bleeding.[44,45]

Hysterectomy is the definitive surgical therapy to control bleeding. Hysterectomy is required if bleeding continues despite ligation of the internal iliac arteries. Subtotal or total hysterectomy is curative in PPH.[46] In cases of uterine rupture, it is the only surgical option, and nonsurgical modalities are only temporizing measures until the patient can be brought to the operating room. Clark and colleagues[47] attempted to identify patients at risk for hysterectomy based on the cause of the PPH and risk factors but found that only 74% of patients requiring hysterectomy were identified before delivery. Forty-three percent of the patients had uterine atony.

COMPLICATIONS

Complications from the bleeding include hematologic abnormalities such as DIC and dilutional coagulopathy from massive fluid resuscitation and/or massive transfusion (greater than 10 units of packed red blood cells). Dilutional coagulopathy occurs when more than 80% of the original blood volume has been replaced. Life-threatening complications of hemorrhagic shock, including renal failure and liver

failure, acute respiratory distress syndrome (ARDS), and Sheehan's syndrome, can occur. Sheehan's syndrome can result from severe PPH that causes permanent hypopituitarism from avascular necrosis of the pituitary gland.[48]

PROGNOSIS

The prognosis of PPH depends on many factors, some of which are directly related to prompt diagnosis and treatment. The cause of bleeding, the duration of bleeding, and the extent of bleeding all affect the likelihood of a good outcome.

ANNOTATED REFERENCES

Alexander J, Thomas P, Sanghera J: Treatments of secondary postpartum hemorrhage. Cochrane Database Syst Rev 2003;(1):CD002867.

The objective of this extensive review was to evaluate the relative effectiveness and safety of the treatments used in the medical and surgical management of secondary PPH. Medical therapies reviewed included antibiotics, oxytocic drugs, and hormone therapy. The authors researched databases, including MEDLINE as early as 1966. In developed countries, 2% of postpartum women are admitted to a hospital with an admission diagnosis of secondary PPH, and 1% undergo surgical evacuation of the uterus, most commonly for retained products of conception. Despite this frequency, there is little documentation in the literature concerning the morbidity and potential mortality of this disorder. The underlying cause of this condition often is not established. Some studies have shown an increase in the frequency of women with primary PPH at the time of delivery or with a previous history of secondary PPH. The administration of ergometrine, precipitous labor, prolonged third stage of labor, multiple gestations, multiparity, and endometritis are some of the risk factors leading to secondary PPH. The authors did not find any systematic reviews or RCTs in the literature to assess the effectiveness of treatments of secondary PPH.

Berg CG, Atrash HK, Koonin LM, et al: Pregnancy-related mortality in the United States, 1987-1990. Obstet Gynecol 1996;88:161.

The objective of this epidemiologic study, using data from the Pregnancy-Related Mortality Surveillance System of the Centers for Disease Control and Prevention (CDC), was to examine the trends of risk factors and causes for maternal mortality and to identify patients at high-risk for death. Since 1979, the CDC and the American College of Obstetricians and Gynecologists have collected information on all maternal deaths in the United States. Results showed that maternal death rates, which had been decreasing annually after 1979, began to increase from 1987 to 1990. The three leading causes of maternal death were hemorrhage, embolism, and hypertensive disorders of pregnancy. The number of deaths due to hemorrhage and anesthesia complications has decreased, but deaths associated with heart disease and infection have increased.

Clark SL, Yeh SY, Phelan JP, et al: Emergency hysterectomy for obstetric hemorrhage. Obstet Gynecol 1984;64:376.

Clark examined the predisposing factors that led to 70 emergency hysterectomies for PPH. The three most common indications were uterine atony (43%), placenta accreta (30%), and uterine rupture (13%). There was a significant association of uterine atony with the presence of chorioamnionitis, cesarean section for labor arrest, oxytocin augmentation of labor, magnesium sulfate infusions, and fetal weight (overdistention of the uterus). The presence of placenta previa or placenta accreta in a patient with a prior cesarean delivery significantly increased the risk of PPH requiring hysterectomy for control of the bleeding. Despite a wide inclusion of predisposing factors for requiring a hysterectomy, only 74% of patients with PPH leading to hysterectomy could be identified before delivery.

Jackson KW Jr, Allbert JR, Schemmer GK, et al: A randomized controlled trial comparing oxytocin administration before and after placental delivery in the prevention of postpartum hemorrhage. Am J Obstet Gynecol 2001;185:873.

The objective of this RCT was to determine the optimal time to administer oxytocin in the third stage of labor. Previous studies had shown a 40% decrease in the incidence of PPH when prophylactic oxytocin was given after fetal or placental delivery. Prior studies had also shown that administration of oxytocin before delivery of the placenta facilitated delivery of the placenta. However, opponents of this practice are concerned about the potential risk of retained placental parts. In this study, 1486 patients were randomly assigned to receive oxytocin either at presentation of the fetal anterior shoulder or with delivery of the placenta. The authors found no difference in frequency of PPH or in duration of the third stage of labor when the oxytocin was given before or after delivery of the placenta. There was no increase in the incidence of retained placenta among those patients who received oxytocin after delivery of the fetus but before delivery of the placenta. Their final recommendation was to proceed with active management of the third stage of labor with controlled cord traction until the placenta is removed. Oxytocin can be given either before or after placental delivery to facilitate uterine contractions.

Ornan D, White R, Pollak J, et al. Pelvic embolization for intractable postpartum hemorrhage: Long-term follow-up and implications for fertility. Obstet Gynecol 2003;102:904.

The objective of this study was to determine the long-term sequelae of pelvic embolization for postpartum hemorrhage and, in particular, its relation to fertility after the procedure. Selective arterial embolization has been performed for intractable PPH unresponsive to standard measures. However, little evidence is available concerning possible long-term sequelae, including the possibility of future pregnancies. These authors did follow-up interviews with 28 patients who had undergone arterial embolization for refractory bleeding after delivery. The average time to follow-up was 11.7 ± 6.9 years. Arterial embolization was successful in all but one of the patients. All patients who had subsequent pregnancies had no difficulties in conceiving and no complications associated with pregnancy or delivery. No significant maternal morbidities were noted in the patients. This study offers evidence that selective arterial embolization as treatment for refractory PPH is a relatively safe procedure in the short term, and in the long term, compared with hysterectomy, it offers the woman the possibility of fertility.

Chapter 184

TRAUMA IN THE GRAVID PATIENT

Samuel A. Tisherman

KEY POINTS

1. Optimal care for the mother provides the best care for the fetus: **"Save the mother, save the fetus."**

2. The initial assessment and resuscitation of the gravid patient should **follow standard protocols**, including radiographic studies, with few exceptions.

3. **Early fetal monitoring and obstetric consultation is critical** if the fetus has reached the point of potential viability.

Trauma is the most common nonobstetric cause of death in pregnant women. In Cook County, Fildes and coworkers[1] found that 46% of deaths among pregnant women were the result of trauma. Of these, 57% were homicides and 9% were suicides. Motor vehicle crashes accounted for 21% of the cases. In contrast, in Iowa, Varner[2] found that motor vehicle crashes were the most common cause of traumatic maternal death. More often, trauma during pregnancy causes death of the fetus, although fetal demise is frequently associated with maternal death.[3,4] Among fetal deaths due to trauma, an analysis of retrospective data from 16 states showed that 82% were secondary to motor vehicle crashes, 6% were related to injuries caused by firearms, and 3% were associated with falls.[5] The most common cause of traumatic fetal death if the mother survives is abruptio placentae. The most common maternal injury that results in fetal death is pelvic fracture, which frequently leads to fetal skull fracture and intracranial injury. Penetrating trauma, often secondary to domestic violence, is caused more often by gunshot wounds than by stab wounds.

The major causes of death from trauma (i.e., head injury and hemorrhage) are similar in gravid and nongravid patients. Patterns of injury are generally similar, based on mechanism of injury.

The outcome from trauma for mother and fetus depends on multiple factors, including the gestational age of the fetus and the mechanism and severity of the injury. According to data analyzed by Scorpio and colleagues,[6] the only independent factors that predict fetal demise in gravid victims of mostly blunt trauma (80% motor vehicle crashes) are injury severity score[7] and admission serum bicarbonate level. The serum bicarbonate concentration or base deficit may be an important marker of occult hypoperfusion in trauma victims, although serum bicarbonate concentration is normally decreased late in pregnancy. The critical factor for the fetus is the extent to which trauma disrupts normal uterine and fetal physiology. Fetal demise occurs in up to 80% of gravid patients who develop hemorrhagic shock.[8] In addition, even minor injuries to the mother can result in abruptio placentae or fetal demise. In one study of interpersonal violence as a cause of trauma in pregnancy,[9] five of eight women with fetal loss had no apparent physical injury.

Any female patient of child-bearing potential could be pregnant at the time of injury. Therefore, a screen for β-human chorionic gonadotropin should be routine during the initial assessment of all such patients. Recognition that a "second" patient is present is essential for the care of both mother and fetus. Optimal management of the pregnant trauma victim is the best way to optimize outcome for the fetus; the dictum is, "Save the mother, save the fetus." To manage the gravid patient, the traumatologist or intensivist must have an understanding of fetal and maternal physiology, as well as the specific complications of trauma that are unique to these patients. Early obstetric consultation should be obtained. If delivery of a viable fetus is imminent, neonatology consultation also may be needed.

FETAL PHYSIOLOGY

During the first week after conception, the conceptus has not yet implanted in the uterus, making it relatively resistant to injury. Soon thereafter, the blastocyst begins implantation and the placenta begins to develop. The embryo attaches to the uterus via anchoring villi. The placenta is not as elastic as the myometrium, potentially leading to shear stresses and disruption of the villi (particularly if intra-amniotic fluid pressure is increased) when force is applied to the uterus. The resulting abruptio placentae rapidly leads to fetal hypoxemia, acidosis, and death.

On the positive side, amniotic fluid is a cushion for the fetus, although the fetus can still suffer injury as a result of rapid compression, deceleration, or contrecoup injury. Late in pregnancy, the head of the fetus typically is in the pelvis, and pelvic fractures can lead to fetal skull fracture and brain injury.[5]

Adequate oxygen delivery to the fetus is critical during pregnancy. Blood flow to the uterus decreases proportionally as maternal systemic blood pressure decreases. In addition, as the mother becomes hypovolemic, peripheral vasoconstriction can further decrease uterine circulation. The placenta is exquisitely sensitive to catecholamines. The ability of the fetus to withstand changes in uterine blood flow or oxygenation is variable. The fetus can redistribute blood flow to the most vulnerable organs, the brain and heart, but the protection afforded by this response (the "diving reflex") is limited. Decreased placental blood flow quickly leads to fetal distress.

ANATOMIC AND PHYSIOLOGIC CHANGES ASSOCIATED WITH PREGNANCY

The gravid patient undergoes a multitude of anatomic and physiologic changes to accommodate the developing fetus.[10] These changes have a significant impact on anatomic injury patterns and the response to injury.

From a respiratory standpoint, maternal tidal volume increases by as much as 40%, causing respiratory alkalosis. Renal compensation maintains a normal arterial pH. The hemidiaphragms are elevated, decreasing functional residual capacity. The gravid patient has little respiratory reserve and desaturates quickly. Failure to recognize the more cephalad location of the hemidiaphragms can lead the operator to place chest tubes into the abdomen.

From a cardiovascular standpoint, heart rate increases by 15 to 20 beats/min during the third trimester. During the second trimester, both systolic and diastolic blood pressure decrease by about 15 mm Hg, then increase to normal levels during the third trimester. Cardiac output increases by 1 to 1.5 L/min by the 10th week in pregnancy due to increased plasma volume and decreased peripheral resistance.

Maternal blood volume increases by almost 50% by 28 weeks, but red blood cell mass does not increase proportionally, resulting in the "anemia of pregnancy." Normal hematocrit late in pregnancy is 31% to 35%. A mild leukocytosis (up to 18,000 cells/mL) occurs during the second trimester. Circulating levels of coagulation factors and fibrinogen increase, whereas plasminogen activator levels decrease during pregnancy, leading to an increased risk of thromboembolism. Trauma to the gravid uterus can lead to release of thromboplastic factors (e.g., amniotic fluid), triggering the development of disseminated intravascular coagulation (DIC). Serum albumin levels decrease to 2.2 to 2.8 g/dL.

Decreased gastric motility and cephalad displacement of the abdominal contents predispose women to gastroesophageal reflux and aspiration. Gallbladder function is also impaired, increasing the risk of stone formation.

The abdominal examination of a gravid woman is complicated by the cephalad displacement of abdominal contents by the enlarging uterus. The urinary bladder is displaced upward, out of the pelvis, and the ureters become dilated after the 10th week of gestation.

The uterus increases in size from 70 to 1100 g during pregnancy; after 12 weeks, it takes on an intra-abdominal position, increasing risk of direct trauma. At 20 weeks, the fundus reaches the umbilicus. By 34 to 36 weeks, the fundus reaches the costal margin. Uterine blood flow increases to 10 times normal. One of the most important consequences of the anatomic changes during the latter half of pregnancy is that the uterus can occlude the inferior vena cava when the patient is in the supine position (supine hypotension syndrome), leading to hypotension from decreased venous return. Positioning the patient with the right side of the torso elevated can increase cardiac output by up to 25%.

The pelvis of the gravid female has relaxed ligaments, causing gait instability and risk of falls. In addition, venous engorgement in the pelvis increases the risk of severe hemorrhage.

From an endocrine standpoint, the hormones of pregnancy (placental lactogen, progesterone, estrogen, parathormone, and calcitonin) lead to insulin resistance and diabetes of pregnancy, decreased lower esophageal sphincter pressure, decreased gastric emptying, and increased calcium absorption. The pituitary gland is increased in size by 135% with increased blood flow demands. Hemorrhagic shock can lead to necrosis of the gland and pituitary insufficiency (Sheehan's syndrome).

Preeclampsia (triad of hypertension, proteinuria, and peripheral edema) can increase the risk of intracranial hemorrhage or seizures. Subsequent neurologic findings may mimic head injury.

INITIAL ASSESSMENT AND RESUSCITATION

Optimal care of the mother maximizes the chances for survival of the fetus. Resuscitation of the gravid patient should follow guidelines for the nongravid patient. Given the exquisite sensitivity of the placenta and fetus to hypoperfusion and hypoxemia, supplemental oxygen and intravenous fluids should be administered early, even before extrication if possible, particularly because the latter may be delayed by anatomic factors. There is no indication for fetal assessment in the field. Use of the pneumatic antishock garment (PASG) for stabilization of fractures or control of hemorrhage is contraindicated, because the resulting increase in intra-abdominal pressure can further decrease venous return in the gravid patient.

Prehospital protocols and interhospital transfer arrangements must account for management of a pregnant trauma victim. The optimal receiving facility has obstetric and neonatology consultants available and may not be the closest trauma center.

The airway of the gravid patient is at risk because of the tendency toward gastroesophageal reflux and aspiration. In addition, the vocal cords are frequently edematous. Ventilation of the gravid patient late in pregnancy can be impeded by the enlarged uterus and cephalad positioning of the abdominal contents. Functional residual capacity may be significantly reduced, leading to more rapid respiratory decompensation, particularly with chest trauma.

Because of the increased blood volume late in pregnancy, the mother may not show typical signs of hypovolemia, even with loss of a large volume of blood (up to 1500 mL). However, uterine perfusion still may be compromised. Uterine blood flow may decrease by up to 30% before the mother demonstrates clinical signs of shock. Aggressive volume replacement is necessary to ensure adequate uterine blood flow. Blood transfusions should be administered according to standard guidelines, but the mother's Rh-antigen status must be considered. If it is unknown, Rh-negative blood should be administered. Invasive hemodynamic monitoring should be considered early during resuscitation to ensure adequate volume resuscitation.

To prevent the supine hypotensive syndrome, patients beyond 20 weeks of gestation should be placed in the left lateral decubitus position to relieve the pressure of the uterus on the inferior vena cava. The uterus also can be manually displaced to the left. If the patient is immobilized on a long board, the entire board can be tilted 15 degrees to the left with a wedge. Vasopressors, which are very rarely indicated in trauma patients, should be avoided unless absolutely necessary because of the risk of decreasing uterine blood flow.

In addition to the standard initial assessment, evaluation of the gravid trauma patient should include a focused history and physical examination related to the pregnancy. The obstetric history should include the date of last menstrual period, expected date of delivery, date of first fetal movement, and status of current and previous pregnancies. The physical examination should include measurement of fundal height. Fetal age can be estimated as 1 week for each centimeter of fundal height above the symphysis pubis. The abdominal examination should assess uterine tenderness and consistency, presence or absence of contractions, and fetal position and movement. Pelvic examination should evaluate the presence of blood or amniotic fluid, cervical effacement, dilation, and fetal station. Amniotic fluid can be identified with the use of Nitrazine paper; a pH of 7 to 7.5 suggests the presence of amniotic fluid. Vaginal bleeding may indicate abruptio placentae. Examination of the fetus beyond 20 weeks should include auscultation of fetal heart tones. The normal range for the fetal heart rate is 120 to 160 beats/min.

Standard laboratory tests should be obtained, including a pregnancy test. In addition, coagulation studies, including fibrinogen level, should be checked, because DIC can occur as a result of release of thromboplastic substances from abruptio placentae or amniotic fluid embolism. Treatment may include urgent delivery of the fetus and blood component therapy.

RADIOGRAPHIC STUDIES

Evaluation of the trauma victim invariably involves multiple radiographic studies. Concern for fetal radiation exposure should not prevent clinicians from obtaining studies needed for optimal care of the mother, although unnecessary duplication of radiographic studies should be avoided.

The effect of radiation during development of the embryo and fetus depends on the dose and timing. Previously, it was believed that any radiation very early in development of the embryo would be injurious. More recent findings, however, suggest that this is not the case and that the fetus is most sensitive at 8 to 15 weeks, when brain development is maximal.[11] Radiation can be teratogenic and can retard growth or cause postnatal neoplasia.

Mann and associates[12] stratified risk of adverse effects of radiation for diagnostic studies. Less than 10 mGy (equivalent to 1 rad) was considered to be low risk; 10 to 250 mGy, intermediate risk; and greater than 250 mGy, high risk. In general, a single exposure for a plain radiograph results in an exposure of 2 mGy, whereas computed tomography (CT) is associated with an exposure of 5 mGy per slice. Fluoroscopy exposes the patient to as much as 10 mGy per minute. Exposure in the low-risk category carries minimal risk of mutations. Though the risk of childhood cancers may be increased, the resultant risk remains less than 0.1%. In the intermediate-risk category, specifically beyond 150 mGy, teratogenic effects may be seen. In the high-risk category, the risk of teratogenic or carcinogenic effects increases substantially, perhaps to 2% to 3% beyond that of the normal population.

The greatest exposure to the fetus occurs when it is in the direct beam of the radiograph. To minimize exposure, the lower abdomen and pelvis of the gravid patient can be shielded with lead. Typical radiation exposure for the shielded fetus during a maternal chest radiograph is less than 0.01 mGy. In contrast, if a pelvic CT scan is performed, the fetus cannot be shielded; this study exposes the fetus to 20 to 80 mGy.[13]

BLUNT TRAUMA

Radiographic evaluation of the gravid victim of blunt trauma should begin with the standard chest, pelvis, and cervical spine radiographs. Additional studies should be chosen based on physical examination findings, the potential benefit to the mother, and the risk to the fetus. If there are acceptable choices for evaluation, the one that entails the least radiation exposure to the fetus should be used. For example, ultrasound or diagnostic peritoneal lavage (DPL) could be used to evaluate the abdomen, instead of CT, although the latter should be performed if necessary. The focused abdominal sonogram for trauma (FAST) may be used in gravid patients, just as in other patients, except that the superior displacement of abdominal organs by the uterus should be considered during probe placement. DPL should be performed cephalad to the umbilicus. If there is a choice between radiographic embolization of a bleeding splenic injury or laparotomy, the operative approach may be the more appropriate choice. Weighing the risks and benefits of radiographic studies is complex. Decisions should be made by the most senior physician involved in the care of the patient.

PENETRATING TRAUMA

Most instances of penetrating trauma to the gravid abdomen are caused by gunshot and knife wounds.[14,15] As gestation progresses, the uterus becomes the most likely organ to be injured. The uterus and amniotic fluid can slow the velocity of missiles, decreasing potential injury to the mother, although not protecting the fetus very well. Fetal mortality is 47% to 71%.[15] Penetrating trauma to the upper abdomen frequently involves multiple loops of bowel, which are compressed above the enlarged uterus, leading to complex injuries. Management of gravid patients with entry wounds below the fundus of the uterus is controversial. Although routine laparotomy is indicated for nongravid victims of penetrating abdominal trauma, particularly gunshot wounds, Franger and coworkers[15] recommended nonoperative management if maternal vital signs and fetal heart rate tracings remain normal, suggesting no evidence of maternal or fetal compromise or intra-abdominal hemorrhage. Radiographic determination of bullet location may be helpful. Intrauterine bullets may be observed. If laparotomy is performed, all of the bowel should be carefully explored and wounds repaired. Wounds to the uterus should also be closed.

OPERATIVE PROCEDURES

Operative intervention in the gravid patient should be based on standard indications for nongravid patients. There is no reason for delay. Anesthetic management with inhalational agents and neuromuscular blockade is considered safe. Local anesthetics should be used with caution, because these agents can cross the placenta.

MEDICATIONS

Medications frequently have different effects on the gravid patient and the fetus than they do on normal, nongravid women. Table 184-1 lists commonly used medications and the current recommendations regarding their use

TABLE 184-1. USE OF MEDICATIONS IN PREGNANT WOMEN

Category	Safe	Use with Caution	Contraindicated
Analgesics	—	Narcotics (fetal respiratory depression) Nonsteroidal anti-inflammatory drugs (prostaglandin inhibition) Acetaminophen (safe for short-term use, liver toxicity)	Aspirin (prolonged labor and increased bleeding, intrauterine growth retardation)
Anesthetics	Inhalational anesthetics Neuromuscular blockers	Local anesthetics (cross placenta)	—
Antibiotics	Penicillins Cephalosporins Erythromycin Clindamycin	Aminoglycosides (fetal ototoxicity) Sulfonamides (neonatal kernicterus) Quinolones (insufficient data) Metronidazole (insufficient data, carcinogen in rats) Azithromycin (insufficient data)	Chloramphenicol (bone marrow suppression) Tetracyclines (inhibit fetal bone growth) Fluconazole (teratogenic)
Anticoagulants	Heparin Low-molecular-weight heparins	—	Coumadin (crosses placenta)
Anticonvulsants	—	Benzodiazepines (fetal respiratory depression) Barbiturates (fetal respiratory depression)	Phenytoin (teratogenic) Valproic acid (congenital malformations, fetal hyperbilirubinemia, neural tube defects)
Antiemetics	Metoclopramide Prochlorperazine Ondansetron	Promethazine (fetal respiratory depression) Droperidol (insufficient data, increased mortality in rats) Trimethobenzamide (limited risk of teratogenicity)	—
Gastric protective agents	Sucralfate Lansoprazole Pantoprazole	Histamine-2 blockers (insufficient data)	—
Sedatives	—	Propofol (fetal depression) Haloperidol (limb malformations, cardiac anomalies)	Benzodiazepines (floppy baby syndrome, withdrawal syndrome)
Vasopressors	Dobutamine	Dopamine, norepinephrine (increased uterine vascular resistance)	—
Other	—	Hydrocortisone (low birthweight, cataracts, cleft palate)	

during pregnancy. Because not all medications, particularly newer ones, have been extensively tested in pregnant women, all medications should be administered with some caution in the gravid patient.

MONITORING

Monitoring of fetal cardiac activity and maternal uterine activity (cardiotocographic monitoring) is indicated if the fetus has reached the point of viability if delivered. Because fetal distress can occur shortly after injury, monitoring should begin as soon as possible. Almost all patients who develop abruptio placentae have frequent uterine contractions (more than 8/hour) during the first few hours after trauma; this is the most frequent finding with abruption. Continuous monitoring of the fetal heartbeat can detect fetal distress quickly. The normal fetal heart rate is 120 to 160 beats/min. Signs of fetal distress include an abnormal baseline fetal heart rate, absence of normal accelerations and beat-to-beat variability, and repetitive decelerations. The duration of monitoring is somewhat controversial. Although delayed abruption has been reported,[16,17] these patients were not monitored immediately after injury. Monitoring is clearly recommended for gravid patients with frequent uterine activity (more than 5 contractions per hour), abdominal or uterine tenderness, vaginal bleeding, rupture of amniotic membranes, or hypotension. Some have suggested that patients who are asymptomatic should be observed for at least 4 hours,[18] and others have suggested that monitoring be carried out for 24 hours.[19]

The utility of ultrasonography of the pelvis during the initial management of the gravid patient is less clear. On the one hand, it is less accurate than cardiotocographic monitoring for detection of abruptio placentae or fetal distress. On the other hand, it can establish gestational age, determine fetal well-being if cardiac monitoring is equivocal, verify the presence or absence of fetal cardiac activity, and estimate the volume of amniotic fluid if rupture of membranes is suspected.

Early obstetric consultation is critical so that, if fetal distress occurs, rapid intervention, including cesarean section, can proceed. Neonatology consultation may also be indicated.

SPECIFIC COMPLICATIONS OF PREGNANCY

FETOMATERNAL HEMORRHAGE

After trauma, fetal blood can cross the placenta and enter the maternal circulation. Fetomaternal hemorrhage occurs in about one in four gravid trauma victims, a rate 4 to 5 times higher than that in uninjured gravid women.[20] The volume can be approximated by measuring the ratio of fetal to maternal red blood cells in the maternal circulation (Kleihauer-Betke test). Complications include Rh sensitization of the mother, neonatal anemia, cardiac arrhythmias in the fetus, and fetal death from exsanguination. Maternal sensitization may be prevented by administration of Rho(D) immune globulin. Because the level required for a positive Kleihauer-Betke test is greater than the amount of fetal hemoglobin that can sensitize the mother, administration of Rho(D) immune globulin is indicated in almost all Rh-negative mothers, unless the injury is relatively minor and far removed from the uterus.

ABRUPTIO PLACENTAE

The most common cause of fetal death with maternal survival is abruptio placentae, a complication that can occur even after minor trauma, particularly late in pregnancy. Patients present with abdominal pain, vaginal bleeding, premature rupture of membranes with leakage of amniotic fluid, uterine tenderness and rigidity, expanding fundal height, and maternal shock. Fetal distress may rapidly follow. If the fetus is viable, cesarean section may be necessary.

AMNIOTIC FLUID EMBOLISM

Trauma to the uterus can result in embolization of amniotic fluid into the maternal circulation, causing a consumptive coagulopathy. Treatment consists of delivery of the fetus and transfusion of platelets and clotting factors, including fibrinogen.

PREMATURE LABOR

Premature uterine contractions associated with cervical dilatation and effacement (i.e., signs of premature labor) are common after trauma. Premature labor is usually self-limited, but some patients require tocolytics. Evidence of abruptio placentae is a contraindication to tocolytic therapy.

UTERINE RUPTURE

Direct trauma to the uterus can result in rupture, which almost always leads to fetal death and significantly increases the risk of maternal death (usually from concomitant injuries). Typical findings include abdominal pain and tenderness with peritoneal signs. If the fetus is out of the uterus, it may lie in a transverse or oblique position. Fetal body parts may be palpable, although the uterine fundus may not be. Fortunately, uterine rupture occurs only in the most seriously injured patients and is rare.

FETAL DEMISE

If fetal demise occurs, labor usually begins within 48 hours. If it does not, induction or cesarean delivery is indicated, as well as observation for evidence of DIC.

CESAREAN SECTION

Depending on the potential for viability based on fetal age, the indications for urgent cesarean section in gravid trauma victims include fetal distress, abruptio placentae, uterine rupture, and fetal malposition with premature labor.

Possible maternal factors include inadequate exposure for control of other injuries and DIC.

CARDIAC ARREST

During resuscitation for maternal cardiac arrest, standard algorithms should be applied initially. The uterus can be displaced manually toward the left side, off the inferior vena cava. Optimization of cardiac output and perfusion of the uterus via left thoracotomy and open cardiac massage along with emergency cesarean section should be considered. By the time the mother has suffered a cardiac arrest from trauma, the fetus has already experienced severe hypoxia. Cesarean delivery may be indicated if it can be performed within 5 to 15 minutes after loss of pulse in the mother[21]—perhaps even later, if fetal vital signs persist. Cardiopulmonary resuscitation must be continued until delivery is accomplished. Delivery has also been reported to allow successful maternal resuscitation. The decision to proceed with postmortem delivery must be made quickly by the traumatologist and obstetrician; hemostasis and antisepsis become secondary issues. Neonatologists must be available.

MATERNAL HEAD TRAUMA

Continuing life support in a gravid patient with severe head trauma but a viable fetus is controversial. Brain-dead patients have been sustained long enough for safe delivery of the fetus.[22] Consultation with obstetricians and ethicists is essential.

PREVENTION

Seatbelt use improves survival after motor vehicle crashes by preventing ejection from the vehicle.[23] The shoulder belt can help dissipate the force of deceleration and prevent severe flexion at the waist. Unfortunately, standard seatbelt and shoulder harnesses were not designed for the gravid patient. The lap belt can ride high, risking direct compression of the uterus. Design of new crash dummies could allow development of better safety restraint systems that not only decrease injury to the gravid patient but also decrease the risk of abruptio placentae.[24]

Violent trauma is a major cause of maternal and fetal death that is most likely underreported.[25,26] Approximately 17% of gravid trauma patients have been injured by another person. Up to 60% of these are cases of repeated domestic violence. Factors that should raise concern about domestic violence include injuries inconsistent with the history, diminished self-image, depression, history of self-abuse or suicide attempts, substance abuse, self-blame for injuries, and frequent visits. Concern should be raised if the partner insists on being present for the examination and monopolizes the conversation.[8] Physicians have a responsibility to identify these injuries and document them with the appropriate authorities.

SUMMARY

The initial assessment and resuscitation of the gravid trauma patient should follow standard trauma management guidelines, recognizing that maternal respiratory reserve may be limited and that the fetus may be compromised even if the mother looks well resuscitated. Maternal and fetal physiology should be kept in mind. Specific complications related to pregnancy should be sought. A viable fetus should be monitored. Early obstetric consultation is needed. Radiographic studies necessary for optimal care of the mother should be obtained. "Save the mother, save the fetus."

ANNOTATED REFERENCES

Mann FA, Nathens A, Langer SG, et al: Communicating with the family: The risks of medical radiation to conceptuses in victims of major blunt-force torso trauma. J Trauma 2000;48:354-357.

From the perspective of the trauma surgeon, this paper provides background information to assist the clinician in discussing honestly with a patient or family the risks of radiologic tests in trauma patients.

Pearlman MD, Tintinalli JE, Lorenz RP: A prospective controlled study of outcome after trauma during pregnancy. Am J Obstet Gynecol 1990;162:1502-1507.

This paper illustrates the utility of early cardiotocographic monitoring of the gravid trauma patient.

Pearlman MD, Tintinalli JE, Lorenz RP: Blunt trauma during pregnancy. N Engl J Med 1990;23:1609-1613.

This classic paper reviews fetal physiology and the anatomic and physiologic changes that occur in the gravid patient. The authors then review the initial assessment of the gravid trauma victim from the perspective of the obstetrician, with emphasis on issues that directly affect the fetus.

Shah AJ, Kilcline BA: Trauma in pregnancy. Emerg Med Clin North Am 2003;21:615-629.

This review examines the management of trauma in a pregnant patient from the emergency medicine perspective, with emphasis on prehospital and emergency department management.

Weiss HB, Songer T, Fabio A: Fetal deaths related to maternal injury. JAMA 2001;286:1863-1868.

This is a retrospective review of fetal deaths related to maternal injury, with data drawn from the death registries from 16 states. A better understanding of the mechanisms of injury based on these data should help targeting of prevention programs.

Section XII

PHARMACOLOGY AND TOXICOLOGY

Chapter 185

GENERAL PRINCIPLES OF PHARMACOKINETICS AND PHARMACODYNAMICS

Richard C. Brundage • Henry J. Mann

KEY POINTS

1. Pharmacokinetics is likely to be useful in treatment when there is a strong relationship between drug concentration in an easily sampled fluid and the pharmacologic response associated with a given drug concentration.

2. **The one-compartment pharmacokinetic model is the most useful model in patient care,** because, although many of the complex underlying principles of drug distribution and elimination are simplified by the model, it can still roughly predict future concentrations of drugs.

3. **Volume of distribution (V)** reflects the resulting concentration from a given drug dose and **is not directly associated with a physiologic space.**

4. **Drug half-life ($t_{1/2}$)** is a measure of how quickly a drug is eliminated from the body; it is related to the first-order elimination rate constant (K) by the equation, $t_{1/2} = 0.693/K$.

5. Clearance (CL) is a primary pharmacokinetic parameter that usually describes the volume of blood completely cleared of drug per unit time.

6. The area under the concentration-time curve (AUC) is a measure of drug exposure; it is determined by the dose of drug and the clearance through the relationship, **AUC = Dose/CL.**

7. In a one-compartment pharmacokinetic model, the change in drug concentration (ΔC) can be predicted by the dose of drug and volume of distribution through the relationship, $\Delta C = Dose/V$.

8. Half-life ($t_{1/2}$) changes in proportion to changes in either V or CL, as reflected by the equation, $t_{1/2} = 0.693 \times V/CL$.

9. Most drugs demonstrate at least two compartments when pharmacokinetics are examined closely; changes in concentration reflect a short distribution phase (α) and a longer elimination phase (β).

10. After five half-lives of either α (the distribution $t_{1/2}$) or β (the elimination $t_{1/2}$), a drug will be 97% distributed throughout the body or eliminated from the body.

11. The extent of drug absorption is termed bioavailability (F); it is generally referenced to the amount of drug available systemically when the drug is given intravenously

12. The **first-pass effect** refers to the elimination of drug that is absorbed orally but then metabolized by enzymes in either the liver or the gut wall before reaching the systemic circulation.

13. Pharmacodynamics is the study of the relationship between the concentration of drug and its pharmacologic effect.

14. The simple Emax pharmacodynamic model demonstrates a hyperbolic relationship between effect and dose that is described by the equation, Effect = (Emax × concentration) ÷ (EC50 + concentration), where Emax is the maximal effect attainable and EC50 is the concentration at which half the maximal effect is observed.

15. Observed **pharmacologic effects often lag behind the serum concentration eliciting the effect,** and in some instances there is a disequilibrium between effects and concentration over time, which can be observed as a hysteresis loop when effect and concentration pairs are connected in a time order.

16. Antagonists may inhibit an effect at a receptor through concentration-dependent competitive blocking or by binding irreversibly to the receptor.

17. Although many drugs are bound to some extent by plasma proteins and their effect is determined by the concentration of the unbound portion of the drug, **changes in protein binding do not have a clinically significant effect in most patient situations.**

18. Nonlinear pharmacokinetics are exhibited when CL changes disproportionately with changes in drug concentration, as reflected by the Michaelis-Menten equation, CL = Vmax ÷ (Km + concentration), in which Vmax is the maximum rate of elimination, Km is the concentration of drug that results in one-half the maximum rate, and C is the concentration of drug.

19. **Elderly patients may have significant changes in V and in CL for a given drug** because of changes in percentage of body fat or decreased function of the kidney or liver with increasing age.

Critically ill patients admitted to ICUs suffer from a variety of physiologic insults that accompany their severe illness. These insults, combined with the rapidly changing physiologic status of the patient, result in significant challenges to appropriate drug dosing. An understanding of the pharmacokinetic implications of these physiologic changes and their subsequent effect on pharmacodynamics is required to properly treat critically ill patients. This chapter reviews the basic principles of pharmacokinetics and pharmacodynamics with an emphasis on how they might be affected by critical illness.

Pharmacokinetics and pharmacodynamics describe, respectively, the amount of drug in the body at a given time and the pharmacologic effects caused by the drug.[1] Pharmacokinetics describes the movement of a drug into, within, and out of the body over time, whereas pharmacodynamics explains the effects the drug has on the body that result in a clinical response. A general understanding of pharmacokinetic parameters, such as clearance, volume of distribution, half-life, steady state, and absorption, along with pharmacodynamic principles such as receptor theory, potency, affinity, tolerance, and minimum effective concentration greatly enhances the clinician's ability to make informed choices in the treatment of the critically ill patient.

GENERAL PRINCIPLES OF PHARMACOKINETICS

Clearance, volume of distribution, half-life, and bioavailability are four pharmacokinetic parameters that allow the clinician to better estimate dosing requirements. If the concentration of a drug in an easily assessable sampled fluid (e.g., plasma, urine, saliva) correlates well with the pharmacologic response (therapeutic or toxic) to the drug, then the application of pharmacokinetics in dosing is likely to be beneficial.[2] Usually, the concentration of a drug cannot be measured at the exact site of action (e.g., a receptor on the cell surface), so it is necessary that there be a predictable relationship between the concentration that is measurable and the concentration at the site of the effect.[3,4] These concentrations do not need to be equal, but they should reflect a similar direction and magnitude of change over time (Fig. 185-1).

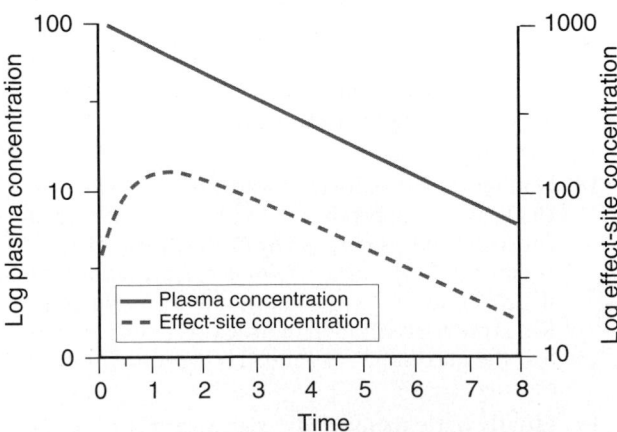

FIGURE 185–1. For concentration monitoring to be useful, there must be a strong relationship between the concentration of the drug measured in an easily accessible fluid and the concentration at the effect site. The concentration at the effect site may be less, more, or equal to the concentration in the sampled fluid.

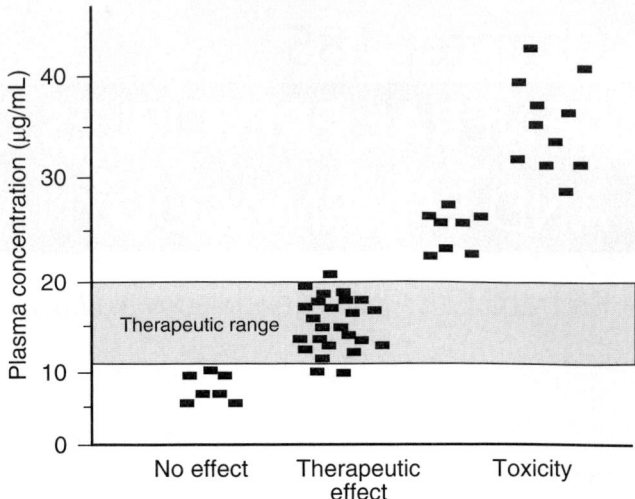

FIGURE 185–2. The therapeutic range represents the concentration at which a desired effect is likely to occur in most patients and an adverse or toxic effect is rare. If such a range cannot be established, then concentration monitoring for the drug is not likely to be of benefit. The therapeutic range is often established by dose-ranging studies during phase 2 drug development and confirmed during the phase 3 trial.

Measurement of the relationship between drug concentration and therapeutic or toxic response in a large number of patients allows the development of a therapeutic range or target concentration for that drug (Fig. 185-2).[5-10] Table 185-1 lists a number of drugs commonly used in the ICU for which therapeutic ranges have been established and for which therapeutic drug monitoring is often recommended (see Table 185-1).[11,12] Critically ill patients have a multitude of host factors (e.g., hemodynamic status, decreased organ function, nutritional status, concurrent disease states) that increase the likelihood that individualized drug dosing based on individualized pharmacokinetic assessment will be beneficial (Fig. 185-3).[13-16] There can be gender-related differences in both pharmacokinetic and pharmacodynamic responses.[17-19] Individual chapters in this text are devoted to many of these agents and their adjustments for dosing in patients with renal or hepatic failure.

PHARMACOKINETIC MODELS

The pharmacokinetic concepts of clearance, volume of distribution, half-life, and bioavailability are based on physiologic

TABLE 185–1. THERAPEUTIC RANGES OF DRUGS COMMONLY USED IN CRITICAL CARE	
Drug	**Therapeutic Range**
Amikacin	Trough, <5 μg/mL
	Peak, <30 μg/mL
Cyclosporine	Whole blood, 150 ng/mL
Digoxin	0.50-2.0 ng/mL
Gentamicin	Trough, <2 μg/mL
	Peak, <10 μg/mL
Lidocaine	1.5-5 μg/mL
Phenytoin	10-20 μg/mL
Quinidine	2-5 μg/mL
Theophylline	10-20 μg/mL
Tobramycin	Trough, <2 μg/mL
	Peak, <10 μg/mL
Vancomycin	Trough, <5 μg/mL
	Peak, <30 μg/mL

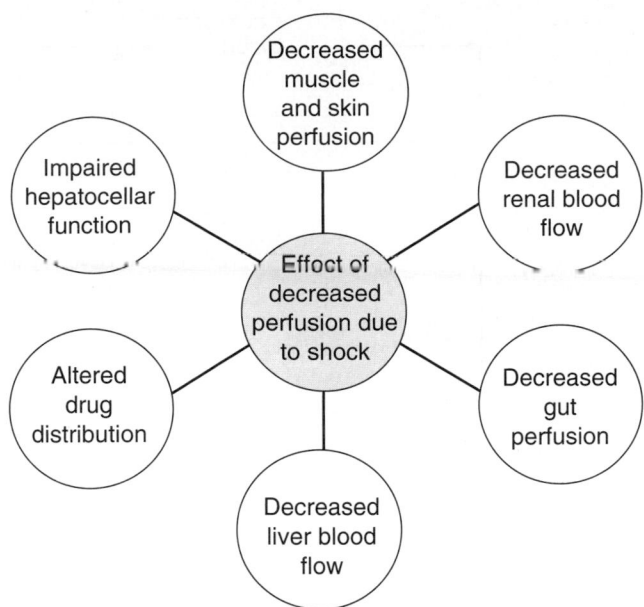

FIGURE 185–3. Example of interacting factors that determine the effect seen after administration of a single drug dose in an individual patient in the intensive care unit. A patient experiencing shock has decreased drug clearance by the liver and kidney; slowed absorption of oral, intramuscular, or topical medications; and a highly variable volume of distribution based on fluid status.

One-Compartment Model

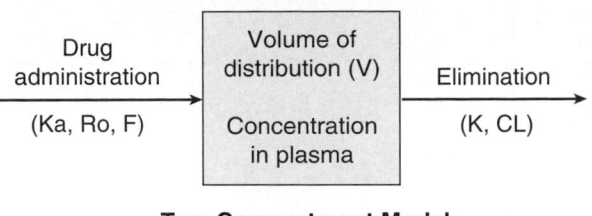

Two-Compartment Model

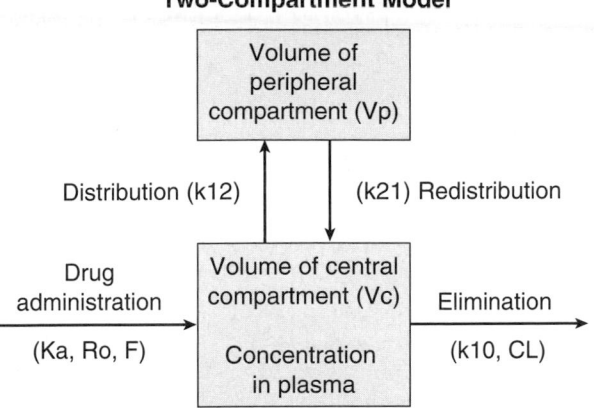

FIGURE 185–4. In the simplest pharmacokinetic model, the body is treated as a single compartment into which drug is delivered and eliminated. The resulting concentration in the compartment defines the apparent volume of distribution. Most drugs follow the more complicated two-compartment model, which assumes a distribution phase between the central or plasma compartment and the tissue. See text for explanation of terms.

principles.[20] The physiologic processes governing these concepts are enormously complex, and many simplifying assumptions need to be made before the mathematics describing drug concentrations become tractable. Although sophisticated computer modeling approaches are available in research settings, most of the clinically useful pharmacokinetic equations are based on one- or two-compartment models (Fig. 185-4).[21]

The simplest model and the most basic equations describe the one-compartment model. When the drug enters the compartment, it is assumed to be instantaneously and completely mixed in a given volume of distribution (V), resulting in a uniform concentration throughout the compartment. The parameter K is the first-order rate constant that reflects the usual situation of elimination being a first-order linear process. The drug is assumed to enter the compartment instantaneously in the case of an intravenous bolus dose. If dosing uses the oral or intramuscular routes, then entry into the compartment is assumed to occur at a rate defined by a first-order absorption rate constant (Ka). Entry into the compartment is assumed to occur at a rate described by a zero-order rate constant (Ro) if the drug is administered by constant intravenous infusion. Bioavailability (F) is defined as the fraction of the administered dose that reaches the systemic circulation.

Clearance (CL) is a primary parameter that can be physiologically associated with a particular organ in the body such as the liver or kidney. Clearance can be calculated according to the equation, $CL = K \times V$, leading to the impression that CL is a function of the parameters K and V. However, this arrangement of the equation is not correct from a physiologic point of view. CL and V are both primary parameters, and K is a secondary parameter. The first-order rate is determined by changes in either CL or V, and the equation is correctly written, $K = CL/V$.

Half-life ($t_{1/2}$) is a useful measure of how quickly a drug is eliminated from the body, and it is related to the first-order elimination rate constant:

$$t_{1/2} = \frac{ln(2)}{K} = \frac{0.693}{K}$$

Specifically, $t_{1/2}$ defines the length of time it takes for the drug concentration to decrease by one-half. In a linear pharmacokinetic system with first-order elimination, the $t_{1/2}$ is a constant, and it takes the same amount of time for the concentration to fall from 100 to 50 arbitrary units as it does to decline from 50 to 25 arbitrary units (Fig. 185-5).

The single-compartment model allows concentration at any point in time to be calculated using the following equation:

$$C2 = C1 \times exp^{-K \times \Delta t}$$

where Δt is the time elapsed between the measurement of two concentrations, C1 and C2. It is the properties of this equation that give rise to the familiar exponentially decreasing concentration-time curve, which becomes linear when plotted on semilog coordinates.

The human body is not a single, well-stirred compartment, and it is amazing that such a simple mathematical model can be so useful in the clinical setting. If the body is conceptualized as consisting of individual tissues and organs, the same mathematical treatment can be applied. The concept of the volume of distribution needs to be somewhat modified to recognize not only the physical size of the organ or tissue but also the fact that drugs accumulate to differing degrees in different tissue spaces.[22,23] For example, lipophilic drugs

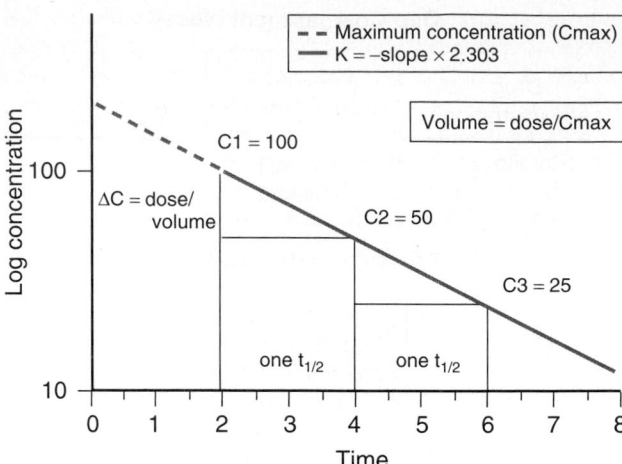

FIGURE 185–5. Log concentration-time curve for a one-compartment model after intravenous administration, illustrating volume of distribution, elimination rate constant (K), and half-life ($t_{1/2}$). C1, C2, and C3 are measured drug concentrations; ΔC is the change in drug concentration between measurements.

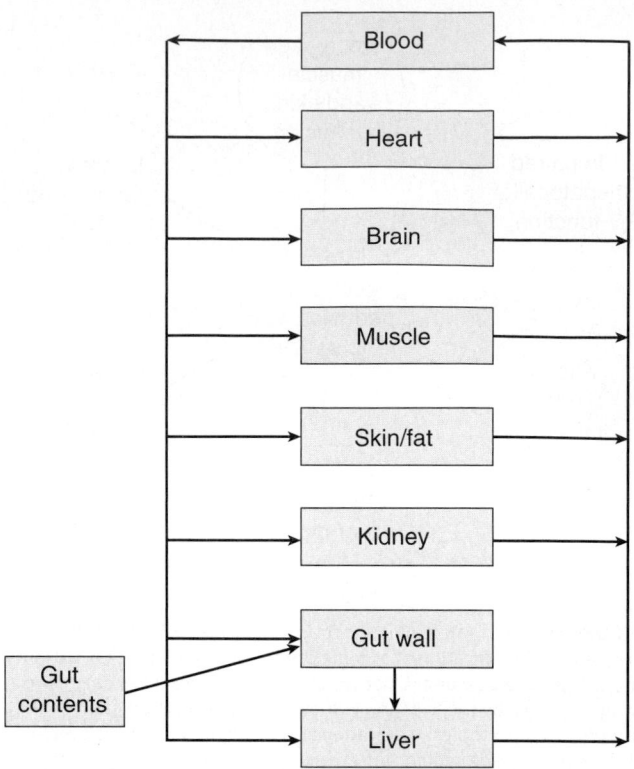

FIGURE 185–6. Physiologically based models allow individual characterization of drug distribution or clearance for each organ or tissue and also describe the mixed volume effects seen when sampling from blood.

have a high affinity for adipose tissue, and this is reflected by a large partition coefficient (R). The time constant associated with each tissue is a function of the rate of blood flow to that tissue (Q), the physical volume of the tissue (V_T), and the partition coefficient, and it determines the rate at which equilibrium is reached. This results in a set of exponential equations with a time constant unique to each tissue:

$$\exp^{-(Q/V_T \times R) \times t}$$

There is a branch of pharmacokinetics, known as physiologically based pharmacokinetic modeling, that uses blood flows, organ volumes, and partition coefficients to characterize concentration-time profiles.[24-27] In this model, each tissue space ultimately contributes to the venous pool (Fig. 185-6). However, the overall shape of the concentration-time profile in the venous blood is controlled not by the number of tissue spaces or their effective volumes but by their time constants. Tissues with similar time constants, Q/VR, produce similar drug profiles in their venous outflows and appear as a single exponent in pooled venous blood. Practically speaking, many tissues and organs reach equilibrium over similar time frames, and often no more than two distinct time constants are observed. Therefore, this situation can be described by a two-compartment model, characterized by a rapidly distributing central compartment and a more slowly equilibrating peripheral compartment (Fig. 185-7). The equation describing the concentration-time profile for the two-compartment model is

$$C = A \times \exp^{-\alpha \times t} + B \times \exp^{-\beta \times t}$$

The distinguishing feature of this biexponential equation is that, when it is plotted on semilog coordinates, the concentrations are the sum of two distinct straight lines. Hence, there are two half-lives. One is known as the terminal or β half-life, and the other is the rapid, distribution, or α half-life. Once the rapid distribution exponential becomes negligible in the equation, all that remains is the slower exponential term, and the concentration-time profile resembles that for a

single-compartment drug. Consequently, the equation

$$C2 = C1 \times \exp^{-\beta \times \Delta t}$$

in which β replaces K, can still be used to predict concentrations as long as both C1 and C2 are in the postdistributive phase. This sum-of-exponentials approach can be extended to three-compartment or even more complex models, but it is difficult to obtain all the concentrations needed to characterize each exponent.

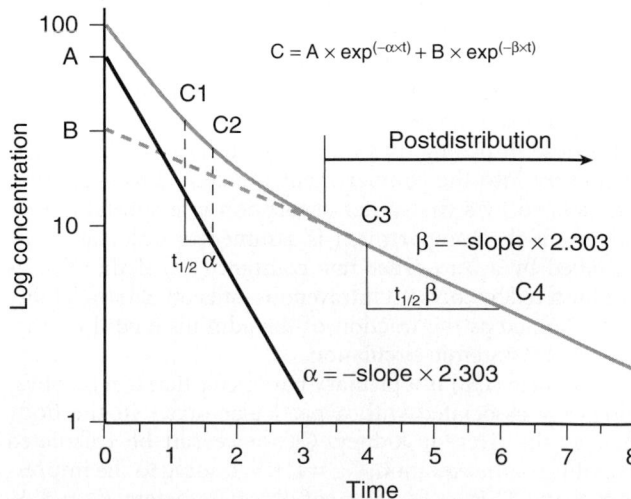

FIGURE 185–7. Log concentration-time curve for a two-compartment model after intravenous push administration, illustrating a distribution period (α) and postdistribution period (β). Concentrations at C1 and C2 are reflective of both distribution and elimination processes, whereas concentrations at C3 and C4 are primarily affected by elimination processes (clearance).

CLEARANCE

Clearance (CL) is a primary pharmacokinetic parameter that measures the ability of the body to eliminate a drug.[28,29] It is often stated that clearance is the volume of blood (plasma) that is completely cleared of drug per unit time. Although this is one way to define clearance, it does not capture the relationship between drug clearance (mL/min) and the rate of drug elimination (mg/hour). In pharmacokinetics, the general concept of clearance is defined as the rate of elimination relative to the concentration. In a first-order pharmacokinetic system, the rate of elimination is proportional to the drug concentration, and clearance is this proportionality constant.

$$\text{Rate of elimination} = \text{CL} \times \text{concentration}$$

Clearance is clinically useful because it can be related directly to the organ of elimination. We can talk about renal clearance, hepatic clearance, or biliary clearance, and the sum of each of the individual clearances is the total body clearance.[30,31] The immediate clinical consequence is the ability to adjust doses in response to changes in specific organ function. For example, a patient with developing renal failure is likely to require a reduction of the dose of a drug that is eliminated by the kidney, but not necessarily a reduction of the dose of a drug that is eliminated by the liver.[32] If the clearance of a drug is known to be 50% renal and 50% hepatic and renal function is decreased by 50%, it is necessary to reduce the dose by only 25% to maintain the same concentration.

The primary clinical utility of clearance is that it is the single pharmacokinetic parameter that determines overall drug exposure. The area under the curve (AUC) on a plot of drug concentration as a function of time is often taken as a measure of drug exposure, and it is determined from the dose and clearance (CL):

$$\text{AUC} = \frac{\text{Dose}}{\text{CL}}$$

This relationship is also observed when the steady-state concentration is considered as the measure of drug exposure. During a continuous intravenous infusion, the steady-state concentration (Css) is solely a function of the infusion rate (Ro) and the clearance (CL):

$$\text{Css} = \frac{\text{Ro}}{\text{CL}}$$

Notice that Css is not a function of the volume of distribution. As counterintuitive as it may seem, doubling the volume of distribution will not result in a halving of Css. The important point to keep in mind is that the equation is predicting the concentration *at steady state*. During a constant infusion at steady state, the rapid doubling of the volume of distribution will only *transiently* decrease the concentration by half. If the infusion rate remains unchanged, the concentration will return to the same steady-state concentration, as long as clearance remains unchanged.

The same principle applies to intermittent intravenous or oral dosing as well as continuous infusion. The challenge with intermittent dosing is in understanding which concentration is being predicted at steady state, because concentrations are going up and coming down over each dosing interval. The average concentration at steady state (Css, avg) is a time-averaged concentration (i.e., the mean of *all* concentrations in the dosing interval); as in the case of a constant infusion, it is a function of clearance and the dosing rate. In the case of oral administration, the dosing rate becomes slightly more complicated, in that it is a function of the dose administered (D), the dosing interval (τ), and bioavailability (F):

$$\text{Css, avg} = \frac{F \times D/\tau}{\text{CL}}$$

As before, overall drug exposure is not influenced by volume of distribution but does change in proportion to changes in clearance or the dosing rate, through changes in F, D, or τ.

VOLUME OF DISTRIBUTION

The volume of distribution (V) is another primary pharmacokinetic parameter that is useful in determining the change in drug concentration for a given dose.[33] After an intravenous bolus dose in a one-compartment pharmacokinetic model, the change in concentration (ΔC) is a function of the dose (D) and the volume of distribution (V):

$$\Delta C = \frac{D}{V}$$

This equation is useful for predicting both the concentration after a first bolus dose and the increase in concentration at any point in time after a bolus dose. If a concentration before administration of a bolus dose is known or can be estimated, the equation can be used to predict the increase in concentration after the dose is administered (see Fig. 185-5). It is not necessary to have a steady-state condition to use this equation, a fact that makes it very useful in critical care.

The value for volume of distribution does not necessarily coincide with any particular physiologic space. This becomes readily apparent with a drug such as digoxin, which has a volume of distribution of approximately 440 L. Clearly, a volume of distribution of that magnitude cannot have a relationship to any physiologic space in a standard-sized human. For this reason, the term "apparent volume of distribution" is often used.

The concept of volume of distribution gets more confusing when more than one compartment is needed to describe the pharmacokinetics of a drug. Mathematically, the volume of distribution is a hypothetical volume that is needed to relate the amount of drug in the body to a measured concentration in a fluid, often in plasma. Unlike the one-compartment model, in which all of the drug in the body is in a single compartment until it is eliminated, drug also circulates through additional compartments in a multicompartment model. In this situation, the volume of distribution must increase as drug distributes to other compartments, until pseudodistribution equilibrium among all compartments is reached. Technically, an infinite number of volumes of distribution are observed as this equilibration process occurs, but only three are commonly defined. The volume of distribution of the central compartment (Vc) is the volume of the usual sampling compartment; it is always the smallest volume term. Immediately after administration of an intravenous bolus, all added drug is in the central compartment and Vc can be used to calculate a change in concentration.

The volume of distribution increases over time until a distribution equilibrium is reached among all compartments. This is the largest value for the volume of distribution. The fact that distribution equilibrium has occurred can be determined from a log-concentration versus time plot (see Fig. 185-7). The curve becomes log-linear when the rate of drug entry into each peripheral compartment equals the rate of exit from each compartment. Because it is often calculated using the clearance and the β or terminal elimination half-life, this volume is often called V_β:

$$V_\beta = \frac{CL}{\beta}$$

The third commonly used volume term is the steady-state volume of distribution (Vss). It is the sum of the volumes of all the compartments in the model. If a drug were infused to steady state, Vss would be the proportionality constant relating the steady-state concentration to the total amount of drug in the body. Practically speaking, Vss is not often used in individualizing drug dosing.

HALF-LIFE

The half-life ($t_{1/2}$) is a pharmacokinetic parameter defined as the length of time it takes to reduce the drug concentration by half (see Fig. 185-5).[33] The half-life is referred to as a secondary parameter because it is a function of the two primary parameters, clearance and volume of distribution:

$$t_{1/2} = \frac{ln(2) \times V}{CL} = \frac{0.693 \times V}{CL}$$

A change in either clearance or volume of distribution results in a proportional change in half-life.

Because the half-life characterizes how rapidly concentration decreases over time, the primary clinical application for this parameter is for determining how often to dose a drug. Drugs with rapid half-lives need to be dosed more frequently than drugs with longer half-lives. The dosing of aminoglycoside antibiotics exemplifies this concept. The half-life for an aminoglycoside is relatively short in patients with good renal function (high clearance), and the drug may need to be dosed every 6 hours. In patients with poor renal function, the half-life is relatively longer, and dosing may be prolonged to 12- or 24-hour intervals to maintain appropriate peak and trough concentrations. In the critical care patient, the development of renal failure can significantly change the aminoglycoside clearance, and the accompanying change in drug half-life will necessitate a change in the dosing interval.

In a one-compartment system with a constant clearance and volume of distribution, it is clear that the drug half-life will also be a constant. However, in a multicompartment model, the volume of distribution increases over time as drug equilibrates into tissue compartments until V_β is reached. According to the previous equation, the half-life also increases over time and eventually reaches a maximum at $t_{1/2}\beta$ (see Fig. 185-7).

In multicompartment models, there is usually one half-life of interest for each compartment. These half-lives are derived from the hybrid time constants associated with each compartment. In a two-compartment model, these two exponentials are typically called α and β and are arbitrarily termed the rapid and slow exponents, respectively. These time constants give rise to the rapid or distribution $t_{1/2}\alpha$ and the slower or terminal $t_{1/2}\beta$. One useful way to think about distribution half-lives is analogous to the standard way of thinking about any half-life. In the one-compartment model, it takes five half-lives for 97% of the drug to be eliminated from the body. The situation is similar for each exponent, but the interpretation is that it takes five distribution half-lives for that exponent to become negligible in the sum of exponentials equation. In other words, it takes five α half-lives before the rapid distribution phase is completed, and the remaining concentration-time profile reflects the elimination or β phase.

All drugs have a rapid distribution phase that could be detected if concentrations were measured frequently enough. Aminoglycosides again are a good illustrative example of this concept, because they have a rapid, although not instantaneous, distribution phase (Fig. 185-8). With a distribution phase half-life of 5 to 10 minutes, it would take approximately 25 to 50 minutes before the log-linear elimination phase could be observed. It is this distribution process that is the basis for the recommendation to wait approximately 1 hour after the end of an infusion before sampling blood to measure the aminoglycoside concentration. Should a blood sample be obtained before this time, the drug will be in the distribution phase, and the concentration measured will lead to underestimation of the drug half-life. In addition, slowly equilibrating compartments have been demonstrated when aminoglycoside concentrations are measured during washout.[34] Aminoglycosides are usually dosed frequently enough so that the slowly equilibrating compartment is not detected.

BIOAVAILABILITY

The extent of drug absorption, termed bioavailability (F), is generally referenced to the amount of drug available

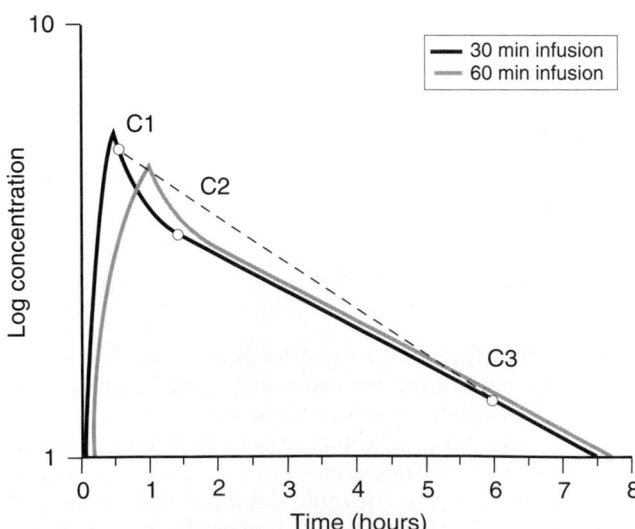

FIGURE 185–8. If an aminoglycoside (tobramycin) is administered by intravenous infusion over 30 minutes, the peak concentration will be higher than with infusion over 60 minutes, but the total area under the curve will be the same. If therapeutic drug monitoring occurs and a sample is taken during the distribution phase (C1) and paired with a concentration obtained during the postdistribution phase (C2 or C3), the calculated half-life will be shorter than if two samples from the postdistribution phase (e.g., C2 and C3) are paired together.

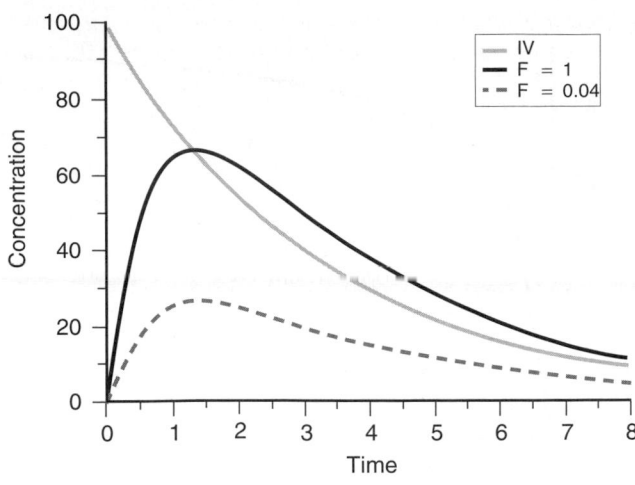

FIGURE 185–9. Bioavailability is determined relative to the area under the concentration-time curve (AUC) after intravenous (IV) administration of drug. An extravascular (e.g., intramuscular, oral, rectal) dose that is 100% absorbed (F = 1) has complete bioavailability (i.e., the extravascular AUC equals the intravenous AUC). A drug dose with 40% bioavailability (F = 0.4) would result in 40% of the drug exposure relative to an intravenous dose.

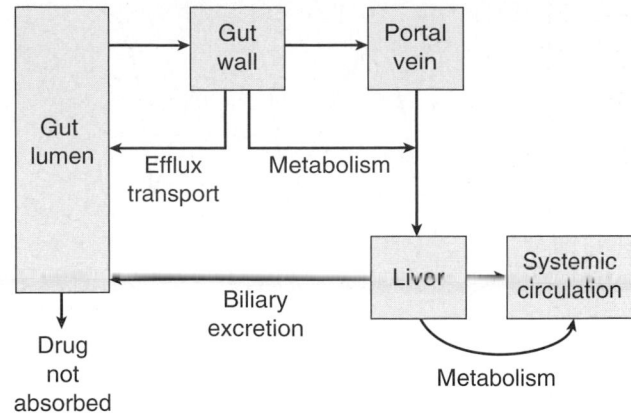

FIGURE 185–10. Drug administered orally must pass through the gut wall and through the liver before becoming available in the systemic circulation. Drug transporters and metabolism in the gut wall, combined with metabolism during the first pass through the liver, can result in significant decreases in bioavailability.

systemically when the drug is given intravenously. This parameter is determined by comparing the AUC of the drug given by intravenous administration to that of the same drug given by another route (Fig. 185-9). The intravenous administration of a drug is said to be 100% bioavailable (F = 1), and other forms of administration (e.g., oral dosing, intramuscular injection) often have a reduced bioavailability fraction (e.g., F = 0.8, or 80% bioavailability). A number of drug formulations as well as individual patient factors determine bioavailability. In essence, however, F is a function of the degree of absorption and the amount of drug metabolized or eliminated before entering the systemic circulation (first-pass effect).[35] Drugs with low bioavailability either cannot be administered by any route other than the intravenous one (e.g., sodium nitroprusside, dobutamine) or require higher doses when given via the oral route compared with the intravenous route (e.g., furosemide, morphine, propranolol). Alternative routes of administration (e.g., rectal, topical, subcutaneous, intramuscular injection) are occasionally used in critically ill patients due to poor oral bioavailability. These routes all suffer from problems with delayed or poorly predictable serum concentrations. Vasoconstriction, hypoperfusion, edema, gastric suctioning, ileus, diarrhea, and enhanced gastrointestinal motility are all common problems in critically ill patients that may further adversely affect bioavailability.

The first-pass effect (Fig. 185-10) refers to the elimination of drug that is absorbed orally but then is metabolized by enzymes in the gut wall or in the liver before reaching the systemic circulation. As a drug is absorbed and passes through the gut wall, it can be acted upon by transport proteins (primarily P-glycoprotein) that actively pump drug molecules back into the lumen of the gastrointestinal tract.[36-40] All drug molecules that are not pumped out enter the hepatic circulation and are subject to metabolism in the liver before their first opportunity to be presented to the systemic circulation.[41] Drugs that have a high hepatic extraction ratio (i.e., are very efficiently removed by the liver) are most likely to show a decreased bioavailability due to this first-pass effect; conversely, they are also subject to increased

bioavailability if liver dysfunction decreases the hepatic extraction ratio.

STEADY STATE

After an infusion is started, drug concentrations increase and eventually reach a concentration that does not change over time (Fig. 185-11).[42] At this point, the amount of drug entering the body is equal to the amount leaving it during a given period of time, and steady-state conditions apply. During intermittent dosing, drug concentrations accumulate over time, and eventually a steady state is attained. Drug concentrations increase as more drug is administered or absorbed and decrease during elimination, but the concentration profile over each interval resembles all the other steady-state profiles (Fig. 185-12). In the clinical setting, measurement of drug concentration is often delayed for a period equal to five half-lives, because at that point the concentration will reflect 97% of the final steady-state concentration.

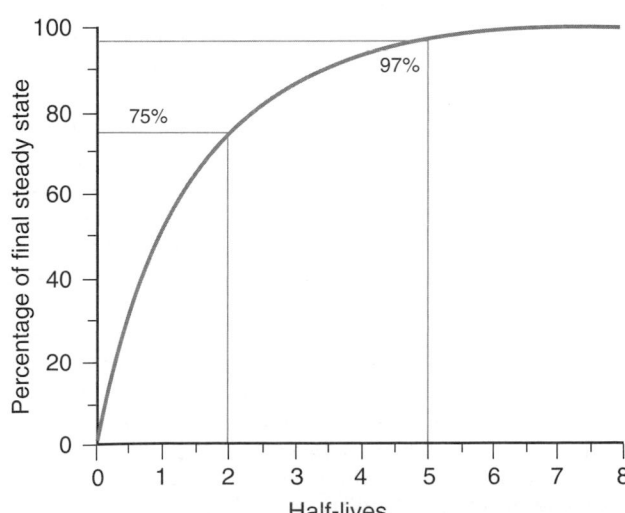

FIGURE 185–11. Concentrations exponentially approach a steady-state value during a constant infusion in a one-compartment model. After five half-lives of a drug, its concentration is at 97% of the final steady-state value.

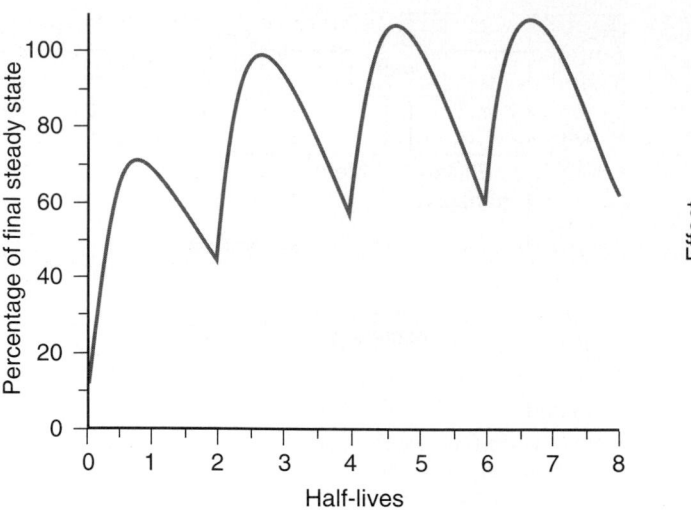

FIGURE 185–12. With intermittent dosing (oral, intravenous, or intramuscular dosing), concentration profiles also approach a steady state, wherein peak and trough concentrations during a given cycle are reproducible in the next cycle.

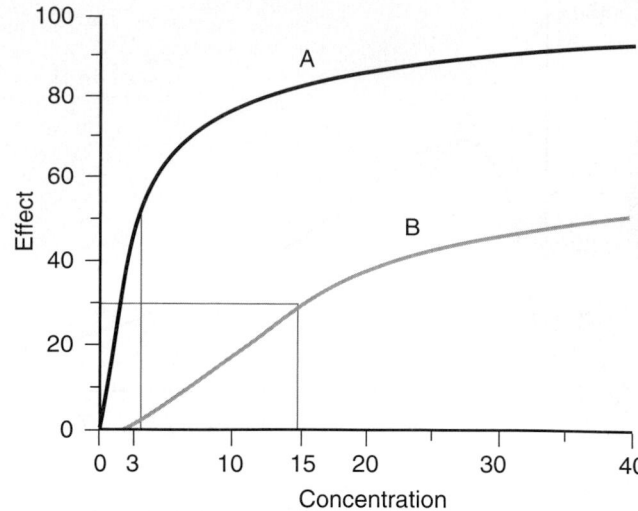

FIGURE 185–13. The Emax pharmacodynamic model illustrates the fact that when drug concentrations exceed the concentration at which half the maximal effect is expected (EC50), there is a decreasing return in terms of effect as the dose is further increased. Drug A has a lower EC50 (3) than drug B (15) and is said to be more potent than drug B.

PHARMACODYNAMICS

Pharmacodynamics is the study of the relationship between the concentration of a drug and its pharmacologic effect.[2] The application of pharmacodynamic models has become routine in the drug development process, where they are used to determine drug-dosing regimens. These models can become quite complex, particularly if they are mechanism-based models.

Although a pharmacodynamic model can involve many linked mathematical submodels, this is not the type of model that is likely to be useful in a clinical setting. The principles underpinning the relatively simple Emax model are often adequate.[43] Mathematically, the equation relating effect and concentration can be described with the Emax equation:

$$\text{Effect} = \frac{\text{Emax} \times \text{concentration}}{\text{EC50} + \text{concentration}}$$

Graphically, this equation has a hyperbolic shape (Fig. 185-13). The parameters of this model are the Emax and the EC50. Emax represents the maximal effect attainable due to the drug. The EC50 is the concentration at which half the maximal effect is observed; it is a measure of drug potency. An important feature of this plot reaffirms the intuitive notion that a dose cannot be continually increased with the expectation that the effect will continue to increase proportionately. In essence, the law of diminishing returns applies: continually smaller increases in effect are observed as the concentration increases. Practically speaking, if the drug concentration is expected to be at the EC50 or lower, increasing the dose will produce a meaningful increase in effect. However, if the concentration exceeds the EC50, then increasing the dose may not be warranted, because only small increases in effect may be expected, and the increased concentrations may place the patient at risk for development of adverse drug-related effects.

Several modifications of the basic Emax model are found in the literature. For example, a baseline can be added to the model, the drug may actually be responsible for inhibiting a given effect, the effect can be reparametized as a percentage change from baseline, or a sigmoidicity term may be added to create an S-shape in the functional relationship. The same basic features of the plot will be observed. In the absence of drug (i.e., when the concentration equals zero), there will be no effect due to the drug. At the other extreme, there will be a maximal effect that can be elicited by the drug. As concentrations increase beyond EC50, the change in effect due to the drug begins to reach a plateau.

Another point to consider is that time does not appear in the effect model. The concentrations are explicitly defined as steady-state concentrations, and the effect resulting from a given concentration is considered to be a steady-state effect. This model applies when drug in the plasma rapidly equilibrates with drug at the site of action, and there is no indirect mechanism between the concentration at the site of effect and the effect. The more common situation is that the effect lags somewhat behind the concentration (Fig. 185-14). If concentrations are going up and coming down over time, as would be expected with an intermittent intravenous or oral dosing schedule, the effect is also expected to go up and down over time, but the time frames may not exactly coincide. For example, the plasma concentration might peak at 1 hour and the effect might peak several hours later. There is a mismatch or disequilibrium between concentration and effect, and a plot of effect versus concentration, with the points connected in time order, yields a hysteresis loop (Fig. 185-15). It can be seen that for any given concentration, there are two levels of effect, one on the upswing of the concentration-time curve and the other on the downswing. Both empiric and mechanistic pharmacodynamic modeling approaches have been developed to allow for this disequilibrium. Although the modeling of effect-time curves is achievable and these models are useful in predicting effects with various dosing regimens, their routine use in clinical settings has been limited.

The pharmacodynamic effects noted with a given drug result from the drug's interaction with receptors and the resultant activation or inhibition of effects mediated by that receptor. These effects may be either the therapeutic action desired or a toxic effect that is unwanted. Generally, it is assumed that the intensity of effect produced by the drug is

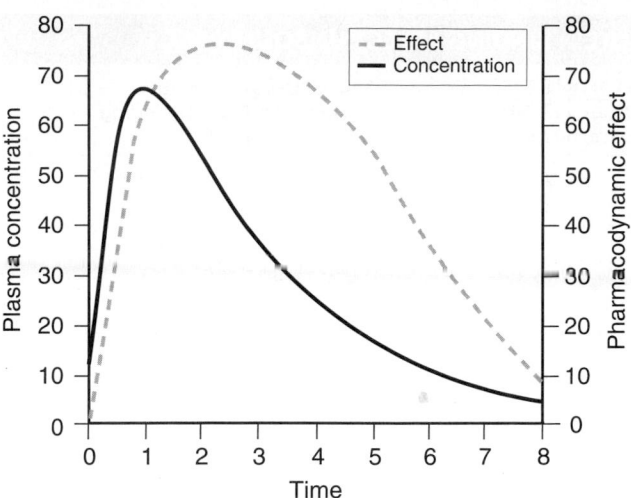

FIGURE 185–14. Pharmacodynamic effects often lag behind the matching pharmacokinetic model. In this instance, the maximum concentration in the blood occurs at 1 hour while the maximal drug effect occurs between 2 and 3 hours.

a function of the quantity of drug at the receptor site, whereas relative potency results from varying degrees of selectivity for the receptor and the receptor's affinity for binding the drug. More potent drugs elicit a given effect at lower concentrations than do less potent drugs.

Drugs that stimulate a response from the receptor are agonists, and those that inhibit a response from the receptor are antagonists. Because antagonists have no effect of their own at the receptor, the net effect depends on both the concentration of the antagonist and that of the agonist that is blocked. The relative concentration of the agonist compared with the antagonist primarily determines the effect observed when an antagonist is competitive for the same binding site as the molecule or drug that stimulates the receptor.

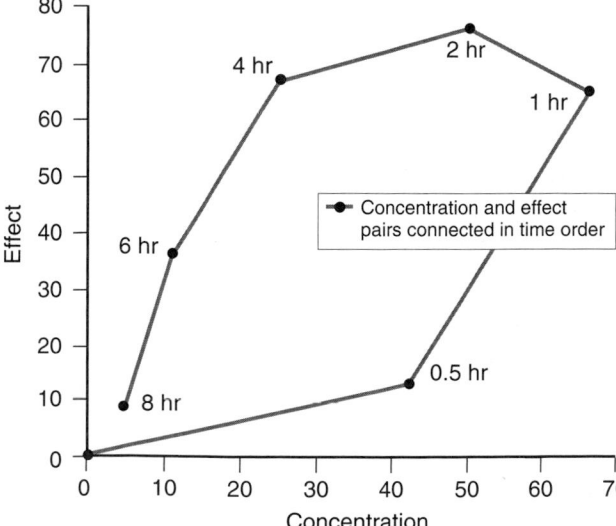

FIGURE 185–15. A counterclockwise hysteresis loop occurs when an effect at a given concentration is less at an early point in time but strengthens at the same concentration later in time. This may be caused by an active metabolite, increased sensitization to the drug, or the need for a distribution period from the sampled fluid to the effect site. The opposite can occur (i.e., a clockwise hysteresis loop) if a given effect decreases over time, as in the development of tolerance to the drug.

Irreversible antagonists, however, either bind with very strong affinity to the receptor so they cannot be displaced or bind to another site on the substrate that interferes with binding at the receptor. The effect of irreversible antagonists is independent of the agonist's concentration and results in a decrease in the maximal effect of the agonist. The duration of effect for irreversible antagonists is determined by the rate of turnover for the receptor.

Tolerance to a drug is seen when the response at a given dose decreases. This may be a result of receptor downregulation (decreased number or sensitivity of receptors) or enzyme induction (increased metabolism). Cross-tolerance occurs when similar drugs act on the same receptor, as is commonly seen with opioids.

PROTEIN BINDING

Many drugs are bound to plasma proteins, and the terms bound drug concentration (Cb), unbound (or free) drug concentration (Cu), total (bound plus unbound) drug concentration (Ctot), and unbound (or free) fraction (fu) are frequently used:

$$Ctot = Cu + Cb$$

$$fu = \frac{Cu}{Ctot}$$

Intuitively, it is clear that when a drug is displaced from its binding sites in the plasma, the increase in unbound drug concentration can lead to adverse reactions. A series of scientific papers published in the mid-1960s set this direction for interpretation of the clinical implications of protein binding. In a study of the interaction between warfarin and phenylbutazone, it was shown that phenylbutazone increases plasma warfarin concentration and also increases prothrombin time.[43a] In addition, warfarin binding was studied in vitro, and it was clearly shown that phenylbutazone displaces warfarin from binding sites. It was concluded that phenylbutazone potentiates the action of warfarin in vivo by displacing warfarin from its binding to plasma albumin, causing more warfarin to be available to specific sites of biologic action. Although it may have been intuitive to relate the in vivo and in vitro observations in a cause-and-effect manner, this is not the correct explanation for the drug interaction. It is now known that the drug interaction is mediated through an inhibition of warfarin metabolic clearance by phenylbutazone.[43b]

The pharmacokinetic concepts concerning the implications of protein binding were reviewed in 2002 by Benet and Hoener.[44] The mathematical approach is not repeated here, but when one assumes physiologically based models for clearance, volume of distribution, and protein binding, changes in plasma protein binding can be shown to have little clinical relevance. These clearance concepts illustrate that physiologic parameters (intrinsic clearance, organ blood flow, and protein binding) have an impact on some pharmacokinetic parameters, and these changes result in changes to the shape of the plasma-concentration time profiles. However, these effects do not necessarily translate into clinically relevant changes in effective concentrations. To better understand this concept, the relationship between drug exposure and pharmacodynamic effect must be considered.

One of the more useful measures of exposure is the AUC. When talking about pharmacologic effects, some statement

TABLE 185–2. CIRCUMSTANCES IN WHICH CHANGES IN PROTEIN BINDING AFFECT UNBOUND AUC

Routes of Administration and Elimination	Effect of Protein Binding Possible		No. of Drugs Meeting Criteria for Protein-binding Effect (N = 456)*
	Drugs with Low Extraction Ratio	Drugs with High Extraction Ratio	
Intravenous			25 (hepatic and nonhepatic)
Hepatic clearance	NO	YES	
Nonhepatic clearance	NO	YES	
Oral			
Hepatic clearance	NO	NO	N/A
Nonhepatic clearance	NO	YES	None

AUC, area under the concentration-time curve.
*Criteria for selection included >70% protein binding and hepatic clearance ≥6.0 mL/min/kg or nonhepatic extraction ratio clearance >0.28 × renal blood flow (>4.8 mL/min/kg).
Modified from Benet LZ, Hoener BA: Changes in plasma protein binding have little clinical relevance. Clin Pharmacol Ther 2002;71:115-121.

is usually made that effect is related to the unbound concentration. This extrapolates directly to saying that the unbound AUC (AUCu) is what is important in determining drug effect.

$$AUCu = fu \times AUC = fu \times F \times \frac{Dose}{CL}$$

where fu is the fraction unbound, F is the bioavailability, and CL is the clearance.

After standard assumptions are made regarding high- and low-clearance drugs, something quite interesting occurs when the appropriate equations for clearance and bioavailability are substituted into the equation for AUCu. For all drugs administered orally and eliminated hepatically, the fu term cancels out of the equation. Overall unbound drug exposure is not a function of fu, and there will presumably be no change in pharmacologic effect with changes in protein binding. Similarly, it can be seen that the AUCu for all drugs with low extraction ratios—whether administered orally or by the intravenous route, and whether eliminated by the liver or nonhepatically—is not a function of fu after the appropriate substitutions are made. Again, changes in protein binding will not result in changes in unbound exposure. The expression for AUCu retains a term for protein binding for all high-clearance drugs administered by the intravenous route (regardless of clearance method), and for high-clearance drugs administered orally that are eliminated by extrahepatic pathways.

To address this issue, Benet and Hoener reviewed pharmacokinetic data on 456 drugs from the literature (Table 185-2). No drug administered orally that had a high elimination ratio and was nonhepatically eliminated met the criterion for significant (greater than 70%) protein binding. Only 25 (5%) of the 456 drugs had high extraction ratios, were not administered by the oral route, and met the criterion for which protein binding may influence drug exposure. However, many of these 25 agents are routinely used in critical care (Table 185-3).

In critically ill patients, protein concentrations can change over time. This is particularly true of the acute phase reactant, α_1-acid glycoprotein (AAG). In addition, some patients (e.g., those undergoing dialysis or cachexia) have altered protein binding.[44a,44b] Although it might seem intuitive to automatically adjust drug doses in response to changes in protein binding, the information in Table 185-2 should be considered. The extent of protein binding, the route of administration, the route of elimination, and the extraction ratio of the drug all should be considered when determining whether a change in binding is likely to result in a change in effect.[45,46]

As a final note on protein binding, care must be taken when evaluating drug concentrations in patients with altered protein binding. Consider the case of phenytoin. The percentage of unbound drug is typically 10%, but is approximately doubled (20%) in patients receiving hemodialysis (Table 185-4). If phenytoin were administered as a standard dose to all patients, there would not be a problem; phenytoin is a low-clearance drug, and protein binding should not influence overall unbound exposure, whether the drug is administered orally or intravenously. However, phenytoin concentrations are often obtained for the purposes of therapeutic drug monitoring, to achieve a commonly accepted therapeutic range of 10 to 20 mg/L. In patients with normal binding, this drug level equates to an unbound therapeutic range of 1 to 2 mg/L. However, in patients with an altered binding of 20%, the desired unbound concentration is still 1 to 2 mg/L, but the total concentration is approximately halved. In such cases, if the dose of phenytoin is increased to bring the total concentration into the therapeutic range,

TABLE 185–3. TWENTY-FIVE DRUGS FOR WHICH CHANGES IN PROTEIN BINDING MAY INFLUENCE CLINICAL DRUG EXPOSURE AFTER INTRAVENOUS OR INTRAMUSCULAR ADMINISTRATION*

Alfentanil	Itraconazole
Amitriptyline	Lidocaine
Buprenorphine	Methylprednisolone
Chlorpromazine	Midazolam
Cocaine	Milrinone
Diltiazem	Nicardipine
Diphenhydramine	Pentamidine
Doxorubicin	Propofol
Erythromycin	Propranolol
Fentanyl	Remifentanil
Gold sodium thiomalate	Sufentanil
Haloperidol	Verapamil
Idarubicin	

*Criteria for selection included >70% protein binding and hepatic clearance ≥6.0 mL/min/kg or nonhepatic extraction ratio clearance >0.28 × renal blood flow (>4.8 mL/min/kg).
Modified from Benet LZ, Hoener BA: Changes in plasma protein binding have little clinical relevance. Clin Pharmacol Ther 2002;71:115-121.

TABLE 185–4. EFFECT OF DECREASED PROTEIN BINDING ON BOUND AND UNBOUND CONCENTRATIONS OF PHENYTOIN (PHT)

Concentration	Concentrations of PHT at Therapeutic Range (mg/L)		Result of Erroneous Increase in PHT Dose in Patient with Decreased Protein Binding*
	Typical Patient	Patient with Protein Binding Decreased by 50%	
Total (Ctot)	20	10	20
Unbound (Cu)	2 (10%)	2 (20%)	4 (20%)
Bound (Cb)	18	8	16

*Because of the altered protein binding, Ctot is less when Cu is in the therapeutic range (i.e., 2 mg/L). During therapeutic drug monitoring, it is the Ctot that is measured. If the decreased protein binding is not taken into account and the PHT dose is increased to achieve a Ctot of 20 mg/L, the actual Cu will be 4 mg/L, twice the desired therapeutic range, and toxic effects could ensue.

toxicities may be observed because the unbound concentration will be approximately twice the desired value.

NONLINEAR PHARMACOKINETICS

The application of pharmacokinetics to therapeutic drug monitoring becomes considerably more difficult with drugs that exhibit nonlinearities. With linear pharmacokinetics, parameters are stable over time and across concentrations. Doubling of the dose results in doubling of the concentration, and a given dose provides the same AUC, regardless of the dosing history and even if it is the first dose. Nonlinear pharmacokinetics is a term used when the principle of superposition no longer holds. An increase in dose may result in an increase in concentration that is more than or less than proportional, or it may result in clearance changes over time (Fig. 185-16). There are several common types of nonlinearities that occur in the clinical setting.[47]

Phenytoin is the classic example for nonlinear elimination. Increases in a phenytoin dose can result in greater than proportional increases in concentration. In any pharmacokinetic system, clearance (CL) is defined as the rate of elimination relative to the concentration (C). Hence, an instantaneous rate of elimination can be defined as follows:

$$\text{Rate of elimination} = CL \times C$$

In a linear elimination process, clearance is constant, and doubling the concentration doubles the rate of elimination. In the case of phenytoin with nonlinear elimination, the rate of elimination does not increase in proportion to the concentration, and clearance is not a constant. This occurs because the metabolic pathway responsible for the elimination of phenytoin is saturable. The enzyme system has a maximum rate of metabolism that can be approached at therapeutic concentrations of phenytoin. These principles can be better understood by considering the rate of elimination described by the Michaelis-Menten equation (Fig. 185-17). It has two parameters, the maximum rate of elimination (Vmax) and the concentration that results in one-half the maximum rate (Km):

$$\text{Rate of elimination} = \frac{Vmax \times C}{Km + C}$$

Although the parameters Vmax and Km are constant, it can be seen that clearance is a function of concentration (C). The clearance of a drug decreases as the concentration increases:

$$CL = \frac{\text{Rate of elimination}}{C} = \frac{Vmax}{Km + C}$$

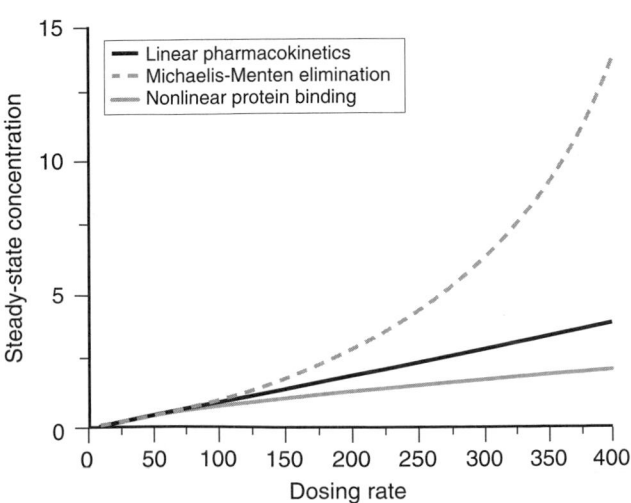

FIGURE 185–16. Drugs with nonlinear characteristics often can be predictable within a given dose range but then exhibit disproportionate increases or decreases in concentration as doses are increased further.

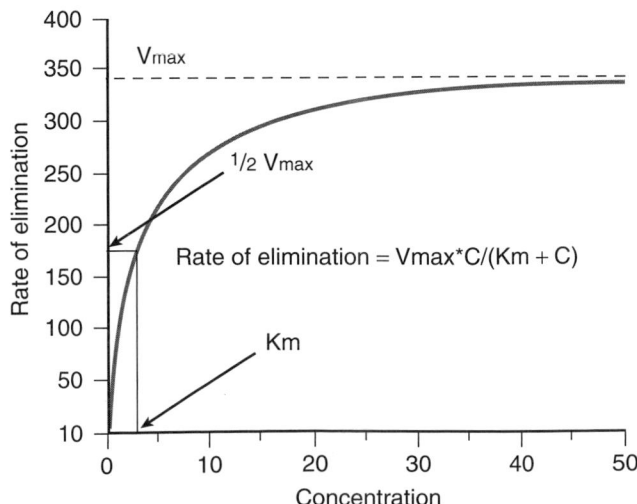

FIGURE 185–17. The Michaelis-Menten model demonstrates elimination as a nonlinear function of concentration, with characteristics including a maximum rate of elimination (Vmax) and a concentration at which one half of the maximum rate of elimination occurs (Km).

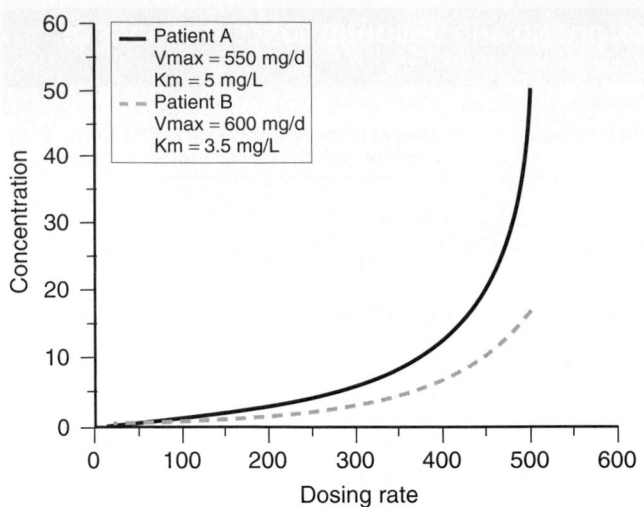

FIGURE 185–18. The same phenytoin dose increase can result in very different steady-state concentrations in patients with differing Vmax and Km parameters. Patient A is likely to have controlled seizures at doses of 350 to 400 mg/day, whereas seizures in patient B would not be controlled in this dose range.

Although enzyme systems do have maximal rates, the usual concentrations attained in the clinical setting produce rates of elimination that are far below the maximal rate of the enzyme. In the last equation, if C is considerably lower than Km (i.e., negligible), the quantity Vmax ÷ (Km + C) is little influenced by concentration, and clearance becomes a constant. Therefore, even though many drugs are metabolized by hepatic enzymes, few drugs of clinical interest display detectable nonlinear elimination.

At steady state, the amount of drug eliminated every day must equal the dose taken, so the elimination rate equals the dosing rate. The equation for the steady-state concentration (Css) is

$$Css = \frac{\text{Dosing rate} \times Km}{Vmax - \text{Dosing rate}}$$

This equation shows that an increase in dosing rate produces a greater than proportional increase in the steady-state concentration. Furthermore, if the dosing rate exceeds Vmax, then a steady-state concentration will never be attained. The nonlinear relationship between phenytoin dosing rate and

I. Absorption ↑ gastric pH ↓ gastrointestinal motility
  ↓ splanchnic blood flow ↓ intestinal absorptive surface

II. Distribution ↑ body fat proportion ↓ lean body mass (LBM)

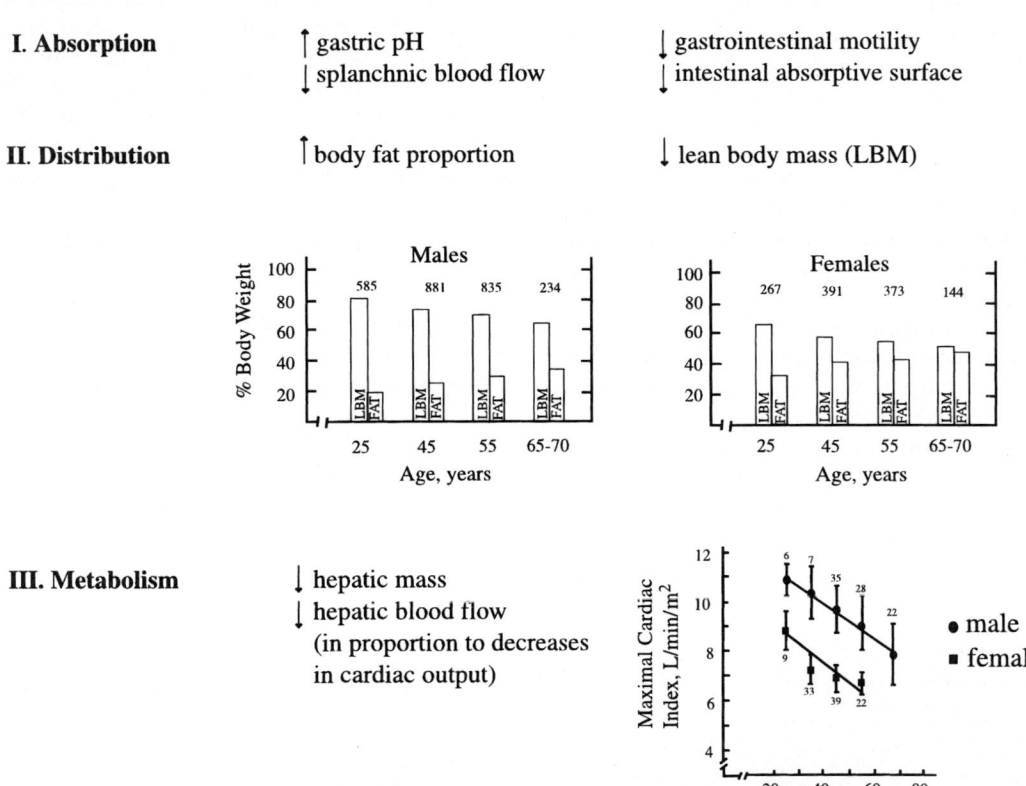

III. Metabolism ↓ hepatic mass
  ↓ hepatic blood flow
   (in proportion to decreases
   in cardiac output)

IV. Elimination

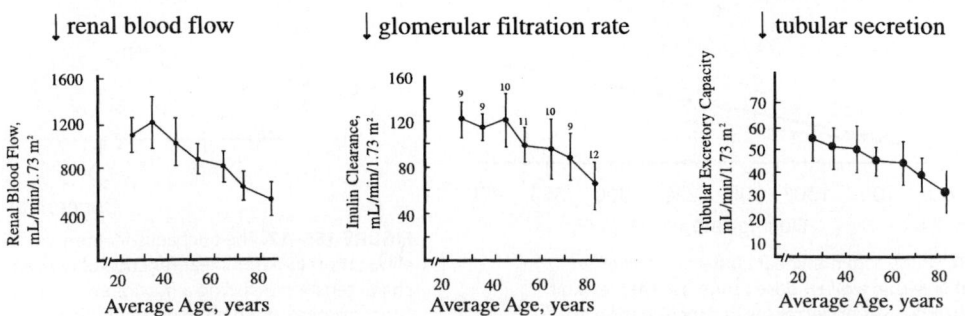

FIGURE 185–19. Physiologic changes with aging that may affect drug distribution are reflected. (From Evans WE, Schentag JJ [eds]: Applied Pharmacokinetics: Principles of Therapeutic Drug Monitoring, 3rd ed. Vancouver, WA, Applied Therapeutics, 1992, pp 9-1–9-43.)

steady-state concentration can be seen for two patients with different Vmax and Km parameters (Fig. 185-18). It is easy to understand the difficulties in dosing nonlinear drugs such as phenytoin. A dose increase that provides a nearly proportional increase in concentration in one patient could produce a much greater concentration in another. These two curves would be straight lines for drugs that displayed linear pharmacokinetics.

Another type of nonlinearity is time-dependent pharmacokinetics. The classic example in this category is the ability of carbamazepine to induce its own metabolism.[47a] This autoinduction causes the clearance of carbamazepine to increase over time. It is important to gradually increase the dose of carbamazepine during the first few weeks of therapy up to the expected maintenance dose, to avoid toxicities related to elevated concentrations.

Protein binding can also become saturable with some drugs. Although it is intuitive to think that this would result in higher unbound drug concentrations available to exert desirable effects and toxicities, it must be kept in mind that the organs responsible for drug clearance are eliminating unbound drug. Unless the clearance of a drug also changes, the steady-state unbound concentration will remain constant in the face of saturable protein binding. The total concentration (Ctot) is a function of the unbound concentration (Cu) and the fraction unbound (fu):

$$Ctot = \frac{Cu}{fu}$$

The fraction unbound does increase at higher unbound concentrations, with the result that total concentrations do not increase in proportion to unbound concentrations. This can be perplexing in therapeutic drug monitoring situations. Increases in dose produce less than expected increases in total concentration. As the dose is pushed higher to reach therapeutic concentrations based on total concentration, toxicities may be observed because saturable binding causes the unbound concentration to be greater than expected.

ALTERATIONS IN THE ELDERLY

The number of people older than 65 years of age is increasing in the United States and in many European countries, and this growth in the elderly population will result in an even greater percentage of ICU beds occupied by older patients. Compared with younger patients, elderly patients typically are taking more drugs, have more underlying organ dysfunction (hepatic, renal, central nervous system), are more likely to be malnourished and to have altered protein binding on this basis, and have reduced or increased responses to some medications.[48] These age-related changes further complicate management of the superimposed critical illness because of large interindividual variations in drug disposition (Fig. 185-19).

Elderly patients may have a decreased rate of drug absorption, although the total amount of drug absorbed is usually unchanged. As the body ages, the percentage of body mass that is fat increases. This change results in greater distribution of lipophilic drug into fat, leading to longer half-lives for drugs such as anesthetics, barbiturates, and benzodiazepines. Clearance of many drugs is decreased in the elderly, because liver and kidney both show decreased function with

TABLE 185–5. EFFECTS OF AGING ON THE CLEARANCE OF SOME OXIDIZED AND CONJUGATED DRUGS

Drug	Effect	Reference
Oxidized		
Chlordiazepoxide	↓↓	Am J Psychiatry 1977;134:559
Desmethyldiazepam	↓↓	Br J Clin Pharmacol 1979;7:119
Erythromycin	↓↓	Eur J Clin Pharmacol 1990;39:161
Haloperidol	↓↓	Neuropsychobiology 1996;33:12
Midazolam	↓↓	Biochem Pharmacol 1992;44:275
Nicardipine	↓↓	Am Heart J 1989;117:256
Nifedipine	↓↓	Br J Clin Pharmacol 1988;25:297
Phenytoin (free)	↓↓	Clin Pharmacokinet 1981;6:389
Propranolol	—	Br J Clin Pharmacol 1979;7:49
Theophylline	↓↓	Eur J Clin Pharmacol 1989;36:29
Verapamil	↓↓	Acta Med Scand 1984;681(Suppl):25
Conjugated		
Acetaminophen	↓	Br J Clin Pharmacol 1990;30:634
Lamotrigine	↓	J Pharm Med 1991;1:121
Lidocaine	↓↓	J Cardiovasc Pharmacol 1983;5:1093
Lorazepam	↓	Clin Pharmacol Ther 1979;26:103
Metronidazole	—	Hum Exp Toxicol 1990;9:155
Morphine	↓	Age Ageing 1989;18:258
Oxazepam	—	Clin Pharmacol Ther 1981;30:805

—, no effect; ↓, minor effect; ↓↓, significant effect.
Modified from Woodhouse K, Wynne HA: Age-related changes in hepatic function: Implications for drug therapy. Drugs Aging 1992;2:243.

increasing age (Table 185-5). This change can lead to a greater incidence of toxicity, because metabolites may accumulate that are associated with adverse effects. Overall, the same careful attention to dosing that is required for all critically ill patients must be extended to the elderly. Drugs should be stopped as soon as possible, and dosage increases should be cautiously applied.

ANNOTATED REFERENCES

Benet LZ, Hoener B: Changes in plasma protein binding have little clinical relevance. Clin Pharmacol Ther 2002;71:115-121.
This manuscript systematically presents the rationale behind the statement that changes in protein binding have little clinical relevance. The physiology and mathematics needed to understand the rationale are presented in an easily understood fashion.

De Paepe P, Belpaire FM, Buylaert WA: Pharmacokinetic and pharmacodynamic considerations when treating patients with sepsis and septic shock. Clin Pharmacokinet 2002;41:1135-1151.
This review article details the pharmacokinetic changes observed during sepsis and septic shock. It provides a good discussion of the relationships between drug clearance and organ function.

Gibaldi M, Perrier D: Pharmacokinetics, 2nd ed. New York, Marcel Dekker, 1982.
This text provides detailed coverage of the mathematical aspects of pharmacokinetics. Most of the equations used in clinical pharmacokinetics, and their derivations, are presented.

Renton KW: Alteration of drug biotransformation and elimination during infection and inflammation. Pharmacol Ther 2001;92:147-163.
This review describes the relationship between cytochrome P450 expression and inflammation. Mechanisms of cytochrome P450 regulation and the impact of cytokines on drug metabolism are presented.

Schulz M, Schmoldt A: Therapeutic and toxic blood concentrations of more than 800 drugs and other xenobiotics. Pharmazie 2003;58:447-474.
This is an excellent reference article that contains an exhaustive compilation of drugs with their therapeutic, toxic, and fatal concentration ranges. The article also provides half-lives and references for each drug.

Chapter 186

POISONING: OVERVIEW OF APPROACHES FOR EVALUATION AND TREATMENT

Donna Seger

KEY POINTS

1. The theory of gastric decontamination is that removal of toxins from the stomach (where absorption is poor), before they move into the small bowel (where absorption is more rapid), decreases the toxicity of the poisoning.

2. Stabilization of the patient always precedes antidote administration. The effects of the toxin may outlast the effects of the administered antidote. Patients receiving antidotes should be observed in a critical care setting.

3. Treating a hypotensive, poisoned patient with large volumes of fluids may predispose the patient to the development of acute respiratory failure.

4. Attempts to prevent acute renal failure (ARF) in the poisoned patient are crucial, because there is no specific therapy once ARF has occurred.

5. An aggressive approach should be taken toward terminating seizures in the poisoned patient. Benzodiazepines are the drugs of choice to quickly terminate seizures, because they are lipophilic and rapidly enter the central nervous system.

6. Administration of sedatives to help the poisoned patient with respiratory distress "tolerate the tube" for endotracheal intubation causes prolonged extubation times and potential complications.

7. The clinical value of analytic toxicology testing depends on the clinician's ability to understand and interpret the results.

GASTROINTESTINAL DECONTAMINATION

The theory of gastric decontamination (GID) is that removal of toxins from the stomach (where absorption is poor), before they move into the small bowel (where absorption is more rapid), decreases the toxicity of the poisoning.

Because of the controversies regarding the role of gut decontamination, senior toxicologists from the American Academy of Clinical Toxicology and the European Association of Poisons Centres and Clinical Toxicologists (EAPCCT) agreed to collaborate on the production of Position Statements on GID treatments. These statements, published in 1997, are systematically developed guidelines founded on a criteria-based critical review of all relevant scientific literature.[1] The Position Statements were updated in 2004. GID Position Statement summaries are presented in this chapter.

IPECAC

Ipecac is prepared form the *Cephalis accuminata* or *Cephalis ipecacuanha* plant. Vomiting within 30 minutes after administration is caused by local irritation of the gastric mucosa, which induces reflex vomiting. Vomiting after 30 minutes is centrally induced.[2]

Position Statement. Syrup of Ipecac should not be administered routinely in the management of poisoned patients. In experimental studies, the amount of marker removed by ipecac was highly variable and diminished with time. There is no evidence from clinical studies that ipecac improves the outcome of poisoned patients, and its routine administration should be abandoned.[3]

GASTRIC LAVAGE

In gastric lavage, a large-bore (36F to 40F or 30 English gauge) orogastric tube is passed, after which small volumes (200 to 300 mL) of liquid are alternately administered and aspirated. Endotracheal intubation should precede this procedure in a comatose patient. An oral airway prevents biting of the tube. The amount of stomach contents removed is highly variable and decreases with time.[4-6] The procedure may actually push stomach contents into the intestine.[7] Contraindications include loss of protective airway reflexes, unless the patient is intubated; ingestion of a corrosive or hydrocarbon; gastrointestinal pathology; and other medical complications that could be compromised by the use of lavage. Complications of the procedure include aspiration, laryngospasm, hypoxia and hypercapnia, mechanical injury, and fluid and electrolyte imbalance in children.[8]

Position Statement. Gastric lavage should not be employed routinely in the management of poisoned patients. It should not be considered unless the patient has ingested a potentially life-threatening amount of a poison and the procedure can be undertaken within 60 minutes after ingestion. Even then, clinical benefit has not been confirmed in controlled studies.[8]

SINGLE-DOSE ACTIVATED CHARCOAL

Activated charcoal is made when coconut shells, peat, wood, or other materials undergo controlled pyrolysis and are subsequently activated by heating in steam or air at high temperatures. Activation creates multiple internal pores and the small particle size necessary for adsorption. The adsorptive surface contains many carbon moieties that adsorb poisons with varying affinities. Although in vitro studies demonstrate adsorption of many drugs to activated charcoal, animal studies reveal variable reduction in marker absorption.[9] Volunteer and clinical studies have not demonstrated that administration of single-dose activated charcoal improves outcome. Contraindications to the administration of activated charcoal include decreased level of consciousness and unprotected airway, ingestion of caustic or hydrocarbon, gastrointestinal pathology, and medical conditions that could be further compromised by the administration of activated charcoal. Complications include aspiration and direct administration of charcoal into the lung.[10]

Because activated charcoal is an inert substance, it has been the belief that lung injury after aspiration of activated charcoal was caused by gastric contents. Aspiration of gastric contents causes neutrophils to release neutrophil elastase, which increases pulmonary vascular permeability.[11] In comparison, intratracheal administration of activated charcoal does not increase elastase in the bronchoalveolar fluid.[12] Activated charcoal may activate alveolar macrophages, which are a potent source of oxygen radicals, proteases, and other inflammatory mediators. Charcoal also causes obstruction of small distal airways that intersperse with unobstructed airways. Overdistention of alveolar segments in areas not occluded by charcoal leads to volutrauma in those areas, which increases microvascular permeability.[13] Although case reports reveal long-term pulmonary pathology after aspiration or instillation of activated charcoal,[14,15] the true incidence of chronic problems after charcoal aspiration is unknown.

Position Statement. Single-dose activated charcoal should not be administered routinely in the management of poisoned patients. The effectiveness of charcoal decreases with time; the greatest benefit is obtained within the first hour after ingestion. Administration of activated charcoal may be considered if a patient has ingested a potentially toxic amount of poison (that is known to be adsorbed to charcoal) not longer than 1 hour before treatment. There is no evidence that the administration of activated charcoal improves outcome.[10,16]

CATHARTICS

Position Statement. The administration of a cathartic alone has no role in the management of the poisoned patient. The routine use of a cathartic in combination with activated charcoal is not endorsed.[17]

WHOLE-BOWEL IRRIGATION

Whole-bowel irrigation consists of administration through a nasogastric tube of an osmotically balanced, polyethylene glycol–based electrolyte solution to decontaminate the entire gastrointestinal tract by physically expelling intraluminal contents. As much as 1500 to 2000 mL/hour may be administered to an awake patient. Negotiations to let the patient attempt to drink the solution only cause delay, because patients are unable to drink at a constant rate. Contraindications include bowel pathology, unprotected or compromised airway, hemodynamic instability, and intractable vomiting. Complications are nausea, vomiting, and abdominal cramps.[18]

Position Statement. Whole-bowel irrigation should not be used routinely in the poisoned patient. Whole-bowel irrigation should be considered for potentially toxic ingestions of sustained-release or enteric-coated drugs. There are insufficient data to support or exclude the use of whole-bowel irrigation for toxic ingestions of lithium, iron, lead, zinc, or packets of illicit drugs.[18]

CLINICAL IMPLICATIONS OF GASTROINTESTINAL DECONTAMINATION

There is no role for syrup of ipecac in the hospital setting. Gastric lavage may be considered in the obtunded patient if it can be administered within 1 hour after the ingestion. Single-dose activated charcoal should not be routinely administered in the patient with mild to moderate poisoning. Whole-bowel irrigation should be considered in an awake patient within the first hours after ingestion of a sustained-release preparation, ionic compounds (e.g., lithium), or packets of illicit drugs.

These guidelines refer to the routine management of poisoned patients. Cellular toxins require special consideration. The physician should always call the Poison Center (1-800-222-1222 in the United States) to discuss a patient with a potentially life-threatening ingestion.

ENHANCED ELIMINATION

MULTIPLE-DOSE ACTIVATED CHARCOAL

Multiple-dose activated charcoal is the repeated oral administration of activated charcoal to enhance drug elimination. If the drug concentration in the gut is lower than that in the blood, the drug will passively diffuse back into the gut. The concentration gradient, intestinal surface area, permeability, and blood flow determine the degree of passive diffusion. As the drug passes continuously into the gut, it is adsorbed to charcoal, a process called "gastrointestinal dialysis." Multiple-dose activated charcoal also interrupts the enterohepatic and enterogastric circulation of drugs. Drugs with a prolonged elimination half-life, a small volume of distribution (less than 1 L/kg), and little protein binding are the most amenable.[19]

The initial dose of charcoal is 50 to 100 g, and this treatment is followed every 1, 2, or 4 hours by a dose equivalent to 12.5 g/hour. More frequent, smaller doses may prevent vomiting. Addition of a cathartic (e.g., sorbitol) may be considered for the initial one or two doses. Continuous use of a cathartic can cause diarrhea and fluid and electrolyte imbalance. Multiple-dose activated charcoal may be continued until the patient improves clinically. Contraindications include an unprotected airway, intestinal obstruction, and an anatomically abnormal gastrointestinal tract. Complications include bowel obstruction and vomiting with subsequent aspiration.[19]

Position Statement. Multiple-dose activated charcoal should be considered if a patient has ingested a life-threatening amount of carbamazepine, dapsone, phenobarbital, quinine, or theophylline. With all of these drugs, data confirm enhanced elimination, although no controlled studies have demonstrated clinical benefit.[19]

URINARY ALKALINIZATION

Urinary alkalinization is the administration of intravenous sodium bicarbonate to produce urine with a pH of 7.5 or higher. The objective of treatment is pH manipulation, not forced diuresis. Hypokalemia is the most common complication. Alkalemia may also occur.[20]

Position Statement. Urinary alkalinization should be considered as first-line treatment in patients with moderately severe salicylate poisoning who do not meet the criteria for hemodialysis and in those with severe 2,4-dichlorophenoxy-acetic acid or mecoprop (MCPP) poisoning. Urinary alkalinization is not recommended as first-line treatment in phenobarbital poisoning because multiple-dose activated charcoal is superior.[20]

SELECTED ANTIDOTES

Stabilization of the patient always precedes antidote administration. The effects of the toxin may outlast the effects of the administered antidote. Patients receiving antidotes should be observed in a critical care setting.

DEXTROSE

Up to 8% of patients with altered mental status are hypoglycemic.[21] Hypoglycemia may be a result of the drug or toxin exposure, nutritional deprivation, or a medical complication (e.g., sepsis, hyperthermia). Glucose should be checked at the bedside for all patients with altered mental status.

NALOXONE

Endogenous and exogenous opiates produce their effects by binding at one or more opiate receptors. Naloxone, nalmefene, and naltrexone are competitive opioid antagonists that bind at the mu (μ), kappa (κ), and delta (δ) receptors and competitively prevent the binding of endogenous and exogenous opiates at these receptors. The duration of action of naloxone is 15 to 90 minutes. Its clinical effects depend on the dose and route of naloxone administration as well as the dose and rate of elimination of the opiate agonist. Naloxone may be administered by intravenous, intramuscular, intratracheal, or sublingual routes. After intravenous administration, naloxone rapidly enters the central nervous system (CNS). In patients with opiate poisoning, consciousness is restored and respiration improved within 1 to 2 minutes. Meiosis, inhibition of baroreceptor reflexes, laryngospasm, and decreased gastrointestinal motility are also reversed.[22]

Certain nonopiate drugs can cause release of endogenous opiates, contributing to CNS and respiratory depression as well as hypotension. Alternatively, nonopiate drugs and naloxone may compete for an unidentified nonopiate receptor that contributes to CNS depression and hypotension. Naloxone may reverse the toxicity caused by such drugs as clonidine, angiotensin-converting enzyme inhibitors, and sodium valproate. Naloxone should be administered to all patients with altered mental status or coma of unknown cause.

Opiate-dependent patients should receive only small doses, in an effort to prevent rapid withdrawal. If a patient is not opiate dependent, a reasonable starting dose is 2 mg, increasing to 10 mg if there is no response. Large doses of naloxone may be necessary to reverse the effects of nonopiate drugs or of opiate drugs with high affinity for the δ and κ opiate receptors.

If respiratory depression returns, the initial dose of naloxone may need to be repeated or a constant infusion of naloxone initiated. The starting dose for a constant infusion of naloxone is hourly administration of about one half to two thirds of the bolus dose that reversed the opiate effects. If withdrawal is precipitated, it is short-lived and not life-threatening. Complications of naloxone administration are very rare.[23]

FLUMAZENIL

Flumazenil competitively antagonizes the pharmacologic effects of drugs that act on the benzodiazepine receptor. Receptor occupancy follows the law of mass action, and antagonism is dose dependent. The duration of action is variable and depends on the type of benzodiazepine ingested, the relative doses of agonist and antagonist, the presence of ongoing benzodiazepine absorption, and the relative receptor binding affinities. Flumazenil also antagonizes the sedative effects of drugs other than benzodiazepines, such as zolpidem (Ambien), cannabis, ethanol, promethazine, chlorzoxazone, and carisoprodol. These drugs may have differing affinities for the γ-aminobutyric acid A (GABA$_A$) receptor, implying that the dose of flumazenil required to reverse the effects depends on the affinity of the specific drug for the receptor.[24]

Flumazenil is safe and effective for reversing conscious sedation after short procedures such as endoscopy. This safety has been generalized to imply that flumazenil is also safe in the patient with a multidrug overdose and that reversal of benzodiazepine-induced sedation prevents morbidity from procedures such as endotracheal intubation and computed tomography. However, many patients have experienced single or multiple seizures after flumazenil administration. Status epilepticus has been precipitated, leading to death. The data are insufficient to determine whether morbidity or mortality is increased as a result of flumazenil-precipitated seizures.[25,26]

Flumazenil administration may precipitate seizures in patients with an overdose who have a history of coingestion of a benzodiazepine and a proconvulsant drug, a history of seizures, chronic benzodiazepine ingestion, a history of head injury, or ingestion of only a proconvulsant drug. Identification of patients at risk for seizure is difficult.[27] At the very least, obtaining an electrocardiogram (to rule out exposure to proconvulsant tricyclic antidepressants) and urine drug screen is reasonable before flumazenil administration. Resedation occurs after 18 to 120 minutes in approximately one half of the patients awakened by flumazenil. Therefore, either continuous intravenous infusion or observation for a number of hours is required.[28]

Administration of flumazenil to the patient with an overdose should be limited to the following situations: iatrogenic overdose with known patient history; obtundation in a toddler secondary to ingestion of benzodiazepine, and reversal of a paradoxical response to benzodiazepine.

PHYSOSTIGMINE

Physostigmine inhibits acetylcholinesterase, the enzyme responsible for the metabolism of acetylcholine (ACH). ACH is an endogenous neurotransmitter that mediates action by binding to muscarinic and nicotinic receptors. Accumulation of ACH stimulates cholinergic nerve endings. In the poisoned patient, physostigmine is most frequently administered to treat anticholinergic toxicity. Clinical signs of anticholinergic toxicity are recognized by the pneumonic "Blind as a bat, Red as a beet, Hot as a hare, Dry as a bone, Mad as a hatter." Physostigmine administration may be considered if life-threatening clinical signs of anticholinergic peripheral effects (hypertension, tachycardia, and seizures) or central effects (painful psychosis) are present. However, it is extremely difficult to balance cholinergic and anticholinergic forces. Complications of cholinergic crises (caused by excess physostigmine) include hypertension, arrhythmia, asystole, bronchorrhea, bronchoconstriction, seizures, and status epilepticus. Contraindications to physostigmine administration include reactive airway disease, peripheral vascular disease, intestinal or bladder obstruction, and treatment with a depolarizing neuromuscular blocking agent (e.g., succinylcholine). An acceptable dose of physostigmine is 2 mg intravenously over 10 minutes. This drug should be administered in the presence of a physician, because of the potential for precipitation of life-threatening cholinergic effects.[29]

HYPOTENSION IN THE POISONED PATIENT

Hypotension in the poisoned patient is most frequently caused by receptor blockade, drug-induced myocardial depression, or drug-induced vasodilatation. It is reflex to treat initial periods of hypotension with fluids; however, unless the poisoned patient is hypovolemic, large volumes of fluid may predispose the patient to the development of acute respiratory failure.

Catecholamines are the pressors of choice for treatment of hypotension in most intensive care unit (ICU) patients who are older, chronically ill, or acutely ill from an infectious process. The causative factors in sepsis-induced vasodilation and myocardial depression/ischemia are different from the factors that cause drug-induced vasodilation, myocardial depression, or ischemia. Treatment approaches must address the cause of the hypotension and not assume that all hypotensive patients may be treated in a similar manner.

The poisoned patient who is young and healthy responds to hypotension with an outpouring of endogenous catecholamines. Adrenergic receptors are sensitive in the young patient. Administration of further catecholamines is unlikely to be of benefit, because all catecholamine receptors are stimulated by endogenous catecholamines. Agents that must be considered for the treatment of hypotension in the poisoned patient are sodium bicarbonate (for a sodium channel–blocking agent), glucagon, and insulin/glucose.

GLUCAGON

The cardiovascular effects of glucagon are mediated by myocardial glucagon receptors, which are catecholamine independent. Stimulation activates adenylate cyclase, leading to increased intracellular levels of the second messenger, cyclic adenosine monophosphate (cAMP). This cyclic nucleotide increases myocardial calcium uptake. Both the slope of phase zero of the action potential and the conduction velocity through the atrioventricular node are increased. Glucagon increases heart rate and stroke volume, thereby increasing cardiac output. After intravenous administration, augmented inotropy is seen within 1 to 3 minutes, with a peak effect in 5 to 7 minutes.[30]

Glucagon should be considered early in the treatment of the hypotensive poisoned patient. Treatment regimens vary. An acceptable regimen is 10 mg of glucagon given over 10 minutes (rapid administration causes vomiting), followed by 1 to 3 mg/hour. If the patient wretches, the hourly dose of glucagon should be decreased. Elderly patients may be more sensitive to the emetic effects of the drug.

INSULIN AND GLUCOSE

Insulin improves contractility in anoxic rat hearts and improves the cardiac index after cardiopulmonary bypass surgery. During drug-induced shock, insulin shifts myocardial fatty acid oxidation to carbohydrate oxidation, which increases contractility, left ventricular pressure, and rate of change of developed pressure. Enhanced fatty acid oxidation, such as occurs after epinephrine administration, transiently increases contractility at the expense of increased myocardial oxygen consumption.[31]

In the hypotensive poisoned patient, a reasonable dose of insulin is 10 units of regular insulin and 50 mL of 50% dextrose solution. This should be followed by infusion of 6 units of insulin per hour, with concurrent administration of sufficient glucose to maintain euglycemia. Hourly serum glucose checks are mandatory, because hypoglycemia occurs frequently.

CARDIAC ARRHYTHMIAS

ICU treatment regimens assume that a diseased heart is the cause of most cardiac arrhythmias. This assumption is invalid in the poisoned patient. Treatment of the arrhythmia must take into consideration the pharmacology of the toxin causing the arrhythmia.

ACUTE RENAL FAILURE

In the poisoned patient, acute renal failure (ARF) is most frequently the result of a decrease in extracellular fluid volume and renal hypoperfusion caused by drug- or chemical-induced vasodilation, drug-induced myocardial depression, or rhabdomyolysis. Attempts to prevent ARF are crucial, because there is no specific therapy once ARF has occurred. Studies evaluating the efficacy of low-dose dopamine (0.5 to 3.0 mg/kg/min) in preventing ARF have not demonstrated any benefit, but the patient populations in these studies consisted of critically ill patients with established ARF or high risk for development of ARF.[32] The efficacy of administration of low-dose dopamine after periods of hypotension in poisoned patients, who typically are younger and without chronic disease, has not been evaluated. When dopamine is administered to normal human subjects, there is a dose-dependent increase in renal blood flow, sodium excretion, and glomerular filtration rate.[33] Low-dose dopamine also limits adenosine triphosphate (ATP) utilization and oxygen requirements in nephron segments at risk for ischemia.[34] In cases of drug-induced hypotension, it seems reasonable to administer low-dose dopamine to previously healthy poisoned patients who have adequate vascular volume and who remain oliguric or anuric despite maximal diuretic therapy.

SEIZURES

Blood pH may be as low as 7.17 at 30 minutes and 7.20 at 60 minutes after resolution of a 30- to 60-second seizure.[35] Acidosis decreases cardiac output, oxygen extraction, and left ventricular end-diastolic pressure and impairs myocardial contractility. If a patient has ingested a cardiotoxic drug (e.g., a tricyclic antidepressant) that causes significant myocardial depression, the consequences of acidosis can increase the toxicity of the drug. Ictal increases in plasma epinephrine levels may add to the potential risk for cardiac arrhythmias. Additionally, airway reflexes are inhibited postictally, which adds to the potential for aspiration.[36]

Whether seizures increase morbidity and mortality in poisoned patients is difficult to ascertain. Deaths of poisoned patients who experience seizures are usually attributed to the toxicity of the drug. Because of the number of variables, it is impossible to know whether the risk for mortality is influenced by the presence of convulsions. Accordingly, the physician should take an aggressive approach toward terminating seizures in the poisoned patient. Benzodiazepines are the drugs of choice to quickly terminate seizures, because they are lipophilic and rapidly enter the CNS.

MECHANICAL VENTILATION AND EXTUBATION

Poisoned patients are endotracheally intubated because they have ingested a drug that causes either respiratory depression or depression of their sensorium, resulting in loss of protective airway reflexes. As the drug is metabolized, its effects abate and the patient's sensorium improves. The patient may become alert slowly or very suddenly. The patient should be extubated if ability to protect the airway is evident and ventilation is adequate for 15 to 60 minutes with minimal respiratory support (e.g., 5 cm H_2O positive end-expiratory pressure and 5 cm H_2O pressure support). Administration of sedatives in an attempt to help the patient "tolerate the tube" causes prolonged extubation times and potential complications.

THE TOXICOLOGY LABORATORY

Urine drug screens are usually obtained in poisoned patients; however, there is no standardized screen. Interpretation of urine drug screen results depends on the clinician's knowledge of which toxins have been screened and whether confirmatory testing (ideally performed by a different analytic method) will follow. The length of time required to receive results varies among hospitals. Quantitative serum drug testing is done when quantitation of a toxin is clinically relevant, as is the case for acetaminophen,

anticonvulsant agents, salicylates, digoxin, ethanol, ethylene glycol, methanol, iron, lithium, and theophylline. The clinician caring for the poisoned patient should discuss drug testing with the analytic toxicologist so that the results of testing can be appropriately interpreted. The clinical value of analytic toxicology testing depends on the clinician's ability to understand and interpret the results.

ANNOTATED REFERENCES

Arnold TC, Willis BH, Xiao F: Aspiration of activated charcoal elicits an increase in lung microvascular permeability. J Toxicol Clin Toxicol 1999;37: 9-16.

The capillary filtration coefficient, a measure of lung microvascular permeability, was determined in rat lungs before and after intratracheal instillation of activated charcoal. There was a marked increase in permeability in those lungs exposed to activated charcoal.

Hoffman R, Goldfrank L: The poisoned patient with altered consciousness. JAMA 1995;274:562-568.

This Medline review of large trials to determine the diagnostic efficacy of antidotes concluded that dextrose and thiamine hydrochloride should be administered to all patients with altered consciousness. Administration of naloxone should be reserved for patients with clinical signs of opiate intoxication. Flumazenil should be reserved for reversal of conscious sedation and selected cases of benzodiazepine overdose.

Kline JA, Raymond RM, Leonova E, et al: Insulin improves heart function and metabolism during non-ischemic cardiogenic shock in awake canines. Cardiovasc Res 1997;34:289-298.

This study examined heart function during insulin treatment of verapamil-induced cardiogenic shock in awake canines. Insulin improved systolic and diastolic heart function during aerobic shock and accelerated in vivo myocardial lactate oxidation.

Mathieu-Nolf M, Babe MA, Coquelle-Couplet V, et al: Flumazenil use in an emergency department: A survey. Clin Toxicol 2001;39:15-20.

This survey reported on 29 patients who received flumazenil in the emergency department. Subsequent expert review considered that flumazenil was indicated in only 18 of these patients. Of the remaining 11 patients, a severe complication occurred in 1. There was no difference in outcome measures between those patients who received flumazenil and those who did not.

Merigian K, Glaho K: Single-dose oral activated charcoal in the treatment of the self-poisoned patient: A prospective, randomized controlled trial. Am J Ther 2002;9:301-308.

A total of 1479 patients with overdose were randomly assigned to receive or not receive activated charcoal. Gastric emptying was not performed. There were no differences between the two groups in length of intubation time, length of hospital stay, or complication rate.

Merigian KS, Woodard M, Hedges JR, et al: Prospective evaluation of gastric emptying in the self-poisoned patient. Am J Emerg Med 1990;8: 479-483.

This was a randomized study of 357 symptomatic overdose patients who underwent gastric emptying (ipecac or gastric lavage, depending on mental status) before administration of activated charcoal. There was no difference between the two groups in length of stay in the emergency department, ICU length of stay, duration of intubation, or incidence of clinical deterioration over the first 6 hours. Gastric emptying was associated with an increased incidence of aspiration pneumonia.

Orringer DE, Eustace JC, Wunsch CD, Gardner LB: Natural history of lactic acidosis after grand mal seizures. N Engl J Med 1977;15:796-799.

This classic article demonstrated that significant acidosis can occur for up to 1 hour after a single 30- to 60-second seizure.

Pond SM, Lewis-Driver DJ, Williams GM, et al: Gastric emptying in acute overdose: A prospective randomized controlled trial. Med J Aust 1995;163: 345-349.

This was a randomized study of gastric emptying versus no gastric emptying. A total of 342 patients underwent lavage or no gastric lavage before administration of charcoal. There were no significant differences between the two groups in incidence of clinical deterioration or improvement during the first 6 hours. However, only 55 patients presented within 1 hour, of whom just 14 were not lavaged.

Saetta J, March S, Gaunt ME, Quinton DN: Gastric emptying procedures in the self-poisoned patient: Are we forcing gastric content beyond the pylorus? J R Soc Med 1991;84:274-276.

Recovery of ingested substances after gastric lavage diminishes with increased time since ingestion. In only 10 of 73 cases were more than 10 therapeutic doses of the ingested drug recovered in the lavage fluid.

Sauvadet A, Rohn T, Pecker F, et al: Arachidonic acid drives mini-glucagon action in cardiac cells. J Biol Chem 1997;272:12437-12445.

Glucagon triggers release of arachadonic acid (AA) and is then processed by cardiac cells into a terminal fragment, mini-glucagon, which is an essential component of the contractile positive inotropic effect. AA and cAMP are both second messengers.

Chapter 187

ETHANOL, METHANOL, AND ETHYLENE GLYCOL

James A. Kruse

ETHANOL INTOXICATION

Ethanol, also known as ethyl alcohol or grain alcohol, is only one of many compounds chemically classified as alcohols, but it is the only one that is legitimately contained in alcoholic beverages. It is a clear, colorless liquid, with a pleasant odor and a burning taste, found in fermented alcoholic beverages. Ethanol also finds wide use in laboratories and in industry as a solvent and synthetic precursor, in pharmaceutical manufacturing as a vehicle for certain medicines (e.g., cough syrups, some intravenous drugs), in food extracts, and in numerous toiletries, including mouthwashes, colognes, and cosmetics. It also serves as a component in various residential and commercial cleaning agents and paint removers, in which case it is usually *denatured*, meaning that it has been intentionally rendered unfit for consumption, usually to comply with governmental regulations. Denaturing is commonly accomplished by the addition of methanol or toxic hydrocarbons. Some versions of the alternative motor vehicle fuel known as *gasohol* consist of a mixture of gasoline and ethanol.

The ethanol content of alcoholic beverages varies, but typical concentrations range from 40% to 55% (volume/volume) in whiskey and related distilled spirits, 10% to 15% in table wines, and 4% to 6% in most beers. The ethanol concentration in distilled spirits is traditionally listed in terms of *proof*. In the United States, this expression represents twice the percentage concentration; for example, 80 proof is equivalent to 40% ethanol by volume.

Ethanol is rapidly absorbed by the gastrointestinal tract and distributed throughout body water.[1] The blood ethanol concentration (in mg/dL) resulting from a one-time dose can be estimated from the volume (in mL) of ingested alcoholic beverage, the fractional concentration of ethanol (by volume) in the beverage, and body weight (in kg), by the following equation:

$$\text{Blood ethanol concentration} = \frac{\text{Volume ingested} \times \text{Ethanol concentration} \times 79}{0.6 \times \text{Body weight}} \quad (1)$$

The denominator coefficient is the fraction of body weight representing total body water volume, approximating the volume of distribution for ethanol, about 0.6 L/kg. The numerator coefficient converts volume units to weight units based on the density of ethanol (0.79 g/mL) and converts the resultant concentration units from g/L to mg/dL. Accordingly, each 1 ounce of 100 proof whiskey, 12 ounces of beer, or 4 ounces of a typical table wine consumed by a 70-kg man should theoretically raise the blood ethanol concentration by approximately 30 mg/dL. Given that the ingestion commonly occurs over time and that metabolism is ongoing, this prediction tends to overestimate the peak blood ethanol level.

METABOLISM

Between 2% and 10% of ingested ethanol is excreted intact by the kidneys and lungs, but the major fraction is metabolized by hepatic alcohol dehydrogenase (ADH) to acetaldehyde by the following reaction[2]:

$$CH_3CH_2\text{-OH} + NAD^+ \xrightarrow{\text{ADH}} NADH + H^+ + CH_3\text{-}\overset{\text{O}}{\overset{\|}{C}}\text{-H} \quad (2)$$

Ethanol   Acetaldehyde

At high blood ethanol levels, a particular isoform of the hepatic microsomal cytochrome P450 enzyme (CYP2E1) provides an additional, albeit normally minor, oxidative pathway for ethanol metabolism:

$$CH_3CH_2\text{-}OH + NADPH + H^+ + O_2 \xrightarrow{CYP2E1} NADP^+$$
$$\text{Ethanol}$$

$$(3)$$

$$+ CH_3\overset{\overset{\displaystyle O}{\|}}{\text{-}C}\text{-H} + 2H_2O$$
$$\text{Acetaldehyde}$$

This alternative pathway is inducible with chronic ethanol exposure. Minor amounts of ethanol can also be metabolized by peroxisomal catalase:

$$CH_3CH_2\text{-}OH + H_2O_2 \xrightarrow{Catalase}$$
$$\text{Ethanol}$$

$$(4)$$

$$CH_3\overset{\overset{\displaystyle O}{\|}}{\text{-}C}\text{-H} + 2H_2O$$
$$\text{Acetaldehyde}$$

Acetaldehyde produced by any of the preceding reactions is converted by hepatic acetaldehyde dehydrogenase (ALDH) to acetate:

$$CH_3\overset{\overset{\displaystyle O}{\|}}{\text{-}C}\text{-H} + NAD^+ + H_2O \xrightarrow{ALDH} NADH$$
$$\text{Acetaldehyde}$$

$$(5)$$

$$+ 2H^+ + CH_3\overset{\overset{\displaystyle O}{\|}}{\text{-}C}\text{-O}^-$$
$$\text{Acetate}$$

Acetate can then enter the tricarboxylic acid cycle and ultimately be metabolized to carbon dioxide (CO_2) and water. Polymorphism in the dehydrogenase enzymes can result in increased production rates or diminished metabolic clearance of acetaldehyde. As a consequence, some individuals experience marked vasodilation, facial flushing, tachycardia, and other unpleasant symptoms after ethanol consumption because of the effects of excessive acetaldehyde accumulation. Alleles leading to this reaction are particularly prevalent in persons of Chinese or Japanese descent but are uncommon in Caucasians.[2]

Metabolic conversion of ethanol to acetaldehyde and acetate by dehydrogenases raises the ratio of reduced nicotinamide adenine dinucleotide (NADH) relative to its oxidized form (NAD^+). This change in intracellular redox state favors conversion of pyruvate to lactate by lactate dehydrogenase (LDH) and can thereby raise the blood lactate concentration:

$$CH_3\overset{\overset{\displaystyle O\ \ O}{\| \ \ \|}}{\text{-}C\text{-}C}\text{-O}^- + NADH + H^+ \xrightarrow{LDH}$$
$$\text{Pyruvate}$$

$$(6)$$

$$NAD^+ + CH_3\text{-}\overset{\overset{\displaystyle HO\ \ \ O}{| \ \ \ \ \|}}{CH\text{-}C}\text{-O}^-$$
$$\text{Lactate}$$

The resulting increase in blood lactate level is usually small, however, and the presence of lactic acidosis should prompt consideration of an alternative cause, such as circulatory shock or seizures.[3]

Ethanol elimination generally follows zero-order kinetics, with elimination rates of 5 to 10 g/hour in nonhabituated subjects, approximately corresponding to a fall in blood ethanol concentration of 10 to 25 mg/dL/hour. This rate can more than double in individuals who are chronically habituated to high daily doses of ethanol.

CLINICAL MANIFESTATIONS

Excessive chronic ingestion of ethanol plays a causative role in a number of important diseases, such as cirrhosis, hepatitis, pancreatitis, cardiomyopathy, and malignancies. Ethanol use can result in gastrointestinal hemorrhage by several mechanisms, including gastritis, ulcers, esophageal varices, and Mallory-Weiss tears.

Acute intoxication can induce cardiac dysrhythmias, particularly atrial fibrillation. As denoted by the descriptive sobriquet, "holiday heart syndrome," this phenomenon frequently occurs during an alcoholic binge. A variety of neurologic abnormalities are associated with chronic alcoholism, including Wernicke-Korsakoff syndrome, chronic cerebellar ataxia, Marchiafava-Bignami syndrome, peripheral neuropathies, organic brain syndrome, and central pontine myelinolysis.[4] Wernicke's encephalopathy can manifest as lethargy, impaired mentation (inability to concentrate, confusion, disorientation), truncal ataxia, and extraocular motor abnormalities (horizontal and vertical nystagmus, internal strabismus, ophthalmoplegia), whereas Korsakoff's dementia manifests as retentive memory impairment, confabulation, and learning deficits.[5]

Acutely, ethanol has well known, dose-dependent inebriating and sedating effects (Table 187-1), although remarkable

TABLE 187-1. RELATIONSHIP BETWEEN BLOOD ETHANOL CONCENTRATION AND CLINICAL MANIFESTATIONS*

Blood Ethanol Concentration (mg/dL)	Clinical Manifestations
<30	Little demonstrable effect
30-50	Mild euphoria, minimal central nervous system effects, subjective sensation of cutaneous warmth
50-80	Relaxation, jocularity, gregariousness, cutaneous flushing, prolongation of reaction time
80-100	Statutory intoxication in many jurisdictions
100-200	Loquacity, animation, exuberance, exaggerated emotional responses, uninhibited behavior, impaired judgment
200-300	Sedation interrupted by periods of boisterous or antisocial behavior, nausea, emesis, dysarthria, horizontal nystagmus, impaired visual pursuit, diplopia, ataxia
300-400	Unstable station and gait, incoherent speech, somnolence, impairment of protective airway reflexes, incontinence, obtundation, stupor
>400	Coma, loss of protective reflexes, respiratory depression, death

*This information serves only as a imperfect guide, because considerable variability and overlap is possible, and individuals with chronic heavy ethanol exposure often develop learned tolerance.

variability in this relationship is observed in some individuals.[4] These central nervous system (CNS) effects appear to be at least partly caused by interference with N-methyl-D-aspartate receptor and perhaps γ-aminobutyric acid receptor function.[4,6,7] The cognitive, behavioral, perceptual, and psychomotor effects of ethanol intoxication play a causative role in a substantial proportion of deaths and injuries involving motor vehicle–related trauma, accidental drownings, residential fires, homicides, and suicides. Most state statutes set the legal driving limit for blood ethanol concentration at 80 or 100 mg/dL. Tachycardia, mydriasis, diaphoresis, hypotension, and either hypothermia or hyperthermia can occur in cases of marked intoxication. Blood ethanol concentrations of approximately 350 mg/dL have been associated with fatal outcomes, although many patients have survived much higher levels, including one subject who reportedly survived a level of 1500 mg/dL.[8]

LABORATORY MANIFESTATIONS

The concentration of ethanol in the blood correlates at least approximately with the manifestations of intoxication (see Table 187-1). In chronic alcoholic subjects, a blood ethanol concentration lower than 250 mg/dL is an unlikely explanation for alterations in consciousness and should prompt a search for an alternative cause.[8] Numerous other blood test abnormalities can be seen in intoxicated subjects, particularly in patients with chronic ethanol abuse, including hyponatremia, hypokalemia, hypomagnesemia, hypophosphatemia, hypoglycemia, hypertriglyceridemia, leukopenia, thrombocytopenia, and coagulopathy. Elevated activities of various circulating enzymes, including amylase, lipase, creatine phosphokinase, transaminases, and γ-glutamyl transpeptidase, can occur as a reflection of alcohol-induced pancreatitis, rhabdomyolysis, hepatitis, or cirrhosis. The latter can also result in hyperbilirubinemia and hypoalbuminemia.

TREATMENT

In the absence of associated illness or injury (Table 187-2), mild to moderate intoxication requires no special treatment other than abstinence and a period of observation. Regardless of the degree of intoxication, withdrawal precautions are recommended for chronic imbibers, particularly those with a history of heavy chronic use or alcohol withdrawal manifestations. The treatment of severe ethanol intoxication is largely supportive. As with any patient who presents to the hospital in an unconscious state, initial empirical treatment should include intravenous thiamine, dextrose, and naloxone, once adequate airway, ventilation, and perfusion are ensured. Gastric lavage and activated charcoal administration are of dubious value for hastening removal of ethanol from the body.[9-12]

The unconscious, stuporous, or delirious patient with ethanol intoxication can present a diagnostic challenge. Historical information is often lacking or inadequate, and the physical examination can be compromised by lack of cooperation. A central concern is that another disorder may be present, in lieu of or in addition to ethanol intoxication. The other disorder may be chiefly responsible for the alteration in consciousness or may require specific, urgent treatment. For example, inebriated subjects are at high risk for trauma (e.g., battery, falls, motor vehicle accidents) and therefore should be evaluated for physical injuries. Subdural hematoma is a particular concern, and any history, physical findings or suspicion of head injury should prompt cranial imaging by computed tomography. Chronic ethanol abuse also predisposes to infection, particularly aspiration pneumonia and *Klebsiella pneumoniae* pneumonia. Pneumococcal or *Listeria* meningitis, although not as common, is a consideration in the intoxicated patient with an altered sensorium, fever, and other compatible findings. Additional potentially confounding problems include concomitant toxic ingestions or drug overdoses, psychiatric disorders, alcohol withdrawal, and, in patients with advanced cirrhosis, hepatic encephalopathy or spontaneous bacterial peritonitis.

A thorough evaluation for common associated illnesses and injuries should include physical and laboratory examinations for evidence of head, neck, and somatic trauma, rhabdomyolysis, pancreatitis, hepatic dysfunction, coagulopathy, blood dyscrasias, and fluid and electrolyte derangements. Accordingly, routine laboratory testing should include a complete blood count (including platelet count); prothrombin and partial thromboplastin times; serum assays for electrolytes (including sodium, potassium, chloride, total CO_2 content, magnesium, and phosphorus); glucose; liver and kidney function tests; and amylase, lipase, transaminase, and creatine phosphokinase activities. Screening for alternative or concomitant intoxications or overdoses is often fruitful.[13] Identification of metabolic acidosis should prompt investigation for alcoholic ketoacidosis, lactic acidosis, renal failure, and relevant toxic ingestions, particularly methanol and ethylene glycol (see later discussion). Microbiologic cultures are indicated if there are signs of serious infection.

TABLE 187–2. CONCOMITANT OR COMPLICATING DISORDERS ASSOCIATED WITH ALCOHOL INTOXICATION OR WITHDRAWAL

Alcoholic hepatitis	Hypoglycemia
Aspiration pneumonitis	Hypothermia
Circulatory shock (due to dehydration or hemorrhage)	Infections (e.g., pneumonia, meningitis)
Cirrhosis	Intracranial hemorrhage (e.g., subdural hematoma)
Coagulopathy	Pancreatitis
Dehydration	Peripheral neuropathy
Drug overdose or other toxic ingestion	Psychosis
Electrolyte derangements	Rhabdomyolysis
Gastrointestinal hemorrhage (due to gastritis, peptic ulcer disease, esophageal varices, hemorrhoids, or Mallory-Weiss tear)	Seizures
	Sepsis
Head injury	Thrombocytopenia
Heat stroke	Vitamin deficiency (folate, thiamine, other B vitamins)
Hepatic encephalopathy	Wernicke-Korsakoff syndrome

Intravenous thiamine and a multivitamin preparation containing folate are routinely administered to hospitalized patients with alcohol intoxication or withdrawal. Parenteral thiamine (50 or 100 mg) is given during the initial phase of management, regardless of the level of sensorium, to prevent or treat Wernicke-Korsakoff syndrome.[5] An argument can be made that folate and vitamin B_{12} administration are better delayed until the complete blood count can be assessed, so that specific vitamin assays may be obtained if macrocytic anemia is present.

Hydration is necessary in some intoxicated patients. Dextrose-containing saline solutions are usually the fluid of choice to correct dehydration and prevent hypoglycemia. Dextrose administration is traditionally preceded by thiamine dosing. Patients with hypoglycemia require rapid intravenous injection of dextrose followed by a continuous dextrose infusion titrated to the results of frequent serial blood glucose tests. Hypokalemia, hypomagnesemia, and hypophosphatemia should be corrected with the use of appropriate oral or parenteral supplementation. Patients with anemia or a suggestive history or physical findings may require further investigation for gastrointestinal hemorrhage. Patients requiring admission to an intensive care unit (ICU) should have a chest radiograph as well as an electrocardiographic evaluation.

Oxygenation may be assessed either by pulse oximetry or by arterial blood gas analysis, and supplemental oxygen should be provided as necessary. Administration of vitamin K, fresh-frozen plasma, or platelet transfusions may be necessary if there is gastrointestinal or other hemorrhage and coagulopathy or severe thrombocytopenia. The level of consciousness should be monitored periodically. Hemodialysis has been employed and is effective at removing ethanol from the body, but in general this modality poses greater risks than simply providing supportive care and allowing physiologic ethanol elimination. Its use could be considered in rare cases of profound, life-threatening ethanol intoxication, or if there are other reasons for dialysis.[14,15]

ALCOHOLIC KETOACIDOSIS

Alcoholic ketoacidosis (AKA) is an uncommon metabolic disturbance that occurs in a small proportion of chronic ethanol abusers for unclear reasons. Although the degree of acidosis can sometimes be severe, the disorder usually has a benign hospital course as long as intravenous dextrose and fluids are provided. Morbidity results chiefly from associated complications of alcohol abuse.

METABOLISM

Although the precise metabolic mechanisms that lead to the development of AKA are incompletely understood, several mechanisms appear to be operative. Abnormal insulin and counterregulatory hormone levels occur,[16] but the disorder is distinct from simple starvation and diabetes mellitus. Ethanol results in inhibition of gluconeogenesis and depletion of glycogen stores, leading to low glucose availability, particularly when coupled with fasting. Hypoglycemia causes release of epinephrine, cortisol, and growth hormone, as well as decreased insulin production; these are all factors that favor ketone synthesis. As shown earlier in equation 5, ethanol metabolism results in a surfeit of acetate and NADH;

these conditions also promote lactate and ketone production. Marked ketonemia results in acidosis and ketonuria. The latter causes an osmotic diuresis, intravascular volume depletion, dehydration, and electrolyte losses. Thus, starvation, dehydration, excessive acetate production, an altered redox state, hormonal imbalances, and perhaps genetic predisposition, are all potentially involved.[17]

The so-called ketone bodies that accumulate in all forms of endogenous ketoacidosis are acetone, β-hydroxybutyrate, and acetoacetate. Acetone is only a minor product, produced by decarboxylation of acetoacetate, either spontaneously or catalyzed by acetoacetate decarboxylase (AAD):

$$CH_3\text{-}\underset{\text{Acetoacetate}}{\overset{O}{\overset{\|}{C}}\text{-}CH_2\text{-}\overset{O}{\overset{\|}{C}}\text{-}O^-} + H^+ \xrightarrow{\text{AAD}}$$

$$\underset{\text{Acetone}}{CH_3\text{-}\overset{O}{\overset{\|}{C}}\text{-}CH_3} + CO_2 \tag{7}$$

Acetone is excreted in the breath and urine, where it may be detected by physical examination or urinalysis, respectively. β-Hydroxybutyrate and acetoacetate are interconvertible by the enzyme β-hydroxybutyrate dehydrogenase (βHD), and the two compounds normally exist in equilibrium:

$$CH_3\text{-}\underset{\text{β-Hydroxybutyrate}}{\overset{OH}{\overset{|}{C}H}\text{-}CH_2\text{-}\overset{O}{\overset{\|}{C}}\text{-}O^-} + NAD^+ \underset{\overrightarrow{}}{\overset{\beta HD}{\rightleftharpoons}}$$

$$NADH + H^+ + CH_3\text{-}\underset{\text{Acetoacetate}}{\overset{O}{\overset{\|}{C}}\text{-}CH_2\text{-}\overset{O}{\overset{\|}{C}}\text{-}O^-} \tag{8}$$

In both AKA and diabetic ketoacidosis (DKA), β-hydroxybutyrate is quantitatively the more important molecule. However, the ratio of β-hydroxybutyrate to acetoacetate tends to be higher in AKA (typically 5:1, but as high as 10:1), compared with DKA (typically 3:1).

CLINICAL MANIFESTATIONS

AKA characteristically develops 24 to 72 hours after an alcoholic debauch, as the blood ethanol concentration is declining, during which time the subject ceases ethanol consumption and has little or no caloric intake. Gastrointestinal symptoms predominate and include anorexia, nausea, epigastric pain, and vomiting.[18,19] The subject usually has a temporary aversion to food and alcoholic beverages and complains of malaise. On physical examination, there is a clear sensorium in most cases. The odor of acetone may be detectable on the subject's breath. Tachypnea or Kussmaul respirations may be evident if there is marked acidemia. Tachycardia and other signs of volume depletion may be apparent. In some cases, manifestations of underlying cirrhosis (e.g., jaundice, ascites, ecchymoses, hemorrhoids) or other disorders commonly associated with chronic alcohol abuse (see Table 187-2) may be present.

LABORATORY MANIFESTATIONS

The key laboratory findings in AKA are metabolic acidosis, ketonemia, and ketonuria in the presence of a normal, low, or only mildly elevated blood glucose concentration. Ethanol may be detectable in the blood, but it is not a requirement for the diagnosis and is frequently not detectable by the time the patient presents to the hospital. If the acidosis is clinically significant, elevation of the serum anion gap is expected. Other causes of metabolic acidosis must be excluded. Simple starvation can cause mild ketoacidosis, but with simple starvation the serum total CO_2 content or bicarbonate concentration generally remains greater than 18 mmol/L. DKA and renal failure are readily excluded by routine blood glucose and creatinine measurements. Lactic acidosis may be suggested by the associated clinical setting or by findings (e.g., seizures, hypotension), but it should be excluded by direct assay. Mild degrees of hyperlactatemia can occur in AKA, but concentrations greater than 3 mmol/L should prompt consideration of occult hypoperfusion, seizures, or another cause. Occult toxic ingestions also require exclusion, particularly ingestions of methanol, ethylene glycol, and salicylate intoxication.[15,20-23] Ingestion of exogenous acetone or isopropanol can cause marked ketosis due to acetonemia, but these intoxications are not associated with anion gap elevation or metabolic acidosis unless the poisoning is severe enough to cause seizures or circulatory shock, thereby resulting in lactic acidosis.

The high ratio of β-hydroxybutyrate to acetoacetate seen in AKA has clinical relevance when interpreting laboratory tests. A common assay for ketone bodies uses the semiquantitative nitroprusside reaction. Nitroprusside reacts colorimetrically with acetone and acetoacetate, but not with β-hydroxybutyrate. As a result, and in comparison with DKA, the degree of ketonemia detectable in AKA is often disproportionately low relative to the degree of metabolic acidosis present. Therefore, severe metabolic acidosis due to DKA is typically associated with marked levels of ketosis, whereas severe acidemia in AKA may appear to be associated with only mild to moderate ketosis by nitroprusside-based testing. In milder cases of AKA, those associated with a mild degree of metabolic acidosis in which the acidosis is due mostly to elevation of β-hydroxybutyrate, the acetoacetate and acetone levels may not be sufficiently elevated to yield detectable ketosis by the nitroprusside test.

Because vomiting and dehydration are frequent manifestations in AKA, metabolic alkalosis can complicate the acid-base derangement. The combination of metabolic acidosis (from ketoacidosis) and metabolic alkalosis (from vomiting and volume contraction) can result in arterial pH and blood gas values that underestimate the severity of one or both of these metabolic disturbances. For example, mild metabolic alkalosis can be obscured by the presence of moderate or severe metabolic acidosis. Rarely, both metabolic processes are present and of approximately equal severity. In this situation, blood pH and bicarbonate concentration can be within normal limits despite the acid-base disturbances.[22] Or, the metabolic alkalosis can predominate and obscure the acidosis. The serum anion gap can aid in detecting these situations. An abnormally high anion gap suggests metabolic acidosis, even if no acid-base disorder is evident by arterial blood gas analysis. In the face of a wide serum anion gap, the quotient of the delta anion gap (i.e., the subject's anion gap minus the average normal anion gap) divided by the delta bicarbonate (i.e., the subject's blood bicarbonate concentration minus the average normal bicarbonate concentration) should equal unity in organic metabolic acidoses, if there is no metabolic alkalosis.[24] A quotient well above unity (e.g., greater than 1.2) is evidence of concomitant metabolic alkalosis.

TREATMENT

Alternative explanations for the metabolic acidosis should be promptly excluded.[23] As in acute alcohol intoxication, the initial assessment should focus on identifying relevant alternative, underlying, or complicating illnesses or injuries that may require specific, urgent therapy. Although patients with AKA sometimes have severe metabolic acidemia, the acid-base disturbance usually responds rapidly to intravenous hydration and ample dextrose administration.[17] Rapid infusion of 50 mL of 50% dextrose is indicated if hypoglycemia is identified. Five percent dextrose in normal saline is infused intravenously (i.v.), at a high rate initially, to correct any hypovolemia or hypoglycemia and to provide substrate for metabolic correction of the ketoacidosis. Thereafter, dextrose containing normal or half-normal saline can be substituted at a high maintenance infusion rate, titrated to ongoing fluid losses. Ample dextrose administration is key to reversing the metabolic acidosis. The blood glucose concentration should be monitored frequently to allow detection of recurrent hypoglycemia or any intolerance to the provided glucose load.

In addition to specific tests related to acid-base imbalances, the same screening laboratory studies listed for acute alcohol intoxication should be evaluated. Serial acid-base and serum electrolyte testing is performed to monitor the response of the acidosis to treatment and to monitor for specific electrolyte abnormalities. Sodium bicarbonate and insulin are rarely, if ever, necessary. Potassium, magnesium, or phosphorus supplementation is provided if a deficiency is found by blood testing. Thiamine and multivitamins are indicated routinely. Because vomiting is common, the patient should be given nothing by mouth initially. Nasogastric intubation is indicated if there is recent or ongoing vomiting, evidence of pancreatitis, or suspicion of gastrointestinal hemorrhage. Ethanol withdrawal precautions are observed.

ETHANOL WITHDRAWAL

Ethanol withdrawal is common among hospitalized patients, either as a primary reason for admission or as a development during hospitalization for some other illness or injury. It is a potentially fatal syndrome that occurs after abrupt discontinuation of ethanol in individuals who regularly consume ethanol-containing beverages. Although in most cases it occurs after complete abstinence, it can also occur in the face of on-going ethanol consumption if the level of ethanol intake is substantially decreased. The pathophysiology is incompletely understood but probably involves changes in neurotransmitter levels and alterations in neurotransmitter receptor function within the CNS, as well as elevated circulating catecholamine levels.[6,7,25,26] A number of disorders should be of particular consideration in the differential diagnosis of alcohol withdrawal (see Table 187-2). The mortality rate associated with advanced stages of alcohol withdrawal can exceed 15%.[27,28]

CLINICAL MANIFESTATIONS

The syndrome is traditionally classified into four stages, although the stages do not always follow the indicated sequence, and not every patient develops every stage.[28] The time of development of each stage is also quite variable, and overlap can occur. A typical temporal sequence is described.

The first stage occurs 6 to 24 hours or more after the last drink or after a somewhat longer period of markedly decreased ethanol intake. Manifestations include anxiety, restlessness, decreased attention, tremulousness, insomnia, and craving for alcoholic beverages. Stage 2, which occurs about 24 hours after the onset of abstinence, is characterized by hallucinations, misperceptions, irritability, and vivid dreams.[29] Hallucinations may be auditory, but more often they are visual or tactile. Formication, the delusional sensation of insects crawling on the skin, and vivid or threatening visual hallucinations are particularly common. During this stage, the patient may appear otherwise lucid or somewhat confused, hypervigilant, and easily startled or misled. In stage 3, which commonly occurs 7 to 48 hours after cessation of drinking, seizures occur, usually of the grand mal variety.[4] The seizures classically manifest as a cluster of brief, tonic-clonic convulsions, at one time referred to as "rum fits." They are more likely to occur in subjects with a history of repeated withdrawal episodes.[30] A relatively lucid interval, ranging from hours to 2 or 3 days, is sometimes seen between stages 3 and 4. Stage 4 manifests 2 to 6 days, or more, after initiation of abstinence and consists of a global confusional state associated with signs of neuronal excitation and severe autonomic hyperactivity. Vernacular usage notwithstanding, the term *delirium tremens* refers specifically to stage 4 of withdrawal. Only a small minority of individuals with alcohol withdrawal develop delirium tremens. Tremors, hallucinations, and seizures are common during this stage. As is characteristic of delirium in general, the degree of confusion and disorientation can wax and wane. Hyperadrenergic manifestations may include diaphoresis, flushing, mydriasis, tachycardia, hypertension, and low-grade fever.[4]

LABORATORY MANIFESTATIONS

There are no specific laboratory manifestations of ethanol withdrawal. Laboratory abnormalities are a reflection of any concomitant or underlying disorders, such as cirrhosis, coagulopathy, gastrointestinal bleeding, infection, pancreatitis, or aspiration pneumonitis. Electrolyte disorders are common, particularly hypokalemia, hypomagnesemia, and hypophosphatemia. Serum creatine phosphokinase activity should be evaluated, because rhabdomyolysis is a common complicating problem and can lead to renal failure or compartment syndrome.

TREATMENT

Early-stage withdrawal with mild symptoms does not generally require treatment in an ICU setting. Full-blown delirium tremens, on the other hand, often requires more vigilant monitoring than can be provided on many general medical or surgical units. Comorbid conditions that should prompt special consideration for ICU admission include acute coronary syndromes, congestive heart failure, severe sepsis, acute gastrointestinal bleeding, pancreatitis, hepatic failure, spontaneous bacterial peritonitis, hypothermia, and hyperthermia. Other factors to consider include advanced age, renal failure, severe electrolyte deficiencies, marked rhabdomyolysis, symptomatic hypoglycemia, recurrent or prolonged seizures, cardiac dysrhythmias, hypotension, and respiratory or airway compromise.

After ensuring an adequate airway, ventilation, oxygenation, and perfusion; establishing intravenous access; and excluding serious coexisting or complicating disorders, treatment focuses mainly on judiciously titrated sedation and vigilant monitoring for progression of the syndrome or development of complications. As with the acutely intoxicated patient, all patients with alcohol withdrawal are given prophylactic multivitamin supplements, including parenteral thiamine and folate, and fluid deficits and electrolyte deficiencies are corrected.[31] Routine administration of magnesium sulfate in the absence of hypomagnesemia has not been shown to be beneficial.[32,33] Prophylactic measures against gastritis and deep vein thrombosis are recommended.

A calm, nonthreatening, protective environment with frequent verbal orientation and reassurance is provided to allay anxiety and fear and to minimize agitation. This approach may suffice in milder cases, but more advanced withdrawal necessitates pharmacologic intervention. The principle underlying this pharmacotherapy is that administration of a cross-tolerant agent to achieve light to moderate sedation will ameliorate the severe manifestations of withdrawal (including autonomic and psychomotor hyperactivity), provide subjective relief, protect the patient from self-harm, and allow specific therapeutic interventions until spontaneous recovery occurs.

The agent of choice is a benzodiazepine, given orally in milder cases or i.v. in more severe withdrawal states.[29,31,34,35] Lorazepam can be administered i.v. in incremental doses, starting with 1 or 2 mg, followed by intermittent (e.g., every 2 to 6 hours) intravenous dosing or a continuous intravenous infusion (e.g., initiated at 1 mg/hour and titrated to effect).[28,36] Alternatively, midazolam can be employed, beginning with 2 to 4 mg by intravenous injection, followed by 2 mg/hour by continuous intravenous infusion, which may be titrated to effect. Diazepam is another option, given initially in titrated doses of 5 to 10 mg, at intervals as frequent as every 10 minutes if necessary, until a calm but awake level of consciousness is achieved. Subsequent dosing at 5 to 20 mg every 4 to 6 hours is typically required with this agent. Prolonged administration of diazepam may lead to a prolonged duration of sedation due to accumulation of the parent drug and an active metabolite, both of which have long half-lives. This effect is less likely to occur with lorazepam.

Oral chlordiazepoxide has been employed commonly in mild cases of withdrawal that do not require intravenous sedation.[29] It may also be used in more serious cases after the severe manifestations have abated and parenteral benzodiazepines are no longer required. Typical oral dosage is 25 to 100 mg every 6 to 12 hours. Intramuscular administration is sometimes employed, but it entails a less predictable dose-response due to erratic absorption, and there is the potential for a depot effect.

Other sedative-hypnotic drugs can be effective but are not considered first-line therapeutic agents.[31,34] Barbiturates have a long history of successful use. The most commonly used agent is phenobarbital, which can be difficult to titrate because of its long duration of action. The shorter-acting barbiturate pentobarbital also has been employed. Oral ethanol and paraldehyde have been used but are discouraged, in part because of the risks of aspiration and gastric irritation, but also because their use can be interpreted as reinforcing the acceptability of using alcoholic beverages, either in general or for treatment of withdrawal symptoms. The latter criticism has also been directed at the use of ethanol administered i.v. for this purpose. Propofol is effective, but it is not a first-line agent and is not recommended unless a cannulating airway (endotracheal tube or tracheostomy tube) is in place and mechanical ventilation is used.[28] Regardless of the specific sedative agent employed, appropriate dose titration is crucial. The goal is to ameliorate the manifestations of withdrawal without causing excessive sedation. Sedation should be titrated with the use of an objective sedation scale, such as the Ramsay Sedation Scale,[37] the Riker Sedation-Agitation Scale,[38] or the Richmond Agitation-Sedation Scale.[39] The goal should be to achieve a calm, awake state or, if that is not feasible, a state of light somnolence from which the patient can easily be aroused and is able to respond verbally.

Clonidine may be administered if hyperautonomic symptoms are prominent.[40,41] Typical oral dosing is 0.1 to 0.2 mg every 6 to 12 hours. β-Adrenergic receptor blockers are not recommended for routine use, but, barring contraindications, they may be considered in selected cases as adjunctive agents for controlling severe hyperadrenergic manifestations. Haloperidol and other neuroleptic agents are not routinely used because they can lower the threshold for seizures. In selected cases, haloperidol may be used in conjunction with benzodiazepines for marked agitation or hallucinations, but this agent or similar drugs should not be used as monotherapy.[34]

Seizure precautions should be used for all patients in withdrawal. Withdrawal seizures are managed primarily with benzodiazepines, which usually are effective at the doses used for sedation.[36] In refractory cases, higher doses may be necessary, but use of higher doses may necessitate endotracheal intubation and mechanical ventilation. Concomitant use of other anticonvulsants also can be considered. Barbiturates may be used for this purpose, but phenytoin is usually ineffective unless the seizures are due to a specific cause other than alcohol withdrawal, such as underlying epilepsy or a complicating acute disorder of the CNS (e.g., meningitis, head trauma).[31,42,43] In such cases, phenytoin is usually the anticonvulsant of choice.

Once severe manifestations have been controlled with parenteral sedation for a period of at least 24 hours, tapering of the dose can be attempted. If tapering of sedation is tolerated, further gradual tapering is attempted, with the goal of substituting oral for parenteral benzodiazepine administration. This process typically takes up to several days, but there is substantial variability.

METHANOL INTOXICATION

Methanol, also known as wood alcohol, is a clear, colorless liquid having a faint, alcoholic odor. It is widely used in laboratories and industry as a solvent and synthetic precursor. It is also a constituent or vehicle in numerous commercially available products for residential use (Table 187-3).[15] Methanol is also used as a denaturant to intentionally render ethanol unfit for consumption. The minimum lethal dose of methanol is highly variable, reportedly ranging from less than 10 mL to more than 500 mL. This variability may result from multiple factors, including the degree of concomitant ethanol intoxication, the presence of folate deficiency, and perhaps other factors.

More than 2000 cases of methanol exposure are reported annually by the American Association of Poison Control Centers, most of which are accidental.[44-46] Intentional ingestion can represent a suicidal gesture or attempt, but it more commonly occurs among desperate alcoholics who have no access to ethanol-containing beverages and are either unaware

TABLE 187-3. COMMON COMMERCIAL PRODUCTS THAT MAY CONTAIN METHANOL

Denatured alcohol
Windshield washer fluids
Windshield de-icers
Sterno ("canned heat")
Antifreeze
Paints and paint removers
Wood stains
Shellacs and varnishes
Lacquer and paint thinners
Furniture refinishers
Dry gas
Gasoline (some forms of gasohol)
Dyes
Duplicating fluids
Carburetor cleaners
Adhesives
Glass cleaners
Dewaxing preparations
Pipe sweetener
Embalming fluids
Various other solvents and cleaners

From Kruse JA: Methanol, ethylene glycol, and related intoxications. In Carlson RW, Geheb MA (eds): Principles and Practice of Medical Intensive Care. Philadelphia, WB Saunders, 1993, p 1714, with permission.

or heedless of the risks of consuming methanol. There are individual cases of surreptitious poisoning in which an individual prepares a small volume of an alcoholic drink intentionally laced with methanol with malice aforethought for the intended victim. More often, malicious intent is absent and the goal is simply illicit production of a small or large volume of alcoholic beverage, with methanol used because of its availability or under a mistaken rationale that it will serve as a more potent, but still potable, inebriant. Sharing or black-market distribution of these illicit concoctions has resulted in periodic epidemics of methanol intoxication, sometimes involving hundreds of unwitting subjects.[47-51] There are also rare reports of dermal or inhalational exposure causing intoxication, but most cases involve oral ingestion.[52]

METABOLISM

Other than its inebriant and mucosal irritant effects, methanol per se is nontoxic. However, it is metabolized slowly to formaldehyde:

$$CH_3\text{-}OH + NAD^+ \xrightarrow{\ ALDH\ } NADH$$

$$\text{Methanol} \qquad + \underset{\text{Formaldehyde}}{H\text{-}\overset{\overset{\text{O}}{\|}}{C}\text{-}H} + H^+ \qquad (9)$$

and then rapidly to formic acid, depicted here as its dissociation products, formate and a hydrogen ion[53]:

$$\underset{\text{Formaldehyde}}{H\text{-}\overset{\overset{\text{O}}{\|}}{C}\text{-}H} + NAD^+ \xrightarrow{\ ALDH\ } NADH$$

$$+ \underset{\text{Formate}}{H\text{-}\overset{\overset{\text{O}}{\|}}{C}\text{-}O^-} + 2H^+ \qquad (10)$$

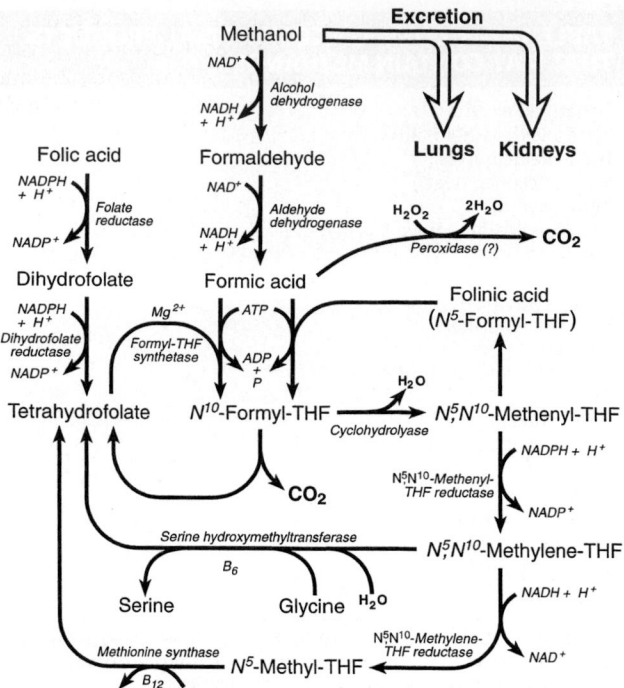

FIGURE 187–1. Metabolic pathways involved in methanol metabolism, showing the role of folate derivatives as enzymatic cofactors operative in the elimination of formic acid. ADP, adenosine diphosphate; ATP, adenosine triphosphate; NAD+ and NADH, oxidized and reduced forms of nicotinamide adenine dinucleotide, respectively; NADP+ and NADPH, oxidized and reduced forms of nicotinamide adenine dinucleotide phosphate, respectively; THF, tetrahydrofolate. (Adapted from Kruse JA: Methanol poisoning. Intensive Care Med 1992;18:391-397, with permission.)

Formic acid production can thus result in metabolic acidosis. Independent of the acidosis, formic acid inhibits cytochrome oxidase and has direct neurotoxic effects, particularly affecting the retina and optic nerves.[51,54-59] Small amounts of methanol are present as congeners in fermented alcoholic beverages.[60] Small amounts are also formed during the metabolism of certain fruits and vegetables and by metabolism of the artificial sweetener, aspartame.[61,62] However, the quantity of methanol available or formed from these sources is small, and there are enzyme systems present in the body that can convert these small amounts of formate to harmless CO_2 (Fig. 187-1).The large amounts of formate produced in serious cases of methanol intoxication overwhelm these enzymes, resulting in toxic accumulation of formate. Certain nonhuman mammalian species have enzymes with much higher activity for metabolism of formate; even large quantities of methanol are nontoxic to these species. Methanol ingested by these species is still converted to formaldehyde and formate, but these toxins are rapidly metabolized to CO_2 so that significant formate accumulation does not occur. The enzymes that convert formate to CO_2 require folate as an obligate cofactor.[53]

CLINICAL MANIFESTATIONS

Like ethanol, methanol has dose-dependent sedating and inebriating effects that manifest shortly after ingestion, but methanol is less potent in this regard. Both alcohols also have similar gastrointestinal irritant effects that can provoke

nausea, vomiting, abdominal pain, gastritis, hematemesis, and pancreatitis, although methanol may be more potent in this regard. Methanol ingestion can lead to additional CNS manifestations that are not observed with ethanol intoxication, which can sometimes provide helpful clinical clues in cases of occult methanol intoxication.[49,51] These more specific manifestations are caused by formate, the end product of methanol metabolism. There is a characteristic delay, usually 12 to 24 hours, between ingestion and development of these manifestations, and this delay is attributable to the relatively slow conversion of methanol to formaldehyde. Delayed CNS manifestations can include cerebral edema, seizures, signs of meningeal irritation, and cerebral infarction (particularly infarction of basal ganglia). However, the most specific clinical findings are ocular and range from mildly blurred vision, to visual field defects or tunnel vision, to complete and sometimes permanent blindness.[49,51] Other possible ocular findings include scotomata, scintillations, papilledema, and loss of pupillary light reflexes. Most survivors recover visual function, but permanent visual deficits occur in as many as one third of patients with serious intoxication. If the metabolic acidosis is severe, it can result in Kussmaul respirations and dyspnea. In the most severe cases of poisoning, profound acidosis, respiratory failure, and circulatory shock intervene. Severe global brain injury and brain death can also occur.

For cases in which the patient offers historical information detailing an obvious toxic ingestion, the diagnosis of methanol intoxication is straightforward. Confirmatory diagnostic studies can be obtained and treatment initiated. In other cases, the diagnosis is not straightforward. Some poisoned patients may be unable to provide any history because of stupor or coma. Alert patients may be unaware that the alcoholic beverages they were provided had been adulterated. Others may be alert and aware that they ingested a toxic substance but unwilling to provide the necessary history because of fear of social stigmatization or legal recrimination, or as a manifestation of irrational or sociopathic behavior.

The presence of methanol may be detectable on the intoxicated patient's breath, but the agent's subtle odor can be difficult to appreciate and may be confused with ethanol. As a corollary, if a patient who appears inebriated has no breath odor of any type of alcohol, suspicion should be raised of methanol or a related toxic ingestion. In some cases, a faint odor reminiscent of formalin may be noticeable on the patient's breath. The obvious presence of ethanol on the breath does not exclude the possibility of methanol ingestion; coingestions involving these two alcohols are frequent.

LABORATORY MANIFESTATIONS

The clinical laboratory can be helpful by providing clues to the diagnosis in cases of occult intoxication and by corroborating cases with a clear history of methanol ingestion. The serum electrolyte panel may show an abnormally low total CO_2 content as a consequence of metabolic acidosis due to formic acid accumulation. The dissociation product of formic acid, formate, is negatively charged and can widen the serum anion gap. Arterial blood gas analysis can corroborate the presence of metabolic acidosis. Metabolic acidosis associated with a wide serum anion gap has a limited number of causes, the most common of which are lactic acidosis, ketoacidosis, and renal failure.[22,23] These other causes of wide-gap metabolic acidosis are easily excluded by measuring blood lactate, ketones, glucose, and creatinine levels.

Certain toxins (e.g., propylene glycol) can result in lactic acidosis by direct metabolic conversion of the parent compound to lactate. More commonly, lactic acidosis can occur in association with any toxic exposure or drug overdose that causes seizures or circulatory shock (e.g., iron, isoniazid). The metabolic acidosis seen in methanol intoxication is mainly due to formic acid, but can also be due in part to lactic acidosis secondary to these mechanisms. Analogous to ethanol metabolism, conversion of methanol to formaldehyde and formic acid leads to a reducing environment in cells, which tends to increase lactate concentration. By inhibiting cytochromes, formate also may interfere with normal aerobic metabolism and lead to an increase in anaerobic glycolysis with resulting lactic acidosis. Therefore, hyperlactatemia does not exclude methanol poisoning. A few other toxic agents besides methanol, notably ethylene glycol and salicylates, can directly cause a wide anion gap metabolic acidosis. Although measurement of plasma formate concentration would seem to be a rational method to confirm the diagnosis of methanol poisoning, this assay is rarely available in hospital laboratories.[63]

Life-threatening methanol poisoning can result in profound metabolic acidosis, which sometimes is refractory to large doses of sodium bicarbonate. However, even with severe methanol exposure, metabolic acidosis may be absent if testing is performed within a few hours after the ingestion.[63] In these cases, the plasma methanol level may be very high, but the slow rate of its metabolism has not allowed for appreciable conversion to formic acid. Therefore, in the presence of a compatible history for toxic alcohol ingestion, the absence of a wide anion gap or hypobicarbonatemia should not be regarded as excluding the possibility of methanol poisoning.

A potentially useful screening test for recognition of methanol exposure early in its course is the serum osmolality gap. Serum osmolality is determined by the concentration of osmotically active solutes, or *osmoles*.[65,66] Osmotic activity is directly proportional to the osmole concentration of a solution, which is directly proportional to the mass concentration (i.e., weight/volume) of the solute and inversely proportional to the solute's molecular weight. Therefore, to have an appreciable effect on osmolality, a solute must be present at relatively high mass concentration and have a relatively low molecular weight. For example, albumin is present at relatively large mass concentrations in serum, normally averaging about 4000 mg/dL, in comparison with urea, which normally averages only about 10 mg/dL. However, albumin has a far higher molecular weight (approximately 69,000 daltons, compared with 60 daltons for urea), making its osmolar concentration less than 1 mOsm/L. The elemental ions sodium and chloride are present in appreciable mass concentration, and their atomic weight is comparatively low (23 and 35 daltons, respectively), making them quantitatively important serum osmoles. Therefore, total serum osmolality normally comprises sodium, low atomic or molecular weight anions, plus urea and glucose; although many other osmoles are present in serum, their collective contribution is comparatively small. Based on these principles, serum osmolality may be estimated by the following formula[66]:

$$\text{Estimated serum osmolality} = 2 \times \text{Na}$$
$$+ \frac{\text{SUN}}{2.8} + \frac{\text{Glucose}}{18} \quad (11)$$

where the serum sodium concentration (Na) is given in mmol/L, and the serum urea nitrogen (SUN) and serum glucose concentrations are in mg/dL. The divisors, 2.8 and 18, are necessary to convert the conventional units of mg/dL to mmol/L. They are based on the molecular weights of the respective compounds.

Because ethanol is osmotically active and may be present in the blood in relatively high concentrations, the formula may be expanded to include a term for ethanol:

$$\text{Estimated serum osmolality} = 2 \times \text{Na}$$
$$+ \frac{\text{SUN}}{2.8} + \frac{\text{Glucose}}{18} + \frac{\text{Ethanol}}{4.6} \quad (12)$$

Here the units for ethanol are mg/dL, and the divisor is based on the molecular weight of ethanol, 46 daltons. These millimolar concentration units technically provide an estimate of serum *osmolarity*; however, for practical purposes, they can be equated to millimolal units and designated *osmolality* (i.e., milliosmoles per kilogram of water). Just as ethanol can appreciably affect serum osmolality, so too can methanol.[64,67] The serum osmolality may be estimated from the formula shown and compared with a more direct measurement of serum osmolality; the difference between the two results affords a method for detecting and crudely quantifying the concentration of exogenous osmoles such as methanol. This is accomplished by means of the following formula:

$$\text{Osmole gap} =$$
$$\text{Measured osmolality} - \text{Estimated osmolality} \quad (13)$$

Measured serum osmolality is determined in most clinical chemistry laboratories by analysis of the freezing point of the sample. Freezing point represents a colligative property of solutions that is depressed in proportion to osmolality regardless of the chemical nature of the osmoles. This method therefore allows an empirical assessment of osmolality. The normal serum osmole gap is typically less than 10 mOsm/kg H_2O with this formula. Appreciable elevation of the osmole gap suggests the presence of an exogenous osmole (e.g., methanol). The only toxins that can appreciably affect the osmole gap are those that have a low molecular weight and can accumulate in relatively high concentration in the blood. A number of other exogenous compounds besides methanol meet these criteria, including ethylene glycol, acetone, isopropanol, propylene glycol, and acetonitrile, all of which have been reported to increase osmolality and the osmole gap.[15,22,65,66]

The constellation of laboratory findings that includes metabolic acidosis along with abnormal widening of both the serum anion gap and the serum osmole gap provides presumptive or corroborative evidence of methanol (or ethylene glycol) poisoning in compatible clinical settings. However, the serum osmole gap is not foolproof, and it has important limitations. False-positive results have been described in cases of circulatory shock, DKA or AKA, the hyperosmolar hyperglycemic nonketotic dehydration syndrome, chronic renal failure, and multiple organ system failure.[66] False-negative results can occur if the ingestion involved a small, but still potentially lethal, volume of methanol. When assessing the serum osmole gap, it is important to ensure that all relevant measurements are made from the same serum specimen, to minimize variability caused by temporal changes in individual analyte concentrations.

Some clinical chemistry laboratories assay serum osmolality by the dew point or vapor pressure method. For technical reasons, this method yields spuriously low osmolality readings in the presence of ethanol, methanol, and other volatile alcohols, and therefore it should not be used to assess the osmole gap.[66]

Methanol assays are available in many clinical chemistry laboratories and provide a direct assessment of methanol concentration in serum samples. This test is not definitive, because patients who present late after methanol intake may have metabolized much or all of the ingested alcohol, although the toxic byproducts may be present in appreciable concentration.[68] The delay between ingestion and presentation represents another factor that may explain the wide range of blood methanol concentrations reportedly associated with fatal outcome.[69] Methanol assay results should be interpreted in conjunction with assessments of acid-base status, serum anion gap, and serum osmole gap, as well as the history and clinical findings.

TREATMENT

As with any toxic ingestion, the patient's airway and ventilation must be immediately assessed; if necessary, adequate airway and respiratory support must be provided. Circulatory shock is treated with fluid resuscitation, inotropic support, and vasopressor agents as appropriate. Whether the patient is initially unstable or not, close monitoring of vital signs, cardiopulmonary status, and neurologic status is indicated. Vomiting should not be induced, because of the risk of aspiration and the lack of demonstrable benefit. Gastric lavage is unlikely to be of value unless the patient presents within 1 hour after ingestion. Activated charcoal is also of dubious benefit unless there is a concomitant toxic ingestant.[9,10,12,70-75] However, cointoxication with another drug or toxin should be considered routinely. Accordingly, naloxone should be administered if the subject is unconscious. Blood and urine samples should be obtained for toxicologic screening. As in acute ethanol intoxication, complicating and occult underlying comorbid disorders must be considered (see Table 187-2).

Specimens should also be obtained for diagnostic laboratory tests. However, because specific toxicologic identification is not available on site at all hospital laboratories, antidotal therapy should not be delayed if there is an obvious history of methanol ingestion.[8,53,75,76] Even if "stat" testing is available, methanol intoxication may not be considered in occult cases until routine laboratory test results are obtained and reveal unexplained metabolic acidosis. In such cases, the preliminary laboratory test results, in conjunction with a compatible setting and perhaps physical findings, may allow a presumptive diagnosis to be made and antidotal treatment to be initiated. That treatment can then be stopped if further studies convincingly argue against methanol intoxication. Symptomatic poisoned patients require ICU admission for frequent monitoring of vital signs and level of consciousness and to provide specific antidotal treatment, which consists of ethanol or fomepizole administration, hemodialysis, and folate administration.

Ethanol has been the conventional form of antidotal pharmacotherapy for methanol intoxication. The principle is that alcohol dehydrogenase and aldehyde dehydrogenase have higher affinity for ethanol than for methanol, and ethanol thereby serves as an effective competitive inhibitor.[77-80] As a result, conversion of methanol to formaldehyde and formate is significantly slowed in the presence of ethanol, allowing methanol to be excreted by the kidneys and lungs, and by hemodialysis if that modality is employed. If inhibition is incomplete, the body may be able to safely eliminate the much smaller amounts of formaldehyde and formate that are metabolically produced from the methanol. Indications for ethanol therapy include a serum methanol concentration greater than 20 mg/dL, or a history or strong clinical suspicion of methanol ingestion in conjunction with either an elevated osmole gap or evidence of metabolic acidosis (e.g., arterial blood pH less than 7.30 and bicarbonate less than 20 mmol/L).

Ethanol can be given orally, by gastric or enteral instillation, or by vein. Oral dosing can be considered in mild cases, if the patient is completely alert and is accustomed to drinking undiluted liquor. The solution is usually prepared from commercially available liquor, available in many hospital formularies, and diluted to a final concentration of 20% ethanol. Even with dilution, subjects who are uninitiated to drinking this quantity of ethanol over a short interval are unlikely to avoid vomiting. This increases the risk of aspiration, particularly when coupled with the sedating effects of the administered ethanol and the potential CNS effects of the ingested methanol. For these reasons, intravenous ethanol administration is usually preferred over the oral route. This can be accomplished with the use of a sterile solution of either 5% or 10% (volume/volume) ethanol in 5% (weight/volume) dextrose. These solutions are markedly hyperosmolar (approximately 2000 mOsm/kg H_2O for 10% ethanol in 5% dextrose and water) and therefore must be administered through a central venous catheter.

A loading dose is given so as to rapidly effect maximal enzyme inhibition. The goal is to achieve a serum ethanol level of 100 to 150 mg/dL. Based on the volume of distribution of ethanol (0.6 to 0.7 L/kg in men, slightly less in women and elderly subjects, and less in obese subjects) and a target serum ethanol concentration of 100 mg/dL, the necessary loading dose is theoretically 600 mg/kg in terms of absolute ethanol. Given the specific gravity of absolute ethanol (0.79), this is equivalent to a dose of 0.76 mL/kg in terms of absolute ethanol. Absolute (i.e., 100%) ethanol is unlikely to be available in a hospital formulary. Oral loading can be accomplished using 100 proof liquor, which is 50% ethanol by volume (equivalent to 40 g/dL), at a dose of 1.5 mL/kg. Alternatively, intravenous loading using a 5% (volume/volume) solution of ethanol in dextrose and water (i.e., an ethanol concentration of 4 g/dL by weight/volume) would require 15 mL/kg, typically administered over 1 hour. The dosing calculations described frequently underestimate the ethanol dose necessary to achieve the target level. Loading doses of 700 mg/kg given i.v., or even higher doses if given orally, are more likely to achieve the goal initially.[1] If the patient's current ethanol concentration is already at or above the targeted level due to coingestion of ethanol, no ethanol loading dose is required. A proportionately lower loading dose is used in patients with a preexisting subtherapeutic blood ethanol concentration.

Maintenance dosing is required to maintain the targeted blood ethanol concentration. For patients with little or no history of ethanol exposure, the average required maintenance dose has been estimated to be about 70 mg/kg/hour, in terms of absolute ethanol. For oral dosing with 100 proof liquor, this is equivalent to 0.18 mL/kg/hour. Hourly oral maintenance doses are necessary and should be diluted to 20% to minimize epigastric pain and emesis. Using intravenous maintenance dosing, a continuous infusion of 5% ethanol solution is administered at 1.8 mL/kg/hour. Subjects who consume ethanol chronically on a regular basis metabolize ethanol at considerably higher rates and therefore require higher maintenance doses. The necessary maintenance dose in such cases depends on the individual's exposure history, but it can be 2 to 3 times higher than the cited dose, or even higher in some cases. If hemodialysis is used during ethanol therapy, it will effectively remove ethanol from the body. Therefore, the maintenance ethanol dose needs to be increased, often doubled or tripled, during dialysis. Accurate prediction of the required ethanol dosing in individual cases is not possible, and maintenance of the desired therapeutic ethanol concentration can be challenging. Serial serum ethanol levels are obtained every 1 to 2 hours to allow the ethanol dosing to be titrated, striving to maintain a serum ethanol level between 100 and 150 mg/dL. Lower serum ethanol concentrations risk incomplete inhibition and toxicity from the products of methanol metabolism. The risks with higher levels are sedation, inebriation, and impairment of protective airway reflexes. Treatment is continued until serum methanol levels are less than 20 mg/dL. Intravenous ethanol therapy can entail large fluid volumes to achieve and maintain the desired blood ethanol level; for this reason, attention to fluid balance is important.

Fomepizole (4-methylpyrazole) is a newer therapeutic alternative to ethanol.[81-84] Like ethanol, fomepizole inhibits alcohol dehydrogenase, but it is considerably more costly than ethanol. Nevertheless, fomepizole has the potential advantage of being easier to dose and titrate, and it has no sedative effects. Frequent serial blood ethanol assays are avoided. Compared with oral dosing of ethanol, there is no risk of nausea, vomiting, gastritis, or abdominal pain with fomepizole. Compared with intravenous ethanol administration, there is less risk of overhydration. The indications for fomepizole use are the same as for ethanol therapy.

Fomepizole is given i.v. as a loading dose of 15 mg/kg, followed by 10 mg/kg every 12 hours for four doses and then 15 mg/kg every 12 hours until the serum methanol concentration is less than 20 mg/dL. Each dose is infused over 30 minutes. Dosing is altered if hemodialysis is employed. If dialysis is initiated, the next slated dose is given immediately if 6 hours or longer has elapsed since the last dose, but no dose is given if it has been less than 6 hours since the last dose. During ongoing hemodialysis, fomepizole is dosed at intervals of 4 hours. At termination of hemodialysis, if less than 1 hour has elapsed since the last dose, no fomepizole is administered; if 1 to 3 hours has elapsed between the last dose and the end of dialysis, half of the next scheduled fomepizole dose is administered; and if more than 3 hours has elapsed, the next scheduled fomepizole dose is given at the end of hemodialysis. Subsequent fomepizole dosing after hemodialysis is every 12 hours.

Severe methanol poisoning can be associated with profound metabolic acidosis in some cases. Traditionally, sodium bicarbonate was a staple part of the treatment for most causes of metabolic acidosis, but lack of demonstrable efficacy has tempered its routine use, particularly in the treatment of lactic acidosis and DKA. There are laboratory animal data and anecdotal clinical reports ascribing benefit to bicarbonate administration in toxic alcohol and glycol poisoning in terms of reversing ocular manifestations and lowering mortality, but controlled clinical trials are lacking. There also is evidence that undissociated formic acid is more toxic than the dissociation product, formate; increasing the

extracellular fluid pH favors conversion of formic acid to formate.[85] Given the potential severity of the acidosis and the likely benefit of alkali therapy, sodium bicarbonate is recommended for subjects with an arterial pH less than 7.30, although intentional alkalemia is not advocated. Sodium bicarbonate dosing is empirical, titrated to serial arterial blood gas and serum CO_2 content assays.

Ethanol and fomepizole minimize conversion of methanol to its toxic metabolites, but these forms of pharmacotherapy do not hasten elimination of methanol from the body. Methanol is excreted by the kidneys and lungs, but only slowly. Hemodialysis can effectively and more rapidly remove methanol and its toxic metabolites from the body. Charcoal or resin hemoperfusion techniques are not effective, and peritoneal dialysis is recommended only if hemodialysis is not available. Hemodialysis is recommended as a supplement to ethanol or fomepizole in patients with serious degrees of methanol intoxication. Serious intoxication is defined by the presence of metabolic acidosis, a serum methanol level greater than 50 mg/dL, any type of subjective or objective ocular findings, or other findings that indicate severe poisoning. Hemodialysis also is recommended if there is renal impairment. As previously noted, fomepizole and ethanol dosing must be altered during hemodialysis. Methods have been described to incorporate ethanol into the dialysate, to facilitate maintaining therapeutic ethanol levels during hemodialysis.[86] The endpoint for dialysis is a serum methanol level less than 20 mg/dL and normalization of the anion gap, indicating clearance of formate. Direct measurement of plasma formate would be a logical method of monitoring if rapid assays were available.

In humans and certain nonhuman primates, formate is only slowly metabolized, allowing the development of acidosis and ocular pathology if substantial amounts of methanol are ingested. Monkeys given large doses of folinic or folic acid before or after methanol administration had lower formate levels and less toxicity than control animals.[87] Based on these and other experimental data, large doses of folic or folinic acid are recommended in clinical methanol poisoning. Typical recommendations are to administer 50 mg of folinic or folic acid i.v. every 4 to 6 hours.

ETHYLENE GLYCOL INTOXICATION

Ethylene glycol is a clear, colorless, almost odorless, sweet-tasting, viscous liquid that is commonly used as the main constituent in most formulations of permanent automotive antifreeze. It also finds use in a variety of commercially available automotive fluids and paint products (Table 187-4), and

TABLE 187–4. COMMON COMMERCIAL PRODUCTS THAT MAY CONTAIN ETHYLENE GLYCOL

"Permanent" antifreeze
Paints and lacquers
Polishes and detergents
Inks
Cosmetics
Hydraulic brake fluids
Solar collector fluids
Car wash fluids

From Kruse JA: Methanol, ethylene glycol, and related intoxications. In Carlson RW, Geheb MA (eds): Principles and Practice of Medical Intensive Care. Philadelphia, WB Saunders, 1993, p 1716, with permission.

it is used industrially as a solvent and synthetic precursor. Like methanol, it is occasionally ingested, either intentionally as an ethanol substitute or accidentally. More than 5000 cases of ethylene glycol exposure have been reported annually by the American Association of Poison Control Centers in recent years.[44,45] Based on limited anecdotal data, the lethal dose in humans has been estimated at 1 to 2 mL/kg, but there are case reports of fatalities after lower doses and survival after higher doses.

METABOLISM

The metabolism of ethylene glycol is more complicated than that of methanol.[88,89] As with methanol, the parent compound possesses only minor toxic potential compared with its metabolites. Also in common with methanol, the initial step in metabolism is catalyzed by alcohol dehydrogenase (Fig. 187-2). This results in the production of glycoaldehyde, which can be converted to glyoxal. Both glycoaldehyde and glyoxal are metabolized first to glycolic acid, then more slowly to glyoxylic acid, and finally to oxalic acid. Glycoaldehyde and glyoxylate have demonstrable nephrotoxicity in isolated rodent renal tubular segments, whereas glycolate, oxalate, and ethylene glycol do not.[90] Glycolate and probably some of the other metabolites are also neurotoxic. Oxalic acid can precipitate as calcium oxalate crystals within various tissues, including notably the renal parenchyma and tubules.

CLINICAL MANIFESTATIONS

The initial effects involve the CNS and typically manifest within 30 minutes to 12 hours after ingestion.[15] These can range from effects that are similar to those seen with acute ethanol intoxication, such as excitement, confusion,

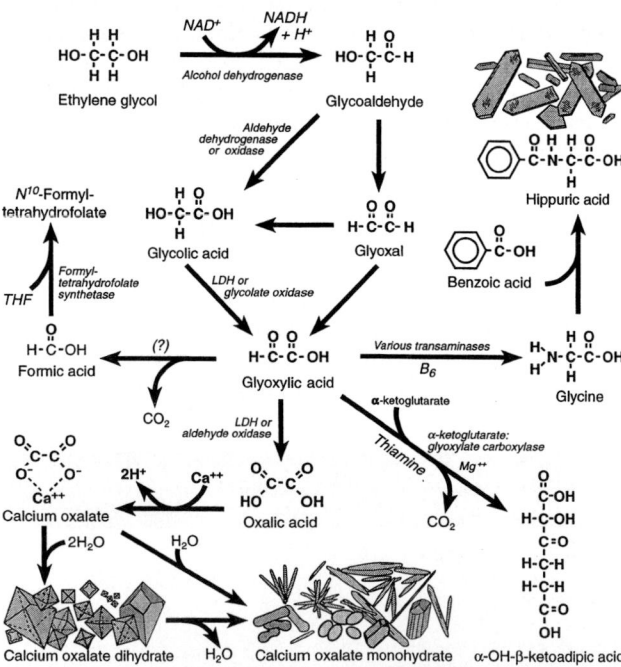

FIGURE 187–2. Metabolic pathways involved in ethylene glycol metabolism, with schematic morphologies of representative urinary crystals. LDH, lactate dehydrogenase; THF, tetrahydrofolate. (Adapted from Kruse JA: Ethylene glycol intoxication. J Intensive Care Med 1992;7:234-243, with permission.)

disorientation, and ataxia, to signs of CNS depression, such as lethargy, stupor, or coma. Nausea, vomiting, myoclonus, and seizures can also occur. Cranial nerve deficits, including nystagmus, ophthalmoplegia, facial palsy, dysarthria, and dysphagia have been reported. There are also rare case reports of pupillary abnormalities and changes in visual acuity, but these are not characteristic; if they do occur, they may be the result of to coingestion of methanol. Classically, the second phase manifests 12 to 24 hours after ingestion and consists of cardiorespiratory effects, which may include dyspnea and a Kussmaul respiratory pattern secondary to metabolic acidosis or pulmonary edema. The latter can result in frank respiratory failure necessitating endotracheal intubation and mechanical ventilation. Tachycardia, hypotension, frank circulatory shock, coma, and death can also occur during this phase. The third phase, which usually takes 1 to 3 days to manifest, consists of renal failure, either oliguric or nonoliguric, due to acute tubular necrosis. Flank pain can also occur. The time course of each phase of intoxication is variable, and overlap is frequent.

LABORATORY MANIFESTATIONS

Laboratory findings are similar to those seen in methanol poisoning. Detection of ethylene glycol in serum provides definitive evidence of the diagnosis. However, if the patient presents late, the assay concentration may not represent the patient's peak ethylene glycol level if significant metabolism has occurred. In a substantial ingestion, metabolic acidosis due to metabolic breakdown of the parent compound occurs during the first phase of intoxication.[68] The acidosis may be severe and is principally caused by glycolic acid accumulation.[91-94] Dissociation of this acid results in the accumulation of glycolate, which leads to an increase in the serum anion gap.

Measurement of the plasma glycolate concentration is a rational method of assessment, but clinical availability of the assay is lacking.[63] The blood lactate concentration may be elevated because of the reducing intracellular milieu induced by ethylene glycol metabolism, or as a manifestation of complicating seizures or circulatory shock. Lactate levels also may be artifactually elevated to a substantial degree, because of the cross-reactivity of glycolate with lactate in certain automated lactate analyzers.[95] The serum osmole gap may be elevated due to high blood levels of ethylene glycol and its metabolites. Because the molecular weight of ethylene glycol (62 daltons) is higher that of methanol (32 daltons), the osmole gap is less affected by a given amount (by weight) of ethylene glycol ingested, or by a given blood level (by weight/volume), compared with methanol.[66] Therefore, the osmole gap is more likely to yield a false-negative result after ingestion of ethylene glycol, compared with a similar mass amount of methanol.

There are two notable laboratory findings that may be seen in ethylene glycol poisoning; these are findings that are not observed in methanol poisoning. The first is calcium oxalate crystalluria. Oxalate produced by ethylene glycol metabolism chelates calcium, forming crystals and potentially producing hypocalcemia in the process (see Fig. 187-2). Two crystalline forms of this organic salt can occur. One is calcium oxalate dihydrate, also known as weddellite. These crystals have a characteristic octahedral shape, making them relatively easy to distinguish from various nonoxalate forms of crystalluria. The second form is calcium oxalate monohydrate, also known as whewellite. These crystals can be polymorphic; they can appear as monoclinic prisms or assume a needle-like, dumbbell-shaped, ovoid, or hempseed-like appearance. Hippurate crystalluria also has been described, but it can be difficult to morphologically discriminate hippurate from some forms of whewellite by light microscopy.[88] The finding of oxalate crystalluria corroborates the diagnosis; however, these crystals can occasionally be seen in the urine in the absence of ethylene glycol exposure, so their presence is not proof of glycol poisoning. On the other hand, because crystalluria does not uniformly occur after ethylene glycol ingestion, its absence does not exclude the diagnosis.

The other potential finding is fluorescence of the urine on exposure to ultraviolet radiation.[96,97] This occurs when the formulation of ethylene glycol ingested contains fluorescein, a fluorescent dye added to many automotive antifreeze solutions to facilitate identification of cooling system leaks and to mitigate accidental confusion with potable liquids. The fluorescein is excreted in the urine and fluoresces yellow-green on exposure to ultraviolet light, such as from a Wood's lamp (commonly used in emergency departments and ophthalmology clinics to detect corneal lesions after topical application of fluorescein to the eye). False-positive results have been described due to other fluorescent substances in urine (e.g., carotene, carbamazepine, niacin, benzodiazepine metabolites) and from certain types of glass or plastic specimen containers that have a high degree of native fluorescence.[96,98] False-negative results may occur if more than 4 hours has elapsed since the ingestion; this is sufficient time for the fluorescein to be excreted, at least by some individuals. A false-negative result is obviously expected if the ingested ethylene glycol formulation did not contain fluorescein or involved a small volume. False-negative results can occur if the urine pH is below 4.5, but this may be circumvented by urine pH testing followed by upward titration of the specimen's pH if necessary. Owing to interfering factors and the limited ability of untrained examiners to detect fluorescence, clinical decision-making should not hinge on this test in isolation.[99]

TREATMENT

With a few exceptions, the treatment of ethylene glycol poisoning is the same as for methanol intoxication. Gastric lavage may have some efficacy, but only if it is performed within 1 hour after the ingestion. Activated charcoal is not effective unless there is an amenable concomitant toxic ingestion.[12,100] Ethanol[80,101,102] or fomepizole[81-84] is administered to slow conversion of the glycol to toxic intermediates; sodium bicarbonate is given if there is significant metabolic acidosis (e.g., arterial pH less than 7.30); and hemodialysis is used in cases of serious intoxication to speed elimination of the parent compound and toxic metabolites. Ethanol or fomepizole is recommended if the serum ethylene glycol concentration is greater than 20 mg/dL. However, ethylene glycol assays are not available at all institutions, and inhibitor treatment should be initiated while awaiting definitive identification of the glycol if there is presumptive evidence of intoxication.[8,76,88] This includes a clear history of recent ethylene glycol ingestion, or strong clinical suspicion of ingestion in conjunction with either an elevated osmole gap, evidence of metabolic acidosis (e.g., arterial blood

pH less than 7.30 and bicarbonate less than 20 mmol/L), or oxalate crystals in the urine. Dosing of ethanol and fomepizole is the same as for methanol intoxication. Fomepizole can be recommended over ethanol if the sensorium is depressed. Inhibitor treatment is continued until the serum ethylene glycol level is less than 20 mg/dL.

Hemodialysis can be even more important in ethylene glycol poisoning than in methanol intoxication because the former can result in severe renal dysfunction, thereby interfering with excretion of the compound and its toxic metabolites. Dialysis is conventionally recommended for all patients with serum ethylene glycol levels greater than 50 mg/dL. Hemodialysis is indicated for all patients with renal dysfunction and for patients with metabolic acidosis or other toxic manifestations. The conventional endpoint for dialysis is a serum ethylene glycol concentration lower than 20 mg/dL in conjunction with normalization of the anion gap, indicating clearance of toxic metabolites.

Although there is some evidence that formic acid may be produced as a minor product of ethylene glycol metabolism, it probably does not play a significant role in the pathophysiology of this form of poisoning. Therefore, folate administration has not been routinely recommended. However, there is more convincing evidence that glyoxylate may be metabolized to nontoxic products by enzyme systems that rely on other vitamin cofactors, specifically pyridoxine (vitamin B_6) and thiamine (see Fig. 187-2). Providing supplements of pyridoxine (e.g., 50 mg i.v. every 6 hours) and thiamine (e.g., 100 mg i.v. every 6 hours) could hasten elimination of toxic intermediates, although evidence of efficacy is quite limited.[88] Given the low toxicity of these vitamins, both are recommended. Magnesium is a necessary cofactor for the enzymatic degradation of glyoxylate, and supplemental magnesium should be given if there is hypomagnesemia.

Routine intravenous administration of calcium salts was advocated at one time as a therapeutic means of lowering oxalate levels in body fluids in cases of ethylene glycol poisoning. However, precipitation of calcium oxalate in vital organs is probably more likely to have harmful effects. Therefore, routine therapeutic administration of calcium to correct hypocalcemia is no longer advised unless the hypocalcemia is severe enough to cause manifestations.

ANNOTATED REFERENCES

Barceloux DG, Bond GR, Krenzelok EP, et al: American Academy of Clinical Toxicology practice guidelines on the treatment of methanol poisoning. J Toxicol Clin Toxicol 2002;40:415-446.
An expert panel provides an extensive review covering the epidemiology, mechanisms of toxicity, clinical and laboratory manifestations, and detailed practice guidelines pertaining to methanol intoxication.

Brent J, McMartin K, Phillips S, et al: Fomepizole for the treatment of ethylene glycol poisoning. N Engl J Med 1999;340:832-838.
This multicenter, open-label study of fomepizole use in patients with ethylene glycol intoxication demonstrated decreases in urinary oxalate, plasma ethylene glycol, and plasma glycolate concentrations after initiation of fomepizole therapy.

Holbrook AM, Crowther R, Lotter A, et al: Meta-analysis of benzodiazepine use in the treatment of acute alcohol withdrawal. CMAJ 1999;160:649-655.
This study analyzed 11 randomized, controlled clinical trials that involved patients with acute ethanol withdrawal and compared benzodiazepine use to placebo or an active control drug. The report concluded that benzodiazepines should remain the drugs of choice for treatment of acute ethanol withdrawal.

Kruse JA, Cadnapaphornchai P: The serum osmole gap. J Crit Care 1994; 9:185-197.

This comprehensive review covers the underlying principles, derivation, clinical utility, and interpretation of the serum osmole gap. The review includes important caveats regarding factors that can lead to false-negative and false-positive findings.

Winter ML, Ellis MD, Snodgrass WR: Urine fluorescence using a Wood's lamp to detect the antifreeze additive sodium fluorescein: A qualitative adjunctive test in suspected ethylene glycol ingestions. Ann Emerg Med 1990;19:663-667.

This study involving healthy volunteers who ingested sodium fluorescein, documents the potential usefulness of exposing urine samples to ultraviolet radiation as a simple means of identifying occult toxic exposure to ethylene glycol–based automotive antifreeze. Various pitfalls and limitations of the technique are described.

Chapter 188

ANTICONVULSANTS IN THE INTENSIVE CARE UNIT

Marek Mirski

KEY POINTS

1. Most anticonvulsants have their action on **hepatic metabolism and affect protein binding,** frequently leading to altered kinetics of other agents. This is especially important when dealing with the critically ill patient. Vigilant monitoring of serum anticonvulsant levels may be required, and altered dosing of other medications may be also necessary.

2. Management of severe toxicity requires comprehensive supportive therapy, which includes **airway management and hemodynamic support.** The use of oral activated charcoal has been an effective therapy for some agents, as has been hemapheresis.

3. **Benzodiazepines** possess nominal overt toxicity, mostly interfering with the neurologic examination because of their γ-aminobutyric acid (GABA)–agonist mechanism of action. It is important to be cognizant of potential dependence or withdrawal symptoms on discontinuation or reduction in dose after prolonged therapy.

4. **Diazepam is not commonly advocated,** because both midazolam and lorazepam possess superior qualities regarding ease of delivery, fewer adverse effects, and superior pharmacodynamics of drug action.

5. **Phenytoin and fosphenytoin** are popular agents for seizure control in the intensive care unit (ICU), despite several key drawbacks. Drug interactions are a major concern, as are the adverse actions of these drugs, such as potential for cardiac dysrhythmias and bone marrow suppression.

6. **Phenytoin** should be reserved only for patients with well-functioning peripheral intravenous or central lines. Fosphenytoin may be administered intramuscularly as well as intravenously.

7. **Carbamazepine,** like phenytoin, is a potent inducer of hepatic enzymes. Altered kinetics of other drugs may be a complicating feature of ICU care.

8. **SIADH is a common adverse event** in patients treated with carbamazepine.

9. **Valproic acid** is available in intravenous and oral forms, providing optimal ICU utility, like phenytoin, phenobarbital, and benzodiazepines. **Hyperammonemia** is a common adverse effect of valproate therapy. **Pancreatitis and hepatic dysfunction** are additional risks with valproic acid.

10. **Propofol** is not an anticonvulsant in low, sedative doses. It terminates seizures via suppression of cortical electroencephalographic activity only. Propofol is not recommended for prolonged control of status epilepticus because of potential myocardial dysfunction and lactic acidosis. Propofol cannot be used for patients who are intolerant of eggs or who have gross hepatic dysfunction or failure. Strict aseptic technique must be observed.

11. **Phenobarbital** remains a drug to be considered for seizure control and termination in the ICU. Aside from hepatic enzyme induction, it is relatively devoid of serious toxicity. Phenobarbital has an extremely long half-life of more than 100 hours.

12. All recently approved anticonvulsants are available **in oral forms only,** limiting ICU utility.

13. **Levetiracetam** possesses few toxicities and drug interactions, making a strong showing in ICU practice as an adjunctive anticonvulsant. Monotherapy in the ICU has not been established but may be effective.

The treatment of seizures in the intensive care unit (ICU) involves two distinct elements: (1) the acute termination of ictal activity and (2) the prevention of further seizures. Many seizures manifest as a single, self-limited episode, which should alert the ICU team, in a dramatic fashion, that a metabolic or structural abnormality exists. Correcting the underlying pathology and initiating prophylaxis may prevent seizure recurrence in such cases. In these instances in the ICU, acute treatment is not necessary. Prophylaxis against recurrence may not be warranted if the precipitating factors have been dealt with in an optimal fashion. However, because of the potential for escalation to refractory seizures, it is common to prescribe seizure prophylaxis for a patient in the ICU once a seizure has been documented. To optimally treat patients in the ICU who have seizures or are at risk for seizures, the risks and benefits of the anticonvulsant must be assessed before initiation of therapy.

ANTICONVULSANTS: GENERAL CONCERNS

An ideal anticonvulsant for use in the ICU would be available for intravenous (i.v.) administration, unlikely to cause phlebitis, highly lipid soluble to promote optimal penetration into the central nervous system (CNS), devoid of sedative effects, able to provide prolonged protection against seizures, free of toxic side effects, characterized by having pharmacologically inactive metabolites, and not dependent on hepatic or renal clearance mechanisms. It is obvious from a cursory review of the drug armamentarium that no available anticonvulsant is ideal.

Individual anticonvulsant medications are primarily selected for use against specific seizure types. Some agents are mostly used for acute or emergency therapy, whereas others are primarily indicated for chronic prophylaxis against seizures. In the ICU, however, additional concerns arise that are related to the potential for drug-induced side effects. Both idiosyncratic and dose-dependent complications of therapy can occur. Various factors are implicated in the development of toxicity secondary anticonvulsant therapy. The following sections describe common metabolic and pharmacodynamic features of anticonvulsants that are important concerns in ICU practice.

PROTEIN BINDING

Drugs such as phenytoin, carbamazepine, and valproic acid are extensively protein bound, yet it is the free drug in the circulation that is the active moiety. Critically ill patients are often catabolic and have reduced plasma protein levels. Accordingly, free drug concentrations may be significantly increased despite normal total serum drug levels.[1] There is often discordance between total and free serum levels in patients with hepatic or renal dysfunction. Routine monitoring of free drug levels is expensive but warranted in these patients. However, most hospital laboratories are unable to provide the clinician with free drug levels for most anticonvulsants; phenytoin is the only common exception to this rule.

SEDATION AND COGNITIVE IMPAIRMENT

Sedation and cognitive impairment are the two most common *dose-dependent* side effects of anticonvulsants. They occur commonly even when the drug level is in the therapeutic range. These complications are particularly common in the elderly and the seriously ill. Significant impairment can be seen with the use of phenobarbital, primidone, phenytoin (if administered rapidly), and topiramate.

METABOLIC DERANGEMENTS

Hyponatremia has been reported in patients given carbamazepine, oxcarbazepine, or other anticonvulsants (rarely), and has been implicated in the development of the syndrome of inappropriate antidiuretic hormone (SIADH) (Table 188-1). Patients at risk for hyponatremia include the elderly, menstruating women, those requiring high fluid intake, those with renal failure, postoperative patients, and those requiring concurrent therapy with medications that also can cause hyponatremia.[2]

DRUG FEVER

The development of a fever coincident with the initiation of anticonvulsant therapy in the ICU setting complicates patient management. Development of drug fever is particularly common with phenytoin and fosphenytoin, but it can

TABLE 188–1. MEDICATIONS ASSOCIATED WITH THE SYNDROME OF INAPPROPRIATE ANTIDIURETIC HORMONE

Barbiturates	Haloperidol
Carbamazepine	Chlorpropamide
Oxcarbazepine	Thioridazine
Thiazides	Imipramine
Vincristine	Monoamine oxidase inhibitors
Cyclophosphamide	Bromocriptine
General anesthetics	Oxytocin
Nicotine	Acetamides
Clofibrate	Tolbutamide
Nonsteroidal anti-inflammatory drugs	

Adapted from Asconape J: Some common issues in the use of antiepileptic drugs. Semin Neurol 2002;22:27.

occur with other anticonvulsants as well.[1] A rise in the peripheral eosinophil count supports the diagnosis of drug fever. However, it is frequently the case that a trial with an alternative anticonvulsant is necessary to firmly diagnose drug-induced fever.

ALTERATION IN NEUROLOGIC EXAMINATION

Ataxia and brainstem dysfunction may be a result of phenytoin or carbamazepine toxicity, and valproic acid can induce tremors. Carbamazepine toxicity can be biphasic, manifesting acutely due to the parent compound and subacutely as a consequence of accumulation of the toxic 10,11-epoxide metabolite.[1]

RENAL DISEASE

Clearance of anticonvulsants can be significantly perturbed when the glomerular filtration rate (GFR) decreases to less than 10 mL/min. Clearance of phenobarbital and carbamazepine are not greatly affected, but phenytoin and valproic acid serum levels can rise or fall as a function of changes in GFR. In these cases, free levels may be a better guide to dosing, because of the high level of protein binding exhibited by these agents.[1] During dialysis, phenytoin levels are not dramatically affected, but phenobarbital levels are.

DRUG INTERACTIONS

Many anticonvulsants have effects on hepatic metabolism and protein binding, leading to altered kinetics of other agents. Phenytoin, carbamazepine, and phenobarbital, for example, are all potent stimulators of hepatic P_{450} enzyme systems (Tables 188-2 and 188-3) and can affect the concentration of other medications (Tables 188-5 and 188-6), including concomitantly administered anticonvulsant drugs (see Table 188-4). Phenytoin can reduce the plasma concentration of carbamazepine and valproic acid, whereas the interaction with phenobarbital is variable. Phenytoin decreases the effectiveness of warfarin and theophylline. Valproic acid inhibits the metabolism of phenobarbital and carbamazepine (including its 10,11-epoxide metabolite), which can increase serum levels of these drugs. Carbamazepine increases the hepatic metabolism of diazepam and valproic acid. Phenobarbital results in decreased levels

TABLE 188–2. METABOLIC PATHWAYS OF ANTICONVULSANT DRUGS

CYP1A2	CYP2C9	CYP2C19	CYP3A4
Carbamazepine*	Phenytoin Phenobarbital Valproate*	Phenytoin* Diazepam	Carbamazepine Tiagabine Zonisamide Ethosuximide Felbamate

*Minor metabolic pathway.
CYP, cytochrome P450.
Adapted from Asconape J: Some common issues in the use of antiepileptic drugs. Semin Neurol 2002;22:27.

TABLE 188–3. ANTICONVULSANT INDUCTION OF HEPATIC METABOLIC ENZYMES

Inducers	Inhibitors	No or Minimal Effect
Carbamazepine Phenytoin Phenobarbital Primidone	Valproate Felbamate	Gabapentin Lamotrigine Topiramate Tiagabine Oxcarbazepine Levetiracetam Zonisamide

Adapted from Asconape J: Some common issues in the use of antiepileptic drugs. Semin Neurol 2002;22:27.

of warfarin, theophylline, and cimetidine.[5] Cimetidine, amiodarone, isoniazid, and chlorpromazine all decrease hepatic metabolism of many drugs, and phenytoin is commonly affected (Table 188–6). Conversely, drugs that can decrease phenytoin levels include digoxin, cyclosporine, corticosteroids, warfarin, and theophylline. Aluminum hydroxide, magnesium hydroxide, and calcium antacids decrease the absorption of enterally administered phenytoin.

IDIOSYNCRATIC REACTIONS

Hypersensitivity is common with phenytoin and carbamazepine. Common features include fever, rash, and eosinophilia.[1] Drugs with a high risk for rash include phenytoin, phenobarbital, primidone, lamotrigine, carbamazepine, oxcarbazepine, and zonisamide (Table 188–7).[3] Transient leukopenia and thrombocytopenia is commonly seen with carbamazepine and valproate. Less common drug effects include hepatic failure, pancreatitis (valproic acid), agranulocytosis, aplastic anemia, megaloblastic anemia (phenytoin), Stevens-Johnson syndrome, and a lupus-like syndrome. Severe hepatic dysfunction, although rare, may occur with valproic acid therapy secondary to a toxic metabolite. This potentially fatal action most often occurs in children younger than 2 years of age who are receiving aspirin and polypharmacy for seizure control.

MANAGEMENT OF ANTICONVULSANT TOXICITY

Management of severe toxicity requires comprehensive supportive therapy, including airway management, hemodynamic support, and oral administration of activated charcoal, which has been especially useful for acute valproate acid intoxication.[6] Concurrent hemoperfusion and hemodialysis to enhance elimination of the anticonvulsant has been described in cases of valproic acid or carbamazepine poisoning in which the patients were hemodynamically unstable and their clinical condition was worsening despite aggressive supportive care.[7]

SPECIFIC ANTICONVULSANT PROPERTIES BY CLASS

BENZODIAZEPINES

For immediate therapy, benzodiazepines are still considered the first line of treatment against most seizures. These drugs are highly lipophilic and are potent agonists for the γ-aminobutyric acid (GABA) receptor on neurons. These agents improve local inhibition of signal transmission. The most commonly used benzodiazepines in the ICU are diazepam, lorazepam, and midazolam. In cases of hepatic failure, oxazepam may be preferred, because it is the one benzodiazepine that is not metabolized by the liver.[8]

There are instances in which where short-acting benzodiazepines (i.e., midazolam, diazepam) may be preferable. Neurologic assessment and management may be seriously confounded in patients receiving anticonvulsants that cause prolonged sedation. If such concerns exist, it may be preferable to initiate treatment of seizures using a short-acting benzodiazepine, followed immediately by a loading dose of a less-sedating medication, such as phenytoin or other maintenance anticonvulsant.

If the seizures have not been brought under control by therapeutic doses of benzodiazepines, additional medications are in order. Tachyphylaxis rapidly develops with the use of

TABLE 188–4. ALTERATIONS IN DRUG PLASMA LEVELS WITH COMBINATION ANTICONVULSANT USE

Added Drug	%*	Effect on Plasma Levels of Primary Agents				
		Phenytoin	Phenobarbital	Carbamazepine	Valproic Acid	Benzodiazepines
Phenytoin	90	—	Variable	↓	↓	—
Phenobarbital	45	↑, then ↓	—	Variable	↓	↓
Carbamazepine	75	Variable	Variable	↓	↓	↓
Valproic acid	90	↓, but ↑ in free levels	↑	Variable or ↑ in 10,11-epoxide	—	↑
Benzodiazepines	—	↓	Variable	—	Variable	—

*Percentage serum protein bound.
↓, Decrease; ↑, increase.
Adapted from Varelas PN, Mirski MA: Seizures in the adult intensive care unit. J Neurosurg Anesthesiol 2001;13:163.

TABLE 188–5. EFFECTS OF ANTICONVULSANT DRUGS ON COMMONLY USED MEDICATIONS

	Effect on Plasma Levels or Clinical Effectiveness of Primary Agent				
Added Drug	*Warfarin*	*Theophylline*	*Corticosteroids*	*Haloperidol*	*Lithium*
Phenytoin	↓	↓	↓	—	—
Phenobarbital	↓	↓	↓	↓	↑

↓, Decrease; ↑, increase.
Adapted from Varelas PN, Mirski MA: Seizures in the adult intensive care unit. J Neurosurg Anesthesiology 2001;13:163.

benzodiazepines, and these agents are not suitable for chronic prevention of seizures. Common **second-line agents**, which are useful because of their efficacy and availability in i.v. formulations, include (1) phenytoin and fosphenytoin, (2) carbamazepine, and (3) valproic acid.

Diazepam

Diazepam (Valium) has been historically popular, although its use has been declining because of the availability of superior agents, namely midazolam and lorazepam. After administration, diazepam, which is highly lipophilic, rapidly redistributes from the plasma into tissues. The anticonvulsant duration is just a few minutes. Diazepam is not water soluble and requires emulsification with a vehicle (propylene glycol) for i.v. administration. Therefore, this drug can irritate veins and should be administered slowly, preferably into a large vein.

Dosing

Adults. The oral dose in adults is 2 to 10 mg, administered two to four times per day; the i.v. dose is 2 to 4 mg and may be repeated in 3 to 4 hours if needed. In status epilepticus, the i.v. dose is 5 to 10 mg every 10 to 20 minutes, up to 30 mg in an 8-hour period.

Elderly. In elderly patients, absorption is more reliable by the oral rather than the intramuscular (i.m.) route; consider a dosage reduction in elderly patients.[9,10]

TABLE 188–6. COMMON DRUG INTERACTIONS WITH PHENYTOIN AND CARBAMAZEPINE

Added Drug	Phenytoin	Carbamazepine
Salicylates	↑	—
Erythromycin	—	↑↑
Chloramphenicol	↑	—
Trimethoprim	↑	—
Isoniazid	↑	↑
Propoxyphene	↑	↑
Amiodarone	↑	—
Diltiazem, verapamil	—	↑
Cimetidine	↑	↑
Ethanol	↓	—
Rifampin	↓	—
Digitoxin	↓	—
Cyclosporine	↓	—
Warfarin	↓	—
Theophylline	↓	—
Glucocorticoids	↓	—

↓, Decrease in plasma levels; ↑, increase in plasma levels; ↑↑, large increase in plasma levels.
Adapted from Varelas PN, Mirski MA: Seizures in the adult intensive care unit. J Neurosurg Anesthesiology 2001;13:163.

Hepatic Impairment. Reduce the dose by 50% in patients with cirrhosis and avoid in those with severe or acute liver disease.

Renal Impairment. Diazepam is not dialyzable; supplemental dosing is not necessary.

Forms Available. Forms available include rectal gel, 5 mg/mL (15 mg, 20 mg); injection solution, 5 mg/mL; oral solution, 5 mg/mL (30 mL); and tablet (2 mg, 5 mg, 10 mg).

Mechanisms of Action. Diazepam binds to GABA-A receptors, resulting in opening of a chloride channel, with resulting hyperpolarization and inhibition of neuronal firing.

Pharmacokinetics

Oral Absorption. Diazepam is 85% to 100% absorbed following oral administration.

Distribution. Diazepam is 98% protein bound.

Elimination. The half-life of the parent drug is 20 to 50 hours; that of the active major metabolite (desmethyldiazepam) is 50 to 100 hours.

Metabolism. Diazepam is metabolized in the liver.

Drug Interactions. Theophylline can antagonize the effects of benzodiazepines. Oral contraceptives can decrease clearance. Therapeutic effects of levodopa may be reduced. Additive sedative effects, respiratory depression, or both may occur with ethanol, barbiturates, and narcotic analgesics. The potential for P_{450} enzyme induction exists with phenobarbital, phenytoin, carbamazepine, rifampin, and rifabutin.[1,4,5]

Adverse Reactions and Toxicities. Hypotension, drowsiness, ataxia, paradoxical excitement or rage, memory impairment, rash, decrease in respiratory rate, and frank apnea all can occur after diazepam administration. All benzodiazepines are associated with dependence or withdrawal symptoms on discontinuation or reduction in dose after prolonged therapy.[11] Acute withdrawal symptoms, including seizures, may be

TABLE 188–7. ANTIEPILEPTIC DRUGS AND RISK OF SKIN RASH

High Risk	Low Risk
Phenytoin	Valproate
Phenobarbital	Topiramate
Primidone	Gabapentin
Carbamazepine	Tiagabine
Oxcarbazepine	Levetiracetam
Lamotrigine	
Zonisamide	

Adapted from Asconape J: Some common issues in the use of antiepileptic drugs. Semin Neurol 2002;22:27.

precipitated in such cases. Administration of the GABA antagonist flumazenil may induce withdrawal symptoms and seizures in patients receiving benzodiazepines for prolonged periods.[12]

Contraindications. Contraindications are narrow-angle glaucoma and pregnancy.

Midazolam

Midazolam has largely replaced diazepam for use as a short-acting benzodiazepine. It is highly lipophilic, and its effects appear rapidly (within one to two circulation times within the CNS).[13] Midazolam is marketed as a water-soluble compound; when injected intravenously, the drug is transformed into a lipophilic compound by virtue of the rapid closure of the diazepine ring. Therefore, the drug is less irritating to veins than diazepam.

Dosing

Adults. The initial i.v. dose is 0.5 to 2 mg; no more than 2.5 mg should be administered over a period of 2 minutes. A total dose greater than 5 mg usually is not required. The maintenance dose is approximately 25% of the dose needed to reach the sedative effect. Consider a decrease in dosage by 30% if narcotics or other CNS depressants are administered concurrently.

Elderly. Consider a dosage reduction based on altered kinetics[14] and sensitivity in elderly patients.

Hepatic Impairment. Reduce the dose by 50% in patients with cirrhosis and avoid in those with severe or acute liver disease.

Renal Impairment. Midazolam is not dialyzable; supplemental dosing is not necessary.

Forms Available. Forms available include injection solution, 1 mg/mL (2 mL, 5 mL, 10 mL) and 5 mg/mL (1 mL, 2 mL, 5 mL, 10 mL); syrup, 2 mg/mL (118 mL) and tablet (2 mg, 5 mg, 10 mg).

Mechanisms of Action. Midazolam binds to GABA-A receptors, resulting in opening of a chloride channel, with resultant hyperpolarization and inhibition of neuronal firing.

Pharmcokinetics

Absorption. The bioavailability of midazolam is 45%.

Distribution. The volume of distribution (V_d) is 0.8 to 2.5 L/kg; midazolam is 95% protein bound.

Elimination. The half-life of the parent drug is 1 to 4 hours.

Metabolism. Midazolam is hepatically metabolized, being biotransformed into two active metabolites: α-hydroxymidazolam (60% potency) and α-hydroxymidazolam glucuronide (10% potency). Less than 1% of the drug is excreted unchanged in the urine, the excreted compounds being glucuronide-conjugated metabolites.[13]

Drug Interactions. Midazolam's drug interactions are the same as those of diazepam.

Adverse Reactions and Toxicities. Modazolam's adverse reactions and toxicities are the same as those of diazepam.

Contraindications. Contradictions are narrow-angle glaucoma and pregnancy.

Lorazepam

Lorazepam is the least lipid-soluble agent among the three commonly used benzodiazepines. As a result, lorazepam has a delayed onset of action and prolonged duration of effect.[15] It is ideally suited for acute therapy together with longer-acting prophylaxis against seizure recurrence. In a 5-year randomized, double-blind, multicenter trial of four i.v. regimens for the treatment of generalized status epilepticus, Treiman and colleagues[16] found that lorazepam (0.1 mg/kg) was successful in 64.9% of patients and was significantly superior to phenytoin ($P = .002$) in a pair-wise comparison. It is important to note that the longer duration of action of lorazepam may adversely affect the neurologic examination for several hours, potentially complicating diagnosis and medical management.

Dosing

Adults. The oral dose is 1 to 2 mg every 30 to 60 minutes for tranquilization of an agitated patient. The i.v. dose is 2 to 4 mg and may be repeated in 3 to 4 hours if needed. In status epilepticus, the i.v. dose is 4 to 8 mg given over 2 to 5 minutes; alternatively, a dose of 0.1 mg/kg may be used. Lorazepam may be given intramuscularly with little discomfort.

Elderly. Consider dosage reduction in elderly patients.

Hepatic Impairment. Reduce the dose by 50% in patients with cirrhosis and avoid in those with severe or acute liver disease.

Renal Impairment. Lorazepam is not dialyzable; supplemental dosing is not necessary. Large doses of the polyethylene glycol emulsion can cause nephrotoxicity.[17]

Forms Available. Forms available include injection solution, 2 mg/mL (30 mL) and tablet (0.5 mg, 1 mg, 2 mg).

Mechanisms of Action. Lorazepam binds to GABA-A receptors, resulting in opening of the GABA chloride channel, with resultant hyperpolarization and inhibition of neuronal firing.

Pharmacokinetics

Absorption. Absorption of lorazepam is rapid in the CNS.

Distribution. Lorazepam is 85% protein bound; the V_d is 1.3 L/kg in adults.

Elimination. Hepatic metabolism is followed by renal excretion.

Metabolism. Hepatic metabolism leads to inactive compounds. Metabolism of lorazepam is inhibited by valproic acid. The drug half-life is 12.9 hours in adults, 15.9 hours in the elderly, and 32 to 70 hours in patients with end-stage renal disease.

Drug Interactions. Lorazepam's drug interactions are the same as those of diazepam.

Adverse Reactions and Toxicities. Lorazepam's adverse reactions and toxicities are similar to those of diazepam. Additionally, use of lorazepam in higher doses and in infusions has been associated with lactic acidosis, hyperosmolar coma, and a reversible nephrotoxicity caused by the solvents, propylene glycol and polyethylene.[17]

Contraindications. Contraindications are narrow-angle glaucoma and pregnancy.

Phenytoin

Phenytoin has been and remains the drug most commonly used in the ICU for seizure prophylaxis, for several reasons: ease of administration, readily available i.v. and oral forms, rare severe toxicity, and efficacy against many seizure syndromes that occur in the ICU setting, including status epilepticus. Phenytoin has been shown to decrease the incidence of seizures during the first week after traumatic head injury by 73% compared with placebo.[18] In light of its non–GABA agonist action, phenytoin is not particularly effective against most drug-induced convulsions, especially those triggered by β-lactam antibiotics. These agents induce seizures through their GABA-antagonist action. Phenytoin is indicated for use against generalized tonic-clonic seizures, focal and complex partial seizures, and prevention of seizures after head trauma or neurosurgery.

Dosing

Adults. For seizure prophylaxis or initial therapy to combat seizures, the loading dose is 15 to 20 mg/kg i.v.; the oral loading dose should be given in three divided doses every 2 hours. For i.v. administration, the drug should be given at a rate of less than 50 mg/min, because the glycol vehicle can cause hypotension and heart block. The maintenance dose of 5 to 6 mg/kg/day orally may given as one dose or in divided doses.

Elderly. Because of the increased likelihood of hypotension and heart block, the administration rate should be decreased in elderly patients (e.g., 20 mg/min).

Hepatic Impairment. Phenytoin should be used with caution in patients with hepatic impairment, because there is decreased clearance of the drug in cirrhosis. Monitoring of liver function tests and free phenytoin levels is advocated.

Renal Impairment. In patients with renal insufficiency, the interpretation of total levels is difficult, because the free fraction is increased due to the reduction of plasma protein concentration. Monitoring of free serum levels is recommended.

Forms Available. Forms available include capsule (30 mg, 100 mg, 200 mg, 300 mg); injection solution, 50 mg/mL (2 mL, 5 mL); oral suspension, 125 mg/5 mL (240 mL); and chewable tablet (50 mg).

Mechanisms of Action. Phenytoin's mechanism is not entirely clear, although the drug blocks sodium channels, which reduces neuronal excitation.

Pharmacokinetics

Absorption. Phenytoin is slowly absorbed orally, and its absorption is even slower when it is given concurrently with enteral feedings. Therefore, tube feedings should be discontinued 2 hours before and 2 hours after each enteral dose of the drug. The bioavailability of phenytoin is form dependent. The reference target range is 10 to 20 μg/mL total; the reference target range for free drug level is 0.1 to 0.2 μg/mL. One should monitor free levels in physiologic states that cause decreased serum albumin concentration (e.g., burns, head injury,[19] hepatic cirrhosis, nephrotic syndrome, pregnancy, cystic fibrosis, hepatic failure, renal failure).

Distribution. The V_d is 0.6 to 0.7 L/kg; phenytoin is 90% to 95% protein bound.

Elimination. After being hepatically metabolized, phenytoin is excreted in the urine as glucuronides with a half-life of approximately 22 hours.

Metabolism. Phenytoin is metabolized by the liver. Phenytoin metabolism obeys dose-dependent capacity-limited (Michaelis-Menten) pharmacokinetics. Serum and free levels can abruptly increase once the capacity for metabolism is exceeded (zero-order kinetics).

Drug Interactions. As isolated phenomena, phenytoin can enhance the hepatotoxicity of acetaminophen, blunt the diuretic effect of furosemide, increase the metabolism of 3-hydroxy-3-methyl-glutaryl coenzyme A (HMG-CoA) reductase inhibitors, decrease the duration of effect of neuromuscular blocking agents, and reduce the metabolism of thyroid hormones.[4,5] Antacids can decrease the absorption of phenytoin, whereas amiodarone can increase its serum concentration. The sedative effects of this anticonvulsant may be additive with those of other CNS depressants.

As an inducing agent for hepatic metabolism, phenytoin increases the clearance of corticosteroids and many anticonvulsants (barbiturates, carbamazepine, ethosuximide, felbamate, lamotrigine, tiagabine, topiramate, and zonisamide).[5] Therefore, anticonvulsant polypharmacy can be frustrated by the addition of phenytoin. However, phenytoin does not affect gabapentin or levetiracetam levels. As would be expected, serum levels of phenytoin may be decreased by concomitant use of other hepatic enzyme inducers (e.g., barbiturates, carbamazepine, ethanol, dexamethasone, rifampin). Because of hepatic P_{450} enzyme induction, the use of phenytoin should be avoided if possible in patients with porphyria.

In contrast, hepatic enzyme CYP3A4 inhibitors (amiodarone, cimetidine, fluvoxamine, some nonsteroidal antiinflammatory drugs, metronidazole, ritonavir, sulfonamides, troglitazone, valproic acid) and the CYP2C19 inhibitors (felbamate, fluconazole, fluoxetine, fluvoxamine, omeprazole) can increase serum phenytoin levels.[3]

Adverse Reactions and Toxicities. Phenytoin has been associated with thrombophlebitis and toxic epidermal necrolysis.[20,21] If phenytoin is administered rapidly (faster than 50 mg/min), it can cause hypotension, bradycardia, and bundle branch block. A phenytoin-induced rash is common (20%).[3] Hyperglycemia, leukopenia, and thrombocytopenia have been reported. Skin necrosis at the infusion site is a strong argument for conversion to fosphenytoin, and this newer agent also should be considered if good venous access is questionable. Small veins can develop phlebitis and can be the source of transient discomfort during infusion, even if no extravasation occurs.

Side effects with long-term use include gingival hypertrophy, cerebellar atrophy, coarsening of facial features, osteoporosis, vitamin D deficiency, and peripheral neuropathy.[1,3,4]

If phenytoin is administered in high doses or high concentrations, nystagmus, diplopia, ataxia, slurred speech, drowsiness, and coma may occur.

Fosphenytoin

Fosphenytoin (Cerebyx) is a phosphate ester prodrug of phenytoin. It is highly water soluble. If administered parenterally (i.v. or i.m.), fosphenytoin is rapidly metabolized into phenytoin. It can be infused up to three times faster than phenytoin (150 mg/min).[22] The time to peak serum effect is similar to that of phenytoin because of enzymatic conversion. Kugler and colleagues[23] suggested that fosphenytoin and phenytoin are likely to have similar times of onset of effect in controlling status epilepticus. The benefits of fosphenytoin are faster administration rate and less problem with adverse effects (hypotension, phlebitis, and soft-tissue injury from extravasation). Although fosphenytoin is a more expensive alternative, the cost of treating the complications from the use of i.v. phenytoin can be substantially higher.[20]

Dosing

Although fosphenytoin is a different drug from phenytoin when initially administered, its dosage is always described as phenytoin equivalents (PE). Because fosphenytoin is water soluble, it can be administered safely by the i.m. route (phenytoin cannot).[24]

Adults. For acute management and in prophylaxis, 15 to 20 mg/kg phenytoin equivalents i.v. is administered at a rate of 100 to 150 mg/min.[22] The maintenance dose is 4 to 6 mg/kg/day i.v. or i.m. Phenytoin is 90% bioavailable when given orally, compared with 100% when given parenterally.

Therefore, a higher dosage may be necessary when converting from parenteral to oral administration. The therapeutic range is the same as for phenytoin, 10 to 20 μg/mL.

Elderly. The geriatric population may be more sensitive to hypotension and sedation associated with higher infusion rates.

Hepatic Impairment. Phenytoin clearance can be markedly reduced in cirrhosis; free levels should be monitored.

Renal Impairment. Free phenytoin levels should be monitored closely. Phenytoin is not significantly dialyzed.

Forms Available. Forms available include injection solution, 75 mg/mL (equivalent to phenytoin sodium, 50 mg/mL).

Mechanisms of Action. Fosphenytoin is the diphosphate ester salt of phenytoin; it acts as a water-soluble prodrug of phenytoin. After administration, plasma esterases convert fosphenytoin to phosphate, formaldehyde, and phenytoin, the active moiety. Phenytoin acts as a sodium channel blocker to reduce neuronal excitability.

Pharmacokinetics

Absorption. The rise in serum concentration of fosphenytoin may be faster compared with phenytoin when fosphenytoin is administered i.v., because of the higher maximal recommended infusion rate (150 mg/min, versus 50 mg/min for phenytoin). However, because of the necessary biotransformation (conversion to phenytoin after i.v. administration takes about 15 minutes), the resulting time required to reach peak serum level of phenytoin is similar for the two agents.[22] The bioavailability of each approaches 100%.

Distribution. Between 95% and 99% of fosphenytoin is bound to albumin. During i.v. administration, fosphenytoin can displace phenytoin and increase the free fraction (up to 30% unbound) during the period required for conversion of fosphenytoin to phenytoin. The half-life of fosphenytoin is 12 to 29 hours.

Elimination. Fosphenytoin is excreted in the urine as an inactive metabolite.

Metabolism. Fosphenytoin is converted via hydrolysis to phenytoin. See phenytoin for further metabolism.

Drug Interactions. The drug interactions of fosphenytoin are the same as for phenytoin.

Adverse Reactions and Toxicities. The most important side effects with i.v. use of fosphenytoin (or phenytoin) are cardiovascular collapse and CNS depression. Paresthesias and pruritus are more common with fosphenytoin than phenytoin, and they occur more often with i.v. than with i.m. administration.[3,4] The drug is contraindicated in patients with sinus bradycardia, sinoatrial block, second- or third-degree atrioventricular block, or Stokes-Adams syndrome. As with phenytoin, it is important to monitor the hematologic profile and liver function tests. Other side effects include gingival hyperplasia, gynecomastia, bone marrow suppression, and vermian cerebellar atrophy.[3,4] Venous irritation is less common with fosphenytoin than with phenytoin.[25]

Contraindications. Fosphenytoin is a pregnancy category D drug.

Carbamazepine

Carbamazepine (Tegretol) is indicated for partial seizures with complex symptomatology (psychomotor, temporal lobe), generalized tonic-clonic (grand mal) seizures, and mixed seizure patterns. The drug is not available for i.v.

administration and therefore is not typically used for acute termination of seizures or prophylaxis against seizures in the ICU. When using carbamazepine, it is recommended that the following parameters be monitored (see later discussion): complete blood count, reticulocyte count, serum iron concentration, liver function tests, urinalysis, serum electrolyte panel, serum drug levels, and thyroid function tests.

Dosing

Adults. Typically, carbamazepine is administered as 200 mg two or three times daily, then increased by 200 mg/day at weekly intervals until therapeutic levels are achieved. The usual therapeutic dose is 800 to 1200 mg/day in three or four divided doses. Dosage must be adjusted according to the patient's response. The target serum concentration 4 to 12 μg/mL.[26]

Elderly. Lower doses typically are used in elderly patients (100 mg one to two times per day). The typical dose is 400 to 1000 mg/day.

Hepatic Impairment. Carbamazepine is hepatically metabolized to an epoxide intermediate, which itself has an appreciable anticonvulsant action.

Renal Impairment. In renal impairment, if GFR is less than 10 mL/min, administer 75% of the typical dose.

Forms Available. Forms available include extended-release capsule (200 mg, 300 mg); oral suspension (100 mg/5 mL); tablet (200 mg); chewable tablet (100 mg); and extended-release tablet (100 mg, 200 mg, 400 mg).

Mechanisms of Action. Like phenytoin, carbamazepine acts as a sodium channel blocker. It also stimulates the release of antidiuretic hormone and is chemically related to the tricyclic antidepressants.

Pharmacokinetics

Absorption. Orally administered doses of carbamazepine are slowly absorbed; the time to peak serum concentration is 4 to 8 hours. Bioavailability approximates 85%.

Distribution. The V_d of carbamazepine is 0.9 L/kg in adults, with 75% to 90% of the drug being protein bound.[26]

Elimination. Carbamazepine is excreted in the urine.

Metabolism. Carbamazepine is hepatically metabolized to a pharmacologically active epoxide metabolite; the half-life is 8 to 60 hours.[27]

Drug Interactions. The oral carbamazepine suspension should not be administered at the same time as other liquid medicinal agents, because it can form a precipitate when combined with chlorpromazine or thioridazine. Barbiturates, benzodiazepines, and phenytoin can decrease carbamazepine levels, owing to induction of hepatic metabolism.[4,5] Conversely, isoniazid, felbamate, danazol, diltiazem, and verapamil can increase carbamazepine levels. Carbamazepine itself can increase the metabolism of warfarin, valproic acid, tricyclic antidepressants (particularly the serotonin-mediated agents), thyroid hormone, theophylline, oral contraceptives, methadone, doxycycline, corticosteroids, calcium channel blockers (except diltiazem and verapamil), cyclosporine, tacrolimus, and ethosuximide.[4]

Adverse Reactions and Toxicities. Like phenytoin, carbamazepine may induce atrioventricular block and other dysrhythmias.[28] Also, sedation, dizziness, ataxia, and rash may occur after carbamazepine administration, although less commonly than is the case with phenytoin. Severe hyponatremia secondary to SIADH is relatively commonly associated with use of carbamazepine.[2] Nausea, aplastic anemia, agranulocytosis, thrombocytopenia, bone marrow suppression, and hepatic failure have all been reported. Carbamazepine is a pregnancy category D drug.

Contraindications. Carbamazepine should not be used concurrently with monoamine oxidase inhibitors, and it should be administered with caution to patients with hepatic, renal, or hematologic disease. Caution should be exercised in patients with increased intraocular pressure, because carbamazepine has mild anticholinergic activity.

Valproic Acid

Valproic acid is indicated as monotherapy and as adjunctive therapy for the treatment of almost all seizures types, including complex partial seizures, absence seizures, generalized tonic-clonic seizures, myoclonic seizures, and other partial seizures. Intravenous valproate was shown to be useful for the treatment of refractory status epilepticus in two European studies.[29,30] More recently, the licensing of an i.v. formulation in the United States has increased the utility of valproic acid in the ICU setting and as a treatment for acute seizures including status epilepticus.

Dosing

Adults. The usual oral adult dose of valproic acid is 10 to 15 mg/kg/day in three divided doses, increased by 5 to 10 mg/kg/day at weekly intervals until therapeutic levels are achieved. The maintenance dose is 30 to 60 mg/kg/day. Sustained-release valproic acid (Depakote ER) is usually given once daily. Conversion to the extended-release formulation may require an increase in the dose by 20%. The i.v. dose is 15 to 20 mg/kg. The drug should be infused no faster than 20 mg/min.

Elderly. The dosing of valproic acid in elderly patients is approximately the same as the adult dosing recommendation.

Hepatic Impairment. A dosage reduction is necessary with hepatic failure, because the clearance of valproic acid is decreased with liver impairment.[1,31] Decreased albumin concentration in hepatic disease is associated with a 2- to 2.6-fold increase in the unbound fraction. Therefore, free concentrations of valproate may be elevated while the total concentrations appear normal.

Renal Impairment. If GFR is less than 10 mL/min, a 27% reduction in clearance of unbound in valproic acid is seen. Hemodialysis reduces valproic acid concentrations by 20%, and the high degree of protein binding hinders the effectiveness of removal by dialysis.

Forms Available. Forms available include capsule (250 mg); capsule/sprinkles (125 mg); injection solution, 100 mg/mL (5 mL); syrup 250 mg/5mL (5 mL, 480 mL); delayed-release tablet (125 mg, 250 mg, 500 mg); and extended-release tablet (250 mg, 500 mg).

Mechanisms of Action. Current data suggest that valproic acid causes an increased availability of GABA or may enhance the action of GABA. It is also thought to act on thalamic (T-type) calcium channels as an inhibitor, and it may also cause sodium channel blockade and enhanced potassium channel conductance.

Pharmacokinetics

Absorption. Enteric forms of valproic acid are rapidly and almost completely absorbed from the gastrointestinal tract. Peak plasma concentrations are observed 1 to 4 hours after ingestion. Therapeutic serum concentrations are 50 to 125 μg/mL.

Distribution. Valproic acid is 80% to 90% protein bound. Hence, at usual concentrations or dosing, the V_d is only slightly greater than plasma volume.

Elimination. Valproic acid is excreted in the urine after hepatic metabolism. Less than 3% of the anticonvulsant is excreted unchanged in the urine, and it is eliminated by first-order kinetics. The half-life of valproic acid is 9 to 16 hours.

Metabolism. Valproic acid is metabolized extensively by the liver via glucuronic acid conjugation and mitochondrial beta and omega oxidation to produce multiple metabolites, some of which are biologically active.

Drug Interactions. Serum levels of valproic acid may be reduced by acyclovir, whereas lamotrigine and phenytoin can enhance metabolism of the drug.[4,5] Valproic acid can increase diazepam, lamotrigine, and carbamazepine concentrations.[32] Macrolide antibiotics and nimodipine can decrease metabolism of valproic acid. Valproic acid use inhibits metabolism of phenobarbital.

Adverse Reactions and Toxicities. The side effects of valproic acid include somnolence, dizziness, insomnia, alopecia, pancreatitis,[33] thrombocytopenia, tremor, weight gain, rash, bone marrow suppression,[34] decreased carnitine levels, hyperammonemia, and SIADH. Additionally, the anticonvulsant has been reported to cause frank hepatic failure. Developmentally, neural tube defects are a recognized toxicity. Valproic acid can stimulate the replication of human immunodeficiency virus and cytomegalovirus in infected patients.

Acute dose-dependent valproic acid intoxication induces mild to moderate lethargy in smaller doses, and coma or fatal cerebral edema in higher toxic amounts.[35] In contrast to either phenytoin or carbamazepine, nystagmus, dysarthria, and ataxia are rarely noted after valproic acid overdose. Valproic acid also can increase serum ammonia levels through interaction with carnitine. In the management of valproic acid intoxication, naloxone occasionally is effective.

Contraindications. Contradictions are pregnancy, urea cycle disorders, and hepatic dysfunction.

PROPOFOL

Typically used for induction or maintenance of anesthesia, propofol is occasionally used for the acute termination of seizures and for management of status epilepticus. Propofol is not a true anticonvulsant, because seizures are only terminated so long as general anesthesia is maintained by the drug. The drug must be used in association with continuous cardiac and blood pressure monitoring, and the patient must be prepared for mechanical ventilation. A major toxicity of propofol is its emulsion formulation. The drug itself acts similar to the ultrashort-acting barbiturates, although with a more rapid time of elimination.

Dosing

Adults. The dosage of propofol must be individualized based on total body weight and titrated to desired effect. As a continuous infusion, the initial sedation dose is usually 1.2 mg/kg/hour (20 μg/kg/min). However, for cessation of seizures, a dose that yields a general anesthetic state or a flat or "burst-suppression" electroencephalogram (EEG) is required. This dose is typically about 7.2 to 14.0 mg/kg/hour (120-240 μg/kg/min).[36] This can be increased by 1 to 2 mg/kg/hour every 5 to 10 minutes until the desired level of sedation or EEG correlate is achieved.

Elderly. Dosing in the geriatric population is reduced because it requires less drug to promote EEG silence or burst-suppression.

Hepatic Impairment. Propofol is hepatically metabolized, and some evidence suggests the existence of potentially toxic metabolic intermediates. These intermediates may accumulate during low-flow states such as hepatic congestion or decreased cardiac output.

Renal Impairment. Propofol is primarily hepatically metabolized, and the conjugated drug is excreted in the urine.

Forms Available. Propofol is available as an emulsion (10 or 20 mg/mL); it contains sodium metabisulfite, egg lecithin, soybean oil, and ethylene diamine tetraacetic acid (EDTA).

Mechanisms of Action. The mechanism of action of this drug appears to mirror that of the ultrashort-acting barbiturates that are GABA receptor agonists . It is a phenolic compound with general anesthetic properties. It is, however, structurally unrelated to the barbiturates, opioids, or benzodiazepines.

Pharmacokinetics

Absorption. The onset of action of propofol is extremely rapid (10 to 15 sec).[37]

Distribution. The drug is highly lipophilic, with a large V_d (2 to 10 L/kg). Propofol is 97% to 99% protein bound while in serum.

Elimination. The duration of action of propofol is approximately 3 to 5 minutes after a single bolus injection. It is excreted in the urine (88% as metabolites, 40% as the glucuronide metabolite). The clearance of propofol is 20 to 30 mL/kg/min, which exceeds liver blood flow.[37] This suggests that there are extrahepatic sites of propofol metabolism to account for the rapid clearance of the drug.

Metabolism. Propofol is metabolized in the liver (and possibly in additional sites) to water-soluble sulfate and glucuronide conjugates.

Drug Interactions. Propofol can potentiate the neuromuscular blockade of vecuronium.[36]

Adverse Reactions and Toxicities. Common side effects include a burning sensation at the injection site, hypotension, and apnea. Propofol can induce respiratory acidosis. The use of propofol can have more severe cardiovascular consequences in patients with severe cardiac disease (cardiac ejection fraction less than 50%). The emulsion can decrease circulating zinc levels due to binding of the cation by the additive, EDTA. Because of the insolubility of the drug, it is delivered as an emulsion that is a potential growth medium for bacteria.[38] EDTA is added to serve as a bacteriostatic agent, but the risk of contamination with bacteria remains a concern. Therefore, strict aseptic technique must be observed with its use, and routine changing of the i.v. delivery lines must be carried out.

Common clinical features of a "propofol infusion syndrome" have been described; findings can include hyperkalemia, hepatomegaly, lipemia, metabolic acidosis, myocardial failure, and rhabdomyolysis.[39] This syndrome was initially described in children who were cared for in the ICU for prolonged periods with high doses of propofol used for sedation.[40-42] It is apparent that adults can also be at risk for development of lactic acidosis and myocardial dysfunction.[39] Recently reported cases suggest an association between propofol infusion and death secondary to myocardial failure. Therefore, the safety recommendation is that propofol for use in the ICU be restricted to doses no greater than 5 mg/kg/hour, and that propofol infusion for sedation of critically ill adults should be limited to 48 hours, at least if high doses are used (general anesthetic depth).

Contraindications. Propofol is relatively contraindicated in patients with hyperlipidemia or also increased intracranial pressure or sepsis unless cerebral perfusion and visceral organ perfusion are supported. Because of the emulsion base, patients who are allergic to egg whites also should not be given this drug. The pregnancy risk factor is B. For seizure control, propofol is absolutely contraindicated in nonintubated patients because it is necessary to induce general anesthesia to terminate seizure activity.

PHENOBARBITAL

Phenobarbital remains a mainstay of anticonvulsant therapy. As a potent GABA agonist, phenobarbital is an effective anticonvulsant against a broad range of seizure types, being most commonly targeted against generalized motor seizures. A favorable feature is its relative lack of serious toxic effects. Additional desirable characteristics for use in the ICU include its broad efficacy, titratability to "burst-suppression" capability,[43-45] availability as an i.v. agent, and ease of transition to oral dosing, if desired. Its chief negative attributes are its long half-life and its ability to potently induce hepatic P_{450} enzymes.

Dosing

Adults. The oral dose is 30 to 120 mg/day in two or three divided doses; in status epilepticus, the loading dose is 15 to 18 mg/kg i.v.[45] The anticonvulsant maintenance dose ranges between 1 and 3 mg/kg/day in divided doses.

Elderly. Phenobarbital is not recommended for use in the elderly, yet it is still used to treat older patients in the outpatient setting.

Hepatic Impairment. Because phenobarbital is primarily metabolized in the liver, increased side effects may occur in patients with severe hepatic disease. The plasma drug levels and liver function tests should be monitored to estimate clearance of this already long-acting agent.

Renal Impairment. If GFR is less than 10 mL/min, it is advisable to administer the drug every 12 to 16 hours. Phenobarbital, unlike phenytoin, is substantively (20% to 50%) dialyzed during hemodialysis.

Forms Available. Forms available include elixir, 20 mg/5 mL; injection solution, 60 mg/mL and 130 mg/mL; and tablet (15 mg, 30 mg, 32 mg, 60 mg, 65 mg, 100 mg).

Mechanisms of Action. Phenobarbital is a classic and potent GABA agonist.

Pharmacokinetics

Absorption. Oral absorption is rapid and almost complete (70% to 90%). The time to peak plasma level is 1 to 6 hours after an oral dose, and approximately 30 minutes after i.v. administration. The serum reference range is 20 to 40 µg/mL.

Distribution. Phenobarbital is 20% to 45% protein bound. Fractional protein binding is less than that of many other anticonvulsants. Because of its relatively low protein binding, phenobarbital is appreciably dialyzed.

Elimination. The drug's half-life in adults ranges between 37 and 73 hours. Most of the drug is excreted in the urine as hepatic metabolites; about 20% to 50% is excreted as the unchanged drug.

Metabolism. Phenobarbital is chemically modified by the liver via hydroxylation and glucuronide conjugation.

Drug Interactions. Barbiturates are enzyme inducers and therefore can reduce the half-life of many agents, as well as increase the toxicity of drugs that form toxic intermediates during hepatic metabolism.[1,4] Therefore, barbiturates can enhance the hepatotoxicity of acetaminophen. Phenobarbital increases the metabolism of certain antiarrhythmics (disopyramide, propafenone, and quinidine), anticonvulsants (ethosuximide, lamotrigine, phenytoin, tiagabine, topiramate, and zonisamide, but not levetiracetam or gabapentin), β-adrenergic blockers, calcium channel blockers, chloramphenicol, cimetidine, corticosteroids, cyclosporine, doxycycline, estrogens, furosemide, methadone, oral contraceptives, tricyclic antidepressants, and warfarin.[4,5] Conversely, the metabolism of barbiturates is inhibited by monoamine oxidase inhibitors and valproic acid. Barbiturates can decrease vitamin D levels.

Adverse Reactions and Toxicities. Phenobarbital, like all barbiturates, retards cerebral excitation and therefore can lead to cognitive dysfunction, sedation, lethargy, ataxia, nystagmus, and, in large doses, coma and respiratory depression.[43-45] Although they are uncommon, hematologic disturbances can occur and include agranulocytosis, thrombocytopenia, and megaloblastic anemia.[1] Activated charcoal and hemoperfusion have been implemented in cases of acute massive phenobarbital poisoning.[46-48]

Contraindications. Because the barbiturates have a significant impact on hepatic function, their use should be questioned for patients with any hepatic impairment. Patients with porphyria are not candidates for this drug. If it is given in large doses (e.g., to arrest active seizures), respiratory depression is a major concern, and airway protection is commonly required. Phenobarbital is not suggested for use during pregnancy, but, considering that all anticonvulsants fall into this category, it appears to be no worse than others, and perhaps devoid of some of the neural tube defects and other malformations distinctly attributed to other agents.

NEWER ANTICONVULSANTS

Several newer anticonvulsants have been introduced into the market during the past 15 years. However, the lack of available i.v. formulations severely limits their use in treating seizures in the ICU. The agents typically are initiated when enteral therapy is considered suitable. Some studies have demonstrated that the oral preparations of some of these agents can still be of some benefit. Topiramate tablets, for example, have been crushed to a powder, mixed with water, and administered via nasogastric tube, and have been shown to be effective in refractory status epilepticus. Agents such as gabapentin, lamotrigine, topiramate, and vigabatrin are often considered more suitable for adjunctive therapy than for monotherapy. Lamotrigine is the only agent approved for monotherapy, but gabapentin and oxcarbazepine may soon also have such an indication.[8,49]

Gabapentin and vigabatrin are excreted unchanged in the urine and are useful in patients with hepatic failure. In patients with renal failure, vigabatrin, gabapentin, and topiramate should be used cautiously and in reduced dosages. Tiagabine's pharmacokinetics are not affected by either renal or hepatic dysfunction. The possibility of drug interactions also is important to know. Lamotrigine used in combination with carbamazepine has resulted in toxicity from the latter agent. Other anticonvulsant drugs have little effect on gabapentin, and it has no substantial influence on the

pharmacokinetics and serum concentrations of other seizure medications.[8,49]

Levetiracetam (Keppra)
Levetiracetam is currently recommended for use as adjunctive therapy against partial-onset seizures. Nonetheless, there is increasing interest in its use within an ICU setting because of the very low toxicity and paucity of drug interactions associated with this agent.

Dosing
Adults. Levetiracetam is available only in oral form; dosing is typically 500 to 1500 mg twice daily; the maximal recommended dose is 3000 mg/day. Higher doses have been used, however.

Elderly. No major changes in dosing have been recommended for elderly patients.

Hepatic Impairment. No adjustment for hepatic impairment is required.

Renal Impairment. The following dosing adjustments of levetiracetam are recommended based on GFR:

1. GFR greater than 80 mL/min: 500 to 1500 mg twice daily
2. GFR 50 to 80 mL/min: 500 to 1000 mg twice daily
3. GFR 30 to 50 mL/min: 250 to 750 mg twice daily
4. GFR less than 30 mL/min: 250 to 500 mg twice daily

Patients with end-stage renal failure who are undergoing hemodialysis should receive 500 to 1000 mg daily and a supplemental dose of 250 to 500 mg after each dialysis treatment. Approximately 50% of levetiracetam is removed during standard hemodialysis.

Forms Available. Levetiracetam is available in oral form as a tablet (250 mg, 500 mg, 750 mg).

Mechanisms of Action. The mechanism for the anticonvulsant action of levetiracetam is as yet unknown.

Pharmacokinetics
Absorption. Following oral ingestion, absorption is both rapid and complete. The time to peak effect is 1 hour, with 100% bioavailability.

Distribution. Levetiracetam is less than 10% protein bound.

Elimination. Levetiracetam has a half-life of approximately 6 to 8 hours, and it is excreted essentially unchanged in the urine.

Metabolism. Levetiracetam is not extensively metabolized.

Drug Interactions. No significant drug interactions have been reported for levetiracetam.

Adverse Reactions and Toxicities. Although levetiracetam is relatively free of side effects, somnolence, weakness, ataxia, and dizziness may occur. Behavioral abnormalities have been reported, although rarely. There is some evidence linking levetiracetam with bone marrow suppression.[3]

Contraindications. The pregnancy category is C.

Gabapentin (Neurontin)
Gabapentin is indicated as adjunctive treatment for partial-onset seizures. It is also widely prescribed for the treatment of neurogenic or neuropathic pain.

Dosing
Adults. Only the oral form is available; the initial dose is 300 mg three times daily, and the maximal dose is 3600 mg/day.

Elderly. Dose reductions of gabapentin may be necessary for elderly patients based on age-related decreases in renal function.

Hepatic Impairment. No dosage adjustment of gabapentin is required.

Renal Impairment. Dose reductions of gabapentin may be necessary based on the patient's GFR. Supplemental doses are commonly administered after hemodialysis.

Forms Available. Forms available include capsule (100 mg, 300 mg, 400 mg); elixir (250 mg/5 mL); and tablet (600 mg, 800 mg).

Mechanisms of Action. The exact mechanism of action of gabapentin remains unknown. It appears not to interact with GABA receptors.

Pharmacokinetics

Absorption. Gabapentin is incompletely absorbed (50% to 60%).

Distribution. Gabapentin's V_d is only 0.6 to 0.8 L/kg, and protein binding is minimal.

Elimination. The drug's half-life is 5 to 6 hours, and it is renally excreted.

Metabolism. There is no appreciable drug metabolism.

Drug Interactions. Gabapentin's interactions with other agents are not as complex as is the case for phenytoin, valproic acid, or phenobarbital. However, the drug is not as free of drug interactions as levetiracetam. Antacids reduce the bioavailability of enteral gabapentin by 20%.[3] Therefore, gabapentin should be taken at least 2 hours after antacid administration. Cimetidine may decrease the clearance of gabapentin. Serum concentrations of gabapentin have been shown to increase with concurrent morphine use. Although phenytoin serum concentrations can be increased by gabapentin, those of valproic acid, carbamazepine, and phenobarbital do not seem to be affected by this drug.[3,4,5]

Adverse Reactions and Toxicities. Although gabapentin usually is very well tolerated, it may induce somnolence, dizziness, ataxia, fatigue, peripheral edema, pruritus, nausea and vomiting, leukopenia, and tremor.[3]

Contraindications. The pregnancy category of gabapentin is C.

ANNOTATED REFERENCES

Asconape J: Some common issues in the use of antiepileptic drugs. Semin Neurol 2002;22:27-39.

In this article, several common clinical situations in the management of patients with epilepsy are presented in the form of case studies. These cases illustrate some current aspects of the use of the anticonvulsants and provide some guidelines to help the treating physician in the increasingly complex process of seizure therapy.

Cramer JA, Fisher R, Ben-Menachem E, et al: New antiepileptic drugs: Comparison of key clinical trials. Epilepsia 1999;40:590-600.

This is a good review of data accrued from clinical trials of five new antiepileptic drugs (AEDs). The efficacy in reducing seizures and self-reported adverse events are incorporated here as a basis of selection among new AEDs. Drawbacks to use of these data also are demonstrated.

Dreifuss FE. Toxic effects of drugs used in the ICU: Anticonvulsant agents. Crit Care Clin 1991;7:521-532.

This is an excellent review of the most common anticonvulsants used in the ICU. Despite its age, the information remains highly useful, especially in light of the fact that most medications used for the treatment of seizures in the ICU setting are the older drugs available in i.v. preparations (except valproic acid, which is more recent).

Mirski MA, Williams MA, Hanley DF: Prolonged pentobarbital and phenobarbitone coma for refractory generalized status epilepticus. Crit Care Med 1995;23:400-404.

This is a case report of a particularly difficult and refractory case of status epilepticus that describes the difficulties of adequacy of control and treatment given the adverse actions of the anticonvulsant drugs. Included are clearly presented problematic issues relating to hepatic enzyme induction, polypharmacy, induced "burst-suppression" coma, hemodynamic and respiratory decompensation, and emergence with control of the primary seizure state. This describes the longest duration of barbiturate coma for the treatment of seizures that has been reported, 53 days, with good outcome.

Treiman DM, Meyers PD, Walton NY, et al: A comparison of four treatments for generalized convulsive status epilepticus. Veterans Affairs Status Epilepticus Cooperative Study Group. N Engl J Med 1998;339:792-798.

This report describes the largest controlled drug trial (384 patients) for the treatment of status epilepticus. It was a 5-year randomized, double-blind, multicenter trial of four intravenous regimens: diazepam followed by phenytoin; lorazepam alone; phenobarbital alone; and phenytoin alone. The study concluded that lorazepam was superior to phenytoin alone (P < .02), and phenobarbital and phenytoin followed by diazepam were similar in efficacy to lorazepam.

Varelas P, Mirski MA: Seizures in the ICU. J Neurosurg Anesthesiol 2001;13:163-175.

This is a recent comprehensive review of seizures occurring in the ICU setting; it includes etiology of seizures (including a review of the ICU iatrogenic causes), diagnosis algorithm, and treatment. Numerous tables of anticonvulsant drug mechanisms, toxicity, and drug-drug interactions are included.

Chapter 189

CALCIUM CHANNEL BLOCKER TOXICITY

Daniel E. Brooks • Kenneth D. Katz

KEY POINTS

1. **An accurate history of ingestion is critical in regard to treatment of the toxicology patient,** and an attempt should be made to elucidate other ingested toxins or medications that could complicate therapy. Family, friends, witnesses, and prehospital employees are excellent sources if the patient cannot provide necessary information.

2. **Patients can rapidly deteriorate after a toxic ingestion of a calcium channel blocker (CCB).** Patients require at least 6 hours of monitoring and observation after the acute ingestion of an immediate-release formulation. Patients who are exposed to a sustained-release medication, and those with any evidence of instability, require admission and observation in a monitored setting.

3. **Gastric decontamination has very limited utility after any toxic ingestion, including CCBs.** The routine use of ipecac, gastric lavage, or cathartics is not recommended. The use of activated charcoal is recommended only within 1 hour after ingestion and provided that continued airway protection can be ensured. The use of whole bowel irrigation should be discussed with a poison control center or medical toxicologist.

4. **After the development of cardiovascular shock, the mainstay of therapy involves the use of vasoactive drugs (i.e., norepinephrine or isoproterenol) to maintain adequate perfusion to vital organs.** Other interventions, such as atropine, calcium salts, and crystalloid fluids, have limited potential for correcting significant toxicity.

5. **Invasive hemodynamic monitoring should be instituted quickly** in patients severely poisoned by CCBs, and it should be continued until resolution of cardiovascular instability.

6. **Pulmonary edema can accompany severe poisoning by CCBs, especially after excessive fluid volume administration.** Physicians should maintain a high clinical suspicion throughout the resuscitation period.

7. **Optimal treatment for individual poisoned patients depends on exact information and unique factors.** Consultation with a regional poison control center (800-222-1222) or medical toxicologist may offer additional information that can assist patient evaluation, management, and disposition.

Calcium channel blockers (CCBs), also referred to as calcium entry-blocking agents or calcium antagonists, are commonly used in the treatment of angina and hypertension. Their use is complicated by adverse side effects, iatrogenic errors, and intentional overdoses. Significant morbidity and mortality can occur after accidental or intentional CCB poisoning. In 2002, the American Association of Poison Control Centers recorded 9585 exposures to CCBs, with 68 reported deaths. As a group, cardiovascular drugs, including CCBs, were responsible for 61,000 calls and 181 deaths reported to national poison centers.[1]

PHARMACOLOGY

CCBs are classified into five groups, based on structure or functional activity. The first group, exemplified by the T-channel blocker, mibefradil, is unique because these agents antagonize T-type calcium channels. The other four groups are divided based on structural differences, and all antagonize L-type calcium channels. These groups include the phenylalkylamines (e.g., verapamil), benzothiazepine (e.g., diltiazem), dihydropyridines (e.g., nifedipine), and diarylaminopropylamine ether (bepridil). Their mechanism of action involves inhibition of calcium influx through voltage-dependent L-type calcium channels.[2,3] This inhibition results in decreased intracellular calcium concentration, relaxation of vascular smooth muscle, decreased systemic vascular resistance, and inhibition of intracardiac nodal excitation.[3,4] Some CCBs, particularly verapamil, have higher binding affinity for myocardial calcium channels, resulting in sinoatrial and atrioventricular nodal inhibiton.[4-8]

The most commonly used CCBs (verapamil, diltiazem, and nifedipine) are well absorbed after oral ingestion, are highly protein bound at therapeutic concentrations, and undergo a variable amount of first-pass metabolism after oral administration.[9-13] There is variability in volumes of distribution (V_d). For example, verapamil's V_d is 5.3 L, yet nifedipine's is just 0.8 L. These characteristics (high protein binding and large V_d) suggest limited utility of hemodialysis for toxicity. After absorption, CCBs are hepatically metabolized by saturable enzymes to metabolites with variable activity.[9,10,12,14] Therapeutic half-lives range from less than 2 hours to longer than 60 hours. After massive ingestion or in patients with congestive heart failure or hepatic dysfunction, decreased metabolism leads to increased concentrations of active compounds and prolonged half-lives.[15-18] Patients with either liver dysfunction or decreased hepatic perfusion may experience decreased elimination of CCBs.[12,19]

All CCBs are pregnancy category C drugs and have been associated with teratogenic and embryocidal effects in animal studies. After therapeutic use, CCBs can be recovered from breast milk and exposed offspring, but the neonatal effects, if any, require further investigation.[20-23]

CLINICAL MANIFESTATIONS OF TOXICITY

The potentially life-threatening effects of CCB intoxication center on the cardiovascular system. The most common clinical manifestations are sinus bradycardia, hypotension, and shock. Clinical effects may vary in mild to moderate poisoning, depending on the specific medication ingested. Phenylalkylamine and benzothiazepine toxicity commonly manifest as bradycardia and hypotension secondary to significant negative inotropic and chronotropic cardiovascular effects.[24,25] Dihydropyridine toxicity, however, may result in hypotension with reflex tachycardia because of the affinity of these agents for the peripheral vasculature.[24,25] In massive overdose, specificity is lost, and all agents can cause bradycardia, depressed cardiac contractility, and cardiovascular collapse.[25] Furthermore, cardiovascular compromise may be compounded by ingestion of other cardiovascular toxins in addition to underlying patient comorbid illness.

Pulmonary toxicity from CCB poisoning includes both cardiogenic and noncardiogenic pulmonary edema secondary to several purported mechanisms: negative chronotropy, excessive fluid resuscitation, increased capillary permeability secondary to drug effect, and increased sympathetic discharge in response to shock.[26]

Neurologic manifestations include myoclonus, dizziness, syncope, focal neurologic deficits, and seizures. These are most likely related to central nervous system hypoperfusion.[25,27]

Gastrointestinal symptoms caused by CCB ingestion are nonspecific and include nausea and vomiting.[25]

CCB toxicity with ensuing shock can cause diffuse organ dysfunction, such as renal failure, secondary to poor tissue perfusion.

Metabolic derangements, including hypokalemia and mild hyperglycemia, may be found due to calcium channel blockade in the pancreatic beta islet cell that impairs insulin release.[28] Metabolic acidosis can be caused by poor tissue perfusion and mitochondrial dehydrogenase inhibition.[29]

Sustained-release preparations can cause delayed-onset toxicity as late as 12 hours after ingestion.[25]

DIFFERENTIAL DIAGNOSIS

The most common agents in the differential diagnosis of CCB poisoning are β-adrenergic antagonists, cardiac glycosides, imidazolines, class 1a and 1c antidysrhythmics, cyanide, organophosphates, and tricyclic antidepressants (late).[25,30] Although the specific diagnosis of CCB toxicity may not be readily discernible at the bedside, the mainstay of therapy is maintenance of a secure airway and cardiovascular support.

Included in the differential diagnosis of CCB poisoning are nontoxicologic entities: acute coronary syndromes, hyperkalemia, myxedema coma, hypothermia, and sepsis.

DIAGNOSTIC TESTING

The diagnosis of CCB poisoning is based predominantly on the history and physical examination. Both routine and comprehensive drug screening assays routinely miss CCBs.[31] Although there are no specific laboratory tests available to diagnose CCB poisoning, some laboratory studies should be obtained to aid clinical management.

A 12-lead electrocardiogram should be obtained to define the cardiac rhythm and intervals. Arterial blood gas measurement offers a rapid assessment of oxygenation, tissue perfusion, and serum potassium. Chest radiography can demonstrate cardiac size and the presence of pulmonary edema. Serum electrolytes, glucose concentration, and markers of renal function are helpful in terms of both diagnosis and treatment. Serum calcium levels generally are not affected by CCBs, but serial levels may be necessary if the patient is treated with parenteral calcium salts.

Serum levels of cardioactive medications with established therapeutic concentrations (e.g., digoxin, procainamide) should be obtained for patients with a suggestive history or physical examination.

TREATMENT

Gastric decontamination plays a limited role in the vast majority of acute poisonings, including CCB poisoning. A single dose of activated charcoal without a cathartic may be administered within 1 hour after ingestion.[32] A patient who presents immediately after a known, massive ingestion may benefit from other gastric decontamination techniques (e.g., whole bowel irrigation) after discussion with a poison control center. Whole bowel irrigation is recommended for ingestion of sustained-release preparations and may supplement ongoing resuscitative therapies.[33,34]

Treatment of the patient poisoned by CCBs focuses on early recognition of shock and aggressive cardiovascular support. Patients who are obtunded, have poor airway protective mechanisms, are hypoxemic, or are in shock should undergo endotracheal intubation. A low threshold should be maintained to initiate invasive monitoring techniques (arterial, central venous, and pulmonary catheters) for both administration of treatments and assessment of clinical responses. All patients should have a urinary bladder catheter to accurately monitor urinary output.

Clinically significant CCB toxicity usually involves bradydysrhythmia or hypotension or both. Treatment in the patient who demonstrates cardiovascular effects should generally be guided by the presence or absence of end-organ dysfunction (e.g., mental status, tissue perfusion, urine output) and not solely by heart rate or blood pressure. For example, a bradycardic patient with normal mental status, normal blood pressure, and no demonstrable acidosis or renal dysfunction may not require further treatment unless clinical deterioration ensues.

Treatment of symptomatic bradycardia enlists an arsenal of therapies, including atropine, external or internal pacing, parenteral calcium salts, glucagon, vasopressors, and even extracorporeal hemodynamic support. None of the treatments has been studied in randomized, controlled human studies, and their use is based on animal studies, human case reports, and case series. Severely poisoned patients may require several concomitant therapies to achieve cardiovascular stabilization.

Intravenous fluids should be administered to hypotensive patients to improve blood pressure and tissue perfusion. A total of 2 L of lactated Ringer's solution or normal saline solution should be given. Care should be maintained not to administer excessive volume to patients poisoned by CCBs because of the risk of pulmonary edema.[26]

Atropine has limited utility in reversing bradycardia, but it may be administered on an emergency basis while other therapies are being prepared.[25,35]

External or internal pacemaker therapy may be attempted in addition to intravenous fluids and atropine to improve symptomatic bradycardia. If capture is achieved, the heart rate should be set at 50 to 60 bpm, with a target systolic blood pressure of 90 to 100 mm Hg to increase tissue perfusion. However, pacemaker therapy is often ineffective in sustaining hemodynamic improvement.[25,35]

Administration of parenteral calcium salts may augment heart rate and blood pressure in the face of CCB poisoning.[35] Calcium chloride contains approximately three times the amount of calcium as the gluconate salt and is the preferred agent.[36] Slow boluses of 1 to 3 g of calcium chloride may be given, and a continuous infusion of 2 to 6 g/hour may be initiated if a favorable hemodynamic response is noted.[37,38] Serum ionized calcium levels should be monitored during parenteral calcium infusions and should be maintained at approximately 2 to 3 mmol/L.[25,36] The use of parenteral calcium salts should be avoided if digoxin toxicity is suspected.[25] Instead, Digibind Fab antibodies should be administered.

Although more commonly associated with β-adrenergic antagonist poisoning, intravenous glucagon may offer another treatment modality by increasing cyclic adenosine monophosphate (cAMP) production to increase cardiac contractility and rate.[24,39] Intravenous boluses of 2 to 10 mg may be administered, and resulting effects should be monitored. A beneficial response should be followed by a constant infusion of 2 to 5 mg/hour. Side effects of glucagon administration include nausea, vomiting, hyperglycemia, and potential phenol toxicity.[25,40] Glucagon always should be prepared in normal saline or 5% dextrose because of the potential toxicity of the phenol diluent.[25]

Although several vasopressors have been used for the treatment of CCB toxicity, there is no optimal agent. Dopamine, epinephrine, isoproterenol, amrinone, and aminophylline all have demonstrated efficacy in animal models and humans series. In general, a patient with severe CCB poisoning should receive a pressor titrated to achieve a perfusing heart rate and blood pressure. In the face of significant hypotension, the choice of vasopressor should be based on the preexisting heart rate. For example, if the patient is hypotensive with reflex tachycardia, an α-adrenergic agonist should be employed. We recommend isoproterenol or epinephrine as an initial agent based on the patient's presenting heart rate and blood pressure, pharmacologic properties and our experiences.

Three investigational therapies are insulin/dextrose infusion, hypertonic saline, and 4-aminopyridine. The use of an insulin/dextrose infusion may correct the state of hypoinsulinemia and impaired cellular glucose uptake found in CCB poisoning.[28] However, this intervention "cannot be recommended due to limited supportive data."[37] Hypertonic saline has been studied only in animals as a potential treatment for verapamil poisoning. The proposed mechanism involves increasing the pH around the calcium channel and reversing potential verapamil-induced sodium channel blockade.[41] The drug 4-aminopyridine blocks the outward rectifying potassium channel, allowing more calcium to enter the myocardial cell.[25] This drug has demonstrated some success in animal models and in a single verapamil-poisoned patient receiving hemodialysis.[42] The routine use of any experimental therapies cannot be recommended without further investigation.

Treatment endpoints are maintenance of oxygenation, heart rate, and blood pressure to sustain adequate tissue perfusion. Meticulous and repetitive measurements of hemodynamic parameters, mental status, urine output, and acid-base status are paramount and guide the clinician as to the effectiveness of instituted therapy.

Patients who remain in cardiovascular collapse despite aggressive resuscitation may be candidates for extracorporeal blood pressure support in the form of cardiopulmonary bypass or intraortic balloon counterpulsation.[24,43]

Table 189-1 presents a summary of pharmaceutical interventions after CCB toxicity.

PATIENT MONITORING AND DISPOSITION

Patients should be observed in a monitored setting for at least 6 hours after an acute ingestion of a regular-release CCB for evidence of cardiovascular instability. Early medical clearance requires the administration of activated charcoal,

TABLE 189-1. PHARMACEUTICAL INTERVENTIONS AFTER CALCIUM CHANNEL BLOCKER TOXICITY

Drug	Dose	Goal
Activated charcoal	1–2 g/kg	Decreased systemic absorption (give within 1 hr after ingestion)
Whole bowel irrigation	500–2000 mL/hr until clear rectal effluent	Decreased system absorption (use after contacting a poison control center)
Intravenous fluids	2 L of normal saline solution or lactated Ringer's solution (limit intravenous fluids unless significantly dehydrated)	Increased BP
Calcium chloride	1 ampule i.v. over 2 min	Increased HR and SVR
Atropine	0.5–1 mg i.v. every 3 min (maximum dose is 3 mg)	Increased HR and CO
Glucagon	5–10 mg bolus, then 2–5 mg/hr infusion	Increased SVR (titrate for effect)
Isoproterenol	Initiate at 2 µg/min	Increased CO (titrate for effect)
Epinephrine	Initiate at 2 µg/min (consider weight-based dosing)	Increased SVR (titrate for effect)
Norepinephrine	Initiate at 0.5 µg/min (consider weight-based dosing)	Increased SVR (titrate for effect)
Ventricular pacing	Achieve ventricular capture at 50–60 bpm	Increased HR and CO (only if other interventions fail)
Intra-aortic balloon pump	Consult cardiologist	Only if refractory to all other interventions
Cardiopulmonary bypass	Consult cardiothoracic surgeon	Only if refractory to all other interventions

BP, blood pressure; CO, cardiac output; HR, heart rate; SVR, systemic vascular resistance.

maintenance of normal mentation and hemodynamics, and exclusion of ingestion of other medications or toxins. Patients ingesting toxic amounts of a sustained-released CCB formulation should be monitored for 24 hours because of the risk of delayed symptoms. Those presenting with any evidence of cardiovascular instability should be admitted to an intensive care unit for further care and monitoring.

After resuscitation, an asymptomatic period of 24 hours is appropriate for medical clearance. As expected, a psychiatrist should evaluate all patients with a history or suspicion of intentional ingestion before ultimate disposition.

CONCLUSIONS

CCBs hold the potential for causing severe and delayed hemodynamic instability. Appropriate evaluation and monitoring of asymptomatic patients, as well as aggressive interventions in those patients with cardiovascular collapse, ensures optimal patient outcomes. Clinicians should initiate catecholamine infusions early in hypotensive patients who fail to respond to moderate fluid resuscitation. Consultation with a regional poison control center (telephone 800-222-1222 in the United States or www.eapect.org in Europe) or a medical toxicologist can offer insight into underlying pathophysiology and assistance with patient management.

ANNOTATED REFERENCES

Albertson TE, Dawson A, Latorre F, et al: TOX-ACLS: Toxicologic-oriented advanced cardiac life support. Ann Emerg Med 2001;37:S78-S90.
A consortium of medical toxicologists and emergency physicians reviews the medical literature in an attempt to provide evidence-based recommendations for the treatment of the acutely poisoned toxicology patient. The uses of both calcium salts and insulin/dextrose in CCB toxicity are critically discussed.

Katz AM, Hager WD, Messineo FC, et al: Cellular actions and pharmacology of calcium-channel blockers. Am J Emerg Med 1985;3(Suppl 6):1-9.
This review article covers the cellular mechanisms of action for CCBs and reviews the physiologic action of calcium. The pharmacology of calcium antagonists is briefly covered.

Kerns W, Kline J, Ford MD: B-blocker and calcium channel blocker toxicity. Emerg Med Clin 1994;12:365-390.
The authors provide a thorough review of the pathophysiology, clinical presentation, and treatment of CCB toxicity. Although written in 1994, it still provides a very good reference for any physician treating a CCB-poisoned patient.

Ramoska EA, Spiller HA, Winter M, Borys D: A one-year evaluation of calcium channel blocker overdoses: Toxicity and treatment. Ann Emerg Med 1993;22:196-200.
The authors collected data from more than 130 CCB-poisoned patients and described the clinical manifestations and treatment efficacies. Although this was not a randomized, controlled trial, it does provide some useful information, especially regarding the utility of commonly recommended "antidotes."

Taira N: Differences in cardiovascular profile among calcium antagonist. Am J Cardiol 1987;59:24B-29B.
This review article compares the inotropic, chronotropic, and dromotropic effects of calcium antagonists and discusses possible mechanisms for the observed differences.

Chapter 190

DRUG DOSING IN THE PATIENT WITH RENAL FAILURE

Gary R. Matzke

KEY POINTS

1. The calculation of creatinine clearance from a timed urine collection with creatinine measurement in serum and urine has been the standard clinical measure of renal function for decades.

2. Clearance of hundreds of drugs is reduced in critically ill patients, especially patients with acute renal failure or chronic kidney disease.

3. Volume of distribution of several drugs is increased significantly in patients with acute renal failure or chronic kidney disease, typically as a result of fluid overload, decreased protein binding, or altered tissue binding.

4. Individualization of therapy for a patient receiving continuous renal replacement therapy depends on the patient's residual renal function and the clearance of the drug by the mode of continuous renal replacement therapy the patient is receiving.

Up to 40% of patients in the ICU develop renal dysfunction,[1] whereas the incidence of acute renal failure on admission to an ICU varies between 5.4% and 25% of patients, depending on how acute renal failure is defined. Renal replacement therapy is required for 5% of all patients admitted to an ICU, one third of whom have chronic kidney disease on admission.[2] Critically ill patients with acute renal failure have higher mean Acute Physiology, Age, and Chronic Health Evaluation (APACHE) III scores, greater hemodynamic instability, longer ICU stays, and higher ICU and hospital mortality than patients without acute renal failure: ICU and hospital mortality is roughly fourfold higher in patients with acute renal failure.[3] Critically ill patients with chronic kidney disease have poorer outcomes than patients with normal renal function, and the presence of chronic kidney disease is a significant predictor of hospital mortality in APACHE score tools.[4,5] Patients with chronic kidney disease who have a similar severity of illness to patients with acute renal failure have a better outcome, however; mortality in chronic kidney disease patients is 50%—still double that of patients without renal dysfunction.[2,3] Renal dysfunction also alters the absorption, distribution, metabolism, and elimination of many pharmacotherapeutic agents used in the treatment of critically ill patients. In this chapter, the drugs affected are tabulated, and the mechanisms responsible for the changes in disposition are discussed. A general construct for the individualization of drug therapy in patients with chronic kidney disease or acute renal failure is presented along with dosage guidelines for the 80 most commonly used ICU medications. Finally, the influence of continuous and intermittent renal replacement therapy on drug clearance is discussed, and dosage guidelines are tabulated for selected drugs for patients with severe chronic kidney disease or acute renal failure.

QUANTITATION OF RENAL FUNCTION

Accurate assessment of renal function in critically ill patients is imperative. Serial estimates or measurements of renal function routinely are recommended to guide individualization of drug dosage regimens to optimize clinical outcomes. The calculation of creatinine clearance from a timed urine collection with creatinine measurement in serum and urine has been the standard clinical measure of renal function for decades. Urine is difficult to collect accurately in the ICU, and the fact that many commonly used medications interfere with creatinine measurement, especially if colorimetric assay methods such as the Jaffé method are used, limits the utility of this approach.[6-8] The administration of radioactive (^{125}I iothalamate, ^{51}Cr-EDTA, or technetium 99m-DTPA) or nonradioactive (aminoglycosides, iohexol, iothalamate, and inulin) markers of glomerular filtration rate, although scientifically sound, is clinically impractical because intravenous or subcutaneous administration of the marker and the collection of multiple timed blood and urine collections make the procedures expensive and difficult to perform.

Estimation of creatinine clearance or glomerular filtration rate requires only routinely collected laboratory and demographic data and is inexpensive and clinically feasible. The Cockcroft and Gault method for creatinine clearance[9] and the Levey method for glomerular filtration rate[10,11] correlate well with creatinine clearance and glomerular filtration rate measurements in individuals with stable renal function.[10,12] These methods lose their predictive performance, however, in patients with liver disease[13-15] or unstable renal function.[6,16,17] Finally, although several methods for creatinine clearance estimation in patients with unstable renal function have been proposed,[8] the accuracy of these methods has not been rigorously assessed, and at present their use cannot be recommended.

ALTERED DRUG DISPOSITION IN CRITICALLY ILL PATIENTS WITH RENAL INSUFFICIENCY

EFFECT ON DRUG ABSORPTION

The absorption of drugs from the gastrointestinal tract is rarely altered in patients with chronic kidney disease or acute renal failure. The systemic availability of some drugs is increased in chronic kidney disease patients as a result of a decrease in metabolism during the drug's first pass through the gastrointestinal tract and liver (Table 190-1).[18,19] Some orally administered drugs that are extensively metabolized before reaching the systemic circulation may have increased bioavailability; the number of drugs for which this has been documented is small.[20,21]

EFFECT ON DRUG DISTRIBUTION

The volume of distribution of several drugs is increased significantly in patients with acute renal failure or severe chronic kidney disease.[19,22,23] Increases may result from fluid overload, decreased protein binding, or altered tissue binding (Table 190-2). The volume of distribution of only a few drugs is decreased in patients with chronic kidney disease, and the mechanism proposed for this change is a reduction in tissue binding. Digoxin and pindolol are two prime examples, and for both of these a significant relationship between the decrease in distribution volume and creatinine clearance has been reported.[24]

EFFECT ON DRUG METABOLISM

In rat models of chronic kidney disease, protein expression in the liver of several cytochrome P_{450} (CYP) enzymes, including CYP3A1 and CYP3A2 (equivalent to human CYP3A4), is reduced by 75%.[25] Enzyme-selective breath test analysis in animals also suggests a differential effect on enzyme activity with CYP2C11 and CYP3A2 being significantly reduced, whereas CYP1A2 activity is unchanged.[26] Preliminary human data suggest a differential effect of chronic kidney disease on cytochrome P_{450} enzyme activity: CYP2C19 and CYP3A4 are reduced, whereas CYP2D6 and CYP2E1 are not affected.[27,28] This differential effect on

TABLE 190-2. EFFECT OF END-STAGE RENAL DISEASE ON DISTRIBUTION VOLUME OF SELECTED DRUGS*

Drug	Normal	ESRD
Increased		
Amikacin	0.20	0.29
Azlocillin	0.21	0.28
Cefazolin	0.13	0.16
Cefonicid	0.11	0.14
Cefoxitin	0.16	0.26
Cefuroxime	0.20	0.26
Clofibrate	0.14	0.24
Cloxacillin	0.14	0.26
Dicloxacillin	0.08	0.18
Erythromycin	0.57	1.09
Furosemide	0.11	0.18
Gentamicin	0.20	0.29
Isoniazid	0.60	0.80
Minoxidil	2.60	4.90
Naproxen	0.12	0.17
Phenytoin	0.64	1.40
Trimethoprim	1.36	1.83
Vancomycin	0.64	0.85
Decreased		
Chloramphenicol	0.87	0.60
Digoxin	7.30	4.10
Ethambutol	3.70	1.60
Methicillin	0.45	0.30
Pindolol	2.10	1.10

*A change of ±25% was considered to be clinically significant.
ESRD, end-stage renal disease.
Data from references 19, and 22-24.

individual enzymes may help to explain some of the conflicting reports of drug metabolism alterations in the presence of severe chronic kidney disease.

The reduction of nonrenal clearance of several drugs reported in patients with severe chronic kidney disease supports the premise that alterations in hepatic cytochrome P_{450} enzymes modify their metabolism (Table 190-3).[19,28] Prediction of the effect of chronic kidney disease on the metabolism of a particular drug is difficult even for drugs within the same pharmacologic class.[29] The reductions in nonrenal clearance for patients with chronic kidney disease are generally proportional to the reductions in glomerular filtration rate.

Critically ill patients with acute renal failure may have a higher residual nonrenal clearance, however, than patients with chronic kidney disease who have a similar creatinine clearance.[30-32] This difference may be the result of less exposure to or accumulation of uremic waste products that alter hepatic function. Because a patient with acute renal failure may have a higher nonrenal clearance than a patient with chronic kidney disease, the resultant plasma concentrations are lower than expected and possibly subtherapeutic if classic chronic kidney disease–derived dosage guidelines are followed.

EFFECT ON RENAL EXCRETION

Renal clearance is the composite of glomerular filtration rate, renal tubular secretion, and reabsorption: renal clearance = (glomerular filtration rate $\times f_u$) + (renal tubular

TABLE 190-1. BIOAVAILABILITY OF DRUGS IN PATIENTS WITH RENAL DISEASE

Decreased	Unchanged	Increased
Xylose	Cimetidine	Bufuralol
Furosemide	Ciprofloxacin	Dextropropoxyphene
Pindolol	Codeine	Dihydrocodeine
	Digoxin	Erythromycin
	Labetalol	Oxprenolol
	Trimethoprim	Propranolol
	Sulfamethoxazole	Tacrolimus
		Tolamolol

TABLE 190–3. EFFECT OF END-STAGE RENAL DISEASE ON NONRENAL CLEARANCE OF SELECTED DRUGS*

Decreased

Acyclovir	Cefsulodin	Imipenem	Procainamide
Aztreonam	Ceftizoxime	Isoniazid	Quinapril
Bufuralol	Cilastatin	Methylprednisolone	Roxithromycin
Captopril	Cimetidine	Metoclopramide	Verapamil
Cefmenoxime	Ciprofloxacin	Minoxidil	Zidovudine
Cefmetazole	Cortisol	Moxalactam	
Cefonicid	Encainide	Nicardipine	
Cefotaxime	Guanadrel	Nimodipine	
Cefotiam	Erythromycin	Nitrendipine	

Increased

Bumetanide
Cefpiramide
Fosinopril
Nifedipine
Phenytoin
Sulfadimidine

*A change of ±40% was considered clinically significant.
Data from references 19, 22-24, and 28.

TABLE 190–4. DRUGS THAT ARE ACTIVELY SECRETED BY THE RENAL TUBULES

Anionic Transport

Acetazolamide	Ceftizoxime	Nitrofurantoin
Amantadine	Cefuroxime	Norfloxacin
Ampicillin	Cephalothin	Prostaglandin E_2
Bumetanide	Cephapirin	Para-aminohippurate
Carbenicillin	Cephradine	Penicillin G
Cefamandole	Ciprofloxacin	Phenolsulfon-
Cefazolin	Clofibrate	phthalein
Cefmenoxime	Dehydroepiandrosterone	Phenylbutazone
Cefmetazole	sulfate	Probenecid
Cefoperazone	Ethacrynic acid	Quinapril
Ceforanide	Folic acid	Sulfamethoxazole
Cefotaxime	Furosemide	Sulfinpyrazone
Cefotiam	Indomethacin	Sulfisoxazole
Cefoxitin	Methotrexate	Thiazides
Ceftazidime	Moxalactam	Uric acid
	NSAIDs	Zidovudine
	Nafcillin	Zomepirac

Cationic Transport

Amiloride	Famotidine	Quinine
Cimetidine	L-carnitine	Ranitidine
Creatinine	Morphine	Triamterene
Digoxin	N-acetyl-procainamide	Trimethoprim
Dipyridamole	Procainamide	Vancomycin
Dopamine	Quinidine	Verapamil

P-Glycoprotein/Multidrug Resistance–Associated Protein Transport

Clarithromycin	Fexofenadine	Reserpine
Cyclosporine	HIV protease inhibitors	Steroids
Digoxin	Losartan	

HIV, human immunodeficiency virus; NSAIDs, nonsteroidal anti-inflammatory drugs.
Data from references 24, 33, and 34.

secretion – renal reabsorption), where f_u is the fraction of the drug unbound to plasma proteins. An acute or chronic progressive reduction in glomerular filtration rate results in a decrease in renal clearance; this historically has been the primary evidence on which drug dosage guidelines for patients with acute renal failure or chronic kidney disease have been predicated. The contribution of a reduction in renal clearance to the degree of change in the total body clearance of a drug is highly dependent, however, on the fraction of the dose eliminated unchanged by the normal kidney, the intrarenal pathways for drug elimination and transport, and the degree of functional impairment of each of these pathways.[24]

Drug elimination by glomerular filtration rate occurs by diffusion, but renal tubular secretion and renal reabsorption are bidirectional processes that involve carrier-mediated renal transport systems and passive diffusion. The important renal transport systems include the organic anionic, organic cationic, nucleoside, and P-glycoprotein transporters, which are involved in the renal tubular excretion of multiple compounds (Table 190-4).[33,34] The clearance of drugs that are extensively renally secreted (renal clearance >300 mL/min) may be reduced significantly in the presence of normal renal function and mild-to-moderate chronic kidney disease secondary to drug or disease interactions with the renal transporter.

STRATEGIES FOR DRUG THERAPY INDIVIDUALIZATION

This section provides a practical approach for drug dosage individualization in critically ill patients with acute or chronic kidney disease and patients receiving continuous renal replacement therapy or intermittent hemodialysis. Basic pharmacokinetic principles (see Chapter 185) combined with the disposition properties of a particular drug and a quantitative measure of the patient's degree of renal function enable the clinician to design an individualized therapeutic regimen.

IMPACT OF RENAL INSUFFICIENCY

Accurate characterizations of the relationship between the pharmacokinetic parameters of a drug and renal function are not always available. Secondary references, such as the *American Hospital Formulary Service Drug Information*,[35] *Drug Prescribing in Renal Failure* by Aronoff and colleagues,[36] and *Goodman and Gilman's The Pharmacological Basis of Therapeutics*,[37] are excellent sources for the pharmacokinetic characteristics of drugs in subjects with normal renal function. These references often do not provide the explicit relationships of the kinetic parameters with creatinine clearance or glomerular filtration rate, however. These relationships, if available, along with the patient's creatinine clearance, enable prediction of the patient's kinetic parameters and the calculation of a therapeutic regimen to attain the desired therapeutic goals as described in Chapter 185.

If the relationship of a drug's total body clearance with creatinine clearance is not known, one can estimate the patient's total body clearance, provided that the fraction of the drug that is eliminated renally unchanged (f_e) in subjects with normal renal function is known. The following approach assumes that the volume of distribution is unchanged and that the change in total body clearance is proportional to creatinine clearance, that renal disease does not alter the drug's metabolism, that the metabolites if formed are inactive and nontoxic, that the drug obeys first-order (linear) kinetic principles, and that it is described adequately by a one-compartment model. If these assumptions are valid, the kinetic parameter/dosage adjustment factor (Q) can be calculated as Q =1 − (f_e [1 - KF]), where KF is the ratio of the patient's creatinine clearance to an assumed normal value of 120 mL/min. The estimated total body clearance (CL_{PT}) can be calculated as follows: $CL_{PT} = CL_{normT} \times Q$, where CL_{normT} is the value in patients with normal renal function (i.e., patients with a creatinine clearance of ≥120 mL/min). The elimination rate constant of the drug can be calculated as the quotient of the estimated total body clearance and volume of distribution. When these three key kinetic parameters are estimated, the individualized dosage regimen can be calculated as described in Chapter 185.

The optimal dosage regimen for an ICU patient with acute renal failure or chronic kidney disease depends on the desired goal. If there is a significant relationship between maximal plasma concentration and clinical response[38] (e.g., aminoglycosides) or toxicity[39] (e.g., quinidine, phenobarbital, and phenytoin), the dose and dosing interval may need to be modified. If the dosing interval is increased, the maximal plasma concentration and minimal plasma concentration are similar to values in individuals with normal renal function, but the desired target concentrations may not be precisely attained. In this case, consultation with a clinical pharmacist/pharmacologist may be warranted to facilitate the design of a revised dosage regimen. If no specific target values for maximal plasma concentration or minimal plasma concentration have been reported, attaining the same average steady-state concentration may be appropriate (e.g., cephalosporins). This goal can be achieved by decreasing the dose ($D_{PT} = D_{NORM} \times Q$) or prolonging the dosing interval (τ) ($\tau_{PT} = \tau_{NORM} \div Q$)*. If the dose is reduced while the dosing interval remains unchanged, the maximal plasma concentration becomes lower and the minimal plasma concentration higher (Fig. 190-1). This dosage adjustment method if taken to the extreme results in the maintenance of the desired average steady-state concentration by the continuous infusion of a parenteral product. These principles have been used to derive dosage recommendations for 80 commonly used drugs in the ICU for patients with mild, moderate, and severe renal insufficiency (Table 190-5).

IMPACT OF RENAL REPLACEMENT THERAPY

Removal of a drug from the systemic circulation by renal replacement therapy involves several processes: movement from the blood across the dialyzer/hemofilter membrane and into the dialysate/ultrafiltrate and potentially adsorption on the membrane. Passive diffusion (i.e., movement from an area of higher concentration [blood] to one of lower concentration [dialysate]) is the primary mode of drug removal. The renal replacement therapy clearance tends to increase when there is an increase in the surface area of the dialyzer/hemofilter, blood and dialysate/ultrafilrate flow rate, or duration of the treatment. Convective transport and clearance, which represent the simultaneous movement of drug within ultrafiltered plasma water, must be considered if ultrafiltration is a significant component of the renal replacement therapy prescription. Renal replacement therapy clearance is

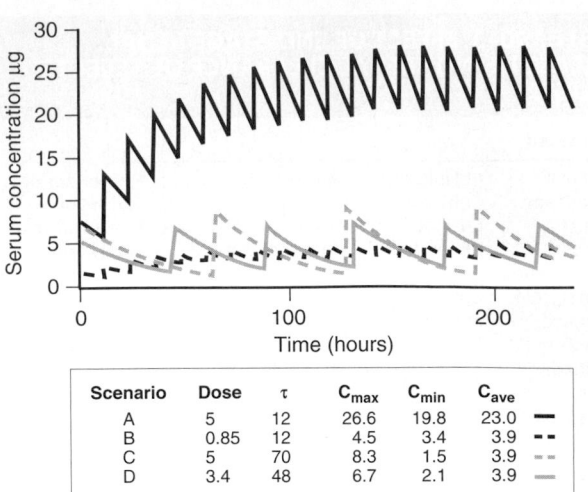

Scenario	Dose	τ	C_{max}	C_{min}	C_{ave}	
A	5	12	26.6	19.8	23.0	—
B	0.85	12	4.5	3.4	3.9	- -
C	5	70	8.3	1.5	3.9	- - -
D	3.4	48	6.7	2.1	3.9	—

FIGURE 190-1. Without a change in dosage regimen, this patient would achieve excessive steady-state serum concentrations (scenario A). Although the average steady-state concentrations (C_{ave}) are identical, the concentration-time profile would be markedly different if one changes the dose and maintains the dosing interval constant (scenario B) versus changing the dosing interval and maintaining the dose constant (scenario C) or changing both (scenario D). C_{max}, maximal concentration; C_{min}, minimal concentration. (From Frye RF, Matzke GR: Drug therapy individualization for patients with renal insufficiency. In Dipiro JT, Talbert RL, Yee GC, et al [eds]: Pharmacotherapy: A Pathophysiologic Approach. New York, McGraw Hill, 2002, pp 939-952.)

higher for drugs that are water soluble, have a low molecular weight, have minimal to no binding to plasma proteins, and have a small volume of distribution.

CONTINUOUS RENAL REPLACEMENT THERAPY

The three primary types of continuous renal replacement therapy are continuous arteriovenous or venovenous hemofiltration, continuous arteriovenous or venovenous hemodialysis, and continuous arteriovenous or venovenous hemodiafiltration. During continuous arteriovenous or venovenous hemofiltration, drugs are removed primarily by convection/ultrafiltration.[40] The clearance of a drug is a function of the permeability of the hemofilter, which is called the sieving coefficient, and the ultrafiltrate flow rate. The sieving coefficient can be approximated by dividing the concentration of the drug in the ultrafiltrate (C_{uf}) by the concentration in the plasma entering the hemofilter (C_a): sieving coefficient = C_{uf}/C_a. The sieving coefficient is often approximated by the fraction unbound to plasma proteins (f_u) because plasma concentrations of the drug of interest may not be readily available. The clearance by continuous arteriovenous or venovenous hemofiltration can be estimated as ultrafiltrate flow rate × f_u. Drug clearance by continuous arteriovenous or venovenous hemodiafiltration can be estimated, provided that the blood flow rate is greater than 100 mL/min and dialysate flow rate is less than 33 mL/min, as (ultrafiltrate flow rate + dialysate flow rate) × (f_u or sieving coefficient). If ultrafiltrate flow rate is negligible (<3 mL/min), as is often the case with continuous arteriovenous or venovenous hemodialysis, continuous or venovenous hemodialysis clearance can be estimated as the product of dialysate flow rate and f_u or sieving coefficient.

Individualization of therapy for a patient receiving continuous renal replacement therapy depends on the patient's residual

---

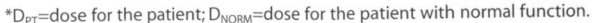

*D_{PT}=dose for the patient; D_{NORM}=dose for the patient with normal function.

TABLE 190–5. DRUG DOSING GUIDELINES FOR PATIENTS WITH RENAL INSUFFICIENCY

Drug	Volume of Distribution (L/kg)	Plasma Protein Binding (%)	Percent Excreted Unchanged in Urine	Regimen for Normal Renal Function	Method	Glomerular Filtration Rate mL/min)*		
						>50	10-50	<10
Acetazolamide	0.2	70-90	100	250 mg q6-12h	IDI	q6h	q12h	Avoid
Acyclovir	0.7	15-30	40-70	5 mg/kg q8h	DD and IDI	5 mg/kg q12-24h	5 mg/kg q24h	2.5 mg/kg q24h
Adenosine	ND	0	<5	3-6 mg i.v. bolus	NC	100%	100%	100%
Alteplase	0.1	ND	ND	60 mg/1 h, then 20 mg/h for 2 h	NC	100%	100%	100%
Amiodarone	70-140	96	<5	800 mg load, then 600 mg q24h	NC	100%	100%	100%
Amoxicillin	0.26	15-25	50-70	250-500 mg q8h	IDI	q8h	q8-12h	q24h
Amphotericin B	4	90	5-10	20-50 mg	IDI	q24h	q24h	q24-36h
Amphotericin B lipid complex	1.7-3.9	90	<1	5 mg/kg q24h	IDI	q24h	q24h	q24-36h
Ampicillin	0.31	0.17-20	60-90	250 mg-2 g q6h	DI	q6h	q6-12h	q12-24h
Atenolol	1.1	20	55	50-100 mg q24h	DD and IDI	100%	50% q48h	30-50% q48-96h
Azithromycin	18	8-50	6-12	250-500 mg q24h	NC	100%	100%	100%
Aztreonam	0.5-1	45-60	75	2 g q8h	DD‡	100%	50-75%	25%
Bumetanide	0.2-0.5	96	33	1-2 mg q8-12h	NC	100%	100%	100%
Cefazolin	0.13-0.22	80	75-95	1-2 g q8h	IDI	q8h	q12-24h	q24-48h
Cefepime	0.3	16	85	2 g q12h	IDI	q12h	q16-24h	q24-48h
Ceftazidime	0.28-0.4	17	60-85	1-2 g q8h	IDI	q8-12h	q24-48h	q48h
Ceftriaxone	0.12-0.18	90	30-65	0.2-1 g q12h	IDI	q12h	q18h	q24h
Cimetidine	0.8-1.3	20	50-70	400 mg q12h	DD	100%	50%	25%
Ciprofloxacin	2.5	20-40	50-70	400 mg q12h	DD	100%	50-75%	50%
Cisapride	2.4	98	5	5-10 mg q8h	DD	100%	100%	50%
Clarithromycin	2-4	70	15-25	0.5-1 g q12h	DD	100%	75%	50-75%
Clindamycin	0.6-1.2	60-95	10	150-300 mg q6h	NC	100%	100%	100%
Colistin	0.5	Low	65-75	2.5 mg/kg q12h	DD	75%	50%	25%
Diltiazem	9-10	98	<10	10 mg q24h	NC	100%	100%	100%
Enalapril	ND	50-60	43	5-10 mg q12h	DD	100%	75-100%	50%
Enoxaparin	0.12	ND	43	Indication dependent	DD	100%	75%	50-75%
Epoprostenol	0.36	ND	<5	2-12 ng/kg/min	NC	100%	100%	100%
Esmolol	ND	ND	<10	Individualize	NC	100%	100%	100%
Etomidate	2-4.5	75	2	0.2-0.6 mg/kg	NC	100%	100%	100%
Famciclovir	1.5	25	50-65	500 mg q8h	DD and IDI	100%	250-500 q24-48h	250 mg q48h
Famotidine	0.8-1.4	15-22	65-80	20-40 mg q24h	DD	50%	25%	10%
Fenoldopam	0.2	ND	<5	0.05-0.1 µg/kg/min	NC	100%	100%	100%
Fentanyl	2-4	80-84	<5	Individualize	DD	100%	75%	50%
Fluconazole	0.7	12	70	200-400 mg q24h	NC	100%	100%	100%
Flucytosine	0.6	10	90	37.5 mg/kg q6h	IDI	q12h	q16h	q24h
Foscarnet	0.3-0.6	17	85	40 mg/kg q8h or 90 mg/kg q12h	DD	70%	37.5%	15%
Gabapentin	0.7	0	90	300-600 mg q8h	DD and IDI	400 mg q8h	300 mg q12-24h	300 mg q48h
Ganciclovir	0.47	ND	90-100	5 mg/kg q12h	IDI	q12h	q24-48h	q48-96h
Glipizide	0.13-0.16	97	4.5-7	2.5-15 mg q24h	DD	100%	50%	50%
Hydralazine	0.5-0.9	87	25	25-50 mg q8h	IDI	q8h	q8-12h	q12-24h
Imipenem†	0.17-0.3	13-21	20-70	0.5-1 g q6h	DD	100%	50%	25%
Insulin	0.15	5	None	Variable	DD	100%	75%	50%
Itraconazole	10	99	35	100-200 mg q12h	DD	100%	100%	50%

Continued

TABLE 190–5. DRUG DOSING GUIDELINES FOR PATIENTS WITH RENAL INSUFFICIENCY—CONT'D

Drug	Volume of Distribution (L/kg)	Plasma Protein Binding (%)	Percent Excreted Unchanged in Urine	Regimen for Normal Renal Function	Method	Glomerular Filtration Rate (mL/min)*		
						>50	10-50	<10
Labetalol	5.6	50	<5	200-600 mg b.i.d.	NC	100%	100%	100%
Lansoprazole	ND	>98	0	15-60 mg q24h	NC	100%	100%	100%
Lepirudin	~0.2	ND	35-45	0.4 mg/kg, then 0.15 mg/kg/h	DD	100%	30-50%	15%
Levofloxacin	1.1-1.5	24-38	67-87	500 mg q24h	DD and IDI	100% q24-48h	250 mg q48h	250 mg q48h
Linezolid	0.93	30	30	600 mg q12h	NC	100%	100%	100%
Lisinopril	0.13-0.15	0-10	80-90	5-10 mg q24h	DD	100%	50-75%	25-50%
Lispro insulin	0.26-0.36	ND	ND	Variable	DD	100%	75%	50%
Lorazepam	3.4	ND	0	1-2 mg q8-12h	NC	100%	100%	100%
Meropenem	0.35	2	65	0.5-1 g q6h	DD and IDI	500 mg q6h	250-500 mg q12h	250-500 mg q24h
Methyldopa	0.5	15	25-40	250-500 mg q8h	IDI	q8h	q8-12h	q12-24h
Methylprednisolone	1.2-1.5	40-60	<10	4-48 mg q24h	NC	100%	100%	100%
Metoprolol	5.5	8	5	50-100 mg b.i.d.	NC	100%	100%	100%
Metronidazole	0.25-0.85	20	20	7.5 mg/kg q6h	DD	100%	100%	50%
Miconazole	ND	90	1	200-1200 mg q8h	NC	100%	100%	100%
Midazolam	1-6.6	93-96	0	Individualize	DD	100%	100%	50%
Milrinone	0.25-0.35	ND	80-85	15-75 μg/kg i.v., then 2.5-1.5 mg q6h orally	DD	100%	100%	50-75%
Morphine	3.5	20-30	0	2-20 mg q4h	DD	100%	75%	50%
Nimodipine	0.9-2.3	98	<10	30 mg q8h	NC	100%	100%	100%
Ofloxacin	1.5-2.5	25	68-80	400 mg q12h	DD and IDI	100%	200-400 mg q24h	200 mg q24h
Omeprazole	ND	95	<5	20-60 mg q24h	NC	100%	100%	100%
Ondansetron	2	75	<5	8-10 mg i.v. q6-12h	NC	100%	100%	100%
Penicillin G	0.3-0.42	50	60-85	0.5-4 million U q6h	DD	100%	75%	20-50%
Phenytoin	0.6-0.9	90	2	1 g load, then 300-400 mg q24h	NC	100%	100%	100%
Piperacillin	0.2-0.3	30	75-90	3-4 g q4h	IDI	q4-6h	q6-8h	q12h
Propofol	8-19	96-99	0.3	2-2.5 mg/kg	NC	100%	100%	100%
Quinupristin/dalfopristin	0.79/0.43	23-32/50-56	15.1/18.7	7.5 mg/kg q12h	NC	100%	100%	100%
Ramipril	1.2	55-70	10-21	10-20 mg q24h	DD	100%	50-75%	25-50%
Ranitidine	1.2-1.8	15	80	150-300 mg q24h	DD	75%	50%	25%
Rifampin	0.9	60-90	15-30	600 mg q24h	DD	100%	50-100%	50-100%
Sodium valproate	0.19-0.23	90	3-7	15-60 mg/kg q24h	NC	100%	100%	100%
Ticarcillin	0.14-0.21	45-60	85	3 g q12h	DD and IDI	1-2 g q4h	1-2 g q8h	1-2 g q12h
Tobramycin	0.22-0.33	<5	95	1.7-2.3 mg/kg q8h	IDI	q12-24h	q24-48h	q48-72h
Trimethoprim	1-2.2	30-70	40-70	100-200 mg q12h	IDI	q12h	q18h	q24h
Urokinase	ND	ND	ND	4400 U/kg load, then 4400 U/kg qh	NC	100%	100%	100%
Valacyclovir, prodrug for acyclovir				500 mg q12h to 1000 mg q8h	DD and IDI	100%	0.5-1 g q12-24h	0.5 g q24h
Vancomycin	0.6-0.9	30-50	90-100	500 mg q6h or 1 g q12h	DD and IDI	1 g q12-24h	1 g q24-96h	1 g q4-7d
Vecuronium	0.18-0.27	30	25	0.1 mg/kg load, then 0.01-0.05 mg/kg q15min	NC	100%	100%	100%

DD, dose reduction method; the percent of the dose for normal renal function to be given at the interval for normal renal function is listed; IDI, increase dose interval method; the interval to be used with the dose for normal renal function is listed; DD and IDI, adjustment of dose and interval; ND, no data; NC, no change.
*The range following glomerular filtration rate (GFR) indicates the use of the dose that corresponds to that range of GFR in patients not on dialysis.
†Seizures in end-stage renal disease.
‡When DD method is employed, the reduced maintenance dose should be preceded by the administration of the standard dose for a patient with normal renal function.
Data from references 35-37 and 39.

renal function and the clearance of the drug by the mode of continuous renal replacement therapy the patient is receiving. The patient's residual drug clearance can be predicted based on the creatinine clearance and the relationship between total body clearance of the drug with creatinine clearance as described previously. The continuous renal replacement therapy clearance, sieving coefficient, and recommended initial dosage regimens of selected drugs that are used frequently in ICU patients receiving continuous arteriovenous or venovenous hemofiltration are listed in Table 190-6.[41,40] Values observed in patients receiving continuous arteriovenous or venovenous hemodialysis or continuous arteriovenous or venovenous hemodiafiltration are listed in Table 190-7. In cases in which specific data on drug clearance are not available and the patient is receiving continuous venovenous hemofiltration, continuous venovenous hemodialysis, or continuous venovenous hemodiafiltration at a dialysate flow rate or ultrafiltrate flow rate of approximately 2 L/h or greater, drug dosing should be initiated at a level consistent with the individual having a creatinine clearance of 30 to 50 mL/min as listed in Table 190-5.

HEMODIALYSIS

Drug-related factors that influence hemodialyzability include the molecular weight, protein binding, and volume of distribution of a drug.[19] The dialysis prescription factors include the composition of the dialyzer, surface area, and blood and dialysate flow rates. The semisynthetic and synthetic dialyzers used in high-flux hemodialysis have the largest ultrafiltration rates and more closely mimic the filtration characteristics of the human kidney. These dialyzers allow the passage of most drugs that have a molecular weight of 15,000 or less.[42] High-molecular-weight drugs, such as vancomycin, are significantly cleared by this mode of dialysis, and the clearance of many smaller drugs is significantly increased as reviewed by Matzke[43] (Table 190-8). A patient receiving high-flux dialysis often requires larger doses than the doses recommended in most reference texts to attain the desired plasma concentrations.

Quantification of the impact of hemodialysis on drug disposition can be calculated in several ways, and this contributes to the variability of values in the literature.[19] The difference between the half-life during dialysis and the half-life of the drug when the patient is off of dialysis provides a crude guide to the impact of dialysis. The half-life during dialysis may not be interpretable in acute renal failure patients because declining plasma drug concentrations during dialysis represent elimination by the patient, which may be considerable. The most accurate means of assessing the effect of hemodialysis is to calculate the dialyzer clearance

TABLE 190–6. CLEARANCE OF DRUGS IN PATIENTS RECEIVING CVVH/CAVH*

Drug	Hemofilter	Ultrafiltration Rate (mL/h)	Half-life (h)	CVVH Clearance (mL/min)	Dosage Recommendation
Amikacin	PS	600	29.7	10.1	IND
	PS	1152	11.4	16.4	
Amrinone	PS	245-576	—	2.4-14.4	None provided
Atracurium	PA	1140	—	8.25	None provided
Ceftazidime	AN69	500-1000	—	7.5-15.6	500 mg q12h
	PMMA	500-1000	—	6.7-12.9	
	PS	500-1000	—	7.6-15.5	
Ceftriaxone	AN69	500-1000	—	4-7.7	300-400 mg q12h
	PMMA	500-1000	—	7.1-11.9	
	PS	500-1000	—	6.9-11.3	
	PA	1200-1800	10.8	16.6	1000 mg q24h
Cefuroxime	PS	850	7.9	11	0.75-1 g q24h
Cilastatin	PS	72-828	13.8	4	NA
Ciprofloxacin	AN69	1000	18.5	12.4	400 mg q24h
Clavulanic acid	PS	NR	2.45	25.2	NA
Fluconazole	AN69	1167	37.7	17.5	400-800 mg q24h
Gentamicin	PS	140-393	34.6	3.47	IND
	PS	322.3	65.4	1.5-12.5	
Imipenem	PS	1000	2.9	13.3	500 mg q6-8h
	PS	1000	3	13.3	
	PS	72-828	2.2	6.6	
Levofloxacin	AN69	1155	26.9	11.5	250 mg q24h
Meropenem	PA	1500-1800	6.37	16.7	0.5-1 g q12h
	PAN	6000-9000	8.7	22	
	PS	2760	2.3	49.7	
	PAN	100-2000	5.9	24.9	
Phenytoin	PS	165	—	1.02	IND
Ticarcillin	PS	NR	4.6	12.3	2 g q8-12h
Tobramycin	PS	140-393	34.6	3.5	IND
Vancomycin	PA	1000	36.5	23.3	750-1250 mg q24h
	AN69	500-1000	—	5.6-11.7	
	PMMA	500-1000	—	6.9-14.4	
	PS	500-1000	—	5.6-11.4	
	S	1000-2000	18.4	6.7-13.3	

*Data are mean or range.
CAVH, continuous arteriovenous hemofiltration; CVVH, continuous venovenous hemofiltration; IND, individualize because desired concentrations may vary markedly depending on patient's condition; LD, loading dose; MD, maintenance dose; NA, not applicable; NR, not reported; PA, polyamide; PMMA, polymethyl methacrylate; PAN, polyacrylonitrile; PS, polysulfone.
Data from references 30-32, 40, and 41.

TABLE 190–7. PHARMACOKINETICS AND CLEARANCE OF DRUGS IN PATIENTS RECEIVING CAVHD/CVVHD*

Drug	Hemofilter	Dialysate Flow Rate (L/h)	Ultrafiltration Rate (mL/h)	Half-life (h)	CVVHD Clearance (mL/min)	Dosage Recommendation
Acyclovir	AN69	0.9-1	65-115	30	NR	5 mg/kg q12h
Ceftazidime	AN69	1-2	448	14.7	13.1-15.2	1 g q24h
	AN69	1-2	30-180	NR	13.5-21.6	0.5-1 g q12h
	PMMA	1-2	30-180	NR	16.6-27.5	
	PS	1-2	30-180	11.9	14.5-24.2	
Ceftriaxone	AN69	1-2	30-180	NR	11.7-13.2	250 mg q12h
	PMMA	1-2	30-180	NR	19.8-30.5	300-400 mg q12h
	PS	1-2	30-180	NR	21.8-29.6	
Cefuroxime	AN69	1-2	448	12.6	14-16.2	750 mg q12h
Cilastatin	AN69	1	500	9.2-14.9	10	NA
Ciprofloxacin	AN69	1-2	434	6.4	16.2-19.9	300 mg q12h
	AN69	1	NR	9.4	37	
	AN69	0.8-1	1044	8.3	21	
Fluconazole	AN69	1	NR	33.8	25	400-800 mg
	AN69	1	1158	23.8	30.5	q12h
Ganciclovir	AN69	1	NR	18.9	12.9	2.5 mg/kg q24h
Gentamicin	AN69	1	420	27	5.2	IND
Imipenem	AN69	1-3	500	1.7-1.9	16-30	500 mg q6-8h
	PS	1.5	NR	3.5	11.6	
Levofloxacin	AN69	1	1110	18.6	21.7	250 mg q24h
Meropenem	PAN	2	NR	4.3	20	1000 mg q8-12h
	PAN	1.6	NR	4.5	30.4	
	PAN	1-1.5	NR	4.4	38.9	
Mezlocillin	AN69 and PS	1-2	0-200	1.1-8.8	11-44.9	2-4gm q24
Piperacillin	AN69	1.5	80-200	4.3	22	4 g q12h
Sulbactam	AN69 and PS	1-2	0-200	4.3-6.4	10.1-22.8	0.5 g q24h
Tazobactam	AN69	1.5	80-200	5.6	17	PIP/TAZO†: 3.375 g q8-12h
Teicoplanin	AN69	1	258-650	99	3.6	LD: 800 mg, then 400 mg q24h × 2; MD: 400 mg q48-72h
Vancomycin	AN69	1-2	570	24.7	12.2-16.6	7.5 mg/kg q12h
	AN69	0.5	474	13.9	4.2	
	AN69	1	162	56.3	8.1	
	AN69	1-2	30-180	NR	10-13.4	
	PMMA	1-2	30-180	NR	14.7-27	1-1.5 g q24h
	PS	1-2	30-180	27.2	1.4-22.1	0.85-1.35 g q24h

*Data are mean or range.
†PIP/TAZO, piperacillin and tazobactam in combination.
CAVHD, continuous arteriovenous hemodialysis; CVVHD, continuous venovenous hemodialysis; IND, individualize because desired concentrations may vary markedly depending on patient's condition; LD, loading dose; MD, maintenance dose; NA, not applicable; NR, not reported; PA, polyamide; PAN, polyacrylonitrile; PMMA, polymethyl methacrylate; PS, polysulfone.
Data from references 30-32, 40, and 41.

of the drug.[19] Because drug concentrations generally are determined in plasma, the calculation of plasma clearance by the dialyzer (CL^p_D) can be calculated as: $CL^p_D = Q_p ([A_p - V_p]/A_p)$ where A_p is the concentration of drug in plasma going into the dialyzer, V_p is the concentration of drug in the plasma leaving the dialyzer, and Q_p is plasma flow, which equals blood flow through the dialyzer (1 − hematocrit). This method accounts for clearance due to diffusion, convection, and adsorption to the dialyzer. The recovery clearance (CL^r_D) approach also has been used for the determination of dialyzer clearance: $CL^r_D = R/AUC_{0-t}$, where R is the total amount of drug recovered unchanged in the dialysate and AUC_{0-t} is the area under the predialyzer plasma concentration-time curve during hemodialysis.[19] This method yields lower clearance values than the previous method if there is a significant degree of binding of the drug to the dialyzer. If adsorption contributes minimally to clearance, the two methods are likely to correlate well.

Drug-dosage regimen individualization can be accomplished by using values of dialyzer clearance, volume of distribution, or half-life during dialysis from the literature. Because clearance terms are additive, the total clearance during dialysis can be calculated as the sum of the patient's residual total body clearance and dialyzer clearance. The half-life during the period between dialysis treatments can be calculated using an estimate of the drug's distribution volume: half-life $=(CL_{PT} + CL_D)/V_D$, where CL_{PT} is the patient's residual total body clearance, CL_D is dialyzer clearance, and V_D is volume of distribution.

The dialyzer clearances for several drugs commonly administered to ICU patients are listed in Table 190-8 along with initial dosage recommendations. Because there is marked variability among dialyzers in the dialyzer clearance of some drugs, it is recommended that dialyzer clearance data for a cellulose dialyzer–drug pair not be extrapolated directly to a synthetic dialyzer. If there are no data regarding high-flux dialysis for a given drug, one should anticipate that the dialyzer clearance by the synthetic dialyzer will be 60% to 100% greater than that of the cellulose dialyzer. If there are no published data on dialyzer clearance or reference

TABLE 190–8. HEMODIALYSIS CLEARANCE BY HEMODIALYSIS*

Drugs	Dialyzer Used	Type of Dialyzer[†]	Hemodialysis Clearance (mL/min)	Dosage Recommendation
Acyclovir	UNK	UNK	113	5-10 mg/kg q24h
	UNK	UNK	UNK	LD: 6 mg/kg; MD: 3 mg/kg q12h
Amikacin	Multiple	CU, CA, RC, PAN	32-125	LD: 5-7.5 mg/kg; MD: IND
Ampicillin/amoxicillin	CDAK 3500	CA	30-60	1000 mg q12-24h
Sulbactam[†]	C-DAK 3500	CA	87.1	0.75-1.5 g q24-48h
Aztreonam	Gambro Lundia	CU	43	LD: 1 g; MD: 0.5 g q12h
Cefazolin	Baxter CT 190	CTA	30.9	15-20 mg/kg q48-72h
	Terumo T175/220	C	20	
	Baxter CA170/210	CA	15.1	
	Fresenius F80	PS	38	1 g q48-72h
Cefmetazole	Baxter CA170/210	CA	86.1	2 g q48-72h
Ceftazidime	Baxter CF 2308	CU	60	1 g q48h
	Fresenius F-60	PS	155	1 g q24h
Cefepime	Baxter CA210/170	CA	158	1-2 g q48-72h
	Fresenius F-60	PS	126.8	
Ceftriaxone	Bellco BL611	H	24	0.5-1 g q24h
	Fresenius E2	CU	31.6	
	Fresenius F40	PS	41.9	
Ceftizoxime	Gambro Lundia	C	44.8	1 g q48h
Clavulanic acid[‡]	Bellco BL 612-M	CU	92.8	100 mg q12-24h
Fluconazole	UNK	UNK	NR	0.2-0.8 g q48h
Ganciclovir	Gambro Lundia IC 3L	CU	48.3	LD: 5 mg/kg; MD: 0.5 mg/kg q48-72h
Gentamicin	Multiple	CA, CU, CR	27-58	LD: 1.7-2.3 mg/kg; MD: IND
	Fresenius F-80	PS	116	
Imipenem/cilastatin	Gambro Lundia 1m2	CU	84/41	0.25-0.5 g q12h
Meropenem	Gambro GFE 11, 15, 18	CU	19	0.5 g q24h
	UNK	CU	22	1 g q48-72h
Metronidazole	Multiple	CA, CU, RC	70-125	0.5-1 g q8h
Mezlocillin	Multiple	CU, C	24-67	2-4 g q8h
Ofloxacin	Gambro IC 3N	CU	59-69	200 mg q24-48h
Phenobarbital	UNK, Fresenius F80	UNK PS	60-174	30 mg q6-8h
Piperacillin	Baxter CF 1511	CU	78.2	4 g q12h
	Baxter CA 210	CA	69.4	
Sulfamethoxazole	Terumo TE-10	CU	42	See Trimethoprim
Tazobactam[§]	Baxter CA210	CA	94.6	PIP/TAZO[¶] 2.25-4.5 g q8-12h
Teicoplanin	Fresenius F8	PS	3.9	6 mg/kg q72h
	Fresenius F60	PS	39.7	LD: 800 mg; MD: 400 mg day 2 3, 5, 12, 19, then IND
Ticarcillin	Baxter UF II	CU	46	3 g q12h
Tobramycin	CDAK 3500	CA, CU	30-55	LD: 1.7-2.3 mg/kg; MD: IND
Trimethoprim	Terumo TE-10	CU	38	5 mg/kg q48-72h
Vancomycin	Baxter CA-210	CA	NR	15 mg/kg q7d
	Fresenius F-80	PS	130.7	LD: 15-25 mg/kg; MD: 7.5 mg/kg q48-72h
	Baxter CT-190	CTA	100.7	
	Hospal Filtral 16	PAN	71.3	

*Data are mean or range.
[†]Used only in fixed-dose combination with ampicillin.
[‡]Used only in fixed-dose combination with amoxicillin or ticarcillin.
[§]Used only in fixed-dose combination with piperacillin.
[¶]PIP/TAZO, piperacillin and tazobactam in combination.
Calculated from author's data.
mL/min/m².
C, cellulose; CA, cellulose acetate; CTA, cellulose triacetate; CR, cuprammonium; CU, cuprophane; H, hemophan; IND, individualize because desired concentrations may vary markedly depending on patient's condition; LD, loading dose; MD, maintenance dose; NR, not reported; PAN, polyacrylonitrile; PMMA, polymethyl methacrylate; PS, polysulfone; RC, regenerated cellulose; UNK, unknown.
Data from references 22, 23, 39, and 43.

sources do not identify the dialyzer that was used, prospective plasma concentration monitoring is recommended to guide therapy.

SUMMARY

The clearance of hundreds of drugs is reduced in critically ill patients, especially patients with acute renal failure or chronic kidney disease. The impact of renal replacement therapy can increase significantly the clearance of many of these agents and necessitate the generation of a revised dosage regimen if one hopes to achieve the desired therapeutic outcomes. The principles in this chapter and the tabulated pharmacokinetic data provide a construct from which clinicians can initiate this process.

ANNOTATED REFERENCES

Aronoff GR, Berns JS, Brier ME, et al: Drug Prescribing in Renal Failure: Dosing Guidelines for Adults, 4th ed. Philadelphia, American College of Physicians, 1999.

This has been the premier clinical reference source for dosage recommendations for patients with reduced renal function for almost two decades. This edition included for the first time dosing guidelines for individuals receiving various modalities of continuous renal replacement therapy. Although it is not designed to precisely individualize therapy, such that desired target plasma drug concentrations are achieved, it remains a sound and reliable tool for initiating drug therapy in critically ill patients.

Levey AS, Greene T, Kusek JW, Beck GJ: A simplified equation to predict glomerular filtration rate from serum creatinine. J Am Soc Nephrol 2000; 11: A0828.

The authors refined their earlier equation to predict GFR from serum creatinine concentration and other factors. It was initially developed by stepwise regression of the results from 1070 of the patients enrolled in the baseline period of the Modification of Diet in Renal Disease (MDRD) Study. The simplified equation provided a more accurate estimate of GFR than measured creatinine clearance or other commonly used equations. It demonstrated accuracy similar to the full equation. This approach has now become the "accepted" method to evaluate renal function in patients with chronic kidney disease.

Matzke GR: Status of hemodialysis of drugs in 2002. J Pharm Practice 2002;15:405-418.

This review article addresses drug dialyzability in a quantitative fashion and outlines the key hemodialysis procedure variables that affect drug removal/dialyzer clearance. It also provides a conceptual framework for the individualization of drug therapy for patients receiving acute or chronic hemodialysis. Drug dosage regimen guidelines are presented for the initiation of drug therapy with many medications commonly utilized for the dialysis-dependent patient. Forty three commonly utilized medications, the majority of which are classically considered to be dialyzable, were reviewed. For 60% of these agents, the data were derived from studies conducted with dialyzers that are no longer commercially available. Data for 17 drugs that were evaluated with new currently available dialyzers as well as those that are no longer commercially available revealed that the clearance by the dialyzer increased by as much as 3-10–fold. The dosage regimens of many drugs for dialysis patients are thus antiquated and likely will result in an excessively conservative approach to therapy.

Mueller BA, Scarim SK, Macias WL: Comparison of imipenem pharmacokinetics in patients with acute or chronic renal failure treated with continuous hemofiltration. Am J Kidney Dis 1993;21:172-179.

Dosing recommendations for the administration of many drugs, including imipenem, to patients with acute or chronic kidney disease are based on the relationship between creatinine and drug clearance in patients with chronic kidney disease. This study confirmed prior observations by this group that the relationship between creatinine and drug clearance of some drugs in critically ill patients with acute kidney disease is different than those observed in patients with chronic kidney disease. The total clearance of imipenem in patients with acute renal failure (108.3 +/– 13.8 mL/min; mean +/– SD) was significantly greater than the total clearance measured in patients with chronic renal failure (64.4 +/– 10.5 mL/min; P <0.02). This increased clearance resulted from a greater nonrenal clearance of the drug. The dosage required to achieve the desired therapeutic outcomes will therefore need to be increased.

Nolin TD, Frye RF, Matzke GR: Hepatic drug metabolism and transport in patients with kidney disease. Am J Kidney Dis 2003;42:906-925.

This review summarizes data available through June 2003 regarding the effect of acute and chronic kidney disease on drug metabolism and renal drug transport. Knowledge of the impact and nature of these alterations associated with kidney disease may facilitate the individualization of medication management in patient populations.

Chapter 191

ANTIDEPRESSANT DRUG OVERDOSE

John W. Kreit

KEY POINTS

1. Antidepressants are the third most common cause of overdose-related death.

2. Antidepressants are most commonly divided into four categories—tricyclic antidepressants (TCAs), selective serotonin reuptake inhibitors (SSRIs), monoamine oxidase inhibitors (MAOIs), and the "atypical" antidepressants.

3. Most antidepressant medications act to increase the extraneuronal concentration of both serotonin (5-HT) and norepinephrine (NE). TCAs and SSRIs prevent the reuptake of these neurotransmitters by inactivating specific transporters in the presynaptic neuron. MAOIs prevent the breakdown of 5-HT and NE after reuptake has occurred.

4. The clinical manifestations of TCA overdose are largely caused by antagonism at α_1-adrenergic and histamine receptors and direct blockade of sodium channels in the His-Purkinje system and ventricular myocardium. Patients typically present with a cholinergic toxidrome that may be complicated by ventricular dysrhythmias, impaired cardiac conduction and contractility, hypotension, seizures, and respiratory failure.

5. A limb lead QRS duration greater than 0.10 second, marked right axis deviation, and an R-wave amplitude greater than 3 mm in lead aVR accurately identify patients who are at risk for development of seizures and ventricular dysrhythmias after TCA overdose. These ECG findings are usually evident at the time of presentation and almost always precede the onset of serious toxicity.

6. MAOI overdose is usually accompanied by mydriasis, flushing, diaphoresis, tachycardia, and hypertension and may cause severe hyperthermia, muscular rigidity, delirium, and seizures.

7. Unlike TCA and MAOI overdose, SSRI ingestion is usually accompanied by little significant toxicity, although seizures, cardiac conduction disturbances, atrial and ventricular dysrhythmias, and serotonin syndrome have occasionally been reported.

8. Treatment of antidepressant drug overdose is largely supportive. Single-dose activated charcoal should be administered to patients who present within 1 hour after ingestion. Gastric lavage *may* be of benefit if performed within 1 hour after a potentially fatal ingestion. Patients with TCA overdose who have signs of cardiac toxicity (i.e., QRS or QT prolongation, ventricular dysrhythmias, heart block, hypotension) should receive intravenous sodium bicarbonate with the goal of achieving and maintaining an arterial pH of 7.50 to 7.55.

Depression is a common and extremely important disease. It has been estimated that 5% to 10% of Americans suffer from depression and that almost one person in five will develop this disease during their lifetime.[1,2] Fortunately, depression usually responds to pharmacologic therapy, and many effective medications are currently available. In patients with refractory depression, however, intentional overdoses of these drugs are common. The American Association of Poison Control Centers recently reported that antidepressants are the third most commonly ingested class of medications, after analgesics and sedatives/hypnotics/antipsychotics.[3] They are also the third most common cause of overdose-related death[3] and are responsible for approximately 8% of all suicides.[4]

Despite the large and ever-growing number of antidepressants, these drugs can be separated into just a few major categories. As shown in Table 191-1, the most commonly used classification scheme divides these medications into tricyclic antidepressants (TCAs), selective serotonin reuptake inhibitors (SSRIs), monoamine oxidase inhibitors (MAOIs), and a miscellaneous group of drugs referred to as "atypical" antidepressants. Although this classification is suboptimal from a pharmacologic standpoint because it mixes structural (TCA) and functional (SSRI, MAOI) drug characteristics, it does provide an effective framework for discussing the clinical manifestations and management of toxic ingestions.

PHARMACOLOGY

Before discussing the actions of the antidepressant drugs, it is important to review the release, reuptake, and metabolism of two monoamine neurotransmitters, which are believed to play a major role in the pathogenesis of depression. Serotonin (5-hydroxytryptamine, 5-HT) and norepinephrine (NE) are each synthesized by specific neurons and packaged into vesicles in the presynaptic nerve terminal. An action potential causes these vesicles to fuse with the nerve membrane, thereby releasing 5-HT or NE into the synaptic cleft. After release, these neurotransmitters bind to specific

TABLE 191–1. CLASSIFICATION OF ANTIDEPRESSANT MEDICATIONS

Generic Name	Brand Name
Tricyclic Antidepressants	
Amitriptyline	Elavil
Amoxapine	Asendin
Clomipramine	Anafranil
Desipramine	Norpramin
Doxepin	Adaptin, Sinequan
Imipramine	Tofranil
Maprotiline	Ludiomil
Nortriptyline	Pamelor
Protriptyline	Vivactil
Trimipramine	Surmontil
Selective Serotonin Reuptake Inhibitors	
Citalopram	Celexa
Escitalopram	Lexapro
Fluoxetine	Prozac
Fluvoxamine	Luvox
Paroxetine	Paxil
Sertraline	Zoloft
Venlafaxine	Effexor
Monoamine Oxidase Inhibitors	
Isocarboxazid	Marplan
Moclobemide*	Manerix
Phenelzine	Nardil
Tranylcypromine	Parnate
Atypical Antidepressants	
Bupropion	Wellbutrin
Mirtazapine	Remeron
Nefazodone	Serzone
Trazodone	Desyrel

*Not available in the United States.

receptors, termed α and β, and each has two major subtypes, referred to as α_1, α_2, β_1, and β_2. After release, the actions of 5-HT and NE are terminated primarily by active reuptake into the presynaptic neuron by amine-specific transporters. There, they are either repackaged into vesicles for future release or inactivated by the mitochondrial-bound enzyme monoamine oxidase (MAO). MAO has the important role of inactivating a wide variety of monoamines and is found in a large number of organs and tissues. There are two enzyme subtypes. MAO-A is found in the CNS, liver, and gastrointestinal tract and inactivates 5-HT, NE, dopamine, epinephrine, and tyramine.[5] MAO-B is found primarily in the CNS and in platelets, and its substrates include dopamine, phenylethanolamine, tyramine, and tryptamine.[5]

PHARMACOLOGIC ACTIONS

Most antidepressant medications, regardless of their classification, act to increase the extraneuronal concentrations of both 5-HT and NE. TCAs and SSRIs prevent the reuptake of these biogenic amines by inactivating their specific transporters in the presynaptic neuron. MAOIs, on the other hand, prevent the breakdown of 5-HT and NE after reuptake has occurred. Most MAOIs, including isocarboxazid, phenelzine, and tranylcypromine, irreversibly inactivate both MAO-A and MAO-B. A newer generation of drugs, most notably moclobemide, competitively inhibit MAO-A; they are often referred to as reversible MAOIs. The atypical group of antidepressants consists of drugs whose mechanisms of action differ from those of the TCAs, SSRIs, and MAOIs. Bupropion acts primarily by inhibiting dopamine reuptake.[5,6] Mirtazapine, nefazodone, and the structurally related trazodone are potent antagonists of postsynaptic 5-HT_{2A} receptors.[5,6]

In general, TCAs preferentially inactivate the NE transporter, and SSRIs, as their name indicates, primarily block 5-HT reuptake. As shown in Table 191-2, however, drugs in both classes have a wide range of potencies and specificities for the 5-HT and NE transporters.[5,6] When considering the TCAs, for example, desipramine is the most potent inhibitor of NE reuptake, whereas clomipramine is the most effective

postsynaptic receptors. Seven serotonin receptor families (designated 5-HT_1, 5-HT_2, and so forth) have been identified, and many contain more than one receptor subtype (e.g., 5-HT_{1A}, 5-HT_{1B}).[5] Each family and each receptor subtype appears to have specific functions and distributions throughout the body, although all are present in the central nervous system (CNS). NE binds to two major families of postsynaptic

TABLE 191–2. POTENCIES OF ANTIDEPRESSANTS FOR BLOCKING NEUROTRANSMITTER REUPTAKE

Drug	Norepinephrine (NE)	Serotonin (5-HT)	Selectivity*
NE-selective drugs			
Desipramine	+++++	++	++
Protriptyline	++++	++	++
Nortriptyline	+++	++	+
Amoxapine	++	+	+
Doxepin	++	+	+
5-HT–selective drugs			
Paroxetine	+	+++++	+++
Clomipramine	+	++++	+++
Sertraline	±	++++	++++
Fluoxetine	±	+++	+++
Citalopram	—	+++	+++++
Imipramine	+	+++	++
Fluvoxamine	—	++	+++
Amitriptyline	+	++	+
Venlafaxine	—	++	+++

The symbol — indicates no effect. Potency increases progressively from ± to +++++.
*Selectivity refers to the difference between a drug's ability to block NE and 5-HT reuptake.

TABLE 191–3. POTENCIES OF ANTIDEPRESSANTS AS RECEPTOR ANTAGONISTS

Drug	Receptors Blocked		
	Cholinergic	Histamine (H_1)	Adrenergic (α_1)
Amitriptyline	+++++	++++	+++++
Protriptyline	+++++	++	++
Clomipramine	+++++	++	++++
Doxepin	++++	+++++	+++++
Imipramine	++++	+++	++
Paroxetine	+++	—	—
Nortriptyline	+++	+++	+++
Desipramine	+++	—	++
Sertraline	+	—	+
Mirtazapine	+	+++++	+
Amoxapine	+	++	+++
Fluoxetine	+	—	—
Citalopram	+	—	—
Fluvoxamine	—	—	—
Venlafaxine	—	—	—
Bupropion	—	—	—
Nefazodone	—	+++	+++++
Trazodone	—	+	++++

The symbol — indicates no effect. Drug potency increases progressively from + to +++++.

serotonin reuptake blocker. Of the SSRIs, paroxetine is the most potent serotonin reuptake inhibitor, but citalopram is the most selective. At present, it is not clear that differences in drug selectivity translate into differences in efficacy, and differences in potency are largely eliminated through dosage adjustments.

In addition to their therapeutic effects on neurotransmitter reuptake, antidepressant drugs also have variable abilities to block α_1-adrenergic, cholinergic, and histamine (H_1) receptors. As shown in Table 191-3, the TCAs are much more effective antagonists than the SSRIs, although potency at each receptor varies widely within this class of drugs.[5,6] Several of the atypical antidepressants are also potent antagonists of H_1 and α_1-adrenergic receptors.[5,6]

ABSORPTION, DISTRIBUTION, METABOLISM, AND EXCRETION

In general, the antidepressants are well absorbed after oral administration, and peak plasma concentrations are usually achieved within several hours. Once absorbed, the TCAs have a very large volume of distribution because they become tightly bound to plasma proteins and accumulate in virtually all tissues and organs. The TCAs, SSRIs, and atypical antidepressants undergo metabolism by the cytochrome P450 microsomal enzymes in the liver.[5,6] This process generates metabolites that are often pharmacologically active. The metabolites can achieve circulating levels that are higher than that of the parent compound or have an elimination half-life that exceeds that of the parent compound, or both. The MAOIs are metabolized primarily by hepatic acetylation, and the rate at which this process occurs varies widely among the population—that is, some people are fast acetylators whereas others are slow acetylators.[5] The duration of action of the antidepressants depends on the clearance rate of the parent compound as well as that of any active metabolites. Table 191-4 demonstrates that the elimination half-life of these drugs varies considerably.[5,6] For example, fluoxetine and its active metabolite norfluoxetine have half-lives of

about 2 and 10 days, respectively, whereas venlafaxine and nefazodone have half-lives of approximately 5 and 3 hours, respectively. Because it takes approximately five half-lives for complete drug elimination to occur, many of the antidepressants can have prolonged effects even after they have been discontinued. Except for moclobemide, which is reversible and short-acting, irreversible enzyme inactivation by the MAOIs causes their effects to last up to 2 weeks after these drugs have been discontinued.[5]

TABLE 191–4. ELIMINATION HALF-LIVES OF ANTIDEPRESSANT MEDICATIONS

Drug	Half-life (hours)*
Tricyclic Antidepressants	
Amitriptyline	16 (30)
Amoxapine	8 (30)
Clomipramine	32 (70)
Desipramine	30
Doxepin	16 (30)
Imipramine	12 (30)
Maprotiline	48
Nortriptyline	30
Protriptyline	80
Trimipramine	16 (30)
Selective Serotonin Reuptake Inhibitors	
Citalopram	36
Escitalopram	30
Fluoxetine	50 (240)
Fluvoxamine	20
Paroxetine	20
Sertraline	24 (65)
Venlafaxine	5 (11)
Atypical Antidepressants	
Bupropion	14
Mirtazapine	24
Nefazodone	3
Trazodone	6

*The numbers in parentheses indicate the elimination half-life of pharmacologically active metabolites.

TOXICOLOGY

TRICYCLIC ANTIDEPRESSANTS

Clinical Features

As shown in Table 191-5, the manifestations of TCA overdose are dominated by neurologic and cardiovascular abnormalities, which can be attributed in large part to the antagonist properties of these drugs. Patients typically present with symptoms and signs of an anticholinergic syndrome (or toxidrome), which may include mydriasis, ileus, urinary retention, fever, flushing, sinus tachycardia, CNS depression that ranges from lethargy to coma, and seizures. Blockade of α_1-adrenergic receptors causes vasodilation that can lead to hypotension. TCAs also cause direct cardiac toxicity by blocking sodium channels in the His-Purkinje system and ventricular myocardium.[7] This effect slows depolarization of the action potential. Consequences can be prolongation of the QRS and QT intervals and development of heart block or ventricular dysrhythmias or both. Inhibition of the sodium current also may lead to decreases in myocardial contractility, stroke volume, and cardiac output. Hypotension and shock can result from vasodilation, impaired contractility, or both.

Diagnosis and Evaluation

The diagnosis of TCA overdose should be strongly suspected in any patient who presents with an anticholinergic toxidrome, especially if the electrocardiogram (ECG) demonstrates characteristic changes (see later discussion). Qualitative urine immunoassays for TCAs may be used to increase the level of suspicion, but they do not distinguish therapeutic from toxic ingestions, and they have relatively low specificity due to cross-reactivity with other drugs, including phenothiazines and diphenhydramine.[8] Quantitative serum assays can be used to confirm a toxic ingestion, but long turnaround time typically limits their clinical usefulness. In patients with a known ingestion, measurement of the TCA concentration is not helpful, because it is a poor predictor of serious toxicity and patient outcome.[9]

An ECG must be obtained for all patients with confirmed or suspected TCA overdose, both to detect conduction

TABLE 191–5. CLINICAL MANIFESTATIONS OF TRICYCLIC ANTIDEPRESSANT OVERDOSE

Central Nervous System

Central nervous system depression
Seizures
Respiratory depression

Cardiovascular System

Sinus tachycardia
Prolonged QRS and QT intervals
Heart block
Ventricular tachycardia/fibrillation
Hypotension/shock

Miscellaneous

Mydriasis
Ileus
Urinary retention
Fever
Flushing

disturbances and dysrhythmias and to assess prognosis. Unlike the serum TCA concentration, several ECG findings have been shown to accurately identify patients at risk for development of seizures and ventricular dysrhythmias. The most commonly cited predictor is a limb-lead QRS duration greater than 0.10 second,[9] although marked right axis deviation and R-wave amplitude greater than 3 mm in lead aVR have been reported to have a higher sensitivity and specificity for serious toxicity.[10-12] These ECG findings are especially useful because they usually are evident at the time of presentation and almost always precede the onset of serious symptoms and signs.[13]

Arterial blood gas measurements are also essential in patients with TCA poisoning, both to assess the degree of respiratory depression and to determine arterial pH. Acidemia reduces TCA-protein binding, thereby increasing the concentration of the free drug and the risk of serious toxicity. Therefore, it is very important to maintain arterial pH within the normal range by administering sodium bicarbonate, adjusting mechanical ventilation, or both. As discussed later, in patients with severe toxic manifestations, sodium bicarbonate should be administered to maintain an alkaline arterial pH.

Management

Prevention of Absorption

Although gastric lavage has long been advocated in the initial management of most drug intoxications, there is little evidence to support its use. In most poisoned patients, including those who have ingested TCAs, gastric lavage fails to significantly reduce drug absorption.[14,15] Furthermore, several randomized trials comparing lavage plus activated charcoal with activated charcoal alone have failed to show an improvement in patient outcome,[16,17] although one study did find that lavage was beneficial when performed within 1 hour after drug ingestion.[18] In a prospective, randomized trial in patients with TCA poisoning, Bosse and colleagues[19] found that gastric lavage did not reduce hospital or intensive care unit (ICU) stay or days of mechanical ventilation. Based on a thorough review of the medical literature, the American Academy of Clinical Toxicology recommends that gastric lavage be *considered* only if it can be done within 1 hour after a potentially *fatal* ingestion.[20] Gastric lavage is performed through a large-bore orogastric tube inserted with the patient in the left lateral/head down position and must be preceded by endotracheal intubation in those with an impaired level of consciousness. It is recommended that small aliquots of saline or water (200 to 300 mL) be used to minimize the risk of vomiting and the movement of gastric contents into the small bowel.[20] Lavage should continue until the effluent is free of particulate matter.

Activated charcoal is an inert, nonspecific adsorbent that irreversibly binds most drugs and toxins and has a time-dependent effect on drug absorption. In volunteer subjects, a single dose of activated charcoal decreases absorption by an average of 69% and 34% when administered within 30 and 60 minutes after drug ingestion, respectively.[21] Studies in animals and human volunteers also demonstrate that the effect of activated charcoal is dose-dependent.[22,23] Accordingly, the dose of activated charcoal should be at least 10 times that of the ingested drug.[24] A standard dose of 50 g should be administered if the dose of the ingestion cannot be quantified.

Despite its proven ability to prevent drug absorption, randomized clinical trials have failed to show that a single dose of activated charcoal improves patient outcome. For example, Hulten and colleagues[25] randomly assigned 77 patients with TCA intoxication to gastric lavage with or without charcoal administration. No difference in symptoms, ICU or hospital stay, need for ventilatory support, or duration of mechanical ventilation was found between the two groups. Based on similar results in patients with a variety of drug ingestions, the American Academy of Clinical Toxicology recommends that activated charcoal be administered only to patients who present within 1 hour after a potentially toxic ingestion.[21]

Enhancement of Drug Elimination

Repeated doses of activated charcoal can increase drug clearance by interrupting enterohepatic circulation and by reducing the concentration of free drug in the intestinal lumen, thereby creating a diffusion gradient from the blood (a process referred to as "gastrointestinal dialysis"). Although multiple doses of activated charcoal increase the clearance of several drugs, including carbamazepine, phenobarbital, and theophylline, studies examining TCA clearance in volunteer subjects have yielded inconclusive and often conflicting results, and no studies have examined this therapy in poisoned patients.[26] For this reason, multiple-dose charcoal is not recommended for patients with TCA intoxication.[26]

Hemodialysis and charcoal hemoperfusion would be expected to be ineffective in removing TCAs and their active metabolites, because avid tissue and plasma protein binding leaves only a small fraction of free drug available for diffusion or adsorption. Although beneficial effects have been reported,[27,28] based on these pharmacokinetic considerations and the lack of efficacy in experimental studies,[29] extracorporeal therapy is not currently recommended for patients with TCA poisoning.

Sodium Bicarbonate

Several controlled trials in animals and case reports and case series in humans have demonstrated that administration of sodium bicarbonate is often effective in shortening the QRS interval, terminating ventricular dysrhythmias, and increasing blood pressure after TCA overdose.[30,31] Three potential mechanisms for these beneficial effects have been proposed.[30] First, alkalinization of the serum increases protein binding of TCAs, thereby reducing the concentration of free drug. Second, by causing drug ionization, alkalinization may reduce the affinity of TCAs for the myocardial sodium channel receptor. Third, an increase in the serum sodium concentration may overcome sodium channel blockade. This final mechanism may explain why hypertonic saline has been reported to reverse cardiac toxicity in some animal studies and in case reports in humans.[32] It may also explain the observation that hyperventilation appears to be less effective than sodium bicarbonate administration.[30] Based on this information, it is currently recommended that patients with evidence of cardiac toxicity (i.e., QRS or QT prolongation, ventricular dysrhythmias, heart block, hypotension) receive sodium bicarbonate with the goal of achieving and maintaining an arterial pH of 7.50 to 7.55.[33]

Treatment of Specific Complications

Dysrhythmias

Ventricular tachycardia and fibrillation accompanying TCA overdose are often refractory to drug therapy, and treatment should focus on the administration of sodium bicarbonate and the correction of acidemia, hypoxemia, and electrolyte abnormalities. Antiarrhythmic drugs categorized as class IA (procainamide), IC (flecainide, propafenone), and III (amiodarone, bretylium, ibutilide, sotalol) are not only ineffective but should be avoided because they, like the TCAs, can prolong depolarization. Case series have described the successful use of both lidocaine[34] and phenytoin[35,36] in patients with cardiotoxicity refractory to sodium bicarbonate therapy, and case reports have suggested that magnesium sulfate may be effective in cases of refractory ventricular dysrhythmias.[37]

Hypotension

Because TCA-induced hypotension may result from vasodilation, impaired cardiac contractility, or both, right heart catheterization is often useful in determining the predominant cause and the most appropriate therapy. Vasodilation resulting from α_1-adrenergic blockade causes a drop in systemic vascular resistance (SVR) and is most effectively treated with volume resuscitation followed, if necessary, by the use of one or more vasopressors. NE may be more effective than dopamine in this setting,[38] and high-dose glucagon has been reported to be beneficial in patients with refractory hypotension.[39] On the other hand, impaired myocardial contractility leads to a fall in cardiac output and a compensatory rise in SVR and responds best to dobutamine and afterload reduction. Sodium bicarbonate administration is often effective in improving hypotension, regardless of the underlying mechanism.

Respiratory Failure

CNS depression or seizures may lead to decreased respiratory drive, hypoventilation, and inability to protect the airway, and patients with severe intoxication often require intubation and mechanical ventilation. In nonintubated patients, serial arterial blood gas measurements must be obtained to evaluate for respiratory (and metabolic) acidosis, and frequent clinical assessment of airway protective reflexes is required.

Seizures

Successful control of seizures has been reported with benzodiazepines, phenytoin, and phenobarbital. Propofol has been effective in patients with refractory status epilepticus.[40]

Clinical Course and Monitoring

Patients with TCA overdose can become critically ill very rapidly, even when initial symptoms or signs are minimal.[41] However, patients who develop major signs of toxicity (coma, seizures, respiratory depression, hypotension, ventricular dysrhythmias) almost invariably do so within 6 hours after presentation, and almost all deaths occur within the first 16 hours.[41] The maximum QRS duration also typically occurs within the first 6 hours[9] and usually returns to normal within 12 to 18 hours.[42] Patients rarely develop seizures or ventricular dysrhythmias after the QRS interval has returned to less than 0.10 second.[9,42] Based on this information, patients should be admitted to an ICU if they have major signs of toxicity or QRS prolongation or if they have been monitored for less than 6 hours in the emergency department. Patients should be transferred from the ICU only after their QRS interval has returned to normal.

SELECTIVE SEROTONIN REUPTAKE INHIBITORS

Clinical Features

The SSRIs have a much more favorable side-effect profile than the TCAs, and overdoses are usually associated with little significant toxicity.[43,44] The most common manifestations are lethargy, diaphoresis, nausea and vomiting, sinus tachycardia, and tremor. Seizures, serotonin syndrome (discussed later), cardiac conduction disturbances (including QRS and QT prolongation), and atrial and ventricular dysrhythmias occasionally have been reported.[45,46] These complications are more likely to occur with venlafaxine than with the other SSRIs.[43,47] Mortality due to SSRI overdose is very uncommon and in most reported cases has been associated with coingestion of other psychotropic agents, benzodiazepines, opiates, or alcohol.[4,43,48] Because of its predilection for more severe toxicity, venlafaxine overdose is associated with the highest mortality rate among the SSRIs.[43,47]

Although uncommon, the most serious toxic manifestation of the SSRIs is a constellation of symptoms and signs referred to as the serotonin syndrome.[49,50] This syndrome may develop during therapy or after overdose and is characterized by the triad of altered mentation, autonomic dysfunction, and neuromuscular hyperactivity. The serotonin syndrome usually develops within 24 hours after the initiation, dose increase, or overdose of the offending medication. Table 191-6 lists the frequency of the clinical manifestations noted in 41 patients diagnosed with this disorder.[49] Laboratory findings are variable and nonspecific and may include leukocytosis and elevations of creatine phosphokinase and the hepatic transaminases.[49,50]

The serotonin syndrome is believed to result from excessive stimulation of $5\text{-}HT_{1A}$ and possibly $5\text{-}HT_2$ receptors; therefore, it can be precipitated not only by SSRIs, but also by any drug that increases the extraneuronal concentration of serotonin.[49] As shown in Table 191-7, excess serotonergic activity may result from several mechanisms, including decreased serotonin metabolism or reuptake, increased release

of serotonin, and the use of 5-HT receptor agonists.[49-52] Although it has been reported with a single agent, the serotonin syndrome almost always occurs in patients taking two or more drugs that increase 5-HT levels. The most commonly implicated drug combinations are an SSRI with a TCA and an SSRI with an MAOI.[49] The serotonin syndrome has also been reported in patients receiving one or more medications that inhibit SSRI metabolism by the cytochrome P450 system.[53]

The diagnosis of serotonin syndrome is based on the presence of typical symptoms and signs, the recent initiation or ingestion of one or more serotonergic medications, and the exclusion of other medical and psychiatric conditions.[49] Neuroleptic malignant syndrome is perhaps the most commonly considered alternative diagnosis, because altered mentation and autonomic and neuromuscular dysfunction occur in both. Several important differences exist, however.[54,55] First, neuroleptic malignant syndrome is an idiosyncratic reaction that usually develops after prolonged exposure to neuroleptic drugs or the withdrawal of dopamine receptor agonists. Second, unlike serotonin syndrome, the clinical manifestations of neuroleptic malignant syndrome usually develop gradually over days or weeks. Finally, neuroleptic malignant syndrome usually is accompanied by marked hyperthermia, severe muscle rigidity, and rhabdomyolysis, but not by mydriasis, diarrhea, hyperreflexia, and myoclonus. It is also important to note that, unlike serotonin syndrome, neuroleptic malignant syndrome is frequently associated with multiple organ failure, and death occurs in as many as 20% of patients.[54,55]

TABLE 191-7. DRUGS THAT INCREASE SEROTONIN ACTIVITY, BY MECHANISM

Increased Serotonin Synthesis

L-tryptophan

Decreased Serotonin Metabolism

Phenelzine
Tranylcypromine
Moclobemide
Isocarboxazid
Selegiline

Serotonin Receptor Agonist

Buspirone
Lithium
Metoclopramide
Sumatriptan
Valproic acid

Increased Serotonin Release

Amphetamines
Cocaine
MDMA (ecstasy)
Reserpine

Inhibition of Serotonin Reuptake

Tricyclic antidepressants
Selective serotonin reuptake inhibitors
Meperidine
Nefazodone
Trazodone
Dextromethorphan
Tramadol
Brompheniramine

TABLE 191-6. CLINICAL MANIFESTATIONS OF THE SEROTONIN SYNDROME

Manifestation	% of Cases
Altered Mentation	
Confusion	41
Agitation	36
Coma	10
Lethargy/obtundation	7
Autonomic Dysfunction	
Diaphoresis	49
Tachycardia	44
Hyperthermia	27
Nausea/vomiting	27
Mydriasis	20
Diarrhea	10
Neuromuscular Hyperactivity	
Myoclonus	49
Hyperreflexia	41
Restlessness	29
Muscle rigidity	20
Tremor	17
Trismus	7

From Callahan M, Kassal D: Epidemiology of fatal tricyclic antidepressant ingestion: Implications for management. Ann Emerg Med 1985;14:29-37.

Management

The treatment of SSRI overdose is primarily supportive. Gastric lavage is almost never indicated, given the low risk of serious drug toxicity. Single-dose activated charcoal may be administered to patients who present within 1 hour after drug ingestion. Because major morbidity and mortality almost always result from the effects of other ingested medications, efforts must be made to identify and treat the toxic manifestations of these drugs.

Treatment of the serotonin syndrome is also largely supportive, although it is essential that all serotonergic agents be identified and discontinued. The serotonin syndrome usually has a benign course, and symptoms and signs typically resolve within 24 hours after discontinuation of the offending medications.[49] Occasionally, however, severe complications occur and require specific therapy; these include marked hyperthermia, rhabdomyolysis, disseminated intravascular coagulation, renal failure, and acute respiratory distress syndrome. Case reports suggest that the serotonin receptor antagonists, cyproheptadine and chlorpromazine, may be useful in severe cases.[56,57]

MONOAMINE OXIDASE INHIBITORS

The symptoms and signs that accompany MAOI overdose are believed to result primarily from a hyperadrenergic state produced by the inability to metabolize and inactivate NE in the central and peripheral nervous systems. Overdose with the irreversible MAOIs is commonly accompanied by life-threatening toxicity, and the mortality rate is similar to that of TCA ingestion.[4,47] Clinical manifestations, which may be delayed for up to 24 hours, include mydriasis, flushing, diaphoresis, tachycardia, hypertension, hyperthermia, muscular rigidity, agitation, delirium, and seizures.[58,59] Hypotension may occur later in the course, probably as the result of depletion of NE stores. As discussed previously, the serotonin syndrome may also develop, especially if MAOIs are combined with another drug that increases CNS serotonin levels. Reversible MAOIs, such as moclobemide, are much less toxic, and even massive overdoses have been accompanied by little morbidity.[60]

Patients with MAOI overdose should undergo gastric lavage and receive activated charcoal, if they present within 1 hour after drug ingestion.[20,21] Severe hypertension is best controlled with sodium nitroprusside, and hypotension usually responds well to NE.[58,59] Dopamine acts largely by releasing stored NE and should be avoided, because it may either worsen the hyperadrenergic state or be ineffective due to endogenous NE depletion.[58,59] Hyperthermia may be severe and may require evaporative cooling techniques. Muscle rigidity usually responds to benzodiazepines but may require the use of neuromuscular blockade. Seizures typically respond to benzodiazepines, phenytoin, and phenobarbital.

ATYPICAL ANTIDEPRESSANTS

Relatively little is known about the consequences of overdose with the atypical antidepressants. Large overdoses of bupropion can cause seizures and QRS prolongation, and rhabdomyolysis and hepatic necrosis have been reported.[61] The major manifestations of nefazodone and trazodone overdose are hypotension and CNS depression, which may progress to coma.[62,63] Mirtazapine ingestion has been accompanied by CNS and respiratory depression.[64] Treatment of overdose with one of the atypical antidepressants is largely supportive. Patients who present within 1 hour after ingestion should undergo gastric lavage and receive single-dose activated charcoal.[20,21]

ANNOTATED REFERENCES

Richelson E: Pharmacology of antidepressants. Mayo Clin Proc 2001;76:511-527.
> This is an authoritative and comprehensive review of the absorption, elimination, and pharmacologic actions of the antidepressants.

Boehnert MT, Lovejoy FH: Value of the QRS duration versus the serum drug level in predicting seizures and ventricular arrhythmias after an acute overdose of tricyclic antidepressants. N Engl J Med 1985;313:474-479.
> This prospective study was the first to demonstrate that ECG changes are much more accurate than serum drug levels in predicting major TCA toxicity.

Blackman K, Brown SG, Wilkes GJ: Plasma alkalinization for tricyclic antidepressant toxicity: A systematic review. Emerg Med 2001;13:204-210.
> This article reviews the mechanisms of action and therapeutic effect of sodium bicarbonate administration in patients with severe TCA toxicity.

Mason PJ, Morris VA, Balcezak TJ: Serotonin syndrome: Presentation of 2 cases and review of the literature. Medicine (Baltimore) 2000;79:201-209.
> This is a comprehensive review of the clinical manifestations, diagnosis, and treatment of serotonin syndrome.

Thorp M, Toombs D, Harmon B: Monoamine oxidase inhibitor overdose. West J Med 1997;166:275-277.
> This article is one of the few published reviews of MAOI intoxication.

Chapter 192
CLINICAL USE OF IMMUNOSUPPRESSANTS

Kristine S. Schonder • Robert J. Weber • John J. Fung • Thomas E. Starzl

KEY POINTS

1. **Allograft rejection** is mediated primarily by the T cell in response to the presence of an antigen, which is processed by antigen-presenting cells (APC) and carried on the major histocompatibility complex (MHC) molecules to the T cell.

2. **The T-cell receptor (TCR)**, in conjunction with accessory molecules such as CD3, CD4, and CD8, interacts with the antigen fragment on the MHC molecule and produces the growth factor interleukin-2 (IL-2) to activate the T cell and stimulate proliferation of the T cell.

3. **During allograft rejection**, cytokines attract various cells into rejecting allografts, stimulate the production of antibodies, and produce inflammation.

4. **Effective immunosuppressive protocols** combine multiple drugs targeted at different sites of the T-cell activation cascade.

5. **Corticosteroids block the early steps of T-cell activation;** they are used in tapering doses during the induction and maintenance phases of immunosuppressive protocols and in high, brief doses for the reversal of acute rejection episodes.

6. **The backbone of immunosuppressive protocols** are the calcineurin inhibitors cyclosporine and tacrolimus, which inhibit IL-2 production and subsequent T-cell activation and proliferation.

7. **Azathioprine and mycophenolate mofetil** inhibit purine synthesis, thereby disrupting the cell cycle and T-cell proliferation.

8. **Sirolimus** blocks the cellular response to IL-2 and inhibits the progression of the cell cycle, inhibiting T-cell proliferation.

9. **Antithymocyte globulin and monoclonal antibodies are potent cytotoxic compounds** that cause rapid, profound, and prolonged T-cell depletion; they are effectively used to reverse acute rejection episodes or as induction therapy before transplantation.

10. **Drug concentration monitoring is necessary** to maximize efficacy in preventing allograft rejection while minimizing the potential for significant adverse effects; monitoring aids in the management of drug interactions, particularly with cyclosporine, tacrolimus, and sirolimus therapy.

Advances in molecular biology and immunology have provided for greater understanding of the mechanisms involved in allograft rejection. Many of the key pathways of organ rejection are targeted by the growing armamentarium of immunosuppressive drugs available today. The vast array of immunosuppressive combinations has dramatically decreased the incidence of acute allograft rejection. However, very little ground has been gained with respect to the impact of chronic allograft rejection on long-term allograft survival. Furthermore, the relative nonselectivity of the current immunosuppressants with long-term use can lead to the development of malignancies and opportunistic infections. As we continue to explore different combinations of immunosuppressants and new immunosuppressive pathways, we will continue to grow in our comprehension of the immune system and come closer to true allograft acceptance.

BASIC PRINCIPLES OF IMMUNOSUPPRESSION

Optimal immunosuppression, as it relates to transplantation, is defined as the level of drug therapy that achieves graft acceptance with least suppression of systemic immunity. By optimizing immunosuppressive therapy, systemic toxicity (i.e., infection and malignancy) and other side effects can be minimized, albeit not entirely eliminated. Because monitoring of blood levels and titration of immunosuppression on this basis is possible with only a few agents, in practice, oversuppression or undersuppression almost invariably becomes apparent only in retrospect. Recently, monitoring of CD3+ cell counts has provided an alternative means of measuring the degree of immunosuppression.

Current immunosuppression protocols typically use multiple drugs, each directed at a discrete site in the T-cell activation cascade.[1] Most immunosuppressive regimens combine drugs, often with differing modes of action and toxicities, allowing lower doses of each drug. Transplantation immunosuppression can be (1) *pharmacologic*, consisting of drugs such as corticosteroids, cytokine suppressive agents, and cell cycle inhibitors, or (2) *biologic*, consisting of monoclonal and polyclonal antilymphocyte antibodies and anticytokine receptor antibodies.[2]

The combination of cyclosporine or tacrolimus with a corticosteroid forms the backbone of most *maintenance immunosuppressive regimens* being used today. An antiproliferative agent may also be added. In general, the early postoperative period calls for the greatest degree of immunosuppression. As time goes on, many patients can maintain graft function with smaller doses of immunosuppressive agents.

If *acute cellular rejection* occurs, it is common to treat with a brief course of high-dose corticosteroid therapy, antilymphocyte antibodies, or both. Generally, high doses of a corticosteroid are used initially to reverse the acute attack on the allograft. Antilymphocyte antibody therapy with monoclonal or polyclonal antibodies is used for more severe rejection or if corticosteroid therapy fails.

Induction therapy, also called *prophylactic therapy*, refers to the use of antilymphocyte antibodies immediately after transplantation. This practice is based on the theory that early incapacitation of the immune system may reduce the likelihood of subsequent rejection. Claimed benefits are delayed onset of acute rejection, fewer episodes of rejection, and no significant increase in infectious complications.[3,4] The related concept of *sequential therapy* was introduced in response to the significant renal toxicity of cyclosporine observed in recipients of liver, heart, and kidney transplants. The practice is to use antibody therapy for the first 1 to 2 weeks after transplantation—the period in which renal injury is most likely to occur from a variety of insults. Cyclosporine therapy is not used during this period but is started later. The impact of this strategy on long-term renal function is much less clear.

This early intensification of immunosuppression is not universally accepted. Some experts voice concern because of the well-known association between antilymphocyte antibody therapy (and immunosuppression in general) and infection and malignancy.[5,6] Others describe no benefit, greater expense,[7] or the successful use of regimens that avoid induction altogether.[8] Intermediate strategies involve the use of induction only in high-risk patients or the use of just one dose of an antilymphocyte agent, followed by early evaluation of renal function.

Although some patients can tolerate complete withdrawal of immunosuppressive therapy without exhibiting rejection,[3] it is best done as a protocol-based strategy with patients under strict supervision. The current general approach is to minimize long-term immunosuppression. Various withdrawal protocols target individual components of the immunosuppressive regimen (e.g., corticosteroids, calcineurin inhibitors) in an attempt to decrease serious complications of immunosuppression; namely, infection, malignancy, and renal dysfunction.

OVERVIEW OF TRANSPLANTATION IMMUNOBIOLOGY

Antigen specificity is determined by an antigen-binding unit on the surface of the T cell called the T-cell receptor (TCR). The specificity and diversity of the TCR binding site result from variations in its amino acid composition among different T cells. The gene sequence coding for the TCR rearranges during development in the thymus, such that each T cell has a different TCR binding specificity. The result is a complex system that enables lymphocytes to discriminate between "self" and "nonself" or foreign antigen.

Once inside tissues or the circulation of the body, foreign antigen is presented to the lymphocytes by antigen-presenting cells (APCs), epitomized by dendritic cells. APCs phagocytose foreign proteins and cleave them enzymatically into small peptides that are 8 to 12 amino acids in length. These peptides are loaded onto a class of specialized carrier molecules, known as major histocompatibility complex (MHC) molecules.

The MHC molecule carries the peptide fragment to the cell surface, where it is displayed to T cells in the host lymphoid organs. Thus, there are three essential requirements for the adaptive immune response known as rejection: (1) the presence of an antigen fragment or protein (a ligand) at the cell surface of the APC, (2) a receptor fit for the ligand, and (3) the activation of T cells.

The migration pattern of the antigen also is a critical factor. The only mobile antigen in organ transplantation consists of passenger leukocytes of bone marrow origin that are present in the graft and that migrate promptly and preferentially to host lymphoid organs.[9-11] These organs or organized heterotopic lymphoid collections provide the unique architectural structure and cellular milieu wherein factors that are necessary for progression from an immunogenic environment to a tolerogenic environment are present in abundance. These factors include cytokines, other molecules, cell–cell proximity, and homing mechanisms that ensure an efficient response to the antigen.[12] In the lymphoid organs, dendritic cells and other APCs that have captured and processed the antigen present the peptide fragment of the antigen to antigen-specific TCRs in the context of their upregulated host MHC peptide.

The efferent (effector) phase begins with the secretion of interleukin-2 (IL-2, or T-cell growth factor) and interferon-α (IFN-α) by activated lymphocytes. The antigen-specific immune activation and clonal expansion is aborted unless there is upregulation by the APCs of "accessory" cell-bound (costimulatory) molecules that sustain accelerated production of IL-2 and foster the secretion of numerous other cytokines (e.g., IL-1, IL-6, IL-9, IL-10, IFNs, tumor necrosis factor-α [TNF-α], TNF-β) and growth factors (granulocyte colony-stimulating factor [G-CSF] and granulocyte-macrophage colony-stimulating factor [GM-CSF]).[13] The sequential nature of the response amplification has been obscured by use of the term "costimulatory" to describe the accessory molecules, implying that the afferent and early effector phases are simultaneous.

The TCR is a cell surface molecule that associates with "accessory" molecules, including CD3, and either CD4 or CD8. The TCR-CD3 complex interacts with the peptide fragment carried by the MHC molecule of the APC. This complex is stabilized by the CD4 or CD8 molecule of the T cell. This interaction produces the signal that initiates activation of the T cell, leading to proliferation of a T-cell clone that recognizes the particular antigen fragments of the foreign protein. The basis for MHC-restricted antigen recognition requires antigen presentation by APCs bearing an MHC molecule specific to the host.

Antigen-directed proliferation of T-cell clones is absolutely essential for an effective immune response. The response is driven by a positive feedback loop. T cells that recognize antigen make the potent growth factor IL-2 and simultaneously become responsive to IL-2 by expressing the IL-2 receptor. This dual synthesis allows the cells to stimulate their own proliferation, as well as the proliferation of other T cells. Lymphocytes recirculate at a rate of 1% to 2% per hour, migrating through all tissues of the body. Specialized cell surface "homing" molecules on T lymphocytes mediate attachment to targeted alien tissues, with a special avidity for the endothelial cells of an allograft's vessels.

During an ongoing immune response, proliferating T cells recruit many other cell types and immune mechanisms into action. The cytokines can attract and activate other leukocytes. For example, cytokines produced by CD4-positive helper T cells attract macrophages and CD8-bearing cytotoxic lymphocytes into rejecting allografts.[14] These cytokines also trigger macrophage activation and CD8+ T-lymphocyte cell maturation. The resulting multicellular tissue infiltration has traditionally been referred to as a *delayed-type hypersensitivity* response. Cytokines released by helper T cells also are responsible for the activation of B cells and thus, indirectly, for the majority of antibody production. Cytokines also upregulate both MHC molecules on tissues and adhesion molecules on endothelium. These events aid in the entry and accumulation of leukocytes. Finally, cytokines activate distant organ responses, such as the hepatic acute phase response, production of phagocytes in the bone marrow, and the hypothalamic-pituitary axis, producing the systemic signs of inflammation.

Once the antigen is consumed or removed, the process downregulates. If antigen removal is incomplete, continuously sensitized ("memory") T cells remain and contribute to a stronger secondary response on rechallenge with the same antigen. However, in some instances, if the antigen cannot be eliminated, the immune response can become exhausted and T cells deleted by mechanisms that are not fully understood but include Fas ligand–mediated apoptosis. Exhaustion-deletion in the first weeks or months after transplantation is never complete, but it can be maintained in a stable state by small numbers of persistent donor leukocytes.

Molecular insights regarding IL-2 gene transcription and the structure of the IL-2 receptor (IL-2R) have led to IL-2R–targeted therapy. As molecular knowledge has advanced, investigators have gained greater understanding of the workings of many immunosuppressants. New strategies guided by this knowledge have resulted in attempts to develop site-directed immunosuppression. Virtually every known step of the immune process can be targeted, and many new drugs are now in various stages of evolution.

SPECIFIC AGENTS

CORTICOSTEROIDS

Corticosteroids are extensively used in brief courses, at high doses, for the reversal of acute rejection episodes. These drugs are also used extensively in clinical immunosuppressive protocols, for both induction and maintenance phases.[15] Five glucocorticosteroids are commonly used in transplantation: hydrocortisone, prednisone, prednisolone, methylprednisolone, and dexamethasone.

Because hydrocortisone has the greatest mineralocorticoid activity per unit of glucocorticoid activity, its routine application in transplantation is relatively limited. The other four agents have more glucocorticoid activity in proportion to their mineralocorticoid activity.

Prednisone has an oral bioavailability of about 80%, and it is metabolized in the liver to its active form, prednisolone. Oral prednisolone has a bioavailability of 100%. The serum half-life of both prednisone and methylprednisolone is 2 to 3 hours.[16] The oral bioavailability of dexamethasone is 61%, with a half-life of 2 hours.[17] However, the clinical activity of corticosteroids (i.e., suppression of cytokine production) persists for 24 hours or longer. In other words, the half-life for biologic activity is much longer than the circulating half-life.

There is no universally accepted fixed dosing regimen for corticosteroids. Rather, the dose is often dictated by local protocol. A preoperative dose of 250 to 1000 mg of methylprednisolone may be given, followed by 20 to 200 mg/day during the first week. Acute rejection may be treated with one to three large doses—250 to 1000 mg of methylprednisolone—or by a regimen starting at 200 mg/day of oral prednisone and tapering to baseline maintenance doses over 3 to 6 days. There is evidence that doses lower than those traditionally used can be equally effective. In combination regimens, steroid doses often can be reduced to 5 or 10 mg/day or less and perhaps given every other day.

Corticosteroids have broad effects on many cell types. These agents interfere with the production of IL-1 and IL-2, blocking the early steps of T-cell activation. Other pharmacologic effects related to immune function include the following:

1. Antagonism of inflammatory mechanisms by stabilization of leukocyte lysosomal membranes, reduction in capillary permeability, and inhibition of histamine release and the kinin and complement systems
2. Drastic reduction of lymphocyte traffic and circulating immunoglobulin levels and reduction in the number of neutrophils and eosinophils
3. Inhibition of leukocyte adhesion to endothelium

Prednisone and prednisolone have much less mineralocorticoid effect than the naturally occurring glucocorticoids do; however, sodium retention, edema, hypertension, potassium loss, and hypokalemic alkalosis can be seen with prolonged use of these drugs. Suppression of the pituitary-adrenal axis can be seen with all corticosteroids, but the magnitude of this effect varies among patients. Acute adrenal insufficiency can develop unexpectedly if patients are stressed, even as long as 12 months after steroids are withdrawn.

The adverse effects of corticosteroids are numerous and cause considerable morbidity. An increased incidence of serious infections is well documented. Impaired fibroblast growth and collagen synthesis contribute to poor wound healing. Hence, surgical wounds and anastomoses are at increased risk for dehiscence, and gastrointestinal ulcers tend to heal slowly, leading to increased risks of perforation and rebleeding. Spontaneous ulceration of the gastrointestinal tract occurs in approximately 2% of patients taking steroids. Because signs of inflammation are suppressed, the diagnosis of intraabdominal infection and peritonitis can be significantly delayed, sometimes with disastrous consequences.

Steroids impair glucose tolerance, often dramatically. For patients receiving large doses of steroids, it often is best to use "sliding-scale" insulin regimens to ensure adequate control of blood sugar levels. Some patients require long-term therapy with oral hypoglycemic agents or insulin to maintain adequate glucose control.

Central nervous system effects, such as euphoria and mood swings, are well known. These adverse effects are generally dose dependent and are seen most frequently early in the postoperative period or with therapy for acute rejection episodes, when higher doses of steroids are used. Central nervous system effects are usually self-limited and do not require treatment.

Long-term use of steroids can cause bone demineralization and lead to osteoporosis. Atherosclerosis may be accelerated. Prolonged administration of glucocorticoids is associated with an increased incidence of cataracts and elevated intraocular pressure (glaucoma). Soft-tissue and dermal changes (e.g., fat redistribution, skin atrophy, "moon face," striae) produce the characteristic cushingoid appearance.

To minimize the development of adverse sequelae, most immunosuppressive protocols attempt to reduce the dose of steroids over time to physiologic levels (equivalent to 5 mg/day or less of prednisone). However, corticosteroid doses must be reduced carefully to minimize side effects while maintaining adequate immunosuppression to prevent acute rejection of the allograft.

CYTOKINE INHIBITORS

Before the introduction of cyclosporine, immunosuppression protocols relied heavily on corticosteroids and cytotoxic drugs. These regimens had the disadvantage of producing broad suppression of the immune and inflammatory cascades. Cyclosporine introduced a new era of immunosuppression, because it provided potent, relatively specific, and noncytotoxic suppression of T-cell activation.

Cyclosporine

Cyclosporine is a lipophilic cyclic polypeptide with 11 amino acids and a molecular weight of 1202. On entering the T cell, cyclosporine binds to cyclophilin, a cytoplasmic immunophilin protein. The cyclosporine-cyclophilin complex inhibits the activity of calcineurin, which, in turn, inhibits transcription of several genes, including those transcribing IL-2, IL-3, IL-4, GM-CSF, IFN-γ, and TNF-α. One key action that results from blockade of calcineurin is inhibition of signaling via nuclear factor of activated T cells (NF-AT), which regulates activation of the IL-2 gene; this effect ultimately prevents the synthesis of IL-2.[18] Inhibition of the synthesis of IL-2, a potent T-cell growth factor, is the crucial activity of cyclosporine.

Cyclosporine is insoluble in water and therefore must be dissolved in an organic solvent. There currently exist two formulations: cyclosporine (Sandimmune, Novartis Pharmaceuticals, East Hanover, NJ) and cyclosporine for microemulsion (cyclosporine, modified; Neoral, Novartis Pharmaceuticals, and Gengraf, Abbott Laboratories, North Chicago, IL). The microemulsion formulation substantially increases cyclosporine absorption; the overall time to peak cyclosporine concentration is reduced, the peak concentration is higher, and the area under the curve (AUC) is increased. The lipophilicity of the conventional cyclosporine formulation is responsible for its variable bioavailability.

Oral bioavailability is about 30%, but there is much individual variability (range, 10% to 60%). Absorption in the small intestine decreases with bowel dysfunction or reduced bile flow.[19] The volume of distribution of cyclosporine is large and variable. Cyclosporine is metabolized in the liver via cytochrome P450 (CYP) 3A4 enzymes. It also is a substrate for the p-glycoprotein efflux pump. The mean terminal half-life with normal liver function is 19 hours. The microemulsion formulation of cyclosporine has superior pharmacokinetics, does not require bile excretion for its bioavailability, and is better dispersed and absorbed compared with conventional cyclosporine. The relative bioavailability of the microemulsion formulation is approximately 60%.[20] The total AUC is increased by 30% compared with the conventional formulation.[21]

At least 17 cyclosporine metabolites have been identified, and at least a few of them are immunosuppressive, although considerably so less than the parent compound. The half-life increases with hepatic failure and is changed significantly by coadministration of a large number of other drugs that can increase or decrease serum levels by induction or competitive

TABLE 192–1. SOME OF THE DRUGS THAT ALTER CYCLOSPORINE AND TACROLIMUS CONCENTRATIONS

Increase	Decrease
Diltiazem	Rifampin
Nicardipine	Carbamazepine
Verapamil	Phenobarbital
Fluconazole	Phenytoin
Itraconazole	Ticlopidine
Ketoconazole	Nafcillin
Clarithromycin	
Erythromycin	
Methylprednisone (in large doses)	
Bromocriptine	
Danazol	
Protease inhibitors	

inhibition of P450 (Table 192-1).[22] For all these reasons, it is essential that levels be monitored regularly and dosage adjusted accordingly.

Monitoring of cyclosporine levels is not straightforward. Different results are obtained when cyclosporine concentrations in blood or plasma are determined by radioimmunoassay and by high-pressure liquid chromatography (HPLC). Neither method is clearly superior, and there are no universally accepted blood levels; target levels vary widely from center to center. Desired levels in serum or plasma, as measured by radioimmunoassay,[23] are 150 to 250 ng/mL at the time of transplantation, tapering to 50 to 100 ng/mL after 3 to 6 months. If the drug is measured in whole blood by HPLC, desired levels are 100 to 300 ng/mL initially, tapering to 80 to 200 ng/mL.

Recent literature suggests that AUC values and peak concentrations measured 2 hours after dosing (C_2) are more sensitive predictors of cyclosporine effects and may be better parameters to guide therapeutic monitoring of the microemulsion formulation of cyclosporine. Decreased bioavailability of cyclosporine has been correlated with acute rejection.[24] The first 4 hours after administration of a dose of cyclosporine represents the period of greatest variability in cyclosporine absorption.[25] Limited sampling techniques, consisting of two to five blood samples drawn within the first 4 hours after cyclosporine administration, are used to determine the AUC. AUC values greater than 4400 μg/L/hour correlate well with a low incidence of allograft rejection.[24,26] One study compared the correlation between the trough concentration, C_2, and the occurrence of rejection and concluded that trough concentrations lack predictive value; however, acute rejection did not occur in patients with C_2 values greater than 1200 μg/L.[27] Because of the convenience of a single blood sample compared with the multiple blood samples necessary for AUC measurements, C_2 monitoring is becoming a preferred way to adjust cyclosporine dosing. C_2 levels should range between 1.5 and 2.0 μg/mL for the first few months after transplantation and should be reduced to 0.8 μg/mL after 6 to 12 months of therapy.[26,28]

The typical daily intravenous dose of cyclosporine is 4 to 5 mg/kg. This amount can be given in two divided doses, each being delivered over 2 to 6 hours. Alternatively, some prefer to use a slow, continuous infusion over 24 hours. The changeover to oral dosing usually requires a dose three times higher, or about 12 to 15 mg/kg/day. Oral cyclosporine should be administered every 12 hours. After 1 to 2 weeks, the dosage can be slowly tapered, once equilibration within body fat stores occurs. In many patients, the dose is tapered to as low as 3 mg/kg/day by 6 months after transplantation. Liver transplant recipients who have a T tube, which diverts some bile flow, require higher oral doses because of decreased absorption. Pediatric patients eliminate cyclosporine faster than adults do, and they require larger doses, typically about 5 to 6 mg/kg/day intravenously and 14 to 18 mg/kg/day orally. Some pediatric patients require doses up to 50% to 100% larger than adult doses.

Several adverse effects can occur early after initiation of cyclosporine therapy. Acute nephrotoxicity and hypertension are major problems. The mechanisms responsible for these adverse effects are controversial.[29,30] Nephrotoxicity may be the result of cyclosporine-induced afferent arteriolar vasoconstriction that results, in part, from an imbalance between the production of prostaglandin E_2, a vasodilator, and that of thromboxane A_2, a vasoconstrictor.[31,32] Other possible factors include endothelin-1–induced vasoconstriction and impaired nitric oxide production.[33] Cyclosporine-induced nephrotoxicity is transient and reversible with a decrease in dosage or discontinuation of the drug.[34] The incidence of nephrotoxicity varies from approximately 25% to 38%.[35]

Neurotoxicity associated with cyclosporine ranges from minor toxicity, manifesting as tremors, to severe complications, such as seizures or encephalopathy.[36] Tremors caused by cyclosporine are common (prevalence, 10% to 55%) and may improve over time without a change in therapy. The causal association between seizures and encephalopathy often is not clear.[36] Several reports have detailed a rare syndrome that is characterized by confusion and cortical blindness in both liver and bone marrow transplantation patients. Hypomagnesemia and hypocholesterolemia are believed to be risk factors for cyclosporine-induced neurotoxicity.[29]

Hypertension occurs frequently and usually begins within weeks after commencement of cyclosporine therapy. The incidence of hypertension varies widely in different patient populations, ranging from 10% to 80%.[35] It is hypothesized[37] that hypertension is caused by cyclosporine-induced vasoconstriction in the renal or systemic circulation, or both, perhaps as a result of antagonism of endothelium-derived relaxation factors or increased synthesis of endothelin-1, a vasoconstrictor. Hypertension responds to sodium restriction. Hypertension is best managed with diuretics or calcium channel blockers.[30]

Cyclosporine is diabetogenic, although analysis of this effect is confounded by the frequent concomitant use of steroids with cyclosporine. Other metabolic effects of cyclosporine include hypochloremic alkalosis and changes in serum concentrations of potassium, magnesium, prolactin, and testosterone. Hepatotoxicity, manifested by cholestatic jaundice, is common,[29] but intrahepatic cholestasis often resolves if the dose of cyclosporine is reduced. Connective tissue side effects of cyclosporine are common and can be distressing to the patient because of the cosmetic manifestations. These changes include hirsutism (seen within 2 to 4 weeks in 20% to 45% of patients receiving cyclosporine), gingival hyperplasia (in 4% to 16% of patients), and coarsening of facial features.[38] Long-term administration of cyclosporine is associated with irreversible nephrotoxicity. The incidence of this serious side effect is estimated to be 15% to 40%.[39] The pathologic lesion resembles nephrosclerosis.[40]

Tacrolimus

Tacrolimus (FK-506; Prograf, Fujisawa Healthcare, Deerfield, IL) is a macrolide antibiotic with immunosuppressive activity produced by the fungus *Streptomyces tsukubaensis*. It is approved by the U.S. Food and Drug Administration (FDA) for liver and kidney transplant recipients. It is also used extensively in small bowel, pancreas, heart, and lung transplantation. The molecular structure of tacrolimus is unrelated to that of cyclosporine, and the two drugs have different cytosolic binding sites.[41,42] Tacrolimus binds to the immunophilin called FK-binding protein-12 (FKBP12).[43] Like the cyclosporine-cyclophilin complex, the tacrolimus-FKBP12 complex binds to and inhibits the activity of calcineurin. As is the case with cyclosporine, inhibition of calcineurin by tacrolimus blocks the transcription of several genes, including the genes transcribing IL-2, IL-3, IL-4, GM-CSF, IFN-γ, and TNF-α. The effect of tacrolimus on TNF-β expression differs from that induced by cyclosporine. Tacrolimus-mediated inhibition of TNF-β expression may play a role in reducing chronic rejection,[43] although no clinical difference has been noted between the two drugs. Like cyclosporine, inhibition of calcineurin disrupts signaling via NF-AT, ultimately inhibiting the synthesis of the potent T-cell growth factor, IL-2; this is the key pharmacologic effect of tacrolimus. The immunosuppressive effects of tacrolimus also may involve other pathways that activate T cells.[44]

Tacrolimus is highly lipophilic and must be dissolved in an organic solvent. Oral bioavailability is highly variable and poor, reportedly ranging from 6% to 56%, with a mean of 25%.[45] The gastrointestinal absorption of tacrolimus, compared with that of cyclosporine, is less dependent on bile flow.[46] Tacrolimus is extensively bound to erythrocytes because of the high concentration of FKBP12 found in the red blood cells. Like cyclosporine, tacrolimus is metabolized in the liver via the cytochrome P450 enzyme system, primarily by CYP3A4, although other enzymes have been reported to be involved as well.[47] Tacrolimus metabolism, like that of cyclosporine, can be significantly altered by liver dysfunction or coadministration of other drugs that induce or competitively inhibit P450; these effects can decrease or increase circulating levels of tacrolimus (see Table 192-1). Tacrolimus is a substrate for the p-glycoprotein efflux pump. The mean terminal half-life of tacrolimus is 12 hours. At least 15 metabolites of tacrolimus have been identified.[43] Some of these metabolites have as much as 10% of the immunosuppressive activity of the parent compound.[47]

Therapeutic monitoring of circulating tacrolimus concentrations is essential for preventing toxicity while maintaining adequate immunosuppression. Plasma and whole-blood trough concentrations correlate with AUC as well as clinical outcomes and toxicities.[48] Because of the extensive binding of tacrolimus to erythrocytes, whole-blood tacrolimus concentrations are 10 to 30 times higher than the corresponding plasma concentrations.[47] The most commonly used tacrolimus assay is the microparticulate enzyme immunoassay, although HPLC and enzyme-linked immunosorbent assays are also readily available.[49] The therapeutic range for tacrolimus levels in whole blood is 5 to 20 ng/mL. Plasma tacrolimus levels should be maintained between 0.5 and 2 ng/mL.

The typical intravenous dose of tacrolimus is 0.05 to 0.1 mg/kg/day. The drug should be administered as a slow, continuous infusion over 24 hours. Oral doses are generally three to four times higher than intravenous doses and range from 0.1 to 0.2 mg/kg/day, administered in two divided doses every 12 hours. Maintenance doses of tacrolimus range from 0.0125 to 0.5 mg/kg/day due to variability among patients with respect to absorption of the drug and requirements for immunosuppression.[47] No decrease in tacrolimus dose is needed when the T tube is clamped after liver transplantation. Tacrolimus clearance is faster in pediatric patients; therefore, larger doses may be required in children compared with adults.[47] Pediatric intravenous doses range from 0.03 to 0.05 mg/kg/day, and pediatric oral doses range from 0.15 to 0.3 mg/kg/day in divided doses.

Tacrolimus has a potential advantage over cyclosporine because of its ability to reverse ongoing acute rejection.[50-53] Experience with tacrolimus was first gained when the drug was used as rescue therapy in liver and kidney transplantation.[54-56] Today, tacrolimus is used as a primary immunosuppressive agent for all types of solid organ transplants.

The toxicity profile for tacrolimus is similar to that of cyclosporine, perhaps because they have a similar mechanism of action (i.e., calcineurin inhibition). As experience has been gained with tacrolimus, it is clear that many of the toxic side effects are dose related and are best managed by reducing the dose. Acute nephrotoxicity induced by tacrolimus is dose related. The incidence is not clearly defined in the literature, but it is similar to that of cyclosporine and most likely results from afferent arteriolar vasoconstriction. Nephrotoxicity resolves after the dose of tacrolimus is reduced or the drug is discontinued. As with cyclosporine, irreversible renal injury can occur after prolonged therapy with tacrolimus.[57]

Neurotoxicity is the most commonly reported adverse effect of tacrolimus. The reported incidence ranges from 3.6% to 32%.[58] This side effect can range from mild toxicity, such as tremors, headaches, paresthesias and insomnia, to severe complications including encephalopathy, coma, seizures, and psychosis. Usually, neurotoxicity associated with tacrolimus responds to a reduction of the dose; however, idiosyncratic reactions may require discontinuation of the drug.

The potential for tacrolimus to induce a diabetic state is similar to that for cyclosporine.[59,60] Increased fasting glucose levels and the development of overt diabetes mellitus are associated with elevated tacrolimus concentrations (greater than 15 ng/mL), acute rejection, and higher body mass index.[61] Tacrolimus-induced diabetes mellitus is reversible.[62]

Hyperkalemia and hypomagnesemia are commonly noted in patients receiving tacrolimus. Acute hyperkalemia can be managed with standard approaches, including administration of insulin and glucose and sodium bicarbonate or a cation exchange agent (sodium polystyrene sulfonate). Chronic hyperkalemia may require therapy with fludrocortisone acetate to increase renal potassium excretion. Hypomagnesemia often requires magnesium replacement to avoid complications.

The incidences of hypertension and hyperlipidemia associated with tacrolimus therapy appear to be lower than those reported with cyclosporine.[63-66] This more favorable adverse effect profile has been reported to translate into a decrease in the number of cardiovascular complications in patients treated with tacrolimus compared with cyclosporine.[66]

Tacrolimus is not associated with the connective tissue side effects seen with cyclosporine; therefore, cosmetic problems are not seen. Alopecia can be problematic for patients receiving tacrolimus, but this problem is reversible and usually does not require dosage adjustments.[67]

CELL CYCLE INHIBITORS

The precise mechanism of immunosuppression mediated by cytotoxic drugs is not known; however, the negative effect of these agents on the proliferation of lymphocytes is believed to inhibit the generation of antigen-specific T-cell clones. As one might expect, an increased risk of malignancies with the long-term use of these agents is a concern.

Azathioprine

Azathioprine (AZA; Imuran, Prometheus Laboratories, Greenville, NC), a thio analog of the purine adenine, inhibits purine metabolism. The parent drug is inactive but is rapidly converted to 6-mercaptopurine (6-MP) in red blood cells and subsequently to 6-thioinosine monophosphate, a purine analog, in vivo.[68] Both the de novo and the salvage pathways of purine synthesis are inhibited by azathioprine. 6-Thioguanine nucleotides interfere with DNA and RNA synthesis, rendering cells unable to function properly and allowing strand breaks in chromosomes. Azathioprine is most toxic to proliferating cells that are making new DNA.

Azathioprine can be used in maintenance immunosuppressive regimens; it has no usefulness for the treatment of acute rejection episodes.[69] The oral bioavailability of azathioprine is approximately 40%. Metabolism of 6-MP involves catabolism by xanthine oxidase in the liver and gut to inactive metabolites that are excreted by the kidneys. The 6-thioguanine nucleotides have a very long tissue half-life (approximately 13 days), permitting azathioprine to be administered by once-daily dosing. The inactive end metabolite is 6-thiouric acid, which is excreted by the kidneys. With congenital deficiency of the enzyme, thiopurine methyltransferase, (incidence, 1 in 300 patients), or with renal failure, accumulation of 6-thioguanine nucleotides causes increased toxicity.

The starting dose for azathioprine is 3 to 5 mg/kg once daily. The drug can be given intravenously at half the dose for brief periods. The typical maintenance oral dosage after transplantation is 2 to 3 mg/kg daily. Tapering of the dose to 1 to 2 mg/kg per day is often possible over time. In combination regimens, azathioprine can be reduced to as low as 0.25 to 0.5 mg/kg/day.

Dose-limiting myelosuppression usually occurs 1 to 2 weeks into therapy. Pancytopenia and thrombocytopenia with megaloblastic anemia is the pattern usually seen. White blood cell counts lower than 3000 cells/mm³ warrant dose reduction or discontinuation of the drug. As with other antiproliferative drugs, nausea, vomiting, and hair loss may occur. Hepatic injury can occur in two patterns. One form is reversible hepatitis. The other form is rare but serious hepatic veno-occlusive disease, which can cause irreversible liver damage. Azathioprine therapy also has been associated with pancreatitis. Because of concerns about hepatotoxicity and pancreatitis, some transplantation experts questioned the value of azathioprine for immunosuppression.[70,71] Hypersensitivity to azathioprine has been reported to cause a variety of manifestations; diagnosis of these disorders is based largely on clinical findings.

Allopurinol inhibits xanthene oxidase, one of the enzymes involved in degradation of azathioprine metabolites, thereby increasing the toxicity of the parent compound. Accordingly, if therapy with allopurinol is indicated, this agent should be added cautiously to an immunosuppressive regimen containing azathioprine. If allopurinol must be used, the dose of azathioprine should be reduced by more than 50%.

Mycophenolate Mofetil

Mycophenolate mofetil (MMF; CellCept, Roche Laboratories, Nutley, NJ) is a prodrug of mycophenolic acid (MPA). MPA noncompetitively inhibits inosine monophosphate dehydrogenase (IMPDH), a key enzyme that regulates the purine nucleotide de novo synthesis pathway.[72] T and B lymphocytes are dependent on IMPDH and the de novo pathway for purine synthesis during proliferation. Other cell lines, including granulocytes, red blood cells, platelets and tissue cells, use both the de novo and the salvage pathways for purine synthesis.[73] For this reason, MPA is more selective for T and B lymphocytes, which results in a more favorable adverse effect profile. MPA also may induce apoptosis in activated T cells, and it may interfere with expression of adhesion molecules in leukocytes and lymphocyte recruitment.[74]

Mycophenolate mofetil is rapidly absorbed after oral administration and undergoes rapid first-pass metabolism in the liver to MPA, the active form of the drug. The bioavailability of MPA is 94%.[72] Maximum concentrations of MPA are reached approximately 1 hour after oral administration.[75] MPA binds to plasma albumin, and free MPA levels can be altered by fluctuations in albumin levels or other medications that compete for albumin binding. Metabolism of MPA occurs by glucuronidation in the liver and renal tubular cells, primarily to an inactive compound, mycophenolic acid glucuronide (MPAG), which is eliminated by the kidneys[72] and to a second acyl glucuronide (M-2), which has in vitro activity.[76]

The dose of mycophenolate needed to prevent rejection in kidney and liver transplant recipients is 2 g/day. Cardiac transplant recipients generally require higher levels of immunosuppression and should receive 3 g/day. The total daily dose should be administered over two dosing intervals. Patients who are unable to tolerate twice daily dosing may benefit from separation of the total daily dose into three or four dosing intervals.

The need for therapeutic monitoring of MPA levels remains controversial. Currently, two assays are available: HPLC and an enzyme-multiplied immunoassay technique (EMIT). HPLC can measure both MPA and metabolite concentrations and is sensitive enough to measure free MPA concentrations.[77] The active metabolite of MPA, M-2, cross-reacts with the EMIT assay, resulting in higher measured concentrations. A correlation between acute rejection and both total MPA AUC and trough MPA concentrations determined by HPLC has been demonstrated.[78] Acute rejection is predicted better by trough levels than by the AUC. However, the risk of adverse effects correlates better with the dose of MPA rather than circulating MPA concentrations.[79] The therapeutic range for total MPA AUC is 30 to 60 mg/h/L.[78] MPA trough levels should be maintained between 1 and 3.5 mg/L.[77] Another monitoring strategy is measurement of the early peak concentration (30 minutes after oral dose [C_{30}]).[80] Further studies are necessary to determine the most appropriate strategy for therapeutic monitoring of MPA.

The most common adverse effects are gastrointestinal. Mild effects include nausea, vomiting, diarrhea, constipation, and dyspepsia. Severe complications, including cholecystitis, large bowel perforation, and pancreatitis, are rare and have not been definitively related to treatment with MPA. Mild gastrointestinal effects usually are transient. Prolonged symptoms can be managed by either reducing the dose of MPA or increasing the number of dosing intervals from twice daily to three or four times daily.[81]

Hematologic adverse effects are rare and are manifested as bone marrow suppression. The most commonly reported features are leukopenia and anemia, but the side effect profile also can include thrombocytopenia and pancytopenia. The onset of myelosuppression typically occurs within the first 6 months after starting MPA therapy and may be dose related. Resolution occurs within 1 week after stopping the drug in most cases.[72]

Infections are frequently cited as adverse effects of MPA, but they are a complication of immunosuppression in general. The reported incidence of opportunistic infections was increased in patients receiving MPA in addition to cyclosporine and prednisone compared with those receiving cyclosporine and prednisone alone[81,83]; however, no difference was reported when the MPA-containing regimen was compared with cyclosporine, prednisone, and azathioprine.[84] Nephrotoxicity and hepatotoxicity have not been reported with MPA.

MPA is effective maintenance therapy for prevention of acute rejection of solid organ allografts in combination with other immunosuppressive agents, such as corticosteroids and cyclosporine[82-84] or tacrolimus.[85] MPA has been used to treat acute rejection of renal transplants[86] and, in refractory rejection, to reduce the use of antilymphocyte therapy.[87] In addition, MPA has been used as rescue therapy for acute and chronic rejection of cardiac transplants.[88] Recent studies have shown promise in combining MPA with sirolimus to eliminate the need for calcineurin inhibitors, thereby reducing the potential for nephrotoxicity.[89,90]

Sirolimus

Sirolimus (rapamycin; Rapa; Rapamune, Wyeth Laboratories, Philadelphia, PA) is a macrolide antibiotic that is structurally related to tacrolimus. Like tacrolimus, it also binds to FKBP12, but sirolimus does not inhibit calcineurin or block cytokine gene transcription in T cells; rather, it inhibits the mammalian targets of rapamycin (mTOR). When stimulated by IL-2 and other growth factors, mTOR activates kinases that translate cytokine messenger RNA, which ultimately progresses the cell cycle from G_1 to the S phase. By blocking mTOR, sirolimus inhibits the cellular response to IL-2 and inhibits progression of the cell cycle, thereby prohibiting T-cell proliferation.[91]

Sirolimus is insoluble in water and must be dissolved in an organic solvent. It has poor bioavailability (15%). Maximum concentrations are reached within 2 hours after oral administration.[92] Because of its high lipophilicity, sirolimus readily enters cells, producing a large volume of distribution. Sirolimus binds extensively to erythrocytes (95%) because of their high FKBP12 content; minimal binding occurs with other plasma proteins.[93] Like cyclosporine and tacrolimus, sirolimus is metabolized primarily in the liver by CYP3A4. Sirolimus is also a substrate for the p-glycoprotein efflux pump. O-demethylation and hydroxylation produce several metabolites. The metabolites of sirolimus have less than 10% of the immunosuppressive activity of the parent compound and are excreted via the bile into feces.[91]

Hepatic metabolism by the CYP3A4 enzymes creates the potential for significant changes in the half-life of sirolimus if other drugs affecting these enzymes are also administered. These changes can decrease or increase serum levels by induction or competitive inhibition of P450. Many of the same drugs that alter cyclosporine and tacrolimus levels can also alter sirolimus levels (see Table 192-1). Coadministration of sirolimus with cyclosporine significantly increases the AUC and trough concentrations for sirolimus. Likewise, sirolimus also significantly increases the AUC and trough concentrations for cyclosporine. To minimize the interaction and potential toxicities of the two drugs, sirolimus administration should be separated from cyclosporine administration by 4 hours.[94]

Its long half-life of approximately 60 hours[95] makes sirolimus suitable for once-daily dosing. The two pivotal trials that led to the FDA-approval of sirolimus capitalized on the interaction that occurs with coadministration of cyclosporine and sirolimus. These studies demonstrated a reduction of acute rejection episodes in kidney transplant recipients when sirolimus was given using either of two fixed dosing regimens: a 6-mg loading dose followed by 2 mg daily or a 15-mg loading dose followed by 5 mg daily.[96,97] These results suggest that therapeutic drug monitoring is not necessary. However, clinical experience indicates that sirolimus therapy is optimized when doses are based on blood concentrations, particularly if sirolimus is used in the absence of cyclosporine synergy.[98]

Therapeutic monitoring of sirolimus should be based on whole-blood concentrations, because large amounts of the drug are sequestered in erythrocytes, resulting in undetectable concentrations in plasma.[99] HPLC with mass spectroscopy and ultraviolet detection are the most commonly used methods to measure sirolimus concentrations. A correlation between the trough level and the AUC for sirolimus has been established.[100,101] Furthermore, there is a strong correlation between the rate and severity of acute rejection and low trough levels, as well as between the occurrence of adverse effects and high trough levels. The therapeutic range is 5 to 15 ng/mL.[101] A microparticle enzyme immunoassay has been developed[102] and may be beneficial for analyzing multiple samples with more rapid turnaround.[103] Frequent monitoring of sirolimus levels is not warranted because of the long half-life of the drug. Sirolimus levels should be evaluated 5 to 7 days after initiation of therapy or a dose change, to allow sufficient time for drug levels to reach steady state.[100]

The adverse effect profile of sirolimus is different from that of other immunosuppressants. Unlike cyclosporine and tacrolimus, sirolimus rarely causes nephrotoxicity or neurotoxicity. Dose-dependent myelosuppression can be seen after initiation of sirolimus therapy. Thrombocytopenia commonly manifests within the first 2 weeks of therapy but improves with continued treatment. Leukopenia and anemia may also manifest shortly after initiation of therapy, but they are transient.[103] Thrombocytopenia and leukopenia are related to sirolimus trough concentrations greater than 15 ng/mL.[101]

Hyperlipidemia is commonly seen in patients receiving sirolimus; the findings are hypercholesterolemia and hypertriglyceridemia. This effect has been reported in virtually all clinical trials.[91] Peak levels of total cholesterol and triglycerides are dose related and usually are reached within 3 months after initiation of sirolimus, but the levels decrease after 1 year.[103] Both changes are reversible with dose reduction or discontinuation.[92] The cause of sirolimus-associated hyperlipidemia is thought to be overproduction of lipoproteins or inhibition of hepatic lipoprotein lipase, leading to decreased lipolysis.[103] Use of antihyperlipidemic agents, such as the 3-hydroxy-3-methylglutaryl coenzyme A (HMG-CoA) reductase inhibitors, is effective for treating hyperlipidemia in patients receiving sirolimus. Analysis of cholesterol values after 1 year of sirolimus therapy in the Framingham Model

indicates that sirolimus should cause only a modest increase in the incidence of ischemic heart disease in kidney transplant recipients (2 to 3 new cases per 1000 persons per year).[103] Therefore, treatment with sirolimus should have only a minimal impact on the risk for cardiovascular disease. It has been proposed that the decreased incidence of hyperlipidemia associated with tacrolimus compared with cyclosporine may lessen the frequency and severity of hyperlipidemia in transplant recipients who receive tacrolimus- and sirolimus-based immunosuppressive therapy.[103]

Mouth ulcers have been reported with sirolimus; they appear to be more pronounced with the liquid formulation and may be dose related. Other adverse effects reported with sirolimus include elevated liver enzymes, lymphocele formation, hypertension, rash, acne, diarrhea, and arthralgia.

Sirolimus is effective as maintenance therapy for the prevention of acute rejection of solid organ allografts in combination with steroids and cyclosporine[96,97] or tacrolimus.[104] It also is effective in steroid-withdrawal regimens[105] or to spare cyclosporine in an attempt to minimize nephrotoxicity associated with this agent.[106,107] It is speculated that sirolimus may reduce the potential for chronic rejection by inhibiting growth factor–mediated cell proliferation and intimal hyperplasia associated with chronic rejection,[103] but longer follow-up is necessary to prove this theory.

BIOLOGIC AGENTS

Antithymocyte Globulin

Antilymphocyte antibodies such as antilymphocytic globulin (ALG) were first produced by immunization of animals against purified lymphocyte preparations, resulting in multispecific polyclonal antibodies. Antibodies that cross-reacted with other cellular molecules in blood were then removed by extensive adsorption to blood components. Because of variability among immunized animals, substantial amounts of ALG were pooled to produce a more homogeneous preparation.

Antibodies to surface molecules on lymphocytes interfere with lymphocyte function in the immune response by several possible mechanisms. Lymphocytes are removed from the circulation rapidly after treatment with antilymphocyte antibodies. In addition, lymphocytes are phenotypically and functionally altered. Thymocytes, unactivated lymphocytes, and T and B lymphoblasts are used to produce the equine polyclonal antibody, antithymocyte globulin (ATG; ATGAM, Pharmacia & Upjohn, Kalamazoo, MI). A newer rabbit preparation, RATG (Thymoglobulin, SangStat Medical Corporation, Fremont, CA), is less immunogenic and may have other advantages over the equine preparation. B lymphocytes are targeted to a lesser extent with RATG than with equine ATG,[108] helping to some extent to preserve infection-induced antibody production. Furthermore, CD4+ T lymphocytes are the predominant target of RATG,[109] and this agent has lesser effects on other leukocytes, compared with equine ATG. RATG-induced lymphocytopenia persists for a much longer time than with former antilymphocyte preparations. Surface molecules that serve as binding sites for RATG include the T-cell antigens, CD6, CD16, CD18, CD38, CD40, and CD58, among others. The result is inhibition of cellular function of other cell lines, including monocytes, thymocytes, natural killer cells, leukocytes, and dendritic cells.

Equine ATG is administered in a single daily dose (10 to 15 mg/kg). The dose of RATG, which is more potent, is 1 to 1.5 mg/kg given as a single daily dose. Therapy for acute rejection usually is continued for 7 to 14 days. Induction therapy with polyclonal antibodies typically uses the same doses for 5 to 10 days of therapy. Polyclonal preparations cause a high incidence of febrile reactions with the first few doses. Antihistamines (usually diphenhydramine, 50 mg), antipyretics (i.e., acetaminophen, 650 mg), and corticosteroids are given as premedications.

Because of the lack of specificity of polyclonal antibodies, therapeutic drug monitoring generally is not useful. In addition, fixed weight-based dosing regimens reduce the need for drug concentration monitoring. Some advocate monitoring the number of CD3+ lymphocytes with flow cytometry as a gauge of immunosuppressive effect.

The effects of ATG on other cell types is the basis for adverse effects associated with these preparations. The most troublesome adverse effect is myelosuppression, manifested by leukopenia, anemia, and thrombocytopenia. These effects are dose related and can be managed by decreasing the dose or discontinuing the drug.

As described previously, the first few doses of ATG preparations are often accompanied by fever, which can be ameliorated with the use of appropriate premedications. Other adverse effects include anaphylactic reactions, hypotension, urticaria, and serum sickness, particularly with equine ATG. After approval of RATG, use of equine ATG declined considerably because of the better side effect profile of RATG and its increased efficacy in reducing acute rejection[110] and preventing rejection as part of induction therapy.[111]

The efficacy of ATGs in reversing solid organ allograft rejection has been well established. ATGs are frequently reserved for steroid-resistant allograft rejections. Prospective, controlled studies have demonstrated equal or superior efficacy for both equine and rabbit ATG in preventing rejection as induction therapy, compared with OKT3.[112,113] High doses of RATG are also being used in T cell–depleting regimens to induce tolerance and to allow for monotherapy after transplantation with subsequent weaning of immunosuppression.[114]

Anti-CD3 Monoclonal Antibody

Efforts to increase the potency and decrease the variability of ALGs led to development of single-specificity monoclonal antibodies. The first of these products was muromonab CD3 (OKT3; Orthoclone OKT3, OrthoBiotech Products, LP, Raritan, NJ). OKT3 is a purified murine-derived monoclonal antibody directed at the ε chain of the CD3 receptor,[115] which is found on all mature human T cells.[116] After administration, OKT3 binds to the CD3 receptor, opsonizing the cells and promoting their rapid removal from the circulation.[116,117]

Elimination of OKT3 occurs in two phases and is principally linked to T-cell binding. The first phase is elimination associated with rapid removal of the T cells bound to OKT3. The second, slower phase occurs days after initiation of therapy. The overall half-life for the agent is 18 hours.[117]

Dosing for OKT3 uses a fixed regimen of 5 mg/day for 10 to 14 days for treatment of acute rejection. Prophylactic induction regimens use the same dose for 7 to 10 days. After the first one or two doses, proinflammatory cytokines are released by opsonized lymphocytes, leading to clinical findings reminiscent of severe sepsis.[117] This *first-dose effect* frequently is associated with fever, chills, tachycardia, nausea, vomiting, diarrhea, bronchospasm, pulmonary edema, and elevation or depression of blood pressure. These effects can be ameliorated if the patient is pretreated with a 1-g intravenous bolus of methylprednisolone 15 to 60 minutes before OKT3 infusion.[118] Premedication often also includes antihistamines, diphenhydramine, and acetaminophen. Anaphylaxis occurs in fewer than 1% of patients; nonetheless, a skin test or test dose is recommended before OKT3 therapy is initiated.

The murine nature of the drug leads to anti-mouse immunoglobulin antibody formation. Individuals vary in the amount of endogenous antibody (directed against the mouse antibody) they form. This antibody production can be decreased by continuing other immunosuppressive treatments during monoclonal antibody administration. Human antimurine OKT3 antibodies usually peak after 1 to 2 weeks of therapy and can decrease the efficacy of future courses of therapy.[117] Repeat treatment with OKT3 is still successful in many cases, if larger doses of antibody are used for subsequent courses. Patients who produce very high antibody titers, probably about 5% to 20% of those receiving OKT3, fail to respond to subsequent doses of the drug even when the dose is increased. Some advocate monitoring of CD3+ T-cell counts with flow cytometry for patients receiving OKT3. If CD3+ cells reach 10%, it is recommended either that the dose of OKT3 be increased (to as much as 15 mg/day) or that treatment be discontinued. Others suggest monitoring anti-OKT3 antibody titers.

As described previously, OKT3 therapy produces a first-dose response that manifests within 45 to 60 minutes and must be managed with premedication. Because of the risk of severe pulmonary edema, fluid status should be evaluated if patients weigh more than 2% more than their usual body weight, and diuresis should be considered before proceeding with OKT3 therapy.

Septic meningitis also has been described as an early complication of OKT3 therapy, manifesting 2 to 7 days after initiation of OKT3. The common symptoms are fever, headache, and photophobia. The phenomenon appears to be self-limited and may be related to the release of cytokines early after OKT3 administration.

The potent suppression of T-lymphocyte populations is associated with an increased incidence of viral infections and lymphoproliferative disorders. It is not clear whether antibody therapy is worse in this regard than other approaches for achieving immunosuppression. Some evidence suggests that problems arise because antibodies are used for too long a time or too late in the course of resistant rejection, when the immunosuppression burden is already high.

The efficacy of OKT3 for treatment of acute rejection and induction strategies is well documented. However, OKT3 use has declined with the availability of better-tolerated antithymocyte preparations (i.e., RATG) that do not induce antibody production against the drug. OKT3 is often reserved as therapy for acute rejection that is resistant to steroids or other antilymphocyte preparations.

Anti–Interleukin-2 Receptor Monoclonal Antibodies

T-cell activation is characterized by the expression of IL-2 and high-affinity IL-2R by T cells. IL-2 exerts its effects on T lymphocytes by binding to the IL-2R. By binding to the α subunit of the IL-2R on activated T cells, anti–IL-2R antibodies inhibit IL-2–mediated T-cell activation and proliferation. Two anti–IL-2R monoclonal antibodies are currently available, daclizumab (Zenapax, Hoffman-LaRoche, Nutley, NJ) and basiliximab (Simulect, Novartis Pharmaceuticals). The important differences between the two drugs relate to the structure of the antibodies and the dosing strategies for each.

Daclizumab is a unique hybrid monoclonal antibody in which the variable region (binding site for the IL-2R) is murine but the remainder of the immunoglobulin molecule is human (immunoglobulin G$_1$). Only 10% of the hybrid molecule is of murine origin. As a result, antibody formation directed against the drug is decreased (e.g., in comparison with OKT3) and half-life is prolonged. Basiliximab is a chimeric anti–IL-2R antibody with a mechanism of action that is the same as daclizumab. In this monoclonal antibody, murine immunoglobulin amino acid sequences represent an even smaller fraction of the protein than is case for daclizumab.

Dosing strategies for anti–IL-2R monoclonal antibodies begin with administration of the first dose, before transplantation. A dose of 1 mg/kg of daclizumab is administered intravenously, and this dose is repeated every 14 days for a total of five doses. Newer dosing strategies use higher doses (2 mg/kg), or abbreviated schedules of two or three total doses, or both.[119] A 20 mg/kg dose of basiliximab is administered intravenously before transplantation, and this dose is repeated once more on day 4.

Anti–IL-2R monoclonal antibodies are effective in preventing acute rejection after transplantation. However, these agents are ineffective for reversing acute cellular rejection. Both drugs are well tolerated, with no differences in adverse effects reported in clinical trials between the drugs and placebo. Daclizumab and basiliximab have the reported beneficial effects of reducing delayed graft function and delaying calcineurin inhibitor use (to decrease nephrotoxicity).[120,121]

Anti-CD52 Monoclonal Antibody

CD52 is a surface marker found on mature T and B lymphocytes. It also is found to varying degrees on monocytes, macrophages, granulocytes, and natural killer cells. Alemtuzumab (Campath, ILEX Pharmaceuticals, LP, San Antonio, TX) is a humanized monoclonal antibody directed at the CD52 antigen that causes complete lympholysis, resulting in significant T-cell depletion. The early experience with alemtuzumab suggest that lower degrees of immunosuppression are needed after T-cell depletion following alemtuzumab infusion. Reports indicate that only single-drug therapy, usually with a calcineurin inhibitor (cyclosporine or tacrolimus) or sirolimus, is necessary after patients receive induction therapy with alemtuzumab.[122-124] Alemtuzumab also has been successfully used to treat acute rejection episodes.[125,126]

The dose of alemtuzumab administered in transplantation is 30 mg intravenously. Significant adverse effects are noted with administration of alemtuzumab, notably rigors, hypotension, fever, shortness of breath, bronchospasms, and chills. Premedication with diphenhydramine, acetaminophen, and corticosteroids is required before alemtuzumab administration to minimize the infusion-related effects. Other adverse effects noted after alemtuzumab therapy include neutropenia, anemia, thrombocytopenia, and pancytopenia.

IMMUNOSUPPRESSIVE AGENTS IN CLINICAL DEVELOPMENT

Everolimus

Everolimus (SDZ-RAD; Certican, Novartis Pharma AG, Basel, Switzerland) is an inhibitor of mTOR that is structurally similar to sirolimus and is currently approved for use in Europe. Everolimus produces the same inhibition of cell cycle progression and ultimate inhibition of T-cell proliferation. Dosing for everolimus is 3 mg daily. The half-life of everolimus is 16 to 19 hours, which is shorter than the half-life of sirolimus.[127] The adverse effects of everolimus are similar to those reported for sirolimus and include hypercholesterolemia, hypertriglyceridemia, and hematologic effects such as thrombocytopenia and anemia.

Mycophenolate Sodium

Mycophenolate sodium (Myfortic, Novartis Pharma AG) is an enteric-coated formulation of the sodium salt of mycophenolic acid that is currently approved for use in Europe. The enteric coating of mycophenolate sodium helps to minimize the gastrointestinal side effects that are associated with mycophenolate mofetil. Once in the small intestine, mycophenolic acid is released directly in the gastrointestinal tract for absorption. The immunosuppressive activity of mycophenolate sodium is identical to that of mycophenolic acid, the activated form of mycophenolate mofetil. The dose of mycophenolate sodium is 1.44 g/day, which is equivalent to 2 g/day of mycophenolate mofetil.

Leflunomide

Leflunomide (Avara, Aventis Pharmaceuticals, Kansas City, MO) is converted to an active metabolite, A77,1726. The latter compound inhibits de novo pyrimidine synthesis in T and B lymphocytes by inhibiting tyrosine kinase activity of the TCR or cytokine receptors. It is currently marketed as a treatment for rheumatoid arthritis. One study investigating leflunomide in liver and kidney transplant recipients administered a loading dose of 200 mg/day for 7 days, followed by a maintenance dose of 40 to 60 mg/day. Concentrations greater than 50 µg/mL allowed for lower doses of prednisone and calcineurin inhibitor, whereas concentrations of less than 80 µg/mL were associated with fewer adverse effects. Adverse effects included skin rash, anemia, and elevated liver enzymes.[128] Leflunomide was effective in reducing acute rejection and may show promise in reversing chronic rejection.[129]

FTY-720

FTY-720 is a novel immunosuppressant that does not affect T-cell activation but alters lymphocyte trafficking by altering the expression or function of adhesion molecules. The effect of treatment with this agent is the sequestration of T cells in secondary lymphoid organs (i.e., not in the allograft), producing peripheral lymphopenia.[130] FTY-720 is being investigated for the treatment and prevention of both acute and chronic rejection.

Mizoribine

Mizoribine is an imidazole nucleoside antibiotic that undergoes phosphorylation to inhibit both IMPDH and guanosine 5-monophosphate synthetase during purine synthesis.[131] The result is inhibition of RNA and DNA synthesis and consequent inhibition of both humoral and cellular immune responses. Limited clinical trials using mizoribine in place of azathioprine and with cyclosporine and corticosteroids have shown decreased graft loss to chronic rejection in renal transplant recipients.[132] Mizoribine has been used as a maintenance agent, in combination with cyclosporine and steroids, primarily in renal transplantation patients.[133] The drug appears to have advantages over azathioprine, in particular less myelotoxicity and hepatotoxicity.[134] Although it has not been compared in clinical trials, it is expected to have efficacy similar to that of mycophenolate mofetil, because the two drugs have similar mechanisms of action.[135]

Mizoribine is administered once daily as an oral dose of 50 to 300 mg/day. Peak blood levels are achieved 2 to 3 hours after an oral dose. The major elimination pathway of mizoribine is renal (85% of the dose is excreted unchanged in the urine), and the half-life is 4 hours.

Brequinar

Brequinar is an antimetabolite with broad antineoplastic activity that has been tested in humans with cancer.[136,137] It inhibits the de novo pathway of pyrimidine synthesis, blocking RNA and DNA synthesis. Dose-limiting toxicities are thrombocytopenia and a severe desquamative dermatitis. The antiproliferative effects of the drug appear to be mediated by depletion of the pyrimidine precursors needed for DNA and RNA synthesis. Brequinar is a potent immunosuppressant in a rat model[138] and appears to act synergistically, at least in vitro, with cyclosporine and sirolimus.[139]

Anti-CD4 Antibody

Antibodies targeted against the CD4 receptor prevent the initiation of the immune response caused by presentation of MHC class II alloantigens. Selective disruption of the MHC class II–CD4 interaction can prolong allograft survival and induce tolerance in animal models.[140] These antibodies reduce synovial inflammation in rheumatoid arthritis and cause profound and long-term immunosuppression.[141] Use of anti-CD4 in conjunction with cytotoxic T lymphocyte-associated antigen 4 immunoglobulin (CTLA4-Ig) has been shown to prolong the survival of hamster liver xenografts in rats.[142] Use of murine OKT4 in cadaveric renal transplantation has not shown promise.[143] A human anti-mouse antibody (HAMA) response of more than 3 times the pretreatment level was observed in 84% of patients. An open-label pilot trial of murine OKT4A in humans produced mixed results.[144] The dose used in the study produced only partial CD4 saturation in all patients and was inadequate to reduce rejection. However, no HAMA response was observed. Other humanized anti-CD4 monoclonal antibodies are being evaluated.[2,144]

Anti-CD45 Antibody

The CD45 epitope plays a role in the regulation of T-cell activation. The CD45RB monoclonal antibody has been shown to effectively prevent allograft rejection in animal models and may have some applicability in humans in the future.

Anti-CD40–Ligand and Anti-CD40 Antibody

CD40 is a costimulatory molecule for MHC class II alloantigens that is present in large amounts on mature dendritic cells. Costimulation is necessary for T-cell sensitization and activation. Use of antibodies to prevent costimulation may induce tolerance by blocking activation of the T cell. In animal models, anti-CD40 or anti-CD40–ligand monoclonal antibodies have been shown to prevent and even reverse acute allograft rejection, leading to prolonged graft survival without the need for chronic maintenance immunosuppression[145,146] and to delayed onset of chronic rejection.[147] Other studies have demonstrated the tolerogenic potential of anti-CD40–ligand in animal models.[148]

Anti–Leukocyte Function–Associated Antigen-1

Leukocyte function–associated antigen-1 (LFA-1) plays an important role in adhesion of leukocytes to endothelial cells and to a variety of targets on T cells during the immune response. The immunosuppressive effect of anti–LFA-1 (anti-CD11a, anti-CD18) monoclonal antibody (odulimomab) was similar to that of RATG as induction therapy in renal allograft recipients.[149] Fewer patients required dialysis in the anti–LFA-1 monoclonal antibody group, possibly due to prevention of endothelial cell activation and the consequent protection of the allograft from ischemic damage. This same effect of protection from renal ischemia has been confirmed in animal models.[150] The combination of anti–intracellular adhesion molecule-1 (ICAM-1) antibody (enlimomab) and anti–LFA-1 monoclonal antibody has been shown to induce tolerance to murine cardiac allografts.[151,152]

Anti-CTLA4-Ig

CTLA4-Ig is a chimeric fusion protein that blocks the B7-CD28/CTLA4 pathway and thereby inhibits T-cell activation and IL-2 production. Development of chronic renal allograft rejection is prevented by CTLA4-Ig in animal models.[153] Current studies are investigating the use of this molecule with other costimulatory modulators, such as anti-CD40 ligand[147] and anti–LFA-1,[154] to induce tolerance in animal models.

Anti–Intracellular Adhesion Molecule-1

ICAM-1 is an immunoglobulin-like molecule that aids adhesion and migration of leukocytes in the vessels and also acts as a costimulatory molecule for T-cell activation. Use of anti–ICAM-1 monoclonal antibody (enlimomab) has not shown promise in reducing the incidence of acute rejection or delayed graft function in renal transplants.[155] However, anti–ICAM-1 in combination with anti–LFA-1 produced tolerance in animal models.[151,152]

FUTURE DIRECTIONS

The number of patients awaiting solid organ transplantation continues to grow each year. However, the number of organs available for donation shows very little change from year to year. Increased organ donation awareness among the public and increased use of organs from living donors have contributed to small annual increases in the number of organs available for transplantation, but the number still falls short of meeting the needs of the more than 80,000 candidates waiting for solid-organ transplants. Other strategies must be explored to try to meet the demand for organ transplantation.

Greater understanding of the way the immune system functions with respect to chronic allograft acceptance is vital to increasing the survival of transplanted allografts. Complete allograft acceptance without immunosuppressive therapy would eliminate the occurrence of long-term sequelae of immunosuppression, such as malignancies and opportunistic infections. Chimerism, a principle that is becoming better understood by transplantation immunologists, allows the donor and recipient leukocytes to stably coexist. Chimerism is essential for complete allograft acceptance with or without immunosuppression.

The principles of allograft tolerance build on the concept of chimerism in that the interaction between donor and recipient leukocytes allows for low-level activation of both populations, resulting in exhaustion of each species.[9,156,157] Tolerance can be induced with the use of T-cell–depleting regimens, followed by low doses of immunosuppressive medications.[114] Current research includes investigation of other means of modulating the immune response to induce tolerance, including modulation of adhesion and costimulation pathways.

A better understanding of tolerance induction with immunosuppressive regimens will play a key role in permitting successful xenotransplantation. Use of xenoallografts can greatly increase the number of donor organs available for transplantation to help match the demand.

ANNOTATED REFERENCES

Bullingham RES, Nicholls AJ, Kamm BR: Clinical pharmacokinetics of mycophenolate mofetil. Clin Pharmacokinet 1998;34:429-455.

The pharmacokinetics of mycophenolate mofetil is emphasized in this article, with an overview of the mechanism of action and pharmacodynamic properties of the drug. Clinical monitoring and the correlation of plasma concentrations with adverse and immunosuppressive effects are highlighted.

Denton MD, Magee CC, Sayegh MH: Immunosuppressive strategies in transplantation. Lancet 1999;353:1083-1031.

This article provides a thorough review of the mechanisms of allograft rejection and the rationale for the selection of agents directed at specific targets in the immune cascade. Various approaches to immunosuppression in transplantation are highlighted, as well as the specific agents used and novel agents currently under investigation.

Dunn CJ, Wagstaff AJ, Perry CM, et al: Cyclosporine: An updated review of the pharmacokinetic properties, clinical efficacy and tolerability of a microemulsion-based formulation (Neoral) in organ transplantation. Drugs 2001;61:1957-2016.

This article provides in-depth review of the pharmacokinetic properties of cyclosporine and its use in various solid organ transplants. In addition to novel approaches to clinical monitoring of cyclosporine, comparisons with other immunosuppressive agents in solid organ transplantation is discussed.

Kahan BD, Camardo JS: Rapamycin: Clinical results and future opportunities. Transplantation 2001;72:1181-1193.

This article provides a review of the pharmacology and pharmacodynamics of sirolimus and its role in solid organ transplantation. Adverse effects, clinical efficacy, and therapeutic monitoring are addressed, as well as immunosuppressive strategies with sirolimus-based therapy.

Scott LJ, McKeage K, Keam SJ, Plosker GL: Tacrolimus: A further update of its use in the management of organ transplantation. Drugs 2003;63:1247-1297.

An extensive review of the pharmacokinetic and pharmacokinetic properties of tacrolimus and its use in various solid organ transplants is presented, with emphasis on the use of tacrolimus for immunosuppressive strategies. Therapeutic efficacy, adverse effects, and place in therapy are addressed.

Chapter 193

DIGITALIS

Emily E. Castelli • Jill A. Rebuck

KEY POINTS

1. Initial loading doses of intravenous digoxin for new-onset atrial fibrillation, approximately 10 µg/kg over a 24-hour period based on lean body weight, should be administered to adequately control ventricular rate in most patients.

2. Renal-impaired patients and elderly patients commonly require 50% less digoxin than do other patients in critical care.

3. The therapeutic range for digoxin administered to control supraventricular tachyarrhythmias is 1 to 2 ng/mL; for heart failure, it is 0.5 to 0.8 ng/mL.

4. Adverse effects of digitalis include nausea, vomiting, diarrhea, visual disturbances, confusion, hyperkalemia, and cardiac arrhythmias.

5. An increase in digoxin concentration may occur with concomitant administration of amiodarone, verapamil, quinidine, spironolactone, clarithromycin, itraconazole, or captopril.

6. A decrease in digoxin concentration may occur with concomitant administration of cholestyramine, colestipol, kaolin-pectin, oral antacids, metoclopramide, neomycin, sulfasalazine, levothyroxine, or rifampin.

7. Digoxin toxicity should be treated by administering activated charcoal to prevent further absorption of the drug and infusing digoxin immune Fab to bind the drug once absorption has occurred. Supportive care with advanced cardiac life support protocols and treatment of hyperkalemia should also be undertaken.

THERAPEUTIC INDICATIONS

Digoxin is indicated primarily for the treatment of congestive heart failure (CHF) and atrial fibrillation, the latter being the predominant reason for use in the critical care setting.[1] In recent investigations, digoxin was shown to be beneficial in patients with CHF because it improved exercise tolerance and reduced hospitalizations without causing an increase in mortality.[2,3] Digoxin is indicated as a useful adjuvant to angiotensin-converting enzyme inhibitor and β-adrenergic blocker therapy in patients with CHF. However, digoxin is not indicated as primary treatment for stabilization of acutely decompensated heart failure.[4,5]

In the critical care setting, digoxin is used mostly to treat atrial arrhythmias, predominantly atrial fibrillation.[6] In chronic atrial fibrillation, digoxin is useful for controlling the ventricular rate in patients with left ventricular systolic dysfunction.[5] In acute atrial fibrillation, digoxin provides effective ventricular rate control and represents a useful therapy for rate control, especially if left ventricular function is compromised.[1,6] The agent does not restore normal sinus rhythm, although occasionally atrial fibrillation spontaneously resolves during initial therapy.[5,7] Digoxin has inotropic, neurohormonal, and vagomimetic effects with a delayed onset of action and a narrow therapeutic window.

MECHANISM OF ACTION

Digoxin is a cardiac glycoside with specific effects on the myocardium. Inhibition of the sodium-potassium adenosine triphosphatase (Na^+,K^+-ATPase) pump increases the intracellular sodium concentration and subsequently increases the intracellular calcium concentration by stimulation of sodium-calcium exchange.[1,8] The pharmacologic effects of digoxin include increased force of systolic contraction (i.e., positive inotropic activity); decreased activation of the sympathetic nervous system and renin-angiotensin system (neurohormonal deactivating effect); and decreased heart rate and conduction velocity within the atrioventricular (AV) node (vagomimetic effect). Neurohormonal effects occur at low dosages, independent of inotropic effects. Hemodynamic improvement is observed in CHF related to both the inotropic and the neurohormonal effects of digoxin. The vagal effects of digoxin result in slowed conduction and prolongation of AV-node refractoriness, which slows the ventricular response in patients with atrial fibrillation. The overall response to digoxin is an increase in cardiac output and reduction in pulmonary artery pressure, systemic vascular resistance, plasma norepinephrine level, and pulmonary capillary wedge pressure. Minimal changes in blood pressure occur with initiation of therapy.[7]

PHARMACOKINETICS

Intravenous preparations are 100% bioavailable, whereas most oral formulations provide only 60% to 85% bioavailability.[1] Capsules containing liquid have increased bioavailability, being about 90% to 100% of the intravenous formulation. Therefore, dosing considerations are important when switching between oral and intravenous preparations. Digoxin absorption occurs primarily in the small intestine. Impaired absorption after oral administration can occur if intestinal function is impaired, although partial gastrectomy or jejunoileal bypass does not affect absorption to an appreciable extent.[1,9,10]

The distribution phase of digoxin metabolism is prolonged after oral or intravenous administration. In attempting to achieve adequate rate control of atrial arrhythmias, the onset of action for digoxin is slower than that of diltiazem.[6,8] For patients started on oral therapy, the onset of action occurs within 0.5 to 2 hours, and peak effects are seen within 6 to 8 hours.[1] After intravenous administration, onset occurs in 5 to 30 minutes, and peak effect is observed within 1 to 5 hours.[11] This delay in pharmacologic effect may be undesirable in the setting of acute atrial fibrillation. Pharmacologic effects typically persist for 3 to 4 days after withdrawal of digoxin therapy.

Approximately 20% to 30% of digoxin is protein bound in patients with normal renal function or uremia.[1] Digoxin is extensively bound to multiple tissues, particularly to Na^+,K^+-ATPase in cardiac and skeletal muscle, and demonstrates a large volume of distribution. The volume of distribution for digoxin averages 6 to 7 L/kg of total body weight in patients with normal renal function. A decrease in the volume of distribution occurs in patients with renal dysfunction or dialysis.

With normal renal function, the elimination half-life is 36 to 48 hours. Elimination is prolonged in patients with renal dysfunction, being about 3.5 to 5 days in anuric patients.[11] Metabolism occurs primarily in the liver, but the drug also is metabolized by bacteria within the large intestine after oral administration.[1] Excretion of digoxin is predominantly in the urine as unchanged drug. The drug is cleared by glomerular filtration and active tubular secretion. Small amounts are excreted in bile and feces. Approximately 30% of the total digoxin load in the body is eliminated daily in patients with normal renal function. The metabolism and excretion of digoxin is not appreciably altered in patients with liver disease if normal renal function is present. Importantly, increased urinary output does not result in enhanced elimination of digoxin, because elimination is dependent on age, gender, and serum creatinine. Estimations of creatinine clearance (CrCl) in milliliters per minute can be calculated from the patient's age (in years) and the serum creatinine concentration (in mg/dL) by the modified Cockroft and Gault equation:

$$CrCl = [140 - age/(serum\ creatinine)]$$

This is the value for a male patient; for a female, multiply the result by 0.85. Given the CrCl, estimates of daily digoxin elimination can be made by the following equation:

$$Daily\ percentage\ of\ digoxin\ eliminated = 14 + [CrCl \div 5]$$

DOSING RECOMMENDATIONS

GENERAL CONSIDERATIONS

Lean body mass should be used to calculate the appropriate digoxin dosage for adult patients in intensive care units (ICUs), because no appreciable amount of digoxin is distributed to body fat.[12] Age, renal function, and weight all need to be considered when calculating both loading and maintenance doses for initiation of digoxin therapy.[1] Digoxin dosages in the pediatric population must be carefully titrated, especially in neonates. For children from infancy to age 10 years, substantially higher dosing is necessary, in comparison with adult patients (see later discussion). In addition, concomitant medications (discussed later) may influence serum digoxin levels and should be considered when initiating therapy.

INITIAL LOADING DOSE

Recent literature does not support initial bolus dosing for patients with CHF.[1] If deemed appropriate, a dose of 8 to 12 µg/kg is suggested for adult patients in heart failure who have a normal sinus rhythm. In the acute setting, administration of an initial loading dose is recommended for the management of supraventricular tachyarrhythmias. Determination of lean body weight (LBW, in kilograms) is necessary in order to calculate digoxin loading and maintenance dosing. Appropriate dosing weight can be calculated from the following equations.

For a male patient,

$$LBW = 50 + [(2.3)(number\ of\ inches\ tall\ over\ 5\ feet)]$$

or

$$LBW = [(0.9)(height\ in\ centimeters)] - 88$$

For a female patient,

$$LBW = 45.5 + [(2.3)(number\ of\ inches\ tall\ over\ 5\ feet)]$$

or

$$LBW = [(0.9)(height\ in\ centimeters)] - 92$$

An initial intravenous loading dose for adults of 10 to 15 µg/kg based on LBW is necessary for adequate ventricular rate control in the setting of atrial fibrillation or atrial flutter. Renally impaired patients and those older than 70 years of age require lower initial loading doses; a 50% dosage reduction is recommended. Typically, the loading dose is administered as approximately one half of the total dose immediately (maximum of 500 µg administration at one time), followed in 6 to 8 hours by 25% of the total dose, with the remaining 25% given after another 6 to 8 hours.[1] For example, a loading dose of 1000 µg should be administered as a 500-µg intravenous bolus, followed by 250 µg intravenously every 6 hours for two doses. A thorough clinical evaluation of the ICU patient should be completed before additional bolus doses are given during the loading dose phase of therapy, to prevent toxicity.

MAINTENANCE DOSING

If the initial loading dose of digoxin was successful at controlling the ventricular response of a supraventricular arrhythmia, a maintenance dose should be initiated.[1] The maintenance dose is also determined by renal function and the patient's LBW. The maintenance dose (in micrograms) needed by patients not previously receiving digoxin therapy can be estimated from the loading dose (in micrograms) and the percentage of drug eliminated each day as follows:

$$Maintenance\ dose = Loading\ dose \times Amount\ eliminated\ daily$$

Typical intravenous maintenance dosages range from 125 to 250 µg/day for patients with adequate renal function. Occasionally, patients require higher dosages to maintain ventricular rate control. In patients with significantly impaired renal function (CrCl less than 10 mL/min), dosages of less than 125 µg/day are necessary to prevent toxicity. Digoxin in these patients is commonly administered as 125 µg every other day.

Patients who are switched from intravenous to oral therapy must have dosage adjustments made as necessary.[1] If changing from intravenous therapy to oral tablets or elixir, the digoxin dosage should be increased by approximately 20% to 25%. However, no dosage adjustment is needed if the oral therapy uses liquid-filled capsules. For example, 100 µg of the intravenous product is approximately equivalent to 100 µg of the liquid-filled capsules (Lanoxicaps) or 125 µg of the tablet (Digitek, Lanoxin) or the elixir formulation.

SPECIAL POPULATIONS

THYROID DYSFUNCTION

Thyroid dysfunction results in an altered pharmacodynamic profile. Hypothyroid patients require decreased digoxin dosages compared to euthyroid ICU patients.[1,9,10] Hyperthyroid patients commonly need increased digoxin dosages, potentially secondary to increased resistance to digoxin therapy. Alterations in absorption, tissue distribution, renal excretion, and sensitivity of digitalis receptors in patients with thyroid disease have been proposed as mechanisms to explain altered serum digoxin concentrations.[9,10]

ELECTROLYTE DISTURBANCES

Hypokalemia enhances the effects of digoxin by increasing the cardiac effects due to depletion of intracellular potassium.[1] Hypomagnesemia requires larger digoxin doses for rate control in the setting of atrial fibrillation.[1] Repletion of potassium and magnesium to adequate levels should be completed before initiation of digoxin therapy to prevent potential proarryhthmic effects. Significant hypercalcemia may result in an enhancement of digoxin toxicity.[1]

HEART DISEASE

For patients with coronary artery disease, cor pulmonale, or extensive myocardial damage including previous myocardial infarction, a reduction of digoxin dosage may be necessary.[1] Digoxin has been reported to increase mortality in patients with acute ischemic syndromes,[13,14] although more recent data do not support this idea.[11] The increase in sensitivity to digoxin based on underlying cardiac disease mandates caution and careful patient monitoring.

GENDER

When used to treat heart failure and decreased left ventricular function, digoxin was found to have different effects on all-cause mortality in men as compared with women.[15] Specifically, digoxin was associated with increased all-cause mortality among women in a population with heart failure and depressed left ventricular systolic function.[15] The impact of gender on the pharmacologic effects of digoxin used to treat supraventricular arrhythmias is currently unknown, and dosage adjustments are not recommended on the basis of gender at this time.

PREGNANCY

Digoxin is a category C medication and should be considered for pregnant patients only if the benefits clearly outweigh the risks and no alternative is available. The impact in terms of fetal harm or reproductive capacity is unknown.[16]

RENAL DYSFUNCTION

The kinetic parameters of digoxin are severely altered in patients with impaired renal function. The elimination half-life is prolonged, and clearance is impaired. In addition, volume of distribution is decreased. The degree of dosage adjustment needed to maintain therapeutic drug levels correlates with the degree of renal insufficiency. Dosage adjustment is necessary to prevent toxicity, because digoxin is primarily excreted by the kidney. Digoxin is not removed to any appreciable extent by either peritoneal dialysis or hemodialysis. The pharmacokinetics of digoxin have not been studied during continuous renal replacement therapy.

PEDIATRICS

Individualized dosing is extremely important in pediatric patients. In newborns, a reduction in renal clearance of digoxin is observed, necessitating dosage adjustments, especially in premature infants.[1] Divided daily dosing is often necessary in infants and those younger than 10 years of age. The elixir formulation is especially suitable for the pediatric population. Loading dosages of the pediatric elixir differ based on age: 20 to 30 µg/kg for premature infants, 25 to 35 µg/kg for full-term newborns, and 35 to 60 µg/kg for children younger than 2 years of age. For children aged 2 to 5 years, oral loading doses of 30 to 40 µg/kg are appropriate, and for those aged 5 to 10 years, the oral loading dose is 20 to 35 µg/kg. Children older than 10 years of age require 10 to 15 µg/kg initially. Maintenance doses for pediatric patients are approximately 25% of the oral loading dose necessary to achieve the optimal therapeutic effect. If intravenous therapy is necessary, the dose is approximately 80% of the total oral elixir requirement.

THERAPEUTIC MONITORING

Measurements of digoxin concentration are useful in certain situations to assist in evaluating the effects of the drug on the disease state being treated and to avoid toxicity.[1] For treatment of supraventricular tachyarrhythmias, the usual therapeutic range for serum digoxin concentration is 1 to 2 ng/mL. However, patients can require serum concentrations as great as 3 ng/mL. The concentration is correlated with effectiveness or toxicity in a particular patient. The same level that is toxic in one patient may be therapeutic in another. Therefore, dose titration should be based on the heart rate and signs or symptoms of toxicity rather than the absolute digoxin concentration.

Evidence to support the use of serum concentrations to ensure efficacy in the treatment of heart failure is lacking. Lower digoxin concentrations (0.5 to 0.8 ng/mL) appear to provide equal or superior efficacy and avoid toxicity.

Gheorghiade and colleagues[17] found that exercise time, heart failure scores, heart rate, and neurohormonal findings were similar among patients with serum digoxin concentrations of 0.67 ± 0.22 ng/mL compared with 1.22 ± 0.35 ng/mL. Mean concentrations of 0.8 ng/mL provided a reduction in rate of hospitalizations and worsening heart failure.[2,18] Rathore and associates[19] demonstrated that patients with digoxin concentrations of 0.5 to 0.8 ng/mL had a reduction in absolute mortality rate of 6.3%, compared with patients who received placebo. However, no reduction in mortality was observed for patients with concentrations of 0.9 to 1.1 ng/mL, compared with the placebo group, and an increase in mortality was found for patients with levels of 1.2 ng/mL or greater.

Measurements of serum digoxin concentrations may be particularly useful when kinetic parameters are changing.[1] For example, in patients with improving or declining renal function or in situations in which a drug interaction could decrease absorption or digoxin clearance, monitoring levels is helpful. Digoxin concentrations can be obtained periodically to detect excessive drug levels and prevent toxicity.

Proper timing of digoxin measurements is critical. Although digoxin is found in the plasma compartment within a brief period after administration, the medication distributes slowly into the heart and other tissues.[20] Because the heart is the site of action, digoxin concentrations measured less than 4 hours after intravenous administration, or 6 hours after oral administration, are misleading. The optimal time to measure digoxin levels is 12 to 24 hours after administration. For patients with normal renal function, digoxin concentrations do not reach steady state for 7 to 10 days in the absence of a loading dose. As renal function declines, clearance of digoxin is impaired and the time to reach steady state is prolonged. In patients with end-stage renal failure, this duration is extended to 15 to 20 days. Levels obtained before the drug has reached steady state can be useful to prevent toxicity or assess a trend. However, these concentrations do not reflect the maximum concentration at steady state.

CONTRAINDICATIONS

Contraindications to the use of digoxin include ventricular fibrillation and hypersensitivity to digoxin or digitalis compounds.[16] The risk of digoxin use is higher in patients with preexisting sinus node disease or incomplete AV block, in those with an accessory AV pathway (Wolf-Parkinson-White syndrome), and in those who have heart failure with preserved left ventricular systolic function (isolated diastolic dysfunction). Patients with sinus node disease can develop severe sinus bradycardia or sinoatrial block. An advanced or complete AV block may develop in individuals with a previously incomplete block. The use of digoxin in patients with an accessory AV pathway may result in an increase in the frequency of anterograde conduction via the accessory pathway, with a rapid ventricular response or atrial fibrillation. Individuals with restrictive cardiomyopathy, constrictive pericarditis, amyloid heart disease, or acute cor pulmonale are particularly susceptible to digoxin toxicity.[16] Digoxin therapy can adversely affect patients with idiopathic hypertrophic subaortic stenosis by causing further obstruction to outflow.

ADVERSE EFFECTS

Noncardiac digoxin toxicities include gastrointestinal effects (anorexia, nausea, vomiting, diarrhea, abdominal pain),

central nervous system abnormalities, and hyperkalemia.[7,21] Possible central nervous system effects include lethargy, confusion, weakness, headache, delirium, psychosis, transient amblyopia, photophobia, blurred vision, scotomata, photopsia, decreased visual activity, and color irregularities such as yellow-green or red-green halos around lights. Hyperkalemia results from excessive blockade of the Na^+,K^+-ATPase pump and is an index for outcome. Acute manifestations of digoxin toxicity are often more severe than are chronic adverse effects.

Numerous cardiac arrhythmias may result from digoxin toxicity.[7,21] Cardiac effects can manifest as an increase in vagal tone causing sinus bradycardia. In the early phase of an overdose or in acute toxicity, the arrhythmia is likely to respond to atropine administration. However, atropine may be ineffective in later phases of acute poisoning or during chronic digoxin administration. Other arrhythmias that may become evident are paroxysmal atrial tachycardia, atrial flutter or atrial fibrillation with AV block, dysfunction of the conduction system, and ventricular ectopic beats.

DRUG INTERACTIONS

Digoxin is a substrate of P-glycoprotein,[22-28] and amiodarone,[22] verapamil,[23] quinidine,[24,25] clarithromycin,[26] itraconazole,[27] and cyclosporin A[28] are potent inhibitors of P-glycoprotein. P-glycoprotein is encoded by the multidrug-resistance (*MDR1*) gene and is found in kidney, liver, colon, jejunum, adrenal glands, blood-brain barrier, placenta, and testis.[23] The role of P-glycoprotein in the body is uncertain. However, one role appears to be to act as an ATP-dependent efflux pump.

Within 5 to 7 days after institution of amiodarone therapy in patients receiving digoxin, amiodarone inhibits P-glycoprotein in kidneys and liver, resulting in a decrease in renal and nonrenal clearance of digoxin.[1,7,22] Renal and nonrenal clearance of digoxin also decreases with concurrent administration of verapamil, resulting in a 70% to 100% increase in serum digoxin concentration.[1,7] Although not as extensively studied, a decrease in digoxin clearance may also occur with concomitant diltiazem use.[29] Administration of digoxin and verapamil or diltiazem should be avoided by selecting an alternative agent. Quinidine decreases renal and nonrenal clearance of digoxin and increases the rate and extent of digoxin absorption. If amiodarone, verapamil, or quinidine is administered to a patient taking digoxin, the digoxin dose should be decreased by 50% and serum digoxin concentrations should be monitored closely.

With the administration of clarithromycin, the oral bioavailability of digoxin increases and nonglomerular renal clearance of digoxin decreases.[26] This results in a 1.8-fold increase in digoxin concentration. By inhibiting P-glycoprotein, itraconazole use decreases the renal clearance of digoxin by approximately 20%, increases oral bioavailability by 30%, and results in a 2-fold increase in digoxin serum concentrations.[27] Renal excretion of digoxin is also inhibited by administration of cyclosporine.[28] Serum digoxin concentrations should be monitored closely when clarithromycin, itraconazole, or cyclosporine therapy is started in a patient receiving digoxin.

In patients with severe heart failure, captopril causes a 1.6-fold increase in peak digoxin concentrations.[30] This effect may not occur in patients with New York Heart Association class II or III heart failure. The mechanism of the interaction is unknown; it may be caused by a decrease in glomerular filtration and tubular secretion of digoxin.

Spironolactone decreases renal[31] and nonrenal[1,7] clearance of digoxin. In addition, spironolactone and canrenone, a metabolite of spironolactone, cross-react with several of the assays used to monitor digoxin concentrations.[32,33] An increase in the apparent digoxin concentration was observed when the drug was assayed by fluorescence polarization immunoassay (FPIA), aca,[32] or Elecsys 2020.[33] In contrast, a decrease in the apparent concentration occurred when the microparticle enzyme immunoassay (MEIA),[32] AxSYM MEIA II,[33] IMx MEIA II,[33] or Dimension Systems[33] were used to measure digoxin levels. Spironolactone did not appear to interact with the chemiluminescent assay (CLIA),[32] EMIT 2000,[33] Tina Quant,[33] or Vitros slides.[33] Interference with the MEIA and FPIA assays was eliminated when free concentrations were measured.[32] Digoxin concentrations should be monitored more frequently after starting spironolactone to avoid accumulation of the medication; however, CLIA, EMIT 2000, Tina Quant, Vitros slides, or free levels should be used to accurately measure digoxin concentrations.

Multiple medications decrease the bioavailability of digoxin and result in lower serum concentrations.[1,7] Cholestyramine, colestipol, kaolin-pectin, and oral antacids decrease the absorption of oral digoxin by binding digoxin in the gastrointestinal tract. These medications should be administered at least 2 hours apart to prevent this effect. Metoclopramide decreases the absorption of digoxin tablets by increasing gastrointestinal motility. The administration of digoxin capsules instead of tablets in patients receiving metoclopramide is suggested to avoid this reaction. Absorption of digoxin is lowered by the concurrent administration of neomycin or sulfasalazine. This interaction should be avoided; however, if a patient needs to receive both medications, the doses should be spaced by approximately 2 hours.

Patients receiving levothyroxine and digoxin should have close monitoring of thyroid hormone levels and digoxin concentrations. Hyperthyroidism was shown to decrease digoxin levels by increasing the volume of the central compartment.[34] In contrast, hypothyroidism may have no effect or may cause an increase in the digoxin concentration.[34,35]

Rifampin administration induces intestinal P-glycoprotein activity.[36] This results in a decrease in digoxin oral bioavailability by approximately 30%, with no apparent change in digoxin renal clearance. Because of the decrease in bioavailability, maximum plasma digoxin concentrations are reduced by 58%.

TREATMENT OF DIGOXIN TOXICITY

The treatment of digoxin toxicity includes several steps, which vary based on the acuteness of the situation. In acute overdoses, prevention of further absorption using activated charcoal should be instituted.[37] The administration of syrup of ipecac, insertion of a gastric tube, and gastric lavage should be avoided, because vomiting induced by these methods intensifies vagal tone.

Supportive care is required to manage electrolyte disturbances and dysrhythmias.[21,37,38] Hyperkalemia should be treated by the standard approaches. Sodium polystyrene sulfonate (Kayexalate) may remove potassium, and, if hyperkalemia is severe, digoxin immune Fab should be administered (see next section). Caution should be used in administering both digoxin immune Fab and sodium polystyrene sulfonate, because hypokalemia may occur.

In the case of life-threatening arrhythmias, digoxin immune Fab should be administered.[21,37] If administration of digoxin immune Fab is delayed or treatment is needed until the onset of the effect of this agent, advanced cardiac life support (ACLS) protocols should be followed.

DIGOXIN IMMUNE FAB

The digoxin immune Fab (ovine) products available in the United States are Digibind and DigiFab. The products are developed by immunizing sheep with a digoxin analog and then isolating the digoxin-specific Fab fragments from ovine blood.[39,40] Digoxin immune Fab is used for the treatment of acute and chronic life-threatening digoxin toxicity or overdose. In addition, digoxin immune Fab is used to bind other digitalis glycosides.[37] The binding affinity of digoxin for digoxin immune Fab is higher than its affinity for the sodium pump receptors. Once the Fab-digoxin complex is formed, the complex is eliminated by the kidneys and the reticuloendothelial system.

Based on an in vivo kinetic study of healthy volunteers, Digibind and DigiFab result in similar reductions in free serum digoxin concentrations.[41] Resolution of gastrointestinal symptoms occurs within minutes after beginning a bolus infusion.[42,43] Within 30 to 60 minutes, hyperkalemia starts to resolve and electrocardiogram abnormalities cease. The effect lasts for several days, requiring the complex and the drug to be cleared renally.[39,40] Digoxin immune Fab is not removed by hemodialysis.

Each vial contains 38 mg (Digibind) or 40 mg (DigiFab) of digoxin immune Fab and binds approximately 0.5 mg of digoxin.[39,40] Adult and pediatric patients who acutely ingest an unknown amount of digoxin or other digitalis glycoside should receive 20 vials of either product. Pediatric patients should be closely monitored for volume overload. Administration of all 20 vials at once is likely to result in a faster onset of action but may increase the risk of an allergic reaction. Alternatively, 10 vials may be administered with careful observation of the patient, after which 10 additional vials may be given if clinically indicated.

Adults who exhibit toxicity secondary to chronic dosing of digoxin, for whom a digoxin level is unavailable, should be given 6 vials of either product.[39,40] One vial should be sufficient for infants and children weighing 20 kg or less.

If an individual acutely ingests a known amount of digoxin, the dose is based on the estimated total body load (in milligrams) for digoxin capsules or digitoxin:

$$\text{Total body load} = (\text{Number of capsules ingested}) \times (\text{Dose of capsules})$$

If digoxin tablets were ingested, the total body load should be multiplied by 0.8 to account for the reduced bioavailability of the product. The number of vials needed can then be calculated by remembering that each vial of digoxin immune Fab binds approximately 0.5 mg of digoxin.

$$\text{Number of vials needed} = (\text{Total body load}) \div 0.5 \text{ mg}$$

Calculation of the digoxin immune Fab dose can also be based on the steady-state digoxin concentration.[39,40] Concentrations obtained in an acute overdose may be misleading and may result in underdosing, because digoxin can continue to be absorbed via the gastrointestinal tract.

Calculation of the number of vials of Fab product required for an adult patient who is experiencing digoxin toxicity is based on the serum digoxin level (in nanograms per milliliter) and the patient's weight in kilograms), as follows:

$$\text{Number of vials} = (\text{Serum digoxin concentration}) \times (\text{Weight}) \div 100$$

For digitoxin, the calculation is as follows:

$$\text{Number of vials} = (\text{Serum digitoxin concentration}) \times (\text{Weight}) \div 1000$$

For infants and children who require small doses of digoxin immune Fab, the vial may be reconstituted to provide a 1 mg/mL concentration by adding 34 mL of sterile sodium chloride to a vial of Digibind, or 36 mL to a vial of DigiFab.

The rate of administration has varied in clinical trials and case reports. Doses are typically given as a bolus over 15 to 30 minutes.[43-45] Schaumann and colleagues[46] evaluated the kinetics of digoxin immune Fab in 17 patients with acute overdose. They concluded that a bolus dose of 160 mg (4 vials) over 30 minutes, followed by an infusion of 0.5 mg/minute over 8 hours, optimally binds digoxin as it rediffuses into the blood from the tissues. Patients experiencing rebound toxicity 8 to 12 hours after the initiation of treatment could be given 0.1 mg/min.

There are no known contraindications to the use of digoxin immune Fab.[39,40] However, allergic reactions and anaphylactic reactions have occurred. Patients at a higher risk for experiencing allergic reactions are those who are allergic to papain, chymopapain, other papaya extracts, pineapple enzyme bromelain, dust mites, or latex. Because the drug is an animal product, individuals who are allergic to sheep or wool are at higher risk. In addition, patients who have previously received digoxin immune Fab are at an increased risk. Skin testing has not been shown to be useful and results in delay of therapy.

Patients must be closely monitored for significant decreases in potassium concentrations, as well as for deterioration secondary to the withdrawal of an inotropic agent in patients with low cardiac output states.[39,40] There is a theoretical risk of development of antibodies to the drug; however, this occurrence has not been reported.

After acute digoxin administration, rebound of free digoxin concentrations was observed 8 to 24 hours after initiation of Fab therapy.[41,46] The cause of this condition is not entirely clear. Proposed mechanisms include a release of free digoxin by metabolic degradation of the Fab-digoxin complex[37] and rediffusion of free digoxin from the tissues into the serum.[46] Patients should be observed closely for indications that a rebound effect is occurring. Monitoring of total serum concentrations is unnecessary, because immune Fab interacts with most assay methods. Free digoxin concentrations in ultrafiltration samples provide the most accurate results.[47]

ANNOTATED REFERENCES

The Digitalis Investigation Group: The effect of digoxin on mortality and morbidity in patients with heart failure. N Engl J Med 1997;336:525-533.
The Digitalis Investigation Group (DIG) trial was a multicenter, randomized study that included patients with an ejection fraction of 45% or less. No difference in mortality was found between the group of patients receiving digoxin and those receiving placebo. There were statistically significant decreases in overall hospitalizations and heart failure–related hospitalizations.

Packer M, Gheorghiade M, Young JB, et al, for the RADIANCE Study: Withdrawal of digoxin from patients with chronic heart failure treated with angiotensin-converting-enzyme inhibitors. N Engl J Med 1993;329:1-7.
Patients with New York Heart Association class II or III heart failure and ejection fraction of 35% or less were randomly assigned to continue digoxin or to change to placebo. Compared with the digoxin group, the placebo group had worsening heart failure, decreased functional capacity, decreased quality of life scores, and decreased ejection fraction.

Rathore SS, Curtis JP, Wang Y, et al: Association of serum digoxin concentration and outcomes in patients with heart failure. JAMA 2003;289:871-878.
This post hoc analysis of men in the DIG trial found that the mortality rate of patients with serum digoxin concentrations between 0.5 and 0.8 ng/mL was lower than that of patients receiving placebo. The mortality rate in the group of patients with serum concentrations between 0.9 to 1.1 ng/mL was not different from that in the placebo group. Those patients with a serum concentration of 1.2 ng/mL or greater had a higher mortality rate that patients in the placebo group.

Rathore SS, Wang Y, Krumholz HM: Sex-based differences in the effect of digoxin for the treatment of heart failure. N Engl J Med 2002;347:1403-1411.
This post hoc subgroup analysis of the DIG trial found in a multivariate analysis that men who received digoxin had a slight reduction in risk of death, compared with men who received placebo. However, there was a significantly increased risk of death for women in the digoxin group, compared with women in the placebo group.

Rich MW, McSherry F, Williford WO, et al: Effect of age on mortality, hospitalizations and response to digoxin in patients with heart failure: the DIG study. J Am Coll Cardiol 2001;38:806-813.
This subanalysis of the DIG study stratified patients with chronic heart failure by age. The reduction in all-cause admissions, heart failure–related admissions, and heart failure–related deaths found in the original study was independent of age.

Chapter 194

HEAVY METALS

Leo J. Sioris

KEY POINTS

1. The dose, chemical compound, route of exposure, and duration of exposure (acute or chronic) all affect the clinical presentation and approach to management, making heavy metal poisoning one of the most difficult and complex areas in toxicology.

2. Lead poisoning should be considered in any patient presenting with unexplained multiorgan system disease.

3. Children absorb up to 50% of ingested lead, whereas adults absorb only about 10% to 30%.

4. Ingestion of 10 to 30 g of a lead salt is sufficient to cause death.

5. A large part of the population is exposed to mercury by the consumption of food and fish contaminated by the industrial release of mercury into the environment and from natural sources.

6. Mercury is rapidly distributed to all organs of the body. The kidney accumulates high concentrations, as does the brain.

7. The most common acute exposure to elemental mercury is by inhalation.

8. The lethal dose of inorganic mercury salts is approximately 0.5 to 4 g, depending on the compound. For mercuric chloride, the lethal dose has been estimated to be 30 to 50 mg/kg.

9. Arsenic is widely distributed in nature in soil, rocks, and water. It accumulates in fish and shellfish as an essentially nontoxic, organic compound. Arsenic is used in a variety of manufacturing processes and industries, including the production of alloys and semiconductors, pigments and glass, and pesticides.

10. Acute ingestion of as little as 100 mg of inorganic arsenic has been reported to cause severe toxicity. Estimates of the amount needed to cause acute toxic effects in humans range from 1 mg to 10 g for various arsenic compounds.

11. The lethal dose of arsenic trioxide is estimated to be in the range of 70 to 300 mg in adults.

12. Inorganic and organic forms of arsenic are well absorbed by inhalation and oral routes.

Lead, mercury, and arsenic poisoning are the most common forms of heavy metal poisoning seen in the ICU. The dose, chemical compound, route of exposure, and duration of exposure (acute or chronic) all affect the clinical presentation and approach to management, making heavy metal poisoning one of the most difficult and complex areas in toxicology.

LEAD

Lead is the most common metal poison and is the oldest known human toxicant.[1] The toxic effects of lead have been known for millennia. No other substance can claim such a long and well-documented history, yet exposures still occur and new cases continue to appear. Lead is not required for any biologic function in the body and excessive exposure and absorption result in toxicity.

Lead is extensively used in industrial, commercial, and consumer products. It is used in batteries, solder, pipes, ceramics, glass, paints, caulks, inks, and bullets. It is also found in various arts and crafts products, gasoline, food containers, moonshine, and traditional folk remedies. Lead-containing paint in older housing is the most common source of exposure in children; lead-containing paint can also expose adults to lead when they are renovating older homes.

PATHOPHYSIOLOGY/KINETICS

Lead exists in a number of inorganic forms, such as lead silicate, carbonate, sulfide, nitrate, and oxide. Tetraethyl lead and tetramethyl lead, used as gasoline additives, are the primary forms of organic lead.

Lead exerts its effects through many different mechanisms. It inhibits sulfhydryl-containing enzymes and interacts with the essential cations of zinc, calcium, and iron, resulting in the inhibition of enzymatic processes. One of the most well researched areas is lead's inhibition of heme biosynthesis. Lead inhibits delta-aminolevulinic acid dehydratase, an enzyme that catalyzes protoporphyrin formation and heme synthesis, and ferrochelatase, which catalyzes iron's inclusion into the porphyrin ring structure. Lead also interferes with vitamin D synthesis in the kidney, steroid metabolism, red blood cell and mitochondrial membrane integrity, neurotransmitter concentrations, and nucleotide metabolism. Taken together, these actions result in a high potential to produce multiple organ system toxicity.

The pathophysiologic model of the absorption, distribution, and elimination of lead is complex and not well understood. Research has shown that lead is widely distributed from blood to soft tissue and bone. Once there, it substitutes for calcium in bone and is retained for decades unless mobilized. The amount of absorbed lead stored in bone is estimated at 90%. Over time, lead is primarily eliminated unchanged by the kidney.

The half-life of lead in the blood following a single ingestion is widely reported to be approximately 4 to 6 weeks. The half-life in bones has been reported to be more than 10 years.[2]

ABSORPTION AND TOXIC DOSES

Ingestion is the primary route of exposure in children. In adults, inhalation exposures may be seen in various occupational and environmental settings. Inhalation occurs through the lungs as a vapor or as very fine particles, where it is well absorbed. Large lead particles and insoluble lead compounds are more poorly absorbed. Inorganic lead is not well absorbed through the skin, whereas organic lead is well absorbed dermally. Infants and children are at the highest risk of poisoning from lead exposure due to increased absorption, decreased elimination rate, and increased sensitivity to the toxic effects of lead.

Children absorb up to 50% of ingested lead, whereas adults absorb only about 10% to 30%. Ingestion of 10 to 30 g of a lead salt is sufficient to cause death.[3] The ingestion of a solid lead object, such as a curtain weight or fishing weight, may result in lead encephalopathy and death, if the object is retained for a long period of time.

PRESENTATION AND TOXICITY

The wide constellation and variable onset of nonspecific symptoms leads to challenges in the diagnosis of lead poisoning. Also, low levels of lead exposure produce subclinical neurobehavioral and biochemical changes that raise serious questions as to indications for pharmacological interventions (Table 194-1).

Acute, single exposure lead poisoning is rare and occurs primarily in adults. The typical picture of lead poisoning is an acute-on-chronic exposure. Children, in particular, exhibit this presentation, when they have ongoing chronic exposure with an acute crisis. Toxicity characteristically manifests with nonspecific gastrointestinal effects, red blood cell hemolysis, liver injury, and effects on the central nervous system (CNS) leading to encephalopathy.[4]

Chronic exposure presents a more varied picture with toxicity possible to a wide variety of organ systems. Clinical signs of chronic exposure often mimic those of other disease states. There is great variability among patients in the development of organ system toxicity and an unpredictable time course is common.

Clinical signs of chronic exposure related to the gastrointestinal tract include nausea, vomiting, colicky abdominal pain, and diarrhea or constipation. A metallic taste may be noted in the mouth, and over a longer term, weight loss may be seen in children.

Hematologic effects lead to anemia, which is initially hypochromic and microcytic, but with prolonged chronicity becomes normochromic and normocytic. Hemolysis, although reported, is not common in chronic exposures. The inhibition of enzymes necessary for the development of hemoglobin leads to increased urinary levels of delta-aminolevulinic acid and coproporphyrin. Basophilic stippling occurs due to blockade of pyrimidine-5′-nucleotidase in erythrocytes; if present, this finding aids diagnosis.[5]

Lead readily crosses the blood-brain barrier, resulting in wide-ranging CNS effects. Clinical signs include headache, lethargy, irritability, confusion, delirium, impaired concentration, seizures, and coma. Low-level exposures in children (diagnosed as whole blood lead levels of 10 μg/dL to 25 μg/dL) may be associated with cognitive and behavioral toxicity and are difficult to diagnose unless a blood lead level is determined. Low-level exposures have been associated with learning disabilities, decreased intelligence, and impaired neurobehavioral development that may be only partially reversed with treatment.[6,7]

Peripheral nervous system involvement occurs as a result of axonal degeneration and segmental demyelination, leading to effects on motor function and weakness of the extensor muscles of the upper extremities. Paresthesias are uncommon.

TABLE 194-1. POISONING TOXICITY PRESENTATION OF LEAD

Acute Presentation	Chronic Presentation

Nonspecific gastrointestinal effects
Red blood cell hemolysis
Liver injury
Central nervous system (CNS) effects
  leading to encephalopathy
	Gastrointestinal tract:
	Nausea, vomiting, colicky abdominal pain, diarrhea or constipation; metallic taste may
	  be noted in the mouth; over longer term, weight loss may be seen in children.
	Hematologic:
	Anemia, hemolysis (not common), increased urinary levels of delta-aminolevulinic acid
	  and coproporphyrin, basophilic stippling
	Central nervous system:
	Headache, lethargy, irritability, confusion, delirium, impaired concentration,
	  seizures, and coma.
	In children, low-level exposures may be associated with cognitive and behavioral toxicity:
	  learning disabilities, decreased intelligence, impaired neurobehavioral development
	Peripheral nervous system:
	Effects on motor function, weakness of the extensor muscles of the upper extremities
	Muscles and joints:
	Pain, arthropathies from a retained bullet
	Kidneys:
	Fanconi-like syndrome in children characterized by glucosuria, phosphaturia, and
	  aminoaciduria; lead nephropathy commonly reported, as is hyperuricemia and gout
	Cardiovascular:
	Hypertension; overall, cardiovascular effects are rare
	Ocular and Auditory
	Reproductive
	Lead crosses the placenta into the fetus, possibility of severe toxicity
	Carcinogenic possibility

Peripheral neuropathy does not usually correlate well with whole blood lead levels or duration of exposure.

Muscle and joint pain are common and lead arthropathies have developed secondary to fragments of lead bullets located near a synovial space. Synovial fluid is more apt to break down lead from a retained bullet and make it available as a toxicant. The potential for development of toxic lead levels is also dependent on the degree of fragmentation of the bullet.

Effects on the kidney include development of a Fanconi-like syndrome in children that is characterized by glucosuria, phosphaturia, and aminoaciduria. Lead nephropathy, presenting as chronic interstitial nephritis or tubular dysfunction, is commonly reported as is hyperuricemia and gout.[8-10]

A variety of other effects have been reported. Hypertension has occurred in cases of chronic exposure with levels greater than 30 µg/dL, but overall, cardiovascular effects are rare.[11,12]

Several ocular and auditory disturbances have been noted.[13,14] Lead can result in numerous effects on the reproductive system and the metal crosses the placenta into the fetus, where it may cause severe toxicity. Lead is considered possibly carcinogenic to humans by the International Agency for Research in Cancer.

Inhalation of leaded gasoline, which contains tetraethyl (organic) lead, presents a different scenario with signs primarily associated with CNS toxicity. Tetraethyl lead is very lipophilic and readily crosses the blood-brain barrier. Manifestations of toxicity include ataxia, peripheral neuropathy, delirium, hallucinations, myoclonus, hyperreflexia, seizures, and coma. Response to treatment is generally poor.

DIAGNOSIS

Lead poisoning should be considered in any patient presenting with unexplained multiorgan system disease. Patients presenting with or without a history of lead exposure with symptoms suggestive of exposure should be evaluated for lead poisoning and a whole blood lead level measured. A free erythrocyte protoporphyrin level may be helpful in the assessment of chronic exposures. A complete blood cell count and a peripheral smear should be evaluated for anemia and basophilic stippling in all patients.

Radiographic evidence of lead exposure is useful in the assessment of lead poisoning in children. Increased density or "lead-lines" may be evident in the metaphyseal areas of the long bones and in the pelvis. Ingested flakes or other lead-containing objects sometimes can be seen on a plain abdominal radiograph. L-line and K-line x-ray fluorescence has been shown to be helpful in determining life-long bone lead accumulation in the assessment of chronic lead exposure.[15]

LABORATORY

Evaluation of whole blood lead levels needs to be done carefully, especially in cases of acute exposure, when blood lead levels may appear unusually high. The relationship between blood lead levels and toxicity is best made in cases of chronic exposure after distribution has occurred and a steady state has been established. Even then, wide variability exists between blood lead levels and clinical findings. Lead levels in chronic exposures do not reflect the total body burden of lead.

The level at which lead is presumed to cause organ system toxicity has changed many times over the years. There is no "normal" whole blood lead level; background levels in the nonexposed population are generally less than 10 µg/dL, and these levels are not expected to result in any significant inhibition of biologic function. Levels greater than 10 µg/dL indicate some level of exposure to lead. Subclinical neurologic effects have been noted in adults beginning at levels of 30 to 60 µg/dL. In children and adults, gastrointestinal, neurologic, and hematologic effects begin at levels of 25 to 40 µg/dL but may not lead to overt symptoms until levels of 60 µg/dL are reached in children and 80 µg/dL in adults. Peripheral neuropathy due to lead poisoning is generally seen at levels greater than 60 µg/dL in both children and adults and encephalopathy at greater than 80 µg/dL in children and 100 µg/dL in adults. Lead nephropathy occurs when levels are more than 40 to 60 µg/dL.

Free erythrocyte protoporphyrin, sometimes referred to as zinc protoporphyrin, is another useful laboratory test for assessing chronic lead poisoning. Inhibition of heme synthesis by lead is reflected by a free erythrocyte protoporphyrin level greater than 35 µg/dL but is not diagnostic for chronic lead toxicity. An elevated free erythrocyte protoporphyrin level (in the absence of a high blood lead level) may be associated with iron deficiency anemia. Lead affects only developing red blood cells, so elevations in free erythrocyte protoporphyrin will be delayed after exposure to lead by a minimum of several weeks. The free erythrocyte protoporphyrin level is normal in cases of acute exposure despite high blood lead levels.

Other diagnostic tests include elevated urinary levels of delta aminolevulinic acid, coproporphyrin, and lead. Urinary levels of aminolevulinic acid and coproporphyrin can help support the diagnosis of lead poisoning but are not accurate as sole indicators and generally are not recommended.[16,17] Urine lead levels are most useful when used to evaluate lead excretion following a lead mobilization test. A 24-hour urine sample is collected and assessed for lead content before and after a single dose of a chelating agent. This test is used to assess whether lead can be mobilized by chelation therapy and excreted when the blood lead level and exposure history are difficult to interpret. Recent research results have questioned the reliability of this test in determining the body burden of lead and the potential for successful chelation therapy.[16-18]

MANAGEMENT

Initial decontamination of patients who have ingested lead-containing liquids or powders should include gastric lavage, regardless of the quantity ingested. Small amounts of lead-containing substances can contain large quantities of lead. The administration of activated charcoal is of questionable efficacy for the management of patients after ingestion of inorganic lead salts. However, charcoal may be of benefit and should be administered in the management of patients after ingestions of organic lead compounds. As with all hazardous chemical exposures, the source needs to be identified and eliminated to avoid repeated exposure.

If there is radiographic evidence of lead substances in the gastrointestinal tract, whole bowel irrigation should be considered. At the very least, repeated doses of cathartics and enemas should be administered until the substance is cleared. To ensure adequate excretion of lead, an adequate urine flow should be established. Owing to the potential for cerebral edema, care should be taken to avoid overhydrating the patient. Supportive care should be administered as appropriate, and seizures treated according to standard guidelines.

Surgical removal of lead-containing objects should be considered in patients with elevated blood lead levels and radiographic evidence that the objects were not removed following whole bowel irrigation or cathartics. Surgical removal of bullets should be considered if they are located near synovial spaces, especially if elevated lead levels are present along with symptoms.

Chelation therapy for lead poisoning has been recommended for years without controlled clinical trials documenting correct dosing or efficacy. Nevertheless, chelating agents remain the mainstay of treatment and have been used safely and successfully to treat patients with lead toxicity or elevated lead body burdens.

Over many decades, the Centers for Disease Control, medical reference texts, and primary articles in the literature have recommended many different threshold blood lead levels that should be used as triggers for instituting various treatments. The following recommendations are reflective of those in current practice and have had the benefit of peer review.

Asymptomatic as well as symptomatic adults with blood lead levels greater than 100 µg/dL should be treated with a chelating agent. A blood lead level greater than 70 µg/dL in a child with or without symptoms is considered a medical emergency and requires immediate hospitalization and chelation therapy.[19] Chelation is recommended in all children with blood lead levels greater than 45 µg/dL, regardless of the presence of symptoms. At levels between 25 and 44 µg/dL, a lead mobilization test should be considered to identify whether lead can be mobilized and eliminated. Although this test is not used as frequently as in the past, it may still be of assistance in certain patients. Close monitoring, but not chelation, is recommended for children with levels between 10 and 24 µg/dL.

The following guidelines include recommendations for treatment based on the presence or absence of symptoms, lead levels, and types of chelators.

Asymptomatic adults and children with blood lead levels of 80 µg/dL or greater and 45 µg/dL, respectively, should be considered for chelation with dimercaptosuccinic acid (DMSA, Succimer). Dosing for both children and adults is initiated at 10 mg/kg three times daily for 5 days and then twice daily for 14 days. Repeated courses, if needed, are administered following a 2-week drug-free period. Chelation therapy may be repeated sooner if blood lead levels warrant it.

Symptomatic patients without encephalopathy should be treated with DMSA as described earlier or calcium disodium edetate (CaEDTA). DMSA is the agent of choice if the patient has no gastrointestinal signs and is able to take oral medications. CaEDTA, eliminated solely by the kidney, is nephrotoxic in high doses and should not be used in the presence of renal failure. CaEDTA is administered at a dose of 20 to 30 mg/kg/24 hours (not to exceed 2 g/day) for adults by continuous slow intravenous infusion at a concentration of 2 to 4 mg/mL in 5% dextrose in water or saline. The dose in children is 1000 to 1500 mg/M²/24 hours administered by continuous intravenous infusion.

Simultaneous administration of dimercaprol (British anti-lewisite, or BAL) with CaEDTA, at the lower dose levels given below, is advocated by some experts.

Dimercaprol should be discontinued once lead levels are less than 45 µg/dL. Administration of CaEDTA should continue for 5 days and therapy re-evaluated following a 48- to 72-hour drug-free period. Repeated courses are administered as needed to reduce the blood lead level to less than 45 µg/dL and until symptoms have largely resolved or cannot be diminished further.

Lead encephalopathy should be considered a medical emergency with monitoring of the patient in an ICU. Symptomatic patients with encephalopathy should be administered CaEDTA at higher dosage ranges for 5 days. CaEDTA primarily chelates lead present in soft tissues, does not cross into the red blood cells, and crosses the blood-brain barrier slowly. Some experts suggest the use of dimercaprol 4 hours before CaEDTA administration, since dimercaprol crosses into the brain and red blood cells and can mobilize lead for elimination.[20,21]

Dimercaprol is given along with the CaEDTA for 3 to 5 days. It is dosed at 3 to 5 mg/kg every 4 hours and is given intramuscularly. After the first 2 days, the dosing interval can be expanded to every 6 to 12 hours, depending on improvement in symptoms and reduction in lead levels. Adverse effects such as pain at the injection site, fever, sterile abscesses, nausea, and vomiting make administration uncomfortable for the patient. Dimercaprol is excreted primarily in the bile; thus, patients with liver disease may have a difficult time tolerating this agent.

For all chelating regimens, blood lead levels should be repeated every few days during chelation to document efficacy. After each course of chelation therapy (5 days for CaEDTA, 19 days for DMSA), the continued need for further chelation is evaluated by monitoring for a rebound in blood lead levels. This rebound effect is caused by re-equilibration of lead from bone and soft tissue to central compartments. Patients with lead levels greater than 45 mg/dL and those with persistent treatable symptoms should receive further courses of chelation.

MERCURY

Mercury, a nonessential element, has a long history of use and toxicity. Even after 2000 years of varied uses and medicinal applications, exposures leading to poisoning continue to occur. Mercury is used in batteries, paints, dyes, switches, jewelry, light bulbs, dental products, thermometers, fungicides, and inks. It is used to produce caustic soda and chlorine, and in plating, fur processing, tanning of hides, mining, and photography. Historically, mercury has been used as an antiseptic, in diuretics, for dermatologic purposes, and as a medicinal agent for syphilis.

Because of the natural occurrence of mercury in the environment, all populations are exposed to low levels of it. A large part of the population is exposed to mercury by the consumption of food and fish contaminated by the industrial release of mercury into the environment and from natural sources. Inorganic mercury can be converted to methylmercury by aquatic organisms and accumulated by large fish (tuna and swordfish) that may be ultimately consumed by humans. Mass epidemics of mercury poisoning have occurred in Japan and Iraq, where thousands were affected because of contamination of water and food supplies, respectively.[22,23]

PATHOPHYSIOLOGY/KINETICS

Mercury occurs in three forms: elemental mercury (Hg⁰), inorganic mercury, and organic mercury. Inorganic mercury is found in either the Hg^{+1} (mercurous) or Hg^{+2} (mercuric) valence states and forms salts. Examples of inorganic mercury-containing salts are mercuric chloride, mercuric bromide, mercuric sulfide, and mercuric cyanide. The organic form is usually found with either aryl or short-to-long chain alkyl groups attached. Organic mercury can be found as methylmercury, phenylmercury, and thimerosal, among other compounds. Similar to other heavy metals, chemical form and valence, along with dose and route of exposure, greatly influence the toxicity and kinetics of mercury compounds.

Mercury is a cellular poison. Toxicity is produced when mercury binds with sulfhydryl groups and a number of other chemical groups, such as amides, amines, carboxyl, and phosphoryl groups.[24] Enzymatic activity and cell metabolism are adversely affected and eventually cell death occurs.

Mercury is considered highly lipid soluble, especially in its elemental and organic forms. It is rapidly distributed to all organs of the body. The kidney accumulates high concentrations, as does the brain.[25] Inorganic forms do not cross the blood-brain barrier well; elemental and organic forms do.

Elemental mercury must be metabolized to mercuric ion to cause toxicity; therefore, symptoms resemble toxicity from inorganic mercury salts. Mercury is then eliminated in both urine and feces. Inorganic mercury is reduced to metallic mercury and exhaled through the lungs as well as through the urine and feces. Aryl mercury compounds (one form of organic mercury) are also metabolized to mercuric ion, but to a much greater extent and faster rate than methylmercury (another form of organic mercury). Consequently, toxicity from aryl mercury compounds resembles that of inorganic mercury salts once metabolism has occurred. Methylmercury is only minimally metabolized to the mercuric ion form, allowing for its distribution and accumulation into the CNS. It is primarily excreted in the feces (>90%), and very little excreted by the kidneys. It undergoes enterohepatic recirculation.[26]

The half-life for elemental mercury is about 60 days. The half-life for the inorganic salts is around 40 days and that of organic mercury compounds ranges from 40 to 105 days.

ABSORPTION AND TOXIC DOSES

Elemental mercury is the only metal that is liquid at room temperature. It sublimates readily into the air (especially when the metal is heated), and mercury vapor can cause toxicity by inhalation. Eighty percent of an inhaled dose is absorbed; the remainder is retained in the lung.[27,28] Elemental mercury is poorly absorbed from the gastrointestinal tract and not readily absorbed from the skin. The lethal dose of elemental mercury has been reported to be 100 g.[29]

Less than 15% of inorganic mercury salts are absorbed from the gastrointestinal tract, whereas absorption is greater than 90% for methylmercury. The lethal dose of inorganic mercury salts is approximately 0.5 to 4 g, depending on the compound. For mercuric chloride, the lethal dose has been estimated to be 30 to 50 mg/kg.[30]

Methylmercury is also well absorbed from the lung through inhalation and also from the skin. The short chain alkyl compounds of organic mercury, e.g., methylmercury, are the most toxic. Ingestion of 10 to 60 mg/kg of methylmercury is reported to be lethal. Phenylmercury is thought to be moderately toxic, being between that of inorganic mercury and the alkyl organic forms. The average lethal dose of organic mercury compounds has been estimated to be 100 mg.[3]

PRESENTATION AND TOXICITY

The most common acute exposure to elemental mercury is by inhalation. Toxicity to the lung results from both a direct irritant effect on the airways and alveoli and its activity as a cellular poison. A variety of pulmonary manifestations of toxicity ensue, ranging from a metal fume fever type of presentation with symptoms of cough, fever, and chills to acute bronchitis, interstitial pneumonitis, pulmonary edema, and respiratory failure. Over time, inhaled vapors of elemental mercury accumulate and are metabolized in the CNS, leading to entrapment of the mercuric ion and eventual neurotoxicity (Table 194-2).

Ingestion of liquid elemental mercury usually does not lead to toxicity. The presence of any bowel irregularities or

TABLE 194–2. POISONING TOXICITY PRESENTATION OF MERCURY

	Acute Presentation	Chronic Presentation
	Acute and chronic organic mercury poisoning are very similar in presentation but vary according to the specific compound involved	
Inhaled	**Pulmonary:** Metal fume fever type of presentation with symptoms of cough, fever, chills, acute bronchitis, interstitial pneumonitis, pulmonary edema, respiratory failure	Inorganic mercury poisoning resembles toxicity from chronic elemental mercury exposure but includes early signs of gingivitis, excessive salivation, dermatitis, tremor, behavioral effects, sensory and motor deficits resembling those of arsenical neuropathy, irritability, headache, pathologic shyness, poor attention span, memory loss.
	Central nervous system: Over time, inhaled vapors lead to eventual neurotoxicity Mercuric chloride most frequently consumed agent	Delirium and hallucinations may occur in severe exposures. **Renal:** Proteinuria, nephrotic syndrome
Ingested	**Gastrointestinal tract:** Blisters and ulcers in the mouth, nausea and vomiting, gastritis, esophageal burns, hemorrhage, ulcerative colitis **Kidney:** Acute tubular necrosis, acute renal failure within several days of exposure. **Laryngeal, tracheal, and pulmonary edema** **Hypotension and hypovolemic shock** primary cause of death. **Neurologic:** Usually limited to tremor, loss of coordination, hyperreflexia, confusion, lethargy **Dermatologic:** Discoloration of the skin, burns or irritation, dermatitis, systemic toxicity	

disease, however, may allow retention and eventual metabolism to organic mercurial forms by bacteria, which are then absorbed and lead to toxicity.

Acute inorganic mercury poisoning most commonly results from ingestion. The accidental or intentional consumption of inorganic salts has occurred throughout the years due to their ready availability. Mercuric chloride is the agent most frequently consumed. Inorganic mercury salts are considered corrosive agents, and poisoning initially affects the gastrointestinal tract. Systemic effects follow; the kidney is the primary organ affected. Gastrointestinal effects range from blisters and ulcers in the mouth to nausea and vomiting, gastritis, esophageal burns, hemorrhage, and ulcerative colitis.[31,32] Aspiration may lead to laryngeal, tracheal, and pulmonary edema. The effect on the kidney usually manifests as acute tubular necrosis and acute renal failure within several days of exposure.[33] Hypotension and hypovolemic shock, from the loss of blood and fluids, is the primary cause of death. Neurologic effects in acute exposures are usually limited to tremor, loss of coordination, hyperreflexia, confusion, and lethargy. Dermatologic exposure may lead to discoloration of the skin, burns or irritation, and dermatitis. Excessive use of mercury-based dermatologic preparations has led to systemic toxicity.[34]

Chronic inorganic mercury poisoning resembles toxicity from chronic elemental mercury exposure but includes early signs of gingivitis and excessive salivation, dermatitis, tremor, behavioral effects, sensory and motor deficits resembling those of arsenical neuropathy, irritability, headache, pathologic shyness, poor attention span, and memory loss.[30,35] Delirium and hallucinations may occur with severe exposures. Renal toxicity may manifest as proteinuria and nephrotic syndrome.

Acute and chronic organic mercury poisoning are very similar in presentation but vary according to the specific compound involved. Symptoms may be delayed for many weeks or months after chronic exposure. Phenyl and long chain alkyl forms produce findings that resemble toxicity from chronic inorganic mercury salts. Short chain alkyl forms, such as methylmercury, result in toxicity that is primarily limited to the CNS. A classic triad of dysarthria, ataxia, and visual field constriction has been described by Hunter and colleagues.[36] Others have described paresthesias, tremor, and spasticity.[37,38] High doses may also lead to dermatitis, electrocardiographic changes, and renal toxicity.

DIAGNOSIS

The diagnosis is dependent on identification of signs and symptoms characteristic of mercury poisoning along with the presence of elevated blood and/or urine mercury levels. A thorough history, including occupation and food consumption, should be taken to confirm an exposure to mercury.

LABORATORY

Complete blood cell count, blood urea nitrogen concentration, serum creatinine concentration, urinalysis, serum electrolyte concentrations, and serum liver enzyme levels should be evaluated in all patients suspected of mercury exposure. If the exposure involves potentially corrosive inorganic mercury salts, blood should be typed and cross-matched for treatment of potential gastrointestinal hemorrhage.

A 24-hour whole blood mercury level is preferred when making an assessment for acute mercury exposure.[39,40]

Urinary levels are also used but are most beneficial in the assessment of chronic exposures and in monitoring the effectiveness of chelation therapy. Blood mercury levels are useful to confirm exposure to elemental, inorganic, and methylmercury, and, because of mercury's rapid distribution, should be obtained as soon as possible after exposure. Consideration should be given to the recent consumption of seafood when assessing blood mercury levels.

In the nonexposed individual, blood levels less than 2.0 µg/dL and urine levels less than 20 µg/L are considered normal; however, there are wide individual and interlaboratory variations. Blood levels of 5 µg/dL or greater are consistent with recent exposure and are more predictably associated with the onset of symptoms and toxicity. Overall, there is minimal correlation of blood or urine mercury levels with toxic effects.[30] Deaths have been reported with methylmercury with levels greater than 60 µg/dL and as low as 40 µg/dL from vaporized elemental mercury.[3]

A 24-hour urine collection is useful for the assessment of chronic exposures to elemental or inorganic mercury and to assess treatment with chelation therapy. This test is not helpful in estimating total body burden. Symptoms arising from toxicity generally begin when urinary mercury levels are greater than 20 µg/L but may not be overtly evident until levels greater than 100 µg/L are reached. Spot sampling may be helpful in quickly identifying an exposure until a 24-hour sample can be taken. Since methylmercury is not excreted to an appreciable extent in the urine, urinary mercury levels are not helpful in assessing acute or chronic methylmercury exposures.[41]

Hair analysis is helpful in confirmation of exposure to organic mercury compounds, especially methylmercury, when environmental exposure cannot be ruled out. Segmental hair analysis may be of help in assessing exposure over time; however, there are numerous difficulties in making these analyses, and their accuracy is unreliable. Overall, hair analysis provides little additional information and is not useful for elemental or inorganic mercury exposures.

Abdominal radiographs may be useful in assessing the ingestion and gastrointestinal transit of elemental and inorganic mercury compounds, although a negative radiographic finding does not necessarily imply that mercury is not present. A chest radiograph may also identify aspirated elemental mercury.

Urinary N-acetyl beta-glucosaminidase has been shown to be an early indicator of renal toxicity in chronic inorganic mercury exposures; however, this assay is not specific for mercury poisoning.[42]

MANAGEMENT

Patients with inhalation exposures to mercury should be monitored closely for the development of pulmonary edema and pneumonitis. The airway should be managed aggressively and supplemental oxygen administered as needed. Further treatment is supportive unless elevated blood or urine mercury levels are measured and found to be elevated, in which case chelation therapy should be considered.

Gastric decontamination is unnecessary for ingestions of elemental mercury, since this form is not absorbed during routine transit through the gastrointestinal tract. Patients with these ingestions should be monitored closely, however, in the event an obstruction occurs or mercury is retained in the bowel. If there is radiographic evidence of retention, whole bowel irrigation with a polyethylene glycol solution should be considered. Follow-up radiographs should be taken to document effectiveness, and clinical status evaluated to determine the need for surgical removal.

Ingestion of inorganic or organic forms of mercury requires aggressive decontamination with gastric lavage, if performed within 1 hour of ingestion; otherwise, activated charcoal should be administered. Care should be taken with gastric lavage after ingestions of corrosive inorganic salts, since there is a risk of perforation. Endoscopy should be considered in these situations to assess the extent of injury before initiating lavage. To facilitate binding of mercury, addition to the lavage fluid of a protein source, such as milk or egg whites, has been recommended by some practitioners. The effectiveness and benefit of this approach have not been adequately evaluated, and its utility should be considered questionable. If there is radiographic evidence of mercury remaining in the gastrointestinal tract after lavage, whole bowel irrigation should be performed and follow-up evaluation of efficacy determined with abdominal radiographs and measurement of whole blood mercury levels.

Induction of emesis should be avoided in cases of ingestion of inorganic mercury salts because of their corrosive nature but could be considered with organic mercurials, provided that ingestion has occurred within the previous 30 minutes.

Activated charcoal effectively binds inorganic and organic forms of mercury and should be administered following lavage. It is not known whether activated charcoal binds elemental mercury. It is the author's opinion that repeated doses of activated charcoal should be considered in cases of methylmercury exposure, since enterohepatic recycling occurs. A polythiol resin has been recommended for repeated dosing in cases of methylmercury poisoning for the same reason.[43,44]

If mercury exposure is highly suspected and there are symptoms suggestive of poisoning, chelation therapy should be started using either DMSA or dimercaprol. Chelation treatment has been recommended when mercury blood levels are greater than 3.5 μg/dL or when urine levels are greater than 100 μg/L.[45] The time needed for mercury blood and urine level analysis means that chelation should be instituted before laboratory results are completed. The immediate initiation of treatment with chelators is believed to be critical to their effectiveness in mitigating toxicity. Once mercury-induced neurotoxicity is established, chelators have little impact on the course of the illness.

DMSA has been shown to be more efficacious and has a wider safety profile than dimercaprol. It is the current agent of choice, although it has not been approved by the Food and Drug Administration for this use.[44,46] DMSA can be used for all types of mercury poisoning, whereas dimercaprol should be limited to use for inorganic mercury exposures. Animal studies have shown that dimercaprol increases the CNS levels of mercury after elemental and organic mercury exposures, and it use, therefore, is contraindicated.[47]

An oral chelator, such as DMSA, should not be used if there are gastrointestinal symptoms, if mercury is present in the gastrointestinal tract, or if hypotension is present (which may lead to decreased mesenteric blood flow and decreased absorption), making dimercaprol the preferred agent under these conditions. For those patients who cannot tolerate DMSA or are allergic to it, D-penicillamine can be used. A dosage regimen similar to that used in the treatment of lead toxicity is used (250 mg capsule four times daily, for adults). Renal function should be assessed prior to initiation

of therapy. Since dimercaprol is mostly excreted into the bile, it is considered the agent of choice in patients with renal failure.

Chelation should continue until symptoms have largely resolved and the whole blood mercury level, at 1 week after the cessation of therapy, is less than 2.0 μg/dL for cases of organic mercury poisoning and the urine mercury level is less than 20 μg/L for cases of elemental and inorganic mercury poisoning. Repeated cycles of chelation may be indicated.

In the case of ingestion of corrosive inorganic salts, where there is a higher risk of perforation and bleeding leading to hypotension and shock, aggressive fluid management is important. Urine output should be monitored carefully and volume losses and maintenance fluids replaced.

Hemodialysis and hemoperfusion do not significantly affect mercury removal unless chelators are administered. Both the dimercaprol and DMSA mercury complexes are dialyzable and, in the presence of acute renal failure, dialysis substantially improves their removal. In the patient with adequate renal function, clearance of these chelator-metal complexes should be adequate and dialysis is of no benefit.

ARSENIC

Arsenic is widely distributed in nature in soil, rocks, and water. It accumulates in fish and shellfish as an essentially nontoxic organic compound. Arsenic is used in a variety of manufacturing processes and industries, including the production of alloys and semiconductors, pigments and glass, and pesticides. Inorganic arsenic compounds are no longer used in agriculture in the United States, but organic arsenic compounds continue to be used as pesticides. Treatment of wood with "chromated copper arsenate" is one of the largest uses of arsenic. This product is also called CCA-, salt-, or arsenic-treated wood. The unrestricted use of CCA-treated wood in residences and recreational areas was stopped in the United States on January 1, 2004.

Dietary intake constitutes the primary source of exposure, but occupational exposures, homeopathic medicines, and suicidal and homicidal acts continue to result in cases of arsenic toxicity. Some areas of the world have very high levels of arsenic in water supplies that have caused mass exposures and illnesses.

PATHOPHYSIOLOGY/KINETICS

Arsenic exists in one of four valences: As^0 (elemental), As^{-3}, As^{+3}, and As^{+5}. Arsenic, in the As^{-3} valence, is found in combination with hydrogen as "arsine." This gas is extremely toxic, but exposure to it is rare. The positive trivalent (+3) and pentavalent (+5) species are the most commonly involved in cases of human exposure. The positive trivalent form is commonly found as arsenic trioxide, sodium arsenite, and arsenic trichloride. The pentavalent form is found as arsenic pentoxide, arsenic acid, and arsenate salts. The toxicity of arsenic varies with the valence: The −3 valence (as AsH_3, arsine) is the most toxic; the +3 valence is somewhat less toxic, but it is still two to 10 times more toxic than the pentavalent form.

Trivalent arsenic interacts with sulfhydryl groups, leading to decreased adenosine triphosphate production, whereas the pentavalent form uncouples oxidative phosphorylation by substituting for phosphate. Both mechanisms negatively affect energy production and cellular metabolism, resulting in cell death.

Following absorption, arsenic is bound to plasma proteins and distributed to organs and soft tissues. Over a period of many weeks, arsenic becomes bound to keratin, the sulfhydryl-rich protein found in nails, hair, skin, and bone. Nonpathognomonic, transverse white bands, called Mees' (or Aldrich-Mees) lines, may form across nails 6 weeks or more following large acute or chronic exposures. The type and time of exposure can be estimated by evaluating the line and distance from the line to the base of the nail.

Inorganic arsenic compounds are metabolized in the liver by methylation to mono-methylarsonic acid and dimethylarsinic acid; the metabolites are eliminated by the kidney. Reduction of pentavalent arsenic to the more toxic trivalent form occurs in vivo, as part of the metabolic process, which leads to methylation.[48] The elimination of arsenic in humans is triphasic. The first phase has a half-life of approximately 2 hours, the second phase has a half-life of around 30 hours, and a slow third phase has a half-life of about 200 hours.[49]

ABSORPTION AND TOXIC DOSES

Inorganic and organic forms of arsenic are well absorbed by inhalation and oral routes. They are not well absorbed dermally unless the skin is denuded (Table 194-3).

Trivalent arsenic compounds are significantly more toxic than their pentavalent congeners. The amount of arsenic reported to cause toxicity and death varies widely in the literature. This dose is dependent on the chemical and physical properties of the arsenic compound. Water-soluble compounds are more toxic than are nonsoluble compounds. Acute ingestion of as little as 100 mg of inorganic arsenic has been reported to cause severe toxicity.[50] Estimates of the amount needed to cause acute toxic effects in humans range from 1 mg to 10 g for various arsenic compounds.[51] The lethal dose of arsenic trioxide is estimated to be in the range of 70 to 300 mg in adults.[52,53]

PRESENTATION AND TOXICITY

Arsenic poisoning has been characterized as one of the "great impersonators" of medicine. It is very difficult to establish the diagnosis without a thorough history and high index of suspicion. Arsenic poisoning can mimic numerous other disease states and lead to an exhaustive and costly diagnostic effort.

Exposure to arsenic can occur by inhalation, skin absorption, or, most commonly, ingestion. The onset of symptoms generally occurs within 30 minutes after an acute ingestion.

TABLE 194–3. POISONING TOXICITY PRESENTATION OF ARSENIC

	Acute Presentation	Chronic Presentation
Ingestion	One of the "great impersonators" of medicine Arsenic poisoning can mimic numerous other disease states. Toxicity can occur in nearly every organ system. Ingestion most common exposure. Garlic-like or metallic taste may be noted in the mouth; stool may develop a garlic odor. **Upper gastrointestinal tract:** Trivalent arsenic compounds often result in burning of the mouth and throat, difficulty swallowing, nausea, severe vomiting, abdominal pain, bloody or rice water-like diarrhea, and hemorrhagic gastritis, inflammatory necrosis in mucosa and submucosa of the stomach and intestine causing "rice-water stool" that may eventually lead to perforation. **Cardiovascular:** Hypotension, tachycardia, hemorrhagic shock, torsades de pointes, ventricular fibrillation, QTc prolongation and T wave changes, myocardial depression. Facial edema, muscle cramping, and fluid and electrolyte disturbances may occur. **Central nervous system:** Stupor and delirium can progress to seizures, coma, and chemical-induced encephalopathy. Death from acute exposure is most commonly a result of shock secondary to volume losses. **Neuropathy:** Symmetrical, develops distally, usually begins on soles of feet, progresses to hands, continues to move proximally. Characterized by paresthesias, sometimes burning type pain Severe muscle weakness and wasting	**Hepatic toxicity:** Liver enlargement, cirrhosis, liver cell injury, elevation of circulating transaminase levels **Hematologic:** Pancytopenia, leukopenia, thrombocytopenia Peripheral vascular disease with symptoms similar to those seen in Raynaud's phenomenon, may progress to endarteritis obliterans. **Cardiovascular:** Arsenic-associated myocarditis, variety of dysrhythmias **Dermatologic:** Skin lesions, flushing, patchy hyperpigmentation, keratosis, diffuse desquamation, exfoliative dermatitis, skin cancers, Mees' lines, keratosis
Inhalation	**Pulmonary:** Acute respiratory failure, as a result of neuromuscular weakness, metal fume fever, noncardiogenic pulmonary edema. **Hematologic:** Hemolysis, anemia, basophilic stippling of red cells, acute tubular necrosis, hematuria, rhabdomyolysis **Dermatologic:** Irritation and corrosive effects at the site of contact, sensitization, vesicular, pustular eruptions	

The presence of food delays absorption, and therefore symptoms, for up to several hours. Depending on the dose and duration of exposure to arsenic, toxicity can occur in nearly every organ system. The literature is replete with the many clinical manifestations seen in cases of arsenic poisoning.

Both acute and chronic effects can occur after a significant acute exposure. After ingestion of arsenic compounds, a garlic-like or metallic taste may be noted in the mouth; the stool may also develop a garlic odor. Trivalent arsenic compounds often result in burning of the mouth and throat, difficulty swallowing, nausea, severe vomiting, abdominal pain, bloody or rice water-like diarrhea, and hemorrhagic gastritis.[54] Inflammatory necrosis occurs in the mucosa and submucosa of the stomach and intestine and causes a "rice-water stool" that may eventually lead to perforation. These upper gastrointestinal findings are not associated with exposure to pentavalent arsenic compounds. Loss of fluid volume and vasodilation eventually lead to hypotension and tachycardia. Other cardiovascular symptoms include hemorrhagic shock, torsades de pointes, ventricular fibrillation, QTc prolongation and T wave changes, and myocardial depression.[55-57] Facial edema, muscle cramping, and fluid and electrolyte disturbances may occur. After ingestion of high doses of arsenic, stupor and delirium can progress to seizures, coma, and a chemical-induced encephalopathy. Death from acute exposure is most commonly a result of shock secondary to volume losses.

Acute respiratory failure, as a result of neuromuscular weakness, has been noted for up to several weeks after ingestion in cases of severe exposures.[58] Acute inhalation of arsenic compounds has resulted in metal fume fever and noncardiogenic pulmonary edema.[59]

The neuropathy of arsenic poisoning begins 1 to 3 weeks after ingestion. The condition is symmetrical and develops distally. It usually begins on the soles of the feet, progresses to the hands, and continues to move proximally.[60] The neuropathy is characterized by paresthesias and sometimes is accompanied by a burning-type pain. Sensory findings are generally more common than motor effects. Nerve conduction velocity is slowed and severe muscle weakness and wasting may occur, potentially leading to permanent disability. These findings may be confused with Guillain-Barré syndrome.[61]

Hepatic toxicity is not common in cases of acute exposure but rather with chronic exposure. Liver enlargement and cirrhosis have been reported as well as liver cell injury and elevation of circulating transaminase levels.[62]

Hematologic effects include hemolysis and anemia. Basophilic stippling of red blood cells may be present.[63] Pancytopenia has been reported in patients with acute exposures, but it is more commonly found in patients with chronic exposures. Leukopenia and thrombocytopenia also have been reported.[64]

Chronic arsenic exposure may cause peripheral vascular disease with symptoms similar to those seen in Raynaud's phenomenon.[65] In some patients, this process may progress to endarteritis obliterans. Arsenic-associated myocarditis and a variety of dysrhythmias have been reported in chronic exposures.[66]

Acute tubular necrosis resulting from red blood cell hemolysis may be seen after exposure to arsine gas and other arsenic compounds. Hematuria and rhabdomyolysis also have been reported after severe acute exposures.[67]

Exposure to trivalent arsenic compounds can cause irritation and corrosive effects at the site of contact. Contact with trivalent and pentavalent forms can result in sensitization; vesicular, pustular eruptions have occurred after acute exposures. With the exception of "acute on chronic" exposures, other dermatologic findings are not common in patients with acute arsenic poisoning. Skin lesions are often the first signs of chronic arsenic exposure and may last for many years.[63] Dermatologic findings include flushing, patchy hyperpigmentation, keratosis, diffuse desquamation, and exfoliative dermatitis.[54,60,68] Skin cancers are frequently associated with these skin findings. Mees' lines and keratosis are more commonly seen in chronic arsenic exposures.

DIAGNOSIS

The diagnosis is dependent upon identification of signs and symptoms characteristic of arsenic poisoning along with the presence of an elevated 24-hour urine arsenic level. Arsenic poisoning should be considered in any patient presenting with multiorgan system disease or with a peripheral neuropathy of unknown origin. Arsenic is radiopaque, and it may be visualized by an abdominal radiograph after an acute ingestion.

LABORATORY TESTS

A complete blood cell count as well as serum electrolyte levels, urinalysis, and liver and renal function tests should be performed in all patients. A 24-hour urine collection is preferred for evaluation of arsenic exposure, but a random spot urine test can be used for screening. A spot urine arsenic level more than 200 µg/L is considered high, but chelation therapy should await confirmation by a 24-hour urine collection. Twenty-four hour arsenic levels greater than 50 to 100 µg/L should be considered elevated because most "non-arsenic exposed" people have urine levels less than 50 µg/L. When urinary arsenic levels are more than 50 µg/L, the contribution from dietary intake must be determined. Fish and shellfish are common sources of dietary arsenic, and consuming these foods should be avoided for 48 hours preceding the collection of a specimen.[69] Urinary arsenic levels resulting from seafood consumption may reach 1700 µg/L within 4 hours of eating.[3] The pentavalent organic form of arsenic found in seafood is arsenobetaine. This compound is not considered toxic. If the source of exposure is unknown or the ingestion of seafood is suspected, arsenic speciation (valence and inorganic versus organic compound) can help clarify the source.

A blood arsenic level provides very little information for diagnosis or treatment but may be of benefit in documenting an acute exposure, if performed quickly before tissue distribution and clearance occurs. Blood levels are of no value in cases of chronic exposure. Arsenic can also be measured in hair and nail samples, but these specimens are of questionable value in the critical care setting.

MANAGEMENT

Gastric lavage is recommended if the patient is seen within 1 hour after acute ingestion. If there is radiographic or other evidence that arsenic is in the lower gastrointestinal tract, whole bowel irrigation should be considered. The use of activated charcoal in these patients is of questionable value, although it is still recommended by some practitioners.

When signs and symptoms of arsenic toxicity are sufficient to require chelation therapy, the patient's volume status should be monitored and treated aggressively. Intravenous crystalloid solutions should be used to treat fluid losses and associated hypotension. Urine output should be maintained at 1 to 2 mL/kg/h, and at 2 to 3 mL/kg/h in those who have developed hemolysis to prevent pigment deposition in the renal tubules. To further prevent deposition of red blood cell breakdown products, alkalinization of the urine in these patients is also recommended.

Chelation therapy should be considered in symptomatic patients with documented elevated body levels of arsenic. If clinically necessary, chelation therapy can be started while waiting for laboratory confirmation. Chelation therapy in asymptomatic patients with elevated levels is controversial, especially when levels are elevated from pentavalent forms of arsenicals. Some authors have suggested that chelation may be warranted as a precautionary measure to prevent toxicity and a delayed peripheral neuropathy.[70] Other authors have noted that there is little evidence to support this premise.[71]

DMSA has been recommended by some authorities as the chelator of choice in individuals who are able to take medications orally. DMSA is considered more efficacious than D-penicillamine and is associated with fewer adverse effects.[72] DMSA is also the agent of choice if long-term therapy is necessary. The dosing regimen of DMSA for arsenic poisoning is unknown; therefore, the manufacturer's recommended dose regimen for lead is generally followed. Initially, a dose of 10 mg/kg every 8 hours for 5 days is administered. The interval is then decreased to every 12 hours and continued for 14 days. Repeated courses of therapy are recommended if symptoms persist and levels remain elevated. A 2-week "drug holiday" between courses is recommended. D-Penicillamine can be used as an alternative in those patients unable to take DMSA. Penicillamine is administered at 100 mg/kg/day, up to a maximum of 2 g daily in four divided doses. In critically ill patients, combined therapy with dimercaprol and D-penicillamine should be considered, as the manufacturer of DMSA does not currently recommend simultaneous use with dimercaprol. Dimercaprol should also be used in patients with gastrointestinal symptoms. Dimercaprol is administered in doses of 3 to 5 mg/kg intramuscularly every 4 to 12 hours, depending on severity of symptoms. Therapy with dimercaprol and D-penicillamine is continued for a 5-day course. This treatment is followed by a 2-day drug holiday during which the need for further chelation is assessed. Subsequent 5-day courses of dimercaprol and/or D-penicillamine therapy are administered as needed. Dimercaprol should be discontinued once oral therapy is tolerated or serious symptoms have diminished. Chelation therapy may be terminated once urinary arsenic levels fall to less than 50 μg per 24-hour collection.[73] Maintenance dosing for dimercaprol and penicillamine should be decreased in the presence of renal failure. Chelation therapy does not have a significant effect on encephalopathy or neuropathy even if started soon after exposure.[60,74] In light of the enhanced efficacy of DMSA over D-penicillamine and its improved safety profile, DMSA should be considered the agent of choice when oral chelation therapy is indicated for arsenic poisoning.

Continuous cardiac monitoring is recommended for all symptomatic patients and arrhythmias is treated with standard agents. Since arsenic prolongs the QT interval, type 1a anti-arrhythmic agents should be avoided. In patients with renal failure, hemodialysis should be performed because arsenic and chelated arsenic are primarily eliminated by the kidney. Dialysis is of questionable benefit in those with normal kidney function.

ANNOTATED REFERENCES

Baselt RC: Disposition of Toxic Drugs and Chemicals in Man, 5th ed. Forest City, CA, Chemical Toxicology Institute, 2000.
> Entries for 482 drugs and chemicals in alphabetical order. Includes pharmacokinetic data and descriptions of occurrence and usage, blood concentrations, metabolism and excretion, toxicity, and analysis. Toxicology section contains concentrations found in various body fluids and tissues reported from fatal poisonings.

Nash D, Magder L, Lustberg M, et al: Blood lead blood pressure, and hypertension in perimenopausal and postmenopausal women. JAMA 2003;289:1523-1532.
> Article examines relationship of blood lead level with blood pressure and hypertension prevalence in a population-based sample of perimenopausal and postemopausal women in the United States.

HSDB: Hazardous Substances Data Bank. Bethesda, MD, National Library of Medicine, National Toxicology Program, 1992.
> Over 4600 records on potentially hazardous chemicals.

Nemery B: Metal toxicity and the respiratory tract. Eur Resp J 1990;3: 202-219.
> Good review of lung disease caused by metal compounds. Looks at occupational exposure to toxic agents.

Donofrio PD, Wilbourn AJ, Albers JW, et al: Acute arsenic intoxication presenting as Guillain-Barre-like syndrome. Muscle Nerve 1987;10:114-120.
> Case report of four patients with subacute onset progressive polyradiculoneuropathy following high-dose arsenic poisoning.

Chapter 195

HYDROCARBONS

F. Kay Seymour • John A. Henry

KEY POINTS

1. **Hydrocarbons** are composed of hydrogen and carbon, although other elements may be included that can markedly alter their properties. Their molecular size varies widely, mainly because of the carbon chain length.

2. Hydrocarbon uses and consequently their **potential for human exposure** range widely. Most cases of toxicity now occur in developing countries.

3. Their **potential for toxicity** varies widely, depending on their physical and chemical properties, in particular their volatility and viscosity. The use of additives rarely affects the toxicity of the final product.

4. Management of toxicity benefits from simplified guidelines that consider the product by its type; management in most cases is symptomatic.

5. **Ingestion often causes little toxicity**, unless pulmonary aspiration occurs. Aspiration can lead to an acute pneumonitis, which may be self-limited, but which may require ventilatory support. The use of corticosteroids in such cases is controversial.

6. After **acute exposure**, other major medical problems can result from systemic absorption; these include central nervous system depression and renal failure.

7. **Local effects** of hydrocarbon toxicity depend on the part of the body exposed but include cutaneous and ocular irritation and gastrointestinal disturbance.

8. **Abuse of hydrocarbons** (including adhesives and gasoline) can lead to loss of consciousness, cardiac arrhythmias, and cerebral damage.

9. **Chronic exposure to hydrocarbons** (notably hexane) can lead to neuropathy, and benzene is considered a human carcinogen. Improved industrial safety measures have made chronic complications a rarity.

Hydrocarbon ingestion is a common form of toxic exposure. Most cases involve children younger than 5 years of age who are attracted to liquid hydrocarbon products with attractive colors or odors. These products are often inappropriately stored in the home, sometimes in beverage bottles, and may be mistakenly ingested by a child who is unaware of the contents. Severe toxicity is unusual.

Industrial workers may be exposed to toxic amounts of hydrocarbons by inhalation, either acutely as a result of an industrial accident, or chronically. Local and systemic effects of exposure to hydrocarbons are reviewed in this chapter, as are immediate assessment and recommended management of acute exposure to petroleum products.

This chapter deals with the acute toxicity of hydrocarbons encountered in the public domain. Hydrocarbons find their way into most people's lives, refined or derivatized as a variety of fuels, lubricants, household and industrial products, medicines, and plastics. Exposure to hydrocarbons results mostly from product use but may occasionally occur because of accidents and failures during manufacture, transportation, use, and disposal. The most important clinical problems are the central nervous system (CNS) depressant effect of volatile hydrocarbons and pulmonary aspiration of low-viscosity products. Prolonged exposure to high concentrations of hydrocarbons by inhalation can cause CNS deterioration. Cutaneous sensitization and irritation are unusual. Defatting of skin can be a problem in chronic exposure situations if good handling practices are not enforced. This chapter concentrates on the medical assessment and management of incidents involving acute exposure.

INFORMATION SOURCES AND RESOURCES

Much of the literature on acute hydrocarbon toxicity dates back to the 1970s, when exposure was more common than now. Since that time, improved safety and preventive measures have markedly reduced the number of cases of severe exposure. This is also apparent from a consideration of the world literature on the topic, which is largely limited to individual case reports.

Poison control centers maintain databases detailing the composition, toxicity, and action to be taken in case of exposure.[1] Hydrocarbon products are manufactured to a performance specification, not a chemical one. Hence, the chemical composition of any product type is generally variable as well as extremely complex (e.g., a gasoline fuel oil typically contains more than 100 different chemicals). Knowledge of the precise chemical composition of petroleum products is of minimal value in the treatment of poisoning. More important are details of the physiologically active ingredients, which determine the likely toxicity and clinical management.[2-4]

Such information is available through an internationally recognized nomenclature system used on additive labels and data sheets; these are the major means of providing information for users and health professionals, respectively.

TABLE 195–1. HYDROCARBONS AND THEIR CHARACTERISTICS

Substance	Synonyms	Uses	Composition/Viscosity
Petrol	Petroleum spirit; gasoline; naphtha	Motor fuel	C4/C12 mixed hydrocarbons and alcohols, SSU <35
Paraffin	Kerosene; barbecue lighter fluid; jet fuel; lamp oil; no. 1 fuel oil	Heating/cooking fuel	C9/C16 paraffinic hydrocarbons, SSU <35
Diesel fuel/gas oil	Automotive gas oil; DERV; domestic fuel oil; heating oil; industrial gas oil; marine diesel; no. 2 and no. 4 fuel oil	Fuel; industrial solvent	C11/C25 mixed hydrocarbons, SSU <60
Lubricating oil	Various branded engine oils and light oils for domestic use	General and specific lubrication	C15/C50 mixed hydrocarbons and additives, SSU >100
Fuel oil	Light/medium/heavy fuel oil; marine fuel oil; no. 6 fuel oil; Black Oil; residual fuel	Industrial and marine engines; industrial heating plants; power generation	Very complex mixtures of hydrocarbons from about C20 upward, SSU 60-6000

SSU, Saybolt Seconds Universal (a common measure of viscosity, in efflux time in seconds).

This system, which has been in use for about 20 years, is fully documented in the TOMES Plus INFOTEXT Information System published by MICROMEDEX, Inc., and held by poison control centers around the world.

PHYSIOLOGICALLY ACTIVE CONSTITUENTS

Consideration of any hydrocarbon product should include the two main groups of constituents: the hydrocarbon fraction and the additives. With the exception of tetraethyl lead and tetramethyl lead, which are no longer allowed as fuel additives in most countries, additives are unlikely to affect the clinical features of hydrocarbon toxicity.

HYDROCARBONS

Hydrocarbons may be considered as aliphatic hydrocarbons, halogenated hydrocarbons, aromatic hydrocarbons, and terpenes. Their toxic properties depend largely on their volatility and viscosity (Table 195-1).

Volatility describes the tendency of a liquid to vaporize. Generally speaking, the lower the molecular weight and the higher the degree of unsaturation or aromaticity, the greater the volatility. Some hydrocarbons are gaseous at ambient temperatures. The more volatile hydrocarbons are more lipid-soluble and therefore more readily absorbed by inhalation or ingestion. They also more readily enter the CNS and other target organs.

Viscosity is the resistance offered by a fluid to flow. It is also an indirect measure of molecular size. It is the single most important physical property influencing the risk of aspiration associated with a liquid. The viscosity of a substance determines not only the likelihood of its entry into the trachea but also the rate and extent of its penetration into the terminal bronchioles and alveoli and, hence, its ability to cause damage to the respiratory system. The lower the viscosity, the greater the risk of pulmonary aspiration.

The gaseous short-chained aliphatic hydrocarbons (methane, ethane, propane, and butane) tend to act as simple asphyxiants. Their presence in the respiratory tract displaces air, which causes hypoxia by lowering the partial pressure of oxygen. Halogenated aliphatic hydrocarbons have at least one hydrogen atom replaced by a halogen atom (bromine, chlorine, fluorine or iodine). The high volatility of these substances means that they are readily inhaled, either accidentally

or as drugs of abuse. Inhalation is their main route of toxicity. Aromatic hydrocarbons (containing one or more benzene rings) are found in many household products. Toluene and xylene, in particular, are commonly abused, because they produce euphoria when inhaled. These agents cause adverse metabolic, CNS, renal, and cardiovascular effects. The fourth group of hydrocarbons are the terpenes, a class of unsaturated, nonaromatic cyclic hydrocarbons that includes pine oil and turpentine. The terpenes are less volatile than other hydrocarbons, and the route of toxicity is more likely to be gastrointestinal absorption than inhalation. The differences in volatility and viscosity among hydrocarbons lead to clear differences in types of exposure and potential for toxicity.

Routes of Exposure and Toxicity
Hydrocarbons with High Volatility and Minimal Viscosity
Simple gases (e.g., methane, ethane, propane, butane, pentane) and light aromatic hydrocarbons (e.g., benzene, toluene) are examples of hydrocarbons with high volatility and minimal viscosity. Inhalation of the simple gases can replace alveolar gas, causing hypoxia. The light aromatic hydrocarbons can easily cross the alveolar-capillary membrane and cause CNS symptoms. The lung is spared injury, but cardiotoxic effects have been reported. Gastrointestinal absorption can be significant.

Hydrocarbons such as toluene and xylene are sometimes used as solvents in pesticides, which are widely available, especially in developing countries. Usually most of the toxicity is caused by the pesticide, but the solvents can be associated with substantial toxicity as well (Table 195-2).

Hydrocarbons with Intermediate Volatility and Low Viscosity
Examples of hydrocarbons with intermediate volatility and low viscosity include gasoline (petrol), naphtha, and hydrocarbon solvents. The primary problem from these agents is pulmonary aspiration. However, they may cause euphoria and CNS depression when inhaled. Effects from gastrointestinal absorption are not significant.

Hydrocarbons with Low Volatility and Low Viscosity
Hydrocarbons with low volatility and low viscosity include diesel and heating oils. The main problem associated with these compounds is aspiration pneumonia. Gastrointestinal absorption is minimal.

TABLE 195–2. PHYSIOLOGIC SYSTEMS AFFECTED BY TOXICITY OF VARIOUS CLASSES OF HYDROCARBONS

Class	Examples	Physiologic system affected
High volatility, minimal viscosity	Simple gases, light aromatic hydrocarbons	Pulmonary—asphyxiation Central nervous system Cardiovascular Gastrointestinal
Intermediate volatility, low viscosity	Gasoline (petrol), naphtha, hydrocarbon solvents	Pulmonary—aspiration Central nervous system
Low volatility, low viscosity	Diesel oil, heating oil	Pulmonary—aspiration
Minimal volatility, high viscosity	Lubricating oils, mineral oil, bitumen	Pulmonary—pneumonia

Hydrocarbons with Minimal Volatility and High Viscosity

Examples of hydrocarbons with minimal volatility and high viscosity include lubricating oils, mineral oil, and bitumen. These materials are highly viscous and are essentially nontoxic but can cause lipoid pneumonia in cases of direct aspiration into the lungs. This form of pneumonia is more localized and less inflammatory than that produced by products with lower viscosity.[5,6]

Local and Systemic Effects of Hydrocarbons

Local effects depend on the part of the body exposed and the duration of exposure, whereas systemic effects relate both to the amount absorbed and to the degree of pulmonary or other organ toxicity caused.

Local Effects

Cutaneous injury appears to be a result of irritant effects and the ability of hydrocarbons to dissolve fat. It is mainly caused by the removal of fat within the layers of the skin—hence the term "defatting." Dehydration of the skin probably also contributes to the damage. The depth of injury is related to the duration of exposure and the concentration of the agent; most commonly, the damage is superficial. The affected area may be erythematous, and blistering may occur. A severe burn appears red and raw, often with a margin of dead skin at the edges. Cutaneous absorption of petroleum products may occur, and systemic toxicity from this route is possible, but with acute exposures its clinical significance is probably negligible.[7]

Ocular exposure usually causes little or no injury, although there may be considerable stinging and discomfort. Photophobia, redness, and transient corneal irritation may be present.

Pulmonary pathology results most commonly from aspiration into the bronchial tree of hydrocarbons with low viscosity. Aspirated hydrocarbons disrupt surfactant and the bronchial epithelial cell barrier, leading to alveolar instability, early distal airway closure, ventilation/perfusion mismatching, and, subsequently, hypoxemia.[8] Initially, cyanosis may result from replacement of oxygen by vaporized hydrocarbons; subsequent hypoxemia is caused by surfactant loss and direct alveolar injury. Bronchospasm may contribute to ventilation/perfusion mismatches.

Gastrointestinal symptoms, although unpleasant, are usually only transient and result from local irritation of the pharynx, esophagus, stomach, and small intestine. Patients may experience symptoms such as nausea, vomiting, and diarrhea. Small areas of fatty infiltration and congestion of the liver have been described, and a single fatality from hepatic failure has been reported in an abuser of butane aerosols.[9]

Systemic Effects

The CNS toxicity occasionally observed after hydrocarbon exposure appears to be indirect and secondary to pulmonary involvement. Experiments using paraffin in baboons suggest that the primate brain is resistant to the direct effects of kerosene and that the most potent cause of CNS damage is hypoxia secondary to pneumonitis.[10] This concept was supported by a large, retrospective study of cases of poisoning in children. The development of neurologic complications correlated with severe pulmonary involvement only. It seems likely, therefore, that CNS complications are mainly caused by hypoxia secondary to pulmonary involvement, rather than a direct neurotoxic effect.[11] Neurologic abnormalities include behavioral changes, movement disorders (resting and action tremor, myoclonus, chorea, ataxia), pyramidal signs, and seizures. In acute cases in which large doses of organic solvents were inhaled, an acute narcotizing response is thought to occur.[12] However, the situation of chronic exposure is less clear. A detailed analysis of 30 cases of presumed toxic encephalopathy found either lack of demonstrable neurologic abnormalities or alternative explanations in all patients.[13]

Cardiac manifestations of hydrocarbons are thought to be responsible for numerous reports of sudden death with abuse by inhalation. The mechanism responsible for the development of dysrhythmias is believed to be sensitization of the myocardium to endogenous catecholamines, often aggravated by hypoxemia due to displacement of oxygen or respiratory depression.

Glomerulonephritis, renal tubular acidosis, and chronic tubulointerstitial nephritis all have been associated with long-term hydrocarbon exposure. Intravascular hemolysis after aspiration of gasoline has been reported in a small number of cases, possibly due to damage to the red blood cell membrane and induction of lipolysis by lipid solubilization.[14] Gasoline also contains a small amount of benzene (less than 1%), which is a human carcinogen (Table 195-3).

ADDITIVES

Fuel products and lubricants contain a wide range of additives and other chemicals. However, apart from lubricants, these chemicals are generally used at such low concentrations that they have no impact on the toxicity of the finished products. Finished lubricants may contain as much as 15% to 20% additives, but most of these are not classified as dangerous or are used at such low concentrations that toxicity is not significantly affected. The additives themselves are commonly manufactured in or diluted with oil products of various kinds, and these may affect the way the additive is classified and labeled. Additives that contain a significant proportion

TABLE 195–3. EFFECTS OF HYDROCARBONS ON BODY SYSTEMS AND FUNCTION

System or function	Effect
Central nervous system	Anesthetic effect—central nervous system depression
	Asphyxiant effect (e.g. petrol vapor)
	Secondary to aspiration and pulmonary hypoxia
Peripheral nervous system	Peripheral neuropathy (u-hexane)
Pulmonary	Aspiration pneumonitis
Cardiovascular	Cardiac sensitization
Renal	Acute tubular necrosis
Hepatic	Fatty infiltration
Hematologic	Acute leukemia
	Aplastic anemia
Cutaneous	Defatting
	Burns
Biochemical	Metabolic acidosis
	Respiratory acidosis
Other effects	Hydrocarbon exposure rarely affects other body systems (endocrine, gastrointestinal, ophthalmic) to cause severe dysfunction
	Burns
	Trauma

of a base oil, if ingested, cause some irritation of the digestive tract and associated symptoms (nausea, vomiting, and diarrhea). If vomiting occurs with additives that contain a sufficient level of a low-viscosity oil product, there is a danger of aspiration into the lungs, causing chemical pneumonitis. A more detailed discussion of additives and their toxicity can be found elsewhere.[15]

DIAGNOSIS AND ASSESSMENT

TRIAGE

Petroleum product toxicity can occur in many ways, from accidental exposure in children to industrial accidents. There are various ways in which these products cause toxicity. Most patients who have ingested hydrocarbons and are asymptomatic may be cared for at home, provided someone responsible is able to observe them. There must be no history of specific toxic components involved, which is generally the case with most commercially available products (e.g., fuels, solvents, cleaning agents). The patient must have rapid access to a hospital in case delayed symptoms develop.

All patients who have had symptoms suggestive of aspiration (choking, coughing, gagging) should be assessed in the emergency department. By the time they come to medical care, most are asymptomatic. Asymptomatic patients should have a chest radiograph and be observed for 6 hours. They can usually be discharged if no abnormality develops.

The main indications for admission are as follows:

- Respiratory signs or symptoms, fever, or lethargy. These usually appear soon after ingestion.
- Ingestion of systemically absorbed substances. Patients should be observed for signs of CNS toxicity.
- Suicide attempt, which requires psychiatric assessment.
- Ingestion as a presenting feature of child abuse. Although this is very uncommon, the diagnosis is not to be missed and should always be considered in any child who presents with a toxic ingestion.

HISTORY

A detailed history must be obtained from the patient or, if necessary, from witnesses. In childhood poisonings, it is often difficult to know whether the patient has ingested the suspected substance or not. Typically, the key information required is the following:

- Age of patient.
- Substances involved or suspected. The container with its label should be brought with the patient. A sample of the product usually is not required, because there is little need to analyze the substance, and in any case this can be done only by a specialized laboratory. However, if the offending item has been stored in an inappropriate container, an informed guess as to the contents can be made.
- Time of exposure and duration of exposure.
- Mode of exposure—ingestion, inhalation, dermal or ocular contact.
- Whether the patient has vomited or had any other symptoms.
- Whether the patient has taken alcohol or other drugs that might affect the clinical presentation.
- Past medical history and current drug treatment.

IMMEDIATE MANAGEMENT

AIRWAY, BREATHING, CIRCULATION

The "ABCs" are first attended to. A clinical history and assessment are made. Fluid administration should be aimed at replacement of losses while taking care to avoid precipitating pulmonary edema by excessive hydration.

RESPIRATORY ASSESSMENT

A patent airway is the first priority. If there is evidence of respiratory involvement, a high inspired oxygen concentration should be provided, and nebulized bronchodilators may be used with caution, if bronchospasm is severe (see later discussion). The next consideration is to decide whether the patient requires mechanical ventilation. Signs of respiratory distress, such as cyanosis, use of accessory muscles, and rate and depth of respiration, should be noted. If there is any doubt, the oxygen saturation and minute volume should be measured. If the minute volume is less than 4 L/min in an adult, endotracheal intubation and mechanical ventilation are likely to be required. Auscultation may demonstrate crepitations or crackles (75% of cases), wheezing, and diminished breath sounds, but abnormal findings may be absent. Lower airway involvement may be present despite a normal chest examination. A typical hydrocarbon odor is often detected, but this finding is not a reliable indicator of significant ingestion or aspiration.

Most patients become symptomatic within 30 minutes after ingestion. Almost immediately after aspiration, there are signs of tracheobronchial irritation, manifested as coughing and choking. These signs may be transient due to the initial volatilization of the petroleum distillates. Aspiration into the lungs is indicated by gasping and more prolonged coughing. Arterial blood gases should be measured in the clinically ill patient. Patients who present with significant respiratory compromise need an urgent chest radiograph, whereas patients with minimal symptoms should be reassessed over a 6-hour period to determine whether radiography is indicated.

Signs and symptoms may progress over the first 24 hours. Initially, most patients with significant exposure become hypocapnic from hyperventilation. Nasal flaring, intercostal retraction, dyspnea, tachypnea, and varying degrees of cyanosis may follow. In severe cases, pulmonary edema and hemoptysis or pink, frothy sputum may be evident, later followed by the development of shock and cardiorespiratory arrest. If death is to occur, it usually does so within the first 24 hours.[16] Otherwise, pulmonary symptoms plateau in about 48 hours, and complete resolution occurs in 3 to 5 days. Derangement of normal pulmonary surfactant properties by aspirated hydrocarbons has led to the suggestion that early use of continuous positive airway pressure (CPAP) or positive end-expiratory pressure (PEEP) may be beneficial. Treatment should be considered for children with severe pulmonary complications. Studies have shown that treatment decreases barotrauma, air leaks, and morbidity. Extracorporeal membrane oxygenation (ECMO) has been used occasionally to oxygenate the patient's blood while allowing lung tissue to heal. ECMO consists of a modified cardiac bypass procedure but does not require that the chest be opened.[17]

Intravenous exposure, although rare, usually causes a chemical pneumonitis, occasionally hemorrhagic in nature.

CARDIOVASCULAR ASSESSMENT

Pulse rate and blood pressure should be recorded and intravenous access secured. Patients with more than mild symptoms should be monitored with pulse oximetry and have an electrocardiogram performed. Myocardial involvement is rare after acute hydrocarbon ingestion. However, dysrhythmias can occur during solvent abuse. The mechanism is believed to be a result of hydrocarbon-mediated sensitization of the myocardium to endogenous catecholamines.[18] Sudden death has been reported, especially with abuse of chlorinated and fluorinated hydrocarbons.[19,20]

SKIN AND EYE ASSESSMENT

After spillages involving skin contact, contaminated clothing should be removed and the affected area washed with soap and plenty of water.

Accurate assessment of the burn surface area and proper fluid management may be required. Contact with petroleum distillates can cause a variety of skin manifestations, ranging from mild erythema to full-thickness skin loss. Features of eczematous dermatitis, such as redness, itching and inflammation, may be seen. A clinical picture resembling toxic epidermal necrolysis with areas of bullae and denuded skin has been described. Compared with thermal and other chemical burns, the latency period before signs and symptoms occur may be longer.

Subcutaneous injection of hydrocarbons may lead to cellulitis and abscess formation. Initial treatment consists of cleansing the wound area, tetanus prophylaxis and use of radiography or ultrasonography to determine the location of material. High-pressure injection injuries (e.g., from pinhole leaks in high-pressure hydraulic equipment) require particular attention, although initially there may be no signs or symptoms. Significant swelling and pain can develop within a few hours. Sterile abscess formation, ischemia, and chronic bone and connective tissue injuries occur.[21-23] Surgical débridement and irrigation is the recommended treatment for any significant high-pressure injection injury. Further discussion of this topic is beyond the scope of this text.

In the case of ocular exposure to volatile substances, it is more appropriate to hold the lids open, allowing the substance to evaporate, than to wash out the eye with water. Ocular exposure generally causes little or no injury, provided there are no abrasions. Considerable discomfort, photophobia, redness, and transient corneal irritation may be present, but these symptoms resolve with conservative management.

GASTROINTESTINAL ASSESSMENT AND DECONTAMINATION

Gastrointestinal symptoms after hydrocarbon ingestion are common but usually are minor. Turpentine is particularly associated with such symptoms. There may be local irritation of the mouth and pharynx. In more severe cases, hydrocarbons can cause nausea, vomiting, abdominal pain, and distention. Diarrhea, hematemesis, and melena are rare.

The ability of hydrocarbons to produce spontaneous vomiting is associated with a high risk for development of aspiration pneumonitis. Any vomit produced should be inspected for evidence of ingestion, and a 20-mL sample should be saved in a universal container.

The traditional methods of gastrointestinal decontamination have been closely reviewed recently, leading to the production of position statements from the American and European toxicology associations.[24,25] However, these statements are of little use in the management of hydrocarbon ingestion, because of the paucity of data and the special properties of hydrocarbons. In general, the risk of aspiration posed by gastric emptying outweighs any potential benefit. The situation may be briefly reviewed as follows:

- Emesis—Although syrup of ipecacuanha is the only substance now available for inducing emesis, it is contraindicated after ingestion of volatile hydrocarbons, because emesis may increase the risk of pulmonary aspiration.
- Gastric lavage—Gastric lavage can be carried out only after endotracheal intubation to protect against aspiration. This requirement reduces its use in practical terms to the patient who is already extremely ill or unconscious after massive hydrocarbon ingestion.
- Activated charcoal—Activated charcoal does not effectively adsorb petroleum distillates, and it may increase the risk of aspiration. However, it may be needed to adsorb a toxic substance (e.g., a pesticide) that is formulated in a petroleum base.
- Catharsis—Cathartics are contraindicated in all toxic ingestions.
- Whole bowel irrigation—There is currently no evidence that whole bowel irrigation is of benefit after the ingestion of hydrocarbons.

NEUROLOGIC ASSESSMENT

Studies show that gastrointestinal absorption of hydrocarbons does not produce pulmonary pathology or major CNS toxicity. However, inhalation of hydrocarbons may be associated with signs of CNS toxicity. This phenomenon may occur as a direct effect on the CNS or secondary to hypoxia.[10,11] Hydrocarbon exposure results in CNS depression;

somnolence, dizziness, and hyporeflexia are common. It is very unusual for convulsions and coma to occur. Unlike the aliphatic hydrocarbons, systemically absorbed aromatic and halogenated compounds can have marked initial excitatory effects leading to euphoria, agitation, delirium, hyperreflexia, and seizures. If consciousness is impaired, the conscious level should be recorded with the use of a coma grading system such as the Glasgow Coma Scale. If altered mental status might also be due to alcohol or drug misuse, patients should receive naloxone, glucose, and thiamine, as appropriate.

OTHER ORGAN SYSTEMS

Transient hepatosplenomegaly and renal and hematologic abnormalities may occur, depending on the exposure and the substance.[26,27] Because petroleum distillates are used as the base for organophosphate preparations, the breath odor of a volatile substance may mask the true diagnosis. A cholinergic crisis must be considered if symptoms such as profuse salivation, lacrimation, diarrhea, bronchorrhea, cramps, miosis, and urinary incontinence are present.

INVESTIGATIONS

In straightforward cases of hydrocarbon exposure, there usually is no point in routinely ordering such tests as full blood count, urea and electrolytes, liver function tests, chest radiograph, and electrocardiogram.[19] However, if the patient is ill enough to require admission to the hospital, a small number of baseline tests are indicated, because deterioration may occur. In addition to continuous monitoring of oxygen saturation, arterial blood gases must be monitored in all patients with respiratory symptoms. Varying degrees of hypoxia without hypercapnia are the most common findings. Occasionally, metabolic acidosis is seen (e.g., in cases of toluene poisoning). The complete blood count may show leukocytosis with left shift, a relatively early finding that can persist for several days. Serum electrolyte concentrations, coagulation studies, urinalysis, and renal and liver function tests are usually abnormal only in cases of chronic exposure.

Measurement of the blood hydrocarbon levels has no place in acute diagnosis or management and is of little value except for forensic, medicolegal, or research purposes. However, it is normal practice to save an anticoagulated blood sample and a urine sample on admission, in case analysis should subsequently be necessary.

Chest radiographic abnormalities correlate poorly with clinical symptoms and may be abnormal in patients who are asymptomatic.[16] Between 70% and 75% of patients hospitalized with suspected hydrocarbon aspiration have chest radiographic signs. Abnormalities may start to appear within 30 minutes, but they more commonly appear later, and they may not develop for up to 24 hours after exposure.[28] The most commonly seen abnormalities are increased bronchovascular markings and bilateral basal shadowing. Upper lobe signs are uncommon. Infiltrates usually reach their maximum in 3 to 4 days and clear within 2 weeks after onset. Other rare findings include pleural effusion, pneumothorax, and pneumomediastinum.[29]

DRUG TREATMENT

CORTICOSTEROIDS

The evidence suggests that corticosteroids are ineffective in altering the acute course of hydrocarbon pneumonitis.[30,31]

Although a single report of a late-treated case suggests that high-dose corticosteroids may produce resolution of lung damage, the evidence from animal studies of combined steroid and antibiotic therapy has not demonstrated any beneficial effect.[32,33] Indeed, corticosteroid-mediated suppression of the immune response may promote bacterial colonization. There is no evidence that bacteria play a role in the pathogenesis of chemical pneumonitis.[34]

SUPERINFECTION

Bacterial superinfection may be difficult to diagnose. Fever and leukocytosis are common in uncomplicated hydrocarbon pneumonitis, and bacterial superinfection is therefore a microbiologic diagnosis. However, despite this diagnostic difficulty, prophylactic antibiotics should not be prescribed routinely.

BRONCHODILATORS

Bronchospasm can exacerbate respiratory distress, and it is tempting to give bronchodilators to wheezy patients, but they should be used with caution. A sympathomimetic agent, such as salbutamol, may be used if there is a decrease in forced expiratory volume, because the risk of precipitating dysrhythmias with this drug is negligible. Epinephrine should be avoided because of the potential risk of myocardial sensitization to catecholamines.

LONG-TERM EFFECTS

Full recovery is the normal outcome of hydrocarbon poisoning. Some researchers have suggested that minor abnormalities of pulmonary function can persist, but their clinical significance is not clear.[35,36]

CHRONIC EXPOSURE AND CARCINOGENICITY

Benzene is a human carcinogen. Acute myelocytic and monocytic leukemias have been reported with chronic benzene exposure, as have lymphoproliferative disorders.[37] Chemicals containing straight chains of six carbon atoms (e.g., n-hexane, methyl-n-butyl-ketone) are also known for their potential to cause peripheral neuropathy. Toluene inhalation over long periods has been associated with renal tubular acidosis and peripheral sensorimotor neuropathy. Discussion of chronic toxicity and carcinogenicity are outside the scope of this chapter, but reviews are available.[38]

PREVENTION

Hydrocarbon products used in the domestic environment are still frequently stored in homes and garages in unmarked containers or beverage bottles. They also may have attractive aromas and be brightly colored. It is not surprising, therefore, that most cases of exposure in the home involve accidental ingestions by young children. Although education in schools is beneficial, a large proportion of childhood poisonings occur in the pre–school-age group. Children younger than 6 years of age accounted for more than 50% of all exposures reported to poison control centers in the United States in 1996, and 2.4% of pediatric poisonings involved hydrocarbons.[39] Parents should be educated to keep potentially toxic materials out of the reach of children. Familiar bottles or containers should never be used for the storage of these products. The companies that supply the domestic market with small quantities of products also have a role to play in developing suitable packaging and labeling of their products. The introduction of child-resistant containers, often required by law, has raised public expectation of suitably safe packaging and presentation, not only of medicines but also of all household and do-it-yourself products. Although steps can be taken to prevent the accidental ingestion of hydrocarbon products by children, a different approach is required against the deliberate inhalational abuse of hydrocarbons, which occurs typically in adolescents.[40,41]

As a result of increasing awareness and the gradual development of regulatory controls, industrial poisoning is rare nowadays. The precautions recommended to minimize adverse health effects are all aimed at limiting exposure. The onus is on both the manufacturer and the user to assess risks and implement workplace standards. Fuels are normally stored and handled in systems that, for the most part, are "closed." Hence, most of the time, exposure and any risk of adverse effects are minimized. However, during certain operations, such as loading or unloading or the maintenance of storage tanks, it is appropriate to take special care to avoid skin contact and excessive inhalation of vapor.

CONCLUSION

Every clinician needs a basic awareness of the presentation and management of acute exposure to petroleum products, especially because the clinical presentation can be acute, requiring urgent action. Once the initial emergency has been dealt with, there are a large number of reliable information sources that can be consulted to provide data on the composition of products and the clinical features and management of individual problems. Much of this information is based on a general knowledge of the chemical properties and potential toxicity of the substance concerned, because the literature is relatively sparse. The paucity of clinical experience

also shows that preventive measures have been increasingly successful. Petroleum products should form a decreasing proportion of the workload of emergency physicians and intensivists, but preparedness is needed for the cases that will still inevitably occur.

ANNOTATED REFERENCES

Anas N, Namasonthi V, Ginsburg CM: Criteria for hospitalising children who have ingested products containing hydrocarbons. JAMA 1981;246:840-843.
This retrospective study reviewed the records of 950 children who ingested products containing hydrocarbons. Only seven children experienced pulmonary complications, all of whom had radiographic evidence of pneumonia and were symptomatic at the time of exposure.

Brent J: Solvent encephalopathy: A critical appraisal (Abstract). J Toxicol Clin Toxicol 2003;41:389-390.
Inhalation of large doses of organic solvents causes an acute narcotizing effect similar to that of general anesthetics. Chronic encephalopathy has been well described with long-term toluene abuse, but it is uncommon with other hydrocarbons.

Majeed HA, Bassyouni H, Kalaawt M, et al: Kerosene poisoning in children: A clinico-radiological study of 205 cases. Ann Trop Paediatr 1981;1:123-130.
This retrospective study reviewed the records of 205 children with kerosene poisoning who were admitted to a pediatrics department over a 4-year period. There was a strong relationship between the severity of pulmonary involvement and the development of neurologic complications, indicating that hypoxia secondary to pulmonary involvement is the main cause of CNS complications.

Schoo MJ, Scott FA, Boswick JA Jr: High-pressure injection injuries of the hand. J Trauma 1980;20:229-238.
This case series and review of 132 case reports of high-pressure injection injuries confirmed that early surgical débridement of the injected part is crucial to prevent necrosis and subsequent fibrosis of the affected area. Early use of steroids and appropriate antibiotics prevents the development of severe infection.

Steele RW, Conklin RH, Mark HM: Corticosteroids and antibiotics for the treatment of fulminant hydrocarbon aspiration. JAMA 1972;2119:1434-1437.
An early but important study in which 20 mongrel dogs were given a median lethal dose of kerosene intratracheally. They were treated with either corticosteroids (dexamethasone phosphate) plus antibiotics or placebo. There were four deaths in the treated group and five in the control group, with no differences in any of the parameters measured between the survivors. This suggests that steroid therapy does not make a difference in outcome following hydrocarbon aspiration.

Chapter 196

LITHIUM

Rasheed A. Balogun • Mark D. Okusa

KEY POINTS

1. Lithium is used widely in the treatment of bipolar disorder and other conditions. Cases of lithium intoxication are common because of the narrow therapeutic index of the drug and various other factors that increase risk of toxicity. **Lithium toxicity can occur even when the drug is used as prescribed.**

2. In adults, a typical dose is 900 to 1800 mg/day in three to four divided doses. The time to peak plasma level is 2 to 4 hours after ingestion, and excretion is primarily renal (excreted unchanged in urine). The therapeutic level of lithium is 0.7 to 1.2 mEq/L, and the toxic level is greater than 1.5 mEq/L (**narrow therapeutic index**).

3. Predisposing factors leading to acute lithium intoxication include chronic kidney disease, surgery, drug interactions, dehydration, and volume depletion.

4. Patients present with **a variety of clinical manifestations, which are mainly neurologic.** Confusion, seizures, and impaired consciousness leading to coma can occur. Cerebellar manifestations include dysarthria, truncal ataxia, broad-based ataxic gait, nystagmus, and varying degrees of incoordination. Electrocardiographic changes occur frequently with lithium intoxication; examples include transient ST-segment depression and inverted T-waves in V4-6.

4. **Treatment of acute lithium intoxication depends on serum level and renal function.** The usual medical measures to support the airway and circulatory system, common to all intoxications, also apply here. For a serum **lithium level greater than 3.5 to 4 mEq/L, most patients require hemodialysis;** for patients who have levels between 2 and 4 mEq/L accompanied by clinical instability and severe neurologic signs (e.g., seizures, stupor, coma), hemodialysis is required. For those with serum lithium levels between 1.5 and 2.5 mEq/L, intravenous fluid therapy or forced diuresis treatment should be recommended only if the patient has early signs of lithium intoxication and normal renal function and it is certain that the serum lithium concentration has been elevated for only a few days and not above 2.5 mEq/L. Dialysis should be instituted in all patients if a serum lithium concentration of 1 mEq/L is not reached within 30 hours.

5. With adequate recognition and treatment, most patients can have a full recovery. Late presentation, delayed treatment, or inadequate treatment may lead to irreversible neurologic deficits or death.

Lithium, as a pharmacologic agent for the treatment of mania, was introduced by Cade in 1949.[1] Despite the frequent occurrence of lithium intoxication, this drug continues to be used. The U. S. Food and Drug Administration (FDA) approved the use of lithium for the treatment of mania in 1970 and for maintenance therapy of bipolar disorder in 1974.[2-6] Lithium is also used for other nonapproved psychiatric and nonpsychiatric disorders.[7] The incidence of lithium intoxication has been increasing, because the drug is being used more frequently and has a narrow therapeutic index. Many factors can increase the risk of toxicity even when the drug is used as prescribed. Lithium toxicity occurs in two main settings: acute ingestion of a large dose (e.g., suicide attempt) or, more commonly, chronic accumulation of the drug during prescribed maintenance therapy. The latter problem can be avoided by a thorough understanding of conditions and drug interactions that increase the risk of lithium toxicity.

Lithium intoxication causes multisystem dysfunction and irreversible neurologic deficits; it is fatal in 9% to 25% of patients.[8] Early detection and treatment are critical to improve outcomes. This chapter emphasizes the pharmacology and physiology of lithium that underlie its toxicity and provides physicians with the foundation to effectively treat lithium intoxication.

PHARMACOLOGY

Lithium is a monovalent cation and, like sodium, potassium, rubidium, and cesium, a group IA alkali metal. Lithium shares some characteristics with sodium and potassium; however, differences in ionic radii among lithium (0.60 Å), sodium (0.95 Å), and potassium (1.33 Å) are responsible for the pharmacologic effects of lithium.[9-11] For example, unlike sodium and potassium, only a small gradient for lithium can be maintained across biologic membranes.

Lithium is usually administered as lithium carbonate or, less commonly, lithium citrate. In adults, a typical dose is 900 to 1800 mg/day in three to four divided doses. Lower doses are recommended in children and the elderly. A dose of 300 mg lithium carbonate contains 8.12 mEq lithium ion. After oral administration, lithium is readily absorbed, with

TABLE 196–1. PHARMACOLOGY OF LITHIUM

Parameter	Value
Molecule	Monovalent cation; radius, 0.6 Å; weight, 7 Da
Dose (adult)	900-1800 mg/day in 3-4 doses (less in sustained-release form)
Therapeutic serum level	0.7-1.2 mEq/L
Toxic levels	>1.5 mEq/L (narrow therapeutic index)
Bioavailability	>95%
Volume of distribution	0.7-0.9 L/kg in steady state
Half-life	12-27 hr after single dose (longer with chronic therapy and in elderly patients)
Time to peak plasma level	2-4 hr after ingestion
Elimination	Primarily renal; excreted unchanged in urine

TABLE 196–2. FACTORS PREDISPOSING TO LITHIUM TOXICITY

1. Infection
2. Volume depletion
3. Gastroenteritis
4. Overdose (e.g., suicide attempt)
5. Chronic kidney disease
6. Surgery
7. Decreased "effective arterial volume"
   a. Congestive heart failure
   b. Cirrhosis
   c. Nephrosis
8. Drugs
   a. Nonsteroidal antiinflammatory drugs
   b. Diuretics
   c. Tetracycline
   d. Cyclosporine
9. Decreased dietary sodium intake
10. Anorexia

complete absorption occurring at approximately 8 hours and peak levels 2 to 4 hours after ingestion.[12] Lithium is not protein bound; it distributes freely in total body water and accumulates in various tissues, with the exception of cerebrospinal fluid. In the steady state, the volume of distribution for lithium is 0.7 to 0.9 L/kg (Table 196-1). Lithium concentration in cerebrospinal fluid is 40% of the plasma level[13] as a result of transport of lithium out of the cerebrospinal fluid by brain capillary endothelium, arachnoid membrane, or both.[14]

The therapeutic level of lithium is 0.7 to 1.2 mEq/L. The toxic level is greater than 1.5 mEq/L; therefore, the drug has a very narrow therapeutic index. The plasma elimination half-life of a single dose is between 12 and 27 hours.[15-17] Elimination takes longer in the elderly; in these patients, the half-life can be as long as 36 hours.[18] Elimination half-life also varies with duration of therapy[19]; it may be considerably longer in patients treated chronically. The longer half-life is caused by intracellular accumulation and inhibition of lithium efflux after chronic lithium therapy.

Approximately 95% of a single dose of lithium is excreted unchanged in the urine; only trace amounts are found in feces.[12] Lithium is not bound to proteins and therefore is freely filtered by the glomerulus; 80% of the filtered load of lithium is reabsorbed, and 20% is excreted in the urine.[20] Renal lithium clearance in normal individuals is 10 to 40 mL/min[15,16,20]; the fractional lithium clearance is estimated to be 0.17 to 0.29.[16,20,21]

Because lithium clearance is proportional to the glomerular filtration rate (GFR), factors affecting the GFR have significant influence on the clearance of lithium. Substantial reductions in lithium dosage must be made in patients with chronic kidney disease. Furthermore, alterations in the proximal reabsorption of lithium can alter the fractional excretion of lithium without significantly affecting GFR. This characteristic of renal lithium handling has important therapeutic implications. Drugs known to inhibit proximal reabsorption of lithium may increase the fractional excretion of lithium and thereby increase lithium removal. Diuretics that alter proximal reabsorption of sodium (e.g., acetazolamide, aminophylline, urea) increase fractional excretion of lithium,[20] whereas other diuretics (e.g., thiazides, ethacrynic acid, spironolactone) act distal to the proximal tubule and have no effect on fractional excretion of lithium.[21] These results suggest that the primary site of lithium reabsorption is in the proximal tubule.

LITHIUM TOXICITY

Patients with lithium intoxication exhibit a variety of clinical manifestations. The severity of symptoms frequently is proportional to the degree of elevation of serum lithium levels.[22] However, symptoms do not always correlate with lithium levels, because symptoms of toxicity have occurred at therapeutic levels[9,11,23-25] and minimal symptoms have resulted from high levels.[9,26] In general, however, serum lithium levels of 1.5 to 2.5 mEq/L at 12 hours after the last dose of lithium usually are accompanied by slight or moderate symptoms of intoxication, values of 2.5 to 3.5 mEq/L are to be regarded as serious, and values greater than 3.5 mEq/L are life-threatening.[9]

The patient's history often reveals associated conditions predisposing to lithium toxicity (Table 196-2). Factors that predispose to toxicity include advanced age,[27] schizophrenia, preexisting brain damage,[28] and rapid rise of serum concentration after an acute overdose. Other conditions, such as diarrhea, vomiting, inadequate fluid therapy after surgery, diuretics, and volume depletion, are associated with states of sodium depletion. Because sodium balance affects the clearance of lithium,[20,29-31] decreased dietary sodium intake[32-35] and chronic therapy with furosemide or a thiazide diuretic[30,36-41] are situations associated with lithium intoxication. These conditions often result in a vicious cycle that potentiates lithium toxicity (Figure 196-1).

A number of drugs are associated with acute lithium toxicity (Table 196-3). Lithium toxicity has been reported with the concomitant use of nonsteroidal antiinflammatory drugs (NSAIDs), including cyclooxygenase II inhibitors.[42-56] Patients with congestive heart failure and volume depletion who depend on endogenous prostaglandin synthesis to maintain renal blood flow and GFR are more susceptible to lithium toxicity when they take NSAIDs. In these patients, prostaglandin inhibition by NSAIDs can markedly reduce GFR and lithium clearance, causing significant lithium toxicity. Long-acting angiotensin-converting enzyme inhibitors[57] and angiotensin receptor blockers[58-65] decrease GFR and fractional excretion of lithium,[20] thereby predisposing patients to lithium toxicity.

CLINICAL FEATURES OF LITHIUM TOXICITY

Patients with lithium toxicity present with a variety of clinical manifestations (Table 196-4). Neurologic symptoms

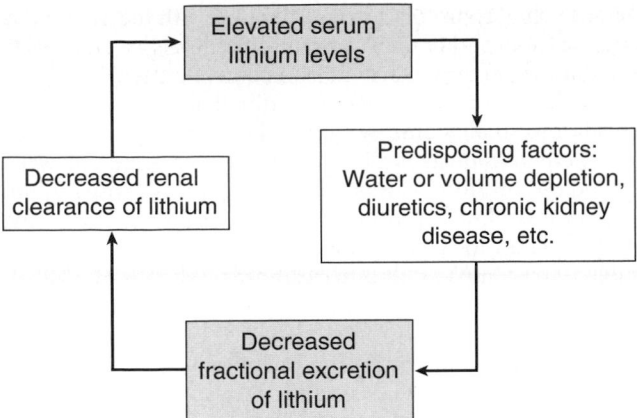

FIGURE 196–1. Vicious cycle of lithium toxicity.

TABLE 196–4. CLINICAL MANIFESTATIONS OF LITHIUM INTOXICATION

1. Central nervous system
   a. State of consciousness (confusion to coma)
   b. Cerebellar symptoms
      1. Dysarthria
      2. Ataxia
      3. Nystagmus
      4. Tremor
   c. Basal ganglia
      1. Choreiform movements
      2. Parkinson-like movements
   d. Seizures
   e. Death
2. Gastrointestinal
   a. Nausea/vomiting
   b. Bloating
3. Cardiac
   a. Syncope
4. Renal
   a. Polyuria
   b. Polydipsia
   c. Renal insufficiency
5. Neuromuscular
   a. Peripheral neuropathy
   b. Myopathy
6. Endocrine
   a. Hypothermia
   b. Hyperthermia

are predominant.[8] Central nervous system symptoms often develop gradually, starting initially with confusion and progressing to impaired consciousness, coma,[8,66] and, occasionally, death.[67] Cerebellar manifestations are often prominent and can include dysarthria,[68] truncal ataxia, broad-based ataxic gait, nystagmus, and varying degrees of incoordination. Other central nervous system manifestations of lithium intoxication are seizures[66 70] and involvement of the basal ganglia, as suggested by choreiform movements[28,71,72] and Parkinson-like movements.[73]

Gastrointestinal side effects of lithium therapy include gastric irritation, epigastric bloating, abdominal pain, nausea, vomiting, and diarrhea.[74] Although these are common findings, gastrointestinal complaints are not prominent manifestations of lithium intoxication.[8]

Electrocardiographic changes are frequently associated with lithium therapy.[74] Lithium intoxication can be associated with transient ST-segment depression or inverted T waves in leads V4-6.[8] Although electrocardiographic changes are common, cardiac symptoms are rarely manifestations of lithium intoxication. Sinus node dysfunction has been reported to be a consequence of lithium intoxication leading to syncope.[75,76]

Polyuria and polydipsia are frequent side effects of lithium therapy; they are estimated to occur in 20% to 70% of patients.[3] The concentrating defect may develop not only in patients who are overtly toxic but also in those with therapeutic levels.[3] Polyuria may lead to volume depletion and decrease the fractional excretion of lithium. The mechanisms responsible for lithium-induced polyuria were summarized by Singer[3]; they include primary polydipsia, central diabetes insipidus, and nephrogenic diabetes insipidus.

Other, less common manifestations of lithium intoxication are hyperthermia,[77] hypothermia,[78] peripheral neuropathy,[79,80] myopathy,[81] and severe leukopenia.[82]

TABLE 196–3. KNOWN DRUG INTERACTIONS OF LITHIUM

Drug	Effect on Serum Lithium Levels
Diuretics	
Thiazides	Increase
Loop diuretics	Decrease
Osmotic diuretics	Decrease
Potassium sparing	Decrease
Methyl xanthine	Decrease
Acetazolamide	Decrease
Angiotensin-converting enzyme inhibitors	Increase
Angiotensin receptor blockers	Increase
Phenothiazines	Increase
Nonsteroidal antiinflammatory drugs	
Indomethacin	Increase
Ibuprofen	Increase
Mefenamic acid	Increase
Naproxen	Increase
Sulindac	None
Aspirin	None
Cyclooxygenase II inhibitors	Increase
Tetracycline	Increase
Cyclosporine	Increase
Fluoroquinolones	Increase

Modified from references 7, 103-105.

TREATMENT

The initial management of lithium intoxication is determined by the degree of intoxication (serum level), a history of acute versus chronic lithium exposure, the clinical symptoms, and the adequacy of renal function.[83] As noted in Table 196-3, patients present with a variety of clinical manifestations from chronic lithium therapy to acute overdose. Those who appear to have severe impairment of consciousness require airway protection and admission to an intensive care unit. Activated charcoal is an ineffective gastrointestinal decontaminant in lithium overdose because it does not absorb strongly ionized chemicals. In contrast, polyethylene glycol (CoLyte, GoLYTELY) has been shown to be effective in acute lithium intoxication.[84]

Volume status should be assessed, because significant volume depletion can occur as a result of urinary concentrating defects. Many of these patients have volume-responsive

TABLE 196–5. LITHIUM REMOVAL

Mode	Lithium Clearance (mL/min)
Renal excretion	10-40
Forced diuresis	0.9-39
Peritoneal dialysis	9-15
Hemodialysis (blood flow, 126-250 mL/min)	70-170
Continuous renal replacement therapies	Variable, about 20.5

decreases in renal function.[8] Therefore, fluid resuscitation is critical in the initial management. Administration of large volumes of isotonic saline should be done carefully, because severe hypernatremia has been associated with such fluid management.[4,8,72,85,86]

After fluid resuscitation, efforts to enhance lithium removal are the next step. Various modalities for lithium removal are listed in Table 196-5. The efficacy of each modality in removing lithium can be assessed by comparing lithium clearance values. Because there are no controlled studies measuring lithium clearance during intoxication, the following data on lithium clearance rely heavily on case reports.

In normal individuals, renal lithium clearance is about 10 to 40 mL/min.[15,16,20] Hansen and Amdisen[8] reported that renal lithium clearance is 0.9 to 18.4 mL/min in patients with lithium intoxication. Of the 23 patients studied by these authors, only 5 had normal renal function (i.e., creatinine clearance greater than 78 mL/min). Therefore, in patients with lithium intoxication, the ability to remove lithium by renal excretion can be limited by poor renal function.

Because 80% of lithium is reabsorbed in the proximal tubule, factors that decrease proximal lithium reabsorption can increase lithium clearance, enabling enhanced lithium removal during states of intoxication. Because sodium balance alters the clearance of lithium,[29-31,87] forced diuresis with isotonic saline has been used as a treatment of lithium intoxication. Because consistent therapeutic benefits have not been achieved with forced diuresis[8,88] and because of the potential for hypernatremia, forced diuresis is not recommended for severe lithium intoxication.[8,18] However, if lithium clearance is impaired as a result of volume contraction, administration of isotonic saline may increase lithium clearance transiently.

The effects of various agents on the clearance of lithium have been studied in humans challenged with a single dose of lithium.[20] Whereas water loading, furosemide, thiazide diuretics, ethacrynic acid, ammonium chloride, and spironolactone did not increase clearance of lithium, sodium bicarbonate, acetazolamide, urea, and aminophylline were effective. Clinical studies employing these agents for lithium removal during intoxication have not been reported.

Peritoneal dialysis is another means of lithium removal. Wilson and coworkers,[89] using 2 L exchanges per hour, attained clearances of 13 to 15 mL/min. Similar results were achieved by O'Connor and Gleeson,[88] who reported lithium clearances of 9 mL/min with frequent 2-L exchanges. Although peritoneal dialysis is no more efficient in removing lithium than forced diuresis, it avoids problems associated with intravenous administration of large volumes of isotonic saline.

Conventional hemodialysis remains the mainstay of therapy in severe lithium intoxication. The decision to use hemodialysis (or other extracorporeal therapies) should be made by the nephrologist in consultation with the intensivist. Specific factors other than serum lithium levels are not always evident to staff at the local poison control center.[90]

Lithium is one of the most readily dialyzable toxins as a result of its small atomic weight and negligible protein binding. Several reports indicate lithium clearances between 70 and 170 mL/min with hemodialysis.[8,91,92] Because lithium clearance is almost proportional to blood flow, increasing the blood flow to 300 mL/min can further enhance clearance. Table 196-5 compares lithium clearance by various modalities, showing the superiority of hemodialysis to other traditional methods.

The duration of hemodialysis should be guided by serial measurements of serum lithium levels. When the levels approach the therapeutic range, dialysis may be terminated; however, subsequent hemodialysis may be necessary, because serum levels may rise after termination of hemodialysis.[8,83,92] This rebound effect occurs as a result of continued absorption of lithium from the gastrointestinal tract, delayed release from long-acting preparations, and redistribution of lithium from intracellular stores.[83] Although serum lithium clearance has been reported to range from 70 to 170 mL/min,[89,91] the extraction or clearance of lithium from intracellular stores, as reflected by red blood cell clearance, is only 10 to 13 mL/min.[91] This slower extraction of lithium from intracellular stores contributes to the rebound effect.

Continuous renal replacement therapy (e.g., continuous arteriovenous hemodiafiltration, continuous venovenous hemofiltration) has been used either as an alternative to conventional hemodialysis or in addition to conventional hemodialysis.[93-97] The combination of conventional hemodialysis followed by continuous renal replacement therapy is very useful for preventing the rebound phenomenon.[83,94,95]

Table 196-6 summarizes the management of lithium intoxication. Initially, the degree of consciousness and volume status should be assessed. The airway should be protected if necessary, and isotonic saline should be administered for volume repletion. After these critical maneuvers, management should focus on lithium removal. The method of lithium removal is determined by the degree of elevation of the serum lithium concentration, severity of symptoms, and duration of intoxication. Although each patient should be evaluated individually, rough guidelines with rational

TABLE 196–6. MANAGEMENT OF LITHIUM INTOXICATION

1. Oral airway protection in those patients with severe impairment of consciousness
2. Volume resuscitation
3. Whole bowel irrigation with polyethylene glycol (CoLyte, GoLYTELY) to prevent continued absorption of lithium
4. Lithium removal
   a. Serum lithium level >3.5-4 mEq/L—Most patients require hemodialysis.[96,97]
   b. Serum lithium levels 2-4 mEq/L—Unstable patients and patients with severe neurologic signs (seizures, stupor, coma) require hemodialysis.[8]
   c. Serum lithium levels 1.5-2.5 mEq/L—Fluid therapy or forced diuresis treatment should be recommended only for patients with early signs of lithium intoxication and normal renal function, and when it is certain that serum lithium has been elevated for only a few days and not higher than 2.5 mEq/L; dialysis should be instituted if a serum lithium concentration of 1 mEq/L is not reached within 30 hr.[8]

therapeutic options can be derived from knowledge of the pharmacokinetics of lithium removal. For those patients with minimal symptoms, normal renal function, and mild elevation of serum lithium levels (less than 2.5 mEq/L), intravenous hydration may be adequate. Urinary electrolytes should be evaluated as a guide to the type of replacement fluid used. This approach avoids hypernatremia, which commonly occurs with forced diuresis. For severe lithium intoxication, hemodialysis is clearly superior to other modalities. Peritoneal dialysis or continuous arteriovenous hemofiltration may be used if hemodialysis is not available.

PROGNOSIS

The outcome after lithium intoxication is favorable; most patients exhibit reversible neurologic deficits.[8] However, long-lasting neurologic sequelae may occur.[98-102] Permanent neurologic changes appear to stem primarily from cerebellar deficits. Prominent manifestations include ataxic scanning articulation, gait and truncal ataxia, inability to perform heel-to-shin and finger-to-nose maneuvers, bilateral adiadochokinesia, nystagmus, hypertonic musculature, short-term memory deficits, and dementia. Concomitant therapy with neuroleptics, associated multisystem organ failure, and alcohol abuse have clouded the interpretation of the literature.

ANNOTATED REFERENCES

Borkan SC: Extracorporeal therapies for acute intoxications. Crit Care Clin 2002;18:393-420.
This is an extensive review of extracorporeal therapies used in treatment of acute drug and substance intoxications in the ICU, including lithium toxicity.

Menghini VV, Albright RC: Treatment of lithium intoxication with continuous venovenous hemodiafiltration. Am J Kidney Dis 2000;36:E21.
This is a report of a case of intentional acute or chronic lithium intoxication in which continuous venovenous hemodiafiltration was successfully used as the sole modality of extracorporeal therapy.

Meyer RJ, Flynn JT, Brophy PD, et al: Hemodialysis followed by continuous hemofiltration for treatment of lithium intoxication in children. Am J Kidney Dis 2001;37:1044-1047.
This is an early report of the use of continuous venovenous hemodiafiltration after conventional hemodialysis to treat acute lithium intoxication in two adolescent patients; the continuous clearance of lithium prevented the rebound phenomenon.

Okusa MD, Crystal LJT: Clinical manifestations and management of acute lithium intoxication. Am J Med 1994;97:383-389.
This is an extensive review of the clinical presentation and treatment of acute lithium toxicity with emphasis on the pharmacology of lithium and comparison of various extracorporeal treatment modalities.

Timmer RT, Sands JM: Lithium intoxication. J Am Soc Nephrol 1999;10:666-674.
This is an extensive review of the clinical presentation and treatment of lithium toxicity.

Chapter 197

THEOPHYLLINE AND OTHER METHYLXANTHINES

Keith M. Olsen

The methylxanthines, theophylline and its water-soluble derivative, aminophylline (theophylline ethylenediamine), have been used in the treatment of acute and chronic asthma for decades. Clinical studies suggest that theophylline offers minimal additional benefit to inhaled bronchodilators and results in a greater frequency of adverse events. More recent data propose that theophylline may have a role in the treatment of acute asthma in critically ill asthmatic patients with impending respiratory failure and in the treatment of severe acute exacerbations of chronic obstructive pulmonary disease (COPD). Theophylline's role in the treatment of pediatric patients also remains controversial. Caffeine, also a methylxanthine and metabolic derivative of theophylline, is indicated in the prevention of neonatal apnea and is a commonly utilized agent in the neonatal ICU.

PHARMACOLOGY

MECHANISMS OF ACTION

Although theophylline has been available for more than 60 years and there have been thousands of published research papers and more than 1800 clinical trials, the specific pharmacologic actions of theophylline in airway disease are not completely known. With the application of new research techniques, the molecular mechanisms of theophylline are slowly emerging. Theophylline has bronchodilator properties, antiinflammatory effects, and extrapulmonary actions. Bronchodilation is caused by weak, nonselective inhibition of phosphodiesterases 3 and 4 (PDE3, PDE4), which increases

the intracellular concentration of cyclic adenosine monophosphate (CAMP).[1] As a consequence, calcium and potassium channels are modulated, leading to relaxation of airway smooth muscle cells. The result is bronchodilation, although the magnitude of the effect is small compared with that induced by β$_2$-adrenergic agonists. In addition, theophylline may have beneficial airway effects on mucociliary clearance by increasing ciliary beat frequency.[2,3]

Theophylline also appears to have antiinflammatory effects in patients with asthma and COPD.[1,4] The antiinflammatory mechanisms appear to be quite diverse and are related to inhibition of PDE isoenzymes in inflammatory cells, adenosine receptor antagonism, promotion of interleukin-10 release, inhibition of apoptosis, and inhibition of tumor necrosis factor (TNF) secretion, among other effects.[5] Evidence for the antiinflammatory effects of theophylline includes reduction in CD4-positive T lymphocytes in airways exposed to allergens, reduction in neutrophil influx in patients with nocturnal asthma, and reduction in the number of eosinophils in bronchoalveolar lavage (BAL) samples obtained from patients with attacks of severe asthma.[6,7] In subjects with COPD, theophylline reduces total neutrophil count and neutrophil chemotactic responses. The antiinflammatory effects of theophylline are observed when circulating levels of the drug are at the lower end of the therapeutic range, suggesting that lower doses may be beneficial in some patients.[1,8,9]

Theophylline has some extrapulmonary effects, including diuresis and a poorly understood action on respiratory muscles. Some investigators have demonstrated increased diaphragmatic muscle contractility and a reversal of fatigue. The clinical application of these latter effects remains controversial.

PHARMACOKINETICS AND PHARMACODYNAMICS

Theophylline is regarded as having a narrow therapeutic spectrum, and toxicity develops when therapeutic serum concentrations are exceeded. Benefits and risks are related to the serum concentration, which is a function of the dose and clearance of theophylline in individual patients. Because theophylline exhibits a dose-response relationship, drug-drug interactions, and variable pharmacokinetics among critically ill subjects, only clinicians who are experienced with dosing and adjustment of infusions should use it. If theophylline is administered intravenously, there usually is a lag of 15 to 60 minutes between achievement of therapeutic serum concentrations and detection of pulmonary airway responses.[10,11] The relationship between the serum concentration of theophylline and bronchodilation, as measured by improvement in forced expiratory volume over 1 second (FEV_1), is linear. FEV_1 improves by 2% for each 1-mg/L increase in serum theophylline concentration.[10-12] When the drug concentration approaches 20 mg/L, the potential benefit of increased bronchodilation is minimal and must be weighed against the possibility of unwanted adverse events. In 1997, an expert panel report from the U. S. National Institutes of Health (NIH) describing guidelines for the diagnosis and treatment of asthma reduced the recommended theophylline therapeutic serum concentrations from between 5 and 20 mg/L to between 5 and 15 mg/L.[12,13-15] Few data are available to support the use of serum concentrations greater than 15 mg/L. Some patients with impending respiratory failure may benefit from serum concentrations approaching 15 mg/L, but the benefit of pulmonary improvement in relation to the risk of adverse events should be carefully addressed. Antiinflammatory properties, prevention of neonatal apnea, and diaphragmatic contractility are seen at concentrations less than 10 mg/L.[1,16,17]

Theophylline distributes readily into fat tissue in both adults and children (mean volume of distribution, 0.45 L/kg). Therefore, total body weight should be used for calculating loading doses and initial intravenous infusion rates. Morbidly obese patients who exceed ideal body weight by more than 50% may be the exception[17]; the initial dose should be approached with extreme caution in this patient population. All methylxanthines are eliminated by hepatic metabolism; renal elimination accounts for up to 10% to 15% of the overall excretion in adults.[17] Neonates have less developed hepatic metabolism, and renal elimination may approach 50%.[17] The primary route of metabolism is mediated via the cytochrome P450 system, and the CYP1A2 microenzyme is the most important pathway for theophylline metabolism.[18] Less than 10% of theophylline is metabolized to caffeine; however, neonates eliminate caffeine in a more predictable fashion, and this agent maybe used in place of theophylline for the prevention of apnea. Theophylline's half-life varies widely (3.4 to 30 hours), depending on age and underlying physiologic factors. Numerous factors affect the metabolic clearance of theophylline in critically ill patients; variations within and among patients of 25% or more have been observed.[18,19] Factors that influence the activity of hepatic enzyme function involved in theophylline clearance, such as gender, age, obesity, diet, and history of tobacco use, may potentially influence metabolism and serum concentrations. Concomitant conditions found in ICU patients that may significantly alter theophylline clearance are listed in Table 197-1. Other drugs that either inhibit or stimulate CYP1A2 can alter clearance of theophylline and lead to life-threatening

TABLE 197–2. DRUGS THAT SIGNIFICANTLY ALTER THEOPHYLLINE CLEARANCE

Decrease clearance	Increase clearance
Erythromycin	Phenobarbital
Diltiazem/verapamil	Phenytoin
Cimetidine	Rifampin
Ciprofloxacin	Ketamine
Propranolol and other β-adrenergic blockers	Isoproterenol
	Allopurinol
	Methotrexate
	Propafenone

adverse events secondary to toxic levels of the drug. Agents known to affect theophylline clearance are outlined in Table 197-2.[20] Clinicians should be vigilant regarding these drug-drug and drug-disease interactions that significantly alter theophylline clearance. Recognition of these factors is essential to minimize toxicity and maximize efficacy. Careful therapeutic monitoring of serum levels is strongly recommended.[21,22]

CLINICAL UTILITY

ACUTE SEVERE ASTHMA

Adult asthmatics with an acute exacerbation usually are admitted to the hospital after presentation to the emergency department. These patients are routinely treated with supplemental oxygen, short-acting inhaled or nebulized β_2-adrenergic agonists, nebulized ipratropium, and intravenous glucocorticoids. The routine use of intravenous aminophylline or theophylline in the management of acute severe asthma has been replaced by the use of high doses of short-acting β_2-adrenergic agonists. The NIH expert guidelines for the management of hospitalized adult patients with severe asthma do not include theophylline as a routine treatment option.[23,24] β_2-Adrenergic agonists offer a better safety profile and appear to have equal or greater efficacy. In a metaanalysis, the addition of aminophylline to other therapies in acute asthma offered little additional efficacy, resulted in a higher morbidity related to adverse events, and required more intense monitoring of serum concentrations with meticulous dose adjustments.[25] More recently, the Cochrane database and others[26,27] concluded that aminophylline does not appear to confer additional benefit. Intravenous theophylline or aminophylline should be considered only in adult asthmatics with severe exacerbations that are not responding to other treatment modalities and in patients with impending respiratory failure.

The role of methylxanthines in the management of acute severe asthma in pediatric patients remains controversial.[28,29] At least seven clinical trials published in the 1990s, all with small sample sizes (range, 21 to 42 subjects), showed no significant benefit when theophylline was added to nebulized albuterol and glucocorticoids in hospitalized patients aged 2 to 18 years.[26,27,30-35] Most of these studies targeted a theophylline serum concentration of 10 to 20 mg/L and measured a primary outcome by improvement in a clinical score or in FEV_1.[28] Two small trials (21 and 23 patients), demonstrated improvement in FEV_1 and clinical symptom score when theophylline was added to albuterol and either hydrocortisone or methylprednisolone.[36,37] Two larger, randomized trials

TABLE 197–1. PHYSIOLOGIC AND ENVIRONMENTAL FACTORS THAT AFFECT CLEARANCE OF METHYLXANTHINES IN CRITICALLY ILL PATIENTS

Factor	Effect on clearance
Hepatic insufficiency	Decreased
Congestive heart failure	Decreased
Fever	Decreased
Age	Decreased
Tobacco/marijuana use	Increased
Congestive heart failure	Decreased
Infection	Decreased or no change
Hypothyroid or hyperthyroid disease	Decreased or increased
Cystic fibrosis	Increased
Hypoxemia	No change

(163 and 47 patients) evaluated intravenous aminophylline in pediatric patients with severe acute asthma that was not responsive to glucocorticoids and nebulized albuterol. Both studies demonstrated improvement in FEV_1 and clinical score, but treatment with aminophylline did not reduce hospital length of stay.[38,39] The addition of theophylline to other therapies in adult or pediatric patients with exacerbations of severe asthma should be weighed carefully, considering the potential benefits, toxicities, and need for intensive therapeutic drug monitoring.

SEVERE EXACERBATION OF CHRONIC OBSTRUCTIVE PULMONARY DISEASE

As in severe acute asthma, the routine use of intravenous methylxanthines in severe exacerbation of COPD is not supported by large, randomized clinical trials.[40] However, several studies have documented the benefits of use of two bronchodilators simultaneously.[41,42] The combination usually consists of a β_2-adrenergic agonist and an anticholinergic drug (e.g., ipratropium). In acute severe exacerbations that require hospitalization, these agents should be continued at the highest doses tolerated. If an inadequate response is observed, the addition of intravenous aminophylline or theophylline should be considered.[43] Patients receiving oral theophylline on presentation to the emergency department (ED) demonstrated deterioration when theophylline is withdrawn.[42] A study that evaluated 143 patients receiving care in the ED demonstrated a trend toward decreased hospitalization rate when aminophylline was added to the treatment regimen.[42] The patients did not demonstrate improvement in FEV_1 but may have been aided by the antiinflammatory effects of the drug and by drug-induced improvements in diaphragmatic muscle strength. As with acute severe asthma, the addition of theophylline to the regimen of a COPD patient should be weighed against the potential risk of toxicities.

OTHER CLINICAL USES

Theophylline has been demonstrated to increase diaphragmatic muscle strength in healthy volunteers. Increased respiratory muscle strength may benefit some patients who are on the verge of needing mechanical ventilation, or it may help wean patients from mechanical ventilation.[1] However, this effect has not been evaluated in a prospective, randomized, clinical trial. Theophylline at therapeutic serum concentrations increases mucociliary clearance in mechanically ventilated ICU patients, but its routine use is discouraged because of the availability of agents with lower incidences of toxicity.[43] Finally, theophylline and caffeine have been used for the prevention of apnea in the neonatal ICU.[44-46]

ADVERSE EVENTS

Systemic adverse events and theophylline serum concentrations are directly related.[46,47] When serum concentration is 10 mg/L or less, adverse events are minimal but may include nausea, vomiting, and diarrhea.[48] When the serum concentration is greater than 10 mg/L, patients often experience tachycardia, tremors, and metabolic abnormalities (electrolytes and glucose). Although these adverse events are generally well tolerated in the outpatient setting, significant morbidity may occur in critically ill patients.

MANAGEMENT OF ACUTE TOXICITY

Despite the declining use of oral theophylline, acute intoxication remains a cause of morbidity and mortality. Significant toxicity may occur if the serum theophylline concentration is greater than 25 mg/L.[49] Clinical responses to acute theophylline overdose may be classified into neurologic, cardiovascular, and metabolic categories.[50,51] Cardiac toxicity, the most common acute manifestation, is evident by the appearance of tachycardia and arrhythmias. Profound hypotension and cardiovascular collapse have been reported with serum concentrations greater than 50 mg/L.[49,51] Seizures are rare unless the serum concentration is greater than 80 mg/L.[49,50] Metabolic abnormalities, including hypokalemia, hypomagnesemia, hypercalcemia, and hyperglycemia, are common and may complicate the treatment of cardiovascular and neurologic adverse events.[48,50,51]

On initial presentation, standard acute overdose therapy should be applied. Initial gastric lavage may be useful. Multidose activated charcoal enhances elimination, because theophylline undergoes significant enterohepatic recirculation. Seizures should be treated with benzodiazepines; if they are refractory, phenobarbital may be effective. Phenytoin may worsen theophylline-induced seizures and should be avoided.[52] Supraventricular arrhythmias and tachycardia may be managed by β-adrenergic blockers or calcium antagonists, and hypotension with fluids that expand vascular volume.[50,53,54] β-Adrenergic blockers should be used cautiously in patients with underlying COPD or asthma. Ventricular arrhythmias are managed with lidocaine and other standard agents.

In a study of 356 patients with theophylline serum concentrations greater than 30 mg/L, the most notable finding was the tolerance of extremely high theophylline concentrations without development of major toxicity.[49] Despite these data, when life-threatening conditions such as refractory seizures, hypotension, or arrhythmias are present or the serum concentration is greater than 80 mg/L, hemodialysis or hemoperfusion with charcoal should be initiated.[49] Institutions that cannot provide charcoal hemoperfusion should institute continuous venovenous hemofiltration, because this intervention results in a rapid reduction of the theophylline serum concentration and is an acceptable alternative.[54] Theophylline serum concentration should be monitored every 2 hours until declining values are confirmed.

SUMMARY

A narrow therapeutic index, frequent toxicities, drug interactions, and complicated dosing issues make the use of methylxanthines problematic in the acute care setting. Potential benefits should be weighed against the risks. Clinicians who are unfamiliar with the dosing of theophylline should consider consulting other experts before initiation of therapy.

ANNOTATED REFERENCES

Bach PB, Brown C, Gelfand BA, McCrory DC: Management of acute exacerbations of chronic obstructive pulmonary disease: A summary and appraisal of published evidence. Ann Intern Med 2001;134:600-620.
   This paper critically reviews the available data on diagnostic evaluation, risk stratification, and therapeutic management of patients with acute exacerbations of COPD.

Global Initiative for Asthma: Global Strategy for Asthma Management and Prevention NHLBI/WHO Workshop Report. NIH Publication 02-3659. Bethesda, MD, National Institutes of Health, National Heart, Lung, and Blood Institute, 2002.

This paper represents a comprehensive evidence-based approach to diagnosis and management of asthma based on the currently available science.

Pauwels RA, Buist AS, Caverley PM, et al: Global strategy for the diagnosis, management, and prevention of chronic obstructive pulmonary disease. NHLBI/WHO Global Initiative for Chronic Obstructive Lung Diseases (GOLD) Workshop summary. Am J Respir Crit Care Med 2001;163:1256-1276.

These guidelines on obstructive lung disease are derived from a consensus expert panel. They are directed toward evidence-documented treatment and provide recommendations for management of various stages and scenarios of obstructive lung disease.

Shannon M: Life-threatening events after theophylline overdose: A 10-year prospective analysis. Arch Intern Med 1999;159:989-994.

This longitudinal cohort study of 356 patients with theophylline overdose identifies major adverse events, their incidence, and their significance after serum concentrations greater than 30 mg/L.

Wrenn K, Slovis CM, Murphy F, Greenberg RS: Aminophylline therapy for acute bronchospastic disease in the emergency room. Ann Intern Med 1991;115:241-247.

This study randomly assigned 135 COPD patients presenting to the ED to receive either intravenous aminophylline or placebo. Aminophylline appeared to decrease hospital admissions by three-fold as compared with placebo.

Chapter 198

ANTIPSYCHOTICS

Mark Dershwitz

KEY POINTS

1. Among the **phenothiazines and butyrophenones,** there is generally an inverse relationship between the degree of sedation and the propensity to cause hypotension on the one hand, and the likelihood of causing extrapyramidal effects on the other.

2. The **atypical antipsychotics** tend to cause little to no extrapyramidal effects. They tend to be sedating and are likely to cause hypotension.

3. **Haloperidol is the primary medication** used in the intensive care unit for managing agitation or delirium. The initial dose is usually low but may be escalated over a short period to control symptoms. An infusion of haloperidol may be used in persons with symptoms that are particularly difficult to manage.

4. **Antipsychotic-induced extrapyramidal effects and hypotension** are treated with specific pharmacologic agents. Other adverse effects of the antipsychotics usually are managed supportively or by discontinuation of the medication, or both.

5. **Deliberate or accidental overdose of antipsychotics** rarely leads to death. Appropriate care of patients who have overdosed is generally supportive.

PHARMACOLOGY OF THE ANTIPSYCHOTICS

The broad class of medications used to treat psychoses is of interest to intensivists for two reasons. First, some of these medications are useful in the management of agitated or delirious patients in the intensive care unit (ICU). Second, intensivists may need to care for patients with accidental or deliberate overdose of such medications, either alone or in combination with other medications.

The antipsychotics may be divided into three categories based on their chemical structure and receptor-binding activities. These three categories are the phenothiazines, the butyrophenones, and the atypical antipsychotics. The prototypical antipsychotic agent in the phenothiazine class is chlorpromazine (Thorazine). Its pharmacology is discussed in detail in this chapter and then compared with that of the newer antipsychotic agents.[1] The structures of some of the commonly used antipsychotics are shown in Figure 198-1.

In terms of the number of the neurotransmitter systems with which it interacts, chlorpromazine is one of the "dirtiest" drugs in pharmacology. It is a competitive antagonist at the dopamine (D_2), muscarinic, cholinergic, histamine (H_1), α-adrenergic, and serotonin (5-HT_2) receptors. It is believed that its primary antipsychotic effect results from dopaminergic blockade, whereas many (but certainly not all) of its adverse effects result from blockade of cholinergic (sedation, dry mouth) and α-adrenergic (orthostatic hypotension) receptors. The relative propensities of some of the antipsychotics to cause sedation, extrapyramidal effects, and hypotension are listed in Table 198-1.

When chlorpromazine is given to a "normal" individual, behavior is diminished and responses to stimuli are fewer, slower, and smaller in magnitude. If it is given in high doses, a catatonic state is induced, although consciousness and memory are preserved. In fact, when the drug wears off, individuals can describe in great detail how bad it made them feel, although they are most unlikely to complain of the dysphoria while it is occurring. This is in distinct contrast to the benzodiazepines, which often produce anterograde amnesia.

When chlorpromazine is given to a psychotic patient, there usually is improvement in the thought disorder. In schizophrenia, the delusions and hallucinations become less pronounced or disappear, and thinking becomes more orderly. Even if some hallucinations remain, the patient is far more likely to recognize them as unreal.

Because of the wide prevalence of dopaminergic neurons in the central nervous system, chlorpromazine has widespread effects. The specific areas of the brain in which the antipsychotic effect occurs remain obscure. Chlorpromazine lowers the seizure threshold and must be used with caution in persons who are prone to seizures. Because dopamine is released by the hypothalamus to inhibit prolactin secretion by the pituitary, chlorpromazine causes an increase in prolactin secretion. Chlorpromazine exerts its antiemetic effect by blocking dopamine receptors in the chemoreceptor trigger zone.

Blockade of dopamine receptors in the basal ganglia leads to extrapyramidal effects: akathisia, dystonia, rigidity, and tardive dyskinesia. Akathisia is an uncomfortable inability to sit still. Patients feel the need to be in constant motion and may appear to be agitated (although they are not). The acute dystonic signs are usually manifested as uncomfortable (and embarrassing) contractions of the muscles of the face and neck. The rigidity that occurs may be clinically indistinguishable from that of Parkinson's disease. All of these effects occur early in the course of treatment with chlorpromazine and are dose related. In addition, they are readily treated by the administration of such anticholinergic medications as benztropine or diphenhydramine (see later discussion).

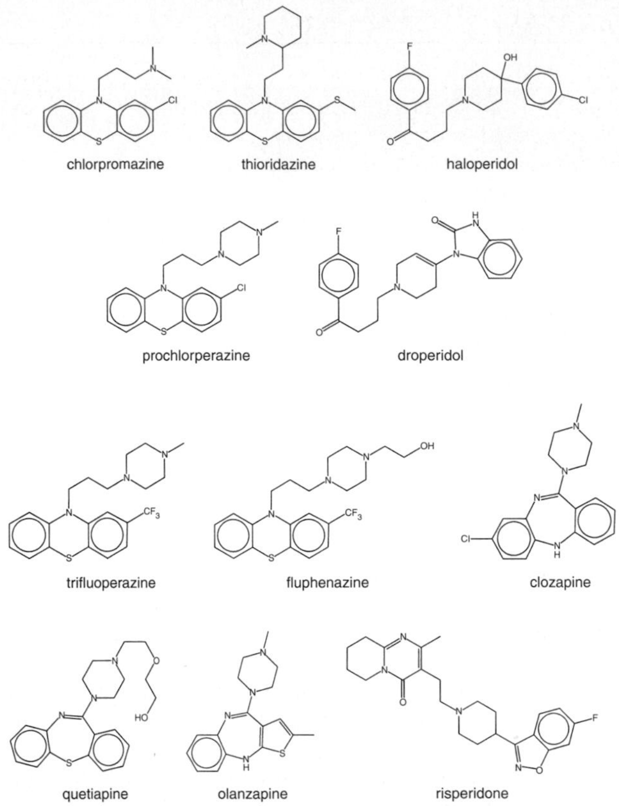

FIGURE 198–1. Structures of the antipsychotics discussed in this chapter.

TABLE 198–1. ADVERSE EFFECTS OF SOME OF THE ANTIPSYCHOTIC MEDICATIONS

Medication	Sedation	Extrapyramidal Effects	Hypotension
Phenothiazines			
Chlorpromazine	+++	++	+++
Thioridazine	+++	+	+++
Trifluoperazine	+	+++	+
Fluphenazine	+	++++	+
Prochlorperazine	+++	++	+++
Butyrophenones			
Haloperidol	+	++++	+
Droperidol	+	++++	+
Atypical antipsychotics			
Clozapine	+++	0	+++
Olanzapine	+	+	++
Quetiapine	+++	0	++
Risperidone	++	++	+++

0, no effect; increasingly strong effects are indicated by the number of + symbols.
Adapted from Baldessarini RJ, Tarazi FI: Drugs and the treatment of psychiatric disorders: Psychosis and mania. In Hardman JG, Limbird LE (eds): Goodman and Gilman's The Pharmacological Basis of Therapeutics, 10th ed. New York, McGraw-Hill, 2001.

Tardive dyskinesia may occur after prolonged therapy with chlorpromazine (although it rarely occurs very early). It is characterized by involuntary, repetitive, stereotyped movements, usually of the face, such as lip smacking, eye blinking, grimacing, or tongue protruding. Paradoxically, the dyskinetic movements may be suppressed by increasing the dose of chlorpromazine. Tardive dyskinesia is often permanent, persisting after the discontinuation of chlorpromazine.

Neuroleptic malignant syndrome is a rare complication of chlorpromazine therapy and is characterized by hyperthermia (due to generalized muscle contracture), stupor, and such metabolic abnormalities as myoglobinemia and elevation of the creatine kinase concentration. It resembles malignant hyperthermia, which is a rare adverse reaction to certain anesthetic medications. The treatment of the neuroleptic malignant syndrome is discussed later in this chapter.

Because chlorpromazine also blocks the muscarinic and α-adrenergic receptors, many of its other adverse effects are readily predicted: orthostatic hypotension, nasal stuffiness, dry mouth, blurred vision, and urinary retention. Chlorpromazine (and many of the other phenothiazines) can cause jaundice. Tolerance does not develop to the antipsychotic effects of chlorpromazine, although tolerance to the sedative effects does occur over a period of a few weeks.

There are many other antipsychotic medications, whose effects differ from those of chlorpromazine primarily on the basis of different degrees of blockade of the various receptor types. In general, those medications with a greater anticholinergic effect are more sedating and less likely to cause extrapyramidal effects. They also tend to cause more orthostatic hypotension due to α-adrenergic blockade. Conversely, those medications with a lesser anticholinergic effect (and which tend to be much more potent dopaminergic

antagonists) are less sedating, cause less orthostatic hypotension, and are more likely to produce extrapyramidal effects.

Other phenothiazines in common use include thioridazine (Mellaril), trifluoperazine (Stelazine), and fluphenazine (Prolixin). Thioridazine has greater sedating and hypotensive effects than chlorpromazine, while causing many fewer extrapyramidal reactions. Trifluoperazine and fluphenazine are less sedating, cause fewer hypotensive effects, and are more likely to cause extrapyramidal reactions than chlorpromazine.

All of the phenothiazine antipsychotics have antiemetic activity. Because many "normal" patients (who happen to be nauseated) would be distressed to be treated with a medication whose primary purpose is the management of psychoses, prochlorperazine (Compazine) is marketed as an antiemetic. Its pharmacology is very similar to that of chlorpromazine. It is available in a multitude of preparations to make administration convenient: tablets, liquid, suppository, and injection.

Haloperidol (Haldol) is in the butyrophenone class. It causes little sedation or hypotension and has high incidence of extrapyramidal effects. Because of its decreased propensity to cause hypotension, especially in the hypovolemic patient, haloperidol is the most commonly used antipsychotic in the ICU for the management of delirium or agitation (see Chapter 2). Droperidol (Inapsine) is pharmacologically very similar to haloperidol and is commonly used by anesthesiologists as an antiemetic.

The atypical antipsychotics are "atypical" in that they have less (or no) antagonistic activity at dopaminergic and cholinergic receptors. Their antipsychotic activity is thought to be due to 5-HT_2 blockade. Because they are also potent α-adrenergic antagonists, orthostatic hypotension is a common problem. However, extrapyramidal effects are much rarer than with any of the older antipsychotic agents. Drugs in this class include clozapine (Clozaril), olanzapine (Zyprexa), quetiapine (Seroquel), ziprasidone (Geodon), and risperidone (Risperdal). Clozapine can cause agranulocytosis and seizures; regular monitoring of the white blood cell count is necessary in patients taking the drug.

For the emergency management of agitation, delirium, or acute psychosis, haloperidol may be given intravenously or intramuscularly, or chlorpromazine, olanzapine, or ziprasidone may be given intramuscularly. Chlorpromazine should rarely be given intravenously because of its profound vasodilating effect, which is especially pronounced in hypovolemic patients.

USE OF ANTIPSYCHOTICS IN THE INTENSIVE CARE UNIT

The most common indication for the use of antipsychotic medications in the ICU is for the treatment of agitation or delirium. Haloperidol is the usual drug of choice for this indication because of intensivists' familiarity with it and because of its substantial safety record.

If the need to begin treatment is not urgent, and if gastrointestinal absorption is expected to be reliable, oral haloperidol may be used at a beginning dose of 0.5 to 1 mg and repeated as needed. As the duration of therapy increases, the interval between doses also increases, because the terminal half-life of haloperidol is about 1 day in normal persons and may be prolonged in critically ill persons. In the urgent management of severe agitation, the intravenous (or less desirably, the intramuscular) route may be used. A reasonable starting dose is 2.5 to 5 mg; if an inadequate response is obtained, additional escalating doses (e.g., twice the previously administered dose) may be given every 5 to 10 minutes. Once reasonable efficacy has been achieved, the last administered dose may then be repeated every 4 to 6 hours. Some critically ill patients require hundreds of milligrams daily for the management of agitation or delirium. One alternative to the frequent administration of bolus injections of haloperidol is administration of haloperidol by continuous infusion. This method may provide better control in some patients and may decrease the nursing effort required to maintain adequate control of the agitation or depression.[2] After steady-state blood concentrations of haloperidol are approached, days are required for the effects to wane after stopping administration.

Chlorpromazine is usually a less desirable alternative in this scenario because of its significant hypotensive effect caused by α-adrenergic blockade. Hypotension due to chlorpromazine is especially pronounced after intravenous administration, and if chlorpromazine must be given by this route, the injection should be made very slowly. In comparison to haloperidol, chlorpromazine is also significantly more sedating, which might be an attractive side effect. In general, the addition of a sedative such as a benzodiazepine or propofol to a haloperidol regimen provides superior effects with fewer hemodynamic effects.

Olanzapine has recently been studied in comparison with haloperidol for the treatment of delirium in the ICU.[3] Overall efficacy was comparable with either medication, and there were fewer extrapyramidal effects with olanzapine. The newer medication is substantially more expensive and has recently become available for intramuscular injection.

All of the phenothiazine and butyrophenone antipsychotic agents have antiemetic activity by virtue of their ability to block the dopamine receptor in the chemoreceptor trigger zone. Antiemetic doses are much lower than the usual antipsychotic doses. The antiemetic with which there is the most experience is droperidol. The usual antiemetic dose is 1.25 mg given two to three times daily. This dose rarely causes sedation or any other adverse effects. If droperidol at this dose does not relieve the emetic symptoms, an antiemetic from a different class (e.g., a 5-HT$_3$ antagonist) should be given.

MANAGEMENT OF ADVERSE EFFECTS

The extrapyramidal effects of the antipsychotics are uncomfortable but rarely hazardous. The exception is an unusual presentation of acute dystonia that is manifested as airway compromise. If the administration of an anticholinergic agent does not provide rapid relief, then paralysis and intubation are required to maintain airway integrity.

For the treatment of extrapyramidal effects caused by an antipsychotic drug, a centrally acting anticholinergic is given, usually intravenously. The usual doses are 1 to 2 mg of benztropine (Cogentin) or 25 to 50 mg of diphenhydramine (Benadryl). Diphenhydramine causes more sedation than benztropine does, which may or may not be advantageous in a particular patient. Because the extrapyramidal effects are dose related, decreasing the subsequent dose may lessen the likelihood of recurrence. Alternatively, changing to a different medication with fewer inherent extrapyramidal effects is also an option (see Table 198-1). However, such a change in therapy is likely to result in greater hypotensive effects from the antipsychotic medication, a factor that must be considered in critically ill patients.

The neuroleptic malignant syndrome is a rare and frequently fatal constellation of symptoms including catatonia, stupor, rigidity, hyperthermia, autonomic instability, and rhabdomyolysis leading to myoglobinemia and elevated creatine kinase. It is more commonly associated with the more potent antipsychotics (e.g., haloperidol), and dopaminergic blockade is thought to be the initial underlying mechanism. However, all of the atypical antipsychotics have been reported to cause neuroleptic malignant syndrome.

Treatment of neuroleptic malignant syndrome requires such supportive measures as cessation of the antipsychotic medication, active cooling, maintenance of blood pressure, and maintenance of urine output. In addition, the duration of the episode and overall mortality are both decreased by the addition of pharmacologic therapy.[4] The dopaminergic agonists amantadine (Symmetrel) and bromocriptine (Parlodel) are both effective. In addition, dantrolene (Dantrium), a muscle relaxant with an intracellular mechanism of action that is also used to treat malignant hyperthermia, decreases heat production in neuroleptic malignant syndrome by decreasing skeletal muscle rigidity. Some clinicians consider neuroleptic malignant syndrome to be primarily a catatonic state and have treated it with electroconvulsive therapy, thereby achieving a decrease in mortality.

Most of the phenothiazine and butyrophenone antipsychotics are thought to increase the incidence of torsades de pointes, a form of ventricular tachycardia that may deteriorate into ventricular fibrillation.[5] Cases of torsades de pointes have also been ascribed to therapy with the atypical antipsychotics, although the incidence is much lower. Torsades de pointes is usually, but not always, preceded by an increase in the corrected QT interval (QTc) on the electrocardiogram. QTc prolongation is a known dose-related effect and is common during therapy with thioridazine, chlorpromazine, haloperidol, and droperidol. Torsades de pointes is more likely when the QTc is lengthened beyond 500 msec or when it is prolonged 60 msec or more beyond its usual baseline value. Discontinuation of the antipsychotic agent decreases QTc and the associated risk of torsades de pointes.

Hypotension due to α-adrenergic blockade often accompanies therapy with the phenothiazines and atypical antipsychotics. The degree of hypotension may be exaggerated in persons with coexisting hypovolemia and in those who are receiving therapy with β-adrenergic antagonists, because the efferent limb of the barostatic reflex is blocked. Infusion of phenylephrine (Neo-Synephrine), a pure α-adrenergic agonist, restores blood pressure without producing other cardiovascular perturbations.

The seizure threshold may be lowered by antipsychotic medications, especially chlorpromazine and clozapine.[6] However, because the effect is dose dependent, large doses of other antipsychotics have also been associated with seizures, both in persons with a known preexisting seizure disorder and in persons with no prior history. The approach to treatment of an antipsychotic-related seizure is similar to that used with other drug-induced or idiopathic seizures: initial measures to maintain airway patency, along with the administration of supplemental oxygen, the administration of an anticonvulsant medication (e.g., diazepam [Valium]) if the seizure does not terminate spontaneously, and the withdrawal or decrease in the dose of the offending medication (if known).

MANAGEMENT OF ANTIPSYCHOTIC OVERDOSE

Patients may accidentally or deliberately administer an overdose of an antipsychotic, either alone or in combination with other medications or alcohol. Such patients may require admission to an ICU. In contrast to other classes of medications that are active in the central nervous system, such as the tricyclic antidepressants, barbiturates, and opioids, all of the antipsychotics have a high therapeutic index (in terms of lethality), and deaths due to overdose are quite rare.[7] When deaths have occurred after overdoses in persons who were found alive and transported to a hospital, the most common cause has been aspiration pneumonitis.

Treatment of the overdose in the ICU is supportive. If the patient is comatose and unable to protect the airway, tracheal intubation should be performed, and the endotracheal tube should be kept in place until consciousness returns. Hypotension is treated with intravenous fluid administration, and infusion of the α-adrenergic agonist phenylephrine may be added if there is an inadequate response to fluids alone.

Continuous electrocardiographic monitoring is continued until the blood concentration of the medication is predicted (or demonstrated) to be subtherapeutic, because of the possibility of torsades de pointes or other ventricular dysrhythmias. There is no demonstrated efficacy (and certainly there is potential toxicity) of the administration of potassium or magnesium to such persons with prolonged QTc. Seizures that do not resolve spontaneously may be treated with diazepam, as described earlier. Extrapyramidal symptoms are treated with diphenhydramine or benztropine, as described earlier. Delirium from excessive central cholinergic blockade should respond to the administration of physostigmine (Antilirium), 1 to 2 mg intravenously. Because antipsychotics have large volumes of distribution and a high degree of protein binding, dialysis has little efficacy in decreasing the blood concentration.

ANNOTATED REFERENCES

Baldessarini RJ, Tarazi FI: Drugs and the treatment of psychiatric disorders: Psychosis and mania. In Hardman JG, Limbird LE (eds): Goodman and Gilman's The Pharmacological Basis of Therapeutics, 10th ed. New York, McGraw-Hill, 2001.
   This is a detailed and comprehensive consideration of the pharmacology of antipsychotic medications, from which the initial section of this chapter was drawn.

Burns MJ: The pharmacology and toxicology of atypical antipsychotic agents. Clin Toxicol 2001;39:1-14.
   This is a detailed and comprehensive review of the adverse effects, their management, and the treatment of overdose with atypical antipsychotic agents.

Caroff SN, Man SC, Keck PE Jr: Specific treatment of the neuroleptic malignant syndrome. Biol Psychiatry 1998;378-381.
   This is a detailed review of the efficacy of the therapies that have been employed for the treatment of the neuroleptic malignant syndrome, including medications and electroconvulsive therapy.

Haddad PM, Anderson IM: Antipsychotic-related QTc prolongation, torsade de pointes and sudden death. Drugs 2002;62:1649-1671.
   This is a detailed and comprehensive review of antipsychotic medications in terms of their propensity to cause torsades de pointes, a potentially life-threatening dysrhythmia.

Pisani F, Oteri G, Costa C, et al: Effects of psychotropic drugs on seizure threshold. Drug Saf 2002;25:91-110.
   This is a detailed and comprehensive review of the pharmacologic effects of antipsychotics on the seizure threshold.

Chapter 199

PRINCIPLES OF NSAID THERAPY IN CRITICAL CARE MEDICINE

Nicole Ansani • Terence Starz

KEY POINTS

1. Although the pharmacokinetic characteristics of nonsteroidal anti-inflammatory drugs (NSAIDs) are similar, pharmacodynamic differences in cyclooxygenase-1 (COX-1) and COX-2 inhibition account for differences in NSAID toxicity.

2. NSAIDs have significant benefit in the management of pain, inflammation, and fever in critically ill patients. All nonselective and COX-2–selective NSAIDs exert similar efficacy for these indications.

3. The most common toxicities associated with NSAIDs are gastrointestinal, cardiovascular, and renal and are related primarily to COX inhibition of prostaglandin production.

4. When NSAID therapy is initiated in the critically ill patient, the patient's risk profile for toxicity must be considered. Patients at high risk for gastrointestinal toxicity should be prescribed a COX-2–selective inhibitor.

Nonsteroidal anti-inflammatory drugs (NSAIDs) are one of the most commonly prescribed classes of medications in the United States.[1-4] More than 110 million NSAID prescriptions and more than 30 billion over-the-counter tablets or capsules are sold yearly in the United States.[5-7] NSAIDs have important clinical uses in critically ill patients, especially for treatment of pain and inflammatory states and reduction of fever. However, certain pharmacologic properties and their mechanism of action can cause serious side effects and can affect other medications used concomitantly. Common toxicities of NSAID therapy include gastrointestinal, cardiovascular, and renal side effects. The pharmacologic characteristics of NSAIDs related to cyclooxygenase-1 (COX-1) and COX-2 enzyme inhibition result in differences among the agents. Patient characteristics and NSAID toxicity profiles are important for the appropriate use of NSAIDs in the critically ill patient.

All NSAIDs have analgesic, anti-inflammatory, and antipyretic properties and have been used since the time of Hippocrates in the 4th century BCE. In 1897, Felix Hoffmann, a chemist for Friedrich Bayer & Co. in Germany, synthesized aspirin by adding acetic acid to sodium salicylate, initiating the modern era of NSAIDs.[1] Beginning in the

1960s, many NSAIDs, including indomethacin, ibuprofen, naproxen, and diclofenac, were introduced and showed therapeutic and toxic effects similar to those of aspirin. More recently, new NSAIDs with less potential for toxicity, including celecoxib, rofecoxib, and valdecoxib, have been developed. Currently, 26 NSAID chemical compounds are available in the United States.[8,9]

NSAID PHARMACODYNAMICS

Although NSAIDs belong to a number of chemical families, including acetic acids, oxicams, propionic acids, salicylates, benzenesulfonamides, and furanones (Table 199-1), all NSAIDs are weakly acidic chemical compounds. Many similarities in pharmacokinetic properties are shared by various NSAIDs.[11] Their absorption is primarily in the large surface area of the small intestine as well as in the stomach.[11] The acidic nature of NSAIDs can cause direct gastrointestinal mucosal injury. Gastrointestinal absorption of NSAIDs normally occurs rapidly, within 15 to 30 minutes. Different product formulations, including enteric-coated and delayed-release preparations, decrease gastric emptying, and altered gastric transit time can delay drug absorption, time to peak effect, and half-life.[12] For example, 4 to 6 hours is required for peak absorption of enteric-coated products.[12] After absorption, NSAIDs are more than 90% bound to plasma proteins, especially albumin, which influences their distribution and drug-drug interaction potential. Unbound drug is responsible for the pharmacologic actions of NSAIDs.[11] Hypoalbuminemia with alcoholic liver disease can result in greater unbound drug and increased risk for NSAID-related adverse events.[12]

NSAIDs are primarily eliminated by renal and biliary excretion.[13] The elimination half-lives of NSAIDs vary from 0.25 to 70 hours, which accounts for differences in dosing schedules (see Table 199-1). Factors that delay NSAID clearance increase their potential for adverse reactions. The dose of NSAIDs should be lowered proportionally in patients with impaired kidney function. Reduced renal function prolongs NSAID half-life and extends the effects on the gastrointestinal tract and kidneys.[11,14] NSAIDs are hepatically metabolized to both active and inactive metabolites, primarily through the cytochrome P450 enzymes, glucuronidase enzymes, or both.[11,13] Certain NSAIDs, such as nabumetone and sulindac, are prodrugs and require metabolism by the liver to generate pharmacologically active metabolites.[11] The hepatic clearance of NSAIDs is dependent on blood flow to

TABLE 199–1. CHARACTERISTICS OF COMMONLY PRESCRIBED NSAIDs

Generic name (*trade name*)	Dose*		Pharmacokinetics	
	Available dosages (mg)	Common dosing intervals	Drug metabolism	Elimination half-life (h)
Nonselective NSAIDs				
Acetic acid group				
Diclofenac DR	25	bid-tid	Oxidation	1-2
(*Voltaren*)	50	qd-bid		
Diclofenac XR	75			
(*Voltaren XR*)	100			
Etodolac	200	bid-tid	Oxidation,	7
(*Lodine*)	300	qd	conjugation	
Etodolac XL	400			
(*Lodine XL*)	500			
	400			
	500			
	600			
Ketorolac IM injection	30	qd-qid	Conjugation	2.5-8.5
(*Toradol IM*)	60			
Indomethacin	25	bid-tid	Oxidation,	4.5-6
(*Indocin*)	50	qd-bid	conjugation	
Indomethacin SR	75			
(*Indocin SR*)				
Nabumetone	500	qd-bid	Oxidation	22-30
(*Relafen*)	750			
Sulindac	150	bid	Oxidation, reduction	16
(*Clinoril*)	200			
Tolmetin	400	tid	Conjugation	5
(*Tolectin*)	600			
Oxicam group				
Meloxicam	7.5	qd	Oxidation	13-20
(*Mobic*)	15			
Piroxicam	10	qd	Oxidation	30-86
(*Feldene*)	20			
Propionic acid group				
Fenoprofen	200	tid-qid	Glucuronidation	3
(*Nalfon Pulvules*)	300			
Flurbiprofen	50	bid-qid	Oxidation	3-6
(*Ansaid*)	100			
Ibuprofen	400	tid-qid	Oxidation	2-2.5
(*Motrin*)	600			
	800			
Ketoprofen	50	tid-qid	Conjugation	2-4
(*Orudis*)	75	qd		3-7
Ketoprofen XR	100			
(*Oruvail*)	150			
	200			
Naproxen	250	bid	Conjugation,	12-15
(*Naprosyn*)	375	qd	oxidation	
(*Naprelan*)	500			
	375			
	500			
Oxaprozin (*Daypro*)	600	qd-bid	Oxidation, conjugation	50-60
Salicylate				
Aspirin	325	bid-qid	Hydrolysis, conjugation,	0.25-0.5
(*Ecotrin, Ascriptin*)	500		glucuronidation	
Choline magnesium	500	bid-tid	Conjugation	2-12
trisalicylate	750			
(*Trilisate*)	1000			
Cyclooxygenase-2 agents				
Benzenesulfonamide group				
Celecoxib	100	qd-bid	Conjugation	11-16
(*Celebrex*)	200			
Valdecoxib	10	qd	Glucuronidation	8-11
(*Bextra*)	20			
Furanone group				
Rofecoxib	12.5	qd	Cytosolic enzymes	16-18
(*Vioxx*)	25			
	50			

NSAID, nonsteroidal anti-inflammatory drug.
*A dosage range exists for each NSAID that must be individualized depending on patient characteristics and disease mechanism.
Data from references 9-11.

the liver, degradation rates by hepatic enzymes, and the amount excreted in the bile. Moderate to severe liver disease impairs NSAID metabolism, increasing the potential for NSAID toxicity. With advancing age, the hepatic clearance of certain NSAIDs, including diclofenac, etodolac, flurbiprofen, ibuprofen, indomethacin, meloxicam, nabumetone, naproxen, oxaprozin, piroxicam, and sulindac, is slower because of decreased hepatic phase I oxidative, reductive, and hydrolytic catalytic reactions.[11]

Until 1971, the mechanism of action of NSAIDs was not well understood.[1] It was then recognized that although NSAIDs have a number of physiologic effects, their principal action is the inhibition of the cyclooxygenase (COX) enzyme. COX is responsible for the production of prostaglandins (PG) and thromboxanes (TX), which are derived from arachidonic acid, an unsaturated fatty acid present in all body cell membranes. PGs and TXs belong to a class of bioactive autocoids called eicosanoids, and they have a number of important physiologic functions in the body. PGs and TXs mediate normal homeostatic functions of the upper gastrointestinal tract, kidneys, and platelets. PG and TX are critical in the inflammatory response because of their influences on vascular permeability, platelet function, and immune reactions. These autocoids are involved in both peripheral and central pain processing and have a role in fever production.[15,16]

There are two isoforms of the COX enzyme: COX-1 and COX-2. Although the COX enzymes are coded on two separate genes, they share 63% structural homogeneity, have similar mechanisms of action, and produce identical compounds from arachidonic acid.[15-18] The expression and regulation of COX-1 and COX-2 differ in various organs and tissues; however, their physiologic effects are overlapping.[2,15,16,19,20] Differences in the structural configurations of COX-1 and COX-2 enzyme side chains determine whether a particular NSAID will inhibit the enzyme. Isoform nonselective NSAIDs (e.g., naproxen, ibuprofen) inhibit both COX-1 and COX-2, thereby decreasing the production of PGs involved in both homeostatic and inflammatory actions. The COX-2–selective agents (celecoxib, rofecoxib, and valdecoxib) have 50-fold greater activity against COX-2 than COX-1 and exert their actions primarily in inflammatory processes.[19,21] Both COX-1 and COX-2 are involved in pain processing.

Differences in modes of COX-1 and COX-2 inhibition allow for comparisons of drug effect.[6] Nonselective NSAIDs exert one of three kinetic models for inhibiting the COX-1 and COX-2 enzymes: (1) rapid, reversible binding (e.g., ibuprofen); (2) rapid, lower-affinity reversible binding followed by time-dependent, higher-affinity, slowly reversible binding (e.g., indomethacin); or (3) rapid, irreversible binding followed by covalent modification (e.g., aspirin). Aspirin is the only NSAID that covalently modifies both COX enzymes, thereby resulting in permanent inhibition of both isoforms.[22] COX-2–selective inhibitors act on COX-2 by a time-dependent, slowly reversible mechanism. They also can affect COX-1 by a freely reversible and competitive mechanism. The result of this two-stage process by COX-2–selective agents is maximal inhibition of COX-2 with minimal inhibition of COX-1.[23] The structural basis for kinetic modeling is not well understood, and variations in the time-dependent inhibition are present among NSAID classes and among agents within the same class.[17]

COX biochemical selectivity of NSAIDs is related to the in vitro drug concentration necessary to inhibit COX-2 activity

completely and COX-1 activity by 50%.[2,16] Other in vitro blood assays of COX-isoform activity were developed based on comparative NSAID effects on production of TXB_2 and PGE_2. However, neither of these measurements predicts clinical differences in NSAID efficacy or toxicity.[2,16] Data from clinical trials demonstrating a decreased incidence of gastrointestinal toxicity and an absence of platelet inhibition with COX-2–selective versus nonselective agents have been the clinical parameters used to distinguish among the various agents.[2]

COX converts arachidonic acid to the inactive precursor PGG_2 and then PGH_2. PGH_2 is metabolized in various tissues to physiologically active products, including PGI_2, PGE_2, and TXA_2. The amounts of the different PGs produced determine their biologic effects on tissues. PGs exert their effects by activating specific cell-membrane receptors of the superfamily of G protein–coupled receptors.[1] PGI_2 has important regulatory effects on renal blood flow, gastric mucosa, uterine smooth muscle, and bronchial smooth muscle. PGI_2 also inhibits platelet aggregation. PGE_2 is an abundant PG with important regulatory effects on fever and of the reproductive, gastrointestinal, neuroendocrine, and immune systems.[24] PGE_2 is present at sites of inflammation as a potent vasodilator in acute and chronic inflammatory diseases and in tissue injury. PGE_2 also can promote labor and dysmenorrhea.[24] TXA_2 promotes platelet aggregation and vasoconstriction. TXA_2 is released with tissue injury and plays a role in cellular responses to inflammation.[20]

PGs produced by COX-1 are primarily involved in "housekeeping" activities, such as maintaining the protective gastrointestinal mucosal barrier in the stomach and intestines, modulating intrarenal hemodynamics, influencing platelet function (especially aggregation), and regulating vascular homeostasis. High levels of COX-1 are present in the gastrointestinal mucosa, renal collecting tubules, vascular endothelium, monocytes, platelets, and seminal vesicles. For example, PGs produced by COX-1 provide gastric protection by reducing gastric acid secretion, stimulating mucus secretion, and promoting gastric mucosa vasodilation. Kidney function is affected by the localization of COX-1 in the collecting ducts and renal vasculature. COX-1 converts PGH_2 to TXA_2, which promotes platelet aggregation. Although the major role of COX-1 is homeostasis, COX-1 may contribute to PG production in certain inflammatory reactions, including those in the synovia of inflamed joints and atherosclerotic plaques.[15,16,19,20]

The primary role of COX-2 is in inflammatory reactions that result in PG production by fibroblasts, macrophages, endothelial cells, and synoviocytes. This enzyme is also important in pain and fever mechanisms.[17] Certain other tissues express COX-2, especially the cortical macula densa, medullary interstitial cells, and the kidney vasculature.[16,20] Small amounts of COX-2 are also found in the small intestine, ovary, uterus, bone, and brain.[15,17,20] Because COX-2 expression is regulated by growth factors, its role in wound repair is under investigation.[17]

CLINICAL IMPLICATIONS AND USES OF NSAIDs IN CRITICALLY ILL PATIENTS

NSAIDs have important analgesic, anti-inflammatory, and antipyretic therapeutic roles in critically ill patients. NSAIDs also have the potential to cause toxic side effects. In addition, they are in widespread use, and patients presenting to the intensive care unit (ICU) frequently are taking either prescription or over-the-counter NSAIDs. NSAIDs must be considered as possible contributors to various disease processes (e.g., gastrointestinal bleeding). NSAIDs often are used therapeutically (e.g., for treatment of postoperative pain or fever), and questions often arise as to whether NSAID therapy should be continued when therapy with other agents (e.g., concomitant anticoagulant use) is considered during the acute illness.

In clinical trials, all nonselective and COX-2–selective NSAIDs in equipotent doses have demonstrated similar efficacy in relieving pain, inflammation, and fever.[25-27] However, there is significant variability in the clinical effects of NSAIDs within and among patients, with approximately 70% to 80% of individuals responding to any particular agent.[28,29] Lack of response to one NSAID does not preclude benefit from another.[28,29] Over time, the efficacy of a given agent may decrease, and changing to another NSAID may be beneficial. Differences in response to various NSAIDs may be related to COX-1 and COX-2 inhibitory pharmacodynamics, because no definite clinical characteristics have been identified in nonresponders, as compared with responders.[11,22] In contrast, toxicity profiles of nonselective and COX-2–selective agents have a defined relationship to the degree of COX-1 and COX-2 inhibition, especially for the development of gastrointestinal adverse events or antiplatelet effects.

USE OF NSAIDs FOR MANAGEMENT OF PAIN AND INFLAMMATION

Pain management is a key issue for critical care clinicians. Ineffective pain relief of critically ill patients may lead to deleterious cardiac, pulmonary, and central nervous system (CNS) responses.[30] Clinical trials comparing efficacy for acute pain among NSAIDs or between NSAIDs and other analgesics come from models of single-dose dental pain, orthopedic and gynecologic surgeries, and dysmenorrhea. Studies of NSAIDs for treatment of chronic pain and inflammation have focused primarily on musculoskeletal disorders, including osteoarthritis, rheumatoid arthritis, and low back pain.

Pain is a complex symptom with sensory and emotional components that signals tissue injury or damage. The body's pain matrix includes pain recognition and pain-generating mechanisms in tissues, synaptic connections of first- and second-order neurons at the dorsal horn of the spinal cord, and central processing in the spinal cord and brain.[31] PGs play an important role in signal transmission and processing of pain at each level of the matrix.

Pain is initiated by activation of tissue nociceptors in various disease states by mechanical, thermal, and chemical stimuli. Surgical trauma and other forms of tissue injury induce expression of COX-2, and to a lesser extent COX-1, resulting in the generation of PGs, especially PGE_2.[31-33] PGs sensitize A-δ and C primary afferent sensory nerve fibers that carry impulses to the dorsal horn of the spinal cord. Glutamate, substance P, and other mediators, along with PGs, are involved in dorsal horn pain processing. PGs have also been identified in the hypothalamus and other areas of the brain; however, their effects in ascending and descending nociceptive pathways are not yet defined.[31] By inhibiting PGs at these different levels of the pain matrix, NSAIDs can have important effects on pain processing. For example, NSAIDs reduce PG-mediated protein kinase A phosphorylation of

sodium channels in nociceptor terminals.[34] At the spinal cord level, inhibition of PGE_2 production by NSAIDs reduces hyperalgesia and allodynia in experimental models.[31] COX-2 is released in spinal cord neurons and other regions of the CNS, resulting in increased PGE_2 production in cerebrospinal fluid. Continuous production of PGs by COX after tissue injury may lead to a hyperalgesic state and is a proposed trigger of chronic pain.[35]

SURGICAL PAIN

Inadequate postoperative pain control has been associated with increased morbidity, increased length of stay, and increased costs for ICU patients.[36] Although opioids are commonly prescribed for surgical and trauma pain and other acute pain states, limitations to their use include acute side effects such as nausea and vomiting, drowsiness, and respiratory depression, which can prolong postoperative recovery and increase costs.[17] NSAIDs are effective in combination with other analgesics in management of the acute pain of tissue injury.[37] For example, the use of NSAIDs in orthopedic and other types of surgeries, including knee arthroscopy, hip replacement, spinal surgery, and gynecologic laparoscopy, decreases postoperative opioid requirements.[28,38-42] In addition, NSAID therapy alone can provide effective postoperative pain relief.[42,43] However, because of the potential for adverse reactions, including gastrointestinal toxicity, platelet inhibition with increased bleeding risk, and renal dysfunction especially with hypovolemia, nonselective NSAIDs currently have a limited role in the management of postoperative pain.[39,40,44] COX-2–selective inhibitors are equally effective in pain relief as nonselective NSAIDs, but they have decreased toxicity because of less gastrointestinal effects and no platelet inhibition.[44] Recent studies of the use of COX-2–selective inhibitors in orthopedic and gynecologic surgeries demonstrated significant reductions in opioid consumption, decreased postoperative opioid side effects including nausea and vomiting, and improved subjective pain assessment on visual analog testing, without differences in postoperative blood loss.[32,39-41,43,45,46] In addition, preoperative use of COX-2–selective agents in knee arthroscopy, compared with postoperative use, can delay the time to first analgesic request and decrease total opioid consumption.[39] The clinical impact of NSAID therapy on wound and bone healing after surgery is unclear.[47-49] NSAIDs, especially indomethacin, have been used perioperatively to reduce heterotopic bone formation after acetabular fracture surgery.[50] Recent data from animal and human trials suggest that NSAIDs may impair bone healing after fractures because of the role of PGs in osteogenesis.[48-51]

Ketorolac is currently the only injectable NSAID available in the United States.[33] Clinical studies comparing injectable ketorolac with morphine in the management of postoperative pain after orthopedic, gynecologic, and major abdominal procedures have shown similar efficacy but slower onset of action with ketorolac.[52] Combination therapy with ketorolac and morphine improves analgesic benefit compared with morphine alone and reduces total morphine consumption.[53] The use of ketorolac in acute pain states is now limited because of postmarketing reports of toxicity, including peptic ulcers, gastrointestinal bleeding, and renal insufficiency.[32,52] In addition, dosing adjustments are necessary for patients with renal dysfunction and elderly patients, and duration of therapy should not exceed 5 days.[54]

REGIONAL INFLAMMATORY STATES

The anti-inflammatory properties of NSAIDs are beneficial in certain acute disease states affecting critically ill patients, including various systemic and regional rheumatic disorders and localized inflammatory conditions such as pleuropericarditis. PGs, especially PGI_2 and PGE_2, are induced by interleukin-1 (IL-1), IL-6, and IL-8. These PGs are important mediators of inflammatory reactions; they influence vascular reactivity and increase vascular permeability.[24,55,56]

Rheumatic diseases, such as rheumatoid arthritis and systemic lupus erythematosus (SLE), present therapeutic challenges to the critical care clinician. There may be concerns about the role of NSAIDs in the causation of the acute problem, especially gastrointestinal bleeding and fluid retention disorders. NSAIDs are an important component of the therapeutic regimen for the synovitis of inflammatory arthritis and for serositis involving pleural or pericardial membranes.[54,57] Discontinuation of NSAID therapy can result in a significant increase in synovitis. The anti-inflammatory effects of NSAIDs often require higher doses than those needed for a chronic analgesic response. No significant differences in effectiveness in suppressing inflammation have been demonstrated among the various nonselective and COX-2–selective agents.[58-61] However, because of their more favorable side-effects profile, COX-2–selective inhibitors have become increasingly used in these rheumatic disease states.

Acute crystal-induced arthritis, including gout and pseudogout, are common problems in critically ill patients. Inflammation, in response to uric acid and calcium pyrophosphate dihydrate crystals, respectively, is induced by immune mediators such as PGs, cytokines, bradykinin, and leukotrienes, which produce capillary dilation, neutrophil migration, and pain stimulation. NSAIDs, especially indomethacin, have been shown to be very beneficial in acute crystal-induced arthritis.[55,56] Aspirin should not be used for gout because it influences renal tubular uric acid excretion, thereby causing fluctuations in serum uric acid levels, potentially aggravating acute gouty arthritis. Because NSAIDs are administered only orally and can be toxic, their use is limited in the critical care setting. Alternative treatments for crystal-induced arthritis include corticosteroids and colchicine for gout.

Occasionally, acutely ill patients require NSAID therapy for its anti-inflammatory and analgesic properties because of concurrent regional musculoskeletal disorders such as shoulder or elbow tendonitis or back problems.[62,63] Finally, NSAIDs have been used to treat pleuropericarditis of nonrheumatic origin, including viral serositis and the postmyocardial infarction (Dressler's) syndrome.

CARDIOVASCULAR PROTECTION

Abnormalities within the cardiovascular system are frequently present in critically ill patients. Because PGs play pathophysiologic roles in coagulation and inflammatory mechanisms involved in cardiovascular diseases, NSAIDs, especially aspirin, have an important therapeutic potential. TXA_2, synthesized by platelets, is produced by COX-1 (together with another enzyme, thromboxane synthase); it promotes platelet aggregation on abnormal vascular endothelium and in areas of vascular stasis, leading to thrombosis. All nonselective NSAIDs inhibit COX-1; however, only aspirin does so irreversibly through acetylation.[64] The U.S. Preventative Services Taskforce reviewed the use of aspirin for the primary prevention of cardiovascular events. The 5-year coronary heart disease risk was stratified based on patient characteristics and included men older than 40 years of age, postmenopausal women, younger persons with diabetes or hypertension, and cigarette users. The Taskforce recommended use of low-dose aspirin (81 to 325 mg/day) for high-risk patients (i.e., 5% risk within 5 years) to reduce cardiovascular events, including nonfatal myocardial infarction, fatal coronary heart disease, and nonhemorrhagic stroke.[65] For those individuals with a lower risk of having a coronary heart disease event, the benefit was negated by the toxic effects of aspirin, including gastrointestinal events and hemorrhagic stroke. For secondary prevention in individuals who have had a myocardial infarction, The American College of Cardiology and the American Heart Association recommend low-dose, long-term aspirin therapy.[64]

Although other nonselective NSAIDs reversibly inhibit the COX-1 enzyme in platelets, they have not been demonstrated to reduce cardiac events and currently should not be used for primary or secondary prevention of vascular disease. Recent reports have shown a reduction in the incidence of myocardial infarction with naproxen use in high-risk patients; however, further data are needed to establish the role of this drug in cardiovascular prevention.[66-69] Another report hypothesized that coadministration of aspirin and ibuprofen may negate the cardioprotective effects of aspirin because of competitive binding at COX-1 catalytic receptor sites.[70] Finally, although COX-2–dependent PG production also occurs at sites of inflammation, including atherosclerotic plaques, clinical trials of celecoxib and rofecoxib have not demonstrated cardiovascular benefits.[71,72]

Aspirin has been compared with adjusted-dose warfarin for the prevention of stroke in atrial fibrillation. The Sixth American College of Chest Physicians (ACCP) Consensus Conference on Antithrombotic Therapy recommended that drug selection in atrial fibrillation be based on risk likelihood: adjusted-dose warfarin for patients with a high risk of stroke, aspirin or adjusted-dose warfarin for those with a moderate risk; and aspirin for those with a low risk.[73,74] The risk for stroke is increased by a history of prior stroke, systemic embolus, hypertension, poor left ventricular systolic function, age greater than 75 years, rheumatic mitral valvular disease, or a prosthetic heart valve.[73] Although both adjusted-dose warfarin and aspirin confer significant stroke reduction with atrial fibrillation, their concomitant use does not impart greater benefit and increases side effects.[73,74]

Aspirin therapy, alone or in combination with dipyridamole, can delay the progression of established arterial occlusive disease in patients with chronic lower-extremity arterial insufficiency.[75] Low-dose aspirin is beneficial in preventing morbidity and mortality from stroke and myocardial infarction in patients with peripheral arterial disease.[65,75,76] In addition, low-dose aspirin is used as prophylaxis and treatment for ischemic cerebrovascular disease, alone and in combination with dipyridamole, and has been demonstrated to reduce the risk of stroke in individuals with transient ischemic attacks or completed ischemic strokes due to thrombosis.[77]

FEVER

The mechanisms of fever involve either the peripheral release of pyrogenic cytokines (IL-1, IL-6, tumor necrosis factor, and interferon-α) from monocytes and macrophages or the presence of circulating endotoxins, which stimulate the central production of PGE_2 via COX-2 in vascular endothelial cells. PGE_2 targets hypothalamic thermoregulatory neurons.[78-80] Knockout mice lacking the COX-2 enzyme are unable to mount a fever when exposed to exogenous pyrogens.[78,79] The COX-1 enzyme is not involved in thermal regulatory control.[78]

Aspirin has long been recognized as an effective antipyretic agent, and it is the "gold standard" with which acetaminophen and other NSAIDs are compared. Studies evaluating the antipyretic properties of NSAIDs are primarily from the pediatric literature. A meta-analysis of adult fever trials has not been possible because of differences in patient populations, NSAID dosing schedules, and outcome measures. However, studies in adults have shown equal or superior antipyretic efficacy of NSAIDs compared with acetaminophen.[79] NSAIDs are more effective in reducing fevers associated with cancer than those caused by infection, although the mechanism is not clear.[79] The duration of action of various NSAIDs in fever is related to drug half-life and to drug concentration in the hypothalamus, a parameter that is determined by drug transport across the blood-brain barrier.[78] There are limited data evaluating the clinical use of COX-2–selective agents for fever; however, a beneficial effect has been demonstrated.[79,81,82] Toxicities of the various nonselective NSAIDs limit their clinical utility compared with acetaminophen, especially in critically ill patients.[79,82]

SEPTIC SHOCK

Septic shock is a clinical syndrome that can occur with bacterial sepsis that results in inadequate tissue perfusion and an associated excessive or dysregulated host inflammatory response.[83] Limited animal data have shown that NSAIDs can significantly decrease the morbidity and mortality associated with sepsis.[84] However, the benefit of anti-inflammatory agents, including NSAIDs, in reducing the mortality associated with sepsis in humans has not been demonstrated in clinical trails.[83] The Ibuprofen in Sepsis Study Group evaluated the impact of ibuprofen on organ failure and mortality in 455 patients with sepsis syndrome. Significant improvements in temperature, heart rate, oxygen consumption, and lactic acidosis were noted, but there was no reduction in organ failure or 30-day mortality compared with standard care. Although ibuprofen and other NSAIDs have some physiologic effects in sepsis, they do not reduce morbidity and mortality in septic shock, except possibly in patients with hypothermia.[84,85]

TOXICITY OF NSAIDs

GASTROINTESTINAL TOXICITY

PGs play a critical role in maintenance of the gastrointestinal mucosal barrier. Beneficial effects include maintenance of epithelial mucus secretion, mucosal blood flow, bicarbonate secretion, and epithelial proliferation. These protective mechanisms may be altered by NSAID-mediated inhibition of PG synthesis and local mucosal damage by the acidic NSAID compounds.[86] The spectrum of gastrointestinal injury includes mucosal irritation and ulceration in the stomach and small intestine with bleeding and perforation.

Gastroduodenal lesions, including erosions on endoscopy and ulceration, have been reported in 20% to 40% of NSAID users who took the medication for 1 month or longer. Serious gastrointestinal complications, including ulceration, perforation, and bleeding, occur in 1% to 2% of short-term NSAID users and in 2% to 5% of patients on chronic NSAID therapy.[87] Gastrointestinal lesions related to NSAIDs frequently are asymptomatic. For example, approximately 40% of patients with endoscopically proven gastritis do not have symptoms.[87,88] Other studies confirm the occurrence of NSAID-induced gastrointestinal toxicities, although the reported incidences vary depending on the characteristics of the study population and the evaluation tools used.[87] The Arthritis, Rheumatism, and Aging Medical Information System (ARAMIS) prospectively evaluated outcomes including adverse effects from NSAID therapy in more than 36,000 patients with osteoarthritis or rheumatoid arthritis from 17 centers in the United States and Canada, accounting for more than 300,000 patient-years.[87] Based on this study population, it was calculated that more than 16,000 NSAID-related deaths could occur yearly in the United States, a number that is similar to the death rate for leukemia and that exceeds the rates for malignant melanoma and asthma.[87]

When a critically ill patient is prescribed either nonselective or COX-2–selective therapy, evaluation of their gastrointestinal toxicity profile is essential. Evidenced-based risk factors for gastrointestinal toxicity with use of nonselective NSAIDs include age greater than 65 years; history of previous upper gastrointestinal ulcers or upper gastrointestinal bleeding, and use of corticosteroids, oral anticoagulants, or high-dose NSAIDs.[89-94] Data have also implicated cigarette smoking, alcohol use, and *Helicobacter pylori* infection as possible risk factors for nonselective NSAID–related gastrointestinal toxicity.[86,95] Although both NSAIDs and *H. pylori* infection influence gastric PG production, the relative gastrointestinal risk is controversial. If a patient is *H. pylori*–positive, consideration for eradication of the infection should be made before NSAID therapy is initiated.[96] Low-dose aspirin increases the occurrence of serious gastrointestinal complications if it is given concomitantly with either nonselective or COX-2–selective NSAIDs because of the COX-1–inhibiting and local effects of the aspirin.

Individuals with an increased likelihood of developing nonselective NSAID–related gastrointestinal toxicities may benefit from COX-2–selective agents, which have demonstrated a more favorable gastrointestinal risk profile.[89-94] Gastrointestinal toxicity with both nonselective and COX-2–selective agents increases in patients older than 50 years of age; however, COX-2–selective agents pose a lower risk.[89] In patients who are at low risk for gastrointestinal toxicities, the preferential use of COX-2–selective agents is not warranted.[89]

The CLASS[97] and VIGOR[98] studies are landmark NSAID safety trials that compared the gastrointestinal side effects of the COX-2–selective agents celecoxib and rofecoxib, respectively, with those of nonselective NSAIDs.[97,98] The primary outcome endpoints of the CLASS study (ulceration, perforation, and bleeding) were similar for celecoxib compared with ibuprofen or diclofenac, whereas the VIGOR trial showed a statistically significant decrease in primary endpoints (ulceration, perforation, bleeding, and symptomatic ulcers) for rofecoxib compared with naproxen. However, after consideration of symptomatic ulcers was added to the primary analysis of CLASS data, a significantly lower incidence of gastrointestinal toxicity was found with celecoxib. In addition, a subanalysis of CLASS that excluded patients receiving concomitant low-dose aspirin therapy revealed a significantly lower rate of gastrointestinal complications with or without inclusion of symptomatic ulcer in the celecoxib group. Nonetheless, the U.S. Food and Drug Administration still requires celecoxib and rofecoxib to carry gastrointestinal warning labeling similar to that required for nonselective NSAIDs. Differences in study methodology (study duration, subject selection, primary and secondary outcome endpoints), patient population (osteoarthritis and rheumatoid arthritis in CLASS, rheumatoid arthritis in VIGOR), and concomitant therapy (no aspirin in VIGOR) precluded making valid comparisons between the CLASS and VIGOR data. With valdecoxib, the most recently introduced COX-2 agent, gastrointestinal endoscopic studies with therapeutic and supratherapeutic doses have demonstrated lower rates of gastroduodenal ulcers compared with nonselective NSAIDs.[99] Currently, there are very limited published data evaluating the clinical gastrointestinal profile of valdecoxib.

For the critically ill patient who is experiencing gastrointestinal problems and taking nonselective or COX-2–selective NSAIDs, proper evaluation of the gastrointestinal tract is imperative and usually requires upper gastrointestinal endoscopy. Furthermore, additive bleeding risks (e.g., heparin, other anticoagulants) and underlying disease-related factors are often introduced in the critical care setting. The mortality rate for NSAID-induced ulceration and bleeding is approximately 10%.[88] The first step in the management of NSAID-related gastrointestinal ulcers is discontinuation of the NSAID therapy.

Pharmacologic treatment options have focused on the inhibition of acid secretion and the replacement of PG deficiency; these options include proton pump inhibitors, histamine$_2$-receptor antagonists, misoprostol, and protective barrier agents.[100-102] Suppression of acid by histamine$_2$-receptor antagonists can effectively heal gastric and duodenal ulcers on discontinuation of the NSAID.[100] If NSAID therapy must be continued, the rate of ulcer healing with histamine$_2$-receptor antagonists is decreased.[88] Proton pump inhibitors markedly suppress acid secretion and are very effective at healing gastric and duodenal ulcers, even if the NSAID is continued.[100] Proton pump inhibitors and misoprostol have been shown to be superior to histamine$_2$-receptor antagonists for gastric ulcer healing.[100,101] However, because misoprostol often is not well tolerated, its role in clinical practice is limited. Comparative studies of omeprazole, ranitidine, misoprostol, and sucralfate demonstrated a therapeutic advantage of the proton pump inhibitor that ranges from 10% to 40%.[100] For NSAID prophylaxis, proton pump inhibitors are superior to histamine$_2$-receptor antagonists in reducing the risk of both gastric and duodenal ulceration.[100,101] Although high doses of misoprostol and proton pump inhibitors are effective for preventing NSAID-induced gastric ulcers, misoprostol compliance is poor due to gastrointestinal side effects such as nausea and diarrhea.[102]

Monitoring for bleeding is another important factor in the critical care setting. The effects of aspirin and NSAIDs on fecal occult blood tests have been evaluated. Aspirin in doses less than 325 mg/day does not interfere with fecal occult blood testing and does not need to be discontinued during stool collection.[103] Typically, NSAID-induced fecal blood loss is dose-dependent and may correlate with the severity of endoscopically detected upper gastrointestinal lesions.[104] Fecal occult blood loss associated with COX-2 inhibitor therapy is reported to be similar to that observed with placebo.[104]

CARDIOVASCULAR AND RENAL TOXICITY

The risk of cardiovascular side effects with COX-2–selective agents compared with nonselective NSAIDs remains controversial. The VIGOR trial[98] reported a significant increase in the incidence of myocardial infarction for rofecoxib compared with naproxen, whereas the CLASS study[97] showed no difference in cardiovascular endpoints between celecoxib and ibuprofen or diclofenac. Differences in methodology between the studies, especially the fact that low-dose aspirin was not permitted in the VIGOR trial, make them difficult to compare. In addition, the antiplatelet effects of the nonselective NSAIDs may have influenced the results.

Both COX-1 and COX-2 are constitutively expressed in the kidney, predisposing to renal problems with either NSAID class. The adverse effects of nonselective NSAIDs and those of COX-2–selective agents on renal function appear to be similar.[105] NSAID-related renal toxicities most commonly include decreased glomerular filtration rate and decreased sodium excretion.[106] The deleterious effects of NSAIDs on renal homeostasis are most pronounced in patients with renal insufficiency and volume depletion. The risk of deleterious effects also is increased in patients with hypertension, congestive heart failure, edema, chronic renal failure, advanced age, or concomitant diuretic therapy.[105,106,108] Less commonly, patients present with NSAID-induced acute interstitial nephritis, which accounts for fewer than 2% of hospital admissions related to drug-induced renal failure.[106] Nephrotic syndrome and papillary necrosis have rarely been associated with chronic NSAID use. Although nephrotic syndrome is generally reversible, papillary necrosis, which occurs most often with NSAID overdose, can result in permanent renal impairment.[106] As with nonselective NSAIDs, the renal adverse effects of COX-2–selective agents tend to occur early in therapy and usually are reversible on discontinuation of the drug.[105,108]

Blood pressure elevation has been associated with both nonselective and COX-2–selective agents. Mean blood pressure increases of 3 to 6 mm Hg have been reported with short-term NSAID therapy, especially in patients with pre-existing hypertension. Patients with cardiovascular disease, hypertension, renal or hepatic insufficiency, or advanced age should be monitored for fluid retention, which can affect blood pressure during therapy with NSAIDs (including COX-2–selective drugs).[106,109] Data from studies of COX-2–selective agents indicate that there is a similar risk of hypertension, leading to labeling precautions for both COX-2–selective and nonselective NSAIDs, with additional precautions for higher doses of rofecoxib.[109,110] In addition, drug-drug interactions of nonselective NSAIDs or COX-2–selective inhibitors with antihypertensive agents, including angiotensin-converting enzyme (ACE) inhibitors, β-adrenergic blockers, and diuretics, may accentuate NSAID-mediated inhibition of renal PG production, thereby lessening antihypertensive efficacy.[13] Monitoring of hypertension, renal function, and edema is recommended for all patients on NSAID therapy, especially those with the risk factors noted previously.[106]

HYPERSENSITIVITY REACTIONS

Hypersensitivity reactions to NSAIDs occur rarely, and they are more common in individuals with nasal polyps or asthma. Allergic reactions, including bronchoconstriction, rhinitis, and urticaria, have been associated with all nonselective NSAIDs and COX-2–selective inhibitors. Recent data suggest a role of altered COX-2 regulation associated with the aspirin-intolerant asthma/rhinitis syndrome.[111] Because of the potential for cross-reactivity, avoidance of all NSAIDs is recommended in patients with a history of bronchoconstriction or allergic reactions to any NSAID. One exception is choline magnesium trisalicylate, which is well tolerated by aspirin-sensitive asthmatic patients.[112]

Various cutaneous reactions have been described with all NSAIDs, especially skin eruptions of a pustular, acneiform nature that are often pruritic. Cessation of NSAID therapy is usually required. Because of their sulfonamide-like chemical structure, celecoxib and valdecoxib should not be used in patients with a history of allergic cutaneous and other hypersensitivity reactions to sulfa drugs.[99,113] Rofecoxib has a sulfonyl structure and does not carry a sulfa cross-reactivity warning.

Other, less common adverse events associated with NSAIDs include hepatic abnormalities with elevated liver function tests, headache, confusion (especially in older individuals), sleep disturbances, and tinnitus. In rare cases, NSAIDs have been implicated in causing aseptic meningitis and, in children, Reye's syndrome.[13,28]

DRUG-DRUG INTERACTIONS

Drug-drug interactions, especially with regard to toxicity, are important considerations when initiating therapy with NSAIDs in the critical care setting or managing treatment in a patient who is already taking an NSAID. Drug-drug interactions with NSAID therapy may result from their pharmacodynamic properties (e.g., inhibition of COX and related effects on gastrointestinal mucosa, kidneys, and platelets) or their pharmacokinetic properties (e.g., protein binding, drug metabolism).

Nonselective NSAIDs affect other antiplatelet agents via additive inhibition of platelet aggregation. The result is an increased bleeding risk with the concomitant use of NSAIDs and other antiplatelet agents, such as heparin, low-molecular-weight heparin, warfarin, clopidogrel, ticlopidine, lepirudin, and argatroban.[13,114] Similarly, concurrent therapy with drotrecogin-α (activated) and NSAIDs must be undertaken cautiously, especially with aspirin at a dose greater than 650 mg or with other NSAID agents.[115] A COX-2–selective NSAID may be administered concurrently with warfarin with caution and appropriate monitoring.

Significant drug-drug interactions have been documented with use of NSAIDs and lithium. Both nonselective and COX-2–selective NSAIDs decrease lithium clearance and increase serum lithium concentrations by inhibiting renal PG production and altering intrarenal blood flow. Serum lithium levels and the clinical signs and symptoms of bipolar disorder should be evaluated in patients with concomitant NSAID use.[13,114]

Data are conflicting regarding the drug-drug interaction potential of ACE inhibitors and NSAIDs. Mixed results of significant drug interactions have been noted in hypertension, coronary artery disease, and congestive heart failure

trials, particularly with doses of aspirin greater than 325 mg/day.[116] In patients with congestive heart failure, ACE inhibitors increase bradykinin production, resulting in increased synthesis of the vasodilating PGs, prostacyclin and PGE_2, which reduces cardiac afterload. By blocking COX and inhibiting the production of PGs, NSAIDs may antagonize the beneficial vasodilatory effects of ACE inhibitors, leading to decreased cardiac output and worsening of heart failure.[118,119] In addition, concurrent use of ACE inhibitors and NSAIDs may reduce the beneficial effects of renal PGE_2 on sodium excretion produced by ACE inhibitors.

Concurrent administration of digoxin and NSAIDs can decrease renal clearance of digoxin, increase plasma drug concentration, and potentate digoxin toxicity.[114]

NSAIDs interact with anticonvulsant agents, such as phenytoin and valproic acid, by displacing the anticonvulsants from their protein-binding sites, which increases the free drug concentration and the potential for anticonvulsant toxicity.[114]

Combination use of corticosteroids and aspirin can increase renal clearance of salicylate and significantly decrease plasma salicylate concentrations. Therefore, a potential for aspirin toxicity exists when tapering high-dose steroids. Appropriate monitoring is warranted, especially for gastrointestinal bleeding, because of increased salicylate concentrations.[114]

OVERDOSE

Despite the common use of NSAIDs in clinical practice, serious acute overdose and adverse sequelae are reported infrequently. The Toxic Exposure Surveillance System (TESS) annual report of poisoning data from the American Association of Poison Control Centers documented 27 deaths due to aspirin overdose in the year 2000.[119] The mechanism of NSAID toxicity in overdose is related to both their acidic nature and their inhibition of PG production.

Although NSAID overdose is uncommon, prompt recognition and management of overdose is important. With salicylate overdose, the severity typically depends on the dose ingested and the salicylate concentration that correlates with the degree of acid-base disturbance. Measurement of salicylate levels is important in all cases of aspirin overdose to guide management.[119-121] Serum salicylate levels should be measured 4 hours after ingestion and repeated in 2 to 4 hours to determine the peak concentration.[119,120] If the acute ingestion was with an enteric-coated product, salicylate levels should be monitored for 12 hours, because of the delay in absorption and time to peak concentration.[120] Generally, salicylate levels of 300 to 600 mg/L are associated with mild toxicity, 600 to 800 mg/L with moderate toxicity, and greater than 800 mg/L with severe toxicity.[119] For nonselective NSAIDs, plasma concentrations are not commonly measured and are less helpful, because the half-life of many of these agents is relatively short.[119]

Although patents with overdoses of aspirin and other NSAIDs may be asymptomatic depending on the amount ingested, common symptoms include nausea, vomiting, abdominal pain, tinnitus, hearing impairment, and CNS depression. With higher-dose aspirin ingestion, metabolic acidosis, renal failure, greater CNS changes (e.g., agitation, confusion, coma), and hyperventilation with respiratory alkalosis occur. The presence of acidemia permits more salicylic acid to cross the blood-brain barrier, with more severe

CNS toxicity.[120] In addition, salicylate toxicity can stimulate the respiratory center, leading to hyperventilation and respiratory alkalosis.[113] With other nonselective NSAID ingestions, symptoms are similar to those occurring with aspirin overdose.[119,121,122]

There is no antidote for salicylate or NSAID poisoning. Management varies depending on the amount of NSAID ingested and is directed at symptomatic support, prevention of further absorption, and correction of acid-base imbalance.[119,120] Appropriate hydration should be administered in all overdose situations. Although evidence is limited for the benefit of absorption therapy in aspirin overdose, activated charcoal is often administered within 1 hour after aspirin ingestion and repeated hourly for four doses until the salicylate levels peak.[93,119,120] Urine alkalinization increases salicylate elimination, especially in adult patients with salicylate levels of 600 to 800 mg/L and in the elderly.[119] Because of the relatively neutral pK of salicylic acid, increasing the urine pH from 5 to 8 is associated with a 10- to 20-fold increase in renal salicylate clearance. Infusion of 1 L of sodium bicarbonate (1.26%) over 3 hours is the recommended regimen for urine alkalinization. The circulating potassium level should also be evaluated because of the acidosis. Consideration of potassium replacement is recommended; however, administration of sodium bicarbonate should not be delayed until potassium levels are stabilized.[119,120] In severe cases of aspirin overdose, hemodialysis is effective at removing salicylate and correcting acid-base imbalances and has been shown to reduce morbidity and mortality. Hemodialysis should be considered in patients with salicylate levels greater than 800 mg/L and in the elderly. Hemodialysis also should be considered in patients with metabolic acidosis refractory to treatment, severe and symptomatic CNS toxicity (e.g., coma, convulsions), acute pulmonary edema, or acute renal failure.[119,120] Urinary alkalinization should be continued while hemodialysis is administered. Figure 199-1 provides a treatment algorithm for management of salicylate toxicity.

In nonaspirin NSAID overdose, management is also directed toward supportive care. In addition, activated charcoal is useful if administered within 1 hour after ingestion to patients who took more than 100 mg/kg body weight of ibuprofen or more than 10 tablets of other NSAIDs.[119] If renal insufficiency occurs with the overdose, NSAID accumulation is more pronounced.[121-123] Hepatotoxicity is more commonly seen with diclofenac overdoses, in female patients, in patients older than 50 years of age, and in patients with pre-existing autoimmune disease.[121]

SUMMARY

NSAIDs are a common class of medications that are used for a variety of pain indications and for fever in critically ill patients. In general, the lowest effective dose of the NSAID should be used for the shortest duration indicated. Before initiation of NSAID therapy, the following factors must be considered: diagnosis, patient characteristics, efficacy, side effects, and cost. Appropriate clinical and laboratory follow-up is necessary, especially for patients with changing organ function and those taking other medications known to increase bleeding potential. If a critically ill patient is receiving NSAID therapy at the time of presentation, appropriate monitoring of efficacy and toxicity is essential. When selecting an NSAID, the efficacy profile should be balanced with the toxicity profile and with patient characteristics to provide the most appropriate, safe, and cost-effective therapy.

ANNOTATED REFERENCES

Bombardier C, Laine L, Reicin A, et al: Comparison of upper gastrointestinal toxicity of rofecoxib and naproxen in patients with rheumatoid arthritis. N Engl J Med 2000;343:1520-1528.

This prospective, randomized, multicenter trial evaluated the gastrointestinal toxicity of rofecoxib and naproxen. Significant reductions in the primary outcome—perforation, ulceration, bleeding, and symptomatic ulcers—were seen with rofecoxib. A significant increase in myocardial infarction was seen with rofecoxib compared to naproxen. Concomitant aspirin use (e.g., cardioprotection) was not permitted in this trial.

Plaisance KI, Mackowiak PA: Antipyretic therapy: Physiologic rationale, diagnostic implications, and clinical consequences. Arch Intern Med 2000;160:449-456.

This review article focused on the role of NSAID therapy in the management of fever. Efficacy of NSAIDs in reducing fever results from their inhibition of the COX-2 enzyme. Studies report similar or improved antipyretic efficacy and similar toxicity with NSAID therapy compared to acetaminophen.

Silverstein FE, Faich G, Goldstein JL, et al: Gastrointestinal toxicity with celecoxib vs nonsteroidal anti-inflammatory drugs for osteoarthritis and rheumatoid arthritis the CLASS study: A randomized controlled trial. JAMA 2000;284:1247-1255.

This prospective, randomized, multicenter study compared the gastrointestinal toxicity (perforation, ulceration, bleeding) of celecoxib with those of ibuprofen and diclofenac. Although there was a trend toward reduction in gastrointestinal endpoints for the primary outcome, a significant reduction in gastrointestinal events was seen with celecoxib for the composite of ulceration, perforation, bleeding, and symptomatic ulcers. Concomitant aspirin use was permitted in this trial.

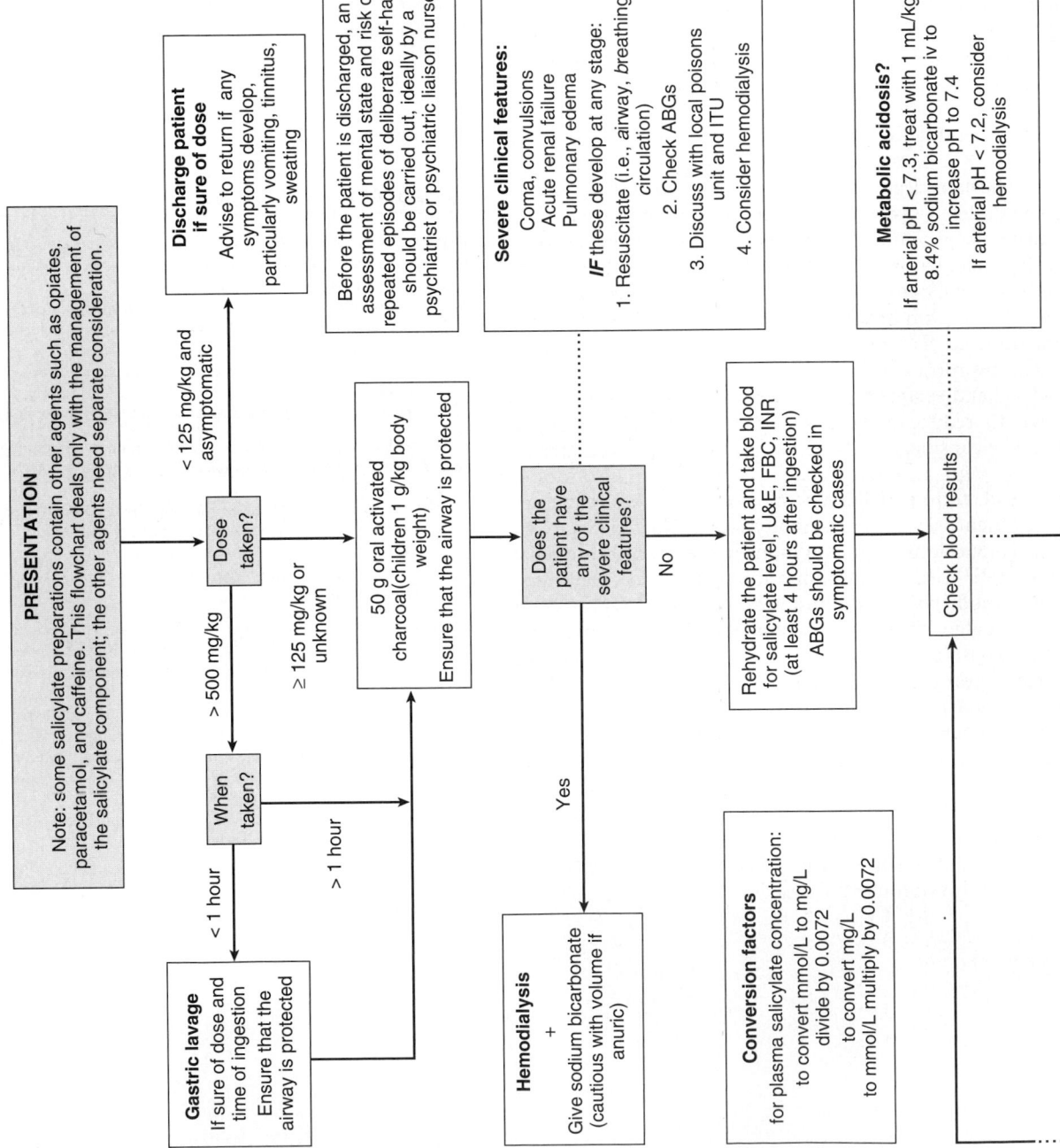

PRESENTATION

Note: some salicylate preparations contain other agents such as opiates, paracetamol, and caffeine. This flowchart deals only with the management of the salicylate component; the other agents need separate consideration.

Gastric lavage
If sure of dose and time of ingestion
Ensure that the airway is protected

When taken?
< 1 hour
> 1 hour

Dose taken?
> 500 mg/kg
≥ 125 mg/kg or unknown
< 125 mg/kg and asymptomatic

Discharge patient if sure of dose
Advise to return if any symptoms develop, particularly vomiting, tinnitus, sweating

Before the patient is discharged, an assessment of mental state and risk of repeated episodes of deliberate self-harm should be carried out, ideally by a psychiatrist or psychiatric liaison nurse

50 g oral activated charcoal(children 1 g/kg body weight)
Ensure that the airway is protected

Does the patient have any of the severe clinical features?
Yes
No

Hemodialysis
+
Give sodium bicarbonate (cautious with volume if anuric)

Severe clinical features:
Coma, convulsions
Acute renal failure
Pulmonary edema
IF these develop at any stage:
1. Resuscitate (i.e., airway, breathing, circulation)
2. Check ABGs
3. Discuss with local poisons unit and ITU
4. Consider hemodialysis

Rehydrate the patient and take blood for salicylate level, U&E, FBC, INR (at least 4 hours after ingestion)
ABGs should be checked in symptomatic cases

Conversion factors
for plasma salicylate concentration:
to convert mmol/L to mg/L divide by 0.0072
to convert mg/L to mmol/L multiply by 0.0072

Check blood results

Metabolic acidosis?
If arterial pH < 7.3, treat with 1 mL/kg 8.4% sodium bicarbonate iv to increase pH to 7.4

If arterial pH < 7.2, consider hemodialysis

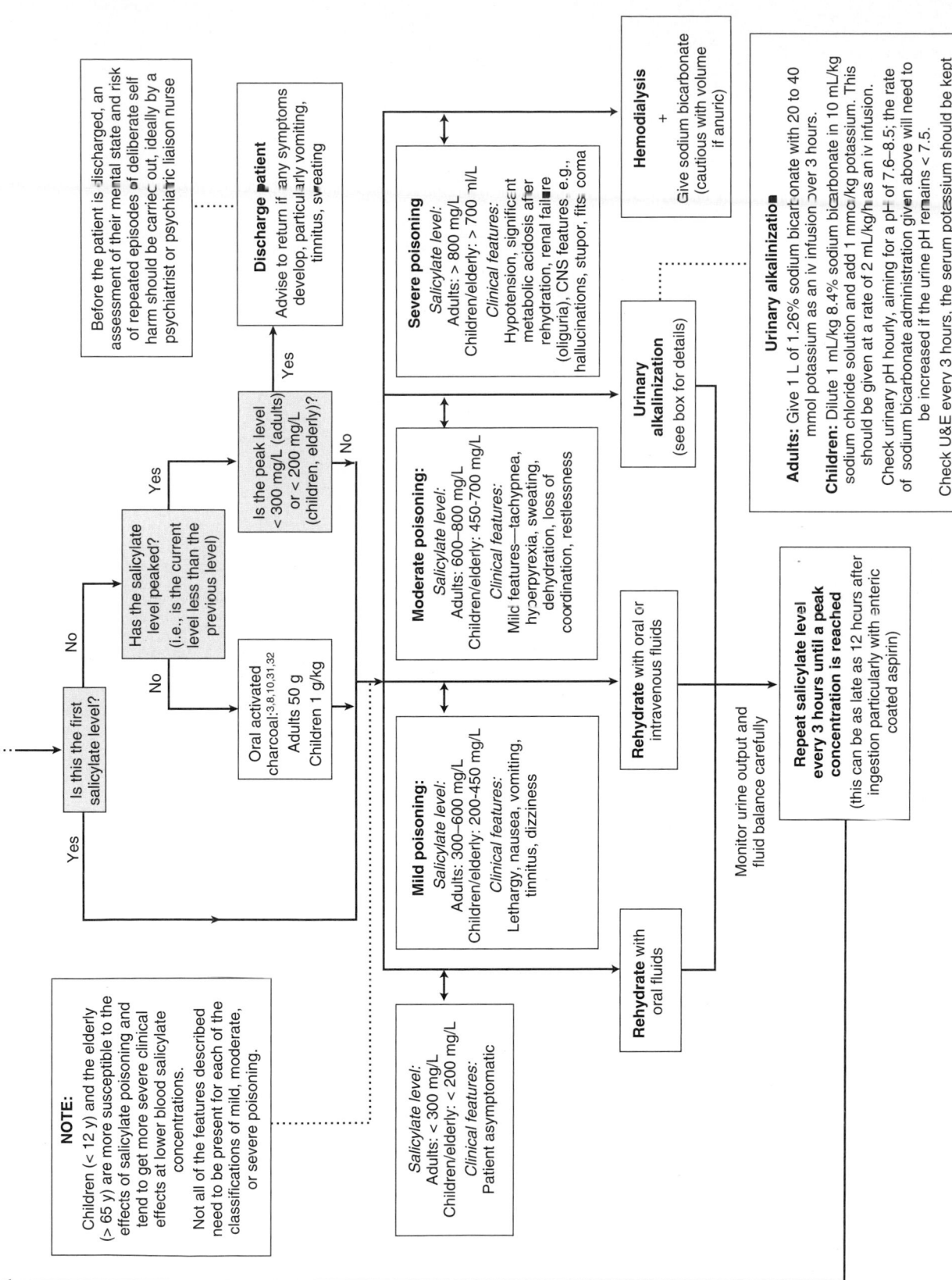

FIGURE 199–1. Evidence-based flowchart for management of salicylate poisoning. (From Dargan PI, Wallace CI, Jones AL: An evidence based flowchart to guide the management of acute salicylate (aspirin) overdose. Emerg Med J 2002;19:206-209, with permission of the BMJ Publishing Group.)

Chapter 200

OPIOIDS

Nicole C. Bouchard • Lewis S. Nelson

KEY POINTS

1. Most opioids and their metabolites are **cleared renally** and require dosing adjustments in patients with renal failure and in the elderly.

2. If tolerance and dependence to opioid analgesics exist, patients may require very large doses to achieve a therapeutic effect. Most patients can be effectively treated **if clinical guidelines for opioid prescription are followed.**

3. **Appropriate use of naloxone to reverse symptoms of respiratory depression** can prevent intubation in most cases of opioid toxicity. The suggested doses are 0.05 mg intravenously (i.v.) rapidly titrated to adequate respirations in tolerant patients and 1 to 2 mg i.v. in nontolerant patients and children.

4. The **empiric use** of high-dose (0.4 to 2 mg) naloxone often precipitates a dramatic antagonist-induced withdrawal in the opioid-tolerant patient. This can be associated with vomiting, aspiration, catecholamine surge, and severe agitation.

5. Opioids can have synergistic effects on central nervous system depression and blood pressure **if used with other sedatives.**

6. **Meperidine should be used with caution, if at all**, because accumulation of its metabolite is associated with seizures. It is also associated with serotonin syndrome in patients taking proserotoninergic medications.

HISTORY

Few medicines have graced history as have opium and its derivatives. Sumerians are said to have used and cultivated the opium poppy as early as the third millennium BC. Further accounts of its religious and medicinal use are recorded in manuscripts dating back to ancient Egyptian, Greek, and Roman times. Opium is obtained from the opium poppy, *Papaver somniferum*. Incision of the mature seedpod yields opium, a brown, sap-like gum. Crude opium contains as many as 20 other alkaloids, including approximately 10% morphine and 0.5% codeine.

In 1806, a German pharmacist, Sertürner, isolated the active alkaloid from opium and named it morphine, after Morpheus, the Greek god of dreams. In 1874, heroin was first synthesized from morphine and subsequently marketed as an opioid more potent than morphine and free of abuse potential. The invention of hypodermic needles revolutionized surgery and created a new avenue for abuse. In 1914, in the United States, the landmark Harrison Narcotic Act was passed, prohibiting the nonmedicinal use of opioids. Opioids have remained a cornerstone of both medical care and the world pandemic of drug abuse.

NOMENCLATURE

The term *opiate* refers specifically to opioids derived directly from the opium poppy, namely morphine and codeine, whereas the broader term *opioid* encompasses a wide range of compounds that display opium-like effects by binding to opioid receptors. The opioids include all of the natural opiates as well as semisynthetic opioids (e.g., oxycodone, heroin) and synthetic opioids (e.g., meperidine, methadone). The term *narcotic* has classically been used in association with illicit drugs of abuse, not necessarily opioids. In the strictest use of the word, "narcotic," derived from the Greek *narcosis,* refers to a drug that induces a somnolent state.

PHARMACOLOGY AND RECEPTOR PHYSIOLOGY

Opioids act as agonists to opioid receptors at presynaptic and postsynaptic sites in various regions of the brain and spinal cord, including the periaqueductal gray area of the brainstem, amygdala, corpus striatum, thalamus, and medulla, as well as the substantia gelatinosa (dorsal/posterior horn) in the spinal cord. Opioid receptors are also found in peripheral tissues at afferent pain neurons, in the smooth muscle of the gastrointestinal tract, and intra-articularly. Agonism at opioid receptors decreases neurotransmission through pain neurons both in the periphery and in the spinal cord. Opioid receptor agonism also diminishes the brain's perception of pain. This reduction in nerve transmission occurs through alteration of the release of neurotransmitters, such as acetylcholine, norepinephrine, dopamine, serotonin (5-HT), glutamate, and substance P. Decreased neurotransmission is thought to be secondary to membrane hyperpolarization or decreased neurotransmitter release from presynaptic vesicles or both.[1]

Three major classes of opioid receptors have been identified: mu, delta, and kappa. All of these receptors are G protein coupled and have seven transmembrane receptors with significant sequence homology. Opioid receptor agonists and antagonists interact with one or more of these receptors with

TABLE 200–1. OPIOID RECEPTOR SUBTYPES AND THEIR ASSOCIATED CLINICAL EFFECTS

Traditional notation	mu_1	mu_2	delta	$kappa_{1,2,3}$
IUPHAR notation	OP_{3a}	OP_{3b}	OP_1	$OP_{2a,b,c}$
Endogenous ligand	Endorphins	Endorphins	Enkephalins	Dynorphins
Effect	Analgesia (supraspinal and peripheral), sedation, euphoria, urinary retention, miosis, hypothermia	Analgesia (spinal), respiratory depression, bradycardia, physical dependence, gastrointestinal effects, pruritus, growth hormone release	Analgesia (spinal and supraspinal), antitussive effect, modulation of mu receptor function, inhibition of dopamine release	Analgesia (spinal and supraspinal) antitussive effect, psychotomimesis, dysphoria, miosis, diuresis

IUPHAR, International Union of Pharmacology.
From Dhawan BN, Cesselin F, Raghubir R, et al: International Union of Pharmacology. XII. Classification of opioid receptors. Pharmacol Rev 1996;48:567-592.

varying affinities.[1,2] This Greek-derived nomenclature is commonly used by most of the scientific community. In 1996, the International Union of Pharmacology (IUPHAR) recommended a new nomenclature for opioid receptors, with the intention of creating consistency in naming with other neurotransmitter systems (Table 200-1). The traditional Greek notations are used in this text. Several other new receptor subtypes have been identified. Their clinical significance and classification are unclear at this time.

PHARMACOKINETICS

ABSORPTION

Most opioids are well absorbed via the subcutaneous and intramuscular routes. Although gastrointestinal absorption tends to be rapid, the oral bioavailability of many opioids is limited by extensive first-pass hepatic metabolism. After large oral doses, first-pass metabolism can become saturated and oral bioavailability can be increased. Codeine and oxycodone are two opioids with very good oral bioavailability. The transdermal application of fentanyl is also used in clinical practice.

DISTRIBUTION

Tissue uptake is variable and depends largely on the drug's lipophilicity. Highly lipophilic compounds, such as fentanyl, readily penetrate the central nervous system (CNS), the dura of the spinal column, and tissue "reservoirs." Opioids exhibit varying degrees of plasma protein binding and typically have large volumes of distribution. Serum concentrations of opioids should not be used as a gauge of clinical effect, because fat, skeletal muscle, lungs, and viscera act as reservoirs after opioid administration. Redistribution from saturated tissue depots can produce persistent or recurrent sedation after discontinuation of prolonged infusions of certain opioids, such as fentanyl.[4,5]

METABOLISM

Hepatic metabolism of opioids, typically by the P450 cytochromes CYP3A4 and CYP2D6, can produce metabolites with either greater or lesser activity than the parent compound. For example, codeine is an active antitussive agent but an ineffective analgesic. The metabolism of codeine to morphine by CYP2D6 reduces its antitussive actions but markedly improves its analgesic properties. Morphine and its

semisynthetic derivatives are converted to polar glucuronide metabolites, some of which are active. Metabolism of certain opioids also occurs by similar mechanisms in extrahepatic sites, especially the kidneys.

ELIMINATION

Most opioids and their metabolites are cleared renally and require dosing adjustments in patients with renal failure. Biliary excretion is limited for most opioids.

CLINICALLY IMPORTANT EFFECTS IN THE INTENSIVE CARE UNT

Analgesia, euphoria, sedation, miosis, and respiratory depression are considered to be the classic opioid effects. In addition, opioids have many more clinically relevant effects, many of which are not typically relevant in the ICU setting; these are summarized by physiologic system in Table 200-2.

ANALGESIA

Opioids are modulators of pain perception both at the level of the CNS and in the periphery. High concentrations of opioid receptors (largely the mu type) are found in areas of the brain that are associated with analgesia. Cortical effects include decreased reception of painful sensory inputs and enhanced inhibitory outflow from the brain to the sensory nuclei of the spinal cord (dorsal root nuclei). In addition, there is decreased neurotransmission from peripheral afferent pain neurons to the spinal cord and from the spinothalamic tract to the brain. The net effect is decreased perception of nociceptive information. Analgesia is mediated by the mu, delta, and kappa opioid receptor subtypes (see Table 200-1). Morphine also appears to be an effective analgesic (via the mu receptor) when administered intra-articularly.[6,7] Tolerance develops to the analgesic effects with repeated use.

Very-low-dose naloxone (0.25 µg/kg/hour) improves the efficacy of morphine analgesia, whereas at higher doses (1.0 µg/kg/hour) analgesia is obliterated by naloxone. The mechanism of this effect is unclear.[8]

EUPHORIA

The euphoric effects of opioids are typically described as pleasant floating sensations accompanied by a decrease in anxiety and distress. Not all exogenous opioids induce the

TABLE 200–2. SUMMARY OF CLINICAL EFFECTS OF OPIOIDS BY PHYSIOLOGIC SYSTEM

System	Clinical Effect
Cardiovascular	Hypotension (vasomotor centers and histamine), bradycardia (first or second degree), dysrhythmias (overdose, propoxyphene), QRS prolongation (propoxyphene), QT prolongation (methadone)
Dermatologic	Urticaria, flushing, pruritus (centrally mediated)
Endocrinologic	Reduced release of antidiuretic hormone (controversial), reduced release of gonadotropin
Gastrointestinal	Nausea, vomiting (5-HT$_2$ mediated), delayed gastric emptying, constipation, increased smooth muscle tone (biliary tract, intestinal, pylorus, anal sphincter)
Genitourinary	Urinary retention, ureteral spasm, decreased renal function and renal blood flow, antidiuresis, priapism (neuraxial use)
Immunologic	Mast cell degranulation/histamine release, cytokine stimulation (IL-1), but true allergic reaction is rare
Maternal/Fetal	Placental transmission, neonatal blood-brain barrier immature, neonatal respiratory depression and opioid dependence, neonatal withdrawal (seizures)
Musculoskeletal	Truncal/chest wall rigidity and myoclonus (fentanyl derivatives)
Neurologic	Analgesia, euphoria, sedation, psychotomimesis, seizures (meperidine, propoxyphene, tramadol, rarely fentanyl)
Ophthalmic	Miosis, normal or dilated pupils (meperidine, pentazocine, diphenoxylate, propoxyphene, severe systemic hypoxia)
Pulmonary	Respiratory depression, antitussive effect, bronchospasm, pulmonary edema

5-HT, serotonin; IL, interleukin.

same degree of euphoria. Activation of the mu/delta receptor complex in the ventral tegmental area,[9] followed by dopamine release in the mesolimbic system, is most likely responsible for these effects.[10,11]

The degree of lipophilicity and CNS penetration is directly proportional to the euphoric properties of the opioid. For example, heroin, which enters the CNS with relative ease, is associated with greater euphoria than is the less lipophilic morphine.[12] Fentanyl produces euphoric effects akin to those of heroin[13] and is occasionally used as an adulterant in illicitly obtained heroin.[14] The apparently enhanced euphoric effect of meperidine may be related to its lipophilicity and its ability to alter serotonergic neurotransmission.

By contrast, pentazocine, an agonist-antagonist opioid (i.e., an agent that is both an agonist at kappa receptors and an antagonist at mu receptors), produces dysphoria and psychotomimesis, an effect that most likely is mediated via kappa$_2$ receptor agonism.[15] It can also induce a withdrawal syndrome in opioid-tolerant individuals secondary to its mu receptor antagonist effects.

SEDATION

Drowsiness and mental clouding are frequent in opioid-using patients. Different opioids are associated with different degrees of sedation despite equianalgesic dosing. Unlike sedative hypnotics, there is little or no associated amnesia unless the patient has been comatose. Electroencephalograms of opioid-sedated patients usually show slow delta waves that resemble sleep.

RESPIRATORY DEPRESSION

All opioid agonists produce dose-dependent depression of ventilation. In fact, at equianalgesic doses all opioid agonists lead to a similar degree of respiratory depression.[16,17] In the absence of secondary causes, death from opioid overdose is almost exclusively caused by respiratory depression.

Medullary mu$_2$ receptors are believed to be responsible for the development of respiratory depression.[18] Their agonism diminishes chemoreceptor sensitivity to hypercapnia, resulting in loss of hypercarbic ventilatory stimulation.[19] They also decrease the central response to hypoxia[19] and inhibit the medullary and pontine respiratory centers that regulate the rhythm of breathing.[17] The combination of these effects leads to prolonged pauses between breaths, periodic breathing, hypopnea, bradypnea, and, in extreme cases, apnea. It is important to note that the initial manifestation of respiratory depression may be a hypopnea, with or without a decrease in respiratory rate.[17]

Patients do not develop complete tolerance to the respiratory depressant effects of the opioids.[20] For example, patients enrolled in methadone maintenance therapy may experience chronic hypoventilation.[21] A ceiling effect on respiratory depression exists with partial agonist and agonist-antagonist opioids.[22]

Elderly and sleeping patients are more sensitive to the ventilatory depressant effects of opioids.[23] A strong painful stimulus can sometimes transiently overcome or prevent respiratory depression. Similarly, when pain is relieved, as in orthopedic reductions, respiratory depression may ensue. Bronchoconstriction can also occur, most likely as a result of histamine release as well as indirect effects on bronchiolar smooth muscle. Depression of ventilation may also occur in patients receiving neuraxial opioid administration; these effects may be delayed and may be accompanied by respiratory depression (see "Neuraxial Opioids").

SEIZURES

Seizures are rare with the therapeutic use of most opioids, the primary exception being tramadol. If they occur in the setting of an acute opioid overdose, they are likely to be secondary to hypoxia. Seizures are associated with meperidine, propoxyphene, and tramadol toxicity. These drugs are further discussed in a later section. In a mouse model, naloxone antagonized the convulsant effects of propoxyphene, but not those of meperidine or normeperidine.[24] Fentanyl-associated myoclonus may resemble seizure activity, but true seizures rarely occur with fentanyl.[25]

MUSCULOSKELETAL EFFECTS: TRUNCAL RIGIDITY AND MOVEMENT DISORDERS

The i.v. use of a number of opioids has been associated with motor abnormalities ranging from an increased tone to overt myoclonus involving the chest wall and other truncal muscles. This complication is seen when large doses of highly lipophilic opioids, such as fentanyl, sufentanil, or alfentanil, are administered rapidly by the i.v. route.[26] Whereas it was previously believed that opioid actions at the level of the spinal cord were responsible for this effect, it now appears that a central dopaminergic effect may be contributory.[27] Both naloxone[28] and neuromuscular blockade can overcome rigidity. Sufentanil (and possibly other agents) can cause closure of the vocal cords, leading to difficult bag-valve-mask ventilation.[29] As noted, myoclonic activity, resembling seizure activity, has been observed in patients receiving high-dose, rapidly-infused fentanyl.[25]

CARDIOVASCULAR EFFECTS

The peripheral arterial and venous dilation caused by opioids appears to be mediated by both central depression of vasomotor centers and histamine release.[30] Hypotension occurs more frequently in stressed individuals and in those with decreased intravascular volume. Histamine release occurs via non–immunoglobulin E–mediated mast cell degranulation.[31] Different opioids produce different degrees of histamine release; for example, meperidine and morphine produce much greater release of histamine than do fentanyl and sufentanil.[32] The severity of histamine response can be reduced by slowing the rate of infusion, and hypotension can be reduced by optimizing intravascular volume. Use of the Trendelenburg position and saline infusion are appropriate initial interventions for opioid-associated hypotension.

Bradycardia is occasionally associated with opioid use and is most often secondary to decreased excitatory stimulation and hypoxia. Primary opioid-induced bradycardia is more rare and is thought to be related to increased vagal nerve activity. Morphine may also exert direct slowing effects on the sinoatrial and atrioventricular nodes.

Overall, there are no consistent effects of opioids on cardiac output or the electrocardiogram. Wide-complex dysrhythmias and impaired contractility are associated with propoxyphene overdose via sodium channel blockade (class Ia antidysrhythmic effect). Illicit opioid use is sometimes associated with cardiac effects secondary to adulterants or co-ingestants; examples are quinine and cocaine ("speedball"), respectively. Chronic high-dose methadone use is associated with prolongation of the QT interval.[33]

EFFECTS ON CEREBRAL CIRCULATION

There are minimal effects on cerebral circulation except in the setting of respiratory depression with hypoventilation and increased arterial partial pressure of carbon dioxide ($PaCO_2$). Increased $PaCO_2$ causes cerebral vasodilatation and increased cerebral blood flow, both of which can increase intracranial pressure. This is of importance in treatment of head injuries or increased intracranial pressure from other causes. In the absence of hypoventilation, opioids actually can decrease cerebral blood flow and possibly intracranial pressure.

SPECIFIC AGENTS

Opioids are among the most widely used drugs in clinical practice. A comprehensive knowledge of their effects and therapeutic applications is essential for any intensive care provider. Table 200-3 summarizes specific agents used in clinical practice.

MORPHINE

Morphine is the prototypical opioid. Its pharmacologic effects are primarily caused by binding to the mu receptor and, to a much less extent, the delta and kappa receptors.

It is a potent analgesic with typical opioid side effects including sedation, respiratory depression, decreased gastric motility, nausea and vomiting, histamine release, and miosis. Despite its efficacy, morphine has relatively poor penetration into the CNS, largely because of its low lipid solubility.

The principal pathway of morphine metabolism is via glucuronidation in the liver and kidneys. The active metabolite, morphine-6-glucuronide, is more potent than morphine and is largely renally excreted.[34,35] Renal failure can lead to accumulation of this active metabolite, with unexpected toxic effects after even low doses.[36-38]

HEROIN

Heroin, also referred to as diacetylmorphine, is a highly lipophilic, semisynthetic opioid produced by acetylation of morphine. Heroin is a prodrug and is devoid of intrinsic opioid effects. It rapidly enters the CNS, where it is deacetylated to the active metabolite monacetylmorphine and morphine. Illicit heroin is typically administered by nasal insufflation, subcutaneous injection (i.e., "skin popping"), smoking, or i.v. injection. The practice of inhaling vapors from heroin heated in aluminum foil is termed "chasing the dragon"; it is associated with a rapidly progressive, irreversible spongiform leukoencephalopathy.[39-41]

MEPERIDINE

Meperidine is a synthetic opioid that acts at both mu and kappa receptors. At equianalgesic doses, its side effect profile is similar to that of morphine, with the exceptions of enhanced euphoria and pronounced orthostatic hypotension from vasodilation and histamine release.

Of special note is meperidine's extensive hepatic metabolism (90%) to normeperidine, a less potent analgesic that is renally eliminated. Normeperidine produces CNS excitation and is associated with myoclonus, delirium, and seizures. Metabolite accumulation occurs primarily in the context of escalating doses and renal failure.[42,43] Meperidine also blocks the reuptake of serotonin by presynaptic neurons in the CNS and by this mechanism may produce serotonin syndrome in patients who are taking monoamine oxidase inhibitors[44] or other proserotoninergic drugs (see "Drug Interactions").[45,46] The potential for these side effects, especially seizures, has led to a decline in the popularity of meperidine in many institutions.

Unique ICU uses for meperidine include suppression of shivering in postoperative patients and in those receiving blood products[47] or amphotericin. This effect is most likely mediated by changes in the shivering threshold.[48,49]

FENTANYL AND SUFENTANIL

Fentanyl, which has a rapid onset and a short duration of effect, is an important drug for use in the ICU. Its peak effect occurs within 6 to 7 minutes after i.v. administration. Its very short half-life results from rapid distribution into inactive tissues such as fat, lungs, and skeletal muscle. Prolonged infusions or massive doses may lead to accumulation of drug within these tissue reservoirs, resulting in prolonged duration of effect after discontinuation of the infusion. Lung uptake of up to 75% of a parenteral dose can occur and is often referred to as first-pass pulmonary uptake. Fentanyl is associated with

TABLE 200–3. SUMMARY OF OPIOIDS USED IN CLINICAL PRACTICE

Agent	Receptor Effect*	Preparations and Routes of Administration	Typical Doses	Comments
Natural and Semisynthetic Opioids				
Codeine[†]	mu > delta, kappa	PO, SC, IM, IV	Antitussive: 15 mg PO Analgesic: 60-120 mg PO	Mild to moderate pain, antitussive
Morphine (MSIR, MS Contin)	mu >> delta, kappa	PO, PR, SC, IM, IV, SR, NA	IR: 10-30 mg PO q4h CR: 30-200 mg PO q8-12h 0.1-0.2 mg/kg IM/SC or slow IV q4h PCA: see guidelines elsewhere in this section	Moderate to severe pain, prototype opioid, prolonged effects with CR formulations
Fentanyl (Oralet, Actiq, Duragesic patches, Sublimaze)	mu	PO (lollipop), transdermal, IV, NA	Lollipop: 5-15 μg/kg PO every dose Transdermal: 25-100 μg/h q72h Analgesia/procedures: 1-2 μg/kg IV General anesthesia: 2-20 μg/kg IV	Severe pain, very-short-acting (<1 h), truncal rigidity if administered rapidly by IV, can accumulate in tissue reservoirs
Sufentanil	mu	IV, NA	Analgesia: 0.1-0.4 μg/kg IV Anesthesia: 10-30 μg/kg IV	Severe pain, ultra-short-acting, vocal cord closure, favorable hemodynamics
Buprenorphine[‡] (Buprenex, Subutex, Suboxone)	partial mu agonist	SL, IM, IV	4-16 mg SL qd 0.3-0.6 mg IM/IV q6-8h	Moderate to severe pain, opioid replacement therapy
Synthetic Opioids				
Hydrocodone[†] (Vicodin, Norco)	mu	PO	2.5-10 mg PO q4-6h	Moderate to severe pain
Hydromorphone (Dilaudid)	mu	PO, SC, PR, IV, NA	2-4 mg PO q4-6h or 3 mg PR q6-8h 0.5-2 mg IM/SC or slow IV q4-6h	Moderate to severe pain
Oxycodone[†] (Percocet, OxyContin)	mu	PO	IR: 5 mg PO q6h CR: 10-40 mg PO q12h	Moderate pain, prolonged effects with CR formulations
Oxymorphone (Numorphan)	mu	SC, PR, IM, IV	1-1.5 mg IM/SC q4-6h 0.5 mg IV q4h	Moderate to severe pain
Propoxyphene[†] (Darvon)	mu, la antidysrhythmic	PO	65 mg PO q4h	Moderate pain, seizures, dysrhythmias, rhabdomyolysis
Meperidine (Demerol)	mu and kappa, 5-HT	PO, SC, IM, IV, NA	Analgesia: 50-100 mg IV q2-4h Shivering: 25-50 mg IV	Moderate to severe pain, treatment of shivering, seizures, serotonin syndrome
Methadone (Dolophine)	mu	PO, SC, IM	Analgesia: 2.5-20 mg PO/SC/IM q3-4h MMST: usually 20-200 mg PO QD	Moderate to severe pain, caution with repeat doses, long-acting (>24 h)
"Nonopioid" Opioids				
Tramadol (Ultram)	weak mu, inhibits NE and 5-HT reuptake	PO, IM, IV	Analgesia: 50-100 mg PO q4-6h Shivering: 1 mg/kg IV	Moderate pain, treatment of shivering, seizures
Dextromethorphan ("DM" cough preparations)	NMDA and 5-HT	PO	10-30 mg PO q4-6h	Antitussive, other psychoactive effects, poor response to naloxone, serotonin syndrome
Opioid Agonist/Antagonist Opioids				
Butorphanol (Stadol)	kappa agonist, mu antagonist	Intranasal, IM, IV	1-4 mg IM or 0.5-2 mg IV q3-4h	Moderate pain
Pentazocine[‡] (Talwin)	kappa agonist, mu antagonist	PO, IM, IV	50 mg PO q3-4h 30 mg IM/IV q3-4h	Moderate pain, dysphoria, opioid withdrawal in tolerant patients
Opioid Antagonists				
Naloxone (Narcan)	mu, kappa, delta antagonist	IM, IV, PO (very limited bioavailability)	Pruritus/analgesia[§]: 0.25 μg/kg/h IV Antidote: 0.05-2 mg IV q2-5min titrated to effect; use very low doses in tolerant patients	Antidote for reversal of opioid effect, use continuous infusions for overdose with CR opioids or body packer
Naltrexone (Trexan)	mu antagonist	PO	50 mg PO qd	Long-acting (>24 h)

CR, controlled release; 5-HT, serotonin; IM, intramuscular; IV, intravenous; IR, immediate release; MMST, methadone maintenance substitution therapy; NA, neuraxial; NE, norepinephrine; NMDA, N-methyl-D-aspartate; PCA, patient-controlled analgesia; PO, per os; PR, per rectum; SC, subcutaneous; SL, sublingual; SR, sustained release.
*Agonism unless specified.
[†]Preparations may also contain acetaminophen or acetylsalicylic acid.
[‡]May contain naloxone in some oral formulations as a deterrent to parenteral use of the drug.
[§]For use with continuous infusions of neuraxial opioids or PCA.

fewer cardiovascular effects and histamine release than either morphine or meperidine.[50] Fentanyl undergoes extensive hepatic metabolism to norfentanyl, an active metabolite that is renally eliminated. Prolonged effects can be seen in the elderly and in patients with renal impairment. Fentanyl-associated myoclonus may resemble seizure activity, however electrocardiograms recorded in these patients failed to show seizure activity.[25]

Sufentanil is a fentanyl analog with 5 to 10 times its analgesic potency. Sufentanil offers the advantage of even greater hemodynamic stability, and it is an analgesic of choice in cardiac surgery.[51-54] After cessation of a prolonged infusion, persistent sedation is not as prominent with sufentanil as it is with fentanyl. Sufentanil should be considered a practical and appropriate analgesic for use in the ICU.

METHADONE

Methadone is a synthetic opioid with high oral bioavailability and a prolonged duration of action (greater than 24 hours). Its most common use is in substitution therapy for opioid dependence. It is also used as an analgesic in patients with chronic pain and in postoperative analgesia. It is hepatically metabolized to inactive metabolites that undergo urinary and biliary excretion. Overall, its side effect profile resembles that of morphine. It is, however, associated with less euphoria and less sedation than other opioids. Tolerance to methadone may require escalating doses when it is used for prolonged period. Methadone at high doses may produce QT prolongation and torsades de pointes.[33]

BUPRENORPHINE

Buprenorphine is a partial agonist that has 50 times greater affinity for the mu receptor than does morphine. It is, therefore, relatively resistant to antagonism by naloxone and can displace other opioids from mu receptors. It is rarely used as an analgesic but is rapidly replacing methadone as the standard agent for substitution therapy in patients with opioid abuse (i.e., Subutex, Suboxone). Because it is a partial mu agonist, there may be less ventilatory depression associated with buprenorphine than with full agonist opioids[22]; in fact, a "ceiling effect" exists, in that no further respiratory depression occurs beyond a certain dose range.

NALOXONE

Naloxone is a pure competitive antagonist at mu, delta, and kappa receptors. It is commonly used in both prehospital and hospital settings to reverse opioid-induced respiratory depression. The typical prehospital use by emergency medical service personnel is in the range of 0.4 to 2.0 mg (intramuscularly or i.v.) for respiratory depression and coma. This extremely high dose often precipitates a dramatic and acute withdrawal in the tolerant individual. Vomiting, aspiration, and severe agitation are common with antagonist-precipitated acute withdrawal (see "Opioid Overdose"). Aspiration is a particular risk after use of naloxone in opioid-dependent patients who have secondary causes for their depressed level of consciousness. In these patients, naloxone produces vomiting but does not fully awaken the patient, predisposing to aspiration.

Some sources recommend the use of low-dose naloxone infusions (0.25 μg/kg/hour) to protect against ventilatory depression and to decrease symptoms of pruritus, nausea, and vomiting in patients receiving continuous opioid infusions, in addition to augmenting analgesia.[8] In the ICU setting, this approach may benefit patients who are receiving patient controlled analgesia (PCA) or neuraxial (i.e., epidural or spinal) analgesia.

Of note, orally administered naloxone has very poor bioavailability because of an extensive first-pass effect and therefore produces minimal if any systemic effects.[55] It is included in some oral analgesic preparations as a deterrent to parenteral abuse (see Table 200-3).

SPECIAL CLINICAL SITUATIONS

TOLERANCE, DEPENDENCE, AND WITHDRAWAL

Tolerance and dependence are inevitable features of chronic opioid use. *Tolerance* refers to decreasing effectiveness and the need for higher doses with repeated use, whereas *dependence* refers to the occurrence of withdrawal symptoms on cessation of the drug. Cross-tolerance exists between various opioids but is imperfect. Tolerance usually takes 2 to 3 weeks to develop with analgesic doses of morphine and can occur without dependence. Some mild degree of physical dependence can occur after as brief a period as 48 hours of continuous medication. This consideration is important in the care of patients using PCA devices and symptomatic heroin body packers.

Although tolerance, dependence, and abuse of opioids for the treatment of pain syndromes can be significant issues in clinical practice, undertreatment in patients with pain for fear of tolerance and dependence is a common mistake made by clinicians. The vast majority of patients can be effectively treated if clinical guidelines for opioid prescription are followed.[56,57] If tolerance and dependence to opioid analgesics exists, patients may require very large doses to achieve a therapeutic effect. Consultation with a pain management specialist may be warranted for such patients.

The opioid withdrawal syndrome comprises a unique cluster of symptoms. The syndrome includes yawning, lacrimation, piloerection, coryza, and restlessness initially, progressing to abdominal cramps, nausea, vomiting, and diarrhea. Altered mental status is only rarely present. The onset and duration of the withdrawal syndrome vary with the duration of effect of the implicated opioid. Although it can be extremely distressing to the patient, opioid withdrawal typically is not life-threatening. The exceptions are acute withdrawal precipitated by large doses of antagonist in dependent individuals and opioid withdrawal in the neonate. Treatment options for opioid withdrawal include supportive care, treatment with antiemetics and clonidine (a centrally acting α₂-agonist that diminishes CNS symptoms), or administration of an opioid agonist, typically methadone. The administration of morphine and/or replacement of the prescribed opioid may be sufficient in a patient who is withdrawing from opioids taken for chronic pain.

OPIOID OVERDOSE

The classic findings in patients with the opioid toxidromes are miosis, diminished bowel sounds, CNS depression, and respiratory depression, with coma and apnea in extreme cases. The major cause of death in opioid overdose is respiratory depression. Other complications are usually secondary to hypoxia (e.g., seizures, dysrhythmias, brain injury). Many patients with opioid overdose require admission to an ICU for monitoring, medical management, or respiratory support.

The appropriate use of naloxone to reverse symptoms of respiratory depression can prevent intubation in most cases. For example, for opioid overdose in an opioid-dependent patient (i.e., user of prescription analgesics, heroin, or methadone), a starting dose of 0.05 mg i.v. is indicated, using ventilatory support and rapid titration to higher doses if necessary. The endpoint of reversal should be adequate respiration, not complete reversal of sedation.[58] High doses of naloxone (e.g., 1 to 2 mg i.v.) may be used safely in children and in nontolerant individuals. Continuous infusions may be appropriate for patients who have overdosed with long-acting opioids.[59] Symptomatic opioid body packers (i.e., people hired to swallow large amounts of tightly wrapped heroin packets and smuggle them across international borders) are likely to require continuous naloxone infusions until the packets are passed or removed. Tolerance and dependence can occur in these patients if "leaking" is protracted. Body packers usually are not opioid users themselves.[60]

There is some suggestion that the catecholamine surge associated with rapid reversal with naloxone in tolerant individuals may precipitate acute lung injury (i.e., acute pulmonary edema). Dog models of opioid overdose suggest that hypercapnia may worsen the catecholamine release associated with naloxone administration hemodynamics.[61,62] Adequate ventilation to normalize $PaCO_2$ before antagonist administration is suggested to prevent hemodynamic instability. However, to date no single mechanism has been described for the development of opioid-associated pulmonary edema, and it is likely that multiple factors are involved. There is certainly an association between naloxone administration and the *diagnosis* of pulmonary edema. The typical clinical presentation is an obtunded patient with profound respiratory depression who awakens either spontaneously or as the result of antagonist administration. In these situations, it is likely that patients with heroin overdose developed acute lung injury as a result of their respiratory depression or apnea and that naloxone administration merely unmasked the effects by restoring spontaneous respirations.[63] This model proposes that hypoxic pulmonary endothelial damage may occur during near-apneic periods.

If acute withdrawal is precipitated, supportive care is recommended. Sedation of an agitated patient in acute withdrawal from naloxone very often leads to an even more profound sedation, requiring intubation when naloxone's effects wane in 30 to 45 minutes.

Many illicit drug users "co-ingest" other drugs of abuse, such as cocaine (i.e., speedball), amphetamines, and benzodiazepines with opioids. These other drugs may complicate the clinical presentation, and their toxic effects may be unmasked after the administration of naloxone. It is important to note that not all opioid-intoxicated patients present with miosis. Severe systemic hypoxia and presence of co-ingestants can produce normal-sized or dilated pupils.

Acetaminophen and acetylsalicylic acid (ASA) are common ingredients in analgesic combinations, and the presence of these drugs in the serum should be actively sought in any patient with a suicide attempt by overdose.

Consultation with a medical toxicologist or Poison Control Center is strongly recommended for all cases of opioid overdose, especially those involving body packers, continuous-release preparations, electrocardiographic changes, or severe respiratory depression.

DRUG INTERACTIONS

Opioids given in combination with either sedative-hypnotics (e.g., benzodiazepines) or propofol can have a synergistic effect on systemic vascular resistance,[64] level of sedation, and respiratory depression.[64-68]

Meperidine and dextromethorphan are associated with serotonin syndrome This syndrome typically develops in patients who are simultaneously taking two proserotoninergic drugs. Some commonly prescribed proserotoninergic drugs include monoamine oxidase inhibitors, selective serotonin reuptake inhibitors (SSRIs), valproic acid, lithium, clonazepam, and buspirone. Patients taking proserotoninergic drugs should not receive meperidine or dextromethorphan.[44-46] Morphine, fentanyl, and methadone are not associated with serotonin syndrome.

NEURAXIAL OPIOIDS

The term *neuraxial opioids* refers to the administration of opioids into the epidural or subarachnoid space ("spinal"). The use of neuraxial opioids is common in the care of postoperative and traumatized patients in an intensive care setting. To exert their clinical effects, opioids need to diffuse across the dura and gain access to the substantia gelatinosa of the spinal cord. Opioid receptors in the spinal cord are of the mu, delta, and kappa type.

Neuraxial opioids tend to be associated with fewer systemic effects when compared with orally or parenterally administered opioids. Some highly lipophilic opioids (e.g., fentanyl, sufentanil) diffuse into the systemic circulation so quickly that their use in neuraxial analgesia may offer little benefit over i.v. use. For other opioids, especially morphine and meperidine, systemic effects are usually caused by a combination of systemic absorption and cephalad migration of drug into the CNS. Typically, 5 to 10 times the dose used for spinal analgesia is required for epidural analgesia. Care should be taken to avoid inadvertent overdose by using epidural analgesia doses in the subarachnoid space.

The common side effects of neuraxially administered opioids are pruritus, nausea and vomiting, urinary retention (via inhibition with sacral spinal cord parasympathetic neurons), and ventilatory depression. Although early ventilatory depression rarely occurs, depression occurring within 2 hours after administration most likely represents systemic absorption of lipid-soluble opioid. Delayed respiratory depression can be seen as long as 6 to 12 hours after neuraxial administration and most likely represents cephalad migration of opioid to the CNS.[69]

In general, neuraxial use of opioids should be considered safe and effective. Care should be taken with their use, because they are not without CNS and systemic side effects. Most side effects respond to parenteral naloxone.

THE PATIENT WITH PAIN

In the ICU, analgesic requirements can be significant, and opioids are often chosen because of their efficacy and predictability. Morphine, hydromorphone, fentanyl, and sufentanil are among the most commonly used opioids in the ICU setting. All modes of delivery are associated with systemic side effects. A more complete discussion of analgesia may be found in Chapter 3.

SUMMARY

The use of opioids in the management of hospitalized and nonhospitalized patients is widespread, as is their abuse in the community. A solid understanding of their physiologic effects in therapeutic and toxic doses is essential for intensive care physicians. Withholding or underdosing of opioid analgesics in patients with pain due to fear of tolerance and dependence is not supported by the medical literature and should be strongly discouraged. Opioid-tolerant and -dependent patients do, however, have different treatment needs and require special attention by the medical staff. The appropriate use of naloxone, a short-acting antagonist, can prevent complications in many cases of opioid toxicity. Buprenorphine, a partial agonist-antagonist, is likely to replace methadone in many outpatient replacement therapy treatment programs, and physicians need to become familiar with its unique properties. Consultation with a medical toxicologist or Poison Control Center is recommended for management of complicated cases of opioid overdose.

ANNOTATED REFERENCES

Bailey PL, Egan TD, Stanley TH: Intravenous opioid anesthetics. In: Miller RD (ed): Anesthesia, Vol 1, 5th ed. Philadelphia, Churchill Livingstone, 2000, 273-376.
This chapter has an in-depth review of opioid physiology, pharmacodynamics, and pharmacokinetics, as well as concepts and applications that are applicable to both anesthesia and critical care settings.

Chaney MA: Side effects of intrathecal and epidural opioids. Can J Anaesth 1995;42:891-903.
This review is a thorough discussion of side effects that can occur with neuraxial opioid use.

Nelson LS: Opioids. In: Goldfrank LR, Flomenbaum NE, Lewin NA, et al (eds): Goldfrank's Toxicologic Emergencies, 7th ed. New York, McGraw-Hill, 2002, 901-917.
The opioid chapter in this text highlights the management of most forms of opioid overdose and features detailed information about the toxic effects of opioids and opioids of abuse. Details regarding proper dosing of naloxone and naloxone infusions are featured.

Reisine T. Opiate receptors. Neuropharmacology 1995;34:463-472.
This article is a classic review of opioid receptors and receptor physiology.

Traub SJ, Hoffman RS, Nelson LS: Body packing: The internal concealment of illicit drugs. N Engl J Med 2003;349:2519-2526.
This is article is a recent, in-depth review of management in opioid body packers.

Chapter 201

PESTICIDES AND HERBICIDES

Rick Kingston

KEY POINTS

1. General principles of management for many of the pesticide toxicities have changed in recent years, most notably related to use of gastric lavage, activated charcoal, and syrup of ipecac for gastric decontamination.
2. Mnemonics aid clinicians in recognizing the constellation of signs and symptoms associated with organophosphate poisoning and include:
   - DUMBELS (*d*iarrhea, *u*rination, *m*iosis, *b*ronchospasm, *e*mesis, *l*acrimation, *s*alivation)
   - SLUDGE (*s*alivation, *l*acrimation, *u*rination, *d*efecation, *e*mesis)
3. Severe poisonings from chlorphenoxy herbicides are rare, and management is aimed at supportive care, as there are no known antidotes.
4. Any ingestion of a concentrated solution of paraquat is potentially life threatening and must be aggressively treated.

The Environmental Protection Agency (U.S. EPA) broadly defines a pesticide as any substance or mixture of substances intended for preventing, destroying, repelling, or mitigating any pest. These agents are typically further classified according to their chemical, physical, or biologic class, or they can be categorized as acting on either animal pests or undesirable plants. In the context of intended use, the categories of *insecticide*, *herbicide*, and *rodenticide* are also commonly used and are often useful for reviewing toxicity profiles of agents most likely to be encountered in critical care medicine.

GENERAL PRINCIPLES OF MANAGEMENT

As with a variety of other toxic exposures, the general principles of management for many of the pesticides have changed in recent years. Most notably these changes have related to gastric decontamination, including use of gastric lavage, activated charcoal, and syrup of ipecac. Ipecac has largely been abandoned for routine use in either the prehospital or hospital care setting.[1,2] Its slow onset of action, incomplete return of toxin, and ability to cause emesis in an unconscious or seizing patient render it unacceptable for gastric decontamination.

Gastric lavage is still a preferred method of decontamination when a substantial amount of pesticide has been ingested and the patient presents within 60 minutes of ingestion.[3] Care must be taken to ensure that the patient's airway is protected with a cuffed endotracheal tube. Lavage should be performed using a large-bore orogastric tube with adequate aliquots of water or saline. Since recovery rates may be low, clinicians should evaluate the risk-to-benefit ratio for each patient. Although activated charcoal is the treatment of choice for most significant toxic ingestions, its value in cases of pesticide poisoning has not been systematically studied or proved.[4] Still, administration of activated charcoal is potentially beneficial, especially with extremely toxic substances, such as paraquat and diquat, or substantial ingestions of long-acting anticoagulant rodenticides. Patients must have active bowel sounds, and adults typically receive 25 to 100 g activated charcoal commercially available and premixed with sorbitol (first dose) or water (subsequent doses). Children and infants receive 25 to 50 g or 1 g/kg body weight of activated charcoal in commercially available and premixed solutions of sorbitol or water. Although repeat doses every 2 to 6 hours have also been used with anecdotal success, the safety of repeat doses containing sorbitol or other cathartics has not been established and care must be taken that electrolyte imbalances do not occur.

Because many pesticides have hydrocarbon diluents or vehicles, gastric decontamination must be cautiously attempted in only those patients likely to receive the greatest benefit. Hydrocarbon aspiration is a real concern, and attempts at most forms of gastric decontamination will likely increase the risk of occurrence.

Skin decontamination in cases of dermal exposure is indicated for all substantial exposures and should be carried out concomitantly with other life-saving measures. Care should be taken to remove contaminated clothing, avoiding contamination of emergency and health care personnel. Full decontamination of all exposed tissue should be carried out, using copious amounts of soap and water. Some agents, such as the fungicide chlorothalonil, are corrosive, and in cases of ocular exposure may require extensive eye washing and evaluation by an ophthalmologist.

SPECIFIC AGENTS

There are more than 3000 different formulations and 25,000 brand names of pesticides registered by the U.S. EPA.[5] A brief listing of those categories of agents most likely to be encountered in critical care medicine include the organophosphates, *N*-methyl carbamates, solid organochlorines, pyrethroids and pyrethrins, chlorophenoxy herbicides, paraquat, diquat, and a limited variety of commonly encountered agents with unique toxicology profiles.

INSECTICIDES

ORGANOPHOSPHATES

The primary toxicologic effects of organophosphate insecticides relate to their ability to phosphorylate acetylcholinesterase, thereby forming an irreversible covalent phosphate linkage with the serine residue of the active site. This inhibition effectively allows unopposed action of acetylcholine at nerve synapses, resulting in sustained depolarization of postsynaptic neurons. This action occurs both in the central nervous system (CNS) as well as the muscarinic sites in the peripheral nervous system, nicotinic sites in the sympathetic and parasympathetic ganglia, and nicotinic sites at neuromuscular junctions. Although organophosphate insecticides registered by the U.S. EPA are relatively selective for the cholinesterase found in insects, these compounds also affect mammalian acetylcholinesterase, especially when there has been exposure to a large amount or high concentration of the insecticide.[6] Acutely poisoned patients present with a range of signs and symptoms, depending on the dose and potency of the agent involved. Significant poisoning results in respiratory failure due to muscle weakness, excessive production of mucous secretions, and noncardiogenic pulmonary edema. Severe poisoning also can cause neurologic effects, including seizures, coma, or delirium, which result from cholinergic input in the midbrain and medulla. Dystonias, choreoathetoid movements, and fasciculations are also noted. Some organophosphates, such as the triaryl phosphates, can produce a delayed peripheral neuropathy, known as organophosphate-induced delayed neuropathy. This syndrome becomes apparent 1 to 2 weeks after acute poisoning.[7,8] A variety of cardiac arrhythmias also have been reported, including tachyarrhythmias, bradyarrhythmias, and torsades de pointes ventricular tachycardia. Diarrhea and vomiting are almost universally seen in cases of severe poisoning, along with excessive secretions of tears, saliva, and sweat. Numerous mnemonics have been devised to help clinicians recall this constellation of symptoms, including DUMBELS (*d*iarrhea, *u*rination, *m*iosis, *b*ronchospasm, *e*mesis, *l*acrimation, *s*alivation) and SLUDGE (*s*alivation, *l*acrimation, *u*rination, *d*efecation, *e*mesis).

An intermediate syndrome or type II toxicity also has been described. Patients with this syndrome exhibit paralysis of proximal limb muscles, neck flexor muscles, motor cranial nerves, and respiratory muscles without significant muscarinic symptoms. These effects are noted 24 to 96 hours after initial signs and symptoms and are believed by some experts to be the result of initial underdosing with the antidote.[9-12]

Diagnosis of organophosphate poisoning typically requires a clinical picture of cholinergic symptoms, onset of symptoms within 12 hours of exposure, a 50% reduction of plasma and red blood cell cholinesterase activity relative to baseline, and clinical improvement of muscarinic signs and symptoms with the administration of atropine.

The most severe cases of poisoning can be rapidly fatal if not aggressively treated. Atropine is the mainstay of treatment, and in some cases extremely large doses (>100 mg/day) are required to reverse muscarinic symptoms. Subsequent treatment with pralidoxime, which regenerates acetylcholinesterase by reversing phosphorylation of the active site on the enzyme, is also warranted in cases of moderate to severe poisoning with respiratory compromise or seizures or coma. Pralidoxime is used in combination with atropine because atropine only blocks the effects of acetylcholine at postsynaptic neurons but does not regenerate acetylcholinesterase. If the patient receives appropriate treatment and survives the first few hours, prognosis is good, even in severe cases of poisoning.

N-METHYL CARBAMATES

N-methyl carbamate insecticides share similar toxicologic effects with organophosphate insecticides in that both inhibit acetylcholinesterase. These insecticides differ from organophosphates in that they cause reversible carbamylation of the acetylcholinesterase enzyme. This carbamyl-acetylcholinesterase combination dissociates more readily than the organophosphate phosphoryl-acetylcholinesterase complex, resulting in a shorter duration of clinical effects, a wider range between doses, causing clinical effects and fatality, and diminished usefulness of blood cholinesterase measurements.

In cases of serious poisoning, patients demonstrate CNS depression with coma, seizures, and hypotonicity. Nicotinic effects, including hypertension and cardiorespiratory depression, are also common. Respiratory effects such as dyspnea, bronchospasm, bronchorrhea, and pulmonary edema, are also likely to be present.[13]

As in severe cases of organophosphate poisoning, treatment should be based on a high index of suspicion or history suggestive of either organophosphate or carbamate exposure and the presence of characteristic symptoms. Therapy should not be delayed, pending confirmation by blood cholinesterase testing. Cholinesterase testing may be of more limited value in patients with carbamate poisoning, depending on the timing of the sampling, because in vitro regeneration of acetylcholinesterase may render the results unreliable in confirming exposure.[14,15]

The initial treatment of choice is atropine, and, as in severe cases of organophosphate poisoning, large doses may be required to reverse symptoms of cholinergic crisis. Although pralidoxime may be relatively contraindicated in cases of carbamate poisoning because it could act as an additional competitive inhibitor of acetylcholinesterase, the risk of adverse effects is small in comparison to the potential benefit in cases of poisoning from an unknown cholinesterase inhibitor.

Prognosis in cases of carbamate poisoning is typically excellent when treatment is prompt and appropriate. In contrast to organophosphate poisoning, delayed or prolonged symptoms are not expected after treatment of carbamate poisoning.

SOLID ORGANOCHLORINES

The use of solid organochlorine compounds as insecticides has been sharply curtailed in recent years, and a number of U.S. EPA registrations have been cancelled. Many agents, including aldrin, dieldrin, benzene hexachloride, chlordane, and DDT, are no longer used. Still, a variety of agents remain on the market, including dicofol, dienochlor, endosulfan, lindane, and methoxychlor. Although serious poisoning from older, more toxic agents is less likely, occasionally, exposures to some residual products occur.

Cases of mild acute poisoning often result in CNS effects, including headache, dizziness, nausea, vomiting, incoordination, tremor, and mental confusion. More severe cases of poisoning cause convulsions but may be limited to myoclonic jerking movements.[16] Symptoms may progress to coma and respiratory depression. Cardiac irritability may result in arrhythmias.

Confirmation of poisoning is more likely to be made from a strong history of exposure because laboratory analysis is not routinely available and the results are difficult to interpret. Although severe cases of exposures may demonstrate correspondingly high blood levels, measurable low levels do not necessarily confirm poisoning.

Treatment of patients with severe poisoning is aimed at controlling convulsions and monitoring for respiratory compromise. Use of atropine, epinephrine, and other adrenergic amines should be used only if absolutely necessary because enhanced myocardial irritability predisposes to ventricular fibrillation.

PYRETHRIN/PYRETHROID

Pyrethrins (e.g., jasmolin, cinerin, pyrethrin) are naturally occurring esters of chrysanthemic and pyrethric acid, extracts of the *Chrysanthemum cinerariaefolium* flower. Pyrethroids (e.g., allethrin, bioresmethrin, cypermethrin, deltamethrin, fenvalerate, permethrin, phenothrin, resmethrin, tetramethrin) are synthetic pyrethrins, chemically modified to increase stability in the natural environment. A variety of different types of formulations are used for the control of insects on animals, in the house and garden, and in agriculture. Pyrethroids and pyrethrins interact with sodium channels in peripheral and central nerve cells to prolong the increase in permeability during the action potential excitatory phase of impulse transmission, resulting in failure of the cell to depolarize. In humans, rapid cleavage of an ester linkage along with oxidation to nontoxic metabolites limits toxicity. Pyrethrins and pyrethroids in their diluted form are poorly absorbed across intact skin and rarely result in toxicity. Despite limited absorption, an additional reason for low toxicity relates to rapid biodegradation by mammalian liver enzymes (ester hydrolysis and oxidation). Unless significant ingestion of more concentrated products occur, serious toxicity is unlikely. In rare cases of exposure to very large amounts, patients must be monitored for the development of neurotoxic effects, such as seizures.

OTHER AGENTS

A variety of other pest management agents registered for use in the United States include insecticides, acaricides, and repellents that have pharmacologic and toxicologic profiles that are distinct from those of carbamates and organophosphates. Agents such as boric acid are commonly involved in exposure but may not necessarily result in serious toxicity. Exposures to other agents including benzyl benzoate, chlordimeform, chlorobenzilate, and cyhexatin rarely result in significant poisoning. Diethyltoluamide (DEET) is used extensively as an effective insect repellent and rarely results in serious systemic poisoning unless large amounts are ingested.

HERBICIDES

CHLOROPHENOXY HERBICIDES

Chlorophenoxy compounds, such as 2,4-dichlorophenoxyacetic acid (2,4-D), MCPA, MCPB, MCPP, and 2-methyl-3, 6 dichlorobenzoic acid, are some of the most widely used herbicides in the U.S. market today. Fortunately, except for cases of massive intentional ingestion, severe poisoning is rare. Typical low-level exposures result in moderate irritation

to skin and mucous membranes and inhalations of sprays cause a burning sensation in the nasopharynx and chest. In cases of large deliberate ingestion, severe poisoning is associated with renal failure, acidosis, electrolyte disturbances, and multiple organ failure. There are no known antidotes, and management is aimed at supporting failed organ systems. Although forced alkaline diuresis has been used successfully, other measures, such as hemodialysis, have not been proved to be of benefit, probably because these compounds are highly protein-bound.

PARAQUAT

Paraquat and diquat are nonselective dipyridyl contact herbicides. Paraquat is a restricted-use herbicide for most applications, although dilute solutions of 0.276% are available to consumers for spot weed killing. Of all registered herbicides, paraquat exposures are the most serious and potentially life threatening. Paraquat affects the gastrointestinal tract, kidneys, liver, heart, lungs, and other organs. Ingestion of as little as 10 to 15 mL of a 20% solution is life threatening. Although inhalation toxicity is rare, ingestions result in systemic toxicity with the lung being the target organ. Both type I and type II pneumocytes appear to accumulate paraquat. Biotransformation of paraquat in these cells results in the formation of free radicals, lipid peroxidation, and cell death.[17-19] Concentrated paraquat is also quite corrosive, and prolonged contact may result in erythema, blistering, abrasion, and ulceration.[20,21] Although absorption across intact skin is slow, once the skin is abraded, eroded, or otherwise damaged, much greater absorption can occur.

Ingestions of more concentrated paraquat solutions produce swelling, edema, and painful ulceration of the oral cavity, pharynx, esophagus, stomach, and intestine. Liver injury may be evident from centrizonal hepatocellular injury with corresponding elevations of circulating levels of aspartate transaminase, alanine transaminase, and lactate dehydrogenase. Kidney damage is also often seen, and evidence of early damage may suggest a grave prognosis, as impaired renal function decreases clearance of paraquat from the body.

Acute poisoning can result in severe pulmonary edema within hours of ingestion, although delayed toxicity manifesting as pulmonary fibrosis typically results in death 7 to 10 days after exposure. Toxic concentrations of paraquat can accumulate in the lung within hours of exposure, which limits the utility of various methods of decontamination or enhanced elimination. Rough estimates of toxicity suggest that ingestion of less than 20 mg/kg body weight of paraquat typically results in recovery, whereas ingestion of more than 40 mg/kg body weight results in 100% mortality within 1 to 7 days.[21]

Treatment includes induction of emesis or gastric lavage immediately after ingestion because even small returns of the substance can be beneficial. Administration of activated charcoal, Robinson's Bentonite, or Robinson's Fuller Earth (dose for adults is 100 to 150 g; dose for children is 2 g/kg) via a nasogastric tube with a cathartic is also warranted. Diagnosis should be confirmed through quantification of paraquat in urine or plasma. Manufacturers of paraquat may be able to aid in obtaining analysis of biologic fluids for the presence of paraquat.

Because the presence of oxygen increases free radical formation, the use of supplemental oxygen should be restricted if possible.[22,23] Patients should be closely monitored for development of acute respiratory distress syndrome and impending respiratory failure. A variety of other measures have been employed to increase elimination of paraquat. Although peritoneal dialysis or hemodialysis may be used in patients developing renal failure, data on benefits are still inconclusive. Hemoperfusion for several consecutive days through a charcoal column can be used but should be started within 24 hours and preferably within 12 hours of ingestion. Although the use of various antioxidants and free-radical scavengers has been postulated to reduce free radical damage, no benefits have been seen in animal studies.

One case reported the use of deferoxamine 100 mg/kg in 24 hours and continuous infusion of N-acetylcysteine at dose of 300 mg/kg per day for 3 weeks to treat an ingestion of 50 to 60 mL of a 20% solution of paraquat in an adult male patient.[24] The patient survived without major sequelae. In another case, a 52-year-old man ingested approximately 50 mL of a solution containing 13% paraquat and 7% diquat and subsequently developed acute respiratory distress syndrome and pulmonary fibrosis. Survival prediction for the corresponding paraquat plasma levels was 30%. Treatment included oral Fuller's Earth, forced diuresis, hemofiltration, N-acetylcysteine, methylprednisolone, cyclophosphamide, vitamin E, colchicine, and delayed continuous nitric oxide inhalation. The patient recovered with preservation of normal pulmonary function. The authors of this case report were unsure which modality accounted for the successful outcome but were encouraged with the use of nitrous oxide.[25]

DIQUAT

Diquat is a dipyridyl compound similar to but less toxic than paraquat. The lower toxicity may be due to the fact that diquat is not selectively concentrated in the lungs. Although lung damage to type I pneumocytes does occur, type II pneumocytes are spared and progressive fibrosis has not been reported.[26,27]

Significant exposures to diquat can result in toxicity to the gastrointestinal tract, brain, and kidneys. Signs and symptoms of CNS toxicity, including lethargy, seizures, and coma, may be seen.[28,29] Treatment of diquat exposure is similar to treatment of paraquat exposure and consists of gastric decontamination and respiratory support. However, there are limited studies documenting the effectiveness of most of the therapeutic modalities that have been employed.

ANNOTATED REFERENCES

Bond GR: Home syrup of ipecac use does not reduce emergency department use or improve outcome. Pediatrics 2003;112:1061-1064.

The usefulness of syrup of ipecac as a home treatment for poisoning and the need to keep it in the home has been increasingly challenged. This study suggests there is no reduction in resource utilization or improvement in patient outcome from the use of syrup of ipecac at home. Although these data cannot exclude a benefit in a very limited set of poisonings, any benefit remains to be proven.

American Academy of Pediatrics Committee on Injury, Violence, and Poison Prevention: Poison treatment in the home. American Academy of Pediatrics Committee on Injury, Violence, and Poison Prevention. Pediatrics 2003;112:1182-1185.

The AAP states that ipecac should no longer be used routinely as a home treatment strategy for child poisoning and that existing ipecac in the home should be disposed of safely. Recently, there has been interest regarding activated charcoal in the home as a poison treatment strategy. After reviewing the evidence, AAP believes that it is premature to recommend the administration of activated charcoal in the home. The first action for a caregiver of a child who may have ingested a toxic substance is to consult with the local poison control center.

Chapter 202
SEDATIVES AND HYPNOTICS

Debra J. Skaar • Craig R. Weinert

XII

1715

KEY POINTS

1. **Unidentified or untreated pain** is an important cause of anxiety in critically ill patients.

2. **Commonly used sedative medications,** in moderate to high doses, lead to comparable changes in patients' level of consciousness and spontaneous muscle activity. Therefore, optimal clinical use is determined more by the process of sedation (goal setting, evaluation, and communication) than by prescription of a specific drug.

3. **Sedatives should be titrated** to defined endpoints, with scheduled efforts to taper doses or perform daily interruption of therapy or both.

4. Sedation goals for critically ill patients should frequently be reassessed by a **sedation assessment tool** acceptable to intensive care practitioners.

5. Implementation of **evidence-based guidelines,** such as a sedation algorithm or protocol, to complement clinical judgment improves outcomes in mechanically ventilated patients.

RATIONALE FOR SEDATIVE USE IN THE INTENSIVE CARE UNIT

Medications are commonly administered to critically ill patients to diminish fundamental activities of the central nervous system (CNS) such as wakefulness, memory, and control of voluntary muscle contraction and to minimize unpleasant symptoms such as dyspnea, anxiety, and fear. This is especially true for mechanically ventilated patients, because they are more likely to receive sedative-analgesics, and in higher doses, than are nonintubated patients.[1] Paradoxically, most patients in intensive care units (ICUs) who receive these potent CNS-active medications are not suffering from acute neurologic diagnoses such as stroke, seizure, or infection. Therefore, this chapter focuses on sedative use in critically ill patients who may have toxic-metabolic encephalopathy or, more likely, no CNS abnormalities at all.

The sedative and analgesic drugs commonly administered to ICU patients are derived from five distinct pharmacologic classes: opiates, benzodiazepines (BZDs), isopropylphenol anesthetics, α_2-adrenoreceptor agonists, and dopamine-blocking antipsychotic medications. This wide-ranging armamentarium allows the intensivist to choose drugs from different classes to treat specific symptoms and avoid overlapping adverse effects, as an oncologist might use chemotherapeutic agents to treat a malignancy. However, at doses commonly given to critically ill patients, these medications induce relatively similar clinical effects, both desirable and adverse. This problem of drug nonspecificity is compounded by use of imprecise language by caregivers to describe patients' behavior and communicate sedative goals to others. Clinicians also have scanty scientific data that define the acceptable level of symptoms or behavior for their patient.

The expression "sedation" or "sedative medications" encompasses elements of sedation, hypnosis, amnesia, analgesia, and muscle relaxation. These words have discrete but related meanings. *Sedatives* create a state of calmness or lack of excitability without necessarily decreasing awareness. *Hypnotics* and *general anesthetics* induce sleep or, more precisely, create the appearance of sleep by reducing the level of consciousness, arousability, or awareness. *Amnestics* impede new memory formation, whereas *analgesics* reduce the symptom of pain by peripheral or central mechanisms. Excessive skeletal muscle contraction or motor activity is a major manifestation of the term "agitation," which, along with level of consciousness, is the primary observable behavior measured by many sedation scales.[2] *Antipsychotics* and *neuroleptics* ameliorate disorganized thinking and inappropriate behavior. Most "sedative" medications have clinical effects in several of these categories. For instance, a drug may have both sedative and hypnotic properties, or both analgesic and hypnotic effects, or both antipsychotic and sedative effects. Although no one sedative has a completely specific effect, medications typically have greater effects in one of the categories, and the thoughtful intensivist can prescribe medication combinations that maximize desired effects while minimizing unwanted effects. Importantly, given in higher doses, almost all of the medications described in this chapter decrease the level of consciousness and reduce unwanted skeletal muscle activity.

GOALS OF SEDATION FOR PATIENTS IN INTENSIVE CARE UNITS

Table 202-1 lists 15 indications for administration of sedative and analgesic medications to critically ill patients. The physician should mentally compare the number of possible indications for use of sedative-analgesics in ICU patients with an analogous list for use of other ICU medications. For example, antibiotics have two indications, to prevent or to

TABLE 202–1. INDICATIONS FOR ADMINISTERING SEDATIVE-ANALGESIC MEDICATIONS TO CRITICALLY ILL PATIENTS

Indication	Comment
Minimize ventilator dysynchrony	Poor synchrony may lead to hypoxemia and dyspnea and is distressing to caregivers. Ventilator adjustment may improve synchrony without medications.
Reduce dyspnea associated with severe acute respiratory failure	Reducing minute ventilation to avoid ventilator-induced lung injury can cause severe dyspnea. Tachypnea with short expiratory times can lead to increased auto-PEEP and hypotension.
Increase tolerance of intubation	A translaryngeal endotracheal tube can cause pain, gagging, and reflexive biting. Local airway anesthesia can reduce the need for sedatives and analgesics.[71]
Reduce anxiety	Acute severe illness possibly leading to disability or death may produce unwanted psychological distress
Reduce recall of ICU symptoms	Recall of distressing symptoms such as severe dyspnea, terror, restraint, or pain can have long-term psychological consequences.[28]
Reduce stress response and oxygen consumption	Reducing unwanted motor activity or respiratory effort can decrease total-body oxygen consumption by 15%.[72]
Reduce elevated intracranial pressure	Coughing, straining, or excessive ventilator dysynchrony can cause dangerous spikes in intracranial pressure.
Reduce pain	Surgical or traumatic wounds, catheter and tube placement, and immobilization usually cause pain.
Prevent removal of life support technology	Removal of an endotracheal tube or vascular catheter can cause death within minutes.
Induce sleep	ICU patients often have abnormal chronobiology cycles associated with delirium and impaired immune function.
Increase efficiency of patient care delivery	Constant visual observation and verbal and tactile patient reassurance may not be possible in understaffed units.
Protect caregivers from violent behaviors	Confused patients can violently assault caregivers.
Adjunct during pharmacologic paralysis	Awareness during pharmacologic paralysis is inhumane and can have long-term psychological consequences.
Treat delirium	Antipsychotics may reduce disorganized thought processes or behavior while the underlying cause of the delirium is treated.
Family considerations	Repeatedly observing the distress of a loved one can cause anguish in family members, who may request that additional sedatives be given to the patient.[23]

ICU, intensive care unit; PEEP, positive end-expiratory pressure.

treat infections, and gastric acid–reducing medications have two indications, to prevent gastrointestinal bleeding and to improve symptoms of esophageal reflux. Much of the art of sedating ICU patients lies in determining which of the many indications applies to the individual patient on a given day and communicating that rationale to other caregivers.

EPIDEMIOLOGY OF SEDATIVE USE IN THE INTENSIVE CARE UNIT AND CONDITIONS REQUIRING SEDATION

ICU practice surveys and studies of pharmacy records have shown that patients who are ventilated or have greater severity of illness (especially respiratory severity) are more likely to receive sedative-analgesic medications.[3] Sedatives are often given in combination, especially opiates and BZDs, and delivered as continuous infusions.[4,5] Propofol was prescribed more frequently in recent studies,[6] whereas antipsychotics and newly licensed sedatives such as dexmedetomidine were used less commonly. In 1994, 78% of ICU patients received an opiate during a 5-day study period; 55% received a BZD, and 7% received an antipsychotic.[7] In a single medical ICU, 65% of ventilated patients received either a continuous sedative-analgesic infusion or intermittent bolus therapy during intubation. Continuous infusion therapy was associated with a markedly prolonged duration of mechanical ventilation.[8] In a clinical trial involving patients with adult respiratory distress syndrome (ARDS), sedatives were administered during 70% of patient ICU days.[9]

What are the clinical consequences of widespread use of potent sedatives? Because there are numerous causes of decreased consciousness in critically ill patients, it is difficult to estimate the independent effect of sedative medications on patients' clinical status. In one study, patient assessments found that one third of subjects were in an unarousable or deeply sedated state; another one third were in a state of moderate to light sedation, and one third were in an alert and calm state.[10] The correlation between sedation level and amount of sedative medication received during the 8 hours before the assessment was weak ($r = -0.13$ to -0.32) across the opiate, BZD, and propofol medication classes. These results suggest that nonmedication factors (e.g., organ failure-associated encephalopathy) influence sedation scale measurement, that pharmacologic effects of sedatives accumulate over days rather than hours, or that dose-effect relationships are nonlinear. All of these effects are likely to be present in ICU patients.

Determining the specific reasons for administration of sedative medications is problematic in clinical studies, but the question can be approached by determining the prevalence of the syndromes, symptoms, or behaviors that may lead to sedative intervention. Between 20% and 60% of patients recalled significant pain during their ICU stay.[11-13] Therefore, caregivers should consider pain as the most likely cause of patient distress or agitation. Delirium was objectively diagnosed in 83% of ICU patients at some time during their illness.[14] However, ICU delirium is often hypoactive, manifested as inattention rather than agitation, and therefore may not lead to sedative administration. Although the expected effects of sedative medications can mimic symptoms of delirium such as inattention, confusion, and fluctuating level of consciousness, sedatives used in the ICU (e.g., BZDs, opiates) are rarely the sole, direct cause of delirium in these patients.

Agitated behavior, as documented by nursing notes, occurred in 71% of ICU patients studied, with two thirds of the episodes judged as being severe or dangerous. In this study, caregivers often identified three or more factors that they believed contributed to the agitated episode.[15] Another study of ventilated patients detected agitation in less than 5% of 1833 separate assessments.[10] The low prevalence of agitation in this study may have occurred because agitation was assessed only during a narrow time interval. If agitation occurred but subsequently resolved (with or without medication administration) between assessment points, the episode would not have been recorded. These results suggest, that because agitation is so visibly apparent and is associated with numerous adverse clinical events, caregivers intervene quickly even if the underlying cause or causes are difficult to identify. Contemporary sedative medications are very potent, and with aggressive dosing caregivers can minimize almost any level of agitation, albeit with an increased risk of other adverse effects.

Anxiety during the acute illness is commonly recalled by ICU survivors,[12] although a sample of 192 awake ventilated ICU patients reported a mean anxiety level during intubation that was only slightly higher than that of nonintubated patients assessed on a general medical-surgical ward.[16] These results imply that, after clinical stabilization, caregivers should not assume that all ventilated patients require anxiolytic medications to treat overwhelming anxiety and fear.

ICU patients recall sleep disruption as a major problem during their ICU stay. Polysomnograms demonstrated that only 40% of critically ill patients exhibited even brief periods of normal rapid eye movement (REM) sleep, because of frequent arousals and severely fragmented sleep architecture.[17] The other 60% of patients, who also, as a group, received more sedative medications, showed no evidence of electrophysiologic sleep but rather had electroencephalograms (EEGs) consistent with diffuse encephalopathy and coma. Environmental interventions to improve sleep quality (e.g., noise and light abatement) have not clearly been successful in improving EEG-documented sleep.[18] Pharmacologic interventions such as increasing propofol infusion rates at night can generate a diurnal pattern of patient arousability, but there is no evidence that propofol, or any other widely used ICU sedative, creates restful, physiologic sleep in ICU patients.[19] In a small trial using wrist actigraphy to estimate sleep quality, nighttime administration of melatonin improved sleep in ICU patients with respiratory failure.[20] The rationale for administration of additional sedation at night is often conceptualized as "resting" patients in preparation for weaning trials in the morning. However, there are few data to support this appealing concept, and one study showed that the reintubation rate was greater in patients with lower sedation scores (i.e., greater sedation) during the shift interval before the planned extubation.[10]

Dyspnea is an important symptom to consider, because many ICU patients have respiratory failure requiring mechanical ventilation.[21] Dyspnea is a complex symptom that arises from both acute and chronic cardiopulmonary conditions but also from constraints imposed by mechanical ventilators. Excessively small tidal volumes, short expiratory times, or slow inspiratory flow rates can worsen dyspnea and lead to potentially injurious ventilator dysynchrony. A newer ventilatory mode that allows spontaneous respiratory efforts throughout the respiratory cycle was found to decrease sedation requirements in patients with ARDS.[22] Opiates are considered first-line medications to relieve dyspnea. However, in patients with communication difficulties, caregivers cannot easily determine whether a little dyspnea is causing a lot of anxiety (in which case BZDs should be used) or a lot of dyspnea is causing a little anxiety (for which opiates should be used).[23] ICU personnel may choose to use continuous-infusion opiate therapy for almost all ventilated patients, reasoning that most critically ill patients are dyspneic or in pain or both.[24]

Although detailed investigations are lacking, patients with more severe respiratory failure clearly receive more sedative medications. However, the number of ICU patient-days with severe respiratory failure (e.g., high positive end-expiratory pressure, high inspired oxygen fraction, prone positioning, permissive hypercapnia) represents a minority of all patient-ventilator days. For example, among patients with acute respiratory failure due to exacerbation of chronic obstructive pulmonary disease or ARDS, 40% of time on the ventilator was spent in the weaning phase.[25] Similarly, one third of all ventilated patients examined during a single cross-sectional time point were in the weaning phase.[21] Therefore, as patients' respiratory support requirements lessen, sedation should also be weaned. When patients become more alert, caregivers may have heightened concern for inadvertent removal of life-support technology. Although sedatives or restraints offer no guarantee against "treatment interference,"[26] fewer than 2% of ventilated patients had unexpected extubations that required reintubation.[25]

Sedatives, especially BZDs, may be given to induce anterograde amnesia of the presumably psychologically stressful ICU experience.[27] This indication is supported by an observational study of ARDS survivors in which patients with a greater number of recalled ICU traumatic experiences were more likely to develop persistent symptoms of post-traumatic stress disorder years later.[28] On the other hand, no one knows the quantity of sedative medication in each class that is required to reliably ensure complete amnesia. At equivalent sedation levels during prolonged ventilatory support, midazolam induced amnesia more reliably than propofol did.[29] In general, intensivists must balance the trial-proven benefits of administering fewer sedative medications (by daily stopping of sedative infusions or use of sedation protocols) against the uncertain adverse effects of unpleasant symptom recall. Indeed, the data suggest that recall of delusional memories (often exacerbated by sedatives) is associated with greater post-ICU psychopathology than is patient recall of unpleasant but real memories.[30]

PHARMACOLOGY AND CLINICAL USE OF SEDATIVES COMMONLY ADMINISTERED IN THE INTENSIVE CARE UNIT

The intensity of sedation required for patients can vary markedly throughout their ICU stay, depending on the course of their disease, the external environment, and the time of day. The ideal sedative possesses a rapid onset of action, is convenient to administer and titrate, produces effective and reproducible sedation to the desired clinical goal, and is free of hemodynamic, cardiac, or respiratory side effects. To simplify extended infusion in the critically ill patient, the ideal sedative should also exhibit linear pharmacokinetics with no clinically significant protein binding or drug interactions. Drug clearance in renal and hepatic impairment should be clearly characterized, and the sedative ideally would not be cleared by dialysis. Finally, the ideal sedative would permit rapid and predictable recovery after discontinuation, with no long-term adverse effects. Although new sedative agents have been added to the armamentarium in recent years, this optimal group of characteristics has yet to be formulated in a single agent. Combination therapy is often used to optimize sedation in critically ill patients, with a BZD or propofol and an opioid analgesic the most common choices.[3,7,31]

OPIOID ANALGESICS

Although opioid analgesics are recognized as the drug class most frequently prescribed for pain management, opioids also have a role in management of anxiety. Unrecognized or inadequately treated pain from pathology or ICU procedures can create anxiety in 20% to 60% of patients.[11-13] Patients who are unable to communicate the source of their distress may suffer from persistent pain. For this reason, early and systematic scrutiny for the presence of pain is crucial to effective management in the visibly anxious ICU patient.

Analgesic agents recommended for use in critically ill patients by the 2002 American College of Chest Physicians/Society of Critical Care Medicine/American Society of Health System Pharmacists Clinical Practice Guidelines[32] (hereafter referred to as the Practice Guidelines) are described in Table 202-2. Differences in analgesic potency, response, and recovery time are associated with the pharmacokinetic properties of each drug as well as their mu and kappa receptor-binding affinity in the CNS. In addition to sedation and analgesia, opioids can produce respiratory depression, constipation, urinary retention, nausea, and confusion. Combined use of opioids and BZDs results in synergistic effects that permit dosage reduction, which may reduce adverse effects and drug accumulation. For patients with chronic pain or previous use of opioids, increased dose requirements due to tolerance should be considered. The use of the opioid antagonist naloxone as a reversal agent is not recommended routinely after prolonged opioid analgesia

because of the risk of withdrawal symptoms and the potential to induce cardiac arrhythmias.[32]

Several analgesics are not recommended for critically ill patients. Meperidine has an active metabolite, normeperidine, that causes CNS excitation associated with delirium and seizures. Because the active metabolite is excreted by the kidneys, patients with renal insufficiency are at high risk for adverse effects. Opioid antagonist-agonists (e.g., nalbuphine, butorphanol, buprenorphine) can reverse other opiate agents and are not recommended for routine use in the ICU. Nonsteroidal anti-inflammatory analgesics offer few advantages for the critically ill and can cause gastrointestinal bleeding, bleeding due to platelet inhibition, and renal insufficiency.[32] Alfentanil, sufentanil, and remifentanil are fentanyl derivatives with higher potency and/or shorter half-lives than fentanyl, but comparative data evaluating these agents for sedation in the ICU are scarce, and they are more expensive than fentanyl.[31,33]

BENZODIAZEPINES

BZDs are widely used as ICU sedatives because they produce anxiolysis and amnesia at lower doses and induce hypnosis at higher doses. BZDs cause anterograde amnesia by blocking the acquisition and encoding of new information and unpleasant experiences. BZDs also exhibit anticonvulsant and muscle relaxant effects that may be desirable in selected ICU patients.

The anxiolytic, amnestic, anticonvulsant, and muscle-relaxing effects of BZDs are mediated through $GABA_A$ binding sites on neuronal γ-aminobutyric acid (GABA) receptors. After binding to the receptor site, BZDs facilitate the GABA-mediated increase in chloride conductance with subsequent membrane hyperpolarization and inhibition of neuronal impulses. The amnestic properties correlate with GABA agonist activity in the limbic system.[34] BZD binding is stereospecific and saturable, and the potency of an individual BZD agent correlates with its receptor affinity. Other ligands act as antagonists (e.g., flumazenil) or inverse agonists. Inverse agonists reduce the efficiency of GABA interaction with the receptor, causing CNS stimulation; drugs with these properties are in development.[35] Table 202-3 describes the comparative pharmacology of selected BZDs and other ICU sedatives.

TABLE 202–2. OPIOID ANALGESICS RECOMMENDED FOR USE IN INTENSIVE CARE UNITS

Drug	Equianalgesic Intravenous Dosage	Half-life (h)	Elimination Glucuronidation	Active Metabolites	Special Considerations
Morphine sulfate	10 mg Infusion: 0.07-0.5 mg/kg/h	2-3	Reduced in cirrhosis, burns, septic shock, and renal failure	Morphine-3 glucuronide, morphine-6 glucuronides	Histamine release can cause hypotension and cardiovascular instability
Fentanyl	200 µg Infusion: 0.7-10 µg/kg/h	From 0.5-1 to 9-16	Oxidation	None	Rigidity is occasionally seen with high doses; preferred for patients with hemodynamic instability, sensitivity to histamine release, or morphine allergy
Hydromorphone	1.5 mg Infusion: 7-15 µg/kg/h	2-3	Glucuronidation	None	Alternative to fentanyl; oral form available

From Jacobi J, Fraser G, Coursin D, et al: Clinical practice guidelines for the sustained use of sedatives and analgesics in the critically ill adult. Crit Care Med 2002;30(1):119-141.

TABLE 202–3. CLINICAL PHARMACOLOGY OF SELECTED SEDATIVES

Drug	Estimated Comparable Sedative Dose	Onset with Intravenous Administration (min)	Half-life (h)	Active Metabolites	Intravenous Dose	Infusion Dosage Range	Relative Cost/day*
Diazepam	5 mg	2-5	20-120	Yes	0.03-0.1 mg/kg q0.5-6h	—	$-$$
Lorazepam	1 mg	5-20	8-15	None	0.02-0.06 mg/kg q2-6h	0.01-0.1 mg/kg/h	$$
Midazolam	2-3 mg	2-5	3-11	Yes	0.02-0.08 mg/kg q0.5-2h	0.04-0.2 mg/kg/h	$$
Propofol	50 µg/kg/min	1-2	26-32	None	—	5-80 µg/kg/min	$$$
Dexmedetomidine	0.5 µg/kg/h	5-10	2-7.5	None	—	0.2-0.7 µg/kg/h	$$$
Haloperidol	—	3-20	18-54	Yes†	0.03-0.15 mg/kg q0.5-6h	0.04-0.15 mg/kg/h	$$

*Based on 2003 average wholesale price and usual dosages: $, less than $10/day; $$, between $10 and $100/day; $$$, greater than $100/day.
†Associated with extrapyramidal symptoms.

Both acute and chronic tolerance to BZDs (associated with decreased receptor activity) has been described. In ICU patients, acute tolerance can occur after just 24 hours.[35] Paradoxical reactions have also been associated with BZDs, most commonly in the elderly and in patients with preexisting CNS disease, substance abuse, or psychiatric disease. Patients who develop a paradoxical reaction to a BZD should be switched to a medication in another drug class, such as propofol or haloperidol.

Diazepam is highly lipophilic. This property promotes rapid distribution to the brain and a prompt onset of action (2 to 5 minutes) when the drug is given intravenously. Diazepam has a volume of distribution averaging 2.9 L/kg in critically ill patients, is highly protein bound, and is metabolized by the cytochrome P-450 (CYP) microsomal enzymes into the active metabolites oxazepam and desmethyldiazepam. The mean half-life of diazepam is 72 hours, with wide interpatient variability. Oxazepam has a half-life of 10 hours and undergoes further conjugation before elimination. Desmethyldiazepam has a half-life between 100 and 200 hours and is eliminated by the kidneys; therefore, sedative effects may be prolonged in patients with renal failure.

The primary metabolic pathway for diazepam, the CYP subfamily CYP2C19, is genetically polymorphic. Isoenzymes of CYP2C19 that are present in 3% to 5% of Caucasians and African-Americans and 12% to 100% of Asian ethnic groups are associated with a significant decrease in diazepam metabolism. Therefore, on occasion, a patient treated with diazepam may experience unexpectedly prolonged sedation.[36] Some drugs commonly used in critically ill patients also inhibit CYP2C19 activity, including amiodarone, fluconazole, omeprazole, and valproic acid. In contrast, cigarette smoking induces hepatic microsomal enzymes. This effect increases the clearance of diazepam and other BZDs.[37] For these reasons, the clinical response to diazepam is often unpredictable in critically ill patients.

Lorazepam has been a preferred agent for ICU sedation in many critical care units since its approval in 1977. Because lorazepam undergoes hepatic glucuronidation to inactive metabolites, its pharmacokinetic parameters are not altered significantly in elderly or critically ill patients except in those with severe renal or hepatic failure. Lorazepam is the least lipophilic of the injectable BZDs; therefore, it crosses the blood-brain barrier slowly, resulting in a delayed onset of action (5 to 20 minutes) and a longer duration of action, with an elimination half-life of 10 to 20 hours.[38] With chronic dosing, lorazepam accumulation and prolonged sedation are less likely than with diazepam. Lorazepam is also 5 to 6 times more potent than diazepam, and the amnestic effect of lorazepam is longer than an equivalent diazepam dose. Lorazepam can be given by intramuscular injection.[35]

Lorazepam is formulated in 18% polyethylene glycol (PEG) and 2% benzyl alcohol in propylene glycol (PG) for injection. Although usual lorazepam doses deliver only minute amounts of PEG and PG, long-term sedation with high doses can lead to patients' receiving substantial doses of PEG and PG. Both the PEG[39] and the PG[40,41] vehicle have been associated with lactic acidosis, hyperosmolar coma, and reversible nephrotoxicity with high doses or lengthy infusions. Although the dosages implicated have not been prospectively defined, lorazepam doses exceeding 18 mg/hour for longer than 4 weeks, or 25 mg/hour for hours to days, should be avoided.[32] Because of poor solubility, precipitation can occur when lorazepam is administered by continuous infusion. On the basis of manufacturer information and clinical recommendations, the manufacturer's vial concentration (either 2 or 4 mg/mL) should be diluted 1:1 with 5% dextrose injection in a glass container, not in polyvinyl chloride bags.[42]

Midazolam, a short-acting, water-soluble BZD prodrug, is approximately 3 times more potent than diazepam. After self-converting to a lipid-soluble form by closure of the diazepine ring at physiologic pH in the bloodstream, midazolam rapidly enters the CNS to produce sedation within 2 to 5 minutes. This property makes midazolam ideal for patients who require immediate control of anxiety or agitation.[32] Initial dosages recommended are 2 to 5 mg intravenously every 5 to 15 minutes. The drug quickly redistributes to peripheral tissues, and effects dissipate if a continuous infusion is not initiated. When infused over days for chronic sedation, the mean elimination half-life of 10 hours may increase to 30 hours as peripheral tissue stores release accumulated midazolam. The pharmacodynamic effects of BZDs often do not correspond well with reported elimination half-lives.[43] In comparing the clinical sedation recovery rate (time to wakefulness) for midazolam versus diazepam, 8 trials reported a faster recovery rate from diazepam, 19 trials reported no difference in sedative recovery time, and only 1 trial demonstrated a faster recovery with midazolam.[32]

Midazolam is metabolized by the CYP3A4 isoenzyme to an active metabolite, α-hydroxymidazolam, which has 60% of the potency of the parent drug. α-Hydroxymidazolam is quickly biotransformed to its conjugated salt, α-hydroxymidazolam glucuronide (10% potency), which does not significantly contribute to the sedative properties of midazolam except in renal failure. Inhibitors of CYP3A4, such as macrolide antibiotics, diltiazem, propofol, and fluconazole, reduce the metabolism of midazolam and prolong its sedative actions.[35] The combined effects of drug interactions, altered protein binding, fluid shifts, altered hepatic metabolism, and renal failure can result in prolonged elimination and an unpredictable time to awakening after midazolam discontinuation when the drug is used for longer than 48 to 72 hours. For these reasons, the Practice Guidelines recommend midazolam for short-term use only.[32]

Several randomized, controlled studies have compared BZD sedatives in critically ill patients. Two unmasked studies in mixed ICU patients reported no difference between midazolam and lorazepam in time until sedation or in time until return to baseline mental status.[44,45] In contrast, a double-masked, randomized comparison of lorazepam versus midazolam using a target-controlled intravenous infusion titrated to maintain a moderate level of sedation for 12 to 72 hours reported a delayed emergence from sedation with lorazepam.[38] Other longer-term studies suggest that lorazepam is easier to titrate to the desired sedation level than midazolam.[46]

Because lorazepam is equally effective and produces less hypotension, it is the BZD recommended in the Practice Guidelines for most ICU patients; it is administered either by continuous infusion or by intermittent i.v. dosing (1 to 4 mg every 2 to 6 hours).[32]

BZDs, particularly midazolam and diazepam, can cause respiratory depression and hypotension due to vasodilation when administered in large doses. If these effects require rapid reversal, flumazenil may be used to antagonize BZD agonists at the GABA receptor–binding site. Flumazenil administered intravenously in doses of 0.2 to 1 mg reverses the sedative and amnestic effects of BZDs immediately. Flumazenil is metabolized rapidly, with a half-life of 1 hour but with a clinical duration of effect often less than 30 minutes; therefore, situations requiring prolonged antagonism may necessitate a continuous flumazenil infusion. Diagnostically, flumazenil has been used to differentiate between BZD-induced unresponsiveness and other CNS pathology. Flumazenil is relatively contraindicated in patients with known BZD dependence and chronic use, because acute withdrawal symptoms and seizures have been reported in these patients.[35]

PROPOFOL

Propofol is a 2,6-diisopropylphenol initially introduced in 1982 as an induction agent in anesthesia. Over the past 20 years, several other useful indications have been identified for this agent. In addition to being an anxiolytic/sedative/hypnotic, propofol has antiemetic, antipruritic, anticonvulsant, bronchodilatory, muscle relaxant, and possibly anti-inflammatory and antiplatelet effects.[47] Propofol has been shown to improve outcome in patients with traumatic brain injury, possibly because of decreases in cerebral metabolism and intracranial pressure.[48] Its anxiolytic properties are thought to result from activation of $GABA_A$ receptors within

the CNS. Studies have not demonstrated a comparable synergistic sedative effect with opioids that the BZDs possess, and propofol may not produce an amnestic effect equivalent to that of BZDs.[29] Because of its high lipophilicity and short half-life, propofol has a rapid onset of action (1 to 2 minutes) and a short duration of action (10 to 15 minutes) compared with other sedative options. For patients receiving propofol infusions for longer than 72 hours, the wake-up time can extend to 30 to 60 minutes. The pharmacokinetic profile of propofol is best described by a three-compartment model with an elimination half-life of 30 to 60 minutes. Propofol has a volume of distribution of 600 to 800 L, suggesting that the drug is rapidly cleared from the central compartment into fatty tissues, and elimination is not appreciably altered by hepatic or renal failure. For these reasons, an intravenous infusion of propofol can be predictably titrated from light sedation to a deeper hypnotic state for patients who require varying levels of sedation throughout the day. Simply stopping the infusion can reverse the sedative effects, usually within 1 hour and often within 15 minutes. The Practice Guidelines recommend propofol as the sedative of choice when rapid awakening is important.[32]

Propofol is a negative inotrope and can cause vasodilation with dose-related hypotension. Patients should be euvolemic before a slow bolus or infusion is administered. Bradycardia and apnea also may occur during bolus administration. When propofol is combined with BZDs or opioids, synergistic cardiovascular and respiratory adverse effects can be seen.

Propofol is available in 1% or 2% concentrations formulated in an oil-in-water emulsion that provides 1.1 kcal/mL from fat. To reduce the possibility of fat overload and hypertriglyceridemia in critically ill patients, the lipid contribution from a propofol infusion should be counted as a calorie source in the daily nutritional plan. Patients receiving propofol infusions for longer than 2 days should have their serum triglycerides monitored.[32]

Reports of infections in patients receiving propofol prompted the addition of ethylenediaminetetraacetic acid (EDTA) to retard bacterial growth. A generic propofol formulation (propofol, Gensia Sicor) is also available that contains sodium metabisulfite (0.025%) as a preservative and has a lower pH than the EDTA formulation; individuals who are sensitive to sulfites should not receive this product. Although the U.S. Food and Drug Administration (FDA) considers these products to be bioequivalent and interchangeable (i.e., AB rated), reports suggest that the generic emulsion is less stable physiochemically and more conducive to microbial growth.[34,49] Caregivers should administer propofol through a dedicated intravenous line to avoid drug incompatibility and should change the bottles and tubing daily to minimize the risk of bacterial contamination.

Prolonged, high-dose infusions of propofol have been associated with a clinical syndrome of metabolic acidosis, bradycardia, hyperlipidemia, dysrhythmias, and cardiac arrest.[50,51] For this reason, propofol is not recommended by the FDA for prolonged sedation of pediatric patients, and it should be used cautiously in adults who develop unexplained metabolic acidosis or cardiac arrhythmias. Alternative sedative agents should be considered for patients receiving high-dose propofol (greater than 75 to 100 µg/kg/min) and for patients who require vasopressors or cardiac inotropes.[32]

Comparing the quality of short-term (less than 24 hours) sedation of cardiac surgery patients, two trials favored propofol over midazolam and seven reported no difference. Time to extubation after sedative cessation was shorter for patients receiving propofol than for those receiving midazolam in five of eight studies, but the overall duration of mechanical ventilation was equivalent in six of seven studies. In surgical or mixed ICUs, three of six trials reported that the quality of sedation was better with propofol, whereas the other three trials found no difference. Time to extubation was less with propofol than with midazolam in all studies assessing this endpoint.[52,53] Hypotension was more frequent with propofol.[29,54]

Fourteen surgical or mixed ICU studies have compared the use of sedative drugs for longer than 24 hours. The quality of sedation was comparable between propofol and midazolam in half of the studies. Midazolam was preferred over propofol in one study, and propofol was superior in two studies. In all four trials reporting time to extubation, the group receiving propofol was extubated sooner after sedation cessation than the midazolam group.[29,52,53,55] Therefore, based on the best scientific evidence, propofol is at least as effective as midazolam in sedation quality and is associated with a shorter time to extubation for patients receiving short- or long-term sedation. Propofol is also associated with more hypotension and higher drug costs than midazolam.

CENTRAL α$_2$-ADRENORECEPTOR AGONISTS

Dexmedetomidine is the first selective α$_2$-adrenoreceptor agonist approved for short-term (less than 24 hours) infusion as a sedative for patients receiving mechanical ventilation. This drug exerts sedative effects via postsynaptic activation of α$_2$-adrenoreceptors in the CNS and analgesic action by inhibiting norepinephrine release presynaptically. In addition, it inhibits sympathetic activity, thereby decreasing blood pressure and heart rate. Dexmedetomidine is eight times more potent than its relative, clonidine, at stimulating α$_2$-adrenoreceptors.

Dexmedetomidine offers several advantages as a sedative in the ICU. First, dexmedetomidine does not cause significant respiratory depression, and it may be the ideal choice for patients nearing extubation, who still require light sedation. Dexmedetomidine has a rapid distribution phase (6 minutes) and an elimination half-life of 2 hours. These pharmacokinetic properties permit easy dose titration in response to fluctuating sedative needs. Another advantage is the low level of sedation that can be achieved with dexmedetomidine. Patients appear comfortably sedated while undisturbed but can easily be awakened.[34]

A trial comparing dexmedetomidine with propofol infusion found equivalent sedation, no difference in arterial pressure, and a similar time interval from cessation of sedation infusion to extubation. Patients in the dexmedetomidine group required less adjunctive opioid analgesia than did patients receiving propofol, and patients receiving dexmedetomidine were easily aroused for evaluation.[56] Another study also documented a reduction in morphine doses by 50% when patients were treated with dexmedetomidine.[34] However, in short-term studies of mild-to-moderate sedation in healthy volunteers, dexmedetomidine did not demonstrate analgesic effects against heat or electrically generated pain.[57a]

In situations in which amnesia is crucial, dexmedetomidine therapy should be combined with low doses of BZDs.

Dexmedetomidine has also been used successfully to ameliorate the hyperadrenergic state of drug withdrawal caused by alcohol, illicit drugs, or long-term sedative-analgesic use in the ICU.[57]

Dosage reduction is recommended with hepatic but not renal impairment. Hypotension or bradycardia appears to be most frequent in patients with cardiac conduction defects or hypovolemia. Some patients cannot tolerate the 1 µg/kg loading infusion of dexmedetomidine; for these patients, therapy may be initiated with a maintenance infusion (0.2 to 0.7 µg/kg/hour) that can be titrated to desired effects. Because dexmedetomidine is approved for use only for 24 hours, further pharmacokinetic, pharmacodynamic, and clinical research is necessary before it can be recommended for long-term use in ICU patients.

HALOPERIDOL

Haloperidol, a butyrophenone neuroleptic, is the preferred agent to treat patients with agitated delirium in the ICU. Neuroleptics antagonize dopamine-mediated neurotransmission in the basal ganglia, ameliorating hallucinations, delusions, and unstructured thought patterns. Haloperidol and other neuroleptic agents also possess sedative effects.

Haloperidol has a fast onset of action (5 to 20 minutes) and a long half-life (18 to 54 hours). In the ICU, haloperidol is commonly administered by intermittent i.v. injection of 2 to 5 mg, followed by repeated doses (sometimes double the previous dose) every 15 to 20 minutes until agitation is controlled. Repeated doses every 4 to 6 hours are usually continued for a few days, after which the drug is tapered as the patient's clinical status permits.

High doses of haloperidol (greater than 400 mg/day) have been associated with QT$_C$ prolongation and an increased risk of ventricular arrhythmias including torsades de pointes; therefore, patients receiving haloperidol should be electrocardiographically monitored. Extrapyramidal symptoms can occur that require neuroleptic discontinuation and treatment with diphenhydramine or benztropine.[32]

OPTIMIZING SEDATION AT THE BEDSIDE

For many sedative-analgesic medications used in the ICU, there is a marked variation in the doses needed to achieve a desired clinical effect. This variability may result from altered drug kinetics, changes in receptor density, or unpredictable postreceptor effects; in addition, the intensity of the underlying symptom (e.g., dyspnea, pain) or behavior (e.g., agitation, ventilator dysynchrony) varies from patient to patient. Therefore, most sedative-analgesic medications are titrated to a desired clinical effect. Effective titration requires that caregivers address several concepts. First, providers must identify the unwanted symptom or behavior and exhaust all feasible nonpharmacologic interventions before administering drug therapy. Second, caregivers should use a rating instrument or scale to reliably measure the level or state of the target behavior. Third, providers should agree on the desired level of the symptom or behavior. Fourth, caregivers should realize that the desired level is likely to change over time and that regular reassessment is required.

Most "sedation scales" are observer-rated assessments of level of consciousness and agitation.[2] More comprehensive scales may assess additional domains such as pain, anxiety, or ventilator synchrony, but multidomain instruments can become unwieldy if documentation requirements are excessive. Scales can report domain scores separately or combine two domains in a single choice scale, thereby assuming that the activity in one domain precludes activity in the other domain, which is not always the case. For instance, agitation can occur in the presence of decreased level of consciousness. Most consciousness scales use a graded stimulation protocol to obtain a standard patient response such as eye opening. Rating agitation is more ambiguous, because patient behaviors (e.g., excessive motor activity, pulling at tubes, striking at staff) are variably graded on intensity, frequency, or probability that the agitation will cause immediate adverse consequences. Consider how "agitated" is an otherwise calm patient who is slowly pulling on his or her endotracheal tube. Sedation scales such as the modified Ramsay sedation scale (RSS), Richmond Agitation and Sedation Scale (RASS), Sedation Agitation Scale (SAS), and Motor Activity and Assessment Scale (MAAS) are similarly constructed and scored, have excellent interrater reliability, and have been validated by correlation with other scales, physiologic variables, or medication exposure. The Vancouver Interaction and Calmness Scale (VICS) differs from other sedation scales because it is a summated rating scale that reports two domain scores separately.[58] As such, VICS is more responsive to subtle changes in a patient's condition but at the cost of increased response burden. The clinical benefit of documenting or targeting very precisely defined sedation states is unknown and may be impractical. In 15 clinical trials in which close attention was paid to achieving and maintaining a predetermined sedation target (usually with the RSS), patients were at the sedation target, on average, only 68% of the time.[53]

Even if sedation effects are reliably measured, determining the optimal sedation state of an ICU patient is based more on clinical opinion than scientific evidence. Titration of medications to achieve a condition such as "lightly asleep but easily arousable" or "calm and cooperative" appears sensible, but a survey of intensivists asked to choose an appropriate sedation level for a patient with severe hypoxemia yielded a remarkably wide range of responses, ranging from unresponsive to awake.[6] Sedation targets for clinical trials are also highly variable: in 19 trials using the six-level RSS, the target sedation level was defined variously as 3, 5, 2-3, 2-4, 2-5, 3-4, or 4-5.[53] One can conclude that, in the absence of compelling data proving that one level of sedation is superior to another, use of relatively imprecise single-item sedation scales is sufficient for clinical purposes.

Monitoring of cortical electrical activity to indicate sedation intensity has long been a goal of intensivists. Multichannel EEG monitoring is the gold standard for evaluating cortical activity, but interpretation remains predominantly qualitative and requires specialized training. Researchers have developed numerous signal-processing algorithms to convert limited EEG data into simpler quantitative output. The Bispectral Index (BIS) algorithm has been one of the most widely studied and yields a score of 0 (isoelectric, no cortical function) to 100 (fully awake). Initially developed to assess the depth of hypnosis during short-term general anesthesia, BIS is also used to monitor long-term ICU sedation.[59] However, studies have identified problems that have slowed the acceptance of this promising technology. First, spuriously high readings (i.e., readings indicating greater wakefulness than actually exists) can result from muscle activity in nonparalyzed patients.[60,61]

Although new electronic filters suppress myographic signals, there can be substantial variability of output even in stable, pharmacologically paralyzed patients.[62] Clinicians using BIS should assess trends in BIS output and integrate other clinical data before making an intervention. Second, there is little evidence that BIS monitoring of general ICU patients has advantages over routine sedation assessment using observer-rated scales. BIS technology is superior in limited situations (e.g., paralysis) in which stimulus-response sedation assessment is inadequate. For instance, medicating to a BIS score lower than about 60 makes awareness and recall unlikely. Similarly, sedation scales cannot score below a "floor" level in which patients exhibit no motor response to painful stimuli, but BIS can distinguish between levels of deep sedation. For instance, BIS scores of 55 and 35, respectively, in two patients who both score at the lowest level of a standard sedation scale suggest that the latter patient has greater suppression of cortical activity. If there is no clinical reason for maintaining the patient at 35, then sedatives could be decreased to allow the BIS to rise. This process of identifying excessively sedated patients might shorten wake-up time and lead to faster weaning; however, this putative advantage has not yet been demonstrated in large ICU studies. Third, the BIS algorithm was designed to correlate with hypnosis (arousability) and recall, but it is not a pain, dyspnea, or anxiety monitor. Postoperative studies have shown that opiate-induced hypnosis can occur before analgesic effects and that seemingly sedated patients can have significant pain when awakened.[63]

Until recently, clinical research in ICU sedation has focused on investigating changes in acute physiology after medication administration or conducting head-to-head medication trials. Two studies suggest, however, that the method of administering sedatives is more important than the specific drug given to patients. In one study, the duration of mechanical ventilation was decreased by more than 50% in ventilated patients who were sedated with a protocol that linked medication dosing to a specified sedation level, compared with patients who were treated without a sedation protocol.[64] The marked decrease in ventilator time was attributable to the protocol, which decreased infusion rates when patients were at target sedation level (RSS 3), thereby minimizing the time during which patients were receiving continuous medication infusions. In another study, a protocol used continuous infusions (midazolam or propofol) but stopped the infusions daily, restarting them (at half the rate) only after patients became awake.[24] Compared with a group that did not have this "stop" intervention, the experimental group used less midazolam but similar amounts of propofol. Nevertheless, in both midazolam and propofol subgroups, the daily interruption of infusions increased the number of days patients were awake, decreased the duration of mechanical ventilation by 2.4 days, and decreased the number of diagnostic tests performed to assess abnormal mental status. These two trials support the following important concept: because there are only slight differences in the effects of sedative medications used in the ICU, the manner in which the medication is administered is likely to be more important than the specific drug is used.

Patients with prolonged ICU stays may be treated with high doses of sedative-analgesic medications for weeks. There is growing evidence that tolerance to opiates, BZDs, and propofol can develop in less than 1 week and that abstinence or withdrawal symptoms can occur if sedative doses are reduced too rapidly.[65] Withdrawal symptoms of anxiety, agitation, gastrointestinal dysfunction, and tachycardia are nonspecific, and intubated patients have difficulty communicating symptoms to caregivers. Because of the altered pharmacokinetics of critically ill patients and the difficulty in identifying withdrawal syndromes, there are few data to guide clinicians in prescribing tapering regimens when withdrawal symptoms are suspected. Logical interventions for patients who have been on prolonged courses of sedative medications include converting continuous infusions to scheduled doses; using longer-acting medications within the same pharmacologic class; reducing the total daily dose by 10% per day; changing the intravenous route to enteral; and prescribing an α_2-adrenoreceptor agonist such as clonidine.[66]

PHARMACOECONOMICS OF SEDATIVES USED IN THE INTENSIVE CARE UNIT

Occupied beds in the ICU consume a disproportionate and growing share of hospital resources. It is estimated that pharmaceutical agents comprise 10% of the cost of an ICU stay and that 15% of drug expenditures are for sedatives. To promote optimal use of critical care resources, evidence for cost-effectiveness in addition to safety and efficacy must be examined for each sedative. Pharmacoeconomics, the global approach of evaluating the net impact of drug selection on the total cost of delivering health care, determines which therapies offer quality care at an acceptable cost.

New drugs cost more than available generic formulations. One comparison of lorazepam, midazolam, and propofol in critically ill trauma patients found lorazepam to be the best choice for continuous sedation, based on 1995 acquisition cost; however, lorazepam acquisition costs were lower because of an available generic formulation.[67] Because the time to extubation was shorter with propofol than with midazolam, overall costs were lower with propofol in a Spanish study even though propofol acquisition costs were three times higher than those of midazolam.[55] Other investigators have compared quality of sedation, safety, and costs of propofol versus midazolam during short-to-medium and long-term sedation with similar results. Propofol provides comparable sedation safety and efficacy at lower health care costs due to earlier extubation and shorter ICU stays.[52] Propofol and midazolam are now both available generically at a lower cost.

Economic analysis must consider dynamic pricing of drugs within the United States and throughout the world. Acquisition costs of drugs represent only one piece of the decision-making process. In the analysis of sedative agents, adequacy of sedation, time to extubation, and time to ICU discharge are important endpoints. Preventable adverse drug effects and increased use of diagnostic and therapeutic resources also affect total hospital costs. Health-related quality of life and post-ICU long-term consequences of ICU sedation should be incorporated into future pharmacoeconomic analysis.

Implementation of clinical practice guidelines can improve outcomes and lower costs. One institution reduced direct drug costs, ventilator time, and length of stay after implementing interdisciplinary sedation guidelines.[68] Evidence-based protocols and practice guidelines should be accompanied by interdisciplinary collaboration and education to ensure that they are positioned as guides, not rigid rules that replace clinical judgment.

Until pharmacoeconomic research provides definitive data on costs and outcomes, the best strategy to optimize sedation at acceptable costs includes selecting a sedative based on current practice guidelines, titrating doses to a patient-specific goal, and frequently reevaluating the defined endpoint with an assessment tool. Scheduled efforts to taper sedative doses or perform daily interruption of therapy (or both), as part of an interdisciplinary sedation plan, may optimize sedative outcomes and reduce costs more than interventions that restrict the use of specific sedative medications.

TOXIC INGESTION OF SEDATIVE-HYPNOTICS

Of the sedative medications discussed in this chapter, BZDs and opiates are most likely to be involved in toxic ingestions, either accidental or intended. Patients with overdoses from either medication class can present with stupor or coma with hypotension (usually mild and responsive to fluid boluses) and hypotonia. Pupil size may be helpful: pupils are pinpoint in opiate ingestion, mid-size in BZD toxicity. Toxicity is usually short-lived and completely reversible unless complications such as anoxic encephalopathy or aspiration pneumonia occur. General principles of toxic ingestion management are paramount: assume that the patient has a polydrug ingestion until conclusive data are obtained; ensure adequate ventilation and airway protection; avoid gastric lavage unless the time of ingestion is very recent; and give activated charcoal for oral ingestions.[69]

Specific antidotes are available for each medication class. Naloxone can be given as both a diagnostic and therapeutic medication; lack of improvement in level of consciousness or respiratory depression after administration of 10 mg of naloxone (starting with 0.4 mg and giving subsequent doses of 2 mg every few minutes) makes opiate toxicity an unlikely cause of the patient's symptoms. If a response is observed, then practitioners should be prepared to administer repeated naloxone boluses every 30 to 60 minutes or to start a continuous infusion at 0.4 to 0.8 mg/hour. Occasionally, a patient with opiate overdose develops pulmonary edema requiring mechanical ventilation, but the edema usually resolves within a few days without specific treatment.

Flumazenil is a specific antidote for BZD toxicity. A patient's symptoms should improve within a minute after a bolus administration of 0.2 mg and subsequent 0.3-mg doses every 30 seconds. Administration of flumazenil to patients receiving chronic BZD therapy may precipitate an unpleasant acute withdrawal syndrome and, theoretically, increase the risk of seizure.[69] However, no seizures were observed after flumazenil treatment in 110 patients with suspected BZD overdose, including many patients with polydrug ingestions (e.g., co-ingestion of tricyclic antidepressants).[70]

ANNOTATED REFERENCES

Brook AD, Ahrens TS, Schaiff R, et al: Effect of a nursing-implemented sedation protocol on the duration of mechanical ventilation. Crit Care Med 1999;27:2609-2615.
Protocol-based, nurse-directed sedation during mechanical ventilation was compared with traditional non–protocol-directed sedation in a medical

ICU in a randomized, controlled trial. Protocol-driven sedation reduced the duration of mechanical ventilation, the length of ICU and hospital stay, and the need for tracheostomy in patients with acute respiratory failure.

De Jonghe, B, Cook D, Appere-De-Veechi C, et al: Using and understanding sedation scoring systems: A systematic review. Intensive Care Med 2000;26:275-285.

This review describes and critiques 25 published sedation scales, with specific attention to 4 scales that demonstrate adequate reliability and validity for clinical use. The justification for the clinical use of sedation scales is reviewed, and areas for improvement in future scale development are suggested.

Jacobi J, Fraser GL, Coursin DB, et al: Clinical practice guidelines for the sustained use of sedatives and analgesics in the critically ill adult. Crit Care Med 2002;30:119-141.

This is a comprehensive update of the ACCP, SCCM, and ASHP practice guidelines for the optimal use of sedatives and analgesics in critically ill patients, including descriptions of new drugs and grading of the scientific evidence that supports the recommendations.

Kress JP, Pohlman AS, O'Connor MF, Hall JB: Daily interruption of sedative infusions in critically ill patients undergoing mechanical ventilation. N Engl J Med 2000;342:1471-1477.

A randomized trial performed in a medical ICU showed that daily awakening of mechanically ventilated patients by interruption of sedative infusions reduced the duration of ventilation, reduced ICU stay, and led to less diagnostic testing compared with no daily awakening. Rates of complications such as unplanned extubations were not different between groups. A follow-up study in these patients showed that patients in the daily awakening group had better psychological adjustment after the ICU experience and less PTSD symptoms.[71a]

Ostermann ME, Keenan SP, Seiferling RA, Sibbald W: Sedation in the intensive care unit: A systematic review. JAMA 2000;283:1451-1459.

This systematic review evaluates and summarizes the strongest comparative studies that address which sedatives are associated with the best level of sedation, shortest time to extubation, and shortest length of ICU stay.

Chapter 203
TOXIC INHALATIONS

Beatrice Nyakonu Schwake • Suzanne J. Tschida

KEY POINTS

1. **Toxic inhalants produce injury by direct respiratory irritation or systemic absorption after inhalation.** The chemical activity, particle size, and solubility of the irritant gas determine the area of pulmonary deposition and degree of absorption.

2. Because of its high water solubility, **low concentrations of ammonia produce severe upper respiratory tract symptoms**, which prompt the individual to evacuate from the site of exposure before more significant toxicity can occur.

3. **Mild exposures to hydrogen sulfide** result in mucous membrane irritation, whereas **higher concentrations** lead to anoxia, metabolic acidosis, cardiac toxicity, and neurologic signs including headache, convulsions, and coma.

4. **Brief exposures to very high concentrations of hydrogen sulfide may result in sudden loss of consciousness**, the so called "knockdown" effect, which is thought to be caused by a direct toxic effect on the brain.

5. **Hyperbaric oxygen and nitrites may be beneficial** in severe cases of hydrogen sulfide toxicity, although data are limited.

6. In the community setting, **exposure to low concentrations of chlorine is common**; however, **in high concentrations, chlorine can produce significant toxicity,** and it was actually used for this purpose in World War I as a chemical war agent.

7. **Patients with significant nitrogen dioxide exposure initially may have mild pulmonary symptoms, followed by pulmonary edema**; some may even progress to severe interstitial lung disease weeks later.

8. **Phosgene toxicity** is thought to consist mostly of oxidant-like lung tissue damage that can lead to pulmonary edema.

9. **Signs and symptoms of carbon monoxide toxicity** may not correlate with blood carboxyhemoglobin concentrations in adult patients with cardiovascular or pulmonary diseases or in pediatric patients.

10. **In carbon monoxide toxicity, the use of hyperbaric oxygen, as opposed to normobaric oxygen, offers three potential benefits:** (1) increased plasma oxygen concentration, (2) decreased plasma carboxyhemoglobin half-life, and (3) enhanced cerebral vasoconstriction potentially reducing intracranial pressure and cerebral edema.

The inhalation of toxic gases and fumes results in a wide spectrum of pulmonary and systemic injuries based on the chemical properties of the gases, the intensity and duration of exposure, and the impairment of host or pulmonary defenses. Most patients with lower levels of exposures to toxic gases (either known or unknown exposure) present with a wide range of vague symptoms, and treatment is usually supportive. In cases of massive acute inhalations, however, the magnitude of the immediate symptoms in conjunction with the history of exposure may aid in early diagnosis and treatment by medical personnel. Identification of the inhaled chemical is not always possible, and the onset of serious symptoms and injury due to inhalation exposure may be delayed for several hours or days, further hindering identification of the offending inhalant and proper treatment.[1] Although emergency medical personnel may be familiar with a few common toxic inhalants, they typically are inexperienced in the diagnosis and treatment of the multitude of chemical exposures that may occur and should consult occupational and/or toxicology specialists early in the care of patients with suspected exposures. The involvement of these specialists is also important for monitoring and documentation of the long-term sequelae of inhalant exposures, which are poorly understood.

Historically, most toxic inhalations are the result of chemical leaks in industrial settings or during transportation of chemicals, so knowledge of the potential toxins in each setting is important. Carbon dioxide and hydrogen sulfide are produced during mining or fermentation processes. Hydrogen chloride and vinyl chloride are byproducts of the production of plastics. Arsine, phosphine, and diborane are toxic gases used in the microelectronics industry. The oxides of metals can produce "metal fume fever" in industrial or recreational welding operations. In the community setting, potential exposures include chlorine gas from cleaning supplies, methylene chloride from paint removers, carbon monoxide from heaters or automobiles, and hydrogen cyanide from fires. Inhalant abuse in the community can result in toluene, benzene, acetone, or Freon toxicity. Lastly, warfare and terrorism are growing arenas for toxic inhalant exposures. A variety of chemical weapons are an impending source of massive human destruction by dermal or inhalant exposure. Gases that might be used in warfare or terrorism include chlorine, phosgene, nerve gases, and mustard gas.

Inhaled toxicants produce injury by two distinct mechanisms (or a combination of both, as in the case of smoke or hydrogen sulfide inhalation). The first mechanism is regional pulmonary injury resulting from inhalation of either a direct respiratory irritant or a gas that invokes an antigen-induced immune response in a sensitized individual (Table 203-1).[1] Exposures to direct respiratory irritants are the most common type of all the toxic inhalations. The chemical activity, particle size, and solubility of the irritant gas determine the area of deposition of the gas in the respiratory tract and the degree of systemic absorption. In general, gases with a larger particle size (greater than 5 μm) particle size and higher water solubility (classified as type I toxic inhalants) dissolve more readily in the mucous membranes of the oral and nasal passages and produce upper airway symptoms such as conjunctival irritation, nasal discharge, laryngospasm, cough, and stridor. The symptoms of these gases in the proximal airways are particularly noxious and may trigger recognition of toxic gas exposure and evacuation of exposed individuals before more devastating exposure and lower airway injury can occur. Gases with moderate particle size (1 to 5 μm) and moderate water solubility (also classified as type I toxic inhalants) include chlorine, chloramine, and bromine. Deposition of these gases occurs primarily in the middle sections of the respiratory tract. Irritant gases with smaller particle size (less than 5 μm) and low water solubility (type II toxic inhalants) deposit in the terminal airways, producing alveolar or parenchymal injury. Nevertheless, these compounds can still cause minor upper airway irritation.[1] Examples of type II gases include the nitrogen oxides, nitric acid, phosgene, and ozone. Toxicity may manifest as dyspnea (acute or delayed), bronchospasm, cyanosis, pulmonary edema (possibly delayed in onset), and, in the case of exposure to nitrogen dioxide, bronchiolitis obliterans. Although the chemical properties of the irritant gas predict the area of lung injury, massive exposure to any irritant gas can produce significant injury at all levels of the respiratory tract.

The second mechanism by which inhaled toxicants produce injury is systemic toxicity, which results from systemic absorption after inhalation. These systemic (type III) toxic inhalants generally produce little or no respiratory symptoms but cause significant central nervous system and cardiac symptoms due to tissue hypoxia. Examples of these gases include asphyxiants, organophosphates, volatile hydrocarbons, and metal fumes (see Table 203-1).[1]

DIRECT PULMONARY IRRITANTS: HIGH WATER SOLUBILITY (TYPE I)

AMMONIA

Ammonia is a colorless, alkaline gas with a pungent, stinging smell detectable at concentrations of 30 to 53 parts per million (ppm). This gas has half the density of air and therefore rises easily.[2-4] Ammonia is used in higher concentrations as an industrial chemical in the synthesis of fertilizers, synthetic fibers, plastics, explosives, dyes, and pharmaceuticals and in lower concentrations in household cleaning and bleaching supplies.[2-4] It is also a commercial refrigerant gas and is produced during the combustion of silk, nylon, wool, and melamine resins.[1-4]

Ammonia easily combines with moisture in the upper respiratory tract to form ammonium hydroxide (NH_4OH), which dissociates to form hydroxyl and ammonium ions and heat, leading, respectively, to irritant alkali effects and thermal injury. The type and magnitude of injury depend on the concentration and duration of exposure (Table 203-2).[1,2,4] Because of its strong odor and the irritation of the eyes and mucous membranes that ammonia causes after exposure to even low concentrations, most patients are able to remove themselves from the exposure and thereby limit significant pulmonary injury. Higher concentrations of ammonia are very irritating to the eyes; penetration can occur within 5 to 7 seconds, leading to irritation, corneal ulceration, and blindness, which may hinder escape of the individual from

TABLE 203–1. TOXIC INHALANTS

Category	Examples
Pulmonary irritant toxic gases	
High water solubility (type I)	Acetic acid, ammonia, formaldehyde, acrolein, hydrogen chloride (muriatic acid), hydrogen fluoride, hydrogen sulfide, sulfur dioxide, sulfuric acid
Moderate water solubility (type I)	Chlorine, bromine
Low water solubility (type II)	Nitrogen oxides, nitric acid, phosgene, ozone
Pulmonary immunologic toxic inhalants	Toluene diisocyanate, formaldehyde, methylene bisphenyl isocyanate, soldering flux, ammonia, chlorine, nitrogen dioxide, miscellaneous dusts
Systemic toxicants or nonirritant gases (type III)	
Asphyxiants	Nitrogen, methane, carbon dioxide, argon, helium, nitrous oxide, hydrogen, hydrogen cyanide, hydrogen sulfide, methylene chloride
Organophosphates	Insecticides, nerve gases
Hydrocarbons	
Aromatic	Benzene, toluene, vinyl chloride
Chlorinated	Trichloroethylene, trichloroethane
Fluorinated	Freon
Metal fumes	Cadmium, mercury, zinc, nickel, chromium

TABLE 203–2. SIGNS AND SYMPTOMS OF AMMONIA TOXICITY

Exposure	Signs and symptoms
Mild exposure	Inflammation of skin, oropharynx, and/or upper respiratory tract, conjunctivitis
Moderate exposure	Burning of skin, nose, and/or oropharynx
	Edema of mucosal passages, soft palate, posterior pharyngeal wall, trachea
	Dyspnea, wheezing, chest tightness, upper airway obstruction.
	Nausea, vomiting
Severe exposure	Upper airway obstruction, pulmonary edema, laryngospasms, stridor, hoarseness, second- or third-degree burns on skin or mucosal membranes, pulmonary edema

the area of exposure.[2] Ammonia is also very irritating to the mucous membranes of the upper respiratory tract and may lead to dyspnea, wheezing, tracheobronchial edema, and airway obstruction.[2,3,5] In most cases, there is complete recovery from the chemical irritant effects of ammonia, but residual bronchiectasis and small airway disease have been reported.[6] Thermal injury of the oropharyngeal wall, larynx, and lower respiratory tract may result from the interaction of ammonia with moisture in the mucosal membranes; the clinical effects depend on the concentration of ammonia and the duration of exposure.[7] In severe exposures, full-thickness burns, liquefaction necrosis of the tissues, and pulmonary edema may be seen. In moderate and severe ammonia exposures, there may be a biphasic clinical response to injury. The initial signs and symptoms of pulmonary edema, congestion, hemorrhage, and atelectasis improve temporarily over 2 to 3 days but are followed by respiratory failure associated with airway obstruction and bilateral infiltrates on chest radiography.[2,3] The mortality rate may be 40% in severe exposures.[1]

The treatment of ammonia inhalation is primarily supportive after evacuation from the exposure and decontamination if necessary. Because of the irritating effects on mucous membranes and the potential for ulceration, it is important to obtain early specialized care for ocular and dermal burns to improve long-term outcomes for the patient.[2] The eye sac should be irrigated with sterile water or saline for 20 minutes or until the pH is less than 8.5.[3,4] To facilitate this irrigation, topical anesthetics may be required.[3] For respiratory support, a nasal or oral tracheal tube with the largest tube possible is recommended to prevent airway obstruction; cricothyrotomy may be necessary if the airway is already obstructed.[3,5] Early intubation can be life-saving in patients with severe symptoms, because they are at high risk for airway obstruction due to the nature of ammonia-related burns.[7] For the management of bronchospasm, oral or inhaled bronchodilators may be helpful. Inhaled or intravenous corticosteroids have been used in cases of severe bronchospasm refractory to bronchodilator therapy, although the use of these agents is controversial.[3-5] There is a high risk of superinfection in severe exposures to any of the toxic inhalants (particularly with chemical warfare) because of damage to the mucosal barrier to infection, altered lung bacterial clearance, and leukocyte function abnormalities.[6] Nevertheless, prophylactic antimicrobial agents should not be routinely administered because of the potential for selection of resistant organisms.[3]

HYDROGEN SULFIDE

Hydrogen sulfide (H_2S) is an irritating, nonflammable, colorless gas that has a distinct "rotten-egg" odor.[8-10] H_2S is encountered in various industrial settings, including the production of natural gas, heavy water, petroleum, metal processing, mining, and paper pulp and in tannery work.[8,9,11,12] It is an intermediate in hydrocarbon manufacture and is also found in municipal sewers and sewer treatment plants, in manure operations, and in any contained spaces where sulfur-containing organic material has decayed.[8,9,11-14] It is also found in crude oil, volcanic gas, and some hot springs.[9,10] Most cases of significant H_2S exposure occur in the industrial setting and are unintentional.[9]

Tissues with exposed mucous membranes and high oxygen concentration are most susceptible to H_2S toxicity. Toxicity is concentration dependent; the effects are generally reversible. Short exposures to very high concentrations are much more toxic than are prolonged exposures to lower concentrations. H_2S is an irritant; in cases of mild exposure, mucous membrane irritation may be seen, with symptoms of nausea, vomiting, pharyngitis, and conjunctivitis. After dissociation of H_2S, sulfide ions bind to ferric ion in cytochrome oxidase, inhibiting mitochondrial utilization of oxygen for oxidative phosphorylation.[10,11,15] After exposure to a high concentration of H_2S, mitochondrial inhibition leads to development of metabolic acidosis.[15] H_2S also causes potassium channel–mediated hyperpolarization of neurons and enhancement of inhibitory neuronal pathways.[16] Patients with H_2S toxicity usually present with neurologic signs varying in severity from headache, weakness, and incoordination to convulsions and coma.[8-10] Olfactory paralysis can occur at concentrations of 100 to 150 ppm and render the victim unaware of the exposure.[16] The "knock-down" effect is a sudden loss of consciousness that occurs after short exposures to very high concentrations (750 to 1000 ppm) of H_2S, followed by complete recovery.[13,15] This happens too quickly to be attributed to the effect of H_2S on mitochondrial function, and it may actually result from a direct toxic effect of H_2S on the brain.[15] Respiratory signs can range from dyspnea, cough, and sore throat to pulmonary edema, cyanosis, and hemoptysis after exposure to higher concentrations.[8-10] After exposure to 100 to 400 ppm H_2S, necrosis of the nasal epithelium followed by exfoliation of ciliated and mucosal cells can occur.[8] Chest radiographs obtained after severe exposures often display pulmonary edema and evidence of aspiration pneumonitis.[9,13] Cardiac toxicity and cardiopulmonary arrest usually occur after exposure to H_2S concentrations greater than 700 ppm due to anoxia or direct cardiac toxicity.[15]

Immediate removal from exposure and administration of high-flow oxygen are the first steps in treatment; intubation and mechanical ventilation should be performed, if needed. Diagnosis of H_2S toxicity is usually made by the history of exposure and signs and symptoms. Sulfhemoglobin levels are not reliable and often are not elevated despite definitive exposure.[16] Sulfide anion concentration can be measured in plasma, but the assay must be done within 2 hours after exposure and analyzed immediately; ultimately, this result will not influence clinical management.[16] Hyperbaric oxygen (HBO) may be beneficial in severe cases to achieve rapid tissue oxygenation, although human experience in H_2S toxicity is limited to case studies.[17,18] HBO supersaturates tissues with oxygen, which competes with H_2S for binding to cytochrome oxidase. HBO also may enhance sulfide detoxification by increasing sulfide oxidation to sulfate or thiosulfate.[16] In several cases, HBO treatment showed benefit when used together with administration of sodium nitrite, which is another proposed treatment for H_2S toxicity.[8,9] Sodium nitrite induces methemoglobin formation, and methemoglobin combines with H_2S to form the nontoxic sulfmethemoglobin, which is subsequently excreted via the kidneys.[9,15] Whether nitrite therapy is beneficial beyond a few minutes after H_2S exposure is questionable given that sulfide oxidation is extremely rapid, so the amount of sulfide bound to cytochrome oxidase is probably marginal by the time a patient is being treated by medical staff.[16]

DIRECT PULMONARY IRRITANTS: MODERATE WATER SOLUBILITY (TYPE I)

CHLORINE

Chlorine is a dense (2.5 times denser than air), yellowish-green gas that has a distinctive irritating odor at a threshold of 0.2 to 3.5 ppm.[6,19-21] It was used as a chemical warfare agent in World War I. Chlorine is moderately soluble in water and is used extensively in the industrial setting for the production of chlorinated chemicals, in bleaching processes, in the manufacture of plastics, and in water or sewage disinfection.[19] Most toxic exposures to chlorine are occur during industrial accidents or transportation of liquid chlorine.[6] In the community setting, liquid chlorine is used as a disinfectant in swimming pools and as a component of many household cleaning and drain-enhancing agents.[6,19,21] In this setting, chlorine toxicity can result from mixing of sodium hypochlorite (household bleach) with vinegar or ammonia.[20]

Chlorine reacts with water in mucous membranes to form hydrochloric and hypochlorous acids, along with elemental chlorine and reactive oxygen species ($Cl_2 + H_2O \rightarrow HOCl + HCl \rightarrow Cl_2 + H_2O_2$).[20] Chlorine gas is more irritating to respiratory mucosa than is hydrochloric acid, but cellular injury is thought to be caused by the reactive oxygen species that are formed.[20-22] Given its moderate water solubility, chlorine can irritate the upper and lower respiratory tracts to various degrees, depending on the concentration and duration of exposure. Immediately after minor exposures, common symptoms include nausea, vomiting, headache, a burning sensation in the eyes or throat, and cough.[6,21] After more significant exposures, patients present with dyspnea, tachypnea, bronchospasm, wheezing, stridor, pneumonitis, hypoxemia, and respiratory distress.[20,21,23-25] In severe exposures, death can occur, usually from toxic pulmonary edema with respiratory failure. Pathologic changes in the respiratory tract include epithelial cell necrosis and sloughing,

inflammation, purulent intraluminal exudate, and interstitial and alveolar pulmonary edema.[20,25,26] Four phases of acute pulmonary toxicity have been described and serve as a model for exposures to many irritant gases (Table 203-3).[27]

Treatment of chlorine gas exposure begins with removal of the patient from the exposure source, followed by assessment of need for early airway support, rest, and other supportive modalities. Symptoms of upper respiratory tract irritation can be alleviated with administration of humidified oxygen, but patients should not be overoxygenated, because this intervention theoretically could aggravate chlorine-induced formation of reactive oxygen species.[19-21] Severe cases might require continuous positive airway pressure or mechanical ventilation. Bronchoconstriction and bronchospasm should be treated with nebulized or inhaled β-adrenergic agonists, and cough should be treated with antitussives.[21] Retrospective, uncontrolled studies have reported that low concentrations of nebulized sodium bicarbonate (3.75% to 5%) relieve symptoms in patients with mild cases of chlorine gas inhalation.[21,24,28] The mechanism of action is postulated to be neutralization of the hydrochloric acid that is formed when chlorine reacts with water.[21] It is unclear whether the findings in these studies reflect the natural clinical resolution of symptoms after chlorine exposure or a true treatment effect of nebulized sodium bicarbonate.[20] Anecdotal case reports have suggested beneficial effects of systemic corticosteroids after chlorine gas exposure.[29] Animal data have also shown a benefit of nebulized corticosteroids administered immediately after chlorine gas injury on oxygenation and cardiovascular function with presumably minimal systemic corticosteroid effects.[25] Animal data also have shown that delayed administration of nebulized corticosteroids 60 minutes after chlorine exposure was less effective than immediate treatment or treatment 30 minutes after exposure.[23]

DIRECT PULMONARY IRRITANTS: LOW WATER SOLUBILITY (TYPE II)

NITROGEN DIOXIDE

Nitrogen dioxide (NO_2) is an insoluble, dense, reddish-brown, powerful oxidant gas with a pungent odor.[30-32] Exposures occur in industrial and occupational settings. NO_2 is produced by ice-resurfacing machines in indoor arenas; in the manufacture of dyes, fertilizers, celluloid, and lacquer; and in acetylene and electric arc welding.[30,31,33] The oxidation of nitrogen-rich fertilizer on crops in silos during the first hours to days of storage generates NO_2, and exposure can result in "silo fillers' disease."[32]

TABLE 203–3. PHASES OF ACUTE IRRITANT GAS PULMONARY INJURY		
Phase	**Time since exposure**	**Symptoms**
I	0-6 h	Choking and coughing, which gradually subside after removal from exposure
II	6 h to 8 d	Oropharyngeal and pulmonary edema, exudative inflammatory bronchitis with plugging of medium and small bronchi, atelectasis, progressive upper and/or peripheral airway obstruction
III	1-4 wk	Gradual improvement of pulmonary function
IV	>4 wk	Continued improvement in airway obstruction, possible persistence of maldistribution of ventilation, possible persistence of severe chronic airway disease

Because of its poor water solubility, little upper airway or ophthalmologic irritation is produced by exposure to NO_2. Instead, the toxic effect of NO_2 is at the level of the alveoli. The low solubility of the gas also contributes to a time delay between initial exposure to NO_2 and development of significant pulmonary problems.[6] The extent of injury depends on the concentration and duration of exposure. Three mechanisms of toxicity have been hypothesized. NO_2 may produce tissue damage as a result of the formation of free radicals, followed by lipid peroxidation and membrane destruction.[30] The injury may be further aggravated by the combination of NO_2 with water, which produces nitric and nitrous acids, causing chemical pneumonitis and pulmonary edema.[1,30] Lastly, NO_2 may be systemically absorbed, resulting in methemoglobinemia.[34]

The pattern of NO_2 toxicity has been described as triphasic.[1,6] Mild symptoms, such as cough, dyspnea, and headache, develop initially after exposure; they typically dissipate over a few hours but may persist for weeks in some cases. This is followed by a delayed phase with pulmonary edema.[1] Some patients progress to the third phase weeks later and develop bronchiolitis obliterans and chronic interstitial lung disease.[1,33]

For patients with hypoxemia due to NO_2 toxicity, supplemental oxygen should be administered.[30,33] The utility of corticosteroids in cases of NO_2 toxicity is unproven. Data from animal models of NO_2 toxicity have shown amelioration of pulmonary tissue damage by corticosteroid administration, whereas other data have failed to shown beneficial effects.[35,36] β_2-Adrenergic agonists should be administered if there is a component of airway obstruction, and diuretics may be used for management of pulmonary edema.[30,33,37]

PHOSGENE

Phosgene ($COCl_2$) is a poorly water soluble, dense, colorless, highly reactive oxidant gas with a characteristic moldy hay or green corn smell.[38,39] It has many industrial sources, because it is used in the synthesis of various resins, aniline dyes, insecticides, and plastics.[38-40] Exposure may occur when paint removers, solvents, or dry cleaning products containing methylene chloride are exposed to heat and produce phosgene gas.[38,41] Phosgene is also produced during the combustion of polyvinylchloride.[6] Historically, phosgene was used as a chemical war gas and was responsible for approximately 80% of gas-related deaths in World War I.[38-40]

With most gases, the victim of a potentially toxic exposure is alerted by ocular and mucous membrane irritation at low inhaled concentrations. In the case of phosgene, irritation occurs only at higher concentrations. Phosgene also causes prompt fatigue of the olfactory system, which is another lost warning sign of exposure.[39] Higher concentrations of phosgene initially produce eye irritation, coughing, chest tightness, tachycardia, tachypnea, and dyspnea, which gradually resolve.[38,39,41] Because of phosgene's low water solubility, inflammation of mucous membranes is indicative of exposure to high concentrations. Deep tissue damage may ensue after higher-dose exposures, and delayed symptoms of pulmonary edema and respiratory failure develop after an asymptomatic period.

Phosgene causes oxidant-like injury by two chemical reactions, acylation and hydrolysis.[39] In the acylation process, phosgene irreversibly reacts with nucleophilic groups of tissue macromolecules, resulting in denaturation

of proteins.[39] Pharmacologic strategies designed to replenish tissue levels of glutathione may diminish phosgene-induced injury.[39] Glycolysis and oxygen utilization by lung cells is inhibited, and tissue concentrations of adenosine triphosphate (ATP) and adenosine monophosphate (ADP) are decreased.[39] These mechanisms cause pulmonary edema due to destruction of cell membranes and increased vascular membrane permeability.[38] Phosgene inhalation also has been shown in animal models to stimulate the synthesis of lipoxygenase products, which may contribute to the development of pulmonary edema by increasing pulmonary vascular permeability.[39,40,42,43] In addition, on moist membranes, phosgene is hydrolyzed to carbon dioxide and hydrochloric acid.[38,39] Given the low water solubility of phosgene, only small amounts of hydrochloric acid are produced after contact with the ocular, nasopharynx, and upper respiratory tract mucous membranes, but the acid formed still can cause immediate irritation after significant exposures to phosgene.

As with the other toxic inhalants, initial management of phosgene exposure includes evacuation from the exposure site; basic resuscitation procedures; decontamination of contaminated skin, eyes, and clothing; and advanced life support measures, including endotracheal intubation for victims of severe exposures and those with evidence of upper airway obstruction or respiratory distress.[39] Supportive care is necessary in cases of mild exposure with symptoms of ocular or upper airway irritation. For more severe exposures, prophylactic treatment may diminish or avert the latent phosgene-induced activation of the inflammatory cascade before the development of pulmonary edema, although human data are lacking.[39] Systemic or inhaled corticosteroids have been recommended for prevention of pulmonary edema.[39,42] Nonsteroidal anti-inflammatory agents (e.g., ibuprofen) also have been shown to prevent the development of pulmonary edema in animal models of phosgene exposure.[44] Another prophylactic treatment that has decreased pulmonary edema in phosgene-exposed animal models is the intratracheal administration of N-acetylcysteine.[40] N-acetylcysteine prevents edema formation by decreasing peptide leukotriene production and lipid peroxidation and promoting the formation of glutathione.[40]

For treatment of established pulmonary edema after phosgene exposures, endotracheal intubation and mechanical ventilation or continuous positive airway pressure may be required. The administration of systemic or inhaled corticosteroids and diuretics has been recommended for treatment of phosgene-induced pulmonary edema, although human data to support the use of these agents are lacking. Intravenous administration of aminophylline to animals with phosgene exposure significantly reduced the development of pulmonary edema.[45]

SYSTEMIC TOXIC INHALANTS (TYPE III)

CARBON MONOXIDE

Carbon monoxide (CO) is a colorless, odorless, nonirritating, toxic gas that is lighter than air.[46,47] It is present in air at a concentration of less than 0.001%.[47] CO is the leading cause of death due to poisoning in the United States, and reported mortality rates have ranged from 1% to 31% in large series.[46,48] The true incidence of CO poisoning is not known, because many nonlethal cases go unreported or undetected.[48]

CO is generated from appliances that use carbon-based fuels, such as motor vehicles, heaters, furnaces, and wood stoves.[46,47] It is a product of incomplete combustion of organic compounds and is usually a component of the gases generated by household fires.[46,47] CO poisoning can also result from inhalation of paint removers containing methylene chloride, which is hepatically metabolized to CO.[46,47]

CO binds preferentially but reversibly to hemoglobin, with an affinity 200 to 300 times greater than that of oxygen, to form carboxyhemoglobin (COHb), thus displacing oxygen and reducing arterial oxygen content.[46,47] Potential mechanisms of CO toxicity include (1) decreased blood oxygen-carrying capacity due to the COHb complex; (2) altered dissociation characteristics of oxyhemoglobin, which cause oxygen to be more tightly bound to hemoglobin and produce hypoxia; (3) inhibition of cellular respiration by binding to heme-containing proteins such as cytochrome oxidase and hyperoxidases; and (4) binding to myoglobin, which causes myocardial and skeletal muscle dysfunction.[46,47]

After exposure, CO dissociates from hemoglobin and is excreted by the lungs. The half-life of COHb after methylene chloride exposure is up to 2.5 times longer than with normal CO exposure, because methylene chloride continues to be metabolized to CO by the liver.[47] A decrease in oxygen delivery to the brain stimulates the ventilatory drive and thus minute ventilation. This leads to more CO inhalation, resulting in respiratory alkalosis. CO binds to cardiac and skeletal myoglobin with a higher affinity than it binds to hemoglobin. CO therefore remains bound to myoglobin, particularly cardiac myoglobin, long after CO is released from hemoglobin. This leads to a rebound effect when CO is finally released from myoglobin and binds to hemoglobin, thereby increasing carboxyhemoglobin concentrations and toxicity symptoms again.[46]

Initial symptoms of acute CO poisoning are headache, lethargy, nausea and vomiting, and difficulty with memory or confusion.[46,47] The severity of CO toxicity symptoms correlates roughly with the COHb blood concentration.[46] Patients usually are asymptomatic if the COHb concentration is less than 10%. As the concentration increases to more than 20%, dizziness, headache, nausea, and confusion may develop. If the COHb concentration is greater than 40%, coma and seizures due to cerebral edema may be seen. Cardiopulmonary dysfunction and death are likely if the concentration is greater than 60%. The presentation and severity of clinical symptoms of CO toxicity do not always correlate with the blood COHb concentration, however.[47] Patients with underlying cardiovascular or respiratory diseases have more severe symptoms of CO toxicity relative to the blood COHb concentration.[47] A person who smokes more than 40 cigarettes daily can have a baseline COHb concentration as high as 18% without significant symptoms of CO toxicity.[47] Children and infants have a higher risk of CO toxicity because of their higher metabolic rates.[49] Fetal hemoglobin binds CO more avidly than does the mother's hemoglobin, and transplacental perfusion for elimination is slower. Therefore, fetal COHb concentrations continue to increase after maternal CO exposure, and they tend to be about 10% higher than those in the mother. Retrospective studies show that fetal mortality may be 36% to 67% after maternal CO exposure.[46,49]

Patients with acute CO toxicity have parenchymal interstitial edema, as evidenced by a "ground glass" appearance on chest radiography, caused by tissue hypoxia or the toxic effects of CO on alveolar membranes, or both.[47] Pulmonary edema and hemorrhage also result from the hypoxic effects of CO on myocardial tissue, resulting in left ventricular failure. Pulmonary edema can also be caused by aspiration of gastric contents, as a result of altered level of consciousness.

The most common long-term sequelae of CO poisoning are neuropsychiatric effects, which can occur immediately after exposure and persist or can be delayed, often developing within 20 days after CO exposure.[46,47,50] These effects do not correlate with the concentration of COHb in the blood at the time of exposure, but they may correlate with the level of consciousness on admission to the hospital.[47,49] Neuropsychiatric effects were noted in 11% to 40% of patients in one study, and they often appeared after a period of apparent recovery.[47] Symptoms include irritability, confusion, cognitive and personality changes, psychic akinesia, parkinsonism, psychotic encephalopathy, amnesia, apathy, dementia, mutism, and urinary and fecal incontinence. These symptoms may occur 3 to 21 days after exposure.[49]

The most important aspect of treatment in any toxic inhalation is to remove the patient from the source of exposure. In the case of CO exposures, keeping the patient close to the ground (because oxygen is heavier than CO) may help to further reduce exposure time.[47] After arrival at the hospital, a blood COHb concentration should be obtained during the initial assessment. Patients with a COHb concentration greater than 25% should be evaluated for admission even in the absence of toxic symptoms.[47] Other situations that warrant admission for evaluation of CO toxicity include the presence of cardiovascular disease with an COHb concentration greater than 15%; pregnancy with a COHb concentration greater than 10%; an abnormal electrocardiogram or ischemic chest pain; and the presence of metabolic acidosis, thermoregulatory difficulties, abnormal neuropsychiatric testing results, hypoxemia (partial pressure of oxygen in arterial blood [PaO_2] less than 60 mm Hg), an abnormal chest radiograph, or a history of unconsciousness.[47]

Treatment of CO toxicity after evacuation from the exposure consists primarily of administration of supplemental oxygen. The goal of oxygen therapy in patients with CO toxicity is to improve the blood oxygen content by increasing the PaO_2.[46] The initial approach is to provide 100% supplemental oxygen, using a tight-fitting mask with nonrebreathing valves. Endotracheal intubation may be necessary in symptomatic patients who require oxygen supplementation but cannot protect their airway.[47] In some cases, transfusion with packed red blood cells can be a source for oxygenated blood. HBO has been used as a method of oxygenation in CO toxicity, particularly in cases of lost consciousness or severe poisoning.[46,47,49,51] HBO increases the dissolved oxygen content in the blood and produces a more rapid reduction in COHb concentrations, compared with normobaric oxygen.[50] The half-life of COHb in a healthy volunteer breathing room air is 4 to 5 hours.[46] The half-life of COHb during administration of 100% oxygen is approximately 90 minutes, and it is less than 30 minutes during administration of HBO at 3 atmospheric pressures (atm).[47,51] HBO may cause cerebral vasoconstriction, thereby reducing intracranial pressure and cerebral edema, and it also may produce a more rapid dissociation of CO from respiratory cyctochromes.[46]

In spite of the potential benefits of HBO in CO toxicity, its use in acute poisonings has been controversial. Risks with HBO therapy include aural barotrauma, hyperoxic seizures, anxiety, and time delay associated with transportation to a treatment center equipped with HBO. There are no studies that have specifically analyzed the risks versus benefits of HBO.[50] A recent study by Weaver and colleagues[50] evaluated the rates of cognitive sequelae in patients with acute, symptomatic CO poisoning treated with HBO versus normobaric oxygen. Patients randomly assigned to HBO received three sessions of treatment, lasting 150, 120, and 120 minutes, respectively. In the first HBO session, patients received oxygen at 3 atm for 75 minutes, followed by 2 atm for another 75 minutes. The second and third HBO sessions were maintained at 2 atm. These sessions were done at intervals of 6 to 12 hours, with the first session being within 24 hours after exposure. HBO therapy was found to reduce cognitive sequelae by 46% at 6 weeks after treatment. Cognitive sequelae at 6 and 12 months were also less frequent in the HBO group than the normobaric-oxygen group.

Reduction of intracranial pressure (ICP) may be necessary. Intracranial hypertension is present in some patients secondary to brain edema.[46,47] The use of corticosteroids has been suggested but not studied.[47] In some cases, hyperosmolar agents, particularly mannitol (0.25 to 2 g/kg as a 20% solution), has been used with ICP monitoring.[47] In these patients, fluid administration should also be reduced to keep the ICP down. Seizures can be one of the presenting symptoms of CO poisoning; it may be treated with diazepam or lorazepam. In some cases, phenytoin has also been used.[47]

CONCLUSION

In summary, there are numerous gases that can cause inhalational toxicity by direct pulmonary injury, systemic toxicity, or a combination of both mechanisms. Occupational exposures and fires are the most common sources of accidental exposure.[1] Prevention of exposure in the workplace by limitation of exposure risks and safety measures is important. Anticipation and preparation for potential industrial exposures in a given geographical setting are also important, and education of medical personnel regarding local chemical use and material safety data sheet availability is good preemptive practice. It is important for medical staff to be aware of the symptomatology of the more common occupational and household potential exposures and to gather in-depth historical information in cases of gas exposure to aid in the identification and proper treatment of the exposure. For most inhalational exposures, decontamination and supportive care are the mainstays of therapy. In more severe gas exposures, other modalities may be useful, and involvement of occupational medicine or toxicology specialists in the case management may be necessary.

ANNOTATED REFERENCES

Bosse GM: Nebulized sodium bicarbonate in the treatment of chlorine gas inhalation. J Toxicol Clin Toxicol 1994;32:233-241.

Nebulized sodium bicarbonate has been used anecdotally in cases of chlorine toxicity with benefit. This is a 2-year retrospective review of 86 cases of chlorine toxicity from 49 medical facilities in which there was no further clinical deterioration after administration of sodium bicarbonate by nebulization. Prospective trials are lacking.

Reiffenstein RJ, Hulbert WC, Roth SH: Toxicology of hydrogen sulfide. Annu Rev Pharmacol Toxicol 1992;32:109-134.

This comprehensive review of hydrogen sulfide discusses the physicochemical properties, mechanisms of injury, clinical manifestations on primary organ systems, and therapeutic management strategies.

Rorison DG, McPherson SJ: Acute toxic inhalations. Emerg Med Clin North Am 1992;10:409-435.

This article provides an excellent overview of the major toxic inhalants, including industrial and community sources of exposure, pathogenesis and determinants of toxicity, and treatment options.

Sciuto AM, Strickland PT, Kennedy TP, Gurtner GH: Protective effects of N-acetylcysteine treatment after phosgene exposure in rabbits. Am J Respir Crit Care Med 1995;151:768-772.

This study provided an excellent overview of the mechanisms of phosgene-induced pulmonary injury and also examines the protective effects of N-acetylcysteine administration after phosgene exposure. Intratracheal administration of N-acetylcysteine prevented pulmonary edema and peptide leukotriene production.

Weaver LK, Hopkins RO, Chan KJ, et al: Hyperbaric oxygen for acute carbon monoxide poisoning. N Engl J Med 2002;347:1057-1067.

In this randomized, double-blind trial, the benefit of hyperbaric oxygen over normobaric oxygen was seen in patients receiving three treatments of hyperbaric oxygen within a 24-hour period after acute CO poisoning. The trial was stopped after the third of four scheduled interim analyses due to significant reduction in risk of cognitive sequelae at 6 weeks and 12 months.

Chapter 204

PHARMACOECONOMICS IN CRITICAL CARE

Joseph F. Dasta • Amy J. Durtschi • Sandra Kane-Gill

KEY POINTS

1. Overall health care costs continue to rise, with ICUs consuming a third of inpatient costs at a daily cost of approximately $3500.

2. Pharmacoeconomic evaluations of pharmaceuticals attempt to identify the value of drug therapy from a clinical, economic, or humanistic perspective.

3. Representative expensive ICU-related conditions in which more effective therapy is needed include acute congestive heart failure, acute renal failure, severe sepsis and sepsis syndrome, ventilator-associated pneumonia, catheter-related sepsis, bloodstream infections, deep venous thrombosis, agitation, and pain.

Pharmacoeconomics is a branch of health economics that analyzes the economic impact and cost-effectiveness of pharmaceuticals.[1] This definition has been broadened to include not only the economic costs, but also the quality-of-life or humanistic consequences of drug therapy. Evaluation of therapeutic protocols and guidelines also is included in pharmacoeconomic studies.[2] It has been suggested that health economics can help answer two fundamental questions: (1) Is a given therapy (or program) worth using when compared with alternatives? (2) Should a portion of available health care resources be allocated to a given therapy or program?[3]

The science of pharmacoeconomics has evolved in complexity and applicability since the term was first used in 1986.[2] Today a considerable amount of research in pharmacoeconomics is being conducted by academic medical centers, pharmaceutical companies, and health services research and consulting companies. Clinicians, administrators, and health care systems are mandating that economic information be added to the clinical effectiveness of new therapies before a drug is added to a formulary. The Academy of Managed Care Pharmacy published "The Format for Formulary Submissions in 2000" with version 2.0 released in 2002.[4] The goal of these guidelines is to ensure that all new products bring added clinical and economic value to the insured population. The Academy wants its members to be able to evaluate new therapies objectively from safety, effectiveness, and economic perspectives compared with current treatments. As such, pharmacoeconomic data can help in making more informed decisions about selecting a particular drug for a patient or health care system.

ECONOMICS OF HEALTH CARE AND INTENSIVE CARE UNIT CARE

One of the catalysts driving the growth of pharmacoeconomics is the staggering cost of health care. In 2001, health care spending in the United States increased 8.7% to a total of $1.4 trillion, which represents 14.1% of the gross domestic product of the United States.[5] Hospital sector spending in the United States increased 8.3% in 2001 to $451 billion. It is projected that health care expenditures in the United States will reach $3.4 trillion in 2013.

Although pharmaceuticals constituted only 9.4% of total health care costs in the United States in 2000, they represented the fastest growing health expenditure category.[6] Between 1990 and 2000, spending on prescription drugs increased by more than 200%. In 2002, pharmaceutical expenditures in the United States are expected to increase about 15% to nearly $200 billion.

The cost of drug therapy is complex and consists of multiple components. Table 204-1 summarizes the components of the cost of the drug product and the cost of complications.[7] It is easy to obtain data on acquisition costs of drugs and materials to prepare and administer drugs. Determining the cost of adverse drug events is far more challenging, however, and often is not considered. These data cannot be ignored because the estimated annual costs of drug-related problems in the United States increased from $77.6 billion in 1995 to $155 billion in 2000.[8]

ICUs consume significant resources in hospitals. The large economic burden of the ICU is out of proportion, however, to the number of ICU beds in the institution. ICU beds account for less than 10% of all inpatient beds in the United States, yet consume about 33% of inpatient costs, or $60 billion annually.[9] The cost of an ICU day is estimated to be three to four times the cost of a ward day.[10] Rapoport and colleagues[11] collected cost data from 751 patients in two

TABLE 204–1. COST OF A DRUG VERSUS COST OF A COMPLICATION

Cost of a drug	Cost of a complication
Acquisition cost	Increased morbidity cost
Associated material preparation and delivery cost	Increased mortality cost
Number of doses per day cost	Increased total cost
Route of administration cost	Increased length of stay
Labor preparation and administration cost	Increased intensity of care
	Decreased patient satisfaction

TABLE 204–2. TOP 10 DRUGS BY COST IN THE INTENSIVE CARE UNIT

Fiscal year 1999	% of ICU drug costs	Fiscal year 2000	% of ICU drug costs	Fiscal year 2001	% of ICU drug costs	YTD fiscal year 2002*	% of ICU drug costs
Albumin	13.2	Albumin	12.9	Propofol	13.2	Albumin	11.2
Propofol	6.8	Propofol	9.4	Albumin	12.3	Propofol	10.8
LAmB	3.6	HBIG	4.7	Mycophenolate	4.6	Mycophenolate	4.9
HBIG	3.4	Piperacillin	3.1	LAmB	3.1	Amiodarone	3.5
Fluconazole	2.4	LAmB	2.8	Fluconazole	2.6	Erythropoietin	3.2
Dialysate	2.2	Dialysate	2.3	Dialysate	2.3	Rabbit antithymocyte globulin	3
Octreotide	2	Fluconazole	2.3	Amiodarone	2.1	LAmB	2.6
Urokinase	2	Amiodarone	1.8	Quinupristin and dalfopristin	1.7	Fluconazole	2.5
Ticarcillin	2	Levofloxacin	1.5	Erythropoietin	1.6	Piperacillin	2.2
IVIG	1.8	Alteplase	1.5	Levofloxacin	1.5	Dialysate	1.9

HBIG, hepatitis B immune globulin; IVIG, intranenous immune globulin; LAmB, liposomal amphotericin; YTD, year to date.
Data are from a partial fiscal year* (July 1, 2001, to May 31, 2002).

ICUs and found the first ICU day was about 4 times more expensive than ward days (after ICU discharge), whereas ICU days after the first day were 2.5 to 3 times as expensive as ward days. Chelluri and associates[12] collected cost data from 813 mechanically ventilated adults at one medical center and reported a median daily ICU cost of $2655 (range $1010 to $13,047). Medical ICU patient costs were lower than surgical ICU patient costs ($2308 versus $2954). Finally, a large database of more than 50,000 patients from 252 ICUs revealed a mean ICU total cost of $19,725.[13] Daily ICU costs were greatest on day 1 (average $7728), decreased on day 2 (average $3872), and stabilized on day 3 and beyond at approximately $3500. Mechanically ventilated patients had the highest ICU costs; use of a ventilator increased average cost by $1522. Therapeutic interventions that can reduce ICU length of stay by even 1 day can have a significant impact on total hospital costs, particularly in patients requiring mechanical ventilation.

Drug costs in the ICU are difficult to quantify because most hospitals are not sufficiently computerized to track these data. Data from one academic medical center were collected over 4 years in 23,000 patients to evaluate costs of drugs used in the ICU.[14] Table 204-2 lists the top 10 drugs by cost used in the ICU over the study period. Approximately 15 drugs accounted for more than 50% of drug costs in the ICU. Drug costs in the ICU averaged 38% of the hospital's total drug costs and increased at a higher rate than non-ICU drug costs over the 4-year period (12.4% versus 5.9%). Fiscal year 2002 data revealed an ICU drug cost of $312 per day compared with $112 per day outside of the ICU; pharmacy charges were 13% of total charges in the ICU. The magnitude of drug usage and the high costs of pharmacotherapy in the ICU, coupled with increasing fiscal awareness and tight budgets, give rise to the ICU being an important area for pharmacoeconomic evaluation.

ECONOMIC EVALUATIONS IN CRITICAL CARE MEDICINE

Although any economic analysis could be performed in a critical care environment, some of the more appropriate are cost-effectiveness analysis, cost benefit analysis, cost minimization analysis, cost utility analysis, and cost of illness. Cost-effectiveness evaluation is discussed in greater depth

because it is the most commonly performed and is the approach recommended by expert bodies.[15]

Cost-effectiveness analysis is a full economic evaluation because costs and outcomes are considered. A drug is evaluated on the basis of cost and outcome in reference to a comparator, which is usually the current standard of care. In a cost-effectiveness evaluation, the most preferred therapy has increased effectiveness at decreased cost.

In 1996, the Panel on Cost-Effectiveness in Health and Medicine (PCEHM) published guidelines for the conduct and reporting of economic analyses.[16] The group's objective was to improve the quality of data and increase the application of cost-effectiveness evaluation in medicine by providing guidelines for the development and analysis of these types of studies. This work resulted in some key points to consider when employing a cost-effectiveness evaluation, including the use of a reference case for comparison, the importance of transparent methods and logic, and the consideration of the perspective being evaluated. Perspective refers to the point of view for the analysis; is it the patient's, the provider's, the payer's, or society's? The PCEHM recommends the societal perspective as being the most comprehensive, and considers workforce and familial aspects of illness. The PCEHM recommends using the following steps when designing a cost-effectiveness analysis:

1. The analysis plan should include the development of a conceptual model describing the intervention and its effects on health outcomes. This plan should incorporate the most fundamental aspects of a cost-effectiveness evaluation: the data collection plan and the analytic plan. The methods used to collect data on costs, health effects, patient preferences, relevant comparators, and perspective should be determined during this phase.

2. The conceptual model should incorporate the schematic of a decision tree, wherein all possible treatment outcomes are considered. It should be constructed to represent health effects and should be used to reflect the cascade of cost implications resulting from an intervention. The model should be an inclusive representation of all possible clinical outcomes. Figure 204-1 depicts a decision tree evaluating a new therapy for heart failure. In the tree, a square indicates a choice is being made, a circle indicates a chance of an outcome occurring, and a triangle indicates the end of a tree branch, commonly referred to

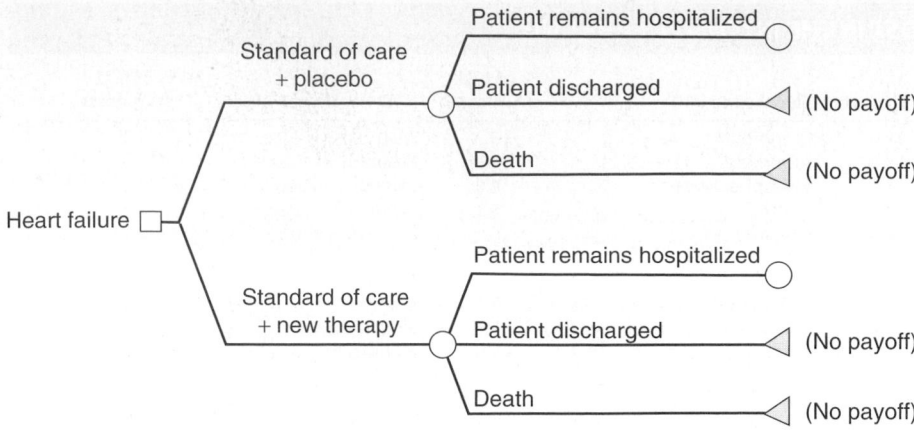

FIGURE 204-1. Example of a decision tree.

as a *terminal node*. Each branch calculates the probability of an event occurring. The terminal node depicts the probability and cost.

3. Collecting appropriate data can be the most challenging aspect of a cost-effectiveness evaluation. The analyst is tasked with considering every aspect of therapy and possible comparators during the first two phases of development. This phase should incorporate a reality check, as the availability of necessary data comes into question. The researcher can use a variety of resources, including experts in the field, published epidemiologic studies, the medical literature, and various cost databases. Data may need to be collected prospectively in a primary cost-effectiveness trial, or data collection can be piggy-backed onto a clinical study. Study protocols must be naturalistic in design, not protocol driven, to capture effectively all costs and outcomes associated with a particular intervention.

4. Computing cost and effectiveness may entail the use of computerized spreadsheets, decision-analysis software, or simulation software. Commonly employed methods include Monte Carlo simulation; state-transition models; and decision tree models from programs such as DATA, Decision-Maker, and SMLTREE.

The American Thoracic Society convened a workshop to address the application of the PCEHM guidelines to a critical care environment.[17] A group of experts compiled key considerations for a cost-effectiveness evaluation in the ICU, including the following: (1) Evidence for the effectiveness of critical care interventions is often lacking; (2) ICU care is often supportive rather than curative; (3) critical illness is a complex process that can occur in a heterogeneous population; (4) many ICU outcome measures are not well suited for cost-effectiveness evaluation; (5) many of the recommended outcomes in cost-effectiveness evaluation (quality of life, utility measures) are difficult to measure in critical illness; (6) valuing the importance of end-of-life care is difficult; (7) the burden of critical illness on family members is not easily captured; and (8) data on the costs of ICU therapies are often derived from sources with different practice patterns. Additionally, determining a single comparator is sometimes a challenge, and it is difficult to assign the societal perspective to an acute care setting. These issues and others must be considered carefully when undertaking a cost-effectiveness evaluation in the ICU.

Cost utility analysis has been called a form of cost-effectiveness evaluation that examines the utility or value of an outcome. Patient, family member, provider, or societal preferences can value health outcomes. Commonly used measures of utility include quality of life and time tradeoff techniques that allow a patient to "value" a current state of health. Cost per quality-adjusted life-year can be measured for alternative therapies by assessing the length of time a patient is in a state of health rated on a scale of 0 to 1, where *1* equals perfect health and *0* equals death.

Cost minimization assumes equal effectiveness for each alternative and evaluates the impact on an identical outcome. If two ICU sedatives produce the same quality of sedation, but one requires a more labor-intensive administration protocol, a decision maker could apply a cost minimization analysis to determine the preferred, less costly drug.

Cost benefit analysis compares the costs and benefits of alternative therapies. This type of economic evaluation rarely is applied to health care interventions. In a cost benefit analysis, all therapy benefits are converted to monetary value. This conversion allows the analysis of treatments for various disease states, a unique feature of cost-benefit analysis.

Cost-of-illness studies describe the economic burden of a specific condition or disease state and are frequently part of epidemiology studies. This type of analysis may take into consideration the workforce and societal impact of illness, in addition to the financial implications for payers and providers. A special type of cost of illness study reflects the cost of acute illness. This analysis is better suited for an ICU patient population because the goal is to assess the costs associated with an acute exacerbation of illness, not the impact of a chronic condition. The costs associated with the development of acute renal failure, for example, could be ascertained with this type of analysis.

DETERMINING COSTS IN THE INTENSIVE CARE UNIT

Three approaches frequently are used to assess the economic burden of a disease state—prospective study design, retrospective analysis, and decision modeling.[18] A prospective study gives the investigator an opportunity to measure important variables completely and accurately. Retrospective database analysis reviews data that already have been assembled and has the advantage of being much less costly and time-consuming than prospective studies with the ability to review many patients easily. Example databases include those from Medicare and the National Center for Health Statistics.

In retrospective studies, the subjects already are assembled, baseline measurements already have been made, and the follow-up period already has occurred. Care must be taken, however, to de-identify patients properly to preserve patient confidentiality. The total direct and indirect costs of a condition may be readily assessed. Total direct costs include the value of all goods, services, and other resources that are consumed in the provision of an intervention or in dealing with the side effects of the intervention or other current or future consequences linked to the intervention.[19] Indirect costs are the costs that are the result of a certain therapy or illness, such as lost wages, workforce replacement, or child care that may be necessary.[17,20]

Patient billing information and summary estimates of department-level expenditures can be used to estimate costs when hospital administrative data are used. With such data, a range of approaches can be pursued. At one extreme, hospital charges can be used as a proxy of costs. This approach may be reasonable in a comparative analysis of interventions, assuming that charges per admission are roughly proportional to economic costs per admission.[19] Another approach is to use the department's cost-to-charge ratio, which has been shown to perform accurately when evaluating average costs per diagnosis-related group.[21]

COST OF INTENSIVE CARE UNIT–RELATED CONDITIONS

The evaluation of the economic consequences of medical conditions is one of several areas of focus since the 1990s in the effort to decrease overall health care spending and identify high-cost diseases to target therapies. Numerous studies have addressed the costs of various treatments and interventions in the ICU.[1]

CONGESTIVE HEART FAILURE

Among the nearly 5 million Americans with congestive heart failure, the number of hospital discharges related to congestive heart failure has increased by 165% in the past 20 years.[22] Acute congestive heart failure is the reason for at least 20% of hospital admissions in patients older than 65 years old and the most expensive admission diagnosis with more than $24.3 billion spent in the United States during 2003.[23] In 1998, the cost per admission of a congestive heart failure patient was $5471, and in 2001, hospitals lost on average $1288 per Medicare patient.[24] These data may underestimate the actual economic burden because one study reported one third of patients with clinical evidence of congestive heart failure did not receive the correct diagnostic code for this condition.[25] More data are needed to better understand the financial impact of acute congestive heart failure.

ACUTE RENAL FAILURE

Acute renal failure is associated with a high mortality rate. Little is known about the costs associated with treating acute renal failure. In one study of 2400 coronary artery bypass graft patients, patients who developed acute renal failure had an almost twofold increase in ICU length of stay and total hospital length of stay.[26] For patients requiring renal replacement therapy, the length of stay in the ICU and the hospital was twice as long as for patients with acute renal failure not needing renal replacement therapy and five times as long as for patients without acute renal failure. It has been estimated that acute renal failure after coronary artery bypass graft surgery in the United States increases total ICU stay by 200,000 days per year and total hospital stay by 400,000 days per year.[26] The incremental health care costs associated with acute renal failure in this population are projected to be in the millions of dollars annually.

A prospective cohort study of 9105 patients involved 490 patients who required renal replacement therapy in five teaching hospitals.[27] The results showed that initiating renal replacement therapy and aggressively treating patients with a poor prognosis is expensive, ranging from $61,900 per quality-adjusted life-year to $274,100 per quality-adjusted life-year (in 1997 dollars), depending on the probability of surviving 6 months. The authors concluded that initiating dialysis was not cost-effective when the therapeutic intervention was applied to acute renal failure patients with an average probability of surviving 6 months.

Another study reviewed post–coronary artery bypass graft patients to determine the average costs for caring for patients who developed postoperative acute renal failure compared with patients who did not develop postoperative acute renal failure.[28] When total hospital costs were calculated for the case and the control groups, the difference attributable to acute renal failure was $21,709. Most of the cost difference (70.3%) was associated with care in the ICU. The incremental costs were related directly to the increase in ICU length of stay in patients with acute renal failure.

INFECTIOUS DISEASES

Ventilator-associated pneumonia is a frequent complication of mechanical ventilation in critically ill patients and is associated with a 20% to 30% mortality rate.[29] Preliminary studies estimated that the cost of ventilator-associated pneumonia ranges from $5365 to $10,062 per patient.[29] Boyce and coworkers[30] reported a median loss to the institution of $15,360 per patient with ventilator-associated pneumonia under a prospective payment system. Neither the Shorr study[29] nor the Boyce study[30] evaluated total costs, however. Another study determined the attributable cost of ventilator-associated pneumonia in a nonteaching U.S. medical center.[31] Compared with noninfected mechanically ventilated patients, patients with ventilator-associated pneumonia had a higher incidence of bacteremia (36% versus 22%), longer ICU length of stay (26 versus 4 days), and greater mortality rate (50% versus 34%). Hospital costs for ventilator-associated pneumonia patients were significantly higher ($70,568 versus $21,620) with a higher proportion of total costs being room, nursing, pharmacy, and respiratory therapy expenses. The cost differences for patients developing early-onset compared with late-onset, ventilator-associated pneumonia were $36,822 versus $60,562. The attributable cost of ventilator-associated pneumonia when adjusted for a wide variety of factors was $11,897 (95% confidence interval $5265 to $26,214). Ventilator-associated pneumonia is an expensive condition that warrants better prevention and treatment strategies. Approaches that provide even a small clinical effect can have a significant economic benefit.[29]

Bloodstream infections occur two to seven times more frequently in ICU patients than in ward patients and are associated with high mortality, particularly in ICU patients, averaging 56% (31% to 82%).[32] A pairwise case-control study of 4000 surgical ICU patients over a 2-year period revealed that 97 patients developed nosocomial bloodstream infection with a crude mortality rate of 50% compared with 35% in control ICU patients.[32] The additional length of hospital stay was 14 days, whereas the additional ICU stay was 8 days. The total excess cost of this condition was $2.8 million, or $33,268 per patient and $40,890 per survivor. In a subsequent study involving 3000 medical ICU admissions, infected patients were matched to controls with respect to several factors, including APACHE III (Acute Physiology, Age, and Chronic Health Evaluation) score.[33] Among the 68 patients developing a nosocomial bloodstream infection, there was no difference in crude mortality between patients and controls. The difference in median hospital and ICU length of stay was 7 and 5 days, and cost difference averaged $23,751, which increased to $34,508 in survivors.

Catheter-related infections occur at an estimated rate of 5.3 per 1000 catheter days and are another major cause of increased morbidity, mortality, and cost to ICU patients.[34] Several studies have calculated the cost per infection, and estimates range from $34,508 to $56,000 for an annual cost of $296 million to $2.3 billion.[34]

SEVERE SEPSIS AND SEPSIS SYNDROME

The incidence of severe sepsis in the United States is estimated to be 751,000 cases per year. The method for identifying this occurrence differs from previous epidemiologic estimates for a single-center study and a multicenter study that excluded pediatric patients.[35,36] The mortality rate associated with severe sepsis is 28.6% and increases to 38.4% in patients older than age 85 years. The average cost per case of severe sepsis is $22,100. The estimated annual cost in the United States is $16.7 billion.

Other studies have been performed in Quebec, Germany, and Austria to estimate the costs associated with caring for patients with severe sepsis or septic shock.[37-39] Many countries are quantifying the incidence, cost, and outcomes of sepsis as a means of understanding the importance of the syndrome and justifying costly treatments.

DEEP VENOUS THROMBOSIS

The average annual incidence of deep venous thrombosis in the United States in 1991 was 48 per 100,000 patients; the in-hospital mortality associated with this condition was 12%.[40] The prevalence of deep venous thrombosis depends on the patient population, being approximately 80% in trauma patients, approximately 23% in patients recovering from total hip arthroplasty, 14.9% in seriously ill medical patients, and 11% in general surgery patients receiving no thromboprophylaxis.[41-43] The cost of deep venous thrombosis varies among these patient populations, being about $1394 in 1993 and $3068 in 2000.[44,45] These cost estimates depend on treatment approaches, institution, year of occurrence, and type of physician providing treatment. Despite the variability in prevalence and cost, deep venous thrombosis is a concern because of its associated mortality.

COST OF PHARMACOTHERAPY IN CRITICAL CARE

ANTIBIOTICS

Use of antibiotics is rampant in ICUs. Studies report 70% to 92% of patients in ICUs receive antibiotics.[46] One component of the impact of antibiotics is their acquisition costs. In 1985, it was estimated that antimicrobials constitute 25% of total drug expenditures; antibiotics were the second and third most expensive class of drugs in the ICUs at the University of Minnesota.[47] Additional cost drivers associated with antimicrobial use include the development of resistant organisms. The annual cost of resistance in 1989 was estimated to range from $100 million to $30 billion.[46] One study reported the impact of methicillin-resistant *Staphylococcus aureus* was a 2.5-fold increase in mortality rate and an incremental cost of $2500 per infection.[48]

Several studies have evaluated strategies to optimize the use of antimicrobials in the ICU to reduce the incidence of resistance and cost of these agents. Therapeutic protocols for antibiotic use reportedly can reduce the emergence of resistant organisms and decrease antibiotic costs.[49,50] Estimated cost savings have ranged from $400 less in charges per patient to a 65% reduction of antibiotic expenditures in the ICU after the implementation of the guidelines.[49,50] Other approaches include the use of restrictive or open antimicrobial formularies, intravenous-to-oral antimicrobial switching programs, and antibiotic stop orders.[46,51] One hospital implemented a comprehensive clinical pharmacy intervention program consisting of streamlining antimicrobial use and discontinuing unnecessary antimicrobials. Their 1993 antimicrobial expenditure was half that of other comparable hospitals.[46]

DROTRECOGIN ALFA (ACTIVATED)

A cost-effectiveness analysis of drotrecogin alfa (activated) was conducted in conjunction with a clinical trial of the safety and efficacy of this recombinant protein as an adjuvant treatment for severe sepsis.[52] The clinical trial reported a 6.1% absolute reduction in mortality in patients receiving drotrecogin alfa (activated). The acquisition cost of a course of drotrecogin alfa (activated) for a 70-kg patient is approximately $7000. The cost-effectiveness study used the PCEHM guidelines, as modified by the American Thoracic Society, whereby lifetime estimates of costs and effects were generated using the U.S. societal perspective.[53] Despite the fact that there were more survivors among patients treated with drotrecogin alfa (activated) compared with placebo, there were no significant differences in costs per patient or resource use, excluding the cost of the drug. The cost per survivor was estimated to be $160,000. Long-term costs and outcomes were modeled, assuming that survivors lived an average of 12.2 years with utility adjusted to 8.4 quality-adjusted life-years. Based on these calculations, the cost per life-year saved was $33,000 per life-year saved and the cost per quality-adjusted life-year was $48,800. These figures are similar to other life-saving therapies and consistent with a cutoff of $50,000 per quality-adjusted life-year for a therapy to be considered cost-effective. Because the clinical benefits of drotrecogin alfa (activated) seem to be most evident in the most severely ill patients, however, costs also were calculated incorporating the assumption that the recombinant protein would be used only in the sickest group of patients with severe sepsis. The cost per quality-adjusted life year in patients with an APACHE II score greater than 25 was $27,400. A decision by the Center for Medicare and Medicaid Services in the United States is expected to help offset the financial burden of drotrecogin alfa (activated) usage in hospitals.[54] Effective October 2002, a new severe sepsis code was established (995.92), and in August 2002, the Federal Register identified drotrecogin alfa (activated) as a new technology with a procedure code (00.11). When use of drotrecogin alfa (activated) is properly coded, hospitals receive 50% (maximum of $3400) of the cost of drotrecogin alfa (activated) for cases of severe sepsis that exceed the diagnosis-related group payment rate. To take advantage of this reimbursement mechanism, hospitals must have surveillance systems in place to code properly patients who receive this drug.

SEDATIVES

Sedatives, commonly used in the ICU to treat agitation, account for 10% to 15% of ICU-related drug costs.[55] At one institution, propofol alone accounted for 10% to 13% of the ICU drug costs.[14] Because of the financial impact of sedatives and the development of guidelines for the use of these agents, it is surprising that only a few studies have evaluated the costs associated with using this class of drugs.

One study compared midazolam and propofol in a prospective, randomized trial.[56] The propofol group spent fewer hours on mechanical ventilation and required less time from discontinuation of drug infusion to extubation. Total costs with propofol averaged $9466, compared with $10,828 with midazolam. Although both drugs were equally effective as sedatives, administration of propofol was associated with shorter weaning times than midazolam, resulting in a more favorable economic profile.

Another study evaluated the impact on costs of implementing a sedation protocol.[57] The investigators carrying out this trial showed that time on the ventilator and length of stay were significantly shorter after implementation of the guidelines. Drug costs were significantly reduced as well. The cost of propofol was $355.82 to $1010.85 before implementation of the guidelines and $123.06 to $460.50 after implementation of the guidelines. Total sedation costs were reduced from $4515 to $1152. Rational use of guidelines for ICU sedation resulted in safe, cost-effective improvements in the provision of care.

Anis and coworkers[58] conducted a multicenter, randomized trial comparing midazolam and propofol in 156 patients. More of the patients in the propofol arm than in the midazolam arm achieved adequate sedation (60% versus 44%). The time between drug discontinuation and extubation was shorter among propofol-treated patients than among midazolam-treated patients (2.5 hours versus 7.1 hours). Overall length of ICU stay was not different, however. One reason proposed to explain these seemingly disparate findings is that although patients often were ready for ICU transfer, beds were not available on the wards to receive them. If a model is developed that assumes the time from extubation until discharge is the same for both drugs, the net savings for choosing propofol rather than midazolam is $403 per patient.

NEUROMUSCULAR BLOCKERS

Studies evaluating the cost associated with neuromuscular blocker therapy commonly focus on acquisition cost of the drug, favoring the older, more familiar agents, such as pancuronium.[59-62] As previously discussed, the total costs of drug use extend beyond simple acquisition costs. In the case of neuromuscular blockers, one should consider costs associated with treatment for prolonged motor weakness.[63,64] Prolonged motor weakness has been estimated to cost $54,632 per patient.[63] Costs for recovery from general anesthesia in a postanesthesia care unit after surgery were compared for patients who received short/intermediate-acting neuromuscular blockers and patients who received long-acting neuromuscular blockers. Use of long-acting neuromuscular blockers was associated with a 41-minute longer recovery time and an excess cost of $91.[64] This amount may not seem to be substantial, but permitting patients to be transferred more quickly out of a busy postanesthesia care unit would permit more rapid turnover of patients, saving other costs.

Train-of-four monitoring reduces recovery time and can lower the risk of prolonged neuromuscular dysfunction, reducing ICU costs. The benefits from monitoring intraoperatively have not precluded the occurrence of residual muscle weakness.[65,66] The implementation of protocols that guide the use of neuromuscular blockers in the ICU is a cost-effective approach to managing patients.[57,67] Studies evaluating the quality of life after prolonged paralysis could aid clinicians in understanding the effects of prolonged neuromuscular dysfunction and the costs from a societal perspective reported in quality-adjusted life-years.

THROMBOPROPHYLAXIS AND DEEP VENOUS THROMBOSIS TREATMENT

The cost of treatment requires identifying costs beyond the drug acquisition price. It is often too difficult to determine the exact amounts attributable to the administration of a drug or the treatment of an adverse drug event. It is sometimes necessary to be resourceful and combine institution-specific data with information available in the literature. Gould and associates[68] compared the costs and clinical outcomes from a societal perspective for two groups of 10,000 hypothetical adult patients with a diagnosis of acute, proximal, lower extremity deep venous thrombosis. The low-molecular-weight heparin group received enoxaparin (1 mg/kg) twice daily for 6 days, and the unfractionated heparin group received a continuous infusion of heparin (30,000 IU/d). Assessing only the inpatient results associated with treatment, the probability differences in outcomes were obtained from a previously published report of results from a clinical trial. The resulting costs were $26,361 for the low-molecular-weight heparin group and $26,316 for the unfractionated heparin group.[69] Although the additional net cost of $155 was related to inpatient treatment with low-molecular-weight heparin, the increase in quality-adjusted life-years by 0.02 for the low-molecular-weight heparin group resulted in a societal cost advantage of $7820 per quality-adjusted life-year. Shorr and Ramage[70] compared the cost-effectiveness of enoxaparin (30 mg every 12 hours) with unfractionated heparin (5000 U every 12 hours) for the prevention of deep venous thromboses after major trauma in a cohort of 1000 hypothetical patients.[70] Cost and consequence data were obtained from the literature and the experience at one institution. The analysis assumed that enoxaparin reduces the incidence of deep venous thrombosis by 50%, increases the chance of a major bleed by 2.3%, and costs seven times more than unfractionated heparin. Under these assumptions, net savings were $391.23 per deep venous thrombosis prevented with enoxaparin.

Another literature-based decision analysis compared the cost-effectiveness of conventional low-dose heparin, dalteparin, and intermittent pneumatic compression devices for thromboprophylaxis with a no-prophylaxis group.[71] In contrast to the results from Shorr and Ramage,[70] the most cost-effective therapy was unfractionated heparin at $86 per complication-free patient. This study included costs that Shorr and Ramage did not,[70] such as the cost of labor and a pulmonary embolism.[71] Other studies have evaluated the use of low-molecular-weight heparin compared with unfractionated heparin for the treatment of myocardial infarction, treatment of thromboembolism, and prevention of deep venous thromboses.[70,72-74] Most of the cost analyses are for prevention, and consistently thromboprophylaxis is more cost-effective than no prophylaxis, although the most cost-effective agent is not clear. Clinicians need to be cautious when interpreting the results of these studies to ensure that all costs and all consequences of the therapy are considered. In addition, clinicians need to ensure that the outcome data are obtained from a variety of reliable resources.

COST OF INTENSIVE CARE UNIT MANAGEMENT

INTENSIVIST-LED MULTIDISCIPLINARY TEAM

Another mechanism to use hospital resources effectively is to manage ICU patients using an intensivist-led multidisciplinary team. There are data to support the view that high-intensity ICU physician staffing can reduce ICU and hospital lengths of stay and reduce hospital and ICU mortality.[75] A pharmacist contributing to ICU rounds also reduces costs and improves outcomes.[76,77] Although the cost reductions associated with critical care nurse and respiratory therapist services have not been evaluated, their impact on clinical outcomes is shown through involvement in sedation protocols and weaning protocols.[78-80] Consistent with the Leapfrog initiative (http://www.leapfroggroup.org/), developing an intensivist-led multidisciplinary team would improve outcomes and use ICU resources efficiently.

ROLE OF THE FOOD AND DRUG ADMINISTRATION

The role of pharmacoeconomics in the view of the U.S. Food and Drug Administration (FDA) is an area of considerable debate. Globally the European Agency for the Evaluation of Medicinal Products and the National Institute for Clinical Excellence, part of the National Health Service in the United Kingdom, are working on guidelines for the inclusion, use, and promotion of data from economic evaluations of new therapies.

The FDA Modernization Act of 1997 addressed the inclusion of pharmacoeconomic and outcomes research in managed care formulary submission. There are currently no federal guidelines in the United States, however, for the use of pharmacoeconomic information in drug promotion and labeling; this includes information on the quality-of-life impact a new drug may have on a patient and family. Consequently, much confusion exists regarding what types of economic claims are appropriate and the level of evidence required.[81] Guidance from the Center of Drug Evaluation and Research suggests that the scientific rigor should be similar to that required for effectiveness studies (i.e., data should come from prospective, randomized, controlled trials with standard-of-care comparisons). Modeling and retrospective database analysis would be taken into consideration, but only if the methods are strict and transparent. The FDA and Division of Drug Marketing, Advertising, and Communications review potential protocols for the possibility of acceptance as supportive documentation. The inclusion of pharmacoeconomic or quality-of-life data that have not been approved by the FDA or Division of Drug Marketing, Advertising, and Communications results in warning letters and notices of violation. From 1997 through 2001, 56 such letters were sent to the pharmaceutical industry. Most claim violations centered on unsupported promotion of effectiveness and improved quality of life.

CONCLUSION

The ICU is a complex environment associated with extensive drug use. Considering the fiscal constraints on the provision of health care, the ICU is an area where pharmacoeconomic evaluation may be the only way to justify the use of selected drugs in various guidelines and protocols. Applying principles of pharmacoeconomics to critical care gives decision makers additional tools to make cost-effective decisions for direct patient care and for health systems. The economic burden of several conditions seen in the ICU and the costs associated with their treatment are beginning to be understood. The data are less than perfect. Clinicians and administrators rely on existing economic literature to assist with their decisions. The generation of additional cost-effectiveness studies of new and existing pharmaceuticals is necessary to make sound decisions. Simply selecting the cheapest therapy or the newest therapy may not be best for patients or society. Current understanding suggests the optimal model for care is an intensivist-led multidisciplinary team that works collectively to develop therapeutic protocols and guidelines based on the latest clinical and economic information.

ANNOTATED REFERENCES

Drummond MF, O'Brien B, Stoddart GL, Torrance GW: Methods for the Economic Evaluation of Health Care Programmes. New York, Oxford University Press, 1997.

This book is considered by many to be a classic in the application of economic theory to health care. Because a drug or treatment is evaluated on the basis of cost and outcome in reference to the current standard of care, cost-effectiveness analysis is the most common technique used. The authors conclude that cost-effectiveness analysis is a full economic evaluation because costs and outcomes are considered, and the results from a cost-effectiveness analysis are a crucial component in the decision to allocate limited resources.

Format for Formulary Submissions (FMCP), v 2.0 Academy of Managed Care Pharmacy and Evidence-Based and Value-Based Formulary Guidelines. Available at: http://www.Amcp.org/Amcp.ark?c=Pr&sc=Link. Accessed September 28, 2004.

This reference and website provides the guidelines and instructions for developing an evaluation of a drug being submitted for National Formulary consideration status at an institution. It is increasingly used by managed care groups as a way of assessing the clinical and economic benefits of a new drug.

Mamdani NM, Weingarten CM, Stevenson JG: Thromboembolic prophylaxis in moderate-risk patient undergoing elective abdominal surgery: Decision and cost-effectiveness. Pharmacotherapy 1996;16:1111-1127.

This study is an example of taking into consideration all consequences, costs, and alternative choices of therapy to aid in making therapeutic decisions. Comparing this study with similar studies may provide varying results depending on the assumption of the model and the method of obtaining cost and consequence data.

Shorr AF: An update on cost-effectiveness analysis in critical care. Curr Opin Crit Care 2002;8:337-343.

This review article provides an overview of economic analysis with a focus on costs and dealing with uncertainty and issues related to outcome assessment on ICU-specific diseases and health care systems pertaining to critically ill patients.

Weber RJ, Kane SL, Oriolo VA, et al: Impact of intensive care unit (ICU) drug use on hospital cost: A descriptive analysis, with recommendations for optimizing ICU pharmacotherapy. Crit Care Med 2003;31:S17-S24.

This article not only reviews issues of assessing drug costs in critical care, but also provides data on drug use and costs at one academic medical center. The unique aspect of this study is that it provides financial information on drugs used while a patient was in the ICU over 4 years in more than 20,000 patients. This type of analysis can be used as a basis of assessing whether certain expensive drugs are being used appropriately in the ICU.

Section XIII

PROCEDURES

Chapter 205

DIFFICULT AIRWAY MANAGEMENT FOR INTENSIVISTS

John J. Schaefer • Rene Gonzales

KEY POINTS

1. **Successful management of complex airways in the ICU** requires not only skill but also planning, communication, cooperation, and understanding between the intensivist and a range of other health care providers.

2. All clinicians involved in airway management must be familiar with the **ASA Practice Guidelines for Management of the Difficult Airway.**

3. **Inadequate ventilation** is defined by:
   a. Absence of detectable exhaled CO_2
   b. Spirometrically measurable exhaled gas flows, breath sounds, or chest movements
   c. Presence of cyanosis
   d. Signs of severe airway obstruction
   e. Gastric air entry or dilatation
   f. Hemodynamic changes associated with hypoxemia or hypercarbia, such as hypertension, tachycardia, or arrhythmia

4. A patient who is **difficult to intubate is not necessarily difficult to ventilate.**

5. Selecting among basic airway management choices is the **most critical step** in management of the difficult airway.

The management of patients with a difficult airway can be one of the most challenging problems in clinical medicine. The following statements apply to airway management in the intensive care setting:

- The patients are very ill patients.
- The clinical stakes are high (i.e., life and death decisions are required).
- The time pressures are intense (the onset of cerebral hypoxia occurs within 2 minutes).
- Difficult airways are a common problem; the immediate environment may be less than optimal (patients arrest in remote sites).
- The intensivist is often involved in such cases as either the primary caregiver or as a consultant, often on an urgent or emergency basis (i.e., as a member of the code team).

Successful management of complex airways in the ICU requires not only skill but also planning, communication, cooperation, and understanding between the intensivist and a range of other health care providers. The reported incidence of "failed intubation" greatly depends on the training and experience of the individual health care provider, ranging from approximately 0.05% of surgical patients (anesthesia care providers) to 10% of prehospital patients (emergency medical technicians or paramedic care providers).[1,2]

There have been several important advances in the field of difficult airway management in the past few years. A large body of literature on this subject has also emerged. These advances are reviewed in this chapter with the goal of familiarizing the intensivist with these new practice guidelines and airway management devices and techniques.

AMERICAN SOCIETY OF ANESTHESIOLOGISTS (ASA) PRACTICE GUIDELINES FOR MANAGEMENT OF THE DIFFICULT AIRWAY

In 1991, the ASA appointed a task force consisting of academic and private-practice anesthesiologists, as well as a research methodologist, to develop practice guidelines to assist anesthesiologists in the management of patients with suspected as well as unanticipated difficult airways. The task force conducted an extensive search of the medical literature (1973 to 1991). The articles collected were reviewed, analyzed, and rated by the task force. Rigorous statistical analysis, including meta-analysis, was performed. The findings based on literature analysis were supplemented by opinions from the task force members as well as 50 consultant anesthesiologists. The Practice Guidelines, including the ASA Difficult Airway Algorithm, were approved by the ASA and published in March 1993 (Fig. 205-1).[3]

Over the past year, the ASA Difficult Airway Practice Guidelines have been extensively publicized and taught at national and regional meetings, in continuing education courses, and in anesthesiology residency programs in the United States. It is important that all clinicians involved in airway management be familiar with the ASA guidelines.

The introduction to the ASA guidelines states that they are recommendations developed to assist the practitioner and patient in making decisions; however, it also emphasizes that the recommendations may be adopted, modified, or

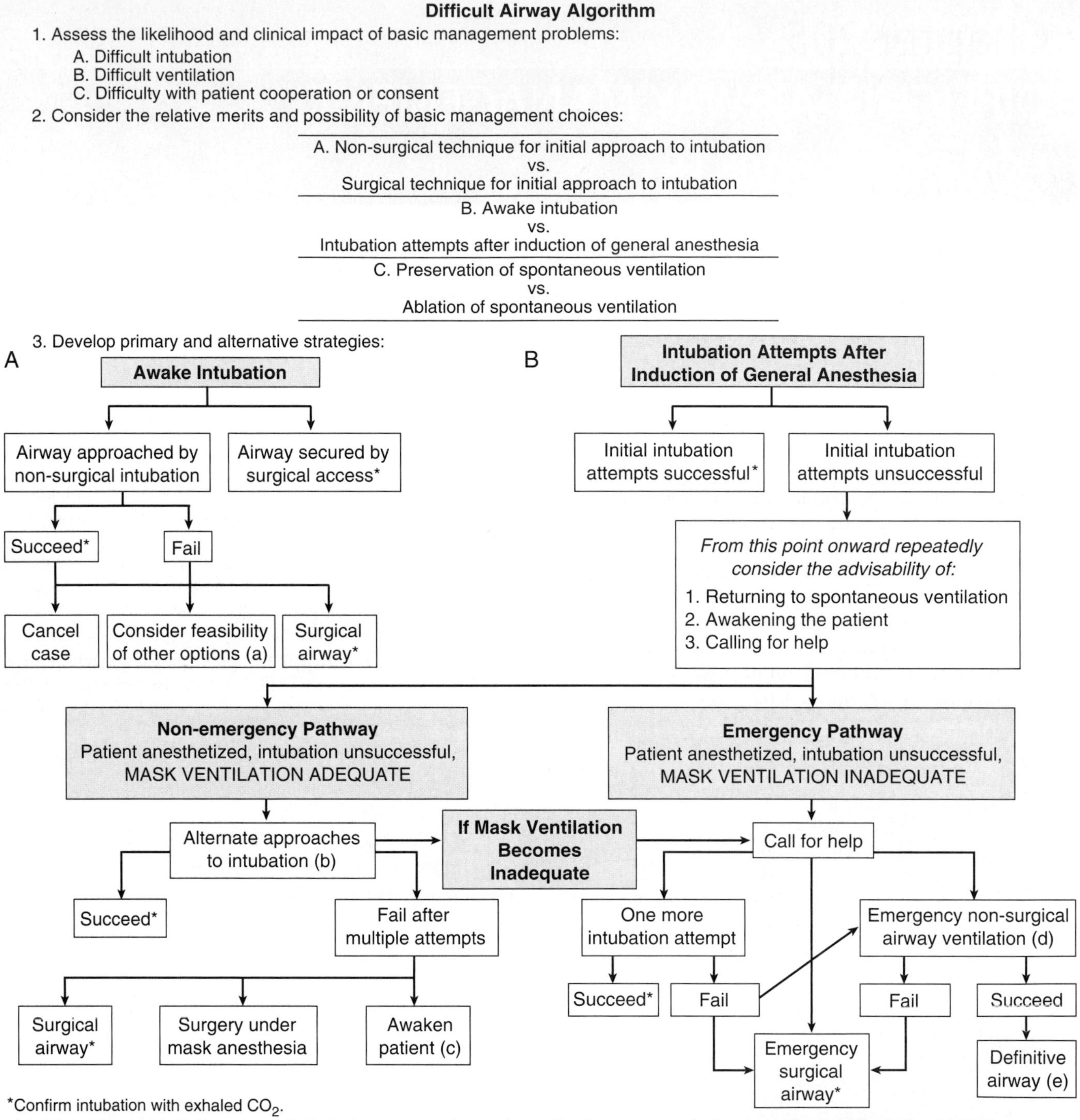

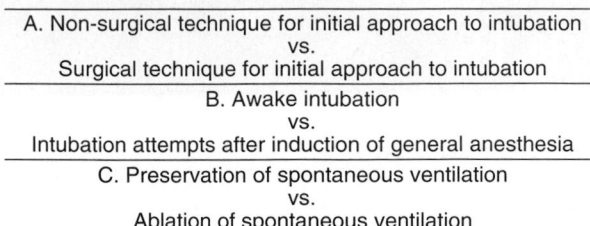

Difficult Airway Algorithm

1. Assess the likelihood and clinical impact of basic management problems:
   A. Difficult intubation
   B. Difficult ventilation
   C. Difficulty with patient cooperation or consent
2. Consider the relative merits and possibility of basic management choices:

| A. Non-surgical technique for initial approach to intubation |
| vs. |
| Surgical technique for initial approach to intubation |
| B. Awake intubation |
| vs. |
| Intubation attempts after induction of general anesthesia |
| C. Preservation of spontaneous ventilation |
| vs. |
| Ablation of spontaneous ventilation |

3. Develop primary and alternative strategies:

A

Awake Intubation

- Airway approached by non-surgical intubation
  - Succeed*
    - Cancel case
  - Fail
    - Consider feasibility of other options (a)
    - Surgical airway*
- Airway secured by surgical access*

B

Intubation Attempts After Induction of General Anesthesia

- Initial intubation attempts successful*
- Initial intubation attempts unsuccessful
  - *From this point onward repeatedly consider the advisability of:*
    1. Returning to spontaneous ventilation
    2. Awakening the patient
    3. Calling for help

Non-emergency Pathway
Patient anesthetized, intubation unsuccessful, MASK VENTILATION ADEQUATE

- Alternate approaches to intubation (b)
  - Succeed*
  - Fail after multiple attempts
    - Surgical airway*
    - Surgery under mask anesthesia
    - Awaken patient (c)

If Mask Ventilation Becomes Inadequate

Emergency Pathway
Patient anesthetized, intubation unsuccessful, MASK VENTILATION INADEQUATE

- Call for help
  - One more intubation attempt
    - Succeed*
    - Fail
      - Emergency surgical airway*
  - Emergency non-surgical airway ventilation (d)
    - Fail
      - Emergency surgical airway*
    - Succeed
      - Definitive airway (e)

*Confirm intubation with exhaled CO_2.

(a) Other options include (but are not limited to): surgery under mask anesthesia, surgery under local anesthesia infiltration or regional nerve blockade, or intubation attempts after induction of general anesthesia.

(b) Alternative approaches to difficult intubation include (but are not limited to): use of different laryngoscope blades, awake intubation, blind oral or nasal intubation, fiberoptic intubation, intubating stylet or tube changer, light wand, retrograde intubation, or surgical airway access.

(c) See awake intubation.

(d) Options for emergency non-surgical airway ventilation include (but are not limited to): transtracheal jet ventilation, laryngeal mask ventilation, or esophageal-tracheal combitube ventilation.

(e) Options for establishing a definitive airway include (but are not limited to): returning to awake state with spontaneous ventilation, tracheotomy, or endotracheal intubation.

FIGURE 205–1. American Society of Anesthesiologists Practice Guidelines for management of a difficult airway.

rejected according to clinical needs or constraints, as well as by the evolution of medical knowledge or technology. It is important to note that the airway management techniques referred to in the guidelines are based on efficacy-based evidence. Accordingly, airway management techniques or devices discussed in this review are limited to those in which bodies of evidence suggest their efficacy of use.

The ASA guidelines recommend that a strategy be preformulated for the management of all difficult airways. The strategy should be tailored to the condition of the individual patient, as well as the skills and preferences of the physician(s). Specific contingency plans, whenever possible, should be part of the management strategy.

DEFINITIONS

Because no standard definition of the difficult airway was previously available in the medical literature, the ASA task force created a working definition. A *difficult airway* is defined as "the clinical situation in which a conventionally trained anesthesiologist experiences difficulty with mask ventilation or tracheal intubation, or both."[3]

The guidelines go on to define *difficult endotracheal intubation* as a situation in which "proper insertion of a tracheal tube with conventional laryngoscopy requires more than three attempts" by a "conventionally trained anesthesiologist." Conceptually this is also a useful clinical definition as a benchmark for when to stop attempting this technique because iatrogenic airway complications including the progression to a "cannot ventilate" clinical situation directly correlate with the number of direct laryngoscopies beyond three attempts.[4] The guidelines also define *difficult mask ventilation.* Inadequate oxygenation is defined as an oxygen saturation (SaO_2) less than 90% by pulse oximetry when 100% inspired oxygen is being used. This is also a critical clinical airway management concept to understand in terms of the basis for making clinical judgments of when and how to proceed. Figure 205-2 demonstrates the rate arterial hemoglobin desaturates with the onset of apnea in different types of patients. Note that once the SaO_2 drops to less than what Benumoff and colleagues[5] describe as the "critical SaO_2" (93%), one enters the steep part of the hemoglobin desaturation curve, leaving 1 to 2 minutes before the patient arrests from hypoxia. In context of airway management, this fact means that when the clinician is faced with a "cannot intubate, cannot ventilate" situation and SaO_2 is less than 93%, the airway manager must rapidly proceed with definitive techniques and abandon consideration of waiting for the patient to return to spontaneous ventilation. *Inadequate ventilation* is defined by the absence of detectable exhaled CO_2, spirometrically measurable exhaled gas flows, breath sounds, or chest movements. It is also defined by the presence of cyanosis, signs of severe airway obstruction, gastric air entry or dilatation, or hemodynamic changes associated with hypoxemia or hypercarbia, such as hypertension, tachycardia, or arrhythmia.

Although these working definitions may seem intuitively obvious, it is important to codify and publicize such definitions, because many of the recommendations in the guidelines are predicated on the clear identification of a given airway as "difficult." The ASA Difficult Airway Guidelines also urge clinicians and authors to use explicit descriptions of the difficult airway when documenting such situations in the medical record and publications. This type of explicit detailed information is more clinically useful and allows for more meaningful analysis of the literature.

PREPARATION

Personnel

In situations in which a difficult airway is suspected in advance, the ASA guidelines recommend that at least one additional individual be immediately available to serve as an assistant in difficult airway management. The intensivist should have help available when dealing with a potentially difficult airway. More important, the intensivist should anticipate and plan for getting assistance at the appropriate skill level. These rules are prompted by the recognition that one may not have much time to get surgical help or other assistance once the SaO_2 decreases to less than 93%. Conceptually, these rules could be extended beyond having the appropriate personnel available to include the "appropriate setting." For example, there are clinical situations in which a difficult airway is best managed in an operating theater rather than the patient's room or even an ICU.

Equipment

The ASA guidelines recommend that at least one portable storage unit that contains specialized equipment for difficult airway management be readily available at all anesthetizing stations. This portable unit is also known in many anesthesiology departments as "the difficult airway cart." The ASA task force's recommended list of specialized airway equipment to be placed on this cart is listed in Table 205-1. Whereas maintaining a "difficult airway cart" fully stocked and immediately

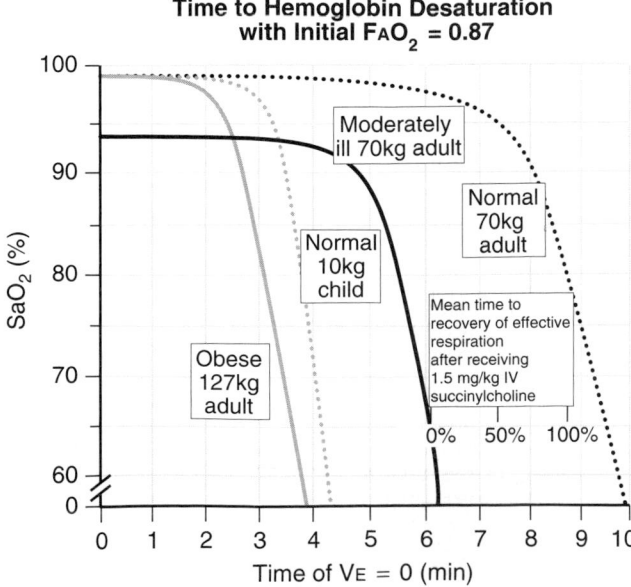

Time to Hemoglobin Desaturation with Initial $F_AO_2 = 0.87$

Moderately ill 70kg adult

Normal 70kg adult

Normal 10kg child

Obese 127kg adult

Mean time to recovery of effective respiration after receiving 1.5 mg/kg IV succinylcholine

0% 50% 100%

SaO_2 (%)

Time of $V_E = 0$ (min)

FIGURE 205-2. Hemoglobin desaturation curve.

TABLE 205-1. SUGGESTED CONTENTS OF A MANAGEMENT CART FOR A DIFFICULT AIRWAY

- Rigid laryngoscope blades of alternate design and size from those routinely used
- Endotracheal tubes of assorted size
- Endotracheal tube guides; examples include semi-rigid stylets with or without a hollow core for jet ventilation, light wands, and forceps designed to manipulate the distal portion of the endotracheal tube
- Fiberoptic intubation equipment
- Retrograde intubation equipment
- At least one device suitable for emergency nonsurgical airway ventilation; examples include a transtracheal jet ventilator, a hollow jet ventilation stylet, the laryngeal mask, and the esophageal-tracheal Combitube
- Equipment suitable for emergency surgical airway access (e.g., cricothyrotomy)
- An exhaled CO_2 detector

Airway Axes Alignment and Exposure of the Glottic Opening

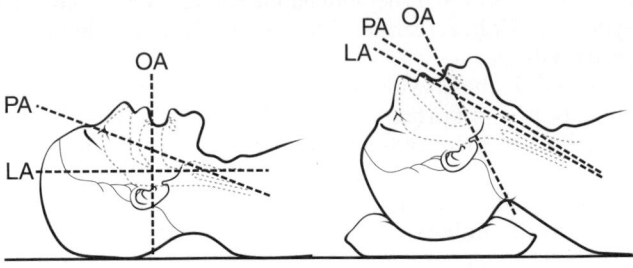

OA = oral axis, PA = pharyngeal axis, LA = laryngeal axis

FIGURE 205–3. Airway axes.

available to operating theaters seems intuitive for anesthesiologists, this concept is directly transferable to the ICU, where difficult airways also are likely to be encountered with some frequency. Although the equipment listed in Table 205-1 is comprehensive for the practicing anesthesiologist, the equipment appropriate to the ICU should include a range of intubation equipment, equipment to support "awake" airway management, equipment for at least one "supraglottic" airway management technique, and emergency equipment for at least one "subglottic" airway management technique (e.g., percutaneous cricothyrotomy). For the code situation in a random location, at least one supraglottic and one subglottic airway management technique or device should be immediately available by virtue of inclusion on a readily available "code cart" or "code bag." Policies and procedures

to maintain and check this type of equipment are critical to ensure its timely availability in critical situations.

Patient Evaluation

The first step and concept in the ASA guidelines (see Fig. 205-1) recommends that "an airway history, physical examination, and review of previous medical records be conducted, whenever feasible, prior to airway management intervention in all patients." The guidelines specifically recommend assessing the patient to anticipate difficulty with (1) intubation, (2) ventilation, and (3) cooperation or consent. This first concept is the one most likely to lead to preventable adverse outcomes in difficult airway management. This point is supported by analysis of the ASA's closed claims project.[6] In this analysis, adverse respiratory events constituted the largest category of claims; three fourths were believed to be preventable, and 85% of the outcomes were either permanent brain damage or death.

Physical Signs of a Potentially Difficult Intubation

Understanding the physics necessary to provide a visual anatomic view of the glottis (Fig. 205-3) basically includes proper alignment of the oral, pharyngeal, and laryngeal axes. Abnormalities in traditional anatomic airway examinations all interfere with aligning these axes. A useful guide to these basic anatomic examinations is included in Table 205-2. To be useful, anatomic examination actually must be carried out and the information gleaned must be factored into the clinical strategy. The Mallampati examination is detailed in Figure 205-4. In addition to anatomic factors specifically related to performing a traditional intubation, identification/palpation of the cricothyroid membrane is recommended before initiating an airway management

TABLE 205–2. RECOMMENDED AIRWAY MANAGEMENT

Preoperative Examination	Acceptable Endpoints	Significance of Endpoints
Length of upper incisors	Qualitative/short incisors	Long incisors: blade enters mouth in cephalad direction.
Involuntary: maxillary teeth anterior to mandibular teeth	No overriding of maxillary teeth anterior to the mandibular teeth	Overriding maxillary teeth: blade enters mouth in a more cephalad direction.
Voluntary: protrusion of mandibular teeth anterior to maxillary teeth	Anterior protrusion of the mandibular teeth relative to the maxillary teeth	Test of temporomandibular joint function: means there is good mouth opening and jaw will move anteriorly with laryngoscopy.
Intercisor distance	>3 cm	A 2-cm flange on blade can be easily inserted between teeth.
Oropharyngeal class (Mallampati exam)	≤Class II	Tongue is small in relation to size of oropharyngeal cavity.
Narrowness of palate	Should not appear very narrow and/or highly arched	A narrow palate decreases the oropharyngeal volume and room for both blade and endotracheal tube.
Mandibular space length (thyromental distance)	=5 cm or +3 ordinary-sized fingerbreadths	Larynx is relative to other upper airway structures.
Mandibular space compliance	Qualitative palpation of normal resilience/softness	Laryngoscopy retracts tongue in the mandibular space. Compliance of the space determines if tongue fits into mandibular space.
Length of neck	Qualitative. A quantitative index is not available.	A short neck decreases the ability to align the upper airway axes.
Thickness of neck	Qualitative. A quantitative index is not available.	A thick neck decreases the ability to align the upper airway axes.
Palpation of cricoid membrane	Cricoid membrane can be readily identified.	If the cricoid membrane cannot be palpated readily, then the ability to perform transtracheal jet ventilation or establish a surgical airway is not available as an option in an emergency.
Cervical range of motion	Neck flexed on chest 35 degrees + head extended on neck 35 degrees = sniff position.	The sniff position aligns the oral, pharyngeal, and laryngeal axes to create a favorable line of sight.

Samsoon and Young Modification of the Mallampati Airway Classification

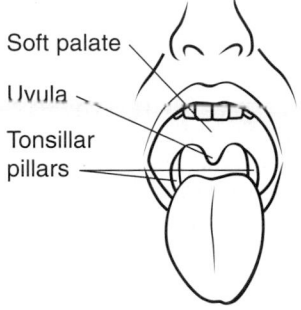
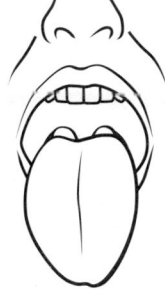
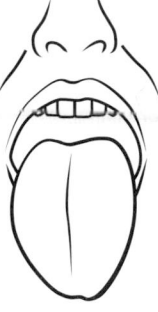
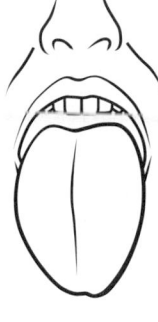

Soft palate
Uvula
Tonsillar pillars

FIGURE 205–4. Samsoon and Young modification of the Mallampati airway classification.

Class I:
Visualize the soft palate, uvula, fauces, anterior and posterior tonsillar pillars

Class II:
Soft palate, fauces, uvula

Class III:
Soft palate, base of uvula

Class IV:
No structures are visible, only hard palate

strategy because the ability to accurately identify this structure is key to successfully implementing subglottic airway management techniques in an emergency. The presence of facial hair should alert the operator of the possibility of difficulty with establishing an effective mask seal.

A number of studies have investigated the sensitivity or predictive value of various physical signs of a potentially difficult intubation.[7-11] No physical finding is completely reliable for predicting a difficult intubation; however, if two or three of the physical signs listed in Table 205-2 are present, then the clinician should have a strong index of suspicion for the possibility of the patient being difficult to intubate. Specific planning for this possibility needs to be carried out.

Physical Signs of Potentially Difficult Ventilation

Compared with predicting whether a patient will be difficult to intubate, it is potentially more important to predict whether a patient will be difficult to ventilate. A patient who is difficult to intubate is not necessarily difficult to ventilate. Although not well defined in the literature, approximately 15% of patients who are difficult to intubate are also difficult to ventilate.[12] This percentage is based on studies of surgical patients being managed by anesthesia caregivers. Anesthesiologists and anesthetists tend to be highly skilled and experienced airway managers. Thus, the percentage of patients who are both hard to intubate and hard to ventilate is likely be higher, if the airway is being managed by less experienced clinicians. Physical signs associated with difficult ventilation include presence of facial hair, obesity, a short thick neck, and a Mallampati 3 or 4 airway.

Other Considerations

Whereas airway evaluation and airway management strategies traditionally focus on anatomic factors, certain important physiologic factors also should be considered in the development of an airway management strategy. The most important physiologic factors are those that determine oxygen supply and demand to critical organs, such as the heart and brain.

Examples of disease states that limit oxygen supply to end organs include severe pulmonary, coronary artery, or cerebrovascular disease. Pathophysiologic states that increase tissue oxygen demands include fever, sepsis, hyperthyroidism, and hyperdynamic cardiovascular states. Despite the administration of supplemental oxygen or even preoxygenation with 100% oxygen, these conditions may diminish the apneic time before hypoxia occurs in certain tissues. Another important and common clinical condition that can accelerate tissue hypoxia is obesity. In the supine position, the obese abdomen encroaches on the thoracic cavity and compresses the lungs. As a result, even after full preoxygenation with 100% oxygen by mask, morbidly obese patients desaturate to dangerously low SaO_2 values much more rapidly than patients of average body weight.[2]

THE ASA DIFFICULT AIRWAY ALGORITHM

The core of the ASA Difficult Airway Practice Guidelines report is summarized in a flow diagram known as the ASA Difficult Airway Algorithm, or simply the Algorithm. This algorithm is presented in its entirety in Figure 205-1. The upper portion of the algorithm, sections 1, 2, and 3A, involves decisions that must be made before the induction of general anesthesia in patients with known or suspected difficult intubation. The rest of the algorithm (Section 3B) deals with the management of the unanticipated difficult airway that becomes manifest after the induction of general anesthesia. It should be noted that this situation quickly branches into either the "can ventilate but cannot intubate" ("nonemergency") pathway, or the "can ventilate but cannot intubate" ("emergency") pathway. The ASA algorithm may be a very useful tool not only for planning but also for teaching and for retrospectively analyzing clinical airway management strategies. At the University of Pittsburgh School of Medicine, we use the guidelines depicted in Figure 205-5. This approach is related to the ASA algorithm, but it is

1. | Consider basic airway management problems: |

    A. Difficult ventilation?
    B. Difficult intubation?
    C. Acute medical care needs
    D. Difficulty related to patient cooperation or consent

2. | Consider basic airway management choices: |

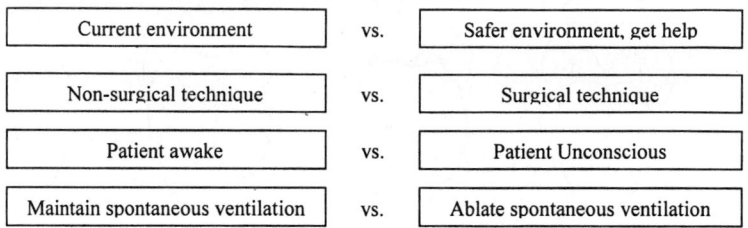

Current environment	vs.	Safer environment, get help
Non-surgical technique	vs.	Surgical technique
Patient awake	vs.	Patient Unconscious
Maintain spontaneous ventilation	vs.	Ablate spontaneous ventilation

3. | Prepare primary and alternative airway management strategies:* |

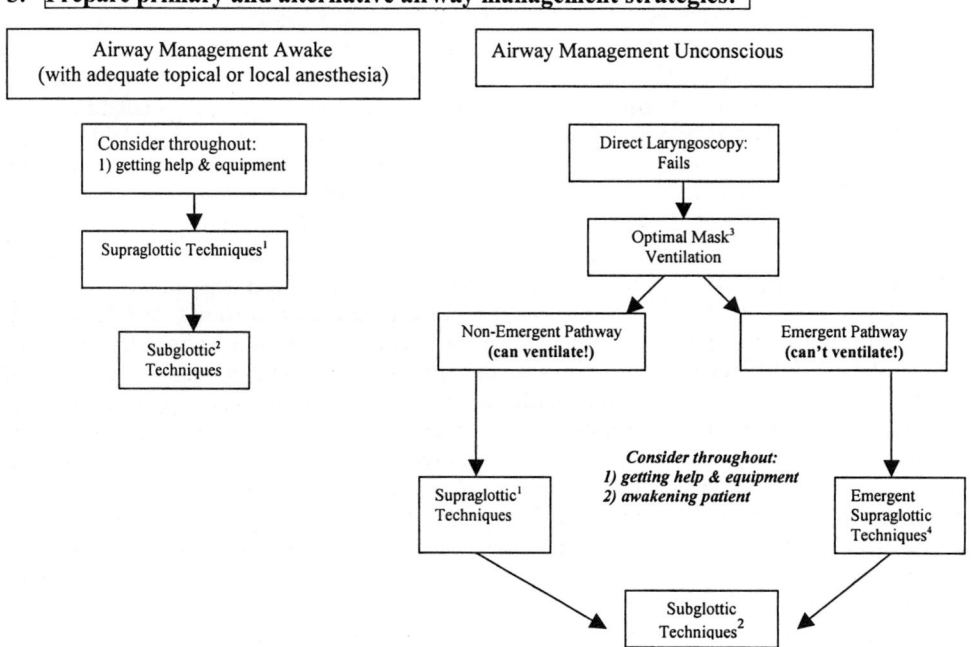

FIGURE 205–5. Universal guidelines for management of a difficult airway. (Copyright University of Pittsburgh and John J. Schaefer III, MD.)

XIII

1748

* Confirm adeq. Ventilation & correct placement with: breathsounds, ETCO2 detection, pulse oximetry, CXR.
1.   Supraglottic Techniques: Fiberoptic bronchoscopy, lighted stylet, retrograde intubation, fast track LMA, bougie
2.   Subglottic Techniques: Cricothyrotomy, tracheostomy, transtracheal jet ventilation
3.   Optimal Mask Ventilation: Use of oral, nasal airway with triple airway maneuvers combined with mask ventilation use of laryngeal mask airway (LMA)
4.   Emergent Supraglotic Techniques: LMA, combitube, fast track LMA

designed for all airway managers and clinical situations. In essence, these guidelines reduce to only three concepts:

1. Assess the airway to inform the subsequent choice of technique(s).
2. Make the appropriate basic airway management choices.
3. Determine the primary and alternative strategies.

CONSIDER BASIC AIRWAY MANAGEMENT PROBLEMS

Factors that could influence the basic choice of airway management include physical signs of potential difficulty in either intubating or ventilating the patient. Other factors can be important as well. For example, the approach toward airway management should be modified if there is a possibility of an unstable cervical spine. One should never skip the initial examination, even if only a very quick and cursory inspection is all that can be carried out.

CONSIDER BASIC AIRWAY MANAGEMENT CHOICES

This is the most critical step in management of the difficult airway. At this stage, the operator answers critical questions regarding initial management of the airway:

1. Should the airway be managed with the patient in the current location or is it wiser to move the patient to a safer environment?

2. Should the airway be controlled using a surgical or a non-surgical approach?
3. Should intubation be performed with the patient awake or is it safer to ablate consciousness?
4. Is it safer to maintain or ablate spontaneous ventilation?

These choices require an intellectually honest inventory of one's own abilities in the various airway management techniques as well as an assessment of what would be the optimal airway management scenario for the patient. In the interests of optimal patient care and safety, it is always prudent to have skilled help and access to alternative airway management equipment when approaching the patient with a difficult airway.

PRIMARY AND ALTERNATIVE AIRWAY STRATEGIES

This portion of the guidelines emphasizes that the operator should always seek to anticipate airway management strategies that are appropriate for the clinical situation. Some fundamental concepts underlying airway management choices at this stage include:

1. Performing more than three laryngoscopies (by an experienced airway manager) increases the incidence of airway complications, particularly conversion of a non-emergency "can ventilate" situation into an emergency "cannot ventilate" one.
2. Once intubation has failed, it is critical to rapidly attempt optimal mask ventilation (using one or two airway managers with placement of an adequately sized oral and/or nasal airway). When one cannot establish adequate mask ventilation, it is critical to rapidly obtain assistance and appropriate equipment, then rapidly and methodically attempt to establish adequate ventilation with either a supraglottic or a subglottic airway management technique.
3. From the onset of difficulty, if unconsciousness has been induced with or without ablation of spontaneous ventilation, one should constantly be considering the advisability of restoring spontaneous ventilation and consciousness for safety reasons. Restoring spontaneous ventilation and consciousness is not always feasible, particularly if the patient is desaturating and one cannot ventilate at all.
4. In the "Emergent Pathway," appropriate airway management techniques include those that conceptually do not take much time to perform (laryngeal mask airway, Combitube, transtracheal jet ventilation, and cricothyrotomy).
5. The "Non-Emergent Pathway" for airway management includes those techniques that can take a substantial amount of time (>5 minutes) to perform, such as fiberoptic assisted intubation, retrograde intubation, and tracheotomy, in addition to utilizing the "Emergent Pathway" techniques previously listed.
6. In general, it is safer (for the patient) to proceed from attempting supraglottic techniques before subglottic techniques, if the clinical situation allows for a choice.
7. With adequate topical application of local anesthetics, almost any technique can be used to obtain an airway in an awake patient (although use of a Combitube is not recommended in awake patients). Nevertheless, the safest route to establishing a directly visualized definitive airway is fiberoptic-guided endotracheal intubation.

8. There is a consensus among anesthesiologists that the most effective overall airway management technique in both the "Awake" pathway or unconscious "Non-Emergent Pathway" is endotracheal intubation guided by using fiberoptic laryngoscopy/bronchoscopy. There is a consensus among anesthesiologists that the most effective overall airway management technique in the "Emergent Pathway" is use of the laryngeal mask airway.

"AWAKE" EXAMINATION OR INTUBATION

In the patient with a known or suspected difficult airway, the ASA Difficult Airway Practice Guidelines recommend that consideration should be given to the merits and feasibility of an examination or endotracheal intubation and, in some cases, even tracheotomy while the patient is conscious or awake.

In the past few years there have been significant refinements in techniques for providing excellent local anesthesia to the upper airway from the mouth or nose to the trachea. Some effective techniques entail multiple sequential steps, using a combination of local anesthetic sprays, jellies, ointments, and solutions.[13] Another single-step technique takes advantage of an inexpensive, commercially available hand-held nebulizer to permit the patient to breath a nebulized local anesthetic.[14] If the equipment is kept readily available, excellent topical anesthesia of the entire upper airway can routinely be achieved in less than 10 to 15 minutes.[15] Excellent upper airway anesthesia can be reliably produced for flexible or even rigid instrumentation and intubation of the airway. Adequacy of local anesthesia is confirmed by the absence of adverse hemodynamic responses (e.g., hypertension, tachycardia, electrocardiographic changes)[16] or by coughing or movement. Adequacy of the local anesthesia is also supported by reports documenting excellent patient acceptance in postoperative interviews, even when little or no sedation has been used. A few minutes of preoperative explanation and psychological preparation of the patient, as well as systematic application of topical anesthesia to the upper airway, permits the use of minimal, titrated sedation. It is important to understand that the goal of sedation at this point is relief of anxiety while maintaining consciousness. Heavy or deep sedation to induce amnesia or offset inadequate suppression of airway reflexes is contraindicated in the setting of a difficult airway.

THE UNCOOPERATIVE PATIENT

The uncooperative patient with a known or anticipated difficult airway presents a special problem. The problem of the uncooperative patient is acknowledged in the ASA Difficult Airway Practice Guidelines. These special and challenging cases require expert judgment, skill, and management. Our approach is to first acknowledge that these are special cases, which may require extensive modification of our airway management strategy or simply more time. A useful first step is to spend a bit more time in the preoperative interview attempting to gauge the underlying reasons for and the predicted degree of lack of cooperation. Frequently, patients who are labeled as extremely uncooperative end up accepting "awake" airway examination or intubation, particularly if the etiology of the problem is fear, lack of understanding, denial of the disease state, or mild or even moderate mental retardation or dementia. At times, modification of the environment (e.g., minimizing operating room personnel and noise) is sufficient to permit an "awake" procedure. In other cases, careful and judicious use of sedation before the application of local anesthesia to the airway will allow successful "awake" intubation. For example, many patients with Down syndrome tolerate awake intubation after being sedated with intramuscular ketamine. This sedative/hypnotic drug depresses respiratory drive and airway patency less than other sedative drugs. Alternatively, careful titration of a short-acting intravenous narcotic (e.g., fentanyl) and a short-acting benzodiazepine (e.g., midazolam) is a rational approach, particularly because rapid-acting and specific reversal agents (antagonists) are currently available for these classes of sedative drugs. Another rational choice is the ultra-short-acting sedative propofol, because its rapid onset and offset facilitate titration if one has sufficient experience with its use.

The ASA guidelines acknowledge that airway management in some uncooperative patients may require an approach (e.g., intubation after induction of general anesthesia) that might not be regarded as a primary approach in a cooperative patient.

STRATEGY FOR EXTUBATION OF THE PATIENT WITH A DIFFICULT AIRWAY

The ASA guidelines also recommend the formulation of a specific strategy (including contingency plans) for extubation of patients with a difficult airway. Consideration should be given to the relative merits of awake extubation versus extubation before the return of consciousness versus elective prolonged intubation or tracheotomy. Consideration should also be given to the use of a device, such as a ventilating tube changer, that can serve as a guide for expedited re-intubation as well as for the transient provision of oxygenation, ventilation, and suctioning of the trachea (see Endotracheal Tube Exchange Catheters). At our institution, consideration is routinely given to the early administration of a single dose of corticosteroid for the purpose of reducing mucosal inflammation in patients, who required multiple intubation attempts. The ASA guidelines recommend that the anesthesiologist inform the patient (or responsible family member) of the airway difficulty that was encountered, and the airway management techniques that were used should also be described in detail in the patient's medical record to guide and facilitate future care. Some investigators have even recommended that patients who have experienced significant difficulty with airway management wear a medical alert bracelet. The Medic Alert Foundation now provides a special "Difficult Airway" bracelet. Finally, patients experiencing airway management problems, particularly needing multiple instrumentations, should be observed and treated for complications such as edema, bleeding, tracheal or esophageal perforation, pneumothorax, aspiration of gastric contents, hypoxic brain injury, or myocardial infarction in an appropriate observation unit when necessary.

FLEXIBLE FIBEROPTIC INTUBATION

Fiberoptically guided endotracheal intubation was initially described in the anesthesiology literature in 1967 (Fig. 205-6). However, its current prominent role in the management of difficult airways was not well established until the 1980s when Ovassapian and coworkers,[15,16] Wang and colleagues,[17]

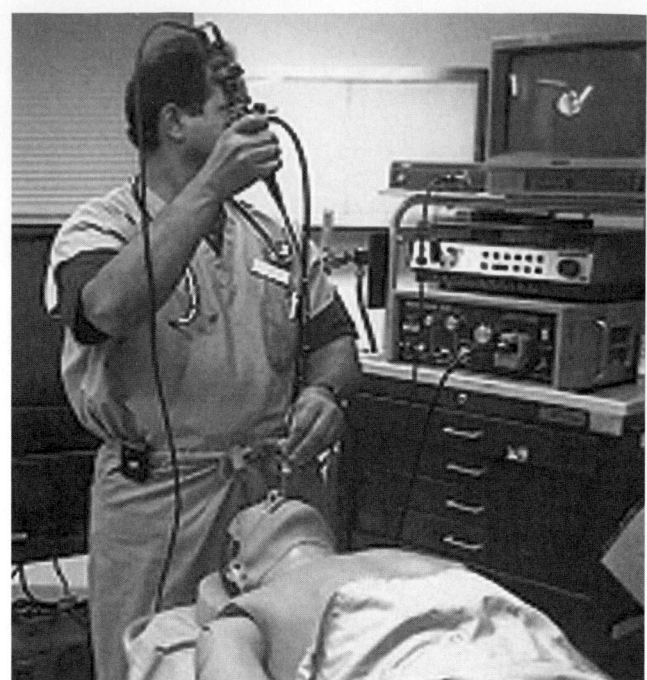

FIGURE 205–6. Fiberoptic bronchoscope–guided endotracheal intubation.

and Patil and associates[18] published reports, series, and studies regarding data indicating that flexible fiberoptically guided endotracheal intubation can be useful in the management of both routine and difficult airways. Several optical equipment manufacturers developed and refined flexible fiberscopes specifically for endotracheal intubation. These flexible "intubating fiberscopes" are more slender than conventional flexible bronchoscopes used in pulmonology, yet they retain excellent optics. Intubating fiberscopes are also available in pediatric sizes that can accommodate very small endotracheal tubes. Fiberoptically guided placement of the endotracheal tube is extremely useful for awake intubation in the spontaneously breathing patient with a known or suspected difficult airway.

The ASA Difficult Airway Algorithm also recommends fiberoptic intubation as one of the options when a "cannot intubate but can ventilate" situation arises after the induction of general anesthesia. Before fiberoptic endoscopy, the endotracheal tube is premounted over the fiberscope (or fiberoptic bronchoscope) and moved as far proximally on the scope as possible. Additionally, oxygen is insufflated through the working channel of the fiberscope to blow secretions away from the optical field. Suction is rarely effective through the working channel of the intubating fiberscope, because the lumen is only 1.2 mm in diameter. Suction also tends to trap viscous secretions in front of the optics, thus interfering with the view seen by the endoscopist. The working channel can also be used for instillation of local anesthesia as the fiberscope is advanced. Fiberoptic endotracheal intubation can be accomplished via the nasal route or the oral route or in combination with percutaneous retrograde passage of a guide wire via the cricothyroid membrane into the working channel of the fiberscope (see Retrograde Intubation). Once the planned route of intubation is determined and topical or general anesthesia is achieved, the endoscope is advanced through the larynx and into the mid trachea. When the endoscope is successfully positioned in the mid trachea, the endotracheal tube is gently advanced to the vocal cords, rotated 90 degrees in a counterclockwise manner, and then advanced. The counterclockwise rotation prevents the bevel of the endotracheal tube from ensnaring a vocal cord and potentially dislocating it. The endoscope is withdrawn after confirming intratracheal positioning of the endotracheal tube. In addition to its indications in the management of many difficult airway situations, fiberoptic endoscopy is very useful for proper positioning of double-lumen endotracheal tubes. It is also quite useful in endotracheal tube changes as well as in the perioperative evaluation of ventilatory problems and endotracheal position. Additionally, in a darkened room, the flexible fiberoptic laryngoscope with a sufficiently bright light source may also be used as a "light wand" to identify the laryngeal inlet by transillumination for endotracheal intubation (see Light Wands). Despite its utility, flexible fiberoptic intubation and visualization do have limitations. Minimal trauma to the fiberoptic scope can break the optical bundles and distort the visual field. The presence of active airway bleeding or other opaque secretions, such as vomitus, can limit the usefulness of the fiberoptic technique. Awake fiberoptic intubation also may be of limited usefulness in uncooperative patients or in patients with inadequate topical anesthesia of the upper airway. Finally, patients with severe restriction of the laryngeal or tracheal caliber by large intrinsic or extrinsically compressive masses may actually experience complete airway obstruction with introduction of the flexible intubating fiberscope.

LIGHT WANDS

The light wand or lighted stylet is simply a malleable stylet with a light source that provides illumination at the distal tip (Fig. 205-7). Many are portable, battery-powered units with a small bulb at the distal tip, although some fiberoptically illuminated units have been introduced. The light wand, with an endotracheal tube premounted over it, is inserted blindly into the hypopharynx. If the tip is directed at the laryngeal inlet, a bright glow should be observed in the anterior neck as the larynx and soft tissues of the neck are transilluminated. It thus can serve as a guide to successful "blind" intubation. In 1957, Macintosh and Richards described an "illuminated introducer" to assist in endotracheal intubation.[19] Over the past 15 years, reports in the medical literature have described success using the light wand when endotracheal intubation using conventional direct laryngoscopy was unsuccessful or impractical.[20,21] The ASA Difficult Airway Algorithm recommends the light wand as one option when intubation is unobtainable by routine direct laryngoscopy in "cannot intubate but can mask ventilate" situations. The technique of intubation with the light wand is simple to teach to individuals with previous experience in basic intubation skills. Successful use by residents in anesthesiology and emergency medicine, and by other emergency personnel, has been noted in the literature.

Before use, the light wand should be lubricated and the endotracheal tube should be premounted over the wand. Depending on the length of the particular light wand chosen, the endotracheal tube may need to be shortened by cutting off a proximal segment. The distal end of the light wand should then be bent to form an approximately 90-degree angle ("hockey stick") or curve to approximate the patient's oropharyngeal anatomy. The light wand/endotracheal tube combination is then inserted over the tongue in the midline and advanced blindly into the hypopharynx. It may be necessary to gently pull the tongue forward or to elevate the mandible. From this point on, the operator observes the anterior neck for the classic midline "bright glow" at the level of the thyroid cartilage emitted from the distal end of the light wand. This signals entrance through the laryngeal structures into the trachea. The endotracheal tube is then advanced as the light wand is gently removed.[22] Proper endotracheal tube position must then be confirmed as in any other intubation sequence. Dimming the ambient lighting will make the process of transillumination more effective with standard commercial light wands. If the illumination glow is dull, diffuse, or absent, this may signal an esophageal intubation. Successful nasotracheal intubation using the light wand has been reported.[23] In the emergency department or the field, use of the light wand may be better than blind nasotracheal intubation in the apneic patient, particularly when a cervical spine injury is suspected or when fiberoptic endoscopy or surgical tracheal access is impractical, because of secretions or lack of training of emergency personnel.

Holzman and colleagues presented their experience with the light wand in 31 children with abnormal airways, including Treacher Collins and Pierre Robin syndromes.[24] Only one child could not be intubated with the light wand. All of these children could be ventilated by mask without any problems. These authors pointed out that the diameter of the encased bulb limited the smallest endotracheal tube that could be used to 5.0 to 5.5 mm. Complications related to the use of the light wand have been documented. However, these occurrences are rare. Two cases of arytenoid dislocation have been reported. Stone and associates reported a case involving separation of the bulb from the stylet, necessitating bronchoscopic retrieval of the object from the patient's right lung.[25] This problem has since been remedied by securely encasing the bulb along with the stylet. Cohn and Joshi reported fracture and separation of the stylet from the handle during management of a difficult airway.[26] This occurred during the withdrawal of the lubricated light wand from the endotracheal tube. Overall, a major advantage of the light wand technique is that it is easy to learn. The device is simple to operate, lightweight, and easily portable. It works well in situations with poor ambient lighting and is applicable when cervical spine and temporomandibular

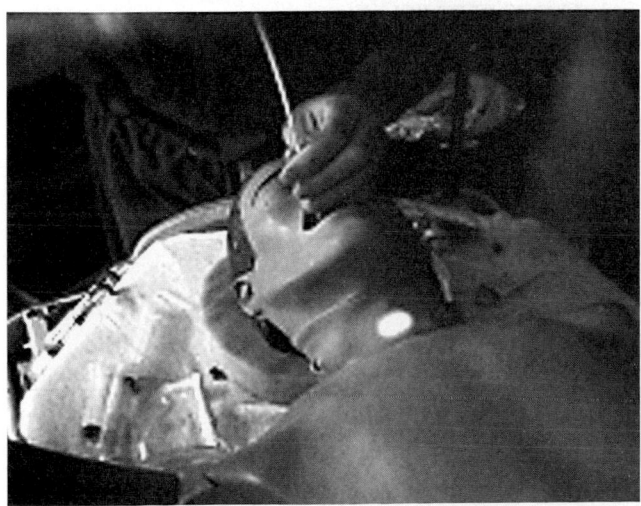

FIGURE 205-7. Lighted stylet–guided endotracheal intubation.

joint mobility is limited. The presence of blood or secretions in the oropharynx do not interfere with the technique. However, there are some situations in which the light wand may not be applicable, including obese patients with thick necks or other patients with anterior cervical pathology that would make it difficult to visualize the illumination and patients with upper airway pathology such as friable tumors that might preclude the use of blind intubation techniques.

RETROGRADE INTUBATION

Retrograde (translaryngeal-guided) intubation techniques have been used for several decades.[27] Retrograde intubation is listed as an option in the nonemergency section ("cannot intubate but can mask ventilate") of the ASA Difficult Airway Algorithm (see Fig. 205-1). Retrograde-guided intubation also has been used electively for awake intubations. Because even in the best of hands the technique requires several steps and, thus, considerable time before oxygenation and ventilation can be initiated, it is probably best reserved for the previously mentioned situations. Reported indications for this technique include trismus, ankylosis of the jaw or cervical spine, and maxillofacial trauma.[28,29]

In the retrograde technique,[28] the cricothyroid membrane is punctured with either a 17-gauge epidural needle or a large-bore intravenous catheter that is directed cephalad (Fig. 205-8). A long, thin, flexible guide (either an epidural catheter or an angiography guide wire at least 70 cm in length) is then fed through until it emerges from the mouth or one of the nares. Occasionally, the guide wire of an epidural catheter must be "fished" out of the oropharynx with a clamp. The distal end emerging from the neck is secured with a clamp. The proximal end of the guide wire can then be used to guide an endotracheal tube directly into the trachea. Alternatively, the guide wire can be fed into the suction channel of an intubating flexible fiberscope with an endotracheal tube premounted on it. Both the scope and the tube can then be directed visually and mechanically into the trachea using the wire as a guide. Potential complications of the retrograde technique include needle or guide wire trauma to the upper airway or other tissues of the neck.

THE ESOPHAGEAL-TRACHEAL COMBITUBE

The Esophageal-Tracheal Combitube (Kendall-Sheridan, Argyle, NY) is an emergency airway management device for patients requiring rapid control of the airway, particularly when poor laryngoscopic visualization of the larynx makes tracheal intubation impossible.[30-34] Because the Combitube has some similarity to an older airway management device known as the "esophageal obturator airway," some clinicians still confuse the two devices. However, the similarities are minimal and superficial. Esophageal obturator airways, because of a variety of problems and limitations, are rarely used or useful. On the other hand, the newer Combitube is currently recommended as one of the acceptable options in the "emergency" (cannot intubate/cannot ventilate) portion of the ASA Difficult Airway Algorithm (see Fig. 205-1). In many cases, this device can provide lifesaving emergency ventilation and oxygenation as a temporary measure until a surgical airway can be obtained and secured. Adequate ventilation and arterial blood gas values have been reported for up to 8 hours in patients who have been emergently intubated with the Combitube.[35]

The Combitube is a double-lumen soft plastic tube that is inserted into the mouth without laryngoscopy and advanced blindly into either the trachea or esophagus (Fig. 205-9; see also Figs. 205-3 and 205-4). One lumen is open distally, like a conventional endotracheal tube. The other lumen has a closed, rounded distal end but has ventilating side-holes more proximally. The Combitube has two inflatable cuffs: a smaller distal cuff similar to that of a conventional endotracheal tube and a larger proximal cuff designed to seal the pharynx.

Because of its design, the Combitube can be used to effectively ventilate the upper airway regardless of whether it is placed into the trachea or esophagus, simply by selecting the appropriate lumen. The proper lumen for ventilation is determined empirically by auscultation of the lungs and stomach and confirmed by capnometric detection of carbon dioxide, when available.

The Combitube has been shown to provide effective oxygenation and ventilation without the need for direct visualization of the airway in a variety of emergency situations. Only minimal training is required to obtain high rates of successful placement.[35] This device has been used emergently in

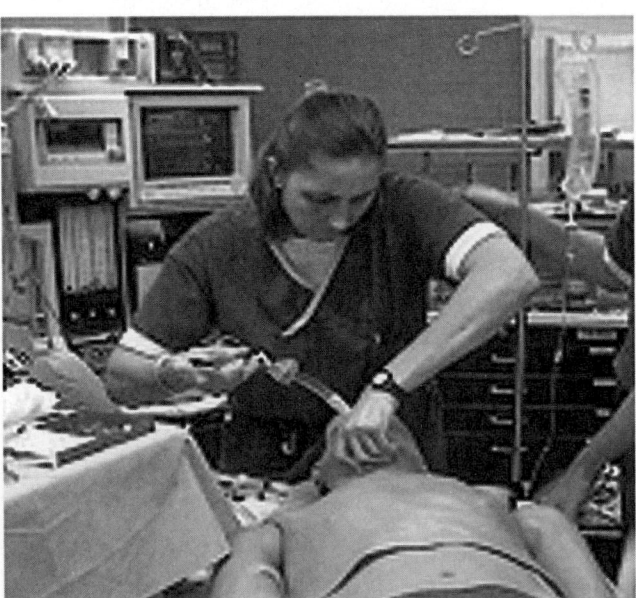

FIGURE 205–9. Esophageal-Tracheal Combitube (Kendall-Sheridan, Argyle, NY).

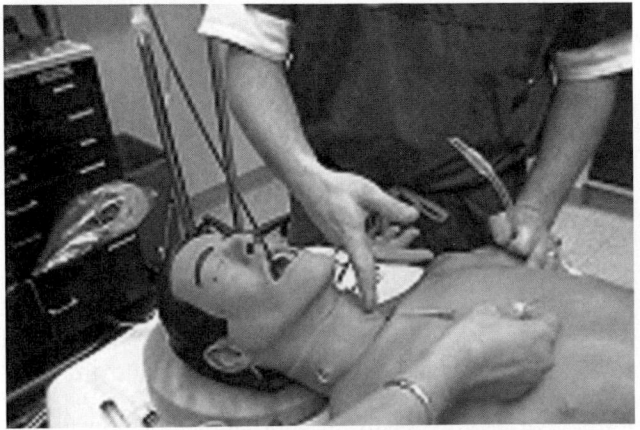

FIGURE 205–8. Retrograde endotracheal intubation.

several cases of expanding neck hematomas when endotracheal intubation was unsuccessful.[36,37]

The Combitube is now available in two sizes: a "regular adult" (41 French or 13.5-mm outer diameter) and a "small adult" (37 French or 12-mm outer diameter). Because of its relatively large size, however, the Combitube is contraindicated in very small adult patients and in pediatric patients. It should be used with caution in patients with upper esophageal pathologic processes. It also may not be effective in patients with upper airway tumors, particularly obstructing tumors or other stenosing lesions of the hypopharynx, larynx, or trachea. Laryngospasm of the vocal cords, as well as foreign bodies in the larynx or trachea, may impair ventilation via the Combitube when it is in the esophageal position.

THE LARYNGEAL MASK AIRWAY

The laryngeal mask airway (LMA) was developed by the English anesthesiologist Brain and his colleagues[38] and has been available in the United States since late 1992 (Fig. 205-10).[39] Worldwide, LMAs have become very popular and have been used over 10 million times.[40] The LMA is useful for both elective, routine anesthetics and for many emergency difficult airway situations.

An LMA resembles a very small anesthesia mask (the "cuff") attached to the distal end of a segment of large diameter endotracheal tube; indeed, the LMA may be considered a hybrid between an endotracheal tube and facemask. No neck movement or laryngoscopy is required for insertion of the LMA. It is inserted by digitally guiding the deflated cuff across the hard palate down to the hypopharynx without the need for direct visualization of the glottis. Insertion is complete when resistance is met. The cuff is then inflated, helping to secure it in place.[39] Six sizes of LMAs are marketed in the United States, making the device applicable for patients from neonates to large adults. An ideally placed LMA will have its distal central lumen over the laryngeal inlet with the distal tip of its cuff covering the upper esophageal opening and the remainder of the cuff positioned in the hypopharynx in contact with the pyriform fossae and the laryngeal surface of the epiglottis (see Fig. 205-7). Successful placement resulting in adequate ventilation and oxygenation is achieved in a very high percentage of elective LMA insertions. Several series

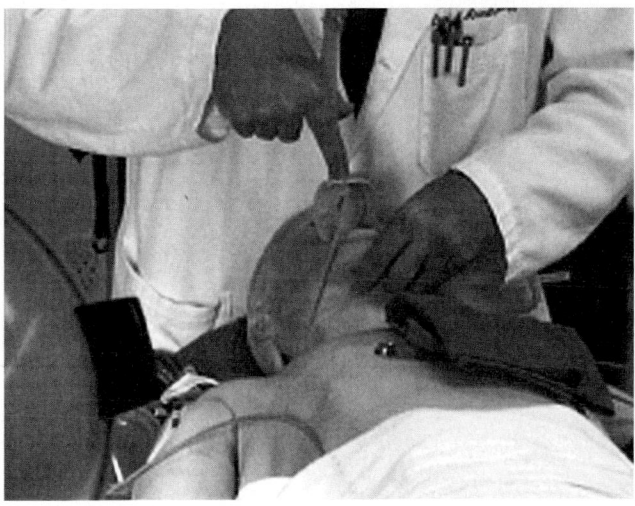

FIGURE 205–10. Laryngeal mask airway.

report success rates in the 95% to 99% range in patients of all ages.[40-44]

The LMA does not require support to stay in place. It was designed to be less labor-intensive than a facemask, allowing ventilation while "freeing up" the anesthesiologist's hands to prepare and administer medications, adjust gas flows, and attend to other aspects of intraoperative patient care.[40]

The LMA is too bulky and short to enter the esophagus or larynx, thus reducing the potential for inadvertent esophageal or mainstem bronchial intubations. These are two major potential problems with endotracheal intubation, especially in pediatric patients. Compared with standard direct laryngoscopy and intubation and mask ventilation, LMA insertion is easier to learn and perform.[43,45,46] With use of the LMA, there are fewer postoperative sore throats,[44] coughing,[48] and minimal potential for laryngeal pathology. There is probably less alteration in cardiovascular status[49] and intraocular pressure[50] than with direct laryngoscopy and intubation. No muscle relaxation is required for LMA insertion. Additionally, LMAs are reusable.

The LMA has two other advantages over endotracheal intubation. First, because of its shape, the LMA is actually easier to insert in many patients in whom routine direct laryngoscopy and intubation would be difficult.[51] Second, ideal positioning of the LMA in the hypopharynx is not required to provide adequate ventilation.[52]

These factors have helped the LMA to achieve popularity for elective anesthetic cases as well as recognition in the "emergency" pathway section ("cannot intubate, cannot ventilate") of the ASA Difficult Airway Algorithm (see Fig. 205-1). In many emergency airway situations, the LMA can be inserted quickly and without laryngoscopy, thereby potentially serving as a lifesaving ventilating measure. Once in place, the LMA can also be used as a guide for either "blind" or flexible fiberoptic intubation through its central channel using a small endotracheal tube.

Because the LMA does not pass into the trachea and does not completely partition the airway from the esophagus, the greatest risk when using an LMA is pulmonary aspiration of regurgitated stomach contents or pharyngeal matter. If used in properly selected patients, however, the risk of aspiration with an LMA approximates that of facemasks or endotracheal tubes.[53]

The LMA cannot provide a definitive airway. Peak inspiratory pressures greater than 20 cm H_2O can displace an LMA and force air down the esophagus.[39,54] Because most forms of controlled ventilation in adults routinely achieve pressures greater than this level, using controlled positive-pressure ventilation through an LMA in ICU patients is not ideal. The LMA is, therefore, best used for the management of spontaneously breathing patients.

The effect of the LMA on pharyngeal mucosa after prolonged use is unclear.[55] There is no consensus regarding effects of the LMA on upper esophageal sphincter tone.[53] The contraindications to using the LMA are similar to those for facemasks and include patients with a "full stomach," hiatal hernia, obesity, emergency surgery, and abdominal surgery. A requirement for controlled ventilation and the necessity for the prone or lateral position are strong relative contraindications for elective LMA use. Additionally, the LMA cannot be used if the mouth cannot be opened.

The LMA also has been used to provide ventilation in patients with abnormal airways secondary to congenital defects such as the Robin sequence.[56] Common sense dictates,

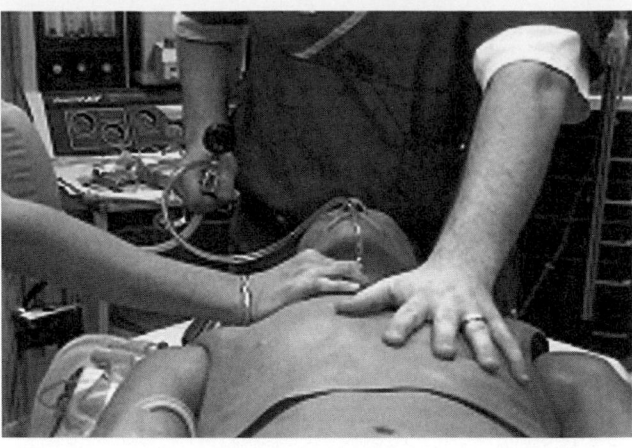

FIGURE 205–11. Transtracheal jet ventilation.

however, that patients with supraglottic/hypopharyngeal lesions, severely hypertrophied tonsils, or marked laryngeal or tracheal deviation from midline might be poor candidates for LMA use.

CRICOTHYROID PUNCTURE AND TRANSTRACHEAL JET VENTILATION

Percutaneous transtracheal jet ventilation (TTJV) using a large-bore intravenous catheter inserted through the cricothyroid membrane is a simple, quick, relatively safe, and often extremely effective treatment of choice for the desperate "cannot intubate/cannot ventilate" situation[28,57] TTJV can serve as a lifesaving temporary measure until a less-hurried, more definitive airway (endotracheal intubation, surgical cricothyrotomy, or tracheostomy) can be obtained.

As depicted in Figures 205-11 and 205-12, TTJV requires only (1) large-bore intravenous catheter (preferably 14 or 16 gauge, 1.25 to 2 inches in length); (2) high pressure oxygen source (preferably 50 pounds per square inch), such as unregulated standard hospital "wall" oxygen; (3) manual jet insufflator or injection device (these are commercially available and relatively inexpensive); and (4) proper connectors (which are part of the commercially available units). Alternatives to unregulated wall oxygen and the manual jet insufflator include connections to a standard hospital flowmeter[58] (provided the flowmeter is opened maximally to greater than 15 L/min) or connection to the breathing circuit or common gas outlet of an anesthesia machine or mechanical ventilator. However, these alternative methods also require proper connectors, which should be preassembled into "kits." A high-frequency jet ventilator, if available, is certainly a suitable alternative source, but it is much more expensive and occupies more space than manual (low-frequency) jet injectors.

The recommended TTJV pattern is 1 second "on" and 1 to 3 seconds "off." The patient's chest should move during inspiration and exhalation. It is imperative to ensure adequate egress of the injected oxygen from the mouth or nose during the expiratory phase of TTJV to prevent excessive build-up of pressure in the lungs. Excessive pressure can lead to barotrauma, manifested by pneumothorax or even tension pneumothorax. Maintaining sufficient upper airway patency to permit egress of gas during the exhalation phase of TTJV may require the jaw thrust or chinlift maneuver, insertion of an oropharyngeal or nasopharyngeal airway, or sometimes even sustained rigid laryngoscopy. Other potential complications from percutaneous TTJV include bleeding or needle injury to the airway or other cervical structures. The intravenous catheter should be directed caudad during insertion and held tightly during jet insufflation to prevent the catheter from dislodging as a result of the high oxygen pressures.

TTJV is one of the recommended options in the "emergency" section ("cannot intubate/cannot ventilate") of the ASA Difficult Airway Algorithm (see Fig. 205-1).

ENDOTRACHEAL TUBE EXCHANGE CATHETERS

Endotracheal tube changers or airway exchange catheters are long narrow catheters that are placed down the central lumen of an endotracheal tube that is already in place in the trachea (Fig. 205-13).[59] The endotracheal tube can be removed, while the tube changer is left in place in the trachea to act as a guide to facilitate rapid reinsertion of a new endotracheal tube, particularly if the original intubation was difficult. Re-intubation thus can be performed quickly, often without laryngoscopy.

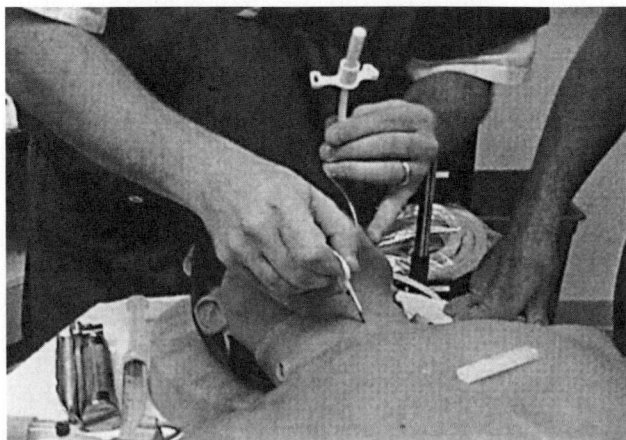

FIGURE 205–12. Percutaneous transtracheal jet ventilation.

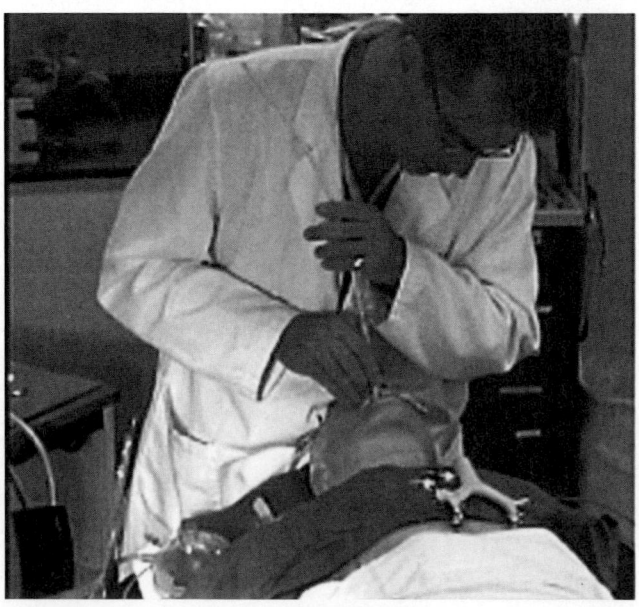

FIGURE 205–13. Endotracheal tube exchangers.

Tube changers are most often used to replace a damaged endotracheal tube with a new one or a smaller endotracheal tube with a larger one. A tube changer also can be of value for a trial of extubation in a patient who was difficult to intubate. In these cases, instillation of local anesthesia via the original endotracheal tube is usually necessary to prevent coughing and bucking produced by irritation of the trachea by the tube changer in an awake patient.

In 1987, Bedger and Chang[59] developed and described a new, modified tube exchange catheter that was hollow and thus permitted emergency ventilation or jet ventilation, if necessary, during a tube change or trial of extubation. A similar ventilating tube changer is now commercially available (Cook Critical Care, Bloomington, IN). This hollow catheter is 90-cm long (approximately three times the length of most conventional adult endotracheal tubes). The catheter is available in adult and pediatric sizes. The latter can be inserted into endotracheal tubes as small as 3.0-mm internal diameter. The catheter comes with two easily attached adapters for connecting it to oxygen sources. One is a standard 15-mm connector that fits any standard anesthesia breathing circuit or breathing bag. The other is a Luer-Lok connector that attaches the device to many jet ventilator assemblies. These adapters allow the Cook airway exchange catheter to function as a ventilatory device, even if placed without an endotracheal tube.

The ASA Difficult Airway Practice Guidelines suggest that tube changers may be a useful part of an extubation plan for a patient who was difficult to intubate. The ASA Difficult Airway Algorithm also lists tube changers as one of several devices that may be useful aids to intubation in the "non-emergency pathway" section ("cannot intubate, but can ventilate") of the algorithm.

Although often extremely useful and even lifesaving,[60] there are several problems that can arise from the use of tube changers. When used for trials of extubation, a tube changer actually can contribute to a failed trial by one of two mechanisms. The first is tracheal irritation leading to excessive coughing or bronchospasm. The second is increased work of breathing by occupying cross-sectional area in an already stenosed airway. The first problem can often be prevented by instillation of local anesthesia via the endotracheal tube before the insertion of the tube changer. The second problem can be avoided by the selection and use of a tube changer of sufficiently narrow gauge.

Another hazard with the use of tube changers is the possibility of dislodging of the catheter from the trachea during removal of the original endotracheal tube. If the tube changer migrates into the esophagus, subsequent intubation can result in esophageal intubation. Selection of a sufficiently long exchange catheter and judicious lubrication of the tube changer may reduce friction with the endotracheal tube and thereby reduce the risk of dislodging.

Because most tube changing catheters are semirigid, there is always a risk of mucosal injury. And finally, jet ventilation via a ventilating tube changer may result in barotrauma and even tension pneumothorax, particularly in patients with poor pulmonary or thoracic compliance and in situations in which there is inadequate egress of gases.

CONCLUSION

There have been significant advances in the subject of difficult airway management for anesthesiologists in the past several years. Many of these concepts and techniques can be used by intensivists, who are often faced with the management of complicated and difficult airways. Knowledge of these changes is important for the intensivist, who often works hand-in-hand with the anesthesiologist in the perioperative management of patients with difficult airways. The ASA Practice Guidelines for Management of the Difficult Airway provide a framework for discussion, teaching, and analysis of the complex topic of airway management. All medical professionals involved in airway management should be familiar with the ASA Guidelines. A primary strategy including contingency plans should be carefully formulated before making any attempts to intubate or extubate patients with a difficult airway. Several new devices to assist in the management of the difficult airway have come into widespread use in the past few years. Most of these devices are extremely helpful and potentially even lifesaving. However, all have limitations, contraindications, and potential complications.

ANNOTATED REFERENCES

Benumof J: Management of the difficult adult airway. Anesthesiology 1991;75:1087-1110.
Comprehensive description of difficult airway management with special emphasis on awake tracheal intubation.

Brimacombe JR, Berry A: The incidence of aspiration associated with the laryngeal mask airway: A meta-analysis of published literature. J Clin Anesth 1995;7:297-307.
Review of 547 publications for analysis of observational studies in which laryngeal mask airway was the main form of airway management.

Gaughan SD, Ozaki GT, Benumof JL: A comparison in a lung model of low- and high-flow regulators for transtracheal jet ventilation. Anesthesiology 1992;77:189-192.
Good study of low-flow pressure-reducing regulator (LFR) versus high-flow regulator (HFR) for producing adequate transtracheal jet ventilation (TTJV).

Mallampati SR, Gatt SP, Gugino LD, et al: A clinical sign to predict difficult tracheal intubation: A prospective study. Can Anaesth Soc J 1985;32:429.
Evaluation in 210 patients of the Mallampati grading system involving preoperative ability to visualize the faucial pillars, soft palate, and base of uvula as predictor of difficulty in laryngeal exposure.

Verdile VP, Chiang JL, Bedger R, et al: Nasotracheal intubation using a flexible lighted stylet. Ann Emerg Med 1990;19:506-510.
Clinical trial of 80 patients undergoing nasotracheal intubation for elective ear, nose, and throat or maxillofacial surgery randomized to be nasotracheally intubated blindly or with a stylet by an emergency medicine resident or anesthesiologist.

Chapter 206
BEDSIDE ULTRASONOGRAPHY

Yanick Beaulieu • John Gorcsan

KEY POINTS

1. As a result of improvements in transthoracic imaging, most ICU patients now can be adequately studied with transthoracic echocardiography (TTE) first.

2. Transesophageal echocardiography (TEE) is particularly useful in the ICU for the assessment of unexplained hypotension, suspected aortic dissection, valvular vegetation, source of cardiac or aortic emboli, prosthetic heart valves (especially mitral), and detection of intracardiac shunts.

3. The use of ultrasound guidance during central venous catheterization has been well shown to reduce the risk of complications, improve the rapidity of catheter placement, and improve the overall success of the procedure.

4. Successful performance of bedside ultrasonography by intensivists has been shown to be feasible and potentially to provide rapid, accurate diagnostic information that can have a dramatic impact on the treatment of critically ill patients.

5. Adequate training and maintenance of competence is crucial for the intensivist to perform bedside ultrasonography safely and efficiently because inappropriate interpretation or application of data gained by a poorly skilled user may result in adverse consequences.

Advances in ultrasound technology continue to enhance its diagnostic applications in daily medical practice. Constantly evolving, this tool has become useful to properly trained cardiologists, anesthesiologists, intensivists, surgeons, obstetricians, and emergency department physicians. Ultrasound can enable rapid, accurate, and noninvasive diagnosis of a broad range of medical conditions. Patients in the ICU present daily diagnostic and therapeutic challenges to the medical team. The availability of ultrasound instrumentation in critical care units has facilitated greatly the evaluation and treatment of patients with a wide spectrum of conditions. Although TEE previously was the principal diagnostic approach using ultrasound to evaluate ICU patients, advances in ultrasound imaging, including harmonic imaging, digital acquisition, and contrast for endocardial enhancement, have improved the diagnostic yield of TTE, which is simpler and safer to perform. Ultrasound devices continue to become even more portable than in the past, and hand-carried devices now are

readily available for bedside applications. This chapter discusses the application of bedside ultrasonography in the ICU. The emphasis is on echocardiography and cardiovascular diagnostics. The use of bedside ultrasound to facilitate central line placement and to aid in the care of patients with pleural effusions and intra-abdominal fluid collections also is addressed.

USE OF BEDSIDE ULTRASONOGRAPHY IN THE INTENSIVE CARE UNIT

GENERAL INDICATIONS

Ultrasonography has become an invaluable tool in the management of critically ill patients. Its safety and portability allow for use at the bedside to provide rapid, detailed information regarding the cardiovascular system[1] and the function and anatomy of certain internal organs. It also can be used by the clinician to assess the pleural and intra-abdominal spaces and to perform some invasive procedures safely. General indications for performance of echocardiography in the ICU are listed in Table 206-1. Table 206-2 lists major indications for performance of primary TEE in the ICU. Other indications for use of bedside ultrasonography by the intensivist in critically ill patients are listed in Table 206-3.

TECHNICAL ASPECTS

Acoustic Window in a Critically Ill Patient

The practical value of bedside ultrasonography in the management of critically ill patients is now widely accepted despite the inherent limitations of the technique.[2] These limitations are related mostly to suboptimal imaging conditions that commonly are encountered when performing studies of critically ill patients. The constrained physical environment of the ICU also can compromise the quality of the images obtained. For an ultrasound study to be deemed adequate, a good acoustic "window" is required to allow accurate analysis. Ultrasonography uses the physical principle that sound is reflected from tissue interfaces, allowing a two-dimensional image of the anatomic structure studied to be constructed.[3] Anything hindering the reflection of this acoustic signal—air, bone, calcium, a foreign body, or another interposed structure—interferes with ultrasound transmission and diminishes the overall quality of the examination. In the ICU, many patients are mechanically ventilated. In these patients, adequate imaging can be limited due to pneumothorax, pneumomediastinum, or subcutaneous emphysema.[2] Other important factors limiting data acquisition in critically ill patients are related to surgical wounds

TABLE 206–1. GENERAL INDICATIONS FOR PERFORMANCE OF AN ECHOCARDIOGRAPHIC EXAMINATION IN THE INTENSIVE CARE UNIT

Hemodynamic instability
  Ventricular failure
  Hypovolemia
  Pulmonary embolism
  Acute valvular dysfunction
  Cardiac tamponade
  Complications after cardiothoracic surgery
Infective endocarditis
Aortic dissection and rupture
Unexplained hypoxemia
Source of embolus

TABLE 206–3. OTHER INDICATIONS FOR USE OF BEDSIDE ULTRASONOGRAPHY BY THE INTENSIVIST

Central line placement
Assessment of pleural effusions and intra-abdominal fluid collections
Urinary bladder scan
FAST
Intra-aortic balloon counterpulsation
Ventricular assist devices

FAST, focused assessment of the trauma patient.

and dressings, tapes, tubing, obesity, and chronic obstructive pulmonary disease. In addition, lack of patient cooperation and the impossibility of moving some patients into the optimal position for the examination contribute to a high prevalence of technically inadequate studies.[2]

Although ultrasonography permits evaluation of the structure and function of the heart and other important organs and structures, acquisition of data and interpretation of results are fraught with potential traps.[4] Performing an ultrasound examination requires a thorough knowledge of anatomy and instrumentation, including attention to gain control, gray scale settings, Doppler velocity settings, and transducer placement.

Preparation of the Patient

Before starting an ultrasound examination at the bedside in the ICU, certain important criteria should be fulfilled. The criteria vary depending on the type of examination being performed (TTE; TEE; vascular, abdominal, or thoracic ultrasound) and on certain patient-related factors (e.g., presence or absence of mechanical ventilation, nasogastric tube, or surgical dressings).

An awake patient should be informed about the importance of the ultrasound investigation and should be provided with an explanation of how the clinician will perform the examination.[3] These steps are especially important when the examination uses the transesophageal route. For this procedure, written informed consent usually is required in most centers.

TABLE 206–2. MAJOR INDICATIONS FOR PERFORMANCE OF PRIMARY TRANSESOPHAGEAL ECHOCARDIOGRAPHY STUDY IN THE INTENSIVE CARE UNIT

Diagnosis of conditions in which the superior image quality is vital (i.e., aortic dissection, assessment of endocarditis and its complications, intracardiac thrombus)
Imaging of structures that may be inadequately seen by TTE (i.e., thoracic aorta, left atrial appendage, prosthetic valves)
Echocardiographic examinations of patients with conditions that prevent image clarity with TTE (i.e., severe obesity, emphysema, mechanical ventilation with high level of PEEP, presence of tubes, surgical incisions, dressings)
Acute perioperative hemodynamic derangements

PEEP, positive end-expiratory pressure; TTE, transthoracic echocardiography.

POSITIONING

Proper positioning of the patient is important for obtaining an adequate image. For performance of TTE and TEE, optimal imaging usually is obtained by having the patient in the left lateral decubitus position. For other types of ultrasound studies, adequate positioning of the patient varies depending on the structures being assessed (e.g., pleural space, peritoneal cavity, vascular structures, or bladder). Care must be taken when positioning a critically ill patient in bed because these patients often have multiple vascular catheters, an endotracheal tube, drains, and other tubes or devices connected to them. When the ultrasound examination is done to localize and mark pleural or abdominal fluid collections for subsequent drainage, it is crucial that the patient remain in the same position used during the marking procedure until the actual drainage of the collection is performed. Risks of perforating surrounding organs (e.g., heart, spleen, liver, lungs, or bowel) and inducing significant morbidity are increased if the drainage is performed in a position different from the one used during marking.

SEDATION

To optimize the ultrasound examination, the patient must be cooperative and nonagitated. Noninvasive procedures such as TTE and abdominal ultrasound usually are well tolerated by patients, and additional sedation rarely is needed to perform these procedures. When performing TEE, however, certain precautions need to be taken. Patients should fast (or have their tube feeds stopped) for at least 4 hours before the procedure. Topical anesthesia of the oropharynx also is helpful before insertion of the TEE probe, especially in patients who are not endotracheally intubated.[3] Even if adequate topical anesthesia is provided, insertion of the TEE probe still can cause significant discomfort and anxiety, so providing adequate sedation and analgesia is important. Frequently used sedative or analgesic agents include intravenous midazolam, fentanyl, and propofol. Dosing should be titrated according to the clinical parameters, including arterial blood pressure, minute ventilation, and arterial oxygen saturation.[3] Sedative-induced hypotension is a frequent problem in patients with depressed ventricular function or decreased systemic vascular resistance, and occasionally patients may require transient support with a vasopressor agent. If the patient is extremely uncooperative, transient paralysis, accompanied by increased sedation, may need to be used to perform TEE safely.

Monitoring During the Procedure

Most ICU patients are monitored continuously, at least for certain respiratory, cardiac, or hemodynamic parameters. It is essential that patients undergoing an ultrasound examination in the ICU be monitored at least with noninvasive recording of blood pressure, pulse oximetry, and electrocardiogram. Even TTE or abdominal ultrasound examinations can be associated with inadvertent pulling of tubes or drains, and anxiety can be encountered during the procedure. Because of its more invasive nature, TEE may induce complications, such as increased agitation, respiratory distress, and pain during insertion of the probe. These effects can be associated with substantial changes in blood pressure and ventilatory status. Administration of sedatives and sometimes paralytic agents can induce further changes in hemodynamic and respiratory status.[3,5]

Safety

Performance of ultrasound examinations in the ICU allows procedures that previously required transport to the radiology suite to be performed at the bedside. This is an important advantage to a critically ill patient because transport out of and back to the ICU is known to be associated with increased risk of complications.[6] Performance of bedside TTE and of other noninvasive ultrasound examinations is safe and not associated with significant risks to the patient. Performance of bedside TEE also is associated with a low incidence of serious complications, (<0.5% in the general population and the elderly).[5] The reported mortality rate associated with TEE is 0.01% to 0.03%.[7] Most patients undergoing TEE examinations in the ICU usually are receiving mechanical ventilation and have continuous monitoring of arterial blood pressure, electrocardiogram, and oxygen saturation.[8] Transient hypotension, typically attributable to administration of sedative medications, usually can be treated with vasopressors or intravenous fluids or both. The risk of injury to the pharynx or esophagus is greater in anesthetized and endotracheally intubated, critically ill patients than in awake patients because anesthetized patients cannot assist with probe insertion by swallowing and do not resist when insertion is difficult.[8] Increased difficulty in directing the TEE probe also can be encountered due to the presence of a nasogastric tube. Coagulopathy and thrombocytopenia, common problems in critically ill patients, can increase the risk of hemorrhage due to mucosal injury during blind insertion of the TEE probe. Daniel and colleagues[9] reported significant complications related to TEE in 18 (0.18%)of 10,218 examinations. In 11 studies reporting on 943 patients undergoing TEE, the rate of complications was 1.7%.[5] Serious complications occurred in only two patients (0.2%). Colreavy and associates[8] studied the safety and utility of TEE performed by ICU physicians in 255 critically ill patients and showed that TEE was associated with a complication rate of only 1.6%. It is reasonable to conclude that TEE is associated with few complications given the high severity of illness among ICU patients.[5] Close monitoring of hemodynamic and oxygenation parameters is essential. Table 206-4 lists specific contraindications to the insertion of a TEE probe.

BEDSIDE ECHOCARDIOGRAPHY IN A CRITICALLY ILL PATIENT

Echocardiography can provide diagnostic information noninvasively regarding cardiac structure and mechanical function. The supplementary information provided by this technique can help determine the cause of hypotension refractory to inotropic support or vasopressor infusions.[3] It also can help in the diagnosis of a wide spectrum of other

TABLE 206–4. CONTRAINDICATIONS TO INSERTION OF TRANSESOPHAGEAL ECHOCARDIOGRAPHY PROBE

Absolute Contraindications

Esophageal pathologies
Stricture
Mass or tumor
Diverticulum
Mallory-Weiss tear
Dysphagia or odynophagia not previously evaluated
Cervical spine instability

Relative Contraindications

Esophageal varices
Recent esophageal or gastric surgery
Oropharyngeal carcinoma
Upper gastrointestinal bleeding
Severe cervical arthritis
Atlantoaxial disease

cardiovascular abnormalities and guide therapeutic management. An adequate understanding of the proper use of echocardiography is a prerequisite for the intensivist. General indications for performance of an echocardiographic examination in the ICU are listed in Table 206-1.

TRANSTHORACIC VERSUS TRANSESOPHAGEAL ECHOCARDIOGRAPHY IN A CRITICALLY ILL PATIENT

Accurate and prompt diagnosis is crucial in the ICU. The easiest and least invasive way to image cardiac structures is TTE.[3] This noninvasive imaging modality is of great value in the critical care setting because of its portability, widespread availability, and rapid diagnostic capability. In the ICU, TTE in certain cases may fail to provide adequate image quality because of different factors that potentially can hinder the quality of the ultrasound signal, as was described previously. The failure rate (partial or complete) of TTE in the ICU has been reported to be 30% to 40%.[10,11] Improvements have been made in transthoracic imaging (e.g., harmonics and contrast and digital technologies), however, resulting in a lower failure rate of TTE in the ICU (10% to 15% in our institution).

TEE is particularly useful for evaluation of suspected aortic dissection, prosthetic heart valves (especially in the mitral position), source of cardiac emboli, valvular vegetations, possible intracardiac shunts, and unexplained hypotension. TEE allows better visualization of the heart in general and especially the posterior structures, owing to the proximity of the probe and favorable acoustic transmission.[1] TEE also has limitations, however. For several areas of the heart and great vessels, TEE may provide limited images. The view of the left ventricular apex often is foreshortened with TEE, and an apical left ventricular clot can be missed. TTE usually is superior for visualization of the apex. Because of interposition of the left mainstem bronchus, the superior portion of the ascending aorta is another important area that may not be well visualized with TEE. With TEE, transducer position and angulation are constrained by the relative positions of the esophagus and heart. The relatively fixed relationship between the position of the probe and the heart often makes it impossible to align the Doppler beam parallel to the flow of interest (e.g., to evaluate the jet of blood resulting from aortic stenosis). In addition, standard anatomic measurements often are more difficult to obtain with TEE due to the two-dimensional image planes.

As a result of the significantly improved technical quality of TTE, most ICU patients can be studied satisfactorily with this modality. Immediate TEE is still preferable, however, in certain specific clinical situations in which TTE is likely to fail or be suboptimal.[11] The major indications for primary TEE in the ICU[12,13] are listed in Table 206-2. Even when TEE is necessary, data from the TTE examination are often essential for the final clinical interpretation.

HEMODYNAMIC EVALUATION

Ventricular Function

Left Ventricular Systolic Function

The evaluation of left ventricular performance by echocardiography is often paramount in the ICU. Accurate and timely assessment of systolic function should be an integral part of the medical management of hemodynamically unstable critically ill patients. *Global* assessment of left ventricular contractility includes the determination of ejection fraction, circumferential fiber shortening, and cardiac output.

The simplest quantitative approach is to measure the mid–left ventricular short-axis dimension at end diastole and end systole for determination of the percent *fractional*

shortening. Fractional shortening is related directly to ejection fraction; normal fractional shortening is 30% to 42%.[1]

$$\text{Fractional shortening} = \frac{\text{end-diastolic dimension} - \text{end-systolic dimension}}{\text{end-diastolic dimension}}$$

In the setting of regional wall motion abnormalities, fractional shortening may underestimate or overestimate global ventricular function and must be interpreted in light of what is seen in all of the two-dimensional imaging planes of the ventricle.[14]

Global systolic ventricular function also can be assessed quantitatively by *fractional area change* (normal value is 36% to 64%)[15] and ejection fraction (normal value is 55% to 75%) (Fig. 206-1):

$$\text{Fractional area change} = \frac{\text{end-diastolic area} - \text{end-systolic area}}{\text{end-diastolic area}}$$

$$\text{Ejection fraction} = \frac{\text{End-diastolic volume} - \text{end-systolic volume}}{\text{end-diastolic volume}}$$

These measurements require good image quality because endocardial border contours need to be traced (see Fig. 206-1).

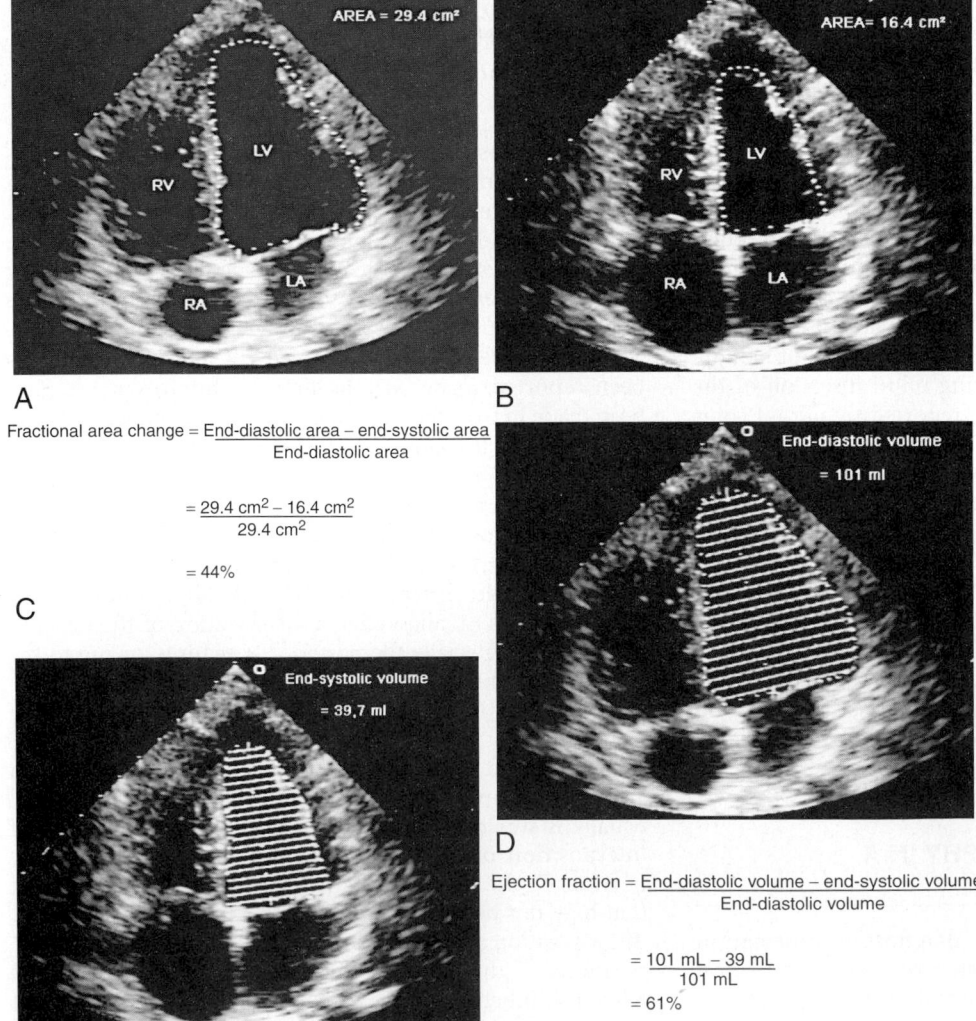

FIGURE 206–1. Fractional area change and ejection fraction calculation. Endocardial contour of the left ventricular cavity is traced at end diastole (A) and at end systole (B) in the transthoracic apical four-chamber view. Machine-integrated software computes the data and gives corresponding end-diastolic and end-systolic areas. Fractional area change can be calculated with these data (C). Normal values are 36% to 64%.[15] Corresponding end-diastolic (D) and end-systolic (E) volumes are computed using the modified Simpson's method. The data are used to calculate the ejection fraction (F). Normal values are 55% to 75%. LA, left atrium; LV, left ventricle; RA, right atrial; RV, right ventricle.

A — End-diastole, AREA = 29.4 cm²

B — End-systole, AREA = 16.4 cm²

$$\text{Fractional area change} = \frac{\text{End-diastolic area} - \text{end-systolic area}}{\text{End-diastolic area}}$$

$$= \frac{29.4 \text{ cm}^2 - 16.4 \text{ cm}^2}{29.4 \text{ cm}^2}$$

$$= 44\%$$

C

D — End-diastolic volume = 101 ml

E — End-systolic volume = 39.7 ml

$$\text{Ejection fraction} = \frac{\text{End-diastolic volume} - \text{end-systolic volume}}{\text{End-diastolic volume}}$$

$$= \frac{101 \text{ mL} - 39 \text{ mL}}{101 \text{ mL}}$$

$$= 61\%$$

F

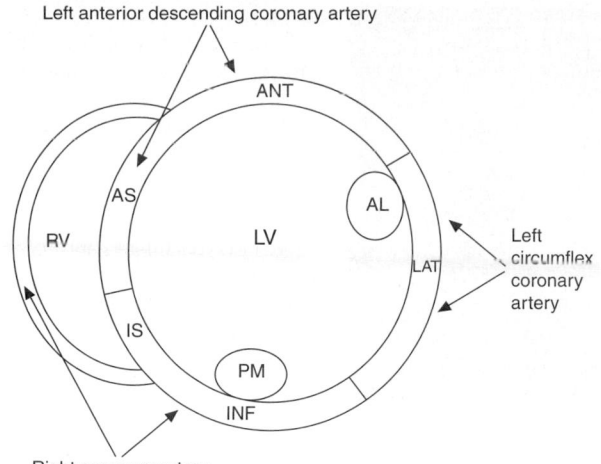

FIGURE 206–2. Transthoracic short-axis echocardiographic view of the left (LV) and right (RV) ventricles at the midpapillary muscle level. In this tomographic view of the heart, areas of myocardium and papillary muscles (AL, anterolateral; PM, posteromedial) supplied by all three major coronary arteries are represented. ANT, anterior; AS, anteroseptal; INF, inferior; IS, inferoseptal; LAT, lateral.

Machine-integrated software computes the data and provides volumes, areas, and the resultant ejection fraction (see Fig. 206-1). In patients with regional wall motion abnormalities, more precise measures of stroke volume can be made by approximating ventricular volumes as a stack of elliptical discs on biplane imaging (*modified Simpson's method*).[1,15]

In the critical care setting, endocardial border definition may be suboptimal because of poor image quality.[10,16,17] In these cases, global ventricular function often is assessed *qualitatively* by visual inspection alone. This method has been found to be reliable when used by experienced clinicians.[18] By simple visualization of the kinetics and size of the cardiac cavities in real time, an experienced intensivist with a sufficient echocardiographic background can establish a functional diagnosis immediately.

Analysis of *regional wall motion* includes a numerical scoring system to describe the movement of the different regions of the left and right ventricle (1 = normokinesia;

2 = hypokinesia; 3 = akinesia; 4 = dyskinesia; 5 = aneurysmal change).[15] Visualized from the short-axis view of the left ventricle, a complete overview of myocardial areas perfused by the three major coronary arteries can be obtained (Fig. 206-2). If the TTE examination is technically difficult and the endocardium is poorly visualized, harmonic imaging and possibly contrast, if needed, can improve endocardial border visualization dramatically and subsequent evaluation of global systolic function (as discussed further later in this chapter). For the remaining few technically challenging cases with suboptimal TTE, performance of TEE allows for a more precise evaluation of ventricular function in most critically ill patients because of the higher image quality that can be obtained with this echographic modality.

Left Ventricular Failure in the Intensive Care Unit

In a critically ill patient with unexplained hemodynamic instability, determination of cardiac function is an integral part of the medical management. Echocardiography is valuable in this setting because the clinical examination and invasive hemodynamic monitoring often fail to provide an adequate assessment of ventricular function. In a study by Fontes and coworkers[19] that compared pulmonary artery (Swan-Ganz) catheterization and TEE, the overall predictive probability for conventional clinical and hemodynamic assessment of normal ventricular function was 98%, whereas for abnormal ventricular function (ejection fraction <40%), it was 0%. Several other studies have reported similar results.[20-22] Assessment of biventricular function is one of the most important indications for performance of echocardiography in the ICU. In a study by Bruch and associates,[23] 115 critically ill patients were studied by TEE. The most common indication for TEE was hemodynamic instability (67% of patients). Of these hemodynamically unstable patients, 20 (26%) were found to have significant left ventricular dysfunction (ejection fraction <30%). In a study by McLean[24] of the use of TEE in the ICU, the most common reason to request a TEE was assessment of left ventricular function. In most patients, left ventricular function was assessed adequately by TTE before TEE. In a study by Vignon and colleagues,[17] TTE allowed adequate evaluation of global left ventricular function in 77% of mechanically ventilated ICU patients. Although TEE was

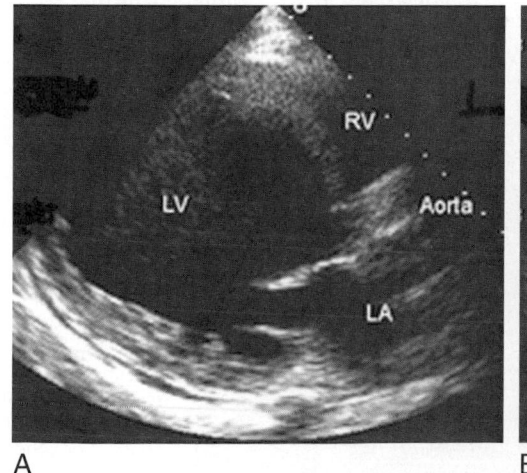

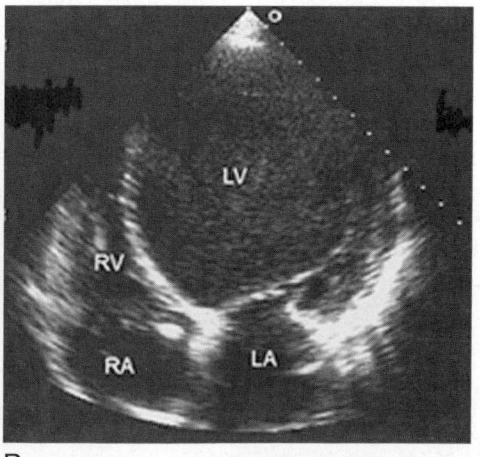

FIGURE 206–3. Dilated cardiomyopathy. Transthoracic examination of a severely dilated left ventricle (LV) in the parasternal long-axis *(A)* and apical four-chamber *(B)* views. The 65-year-old patient presented with flash pulmonary edema and later was found to have severe diffuse coronary artery disease. LA, left atrium; RA, right atrium; RV, right ventricle.

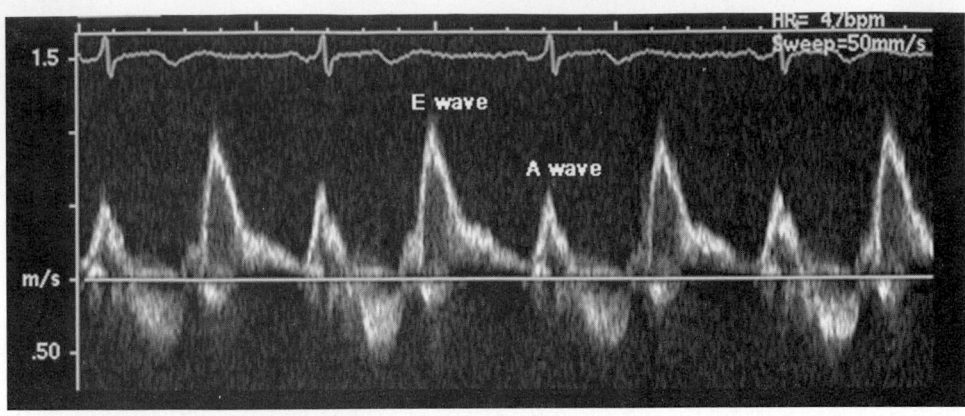

FIGURE 206–4. Normal mitral inflow profile as measured by transthoracic pulsed wave Doppler at the tips of the mitral leaflets. It is characterized by an early filling phase (E wave) followed by atrial systole (A wave), which results in additional filling. These filling parameters are related to intrinsic diastolic myocardial properties and can be influenced by many different factors (see text).

needed for most other indications, TTE was shown to be an excellent diagnostic tool for assessment of left ventricular function in the ICU (Fig. 206-3), even when positive end-expiratory pressure is present.

Several important points should be emphasized: (1) Significant left ventricular dysfunction is common in critically ill patients; (2) ventricular function should be assessed in all patients with unexplained hemodynamic instability because this information is particularly important for guiding resuscitation and informing decisions regarding subsequent medical or surgical management; (3) it is now possible to obtain adequate information about ventricular function in most ICU patients using TTE, but TEE provides better accuracy in patients with suboptimal imaging by TTE.

Sepsis-Related Cardiomyopathy

Classically, septic shock has been considered a "hyperdynamic" state characterized by normal or high cardiac output. Echocardiographic studies indicate that ventricular performance often is markedly impaired in patients with sepsis.[25,26,27] Parker and associates[28] were the first to describe left ventricular hypokinesis in septic shock. They reported that survivors manifested severely depressed left ventricular ejection fraction, but that adequate left ventricular stroke output was maintained as a result of acute left ventricular dilation.[29] Jardin and coworkers[25] studied 90 patients with septic shock and performed daily bedside assessments of left ventricular volume and left ventricular ejection fraction using TTE. They observed that left ventricular ejection fraction was significantly depressed in all patients, resulting in severe reductions in left ventricular stroke volume. Of these patients, 34 (38%) eventually were weaned from hemodynamic support and showed gradual improvement in left ventricular ejection fraction and ultimately recovered.

The remaining 56 patients (62%) eventually died (of early circulatory failure or late multiple organ failure). In this subset, the degree of left ventricular dysfunction was less than in survivors, but failed to improve over time. The severity of left ventricular dysfunction does not predict outcome. A paradoxical relationship between the degree of left ventricular dysfunction and the likelihood of recovery also has been described by others.[25,28,30,31] Among patients who survive, left ventricular dilation and systolic dysfunction usually are reversible.

Left ventricular ejection fraction might not be a reliable index of left ventricular systolic function in patients with early septic shock because this is a state characterized by low systemic vascular resistance that unloads the left ventricle.[25] Normal or supranormal ejection fraction in early sepsis might lead clinicians to make the wrong inference about cardiac reserve because left ventricular ejection fraction might decrease if afterload is increased by the administration of vasopressor agents.

Left Ventricular Diastolic Function

In the ICU, diastolic dysfunction should be suspected when ventricular filling pressure (pulmonary capillary wedge pressure) is elevated and ejection fraction is normal or supranormal.[1] The diastolic properties of the ventricle often are assessed by evaluating Doppler echocardiographic mitral inflow and pulmonary venous flow patterns. Mitral inflow, as measured by pulsed wave Doppler at the tips of the mitral leaflets, is characterized by an early filling phase (E wave) followed by atrial systole, resulting in additional filling (A wave) (Fig. 206-4). The transmitral Doppler pattern always should be interpreted in conjunction with pulsed wave Doppler of the pulmonary venous flow, which is characterized by a systolic phase (S), a diastolic phase (D), and an

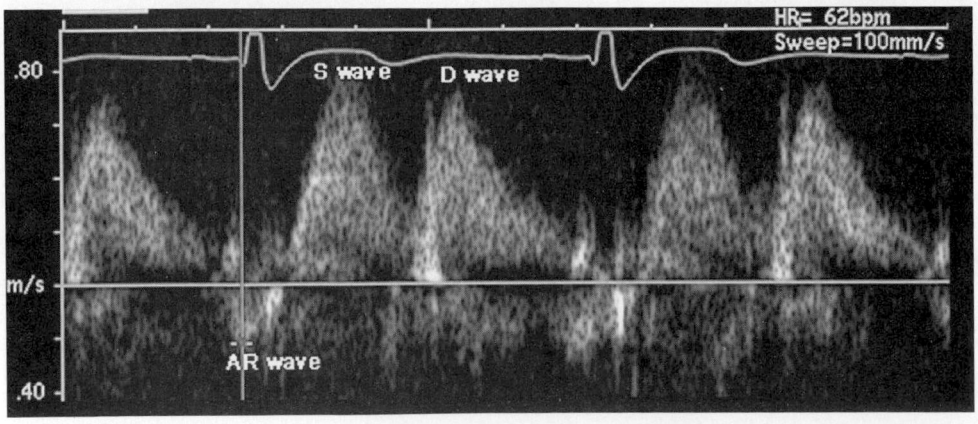

FIGURE 206–5. Normal pulmonary venous flow profile as measured by transthoracic pulsed wave Doppler with the sample volume placed in the right superior pulmonary vein. It is characterized by a predominant systolic wave (S), a diastolic wave (D), and an atrial wave (AR) (from reversal of flow into the pulmonary veins occurring during atrial contraction). The pulmonary venous flow profile always should be interpreted in conjunction with the transmitral Doppler pattern to have a more complete assessment of diastolic function.

atrial phase (AR) from reversal of flow into the pulmonary veins during atrial contraction (Fig. 206-5). These filling patterns are related to the intrinsic diastolic properties of the myocardium and are influenced by many different factors, particularly left atrial pressure, heart rate, ischemia, ventricular hypertrophy, and valvular pathologies. Only modest correlation has been found between Doppler indices of diastolic function and parameters measured using more invasive means.[32,33] Integrated interpretation of mitral and pulmonary venous flow patterns may be useful for diagnosing abnormal myocardial relaxation (e.g., owing to hypertensive heart disease, hypertrophic cardiomyopathy, or coronary ischemia) or restrictive pathology (e.g., owing to cardiomyopathy, constrictive pericarditis, coronary artery disease, cardiac transplantation, or dilated cardiomyopathy). Nevertheless, these findings must be interpreted with caution when caring for critically ill patients, given the many different factors that can acutely influence flow patterns in this population of patients.

Right Ventricular Function and Ventricular Interaction

Abnormal right ventricular function often plays an important and sometimes underestimated role in the pathogenesis of critical illness.[34-36] Based on an echocardiographic definition,[37] massive pulmonary embolism and acute respiratory distress syndrome are the two main causes of acute cor pulmonale in adults.[38] In the critical care setting, right ventricular function also can be altered by any other perturbations that increase right ventricular afterload, such as positive end-expiratory pressure or increased pulmonary vascular resistance (from vascular, cardiac, metabolic, or pulmonary causes). Depressed right ventricular systolic function also often is associated with right ventricular infarction, most commonly in the setting of inferior myocardial infarction. Acute sickle-cell crisis, air or fat embolism, myocardial contusion, and sepsis are other causes of acute right ventricular dysfunction.

Adequate assessment of right ventricular function is important when caring for hemodynamically unstable critically ill patients, specifically patients with massive pulmonary embolism and acute respiratory distress syndrome, because the diagnosis of concomitant significant right ventricular dysfunction may alter therapy (e.g., fluid loading, use of vasopressors, use of thrombolytics) and provide information about prognosis.[38,39] Echocardiographic examination of the right ventricle requires primarily an assessment of the *size* and *kinetics* of the cavity and septum.[37,40] Normally the right ventricle appears relatively flat. As it dilates, the apical region of the right ventricle becomes more rounded (Fig. 206-6). In the short-axis view, the right ventricle, which usually has a crescentic shape, becomes oval because of septal displacement and bulging of the right ventricular free wall (see Fig. 206-6).[1] Right ventricular size and function generally are evaluated by visual comparison with the left ventricle. Right ventricular diastolic dimensions can be obtained by measuring right ventricular end-diastolic area in the long axis, from an apical four-chamber view, using either TTE or TEE.

Because pericardial constraint necessarily results in left ventricular restriction when the right ventricle acutely dilates (i.e., there is ventricular interaction), one of the best ways to quantify right ventricular dilation is to measure the *ratio* between the right ventricular and left ventricular end-diastolic areas, an approach that cancels out individual variations in cardiac size.[37,40] Moderate right ventricular dilation corresponds to a diastolic ventricular ratio greater than 0.6; severe right ventricular dilation corresponds to a ratio greater than or equal to 1.[37,40] Right ventricular diastolic enlargement usually is associated with right atrial dilation, inferior vena caval dilation, and tricuspid regurgitation. When pressure in the right atrium exceeds pressure in the left atrium, the foramen ovale may open. Pressure and volume overload of the right ventricle can lead to distortion of left ventricular geometry and abnormal motion of the interventricular septum. With conditions of high strain imposed on the right ventricle (volume or pressure overload or both), the interventricular septum flattens, and the left ventricle appears to have a "D" shape (see Fig. 206-6).[4,37] This "paradoxical" septum motion also is seen at the interatrial level.

Because the two ventricles are enclosed within the relatively stiff pericardium, the sum of the diastolic ventricular dimensions has to remain constant.[41] Acute right ventricular or left ventricular dilation can occur only if it is associated with an acute and proportional reduction in left ventricular or right ventricular diastolic dimension (i.e., ventricular interaction). With acute right ventricular dilation, septal displacement impairs left ventricular relaxation; the opposite occurs with acute left ventricular dilation. In these situations, the pressure-volume relationships of the left and right heart chambers are altered, and information obtained from a pulmonary artery catheter could be misleading (e.g., high filling pressures are recorded despite normal or even low circulating volume).

Pulmonary Embolism

Hemodynamic instability from acute cor pulmonale as a consequence of massive pulmonary embolism is a relatively common occurrence in critically ill patients. Until more recently, contrast pulmonary angiography generally was regarded as the gold standard for the diagnosis of pulmonary embolism. Angiography is an invasive procedure, however, and carries the risk of major complications in patients with circulatory failure.[42] Contrast-enhanced helical computed tomography (CT) is an accurate and noninvasive test that has replaced angiography for the diagnosis of pulmonary embolism. Even CT requires transportation of patients to a location outside of the ICU, however, and transport alone is associated with significant risks. Echocardiography is well suited for diagnosis of pulmonary embolism because it can be done within minutes at the bedside. The diagnosis of acute cor pulmonale at the bedside with TTE has good positive predictive value for massive pulmonary embolism.[43,44] This technique can detect acute right ventricular dilation and dysfunction resulting from a large pulmonary embolism. The finding of right ventricular dilation and dysfunction is not specific, however, for pulmonary embolism because these findings may be observed with a variety of other conditions associated with increased right ventricular strain. In a study by McConnell and associates,[45] patients with acute pulmonary embolism were found to have a distinct *regional* pattern of right ventricular dysfunction with akinesia of the mid-free wall but normal motion at the apex by TTE. These findings contrasted with findings obtained in patients with primary pulmonary hypertension, who had abnormal wall motion in *all* regions. Regional right ventricular dysfunction had a sensitivity of 77% and a specificity of 94% for the diagnosis of acute pulmonary embolism; positive predictive value was 71%, and negative predictive value was 96%. The presence of

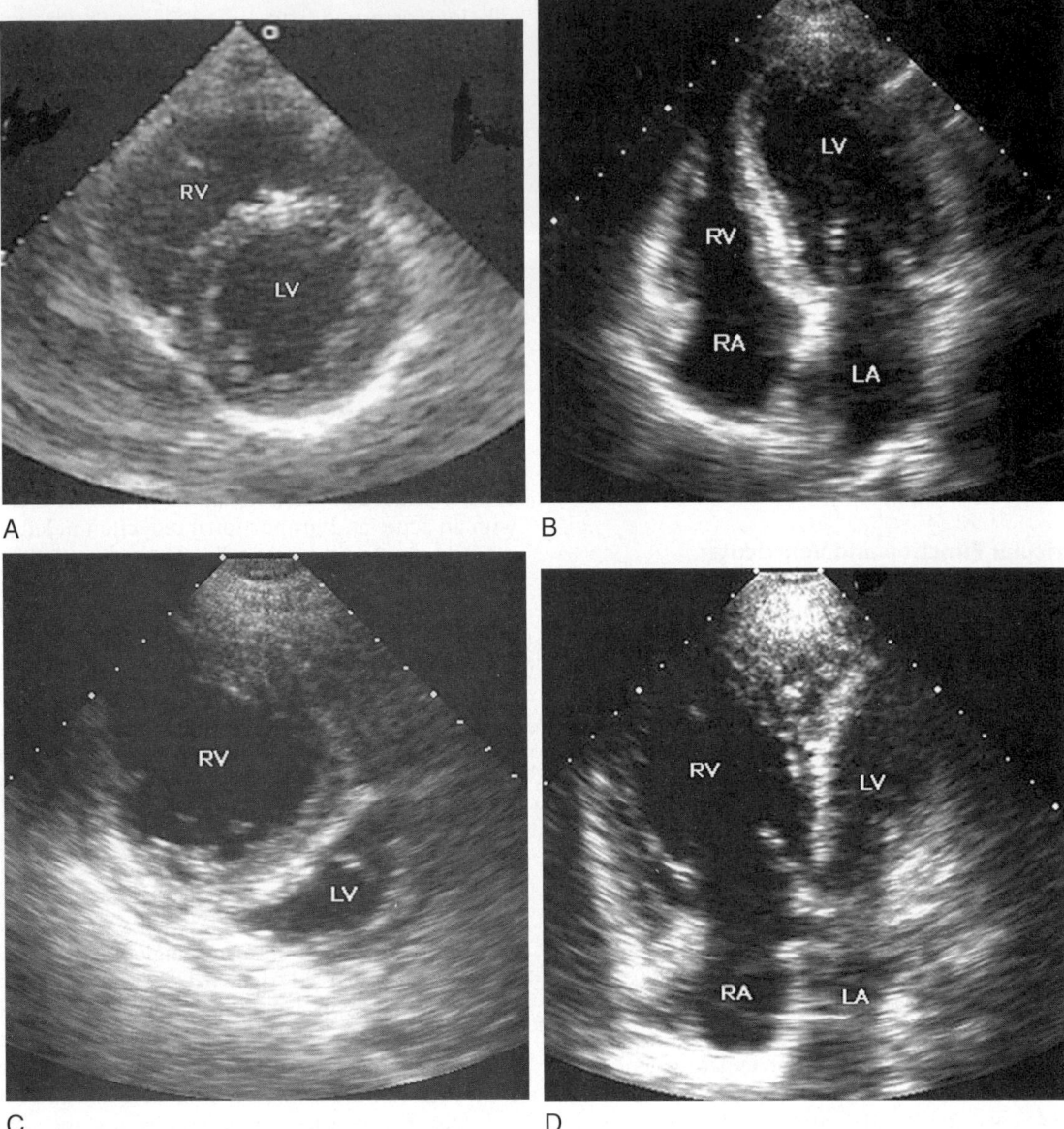

FIGURE 206–6. Severe right ventricular failure and dilation. *A*, Normal transthoracic parasternal short-axis view of the left (LV) and right (RV) ventricles at the midpapillary muscle level. *B*, Normal transthoracic apical four-chamber view of the left ventricle and right ventricle. These pictures of a normal heart depict the relationship between the left ventricle and right ventricle, with the left ventricle being normally larger than the right ventricle and the interventricular septum bulging slightly toward the right ventricle. *C*, Transthoracic parasternal short-axis view of the left ventricle and right ventricle in a patient with severe right ventricular failure and dilation. The right ventricular cavity is seen to be much larger than the left ventricular cavity. Because of the high volume and pressure in the right ventricle, the interventricular septum is bulging toward the left. This gives the left ventricle a characteristic "D" appearance. *D*, Transthoracic apical four-chamber view of the same patient shows the inverse relationship between the left ventricular and right ventricular sizes. The right ventricular dilation can occur only if associated with a proportional reduction in left ventricular diastolic dimension ("ventricular interaction"). This reduction in left ventricular diastolic dimension significantly impairs left ventricular relaxation and changes the pressure-volume relationship of the left heart chambers. LA, left atrium; RA, right atrium.

regional right ventricular dysfunction that spares the apex should raise the level of clinical suspicion for the diagnosis of acute pulmonary embolism.

Central pulmonary emboli are present in half of patients with symptoms of pulmonary embolism and acute cor pulmonale on TTE.[5] Emboli lodged in the proximal pulmonary arteries usually cannot be visualized using TTE.[5] Because other clinical conditions can produce acute cor pulmonale in the ICU, better visualization of the pulmonary arteries is needed to achieve high accuracy for the diagnosis of pulmonary embolism. This goal can be achieved by using TEE.

TEE has a good sensitivity for detecting emboli that are lodged in the main and right pulmonary arteries but is limited for the detection of more distal or left pulmonary emboli.[5,46,47] If an embolus is visualized, the diagnosis is made. If the study is negative when the index of suspicion for pulmonary embolism is high, however, TEE must be followed up by a more definitive test, such as angiography or helical CT. Also, when there is high clinical suspicion for pulmonary embolism but no emboli are visualized using TEE, the potential for nonthrombotic causes of pulmonary embolism, such as air or fat emboli, must be kept in mind.

The demonstration of acute cor pulmonale with echocardiography has important prognostic and therapeutic implications.[48,49] The presence of cor pulmonale with massive pulmonary embolism is associated with increased mortality, whereas the absence of right ventricular dysfunction is associated with a better prognosis.[39] There is no consensus on the precise indications for administration of thrombolytics in massive pulmonary embolism complicated by acute cor pulmonale.[50,51] A safe and reasonable strategy for managing critically ill patients with suspected massive pulmonary embolism is as follows:

1. Initially perform bedside TTE, looking for the presence of regional right ventricular dysfunction as described earlier. If the TTE examination is suboptimal, TEE should be performed.
2. If echocardiography is inconclusive or negative and the clinical suspicion of a pulmonary embolism remains high, a definitive confirmatory radiologic test (preferably helical CT) should be performed.

Assessment of Cardiac Output

Measurement of cardiac output remains a cornerstone in the hemodynamic assessment of critically ill patients. Thermodilution is considered the gold standard approach for determining cardiac output in most ICUs. Measurement of cardiac output using thermodilution requires placement of a pulmonary artery catheter (or at least central venous and arterial catheters) and, although a useful technique, is invasive and potentially inaccurate. Unreliable values are particularly common in the presence of triscuspid regurgitation related to high pulmonary artery pressure. Several methods for determining cardiac output have been described using two-dimensional and Doppler echocardiography. With this technique, stroke volume and cardiac output can be determined directly by combining Doppler-derived measurements of instantaneous blood flow velocity through a conduit with the cross-sectional area of the conduit. Blood flow can be calculated through various cardiac structures, including the pulmonary valve,[52] the mitral valve,[53,54] and the aortic valve.[55-58] In the absence of intracardiac shunts, blood flow through these structures should be the same (continuity equation).[59] Of these methods, the one using the left ventricular outflow tract and aortic valve as the conduit is probably the most reliable and most commonly used. There is excellent agreement with thermodilution in most situations.[55-58] The left ventricular stroke volume is obtained by measuring the cross-sectional area of the left ventricular outflow tract (area [cm^2] = (left ventricular outflow tract diameter [cm^2]) $\times$ ($\pi/4$), assuming that just below the aortic annulus, the left ventricular outflow tract is circular) multiplied by the transaortic flow velocity time integral derived from a spectral Doppler tracing. The stroke volume obtained is multiplied by the heart rate to give the cardiac output: cardiac output = cross-sectional area $\times$ velocity time integral $\times$ heart rate (Fig. 206-7).

With TTE, the left ventricular outflow tract diameter usually is obtained from the parasternal long-axis view, just below the insertion of the aortic valve leaflets. The Doppler interrogation is performed through the aortic valve from the apical view (see Fig. 206-7). With TEE, the left ventricular outflow tract diameter usually is obtained from the five-chamber view of the left ventricle. The transgastric view usually is used to obtain an apical long-axis view of the aortic valve through which Doppler interrogation is performed.[60]

With either TTE or TEE, obtaining an accurate left ventricular outflow tract diameter and Doppler signal is essential to have an accurate cardiac output calculation. Because the measure of the left ventricular outflow tract diameter has a second-order relationship with the cross-sectional area (see previous formula), it is crucial that this measure be determined precisely. For the Doppler signal to be reliable, the Doppler sample must be parallel to the transaortic flow with an angle of incidence not exceeding 20 degrees to avoid underestimation of transaortic velocity. Using TTE, McLean and coworkers[61] showed an excellent correlation ($r = 0.94$) between cardiac output determined by the left ventricular outflow tract Doppler method and the thermodilution method in critically ill patients. Other studies have shown similar results.[55] In a study by Feinberg and colleagues,[58] cardiac output determined by TEE Doppler imaging was obtainable in 88% of 33 critically ill patients, and there was good correlation ($r = 0.91$) with the thermodilution method. Descorps-Declere and associates[60] also showed transgastric pulsed Doppler measurement across the left ventricular outflow tract with TEE to be a clinically acceptable method for cardiac output measurement in critically ill patients ($r = 0.975$ compared with the thermodilution method).

Another promising ultrasound-based technology to estimate cardiac output noninvasively in adults uses a small transesophageal Doppler probe to measure blood flow velocity waveforms in the descending aorta combined with a nomogram (based on height, weight, and age) for estimation of aortic cross-sectional area. This minimally invasive esophageal probe can be inserted easily in sedated patients and left in place safely for several days to provide continuous monitoring of cardiac function.[62,63] Several technical problems can limit the accuracy of cardiac output measurements by esophageal Doppler monitoring,[62] however, and although initial results are promising,[64-66] more studies are needed to make a decision regarding the accuracy of this technique in critically ill patients.

Assessment of Filling Pressures and Volume Status

Adequate determination of preload and volume status is important for proper management of critically ill patients. Invasive pressure measurements to assess left ventricular filling are commonly used at the bedside to make inferences regarding left ventricular preload. These pressure measurements correlate only weakly with left ventricular volume, however.[67] Data from invasive monitoring using pulmonary artery catheterization may be misleading because ventricular compliance is altered secondary to numerous factors.[68,69] Differences in diastolic compliance among patients may account for the weak correlation between pressure and volume and may limit the ability to use pressure measurements alone to derive information concerning left ventricular preload.[14] Echocardiography can be helpful for adequately assessing preload. Parameters that can be measured using two-dimensional imaging are left ventricular end-diastolic volume and left ventricular end-diastolic area. Using Doppler interrogation, additional information—mainly transmitral diastolic filling pattern and pulmonary venous flow—can be obtained.

Two-Dimensional Imaging

Echocardiography has been validated for left ventricular volume measurements.[15] Subjective assessment of left ventricular volume by estimating the size of the left ventricular

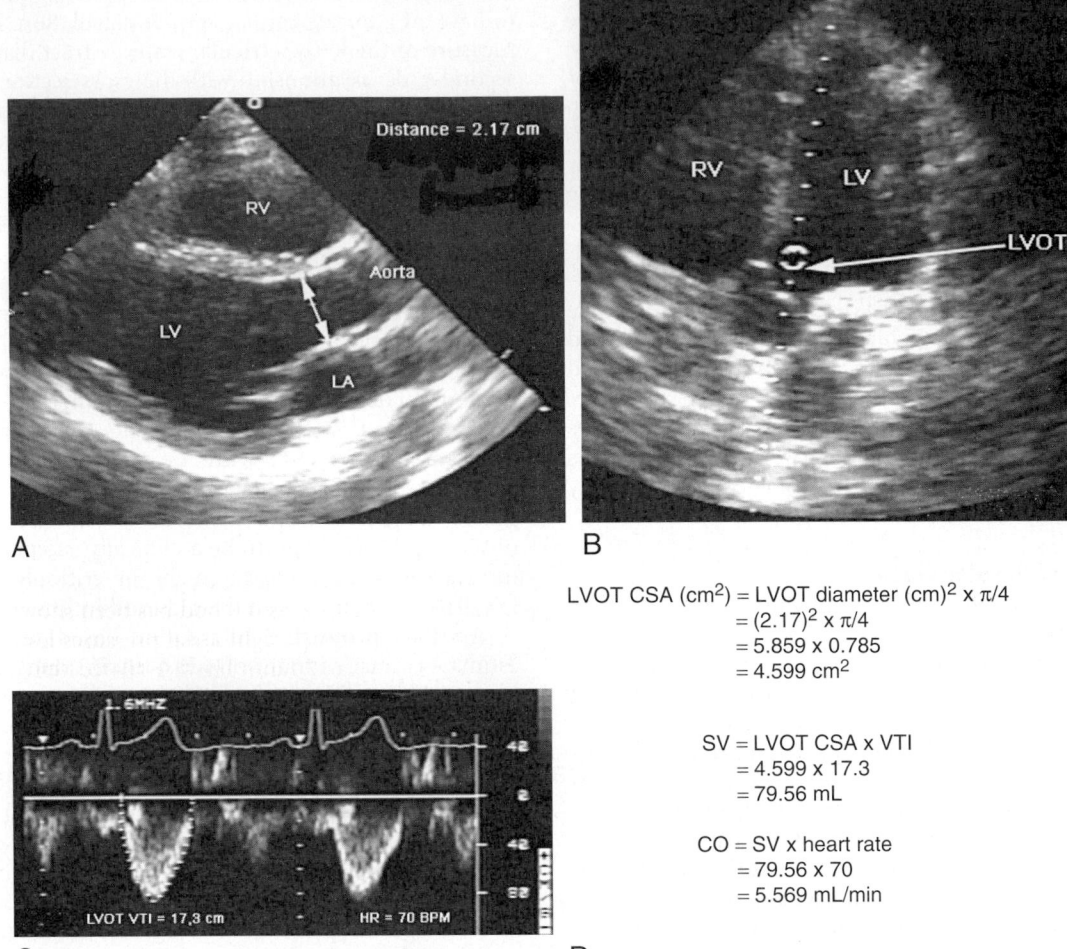

LVOT CSA (cm^2) = LVOT diameter (cm)^2 x π/4
= (2.17)^2 x π/4
= 5.859 x 0.785
= 4.599 cm^2

SV = LVOT CSA x VTI
= 4.599 x 17.3
= 79.56 mL

CO = SV x heart rate
= 79.56 x 70
= 5.569 mL/min

FIGURE 206–7. Calculation of the stroke volume and cardiac output from the left ventricular outflow tract (LVOT). *A,* Left ventricular outflow tract diameter obtained from the transthoracic parasternal long-axis view, just below the insertion of the aortic valve leaflets. In this example, the left ventricular outflow tract diameter is 2.17 cm. *B,* Doppler interrogation (with pulsed wave Doppler) is performed from the apical view with the sample volume being placed in the left ventricular outflow tract, just below the aortic valve. *C,* Spectral Doppler tracing from the left ventricular outflow tract from which the transaortic flow velocity time integral (VTI) is derived. In this example, the VTI is 17.3 cm. *D,* The left ventricular stroke volume (SV) is obtained by measuring the cross-sectional area (CSA) of the left ventricular outflow tract (area [cm^2] = left ventricular outflow tract diameter [cm^2] × π/4) and multiplying by the transaortic VTI derived from the spectral Doppler tracing. The stroke volume obtained is multiplied by the heart rate to give the cardiac output (CO). LA, left atrium; LV, left ventricle; RV, right ventricle.

cavity in the short-axis and long-axis views is often adequate to guide fluid volume therapy at the extreme ends of cardiac filling and function. More precise, quantitative values are desirable, however, and can be obtained by using endocardial border tracing (as described earlier). The normal left ventricular end-diastolic volume as determined by echocardiography is 80 to 130 mL,[15] and the normal left ventricular end-diastolic volume index is 55 to 65 mL/M^2.[15] Left ventricular end-diastolic area measured in the left parasternal short-axis view at the level of the midpapillary muscle is commonly used to estimate volume status (Fig. 206-8). The normal values for left ventricular end-diastolic area in the short-axis view are 9.5 to 22 cm^2.[15]

Two-dimensional TTE evaluation of ventricular dimensions has been found to be useful in assessing preload and optimizing therapy of ICU patients.[25,70] Nevertheless, image quality may be suboptimal and preclude adequate visualization of the endocardial border by TTE. This potential limitation of TTE has been partly circumvented in recent years with the advent of harmonic imaging and contrast echocardiography (see later). In cases in which endocardial border visualization remains suboptimal, TEE is the modality of choice. With TEE, left ventricular volume can be estimated rapidly by subjective assessment of the left ventricular size. Quantitatively, it is estimated most often by determining left ventricular cross-sectional area at the end of diastole, most commonly using the transgastric short-axis view at the level of the midpapillary muscle. This section is used because of the reproducibility of the view and because changes in left ventricular volume affect the short axis of the ventricle to a greater degree than the long axis.[14] The end-diastolic area must be measured consistently from the same reference section. End-diastolic area measured with TEE correlates with left ventricular volume determined by radionuclide studies.[70]

Systolic obliteration of left ventricular cross-sectional area accompanies decreased end-diastolic area and is considered to be a sign of severe hypovolemia (Fig. 206-9). Although a small end-diastolic area generally indicates

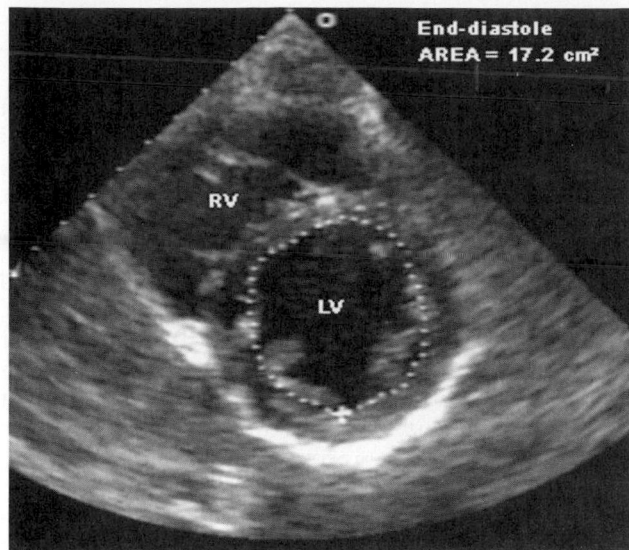

FIGURE 206–8. Calculation of left ventricular end-diastolic area in the transthoracic short-axis view at the level of the midpapillary muscle by endocardial contour tracing. Values of normal left ventricular end-diastolic area in the short axis range from 9.5 to 22 cm².[15] The level of the midpapillary muscle is used because of the reproducibility of the view and because changes in left ventricular volume affect the short axis of the ventricle to a greater degree than the long axis. LV, left ventricle; RV, right ventricle.

hypovolemia, a large end-diastolic area does not indicate adequate preload in patients with left ventricular dysfunction. Also, when systemic vascular resistance is low, as in early sepsis, left ventricular emptying is improved because of the lowered afterload. In these situations, it may be difficult to differentiate hypovolemia from low systemic vascular resistance by echocardiography alone because both conditions are associated with decreased end-diastolic area.

Knowledge of left ventricular end-diastolic volume or absolute preload does not allow for accurate prediction of the hemodynamic response to alterations in preload.[71] Tousignant and associates[72] investigated the relationship between left ventricular stroke volume and left ventricular end-diastolic area in a cohort of ICU patients and found only a modest correlation ($r = 0.60$) between single-point estimates of left ventricular end-diastolic area and responses to fluid loading. Based on the assumption that changes in end-diastolic area occur because of changes in left ventricular volume, the determination of this area and its subsequent degree of variation after a fluid challenge could help better assess *preload responsiveness*. Studies have shown that changes in end-diastolic area measured by TEE using endocardial border tracing are closely related to changes in cardiac output and are superior to measurements of pulmonary artery occlusion pressure for predicting the ventricular preload associated with maximal cardiac output.[73]

Circulating volume status also can be assessed by two-dimensional echocardiography by indirectly estimating right atrial pressure; this is often done by assessing the diameter and change in caliber with inspiration of the inferior vena cava (Fig. 206-10). This method has been shown to discriminate reliably between right atrial pressures less than 10 mm Hg or greater than 10 mm Hg.[74] A dilated vena cava (diameter >20 mm) without a normal inspiratory decrease in caliber (>50% with gentle sniffing) usually indicates elevated right atrial pressure. In mechanically ventilated patients, this measure is less specific because of a high prevalence of inferior vena cava dilation.[75,76] A small vena cava reliably excludes the presence of elevated right atrial pressure in these patients.[75,76]

Doppler Flow Patterns

Information obtained by analysis of the Doppler signal at the level of the mitral valve and pulmonary vein offers additional information about preload.[77,78] These Doppler

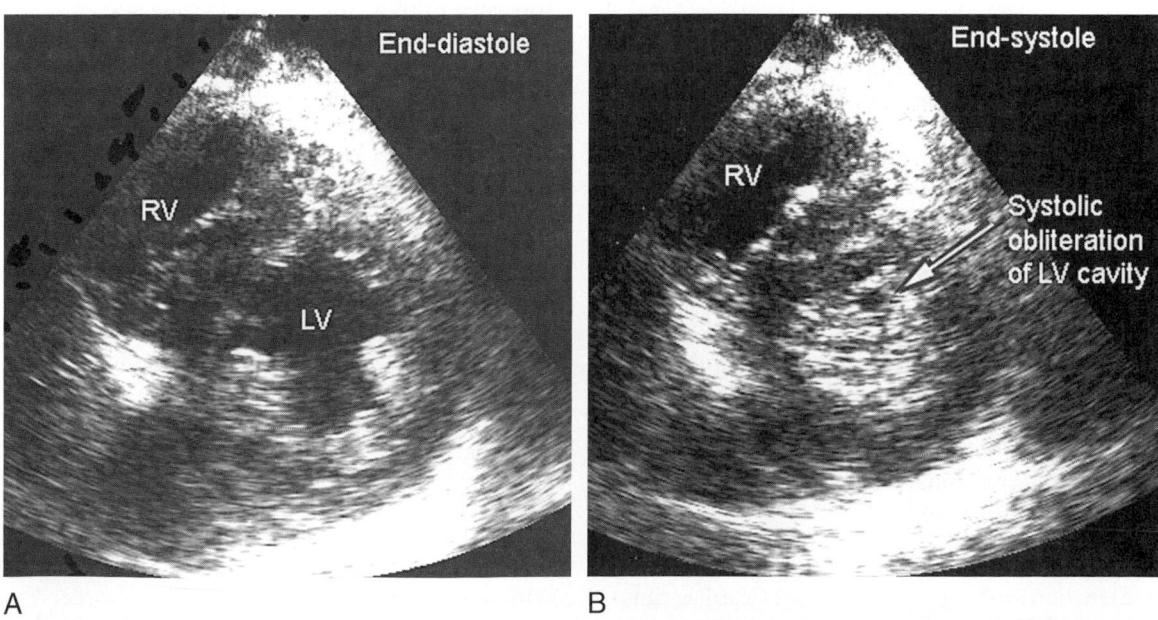

A B

FIGURE 206–9. Systolic obliteration of the left ventricle (LV) in a patient with severe left ventricular hypertrophy and dehydration. This transthoracic parasternal short-axis view shows the left ventricle at end diastole *(A)* and at end systole *(B)*. Nearly complete obliteration of the left ventricular cavity is seen at end systole. Systolic obliteration of the cross-sectional area accompanies decreased end-diastolic area and is considered to be a sign of severe hypovolemia. In this case, the patient presented with hypotension and was found to be severely dehydrated because of a viral gastroenteritis. RV, right ventricle.

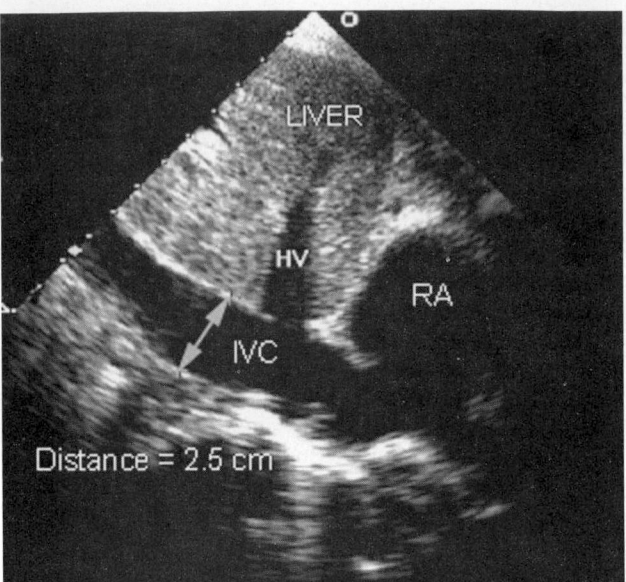

FIGURE 206–10. Indirect assessment of circulating volume status on two-dimensional echocardiography by assessing the diameter and change in caliber with inspiration of the inferior vena cava (IVC). This method has been shown to discriminate reliably between right atrial pressures of less than or greater than 10 mm Hg. A dilated vena cava (>20 mm) without the normal inspiratory decrease in caliber (>50% on gentle sniffing) usually indicates elevated right atrial pressure. A small vena cava reliably excludes elevated right atrial pressure in these patients. In this case, the IVC was dilated at 2.5 cm with minimal respiratory variation in a patient spontaneously breathing. The right atrial pressure was estimated to be approximately 10 to 15 mm Hg. Images were obtained in the subcostal view. HV, hepatic veins; RA, right atrium.

profiles can be obtained by either TTE or TEE. Transmitral parameters that have been studied include the relation of early to late transmitral diastolic filling (E/A ratio), isovolumetric relaxation time, and the rate of deceleration of early diastolic inflow (deceleration time).[1]

A decrease in preload causes a significant reduction in the E wave (early filling flow wave) velocity at the mitral level in conjunction with a decrease of the S wave (systolic flow wave) in the pulmonary vein. In clinical practice, the E/A ratio is easy to assess; the normal value of this ratio is approximately 1.[1,3] In conjunction with normal left ventricular contractility, a low E/A ratio is usually a characteristic sign of inadequate preload.[79]

Pulmonary venous flow also can be used to assess left atrial pressure. A normal pulmonary venous flow pattern, showing a predominance of flow during systole (S phase) compared with early diastole (D phase), usually indicates that left atrial pressure is less than 8 mm Hg, whereas the opposite predominance of flow (in the absence of significant mitral regurgitation) usually indicates elevation of left atrial pressure.[1]

Transmitral and pulmonary vein Doppler patterns strongly depend on intrinsic and external factors and are not affected purely by the loading conditions of the left ventricle. It is crucial that interpretation of Doppler parameters be done in conjunction with a global analysis of cardiac function and other available hemodynamic or anatomic variables.

Hypovolemia in the Intensive Care Unit

Precise and rapid assessment of volume status is crucial when caring for hemodynamically unstable ICU patients.

Hypovolemia is one of the most common causes of hypotension in the ICU. As was discussed in detail earlier, bedside echocardiography offers a quick and reliable way of estimating volume status by evaluating cardiac dynamics and left ventricular dimensions and area. In general, TTE has good sensitivity for diagnosing the presence of a small, hyperdynamic left ventricle, the most typical finding in hypovolemic patients with underlying normal cardiac function.

When dynamic left ventricular obstruction is present, cardiac output is low, and even in the presence of marked hypovolemia, pulmonary artery occlusion pressure is high. Paradoxical worsening of hypotension after intravascular volume loading may be the first clue to dynamic left ventricular obstruction in critically ill patients. It is important that this entity be recognized early and that the pathophysiologic process be well understood because inadequate management of this condition can lead rapidly to worsening of hemodynamic status and death. Dynamic obstruction of the left ventricle can present in different forms. One of these forms is *dynamic left ventricular outflow tract obstruction*. Although dynamic left ventricular outflow tract obstruction is seen often in association with asymmetrical septal hypertrophy, it also can occur in other situations.[80,81] Dynamic left ventricular outflow tract obstruction is thought to be caused by the Venturi effect. This effect results when excessive acceleration of blood through a conduit produces a decrease in pressure. In the left ventricular outflow tract, such a decrease in pressure leads to a suction phenomenon that draws the anterior mitral leaflet and chordae inward toward the interventricular septum.[82] This systolic anterior motion of the mitral valve leads to contact between the mitral leaflet and the septum that creates an obstructive subaortic pressure gradient and distortion of the mitral valve leaflet coaptation (Fig. 206-11).[82] By two-dimensional echocardiography, the left ventricle appears to be small and hyperdynamic, and there is motion of the anterior leaflet (or chordae or both) toward the septum in systole (see Fig. 206-11). With color Doppler, a "mosaic" pattern of flow is seen in the left ventricular outflow tract owing to the high velocity and turbulence. Variable degrees of asymmetrical mitral regurgitation also may be present (see Fig. 206-11). Continuous wave Doppler shows the presence of a significant gradient in the left ventricular outflow tract. Dynamic left ventricular obstruction also can be present without systolic anterior motion. In the presence of reduced afterload, dehydration, or significant catecholaminergic stimulation, patients with a small, hypertrophied left ventricle (typically seen in elderly patients with chronic hypertension) can develop midventricular obstruction because of hyperdynamic systolic obliteration of the left ventricular cavity (see Fig. 206-9).[83] These physiologic factors may predict development or worsening of left ventricular dynamic obstruction. Interplay of these factors, with preexisting ventricular hypertrophy, predisposes the patient to develop cardiogenic shock from this combined loss of preload and presence of dynamic left ventricular obstruction. Dynamic left ventricular obstruction also has been described in patients with acute myocardial infarction, mostly in association with apical infarction.[81,84,85]

In a study by Chenzbraun and coworkers[85] in ICU patients, four patients with hemodynamic instability were found to have a small hyperdynamic ventricle on TEE. Of these four patients, three had pulmonary artery occlusion pressure greater than 20 mm Hg. A study by Poelaert and associates[20] that evaluated the diagnostic value of TEE

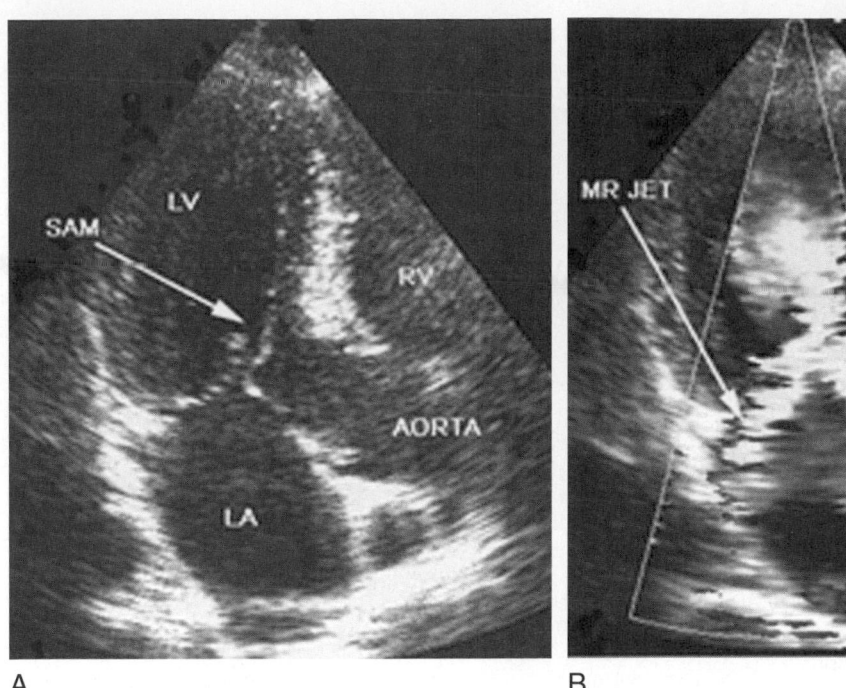

FIGURE 206–11. Systolic anterior motion (SAM) of the mitral valve in a patient with asymmetrical left ventricular hypertrophy and dehydration. Two-dimensional transthoracic apical long-axis view shows movement of the anterior leaflet of the mitral valve *(arrow)* toward the interventricular septum during systole *(A)*. This creates a subaortic dynamic obstruction. The resulting high velocity and turbulence in the left ventricular outflow tract (LVOT) gives a "mosaic" pattern of flow on color Doppler *(B)*. A variable degree of asymmetric mitral regurgitation (MR) also may be present secondary to the systolic anterior motion as shown in this example *(B)*. LA, left atrium; LV, left ventricle; RV, right ventricle. (See Color Section in this text.)

compared with pulmonary artery catheterization showed that pulmonary artery catheterization failed to diagnose the presence of hypovolemia in 44% of patients when TEE showed systolic obliteration of the left ventricular cavity, supporting a diagnosis of hypovolemia. TTE and TEE have been shown to play a key role in making the diagnosis of hypovolemia and left ventricular dynamic obstruction, leading to a dramatic impact on therapy.[19,21,22,82-85]

Assessment of Pulmonary Artery Pressure

Pulmonary hypertension is common in critically ill patients and is a manifestation of various pulmonary, cardiac, and systemic processes. Pulmonary hypertension is said to be present when systolic pulmonary pressure is greater than 35 mm Hg, diastolic pulmonary pressure is greater than 15 mm Hg, and mean pulmonary pressure is greater than 25 mm Hg.[59] Many echocardiographic methods have been validated for noninvasive estimation of pulmonary artery pressure.[59,86] These methods can be helpful in the ICU. Systolic and diastolic pulmonary artery pressures are determined from the tricuspid and pulmonary regurgitation velocities (some degree of regurgitation is essential to be able to obtain a Doppler signal and subsequently determine pulmonary artery pressure). Tricuspid regurgitation is present in more than 75% of healthy adults[59] and in approximately 90% of critically ill patients.[87] Peak tricuspid regurgitation velocity, usually obtained by continuous wave Doppler from the right ventricular inflow or the apical four-chamber view position, reflects the pressure difference during systole between the right ventricle and the right atrium (Fig. 206-12).[88-90] Peak systolic pulmonary artery pressure is determined from the peak tricuspid regurgitation Doppler velocity using the modified Bernoulli equation[91]: $\Delta P = 4 \times$ (peak tricuspid regurgitation velocity)^2. To this peak

systolic pressure gradient between right ventricle and right atrium is added the estimated right atrial pressure (see previous section) to obtain the peak right ventricular systolic pressure. In the absence of pulmonic stenosis or right ventricular outflow obstruction, peak right ventricular systolic pressure is equal to systolic pulmonary artery pressure (see Fig. 206-12). Echocardiography also can determine diastolic pulmonary artery pressure by applying the modified Bernoulli equation using the regurgitant Doppler velocity of the pulmonary valve to obtain the gradient between the pulmonary artery and the right ventricle at end diastole. To this is added the estimated right atrial pressure (equivalent to right ventricular end-diastolic pressure in the absence of tricuspid stenosis) to obtain end-diastolic pulmonary artery pressure: end-diastolic pulmonary artery pressure = 4 × (peak pulmonary regurgitation velocity)^2 + estimated right atrial pressure. Approximately 70% of critically ill patients have an adequate Doppler signal of pulmonic insufficiency for this calculation.[92] Tricuspid and pulmonary regurgitation are present at the same time in more than 85% of subjects.[93]

Assessment of Valvular Function and Integrity

Attention has been drawn to the limitations of the physical examination for the detection of cardiovascular abnormalities.[94,95] This problem is enhanced in acutely ill patients in the ICU, and many cardiovascular abnormalities may be concurrent with noncardiac illness without being clinically suspected.[96] Significant valvular abnormalities are a good example of such cardiovascular pathologies that can be present in a critically ill patient without being clinically recognized.[96] Even in the presence of invasive monitoring, significant valvular pathologies may be missed.

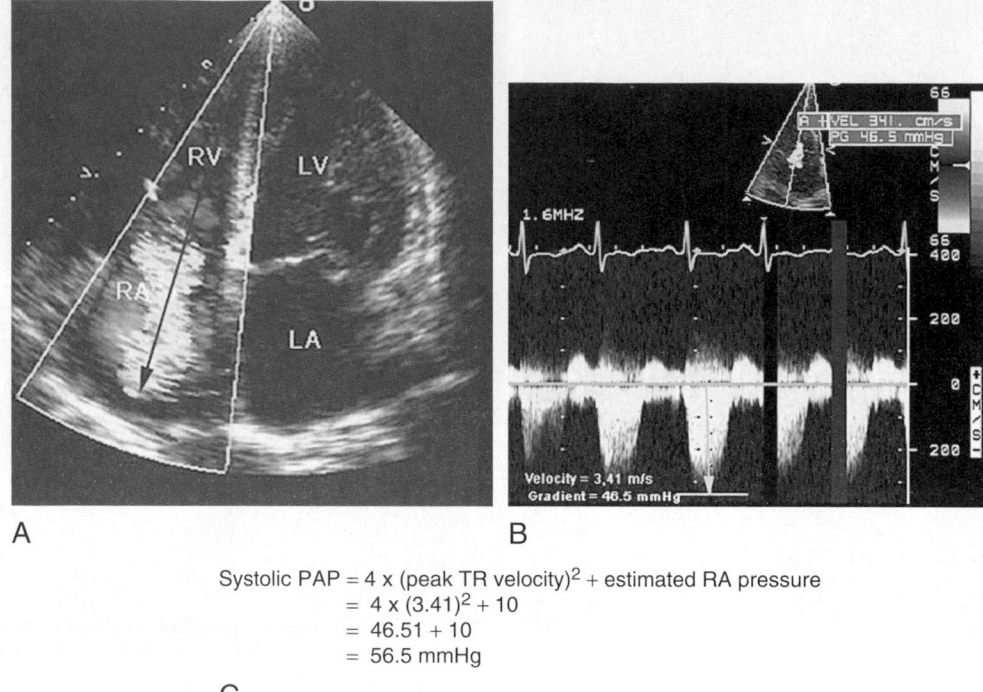

$$\text{Systolic PAP} = 4 \times (\text{peak TR velocity})^2 + \text{estimated RA pressure}$$
$$= 4 \times (3.41)^2 + 10$$
$$= 46.51 + 10$$
$$= 56.5 \text{ mmHg}$$

C

FIGURE 206–12. Calculation of systolic pulmonary artery pressure (PAP). *A,* Color Doppler transthoracic apical four-chamber view showing a significant tricuspid regurgitation (TR) jet from right ventricle (RV) to right atrium (RA). The peak tricuspid regurgitation velocity is measured by placing the continuous wave Doppler in the center of the tricuspid regurgitation jet *(arrow). B,* Spectral continuous wave Doppler profile of the tricuspid regurgitation jet. Peak tricuspid regurgitation velocity (3.41 m/s) and peak systolic pulmonary artery pressure gradient (46.5 mm Hg) can be obtained with this modality. *C,* Peak systolic pulmonary artery pressure also can be determined from the peak tricuspid regurgitation Doppler velocity using the modified Bernoulli equation: $\Delta P = 4 \times (\text{peak tricuspid regurgitation velocity})^2$. To this peak systolic pressure gradient between right ventricle and right atrium is added the estimated right atrial pressure (determined to be 10 in this example) to obtain the peak right ventricular systolic pressure. In the absence of pulmonic stenosis or right ventricular outflow obstruction, peak right ventricular systolic pressure is equal to systolic pulmonary artery pressure. LA, left atrium; LV, left ventricle. (See Color Section in this text.)

Precise evaluation of the valvular apparatus often may be warranted in the ICU. The most common indications for bedside echocardiography for evaluation of valvular apparatus in this patient population are for suspected endocarditis,[8,24] acute aortic or mitral valve regurgitation,[97,98] and prosthetic valve dysfunction.[16] Echocardiography is uniquely suited to the evaluation of valvular heart disease because of its ability to provide information regarding the etiology and severity of valvular lesions. In the ICU, TTE can provide valuable information concerning valvular integrity and function,[16] but it may be suboptimal and not sensitive enough to detect endocarditis, a dysfunctional mitral valve, or prosthetic valve dysfunction. TEE is often warranted.

Valvular Regurgitation and Prosthetic Valve Dysfunction

In a patient with unexplained hemodynamic instability and a grossly normal TTE examination, performance of subsequent TEE is important to rule out the presence of significant undetected valvular pathology. Common valvular pathologies that can be missed are mitral regurgitation and prosthetic valve dysfunction. In some situations, TTE may provide better imaging than TEE for evaluation of anterior structures such as the aortic valve (native or prosthetic) and for Doppler measurements. TEE is clearly superior to TTE for evaluation of mitral valve pathologies (native and prosthetic). In a study of ICU patients by Alam,[16] TTE compared with TEE was shown either to miss or to underestimate the severity of regurgitation of St. Jude and bioprosthetic valves in the mitral but not in the aortic position.

With acute severe mitral regurgitation, the diagnosis may be clinically difficult because the murmur is often of short duration and low intensity (because of rapid pressure equalization between the left ventricle and the relatively noncompliant left atrium). By TTE, the size of the regurgitant jet in acute mitral regurgitation may appear small and lead to underestimation of severity.[99] Because of its close anatomic proximity, TEE provides a much more precise evaluation of the degree of mitral regurgitation (Fig. 206-13) and provides crucial diagnostic information regarding the cause for mitral regurgitation. The diagnosis of acute mitral regurgitation represents a medical emergency that may necessitate urgent surgery, and so the threshold to perform a TEE when this entity is suspected should be low.[8,10,97] Also, several investigators have confirmed the superior accuracy, sensitivity, and reliability of TEE over TTE for dysfunction of mitral prostheses, in which ultrasonic shadowing of the left atrium often occurs with the standard transthoracic studies.[100-103]

Traumatic Valvular Injuries

Traumatic valvular injuries associated with myocardial injury may present as acute regurgitation. Bedside exclusion of major trauma to the aorta, valves, and myocardium is important in the post-trauma context.[104,105] Valvular injuries may occur as a consequence of blunt or penetrating trauma. Most frequently the aortic valve is injured; less commonly

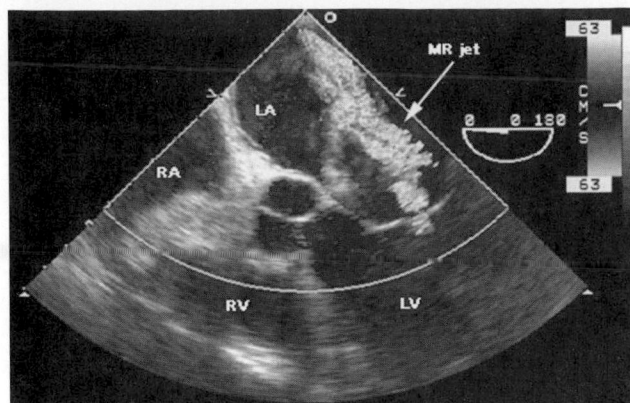

FIGURE 206–13. Severe mitral regurgitation (MR). Transesophageal five-chamber view shows severe mitral regurgitation with a large regurgitant jet *(arrow)* going far posteriorly in the left atrium (LA). In this case, systolic flow reversal in the pulmonary veins (another echocardiographic sign of severe mitral regurgitation) also was present (not shown on this picture). Because of its close anatomic proximity, transesophageal echocardiography is an excellent tool for the precise evaluation of the degree of mitral regurgitation. LV, left ventricle; RA, right atrium; RV, right ventricle. (See Color Section in this text.)

the mitral and tricuspid valves are injured.[106] Valvular dysfunction is usually due to a torn leaflet or rupture of a papillary muscle or chordae.[106] In trauma patients, TEE is the bedside imaging modality of choice to detect these pathologies.[104,105] In a study by Chirillo and coworkers assessing the usefulness of TTE and TEE in recognition and management of cardiovascular injuries after blunt chest trauma, TTE provided suboptimal imaging in 62% of patients, and the bad quality of images obtained was the main cause for the low sensitivity of TTE compared with TEE.

Evaluation of the Pericardial Space

Echocardiography is an essential instrument for the diagnosis of pericardial disease. In the ICU, the most common clinical indication for assessment of the pericardial space is suspected tamponade. The pericardium is a potential space that can become filled with fluid, blood, pus, or, uncommonly, air. Presence of fluid in this space is detected as an echo-free space. Pericardial fluid usually is detected easily with TTE. The parasternal long-axis and short-axis views and the apical views usually reveal the effusion (Fig. 206-14). In many critically ill patients with suboptimal TTE image quality, the subcostal view is often the only adequate window available to detect the presence of a pericardial effusion. In these ICU patients with poor acoustic windows and in the post–cardiac surgical setting, TEE may be needed to assess the pericardial space adequately.

In addition to assisting in the diagnosis of pericardial effusion and tamponade, two-dimensional echocardiography can assist in its drainage, as pericardiocentesis can be performed safely under two-dimensional echocardiographic guidance.[107,108] By determining the depth of the effusion and its distance from the site of puncture, it is possible to optimize the needle placement. Echocardiography also can be used for immediate monitoring of the results of the pericardiocentesis.

Cardiac Tamponade in the Intensive Care Unit

The most common causes of cardiac tamponade in the ICU are listed in Table 206-5. Echocardiographic two-dimensional

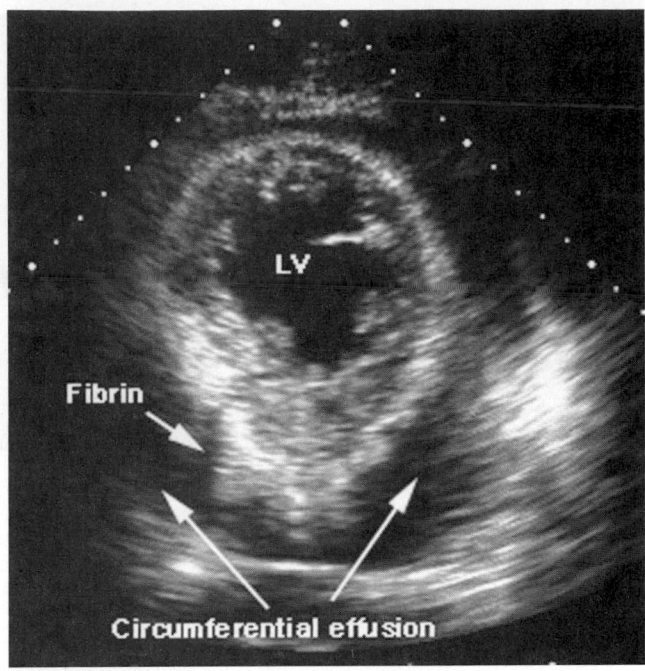

FIGURE 206–14. Large pericardial effusion. Transthoracic parasternal short-axis view shows a large, predominantly echo-free space around the left ventricle (LV). This space represents fluid in the pericardium. In this case, the large circumferential pericardial effusion was bloody at pericardiocentesis. Particulate matter (e.g., fibrin and clots) can be visualized as denser echos around the heart and floating in the effusion.

signs of tamponade are a direct consequence of increased pericardial pressure, leading to diastolic collapse of one or more cardiac chambers (usually on the right side first) (Fig. 206-15). Usually, collapse of the right ventricular free wall is seen in early diastole, and right atrial wall collapse is seen in late diastole.[14] This latter sign is sensitive but not specific for tamponade. It is, however, specific for a hemodynamically significant effusion, if the right atrial collapse lasts longer than one third of the R-R interval.[14,109] In the presence of a massive effusion, the heart may have a "swinging" motion in the pericardial cavity. This finding is not always present in cardiac tamponade because the amount of fluid in the pericardial space may be small but still cause a tamponade physiology, depending on the acuity with which the effusion accumulates and the compliance of the pericardium. In poststernotomy patients, tamponade may be missed by TTE (even in cases in which imaging quality seems adequate) because hematomas causing selective cardiac chamber compression are often in the form of loculated clots, located

---

TABLE 206–5. MOST COMMON CAUSES OF CARDIAC TAMPONADE IN THE INTENSIVE CARE UNIT

Myocardial or coronary perforation secondary to catheter-based intervention (i.e., after intravenous pacemaker lead insertion, central line placement, or percutaneous coronary interventions)
Compressive hematoma after cardiac surgery
Proximal ascending aortic dissection
Blunt or penetrating chest trauma
Complication of myocardial infarction (e.g., ventricular rupture)
Uremic or infectious pericarditis
Pericardial involvement by metastatic disease or other systemic processes

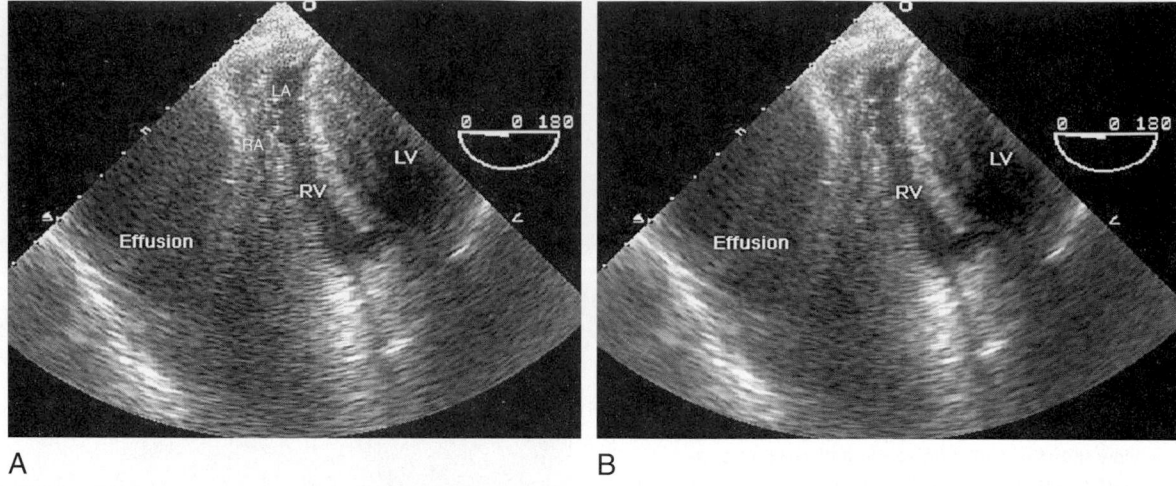

A   B

FIGURE 206–15. Cardiac tamponade. Transesophageal four-chamber view *(A)* shows the presence of a large effusion that severely compresses the right atrium (RA) and right ventricle (RV), which appear slitlike. The left ventricle (LV) also is small because of indirect compression and underfilling. Transgastric short-axis view *(B)* of the same patient shows the large pericardial effusion and severely compressed ventricular chambers. This postcardiotomy patient was in profound shock and was brought back to the operating room emergently for re-exploration and drainage of the effusion. LA, left atrium.

in the far field of the ultrasound beam in the posterior heart region (even when the anterior pericardium is left open).[110] The right atrium and right ventricle may be spared in such cases secondary to postoperative adhesions or tethering of the right ventricle to the chest wall anteriorly.[110]

Another (indirect) sign of a hemodynamically significant pericardial effusion on two-dimensional imaging is plethora of the inferior vena cava with blunted respiratory changes.[1] The latter sign is less valuable in mechanically ventilated patients because they often have a stiff dilated inferior vena cava, even in the absence of a pericardial effusion.

Doppler findings of cardiac tamponade are based on characteristic changes in intrathoracic and intracardiac hemodynamics that occur with respiration. Because of the principle of ventricular interaction, mitral inflow velocity (E wave) decreases after inspiration and increases after expiration. Reciprocal changes occur with respect to tricuspid inflow velocity. With tamponade, the exaggerated inspiratory-expiratory variation of the inflow velocity (E wave) over one respiratory cycle should be greater than 40% on the left and greater than 80% on the right.[111] In critically ill patients, however, mechanical ventilation, bronchospasm, significant pleural effusion, and respiratory distress can alter intrathoracic and intracardiac hemodynamics and make these Doppler findings less reliable. A significant pleural effusion sometimes causes significant respiratory Doppler variations of the inflow velocities that disappear when the effusion is drained.[112] The presence of arrhythmia also makes the Doppler findings difficult to interpret. In some circumstances, echocardiographic signs of tamponade may be subtle or absent, so one must keep in mind that the diagnosis of tamponade remains a clinical one and that the echocardiographic signs must be analyzed in conjunction with the clinical findings.

Complications After Cardiac Surgery

Bedside echocardiography has proved to be of particular value in the critical care management of patients with hemodynamic instability after cardiothoracic operations.[7,8,83,113-115] TTE is often severely limited in this group of patients.[5,8]

TEE is the modality of choice in this setting because it provides detailed information that can help determine the cause of refractory hypotension. The most frequent echocardiographic diagnoses encountered in these patients are left ventricular or right ventricular failure, tamponade, hypovolemia, and valvular dysfunction. Schmidlin and colleagues[116] studied 136 patients after cardiac surgery and showed that a new diagnosis was established or an important pathology was excluded in 45% of patients undergoing TEE. A therapeutic impact was found in 73% of cases. The main indications for TEE in this study were control of left ventricular function (34%), unexplained hemodynamic deterioration (29%), suspicion of pericardial tamponade (14%), cardiac ischemia (9%), and "other" (14%). Reichert and associates[113] performed TEE in hypotensive patients after cardiac surgery. Left ventricular failure was found in 27% of patients; hypovolemia, in 23%; right ventricular failure, in 18%; biventricular failure, in 13%; and tamponade, in 10%. Comparison with hemodynamic parameters showed agreement on diagnosis (hypovolemia versus tamponade versus cardiac failure) in only 50% of the cases. Echocardiography identified two cases of tamponade and six of hypovolemia that were not suspected based on standard hemodynamic data. In five patients with hemodynamic findings suggesting tamponade, unnecessary reoperation was prevented because TEE ruled out this diagnosis. Costachescu and colleagues[22] also showed the superiority of TEE compared with conventional monitoring with pulmonary artery catheterization in diagnosing and excluding significant causes of hemodynamic instability in postoperative cardiac surgical patients.

Descriptions of the echocardiographic findings of left ventricular dysfunction, tamponade, hypovolemia, and valvular dysfunction were described earlier in this chapter.

INFECTIVE ENDOCARDITIS

Occurrence of infective endocarditis in patients hospitalized in an ICU is common. It is often in the differential diagnosis of febrile patients in the ICU. Infective endocarditis was the second most common indication for performance of an echocardiogram among centers reporting their experience, as summarized in a review article by Heidenreich.[5] Nearly all critically ill patients are at risk for iatrogenic infection, bacteremia, and subsequent endocarditis because of the presence of multiple indwelling catheters, severe underlying diseases, malnutrition, and prolonged mechanical ventilation. Classic clinical findings suggesting endocarditis[106] are uncommon in this patient population. Echocardiography is the test of choice for the noninvasive diagnosis of endocarditis. Fowler and coworkers[117] studied patients with *Staphylococcus aureus* bacteremia referred for TEE and showed that endocarditis ultimately was diagnosed in 25%. Only 7% of these patients had physical findings suggesting endocarditis before TEE. Absence of clinical stigmata is especially likely if the infection presents acutely. Because the consequences of untreated endocarditis are devastating and often ultimately fatal, it is important that the infection and its complications be recognized promptly and treated appropriately.[59]

The echocardiographic features typical for infective endocarditis are[59,118] (1) an oscillating intracardiac mass on a valve or supporting structure or in the path of a regurgitant jet or an iatrogenic device, (2) abcesses, (3) new partial dehiscence of a prosthetic valve, or (4) new valvular regurgitation. Sensitivity for the echographic diagnosis of endocarditis is 58% to 62% for TTE and 88% to 98% for TEE.[119,120] TEE is particularly useful for detecting small vegetations[121] and detecting vegetations on prosthetic valves. TEE also has been shown to be superior to TTE for diagnosing complications of endocarditis, such as aortic root abscess, fistulas, and ruptured chordae tendineae of the mitral valve.[16] Among ICU patients, sensitivity of TTE for the diagnosis of endocarditis is often poor because the quality of the transthoracic study is commonly suboptimal. The sensitivity of TEE for suspected infective endocarditis usually is excellent in the ICU (Fig. 206-16). In a study by Font and colleagues,[97] a search for vegetations was the indication for 51 (46%) of 112 TEE studies performed for critically ill patients. TEE increased the detection rate by 27% compared with TTE. Suspicion of endocarditis represented 29% of the

indications for TEE in a study of ICU patients by Chenzbraun and associates.[85] Nine (27%) of 31 patients with suspected infective endocarditis had a positive study for endocarditis. All positive studies were in patients who had an increased likelihood for infective endocarditis before the examination, as indicated by the presence of fever, positive blood cultures, new-onset murmur, prosthetic valve, or new-onset heart failure (alone or in combination). None of the patients with native valves and no clinical features of endocarditis had a TEE study diagnostic of infective endocarditis and in none of them was the diagnosis of infective endocarditis made later. The findings from this study indicate that TEE is not useful as a screening procedure for infective endocarditis in septic patients without high clinical likelihood for endocarditis. The low yield of TEE when the clinical likelihood of infective endocarditis is low has been confirmed by other authors.[8,16]

As concluded by Colreavy and colleagues,[8] performance of TEE in the ICU for suspicion of infective endocarditis should be (1) for cases associated with a clinical likelihood of endocarditis and a negative TTE examination, (2) for suspected prosthetic valve endocarditis, (3) for assessment of complications in known cases of endocarditis, and (4) for cases of *S. aureus* bacteremia when the source is unknown or blood cultures remain positive despite antibiotic therapy. When assessing a patient for infective endocarditis by echocardiography, one must keep in mind the noninfectious causes of vegetations that may result from tumors, myxomatous degeneration, marantic endocarditis, Lambl's excrescences, valve thrombus, and suture material in patients with repaired native or prosthetic valves.

ASSESSMENT OF THE AORTA

In the ICU, use of bedside echocardiography for assessment of suspected aortic pathologies provides many advantages over CT or aortography: There is no need for intravenous contrast administration, there may be less time delay, there is no need for transportation of a critically ill patient, and cardiac morphology and function can be evaluated at the same time.[3] For many years, aortography has been the gold

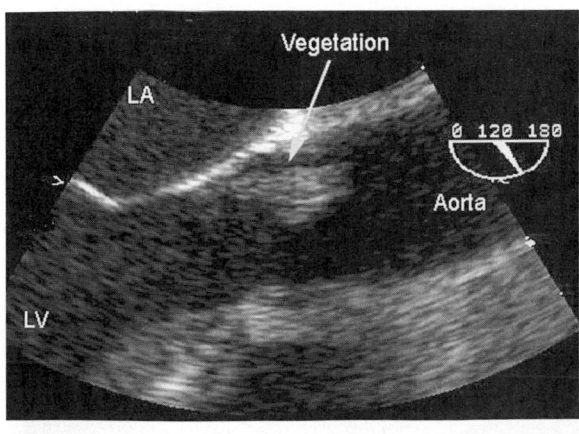
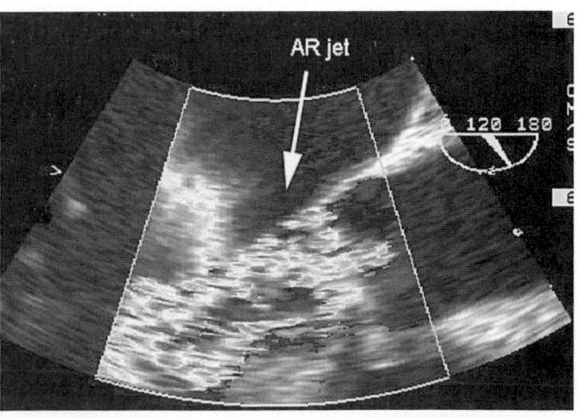

FIGURE 206-16. Infective endocarditis of the aortic valve. A 55-year-old patient was admitted to the ICU with fever, chills, hypotension, and respiratory distress for which he had to be intubated. He had 4/4 positive blood cultures for *Staphylococcus aureus*. Transthoracic echocardiography was performed initially, but the quality was suboptimal, and no definite conclusion could be reached. Subsequent transesophageal echocardiography revealed a large vegetation on the left aortic coronary cusp as seen in the midesophageal view at 120 degrees (A). Color Doppler examination (B) revealed the presence of associated severe aortic regurgitation (AR). The patient was treated with antibiotics and emergent aortic valvular surgery. LA, left atrium; LV, left ventricle. (See Color Section in this text.)

standard for the investigation of suspected injuries of the aorta.[3] The advent of noninvasive modalities such as CT, magnetic resonance imaging, and TEE with their excellent sensitivity and specificity to diagnose aortic pathologies has decreased the need for aortograms.

Suspected aortic pathologies can be encountered in different ICU settings. The aorta may need to be imaged to rule out dissection, rupture, aneurysm, aortic debris, or aortic abscess. TTE is a good initial imaging modality for evaluation of the proximal aorta (ascending aorta and arch).[59] The descending thoracic aorta cannot be adequately assessed and visualized, however, with this modality. Because of the close anatomic relationship between the thoracic aorta and the esophagus, TEE allows optimal visualization of the entire thoracic aorta (Fig. 206-17). As described earlier, there exists a "blind spot" in the distal portion of the ascending aorta and the proximal portion of the transverse aorta where imaging can be suboptimal.[122,123]

Aortic Dissection and Rupture

Patients presenting with suspected aortic dissection need emergency diagnosis and treatment. Different noninvasive tests have been advocated for evaluation of suspected aortic dissection, including TEE, CT, and magnetic resonance imaging.[5,124] Nienaber and coworkers[124] compared all three modalities and found that they had similar sensitivities (98%). Magnetic resonance imaging had higher specificity than TEE (98% versus 77%). A limitation of the study was that single-plane TEE was used. With multiplane TEE, specificity is improved to greater than 90% (see Fig. 206-17).[122] TEE was compared with CT and aortography in a multicenter European cooperative study,[125] and it was shown that TEE was superior compared with both modalities for the diagnosis of aortic dissection (sensitivity 99%). Other studies have confirmed the high accuracy of TEE.[125-128] A negative TEE examination for the diagnosis of aortic dissection, even in a high-risk population, has high negative predictive value.[129]

Another common indication to perform emergency aortic imaging in the ICU is assessment of patients with blunt or penetrating chest trauma.[3] These patients are at high risk of life-threatening aortic injuries, such as traumatic

dissection and rupture, and prompt diagnosis and treatment are required. Exclusion of major trauma to the ascending and descending aorta at the bedside is important in this context.[105] The value of TEE on admission for trauma patients with enlarged mediastinum and hemodynamic instability, with or without a combination of several other symptoms (e.g., pleural effusion, decreasing hematocrit, thoracic vertebral fracture), has been stressed by many authors.[130-133] Patients usually have a contained hematoma around the aortic dissection.[131] Transection of the thoracic aorta usually is seen at the level of the ligamentum arteriosum.

Additional helpful features of TEE in the evaluation of aortic pathologies are the ability to detect or assess extension of dissection into the proximal coronary arteries; the presence of pericardial or mediastinal hematoma or effusion; the presence, severity, and mechanism of associated aortic valve regurgitation; the point of entry and exit between the true and false lumens; the presence of thrombus in the false lumen; and ventricular function.[16] When TEE findings are equivocal or negative in cases of suspected thoracic aortic disease, other imaging modalities, such as aortography, CT, or magnetic resonance imaging, should still be performed.

ASSESSMENT FOR INTRACARDIAC AND INTRAPULMONARY SHUNTS

In critically ill patients, clinical suspicion for an intracardiac or intrapulmonary shunt most often is raised in the context of unexplained embolic stroke or refractory hypoxemia. In such cases, the presence of a right-to-left shunt needs to be excluded. Common origins of right-to-left shunt are atrial septal defect or patent foramen ovale at the cardiac level[5] and arteriovenous fistula at the pulmonary level.[5] To be able to detect the presence of such a shunt at the bedside, a contrast study often is needed because the shunt is usually not well visualized with two-dimensional echocardiography alone. Color-flow imaging increases the detection rate of intracardiac shunt to some extent, but usually only when the shunt is large. Accordingly a contrast study should be performed routinely as part of a TEE or TTE examination when evaluating a patient with unexplained embolic stroke or

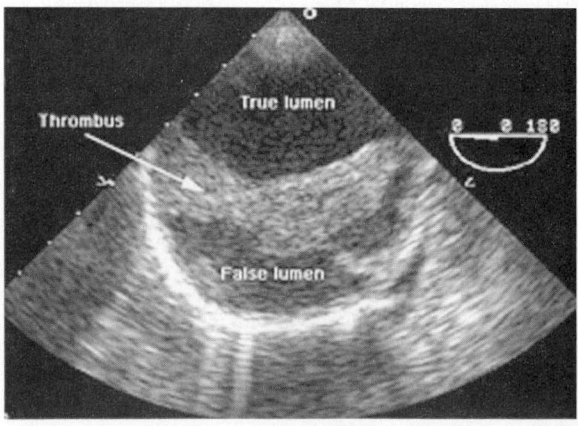
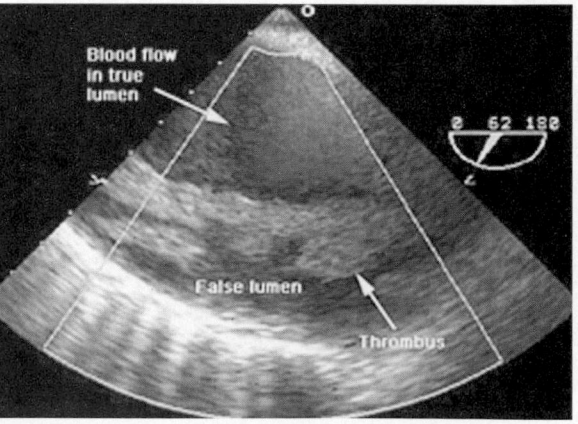

A   B

FIGURE 206–17. Dissecting thoracic aortic aneurysm. A 65-year-old patient presented to the emergency department with severe ripping chest pain radiating to the back. The initial electrocardiogram was unremarkable, and the chest x-ray showed a widened mediastinum. The patient underwent transesophageal echocardiography, which revealed the presence of a large dissecting aneurysm of the descending thoracic aorta. The short-axis view (A) revealed the presence of a large aneurysm with a true and a false lumen. The false lumen was filled with thrombus (arrow). On the longitudinal view with color Doppler (B), blood flow in the true lumen is visualized. The patient was taken emergently to the operating room. (See Color Section in this text.)

refractory hypoxemia in the ICU. For this purpose, agitated saline contrast is usually used. Approximately 0.5 mL of air is mixed with 10 mL of normal saline and is vigorously agitated back and forth between two syringes connected to the patient by a three-way stopcock. After an adequate echocardiographic view of the right and left atrial cavities has been obtained, the agitated saline is forcefully injected intravenously. After injection, the contrast is seen in the vena cava, right atrium, right ventricle, and pulmonary artery. In the absence of a shunt, only a minimal amount of contrast should be seen in the left-sided cavities because most of the microbubbles from the agitated saline are not able to pass through the pulmonary capillaries. If an intracardiac shunt is present, such as an atrial septal defect or patent foramen ovale, left-sided contrast is observed immediately after right-sided opacification, and the contrast is seen going through the interatrial septum (Fig. 206-18). Performance of a Valsalva maneuver by the patient during contrast injection increases the sensitivity of the bubble study to detect right-to-left shunting. In mechanically ventilated patients, a maneuver equivalent to a Valsalva may be performed, by inducing sudden release of sustained airway pressure previously achieved by inflating the lungs manually. This maneuver reverses the atrial transseptal gradient and may help uncover a patent foramen ovale that would not have been seen otherwise. Right-to-left shunting also can be caused by the presence of pulmonary arteriovenous fistulas. These often are associated with end-stage liver disease (hepatopulmonary syndrome). With this type of shunt, contrast is seen to appear in the left atrium from the pulmonary veins instead of through the atrial septum; this finding is best detected by TEE, which usually permits visualization of all four pulmonary veins. The characteristic of intrapulmonary versus intracardiac shunt is that there is a longer delay (three to five cardiac cycles) between the appearance of contrast from the right-sided to left-sided cavities in the presence of an intrapulmonary shunt.[5] Agitated saline is a simple and easy way to use contrast at the bedside.

Other types of intracardiac shunts also can be encountered in the ICU. After myocardial infarction, patients can develop cardiogenic shock because of acute development of a ventricular septal defect and resultant left-to-right shunt. Physical examination and invasive hemodynamic monitoring (pulmonary artery catheterization) sometimes can miss this diagnosis. Echocardiography reveals a disrupted ventricular septum with a high-velocity, left-to-right shunt. This kind of shunt usually is well visualized without use of contrast. The diagnosis can be established by two-dimensional and Doppler TTE in approximately 90% of cases.[134] Penetrating cardiac trauma often is associated with intracardiac and extracardiac shunts, and TEE is becoming the obvious tool for perioperative early identification of occult shunts.[14] Identification of these shunts is paramount in these critically ill patients because missing them may lead to cardiac tamponade and rapid death. TEE has been shown to be superior to angiography and TTE to visualize these lesions.[135-137]

Unexplained Hypoxemia

Patent foramen ovale is present in 25% to 30% of healthy individuals.[59,106] Usually, it allows only minimal and intermittent right-to-left shunting. When the right atrial pressure is increased and exceeds left atrial pressure, the patent foramen ovale can widen and significantly increase the importance of the right-to-left shunt with resultant significant hypoxemia. In a critically ill patient, this increase in right-sided pressure can occur from pulmonary hypertension, secondary to acute respiratory distress syndrome or pulmonary embolism, right ventricular failure (from infarction or pulmonary hypertension), or severe tricuspid regurgitation, which is often seen in the ICU for a variety of reasons. In critically ill patients, TEE is in general more useful than TTE for evaluation of patent foramen ovale, atrial septal defect (see Fig. 206-18), and pulmonary arteriovenous fistula[138] because of the close proximity of the lesion to the ultrasound transducer.

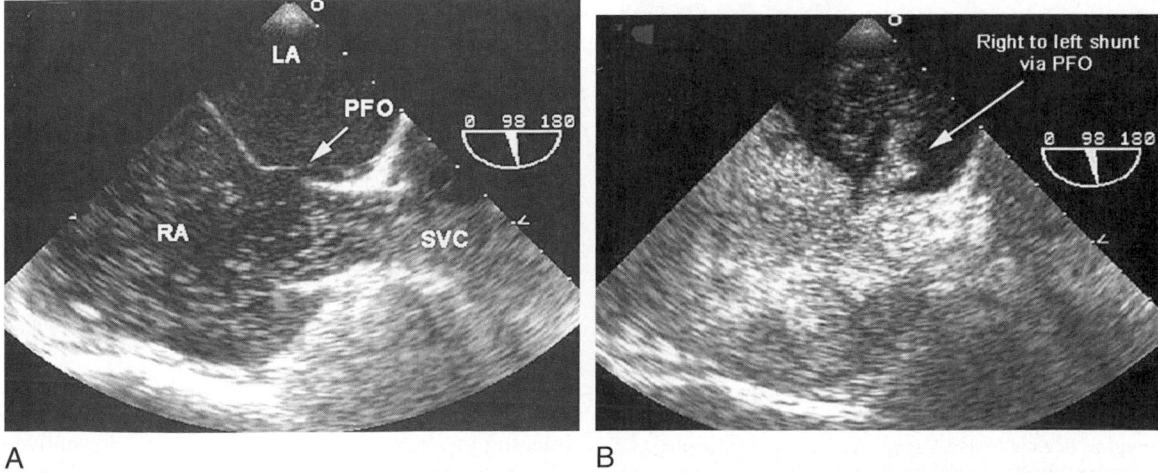

FIGURE 206–18. Positive bubble study shows the presence of a right-to-left shunt via a patent foramen ovale (PFO). Transesophageal echocardiography was performed in a patient hospitalized in the ICU for pneumonia. He presented with refractory hypoxemia that was out of proportion to the underlying minor pulmonary process. Transesophageal echocardiography was obtained (multiplane transducer at 98 degrees) and showed the presence of a patent foramen ovale with a significant right-to-left shunt because of elevated right atrial pressure. Soon after contrast injection *(A)*, the bubbles are seen arriving in the right atrium (RA) from the superior vena cava (SVC). A few seconds later, a complete opacification of the right atrium is reached, and the bubble contrast is clearly seen shunting through the patent foramen ovale from the right atrium to left atrium (LA) *(B)*.

Patients with patent foramen ovale and persistent refractory hypoxemia despite ventilator and hemodynamic manipulation sometimes may need to have catheter-based septal defect closure devices inserted. TEE is crucial to assist in the performance of this procedure.[139]

SOURCE OF EMBOLUS

In the setting of acute unexplained stroke, echocardiography often is required to determine if a potential embolic source of cardiac origin is present. TEE is the modality of choice for this purpose. Possible cardiac sources of emboli to the arterial circulation include left atrial or appendicular thrombus, left ventricular thrombus, thoracic atheromatosis, and right-sided clots (right atrium, right ventricle, vena cava) combined with a right-to-left intracardiac shunt (leading to a paradoxical embolus). Cardiac tumors and vegetations are other potential sources of emboli from cardiac origin that need to be considered.

In a critically ill patient with atrial fibrillation or flutter when cardioversion is considered, performance of TEE is helpful for evaluating the left atrium and appendage for the presence of thrombus (Fig. 206-19). If no intracardiac clots are documented, cardioversion can be performed with minimal embolic risks.

USE OF CONTRAST AND HARMONIC TECHNOLOGY TO ENHANCE TRANSTHORACIC EXAMINATIONS WITH POOR IMAGE QUALITY IN A CRITICALLY ILL PATIENT

Using standard echocardiographic methods, endocardial delineation is suboptimal in approximately 30% of cases.[140]

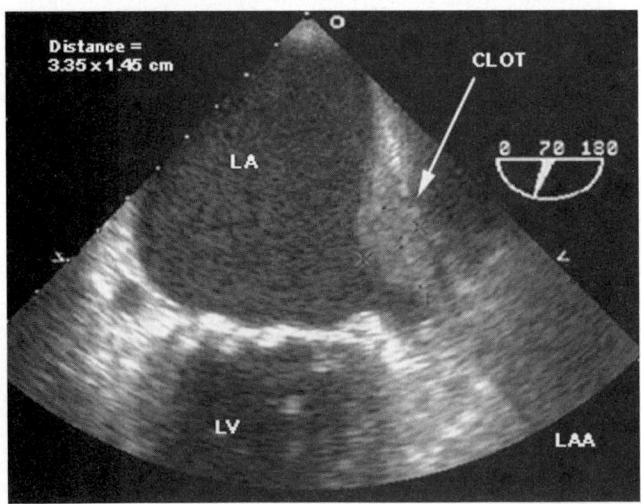

FIGURE 206–19. Large clot in the left atrial wall and left atrial appendage (LAA). A 72-year-old patient hospitalized in the ICU for urosepsis developed rapid atrial fibrillation. She was initially anticoagulated and rate-controlled. Despite resolution of the septic picture, she remained in atrial fibrillation 4 days after its onset. The patient underwent transesophageal echocardiography before undergoing a planned electrical cardioversion. The midesophageal view with multiplane transducer at 70 degrees revealed the presence of a large clot (3.35 × 1.45 cm) in the posterolateral wall of the left atrium (LA) extending into the LAA. With these findings, the patient's anticoagulation regimen was intensified, and the cardioversion was not performed. LV, left ventricle.

Two developments in ultrasound have improved the quality of endocardial border definition, however: *harmonic imaging* and *intravenous contrast echocardiography*.[141] Dramatic improvements in image quality have been achieved with the development of harmonic imaging. This technology exploits the formation of ultrasound signals that return to the transducer at a multiple of the transmitted (fundamental) frequency, referred to as the *harmonic frequency*.[1] Signals are received by the ultrasound transducer at twice the transmitted frequency. This "second harmonic imaging" results in images with better contrast between the myocardium and cardiac chambers and improved endocardial definition compared with fundamental imaging.[142-144] Nowadays, most ultrasound equipment includes harmonic imaging as a standard feature.

In critically ill patients with poor acoustic windows, endocardial visualization still may be inadequate despite the use of second harmonic imaging.[140] In these patients, contrast agents, capable of producing left ventricular cavity opacification with an intravenous injection, can be helpful in delineating endocardial borders. Several contrast agents are currently available that contain albumin microspheres filled with perfluorocarbon gas, allowing for the passage of contrast through the lungs with appearance of contrast in the left venticle.[1] The chamber is opacified by the contrast agent within 1 minute of administration and allows improved endocardial border detection. The presence of contrast also enhances Doppler signals.[145] Studies have examined the impact of these newer modalities of harmonic imaging and contrast in the ICU. Reilly and coworkers[146] assessed the benefits of contrast echocardiography for the evaluation of left ventricular function in 70 unselected ICU patients. Twenty-two patients (31%) were receiving mechanical ventilation. Left ventricular ejection fraction could not be obtained at all in 23% of patients with standard imaging. When harmonic imaging was employed, left ventricular ejection fraction was unobtainable in only 13% of patients. When contrast imaging was employed, left ventricular ejection fraction was measurable in all of the patients. Ejection fraction was confidently determined in 56%, 62%, and 91% of patients with standard imaging, harmonic imaging, and contrast imaging. In this study, contrast imaging was safe and dramatically improved the capacity to evaluate left ventricular ejection fraction and regional wall motion reliably compared with fundamental and harmonic imaging. Yong and associates[141] extended these observations by comparing the results of harmonic and contrast imaging with an independent standard (i.e., TEE) in 32 consecutive critically ill patients who were considered technically very difficult. Estimation of ejection fraction was possible in 31%, 50%, and 97% with fundamental imaging, harmonic imaging, and contrast imaging. Quantification of ejection fraction by contrast enhancement correlated best with TEE ($r = 0.91$).

In critically ill patients with suboptimal TTE image quality, contrast echocardiography combined with harmonic imaging provides a noninvasive and safe alternative to TEE for determination of regional and global left ventricular function (Fig. 206-20).[140] It is a rapid and simple technique that can be performed at the bedside in the ICU with positive impact on interpretation of left ventricular function. Before using TEE, this technique should be considered in critically ill patients when TTE is inadequate for evaluation of left ventricular function.[140]

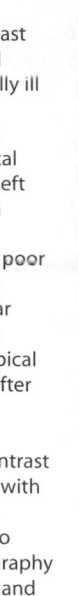
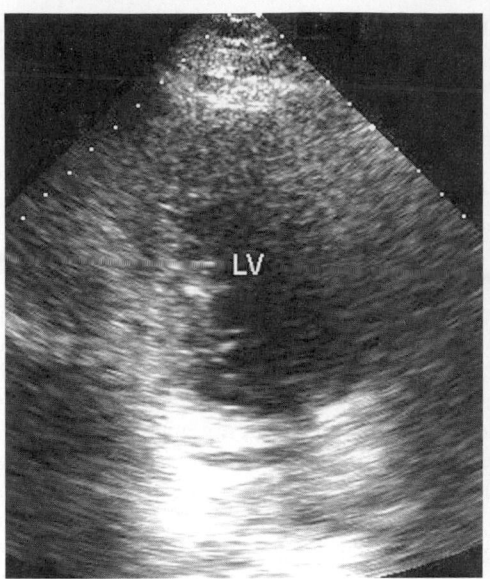
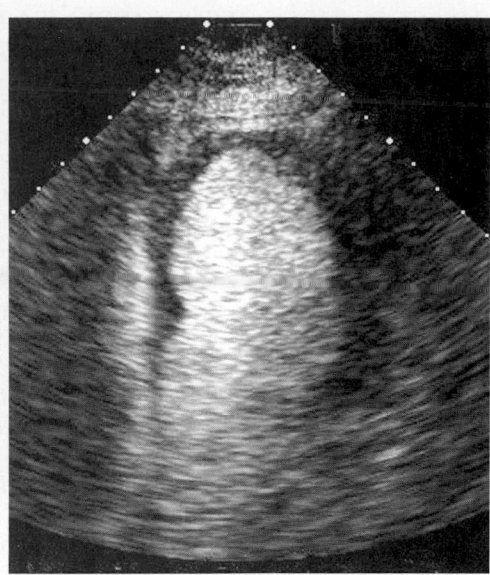

FIGURE 206–20. Use of contrast agent to improve endocardial border delineation in a critically ill patient with suboptimal transthoracic image quality. A suboptimal transthoracic apical two-chamber view (A) of the left ventricle (LV) obtained from a ventilated ICU patient with hemodynamic instability. The poor endocardial resolution makes regional and global ventricular function hard to assess. Same transthoracic two-chamber apical view (B) in the same patient after contrast injection. A dramatic improvement in endocardial border definition is noted. Contrast echocardiography combined with harmonic imaging provides a noninvasive, safe alternative to transesophageal echocardiography for determination of regional and global left ventricular function.

A

B

COMPARISON BETWEEN BEDSIDE ECHOCARDIOGRAPHY AND PULMONARY ARTERY CATHETER IN THE INTENSIVE CARE UNIT

Since its introduction into clinical practice in 1970, pulmonary artery catheterization has been the standard hemodynamic monitoring technique for critically ill patients in the ICU.[147-149] Pulmonary artery catheterization provides clinicians with indices of cardiovascular function to assist in therapeutic decision-making. Pulmonary artery catheterization can be a useful diagnostic tool, aiding in the management of critically ill patients. Nevertheless, poor interpretation of the data it provides can lead to excessive morbidity and mortality.[63,147,150,151] Conventional monitoring using a pulmonary artery catheter has been shown to be limited in the evaluation of global ventricular function,[19,21] and echocardiographic studies have established that pulmonary artery occlusion pressure often does not allow accurate assessment of left ventricular preload.[26,152,153] The frequent changes in ventricular compliance and loading conditions occurring in critically ill patients can affect systolic and diastolic function. In such cases, conventional monitoring does not enable early detection of acute changes in function, and it does not allow the clinician to discern systolic from diastolic changes.[19]

In critically ill patients, echocardiography, particularly TEE, has the ability to clarify diagnosis and define pathophysiologic process more precisely than pulmonary artery catheterization. In a prospective study of limited scope, Benjamin and colleagues[21] found that TEE-derived data disagreed with the pulmonary artery catheterization evaluation of intracardiac volume in 55% of cases and with the pulmonary artery catheterization assessment of myocardial function in 39% of cases. These authors also showed that the post–pulmonary artery catheterization therapeutic recommendations were different from the post-TEE therapeutic recommendations in 58% of patients. In a retrospective analysis of 108 critically ill patients who underwent a TEE, Poelaert and coworkers[20] found that of 64% of patients with pulmonary artery catheterization, 44% underwent therapy changes after TEE (41% in the cardiac and 54% in the septic subgroup). Also, these investigators found that in 41% of patients without pulmonary artery catheterization, TEE led to a change in therapy. They concluded that TEE produced a change in therapy in at least one third of ICU patients independent of the presence of pulmonary artery catheterization.[20]

Another significant advantage of echocardiography in the ICU is the speed with which it can be performed relative to pulmonary artery catheterization. In the study by Benjamin and colleagues,[21] TEE was performed in 12 ± 7 minutes versus 30 minutes or more for pulmonary artery catheterization insertion. In a study by Kaul,[154] the average time required to place a pulmonary artery catheter and record the data was 63 ± 45 minutes versus 19 ± 7 minutes to perform bedside TEE. Reported complications of pulmonary artery catheterization include pneumothorax, hemothorax, bacteremia, sepsis, cardiac arrhythmias, pulmonary artery rupture, cardiac perforation, and valvular damage.[21] Compared with pulmonary artery catheterization, bedside echocardiography has a better safety profile, as reported previously in this chapter.

A major advantage of pulmonary artery catheterization versus TEE is that the catheter can more easily serve as a continuous monitoring technique to assess the response to a therapeutic intervention.[21] This potential advantage may provide little benefit, however, in patients in whom the information is misinterpreted or inadequate. In some ICUs, TEE has completely replaced pulmonary artery catheterization for assessment of circulatory status of mechanically ventilated patients.[38]

Despite having multiple limitations, pulmonary artery catheterization still has a role in the ICU and remains a useful diagnostic tool when used by physicians who have extensive experience with it.[20,155] A combination of invasive pressure monitoring and TEE probably offers the most complete evaluation at the bedside of morphology and intracardiac hemodynamics and provides a more precise pressure-volume evaluation of left ventricular and right ventricular function and filling.[20,22]

IMPACT OF BEDSIDE ECHOCARDIOGRAPHY ON DIAGNOSIS AND MANAGEMENT IN A CRITICALLY ILL PATIENT

Echocardiography often provides unexpected diagnoses in critically ill patients. Compared with TTE and invasive hemodynamic monitoring, TEE frequently provides different or additional information. This information often is important for adequate and optimal adjustment of therapy. Several studies have examined the impact of bedside echocardiography, particularly TEE, on the management of critically ill patients. Published studies have reported changes in management after TEE in 30% to 60% of patients,[17,20,156,157] leading to surgical interventions in 7% to 30%.[17,98,157,158] Impact varies depending on the type of ICU population being studied. Several studies have reported the clinical impact of urgent TEE in hemodynamically unstable patients.[157,159,160] In a prospective study of surgical ICU patients by Bruch and associates,[23] echocardiography altered management in 50 (43%) of 115 patients. Alterations in medical management induced by TEE included administration of fluids and initiation or discontinuation of inotropic agents, anticoagulants, or antibiotics. These findings are similar to findings reported in patients in medical or coronary care ICUs.[10,158] In a retrospective study done by Colreavy and associates[8] of a mixed medical and surgical ICU population, TEE findings led to a significant change in management in 32% of all studies performed. In a prospective study by Heidenreich and coworkers[161] of 61 critically ill patients with unexplained hypotension, new diagnoses not made with TTE were made in 17 patients (28%), leading to surgical intervention in 12 (20%). Prospective randomized trials to study the ultimate impact of bedside echocardiography on mortality and morbidity in the ICU are needed. Such studies would be difficult to do, however, given the growing use and importance of this technology in the critical care setting.

OTHER APPLICATIONS OF BEDSIDE ULTRASONOGRAPHY IN THE INTENSIVE CARE UNIT

CENTRAL LINE PLACEMENT

Central venous catheterization is performed frequently in critically ill patients. Placement of a central venous catheter is not without risk and can be associated with adverse events that are hazardous to patients and expensive to treat.[162-164] Complications can be seen in 15% to 20% of cases.[165-167] As described in a review by McGee and Gould,[168] complications related to central venous line placement are most often mechanical (arterial puncture, local hematoma, hemothorax, pneumothorax), infectious (catheter colonization and related bloodstream infection), and thrombotic. Complications are influenced by patient factors (obesity, coagulopathy, previous failed catheterization), site of attempted access, and operator experience.[169] As previously reported, only approximately 38% to 65% of patients are cannulated on the first attempt using a blind method.[170,171]

The use of ultrasound guidance during central venous catheterization has been well shown to reduce the risk of complications, mostly so for the internal jugular route. Ultrasound guidance also speeds catheter placement, decreases the number of attempts before successful placement, and

improves the overall rate of successful placement. Ultrasound can be used to help localize and define the anatomy of the vein with subsequent placement of the central venous catheter by the standard use of anatomic landmarks, at the site identified by ultrasound, with the knowledge that a vein is present, patent, and of adequate size. Ultrasound also can be used to provide real-time, two-dimensional ultrasound guidance to locate the vein and subsequently introduce the needle through the skin and into the vessel. Multiple studies have reported the superiority of ultrasound-assisted cannulation of the internal jugular vein in ICU patients compared with the external landmark–guided technique.[170-172] Trials looking at ultrasound guidance after failure by the landmark method reported success rates ranging from 33% to 100%.[169,173-175] A meta-analysis[175] of the literature comparing guidance using anatomic landmarks only versus guidance using ultrasound for the placement of central venous catheters indicates that ultrasound guidance significantly decreases placement failure by 64%, decreases related complications by 78%, and decreases the need for multiple placement attempts by 40%. Data showing superiority of the ultrasound guidance technique are consistent and strong for the internal jugular vein approach but less so for subclavian venous catheterization.[175-177]

Some patients can be identified in whom cannulation may be more difficult or in whom consequences of a complication could be more serious.[169] In these patients (Table 206-6), central venous cannulation may be laborious and risky, and ultrasound guidance should be considered. Hatfield and Bodenham[169] showed the benefit of portable ultrasound when central venous access was difficult. As suggested by this study and others,[178] ultrasound guidance is particularly beneficial when used in difficult cases or when a competent operator fails after a few attempts using surface landmarks.

Ultrasound guidance is useful for operators with varying levels of experience.[169,175] The technique is easy to learn and can be self-taught with some practical assistance from radiologists or other experienced sonographers.[169,179,180] Familiarity with the anatomy and equipment is easy to obtain safely at the bedside.

Most large vessels that are catheterized usually can be imaged by ultrasound. Different types of ultrasound modalities can be used to help guide central vessel cannulation, including two-dimensional ultrasound, Doppler transducer, Doppler with the probe in the needle, and fingertip pulse Doppler. With two-dimensional imaging, fluid, such as blood in vessels, is black because there is nearly complete

---

TABLE 206–6. CRITERIA FOR DIFFICULT CENTRAL VENOUS ACCESS

Limited access sites for attempts (e.g., local infection, other catheters present)

Difficult to identify surface landmarks (e.g., local swelling or deformity, severe obesity)

Previous complications (e.g., pneumothorax, arterial puncture)

Previous catheterization difficulties (e.g., multiple sites attempted, failure to gain access, >3 punctures at one site)

Uncorrected coagulopathy (APTT >1.5 ×; INR >>1.8; platelets <50,000/μL)

Patient unable to tolerate supine position

Known underlying vascular anomalies

APTT, activated partial thromboplastin time; INR, international normalized ratio.

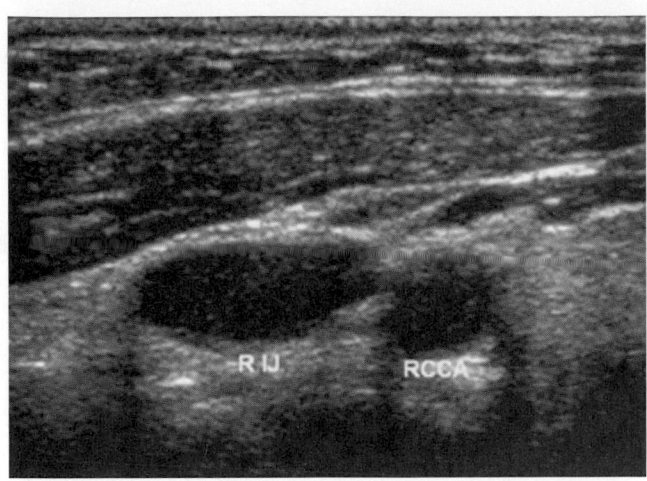

FIGURE 206–21. Transverse view of normal anatomy of the right internal jugular (RIJ) vein and right common carotid artery (RCCA). Ultrasound examination helps determine the anatomic relationship, size, and patency of the vessels. Knowledge of these important vessel characteristics helps determine if the anatomy is suitable for central vein catheterization at a low risk. If the vessel anatomy is normal and the operator is experienced, subsequent venous catheterization can be done by the surface landmark technique or under real-time ultrasound guidance. If high-risk characteristics are identified (see Table 206-6), however, real-time ultrasound guidance (or selection of a different access site) would be preferred. (Courtesy of Dr. Kurian Puthenpurayil.)

another (Fig. 206-21). The transverse and longitudinal views enable the sonographer to monitor in real time the passage of the needle through the skin and the anterior vessel wall. Ultrasound guidance also ensures detailed and accurate control of the needle (Fig. 206-22).[169]

During vessel examination, the sonographer specifically should assess the presence and patency of the vein (Fig. 206-23), the distensibility and compressibility of the vein, the position of the vein relative to the surrounding arteries (Fig. 206-24), and the presence of a thrombus in the vein (Fig. 206-25).[169] Ultrasound identification of certain anatomic characteristics, such as small vessel size (<5 mm), intraluminal thrombus, and anterior location of the artery relative to the vein, helps the physician to identify unfavorable vessel anatomy and so choose another catheterization site. A study by Levin and colleagues[182] showed that two-dimensional ultrasound guidance for the insertion of radial artery catheters was easy to use and increased the rate of success of insertion at first attempt. It was determined to be a useful adjunct to arterial catheter insertion. More studies are needed in the use of ultrasound for cannulation of peripheral arterial conduits.

transmission of ultrasound.[169] Color Doppler mode helps to delineate the flow patterns in the vessels. Doppler-only equipment that provides no images has shown equivocal results in studies of vascular access.[176,181]

With two-dimensional imaging, arteries are characteristically small, pulsatile, and difficult to compress with the probe.[169] Veins are usually larger, are nonpulsatile (except in the presence of severe tricuspid regurgitation), are easily compressible, and distend when the patient is placed with the head down or when a Valsalva maneuver is performed.[169]

Vessels can be examined in the transverse and longitudinal views. The transverse view permits identification of the vein and arteries based on the sonographic characteristics mentioned earlier and clarifies their positions relative to one

ASSESSMENT OF PLEURAL EFFUSIONS AND INTRA-ABDOMINAL FLUID COLLECTIONS

In critically ill patients, atelectasis and pleural effusions are frequent and often are present at the same time. Patients in the ICU are most often supine, and chest x-rays performed in this position offer limited sensitivity for the diagnosis of pleural effusion.[183] In many instances, neither atelectasis nor infiltration can be differentiated from pleural effusion. An alternative diagnostic method is needed to provide better results. Decubitus chest radiographs may show if fluid is free flowing, but this approach cannot localize or characterize the effusion precisely. CT of the chest shows the amount and distribution of fluid and is superior to plain lateral decubitus films. CT also can differentiate fluid from atelectasis and reveal information about the lung parenchyma. Chest CT requires transport to the radiology suite, however, which can be hazardous in unstable critically ill patients. Ultrasound examination of the pleural space has proved to be valuable

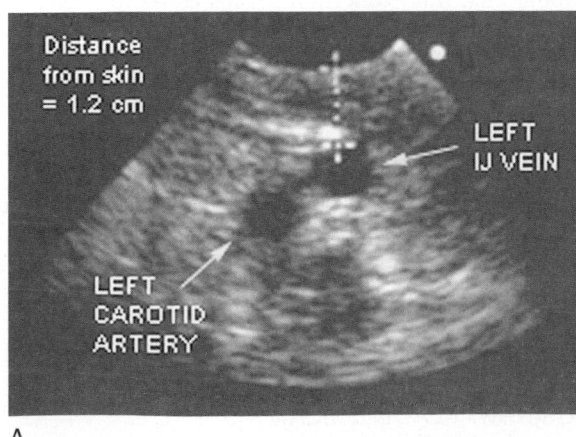

A

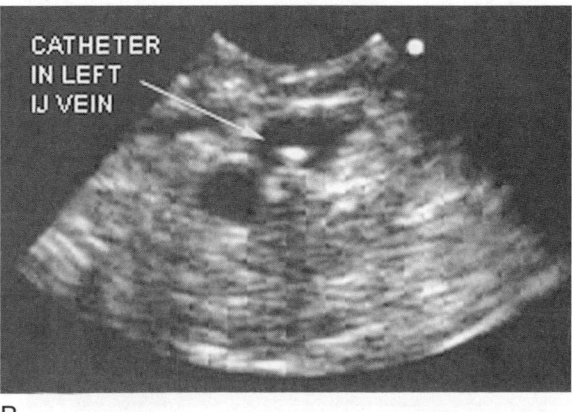

B

FIGURE 206–22. Transverse view of left carotid artery and left internal jugular (IJ) vein. The distance from the skin to the anterior wall of the vein is measured before insertion of a central venous catheter (A). Knowledge of this distance prevents the operator from going too deep with the needle when searching for the vein; this helps decrease the incidence of pneumothorax. After insertion, the catheter position in the jugular vein is confirmed (B).

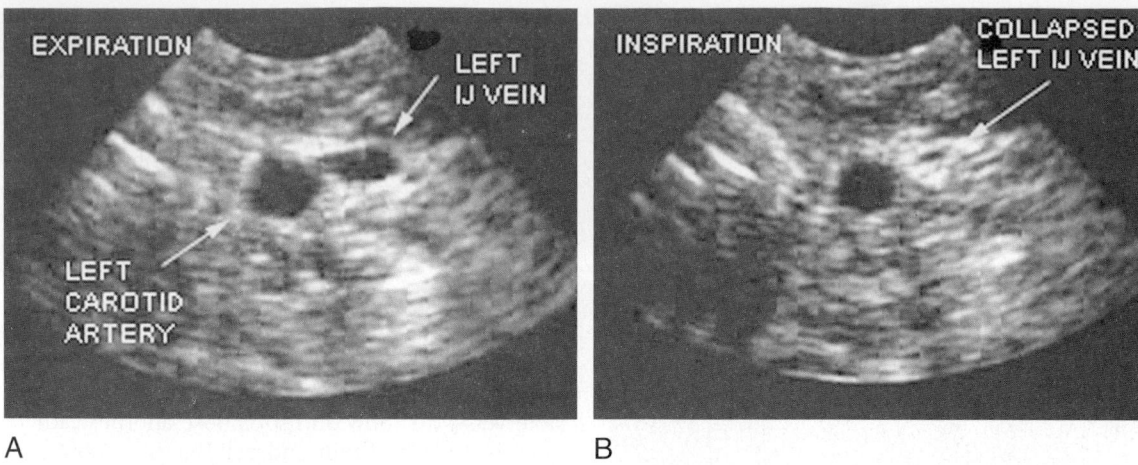

FIGURE 206–23. Transverse view of the left carotid and internal jugular (IJ) vein in a spontaneously breathing patient sitting in bed at a 30-degree angle. The patient was febrile and dehydrated. A near-total collapse of the vein (which is of small caliber) can be appreciated on inspiration *(B)* compared with expiration *(A)*.

for diagnosis of effusion.[184-188] The value of ultrasound for localizing fluid before catheter drainage or simple thoracentesis is well recognized. Ultrasound is especially valuable for localizing loculated or small effusions before a drainage procedure. In mechanically ventilated patients, blind thoracentesis can be hazardous, especially if the effusion is small or if the patient is on a high level of positive end-expiratory pressure.[189] Lichtenstein and coworkers[189] evaluated the feasibility and safety of ultrasound-aided thoracentesis in 40 mechanically ventilated patients. No complications occurred in the 45 ultrasound-aided thoracenteses, all performed by ICU physicians.

Basic skill required to detect a pleural effusion may be acquired in minutes and improves with experience.[190] In most instances, the pleural tap does not have to be done under real-time ultrasound guidance. A critically ill patient first must be positioned adequately on the back or on the side. Scanning of the pleural space is performed with the ultrasound probe. The probe must be oriented upward and downward, laterally and medially, and anteriorly and posteriorly so as to obtain a complete anatomic assessment of the area. The pleural fluid is usually hypoechogenic and appears black. The surrounding solid structures (soft tissue, diaphragm) and organs (lung, liver, heart, spleen) are visualized as structures with different degrees of echogenicity around the effusion (Fig. 206-26). The presence of aerated lung causes airy artifacts. Ribs usually yield artifactual anechoic images. When the effusion has been well assessed, one must determine the feasibility of safely doing a thoracentesis. One must check for the absence of interposition of lung, heart, liver, or spleen during the respiratory cycle[189] to avoid puncturing these organs, which potentially can cause catastrophic complications. When an optimal and safe position for thoracentesis has been determined, the skin should be marked and disinfected, and the patient should remain in the exact same position as was used during the ultrasound examination. Optimally the puncture should be done within seconds to minutes of the marking.

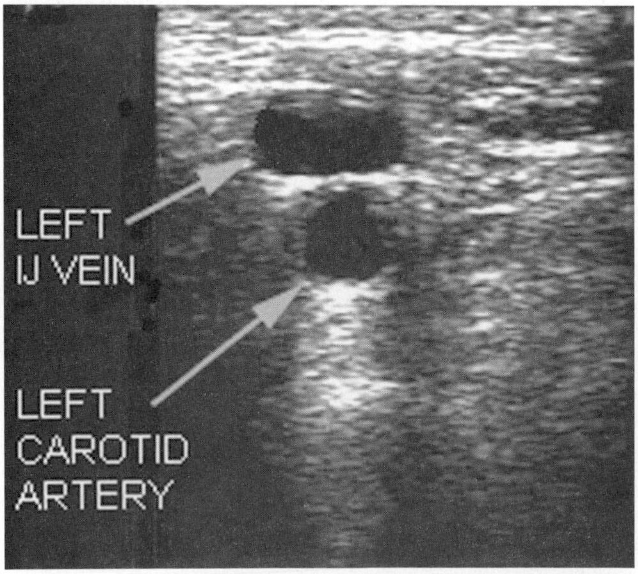

The same diagnostic and therapeutic procedures described earlier can be applied for intra-abdominal fluid collections in a critically ill patient. Evaluation for intra-abdominal fluid collection or abscess is restricted to areas that are not impeded by gas-filled structures[191] and include the regions around the liver and gallbladder, spleen, kidneys and lateral retroperitoneal areas, and pelvis around the uterus and bladder.[191] Fluid that does not change shape with probe pressure or patient positioning most likely represents a loculated collection.[191] Echogenic material and diffuse echoes on ultrasound within a fluid collection suggest the presence of particulate matter (e.g., fibrin or clots) and may represent an exudate or blood collection. As with pleural effusions, intra-abdominal fluid collections can be percutaneously sampled or drained safely at the bedside under real-time ultrasound guidance (Fig. 206-27).

URINARY BLADDER SCAN

Bladder-scanning devices are portable units that can provide a measurement of urine volume in the bladder (Fig. 206-28) and avoid bladder overdistention and reduce the need for unnecessary catheterization.[191,192] Studies have shown that

FIGURE 206–24. Transverse view of left internal carotid artery and left internal jugular (IJ) vein. Notice the relative position of the jugular vein directly overlying the carotid artery. This type of anatomy is common on the left side and, when present, significantly increases the risk of procedure failure or arterial puncture.

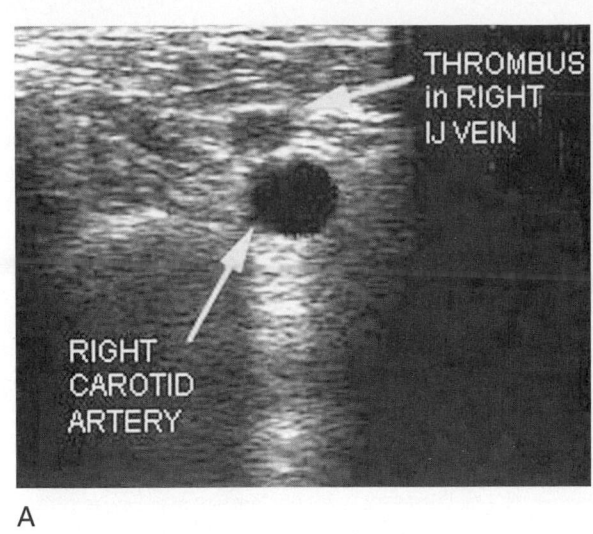

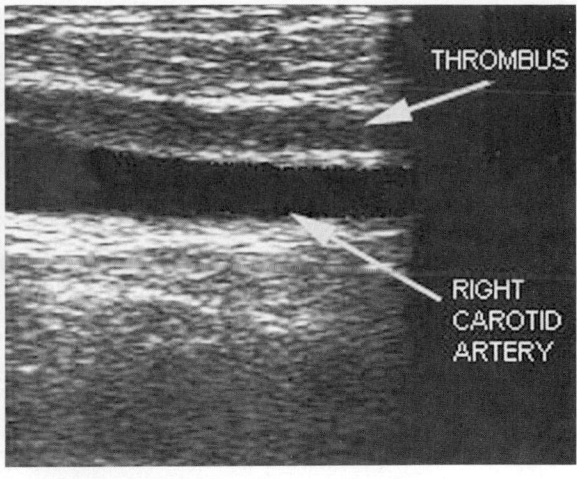

FIGURE 206–25. Transverse *(A)* and longitudinal *(B)* views of the right carotid artery and right internal jugular vein. Complete thrombosis of the right internal jugular (IJ) vein can be appreciated. Notice the small caliber of the thrombosed vein and the increased echogenicity of the thrombotic material within it. The vessel could not be compressed by probe pressure.

frequent catheterization is a major risk factor for urinary tract infections that can be costly to medical centers.[193-195] Use of a portable bladder-scanning device to reduce the incidence of nosocomial urinary tract infections was described by Moore and Edwards.[196] Bedside ultrasound assessment of volume in the urinary bladder also can be helpful in the evaluation of oliguria or anuria to rule out obstruction of the urinary catheter.

FOCUSED ASSESSMENT OF THE TRAUMA PATIENT

Since the early 1990s, bedside ultrasound has been used in the United States as an additional diagnostic modality for use in determining the presence of intra-abdominal injury after blunt trauma.[197] It is performed in the trauma bay during the secondary survey (as described in Advanced Trauma Life Support) or as part of the primary survey in hemodynamically unstable patients.[191,198-202] The focused assessment for sonographic examination of trauma (FAST) should be done with a specific purpose, usually identification of hemoperitoneum, hemothorax, or tamponade.[191] FAST seeks to determine the presence of fluid in four areas: (1) the subxiphoid region in the pericardial sac, (2) the right upper quadrant in Morison's pouch, (3) the left upper quadrant in the splenorenal recess, and (4) the pelvis in the pouch of Douglas or rectovesical space (Fig. 206-29).[19] Because the FAST examination is noninvasive and quickly

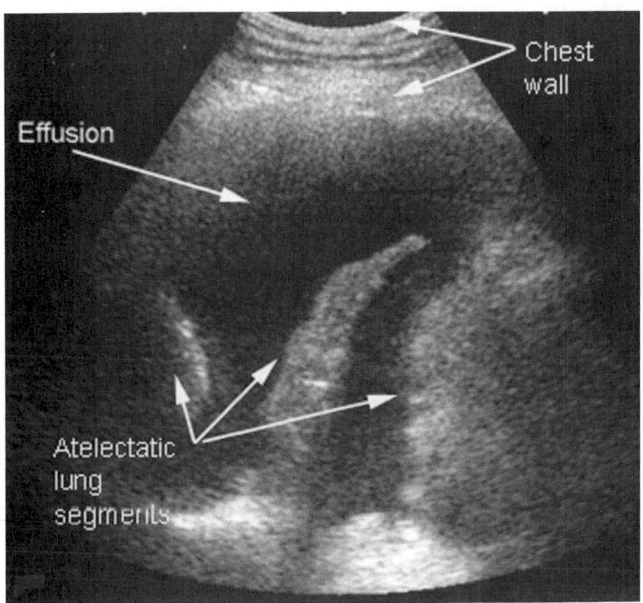

FIGURE 206–26. Transverse view of a right pleural effusion. Collapsed atelectatic lung is well visualized "floating" in the effusion. (Courtesy of Dr. Kurian Puthenpurayil.)

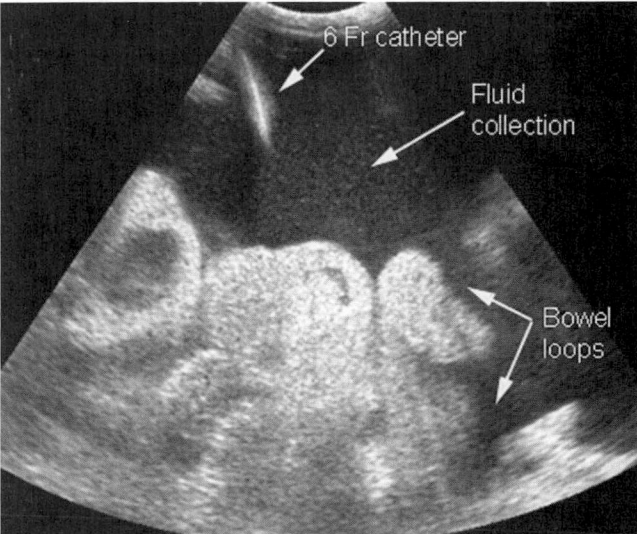

FIGURE 206–27. Transverse view of a left lower quadrant abdominal collection. Echogenic, particulate material can be seen floating in the collection. Loops of bowel also are well visualized. A 6 Fr catheter was inserted under ultrasound guidance to drain the collection, which was found to be chylous. Fluid collection with echogenic material and diffuse echoes on ultrasound are suggestive of particulate matter (e.g., fibrin or clots) and may represent an exudate or blood collection. (Courtesy of Dr. Kurian Puthenpurayil.)

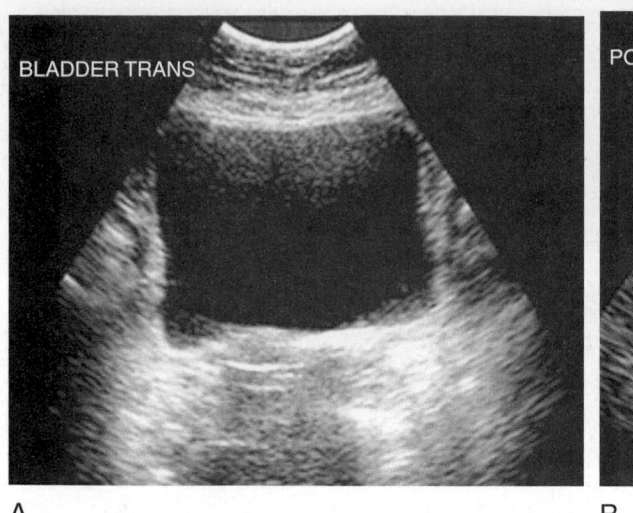

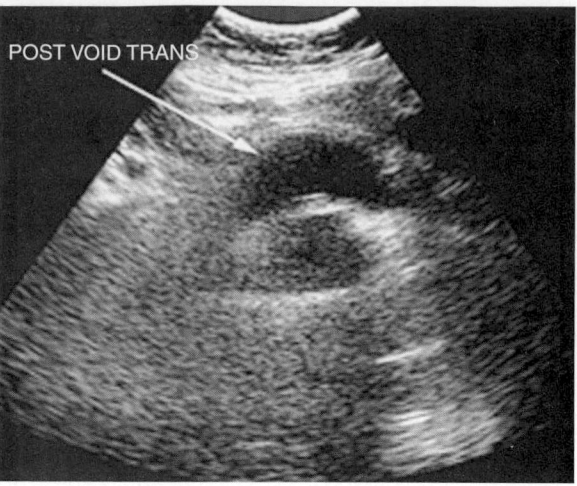

A   B

FIGURE 206–28. Urinary bladder. Suprapubic transverse view of a full urinary bladder *(A)*. This "square" appearance of the bladder with a concave superior wall is typical of a moderately full bladder. When overdistended (i.e., in the presence of a low urinary tract obstruction), the bladder is large and adopts a round, globulous shape (not shown). Suprapubic transverse view of an empty bladder *(B)*. When empty, the bladder can become small and commonly may be difficult to identify. (Courtesy of Dr. Kurian Puthenpurayil.)

performed at the bedside, it is ideal for detecting intra-abdominal injury in the resuscitation area. It has now been incorporated in the trauma resuscitation algorithm of most Level I trauma centers in the United States.[191,203]

Use of the FAST examination has been shown to diminish the need for more invasive diagnostic measures, such as diagnostic peritoneal lavage and subsequent exploratory laparotomy.[204,205] The FAST examination has been shown to be most accurate when performed for evaluation of hemodynamically unstable patients.[203,206-208] Studies have suggested that its use as a screening tool for blunt abdominal injury in hemodynamically stable trauma patients may result in underdiagnosis of intra-abdominal injuries.[202,203,209]

FIGURE 206–29. Focused assessment for sonographic examination of trauma (FAST). The FAST examination seeks to determine the presence of fluid in four areas: (1) the subxiphoid region in the pericardial sac, (2) the right upper quadrant in Morison's pouch, (3) the left upper quadrant in the splenorenal recess, and (4) the pelvis in the pouch of Douglas or rectovesical space.

INTRA-AORTIC BALLON COUNTERPULSATION

Bedside TEE may be helpful in different aspects of intra-aortic ballon counterpulsation management. Before insertion, TEE can rule out the presence of significant aortic regurgitation, which would represent a contraindication to intra-aortic ballon counterpulsation use. After insertion, TEE can confirm the position of the intra-aortic catheter in the descending thoracic aorta, ensure correct functioning of the balloon (visualization of inflation and deflation), and rule out the presence of important complications of aortic catheter insertion (e.g., aortic dissection). TEE also may be used for monitoring of the ventricular function while separating the patient from the intra-aortic ballon counterpulsation device.

VENTRICULAR ASSIST DEVICES

Different complications are likely to occur after ventricular assist device implantation, such as bleeding and hemodynamic instability. Maintenance of ventricular assist device flow is a key indicator of the overall status of the system. In the postoperative period, low ventricular assist device flow is usually due to hypovolemia and right ventricular dysfunction. TEE can be helpful for the diagnosis and monitoring of both of these conditions. Right ventricular failure has been shown to occur in approximately 20% to 25% of patients being supported with an isolated left ventricular assist device.[210] With prosthetic circulatory support devices, there can be dramatic changes in ventricular volumes and hemodynamic conditions and substantial direct and indirect changes to the contralateral ventricle due to ventricular interactions. TEE can help the clinician monitor and understand these ventricular interactions.[211] It also can help assess adequacy of flow and the patency of the inflow and outflow cannulas to eliminate the presence of a thrombus and collapse or displacement of the cannulas. It also can motivate an urgent return to the operating room if a cardiac tamponade is diagnosed. If hypoxemia supervenes in the ICU, the presence of a patent foramen ovale needs to be ruled out.

For patients placed on extracorporeal membranous oxygenation support, bedside TEE also can be used to monitor ventricular function during weaning of the circulatory assistance.

PERFORMANCE OF BEDSIDE ULTRASONOGRAPHY BY THE INTENSIVIST

In acute situations in the ICU, it may be difficult to have a cardiologist or sonographer available on immediate call on a 24-hour basis to perform a bedside ultrasound examination. The value of immediate bedside echocardiography for aiding in diagnosis and management of acute hemodynamic disturbances has been well shown in the literature in the ICU and the emergency department.[212,213]

Ultrasound technologies are not exclusive to the radiologist or cardiologist. Appropriately trained emergency department physicians, surgeons, anesthesiologists, and ICU specialists have been using ultrasound devices with great success. Anesthesiologists were instrumental in many of the pioneering studies of TEE in the operating room and the ICU.[4,22,214,215] Successful performance of bedside echocardiography by noncardiologist intensivists also has been well shown in the literature.[8,21,216] A study by Benjamin and colleagues[21] showed that a limited TEE examination performed and interpreted by intensivists (after training under the supervision of two cardiologists) is feasible and provides rapid, accurate diagnostic information that can have a dramatic impact on the treatment of critically ill patients.[21] The safety and utility of performance of bedside ultrasound by the intensivist for various other purposes in the ICU (central venous cannulation, thoracentesis, paracentesis) also have been well shown.[170-172,189]

With the increasing popularity of ultrasound devices, particularly lightweight, portable, hand-held devices, there is controversy regarding the advisability and the use of noncomprehensive "goal-directed" examinations performed by clinicians without cardiology or radiology training.[104] Studies with these portable devices, which provide basic two-dimensional and Doppler flow imaging, showed that they can provide important anatomic information,[216-220] but that, even in highly skilled hands, they may provide suboptimal imaging or diagnostic capabilities in the ICU.[218] Inappropriate interpretation or application of data gained by a poorly skilled user may result in adverse medical, ethical, and social consequences.[104] To avoid misusing the technology, adequate training is essential.

The era of a technology-extended physical examination[219] seems to have arrived, and there seems to be a role for a user-specific, focused ultrasound examination.[104,221] An examination said to be "targeted," "focused," and "limited" may often equate with "incomplete," "inadequate," or "inaccurate." Training must be individualized and tailored to specific needs, and appropriate user-specific application depends directly on the training and expertise of the user.[104] Provided that adequate expert back-up is available, the training of intensivists in performing "focused" or more comprehensive bedside ultrasound examinations is not only feasible, but also can be done safely and rapidly and yield information pertinent to the management of critically ill patients. General guidelines in training for TTE and TEE have been developed by the American Society of Echocardiography in association with the American Heart Association and the American College of Cardiology.[222] Since 1996, the American Society of Anesthesiologists and Society of Cardiovascular Anesthesiologists also have developed practice guidelines for perioperative TEE.[223] The importance of adequate training and subsequent maintenance of competence cannot be overemphasized because inappropriate use or misapplication potentially could temper the acceptance and limit the value of performance of bedside ultrasonography by the intensivist.

Training of intensivists and emergency department physicians in performance of emergency bedside ultrasonography should provide rapid answers to clinical questions that may strongly affect medical and surgical management decisions. As has been mentioned by different authors,[190,224] training in echocardiography and general ultrasonography should be incorporated in the critical care fellowship with special emphasis on TEE as part of the training program. It is hoped that critical care and echocardiographic societies will credential such additional training in the near future.

ANNOTATED REFERENCES

Benjamin E, Griffin K, Leibowitz AB, et al: Goal-directed transesophageal echocardiography performed by intensivists to assess left ventricular function: Comparison with pulmonary artery catheterization. J Cardiothorac Vasc Anesth 1998;12:10-15.

This prospective, blinded study shows that intensivists can be trained to perform limited-scope, goal-directed TEE rapidly and safely that can yield pertinent data for the management of a critically ill patient.

Colreavy FB, Donovan K, Lee KY, et al: Transesophageal echocardiography in critically ill patients. Crit Care Med 2002;30:989-996.

This retrospective study shows the safety and utility of TEE in the ICU when performed by appropriately trained intensive care physicians.

Goldhaber SZ: Echocardiography in the management of pulmonary embolism. Ann Intern Med 2002;136:691-700.

This article reviews the different utilities and limitations of echocardiography in the management of pulmonary embolism.

Lichtenstein D, Hulot JS, Rabiller A, et al: Feasibility and safety of ultrasound-aided thoracentesis in mechanically ventilated patients. Intensive Care Med 1999;25:955-958.

This prospective study done in critically ill patients illustrates that ultrasound localization makes thoracentesis a safe and easy procedure in patients on mechanical ventilation when a few basic rules are followed.

Yong Y, Wu D, Fernandes V, et al: Diagnostic accuracy and cost-effectiveness of contrast echocardiography on evaluation of cardiac function in technically very difficult patients in the intensive care unit. Am J Cardiol 2002;89:711-718.

This article compares use of harmonic imaging alone or in combination with contrast material with TEE in critically ill patients who were considered technically very difficult. It illustrates the significant impact of the use of contrast imaging in the ICU.

Judith Pepe

KEY POINTS

1. Multilumen catheters are not associated with an increased risk of infection compared with single-lumen catheters and can be used safely when infusion of multiple agents is required.

2. Peripherally inserted central catheters are becoming more useful in the care of critically ill patients, but their effectiveness compared with centrally inserted central venous catheters (CVCs) in this patient population needs to be determined.

3. Proper selection of catheter type and insertion site, operator experience, and vigilant attention to the details of insertion technique minimize the morbidity and mortality associated with CVCs.

4. The use of ultrasound to assist in the insertion of CVCs decreases complication rates associated with CVCs, particularly for less experienced operators and in sites other than the subclavian vein.

5. Antibiotic-coated catheters decrease the incidence of catheter colonization and catheter-related bloodstream infection.

Physicians in the United States perform central venous catheterization more than 5 million times every year.[1] Central venous catheterization has become one of the most frequent bedside procedures performed in ICUs, and complications related to it can be responsible for significant morbidity in a critically ill patient. It is estimated that 8% of all hospitalized patients have a CVC placed.[2] Strict adherence to the proper selection of appropriate patients, catheters, and insertion sites and the use of a systematic approach to catheter placement and management help minimize the complication rate, which has been reported to be 26%.[3]

INDICATIONS

To avoid complications, the placement of a CVC should occur only if the perceived goal of the procedure cannot be accomplished with peripheral catheters. A CVC may not be required if the only goal is volume resuscitation. Intravenous fluid can be infused more rapidly through a 2.5-inch, 16-gauge catheter than through a similar-diameter central catheter,[4] although an 8.5-Fr. catheter is most appropriate for rapid, massive volume resuscitation owing to the high flow rates achievable with this catheter. Placement of a peripheral venous catheter may be difficult in patients with hypovolemic and cardiogenic shock because of peripheral vasoconstriction. Volume resuscitation for shock and hypovolemia may be an indication for CVC placement in some patients. During cardiopulmonary resuscitation, administration of drugs peripherally is less effective than central administration,[5] and so CVC access is indicated in this instance. The infusion of agents that may irritate and sclerose peripheral veins, such as concentrated potassium chloride solutions, total parenteral nutrition solutions, parenteral chemotherapy agents, and vasopressors, should be administered through a CVC. Central venous pressure monitoring, pulmonary arterial pressure monitoring, emergency transvenous pacemaker insertion, hemodialysis, and plasmapheresis also are indications for the establishment of central venous access.

CONTRAINDICATIONS

There are no absolute contraindications to the establishment of central venous access in a patient as long as there are no restrictions on the choice of site to minimize potential complications. In the presence of severe coagulopathy or thrombocytopenia, the femoral vein is the preferred site because bleeding at this location is controlled easily with manual pressure. A peripherally inserted central catheter is also an alternative because of the ease with which bleeding can be controlled in the antecubital region. The subclavian vein should be avoided in coagulopathic patients because this vessel cannot be compressed manually. Although bleeding from the internal jugular vein can be easy to control, a large hematoma may result from multiple attempts at cannulation of this vein, and the airway can be compromised as a result. When the preferred sites are not accessible, reversal of the coagulopathy or thrombocytopenia with blood products allows for the safe cannulation of the subclavian or internal jugular veins.

Other relative contraindications to placement of a CVC include infection at the chosen site, the presence of an ipsilateral arteriovenous fistula for hemodialysis, venous thrombosis at or near the chosen site, and presence of an inferior vena cava filter.[6] If care is taken to avoid passage of the guidewire beyond 20 cm, entanglement with the inferior vena cava filter usually can be avoided.

TYPES OF CATHETERS

Several types of catheters are available for the purpose of central venous catheterization. CVCs can be single-lumen or multilumen, centrally inserted or peripherally inserted, coated with antibiotics, and temporary or long-term. Most long-term catheters, such as implantable ports and Groshong or Hickman catheters, are placed surgically and tunneled subcutaneously. These devices do not have a role in the acute care of critically ill patients. Subcutaneous tunneling, which is known to decrease the rate of catheter infection, is not practiced routinely for the placement of the temporary, shorter, percutaneously placed catheters commonly used in the ICU. Tunneling was shown to be ineffective for decreasing the rate of infection in short-term catheters.[7]

Because of the complexity of most critically ill patients, catheters with multiple lumens generally are required for the infusion of multiple agents that often are not mutually compatible. Centrally delivered total parenteral nutrition solutions require a dedicated port and typically are delivered through a triple-lumen catheter. Because multilumen catheters have more hubs and are subject to more manipulations than single-lumen catheters, it is surmised that they are associated with a higher risk of catheter-related bloodstream infection. Several clinical trials that have directly compared rates of catheter-related bloodstream infection between single-lumen and multilumen catheters have reported mixed results, however.[8-11] A meta-analysis found that catheter-related bloodstream infection was more common with multilumen catheters.[12] When the authors eliminated the lower quality studies, however, multilumen catheters were not found to have a statistically significant higher rate of catheter-related bloodstream infection.

Cardiologists have used peripherally inserted central catheters since the 1940s.[13] Typically, these catheters are inserted by radiologists or specially trained nurses via the basilic or cephalic veins in the antecubital fossa. Their use was expanded to patients who needed long-term access for chemotherapy or parenteral nutrition.[14,15] These catheters were recognized for their potential for causing thrombosis, and subsequently interest in their application waned.[16] To reduce costs and the mechanical complications associated with centrally inserted central catheters, peripherally inserted CVCs again gained favor.[17,18] These catheters now are made of polyurethane and have been reported to have relatively lower thrombogenicity than in the past. A report of 1273 peripherally inserted central catheters placed in non-ICU patients showed a 2.8% incidence of thrombosis and an overall complication rate of 4.7%.[19] Smith and colleagues[13] challenged the superiority of peripherally inserted central catheters over CVCs, however, because of higher rates of thrombosis and other complications with the former. These data were obtained in a retrospective study and compared surgically placed, tunneled catheters in non-ICU patients with peripherally inserted central catheters. Because of their ease of placement and lower rate of pneumothorax, peripherally inserted central catheters are gaining popularity as an alternative to centrally placed CVCs in critically ill patients.[20] Whether peripherally inserted central catheters should supplant centrally placed CVCs is not known. The advantages and disadvantages of peripherally inserted central catheters are listed in Table 207-1.

A variety of adaptations in the composition of catheters have been marketed as ways to decrease the incidence of catheter-related bloodstream infection. Migration of skin organisms along the catheter has long been recognized as a significant source of infection. An attachable subcutaneous

TABLE 207–1. ADVANTAGES AND DISADVANTAGES OF PERIPHERALLY INSERTED CENTRAL CATHETERS

Advantages	Disadvantages
Low complexity of placement	Inadequate for central pressure monitoring
Quick	
Can last for weeks to months	Inadequate for rapid bolus injection
Low infection rate	
Low complication rate	Inadequate for rapid fluid resuscitation
Can be used in ambulatory setting	
Low cost	
High patient tolerance	
Obviates need for multiple peripheral catheters	

cuff made of biodegradable collagen impregnated with bactericidal silver (Vita Cuff; Vitaphore Corp, Menlo Park, CA) was developed to address this. Results in prospective, randomized trials have been mixed,[21,22] and its use never truly became widespread. Antibiotic-coated and antibiotic-impregnated CVCs also were introduced as means to decrease catheter-related bloodstream infection. The commercially available CVCs of this type now are treated intraluminally and extraluminally with either chlorhexidine/silver sulfadiazine (ARROWgard Blue; Arrow International, Reading, PA) or rifampin/minocycline (Cook Bio-Guard Spectrum; Cook Critical Care, Bloomington, IN). This treatment of the CVC addresses the mechanism of hub contamination and skin contamination at the insertion site. Most clinical trials with chlorhexidine/silver sulfadiazine–coated catheters have shown a significant reduction in colonization and reduced rates of catheter-related bloodstream infection compared with nontreated catheters.[23-25] Only one study showed a statistically significant decrease in catheter-related bloodstream infection.[26] A meta-analysis of 13 randomized trials comparing chlorhexidine/silver sulfadiazine–coated catheters with noncoated catheters showed a statistically significant advantage of the coated catheters, however, with respect to the reduction of catheter-related bloodstream infection.[27] Catheters coated with rifampin/minocycline also are effective in preventing catheter-related bloodstream infection and catheter colonization.[28,29] When these two types of antibiotic-coated catheters were compared with each other, there was a statistically significant improvement in the rates of catheter colonization and of catheter-related bloodstream infection and cost effectiveness with the rifampin/minocycline–coated catheter.[29-32] This difference is likely due to internal and external coating of this catheter, whereas the chlorhexidine/silver sulfadiazine–coated catheter only more recently has been treated internally and externally and has not yet been subjected to a trial comparing it with the rifampin/minocycline catheter. Although development of bacterial resistance has not been problematic, there have been sporadic case reports of anaphylactic reactions in patients with unsuspected allergies to chlorhexidine who received chlorhexidine/silver sulfadiazine–coated catheters.[33,34] The use of these specially treated catheters probably is best limited to patients at high risk for developing catheter-related bloodstream infection and in whom the anticipated length of catheterization is greater than 7 to 10 days.

INSERTION TECHNIQUE

The insertion of CVCs can be accomplished by a cutdown approach or percutaneously. The cutdown approach uses the cephalic, external jugular, internal jugular, or femoral veins for central access. Surgical cutdown also can be performed on the veins of the antecubital fossa to establish central venous access peripherally. Although direct access to the vein via cutdown virtually eliminates complications such as pneumothorax, hemothorax, and chylothorax,[35] a surgeon and costly operating room time are required for this approach, and the risk of such complications is so low with today's percutaneous approach that most practitioners access the central veins percutaneously. The first report of using the percutaneous method to access the central veins came from Aubaniac,[36] who, in 1952, described the use of CVCs for rapid fluid resuscitation of injured soldiers during World War II. The Seldinger technique has become the standard approach for percutaneous central venous catheterization. This technique, in which a guidewire placed through the access needle guides the passage of a catheter into the vein, was first described by Seldinger as a means of obtaining arterial access for angiography.[37]

When it has been established that the chosen catheter type is indicated, the operator should obtain informed consent from the patient or the health care proxy based on a discussion of the benefits, risks, and alternatives to percutaneous central venous catheterization. Distinct consent for this procedure may not be necessary if the procedure falls under the hospital's global consent obtained on admission. Obtaining separate informed consent is not always possible when emergency central venous access is required. Ideally the most experienced physician of the team should perform the procedure because mechanical complications are diminished with increased experience with the procedure.[38,39] Proper site selection is also paramount for minimizing the risk of mechanical complications associated with the procedure. Common sense dictates that sites where previous access attempts have failed or where there is skeletal deformity, previous surgery, radiation, or scarring should be avoided if possible.[39]

It is not clear whether any of the centrally located access sites are superior in decreasing the risk of mechanical complications. A meta-analysis comparing the internal jugular approach with subclavian access showed that internal jugular access was associated with significantly more arterial punctures but fewer problems related to malpositioning of the catheter.[2] There were no valid randomized trials that could be included in this analysis, however. No differences in the rate of mechanical complications were found in a study that compared femoral vein cannulation with subclavian vein cannulation,[40] but catheters placed via the femoral vein may have a higher incidence of malpositioned catheters.[41] The safest approach is to consider the clinician's own experience and comfort with the chosen site, along with the patient's body habitus and clotting ability. The use of ultrasound to guide insertion may be beneficial in improving rates of successful cannulation, particularly when accessing the internal jugular vein[42-45] or when operators are inexperienced.[44,45] For experienced operators placing subclavian catheters it may not be helpful and may add significantly to the length of the procedure.[46,47]

For catheter placement, the patient is positioned supine. Placement of a roll vertically between the shoulder blades for subclavian access is recommended because it opens up the deltopectoral triangle and allows more parallel access to the vein. A roll should be placed horizontally across the shoulder blades for internal jugular access to hyperextend the neck, which makes the vein easier to access. Slight Trendelenburg positioning to 10 or 15 degrees also is helpful to dilate the central veins. The reverse Trendelenburg position may be helpful for femoral vein access and may facilitate central chest or neck vein access in a morbidly obese patient because it allows the chest wall to fall away from the insertion site. It is not recommended to use reverse Trendelenburg positioning for central neck or chest vein access in a hypovolemic morbidly obese patient, however.

The entire procedure should be done under sterile conditions using maximal barrier precautions because this has been shown to decrease significantly the rate of catheter infection.[48] The literature convincingly supports the recommendation that the operator should always don gown, mask, cap, and gloves and carry out meticulous sterile preparation of the area, preferably with 2% chlorhexidine.[49] Towels are used to square off the sterile area, and a larger sterile area should be established with the use of large drapes. The use of the single, small, paper drape with a central opening as the sole means of establishing the sterile field is strongly discouraged.

The Seldinger technique is the standard approach used regardless of catheter type or site of insertion. The approach for each site is depicted in Figures 207-1 through 207-5. After adequate local anesthesia has been established, the needle is inserted slowly at the appropriate landmark for the chosen site (Table 207-2), while maintaining slight negative pressure on the syringe barrel. Using a smaller finder needle first is often helpful for the internal jugular vein, but a small needle is usually too short to be used for the approach to the subclavian vein. A flash of venous blood into the syringe confirms the entrance of the needle into the vein. The syringe is removed from the needle, and a guidewire is passed through the needle into the vein to a maximal length of 20 cm (corresponding approximately to the atriocaval junction). Most guidewires are marked at this point. The needle should be introduced with the beveled edge downward to encourage the caudad passage of the wire when accessing the subclavian vein. The needle is removed carefully over the wire, leaving the guidewire in place. The operator maintains manual control of the wire at all times.

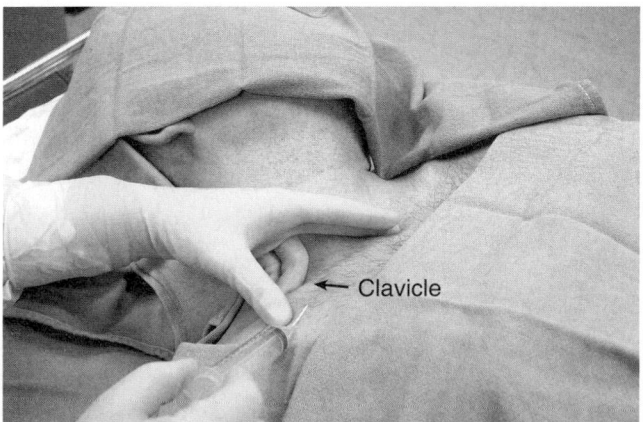

FIGURE 207–1. Infraclavicular approach to subclavian vein.

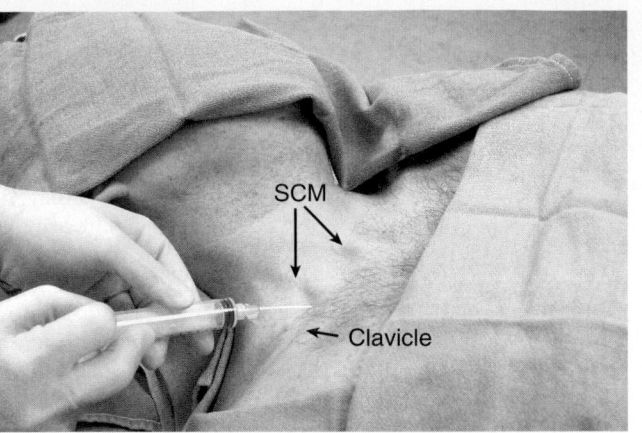

FIGURE 207-2. Supraclavicular approach to subclavian vein. SCM, sternocleidomastoid.

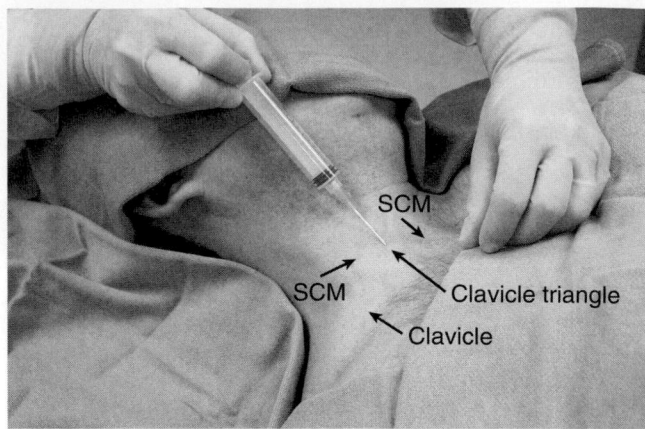

FIGURE 207-3. Middle approach to internal jugular vein. SCM, sternocleidomastoid.

A 0.5-cm skin incision is created with a No. 11 blade at the wire insertion site, followed by the passage and withdrawal of a dilator. Bleeding from the site can occur after this step, and intermittent control with gauze may be necessary. The catheter is inserted into the vein over the guidewire up to a maximal distance of 20 cm, then the guidewire is withdrawn. The distance the catheter should be inserted to ensure placement at the atriocaval junction depends on the site of cannulation.[50] Table 207-3 lists the proper maximal distances according to insertion site. Placement of the catheter into the vein should stop any bleeding that may have emanated from around the guidewire. If a Cordis catheter is being placed, the dilator and the catheter are introduced over the guidewire simultaneously because the Cordis catheter by itself is too flexible for successful placement. Aspiration of blood from all ports of the catheter confirms its intravenous location. Connecting a short length of transducer tubing to the needle prior to inserting the Seldinger wire while observing a central venous pressure wave is another way to confirm the intravenous position of the catheter. Rapid capping of all ports must occur to prevent air embolus. All ports are flushed with saline or heparin solution, and the catheter is secured to the skin with sutures. Finally, a dressing of either sterile gauze or sterile, transparent, semipermeable bandage is placed to minimize the incidence of catheter-related infection.[51] A chest x-ray should be obtained to confirm proper catheter position at the atrial-caval junction and to rule out any intrathoracic complications.

COMPLICATIONS

According to the U.S. Food and Drug Administration, overall reported complication rates of CVCs are 10%.[52] Factors that are known to influence complication rates include site of catheter insertion, side of insertion, intravascular volume depletion, emergency placement, coagulopathy, and distortion of normal anatomic landmarks. Complications can be grouped into three categories: mechanical, infectious, and thrombotic/embolic (Table 207-4).

Mechanical complications are usually the direct result of the procedure and can be recognized within a short time of catheter placement. One of the most common complications reported is atrial arrhythmia; the incidence of this complication is 41%.[53] Most arrhythmias are clinically inconsequential, and the incidence of malignant ventricular arrhythmias is low. This complication is preventable because it is the direct result of the guidewire or catheter being advanced too far.

Arterial puncture is another commonly reported mechanical complication and occurs most often with femoral and internal jugular vein cannulation.[3] Approaching the subclavian vein too far laterally along the clavicle increases the risk of subclavian artery puncture. Bleeding from the subclavian

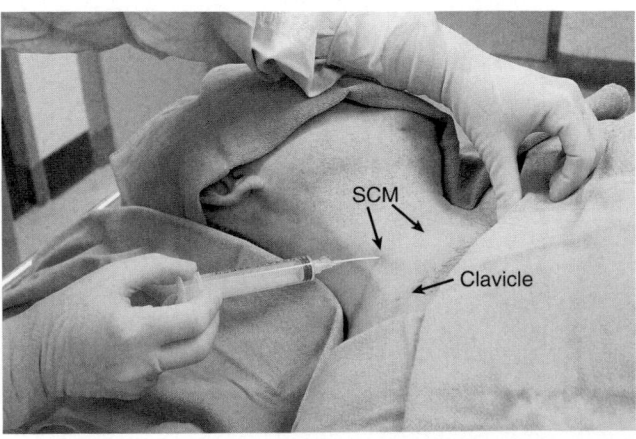

FIGURE 207-4. Posterior approach to internal jugular vein. SCM, sternocleidomastoid.

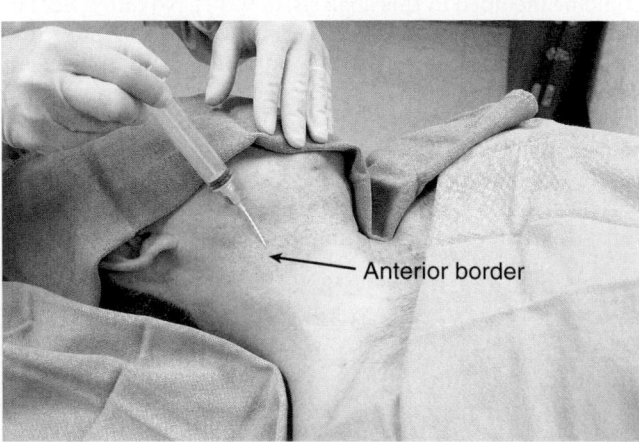

FIGURE 207-5. Anterior approach to internal jugular vein.

TABLE 207–2. LANDMARKS AND TECHNIQUES FOR CENTRAL VENOUS CATHETERIZATION

	Subclavian		Internal jugular			Femoral
	Infraclavicular	Supraclavicular	Anterior	Middle	Posterior	
Position	Trendelenburg Head turned to opposite side Ipsilateral arm adducted	Trendelenburg Head turned to opposite side Ipsilateral arm adducted	Trendelenburg Head turned to opposite side	Trendelenburg Head turned to opposite side	Trendelenburg Head turned to opposite side	Supine with thigh in slight abduction
Needle insertion	2 cm inferior to midportion of clavicle, "walk" down clavicle and advance just deep to clavicle	Just above clavicle lateral to clavicular head of SCM	Anterior border of SCM midway between angle of mandible and clavicle	Apex of triangle formed by two heads of SCM	Posterior border of SCM midway between angle of mandible and clavicle	Medial to femoral artery pulsation at junction of middle and distal thirds of distance between pubic tubercle and ASIS
Angle of needle	Advance needle under clavicle toward sternal notch	Advance needle at 45-degree angle just under clavicle toward contralateral nipple	Advance needle toward medial aspect of ipsilateral nipple at 30- to 45-degree angle	Advance needle toward ipsilateral nipple at 30- to 45-degree angle	Advance needle toward sternal notch at 30-degree angle	Advance needle toward umbilicus at 30- to 45-degree angle

ASIS, anterior superior iliac spine; SCM, sternocleidomastoid.

artery is difficult to control with direct pressure. A large extrapleural hematoma or clinically significant hemothorax may result from subclavian artery injury. Control of carotid or femoral artery injury usually is accomplished with direct pressure. If the injury is due to the placement of a large-bore catheter (>8 Fr.) or if coagulopathy exists, surgical control may be necessary. A large, rapidly expanding hematoma in the neck may cause airway compromise as well. The incidence of pneumothorax is 1% to 3% in published reports.[2,39,40] Most pneumothoraces due to central venous catheterization are small (<30%) and, unless the patient is receiving positive-pressure mechanical ventilation, can be managed expectantly with close observation and a follow-up chest x-ray. Pneumothorax occurs less often from internal jugular compared with subclavian vein cannulation and is more likely to occur after left subclavian vein attempts owing to the more cephalad position of the apex of lung on that side. Mediastinal or subcutaneous air may be the only indication that there has been violation of the pleura. In the setting of mechanical ventilation, pneumothorax can be deadly. Any hemodynamic instability that occurs during placement of an internal jugular or subclavian venous catheter should raise the suspicion of tension pneumothorax, and thoracic decompression should be accomplished without delay.

Air embolus is rare with a reported incidence of 0.1%[54] and can occur on catheter insertion or removal or during opening of the catheter hub to air. This potentially devastating complication is preventable if care is taken to use the Trendelenburg position, preflush the catheter with saline, and cap off any unused ports before insertion. Using the head-down position and rapid occlusion of the exit

site helps minimize air embolus during catheter removal. Maneuvers to perform in cases of suspected venous air embolism include placing the patient in steep Trendelenburg position with the left side down, administering 100% oxygen, and providing hemodynamic support, if necessary. Aspiration of air from the catheter in situ may be attempted, but it may not be successful.

Catheter malposition, defined as inappropriate position of the catheter tip, can be detected if present in 100% of cases if a chest x-ray is always taken postprocedure. When catheter malposition is detected, it must be remedied either by pulling the catheter back and resuturing it or exchanging the catheter at the bedside over a guidewire (possibly with fluoroscopic guidance). Catheter occlusion, venous thrombosis, venous embolism, venous perforation with hemothorax or infusion of intravenous solution into the mediastinum, or right atrial perforation with tamponade may occur if the catheter tip does not lie properly parallel within the lumen of the superior vena cava. Venous or cardiac perforation also

TABLE 207–3. LENGTH OF CATHETER INSERTION

Site	Distance from skin insertion site (cm)
Right internal jugular	16
Right subclavian	18
Left internal jugular	19
Left subclavian	20

TABLE 207–4. COMPLICATIONS OF CENTRAL VENOUS CATHETERS

Mechanical	Infectious	Thrombotic/embolic
Atrial arrhythmia	Septic thrombophlebitis	Deep venous thrombosis
Ventricular arrhythmia	Catheter-related infection	Pulmonary emboli
Arterial puncture	Catheter-related sepsis	Systemic emboli
Hematoma		Catheter occlusion
Hemothorax		
Pneumothorax		
Air embolus		
Catheter malposition		
Venous perforation		
Cardiac perforation		
Cardiac tamponade		
Thoracic duct injury		
Chylothorax		
Arteriovenous fistula formation		
Tracheal injury		
Nerve injury		

can occur during the procedure. Perforation of a vessel usually is caused by the stiffer dilator or sheath's failure to follow the course of the guidewire. Ensuring that the wire always moves easily within the dilator or sheath can help prevent this complication.

Femoral, subclavian, and internal jugular vein wires can become entangled with vena caval filter devices.[55] The thoracic duct, which enters the venous system near the junction of the left subclavian and left internal jugular veins, can be injured during cannulation of these veins on the left side. Injury usually goes unnoticed until a pleural effusion, representing a chylothorax, becomes evident on subsequent chest x-rays. This complication usually is managed with drainage and dietary restriction but may require surgical ligation for definitive control. Other mechanical complications include arteriovenous fistula formation and injury to the trachea or nerves such as the brachial plexus and femoral, phrenic, vagus, and cranial nerves.

Thrombosis and embolus can occur as a result of catheter placement. Most of the data known about catheter-related thrombosis come from studies about surgically placed, tunneled CVCs in oncologic and pediatric patients. In patients with malignancies, the rate of catheter-related thrombosis has been reported to be 36%.[35] Upper extremity deep venous thrombosis represents 15% of deep venous thromboses in the ICU; virtually all are related to subclavian or internal jugular venous cannulation.[56] The risk of deep venous thrombosis is much greater with femoral and internal jugular vein catheters than with subclavian vein catheters,[40,57] although reports of higher incidence in subclavian veins also exist.[58] Risk factors for the development of catheter-related thrombosis include internal jugular route, absence of systemic heparinization, and infusion of a lipid emulsion.[57] Even though most catheter-related thrombosis may be asymptomatic,[58] it is still important to make the diagnosis and treat it because of the associated 10% risk of pulmonary embolism.[35] Catheter-related thrombosis in surgically placed, tunneled catheters may not necessitate removal of the catheter, but rather can be managed by infusing thrombolytic agents.[35,59] For a critically ill patient, systemic anticoagulation should be initiated, and the offending catheter should be removed unless no other site exists for CVC replacement. In such cases, serial duplex scanning may be useful to detect propagation of the clot, a finding that would necessitate catheter removal. Malpositioning of the catheter tip also is associated with deep venous thrombosis, most likely related to repeated local injury to the venous endothelium or proximal positioning, where venous flow is slower. Other catheter-related factors affecting the risk of deep venous thrombosis include catheter material, catheter diameter, and site of entry. Older polyethylene catheters were stiffer and more thrombogenic than the polyurethane and silicone catheters used today.[60]

SUMMARY

CVCs play an important role in the management of critically ill patients. Safe placement is maximized by the proper choice of patient, site, and catheter type and strict adherence to a systematic approach to insertion. Vigilance toward detection of complications minimizes morbidity.

ANNOTATED REFERENCES

Darouche RO, Raad II, Heard SO, et al: A comparison of two antimicrobial-impregnated central venous catheters. N Engl J Med 1999;340:1-8.

This prospective, randomized, multicenter study showed that use of CVCs impregnated with minocycline and rifampin results in lower catheter colonization and catheter-related bloodstream infection rates than use of catheters impregnated with chlorhexidine and silver sulfadiazine. The superiority of the minocycline/rifampin catheter may be due to its dual coating of the internal and external surfaces, whereas the chlorhexidine/silver sulfadiazine catheter used in the study was coated only on its external surface.

McGee DC, Gould MK: Preventing complications of central venous catheterization. N Engl J Med 2003;348:1123-1133.

This review article details the types of catheters, insertion sites, and insertion techniques that should be used to minimize the complications that can occur as a result of central venous catheterization. To minimize mechanical complications, the authors recommend an experienced operator, use of ultrasound guidance, and avoidance of routine catheter changes.

Merrer J, DeJonghe B, Golliot F, et al: Complications of femoral and subclavian venous catheterization in critically ill patients: A randomized controlled trial. JAMA 2001;286:700-707.

This prospective, randomized, multicenter study of 289 patients showed similar mechanical complication rates in femoral and subclavian venous catheters. The femoral catheters had a statistically significantly higher rate of thrombotic and infectious complications.

Randolph AG, Cook DJ, Gonzales CA, et al: Ultrasound guidance for placement of central venous catheters: A meta-analysis of the literature. Crit Care Med 1996;24:2053-2058.

This meta-analysis of eight randomized, controlled trials on the use of ultrasound guidance for the placement of CVCs showed that ultrasound significantly reduced the number of complications and catheter placement attempts compared with the landmark technique. Most of the studies were of internal jugular catheter placements.

Ruesch S, Walder B, Tramer MR: Complications of central venous catheters: Internal jugular versus subclavian access—a systematic review. Crit Care Med 2002;30:454-460.

This meta-analysis of 2085 internal jugular catheters and 2428 subclavian catheters from 17 prospective, nonrandomized trials showed the internal jugular approach to have more arterial punctures but fewer catheter malpositions. There was no difference in the rates of hemothorax or pneumothorax between the two approaches. Selection bias may be a factor in these findings, and caution is urged before using these results as the sole basis to dictate clinical practice.

Chapter 208

ARTERIAL CANNULATION AND INVASIVE BLOOD PRESSURE MEASUREMENT

Phillip D. Levin • Yaacov Gozal

KEY POINTS

INSERTION SITE AND EQUIPMENT

1. The common sites of arterial line insertion are the radial, femoral, and dorsalis pedis arteries. These arteries are superficial, covered only by skin, fascia, and fat and are easily compressible.

2. The arterial line can be inserted using a simple catheter-over-needle arrangement (with or without a guidewire) or a set based on the Seldinger technique.

3. Guidewires should only be used when back flow of blood is present to avoid arterial damage.

4. Doppler or ultrasound can be helpful for difficult line insertion.

5. Errors in pressure measurement can arise from incorrect zeroing, overshoot, or damping.

6. When zeroing, the height difference between the arterial puncture site and the transducer must be taken into account.

7. Overshoot and damping affect the systolic blood pressure more than the diastolic or mean pressure.

8. The fast flush test can be used to assess underdamping or overdamping.

9. Low-concentration heparin is the most common arterial line flush solution. Sodium citrate, papaverine, and saline have been used.

VASCULAR AND LOCAL COMPLICATIONS

1. Arterial obstruction is very common after catheter insertion, although rarely detrimental.

2. Obstruction may be mechanical from the catheter or result from thrombosis.

3. Small arteries, female gender, and shock are risk factors for thrombosis.

4. Pain, weakness, changes in sensation, pallor, or decreased temperature should prompt immediate catheter removal.

ERRONEOUS BLOOD TESTS

1. The majority of blood tests obtained from the arterial line will be accurate.

2. The type of flush solution used may interfere with certain tests.

3. Particular care should be taken when interpreting the activated partial thromboplastin time and blood culture results in samples drawn from the arterial line.

4. Five to six times the deadspace volume might be required for accurate tests, which may be reinfused with appropriate precautions.

ANEMIA, HEPARIN-INDUCED THROMBOCYTOPENIA, AND INFECTION

1. Anemia can result from the volumes of blood drawn from the arterial line. Simple steps can reduce this blood loss.

2. Heparin-induced thrombocytopenia (HIT) is a syndrome defined by thrombocytopenia and thrombotic events in the presence of heparin/platelet factor 4 (PF4) complex antibodies.

3. Even very small doses of heparin can induce or maintain HIT. All sources of heparin should be removed if HIT is suspected, including from arterial line flush.

4. The rate of bloodstream infections related to the arterial line has been estimated to be 2.9 per 1000 catheter-days, whereas 1.5 in 100 arterial catheters cause infection.

5. Insertion technique, duration of cannulation, site, insertion site, and frequency of set changes have all been related to an increased infectious risk.

6. Comparisons of studies relating to infectious risk are difficult owing to differing definitions of infection and study methodology.

7. The Centers for Disease Control and Prevention recommends: Use a 2% chlorhexidine solution for skin cleaning, do not change arterial catheters routinely, change the pressure monitoring sets and transducers every 96 hours, and do not use dextrose-containing flush solution.

Peripheral artery cannulation is one of the most commonly performed invasive procedures in the ICU,[1] and the resulting arterial line is an integral part of intensive care patient management. There are three main indications for arterial line insertion: (1) to allow continuous beat-to-beat monitoring of blood pressure; (2) to provide pain-free, convenient, and repeated access to arterial blood for the assessment of pulmonary and cardiovascular function; and (3) to provide a source of blood for blood tests as required without the need for repeated venipuncture. A review of the relevant anatomy, equipment, and techniques for arterial line placement is provided in this chapter along with some of the more common complications.

SITES OF INSERTION

An arterial line can be inserted into almost any palpable peripheral artery. The most common sites in clinical practice are the radial artery (employed in up to 78% of ICU patients[2,3]), the femoral artery (employed in up to 45%[2,3]), and the dorsalis pedis artery. Axillary and ulnar artery cannulation are performed somewhat more rarely; brachial and temporal artery cannulation is not recommended. Cannulation of the carotid arteries is absolutely contraindicated for obvious reasons. Each arterial site has advantages and disadvantages.

THE RADIAL AND ULNAR ARTERIES

The radial artery originates in the antecubital fossa at the level of the neck of the radius as a terminal branch of the brachial artery. The artery runs down the length of the forearm laterally. For the distal part of its course it is covered only by fascia and skin and lies above the radius, where it is easily palpated. At the level of the wrist the artery winds laterally around the radius and enters the posterior aspect of the hand. It terminates by dividing into the superficial and deep palmar arches, which are anastomoses with the ulnar artery. The radial artery lies near the superficial branch of the radial nerve in its distal course.

The ulnar artery is the other terminal branch of the brachial artery, also originating in the antecubital fossa at the level of the radial neck. It is usually larger than the radial artery. The ulnar artery runs medially along the length of the forearm. As opposed to the radial artery, for most of its course the ulnar artery lies deep to the muscles of the forearm, becoming superficial only toward the wrist. The ulnar artery lies close to the ulnar nerve in its distal course.

When compared with the ulnar artery, the radial artery is superficial for a longer part of its course, is easily palpated above the radius, and is less closely associated with neural structures. It is, however, a smaller artery. The radial artery is cannulated within a few centimeters of the anterior wrist creases, where it lies conveniently over the radius.

Advantages. Advantages of radial artery cannulation include huge experience and safety, peripheral position, double blood supply to the dependent territory (by the ulnar artery), and easy compression in the event of bleeding.

Disadvantages. Disadvantages include technical difficulties owing to the small size of the vessel or vasoconstriction (the radial artery pulse may not be palpable when blood pressure is less than 80 mm Hg) and inaccurate blood

pressure measurements (when compared with the central circulation).[4-6]

The modified Allen test has been proposed as a screening tool prior to radial artery cannulation to ensure the presence of adequate distal collateral circulation.[7,8] The Allen test has, however, been found to have high interobserver variability[9] and to lack sensitivity and specificity.[10,11] It is not widely used. It is prudent, however, to avoid insertion of an arterial catheter into the radial or ulnar artery when the other artery is known to be absent or occluded.

Positioning for Cannulation. The forearm should be supine and the wrist slightly extended and supported.

THE AXILLARY AND BRACHIAL ARTERIES

The axillary artery is a continuation of the subclavian artery beginning at the outer border of the first rib. The artery is surrounded by the cords of the brachial plexus. Its position relative to the other structures of the axilla varies according to the position of the arm. The artery ends at the inferior border of the teres major muscle, where it becomes the brachial artery. The brachial artery runs down the upper arm to the elbow. Initially, it is medial to the humerus, but distally it spirals anteriorly to end as the radial and ulnar arteries approximately 1 cm distal to the elbow. The brachial artery lies near the ulnar and median nerves in its proximal course and near the median nerve in its distal course.

Advantages. The axillary artery is a large artery, and pressure measurements reflect the central circulation.

Disadvantages. The arm position required for axillary artery cannulation may be contraindicated or difficult for some patients. Care should be taken if a long catheter is used, because its tip might be proximal to the origin of the brachiocephalic artery/left common carotid artery. In this case embolic material from the line (i.e., air bubbles or thrombus) could be introduced into the brain. The risk of line infection may also be higher relative to other sites.[12]

Positioning for Cannulation. For axillary artery cannulation the arm should be bent at the elbow and raised above the head (abducted and flexed to 90 degrees). The pulse can then be palpated in the axilla.

The brachial artery is punctured where it is palpable medially on the anterior aspect of the elbow. Generally, cannulation of the brachial artery is not recommended, because it is associated with specific and potentially severe complications (see later).

THE FEMORAL ARTERY

The femoral artery originates as a continuation of the external iliac artery at the level of the inguinal ligament. At the level of the inguinal ligament, it lies midway between the anterior superior iliac spine and the symphysis pubis. Distal to the inguinal ligament, the artery lies medial to the femoral nerve and lateral to the femoral vein and is superficial, being covered only by fascia, fat, and skin. The femoral artery runs down the thigh and terminates as the popliteal artery in the knee.

Advantages. The femoral artery is a large artery that is easier to locate and puncture than the radial artery.[13] Blood pressure measurements reflect central blood pressure, and the femoral artery is palpable at a lower blood pressure than the radial artery. The femoral arterial line has a lower rate of catheter malfunction and greater longevity (compared with the radial artery).[3]

Disadvantages. In obese subjects, adipose tissue and skin folds may create difficulties in the approach to the groin. The skin over the puncture site also can be compromised by chronic inflammatory changes or fungal infections, and the artery itself may be very deep and difficult to locate. The insertion site also may be difficult to keep clean and well dressed. The risk of hemorrhage into the retroperitoneal space (which may initially be undetectable clinically) is unique to this site. The femoral artery is a common site for vascular surgery in the leg, and this represents a strong relative contraindication to arterial cannulation.

Position for Cannulation. In a supine patient, assistance may be required in retracting abdominal and thigh adipose tissue to allow access to the groin.

DORSALIS PEDIS

The dorsalis pedis artery begins anterior to the ankle as a branch of the anterior tibial artery. The artery runs distally in the foot between the tendons of the extensor digitorum longus and extensor hallucis longus. It terminates as it turns in to the foot toward the sole between the first two metatarsal bones. During its course over the foot the artery is covered only by fascia and skin and is easily palpable.

Advantages. The dorsalis pedis is an easily accessible, compressible small artery.

Disadvantages. This artery is the most distant from the central circulation. Vasoconstriction can affect the quality of the arterial signal. In addition, the distance from the central circulation may result in an artificially elevated systolic pressure reading resulting from interaction of the arterial pressure wave on smaller and smaller arteries.[14]

Position for Cannulation. The foot is placed in a neutral position with slight extension of the ankle.

ADDITIONAL CONSIDERATIONS

From this discussion of relative anatomy the features of the arteries commonly used for monitoring become clear: all are superficial, covered only by fascia and skin, easily palpable, and easily compressible. The specific artery chosen for insertion of an arterial line should be influenced by the experience of the operator, ease of palpation, contraindications, and limitations in positioning.

After adequate positioning, the chosen arterial line insertion site should be cleaned and sterilized. The operator should don a mask, sterile gown, and gloves, and drapes should be used to create a sterile field around the insertion site, although the efficiency of these measures has been questioned.[15] Local anesthesia (approximately 1 mL of 1% to 2% lidocaine *without epinephrine*) should be infiltrated around the insertion site using a small-gauge (24- to 26-gauge) needle. Epinephrine should be avoided as an additive to the local anesthetic in order to prevent arterial spasm.

EQUIPMENT

Before actually inserting the arterial cannula, the monitoring equipment, cables, arterial line setup, and adhesive tape/sutures should all be prepared and checked. Beyond the arterial cannula, the arterial line setup consists of noncompliant tubing; three-way taps (stopcocks), a pressure-transducing device, a flush system, and the monitor. The arterial cannula is connected to a short length of tubing and then to at least one three-way tap. This tap is used for blood sampling and may also be used for zeroing the setup. The three-way tap is, in turn, connected to the pressure-transducing device, which is connected to the monitor. The pressure transducer is also connected to the flush system. The flush system consists of a bag of intravenous fluid under pressure from which all air has been removed. The fluid bag is compressed to a pressure greater than the arterial pressure using a pressure bag or cuff. The flush system maintains a continuous but slow (3 mL/h) flow of fluid through the system and into the artery to maintain cannula patency. The arterial line system may include additional three-way taps, connections to other pressure monitoring sites (e.g., central venous pressure), and damping devices as required.

SETS FOR ARTERIAL CANNULATION AND INSERTION TECHNIQUE

A multiplicity of arterial cannulation sets exists, falling into three main groups: sets based on a cannula-sheathed needle (equivalent to the normal intravenous catheter) with or without an additional wire, sets based on the Seldinger technique, and sets used for direct arterial cutdown techniques.

The simplest technique for arterial line insertion employs a 20-gauge catheter-over-needle arrangement: a simple 20-gauge intravenous cannula can be used, although catheters specifically made for arterial puncture are available. Such a catheter is suitable for the smaller arteries described earlier (radial or dorsalis pedis). After appropriate positioning, the patient's pulse is palpated with the nondominant hand and the cannula inserted at an angle of 45 to 60 degrees to the skin and into the artery using the dominant hand. The cannula and needle may be advanced until blood flashback is seen in the needle, and then the cannula is threaded into the artery (in a manner similar to intravenous insertion), or a through-and-through technique can be employed. In the through-and-through technique the needle and cannula are inserted directly through both the front and back walls of the artery without seeking blood flashback. The needle is withdrawn partially or fully from the cannula. The cannula is then slowly drawn back until the blood flashback is seen and subsequently threaded into the artery. In the event that blood flashback is not seen, the needle should not be reinserted into the cannula because it may perforate the side or cut off a distal segment.

Occasionally, difficulty may be found in inserting the cannula despite good back-flow of blood through it. In this circumstance, the arterial line wire may be of use. The wire fits through the cannula (after the needle has been removed) and may be manipulated into the artery. The wire need only be inserted a few centimeters beyond the catheter tip (into the artery), and the cannula can then be threaded. As a precondition to wire insertion, good back-flow of blood must be noted through the cannula, and under no circumstances should the wire be inserted with force, because this can lead to perforation or dissection of the artery.

Some cannula-over-needle sets exist that include a wire that is preconnected to the needle/cannula apparatus. These sets are available for both smaller and larger arteries and represent a combination of the guidewire and Seldinger techniques. The artery is punctured by one of the techniques described earlier using the needle and cannula assembly. Blood flashback is seen in the tube housing the wire. Once blood is seen to return, the wire is advanced through the needle while it is still (at least partially) within the cannula and into the artery. The cannula is then advanced over the wire into the artery.

For larger or deeper arteries (femoral and axillary), set types based on the Seldinger technique are available. Using this technique, the artery is sought and punctured with a needle, the wire is inserted through the needle, the needle is removed, and the catheter is inserted over the wire. This differs from the wire technique described earlier, because the wire is inserted through the needle and then the needle is removed before the cannula is inserted. In the guidewire procedure described earlier, the wire is either inserted through the cannula once the needle has been removed or inserted through the needle and cannula together.

Arterial cannulation can be very challenging, especially in patients with severe peripheral vascular disease or low blood pressure. Under these circumstances, additional equipment may be required to help locate the artery. Both Doppler and ultrasound probes may be useful.

The Doppler probe provides an auditory signal corresponding to blood flow. The characteristic arterial pulse form is easily distinguished from venous blood flow. The point of maximal Doppler response lies directly above the artery and may help in directing the needle to localize the artery.[16]

By using small mobile ultrasound devices with high-frequency probes the artery may actually be visualized. It is seen as a pulsating echogenic (white) ring on cross section. The arterial catheter needle can also be seen on ultrasound (as a straight echogenic line) and can thus be directed into the artery. Use of ultrasound has been shown to increase success at the first attempt of arterial line insertion.[17]

Cutdown techniques are rarely required in adults. This issue for pediatric patients is addressed in Chapter 228.

Once inserted, the arterial cannula should be well fixed to the patient to prevent accidental removal and connected to the flush/pressure transduction system. Fixation can be achieved either with tape or with sutures. Once the presence of an adequate waveform on the monitor has been confirmed, the next step is to zero the system.

ZEROING

The importance of accurate zeroing cannot be overstated—zeroing problems reflect one of the most common sources of error in pressure-transduction systems. Zeroing has two main functions: the first is to equilibrate the monitor, and the second is to correct for the contribution of the fluid column in the pressure-transduction system between the patient and the pressure transducer.

The pressure transducers in use today are rugged, inexpensive, and accurate.[18] They convert pressure applied from the artery via the fluid-filled tubing to the transducer into electrical energy. The electrical signal generated by the transducer is then amplified in the monitor to produce a waveform on the screen and a numerical measure of blood pressure. To carry out this conversion of mechanical pressure into an electrical signal, the transducer also requires an "excitation voltage" to be provided by the monitor. The standard responsiveness of the transducer is 5 μV/V excitation voltage/mm Hg,[18] and atypical excitation voltage is 6 V. Therefore, the pressure transducer produces 30 μV/mm Hg pressure applied from the artery. Typically, this signal is amplified 1000 times by the monitor, so that for each 100 mm Hg of

blood pressure the monitor output is 3 V.[18] Before their first use, and periodically during their use, the interaction of the excitation current, the transducer response, and the monitor amplification requires resetting—in the first instance to standardize the system and thereafter to compensate for any drift. This calibration is achieved by zeroing or standardizing the measurement to atmospheric pressure, which thereafter is the zero reference point for further measurement. With current semiconductor equipment, calibration to a mercury manometer is not required.[18]

The arterial line is zeroed by exposing the pressure transducer to atmospheric pressure, for example by turning one of the three-way taps such that it is closed to the patient and the transducer is open to room air. The zero procedure is activated on the monitor and the system left untouched for a few seconds until a flat line appears on the arterial monitor tracing and the monitor reads zero. The three-way tap is then closed to air and opened to the patient, and blood pressure can be measured. The zero point (the three-way tap used for zeroing) can be near to the patient or near to the transducer. It is important to consider that the pressure measured by the monitor will represent the patient's arterial pressure plus any contribution made by the column of fluid in the pressure tubing between the patient and the zero point.

To illustrate this point, consider the change in pressure reading if the pressure transducer is lowered by 100 cm to the floor. In addition to the patient's blood pressure acting on the pressure transducer, a column of water 100 cm long is also present and contributes to the pressure reading. The blood pressure reading is in millimeters of mercury, so it will increase by 100/1.36, or by 73 mm Hg. If the pressure transducer is raised relative to the patient, then the pressure recorded by the monitor will decrease in a similar manner. Appropriate zeroing of the pressure transducer can compensate for these differences. Continuing the example above, while the transducer is 100 cm lower than the patient, the three-way tap near the patient's radial artery is closed to the artery and opened to room air. The monitor is re-zeroed. Now the zero incorporates the contribution made by the 100 cm column of water in the tubing; and when the arterial pressure is measured again, it will once more be accurate. Although this example is extreme, smaller changes in relative position are common; the transducer is attached to the patient at the level of his shoulder while he is supine. The patient is subsequently repositioned from supine to sitting. His shoulder is raised by 20 cm relative to his femoral artery, and the pressure recorded on the monitor decreases by 20/1.36 = 15 mm Hg. This change might not cause a change of therapy if arterial pressure is being measured. However, if intracranial pressure (ICP) or central venous pressure (CVP) is being measured, a 15-mm Hg inaccuracy in the measurement could be critical. By convention, for arterial pressure measurement, the zero point is set at the height of the right atrium (i.e., the midaxillary line in the supine patient).

DAMPING

Another potential source of error in the measurement of blood pressure using the arterial line results from the interaction between the arterial pressure wave and the physical properties of the arterial line setup. This interaction can lead to underdamping (resonance or overshoot) and a spuriously high blood pressure reading or overdamping with a spuriously low blood pressure.

The arterial pulse waveform can be described as a summation of component sine waves with frequencies that are mainly in the range of 3 to 5 Hz. The arterial line set tubing has a natural frequency that is usually greater than 20 Hz. If the natural frequency of the arterial line set is decreased, it can approach the component frequencies of the arterial pulse waveform and resonance may occur or increase. Resonance modulates the pressures measured. The main effect will be an increase in the recorded systolic blood pressure. A decrease in the recorded diastolic blood pressure may also occur while, typically, mean blood pressure will not be affected. Perhaps the most common cause of underdamping is the use of an excessive length of pressure tubing between the arterial insertion site and the pressure transducer. Underdamping also may be a problem when measuring central arterial pressures and in the presence of severe vasoconstriction.

Overdamping decreases the transfer of energy from the artery to the pressure transducer. Damping results from the absorbance of energy by the fluid contents of the arterial set tubing and the tubing wall itself and from the friction between them. Damping is quantified by the damping coefficient (zeta), a measure of the time required for the system to come to rest after activation. Increased damping decreases the recorded systolic pressure and, to a lesser extent, increases the recorded diastolic pressure; mean pressure is affected the least. Damping is increased by the use of compliant, kinked, or partially occluded tubing and by loose connections and leaks (Table 208-1).

To obtain an accurate measure of the blood pressure from the arterial line, the system must be properly balanced. One method to assess balance utilizes the "fast flush test."[19,20] This test is performed by activating the flush device for a few seconds and then releasing it. On activation of the flush device, the pressure measured rises to a plateau. After release, the pressure waveform drops abruptly and small sharp waves may be seen (Fig. 208-1). In a balanced system, there should be only one such sharp wave. Figure 208-1A shows a system that is underdamped; there are multiple sharp waves after release of the flush. The reason for the underdamping in this case was the use of an excessive length of pressure tubing. Figure 208-1B shows the effect of removing the excess length of pressure tubing. Only one sharp wave follows the flush, indicating that the system is now well balanced. An alternative

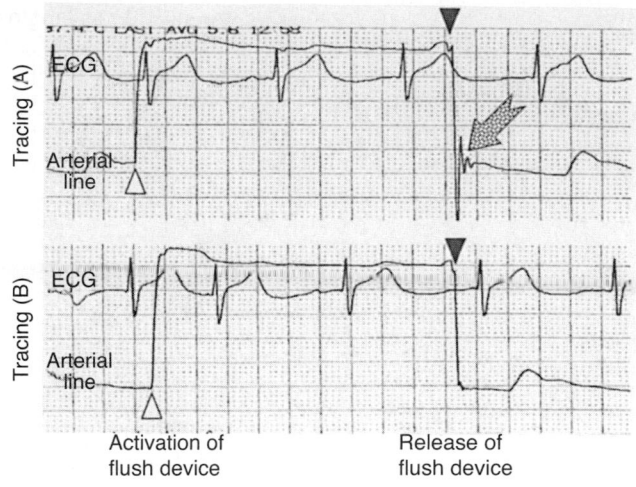

FIGURE 208–1. The fast flush test, electrocardiogram, and arterial line tracings. Tracing A shows underdamping or overshoot with multiple sharp waves following the release of the flush device (*speckled arrow*). Tracing B shows a balanced system, with only one sharp wave following flush release. The *white arrowheads* indicate the beginning of the system flush, whereas the *black arrowheads* represent its termination.

correction that could have been applied (if the tubing length was required) might have been to increase the damping coefficient with the aid of a dampening device. Using this device is similar in effect to introducing a small air bubble into the arterial line tubing; however, its use does not incur the risk of air embolus.

Figures for the natural frequency and damping coefficient of an arterial line setup can be approximated from a tracing of the fast flush test.[20] The natural frequency of the arterial line setup can be calculated from the cycle length of the sharp waves, whereas the damping coefficient can be calculated from the rate at which the waves decline in amplitude. Figure 208-2 shows an enlargement of the flush release in the underdamped arterial line tracing in Figure 208-1A and illustrates the calculation. Based on this tracing, the natural frequency was calculated at 22.7 Hz, while the damping coefficient was 0.34. Removal of the excess tubing (producing the tracing in Fig. 208-1B) resulted in a natural frequency of 50 Hz, while the damping coefficient was unchanged.

FLUSH SOLUTIONS

To maintain patency and prevent thrombosis of the arterial catheter, it must be continually flushed. Numerous additives have been proposed to achieve this aim, including heparin (the most commonly used), sodium citrate, papaverine, and normal saline. The infusion of heparin through the arterial catheter has been repeatedly shown to be more effective than normal saline in maintaining patency and/or arterial pressure measurements.[21-25] The concentration of heparin used in the arterial line flush is usually less than 10 units/mL, with 1 unit/mL being common. Concentrations as low as 0.25 unit/mL, infused at 3 mL/h, are efficacious.[26]

Sodium citrate (1.4% solution) has been suggested as a flush solution that avoids the potential complications

TABLE 208–1. CAUSES OF UNDERDAMPING (OVERSHOOT) AND OVERDAMPING

Causes of Underdamping

Central pressure measurement
Long pressure tubing
Marked vasoconstriction

Causes of Overdamping

Air in tubing
Blood clots
Complaint tubing (not stiff-walled pressure tubing)
Kinked arterial catheter
Leaks in system (hole in tubing)
Loose connections

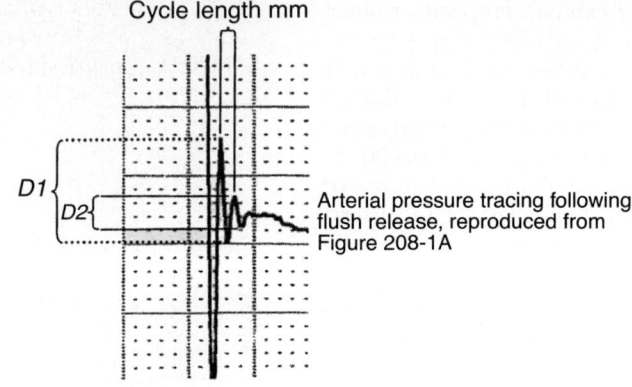

Cycle length mm

D1

D2

Arterial pressure tracing following flush release, reproduced from Figure 208-1A

$$\text{Natural frequency} = \frac{\text{Paper speed (mm/sec)}}{\text{Cycle length (mm)}} = \frac{25}{1.1} = 22.7 \text{ Hz} \qquad (Equation\ 1)$$

$$\text{Damping coefficient} = \sqrt{\frac{\left(\ln \frac{D2}{D1}\right)^2}{\pi^2 + \left(\ln \frac{D2}{D1}\right)^2}} \qquad (Equation\ 2)$$

Inserting values from the figure above:
D2 = 2.5 mm   D1 = 7.8 mm   D2/D1 = 0.32,
And from the graph below, or the calculation, damping coefficient = 0.34

Graphic representation of (Equation 2)—
the relation between D2/D1 and the damping coefficient

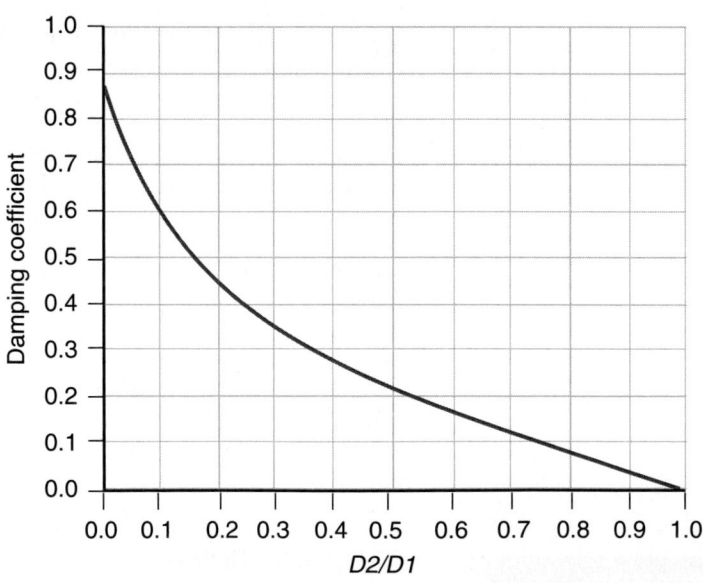

FIGURE 208-2. Calculation of natural frequency and damping coefficient. (Adapted from Gardner RM: Direct blood pressure measurement—dynamic response requirements. Anesthesiology 1981;54:227-236.

associated with the use of heparin and has been found to be equally effective.[27] Papaverine is an additional alternative.[28,29] Dextrose-containing solutions are not recommended for flushing the arterial line.[30]

The use of flush solutions, although beneficial, is associated with potential complications, mainly in their effect on blood test samples obtained through the arterial line.

COMPLICATIONS

The cumulative experience with arterial lines in patients in ICUs is huge; therefore, there is a considerable body of literature concerning complications. Complications are associated with the introduction and maintenance of a cannula in the artery and with its use. Common complications have been collected into series, whereas individual case reports describe a wide spectrum of rarer occurrences. The more common complications are described.

VASCULAR AND LOCAL COMPLICATIONS

Vascular and local complications vary from the clinically mild (small hematoma formation, insignificant bleeding) to catastrophic (permanent ischemic limb damage). A summary of 78 studies concerning the incidence rates for vascular and local complications of radial, femoral, and axillary arterial lines has been published and is summarized in Table 208-2.[31] Temporary arterial occlusion is common for all sites; the smaller radial artery is at greater risk than the larger femoral and axillary arteries. Arterial occlusion occurs in part as a result of mechanical obstruction of the artery by the cannula and in part by the formation and propagation of thrombus. Despite its high incidence, arterial occlusion is not detrimental in the majority of cases.[10,31,32] The arteries recannulize rapidly (within a week),[8,10,32-34] and permanent ischemic sequelae of arterial cannulation are fortunately rare.[31,32] Attempts have been made to correlate a wide variety of factors with increased risk of arterial obstruction, and some of these are summarized in Table 208-3. The use of Teflon catheters has been associated with a decreased risk of arterial thrombosis,[33,35,36] whereas outcome is independent of the age of the patient.[37,38]

Catheterization of the brachial artery is generally not recommended due to potentially severe complications. These include forearm ischemia (secondary to mechanical obstruction of the artery by the catheter and/or thrombus), compartment syndrome (described in case reports[39-41]), and damage to the median nerve (from either ischemia, direct mechanical trauma, or pressure secondary to a hematoma[42]). Anticoagulation has been associated with a number of these complications[39,43,44] and represents a relative contraindication.

Despite the widespread recommendation not to cannulate the brachial artery, its use has been reported in 3% of ICU patients.[2] Wider experience has been described in other specialties (for example, angiography, single puncture for blood gases,[45] and long-term access to the arterial circulation), and provides an indication of potential complication rates. In a study of 10,500 patients undergoing cardiac angiography via the brachial artery, surgical intervention was required for 0.57%, most commonly due to hand ischemia.[46] The incidence of median nerve damage after cardiac catheterization via the brachial artery is 0.2% to 1.4%,[42] whereas vascular angiography performed through the

TABLE 208-3. FACTORS ASSOCIATED WITH INCREASED RISK OF ARTERIAL OBSTRUCTION

Use of smaller arteries (radial and dorsalis pedis vs femoral or axillary[31])
Large catheter size[33,105]
Multiple insertion attempts[33,37]
Presence of hematoma[10]
Female sex[10,33,38]
Preexisting peripheral vascular disease[32]
Prolonged shock[32]
Use of vasoconstrictor drugs[32]

brachial artery in 1326 patients was associated with a brachial artery thrombosis rate of 0.28% for men and 1.24% for women.[47] Long-term cannulation of the brachial artery has been described in a study of 225 transbrachial intrahepatic cannulas (in situ for up to 14 months) and seems to be associated with a higher incidence of vascular complications.[48] In this study, radial pulses were found to be diminished in 88 (39%) patients and ischemic symptoms of the forearm developed in 16 patients (8%). Brachial artery thrombosis had an incidence of 1.7%.

In clinical practice the territory supplied by an artery that has been cannulated should be closely monitored. Pain, weakness, changes in sensation, pallor, or decreased temperature all suggest compromised arterial blood flow and should prompt the immediate removal of the arterial cannula. Usually removing the catheter will be sufficient to restore adequate blood flow.

ERRONEOUS BLOOD TEST RESULTS

The arterial line is used as a convenient source of blood for laboratory examination in the ICU patient, and most samples so obtained will be reliable. Possible sources of error should, however, be considered. The most common cause of an unreliable blood test result is either dilution or contamination of the sampled blood with flush fluid. Removal of inadequate "deadspace" from the arterial line setup before obtaining blood for hemoglobin estimation, for example, may lead to a diluted sample and a falsely low hemoglobin level. If heparin from the flush solution is introduced into a test of the activated partial thromboplastin time (aPTT), this test will be markedly prolonged. Heparin in higher concentration may also artifactually decrease the pH and P_{CO_2} measurements.[49-51] If sodium citrate is used in the flush solution and inadvertently introduced into blood samples,

TABLE 208-2. VASCULAR COMPLICATIONS OF ARTERIAL LINES PER SITE

Site	Temporary Occlusion	Hematoma	Bleeding	Permanent Ischemic Damage	Pseudoaneurysm
Radial					
%	19.7	14.4	0.53	0.09	0.09
N	4217	2903	375	4217	15623
Femoral					
%	1.45	6.1	1.58	0.18	0.3
N	688	461	316	1664	2100
Axillary					
%	1.18	2.28	1.41	0.2	0.1
N	930	744	711	989	1000

then spurious hypocalcemia and a low pH might be reported along with increased glucose.[51]

The solution to the problem of flush contamination lies in the withdrawal of an adequate "deadspace" of flush solution and diluted blood before obtaining the blood for testing. The interaction between heparin in the flush solution and the measurement of aPTT is particularly problematic and has been repeatedly studied in an attempt to determine the minimum deadspace volume required to obtain a reliable test result.[52-57] Five to six times the tubing volume from the artery to the sampling three-way tap (i.e., the deadspace volume) should be withdrawn before the blood for this test to obtain a reliable result.

Whether this deadspace volume should be discarded or returned to the patient depends mainly on maintenance of sterility and speed of sampling. Sterility can be maintained using a closed system, such that the deadspace blood is maintained in an internal reservoir. Specially designed systems exist with internal reservoirs[58,59]; however, a simpler double-tap arrangement has also been described.[60] In this system, an extra three-way tap is added distal (i.e., further away from the patient) to the sampling port. A syringe is attached to the extra three-way tap. The deadspace blood is drawn into this syringe, and the blood sample is taken from the more proximal (i.e., closer to the patient) tap. After blood sampling, the deadspace blood can be returned.

Blood cultures obtained from the arterial line represent another test in which results might be compromised. The sensitivity of cultures drawn in this way is similar to or slightly higher than that of blood cultures obtained by venipuncture; specificity, however, is lower.[61,62] The lower specificity presumably reflects introduction of organisms into the culture bottles from the three-way tap or the catheter itself.

ANEMIA

The ease with which blood specimens can be obtained from the arterial line, and the requirement for frequent testing in critically ill patents, may lead to the removal of considerable volumes of blood. In one study, the mean volume removed daily was 41.1 ± 39.7 mL.[63] Phlebotomy contributes to the development of anemia among ICU patients and has been implicated as a cause for blood transfusions.[64,65] Relatively simple steps can reduce the blood loss associated with tests. Such steps include return of deadspace blood (as described earlier)[58,60]; use of pediatric-sized sample tubes[66,67]; communication with the various laboratories to define the minimal blood volume required for various tests[68]; and point-of-care testing.[69] Despite their simplicity, these steps are infrequently employed.[70]

HEPARIN-INDUCED THROMBOCYTOPENIA

The use of heparin can be associated with a syndrome of thrombocytopenia and thrombotic events usually appearing after approximately 5 days of heparin therapy.[71] This HIT is thought to be mediated by IgG antibodies that develop in response to immunization against the heparin/platelet factor 4 (PF4) complex; these are called HIT antibodies.[71] The attachment of these antibodies to the heparin/PF4 complex on the platelet surface activates the platelets and induces thrombosis. Both venous and arterial thrombi can occur.[72] The presence of HIT antibodies does not, however,

inevitably lead to thrombotic episodes. For example, up to 50% of cardiac surgery patients develop HIT antibodies but thrombotic events are relatively rare (2% to 3%).[73-75] The diagnosis of the HIT syndrome is therefore based on the presence of the antibodies, thrombocytopenia, and thrombotic events.[71]

The overall incidence of this syndrome is reported to be approximately 5%. It is more common in women than men[71] and in surgical[76] as compared with medical[72,77] or obstetric patients[78] and is also more common after the use of unfractionated heparin than low-molecular-weight heparin.[76] A single dose of heparin is sufficient to induce HIT,[79] and the presence of as little heparin as that found bound to heparin-coated central venous catheters may be sufficient to sustain the immune response.[80] The development of HIT antibodies has been linked with the administration of heparin in intravascular device flushes[81-83] and also with low doses of heparin used in arterial flush solutions.[84]

Treatment for the HIT syndrome includes the cessation of administration of all sources of heparin, including those in the line flush solutions. The use of other anticoagulants for thrombotic episodes is recommended. Removing heparin from flush solutions also may be indicated in the presence of HIT antibodies and thrombocytopenia before any thrombotic events.[71]

After the decline in HIT antibody levels, the short-term use of heparin for certain indications (e.g., cardiac surgery) is considered acceptable.[71] It is prudent, however, to avoid heparin in the arterial line for patients with a history of HIT until further evidence of the risk of repeated episodes of HIT becomes available.

INFECTION

A patient may develop a bloodstream infection from the arterial line by one of three main routes. Infections have been introduced via infected equipment, such as reusable transducer domes[85] or infected flush solutions[86]; however, with the advent of disposable equipment and improved flush systems, the significance of this route of infection has declined. Two potential routes of infection remain: from the skin puncture site along the catheter and through the three-way taps.[30,87-91] The predominant organisms associated with arterial line infection are gram-positive cocci (*Staphylococcus aureus* and *S. epidermidis*), although gram-negative rods may also be found.[13,34,92]

Defining a precise rate of infection for the arterial line is not straightforward, because a multiplicity of definitions of catheter-related bloodstream infection are used in different studies and variables have not been standardized among studies. Clinical, research, and surveillance criteria exist for defining catheter-related infection. Clinical criteria include presence of signs of infection (e.g., fever, increased white blood cell count) associated with an arterial line in place longer than 96 hours with signs of local infection and no other source of sepsis. Whereas these criteria might be useful in clinical practice, they are too broad for research purposes. Surveillance criteria, such as those defined by the Centers for Disease Control and Prevention, include any significant bloodstream infection in the presence of a vascular catheter and no other source of sepsis.[30] This definition overestimates the incidence of catheter-induced bloodstream infection because it includes bloodstream infection from occult sources other than intravascular lines.[30]

TABLE 208-4. FACTORS POTENTIALLY ASSOCIATED WITH A CHANGE IN THE INFECTIOUS RISK OF THE ARTERIAL LINE

Increased Risk
Cut down technique vs percutaneous insertion[94]
Duration of cannulation >96h[12,13,94,95,103]
Axillary artery site[12]
Frequent arterial line set changes[106]

Decreased Risk
Teflon catheters (vs polyvinyl chloride)[107]
Heparin (in central venous pressure and pulmonary artery catheters)[23]
Use of chlorhexidine-containing skin preparation solutions[96,97]
Factors not associated with a change in infectious risk
Femoral vs. radial artery insertion site[2,13,37]
Dorsalis pedis vs. radial artery insertion site[34]
Duration of catheterization >96h[37,92]
Systemic antibiotic prophylaxis before arterial[94] or central line insertion[102,108,109]

Research criteria can include the use of arterial line tip cultures (often quantitative or semiquantitative[93]) usually correlated to venous blood culture results.[12,94,95] Combinations of these definitions have been employed.[34,96]

With regard to arterial line variables, virtually every aspect of line insertion and maintenance (for either central venous or arterial catheters) has been examined for an effect on infection rate. Factors that have been evaluated include type of skin preparation solution used[96-98]; insertion site; dressing type and care[30,90,91,99,100]; arterial catheter length; site of insertion; catheter material; type of flush solution; and frequency of set changes (Table 208-4). Consistency is not found in the results of all these studies, and not all these factors have been standardized from study to study, possibly confounding direct comparisons.

Despite this variability, a meta-analysis of four arterial line studies reported that the rate of bloodstream infections related to arterial lines was 2.9 infections/1000 catheter-days and that 1.5 per hundred arterial catheters were found to cause a bloodstream infection.[91,101] These rates compared to 2.2 infections/1000 catheter-days and 3.6 infections/100 catheters for unmedicated central venous catheters (CVCs), 0.2 and 0.2 for antiseptic-coated CVCs, and 2.5 and 4.3 for antibiotic-coated CVCs.[91,101] The implication of this study is that the infection rate associated with arterial catheterization is higher than generally assumed and may be higher than for the newer types of CVCs. Additional studies have reported the proportion of arterial catheters that cause bloodstream infections to range from 0% to 5.5%,[2,3,13,92,94,102-104] whereas the rate of arterial line colonization can be as great as 44%.[12,89,102]

The Centers for Disease Control and Prevention summarized these diverse findings into these recommendations: use a 2% chlorhexidine solution for skin cleaning; do not change arterial catheters routinely; change the pressure monitoring sets and transducers every 96 hours; do not use dextrose in the flush solution.[30]

In clinical practice it is unlikely that an arterial cannula present for less than 96 hours is the cause of an infection. If the arterial line has been present for more than 96 hours, and no other source of sepsis is identified, strong consideration should be given to removing or replacing the arterial catheter. The presence of redness or pus at the arterial cannula introduction site should further increase the index of suspicion of an arterial line–related infection.

ANNOTATED REFERENCES

Gardner RM: Direct blood pressure measurement—dynamic response requirements. Anesthesiology 1981;54:227-236.
   A description of natural frequency and damping as related to the arterial line. Also included are a description of the fast flush test and its interpretation. Graphs, formulae, and recommendations are provided to obtain a well-balanced system and accurate blood pressure readings.

Martin C, Saux P, Papazian L, et al: Long-term arterial cannulation in ICU patients using the radial artery or dorsalis pedis artery. Chest 2001;119: 901-906.
   A prospective observational study examining the complications of dorsalis pedis (DPA) (131 patients) versus radial artery (RA) cannulation (134 patients) in consecutive groups of patients. The study showed that arterial occlusion was very common (present to some degree in 63% of the DPA patients and 76% of the RA patients) but clinically asymptomatic.

O'Grady NP, Alexander M, Dellinger EP, et al: Guidelines for the prevention of intravascular catheter-related infections. Centers for Disease Control and Prevention. MMWR Recomm Rep 2002;51:1-29.
   An overview of catheter-related infections, both venous and arterial, including epidemiology, pathogenesis, strategies for prevention, and specific recommendations from the CDC.

Vincent JL, Baron JF, Reinhart K, et al: Anemia and blood transfusion in critically ill patients. JAMA 2002;288:1499-1507.
   An investigation of anemia and blood transfusion in ICU patients including an examination of phlebotomy for blood tests. A total of 41.1 ± 39.7 mL (mean ± SD) blood was withdrawn per day from ICU patients on 4.6 ± 3.2 occasions. There was a correlation between severity of illness and quantity of blood drawn.

Warkentin TE: Heparin-induced thrombocytopenia: Pathogenesis and management. Br J Haematol 2003;121:535-555.
   A recent broad review of the pathophysiology, epidemiology, clinical features, and treatment of HIT.

Chapter 209

BEDSIDE PULMONARY ARTERY CATHETERIZATION

Karen Ashworth • Michelle Hayes

KEY POINTS

1. Assess risk/benefits to patients before catheter insertion.
2. Measurements should be performed and interpreted by an experienced practitioner.
3. Benefits of bedside pulmonary artery catheterization remain controversial.

Although cardiac catheterization was described over a century ago, the placement of right-sided heart catheters in humans first took place in the 1920s and 1930s. Over the following decades many advances were made, leading to the first description of a use of the pulmonary artery catheter at the bedside in 1964.[1] The validation of cardiac output measurement by thermal dilution followed in 1968,[2] and in 1970 Swan and his colleagues reported the use of a flexible, balloon-tipped catheter that allowed pulmonary artery catheterization without radiographic guidance.[3]

In the following 20 years pulmonary artery catheterization became the gold standard for cardiovascular monitoring in intensive care patients. More than 1 million per annum were used in the United States, and more than 300,000 were used yearly in Europe by the 1990s. Data from the EPIC study published in 1995 revealed that 12.8% of intensive care patients underwent placement of a pulmonary artery catheter (PAC).[4]

Although controversy concerning the safety and efficacy of the PAC had appeared in the literature over the previous decade,[5,6] it was not until 1996 that concern really increased. Published that year was an observational study of 5735 critically ill patients, demonstrating that right-sided heart catheterization was associated with an increased mortality and increased use of resources.[7] Publication of this study led to immediate calls for either appropriate randomized trials to be undertaken or imposing a moratorium on use of the PAC.[8] To date, however, despite further work, there remains no consensus on whether use of the PAC is either beneficial or harmful for critically ill patients.

INDICATIONS

There are potential complications associated with the insertion of a PAC. Therefore, it is important to consider whether the data that can be obtained contribute to management or whether less invasive technique would give the same information. It is also important to ensure that the patient is in an appropriate setting and that there are experienced practitioners available to interpret the data.

Recommendations for clinical practice were made by the Society of Critical Care Medicine in 1997[9] and the American College of Cardiology in 1998.[10] These recommendations are not intended to be absolute indications but rather situations in which the PAC may be beneficial and are summarized in Table 209-1.

INSERTION

THE CATHETER

The standard pulmonary artery catheter is made of radiopaque, flexible plastic. It is 110 cm long and 7-Fr gauge with 10-cm markings along its length. At the distal end there is a latex balloon with a volume of 1.5 mL, and there is also a thermistor 4 cm from the catheter tip. At the proximal end of the catheter there are four ports. One is proximal, one is distal, one is for balloon inflation, and one is for external connection to the thermistor. The proximal port is 30 cm from the catheter tip and is used to measure right atrial (RA) pressure; it can also be used for injection of fluid to determine cardiac output. The distal port is for measurement of RA, right ventricular (RV), pulmonary artery (PA), and pulmonary artery wedge (PAWP) pressures as the catheter is passed through the chambers of the heart. This port is also used for sampling mixed venous blood.

Under sterile conditions, the PAC is passed through a 7.5- to 9-Fr gauge introducer, which has a hemostatic valve at its proximal end to prevent air embolism and blood leakage. It also has a side-arm port for infusion. The introducer is inserted by the Seldinger technique into a central vein, most commonly the internal jugular or subclavian. Femoral and antecubital routes can also be used, but these sites are often associated with difficulty in insertion.

PREPARATION

1. Check the patient's electrocardiogram (ECG), coagulation profile, and serum electrolyte panel. If there is left bundle branch block on the ECG, insertion may cause complete heart block and a catheter with a pacing facility is recommended. Clotting disorders should be corrected, if possible. If coagulopathy cannot be corrected, then use of the femoral or antecubital route should be considered. If the patient has a pacemaker already, the catheter should be placed under radiographic guidance to avoid dislodging the device. Low serum potassium and magnesium levels should be corrected.

TABLE 209–1. RECOMMENDATIONS FOR PAC INSERTION

Cardiovascular disease

Myocardial infarction
- Complicated by cardiogenic or hypovolemic shock when initial therapy with volume expansion or inotropes has failed
- Short-term guidance of management in acute mitral regurgitation or ventricular septal rupture before surgery
- Right ventricular infarction not responding to therapy
- Acute pulmonary edema not responding to therapy

Heart failure
- Differentiation between causes of pulmonary edema and guidance of therapy when there has been a lack of response to treatment
- Guidance of perioperative management in patients with decompensated heart failure undergoing high-risk cardiac surgery
- Detection of pulmonary vasoconstriction and determination of reversibility in patients being considered for heart transplantation

Cardiac surgery
- Differentiation of causes of low cardiac output when clinical/echocardiographic assessment inconclusive
- Guidance of management of low cardiac output
- Differentiation of right and left ventricular dysfunction and pericardial tamponade when clinical/echocardiographic assessment is inconclusive
- Diagnosis and guidance of management of pulmonary hypertension in patients with systemic hypotension and evidence of inadequate organ perfusion

Primary pulmonary hypertension
- Diagnosis, assessment of severity, and guidance of therapy
- Assessment of hemodynamic variables before lung transplantation

Respiratory failure

- May alter treatment and correct misdiagnosis
- May benefit patients with acute lung injury and ARDS who are hypotensive or have evidence of poor end-organ perfusion and those refractory to diuretic therapy

Trauma

- To ascertain status of underlying cardiovascular performance
- To direct therapy when noninvasive monitoring is inadequate or misleading
- To assess response to resuscitation
- To potentially decrease secondary injury in severe closed-head or acute spinal cord injuries

Septic shock

- In patients unresponsive to fluid resuscitation and vasopressors, if the information from the PAC prompts a change in therapy

Perioperative period

- Cardiac surgery: see above
- Peripheral vascular surgery: may lead to fewer complications
- Aortic surgery: may be useful in patients at high risk (e.g., suprarenal surgery, left ventricular dysfunction ± coronary artery disease)

Critically ill pediatric patients

- Pulmonary hypertension
- Shock refractory to fluid resuscitation ± vasoactive agents
- Severe respiratory failure requiring high airway pressures
- Multiple organ failure

---

2. Inflate the balloon to check for symmetry and leaks, and then deflate it before insertion.
3. Connect the distal lumen to the pressure-monitoring system and flush all lumens with sterile saline solution.
4. Zero-reference the pressure transducer and perform the fast flush test to confirm frequency response and degree of damping.
5. Slide the protective sleeve onto the catheter to maintain sterility if further manipulation is required at a later date.

INTRODUCING THE CATHETER (FIG. 209-1)

1. Pass the catheter through the hemostatic valve of the introducer.
2. Inflate the balloon once the catheter tip has passed through the end of the introducer. A central venous pressure (CVP)/RA waveform should appear after insertion of 15 to 20 cm of catheter when using the subclavian or internal jugular route, after 30 cm for the femoral route, and after 50 cm for the antecubital route.
3. Advance the catheter farther another 10 cm. It should pass into the RV and give an RV pressure waveform.

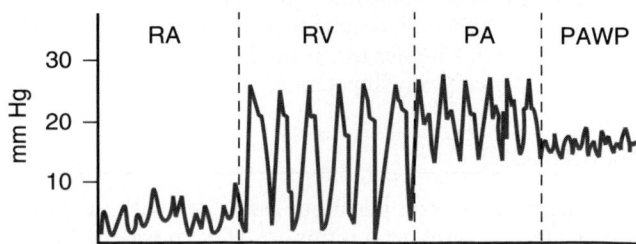

FIGURE 209–1. Trace demonstrating the change in pressures as a pulmonary artery catheter passes through the chambers of the heart to the pulmonary artery.

4. Advance the catheter another 10 cm to pass into the PA.
5. Advance it 10 cm farther to obtain a PAWP waveform.
6. Once a PAWP waveform has been obtained, deflate the balloon to check there is a return to a PA waveform.
7. Lock the proximal protective sleeve onto the catheter and the distal protective sleeve onto the hemostatic valve of the introducer.
8. Once the catheter is in place, check the position with a chest radiograph. In 90% of cases the tip is in the right lung. The tip should be within 2 cm of the cardiac shadow.
9. The catheter tip should be in West zone III. This is the region characterized by the pulmonary artery pressures that are greater than alveolar pressures. If the tip is in zone I or II, then the PAWP may reflect alveolar pressure rather than left atrial (LA) pressure. Zone III conditions occur in the dependent part of the lung and can be assumed if the criteria shown in Table 209-2 apply.
10. All pressures should be measured at end expiration when alveolar pressure should be closest to atmospheric pressure.

MANAGEMENT OF THE CATHETER

1. Always have the PA trace displayed on the monitor.
2. Never withdraw the catheter without first deflating the balloon.
3. Do not insert large lengths of catheter without observing a pressure change, because this maneuver may lead to looping and knotting of the catheter.
4. There may be difficulties in reaching the RV or PA owing to RA or RV dilatation, tricuspid regurgitation, atrial myxoma (rare), entry into the coronary sinus (rare), or abnormalities of the central veins. Solutions may include advancing the catheter with the balloon partially deflated during inspiration, repositioning the patient in a head-up or right lateral position, or flushing the catheter with iced saline to make it more rigid.
5. If the PAWP trace is obtained when the balloon is inflated with less than 0.8 mL of air or if there is a progressive elevation of pressure when the balloon is inflated, the catheter tip is too peripheral and should be withdrawn slightly to decrease the risk of PA rupture/infarction. This condition is called "overwedging" and indicates occlusion of the distal lumen by an overinflated balloon.
6. Daily monitoring of the position of the PAC is required. Routine daily chest radiographs are not necessary as long as 1.25 to 1.5 mL of air is required to inflate the balloon to obtain a PAWP tracing and the PAC has not migrated by more than 1 cm from its original position.[11]

7. The catheter should be removed immediately when it is no longer required for patient care or if the patient has an unexplained fever. The time until PAC replacement can be extended to 7 days if there is no evidence of catheter-related infection.[12]
8. Balloon rupture can be identified by failure to wedge and by failure of the syringe plunger to spontaneously deflate the balloon.

MEASUREMENT OF THE PAWP (TABLE 209-3)

In uncomplicated cases, the CVP provides a reasonable guide to the filling pressures of both sides of the heart. In critically ill patients, however, there is often a disparity between right and left ventricular function. The PAWP is an indirect measure of left ventricular filling pressure.

The inflated balloon of the PAC prevents blood flow through an individual branch of the pulmonary artery (Fig. 209-2). The distal lumen of the PAC thus measures the pressure downstream. It is assumed that there is a continuous column of blood between the distal lumen and the left ventricle, and therefore PAWP is equal to left ventricular end-diastolic pressure (LVEDP). Further, it is assumed that LVEDP is proportional to left ventricular end-diastolic volume (LVEDV), but this assumption is not always valid.

PAWP actually reflects the pressure where the nonflowing blood rejoins the blood flowing from the nonoccluded branches of the pulmonary artery. This region is called the j point. Thus, PAWP is intermediate between pulmonary capillary pressure and left atrial pressure. There are many conditions, however, in which this theoretical continuous column of blood is interrupted, and in these circumstances PAWP can no longer be assumed to equal LVEDP (Table 209-4).

INTERPRETATION OF THE MEASURED PRESSURES AND WAVEFORMS

The pulmonary artery waveform has a systolic and diastolic pressure with a dicrotic notch, corresponding to closure of the pulmonary valve. The PAWP, like the CVP, has a venous waveform with a, c, and v waves, corresponding to left atrial contraction, closure of the mitral valve, and passive left atrial filling, respectively.

The a wave coincides with the point of maximal filling of the left ventricle and is therefore the value that should be used for measurement of LVEDP. A large-amplitude a wave with an increase in measured PAWP suggests left ventricular ischemia and decreased ventricular compliance. A large v wave on the PAWP trace represents mitral regurgitation or an acute volume load to the left atrium as occurs with

TABLE 209–2. CRITERIA FOR ZONE III CONDITIONS

- Respiratory oscillations should occur.
- PAWP should be less than diastolic pulmonary artery pressure.
- Morphology of the PAWP should be that of an atrial pressure tracing and have a and v waves.
- The lateral radiograph should show the catheter tip below the LA.
- Blood aspirated from the distal lumen while the balloon is fully inflated should have an oxygen saturation approximating arterial blood.
- Change in PAWP should be less than half the change in PEEP during alterations in PEEP.
- Respiratory swings in PAWP should be less than half of the respiratory swings in alveolar pressure.

TABLE 209–3. PRESSURES MEASURED USING THE PULMONARY ARTERY CATHETER

Measured Pressures	Normal Range (mm Hg)
Right atrium (mean)	0-8
Right ventricle (systolic)	15-25
Right ventricle (diastolic)	0-8
Pulmonary artery (systolic)	15-25
Pulmonary artery (diastolic)	8-15
Pulmonary artery (mean)	10-20
Pulmonary artery wedge pressure	6-15

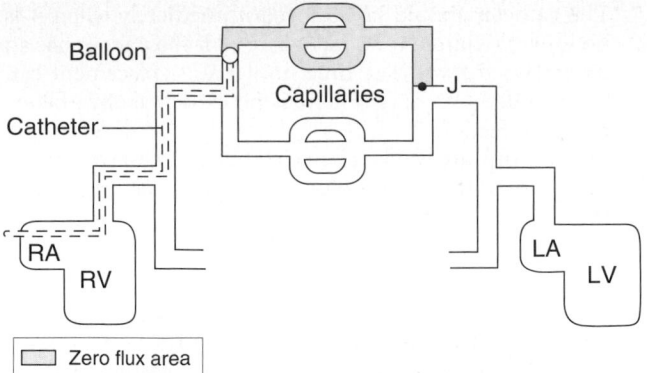

FIGURE 209–2. Illustration of the pulmonary artery catheter in a wedged position to explain relationship to left ventricle. (From Perret C, Tagan D, Feihl F, Marini JJ: The Pulmonary Artery Catheter in Critical Care: A Concise Handbook. London, Blackwell Science, 1996.)

TABLE 209–4. CIRCUMSTANCES IN WHICH PAWP CAN NO LONGER BE ASSUMED TO EQUAL LVEDP

PAWP > LVEDP	PAWP < LVEDP
Pulmonary venous obstruction: atrial myxoma, pulmonary fibrosis, vasculitis	Decreased left ventricular compliance
Valvular heart disease: mitral stenosis, mitral regurgitation	Aortic regurgitation
Elevated alveolar pressure: catheter tip outside West zone III, high inflation pressures, intrinsic PEEP, airway obstruction	Decreased pulmonary vascular bed: pneumonectomy, massive pulmonary embolism

septal rupture. Large v waves can be interpreted as an unwedged trace, prompting the operator to insert the catheter farther, risking rupture of the pulmonary artery. The right atrial pressure waveform can look like an RV waveform if there is significant tricuspid regurgitation. In cardiac tamponade, the right atrial pressure, pulmonary artery pressure, and PAWP are all abnormally high and similar as they equilibrate with pericardial pressures. A "dip and plateau" waveform may be seen in the right ventricular pressure tracing in constrictive pericarditis, restrictive cardiomyopathy, right ventricular infarction, and massive pulmonary embolism. This pattern is due to impaired ventricular filling during diastole. In massive pulmonary embolism, the pulmonary artery waveform may resemble the right ventricular pressure tracing owing to loss of arterial distensibility secondary to pulmonary hypertension. Causes of an increase in the measured pressures are documented in Table 209-5.

Pulmonary capillary pressure is the effective hydrostatic pressure in the pulmonary capillaries and is greater than the PAWP. It is of theoretical rather than practical interest.

MEASUREMENT OF CARDIAC OUTPUT

Thermodilution is the standard method for the measurement of cardiac output. Measurement is based on the indicator dilution principle, which states that when an indicator substance is added to a stream of flowing blood, the flow rate is inversely proportional to the mean concentration of the indicator at a downstream site. In the case of thermodilution, the indicator used is temperature, using either a bolus of cold injectate (cold thermodilution) or a thermal filament to generate heat (warm thermodilution).

COLD THERMODILUTION

The indicator used is usually a 10-mL bolus of room-temperature 5% dextrose solution or normal saline. It is not necessary to use ice-cold fluid. It is important to ensure that the balloon is fully deflated and that the pulmonary artery waveform is being monitored before performing the cardiac output measurement. The indicator is injected as a bolus within 4 seconds through the proximal port of the PAC and mixes with blood in the right ventricle. The thermistor proximal to the balloon then records the temperature change in the pulmonary artery and a temperature-time curve is displayed.

The average of three curves should be obtained, and any curves with an unstable baseline, a jagged profile, or an absence of return to baseline should be omitted. The area under the curve is inversely proportional to the flow rate in the pulmonary artery, which is assumed to be equal to the cardiac output.

The computer then derives the cardiac output by using a modification of the Stewart-Hamilton equation (Table 209-6). The computation constant represents the product of the specific heat and gravity of both injectate and blood and the dead space volume in the intravascular portion of the catheter.

Causes of error are shown in Table 209-7.

WARM THERMODILUTION

This is a semi-continuous method in which a thermal filament is mounted on the PAC 14 to 25 cm from the tip.

TABLE 209–5. CAUSES OF AN INCREASE IN THE MEASURED PRESSURES

Right Atrial Pressure	Right Ventricular Pressure	Pulmonary Artery Pressure	PAWP
RV infarction or ischemia	RV infarction or ischemia	Volume overload	Any increase to left ventricular filling
Pulmonary hypertension	Pulmonary hypertension	Raised pulmonary vascular resistance	Mitral stenosis
Pulmonary stenosis	Pulmonary stenosis	Primary lung disease	LV systolic or diastolic dysfunction
Left-to-right shunts	Pulmonary embolism	Primary pulmonary hypertension	LV volume overload
Tricuspid valvular disease	Cardiac tamponade	Pulmonary embolism	Myocardial ischemia or infarction with decreased
			LV compliance
Cardiac tamponade	Constrictive pericarditis	Hypoxic pulmonary vasoconstriction	Cardiac tamponade
Constrictive pericarditis	Restrictive cardiomyopathy	Left-to-right shunt	Constrictive pericarditis
Restrictive cardiomyopathy		Mitral valve disease	Restrictive cardiomyopathy
Volume overload			

TABLE 209–6. STEWART HAMILTON EQUATION

$$\text{Cardiac output} = \frac{\text{Injecte volume} \times (\text{blood temp.} - \text{injecte temp.}) \times \text{computation constant}}{\text{Area under the curve}}$$

TABLE 209–7. CAUSES OF ERROR

- Irregular or lengthy injection
- Insufficient mixing in the right ventricle (tricuspid regurgitation, which underestimates cardiac output, or in intracardiac shunts, which overestimate cardiac output)
- Contact between vessel wall and thermistor
- Abrupt variation in heart rate during measurement
- Respiratory fluctuations
- Rapid infusion of fluid through side-arm ports.

The filament intermittently generates pulses of heat, and the temperature change is recorded by the thermistor in the pulmonary artery. These pulses of heat are pseudo-random to minimize the influence of other sources of temperature change such as infusions or respiratory fluctuations. The cardiac output is updated every 30 to 60 seconds and is time averaged over the previous 3 to 6 minutes.

These newer catheters are usually combined with a facility for continuous monitoring pulmonary artery oxygen saturation by fiberoptic reflective spectrophotometry (Table 209-8).

COMPLICATIONS

Complications that are unique to the PAC and not just due to insertion of a central venous catheter can be divided into those caused by placement and the longer-term complications due to its presence.

Placement

The most commonly occurring arrhythmias are premature atrial or ventricular contractions that are self-limiting and can occur on insertion or withdrawal of the catheter. Sustained ventricular arrhythmias have been reported in up to 3% of patients and are most likely to occur in the presence of hypothermia, hypoxemia, acidosis, electrolyte disturbance, myocardial ischemia, or infarction and when there is a prolonged insertion time.[13] Right bundle branch block can occur in up to 5% of patients,[14] and this can potentially lead to complete heart block in patients who have preexisting left bundle branch block. It is advisable in these cases to use a PAC with pacing capabilities or to have a spare lumen available for rapid pacemaker placement.

If the catheter is allowed to pass the recommended intervals without a pressure change, looping and knotting of the catheter can occur. Knotting also can occur if there are multiple catheters in the heart. The knot generally can be removed by placing a guidewire through the PAC to undo the loop or by pulling the loop tight against the introducer sheath and removing the whole unit. Occasionally,

thoracotomy may be necessary. Tricuspid pulmonary regurgitation or chordae tendineae rupture can occur if the catheter is withdrawn with the balloon inflated.

Presence of the Catheter

Pulmonary artery rupture is the most serious complication, with a mortality of greater than 30%.[15] Fortunately it occurs in less than 0.1% of cases.[15] Any hemoptysis, hypoxemia, or shadowing on the chest radiograph should alert the physician. Diagnosis is confirmed by pulmonary angiography. Treatment consists of embolization[16] or thoracotomy. Factors increasing the risk of rupture include pulmonary hypertension, age, hypothermia, coagulation disorders, and distal positioning of the catheter.[15]

Pulmonary infarction may be due to catheter-related thromboembolism or obstruction of the pulmonary blood flow by the catheter tip or prolonged inflation of the balloon. Diagnosis should be considered when there is hemoptysis or a wedge-shaped opacity on the chest films.

The risk factors for catheter-related infections include prolonged catheterization, colonization of the catheter site, use of the internal jugular route when compared with the subclavian route, and frequent manipulations.[17] Endocarditis occurs in less than 2% of cases.[18]

The catheter may act as a nidus for thrombus formation or can induce mural thrombi by damage to a vessel wall. These complications can occur in up to 30% of cases[19] and may be reduced with the use of heparin-bonded catheters.

CONTROVERSIES

Although there does appear to be evidence that the PAC is helpful in the management of circulatory disorders, there is, unfortunately, a lack of randomized, controlled studies looking at its impact on survival. Anxieties regarding the PAC have

TABLE 209–8. NORMAL RANGE OF CARDIAC OUTPUT AND DERIVED VARIABLES

Variables	Formula	Normal Range
Cardiac output (L/min)		4-7
Cardiac index (L/min/M²)	CO/BSA	2.8-4.5
Stroke volume (mL)*	CO/HR	60-100
Systemic vascular resistance (dynes • sec/cm⁵)*	$(\text{MAP} - \text{CVP}) \times 80/\text{CO}$	900-1400
Pulmonary vascular resistance (dynes • sec/cm⁵)*	$(\text{MPAP} - \text{PAWP}) \times 80/\text{CO}$	60-120
Left ventricular stroke work index (g/M²)	$\text{SVI} \times (\text{MAP} - \text{PAWP}) \times 0.0136$	43-61
Right ventricular stroke work index (g/M²)	$\text{SVI} \times (\text{MPAP} - \text{CVP}) \times 0.0136$	7-12
Oxygen delivery (mL/min)*	$10 \times \text{CaO}_2 \times \text{CO}$	850-1050
Oxygen uptake (mL/min)*	$10 \times (\text{CaO}_2 - \text{CvO}_2) \times \text{CO}$	180-300

$\text{CaO}_2 = (\text{Hb} \times \text{SaO}_2 \times 1.34) + (\text{PaO}_2 \times 0.003/\text{mmHg})$.
*These variables can also be indexed to body surface area.

been fueled by studies that have associated use of the PAC with an increased mortality.[5-7] These studies, however, were observational, and it is possible that the increased mortality was due to physician bias. Other concerns relate to misinterpretation of the data obtained from the catheter and the possible misuse of data obtained. Clearly, benefits of the PAC may be greater when used by physicians who are more experienced at interpreting the data.

Of the randomized controlled trials that have been performed over the years, there is some evidence to support the use of PAC-guided goal-directed therapy in high-risk surgical patients.[20] The most recent study randomized almost 2000 high-risk surgical patients to PAC-based or CVP-based monitoring and found no difference in outcome.[21] It is possible that these patients had a lower risk of death than those in previous studies.

Concerns regarding the PAC have stimulated research into less invasive methods of cardiac output measurement. It is likely that these will gain popularity owing to their ease of use; however, it is imperative that these methods be validated before they are adopted as an alternative.

ANNOTATED REFERENCES

Brainthwaite MA, Bradley RD: Measurement of cardiac output by thermodilution in man. J Appl Physiol 1968;24:434-438.

The first report of the successful use of the thermal dilution technique to measure cardiac output in man.

Connors AF Jr, Speroff T, Dawson NV, et al: The effectiveness of right heart catheterization in the initial care of critically ill patients. SUPPORT Investigators. JAMA 1995;274:639-644.

An observational study involving 5735 patients that demonstrated that outcome was worse in those who underwent pulmonary artery catheterization. This landmark paper increased concern about the safety and efficacy of the pulmonary artery catheter.

Perret C, Tagan D, Feihl F, Marini JJ: The Pulmonary Artery Catheter in Critical Care: A Concise Handbook. London, Blackwell Science, 1996.

A detailed book covering the theoretical and practical knowledge necessary for safe use of the pulmonary artery catheter.

Sandham JD, Hull RD, Brant RF, et al: A randomised, controlled trial of the use of the pulmonary artery catheter in high-risk surgical patients. N Engl J Med 2003;348:5-14.

A recent study of 1994 elderly, high-risk surgical patients that showed no benefit when therapy was directed by a pulmonary artery catheter compared with standard care.

Swan H, Ganz W, Forrester J, et al: Catheterisation of the heart in man with use of a flow-directed balloon tipped catheter. N Engl J Med 1970;283:447-451.

The development of the Swan-Ganz catheter and its introduction into clinical practice was a pivotal event in critical care. It allowed rapid, safe catheterization of the pulmonary artery without the need for radiographic guidance.

Williams G, Grounds M, Rhodes A: Pulmonary artery catheter. Curr Opin Crit Care 2002;8:251-256.

An up-to-date review of the evidence for and against pulmonary artery catheter efficacy and safety.

Chapter 210

CARDIOVERSION AND DEFIBRILLATION

Raúl J. Gazmuri • Vasundhara Vidyarthi

The term *electrical shock* (or *countershock*) is used to describe the delivery of an electrical current across the heart through electrodes placed directly on either the epicardial or the endocardial surface of the heart or indirectly through electrodes placed on the chest wall with the aim of terminating a wide variety of atrial or ventricular tachyarrhythmias. The term *cardioversion* refers to the delivery of electrical shocks synchronized with the R-wave of the electrocardiogram. The term *defibrillation* refers to the delivery of unsynchronized shocks when no recognizable R-waves are present (usually for the treatment of ventricular fibrillation), or when the urgency of the indication requires immediate action. In this chapter, after brief historical remarks, we discuss the rationale, indications, techniques, and complications of electrical cardioversion and electrical defibrillation.

HISTORICAL REMARKS

In 1947, Claude Beck, a pioneering cardiovascular surgeon at the University Hospitals of Cleveland, successfully defibrillated a 14-year-old boy who developed ventricular fibrillation at the completion of sternal resection for a congenital funnel chest. The chest was reopened and defibrillation attempted using a custom-made defibrillator. The unit had a resistance adjustable between 10 and 35 ohms and was powered by 110 volts alternating current (AC). The patient was successfully defibrillated after prolonged direct manual cardiac massage.[1] His prototype defibrillator followed animal experiments by Carl J. Wiggers, Professor of Physiology at Western Reserve University. Almost 10 years later, Dr. Paul Zoll and colleagues, also using AC shocks, reported the successful termination of ventricular fibrillation by transthoracic delivery of shocks in four patients, with only one survivor.[2] In subsequent studies, Zoll and colleagues[3] extended their initial observations, demonstrating the capability of AC shocks to convert ventricular tachycardias into sinus rhythm. However, it was soon recognized that AC shocks were inconsistently effective and hazardous, causing serious injury to the underlying skin and skeletal muscle.[4,5] Moreover, AC shocks often precipitated episodes of atrial and ventricular fibrillation and injured the myocardium. These observations propelled the search for more effective and safer electrical currents, culminating in the clinical introduction of direct current (DC) cardioversion and defibrillation.

The history of DC cardioversion/defibrillation goes back to the 18th century when Abilgard, using a Leyden jar (a capacitor built in the mid-1700s at the University of Leyden, Holland that used static electricity), first shocked a chicken into lifelessness and upon repeating the shock (hence the term *countershock*) revived the chicken.[6] It was not until the early 1960s, however, that DC shocks were introduced into clinical practice. In 1962, Lown and colleagues[7] demonstrated the clinical effectiveness of synchronized DC shocks using underdamped monophasic waveforms in nine episodes of ventricular tachycardia. The same year, Jude and colleagues[8] reported the successful use of a battery-operated portable defibrillator built with two capacitors that delivered biphasic waveform shocks. In the subsequent years, portable defibrillators continued to be developed, but these devices used monophasic waveforms, predominantly monophasic damped sine or monophasic truncated exponential waveforms (Fig. 210-1).

The introduction of implantable cardioverter-defibrillators affected waveform technology. The initial implantable cardioverter-defibrillators used monophasic truncated exponential waveforms; however, the need for lighter and more efficient defibrillators spearheaded the development of defibrillation using biphasic truncated exponential waveforms. These waveforms have been shown to terminate ventricular fibrillation at lower energy levels.[9] Soon, the use of biphasic waveforms was also extended to external defibrillators, gradually displacing monophasic waveforms for cardioversion and defibrillation.

MECHANISMS

The mechanism by which electrical shocks terminate ectopic rhythms is in part linked to the underlying pathophysiology of arrhythmias. As discussed elsewhere in this textbook,

Monophasic Damped Sine (MDS)

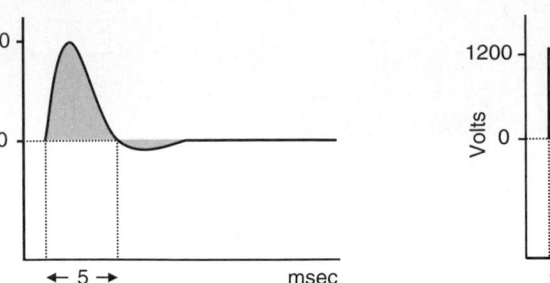

← 5 →   msec

Monophasic Truncated Exponential (MTE)

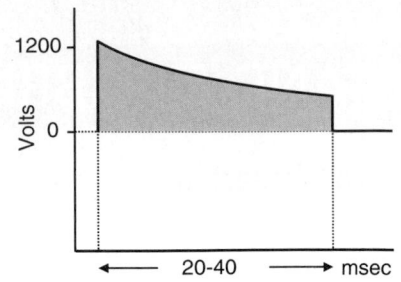

← 20-40 → msec

Biphasic Truncated Exponential (BTE)

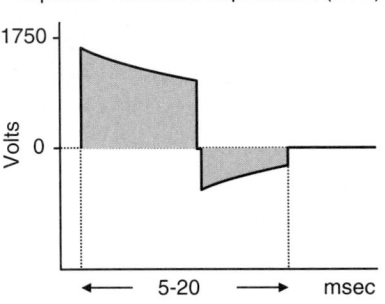

← 5-20 → msec

FIGURE 210–1. Main waveforms used for cardioversion and defibrillation. The energy of the shock (volts) is shown in the y-axis and its duration (milliseconds) in the x-axis. With monophasic waveforms, the current travels in only one direction. Damped sine waveforms return gradually to baseline, whereas truncated exponential waveforms do so abruptly. With biphasic waveforms, the current reverses course during the pulse. Note the very short duration and high peak energy of the monophasic damped sine waveform compared to the monophasic and biphasic truncated waveforms.

ectopic rhythms result from abnormalities in impulse formation, impulse conduction (reentry), or a combination of both.[10,11] Electrical shocks are effective in terminating tachyarrhythmias perpetuated by re-entry mechanisms. One of the essential requirements for reentry is that the leading edge of the "circling" impulse finds myocardial tissue in its excitable state, which is also known as the excitable gap between the leading edge and the trailing tail. A shock capable of depolarizing the excitable gap terminates the arrhythmia by interrupting the reentry circuit. This allows resumption of normal pacemaker activity. Electrical shocks, however, are not effective when ectopic rhythms are the result of abnormalities in impulse formation (i.e., automatic rhythms) such as parasystole, accelerated idioventricular ventricular tachycardias, atrioventricular junctional tachycardias, and automatic atrial tachycardias. For similar reasons, minimizing the likelihood of recurrence requires that triggering and maintaining conditions are also managed (i.e., efforts are made to correct persistent electrolyte abnormalities, unresolved ischemia, inflammation, accessory pathways, and other problems).

The mechanism underlying defibrillation is less well understood. It is generally accepted that ventricular fibrillation reflects continuous re-entrant excitation.[12] Successful defibrillation requires that depolarizing wavefronts be extinguished without precipitating new ones. It was initially postulated by Wiggers that simultaneous depolarization of the entire myocardium was required to halt all activation wavefronts and thus terminate ventricular fibrillation.[13] However, studies in dogs by Zipes and colleagues[14] suggested that depolarization of every ventricular cell was not necessary and that successful defibrillation could be accomplished by depolarizing only a "critical mass." A similar concept was proposed by Mower and colleagues.[15] These investigators suggested that even weaker shocks could achieve defibrillation, provided that the activation wavefronts were halted in a critical mass of myocardium. These concepts assume that the remaining wavefronts occupy a relatively small myocardial mass incapable of sustaining fibrillation.

Many additional complex concepts need to be addressed, however. For example, contingent on myocardial refractoriness, shocks could have the potential for terminating as well as initiating ventricular fibrillation. The concept of "upper limit of vulnerability" deals with this possibility. Shocks must be of sufficient strength not only to halt activation wavefronts but also to prevent reinitiation of fibrillation.[16,17] Tovar and Jones[18] proposed that successful defibrillation is achieved by shocks that prolong the refractory period so that incoming ventricular fibrillation wavefronts are not able to reinitiate fibrillation. More recently, Dillon and Kwaku have proposed the concept of "progressive depolarization," meaning that the same electrical shock is able to depolarize myocardium that is refractory to a normal impulse and thus prevent the post-shock wavefronts from reinitiating ventricular fibrillation.[19-21] Karagueuzian and Chen[22-24] introduced the "propagated graded response cellular depolarization hypothesis." The fundamental principle is that a stimulus can induce a graded response whose amplitude and duration progressively increases (progressive depolarization) as the stimulus strength increases. Strong stimuli prolong refractoriness in such a manner that sites of unidirectional block are converted to bidirectional block. This hypothesis is consistent with the greater efficacy of biphasic shocks.

DIFFERENCE BETWEEN CARDIOVERSION AND DEFIBRILLATION

Cardioversion refers to the delivery of electrical shocks for terminating organized tachyarrhythmias, usually in patients who are hemodynamically stable (i.e., atrial fibrillation, atrial flutter, ventricular tachycardia). For cardioversion, shocks are synchronized to avoid delivery during the so-called ventricular vulnerable period. This refers to an interval during repolarization when shocks can trigger ventricular fibrillation.[25]

Data from recent studies of patients with underlying structural heart disease undergoing implantation of implantable cardioverter-defibrillators indicate that the vulnerable period extends from 60 to 80 msec before to 20 to 30 msec after the apex of the T wave.[26] Interestingly, the timing of the chest wall impact associated *commotio cordis* (sudden cardiac death produced by nonpenetrating chest wall impact) also coincides with this vulnerable period.[27,28]

To synchronize shock delivery, a lead is chosen where the R waves of the electrocardiogram can be readily identified. Proper identification of these waves by the cardioverter unit is seen on the monitor as highlights marking the peaks of the R waves. Once the discharge button is pressed, a time-release function is activated and the shock is delivered coincident with the QRS complex (ventricular depolarization).

Defibrillation refers to the delivery of unsynchronized electric shocks intended to terminate ventricular fibrillation (hence the term). However, unsynchronized shocks are also appropriate for life-threatening rhythms such as pulseless ventricular tachycardia, ventricular flutter, and torsades de pointes when the urgency of the event precludes synchronization or when QRS complexes cannot be readily identified. Shocks are delivered as soon as the defibrillator's capacitor is fully charged. The defibrillator/cardioverter unit must be in the unsynchronized mode; otherwise, it may not deliver a shock, because it is awaiting recognition of the QRS complex. Modern devices can be programmed by the user to default to the unsynchronized or the synchronized mode when turned on and after delivering a shock.

CARDIOVERSION

Electrical cardioversion is indicated when restoration and maintenance of a sinus rhythm is both desirable and feasible. Factors that should influence the decision of whether to use cardioversion include the effectiveness, safety, and availability of alternative pharmacological and mechanical treatments (i.e., agents for rhythm or rate control and ablation procedures). The time of cardioversion is dictated by several factors. Most important are the hemodynamic status of the patient and the presence or absence of concomitant myocardial ischemia or heart failure. Indications for cardioversion[29] are listed on Table 210-1 based on the following three classes.

Class I. Conditions for which there is strong scientific evidence based on randomized clinical trials or general agreement that the procedure should be performed. Class I includes most emergency conditions in which atrial or ventricular tachyarrhythmias prompt hemodynamic instability, myocardial ischemia, or congestive heart failure. These indications commonly include ventricular tachycardias, atrial fibrillation or flutter with rapid ventricular response, and wide or narrow complex supraventricular tachycardias with hemodynamic instability.

Class II. Conditions for which controversy exists regarding the necessity and effectiveness of the procedure. This class includes asymptomatic atrial fibrillation or atrial flutter with slow ventricular response and supraventricular tachyarrhythmias associated with sick sinus syndrome or conduction system disease in which the mainstay of treatment is atrial or dual-chamber pacemaker placement. In this setting, electrical cardioversion may result in severe bradyarrhythmias, and a pacemaker capability is required.[30] Torsades de pointes, which typically occurs in patients with congenital or acquired long QT syndrome, and bradycardia may be terminated by

---

TABLE 210–1. RECOMMENDATIONS FOR ELECTIVE AND EMERGENCY CARDIOVERSION

Class I

Emergency cardioversion for reentrant arrhythmias associated with:
   Hemodynamic instability
   Myocardial ischemia
   Congestive heart failure
   Ventricular tachycardia
Atrial fibrillation or flutter associated with:*
   Hemodynamic compromise
   Difficult control of ventricular rate
   Persistence after removal of initiating and maintaining factors
   Duration of < 1 year
Wide or narrow complex supraventricular tachycardia with
   hemodynamic instability

Class II

Torsade de pointes
Ventricular flutter
Atrial fibrillation or flutter associated with:
   Duration > 1 year
   Large left atrium (> 45 mm diameter)
   Intolerance to antiarrhythmic agents
   Recurrence after previous cardioversion
Stable atrial fibrillation in sick sinus syndrome

Class III

Atrial fibrillation with slow ventricular response in the absence of
   digitalis, beta-blockers, or calcium channel blockers
Digitalis toxicity
Infrequent atrial fibrillation with spontaneous conversion
Chaotic atrial tachycardia
Severe conduction system disease

---

*Recommendations for cardioversion of atrial fibrillation are likely to be further limited in view of recent studies showing that rate control offers comparable or superior clinical outcomes.[52,55]
Adapted from Greene TO, Mittleman RS: Cardioversion and defibrillation. In Rippe JM, Irwin RS, Fink MP, et al (eds): Procedures and Techniques in Intensive Care Medicine. Boston, Little, Brown and Company, 1995, pp 81-92.

---

cardioversion (or defibrillation); however, effective treatment of these dysrhythmias usually requires treatment of predisposing conditions and temporary or permanent atrial or ventricular pacing.[31] Very rapid ventricular tachycardia (>200 beats/min) or ventricular flutter displaying a sawtooth configuration with tall peaked T waves may preclude proper synchronization. The T wave could be mistaken for an R wave, increasing the risk of triggering ventricular fibrillation. Under these circumstances, nonsynchronized delivery of electrical shocks is preferable.

Class III. Conditions for which there is general agreement that the procedure is either unnecessary or the risks outweigh the potential benefits. In patients with unstable atrial tachyarrhythmias and in those with disease of the conduction system, atrial fibrillation may be the most stable rhythm attainable and therefore cardioversion is not indicated. Patients with recurrent episodes of atrial fibrillation that spontaneously reverse to sinus rhythm may not benefit from cardioversion. Digoxin toxicity may present with atrioventricular conduction blocks and various types of tachyarrhythmias including supraventricular tachycardia, atrial fibrillation, and ventricular tachycardia. Treatment with digoxin-specific antigen-binding antibody fragments (Digibind) is considered first-line treatment for severe digoxin toxicity.[32,33] Cardioversion is generally reserved for the treatment of unstable and refractory tachyarrhythmias. If cardioversion is needed, the lowest possible energy level (10-25 J) should be used to minimize risk of inducing intractable ventricular fibrillation.

PROCEDURES FOR CARDIOVERSION

The following section describes the procedures for elective cardioversion. Many of the steps may need to be shortened or circumvented in hemodynamically unstable patients requiring rapid termination of a life-threatening arrhythmia. However, even in emergency situations, efforts should be made to secure some degree of sedation to minimize discomfort and avoid patient recollection of the procedure.

PATIENT PREPARATION

The procedure should be performed in hospital areas equipped with capability for monitoring cardiac rhythm, oxygenation, and vital signs along with capability for airway management and cardiopulmonary resuscitation. The patient should be fasted overnight or for at least 6 to 8 hours and the procedure thoroughly explained to ease fear or anxiety. Informed consent should be obtained from the patient or the legal surrogate decision-maker. If anticoagulation is being provided (e.g., for management of atrial fibrillation), verification of proper anticoagulation is imperative to minimize the risk of procedure-related embolic complications (see Complications). In patients taking digoxin, measurement of circulating digoxin concentration is recommended if toxicity is suspected. Initiation of antiarrhythmic drugs may be considered 24 to 48 hours prior to the procedure. An electrocardiogram should be obtained before and after cardioversion.

SEDATION AND ANESTHESIA

Cardioversion is best performed using a short-acting anesthetic agent under the supervision of an anesthesiologist and a respiratory therapist. At the time of cardioversion, the patient should be unresponsive to simple verbal stimuli. Traditionally, a short-acting barbiturate or a benzodiazepine (such as diazepam) has been used. Recently, shorter acting agents, such as midazolam, propofol, and etomidate, are gaining popularity. In a recent study that evaluated these agents for sedation prior to cardioversion in an emergency department,[34] midazolam had the longest awakening time (median 21 minutes, although this effect could be shortened by flumazenil), followed by etomidate (9.5 minutes) and propofol (8 minutes). However, almost half of the patients treated with etomidate developed myoclonus. Propofol appeared to offer the best combination of effectiveness and safety.

Conscious sedation (in which the patient maintains consciousness but in a somnolent state) represents an alternative to anesthesia with the advantage that it can be given by trained physicians without supervision by an anesthesiologist.[35] The safety and efficacy of conscious sedation using midazolam was reported by Raipancholia and colleagues[36] in 149 consecutive patients undergoing elective cardioversion.

ENERGY OUTPUT AND SETTINGS

The success of cardioversion is largely contingent on the amount of current delivered for the specific type of arrhythmia.

Organized rhythms with a simple re-entry circuit, such as atrial flutter and monomorphic ventricular tachycardia, usually require less current than more complex rhythms, such as atrial and ventricular fibrillation (see later). The amount of current delivered is determined by the device's energy output and the patient's impedance. The energy output, expressed as watt-seconds or Joules (J), is determined by the power (volts × amperes) and duration of the impulse and is selected by the operator within a range of 10 to 360 J, contingent mainly on the presenting rhythm, duration of the arrhythmia, conditions of the myocardium, use of antiarrhythmic agents, and type of waveform chosen. Transthoracic impedance is affected by factors such as the energy selected, electrode size, electrode-skin coupling material, number and time interval of previous shocks, phase of ventilation, distance between electrodes (chest width), and paddle electrode pressure.[37-39] Maximal reduction in thoracic impedance can be attained by using a large electrode size (i.e., 13- rather than 8.5-cm paddles), coupling the paddles to the skin with a salt-containing gel, applying a force of about 12 kg on both paddles,[40] and delivering the shocks during expiration. Male patients with a hirsute chest may have poor electrode-to-chest wall contact, requiring shaving of the area prior to electrode placement.

ELECTRODE POSITION

Location of the electrodes is important to maximize the amount of myocardial mass within the current path. Electrodes should be placed directly against the chest wall, avoiding breast tissue. For most emergency procedures, both electrodes are positioned on the anterior chest wall with one immediately to the right of the sternal border, below the clavicle, and the other to the left of the nipple with the center of the electrode in the midaxillary line. For elective cardioversion, the electrodes can be placed in an anteroposterior position. The anterior electrode is placed over the precordium and the posterior electrode in the right infrascapular location.[41] However, the superiority of one electrode position over another has not been firmly established.[42,43] Regarding polarity, the standard approach is to place the cathode (negative electrode) closer to the heart. This approach has been shown in some[44] but not other[45] studies to improve the efficacy of cardioversion when compared to the reverse polarity configuration. The electrodes should be properly separated and the coupling gel should not be smeared over the chest wall to prevent current from traversing superficially through the chest. Self-adhesive electrode pads are also effective and can be used in any of the aforementioned configurations.[43]

In patients with permanent pacemakers or implantable cardioverter-defibrillators, the electrodes should not be placed near the device generator because electric shocks can cause malfunction of the device and interfere with adequate current delivery to the myocardium. Reevaluation of the pacing thresholds in patients with permanent pacemakers and interrogation of the implantable cardioverter-defibrillator function is recommended after cardioversion.[46]

SYNCHRONIZATION

As discussed earlier, close attention should be paid to the synchronization mode. Delivery of unsynchronized shocks during an organized rhythm risks the development of

TABLE 210–2. KEY STEPS FOR ELECTIVE (AND EMERGENCY) CARDIOVERSION

Provide sedation.

Turn on the cardioverter ("defibrillator") unit.

Attach monitor leads to the patient and ensure proper display of the patient's rhythm.

Engage the synchronization mode (press "synch").

Identify markers on the R waves indicating adequate synchronization. If necessary, adjust the gain of the monitor until markers appear with each R wave.

Select the energy level for the specific arrhythmia.

Place self-adhesive pads on the chest, or position hand-held paddles after applying salt-containing conducting gel (see text for proper position).

Press charge button on the unit, or on the apex (right hand) paddle.

Apply approximately 12 kg pressure on both paddles.

Press the discharge button on the unit or the discharge buttons on the paddles simultaneously.*

Check the monitor. If the arrhythmia persists, increase the energy level according to protocol for the specific rhythm (see text).

Reset the synchronization. Most units default to the unsynchronized mode (allowing immediate defibrillation if ventricular fibrillation ensues).

Repeat the shock until conversion of the arrhythmia or completion of the protocol.

*The operator must ensure that no one is touching the patient at the time of shock delivery. A routine "chant" is recommended in which the operator first announces *"Charging defibrillator – stand clear!"* When the cardioverter/ defibrillator is charged the operator states, *"I am going to shock on three." "One, I am clear"; "Two, you are clear";* and *"Three, everybody is clear"* followed by shock delivery.

Modified from Guidelines 2000 for Cardiopulmonary Resuscitation and Emergency Cardiovascular Care. Part 6: advanced cardiovascular life support: 7D: the tachycardia algorithms. The American Heart Association in collaboration with the International Liaison Committee on Resuscitation. Circulation 2000;102:I158-I165.

ventricular fibrillation if the shock occurs during the ventricular vulnerable period. The synchronization mode should be off when the device is used for defibrillation; otherwise, it may fail to discharge because it fails to detect an "R-wave." The key steps for cardioversion are listed on Table 210-2.[47]

SPECIFIC ARRHYTHMIAS

VENTRICULAR TACHYCARDIA

Cardioversion is a highly effective method for terminating sustained ventricular tachycardias; successful cardioversion is achieved in 95% to 100% of cases.[5,48] Monomorphic ventricular tachycardias typically require less energy than polymorphic ventricular tachycardia. The recommended

initial energy level is 100 J, escalating to 200 J, 300 J, and 360 J if subsequent shocks are necessary.[47]

Defibrillation (unsynchronized shocks) should be considered in life-threatening situations associated with marked hemodynamic compromise and insufficient time for synchronization. When ventricular tachycardia is a manifestation of digitalis toxicity, the use of Digibind or overdrive pacing are preferred choices to avoid the risk of intractable ventricular fibrillation. Polymorphic ventricular tachycardia should be treated as ventricular fibrillation with the delivery of unsynchronized shocks starting at 200 J and escalating if necessary to 300 J and 360 J.

ATRIAL FIBRILLATION

Atrial fibrillation is the most common arrhythmia for which cardioversion is used. The prevalence of atrial fibrillation is about 0.4% in the general population and exceeds 4% in individuals 65 years of age and older (Fig. 210-2).[49-51] It is commonly associated with hypertension, coronary artery disease, cardiomyopathy, and valvular heart disease[52] and predisposes patients to embolic strokes.[53] The atrial rate ranges from 300 to 600 beats/min. However, the atrioventricular node limits the impulses that can be transmitted, yielding lower ventricular rates, which can be further reduced by agents that slow conduction such as digitalis, calcium channel blockers, and beta-adrenergic blockers, often enabling rates to remain within the physiologic range (<80 beats/min at rest and <110 beats/min after a 6-min walk).

The decision to cardiovert atrial fibrillation is usually elective and follows careful consideration of risks and benefits. Reasons given for cardioversion include reduction in the risk of systemic embolization and improved cardiac function. However, recent randomized clinical trials have failed to demonstrate that rhythm control is superior to rate control.[52,54,55] Rhythm control usually requires long-term administration of antiarrhythmic agents, such as amiodarone, sotalol, or propafenone, and use of these drug carries the risk of toxicity. There is also a tendency to discontinue anticoagulation, which has been associated with occlusive strokes.[55] In one of the studies, patients randomized to rhythm control had higher rates of hospitalization and more adverse drug effects.[52] Rate control is usually attained by using digitalis, non-dihydropyridine calcium channel blockers, or a beta-adrenergic blocker; these agents tend to be less toxic than the drugs that are used to provide rhythm control. However, restoration of a sinus rhythm may be reasonable after the first episode of atrial fibrillation, especially for patients with persistent angina and coronary artery disease or congestive

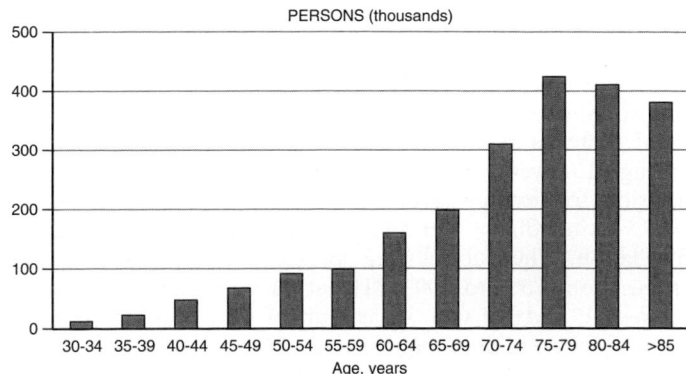

FIGURE 210–2. Prevalence of atrial fibrillation in relation to age in the United States. Study based on four population-based surveys. The median age of patients with atrial fibrillation is approximately 75 years, with 70% of the population between the ages of 65 and 85. (Adapted from Feinberg WM, Blackshear JL, Laupacis A, et al: Prevalence, age distribution, and gender of patients with atrial fibrillation: Analysis and implications. Arch Intern Med 1995;155: 469-473.)

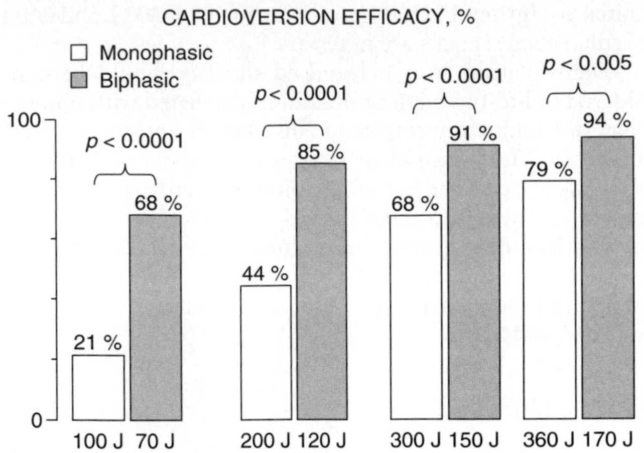

CARDIOVERSION EFFICACY, %

FIGURE 210–3. Randomized trial demonstrating increased efficacy of rectilinear biphasic shocks (70, 120, 150, and 170 J escalating shocks, in 588 patients) compared with damped sine wave monophasic shocks (100, 200, 300, and 360 J escalating shocks, in 577 patients) in patients with atrial fibrillation. (Adapted from Mittal S, Ayati S, Stein KM, et al: Transthoracic cardioversion of atrial fibrillation: Comparison of rectilinear biphasic versus damped sine wave monophasic shocks. Circulation 2000;101:1282-1287.)

heart failure.[56,57] Cardioversion may be performed without the use of antiarrhythmic drugs, thereby avoiding potential side effects, with a plan to shift the strategy to rate control, if there is recurrence. Once a decision to cardiovert has been made, electrical cardioversion is the usual procedure.

The energy for cardioversion is initially set at a level of 100 J and increased, if necessary, by increments of 100 J up to a maximum of 400 J. Some authorities recommend starting with higher energies to reduce the number of shocks (and thus the total energy) delivered. Biphasic waveforms may yield higher conversion rates using lower energy levels.[58] In a recent study,[59] rectilinear biphasic shocks were shown to have greater efficacy and to require less energy than monophasic damped sine shocks (Fig. 210-3). Cardioversion may fail in 5% to 30% of the cases. Failure has been associated with atrial fibrillation of long duration, greater body weight, low ejection fraction, and the presence of idiopathic dilated cardiomyopathy.[60]

ATRIAL FLUTTER

Atrial flutter may manifest with atrial rates ranging between 200 and 300 beats/min (type I) or rates between 320 and 430 beats/min (type II). However, because the atrioventricular node limits conduction, atrial flutter typically manifests with ventricular rates near 150 beats/min (reflecting 2:1 conduction). With drugs that slow conduction (as in atrial fibrillation), the ventricular rate can be reduced to 75 beats/min (4:1 conduction) or 60 beats/min (5:1 conduction). Type I atrial flutter is amenable to conversion by overdrive atrial pacing. However, type II usually requires cardioversion. The decision to attempt cardioversion as opposed to simply achieve rate control falls along the same lines as for atrial fibrillation. The success rate for electrical cardioversion ranges from 75% to 100%. The starting energy is usually between 25 and 50 J, with a maximum of 200 J. Cardioversion of atrial flutter seldom requires more than 200 J.

SUPRAVENTRICULAR TACHYCARDIAS

Any tachycardia greater than 160 beats/min in a resting individual is unlikely to be sinus tachycardia, and a diagnosis of supraventricular tachycardia should be considered. Supraventricular tachycardias typically manifest with heart rates ranging between 150 and 250 beats/min but can be converted to sinus rhythm by maneuvers that elicit vagal responses or by use of adenosine or verapamil with success rates of 75% to 80%. Electrical cardioversion is reserved for supraventricular tachycardias that are refractory to pharmacologic intervention, when there is contraindication to the use of these agents (i.e., severe bronchospasm for adenosine or severe left ventricular dysfunction for calcium channel blockers), or when there is need for immediate restoration of a sinus rhythm (i.e., myocardial ischemia, life-threatening hypotension). The starting energy is 50 to 100 J, and the energy level should be increased by increments of 100 J up to 360 J.

WOLFF-PARKINSON-WHITE SYNDROME

Patients with the Wolff-Parkinson-White syndrome with history of reciprocating atrial tachycardia (40-80%) and atrial fibrillation (14-20%)[61] are at risk for development of ventricular fibrillation. These patients demonstrate rapid conduction over an accessory pathway during atrial fibrillation and have multiple accessory pathways.[62] The development of atrial fibrillation with antegrade conduction over an accessory pathway is considered an emergency because the normal rate-limiting effect of the atrioventricular node is circumvented and the excessive ventricular rates can trigger ventricular fibrillation. Medical therapy must be used cautiously because drugs that block the atrioventricular node may "force" conduction through the accessory pathway. Therefore, digoxin and calcium channel blockers are contraindicated in the management of atrial fibrillation complicating Wolff-Parkinson-White syndrome. Class Ic drugs and procainamide are effective but can provoke or aggravate hypotension because of their negative inotropic action. If the patient is hemodynamically unstable, prompt electrical cardioversion is the treatment of choice.

ANTICOAGULATION

Because of the increased incidence of systemic embolization, anticoagulation is recommended for atrial fibrillation and atrial flutter lasting more than 48 to 72 hours (or when the duration is unknown). Previous guidelines recommended that anticoagulation be started 3 to 4 weeks before and continued for a minimum of 4 weeks after cardioversion.[63] However, because prolonged anticoagulation increases the risk of bleeding and prolonged atrial fibrillation may reduce the rate of successful cardioversion, some authors have proposed cardioversion without the preceding 3 to 4 weeks of anticoagulation if transesophageal echocardiography excludes intracavitary thrombi.[64] Transesophageal echocardiography has excellent sensitivity for detecting thrombi formed in the left atrial appendage that can embolize after cardioversion. This strategy is especially useful when atrial fibrillation is of recent onset and when there is need to expedite cardioversion. Anticoagulation after cardioversion is still recommended for a minimum of 4 weeks. However, recent data suggest that the risk of occlusive strokes persists after this interval, so that anticoagulation may be required for a longer interval.[52,55]

DEFIBRILLATION

Ventricular fibrillation is the underlying rhythm responsible for most episodes of sudden cardiac death.[65] Restoration of spontaneous circulation and subsequent survival is inversely related to the time elapsed between the onset of ventricular fibrillation and the first defibrillation attempt, and it may be as high as 74% if defibrillation is attempted within 3 minutes.[66] However, with each subsequent minute, the chance of survival drops by approximately 10%, such that after a 10-minute delay the possibility of successful resuscitation, using current resuscitation techniques, is almost nil.[67] Although defibrillation as the initial intervention is highly effective when delivered within a relatively short interval after the onset of ventricular fibrillation (i.e., < 4 min), after longer intervals of untreated ventricular fibrillation, a period of chest compression before attempting defibrillation may improve immediate and long-term outcomes.[68-71] This period of chest compression has been shown experimentally to increase myocardial high-energy nucleotides and to restore ventricular fibrillation waveform characteristics to those present shortly after the onset of ventricular fibrillation.[70,72,73]

Current American Heart Association guidelines recommend the initial delivery of up to three shocks using 200 J for the first, between 200 and 300 J for the second, and 360 J for the third shock.[74] If ventricular fibrillation persists, additional 360 J shocks should be delivered after a period of closed-chest resuscitation and administration of a vasopressor agent such as epinephrine (1 mg bolus every 3 to 5 min) or vasopressin (single bolus dose of 40 IU). For shock refractory ventricular fibrillation or pulseless ventricular tachycardia, amiodarone (300 mg bolus, which can be followed by a 150 mg bolus) has been shown to help restore spontaneous circulation.[75,76] The energy recommendations for defibrillation apply specifically to monophasic waveforms. Recent laboratory and clinical data demonstrate that biphasic waveforms can be more effective for terminating ventricular fibrillation using less energy and securing better post-resuscitation myocardial function (Fig. 210-4).[77-80] Biphasic waveforms allow successful defibrillation with lower peak current, which is thought to be an important determinant of myocardial injury.[79,80] More recent animal data suggest that triphasic waveforms may be even more favorable than biphasic waveforms, promoting higher rates of successful defibrillation with fewer episodes of post-shock ventricular tachycardia and asystole.[81]

REPETITIVE DEFIBRILLATION

Multiple shocks are often required to terminate ventricular fibrillation. Yet, it has been shown experimentally that repetitive delivery of electrical shocks may cause myocardial injury,[82-85] leading to conduction abnormalities and worsened post-resuscitation myocardial dysfunction. Thus, strategies for limiting the number of shocks required are warranted. Previous studies have recognized the value of measuring the amplitude and frequency characteristics of ventricular fibrillation waveforms to estimate the duration of untreated ventricular fibrillation,[86] assess myocardial energy metabolism,[87] and predict the response to defibrillation attempts.[88,89]

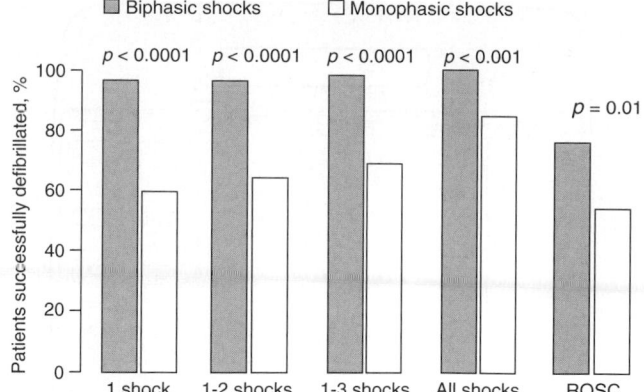

FIGURE 210–4. Fixed 150 J impedance-compensating biphasic truncated exponential waveforms compared with monophasic (truncated exponential or damped sine) waveforms in 115 victims of out-of-hospital ventricular fibrillation. The cumulative percentage of patients in whom ventricular fibrillation was terminated after the delivery of shocks is shown along with the rate of restoration of spontaneous circulation (ROSC). There were also numerical but statistically insignificant higher survival to hospital admission (61% vs 51%) but not higher survival to hospital discharge (28 vs 31). (Adapted from Schneider T, Martens PR, Paschen H, et al: Multicenter, randomized, controlled trial of 150-J biphasic shocks compared with 200- to 360-J monophasic shocks in the resuscitation of out-of-hospital cardiac arrest victims. Optimized Response to Cardiac Arrest (ORCA) Investigators. Circulation 2000;102:1780-1787.)

Waveform analysis that incorporates amplitude and frequency on a single index has been demonstrated experimentally to have better positive and negative predictor power than amplitude and frequency alone.[90,91] Technology incorporating real-time electrocardiographic analysis to guide the delivery of electrical shocks during cardiac resuscitation is awaited.

EQUIPMENT AND PROCEDURES

The technical aspects of defibrillation are similar to those for cardioversion, with the obvious exception that there is no time for sedation. However, because defibrillation occurs in the context of cardiac arrest, attention should be paid to all aspects of cardiac resuscitation. To this end, modern battery-operated portable defibrillators have evolved into highly sophisticated devices with a multiplicity of useful functions with which rescuers should be familiar. A rendition of one of many commercially available devices is shown in Figure 210-5.

AUTOMATED EXTERNAL DEFIBRILLATORS

A crucial milestone in the fight against the scourge of sudden cardiac death was the development of automated external defibrillators (AEDs) in the mid-1970s.[92-94] AEDs were primarily designed for use by medical and non-medical personnel with minimal or no training. AEDs have built-in "intelligence" that allows recognition of "shockable" rhythms and features (usually voice and screen commands) to guide the rescuer through the process of shock delivery. The AEDs analyze short segments of the patient's electrocardiogram, typically 3 to 5 sec long, and assign a simple shock or no-shock decision to each segment. For a shock to be advised, multiple positive shock decisions must be detected. Failure to identify shockable rhythms prompts the AED to indicate that shock is not advised and to start or resume cardiopulmonary

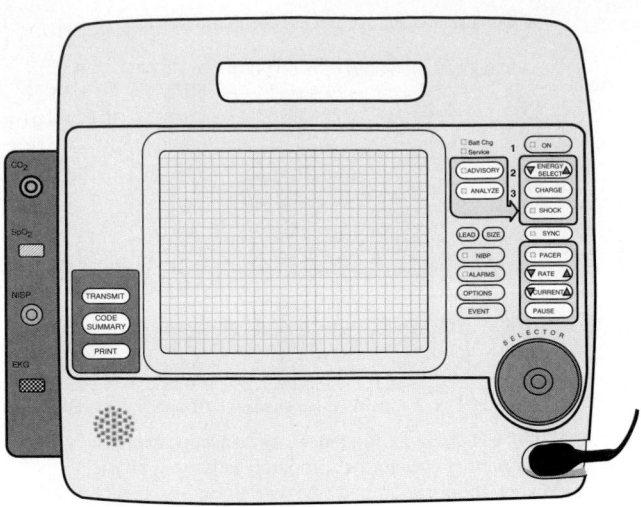

FIGURE 210–5. Rendition of a portable cardioverter/defibrillator (LifePak 12, Medtronic, Physio-Control) with capability for functioning as AED or manually operated defibrillator as well as a transcutaneous pacer. The equipment has also built-in capability for capnography (CO_2), pulse oximetry (SpO_2), noninvasive blood pressure monitoring (NIBP), and 12-lead electrocardiography (ECG) along with electronic data recording and data sharing capability.

resuscitation. Initial AEDs were built to deliver monophasic damped sine and monophasic truncated exponential waveforms. However, subsequent models have incorporated biphasic waveforms. The first biphasic AED defibrillator was marketed in the United States in 1996. Currently, all newly manufactured AEDs use biphasic waveforms.

AEDs are now available in public venues where a large number of people are expected (i.e., planes and airports, sport arenas, hospitals, public building, casinos, gated communities). AEDs have become increasingly more popular and save lives by allowing early defibrillation by bystanders with and without prior training before the arrival of emergency medical personnel.[95,96] Deployment of AEDs within less than 3 minutes in victims of ventricular fibrillation can dramatically increase survival from ventricular fibrillation.[66] A representative tracing of a successful defibrillation is shown in Figure 210-6.

The concept of automated defibrillation has also extended to hospital settings for use in medical and non-medical areas.[97] AEDs have even substituted manual defibrillators in crash carts to be used in noncritical care areas by medical personnel not trained in the recognition and treatment of cardiac arrhythmias. It is important to recognize that AEDs are exceptionally useful devices for use by individuals without training for rhythm recognition. However, AED operation requires frequent interruptions of chest compression for rhythm analysis and shock delivery, and this has been shown experimentally to compromise resuscitability.[98,99] Thus, manually operated defibrillators should be used as soon as trained personnel become available.

COMPLICATIONS

Delivery of electrical shocks using established indications, protocols, and modern technology is safe and effective and carries low risk of complications. Awareness of these complications, however, is important, for they can be minimized.

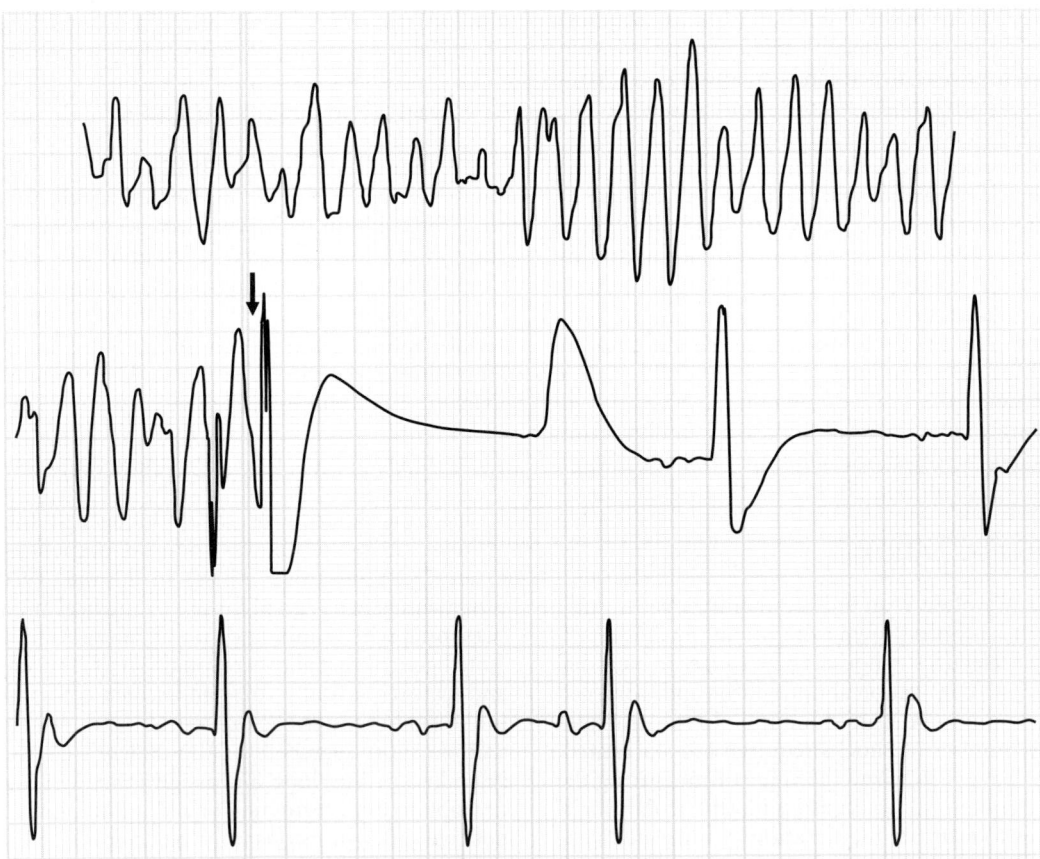

FIGURE 210–6. Representative recording of a successful electrical shock converting ventricular fibrillation into a sinus rhythm. (Adapted from Liddle R, Davies CS, Colquhoun M, Handley AJ: ABC of resuscitation: The automated external defibrillator. BMJ 2003;327:1216-1218.)

THROMBOEMBOLIC EVENTS

Embolization of thrombi formed within the cardiac chambers, most commonly inside the left atrium in patients with atrial fibrillation or atrial flutter, is among the most serious complications of cardioversion. The risk is greatest during the first 3 to 4 weeks after the procedure and is in part related to the development of atrial contractile dysfunction, "atrial stunning," after cardioversion, mostly in patients with atrial fibrillation of greater than 48-hour duration. Atrial stunning may last weeks and predispose to the formation of intracavitary thrombi and embolization.[100,101] In a recent retrospective study, Gallagher and colleagues reviewed the records of 1950 patients who underwent 2639 cardioversion attempts for atrial fibrillation and atrial flutter. In 443 instances, cardioversion was performed within 2 days of the apparent onset of the arrhythmia and only one embolic episode occurred, even though anticoagulation was provided in only 20% of the cases. In most of the instances (n = 1932), however, cardioversion was preceded by warfarin therapy for 3 or more weeks. No embolic complications occurred in 779 attempts when the INR was 2.5 or greater (95% confidence limits, 0-0.48) but in 9 of 756 instances when the INR either was less than 2.5 or was not measured. Embolism was significantly more common when the INR was between 1.5 and 2.4 than when the INR was 2.5 or greater (0.93% vs. 0%; $P = 0.012$). The incidence of embolism was similar after conversion of atrial flutter or atrial fibrillation. The authors of this study recommended that the INR be 2.5 or greater at the time of cardioversion for atrial fibrillation or atrial flutter of uncertain or greater than 2 days' duration.

RESPIRATORY COMPLICATIONS

The brief period of sedation and anesthesia required for cardioversion creates a risk for losing airway patency and for aspiration of gastric contents. These predictable complications can be avoided, especially in elective procedures, by adhering to existing protocols (i.e., fasting before the procedure), by providing careful monitoring of vital signs before, during, and after the procedure, and by having qualified personnel competent in the administration of sedatives and anesthesia present during the procedure.

PULMONARY EDEMA

Pulmonary edema is an infrequent but serious complication that may develop after cardioversion.[102,103] In a recent review of the literature, Gowda and colleagues[103] found that the underlying rhythms were atrial fibrillation (69%), atrial flutter (24%), supraventricular tachycardia (4%), and ventricular tachycardia (4%). The duration of the arrhythmia before cardioversion varied from 1 day to 13 years. Close to 90% of the patients had concomitant cardiovascular disease, including coronary artery disease (38%), rheumatic heart disease (23%), cardiomyopathy

(23%), and hypertension (8%). Pulmonary edema developed within a window of 96 hours, but most of the cases occurred within the first 24 hours. The mechanism responsible for post-cardioversion pulmonary edema is poorly understood but may be in part related to the underlying cardiac condition and use of agents for sedation and anesthesia that depress myocardial function. Nearly one third of patients have a low cardiac output after cardioversion for atrial fibrillation that resolves gradually over a period of several weeks.[104] The recovery of cardiac function in this population has been related to the resolution of atrial stunning.

RELEASE OF ENZYMES

Although high-energy and repetitive shocks can cause variable degrees of myocardial injury, the level of energy and number of shocks typically required for cardioversion is not likely to cause injury. Measurements of specific markers of cardiac injury such as creatine kinase-MB and troponins have consistently been shown not to increase following cardioversion.[105-108] Although prominent increases in total creatine kinase may occur, this typically indicates skeletal muscle injury. Elevation of markers of cardiac injury should therefore point to a possible underlying myocardial process, most likely ischemia.

ANNOTATED REFERENCES

Lown B: Defibrillation and cardioversion. Cardiovasc Res 2002;55:220-224.
Insightful editorial by Dr. Bernard Lown—pioneer of electrical cardioversion—describing the work that led to the development of concepts and equipment for cardioversion. Special reference is made to cardioversion of ventricular tachycardia and atrial fibrillation.

Schneider T, Martens PR, Paschen H, et al: Multicenter, randomized, controlled trial of 150-J biphasic shocks compared with 200- to 360-J monophasic shocks in the resuscitation of out-of-hospital cardiac arrest victims. Optimized Response to Cardiac Arrest (ORCA) Investigators. Circulation 2000;102:1780-1787.
Study demonstrating the greater initial efficacy of biphasic waveform defibrillation compared with monophasic waveform defibrillation in patients with out-of-hospital cardiac arrest.

White RD: New concepts in transthoracic defibrillation. Emerg Med Clin North Am 2002;20:785-807.
Authoritative and comprehensive review of mechanisms underlying electrical defibrillation.

Wik L, Hansen TB, Fylling F, et al: Delaying defibrillation to give basic cardiopulmonary resuscitation to patients with out-of-hospital ventricular fibrillation: A randomized trial. JAMA 2003;289:1389-1395.
Study demonstrating that a period of cardiopulmonary resuscitation before attempting defibrillation in patients with prolonged out-of-hospital ventricular fibrillation improves immediate and long-term outcomes.

Wyse DG, Waldo AL, DiMarco JP, et al: A comparison of rate control and rhythm control in patients with atrial fibrillation. N Engl J Med 2002; 347:1825-1833.
van Gelder IC, Hagens VE, Bosker HA, et al: A comparison of rate control and rhythm control in patients with recurrent persistent atrial fibrillation. N Engl J Med 2002;347:1834-1840.
Studies demonstrating that the traditional strategy of rhythm control may not be superior to rate control in patients with atrial fibrillation.

Chapter 211

TRANSVENOUS AND TRANSCUTANEOUS CARDIAC PACING

Raúl J. Gazmuri • Iyad M. Ayoub

KEY POINTS

1. Cardiac pacing may be considered for the treatment of symptomatic bradyarrhythmias, termination of supraventricular and ventricular tachyarrhythmias, prevention of bradycardia-induced tachyarrhythmias, and improvement of pump function by sequential atrioventricular (AV) pacing.

2. Transcutaneous pacing is especially useful for emergency pacing, standby during acute myocardial infarction, and intraoperative pacing in anesthetized patients.

3. The preferred vascular access sites for emergency transvenous pacing are the right internal jugular vein (first choice) and the left subclavian vein (second choice).

4. Transvenous pacing catheters may be "floated" without use of fluoroscopy, guided by electrocardiographic monitoring and ability to capture; this is facilitated by use of a balloon-tipped pacing catheter advanced through the right jugular vein.

5. Pacing for out-of-hospital asystolic cardiac arrest has not been shown to improve outcome.

6. Complications of transvenous pacing include arrhythmias at the time of insertion, need for subsequent lead repositioning, cardiac perforation, sepsis, phlebitis, and site-specific complications such as pneumothorax and arterial puncture.

Electrical pacing of the heart to substitute or override its native pacemaker activity is an important—and often lifesaving—intervention that should be available in every critical care setting. Indications for cardiac pacing arise from abnormalities in impulse generation and impulse conduction predisposing to serious bradyarrhythmias or tachyarrhythmias or both. Various techniques are available, including transcutaneous pacing,[1,2] transvenous pacing using dedicated[3,4] or multipurpose pulmonary artery catheters,[5] transesophageal pacing,[6,7] transgastric pacing,[8] and direct pacing of the myocardium by the transthoracic approach during cardiac arrest[9] or the open-chest approach during cardiac operations (Table 211-1).[10,11] The choice of the technique depends on the clinical setting (i.e., operating room

versus emergency department), indication (i.e., complete AV block versus prevention of torsades de pointes), urgency (i.e., asystole versus prophylaxis in acute myocardial infarction), chamber(s) to be paced (i.e., ventricular versus sequential AV pacing), lead stability (i.e., persistent bradyarrhythmias versus override pacing for tachyarrhythmias), operator's experience (i.e., vascular access for transvenous versus transcutaneous pacing), and patient's comfort (i.e., transcutaneous versus transvenous pacing in a nonanesthetized patient). The most common methods for closed-chest pacing are transvenous and transcutaneous, and these are discussed in this chapter.

HISTORICAL BACKGROUND

The first successful human cardiac pacing was reported by Zoll in 1952.[12] Using "stimulating electrodes" attached to subcutaneous needles placed in the chest wall of two patients who presented with ventricular asystole, "electric shocks" were successfully delivered, which promoted ventricular beats for extended periods. Two years later, Zoll and colleagues[13] reported on 14 additional patients, most of them presenting with Stokes-Adams syndrome.[13] In 1985, Zoll and colleagues[1] described an even larger group of 134 patients, who were paced in emergency departments, cardiac special care units, and regular wards at various hospitals. In these studies, pacing was delivered using large patch electrodes attached to the precordium and back for "emergency" treatment or "expected" cardiac arrest. Pacing electrodes also were applied prophylactically (i.e., in standby mode) or for termination of various tachyarrhythmias. Transcutaneous pacing was well tolerated in 73 of 82 conscious patients and successfully evoked electrocardiographic responses in 105 patients. There were 29 failures that were attributed to prolonged hypoxia or severe discomfort. Historical footage of the first patients treated with transcutaneous pacing is available at http://www.hrsonline.org/ep-history/topics_in_depth/default.asp#zollfilm.

Another stepping stone was the development of transvenous pacing by Furman and Robinson[3] at Montefiore Medical Center in New York in 1958. Furman devised a technique for right ventricular pacing, using a stimulating catheter electrode of his own design. On July 16, 1958, he successfully paced for 2 hours a patient with complete heart block undergoing colon resection. A second patient was paced for about 4 weeks and thereafter survived for 3 years. These experiences provided the impetus for the further

TABLE 211–1. TECHNIQUES FOR TEMPORARY PACING

Method	Chamber Paced	Uses
Transcutaneous	RV	Arrest, intraoperative,* prophylaxis†
Transesophageal	LA	Prophylaxis atrial, intraoperative
Transgastric	Ventricle	Intraoperative, maintenance
Transvenous, semirigid	RA and/or RV	Arrest, intraoperative, prophylaxis, maintenance
Transvenous, flow-directed	RV	Arrest, intraoperative, prophylaxis, maintenance
Multipurpose PAC	RA and/or RV	Arrest, intraoperative, prophylaxis, maintenance
Transthoracic	Ventricle	Arrest only (infrequently used)
Myocardial	Atrium and/or ventricle	Intraoperative, prophylaxis, maintenance

*Treatment of intraoperative bradycardia associated with low-flow states and bradycardia-induced tachyarrhythmias (i.e., sick sinus and long Q-T syndrome).
†For conditions that may progress to complete atrioventricular block, such as acute myocardial infarction and infective endocarditis.
LA, left atrium; PAC, pulmonary artery catheter; RV, right ventricle.

development of temporary and permanent transvenous cardiac pacing.[4]

INDICATIONS

Temporary cardiac pacing is indicated for therapeutic and prophylactic reasons (Table 211-2). Therapeutic indications arise primarily from abnormalities in impulse generation or conduction causing hemodynamically significant reductions in heart rate (including asystole and symptomatic second-degree or third-degree AV block) and for which medical

TABLE 211–2. GENERAL INDICATIONS FOR TEMPORARY CARDIAC PACING

Conduction Disturbances

Asystole*
Sinus dysfunction with hemodynamically significant bradycardia
Symptomatic and medically refractory second-degree and third-degree AV block
Complete AV block with wide QRS escape rhythm or ventricular response <50 beats/min
Acute myocardial infarction

Rate Disturbances

Termination of recurrent supraventricular and ventricular tachycardia
Suppression of bradycardia-related ventricular tachycardia
Suppression of torsades de pointes

Pump Failure

Sequential AV pacing

Prophylaxis

Pulmonary artery catheterization or right-sided myocardial biopsy in patients with preexisting left bundle-branch block
Cardioversion in patients with sick sinus syndrome
Acute myocardial infarction†
New AV or bundle-branch block in patient with acute endocarditis
Pharmacologic treatment with agents that may exacerbate bradyarrhythmias
Intraoperative in patients with underlying conduction abnormalities predisposing to bradyarrhythmias or tachyarrhythmias

*Shown not to be effective for out-of-hospital asystolic cardiac arrest or for asystole that develops after electrical defibrillation.[28] Should be considered for witnessed asystole.
†For indications during acute myocardial infarction, see Tables 211-3 and 211-4.
AV, atrioventricular.

treatment is either ineffective or not indicated.[14-17] These abnormalities may be the result of disease processes that affect the conduction system (e.g., acute myocardial infarction, sick sinus syndrome, infective endocarditis, Lyme disease), extracardiac abnormalities (e.g., hypoxemia, hyperkalemia, hypothyroidism, intracranial hypertension, vasovagal reactions), or drug toxicity (e.g., due to digitalis, calcium channel blockers, β-adrenergic blockers).[16] Pacing also may be used to terminate supraventricular or ventricular tachycardias by override pacing,[18-20] or for the prevention of bradycardia-induced ventricular tachyarrhythmias (e.g., torsades de pointes). These indications for pacing are particularly appropriate for the management of recurrent tachyarrhythmias when repetitive intervention is required.[18] Placement of a pacing device on standby for prophylaxis is recommended for conditions associated with increased risk of advanced AV block (e.g., acute myocardial infarction, infective endocarditis, surgery in patients with underlying conduction defects). Single-chamber pacing of the right ventricle is the most common and readily available technique. Atrial or sequential AV (dual-chamber) pacing may be required, however, in patients with ventricular dysfunction in whom properly timed atrial contraction may help improve pump function.[21,22]

Temporary cardiac pacing should be provided in an intensive care environment with capability for continuous electrocardiogram monitoring. The staff must be trained to pay close attention to sterility of the access site, stability of the pacing leads, and settings of the pulse generator (rate, output, and sensing). Temporary pacing should be carried out only where there is readiness for the diagnosis and treatment of potentially serious complications. Pacing is indicated in many clinical situations, but acute myocardial infarction and cardiac arrest merit special consideration.

ACUTE MYOCARDIAL INFARCTION

Therapeutic or prophylactic temporary cardiac pacing may play an important role in the management of patients during the acute phase of myocardial infarction. This diagnosis constitutes one of the most frequent indications for closed-chest pacing in nonsurgical patients.[16,23-26] Acute coronary occlusion promotes conduction abnormalities that may lead to complete AV block with variable degrees of hemodynamic compromise. The mechanism and severity of such abnormalities is contingent on the location of the occlusion and preexisting conduction abnormalities. Occlusion of the right coronary artery characteristically affects the sinoatrial node and the AV node and may precipitate transient sinus bradycardia and variable degrees of AV block in addition to inferior or posterior wall infarction. Complete AV block occurs in approximately 12% of patients[23,24] and is associated with increased incidence of left ventricular dysfunction and higher in-hospital mortality (24% versus 6%), but comparable long-term outcome.[23] The escape rhythm originates typically above the bifurcation of the bundle of His, and the morphology of the QRS complex on the electrocardiogram is narrow. Pump dysfunction may develop as a result of concomitant right ventricular infarction. If marked sinus bradycardia or complete AV block accompanies right ventricular dysfunction, increases in heart rate by single-chamber right ventricular pacing may not be effective. Selective atrial pacing or sequential AV pacing—if complete AV block is present—can markedly increase cardiac output.[21,27]

The mechanism of pump failure relates to a conflict of space within the semirigid pericardial sac. Right ventricular dysfunction leads to dilation of this chamber. The dilated right ventricle "squeezes" the left ventricle during diastole, precluding normal left ventricular filling. Atrial contraction (which occurs during the interval of ventricle filling) not only contributes to active filling, but also reduces atrial volume, allowing more space within the pericardial sac for ventricular filling. Atrial or sequential AV pacing is provided by placing a right atrial and a right ventricular pacing lead. Alternatively a multipurpose pulmonary artery catheter with leads for atrial and ventricular pacing may be used, allowing concomitant hemodynamic monitoring.

Occlusion of the left coronary artery also may lead to conduction abnormalities and complete AV block. The underlying mechanism involves injury to the left or right bundle branches (or both) as part of widespread myocardial injury and signals a poor prognosis. The incidence of complete AV block is about 5%, but this condition is associated with high in-hospital mortality (47% versus 12%).[24] Although pacing has not been shown to improve outcome, there is consensus that prophylactic and therapeutic pacing should be considered. Tables 211-3 and 211-4 list the recommendations made by the American College of Cardiology and the American Heart Association in 1999 for transvenous and transcutaneous pacing during an acute myocardial infarction.[25] Emphasis is placed on transcutaneous pacing, especially in patients not requiring immediate pacing and in patients at only moderate risk for complete AV block. Transcutaneous pacing also is appropriate in patients receiving thrombolytic therapy, reducing the need for vascular intervention.

CARDIAC ARREST

Emergent pacing using the transcutaneous or transvenous technique has been attempted during cardiac arrest with disappointing results. This is particularly true in instances of out-of-hospital asystolic cardiac arrest or when asystole develops after electrical defibrillation. In a study by Cummins and colleagues,[28] 278 victims of out-of-hospital cardiac arrest were treated by first responders with capability for transcutaneous pacing, and 368 victims were treated by first responders without such capability. Survival to hospital discharge was dismal, averaging about 2% regardless of whether or not pacing was attempted. In this study, the median time from collapse to pacing was 9 minutes. Smaller series have suggested, however, that some cardiac arrest victims may benefit if emergency transvenous or transcutaneous pacing is

TABLE 211–3. RECOMMENDATIONS FOR PLACEMENT OF TRANSCUTANEOUS PATCHES AND FOR ATTACHING THE PATCHES TO THE PACING SYSTEM IN THE STANDBY OR DEMAND MODE DURING AN ACUTE MYOCARDIAL INFARCTION

Class I (indicated)

Sinus bradycardia (rate <50 beats/min) with symptoms of hypotension (systolic blood pressure <80 mm Hg) unresponsive to drug therapy
Mobitz type II second-degree AV block
Third-degree heart block
Bilateral BBB (alternating BBB, or RBBB and alternating LAFB and LPFB) (regardless of time of onset)
Newly acquired or age-indeterminate LBBB, LBBB and LAFB, RBBB and LPFB
RBBB or LBBB and first-degree A-V block

Class IIa (probably indicated)

Stable bradycardia (systolic blood pressure >90 mm Hg, no hemodynamic compromise, or compromise responsive to initial drug therapy)
Newly acquired or age-indeterminate RBBB[1]

Class IIb (possibly indicated)

Newly acquired or age-indeterminate first-degree AV block

Class III (not indicated)

Uncomplicated acute myocardial infarction without evidence of conduction system disease.

BBB, bundle-branch block; LAFB, left anterior fascicular block; LBBB, left bundle-branch block; LPFB, left posterior fascicular block; RBBB, right bundle-branch block.
Data from Ryan TJ, Antman EM, Brooks NH, et al: 1999 update: ACC/AHA guidelines for the management of patients with acute myocardial infarction. A Report of the American College of Cardiology/American Heart Association Task Force on Practice Guidelines (Committee on Management of Acute Myocardial Infarction). J Am Coll Cardiol 1999;34:890-911.

instituted very early in the course of cardiac arrest.[14,15,17] Patients who respond with return of a pulse usually have some form of spontaneous electrical activity at the time of pacing.

Transcutaneous pacing is technically more feasible than transvenous pacing and can be deployed with minimal delay. Transvenous pacing requires blind insertion and is associated with a low success rate for achieving capture, in part because right ventricular lead placement during ongoing resuscitation is difficult. In one study, right ventricular placement occurred in no more than 30% of the instances.[29] A higher success rate can be attained, however, when using the right internal jugular vein. Blind use of the right subclavian vein is associated with a high percentage of right atrial placement.[29] Another approach is direct transthoracic pacing during cardiac arrest.[9] The technique is more invasive and is used infrequently, especially because of the widespread availability of transcutaneous pacing.

MECHANISM OF PACING

Pacing refers to the induction of a self-propagating wave of depolarization within the myocardium, usually by electrical stimulation; depolarization also may be induced manually by cardiac percussion.[30] Pacing requires that an energy threshold be exceeded, which is a function of the duration and amplitude of the stimulating pulse delivered outside the refractory period of the action potential.

TABLE 211–4. RECOMMENDATIONS FOR TEMPORARY TRANSVENOUS PACING DURING AN ACUTE MYOCARDIAL INFARCTION

Class I

Asystole
Symptomatic bradycardia (includes sinus bradycardia with hypotension and type I second-degree AV block with hypotension not responsive to atropine)
Bilateral BBB (alternating BBB or RBBB with alternating LAFB and LPFB) (any age)
New or indeterminate-age bifascicular block (RBBB with LAFB or LPFB or LBBB) with first-degree AV block
Mobitz type II second-degree AV block

Class IIa

RBBB and LAFB or LPFB (new or indeterminate)
RBBB with first-degree AV block
LBBB, new or indeterminate
Incessant ventricular tachycardia, for atrial or ventricular overdrive pacing
Recurrent sinus pauses (>3 sec) not responsive to atropine

Class IIb

Bifascicular block of indeterminate age
New or age-indeterminate isolated RBBB

Class III

First-degree heart block
Type I second-degree AV block with normal hemodynamics
Accelerated idioventricular rhythm
BBB or fascicular block known to exist before acute myocardial infarction

AV, atrioventricular; BBB, bundle-branch block; LAFB, left anterior fascicular block; LBBB, left bundle-branch block; LPFB, left posterior fascicular block; RBBB, right bundle-branch block.
Data from Ryan TJ, Antman EM, Brooks NH, et al: 1999 update: ACC/AHA guidelines for the management of patients with acute myocardial infarction. A Report of the American College of Cardiology/American Heart Association Task Force on Practice Guidelines (Committee on Management of Acute Myocardial Infarction). J Am Coll Cardiol 1999;34:890-911.

Most modern pulse generators are built to deliver monophasic square wave pulses with a constant current (mA). Use of biphasic waveforms—important for defibrillation—has not been found to offer additional advantages for pacing and may increase the threshold when pulses of short duration are used.[31]

Pacing leads may be bipolar or unipolar. Bipolar leads have two electrical poles: a negative pole (cathode) located at the distal end of the pacing lead and a positive annular pole (anode) located proximal to the distal pole. The cathode is the electrode through which the stimulating pulse is delivered. Unipolar leads have a single distal pole (cathode); the positive pole (anode) is attached to the patient through skin electrodes with a surface area greater than 50 mm^3. Bipolar leads are characterized by relatively small spikes on the paced electrocardiogram.

PACING NOMENCLATURE

A five-letter code has been developed to describe the features of pacemakers. The first three letters are the most important and applicable to temporary pacing. The first letter indicates the chamber being paced (*A*, atrium; *V*, ventricle; and *D*, dual [atrium and ventricle]). The second letter indicates the chamber being sensed (*A*, atrium; *V*, ventricle; *D*, dual

[atrium and ventricle]; and *O*, none). The third letter indicates the response after sensing (*I*, pacing is inhibited; *T*, pacing is triggered; *D*, dual [there is inhibition and triggering]; and *O*, none). The fourth and fifth letters apply to permanent pacemakers and refer to programmability (*P*, rate and output; *M*, multiprogrammable; *C*, communicating; *R*, rate adaptive; and *O*, none) and arrhythmia control (*P*, pacing; *S*, shock; *D*, dual [pacing and shock]; and *O*, none). *VVI* indicates that the ventricle can be paced and sensed and that pacing is inhibited if a beat is sensed; *DDD* indicates that atrium and ventricle can be paced and sensed and that pacing is triggered in each chamber if a beat is not sensed.

TECHNIQUES

TRANSVENOUS PACING

Transvenous pacing is a highly reliable technique with excellent patient tolerability that permits atrial or ventricular pacing (or both) but requires experience and is not without complications (see later).

Vascular Access

Various vessels have been used for vascular access, including the brachial (antecubital), femoral, internal jugular, and subclavian veins. The choice must take into account the urgency of the indication, the importance of pacing stability, the expected duration that pacing will be needed, the experience of the operator, and the risk of site-specific complications. The antecubital and femoral routes were the prime access routes in the 1970s and 1980s.[32] The relatively high incidence of pacemaker failure and complications along with the development of techniques for direct central venous catheterization has made these sites no longer the preferred routes (Fig. 211-1). Central vascular access through the jugular and the subclavian veins provides a much more direct route to the heart and offers greater stability with a lower incidence of pacemaker failure and complications. The currently preferred routes are the right internal jugular vein (first choice) and the left subclavian vein (second choice). These more direct vascular approaches permit rapid catheter placement, which is especially important in emergency situations. The right subclavian can be used, but there is a sharper angle to be negotiated between the subclavian

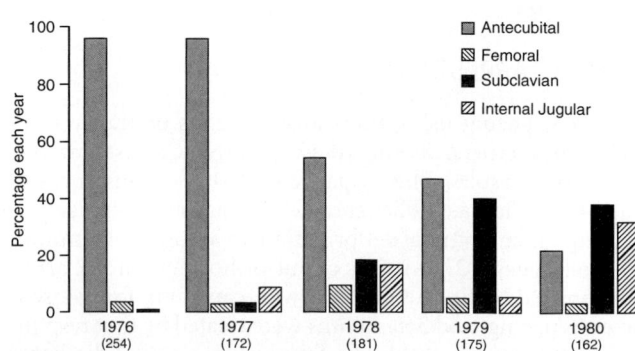

FIGURE 211–1. Changes over a 5-year period at Mayo Clinic on the preferred vascular accesses for transvenous pacing. Numbers in parentheses indicate pacing catheters placed each year. (Data from Hynes JK, Holmes DR Jr, Harrison CE: Five-year experience with temporary pacemaker therapy in the coronary care unit. Mayo Clin Proc 1983;58:122-126.)

vein and superior vena cava. In addition, the need for fluoroscopy may be obviated, especially when using the right jugular vein or when advancing a balloon-tipped pacing catheter. In the event of severe bleeding diathesis, one may consider using the brachial or femoral veins for access, especially if other methods (i.e., transcutaneous, transesophageal) are not available or suitable.

An alternative access is using the right supraclavicular subclavian route. Laczika and colleagues[33] reported a high success rate with a low incidence of complications. Critical care providers are less familiar with this approach, yet the experience in various other settings is favorable.[34,35] The vein is accessed through the angle formed between the junction of the clavicular head and the right sternocleidomastoid muscles with the patient in supine position and the head tilted to the left. The needle is advanced caudally at an angle of 30 to 40 degrees right to the sagittal plane and 10 to 15 degrees anterior to the coronal plane; the vein is typically found 2 to 4 cm deep to the skin.

Catheter Design

Catheters ranging in size from 3 Fr. to 6 Fr. are available in different designs and material reflecting their intended use. Catheters designed for use under fluoroscopy are semirigid (usually made of woven polyester) to facilitate steering into position. They may be straight for right ventricle pacing or have a J tip for right atrial placement. Newer catheters designed for right ventricle placement have a balloon at the tip and can be floated into position. In addition to these dedicated catheters, pacing can be accomplished by using multipurpose pulmonary artery catheters built with up to five electrodes for right atrial and right ventricular pacing.

Positioning

Guiding the pacing catheter into proper position is best accomplished under fluoroscopy. For right atrial pacing, a J-tipped catheter is advanced into the right atrial appendage to provide stable position. The tip of the curvature is oriented superiorly, anteriorly, and slightly medial.[18] For right ventricular pacing, the tip is advanced from the right atrium through the tricuspid valve into the right ventricle. The tip is positioned in the apex, which is visualized left of the spine near the cardiac border with the tip pointing inferiorly and anteriorly. A study has shown that under fluoroscopy, use of balloon-tipped catheters allows better final positioning with less procedure time than semirigid catheters.[36]

When fluoroscopy is not available, the pacing catheter may be advanced "blindly," guided by the electrocardiogram and the position confirmed by successful capturing. Blind placement is facilitated by using flow-directed, balloon-tipped catheters, preferably through the right jugular vein. This approach is gaining popularity, especially in emergency situations when time to initiation of pacing is critical. A V_1 lead of a conventional electrocardiogram is connected to the distal pole (cathode) and used to monitor a unipolar intracavitary electrogram continuously. The tip of the catheter is advanced into the superior vena cava, the balloon inflated, and the catheter advanced further until a right ventricular intracavitary electrogram is recognized (Fig. 211-2). The balloon is deflated and the catheter advanced a few centimeters more to position its tip in the right ventricular apex. Endocardial contact is indicated by the development of an "injury" current characterized by prominent ST-segment elevation. The magnitude of the elevation relates in part to

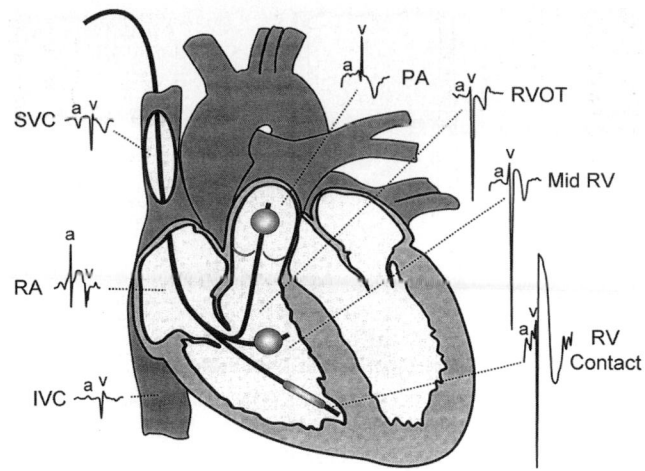

FIGURE 211–2. The distinct morphologies of a unipolar electrogram obtained in various intracavitary positions may be used to guide the placement of a temporary pacing catheter. Note the prominent ST-segment elevation that occurs on contact with the right ventricular endocardium. a, atrial electrogram; IVC, inferior vena cava; PA, pulmonary artery; RA, right atrium; RV, right ventricle; RVOT, right ventricular outflow tract; SVC, superior vena cava; v, ventricular electrogram. (Individual electrograms reproduced with permission from Ellenbogen KA [ed]: Cardiac Pacing. Oxford, Blackwell Scientific Publications, 1992, pp 162-210.)

the pressure applied to the endocardium and is not indicative of better position.[37] It has been recommended that ST-segment elevation be less than 2 mV for right ventricle pacing. In instances of right atrial pacing, the PR-segment elevation is recommended to be less than 0.5 mV. The pacing electrode is connected to the pulse generator and used in unipolar or bipolar configuration.

In emergency situations when pacing is immediately required (extreme bradycardia or asystole), the pacing lead may be advanced with the pulse generator on, set to its maximum output, and in the asynchronous mode at a rate of 70 to 100 ppm. A defibrillator should be available during insertion and afterward because life-threatening ventricular tachyarrhythmias may develop, especially if the pacing lead moves within the ventricular cavity.

An anteroposterior and lateral chest x-ray should be obtained after completion of the procedure to verify proper placement and to exclude possible complications (e.g., pneumothorax). A sterile sleeve should be placed around the catheter (available with most commercially available introducer kits) to facilitate subsequent repositioning if required.

Pulse Generator

Pulse generators typically are designed for ventricular, atrial, and sequential pacing. The basic features of a single-chamber unit are shown in Figure 211-3 and include controllers for output, sensitivity, and pacing rate along with indicators for when the unit is pacing, sensing, and low in battery charge. The generator delivers a pulse of brief duration (e.g., 1.8 msec) with a current ranging from 0.1 to 20 mA (Model 5348, Medtronic). The proper output is set by first determining the pacing threshold. For this purpose, the rate is set to exceed the spontaneous heart rate by at 10 to 20 beats/min, and the output is set to a level expected to capture 100% of the beats (i.e., 6 mA). Capture is verified on the electrocardiogram by identifying the presence of a spike (pulse)

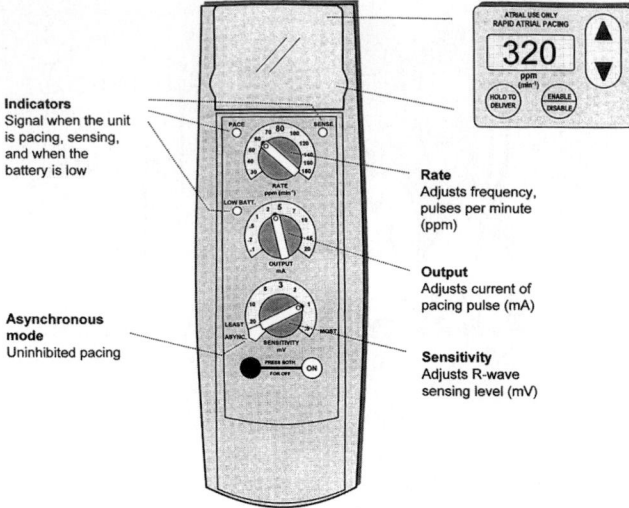

FIGURE 211–3. Rendition of the single-chamber external pulse generator (model 5348, Medtronic) designed for ventricular and atrial pacing.

followed by a wide QRS complex, which, in the case of right ventricular pacing, displays a left bundle-branch block morphology (Fig. 211-4). The output is reduced gradually until beats are no longer captured and increased again to identify the minimal level at which 100% of the beats are paced; this is the threshold output. This threshold level should be less than 1 mA for ventricular pacing and less than 2 mA for atrial pacing, in the unipolar and the bipolar configurations; otherwise, the lead needs to be repositioned. The output is set at about three times the threshold level for reliable capture.

The sensitivity control (range 0.5 to 20 mV) allows the native R-wave to inhibit the pacemaker impulse when the generator is set in *synchronous* mode. In the *asynchronous* mode, the rate is fixed, and the pacer does not sense atrial or ventricular myopotentials. To set the sensitivity, the output is first set to its minimal level (i.e., 0.1 mA), and the pacing rate is set to a value below the spontaneous heart rate. Starting from maximal sensitivity (the lowest value, i.e., 0.5 mV), the sensitivity is gradually decreased (increasing its value) until the unit stops sensing the R-wave. For reliable inhibition, the sensitivity is set at about three times the sensitivity threshold (e.g., if the threshold is 3 mV, the level is set at 1 mV).

The pacing rate for bradyarrhythmias is set according to physiologic needs, usually between 60 and 75 beats/min. Higher rates (800 beats/min) are available for override pacing of ventricular or supraventricular tachyarrhythmias.

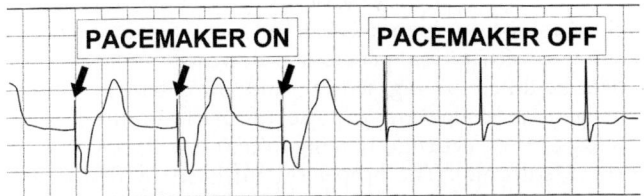

FIGURE 211–4. Pacing is characterized by a sharp spike followed by a wide-complex ventricular beat, which acquires left bundle-branch morphology when the stimulus is delivered to the right ventricle. Normal, atrial paced, narrow-complex ventricular beats are seen after the pacemaker is turned off.

Sequential atrioventricular pacing requires the placement of an additional lead or use of multipurpose pulmonary artery catheters along with a dual-chamber pulse generator. The individual chamber specifications for dual-chamber generators are similar with the option of setting the AV pacing interval between 20 and 300 msec.

TRANSCUTANEOUS PACING

Transcutaneous pacing is a noninvasive and exceedingly safe alternative for ventricular pacing that can be implemented with ease and minimal delay. It is especially attractive for prophylactic pacing,[1] use in emergency settings while preparing for more definitive therapy,[14,17] and under general anesthesia in patients undergoing surgical procedures.[2] The main drawbacks are that pacing is limited to the ventricles (with minimal capability for atrial pacing), capture is not always attained, and tolerability may be poor.

Pulse generators are designed to deliver much higher current levels (200 mA) with a longer pulse duration (20 to 40 msec) to facilitate capture and minimize patient discomfort. The external patches are large (8 cm diameter), self-adhesive, and manufactured to allow electrocardiographic monitoring and defibrillation. The location of the electrodes is important to optimize capture and patient comfort by directing the current path through myocardial tissue. Both patches can be placed on the anterior chest wall or in an anteroposterior configuration. The negative electrode (cathode) is placed anteriorly and close to the heart (typically over the palpable cardiac impulse or centered on a V_3 lead) to minimize the capture threshold. The positive electrode (anode) can by placed over the right upper region of the chest or the posterior chest wall, between the bony spine and the inferior border of either the left or right scapula (Fig. 211-5). The pacing threshold is determined as for transvenous pacing (see earlier), bearing in mind that the pacing threshold is much higher (20 to 140 mA), particularly in patients with emphysema, patients with pericardial effusion, and patients undergoing positive pressure ventilation.[1] The pacing output is set 5 to 10 mA above the threshold. Transcutaneous pacing has been used with moderate success for the treatment of ventricular and atrioventricular reentrant tachycardias by overdrive pacing.[38]

COMPLICATIONS

Pacemaker malfunction, defined as failure to sense, failure to capture, or both, is a relatively frequent occurrence. The actual incidence is influenced by the method of pacing. With transcutaneous pacing, the capture percentage is highly variable, ranging from 10% to 93% contingent on clinical variables.[38-40] Transvenous pacing provides greater reliability than other approaches; nevertheless, malfunction as a result of dislodgment has been reported to occur in 18% to 43% of cases when using the more distal brachial (antecubital) and femoral routes.[32,41,42] Use of the more central jugular or subclavian veins provides greater catheter stability and is associated with a lower incidence of pacemaker malfunction.

Additional complications include ventricular dysrhythmias at the time of insertion, perforation of the myocardium with risk of cardiac tamponade, diaphragmatic stimulation, phlebitis, pneumothorax, arterial puncture,

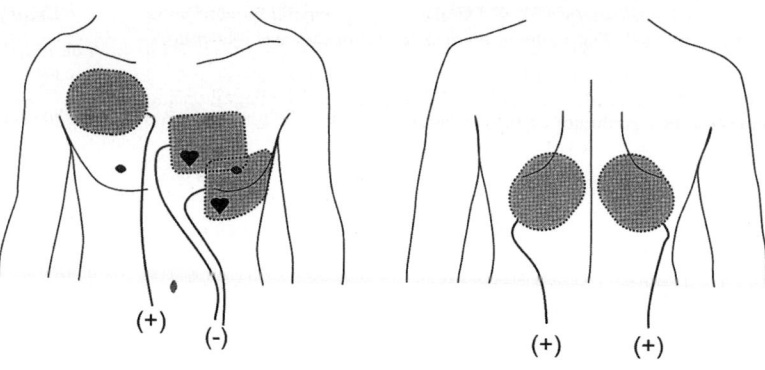

FIGURE 211–5. Placement of skin patches for transcutaneous pacing. The cathode (negative) electrode is identified by a small heart and is placed over the apex (point of maximal impulse) or centered over a V_3 electrocardiographic lead. The anodal (positive) electrode is positioned anteriorly in the right infraclavicular area *(left)* or posteriorly between the spine and either scapula *(right)*. For proper contact, the skin should be cleansed thoroughly with alcohol to remove salt deposits and skin debris, which may contribute to painful pacing and elevated thresholds.

brachial plexus injury, pulmonary embolism, and sepsis.[26,43] Ventricular dysrhythmias may necessitate emergent cardioversion or defibrillation. In a series reported by Jowett and colleagues[16] that included 137 patients who had transvenous pacing for complete AV block complicating an acute myocardial infarction, the most frequent complications were dysrhythmias at the time of insertion (9.2%), need for subsequent lead repositioning (7.4%), cardiac perforation (1.8%), and pneumothorax associated with subclavian vein access (1.2%). Making the diagnosis of cardiac perforation with subsequent cardiac tamponade requires a high index of suspicion. Table 211-5 lists the various signs and symptoms associated with cardiac perforation.[44] Traumatic complications seem to occur more commonly when using brachial and femoral routes, possibly as a result of greater motion of the pacing lead and the use of more rigid pacing catheters.

CONSIDERATIONS

Cardiac pacing by any modality should be avoided if possible in the setting of severe hypothermia, when mechanical or electrical cardiac stimulation may induce refractory ventricular fibrillation. Bradycardia associated with hypothermia may be physiologically appropriate, and treatment may not be indicated. Cardiac pacing may not need to be instituted under conditions of prolonged refractory asystolic cardiac arrest, in which the likelihood of successful resuscitation is nil. A relative contraindication is digitalis toxicity with recurrent ventricular tachycardia. The presence of bleeding diathesis should prompt careful consideration of the indication, method to be used, and route for venous access, if the transvenous approach is to be used. The presence of a mechanical tricuspid valve is a relative contraindication for the transvenous method unless placement in the coronary sinus is contemplated.

Cardiac pacing may be lifesaving and should be used whenever appropriate. It is important to minimize the associated risks, however, by paying close attention to the indications, pacing modalities, access routes, techniques, and duration of pacing and by providing proper follow-up to secure adequate functioning and early identification and treatment of complications if they emerge.

ANNOTATED REFERENCES

Cummins RO, Graves JR, Larsen MP, et al: Out-of-hospital transcutaneous pacing by emergency medical technicians in patients with asystolic cardiac arrest. N Engl J Med 1993;328:1377-1382.
This clinical study shows lack of benefit of transcutaneous pacing by first responders in victims of out-of-hospital asystolic cardiac arrest.

Hynes JK, Holmes DR Jr, Harrison CE: Five-year experience with temporary pacemaker therapy in the coronary care unit. Mayo Clin Proc 1983;58:122-126.
This large series reports a 5-year experience with transvenous pacing showing advantages and disadvantages of various sites for venous access.

Ryan TJ, Antman EM, Brooks NH, et al: 1999 update: ACC/AHA guidelines for the management of patients with acute myocardial infarction. A Report of the American College of Cardiology/American Heart Association Task Force on Practice Guidelines (Committee on Management of Acute Myocardial Infarction). J Am Coll Cardiol 1999;34:890-911.

TABLE 211–5. FEATURES ASSOCIATED WITH MYOCARDIAL PERFORATION BY A TEMPORARY PACING CATHETER

Symptoms

Pericardial chest pain, skeletal muscle stimulation, dyspnea (with tamponade), shoulder pain

Signs

Pericardial rub, intercostals or diaphragmatic pacing, presystolic pacemaker "click" on cardiac auscultation, failure to sense and/or pace, manifestations of tamponade, including hypotension, pulsus paradoxus, and jugular vein distention

Electrocardiogram

Change in paced QRS axis and/or morphology, pericarditis pattern

Chest x-ray

Change in lead position, extracardiac location of lead tip,* new pericardial effusion

Echocardiography

Extracardiac position of lead tip,* pericardial effusion, loss of paradoxical anterior septal motion or rapid initial left posterior septal motion characteristic of right ventricular apical stimulation

Intracardiac Electrograms

Biphasic or predominantly positive unipolar ventricular electrogram recorded from lead tip, change in unipolar electrogram morphology from biphasic R or Rs pattern to rS or S pattern with ST-segment elevation during catheter withdrawal*

*Diagnostic of perforation.
Adapted from Wood MA: Temporary cardiac pacing. In Ellenbogen KA, Kay GN, Willkoff BL (eds): Clinical Cardiac Pacing. Philadelphia, WB Saunders, 1995, pp 687-700.

Updated guidelines are presented for the management of acute myocardial infarction, including recommendations for transcutaneous and transvenous pacing.

Santini M, Ansalone G, Cacciatore G, Turitto G: Transesophageal pacing. Pacing Clin Electrophysiol 1990;13:1298-1323.

This is a comprehensive review article on transesophageal pacing.

Zoll PM, Zoll RH, Falk RH, et al: External noninvasive temporary cardiac pacing: Clinical trials. Circulation 1985;71:937-944.

This large series reports the experience of transcutaneous pacing in various clinical settings.

Chapter 212

VENTRICULAR ASSIST DEVICES

Amit N. Patel • Robert L. Kormos

KEY POINTS

1. Two major categories of ventricular assist device (VAD) systems have been used clinically with significant success in the United States: (a) pneumatic or electrically driven paracorporeal or implantable systems and (b) a centrifugal bypass pump system.

2. Most cardiac surgery programs operate on the premise that temporary ventricular support will allow the heart to recover from potentially reversible injury.

3. The principles of ventricular support include reducing ventricular afterload, preload, and ventricular wall stress and, ultimately, myocardial V_{O_2}; augmenting myocardial perfusion; and maintaining a physiologic systemic cardiac output.

4. The successful use of a VAD depends on careful patient selection.

5. Patients with normal acid-base balance and electrolyte levels, who remain in cardiac failure after placement of an intra-aortic balloon, should be considered for placement of a left ventricular assist device (LVAD).

6. Biventricular support may be required in the acute setting for large acute myocardial infarction with left ventricular dysfunction and severe arrhythmias, biventricular failure, viral myocarditis, and postpartum heart failure.

7. The treatment options leading to right ventricular support are similar to those for left ventricular support and include treatment of associated left ventricular failure, volume loading, physiologic pacing, and insertion of an intra-aortic balloon.

BACKGROUND

The use of mechanical circulatory support is required in a small but increasing proportion of the critically ill patient population with cardiopulmonary disease. Patients may require circulatory support before or after an open cardiac procedure. After acute myocardial infarction, it has been estimated that 10% to 15% of patients with subsequent cardiogenic shock require implantation of a mechanical circulatory support device before definitive corrective therapy can be performed.[1] Patients undergoing cardiac surgery have benefited from the many improvements in surgical technique and perioperative myocardial preservation. However, a proportion of these patients undergoing cardiac surgery are at risk of developing postoperative low output syndrome. One to 5 percent of patients undergoing cardiac surgery cannot be weaned from cardiopulmonary bypass despite adequate volume loading, metabolic stabilization, physiologic pacing, and full inotropic or intra-aortic balloon support.[2] These patients along with up to 30% of patients awaiting cardiac transplantation may be candidates for more extensive means of circulatory support.[3]

It has been 50 years since the introduction of the cardiopulmonary bypass system in cardiac surgery by Gibbon.[4] Many systems of full or partial bypass, relying on atrial or ventricular decompression along with aortic, pulmonary, or femoral artery return, have been developed for use as mechanical circulatory support.[5-8] Clinical evidence for the usefulness of a ventricular assist device (VAD) was initially anecdotal. Patients who could not be weaned from cardiopulmonary bypass recovered after further periods of bypass. As early as 1958, venoarterial bypass was proposed for acute cardiogenic shock.[8] The need for full heparinization and the degree of trauma to blood elements produced by the presence of a bubble oxygenator prompted the search for better methods of support.

The concept of arterial counterpulsation was first proposed in 1961 by Clauss and associates,[6] who developed a pump that could withdraw blood from the arterial circuit during systole and return it during diastole. This system, however, failed to provide adequate support, especially in the setting of hypotension. Using a transatrial septal approach to the left atrium from the jugular vein that allowed partial decompression of the left atrium and returned oxygenated blood to the femoral artery eliminated the need for an oxygenator.[9] This system still required full heparinization and was very traumatic to the blood elements owing to the need for a roller pump. Therefore, a cup was developed by Anstadt and associates in 1966[10]; this cup fit around the ventricles and functioned as a mechanical form of cardiac compression. However, it proved too damaging to the myocardium, especially in the setting of prosthetic valves, and to aortocoronary bypass grafts. Similarly, the intraventricular balloon[11] was too invasive and traumatic to the ventricle, although it did provide some support in the experimental setting. Although noninvasive, an external counterpulsation device, worn around the lower part of the body,[12] increased both preload and afterload and resulted in severe leg pain and cranial venous congestion after several hours' use.

The systems designed around a roller pump required a reservoir; thus, anticoagulation resulted in damage to the

TABLE 212–1. CHARACTERISTICS OF AN IDEAL MECHANICAL CIRCULATORY SUPPORT SYSTEM

- Is capable of producing blood flow of 5 to 6 L/min
- Unloads the left side of the heart by direct drainage from the left atrium or ventricle
- Produces minimal damage to the blood elements and myocardium
- Is not a cause of thromboembolism
- Is capable of reliable function for at least 7 days
- Is easy to set up, easy to use, and safe
- Requires minimal or no heparinization
- Is portable
- Is inexpensive

pump tubing and blood elements. The occlusive nature of the roller pump can lead to an entrance of air under conditions of low preload or bursting lines when pumping against high afterload. The intra-aortic balloon has the advantage of being less invasive but fails to provide adequate unloading to appreciably decrease myocardial work. The Anstadt cup and the intraventricular balloon are too invasive whereas the external counterpulsation device produces severe pain and cranial venous congestion.

The characteristics of an ideal left ventricular assist device (LVAD) are listed in Table 212-1. Most of the available systems are able to provide a wide range of required flows by decompressing the left atrium or ventricle. With the exception of the roller pump, these systems have been designed to produce minimal trauma to blood elements and require minimal or no heparin postoperatively. There are two major categories of VAD systems that have been used clinically with significant success in the United States: (1) pneumatic or electrically driven paracorporeal or implantable systems and (2) centrifugal bypass pump systems.

PHYSIOLOGIC BASIS FOR VAD USE

Many cardiac surgery programs throughout the United States have adopted the use of various types of mechanical support devices.[13-22] Most of these programs operate on the premise that temporary ventricular support will allow the heart to recover from potentially reversible injury. The mechanical support is provided by decompressing the atrium or ventricle and returning blood to the aorta for left ventricular support and to the pulmonary artery for right ventricular support. The devices function using either an electrically or a pneumatically driven pump. The goal of these devices in some cases is to decompress the heart so that recovery may occur after myocardial ischemia. This theory is based on the existence of a border zone of ischemia around established infarction.[23] Recovery may occur in this border zone if the self-perpetuating cycle of ischemia, low output, progressive and irreversible damage, and shock can be halted.[24] The etiology of ischemic injury after cardiopulmonary bypass is usually attributed to poor myocardial protection, but it may also result from overdistention of the ventricle, metabolic abnormalities, incomplete revascularization, coronary spasm, and embolism of air or particulate matter into these vessels. These insults result in an imbalance between oxygen supply and demand, with a subsequent depletion of adenosine triphosphate stores[25] leading to cellular and interstitial edema, increased regional stiffness, and ventricular dysfunction. In most patients requiring mechanical support there is

increased myocardial oxygen consumption (Vo_2). This increases the strain on the myocardium. To obtain balance between oxygen supply and demand, the goal must be to reduce myocardial Vo_2. The principal determinant of myocardial Vo_2 is ventricular pressure work,[26] whereas volume work, preload, and heart rate are less important. Graham and coworkers[27] demonstrated that myocardial Vo_2 depends on left ventricular peak wall stress and the intrinsic contractility of the muscle. Because contractility is already depressed in the low-output syndrome, one can only reasonably reduce myocardial Vo_2 by decreasing peak ventricular wall stress.

The principles of ventricular support include reducing ventricular afterload, preload, and ventricular wall stress and, ultimately, myocardial Vo_2; augmenting myocardial perfusion; and maintaining a physiologic systemic cardiac output. The more complete the reduction in afterload and ventricular tension-time index, the greater the reduction in myocardial Vo_2 and, therefore, infarct size. This approach is more physiologic than using inotropic drugs, which increase contractility, cardiac output, and mean blood pressure at the expense of increasing myocardial Vo_2. Some argue that these goals are achieved with the intra-aortic balloon.[28] There are multiple studies[29-31] that demonstrate that subendocardial perfusion is not maintained and infarct size is not reduced by the intra-aortic balloon because it is able to reduce myocardial Vo_2 by only 50% of that achieved by left ventricular assistance.[32] Also, the intra-aortic balloon can support a ventricle only if that ventricle is functioning at least marginally. Therefore, by supporting the failing ventricle one can arrest the cycle of low output and ischemia and allow for functional recovery in areas not totally infarcted while supporting the systemic circulation.[24] There is, in fact, ample evidence that myocardial infarct size can be limited and myocardial function restored by supporting the ventricle with a VAD.[33-37]

IMPLANTATION CRITERIA

Many potential candidates are assessed for mechanical circulatory support; however, most are not suitable for the rigors of long-term bypass. The successful use of a VAD depends on careful patient selection. In general, it is safe to assume that most patients who would not be considered a candidate for cardiac transplantation should not be placed on a VAD. Patient selection for a VAD can be based on modified Norman's criteria (Tables 212-2 and 212-3).[38-41] Patients who are post cardiotomy require a number of weaning steps from bypass to be performed before the true necessity for and the potential benefits of VAD support can be determined. A device should be implanted as soon as the failure to wean using traditional means is detected. However, the

TABLE 212–2. GENERAL SELECTION CRITERIA FOR MECHANICAL CIRCULATORY SUPPORT

- Patients who develop acute cardiogenic shock after myocardial infarction
- Patients, after technically successful cardiac surgery, who cannot be weaned from cardiopulmonary bypass with conventional methods
- Patients who, within 48 hours of technically successful cardiac surgery, develop low output syndrome and cannot be supported by conventional methods
- Patients suffering from a potentially reversible metabolic cause for cardiac failure (e.g., digitalis overdose, hyperkalemia)

TABLE 212–3. CRITERIA FOR USE OF A MECHANICAL CIRCULATORY SUPPORT DEVICE IN PATIENTS WHO CANNOT BE WEANED FROM CARDIOPULMONARY BYPASS

- Age between 10 and 65 years
- Patients should have good general health except for cardiac disease.
- The cardiac procedure must have been technically satisfactory except for the inability to wean from cardiopulmonary bypass.
- The following must be corrected: acidosis, alkalosis, hypovolemia, hypervolemia, inadequate rate or rhythm, and residual hypothermia. Surgically correctable problems should be dealt with appropriately (e.g., incomplete revascularization, residual valvular defects).
- If a satisfactory rate, rhythm, and blood pressure cannot be established using small doses of inotropic agents (dopamine <10 µg/kg/min) within 30 minutes of the failure of the first attempt at weaning, an intra-aortic balloon should be inserted.
- Failure to wean the patient from cardiopulmonary bypass with the intra-aortic balloon within 45 minutes constitutes failure at this phase and maximum inotrope support should be attempted.
- Failure to wean with the aid of the intra-aortic balloon in conjunction with maximally tolerated inotropic support (doses of dopamine higher than 20 µg/kg/min or an intolerable rhythm response) within 60 minutes of the start of resuscitation is an indication for support with a left ventricular assist device.
- If hypotension and low output syndrome develop in the ICU within 48 hours of cardiac surgery, standard resuscitative efforts are carried out. Pharmacologic agents and intra-aortic balloon support are used. If after 30 minutes of these intense measures the patient has not stabilized, the patient becomes a candidate for support with a left ventricular assist device.

surgeon should not deviate from the normal progression of less invasive therapies that are available (Table 212-4). One of the most crucial steps in successful VAD implementation is timing. The quicker one determines that a VAD is required after cardiotomy, the better the outcome.

INDICATIONS FOR LEFT VENTRICULAR ASSISTANCE

Patients with persistent severe cardiac dysfunction, despite volume loading and pharmacologic support, are eligible for insertion of an intra-aortic balloon for counterpulsation. This intervention decreases the left ventricular afterload and increases myocardial perfusion, which in turn increases the cardiac index by about 0.8 L/min/M^2. Patients with normal acid-base balance and electrolyte levels, who remain in cardiac failure after placement of an intra-aortic balloon, should be considered for LVAD placement. Failure to wean from bypass owing to left ventricular failure is defined by the presence of a systolic arterial blood pressure less than 80 mm Hg or a cardiac index less than 1.8 L/min/M^2 and urine output less than 20 mL/h in the presence of left atrial pressure greater than 25 mm Hg and central venous pressure (CVP) less than 20 mm Hg.

TABLE 212–4. CONVENTIONAL INTRAOPERATIVE THERAPY FOR VENTRICULAR FAILURE

- Optimal volume loading
- Increased reperfusion period
- Inotropic support ± afterload reduction
- Atrioventricular pacing
- Intra-aortic balloon support

These criteria for failure remain the same at each increasingly invasive stage of intervention during the weaning process.

INDICATIONS FOR RIGHT VENTRICULAR ASSISTANCE

Right ventricular failure can be seen either primarily, as a result of poor myocardial protection during bypass or incomplete revascularization, or secondarily, as a consequence of severe left ventricular failure. Isolated right ventricular failure is unusual but can be characterized by CVP greater than 25 mm Hg in conjunction with left atrial pressure less than 10 mm Hg and an inability to volume-load the left ventricle despite an elevated CVP. The limiting factor in the medical therapy for isolated right ventricular failure is usually the development of arrhythmias (including tachycardia), owing to the high doses of inotropic agents used. Occasionally, right ventricular failure may be noticed during the use of left ventricular support; it is characterized by an inability to provide adequate flow owing to low left atrial filling pressure in association with a high CVP. The treatment options leading to right ventricular support are similar to those for left ventricular support and include treatment of associated left ventricular failure, volume loading, physiologic pacing, and the insertion of an intra-aortic balloon. In some cases, pulmonary vascular afterload reduction and right ventricular inotropic support may be provided by the use of isoproterenol, milrinone, and, in cases of severe reactive pulmonary vascular hypertension, prostaglandin E$_1$.

INDICATIONS FOR BIVENTRICULAR ASSISTANCE

Biventricular support may be required in the acute setting for large acute myocardial infarction[42] with left ventricular dysfunction and severe arrhythmias, biventricular failure, viral myocarditis, and postpartum heart failure. In general, the more common patients requiring biventricular assist devices (BIVAD) are patients with LVADs who develop right ventricular failure. The maximum output of the LVAD is directly dependent on the maximum flow achieved by the right ventricle. In some cases, passive flow through the pulmonary bed may be accomplished by increasing the CVP and by using inotropic agents, such as isoproterenol. However, these interventions can lead to peripheral venous hypertension and edema. Mild right ventricular failure can be managed with pharmacologic agents and volume loading, but if the CVP is persistently greater than 25 mm Hg and the LVAD flow rates are less than 1.8 L/min/M^2, a BIVAD or the addition of a right ventricular assist device (RVAD) is indicated. Contraindications to mechanical circulatory support are relative, but some guidelines are outlined in Table 212-5.

DEVICES AVAILABLE FOR VENTRICULAR ASSISTANCE

Once it has been determined that the patient requires mechanical circulatory support there are number of devices available in the United States.[43-47] The type of device implanted is based on a number of factors. The potential need for short- versus long-term and univentricular versus biventricular support should be assessed. If unsure as to the true ventricular support required, a short-term device may

TABLE 212–5. CONTRAINDICATIONS TO THE USE OF A CIRCULATORY ASSIST DEVICE

- Metastatic carcinoma
- Pulmonary hypertension (>6 Wood units or pulmonary systolic pressure >60 mm Hg or transpulmonary gradient >15 mm Hg) for left ventricular assist devices
- Severe peripheral vascular or cerebrovascular disease
- Peptic ulcer disease
- Morbid obesity
- Recent or unresolved pulmonary infarction or pulmonary infiltrate (other than edema)
- Active infection
- Severe hepatic disease
- Blood dyscrasia

be implanted and then upgraded to something more permanent when required.

SHORT-TERM SUPPORT

Centrifugal Bypass Systems

The Biomedicus (Biomedicus Inc., Minnetonka, MI) centrifugal pump is relatively inexpensive and is relatively simple to apply for patients with both univentricular and biventricular failure.[47,48] The Biomedicus pump consists of rotating cones that impart a centrifugal force to the blood, moving it through a constrained vortex. Its nonocclusive nature results in less trauma to blood elements and tubing; because of the negative charge on its internal surfaces along with its unique shape, it can be used with minimal heparin. It adjusts automatically to downstream conditions by reducing its output in the presence of increased afterload due to arterial flow obstruction, even though the pump continues to rotate. Similarly, air cannot be pumped into a patient in large amounts, because the presence of air prevents the centrifugal pump from propelling blood; the presence of air in the system almost completely stops its pumping function. Overall, these characteristics result in less microembolization and lower plasma-free hemoglobin levels than with other systems. The pump is compact and easily portable within a hospital setting. A reservoir and heat exchanger are not required but may be spliced into the circuit. Reliable function can be expected from a pump head for at least 72 hours before it should be changed, owing to potential bearing wear, an occurrence that can lead to overheating at the base of the rotor and subsequent accumulation of thrombus in this area of the pump. However, the Biomedicus pump has been used in conjunction with minimal heparinization for as long as 4 days with no evidence of pump component failure or thromboembolic events. There are a number of limitations of the Biomedicus pump.[48] Once implemented in the operating room or ICU, the patient is bedridden and tied to mechanical ventilatory support. However, use of the device may aid in determining if a more permanent device is required or if the patient may be weaned off the device due to myocardial recovery. The device may be used for a short duration before the risks of intracranial bleeding, infection, and thromboembolic events increase.

Another short-term VAD is the Tandem Heart AB-180 (Cardiac Assist Technologies, Inc, Pittsburgh, PA).[49] The AB-180 is a centrifugal flow VAD that weighs approximately 280 g and has a priming volume of 7 mL. The pump is powered by a stationary electromagnetic motor that drives a magnetic rotor and an impeller, which rotates at 2700 to 4700 rpm. The device has a built-in anticoagulation system to deliver heparin directly to the impeller site to decrease thrombus formation. When placed in the cardiac catheterization laboratory, the inflow cannula is placed transseptally into the left atrium via the femoral vein. The outflow cannula is placed into the femoral artery. The device can pump up to 6 L/min at a mean arterial pressure of 60 to 90 mm Hg provided there is adequate left atrial pressure (>5 mm Hg) to fill the pump. This device is approved by the U.S. Food and Drug Administration (FDA) for 72 hours of use as a bridge to a more long-term VAD or as temporary support, which may be weaned once the heart recovers from acute injury. There are some limitations with this device, as with other centrifugal pumps. There is significant pump output to assist in maintaining systemic blood pressures. However, there is little reduction in the V_{O_2} and wall stress of the left ventricle, but this is still better than the Biomedicus pump. Also, the Tandem Heart is limited by the inflow from the left atrium, which may be reduced in the case of right ventricular failure. Therefore, this device is better suited for left ventricular dysfunction. It still requires the patient to be bedridden and on ventilatory support.

Pneumatic Short-Term VAD

In 1992, the FDA approved use of the ABIOMED BVS 5000 (Danvers, MA) external pulsatile pump. This device is pneumatically driven[50] and can operate one or two blood pumps independently and provide support to one or both ventricles. The BVS 5000 is typically used for short-term mechanical support in postcardiotomy patients with cardiogenic shock or in other situations when myocardial recovery is expected. Biventricular support can be performed without any specialized bedside personnel. This assist device is relatively low in cost and can be instituted without cardiopulmonary bypass (CPB). Theoretically, avoiding CPB may result in less end-organ damage. Various types of cannulas for blood drainage from and blood return to the patient may be used to accommodate differences in anatomy, facilitating simple and efficient insertion. The device consists of a polyurethane chamber in a polycarbonate housing. The atrium of the pump is filled by gravity and empties passively after the ventricle contracts. It supplies blood to a ventricle from which it is separated by a one-way valve. When the ventricle fills with 80 mL of blood, it generates a pressure that is sensed by the console that immediately sends compressed air back to the pumping chamber, causing the bladder to eject its volume. Unidirectional flow is ensured by the presence of one-way valves similar to a human heart. Left ventricular assist may be achieved by using a cannula graft with an extension sewn onto the aorta. The ascending aorta graft is sewn by placing a side-biting clamp on the aorta after heparin is given to achieve an activated clotting time of 300 seconds if the procedure is performed off CPB. Previous coronary grafts are carefully preserved. The inflow cannula may be placed into the left atrium via the right superior pulmonary vein, or into the left ventricular apex while on CPB. The cannulas are positioned away from the heart and tunneled through the abdominal wall to allow for chest closure without compression of the right ventricle.

Once left ventricular assist is started, flows are targeted to be greater than 5 L/min and the decision to start right ventricular assist is made. Inhaled nitric oxide may be used to achieve pulmonary vasodilation if the mean pulmonary artery pressure is more than 25 mm Hg. If needed, an RVAD may be implanted using a the pulmonary artery and the right atrium. RVAD placement may also be performed without CPB as well. Activated clotting time is set at 180 seconds using a heparin infusion usually started 12 hours postoperatively. In some patients, hemodynamic instability during implantation dictates the use of CPB. The device's internal rate is set by cyclic filling and it self-adjusts to maintain a stroke volume of 80 mL. The blood chambers are suspended on a pole so that preload and afterload can be optimized for maximal output, which is usually greater than 5 L/min. In the ICU, filling pressures are adjusted to 8 to 12 mm Hg. Afterload is controlled with vasodilators. Postoperatively, patients may be weaned off mechanical ventilation, and ambulation is possible within the ICU with assistance.

Intermediate-Term Pneumatic VAD

The Thoratec VAD System (Thoratec Corporation, Pleasanton, CA), formerly known as the Pierce-Donachy paracorporeal system,[43] employs a pneumatically activated polyurethane pumping chamber with a polysulfone case. The blood sac is made from Thoralon, a biopolymer that gives blood and tissue compatibility, along with thromboresistance. The chamber has Björk-Shiley (Shiley, Inc., Irvine, CA) inlet and outlet valves and has a stroke volume of 65 mL, with pump rates ranging from 20 to 110 beats/min and flow outputs ranging from 1.3 to 7.2 L/min. It can operate at either a fixed rate that is determined by the user, a fill-to-empty (the heart ejects when a switch is tripped by the chamber being filled), or a mode synchronized to the R wave of the electrocardiogram. This device lies outside the abdominal wall; two percutaneous cannulas drain the left atrium or ventricle and return the blood to the aorta. The device can be used either for left or right or for biventricular support (using two pumps).[51] The Thoratec VAD is FDA approved as a bridge to cardiac transplantation and postcardiotomy recovery of the native heart. This device decreases the Vo₂ of the ventricle by allowing enough decompression resulting in the semilunar valve not opening during systole. The relaxation of the ventricle results in decreased wall stress and allows recovery of the injured myocardium. Patients with the Thoratec VAD benefit from pulsatile flow and may be discharged home until transplantation or weaning of the device. Systemic anticoagulation is still required, which may still lead to bleeding and thromboembolic complications. There is also an inherent risk of cannula tunnel infections, because the VAD is paracorporeal. However, a newer version of the device is an implantable ventricular assist device (IVAD), which may reduce the risk of infections and be more portable.

LONG-TERM SUPPORT

The HeartMate Left Ventricular Assist System (LVAS) (Thoratec Corporation, Pleasanton, CA), formerly the Thermedics device,[44] can be implanted as either a vented electric (XVE) or an implantable pneumatic (IP) LVAD.[17] Both LVADs are designed to assist the pumping function of the left ventricle of the native heart and have a unique textured titanium blood-contacting surface that eliminates the need for systemic anticoagulation. It employs a pusherplate and blood sac with a stroke volume of 85 mL. This system is designed only for left ventricular support, because it requires insertion through a Teflon sewing ring into the ventricular apex with return to the ascending aorta. It employs inflow- and outflow-valved Dacron conduits. This device can be operated in a synchronized counterpulsation mode, at a fixed rate, or in an automatic mode, which is rate responsive to the patient's volume demands. The HeartMate XVE is powered by wearable batteries that allow the patient to be mobile, whereas the IP is powered by an external drive console. Both devices are fully implanted alongside the native heart and are designed to assist the pumping function of the left ventricle. The HeartMate LVAS allows a patient to be discharged home without the risks associated with systemic anticoagulation. It decreases left ventricular myocardial Vo₂. Both devices are approved by the FDA as a bridge to cardiac transplantation. However, the HeartMate LVAS is restricted because it can only be used as an LVAD and must be implanted in the preperitoneal space or abdominal cavity. This means that patients with a small body habitus cannot have this device because of anatomic limitations.

Finally, the Novacor Left Ventricular Assist System (LVAS) (World Heart Corporation, Oakland, CA), an electric VAD,[45] uses a pusherplate and sac blood pump with two Carpentier-Edwards bioprosthetic valves and a fiberglass/polyester-encased solenoid energy converter. Dacron conduits connect the pump to the left ventricular apex and ascending aorta. The energy converter is connected via percutaneous leads to the console. This device can also operate in a fixed rate or counterpulsed mode or can be synchronized to the ECG. The Novacor system is designed to be used only for left ventricular support. Implantation and function are similar to the HeartMate XVE. However, the Novacor LVAS requires systemic anticoagulation.

Many complex and expensive implantable and paracorporeal systems exist for use as VADs. These devices evolved as offshoots from the development of total artificial hearts. Most of these units require full anticoagulation, and not all are adaptable for the right as well as the left ventricle. Centrifugal pumps, on the other hand, are simple to use, are less expensive, and can be used to support either or both ventricles. Although it is stated that minimal anticoagulation is required for its operation, the drive heads of the Biomedicus pump have been found to contain small thrombi beneath the rotor and along its internal struts. Thus, it is necessary to change the pump head at least every 4 days. In addition, thrombi have been found on the cannula tips under conditions of low heparinization. Nevertheless, this device holds the most attraction for many centers where the low output syndrome needs to be tackled without the investment in time and money for the more complex devices.

DESTINATION THERAPY

There are a growing number of patients with heart failure who are not transplant candidates. However, these patients with isolated left ventricular failure may benefit with permanent LVAD therapy, as demonstrated in the REMATCH trial.[52-58] The HeartMate XVE is approved by the FDA for destination therapy. Patients may receive permanent implantation of a LVAD. There are many concerns as to how to select and care for these patients long term. The option is available, but further trials are necessary to determine the best patients for permanent VAD therapy. The criteria for permanent VAD therapy closely resemble those for heart transplantation: New York Heart Association class IV heart failure, left ventricular ejection fraction less than 25%, either peak oxygen consumption less than 12 mL/kg/min or dependence on intravenous intotropic support. The REMATCH study found that mortality at 1 year was 76% in the medical therapy group versus 51% in the LVAD group. The survival at 1 year was 24% in the medical therapy group versus 49% in the LVAD group. These were very dramatic findings that led to the approval of permanent LVAD therapy for patients who were not transplant candidates for various reasons but who met most of the medical criteria for transplantation. Currently, destination therapy is available in the United States only at medical centers that perform heart transplantation, have a VAD program, and are approved by the federal government.

INSTITUTION OF AN LVAD

Once the decision to use the VAD has been made, the following monitoring lines are essential: (1) an arterial pressure line and (2) a pulmonary artery catheter to measure CVP and pulmonary artery pressure. The presence of an atrial septal defect or patent foramen ovale results in immediate desaturation of blood on starting the LVAD. This problem must always be anticipated and dealt with by opening the right atrium to repair the defect. In the early stages of recovery after VAD implantation, it is advised to keep the LVAD flow at 75% of the patient's predicted cardiac output to prevent the development of right-sided heart failure. One should avoid volume overload in an effort to increase cardiac output, because volume overload produces filling pressures that are too high. The high LVAD flow rates that are required to adequately decompress the left atrium subsequently increase the right-sided filling pressures and increase the probability of right-sided heart failure. It is usually safe to volume-load the patient up to a CVP of 15 mm Hg. Patients who cannot raise their left atrial pressure after volume loading to a right atrial pressure of 25 mm Hg are defined as having right ventricular failure. These patients will need support with isoproterenol or right ventricular bypass with a second pump from the right ventricle to the pulmonary artery.

Immediately postoperatively, one should not hesitate to give fresh frozen plasma as well as platelet concentrates to correct any coagulation abnormalities. The intra-aortic balloon is left in place and functioning during the period of LVAD support. The balloon pump produces pulsatile flow with peaks during diastole, thus augmenting coronary blood flow in VADs without native pulsatile flow. If the heart is not too edematous, the sternum is usually closed along with the subcutaneous tissue and skin to reduce the risk of infection and wound dehiscence with long-term ventilation.

CARE OF THE PATIENT IN THE CARDIOVASCULAR ICU

Care of the patient on a mechanical circulatory assist device in the ICU demands close cooperation among perfusionists, nurses, surgeons, intensive care physicians, and family members.

GENERAL PRINCIPLES OF CARE

The patient with a VAD should be cared for just like any other sick patient who has undergone cardiovascular surgery. Arterial pressure, pulmonary artery pressure, and CVP are

monitored continuously. Mechanical ventilation is continued until it is no longer required; routine postoperative analgesics and antibiotics are used. Chest tubes are removed on the first or second postoperative day as determined clinically. Dressings are changed once daily, and the incision and all cannula entry sites are cleaned with antiseptic solution.

HEMODYNAMIC SYSTEM

The cardiac output of the pump is maintained for the first 24 hours at a level comparable to 75% of the patient's last natural cardiac output. This avoids the development of right-sided heart failure and also prevents overperfusion of the kidneys and the brain. Because the left atrial pressure can be altered at will by the LVAD flow rate, the volume status of the patient will be indicated by the CVP. If the CVP is more than 25 mm Hg, right ventricular failure must be considered as the cause of poor left atrial filling. If the CVP is less than 10 mm Hg, volume should be added unless the systemic vascular resistance index is less than 1000 dynes • sec/cm^{-5}/M^2. The ideal systemic vascular resistance index should be in the range of 800 to 1200 dynes • sec/cm^{-5}/M^2, and this can be achieved with the use of a carefully titrated combination of Neo-Synephrine, dopamine, and sodium nitroprusside. The objective is to avoid severe postoperative edema from excessive volume loading yet maintain a sufficient blood pool to avoid wide fluctuations in LVAD flow rates. The LVAD flow rate is gradually increased to achieve a flow of 2.2 L/min/M^2. In patients with prosthetic valves, the pump flow should be decreased by 500 mL/min for 5 to 10 seconds every 2 to 3 hours to ensure that the valve leaflets are opening and closing, thus minimizing thrombus formation. Prosthetic valve function should be verified by echocardiography at least every 2 days. In patients undergoing valve replacement, fusion and thrombosis of the tissue valve leaflets have been seen in low-output states in LVAD patients. The inherent circumferential insufficiency of tilting disk valves makes them less likely to develop this complication.

HEMATOLOGIC SYSTEM

Anticoagulation is started 12 hours after surgery (as long as blood loss from the chest tube is less than 50 mL/h) with intravenous heparin. The platelet count is maintained at more than 50,000/mm^3 with platelet transfusions. Most patients requiring a VAD are potential candidates for cardiac transplantation. Multiple blood transfusions may result in elevated levels of preformed antibodies, making rejection more likely. Therefore, only leukocyte-depleted packed red blood cells should be given for a hemoglobin value less than 9 g/dL. A panel reactive antibody level should be determined on every patient who is considered as a transplant candidate to assess the likelihood of post-transplant rejection.

RENAL SYSTEM

The CVP should be kept at less than 15 mm Hg to avoid renal venous hypertension, and pump flows should be adjusted to prevent hyperperfusion. Broad-spectrum antibiotics should be continued for 4 to 5 days. Keeping the Pco$_2$ in a normal range also has a protective effect on renal function. The urinary catheter should be removed as soon as possible to prevent sepsis. If mild postoperative renal dysfunction develops, continuous veno-veno hemodialysis may be required. It results in a more gradual removal of volume than does conventional hemodialysis, leading to fewer episodes of hemodynamic instability.

PULMONARY FUNCTION AND PHYSIOTHERAPY

It is important that the patient receive the normal postoperative chest physiotherapy and that nursing staff are reassured that no harm can be done to the patient or the pump lines by turning the patient periodically. Active physiotherapy should be carried out, even if only to provide passive range of motion exercises. Any rise in intrathoracic pressure will immediately reduce the flow of blood through the pulmonary circuit and thereby the filling of the left atrium. Airway obstruction, bronchospasm, or tension pneumothorax result in a dramatic drop in the VAD flow rate and must be avoided. Pulmonary toilet is essential with airway suctioning when required as long as the patient remains intubated. Frequent deep breathing after extubation using sustained maximal inhalation techniques (incentive spirometry) is helpful in an effort to avoid formation of atelectasis and pneumonia by stimulating cough and bringing up thick bronchial secretions.

NUTRITIONAL AND GASTROINTESTINAL SYSTEMS

Due to the increased metabolic demands that result from a stress response after surgery and long-term cardiopulmonary support, multiorgan failure often complicates the course of these patients. Therefore, nutritional management is an important component in the care of the VAD patient. The high caloric requirements preferably should be met using a patient's own gastrointestinal tract; occasionally intravenous nutritional support is also required to avoid excessive protein breakdown. Stomach acidity should be reduced with conventional antacid therapy.

COMPLICATIONS OF VAD SUPPORT

There are numerous potential complications that may arise during the course of therapy for heart failure. Once VAD support is implemented, the patient's underlying health status plays a significant role in postoperative recovery and complications. Patients who require preoperative ventilation are at an increased risk for pulmonary complications once VAD support is begun. Also, the device itself triggers a systemic inflammatory response, which may lead to complications with coagulation due to early consumption of blood products. Overall incidence of infection is around 35%. Sites of infection include the pulmonary subsystem, blood, urine, the pump pocket, and the driveline. Most infections are treated with standard antibiotics. However, device-related infections may require early removal of the VAD or treatment with muscle flaps with the aid of plastic surgical approaches. Device-related infections have also been shown to increase the risk of neurologic events in our VAD patients. Neurologic events occur in approximately 5% to 10% of patients. Most are transient in nature, but there are a few that are catastrophic. Therefore, close monitoring of fevers and surgical sites and use of anticoagulation are required to decrease the risk of adverse events.[59-64]

MAINTAINING A SATISFACTORY LIFESTYLE

The patient should be kept pain free but not in deep sedation beyond 24 hours after surgery. It is especially important to avoid pharmacologic paralysis, because this will remove the clinical indicators of cerebral thromboembolism (should it occur). In most circumstances, the patient on a VAD will be conscious and wishing to communicate by 48 hours after surgery. The family must be fully informed of the patient's status and encouraged to support the patient, especially if the device is required for a period of time longer than 48 hours. The patient's anxieties about the device must be recognized and responded to. Regular meetings with nursing and medical staff should be held to answer questions that arise and to aid in effective and consistent communication with the patient and family members.

PATIENT MONITORING IN THE CARDIOVASCULAR ICU

Monitoring of hemodynamic, hematologic, and biochemical variables is carried out according to normal postoperative routines with emphasis on indices of infection, thrombosis, anticoagulation, and hemolysis. Ventricular function is ideally assessed daily by echocardiography. As the ventricle improves, one sees that the left atrial pressure or CVP will rise less as the pump flow is turned down and the pulmonary artery and cardiac output drops lower, thus signifying that the pump contributes less to the total cardiac output. In addition, one will often see a competition for left atrial blood between the recovering native heart and the pump, in that it becomes hard to maintain pump output while the cardiac output remains elevated.

WEANING FROM LVAD

After the first 24 to 36 hours (during which time no attempt is made to wean the LVAD), the pump flow is reduced by 25% and hemodynamic measurements are made. If the cardiac index can be maintained at more than 2.0 L/min/M^2, in association with a systolic blood pressure greater than 80 mm Hg and a pulmonary artery diastolic pressure less than 20 mm Hg, the flow is reduced another 25% and measurements are then repeated. Successive 25% flow reductions can be made every 4 to 6 hours as long as the cardiac index, blood pressure, and pulmonary artery diastolic pressure criteria that were previously defined are met. Weaning is performed under the guidance of echocardiography to assess real-time return of myocardial function.[65] Once a flow of 500 mL/min is tolerated and the just-listed hemodynamics are maintained, the LVAD may be removed. If the hemodynamic status is stable for 24 hours after LVAD removal (as defined by the previous criteria), the intra-aortic balloon pump is removed. In most cases, patients who can be weaned from LVAD demonstrate recovery of function within 48 to 72 hours and recovery from RVAD in somewhat less time. Patients on simultaneous right and left ventricular support usually show recovery of the right ventricle first, followed by the left. If after 7 days of LVAD support the patient cannot be weaned from the device, a condition of pump dependency may have developed. At this point, three possible alternatives exist and the family of the patient should be so informed. The three options are (1) continued prolonged support; (2) referral to a center where cardiac transplantation or an artificial heart can be offered; or (3) gradual weaning of the device despite a lack of evidence indicating native cardiac function. The responsible physician should provide his or her recommendation regarding the best choice, realizing that the right to decide rests with the competent patient. If the patient lacks the capacity to decide, the family normally is expected to make this decision as advised by the surgeon and the appropriate consent should be obtained to proceed accordingly.

LVAD REMOVAL

Removal of the LVAD is performed under general anesthesia in the operating room. The sternotomy wound is opened carefully and any old hematoma is washed out. The pump is turned off, and the lines are clamped with tubing clamps. The pursestring sutures are cut, and all cannulas are removed. The arterial cannula is removed first. The atrial cannula is removed under prolonged inflation of the lungs with positive pressure. This flush of blood presumably expels any thrombus that may have accumulated near the cannulation site and prevents entrance of air into the atrium. Once hemostasis has been verified, mediastinal drainage tubes are inserted and the sternotomy incision is closed in the usual manner.

RESULTS OF VENTRICULAR SUPPORT

The results of ventricular support appear to be influenced by any delay in insertion of the device, the presence or development of biventricular failure, and the presence of completed myocardial infarction at the time of insertion of the device. There have been many studies trying to assess the risk of VAD implantation and the potential risks after transplantation.[66-69] Complications due to the use of assist devices most commonly are bleeding, infection, and thromboembolism (Table 212-6). It is a delay in the insertion of these devices once the diagnosis of intractable failure is made that results in poor recovery. This is primarily related to the development of completed myocardial infarction, compromised end organ dysfunction, and the development of biventricular failure. The results of early LVAD programs were probably affected by this factor of delayed insertion.

The results of univentricular failure treated with VADs are encouraging. Isolated right ventricular failure has a weanability rate of nearly 100% and equally impressive survival; however, it is a relatively rare phenomenon. Isolated left ventricular failure, when treated early, results in a weanability rate of 50% to 75% with survival rates in the range of 20% to 60%; however, the recovery rate drops to 0% in the presence of biventricular failure treated with LVAD alone. It is only when biventricular failure is treated with concomitant right and left ventricular support that a 50% ability to wean and 30% survival rate can be achieved.[17,18,42,57,69,70] The causes of death in patients undergoing ventricular support are most commonly bleeding, infection, myocardial infarction after device removal, and progressive multiorgan dysfunction in the face of compromised flow. Less common causes are device component failure or problems with cannula position and drainage of the ventricle. Once again, the failure of functional recovery while on support probably has

TABLE 212–6. COMPLICATIONS OF CIRCULATORY SUPPORT SYSTEMS

- Tissue ingrowth at areas where conduits join the heart
- Clot formation and embolization
- Infection at sites of anastomosis, tissue ingrowth, or skin penetration
- Bleeding
- Hemolysis
- Device failure (e.g., valves, flexing membranes, control circuit)
- Progressive multiorgan failure

something to do with completed infarction of the ventricle. Myocardial necrosis that is diagnosed by biopsy at the time of implant of the device is present in 86% of patients who fail support and only in 25% of those who recover. Patients placed early on VADs after an acute coronary event may be weaned or bridged to transplant. A small but growing number of patients who are not transplant candidates may benefit from destination therapy.

CONCLUSION

Mechanical circulatory support that provides maximum preload and afterload reduction of a ventricle that cannot be recovered with traditional therapy is feasible. The level of sophistication of these devices varies, but the principles of function remain the same and appear to provide similar results. Recovery of function appears to be related more to the correct timing of insertion of these devices and to the extent that both ventricles are involved. A weanability rate of 50% to 75% with survival around 30% is achievable for left ventricular assistance after cardiotomy. However, with acute myocardial infarction the survival rates are even better. Careful patient selection is important, and specific institutional protocols must be developed for selection and management of this rare but very ill group of patients to have successful outcomes.

ANNOTATED REFERENCES

Loebe M, Soltero E, Thohan V, et al: New surgical therapies for heart failure. Curr Opin Cardiol 2003;18:194-198.
Excellent review detailing several new surgical techniques developed for heart failure patients.

Rose EA, Gelijns AC, Moskowitz AJ, et al: Long-term mechanical left ventricular assistance for end-stage heart failure. N Engl J Med 2001;345:1435-1443.
Findings from the Randomized Evaluation of Mechanical Assistance for the Treatment of Congestive Heart Failure (REMATCH) Study Group. The use of a left ventricular assist device in patients with advanced heart failure resulted in a clinically meaningful survival benefit and an improved quality of life. A left ventricular assist device is an acceptable alternative therapy in selected patients who are not candidates for cardiac transplantation.

Oz MC, Gelijns AC, Miller L, et al: Left ventricular assist devices as permanent heart failure therapy: The price of progress. Ann Surg 2003;238;577-583.
The REMATCH trial evaluated the efficacy and safety of long-term left ventricular assist device (LVAD) support in stage D chronic end-stage heart failure patients. This paper addresses the cost of hospital resource use, and its predictors, for long-term LVAD patients. It concludes that the cost of long-term LVAD implantation is commensurate with other life-saving organ transplantation procedures like liver transplantation, but as it is an evolving technology, there are a number of opportunities for improvement that will likely reduce costs in the future.

Chapter 213
PERICARDIOCENTESIS

Stefano Maggiolini • Giovanni Vitale • Alessandro Bozzano

KEY POINTS

1. **Pericardiocentesis** is a technique that allows the removal of fluids accumulating in the pericardial space. It is useful in the diagnosis and treatment of pericardial effusive diseases.

2. Pericardial space can accommodate from a few milliliters of fluid to substantial amounts, according to the rate of accumulation. **Cardiac tamponade** occurs when intrapericardial pressure equalizes and opposes atrial and ventricular pressures, thus limiting diastolic filling and reducing stroke volume, cardiac output, and arterial pressure.

3. **Clinical signs** of cardiac tamponade include increased central venous pressure, hypotension, tachycardia, and pulsus paradoxus.

4. The effect of pericardiocentesis is immediate. **The drainage of few milliliters of fluid relieves clinical and hemodynamic signs of cardiac tamponade** and avoids progression to cardiac arrest and pulseless electrical activity.

5. Several diagnostic methods, chest radiography, computed tomography (CT), and magnetic resonance imaging (MRI), can detect the presence of a pericardial effusion. **Transthoracic echocardiography** is the most simple and accurate method to diagnose the presence of pericardial fluid and also its hemodynamic consequences, such as collapse of cardiac chambers and the impairment of intracardiac flows.

6. Indication for emergency pericardiocentesis is limited to overt cardiac tamponade. **Elective pericardiocentesis** is warranted when purulent pericarditis is suspected, and it may be indicated when a very large effusion is detected. Thrombocytopenia, bleeding disorders, and anticoagulant therapy contraindicate elective procedures.

7. Blind or electrocardiographic needle monitoring approaches to pericardiocentesis are no longer justified. **Echocardiographically guided pericardiocentesis** is the most simple and safe technique. It can be performed with or without continuous visualization of the needle tip. The needle is most commonly inserted in the area where the pericardial space is closest to the probe and the fluid accumulation is maximal.

8. **Medical management** of critical patients while preparing for pericardiocentesis includes fluids and vasoactive amines.

9. Possible **complications** include lesions of intrathoracic structures. Major complications are rare when pericardiocentesis is performed with an echocardiographically guided technique.

10. **Pericardial drainage** for 24 to 72 hours is effective in preventing recurrence of effusion in most cases. In case of pericardial effusion reaccumulation, which is frequently observed with underlying malignancies, a pleuropericardial window may be created using percutaneous balloon pericardiotomy.

11. **Percutaneous balloon pericardiotomy** is a nonsurgical alternative technique to surgical pericardial window. It may be performed under fluoroscopic guidance using one or two balloons. This technique has a low complication rate.

Pericardiocentesis is a valuable technique in the diagnosis and treatment of patients with pericardial effusion and cardiac tamponade. A blind approach using the trocar-and-cannula method was described at the beginning of the 19th century. The subxiphoid approach was first described in 1911.[1]

PATHOPHYSIOLOGY

The pericardial space normally contains 25 to 50 mL of fluid in adults. If the amount of fluid increases, the pericardium is not immediately distensible, even though stress relaxation may occur within minutes from the beginning of the increase in pericardial pressure.[2] If the fluid accumulates slowly, over weeks or months, the pericardium can increase in size to a maximum capacity of 1 to 2 L. As the volume of the effusion increases, intrapericardial pressure increases too, and the pressure is transmitted to the atrial, ventricular, caval, and pulmonary venous walls. Cardiac tamponade occurs when the amount of pericardial fluid limits diastolic filling and reduces stroke volume, cardiac output, and arterial pressure (Fig. 213-1). Tamponade is a continuum because a small increase in pericardial content couples the pericardium to the heart, significantly increasing atrial and especially ventricular interaction, phenomena that exaggerate the normal reciprocal respiratory effects on the right and left sides of the heart.[3] Once a critical volume is reached, very small increases

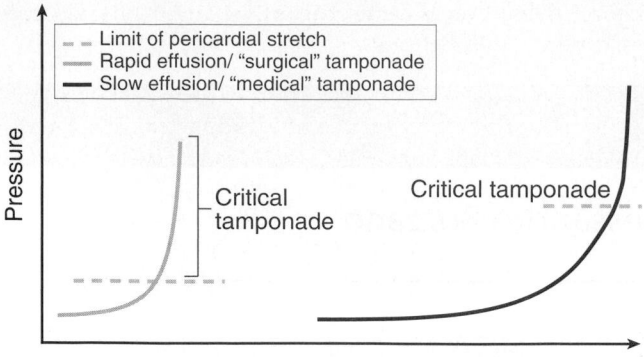

FIGURE 213–1. Pericardial pressure-volume curves with different rates of fluid accumulation. **Left,** Rapidly increasing pericardial fluid fills the pericardial reserve volume, then rises sharply to exceed the limit of parietal pericardial stretch; smaller fluid increments disproportionally increase the pericardial pressure. **Right,** A slower rate of pericardial filling allows more volume to exceed pericardial stretch limit. (From Spodick DH: Pericardial disease. In Braunwald E, et al [eds]: Heart Disease: A Textbook of Cardiovascular Medicine. Philadelphia, WB Saunders, 2001, pp 1841-1876.)

significantly compromise hemodynamic status. As stroke volume decreases, sympathetic tone increases, increasing heart rate and promoting arterial vasoconstriction. Initially, such compensatory mechanisms are effective, and adequate cardiac output and blood pressure are maintained.

Increases in intracardiac pressure and diastolic equalization are the main hemodynamic features of cardiac tamponade. Most patients with cardiac tamponade show a central venous pressure (CVP) greater than 12 to 14 mm Hg. Severe tamponade occurs when intrapericardial pressure reaches 15 to 20 mm Hg.[4] A "pressure plateau" occurs when right atrial pressure, right ventricular diastolic pressure, pulmonary artery diastolic pressure, and pulmonary capillary wedge pressure are identical (difference < 5 mm Hg).[3] At this point, the right ventricle collapses and hypotension becomes severe. During this phase, bradycardia is common. Only an immediate decrease in intrapericardial pressure (as the result of pericardiocentesis) can avoid the otherwise inevitable progression to cardiocirculatory arrest and pulseless electrical activity.

Clinically, *cardiac tamponade* is defined as the decompensated phase of cardiac compression resulting from increased intrapericardial pressure. The clinical signs include elevated jugular venous pressure, hypotension, tachycardia, and pulsus paradoxus. The classic triad of acute compression was described by Beck in 1935[5] and consists in high CVP, decreased arterial pressure, and muffled heart sounds. In the case of a traumatic effusion, only one third of patients present with the complete triad, even though 90% have at least one of the three signs.[6] Pulsus paradoxus is one of the characteristic signs of tamponade. Conventionally, it is defined as a greater than 10-mm Hg fall in systolic arterial pressure during inspiration. Detection of pulsus paradoxus is of fundamental importance in making the diagnosis of cardiac tamponade since most patients with slowly developing cardiac tamponade do not have the classic physical findings described by Beck. It should be noted that conditions other than tamponade (e.g., obesity, cardiac failure, pulmonary emphysema, asthma, pulmonary embolism, constrictive pericarditis and cardiogenic shock) can be associated with pulsus paradoxus.[6-8] Furthermore, the absence of pulsus paradoxus does not exclude the diagnosis of cardiac tamponade. The sensitivity and specificity of pulsus paradoxus as an indicator of tamponade have been reported to be 79% and 40%, respectively.[9]

The intravascular volume status of the patient can influence the clinical presentation. Hypovolemia contributes to a low cardiac output, and in this condition the diagnosis may be more difficult because a significant increase in CVP does not occur. In those rare cases in which tamponade is suspected but CVP is low, a fluid challenge will help clarify the situation and will also improve cardiac output as well, at least temporarily.[10]

Spontaneous versus mechanical ventilation and $PaCO_2$ levels significantly influence the evolution of pericardial tamponade. Pericardial pressure decreases 3 to 6 mm Hg when $PaCO_2$ decreases to 24 mm Hg; conversely, pericardial pressures increase 2 to 4 mm Hg when $PaCO_2$ reaches 57 mm Hg.[11] Increased intrathoracic pressures during the inspiratory phase of mechanical ventilation can decrease cardiac output up to 25% in patients with tamponade.[12] Patients with suspected cardiac tamponade, therefore, should not receive positive-pressure ventilation unless absolutely necessary to avoid further hemodynamic compromise.

EFFECT OF PERICARDIOCENTESIS

The effect of pericardiocentesis is often immediate, because during critical tamponade the heart operates on the steep portion of its pericardial pressure-volume curve (see Fig. 213-1). Drainage of a few milliliters of the effusion significantly increases stroke volume, reduces intrapericardial and atrial pressures, and permits separation between right and left filling pressures. Tachycardia and dyspnea are reduced, while arterial pressure increases and pulsus paradoxus disappears. If elevated and equalized right and left ventricular diastolic pressures persist after pericardiocentesis, and a prominent y descent becomes apparent in the right atrial pressure tracing, then the findings strongly suggest the presence of constricting pericardium due to effusive-constrictive pericarditis.[3]

DIAGNOSTIC CONSIDERATIONS

Pericardial effusions may be diagnosed with different methods, even though their accuracy may vary. Although ECG alterations, including PR-segment depression, low-voltage QRS complex, and electrical alternans, suggest the presence of a significant amount of pericardial fluid, the sensitivity of these findings is too low for clinical utility.[7] Reduction in QRS voltage also can be caused by pulmonary disease and obesity.

Diagnostic information about pericardial effusion can be provided by chest radiography, CT, MRI, and echocardiography. The chest radiograph may show enlargement of the cardiac silhouette, which resembles a "water bottle," without signs of lung congestion. Chest CT and MRI are sensitive and specific techniques that are able to detect the presence and the amount of the effusion and also diagnose related concomitant pathologic entities. These studies also can provide physiologic information in addition to anatomic data. These techniques, however, are difficult to apply in the management of unstable critically ill patients.

Transthoracic echocardiography is the most accurate noninvasive bedside method for establishing the presence of an effusive pericardial disease and for evaluating its hemodynamic effects on the heart, such as abnormal movement of the interventricular septum, diastolic collapse of the right atrial or ventricular walls, and reduced respiratory variation of the diameter of the inferior vena cava.[13-15] During inspiration, the right ventricle (RV) normally dilates owing to the increase in venous return. When cardiac tamponade occurs, movement of the free wall of the RV is limited by the increased pericardial pressure. Consequently, the interventricular septum protrudes into the left ventricle (LV), leading to a reduction of LV size during inspiration. These echographic findings correspond to the clinical sign of pulsus paradoxus.[16] Diastolic collapse of the right atrium (RA) is a more sensitive, although less specific, sign of cardiac tamponade than RV collapse.[13,14] When collapse of at least one right cardiac chamber is considered, sensitivity of tamponade detection is 90% but specificity remains low (65%). Nevertheless, there is good correlation between absence of collapse and absence of tamponade.[15] A "swinging heart" inside the pericardial effusion indicates the presence of a relevant amount of fluid even though it does not necessarily imply hemodynamic compromise. Doppler evaluation of intracardiac flows and their relationship to respiration provides further insights into the pathophysiology of this condition and can play a useful role in the diagnosis of cardiac tamponade. The measure of variation in transvalvular flow with respiration is the most frequently used technique. Normally, the velocity of early rapid ventricular filling (E wave) does not vary significantly with respiration. In the presence of cardiac tamponade, however, early diastolic flow rate through the mitral and aortic valves decreases during inspiration and increases through the tricuspid and pulmonary valves. A greater than 25% reduction of the peak velocity of the E wave in transmitral flow during inspiration suggests the presence of cardiac tamponade.[17] Chronic obstructive pulmonary disease, constrictive pericarditis, pulmonary embolism, and RV infarction may give Doppler images similar to cardiac tamponade.

Evaluation of superior vena cava Doppler flow velocity pattern may provide important data for the diagnosis of tamponade because abnormal venous flow correlates well with tamponade (specificity 91%). Usefulness of this finding is limited, however, because venous flow cannot be evaluated in more than 30% of cases.[15]

INDICATIONS

All causes of acute pericarditis can be associated with pericardial effusion. Other causes of pericardial effusion are neoplasia, myxedema, renal insufficiency, pregnancy, aortic or cardiac rupture, trauma, bleeding diathesis, thrombolytic therapy, nephrotic syndrome, and hepatic cirrhosis.[3,18] Pericardial tamponade can occur after catheter-based procedures and as sequela of cardiac surgery. In a series of 1127 cases of pericardiocentesis, pericardial effusions necessitating pericardiocentesis were due to postoperative effusion, malignancy, and cardiac perforation associated with catheter-based procedures in about 70% of cases.[19] Among the causes of effusions, a significant increase over time in the proportion of cases that were postoperative and secondary to cardiac perforation from catheter-based procedures has been observed (Table 213-1).

Pericardiocentesis is the first treatment option in patients with overt tamponade because only the removal of fluid allows normal ventricular filling and restores adequate cardiac output.

The optimal management of chronic large pericardial effusion without signs of cardiac tamponade is controversial. Some authors suggest that pericardiocentesis should be performed to avoid unexpected progression to cardiac tamponade and also to allow diagnostic tests on the fluid.[20,21] More recently, in a series of 71 patients with clinically significant pericardial effusions without cardiac tamponade, examination of pericardial fluid had a diagnostic yield of only 7%.[22] Accordingly, purely diagnostic pericardiocentesis should be limited to selected cases. Pericardial drainage may be indicated for severe pericardial effusions as defined by Weitzman and coworkers[23] (anterior plus posterior echo-free spaces greater than 20 mm during diastole);[24] in other cases, medical therapy and echocardiographic monitoring may be used as the initial approach.[22]

Elective pericardiocentesis is warranted in patients with suspicion of purulent pericarditis. This is a rare disease, but rapid diagnosis and treatment is essential to prevent serious morbidity, especially in children and immunocompromised patients. Among patients treated only with antibiotics

TABLE 213–1. ETIOLOGY OF EFFUSION STRATIFIED BY TIME

Etiology	Period, No. (% of Group)			P Value
	1 (2/1979-1/1986)	2 (2/1986-1/1993)	3 (2/1993-1/2000)	
Malignancy	91 (41)	159 (39)	125 (25)	<.001
Postoperative	46 (21)	92 (22)	139 (28)	.02
Cardiac perforation from invasive procedure	9 (4)	36 (9)	71 (14)	<.001
Infection	16 (7)	16 (4)	32 (7)	.93
Connective tissue disease	13 (6)	14 (3)	22 (4)	.58
Idiopathic	20 (9)	31 (8)	39 (8)	.69
Ischemic heart disease related	4 (2)	19 (5)	8 (2)	.40
Other*	22 (10)	45 (11)	58 (12)	.68

*Drug-related (including anticoagulation, renal failure, coagulopathies, post radiation therapy, and chest trauma.
Note: A significant increase over time has been observed in the proportion of postoperative effusions and of effusions secondary to cardiac perforation during catheter-based procedures. *P* value expresses the significance of trends over time, as tested by logistic regression analyses.
From Tsang TSM, Enriquez-Sarano M, Freeman WK, et al: Consecutive 1127 therapeutic echocardiographically guided pericardiocentesis: Clinical profile, practice patterns, and outcomes spanning 21 years. Mayo Clin Proc 2002;77:429-436.

without pericardial drainage, purulent pericarditis carries a mortality rate of 70%.[25] Therefore, when a purulent effusion is suspected, pericardiocentesis is indicated. Usually, purulent pericarditis originates from a severe infectious disease. Pneumonia and osteomyelitis are the most common causes, and gram-positive cocci are the most common causative organisms.[26,27] A relative and absolute increase in infections from multiple and gram-negative organisms (usually hospital acquired) has been reported, particularly in immunocompromised patients and after thoracotomy.[3] Other conditions associated with purulent pericarditis include mediastinitis, empyema, prior pericardiotomy, endocarditis, or burn injury.[28] After confirmation of diagnosis, treatment consists of systemic antibiotic therapy and complete evacuation of the effusion. Surgical drainage usually is required, because percutaneous drainage alone is not able to completely evacuate the effusion, which is often rich in fibrin and can be loculated and associated with dense adhesions. An alternative and less invasive method, which can be used to completely evacuate purulent effusions, thus controlling sepsis and avoiding the evolution to constrictive pericarditis, consists of pericardial drainage associated with intrapericardial infusion of streptokinase. Fibrinolytic therapy can enhance the removal of material that would otherwise be too viscous or particulate to be removed by tube drainage. This treatment should be considered before undertaking surgery.[27]

Patients with renal failure and pericardial effusion can be successfully treated with dialysis; in the majority of cases, there is no need to use invasive techniques and pericardiocentesis should be reserved for patients who do not improve after 10 to 14 days of intensive hemodialysis.[29] Monitoring is important in these patients. Because preload is reduced during hemodialysis, the risk of rendering an asymptomatic effusion hemodynamically significant is real.

In cases of hemorrhagic effusion secondary to trauma, aortic dissection, or cardiac rupture, pericardiocentesis is not definitive treatment. Thoracotomy is required to evaluate and repair the injury that caused pericardial bleeding. In these patients, aspiration of a limited amount of fluid can resolve the shock state, but complete aspiration of intrapericardial blood is not indicated, because greatly decreasing intrapericardial pressure can itself increase the risk of rebleeding. False-negative results from pericardiocentesis are obtained in 20% to 40% of cases of traumatic effusion, even when pericardial puncture can be performed without delay.[30,31] False-negative results can be caused by the rapid formation of clots, which impede aspiration of blood. Therefore, failure to aspirate blood in cases of traumatic chest injuries should not exclude the possible diagnosis of hemorrhagic effusion, delaying evacuation.

CONTRAINDICATIONS

There are no absolute contraindications to pericardiocentesis when cardiac tamponade and shock occur. Thrombocytopenia (platelet count < 50,000/mm³), presence of bleeding disorders, and concomitant anticoagulant therapy are contraindications for elective procedures.[32] Coagulopathy may be corrected transfusing fresh frozen plasma or platelets, but this strategy may be time consuming and is associated with the risks of blood transfusion. The infusion of recombinant human factor VIIa may be a new and effective strategy to correct such conditions in a shorter time.[33]

PREPARATION OF THE PATIENT

When the decision to perform pericardiocentesis is reached, it is important to ensure that a central venous catheter is in place. The catheter is essential for monitoring right atrial pressure and permitting the rapid infusion of fluids and drugs, as indicated. Right-sided heart catheterization, which allows monitoring of filling pressures, is advised only when an uncertain diagnosis needs confirmation. Continuous arterial pressure monitoring is indicated to detect the presence of pulsus paradoxus and to rapidly detect and correct sudden hemodynamic instability. If time permits, the patient's blood should be typed and crossmatched before the procedure. Supplemental oxygen always is required.

TECHNIQUE

Percutaneous pericardiocentesis has been performed for many years using the blind subxiphoid approach. This technique is associated with high incidence of morbidity and mortality, and using fluoroscopic guidance or electrocardiographic needle monitoring does not lead to significantly better outcomes.[29,34,35] Accordingly, blind approaches are no longer justified.[36]

CT-guided pericardiocentesis is a safe and valuable technique for pericardiocentesis.

The pericardiocentesis is carried out with a stereotactic device. The pericardium is punctured with a 0.9-mm needle, and a guidewire is introduced through the needle. An indwelling catheter is introduced over the guidewire and is left in the pericardium. Both the subxiphoid and parasternal approaches can be used.[37] The limitation of this approach is that it cannot be performed at the bedside and thus the need for transport may delay the treatment.

Echocardiographically guided pericardiocentesis is a safe and easier technique.[38,39] If the clinical situation allows, both a two-dimensional and Doppler study are performed to assess the size, distribution, and hemodynamic effect of the effusion. The patient is placed in the semireclining position, slightly rotated leftward to enhance fluid collection in the inferoanterior part of the chest. After the pericardial effusion is located, it is important to define the ideal entry site and needle trajectory for pericardiocentesis. The proper landmark for needle insertion corresponds to the area where the pericardial space is closest to the probe and the fluid accumulation is maximal; this site is para-apical more often than subcostal. After appropriate disinfection of the operative field, local anesthesia of the skin is obtained by injecting with 2% lidocaine subcutaneously. The proper trajectory of the needle is defined by the angulation of the transducer. A straight trajectory that avoids puncturing vital structures, including the liver, myocardium, and lung, is chosen. Because ultrasound does not penetrate air-filled spaces, the lung is effectively avoided. The operator should select a site that avoids the internal mammary artery (3 to 5 cm from parasternal border) and the vascular bundle at the inferior margin of each rib. The optimal needle trajectory should be transfixed in the operator's mind and then a 14- to 16-gauge Teflon-sheathed needle with an attached saline-filled syringe is advanced in the direction of the fluid-filled space. On entering the fluid, the needle should be advanced approximately 2 mm farther. The sheath should be advanced over the needle and the steel core withdrawn. If bloody fluid has been aspirated or if the position of the sheath is questionable, then position of the catheter can be confirmed by injecting 5 mL of agitated saline through the sheath. The bubbles in the solution provide a contrast effect that can be observed by two-dimensional echocardiography. Thus, if contrast agent appears in the pericardial space, the procedure can be continued. A guidewire should be advanced through the sheath, and then the sheath should be removed over the guidewire. A small incision of the skin should be made at the entry site, followed by introduction of a dilator (6 to 8 Fr.) over the guidewire. Predilatation of the chest wall passage facilitates subsequent insertion of the introducer sheath-dilator (6 to 8 Fr). The guidewire and the dilator should be removed and only the sheath left in the pericardial sac. A pigtail angiocatheter should be inserted through the introducer sheath and the fluid aspirated.

A different approach utilizes a needle carrier mounted on the transducer to advance the needle to the pericardial space under continuous visualization.[40,41] A bracket is mounted on the probe to support the needle-guide kit. The bracket supports the needle with two different angles, and the operator can choose between a closer angle for the subcostal approach and a wider angle for the apical approach. The probe is covered with the sterile sheath. The needle-guide kit is then mounted on the sheathed probe (needle guide-cover kit CIVCO USA, Kalona, IA) (Figs. 213-2 and 213-3).[40] In other models, the needle is set at an unchangeable angle to the probe, so the path of the puncture is chosen by adjusting the patient-probe angle[41]; this technique has been described only for the subcostal approach. Once placement and direction of the needle are chosen, as just described, the needle (SDN 18-gauge, 9-cm Cook for apical approach, and Angiocath 14-gauge, 133-mm B-D USA for subxiphoid approach) is connected to a syringe for constant gentle aspiration and is slowly introduced through the tissues until there is echographic visualization of the tip (Fig. 213-4A to C). When the pericardial effusion is reached and the placement of the needle inside the pericardial space is echographically confirmed, a J-tipped guidewire is introduced into the pericardial space (see Fig. 213-4D). The technique is summarized in Figure 213-5. If the amount of drained effusion is small or the drained fluid is bloody, previously shaken saline solution is injected and visualization of microbubbles is sought to exclude intracardiac placement of the needle.

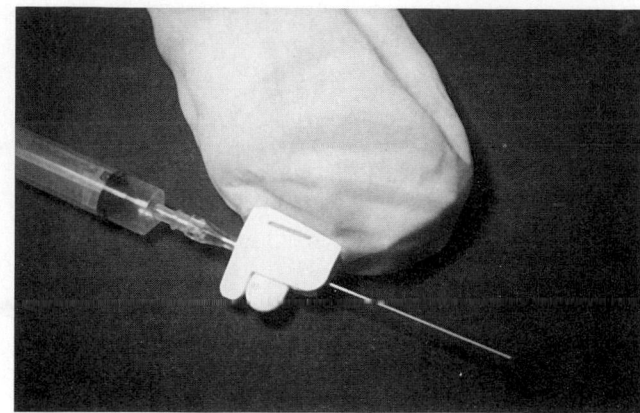

FIGURE 213-3. After bracket is mounted, probe is protected by sterile wrap. (From Maggiolini S, Bozzano A, Russo P, et al: Echocardiography-guided pericardiocentesis with probe-mounted needle: Report of 53 cases. J Am Soc Echocardiogr 2001;14:821-824.)

The needle is then removed and a small skin incision is made at the site of insertion. The drainage catheter (a pigtail angiocatheter 5 to 6 Fr or pericardiocentesis set CORDI-CAN 5213061 BRAUN) is subsequently introduced along the guidewire, according to the Seldinger's technique, immediately or, in case of subcostal approach, after introducing a 5- to 6-Fr dilator over the guidewire. The pericardial effusion is aspirated completely by syringe suction, and the catheter is connected to a disposable flushing system that infuses saline solution at a rate of 3 mL/h to maintain the patency of the system. Aspiration by syringe is repeated every 4 to 6 hours. The catheter is removed once the drainage has decreased to less than 25 to 30 mL in 24 hours. A complete echocardiographic study is performed in all patients before removing the catheter and before discharge from the ICU or coronary care unit. After the procedure, all patients undergo chest radiography to exclude the presence of pneumothorax. The entire procedure can be done by a single physician. However, in our experience, the presence of two operators, one performing the echocardiogram and the other performing the puncture and drainage, seems preferable.

MEDICAL MANAGEMENT

In the unstable patient, during preparation for pericardiocentesis, measures aimed to stabilize the patient should be instituted. Intravenous fluid administration is the best treatment option before and during drainage.[42] An increase in circulating volume, increases transmural pressure in both ventricles, and this improvement in preload should improve stroke volume. An intravascular volume load can be infused even in patients with high central venous pressure, because tamponade is not initially associated with impaired myocardial contractility and the heart can handle the volume challenge. Both animal[43] and human studies[10] show hemodynamic improvements after fluid challenge when tamponade physiology is present. Nevertheless, improvement in cardiac output after fluid infusion may be negligible and fluid infusion cannot substitute for pericardiocentesis.[44] In the case of penetrating cardiac injury, the response to fluid resuscitation may produce improvement or deterioration, depending on the effect that the infusion exerts on eventual rebleeding.[45] Dextran solutions, Hextend, and 5% albumin are reasonable fluids for volume expansion.

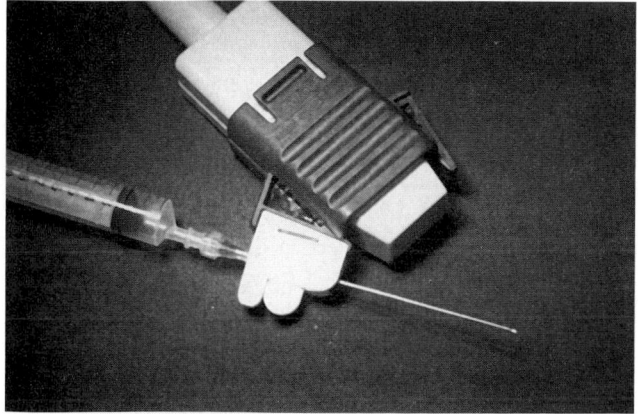

FIGURE 213-2. Echocardiographic probe with bracket, needle guide, and syringe. (From Maggiolini S, Bozzano A, Russo P, et al: Echocardiography-guided pericardiocentesis with probe-mounted needle: Report of 53 cases. J Am Soc Echocardiogr 2001;14:821-824.)

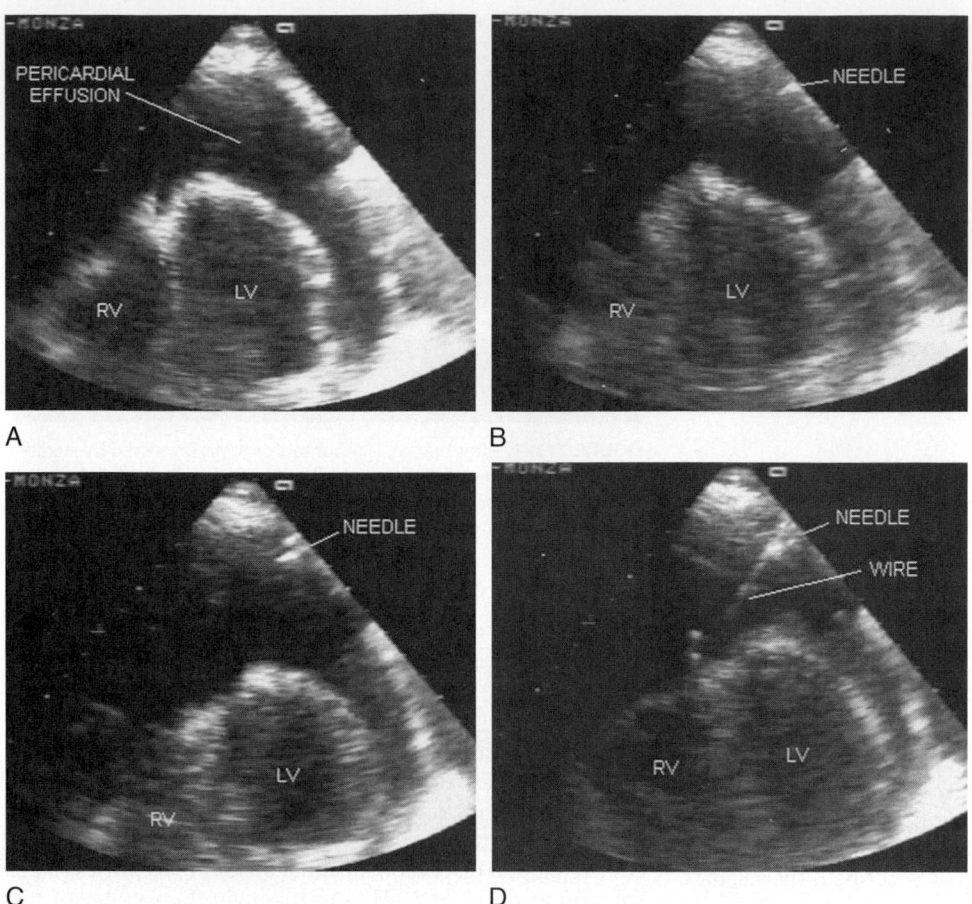

FIGURE 213–4. Two-dimensional echocardiographic image (apical four-chamber view) during needle introduction through tissues. **A,** Detection of pericardial effusion. **B,** Visualization of needle tip. **C,** Needle is advanced through tissues. **D,** Needle enters pericardial space and guidewire is introduced. LV, left ventricle; RV, right ventricle. (From Maggiolini S, Bozzano A, Russo P, et al: Echocardiography-guided pericardiocentesis with probe-mounted needle: Report of 53 cases. J Am Soc Echocardiogr 2001;14:821-824.)

Rarely, pulmonary edema will develop after pericardial drainage, probably as a result of the sudden increase of RV output and pulmonary capillary pressure.[46]

The use of vasodilators has been proposed; infusion of sodium nitroprusside plus blood transfusion improved cardiac output in an experimental animal setting, and

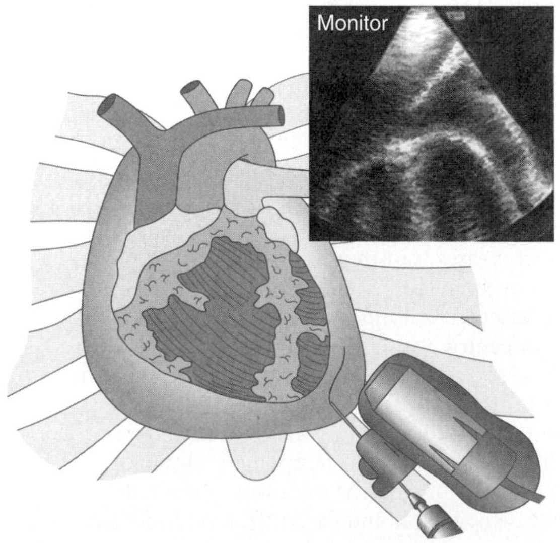

FIGURE 213–5. Representation of pericardiocentesis using the apical approach. The pericardial needle is continuously monitored by apical four-chamber echocardiographic view while entering the pericardial space. When the pericardial effusion is reached, a guidewire is introduced in the pericardial space.

hydralazine plus volume infusion raised cardiac output and blood pressure.[43] Administration of vasodilators, however, is highly risky in hypotensive patients, and in our experience use of these agents is to be avoided. In clinical studies of tamponade patients, nitroprusside failed to show benefits.[44]

Other drugs may be used for obtaining transiently favorable effects. Isoproterenol, norepinephrine, dopamine, and dobutamine can support blood pressure and cardiac output and may permit additional pericardial stretching. Norepinephrine was effective in animal studies, but it did not increase cardiac output in tamponade patients.[47] Both dopamine and dobutamine improved hemodynamics in cardiac tamponade; dobutamine has greater beta activity and therefore it may be considered preferable.[47] The usefulness of inotropes is generally limited because endogenous adrenergic stimulation is already great under tamponade conditions, and ejection fraction is preserved, but stroke volume is critically depressed. Bradycardia and other vagally mediated reflex phenomena during tamponade can be treated with atropine.

Supportive treatment includes correction of metabolic acidosis, because acidosis exerts a depressant effect on the response to endogenous and exogenous catecholamines. New atrial arrhythmias may, in theory, severely impair cardiac output even after drainage of pericardial fluid, because diastolic compliance of the cardiac chambers may remain abnormal for some period of time. Prophylactic use of antiarrhythmic drugs, such as digitalis, has been suggested.[28] However, arrhythmias are relatively rare. Duvernoy and coworkers reported 1 case of atrial fibrillation in a series of 322 patients,[35] and in a series from the Mayo Clinic of 1127 cases, only 2 of nonsustained supraventricular tachycardia were reported, and neither required any specific intervention.[19] Because a prophylactic effect of digitalis on these arrhythmias is not documented, and because brady-arrhythmias requiring atropine may occur in overt tamponade, we do not recommend prophylactic use of digitalis.

COMPLICATIONS

The efficacy and safety of echocardiographically guided pericardiocentesis is well documented. Possible complications include puncture of cardiac chambers, laceration of coronary arteries or intercostal vessels, pneumothorax, pleuropericardial fistulas, arrhythmias, and bacteremia. Only one death attributed to this procedure has been reported in international trials.[19,48,49]

The success rate for the procedure is 97% with a total complication rate of 4.7% (major 1.2%; minor 3.5%).[19] In a series of 53 pericardiocenteses performed under continuous echocardiographic visualization, no major complications occurred, no perforations or ruptures of cardiac chambers were reported, and the incidence of minor complications was 3.7%.[40]

PREVENTION OF CARDIAC TAMPONADE

Pericardial drainage for 24 to 72 hours is sufficient to avoid recurrence of pericardial tamponade in the majority of cases. The recurrence rate after the initial procedure is 27% to 55% for patients who undergo simple pericardiocentesis and 14% to 24% for those who have extended drainage.[19,50] The omission of extended catheter drainage is an important independent predictor of recurrence.[19,50] It is important to empty the pericardial sac as completely as possible, leaving the catheter in place up to 72 hours or more if the fluid has a rate of accumulation greater than 30 mL in 24 hours. Complications associated with the use of a pericardial catheter are rare. Only one case of bacteremia has been reported in 690 cases in which this method has been used.[19,40]

Reaccumulation of pericardial fluid is common in patients with malignant pericardial effusions. In these patients, several procedures have been suggested to prevent recurrence of tamponade. These approaches include repeated pericardiocentesis, which is probably the procedure of choice in patients with end-stage disease, intrapericardial sclerosis, systemic chemotherapy, radiation therapy, surgical intervention, or percutaneous balloon pericardiotomy (Fig. 213-6).[50]

PERCUTANEOUS BALLOON PERICARDIOTOMY

Percutaneous balloon pericardiotomy (PBP) is a nonsurgical alternative technique to surgical creation of a pericardial window. The procedure can be performed either in the catheterization laboratory or at the bedside in the ICU. Generally, in patients with malignant pericardial effusions, reduced life expectancy and the high risk of complications are contraindications to surgical treatment. In these patients, percutaneous pericardiotomy with single (SBP)[51] or double balloon (DBP)[52] is preferable. SBP was described by Zinskind and colleagues in 1993,[51] and the variant with a double catheter was described by Hsu and coworkers in 1997.[52]

CONTRAINDICATIONS

Percutaneous balloon pericardiotomy is contraindicated in patients with loculated effusions, bleeding diatheses, or immunodeficiency states. Respiratory failure and pneumonectomy are considered contraindications owing to the risk of significant pleural effusion associated with the technique. The development of pleural effusion may compromise the remaining lung function in these patients. In patients with, or at high risk for, bacterial or fungal infections this technique may favor the spread of infections to the pleural space.

SINGLE-BALLOON PERICARDIOTOMY TECHNIQUE

Single-balloon pericardiotomy is performed via a subxiphoid approach after induction of local anesthesia and conscious sedation. The procedure is performed under fluoroscopic control. It can be performed immediately after pericardiocentesis or postponed in patients with a drainage catheter in situ. A 0.038-inch guidewire with a preshaped

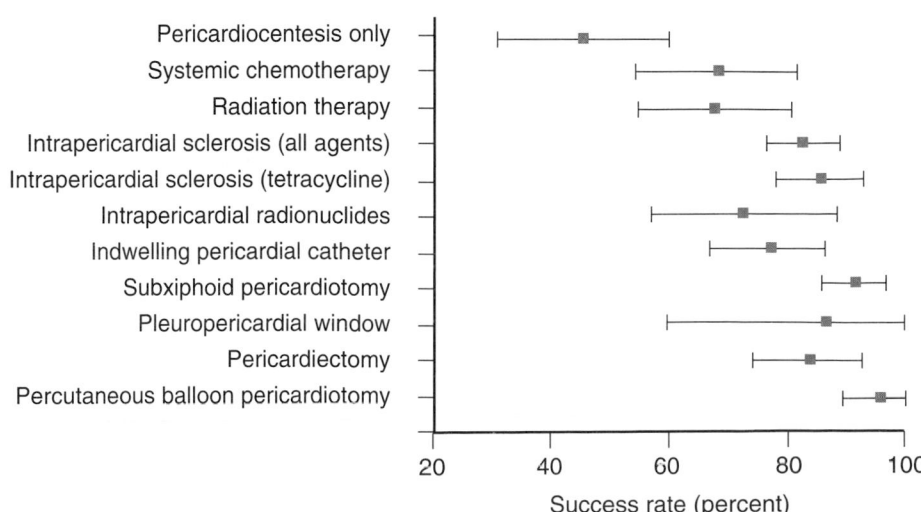

FIGURE 213–6. Success rate with 95% confidence intervals for different treatment modalities of malignant pericardial effusion. (From Vaitkus PT, Herrmann HC, LeWinter MM: Treatment of malignant pericardial effusion. JAMA 1994;272:59-64. Copyright 1994, American Medical Association.)

curve at the tip is advanced into the pericardial space through a drainage catheter. The catheter is then removed, leaving the guidewire in the pericardial space. Its position is confirmed fluoroscopically. After predilation along the track of the wire with a 10-Fr. dilator , a 20-mm diameter × 3-cm long balloon dilating catheter (Boston Scientific, Watertown, MA) is advanced over the guidewire and positioned to straddle the parietal pericardium. The balloon is inflated manually until the waist produced by the parietal pericardium disappears. Biplane fluoroscopy is useful to ensure the correct position of the balloon straddling the parietal pericardium, and a small amount of iodine-containing radiographic contrast agent can be helpful to identify the margins. Two or three inflations are performed to ensure an adequate opening of the pericardium. The balloon-dilating catheter is removed, leaving the guidewire in the pericardial space. A new pigtail catheter is then advanced over this guide and placed into the pericardial space. The drainage catheter should be aspirated every 6 to 8 hours and flushed with heparinized saline solution (5 mL, 100 U/mL) recording drainage volumes. The catheter can be removed when there is less than 50 to 75 mL of pericardial drainage in 24 hours.

DOUBLE-BALLOON PERICARDIOTOMY TECHNIQUE

Two 0.035-inch 150-cm-long J-tip guidewires are advanced through a 7-Fr sheath previously placed in the pericardial space. Once the sheath is removed, an 8- to 12-mm × 2-cm balloon (Meditech; Boston Scientific Cooperation; Watertown, MA), and an 8- to 12-mm × 4-cm balloon (Smash; Schneider Europe, Bülach, Switzerland) are advanced into the pericardial cavity using each guidewire. The guidewires separate from each other after they have passed through the subcutaneous tissue and entered the pericardial cavity. Under fluoroscopy, this crossover point between the two guidewires can be identified, indicating the pericardial border. While partially inflated, the two balloons are positioned at the pericardial border. The two balloons are inflated simultaneously until their waists disappear. Then the longer balloon is held still, while the shorter one is pushed and pulled across the pericardium several times to ensure the creation of an adequate pericardial window, opening into the pleural cavity. Both balloons are then removed, and a pigtail 6-Fr. catheter is positioned in the pericardial space for complete drainage of the effusion. The catheter is kept in place until the daily drainage is less than 100 mL in 2 days.

Until catheter removal, antibiotic prophylaxis may be indicated.

A successful result, defined by the absence of recurrence of pericardial effusion requiring surgical drainage, was reported in 85% of cases in a multicenter PBP registry of 123 patients undergoing percutaneous pericardial window between 1987 and 1994 in 16 centers.[53]

Surgical drainage is preferable when contraindications to PBP exist and when it is important to obtain a specimen of pericardial tissue for histopathologic analysis.

COMPLICATIONS

Clinical trials did not report any deaths associated with this technique.[53] A 13% rate of minor complications has been reported. Fever was frequent, but bacteremia was not documented in any patients. A left pleural effusion develops in the majority of patients during the 24 to 48 hours after the procedure. In the majority of cases, the effusion resolves spontaneously. Thoracocentesis or placement of a chest drainage tube was required in 17% of patients with a preexisting pleural effusion and in 13% of patients without a preexisting effusion to improve the clinical condition.[53] To limit the amount of fluid that can accumulate into the pleural space, it is better to remove the pericardial effusion as much as possible before creating a pleuropericardial window.

ANNOTATED REFERENCES

Maggiolini S, Bozzano A, Russo P, et al: Echocardiography-guided pericardiocentesis with probe-mounted needle: Report of 53 cases. J Am Soc Echocardiogr 2001;14:821-824.

> This study describes a technique of echocardiographically guided pericardiocentesis in which the needle tip is advanced under continuous visualization. Landmarks, materials, and complications are reported and discussed.

Mercè J, Sagristà-Sauleda J, Permanyer-Miralda G, et al: Correlation between clinical and Doppler echocardiographic findings in patients with moderate and large pericardial effusion: Implication for the diagnosis of cardiac tamponade. Am Heart J 1999;138:759-764.

> This prospective study demonstrates that echo-Doppler measurements suggestive of increased pericardial pressure are common in patients with important pericardial effusion without clinical sign of cardiac tamponade. These observations are important for their implications in diagnosis and clinical management of echocardiographic findings suggestive of hemodynamic compromise.

Tsang TS, Enriquez-Sarano M, Freeman WK, et al: Consecutive 1127 therapeutic echocardiographically guided pericardiocentesis: Clinical profile, practice patterns, and outcomes spanning 21 years. Mayo Clin Proc 2002; 77:429-436.

> This is the largest study on echocardiographically guided pericardiocentesis. It provides extensive data on safety and efficacy of this technique. The study shows that the clinical presentation of patients undergoing pericardiocentesis has modified over a 21-year period.

Vaitkus PT, Herrmann HC, LeWinter MM: Treatment of malignant pericardial effusion. JAMA 1994;272:59-64.

> This is an excellent review that describes the success rate of different therapeutic options for the treatment of malignant pericardial effusions.

Ziskind AA, Pearce AC, Lemmon CC, et al: Percutaneous balloon pericardiotomy for the treatment of cardiac tamponade and large pericardial effusions: Description of technique and report of the first 50 cases. J Am Coll Cardiol 1993;21:1-5.

> This paper describes in details the technique used for percutaneous balloon pericardiotomy and demonstrates the feasibility and the efficacy of a nonsurgical alternative for the treatment of recurrent pericardial effusions.

Chapter 214

PARACENTESIS AND DIAGNOSTIC PERITONEAL LAVAGE

Louis H. Alarcon

KEY POINTS

PARACENTESIS

1. **Abdominal paracentesis for ascitic fluid analysis** should be part of the evaluation of patients with new onset of ascites.

2. **Large-volume paracentesis may be therapeutic in patients with refractory ascites,** but it does not address the underlying pathophysiology of this disease and may not affect outcome. In these patients, transjugular intrahepatic portosystemic shunts improve survival without liver transplantation compared with large-volume paracentesis.

3. **The incidence of complications associated with paracentesis is low.** The use of ultrasonography to localize the ascites may be useful and reduces complications. Significant hemorrhage after paracentesis is uncommon, despite the fact that most cirrhotic patients have clotting parameter abnormalities. It is usually not necessary to normalize the prothrombin time before this procedure.

DIAGNOSTIC PERITONEAL LAVAGE

1. **Diagnostic peritoneal lavage (DPL) is primarily useful in detecting hemoperitoneum from blunt solid organ injury,** but it may also be helpful for the diagnosis of hollow viscus injury. The finding of hemoperitoneum in stable patients, however, does not mandate laparotomy, because 30% of these patients would undergo nontherapeutic laparotomy.

2. **For hemodynamically *stable* patients after blunt abdominal trauma with an equivocal abdominal examination,** associated neurologic injury, or painful injuries, abdominal computed tomography (CT) is recommended as the diagnostic modality of choice.

3. **For hemodynamically *unstable* patients after blunt abdominal trauma,** focused abdominal sonography for trauma (FAST) and DPL are the preferred tests, with FAST rapidly gaining acceptance over DPL in many trauma centers as the preferred initial diagnostic modality. These patients should not be subjected to CT.

4. **The use of DPL in the evaluation of patients with penetrating abdominal wounds remains controversial.** Using a low red blood cell (RBC) threshold (1000/mm³) has been described in an attempt to overcome this shortfall.

PARACENTESIS

Paracentesis is the insertion of a needle or catheter into the peritoneal cavity for the purpose of aspirating peritoneal fluid. It is most often indicated for the diagnostic or therapeutic evacuation of ascites. The development of ascites is a common complication of cirrhosis, being more frequent than either encephalopathy and variceal hemorrhage in these patients. The median survival of cirrhotic patients with ascites is 2 years.[1] Other causes of ascites besides cirrhosis include malignancy, heart failure, tuberculosis, renal failure, and pancreatic disease.

The determination of the etiology of ascites is based on the history, physical examination, liver function tests, ultrasonography, and ascitic fluid analysis. Abdominal paracentesis and ascitic fluid analysis should be an early step in the workup of patients with new onset of ascites. Paracentesis is also important to diagnose infection of ascitic fluid, that is, peritonitis.

The mainstays of treatment of ascites secondary to cirrhosis involve dietary sodium restriction (2 g/day) and oral diuretics (spironolactone and furosemide). The underlying etiology of liver disease should be corrected when possible, and ethanol consumption should be strongly discouraged. Abstinence from ethanol can normalize portal venous pressures in some patients with early ethanol-induced liver disease.[2] Patients with early cirrhosis and diuretic-responsive ascites should not be managed by serial paracentesis; rather, medical management should be employed. In the majority of patients, ascites can be controlled with medical management.

In 5% to 10% of patients, ascites becomes resistant to medical treatment. The standard of care for the management of refractory ascites is therapeutic paracentesis. This can be performed as often as every 2 weeks to control symptomatic ascites. Other options for the management of refractory ascites include transjugular intrahepatic portosystemic shunt (TIPS) and liver transplantation. In a randomized trial of 60 patients comparing TIPS with repeated therapeutic paracentesis, the probability of survival without liver transplantation at 2 years was 58% in the TIPS patients as compared with 32% in the paracentesis patients.[3] A smaller study of 25 patients randomized to TIPS or paracentesis showed the opposite: mortality was higher in the TIPS group.[4] Surgical portosystemic shunts and peritoneovenous shunts have fallen out of favor owing to high incidence of morbidity and mortality and to the development of hepatic encephalopathy.

For patients with tense ascites, large-volume paracentesis rapidly relieves intra-abdominal pressure. A single 4- to 6-L paracentesis can be performed safely and often does not require the infusion of colloids.[5] However, paracentesis does nothing to correct the etiology of the ascites, and ascites will recur if sodium restriction and diuretics are not instituted or fail. Referral for liver transplant evaluation should be considered in eligible patients with cirrhosis and refractory ascites.

Infection of ascitic fluid often occurs in cirrhotic patients. When there is no surgically correctable etiology such as perforated viscus, the term *spontaneous bacterial peritonitis* is used. This diagnosis is made when there is a positive ascitic fluid culture or an ascitic fluid polymorphonuclear (PMN) cell count greater than 250 cells/mm^3 in the correct clinical scenario without any evidence for an intra-abdominal, surgically correctable etiology. The infection is usually monomicrobial. Polymicrobial infection suggests secondary peritonitis. Consideration of the diagnosis mandates paracentesis and evaluation of the ascitic fluid; a clinical diagnosis without paracentesis is inadequate.

TECHNIQUE

The patient should be supine. Bedside ultrasonography can be a valuable aid for localizing the largest collection of ascites and avoiding injury to the bowel. The patient should void or have a urinary bladder drainage tube inserted before the procedure. The area is cleansed, draped, and anesthetized. When a small volume of ascitic fluid is needed for diagnostic studies, an 18- or 20-gauge, 2- to 3-inch needle, attached to a 20- to 50-mL syringe is inserted into the abdomen lateral to the rectus muscle in the lower quadrant midway between the umbilicus and the anterior superior iliac spine, avoiding prior surgical incisions. The skin is retracted caudad while inserting the needle. When fluid is aspirated, the needle is stabilized and the fluid sample is obtained by syringe. After removal of the needle, the skin is released, causing the entrance and exit needle sites to form a "Z-tract" that reduces the chance of ascitic fluid leakage. For large-volume paracentesis, a 14- to 16-gauge cannula-over-needle is employed. Once fluid is aspirated in the syringe, the needle is removed, leaving the plastic catheter in place, which is attached to plastic tubing and to a vacuum canister. Usually 4 to 6 L of ascites can be safely removed, although larger volumes have been removed also. When it is necessary to place a catheter into the peritoneal cavity, a guidewire should be inserted into the peritoneal cavity through the needle; an 8.5-Fr. 40-cm polyurethane pigtail catheter should be guided into the peritoneal cavity over the wire and sutured in place.

The aspirated fluid should be submitted for cell count, absolute polymorphonuclear neutrophil count, albumin, total protein concentration, Gram stain, and cultures. Optional studies, based on clinical suspicion, may include glucose concentration, amylase concentration, lactate dehydrogenase concentration, bilirubin concentration, and cytology.

COMPLICATIONS

Paracentesis has been associated with peritonitis, bowel injury, bleeding, injury to the bladder, injury to the epigastric vessels, oliguria, and hypotension. The incidence of significant hemorrhage from this procedure is about 1%, despite the fact that over 70% of patients have clotting parameter abnormalities.[6] Therefore, it is usually not necessary to normalize the prothrombin time before proceeding.[7] Serious complications, such as hemoperitoneum and bowel perforation, are rare (0.1%).[6]

Hypotension after paracentesis in cirrhotic patients can be associated with worsening of arteriolar vasodilation.[8] In the first few hours after large-volume paracentesis there is a reduction in the plasma levels of renin and aldosterone, an increase in atrial natriuretic peptide concentration, a reduction in cardiac filling pressures, and an increase in cardiac index. However, after 12 to 24 hours, these changes reverse, reflecting effective hypovolemia. Infusion of intravenous colloids, specifically albumin, has been shown to attenuate the hemodynamic consequences of paracentesis and the associated neurohumoral alterations.[9] However, no large randomized study has shown that routine expansion of plasma volume with a colloid solution confers a survival advantage.

DIAGNOSTIC PERITONEAL LAVAGE

The evaluation of the abdomen is a critical component in the assessment of injured patients. Failure to identify intra-abdominal injury results in preventable morbidity and mortality in trauma patients. The physical examination for abdominal injury is often hampered by alterations of the sensorium by substances such as ethanol and illicit drugs, injury to the central nervous system, or pain from other injuries. Also, a significant amount of blood can be present in the peritoneal cavity without obvious abdominal distention or peritoneal signs.

DPL, CT, and ultrasonography have emerged as the main diagnostic modalities to evaluate trauma patients and currently have complementary roles. DPL was introduced by Root and colleagues in 1965 for the evaluation of abdominal trauma.[10] In the era before CT and ultrasonography, DPL was the first well-established method to identify hemoperitoneum in trauma patients. DPL is primarily useful in diagnosing hemoperitoneum from blunt solid organ injury, but it can also be helpful for the diagnosis of hollow viscus injury.

For hemodynamically stable patients with an equivocal abdominal examination, associated neurologic injury, or painful injuries, abdominal CT is recommended as the diagnostic modality of choice. CT is also the preferred diagnostic method for determining whether nonoperative management of a solid organ injury is appropriate. Furthermore, in stable patients with a positive DPL, follow-up abdominal CT should be considered. Thus, CT and DPL play complementary roles in the evaluation of stable patients after blunt abdominal trauma.

For hemodynamically unstable patients, focused abdominal sonography for trauma (FAST) and DPL are the preferred tests, with FAST rapidly gaining acceptance over DPL in many trauma centers as the preferred initial diagnostic modality. FAST and DPL are used to rule out hemoperitoneum as the cause of hemodynamic instability. In contrast to DPL, FAST can be used to identify pericardial tamponade.

These tests can be performed expeditiously, and ongoing efforts at resuscitation and evaluation can occur simultaneously with the performance of the test. Because resuscitation is difficult during CT, CT is contraindicated when patients are hypotensive or hemodynamically unstable.

DPL is also useful in certain clinical scenarios. Consider, for example, a head-injured patient needing an emergency craniotomy. DPL can be performed in the operating room at the same time as the craniotomy without interfering with the neurosurgical procedure.

Controversy exists regarding the best way to manage blunt trauma patients with isolated evidence of free intra-abdominal fluid by CT but without evidence of solid organ injury. In a review of the literature, isolated free fluid was seen in 2.8% of over 16,000 blunt trauma patients studied with CT.[11] Of these, only 27% underwent a therapeutic laparotomy. Thus, some experts recommend serial abdominal examinations whereas others recommend surgical exploration to rule out hollow viscus injury. DPL can be useful in the evaluation of patients with suspected perforated viscus. Very early after bowel perforation, the white blood cell (WBC) count in the lavage fluid may be low; however, within a few hours after injury, the degree of inflammation is usually sufficient to increase the WBC count in lavage fluid greater than 500 cells/mm³. The presence of bile, amylase, bacteria, or food particles in lavage fluid also confirms intestinal perforation.

The use of DPL in the evaluation of hemodynamically stable patients with penetrating abdominal wounds remains controversial. A significant number of missed injuries remain undetected by this method. For example, Kelemen and colleagues[12] reported a 21% false-negative rate for stable patients with abdominal gunshot wounds. Using a low red blood cell (RBC) threshold (1000/mm³) has been described in an attempt to overcome this shortfall.[13]

The only absolute contraindication to performing a DPL is clinical condition of the patient mandating immediate laparotomy. Relative contraindications include previous abdominal surgery, cirrhosis, obesity, and coagulopathy. In patients with pelvic fractures or pregnancy, a supraumbilical incision should be performed.

TECHNIQUE

The patient should be in the supine position. Gastric and bladder decompression tubes should be inserted to minimize the risk of injury to these organs. The periumbilical skin should be prepped and draped sterilely. Local anesthesia is injected into the site.

DPL can be performed with an open, semi-open, or closed technique. The open technique employs a midline infraumbilical abdominal incision 2 to 5 cm in length; the incision should be supraumbilical if the patient has a pelvic fracture or if the patient is pregnant. A small incision is made in the midline abdominal fascia and peritoneum. An 8- to 9-Fr. 25-cm lavage catheter with side holes is inserted under direct visualization toward the pelvis. The closed method uses a Seldinger technique. A 16-gauge, 3-inch needle is inserted through a skin puncture and into the peritoneal cavity. A guidewire is passed through the needle into the peritoneal cavity. The lavage catheter is inserted over the wire. The semi-open technique involves incising the skin and fascia and then using a guidewire technique for inserting the catheter into the peritoneal cavity.

Proponents of the open technique argue that it is safer, whereas proponents of the closed and semi-open methods argue that these approaches are more expeditious and can be safely performed by appropriately trained individuals. A large meta-analysis that aggregated results from 1126 patient trials showed that the incidence of major complications is not different for the different DPL techniques.[14] Failure to properly place the catheter and technical difficulties were more likely with the closed method, whereas procedure time was shorter with the open method (17.8 vs. 26.8 minutes, respectively). Sensitivity, specificity, and accuracy were not different between the methods of catheter insertion.

Once the catheter is placed, aspiration should be attempted with a syringe. If 10 mL of blood is aspirated, the DPL is considered "positive" and appropriate surgical intervention undertaken. Otherwise, 1 L of crystalloid solution is infused (10 mL/kg in pediatric patients) and then retrieved by gravity and sent to the laboratory for analysis. In general, the DPL is considered positive in blunt trauma patients if the RBC count is greater than 100,000/mm³, WBC count greater than 500/mm³, or the amylase concentration greater than 100 IU/L. Other "positive" findings include presence of bile or food particles or drainage of lavage fluid from the bladder drainage catheter, gastric tube, or thoracostomy tube. However, using these criteria, an unnecessary laparotomy rate of 24% to 30% has been reported.[15,16] The sensitivity and specificity of the test are dependent on the threshold criteria for determining a positive test result. If the lavage is negative but there is a high index of suspicion for intra-abdominal pathology, the DPL catheter can be left in place for re-lavage to rule out delayed hemoperitoneum or intestinal perforation.

One of the major problems with DPL is that the test is too sensitive. Only about 30 mL of blood in the peritoneal cavity is necessary to produce a positive DPL. In this era of selective management of solid-organ injuries, a significant number of nontherapeutic laparotomies would be performed on the basis of these DPL results, unless diagnostic evaluation includes other modalities as well.

COMPLICATIONS

The main complications of DPL are technical. Bowel or vascular injury occurs in less than 1%.[16] Other complications include bladder injury, bleeding (cause for a false-positive DPL result), and wound infection. More frequent than the technical complications are inaccuracies in the test. False-positive DPL, leading to unnecessary laparotomy as discussed earlier, may occur in as many as 30% of cases.[16] This problem can be reduced by using CT as a complementary test in stable patients. The false-negative rate, that is, failure to diagnose hemoperitoneum, is low. However, DPL is unable to detect retroperitoneal injuries (CT is the preferred test to detect retroperitoneal injuries for the stable patient) and is insensitive for detecting early hollow viscus and diaphragmatic injuries.

ANNOTATED REFERENCES

Gonzalez RP, Turk B, Falimirski ME, Holevar MR: Abdominal stab wounds: Diagnostic peritoneal lavage criteria for emergency room discharge. J Trauma 2001;51:939.

This prospective study of DPL in hemodynamically stable patients with abdominal stab wounds demonstrated that patients with a lavage red blood cell count less than 1000/mm³ could be safely discharged to home from the emergency department.

Hodgson NF, Stewart TC, Girotti MJ: Open or closed diagnostic peritoneal lavage for abdominal trauma? A meta-analysis. J Trauma 2000;48:1091.

This meta-analysis of seven randomized trials comparing open to closed technique for DPL demonstrated comparable rates of major complications. The closed technique was associated with more technical failures in placing the catheter but shorter procedural time compared with the open technique.

Rodriguez C, Barone JE, Wilbanks TO, et al: Isolated free fluid on computed tomographic scan in blunt abdominal trauma: A systemic review of incidence and management. J Trauma 2002;53:79, 2002.

This systematic literature review showed that isolated free fluid without solid organ injury on CT was found in only 2.8% of over 16,000 patients with blunt abdominal trauma. Only 27% of patients with isolated free fluid on CT underwent therapeutic laparotomy. These authors recommend that serial physical examinations be performed in alert patients with isolated free fluid on abdominal CT, whereas patients with altered mental status should undergo diagnostic peritoneal lavage.

Rossle M, Ochs A, Gulberg V, et al: A comparison of paracentesis and transjugular intrahepatic portosystemic shunting in patients with ascites. N Engl J Med 2000;342:1701.

This prospective, randomized trial demonstrated that in patients with refractory ascites and Child class B or C cirrhosis, transjugular intrahepatic portosystemic shunts improved survival without liver transplantation compared with large-volume paracentesis.

Chapter 215

THORACENTESIS

Peter Doelken • Steven A. Sahn

KEY POINTS

1. **Pleural effusions are common in the critically ill and frequently accompany edematous states and the acute respiratory distress syndrome (ARDS).** Many pleural effusions are undetected and resolve with the underlying disease process. Large effusions or effusions thought to be a possible source of infection should be investigated with thoracentesis and pleural fluid analysis.

2. **Imaging is required for the diagnosis of a pleural effusion in the critically ill.** The standard anteroposterior chest radiograph is sufficient for the diagnosis of moderate to large effusions. Ultrasonography or computed tomography (CT) is required to diagnose smaller effusions and to provide image guidance for thoracentesis in patients on mechanical ventilation.

3. **Bedside ultrasonography is the preferred modality for image-guided thoracentesis.** It eliminates transport risk, and the procedure can be performed in virtually any position. Identification of an accessible pleural effusion requires identification of the anatomic boundaries, detection of dynamic fluid signs, and the presence of an access window not compromised by intervening vital structures.

4. Identification of the upper margin of a rib with a small-gauge needle is required before the introduction of a larger-bore thoracentesis catheter. **If fluid cannot be obtained with a small- gauge needle no attempts at placement of a thoracentesis catheter should be made.**

5. **Contraindications to thoracentesis** include lack of operator expertise, severe uncorrectable coagulopathy or thrombocytopenia, and azotemia-induced platelet dysfunction.

6. **Major complications of thoracentesis** include pneumothorax, intercostal artery laceration, and hypotension.

Pleural effusions are common in the critically ill. Most of these effusions are small and do not require investigation or treatment because the cause is often clinically obvious, such as congestive heart failure (CHF) or atelectasis.[1] Many effusions go unrecognized unless ultrasonography is performed or the patient undergoes chest or abdominal CT. The effusions commonly accompany edematous states due to heart failure or volume overload, pneumonia, or ARDS. If a pleural effusion is large or a possible source of infection, the effusion becomes a target of investigation or therapy and diagnostic or therapeutic pleurocentesis should be performed.[2] The pleural fluid obtained should be sent for analysis to guide management. Thoracentesis remains the initial procedure of choice in most cases unless complicating factors are discovered during the evaluation of the effusion and primary thoracostomy tube placement is performed. Thoracentesis has an excellent safety record when performed under ultrasound-guidance by skilled individuals, even in mechanically ventilated patients. Sonographic imaging capabilities have become increasingly available in ICUs and allow the procedure to take place at the bedside, thus eliminating risks associated with transport. If bedside imaging is unavailable and the patient is receiving mechanical ventilation, thoracentesis should be performed in an appropriately equipped radiology suite with personnel skilled in the treatment of tension pneumothorax.

DETECTION OF A PLEURAL EFFUSION

The physical examination is unreliable for the detection of pleural fluid in critically ill patients, especially those receiving mechanical ventilation. It is often impossible to position the patient upright. In addition, peripheral edema, lung consolidation, atelectasis, as well as abdominal distention displacing abdominal organs cephalad increase the likelihood that the examiner will misinterpret physical findings. Therefore, physical examination as the sole modality cannot be used to diagnose a pleural effusion with the degree of confidence required to proceed to thoracentesis with its possible complications. Imaging is therefore indispensable.

The most commonly performed radiologic study in the ICU is the anteroposterior chest radiograph, which is often performed with the patient in a supine or semirecumbent position. Unfortunately, pleural effusion may result in only subtle abnormalities on these radiographs unless the effusion is large. Because of the posterior layering of free flowing pleural fluid, the only abnormality seen on the anteroposterior chest radiograph may be a "veil-like" opacity superimposed on the lung fields. This opacity may be homogeneous in the supine patient or with a gradient of increasing opacity toward the base in the patient in a semirecumbent position. The pleural effusion may displace lung from the costophrenic angle or posterior to the heart, resulting in disappearance of lung markings projected over the dome of the diaphragm or heart shadow. However, these markings are commonly absent in the critically ill for reasons other than pleural effusion,

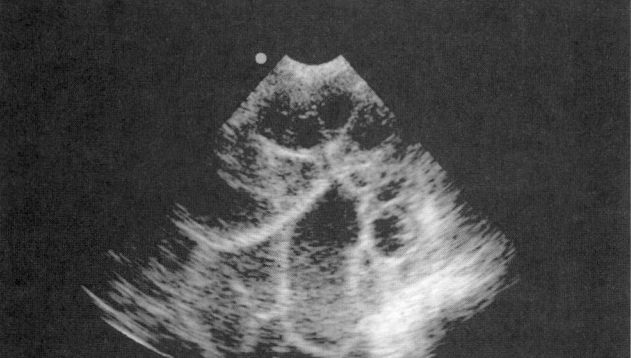

FIGURE 215–1. Anechoic effusion on the left side. The boundaries of the anechoic area are diaphragm, chest wall, and partially aerated lung. The effusion is marked for access.

TABLE 215–1. INDICATIONS AND CONTRAINDICATIONS OF THORACENTESIS IN THE CRITICALLY ILL

Indications

- Effusion not explained by the clinical presentation
- Massive effusion
- Suspected infection
- Suspected complication of pneumonia (empyema)
- Suspected hemothorax

Contraindications

Absolute
- Lack of expertise
- Severe uncorrectable coagulopathy
- Azotemia (creatinine >6 mg/dL)

Relative
- Operator dependent and of technical nature

most notably atelectasis and consolidation. Soft tissue, such as breast tissue, also results in a veil-like opacity on the chest radiograph and should not be interpreted as evidence of pleural effusion. The most common cause of unilateral veil-like opacity is the oblique projection that commonly occurs with anteroposterior chest radiographs. For example, a right posterior oblique view places the right posterior aspect of the chest closer to the cassette and results in increased penetration of the right side. Consequently, the left side appears to have a superimposed, homogeneous, veil-like opacity when compared with the right. Obviously, if a right effusion is present, a right posterior oblique view will result in attenuation of the right veil-like opacity and a pleural effusion may be missed if obliquity is not considered. These factors are most important for small to moderate effusions, because large effusions typically can be easily recognized by the appearance of a peripheral rim of fluid around the lung, a meniscus, and contralateral shift of the mediastinum.[3-5]

Compared with the difficulty of correctly identifying small to moderate pleural effusions on standard anteroposterior chest radiographs, sonography of the pleural space is simple and accurate.[6,7] In addition, there is the capability for image guidance at the bedside, enabling the practitioner to proceed to thoracentesis without delay. These attributes make pleural ultrasonography the modality of choice for the evaluation of pleural disease in the ICU. Sonography for the detection of pleural fluid requires the identification of organs, such as heart, liver, spleen, kidneys, and diaphragm. The lung must be recognized either directly, when it is collapsed or otherwise not aerated, or indirectly, by observation of lung sliding and air artifacts such as the curtain effect and comet tail artifacts. Lung sliding is a misnomer and actually means the sliding movement of the visceral pleural reflection relative to the chest wall with respiration. The aerated lung cannot be visualized directly because air is impenetrable to ultrasound. However, an intermittent obscuration of underlying structures in a curtain-like fashion may be observed. A similar effect may be seen in the presence of a hydropneumothorax, when the pneumothorax intermittently blocks ultrasound transmission. The comet tail artifact is a ray-like air artifact; the rays project from the point of origin to the outer limits of the image. Comet tails seen during chest imaging usually indicate an aerated lung.[8,9] Fluid usually appears as an anechoic, black area on the image that is bounded by chest wall, mediastinum, diaphragm, lung, and pericardium (either all at once or in some combination). Definition of these boundaries locates the anechoic structure in the pleural space. Once that is accomplished, the dynamic character of the anechoic structure is assessed. Dynamic signs of fluid due to

TABLE 215–2. COMPLICATIONS OF THORACENTESIS IN THE CRITICALLY ILL

Major

- Pneumothorax
- Tension pneumothorax
- Arterial laceration
- Hemothorax
- Reexpansion pulmonary edema
- Hypotension

Minor

- Pain at puncture site
- Seroma at puncture site
- Hematoma at puncture site
- Cough
- Vasovagal reaction

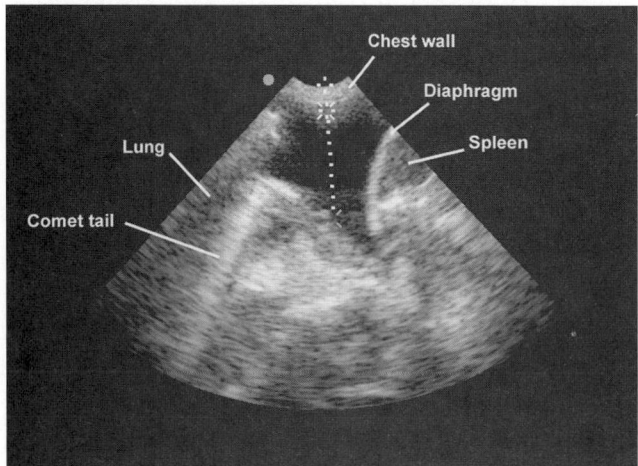

FIGURE 215–2. Fully developed complex septate effusion.

cardiac or respiratory motion are (1) flapping motion of the lung; (2) change of shape; and (3) a swirling or undulating movement of fibrin debris and fronds. At this point, the investigated structure has been located in the pleural space; and if one or more dynamic fluid signs are present, then the liquid nature has been established and pleurocentesis can be performed. The presence of internal echoes in a fluid collection, either homogeneous or heterogeneous, suggests an exudative effusion.[6,7,10-12] In these cases, initial small-bore catheter drainage may be considered in lieu of thoracentesis. The catheters can be chosen in a size only minimally larger than the thoracentesis catheter and may remain in place for continued drainage or removed once pleural fluid analysis provides data that continued drainage is not required.

TECHNIQUE

Thoracentesis in the critically ill, especially the mechanically ventilated patient, should be performed under image guidance. Either CT or ultrasound guidance may be used. Uncooperative subjects must be adequately sedated for the procedure. Standard positioning is not required with image guidance. However, CT-guided accession must be performed with the patient lying supine, prone, or in a lateral decubitus position. With ultrasound guidance, any position may be used. For small, free-flowing effusions, hemodynamically stable patients, even while on mechanical ventilation, may be placed in a sitting position to collect fluid in the costophrenic angle. For moderate or large effusions, the patient should be moved toward the edge of the bed with the head of the bed elevated to a 30- to 45-degree angle, allowing a posterolateral approach. Loculated effusions require individualized positioning, depending on the localization of the collection. Once the patient is positioned appropriately, the location of the effusion is confirmed by imaging and the needle can be inserted. The operator should be familiar with decompression of a tension pneumothorax and insertion of a thoracostomy tube, if thoracentesis is performed in patients on positive-pressure ventilation. The necessary equipment for the management of pneumothorax should be available on short notice, so that treatment can be instituted expeditiously. A tension pneumothorax can quickly become life threatening in mechanically ventilated patients.

After locating a suitable access area and determining the access angle using either CT or ultrasound images, the upper margin of the rib immediately below the access area should be defined by palpation. The area should be disinfected with an iodophor- or chlorhexidine-containing antiseptic before inserting a needle for infiltration of a local anesthetic. The entire procedure should be performed under sterile conditions. In the obese individual, palpation of a rib is often not possible and the rib should be sought with a 21-gauge or smaller needle while infiltrating the area with local anesthetic. Spinal needles may be necessary in very obese patients. Once the upper margin of a rib has been identified, the needle should be advanced over it while injecting more local anesthetic. Accessing the pleural space over the upper margin of a rib places the needle path at a greater distance from the intercostal vessels and nerve. Image guidance does not protect from intercostal vascular injury, and proper technique must always be used. While moving the needle slowly toward the pleural space, intermittent suction should be applied. Once pleural fluid is obtained, the needle depth should be noted and the needle withdrawn under aspiration until fluid flow ceases. When the needle tip is outside the pleural space, the syringe should be exchanged with a new syringe not contaminated by local anesthetic. The needle should then be advanced to the previous depth where fluid was obtained, and a sufficient sample should be aspirated. If therapeutic thoracentesis is desired, the needle is withdrawn after local anesthesia is completed and pleural fluid has been obtained. A suitable drainage catheter should then be inserted through a small skin incision at the same angle over the upper margin of the rib as the finder needle.

The procedure for a catheter-over-needle system is most commonly used today. A thoracentesis catheter should never be inserted if fluid cannot be obtained with a small-bore needle. The catheter should be advanced into the pleural space under continuous application of suction. Once pleural fluid is obtained, the catheter usually needs to be advanced farther by approximately 1 cm to place the catheter with its maximum diameter into the pleural space. If the catheter is not advanced by an additional distance, resistance and catheter damage may occur during advancement of the catheter over the inner cannula of the assembly. There are several low-cost, catheter-over-needle thoracentesis kits commercially available. Some minor features differ among manufacturers; however, the insertion procedure as described earlier applies to all. These commercial kits include drainage bags and a double one-way valve assembly for convenient evacuation of fluid. Throughout the procedure attention should be focused on avoiding entry of air into the needle or catheter while the tip is positioned in the pleural space. If air is introduced into the pleural space, the resulting pneumothorax may lead to unnecessary placement of a thoracostomy tube, although no pulmonary parenchymal injury has occurred. We routinely obtain a chest radiograph after thoracentesis in mechanically ventilated patients.[13]

INDICATIONS AND CONTRAINDICATIONS

An important indication for thoracentesis in the ICU relates to infection of the pleural space. The problem may be primary, such as when patients are admitted with pleural sepsis. Alternatively, the investigation may be prompted to diagnose a possible complication of pneumonia acquired during the ICU stay. Patients with massive pleural effusions and impending respiratory failure may require urgent drainage. In these cases, the pleural effusion usually is only one factor contributing to respiratory failure. Intuitively attractive is the removal of moderate to large effusions in patients on mechanical ventilation to facilitate liberation from the ventilator. However, no evidence exists to support the practice on a routine basis, and the decision to proceed with drainage has to be individualized. Most pleural effusions in the ICU resolve spontaneously, once the underlying disease process is controlled and volume status has normalized. In most patients without suspicion of infectious pleuritis but persistent effusion, diagnosis and management of pleural effusion can be deferred until their conditions are stable and they have been discharged from the ICU.[1,2]

Absolute contraindications to thoracentesis include an uncooperative patient; lack of operator expertise; and severe, uncorrectable bleeding disorders, including uremic platelet dysfunction. Relative contraindications are mainly technical and vary with the degree of operator experience and confidence. They include single lung, severe hypoxemic respiratory failure, and severe emphysema. Risk and benefit should be established on a case-by case basis depending on the predicted value of pleural fluid analysis and its effect on clinical outcome.

COMPLICATIONS

Thoracentesis can have a high complication rate if performed with poor technique and by unskilled personnel. In contrast, thoracentesis is extraordinarily safe in expert hands. The conclusion from the divergent reports of complications of thoracentesis is that only trained staff should perform the procedure. The reputation of thoracentesis as a simple and safe procedure not requiring expertise is undeserved.[14,15] Image-guided thoracentesis in the critically ill has a documented excellent safety record. By using bedside ultrasound, transport risk is eliminated.[16,17] The rate of pneumothorax in clinically guided thoracentesis has been reported to be as high as 30%. This rate is unacceptable, especially when compared with ultrasound-guided thoracentesis, which has a pneumothorax rate consistently reported between 0% and 3%.[14-21]

Pneumothorax due to thoracentesis, in the absence of penetrating chest trauma or preexisting bronchopleural fistula, occurs in three instances. First, the lung can be lacerated by the needle. This complication is largely avoidable with proper image guidance. Second, air can be introduced inadvertently through the needle or catheter system. This complication is avoidable by employing proper technique. Third, the lung may fail to expand because of either bronchial obstruction or visceral pleural restriction causing lung entrapment. During large volume thoracentesis in the presence of an unexpandable lung, extreme negative pressures may be created in the pleural space. This pressure change is not detectable by the operator. If an unexpandable lung is suspected, large-volume thoracentesis should be avoided unless pleural liquid pressure monitoring is available. Small-volume thoracentesis for diagnostic purposes may be performed safely. If complete drainage of a pleural effusion is necessary and an unexpandable lung is suspected, a small-bore thoracostomy should be performed and the effusion drained using a standard three-bottle system. This system operates through a combination of controlled suction and gravity drainage. If an unexpandable lung is present and such a system is used, air will enter the chest through the thoracostomy tube by gravity exchange of fluid and air. If pneumothorax due to unexpandable lung is found after standard large-volume thoracentesis, the air may have entered the pleural space through a bronchopleural fistula created by excessively negative pressure. This condition usually does not require treatment in the spontaneously breathing patient.

However, mechanically ventilated patients may be at risk for the development of a tension pneumothorax, and precautionary placement of a large-bore thoracostomy should be considered.[22]

Image guidance does not reduce the rate of intercostal vascular injury, but proper technique will reduce the risk. Intercostal artery injury may occur because of tortuous vessels, which are more commonly found in the elderly, and laceration can be a lethal event. Treatment usually requires thoracotomy with ligation of the vessel.

Reexpansion pulmonary edema may occur if a large volume of fluid is evacuated from a chronic effusion. This complication is undoubtedly rare; however, the true incidence is unknown. Vagal reactions can be treated with atropine. Hypotension may occur if very large volumes of fluid are withdrawn and may require hours to develop. Hypotension should initially be treated with intravascular volume expansion. Minor complications include hematoma and seroma at the puncture site. Cough is common during large volume thoracentesis and is usually self-limited. Cough without chest pain is probably due to airway irritation during reexpansion of previously collapsed lung. Pleuritic chest pain and pain at the puncture site may occur.

ANNOTATED REFERENCES

Lichtenstein D, Hulot JS, Rabiller A, et al: Feasibility and safety of ultrasound-aided thoracentesis in mechanically ventilated patients. Intensive Care Med 1999;25:955-958.
Report of a series of 45 ultrasound-guided thoracenteses in mechanically ventilated patients. Positive identification of organs adjacent to the suspected effusion was required, and fluid was identified by lung flapping and change of the thickness of the region between lung and chest wall. No complications occurred.

Lomas DJ, Padley SG, Flower CDR: The sonographic appearance of pleural fluid. Br J Radiol 1993;66:619-624.
A case series of 93 pleural effusions with "atypical clinical or radiographic appearance" referred for ultrasound-guided aspiration. Lung flapping, swirling motion of debris or movement of internal septa were used as reliable signs for the presence of pleural fluid and were found in 83% of cases. No major complications resulting from thoracentesis occurred in this series of sonography-guided thoracenteses.

Mayo PH, Goltz HR, Tafreshi M, et al: Safety of ultrasound-guided thoracentesis in patients on mechanical ventilation. Chest 2004;125:1059-1062.
Report of a series of 232 pleural drainage procedures in mechanically ventilated patients performed by intensivists. The physicians were trained in focused sonography of pleural effusion. The dynamic signs accepted as reliable indicators of pleural fluid were lung flapping, swirling motion of debris, or change in shape of the collection during respiration. Positive identification of adjacent organs and a suitable sonographic window were also required to proceed with the intervention. Three (1.3%) procedures were unsuccessful, and three (1.3%) were pneumothoraces.

Chapter 216

CHEST TUBE PLACEMENT, CARE, AND REMOVAL

Gregory A. Watson • Brian G. Harbrecht

Hippocrates was one of the first physicians to perform therapeutic drainage of the pleural space when he described incision, cautery, and the insertion of metal tubes to drain empyema.[1] In the mid 1800s, Hunter designed a hypodermic needle for insertion into and drainage of the pleural space.[2] Playfair placed a drainage tube under water to prevent the retrograde flow of air in 1872, and 4 years later Hewitt described closed-tube drainage of an empyema.[3,4] Drainage of the pleural space in the early 20th century was most frequently performed to drain postinfluenza empyema, but Lilienthal described its use in postoperative thoracic surgical care in 1922.[5,6] By World War II, tube thoracostomy was used regularly after elective thoracotomy, but it was not until the Korean War that emergency tube thoracostomy for penetrating thoracic trauma was performed.[7,8]

Tube thoracostomy, or chest tube placement, is performed to evacuate air and/or fluid from the pleural space. Air in the pleural space, or pneumothorax, can occur spontaneously, but in the critically ill patient it is usually associated with underlying pulmonary disease, penetrating chest trauma, blunt multisystem trauma, invasive procedures (central line insertion), or barotrauma. Pleural effusion simply refers to fluid in the pleural space. It can be serous, sterile, and free-flowing (transudative), viscous and complex (exudative), purulent (empyema), bloody (hemothorax), or chylous (chylothorax). In this chapter, we discuss the basic components of a pleural drainage system, indications for chest tube placement, insertion technique, complications, and common management issues.

COMPONENTS OF A CHEST DRAINAGE SYSTEM

Initial surgical procedures to evacuate the pleural space of infected material relied on open, gravity-dependent drainage or the insertion of metal tubes. Modern chest tubes are made of clear, pliable plastic (polyvinylchloride or silicone) and are configured to facilitate placement into the desired portion of the pleural space. Nearly all forms of chest tubes contain distance markers, multiple drainage holes, and a radiopaque stripe outlining the location of the last drainage hole.[8] The internal diameter ranges in size from 20 to 40 French (Fr) for adult patients (5 to 11 mm) to 6 to 26 Fr for pediatric patients (2 to 6 mm). The tubes may be straight or curved into a right angle (Fig. 216-1). The distal end of the tube (collection system side) is slightly beveled and flared to facilitate connection to accessory tubing and the collection system. A plastic connector of at least 0.25-inch diameter should be used to connect the chest tube to accessory tubing from the collection system. The interface between the chest tube itself and the collection system is often the component of the system with the narrowest diameter, and so the use of

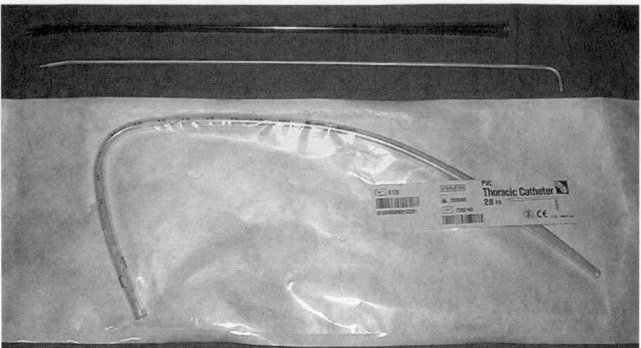

FIGURE 216–1. Standard straight chest tube *(top)* with metal trocar *(middle)* and angled chest tube without trocar *(bottom).*

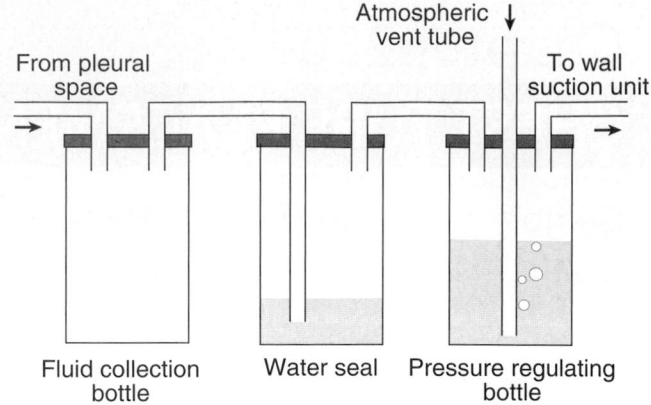

FIGURE 216–2. Schematic of the three components of a modern chest drainage system. (Redrawn from Bar-El Y, Ross A, Kablawi A, et al: Potentially dangerous negative intrapleural pressures generated by ordinary pleural drainage systems. Chest 2001;119:511-514.)

a large, clear connector will minimize obstruction by blood, fluid, or tissue.[8] When multiple tubes are placed in the same hemithorax, a Y connector is often used to simplify nursing care and reduce the number of collection devices. Unfortunately, if the Y connector becomes occluded at the common channel, both chest tubes become nonfunctional. To ensure reliable pleural decompression, each chest tube should be connected to its own individual collection system.

Standard tubing used to connect a chest tube to a collection system is generally 0.5 inch in diameter and 6 feet long. The flow rate through the tubing is inversely proportional to the length of the tubing and directly proportional to the radius. Because pleural fluid frequently may be thick and viscous (empyema, hemothorax), effective drainage may depend on selecting the proper size chest tube and connection tubing. Most standard tubes are capable of flows of 50 to 60 L/min. The tubing itself should be clear enough to permit visualization of fluid and/or air bubbles and flexible and strong enough to avoid iatrogenic injury and withstand the rigors of patient transport and daily care.

A variety of collection systems or devices may be utilized. For patients with a large pneumothorax or one under tension, providing an opening into the pleural space to allow egress of pleural air and restore intrathoracic pressures will be the primary therapeutic maneuver. In these circumstances, a collecting system will prevent two-way air movement through the chest tube and evacuate the pleural space until the injury to the pulmonary parenchyma seals, air leakage stops, and the lung remains fully expanded. For the evacuation of fluid, collection systems provide for the application of negative pressure to assist in fluid removal, prevent two-way air flow through the system, and allow the quantification of the volume of drainage to assist clinical decision making. Connecting a chest tube to a simple gravity-dependent system may permit the immediate drainage of large volumes of fluid but may be unsatisfactory for long-term management. Chronic drainage of small volume collections or persistent air leaks may be performed with specialized devices that facilitate patient mobility while preserving one-way flow of drainage from the pleural space (Heimlich valve).

Generally, however, chest tubes are connected to a modern drainage system using three components consisting of a trap, water seal, and manometer compartments (Fig. 216-2).[8,9] These components are combined into a single transportable unit that permits adjustment of negative pressure, provides for increased patient mobility, and is user-friendly from a nursing perspective. The chest tube with its accessory tubing is connected to the trap portion of the drainage system.

This portion of the drainage system serves as the collection area where fluid from the pleural space fills graduated columns for quantification of the drained volume. The water seal portion of the drainage system allows air and/or fluid to drain from the chest and prevents air from re-entering the pleural space. The manometer portion of the system contains input and output tubes and a central vent, as well as a control that allows regulation of the amount of negative pressure applied. The manometer is connected to a standard wall vacuum source. Most drainage systems also contain a leak meter, with seven chambers of varying size and resistance that allow reliable and accurate quantification of the magnitude of air leaks from the pulmonary parenchyma or through the system (Fig. 216-3).[10]

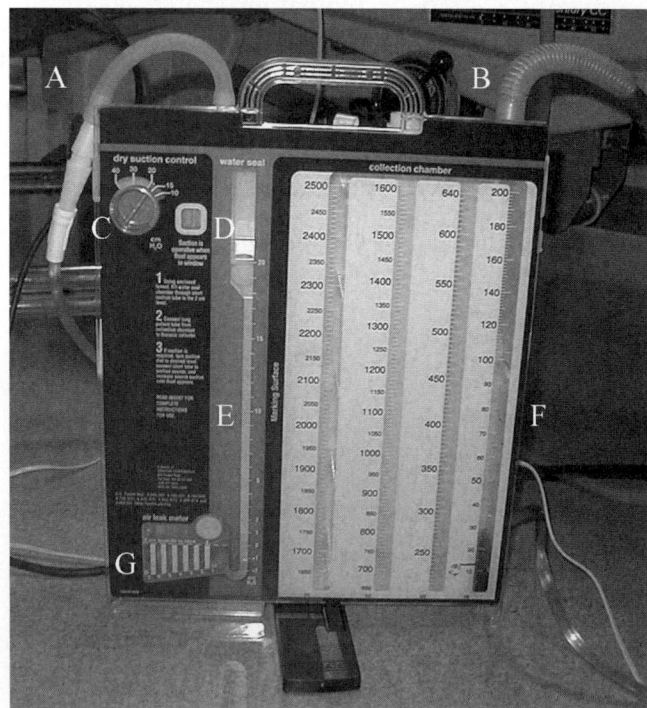

FIGURE 216–3. Modern chest drainage system. A, Accessory tubing to wall suction; B, accessory tubing to chest tube/patient; C, suction control; D, float indicating that suction is operative; E, water seal chamber; F, collection chamber; G, air leak meter.

INDICATIONS FOR TUBE THORACOSTOMY

Placement of a chest tube can be both a diagnostic and a therapeutic maneuver. Chest tube insertion will identify the presence of air or fluid in the pleural space, the character of a pleural effusion (bloody, purulent, serous), and the quantity of fluid in addition to providing the means for its evacuation. Most pleural space collections are adequately treated by simple tube thoracostomy, and thoracoscopy, thoracotomy, or other forms of open surgical drainage are infrequently required.

A variety of conditions may require chest tube placement in the ICU. As already discussed in earlier chapters, these are conditions that lead to the presence of symptomatic or potentially symptomatic air and fluid collections in the pleural space and include pneumothorax from any cause, hemothorax, pleural effusions, and infected pleural fluid collections. The evaluation and management of most of these conditions have been discussed in other chapters (see Chapter 245) and will not be repeated here. Simply put, the need to drain the pleural space or to determine the nature of a pleural collection represents an indication for tube thoracostomy.

TECHNIQUE OF INSERTION

A number of clinical factors should be evaluated before performing tube thoracostomy, including the indication for placement, location of the material to be drained, and general status of the patient. Some authors have recommended placement of the chest tube into a specific location depending on the nature of the material to be drained (anteriorly and apically for the evacuation of air; dependently or posteriorly for the evacuation of fluid).[8] In the absence of pleural adhesions from prior pleural space disease, intrinsic parenchymal disease, or previous surgery, the pleural space for most patients should be readily drainable without specialized placement and entry into the pleural space should generally be gained via a location based on safety and avoidance of complications. Exceptions to this general rule can occur and may merit specialized placement if the fluid is loculated. Loculated fluid may require a tube to be placed by a skilled operator such as a surgeon or with radiologic guidance.[8]

Selection of the proper size tube for pleural drainage is important. A simple pneumothorax or free-flowing serous effusion can be adequately drained with a small-caliber tube (16 to 28 Fr) but blood, pus, or viscous fluid requires a larger tube (32 to 40 Fr chest tube). It is possible that effective drainage of air or fluid can be done with smaller catheters (Fig. 216-4).[11,12] Some investigators have suggested that the increase in flow through a tube of fixed diameter is negligible once the catheters are larger than 7 Fr.[11] Smaller drainage catheters are more likely to occlude, but flushing the drain several times a day or using thrombolytics can help maintain patency.[13] The apparent success of these smaller catheters may be related more to precise placement than is possible with image guidance.[11] Reports of malpositioned chest tubes placed without imaging have varied from 1% to 26%, but how precisely a chest tube must be positioned to provide satisfactory, successful drainage has not been rigorously defined.[11,14]

Once the need for tube thoracostomy has been defined, the proper tube selected, and the necessary equipment obtained for insertion, the relevant patient anatomy should

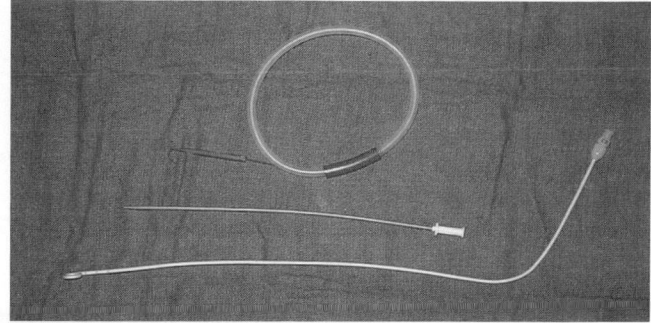

FIGURE 216–4. Pigtail catheter showing the guidewire *(top)*, dilator *(middle)*, and catheter *(bottom)*.

be reviewed. The operator should review the appropriate radiographic studies to ensure that the proper hemithorax in the correct patient is being addressed. After confirming the pleural space requiring drainage, the patient should be positioned supine or with the head of the bed slightly elevated and the ipsilateral arm placed behind the head or abducted. The bed should be at a comfortable height for the physician, and lighting should be adequate. As discussed earlier, placement of a chest tube into a specific location in the pleural space is infrequently required. The site of insertion will usually be chosen based on ease of access to the pleural space (i.e., avoidance of pectoralis major, latissimus dorsi, and breast parenchyma) and avoidance of complications (i.e., injury to major vessels or diaphragm). The American College of Surgeons Committee on Trauma recommends drain placement between the anterior and posterior axillary lines, below the axillary vessels, at a level just above the fifth intercostal space (nipple level in males). The tube should pass just above the superior surface of the rib.[15] The pectoralis major muscle should be avoided because chest tube placement through the pectoral muscles is technically challenging, requires deeper dissection, makes guiding the direction of tube placement within the pleural space difficult, and precludes basal drainage.[16] The proposed site should be identified, the skin cleansed, and local anesthetic infiltrated at the selected intercostal space. Patient education, liberal use of local anesthesia, and premedication with a narcotic or anxiolytic can lessen pain and anxiety.[17] The deeper tissues should likewise be infiltrated, being certain to angle the needle slightly cephalad to anesthetize the periosteum of the appropriate rib. Several passes may be required to cover an area 1 to 2 cm in diameter, and aspiration should be applied intermittently repetitively as the anesthetic is injected. If air or fluid is aspirated, retract the needle while still aspirating until it ceases and then inject additional local anesthetic to anesthetize the parietal pleura.

The chest should be prepared with skin antiseptic and the field draped with sterile towels. The operator should perform a hand scrub, use sterile technique, and practice universal precautions at all times (i.e., the operator should wear a cap, mask, gown, and gloves). All equipment should be available before starting the procedure. Whereas a variety of instruments frequently are present on prepackaged trays available in most emergency departments or ICUs, tube thoracostomy can be readily performed with just a scalpel and a clamp (a large Kelly clamp or small hemostat). The skin and subcutaneous tissues should be incised with a scalpel. While a variety of techniques have evolved to minimize the size of the incision for tube thoracostomy, the smaller the incision the less control the operator has in safely and securely placing the chest tube. An incision large enough to accommodate the operator's index finger and chest tube at the same time is recommended for optimal safety and to minimize complications from insertion. Some recommend placing sutures at this point, with one simple suture at one end of the wound to secure the drain and a vertical mattress suture in the center of the wound to close it after drain removal.[16] Purse-string sutures should be avoided because they do not close the wound along the length of the incision.

Blunt dissection using the index finger and Kelly clamp should be performed to create a subcutaneous tunnel to the appropriate intercostal space (Fig. 216-5).[8] An oblique path angled slightly superiorly between the incision and the entry site into the pleural space will lessen the chances of infection, decrease the risk of air entry on tube removal, and aid wound closure.[8] In situations in which immediate pleural decompression is required, the straightest and fastest path to the pleural space may be more appropriate. The pleural space should be gently entered with the tip of the clamp, and care should be taken to avoid excessive clamp insertion into the pleural space or deeper structures (i.e., pulmonary parenchyma, heart, diaphragm) that could be injured. The clamp may need to be opened slightly to sufficiently enlarge the opening into the pleural space. If the patient is on a ventilator, disconnecting the patient from positive airway pressure before entering the pleural space may minimize the risk of inadvertent injury to lung parenchyma.[18,19] Entry into the pleural space will frequently be confirmed by the immediate return of air or fluid, depending on the indication for chest tube insertion. The index finger should be inserted to confirm entry into the pleural space. One should be able to digitally palpate parietal pleura; often it is also possible to palpate the lung. The index finger should be gently swept around the pleural space to identify the presence of any adhesions, which may be present in up to 15% of cases.[20] The chest tube should then be inserted into the pleural space. The previously used clamp or hemostat can assist in proper tube placement. The clamp can be used to grasp the end of the tube and guide it through the subcutaneous

tissues into the pleural space. The tip of the operator's index finger, inserted alongside the tube, can be used to safely guide the chest tube away from the pulmonary parenchyma. Some prefer that the tip be directed anteroapically for a pneumothorax and posterobasally for fluid. The index finger placed alongside the tube can also be used to ensure that the last drainage hole is placed well within the pleural space because the presence of side holes in the subcutaneous tissue may interfere with proper chest tube function. After the chest tube is advanced into proper position, it should be immediately connected to a drainage system.[16] Most individually wrapped, nonangled chest tubes are packaged with a metal trocar that may be used to assist with placement (see Fig. 216-1). We generally recommend that the trocar be immediately discarded and not used for insertion, owing to the increased risk of lacerating the lung or other important structures.[8] The use of trocars for tube thoracostomy should be discouraged for all but the most experienced of operators. After the chest tube has been inserted, it should be secured to the skin at the exit site with sutures to prevent inadvertent dislodgment. The manner in which the chest tube is secured in place is probably less important than the fact that it is held in place securely and not able to be repositioned by patient movement, patient mobilization, or transport.

The tube should be connected immediately to the collecting system; and if suction is desired, it should be adjusted to provide slow, constant bubbling. Typically, the collection system will be connected to suction to generate negative pressure to facilitate complete pleural drainage. The concern that routine suction after chest tube placement may perpetuate air leaks should be an infrequent concern. Because the amount of suction that is applied to the chest tube may be poorly controlled by simply adjusting the vacuum generated from wall suction devices, the use of slow, consistent bubbling should be used; it will generate the desired pressure without being excessive.[9]

After the drain suture is securely tied to the tube, the wound should be covered with dry gauze and tape. Some use petrolatum gauze to cover the wound, but this could macerate the skin and predispose to infection.[8] A chest radiograph should be obtained to document proper placement, evaluate expansion of the lung, and look for residual pleural fluid or air. Failure to expand the lung on chest radiography after chest tube placement should prompt reevaluation of the patient, and a cause should be sought. Common reasons for failure to expand the lung properly include improper chest tube placement (subcutaneous or extrapleural placement), large pulmonary parenchymal air leaks, improperly functioning collection devices, or leaks within the system.

The accessory tubing should be positioned in a straight or coiled position for optimal drainage. Only a few studies have looked at the positioning of the accessory tubing and its effect on the efficiency of drainage. In both in vitro and in vivo animal studies, chest drainage is optimal when the tubing is in a straight or coiled position compared with placement with a dependent loop.[21,22] However, if a dependent loop cannot be avoided, lifting the tubing and draining it every 15 minutes maintains adequate removal.

Some authors have described variations of the procedure listed earlier for tube thoracostomy, utilizing principles of the Seldinger technique for catheter insertion. A J-type guidewire or a smaller catheter has been used to enter the pleural space initially, followed by placement of a chest tube over the wire.[23,24] The authors claim the incision is smaller, less painful, more cosmetic, and less likely to leak around

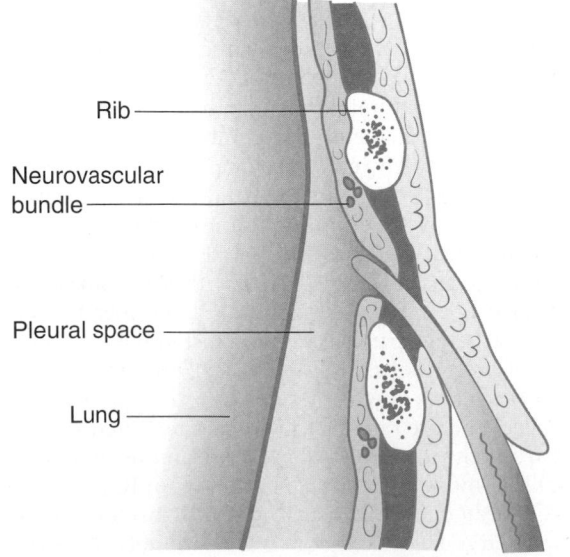

Rib

Neurovascular bundle

Pleural space

Lung

FIGURE 216–5. Use of a Kelly clamp to enter the pleural space. (Redrawn from Miller KS, Sahn SA: Chest tubes: Indications, techniques, management, and complications. Chest 1987;91:258-264.)

the tube. Use of small-bore catheters and the Seldinger technique may be useful for image-guided drainage of localized fluid collections, isolated pneumothoraces, or serous, easily drainable effusions. The small diameter of the tubes used in this technique is frequently inadequate for drainage of viscous or bloody pleural collections, for which large-bore tubes are required.

MANAGEMENT AND TROUBLESHOOTING

At all times, the water level in the system should be maintained, the system should remain upright, and the collection device should be kept below chest level. Daily assessment for the amount of drainage, presence of bubbling, and respiratory variation should be performed.[16] Observation of synchronous motion of fluid in the water seal chamber with respiration suggests that the tube is still functioning in the pleural space and that all connections are tight. If the tube is not functioning and occlusion of the drainage holes is suggested, the tube can be disconnected and flushed with saline.[8] If this fails, fibrinolytics may be an effective alternative, particularly in parapneumonic effusions.[13] Streptokinase, 250,000 units qd, or urokinase, 100,000 units qd, are equally efficacious, although fibrinolytics should be avoided in patients with contraindications (sensitivity, bleeding diatheses, recent hemorrhagic stroke, intracranial neoplasm, or head trauma). If an air leak within the system is suggested, sequential clamping of the accessory tubing with distal suction can be used to identify the sight of the leak. Drainage (bubbling) through the water seal when a clamp is placed just proximal to the point in question that disappears when the clamp is moved distally identifies the location of the leak, which then can be addressed. If this procedure does not identify the location of a leak within the accessory tubing or any of the connections, a major airway injury or bronchopleural fistula may be the problem. A momentum or "swing" leak can be misinterpreted as an air leak, because the patient is capable of generating a large pressure change with inspiration and expiration. Adding fluid to the collection device will frequently resolve this problem.[10] If air is heard at the site of insertion, the incision may be too large and may require an additional suture, a large air leak may exist that requires placement of an additional chest tube, or alternatively the side drainage holes of the chest tube may be outside the pleural space.[16]

Chest tube management, such as when to use suction or water seal, when it is safe to remove the tube, how to remove the tube, and when to obtain a chest radiograph, was largely a matter of personal preference until recently. Simply stated, chest tubes should be removed when the indication for tube thoracostomy has resolved. Management will be slightly different for lung resection patients, trauma patients, patients with iatrogenic pneumothorax, patients with effusions, and patients with empyema. Lung re-expansion without an air leak, negligible fluid output, and resolution of an infectious process are indications for removal.

In patients with simple pneumothorax or hemothorax, the decision to manage the chest tube with suction or water seal has not been well studied. Generally, we place all chest tubes to suction initially to assist in re-expansion of the lung and/or evacuation of fluid. The chest tube remains on suction until the air leak has ceased and the lung is fully expanded. At this point, the chest tube can be converted to water seal and removed when drainage is negligible. Whether the routine use of suction in patients with an uncomplicated

pneumothorax potentiates air leaks is unclear. Martino and colleagues studied whether management without a trial of water seal before chest tube removal allowed for a shorter duration of chest tube use.[25] Two-hundred and five trauma patients with a combination of blunt and penetrating injuries were enrolled in the study, and patients younger than age 15 or on the ventilator for longer than 24 hours were excluded. Criteria for removal included drainage less than 150 mL/day, absence of a significant pneumothorax, and lack of an air leak. Patients were randomized to a no-water-seal group or to water seal. The no-water-seal group had their chest tubes disconnected from suction and pulled immediately, whereas the other group was on water seal for 6 to 8 hours, had a chest radiograph performed, and then had the chest tube removed if no pneumothorax had developed after being placed on water-seal. All tubes were removed at end inspiration with a Valsalva maneuver, and a chest radiograph was obtained after removal. Any patients with a pneumothorax in the water-seal group before tube removal (n = 4) were considered treatment failures. Recurrent pneumothorax occurred in 13 patients in the water-seal group versus 9 in the suction group, but 7 of the nine patients in the suction group required repeat chest tube insertion as opposed to only one in the water-seal group ($P < .05$). Overall, there was no difference in the length of stay or duration of chest tube insertion between the two groups, but replacement of a chest tube did double the length of stay. They concluded that a short trial of water seal before removal should be performed.

In lung resection patients, placement of sutures or a staple line across a lobar bronchus or pulmonary parenchyma may predispose to the development of an air leak or bronchopleural fistula to a much greater extent than that in patients with other indications for tube thoracostomy. Managing chest tubes in postoperative thoracic surgical patients may therefore be more complicated. Cerfolio described a system for classifying the quantity and quality of air leaks after pulmonary resection.[10] This system has been used to predict which patients will do well on water seal, who will require suction, and who will have a prolonged air leak. An air leak is classified based on when it occurs in the respiratory cycle as continuous (C), inspiratory (I), expiratory (E), or forced expiratory (FE). The leak meter on the drainage container is used further to grade the leak along a continuum as small (1) to large (7). This classification also distinguishes between bronchopleural fistula and alveolopleural fistula. Bronchopleural fistula is defined as a communication between a mainstem, lobar, or segmental bronchus and the pleural space, cannot occur unless the patient had a pneumonectomy, lobectomy, segmentectomy, or iatrogenic/traumatic injury, usually manifests as a continuous or inspiratory leak, and almost always requires operation.[10] Alveolopleural fistula, on the other hand, is the most common leak after pulmonary resection or pneumothorax, usually manifests as an expiratory or forced expiratory leak, and almost always seals with tube thoracostomy.[10]

A brief period of suction may be all that is necessary to allow lung expansion in lung resection patients, and longer periods of suction may be harmful. An initial trial by Cerfolio and colleagues randomized thoracotomy patients to suction or water seal on postoperative day 3, and it showed that water seal seemed superior to suction for resolving air leaks.[26] A second prospective study randomized patients to suction or water seal on postoperative day 1, and it showed that 67% of leaks treated with water seal resolved by postoperative day 3. Water seal was superior to suction at stopping air leaks, although a subset of patients were identified who developed pneumothorax or subcutaneous emphysema on water seal. These patients all had an expiratory 4 (E4) leak or larger, and returning the tube to a minimum amount of suction (−10 cm H_2O) resolved the problem.[27] Even shorter periods of suction may be well tolerated and perhaps beneficial. Marshall and associates enrolled 68 patients in a prospective, randomized, controlled trial comparing suction to water seal after pulmonary resection.[28] There were 34 patients in each group, and 15 in each group had an air leak after surgery. The duration of leak was shorter in the water-seal group (1.5 vs. 3.2 days), and it was even more dramatic when they corrected for the length of the staple line. The mean duration to chest tube removal was also less in the water-seal group (3.3 vs. 5.4 days). All patients received between 5 and 30 minutes of suction in the initial postoperative period, and then were randomized to one of two groups. In the suction group, suction was discontinued when no air leak was present and all tubes were removed when drainage was less than 300 mL/day. Pneumothorax did not occur in the suction group, but four patients in the water-seal group developed a pneumothorax greater than 25%. They were placed on −10 cm H_2O suction, with resolution within 24 hours and return to water seal. The seal group also had a trend toward a shorter hospital stay. The authors hypothesized that the staple line was the most likely source of leak and that suction likely makes the leaks larger by keeping the defect open.

If a large (E6/7) leak is encountered on postoperative day 1, it is not going to resolve by postoperative day 4, and these patients can be managed successfully as an outpatient with a Heimlich valve. Cerfolio used suction initially in all his patients to remove residual air from the surgery and to prevent clot formation in the chest drain, which can lead to a local consumptive coagulopathy.[29] He cautioned, however, that the early application of suction can be detrimental in patients with a large air leak on positive-pressure ventilation, because it may effectively reduce their tidal volume.[29] In his experience, suction more negative than −30 cm H_2O is almost never needed. Very high suction should be employed only for selected patients: those with hypoxia and a functioning chest tube without an air leak and an expanding pneumothorax or subcutaneous emphysema that is worsening on −20 cm H_2O suction.

Patients often have two chest tubes placed after lung resection; one is positioned anteroapically to evacuate air and the other is positioned posterobasally to evacuate fluid. If there is no air leak, the lung is fully expanded and drainage is less than 400 mL/day, the posterior chest tube may be removed on postoperative day 2 and the anterior chest tube removed on postoperative day 3.[29] After resection, it is possible that the lung will not entirely fill the hemithorax and appear as a pneumothorax on chest radiography. If there is no air leak and the pneumothorax is stable, the tube usually can be safely removed. If drainage remains greater than 400 mL/day by postoperative day 3, the presence of hemothorax, chylothorax, or rarely cerebrospinal fluid (from inadvertent entry into the subarachnoid space) should be excluded. The drainage should be examined for the presence of triglycerides or blood, and if pneumocephalus is a possibility, computed tomography of the head should be performed. If these studies are negative, the tube probably can be removed safely because the pleura is capable of resorbing

most reactive fluid.[29] Some authors would recommend a trial of chest tube clamping, although we generally do not recommend this, and it should be reserved for only the most experienced clinicians.

The volume of drainage that is considered "safe" for proceeding with chest tube removal has not been clearly defined, and few studies have been done. Frequently, the maximal chest tube output allowed for removal will vary according to the indication for chest tube insertion. Younes and associates performed a prospective randomized trial, looking at drain output in postoperative patients.[30] One-hundred thirty-nine patients were randomized to have their tubes removed when drainage was less than 100 mL/day, 150 mL/day, or 200 mL/day. There was no significant difference in drainage time, hospital stay, or reaccumulation rates among the groups, and they recommended that 200 mL/day could be safely used for chest tube removal if the fluid is not infected. Further study may clarify if larger volumes of drainage are also safe. Empyema is an exception, because chest tubes may remain in place for prolonged periods even with minimal drainage. When managing an empyema, the chest tube is left in place until the patient is afebrile, drainage is scant and serous, and imaging studies show minimal pleural fluid and lack of an empyema cavity.[8] At times, chest tubes used to drain an empyema may remain in place for several weeks.

The timing of chest tube removal relative to the respiratory cycle does not appear to be important. Bell and associates randomly assigned 102 trauma patients to chest tube removal at end inspiration or end expiration to determine the recurrent pneumothorax rate.[31] Proponents of end inspiration claim the lung is maximally expanded and the pleural surfaces opposed, but proponents of end expiration claim the pressure difference between the atmosphere and pleural space is minimized, lessening the risk of inadvertent air entry. Criteria for removal in this study included resolved or small but stable pneumothorax, lack of an air leak on water seal, and output less than 200 mL/day. All patients performed a Valsalva maneuver during removal. Ventilator-dependent patients were included in the end-inspiration group. Recurrent pneumothorax rates were similar with 8% in the end-inspiration group and 6% in the end-expiration group. There were no recurrent pneumothoraces in the ventilator-dependent patients, and the authors concluded that either method was safe.

We routinely perform chest radiography after chest tube removal to confirm that the lung remains fully expanded and to identify potential complications introduced by the chest tube removal process. To determine the appropriate time interval between removing a chest tube and obtaining a chest radiograph, Pizano and coworkers prospectively analyzed 75 trauma patients who were undergoing positive-pressure ventilation.[32] All patients had a solitary chest tube, drainage less than 150 mL/day, no air leak, and no pneumothorax on the previous chest radiograph. They were on water seal for at least 12 hours. Tubes were removed at the end of a ventilated breath, and radiographs were obtained at 1 to 3 hours, 10 hours, and 36 hours after removal. Recurrent pneumothorax occurred in nine patients (12%), and all of the pneumothoraces were detected at the time of the initial chest radiograph. Seven patients had a small (<10%) pneumothorax that remained stable or resolved on subsequent chest radiographs and required no intervention. Two patients (3%) required intervention owing to the size of the pneumothorax. One patient with a 10% to 20% pneumothorax was treated with needle aspiration alone, but the other patient had complete collapse of the lung and required repeat tube thoracostomy. They concluded that a radiograph taken 1 to 3 hours after chest tube removal identifies pneumothorax in ventilated patients.

Routine chest radiography after chest tube removal is not a universal practice. Palesty and coworkers performed a 5-year retrospective study of 73 patients with tube thoracostomies performed in a level II trauma center's ICU to determine if routine chest radiographs obtained after removal impact clinical management.[33] The indications for tube thoracostomy were diverse and included iatrogenic and spontaneous pneumothorax, traumatic hemothorax and hemopneumothorax, malignant and nonmalignant pleural effusions, chylothorax, and postoperative drainage. The tubes were connected to suction and water seal for various periods of time. All chest tubes were removed at end inspiration and with a Valsalva maneuver. Chest radiographs were obtained between 4 and 24 hours after removal. Eight patients had a radiography report that differed from the one obtained before removal, and six of them showed recurrence of pneumothorax or effusion. The other two patients became symptomatic after removal and were managed based on clinical grounds before radiographic results were available. These authors concluded that routine chest radiographs after tube removal are not justified and should be obtained at the discretion of the surgeon. The limitations of this study include the small number of patients involved, the heterogeneous nature of conditions leading to chest tube insertion, and the inherent difficulty in attempting to demonstrate the absence of a benefit with a specific clinical intervention. While the reinsertion rate after tube thoracostomy removal is low, the presence of a small pneumothorax frequently alters management and we continue to obtain routine chest radiographs after chest tube removal.

Thoracostomy tube management clearly has been a matter of individual preference for quite some time and individual practices within an institution often vary widely. Implementing a chest tube practice guideline may help streamline patient management. Adrales and associates investigated the effect of a thoracostomy tube practice guideline on the efficiency of thoracostomy tube management in trauma patients.[34] Sixty-one patients were part of this cohort study, with 14 in the pre-guideline group and 47 in the post-guideline group. The groups were similar, and the algorithm included one dose of a first-generation cephalosporin before insertion that was continued for 24 hours. All patients had a 36-Fr tube placed under sterile conditions and were placed immediately on −20 cm H_2O water suction. Radiographs were obtained within 4 hours. If no air leak was present and drainage was less than 200 mL/day, suction was discontinued and the tubes were placed to water seal. If no leak was present after 6 hours of water seal, the tubes were removed at end inspiration with a Valsalva maneuver. No radiograph was done on water seal, but a radiograph was obtained 4 hours after removal. The post-guideline group averaged three fewer days of tube thoracostomy therapy, and they saved about $3,000 in radiology fees. Complication rates were not different between the two groups. The authors concluded that implementation of a practice guideline did improve efficiency in chest tube management.

As discussed in this section, few aspects of chest tube management have been subjected to rigorous study or are

TABLE 216–1. GUIDELINES FOR TUBE THORACOSTOMY MANAGEMENT

1. Review indications for insertion and chest radiograph before chest tube placement.
2. After insertion, place chest tube to collection device and establish −20 cm H_2O suction.
3. Obtain chest radiograph after insertion.
4. Once the air leak has resolved and the lung is maximally expanded, convert to water seal.
5. Obtain chest radiograph on water seal to confirm maintenance of lung expansion.
6. When drainage is less than 150 to 200 mL/day, remove chest tube.
7. Obtain chest radiograph to confirm lung expansion after chest tube removal.

standardized. The diverse nature of indications for chest tube placement may contribute to this problem because chest tube management for a patient with an empyema will be different from that of a patient with a post-traumatic hemothorax or a postoperative lung resection patient. Some general guidelines are presented in Table 216-1 that may be applicable to most uncomplicated patients.

COMPLICATIONS OF TUBE THORACOSTOMY

The complication rate of chest tube insertion has been reported to be as low as 2% and as high as 21%.[35,36] Use of improper insertion technique, operator inexperience, and forceful use of sharp trocars are avoidable errors that account for many of the complications associated with chest tube placement. The list of complications is extensive and includes injury to virtually every intrathoracic and upper abdominal organ. Long thoracic nerve injury leading to winging of the scapula, puncture of silicone breast implants leading to intrathoracic silicosis, and re-expansion pulmonary edema are also known complications.[16] Compression injuries can result in intercostal neuralgia, Horner's syndrome, phrenic nerve palsy, and delayed esophageal rupture.

Injury to the lung can manifest as hemothorax or persistent air leak with constant bubbling in the leak meter, residual pneumothorax, or spreading subcutaneous emphysema. Expanding subcutaneous emphysema after chest tube placement can be secondary to air leak that is not controlled by the chest tube or because the lung has become adherent to the parietal pleura and the parenchymal leak is not communicating with the chest tube. These patients may require additional tube thoracostomy or surgery to lyse adhesions and reestablish a freely communicating pleural space. If the emphysema is severe, a 3-mm incision above the clavicle can serve as a popoff valve.[29]

Bleeding may be related to the presenting pathology, as in hemothorax secondary to trauma, or may be related to drain placement. Perforation of the heart or great vessels usually manifests as brisk, pulsatile bleeding and hemodynamic instability that requires emergency surgery.[37,38] Bleeding that is less brisk can be due to injury to the intercostal vessels. At times, bleeding may be mild or delayed. A case of subclavian artery injury from tube thoracostomy has been described in a young man with spontaneous pneumothorax that was only discovered days later when the tube was removed in

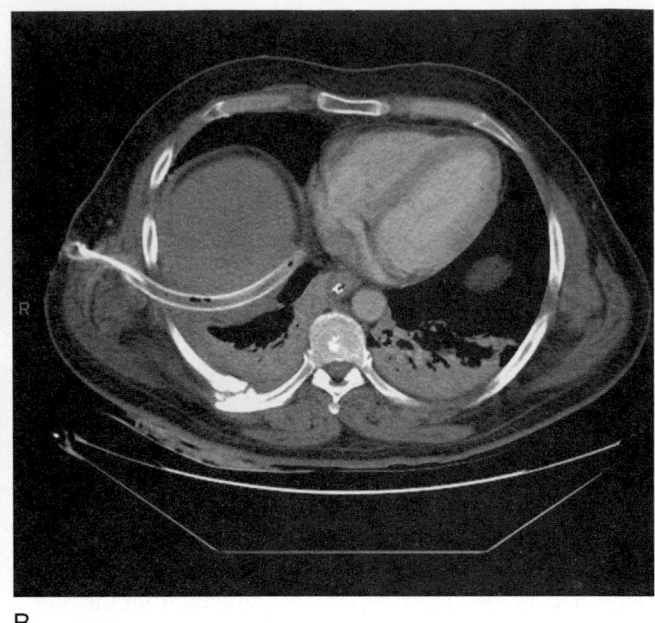

FIGURE 216–6. A, Chest radiograph demonstrating right chest tube placement below the diaphragm. **B,** Computed tomographic scan demonstrating right chest tube placement and above the dome of the liver.

the operating room at the time of a planned bullectomy.[39] Bleeding after tube thoracostomy secondary to injury to the intercostal vessels or other sources may require surgical control. Bleeding also can lead to undrained pleural fluid collections (retained hemothorax) that may require surgical evacuation (via thoracoscopy or thoracotomy) or that may become secondarily infected. Injury to the diaphragm (Fig. 216-6), liver, spleen, or stomach can also manifest as bleeding, as well as drainage of enteric contents through the tube, and has been described in cases of diaphragmatic rupture.[40]

Infectious complications associated with chest tube placement include insertion site (wound) infections and pleural space infections (empyema). Reported empyema rates vary from 1% to 11%.[14,41-43] Infections may be related to the use of poor sterile technique, the urgency in which the tube is inserted, the number of times the procedure is performed, the presence of undrained collections, or the underlying anatomic injury. Bacteria may be introduced into the pleural space from external contamination (penetrating object or the chest tube itself) or from the pulmonary parenchyma. Most often, the offending organisms are grampositive *(Staphylococcus, Streptococcus)* or anaerobic organisms.[44] The presence of undrained fluid, particularly blood, provides an excellent environment for bacterial proliferation. Many clinicians routinely recommend prophylactic antibiotics for tube thoracostomy in an effort to minimize infectious complications, but no true consensus exists regarding the use of prophylactic antibiotics for tube thoracostomy (see later).

Horner's syndrome, characterized by ipsilateral miosis, ptosis, enophthalmos, anhidrosis, and vascular dilation can result from the tip of the chest drain sitting too high in the apex, causing compression of the first thoracic (stellate) ganglion.[45] The majority of these cases will respond to removal or repositioning of the chest tube. Another unusual complication is chest wall arteriovenous malformation,

which has been reported several months after chest drain removal.[46]

Re-expansion pulmonary edema should be considered in a patient who has undergone tube thoracostomy for a large pneumothorax or effusion, has had the lung satisfactorily re-expanded, and suddenly develops dyspnea in the absence of collapse. This is a relatively uncommon complication, but in one series it was reported to occur in 5% of tube thoracostomies.[47] It can be fatal and may be more likely to occur in cases of chronic lung collapse, endobronchial obstruction, trapped lung, rapid removal of air or fluid, and use of high negative pressure for suction.[8] A chest radiograph reveals ipsilateral pulmonary edema, and therapy includes supplemental oxygen, assessment of volume status, diuresis, and possibly mechanical ventilation. Some authors suggest slow removal of large effusions, with removal of less than 1 L in the first 30 minutes, to minimize this risk.[8]

Complication rates may be related to the location in the hospital where the tube was inserted. Chan and associates retrospectively reviewed all chest tubes placed at a university-based level I trauma center over 1 year (n = 352), and they defined complications as empyema, unresolved pneumothorax, persistent effusion, or incorrect placement (Fig. 216-7).[14] The overall complication rate for chest tubes placed in the emergency department (ED) was 14%. The complication rate was 9.2% for chest tubes placed in the operating room (OR) and 25.3% for chest tubes placed on inpatient wards (IW). There was a significant difference in the complication rates for tubes placed in the ED or OR when compared with the wards. The most common complication was unresolved pneumothorax (ED, 13%; OR, 7%; and IW, 21%); malpositioning occurred in 1.1% overall (none in the ED or OR). The authors of this study did not comment on the experience level of the operators, and so it is not clear if location in this study was a surrogate for differences in technique of insertion, urgency of the procedure, or some other variable.

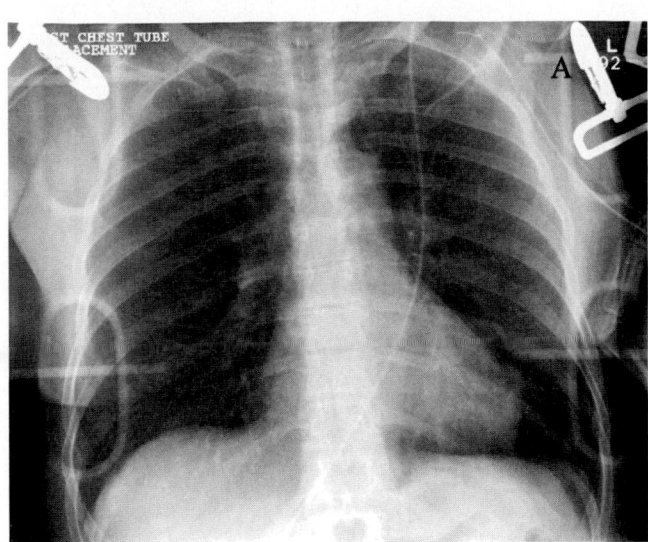

FIGURE 216–7. Chest radiograph demonstrating left chest tube placement in the subcutaneous tissues of the thorax.

PROPHYLACTIC ANTIBIOTIC USE

No clear consensus exists concerning the use of prophylactic antibiotics for tube thoracostomy, and most of the available literature deals with its use in the trauma population. Mandal and colleagues published a retrospective review of 5474 trauma patients managed with tube thoracostomy over 24 years.[42] Prophylactic antibiotics were not administered, and antibiotics were given only to patients who required emergent thoracotomy or had extensive chest wall destruction by shotgun blasts, lung contusion with hemoptysis, associated abdominal trauma requiring laparotomy, or open fractures. Empyema developed in 1.6%, and the majority (91%) were treated without thoracotomy. The authors concluded that prophylactic antibiotics are not justified because of the low incidence of empyema. Aguilar and colleagues reported a 4% incidence of empyema in a retrospective review of 584 trauma patients requiring tube thoracostomy.[44] No patients received prophylactic antibiotics for tube thoracostomy, but 7% received antibiotics at the time of chest tube insertion for other indications. These authors found that antibiotic use was not predictive of empyema development.

Nichols and coworkers performed a randomized, double-blind clinical trial of antibiotics for chest tube placement, enrolling 119 patients requiring tube thoracostomy for isolated chest trauma due to blunt (n = 6) or penetrating (n = 113) injuries.[41] Chest tube placement was performed in the ED using sterile gloves and mask, and the site was prepared using povidone-iodine scrub. Patients were administered either placebo (5% dextrose in water) or 1 g of cefonicid intravenously daily until tube removal. Empyema, pneumonia, or a combination of the above occurred in 10.7% of the placebo group and none of the antibiotic group. No significant differences were noted with respect to duration of tube thoracostomy, peak white blood cell count, peak temperature, or length of stay. However, patients with infectious complications had a longer hospitalization compared with patients without infectious problems (average

length-of-stay increase of 8 days). These investigators concluded that antibiotics significantly reduced the rate of infection.

Gonzalez and associates also completed a randomized, double-blind trial of patients with isolated chest trauma.[48] Both blunt and penetrating mechanisms were included. All tubes were placed by physicians wearing sterile gown, gloves, and mask, and the skin was prepared with povidone-iodine solution. The majority of tubes were placed in the ED. Patients were randomized to receive 1 g of cefazolin intravenously or placebo (albumin) before and every 8 hours after insertion; treatment was continued until removal of the tube. Treatment failure was defined as a thoracic complication that required additional antibiotic therapy, surgical intervention for infection, empyema requiring drainage, or pneumonia. Seven complications occurred in the antibiotic arm (one pleural effusion, two chest tube reinsertions, four additional chest tubes), but none were infectious. In the placebo group, seven complications occurred and four were infectious (two empyemas, two pneumonias). *Staphylococcus aureus* was the most common pathogen responsible, although *Streptococcus pneumoniae* and *Haemophilus influenzae* were also present. The difference was statistically significant ($P < .05$), and the authors concluded that patients who suffer isolated chest trauma and require tube thoracostomy would benefit from antibiotic prophylaxis with a first-generation cephalosporin during the insertion period. Cant and colleagues found similar results (5% infection rate in placebo, none in antibiotic arm) using cefazolin for only 24 hours.[49] Trauma patients may represent a high-risk subpopulation owing to the emergent nature of tube thoracostomy in most circumstances. It is unclear if prophylactic antibiotic use is warranted in other patient populations that may require treatment with tube thoracostomy.

ANNOTATED REFERENCES

Cerfolio RJ: Advances in thoracostomy tube management. Surg Clin North Am 2002;82:833-848.
   This excellent article summarizes several studies utilizing randomized trials or predetermined algorithms for chest tube management. It also describes a classification system for air leaks and when to use water seal versus suction, particularly as it pertains to lung resection patients.

Etoch SW, Bar-Natan MF, Miller FB, et al: Tube thoracostomy: Factors related to complications. Arch Surg 1995;130:521-526.
   This retrospective study in trauma patients highlights the potential morbidity of chest tube insertion and the association of chest tube complications with operator inexperience.

Miller KS, Sahn SA: Chest tubes: Indications, techniques, management, and complications. Chest 1987;91:258-264.
   This excellent review article describes common indications for tube thoracostomy and a safe technique for insertion, as well as common management strategies and complications.

Peek GJ, Firmin RK, Arsiwala S: Chest tube insertion in the ventilated patient. Injury 1995;26:425-426.
   This brief article stresses the importance of disconnecting patients from positive-pressure ventilation before chest tube insertion and describes cases of iatrogenic lung injury caused by tube insertion in patients on positive-pressure ventilation.

Tomlinson MA, Treasure T: Insertion of a chest drain: How to do it. Br J Hosp Med 1997;58:248-252.
   This review article also describes a safe technique for tube thoracostomy with emphasis on anatomic factors that help determine the ideal location for insertion.

Chapter 217

FIBEROPTIC BRONCHOSCOPY

Massimo Antonelli • Giuseppe Bello

KEY POINTS

1. **Fiberoptic bronchoscopy** is a highly versatile technique in diagnosis and managing various pulmonary conditions in critically ill patients.

2. **Bronchial and parenchymal samples** can be obtained at bronchoscopy by bronchoalveolar lavage (BAL), protected specimen brushing (PSB), transbronchial lung biopsy (TBLB), and transbronchial needle aspiration.

3. **The major diagnostic indications** for bronchoscopy in patients admitted to the ICU include hemoptysis, diffuse lung diseases, infections, traumatic airway injuries, acute inhalation injuries, and assessment of optimal positioning of endotracheal tube or intubation damage.

4. The fiberoptic bronchoscope can also be used for **therapeutic interventions,** such as hemostasis in patients with hemoptysis, clearance of retained secretions, removal of aspirated foreign bodies, endotracheal intubation or tube exchange, closure of bronchopleural and tracheoesophageal fistulas, and management of a large airway stenosis.

5. With appropriate care, bronchoscopy is a safe procedure. **Complications** include toxic side effects of sedatives and local anesthesia, airway problems, cardiovascular events, bleeding, pneumothorax, and bacteremia.

6. The absolute **contraindications** to bronchoscopy are the patient's refusal for the procedure and the absence of trained personnel.

7. **Skillfulness** in airway management, mechanical ventilation, and monitoring of critically ill patients is needed to perform bronchoscopy safely at the patient's bedside in the ICU.

Fiberoptic bronchoscopy (FB) is an essential tool for the management of a wide range of pulmonary disorders in critically ill patients. The bronchoscopist must have familiarity with the indications, contraindications, and potential complications of FB to complete the procedure safely and obtain clinically useful results. Knowledge about the upper and lower airway anatomy and the technical aspects of the procedure is also needed.

Since its commercial introduction in 1967,[1] flexible FB has rapidly replaced rigid FB in the diagnosis and treatment of most infectious and noninfectious diseases of the chest.[2] In contrast to rigid bronchoscopy, flexible FB is associated with fewer major complications[3] and offers enhanced visualization of the proximal airways, the upper lobes, and distal orifices.[4] Rigid bronchoscopy, however, remains the modality of choice in several situations, including massive hemoptysis, large foreign body aspiration, endoscopic laser therapy, resection of endobronchial granulation tissue, and placement of airway stents.

The areas covered in this chapter include the bronchoscopic techniques of sampling, the major indications for FB in patients admitted to the ICU, the complications and contraindications to the method, and some procedural considerations.

SAMPLING TECHNIQUES

Fiberoptic bronchoscopy provides direct access to the lower airways for sampling bronchial and parenchymal tissue. Samples are commonly obtained by bronchoalveolar lavage (BAL), protected specimen brushing (PSB), transbronchial lung biopsy (TBLB), and transbronchial needle aspiration (TBNA).

When BAL or PSB is performed, the sampling area is selected based on the location of the new or progressive infiltrate on chest radiograph or the segment visualized during FB as having purulent secretions.[5-7] Data are lacking for the optimal sampling site in patients with diffuse lung infiltrates.

BRONCHOALVEOLAR LAVAGE

Bronchoalveolar lavage allows the recovery of both cellular and noncellular components from the epithelial surface of the lower respiratory tract. The tip of the bronchoscope is wedged as far as possible into a distal airway—generally a fourth- or fifth-order bronchus—and sterile saline solution is instilled through the bronchoscope and then aspirated into a sterile trap. Aliquots of 20 to 60 mL are injected and aspirated back after each instillation. The total amount of fluid used to perform BAL ranges from 140 to 240 mL.[5-7] In the supine patient, BAL fluid recovery is best from the right middle lobe or lingula. At least 5 mL of retrieved fluid is needed for adequate microbiologic analysis.[5]

The first aliquot of aspirated fluid is likely to contain a large amount of material from the proximal airway and must be analyzed separately from the rest.[5] The recovery of more than 5% squamous epithelial cells in the BAL specimen indicates tracheobronchial proximal contamination.[2] When bronchoscopy is performed in awake patients, local anesthesia of the upper and lower airways is needed. Because lidocaine has bacteriostatic properties, use of this local anesthetic could alter microbiologic results. Nevertheless, the use of 2 mL of a 1% lidocaine solution to anesthetize a lobe before BAL is not likely to inhibit bacterial growth.[8]

PROTECTED SPECIMEN BRUSH

To obtain a lower respiratory tract specimen that is not contaminated by proximal airway organisms, PSB can be employed. This technique is performed using a retractable brush within a double-sheathed catheter device with a distal dissolvable plug occluding the outer catheter.[9] The tip of the bronchoscope is positioned close to the sampling area. The catheter is then inserted through the working channel and advanced 1 to 3 cm beyond the distal end of the bronchoscope to avoid the collection of pooled secretions around the distal tip of the instrument. The inner catheter containing the brush is advanced to eject the distal plug into a large airway, and the brush is advanced under direct vision into the desired subsegment. Once the sample is obtained, the brush is retracted into the inner catheter, which is then withdrawn into the outer sheath; and the entire unit is finally removed from the bronchoscope. The distal ends of the outer and inner catheter are sequentially wiped with alcohol, cut with sterile scissors, and discarded. The brush is then advanced beyond the remaining inner catheter, cut with sterile scissors, and placed into 1 mL of transport medium to avoid drying. The specimen is submitted for quantitative culture within 15 minutes. A small quantity of brush secretions may be smeared on a sterile glass slide for a Gram stain and to assess the cellular count.

TRANSBRONCHIAL BIOPSY

Histologic samples of bronchial mucosa, bronchial wall, lung parenchyma, and alveoli may be obtained using TBLB. In patients with diffuse or localized parenchymal disease, TBLB may be a useful and less invasive alternative to open lung biopsy.

When performed by an experienced physician, this procedure has a good diagnostic yield, causes little patient discomfort, and is associated with few complications. In diffuse lung disease, the biopsy specimen should be taken from a peripheral airway, preferably the lower lobe.[10] In this way, alveolar tissue collection is more likely and the danger of significant bleeding may be reduced, owing to the smaller caliber of the distal bronchial vessels. The number of biopsies needed for TBLB is not standardized. However, seven to eight biopsy specimens have been proposed for localized lung lesions, whereas five TBLB samples from one lung seem to ensure a high diagnostic yield for most diffuse lung diseases.[11] A combination of BAL, PSB, and TBLB is recommended in cases of endoscopically visible tumor.[12]

The major risks of TBLB are bleeding and pneumothorax.[13] Saline lavage or a 2- to 3-mL bolus of 1:10,000 epinephrine before biopsy may be used to decrease this risk.[13] When TBLB is performed to evaluate peripheral lung masses, BAL is a useful adjunct to enhance the yield for malignancy and decrease the risk of bleeding.[12] A chest radiograph should be obtained at least 1 hour after TBLB to exclude a pneumothorax.[14] The risk of pneumothorax is higher when TBLB is performed while the patient is receiving positive-pressure ventilation.[15]

Fluoroscopy appears to be unnecessary in patients with diffuse lung disease but is advisable for localized lesions.[14]

TRANSBRONCHIAL NEEDLE ASPIRATION

Tissue samples from paratracheal, hilar, and peribronchial areas may be obtained by TBNA. For visible tumors, the yield from TBNA and forceps biopsy is similar.[16]

A protected transbronchial needle is passed through the working channel of the bronchoscope and positioned with the needle perpendicular to the endobronchial wall.[17]

The tracheal wall, carina, mainstem bronchus, or major spur is pierced with a quick thrust. A suction is then applied to the proximal end of the needle sheath with a 20-mL syringe containing 2 mL of saline solution. The needle and sheath are removed from the bronchoscope and the specimen is collected into a container for cytologic analysis. If a dry syringe is used, the specimen is smeared into a glass slide before examination.[18] At each biopsy site, two or three punctures are commonly made, employing a new needle for each location.

DIAGNOSTIC INDICATIONS

HEMOPTYSIS

Fiberoptic bronchoscopy plays a central role in the evaluation of hemoptysis. The techniques help the clinician localize the specific site and identify the causes. When performed early, during bleeding, or within 48 hours after cessation of hemorrhage, the procedure has a higher likelihood of success.[19,20] Patients with massive hemoptysis (defined as more than 600 mL of blood loss in a 48-hour period[21]) should be intubated to improve gas exchange, allow suctioning, and decrease the risk of sudden cardiorespiratory arrest. If the amount of blood makes it impossible to see the airway and identification of the site of bleeding, rigid FB is the endoscopic procedure of choice.[22] Nevertheless, some clinicians advocate using FB even to evaluate patients with severe hemoptysis.[23]

DIFFUSE LUNG DISEASE

TBLB and BAL are the most common procedures used for the diagnosis of diffuse lung diseases. When diffuse pulmonary infiltrates suggest sarcoidosis or carcinomatosis, TBLB should be considered initially because this procedure has a high diagnostic yield in these disorders.[24,25] TBLB can also be a valid diagnostic tool when a diffuse infectious process is suspected.[26] In cases of idiopathic pulmonary fibrosis (IPF) or other causes of pulmonary fibrosis, TBLB sampling is usually insufficient to obtain a specific histologic diagnosis.

When inorganic pneumoconiosis or pulmonary vacuities are suspected, surgical lung biopsy is the procedure of choice, because this is the only procedure that yields an adequate amount of tissue.[11,27] BAL has a diagnostic specificity only in a few causes of interstitial lung disease, such as alveolar proteinosis,[28] but it is very useful for the diagnosis of eosinophilic pneumonia, malignancy, and several infections associated with diffuse infiltrates, including those caused by *Pneumocystis carinii, Mycobacterium tuberculosis*, various fungal species, *Legionella*, and *Nocardia*.[29-33]

A high percentage of lymphocytes or an increased CD4:CD8 ratio among cells in the BAL fluid supports the diagnosis of sarcoidosis[34,35] even though these findings lack specificity.[34,36,37]

Increased numbers of neutrophils, eosinophils, alveolar macrophages, cytokines, growth factors, and immune complexes have been noted in BAL samples from patients with IPF.[38] These findings are seen in a wide variety of fibrosing lung conditions, however, and cannot be used to establish a definitive diagnosis. Also, the clinical value of BAL to stage or monitor IPF is limited. In cases of IPF, finding a large number of lymphocytes in BAL fluid seems to be associated with a favorable prognosis and a greater responsiveness to corticosteroids.[39]

BAL fluid eosinophilia, in contrast, tends to predict a poor prognosis.[40] Data do not justify serial FB with BAL in the clinical management of patients with IPF.[41]

INFECTION

The high reliability of FB in the diagnosis of pulmonary infections has been widely demonstrated. A prompt diagnosis of ventilator-associated pneumonia (VAP), including specific identification of the bacterial pathogen, is a common challenge in the ICU. Quantitative PSB and BAL have been extensively investigated and have shown a high diagnostic yield for identifying VAP.[5,42]

Quantitative cultures of the collected specimen differentiate colonization from infection. Pneumonia is diagnosed when a quantitative culture identifies more than 10^4 colony-forming units (CFUs) of bacteria per milliliter in the BAL fluid. A value equal to or higher than 10^3 CFUs/mL in the PSB specimen is the cutoff for the diagnosis of nosocomial pneumonia.[5,43,44]

BAL provides a yield of 95% for the diagnosis of P. carinii pneumonia. TBLB has a similar diagnostic yield[45] but may cause pneumothorax; this risk is higher in individuals with human immunodeficiency virus infection.[46] BAL of several bronchial segments has been found to increase the sensitivity for P. carinii identification.[47]

Information is not clear about the best sampling technique for the diagnosis of M. tuberculosis infection. Both TBLB and BAL are effective methods to diagnose M. tuberculosis.[48] The analysis of bronchoscopic secretions or washings is also an option for detecting mycobacterial disease.[49]

Bronchoscopic sampling is commonly used for detecting fungal infections. In immunosuppressed patients, the recovery of Aspergillus or Cryptococcus is predictive of invasive disease and indicates the need for treatment.[50,51] The identification of characteristic hyphae in lavage fluid is more sensitive than fungal cultures for detecting Aspergillus.[51] Radiologic examination, analysis for the presence of Aspergillus antigen, and the polymerase chain reaction (PCR) test may enhance the rate of success.[52-54]

Legionella pneumoniae may be sought in lavage fluid by direct immunofluorescence staining and cultures.[55] PCR is a reliable method for the detection of Legionella species from BAL samples.[56]

The finding of cytomegalovirus (CMV) bronchoscopic specimens may reflect simple colonization of the lungs or pulmonary infection, depending on the clinical presentation.[57] Several methods may be used to identify CMV pneumonia, including cultures, immunofluorescent staining, analysis for intracellular inclusions, and PCR amplification of CMV DNA.[58-61] BAL also may be used for recovering herpesviruses and other pathogenic viruses, including influenza and adenovirus.[62]

TRAUMATIC AIRWAY INJURY

Flexible FB has a role for diagnosing tears and disruptions in the trachea or mainstem bronchi after major chest trauma.[63] Major airway injury should be suspected in the presence of suggestive physical and radiographic findings, such as pneumothorax, subcutaneous emphysema, lung contusion, hemothorax, mediastinal emphysema, flail chest, atelectasis, and hemoptysis. FB performed within the first 3 days of trauma to the chest and upper airway has a diagnostic yield of 53% and may reveal lesions such as tracheal or bronchial transections or lacerations, contusions, distal hemorrhage, and supraglottic lesions.[64]

ACUTE INHALATION INJURY

In acute smoke inhalation, FB examination of the upper airway may be crucial to assess the anatomic level and severity of the injury.[65] Injury to the airways should be suspected in patients who have been exposed to smoke and who have facial burns, soot in the nares or sputum, singed nasal hairs, or hoarseness.[66] Before examining the airways, an endotracheal tube may be placed over the bronchoscope to allow prophylactic intubation in case of symptoms of upper airway obstruction. Signs of severe inhalational injury include mucosal edema, redness or ulceration in the subglottic region, and deposition of carbon particles in the airways. The size of cutaneous burns and burns of the face and neck correlate well with the anatomic and physiologic abnormalities of the upper airway.[67] Before extubation, bronchoscopic examination should be performed to evaluate airway patency and resolution of injuries.

ASSESSMENT OF OPTIMAL POSITIONING OF ENDOTRACHEAL TUBE AND INTUBATION DAMAGE

Fiberoptic bronchoscopy is helpful to ensure the correct endotracheal tube position in the trachea. When a double-lumen tube is used, as in patients with massive hemoptysis or airway trauma, the correct position of the distal cuff may be checked bronchoscopically.[68]

FB is used to identify complications associated with endotracheal intubation, including tracheal damage, tube displacement, edema, or tracheomalacia. With the bronchoscope placed in the endotracheal tube, the balloon is deflated and the tube withdrawn over the instrument, allowing inspection of the subglottic, glottic, or supraglottic regions. This method is particularly helpful in the management of patients undergoing reintubation. If upper airway obstruction occurs during the procedure, the patient may be reintubated simply by readvancing the tube over the bronchoscope.

THERAPEUTIC INDICATIONS

HEMOPTYSIS

Once the bleeding site is identified, local hemostasis can be obtained by irrigating cold normal sterile saline solution.[69] If persistent bleeding occurs, the patient should be turned onto the side of the bleeding and small amounts of 1:10,000 epinephrine solution should be instilled.[14] Further therapeutic measures that can be attempted to stop the bleeding include direct application of a thrombin solution or fibrinogen-thrombin combination[70] or the use of a Fogarty balloon-tipped catheter passed through the bronchoscope into the bleeding lobar orifice.[71] Endobronchial tamponade may stop the bleeding or stabilize the patient's condition before bronchial artery embolization or emergency surgical resection.[72] Another useful technique for control of bleeding is laser photocoagulation therapy performed through the bronchoscope.[73]

RETAINED SECRETIONS AND ATELECTASIS

Fiberoptic bronchoscopy is effective for removing retained secretions and resolving atelectasis in ICU patients. Success rates are as high as 79% to 89% in the most favorable patient populations.[74-77] Patients with lobar atelectasis seem to respond better than those with subsegmental atelectasis or retained secretions.[76,77]

With the exception of obstructing central airway mucus plugs, the radiographic response to successful removal of secretions is delayed by 6 to 24 hours and follows physical examination and gas-exchange evidence of improved aeration.[78] The presence of air bronchograms on the initial chest radiograph predicts delayed resolution of atelectasis.[79] The results of FB are equivalent to those of an aggressive chest physiotherapy regimen.[79] Therapeutic FB should not be delayed in patients with acute life-threatening lobar or whole lung collapse or in those for whom less invasive measures have failed.[80] Even when FB has been successful, chest physiotherapy should be continued, to prevent new airway obstructions.

Other patients that may also benefit from bronchoscopic removal of secretions are those with neuromuscular diseases and those with head or spinal cord injuries.[81] Occasionally, direct instillation of acetylcysteine or DNase through the bronchoscope is necessary to loosen thick and tenacious secretions. Removal of mucus plugs in mechanically ventilated patients may allow weaning from mechanical ventilation.[82]

FOREIGN BODY REMOVAL

Fiberoptic bronchoscopy has an acceptable success rate for the removal of foreign bodies from the tracheobronchial tree.[83-85] The technique is performed by passing a number of extraction tools, such as forceps, wire basket, claw, or inflatable balloon catheter, through the working channel of the bronchoscope. Rigid bronchoscopy or FB may be used, depending on the skill of the operator, and the location and characteristics of the object. If the inhaled object is difficult to remove or is too large to be retrieved through the endotracheal tube, then rigid bronchoscopy should be considered.[85] In these cases, the larger internal diameter of the rigid bronchoscope improves the possibility of removal and provides better control of the airway.

Flexible FB may be helpful when foreign bodies are too distal for access with a rigid bronchoscope or if cervical abnormalities preclude the neck hyperextension. Larger foreign bodies may be retrieved by applying suction and withdrawing the entire bronchoscope with the aspirated object adhering to the tip.

ENDOTRACHEAL INTUBATION AND TUBE EXCHANGE

Fiberoptic bronchoscopy is a useful adjunct to performing endotracheal intubation in various conditions, including stiffness of the cervical spine, acute epiglottitis, trismus, and whenever a difficult intubation is suspected.[86,87] The bronchoscope may be passed transnasally or transorally through the vocal cords into the trachea. Then the endotracheal tube is slipped over the instrument. FB also may be useful for replacing an endotracheal tube in intubated patients.[88,89] Patients who are known to be difficult to intubate and those with an unstable cervical spine are good candidates for fiberoptic tube exchange. The bronchoscope is advanced into the larynx and trachea alongside the existing tube. The cuff of the tube is deflated, and the tip of the bronchoscope is placed 2 to 3 cm above the carina. The tube is retrieved, and the new tube is threaded over the bronchoscope into the trachea. The endoscope is removed and ventilation reinstituted.

BRONCHOPLEURAL AND TRACHEOESOPHAGEAL FISTULAS

In patients who cannot tolerate surgery, fiberoptic techniques are often successful in the treatment of persistent bronchopleural fistulas.[90,91] After placement of a chest tube with a water valve, FB may help the clinician detect the segmental airway responsible for the air leak. Treatment is performed by wedging the tip of the instrument within the segment tributary of the peripheral fistula. Then, a sealing material is injected through the bronchoscope to occlude the distal airway. Multiple agents have been used for this purpose, including tetracycline and doxycycline, followed by autologous blood instillation, absorbable gelatin sponge, fibrin glue, tissue adhesive, lead shot, silver nitrate, and detachable balloons.

FB also should be considered in the management of fistulas between the gastrointestinal tract and tracheobronchial tree. Definitive therapy by the bronchoscopic application of a sealing agent to occlude tracheoesophageal fistulas may be used, particularly in poor surgical candidates.[92]

LARGE AIRWAY STENOSIS

Fiberoptic bronchoscopy has an important role in laser therapy, cryotherapy, placement of airway prostheses, and balloon dilatation to relieve airway obstruction caused by malignant and benign airway lesions.[93] Endobronchial stents in central obstructive lesions may be applied to facilitate weaning from ventilation and prevent impending respiratory failure.[94] Rigid FB is commonly used for stent positioning.

COMPLICATIONS

If basic precautions are taken, FB is a safe procedure. Major complications requiring surgical intervention or resuscitative measures are significantly more likely with rigid bronchoscopy as compared with FB.[95] Flexible FB is associated with a 0.3% incidence of major complications and a mortality rate of 0.02%.[96] Both major and minor complications include periprocedural anesthetic complications, airway problems, cardiovascular events, bleeding, pneumothorax, and bacteremia.[97]

Topical anesthetics can cause problems. The major toxic side effects of topical lidocaine include seizures and cardiac suppression. The total dose of lidocaine should not exceed 8.2 mg/kg.[98] Extra caution regarding the use of lidocaine should be used in patients with hepatic or cardiac insufficiency in whom lidocaine metabolism may be impaired. However, the dose of lidocaine should always be the minimum necessary to provide adequate local anesthesia.[14]

Hypoxemia commonly occurs during FB.[99] The insertion of a bronchoscope into the airways decreases the cross-sectional area available for airflow and hence decreases tidal volume and increases the work of breathing.[100] Continuous suctioning through the instrument evacuates respiratory gases and decreases functional residual capacity, leading to the development of hypoxemia.[100] PaO_2 may decrease substantially during FB. This effect may last a few minutes to several hours after removal of the bronchoscope.[100,101]

In critically ill and mechanically ventilated patients undergoing FB, PaO_2 decreases about 26% from the baseline value.[102] Hypoxemia may be more severe after BAL owing to ventilation-perfusion abnormalities induced by instillation of saline solution.[102,103] In hypoxemic patients requiring FB and BAL, noninvasive positive-pressure ventilation via a facemask can be used to prevent deterioration of gas exchange.[104,105] Hemodynamic effects including arrhythmias and cardiac arrest may be observed during FB in 40% of patients.[106,107]

The risk of arrhythmias is greatest during the passage of the bronchoscope through the vocal cords in nonintubated patients, especially if hypoxemia is present.[107] Significant bleeding, defined as more than 50 mL of blood loss,[108] is a rare event during FB.[97] The likelihood of hemorrhage from FB increases when biopsy or brushing procedures are performed.[109] Patients at higher risk of bleeding include those with uremia, immunosuppression, pulmonary hypertension, liver disease, coagulation disorders, or thrombocytopenia.[110] Pneumothorax is very uncommon after FB but has an incidence of 14% in intubated patients having TBLB.[15]

Fever occurs rarely after FB (1.2%)[97] but occurs more commonly (10% to 30% of cases) after BAL.[111] Fever is thought to be caused by the release of proinflammatory cytokines from alveolar macrophages.[112]

There is controversy regarding the incidence of bacteremia associated with FB. In one study, the bacteremia rate was 6.5%.[113] Prophylactic antibiotics are recommended for rigid but not for flexible FB, except in patients who are asplenic, have a prosthetic valve, or have a previous history of endocarditis.[114] Patients with preexisting reactive airway disease have an increased risk for developing bronchospasm or laryngospasm.[115]

CONTRAINDICATIONS

There are only a few absolute contraindications to FB in the critically ill patient.[14,116]

Flexible FB should not be performed in the following conditions: (1) absence of consent from the patient; (2) lack of trained personnel; (3) refractory hypoxemia; (4) inability to normalize platelet count and coagulation if biopsy or PSB is needed; (5) unstable cardiac disease; and (6) uncontrolled bronchospasm.

For rigid FB, additional contraindications should be considered, including unstable cervical spine, severely ankylosed cervical spine, and restricted temporomandibular joint mobility.[14,116] The risks of FB are thought to be reduced 4 to 6 weeks after myocardial infarction.[117]

The presence of chronic obstructive pulmonary disease (COPD) increases the complication rate of FB.[118] In spontaneously breathing patients with COPD, oxygen supplementation as well as intravenous sedation should be avoided or given with extreme caution to prevent an increase in the arterial carbon dioxide level.

In patients with brain injury, FB increases intracranial pressure (ICP) by at least 50% in 88% of patients, despite the use of sedation, analgesia, paralysis, and tracheal anesthesia.[119] However, concomitant increases of mean arterial pressure tend to maintain adequate cerebral perfusion. The ICP usually returns to basal levels after the procedure.[120] Only a low risk has been described when FB is performed in the presence of an elevated ICP.[121] Although no significant neurologic complications have been noted in patients with brain injury during FB, close monitoring of cerebral pressures is recommended.

PROCEDURE

BASIC CONSIDERATIONS

Before starting FB, informed consent for the procedure should be obtained. Enteral feeding or oral food intake should be suspended 4 hours before and 2 hours after the procedure.[14] Intravenous access must be established in all patients.

Asthmatic subjects should be premedicated with a bronchodilator before the procedure. Platelet count and coagulation times should be checked before performing FB in all patients if a biopsy is anticipated but only in patients with risk factors for bleeding otherwise.

When biopsy specimens are needed, oral anticoagulants should be stopped at least 3 days before FB, or they should be reversed with low doses of vitamin K. If anticoagulants cannot be withdrawn, the International Normalized Ratio (INR) should be maintained at less than 2.5 and heparin should be started.[14] An antibiotic prophylaxis should be considered before FB in patients with splenectomy, presence of a heart valve prosthesis, or previous history of endocarditis.[114]

MONITORING

A full range of physiologic monitoring is necessary during the procedure, including electrocardiogram, pulse oximetry, and continuous intra-arterial blood pressure or intermittent cuff blood pressure measurement at least every 5 minutes. Monitoring ICP is essential in patients with serious head injury. Monitoring end-tidal PCO_2 in such patients may be useful.[120]

BRONCHOSCOPE SIZE

The choice of a bronchoscope varies according to the indication. A scope with a small caliber permits great visualization of the airways, whereas a larger instrument with a wider working channel provides better suctioning and permits the passage of larger bronchoscopic tools. The outer diameter of the bronchoscope should be at least 2 mm narrower than the lumen of the endotracheal tube to prevent excessive increases in airflow resistance and decreases in tidal volume.[100] Lubrication is essential to facilitate passage of the bronchoscope.

SEDATION AND ANALGESIA

The type and level of sedation required depends on the clinical status of the patient. Unstable hypoxic patients with ARDS and those with brain injury may require deep sedation, analgesia, or even neuromuscular blockade.[102,119] Synthetic narcotics such as alfentanil or fentanyl will suppress the cough reflex and provide analgesia. Sedation can be obtained with incremental doses of a benzodiazepine or propofol. If only light sedation is required for comfort during mechanical ventilation, supplemental topical anesthesia with lidocaine injected through the bronchoscope is advisable.[14] Great care must be given when administering anesthetics to patients with renal dysfunction, liver disorders, or congestive heart failure.

VENTILATOR SETTINGS

In patients under mechanical ventilation, the FIO_2 must be increased to 100% before FB and then maintained at this level during the procedure and in the immediate recovery period. Every effort must be made to maintain oxygen saturation above 90% during the entire procedure. It is preferable to adjust the ventilator to a mandatory setting. Positive end-expiratory pressure should be reduced.[100] The ventilator pressure limit should be increased to ensure adequate tidal volume during each respiratory cycle. The ventilator rate may be increased if necessary. Tidal volume and minute ventilation should be monitored.[14] A special swivel connector with a perforated diaphragm, through which the bronchoscope can be passed, prevents loss of the delivered respiratory gases, allowing adequate ventilation.[122]

ANNOTATED REFERENCES

Antonelli M, Cicconetti F, Vivino G, Gasparetto A: Closure of a tracheoesophageal fistula by bronchoscopic application of fibrin glue and decontamination of the oral cavity. Chest 1991;100:578-579.

A tracheoesophageal fistula may be successfully closed with a fibrin adhesive applied by means of a fiberoptic bronchoscope, instead of by esophagoscopy. The procedure is proposed as an alternative to surgery for critically ill patients.

Antonelli M, Conti G, Riccioni L, Meduri GU: Noninvasive positive-pressure ventilation via facemask during bronchoscopy with BAL in high-risk hypoxemic patients. Chest 1996;110:724-728.

Application of noninvasive positive-pressure ventilation via a facemask during fiberoptic bronchoscopy is a safe and effective alternative to intubation for maintaining adequate gas exchange in high-risk hypoxemic patients (PaO_2/FIO_2 ratio ≤ 100).

Antonelli M, Conti G, Rocco M, et al: Noninvasive positive-pressure ventilation vs. conventional oxygen supplementation in hypoxemic patients undergoing diagnostic bronchoscopy. Chest 2002;121:1149-1154.

In hypoxemic patients (PaO_2/FIO_2 ratio ≤ 200), noninvasive positive-pressure ventilation is superior to conventional oxygen supplementation in preventing gas-exchange deterioration during fiberoptic bronchoscopy with better hemodynamic tolerance.

Antonelli M, Lenti L, Bufi M, et al: Differential evaluation of bronchoalveolar lavage cells and leukotrienes in unilateral acute lung injury and ARDS patients. Intensive Care Med 1989;15:439-445.

Bronchoalveolar lavage fluid from ARDS patients shows a similar picture to that obtained from the affected lung of patients with unilateral acute lung injury in terms of cell count and levels of leukotrienes.

Antonelli M, Pennisi MA, Conti G, et al: Fiberoptic bronchoscopy during noninvasive positive-pressure ventilation delivered by helmet. Intensive Care Med 2003;29:126-129.

Noninvasive positive-pressure ventilation through the helmet allows a safe diagnostic fiberoptic bronchoscopy with BAL in patients with hypoxemic acute respiratory failure, avoiding gas exchange deterioration and endotracheal intubation.

Chapter 218

BRONCHOALVEOLAR LAVAGE AND PROTECTED SPECIMEN BRONCHIAL BRUSHING

Jean Chastre • Jean-Yves Fagon

KEY POINTS

1. **Invasive diagnostic methods,** including bronchoalveolar lavage and protected specimen bronchial brushing, could improve the identification of patients with true bacterial pneumonia and facilitate decisions whether to treat, thus affecting clinical outcome.

2. Both methods permit the **collection of distal pulmonary secretions with minimal or no upper airway contamination,** either through a fiberoptic bronchoscope or blindly, using an endobronchial catheter wedged in the tracheobronchial tree.

3. Owing to the inevitable oropharyngeal bacterial contamination that occurs during the collection of all respiratory secretion samples, quantitative culture techniques are needed to differentiate oropharyngeal contaminants present at low concentrations from higher-concentration infecting organisms.

4. Because even a few doses of a new antimicrobial agent can negate the results of microbiologic cultures, **pulmonary secretions in patients suspected of having pneumonia should always be obtained before new antibiotics are administered.**

5. Although appropriate antibiotics may improve survival in patients with bacterial pneumonia, **use of empirical broad-spectrum antibiotics in patients without infection is potentially harmful,** facilitating colonization and superinfection with multiresistant microorganisms.

6. **Bronchoalveolar lavage may also provide useful clues in the diagnosis of other forms of respiratory failure,** such as pulmonary hemorrhage or other types of infections, especially in immunocompromised patients.

The diagnosis of bacterial pneumonia in severely ill patients represents a difficult challenge for clinicians. Concern about the inaccuracy of clinical approaches to recognizing bacterial pneumonia had led numerous investigators to postulate that "invasive" diagnostic methods, including bronchoalveolar lavage (BAL) and the protected specimen brush (PSB) technique, could improve the identification of patients with true bacterial pneumonia and facilitate decisions whether to treat, thus affecting clinical outcome.[1-5] Both methods permit sampling of distal pulmonary secretions with minimal or no upper airway contamination. One approach uses a fiberoptic bronchoscope, and the other uses an endobronchial catheter wedged in the tracheobronchial tree. Both methods use quantitative culture techniques to differentiate between airway colonization and true parenchymal pulmonary infection. However, these procedures require rigorous adherence to microbiologic techniques and are not universally available; for these reasons, their use in everyday practice remains controversial.[6]

SPECIMEN TYPES AND LABORATORY METHODS

PROTECTED SPECIMEN BRUSH TECHNIQUE

The methodology for PSB sampling was originally described by Wimberley and colleagues.[7] This method combines three different techniques: a double-lumen catheter-brush system with a distal occluding plug to prevent secretions from entering the catheter during its passage through the proximal airways; a brush to calibrate the volume of secretions retrieved; and quantitative culture techniques to aid in distinguishing between airway colonization and severe underlying infection, using a cutoff point of 10^3 colony-forming units per milliliter (CFU/mL) to make this distinction. In an in vitro study, this system proved to be the most effective among seven different types tested. Catheters containing a protected brush were passed through a fiberoptic bronchoscope heavily contaminated with saliva to reach the distal sample—a Petri dish containing a known number of organisms.[7] Single-sheathed catheter brushes and telescoping plugged catheter tips with or without distal plugs are also available and have been used for the diagnosis of pneumonia, although neither has been subjected to the rigorous evaluation reported for the PSB.[8,9]

BRONCHOALVEOLAR LAVAGE

BAL requires careful wedging of the tip of the bronchoscope or of a large catheter into an airway lumen, isolating that airway from the rest of the central airway. Infusion of at least 120 mL of saline in several (three to six) aliquots is needed to sample secretions in the distal respiratory bronchioles and alveoli.[10,11] It is estimated that the alveolar surface area distal to the wedged bronchoscope or catheter is 100 times greater than that of the peripheral airway and that approximately 1 million alveoli (1% of the lung surface) are sampled and approximately 1 mL of actual lung secretions is retrieved in the total lavage fluid.[12] The fluid return on BAL varies greatly and may affect the validity of results. In patients with emphysema, collapse of airways with the negative pressure needed to aspirate fluid may limit the amount of fluid retrieved. A very small return may contain only diluted material from the bronchial rather than the alveolar level and thus give rise to false-negative results.[12]

SPECIMEN HANDLING

Regardless of the technique used, rapid processing of specimens for culture is desirable to prevent loss of viability of pathogens or overgrowth of contaminants. For PSB, it is recommended that the brush be aseptically cut into a measured volume (1 mL) of sterile diluent, usually nonbacteriostatic saline or lactated Ringer's solution.[7,11] For BAL, transport in a sterile, leakproof, nonadherent glass container is recommended to avoid loss of cells before direct cytologic assessment. The initial aliquot, which is usually considered to be representative of distal bronchi, should be either discarded or transported separately from the remaining pooled fractions. Although no absolute guideline exists, it is generally accepted that no more than 30 minutes should elapse before specimens are processed for microbiologic analysis.[10,13] According to some investigators, refrigeration may be used to prolong transport time, permitting the procedure to be performed even when the microbiology laboratory cannot immediately handle the specimens (e.g., during weekends or night shifts).[13,14]

Once specimens are received in the laboratory, they should be processed according to clearly defined procedures (see reference 13 for a complete description). Owing to the inevitable oropharyngeal bacterial contamination that occurs during the collection of all respiratory secretion samples, quantitative culture techniques are needed to differentiate infecting organisms from oropharyngeal contaminants present at low concentrations. In patients with pneumonia, pathogens are present in lower respiratory tract inflammatory secretions at concentrations of at least 10^5 to 10^6 CFU/mL, whereas contaminants are generally present at concentrations of less than 10^4 CFU/mL.[15-20] The diagnostic thresholds proposed for PSB and BAL are based on this concept. Because PSB collects between 0.001 and 0.01 mL of secretions, the presence of greater than 10^3 bacteria in the originally diluted sample (1 mL) actually represents 10^5 to 10^6 CFU/mL of pulmonary secretions. Similarly, 10^4 CFU/mL for BAL, which collects 1 mL of secretions in 10 to 100 mL of effluent, represents 10^5 to 10^6 CFU/mL.[11]

Although PSB samples can be subjected to direct microscopy, the optimal method for smear preparation has not been established. For BAL, it is recommended that a total cell count be performed to assess adequacy and a differential count be performed to assess cellularity. For quality assessment, the percentages of squamous and bronchial epithelial cells may be used to predict heavy upper respiratory contamination. Although only a few studies have directly assessed this factor, it is proposed that the sample be rejected if more than 1% of the total cells are squamous or bronchial epithelial cells.[21] Modified Giemsa staining (e.g., Diff-Quik, Scientific Products, McGraw Park, IL) is recommended, as it offers a number of advantages over Gram staining, including better visualization of host cell morphology; improved detection of bacteria, particularly intracellular bacteria; and detection of some protozoan and fungal pathogens (e.g., *Histoplasma*, *Pneumocystis*, *Toxoplasma*, and *Candida* spp.).[11,22]

BRONCHOSCOPIC VERSUS NONBRONCHOSCOPIC TECHNIQUES

FIBEROPTIC BRONCHOSCOPY

Bronchoscopy provides direct access to the lower airways for sampling bronchial and parenchymal tissues at the site of lung inflammation. To reach the bronchial tree, however, the bronchoscope must traverse the endotracheal tube and proximal airways, where contamination is likely to occur. BAL and PSB with quantitative cultures are used to control for this contamination, as discussed earlier. However, poor technique during bronchoscopy can negate the benefit of these modifications. Therefore, to obtain meaningful results with fiberoptic bronchoscopy, it is important to follow a precise methodology, as summarized in the 1994 Memphis International Consensus Conference report (Table 218-1).[10]

One major technical problem with all bronchoscopic techniques is proper selection of the sampling area in the tracheobronchial tree. Almost all intubated patients have purulent-looking secretions, and the first secretions seen may represent those aspirated from another site in gravity-dependent airways or upper airway secretions aspirated around the endotracheal tube. Usually, the sampling area is selected based on the location of the infiltrate on the chest radiograph or the segment visualized during bronchoscopy as having purulent secretions.[10] In patients with diffuse pulmonary infiltrates or minimal changes in a previously abnormal chest film, determining the correct airway to sample may be difficult. In these cases, sampling should be directed to the area where endobronchial abnormalities are maximal. However, when in doubt, and because autopsy studies indicate that pneumonia in ICU patients frequently involves the posterior portion of the right lower lobe, this area should probably be sampled as a first priority.[16,23-25] Although bilateral sampling has been advocated in immunosuppressed hosts with diffuse infiltrates, there is no convincing evidence that multiple specimens are more accurate than single specimens for diagnosing ventilator-associated pneumonia.[26]

The risk inherent in fiberoptic bronchoscopy appears to be slight, even in critically ill patients requiring mechanical

---

TABLE 218–1. PROTECTED SPECIMEN BRUSH METHODOLOGY WHEN USING BRONCHOSCOPY

In intubated patients, sedation and a short-acting paralytic agent are recommended.

Do not administer lidocaine through the suction channel of the FOB, and avoid suction of upper airway secretions.

Position the FOB close to the orifice of the bronchus, draining the segment with new or increased infiltrate as seen on the chest radiograph.

Advance the PSB catheter 3 cm out of the FOB into the desired segment, and eject the distal plug.

Advance the brush, and wedge it into a peripheral position to sample distal secretions.

Retract the brush into the inner cannula and the inner cannula into the outer cannula, and remove it from the FOB.

Separately and sequentially wipe the distal portions of the outer and inner cannulas clean with 70% alcohol, cut, and discard.

Extrude the brush and sever it into a receptacle containing 1 mL of saline or Ringer's solution.

Submit the sample for quantitative culture within 15 min.

FOB, fiberoptic bronchoscope; PSB, protected specimen brush.
Adapted from Meduri GU, Chastre J: The standardization of bronchoscopic techniques for ventilator-associated pneumonia. Chest 1992;102:557S-564S.

ventilation, although the associated occurrence of cardiac arrhythmias, hypoxemia, or bronchospasm is not unusual, even when high levels of oxygen are provided to the ventilator and gas leaks around the endoscope are minimized by a special adapter.[27-30] Careful attention to the anesthesia protocol, including administration of a short-acting neuromuscular blocking agent, and the monitoring of patients during bronchoscopy should permit rapid correction and more frequent prevention of hypoxemia in this setting and, therefore, further decrease the morbidity of this procedure. In a large study, only 5% of patients with acute respiratory distress syndrome had arterial oxygen saturation less than 90% during bronchoscopy, despite severe hypoxemia before bronchoscopy in many patients.[28]

The bleeding risk observed with the PSB technique is particularly high in patients with thrombocytopenia or coagulopathy.[10] Pneumothorax is a potential complication of PSB, although it can occur after BAL alone in mechanically ventilated patients. Although bacteremia does not appear to occur after PSB, release of the cytokine tumor necrosis factor has been documented in patients undergoing BAL.[31] Transbronchial spread of infection is also an extremely remote possibility.[10,13,31]

NONBRONCHOSCOPIC TECHNIQUES

The use of nonbronchoscopic techniques is limited to mechanically ventilated patients, because the endotracheal tube, which bypasses the proximal airways, permits easy access to the lower airways. At least 15 studies have described a variety of nonbronchoscopic techniques for sampling lower respiratory tract secretions; results were similar to those obtained using fiberoptic bronchoscopy.[32] For example, a study of 78 suspected episodes of nosocomial pneumonia in 55 patients found that a protected telescoping catheter gave results similar to those obtained with the PSB technique in 74% of cases.[8] Compared with PSB, nonbronchoscopic techniques are less invasive, can be performed by clinicians not qualified to perform bronchoscopy, have lower initial costs, avoid potential contamination by the bronchoscopic channel, are associated with less compromise of gas exchange during the procedure, and can be performed even in patients intubated with small endotracheal tubes.

Disadvantages include the potential sampling errors inherent in a blind technique and the lack of airway visualization. Although autopsy studies indicate that pneumonia in ventilator-dependent patients has often spread into every pulmonary lobe and involves predominantly the posterior portion of the lower lobes,[16,23,25,33] two clinical studies on ventilated patients with pneumonia contradict those findings, as some patients had sterile cultures of PSB specimens from the noninvolved lung.[34,35] Further, although the authors of most studies concluded that the sensitivities of nonbronchoscopic and bronchoscopic techniques were comparable, the overall concordance was only approximately 80%, emphasizing that, in some patients, the diagnosis could be missed by a blind technique, especially in the case of pneumonia involving the left lung, as demonstrated by Jorda[36] and Meduri[35] and their associates.

DIAGNOSTIC ACCURACY

PROTECTED SPECIMEN BRUSH TECHNIQUE

The potential contribution of the PSB technique to evaluate ICU patients suspected of having bacterial pneumonia has been extensively investigated in both human and animal studies, including eight investigations in which the accuracy of this culture technique was determined by comparison of both histologic features and quantitative cultures from the same area of the lung.[16,18-20,23,24,37,38] Despite the need for cautious interpretation, the results of those studies indicate that the PSB technique offers a sensitive and specific approach to identifying the microorganisms involved in pneumonia in critically ill patients and can differentiate between colonization of the upper respiratory tract and distal lung infection. Pooling the results of the 18 studies evaluating the PSB technique in a total of 795 critically ill patients shows that the overall accuracy of this technique for diagnosing pneumonia is high; sensitivity is 89% (95% confidence interval, 87% to 93%), and specificity is 94% (95% confidence interval, 92% to 97%).[39,40]

BRONCHOALVEOLAR LAVAGE

Although it provides a broader image of lung content than PSB, BAL is subject to the same risk of contamination as protected bronchial brushings. Many groups have now investigated the value of quantitative BAL culture for the diagnosis of pneumonia in ICU patients.[37,39,41] Although some investigators have concluded that BAL provides the best reflection of the lung's bacterial burden, both quantitatively and qualitatively, others have reported mixed results, with BAL fluid cultures having poor specificity for patients with high tracheobronchial colonization. When the results of the 11 studies evaluating BAL fluids from a total of 435 ICU patients suspected of having nosocomial pneumonia were pooled, the overall accuracy of this technique was found to be very close to that of PSB; the Q value was 0.84 (Q represents the intersection between the summary receiver operating characteristics [ROC] curve and a diagonal from the upper left corner to the lower right corner of the ROC space).[39] Similar conclusions were drawn in another meta-analysis when the results of 23 studies were pooled.[41] These data indicate that the sensitivity and specificity of BAL are $73 \pm 18\%$ and $82 \pm 19\%$, respectively.[41]

Because BAL harvests cells and secretions from a large area of the lung, and specimens can be microscopically examined immediately after the procedure to detect the presence or absence of intracellular or extracellular bacteria in the lower respiratory tract, it is particularly well suited to the rapid identification of patients with pneumonia. Several studies have confirmed the diagnostic value of this approach.[3,22,37,42-49] In each study, either Giemsa or Gram stain was positive (>1% of BAL cells containing intracellular bacteria) for most patients with pneumonia and negative for those without pneumonia. Further, in patients with pneumonia, the morphology and Gram staining of these bacteria were closely correlated with bacterial culture results, enabling early formulation of a specific antimicrobial therapy before the culture results became available (Fig. 218-1). However, assessment of the degree of qualitative agreement between Gram stains of BAL fluid and PSB quantitative cultures for a series of 51 patients with ventilator-associated pneumonia showed the correspondence to be complete for 51%, partial for 39%, and nonexistent for 10% of the cases.[44]

PATIENTS ALREADY RECEIVING ANTIMICROBIAL THERAPY

Prior antimicrobial treatment in patients clinically suspected of having pneumonia is frequently cited as a major limitation

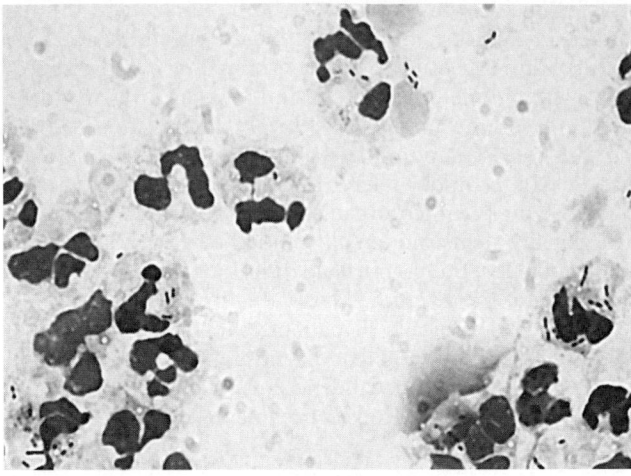

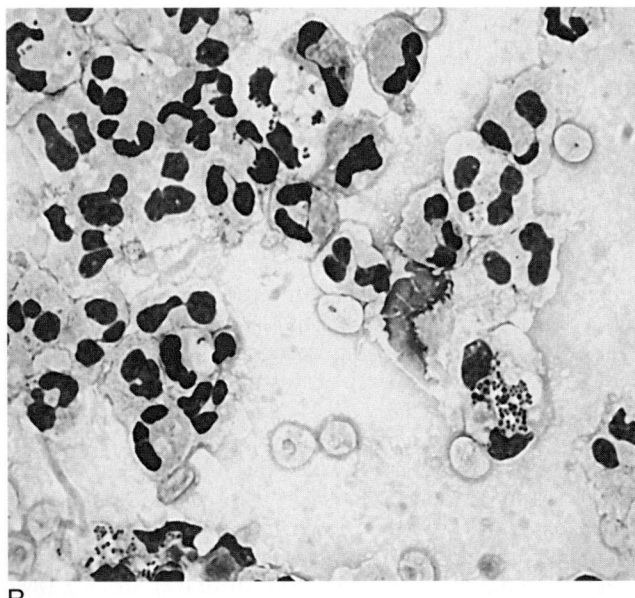

FIGURE 218–1. Light micrographs of neutrophils recovered by bronchoalveolar lavage (BAL) from a patient with pneumonia due to *Klebsiella pneumoniae (A)* and a patient with pneumonia due to *Staphylococcus aureus (B)*. In each patient, the morphology and Gram staining of extra- and intracellular bacteria closely correlated with the results of BAL bacterial cultures.

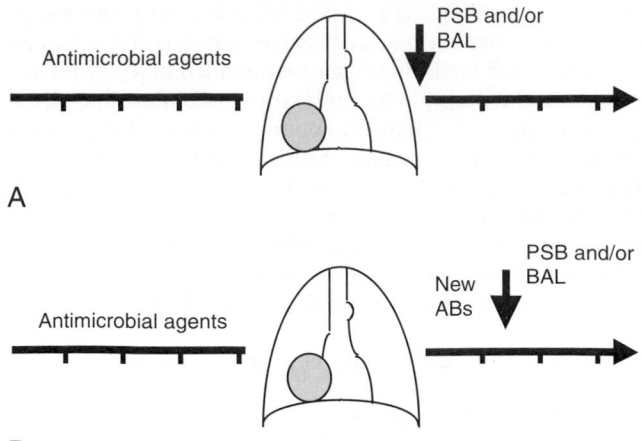

FIGURE 218–2. *A*, When pneumonia develops as a superinfection in a patient who has been receiving antimicrobial agents for several days before the appearance of new infiltrates, and protected specimen brush (PSB) techniques or bronchoalveolar lavage (BAL) is performed immediately, without any modification of the treatment, bacteria responsible for the new infection are mostly resistant to the antibiotics given previously, and culture results will not be modified. *B*, In contrast, when PSB or BAL is done after the introduction of new antimicrobial agents, bacteria responsible for the infection are frequently sensitive to the new antibiotics given, and culture results are negative in a high number of cases. AB, antibiotic; MV, mechanical ventilation.

threshold to define a positive PSB or BAL result in such a setting may be inaccurate, because follow-up cultures can be completely negative in at least 40% of true cases of bacterial pneumonia.[50,53] From a practical point of view, it should be kept in mind that a diagnostic method based on microbiologic culture techniques only documents, qualitatively and quantitatively, the bacterial burden present in the lung tissue that was sampled. In no way can these techniques retrospectively identify resolving pneumonia or determine when antimicrobial treatment and lung antibacterial defenses might have been successful in suppressing microbial growth in lung tissue.[25,33,54-56] Pulmonary secretions therefore need to be obtained before new antibiotics are administered, as is the case for all microbiologic samples.

POTENTIAL LIMITATIONS

Even when PSB and BAL are performed before any antimicrobial treatment has been given for suspected pneumonia, there are three major drawbacks to these techniques. First, even using the most accurate threshold of 10^3 to 10^4 CFU/mL to distinguish patients with airway colonization from those with deep lung infection, a small number of false-positive results may be observed.[57] Second, results of such cultures require 24 to 48 hours; therefore, no information is available to guide initial decisions concerning the appropriateness of antimicrobial therapy and which antibiotics should be prescribed. Finally, BAL and PSB can yield negative results in patients with pneumonia in the following situations: (1) fiberoptic bronchoscopy is performed at an early stage of infection, when the bacterial burden is below the concentration necessary to reach diagnostic significance; (2) specimens are obtained from an unaffected segment; (3) the specimens are processed incorrectly; and (4) the specimens are obtained after initiation of a new class of antimicrobial agents (as described earlier).

to accurate diagnosis, because it may lead to a high number of false-negative results. However, as demonstrated by several investigative teams, the results of respiratory secretion cultures are usually not modified when pneumonia develops as a superinfection in patients who have been receiving systemic antibiotics for several days before the appearance of the new pulmonary infiltrates, because the bacteria responsible for the new infection have become resistant to the antibiotics being given (Fig. 218-2*A*).[16,50,51]

Cultures of pulmonary secretions for diagnostic purposes after the initiation of new antibiotic therapy in patients suspected of having nosocomial pneumonia can clearly lead to a high number of false-negative results, regardless of the method used for sampling secretions (see Fig. 218-2*B*). In a series of 63 episodes of suspected pneumonia in patients in whom therapy had recently been initiated, the sensitivities of the invasive diagnostic methods using traditional thresholds were only 38% for BAL and 40% for PSB.[52] Using a lower

Several investigators have evaluated PSB and BAL reproducibility and concluded that, although in vitro repeatability is excellent and in vivo qualitative recovery is 100%, quantitative results are more variable.[58-60] This variability presumably reflects both the irregular distribution of organisms in secretions and the small volume actually sampled by PSB and BAL. Therefore, as with all diagnostic tests, borderline PSB and BAL quantitative culture results should be interpreted with caution, and the clinical circumstances must be considered before any therapeutic decision is made. Sampling should be repeated in persistently symptomatic patients with an initially negative ($<10^3$ to 10^4 CFU/mL) concentration.[61]

POTENTIAL ADVANTAGES

There are several potential advantages of using PSB or BAL for diagnosing bacterial lung infections in the ICU. First, obtaining distal pulmonary specimens from the suspected area in the lung using PSB or BAL helps direct the initial antibiotic therapy, in addition to confirming the actual diagnosis of bacterial pneumonia. When culture results are available, these methods allow precise identification of the offending organisms, as well as their susceptibilities to antimicrobial agents. These data are invaluable for optimal antibiotic selection and antibiotic streamlining.[62] These data also increase the confidence and comfort levels of health care workers in managing patients with suspected pneumonia.

Second, lavage can provide useful clues for the diagnosis of other forms of respiratory failure, such as pulmonary hemorrhage, or other types of infections, especially in immunocompromised patients.[13] Clearly, the absence of detectable bacteria in BAL cells and negative quantitative PSB and BAL cultures in a patient with no recent changes in antimicrobial therapy should prompt a search for alternative explanations for respiratory dysfunction and fever.[2]

Despite broad clinical experience with the PSB and BAL techniques, it remains unclear which one should be used in clinical practice. The two methods are similarly accurate. Most investigators prefer to use BAL rather than PSB to diagnose bacterial pneumonia because BAL:

1. Has a slightly higher sensitivity to identify microorganisms that can cause ventilator-associated pneumonia.
2. Enables better selection of an empirical antimicrobial treatment before culture results are available.
3. Is less dangerous for many critically ill patients.
4. Is less costly.
5. May provide useful clues for the diagnosis of other types of infections.

However, it must be acknowledged that a very small return on BAL may contain only diluted material from the bronchial rather than the alveolar level and thus give false-negative results, particularly for patients with severe chronic obstructive pulmonary disease. In these patients, the diagnostic value of BAL is greatly diminished, and the PSB technique is preferred. Therefore, the choice of procedure may depend on the preferences and experiences of individual physicians and the patient's underlying disease.

ANNOTATED REFERENCES

de Jaeger A, Litalien C, Lacroix J, et al: Protected specimen brush or bronchoalveolar lavage to diagnose bacterial nosocomial pneumonia in ventilated adults: A meta-analysis. Crit Care Med 1999;27:2548-2560.

The authors conducted a meta-analysis by using summary receiver operating characteristic curves to compare the diagnostic value of quantitative culture of respiratory secretions collected with a bronchoscopic PSB and BAL. Results clearly document that both PSB and BAL are reliable for diagnosing bacterial nosocomial pneumonia.

Fagon JY, Chastre J, Wolff M, et al: Invasive and noninvasive strategies for management of suspected ventilator-associated pneumonia: A randomized trial. Ann Intern Med 2000;132:621-630.

This prospective, randomized, open, multicenter study showed that compared with a noninvasive management strategy, an invasive management strategy based on quantitative culture results of specimens obtained by fiberoptic bronchoscopy was associated with fewer deaths at 14 days, earlier attenuation of organ dysfunction, and less antibiotic use in patients suspected of having ventilator-associated pneumonia.

Johanson WG Jr, Seidenfeld JJ, Gomez P, et al: Bacteriologic diagnosis of nosocomial pneumonia following prolonged mechanical ventilation. Am Rev Respir Dis 1988;137:259-264.

In this landmark study in which cultures of tracheal secretions, BAL, PSB, and direct lung aspirates were compared with cultures of lung homogenates and histologic findings in 35 baboons after 7 to 10 days of mechanical ventilation, the authors demonstrated that BAL provided the best reflection of the lung's bacterial burden, both quantitatively and qualitatively.

Souweine B, Veber B, Bedos JP, et al: Diagnostic accuracy of protected specimen brush and bronchoalveolar lavage in nosocomial pneumonia: Impact of previous antimicrobial treatments. Crit Care Med 1998;26:236-244.

To determine whether the diagnostic accuracy of bronchoscopic samples is affected by prior antibiotic treatment for a previous infection or by antibiotic treatment recently started to treat suspected pneumonia, 63 episodes of suspected ventilator-associated pneumonia were prospectively evaluated. Data confirmed that recently initiated treatment, even after only a few hours of activity, significantly decreases the sensitivity of PSB and BAL specimens. In contrast, current antibiotic treatment prescribed for a prior infectious disease does not modify the diagnostic accuracy of PSB or BAL.

Chapter 219

PERCUTANEOUS DILATATIONAL TRACHEOSTOMY

Daniel R. Margulies • M. Michael Shabot

KEY POINTS

1. **Percutaneous dilatational tracheostomy (PDT) offers most patients** a safe and improved alternative to open tracheostomy.

2. **PDT is usually performed in the intensive care unit** (ICU) rather than the operating room.

3. **PDT is performed by a PDT operator,** who punctures and dilates the trachea and places the tracheostomy tube; **an upper airway endoscopist,** who manages the endotracheal tube and monitors the procedure with a bronchoscope; and **an ICU nurse and a respiratory therapist.**

4. **Use of a well-defined institutional protocol is required to ensure the safety and effectiveness of the procedure.** This includes policies and procedures for conduct of the PDT procedure and privileging and proctoring for PDT operators and endoscopists.

5. **Careful selection of patients for PDT is crucial.** Patients who cannot be intubated or who otherwise require an emergency airway are better suited for cricothyrotomy. Patients with indistinct or difficult neck anatomy should receive an open tracheostomy.

6. **Because the airway is involved, speed and precision in completing the PDT procedure is crucial.** All medications and supplies must be in the room, and the PDT operator and upper airway endoscopist must be either fully trained in the procedure or proctored by fully trained physicians.

Percutaneous dilatational tracheostomy (PDT) is an elective percutaneous procedure that uses the Seldinger technique to place a temporary or permanent tracheal airway. The procedure may be performed in a hospital area appropriate for procedures requiring moderate sedation, such as an intensive care unit (ICU) or operating room. PDT is designed for nonemergency use in patients who have an endotracheal tube in place and who require long-term ventilatory support.

HISTORY OF THE PROCEDURE

Percutaneous tracheostomy (PT) was first described by Sheldon and colleagues[1] in 1955. This initial technique did not involve dilatation; instead, it involved blind and sharp instrumentation of the trachea and was associated with a high complication rate. Since that time, numerous modifications have been introduced to decrease the morbidity and mortality associated with the procedure. Ciaglia and associates[2] introduced the modern percutaneous dilatational tracheostomy (PDT) procedure in 1985. Their technique involved placement of an intratracheal guidewire and dilatation of the tracheostomy tract using the Seldinger technique. Intraoperative bronchoscopy was contributed by Marelli and associates[3] as an additional safety element. The most recent modification was the introduction of a single, tapered dilator. This eliminated the multiple dilators required in the original Ciaglia technique and markedly decreased the number of tracheal manipulations and the potential for complications. The surgical and critical care literature is replete with reports of significant morbidity and mortality from PDT.[4-10] This chapter provides the information necessary to safely initiate and maintain a PDT program.

ADMONITION

Because PDT involves manipulation and total control of the airway, the potential for misadventure is always present. In particular, the airway is unforgiving of errors in patient selection, equipment, ancillary support, operator judgment, technique, and skill. Patients requiring a tracheostomy are already seriously ill and under the best of circumstances can tolerate little more than 3 minutes without oxygen before suffering an anoxic cardiac arrest. For that reason, PDT is much more than a simple procedure. It is an ICU technique that requires written and explicitly followed policies that define which patients are appropriate for the procedure, how the procedure is to be performed, which physicians are privileged to do it, the roles they can play, the ancillary support they require, and the equipment they will use. If it is performed casually, "like any other ICU procedure," it will only be a matter of time before a serious misadventure occurs. PDT must be approached the way a military pilot approaches an aircraft carrier landing: with a combination of training, preparation, assistance, instruments, and skill that ensures a safe landing every time. Nothing can be left to chance. This chapter describes both the technique of successful PDT and the circumstances in which the procedure can safely be performed.

ADVANTAGES

Bedside PDT offers many advantages over standard open tracheostomy. PDT is generally performed in the ICU, thus eliminating the need to transport critically ill patients to the operating room. This removes the dangers associated with the transport of critically ill patients, including accidental dislodgement of numerous catheters, drains, and the endotracheal tube itself. It eliminates operating room costs and minimizes scheduling difficulties, thereby reducing delays.

INDICATIONS

The indications for PDT are the same as for open tracheostomy. Appropriate patients include those who require a temporary or long-term artificial airway for mechanical ventilation, management of secretions, and nonemergency airway obstruction. Patients appropriate for PDT already have an endotracheal tube in place, such that the PDT procedure can be performed electively in a nonemergency fashion. Patients who cannot be intubated or who require an emergency airway are better suited for cricothyrotomy or open tracheostomy.

CONTRAINDICATIONS

It is important to exclude patients who have contraindications to PDT to ensure that the procedure can be safely completed. Contraindications include the following:

- Inability to clearly palpate and identify tracheal landmarks
- Enlarged thyroid or other neck mass
- Active infection at the site
- Emergency need for airway
- Positive end-expiratory pressure (PEEP) greater than 20 cm H_2O

Relative contraindications include previous tracheostomy, previous surgical scar, bleeding, increased intracranial pressure, and clinically significant coagulopathy.

In addition, we do not perform the procedure in patients younger than 16 years of age, because of the scarcity of experience reported in pediatric patients.

THE PDT TEAM

PDT cannot be safely and routinely performed with only one or two physicians, regardless of their skill level. PDT is an ICU-team procedure, and the makeup of the team is critically important. Members of the PDT team should include the following:

- One physician with privileges as the PDT operator. The PDT operator performs the PDT procedure.
- One physician with privileges as a PDT upper airway endoscopist. The upper airway endoscopist manages the bronchoscope and, together with the respiratory therapist, manipulates and positions the endotracheal tube so that the PDT procedure can be performed. (Our institution requires that one of the two physicians present be privileged to perform open tracheostomy should that procedure be required emergently in the course of the PDT procedure.)
- The ICU registered nurse. The nurse monitors the patient's vital signs and other physiologic conditions and administers sedatives and other medications.
- The respiratory therapist. The respiratory therapist manages the ventilator and assists the upper airway endoscopist in holding the endotracheal tube during the procedure.

The requirement that one of the physician team members be privileged to perform open tracheostomy is controversial. Some centers have reported that emergency open tracheostomy is rarely required during attempted PDT and have dropped that requirement.[11] However, unless a surgeon privileged to perform open tracheostomy can be at the patient's bedside within a few seconds, death is a possible outcome, especially if the patient cannot be rapidly reintubated and ventilated. We do not recommend performing PDT without a qualified surgeon at the bedside.[12]

A variety of physicians would appear to have the training and experience and to serve as the upper airway endoscopist during PDT, including ICU intensivists, anesthesiologists, pulmonologists, otolaryngologists, and thoracic surgeons. However, the technique of positioning and maintaining the bronchoscope and endotracheal tube for the PDT procedure (described in detail later) is unlike anything in the prior experience of most anesthesiologists and pulmonary specialists. In most cases, an ICU intensivist serves as the upper airway endoscopist.

PREPARATION FOR THE PROCEDURE

EQUIPMENT REQUIRED AT BEDSIDE

Equipment required at the bedside to perform the PDT procedure includes the following:

- PDT introducer set (Ciaglia Blue Rhino Percutaneous Tracheostomy Introducer Set #C-PTIS-100-HC, Cook Critical Care, Bloomington, IN)
- Bronchoscope with video monitor display and bronchoscopy endotracheal tube adapter
- Continuous electrocardiographic (ECG) monitor
- Blood pressure monitoring device
- Pulse oximeter
- Free-flowing intravenous catheter
- Mechanical ventilator
- Suction
- Resuscitation ("crash") cart
- Open tracheostomy instrument tray (unopened)

The choice of PDT introducer set may vary by institution; ours includes the set listed only because we have significant experience with it. However, it is critical that only one type of PDT introducer set be in use in an institution at any given time. To ensure maximum safety, every aspect of this procedure must be standardized, especially the equipment used. The PDT operator and upper airway endoscopist must be completely familiar and experienced with the equipment they are using. Because of the risk of losing the airway, there is no "extra" time available during the procedure to figure out how to use unfamiliar or nonstandard equipment. A hospital can change the equipment it uses for PDT from time to time to take advantage of new technical developments or cost savings. However, changes must be done with the utmost care, including planning, experience, training, and mentoring of operators to ensure maximal patient safety during the transition.

SUPPLIES AT THE BEDSIDE

Supplies required at the bedside include the following:

- Povidone-iodine or other solution for skin preparation
- 4- × 4-inch bandages

- Syringes and needles
- Sterile gowns and gloves
- Tracheostomy tube
- Kelly clamp
- Sterile saline solution

MEDICATIONS AT THE BEDSIDE

Medications required at the bedside include the following:

- 1% Xylocaine with epinephrine 1:100,000
- Midazolam 1 mg/mL injectable or other appropriate sedative
- Morphine 10 mg injectable or other appropriate narcotic
- Vecuronium injectable or other appropriate paralyzing agent
- Sterile normal saline flush solution
- Other medications at the discretion of the PDT operator

CONDUCT OF THE PROCEDURE

As noted earlier, we use a single, tapered PDT dilator and kit with simultaneous intraoperative bronchoscopy. All the equipment and supplies listed must be present at the bedside, because there is no time to go looking for supplies if an airway emergency occurs during the procedure. Two teams are used simultaneously. One team manages the endotracheal tube, and the other manages the placement of the tracheostomy tube. The patient's physiologic parameters, including arterial oxygen saturation, are monitored continuously throughout the procedure by the ICU nurses and respiratory therapist. Intravenous sedation and paralytic agents are administered as required, and the patient is fully ventilated via an endotracheal tube.

The patient is positioned with the neck slightly extended and a pillow under the shoulders. The Blue Rhino tracheal dilator is dipped in sterile saline to enhance its lubricant coating, and the tracheostomy tube is prepared by inflating the balloon to ensure integrity and then collapsing the balloon by withdrawing all air. The PDT operator reconfirms and verifies the patient's neck anatomy, starting with palpation of the thyroid notch and cartilage, then moving down to the cricothyroid membrane and cartilage and the tracheal rings (Fig. 219-1). If the first two tracheal rings cannot be distinctly identified, the procedure is aborted and an open tracheostomy is performed. The neck is prepared with a povidone-iodine solution. The dermis and subcutaneous tissues are infiltrated with 1% lidocaine with epinephrine.

At this time, the upper airway endoscopist introduces the bronchoscope into the endotracheal tube. The endotracheal tube is untaped and withdrawn until the tip lies just below the vocal cords. Indentation of the trachea by the PDT operator with repeated light finger pressure on the anterior neck helps the bronchoscopist identify when the endotracheal tube has been pulled back far enough. The utmost care is taken to avoid withdrawing the endotracheal tube too far. It is important that a video monitor be used so that the PDT operator can see the endoscopic view. A 2-cm vertical skin incision centered between the first and second tracheal rings is made, and the midline subcutaneous tissues are dissected bluntly with a hemostat until the pretracheal fascia is exposed. The anatomy is confirmed with digital palpation of the cricoid cartilage, because it is essential that the tracheal

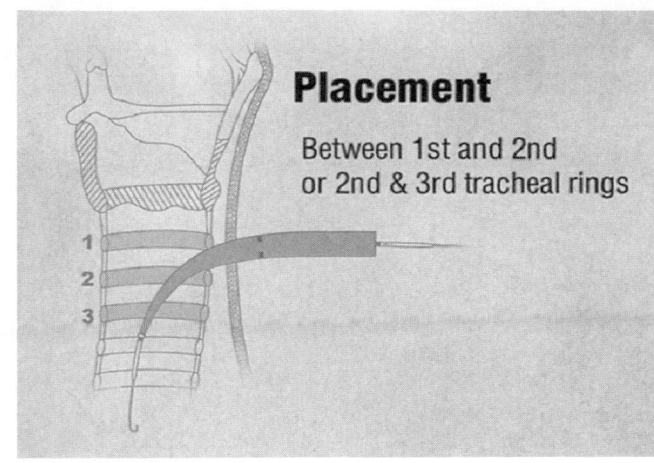

FIGURE 219–1. Essential anatomic landmarks. (From Cook Critical Care, Inc., with permission.)

puncture be made inferior to this landmark. Once again, bronchoscopic visualization of the indentation on the anterior trachea by the PDT operator is essential in determining proper placement of the endotracheal tube for the next step of the procedure.

The PDT operator reconfirms the tracheal anatomy by direct palpation through the incision. The trachea is then punctured between the first and second tracheal rings with a 14-gauge cannula-over-needle from the PDT kit (Fig. 219-2). Tracheal penetration is confirmed by visualization with the bronchoscope as well as aspiration of air from the needle. We recommend that the bronchoscope remain near the tip of the endotracheal tube, but entirely within it, to visualize the trachea through the end and sides of the tube, while protecting the bronchoscope from damage by the puncture needle. A J-tip guidewire is then introduced into the trachea through the cannula and visualized with the bronchoscope. The puncture cannula is then withdrawn, and a stiffer guide cannula is inserted over the guidewire into the trachea. Both the guide cannula and the guidewire are left in place for subsequent dilatation. A small dilator is introduced over the cannula and guidewire to widen the tracheal opening. It is withdrawn, and the lubricated Blue Rhino

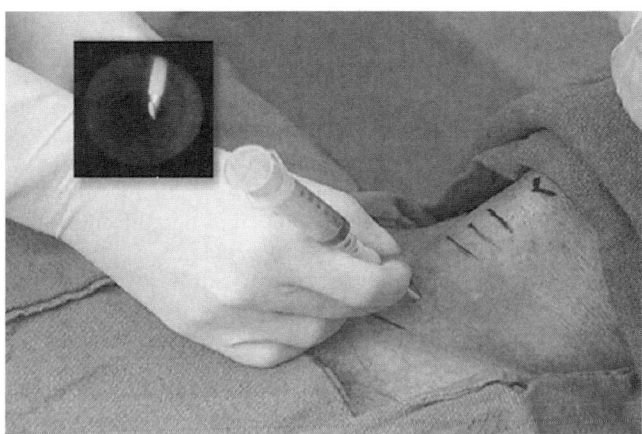

FIGURE 219–2. Tracheal puncture with 14-gauge cannula-over-needle (inset: bronchoscope view). (From Cook Critical Care, Inc., with permission.)

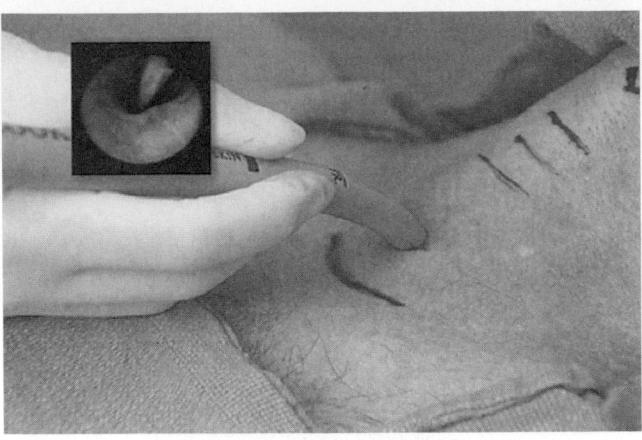

FIGURE 219–3. Insertion of Blue Rhino dilator over the guide cannula (inset: bronchoscope view). (From Cook Critical Care, Inc., with permission.)

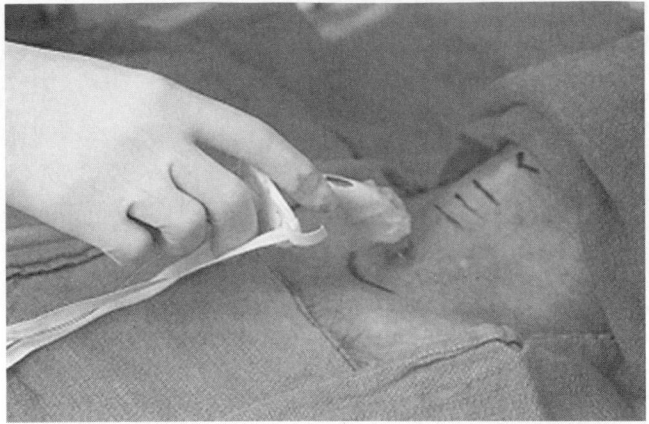

FIGURE 219–4. Insertion of tracheostomy tube over an introducer dilator threaded over the guide cannula. (From Cook Critical Care, Inc., with permission.)

tracheal dilator is then passed over the cannula and guidewire and into the trachea to fully dilate the tract (Fig. 219-3). This requires forceful pressure to accomplish smoothly. The tracheal dilator is then withdrawn, but the guide cannula and guidewire remain in place. The tracheostomy tube is placed onto an introducer dilator, which is then threaded over the guide cannula and guidewire and inserted into the trachea as one (Fig. 219-4). The introducer, guide cannula, and guidewire are then withdrawn, leaving the tracheostomy tube in place. The tracheostomy tube is sutured to the neck with 0-gauge nylon sutures and is also secured around the neck with umbilical tape.

POSTPROCEDURE CARE

A simple 4- × 4-inch gauze dressing is partially slit and placed between the tracheostomy wings and the skin. A chest radiograph is optional, and we do not routinely obtain one. Close observation by the nursing staff is required to detect bleeding externally at the tracheostomy site or internally into the airway. Bleeding must be immediately reported to the PDT operator and ICU physician and must be carefully evaluated and controlled. Bleeding into the airway can lead to formation of an obstructing clot at the carina, with fatal consequences.

Patients with coagulopathy are at higher risk for bleeding after the procedure, either externally from around the stoma or internally into the airway. For such patients, some may prefer to perform the tracheostomy under direct vision, with an open technique. However, we have found that there is a favorable tamponade effect of the dilatational technique used in the percutaneous method. To maximize the benefits of the procedure in the coagulopathic patient, minimal blunt dissection must be used; in this manner, the end result is that the tracheostomy tube compresses the surrounding tissues, controlling local hemorrhage. Similarly, the physician must be careful to perform only one pass with the needle, so that this effect is maximized.

REPORTED COMPLICATIONS

A number of reports have claimed that PDT is a safe procedure with morbidity and mortality rates equivalent to or lower than those of open tracheostomy.[4-6,13] Numerous studies have reported the morbidity of PDT to be between 3% and 19%, compared with a complication rate of 26% to 63% for open tracheostomy.[7,14] Most complications of PDT are minor. They include bleeding that does not require transfusion or operative repair, subcutaneous emphysema, extratracheal cannulation, brief episodes of hypoxia, and stomal infections. Major complications have been reported, including loss of airway, conversion to open tracheostomy, and death.[8] Complication rates have decreased as providers have gained experience with the procedure.

One complication of PDT is bleeding. Bleeding from PDT appears to be comparable to or lower than it is in open tracheostomy. In a study comparing 94 PDT procedures with 252 open tracheostomies, one patient receiving PDT required operative revision (1.1%), compared with four patients (1.6%) undergoing the open procedure.[14] Fewer bleeding problems have been reported since introduction of the single-dilator technique. Tracheoarterial fistula has not been observed with PT; it may be that placement of the tracheostomy above the third tracheal ring reduces the risk of fistula formation.

Stomal infection occurs in approximately 1% of cases. Stomal infections are usually treated with local wound care and antibiotics. A skin incision that is excessively tight or constricting around the tracheostomy tube increases the incidence of infection. It appears that stomal infection rates are also lower in the PT than in open cases, possibly because of the smaller incisions used. Perioperative mortality is low with PDT and is less that 1% in most series. Loss of airway has been reported as a cause of mortality in early series.

Several unique features of PDT may contribute to the lower morbidity reported in these studies. First, the small incision and the relatively atraumatic dilatation expose a small area of soft tissue and few blood vessels. This factor may be responsible for lower rates of bleeding and infection with PDT. The snug fit of the tracheostomy tube along the tract may also tamponade potential postoperative bleeding sites. In contrast to open tracheostomy, PDT can be safely performed in the ICU without electrocautery.[16,18-20] Several authors have reported that PDT can be readily performed with a low complication rate in the monitored ICU setting.[10,15,21] This eliminates the need to transport patients to an operating room for tracheostomy.

In summary, PDT offers most patients a safe and improved alternative to open tracheostomy. Using a well-defined institutional protocol with policies and procedures that cover privileging and proctoring, PDT can be safely performed in ICUs for carefully selected patients.

ANNOTATED BIBLIOGRAPHY

Ciaglia P, Firsching R, Syniec C: Elective percutaneous dilatational tracheostomy: A new simple bedside procedure. Preliminary report. Chest 1985;87:715-719.
This is the first report of a new technique of inserting a tracheostomy tube using the Seldinger technique with a tracheal puncture and tapered dilators over a J-wire and guide cannula.

Fernandez L, Norwood S, Roettger R, et al: Bedside percutaneous tracheostomy with bronchoscopic guidance in critically ill patients. Arch Surg 1996;131:129-132.
This study reported the clinical and financial results of 162 PDT procedures performed with bronchoscopic guidance. Complications including mortality were similar to open tracheostomy, but PDT was performed at a significantly lower cost.

Khalili TM, Koss W, Margulies DR, et al: Percutaneous dilatational tracheostomy is as safe as open tracheostomy. Am Surg 2002; 68:92-94.
This study compared complications and survival in 346 patients undergoing either PDT or open tracheostomy at a single institution over a 16-month period. There were no significant differences in complications or survival.

Marelli D, Paul A, Manolidis S, et al: Endoscopic guided percutaneous tracheostomy: Early results of a consecutive trial. J Trauma 1990;30:433-435.
This report added bronchoscopic guidance to the PDT procedure. Endoscopic visualization of the tracheal puncture, guidewire, and tracheal dilators was believed to increase the safety of the procedure.

Suh, RH, Margulies DR, Hopp ML, et al: Percutaneous dilational tracheostomy: Still a surgical procedure. Am Surg 1999;65:982-986.
This prospective study showed that a program to perform PDT in ICUs can be safely implemented with good clinical results.

Chapter 220

BALLOON TAMPONADE

Howard R. Doyle

KEY POINTS

1. **Balloon tamponade is a temporizing measure**, used when endoscopic management has failed or in the case of bleeding fundal varices.

2. **Balloon tamponade has significant morbidity and mortality** and should be performed by experienced operators (or under their close supervision).

3. **Endotracheal intubation** should always precede placement of a balloon tube.

4. **Radiographic confirmation of correct tube placement** should always precede full inflation of the gastric balloon.

Variceal hemorrhage complicates up to 30% of cases of portal hypertension; more than 80% of patients with cirrhosis and gastrointestinal bleeding prove to be bleeding from varices.[1] Although less than 50% of these patients are still bleeding by the time of the initial endoscopy,[2] variceal sclerosis fails to effect immediate control of bleeding in 15% of cases, and pharmacologic therapy alone fails in 17%.[3] Rebleeding rates are close to 22%.[3] In practice, most patients are treated with a combination of pharmacologic and endoscopic interventions, an approach that substantially lowers the risk of rebleeding.[4] This approach still leaves a small but problematic group of patients who fail therapy and require other measures to obtain temporary control of the bleeding while alternative therapeutic options are considered. Balloon tamponade can be lifesaving in these difficult situations.

The idea of using balloon tamponade to achieve hemostasis in cases of variceal hemorrhage dates back to 1930, when Westphal reported the successful use of a Gottstein dilator in two patients with bleeding esophageal varices.[5] Balloon tamponade was maintained for 24 and 29 hours, respectively, and both patients survived the bleeding episode. Seventeen years later, Rowntree and colleagues used a modified Miller-Abbott tube (with all the perforations occluded, except for the distal three, and a latex bag attached to the distal end) to stop exsanguinating hemorrhage in a patient with alcoholic cirrhosis.[6] The tube was removed 4 days later, having achieved temporary control of the bleeding (the patient rebled 2 months later, necessitating a second round of balloon tamponade). Interestingly, three of the authors later tested versions of their makeshift apparatus on themselves, but these observations were never published.

The following year, Tocantins published a paper reporting the successful management of profuse bleeding from esophageal varices using a modified Miller-Abbott tube.[7] In contrast to the approach in the previously reported cases—inflation of a balloon in the distal esophagus to exert direct pressure on the esophageal varices—Tocantins inflated a balloon in the stomach and then pulled the tube against the cardia to exert pressure on the gastroesophageal junction. Shortly thereafter, separate case reports described the successful use of balloon tamponade using direct pressure on either the distal esophagus[8] or the gastroesophageal junction.[9] The idea of using gastroesophageal junction tamponade to control bleeding esophageal varices was further advanced by Linton, who used it as part of a two-stage approach to variceal hemorrhage (balloon tamponade followed by transthoracic ligation of the varices),[10] and later Nachlas, who emphasized use of the tube to establish the source of bleeding in relation to the diaphragm.[11]

The single-balloon approach, however, had shortcomings. Maintaining the correct position when attempting to provide direct tamponade of esophageal varices was, at best, problematic,[12] and applying pressure on the gastroesophageal junction was not always successful at stopping the bleeding.[11] To overcome these problems, Patton and Johnston modified a double-lumen intestinal tube by attaching to it a distal (spherical) rubber balloon and, immediately proximal to this balloon, a second balloon fashioned from a condom.[12] After the tube was inserted, the distal balloon was inflated in the stomach, and the tube was pulled back until it engaged the gastroesophageal junction, thus ensuring correct placement of the second balloon. The following year, Sengstaken and Blakemore described what would become their eponymous double-balloon tube, made of rubber and fitted with two latex balloons (the distal portion of the esophageal balloon was reinforced, to prevent prolapse into the stomach after inflation).[13] The report was a distillation of their experience with 30 patients over the course of several years (including one hardy individual who had the tube in place for 7 weeks before being discharged alive from the hospital).

A final improvement to the double-balloon tube was described in 1968 by Edlich and colleagues from the University of Minnesota.[14] To decrease the incidence of aspiration pneumonia, the Minnesota tube had an esophageal suction port added to aspirate blood and other secretions that tend to collect proximal to the esophageal balloon. The capacity of the gastric balloon was also increased significantly to 500 to 700 mL,[14] making it more effective in the presence of gastric varices than the Sengstaken-Blakemore tube, whose gastric balloon has a capacity of only 150 to 200 mL.[13] Figure 220-1 shows the "anatomy" of the Minnesota tube.

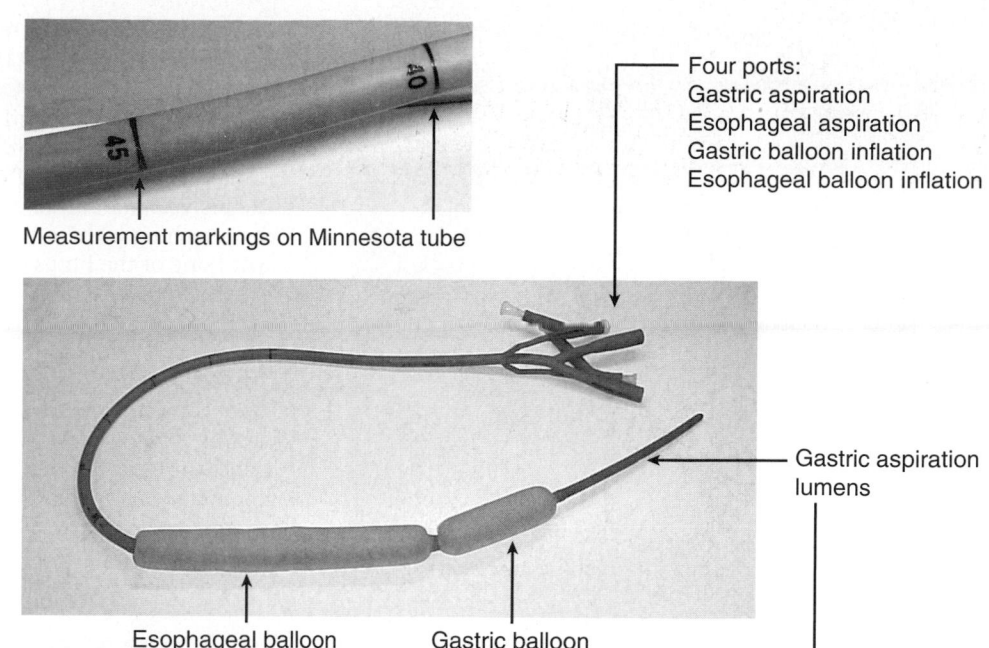

FIGURE 220–1. Anatomy of the Minnesota tube.

Four ports:
Gastric aspiration
Esophageal aspiration
Gastric balloon inflation
Esophageal balloon inflation

Measurement markings on Minnesota tube

Gastric aspiration lumens

Esophageal balloon

Gastric balloon

INDICATIONS AND RESULTS

Balloon tamponade is a temporizing measure. Its use is limited mostly to cases in which sclerotherapy or banding has been unsuccessful or is not feasible, such as when the bleeding is from fundal varices. Balloon tamponade is also used when a transjugular intrahepatic portosystemic shunt has failed to control hemorrhage. Balloon tamponade may make it possible to transfer a patient who is bleeding profusely when the treating institution does not have the resources to manage the case.

The effectiveness of balloon tamponade in securing hemostasis after endoscopic measures have failed is not known, nor is it likely to be determined in the foreseeable future, given the increasing rarity of its use. The available literature on the use of balloon tamponade for primary hemostasis reports success rates from as low as 40%[15] to as high as 100%.[16]

Chojkier and Conn reported the lowest success rate (40%) in obtaining primary hemostasis (defined as control of hemorrhage for at least 24 consecutive hours) in patients with bleeding varices.[15] These poor results can be explained, at least in part, by the fact that the site of hemorrhage (esophageal versus gastric) did not determine the choice of tube (Sengstaken-Blakemore or Linton), the procedures were carried out by junior house officers with varying degrees of supervision, and the source of bleeding was confirmed in only 20% of cases.[15] At the other end of the spectrum is the study of Terblanche and coworkers, who reported a 100% success rate in the initial control of variceal bleeding by means of balloon tamponade.[16] These authors obtained endoscopic confirmation of the bleeding site in every patient, and the Sengstaken-Blakemore tube was placed using a predefined protocol.[16,17] Most studies report that primary hemostasis can be achieved in about 90% of cases.[18-32]

Balloon tamponade can be associated with severe morbidity and mortality, a fact recognized soon after its use became widespread.[33] Early reports of aspiration pneumonia[14,33] and airway obstruction (sometimes fatal)[33,34] led to a universal policy of protecting the airway by means of endotracheal intubation in all patients needing balloon tamponade.[14] Since the adoption of mandatory endotracheal intubation, esophageal perforation is now the most dreaded complication of this procedure, being uniformly fatal in this patient population.[35-37] The likelihood of encountering this catastrophe can be minimized by never inflating the gastric balloon without first obtaining radiographic confirmation of proper tube placement.

PROCEDURE

Attention to detail is paramount to prevent the severe morbidity that can accompany placement of a Minnesota tube.

1. Balloon tamponade should never be attempted with an unprotected airway. If this has not been achieved already, the first step should be endotracheal intubation.
2. After testing and completely deflating the balloons, the lubricated tube is passed transnasally to the level of the aspiration-inflation ports. If the transnasal route cannot be used, transoral insertion is also acceptable.
3. Inflate the gastric balloon with 30 to 50 mL of air, and obtain a chest radiograph to ascertain that the balloon is below the diaphragm. Once correct positioning has been confirmed, finish inflating the gastric balloon to its

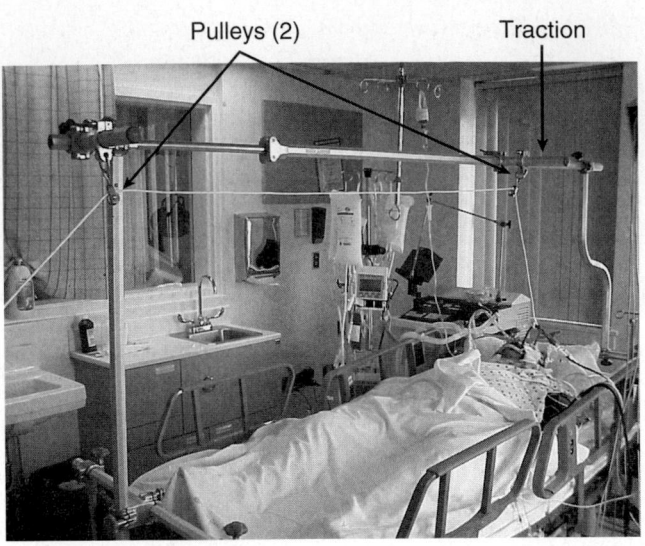

Pulleys (2)   Traction

FIGURE 220–2. Two-pulley and overhead frame for applying traction during placement of a Minnesota tube.

desired final volume. Resist the urge to fully inflate the gastric balloon before radiographic confirmation of proper placement has been obtained (omitting the chest film can be quite tempting when one is managing a patient who is bleeding profusely).

4. Pull the tube back slowly, until resistance is met. Traction can then be applied in a number of ways: with an overhead frame-pulley system, by securely taping the tube to the nose, or, more creatively, by fitting the patient with a football helmet[28] or a catcher's mask.[38] Although the last method may be a good way of maintaining traction while transporting the patient, my preference is to use an overhead frame and two pulleys (Fig. 220-2). The recommended traction weight varies widely; my practice is to use 1 kg. A 1-kg force can be exerted quite conveniently by attaching to the pulley a 1-L bag of any readily available crystalloid solution. The first pulley should be placed at such a distance that the tube makes a relatively acute angle in relation to the face, so as to not put pressure on the nose.

5. Connect the gastric and esophageal suction ports, separately, to suction, and monitor the output. If blood continues to come out of the esophageal port, inflate the esophageal balloon to 25 to 35 mm Hg (this is best done by attaching a three-way stopcock to the inflation port, with one of the limbs connected to a transducer for continuous pressure monitoring).

How long balloon tamponade can be maintained is an open question. Definitive steps to control the bleeding should be taken as soon as the patient has been adequately resuscitated—ideally, within 24 to 48 hours. To discontinue balloon tamponade, the steps are reversed. First, deflate the esophageal balloon, keeping the gastric balloon on traction. If bleeding does not resume, one can proceed to discontinue the traction while keeping the gastric balloon fully inflated. Finally, the gastric balloon is deflated, and the tube is removed.

ACKNOWLEDGMENTS

The author thanks Ake Grenvik, MD, for translating reference 5 from the original German, and William Schwer, RN, for providing the illustrations.

ANNOTATED REFERENCES

Sengstaken R, Blakemore A: Balloon tamponade for the control of hemorrhage from esophageal varices. Ann Surg 1950;131:781-789.
For the historically inclined, this is a readable account of Sengstaken and Blakemore's initial description of the device that bears their name.

Terblanche J, Yakoob HI, Bornman PC, et al: A five-year prospective evaluation of tamponade and sclerotherapy. Ann Surg 1981;194:521-530.
This is a detailed description of the use of balloon tamponade followed by sclerotherapy in 66 patients having 137 separate bleeding episodes. Like most papers about this topic, the approach described has been rendered obsolete by current management, which emphasizes initial endoscopic intervention. However, it provides a good account of the efficacy and safety of balloon tamponade in experienced hands.

Chapter 221

PLACEMENT OF FEEDING TUBES

Eric L. Marderstein • Juan B. Ochoa

KEY POINTS

1. Enteral feeding is generally superior to intravenous total parenteral nutrition, and delivery of nutrition directly to the intestine should be pursued whenever feasible.

2. A plan to provide patients with nutrition is a required part of daily ICU rounds and an important aspect of intraoperative decision-making.

3. Proper evaluation of the patient prior to attempting tube placement is essential to prevent complications. This evaluation should include assessment for any abnormalities of the head and neck anatomy or abnormal laboratory parameters, especially coagulation studies.

4. Having expert supervision at the bedside while learning how to place feeding tubes ensures that the proper technique is mastered and increases the likelihood that the procedure will be successful.

5. Recognizing the tactile feedback from encountering the various anatomic landmarks during placement is important to success.

6. In difficult cases, direct laryngoscopy, fluoroscopy, or endoscopy can be helpful adjuncts to assist with feeding tube placement.

7. Feeding tube placement can result in life-threatening complications such as epistaxis or tension pneumothorax. The presence of an endotracheal tube or a tracheostomy does not protect against feeding tube passage into the airway.

8. Taking a chest radiograph after 35 cm tube passage to verify intraesophageal tube position is a safety measure that has been shown to decrease the incidence of procedure-related pneumothorax.

9. Ideally, patients should be fed into the small bowel, but each patient requires an individual assessment as to risk of aspiration from intragastric feedings.

BENEFITS OF ENTERAL ACCESS VERSUS TOTAL PARENTERAL NUTRITION

Malnutrition in hospitalized patients is associated with an increased risk of complications, prolonged need for mechanical ventilation, and increased chance of mortality.[1]

Although total parenteral nutrition (TPN) can provide nutritional support for selected malnourished critically ill patients, enteral nutrition is considered to be superior. TPN carries the risk of the procedure required for central venous access, and it has been hard to show that using TPN decreases the rate of mortality or the incidence of major complications in critically ill patients.[2]

When compared with TPN, enteral nutrition is more physiologic and less invasive. In addition, enteral nutrition provides trophic support to maintain normal intestinal barrier function.[3] Even in patients with conditions such as pancreatitis or trauma that were formally regarded as contraindications to the use of enteral nutrition, use of the gut for feeding has been shown to result in a better outcome than is achieved by using TPN.[4][5] Additionally, early (as compared to delayed) institution of enteral nutrition in critically ill patients is associated with a decreased incidence of infectious complications, a shorter length of hospital stay, and a trend toward decreased mortality.[6]

INDICATIONS FOR A FEEDING TUBE

A plan to provide critically ill patients with nutrition must be a part of daily routine care in the intensive care unit. Memory aids for the care team in the form of signs, clipboard checklists, or other devices can be helpful to ensure that this consideration is not forgotten.

Adequate fluid resuscitation with stabilization of vital signs and normalization of the base deficit improve the likelihood of success of enteral feeding.[7] Starting or escalating the dose of vasopressors in a previously stable patient are relative contraindications to enteral feeding.[8] During a laparotomy, consideration should be given to access for enteral nutrition and placement of a nasoenteric feeding tube carried out while the patient is still in the operating room. The tube can be placed while the patient is under anesthesia, and its positioning facilitated and confirmed while the abdomen is open.

HISTORICAL PERSPECTIVE AND DESIGN OF STANDARD TUBE

Large-bore nasogastric tubes were first used for feeding with a blenderized house diet that was difficult to administer. In 1976, Dobbie and Hoffmeister published their landmark article describing the use of the Dobhoff narrow-bore polyurethane tube with a metal weighted tip to aid passage into the small bowel.[9] Initially, mercury was utilized as the metal, but tungsten was ultimately deemed safer. Additional innovations included continuous pump delivery of the tube-feeding formula and creation of specialized nutritional formulations. In 1980, Brooks and Dixon reported the use of a metal guidewire to stiffen the tube and facilitate passage.[10] Currently, a wide variety of tubes are available in various diameters and lengths. Newer tubes with design modifications such as "wings" at the tip to facilitate spontaneous advancement through the bowel are now appearing in hospitals.

Generally, tubes range from 5 French (FR) to 14 FR in caliber and from 56 cm to 170 cm in length. Some tubes have ruled markings noting distance inscribed on the catheter. Polyurethane is the most commonly used material, but other plastics, such as polyvinyl chloride, are also used. Most, but not all, tubes are weighted at the tip. Many are self-lubricating at the tip and include a metal guidewire to simplify passage. Radiopaque markings combined with the metal tip and guidewire facilitate identification of the location of the tube (and its tip) under fluoroscopy or on plain radiographs. Many tubes include a second port that can be used for flushing the device to help manage clogging of the tube.

EVALUATION OF THE PATIENT

Evaluation of the patient who is to receive a nasoenteric feeding tube must be focused and complete. The anatomy of the patient is checked to identify factors that will affect the ease of placement. It is important to note whether other tubes, such as a nasogastric tube or an endotracheal tube, are present in the nose or mouth. Despite the presence of balloons designed to protect the airway, endotracheal tubes and tracheostomy tubes increase the risk of intrabronchial placement of feeding tubes, because the newly introduced feeding tube tends to follow the path of the other intrapharyngeal tubes.[11] Surgical fusion of the neck, the presence of a cervical collar, and masses of the neck make placement more difficult. Fracture of the cribriform plate creates the possibility for placement of a nasal tube into the cranium. Esophageal diseases such as varices, cancer, stricture, or diverticulum must be noted, because these conditions can make passage of a feeding more difficult and increase the likelihood of iatrogenic complications.

Alterations of the function and rearrangements of the anatomy of the gastrointestinal tract are important as well. Mechanical bowel obstruction is an absolute contraindication to placement of a feeding tube.

It is reasonable to check the patient's coagulation profile and platelet count. Coagulopathy is not an absolute contraindication to feeding tube placement, but even transient correction of abnormal clotting parameters may increase the safety of the procedure. At the very least, identification of coagulopathy allows the clinician to proceed with caution so that problematic bleeding, especially epistaxis, is not precipitated by tube placement.

A discussion with the patient, or a surrogate if the patient is not able to comprehend, should precede the procedure. The discussion should include the indications for the procedure and its desired benefits, a narrative description of the method of placement, possible complications (listed elsewhere in the chapter), and therapeutic alternatives. The patient or surrogate should be given the opportunity to ask questions and consent to the procedure in the presence of a witness.

PREPARATION FOR AND PERFORMANCE OF THE PROCEDURE

Ideally, didactic instruction followed by simulator repetitions would be optimal training for this procedure. Knowledge of the anatomy of the oropharynx, larynx, esophagus, stomach, and small bowel are important in comprehending the pitfalls that can affect successful feeding tube placement. As with any procedure, it is critical to assemble materials in advance and have expert supervision during the learning stages of a procedure. Often an expert can convey small modifications that are vital to the success of the procedure that are not appreciated by the novice. An expert also has the experience to safely troubleshoot and complete a procedure that a novice might deem unsuccessful. Worse yet, a novice may make adjustments that unknowingly are dangerous in an effort to "get the job done." Regarding this procedure in particular, one study demonstrated that successful tube placement correlates with level of training, a surrogate for experience.[12]

Once the materials are assembled (Table 221-1), don a pair of gloves, gown with long sleeves, and eye protection. Next, position the patient optimally. The seated position is ideal, but even elevating the head of the bed to 30 to 40 degrees is helpful. To facilitate passage through the pylorus, having the patient in the right lateral decubitus position can be helpful. Stand on the right side of the patient with the left hand grasping the lower portion of the feeding tube and the right hand grasping the feeding tube roughly 10 cm from the tip. It is not necessary to use lubricant for the tip because of the narrow caliber of most tubes, but some clinicians prefer to do so. Introduce the tip of the feeding tube into the nostril. Sometimes it is helpful to take a short pause at that point to allow the patient to become used to the sensation of the tube in the nose. Lidocaine jelly may be helpful in decreasing discomfort and increasing patient cooperation.

Gradually advance the tube. The next tactile feedback you will get is when the tube encounters the back of the throat. A gentle push here is often enough to allow the tube to begin to move caudad toward the upper esophageal sphincter. Having the patient flex at the neck voluntarily or having an assistant flex the patient's neck can be helpful at this point in the procedure. It is important that coughing be minimized as much as possible until the tube has passed into the esophagus. Coughing tends to expel the tube.

Once the tube is pointed caudad, it can be advanced several more centimeters before the larynx is encountered. Experience plays a role here, as the location of the larynx becomes anticipated better with repetition. Ideally, the patient will swallow at this point, but some patients do not cooperate. The epiglottis blocks the entrance to the trachea during swallowing and prevents misplacement of the feeding

TABLE 221–1. MATERIALS REQUIRED FOR FEEDING TUBE PLACEMENT
Feeding tube
10-mL syringe
Tape
Sterile water
Stethoscope
Lubricant
Latex gloves (or alternative in case of latex allergy)
Eye protection

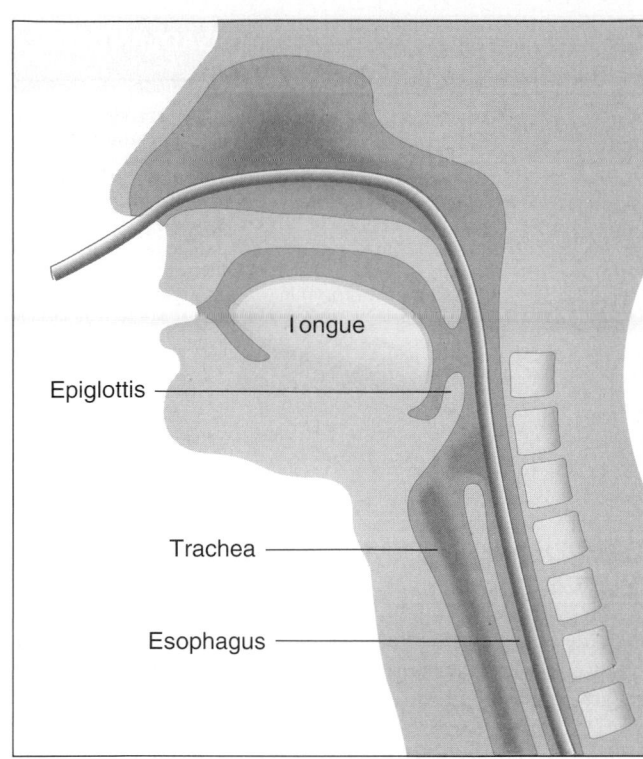

FIGURE 221–1. Anatomy of upper aerodigestive tract.

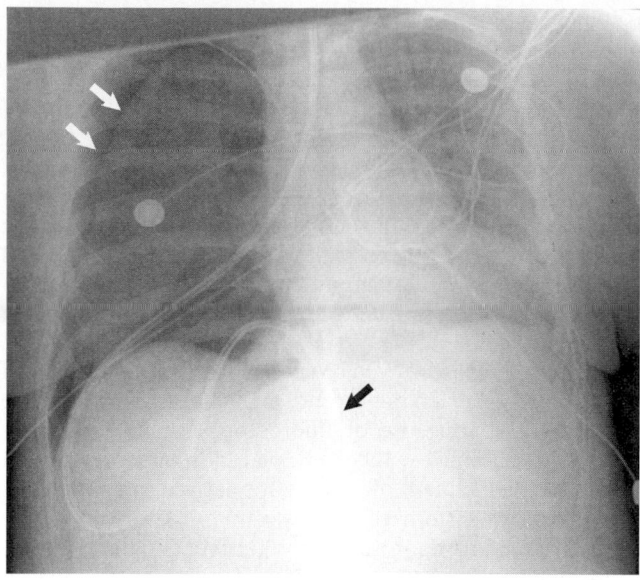

FIGURE 221–2. Pneumothorax caused by feeding tube placement.

tube into the lung (Fig. 221-1). Often with a sense of feel and expectation, the tube is advanced through the pharynx and into the esophagus. Generally, success is more frequent when the larynx is sensed, then a short fast series of pushes (approximately 10 cm total) performed to intubate the esophagus. Many patients will cough if the tube is advanced into the trachea, but patients with a diminished cough reflex due to sedation, encephalopathy, or coma will not cough appropriately despite translaryngeal intubation. In awake and appropriate patients, it can be helpful to have the patient sip water with a straw to facilitate passage into the esophagus.

Once the tube is believed to be in the esophagus, it is advanced to 35 cm and a radiograph taken at our institution to exclude intrabronchial placement. This maneuver is important, since it prevents inadvertent advance of the feeding tube distally into the lungs and the potentially disastrous consequences, such as pneumothorax (Fig. 221-2). Once placement in the esophagus is confirmed radiographically, the feeding tube is advanced into the stomach. In adults, the gastroesophageal junction is about 40 cm from the incisors and the pylorus is about 55 to 60 cm from the teeth (Fig. 221-3). It is often helpful during the procedure to try to pull the guidewire back approximately 2 cm and then restore it again to its previous position. If the tube is kinked, then the guidewire will not be easy to manipulate. In this case, the tube should be pulled back until it is in a position where the guidewire moves easily back and forth, and then the tube can once again be advanced. Once the tube is in satisfactory position, tape is used to affix the tube to the nose of the patient and the procedure is concluded.

Intraesophageal placement can be confirmed with several techniques. A radiograph at 35 cm will determine the position of the tube. At 35 cm, even if the tube is in a bronchus, it has not been inserted far enough to cause a pneumothorax.[13] If the tube is fully inserted before a radiograph is obtained,

intrabronchial placement is more likely to result in pneumothorax.

The "corkscrew" technique has been proposed to facilitate passage of the feeding tube into the small bowel.[14] After intragastric placement is confirmed by auscultation of air, the guidewire is removed, a bend is placed in the guidewire, and the wire is replaced. By twisting the tube as it is advanced, the tactile feedback to the operator is increased and the ability to pass through the pylorus is improved.

Promotility agents have been proposed as a method to facilitate passage of feeding tubes from the stomach into the small bowel. Erythromycin and metoclopramide are

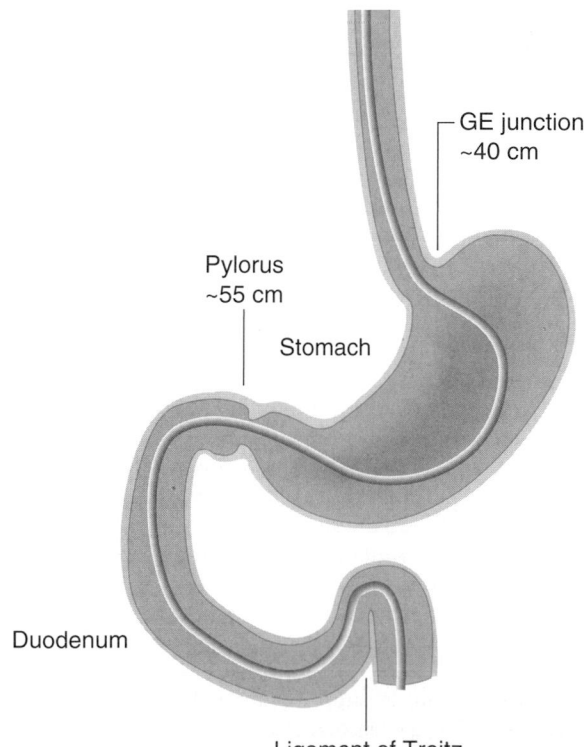

FIGURE 221–3. Proper placement of a feeding tube.

somewhat effective but carry the risk of side effects.[15] Newer agents for this purpose are under development.

ADJUNCTS TO AID PLACEMENT

If it is a struggle to get the feeding tube in the esophagus and the patient is sufficiently sedated, direct laryngoscopy can be utilized to pass the tube under direct vision. In coagulopathic patients or in those patients who have developed some nasal bleeding from prior attempts, the mouth can be used in place of the nose as a site to introduce the tube in sedated patients.

Bedside fluoroscopy can be used to facilitate placement of the feeding tube. Taking care to shield the patient and the clinician, judicious use of fluoroscopy can be especially helpful in enabling the tube to be placed in optimal position well past the ligament of Treitz. Alternatively, a tube that is placed into the stomach already can be advanced to the optimal position fluoroscopically. Drawbacks of this technique include its costs, limited availability, and radiation exposure.

Endoscopy can be helpful for placing and advancing a feeding tube. The tube can be directly visualized with the endoscope. A grasping instrument passed through the working channel of the endoscope can be used to pull the feeding tube into proper position. Some feeding tubes have a suture at their distal end to facilitate endoscopic advancement. However, care must be taken when withdrawing the endoscope so that the feeding tube is not also pulled back out of position. A simple technique of advancing the feeding tube while withdrawing a well-lubricated endoscope suffices to prevent pulling the tube back.

ADVANTAGES AND DISADVANTAGES OF A NASOENTERIC FEEDING TUBE COMPARED WITH A GASTROSTOMY OR JEJUNOSTOMY TUBE

Nasoenteric feeding tubes have advantages and disadvantages when compared to gastrostomy or jejunostomy tubes. Nasoenteric feeding tubes are inexpensive and can be placed at the bedside without anesthesia. However, these tubes can become dislodged, requiring replacement. Even though their caliber is small, the presence of the tube in the nose and throat can cause an awake patient some discomfort. Anatomic problems or underlying disease processes in the nose, pharynx, neck, or esophagus may prohibit nasoenteric feeding tube placement.

Gastrostomy and jejunostomy are surgical procedures. Traditional techniques require open laparotomy. Minimally invasive techniques have decreased the morbidity of these procedures, but they still entail creation of an enterotomy. The devastating complication of the bowel pulling away from the anterior abdominal wall with leakage of enteral contents and nutritional formula into the peritoneal cavity remains a possibility. Additionally, the anatomy of certain patients may make it technically challenging and difficult to place a surgical tube.

Patient factors such as underlying disease, anatomy, and expected duration of support guide the choice of enteral access (Table 221-2). Nasoenteric feeding tubes can be left in place for 6 to 8 weeks routinely, and some patients have had their tubes in place for months.

TABLE 221–2. ADVANTAGES AND DISADVANTAGES OF NASOENTERIC FEEDING TUBES

	Nasoenteric Feeding Tube	Gastrostomy or Jejunostomy
Advantages	Can be placed at bedside	Less easily dislodged
	Easy to remove when not needed	Can access small bowel easier
	No incisions needed	Can be permanent if needed
	Inexpensive	
Disadvantages	Can be uncomfortable in nose	Requires surgical procedure
	Frequent need for replacement	Fistula must heal when removed
	May increase aspiration	Feedings can leak into abdomen
		Some patients are not a candidate

COMPLICATIONS OF FEEDING TUBE PLACEMENT

Feeding tube placement is often taken for granted as a benign undertaking without any real risks to the patient. In reality, this procedure can be associated with serious, even life-threatening, complications.

The placement of the feeding tube, especially in a coagulopathic patient, can precipitate epistaxis. In a patient with a skull fracture, the tube can be placed into the brain through the cribriform plate. If too much pressure is applied when resistance is met in the pharynx, there can be a perforation of the hypopharynx. When esophageal strictures or tumors are present, too much pressure applied may result in perforation at these sites as well.

Unplanned removal of the feeding tube, by either the patient or the caregivers, is a bothersome and common problem. At our institution, 11.3% of all nasoenteric feeding tubes required replacement for unplanned removal (Marderstein EL, Szelc B, Ochoa JB: Unpublished observations, 2002-2003). Replacement of a feeding tube represents an additional expense and a waste of clinicians' time. Moreover, unplanned removal interrupts the provision of nutritional support and exposes the patient to the risk of an additional placement procedure.

Placement of the nasoenteric feeding tube into the lung with subsequent pneumothorax is a surprisingly common and morbid complication of feeding tube placement. Case reports of this complication indicate that tracheostomy or endotracheal intubation and impaired mental status are risk factors.[11,13,16,17] Some of these complications are lethal, being associated with tension pneumothorax or infusion of a nutrient solution into the thorax.[11] A well-designed prospective study found that 2% of all tubes placed were malpositioned in the bronchus and 0.7% were associated with a major complication.[11]

After a series of adverse events at our medical center, we dramatically decreased our incidence of procedure-related pneumothorax by instituting a protocol that mandated a radiograph for verification of intraesophageal placement after passing the feeding tube to 35 cm.[18] An analysis of the cohort of patients experiencing intrabronchial placement demonstrated that 39% were intubated and 33% had tracheostomies, supporting the view that the presence of a cuffed endotracheal or tracheostomy tube provides no protection against passage of a feeding tube into the airway.

TABLE 221–3. MISPLACEMENT OF TUBE*

Number of Misplacements	Patients, n	Pneumo-thorax, n	Misplacements Resulting in Pneumothorax, % [†]
0	3356	0	0.0
1	47	3	6.4
2	17	2	11.8
3 or more	11	4	36.4

*Intrabronchial misplacement is a risk factor for future misplacement. Increasing number of misplacements correlate with development of pneumothorax.
[†]$P < 0.001$ for test of trend of odds and $P < .05$ for test of trend of odds without "Number of misplacements = 0."

Interestingly, 33% of these patients had multiple intrabronchial placements. As illustrated by the findings shown in Table 221-3, patients who experience one intrabronchial placement are at increased risk for future misplacements and an increasing number of misplacements correlates with the risk for pneumothorax.

Additionally, we established and trained a specialized team of nurses to respond to requests for feeding tubes in our intensive care units and place them in accordance with institutional protocols. The aptitude gained from repeated experience with the procedure is evident, as the team has not had a single pneumothorax after more than 500 tube placements and more than two-thirds of the tubes are passed into the small bowel (Marderstein F.I., Szelc B, Ochoa JB: Unpublished observations, 2002-2003).

ASPIRATION AND TOLERANCE OF ENTERAL FEEDS

Patients with a feeding tube often have multiple risk factors for aspiration, including the device itself, which may interfere with normal airway protective mechanisms. All patients receiving enteral tube feeding must be monitored to detect aspiration of the formula. A clinical assessment at the bedside is useful. Evaluation by a speech pathologist can be helpful. Measurement of a low gastric residual volume does not guarantee that the feedings are being tolerated and a large gastric residual volume does not necessarily mean that feedings should be stopped.[19]

Ideally, the feeding tube will traverse the pylorus and its tip will be positioned distal to the ligament of Treitz. Intuitively, a distal placement of the feeding tube should reduce the incidence of gastroesophageal reflux, regurgitation, aspiration, and aspiration pneumonia. However, no single study has provided clear evidence that post-pyloric tube placement (as compared with intragastric tube placement) decreases the incidence of aspiration or aspiration pneumonia.[20] When the results from smaller studies are analyzed collectively, however, feeding into the small bowel is associated with lower rates of aspiration and ventilator-associated pneumonia and increased rates of delivery of nutrients.[21]

Patient-specific and institution-specific factors should guide the decision to seek distal or gastric tube placement. Additional effort to achieve placement of a tube into the small bowel is warranted for patients at high risk for intolerance of enteric feeding (e.g., those requiring infusion of inotropic or vasoactive drugs) or those who have already demonstrated intolerance. The availability of clinicians with expertise in blind small bowel placement and the availability of adjunctive fluoroscopic or endoscopic services will influence the choice to use small bowel feedings as opposed to gastric feedings. For most patients, intragastric feeding is certainly better than no feeding, although small bowel feeding is preferable. Certainly, starting a patient on intragastric feedings while the tube is being manipulated into the small bowel is appropriate, and delays in nutrient delivery because "the tube is not in the small bowel" are generally inappropriate.

CONCLUSION

Enteral tube feeding is generally superior to parenteral nutrition, and early institution of enteral feeding is beneficial. Proper placement of a nasoenteric feeding tube begins with proper evaluation of the patient and an understanding of the anatomy of the mouth, neck, esophagus, stomach, and intestine. Adjuncts such as fluoroscopy, endoscopy, or promotility agents can help passage of the tube into the small bowel, but experience with the procedure and patience at the bedside is critical. Nasoenteric feeding tubes are relatively inexpensive, easy to place, and less invasive than surgical enteral access. The most important complication of placement is pneumothorax. The risk for this complication can be virtually eliminated if the tube is inserted to 35 cm and a radiograph is obtained to confirm intraesophageal position. A specialized team devoted to the placement of nasoenteric feeding tubes can reduce procedure-related complications. Aspiration remains a clinical problem for patients on enteral tube feeds, and tube placement in the small bowel in addition to directed nursing measures might be of benefit.

ANNOTATED REFERENCES

Dobbie RP, Hoffmeister JA: Continuous pump-tube enteric hyperalimentation. Surg Gynecol Obstet 1976;13:273-276.
> In this classic paper, the authors describe their innovative "Dobhoff" small-bore feeding tube with a weighted tip that was named for its inventors.

Heyland DK, Drover JW, Dhaliwal R, Greenwood J: Optimizing the benefits and minimizing the risks of enteral nutrition in the critically ill: Role of small bowel feeding. JPEN 2002;26:S51-S57.
> This meta-analysis of randomized trials concludes that feeding patients into the small bowel is associated with a decrease in gastroesophageal regurgitation, an increase in nutrient delivery, a shorter time to achieve desired target nutrition, and a lower rate of ventilator-associated pneumonia as compared to feeding patients into the stomach. There was no difference in mortality rate between these groups.

Marderstein EL, Simmons RL, Ochoa JB: Patient safety: Effect of institutional protocols on the incidence of pneumothorax after feeding tube placement in the critically ill. American College of Surgeons Papers Session. J Am Coll Surg 2004;199:39-47.
> This retrospective review of more than 4000 feeding tube placements provides evidence that taking a radiograph after 35 cm of tube passage to ensure intraesophageal placement decreases the incidence of pneumothorax after feeding tube placement. In addition, it demonstrates that once a feeding tube is placed into the bronchus, the patient is at greatly increased risk of recurrent misplacements on subsequent attempts.

McClave SA, DeMeo MT, DeLegge MH, et al: North American Summit on Aspiration in the Critically Ill Patient: Consensus Statement. JPEN 2002;26:S80-S85.
> This expert consensus statement provides an excellent overview of the reasons for aspiration in critically ill patients, clinical monitors for aspiration, and evidence-based recommendations for prevention.

Zaloga GP: Bedside method for placing small bowel feeding tubes in critically ill patients. Chest 1991;100:1643-1646.
> This single institution review of feeding tube placement provides rich detail concerning the technical aspects of the procedure performed by the authors. Their methods are particularly effective at passing the tube beyond the pylorus into the small bowel.

Chapter 222
LUMBAR PUNCTURE

Sarice L. Bassin • Thomas P. Bleck

KEY POINTS

1. Lumbar puncture is a **critical adjunctive test** for the diagnosis of many infectious, inflammatory, and neurovascular conditions.

2. Lumbar puncture is usually **performed with the patient in the lateral decubitus position.** The knees are flexed to the abdomen, and the head is flexed with the chin toward the chest. The patient's back is positioned as close as possible to the edge of the bed nearest the examiner.

3. If the patient cannot lie in the lateral decubitus position, then lumbar puncture **can be performed with the patient sitting on the side of the bed leaning forward over a bedside table.** However, once free cerebrospinal fluid (CSF) flow occurs, the patient should be returned to the recumbent position for accurate pressure measurements.

4. By walking the fingers down the spinous processes, **the examiner should be able to identify the L4-L5 and L5-S1 interspaces and mark them on the skin.**

5. Before performing lumbar puncture, **the physician must be certain that the patient does not have an intracranial or spinous (especially intramedullary) mass.**

6. **Coagulopathy and thrombocytopenia are relative contraindications** to lumbar puncture, because epidural hematomas can develop at the puncture site.

All critical care specialists should be adept at performing lumbar puncture. In conjunction with the history and physical examination, it is a critical adjunctive test for the diagnosis of many infectious, inflammatory, and neurovascular conditions.

Lumbar puncture is usually performed with the patient in the lateral decubitus position. The knees are flexed to the abdomen, and the head is flexed with the chin toward the chest. The patient's back is positioned as close as possible to the edge of the bed nearest the examiner. Before preparing the skin, the site of intended puncture should be determined. The interspace between the third and fourth lumbar vertebrae (L3 and L4, respectively) can be located by drawing an imaginary line between the posterior iliac crests. This is usually the most rostral space employed, because the adult spinal cord ends at L2. By walking the fingers down the spinous processes, the examiner should be able to identify the L4-L5 and L5-S1 interspaces and mark them on the skin.

The skin should then be prepared with chlorhexidine or povidone-iodine. The preparation should proceed outward in a spiral and cover several interspaces, in case multiple attempts are necessary. A sterile sheet with an opening for the prepared area should drape the patient's back and be adjusted so that it covers the posterior iliac crest. The skin is anesthetized with 1% lidocaine, using a 25-gauge needle, which is then exchanged for a longer 22-gauge needle to reach deeper tissues.

A 20- or 22-gauge spinal needle is adequate for most lumbar punctures. The needle always should be advanced with the stylet in place to avoid introduction of epidermal cells into the subarachnoid space. The bevel of the needle should be directed upward to separate the fibers of the ligamentum flavum. The needle should be angled 15 degrees cephalad and slightly downward toward the bed. When the dura is punctured and a slight "pop" is felt, the stylet should be withdrawn. If free flow of CSF does not occur, the needle can be rotated or may need to be advanced (after replacing the stylet). Once free flow of CSF is obtained, a manometer should be attached to the spinal needle, usually by way of a stopcock. CSF should rise steadily in the manometer until the opening pressure is reached and respiratory fluctuation can be visualized in the fluid column. The patient's legs should be carefully extended and relaxed for an accurate pressure reading, because abdominal compression transmits pressure to the subarachnoid space.

Once the opening pressure is recorded, four tubes of CSF (3 mL of fluid in each) are usually collected and sent for appropriate studies. It is wise to check with the laboratory before the procedure if any unusual tests are being performed, because an additional tube or larger volumes of CSF may be required, or CSF may need special handling.

After the fluid is obtained, the needle is withdrawn and pressure applied to the puncture site. Most clinicians replace the stylet before withdrawing the needle to minimize the possibility of pulling a nerve root through the dura as the needle is removed. The patient should lie flat for 1 to 3 hours after the procedure to minimize the risk of post-lumbar puncture headache. Considerable argument persists regarding the value of prone or supine positioning on the incidence of headache and about the use of varying sizes and types of needles.

If the physician cannot enter the subarachnoid space with this technique, or the patient cannot lie in the lateral decubitus position, then lumbar puncture can be performed with the patient sitting on the side of the bed leaning forward over a bedside table. However, once free CSF flow occurs, the patient should be returned to the recumbent position for accurate pressure measurements.

If a patient is unable to bend one leg (e.g., after an angiographic procedure), lumbar puncture can be attempted in the lateral position, with the bottom leg held straight and the top leg bent into the abdomen and supported with a pillow. When lumbar spine disease, the question of a spinal mass, or overlying skin infection prevents the lumbar approach, a lateral cervical approach can be performed by a physician trained in this technique.

Before performing lumbar puncture, the physician must be certain that the patient does not have an intracranial or spinous (especially intramedullary) mass. If there is any concern, an imaging study should be performed before the procedure. A rapid drop in pressure from withdrawal of CSF could precipitate herniation or worsening of spinal cord function if a mass lesion is present. If a lumbar puncture is delayed for imaging in a suspected case of bacterial meningitis, empirical antibiotics should be given as cultures can be obtained up to 4 hours after starting treatment.

Coagulopathy and thrombocytopenia are relative contraindications to lumbar puncture, because epidural hematomas can develop at the puncture site. Fresh frozen plasma and platelets should be infused to correct hematologic abnormalities before the procedure. The role of recombinant factor VIIa has yet to be determined. If a coagulopathy is discovered after the procedure, therapy should still be given because bleeding can occur for many hours.

If a lumbar puncture is being performed to evaluate a patient for aneurysmal subarachnoid hemorrhage, one should withdraw the smallest possible amount of CSF to obtain the necessary laboratory tests. Lowering the CSF pressure could increase the transmural pressure across the aneurysm and precipitate rebleeding.

ANNOTATED REFERENCES

Bleck TP: The clinical use of neurologic diagnostic tests. In Weiner WJ, Goetz CG (eds): Neurology for the Non-neurologist, 4th ed. Philadelphia, Harper & Row, 1999, pp 27-37.

Nathan BR: Cerebrospinal fluid and intracranial pressure. In Goetz CG (ed): Textbook of Clinical Neurology, 2nd ed. Philadelphia, WB Saunders, 2003, pp 511-529.

Roos KL: Lumbar puncture. Semin Neurol 2003;23:105-114.
    These publications are excellent references on the mechanics of lumbar puncture and the potential pitfalls of lumbar puncture.

Chapter 223

JUGULAR VENOUS AND BRAIN TISSUE OXYGEN TENSION MONITORING

Roman Hlatky • Claudia S. Robertson

KEY POINTS

1. **Measures of cerebral oxygenation,** such as jugular venous oxygen saturation ($SjvO_2$) or brain tissue oxygen tension ($PbtO_2$), **have been used in place of quantitative cerebral blood flow (CBF) measurements,** because they give an indicator of the **adequacy of CBF** relative to cerebral metabolic requirements.

2. **When CBF is low (25 to 30 mL/100 g per minute),** it can be difficult to decide whether this is an appropriate response to lower cerebral metabolic requirements or whether the brain is hypoperfused. A measure of cerebral oxygenation can be helpful in making this distinction.

3. Although blood in the jugular bulb is derived from both cerebral hemispheres, **it is generally accepted that most patients have a dominant side of venous drainage,** usually the right.

4. **If the monitoring strategy is to use $SjvO_2$ as a monitor of global oxygenation,** then cannulation of the dominant jugular vein is the most logical approach, because the values obtained will be the most representative of the whole brain. However, **if the strategy is to identify the most abnormal** oxygen saturation, then probably the side of interest should be cannulated.

5. **The depth of $SjvO_2$ catheter insertion is approximately equal to the distance from the point of insertion to the level of the mastoid process.** Complications of $SjvO_2$ monitoring are uncommon and are related to catheter insertion. Complications include carotid artery puncture, pneumothorax, nerve injury, infection, and thrombosis.

6. Only a few studies have examined the $SjvO_2$ threshold associated with depletion of energy stores in animals or with loss of consciousness or electroencephalographic changes during anoxia in normal humans. From these studies, **it appears that normal brain metabolism can be altered at $SjvO_2$ values lower than 50% but that values lower than 20% are required for irreversible ischemic injury.**

7. **$SjvO_2$ monitoring** may be useful to guide decisions for optimizing hyperventilation therapy, guiding fluid management and oxygenation, optimizing

perfusion pressure, and detecting arterial-venous fistulas.

8. **Physiologic determinants of the oxygen probe** include the number, diameter, and spatial distribution of capillaries in the local microvasculature. Tissue oxygenation results from diffusion at the capillary interface as well as from direct diffusion to cells along the vessels.

9. **Normal values for $PbtO_2$ are 20 to 40 mm Hg,** and critically low values are 8 to 10 mm Hg.

10. **The likelihood of death in patients with traumatic brain injury increases with increasing duration of $PbtO_2$ values lower than 15 mm Hg.** A $PbtO_2$ value of 10 to 15 mm Hg is currently accepted as the critical limit in traumatic brain injury.

11. **Opinions vary as to whether $PbtO_2$ monitoring should be performed in a relatively undamaged part of the brain,** in which case information is provided on the more global balance between oxygen delivery and demand in the brain tissue, or in the penumbra of an intracranial lesion or vascular territory. Advocates of the latter option emphasize the importance of saving potentially viable tissue.

CEREBRAL BLOOD FLOW ADEQUACY

Measures of cerebral oxygenation, such as jugular venous oxygen saturation ($SjvO_2$) or brain tissue oxygen tension ($PbtO_2$), have been used in place of quantitative cerebral blood flow (CBF) measurements because they give an indicator of the adequacy of CBF relative to cerebral metabolic requirements. Because cerebral metabolic requirements may be reduced after traumatic brain injury, normal CBF values may not apply. When demand exceeds supply, the brain extracts a greater amount of oxygen, resulting in decreased jugular bulb oxygen saturation. As the CBF decreases progressively, a point is eventually reached at which the brain can no longer completely compensate for decreased CBF by a further increase in oxygen extraction. At this point, oxygen consumption decreases and anaerobic metabolism with lactate production ensues. When cerebral oxygen supply exceeds demand, the oxygen saturation of jugular bulb blood is increased.

Cerebral oxygen delivery (DO_2) is described by the following equation: $DO_2 = CBF \times CaO_2$, where CaO_2 is arterial oxygen content. Cerebral oxygen consumption ($CMRO_2$) is described by the equation, $CMRO_2 = CBF \times (CaO_2 - CjvO_2)$, where $CjvO_2$ is the oxygen content of jugular venous blood. The difference in oxygen content between arterial and jugular venous blood is expressed by the term, $(CaO_2 - CjvO_2)$, or $AVjDO_2$. From these equations, it is apparent that $AVjDO_2 = CMRO_2/CBF$.

Normally, $AVjDO_2$ is stable at 4 to 8 mL oxygen per 100 mL blood.[1,2] If $CMRO_2$ remains constant, changes in $AVjDO_2$ should reflect changes in CBF. If $AVjDO_2$ is less than 4 mL oxygen per 100 mL blood, it is assumed that oxygen supply is greater than demand. If $AVjDO_2$ is greater than 8 mL oxygen per 100 mL blood, this parameter suggests that demand exceeds supply.

When CBF is low (25 to 30 mL per 100 g per minute), it can be difficult to decide whether this is an appropriate response to lower cerebral metabolic requirements or whether the brain is receiving less blood flow than is required to meet metabolic demands. A measure of cerebral oxygenation can be helpful in making this distinction. If the brain is ischemic, oxygen extraction will be increased, and $SjvO_2$ will be reduced. On the other hand, if CBF is appropriate for the brain's metabolic requirement, then $SjvO_2$ will be normal. Often this information is more clinically useful than the absolute CBF.

Currently, measurements of $SjvO_2$ and $PbtO_2$ provide an indirect assessment of cerebral oxygen use and are used to guide physiologic management decisions in a variety of clinical settings.[3,4]

JUGULAR OXIMETRY

HISTORICAL ASPECTS

When $SjvO_2$ was first sampled in the 1930s and 1940s, the jugular bulb was directly punctured by a needle that was inserted 1 cm below and 1 cm anterior to the mastoid process.[5] More recently, placement of an internal jugular vein catheter, similar to the type used for central venous pressure monitoring but directed cephalad into the jugular bulb, has allowed repetitive sampling of $SjvO_2$ without repeated needle punctures.[6,7] Currently, fiberoptic catheters allow continuous monitoring of $SjvO_2$ without the need for sampling of blood, except for calibration purposes.[8-10]

Fiberoptic oximetry is based on the unique light absorption spectrum of oxyhemoglobin. One system (Edslab Sat II, Baxter Edwards Critical Care Division, Irvine, CA) uses two wavelengths of light for reflectance spectrophotometry and is calibrated against a sample of the patient's blood. Another system (Opticath Oximetrix, Abbott Critical Care System, Abbott Park, IL) uses three wavelengths of light and can be precalibrated before insertion. An $SjvO_2$ catheter contains two optical fiber bundles. Light is directed into the blood by one of the fiber bundles. The reflected light is transmitted to a photosensor via the second fiber bundle. The photosensor measures the absorption of the reflected light at various wavelengths. $SjvO_2$ is displayed as a percentage of oxygenated hemoglobin relative to total hemoglobin. For $SjvO_2$ catheters using two wavelengths of light, the patient's hemoglobin concentration must be manually entered. The validity of the $SjvO_2$ value depends on the accuracy of the entered hemoglobin concentration. For catheters using three

wavelengths, the hemoglobin concentration is calculated from the absorption spectrum, allowing continuous, real-time monitoring of $SjvO_2$.

SIDE OF CATHETERIZATION

Although blood in the jugular bulb is derived from both cerebral hemispheres (approximately 70% ipsilateral and 30% contralateral),[11-13] it is generally accepted that most patients have a dominant side of venous drainage, usually the right.[7,14] Sinuses that drain to the jugular bulbs differ in size in 88% of patients,[15] and mixing of cerebral venous blood within the sinuses is incomplete.[16,17] The dominant side may be determined by comparing the intracranial pressure increase caused by manual compression of each internal jugular vein,[18] by assessing jugular foramen size (using computed tomography),[19] or by comparing internal jugular vein size using ultrasonography.[20]

Early studies suggested that either jugular bulb would provide similar $SjvO_2$ information in most normal people. However, as early as 1945,[12] it was observed that patients who have focal lesions might have a significant difference in oxygen saturation obtained in the right versus the left jugular bulb.

In patients with bilateral brain injury, the catheter usually is placed in the internal jugular vein on the side of dominant drainage, usually the right.[7,21] In the presence of a focal brain injury, it is controversial whether the catheter should be placed on the side ipsilateral to brain injury or on the dominant side, if different. Stochetti and colleagues[19] noted that the proportion of head-injured patients with relevant discrepancies of $SjvO_2$ between the jugular veins is quite high: 15 of 32 patients showed oxygen saturation differences greater than 15% between the two jugular veins, and only 8 patients had consistent differences of less than 5%. Beards and associates[14] proposed that asymmetry of $SjvO_2$ values greater than 10% occurs 65% of the time. If the monitoring strategy is to use $SjvO_2$ as a monitor of global oxygenation, then cannulation of the dominant jugular vein is the most logical choice, because the data thereby obtained will be the most representative of the whole brain. However, if the strategy is to identify the most abnormal oxygen saturation, then probably the side of interest should be cannulated.

CATHETER PLACEMENT

Contrary to catheterization of the internal jugular vein for central line purposes, for cannulation of the jugular bulb the needle, guidewire, and catheter are advanced in a cephalic direction.[3,4,22-24] The guidewire should be advanced 2 to 3 cm beyond the needle insertion site. Then, the catheter should be advanced until resistance is felt; this distance is usually about 13 to 15 cm and indicates positioning in the jugular bulb. At this time, an awake patient may note a sensation in the jaw or ear as the catheter touches the base of the skull, indicating that the tip of the catheter is in the jugular bulb. The catheter is then pulled back 0.5 to 1.0 cm to minimize the cephalic vascular impact with head movement. The distance of catheter insertion is approximately equal to the distance from the point of insertion to the level of the mastoid process.

Relative contraindications to $SjvO_2$ monitoring are cervical spine injury, presence of a tracheostomy, and coagulopathy. Routine maneuvers to aid placement of a catheter into the internal jugular vein, such as Trendelenberg's position or head rotation, may lead to an increase in intracranial pressure or cervical spine injury.[23,25] The internal jugular vein may be absent, occluded, or in an unusual configuration in approximately 10% of patients.[26,27] Complications of $SjvO_2$ monitoring are uncommon and are related to catheter insertion. Complications include carotid artery puncture, pneumothorax, nerve injury, infection, and thrombosis. Subclinical internal jugular vein thrombosis occurred in 8 of 20 patients who were monitored closely with ultrasonographic examinations while a jugular bulb catheter was in place, but symptomatic thrombosis is very uncommon.[28] The concern that a jugular catheter might obstruct venous return and increase intracranial pressure appears to be unfounded.[29,30]

Lateral cervical spine radiography should be used to confirm catheter tip placement.[31] The catheter tip should be cephalad to the lower border of C1.

METHODOLOGIC CONSIDERATIONS

Historically, a limiting factor in the acceptance of $SjvO_2$ monitoring has been a relatively poor correlation between simultaneous measurements obtained from a cerebral oximetry catheter and $SjvO_2$ measurements made with the use of a co-oximeter.[32] The original oximetry catheters were designed for use in the umbilical arteries of neonates. When they were used in the venous system with nonpulsatile, retrograde flow and a vessel wall that is susceptible to catheter abutment, there were limitations in the correlation of the online saturation value with oxygen saturation values measured by a co-oximeter.[34] These concerns, although still present, have been addressed by recent advances in technology.[32-34]

A second limiting factor concerns the possibility of contamination of blood in the internal jugular vein bulb with venous blood from extracerebral sources. If blood is sampled at a site within 2 cm of the jugular bulb and at a rate of less than 2 mL/minute, there is negligible (approximately 3%) extracerebral contamination.[11,35,36] However, as CBF decreases, the relative contribution of extracerebral venous blood to the $SjvO_2$ reading increases.

A final technologic issue is the concern of catheter migration and abutment against the vessel wall. Change in the light intensity signal together with triggering of the light intensity alarm informs the clinician about this problem. Distinguishing a "desaturation reading" resulting from a change in position of the catheter tip from a pathologic desaturation can be problematic. Slight repositioning of the catheter or the patient's head may be all that is needed to achieve an acceptable light signal. Because of these concerns, it is recommended that cerebral oximetry catheters be routinely calibrated against a control sample assayed with the use of a co-oximeter.

NORMAL VALUES

Gibbs and coworkers[5] studied 50 normal young men and observed that their $SjvO_2$ ranged from 55% to 71% (mean, 61.8%). Data from a recent study of patients with pituitary microadenomas, who underwent selective bilateral venous sampling, suggest that the normal jugular bulb oxygen saturation may be as low as 44% (mean, 57%).[37] In the latter study, optimal placement of the catheter in the jugular bulb was ensured by the use of fluoroscopic control; however,

arterial blood gases were not measured. Without this information, mild hyperventilation cannot be ruled out as a cause for the lower values of $SjvO_2$.

These values for SjvO2 are lower than normal mixed venous oxygen saturation, indicating that the brain normally extracts oxygen more completely from arterial blood, compared with many other organs. Simultaneous measurements of oxygen saturation in the jugular bulb and in the pulmonary artery have shown that $SjvO_2$ cannot be predicted from mixed venous oxygen saturation.[38]

Experimental studies have examined the ischemic thresholds for CBF. Only a few studies have examined the $SjvO_2$ threshold associated with depletion of energy stores in animals or with loss of consciousness or electroencephalographic changes during anoxia in normal humans.[39-42] From these studies, it appears that normal brain metabolism can be altered when the $SjvO_2$ is less than 50% but that values less than 20% are required for irreversible ischemic injury.

CLINICAL APPLICATIONS

Jugular venous oximetry is most often used in patients with head injuries, during neurosurgical procedures, and during cardiovascular procedures.

Head Injury

$SjvO_2$ monitoring may be useful to guide decisions for optimizing hyperventilation therapy,[43-47] guiding fluid management and cerebral oxygenation,[43,47,48] optimizing perfusion pressure,[9,49,50] and detecting arterial-venous fistulas.[51,52] Used together with a transcranial Doppler ultrasonography, $SjvO_2$ can help differentiate hyperemia from vasospasm. With high flow velocity detected by transcranial Doppler ultrasonography, $SjvO_2$ is increased during hyperemia and normal or low if cerebral vasospasm is present.

Routine hyperventilation after traumatic brain injury is not currently recommended.[53] Rather, contemporary guidelines recommend "optimal hyperventilation" guided by $SjvO_2$ monitoring, thus identifying those head-injured patients with the potential for an ischemic response to hypocarbia.[53] Moreover, $SjvO_2$ monitoring is also useful in evaluating the prognosis for head-injured patients.[54]

Cardiovascular and Neurologic Surgery

Neurologic dysfunction is not uncommon after cardiac surgery with cardiopulmonary bypass and has been attributed to the adverse effects of nonphysiologic modes of perfusion.[55] A particularly critical period is the rewarming phase after hypothermic cardiopulmonary bypass. Rewarming has been associated with frequent $SjvO_2$ desaturation events, and these changes have been associated with postoperative neurocognitive deficits.[56-58] Accordingly, some experts suggest that $SjvO_2$ monitoring can be useful during adult[59] and pediatric[60] cardiac surgery.

The potential applications of $SjvO_2$ monitoring during neurosurgical procedures were studied by Matta and colleagues.[61] They demonstrated that the $SjvO_2$ catheter could be placed quickly and could detect critical episodes of $SjvO_2$ desaturation that would otherwise have remained untreated. During intracranial aneurysm surgery, $SjvO_2$ monitoring has been used to determine the minimal blood pressure that should be maintained to avoid hypoperfusion.[62] In patients undergoing carotid endarterectomy under local anesthesia (i.e., while awake), a 25% decrease in $SjvO_2$

correlated with the development of neurologic signs of ischemia.[63] This form of monitoring might be useful as an indicator of the need for selective shunting when patients undergo carotid endarterectomy under general anesthesia.

SUMMARY

$SjvO_2$ is a measure of global cerebral oxygenation and is not particularly sensitive to small areas of focal ischemia. Accordingly, the likelihood of a false-negative value during an episode of focal ischemia depends on the area of ischemia and the capacity of the surrounding "normal" brain tissue to mask or average-out the ischemic tissue. In addition, it is still not clear which jugular vein to cannulate. Because 70% of the cerebral venous blood drains via the ipsilateral jugular veins, some clinicians advocate cannulating on the side of injury. However, in the case of diffuse cerebral injury, most clinicians monitor the right side, because it is commonly dominant. Some clinicians advocate monitoring the side of dominant flow in all situations. More study is needed to definitively determine whether there is an optimal side for $SjvO_2$ monitoring.

Despite the limitations of $SjvO_2$ monitoring, there is no better, commercially available, continuous, relatively low-cost, bedside monitor to assess the adequacy of cerebral oxygenation. $SjvO_2$ provides information on global brain oxygenation and is recommended in the treatment of patients with head injury, especially those receiving hyperventilation therapy.

BRAIN TISSUE OXYGEN TENSION

The major limitation of $SjvO_2$ as a monitor of CBF adequacy is that regional ischemia is not identified. In circumstances in which regional differences in CBF may occur (e.g., brain trauma), $PbtO_2$ as a monitor of cerebral oxygenation may have an important advantage.

HISTORICAL ASPECTS

The principle that an electrode could measure oxygen tension polarographically in blood or tissue was described by Clark in 1956.[64] The diffusion of oxygen molecules through an oxygen-permeable membrane into an electrolyte solution causes depolarization at the nearby cathode, inducing an electrical current that is proportionally related to the amount of oxygen. The earliest direct measurements of $PbtO_2$ in humans were done either intraoperatively or in ventricular cerebrospinal fluid along with a pressure monitor.[65,66] Parenchymal tissue oxygen tension is more commonly monitored now because this parameter responds more rapidly to physiologic events.

METHOD

One available tissue oxygen tension catheter uses the Clark electrode technology (Licox pO_2 probe, Integra Neurocare, San Diego, CA) and is widely used for intracerebral monitoring of $PbtO_2$. This device also can be used for measurements of oxygen tension in other tissues. The catheter has a diameter of 0.5 mm, and the measurement area is 5 mm long. Stable measurements are obtained less than 2 hours after insertion.[67,68] Because the electrode requires temperature correction, a temperature catheter is placed concurrently.

Another catheter that is available for monitoring of tissue oxygen tension (Neurotrend, Codman/Johnson & Johnson, Raynham, MA) uses fluorescence technology. The measurement area of the probe is 2 cm, and its diameter is 0.5 mm. Temperature is measured by an incorporated thermocouple. This catheter offers an additional benefit of measuring pH and partial pressure of carbon dioxide (Pco_2).[69]

These catheters may be introduced through a dedicated two-way or three-way bolt, permitting introduction of catheters for monitoring of intracranial pressure, $PbtO_2$, or temperature. Access also can be used for microdialysis. Alternatively, the probes may be tunneled and positioned locally in the penumbra of a lesion after intracranial surgery.

METHODOLOGIC CONSIDERATIONS

Introduction of any catheter into tissue causes some local damage. Minimal local damage and unchanged diffusion of oxygen toward the catheter were demonstrated for $PbtO_2$ sensors.[70,71] Small microhemorrhages were observed around the catheter tip. The position of the catheter should be controlled by computed tomographic examination, and the catheter should be tested by determining whether there is an increase in $PbtO_2$ in response to a brief increase in the fraction of inspired oxygen (FIO_2).

In a study of 101 patients with traumatic brain injury, van den Brink and coworkers[67] reported a mean zero display error of 0.42 ± 0.85 mm Hg and a room air error of $0 \pm 6\%$. No adverse events or complications related to monitoring were observed. Dings and associates[68] reported a mean zero display error of 1.4 ± 1.3 mm Hg and a room air error of $-6.9 \pm 13.2\%$ using 118 Licox catheters in 101 patients. These authors detected small iatrogenic hematomas in two patients (1.7%). The infection rate was zero.

Physiologic determinants of $PbtO_2$ include the number, diameter, and spatial distribution of capillaries in the local microvasculature. Tissue oxygenation results from diffusion at the capillary interface as well as from direct diffusion to cells along the vessels.[72,73] Measured oxygen tension values are influenced by vascular diameter and the degree of functional shunting. At increased arterial oxygen tension values, these factors may bias the electrode toward higher values.[72] Additionally, measured values may be influenced by the relative contributions of gray versus white matter and by contused or infarcted tissue in the vicinity.[67,68,71,74-76] Interpretation of absolute critical threshold values should be based on changes over time.

BRAIN TISSUE OXYGEN TENSION VALUES

The normal value for $PbtO_2$ is 20 to 40 mm Hg, and $PbtO_2$ is critically low if the value is 8 to 10 mm Hg.[77-80] Hoffman and colleagues[69] found the $PbtO_2$ in patients with ischemia by single photon emission computed tomography (SPECT) scanning to average 10 ± 5 mm Hg, compared with 37 ± 12 mm Hg in normal brain. Valadka and associates[81] found that the likelihood of death after a severe head injury increased with increasing duration of time with a $PbtO_2$ less than 15 mm Hg, and with any occurrence of a $PbtO_2$ less than 6 mm Hg. Kiening and colleagues[82] correlated serial measurements of both $SjvO_2$ and $PbtO_2$ and found that an $SjvO_2$ of 50% tended to correspond to a $PbtO_2$ of 8.5 mm Hg.

CLINICAL APPLICATIONS

Head Injury

PbtO$_2$ monitoring is probably most frequently performed as part of the management of traumatic brain injury.[67,81-87] Low PbtO$_2$ values have been reported in more than 50% of patients during the first 24 hours after injury. The most critical period appears to be the first 8 to 12 hours, a finding that is consistent with results of CBF studies. Depth and duration of tissue hypoxia in traumatic brain injury are related to outcome and are independent predictors of both unfavorable outcome and death.[67,81,82,88] The likelihood of death increases with increasing duration of PbtO$_2$ values lower than 15 mm Hg. A PbtO$_2$ value of 10 to 15 mm Hg is currently accepted as the critical limit in traumatic brain injury. It is necessary to point out that measured values are influenced by the technology used and by heterogeneity of tissue oxygenation.

Subarachnoid Hemorrhage

The relationship between depth of tissue hypoxia and severity of hemorrhage has been documented in patients with aneurysmal subarachnoid hemorrhage.[89-91] Placement of the oxygen tension probe in the area of the brain most likely to be involved in cerebral vasospasm after subarachnoid hemorrhage may provide useful information for guiding hypervolemic, hypertensive therapy.[92]

Other Acute Neurologic Disorders

PbtO$_2$ measurements have been used for the management of primary and secondary brain tumors, arteriovenous malformations, and stroke. There is considerably less experience with PbtO$_2$ monitoring in these situations than in brain trauma. Low oxygen tension was documented in areas adjacent to gliomas and metastatic lesions.[93,94] Decreased baseline tissue oxygenation values, decreased oxygen reactivity, and increased carbon dioxide reactivity have been reported in patients undergoing an operation for an arteriovenous malformation.[95,96]

SUMMARY

Continuous measurement of cerebral oxygenation with an intraparenchymally introduced oxygen sensor is a technically reliable, clinically applicable, and safe technique.

Stabilization of the probe tissue interface can be obtained within a maximum of 2 hours after placement of the catheter. Opinions vary as to whether monitoring should be performed in a relatively undamaged part of the brain, in which case information is provided on the more global balance between oxygen delivery and demand in the brain tissue, or in the penumbra of an intracranial lesion or vascular territory. Advocates of the latter option emphasize the importance of saving potentially viable tissue.

CONCLUSION

Implementation of jugular oximetry or brain tissue oxygen tension monitoring into a treatment protocol must be based on adequate knowledge of the method. The major consideration is whether to use a local sensor or more global monitoring. This decision must be based on an assessment of the heterogeneity of the brain injury. If the injury is diffuse, then a global monitor, such as a SjvO$_2$ catheter, should suffice. If significant regional pathology exists, then a PbtO$_2$ monitor may be useful as a local monitor near the hypoperfused area.

ANNOTATED REFERENCES

Dings J, Meixensberger J, Jager A, et al: Clinical experience with 118 brain tissue oxygen partial pressure catheter probes. Neurosurgery 1998;43:1082-1095.

In this study, the authors documented that PbtO$_2$ monitoring is a safe and reliable technique for monitoring cerebral oxygenation. Excluding the first hour after insertion, data are reliable, with almost 100% good data quality.

Gopinath SP, Robertson CS, Contant CF, et al: Jugular venous desaturation and outcome after head injury. Psychiatry 1994;57:717-723.

The percentage of patients with a poor neurologic outcome was 90% in patients with multiple episodes of desaturation and 74% in those with one desaturation, compared to 55% in patients with no episodes of desaturation.

Kiening KL, Hartl R, Unterberg AW, et al: Brain tissue pO$_2$-monitoring in comatose patients: Implications for therapy. Neurol Res 1997;19:233-240.

The authors concluded that a cerebral perfusion pressure greater than 60 mm Hg emerged as the most important factor determining sufficient brain tissue oxygen tension. Any intervention used to further elevate cerebral perfusion pressure did not improve PbtO$_2$; to the contrary, hyperventilation even bore the risk of inducing brain ischemia.

Robertson CS, Narayan RK, Gokaslan Z, et al: Cerebral arteriovenous oxygen difference as an estimate of cerebral blood flow in comatose patients. J Neurosurg 1989;70:222-230.

These studies suggest that reliable estimates of CBF may be made from AVDO$_2$ and arteriovenous difference of lactate (AVjDL) measurements, which can easily be obtained in the intensive care unit.

Chapter 224

INTRACRANIAL PRESSURE MONITORING

Sarice L. Bassin • Thomas P. Bleck

KEY POINTS

1. The risk of a hemorrhagic complication from placement of an intracranial pressure (ICP) monitor ranges from approximately 0.5% to 10%, depending on monitor type. The risk of hemorrhage increases dramatically with coagulopathy. Therefore, all patients should be screened for bleeding abnormalities and the abnormalities corrected prior to placement of an intracranial device.

2. The rate of infection associated with ICP monitors correlates with duration of placement, the presence of a cerebrospinal fluid leak, and concurrent systemic infection. The utility of prophylactic antibiotics and daily surveillance of cerebrospinal fluid cultures is highly controversial.

3. Meticulous care must be taken to ensure that pressure monitors are properly zeroed. External ventricular drains are fluid-coupled to an external transducer, which must be kept at the level of the external auditory meatus at all times. Fiberoptic or strain-gauge pressure monitors are not fluid-coupled; therefore, they are zeroed prior to insertion into the intracranial compartment and not affected by patient position or bed height.

Intracranial pressure (ICP) monitoring is a fundamental element of care for many patients in the ICU, including those with traumatic brain injury, subarachnoid hemorrhage, and hepatic encephalopathy. Although only clinicians with special training should place the device used to monitor ICP, all critical care specialists should be familiar with the benefits and limitations of various techniques of ICP monitoring.

There are two major complications associated with monitor placement: bleeding and infection. The incidence of complications varies depending on the type of monitor. The incidence of intracranial hemorrhage is 0.5% to 10% after placement of a fiberoptic probe[1-4] and is approximately 1% to 6% after placement of an intraventricular drain.[1,4] Coagulopathic patients are at increased risk of complications due to bleeding[1]; therefore, all patients should be screened for coagulopathy, and clotting abnormalities should be corrected prior to placement of any intracranial device. Although data from several studies indicate that intraventricular monitors are associated with a higher risk of infection than intraparenchymal monitors, these results are probably due in part to factors other than the catheter itself.[1,5-7] The rate of infection correlates with duration of placement,

the presence of a cerebrospinal fluid leak, and concurrent systemic infection.[1,5,8-10] The utility of prophylactic antibiotics and daily surveillance of cerebrospinal fluid cultures is highly controversial.[5,11,12]

Monitoring of the ICP by ventriculostomy is widely accepted as the gold standard. In addition to the diagnostic data provided, ventriculostomy permits periodic drainage of cerebrospinal fluid, a treatment that can be used to help manage intracranial hypertension. There are two approaches for placement: frontal or posterior. For placement of a frontal ventriculostomy, the patient is positioned supine with the head of the bed raised to approximately 20 degrees. The appropriate areas on the hemicranium ipsilateral to the entry point and the contralateral frontal region are shaved or clipped.

The entry point, which is located in the superiorly directed midpupillary line, 3 cm lateral to the sagittal suture and 2 cm anterior to the coronal suture on the right, should be marked on the scalp with a pen and ruler (Fig. 224-1). This is the most commonly chosen site because it sits anterior to the motor strip, is lateral to both the superior sagittal sinus and the large bridging veins, and is on the nondominant

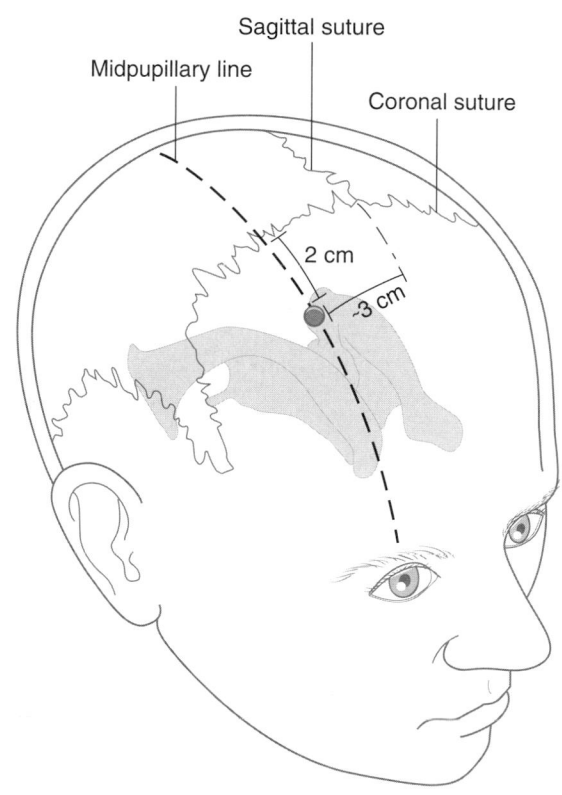

FIGURE 224–1. Landmarks used for frontal ventricular catheter placement.

hemisphere in most patients. However, the standard landmarks may not be reliable in patients with mass lesions due to distortion and shift of the ventricles. For this reason, all patients should receive a radiographic scan of the brain prior to insertion of any pressure-monitoring device.

The shaved area is prepared with chlorhexidine-alcohol solution and covered with a clear drape. The rest of the patient's body is covered with a full-length drape. The operator and assistant should wear gowns, gloves, masks, and head covers. One percent lidocaine solution is injected into the skin and subcutaneous tissue at the planned entry site, and a 1-cm incision is made with the scalpel and taken down to the bone. A hand-held twist drill is held perpendicular to the skull to make a burr hole. The operator must take care during the drilling not to plunge into the brain parenchyma. Once the burr hole is irrigated, a spinal needle is inserted through the dura to verify that the incision is large enough to accommodate the catheter.

The ventricular catheter with stylet in place is advanced through the burr hole perpendicular to the brain parenchyma. The first pass should be attempted with the tip of the catheter aimed toward the inner canthus of the ipsilateral eye. The catheter is inserted to a depth of approximately 6 cm to enter the frontal horn of the lateral ventricle. If cerebrospinal fluid is encountered before a depth of 6 cm, the stylet should be withdrawn and the catheter advanced the remaining distance. If cerebrospinal fluid flow is not obtained at 6 cm, additional passes can be made. The catheter should be removed, flushed, and then reinserted with the stylet in place. For the next attempt, the catheter tip usually should be directed more medially (i.e., toward the bridge of the nose or the inner canthus of the contralateral eye).

The external end of the catheter should be tunneled under the scalp to exit through a separate incision approximately 5 to 6 cm from the entry point. The distal end of the catheter should be connected to an adapter, which is attached to a pressure transducer and/or drainage system. The incision wound should be closed with sutures and the catheter secured to the scalp with nylon suture. A sterile, nonocclusive dressing should be applied to minimize the risk of infection.

Using the posterior approach, the patient is either prone or positioned with a shoulder roll under the ipsilateral shoulder and the head turned to the contralateral shoulder. The entry point is 6 cm from the inion and 3 cm lateral to midline. The ventricular catheter and stylet are passed through the burr hole with the tip aimed toward center of the forehead and advanced to a depth of 6 cm. When CSF flow is encountered, the stylet is held in place and the catheter alone is advanced to a depth of 8 to 12 cm. The same sterile technique described above for the frontal approach should be employed again. A posteriorly placed catheter should also be tunneled under the scalp.

Meticulous care must be employed to ensure reliable ventricular catheter measurements. Since the pressure transducer is zeroed at the level of the external auditory meatus, if the height of the bed or position of the head changes, the transducer needs to be adjusted accordingly. Furthermore, air bubbles, blood clots, or other material can occlude the tubing, leading to inaccurate measurements and making drainage of cerebrospinal fluid problematic. Examination of a well-functioning catheter should reveal pulsations correlating with the patient's pulse in the cerebrospinal fluid column.

Monitoring of the ICP from the subarachnoid space can be performed using a subarachnoid bolt. The device is inserted using the same location and technique described above for burr hole placement. Once the burr hole is drilled, the dura and arachnoid are opened, and the threaded bolt is screwed into the skull. Continuous fluid coupling between the subarachnoid space and an external pressure transducer is recorded through rigid tubing that is attached to the top of the bolt. The main drawback of this system is that swollen parenchyma or a dural flap can occlude the lumen of the bolt, giving erroneous readings.

Several companies manufacture non-fluid-coupled ICP monitors. Pressure measurements are made from either a microchip pressure sensor at the tip of a flexible nylon cable (Codman) or a fiberoptic sensor (Camino). The placement and tunneling of the device is similar to that of a ventriculostomy, but the depth of insertion depends on the compartment being monitored (subdural space, parenchyma, or ventricular system). The device permits continuous monitoring of the ICP in the compartment in which the tip of the probe is placed. Because the fiberoptic monitor does not use a hydrostatic zero level, pressure measurements are not affected by changes in patient position or bed height. The major limitation of the strain gauge and fiberoptic monitors is that zeroing takes place before the transducer is inserted into the skull. Therefore, rezeroing cannot be performed once the monitor is installed. Recalibration after initial implantation, even using sterile technique, is strongly discouraged. Drift is an inherent property of both the miniature strain gauge and fiberoptic ICP monitors, raising concerns about the possibility of over- or underestimating ICP. Evaluation of the strain gauge transducer measured an average drift of 0.2 ± 0.5 mm Hg.[13] The drift of fiberoptic transducers has been reported to average 0.6 to 2 mm Hg/day.[13,14] Over several days, this amount of drift could become clinically significant. For this reason, some authors recommend placing a new fiberoptic catheter if use is prolonged (greater than 5 to 7 days).[1,3] Many of these devices are compatible with magnetic resonance imaging, as long as the extracranial portion of the catheter is not coiled when it is secured to the scalp.

ANNOTATED REFERENCES

Hader WJ, Steinbok P: The value of routine cultures of the cerebrospinal fluid in patients with external ventricular drains. Neurosurgery 2000; 46:1149-1153.

This retrospective analysis of 157 patients from a pediatric neurosurgical center found that routine daily cultures failed to identify catheter-related infections before clinical changes occurred. All infected patients had fever and peripheral leukocytosis on the day the infection was identified, and one had a change in cerebrospinal fluid appearance.

Lyke KE, Obasanjo OO, Williams MA, et al: Ventriculitis complicating use of intraventricular catheters in adult neurosurgical patients. Clin Infect Dis 2001;33:2028-2033.

A prospective analysis of ventriculostomy-related infections in 157 patients found an infection rate of 5.6%. Risk factors for intraventricular catheter–related infection included length of intraventricular catheter placement and cerebrospinal fluid leakage near the intraventricular catheter.

Zabramski JM, Whiting D, Darouiche RO, et al: Efficacy of antimicrobial-impregnated external ventricular drain catheters: A prospective, randomized, controlled trial. J Neurosurg 2003;98:725-730.

This prospective, randomized, multicenter trial examined the efficacy of external ventricular drain catheters impregnated with minocycline and rifampin in preventing catheter-related infections. The antibiotic-impregnated catheters were about 50% less likely to become colonized than the control catheters, and positive cerebrospinal fluid cultures were seven times less frequent in patients with antibiotic-impregnated catheters than in those in the control group. Variables associated with an increased likelihood of catheter-related cerebrospinal fluid infection included placement of the catheter in the emergency room and presence of other infection.

Chapter 225

INDIRECT CALORIMETRY AND METABOLIC MONITORING

Pierre Singer • Jonathan D. Cohen

KEY POINTS

1. Bedside indirect calorimetry can be proposed to critically ill patients in the following conditions: fractional inspired oxygen less than 0.65, hemodynamic and respiratory stability for at least 10 minutes, and no air leak (deflated cuff, chest drains).

2. **Negative energy expenditure is associated with increased morbidity.**

3. No available equation is adequate to predict resting energy expenditure. **Avoiding negative energy balance is achieved by daily measurements of resting energy expenditure and nutritional intake. Nutrient administration can be tailored.**

4. Measurements of oxygen consumption (VO_2) can diagnose sepsis, evaluate efficacy of sedation, and assess efficacy of fluid therapy.

5. Metabolic monitors should be adequately calibrated before use.

Awareness is increasing of the importance of nutrition in the management of critically ill patients. However, adequate nutritional support is rarely achieved in daily practice. The administration of parenteral nutrition is often associated with overfeeding, resulting in hyperglycemia and other complications.[1,2] Overfeeding also can promote inflammation and infections, liver function abnormalities, and carbon dioxide retention.[3] On the other hand, administration of enteral feeding is often associated with gastric intolerance.[4] High gastric residuals may lead to reflux, emesis and aspiration, abdominal distention, and diarrhea.[5] The result is frequent interruptions of feeding and undernutrition that can lead to an increase in complications and higher mortality, especially among patients at risk for multiple organ failure.[6] In view of these considerations, it is important to individualize nutritional support according to each patient's particular requirements. However, this task is one of the most difficult in the management of critically ill patients, because energy requirements are dependent on multiple factors.[7] As an example, consider burn victims. In the 1980s, energy expenditure and requirements in burn victims were reported by Elwyn and colleagues[8] to be markedly elevated, and their recommendations for feeding were widely reproduced in textbooks. However, by providing adequate analgesia, carrying out early excision and skin grafting, and preventing sepsis, modern clinical care of burns has decreased reported measurements of resting energy expenditure (REE) in patients with the same burn surface area.[9]

MEASUREMENT OF RESTING ENERGY REQUIREMENTS

INADEQUACY OF PREDICTING FORMULAS

Since the beginning of the last century, the Harris-Benedict equation has been used to predict REE on the basis of anthropometric parameters.[10] However, the weight of the patient influences the reliability of the formula. Recent studies of young, healthy women have shown that REE is best predicted by the Owen equation for subjects of normal weight, whereas the Bernstein equation is preferred for overweight subjects and the Robertson and Reid equations are most predictive for obese subjects.[11] In a study of critically ill patients, MacDonald and associates[12] compared REE estimates based on five different published equations with results obtained by indirect calorimetry over 24 hours.[12] Patients were divided into two groups, those with a body mass index of less than 25 kg/m^2 and those with a body mass index of less than 30 kg/m.^{2} These authors showed that the Frankenfield equation overestimated energy needs, whereas the Penn State and Ireton-Jones equations underestimated energy needs. The Harris-Benedict equation, multiplied by a stress factor of 1.6, predicted REE within 20% of the value obtained with the use of indirect calorimetry 80% of the time. The authors concluded that none of the equations predicted REE accurately in all patients all of the time. Most of the equations were more accurate at the lower range of basal metabolic index. In children, standard equations fail to accurately predict measured energy expenditure, which has led investigators to devise new predictive formulas.[13]

IMPORTANCE OF ACCURATE MEASUREMENT

The accuracy and precision of indirect calorimetry were evaluated by Wells and Fuller in 1998.[14] Some of the metabolic monitors tested had coefficients of variation of less than 1%, and accuracy within 3% for oxygen consumption (VO_2), carbon dioxide production (VCO_2), and REE. However, many factors can affect the accuracy of indirect calorimetric measurements. Small errors in the measurement of expired gas volumes can produce large errors in calculated values; therefore, it is crucial to detect and eliminate all leaks. This issue is of particular concern if high airway pressures are being used. In addition, high concentrations of inspired oxygen (fractional inspired oxygen [FIO_2] greater than 0.6)

TABLE 225–1. PARAMETERS THAT MODIFY RESTING ENERGY EXPENDITURE (REE)

Factors that Increase REE	% Change	Factors that Decrease REE	% Change
Body size	—	Age >18 y	—
Fever	13% per degree of increase	Hypothermia	13% per degree of decrease
Shivering	100%	—	—
Work of breathing	Up to 25%	Adapted ventilation	15%
Pain, stress, visits	—	Sedation	50%
Chest physiotherapy	—	—	—
Sepsis	—	Multiorgan failure	—
Nutrition	9- 22%	Starvation	10%
Dobutamine	—	β-Blockers	—

can render measurements invalid. Calculation of the respiratory quotient can act as a quality control tool.[15] If the value for respiratory quotient is out of the normal range (i.e., 0.65 to 1.15), then the measurement should be considered invalid.

INDIRECT CALORIMETRY: TECHNIQUES AND CONTINUOUS MEASUREMENT

The period of measurement required to provide accurate information varies in the literature. Smyrnios and associates[16] compared results obtained by making multiple measurements over 30-minute periods (341 30-minute intervals) with the results obtained by averaging data obtained over a 24-hour period of observation.[16] The mean difference was 0 ± 209 kCal/day. The values obtained from the 30-minute studies were within 20% of the values obtained from the 24-hour measurements for 90% of the intervals. It appears, therefore, that 30-minute measurements are acceptable. Cunningham and colleagues[17] reduced the measurement period even further and showed that the difference between a short (5-minute) and a longer (31-minute) measurement interval was less than 5% in 42 of 47 patients in intensive care units (ICUs).[17] The difference was greater than 10% in only 2 patients. These investigators concluded that a 5-minute period of measurement was sufficient if variations during that interval were less than 5%. Greater minute-to-minute variability mandates a longer period of measurement. These findings have been confirmed by others.[18] McClave and coworkers[19] compared measurements obtained during a short-term "snapshot" REE measurement and a 24-hour measurement of total energy expenditure. Periods of steady state were defined by episodes when VO_2 or VCO_2 varied by less than 10%. The coefficient of variation was calculated, and for the unstable patients this parameter was helpful in determining the necessary duration of measurement.

Continuous monitoring has been developed and compared with a standard metabolic monitor.[20] Limits of agreement were wide: -13 ± 30 mL/minute for VCO_2 and -7 ± 50 mL/minute for VO_2 at $FIO_2 = 0.3$. When FIO_2 was increased, these limits of agreement were even worse, especially for VO_2. Using the standard deviation of measurements made over time within individual patients as a measure of reproducibility, the authors found that the continuous system was more reliable at high FIO_2 values, whereas at lower FIO_2 values noncontinuous monitoring using the Deltatrac device (Datex-Ohmeda, Helsinki, Finland) was superior.

There is a large amount of day-to-day variability in energy expenditure.[21] In a study of 60 mechanically ventilated, critically ill patients assessed over 2- to 7-day periods, day-to-day variation was very large and was significantly ($P < .001$) influenced by temperature, but not by illness severity

score (Table 225-1). Day-to-day differences can be as great as 35%. Accordingly, accurate energy balance assessments depend on daily metabolic measurements.

VALUE OF ENERGY BALANCE

Only a few prospective, randomized studies have evaluated the effects of energy balance on outcome. In a prospective trial of 67 ICU patients carried out by Mault and associates,[22] a control group received nutritional support according to predictive equations, and an experimental group had nutritional support guided by indirect calorimetry measurements. In this study, a negative energy balance in excess of 10,000 kCal was associated with a longer duration of mechanical ventilation and a longer ICU stay. Another study in a nursing care center showed a correlation between cumulative negative energy balance and the development of pressure sores ($P = .08$, $r = -.064$).[23]

Our group prospectively measured daily energy expenditure using indirect calorimetry in 50 critically ill patients and related morbidity and mortality to the energy balance derived by the difference between REE and caloric intake.[24] A computerized bedside information system enabled precise calculation of caloric intake from both enteral sources (usually nasogastric feeding) and parenteral sources (usually dextrose-containing fluids). The mean cumulative energy balance was -4747 kCal (range, $+4747$ to $-17,274$ kCal) over a mean period of 12 days (range, 5 to 44 days). Although energy balance and mortality were not correlated, negative energy balance was strongly correlated with the incidence of complications ($r = -.76$, $P < .001$; Fig. 225-1). The main

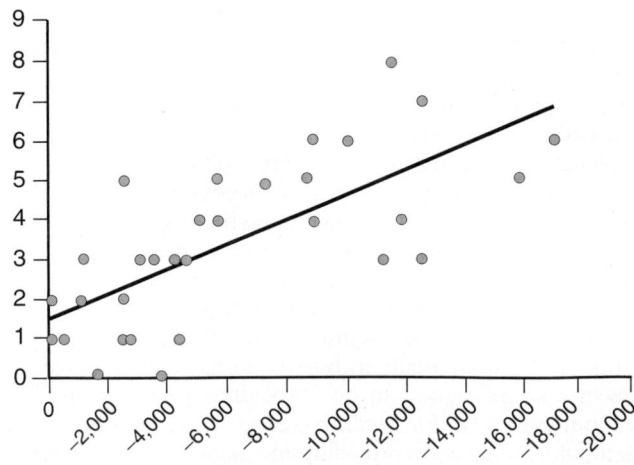

FIGURE 225–1. Correlation between negative calorie balance and number of complications.

complication associated with negative energy balance was renal failure. Other complications included acute respiratory distress syndrome, sepsis, hemodynamic instability, and pressure sores. Barlett and coworkers[6] reported that a cumulative negative energy balance of less than 10,000 kCal during ICU hospitalization was associated with a mortality rate greater than 80%, compared with a mortality rate of 20% among patients with a positive cumulative energy balance.[6]

Although the gastrointestinal tract is the preferred route for providing nutrition,[25,26] enterally fed patients in the ICU are often significantly underfed,[27] and enteral feeding may be associated with appreciable morbidity. In such cases, parenteral nutrition has been used to supplement enteral feeding, and the two therapies should not be regarded as being mutually exclusive.[28] Combined therapy may lead to faster recovery.[29] Indirect calorimetry is an excellent tool to avoid overfeeding and ensure appropriate energy balance in these patients. We suggest that efforts made to achieve accurate measurements using indirect calorimetry should be matched by equal efforts to meet energy and protein requirements with aggressive nutritional support. More studies are still required to provide convincing proof that this strategy can truly improve outcome.[30]

METABOLIC MONITORING IN VARIOUS CLINICAL CONDITIONS

In conditions of stress, defined by the systemic inflammatory response syndrome (SIRS), REE and VO_2 are higher than under control conditions.[31] REE and VO_2 are even greater in patients with sepsis or after trauma.[32,33] However, REE decreases in patients with septic shock[34] and is lower in patients with multiple organ dysfunction syndrome (MODS) who ultimately die, compared with patients with MODS who ultimately survive (Fig. 225-2).[35] Additional studies using serial measurements of REE and VO_2 over time are still needed to adequately characterize the metabolic response to critical illness.[36] Sepsis can increase energy expenditure through sympathetic stimulation, increased temperature, and increased motor activity. REE also can be increased by nutrition through the thermic effect of food. In addition, mitochondrial uncoupling and inefficient metabolism can increase energy demand. On the other hand, hypothermia, starvation, sedation, and decreased level of consciousness can decrease REE (see Table 225-1).

Hayes and colleagues[37] studied patients with sepsis syndrome or septic shock who received fluids and norepinephrine, with or without dobutamine, titrated to cardiac index and oxygen consumption. These investigators showed that non-survivors had reduced cardiac reserve, failed to increase VO_2 after resuscitation, and manifested decreased oxygen extraction after aggressive inotropic support. These observations prompted Kelly[38] to suggest that increasing oxygen delivery and VO_2 may improve outcome. A recent study by Rivers and associates[39] suggested that resuscitating patients with severe sepsis in the emergency department to increase mixed venous oxygen saturation (but not VO_2) improves survival.[39]

In children, metabolic monitors appear to be very accurate even for low levels of VO_2 and VCO_2 during mechanical ventilation. However, as noted earlier, an increase in the standard deviation for VO_2 measurements is observed as FIO_2 increases up to 0.55.[40] Puhakka and coworkers[41] described the metabolic response to stress during recovery from cardiac operations for patients with various congenital heart defects. A minimal response to stress was observed, limited to changes in temperature. Our group studied REE and VO_2 before and after surgery in cyanotic and noncyanotic children with congenital heart disease.[42] REE and VO_2 were similar before and after surgery in both groups, showing that the partial pressure of oxygen (PaO_2) was not a major determinant of VO_2. In mechanically ventilated children, any endotracheal tube leak can lead to large errors, and a modification to the technique should be used when assessing the expired gas lost.[43]

In brain-dead patients, VO_2 and REE are $25 \pm 9\%$ lower than the basal metabolic rate.[44] In contrast, head trauma patients have increased REE, being $21 \pm 11\%$ greater than the basal metabolic rate. Serial studies using transcranial Doppler measurements and indirect calorimetry have revealed a significant correlation between REE and cerebral blood flow ($r = -0.77$, $P < .0001$). It seems that REE is related to cerebral metabolism and not to hypothermia in these patients.

CONCLUSIONS

Many diseases, such as sepsis or burn injury, significantly increase energy expenditure in critically ill patients, whereas other interventions (sedation, hypothermia, administration of β-blockers) can decrease the metabolic response. The only way to provide adequate nutritional support is to measure energy expenditure by indirect calorimetry. This technique allows caregivers to administer adequate energy supplies while avoiding overnutrition or undernutrition that can affect outcome.

ANNOTATED REFERENCES

MacDonald A, Hildebrandt L: Comparison of formulaic equations to determine energy expenditure in the critically ill patient. Nutrition 2003;19:233-239.
> *This paper summarizes the various equations available for predicting REE in critically ill patients and shows their limitations.*

MacLellan S, Walsh T, Burdess A, Lee A: Comparison between the Datex-Ohmeda M-COVX metabolic monitor and the Deltatrac II in mechanically ventilated patients. Intensive Care Med 2002;28:870-876.
> *This is an in vivo study on the accuracy and bias of a continuous metabolic monitor compared with the gold standard measurement tool.*

Moriyama S, Okamoto K, Tabira Y, et al: Evaluation of oxygen consumption and resting energy expenditure in critically ill patients with systemic inflammatory response syndrome. Crit Care Med 1999;27:2133-2136.
> *This paper presents the variations of VO_2 and REE from SIRS to sepsis, severe sepsis, septic shock, and multiorgan failure.*

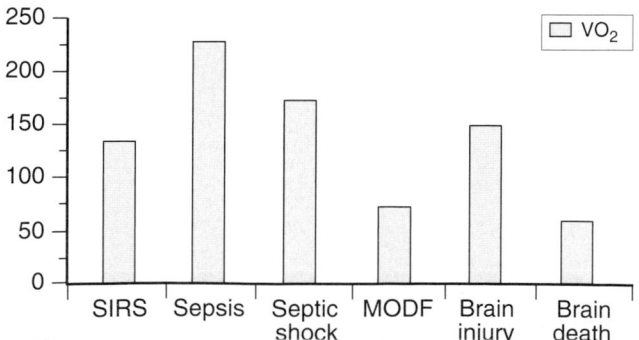

FIGURE 225–2. Oxygen consumption (in milliliters per minute per kilogram body weight) in critically ill patients according to clinical conditions. (Data from references 32 through 36.)

Chapter 226

CANNULATION FOR EXTRACORPOREAL MEMBRANE OXYGENATION

Kenneth R. McCurry • M. Charlene Fabrizio

KEY POINTS

1. **Extracorporeal membrane oxygenation** (ECMO), or **extracorporeal life support** (ECLS), as it is also known, is now a widely applied therapy in the intensive care unit for a variety of cardiac and respiratory ailments.

2. The **cannulation requirements for ECLS** depend on the type of ECLS support used, venoarterial or venovenous, and the manner in which it is applied.

3. Under circumstances of adequate preload, the **main determinant of circuit flow**, and hence the ability to adequately support the patient, is the resistance to flow through the venous drainage cannula.

4. The **resistance to flow through a cannula** is directly proportional to the length of the cannula and inversely proportional to the fourth power of the internal luminal radius.

5. **Modern wire-reinforced cannulas** have superior hemodynamics than older cannulas due to the thinner wall construction and the resulting greater ratio of internal luminal to outer luminal diameter.

6. Adequately sized wire-reinforced cannulas for ECLS can be safely inserted with the use of percutaneous techniques, but this **should be performed only by surgeons experienced with vascular techniques,** because life-threatening complications can occur.

Extracorporeal life support (ECLS), or extracorporeal membrane oxygenation (ECMO), as it is also known, has become an accepted management technique for neonatal, pediatric, and adult patients with cardiac or pulmonary failure of various causes.[1-3] ECLS is used to support neonatal patients with respiratory failure, adult and pediatric patients with postcardiotomy failure, and adult and pediatric patients with primary respiratory failure. It also is used as a resuscitative measure for patients in cardiac arrest, as a bridge to heart or lung transplantation, and for management of lung or heart transplant graft dysfunction after transplantation, in addition to other indications. At its core, ECLS involves the use of a modified heart-lung machine to support cardiac, pulmonary, or cardiopulmonary function (depending on

sites of cannulation and form used) while management strategies are directed at improving cardiac and respiratory function. The technique requires insertion of large-bore venous or venous plus arterial cannulas to drain and return blood to the patient. The type of support needed dictates the requirements for cannulation (see later discussion), and the circumstances and ease of access dictate whether intrathoracic (primarily for postcardiotomy support in the operating room) or extrathoracic cannulation is used. The indications for ECLS and management strategies are discussed elsewhere in this text. This chapter focuses on peripheral cannulation strategies and techniques that can be achieved in the intensive care unit and discusses the authors' preferred circuit for ECLS support and its components.

FORMS OF EXTRACORPOREAL LIFE SUPPORT

ECLS/ECMO involves the use of modified cardiopulmonary bypass in venoarterial or venovenous forms (Table 226-1). There are two types of venovenous support. The first traditionally has been called venovenous (VV) ECLS, and the second has been termed extracorporeal carbon dioxide removal (ECCO$_2$R). Table 226-1 outlines the differences between these forms of extracorporeal support. They differ in the type of support provided (gas exchange only or gas exchange and cardiac support) and in the quantity of desired gas exchange achieved by the circuit.

Venoarterial (VA) ECLS provides both cardiac and pulmonary support and is generally reserved for patients with primary cardiac dysfunction (after cardiotomy, myocardial infarction, or cardiac arrest) and those with respiratory failure and associated hemodynamic instability. VA ECLS requires placement of cannulas for both venous drainage and return of blood to the arterial system. Because total or near-total hemodynamic support is usually necessary, adequate venous drainage is needed to achieve the required flow rate (i.e., 80% to 100% of normal cardiac output). In general, venous access is achieved via a femoral vein. If greater venous drainage is needed than can be achieved with a single femoral venous cannula, a second cannula may be inserted in the internal jugular vein (usually the right) and connected by a "Y" connector to the femoral venous line. Although arterial access in neonates is commonly achieved by cannulation of the common carotid artery, in adults it can be achieved via cannulation of a femoral artery or the right common carotid artery.

TABLE 226–1. COMPARISON OF VARIOUS FORMS OF ADULT EXTRACORPOREAL LIFE SUPPORT (ECLS)

	Venoarterial ECLS	Venovenous ECLS	Extracorporeal carbon dioxide removal
Type of support	Cardiac and pulmonary	Pulmonary	Pulmonary
Goal for circuit	Up to full cardiac and respiratory support as necessary	Near-total pulmonary support (CO_2 and O_2)	Removal of CO_2 (oxygenation achieved through native lungs)
Circuit flow	High (80-100% of cardiac output)	High (80-100 mL/kg/min)	Medium (20-30% of cardiac output)
Cannulation sites	Venous: femoral, internal, jugular, saphenous, or combinations Arterial: femoral artery most common in adults	Femoral, internal jugular, saphenous, or combinations	Femoral, internal jugular, saphenous, or combinations

For most patients with respiratory failure necessitating ECLS, VV support is the preferred methodology. The techniques used include VV-ECLS and $ECCO_2R$. Although both techniques drain blood from the venous system and return blood to the venous system, they differ in the strategy used to achieve gas exchange (see Table 226-1). VV-ECLS uses a strategy of high mass transport of oxygen and carbon dioxide through the circuit and therefore requires little gas exchange through the patient's own lungs. VV-ECLS is inherently inefficient, because oxygenated blood mixes with deoxygenated blood (i.e., there is recirculation). For this reason, some gas exchange by the lungs is frequently necessary (although this goal typically can be achieved with the ventilator set to provide relatively low tidal volumes at relative low rates, thus minimizing barotrauma). To achieve the goal of VV-ECLS, the flow rate through the circuit typically is 80 to 100 mL/kg/minute. For infants and small children, VV-ECLS can be accomplished through a double-lumen cannula[4] or a single-lumen catheter using tidal flow[5] inserted into the jugular vein. Larger children and adults require access to at least two major veins. Frequently, adequate drainage can be achieved via a single cannula, assuming resistance to flow is low enough (see later discussion), with inflow through a second cannulation site. The most common combination of sites is a jugular and a femoral vein (see later discussion).

In contrast to VV-ECLS, the goal of $ECCO_2R$ is removal of carbon dioxide via the circuit, with the majority of oxygen exchange occurring via the native lungs.[6] Carbon dioxide removal is achieved with a much lower circuit flow rate (approximately 1 L/minute) than is required for VV-ECLS. Arterial oxygenation is achieved by mechanical ventilation using high positive end-expiratory pressure (PEEP) and low frequency (i.e., a lung-protective strategy). Vascular access requires cannulation of two veins, although, because of the lower flow requirements, there is less concern about inserting large enough cannulas (see Table 226-1). Common cannulation sites are similar to those used for VV-ECLS.

TECHNICAL CONSIDERATIONS

CANNULA RESISTANCE AND SIZE

An ECLS circuit is a modified, closed cardiopulmonary bypass circuit consisting of drainage and return vascular access cannulas, circuit tubing, an oxygenator (hollow fiber or membrane), a pump (usually roller or centrifugal), and a heat exchanger. The flow that is achievable through a circuit is a function of both patient-related and circuit-dependent factors. The most important patient-related factor is the

patient's intravascular volume status or cardiac preload. Inadequate preload leads to diminished circuit flow as a result of decreased venous return to the pump. This is a dynamic variable that can be altered by infusing fluids to expand circulating volume.

In the setting of adequate preload, circuit flow is limited by the resistance to flow through the venous drainage cannula. The resistance of a cannula is directly proportional to the length of the cannula and inversely proportional to the fourth power of its internal luminal radius. Small variations in the internal luminal radius have dramatic effects on the resistance to venous drainage and greatly impact achievable flow. The length of the cannula also affects flow, but to a lesser extent. Catheter size commonly is based on external diameter. Large differences in wall thickness of the tubing used for cannula construction can result in dramatic differences in inner diameter, and consequent resistance to flow, among cannulas that are nominally "the same size." The cannulas most commonly used today are wire reinforced, which allows the cannula wall to be thinner. As a result, the inner luminal diameter is large relative to the outer luminal diameter, resulting in a lower resistance.

In an effort to standardize assessment of cannula resistance, Bartlett and coworkers[7] developed a standardized number, termed the "M-number," to designate the resistance of a cannula. The M-number is determined based on testing of pressure/flow relationships for each cannula. Based on their assessment of current wire-reinforced cannulas, flow through a 27 Fr cannula 50 cm long is equivalent to flow through a 23 Fr cannula 25 cm long when the pressure gradient across the cannula is 100 cm H_2O.[8] Each of these cannulas provides 6.5 L/minute of flow. However, such differences in diameter can have significant impact on the ease of cannula insertion, particularly if a percutaneous technique is being used (see later discussion). Therefore, when selecting a cannula size for venous drainage, one should consider the type of support and flow necessary, the type of cannula to be used and its resistance, and the patient's size (i.e., the size of the vein into which the cannula will be inserted). In most ECLS programs today, modern wire-reinforced cannulas are used exclusively because of their superior hemodynamic characteristics.

ATRIOFEMORAL VERSUS FEMOROATRIAL FLOW IN VENOVENOUS EXTRACORPOREAL LIFE SUPPORT

As described earlier, VV-ECLS is achieved by drainage and reinfusion into systemic veins (commonly the right internal jugular and common femoral systems). Accordingly, there is inherent inefficiency with VV-ECLS, because some portion of the oxygenated blood from the reinfusion cannula returns to the circuit via the drainage cannula. Traditionally, many ECLS programs placed the venous drainage cannula into the right internal jugular vein, positioning the tip of the catheter in the right atrium; reinfusion was carried out using a cannula in the femoral vein (atriofemoral flow) in a VV system.[8] The rationale for this approach was that the right atrium is a large-capacity structure that should allow greater drainage and a higher flow rate than could be achieved via drainage from the smaller common femoral vein and distal inferior vena cava (femoroatrial flow). The wisdom of this approach was questioned by Rich and colleagues at the University of Michigan.[9] Using a modified circuit that allowed them to switch between atriofemoral and femoroatrial flow, these investigators studied ECLS support provided by each flow direction in 10 patients. Their results demonstrated that femoroatrial directional flow provided higher circuit flow and higher pulmonary artery saturation; for any given value of pulmonary artery saturation, less flow was required with femoroatrial flow than with atriofemoral flow. On the basis of these data, flow in the femoroatrial direction became the preferred method of VV-ECLS support at the University of Michigan. At the University of Pittsburgh, we continue to use this strategy as well.[10]

EVOLUTION OF EXTRACORPOREAL LIFE SUPPORT CANNULATION TECHNIQUES

ECLS was first used for respiratory failure in neonates in the 1960s. In 1976, Bartlett and associates[11] described a series of neonates supported with VA-ECLS in whom cannulation involved insertion of catheters into the right internal jugular vein and common carotid artery via surgical cutdown. After recovery of pulmonary function, the cannulas were removed and the vessels ligated. In the first report of VV-ECLS, in 1979, Gattinoni and colleagues[6] described a complex method of cannulation involving surgical cutdown with proximal and distal drainage of the common femoral vein, distal drainage of the jugular vein, and reinfusion into the proximal jugular vein. The technique was difficult and time-consuming. In 1990, this same group was the first to report the technique of percutaneous placement of wire-reinforced cannulas for VV-ECLS.[12] This technique is now widely used by practitioners who are experienced in large-bore venous cannula insertion for ECLS. However, surgical cutdown using standard surgical techniques is still commonly used and should be used if percutaneous insertion is deemed to be unsafe due to anatomic constraints or if percutaneous insertion fails. Percutaneous insertion of venous cannulas is our preferred approach when it is feasible.

There are numerous advantages of percutaneous venous insertion over surgical cutdown. Following insertion via cutdown, bleeding from the wound is a common problem due to thrombocytopenia as well as the requisite anticoagulation required to prevent thrombosis in the circuit. Any bleeding that is encountered around the cannulation site after percutaneous insertion can easily be controlled with a pursestring suture. Percutaneous cannulation is generally less time-consuming than surgical cutdown, and speed is obviously advantageous when ECLS is instituted on an emergency basis. Percutaneous cannulation does not require the presence of a surgical nursing team. In addition, removal of the cannula is much easier after percutaneous cannulation. Cannula removal after cutdown insertion requires opening of the wound and surgical repair of the previously cannulated vessel, whereas removal after percutaneous insertion is accomplished by removing the cannula and then applying direct pressure over the site for 10 to 20 minutes (depending on the size of the cannula).

The largest reported series of adult patients undergoing percutaneous cannulation for VV-ECLS is from the group at the University of Michigan.[8] Their report included 94 patients and demonstrated a 94% success rate for achieving percutaneous cannulation safely. The size of the cannulas placed ranged from 19 Fr to 23 Fr. Cannulas were placed in the right internal jugular vein and in either the right or the left common femoral vein. There were three arterial injuries that required surgical cutdown for repair and one death resulting from perforation of the superior vena cava during cannulation. Only six patients (6%) had cannula site bleeding that required intervention. In all six cases, bleeding was managed with simple pursestring suture placement. Based on their experience, the team at the University of Michigan concluded that percutaneous venous cannulation for ECLS can be achieved safely but that it should be performed only by surgeons, who have the skills necessary to surgically expose and repair a vessel should an inadvertent injury occur. Our experience at the University of Pittsburgh is similar to the experience at the University of Michigan. In addition, we strongly reinforce the recommendation that this procedure should only be performed by surgeons with vascular experience. The University of Michigan group also has reported their experience with percutaneous cannulation in pediatric patients requiring VV-ECLS support, with similar results.[13]

TECHNIQUE OF PERCUTANEOUS VENOUS INSERTION

Cannulation is usually performed at the patient's bedside with the assistance of nursing staff. Percutaneous venous cannulation for ECLS is achieved with the use of a modified Seldinger technique. The right neck and the appropriate groin region are prepared and draped in a sterile fashion, and anesthesia is achieved with a local anesthetic. Unless contraindicated by immediate postoperative status, all patients receive a bolus of 5000 units of heparin (or 100 units/kg) for the cannulation procedure (percutaneous or open). The vein (femoral or jugular) is accessed at an angle of approximately 30 degrees with the skin, and the guidewire is passed through the needle. As for any percutaneous technique, the guidewire should pass unimpeded. Occasionally, the onset of cardiac ectopy provides evidence regarding the location of the wire's tip. We commonly temporarily replace the wire with an Angiocath or small dilator to verify that the access achieved is venous and not arterial. The wire is then replaced, and, using it a guide, sequentially larger dilators are passed. Manual compression of the insertion site is used to prevent excessive bleeding as the dilators are sequentially removed and reinserted. It is very important to ensure that the wire moves freely during dilatation as well as cannula insertion. Free movement of the guidewire indicates that the dilator or cannula is following the path of the wire and not kinking and taking an alternative path, such as through the vessel wall. Kinking can be prevented by gentle traction on the wire applied by an assistant as the dilator or cannula is passed. Creation of a skin incision slightly smaller than the cannula being inserted facilitates passage of the cannula while still providing good hemostasis.

Occasionally, difficulty is encountered with passage of the cannula under the inguinal ligament or through the dilated opening in the vessel wall. Redilatation with a smaller dilator can facilitate passage. Occasionally, we have passed a hemostat along the path of the wire and manually dilated the tract. This maneuver should be performed with great caution, however, and it is not recommended for the inexperienced. Chen and colleagues[14] described a similar technique using guidewire dilating forceps that were originally designed for percutaneous tracheostomy.[14] These forceps have a groove in the distal aspect to ensure that the forceps follow the path of the guidewire. It should be emphasized that if significant difficulty is encountered or a complication is suspected, percutaneous attempts should be aborted and cannulation should be achieved via surgical cutdown. After cannulation, it is important to assess cannula position by obtaining a radiograph.

We use wire-reinforced cannulas (BioMedicus, Medtronic Inc., Minneapolis, MN) that are heparin bonded (Carmedabonded [CB]) (see later discussion). As outlined earlier, an arterial BioMedicus cannula is shorter than a venous cannula. Based on Bartlett's data, a 23 Fr arterial cannula provides drainage equivalent to that of a 27 Fr venous cannula and should be easier to insert in a percutaneous fashion. In years past, we commonly used 25 Fr to 29 Fr BioMedicus venous cannulas (50 cm), advancing the tip to the right atrium. It can sometimes be difficult to insert this large cannula because of resistance encountered either at the inguinal ligament or at the site of entry into the vein. Following the lead of the University of Michigan group, we now favor a shorter arterial BioMedicus cannula (23 Fr 37 cm) for venous drainage. Smaller cannulas may be used for smaller patients.

ARTERIAL CANNULATION

Arterial cannulation, if necessary, is most often achieved via surgical cutdown. In selected large individuals, we have used a percutaneous insertion technique into a femoral vessel, placing a 19 Fr to 21 Fr arterial BioMedicus cannula. This procedure should be performed only by experienced surgeons, who can address complications if necessary.

Surgical (as well as percutaneous) insertion of arterial cannulas in the femoral artery can sometimes be complicated by malperfusion of the distal extremity. This complication may be addressed in several fashions but should be dealt with expeditiously to avoid severe injury. We prefer the insertion of a modified, cut high-pressure monitoring line (arterial line tubing) down the femoral artery of the affected limb. This can be achieved in the open wound just distal to the reinfusion cannula insertion site or, in the case of a percutaneous cannula, via an incision at a separate site. The tubing is connected to a CB 3/8 × 3/8-inch connector with a luer lock between the arterial cannula and the ECMO arterial pump tubing. An alternative method to avoid ischemia is surgical anastomosis of a graft end-to-side to the femoral artery, with cannulation of the graft.[15]

UNIVERSITY OF PITTSBURGH PREFERRED CIRCUIT SYSTEM

At the University of Pittsburgh, we prefer to use a heparin-bonded ECMO system (Medtronic Carmeda Bio-Active Surface). This system allows for a lower level of anticoagulation, which can be desirable, particularly if ECMO support is required in the postsurgical situation. This system is also easier and quicker to prime than the conventional, nonheparin-bonded Medtronic Avecor silicone membrane oxygenator.

The CB system consists of a CB Medtronic Affinity hollow-fiber oxygenator, a Medtronic CB BioMedicus BP-80 centrifugal pump, and a CB 3/8-inch flow probe, all CB 3/8-inch interior diameter and 3/32-inch wall thickness medical grade tubing, monitoring sites, and extra access sites. The only components in this system that are not heparin bonded are the Walrus high-flow stopcocks with luer-lock extensions (Medical Parameters, Woburn, MA) and the Gish pressure monitoring isolators (Gish Biomedical, Irvine, CA). These components are aspirated and flushed with saline on a timely basis to prevent formation of clots in relatively stagnant areas.

The CB system is more costly to use than a nonheparin-bonded circuit. Also, although the hollow-fiber Affinity oxygenators have plasma resistant fibers, they may become porous (depending on patient condition), leading to a plasma leak. A plasma leak results in leakage of plasma proteins into the gas phase of the oxygenator and out the oxygenator gas exit ports. Not only is this exudate a potential hazard to health care workers and the patient's visitors, but the patient's plasma protein concentration and the gas exchange capability of the oxygenator also may be adversely affected, ultimately leading to oxygenator failure. Typically, oxygenator failure is gradual, allowing for oxygenator change as the plasma leak progresses and before complete oxygenator failure.

The ECMO system is assembled using a Medtronic Portable Bypass System cart or a Sarns Per Cart (Terumo Corporation, Ann Arbor, MI), both of which are compact, portable systems. The perfusate is kept at the desired temperature with a BioCal 370 temperature controller. The Bio-Console is positioned alongside the BioCal 370 temperature controller. A compartment or drawer is available for supplies and has a separate area for two E cylinders of oxygen. A medical air/oxygen blender is placed on one of the two intravenous poles, which can also accommodate a cardiotomy reservoir if necessary. Both systems have a main power cable connected to an integrated power strip that supplies power to the pump, heater-cooler, gooseneck halogen lamp, and activated clotting time (ACT) determinant device. A Medtronic centrifugal pump external drive device and swivel bracket are used to facilitate shortening of patient lines and to aid in transport of the patient and ECMO device.

At our institution, all patients to be managed with ECMO are placed on the Carmeda oxygenator system initially. Although the purchased system comes preassembled from the manufacturer, specific modifications are made to the system. The advantage of lower heparin requirements and anticoagulation levels, especially in the presence of active bleeding, may benefit the patient. The anticoagulation levels are assessed with the use of a Hemochron Celite ACT device (International Technidyne Corporation, Edison, NJ) and are maintained greater than 180 seconds unless active bleeding is present. In the presence of persistent and unusual bleeding, heparin administration may be decreased or stopped completely if the ECMO flows are deemed to be adequate to prevent stagnation in the system, especially in the oxygenator. Flows greater than 3 L/min are generally considered to be adequate to permit use of lower ACT values.

The system is primed with a balanced electrolyte crystalloid, Plasmalyte-A (Baxter Healthcare, Deerfield, IL), which is then displaced with 2 units of red blood cells, 50 mEq sodium bicarbonate, and 500 mg calcium chloride, added carefully. The blood prime is recirculated, warmed, and briefly ventilated with medical air to correct pH and carbon dioxide tension. The total priming volume is approximately 1000 mL.

THE CIRCUIT

Initially, the ECMO pack is modified by the perfusion staff to accommodate priming with a cardiotomy reservoir in the main circuit. After crystalloid priming and blood priming are completed, the cardiotomy reservoir is taken away from the main ECMO circuit but is left with a Medtronic DLP 3/8-inch perfusion adaptor at its tip to allow for rapid infusion of fluids into a Luer connector on the negative venous line, if necessary. The lines that originally had included the cardiotomy reservoir are joined together, and the system is complete: venous line to centrifugal pump to oxygenator to arterial line. The cardiotomy reservoir is taken away from the circuit after the patient stabilizes, or after 6 hours, whichever occurs first. It may be replaced, if necessary.

Pressure-monitoring lines include negative, oxygenator inlet, and oxygenator outlet sites. Gish pressure isolators are used with Walrus stopcock high-flow extensions to connect to 3/16-inch male adaptors at a manifold site at the Medtronic BioPump transducer. The pressure-monitoring sites should be at the level of the patient for correct pressure information. The monitoring devices are completely filled with fluid.

Because we use a centrifugal pump, negative pressure generated by the pump is periodically assessed. Venous drainage is assessed with the use of the negative pressure reading on the inlet side of the centrifugal pump. Optimally, the negative inlet pressure is less than 75 mm Hg. If readings are 75 mm Hg or higher, the venous drainage, cannula position and size, volume status, flow rates, and hemodynamic status are reassessed. Central cannulation should have lower negative pressure readings than peripheral cannulation. The negative pressure is read only intermittently and with caution, because constant negative pressure may pull air out of solution. Knowledge of inlet pressure is critical, however, to optimal ECMO with a circuit containing a centrifugal pump.

The pressure drop across the oxygenator is assessed with the proximal and distal readings. Greater pressure drops are observed with the Avecor oxygenator than with the Affinity oxygenator. Increasing pressure drops not associated with higher flows may be indicative of thrombus formation.

A dry, prepared circuit is always available. It is kept covered and out of high-traffic areas.

ARTERIAL-VENOUS BRIDGE AND RECIRCULATION LINE

This ECMO pack contains an arterial-venous bridge for weaning purposes. Because stagnant blood may initiate clot formation, blood flow through this area is permitted to be about 250 to 300 mL/minute. A 9/16-inch Keck red roller clamp (Cole-Parmer, Chicago, IL) is placed on the bridge. The roller clamp allows for washing of the entire lumen of the bridge, whereas placing a tubing clamp on a portion of the bridge does not, and the latter may permit clot to form in stagnant areas. Flows are checked hourly by clamping the

bridge and checking the change in the centrifugal pump flow. The Keck clamp is physically moved on a timely basis to alleviate deformation on the inside of the tubing.

The Affinity oxygenator contains a 1/4-inch port that is sometimes used for cardioplegia delivery or recirculation in conventional bypass procedures. In the ECMO situation, if the port is permitted to sit stagnant, clot may form. An 18- to 22-inch piece of 1/4-inch CB tubing is connected to that port and then to a Walrus high-flow stopcock with extension tubing to the venous line via a 1/4-inch DLP perfusion adaptor. Flows are limited to 200 mL/minute with a 3/8-inch Keck blue roller clamp in this area. Flows are checked at least hourly, and the clamp is moved on a timely basis.

Hollow-fiber membrane oxygenators may become porous and leak plasma proteins. Oxygenator change is essential, although the patient's condition may be compromised with this action. If foaming at the gas ports becomes obvious, biohazard bags are placed around the effluent ports until change-out is accomplished. A new oxygenator with CB tubing is primed. If active anticoagulation is available, an Avecor silicone oxygenator is desired because of the nonleaking. If active anticoagulation is not desirable, a CB Affinity oxygenator is used. The new circuit is brought to the bedside. The patient's ventilator is set at 1.0 FIO$_2$ and 12 to 18 breaths per minute. A critical care medicine physician is at the bedside during the oxygenator change-out to assess the patient's responses and to manage resuscitation if necessary. At least three staff members (two or three perfusionists and one nurse) are available for change-out for disconnection of the failing oxygenator and managing syringes of fluid for filling and connection of lines for the new oxygenator. Masks are worn, and this procedure is performed in as aseptic fashion as possible.

To moderate the patient's responses to temporary cessation of ECMO flow during oxygenator change-out, the new oxygenator is set at 1.0 FIO$_2$ with blender sweep of 1:1 to blood flow until an arterial blood gas sample is analyzed to ensure acceptable blood gas and oxygenator performance.

HEMOFILTRATION/HEMODIALYSIS

If hemofiltration/hemodialysis is necessary, a Fresenius 7 dialyzer (Fresenius Medical Care, N.A., Lexington, MA) is used. On occasion, a Jostra Baxter HQ 7000 (Jostra AG, Hirrlinger, Germany) hemoconcentrator is used for removing plasma water. The Fresenius device must be prerinsed with at least 2 L of saline. These devices must be totally primed with fluid on both the blood side and the effluent side. Custom tubing may be necessary to accommodate both the blood phase and the fluid side.

The filter is connected into the ECMO circuit with its inflow on a Walrus high-flow stopcock and extension Luer device just distal to the centrifugal head for maximal driving pressure and flow. The hemofilter blood outflow is connected to a Walrus high-flow stopcock with extension Luer port on the negative inlet of the centrifugal pump.

The blood flow is never stopped, because the filters are not heparin-bonded and will clot in the lower anticoagulation levels. If heparin is not being used systemically, 50-mL flushes of saline may be performed every half-hour through the device. This fluid must be considered and added to the total volume-in/volume-out calculation. Both sides of the filter should be observed for thrombus formation. Small amounts of heparin may be infused at the proximal end of the kidney with an intravenous pump to help prevent thrombus formation. Systemic ACT must be observed for effect.

To control dialysate flow and effluent waste flow, an intravenous pump must be used. Currently, the Baxter 6301 or the Baxter Colleague pump (Baxter Healthcare, Round Lake, IL) is used to control inflow and outflow. Baxter intravenous tubing that is approximately 100 inches in length and does not contain one-way valves or needle drop is acceptable. This tubing must be appropriately placed and keyed within the Baxter devices to prevent free flow.

The maximum flow on the Baxter 6301 is 1999 mL/hour. If three pumps are used with the Colleague pump, a flow of 3000 mL/hour may be obtained for either inflow or outflow. Stopcocks set in manifold fashion on both sides of the filtration device are used with the Colleague pump. The effluent is allowed to drain into a urine collection bag and is measured every hour. Renal physicians are responsible for calculation of dialysate components and volume to be removed from the patient. Volume unloading alone is performed by merely connecting the intravenous tubing to the urine collection bag. Observation of patient status with arterial pressure and venous pressure, if available, is necessary.

TRIAL/WEANING

Trial and wean in a VV system is a matter of reducing or turning off gas flows. The ventilator is adjusted for trial settings, and ECMO gas flows are either reduced or totally turned off (disconnected). Pump flows may remain the same, because lung recovery is the issue and cardiac function is not of consequence. Arterial saturations are observed and blood gas analyses are performed at timely intervals. If VV bypass is being used and a venous saturation measurement is desired, one must remember, depending on the site of drawing of the sample, to temporarily clamp the arterial-venous bridge, recirculation line, hemofilter lines, or any arterial effect on the ECMO venous circuit before drawing a venous gas sample from the circuit.

Trial or wean with a VA system is very different. The arterial-venous bridge is used. The ventilator is set at optimal setting. Additional heparin is given to achieve an ACT of 300 seconds. Flow may be reduced by 1 L/min at intervals. ECMO gas flows are reduced accordingly. Observations of the patient's blood pressure and arterial saturation are critical. When it becomes apparent that the patient may be ready to be taken off ECMO, the patient inflow line and patient drainage lines are clamped between the patient and the arterial-venous bridge, and the bridge is opened. There should be a flow of at least 3 L through this circuit to maintain a deposition-free system. At this time, there should be no gas flow to the oxygenator to affect the patient's blood gas readings, which are taken from time to time during the trial/wean to assess the status of the patient.

Depending on the ACT, the patient lines and cannulas should be "flashed" for 5 to 10 seconds every few minutes to keep them free of deposition. The bridge is clamped and patient arterial and venous lines are unclamped for that 5 to 10 seconds. The patient inflow line is then reclamped, the patient venous line is reclamped, and the bridge reopened. During the time of trial/wean, the patient's ACT should be monitored.

ANNOTATED REFERENCES

Alpard SK, Zwischenberger JB: Extracorporeal membrane oxygenation for severe respiratory failure. Chest Surg Clin North Am 2002;12:355-378.
> This review article describes the current state of the art for ECLS therapy.

Bartlett RH, Roloff DW, Custer JR, et al: Extracorporeal life support: The University of Michigan experience. JAMA 2000;283:904-908.
> This seminal article describes the experience at the University of Michigan with the largest series of patients in the world treated with ECLS. It describes the experience with adult and pediatric patients and discusses the evolution of ECLS from the bench to the bedside.

Pranikoff T, Hirschl RB, Remenapp R, et al: Venovenous extracorporeal life support via percutaneous cannulation in 94 patients. Chest 1999;115:818-822.
> This article describes the experience with percutaneous cannulation in the largest series of adult patients published. It includes a good discussion of the technique as well as outcomes.

KEY POINTS

1. **The acute abdomen is a notorious dilemma in the critically ill patient.** Symptoms are unreliable, are nonspecific, are often delayed in presentation, and are out of proportion to the severity of the offending problem. Expeditious diagnosis is difficult but essential for outcome.[1]

2. **Intrahospital transport for diagnostic studies carries a risk** for added morbidity in the critically ill.

3. **Dependence on special procedure units** results in delays in diagnosis and treatment.

4. **Bringing diagnosis and treatment to the intensive care unit bedside** expedites diagnosis and treatment, is more cost effective, and carries the potential for positively affecting outcome.

5. If the appropriate patients are chosen and the effects of peritoneal insufflation appreciated, **bedside laparoscopy in the ICU can be a valuable adjunct in the diagnostic evaluation of the difficult abdomen.**

Procedures used to be performed at the bedside on large open wards. The progression to more complex, more invasive procedures requiring specialized equipment and personnel led to the establishment of special procedure suites. Specialized rooms were used for simple interventions such as dressing changes to formal major operations. This reliance on special rooms led to delays based on limited availability for both diagnostic and therapeutic procedures and the potential for negative impact on outcome. Use of specialized procedure rooms also carries risks associated with intrahospital transport of the critically ill patients, and the use of special procedure suites adds cost for both transport and maintenance of the rooms. These considerations have prompted clinicians caring for critically ill patients to consider conducting more procedures at the bedside in the ICU.

Three important elements have made this more efficient approach possible: (1) multidisciplinary critical care team concept with easy availability of a wide range of specialty experience; (2) portability of essential equipment; and (3) availability of effective continuous intravenous sedation/analgesia. Bedside laparoscopy is an especially attractive example of this management concept. In the past, evaluation of the abdomen for sepsis, perforated viscus, hemorrhage, cholecystitis, or intestinal ischemia required transport of the patient to the radiology suite for computed tomography (CT) (often with equivocal findings) or to the operating room for a formal exploratory laparotomy (often nondiagnostic or nontherapeutic). Laparoscopy, on the other hand, is a cost-effective, sensitive, and specific diagnostic tool that is readily available at the bedside.[2] With today's instruments in experienced hands it carries a low procedural risk, and minor therapeutic maneuvers can be simultaneously accomplished as well.

PHYSIOLOGIC CONSIDERATIONS

Although considered minimally invasive surgery, laparoscopy is nevertheless invasive. The effects of peritoneal insufflation are the most important consideration. To provide the necessary working space, the peritoneal cavity must be insufflated with gas. Carbon dioxide (CO_2) is the gas of choice. CO_2 is nonflammable, so cautery can be used. CO_2 is highly soluble, so gas embolism is rare. CO_2 is inert, and it is cheap. The only potential drawback associated with the use of CO_2 is hypercapnia.[3,4]

The main concern is elevated abdominal pressure caused by the CO_2 insufflation. The adverse effects of elevated intra-abdominal pressure are intensified with higher pressures and longer procedure times. The physiologic alterations caused by pneumoperitoneum affect mostly the cardiac, pulmonary, and vascular systems.

CARDIAC

Increased intra-abdominal pressure impedes venous return and simultaneously elevates central venous pressure (CVP). Thus, during laparoscopic procedures, CVP is useless for estimating the adequacy of intravascular filling. Stroke volume is decreased by pneumoperitoneum, but because heart rate is increased the resulting cardiac output is decreased to a lesser degree.[4,5] Systemic vascular resistance (SVR) and cardiac afterload increase, possibly because of increased sympathetic tone due to hypercarbia.[4,5] These changes can lead to either hypotension or hypertension, depending on the relative changes in stroke volume and SVR. Cardiac arrhythmias can occur. Overall, the workload and oxygen demand of the heart are increased.[4,5] **Close hemodynamic monitoring** and immediate management of significant changes are vital.

PULMONARY

Functional residual capacity and lung compliance are decreased by pneumoperitoneum; airway pressure and airway resistance are increased.[3-6] These changes increase the work of breathing, a phenomenon that is exacerbated by the increased minute ventilation that is needed to remove the CO_2 load imposed by the gas absorbed from peritoneal surfaces. Hypoxia due to both compression atelectasis and CO_2 retention occur, if minute ventilation cannot increase sufficiently. These adverse effects can be further aggravated if the patient is placed in reverse Trendelenburg position. This positioning, which is used to improve exposure of the upper abdomen viscera, permits the weight of the intra-abdominal organs to add to the pressure increase.[3-6] A precipitous drop in end-tidal CO_2 is indicative of air embolism. **Frequent monitoring of both arterial P_{CO_2} and O_2 saturation is indicated throughout the procedure.** A pneumothorax can develop if CO_2 tracks through gaps in the diaphragm into the pleural space.

VASCULAR

The deleterious effects of increased intra-abdominal pressure on visceral organ perfusion are well known.[7] The kidneys are especially sensitive in this regard. Decreased renal perfusion decreases urine output, and oliguria can persist for a prolonged period after the evacuation of the pneumoperitoneum and restoration of baseline intra-abdominal pressure. Acute volume overload and pulmonary edema can result after acute release of pneumoperitoneum, especially if cardiac output was maintained during the procedure by infusion of large amounts of intravenous fluids.[8] Prolonged procedures, coupled with prolonged impaired venous blood return and perioperative hypercoagulability, can increase the risk for deep vein thrombosis.[5]

INTRACRANIAL PRESSURE

Increased intra-abdominal pressure can increase intracranial pressure (ICP) as a result of both chemical and mechanical mechanisms.[3-6] Intra-abdominal hypertension impedes venous drainage from the central nervous system and increases cerebrospinal fluid pressure. These adverse effects are partially mitigated by reverse Trendelenburg positioning. Hypercarbia causes cerebral vasodilation, further worsening the problem. However in an animal model, elevated ICP due to pneumoperitoneum had little effect on cerebral perfusion pressure or jugular vein oxygen saturation.[9,10] Thus, clinical implications of ICP elevation secondary to pneumoperitoneum are not yet known.[9,10] My experience with diagnostic laparoscopy in brain-injured patients has been good. By using low insufflation pressures (~10 mm Hg) and keeping procedure times short (~20 minutes), related problems have been minimized.

ABDOMINAL WALL

In laparoscopic procedures, the abdominal wall is penetrated blindly and there is a risk of injury to intra-abdominal vascular structures. In the absence of portal hypertension, the only vascular structure in the abdominal wall of any consequence is the inferior epigastric artery. Inadvertent puncture of a solid or hollow intra-abdominal organ or a major vascular structure is, of course, potentially a very serious complication.

Despite the potential adverse effects discussed in the preceding paragraphs, laparoscopy is tolerated well by high-risk patients, such as patients with impaired cardiac or pulmonary function, the elderly, the critically ill, and the

multiply injured.[11-17] But it is better to stay out of trouble than get out of trouble, and knowing the potential negative effects of laparoscopy facilitates optimal patient selection, conduct of the operation, and monitoring.

TECHNICAL CONSIDERATIONS

The patient remains in a neutral, supine position and is prepped and draped as for an exploratory laparotomy to allow access to all four abdominal quadrants. Blood pressure, pulse rate, respiratory rate, tidal volume and peak inspiratory pressure, oxygen saturation, and end-tidal P_{CO_2} should be monitored continuously. Recommended basic equipment is listed in Table 227-1.

In the very sick patients, the safest approach for inserting the laparoscope is the open approach originally described by Hasson.[18] This technique allows placement of fascial sutures under direct vision at the beginning of the procedure. As a result, the inserted port for the laparoscope is better stabilized, and the fascial closure at the completion of the procedure is more secure. Prior decompression of the stomach with a nasogastric tube and the bladder with a Foley catheter is advisable. The incision is traditionally placed just cephalad or caudad to the umbilicus. A vertical incision in the midline that can be easily extended is preferable in case a formal laparotomy is necessary later. Under direct vision, the fascia is opened through the linea alba and on each side a size 0 suture is placed. The peritoneum is incised under direct vision, and the operator inserts a finger to ensure safe entry into the peritoneal cavity. Then the cannula is inserted and the two fascial sutures are looped around it in the provided grooves for stabilization. Carbon dioxide is insufflated slowly to minimize adverse effects on respiratory function and hemodynamics. For diagnostic purposes, it is sufficient

TABLE 227–1. RECOMMENDED BASIC EQUIPMENT FOR BEDSIDE LAPAROSCOPY

Optic Equipment

10-mm laparoscope
Computer chip video camera
Light source
Video monitor—one sufficient
Video recorder—optional

Abdominal Access Equipment

Insufflator with pressure monitor
CO_2 gas tank
10-mm Hasson cannula
One to two 5-mm trocar cannulas

Laparoscopic Instruments

One to two atraumatic graspers
Suction irrigator
Blunt probe

Optional Equipment

Coagulation forceps, clip applier/clips, needle holder/sutures, scissors, dissectors

Miscellaneous Items

Sterile drapes and prepping solution
Fascial and subcutaneous skin sutures
Steri-strips, Band aids
4 × 4-inch gauze sponges

to increase intraperitoneal pressure to 10 mm Hg. When percutaneous, blind insufflation with a Veress needle is deemed safe, a 5-mm 30-degree angle scope is an excellent alternative for diagnostic laparoscopy. This choice allows for a smaller incision and insertion of a smaller 5-mm port. An additional 5-mm port can be placed in the right and/or left hemiabdomen under direct vision. This port permits the insertion of a grasper or two to manipulate structures in order to facilitate inspection of intraperitoneal organs. At the end of the procedure, the previously placed midline fascial sutures are tied. For the smaller side ports, skin closure alone is sufficient. **With complete preparation before starting, the procedure can be performed safely with the following personnel:**

- One person dedicated to providing sedation, analgesia, and respiratory and hemodynamic stability. Ideally, this individual is an anesthesiologist, but an intensivist who is credentialed with training and experience in continuous intravenous sedation can perform this function.
- The laparoscopist
- A circulating nurse to obtain necessary equipment and medications
- A respiratory therapist on standby

Sedation and analgesia should be provided intravenously. A short-acting narcotic (e.g., fentanyl, 100 to 200 μg), combined with a short-acting sedative works well. Rarely, supplementation with a short-acting nondepolarizing neuromuscular blocking agent (cis-atracurium, 5 to 10 mg) is required as well. Diagnostic laparoscopy has been done successfully using only local anesthesia and a mild sedative.[23] But, for complex ICU patients with suspected intra-abdominal pathology, using local anesthesia would not be optimal.

INDICATIONS

It is important to distinguish between **diagnostic** and **therapeutic** laparoscopy. Diagnostic laparoscopy requires lower insufflation pressure, a shorter procedure time, fewer trocar sites, and a neutral patient position. Thus, diagnostic laparoscopy is less invasive and physiologically less challenging for the patient than is therapeutic laparoscopy. **Two major groups** of patients are potential candidates for bedside laparoscopy in the ICU. The larger group consists of critically ill patients with a suspected intra-abdominal process. Physical findings are usually unreliable in these patients, and usually they are unable to communicate. Other portable diagnostic modalities such as plain radiographs, ultrasound, and even peritoneal lavage have only limited usefulness. The second group consists of hemodynamically stable victims of blunt or penetrating trauma with possible intra-abdominal injuries based on mechanism of injury. Ultrasound and CT, although useful for detecting hemoperitoneum and injuries of the spleen and liver, are less sensitive for diagnosing diaphragmatic and hollow viscus injuries. Both of those carry the potential for significant morbidity if diagnosis and treatment are delayed.

Data from several large series support the idea that laparoscopy is a sensitive and specific approach for diagnosing significant intra-abdominal pathology in critically ill patients while avoiding the morbidity associated with an unnecessary negative formal laparotomy.[19-21] In two of these series, indicated therapeutic interventions were accomplished laparoscopically at the bedside in the majority of cases.[19,20] Thus, even when a therapeutic procedure is needed, formal (open) laparotomy can often be avoided. However, all three of the series cited reported the results of diagnostic laparoscopy performed in the operating room. The first reported case describing the utility of bedside laparoscopy in the ICU was authored by Iberti and colleagues.[22] This report showed that bedside laparoscopy is technically feasible, even in a patient with a fresh abdominal incision. This idea has received further support in an article by Pecaro.[23] Four of the 11 patients in this series had recent laparotomies. In 6 of the 11 patients studied, the use of bedside laparoscopy avoided nontherapeutic open laparotomy. The procedures were carried out under local anesthesia supplemented with midazolam or propofol. There were no procedure-related complications. The largest series of cases of bedside diagnostic laparoscopy in the ICU was reported by Kelly and colleagues.[24] In 16 of 17 cases, laparoscopy was performed successfully without procedure-related complications. All of the procedures were performed to evaluate patients with sepsis of unknown origin. In one patient, insufflation and therefore laparoscopy was not possible owing to preexisting high intra-abdominal pressures. Ten of the completed procedures were negative. Four patients had intestinal ischemia, and two had cholecystitis. Among the 16 completed procedures, the operative diagnosis was confirmed by laparotomy in six cases, at autopsy in three cases, and by clinical recovery in five cases; thus, the reported accuracy was 100%. Nine of the 14 patients studied had abdominal CT performed before laparoscopy. Abdominal CT in these patients was accurate in only 33%.

In the evaluation of trauma victims, laparoscopy has been used for three main reasons. First, diagnostic peritoneal lavage (DPL) is too sensitive and lacks specificity. Second, negative or nontherapeutic laparotomy for trauma carries a significant morbidity.[25-28] Third, both DPL and CT are unreliable in diagnosing diaphragmatic and hollow viscus injuries. Early studies showed that diagnostic laparoscopy was safe and accurate and avoided nontherapeutic laparotomy[25-28] in hemodynamically stable patients with penetrating trauma. Moreover, diagnostic laparoscopy seemed to shorten hospital stay and save costs. Diagnostic laparoscopy has proven to be especially helpful for evaluating patients with penetrating wounds to the flank or thoracoabdominal area.[25-28] The use of diagnostic laparoscopy has expanded to evaluating selected victims of blunt trauma (e.g., hemodynamically stable children with suspected seatbelt related injuries) with similar good results.[29] Initially, many clinicians believed that laparoscopy offered few advantages relative to DPL or CT.[30-35] However, with the advent of more advanced instruments and improved technical skills, recent publications have been enthusiastic about the advantages of laparoscopy for diagnosis and also treatment of hemodynamically stable blunt trauma patients.[32-40] Laparoscopy is only appropriate for selected blunt trauma victims. Key selection criteria include absence of an absolute indication for expeditious abdominal exploration; hemodynamic stability; and absence of associated injuries requiring immediate attention.

LIMITATIONS

Absolute contraindications to bedside laparoscopy include high preexisting intra-abdominal pressure, known intraperitoneal adhesions, and the presence of an open abdomen or recent dehiscence. Recent laparotomy with incisional closure is not a contraindication. Accordingly, diagnostic laparoscopy is useful for so-called second-look procedures.

ANNOTATED REFERENCES

Brandt CP, Priebe PP, Eckhauser ML: Diagnostic laparoscopy in the intensive care unit: Avoiding the nontherapeutic laparotomy. Surg Endosc 1993;7:168-172.

This is the first case study, to our knowledge, that reports in detail the advantages of bedside laparoscopy in the ICU.

Crist DW, Shapiro MB, Gadacz TR: Emergency laparoscopy in trauma, acute abdomen and intensive care patients. Baillieres Clin Gastroenterol 1993;7:779-793.

This is a very comprehensive case series, describing the utility of bedside laparoscopy in the emergency setting.

Gajic O, Urrutia LE, Sewani H, et al: Acute abdomen in the medical intensive care unit. Crit Care Med 2002;30:1187-1190.

This recent retrospective cohort study outlines in a comprehensive manner the diagnostic dilemma with this entity and the negative impact on outcome, when recognition and intervention are delayed. This emphasizes the utility of bedside laparoscopy.

Pecaro AP: The routine use of diagnostic laparoscopy in the intensive care unit. Surg Endosc 2001;15:638-641.

This recent case series reports the success with bedside laparoscopy under local anesthesia coupled with continuous intravenous sedation only.

Wolf SJ, Stoller ML: The physiology of laparoscopy: Basic principles, complications and other considerations. J Urol 1994;152:294-302.

This review article is a complete description of the impact of the peritoneal insufflation, which is necessary to inspect the peritoneal cavity laparoscopically. It is absolutely mandatory for any laparoscopist to be aware of these effects when selecting suitable patients and to respond to them during the procedure.

Chapter 228

PEDIATRIC INTENSIVE CARE PROCEDURES

Michele Moss • Adriana M. Lopez • Brian K. Eble • Dennis E. Schellhase

KEY POINTS

1. To provide safe, adequate sedation and pain relief for pediatric patients undergoing invasive procedures as well as to more safely and expeditiously perform the procedure, **knowledge of a variety of sedatives and analgesics** is imperative.

2. Because of **differences in the pediatric airway** when compared with the adult airway, management of the pediatric airway can be more difficult.

3. **Intraosseous access in infants and children is an expeditious technique to establish vascular access** in critically ill children in whom obtaining vascular access would be so time consuming as to delay necessary therapy.

4. **Central venous access is a common, relatively safe procedure** in pediatric patients who need stable vascular access for pressor infusions, frequent blood sampling, central venous pressure monitoring, and infusions of hypertonic or sclerosing solutions.

5. **Monitoring of pulmonary arterial pressure is an important part of management** of pediatric patients with presumed or proven pulmonary hypertension, severe shock unresponsive to fluid and pressor therapy, and respiratory failure and cardiac output compromise.

6. Arterial catheters are used in pediatric patients primarily for **continuous blood pressure monitoring and arterial blood gas access.**

7. In pediatric patients there is a reported **frequency of ventricular fibrillation of 11% to 19%** in patients with out-of-hospital arrests; therefore, defibrillation is required in the pediatric arrest scenario including the use of automated external defibrillators.

8. **Multiple techniques of temporary pacing are useful in pediatric patients** who have developed symptomatic bradycardias; transvenous pacing is the best method for patients who need stabilization before having a permanent system installed.

9. **Transesophageal echocardiography** is useful in pediatric patients, most commonly those with congenital cardiac defects, to better delineate their anatomy and to search for valvular insufficiency, residual shunts or obstruction, thrombi, and myocardial dysfunction.

10. Flexible airway bronchoscopy, best performed in critically ill children by an experienced pediatric bronchoscopist, can provide significant information, including the **quality of the distal airways and presence and type of infections.**

11. Thoracentesis and tube thoracostomy are indicated for diagnosis and management of **transudative, chylous, and purulent effusions as well as for pneumothoraces.**

12. **Cardiac tamponade due to pericardial effusions** from trauma, idiopathic pericarditis, postoperative cardiac surgery, chylous effusions, or other causes of pericarditis must be treated emergently with pericardiocentesis by needle or tube placement.

13. Monitoring of intracranial pressure in children, **indicated in traumatic brain injury and diffuse cerebral edema,** is most commonly performed using an intraventricular cannula or tissue monitor.

14. Measurement of jugular bulb venous oxygen saturation in patients with increased intracranial pressure allows some **insight into the adequacy of cerebral blood flow,** which is frequently altered by the disease process or injury and by therapeutic maneuvers.

Critically or potentially critically ill and injured pediatric patients frequently require invasive procedures to adequately maintain and care for them as well as monitor their status. In general, the same techniques apply to children as to adults, with often minor variations due to size and anatomy.

One major difference is the almost ubiquitous requirement for adequate sedation and analgesia when performing the procedure owing to the importance of providing pain relief and sedation and to the rare ability of the pediatric patient to cooperate or understand the procedure. The procedure generally is safer and more expeditious to perform if the patient is adequately sedated. Pediatric patients become just as anxious about procedures as adult patients, and even the most immature neonate feels pain.[1,2]

Another major difference is the need for adequate securing of any device left in place as well as the need for restraining the patient, either mechanically or chemically, to prevent inadvertent or intentional removal of an indwelling device. Inadvertent removal can have devastating consequences, such as inadvertent extubation, so restraint is often justified to avoid harm to the patient.

LOCAL ANESTHETICS

Lidocaine in a 1% concentration is the most commonly used local anesthetic in pediatric patients. It is generally safe and effective. Care must be taken, however, to use it judiciously because of the risk of overdosing a small pediatric patient who needs multiple procedures performed or because a large area needs to be locally anesthetized. It is toxic at a blood level of 6 μg/mL. Infants may be at greater risk because they lack the microsomal enzymes needed for metabolism. Also, lidocaine is less protein bound in infants, increasing the likelihood of toxicity at a given dose per kilogram.[3]

Local anesthetic creams such as EMLA (which is made of prilocaine and lidocaine) are very useful in preparing for an elective procedure. EMLA takes 60 minutes for adequate local anesthesia so it is not indicated for emergent procedures. Newer formulations such as Elomax, which is a lidocaine preparation, are formulated for faster anesthesia (as short as 10 minutes), making it more useful for immediate procedures. These creams can provide enough local anesthesia to relieve the pain from needle punctures.

SEDATION AND ANALGESIA

Callahan describes the ideal drug as being easy to administer with a quick and predictable onset of action, predictable duration of action, and a rapid recovery period.[4] No ideal sedative or analgesic yet exists, but several have many of these characteristics. It is important to assess whether the combination of a sedative with local anesthesia is sufficient (e.g., for placing a peripheral arterial catheter) or whether analgesia is also needed (e.g., for chest tube placement) or if both are needed with neuromuscular blockade (e.g., for intubation). The goal is to use the minimal amount of drug necessary to adequately sedate and/or relieve pain. Appropriate monitoring must also be in place when these drugs are administered. The American Academy of Pediatrics has outlined guidelines for monitoring of pediatric patients during procedural sedation.[5,6] There are several additional drugs available for sedation and/or analgesia than the ones discussed here, many with years of use in pediatric patients. It is important to become familiar with a regimen of drugs and their pharmacodynamic profiles.

Midazolam is a benzodiazepine that has found wide use for procedural sedation because of its rapid onset of action, relatively short duration of action, reasonable predictability, and ease of administration. It can be given intravenously, intranasally, or orally, although the onset of action is longer and it is less predictable when given orally or intranasally. Midazolam provides deeper sedation and better amnesia than other benzodiazepines. Respiratory depression can be a complication especially when it is combined with analgesic agents or when it is administered rapidly. The dosage range reported is wide, from 0.02 to 0.2 mg/kg. Generally, a starting dose of 0.05 mg/kg is used and titrated slowly upward to effect stopping at 0.2 mg/kg. If sedation is inadequate at that dose, another drug should be considered. For patients needing ongoing sedation, such as with mechanical ventilation, midazolam can be delivered as a continuous infusion with a starting dose of 0.05 to 0.1 mg/kg/hr. A higher dose may be required for some patients.

For procedural analgesia, opiate derivatives such as morphine or fentanyl are widely used. Morphine is the standard for analgesia by which all other analgesics are compared. It can be given intravenously, intramuscularly, or orally, but the latter is poor for procedural analgesia. Intravenous administration is preferred. Morphine provides both analgesia and some sedation but may need to be combined with midazolam. The dose of morphine is 0.05 up to 0.2 mg/kg with an onset of action that is immediate, peaks at about 20 minutes, and lasts up to 4 hours. This makes morphine a good choice if the pain from the procedure may persist after the procedure. If ongoing pain relief is needed, morphine can be delivered either in repeated bolus dosing or as a continuous infusion. The starting dose for an infusion is from 0.05 to 0.1 mg/kg/hr. For patients who are conscious and old enough, morphine can be delivered with a patient-controlled analgesia pump. Morphine also can depress respirations. It also can cause release of histamine with redness, wheal, and flare along the intravenous catheter site. Other complications include constipation, urinary retention, miosis, nausea and vomiting, and pruritus.[7,8]

Fentanyl is a synthetic opioid agonist also frequently used for procedural analgesia because of its rapid onset of action, predictable response, and relatively short duration of action. It has a short half-life of only 20 minutes with a duration of action of 30 to 40 minutes. The dose range is 1 to 2 mg/kg because it is about 100 times more potent than morphine. It, too, can cause respiratory depression. There is some evidence that the respiratory depression is more pronounced in infants younger than 3 months of age.[9] Another uncommon side effect that is of concern is "rigid chest syndrome," in which the patient is difficult to ventilate. The glottis may close, making bag-valve-mask ventilation difficult. For severe responses neuromuscular blockade may be needed with subsequent intubation. This response seems to occur with the high doses of fentanyl given for general anesthesia and not procedural sedation. However, one must be prepared for the possibility of this complication if using the drug.

Ketamine is an anesthetic that can be administered in subanesthetic doses, resulting in conscious sedation, analgesia, and amnesia.[10] It may be given either intravenously or intramuscularly. The onset of action when given intravenously is rapid with a short duration of 15 to 20 minutes. Intramuscular administration prolongs the onset and duration of action. The starting doses are 1 to 2 mg/kg when given intravenously and 2 to 4 mg/kg intramuscularly. Some advantages of ketamine are that it produces minimal reparatory depression and, through indirect stimulation of the sympathetic nervous system, increases heart rate and blood pressure. In children with tenuous hemodynamics, ketamine may be a good choice. Because of its systemic vasoconstrictive properties, it is frequently used in patients with cyanotic congenital heart disease because it can maintain pulmonary blood flow. Additionally, it has some bronchodilator properties that make it useful in patients with bronchospasm who need procedures. It does have several side effects of note. In older children and adults, ketamine can produce unpleasant dysphoric dreams and hallucinations during emergence. This reaction can be attenuated by the concurrent use of benzodiazepines. Ketamine also increases secretions, making clearing the airway more difficult. In patients who already may have copious or thick secretions, ketamine may be contraindicated. Ketamine is believed to be contraindicated in patients with head injuries because it may increase intracranial pressure.

Propofol has been safely and effectively used for procedural sedation and anesthesia in pediatric patients.[11] It has a rapid onset of action, predictable response, and short duration of action of 5 to 10 minutes. This makes it useful for short procedures. It can produce respiratory as well as marked cardiovascular depression. Propofol does not have analgesic properties, so an analgesic may also be needed for painful procedures. The initial bolus dose is 2 mg/kg, with an infusion of 50 to 200 µg/kg/min during the procedure. Propofol has been used for continuous sedation in pediatric patients, but because of a disturbing side effect of metabolic acidosis and even death in some patients it is not recommended for continuous sedation in pediatric patients.[12-14] The cause for this metabolic acidosis may be impaired fatty acid metabolism, but it is unclear at what dose this may occur or which patients may be at risk.[15] It does not appear to be a complication of propofol use in adults.

Etomidate is an anesthetic agent that is commonly used in rapid-sequence intubation in adults and is becoming more widely used in pediatrics for the same indication. It has a rapid onset of action and relatively short duration. Etomidate has less adverse hemodynamic effects than other sedative/analgesic drugs, making it attractive for use in patients with cardiovascular compromise. The recommended intravenous dose is 0.3 mg/kg. It has been reported to rarely cause adrenal insufficiency. In one retrospective review and one prospective study of its use in children younger than 10 years old there was no evidence of hemodynamic compromise or adrenal insufficiency when it was use for rapid-sequence intubation.[16,17]

AIRWAY MANAGEMENT

NORMAL ANATOMY OF THE PEDIATRIC AIRWAY

The pediatric airway differs from the adult airway in many aspects.[18,19] Understanding these differences is important for patient management. The larynx in children is located higher in the neck at the level of C3-C4 as opposed to the adult, where the larynx is at C4-C5. This more superior position of the larynx creates more acute angulation during laryngoscopy and can make visualization of the glottic opening more difficult. Also, the tongue is located more superiorly and closer to the palate in children than in adults, potentially causing airway obstruction. The narrowest portion of a child's airway is the subglottic region, whereas the narrowest portion of an adult airway is the vocal cords. This difference allows for uncuffed tracheal tubes to be used in infants and young children. Another major difference is that children have a more protuberant occiput, which may cause excessive neck flexion. Finally, the infant's nares are smaller. Because infants are obligate nasal breathers for the first 6 months of life, occlusion of the nasal passages with secretions, edema, or blood can cause significant resistance to airflow and significantly increase the work of breathing.

MANUAL MANEUVERS FOR OPENING THE AIRWAY

Blood secretions and or vomitus may potentially obstruct the airway and, therefore, must first be removed. The chin lift is the most effective maneuver for opening an obstructed airway. Placing one hand on the forehead to maintain a neutral sniffing position performs this maneuver. The head should be extended slightly if necessary. The fingers of the other hand should be placed on the bony portion of the chin and the mandible lifted upward.[20] To perform the triple airway maneuver, two or three fingers of each hand should be placed at the angle of the mandible. The mandible should then be manipulated so that the mandible and the lower teeth are anterior to the upper jaw and teeth.

INSERTION OF ORAL AND NASOPHARYNGEAL AIRWAYS

Oral and nasopharyngeal airways can sometimes be useful in infants and children to relieve airway obstruction. Oropharyngeal airways should be used only in unconscious patients because they can induce emesis in a patient with an intact gag reflex. The airway should be placed by holding the tongue to the floor of the mouth with a tongue depressor and advancing the airway into position.[21] It should then be taped to prevent expulsion by the tongue.

The nasopharyngeal airway is inserted through the nasal passages and extends to the posterior pharynx and beyond the base of the tongue. It often adequately relieves obstruction and is well tolerated. The appropriate-sized airway extends from the nares to the tragus of the ear. The diameter should be large enough that it does not cause obstruction and not so large that it causes blanching of the alae nasi, causing necrosis.[22] It should be well lubricated before placement and advanced along the floor of the nasopharynx until the flared end rests at the nasal orifice. Risks of nasopharyngeal airways include nasal ulceration, bleeding, laryngospasm, and perforation of the cribriform plate in patients with basilar skull fractures. Contraindications to a nasopharyngeal airway include coagulopathies, cerebrospinal fluid leaks, and basilar skull fractures.

EQUIPMENT FOR AIRWAY MANAGEMENT

It is essential that appropriate equipment be readily available and organized in advance for the management of the pediatric airway.

Oxygen is one essential drug and may be administered via a nasal cannula, hood, or a mask. The mask must fit well, sitting on the bridge of the nose and the bony prominence of the chin.[21] Other essential equipment includes a bag for manual ventilation, a laryngoscope, a variety of blades, appropriately sized tracheal tubes, suction catheters, and a means for securing the tracheal tube. The appropriate-sized tracheal tube for infants and children can be estimated using the following formula:

$$(Age + 16)/4 = Endotracheal\ tube\ size$$

Additional tubes 0.5 mm smaller and 0.5 mm larger should also be available. Uncuffed tracheal tubes are generally recommended for children who are younger than 8 years old. An appropriate-sized endotracheal tube will allow for an audible air leak when the peak inflation pressure is greater than 20 cm H_2O

PHARMACOLOGIC AGENTS

Although intubation is possible without the use of pharmacologic agents, it is advantageous and beneficial to minimize any discomfort and anxiety caused by such a noxious procedure. It is imperative that a highly skilled technician be present because loss of an airway may be catastrophic.

Anticholinergic Agents

Anticholinergic agents such as atropine decrease oral secretions and prevent bradycardia during laryngoscopy, particularly in young infants. Bradycardia may be caused by hypoxemia, succinylcholine, or vagal stimulation during laryngoscopy.[23]

Sedative Agents

Most children benefit from the use of sedatives, including intravenous anxiolytics, narcotics, and anesthetics. Selection of sedatives must be done on an individual basis with consideration given to the hemodynamic status, presence of increased intracranial pressure, age, underlying medical conditions, and disease process.[23] One should be familiar with the variety of drugs available, including side effects, indications, and contraindications.

NEUROMUSCULAR BLOCKADE

The purpose of neuromuscular blocking agents is to provide complete muscle relaxation to facilitate tracheal intubation. These agents should not be used if there is any uncertainty of securing the airway, especially in patients with upper airway obstruction.

TRACHEAL INTUBATION

It is important to have all equipment ready before tracheal intubation. The airway should be opened and cleared to also help facilitate the process. The child may continue to breath spontaneously throughout preparation for the procedure and should be allowed to do so while being preoxygenated and while pharmacologic agents are given. As sedation is given, spontaneous respirations may decrease and the child may require manual ventilation. It is important to confirm that a patient can be manually ventilated before the use of neuromuscular blocking agents. If the child cannot be manually ventilated, neuromuscular blockers should not be used. The child should be placed supine in the sniffing position with the neck slightly flexed and the shoulders and the head slightly extended.

In a patient who has received a neuromuscular blocking agent, the mouth may easily be opened by using the thumb and index finger in a scissor-like fashion between the teeth. The laryngoscope is held in the left hand and placed in the right corner of the child's mouth. The blade is then swept toward the center of the mouth while moving the tongue to the left side of the mouth for better visualization. Structures including the tonsillar pillars and the epiglottis should be visualized as the laryngoscope is advanced. The tip of the laryngoscope is then placed in the vallecula or onto the epiglottis itself. To visualize the larynx, lift the mandible by lifting the laryngoscope blade toward the ceiling at a 45- to 60-degree angle to the child's chest. Avoid "cranking" the laryngoscope back as if on a fulcrum because this can cause injury to the lips and teeth. After visualizing the cords the tracheal tube is placed in the right corner of the mouth beside the laryngoscope blade and advanced through the vocal cords. The tube should be advanced with the vocal

cord mark just past the vocal cords to avoid right mainstem intubation. Ensure the correct position with an end-tidal CO_2 detector, observing equal bilateral chest excursion, maintenance of appropriate oxygen saturation, and auscultation of bilateral breath sounds. CO_2 detection should be maintained after six breaths except in the cases of cardiopulmonary arrest.[21] If a cuffed tracheal tube is used, use the least amount of volume necessary to prevent a leak around the tracheal tube because overinflation of the cuff may lead to injury of the tracheal mucosa and cartilage. The tube should then be secured and the correct position be confirmed by a chest radiograph.

NASOTRACHEAL INTUBATION

Indications for nasotracheal intubation include comfort secondary to minimization of gagging, decreased secretions, and presence of mouth abnormalities. Contraindications include coagulopathy, maxillofacial trauma, and basilar skull fractures.

Like oral tracheal intubation the patient should be positioned in the sniffing position. Use of a topical vasoconstricting agent such as phenylephrine will minimize bleeding from local trauma. Lubricate the tracheal tube and advance it gently posteriorly along the floor of the nasal cavity into the nasopharynx. Use a laryngoscope as described earlier to move the tongue to the left side of the mouth to obtain a direct view of the vocal cords. Identify the tracheal tube in the posterior pharynx and use Magill forceps to maneuver the tip of the tube until it is positioned just above the vocal cords. An assistant can advance the tracheal tube through the vocal cords.

LARYNGEAL MASK AIRWAY

There will be pediatric patients with difficult airways who need immediate airway access. In such circumstances when the patient can neither be mask ventilated nor tracheally intubated, a temporary airway should be used. A laryngeal mask airway (LMA) can be used safely and effectively in infants and children.[24] The LMA consists of a wide-bore tube with a standard 15-mm adapter at the proximal end for attachment to the circuit or resuscitation bag. The distal end is an elliptical mask that can be inflated and conforms to the shape of the larynx. It provides a low-pressure seal for ventilation at the level of the larynx.

LMAs can effectively bypass supraglottic structures and can serve as an effective conduit for placement of a fiberoptic bronchoscope into the trachea because the LMA opening is at the entrance of the glottis. LMAs come in a variety of sizes. They do not provide airway protection from aspiration of gastric contents. Insertion of LMAs may cause coughing, gagging, and laryngospasm.

VASCULAR ACCESS

INTRAOSSEOUS INFUSION

Because vascular access may be very difficult to establish in a critically ill infant or child, intraosseous infusion offers a relatively quick short solution to vascular access. It should be reserved for extreme situations in which vascular access cannot be established within a reasonable time frame for the severity of illness of the patient. The bone marrow is made of sinusoids that drain into medullary venous channels where nutrient and emissary veins direct blood flow into the systemic venous circulation. Infusion of fluids or medications into the marrow allows for complete absorption.[25,26]

Indications

Intraosseous infusion is indicated in life-threatening situations such as cardiopulmonary arrest, severe shock from all causes, and status epilepticus when rapid intravascular access cannot be obtained.[27] Multiple medications have been reported to be effective when given by this route although some drugs (gentamicin, vancomycin) may not reach therapeutic levels. Medications can be delivered both as bolus or continuous infusions. The bone marrow aspirated before any infusions may also be analyzed for laboratory studies with good correlation to venous blood.

Contraindications

There are relatively few contraindications because this is an emergency procedure. However, in the event of a fracture or previous unsuccessful attempt the opposite extremity should be used. Avoid performing intraosseous infusion through infected or burned areas.

Equipment and Procedure

Specially designed intraosseous infusion needles are available, but any Jamshidi-type bone marrow needle can be used. Although a needle with a stylet is preferable to prevent occlusion of the needle with bone fragments, any butterfly or standard hypodermic needle can be used.[28] The preferable site for insertion is the anterior tibia 1 to 2 cm below the tibial tuberosity on the medial aspect of the tibia. Other sites include the distal femur, the medial malleolus, and the anterior superior iliac spine. These sites are useful in pediatric patients from preterm neonates to adolescents. A sternal access system is now available for adult patients.[29]

When placing the intraosseous needle, prepare the site using sterile technique. Carefully identify the tibial tuberosity and identify the flat part of the tibia 1 to 2 cm below it. It is important to twist the needle as it is advanced rather than simply push it into the bone. When there is a sudden decrease in resistance to advancing the needle, the marrow has been entered. Remove the stylet and aspirate. If aspiration is successful, then the needle should be flushed. If no marrow is aspirated, attempt to flush 5 to 10 mL of saline. If the flush proceeds without resistance, the marrow probably has been entered. Continue to observe the area around the needle for evidence of infiltration. If using a site other than the anterior tibia, aim the needle away from the nearest joint space to avoid injury to the epiphysis.

Complications

Complications are rare with this procedure.[30] The most common complications are extravasation of fluid with penetration of the posterior cortex, incomplete cortex penetration, extravasation through a nutrient vessel foramen, or extravasation through a bony defect.[31] Prolonged infusions, infusions under pressure, or catecholamine infusions have increased risk of either extravasation or tissue injury. Infectious complications including osteomyelitis have been reported.[32] There is theoretical concern with fat emboli, and they have been seen in animal models; however, no clinically significant fat embolic events have been reported.

CENTRAL VENOUS CATHETERIZATION

Catheterization of the central veins is a common procedure in seriously ill and injured infants and children. With skilled operators central venous access can be achieved safely and relatively expeditiously. The best location for access is dependent on the skill and experience of the operator and the clinical condition of the patient. Femoral venous access is believed to be preferable for most patients, followed by internal jugular venous access. Subclavian venous access is also used in pediatric patients but has a higher incidence of complication, particularly during catheter insertion, so should be reserved for experienced operators.

Indications

There are many indications for insertion of central venous catheters in pediatric patients, and often multiple indications coexist. Because there is risk associated with both the insertion and the maintenance of these catheters, it is imperative that a true indication for placement be met. Certainly if more than one indication exists then the risk:benefit ratio falls in favor of catheter placement. The indications include monitoring of central venous pressure in hemodynamically unstable patients and for delivery of hypertonic solutions such as total parenteral nutrition or medications with risk of infiltration such as pressor infusions or chemotherapy. Central venous access may also be indicated in patients with poor peripheral venous access in need of ongoing or multiple intravenous catheters. Also, central venous access is used for patients needing frequent phlebotomy. Access of central veins may also be necessary for procedures such as continuous renal replacement therapy, plasmapheresis, plasma exchange, or hemodialysis.

Contraindications

All the contraindications to central venous access are relative. As with all procedures the risks and benefits of the procedure must be weighed carefully. Because bleeding is the most common complication, performing the procedure in a patient with a coagulopathy should be avoided if possible. Correction of the coagulopathy with appropriate blood products should be attempted before the procedure if the acuity of the situation allows. The skin at the insertion site should be clean and free of infection, including lack of diaper dermatitis in the groin. Other relative contraindications include avoiding the use of femoral catheters in patients with traumatic abdominal catastrophes and avoiding placing the catheter close to an artificial foreign body such as a ventriculoperitoneal shunt.[33]

Procedure and Equipment

Appropriate-sized catheters for infants and children are readily available. They are generally made of plastic or a silicone polymer, come in multiple sizes as small as 2.5 French and multiple lengths, and may have multiple ports. Catheters also may be impregnated with antiseptics, antibiotics, or heparin. The choice of catheter depends on the use of the catheter, the condition of the patient, and the site of insertion. For example, a patient needing multiple drug infusions and central venous pressure monitoring would benefit from a multiple-lumen catheter long enough for the tip to be in the central venous circulation. A patient needing only plasmapheresis would be served best with a dialysis-type catheter that is relatively short with two large-bore lumens to optimize blood flow.

The most common technique for accessing the central venous circulation in infants and children is the Seldinger guidewire technique. This technique can be safely used in all of the common locations for accessing the central circulation. With ultrasound guidance, this technique can also be used to access peripheral veins and the catheter directed centrally—the peripherally inserted central catheter.

Direct visualization of a vein for central access, or cutdown, is not commonly used but may be necessary in extreme situations. A catheter placed by cutdown on the greater saphenous vein at the groin is easily directed into the femoral vein and central venous circulation. Cutdown on antecubital or axillary veins can also lead to central access. All of these techniques require experience and some surgical skill.

The selection of the site for insertion is based on the skill and experience of the operator and the patient's condition and size. The femoral veins are relatively easily accessible in nearly all pediatric patients. Although a risk with any site, bleeding is more easily controllable with femoral catheterization. With skilled nursing care there is no greater risk of catheter infection at this site in pediatric patients. The use of the internal jugular vein is also relatively safe in most patients. The right internal jugular is associated with fewer complications than the left. Subclavian venous access is noted to have higher complications at the time of insertion, but the catheter is more easily secured and more comfortable for a mobile patient.

Access for the femoral vein in pediatric patients is similar to that in adults. The pulsations of the femoral artery are located below the inguinal ligament, and the vein is accessed medial to the artery and about 1 cm below the inguinal ligament. If pulsations are not palpable, then the site can be located halfway between the symphysis pubis and the anterior superior iliac spine. The right femoral vein is generally the preferred site because entry into the inferior vena cava is straighter with the catheter less likely to enter other minor veins. For right-handed operators there is more success of entry. Left-handed operators may choose the left femoral vein for easier access.[34]

For internal jugular access the patient is placed supine in Trendelenburg position about 30 degrees head down. The head is turned away from the side to be catheterized. The right side is preferable because of decreased complications and minimal manipulation to enter the superior vena cava. There are three techniques for entry to the internal jugular veins in children. It is recommended to become proficient at one rather than to attempt all three.[34] The anterior approach is most common. First, identify the carotid artery and the anterior border of the sternocleidomastoid muscle. The insertion site is at the midpoint of this anterior border. The needle should be introduced at a 30-degree angle and aimed at the ipsilateral nipple. The patient is placed in the same position for the subclavian approach with the head turned away from the site of insertion. The suprasternal notch, and the clavicle are identified. The needle is inserted below the lateral two thirds of the clavicle and aimed at the suprasternal notch.

Complications

Bleeding, infection, thrombosis, catheter erosion, and pneumothorax or hemothorax are the most common complications of central venous catheters. Bleeding is the most common complication and occurs generally at the time of insertion. Needle puncture of the related artery or perforation of the vein is generally the cause. The bleeding may result in a minor hematoma but can also result in a significant hematoma with airway compression from an internal jugular approach, bladder compression or retroperitoneal hematoma from a femoral approach, or a hemothorax from the subclavian or internal jugular approach. The risk of bleeding is higher in patients with coagulopathy. Bleeding is best controlled with direct pressure. This may not be possible with the subclavian approach. When using direct pressure, patience of the operator is required to adequately maintain pressure long enough to stop bleeding. When applying pressure to the groin, it may be helpful to stabilize the groin with a firm board such as an arm board placed behind the leg and buttocks to maximize the effect of maintaining pressure.

Infection is a common complication of catheters, generally those that have been in place for several days. Central catheter–associated infections can present at the insertion site (more commonly with the cutdown approach), as bloodstream infections, or as septic thromboemboli, endocarditis, or other embolic infections such as lung abscess.[35] The rate of infection as determined by pooled data from 1995 to 2000 from pediatric ICUs that report to the National Nosocomial Infection Surveillance program is 7.7 per 1,000 catheter days. For neonatal ICUs, the data ranged from 11.3 per 1,000 catheter-days for infants weighing less than 1000 g to 4.0 per catheter-days in infants with birth weight greater than 2500 g. The organisms most commonly causing the catheter-related infections are coagulase-negative staphylococci, followed by gram-negative bacteria, enterococci, and *Candida* species.[36]

Multiple aspects of catheter insertion and care have been associated with infection. Following aseptic care techniques, ensuring insertion and maintenance by experienced staff members, and maintaining nurse staffing ratios above certain levels reduce the risk of infections from central venous access.[35,37,38] Unlike in adults, in pediatric patients the femoral site for insertion has not been shown to have a higher risk.[39,40] The use of aseptic technique during catheter insertion has long been recommended, and now the use of full barrier precautions and skin preparation with 2% aqueous chlorhexidine gluconate is recommended.[35,41,42] Prospective studies of these techniques specifically in pediatric patients have not been performed, but the assumption is that both should also be effective and safe in this population. Chlorhexidine is safe even in neonates. The use of antibiotic- or antiseptic-impregnated catheters also decreases the risk of infection. Although the prospective studies have been conducted in adults and not yet in pediatric patients, the catheters are available and approved by the U.S. Food and Drug Administration (FDA) for use in infants as small as 3 kg. Because pediatric patients have limited central venous access sites and a site frequently cannot be reused, regular rotation of catheter sites is not possible. One study evaluating the risk of complications with central venous catheters in pediatric patients showed that the catheters remained uninfected a median of 23.7 days. There did not appear to be a relationship between the daily probability of infection and the duration of catheterization, so it was concluded that routine replacement of central venous catheters in children was not indicated.[43]

Thrombosis can occur in the catheter as well as the vein where the catheter resides. Catheter thrombosis can be safely and effectively treated with thrombolytic drugs such as alteplase. Venous thrombosis can be asymptomatic but may cause veno-occlusive symptoms such as superior vena caval syndrome. Treatment with systemic anticoagulation is indicated in those cases. Certain medical conditions such as diabetic ketoacidosis (even in children) are associated with an increased risk of venous thrombosis to the extent that avoidance of central venous catheterization is recommended if possible.[44]

Because of the proximity of the apices of the lungs to the subclavian veins, pneumothorax is a known complication of catheter insertion at that site. Pneumothorax can also occur with catheter insertion into the internal jugular vein. The left lung apex is higher than the right and, therefore, pneumothorax is more common with left-sided access. A chest radiograph should always be obtained after both successful catheter and unsuccessful catheter insertion at these sites to examine for a pneumothorax. Erosion and perforation of the catheter through a vascular structure or the heart is a known complication of central venous access. Often it is noticed that a collection of fluid such as a pleural or pericardial effusion has developed and the catheter no longer aspirates blood. Immediate radiologic evaluation is indicated in those circumstances. Cardiac tamponade has been reported.[45,46]

PULMONARY ARTERY CATHETERIZATION

In pediatric patients, two techniques are used for measurement of pulmonary artery (PA) pressure—the standard balloon-tipped catheter placed percutaneously at the bedside and a single-lumen catheter placed directly at the time of cardiac surgery. The latter is very common in infants and children with congenital heart disease for which postoperative pulmonary hypertension is a known or predicted problem. This monitoring has been especially helpful when inhaled nitric oxide is used to guide therapy. The flow-directed balloon-tipped catheter, most commonly the Swan-Ganz catheter, has found a role in the management of critically ill pediatric patients, but its use is not as widespread as in adult patients.[47-49]

Indications

For pediatric patients the accepted indications include the following: (1) pulmonary hypertension, either primary or secondary, (2) severe shock unresponsive to fluid resuscitation and vasoactive infusions, and (3) severe respiratory failure requiring high positive airway pressures with associated hemodynamic compromise.[50] Studies showing improved outcomes in critically ill pediatric patients due to the use of the PA catheter are not available.

Pulmonary hypertension in the postoperative patient with congenital heart disease is the most common indication for direct measurement of PA pressure. The preoperative physiology of many unoperated congenital heart defects predisposes the patient to ongoing pulmonary hypertension or episodic pulmonary hypertension in the postoperative periods. Many of these lesions are associated with significant left-to-right shunts, such as large ventricular septal defects, complete atrioventricular (AV) septal defects, and truncus arteriosus. Patients with total anomalous pulmonary venous return with obstruction have severe pulmonary hypertension preoperatively. With changes in ventilation, oxygenation, and pain, wide swings in the PA pressure can occur and can be life threatening. Monitoring PA pressure postoperatively can help guide prevention strategies and therapy.[51-55]

Use of a Swan-Ganz PA catheter in patients with shock, especially septic shock, can allow better definition of their frequently volatile hemodynamic profile patients. One study of patients with septic shock showed they had a higher mortality when their PA occlusion pressure was 8 mm Hg or less, suggesting that placement of a Swan-Ganz catheter in these patients would guide more aggressive fluid resuscitation.[56,57] As in adult patients high ventilatory pressures in children with acute respiratory failure can lead to hemodynamic compromise. In some patients the hemodynamic profiles generated from a Swan-Ganz catheter can help diagnose the cause of the circulatory compromise—whether it is volume restriction or poor cardiac performance. Patients with severely restricted oxygen delivery may benefit from close measurement of their oxygen delivery using variables measured using the Swan-Ganz catheter.[58]

Contraindications

There are no specific contraindications to placing a PA catheter, but there are some relative contraindications. As in the placement of any vascular catheter, the presence of a coagulopathy can increase the risk of placement due to vascular hemorrhage. The presence of significant tricuspid or pulmonary insufficiency as can be seen in patients with structural heart disease can make bedside placement of the catheter very difficult because the flow-directed balloon will not easily advance against the regurgitant jet. However, percutaneous placement using fluoroscopy may still be possible but the catheter will be predisposed to becoming dislodged back into the ventricle. The presence of an intracardiac catheter can cause patients with unstable cardiac arrhythmias—either atrial or ventricular—to experience a deterioration of their condition because of the ongoing electrical irritability from the catheter. Also, the presence of intracardiac shunts, tricuspid insufficiency, or pulmonary insufficiency can make the data obtained particularly from the measurement of cardiac output by the thermodilution technique uninterpretable.

Procedure and Equipment

The single-lumen PA catheter can be of several types, but using a very small gauge (i.e., 20-gauge internal diameter) decreases the risk of intrapulmonary thrombosis. These catheters are placed by direct inspection by the cardiac surgeon at the time of the surgical procedure. They are then tunneled externally for continuous measurement and blood sampling.

The Swan-Ganz type PA catheter is placed percutaneously or rarely by venous cutdown at the bedside. The catheters are available in two sizes: 5 Fr and 7 Fr for pediatric patients. In general, patients weighing less than 15 kg would need the 5-Fr catheter and those weighing more than 15 kg would need the 7-Fr catheter. Because of its size limitation the 5-Fr catheter has only four channels: the distal lumen for measuring PA and pulmonary occlusion pressure, the proximal lumen for measurement of right atrial or central venous pressure and injecting for thermodilution measurement, the thermistor at the tip, and the balloon inflating channel. The 7-Fr catheter is also used in adults. The distance between the proximal and distal ports is important to note in pediatric patients. Ideally, the proximal port sits in the right atrium. The distance between the right atrium and the pulmonary artery varies in the patient based on the patient's size rather than weight. The catheters come with standard distances of 10, 15, 20, and 30 cm difference between the ports. Borland determined the distance between the right atrium and pulmonary artery in a sample of pediatric patients. These data can be helpful in guiding the appropriate choice of catheter.[59]

As in adults the catheters are placed through an introducer sheath generally one size larger than the catheter. This introducer sheath is placed using the Seldinger technique. A catheter or sheath can be place directly into the vein via a cutdown technique, but this is not desirable because it decreases the ability to manipulate the catheter. The percutaneous technique is far preferable.

The site of placement depends on many factors, including the skill of the operator, the size of the patient, the presence of a coagulopathy, the medical condition of the patient, and the accessibility of the vein. The sites most commonly used are the femoral veins, the internal jugular veins, and the subclavian veins. Although any of these sites will allow passage of the catheter into the right atrium and on into the right ventricle and pulmonary artery, less manipulation of the catheter is needed using the right internal jugular vein or the left subclavian vein. However, the right femoral vein also requires less manipulation and is very commonly used due to its easier accessibility and less complications in patients with bleeding diatheses and essentially no risk of pneumothorax in patients with severe lung disease. Other veins at these locations can also be used, but more manipulation may be necessary with bedside access.

The catheter is inserted using sterile technique, and full barrier precautions are recommended. During insertion the transduced pressure tracing is carefully monitored as the catheter courses through the heart. The major difference in passing the catheter in pediatric patients is that the turns and torques of the catheter must be made with more finesse because the distances are shorter and the cavities of the right atrium and ventricle are smaller.

Data Acquisition and Interpretation

As in older patients, much data and information can be obtained using a Swan-Ganz type catheter. Hemodynamic pressures including right atrial and PA pressure can be monitored continuously. PA occlusion pressure (also known as the pulmonary capillary wedge pressure) can be obtained intermittently when the balloon at the tip of the catheter is inflated and floated into the wedge position. Because of the risk of pulmonary infarction, care is taken to maintain the catheter out of the wedge position until the balloon is actively inflated. Because the catheter generally floats to the zone of the lung with the greatest blood flow, it generally will be in area consistent with West Zone III, where arterial pressure is higher than both venous and alveolar pressure. In pediatric patients the best position of the transducer is at the level of the left atrium. This level can be found at the fourth intercostal space in the midaxillary line while the patient is supine. $S\bar{v}O_2$ can also be measured using intermittent sampling from the distal port of the catheter or, if the catheter has an oximeter, can be monitored continuously. Only the larger catheters have that availability. The $S\bar{v}O2$ reflects tissue oxygen utilization and oxygen extraction.

With the use of the thermistor at the tip of the catheter, cardiac output can be measured using the thermodilution technique, a variation on the Fick method.[60] A known volume of fluid at a lower temperature than blood (either iced or room temperature) is injected into the proximal port of the catheter, and the temperature change at the thermistor is noted. The amount of heat loss allows for calculation of flow. A smaller volume of injectate is used in the 5-Fr catheter to avoid fluid overload of the patient. Additionally if iced injectate is used repeatedly, the patient's temperature can be affected. Thus, room temperature injectate is recommended for the smaller pediatric patient. The type of fluid injected also must be taken into consideration for the pediatric patient if repeated measures are to be made. Generally three injections should be made during each measurement period, and with repeated measurements that volume can potentially affect the electrolytes of the pediatric patient. The cardiac output measured in this way is reported divided by the patient's body surface area as the cardiac index.

The catheter is maintained in sterile fashion as with any central venous catheter. The catheter and sheath should have a sterile dressing that is changed according to the protocol for the ICU. The catheter should remain in a sterile sleeve to allow further catheter manipulation while maintaining sterility. The distal port is continuously monitored to detect any change in catheter position such as the appearance of a wedge pressure tracing indicating the catheter has spontaneously advanced or the appearance of a ventricular trace if the catheter falls back into the right ventricle. The electrocardiogram (ECG) must also be continuously monitored to detect arrhythmias secondary to the catheter.

Complications

Complications can occur during three periods: at the time of accessing the vein, during the passage of the catheter, and with prolonged use. Complications occurring during accessing the vein are the same as placing any central catheter. The most common problem during catheter passage is the development of arrhythmias, most of which are benign and self-limited. A caregiver other than the operator must monitor the ECG during placement of the catheter and notify the operator of the presence and type of arrhythmias. Rarely, pharmacologic or electrical intervention would be necessary to control the arrhythmias. The arrhythmia usually resolves with a change in catheter position. For long-term catheter use, the complications included infection or thrombosis. Infection can result not only in sepsis but also in endocarditis.[61] Frequently there is some trauma to the tricuspid and possibly pulmonary valves that would predispose them to endocarditis should a bloodstream infection occur. Thrombosis is another complication seen with these catheters. Pediatric patients may be at greater risk because of the large catheter to vessel size. Other complications can include rupture of the pulmonary artery if the balloon is inflated with the tip already in the wedge position. This can be prevented by careful observation of the pressure tracing to be sure a PA, not wedge, trace is present.

ARTERIAL CATHETERS

Arterial catheterization is performed in pediatric patients using the peripheral and femoral arteries to continuously monitor arterial blood pressure and to sample arterial blood. For neonates the umbilical artery is used. The peripheral arteries most commonly used in pediatrics are the radial, dorsalis pedis, and posterior tibial arteries. Ulnar arteries can also be used, but attention should be paid to the patency of the radial artery.

Indications

The indications for arterial catheterization include continuous arterial blood pressure monitoring in patients who are hemodynamically unstable or who have severe hypertension. Patients who need frequent assessment of arterial blood gases also benefit from having an arterial catheter. Occasionally, patients who need frequent blood sampling and who have relative contraindications to central venous access such as a patient with diabetic ketoacidosis may also benefit from an arterial catheter to use for sampling.

Contraindications

The most important contraindication to arterial catheterization is the situation in which the perfusion of the extremity distal to the arterial catheterization site would be embarrassed by catheter placement. In that situation another site must be chosen. Use of Allen's test before insertion of a radial or ulnar catheter can determine patency of the artery not being used for insertion. As with any procedure, coagulopathy is a relative contraindication.

Procedure and Equipment

Arterial catheters are placed most commonly using the percutaneous approach. As in adults, for peripheral catheters direct insertion of a intravenous-type catheter into the artery is the most common and most successful technique. The Seldinger technique is used for femoral arterial catheterization. Recently, smaller gauge wires (0.15 cm) have been developed. Using a small-gauge butterfly needle and one of these small wires, the Seldinger technique can also be used for peripheral arterial access when direct puncture is not successful. The size catheter for peripheral insertion depends on the size of the patient, with 24-gauge catheters being used for the smaller infants up to 20-gauge catheters for adolescent patients. Larger-gauge catheters are not indicated for peripheral insertion because smaller ones are adequate. Too short a catheter, however, may become dislodged easily. For femoral access the catheter should be long enough to sufficiently enter the artery but of small gauge to prevent occlusion of the artery. A 3-French catheter placed using the Seldinger technique is safe and useful in most pediatric patients except extremely small infants in whom a 20-gauge intravenous catheter can be used.

A cutdown technique can be used if percutaneous access is not possible. This is most easily performed in the radial or posterior tibial artery. Although the femoral artery can be accessed via cutdown, this technique is difficult and requires considerable experience to perform successfully without injuring the artery.

Complications

Bleeding at the time of insertion is a relatively minor complication when using the peripheral arteries, but it may be problematic when accessing the femoral arteries. However, exsanguination can occur if any part of the arterial catheter system becomes disconnected. Continuous monitoring with appropriate alarms can detect immediately when the arterial catheter becomes disconnected. But frequent observation and checking of the system should also occur. Ischemia distal to the arterial catheter can occur even when collateral blood flow is present. Embolic debris or thrombotic occlusion of the vessel can cause the injury. The injuries can be dramatic, resulting in loss of toes, fingers, feet, hands, or even legs. Infection is less of a problem than with central venous

catheterization, most likely owing to the high rate of arterial blood flow.[62,63]

Although occurring less commonly than in adults, symptomatic cardiac arrhythmias do occur in the pediatric patient. Atrial arrhythmias are more common, especially supraventricular tachycardia, which is the most common symptomatic cardiac arrhythmia in children. Atrial flutter and atrial fibrillation also occur in pediatric patients but are more common in patients with underlying heart disease. Ventricular arrhythmias also are seen but are much less common than atrial arrhythmias. In one study from an emergency department, the incidence of symptomatic cardiac arrhythmias was 22.5 per 100,000 in patients younger than 18 years old.[64] Of those, 50% were sinus tachycardia and the rest were supraventricular tachycardia, bradycardia, and atrial fibrillation. Four patients had out-of-hospital arrest during the study period. All of those were documented to have ventricular fibrillation (VF).

Most prehospital cardiac arrests in infants and children are due to respiratory causes with progression of hypoxemia and hypercapnia. The terminal rhythm is most commonly bradycardia with widening of the QRS complex followed by asystole.[65] However, there is a reported frequency of VF ranging from 11% to 19%. The variation appears due to differences in determining the population of arrest victims.[66] In one study it was noted that pediatric patients who do have prehospital VF can be successfully defibrillated (93%) and in this one study had a better outcome than patients with asystole or pulseless electrical activity.[67] In hospital arrests in pediatric patients, VF or ventricular tachycardia is the initial rhythm in 12% and in 25% occurs at some point during the arrest, according to data submitted to the National Registry of Cardiopulmonary Resuscitation.[68]

PROCEDURES FOR ARRHYTHMIAS

DEFIBRILLATION

Indications

In pediatric patients, defibrillation is indicated for documented or suspected VF or pulseless ventricular tachycardia. VF should be suspected when there is a "sudden witnessed collapse."[69] Several clinical scenarios have been associated with VF in pediatrics, including the following: underlying cardiomyopathy or myocarditis, drug intoxication, underlying congenital heart disease, prolonged QT syndrome, a blow to the chest such as from a baseball, electrical shock, and electrolyte abnormalities including hypokalemia. As with adults the more rapid the attempt at defibrillation the more likely restoration of a perfusing rhythm will occur.

Contraindications

There are no contraindications to defibrillation in a patient with proven or suspected VF.

Procedure and Equipment

Although the types of defibrillators are the same for adult and pediatric patients, there are several notable differences, including the energy dose, the size and shape of the child's chest, and the paddle or electrode pad size. The types of defibrillators include the older monophasic type defibrillators, the lower-energy biphasic types, and automatic external defibrillators (AEDs). Although monophasic technology has been used for many years and has proven successful, the newer biphasic technology appears to be favorable. In infant and child animal models the biphasic technology was shown to be more successful in converting VF at a significantly lower energy dose.[70] Animal data have suggested that myocardial damage can result from using excessive energy.[71,72] For the monophasic defibrillator there is no energy dose for infants and children established that relates the dose to successful defibrillation. Gutgesell and associates retrospectively analyzed attempts at defibrillation using the dose of 2 J/kg.[73] They found that when the dose of energy delivered was within 10 J of the 2-J/kg dose, VF was successfully terminated in 91% of shocks. From these data come the recommended dose of 2 J/kg for the starting dose followed by 2 to 4 J/kg and, if necessary, a third dose of 4 J/kg.[69] For the biphasic defibrillators, the energy dose is presumed to be less than the dose for the monophasic defibrillators; however, the dose has not been established. Animal models have shown lower doses to be successful.[70,74]

Transthoracic impedance determines how much energy is required to deliver an adequate shock to the heart for electrical stunning, or defibrillation, of the heart to occur. Impedance is determined by the dose of energy, pad or paddle size, electrode-skin interface, number and intervals of shocks, and pressure of the paddle or pad to the chest. The size of the pad or paddle helps determine impedance. In general, the larger the pad or paddle the lower the impedance. Using too large a pad or paddle may decrease the contact to the chest. Also, if the pads or paddles are too large the contact gel may touch, causing an electrical arc where the energy goes from one pad to another and not through the heart. The smaller, or infant, pad or paddle should be used in patients up to 1 year of age or approximately 10 kg in weight. For larger infants and children, the adult pads or paddles are used.

The placement of the pads or paddles is essentially the same as for adults. One is placed on the upper right side of the chest and the other at the apex of the heart, directly over the heart and to the left of the left mid clavicular line. For some infants because their chest is so small the pads/paddles may still touch in this location. In this case, the pads/paddles may be placed in an anterior/posterior position.

AEDs have been placed in public areas such as airports and sporting venues for expeditious use in the event of VF. The users are often the lay public. This broader potential use of AEDs is intended to decrease the time to defibrillation, which in adults if less than 3 minutes results in a 50% survival rate.[75] Initially, these AEDs were intended for use in adults with their programmed "rhythm libraries" designed for adult rhythms and the dose of energy delivered appropriate for adults. These AEDs were appropriate for larger children, those older than age 8 years. Recent studies have shown that for two AEDs from different manufacturers the rhythm analysis program in each was appropriate for pediatric rhythms.[76,77] Also recently, AED manufacturers have developed pediatric pad and cable systems that effectively raise the impedance in the system, decreasing the dose of energy delivered. The dose may be decreased as much as 50 to 75 J. The FDA has approved these modifications to use in children younger than 8 years. There are currently insufficient clinical data regarding the use of these pediatric pad and cable systems especially in young infants. Because of this information, the International Liaison Committee on Resuscitation (ILCOR) makes the following recommendations regarding the use of AEDs in children:

1. AEDs may be used for children 1 to 8 years old with no signs of circulation preferably with the pediatric pad/cable system adaptations. The adult AEDs may be used for children older than 8 years old. The specific device should have an arrhythmia detection algorithm with a high specificity for pediatric shockable rhythms.
2. The evidence is insufficient to support the use or nonuse of AEDs in children younger than 1 year old.
3. It is still recommended for a lone rescuer to perform 1 minute of CPR before any other action, including attaching an AED or activating EMS.
4. Defibrillation remains recommended for documented VF or pulseless ventricular tachycardia.

Complications

The most important complication would be the failure to successfully return to a perfusing rhythm after defibrillation. Failure to do so can result in either prolonged asystole with no return of cardiac automaticity or in further VF with ultimate development of terminal asystole. There is concern as noted earlier with myocardial damage owing to excessive energy dose but most of that concern is based on animal models and not clinical evidence.

CARDIOVERSION

Synchronized cardioversion is recommended for hemodynamically unstable atrial tachycardias. Most types of atrial tachycardias are amenable to synchronous cardioversion including supraventricular reentry tachycardias via the AV node or via an accessory pathway (Wolff-Parkinson-White), atrial flutter, and atrial fibrillation. It is also recommended for use under elective conditions when medical management of these rhythms has failed. However, certain ectopic arrhythmias will not be converted with cardioversion, including atrial ectopic tachycardia or junctional ectopic tachycardia.

Contraindications

Two areas of concern exist with cardioversion, although this is generally a safe and well-tolerated procedure. The first is patients on digoxin. They have a lowered threshold of VF and have been known to develop it due to cardioversion. So, for patients on digoxin, it is recommended to use lidocaine (1 mg/kg i.v.) before cardioversion. Additionally, one must be prepared to defibrillate the patient should VF occur.

The second area of concern is for patients with atrial fibrillation or atrial flutter. If these rhythms have been chronic and not of acute onset, there is risk of embolism of thrombi occurring in the left atrium. Currently, transesophageal echocardiography can be performed to detect thrombi. However, for patients with a history consistent with chronic atrial tachycardia, anticoagulation for several weeks before cardioversion is recommended to decrease the risk of thromboembolism.

Procedure and Equipment

Because of the discomfort associated with this procedure sedation and analgesia should be provided if the situation allows. In infants with poor perfusion, establishing intravenous access for sedation may delay therapy unnecessarily. Certainly for elective cardioversion, the patient can be prepared for deep sedation by being kept NPO for a prolonged period of time and have adequate intravenous access. The dose used for synchronous cardioversion is much less than for defibrillation. Generally, the initial dose is 0.5 to 1 J/kg, with the second dose being 1 to 2 J/kg. Often because the infant is quite small, the lowest dose on the defibrillator is used. As with synchronous cardioversion in adults, the ECG must be attached to the defibrillator, the defibrillator must be in "sync" mode, and the discharge button must be held until the dose of energy is delivered that requires the machine to detect at least two to three QRS complexes.

As with defibrillation appropriate-sized pads or paddles should be used. The "pediatric" pads or paddles would be used for patients weighing less than 10 kg or younger than 1 year old.

Complications

The most common complication is the development of other arrhythmias such as ventricular tachycardia or, in the patient taking digoxin, VF. Atrial tachycardias may also deteriorate into other atrial tachycardias like atrial flutter or fibrillation. Transient bradycardias such as sinus bradycardia or atrioventricular block may also develop. Thromboembolic complications can also rarely occur, as noted earlier. Theoretically, myocardial injury can occur but with the lower doses of energy needed for cardioversion it is unlikely.

TEMPORARY CARDIAC PACING

Although bradyarrhythmias are unusual occurrences in the pediatric population in general, they are not uncommon in patients with congenital heart disease, particularly in the postoperative period, congenital complete heart block, other forms of heart block, and with ingestions of drugs that can produce bradycardia. When the bradycardia becomes symptomatic or concern exists that it may progress to become symptomatic, then temporary cardiac pacing may be indicated. In general, in emergent situations, the pacing should be ventricular to restore and stabilize cardiac output. Therefore, most temporary systems were designed for ventricular pacing. However, in some instances of bradycardia where AV conduction remains intact, then temporary atrial pacing may be preferred. Maintenance of AV synchrony has been shown to be optimal for cardiac output.

Five types of temporary cardiac pacing are available to pediatric patients: transvenous pacing, transesophageal pacing, epicardial pacing, transcutaneous pacing, and transthoracic pacing. The type of pacing chosen depends on the acuity of the clinical situation, the type of clinical scenario, whether ventricular or atrial pacing is needed, the presumed length of time that temporary pacing will be necessary, and the skill of the operator.

Indications

Symptomatic bradycardia is the ultimate reason for needing temporary cardiac pacing. The type of rhythm and the underlying condition of the patient generally determine if the patient is symptomatic. For the most part, sinus bradycardia is not symptomatic. Because airway, ventilation, and oxygenation abnormalities are the most common cause for sinus bradycardia in children, stabilization of the airway and adequate ventilation and oxygenation usually improves the bradycardia. For other causes, pharmacologic management often with beta-adrenergic agonists can be successful.

Patients with symptomatic advanced-grade heart block need to have pacing. Temporary pacing is indicated while plans are made for permanent pacing. The cause of the heart block usually is cardiac disease such as congenital complete heart block or postoperative heart block. Ingestions of certain medications, especially cardiac medications such as beta blockers, digoxin, or calcium channel blockers, can result in symptomatic bradycardias in children. These patients can often be adequately stabilized with temporary pacing until the drug effects wear off. Pacing, usually transcutaneous or transthoracic pacing, during cardiac arrest is generally futile.

Transvenous Pacing

To achieve transvenous pacing, a pacing catheter is passed into the right atrium and on into the right ventricle, which is then paced. The choice of vein depends on the skill of the operator and the acuity of the situation. The most appropriate vein is the right internal jugular because there is a more direct route into the right ventricle, less manipulation is needed to enter the right ventricle, and the catheter is easier to secure and stabilize in the ventricle. But other central veins can be used, including the subclavian veins, left internal jugular, and femoral veins. Although venous access in children is often easier with the femoral veins, the catheter is more difficult to manipulate into the right ventricle without fluoroscopy and is more difficult to secure in the ventricle. The left subclavian vein should be avoided if the child is large enough to be considered for permanent transvenous pacing, usually above 20 kg.

Contraindications

The only absolute contraindication for temporary transvenous ventricular pacing is the presence of a prosthetic tricuspid valve because damage can occur to the valve necessitating replacement. Severe hypothermia is considered to be a contraindication of internal venous pacing because of the high risk to VF as rewarming occurs. Several relative contraindications have also been reported, including digitalis toxicity, which can also predispose to ventricular arrhythmias and sepsis. Coagulopathy, as with any venous access procedure, is a relative contraindication. Placement is associated with increased risk owing to bleeding, but in emergent situations that risk may be acceptable.

Procedure and Equipment

There are multiple different types of transvenous pacing catheters as small as 5 Fr that can be placed in most infants and children. The lengths of the catheters are variable but generally adequate for most pediatric patients. The pacing catheters are either straight or balloon tipped for flow-directed passage. The electrodes are bipolar electrodes and are located at the tip of the catheter for ventricular pacing. Some catheters also have proximal electrodes that would sit in the right atrium and allow for dual-chamber pacing.

Bedside placement of temporary pacing catheters is possible and more successful if a balloon-tipped catheter is used. If time allows and the personnel are available, the use of fluoroscopy allows for safer and quicker catheter placement. Confirmation of the catheter location is improved with fluoroscopy. If it is unavailable the echocardiography can confirm the catheter location.

Under sterile conditions the vein would be accessed using the Seldinger technique and an introducer sheath placed. Before insertion the pacing catheter should be passed through the sheath to ensure that it is the correct size. Once the sheath is secured in place the pacing catheter is placed into the sheath. The catheter connector pins can be connected to the bedside ECG to aid in passing the catheter. The pin labeled "D" or "1" should be connected to the "right arm lead," and the pin labeled "2" should be connected to the "left arm lead." This allows for an electrogram appearing on the ECG. As the catheter passes from the atrium which a tall atrial electrogram will appear to the ventricle, the tracing will change to a ventricular electrogram. There can be ventricular ectopy when the catheter enters the ventricle but this resolves as the catheter becomes seated in the ventricle. The thresholds are then tested and an optimal position noted. The catheter should then be secured carefully to avoid any movement. Usually a clear adhesive dressing placed over a long length of the catheter will prevent it from becoming dislodged. Catheter position is then confirmed by fluoroscopy, if possible, a chest radiograph, and/or an echocardiogram.

Complications

Complications can occur due to venous access, the mechanical effects of the leads, electrical performance of the leads, infection, and thromboembolism.[78] Venous access complications were previously discussed. The leads themselves can cause ventricular arrhythmias, some of which may be symptomatic. Perforation of the right ventricular lead into the pericardium or into the left ventricle can occur. Pericardial entry may be noted by chest pain if the patient is not sedated, development of a pericardial friction rub, or symptoms of cardiac tamponade. The paced complex should be of a left bundle branch block pattern when the right ventricle is being paced. If the catheter perforates the right ventricular free wall or the septum, then a change in electrocardiographic morphology to a right ventricular bundle branch block pattern may be noted. An echocardiogram can diagnose myocardial perforation and the location of the catheter. Failure to pace is another complication. The location of the catheter should be confirmed if pacing had occurred then ceased. Pacing thresholds are determined by several factors, including the underlying disease, the patient temperature, the electrolyte status of the patient, and concomitant drug therapy. Thresholds should be determined initially and the pacer set at twice the voltage of the threshold. If the original threshold is above 10 mA, consider repositioning the catheter to find an area with a lower threshold. The threshold should be checked every day. In the case of loss of capture, always check the equipment for failure, including battery life and connection of pacing catheter to pacemaker. If the pacemaker is oversensing the patient's underlying rhythm, that can appear as pacemaker failure but can be checked by making the pacemaker insensitive. If pacing still is not occurring, replacement of the catheter may be in order. The longer the catheter is in place the more likely failure to sense or to capture will occur.[79]

Transthoracic Pacing

Transthoracic pacing is rarely indicated; if it is, the situations are desperate. A catheter is placed through the chest wall and directly into the right ventricle when other access to ventricular pacing has failed. In one study of patients with asystole, although capture was achieved in 33% of patients there were no survivors.[80] However, there are several anecdotal stories of successful pacing with survivors.

Contraindications

Because this technique is reserved for extreme circumstances the contraindications are all relative. Before performing this procedure, reevaluation of the situation needs to occur to determine if there are any alternatives to pacing the patient and whether the situation is futile.

Procedure and Equipment

The equipment needed would be a long introducer needle, a bipolar pacing catheter, slip-tipped syringe, and sterile drapes. A kit is commercially available (Elecath) that has all equipment necessary for this procedure. Although it comes in only one size the size would be adequate for all but the smallest patients. The catheter is placed percutaneously via the introducer needle placed at the left xiphocostal angle, 30 degrees to the skin. The needle is aimed and advanced toward the left shoulder while aspirating with the syringe. When blood is obtained, the pacing wire is advanced into the right ventricle. The catheter is then connected to the temporary pacing box, and the highest output is used. Once pacing occurs the needle can be withdrawn and the catheter secured. Catheter position can then be confirmed with a chest radiograph and echocardiogram. The patient must be kept still at bed rest until more secure pacing can be arranged.

Complications

Cardiac tamponade is common. The risk of injury to surrounding structures is quite high, including injury to the heart and major blood vessels, pneumothorax or hemothorax, coronary artery laceration, and liver or lung laceration.[81] The pediatric experience has not been reviewed, but because of the small size of patients the risk of injury to surrounding structures can be assumed to be as high or higher.

Transcutaneous Pacing

Transcutaneous pacing is reserved for emergency pacing of severe symptomatic bradycardia. It is very painful and, hence, best tolerated in those with altered levels of consciousness or those who are sedated. Although the overall outcome for transcutaneous pacing is poor, there is evidence that in certain situations it may be lifesaving.[82] This modality has not been shown to be efficacious in out-of-hospital arrests in pediatric patients.[83] Transcutaneous pacing has its best use in witnessed or in-hospital arrests and severe bradycardia before arrest.

Contraindications

The only true contraindication is in patients with severe chest trauma who do not have enough chest wall to allow the patches to be applied. There are several instances in which transcutaneous pacing will be less effective and pacemaker capture may not be possible. These include extreme obesity, pericardial or pleural effusions, or increased thoracic capacity.[84,85]

Procedure and Equipment

The system is the same for pediatric patients as for the adult system with two electrode patches and the external pacing unit except there are two sizes of patches available. For children weighing less than 15 kg, the pediatric patches are recommended, whereas for children weighing more than 15 kg, the adult patches are used. The patches are marked "front" and "back" so that the negative electrode is anterior and the positive electrode is posterior. This allows for the current to pass from anterior to posterior. The patches can also be placed with the positive electrode on the right chest and the negative on the left side in the midaxillary line, again with the negative electrode over the apex of the left ventricle.[69]

Because the pacing current must traverse the chest wall to reach the heart, the output needed is quite large. These pacing units have a range of 0 to 200 mA with a wider pulse width of 20 or 40 msec. When pacing the patient, the pacing unit is turned to maximal output and adjusted downward as possible. Pediatric patients tend to need lower outputs than adults but that varies with patch size. The PALS course recommends starting with a rate of 100 beats/min and is adjusted as needed.[69] If the patient has some intrinsic rhythm, then the pacer can pace using a ventricular inhibited mode so that the pace does not fire when an intrinsic beat is sensed. If there is no underlying rhythm, then the pacemaker paces continually at a fixed rate.

Complications

The major complication if the system works is pain for the patient, and therefore pain medications with or without other sedation may be necessary.

Epicardial Pacing

Epicardial pacing is performed by the cardiac surgeon placing temporary pacing leads directly on the atrium or ventricle or both at the time of cardiac surgery. In postoperative pediatric cardiac patients, pacing may be necessary in the event of AV dissociation, true AV block, or relative sinus bradycardia. At times, pacing will be needed to suppress other ectopic rhythms. Repair of certain cardiac defects is associated with the potential for AV block, including AV canal, ventricular septal defect, and tetralogy of Fallot. Also, patients with "corrected transposition" are at risk for complete heart block. The AV block seen postoperatively may be temporary owing to edema in the region of the conduction system but may be permanent and ultimately require a permanent system. Generally, several days are allowed to pass to give the edema time to resolve before a decision is made on a permanent system. In the immediate postoperative period, if AV conduction is intact then only atrial pacing is used to maintain AV synchrony, which is important in maintaining cardiac output in the postoperative patient. If, however, there is poor or absent AV conduction, then dual-chamber pacing is preferred. The pacing leads can also be used to diagnose abnormal rhythms; the atrial leads are particularly used in diagnosing atrial or junctional tachycardias. Recently, studies have suggested that pacing both ventricles, a technique called resynchronization pacing, in the postoperative low cardiac output syndrome helps improve systemic blood pressure.[86]

Contraindications

There are no absolute contraindications to the placing of temporary epicardial wires. There may be situations in which there is dense fibrous scar tissue on the heart so that a place on the heart with a low threshold is difficult to find, but that is not a contraindication. Wires still can be placed, realizing that the threshold may be high.

Procedure and Equipment

The wires are placed by the surgeon, generally at the conclusion of the operation. Conventionally, one bipolar lead is placed on the atrium and one on the ventricle. If resynchronization pacing is to be used, then bipolar leads are placed on each ventricle. The wires are then tunneled through the skin. Generally, the ventricular wire is passed to the left of the sternum and the atrial wire to the right of the sternum. This technique may vary by institution but exists to improve wire identification in the ICU. The wires can then be connected to the temporary pacemaker if needed. If pacing is needed, then the thresholds will be tested and appropriate pacing started. The thresholds frequently will increase over several days and the wires are often not useful past 5 to 7 days. In high-risk situations the surgeons may choose to place additional sets of wires as backup.

Complications

This form of temporary pacing is generally very safe. Removal of the wires occurs just with gentle traction. Rarely are there problems with bleeding post removal. Infection of the site of insertion can occur if they are left in for extended periods, but because they are not an "open" system like catheters, the risk for infection is much lower.

Transesophageal Pacing

Transesophageal pacing is a relatively easy technique for both pacing and recording the atrium. It is not useful for ventricular pacing. Like transcutaneous pacing, it is fairly uncomfortable. For this technique a pacing catheter is passed through the nose or mouth of the patient and into the esophagus.

Contraindications

This technique is contraindicated if the patient has AV conduction block because the ventricle cannot be paced. Also, after cardiac transplant, patients cannot be paced using this technique because the transplanted heart lies in front of the esophagus and the tissue being paced is the native atrial tissue. This tissue will not conduct to the new heart. Patients who have esophageal abnormalities such as from recent surgery should not have a transesophageal pacing catheter placed because of the risk of perforation.

Procedure and Equipment

A standard transvenous pacing catheter, usually not balloon tipped, is used with a standard temporary pacemaker. The lead is passed through the nose after applying lubricant. It is passed to the level of the atrium and distal esophagus and attached to the pacemaker. As it is passed it can be connected to an ECG to follow the atrial electrogram. The location where the electrogram is tallest should be the place where pacing will be most effective. The catheter may need to be manipulated to determine the area with the lowest pacing threshold.

Complications

The most common problem with transesophageal pacing is chest pain so pain medication may need to be provided. Perforation of the esophagus is also possible but very rare.

OTHER PROCEDURES

TRANSESOPHAGEAL ECHOCARDIOGRAPHY

Because the transthoracic echocardiographic windows of pediatric patients are often superior to those of adults, the development of transesophageal echocardiography (TEE) in children initially lagged behind its development in adults. Presently, however, TEE has assumed a critical role in the evaluation of children with congenital and acquired heart disease.[87]

Indications

TEE is indicated for pediatric patients who require echocardiographic evaluation but in whom the transthoracic examination is technically inadequate or nondiagnostic. Common examples include the evaluation of patients with intra-atrial baffles, suspected thrombus or vegetation on intravascular devices or heart valves, aortic dissection, or recent postoperative patients with poor transthoracic imaging windows. TEE is frequently used preoperatively to more specifically characterize congenital heart disease and postoperatively after weaning from cardiopulmonary bypass to evaluate for residual defects such as shunts, valvular insufficiency, residual obstruction, and myocardial dysfunction. Recent studies demonstrated that 2% to 14% of planned cardiac surgical procedures were significantly changed based on the results of the intraoperative TEE.[88,89] Pediatric TEE is also useful in the cardiac catheterization laboratory during interventions such as atrial and ventricular septal defect occluder devices, balloon valvuloplasty procedures, stenting procedures, and endomyocardial biopsies.[90]

Contraindications

Contraindications to TEE in pediatric patients include unrepaired tracheoesophageal fistula, recent esophageal surgery, esophageal obstructive lesions, active gastrointestinal bleeding, and perforated viscus. Because neck flexion and extension are frequently required for probe placement, cervical spine abnormalities should be ruled out before the procedure. For patients who require anticoagulation, parameters should be maintained at the lower end of the therapeutic range.[87]

Procedure and Equipment

Because the size of the probe relative to the size of the esophagus and adjacent structures is larger in pediatric patients, and because patients must be cooperative for the procedure to be performed safely, TEE in pediatric patients is generally performed under deep sedation or, more commonly, general anesthesia. Endotracheal intubation for airway protection and controlled ventilation is recommended for smaller patients at increased risk of mechanical airway compromise, children with systemic illnesses that increase their risk of respiratory depression with sedation, children at increased risk of aspiration or impaired airway control, and children with poor underlying cardiorespiratory status, such as severe cyanosis or poor ventricular function.[87] The greatest strength of TEE lies in its ability to image the heart and great vessels not adequately accessible through transthoracic windows, especially the more posterior cardiac structures. These include delineation of atrial anatomy, pulmonary veins, and systemic venous return, both in patients with unrepaired congenital heart disease and in patients after intra-atrial baffle procedures. TEE may also be useful in examining the AV valves, the left ventricular outflow tract, levels of pulmonary outflow tract obstruction, the PA confluence, and proximal branch pulmonary arteries. Limitations to TEE include imaging structures obstructed by bronchial air and limited imaging planes available from the esophageal window.[87]

Commercially available pediatric TEE probes include a biplane transducer with a tip diameter of 9 mm and a multiplane transducer with tip dimensions of 10.7 × 8.0 mm. The smallest probes are recommended by the manufacturer for children as small as 3 kg.[91] Mart and colleagues reported successful intraoperative TEE performed on a 1.4-kg infant, using an 8 × 9-mm probe after predilating the esophagus with a suction catheter.[92]

Complications

Complications of pediatric TEE are relatively rare. The most common complications include inability to successfully intubate the esophagus, airway compromise likely related to compression of the membranous trachea, and compression of posterior vascular structures such as the descending aorta or pulmonary veins.[87] Mild mucosal injury is common after TEE.[93]

FLEXIBLE AIRWAY BRONCHOSCOPY

Flexible bronchoscopes have been utilized for diagnostic and therapeutic procedures in children since 1978.[94] Since then, significant refinements of the procedure and additional clinical applications have been reported and several reviews[95-98] and a guideline[99] have been published. Under most circumstances, flexible airway endoscopy in critically ill children should only be undertaken by an experienced pediatric bronchoscopist. Successful application of flexible airway endoscopy in the pediatric ICU presupposes a basic knowledge of pediatric airway anatomy and management, available bronchoscopes and video documentation, sedation and monitoring, indications, contraindications, specific pediatric procedure-related considerations, as well as potential complications.

Pediatric Airway Anatomy and Management

In addition to obvious size differences between pediatric and adult airways, there are anatomic differences that predispose the infant and young child to airway obstruction with respiratory illness or manipulation. These include a relatively larger tongue in proportion to the oral cavity, more superior position of the larynx in the neck, a narrower and omega-shaped epiglottis that is angled away from the tracheal axis, larger and more redundant arytenoids, a cricoid ring (subglottic space) that is the narrowest portion of the larynx, as well as more compliant and delicate laryngeal and tracheal structures.[100] Thus, in nonintubated children specific techniques that take into account these anatomic differences may be required to maintain airway patency and prevent airway injury. During flexible airway endoscopy, jaw thrust with the head in a neutral "sniffing" position is an effective method of maintaining airway patency in non–critically ill young children without adenotonsillar hypertrophy or cervical injury.[101] In children with adenotonsillar hypertrophy (and without cervical injury) continuous positive airway pressure with either chin lift or jaw thrust may be required.[102] Critically ill children may require additional adjunctive techniques to maintain airway patency, oxygenation, and ventilation (see later).

Available Flexible Bronchoscopes and Video Documentation

There are a number of directable flexible bronchoscopes that are available for pediatric use, including older fiber and newer video bronchoscopes (Table 228-1). Each instrument has unique characteristics and limitations. In nonintubated

TABLE 228–1. DIRECTABLE FLEXIBLE BRONCHOSCOPES FOR USE IN CHILDREN

	Effective outer diameter (mm)	Channel diameter (mm)	Biopsy forceps	Cytology brush	ETT outer diameter* (mm)
Fiber scopes					
Olympus					
BF-XP40	2.8	1.2	Yes	Yes	3.5
BF-3C40	3.6	1.2	Yes	Yes	4.5
BF-P40	5.0	2.2	Yes	Yes†	6.5
Pentax					
FB-8V	2.7	1.2	Yes	Yes	3.5
FB-10V	3.4	1.2	Yes	Yes	4.5
FB-15V	4.9	2.2	Yes	Yes†	6.5
Video scopes					
Olympus					
BF-XP160F	2.8	1.2	Yes	Yes	3.5
BF-3C160	3.8	1.2	Yes	Yes	5.0
BF-P160	4.9	2.0	Yes	Yes†	6.5
Pentax					
EB-1530T3	5.1	2.0	Yes	Yes†	6.5

ETT, Endotracheal tube.
*Recommended smallest ETT that will safely accept particular flexible bronchoscope.
†Protected cytology brush available for particular flexible bronchoscope.

infants and children younger than 2 years of age and children intubated with 3.5- to 4.5-mm endotracheal tubes, the 2.7- to 2.8-mm fiber bronchoscopes are especially useful and are less prone to obstruct the airway than larger instruments. In nonintubated children age 2 to 10 years or children intubated with 5.0- to 6.0-mm endotracheal tubes, the 3.4- to 3.8-mm fiber or video bronchoscopes can be utilized. In older children or children intubated with 6.5-mm or larger endotracheal tubes, the small adult fiber or video bronchoscopes can be utilized. Ancillary equipment including a light source, video camera and recorder, and high-resolution television monitor placed on a mobile cart are particularly helpful in the pediatric ICU. The importance of video documentation during pediatric procedures should not be underestimated. In critically ill children, time in the airway is minimized to avoid airway obstruction and subsequent complications. Video documentation allows shorter procedure times and review in slow motion or frame by frame of airway findings not only by the bronchoscopist but also the intensivist and, if necessary, the airway surgeon.

Sedation and Monitoring

In children undergoing flexible airway endoscopy, sedation is almost always required to obtain useful information and avoid discomfort and airway trauma. Specific sedation recommendations are discussed elsewhere. Appropriate monitoring of critically ill children undergoing flexible airway endoscopy includes the presence of a second physician (intensivist preferred), continuous monitoring of oxygen saturation, respiratory rate, and cardiac rate and rhythm, as well as intermittent (or continuous) monitoring of blood pressure. Careful monitoring should occur during and for a period of time after the procedure, at least until the child has returned to pre–flexible airway endoscopy neurologic and cardiopulmonary status. Intravenous access during the procedure is required. The ability to rapidly re-intubate the patient is essential. In the child with brain injury, flexible airway endoscopy should be performed with caution because

intracranial pressure may transiently but significantly increase during the procedure.[103]

Indications

Upper airway indications for diagnostic flexible airway endoscopy in nonintubated critically ill children include smoke inhalation, airway trauma, acute or postextubation stridor, suspected upper airway obstruction, evaluation of suspected upper airway mass lesions, cyanotic episodes, and severe obstructive sleep apnea. Central or lower airway indications for diagnostic flexible airway endoscopy in nonintubated or intubated critically ill children include smoke inhalation, airway trauma, evaluation of suspected central airway mass lesions, wheezing unresponsive to medical therapy, acute suppurative pulmonary disorders, persistent pulmonary infiltrates or atelectasis, lobar hyperinflation, suspected central airway obstruction, and minor or moderate hemoptysis. Additional indications for diagnostic flexible airway endoscopy in critically ill children with artificial airways include suspected artificial airway obstruction or tracheal injury as well as evaluation before tracheostomy decannulation.[95-98,104-111]

Both bronchoscopy-directed and nonbronchoscopic (blind) bronchoalveolar lavage (BAL) are useful additional diagnostic techniques to obtain airway and alveolar fluid for total and differential cell counts, cytology, histopathology, immunofluorescence and molecular methods of pathogenic organism identification, and cultures for bacteria, fungi, mycobacteria, and viruses.[112,113] Common indications for BAL in the pediatric ICU include evaluation of acute suppurative pulmonary disorders, aspiration, hemoptysis, and new or persistent pulmonary infiltrates or atelectasis in both immunocompetent and immunocompromised critically ill children.[95-98] Bronchoscopy-directed BAL in critically ill intubated children is limited primarily by artificial airway size (see Table 228-1). Nonbronchoscopic BAL is limited by inability to examine the airway for evidence of inflammation or obstruction, direct the catheter to focal airway or parenchymal lesions, and assess placement or obstruction of the artificial airway. Transbronchial biopsies and protected-brush specimens are infrequently obtained in critically ill children, primarily owing to the size of available biopsy forceps and protected cytology brushes and thus resultant requirements for a larger bronchoscope (with channel size of at least 2 mm) and/or larger artificial airway (see Table 228-1). Therapeutic indications for flexible airway endoscopy in critically ill children include intubation of the difficult airway, selective bronchial intubation, removal of large airway obstructive mucus plugs, removal of bronchial casts, and instillation of recombinant human DNase in refractory atelectasis and surfactant in refractory acute lung injury.[95-98,114-116] Although flexible airway endoscopy for foreign body removal has been described in children,[117] rigid-airway endoscopy remains the procedure of choice in most institutions.

Contraindications

In general, flexible airway endoscopy should only be performed if diagnostic or therapeutic benefits outweigh potential risks, however small.[118,119] Significant and potentially absolute contraindications include airway size too small for the available bronchoscope, massive hemoptysis, and marked cardiovascular instability. Relative contraindications include severe upper airway obstruction, profound hypoxemia despite 100% oxygen supplementation, severe pulmonary hypertension, shock, difficult to correct coagulopathy, and significant risk of cerebral herniation.[96,98,99,103,119] Rigid, rather than flexible, airway endoscopy by an experienced pediatric otolaryngologist or airway surgeon should be considered in critically ill children with massive hemoptysis or a suspected foreign body.[99,111]

Specific Pediatric Procedure-Related Considerations

There are several patient, procedure, and study-related considerations when performing flexible airway endoscopy in critically ill children. Before the procedure, communication between the critical care team and bronchoscopist is essential to establish whether flexible airway endoscopy is the most appropriate approach for evaluation and/or management of the patient's airway or pulmonary problem, what procedure should be performed, and what additional preprocedure evaluation of the patient is required. In general, the bronchoscopist should evaluate the patient's cardiopulmonary stability, review metabolic, hematologic, and coagulation laboratory, review chest radiographs, determine the size, if present, of any artificial airways and know or estimate the patient's body weight in kilograms. If possible before the procedure, shock and significant metabolic and coagulation abnormalities should be at least partially corrected. Informed consent should be obtained in all but emergent situations. Both nonintubated and intubated children require adequate sedation, and intubated children may require neuromuscular blockade. Topical anesthesia of the upper and central airways with lidocaine is helpful not only for comfort but also to decrease occurrence of laryngospasm and cough. Total dosages of topical lidocaine should not exceed 8 mg/kg.[120] Topical 1:10,000 epinephrine for management of airway bleeding to be administered via the bronchoscope channel in 0.5- to 1-mL dosages should be available for procedures involving airway brushing or biopsy and transbronchial biopsy. Procedures should be at least transiently discontinued if there are serious complications (see later).

In the face of serious complications, decisions to forgo the procedure should be deferred to the critical care team.

Ancillary equipment that should be available before and during flexible airway endoscopy in critically ill children includes two wall-mounted suction units (one for the bronchoscope), tonsil suction tips, appropriate-size flexible suction catheters, appropriate-size ventilation facemask and bag, as well as resuscitation drugs and equipment. Transnasal insertion of the bronchoscope can be considered in nonintubated relatively stable children without coagulopathy. In children with coagulopathy, transoral insertion or insertion through an endotracheal tube should be considered. During transoral insertion or insertion through an oral endotracheal tube, an appropriate-size bite block should be utilized to minimize potential damage to the bronchoscope.[121] In nonintubated children a clear airway endoscopy mask (VBM Medizintechnik, Germany) that allows simultaneous insertion of the bronchoscope through a side port and delivery of continuous positive airway pressure or ventilation bag breaths may be helpful.[101,102,122] In nonintubated but potentially unstable children, a laryngeal mask airway may be utilized as an alternative to endotracheal intubation to maintain airway patency.[123] However, utilization of a laryngeal mask airway requires deep sedation or general anesthesia and should be performed only by an anesthesiologist skilled in its use in children. In intubated children, an unsealed "T-piece" that does not allow for maintenance of airway pressure is insufficient for maintaining oxygenation or ventilation during flexible airway endoscopy or nonbronchoscopic BAL.[124] Preoxygenation and the use of an adapter attached to the ventilator circuit and endotracheal tube with an aperture that seals around the bronchoscope or catheter (e.g., Ported Double Swivel Elbow, DHD Healthcare, Wampsville, NY) may better maintain oxygenation and ventilation during flexible airway endoscopy or nonbronchoscopic BAL.

The procedure for bronchoscopy-directed and nonbronchoscopic BAL in children is not standardized. The number and size of nonbacteriostatic saline aliquots instilled remains controversial, but typically 2 to 5 aliquots of 0.5 to 1 mL/kg, usually not exceeding 20 mL/aliquot, are utilized. In most situations, the total volume of instilled fluid (all aliquots) should not exceed 10% of functional residual capacity or about 3 mL/kg, with a maximum total in older children or adolescent patients of 300 mL.[26] The usual return of BAL fluid is 40% to 60%. In most clinical laboratories a minimum of 5 to 10 mL of BAL fluid is usually required to perform total cell and differential counts as well as standard pathologic and microbiologic studies. The importance of total and differential cell counts and pathologic evaluation of BAL fluid should not be underestimated. Unusual pulmonary disorders and infections may be missed if these studies are not obtained.[112,113,125,126] Consultation with an infectious disease specialist, pathologist, and/or the microbiology laboratory may be helpful in prioritizing studies and improving diagnostic yield of BAL fluid studies, protected-brush specimens, and airway and transbronchial biopsies. In certain pulmonary disorders such as interstitial lung disorders, invasive fungal pneumonia, and other unusual infections, diagnostic yield from BAL fluid studies, protected-brush specimens, and/or airway and transbronchial biopsies may be inadequate.[127-129] Negative invasive flexible airway endoscopy studies do not obviate the need for further more invasive diagnostic studies, such as open lung biopsy, particularly in critically ill children who are not responding to empirical antimicrobial or other therapy.

Complications

Serious complications of flexible airway endoscopy in non–critically ill children are unusual. In a recent review, serious complications, including significant oxygen desaturation, laryngospasm, excessive coughing, bronchospasm, pneumothorax, and high fever, occurred in less than 2% of procedures.[130] Airway hemorrhage has been reported to occur rarely in children undergoing transbronchial biopsies.[131,132] Fortunately, death associated with pediatric flexible airway endoscopy is distinctly unusual, although two have been reported.[133,134]

Serious complications of flexible airway endoscopy or nonbronchoscopic BAL in critically ill children have not frequently been reported but have included hypoxemia, bradycardia, airway hemorrhage, increased ventilatory requirements, and fever.[110,124,135-137] Factors that may be associated with increased risk of complications include need for mechanical ventilation with high airway pressures, profound hypoxemia, cardiovascular instability, severe coagulopathy, and brain injury. Risk of complications due to flexible airway endoscopy in critically ill children may potentially be decreased by at least partial correction of metabolic, coagulation, and cardiovascular abnormalities, appropriate monitoring, adequate sedation, use of adjunctive airway techniques, use of the smallest flexible bronchoscope appropriate for the diagnostic or therapeutic intervention, and limitation of more invasive flexible airway endoscopy procedures (airway brushing and biopsy, transbronchial biopsy, instillation of medications) to appropriately selected patients.

Summary

There are a number of diagnostic and therapeutic applications of flexible airway endoscopy in critically ill children. Maximizing diagnostic and therapeutic yield and minimizing serious complications can be accomplished by careful patient selection, stabilization of the patient as much as possible before the procedure, careful monitoring, adequate sedation, use of adjunctive airway techniques, presence of a pediatric intensivist during the procedure, and performance of the procedure by an experienced pediatric bronchoscopist.

THORACENTESIS AND THORACOSTOMY

Because of the frequent occurrence of several predisposing conditions such as complex pneumonias, postoperative effusions, and barotrauma, needle thoracentesis and tube thoracostomy are not uncommon procedures in pediatric patients. Needle thoracenteses are performed frequently to drain pleural effusions for diagnosis or treatment and to emergently relieve tension from a pneumothorax while preparations are made for chest tube insertion. Chest tube placement is indicated for ongoing relief of pneumothoraces and for drainage of large effusions or empyemas.

Indications

Tube thoracostomy is needed when collections of either air or fluid need to be drained. The fluid may be a transudative, chylous, or exudative effusion. The indications to place a chest tube for an effusion generally are large size of the effusion, apparent respiratory embarrassment from the effusion, or the concern that the effusion is purulent. In the latter

instance, a limited thoracotomy or thorascopy often is needed to decorticate and drain the empyema. Chest tube placement is also indicated for drainage of pneumothoraces, especially those under tension or in patients on positive-pressure ventilation who are at high risk for developing tension. Pneumothoraces can occur spontaneously but more often are secondary to diffuse lung injury resulting from infectious pneumonitis or chemical pneumonitis such as with hydrocarbon or gastric acid aspiration. They may be due to barotrauma, usually caused by excessive pressure with mechanical ventilation or bag-to-tube ventilation. Although barotrauma most often occurs in patients with underlying lung injury altering the compliance of the lung, it can occur in patients with normal lungs when excessive pressure occurs.

Needle thoracenteses are needed mostly for emergent drainage of a pneumothorax or for diagnosis of a pleural effusion. The definitive treatment of a pneumothorax is tube thoracostomy, but needle drainage may be needed in emergency situations. One scenario would be the development of a tension pneumothorax during air transport of a trauma patient where tube insertion would be difficult but needle drainage can quickly be performed. Needle thoracentesis is also performed when a pleural effusion needs drainage to examine the fluid to make a diagnosis of the cause of the fluid. The pleural effusion undergoing needle thoracentesis can be a transudate from underlying pneumonia often due to bacteria or *Mycoplasma*, oncologic disease such as lymphoma, or collagen vascular disease with associated pleuritis such as lupus erythematosus. Effusions in patients with bacterial pneumonias may require a diagnostic thoracentesis. This is most often needed in patients whose pneumonias are not responding to therapy or in immunocompromised patients who may have pneumonia of unusual etiology.

Contraindications

With coagulopathy elective needle thoracentesis may be contraindicated because of the risk of bleeding. Correction of the coagulopathy with blood products should be attempted. Also, patients with abnormal anatomy (i.e., severe scoliosis) may be at risk for lung (or other organ) puncture with this technique. Generally, these patients benefit from an ultrasound-guided thoracentesis. For a patient with a tension pneumothorax and hence hemodynamic compromise, there are few, if any, contraindications to either needle thoracentesis or chest tube placement

Procedure and Equipment

Thoracenteses are usually performed with a styleted needle such as an intravenous catheter or spinal needle. The advantage of the intravenous catheter is that once the stylet is removed the catheter is relatively soft and less likely to lacerate the lung. Selection of catheter gauge depends on patient size and the potential viscosity of the fluid. If purulent fluid is suspected, then a larger-bore catheter is recommended. Even a 14-gauge catheter can be readily inserted into the intercostal space of an infant. The length of the catheter required again depends on the size of the patient. In small infants and children a catheter greater than 2 cm in length is rarely required. However, larger adolescents or obese children may need catheters 3 to 4 cm in length to enter the pleural space.

The position of the patient for needle thoracentesis again depends on the location of the fluid and on the age, size, and stability of the patient. An older child who is stable can be seated during the procedure, allowing a posterior approach, which for most nonloculated effusions is optimal. However, unstable children or smaller infants should be placed in a supine or in a slight decubitus position. If the fluid volume is small or loculated, an ultrasound of the chest can be performed to identify the best location for draining the fluid.

To drain a tension pneumothorax either at the second intercostal space, midclavicular line or the fourth intercostal space, an anterior axillary line is acceptable. The patient should be placed in the supine position for either approach. To drain fluid, the fourth intercostal space at the anterior axillary line should be used unless an ultrasound evaluation suggests an alternate approach.

Infants and children undergoing thoracentesis should be given adequate sedation and analgesia. As with adults the area is prepared in a sterile fashion and local analgesia is infiltrated. Care must be taken to instill local anesthetics into the subcutaneous tissues down to the intercostal muscle, over the rib, and onto the pleura itself. The catheter is then inserted over the superior aspect of the rib to avoid the intercostal vessels and directed into the pleural space. Often a cough response is elicited when the pleura is disturbed and/or after the fluid is drained and the lung expands. The fluid is removed in sterile fashion and sent for appropriate studies, including culture. Once the catheter is removed a small occlusive dressing is applied to prevent aspiration of air into the pleural space.

Placement of a chest tube in a child is a particularly painful bedside procedure, so sedation and analgesia are imperative. Analgesia may also be required after the procedure while the tube remains in place. Several techniques are available for chest tube insertion in pediatric patients depending on the indication for tube placement, the anticipated length of time the tube is to be needed, and the skill of the operator. Standard chest tubes as well as softer, pigtail catheters are available.

The standard procedure requires sterile preparation and instillation of local analgesia followed by a small incision. Mosquito-type forceps are inserted through the incision and tunneled up one rib space then rotated so that the points of the forceps are aiming toward the pleura. They are then advanced over the superior aspect of the rib and through the pleura. Generally, the pleura will give, often with a "pop." The chest tube is then guided through the defect in the pleura and into the pleural space. Posterior placement of the chest tube is generally optimal for drainage of fluid. Anterior placement, in a patient lying supine, is generally optimal for drainage of a pneumothorax. Occasionally for patients with severe ongoing air leaks requiring prone and supine positioning, placement of anterior and posterior chest tubes may be needed to provide adequate continuous drainage of the pneumothorax.

The chest tube is secured with suture and the incision closed with a pursestring closure with the suture wrapped around the chest tube. The tube should also be secured to the child's side with either tape or a chest tube securing device (commercially available) to prevent the tube from being pulled out when the child becomes more active. The site should be kept clean and povidone-iodine may be used. A clean dressing may be applied. The site should be checked for signs of infection or tissue fatigue.

Two other techniques are available for chest tube placement. Smaller chest tubes are available with a pointed trocar

in the tube that can be placed percutaneously. The site is prepared in the same sterile fashion as in the previous technique, and local analgesia is again infiltrated in the same manner. The chest tube with the trocar is then passed superiorly over the rib and through the pleura into the pleural space. As soon as the pleural space is entered then the trocar must be removed to avoid lacerating the lung or pulmonary vessels. The chest tube is then manipulated into proper position. This technique is most often used in neonates and small infants because their chest wall is thinner and easier to enter with this device. This technique has been associated with laceration of the heart or pulmonary vessels with the trocar and so must be used with great care.

For transudative or chylous effusions, placement of a pigtail drainage catheter into the pleural space is usually sufficient. For very viscous fluid collections these catheters may not have an adequate internal diameter to drain the fluid, and a standard chest tube is indicated. Pigtail catheters have also been shown to effectively drain pneumothoraces.[138] Roberts and colleagues reviewed the experience in one pediatric ICU using pigtail catheters and found the catheters were highly efficacious for draining serous and chylous effusions, slightly less efficacious for draining pneumothoraces and hemothoraces, and poor for draining empyemas.[139] Pigtail catheters were more effective in draining pneumothoraces in smaller infants and children than older children. Complications due to catheter placement occurred in less than 5% of patients but could be serious. One of the advantages of the pigtail catheter is that it is smaller and softer than a conventional thoracostomy tube and hence more comfortable.[138] For patients who are mobile, these tubes may be preferred. The catheters are available in a variety of sizes but one commercially available kit carries an 8.5 Fr catheter that is adequate for even small infants. The tube is placed after a sterile skin preparation and analgesia is administered. The Seldinger technique is used for tube placement. An introducer needle is advanced into the pleural space while being aspirated by the operator using a slip-tip syringe. Once the fluid or air is entered by the needle, a wire is passed through the needle. The needle is then removed and a stiff introducer dilator is passed over the wire and into the pleural space to dilate the subcutaneous tissues and open the pleura. The wire is left in place and the dilator is removed. The catheter is then passed over the wire and into the pleural space. The wire is removed, and the catheter is connected to a Pleur-Evac. The catheter is secured at the site with suture and to the patient with tape or a tube holder. This technique is particularly useful if the fluid is loculated and can be localized using ultrasound. The needle can then be directed toward the fluid collection.

The Seldinger technique can also be used to place standard chest tubes. This technique can be used to drain either fluid or a pneumothorax. Directing the needle toward the air collection can help in placing the tube more precisely into the pneumothorax. As opposed to the pigtail technique where one dilator is used, a series of dilators of increasing size are needed before placing the chest tube itself. The Seldinger technique has been shown to be faster, with a similar complication rate as placement using standard technique in pediatric patients.[140]

Complications

Laceration of the lung or intrapulmonary tube placement may occur with any of these techniques. A bronchopleural fistula can be created with an intrapulmonary chest tube insertion. Bleeding from the lung or chest wall can occur in patients with or without a coagulopathy with any of these techniques. Injury to the diaphragm, liver, or spleen can occur.[141] The heart and pulmonary vessels can be lacerated or entered with a chest tube by any technique, but the standard technique of using a small incision and controlled entry into the pleural space is considered safer in this regard. Mechanical problems that can occur with the chest tube include (1) side holes being placed outside the pleural space, (2) the tube itself being placed into the subcutaneous tissue and not the pleural space, (3) kinking of the tube, and (4) occlusion of the tube due to fibrin or pus. Failure of the drainage system can also result in either failure to drain a pneumothorax or reaccumulation of the air.[142]

PERICARDIOCENTESIS

In the pediatric population, pericardiocenteses are performed most commonly for the relief of cardiac tamponade or impending tamponade and rarely for diagnosing the etiology of a pericardial effusion. The procedure is best performed under controlled circumstances using echocardiography or fluoroscopy. However, in emergency circumstances it can be performed without guidance. The fluid can be drained with either a simple needle or a catheter placed in the pericardium using the Seldinger technique. The latter is preferable if ongoing fluid accumulation is believed to be a potential problem.

Indications
When cardiac tamponade is present, drainage of the fluid is essential. In some instances surgical drainage may be more expeditious or more successful such as in the immediate postoperative cardiac patient whose previous incision can easily be opened to relieve the tamponade. Surgical drainage may also be indicated if the fluid appears purulent by echocardiogram. However, even in those patients a pericardiocentesis may sufficiently relieve the pressure to stabilize the patient before surgery. Most effusions will be amenable to nonoperative drainage with a needle or catheter. Often a large effusion will need to be drained even if overt tamponade is not present. Small infants who are mechanically ventilated and develop a pneumopericardium may require a pericardial tube if hemodynamic compromise is present. Often, pneumopericardium is well tolerated or spontaneously drains into the mediastinum.

Contraindications
There is no contraindication to pericardiocentesis when acute cardiac tamponade is present. Open drainage is the method of choice when there is traumatic tamponade and the patient is in cardiac arrest.[143] The presence of coagulopathy is a relative contraindication in patients needing elective pericardial drainage. Other relative contraindications include inexperience of the operator when the procedure is elective, loculation of the effusion making it difficult to reach percutaneously, and abnormal anatomy of the patient such as severe scoliosis.

Procedure and Equipment
If there is an indication that pericardial fluid could continue to accumulate, then a catheter should be left in place if possible. If the fluid is being drained solely for diagnostic studies, simple needle drainage is adequate.

Both needle drainage and catheter placement are performed under sterile conditions. The patient should be placed supine with the head elevated 30 degrees. The patient should be sedated for both comfort and safety, because inadvertent movement could result in injury to the heart.

To perform simple needle drainage an appropriate needle is chosen. Use of an intravenous catheter with a stylet that can be removed is preferable. This decreases the risk of cardiac laceration. The size of the catheter is dependent on the size of the child and the viscosity of the fluid being drained. Generally, some indication of viscosity is noted by echocardiography. If the fluid has fibrin strands present or there is concern that it may be purulent, a larger-bore catheter should be used. Even a 14- or 16-gauge catheter can be used in a small infant if the fluid is believed to be viscous. The length of the catheter is also important in that even in infants, catheters of at least 1 inch and preferably longer may be necessary to access the fluid. Care must be taken, however, to stop advancing the catheter as soon as fluid is accessed to avoid injury to the heart.

For placement of a catheter for prolonged drainage, the Seldinger technique is used. The catheters are generally soft with multiple side holes for optimal drainage and a pigtail configuration to decrease the risk of cardiac puncture by the catheter. Several catheters and catheter kits are commercially available in sizes amenable to small patients. Generally, catheters of 5 to 8 Fr are appropriate for most pediatric patients. The fluid is accessed using a steel introducer needle or an intravenous catheter. Then a flexible J wire is passed through the needle and the needle removed. A somewhat stiff dilator is then carefully advanced into the pericardial space to enlarge the tract. The dilator is exchanged for a soft, pigtail catheter. The catheter is then attached to a drainage bag after a sample of fluid is sent for studies. The landmarks for entry are similar in children and adults. The needle is introduced at the junction of the xiphoid and left costal margin, inserted at a 30- to 45-degree angle, and directed toward the left clavicle. Echocardiography can be helpful in directing the needle and noting its presence in the pericardial space, although easy aspiration of pericardial fluid must be present to confirm the needle is in proper location.

Complications
The most concerning complications of pericardiocentesis are myocardial perforation and/or coronary laceration. Myocardial perforation may not result in any significant injury if the ventricle is entered. However, a laceration could occur, resulting in bleeding into the pericardial sac, causing or worsening tamponade. Laceration of a coronary artery can result in ischemic injury to the myocardium. Injuries to other organs such as the liver, spleen, stomach, intestines, and diaphragm have been reported. Hemoperitoneum, pneumoperitoneum, hemothorax, and pneumothorax have all been reported. Cardiac arrest and death can also occur.[144,145] In a study of complications of pericardiocentesis in children, five complications occurred in 43 procedures (including myocardial perforation) with no hemodynamic alteration, pneumopericardium, or ST-segment elevation.[146] Myocardial perforation occurred in one critically ill neonate that resulted in death.

NEUROLOGIC PROCEDURES

INTRACRANIAL PRESSURE MONITORING

Increased intracranial pressure (ICP) is a common cause of morbidity and mortality in the pediatric population. The most common causes of increased ICP include brain injury from accidental or intentional trauma, central nervous system lesions such as brain tumors or hemorrhage, cerebral hypoxic-ischemic injury, and cerebral edema from metabolic or infectious diseases. The continuous measurement of ICP may be indicated when the increased pressure cannot expeditiously be relieved by surgical means, as in the relief of hydrocephalus associated with brain tumors. By measuring the ICP, the cerebral perfusion pressure (CPP) can be calculated and appropriately treated.

Indications

The indications for placement of an ICP monitor in children include severe traumatic brain injury and cerebral edema from medical causes. In traumatic brain injury ICP monitoring is indicated after severe injury, which in infants and children is defined as a Glasgow Coma Scale score of 3 to 8.[147] In addition, the presence of open fontanels and/or suturing in an infant does not preclude the development of intracranial hypertension or negate the utility of ICP monitoring.

ICP monitoring has been used in metabolic encephalopathies such as diabetic ketoacidosis and Reye's syndrome. ICP monitoring was an important part of therapy in pediatric patients with the diffuse cerebral edema associated with Reye's syndrome.[148] Although the incidence of Reye's syndrome has decreased, monitoring of ICP in other hepatic or metabolic causes of cerebral edema may be indicated. In cases of meningitis or encephalitis when there is evidence of increased ICP either by physical examination or radiologic imaging, monitoring of ICP may help guide therapy. The use of ICP monitoring in global hypoxic-ischemic injury such as pediatric near drowning is believed to be less useful.[149,150]

Contraindications

The most important contraindication to placement of an ICP monitor is the presence of a coagulopathy, which can be seen in children with multiple trauma, or from massive brain tissue injury or hepatic failure.

For placement of an intraventricular catheter in children, massive cerebral edema may severely impinge on the ventricles and prevent entry of the catheter into the slit-like ventricles. In those cases, a tissue pressure monitor represents a reasonable alternative.

Procedure and Equipment

The available monitoring systems are discussed in detail in Chapter 48 on central nervous system monitoring in adults. Specific pediatric data on the advantages or disadvantages of these systems are lacking. No matter which monitoring system is used, a neurosurgeon skilled in pediatric procedures should perform the catheter placement. Depending on the level of consciousness of the child, additional procedural sedation should be used. Guidelines for preparation and placement of the catheter follow those for the technique used in adults.

Interpretation

The normal ICP in children should be less than 10 mm Hg. CPP is another valuable parameter and is easily calculated as the mean arterial pressure minus the mean ICP. In children,

mortality rate increases when the CPP is consistently below 40 mm Hg.[151] One retrospective study of patients between the ages of 1 and 5 years by Kaiser and colleagues[152] showed that all survivors had CPP greater than 50 mm Hg. Optimal CPP in infants and children has not been adequately determined and probably is age dependent and possibly dependent on disease process.

Complications

Overall, complications with ICP monitoring are infrequent.[153] Infection is the most common complication but is relatively uncommon. The risk of infection increases with the length of time the monitor is in place. Cerebrospinal fluid studies for cell count and culture can be followed daily to detect early evidence of infection. Bleeding can also be a complication, especially if a coagulopathy exists. Bleeding can occur at the time of insertion or may develop over several days. It can develop in either the brain parenchyma or the ventricles. Narayan and associates[154] reported that bleeding at the time of insertion occurred in less than 2% of adults. In a retrospective study of radiographic studies in pediatric patients who had previous intracranial pressure monitors, hemorrhage was found in about 10% of the patients.[155] Tiny punctate hemorrhages were the most common finding, but hemorrhages were clinically silent.

JUGULAR VENOUS MONITORING

The clinical value of jugular venous monitoring in adults is discussed in Chapter 223. Data on the merits of this technique in infants and children are limited.[156]

Indications

The most common indication for placement of a jugular venous bulb catheter is in patients with traumatic brain injury and metabolic cerebral edema. In some pediatric centers the catheters are placed for other critical neurologic situations such as status epilepticus and cerebral arteriovenous malformations.[157] In general this technique is used in situations where cerebral blood flow may be altered in relation to metabolic demands. Cerebral blood flow or metabolism may be altered from the underlying neuropathology, from medications used to manage ICP such as barbiturates, from the use of other therapies (e.g., hypothermia), or from other extracerebral factors (e.g., respiratory compromise).

Contraindications

The technique is contraindicated if the jugular vein is not accessible. Coagulopathy is a relative contraindication. Also this modality is theoretically less useful in focal versus global brain injury in children.

Equipment and Technique

Sampling of jugular venous blood for measurement of oxygen saturation can be intermittent through a standard central venous catheter placed in the jugular bulb or can be continuous using a fiberoptic catheter. The latter technology is available on catheters as small as 4 French, making this approach useful for most children including smaller infants.

Placement of the catheter at the bedside in pediatric patients has been shown to be safe and practical.[158] The side of insertion most commonly is the right jugular vein because it is larger with higher flow. It is also the vein of choice for right-sided lesions or injury and in diffuse bihemispheric disease.

The left internal jugular is chosen with left-sided lesions or if other contraindications to using the right side are present (e.g., ventriculoperitoneal shunt, local trauma, or infarction). There are two basic techniques for placing the catheter into the internal jugular vein: the horizontal supine head-turn technique and placement with the patient in the head-up position.[159] The latter technique is used mostly in the cases with confirmed or suspected cervical trauma.

To use the horizontal supine head-turn technique a towel is placed behind the shoulders to extend the neck and the head is turned in the direction opposite to catheter placement. An imaginary line is drawn from the suprasternal notch to the tip of the mastoid process. The carotid artery is palpated at the midpoint of this line and displaced medially. One centimeter lateral to this midpoint is the entry site for the needle. A local anesthetic can be infiltrated followed by the introducer needle. Standard Seldinger technique can then be followed. The guidewire is passed cephalad until it meets resistance in the jugular bulb. Care must be taken to note that the wire has passed beyond the tip of the needle. After the wire is exchanged for the catheter, the catheter is passed until it meets resistance in the jugular bulb and secured there if blood can be easily withdrawn. Jugular venous samples can be intermittently obtained or, if a fiberoptic catheter was placed, then continuous jugular venous oxygen monitoring can commence. A lateral skull film should be obtained to confirm the proper position of the catheter at the base of the skull.

The head-up technique is reserved for patients with contraindications to movement of the head and neck. The carotid pulsation is found at the level of the inferior border of the thyroid cartilage. The puncture site is slightly lateral to this pulsation. The artery need not be displaced to enter the vein.

Interpretation

The jugular venous oxygen saturation is a reflection of the tissue utilization of oxygen when the arterial content of oxygen is adequate. A decrease in the jugular venous oxygen saturation when arterial oxygen content is normal indicates either absolute or relative cerebral ischemia. When ICP is manipulated by therapeutic interventions, a stable jugular venous oxygen saturation suggests that tissue oxygenation has remained stable, presumably owing to adequate cerebral blood flow. However, decreases in jugular venous oxygen saturation during hyperventilation or barbiturate administration suggest that cerebral blood flow may be inadequate. A threshold value of 50% saturation has been shown to be associated with increased mortality rate in adults with severe traumatic brain injury (see Chapter 55).

Complications

Complications of the jugular bulb catheter are similar to complications of any central venous catheter, including infection and thrombosis. Complications during insertion include inadvertent puncture of the carotid artery (seen in about 15% of infants and children) and venous and arterial hematomas.[160] Gayle and coworkers[160] reported no effect of jugular venous bulb catheterization on ICP in 26 infants and children. The catheters can be malpositioned into smaller veins such as the facial vein. In a study of adult patients with jugular venous catheters, routine ultrasound of the vein noted asymptomatic thrombus formation in 40% of patients. No single clinical factor was associated with thrombus formation, and none became symptomatic.[161]

ANNOTATED REFERENCES

Adelson PD, Bratton SL, Carney NA, et al: Guidelines for the acute medical management of severe traumatic brain injury in infants, children, and adolescents. Pediatr Crit Care Med 2003;4(3 Suppl):S72-S75.

This extensive review uses evidence-based methodology in evaluating all therapies currently available for the management of acute traumatic brain injury in pediatric patients.

Dieckmann RA, Fiser DH, Selbst SM (eds): Illustrated Textbook of Pediatric Emergency and Critical Care Procedures. St. Louis, Mosby-Year Book, 1997.

The authors discuss in depth the indications and techniques for performing a wide variety of emergency and critical care procedures in children. Accompanying the discussion are illustrations showing the appropriate landmarks and procedures for use in infants and children.

O'Grady NP, Alexander M, Dellinger EP, et al: Guidelines for the prevention of intravascular catheter-related infections. Pediatrics 2002;110(5):e51.

These guidelines present an extensive review of the issues involved in catheter-related infections in both pediatric and adult patients. They cover all types of intravascular catheters, including placement of central lines, which is one of the most common invasive procedures in pediatrics and one with a significant number of complications, including infections.

Samson RA, Berg RA, for the American Heart Association and Bingham R for the European Resuscitation Council: Use of automated external defibrillators for children: An update—An advisory statement from the Pediatric Advanced Life Support Task Force, International Liaison Committee on Resuscitation. Pediatrics 2003;112:163-168.

A review of the issues involved with defibrillation in pediatric patients includes the incidence and outcome of ventricular fibrillation as well as the technologic differences in defibrillation in pediatric patients compared with adults. The issues regarding the use of automated external defibrillators in pediatric patients as young as 1 year old are also discussed.

Schellhase DE: Pediatric flexible airway endoscopy. Curr Opin Pediatr 2003; 14:327-333.

An extensive review of the use of bronchoscopy in pediatric patients is presented including the experience in evaluation and management of airway and pulmonary diseases as well as research advances using biopsy and lavage specimens from bronchoscopy.

Section XIV

SURGERY AND TRAUMA

Section XVII

SURGERY AND TRAUMA

Chapter 229

RESUSCITATION OF HYPOVOLEMIC SHOCK

Juan Carlos Puyana

KEY POINTS

1. The bleeding trauma patient requires simultaneous efficient evaluation and rapid treatment to ensure adequate tissue perfusion and successful outcome.

2. Resources such as thermally efficient fluid warmers, effective transfusion services, and rapid availability of coagulation tests are practical aspects of trauma resuscitation that require attention to detail.

3. Preventing hypothermia and recognizing other complications of massive transfusion, as well as following trends in vital signs, peripheral tissue perfusion, urinary output, central venous pressures, and arterial and central venous blood gas analysis, are of vital importance to managing patients with hemorrhagic shock.

Fluids have been given intravenously for the management of fluid deficits for more than 100 years. In 1883, the English physiologist Sidney Ringer discovered that calcium-containing tap water was better than distilled water for maintaining the viability of tissues from animals in vitro.[1] The understanding of the circulatory system and the importance of maintaining adequate circulatory volume were realized long ago. Furthermore, the desired elements and their approximate concentrations in intravenous fluids for plasma substitution have been known for many years.

The first reported intravenous transfusion occurred in 1492.[2] In a desperate attempt to save a dying pope, blood was transfused from three youngsters, using a vein-to-vein anastomosis. Both the patient and the three donors died. The first known successful animal-to-animal transfusion was carried out in 1667. In 1818, Dr. James Blundell performed the first successful transfusion on a patient suffering from hemorrhage during childbirth. In 1830, the gold-plated steel needle for intravenous use was invented. In 1831, a paper published by O'Shaughnessy[3] described the need for administering salts and water to cholera victims, an idea that was put into practice by Thomas Latta soon thereafter. During the 1930s, Baxter and Abbott produced the first commercial saline solutions. In the 1950s, plastic intravenous tubing replaced rubber tubing, and soon thereafter, the central venous approach for venous access was described by a French military surgeon.[4] This approach represented a breakthrough for estimations of the state of hydration (central venous pressure [CVP] measurements) and the need for volume support.

Blalock's fundamental work on shock showed that injury precipitated obligatory local and regional fluid losses, the effects of which could be ameliorated by vigorous restoration of intravascular volume. This concept became a cornerstone to the understanding of the pathophysiology of shock and provided the fundamental rationale for intravenous therapy for hemorrhage and hypovolemia.[5]

The introduction of blood transfusions as the result of noteworthy contributions made by surgeons during World War I and World War II dramatically changed the outcome in cases of severe hemorrhage and traumatic shock. During the Korean War, fluid overload became a common and lethal side effect of resuscitation, owing to a lack of knowledge about how infusates disperse and are eliminated during trauma. Between the Korean conflict and the Vietnam War, Shires and colleagues described the shifts of fluid and electrolytes into cells after severe hemorrhagic shock.[6] As a consequence, the treatment of patients with shock was altered during the Vietnam conflict, leading to better outcomes and a lower incidence of acute renal failure.

EPIDEMIOLOGY OF SEVERE HEMORRHAGIC SHOCK

Traumatic injury is the leading cause of death for individuals younger than 44 years of age in the United States.[7] Overall, trauma results in approximately 150,000 deaths per year, and severe hypovolemia due to hemorrhage is a major factor in nearly half of those deaths.[7-9] Approximately one third of trauma deaths occur out-of-hospital, and exsanguination is a major cause of deaths occurring within 4 hours of injury.[10] The distribution of battlefield injuries in the Vietnam War showed that 25% of the deaths occurred as a result of massive exsanguination and that the victims were not salvageable. An additional 19% of deaths occurred in cases that were deemed salvageable, and these were the result of torso exsanguination (10%) and peripheral exsanguination (19%).[11] As evidenced recently in the Iraq campaign, the fighting of the future is likely to involve terrorists and guerrilla interdictions and will be fought by small groups of combatants over shorter time periods with smaller numbers of casualties at any point in time. However, because of the likely locations of these conflicts, evacuation by air may be difficult or impossible, as was the case in Somalia in 1993.[12] As a result, immediate and even ongoing treatment of casualties may be significantly extended. Shock and ensuing circulatory failure, therefore, may result from a variety of different trauma scenarios. Therapies used in the field may vary depending on the time frame from injury to medical evacuation, the skills and resources of the first responders, and the field site of combatant injury. The incidences of blunt trauma and head injury vary among civilian trauma centers because of geographical reasons. The mechanisms of injury and the severity of blood volume lost, as well as the effectiveness of prehospital intervention, vary widely among trauma centers in regions with mostly rural trauma compared to trauma centers in large inner city scenarios. Controversial issues regarding optimal blood pressure for patients with penetrating injury or with blunt trauma and head injury remain.[13] In the case of civilian trauma, exsanguination also plays a major role even though transport times are shorter and that time at the scene is by average less than in military casualties. The number of preventable deaths due to hemorrhage, however, are significant, and although there is a greater percentage of patients with exsanguination arriving alive to civilian trauma centers, definitive control of hemorrhage and appropriate fluid resuscitation remains the cornerstone of management.[9,14]

CURRENT STATE OF KNOWLEDGE ABOUT INADEQUATE OR INCOMPLETE RESUSCITATION IN HEMORRHAGIC AND HYPOVOLEMIC SHOCK

It has long been recognized, based on the early research of Wiggers, that an animal could be bled to a hypotensive state for a period of time after which the re-infusion of the shed blood would not save the animal's life.[15] This phenomenon was termed *irreversible shock*. Theories about the cause of this state included relaxation of precapillary arteriolar sphincters, injury to the heart, and elaboration of circulating myocardial depressant factors. However, the concepts leading to or facilitating the possibilities of irreversible shock are rarely discussed in the literature at present. Some clinicians now believe that patients in most shock states can be resuscitated with more volume, with correction of hypothermia, and by infusing inotropic agents. Yet many patients continue to die, if not acutely from irreversible shock, then later from events initiated by severe and prolonged shock. Clinically, however, circulatory collapse associated with irreversible shock is the common pathway of progressive deterioration precipitated by trauma, hemorrhage, and severe hypovolemia.

The mechanism of injury, the availability of immediate medical and surgical care, and the ability to provide adequate resuscitation determine how fast and how long the process of circulatory collapse requires. If patients suffering from severe penetrating trauma to the chest or abdomen, with major injuries to the thoracic or intra-abdominal vessels, do not die at the scene, they undergo aggressive interventions that may include an emergency thoracotomy and massive transfusions of packed red blood cells and asanguineous fluids equaling many times their blood volume. These patients may ultimately require damage control interventions and manifest severe hypothermia and coagulopathy as well as circulatory failure even after hemorrhage has been controlled.[16] In contrast, patients with blunt trauma or slow but persistent bleeding from relatively vascular injuries involving smaller arteries or veins may manifest a more protracted, yet equally lethal, form of irreversible shock. These patients may receive

some type of resuscitation but may take hours to arrive to a facility where definitive care can be provided. These patients may not undergo massive transfusion but still ultimately suffer from severe acidosis and hypothermia before dying. Similarly, patients with severe dehydration, or patients with more cryptic forms of shock (e.g., tissue hypoperfusion in the absence of systemic arterial hypotension) may also go on to a more protracted form of organ dysfunction and death. If the resuscitative interventions are provided late, some of the hemodynamic and metabolic abnormalities may improve before death occurs.

HEMODYNAMIC PHASES OF IRREVERSIBLE SHOCK

There are several distinct phases of irreversible shock. In phase I, there is a nonhypotensive period of hemorrhage, which persists through the loss of approximately 20% of blood volume. During phase I, there is a reduction in cardiac output for subjects resting comfortably, and, in animal models, neither administration of beta-adrenergic blockers nor cardiac denervation alters the host's responses.[17] In phase II, with further hemorrhage, mean arterial blood pressure decreases, often abruptly, due to an inappropriate reduction in sympathetic tone, known as the Bezold-Jarisch, or empty-ventricle, reflex.[18] To a first approximation, the Bezold-Jarisch reflex occurs at a predictable level of hypovolemia, roughly 20% of blood loss, although there are important variations among individuals. These variations have been demonstrated in studies involving human volunteers subjected to lower-body negative pressure.[19] In animal models, this reflex is also modulated by the degree of external stress and pain.[20,21] Arterial blood pressure usually stabilizes for a time at approximately 60 mm Hg in phase III, as reduced perfusion to the brain triggers a final intense vasoconstriction of all nonessential organs (i.e., organs other than the brain or heart). Severe hemorrhage causes a decrease in cardiac output and compensatory arteriolar constriction in certain vascular beds, particularly in the splanchnic region. This vasoconstriction diverts blood to the brain and heart and is a physiologic adaptation to low blood pressure and flow associated with hemorrhagic shock. If hypovolemia is not corrected, the vasoconstriction leads to an irreversible state of shock in phase IV, which is usually lethal. In addition, hemorrhagic shock is associated with increased adhesion of polymorphonuclear neutrophils to endothelial surfaces, leading to leukosequestration in the microcirculation, and therefore signals the onset of inflammation.[22] These processes (decreased cardiac output, regional arteriolar vasoconstriction, and leukosequestration) all work together to impair tissue perfusion during hemorrhagic shock and even after resuscitation. At this stage, tissues are severely hypoperfused, lactic acid and inflammatory mediators build up, and there are a number of processes that, along with any further hemorrhage, lead to eventual cardiovascular collapse. These processes include progressive cardiac dysfunction,[23] losses of intravascular fluid to the peripheral tissues, and loss of the ability of arterioles to constrict.[22]

COMPONENTS OF THE HOST RESPONSE TO SHOCK

If the magnitude of the initial insult is sufficiently great or the resuscitative interventions are late or inadequate, then the main driver of overall damage to the host is the hemo-dynamic/metabolic failure associated with hypovolemia itself. Although inflammation ensues as well, the damage/dysfunction caused by inflammation is only seen later. However, if the patient is resuscitated to some degree (as often happens in civilian clinical practice or on the battlefield), then inflammatory damage begins to predominate, extending the insult to the patient and eventually leading to multiple organ failure syndrome (MODS) and death. However, it is imperative to understand how the exact nature of the initial interaction between insult and inflammation will determine the patient's outcome.

CARDIOVASCULAR AND HEMODYNAMIC RESPONSE

Shock is defined as inadequate delivery of O_2 to metabolically active tissues. Severe shock is characterized by acute generalized failure of O_2 delivery that manifests itself as acute organ dysfunction and ischemic tissue injury.[24] Consequent circulatory collapse may be the result of a multitude of factors, all acting simultaneously to ultimately induce a total failure of the circulation. Because the characteristics of circulatory shock change at different degrees of severity, shock was divided into three major stages by Guyton.[25] First is the *nonprogressive stage* or *compensated shock*. In this stage, compensatory mechanisms prevent irreversible organ damage and the individual will achieve full recovery with relatively minimal interventions. Next is the *progressive stage* or *decompensated shock*. In this stage, a substantial fraction of individuals will die if aggressive resuscitation is not provided. Last is the *irreversible stage*. In this stage, shock has progressed to such an extent that all forms of known therapy are inadequate and the individual may linger for several hours until death.[23] Guyton demonstrated that there is progressive deterioration of cardiac output as a component of irreversible shock.[14] However, there is often a dissociation between *total blood flow* (cardiac output) and *effective blood flow* to metabolically active tissues.[26] There is also a poor correlation between changes in cardiac output and systemic blood pressure during progressive shock.[27]

NEUROENDOCRINE RESPONSE

Pressure and stretch receptors in the aortic arch and carotid bodies serve a key role in detecting blood volume and pressure changes and maintaining perfusion to the brain and the heart. The mechanisms involved in maintaining blood pressure homeostasis are autonomic control of cardiac contractility and peripheral vascular tone, hormonal responses to stress and volume depletion, and organ-specific microcirculatory mechanisms that regulate regional blood flow. The magnitude of the neuroendocrine response to hemorrhage is based on the magnitude and rapidity of onset of the decrease in effective circulating blood volume.[28]

The nervous system responds immediately to loss of circulating blood volume with sympathetically mediated arteriolar and venous vasoconstriction.[29-31] This vasoconstriction promptly reduces the capacitance of the circulatory system. High-pressure baroreceptors in the aortic arch and carotid sinus respond instantly to changes in blood pressure by adjusting sympathetic tone. The arterial baroreceptors sense decreased stretch of the arterial wall. The low-pressure

atrial stretch receptors are sensitive to both stretch and pressure. Afferent vagal fibers typically carry signals that tonically inhibit central processors. A decrease in the effective circulating blood volume or blood pressure causes release of the chronic inhibition imposed by the baroreceptors.[32] This message ascends to the nucleus tractus solitarius in the medulla oblongata, resulting in loss of the tonic inhibition of heart rate and up-regulation of sympathetic outflow. With greater blood loss, the role played by the arterial baroreceptors increases. Flow to the heart and brain is maintained until all compensation fails. Intense triggering of sympathetic signals is activated when the arterial blood pressure decreases to less than 50 mm Hg and is maximally stimulated when the systolic blood pressure is less than 15 mm Hg.[25] Blood flow to other (nonvital) tissues decreases markedly. For example, renal blood flow may be reduced to 5% to 10% of normal with acute hypovolemia.[33] Flow to the splanchnic circulation, skin, and skeletal muscle also decreases significantly. These constrictor responses in hypovolemic shock are mediated by epinephrine and norepinephrine, which are released from the adrenal medulla and sympathetic nerve terminals in the walls of blood vessels.

Acute hypovolemia initiates multiple endocrine responses. The nucleus tractus solitarius signals the hypothalamus to release corticotropin-releasing factor and vasopressin. Consequently, plasma levels of adrenocorticotropic hormone, cortisol, vasopressin, and glucagon all increase.[28,32] The renin-angiotensin-aldosterone axis is stimulated with release of the vasoconstricting autocoid angiotensin II.[34] Similarly, release of vasopressin increases water reabsorption in the distal tubule of the kidney and induces splanchnic vasoconstriction. Growth hormone and glucagon oppose the effects of insulin by promoting gluconeogenesis, lipolysis, and glycogenolysis, all aimed at increasing the supply of substrate to support energy production. On the other hand, epinephrine and norepinephrine promote insulin resistance and decrease substrate availability.[35,36]

The sympathetic vasoconstrictor mechanisms are augmented by these hormonal effects in response to hypovolemia. Further loss of fluid or salt through the kidneys is also limited by hormonal effects. The summation of the neuroendocrine response is to maximize cardiac function, conserve salt and water for the maintenance of circulating blood volume, and provide nutrients and oxygen to the brain and the heart.[37]

METABOLIC RESPONSE

If hemorrhage is massive, the compensatory mechanisms designed to spare blood flow to the brain and heart may be overwhelmed, as occurs in cases of irreversible shock. However, if the hemorrhage is controlled or fluid replacement therapy is initiated promptly, the patient may enter a phase described as *compensated shock*.[38] *Circulatory collapse* can occur later if the compensated phase of shock is not recognized or if there is continuous uncontrolled bleeding. In either circumstance, the victim progressively deteriorates and death ensues in minutes to hours, depending on the magnitude of the combined insults (i.e., the *degree* and *duration* of hypovolemia). Recent observations in severely injured patients suggest that continuous monitoring of oxidative metabolism and tissue pH in peripheral organs may be used as indicators of cellular stress and impaired tissue perfusion.[39,40] Minimally invasive assessment of cellular stress—using interstitial pH, tissue P_{CO_2}, and NADH autofluorescence (marker of cellular redox state) as read-outs—may reflect anaerobic metabolism and dysoxia.[41,42] These measurements have been obtained from the gut mucosa, skeletal muscle, subcutaneous tissue, and several other organs.[43,44] Measurements such as tissue PCO_2, PO_2, and pH in these organs have been correlated with specific measurements of cellular dysfunction specific to those organs.[45]

As a consequence of the stoichiometry of the reactions responsible for the substrate level phosphorylation of adenosine diphosphate (ADP) to form adenosine triphosphate (ATP), anaerobic metabolism is inevitably associated with the net accumulation of protons.[46,47] Accordingly, determination that tissue pH is not in the acid range should be sufficient to conclude that perfusion (and therefore arterial oxygen content) are sufficient to meet the metabolic demands of the cells, even without knowledge of the actual values for tissue blood flow or oxygen delivery.[46] By the same token, the detection of tissue acidosis should alert the clinician to the possibility that perfusion is inadequate. It seems likely that monitoring tissue PCO_2 (tissue capnometry) will play a role in establishing thresholds for and transition points into the metabolic failure associated with circulatory collapse.[48] By eliminating the potentially confounding effects of systemic hypocarbia or hypercarbia, calculating and monitoring the gap between tissue PCO_2 and arterial PCO_2 may prove to be even more valuable than simply following changes in tissue PCO_2.[47,49]

Weil and associates[50] described a sublingual PCO_2 sensor and demonstrated that changes in sublingual PCO_2 are more sensitive to changes in cardiac output and blood pressure than any other parameter currently used to quantify hypoperfusion. Shoemaker and associates[39,51] described the use of transcutaneous oxygen tension ($PtcO_2$) and CO_2 tension ($PtcCO_2$) as early warning signals of tissue hypoxia and hemodynamic shock in trauma patients. These authors proposed the use of transcutaneous sensors for the assessment of $PtcO_2$ and $PtcCO_2$ that have been used for years in neonatal medicine as a surrogate measure of arterial blood gases. They showed that, compared with survivors, patients who died had significantly lower $PtcO_2$ and higher $PtcCO_2$ values, beginning with the early stage of resuscitation. Periods of $PtcO_2$ at less than 50 mm Hg for more than 60 minutes or $PtcCO_2$ at greater than 60 mm Hg for more than 30 minutes were associated with 90% mortality and 100% morbidity rates.[51]

McKinley and colleagues[39,52] have demonstrated a correlation between skeletal muscle PCO_2, PO_2, and pH with hemorrhagic shock using fiberoptic sensor technology that allows for continuous monitoring. Both skeletal muscle and gastric mucosa respond similarly to hypotension, and the magnitude of this response is similar for gastric intramucosal pH (pHi) and muscle pH. Skeletal muscle parameters (PO_2, PCO_2, and pH), however, appear to indicate a greater severity of shock and more prolonged recovery than mixed venous measurements or gastric mucosal parameters. Muscle PO_2 may also provide information that is comparable to other more elaborate calculations of O_2 delivery and utilization.[53] In one case report, the continuous monitoring of skeletal muscle pH, PCO_2, and PO_2 was able to detect ongoing hemorrhage of a severely injured trauma patient in the setting of "normal" systemic variables.[39] Although preliminary, these findings suggest that the continuous monitoring of skeletal muscle pH and related parameters may provide a minimally invasive and more sensitive way of following the resuscitative effort.

ACUTE INFLAMMATORY RESPONSE TO SEVERE HEMORRHAGE

Hemorrhage, trauma, and associated hypovolemia may induce an acute inflammatory response that involves a coordinated mobilization of numerous cells, hormones, and molecules of the innate and adaptive immune systems, the neurologic system, and the endocrine system, with repercussions for all organ systems.[54,55] When appropriately controlled and contained, the inflammatory response restores the body to healthy function following clearance of the offending agents and appropriate tissue repair. In more severe settings, however, inflammation remains persistently activated and leads to the detrimental consequences described earlier.

Immune cells, such as macrophages and neutrophils, react to damaged or dysfunctional tissue.[56] Macrophages are present in almost all body tissues and can directly detect bacterial lipopolysaccharide through genetically encoded pattern recognition receptors.[57-59] Adhesion of neutrophils to damaged or dysfunctional endothelium (a consequence of most types of ischemia-reperfusion injury, including hemorrhagic shock[60,61]) leads to microvascular "plugs" that contribute to the "no reflow" state and progressive hypoperfusion.[62,63] Additionally, neutrophils reach other capillary beds by detecting specific signals on vascular endothelium and navigate to their target by following chemoattractants.[64-66] Tissue injury also activates the complement pathway that further stimulates macrophages and neutrophils.[54,67,68]

Once activated, macrophages and neutrophils produce and secrete cytokines, peptide hormones that play a crucial role in mounting successful immune and tissue healing responses. Cytokines regulate the activation of macrophages, neutrophils, and lymphocytes, as well as the production of other cytokines. Cytokines often have varied and overlapping functions.[56,69] Proinflammatory cytokines, such as tumor necrosis factor, interleukin (IL)-1, and IL-6, are produced at various stages of the inflammatory response and promote immune cell activation.[70] The production of these proinflammatory cytokines is counterbalanced by the production of anti-inflammatory cytokines, such as IL-10 and transforming growth factor beta (TGF-β1), that serve to restore homeostasis and promote tissue repair.[71,72]

Proinflammatory cytokines also induce macrophages and neutrophils to produce reactive oxygen and nitrogen species (e.g., nitric oxide [NO], superoxide [O_2^-], hydroxyl radical [OH•], and hydrogen peroxide [H_2O_2]), that are directly toxic to tissue.[68,73,74] With the exception of NO, which may also help to protect the body's cells from damage under certain settings,[75] these molecules are toxic to cells, and the induced dysfunction can incite more inflammation.[76] For example, reactive oxygen species have been implicated in the pathology of ischemia-reperfusion injury,[77] whereas NO can reduce blood pressure and is the major agent implicated in the hypotension characteristic of decompensated hemorrhagic shock.[78] NO appears to be especially relevant to the pathophysiology of irreversible shock: the inducible nitric oxide synthase (iNOS) and its products were found only during the irreversible phase of hemorrhagic shock in rats.[79]

DESIGNING RESUSCITATIVE STRATEGIES

Understanding of the effectiveness of resuscitative fluid therapy can be greatly enhanced if a number of basic principles regarding fluid dynamics, body compartments, and membrane behavior are well understood. These concepts are not only necessary to understand the effects of volume expanders on the circulation but are also required to appropriately interpret conflicting results frequently seen in studies on fluid replacement therapy. These principles predict well what is observed when specific fluid-based therapeutic interventions are applied in the trauma room, the operating room, the ICU, or the wards.

Severe fluid losses and/or fluid deficits can result from a variety of clinical conditions. Furthermore, a myriad of conditions that are characterized by circulatory failure can trigger a complex inflammatory response that has been associated with the ensuing MODS and death. Therefore, a fundamental knowledge of the physiologic bases of fluid therapy is necessary to prevent and minimize the consequences of severe fluid losses and shock.

BODY WATER COMPARTMENTS

There are three body water compartments: the intravascular or plasma volume, the interstitial volume, and the intracellular volume. Under normal circumstances, the interstitial volume is three times the intravascular volume, and the intracellular volume is about 2.5 to three times the interstitial volume. The intracellular volume, therefore, is seven to nine times as large as the intravascular volume (Fig. 229-1). The intravascular volume is well defended by the body. Significant changes in the intravascular volume are not well tolerated. Losses of 30% to 40% of the intravascular volume lead to severe hypovolemia and profound hypotension. Cardiac arrest usually occurs after 50% to 60% of the blood volume is lost. Hypervolemia of 20% to 30% leads to pulmonary edema.[80]

FLUID MAINTENANCE AND REGULATION

The interstitial volume is in continuous equilibrium with the intravascular volume; indeed, the interstitial volume acts like a large capacitor, buffering increases or decreases in intravascular volume. The interstitial volume has two important characteristics. First, it is not as extensively defended a reflex mechanism as the intravascular volume is; therefore, interstitial volume fluctuates widely under normal as well as pathophysiologic circumstances. Second, the interstitial compartment can expand virtually without limitation. The compliance of the interstitial compartment is extraordinarily high, and until the interstitial compartment is filled to about three times its normal volume, the interstitial pressure remains low.[81]

It is important to understand the properties of the membranes that separate the body water compartments to predict the effects of a specific volume expander. These membranes are quite different, and the events that rule fluid exchange are also different in each of these compartments. The intravascular and interstitial compartments are separated by the capillary endothelium, a boundary layer that behaves differently within the various organs of the body. The capillary endothelium is much more permeable, for example, in the lung and the liver than it is in peripheral tissues, such as muscle, skin, and subcutaneous fat.[82] These differences in permeability give rise to dramatically different effects in the behavior of organs in response to hemodilution. The greater the permeability in a capillary bed, the less it is affected by hemodilution. The interstitial concentration of protein is already much higher in tissues, such as the lung, that are supplied by capillary beds with more permeable as compared to less permeable endothelial layers.[83] The capillary endothelium is a very permeable membrane; it allows small molecules to pass through essentially unhindered. Sodium, potassium, water, chloride, and bicarbonate all move freely through the capillary endothelium. Larger molecules such as albumin, however, are restricted to varying degrees from traversing the capillary endothelium.

The leakage of albumin across the endothelium varies depending on the endothelial characteristics of the tissue. In the lung, for example, albumin leakage under normal circumstances is so high that the interstitial concentration of this protein is about 70% to 80% of the plasma concentration.[84] Therefore, the relative protein gradient across the pulmonary capillary for albumin is relatively minor. The permeability to albumin of the liver endothelium is only slightly less than that of the lung; thus, the interstitial concentration of albumin is about 60% of the concentration in plasma. In contrast, peripheral tissues, specifically muscle and fat, leak albumin to the extent that the interstitial concentration is only 20% to 30% of the plasma concentration.[85]

The cell surface membrane is impermeable to proteins (Fig. 229-2). The sodium-potassium pump (Na^+,K^+-ATPase) is the active mechanism that operates at the cell surface, ejecting sodium from the cells and transporting potassium into the cells. The cell membrane is permeable to water. Bicarbonate and chloride also cross relatively freely.

There are crucial differences between the capillary endothelial barrier and the cytosolic membrane barrier. Functioning of the capillary endothelial barrier is relatively independent. The capillary endothelium continues to function for an extended period of time after oxygen delivery ceases and ATP production is compromised. Functioning of the cell surface barrier is energy-dependent. As soon as ATP production is impaired, for example during severe shock, the Na^+,K^+-ATPase stops working. When it stops working, there is passive diffusion of sodium ion into cells, increasing the intracellular osmotic pressure; water flows down the osmotic gradient, leading to cellular swelling, a phenomenon that was described by Shires and associates in animal models of severe irreversible shock.[86]

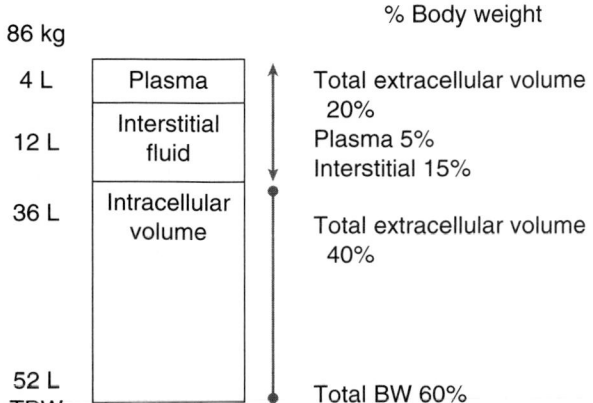

Body Composition

% Body weight

86 kg

4 L — Plasma — Total extracellular volume 20%
Plasma 5%
Interstitial 15%

12 L — Interstitial fluid

36 L — Intracellular volume — Total extracellular volume 40%

52 L — Total BW 60%
TBW

FIGURE 229–1. Total body composition volume compared to percentages of intracellular and extracellular volume.

Membrane Characteristics of Body Water Compartments

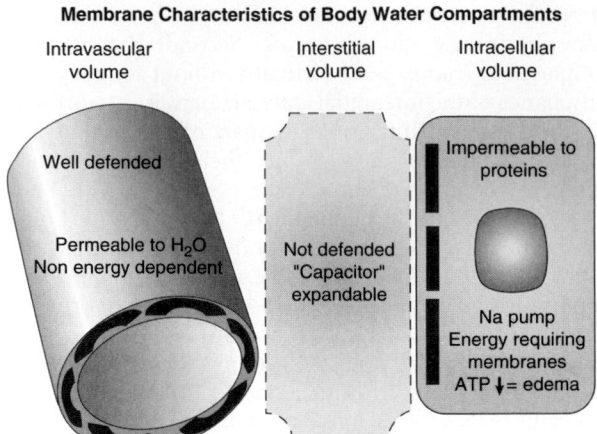

FIGURE 229–2. Membrane characteristics of body water compartments.

VOLUME EXPANDERS AND RESUSCITATION

Resuscitation with Crystalloids

The following is an analysis of the effects of infusing 2 L of a balanced salt solution (such as Ringer's lactate solution) on the intravascular, interstitial, and intracellular volumes. Thirty minutes is allowed for equilibration after infusion into the intravascular space. The crystalloid distributes between the intravascular and the interstitial spaces in proportion to their starting volumes (Fig. 229-3). Because all the components of a balanced salt solution cross the capillary endothelium freely, the capillary endothelium in no way restricts the movement of a balanced salt solution between the intravascular and interstitial compartments. If their starting volumes are in a 1:3 ratio, as is normal in a healthy individual, then the fluid distributes in the same 1:3 ratio (see Fig. 229-1). Thus, in the present example, 500 mL remains in the intravascular compartment and 1500 mL moves into the interstitial space. Since the solution is iso-osmotic with plasma and the intracellular compartment, no osmolar gradient is produced and there is no net movement

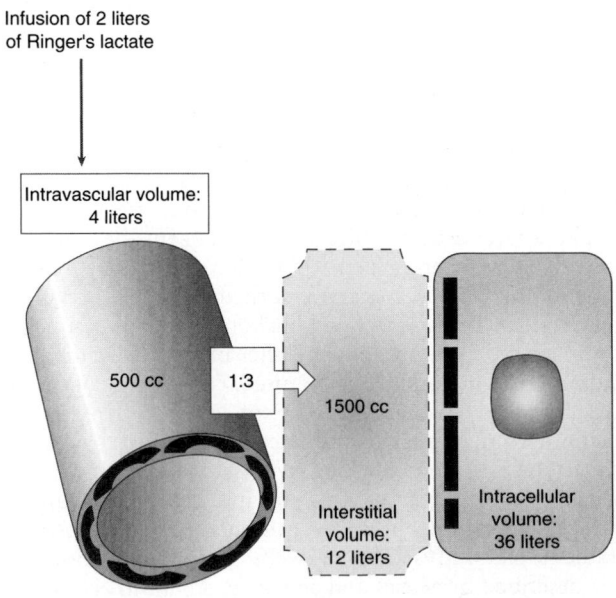

FIGURE 229–3. Infusion of 2 L of Ringer's lactate solution.

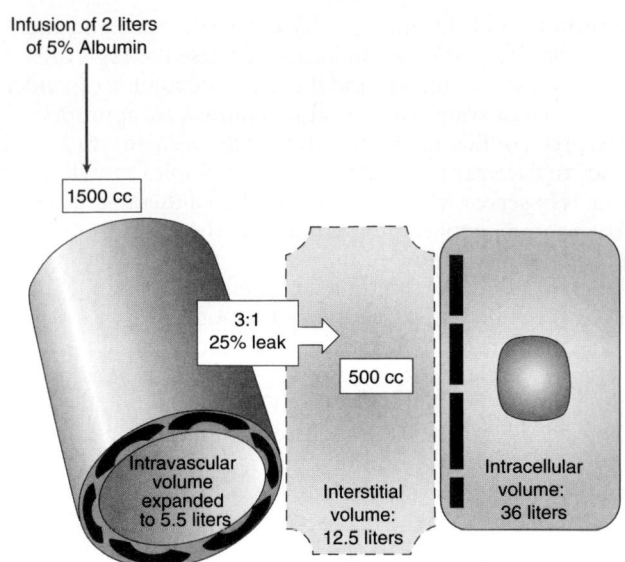

FIGURE 229–4. Infusion of 2 L of 5% albumin.

of water across the cell surface membrane. The volume of the intracellular compartment is, therefore, unchanged.

Resuscitation with Colloids

If, in the above example, we substitute a colloid solution, such as 5% albumin in normal saline, for Ringer's lactate solution and infuse it into the intravascular compartment, the relative leakage of the albumin solution out of this space will be proportional to the net albumin leakage in the body, approximately 25% to 35% (Fig. 229-4).[85] As a result of this effect, an iso-oncotic solution given into the intravascular compartment leaks into the interstitial compartment in rough proportion to the leakage of albumin; that is, about 25% to 35% of the administered volume moves from the intravascular space into the interstitial space. Thus, if 2 L of 5% albumin solution (in normal saline) is infused, 500 mL equilibrates into the interstitium and 1500 mL is retained in the intravascular compartment. Because it is iso-osmotic, there is no net gradient across the cytosolic membrane and intracellular volume remains constant (see Fig. 229-4). A comparison of the net effects of 2 L Ringer's lactate solution and 2 L 5% albumin in normal saline reveals that one fourth of the balanced salt solution (500 mL) remains in the intravascular space whereas three fourths of the colloid solution (1500 mL) remains in the intravascular space. Therefore, there is a ratio of intravascular filling of 3 to 1 between the colloid and crystalloid solutions.

Resuscitation with Hypertonic Saline

The use of hypertonic saline is a topic of great interest, in part because of its potential utility as a pre-hospital resuscitation fluid. Using the above theoretical construct, it is possible to describe the effects on volume re-expansion expected when a 7.5% saline solution is infused into the intravascular compartment. A solution containing 7.5% (weight/volume) sodium chloride exerts eight times the normal osmotic pressure of the body; therefore, as soon as 7.5% saline is introduced into the intravascular space, the resulting increase in osmotic pressure pulls water from the intracellular space. No water is recruited from the interstitial space, because the capillary endothelial barrier is freely permeable to small ions, such as sodium and chloride (Fig. 229-5).

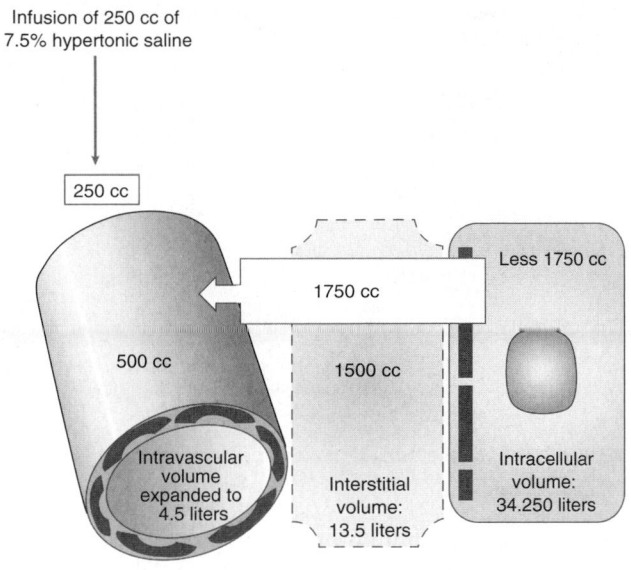

FIGURE 229–5. Infusion of 250 mL of 7.5% hypertonic saline.

Whereas equilibration of a colloid, such as albumin, takes several minutes (10-30), equilibration of hypertonic saline takes only seconds. If 250 mL of 7.5% saline solution is infused intravascularly, it recruits 1750 mL of water from the intracellular space, resulting in a net increment of 2000 mL. Since the salt in the hypertonic saline distributes instantaneously from the intravascular to the interstitial spaces (as noted above), the 2000 mL of water recruited from the intracellular compartment must redistribute into *both* the intravascular and interstitial compartments (in proportion to ratio of the starting volumes of these two spaces).

VOLUME REPLACEMENT AFTER ACUTE BLOOD LOSS

The objective of fluid replacement therapy is to restore intravascular euvolemia. Therefore, we could calculate the theoretical volume of fluid that must be infused to compensate for 1000 mL of blood loss. According to our analysis, if blood loss is replaced with a colloid (5% albumin) solution, then it is necessary to provide 1333 mL to effectively re-expand the intravascular volume (Fig. 229-6B). If the fluid is a balanced salt solution, then the necessary volume will be 4 L (Fig. 229-6A). Finally, if 7.5% saline solution is used, then the volume required to replace the volume losses of 1 L of blood should be 500 mL of hypertonic saline. In clinical practice, however, a 500-mL bolus of 7.5% saline will not be tolerated because it will induce marked hypernatremia and possibly cause seizures. The largest volume of 7.5% saline that can be administered safely is about 250 mL.[87]

EFFECTS OF SEVERE HEMORRHAGE ON THE INTRACELLULAR SPACE AND IMPLICATIONS FOR FLUID REPLACEMENT

Shires and associates[88] demonstrated the need for volume re-expansion in a classic model of hemorrhagic shock in dogs. Animals that were given volume replacement with blood alone had the highest rate of mortality. Survival improved if the animals were treated with both blood and plasma. The group resuscitated with blood plasma and crystalloid solution

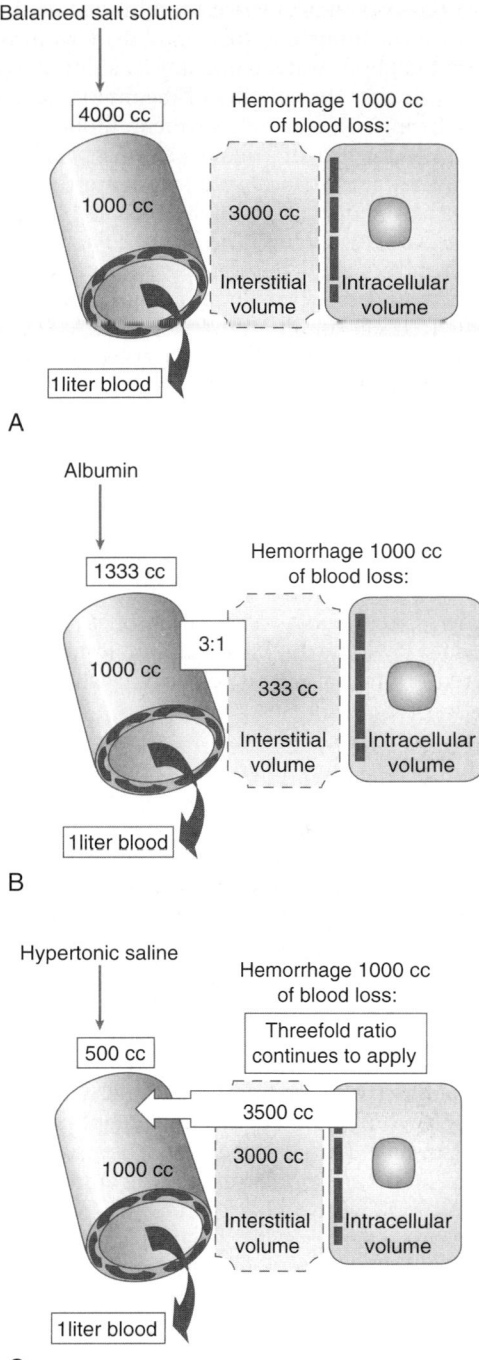

FIGURE 229–6. *A-C,* Volume replacement after acute blood loss.

(Ringer's lactate solution) exhibited the greatest 14-day survival rate in the post-shock period. Extracellular volume was shown to be severely contracted after the hemorrhagic insult.[88] When blood loss reached 25% of total blood volume, extracellular volume decreased by 18% to 26%. Based on these findings, Shires and associates proposed that shock leads to intracellular swelling.

Subsequently, Lewis and collaborators assessed changes in body water compartments in healthy human volunteers and a series of severely traumatized patients, beginning on day 2 after injury. All of these patients were hemodynamically stable in an ICU.[89] Volumes of the three body water compartments were measured using an indicator dilution technique. Indocyanine green dye was used to measure the volume of the intravascular space, bromine was used to assess the volume of the interstitial space, and deuterium was used to measure total body water content.[90] By subtraction, it was possible to calculate the volumes of the interstitial compartment and the intracellular compartment. Blood volume was assessed as a function of colloid osmotic pressure. There were no differences in blood volume among these patients, suggesting that by day 2 in the ICU they had been resuscitated to the same endpoints. The intracellular volume, however, was found to be slightly but significantly decreased in the patients who were severely traumatized and resuscitated with a balanced salt solution.

These data contrasted with the observations made using a canine hemorrhagic shock model by Shires and colleagues, who reported an expansion of the intracellular space. The differences between these two studies might be explained by differences in the timing of the observations relative to the period of hemorrhage. The animal data indicate that cellular swelling occurs during the acute phase of hypotension and severe oxygen depletion, whereas the data from humans indicate that intracellular volume is slightly contracted during the subacute post-resuscitation phase. Interestingly, data obtained by Shire and colleagues indicates that cellular volume returns to normal in subjects in whom the shock period is less than 2 hours.[91]

Cellular edema might result from irreparable damage of the ion pumping machinery of the cytosolic membrane. Alternatively, in some patients, there may be an unrecognized ongoing energetic deficit, despite normal or close to normal clinical parameters, such as blood pressure, heart rate, and urinary output. These circumstances may occur more often than expected and may eventually generate a more protracted form of cellular dysfunction that ultimately becomes apparent as MODS.

When a large volume of resuscitation fluid is required to restore normal hemodynamic parameters, patients often exhibit the effects of massive expansion of interstitial space. In these patients, the interstitial space may have increased by a factor of two or three on the second or third day after injury or surgery. Thus, the normal 3:1 ratio between the volumes of interstitial and intravascular compartments may no longer be valid; rather, the ratio may be 4:1, 5:1, or 6:1 or even greater. Hence, crystalloid solutions will become progressively less effective for expanding intravascular volume (Fig. 229-7). In these cases, a colloid solution, because of its greater effectiveness for expanding the intravascular compartment, is the preferred fluid.

INHERENT COMPLICATIONS OF COMMONLY USED FLUID REPLACEMENT SOLUTIONS

Over the last 10 years, we have seen a plethora of reports describing more specific findings about several of the solutions used for fluid replacement therapy and their many physiologic and biochemical effects. Furthermore, recent reports in animal models as well as meta-analyses of clinical trials have provided new and intriguing data.

ALBUMIN

The use of albumin in critically ill patients was analyzed in a Cochrane report.[92,93] The authors carried out a systematic review of randomized controlled trials comparing

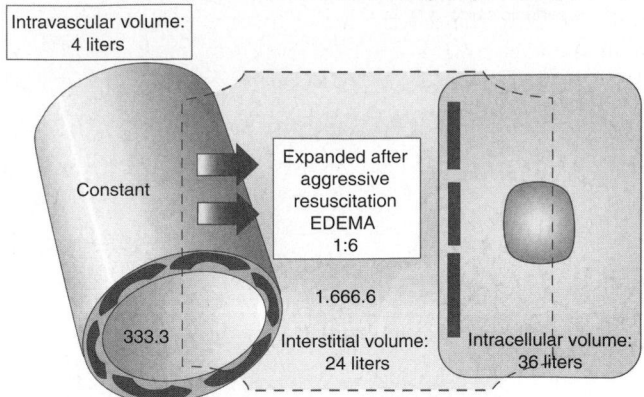

86 Kg man => Water = 60% of body weight = 52 Kg

Intravascular volume: 4 liters

Constant

Expanded after aggressive resuscitation EDEMA 1:6

1.666.6

333.3

Interstitial volume: 24 liters

Intracellular volume: 36 liters

FIGURE 229–7. Volume expansion with crystalloid solution.

administration of albumin or plasma protein fraction with no administration or administration of crystalloid solution in critically ill patients with hypovolemia, burns, or hypoalbuminemia. A total of 1419 patients from 30 separate trials were studied. For each patient category, the risk of death in the albumin-treated group was higher than in the comparison group. For hypovolemia, the relative risk of death after albumin administration was 1.46 (95% confidence interval, 0.97-2.22), for burns the relative risk was 2.40 (95% CI, 1.11-5.19), and for hypoalbuminemia it was 1.69 (95% CI, 1.07-2.67). This review, however, was based on relatively small trials in which there were only a small number of deaths. Therefore, these results must be interpreted with caution.

The analyses suggest that the use of human albumin in the management of critically ill patients should be reviewed. Interestingly, a recent abstract reported the results of a study comparing the safety and efficacy of 5% albumin solution and Ringer's lactate solution for resuscitation of adult ICU patients with shock.[94] This was an open-label randomized multicenter controlled trail. Nineteen patients were treated with albumin and 23 with Ringer's lactate solution. There were no statistically significant differences between groups with respect to days on mechanical ventilation, oxygenation failure, length of ICU stay, or 28-day mortality rate. The incidence of bacteremia was significantly lower in the albumin group ($P = 0.023$). The authors requested access to the Cochrane database and added the results of this trial to the meta-analyses for the burn patients subgroup. When the results from a recent trial were added, the relative risk for death was no longer significant when comparing albumin versus crystalloids.[94] Finally, the SAFE trial carried out in Australia and New Zealand (The Saline versus Albumin Fluid Evaluation [SAFE] Study is a collaboration of the Australian and New Zealand Intensive Care Society Clinical Trials Group), recently published, indicated that there is no difference between albumin and saline in a double-blind randomized population of close to 7000 patients.[95] Of the 6997 patients who underwent randomization, 3497 were assigned to receive albumin and 3500 to receive saline; the two groups had similar baseline characteristics. There were 726 deaths in the albumin group, as compared with 729 deaths in the saline group (relative risk of death, 0.99; 95% CI, 0.91 to 1.09; $P = 0.87$). The proportion of patients with new single-organ and multiple-organ failure was similar in the two groups ($P = 0.85$). There were no significant differences between the groups in the mean (±SD) numbers of days spent in the ICU (6.5±6.6 in the albumin group and 6.2±6.2 in the saline group, $P = 0.44$), days spent in the hospital (15.3 ± 9.6 and 15.6 ± 9.6, respectively; $P = 0.30$), days of mechanical ventilation (4.5 ± 6.1 and 4.3 ± 5.7, respectively; $P = 0.74$), or days of renal-replacement therapy (0.5 ± 2.3 and 0.4 ± 2.0, respectively; $P = 0.41$).

Epidemiologic evidence suggests that there is an increase in mortality among patients with burns, hypoalbuminemia, and hypotension treated with albumin solutions. In critical illness, hypoalbuminemia is a result of transcapillary leak, decreased synthesis, large-volume body fluid losses, and dilution caused by fluid resuscitation. When treating patients with hypoalbuminemia, efforts must be centered around correction of the underlying disorder rather than reversal of hypoalbuminemia.[96]

RINGER'S LACTATE SOLUTION

It is somewhat surprising that after having used Ringer's lactate as a volume expander and resuscitation fluid for more than 70 years, only recently have investigators described the immunologic and proinflammatory effects of this solution on neutrophils and other cells involved in host defense mechanisms. Rhee and associates described neutrophil activation caused by hemorrhagic shock and resuscitation. Using a swine model of shock, they compared the effects of fluid resuscitation in three separate groups: group I received Ringer's lactate solution; group II, shed blood; and group III, 7.5% hypertonic saline solution. Neutrophil activation was measured in whole blood using flow cytometry to detect intracellular superoxide burst activity. They found that neutrophil activation increased significantly immediately after hemorrhage, but it was greatest after resuscitation with Ringer's lactate solution. Animals that received shed blood or hypertonic saline had neutrophil activity return to baseline state after resuscitation.[97] Furthermore, the same group later described how different resuscitative fluids may immediately affect the degree of apoptosis after hemorrhagic shock. In a study in rats, they described how resuscitation with Ringer's lactate solution resulted in a significant increase in small intestinal epithelial and smooth muscle cell and hepatocyte apoptosis.[98]

MANAGEMENT OF HEMORRHAGIC SHOCK

Clinical and Practical Aspects

Severe hemorrhagic shock is characterized by cool, moist, pallid, or cyanotic skin. The patient is tachycardic and hypotensive, and the severity of these clinical manifestations may vary from patient to patient depending on age, underlying cardiovascular disease, and the presence of medications or associated toxic compounds such as drugs or alcohol. The magnitude of the blood volume deficit and the identification of ongoing blood loss are the two key variables that determine success of the resuscitative interventions. The major goal in resuscitation is to stop the bleeding and replete intravascular blood volume to maximize tissue oxygen delivery. Cardiac output, blood pressure, and oxygenated blood flow to vital organs are important determinants of outcome. Management priorities in the trauma patient who is bleeding acutely include airway control, ventilation, and oxygenation. Measurement of blood pressure may not be feasible and is not a necessary requirement to initiate therapy during the primary survey. In fact, a quick global assessment of

adequacy of perfusion can rapidly be obtained by examining the characteristics of the pulse. Obvious signs of shock are sufficient to establish the diagnoses and determine the severity of blood volume. Additional information such as blood pressure measurement, ECG, pulse oximeter, and capnograph may be useful. Adequate intravenous access for infusion of normothermic fluids is the next priority while other causes of severe hypotension and shock are being ruled out.

Ideally any fluid therapy must be accompanied by efforts to control bleeding. An estimate of blood volume deficit after blunt trauma may be obtained by estimating blood losses associated with specific injuries. A unilateral hemothorax may contain 3000 mL of blood, and the abdomen can hold up to 2000 to 5000 mL without noticeable abdominal distension. Other injuries that can be associated with massive hemorrhage include pelvic fractures and retroperitoneal trauma. A femur fracture can lead to the loss of a liter or more of blood, and a tibia fracture can be associated with the loss of 350 to 650 mL of blood.

Vascular Access for Patients with Severe Hemorrhage

In the trauma patient presenting with multiple serious injuries and hemorrhagic shock, vascular access is necessary to restore circulatory volume rapidly. The most important factor in considering the procedure and route for vascular access is anatomic location and magnitude of injuries and the individual physician's level of skill and expertise.

Venous access must never be initiated in an injured limb. In patients with injuries below the diaphragm, at least one i.v. line should be placed in a tributary of the superior vena cava, as there may be vascular disruption of the inferior vena cava. In patients with severe multiple trauma when thoracoabdominal damage is suspected, it is prudent to place one i.v. access site above the diaphragm and one below the diaphragm. Short large-bore catheters should be used. Doubling the internal diameter of the cannula increases flow by 16-fold. A 14-gauge, 5-cm catheter in a peripheral vein infuses fluid twice as fast as a 16-gauge, 20-cm catheter passed centrally. When using 8.5 Fr pulmonary artery catheter introducers, the side port should be removed, as this structure increases resistance roughly four-fold.

ATLS guidelines recommend rapid placement of two large-bore (16-gauge or larger) i.v. catheters in the patient with serious injuries and hemorrhagic shock. The first choice for i.v. insertion should be a peripheral extremity vein. The most suitable veins are at the wrist, on the dorsum of the hand, at the antecubital fossa in the arm, and on the saphenous in the leg. Less preferable sites are the external jugular and femoral veins. The complication rate of properly placed i.v. catheters is low. Intravascular placement of a large-bore i.v. catheter should be verified by checking for backflow. An i.v. site should infuse easily under gravity alone. Intravenous fluids can leak into soft tissues when pumped under pressure, and can lead to development of compartment syndrome. Patients with absent pulses may need to undergo cutdown to cannulate the femoral vein under direct vision to obtain i.v. access.

Subclavian and internal jugular vein catheterization should not be used routinely in hypovolemic trauma patients. The incidence of complications is higher and the rate of success is low due to venous collapse. Rapid peripheral percutaneous i.v. access may be difficult to achieve in patients with hypovolemia and venous collapse, edema, obesity, scar tissue, history of i.v. drug abuse, or burns. Under such circumstances, central access with large-bore catheters may be attempted by percutaneous femoral puncture or cutdown. Subclavian catheterization provides rapid and safe venous access in experienced hands. The most frequent complication of subclavian venipuncture is pneumothorax. Pneumothorax is more likely to occur on the left side because the left pleural dome is anatomically higher. Subclavian and internal jugular catheters should be inserted on the side of injury in patients with chest wounds, reducing the chances of collapsing the uninjured lung. A simple pneumothorax may result in respiratory compromise in individuals with pulmonary contusions or a pneumothorax in the contralateral hemithorax. It is extremely rare that subclavian catheterization is the primary site for i.v. access in the trauma bay. Regardless of the site of insertion, it is extremely important not to force the wire or the introducer if resistance is encountered. Forcing the introducer can result in perforation of large veins or arteries. Venous air embolism is another complication of central line insertion. Any lines placed during resuscitation of a trauma patient without strict aseptic technique should be removed as soon as the patient's condition permits. Although percutaneous placement of an internal jugular catheter is an excellent means for rapidly attaining access, this site is rarely used in trauma victims because of the possibility of cervical trauma and the need for cervical immobilization with a collar.

Femoral vein cannulation is another alternative for line placement and is associated with fewer acute complications. Bowel perforation can occur, especially in patients with a femoral hernia. Penetration of the hip can result in septic arthritis. Thrombophlebitis occurs more often with femoral than with internal jugular or subclavian catheters; however, this complication is most likely with prolonged use. Venous cutdowns can be performed when rapid, secure, large-bore venous cannulation is desirable, such as in hemodynamic shock and when percutaneous peripheral or central access is either contraindicated or impossible to achieve. Strict aseptic technique should be used. Surgical masks and caps should be worn. Venous cutdown has a low potential for anatomic damage. Cutaneous nerve injury is the most common problem. Venous cutdown catheters should be removed as soon as it is possible to achieve i.v. access through standard percutaneous i.v. catheters or a central venous catheter.

Red Cell Transfusion

If the patient has lost large amounts of blood and is in moderate to severe shock as defined by weak pulses, cold and diaphoretic skin, mental status changes, and hypotension, then administration of packed red blood cells is required. Hematocrit should not be used to guide transfusion, because this parameter does not reflect red cell mass during acute blood loss. The early identification of severe injuries with a high likelihood of hemorrhage and the initial assessment of the patient should suffice for the trauma team leader to alert the blood bank in advance. Protocols for massive transfusion should be established and the blood bank should automatically begin preparation of fresh-frozen plasma and platelet packs, if massive bleeding is anticipated.

Available options are type O-negative, type-specific, typed and screened, or typed and cross-matched packed red blood cells. The initial choice depends on the degree of hemodynamic instability. Type O-negative red cells have no major antigens and can be administered safely to patients with any blood type. Unfortunately, only 8% of the population has O-negative blood, and blood bank reserves of O-negative, low-antibody-titer blood are usually low. For this reason, O-positive red cells are frequently used. This is a reasonable approach in males but may be a problem in Rh-negative females with reproductive potential.

If 50% to 75% of the patient's blood volume has been replaced with type O blood (e.g., ~10 units of red cells in an adult patient), one should continue to administer type O red cells. Otherwise, the risk of a major cross-match reaction increases, since the patient may have received enough anti-A or anti-B antibodies to precipitate hemolysis if A, B, or AB units are subsequently given. Obtaining type-specific red cells requires 5 to 10 minutes in most institutions.

When blood is typed and screened, the patient's blood group is identified and the serum is screened for major blood group antibodies. A full cross-match generally requires about 45 minutes and involves mixing donor cells with recipient serum to rule out antigen/antibody reactions.

COAGULATION FACTORS, PLATELETS AND COAGULOPATHY

Severe and uncontrolled hemorrhage is a major cause of death in trauma victims, accounting for close to 40% of mortality in both military and civilian trauma.[9,99] Severe bleeding, surgery, and massive resuscitation interact synergistically to generate the classical lethal triad: hypothermia, acidosis, and coagulopathy.

Failure of coagulation in trauma is multifactorial and is characterized by the combined presence of (1) coagulation abnormalities resembling disseminated intravascular coagulation (DIC), caused by systemic activation of coagulation and fibrinolysis[100]; (2) excessive fibrinolysis (most probably caused by release of tissue plasminogen activator [TPA] from damaged tissues)[100-102]; (3) dilutional coagulopathy caused by excessive fluid treatment[103]; and (4) massive transfusion syndrome resulting in dilution of coagulation factors and impairment of platelet number and function.[104]

The repetitive cycle of added hypothermia, mainly related to bleeding and hypotension,[105] causes slowing of the enzymatic activities of the proteins in the coagulation cascade[106] as well as dysfunction of platelets.[107] Ideally, the introduction of an effective hemostatic agent that could act only at the site of injury, without induction of systemic activation of coagulation, could improve hemorrhage control and reduce hemorrhage-related mortality and morbidity in both military and civilian trauma victims.[108] A number of agents are being used to achieve hemostasis. Such agents may be used topically or systemically. Topical hemostatic agents include vasoconstrictive agents, such as epinephrine, and procoagulant agents, such as thrombin, hemostatic fibrin, gelatin, and spongostan. Systemically administered hemostatic agents include coagulation factors in the form of cryoprecipitate and fresh-frozen plasma. A general hemostatic agent may be one that enhances full thrombin generation and thereby the formation of a stable, tight fibrin hemostatic plug resistant to premature fibrinolysis.

USE OF RECOMBINANT FACTOR VIIa (rFVIIa) AS AN ADJUVANT FOR RESUSCITATION IN THE COAGULOPATHIC PATIENT

Patients with profuse bleeding due to extensive surgery or trauma often develop a complex coagulation pattern that includes reduced levels of fibrinogen, factors VIII and V, and platelets. Low levels of fibrinogen result in the formation of a loose fibrin structure and to a decreased activation factor XIII, the fibrin-stabilizing factor.[109]

Trauma patients with massive bleeding thus may benefit from intravenous rFVIIa in order to help to generate a thrombin peak, which may be enough to form a firm, stable fibrin hemostatic plug and thereby decrease the bleeding.[110] Since thrombin has such a crucial role in providing hemostasis, any agent that enhances thrombin generation in situations with impaired thrombin formation may be characterized as a general hemostatic agent.

Mechanism of Action

Hemostasis is initiated by the formation of a complex between tissue factor (TF), exposed as a result of a vessel wall injury, and activated factor VII (FVIIa) that is normally present in circulating blood. The TF-FVIIa complex converts factor X into FXa on the TF-bearing cell. FXa then activates prothrombin into thrombin. This limited amount of thrombin activates FVIII, FV, FXI, and platelets. Thrombin-activated platelets change shape, resulting in exposure of negatively charged phospholipids, which form a template for thrombin generation involving FVIII and FIX. Full thrombin generation is necessary for complete activation of FXIII and thrombin activatable fibrinolytic inhibitor, TAFI to occur. Furthermore, full thrombin generation is important for the fibrin structure of the hemostatic plug.[111]

The addition of rFVIIa to FVIII- or FIX-deficient plasma has been shown to increase thrombin generation in a cell-based in vitro model. Furthermore, extra rFVIIa was found to normalize fibrin clot permeability in vitro and to tighten the fibrin structure as studied by 3D confocal microscopy. These findings indicate that administration of rFVIIa can compensate for the lack of FVIII and FIX. Accordingly, the administration of exogenous rFVIIa has been found to stop bleeding in hemophilia patients and, provided it is given in doses high enough, to allow major surgery to be performed in severe hemophiliacs with inhibitors. As rFVIIa enhances thrombin generation on already activated platelets, it has been suggested that rFVIIa may also help to improve hemostasis in other situations involving impaired thrombin generation, such as platelet disorders (thrombocytopenia and functional platelet defects). High doses of rFVIIa (90-120 μg/kg) massively increased the level of FVIIa above the physiological normal state. The immediate result is an increase in the generation of thrombin. Furthermore exogenous rFVIIa induces hemostasis independently of tissue factor and factors VIII and IX by binding directly to activated platelet surfaces with low affinity to generate thrombin in a dose-dependent manner.[112]

Pharmacology

Intravenous administration of rFVIIa does not induce systemic activation of coagulation. Administration of rFVIIa shortens PT and PTT, but does not affect levels of thrombin, fibrinogen, or platelet count. The half-life of rFVIIa is 2.7 and 1.3 for children <15 years; however, there is considerable variation among individuals. Initial work in humans indicates that a dose of 90 to 110 μg/kg of rFVIIa (given as a bolus) should be repeated every 2 hours over a 24-h period. Intervals may be increased thereafter, according to the response and the severity of bleeding.[113]

Safety

Since TF is expressed under pathologic conditions such as atherosclerosis, sepsis, or cancer. Accordingly, there is a theoretical risk of thromboembolic complications, such as stroke or myocardial infarction, when rFVIIa is administered to patients with these conditions. According to the manufacturer's information,[111] rFVIIa has been administered to more than 7000 patients. So far, there have been seven reported strokes, eight myocardial infarctions, and one patient with myocardial ischemia. Other reported and possible adverse events include DIC, acute renal failure, and DVT.

Studies on rFVIIa in Trauma and Surgery

Martinowitz and associates reported that administration of rFVIIa caused a cessation of the diffuse bleeding and normalization of coagulation parameters in seven trauma victims with uncontrolled bleeding. Although definitive studies remain to be performed, advocates for the use of rFVIIa in trauma patients suggest that there may be two conceptually different indications for rFVIIa: a prehospital or battlefield indication when rFVIIa should be given in the ambulance before arrival to the trauma center., and the second indication would be at the trauma center as an adjuvant to damage control management.

ANNOTATED REFERENCES

Freeman BD, Natanson C. Anti-inflammatory therapies in sepsis and septic shock. Expert Opin Investig Drugs 2000;9(78):1651-1663.
   Good review of anti-inflammatory treatments: inconsistent efficacy of glucocorticoids and recent clinical trials on pre-inflammatory mediators.

Baldwin AL, Thurston G. Mechanics of endothelial cell architecture and vascular permeability. Crit Rev Biomed Eng 2001;29(2):247-278.
   Good review of mechanisms of endothelial gap formation.

Moore FA, McKinley BA, Moore EE. The next generation in shock resuscitation. Lancet 2004;363(9425):1988-1996.
   Excellent review article and tutorial discussing advances in shock resuscitation and proposal of common protocols for resuscitation among trauma centers.

Chapter 230

MEDIASTINITIS

Barry G. Crowe • Robert G. Johnson

KEY POINTS

1. Infections of the anterior and middle mediastinum most frequently occur as a complication of cardiac surgery.

2. Infections of the posterior mediastinum most frequently occur secondary to esophageal pathology or injury.

3. The diagnosis and treatment are distinctly different for anterior and posterior mediastinal infections.

4. The depth of anterior mediastinal infection is the primary determinant of treatment options, but the interval since antecedent operation and the acuity of the patient are also important in selecting the most appropriate therapy.

5. A variety of imaging techniques can be helpful in determining the anatomic extent of involvement in late-appearing anterior mediastinal infections.

6. Prompt drainage and débridement, associated with appropriate antibiotic therapy, combine to form the cornerstone of treatment of anterior mediastinitis.

7. Multiple options exist for management of the mediastinum after drainage and débridement, but vascularized tissue coverage and vacuum-assisted wound drainage are most commonly employed successfully.

8. Posterior mediastinal infections are most commonly associated with cervical/chest pain, fever, and a recent history of an iatrogenic intervention, dysphagia, retching, or esophagitis.

9. Computed tomography, generally with water-soluble contrast medium enhancement, is an integral part of establishing the diagnosis and treatment options for posterior mediastinal infections.

10. Posterior mediastinitis requires appropriate drainage and antibiotics and, depending on the extent and duration of infection, may benefit from diversion and/or primary esophageal repair.

11. Descending necrotizing mediastinitis can be difficult to diagnose, and successful treatment requires not only appropriate antibiotics and open drainage but also vigilant subsequent imaging to identify any residual abscesses.

Mediastinitis includes a variety of thoracic infections that occur from the sternum to the spine and occur from causes ranging from dental infections to esophageal disease or injuries. Clinically, the diagnosis, treatment, and prognosis of these infections are determined by their location and etiology. The mediastinum is divided anatomically into three compartments: anterior (between the posterior sternum and the anterior pericardium), middle (the intrapericardial contents), and posterior (bounded by the posterior pericardium anteriorly and the spine posteriorly). The pleural cavities are the lateral boundaries for each of these mediastinal spaces. With respect to etiology, mediastinitis can be either primary, arising without prior intervention, or secondary, occurring after intervention. Clinically, one can essentially lump the anatomic anterior and middle compartments together because mediastinitis occurs most commonly in those combined spaces secondarily, as a postoperative complication of commonly performed cardiac operations. Esophageal pathology, primary or secondary to iatrogenic intervention, accounts for the overwhelming majority of mediastinal infections in the posterior compartment.

The diagnosis and treatment are distinctly different for anterior and posterior mediastinal infections. Other more unusual forms of mediastinal infections or inflammations include those that descend via the neck's pretracheal or retropharyngeal spaces from the oral cavity, those that are more indolent than acute, and those that are characterized by fibrosis.

ACUTE ANTERIOR MEDIASTINITIS

Infections of the anterior and middle mediastinum most frequently occur as a complication of cardiac surgery.

Rarely, acute anterior mediastinitis occurs without antecedent median sternotomy (e.g., after traumatic sternal fracture).[1] By far the most common form of acute mediastinitis occurs after sternotomy for a cardiac operation.

Employment of the term *mediastinitis* after cardiac operations varies in the literature and often at the local, institutional, level. Strictly defined, mediastinitis would be diagnosed in those patients who have infection involving the space behind the sternum. More broadly, postoperative infections after cardiac surgery with median sternotomy include those that are superficial or subcutaneous, without associated sternal pathology. A far more subtle distinction and rare entity is the designation of sternitis, or sternal osteomyelitis, without infection behind the sternum. For the purposes of the following discussion, we will assume that any infection posterior to the sternum is an infection of the mediastinum. This category includes patients with deep sternal infections, because no impervious anatomic barrier exists between the posterior cortex of the sternum and the space behind it. Deep sternal infection can be considered one end of the spectrum of mediastinitis; the other end is gross pus in the anterior mediastinum and pericardium. Some patients have sterile sternal dehiscence with no evidence of infection. When there is drainage through the wound, if the wound cannot be closed while it is still uninfected, there is a real opportunity for retrograde infection. Clinically, especially in more obese patients, it is sometimes initially unclear as to whether one is dealing with a superficial problem, a sterile dehiscence, or a deeper infection. Any sternal instability or evidence of separation, such as broken wires on a chest radiograph, suggests the need for re-exploration and appropriate closure. The depth of anterior mediastinal infection is the primary determinant of treatment options, but the interval since antecedent operation and the acuity of the patient are also important in selecting the most appropriate therapy.

INCIDENCE, PATHOLOGY, AND PREVENTION

For at least two reasons, the incidence of mediastinitis is not well established. Various definitions of mediastinitis, sternal osteomyelitis, and deep sternal wound infection are used in the literature and at the local level. Accordingly, the literature is not consistent about the definition of this complication. In addition, the diagnosis is sometimes made weeks or months after hospital discharge, and, hence, the complication is occasionally not noted in the records for the institution where the operation was originally performed. Mediastinitis after sternotomy is reported to complicate 0.4% to 2.0% of cardiac operations.[2] In one very large review of more than 15,000 prospectively registered patients from several institutions, the incidence of "deep sternal wound" infection occurring during the period after hospitalization for coronary artery bypass graft surgery was 1.25%.[3] Another recent series with over 10,000 patients reported an incidence of 1.44%[4] and a decade long experience from a single institution reported an incidence of 0.25%.[5] Increasingly, as the postoperative length of stay decreases, mediastinal infections are diagnosed from days to months after hospital discharge, and these cases may not be captured in some reported series.

Whereas some suggest that postoperative mediastinal infections may be avoided entirely, no substantial data corroborate that hope.[5] Rather, there are a number of host factors that increase the risk of mediastinitis after cardiac operations. Preoperative characteristics associated with an increased incidence include diabetes mellitus, increased body mass index, older age, renal failure, prolonged preoperative hospitalization, chronic obstructive pulmonary disease, and cigarette smoking.[3,4,6] Obviously, most of these host-related conditions cannot be manipulated in a given patient and serve only to suggest an increased risk for mediastinal infection.

As with most infection rates, the occurrence of mediastinitis is influenced by a host of technical and management details. In addition to the host factors mentioned earlier, there are intraoperative factors that influence the risk for mediastinal infection. An increased incidence of deep sternal wound infection has been associated with bilateral internal mammary use, prolonged operative time, and use of the intra-aortic balloon pump.[4,6] Postoperative factors that increase the risk of deep sternal infection include increased blood glucose level (>200 mg/dL),[7] re-exploration, and prolonged

mechanical ventilation.[4,6] Undoubtedly, various factors, such as method of skin preparation, electrocautery use, glove changes, and attention to a host of other details, account for some of the variation in infection rates from surgeon to surgeon and institution to institution. Avoiding sternotomy entirely, as can be done with less chest wall–invasive approaches, appears to drastically reduce or eliminate the risk of mediastinal infection after cardiac operations.[4]

Postoperative tracheostomy is required in some patients, and many of these patients have some of the risk factors for deep sternal wound infection. Open tracheostomy for patients with prolonged ventilator dependence was once deferred for 2 or more weeks after sternotomy for fear of contaminating the anterior mediastinal space. Recently, however, adoption of percutaneous tracheostomy has not been associated with an increased incidence of subsequent mediastinal infection. This technique may allow an earlier, safer switch from an oral to a cervical airway[8-10] in patients requiring prolonged mechanical ventilation.

Most post-sternotomy deep wound infections are caused by staphylococcal species. Mediastinal infections in patients who have been hospitalized for a long time often grow out coagulase-negative staphylococci that are resistant to multiple antibiotics.[11] Gram-negative organisms are sometimes cultured from mediastinal infections, particularly from diabetics, patients with gram-negative pneumonia before operation, or those needing re-exploration.[12]

Given the serious consequences of mediastinitis after cardiac operations, the use of prophylactic antibiotics for clean cardiac operations has long been an established practice. Given the most common organisms in these infections, administration of a first-generation cephalosporin (e.g., cefazolin) is still the most accepted strategy for prophylaxis. Vancomycin is substituted in patients with penicillin allergy, in deference to the possibility of cross-reactivity, and it may be used routinely for an interval in institutions experiencing an outbreak of methicillin-resistant staphylococci. Topical vancomycin has been shown to be effective in decreasing the incidence of sternal infections.[13] Although this approach is used routinely in some institutions, development of vancomycin-resistant staphylococci is a genuine concern.[14]

DIAGNOSIS

Patients with mediastinitis after sternotomy generally have clinical signs. On examination, purulent wound drainage and sternal instability are the most obvious findings, but neither may be present initially. A spiking fever and an acutely elevated leukocyte count are common. Some patients manifest signs of sepsis with mental status changes and hemodynamic instability. Mediastinitis can appear as early as 1 day after operation or as remotely as months after an operation. Rarely it has an indolent course, presenting many months after operation, and there may be isolated involvement of deep tissues, with infection tracking down to the aorta and/or involving some artificial material, such as a pledget or a braided suture. A variety of imaging techniques can be helpful in determining the anatomic extent of involvement in late-appearing anterior mediastinal infections.

The gravity of the diagnosis and the variability of its clinical presentation have encouraged the use of imaging techniques to confirm or refute the possibility of deep sternal or mediastinal infection. Unfortunately, the diagnostic accuracy of most of these techniques permits findings obtained by using them to be supportive[15] but rarely, if ever, definitive in the diagnosis of deep infection. Fluid collections and mediastinal soft tissue changes are common, if not universal, but are not specific for infection.[16] Radionuclide scans using ^{99m}Tc-hexamethylpropylene amine oxime (HMPAO)-labeled leukocytes have also been used in the evaluation of late-presenting, indolent cases in an attempt to separate sternal involvement from infections superficial to it.[17] All these imaging studies are, of course, confounded by changes that one can expect following the operative procedure itself. Blind retrosternal, subxiphoid needle aspiration has been employed, and aspiration with ultrasound guidance has been reported after cardiac transplantation.[18]

TREATMENT

Whereas the need for operative treatment in anterior mediastinitis is firmly established, the techniques successfully employed vary greatly. Some of this variation is explained by the timing of diagnosis (interval since antecedent operation), the depth of the infection, and the acuity of the patient. The experience and choice of the treating surgeon is also a factor in the technique used to manage a deep infection. In patients with suspected infection when there is drainage and some sternal instability, expeditious re-exploration with débridement of the sternal edges and surrounding soft tissues, accompanied by irrigation and drainage, may permit sternal rewiring.[19] For patients with sepsis or gross retrosternal purulence, a staged approach or immediate tissue coverage may be employed. Prompt drainage and then débridement, associated with appropriate antibiotic therapy, combine to form the cornerstone of treatment of anterior mediastinitis.

If sternal re-closure is elected after débridement, an alternative wiring technique, either a variation of the Robicsek[20] weave or a commercially available plate fixation device, is generally used. Cultures obtained at operation dictate the ultimate choice of systemic antibiotics, but initial coverage should include a first-generation cephalosporin and an agent active against gram-negative organisms until Gram stain or culture results are definitive. A variety of irrigation solutions and protocols have been employed in these patients. Diluted antibiotic-containing, povidone-iodine,[19] and aqueous acid solutions have been reported.[21] The duration of irrigation has varied from 3 days to a week, while systemic antibiotics are continued, as would be the case for other bone infections. Unfortunately, primary sternal closure fails in 20% to 40% of the patients.[22] Although débridement with re-closure and irrigation may be viewed as a first-stage procedure, the incidence of recurrence dictates that this approach be considered primarily for patients without gross infection. A true staged approach involves an interval when the sternum and skin are left open and packed. More than two decades ago, before the description of soft tissue coverage by transposition, an open sternotomy was packed with the intention of secondary closure. A number of those patients had bleeding from exposed grafts, the aorta, or right ventricle. Even today some sternotomies are left open for a short period of time in preparation for a second operation to achieve soft tissue coverage. During this interval, dramatic hemorrhage occasionally occurs, usually from a right ventricular injury caused by the overriding sternal edge.[23,24] For this reason, it is recommended that patients with open sternotomies have their right sternal edge

débrided aggressively and that they remain mechanically ventilated until coverage can be achieved.

Whether used as an initial single-stage procedure, or as a secondary procedure, tissue transposition into the anterior mediastinum has dramatically changed the prognosis of this once commonly fatal complication.[25] Either omentum or muscle can be used. Tissues that can be used for muscle flaps include the pectoralis major (detached from its humeral insertion, leaving intact the muscle's origin and blood supply) or the pectoralis major (detached from its precordial origin, thereby maintaining its lateral blood supply). If the ipsilateral mammary artery has not been used as a blood supply for the coronary circulation, the rectus abdominis muscle can be detached distally and rotated on its cephalad attachment into the anterior mediastinal space. The omentum may be based on the right gastroepiploic artery or mobilized leaving the gastroepiploic artery intact. The sternum may be left open with the tissue flap between the remnant edges, or occasionally it may be closed over the flap. Either way, closed suction drains are required for the large mobilized skin flaps and sometimes beneath the transposed tissue flap. Multiple options exist for management of the mediastinum after drainage and débridement, but vascularized tissue coverage and vacuum-assisted wound drainage are most commonly employed successfully.

The choice of omentum versus a muscle flap is sometimes limited by availability (e.g., in patients with prior laparotomies), but, when the option exists, omentum may be preferable to muscle.[26,27] Omentum also has been employed successfully for managing infections after ascending aortic replacement.[28]

Skin coverage over the transposed flap may be accomplished by primary presternal skin reapproximation or split-thickness skin grafting or, with the rectus muscle, a skin paddle may be transposed as well. Recently, débrided sternal wounds have been successfully treated using a closed high-pressure vacuum system.[29-31] In this approach, polyurethane foam (400 to 600 μm pore size) is cut to fit the anterior mediastinal space and sealed to the skin permitting a vacuum (negative 75 mm Hg) to be generated over the entire wound surface. The device is changed regularly to avoid tissue ingrowth. Wounds heal secondarily, with obliteration of the space over a period of weeks.

PROGNOSIS

The mortality rate for mediastinitis has improved dramatically over the past two and one-half decades. The improvement in outcome is due to earlier detection and expeditious operative débridement and tissue coverage. Still, the acute mortality rate for post-sternotomy mediastinitis ranges from 14% to 47%.[2] Patients may die of sepsis or hemorrhage, either as a consequence of direct cardiac injury or secondary to an infected graft or foreign body. More often, death occurs from associated complications. Patients, who develop mediastinitis, often have multiple comorbidities that can negatively influence chances for survival. In a study from the Northern New England Cardiovascular Disease Study Group that adjusted for these various comorbidities, the 4-year mortality rate for patients with postoperative deep sternal infections was three times greater than it was for those without this complication.[3]

POSTERIOR MEDIASTINITIS

Infections of the posterior mediastinum most frequently occur secondary to esophageal pathology or injury. Acute infections that arise in of the posterior mediastinum generally result from esophageal disease that may be primary to the esophagus or, more commonly in the United States, secondary to some intervention. Primarily, esophagitis (e.g., in immunocompromised patients with fungal or viral organisms) may extend through the esophagus, resulting in mediastinitis. More commonly, infection of the posterior mediastinum is the result of instrumentation (scopes, probes, tubes, or dilators) or associated with an anastomotic leak after an esophageal operation. Traumatic injuries to the trachea, proximal bronchi, or esophagus may result in contamination of this space as well. Other causes of posterior compartment mediastinitis include Boerhaave's syndrome, which is rupture of the lower esophagus due to retching, and, more rarely, erosion of a broncholith from a partially or completely obstructed bronchus.[32]

DIAGNOSIS

Clinicians should suspect the diagnosis of mediastinitis when patients present with cervical and/or chest pain and high fever in the context of a history of dysphagia, retching, esophageal instrumentation, or a history of esophagitis. Posterior mediastinal infections are most commonly associated with cervical/chest pain, fever and a recent history of an iatrogenic intervention, dysphagia, retching, or esophagitis.

On examination, supraclavicular crepitus may be identified in patients with upper mediastinal pathology, but this finding is generally absent in patients with middle or lower esophageal disease. Leukocytosis is often the only early laboratory abnormality. Depending on the underlying pathology and duration of contamination, sepsis with mental status changes and hypotension may occur. In some cases, the plain chest film reveals a pleural effusion, and, more rarely, air is seen in the retropharyngeal space or other abnormal locations along the length of the mediastinum posterior to the pericardium. Computed tomography of the chest can more clearly demonstrate any abnormal air or fluid collections along the esophagus or near the esophagogastric junction, and enteric administration of a water-soluble contrast agent can diagnose the presence of an esophageal leak. A more indolent, subacute presentation might be accompanied by an abscess in the mediastinum. Transesophageal ultrasonography and fine-needle aspiration have been jointly used to diagnose a variety of periesophageal infections[33]; and this bedside technique, especially valuable for critically ill patients, may improve diagnostic accuracy relative to standard computed tomography, which, generally with water-soluble contrast medium enhancement, is an integral part of establishing the diagnosis and treatment options for posterior mediastinal infections.

TREATMENT

Some degree of mediastinitis accompanies any transmural disruption of the esophagus. Nevertheless, if it is diagnosed within a few hours after the inciting event, contained esophageal disruption (usually the result of instrumentation) can be managed successfully by serial clinical evaluation, limited oral intake, antibiotic therapy, and repeat imaging.[34]

Operation with primary repair and drainage is most often indicated for the management of patients with mediastinal contamination that is not confined to the site of local perforation but is identified within the first 24 hours.[35] If the time since perforation is sufficiently short, and the injury sufficiently small, the local extent of inflammation will be limited and primary repair of a disruption with or without viable tissue buttressing can be successfully employed. Image-guided nonoperative drainage with antibiotics has been successfully employed in selected cases, when a collection or abscess can be identified.[40]

Drainage with or without some form of diversion should be employed to manage patients with extensive local inflammation, those diagnosed more than 24 hours after perforation, and those with marked manifestations of systemic sepsis. Posterior mediastinitis requires appropriate drainage and antibiotics and, depending on the extent and duration of infection, may benefit from diversion and/or primary esophageal repair.

A variety of procedures for upper alimentary tract diversion have been described, ranging from simple nasogastric suction to cervical esophagostomy with gastrostomy. If the diagnosis of posterior mediastinal infection is made sufficiently early, before the development of sepsis, adequate local drainage and antibiotic therapy are sufficient. In such situations, some have advocated resection of the involved esophagus with appropriate diversion and drainage. Alimentary continuity can be restored after recovery from the mediastinal infection.[36] Continued sepsis and multiple organ failure are the most common causes of death among these patients.

MIGRATORY AND CHRONIC MEDIASTINAL INFLAMMATION

The mediastinum may be infected secondarily from contiguous acute infections involving adjacent anatomic spaces. Pleural or pulmonary processes may transgress the mediastinal envelope, as can infections involving the spine, particularly the vertebral bodies. Mediastinitis can be a complication of intra-abdominal processes, such as subdiaphragmatic abscesses or retroperitoneal extensions from colonic infections. Perhaps the most dramatic and well-described of the migratory mediastinal infections are those that descend from the neck; these are called descending necrotizing mediastinitis. These processes can originate from dental abscesses or Ludwig's angina. Gravity and the negative pressure of the thoracic cavity have been cited as reasons for descent of the infection through the pretracheal space into the upper posterior mediastinum. Descending necrotizing mediastinitis can be difficult to diagnose, and successful treatment requires not only appropriate antibiotics and open drainage but also vigilant subsequent imaging to identify any residual abscesses.

The patients are often young and may have a history of an odontogenic infection. Cervical pain, cellulitis, necrosis, and abscess formation may occur; CT can be diagnostic. Treatment with broad-spectrum antibiotics is essential and must be accompanied by cervical and mediastinal drainage directed by the clinical and radiologic findings. Drainage may be accomplished in a variety of ways including right thoracotomy, left-sided video-assisted thoracoscopy, or an anterior clamshell incision. The mortality of this condition ranges from 20% to 40% and increases directly with the interval between the onset of symptoms and diagnosis. Aggressive imaging surveillance and a commitment to achieving and maintaining drainage may improve the survival of this relatively rare, life-threatening disorder.[37]

Mediastinal fibrosis is a chronic condition that may present precipitously when the process constricts a mediastinal structure compromising its lumen. Pulmonary vein, caval, and tracheal stenoses are seen most commonly. The diagnosis is generally established by computed or magnetic resonance imaging. These studies reveal a diffusely infiltrating, sometimes calcified, mass. The fibrosis is a benign, acellular, proliferation of fibrous, collagenous tissue that is idiopathic or may be an immunologic sequela of a mycotic infection (*Histoplasma capsulatum* is the most common organism involved).[38,39]

ANNOTATED REFERENCES

Bitkover CY, Gardlund B: Mediastinitis after cardiovascular operations: A case-control study of risk factors. Ann Thorac Surg 1998;65:36-40.

This small, controlled study identifies some of the patient and iatrogenic factors that are associated with an increased incidence of this dreaded complication. No such paper is definitive, because similar works are contradictory about specific factors and their risk. For example, this study finds obesity to be associated with increased incidence of infection and other studies find a similar parameter, increased body mass index, to be associated with a lower incidence of infection.

Bladergroen MR, Lowe JE, Postlethwait RW: Diagnosis and recommended management of esophageal perforation and rupture. Ann Thorac Surg 1986;42:235-239.

This classic work is cited because of its age, for despite the fact that there are more recent excellent experiences and reviews, this article demonstrates truths that have not changed for nearly 20 years. Most important among these is that the a shorter time from perforation to treatment is intimately linked to an increased likelihood of survival. A corollary of this is that spontaneous or primary perforations are associated with a poorer outcome. Above all it is not unremarkable how similar are the treatment and overall survival from the this series to contemporary ones.

Bufkin BL, Miller JI, Mansour KA: Esophageal perforation: Emphasis on management. Ann Thorac Surg 1996;61:1447-1451.

These authors present a reasonably large single institution's experience in treating patients with esophageal perforation. They again establish that the majority of these occur in association with diagnostic or therapeutic interventions, but a number occur primarily. The real, albeit limited, role of nonoperative treatment in successfully managing perforations is also nicely addressed. They note an overall mortality of 25%, which is rather consistent in such series over the years and throughout the literature.

Freeman RK, Vallieres E, Verrier ED, et al: Descending necrotizing mediastinitis: An analysis of the effects of serial surgical débridement on patient mortality. J Thorac Cardiovasc Surg 2000;119:260-267.

Experienced surgeons in large, single institutions describe their treatment of 10 patients over 18 years of age and in so doing demonstrate that excellent results can be obtained by thoughtful drainage procedures with aggressive imaging follow-up (a mean of six CT scans, four transcervical drainage procedures, and two transthoracic drainage procedures per patient) without a death. The authors also provide a useful, contrasting review of the literature.

Oakley RE, Wright JE: Current reviews—postoperative mediastinitis: Classification and management. Ann Thorac Surg 1996;61:1030-1036.

This is a well-referenced review of the English literature on post-sternotomy mediastinal infections, including the incidence and variety of treatments for infection according to depth and extent of involvement.

Shackcloth MJ, Edwards J, Griffiths EM: Management of sternal wound complications by high-pressure suction drainage via a polyurethane foam. Ann Thorac Surg 2001;72:984.

These authors nicely describe the technique of foam-covered vacuum drainage treatment for post-sternotomy infections after appropriate débridement. They found a higher rate of treatment failure in a group of historical controls treated with closed suction and continuous irrigation. Although no paper has established an absolutely superior way to manage all post-sternotomy wounds after débridement, clearly the wound vacuum system can be added to the armamentarium of tissue coverage and perhaps replaces closed drainage and irrigation. Another vacuum system is cited in the article by Berg and colleagues.[30]

Zerr KJ, Furnary AP, Grunkemeier GL, et al: Glucose control lowers the risk of wound infection in diabetics after open heart operations. Ann Thorac Surg 1997;63:356-361.

The first of at least four studies by this group on this topic, this seminal large, retrospective report demonstrates the increased incidence of post-sternotomy infection among diabetics and, then, a decrease in that incidence after instituting a protocol for continuous insulin infusion to maintain serum glucose levels less than 200 mg/dL.

Chapter 231

EPISTAXIS

Karen Calhoun

KEY POINTS

1. Epistaxis ranges from a few flecks of blood in the mucus when blowing the nose to life-threatening hemorrhage.

2. In the ICU setting, with the patient supine, and often with diminished alertness, blood from a nasal source may drain under the influence of gravity back into the nasopharynx, pooling there and first being noticed as blood from the mouth.

3. Most epistaxis in the ICU setting is mild and responds to pressure, topical decongestants, fibrin glue, or chemical cautery.

4. It is almost inevitable that patients hospitalized in the ICU will undergo procedures or treatments that traumatize the nasal airway. Measures that can minimize this trauma include:

   a. Gentle technique

   b. Good understanding of nasal anatomy

   c. Generous use of topical vasoconstrictors, lubricants, and humidified air

   d. Use of the softest acceptable materials for passage through the nasal cavity

Epistaxis is a nosebleed. It ranges from a few flecks of blood in the mucus when blowing the nose to life-threatening hemorrhage. The focus in this chapter is on prevention, diagnosis, and management of the types of epistaxis that occur commonly in an ICU setting. Almost all of these occur incidentally in patients hospitalized for other reasons, and a significant proportion of ICU nosebleeds are iatrogenic.

ANATOMY AND PHYSIOLOGY

INTERNAL NASAL ANATOMY

The interior of the nose is divided in half by the bony carti-laginous septum and its mucoperichondrial covering. The septum thus makes up the medial wall of each nasal vault. The floor of the nose is formed by the palatal bone, sloping slightly downward as it goes back. The nasal cavity roof is made up of the sphenoid bone posteriorly, the cribriform plate (ethmoid bone), and the frontal bone anteriorly. Anteroinferiorly, the nostril opens into the nasal vault. The first 8 to 10 mm of nasal lining, going posteriorly from the nostril, is hair-bearing skin. The rest of the nose is lined with respiratory mucosa. The posterior extent of the nasal vault is the choana, or posterior nasal aperture, opening into the nasopharynx.

The most complex nasal anatomy occurs on the lateral wall of each vault, with three bony protrusions, the turbinates, extending into the nasal vault. The inferior turbinate is the biggest, and the superior one, the smallest. The nasolacrimal duct opens into the nasal cavity under the inferior turbinate. The maxillary, anterior ethmoidal, and frontal sinuses drain into the ethmoidal infundibulum, which opens under the middle turbinate. Posterior ethmoidal sinus cells open into the nose under the superior turbinate, and the sphenoidal sinus opens into the nose above and behind the superior turbinate.

VASCULAR ANATOMY

Internal nasal tissue derives blood supply from both the internal and external carotid systems. The internal carotid artery supplies the anterior and posterior ethmoidal arteries via the ophthalmic artery. The external carotid artery sup-plies the nose via the internal maxillary artery and the facial artery. The sphenopalatine artery (branch of the internal maxillary), the superior labial artery (branch of the facial artery), and the anterior ethmoidal artery (branch of the ophthalmic artery) together supply Kiesselbach's plexus in Little's area of the anteroinferior septal mucosa. This rich vascular supply ensures plentiful bleeding when the mucosa is irritated or breached, resulting in epistaxis.

NASAL PHYSIOLOGY

The nose's primary function is conditioning inspired air and conducting this air into and out of the pharynx. In a normal nose, air is warmed, humidified, and filtered of particulate matter before reaching the nasopharynx. The nose also contains sensor cells for olfaction in the superior nasal vault and improves vocal resonance.

HEALTH CARE PERSONNEL SAFETY

The patient with epistaxis is often scared, snorting or blow-ing out blood in attempts to clear the nasal or pharyngeal airway. Blood droplets can be widely and forcefully scattered. Any physician or other health care worker caring for a patient with epistaxis must observe the universal precau-tions. The caregiver should be gowned and gloved and wear eye protection and facial mask.

LOCATION OF BLEEDING

Otolaryngologists refer to nosebleeds as anterior or posterior. This is both an anatomic and a management differentiation.

Most "spontaneous" bleeding in the anterior half of the nose comes from Kiesselbach's plexus, an area easily seen with a nasal speculum and headlight. This area can be irritated by wiping the nose with a tissue, picking the nose, breathing dry or cold air, or being exposed to environmental factors such as cigarette smoke and other airborne irritants and chemicals. Most "spontaneous" bleeding in the posterior part of the nose originates from the sphenopalatine artery, often near the posterior end of the inferior turbinate. Iatrogenic bleeding can occur anywhere in the nose where mucosa is traumatized.

DIAGNOSIS

The basic diagnosis of epistaxis sounds easy; epistaxis is present when there is blood coming out of the nose. In the ICU setting, however, with the patient supine, and often with diminished alertness, blood from a nasal source may drain under the influence of gravity back into the nasopharynx, pooling there and first being noticed as blood from the mouth. Looking in the nose and nasopharynx of patients bleeding from the mouth may lead to rapid identification of a bleeding source. After determining that bleeding is originating in the nose, the next steps in diagnosis are determining exactly where in the nose the bleeding is coming from, how much bleeding there is, and whether it is tapering off or continuing unabated.

Anterior speculum examination with a good headlight and suction usually permits identification of focal anterior bleeding. The exact site of more posterior bleeding, if intermittent or slow, can be determined with a rigid sinonasal endoscope with gentle suction and irrigation. Topical decongestant/anesthetic spray is instilled into the nose before this examination for control of bleeding and patient comfort.

Sometimes, even with the endoscope, a specific source of the bleeding cannot be identified. The two most common causes of this are (1) generalized mucosal ooze in a patient with systemic coagulopathy and (2) bleeding copious enough that even with irrigation and suction clear visualization through the endoscope is obscured.

TREATMENT

FOCAL ANTERIOR BLEEDING

For "spontaneous" anterior bleeding from Little's area, pinching the anterior nose firmly between the thumb and finger provides pressure that often controls the bleeding. Firm pressure is applied for 5 minutes without interruption and then is gently released. If bleeding persists, pressure should be applied for an additional 5 minutes. Pressure can be combined with a topical decongestant, such as oxymetazoline, which causes vasoconstriction, aiding bleeding cessation.

If there is a single identifiable anterior source, such as a small laceration or varicosity, cautery with a silver nitrate stick or electrocautery may provide permanent cessation. For cautery, additional topical or injected anesthetic will make the patient more comfortable. This can be done by saturating a small cotton ball or pledget with the decongestant/anesthetic solution and leaving it inside the anterior nasal cavity for 5 to 10 minutes. After application of the topical anesthetic, lidocaine with epinephrine can be injected into the mucosa under direct or endoscopic visualization, without causing the patient much discomfort, if additional anesthesia is needed.

If silver nitrate cautery is used, the stick is applied directly to the oozing mucosa, cauterizing only the actively bleeding area. The mucosa touched by silver nitrate becomes black immediately. Once bleeding is well controlled, the mucosal area is gently rinsed with saline solution. If electrocautery is used, the grounding pad (if necessary with the unit) is applied to the patient and the oozing area cauterized. With both techniques, the "dose" of cautery used should be the minimum required to control bleeding, avoiding damage to nearby normal mucosa. A small piece of Gelfoam can be applied to the cauterized area. Antibiotic ointment is applied to the area twice a day for 3 to 5 days.

A commercially available "pack" can also control anterior bleeding. These packs do not conform as well to the entire shape of the nasal vault in the way packing can and so may be less effective (depending on the exact site of bleeding). They are, however, quicker and easier to place than anterior packing, which is an acquired skill. Nasal tampons such as Merocel (Xomed) are inserted into the nasal cavity dry and compressed after generously coating them with lubricant. After the tampon is in place, it is expanded with saline to exert pressure on the nasal mucosa.

MIDDLE NOSE: FOCAL OR GENERALIZED OOZE

If bleeding originates slightly more posteriorly but still within the anterior zone, or if there is a generalized mucosal ooze, anterior packing can be used. The nasal cavity is firmly packed with ribbon gauze coated with petroleum jelly or BIP ointment (bismuth subnitrate, iodoform, paraffin). This approach applies pressure from inside the nose against the bleeding mucosa, much as bleeding from a facial laceration is controlled by holding pressure on the bleeding area.

Other options for controlling middle vault bleeding or generalized oozing include variations on anterior packing. The Rhino Rocket (Shippert Medical, Englewood, CO) is rolled polyvinyl alcohol foam on a tampon-like inserter. It unfurls when released in the nose and has a string that remains outside to the anterior nose, facilitating later removal.

POSTERIOR BLEEDING: GENERALIZED OR UNIDENTIFIABLE SOURCE

The source of bleeding from the posterior half of the nose is more difficult to visualize. Direct digital pressure, which works well in the anterior nose, is not effective within the posterior bony nasal vault. So, if bleeding is significant and sustained, if no nasal endoscope is available, or if blood flow obscures the endoscopic view, posterior/anterior packing is usually the first step.

Posterior bleeding cannot be controlled by anterior packing alone, because it is impossible to apply sufficient pressure. Trying to pack gauze into the posterior part of the nose is like trying to stuff a doughnut hole, so that as one packs more from the front the gauze begins to fall out the back (i.e., into the nasopharynx). This is why posterior packing is used for a posterior hemorrhage.

Posterior packing provides a stable platform in the nasopharynx against which the packing inserted from anteriorly can be firmly placed. Traditionally, this is a roll of gauze placed through the mouth that is guided into place in the nasopharynx by strings brought out through the nose, which then pull this pack into position and are tied around the columella.

When a patient is endotracheally intubated, firm pharyngeal packing can be used as a posterior nasal pack. Other alternatives to a posterior gauze pack include a Foley catheter and various nasal balloon devices. A Foley catheter placed transnasally into the nasopharynx and inflated can provide a similar firm nasopharyngeal platform. The commercially available balloon devices for posterior packing generally have two balloons that are inflated separately, one for the nasal vault and the other for the nasopharynx.

AFTER PACKING THE NOSE

Even anterior packing of one nostril compromises nasal respiration and blocks sinus drainage into that nasal cavity. A posterior pack blocks both nasal cavities. If seen as outpatients, all patients with posterior packs are admitted to the hospital for bed rest, oxygen supplementation (by facemask or face tent, not nasal cannula), hydration, and antibiotic therapy (to prevent development of sinusitis or toxic shock syndrome). In the ICU setting, these supportive therapies should be provided for any patient requiring a nasal pack.

When a posterior gauze pack, Foley catheter, or other posterior packing material is secured at the anterior nares, traction where these are secured at the columella carries the risk of columellar irritation and necrosis. Careful padding or devising methods of securing the packing that do not cross the columella will prevent this complication. The key is spreading out the pressure over the columella, rather than having a narrow string crossing the columella. Padding can be provided by folded gauzes, cotton rolls, and so on. Alternately, these ties can be attached to another tie that goes across the entire upper lip, over the ears, and behind the head. Umbilical clamps at the nasal openings can also be used to maintain the forward pressure on the posterior packs. For a critically ill patient, to maintain pressure one can also consider suspending the packing material either to a halo device or other external fixed point (e.g., trapeze frame, ceiling, intravenous line stands)

GENERALIZED MUCOSAL OOZE

When there is generalized mucosal oozing, it is usually because of a systemic clotting problem. In the critical care setting, clotting can be deranged on the basis of a coagulopathy (e.g., secondary to leukemia, an inherited disorder, or anticoagulation medications, disseminated intravascular coagulopathy, post-transfusion coagulopathy) or a systemic illness (e.g., renal or hepatic disease). If the systemic problem is easily correctable (i.e., stopping anticoagulants), nasal packing as described earlier can be used. If, however, the coagulopathy is ongoing, nasal packing can be a self-defeating approach. Although the bleeding stops when the pack is in place, the mucosal microtrauma of pack removal reinitiates the bleeding. Use of absorbable hemostatic agents (Gelfoam, Surgicel, Avitene) or fibrin glue can be helpful.

ADDITIONAL TREATMENT OPTIONS

If a bleeding point is identified but is too far posterior to cauterize at the bedside, the patient can be given general anesthesia in the operating suite. Endoscopically guided suction-cautery can be performed as far back as the choana. Sometimes infracture of the inferior turbinate is required to access a posterior bleeding point.

If bleeding is not controlled by packing, or if it recurs after packing is removed, control by arteriography and embolization or surgery is recommended. Surgical options include transnasal sphenopalatine artery ligation, anterior ethmoidal artery ligation, transantral internal maxillary artery ligation, and ligation of the external carotid artery in the neck.[1-4]

SPECIFIC ICU SITUATIONS

OXYGEN BY NASAL CANNULA

Oxygen supplied by nasal cannula dries the nasal mucosa. The dried mucosa is fragile and bleeds easily. Replacing the oxygen by nasal cannula with humidified oxygen via facemask or face tent will prevent this problem.

Once bleeding has occurred in this situation, the bleeding site can usually be identified on the anterior septum with a nasal speculum and headlight. If the bleeding consists of occasional spotting without active ongoing bleeding, gentle application of petrolatum or antibiotic ointment to this area several times a day will allow the mucosa to heal. If there is active bleeding, chemical or electrical cautery is sometimes needed.

NASAL INTUBATION

The largest cross-sectional diameter in the nasal vault occurs along the floor of the nose, which goes straight back from the nares. The best angle for passing a tube through the nose is found by elevating the nasal tip and passing the tube straight back. For smaller tubes such as nasogastric tubes, lubrication is usually all that is required for smooth passage through the nose.

Nasotracheal intubation is a common cause of epistaxis. Most such bleeding is mild and self-limited. If bleeding occurs during fiberoptic nasal intubation, it can obscure the endoscopic view. Measures that enhance smooth passage of the endotracheal tube through the nose and minimize bleeding include using a topical decongestant on the nasal mucosa before tube passage, generous lubrication of the tube, and thermo-softening of the tube in warmed water. Inspection of the internal nasal passages with a speculum or endoscope allows choosing of the larger side, the one with minimal narrowing by septal deviation, septal spurs, or turbinate hypertrophy. Passage of successively larger soft nasal trumpets can assist with dilating the nasal passage (i.e., compressing the internal soft tissue) before intubation.

POSTOPERATIVE EPISTAXIS

Bleeding from the nose occurring after nasal or facial surgery must be reported immediately to the surgeon. Topical decongestants, pressure, cautery, absorbable hemostatic agents, or nasal packing may be required to control such bleeding. Occasionally the patient will need to return to the operating suite for vessel ligation.

MASSIVE FACIAL TRAUMA

The occurrence of multiple facial fractures can cause epistaxis. Usually this type of bleeding ceases with nasal packing. Occasionally a displaced fracture tents open a lacerated vessel and fracture reduction is required to stop the bleeding. Asch and Rowe forceps are used for this reduction, and a general anesthetic is usually required.

VESSEL PROBLEMS

Rarely, massive epistaxis results from rupture of carotid aneurysms or carotid-cavernous sinus fistulas. Cerebral arteriography and embolization are required to control such bleeding.

CONCLUSION

Because the nose provides a major route for reaching the digestive tract and the airway, it is almost inevitable that patients hospitalized in the ICU will undergo a procedure or treatment that traumatizes the nasal airway. Measures that can minimize this trauma include gentle technique, good understanding of nasal anatomy, generous use of topical vasoconstrictors, lubricants, and humidified air, and use of the softest acceptable materials for passage through the nasal cavity.

Most epistaxis in the ICU setting is mild and responds to pressure, topical decongestants, fibrin glue, or chemical cautery. Because most ICUs are in tertiary care hospitals with medical specialists readily available, an otolaryngologist should be consulted for assistance in the diagnosis and treatment of epistaxis requiring more intervention.

ANNOTATED REFERENCES

Kumar S, Shetty A, Rockey J, Nilssen E: Contemporary surgical treatment of epistaxis: What is the evidence for sphenopalatine artery ligation? Clin Otolaryngol 2003;28:360-363.

Scaramuzzi N, Walsh RM, Brennan P, Walsh M: Treatment of intractable epistaxis using arterial embolization. Clin Otolaryngol Allied Sci 2001;26:307-309.

Spafford P, Durham JS: Epistaxis: Efficacy of arterial ligation and long-term outcome. J Otolaryngol 1992;21:252-256.

Strong EB, Bell DA, Johnson LP, Jacobs JM: Intractable epistaxis: Transantral ligation vs. embolization: Efficacy review and cost analysis. Otolaryngol Head Neck Surg 1995;113:674-678.

These references can be consulted for further reading.

Chapter 232

MANAGEMENT OF THE POSTOPERATIVE CARDIAC SURGICAL PATIENT

Daniel Talmor • Alan Lisbon

KEY POINTS

1. Recent developments in interventional cardiology have led to **older and sicker populations being referred for cardiac surgery.**

2. Much of the **care of cardiac surgical patients** should be protocol driven and conducted in specialized units.

3. Most patients undergoing cardiac surgery require **only a short stay in the intensive care unit.**

4. **Patients may be extubated** once hemodynamic stability is achieved and mediastinal bleeding is deemed to be under control.

5. **Low cardiac output after surgery** should be treated based on the components of the cardiac output: rate, rhythm, preload, afterload, and contractility.

6. **Atrial fibrillation continues to be a cause of significant morbidity.**

7. **Tight blood glucose control has been shown to significantly improve outcomes.**

The first days of care for the cardiac surgery patient present multiple challenges for the intensivist. The intensive care unit (ICU) stay for most cardiac surgery patients lasts for only 24 to 48 hours. However, during this period, life-threatening problems, such as low cardiac output (CO), arrhythmias, and coagulopathy, may become apparent. After 48 hours in the ICU, the problems encountered by postoperative cardiac surgery patients tend to become more like those experienced by other groups of critically ill patients.

THE CARDIAC SURGERY PATIENT IN THE INTENSIVE CARE UNIT

HISTORY OF CARDIAC SURGERY LINKED TO THE HISTORY OF INTENSIVE CARE

The development of modern cardiac surgery has been intimately related to the development of the ICU. This relationship has worked in both directions. Until the 1950s, cardiac surgery was limited to control of traumatic injuries and the closed repair of valves. Development of the extracorporeal pump oxygenator in 1953 by Gibbon ushered in the era of open-heart surgery.[1] Heart valve replacement then became possible. Subsequently, in the 1960s, coronary artery bypass grafting (CABG) for ischemic heart disease was developed and rapidly popularized.[2]

These increasingly complicated cardiac procedures required the development of sophisticated postoperative care. The skills required for postoperative care of these patients led to the development of dedicated ICUs. Several studies have demonstrated that risk-adjusted mortality rates after CABG vary significantly among surgeons and hospitals and that mortality is related both to the number of surgeries performed by each surgeon and the total volume of procedures performed at the hospital.[3-5] For high-risk surgical patients, survival is also related to the characteristics of the ICU care.[6] It is likely that at least some of the mortality advantage seen in high-volume cardiac surgery centers is related to the presence of highly experienced critical care teams.

THE CHANGING EPIDEMIOLOGY OF CARDIAC SURGERY

Over the last decade, the population of patients treated with cardiac surgery has changed dramatically. Advances in cardiology, including reperfusion therapy, angioplasty, stenting, and drug-eluting stents, have obviated the need for surgical approaches to treatment except for particularly complex problems or after failure of other, less invasive modalities. In the year 2000, 561,000 patients in the United States underwent percutaneous transluminal coronary angioplasty (PTCA), an increase of 262% relative to 1987. In the same year, 314,000 patients underwent CABG. Multiyear trends, represented in Figure 232-1, show a leveling off and subsequent decrease in the overall number of patients undergoing CABG.[7] The recently developed sirolimus-coated coronary stent has been associated with even better results.[8,9] It can be expected that these further developments in interventional cardiology will continue to decrease the number of CABG operations being performed.

Even as younger patients are being treated with interventional techniques, the elderly are increasingly referred for operation. Although these operations are successful even in most octogenarians, they are associated with increased hospital mortality and longer ICU and hospital stays. It is clear, however, that good results in terms of long-term survival and quality of life are acheivable.[10]

ALTERNATIVE TECHNIQUES FOR CARDIAC SURGERY

The increasing age of patients undergoing cardiac surgery and the relatively high incidence of adverse effects related to

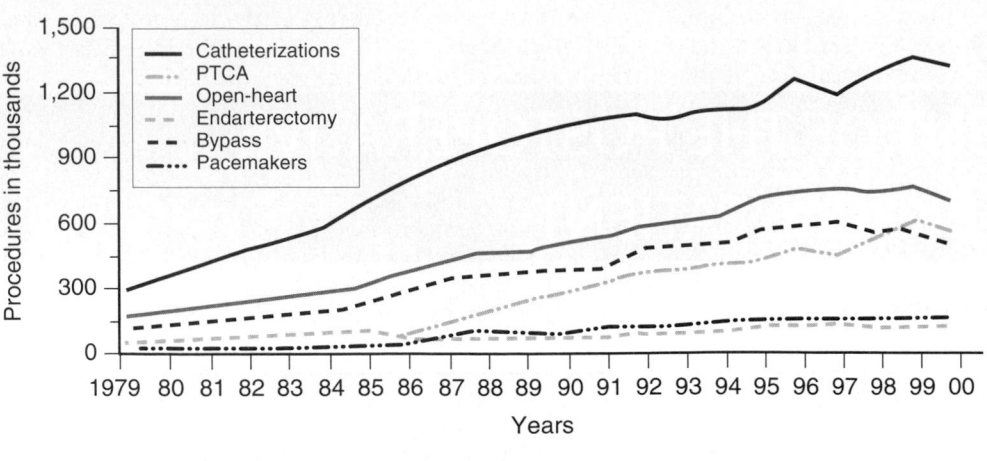

FIGURE 232–1. Trends in cardiovascular operations and procedures in the United States, 1979-2000. PTCA, percutaneous transluminal coronary angioplasty. (From American Heart Association: Heart Disease and Stroke Statistics—2003 Update. Dallas, TX, AHA, 2003.)

cardiopulmonary bypass (CPB) in these patients have led to the development of less invasive cardiac surgical techniques. These techniques are intended to decrease postoperative morbidity, reduce hospital length of stay, reduce costs, and hasten recovery of lifestyle (Table 232-1). Three major techniques have been proposed.

Minimally invasive direct coronary artery bypass (MIDCAB) differs from conventional CABG mainly in the type of incision used for access. In place of the conventional median sternotomy, access is obtained via a left or right thoracotomy, a parasternal incision, or a partial sternotomy. The proposed benefit of such an approach is the reduction in morbidity related to median sternotomy. This proposed advantage has not been demonstrated. MIDCAB grafting is a challenging technique and should be performed only in selected patients with favorable coronary anatomy.

Off-pump coronary artery bypass (OPCAB) is performed on a beating heart without benefit of CPB. The proposed benefit of this procedure is the reduction of morbidity related to hypothermia and CPB. The procedure is undertaken using partial to full heparinization. Extubation may be achieved earlier in these patients, because they do not require rewarming and are less coagulopathic. A subset of patients cannot tolerate the extent of retraction of the heart required for the surgery and need to be urgently placed on CPB. These patients may suffer ischemic myocardial injury and

TABLE 232–1. COMPARISON OF MINIMALLY INVASIVE CARDIAC SURGERY TECHNIQUES

Technique	Incision Site	Cannulation Site	Advantages	Disadvantages
Conventional CABG	Median sternotomy	Ascending aorta Right atrium	Excellent exposure Stable closure Extensive experience	Mediastinitis Slow recovery of upper-extremity function Postoperative cough limited by pain
MIDCAB	Left thoracotomy, *or* Paramedian or right thoracotomy, *or* Partial sternotomy	Ascending aorta Right atrium	Avoids median sternotomy Useful for redo procedure Hastens recovery of upper-extremity function*	Limited exposure No cost savings May require multiple incisions
Port-access	Right anterior thoracotomy, *or* Paramedian or left thoracotomy	Ascending aorta via right paramedian port Femoral vein	Avoids median sternotomy Avoids atriotomy Access to mitral valve Smaller skin incision Decreases hospital stay* Decreases atrial fibrillation incidence* Decreases transfusion* Decreases rehabilitation time*	Increased cost of equipment Contraindicated in patients with ascending aortic pathology Limited operative exposure Significant learning curve unlikely to decrease cerebral emboli
OPCAB	Median sternotomy, *or* Right or left thoracotomy, *or* Partial sternotomy	None	Avoids aortic manipulation Avoids atriotomy and CPB Normothermia Decreases atrial fibrillation incidence* Decreases transfusion* Decreases neurologic morbidity† Decreases pulmonary morbidity†	Cost of equipment Slow recovery of upper-extremity function Mediastinitis Increases intraoperative ischemia Undetermined graft longevity

CABG, coronary artery bypass grafting; CPB, cardiopulmonary bypass; MIDCAB, minimally invasive direct coronary artery bypass; OPCAB, off-pump coronary artery bypass.
*Limited supporting evidence exists.
†Proposed benefit.
Adapted from Reves J, Hill SE, Sum-Ping ST, et al: Perioperative Management of the Cardiac Surgical patient. In Murray, Coursin, Pearl, Prough: Critical Care Medicine: Perioperative Management. Philadelphia, Lippincott Williams & Wilkins, 2002, p 356.)

require support with inotropes or intra-aortic balloon pumping (IABP) during the postoperative period. A retrospective study of 1398 patients showed that use of the OPCAB technique for multivessel myocardial revascularization in high-risk patients significantly reduced the incidence of perioperative myocardial infarction (MI) and other major complications, length of stay in the ICU, and mortality.[11] Others have found a significant improvement in postoperative neurocognitive function, which may, in turn, lead to better quality of life.[12]

A third method of minimally invasive cardiac surgery is the port access technique. This operation entails obtaining access for CPB with the use of endovascular catheters. This allows surgery to be performed using CPB via either a left or a right thoracotomy. The technique is particularly useful for mitral valve replacement through a right thoracotomy and for redo CABG (avoiding the complications associated with repeat sternotomy). The port-access technique has been shown to be safe and is associated with shorter lengths of stay, reduced transfusion requirements, fewer infections, decreased incidence of renal failure, and less atrial fibrillation when compared with conventional techniques.[13,14] Widespread adoption of this technique has been limited by the technical complexity of placing the required catheters, which requires both extra time and a specially trained and skilled operative team.

The techniques of minimally invasive cardiac surgery are still evolving. The intensivist caring for cardiac surgical patients must continue to keep abreast of these new methods.

ORGANIZATION OF THE POSTOPERATIVE CARDIAC SURGERY UNIT

Optimal results from cardiac surgery require a skilled, dedicated, and multidisciplinary ICU team. Patients undergoing cardiac surgery are usually admitted to the hospital on the day of surgery. They arrive in the ICU directly from the operating room (OR). The typical patient is transferred to a step-down unit on the morning after surgery. This unit allows continued monitoring with telemetry for an additional 24 to 48 hours. The increasing age and comorbidity of the population of cardiac surgical patients have led to increasing length of stay in the ICU. Patients remaining in the ICU beyond 48 hours tend to become similar to a standard ICU population as they develop secondary complications such as sepsis, pneumonia, and acute respiratory distress syndrome (ARDS).

Guidelines developed by the American Heart Association and the American College of Cardiology outline the requirements for cardiac surgical ICUs.[15] These include the development of protocol-driven care, a minimum number of cardiac surgical ICU beds that is half the number of surgeries performed per week, and one-to-one nursing care during the first night in the unit. ICU coverage by a dedicated intensivist has been shown to improve outcomes in other types of major surgery and should be recommended after cardiac surgery as well.[6]

SEPARATION FROM CARDIOPULMONARY BYPASS AND THE END OF SURGERY

Successful management of the postoperative cardiac surgery patient begins by understanding what occurs in the OR. Problems encountered in the OR often persist after transfer to the ICU. An understanding of the technical and pathophysiologic aspects of CPB can help the intensivist better manage cardiac surgical patients in the ICU.

CARDIOPULMONARY BYPASS

The goal of CPB is to separate the heart and lungs from the systemic circulation so that the heart can be arrested while the surgical repair is constructed. Blood is drained from the right side of the heart, either by gravity or with vacuum assistance, via a cannula in the right atrium directly or via a cannula in the femoral vein that is advanced into the right atrium. The blood is collected in a reservoir and then pumped through an oxygenator that contains a membrane, where the blood is oxygenated and carbon dioxide is removed (Fig. 232-2). The perfusionist controls both the fraction of inspired oxygen and the rate of oxygen flow through the circuit, thereby controlling the patient's arterial oxygen and carbon dioxide levels, respectively. The treated blood then passes through an air filter and is returned to the patient via an arterial cannula placed in either the ascending aorta or the femoral artery. The perfusionist controls the amount of flow provided to the patient (i.e., CO). Mild to moderate systemic hypothermia (28° to 34°C) is used during bypass to minimize oxygen consumption by both the body and the brain. After adequate CPB is established, an aortic cross clamp is applied to the ascending aorta, between the aortic cannula and the heart. The interval when the cross clamp is applied is referred to as "ischemic" time, because no blood is circulated through the heart during this period. The heart is arrested by infusion of a high-concentration potassium solution into the native coronary arteries (antegrade cardioplegia) via a cannula placed between the aortic cross clamp and the heart. Cardioplegia may also be given "backwards," through the venous system of the myocardium (retrograde cardioplegia), via a catheter placed in the coronary sinus. Potassium is used as the arresting agent because it stops the heart from beating and minimizes myocardial oxygen consumption.

MYOCARDIAL PROTECTION

Several measures are taken to protect the heart during ischemic time, because irreversible myocardial damage may otherwise occur. Electomechanical arrest is the most important protective measure, because the beating action of the heart accounts for about 85% of the heart's total oxygen consumption. The heart is usually cooled to about 10°C with a cold cardioplegia solution (4°C) supplemented with topical ice slush. Additionally, the left ventricle is "vented" to prevent distention, which could lead to subendocardial ischemia. Finally, various additives are included in the cardioplegia solution to minimize myocardial edema, maintain normal intramyocardial pH, and provide substrates for anaerobic metabolism. The adequacy of intraoperative myocardial protection is critical for determining the subsequent course and final outcome of the patient

SEPARATION FROM CARDIOPULMONARY BYPASS

Weaning from CPB is the process whereby cardiopulmonary function is transferred from the bypass system back to the

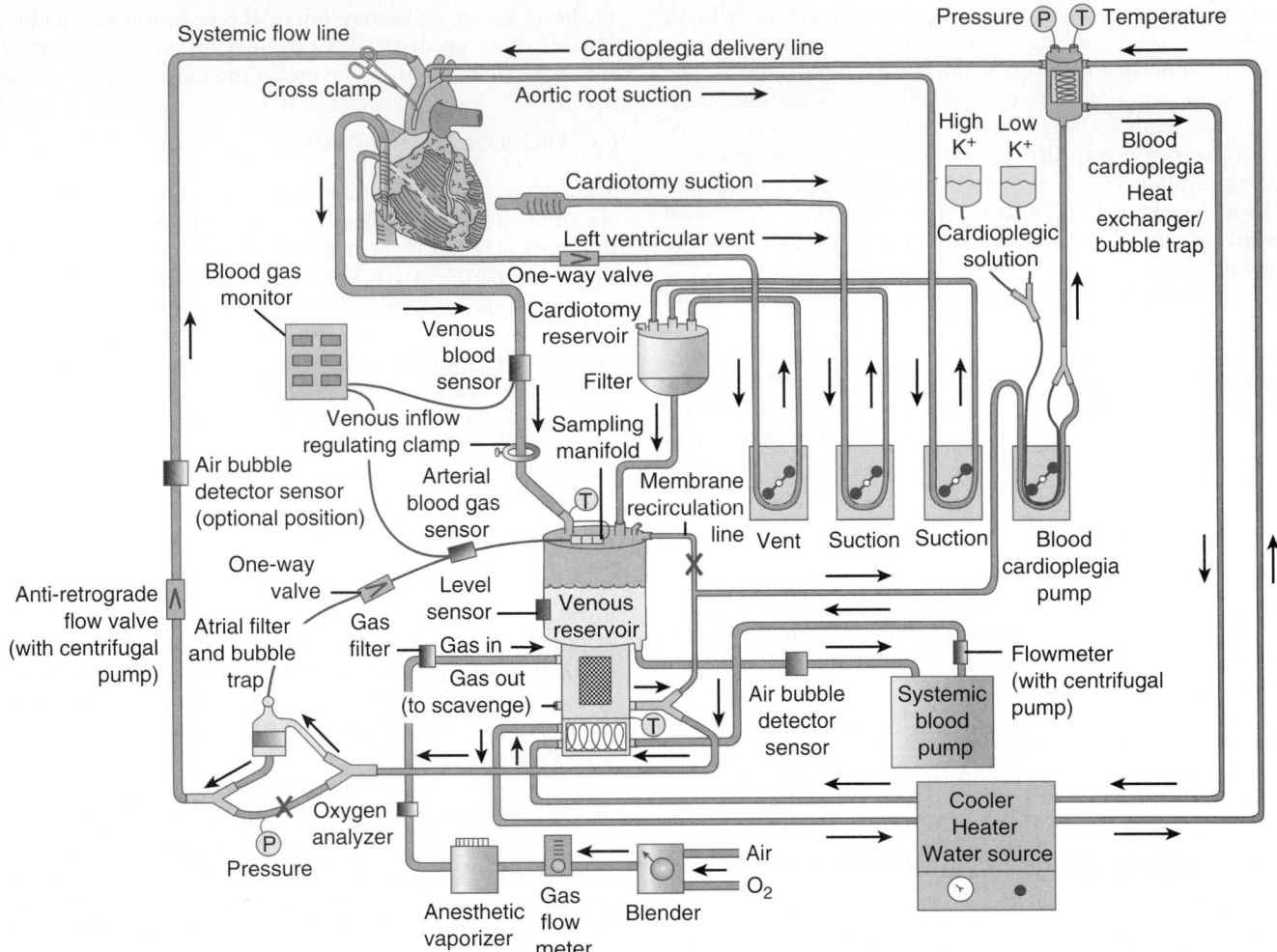

FIGURE 232–2. Cardiopulmonary bypass circuit. (Adapted with permission from Gravlee GP, Davis RF, Kurusz M, Utley JR (eds): Cardiopulmonary Bypass: Principles and Practice, 2nd ed. Baltimore, Lippincott Williams & Wilkins, 2000, p 70.)

patient's own heart and lungs. Successful separation from CPB requires that the metabolic, cardiac, and respiratory parameters are as close to normal as possible. Separation from CPB implies that the native circulation will be required to support the body's metabolic demands. The surgical team manipulates the heart rate and rhythm, preload, afterload, and myocardial contractility to achieve this goal.

In most cases, normal sinus rhythm is restored after discontinuation of cardioplegia and rewarming of the heart. Occasionally, discontinuation of cardioplegia and rewarming leads to the onset of ventricular fibrillation; in such cases, electrical defibrillation is required. Other dysrhythmias that are commonly encountered are atrioventricular disassociation and atrial fibrillation. An attempt should be made to convert these to sinus rhythm by pharmacologic means. Bradyarrhythmias are treated by pacing, using temporary epicardial wires placed by the surgeon after completion of the repair. A heart rate of 70 to 90 beats/min usually is optimal. Pharmacologic support of the circulation may be needed to provide appropriate afterload or systemic vascular resistance (SVR) during separation from CBP. Most patients are vasodilated to some extent, possibly as a result of a systemic inflammatory response to CPB or the effects of rewarming, or both. As a consequence, infusion of a vasoconstrictor is often required. Care must be taken to strike a

proper balance so that increased SVR maintains adequate arterial blood pressure without excessively increasing left ventricular afterload and compromising CO.

Most often, myocardial function is adequate and infusion of an inotrope is not necessary. However, inotropic support often is needed for patients with a poor preoperative ventricular function or inadequate myocardial protection or revascularization during CPB. The optimal inotrope in this situation is a matter of considerable debate, and data are lacking to support a strong recommendation for a specific agent. Epinephrine, norepinephrine, dopamine, dobutamine, amrinone, and milrinone have all been used successfully. Intraoperative monitoring using transesophageal echocardiography (TEE) is particularly useful for titration of inotropic therapy.

Once all preparations for separation have been made, the perfusionist begins to wean the patient from bypass. This is done by slowly decreasing the amount of blood drained from the right atrium while simultaneously reducing flow into the aorta. Once the patient is off bypass (i.e., no blood is being drained from the right atrium into the CPB circuit), the perfusionist, at the direction of the anesthesiologist or the surgeon, may continue to infuse through the aortic cannula. This maneuver allows optimization of ventricular filling or preload. Care must be taken, however, not to overdistend the heart; again, during this period, TEE is extremely useful.

REVERSAL OF ANTICOAGULATION

After weaning from CPB, protamine is given to neutralize any residual heparin. Dosing can be based on the patient's weight, the total amount of heparin given, or an assay of residual heparin activity. Institutional preference governs the technique that is employed, and all have been proven effective. Several adverse responses to protamine administration are possible, including histamine-induced systemic hypotension, immunoglobulin E–mediated allergic reactions, and complement-mediated catastrophic pulmonary hypertension.

TRANSPORT AND ADMISSION TO THE INTENSIVE CARE UNIT

After chest closure, confirmation of hemodynamic stability, and adequate medical and surgical hemostasis, the patient may be transferred to the ICU. Transport of a critically ill patient is a potentially dangerous process and requires extreme vigilance. Transport between the operating room and the ICU should be done with the same degree of monitoring as would be available at either end. This usually includes continuous monitoring of arterial blood pressure, pulmonary artery pressure and/or central venous pressure (CVP), electrocardiogram (ECG), and pulse oximetry. The transport bed should be equipped with a full oxygen tank, Ambu bag and mask, intubation equipment, resuscitation drugs, and a defibrillator. Care must be taken to ensure that infusions of vasoactive drugs are not interrupted.

On arrival in the ICU, the ICU team assumes care of the patient. A detailed sign-out from the operative team ensures continuity of care. The sign-out should include a detailed history, including an assessment of preoperative cardiac functional status, a list of preoperative medications, and a detailed description of the surgery. Key facts are the type of repair performed, target vessels (if the patient has undergone CABG), duration of CPB and cross clamping, difficulties encountered in separation from CPB, presence of abnormal bleeding, and postoperative assessment of cardiac function. All treatments administered in the OR should be detailed, in particular, fluids, blood products, and vasoactive drugs.

Once care has been handed over to the ICU team, a thorough examination of the patient should immediately follow. This examination should include verification of endotracheal tube placement, type and position of arterial or central venous lines, chest tube position and patency, and the presence and location of any epicardial pacing wires.

MONITORING THE POSTOPERATIVE CARDIAC SURGERY PATIENT

HEMODYNAMIC MONITORING

All patients admitted to the ICU after cardiac surgery will have their blood pressure continuously monitored using an intra-arterial line. This is usually placed in either a radial or a femoral artery. Accuracy of the measurements depends on strict attention to calibration, leveling, and removal of air from the tubing. After CPB, femoral arterial pressure may more accurately reflect central aortic pressures,[16] but this

problem has usually resolved by the time the patient arrives in the ICU. If the radial artery is cannulated, the hand should be examined for signs of ischemia.[17] Vascular complications of femoral arterial lines are extremely rare, but femoral catheters may be associated with an increased incidence of infection.[18]

Central venous access is required in all patients for drug administration and hemodynamic monitoring. In the low-risk patient, a CVP catheter may be all that is needed, particularly if echocardiography is available as a backup. Pulmonary artery catheters have the advantage of allowing measurement of pulmonary artery occlusion pressure (PAOP), thermodilution, and CO, as well as sampling of the mixed venous blood saturation (SvO_2). Use of the pulmonary artery catheter remains controversial. Improved outcome due to use of a pulmonary artery catheter for monitoring of cardiac surgical patients has not been demonstrated.[19] Some studies showed an increased risk of death or adverse outcome when treatment was guided by the use of a pulmonary artery catheter.[20,21] However, many of these studies have been criticized on methodologic grounds, and use of the catheter in cardiac surgery is widespread.[22] Current guidelines recommend use of the pulmonary artery catheter in high-risk patients undergoing surgery in an appropriate practice setting.[23] Such a setting is one in which the physician and nursing staff are familiar with the catheter and trained to properly interpret the information obtained. If echocardiography is readily available, then it is possible to manage even high-risk patients using a CVP catheter.

ELECTROCARDIOGRAPHY

On admission to the ICU, the patient is connected to a continuous ECG monitor and a formal 12-lead ECG is obtained. The cardiogram is examined for rate, rhythm, QRS complex morphology, and signs of myocardial ischemia. For patients who are being paced postoperatively, the type of pacing and the degree of capture should be assessed.

Continuous ECG monitoring allows detection of arrhythmias. If an arrhythmia is detected, a 12-lead ECG should be obtained and serum electrolyte concentrations should be measured. Treatment of arrhythmias should be carried out using established protocols.[24] If a malignant arrhythmia occurs, myocardial ischemia should be considered as a possible precipitating cause.

Monitoring of trends in ST-segment elevation or depression allows early detection of postoperative myocardial ischemia. Although transient ST segment changes are relatively common and of unclear significance, persistent changes should be investigated by obtaining a 12-lead ECG and measuring circulating levels of creatine kinase myocardial band (CK-MB), troponin-T, or troponin-I.[25,26] If ischemia is strongly suspected, then echocardiography followed by coronary angiography should be considered. Findings from these studies may indicate the need for further coronary revascularization.

CHEST RADIOGRAPHY

The postoperative chest radiograph should be systematically evaluated. Proper placement of the endotracheal tube and any central lines inserted should be confirmed. If a pulmonary artery catheter is place, the location of its tip should be noted and adjusted as needed. The lung fields should be examined for the presence of pneumothorax or collapse. Additional air may be noted as subcutaneous emphysema or as pneumopericardium, although these findings are of little clinical significance. Further examination of the lung fields commonly shows small areas of atelectasis and pleural effusion. The cardiac silhouette is often enlarged after surgery as a result of myocardial edema and accumulation of fluid in the open pericardial sac. Increasing size of the cardiac silhouette or pleural effusions on serial chest radiographs may be evidence of ongoing mediastinal bleeding.

ECHOCARDIOGRAPHY IN THE INTENSIVE CARE UNIT

Echocardiography is an excellent tool for evaluating chamber size and function and the adequacy of valve repair or replacement. Indications include postoperative assessment of left ventricular function; assessment of unexplained, sudden hemodynamic deterioration; evaluation to rule out pericardial tamponade; and workup of new cardiac ischemia. Limitations to transthoracic echocardiography (TTE) include inadequate windows early after operation due to air and edema in the soft tissues and wound dressings.

TEE is being used more and more by intensivists as a tool to facilitate decision-making in the management of critically ill patients, including cardiac surgical patients. In the cardiac surgical ICU, this modality may have a particularly high yield when it is used to establish the cause of postoperative hypotension.[27] In one large series, a new diagnosis was established or an important pathology was excluded in 45% of TEE examinations performed in the ICU. Pericardial tamponade was diagnosed in 34 cases (11%) and excluded in 36 cases (12%). Other diagnoses included severe left ventricular failure and presence of large pleural effusions. The results of TEE had an impact on therapy in 220 cases (73%) by leading to a change of pharmacologic treatment and/or fluid administration, reoperation, or a decision that reoperation was unnecessary.[28]

CLINICAL MANIFESTATIONS OF THE POSTBYPASS PERIOD

THE NORMAL COURSE

Patients are typically admitted to the ICU intubated and ventilated. Sedation with a short-acting agent, typically propofol, is continued until the patient is ready for extubation. Once hemodynamic stability is ascertained and chest tube drainage is judged to be under control, the patient is allowed to awaken. There is no need for prolonged weaning from mechanical ventilation. A short trial of spontaneous ventilation is sufficient to determine whether respiration will be adequate without mechanical support. The rapid shallow breathing index (RSBI) has been shown to be a sensitive way to assess the likelihood of successful extubation.[29] The RSBI is calculated by dividing the respiratory rate (in breaths per minute) by the tidal volume (in liters). A value of lower than 105 predicts successful extubation. Chest tubes are commonly removed on the first postoperative day. The pulmonary artery catheter, if present, is discontinued, and the patient may be transferred to a step-down unit.

Fast-tracking of cardiac surgical patients refers to a comprehensive program designed to reduce both length of stay and hospital costs.[30,31] As a part of this program, multiple anesthetic techniques, designed to allow earlier postoperative extubation, have been proposed, studied, and shown to be safe. These techniques may allow extubation in the OR. The key to proper use of this technique is patient selection. Although the criteria are expanding, patients with unstable angina or a high degree of congestive heart failure are generally not appropriate candidates for fast-tracking. Because these patients still need to be admitted to the ICU, the cost savings associated with fast-tracking may be less then anticipated.[32]

LOW CARDIAC OUTPUT

Low CO is the most common problem encountered in the postoperative cardiac surgical patient. A hallmark of low CO is low blood pressure. However, a patient may have a low CO with tissue hypoperfusion and still maintain what appears to be an adequate blood pressure. In the postoperative state, the physician must continuously examine and monitor the patient for signs of hypoperfusion. Physical signs of inadequate tissue perfusion include altered mental status; cool, pale, or even cyanotic extremities; diaphoresis; and low urine output. Global measures of hypoperfusion include increasing base deficit, elevated blood lactate concentration, and decreased SvO_2. Although the clinician must consider CO in terms of adequacy of perfusion, blood pressure per se is still important. Both the brain and the kidneys depend on adequate blood pressure to maintain tissue perfusion. Additionally, coronary artery blood flow is dependent on a diastolic blood pressure, a key determinant of coronary artery perfusion pressure.

When assessing a patient with hypotension or signs of hypoperfusion, it is useful to consider the problem in relation to the components of CO; namely, preload, contractility, afterload, and rate and rhythm.

Preload
Preload refers to the stretch of the left ventricle at the end of diastole. Preload is determined by the extent of ventricular filling during diastole. Adequate filling is required to ensure ejection in the subsequent systole. The most common cause of inadequate preload in postoperative patients is hypovolemia. Intravascular volume status should be continually monitored by assessing changes over time with respect to physical examination, chest tube output, and filling pressures (CVP, PAOP, or pulmonary artery diastolic pressure). Because none of the clinically measured filling pressures correlates perfectly with actual ventricular preload (i.e., end-diastolic volume), and correlation is particularly poor when the heart is diseased, it is often useful to obtain a "snapshot" of ventricular filling using echocardiography. By this means, it is possible to assess the relationship between measured filling pressures and actual preload in a specific patient. Preoperative catheterization data also can be helpful for determining this relationship. Hypovolemia should be treated with fluid replacement. Crystalloids are generally used. Surprisingly, there is no generally accepted hemoglobin concentration or hematocrit that should be used as a trigger for ordering transfusion of packed red blood cells.

In some cases, low preload is not caused by absolute hypovolemia but by relative or distributional hypovolemia.

CPB and subsequent rewarming may lead to vasodilatation and a subsequent hypotension. Intravascular volume expansion may be required to maintain perfusion. An acceptable alternative is administration of a low dose of vasopressor, such as phenylephrine or norepinephrine, to maintain an adequate perfusion pressure. Recently, vasopressin, in doses between 0.01 and 0.1 units/min, has been demonstrated to be effective in this situation.[33,34] Vasodilatation is usually a transient problem that resolves during the first several hours after separation from CPB. Continued vasodilatation after this period should prompt a search for another cause, particularly infection.

Pump Failure

Either or both ventricles may fail postoperatively. Decreased myocardial contractility may be caused by impaired preoperative function, inadequate revascularization at surgery, post-CPB reperfusion injury, or perioperative myocardial ischemia or MI. The incidence of infarction is approximately 5% in large series.[35] Preoperative myocardial function and the adequacy of revascularization at surgery should be clear from the history. Determination of circulating levels of CK-MB or troponin postoperatively can provide evidence of perioperative ischemia or infarction.[25,26] Often, diminished contractility after operation is caused by inadequate myocardial protection during surgery. Decreased myocardial contractility secondary to inadequate myocardial protection usually resolves within the first 24 hours postoperatively. ECG changes are nonspecific.

Persistent new myocardial dysfunction associated with ECG changes and echocardiographic evidence of new wall motion abnormalities should raise suspicion that the problem is an occluded graft and MI. Measurements of CK-MB in serum are of limited usefulness, because levels of this enzyme are commonly elevated after surgery due to manipulation of the heart and incision of the atria, structures that are rich in the enzyme. If CK-MB levels are very high, greater than 80 mg/dL, then perioperative MI is likely.[36] Cardiac troponins are more specific for the diagnosis of perioperative infarction. A comparison of CK-MB, troponin-T and troponin-I showed that a troponin-I level of greater than 5 μg/L was the most accurate indicator of MI, being superior to either troponin-T or CK-MB.[37] Elevated serum concentrations of troponin-I are associated with a cardiac cause of death and with major postoperative complications.[38] In addition, troponin-T concentrations measured after surgery are an independent predictor of in-hospital death after cardiac surgery.[26] If ischemia or MI is diagnosed, the patient may be taken for angiography or reexploration and revascularization.

Postoperative valvular insufficiency can occur not only in patients with preexisting valvular lesions but also as a result of injury during surgery. The mitral valve is most commonly affected. Ischemia of the papillary muscles, due to inadequate myocardial protection or perioperative MI, can lead to acute mitral regurgitation in the postoperative period. Diagnosis is often made by TEE in the OR, but inadequate CO and a new systolic murmur should prompt echocardiographic evaluation.

Rate and Rhythm

CO is the product of HR times stroke volume (SV). Many dysrhythmias can adversely affect CO. If the heart rate (HR) is too low, CO can be compromised. If HR is too fast, ventricular filling during diastole can be impaired, decreasing CO. Rhythm disturbances are common after cardiac surgery and may be divided into bradyarrhythmias and tachyarrhythmias; these categories are further divided into atrial and ventricular arrhythmias.

Bradycardia can lead to ventricular distention, increasing wall tension, and decreasing coronary perfusion pressure, factors that can promote development of ischemia and failure. An HR of 80 to 90 appears to be optimal, allowing adequate filling and preventing overdistention but not causing rate-related ischemia. Bradycardia can be corrected by pacing. In general, epicardial pacing wires are left in place after chest closure and are attached to an external pacemaker in the immediate postoperative period. If the dysrhythmia is sinus bradycardia, then atrial pacing is usually optimal. The second most common cause of bradyarrhythmia after cardiac surgery is atrioventricular dissociation. The combination of atrial and ventricular leads allows atrioventricular pacing for management of disassociation. Synchronization of the atrioventricular interval between 0.1 and 0.225 second optimizes CO.[39]

Atrial fibrillation is the most common tachyarrhythmia. It occurs in 10% to 35% of patients after cardiac surgery, usually on the second or third postoperative day. Postoperative atrial fibrillation is associated with increased morbidity and mortality and with longer, more expensive hospital stays.[40] The MultiCenter Study of Perioperative Ischemia (McSPI) group examined 2417 patients undergoing CABG with or without concurrent valvular surgery.[41] The overall incidence of postoperative atrial fibrillation was 27%. Independent predictors of postoperative atrial fibrillation included advanced age, male sex, a past history of atrial fibrillation, a past history of congestive heart failure, and a pre-CPB heart rate greater than 100 beats/min. Surgical practices such as pulmonary vein venting, bicaval venous cannulation, postoperative atrial pacing, and longer cross-clamp times also were identified as independent predictors of postoperative atrial fibrillation. Patients who developed postoperative atrial fibrillation had longer lengths of stay, both in the ICU and in the ward, compared with patients who did not develop the complication.

Although premature ventricular contractions (PVCs) are common, sustained ventricular arrhythmias are far less frequent. Severe ventricular arrhythmias occurring after cardiac surgery are related to ischemia, hypoxemia, hypovolemia, electrolyte abnormalities, the effects of vasoactive drugs, or an underlying preexisting cardiomyopathy.[42] In a series of 2100 cardiac operations, only 16 patients (0.8%) developed ventricular fibrillation or a sustained ventricular tachycardia during the interval from 3 days to 3 weeks after surgery. Ten of these patients had undergone valve surgery.[43] Prognosis in these patients is dependent on the preoperative ventricular prognosis; it is excellent in those with good function. In those with a left ventricular ejection fraction of less than 40%, the mortality rate may be as high as 75%.[44]

Afterload

Ventricular afterload is the impedance to ventricular ejection during systole. Hypertension develops in as many as 60% of patients after surgery. Increased arterial blood pressure occurs even among patients without a preoperative history of hypertension. Predisposing factors include hypoxemia, hypercapnia, inadequate rewarming, pain, fluid overload, and increased sympathetic tone. Perioperative discontinuation of β-adrenergic blockers also may contribute to the development of postoperative hypertension.

Hypertension and increased afterload can lead to myocardial ischemia by augmenting ventricular stroke work. Additionally, hypertension may lead to bleeding from surgical sites, aortic dissection, and increased risk of stroke.

Tamponade

Tamponade refers to the hemodynamic consequences of a collection of blood or other fluid in the pericardial sac. In postsurgical patients, the presentation of tamponade may be subtle and may differ significantly from classic descriptions. Equilibration of filling pressures typically is not seen. More commonly, patients present with isolated elevation of right atrial pressure due to compression of the right atrium and superior vena cava. After cardiac surgery, as many as 66% of pericardial fluid collections are loculated posterior effusions.[45]

Bleeding from the atrial cannulation site is a common cause of tamponade. As the pressure on the right atrium increases, ventricular filling is impaired and CO decreases. Diagnosis of tamponade is made difficult by the high overall frequency of pericardial effusions after surgery. Echocardiographic studies have shown that moderate effusions are present in 30% of patients on the eighth postoperative day, with 2% of patients having large effusions.[46]

Diagnosis of tamponade in the postoperative patient requires a high index of suspicion and prompt intervention. Any hemodynamic instability should be assessed for tamponade. Low CO, hypotension, and tachycardia accompanied by an elevation of the left, the right, or both atrial pressures should lead to a prompt echocardiogram. Other signs that may be present include a widened mediastinum on chest radiography, dysrhythmias, and decreased ECG voltage. Because of the influence of positive pressure ventilation, the classic sign of pulsus paradoxus may not be present.

If time permits, the diagnosis of tamponade can be confirmed with the use of echocardiography. Although effusions are common, signs of compression or collapse of either atrium or of the right ventricle are diagnostic.[47-49] It is important to remember that the diagnosis may be made on clinical suspicion alone and that treatment should not be withheld to await confirmation. Once tamponade is diagnosed, volume transfusion may temporize the situation. Pericardiocentesis is not effective in this situation, and prompt re-exploration for hemostasis and evacuation of clot is indicated.

RESPIRATORY COMPLICATIONS

Patients undergoing cardiac surgery are at risk for multiple pulmonary complications. These include pneumothorax and pleural effusion in the immediate postoperative period. After the first 24 hours, patients sometimes develop acute lung injury (ALI), ARDS, or pneumonia. Diaphragmatic dysfunction secondary to phrenic nerve injury can occur.

Residual pneumothorax is often seen on the initial postoperative chest radiograph. The pneumothorax is commonly on the left side, and it is a result of opening of the left parietal pleura during dissection of the left internal mammary artery. The pneumothorax usually resolves spontaneously as the chest tubes are placed on suction. Occasionally, a pneumothorax is seen on the right side as a result of accidental incision of the right parietal pleura. Right pneumothorax can progress to tension pneumothorax and significant hemodynamic deterioration. This diagnosis should be considered in any unstable patient. Treatment consists of insertion of an additional chest tube.

Pleural effusion in the first 24 hours after cardiac surgery should raise the suspicion of hemothorax. Effusions should be watched carefully for expansion and correlated with other signs and symptoms of continued bleeding. Massive, expanding hemothorax is an indication for re-exploration and hemostasis. Pleural effusion after the first 24 hours is generally a benign process. Most pleural effusions resolve spontaneously. Thoracocentesis should be performed only if the effusion occupies more than 50% of the lung field on radiography or if the patient has significant impairment of respiratory function.

ALI and ARDS are rare complications after cardiac surgery, CPB, and blood transfusion. In one retrospective study of 3278 cardiac surgical patients, only 13 (0.4%) developed ARDS during the postoperative period. The mortality rate associated with this complication was 15%. Another study reported a much higher mortality rate (70%).[50] The patients who developed ARDS were more likely than their matched controls to have had previous cardiac surgery. During the postoperative period, patients with ARDS received more blood products and developed shock more frequently than patients without ARDS.[51]

Nosocomial pneumonia can complicate any ICU stay. Patients who require mechanical ventilation for longer than 48 hours are at particular risk. These pneumonias are usually caused by aspiration of oral or gastric secretions into the lungs. The incidence of nosocomial pneumonia can be reduced by diligent mouth care to prevent pooling of secretions and elevation of the head of the bed to greater than 30 degrees. Nosocomial pneumonia carries a mortality rate of 24% to 50% and warrants appropriate broad-spectrum antimicrobial chemotherapy.[52] The antibiotic prescription can be tailored once the results of sputum cultures are available.

Diaphragmatic dysfunction is usually caused by cold-induced injury of the phrenic nerve due to application of ice slush to the heart as part of the cardioplegia regimen. This complication occurs in up to 2% of patients undergoing cardiac surgery with topical hypothermia; more rarely, it can occur even if topical cooling was not applied.[53,54] While the patient is being ventilated with positive pressure, this injury will not be apparent. If preoperative pulmonary function was normal, then unilateral diaphragmatic paralysis usually is well tolerated. Pulmonary function can be severely compromised, however, if pulmonary problems were present preoperatively or, in rare instances, if bilateral diaphragmatic injury occurs.[55] These patients are at increased risk for development of nosocomial pneumonia, failure to wean from the ventilator, and death. Diaphragmatic dysfunction usually resolves spontaneously within 3 to 4 months.

CONTINUED BLEEDING

Continued bleeding is a common problem and requires immediate and aggressive management before the onset of further complications. The reasons for continued bleeding are often multifactorial and include inadequate surgical hemostasis, platelet dysfunction, coagulopathy, and inadequate heparin reversal. Often these factors occur in combination. Patients undergoing valve replacement are at increased risk.[56]

Multiple clotting abnormalities are possible, most of which result either directly or indirectly from the use of CPB.[57] The tubing, blood reservoir, and oxygenator membrane are all foreign surfaces that can activate the clotting cascade. Because the pump must be primed with either normal saline or lactated Ringer's solution, the priming process leads to substantial dilution of all blood components, including red cells, platelets, and clotting factors. After CPB, the platelet count is decreased and the remaining platelets are functionally deranged.[58,59] There is sequestration of platelets in the liver, in the spleen, and in the CPB circuit itself. Systemic fibrinolysis occurs due to activation of this system by the CPB circuit.

Inadequate reversal of heparin should be diagnosed at the bedside by the activated coagulation test (ACT) or by measurement of the activated partial thromboplastin time (aPTT). Because the half-life of heparin is longer than that of protamine, heparin-induced anticoagulation can rebound in the immediate postoperative period. The treatment is administration of additional protamine.

RENAL DYSFUNCTION

Mild renal dysfunction is a common postoperative event. One multicenter study demonstrated significant worsening of renal function in 7% of patients undergoing myocardial revascularization.[60] Approximately 1% of patients with postoperative acute renal failure (ARF) require renal replacement therapy. These patients have increased morbidity and mortality. Development of ARF can prolong ICU length of stay as much as fivefold.[60]

A multicenter study of 2222 patients undergoing CABG identified five independent preoperative predictors of renal dysfunction: age 70 to 79 years or age 80 to 95 years, congestive heart failure, previous myocardial revascularization, type 1 diabetes mellitus, or preoperative serum glucose levels exceeding 300 mg/dL and preoperative serum creatinine levels of 1.4 to 2.0 mg/dL. Independent perioperative factors that exacerbated risk were CPB lasting 3 hours or longer and various measures of ventricular dysfunction.[60] The predominant predisposing factor appears to be low CO. This factor may be exacerbated by concurrent use of vasopressors, such as phenylephrine.[61]

Renal dysfunction tends to follow one of three main patterns.[62] Abbreviated ARF is a transient event, most probably related to intraoperative renal ischemia. The serum creatinine concentration can be expected to peak on day 4 after surgery. Overt ARF occurs when the duration of the predisposing insult, usually low CO, is longer. The serum creatinine concentration peaks at a higher level than with abbreviated ARF and then decreases over a period of several weeks. Protracted ARF occurs when a second insult, commonly sepsis or hypotension, is superimposed on the resolving renal function. This event triggers a further, often irreversible, decrease in renal function.

NEUROLOGIC COMPLICATIONS

Neurologic sequelae of CPB range from subtle neurocognitive deficits (appearing in up to 80% of patients) to stroke. In order to estimate the relative risks of neurologic sequelae associated with various clinical factors, a logistic regression model was applied to prospectively collected data from 273 patients enrolled at 24 American medical centers.[63] Adverse cerebral outcomes occurred in 16% of patients and were almost equally divided between type I outcomes (8.4%; 5 cerebral deaths, 16 nonfatal strokes, and 2 new transient ischemic attacks) and type II outcomes (7.3%; 17 new cases of intellectual deterioration persisting at hospital discharge and 3 cases of newly diagnosed seizure disorder). Resource utilization for these patients was significantly increased; median ICU stay was prolonged from 3 days to 6 to 8 days. Total duration of hospitalization was increased by 50% (type II, $P = .04$) to 100% (type I, $P < .001$). After discharge from the acute care setting, specialized care was required for 69% of the patients with adverse neurologic sequelae. Risk factors for type I outcomes related primarily to embolic phenomena, including proximal aortic atherosclerosis, intracardiac thrombus, and intermittent clamping of the aorta during surgery. Risk factors for type II outcomes included, in addition to these factors, a preoperative history of endocarditis, alcohol abuse, perioperative dysrhythmia, poorly controlled hypertension, and low CO after CPB.

GASTROINTESTINAL COMPLICATIONS

Acute abdominal complications are relatively rare after cardiac surgery. If they do occur, they are associated with extremely high rates of morbidity and mortality. One prospective study of 1116 patients undergoing CPB found that abdominal complications occurred in 23 (2.1%). Ten of these patients underwent subsequent abdominal surgery, and 20 died. Early complications occurred on postoperative days 6 and 7 and consisted of bowel ischemia or hepatic failure. These complications are probably related to perioperative hypotension and low CO.[64] Late complications consisted of pseudomembranous colitis, cholecystitis, pancreatitis, and rupture of a septic spleen.[65]

Mild transient increases in circulating levels of hepatocellular enzymes are common after surgery. These changes are generally of no consequence; however, increased serum transaminase levels, if sustained or very high (e.g., serum alanine aminotransferase concentration greater than 500 IU/L), may represent evidence of severe ischemic injury of the liver. Severe ischemic liver injury after cardiac surgery carries a high mortality and is strongly associated with low CO and increased filling pressures, suggesting that liver ischemia is induced by a combination of decreased perfusion and congestion.[66]

MANAGEMENT OF COMMON POSTOPERATIVE PROBLEMS

OPTIMIZATION OF CARDIAC OUTPUT

Treatment of hypotension and low CO must be tailored to the cause. Again, it is useful to consider treatment in terms of preload, contractility, afterload, and rate and rhythm. Inadequate filling pressures are treated with volume infusion. The intravascular volume expander may be a crystalloid solution, a colloid solution, or packed red blood cells, if hematocrit is low or there is evidence of ongoing bleeding. It is important to remember that inotropic therapy is ineffective and possibly detrimental if adequate blood volume is not restored.

If CO or blood pressure remains low despite intravascular volume resuscitation, then it is necessary to institute inotropic or vasopressor support. No single agent is optimal in all cases. Rather, selection of the agent should be based on the

TABLE 232–2. COMPARISON OF RELATIVE ACTIVITY OF AVAILABLE VASOACTIVE AGENTS

Agent	α1	β1	β2	Phosphodiesterase Inhibition	Dose (μg/kg/min)
Epinephrine	++	+++	+	–	0.02-0.15
Norepinephrine	++++	+++	+	–	0.02-0.2
Dopamine	++	++	+	–	2-20
Dobutamine	+	+++	+	–	2-20
Phenylephrine	+++	–	–	–	0.3-5
Milrinone	–	–	–	+++	0.35-0.75

–, no activity; +, mild activity; ++, moderate activity; +++, strong activity.

suspected cause of low CO or hypotension and knowledge of the pharmacologic effects of the various inotropic and vasopressor drugs that are available (Table 232-2). If the primary cause of hypotension appears to be vasodilatation, administration of a vasoconstrictor (e.g., phenylephrine, norepinephrine, vasopressin) is indicated. If hypotension is related to inadequate ventricular ejection, then inotropic therapy with a β-adrenergic agent should be instituted. Epinephrine, norepinephrine, dopamine, and dobutamine are all reasonable choices. In patients with chronic systolic dysfunction, response to these agents may be impaired. Chronically elevated levels of circulating catecholamines deplete myocardial norepinephrine stores and down-regulate expression of myocardial β-adrenergic receptors. In these patients, tachyphylaxis to β-adrenergic agonists can develop rapidly. Addition of a phosphodiesterase inhibitor, such as amrinone or milrinone, is often effective in these patients.[67,68] In all cases, agents should be titrated to achieve adequate perfusion.

MECHANICAL SUPPORT OF THE CIRCULATION

Failure to respond to appropriate inotropic therapy may necessitate mechanical support of the circulation. IABP is the most commonly used method. The balloon is positioned in the aorta just distal to the take-off of the left common carotid artery. Inflation of the balloon during diastole increases diastolic pressure, thereby increasing coronary perfusion pressure. Deflation during systole decreases left ventricular afterload. This combination of hemodynamic effects ameliorates myocardial ischemia and improves CO.

Ventricular assist devices (VADs) are more effective than IABP for maintaining CO. Either the left ventricle, the right ventricle, or both can be supported with VADs. Currently, VADs may be used either as a bridge to transplantation or as a bridge to recovery. Either situation assumes that the VAD is a time-limited intervention. There are some data to support the view that resting the heart through the use of a VAD can allow some recovery of acutely injured myocytes, permitting eventual withdrawal of mechanical support. One case series showed that, when VAD was used as a bridge to recovery, 66% of patients were eventually able to wean from support and be discharged home.[69] If the heart is chronically diseased, there is little hope of recovery and the VAD serves to support the patient until transplantation becomes possible.[69,70]

Ongoing clinical trials are investigating the use of VADs as definitive therapy rather than as a bridge to transplantation. Implantation of these devices may increase the long-term survival of patients with end-stage heart failure.[71]

CORRECTION OF ARRHYTHMIAS

Atrial fibrillation is the most commonly encountered arrhythmia after cardiac surgery. Prophylactic use of β-adrenergic blockers reduces the incidence of postoperative atrial fibrillation, and they should be administered after cardiac surgery to all patients, unless specific contraindications are present.[72] Prophylactic treatment with amiodarone and atrial overdrive pacing should be considered for patients who are at high risk for postoperative atrial fibrillation (e.g., those with a history of previous atrial fibrillation or mitral valve surgery).[40,73]

If atrial fibrillation develops after cardiac surgery, the intensivist needs to determine whether the primary strategy should be to control the ventricular rate or to restore normal sinus rhythm. If atrial fibrillation is associated with hemodynamic instability or anticoagulation is contraindicated, rhythm management, using electrical cardioversion, amiodarone, or ibutilide, is preferred.[74,75] Overdrive pacing using atrial pacing wires also can be effective. The appropriate strategy for most stable patients may be control of ventricular rate, because most will spontaneously revert to sinus rhythm within 8 weeks after discharge.[76,77] Appropriate agents to achieve ventricular rate control include intravenous or oral β-adrenergic blockers or calcium-channel blockers. All patients with atrial fibrillation persisting for longer than 24 to 48 hours should be anticoagulated, unless there is a specific contraindication. Long-term outcomes are similar regardless of whether the rate control strategy or the rhythm control strategy is selected.[78,79]

Postoperative ventricular arrhythmias should be treated immediately according to current Advanced Cardiac Life Support (ACLS) protocols.[24] Any postoperative ventricular arrhythmia should prompt a search for an underlying cause. Importantly, ischemia should be ruled out. Patients with sustained ventricular arrhythmias should undergo electrophysiologic testing before long-term antiarrhythmic therapy is instituted. The implantable cardioverter-defibrillator (ICD) device has been shown to be superior to drug therapy for patients with hemodynamically significant arrhythmias.[80]

HYPERTENSION IN THE POSTOPERATIVE PERIOD

Hypertension leading to an increase in ventricular afterload is a common cause of decreased CO. Hypertension can be controlled by an intravenous infusion of sodium nitroprusside, nitroglycerin, β-adrenergic antagonists, or calcium-channel blockers. These agents should augment CO by reducing blood pressure and afterload in the hypertensive patient. Frequently, acute hypertension resolves within 24 to 48 hours postoperatively. If hypertension persists beyond this initial period of recovery, intravenous agents should be weaned and oral therapy initiated. Both β-adrenergic blockers and angiotensin-converting enzyme (ACE) inhibitors have been shown to confer a long-term mortality benefit and should be started. If hypertension was not a problem

TABLE 232–3. EVALUATION AND TREATMENT OF POSTOPERATIVE COAGULOPATHY

Coagulation Test	Normal Range	Suggested Treatment
Body temperature	—	If less than 35.5°C, the patient should be actively rewarmed
Prothrombin time (PT)	11-13.3 sec	Administer fresh-frozen plasma
Partial thromboplastin time (PTT)	21-32 sec	Consider additional protamine*
Platelets	140,000-440,000/μL	If <100,000, transfuse platelets
Fibrinogen	150-360 mg/dL	If <100, transfuse cryoprecipitate
Bleeding time	2.5-9.5 min	If prolonged and platelet count is normal, consider platelet dysfunction and treat with desmopressin acetate (DDAVP) and/or cryoprecipitate
Activated coagulation test (ACT)	90-120 sec	Consider additional protamine*

*Excessive protamine may itself cause bleeding.[102]

preoperatively, then prolonged antihypertensive therapy postoperatively usually will not be necessary.

CORRECTION OF COAGULOPATHY

Postoperative coagulopathy can promote bleeding and accumulation of blood in the chest or pericardial cavity. Aggressive measures must be used to correct the coagulopathy. A systemic approach to the evaluation and treatment of continued bleeding is needed; one such approach is outlined in Table 232-3. Hypothermia can contribute to coagulopathy. Therefore, profoundly hypothermic ICU patients must be actively rewarmed with the use of a warm air device. Laboratory evaluation of suspected coagulopathy should include measurements of platelet count, prothrombin time (PT), aPTT, ACT, and bleeding time.

POSTOPERATIVE BLEEDING

Bleeding that continues after correction of coagulopathy needs to be aggressively treated. Venous bleeding in the chest can be partially controlled by application of positive end-expiratory pressure (PEEP).[81,82]

Continuing mediastinal hemorrhage, or the suspicion of cardiac tamponade, is an indication for immediate re-exploration. Exsanguinating hemorrhage or impending arrest from tamponade may require that re-exploration be carried out at the bedside in the ICU. Bleeding that is unresponsive to medical therapy and requires re-exploration is usually associated with a surgical source. Accepted guidelines for re-operation include bleeding rates of 500 mL/hour for 1 hour, 400 mL/h for 2 hours, or 300 mL/hour for 3 hours. A sudden decrease or total cessation of drainage from mediastinal tubes may be equally ominous. Cessation of drainage from a mediastinal or chest tube can be caused by clotted blood occluding the tube. If bleeding persists but drainage ceases, the result can be tamponade.

Re-exploration is associated with increased morbidity and mortality. However, this increased mortality and morbidity may be partially explained by delays in the decision to re-explore that lead to avoidable open-chest resuscitations in the ICU.[56,83,84]

POSTOPERATIVE RENAL FAILURE

The cornerstone of prevention and treatment of renal failure in the cardiac surgical patient is the maintenance of adequate renal perfusion. This goal is best achieved by optimizing circulating blood volume and CO. Multiple pharmacologic regimens for renal protection have been described. Dopamine at low "renal" doses (1 to 3 μg/kg/min) has been used. The rationale for this strategy is that dopamine activates type 1 dopaminergic (DA1) receptors, leading to renal artery dilation, natriuresis, and diuresis. However, numerous human studies have failed to show that low-dose dopamine prevents renal failure or improves survival.[85] Even low doses of dopamine increase CO, and this may be the basis for any increase in urine output that is observed.[86] Fenoldapam[87] and dopexamine[88] are DA1 receptor antagonists that also have been proposed as renal protective agents and used with mixed success.[89]

Loop diuretics, such as furosemide, have been proposed as renal protective agents, not only because of their ability to produce diuresis and natriuresis, but also because these drugs may reduce medullary tubular oxygen consumption. Mannitol, an osmotic diuretic, been used to prevent development of ARF. Neither mannitol nor furosemide has been shown to improve outcome for patients with ARF.[60] Indeed, these drugs may be deleterious, because of their ability to promote diuresis and thus exacerbate hypovolemia and inadequate renal perfusion. Some success has been reported with the combination of mannitol, furosemide, and dopamine.[90] Infusion of a solution containing these three agents promoted diuresis in patients with acute postoperative ARF and adequate CO and significantly decreased the need for dialysis in the majority of patients.[88] Early administration of this solution in ARF caused early restoration of renal function to normal or baseline status.[90]

The failure of pharmacologic means of preventing and treating renal failure has led to interest in other methods. Early and intensive use of continuous veno-venous hemofiltration achieved a better than predicted outcome in a series of 65 consecutive patients with severe ARF who underwent cardiac operations.[91]

GLUCOSE CONTROL

Recent studies have shown that tight control of blood glucose level in the ICU is associated with improved morbidity and reduced mortality (Table 232-4).[92] Hyperglycemia and insulin resistance are common in critically ill patients, even those who have not previously had diabetes. A prospective, randomized, controlled study in which 1548 mechanically ventilated, adult patients were randomly assigned to receive either intensive insulin therapy (maintenance of blood glucose concentration between 80 and 110 mg/dL) or

TABLE 232–4. PROTOCOL FOR BLOOD SUGAR CONTROL IN THE POSTOPERATIVE PERIOD

Decision to initiate IV insulin
↓
If BG <200 mg/dL, begin D$_5$ ½ NS at 60-100 mL/h
If BG >300 mg/dL, give stat dose of IV insulin, 0.1 U/kg body weight
↓
Initiate an hourly rate (total daily dose of insulin divided by 24)
For patients who have never taken insulin, give 0.02 U/kg body weight per hour*
↓
Check BG hourly and adjust according to table below
Recheck BG hourly
↓
If in desirable range (101-150 mg/dL), continue to check BG every 2 h and adjust as necessary

Current BG (mg/dL)	Previous BG (mg/dL)								
	<60	60-80	81-100	101-150	151-200	201-250	251-300	301-400	>400
<60	Withhold drip and give 1 ampule of 50% glucose; check BG every 30 min until >100 mg/dL, then reinitiate drip at 50% of previous rate								
60-80	Withhold drip; check BG every 30 min until >100 mg/dL, then reinitiate drip at 50% of previous rate								
81-100	↓ rate by 1 U/h	No change		↓ rate by 25% or 0.5 U/h†		↓ rate by 25% or 1 U/h†		↓ rate by 50% or 2 U/h†	
101-150	No change				↓ rate by 25% or 1 U/h†				
151-200	↑ rate by 1 U/h	↑ rate by 0.5 U/h		↑ rate by 25% or 1 U/h†		No change		↓ rate by 25% or 1 U/h†	
201-250	↑ rate by 25% or 2 U/h†		↑ rate by 25% or 1 U/h†			↑ rate by 1 U/h		No change	
251-300	↑ rate by 33% or 2.5 U/h†	↑ rate by 25% or 1.5 U/h†	↑ rate by 25% or 1 U/h†	↑ rate by 1 U/h†		↑ rate by 1.5 U/h†	↑ rate by 25% or 2 U/h†	No change	
301-400	↑ rate by 40% or 3 U/h†								
>400	↑ rate by 50% or 4 U/h†								

Before discontinuing insulin infusion:
Ensure that patient is able to tolerate oral intake
Write orders for alternative glycemic management
Precede discontinuation by 1-2 h with subcutaneous dose of very rapid or rapid insulin. If patient has never taken insulin, use a dose equal to twice the hourly rate of IV insulin. Otherwise, use the dose of insulin or oral agent given before surgery/admission.

BG, blood glucose concentration; D$_5$ ½ NS, 5% dextrose in half-normal saline; IV, intravenous.
*For patients undergoing major surgery (e.g., cardiothoracic surgery, transplantation), higher doses may be necessary.
†Whichever is greater.

conventional treatment (infusion of insulin only if the blood glucose level exceeded 215 mg/dL and maintenance of blood glucose concentration between 180 and 200 mg/dL) has recently been reported. At 12 months, the intensive insulin therapy group had reduced ICU mortality, from 8.0% to 4.6% ($P < .04$). This benefit of intensive insulin therapy was attributable to its effect on mortality among patients who remained in the ICU for longer than 5 days (20.2% with conventional treatment versus 10.6% with intensive insulin therapy; $P = .005$). The greatest reduction in mortality involved deaths due to multiple-organ failure with a proven septic focus. Intensive insulin therapy also reduced overall in-hospital mortality, bloodstream infections, ARF requiring dialysis or hemofiltration, median number of red blood cell transfusions, and critical illness polyneuropathy. Patients receiving intensive therapy were less likely to require prolonged mechanical ventilation and intensive care. Sixty percent of the patients involved in this study were postoperative cardiac surgical patients, and the results may be particularly relevant in this population.

MECHANICAL VENTILATION

In uncomplicated recoveries, patients require only a short period of mechanical ventilation. Typically, volume-controlled ventilation is used until sedation is discontinued and the patient awakens. Once the patient is awake, hemodynamically stable, and without evidence of bleeding, a short trial of spontaneous ventilation is performed. If the weaning trial is successful, the patient is extubated. If continued mechanical ventilation is required because of respiratory failure or hemodynamic instability, either conventional volume-controlled ventilation or pressure support ventilation can be employed.

A small number of patients develop ALI or ARDS. In a large prospective trial of medical and surgical patients with ARDS or ALI, it was clearly beneficial to employ a lung-protective strategy or mechanical ventilation, limiting tidal volume to 6 mL/kg.[93] No such study has been performed in cardiac surgical patients, but it seems reasonable to adopt the same guidelines. These recommendations apply only to patients with established ALI/ARDS; use of low tidal volumes has not been shown to be effective when used prophylactically.

Patients with ALI or ARDS typically require increasing levels of PEEP to support oxygenation. The effect of PEEP on ventricular output is controversial. There is evidence that the application of PEEP up to 30 cm H$_2$O decreases CO by reducing ventricular preload and displacing the interventricular septum toward the left, which restricts left ventricular filling.[94] Other studies have not supported this view. When adult patients with normal preoperative respiratory status were randomly assigned to treatment with graded degrees of PEEP between 0 and 10 cm H$_2$O during mechanical ventilatory support, there were no significant differences in cardiac index among the groups.[95] It is likely that the effects of PEEP on the circulation are widely variable among patients and that the appropriate strategy is upward titration of PEEP under close monitoring.

OUTCOMES OF CARDIAC SURGERY

Increasingly, health care is being driven by outcome data. Cardiac surgery has been one of the leading specialties in this field. It is difficult to assess results from crude mortality data, because these do not take into account case complexity and differing preoperative risks among patients. Crude comparisons of death rates can be misleading and may encourage surgeons to practice risk-averse behavior. Death rates should be stratified by risk. It is, however, possible to make some generalizations. Among low-risk patients undergoing CABG, mortality rates lower than 2% are achievable.[96] Higher mortality rates are to be expected in selected subgroups of patients with major preoperative risk factors (e.g., poor ventricular function, advanced age, comorbid conditions) or major operative risk factors (e.g., reoperative surgery, complex operations).

A prospective cohort of 27,239 consecutive patients undergoing isolated CABG was examined to determine risk factors for hospital mortality. After adjustment for patient and disease characteristics, the following comorbid conditions were found to be related to postoperative mortality: diabetes, vascular disease, chronic obstructive pulmonary disease, peptic ulcer disease, and dialysis-dependent renal failure.[97]

Cardiac surgery is being performed more frequently in patients 80 years of age and older. In one study, the 30-day mortality rate for patients age 65 to 75 years was 3.4%, and for those older than 80 years of age it was 13.5%. Older patients had longer ICU and postoperative lengths of stay. Total direct costs were $4,818 higher in the octogenarian group. Although emergency operations and complex procedures carry high risks for the octogenarians and increasing costs for society, most of these patients can be offered operation with short-term morbidity, mortality, and resource use that only modestly exceed those of younger patients.[98] Once discharged from the hospital, older patients report a high quality of life.[99]

Overall, fewer than 10% of cardiac surgical patients spend more than 48 hours in the ICU. Most survive and eventually report improved functional status and a reasonable quality of life.[100,101]

SUMMARY

Most cardiac surgical patients can be discharged from the ICU to a step-down unit within 24 to 48 hours after operation, but an increasing number cannot. Patients who require longer and more intensive services in the ICU are typically older and sicker preoperatively. Adherence to best practices in the ICU optimizes the opportunity for even these high-risk patients to survive their operation and achieve a good quality of life after their hospitalization.

Ongoing development of less invasive techniques in cardiology and cardiac surgery will, paradoxically, bring about a further increase in the complexity of cases treated in the cardiac surgical ICU as patients who are less sick are treated elsewhere. This trend will lead to increasing challenges for intensivists working in these units and allow them to continue to be at the forefront of critical care medicine.

ANNOTATED REFERENCES

American Heart Association: Heart Disease and Stroke Statistics—2003 Update. Dallas, TX, AHA, 2003.
   This is an authoritative overview of the epidemiology of cardiac disease in the United States. It gives a clear picture of the changing role of cardiac surgery in the treatment of ischemic heart disease.

Bashour CA, Yared JP, Ryan TA, et al:. Long-term survival and functional capacity in cardiac surgery patients after prolonged intensive care. Crit Care Med 2000;28:3847-3853.
   Of those patients requiring ICU stays longer than 10 days after cardiac surgery, more then 50% will be alive at 1- year follow-up. Although these patients are extremely costly in terms of resources expended, they are salvageable.

Eagle KA, Guyton RA, Davidoff R, et al:. ACC/AHA Guidelines for Coronary Artery Bypass Graft Surgery: A Report of the American College of Cardiology/American Heart Association Task Force on Practice Guidelines (Committee to Revise the 1991 Guidelines for Coronary Artery Bypass Graft Surgery). American College of Cardiology/American Heart Association. J Am Coll Cardiol 1999;34:1262-1347.
   These are up-to-date guidelines for management of the cardiac surgical intensive care unit.

Jacka MJ, Cohen MM, To T, Devitt JH, Byrick R: The use of and preferences for the transesophageal echocardiogram and pulmonary artery catheter among cardiovascular anesthesiologists. Anesth Analg 2002;94:1065-1071.
   TEE is now the standard of care in the cardiac surgical OR. This paper demonstrates the utility of TEE in diagnosis and decision-making for the postoperative cardiac surgical patient in the ICU.

Montes FR, Sanchez SI, Giraldo JC, et al: The lack of benefit of tracheal extubation in the operating room after coronary artery bypass surgery. Anesth Analg 2000;91:776-780.
   Fast-tracking of cardiac surgical patients remains an intriguing concept. However, this paper shows no advantage for the routine extubation of patients in the OR.

van den Berghe G, Wouters P, Weekers F, et al: Intensive insulin therapy in the critically ill patients. N Engl J Med 2001;345:1359-1367.
   This is a seminal paper showing the effects of tight control of blood sugar in the ICU on morbidity and mortality. The majority of patients enrolled in this study were postoperative cardiac surgical patients.

Arthur J. Boujoukos

KEY POINTS

1. Patients undergoing living-donor lobar lung transplantation are typically kept sedated on mechanical ventilatory support for at least 72 hours to optimize expansion of the lobes.

2. Management strategies for single-lung transplantation using only a single ventilator to provide ventilation include reducing positive end-expiratory pressure, reducing tidal volume, and accepting a modest level of respiratory acidosis.

3. Ischemia-reperfusion injury is the leading cause of respiratory failure and morbidity early after transplantation.

4. The most severe postoperative lung injuries are associated with severe noncardiogenic pulmonary edema; patients who appear to have a complete loss of epithelial and endothelial integrity can be successfully managed with conventional strategies, the most severe cases requiring support with extracorporeal membrane oxygenation.

5. Acute cellular rejection occurs in nearly all patients at some time in the first year after transplantation. Patients typically present with allograft infiltrates, worsening hypoxemia, and dyspnea.

6. After orthotopic heart transplantation, patients return intubated and mechanically ventilated to the ICU. Inotropic and chronotropic support perioperatively is standard and includes dobutamine, isoproterenol, or epinephrine.

LUNG TRANSPLANTATION

Lung transplantation offers hope for improved survival and quality of life for selected patients with end-stage lung disease. The availability of suitable donor organs and preservation injury remain the initial limiting factors to successful transplantation. As with other transplants, rejection and infection as well as organ system dysfunction associated with the perioperative course remain challenges. However, experience over 40 years has led to substantial improvements in early outcome. Nevertheless, obliterative bronchiolitis resulting from chronic rejection limits the long-term quality of life and is largely responsible for the 45% 5-year mortality rate for lung transplantation.[1]

Indications for lung transplantation in adults are emphysema and alpha-1 antitrypsin deficiency (48%), idiopathic pulmonary fibrosis (17%), cystic fibrosis (16%), and primary pulmonary hypertension (5%).[1] Small numbers of patients have undergone transplantation for sarcoidosis, scleroderma, and other autoimmune syndromes as well as other indications, including retransplantation. Transplantation options include single lung transplantation, double-lung transplantation, heart-lung transplantation, and living-donor lobar lung transplantation. Removal of all native lung tissue and replacement with either double-lung transplantation or living-donor lobar lung transplant is mandatory for all patients with septic lung disease. Patients undergoing living-donor lobar lung transplant, most of whom are cystic fibrosis patients, receive a left and a right lower lobe, each from different donors.[2] Single-lung transplantation is an option for all cases of nonseptic lung disease. The trend toward double-lung transplantation for patients with pulmonary hypertension and even some patients with emphysema reflects a bias at some centers that this procedure delays development of symptomatic obliterative bronchiolitis (due to the greater mass of transplanted lung tissue) and this attribute outweighs the smaller number of patients who can receive transplants when this strategy is adopted.

Donor selection, procurement, and lung preservation protocols tend to be individualized on an institutional basis. The limited availability of donor lungs, however, has increased the scrutiny with which organs are judged to avoid rejecting them inappropriately. Significant lung contusion, smoking-related lung damage, pneumonia, pulmonary edema, and significant aspiration are prime concerns in evaluating the suitability of donor organs. Procurement and lung preservation protocols often include administration of anti-inflammatory agents, pulmonary vasodilators, and antioxidants.

The surgical technique involves a thoracotomy for single-lung transplantation or a clamshell incision for double-lung transplantation and living-donor lobar lung transplants. The surgical procedure includes anastomoses of the pulmonary artery, atrium, and bronchus. Cardiopulmonary bypass is avoided in the case of single-lung transplantation and double-lung transplantation unless preexisting pulmonary hypertension precludes cross-clamping of the pulmonary artery or if cardiorespiratory stability cannot be otherwise maintained. At the completion of the operation, the double endotracheal tube is exchanged for a standard endotracheal tube unless allograft function appears tenuous or there is evidence of air trapping. Heart-lung transplants are performed with either a clamshell incision or a sternotomy. Cardiopulmonary bypass is obviously a requirement in these patients. The vascular anastomoses include the aorta and a cuff of right atrium, including both vena cavae. Bibronchial airway anastomoses are performed that are associated with less dehiscence than a single tracheal anastomosis.

PERIOPERATIVE ICU MANAGEMENT

On transfer to the ICU, patients are often managed with a lung protective strategy that limits tidal volumes to 3 mL/kg per allograft and plateau pressure to less than 32 cm H_2O. Ten centimeters of positive end-expiratory pressure (PEEP) are applied to the allograft and fractional inspired oxygen concentration (FiO_2) is set initially at 0.30 and titrated higher if arterial oxygen saturation (SaO_2) is less than 90%. Left-sided endobrochial tubes are often still in place, but the tip of the left tube is pulled back to the carina and the bronchial balloon is deflated; thus, the tube functions as an endotracheal tube. If there is minimal evidence of postoperative allograft dysfunction, liberation from ventilation can proceed expeditiously once the patient has recovered from general anesthesia. Using 10 cm H_2O of pressure support in the continuous positive airway pressure mode of mechanical ventilation counteracts the airway resistance of the endobronchial tube during weaning. Patients undergoing living-donor lobar lung transplant are typically kept sedated on mechanical ventilatory support for at least 72 hours to optimize expansion of the lobes.

HYPERINFLATION

In cases of single-lung transplantation with emphysema, the transplanted lung can be relatively noncompliant. As a result, the native lung may be hyperinflated. This problem becomes even more apparent when higher levels of PEEP are needed due to allograft dysfunction. Hyperinflation of the native lung leads to mediastinal shift, deterioration in gas exchange, and hemodynamic instability. Although inserting an expiratory pause into the ventilator cycle can be used to assess the level of intrinsic PEEP ("auto-PEEP"), excessive air trapping is easily diagnosed by disconnecting the patient's endotracheal tube from the ventilator tubing for 5 to 10 seconds. In patients with significant air trapping and hyperinflation, this action ("popping the patient off") leads to a significant improvement in blood pressure and oxygenation. Management strategies using only a single ventilator to provide ventilation include reducing PEEP, reducing tidal volume, and accepting a modest level of respiratory acidosis. Alternatively, conversion to independent lung ventilation may be appropriate, particularly in the setting of significant allograft dysfunction and high PEEP requirements. To switch to independent lung ventilation, the double endotracheal tube is advanced into the left mainstem bronchus and the bronchial balloon is inflated. Positioning can be verified by measuring tidal volumes delivered to and returned from each lumen of the double endotracheal tube. Bronchoscopy with a small-caliber bronchoscope is appropriate to verify that (1) the left bronchial balloon is distal to the carina and (2) the end of the left endobronchial tube does not protrude too far distally into the left lung, compromising flow to either the upper or lower division bronchi. Ventilator settings are adjusted for each machine individually. Initially, PEEP for the allograft is set at 10 cm H_2O, tidal volume is set at 3 mL/kg, and rate is set at 20 to 25 breaths/min. Initial settings for the emphysematous native lung typically use a larger tidal volume and a slower rate with 0 to 2.5 cm PEEP. There is no need to synchronize the ventilators.

EARLY POSTOPERATIVE RESPIRATORY COMPLICATIONS

Airways are affected variably by the ischemic/implantation insult. Anastomotic dehiscences are rare, although a recent report suggests that the incidence of this complication is increased when sirolimus is used as an immunosuppressive agent.[3] Anatomically, the transplanted bronchus derives its blood supply from the lung and pulmonary blood flow, since the bronchial arteries are not anastomosed. The longer left mainstem bronchus, particularly adjacent to the anastomosis, is at higher risk for ischemic injury compared with the right bronchus, which generally is anastomosed adjacent to the right upper lobe take-off. Early bronchoscopy often demonstrates relatively normal epithelium. However, more severe airway injury patterns can become apparent over the next several days. The earliest findings are patchy areas of subepithelial hemorrhage that can become confluent. In more severe cases, white plaques can form and frank areas of desiccated, sloughed epithelium become evident. In the most severe cases, eschar is evident and bronchial cartilage may be exposed. Severe airway injury poses the risk of infection and bronchomalacia. The infections are typically due to *Candida* and *Aspergillus* species.[4] In many centers, lung transplant recipients are treated prophylactically with antifungal agents, such as inhaled amphoteracin (50 mg inhaled qd), fluconazole (400 mg p.o. qd), or voriconazole (200 mg p.o. qd). This strategy seems to reduce the rate of airway infection.[5,6] If suspicious plaques are evident bronchoscopically, we perform bronchial biopsy to exclude invasive disease. Inhaled amphotericin B (50 mg bid) is generally administered to patients with severe airway injury and those with cultures demonstrating growth of fungus. Bronchomalacia is generally a long-term complication, although in some cases, this complication can become evident within the first 6 weeks after transplantation. Dynamic airway collapse or fixed stenosis is diagnosed by bronchoscopy. Expandable stents are effective tools to optimize airflow in patients with this complication.[7]

Ischemia-reperfusion injury is the leading cause of respiratory failure and morbidity early after transplantation.[8,9] More than 95% of patients have infiltrates in the allograft by chest radiograph during the first 72 hours.[10] Although edema and atelectasis contribute to these early changes, worsening or persistent infiltrates most likely reflect diffuse alveolar damage secondary to ischemia-reperfusion injury. Mild reperfusion injury often responds to diuresis and additional ventilatory support over 24 to 48 hours. Although many cases of reperfusion injury are evident on chest radiographs obtained on the first postoperative day, in some cases ischemia-reperfusion injury does not become apparent radiographically or physiologically for up to 72 hours posttransplant. In some cases, patients will be successfully extubated only to deteriorate 24 hours later. The most severe episodes of ischemia-reperfusion injury are described as primary graft failure and occur in about 15% of cases of transplantation.[11] These patients develop dense infiltrates within 72 hours, have a markedly widened alveolar-arterial (A-a) oxygen tension gradient, and require prolonged ventilatory support. The management of ischemia-reperfusion injury is supportive, using a lung protective strategy as with acute respiratory distress syndrome (ARDS). Improvement is variable lasting from days to weeks depending on the degree of diffuse alveolar damage. Aggressive diagnostic efforts are made, employing bronchoscopy, bronchoalveolar lavage (BAL), and biopsy, to exclude superimposed infection or rejection. Independent lung ventilation is an effective adjunct in cases of single-lung transplantation with severe ischemia-reperfusion injury. Inhaled nitric oxide also has been utilized in the setting of ischemia-reperfusion injury. Its physiologic effect is to reduce pulmonary vascular resistance and pulmonary arterial pressure and improve oxygenation in those patients with wide A-a gradients.[12] However, an outcome benefit has not been demonstrated, and this therapy is quite expensive; accordingly, inhaled nitric oxide cannot be recommended as standard therapy in patients undergoing lung transplantation any more than it can be for the management of ARDS.[13] When conventional therapy is inadequate to support oxygenation, inhaled nitric oxide is a reasonable adjunct to therapy in an effort to avoid extracorporeal membrane oxygenation (ECMO).

The level of respiratory dysfunction secondary to ischemia-reperfusion injury depends on the extent of the injury and the residual lung reserve. The latter factor is particularly important in single-lung transplantation for emphysema, since the remaining native lung may have substantial residual function. The functional capacity of the native lung often allows the transplant recipient to tolerate a significant degree of allograft dysfunction.[14] Such is typically not the case for IPF patients or recipients with significant pulmonary hypertension, since perfusion to the native lung is minimal once a donor lung with low pulmonary vascular resistance is implanted.

The most severe postoperative lung injuries are associated with severe noncardiogenic pulmonary edema. These patients appear to have a complete loss of epithelial and endothelial integrity. Although some of these patients can be successfully managed with conventional strategies, the most severe cases require support with ECMO. Venovenous ECMO is favored in this circumstance, since venoarterial ECMO shunts blood flow away from the newly implanted lungs. Survival rates to discharge requiring perioperative ECMO are about 50%.[15] If pulmonary edema is unilateral, a diagnosis of pulmonary venous obstruction must be entertained. Although the incidence of this problem is extremely low, a transesophageal echocardiogram should be performed to exclude unilateral venous obstruction.

Muscular weakness or mechanical issues can embarrass postoperative respiratory function. Patients requiring delayed closure of the clamshell incision, which is required in some patients with excessive bleeding, are at higher risk for respiratory dysfunction on this basis. Preoperative muscle wasting is a major contributing factor in most cases. Clinically significant phrenic nerve injury is rare. However, when dissection of the native lungs was difficult due to dense pleural adhesions, phrenic nerve injury can be present and significantly prolong the weaning process. Postoperative neuromuscular blockade should be avoided because of synergistic adverse effects on long-term neuromuscular function that have been associated with simultaneous administration of corticosteroids (a component of most immunosuppressive regimens) and neuromuscular blocking agents.[16] If the patient has difficulty clearing secretions, tracheostomy or minitracheostomy should be performed early.

Patients are treated with antibiotics perioperatively. In patients without suppurative lung disease, antibiotics are stopped within 72 hours if samples from the donor trachea and from the explanted lung are without pathogens. If cultures are positive for potential pulmonary pathogens, a directed course of antibiotics is continued for 7 to 10 days. In patients with septic lung disease, an antibiotic regimen based on preoperative cultures is continued for a minimum of 2 to 3 weeks. Patients also may be treated with prophylactic regimens to prevent cytomegalovirus infection with valganciclovir (450 to 900 mg p.o. qd) and *Clostridium difficile* colitis perioperatively (metronidazole, 250 mg p.o. tid). Pulmonary emboli are common in this population and aggressive prophylaxis against deep vein thrombosis is mandatory.[17] At our center, critically ill transplant patients are screened liberally for deep vein thrombosis with lower extremity Doppler ultrasonography examinations. Our policy advocates a low threshold for placement of an inferior vena caval filter when deep vein thrombosis is diagnosed despite adequate prophylaxis (heparin, 5000 to 8000 units subcutaneously bid).

NEW PULMONARY INFILTRATES

Development of new infiltrates on the chest radiograph after lung transplantation mandates diagnostic evaluation using fiberoptic bronchoscopy with BAL and transbronchial biopsy. If bacterial pneumonia is strongly suspected, particularly if biopsy is thought to be excessively risky, bronchoscopy with BAL and empirical antibiotic therapy is an acceptable alternative. If the Gram stain is unremarkable and distal airways lack evidence of bacterial or fungal infection, transbronchial biopsy is necessary to exclude acute rejection or cytomegalovirus infection.

Conditions other than ischemia-reperfusion injury can lead to diffuse alveolar damage as determined by transbronchial biopsy. Diffuse alveolar damage can result from pneumonia, rejection, cytomegalovirus infection, systemic sepsis, or even BAL. The management of diffuse alveolar damage is supportive, consisting of lung protective ventilation as for ARDS. Management in severe cases can include administration of corticosteroids (e.g., prednisone 2 to 3 mg/kg/day) tapered over 2 to 3 weeks. Corticosteroids may be particularly valuable if the biopsy shows evidence of fibroproliferative changes. However, data from controlled clinical trials are lacking to support this approach.

Because the transplanted lung is in close contact with the external environment, the risk for infection is higher than is the case for other forms of organ transplantation. Accordingly, aggressive diagnostic efforts are the key to the management of graft dysfunction after lung transplantation. Bacterial infections with traditional nosocomial pathogens are most common in the first 30 days.[18] Subsequently, bacterial pneumonia is still responsible for the bulk of new infiltrates, although other causes must be considered as well. Cytomegalovirus infection, causing pneumonia among other problems, occurs in a large fraction of cases. Prophylactic and surveillance strategies to deal with cytomegalovirus infection vary from center to center. Some institutions carry out weekly assays, seeking to detect cytomegalovirus antigen in the bloodstream, and only institute early preemptive therapy with ganciclovir when the antigen is present. Other centers provide prophylaxis using ganciclovir (5 mg/kg i.v. qd) or valganciclovir (900 mg p.o. qd) for 3 months. Other viruses, such as adenovirus, parainfluenza virus, influenza virus, and respiratory syncytial virus, are community-acquired pathogens that can cause significant morbidity and mortality.[19,20]

Fungal pneumonia with *Aspergillus* species occurs but is rare. Far more common is the colonization of airways with *Aspergillus*. Distinguishing between infection and colonization requires computed tomography scan and bronchoscopic evaluation with directed biopsy to areas suspicious for invasive fungal disease. Successful treatment requires appropriate antifungal therapy and reduction in immunosuppression to the lowest levels tolerable. *Candida albicans* in the airway almost always reflects colonization; pneumonia caused by this organism is exceedingly rare. *Pneumocystis carinii* pneumonia is unusual, especially when patients are treated perioperatively with trimethoprim/sulfamethoxazole (160/800 mg p.o. 3 ×/week) as prophylaxis. Infections with *Toxoplasma*, *Nocardia*, *Histoplasma*, *Coccidioides*, *Cryptococcus*, and *Mycobacteria* are quite rare but do occur.

Acute cellular rejection occurs in nearly all patients at some time in the first year after transplantation. Patients typically present with allograft infiltrates, worsening hypoxemia, and dyspnea.[21] Fever and pleural effusion may occur and pulmonary secretions are uncommon. Clinical findings have been shown to be inadequate for diagnosing acute cellular rejection; establishing the diagnosis requires transbronchial biopsy. Maintenance immunosuppression in most centers is based on a three-drug regimen, including either cyclosporin or tacrolimus, prednisone (5 mg p.o. qd), and either mycophenolate (1000 to 1500 mg p.o. bid) or azathioprine (1 to 3 mg/kg p.o. pd). Episodes of significant acute rejection are treated with methylprednisolone (10-15 mg/kg IV qd x 3 days). Response usually occurs within 24 to 72 hours. Failure to respond should prompt rebiopsy to exclude refractory rejection.

Chronic rejection manifests more insidiously. Findings are increased dyspnea, worsening pulmonary function test results, and sometimes cough. Pathologically, patients with chronic rejection manifest findings of obliterative bronchiolitis with a lymphocytic infiltrate in the submucosa and epithelium plus submucosal fibrosis. These findings, however, can be missed on transbronchial biopsy. Obliterative bronchiolitis also can develop in the wake of other insults, such as acute rejection, airway ischemia, lymphocytic bronchitis, and certain infections such as cytomegalovirus infection.[22] More than 60% of lung transplant recipients surviving 5 years develop obliterative bronchiolitis, and the outcome, once obliterative bronchiolitis is apparent, is poor.[23] Patients with obliterative bronchiolitis, in addition to developing progressive deterioration of lung function, are also at high risk for bacterial pneumonia and acute-on-chronic bouts of respiratory failure. Pneumonia is commonly caused by *Staphylococcus aureus* or *Pseudomonas aeruginosa*. Pneumonia and respiratory failure is a common reason for ICU readmission and is the most common cause of death in patients more than 6 months after transplantation.[23]

NONPULMONARY ORGAN SUPPORT AND COMPLICATIONS

Hemodynamic management of patients after lung transplantation is similar to that of other ICU patients, with the exception of volume administration. Given the lack of lymphatics in the allograft and potential ischemic injury of pulmonary endothelium and epithelium, pulmonary edema occurs at lower filling pressures. For that reason, lung transplant recipients should be maintained "on the dry side" using vasopressors or inotropes as needed to support blood pressure and cardiac output. Patients have been screened preoperatively for coronary artery disease, and ventricular dysfunction and ischemia or congestive heart failure should rarely be complicating factors in lung transplant recipients. Atrial arrhythmias are common and can effectively be managed with beta-adrenergic blockade or sotalol in most cases. Amiodarone should be avoided because of its pulmonary toxicity.[24] Diltiazem can unpredictably and markedly affect tacrolimus and cyclosporine levels [25,26] and should be used cautiously.

Patients with preexisting pulmonary hypertension will enjoy a 30% to 40% reduction in pulmonary artery pressure after single-lung transplantation and normalization of pressures with a double-lung transplantation.[27] Postoperative pulmonary hypertension in patients with preexisting pulmonary hypertension is generally well tolerated since the right ventricle (RV) is conditioned and transplantation reduces RV afterload. Only patients with pulmonary hypertension and evidence of low output and high central venous pressure (CVP) require specific therapy. Inotropic agents may be needed for support for a short time after cardiopulmonary bypass.

Renal dysfunction is common, and some patients require renal replacement therapy. In these patients, bicarbonate should be aggressively supplemented enterally to reduce the need for pulmonary compensation for metabolic acidosis. Because transplanted lungs are so sensitive to excessive intravascular volume, ultrafiltration may be required more frequently than is typical for general ICU patients. Tacrolimus or cyclosporine should be maintained at lower levels (8 to 10 ng/mL for tacrolimus, 100 to 150 ng/mL for cyclosporine) in the setting of renal failure in the absence of rejection to optimize chances for early renal recovery. Other nephrotoxins, such as nonsteroidal anti-inflammatory agents, must be completely avoided and computed tomography scans should be performed without intravenous contrast unless absolutely necessary.

Gastrointestinal problems include gastritis and ulcers, ileus, *C. difficile* colitis, and cytomegalovirus enteritis. In some centers, all patients receive an H_2 blocker during their initial hospitalization as well as enteral metronidazole (250 mg p.o. tid) and lactobacillus (1 g p.o. qid) (as prophylaxis against *C. difficile* infection). Cytomegalovirus enteritis can be difficult to diagnose, since tests for circulating cytomegalovirus antigen can have negative results in patients with disease localized to the gastrointestinal tract. Endoscopy with biopsy is appropriate, particularly if thickened bowel is identified radiographically. Patients with cystic fibrosis should be placed on a bowel regimen with lactulose (10 mg p.o. bid) or polyethylene glycol (17 g p.o. bid) to prevent mucous impaction. Gastroesophageal reflux disease is common after lung transplantation and there is evidence that effective treatment can improve lung function in some patients.[28] Pancreatitis, bowel perforation, and cholecystitis are uncommon gastrointestinal problems. These issues should be addressed in the standard manner.

Neurologic sequelae after lung transplant include tremors, seizures, encephalopathy, myopathy, and neuropathy. Drugs, such as tacrolimus and cyclosporine, antibiotics, corticosteroids, and perioperative neuromuscular blocking agents, can be contributing factors. Hyperammonemia after lung transplantation has been reported as a cause of neurologic dysfunction in a small number of cases; the associated mortality rate is high.[29]

HEART TRANSPLANTATION

Heart transplantation has been performed for 35 years for end-stage heart disease. In 2001, 3122 heart transplantations were performed worldwide.[1] Diseases resulting in transplantation include ischemic heart disease (46%) and cardiomyopathy (45%) with congenital disease, valvular disease, amyloidosis, sarcoidosis, retransplant making up much of the remainder. Indications include end-stage cardiomyopathy resulting in New York Heart Association class IV symptoms. Donor availability still remains a primary deterrent to more widespread use of cardiac transplantation. Survival after transplantation exceeds 80% in the first year, 68% at 5 years, and 48% at 10 years.[1]

Heterotopic transplantation is an uncommon procedure that entails implantation of a donor heart in parallel with the failing native heart to reduce postoperative right heart failure in the setting of preoperative pulmonary hypertension. The donor heart is implanted in the right chest with side-to-side anastomoses of the right atrium to right atrium and left atrium to left atrium. The transplanted aorta is anastomosed end-to-side to the recipient aorta and the pulmonary artery of the transplant is joined to the main pulmonary artery of the patient via a graft. The donor left ventricle (LV) provides the bulk of systemic cardiac output while the native RV provides enough support for the unconditioned donor RV to avoid right heart failure in the setting of high pulmonary vascular resistance (greater than 8 Wood units). Overall results are inferior to those of orthotopic transplantation.[30] Additional issues include compromise of right lower lobe function and need for chronic anticoagulation. Orthotopic heart transplant entails the removal of the native heart via sternotomy and replacement with a donor heart with anastomoses of the pulmonary artery, ascending aorta, left atrium, and usually bicaval anastomoses of the right atrium.

HEMODYNAMIC SUPPORT

After orthotopic heart transplantation, patients return intubated and mechanically ventilated to the ICU. Inotropic and chronotropic support perioperatively is standard and includes dobutamine, isoproterenol, or epinephrine. Due to denervation of the transplanted heart, sinus bradycardia and atrioventricular nodal block are common problems in the early postoperative period. An adequate heart rate (80-100 beats/minute) is generally maintained with catecholamine infusions, temporary epicardial pacing, and occasionally the use of oral agents, such as theophylline (50 mg p.o. bid) or isoetharine (5 mg p.o. tid). A small minority of patients require placement of a permanent transvenous pacemaker.

In occasional patients with excessive systemic vasodilation, norepinephrine or vasopressin (0.04 µg/kg/min) may be appropriate adjuncts perioperatively. Inotropic support is weaned over the first few days in most cases. Patients with preexisting pulmonary hypertension may require more

prolonged inotropic support of the unconditioned RV. The addition of milrinone (0.25 to 0.5 µg/kg/min), inhaled nitric oxide (20 to 40 ppm), or inhaled prostaglandin E_1 or I_2 may be appropriate adjuncts immediately postoperatively in the setting of RV failure (high CVP, low stroke volume, and low cardiac output). RV failure generally becomes apparent in the operating room when the chest is still open, but in some cases, increasing CVP and decreasing cardiac output will necessitate evaluation by transesophageal echocardiography. RV failure is confirmed by visualizing the absence of tamponade, a hypokinetic and distended RV, and underfilling of the LV. Humoral (hyperacute) rejection must be ruled out in such cases, particularly if pulmonary vascular resistance is only minimally elevated. RV dysfunction in the setting of relatively normal pulmonary vascular resistance suggests that the primary problem is myocardial dysfunction rather than excessive afterload. When the RV is strained by high pulmonary vascular resistance, care must be taken to avoid overdistention of the chamber. Diuretics and ultrafiltration are employed as early as 8 hours postoperatively if hemodynamically tolerated to keep CVP less than 20 cm H_2O. Nesiritide (0.01 to 0.3 µg/kg/min) can also be added in tandem with diuretics to aid in diuresis in this setting prior to the decision to pursue ultrafiltration.

Arrhythmias are common in the early postoperative period. Bradycardia is most common. Atropine has no effect on the denervated heart. Atrial fibrillation is much more common than other forms of supraventricular tachycardia. Atrial fibrillation is managed with amiodarone (150-mg bolus, 1 mg/min × 6 hours, then 0.5 mg/min infusion). Since digoxin decreases atrioventricular conduction primarily by increasing vagal tone, this drug has little use in the acute management of atrial fibrillation in heart transplant recipients. Beta-adrenergic blockers are generally avoided in the early postoperative period. Diltiazem can be used for acute rate control, but its effects on cyclosporine and tacrolimus metabolism render this drug a second-line agent.

Respiratory complications are similar to those seen with other types of cardiac surgery. In cases in which bleeding is excessive due to redo sternotomy, multiple transfusions pose a risk of acute lung injury. Additionally, several reports suggest a higher incidence of postoperative lung injury in surgical patients on amiodarone, a frequent component of the recipient's preoperative medical regimen.[31] Renal, gastrointestinal, and neurologic complications are similar to those of lung transplant recipients.

REJECTION

Cardiac allograft rejection can occur early in the post-transplantation period. Three-drug regimens similar to those used in cases of lung transplants are the mainstays of maintenance therapy. Induction therapy using Thymoglobulin, OKT3, or an interleukin-2 receptor antagonist is given to about 45% of patients to minimize renal toxicity caused by calcineurin inhibitors in patients with preexisting renal disease.[1] Acute cellular rejection may manifest as arrhythmias, congestive heart failure, fatigue, abdominal pain, low cardiac output, or hypotension. Surveillance endomyocardial biopsies and right heart catheterizations are performed weekly in the early postoperative period. Methylprednisolone (1000 mg IV daily for 3 days) is the standard treatment for acute cellular rejection. A particularly aggressive form of rejection is called *hyperacute rejection* and is mediated primarily by humoral factors. Myocardial biopsy reveals vascular deposition of immunoglobulin and complement with evidence of vascular injury in the absence of a mononuclear cell infiltrate. Treatment includes therapy with corticosteroids, urgent plasmapheresis, and immunoglobulin infusion, but the prognosis is poor.[32] Patients undergoing retransplantation, multiparous women, and patients who have received multiple blood transfusions are at particular risk for hyperacute rejection. In most programs, a negative prospective cross-match or an induction regimen including preoperative plasmapheresis is undertaken before proceeding with transplantation.

INFECTIONS

Infectious complications include routine nosocomial infections, such as pneumonia, catheter-related sepsis, and mediastinitis. Patients who have been bridged to transplant with a ventricular assist device and whose course has been complicated by infection of the ventricular assist device pocket or driveline are more prone to wound infections following removal of the device and transplantation. Cytomegalovirus infection occurs in 10% to 25% of transplant recipients.[33,34] Cytomegalovirus-negative recipients who receive a cytomegalovirus-positive organ are at the highest risk. Surveillance with serum cytomegalovirus antigen assays are the mainstay of management. Some centers employ prophylactic regimens with ganciclovir (5 mg/kg i.v. bid or qd) or valganciclovir (900 mg p.o. qd) for 3 to 6 months. *Toxoplasma* and *P. carinii* (trimethoprim/sulfamethoxazole 160/800 mg p.o. 3 ×/week) prophylaxis are also standard.

LONG-TERM COMPLICATIONS

The bulk of early mortality is caused by primary graft failure (40%), multiple organ dysfunction syndrome (14%), and infection (14%).[1] Late complications of heart transplantation include hypertension (94%), renal dysfunction (31%), hyperlipidemia (82%), diabetes mellitus (32%), and coronary artery vasculopathy (32%).[1] Malignancy, including lymphoma, is responsible for 24% of the deaths 5 years or more after transplantation.[34] Coronary vasculopathy is the "obliterative bronchiolitis" of heart transplantation and leads to deterioration in cardiac allograft function after transplantation.[35] Endothelial cell injury can be triggered by graft ischemia, rejection, viral infections, and hyperlipidemia.

Endothelial injury or activation leads to concentric, distal coronary intimal proliferation, ultimately occluding coronary flow.[36] The absence of cardiac re-innervation in most heart transplant recipients precludes warning symptoms of angina. New onset of congestive heart failure, myocardial infarction, angina, electrocardiographic changes, or syncope, particularly in patients several years post-transplant status, are indications for cardiac catheterization. Stents may be of value in selected cases. Retransplantation is an option, although retransplantation as an indication for transplant carries with it a significantly inferior outcome.[1]

Although coronary vasculopathy impairs long-term results, heart transplantation nevertheless provides a durable treatment for patients with end-stage heart disease. Patients enjoy 50% survival at 9 years.[1] Ninety percent of patients report no limitations on their physical activity at 5 years. Donor availability remains the major limitation to more widespread treatment and success.

ANNOTATED REFERENCES

Chatila WM, Furukawa S, Gaughan JP, Criner GJ: Respiratory failure after lung transplantation. Chest 2003;123:165-173.

This retrospective clinical analysis in a tertiary care transplantation center found that respiratory failure after lung transplantation is common and is associated with high morbidity and mortality. Respiratory failure often occurred in patients with operative technical complications, cardiovascular events, and postoperative ischemia/reperfusion lung injury (IRLI), which were observed most in patients requiring cardiopulmonary bypass because of right ventricular dysfunction.

Christie JD, Bavaria JE, Palevsky HI, et al: Primary graft failure following lung transplantation. Chest 1998;114:51-60.

This retrospective review of 100 consecutive patients undergoing lung transplantation at the University of Pennsylvania Medical Center analyzed the incidence of primary graft failure (PGF) following lung transplantation and characterized its effect on outcomes. PGF occurred in 15% of patients in their series and was associated with a high mortality rate, lengthy hospitalization, and protracted and often compromised recovery among survivors.

Thabut G, Vinatier I, Stern JB, et al: Primary graft failure following lung transplantation: Predictive factors of mortality. Chest 2002;121:1876-1882.

Primary graft failure (PGF) following lung transplantation is a frequent event, with significant ICU morbidity and mortality. This retrospective cohort analysis of 259 patients attempted to assess incidence, outcome, and early predictors of mortality for patients with PGF and to develop an ischemia/reperfusion injury severity score able to accurately predict ICU mortality for these patients. They identified four factors that allow prediction of ICU mortality with good accuracy: age, degree of gas exchange impairment, graft ischemic time, and severe early hemodynamic failure.

Chapter 234

MANAGEMENT OF PATIENTS WITH KIDNEY, PANCREAS, OR KIDNEY/PANCREAS TRANSPLANTATION

Gregory J. Beilman

KEY POINTS

1. **New development of low urine output in the immediate postoperative period** after kidney transplant mandates rapid evaluation for the cause of the oliguria.

2. The incidence of **wound infection after pancreas transplant** is significant (10% to 40%) and is a major cause of postoperative morbidity.

3. **Respiratory failure after kidney and/or pancreas transplant** can be related to any one of a number of serious causes, including infection, cardiac failure, renal failure, and pulmonary emboli. It is important to determine the etiology and initiate therapy rapidly for respiratory failure after kidney and/or pancreas transplantation.

4. **Immunosuppressive agents** have significant side effects and predispose patients to development of infection.

5. **Immunosuppression** must be reduced or discontinued in renal and pancreas transplant patients suspected of harboring severe infection.

6. **Cytomegalovirus infection** is common in renal and pancreas transplant patients and is the cause of significant morbidity

The first successful long-term functioning kidney transplant was performed by Joseph Murray in 1954 between two monozygotic twins, avoiding the problem of rejection. The recipient lived 8 years, dying of a cause unrelated to her renal failure. Critical care practitioners played an important role in the development of transplantation with the development of brain death criteria and the ability to care for patients after brain death, allowing recovery of viable organs to be used for transplantation. The success of organ transplantation has improved with the development of more effective preservation solutions, such as the University of Wisconsin solution in the late 1980s, and with the availability of more effective immunosuppressive agents.

BACKGROUND

KIDNEY TRANSPLANTS

Kidneys are the most frequently transplanted organ; more than 175,000 transplants were performed through 2003 (Table 234-1). Numerous causes of chronic renal failure result in the need for transplantation, the most common being diabetes mellitus and glomerular disorders (Table 234-2). The source of donors for renal transplantation are both cadavers and living donors. In 2001, there were 8200 cadaveric donor transplants and 6000 living donor transplants.[1,2] The living donor pool consists of both living related donors, who have a higher likelihood for a favorable crossmatch, and living unrelated donors. Recent surgical innovations, such as using laparoscopy to obtain the donor kidney, have decreased morbidity for donors, increased the number of potential donors,[3] and decreased costs.[4]

In most cases, the renal transplant operation is done through a retroperitoneal flank incision. An anastomosis is created between the recipient's iliac artery and the donor kidney's renal artery. Another anastomosis is fashioned between the iliac vein and the renal vein. The donor ureter is connected either to the recipient's bladder using a ureteroneocystostomy or to the recipient's ureter via ureteropyelostomy.

PANCREAS TRANSPLANTS

Pancreas transplantation for control of diabetes was first successfully reported by Lillehei and colleagues in 1970.[5] The major indication for transplantation of this organ is diabetes mellitus. Because of the significant morbidity associated with immunosuppression, transplantation of this organ in isolation is uncommon; most pancreatic transplants are carried out in conjunction with a simultaneous or previous kidney transplant. In 2001, there were 886 simultaneous kidney-pancreas transplants, 305 pancreas after kidney transplants, and 163 solitary pancreas transplants.[2] Isolated pancreatic islet cell transplantation (autotransplantation) has been utilized as an adjunct to total pancreatectomy for patients with intractable pain due to chronic pancreatitis and is an active area of research using human and genetically modified animal islet cells to produce insulin while minimizing the risks of immunosuppression. However, these techniques are difficult to apply outside of specialized centers.

The surgical technique for pancreas transplantation involves anastomosis of the pancreatic vascular supply to the iliac artery and vein. A major issue in pancreatic transplantation is ensuring safe drainage of exocrine secretions. The two options employed are drainage of the pancreatic duct into the bladder and drainage of the duct into the small intestine. Bladder drainage has a lower infection rate, but it is associated with metabolic acidosis caused by bicarbonate losses in the urine and cystitis, urethral stricture, and hematuria.

TABLE 234–1. KIDNEY, PANCREAS, AND KIDNEY-PANCREAS TRANSPLANT STATISTICS

Organ	No. of Transplants, 2002	Total Transplants through July 31, 2003	Median Days on Waiting List	1/5 Year Graft Survival (%)	1/5 Year Patient Survival (%)
Kidney*	14,772	175,337	1,144	88/63[†] 94/77[‡]	94/80[†] 98/90[‡]
Pancreas	553	3,346	343	78/45	96/77
Kidney-pancreas	905	10,919	546	92/73[§] 84/69[¶]	95/83

*Both living and cadaver donors.
[†]Cadaver donor.
[‡]Living donor.
[§]Kidney graft survival.
[¶]Pancreas graft survival.
Data from the 2002 Annual Report of the U.S. Scientific Registry of Transplant Recipients and the Organ Procurement and Transplantation Network. Rockville, MD and Richmond, VA: HHS/HRSA/OSP/DOT and UNOS; and from http://www.optn.org/data.

Compared with other solid organ transplant operations, rejection is more difficult to diagnose in pancreas transplantation for a number of reasons. Hyperglycemia is not manifested until a significant portion of the graft is lost. For grafts drained into the bladder, decreases in urinary amylase concentrations sometimes suggest that rejection is occurring, although this test is not very sensitive. Unfortunately, percutaneous biopsy of the pancreas graft is associated with a high complication rate.[6] The problem of detecting rejection of pancreatic grafts has prompted efforts to carry out simultaneous pancreatic and kidney transplants, using the kidney as a "canary" to detect rejection of both organs. This indicator of rejection is not as effective in pancreas-after-kidney transplants because the two organs are immunologically distinct, as evidenced by higher pancreas graft loss rates after pancreas-after-kidney procedures as compared with simultaneous transplants (16% vs. 5%).[7] The advantage of early identification of rejection must be balanced against the increased risk of perioperative complications as a consequence of the more challenging simultaneous operation.

ETHICAL ISSUES

A number of ethical issues are related to transplantation. Unstated (and/or unintended) coercion to donate can be overwhelming for the family members or loved ones of a patient with renal failure. The physician must act as an advisor, not only for the recipient but also for potential donors. The risk mortality for donors, while low (0.03%),[8] is still an issue that should be addressed before donation. There is some evidence that renal donors are at slightly increased risk for late renal failure after donation.[9]

Another ethical issue that arises relates to transplanting a pancreas without performing a kidney transplant in a patient with diabetes mellitus without renal insufficiency. In most patients with normal renal function, the benefits of being insulin free do not outweigh the long-term risks of immunosuppression. It is reasonable to consider pancreas transplant alone in diabetics without end-stage renal failure if there is evidence of early diabetic nephropathy or problems related to blood glucose control are disabling (e.g., lack of awareness of hypoglycemia) or in patients when two or more secondary diabetic complications are present.

A third ethical issue frequently encountered by critical care physicians relates to the decision to reduce temporarily or to discontinue immunosuppression when a transplant recipient presents with a proven or suspected infection. Tension can exist among the critical care team, the transplant team, and the patient surrounding this issue. On the one hand is the possibility of death from uncontrolled infection, and on the other hand is the loss of a kidney or pancreas graft that would provide considerable improvement in the quality of life.

CURRENT IMMUNOSUPPRESSIVE AGENTS/REGIMENS

The field of immunosuppression has undergone many changes over the past decade driven by a much better understanding of the immune system, allowing the development of targeted therapies. Most patients will receive a combination of agents to prevent rejection. These agents include calcineurin antagonists (cyclosporine, tacrolimus), proliferation signal inhibitors (sirolimus, rapamycin, or everolimus), proliferation inhibitors (azathioprine, mycophenolate mofetil), and corticosteroids. Other agents frequently used to combat rejection include antilymphocyte antibodies. A summary of these agents and mechanisms of action is provided in Table 234-3.

Most of the immunosuppressants have significant side effects and toxicities and significant drug interactions. For a complete discussion of this issue please see Chapter 192.

TABLE 234–2. COMMON INDICATIONS FOR KIDNEY TRANSPLANT*

Diabetes mellitus
Glomerular diseases
Hypertensive nephrosclerosis
Retransplant/graft failure
Polycystic kidney disease
Tubular/interstitial diseases
Renovascular and other vascular diseases
Congenital, rare, familial, and metabolic disorders
Neoplasm

*Includes both living and cadaver donors, listed in order of frequency of transplant.
Data from the 2002 Annual Report of the U.S. Scientific Registry of Transplant Recipients and the Organ Procurement and Transplantation Network. Rockville, MD and Richmond, VA: HHS/HRSA/OSP/DOT and UNOS; and from http://www.optn.org/data.

TABLE 234–3. IMMUNOSUPPRESSIVE AGENTS AND MECHANISM OF ACTION

Class of Agent	Uses	Mechanism of Action
Corticosteroids Methylprednisolone, prednisone	Induction, maintenance, rejection	Redistribution of lymphocytes Block T-cell proliferation, IL-2 synthesis
Antilymphocyte antibodies Antithymocyte globulin OKT-3	Induction, rejection	Lymphocyte depletion
Humanized antibodies Basiliximab, daclizumab	Induction, rejection	Specific targets: IL-2 receptor
Calcineurin inhibitors Cyclosporine, tacrolimus	Maintenance, rejection	Inhibit IL-2 production
Proliferation signal inhibitors Sirolimus (rapamycin), Everolimus	Maintenance	Block cytokine-driven cell cycle progression
Antimetabolites (antiproliferative agents) Azathioprine, mycophenolate mofetil	Maintenance	Inhibit RNA/DNA synthesis

IL-2, interleukin-2.

Common side effects of immunosuppressive agents are summarized in Table 234-4.

COMMON RELATED DISEASES AND CONDITIONS

The vast majority of patients receiving kidney and/or pancreas transplants do not require admission to the ICU. For those patients who do require admission, most are admitted because of perioperative difficulties, which are frequently related to an underlying medical disorder (Table 234-5). A number of medical illnesses are more common in patients with chronic renal failure, including atherosclerotic heart disease, hypertension, congestive heart failure, diabetes mellitus, chronic obstructive pulmonary disease, peripheral vascular disease, and cerebrovascular disease. Discussions with the patient or family often will reveal a history of one or more of these illnesses, allowing evaluation and treatment to be tailored appropriately for the patient.

ROUTINE PERIOPERATIVE CARE: KIDNEY OR KIDNEY/PANCREAS TRANSPLANT

For typical kidney transplant recipients without acute tubular necrosis, a brisk diuresis begins within minutes of revascularization of the kidney graft. This diuresis is due to a number of factors, including intraoperative administration of diuretics, proximal tubular damage related to allograft ischemia, fluid and electrolyte disturbances due to chronic renal failure, and osmotic factors related to uremia. In patients after kidney-pancreas transplantation, the diuresis

also can be related to hyperglycemia. Tight control of blood glucose concentration should be achieved using an insulin infusion. Many patients who were euglycemic before transplantation become hyperglycemic after transplantation, owing to the effects of corticosteroids (administered to prevent rejection) and the stress of surgery. Recent evidence shows benefit of tight glucose control in ICU patients.[10] Our current practice is to maintain blood glucose concentration at 80 to 140 mg/dL. An example of an insulin drip protocol is noted in Figure 234-1. Urinary losses should be corrected with a hypotonic solution; a common prescription is 2.5% dextrose in 0.2% saline infused at a rate of 1 mL per milliliter of urinary output for the first 12 to 24 hours after transplantation. Sodium bicarbonate and potassium chloride should be added as needed, based on frequent measurements of serum electrolyte concentrations. Urine volumes of less than 100 to 200 mL/h within the first 12 h after renal transplant may represent a problem with the graft, and this finding should be immediately communicated to the transplant service (Table 234-6).

Immunosuppression is typically initiated in the operating room and continued postoperatively. At most transplant centers, the dosing of the immunosuppressive agents is protocol driven and determined by the transplant service. Examples of standard protocols for kidney transplant and simultaneous kidney-pancreas transplant patients are illustrated in Table 234-7.

Prophylactic antibiotics appropriate to cover skin and genitourinary flora should be given for 24 to 48 hours. Potential agents include ampicillin/sulbactam (1.5 to 3 g i.v. q6h), ertapenem (1 g i.v. daily), ceftriaxone (1 g i.v. daily), and gatifloxacin (40 mg i.v. daily). There is no evidence to

TABLE 234–4. SIDE EFFECTS OF COMMON IMMUNOSUPPRESSIVE AGENTS

Antithymocyte globulin	Fever, leukopenia, thrombocytopenia, serum sickness
Azathioprine	Leukopenia, thrombocytopenia, anemia, hepatotoxicity, pancreatitis
Basiliximab, daclizumab	Hypersensitivity (anaphylaxis), fever,
Corticosteroids	Hyperglycemia, osteoporosis, impaired wound healing, cushingoid facies, addisonian crisis (from rapid withdrawal)
Cyclosporine	Nephrotoxicity, neurotoxicity, drug interactions, hypertension, hyperkalemia, hirsutism, gingival hyperplasia
Sirolimus	Hyperlipidemia, myelosuppression, impaired wound healing, diarrhea, arthralgia
Tacrolimus	Nephrotoxicity, neurotoxicity, drug interactions, hypertension, hyperkalemia, diarrhea
OKT-3	Pulmonary edema, fevers, rigors, diarrhea, headache, bronchospasm, increased cytomegalovirus infection, risk of post-transplant lymphoproliferative disorder

FUMC ICU Insulin Continuous Infusion

GOAL: Maintain glucose level between 80–40 mg/dL. Start protocol only if glucose >140 mg/dL × 2

GENERAL

☑ Discontinue all currently active insulin orders.

☑ Insulin infusions will be provided as 1 unit of regular insulin/mL in 0.9% Normal Saline, in 30 mL syringes, unless otherwise requested.

☑ If patient is on Parenteral Nutrition / Enteral Feeding, and they are held or cycled, contact MD for specific instructions regarding the insulin infusion.

☑ If subcutaneous insulin (sliding scale or scheduled) is ordered, discontinue the insulin infusion 1 hr after the 1st dose of SQ insulin.

☑ Discontinue this protocol when the patient is transferred out of the ICU.

GLUCOSE MONITORING

☑ Bedside glucose monitor (whole blood glucose) Q1H until glucose stable within 80–140 mg/dL × 4, then Q2H until insulin infusion is discontinued. If subsequent glucose values are outside the 80–140 mg/dL range, measure glucose Q1H.

☑ Obtain a STAT plasma glucose for changes in mental status, diaphoresis, or unexplained tachycardia.

INITIATION OF CONTINUOUS INSULIN INFUSION

STEP ONE   For initial glucose value, start insulin infusion according to scale below:

Initial glucose value	Action taken
141–175 mg/dL	Start insulin infusion @2 units/hr
176–220 mg/dL	Give 2 units IV bolus of regular insulin and start insulin infusion @2 units/hr
221–300 mg/dL	Give 4 units IV bolus of regular insulin and start insulin infusion @3 units/hr
301–400 mg/dL	Give 10 units IV bolus of regular insulin and start insulin infusion @4 units/hr

STEP TWO   For 2nd blood glucose value, adjust insulin infusion according to scale below:

Second glucose value	Action taken
<80 mg/dL	Follow instructions for blood glucose value in Step Three
80–140 mg/dL	No changes. Continue current infusion rate.
141–400 mg/dL	Increase insulin infusion **BY** 2 units/hr
>400 mg/dL	**Notify MD**

STEP THREE   For all blood glucose values after the 2nd reading, adjust insulin infusion according to scale below:

Blood glucose value	Action taken
<40 mg/dL	Hold insulin infusion. Notify MD. Give 50 mL IV of Dextrose 50%. Recheck blood glucose in 15 min. If <80 mg/dL, repeat 50mL Dextrose 50%. If recheck glucose >80 mg/dL, then restart insulin infusion at half previous rate.
40–59 mg/dL	Hold insulin infusion. Give 25 mL IV of Dextrose 50%. Recheck blood glucose in 15 minutes. If <80 mg/dL, repeat 25 mL of Dextrose 50%. If recheck glucose >80 mg/dL, then restart insulin infusion at half previous rate.
60–79 mg/dL	Hold insulin infusion. Recheck blood glucose in 1 hour. If <80 mg/dL, follow STEP 3 protocol. If recheck glucose >80 mg/dL, then restart infusion at half previous rate.
80–140 mg/dL	No changes if blood glucose stable within range. If blood glucose is fluctuating within range, titrate in 0.5 unit increments based on patient response to keep within range.
141–175 mg/dL	Increase insulin infusion **BY** 0.5–1 unit/hour
176–220 mg/dL	Increase insulin infusion **BY** 1–2 units/hour
221–260 mg/dL	Increase insulin infusion **BY** 2–3 units/hour
261–300 mg/dL	Increase insulin infusion **BY** 4 units/hour
301–350 mg/dL	Increase insulin infusion **BY** 5 units/hour
351–400 mg/dL	Increase insulin infusion **BY** 6 units/hour
>400 mg/dL	**Notify MD**

MD SIGNATURE:_____ PAGER #: _____ DATE:. _____

FAIRVIEW UNIVERSITY MEDICAL CENTER–PHYSICIAN ORDERS
INSULIN CONTINUOUS INFUSION ICU

FIGURE 234–1.

TABLE 234–5. COMMON PREEXISTING ILLNESSES COMPLICATING POSTOPERATIVE CARE IN RENAL ALLOGRAFT RECIPIENTS

Atherosclerotic heart disease
Hypertension
Congestive heart failure
Diabetes mellitus
Chronic obstructive pulmonary disease
Peripheral vascular disease
Cerebrovascular disease

TABLE 234–6. CAUSES OF OLIGURIA AFTER KIDNEY TRANSPLANT

Clots in bladder
Acute tubular necrosis
Arterial/venous thrombosis
Acute rejection
Ureteral/bladder anastomotic leak

support longer courses of antibiotics in kidney transplant recipients. Trimethoprim/sulfamethoxazole (80 mg trimethoprim/40 mg sulfamethoxazole by mouth daily) is used routinely at most centers for prophylaxis against *Pneumocystis jiroveci* and *Nocardia* species.

Several specific issues should be considered in pancreas transplantation aside from the usual management of kidney transplantation. The first of these is related to the high rate of graft loss in pancreas transplants owing to portal venous thrombosis. Many centers use a low-dose anticoagulation regimen of unfractionated heparin (100 to 500 units i.v. hourly as a continuous drip) in an effort to reduce graft loss from this complication. Systemic anticoagulation increases the risk of postoperative hemorrhage. Second, there is a relatively high incidence of wound and intra-abdominal infections after pancreas transplantation, being as great as 33% in some centers.[11] Some centers advocate longer courses of broad-spectrum antibiotics because of concerns about infection, although data to support this practice are not very convincing.[11,12]

POST-TRANSPLANT COMPLICATIONS

Post-transplant issues requiring ICU admission can be divided into those occurring immediately post-transplant and those occurring at some time remote to the perioperative period. Common postoperative complications after kidney and/or pancreas transplantation are listed in Table 234-8.

POSTOPERATIVE RESPIRATORY FAILURE

The majority of kidney and/or pancreas transplant patients admitted with this diagnosis after surgery have a self-limited form of respiratory failure secondary to the residual effects of general anesthesia. These patients can be extubated when awake, and recovery from the effects of neuromuscular blocking agents is complete or nearly so. Other causes of immediate postoperative respiratory failure include congestive heart failure from perioperative myocardial infarction, pulmonary edema due to intravascular volume overload secondary to acute tubular necrosis, preexisting pneumonia, aspiration pneumonitis, pulmonary embolus, or, rarely, acute respiratory distress syndrome secondary to intraoperative events or post-transplant pancreatitis. In this setting, it

TABLE 234–7. EXAMPLES OF IMMUNOSUPPRESSION PROTOCOLS FOR KIDNEY TRANSPLANT AND SIMULTANEOUS PANCREAS-KIDNEY TRANSPLANT IN THE IMMEDIATE POSTOPERATIVE PERIOD*

a. Kidney Transplant: Non-HLA-identical living recipients and all cadaver recipients with immediate graft function (1st and 2nd transplant) (MMF, mycophenolate mofetil; PRED, prednisone; TMG, thymoglobulin)

Days	Neoral	MMF	PRED	TMG
0		1 g to 1.5 g intraoperatively	500 mg i.v.	1.25 mg/kg intraoperatively
1	Begin Neoral	1 g to 1.5 g bid	1 mg/kg/day	1.25 mg/kg/day for 4 days
2	Twice a day dosing	Continue	0.5 mg/kg/day	
3		Non-African Americans	0.5 mg/kg/day	
4	Maintain levels	Receive 1 g bid	0.25 mg/kg/day	
5	Between 150 and 200	African Americans	0.25 mg/kg/day	
6	HPLC	Receive 1.5 g bid	DC	

b. Simultaneous Kidney-Pancreas Transplant (Campath, alemtuzumab; CellCept, mycophenolate mofetil).

Campath

30 mg i.v. intraoperatively
30 mg i.v. on postoperative day 2, 2 weeks and 6 weeks
30 mg i.v. monthly for 1 year (only if ALC ≥200/mm³)
Give Solu-Medrol 500 mg before 1st dose and 100 mg before each subsequent dose

Thymoglobulin

1.25 mg/kg i.v. on postoperative day 4
Give Solu-Medrol 100 mg i.v. prior to dose

CellCept

Start postoperatively
1.5 g p.o. bid

*Please note that immunosuppressive regimens at most institutions undergo frequent change and vary by recipient status, crossmatch, graft function, and other variables.

TABLE 234–8. COMMON POSTOPERATIVE COMPLICATIONS: KIDNEY, KIDNEY-PANCREAS, PANCREAS TRANSPLANT

Early	Late
Myocardial Infarction	Myocardial infarction
Renal failure	Renal failure
Hyperglycemia	Transplant artery stenosis
Graft thrombosis	Respiratory failure
Hemorrhage	Post-transplant infection (immune-compromised host)
Wound infection	
Respiratory failure	Post-transplant lymphoproliferative disorder
Post-transplant infection (hospital acquired)	Graft pancreatitis
Deep venous thrombosis	Acute and chronic rejection
Metabolic acidosis	
Graft pancreatitis	
Hyperacute and acute rejection	
Bladder leak	
Pseudomembranous colitis	

is key to perform a rapid and thorough diagnostic workup to determine the etiology of more serious causes of respiratory failure. This evaluation should include electrocardiography, determination of circulating levels of cardiac enzymes, chest radiography, arterial blood gas analysis, and measurements of serum electrolytes and blood urea nitrogen/creatinine concentration. Based on findings from history, physical examination, and the results of these initial tests, the clinician can obtain additional tests as needed to establish a diagnosis. Additional tests that may be helpful include duplex ultrasound scans of the lower extremities for deep venous thrombosis, spiral computed tomography (CT) of the chest to evaluate for pulmonary embolus, cardiac echocardiography, diagnostic bronchoscopy, and transplant ultrasound and/or biopsy.

RESPIRATORY FAILURE DISTANT TO TRANSPLANT

Occasionally, patients are admitted to the ICU with respiratory insufficiency or failure weeks or years after pancreatic and/or renal transplantation. The differential diagnosis is broadened in these patients because of the increased risk of infection associated with immunosuppression. The differential diagnosis for respiratory failure includes infectious causes, cardiogenic causes, and renal failure. It is important to glean from the patient, family, or records any features, such as cytomegalovirus (CMV) status of the patient and donor, past history of cardiac disease, and recent changes in transplantation medications. A rapid workup should take place to evaluate the cause of decompensation. It is frequently necessary to intubate the patient, even in the absence of overt respiratory failure, to perform bronchoscopy for diagnostic evaluation. Initial evaluation should include chest radiography; complete blood cell count; determination of serum electrolytes, blood urea nitrogen/creatinine and cardiac enzymes; sputum sampling; and electrocardiography. It is also prudent to include a rapid screen for CMV in this evaluation. Other tests, including diagnostic bronchoscopy, CT of the chest, echocardiography, and lower extremity Doppler examinations, should be carried out as clinically indicated. Typically, the noninfectious causes of respiratory

failure, such as renal failure with fluid overload and myocardial dysfunction causing congestive heart failure, are more readily identified and treated, leaving the more subtle causes to sort through over the next several days of the patient's ICU course. Exclusion of cardiac and renal failure mandates strong consideration for the possibility of an infectious cause of respiratory compromise.

Initial treatment for post-transplant respiratory failure distant to surgery requires broad-spectrum antibacterial, fungal, and viral therapy until a definitive diagnosis is reached. It is not unusual in such circumstances to have patients on agents that will cover common bacterial organisms, *Candida* and *Aspergillus,* and CMV. (See also Chapter 155.) Common regimens include broad-spectrum antibiotic agents with antipseudomonal and antianaerobic activity, an agent with gram-positive activity, a broad-spectrum antifungal agent, and gancyclovir to provide antiviral coverage for cytomegalovirus and other members of the herpesvirus family. A number of appropriate agents for this purpose are listed in Table 234-9. In situations where pseudomonas is strongly suspected, an additional agent should be added to provide double coverage of this organism. In situations where the patient has high risk for or has known vancomycin-resistant *Enterococcus faecium,* one of the new gram-positive agents should be chosen. Another key component of treatment in this setting is strong consideration for short-term discontinuation of most immunosuppressive medications. The practice at my institution is to hold all but maintenance doses of corticosteroids when infection is suspected strongly. It is frequently possible to tailor antimicrobial therapy as results return. For instance, in the setting of a patient with a low white blood cell count, diffuse pneumonitis, and positive screen for CMV, it is not unreasonable to discontinue antifungal therapy. It is important for the intensivist to be willing to revisit the diagnosis on at least a daily basis, especially if the clinical course is not consistent with the working diagnosis.

POSTOPERATIVE OLIGURIA

Postoperative oliguria (see Table 234-6) is a frequent problem in the renal transplant patient. Common causes include blood clots in the bladder causing outflow obstruction, acute tubular necrosis, arterial or venous thrombosis, and acute rejection. Many patients present in the immediate postoperative period with oliguria and suspected acute tubular necrosis (also called "delayed graft function" in this context). In these patients, it is important to monitor fluid balance closely; many will require urgent dialysis for fluid overload or hyperkalemia. Most patients with acute tubular necrosis in the early postoperative period recover adequate renal function and become able to function without dialysis, albeit with less renal reserve than those patients with immediate graft function.[13] Recovery can be delayed for as long as 3 months.

Decreased urine output within several hours of arrival to the ICU mandates a rapid evaluation. Steps should include irrigation of the Foley catheter to exclude outflow obstruction due to clots and optimization of hemodynamic status to maintain adequate renal perfusion. The transplant service should be immediately notified for a significant change in urine output. After irrigation of the catheter to ensure patency, initial evaluation should include complete blood cell count, determination of serum electrolytes and blood urea nitrogen/creatinine, and transplant ultrasound to assess

TABLE 234–9. EMPIRICAL AGENTS FOR EARLY TREATMENT OF INFECTION IN KIDNEY/PANCREAS TRANSPLANT PATIENTS

Class of Agent	Agent	Dose*
Broad-spectrum antibiotic agents[†]	Imipenem/cilastatin	0.5-1 g i.v. every 6-8 h
	Meropenem	0.5-1 g i.v. every 8 h
	Piperacillin/Tazobactam	3.375 g i.v. every 6 h
Gram-positive agents[‡]	Vancomycin	1-1.5 g i.v. every 12-24 h
	Daptomycin[§]	4-6 mg/kg i.v. daily
	Quinupristin/dalfopristin	7.5 mg/kg i.v. every 8 h
	Linezolid	600 mg i.v. every 12 h
Antifungal agents	Liposomal amphotericin B	3-10 mg/kg i.v. daily
	Voriconazole	6 mg/kg i.v. every 12 h × 2, then 4 mg/kg i.v. every 12 h
	Caspofungin	70 mg load, 50 mg i.v. daily
Antiviral agents[¶]	Ganciclovir	2.5-5 mg/kg i.v. every 12 h
	Foscarnet	90 mg/kg i.v. every 12 h

*Please note that doses given do not account for renal or hepatic insufficiency common in critically ill patients. Prior to choosing an empirical antibiotic regimen, the clinician should carefully consider the patient scenario and medication side effects related to the specific patient.

[†]Rather than a single agent, combination agents covering both gram-negative organisms and anaerobes may be chosen (e.g., fluoroquinolone plus clindamycin or metronidazole). For cases with a strong suspicion for *Pseudomonas aeruginosa* infection, additional *Pseudomonas* coverage should be added (e.g., fluoroquinolone or aminoglycoside).

[‡]When vancomycin-resistant *Enterococcus faecium* infection is suspected, one of the latter 3 choices should be employed.

[§]Daptomycin is not indicated for treatment of pneumonia (package insert).

[¶]Antiviral agents directed toward herpesvirus family (most commonly CMV). Adjust for other viruses.

for blood flow to the kidney and fluid collections. A radioisotope renal scan is occasionally helpful to exclude a urinary anastomotic leak or obstruction of the transplanted ureter. A decrease in hemoglobin concentration suggests the possibility of surgical bleeding and may indicate a need for return to the operating room.

Among patients who underwent transplantation in the more distant past, the likely causes of oliguria are quite different and include acute or chronic rejection, renal artery stenosis, and toxic effects of medications, especially calcineurin inhibitors. Major causes of graft loss after kidney and/or pancreas transplant are listed in Table 234-10.[14] Important studies, in addition to baseline laboratory assays, should include drug levels of calcineurin inhibitors, Doppler ultrasound of the transplant, and radioisotope scan. Renal biopsy and angiography also may be indicated. Ultrasound is an excellent noninvasive way to screen for vascular complications, including renal artery stenosis, arteriovenous fistulas, and pseudoaneurysms. Radioisotope scans are a very useful noninvasive modality for assessment of renal function.[15] Management depends on diagnosis but requires careful titration of intravenous fluids on clinical assessment of intravascular volume status and control of hypertension. Renal artery stenosis is typically treated successfully with angiographic stent placement.

HYPERTENSION

Hypertension is common both immediately post-transplant and long term. There is evidence that early postoperative hypertension is associated with delayed graft function,[16,17] making perioperative control of hypertension an important feature of postoperative care. Acute management of hypertension in the intensive care unit consists of appropriate parenteral antihypertensives, including beta-adrenergic blockers or hydralazine.[18] There are no specific guidelines for appropriate agents in transplant patients. My practice is to use an intermediate-acting beta-blocker, such as labetalol (10 to 20 mg i.v. every 4 to 6 hours), until heart rate is less than intravenous hydralazine (10 to 20 mg i.v. every 4 to 6 hours) as needed. A continuous infusion of esmolol offers the benefits of rapid titration. Sodium nitroprusside is reserved for hypertension not controlled with other measures, because of concerns about cyanide toxicity. It is important in this population to titrate blood pressure so that perfusion pressure to the transplanted organ is maintained.

Tacrolimus and cyclosporine are associated with development of new hypertension in patients after renal transplant (25% and 35% of cases, respectively).[17] Long-term control of hypertension after renal transplantation can be managed with a number of classes of agents, including calcium channel blockers, angiotensin-converting enzyme inhibitors, angiotensin-II type-1 receptor blockers, diuretics, and beta-adrenergic blockers. Many authors suggest use of a calcium channel blocker as first-line therapy for chronic use owing to evidence that these agents can reduce cyclosporine-induced renal damage.[18]

MYOCARDIAL INFARCTION

Patients receiving chronic dialysis and those with diabetes mellitus are at increased risk of myocardial infarction. In a single-center study of approximately 2700 kidney transplant recipients, the incidence of perioperative cardiac

TABLE 234-10. MAJOR CAUSES OF GRAFT LOSS AFTER KIDNEY TRANSPLANT

Cause	Incidence*		
	<1 yr	1-5 yr	>5 yr
Thrombosis	25%	0%	0%
Acute rejection	15%	2%	0%
Chronic rejection	6%	28%	25%
Death with function	41%	52%	57%
Noncompliance	4%	9%	11%

*Percent of grafts lost during time period.
(Modified from Matas AJ, Humar A, Gillingham KJ, et al: Five preventable causes of kidney graft loss in the 1990s: A single-center analysis. Kidney Int 2002; 62(2):704-14.)

complications was 6.1%.[19] Preoperative cardiac evaluation in this population can help to reduce the perioperative risk of myocardial infarction. Perioperative beta-adrenergic blockade and aspirin may reduce the risk further. The diagnosis of myocardial infarction is difficult in many cases because of perioperative pain.[20] It is prudent to evaluate at-risk patients with perioperative measurements of circulating troponin levels. Cardiac screening should be considered in diabetics, in patients with a history of cardiac disease, and in patients with intraoperative hypotension. Elevated circulating troponin levels should be followed by transthoracic echocardiography to evaluate for new wall motion abnormalities in addition to electrocardiographic testing. Treatment of myocardial infarction in the early perioperative patients cannot include thrombolytic therapy because of concerns about surgical hemorrhage. This factor and the different pathophysiology of perioperative myocardial infarction contributes to reported mortality rates as high as 25%.[21] For hemodynamically stable patients with only slight increases in circulating troponin levels and new wall-motion abnormalities on echocardiography, the most prudent course may be medical therapy consisting of aspirin and beta-adrenergic blockade with or without systemic heparinization. Invasive intervention may be indicated for patients with hemodynamic instability or other signs of progression of myocardial infarction. Because it is frequently difficult to clinically determine volume status in a patient with chronic renal failure and a new renal transplant and postoperative polyuria, pulmonary artery catheterization can be helpful to titrate volume therapy.

GASTROINTESTINAL PROBLEMS

Appropriate management of abdominal complications in transplant recipients requires a high index of suspicion because immunosuppression can mask many of the early signs of peritonitis. CT of the abdomen should be performed early in the process of evaluation of new or changing abdominal pain in renal or pancreatic transplant recipients.

The transplant population is at risk for development of upper and lower gastrointestinal tract involvement with CMV, leading to abdominal pain, bleeding, and, rarely, perforation. CMV will most commonly occur the first time within about 6 months of transplantation, correlating with the highest immunosuppressive load. CMV infections are more common in patients when the recipient was serologically negative but the donor was CMV positive. CMV-related problems are also more common among those patients with known CMV infection and those treated with relatively high doses of immunosuppression.[22] Diagnostic endoscopy should include tissue biopsies of the stomach or colon to determine whether CMV is present. Initial treatment consists of intravenous ganciclovir or foscarnet, with a switch to maintenance therapy by oral agents as tolerated for a period of weeks to months (see Table 234-9 for initial i.v. dosing).

Colon perforation and lower gastrointestinal hemorrhage are the most common lower tract complications in kidney transplant recipients. Immunosuppressive therapy can mask the signs and symptoms of peritonitis, delaying the diagnosis of perforation. Colonic perforation can be due to pseudomembranous enterocolitis, acute colonic pseudo-obstruction (Ogilvie's syndrome), diverticulitis, ischemic colitis, stercoral perforation, fecal impaction, or other forms of colitis. Diverticulitis may be more common in patients with polycystic kidney disease (20% versus 3% in one small retrospective analysis),[23] and this group of patients also had a higher incidence of gastrointestinal surgical complications.[24] Colonic perforation is an infrequent complication post-transplant (8 of 1530 transplants at one center), with many of these perforations presenting within 14 days of transplant (5 of 8 cases).[25] Surgical therapy for perforated diverticulitis typically includes colostomy, because a fresh anastomosis in this setting is more likely to leak. Perioperative therapy should include broad-spectrum antibiotics directed at gram-negative and gram-positive aerobes, anaerobes, and fungi. Stress-dose corticosteroids should be administered as clinically indicated.

PSEUDOMEMBRANOUS COLITIS

Psuedomembranous colitis due to *Clostridium difficile* should be suspected in any transplant patient presenting with diarrhea. Risk factors for development of pseudomembranous colitis include previous antibiotic therapy and immunosuppression. Pseudomembranous colitis is diagnosed by detecting *C. difficile* toxin in stool. Controversy exists regarding the need for treatment in patients who are *C. difficile* culture positive but *C. difficile* toxin negative, because *C. difficile* may be present but not pathogenic. The development of serious complications due to *C. difficile*, such as toxic megacolon, are directly related to the time from onset of symptoms to the time of initiation of therapy. Empirical therapy should be started when the diagnosis is considered and then discontinued if stool samples are negative for *C. difficile* toxin. Therapy for *C. difficile* enterocolitis consists of either metronidazole (250 mg p.o. q6h for 10 days) or vancomycin (125 mg p.o. q6h for 10 days). Vancomycin has not been demonstrated to be superior to metronidazole and is significantly more expensive.[26]

REJECTION

Rejection is classified according to its temporal relation to the transplant and includes hyperacute, acute, and chronic rejection. Each of these types is mediated via different immunologic mechanisms. Hyperacute rejection occurs within minutes to hours of the transplant and is caused by preformed antibody directed against the transplanted organ. This type of rejection is very uncommon owing to appropriate pretransplant tissue typing. Acute rejection is the most common type of rejection in current clinical transplantation (occurring in 15% to 60% of renal transplant patients).[27] This type of rejection is most frequent within the first 6 weeks to 6 months after transplantation and is the result of activation of host T lymphocytes by antigens in the transplanted organ. Chronic rejection is common in transplanted organs, developing typically over years to decades. Its etiology is less well understood, but it appears to be related to accumulation of microvascular injury over time.

DIAGNOSIS OF REJECTION

Acute rejection of a renal allograft is typically suspected when the serum creatinine and blood urea nitrogen concentrations increase. Other causes should be considered as well, including hypovolemia, drug toxicity, ureteral obstruction, lymphocele, or vascular anastomotic complications. Diagnosis of acute rejection is confirmed by percutaneous biopsy and histopathologic examination, which show edema and focal infiltration of the interstitium and peritubular capillaries by lymphocytes. Another characteristic finding of acute rejection is invasion of tubular epithelial cells by lymphocytes. Diagnosis of pancreas allograft rejection is more problematic. Increased rates of rejection have been reported after simultaneous kidney-pancreas transplant compared with kidney transplant alone.[28] Hyperglycemia is a late finding and occurs after loss of significant islet cell mass. For simultaneous kidney-pancreas grafts, increases in the serum creatinine concentration may prompt suspicion of pancreatic rejection as well. If the pancreatic duct has been anastomosed to the bladder, a decrease in urinary amylase concentration may be helpful as a marker of graft rejection.[29] Biopsy of the pancreas graft is performed either percutaneously or via cystoscopy to confirm the presence of rejection. This procedure has a complication rate of 2.8%.[30] Because the incidence of venous thrombosis is high in pancreas transplantation, Doppler ultrasound should be performed to evaluate this possibility.

Treatment of acute rejection varies between transplant centers. A common initial approach is bolus therapy with high-dose methylprednisolone, at a dose of 500 mg to 1 g i.v. daily. Severe rejection is more commonly treated with antibody therapy consisting of OKT3 or one of the newer antibodies. These treatments are beyond the scope of the present discussion and have been recently reviewed.[31-35] Treatment of acute rejection is usually successful and is typically followed by adjustment of immunosuppression with a switch to different agents.

GRAFT THROMBOSIS

Arterial or venous thrombosis of the kidney allograft should be considered promptly if an established diuresis abruptly ceases in the immediate postoperative period. The transplant service should be immediately notified, because prompt reoperation provides the only opportunity for salvage. The diagnosis can be rapidly established either by Doppler ultrasound or by inspection at the time of reoperation. Pancreatic allograft thrombosis may be related to either technical problems or high vascular resistance in the graft from preservation-related or immunologic injury. The incidence of graft thrombosis for pancreas allografts is 6%.[2] Many centers routinely administer low-dose heparin, dextran, or antiplatelet agents to prevent this complication (e.g., unfractionated heparin, 100 to 300 units i.v./hour; aspirin, 325 mg p.o./day). The use of anticoagulant and/or antiplatelet therapy in this population is not associated with an increased risk of bleeding complications.[36] Signs of pancreatic graft thrombosis include hematuria, tenderness, and swelling of the graft. Treatment for this condition is removal of the graft.

DEEP VENOUS THROMBOSIS

Deep venous thrombosis is a common complication of most major surgical procedures, including kidney or pancreas transplantation.[37] After these procedures patients should receive standard prophylaxis consisting of low-dose fractionated or unfractionated heparin (unfractionated heparin, 5000 units s.c. twice daily; Lovenox, 0.5 mg s.c. twice daily), or application of sequential compression devices.

Iliofemoral thrombosis occasionally follows renal or pancreas transplant, presumably owing to injury of the vein at the time of transplantation. Typically these thromboses respond to standard-dose anticoagulation. Thrombolytics may be considered, especially in the patient who is more than 2 to 3 weeks out from surgery. The use of vena cava filters for patients with proximal deep venous thrombosis, persistent pulmonary embolus, or bleeding complications of anticoagulation is potentially an issue due to the theoretical risk of occlusion of the transplanted renal or portal vein. However, compromised transplant function is rare after placement of a vena caval filter,[38] and it is my practice to place a vena cava filter in this situation.

TRANSPLANT-ASSOCIATED INFECTIOUS DISEASE

The price of success in transplantation is increased susceptibility to infections due to the need for suppression of the host's immune response (see also Chapter 155). As many as 70% of solid-organ transplant recipients experience an infectious complication within the first year of transplant.[39] The risk of infection is highest during the period of most intensive immunosuppression (typically the first 6 to 12 months) and increases with treatment of rejection. The most frequent infections seen early and late after transplantation are presented in Table 234-11.[40] Infectious complications in the first month after transplantation are frequently caused by those organisms likely to cause disease in immunocompetent hosts. The time of greatest immunosuppression (1 to 6 months posttransplant) is the time when the majority of opportunistic infections occur. These infections include a number of viral infections (most commonly CMV) and opportunistic fungal infections (most frequently *Candida* and *Aspergillus*).[40] A high index of suspicion for the presence of infection should be maintained when evaluating transplant patients in the ICU. A key component to treatment of infection in transplant patients is decreasing immunosuppression, because many infections will not be successfully treated without this step.

Bacterial infections are common in the first 30 days after transplant and are related both to the site of surgery and the presence of indwelling lines and catheters. Infection of the surgical site is uncommon in the renal transplant recipient (1% to 2%) and is comparable to the incidence seen in surgery of immunocompetent patients. Pancreas transplantation, on the other hand, is associated with a 10% to 40% incidence of wound infection.[41] Infections from these wounds reflect skin flora, flora of the duodenum and bladder, and flora associated with previous exposure to antibiotics.[41,42]

FUNGAL INFECTIONS

The immunosuppression associated with solid organ transplantation increases the risk of fungal infection. The incidence of these infections also may be increased because of the use of broad-spectrum antibacterial agents. Agents that are useful for treating fungal pathogens include amphotericin B, azoles, and echinocandins. Amphotericin B acts to prevent fungal growth and kills fungi by binding to fungal cell wall sterols and causing cell death via lysis. Azoles inhibit the cytochrome P450 enzyme responsible for ergosterol synthesis. Echinocandins inhibit glucan synthesis, disrupting cell wall structure. The different mechanisms of action of the echinocandins and azoles make consideration of dual

TABLE 234–11. RISK OF INFECTION AFTER TRANSPLANT WITH RESPECT TO TIME AFTER TRANSPLANT

Within 6 Weeks	6 Weeks to 6 Months	Greater Than 6 Months
Viral		
Herpes simplex	Cytomegalovirus (pneumonia)	Cytomegalovirus (retinitis, colitis)
Hepatitis B, C	Hepatitis B, C	Hepatitis B, C
	Epstein-Barr virus	Papillomavirus
	Varicella zoster	Post-transplant
	Influenza	lymphoproliferative disorder
	Respiratory syncytial virus	
	Adenovirus	
Bacterial		
Nosocomial infection (e.g., line, pneumonia, wound, urinary tract infection)	Nocardiosis	Listeriosis
	Listeriosis from *Listeria monocytogenes*	Tuberculosis
	Tuberculosis	
Fungal		
Candidosis	Candidosis	Cryptococcosis
	Aspergillosis	Coccidioidomycosis
	Cryptococcosis	Histoplasmosis
	Coccidioidomycosis	
	Histoplasmosis	
Parasitic		
	Pneumocystis jiroveci infection	*P. jiroveci* infection
	Strongyloidosis	Strongyloidosis
	Toxoplasmosis	
	Leishmaniasis	
	Trypanosoma cruzi infection	

Modified from Snydman DR: Epidemiology of infections after solid-organ transplantation. Clin Infect Dis 2001;33(Suppl 1):S5-S8.

therapy attractive, although combination therapy has yet to be reported in randomized trials.

The most common fungal pathogens seen are *Candida* species. The widespread use of fluconazole has likely contributed to the increased isolation of *Candida* species resistant to fluconazole. Treatment of suspected fungal infection in the transplant patient in the ICU should, therefore, consist of an agent with more broad-spectrum antifungal activity, such as amphotericin B (most commonly one of the liposomal forms), caspofungin (an echinocandin), or voriconazole (an azole with broader antifungal activity). *Aspergillus* infection occurs in approximately 1% of transplant patients and should be considered in patients failing to respond to appropriate initial antimicrobial therapy. The diagnosis of aspergillosis is frequently difficult, and the intensivist may need to empirically initiate therapy well before a final diagnosis is established. Newer diagnostic methods such as galactomannan assay or real-time polymerase chain reaction for aspergillus in the serum may allow an earlier diagnosis, although the specificity of these results is currently not known.[43,44] The high mortality associated with invasive aspergillosis in this population (60%)[45] mandates early empirical therapy.

Viral infections are important causes of morbidity and mortality in the renal and pancreas transplant recipients. Endemic viruses of little concern to the immunocompetent population may produce life-threatening infection in the immunosuppressed host. Common viral pathogens in the kidney and pancreas transplant patient include members of the human herpesvirus family, most notably cytomegalovirus CMV. Infection with this agent affects nearly 50% of kidney and transplant patients; infection occurs during the period from 2 weeks to 3 months after transplantation.[46] The major

risk factors for CMV infection include CMV seronegativity when the donor is seropositive, need for higher doses of immunosuppression, or repeated treatment for rejection.[22] The range and severity of infection with CMV is broad. The most commonly affected organs are the lungs, gastrointestinal tract, liver, retina, and pancreas. The diagnosis of CMV has been recently enhanced by assays identifying CMV antigen in blood or body fluid.[47,48] The primary treatment of CMV infection is prevention, and many transplant centers include ganciclovir or other antiviral therapy in their protocols (valganciclovir, 900 mg once daily, or oral ganciclovir, 1000 mg three times daily within 10 days of transplant and continued through 100 days).[49] Treatment of suspected or identified CMV infection typically consists of intravenous followed by oral ganciclovir (Table 234-9).

PNEUMOCYSTIS JIROVECI (PREVIOUSLY CARINII)

Pneumocystis carinii is a common cause of pneumonia in immunosuppressed patients and should be considered in any patient presenting with respiratory illness who has had prophylactic therapy (trimethoprim/sulfamethoxazole or dapsone) interrupted. Recent work has led to the reclassification of pneumocystis as an unusual fungus,[50] although some authors have disputed this reclassification.[51] Empirical therapy with intravenous trimethoprim/sulfamethoxazole (15 mg/kg of the trimethoprim component per day given in 3 divided doses) or pentamidine (4 mg/kg/day) should be initiated before established diagnosis in this patient population due to the high mortality rate of the untreated disease.

POST-TRANSPLANT LYMPHOPROLIFERATIVE DISORDER

Post-transplant lymphoproliferative disorder (PTLD) includes a broad range of conditions, ranging from simple lymphoid hyperplasia to lymphoma. The etiology of this disorder in the transplant patient is closely related to infection with Epstein-Barr virus (EBV). PTLD typically occurs during times of most intensive immunosuppression. The incidence of PTLD is low in renal and pancreas transplantation compared with other solid organ transplants (2.6% at 10 years).[1] The clinical presentation of this disorder varies widely, and many patients present with nonspecific symptoms such as malaise, fever, and weight loss. Occasionally, patients present to the ICU acutely ill with a markedly elevated blood lactate level that is unresponsive to aggressive fluid resuscitation. Evaluation for suspected PTLD should include imaging of the brain, chest, and abdomen, with targeted biopsies to provide a tissue diagnosis. Treatment of patients with PTLD has not been well codified but may include reduction of immunosuppression, administration of interferon-alfa, antiviral therapy, chemotherapy, and treatment with an anti–B-cell antibody (rituximab).[52-54]

PANCREAS TRANSPLANT

A number of issues are specific to pancreas transplantation, including metabolic acidosis, bladder leak, and graft pancreatitis. Wound infection is more common after pancreas transplantation than after kidney transplantation and should be aggressively treated with appropriate wound care, débridement, and antibiotics. In addition, the pancreas allograft is more likely to suffer thrombosis leading to graft loss.

Metabolic acidosis in pancreas transplant patients is a consequence of using the bladder to drain bicarbonate-rich pancreatic exocrine secretions. To prevent this problem, patients are typically started on oral therapy with sodium bicarbonate (1300 mg by mouth 2 to 3 times daily) to replace losses of the anion via the bladder.

Bladder leak is most commonly from the duodenal segment of the donor pancreas due to devascularization during the graft preparation process or during placement of the graft. This frequent complication (10% of cases) is most common during the first several weeks after transplantation.[55] Diagnosis is aided by having a high index of clinical suspicion and may be confirmed with a high degree of accuracy by CT of the area using contrast agent instilled into the bladder.[56] Treatment for smaller leaks consists of prolonged Foley catheter drainage, whereas larger or chronic leaks require operative intervention.

Graft pancreatitis occurs in 16% of pancreas transplant patients and is a significant cause of graft loss.[57,58] Graft pancreatitis early after transplantation is due to preservation-related or ischemic injury to the pancreas and typically is self-limited. However, the development of peripancreatic fluid collections necessitates evaluation for infection and may require operative intervention ranging from opening a deep abscess to débridement of the involved portions of the pancreas to removal of the entire pancreatic allograft. Removal, if necessary, is best performed early before development of established organ dysfunction.[58] Late graft pancreatitis is related to reflux from the bladder or CMV infection and can be treated by conversion to enteric drainage[59] or specific antiviral therapy,[60] respectively.

ANNOTATED REFERENCES

Geddes CC, Church CC, Collidge T, et al: Management of cytomegalovirus infection by weekly surveillance after renal transplant: Analysis of cost, rejection and renal function. Nephrol Dial Transplant 2003;18:1891-1898.
This single-center study performed an analysis of the cost of routine surveillance for CMV infection after renal transplant compared with prophylactic therapy with ganciclovir. The authors noted a slightly lower cost for a surveillance strategy compared with routine prophylaxis. However, this cost was at the expense of a significantly decreased renal function (nearly 50%) and increased incidence of rejection.

Humar A, Johnson EM, Gillingham KJ, et al: Venous thromboembolic complications after kidney and kidney-pancreas transplantation: A multivariate analysis. Transplantation 1998;65:229-234.
This large single-center study examined incidence and risk factors for thromboembolism in 2100 kidney and kidney/pancreas transplantation over a 10-year period. They identified an incidence of deep venous thrombosis (DVT) of 6.2%. Risk factors for DVT included pancreas allograft, age older than 40 years, previous DVT, and diabetes mellitus. Pulmonary embolus occurred in 2.1% of patients.

Humar A, Kerr SR, Ramcharan T, et al: Perioperative cardiac morbidity in kidney transplant recipients: Incidence and risk factors. Clin Transplant 2001;15:154-158.
This large single-center study of 2694 renal transplant recipients evaluated the incidence of perioperative cardiac morbidity within the first 30 days after transplant. They identified perioperative cardiac morbidity in 6.1% of patients, with complications including arrhythmia (2.7%) and myocardial infarction (1.6%) the most common cardiac morbidities. Risk factors for myocardial infarction included age older than 50 years, preexisting cardiac disease, and diabetes mellitus.

Matas AJ, Humar A, Gillingham KJ, et al: Five preventable causes of kidney graft loss in the 1990s: A single-center analysis. Kidney Int 2002; 62:704-714.
This large single-center review identified five major causes of renal graft loss in the 10 years 1990-1999 in the 1467 primary renal transplants performed at this institution. These causes included thrombosis, acute rejection, chronic rejection, death with function, and noncompliance. Death with function and thrombosis were the most common causes of graft loss in the first year after transplant.

Singh N, Avery RK, Munoz P, et al: Trends in risk profiles for and mortality associated with invasive aspergillosis among liver transplant recipients. Clin Infect Dis 2003;36:46-52.
This single-center study compared two cohorts of liver transplant patients affected with invasive aspergillosis at their institution during 1990-1995 and 1998-2001. They found that in the latter cohort, invasive aspergillosis was occurring later after liver transplant, was associated with less central nervous system infection and had a lower mortality rate (60%).

Thomas MC, Mathew TH, Russ GR, et al: Perioperative blood pressure control, delayed graft function, and acute rejection after renal transplantation. Transplantation 2003;75:189-195.
This single-center study evaluated the relationship of perioperative blood pressure control to delayed graft function and acute rejection and identified a significant relationship between better blood pressure control and reduced rejection and improved graft function.

Chapter 235

LIVER TRANSPLANTATION

David J. Kramer

KEY POINTS

INNOVATIONS IN TRANSPLANT CRITICAL CARE

1. The growing imbalance between the number of donated organs and the number of potential recipients has led to **expansion** of the potential **donor pool** by the use of organs previously considered risky. In particular, donor **age** is no longer an exclusion criterion. Programs with pediatric components have routinely **split livers,** providing a left lobe for pediatric recipients and a right lobe for adult recipients. The development of **in-vivo** splitting has improved graft function. **Live-donor liver transplantation** has moved into the forefront. Left lobe donation has met the needs of many pediatric recipients, and right lobe donation for adults has improved the outlook for many who might not be eligible for a timely cadaveric liver transplant.

2. Advances in general critical care have found application in management of critically ill patients with liver disease, before and after transplantation. **Daily awakening** of patients sedated for mechanical ventilation results in earlier liberation from the ventilator and has direct application to patients with liver disease who metabolize sedatives and analgesics unpredictably. **Tight glucose control** results in a lower infection rate. Infection is a major cause of morbidity and mortality in ICU-bound patients with liver disease, and stress, corticosteroids, and the diabetogenic effects of calcineurin inhibition result in insulin resistance. Renal insufficiency is common in liver failure. Strategies to preserve renal function such as **calcineurin-inhibitor–sparing** immunosuppression regimens are under active investigation. For critically ill patients with renal failure, **intensive dialytic therapy** such as daily dialysis or continuous renal replacement offers ways to reduce infectious complications.

"FAST TRACK" MANAGEMENT OF LIVER TRANSPLANT RECIPIENTS— WITHOUT THE ICU

3. ICU admission is needed for liver transplant recipients for evaluation and management of organ system dysfunction or incipient dysfunction. However, patients who recover from surgery sufficiently that they are awake, hemodynamically stable, extubated and well-saturated and able to cough and cooperate with breathing exercises, and have good graft function do not require admission to the ICU. **These patients can be "fast tracked" with recovery from anesthesia in the postanesthesia care unit (PACU) and transfered directly to the ward.** The care process needs to change significantly to accommodate this approach—to make it safe and fiscally sound.

4. The acuity of such patients exceeds that typical for medical and surgical wards. **Nursing support must be flexible enough to provide ongoing assessment and intervention, which is protocol driven with physician backup.** Support from the intensivists and ICU staff add a safety net if the patient's condition deteriorates.

5. The perspective of the anesthesiologist must change and more closely mimic the approach to induction, maintenance, and emergence from anesthesia that characterizes less demanding procedures. Selection of short-acting analgesics, amnestics, and muscle relaxants must be accompanied by greater use of volatile anesthetics, particularly isoflurane. **Although the exact time will vary, the costs of PACU recovery versus ICU admission probably intersect at 6 hours of PACU care.** Caution must be taken that patients are fully recovered from muscle relaxation.

6. The selection of patients for fast tracking is extremely important. A huge commitment of health care resources has been committed to the transplant recipient at considerable expense. This should not be jeopardized in the effort to "optimize" health care delivery. **Patients with low MELD scores, low intraoperative blood transfusion requirements, short operations, and little extrahepatic organ dysfunction are ideal candidates for "fast tracking."** The transplant intensivist should be kept in the loop so that changes in clinical status can be brought to his or her attention and action can be taken before serious injury occurs.

IMMUNOSUPPRESSION

7. The transplanted liver is much better tolerated and is less immunogenic than other solid organs. **Consequently, acute rejection is less problematic, more**

easily treated, and less closely related, if at all, to chronic rejection. Consequently, efforts to reduce toxicity of immunosuppressive agents have become paramount.

8. Calcineurin inhibitors, cyclosporine, and tacrolimus, cause nephrotoxicity and neurotoxicity that is worse when they are administered intravenously. Thus these agents should be prescribed for enteral administration. Tacrolimus is absorbed throughout the proximal gut and can be given with a nasogastric tube. Absorption is not affected by bile. Tube feedings may interfere with absorption of tacrolimus. The absorption of Neoral, a newer formulation of cyclosporine, does not require bile, and levels do not change after clamping biliary drains.

9. Delayed initiation of calcineurin inhibition can be considered in patients at very low risk for rejection. In others, induction therapy with interleukin-2 receptor (IL-2r) antagonists, such as basiliximab and daclizimab or T cell–depleting agents such as thymoglobulin or alemtuzumab (Campath), allows for much lower doses of calcineurin inhibitors. It may also be steroid sparing. Although the benefits in terms of less nephrotoxicity and less neurotoxicity are clear, the impact of these strategies on rejection rates and re-infection with viral hepatitis remains to be defined.

10. Account must be taken of the small graft size for some recipients with particular attention to lower dose and greater interval between doses in adult recipients of right lobes, pediatric grafts, and recipients of grafts from "marginal" donors.

LIVER-LUNG INTERACTIONS

11. The anatomic relation of the lung to the liver is such that both the effluent from the liver and the blood that bypasses the liver in portosystemic shunting is directed to the lung. Evidence of graft dysfunction may be found in subtle changes in lung function. Indeed, patients may develop **intrapulmonary shunting or pulmonary hypertension or lung injury (acute respiratory distress syndrome [ARDS])** as a consequence. The mortality of liver-associated ARDS exceeds 90% unless liver function can be restored.

12. **Hepatopulmonary syndrome (HPS)** is hypoxemia in the setting of liver disease in which intrapulmonary shunting can be demonstrated with a contrast echocardiogram. Clinical characteristics include dyspnea and oxygen desaturation with standing, platypnea, and orthodeoxia. Despite this echocardiographic finding, the dominant problem is ventilation-perfusion mismatch because most patients will resolve hypoxemia with inhalation of 100% oxygen. Patients with HPS usually resolve their hypoxemia within days or weeks of normalization of graft function. Morbidity, and perhaps mortality, is higher in the patients who have a PaO_2 of less than 200 mm Hg on 100% oxygen. In such patients a fixed intrapulmonary shunt should be sought and embolization considered.

13. Patients with liver disease are six times more likely to develop **pulmonary hypertension.** This is astonishing because nitric oxide production increases with advancing liver failure. Pulmonary hypertension is associated with portal hypertension and may worsen with portosystemic shunting (e.g., with a transjugular intrahepatic portosystemic shunt [TIPS]). Severe pulmonary hypertension is defined as pulmonary artery systolic pressures in excess of 60 mm Hg with elevated pulmonary vascular resistance. Although pulmonary artery pressures may be estimated by echocardiography, pulmonary artery catheterization is required in patients with estimates of elevated pressures. This requires careful measurement of oxygen saturation in the superior vena cava, right atrium, and right ventricle to define a left-to-right shunt. In addition, measurement of the response to a pulmonary vasodilator such as epoprostenol (Flolan) is indicated because preoperative management requires reduction of the pressures and restoration of normal right ventricular function.

Orthotopic liver transplantation (OLTX) is the definitive therapeutic option for patients with end-stage liver disease (ESLD). It affords the opportunity for a disabled person to return to a full and active life. Although expensive, OLTX may well be more cost effective than the routine medical care of terminally ill patients with liver failure.[1,2] The first OLTX in humans was performed by Starzl in 1963.[3] However, significant progress did not occur until the advent of potent immunosuppressive agents, specifically the introduction of cyclosporine in 1981.[4] Technical improvements in surgical approach and organ preservation, combined with increasingly sophisticated anesthetic and intensive care management, have provided 1-year survival rates of nearly 90%.

In this chapter, I outline the many developments that have occurred in this field. Major advances in defining risk categories for candidates and managing patients with cirrhosis and pulmonary hypertension and novel immunosuppressive strategies are described. In recent years, organ allocation has been prioritized such that the sickest patients, those most likely to die, undergo transplants first. This optimizes both aggregate benefit, by improving overall survival of patients with end-stage liver disease, and individual benefit. The latter is manifested by the full recovery of a very sick patient. Conversely, the individual who is not so ill will not bear the risks of surgery. Since February 2002 all patients listed in the United States for liver transplantation have been prioritized by their score on the Model for End-stage Liver Disease (MELD).[5,6]

CANDIDATE SELECTION

Optimal candidates are those for whom the risk of surgery is far outweighed by the potential improvement in their quality of life. Furthermore, the risk of recurrence of the primary disease should be low.[7,8] Not surprisingly, those who are at

TABLE 235–1. CONTRAINDICATIONS TO LIVER TRANSPLANTATION

Absolute	Relative
Extrahepatic malignancy	Cholangiocarcinoma, hepatocellular carcinoma larger than UCSF modification of Milan criteria (see text)
AIDS	HIV infection (in the absence of AIDS)
Hepatitis B with active replication	
Low cerebral perfusion pressure (sustained < 40 mm Hg or cerebral blood flow < 10 mL/min/ 100 g) in fulminant hepatic failure	Low cerebral perfusion pressure (sustained < 60 mm Hg or cerebral blood flow < 20 mL/min/100 g) in fulminant hepatic failure
Infection (extrahepatic)	Portal vein and superior mesenteric vein thrombosis
	Extrahepatic organ system failure not related to the ESLD
Pulmonary hypertension (systolic PA > 60 mm Hg, decompensated RV function)	Pulmonary hypertension (systolic PA < 60 mm Hg, preserved RV function)
Hepatopulmonary syndrome (PaO_2 < 100 mm Hg with FiO_2 = 100%)	Hepatopulmonary syndrome (PaO_2 < 200 mm Hg with FiO_2 = 100%)

HIV, human immunodeficiency virus; AIDS, acquired immunodeficiency syndrome; ESLD, end-stage liver disease; PA, pulmonary artery; RV, right ventricular.

the highest risk with surgery also achieve the greatest gains when they survive. Unfortunately, such patients have a higher mortality and require significantly greater resources, particularly intensive care and rehabilitation. There are few absolute contraindications to OLTX. However, factors have been identified that significantly increase the risk and should be recognized as relative contraindications (Table 235-1). From the surgical perspective, prior right upper quadrant abdominal surgery, particularly biliary reconstruction, results in a technically more difficult procedure. Patients who are sicker with higher MELD scores or U.S. United Network Organ Sharing (UNOS) Status 1,[9] particularly those with fulminant hepatic failure, fare worse. Patients with higher Acute Physiology and Chronic Health Evaluation (APACHE) II scores, who are in the ICU and require mechanical ventilation or hemodialysis, have lower survival. Of course, medical therapy in such circumstances is even less successful and APACHE II models hospital outcome well. However, after transplantation, mortality does not rise linearly as a function of recipient acuity. Patients with high APACHE II scores have a higher post-OLTX mortality than recipients with very low preoperative scores. However, there is a plateau of approximately 25% for recipients with preoperative APACHE II scores greater than 20 (Fig. 235-1). This observation suggests that carefully selected but very ill patients benefit from OLTX.

Patients with cirrhosis and underlying hepatocellular carcinoma are candidates for OLTX if the disease is limited to the liver and the lesions are small, there is no evidence for major intrahepatic venous invasion, and nodal disease is absent. The widely accepted Milan criteria (1 lesion less than 5 cm or 3 lesions each less than 3 cm) have been modified and established as the University of California at San Francisco (UCSF) criteria (1 lesion = 6.5 cm or three or fewer nodules with the largest = 4.5 cm and the total tumor diameter = 8 cm without gross vascular invasion); survival

is more than 80% for these patients.[10] Extensive radiologic staging of these patients to stratify them into tumor stages is imperative so that the risk of postoperative recurrence can be estimated. Patients with biliary tract malignancy, such as cholangiocarcinoma, have a very high rate of recurrence.[11,12] It seems doubtful that more extensive resection, including the liver, a portion of small bowel, and pancreas, will be more successful in controlling recurrence of these tumors.[13,14] Preoperative chemotherapy and irradiation may improve outcome after liver transplantation and is under investigation.[15]

The risk for recurrence of viral hepatitis in the transplanted organ differs for hepatitis A (HAV), hepatitis B (HBV), and hepatitis C (HCV). HAV is an acute illness that may cause fulminant hepatic failure and does not recur after transplantation. Recurrence of HBV, once a near universal problem[16] except after transplantation for fulminant HBV, has been greatly reduced by the routine use of lamivudine and hepatitis B immune globulin (HBIG) titrated to levels of anti-HBV surface antigen antibody (HbsAb). Active HBV replication, documented by the presence of HBV-DNA, must be suppressed with lamivudine or adefovir before surgery.[17-22] For reasons that are unclear, patients transplanted with HBV fare worse at each postoperative stage than those with other causes of ESLD.[24] Some have speculated that this is a systemic disease accounting for both the high rate of re-infection in the absence of prophylaxis and the decreased survival. Hepatitis C presents a more complicated conundrum. Re-infection of the transplanted organ is nearly universal. Currently there is no effective prophylaxis. Clinical progression is highly variable and not easily predicted. Some patients experience rapid deterioration with graft failure within the first year, but others have little histologic damage several years after liver transplantation. Treatment after transplantation with pegylated, recombinant interferon alfa-2b and ribavirin is possible but variably tolerated. Sustained suppression of HCV at the end of therapy is reported to be approximately 26% but sustained in these responders for 3 years.[24] The effect of targeted immunosuppression, particularly reduced corticosteroid dosage, on recurrence of HCV and progression to fibrosis is under investigation.[25]

In view of the need to use additional immunosuppressive drugs to treat the viral illness, one might expect a disastrous course for patients who are infected with the human immunodeficiency virus (HIV) at the time of OLTX. Remarkably, however, this outcome has not been observed. Indeed, in the era of highly active antiretroviral therapy (HAART), survival after OLTX is only slightly lower for HIV-positive patients than it is for HIV-negative patients.[9,26-28]

Patients with thrombosed portal veins present a formidable surgical challenge. Patency of the superior mesenteric vein should be demonstrated by ultrasonography or magnetic resonance imaging (MRI) or angiography before surgery. Occlusion of the superior mesenteric vein usually precludes OLTX, although an innovative approach is to anastomose the donor portal vein to the recipient inferior vena cava with a proximal caval ligature placed to sustain portal flow. Mesenteric venous hypertension is not addressed directly, but portal decompression and improved coagulation reduce the risk of bleeding. Combined hepatic and intestinal transplantation or multivisceral transplantation are alternatives.[29]

Fulminant hepatic failure (FHF) is liver failure with encephalopathy that develops in patients without prior liver disease within an 8-week period or less.[30] Mortality is high

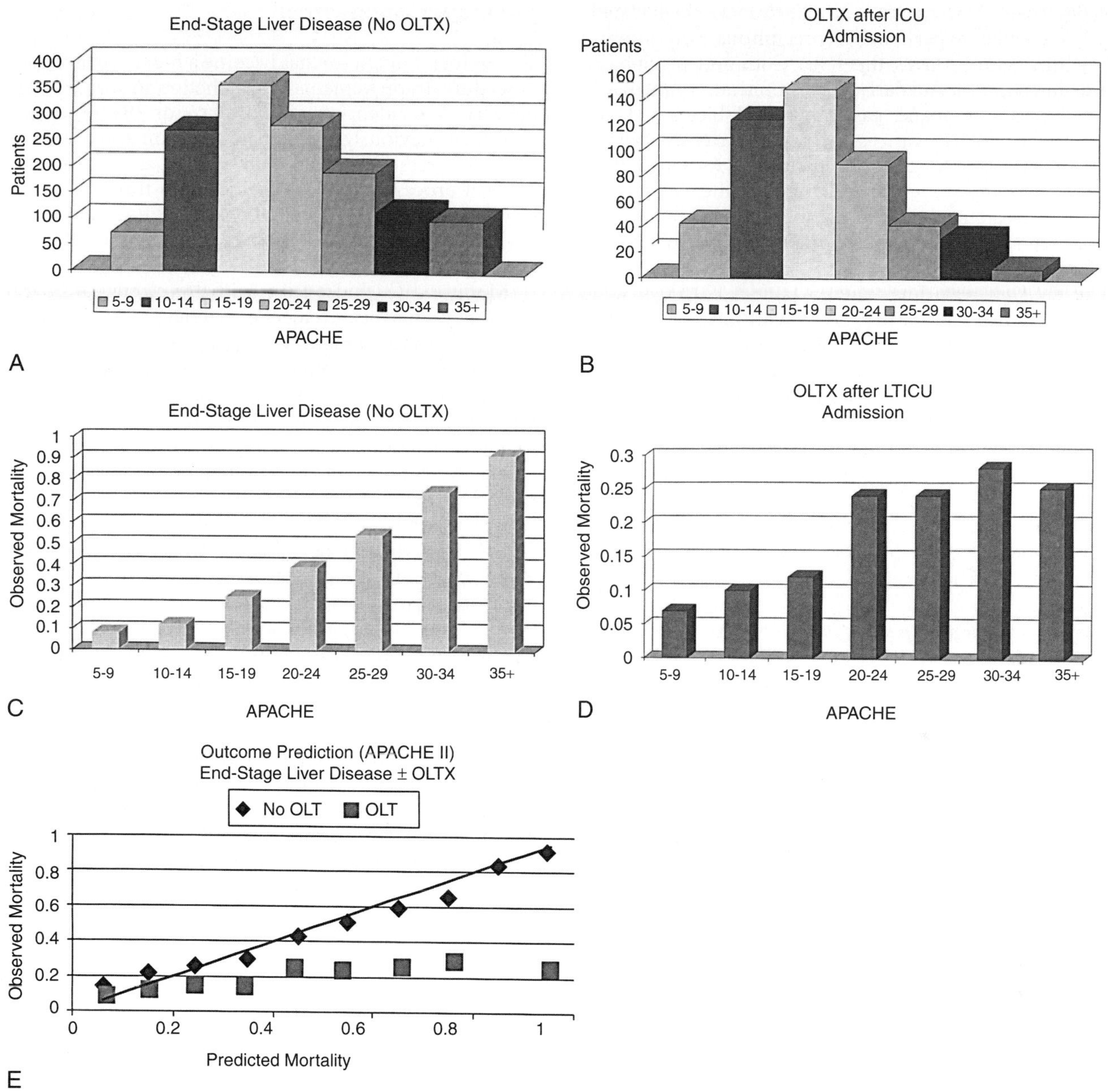

FIGURE 235–1. APACHE II model applied to patients with end-stage liver disease (ESLD) who require ICU admission: 1381 patients did not undergo liver transplantation during that hospitalization (No OLTX) and 489 patients were transplanted during that hospitalization (OLTX). **A,** Distribution of scores in patients who were not transplanted. **B,** Distribution of scores in those transplanted. **C,** Mortality by APACHE II score in those not transplanted. **D,** Mortality by APACHE II score in those transplanted. **E,** Observed mortality as a function of predicted mortality based on APACHE II scores in both the group of patients not transplanted (which tracks the line of identity) and those transplanted.

and predictable.[31] Liver transplantation is the only therapeutic option for patients with a predicted high mortality. With this surgical option, survival has improved from 20% to 75%.[32,33] Such patients are critically ill at the time of transplantation. They require intensive hemodynamic and neurologic monitoring preoperatively, including measurement of intracranial pressure (ICP)[34-38] and cerebral blood flow (CBF). Some patients improve with supportive care (e.g., patients with acetaminophen intoxication, *Amanita* poisoning, or hepatitis A), but most experience a deterioration in their conditions. Progressive encephalopathy with sustained intracranial hypertension results in inadequate cerebral perfusion and precludes successful OLTX because brain death

occurs.[39] Such patients are also prone to the development of pancreatitis, which, when severe, makes OLTX unacceptably risky. Cardiovascular instability,[40] atrial and ventricular arrhythmias,[41] and respiratory insufficiency are common complications of FHF and substantially increase operative risk. If high doses of vasopressors (e.g., >1 µg/kg/min of epinephrine) are needed to maintain adequate blood pressure, then operative risk is unacceptable. Similarly, operative risk is excessive when severe acute respiratory distress syndrome (ARDS) is present (e.g., maintenance of adequate arterial oxygenation requires >10 cm H_2O of positive end-expiratory pressure [PEEP] or fraction of inspired oxygen [FIO_2] >70%).

Patients with ESLD severe enough to make them eligible for OLTX often experience a precipitous deterioration and require admission to the ICU. Common precipitants include infection (particularly pneumonia and spontaneous bacterial peritonitis) and gastrointestinal bleeding (from esophageal or gastric varices, portal hypertensive gastropathy, or gastric or duodenal ulceration). Although these events herald the impending demise of the patient and intensify the search for a donor organ, they also further compromise the potential recipient and may lead to multiple organ dysfunction syndrome (MODS) and death.

The decision regarding when a patient is "too sick" to undergo OLTX is complex. Patients with unresolved extrahepatic infection should not undergo transplantation. Similarly, patients requiring high doses of vasopressors to support blood pressure also should not undergo transplantation. Although they might survive the operation, the graft is likely to fail quickly, resulting in death. Short of this disastrous scenario, my colleagues and I have successfully managed patients after OLTX despite dialysis for renal failure, mechanical ventilation, severe encephalopathy (grade IV), profound coagulopathy, and MODS. Usually, with good hepatic graft function, MODS resolves.

DONOR SELECTION AND OPERATION

The prediction of graft function in a recipient by analysis of donor characteristics remains inexact. No biochemical or physiologic test performs better than the operating surgeon's assessment of suitability of the organ for transplantation. Potential donors, who have malignancy or are infected with HIV or hepatitis B, are eliminated. Hepatitis B core antibody (HbcAb)–positive donors and hepatitis C–positive donors without evidence of fibrosis or cirrhosis may be suitable for recipients with these disease processes. Other considerations include age greater than 65 years (although many grafts from older donors function acceptably) and direct hepatic trauma. Evidence of chronic liver disease in the donor should be sought but often may not be evident until gross inspection or after procurement. Steatotic livers may not function well, but this is difficult to predict. Liver function tests are not sufficiently discriminating to use to refuse a graft. Other measures such as lidocaine clearance[42,43] are not routinely available within a short enough time frame. Liberalization of criteria for donated organs deemed acceptable expands the donor pool. However, it invites more selective matching of donors and recipients. For example, liver function in HCV-positive recipients is worse when the donor is older than 60 years of age.[44]

Brain death results in marked changes in homeostasis for the donor. Hemodynamic instability is common and may result, in part, from massive free water deficits caused by diabetes insipidus. Correction of diabetes insipidus with desmopressin and adequate hemodynamic monitoring and intervention are essential to preserve vital organ function. Anesthesia blunts the response to surgical stimulation. A skilled surgical dissection with rapid identification of the hepatic vessels,[45] cannulation and perfusion with University of Wisconsin (UW) solution, and rapid cooling are essential for graft preservation. Although a cold ischemia time less than 16 hours is preferable, cold preservation time of less than 24 hours is compatible with adequate graft function.[46]

RECIPIENT OPERATION

The recipient operation has become a highly refined surgical procedure. Improvements in anesthetic and surgical practice have made evident the importance of the other factors described previously—candidate selection and donor organ quality—in the eventual outcome for the recipient. The surgical procedure may be divided into three stages: hepatectomy, anhepatic phase, and post-reperfusion phase. Each involves special consideration by the anesthesiologist and surgeon.

Monitoring includes pulse oximetry, electrocardiography, and continuous measurement of arterial pressure (often from two vessels) and pulmonary arterial pressure. Maintenance of large-bore central venous catheters (e.g., two 8.5-French introducers) and the ability to infuse whole blood at rates as high as 2 L/min with a rapid infusion system are essential to maintain hemodynamic stability during occasional episodes of massive hemorrhage. More extensive monitoring is indicated in selected cases. Right ventricular function may be compromised by the presence of pulmonary hypertension, a complication that can develop acutely during reperfusion.[47-50] Right ventricular ejection fraction and end-diastolic volume are more sensitive guides to cardiac preload than are central venous and pulmonary artery occlusion pressures. These values may be obtained by use of the oximetric pulmonary artery (Edwards) catheter.[1] Additional cardiovascular assessment is provided by the frequent use of transesophageal echocardiography. This tool provides a dynamic online picture to the anesthesiologist, allowing him or her to assess the adequacy of resuscitation. In patients with FHF and intracranial hypertension, ICP monitoring is essential. Although CBF measurements are difficult to obtain in the operating room, the arterial-jugular venous oxygen content difference may be used as a surrogate. CBF also may be assessed, using transcranial Doppler ultrasound to measure the velocity of flow in the middle cerebral artery. Continuous electroencephalography (EEG) and compressed spectral array are under investigation as monitoring techniques in this setting.

Anesthesia is often induced with etomidate and maintained with a balanced technique of volatile anesthetics (isoflurane), muscle relaxation (cisatracurium, vecuronium), and judicious use of narcotics (fentanyl) and benzodiazepines (midazolam).[51]

Monitoring of the coagulation capacity of the recipient is complicated because clotting is usually markedly deranged and it is necessary to rapidly correct problems. Depletion of coagulation factors and thrombocytopenia are common. Excessive fibrinolysis, which may be evident early in the procedure but is not of clinical importance at this time point, may become a significant factor after blood loss and at the time of reperfusion. Standard measures of coagulation-prothrombin time (PT), activated partial thromboplastin time (aPTT), and platelet count are very sensitive. However, attempts to correct these values results in excessive transfusion of blood products. There is often significant delay between the time blood is sampled and the results from clotting assays are reported. Finally, standard measures of coagulation provide little information about platelet function and the presence of fibrinolysis. Kang and colleagues introduced the thromboelastograph for routine use during OLTX.[52] This test provides the anesthesiologist with a rapid assessment of coagulation status, the presence or absence of fibrinolysis, and the effects of intervention with protamine or epsilon-aminocaproic acid, an inhibitor of fibrinolysis.[52-54]

The surgical procedure involves meticulous dissection, which is often hampered by severe portal hypertension and substantial bleeding from venous collaterals. Insufficient control results in significant blood loss. Identification of the hilar structures may be complicated by adhesions from prior biliary tract surgery. Patency of recipient vessels and adequacy of blood flow must be assessed before placing the graft into the surgical field. An arterial graft for the hepatic artery may be chosen when the recipient anatomy is anomalous or the caliber of the vessels is too small or when atherosclerosis narrows the celiac trunk or native hepatic artery. Other indications for an arterial graft include a marked size discrepancy between the recipient and donor vessels and inadequate length of the donor artery. Portal venous thrombosis may be managed with a "jump" graft from the superior mesenteric vein if the portal vein cannot be thrombectomized.[55] The donor and recipient caval veins are usually anastomosed end-to-end caudad and cephalad to the liver.

Preservation of blood flow in the inferior vena cava (caval preservation) with or without portal drainage is an alternative technique also known as a "piggyback"[56-58] and may be preferred when there is marked hemodynamic instability. Venovenous bypass was used routinely in the past, because it afforded greater hemodynamic stability and reduced mesenteric congestion (Fig. 235-2).[59] However, the "piggyback" approach requires one less anastomosis and no dissection of the groin or axilla, decreasing the time for surgery by 1 hour. The biliary anastomosis is fashioned after the vascular anastomoses are completed and the graft reperfused. Two options are used: choledochocholedochostomy or mid-jejunal Roux-en-Y limb with choledochojejunostomy. The former procedure requires less dissection and is restorative. Unfortunately, the stenosis rate is quite high. Diseases such as sclerosing cholangitis, which involve the extrahepatic bile ducts, require resection of the bile duct and creation of a choledochojejunostomy. Stenting of the biliary anastomosis—once routine with a tracheostomy tube—is now controversial. One innovative approach is cannulation of the donor cystic duct after donor cholecystectomy, which provides a noninvasive route for cholangiography as well as daily inspection of the bile.

In approximately 10% of patients, reperfusion is accompanied by cardiovascular collapse.[60] Although, the exact mechanism is undefined, marked shifts occur in the concentrations of circulating electrolyte (hyperkalemia and hypocalcemia) and temperature, perhaps in reaction to the preservative solution. A hypocontractile left ventricle complicates the loss of vasomotor tone. Volume resuscitation and inotropic support (epinephrine) with replenishment of calcium guided by ionized calcium analysis are usually sufficient to restore hemodynamic stability. Fortunately, this event is usually short lived. However, significant insults to the graft, heart, kidneys, and brain may occur and require postoperative attention.

POSTOPERATIVE MANAGEMENT

As might be surmised from the preceding discussion, the postoperative management of the OLTX recipient is largely governed by the patient's preoperative condition, the adequacy of the donor organ, and the operative success of the surgical and anesthetic teams. Indeed, the function of the graft is the dominant factor in the recovery of the patient.

LIVER ALLOGRAFT FUNCTION

Early graft function is usually assessed by measuring circulating concentrations of total bilirubin, aminotransferases, canalicular enzymes, and clotting factors. The scheme shown in Table 235-2 is useful for assessing graft function according to these parameters.[61] Other parameters, such as arterial ketone body ratio (AKBR)[62] and oxygen

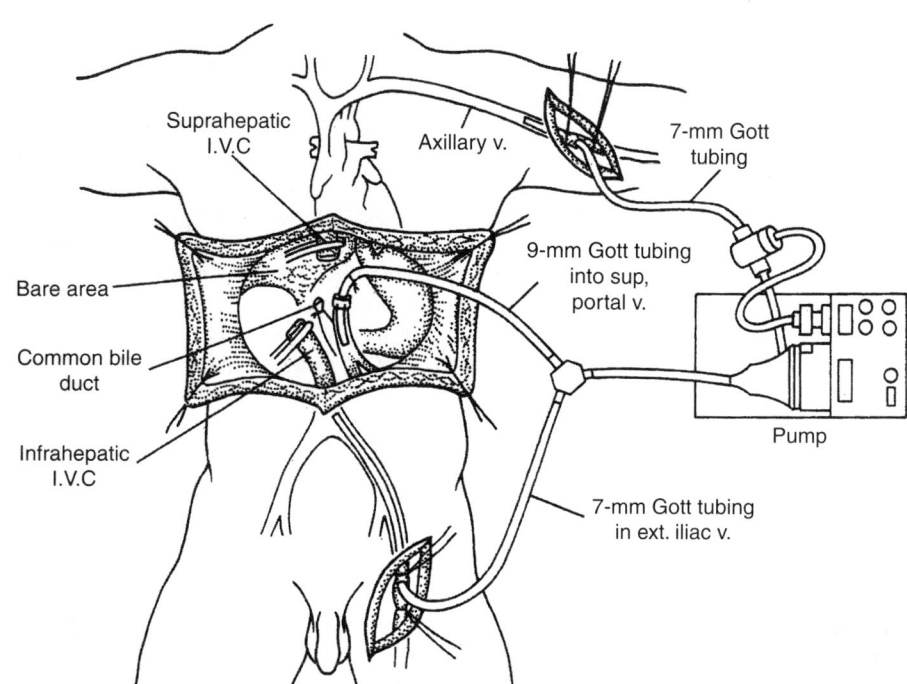

FIGURE 235–2. Venovenous bypass. I.V.C., inferior vena cava; ext. iliac v., external iliac vein. (From Starzl TE, Griffith BP, Shaw BW Jr, et al: Veno-venous bypass without systemic anticoagulation for transplantation of the human liver. Surg Gynecol Obstet 1985;160:270, by permission of Surgery, Gynecology, & Obstetrics.)

Suprahepatic I.V.C

Axillary v.

7-mm Gott tubing

9-mm Gott tubing into sup, portal v.

Bare area

Common bile duct

Infrahepatic I.V.C

Pump

7-mm Gott tubing in ext. iliac v.

TABLE 235–2. CLASSIFICATION OF GRAFT FUNCTION AFTER ORTHOTOPIC LIVER TRANSPLANTATION

Variable	Grade I	Grade II	Grade III	Grade IV
AST ALT	<1000	>1000 initially <1000 at 48 h	>2500 for ≥48 h	>2500 and rising
PT	Normal	Mild prolongation	Very abnormal	Severe coagulopathy
Bile	>40 mL/d	<40 mL/d	Minimal	None

AST, aspartate aminotransferase; ALT, alanine aminotransferase; PT, prothrombin time.
Data from Greig PD, Woolf GM, Sinclair SB, et al: Treatment of primary liver graft nonfunction with prostaglandin E₁. Transplantation 1989;48:447-453.

consumption,[63] also correlate with graft survival. However, in a retrospective review, Doyle and colleagues were unable to identify a unique parameter with adequate sensitivity and specificity to be useful for predicting graft survival in individual OLTX recipients.[64] Other techniques, such as neural network modeling, are under active investigation.[65] An alternative approach is to use a composite acuity score to predict graft and patient survival. For example, Angus and associates showed that the APACHE II score, a widely used severity-of-illness indicator designed for general ICU patients, was useful for predicting both hospital survival and survival at 1 year for liver transplant recipients if the model was recalibrated.[66,67]

Typically, elevated serum bilirubin levels during the first few days after transplantation reflect preoperative values and the consequences of procurement. In the absence of severe procurement injury, serum total bilirubin concentration typically falls to normal during the first week. An injury pattern is evidenced by elevated serum aminotransferase levels. Aspartate aminotransferase (AST) and alanine aminotransferase (ALT) peak during the first 3 days and return toward normal slowly thereafter. Canalicular enzymes (gamma-glutamyl transpeptidase and alkaline phosphatase) typically rise to four or five times normal and return toward normal over the course of the next few weeks. If the liver was injured during procurement, the biochemical changes are greater and last longer. Thus, the peak concentrations for ALT and AST are higher and the serum total bilirubin concentration remains abnormal for a prolonged period, sometimes for weeks, as do circulating levels of canalicular enzymes. Unless the liver is irreversibly damaged, synthetic function normalizes after the third day and the AKBR returns toward 1.0. Although the values may normalize, occasionally graft dysfunction may be evidenced only by the patient's failure to thrive. In particular, MODS may develop or fail to resolve. Re-transplantation may be the only option.

Knowledge of the details of procurement and implantation should color the interpretation of liver function abnormalities in the early postoperative period. Technical problems should always be considered before an immunologic mechanism is implicated. Even with the widespread use of percutaneous liver biopsy, a diagnosis based solely on histology is likely to be incorrect when a vascular or biliary drainage problem is present. Furthermore, if a technical problem is not recognized and impaired liver function is treated as being caused by rejection, then the immunosuppressive regimen will be intensified unnecessarily, placing the patient at grave risk for infectious complications.

The diagnostic work-up for a patient with liver function abnormalities in the perioperative period should include a Doppler ultrasound examination to determine patency of all pertinent vessels. Concern about the adequacy of flow should prompt an angiogram or MR angiogram (MRA). Early occlusion of the hepatic artery should prompt immediate re-exploration, which can result in a nearly 50% graft salvage rate.[68] Early hepatic artery thrombosis may present as a precipitous deterioration in hemodynamics, abrupt development of ARDS, severe coagulopathy, and markedly elevated serum aminotransferase concentrations. Bacteremia is common. Delayed hepatic artery thrombosis is often less dramatic in its presentation.[69] Indeed, some patients are asymptomatic. Others show destruction of the biliary duct system with multiple intrahepatic strictures, bile collections, and intrahepatic abscesses. Recurrent bacteremia, in the absence of another source, may be the only indication of hepatic artery thrombosis.

The presentation of portal venous thrombosis is usually much less dramatic. In the early postoperative period the most frequent manifestation is persistent ascites. Enteric congestion and bleeding as a consequence of portal hypertension may also occur. Later, portal vein thrombosis should be considered in the differential diagnosis, if the patient develops variceal hemorrhage. Although occlusion of the inferior vena cava (IVC) related to retrohepatic caval thrombosis can occur, it is uncommon. Anastomotic strictures are more common. Stenosis at the lower anastomosis of the IVC presents as lower extremity edema and renal dysfunction. Stenosis at the upper anastomosis presents findings similar to those that occur in the Budd-Chiari syndrome, including passive congestion of the liver, ascites, lower extremity edema, and renal failure. The diagnosis may be suggested by ultrasound examination, but more commonly the clinical picture prompts measurements of IVC pressures above and below the anastomoses using a fluoroscopically guided catheter. When strictures are diagnosed, treatment is commonly surgical, but balloon dilatation has been accomplished in some cases.

Patency of the biliary tract should be confirmed using cholangiography, which is simple when a tracheostomy tube or cystic duct tube stents the choledochocholedochostomy. However, this study must be performed percutaneously in patients with choledochojejunostomy, unless a cystic duct tube was used. Disruption of the biliary anastomosis is a rare complication that typically occurs near the end of the first week. Development of this complication may indicate thrombosis of the hepatic artery, which interrupts the blood supply to the donor portion of the common bile duct.

Graft rejection may occur at any point after OLTX. Hyperacute rejection is very rare, if it occurs at all, after OLTX. Nevertheless, a humoral component of rejection may be evidenced by antibody deposition in the arterial endothelium and by persistence or recrudescence of a positive crossmatch.[70] Acute cellular rejection (ACR) is more common and develops in approximately 40% of liver transplant recipients. It typically presents after the first week but can present within the first few days after transplant or present years later. Thus, its usual description as "acute" is a misnomer. The histologic criterion for the diagnosis of ACR is a periductal lymphocytic infiltrate associated with a cellular infiltrate around the central veins.[71] Nevertheless, these changes may be evident to a lesser degree even in the absence of clinical abnormalities. In a graft with stable function, rejection is typically associated with a rise in serum total bilirubin concentration associated with elevations in the circulating levels of aminotransferases and canalicular enzymes. Other clinical findings include signs of the sepsis syndrome, diarrhea, suddenly increasing ascites, eosinophilia, thrombocytopenia, and laboratory evidence of hemolysis. Chronic rejection, also a misnomer because it may occur at any point, is manifested by arteriopathy and vanishing bile ducts. Its presentation is insidious, and signs of terminal liver disease may develop slowly.

IMMUNOSUPPRESSION

The approach to rejection is divided into two phases: prophylaxis and treatment.[72] Prophylaxis is achieved by administering a combination of corticosteroids and cyclosporine (Neoral) or tacrolimus. These agents inhibit IL-2 expression and block T-cell recruitment. They offer a selective approach to immunosuppression in solid organ transplantation. Prospective, randomized trials comparing tacrolimus-based and cyclosporine-based regimens demonstrate that tacrolimus affords better rejection prophylaxis, is associated with less steroid-resistant rejection and need for OKT3,[73,74] and is less costly when medical care in the first post-transplant year is considered.[75]

Azathioprine, used before the advent of newer immunosuppressive agents, is reserved for patients with recurrent rejection episodes or for those unable to tolerate the newer agents. Mycophenolate mofetil is hydrolyzed in vivo to mycophenolic acid. This compound inhibits inosine monophosphate dehydrogenase, resulting in selective inhibition of T- and B-cell proliferation.[76] Mycophenolate mofetil

is more expensive than azathioprine and has gastrointestinal side effects (diarrhea) but less bone marrow toxicity. Data from a prospective randomized trial that enrolled liver transplant recipients indicates that combined tacrolimus, prednisone, and mycophenolate is no more toxic than tacrolimus and prednisone and that the three-drug cocktail may facilitate a reduction in tacrolimus dose.[77] Newer immunosuppressive agents and techniques are under development. The current regimen at Mayo Clinic Jacksonville for prophylaxis is outlined in Table 235-3. Calcineurin inhibition with tacrolimus or cyclosporine is the cornerstone of treatment. Corticosteroids are administered intraoperatively and throughout the early postoperative period. Early introduction of mycophenolate allows a reduction in tacrolimus dose.[78] Sirolimus has been associated with delayed wound healing and hepatic artery thrombosis when administered in the early postoperative period. When introduced later in the transplant course it enables reduction or elimination of the calcineurin inhibition. Thymoglobulin and IL-2 receptor (IL-2r) antagonists may be used for induction of immunosuppression, which allows for delayed introduction of calcineurin inhibitors and is particularly useful in patients with renal impairment at the time of transplantation.

Protocol-driven liver biopsy samples are obtained on day 7. Moderate to severe rejection is treated initially with corticosteroids: 1000 mg of methylprednisolone is administered over a 4-day period (day 0, 500 mg; day 2, 250 mg; day 4, 250 mg). A follow-up liver biopsy is performed on the fifth day. If rejection persists, treatment with 2000 mg of methylprednisolone is given over the next 4 days (day 0, 1000 mg; day 2, 500 mg; day 4, 500 mg). Persistent rejection is deemed "steroid resistant," and treatment with thymoglobulin or OKT3 is indicated.[79-83]

The major side effects of cyclosporine and tacrolimus are similar: both cause significant nephrotoxicity and neurotoxicity.[84] More than 90% of patients[85] sustain some degree of renal injury, which is manifested clinically as azotemia. Renal dysfunction is a consequence of the hemodynamic insults of the procedure and/or the side effects of the calcineurin inhibitors. Ten percent of OLTX patients require some form of renal replacement therapy postoperatively, and a few require

TABLE 235–3. STANDARD IMMUNOSUPPRESSION FOR LIVER TRANSPLANT RECIPIENTS (MAYO CLINIC JACKSONVILLE)

Agent	Initiate	Dose	Target Level	Comments
Tacrolimus	Day 1	0.05 mg/kg p.o. bid	8-12 (days 0-21) 6-10 (days 22-365)	Adjust for renal dysfunction: half dose Cr 1.5-2.0; hold Cr >2.0
Mycophenolate mofetil	Day 0	1000 mg bid start before surgery		Cancer: discontinue once tacrolimus therapeutic
Methylprednisolone	Intraoperative	500 mg		Additional 500 mg if >7 RBCs transfused intraoperative
Methylprednisolone	Day 0	50 mg i.v. bid		
Prednisone	Day 1	25 mg p.o. bid		Taper by day 15 if recurrent hepatitis C virus
	Day 2-3	20 mg p.o. bid		
	Day 4-6	15 mg p.o. bid		
	Day 7-14	10 mg p.o. bid		
	Day 15-20	15 mg p.o. qd		
	Day 21-29	10 mg p.o. qd		
	Day 30-60	7.5 mg p.o. qd		
	Day 61-90	5 mg p.o. qd		
	Day 91-119	2.5 mg p.o. qd		
	Day 120	Discontinue		

long-term hemodialysis. Neurotoxicity is more evident in the elderly and is compounded by serum electrolyte disturbances, particularly hyponatremia and hypomagnesemia.[86] Neurologic dysfunction ranges from a mild expressive aphasia to tremors, confusion, coma, and seizures. Other side effects of cyclosporine, such as hypertension and hirsutism, occur less commonly with tacrolimus. Because tacrolimus is a more potent agent, many patients are able to have the dose of corticosteroids tapered, if not completely discontinued.[87,88]

Abnormal liver function can be a complication of serious systemic illness. For example, hyperbilirubinemia can occur in patients with sepsis and is known as cholestasis lenta. However, jaundice may occur with the development of pneumonia or may herald the presence of an abscess. Other systemic processes, such as disseminated fungal infections (caused by *Candida* species or *Aspergillus*) and herpesvirus infections, such as those caused by herpes simplex or herpes zoster virus, may result in profound derangements of liver function. Another systemic process that can affect the liver is lymphoma. Non-Hodgkin's lymphomas can develop after solid organ transplantation; these malignancies are called post-transplant lymphoproliferative disease. This disease is a function of T-cell suppression mediated by Epstein-Barr virus and may respond to reduction in immunosuppression and antiviral therapy. The transplanted liver may be involved.

HEMODYNAMIC CHANGES

The characteristic hemodynamic changes of ESLD resolve slowly after OLTX. The exact timing is unresolved, and the controversy likely reflects the preoperative state of some of the patients. Thus, problems resolve more slowly in patients with profoundly deranged liver function and MODS than in recipients, who are less ill at the time of transplantation. A vasodilated hyperdynamic state is typical of liver failure[89-93] and rarely normalizes in the immediate postoperative period. Patients who are unable to mount a hyperdynamic response fare worse. Some recipients have preexisting cardiac dysfunction owing to ischemic damage or restrictive cardiomyopathy secondary to amyloidosis or hemochromatosis; these patients are unable to increase stroke volume and cardiac output in response to vasodilation. Similarly, patients with sepsis have a higher mortality if they fail to increase ventricular end-diastolic volume to preserve stroke volume as ejection fraction falls and increase heart rate to increase cardiac output.[94] Elevated central venous pressures are transmitted to the hepatic vein and through the liver. Hepatic congestion results in impaired clearance of bacteria, endotoxin, and cytokines. Elevated hepatic venous pressures are reflected in elevated portal pressures, which increase bacterial translocation and endotoxemia, further compromising graft function. Resuscitation must be guided by measurement of central venous pressure. The etiology of hypotension should be classified as cardiac—a consequence of inadequate preload or impaired contractility—or loss of arterial tone.

Management of hypotension requires immediate restoration of adequate circulating volume, usually to a central venous pressure of less than 12 mm Hg. Inotropic support, using dobutamine or epinephrine, should be added if cardiac output remains low despite volume loading. More typically, patients with liver failure are hyperdynamic and vasodilated. In the distributive shock of liver failure, as in septic shock, norepinephrine restores regional blood flow more effectively than dopamine. Low dose vasopressin (0.04 unit/min) effectively restores perfusion pressure in patients with liver failure. However, vasopressin reduces portal flow and, hence, hepatic perfusion; these effects obviously might be undesirable in transplant recipients with compromised portal flow. Right ventricular function may be gauged using echocardiography or estimating ejection fraction. Then calculate the end-diastolic volume with a pulmonary artery catheter equipped with a rapid response thermistor (Edwards Lifesciences Corp., Irvine, CA). Marked arterial vasodilation requires treatment with vasopressors, particularly when it occurs in the presence of improving graft function. Marked vasodilation, however, also should prompt an evaluation to exclude a focus of inflammation, infection, pancreatitis, or graft rejection.

Cardiac tamponade should be considered in the differential diagnosis of low cardiac output associated with high filling pressures. There are surgical and medical factors that increase the potential for tamponade. Surgical considerations include the superior aspect of the "Mercedes" incision, which can violate the pericardial parietal reflection, and unintentional inclusion of the right atrium in the superior anastomosis to the inferior vena cava. Medical considerations include impaired coagulation, thrombocytopenia, and renal failure. When tamponade develops in the setting of a hyperdynamic and vasodilated state, cardiac output, calculated systemic vascular resistance, and arterial-venous oxygen content difference all may be deceptively normal.

Although hypotension is a more common problem, arterial hypertension may occur in the postoperative period. It commonly reflects inadequate analgesia or sedation,[16] impaired gas exchange, or hypoglycemia. However, hypertension may persist once these factors are addressed, and attention should then focus on the toxic side effects of cyclosporine[95,96] and tacrolimus. Both drugs are vasoconstrictors and may promote hypertension by activating the renin-angiotensin pathway. This complication occurs more commonly with cyclosporine (30% of cases) than with tacrolimus (10% of cases), and cyclosporine-induced hypertension is more resistant to antihypertensive therapy.[97-99] Antihypertensive therapy should be initiated when systolic blood pressure is greater than 160 mm Hg or diastolic blood pressure is greater than 95 mm Hg. I favor combined alpha- and beta-adrenergic receptor blockade with labetalol. Long-term management rests on a combination of angiotensin-converting enzyme (ACE) inhibition, alpha-adrenergic blockade, and calcium channel blockade. Hypertension resistant to the first-line agents is usually managed in the ICU with potent vasodilators, such as sodium nitroprusside, perhaps in combination with an alpha-adrenergic blocking agent.

PULMONARY CONSIDERATIONS

Pulmonary complications of ESLD are common.[99] Atelectasis, pleural effusion, reduced functional residual capacity, and limited vital capacity, due to ascites and chest wall edema, are often present preoperatively. The operative procedure in the upper abdomen, placement of a "normal" sized graft in the site of a shrunken, cirrhotic liver, and postoperative ileus can further decrease vital capacity. Inadequate pain control results in splinting and atelectasis and increases the risk of pneumonia. However, long-term pulmonary sequelae are rare, and most patients have improved pulmonary function tests when studied more than 1 year after OLTX.

Pulmonary infiltrates in patients with liver disease warrant immediate evaluation. Pulmonary infection should be considered, but many pulmonary infiltrates have a noninfectious cause. Pulmonary edema, on the basis of a hydrostatic or a nonhydrostatic mechanism, is common. Nonhydrostatic pulmonary edema (i.e., ARDS) when associated with decreased lung compliance and a requirement for increased FiO_2 to maintain adequate oxygenation, may result from a primary pulmonary infection but more commonly is associated with intra-abdominal inflammation, such as peritonitis and pancreatitis. Graft failure, whether caused by rejection or primary nonfunction or vascular catastrophe (e.g., hepatic artery thrombosis) may also lead to development of ARDS. When liver failure per se is the cause, ARDS usually resolves after successful transplantation.[100] ARDS also may develop during treatment of rejection with OKT3.[101]

Bronchoscopic techniques are used routinely to aid the clinical assessment of pulmonary infiltrates and to establish the diagnosis of pneumonia.[102] Despite the severe coagulopathy that often is present, bronchoalveolar lavage may be performed without significant risk of hemorrhage. Quantitative cultures are obtained and the presence of bacteria at more than 100,000 colony-forming units (CFU)/mL is considered diagnostic of pneumonia. Bronchoalveolar lavage is sensitive but lacks specificity. In selected cases when the identity of the primary offending agent is required, a protected-brush specimen can be collected in a "blind" (i.e., nonbronchoscopic) fashion. Quantitative cultures are obtained; a finding of more than 1000 CFU/mL is considered positive. Complications are rare, but I have avoided this technique in patients with severe coagulopathy. In a study carried out by Chaparala and colleagues, bronchoscopic confirmation was obtained for only one third of cases of suspected pneumonia.[103] Although antibiotic administration confounds the results in some patients, in most cases negative results force an evaluation for other sites of infection or inflammation.

Matuschak and associates have described liver-lung interactions.[104,105] Acute lung injury is common in advanced liver failure.[106] Patients with liver failure and ARDS are at high risk for mortality and are usually eliminated as candidates for liver transplantation. However, in highly selected patients with liver failure and ARDS, lung injury resolves quickly after successful OLTX.[107]

Two additional pulmonary complications—the hepatopulmonary syndrome and pulmonary hypertension—also may develop in patients with liver disease. Cyanosis sometimes occurs in patients with cirrhosis.[108] Several explanations have been tendered. Anatomic right-to-left shunts have been described within the pulmonary circulation[109,110] and between the portal venous system and the pulmonary veins via esophageal veins.[111] Increased closing volume, resulting in air trapping, has been observed. A leftward shift of the oxyhemoglobin saturation curve also has been reported.[112] Most important, many patients have a diffusion defect. Furthermore, hypoxic pulmonary vasoconstriction is impaired. These findings correlate with anatomic studies showing dilated intrapulmonary capillaries.[113] Additionally, studies using inert gas washout techniques have demonstrated that hepatic dysfunction is associated with significant ventilation-perfusion mismatching rather than pure shunt. Patients with the hepatopulmonary syndrome have dilated pulmonary capillaries, which lead to diffusion impairment. Furthermore, increased dispersion in the ventilation-perfusion relationship results in mismatching such that many poorly ventilated units are excessively perfused.[114] Ventilation-perfusion mismatching does not constitute a true right-to-left shunt, which explains the observation that hyperoxia results from prolonged exposure to high FiO_2. The most useful preoperative test is contrast echocardiography, using tiny air bubbles as the contrast agent ("bubble study"). Normally, no contrast agent appears on the left side of the heart after venous injection of the bubbles. The appearance of contrast agent immediately after injection suggests an intracardiac shunt (i.e., patent foramen ovale); contrast agent that appears later (i.e., third to the sixth cardiac cycle) suggests intrapulmonary shunting.[115] Hypoxia usually resolves within the first month, but sometimes resolution is delayed for as long as year after transplantation. Patients who fail to improve should be investigated with pulmonary angiography to identify a single shunt large enough to be embolized.[116]

Pulmonary hypertension occurs more commonly in patients with cirrhosis than in controls and is called portopulmonary hypertension.[117] Other than cirrhosis, no predisposing factor has been identified. The histopathologic abnormalities in the lungs are typical of primary pulmonary hypertension. Secondary causes of pulmonary hypertension, particularly left ventricular failure, left-to-right intracardiac shunting with increased cardiac output, autoimmune disease, and pulmonary embolism, should be eliminated from consideration and both portal and pulmonary hypertension confirmed for the diagnosis of portopulmonary hypertension to be established. In an advanced state it may be difficult to distinguish portopulmonary hypertension from primary cardiac failure with secondary venous congestion and hepatic failure. Portal hypertension can be diagnosed on clinical grounds by the presence of varices, splenomegaly, and ascites or can be measured directly by hepatic vein catheterization and measurement of free and wedged pressures, the latter being an estimate of presinusoidal portal pressure. Echocardiography allows estimation of pulmonary pressures by measuring the regurgitant flow velocity through the tricuspid valve. However, confirmation with pulmonary artery catheterization is necessary. Severe pulmonary hypertension recognized only at the start of the OLTX warrants cancellation of the procedure. In contrast to patients with primary pulmonary hypertension, patients with portopulmonary hypertension benefit minimally from acute pharmacologic interventions directed at reducing the pulmonary arterial pressures. Therapeutic measures such as organic nitrates, sodium nitroprusside, or calcium channel blockers fail to reduce pulmonary artery pressure and can lead to systemic hypotension. Low systemic arterial pressure, in turn, can promote right ventricular ischemia and impair right ventricular function. Initial studies suggested that patients with portopulmonary hypertension are unresponsive to inhaled nitric oxide.[118] Subsequent experience suggests that inhaled nitric oxide ameliorates pulmonary hypertension and improves arterial oxygenation in some patients.[119,120]

An alternative approach borrows from the experience gained by clinicians using continuous infusions of epoprostanil (Flolan) to lower pulmonary artery pressure in patients with primary pulmonary hypertension. Prolonged infusion of the drug over weeks or months allows gradual upward titration of the dose,[121] a tactic that ameliorates pulmonary hypertension without causing systemic hypotension. Cardiac remodeling ensues, leading to improved cardiac output, reduced tricuspid regurgitation, and normalization

TABLE 235–4. PULMONARY HYPERTENSION AND LIVER DISEASE

Category	Mean PA Pressure (mm Hg)	Systolic PA Pressure (mm Hg)
Mild	25-34	35-44
Moderate	35-44	45-59
Severe	45-75	60-100
Very severe	>75	>100

PA, pulmonary artery.

of central venous pressure. The goal of treatment with epoprostanil is a systolic pulmonary artery pressure (PAP) of less than 60 mm Hg (mean < 40 mm Hg), low central venous pressure, elevated cardiac output, and normal response to fluid challenge (i.e., slight increase in PAP, central venous pressure, and right ventricular end-diastolic volume and a large increase in cardiac output). The change in PAP during exercise may provide additional insight into the assessment and management of patients with portopulmonary hypertension. Pulmonary hypertension resolves in some patients after successful OLTX.[122,123] Patients treated with epoprostanil require continued infusion during the immediate postoperative period but usually can be weaned off the drug over the course of several weeks. Although patients with mild pulmonary hypertension (see Table 235-4 for definitions) can tolerate OLTX without significant complications, the picture is bleak for those with moderate to severe pulmonary hypertension (systolic PAP > 60 mm Hg). Most transplant recipients with severe pulmonary hypertension die of right-sided heart failure during reperfusion or during the early recovery phase. These patients tolerate massive fluid shifts poorly. Right ventricular overload and failure develop abruptly, compromising the viability of the graft and resulting in massive hepatic and mesenteric congestion. Low cardiac output results in graft ischemia. These patients succumb quickly, owing to development of MODS, and they are not currently considered candidates for liver transplantation.

Pulmonary hypertension that develops de novo during or acutely after liver transplantation may result from embolic phenomena at the time of transplantation that may be evident on intraoperative transesophageal echocardiography. Patients should be managed with attention to sustaining right ventricular coronary perfusion by maintenance of adequate mean arterial pressure and avoidance of central venous hypertension. Pulmonary hypertension can develop late after liver transplantation. This problem is not always directly related to portal hypertension, because liver function may be normal and the transhepatic venous pressure gradient (pressure difference between wedged and free hepatic venous pressures) may be normal.[124]

Alternative strategies to reduce pulmonary pressure in patients with portopulmonary hypertension are less well documented. Endothelin inhibitors such as bosentan increase the 6-minute walk distance but cause reversible cholestasis. A therapeutic trial of bosentan may still be warranted, but the drug should be discontinued if liver function tests fail to improve on therapy. Despite clinical improvement, a significant decrease in pulmonary artery pressures has not been demonstrated such that OLTX might be considered with this agent alone. Phosphodiesterase-5 inhibitors, such as sildenafil, lower PAP and may serve as an adjunct to epoprostanil. In liver failure, calcium channel blockade results in systemic hypotension before significantly decreasing PAP. However, once systemic hemodynamics normalize after OLTX, treatment with calcium channel blockers is better tolerated.

Mechanical ventilatory support is often required preoperatively for patients with ESLD. Intubation to minimize aspiration is required when the patient cannot protect the airway because of encephalopathy or massive upper gastrointestinal hemorrhage. Respiratory failure can be precipitated by volume overload and pulmonary edema, infection, or profound muscle weakness. These same factors affect the timing of extubation. One must balance the risk of pulmonary infection associated with an endotracheal tube and impaired clearance of secretions with the risks of aspiration and infection resulting from poor cough after extubation. The patient should have a clear mental state and improving liver function values before extubation. Previously, the median duration of intubation after transplantation was 2 days. Recent changes in anesthetic techniques allow many patients to be extubated in the PACU. Now the median duration of intubation for patients who require ICU admission is less than 24 hours. Early extubation postoperatively is the goal, and immediate postoperative extubation is possible in those having an uncomplicated intraoperative course and no life-threatening premorbid extrahepatic organ dysfunction.[125,126]

RENAL CONSIDERATIONS

Renal dysfunction in patients with liver disease is frequently unrecognized. Liver dysfunction and malnutrition make elevations in blood urea nitrogen and serum creatinine concentration unimpressive, despite a significant decrease in glomerular filtration rate. In the post-transplant period, several factors conspire to impair renal function. These factors include preoperative renal failure (hepatorenal syndrome), episodic arterial hypotension resulting in tubular damage, medications (e.g., cyclosporine, tacrolimus, and vasopressors) that cause renal arterial vasoconstriction, and amphotericin, which causes tubular damage.[127] Furthermore, liver allograft dysfunction leads to functional renal impairment—the hepatorenal syndrome. Renal replacement therapy is required for approximately 10% of patients. Continuous renal replacement offers greater hemodynamic stability. This mode of renal replacement results in less complement activation and possibly less end-organ damage and earlier recovery of renal function. The putative renal protective effects of dopamine, calcium channel blockers, and prostaglandin E_1 remain to be demonstrated convincingly in this population.

GASTROINTESTINAL CONSIDERATIONS

Enteral nutrition may be started early in the postoperative period in patients with a choledochocholedochostomy, whereas it is usually deferred for 72 hours in patients with a choledochojejunostomy, because these patients also have undergone jejunojejunostomy (Fig. 235-3). When parenteral nutrition is required, I use crystalline amino acids and supply one third of the nonprotein calories as fat. This approach minimizes glucose intolerance, which is common in the early post-OLTX period.

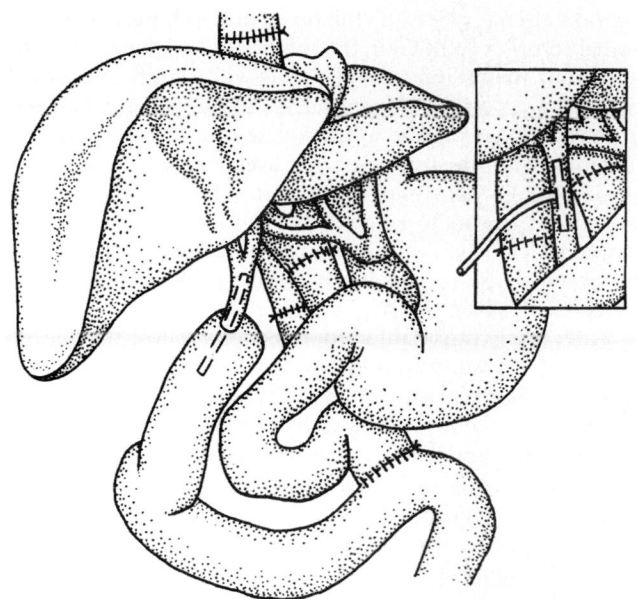

FIGURE 235–3. Choledochojejunostomy and choledochocholedochostomy. (Reprinted with permission from Starzl TE, Demetrius AJ, Van Thiel D: Liver transplantation. N Engl J Med 1989;321:1014, 1092.)

Upper gastrointestinal bleeding in the OLTX recipient is uncommon, but prompt investigation is mandatory when it occurs. Gastritis and stress ulceration are common causes. Recurrence of esophageal and gastric varices often reflects diminished portal vein blood flow or complete thrombosis. Bleeding distal to the ligament of Treitz may be from the site of the jejunojejunostomy. Visualization may require a pediatric colonoscope. Revision of the anastomosis may be unnecessary in most patients by correction of coagulation.

Bleeding from the gastrointestinal tract weeks or months after surgery should prompt a work-up for infectious causes, such as cytomegalovirus (CMV) infection or *Clostridium difficile* enterocolitis. Bleeding may be a manifestation of neoplastic gastrointestinal involvement with lymphoma. Mesenteric and splenic artery aneurysms are associated with portal hypertension and may rupture postoperatively. These lesions are usually recognized at postmortem examination. However, some patients develop an arterioenteric fistula and present with massive gastrointestinal hemorrhage. Angiography can confirm the diagnosis in more stable patients but should not delay exploration because rapid surgical repair is mandatory.

Pancreatitis is a feared complication of OLTX. Although nearly 20% of patients demonstrate biochemical abnormalities, such as elevated serum amylase or lipase levels, only 5% have clinically significant pancreatitis.[128] Conservative measures are usually effective in mild cases. Management of severe pancreatitis is as controversial in this setting as it is in patients without OLTX. The roles of somatostatin and operative débridement with continuous lavage remain to be defined.

NEUROLOGIC CONSIDERATIONS

Patients with minimal pretransplant hepatic encephalopathy who have an uncomplicated operation and receive a well-functioning graft recover rapidly from anesthesia. Changes in mental status require a thorough evaluation. Most commonly, the side effects of immunosuppressive agents, such as

cyclosporine and tacrolimus, may be incriminated but resolved with adjustment of doses. The presence of focal deficits should prompt concern about the possibility of embolic or hemorrhagic complications. Intracranial infection is rare in the early postoperative period but should be considered in patients with headache and confusion.

Patients with early graft dysfunction also often have changes in mentation. Graft swelling may result in portal congestion and portosystemic shunting. Administration of flumazenil may produce a more awake but still encephalopathic patient. The exact mechanism for encephalopathy due to graft dysfunction remains to be elucidated. Side effects of medications assume a much greater role in such patients. Clearance of commonly used immunosuppressive agents, analgesics, sedatives, and hypnotics is impaired. The amnestic effects of some agents may compound the problem. I favor short-acting narcotics, such as fentanyl, for analgesia and propofol[129] or short-acting benzodiazepines, such as midazolam, for sedation. Severe agitated delirium responds best to haloperidol.

The seizure threshold is lowered by several medications used in liver transplant recipients, including cyclosporine, tacrolimus, OKT3, and haloperidol.[130,131] Electrolyte abnormalities, such as hyponatremia and hypomagnesaemia, are common and further lower the seizure threshold. Hypoglycemia also must be considered and rapidly treated.

Nonconvulsive or akinetic seizures, although rare, are more common in this ICU population and should be considered in the differential diagnosis of the comatose patient. Continuous electroencephalography allows seizure detection as well as assessment of the effectiveness of treatment. To minimize the complications of therapeutic coma, it is better to titrate doses of pentobarbital or propofol to burst suppression of 5 to 10 seconds rather than use fixed infusion rates or rely on serum levels.

Patients with FHF require special neurologic consideration. These patients have encephalopathy that is mediated, at least in part, by gamma-aminobutyric acid, as is the case for patients with the portosystemic encephalopathy of chronic liver disease,[132] but they also have intracranial hypertension and cerebral edema.[133] Patients in grade III and grade IV coma should have ICP monitored either with a parenchymal monitor, such as the Codman or Camino devices, or with a combined ventriculostomy and ventricular pressure monitor, such as the Aesculap system. The latter allows drainage of cerebrospinal fluid to directly reduce ICP. The more invasive systems are associated with a higher incidence of complications, including infection and bleeding. CBF can be measured with xenon-133 or with cold xenon as contrast for computed tomographic (CT) scanning. Cerebral oxygen consumption can be determined after placement of a jugular bulb catheter.[122] Cerebral metabolic rate ($CMRO_2$) is related to the product of the CBF and arterial-venous oxygen content difference ($AJVdO_2 = CaO_2 - Cj\overline{v}O_2$), according to the following formula:

$$CMRO_2 = CBF \times AJVdO_2/100.$$

Intracranial hypertension may result from increased CBF or cerebral edema. Elevated CBF with normal oxygen consumption is associated with narrow $AJVdO_2$, whereas cerebral edema is associated with decreased CBF and large $AJVdO_2$. Elevated CBF often heralds increasing ICP.[134] The appropriate approach for treatment of intracranial hypertension depends on the underlying pathophysiology. Elevated ICP with increased CBF responds to hyperventilation, reducing intravascular volume and hypothermia. However, intracranial hypertension with depressed CBF must be treated by increasing mean arterial pressure and administering osmotic agents, such as mannitol, so long as renal function is preserved or continuous renal replacement therapy has been initiated. Hypothermia and therapeutic coma with propofol using continuous EEG monitoring are useful adjuncts in this latter group as well. Patients are considered viable candidates for OLTX as long as EEG activity is preserved and adequate cerebral perfusion pressure and CBF can be maintained. Intraoperative monitoring includes these measures, combined with transcranial Doppler measurements of flow velocity contour in the middle cerebral artery,[135] which facilitate moment-to-moment titration of anesthetics and vasopressors. Although the initial period of graft reperfusion is the most hazardous, cerebral hyperemia and intracranial hypertension may persist for several days postoperatively. These abnormalities usually resolve with good graft function.

Liver transplant recipients are at risk for neuromuscular dysfunction. In a prospective study of 100 liver transplant recipients, my colleagues and I used electromyography and muscle biopsy to supplement the physical examination in patients with muscle weakness. Clinically relevant weakness, defined as weakness requiring prolonged mechanical ventilatory support, occurred in 7% of patients. Electromyography demonstrated that weakness was due to a myopathic rather than neuropathic process, and diffuse myocyte necrosis was evident on muscle biopsy specimens taken from five patients.[136] Predisposing factors included patient acuity postoperatively, as judged by the APACHE II score, poor graft function at 1 week, a requirement for renal replacement therapy, and higher doses of corticosteroids. Patients requiring early retransplantation seemed to be at particular risk.

INFECTIOUS COMPLICATIONS

Rejection of the allograft is treated aggressively when it develops. These measures are often complicated by the parallel development of infections. Heavily immunosuppressed patients die not of rejection but of infection. The paradigm is that immunosuppression sufficient to eliminate rejection results in a defenseless host susceptible to many infections. Solid organs vary in their propensity to stimulate rejection. The liver is relatively less immunogenic; accordingly, immunosuppression can be less intensive but still be effective. In the early postoperative period, bacterial and fungal infections are common. The most frequently involved areas are the operative site and the lungs. Perioperative antimicrobial prophylaxis targets gram-negative rods and enterococci and consists of a second- or third-generation cephalosporin or ampicillin-sulbactam and is continued for 48 hours. Prophylactic regimens vary among centers. Unfortunately, antimicrobial resistance is common and isolates in patients who die of an infectious process are occasionally resistant to all known antimicrobial agents.[137]

Fungal colonization is also common. Patients requiring a prolonged, difficult surgical procedure and multiple transfusions of blood products are at higher risk for fungal infection as are patients undergoing retransplantation.[138,139] Prophylactic antifungal therapy reduces the incidence of both superficial and deep fungal infections. Options include fluconazole,[140] amphotericin (10 to 20 mg daily for the first 2 weeks after surgery), or full doses of amphotericin B liposomal complex (ABLC) in the subgroup at highest risk of filamentous fungal infection. Patients with significant growth of Candida species on quantitative culture of bronchoalveolar lavage often require a full course of amphotericin.[141,142] The outcome has improved for liver transplant recipients who develop Aspergillus infection. This previously fatal infection[143] seems to respond better to liposomal forms of amphotericin, such as ABLC, and I have followed prolonged intravenous use of this agent with a prolonged course of itraconazole given orally.

Later after transplantation, infections reflect the specific effects of immunosuppressive agents on T-cell function. Although bacterial and fungal infections occur, viral infections and infections caused by opportunistic pathogens become more important. Pneumonia caused by *Pneumocystis carinii* was common before the advent of routine prophylaxis with trimethoprim-sulfamethoxazole. Its occurrence now is limited to those for whom prophylactic measures have been stopped.

CMV infections are common in the transplant population.[144,145] However, the clinical severity of infection is quite variable. Some cases are asymptomatic. Others present as a viral syndrome, involve only one organ such as the lungs, gastrointestinal tract, or liver, or involve multiple organs. The patients at highest risk for CMV infection are those who were seronegative before OLTX and received an organ from a seropositive donor. It is debatable whether patients who were seropositive before OLTX experience reactivation of latent virus or are infected by another CMV strain. In addition to the morbidity and mortality attributed directly to CMV, patients with CMV disease also have a higher frequency of bacterial and fungal infections. Increased susceptibility to bacterial and fungal infections may be a function of the CMV infection per se or reflect the effects of more aggressive immunosuppression (e.g., treatment with OKT3) that is a risk factor for CMV infection. Seroconversion may not occur until T-cell immunosuppression is withdrawn.[146]

Prophylactic measures to prevent symptomatic CMV disease are under investigation. One study compared a 2-week course of ganciclovir followed by high-dose acyclovir to high-dose acyclovir alone.[147] At 24 weeks, CMV infection was evident in 60% and disease in 40% of those treated with acyclovir alone, but in the ganciclovir group the rate of infection was only 28% and the rate of disease was only 12%. Surprisingly, these benefits were not realized in the highest risk group (i.e., donor positive, recipient negative). Additional measures, such as CMV immunoglobulin administration, are under investigation.[148,149]

An alternate strategy is to monitor patients closely for evidence of CMV disease. This approach minimizes unnecessary treatment of patients who will not develop CMV disease but also minimizes the delay in those who require treatment. CMV viremia can be recognized very early using the pp65 antigen.[150] Serial determinations in transplant recipients with a sufficiently low threshold of 10 positive cells per 200,000 white blood cells counted in seropositive recipients and any positive cells in seronegative recipients has resulted in good sensitivity and specificity. I treat with ganciclovir until the pp65 antigen test becomes negative. I use foscarnet in cases of clinical progression despite adequate ganciclovir treatment or when pancytopenia is resistant and reflects drug toxicity rather than a primary effect of the CMV infection.

ENDOCRINE CONSIDERATIONS

Hyperglycemia is common in the early postoperative period and reflects the combination of stress and administration of corticosteroids. Patients are routinely managed with continuous infusions of insulin. The dose of insulin is adjusted according to a sliding scale: units of insulin per hour = 0.03 × (blood glucose concentration [mg/dL] − 60 [mg/dL]) with hourly bedside glucose measurements. Conversion to six doses daily and then to twice-daily therapy with regular and NPH insulin is achieved after discharge from the ICU for patients with glucose intolerance. Although lower doses of corticosteroids are possible with cyclosporine and tacrolimus, both of these drugs also impair glucose tolerance. The recognition that increased atherosclerosis occurs in transplant recipients makes tight control of the blood glucose level desirable. Unfortunately, hypoglycemia may be precipitated by liver allograft failure because gluconeogenesis is impaired. The sudden development of marked hyperglycemia or symptomatic hypoglycemia, which is not iatrogenic, should prompt an evaluation for infection.

Adrenal insufficiency is well recognized in patients receiving corticosteroids. An additional factor to consider in these patients is that the right adrenal gland is often sacrificed during the transplant procedure. Adrenal gland infection may be caused by CMV. Adrenal hemorrhage has been observed in patients with profound coagulopathy and in those with gram-negative sepsis. A depressed cortisol response to the corticotropin analog cosyntropin has been a useful diagnostic adjunct for the clinical decision whether to maintain corticosteroid supplementation.

Thyroid dysfunction, particularly hypothyroidism, is common in patients with primary biliary cirrhosis and in autoimmune hepatitis. Sometimes this diagnosis is not considered preoperatively and becomes apparent in the postoperative period as changes in mental status, depressed cardiac output, and arrhythmias prompt evaluation. As with other critical illness, the euthyroid sick syndrome is commonly identified in OLTX patients when a low thyroxine and normal thyroid-stimulating hormone are noted. When newly diagnosed and treated, an addisonian crisis can be averted with adequate corticosteroid replacement.

CONCLUSION

Patients with terminal liver disease can undergo successful transplantation. Critically ill patients with ESLD have dramatic improvement in their quality of life. Intensive care of such patients is demanding but highly rewarding. The acuity of patients and the likelihood of success with liver transplantation for the critically ill must be gauged. The transplant intensivist provides support and guidance for "fast-tracked" patients who can be managed outside the ICU. Developments in the future will focus on optimal candidate selection and more precise immunosuppression.

ANNOTATED REFERENCES

Viral Hepatitis

Grellier L, Mutimer D, Ahmed M, et al: Lamivudine prophylaxis against reinfection in liver transplantation for hepatitis B cirrhosis. Lancet 1996;348:1212.

Prophylaxis against recurrent hepatitis B virus infection has dramatically altered the prospects for these patients after transplantation.

Fulminant Hepatic Failure

O'Grady JG, Gimson AES, O'Brien CJ, et al: Controlled trials of charcoal hemoperfusion and prognostic factors in fulminant hepatic failure. Gastroenterology 1988;94:1186.

O'Grady JG, Alexander GJM, Hayllar KM, et al: Early indicators of prognosis in fulminant hepatic failure. Gastroenterology 1989;97:439.

These two papers set the standard for evaluation of liver support devices. It was not until a randomized controlled prospective study of charcoal hemoperfusion demonstrated no benefit that the field was able to move forward and consider alternative approaches. To date, no subsequent study of support devices has been as robust.

Thromboelastography

Kang YG, Martin DJ, Marquez J, et al: Intraoperative changes in blood coagulation and thromboelastographic monitoring in liver transplantation. Anesth Analg 1985;64:888.

This paper presents the value of an old approach to assessment and monitoring of coagulation that lends itself to point-of-care testing in the ICU and the operating room.

Outcome Prediction

Angus DC, Clermont G, Kramer DJ, et al: Short- and long-term outcome prediction with the APACHE II system after orthotopic liver transplantation. Crit Care Med 2000;28:150-156.

Kamath PS, Wiesner RH, Malinchoc M, et al: A model to predict survival in patients with end-stage liver disease. Hepatology 2001;33:464-470.

Determination of the acuity of recipients allows distribution of organs to the most ill recipients. It also enables comparison among programs for quality control. However, recipient scoring only accounts for part of the outcome variability because donor characteristics and surgical technique are independent factors.

Immunosuppression

European FK506 Multicentre Liver Study Group: Randomised trial comparing tacrolimus (FK506) and cyclosporin in prevention of liver allograft rejection. Lancet 1994;344:423-428.

The U.S. Multicenter FK506 Liver Study Group: A comparison of tacrolimus (FK 506) and cyclosporine for immunosuppression in liver transplantation. N Engl J Med 1994;331:1110-1115.

Lake JR, Gorman KJ, Esquivel CO, et al: The impact of immunosuppressive regimens on the cost of liver transplantation—results from the U.S. FK506 multicenter trial. Transplantation 1995;60:1089-1095.

These are key papers that present the comparison of these two critical immunosuppressants for both clinical and fiscal interests. They are well done and have yet to be replicated with newer immunosuppressants. They demonstrate that for liver transplantation tacrolimus is more effective and less expensive than cyclosporine. Furthermore, although there are significant differences in the side effect profiles of these medications, they are similar with regard to nephrotoxicity and neurotoxicity.

Portopulmonary Hypertension

Krowka MJ, McGoon MD: Portopulmonary hypertension: The next step. Chest 1997;112:869.

Kuo PC, Johnson LB, Plotkin JS, et al: Continuous infusion of epoprostenol for the treatment of portopulmonary hypertension. Transplantation 1997; 63:604.

Portopulmonary hypertension has excluded many patients from liver transplantation and many more died of complications directly related to right-sided heart failure. These papers outline differences between primary pulmonary hypertension and portopulmonary hypertension and the benefit of therapeutic intervention.

Cytomegalovirus

Grossi P, Kusne S, Rinaldo C, et al: Guidance of ganciclovir therapy with pp65 antigenemia in cytomegalovirus-free recipients of livers from seropositive donors. Transplantation 1996;61:1659.

This paper emphasizes the value of determining at-risk patients, those with cytomegalovirus viremia, and treating them effectively before they develop organ dysfunction such as gastroenteritis, pneumonitis, or hepatitis.

Chapter 236

INTESTINAL AND MULTIPLE ORGAN TRANSPLANTATION

George Mazariegos • Jorge Reyes • Kareem Abu-Elmagd • Thomas E. Starzl

KEY POINTS

1. Causes of short gut syndrome involve both surgical causes (e.g., volvulus, necrotizing enterocolitis, mesenteric thrombosis) or functional causes such as motility disorders (e.g., intestinal pseudo-obstruction) and absorptive insufficiencies such as microvillous inclusion disease.

2. Indications for intestinal transplantation approved by Medicare in 2000 include (1) evidence of liver dysfunction or failure; (2) loss of major venous access; (3) frequent central line–related sepsis; (4) recurrent episodes of severe dehydration despite intravenous fluid management.

3. Recipient operations should be tailored to the specific indications of each patient and include isolated intestinal transplantation, combined liver-intestinal transplantation, and multivisceral transplantation, including the stomach.

4. Immunosuppression for intestinal transplantation is based on tacrolimus and steroids. Current modifications in intestinal transplantation include pretreatment of the recipient with antilymphocyte antibody such as antithymocyte antibody to allow for the elimination of maintenance steroid use postoperatively.

5. Sepsis after intestinal transplantation should prompt a rapid examination for technical reasons (e.g., intra-abdominal abscess, anastomotic dehiscence), immunologic events (rejection may lead to bacterial translocation), or Epstein Barr virus–mediated viremia or post-transplant lymphoproliferative disease.

The evolution of intestinal transplantation has distantly paralleled that of kidney and liver transplantation. Although the introduction of cyclosporin A made other organ transplants a clinical reality, success with intestinal transplantation remained almost nonexistent due to a high incidence of graft loss from rejection, infection, and technical complications.[1]

The experimental studies on intestinal transplantation reported by Lillehei and colleagues in 1959 as an isolated organ graft in dogs,[2] and subsequently by Starzl and colleagues with the multivisceral graft in dogs (liver, stomach, pancreatico-duodenal complex, small and large intestine)[3] supported a unidirectional paradigm of transplantation and immunology similar to that found after bone marrow transplantation.[4] These experiments predicted that graft-versus-host disease would be precipitated by immunocytes in lymphoid cell–rich intestinal allografts differing from the recipient across a major histocompatibility complex barrier.[5]

Numerous attempts at clinical intestinal transplantation performed after 1964 under azathioprine/steroid and subsequently cyclosporine immunosuppression were largely unsuccessful. In 1987, a 3-year-old girl received a multivisceral abdominal graft that included the stomach, duodenum, pancreas, small bowel, colon, and liver; she survived for 6 months with good intestinal graft function.[6] A modified application of this operation was the transplantation of a "cluster" of organs in 1989.[7] The allograft consisted of the liver and the pancreaticoduodenal complex (Fig. 236-1). Viability of varying lengths of intestine with these clusters was proven, as was evidence of regeneration after severe rejection-induced injury. The inclusion of the liver in this type of graft was believed to protect the other transplanted organs from the same donor against rejection.[8,9] A recipient of a liver and small bowel graft treated by Grant and associates survived for more than 1 year.[10] Until 1990, there were only two survivors of isolated cadaveric intestinal grafts.[11,12]

The new immunosuppressant, tacrolimus (FK506, Prograf), permitted successful transplantation of human intestinal grafts (alone or as part of a multivisceral graft).[13,14] Successful intestinal transplantation then led to appreciation of the two-way paradigm of transplantation immunology[15]; it was postulated that two cell populations (one of recipient and the other of donor origin) reciprocally modulate immune responsiveness (host-versus-graft and graft-versus-host), including the induction of mutual nonreactivity with consequent organ allograft acceptance.[16]

INDICATIONS

Causes of loss of intestinal function may be acute (e.g., necrotizing enterocolitis, volvulus, mesenteric thrombosis) or chronic (e.g., Crohn's disease, radiation enteritis). Diseases associated with loss of intestinal function also can be divided into surgical (short gut) and nonsurgical causes. Patients with surgical causes generally suffer from loss of bowel length after resections for atresia, infarction (e.g., due to volvulus, vascular catastrophes, necrotizing enterocolitis), or strictures and fistulas as with Crohn's disease. With nonsurgical causes of intestinal failure, the anatomic length and gross morphology of the intestine may be normal.

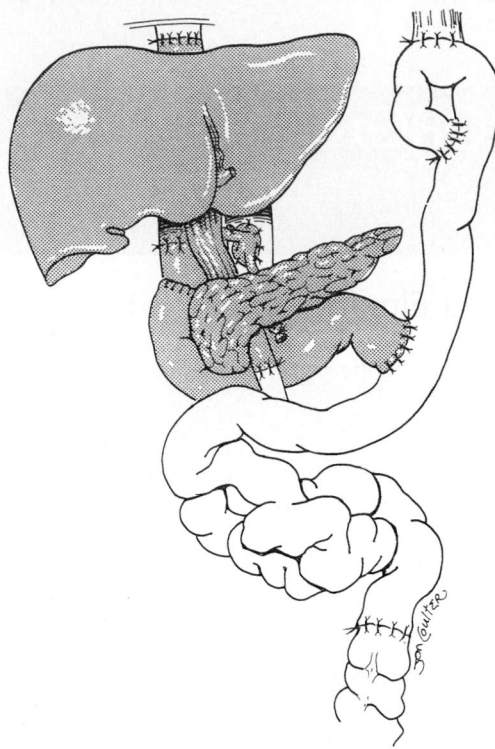

FIGURE 236–1. Cluster allograft (shaded portion), including the liver, pancreas, and duodenal segment of small intestine. (From Starzl TE, Todo S, Tzakis A, et al: Abdominal organ cluster transplantation for the treatment of upper abdominal malignancies. Ann Surg 1989;210:374-386.)

Nonsurgical causes of intestinal failure include motility disorders (e.g., intestinal pseudo-obstruction, Hirschsprung's disease), absorptive problems (e.g., microvillus inclusion disease), polyposis syndromes, and "incarcerating" desmoid tumors. Table 236-1 lists the indications for transplantation in the case experience at the University of Pittsburgh.

Total parenteral nutrition (TPN) is the standard of care for patients who are unable to maintain a normal nutritional state by use of the gastrointestinal tract alone (intestinal failure).[17] Transplantation of the intestine either alone or accompanied by other intra-abdominal organs (liver, stomach, pancreas) may be beneficial in patients who fail this therapy. The stability and duration of TPN support is variable, and failure of TPN can be manifested by complications such as infection, metabolic disorders, difficulty with vascular access (from extensive venous thrombosis), and liver cirrhosis with end-stage liver disease.

The decision regarding allograft composition focuses on the integrity of the remaining gut and other abdominal organs, both functionally and anatomically. Guidelines used in substantiating the need for concomitant liver replacement in these intestinal transplantation candidates are biochemical dysfunction (hyperbilirubinemia, transaminase abnormalities, hypoalbuminemia, and coagulopathy), pathologic processes (fibrosis or cirrhosis on liver biopsy), and the clinical presence of portal hypertension as manifested by hepatosplenomegaly, ascites, or esophageal varices and portal hypertensive gastroenteropathy. Patients deficient in protein S, protein C, and antithrombin III (liver-derived anticoagulation proteins) may be candidates for a combined liver–small intestine allograft in the absence of clinical liver disease.[18] Recipients lacking these substances develop diffuse thromboses within the splanchnic system and undergo transplantation for mesenteric venous hypertension rather than for intestinal failure. Patients with motility disorders or neoplasms that involve extensive lengths of the gastrointestinal tract are also candidates for replacement of this entire system (see Table 236-1).

In October 2000, the Center for Medicare and Medicaid Services approved intestinal, combined liver-intestine, and multivisceral transplantation as a standard of care for patients with irreversible intestinal failure who could no longer be maintained with total parenteral nutrition. Based on the available data, the approved indications for intestinal transplantation included (1) impending liver failure, as manifested by elevated circulating levels of liver enzymes, clinical findings (splenomegaly, varices, coagulopathy), history of stomal bleeding, or hepatic cirrhosis on biopsy; (2) loss of major venous access defined as more than two thromboses in the great vessels (subclavian, jugular, and femoral veins); (3) frequent central line–related sepsis consisting of more than two episodes of systemic sepsis per year, or one episode of line-related fungemia associated with septic shock or acute respiratory distress syndrome; (4) recurrent episodes of severe dehydration despite intravenous fluid management.[19,20]

ABDOMINAL VISCERAL PROCUREMENT

The safe procurement of multiple visceral organs, either en bloc or as separate components, hinges on a few fundamental precepts. Conceptually, the focus is to isolate and cool the organs, thus preserving their vascular and parenchymal anatomy and function. Multivisceral en bloc retrieval, including the stomach, duodenum, pancreas, liver, and small intestine, is the parent operation, and the assembled components have been likened by Starzl and colleagues to a large clump of individual grapes from the whole.[21] An appreciation of the fundamental strategy of multivisceral organ retrieval leads to an understanding of the lesser variant operations[22]—that is, procurement of the liver, small intestine, and the liver and small intestine together.

RECIPIENT OPERATIONS

Most patients who need intestinal or multiorgan replacements have had multiple forays into the abdominal cavity

TABLE 236–1. INDICATIONS FOR COMPOSITE AND ISOLATED INTESTINAL TRANSPLANTATION AT THE UNIVERSITY OF PITTSBURGH AND CHILDREN'S HOSPITAL OF PITTSBURGH	
Pediatric Patients	**Adult Patients**
Volvulus	Trauma
Gastroschisis	Superior mesenteric artery thrombosis
Necrotizing enterocolitis	Crohn's disease
Intestinal atresia	Desmoid tumor
Pseudo-obstruction	Volvulus
Microvillus inclusion disease	Familial polyposis
Intestinal polyposis	Gastrinoma
Hirschsprung's disease	Budd-Chiari disease
Trauma	Intestinal adhesions
	Pseudo-obstruction
	Inflammatory bowel disease
	Radiation enteritis

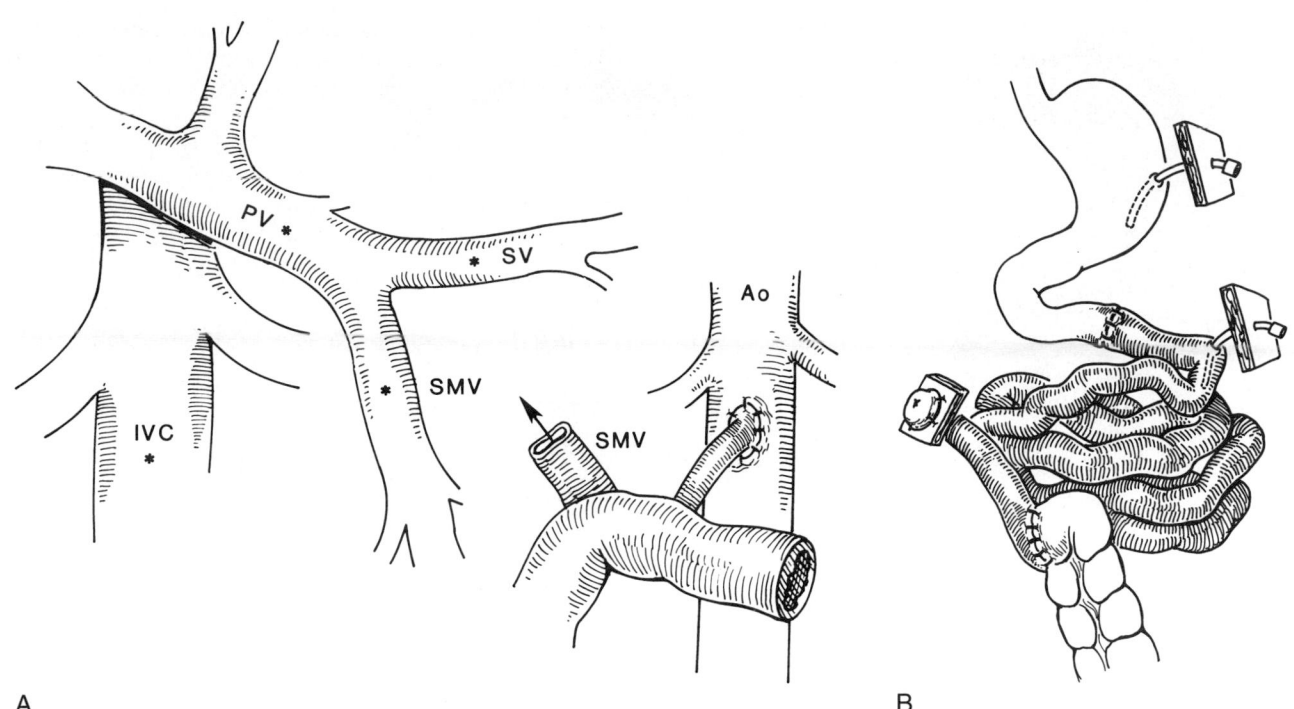

FIGURE 236–2. (A) Arterialization and potential venous drainage options of the isolated small intestine allograft. (B) Illustration of an isolated small bowel graft; the distal ileal chimney allows easy access to bowel mucosa. Ao, aorta; IVC, inferior vena cava; PV, portal vein; SMV, superior mesenteric vein; SV, splenic vein. (From Reyes J, Bueno J, Kocoshis S, et al: Current status of intestinal transplantation in children. J Pediatric Surg 1998;33:243-254.)

for intestinal resections, lengthening procedures, and treatment of complications. This results in volume contraction of the abdominal cavity and severe adhesions. Consequently, the organs of the donor usually need to be smaller than those of the recipient to ensure proper abdominal closure.

In an effort to maximize organ utilization and improve abdominal closure in children undergoing intestinal transplantation, intestinal reduction with or without liver reduction has been used. For example, between July 2002 and September 2003, 31 children received consecutive intestinal transplants consisting of 14 isolated intestinal transplants, 11 liver/intestinal transplants, 4 multivisceral transplants, and 2 modified multivisceral transplants without liver. Reduction of the liver and intestine has been carried out in 17 of 31 cases (55%). A mean length of 1.3 meters of bowel has been reduced in these children, leaving a mean of 2.2 meters (range: 1.1 to 3 meters). Based on these initial results, a donor weight to recipient weight ratio of up to 4:1 has been a practical guideline to use in selection of donors larger than recipients.

Previous operations may complicate the removal of the recipient's organs, especially if cirrhosis, portal hypertension, or inferior vena caval thromboses are present. All of these conditions can be sequelae of the original disease or of prior operations. The recipient operation consists of removal of the failed organs with exposure of the vascular anatomy and, finally, allograft implantation. Following is a brief description of the salient features of the recipient operations.

ISOLATED SMALL BOWEL

In cases of surgical short gut, the proximal and distal remnants of the intestine are identified; when there is functional disease or neoplasm, the recipient's diseased small intestine is removed. The superior mesenteric artery of the donor

bowel is sewn to the infrarenal aorta, and the donor superior mesenteric vein is anastomosed to the recipient portal vein, superior mesenteric vein, splenic vein, or inferior vena cava (Fig. 236-2A). The anastomosis can be facilitated by the use of an interposition venous graft. Reperfusion of the intestinal graft is effected after the vascular anastomoses. Intestinal continuity is completed with proximal and distal anastomoses, and access to the ileum for endoscopic examination is provided by a temporary chimney ileostomy (Fig. 236-2B).[23]

Cold ischemia time refers to the time between procurement and implantation of the allograft and should be less than 10 hours. *Warm ischemic time* for the allograft (sewing-in time) is about 30 minutes and is also a determinant of preservation injury to the intestine. In an attempt to reduce graft dysmotility, a segment of large intestine was included in 32 allografts. This practice was abandoned after 1994.

LIVER–SMALL BOWEL

Liver and small intestine are removed in these patients, but the remainder of the foregut (stomach, duodenum, pancreas) is retained. When possible, the liver is removed with the retrohepatic vena cava preserved in situ ("piggyback").[24] After the enterectomy, the composite allograft is implanted by anastomosing the suprahepatic vena cava of the donor (including the hepatic veins) end-to-side to the recipient's vena cava. The donor infrahepatic vena cava can then be ligated (Fig. 236-3A). The double arterial stem of the celiac and superior mesenteric arteries (using the Carrel patch technique) are connected to the infrarenal aorta (using an aortic conduit or iliac artery homograft), followed by graft reperfusion. Since the axial stem of the portal vein between the donor organs is removed intact, all that is required for the completion of portal flow is attachment of the portal vein of the remnant foregut in the recipient to the intact portal stem

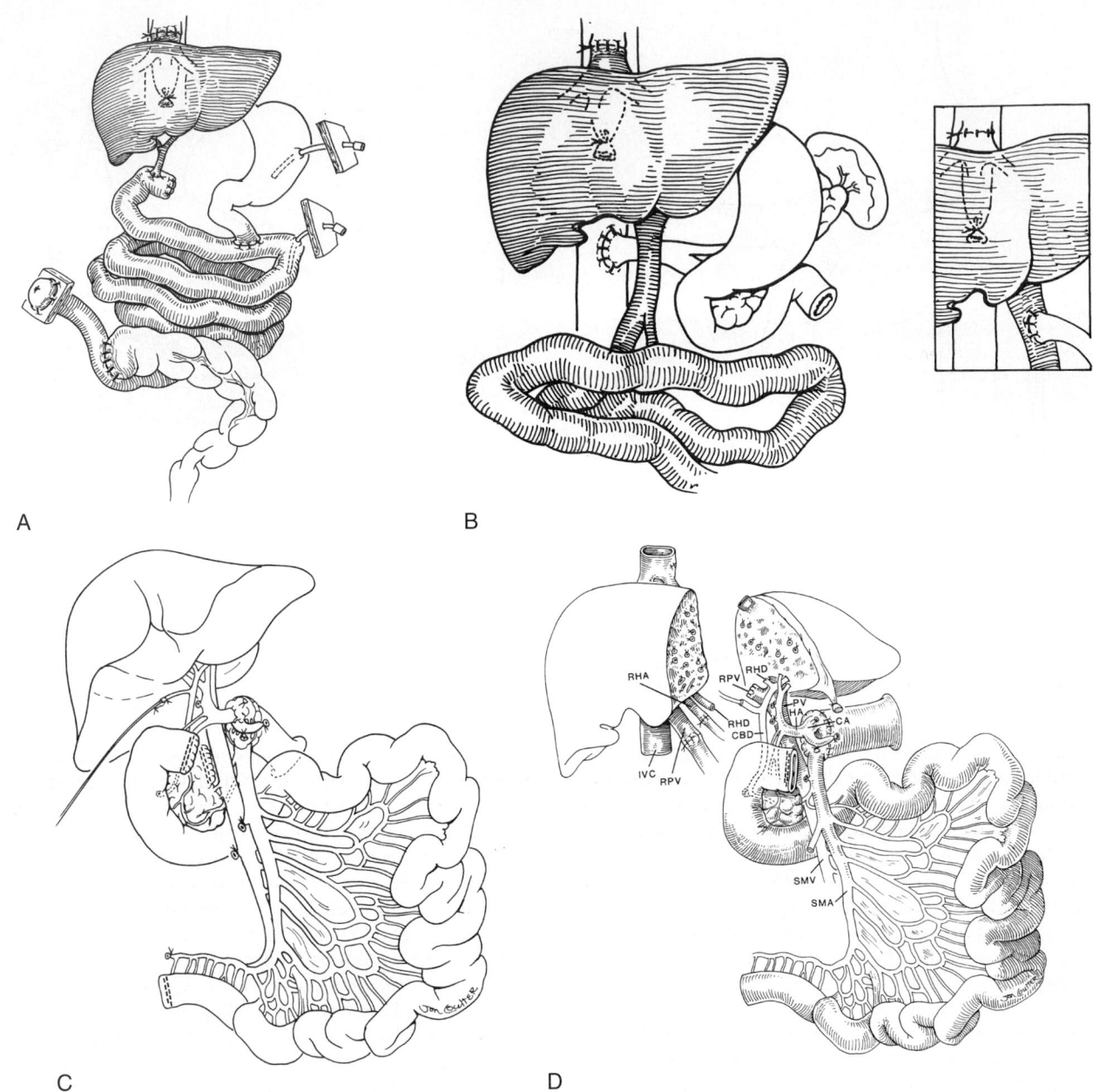

FIGURE 236–3. (*A*) Modification of the liver/small intestinal allograft. (*B*) Combined liver-small intestinal allograft. Systemic portacaval shunt, or recipient portal vein to donor portal vein shunt (inset) allows venous outflow of retained pancreas and stomach from recipient. (*C*) Composite liver and intestine graft with preservation of the duodenum in continuity with the graft jejunum and hepatic biliary system. The allograft pancreas is transected to the right of the portal vein. (*D*) In situ split liver graft, maintaining the left lateral segment in continuity with the hepatic hilus and duodenum, with transection of allograft pancreas. (*B*, from Reyes J, Bueno J, Kocoshis S, et al: Current status of intestinal transplantation in children, J Pediatric Surg 1998;33:243-254; *C*, from Abu-Elmagd K, Reyes J, Todo S, et al: Clinical intestinal transplantation: New perspectives and immunologic considerations. J Am Coll Surg 1998;186:512-527; *D*, from Reyes J, Fishbein T, Bueno J, et al: Reduced sized orthotopic composite liver-Intestinal allograft: Rationale and in situ split technique in an initial experience. Transplantation 1998;66:489-492.)

of the donor. This may not be possible, however, because of a size discrepancy or difficult anatomic relationships between donor and recipient portal veins. In this case, a permanent portacaval shunt is performed (Fig. 236-3B). The intestinal anastomoses are then completed with a proximal jejunojejunostomy, ileocolostomy, a temporary distal ileostomy, and a Roux-en-Y biliary anastomosis. To avoid a biliary anastomosis (with its potential for complications), a modification of the original "cluster" allograft, as depicted in Figure 236-1, has been applied to the liver–small bowel allografts.[25] In the modification, the allograft duodenum remains in continuity with the allograft biliary system and

varying lengths of allograft jejunum/ileum (Fig. 236-3C). In one such graft, a reduced segment of allograft liver (the left lateral segment) was successfully used after an in situ split was performed to overcome a donor–recipient size mismatch in a critically ill pediatric recipient (Fig. 236-3D).

MULTIVISCERAL TRANSPLANTATION

After abdominal exenteration and exposure of the retroperitoneal aorta and inferior vena cava, the multivisceral graft (Fig. 236-4A) is connected by its vascular attachments. First, the suprahepatic attachment is completed, then the

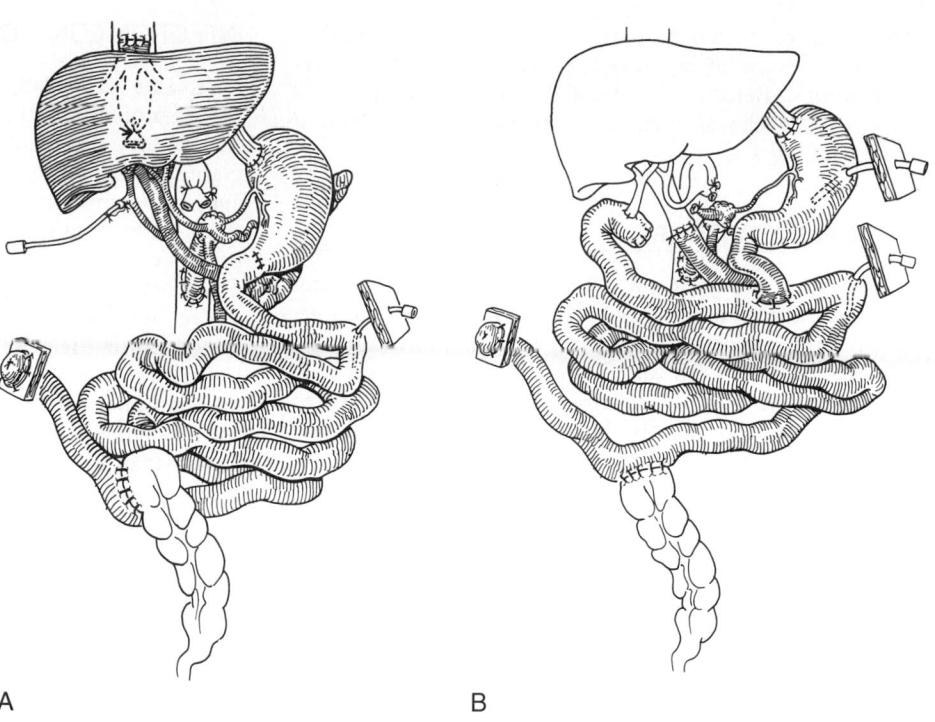

FIGURE 236–4. Diagrams of multiviseral donor organs: complete multivisceral (*A*), modified multivisceral (*B*). (From Reyes J, Bueno J, Kocoshis S, et al: Current status of intestinal transplantation in children. J Pediatr Surg 1998;33:243-254.)

A   B

infrahepatic vena caval connections (or "piggyback" to the skeletonized recipient vena cava) are performed. Finally, the arterioaortic anastomosis (using an aortic interposition homograft) is completed. The recipient's portal vein and its inflow organs (gastrointestinal tract, pancreas, and liver) are removed with the enterectomy. The donor portal vein retains its continuity via the liver in the procurement of the allograft; thus, no portal vein anastomosis is required in this procedure. Patients with a normal native liver can receive a modified multivisceral procedure that excludes the allograft liver as part of the composite of organs. In this modification, portal venous return is directed into the recipient's portal vein (Fig. 236-4B).

Restoration of intestinal continuity requires an esophago-gastric anastomosis and a coloenteric anastomosis with the distal ileum allograft. Initially, the patient also receives an ileostomy. Takedown of the ileostomy can be performed after several months, when oral nutrition is consistently adequate, a stable immunosuppressant regimen has been achieved, and there is no further need for frequent endoscopic surveillance.

IMMUNOSUPPRESSION

Traditionally, immunosuppression for intestinal transplantation has been based on tacrolimus and corticosteroids. Over time, however, the immunosuppressive regimen has evolved. From 1990 to 1995, the regimen used tacrolimus and corticosteroids for induction and maintenance. Induction therapy with cyclophosphamide was used from 1995 through 1997. Daclizumab was used for induction from 1998 through 2001. Preconditioning with Thymoglobulin during induction therapy and tacrolimus monotherapy (without steroids) after transplantation have been in use since 2001 (Table 236-2). The therapeutic principles of the current immunosuppression regimen are pretreatment of the recipient with a lymphocyte-depleting agent to precondition the recipient, and then use

of the lowest possible amount of post-transplant immuno-suppression to prevent frequent rejection episodes yet allow for the tolerogenic effect of the preconditioning to occur.[26]

In this management strategy, Thymoglobulin is given as an initial one-time dose of 5 to 10 mg/kg intravenously in adults or as 5 to 10 mg/kg in divided doses of 3 mg/kg pre-perfusion and 2 mg/kg post-perfusion in children. Subsequent to preconditioning, administration of tacrolimus is begun, using the enteral route. The target steady-state whole blood level of tacrolimus is between 15 and 20 ng/mL. Using the preconditioning regimen as outlined above has allowed the elimination of routine steroid use. Methylprednisolone is given as a bolus at perfusion and as premedication for the lymphocyte-depleting agent, but this drug is not used routinely. The dose is 1 g for adults and 10 mg/kg for children. The goal of tacrolimus monotherapy has been achieved without an increase in rejection rates and with the resulting ability to achieve spaced dosing of tacrolimus to once a day, or even every other day. Prostaglandin E$_1$ (Prostin) is administered at 0.003 to 0.009 µg/kg/min for the first 5 postoperative days. This drug is given for its beneficial effects on renal perfusion as well as its

TABLE 236–2. INTESTINAL TRANSPLANTATION: IMMUNOSUPPRESSION BY ERA

Years	Drug	Cases, n
1990-1995	Tacrolimus/steroids	70
1995-1997	Tacrolimus/steroids /cyclophosphamide	24
1997-1998	Tacrolimus/steroids	13
1998-2001	Tacrolimus/steroids /daclizumab	62
2002-2003	Thymoglobulin preconditioning protocol	81
TOTAL		250

Pre 2002 Base-line Immunosuppression = tacrolimus + prednisone + azathioprine (n = 16), mycophenolate mofetil (n = 2), or sirolimus (n = 16)

prevention of microvascular thrombosis, a key patho-physiologic event in acute cellular rejection and procure-ment injury. Rejection is treated with optimization of tacrolimus levels, supplemental corticosteroids, and, if necessary, OKT3.

POSTOPERATIVE CARE

Recipients of multivisceral, liver–small bowel, or cluster grafts commonly suffer from severe liver failure. Therefore, the care with respect to pulmonary function, infection sur-veillance, and liver graft function is similar to that provided for routine liver transplant recipients. Recipients of isolated small bowel transplants who have stable liver function have a lesser preoperative medical acuity.

VENTILATORY MANAGEMENT

Extubation often can be accomplished within 48 hours of transplantation. Unusual circumstances, such as graft malfunction, sepsis, inability to close the abdominal wall, or severe preoperative hepatic failure, may prevent early extu-bation. Since the operation may be long (8 to 18 hours) and the patients are often in a weakened nutritional state pre-operatively, a careful assessment of weaning parameters is required. Incisional pain, ascites, and pleural effusions may compromise ventilation and the ability to cough. Other fac-tors that can contribute to respiratory dysfunction include muscle wasting and malnutrition, partial or complete paral-ysis of the right hemidiaphragm,[27] and increased intra-abdominal volume with compression of the thoracic cavity due to a discrepancy between the size of the donor and the recipient. These patients often require low doses of intra-venous narcotics, repeated thoracentesis and paracentesis, and supplemental extensive respiratory therapy if they are to avoid the need for reintubation. Patients may require tra-cheostomy, because of the need for prolonged ventilatory support, although this is unusual in children. Rarely, severe rejection of an isolated small intestine allograft with sys-temic venous drainage into the inferior vena cava is heralded by respiratory insufficiency and a clinical picture consistent with acute respiratory distress syndrome.

RENAL FUNCTION

Most intestinal transplant candidates have some degree of renal dysfunction due to multiple episodes of infection, the toxic effects of antibiotics, and hepatic dysfunction. Early after transplantation, there is significant accumulation of interstitial fluid into the graft, lungs, and peripheral tissues; this accumulation peaks at 48 to 72 hours. Extensive volume shifts into the transplanted bowel (related to preservation injury) and marked ascites production (related to mesenteric lymphatic leakage) lead to intravascular volume depletion that can exacerbate the nephrotoxicity of tacrolimus and certain antibiotics. Continuous central venous pressure measurement, often for weeks after transplantation, provides important information for maximizing graft perfusion and preserving the integrity of the kidneys. Two children have had inclusion of an allograft kidney with their primary intestine transplant, and one long-term pediatric survivor required sequential kidney transplantation.

INFECTION CONTROL

Recipients of isolated or composite small bowel grafts receive prophylactic, broad-spectrum intravenous antibiotics. Any history of recent nosocomial infections before trans-plantation should be addressed with the administration of appropriate specific antibiotics. Colonizing organisms growing from enterocutaneous fistulous tracts should be treated perioperatively.

All recipients are given a pre- and postoperative "cocktail" of oral nonabsorbable antibiotics every 6 hours for 2 weeks; the mixture includes amphotericin B, gentamicin, and polymyxin E and is intended to achieve selective bowel decontamination.[28] Surveillance stool cultures are performed weekly. When organisms grow in quantitative cultures to greater than 10^8 colony-forming units/mL in the presence of signs of systemic sepsis or ongoing acute cellular rejection of the allograft, specifically directed intravenous antibiotics are added to the regimen to treat the presumed translocating organisms. Evidence of translocation most commonly occurs during episodes of acute rejection, when the mucosal barrier of the allograft has been immunologically damaged; however, it also can be seen with enteritis associated with Epstein-Barr virus infection.[29]

The antiviral prophylactic strategy has evolved during the past several years. The currently recommended regimen includes a 2-week course of intravenous ganciclovir with concomitant administration of cytomegalovirus-specific hyperimmune globulin (Cytogam).[30] The dose for ganci-clovir is 5 mg/kg twice daily i.v. The dose for Cytogam is 150 mg/kg i.v. in donor CMV (+) to recipient CMV (−) mis-match 2, 4, 6, and 8 weeks after transplant and 100 mg/kg/dose i.v. at 12 and 16 weeks after transplant. Oral administration of trimethoprim-sulfamethoxazole (80 mg p.o. three times weekly) is used for the lifetime of the patient as prophylaxis against *Pneumocystis carinii* pneumonia.

NUTRITIONAL SUPPORT

Full nutritional support is initially provided via standard total parenteral nutrition. This is tapered gradually as oral or enteral feedings (via gastric or jejunal tube) are advanced. Tube feedings are initiated with isotonic formulas tailored to meet specific patient requirements. Most patients do not vol-untarily eat adequate amounts early after the operation. Resistance to resumption of oral feedings is particularly notable in pediatric recipients.[31] Therefore, enteral supple-mentation is required when the intestinal tract becomes functional. This management must be individualized, since the simplicity of an uneventful post-transplant course may suddenly change with any surgical or immunologic complication.

ASSESSMENT OF GRAFT STATUS

A judgment of the anatomic and functional integrity of the graft begins in the operating room. The normal intestine is pink and nonedematous and occasionally demonstrates contractions. Alterations from this appearance can be observed in the operating room and in the ileal stoma postoperatively.

Surveillance for intestinal graft rejection focuses on clinical evaluation and gross morphologic examination of the stoma and the distal ileum. Frequent routine entero-scopic surveillance has been shown to be the most reliable tool for the early diagnosis of intestinal rejection.[32] Endoscopic evaluations are performed routinely twice a week through the allograft ileostomy; upper endoscopy is performed when clinical changes are not elucidated by distal allograft evaluation. Grossly, the bowel reacts to insults in nonspecific ways with edema, cyanosis, congestion, and increased stomal output; these alterations should signal a broad differential diagnosis that includes preservation injury, systemic sepsis, rejection, and enteritis.

The stomal output is assessed for volume, consistency, and the presence of reducing substances, which can be seen in the event of rejection, bacterial overgrowth, or malabsorption. Typically, within the first week of implantation, stomal output is 1 to 2 L/day (for adults) or 40 to 60 mL/kg/day (for children) of clear, watery effluent. If these volumes are exceeded and no significant pathology is present, paregoric, loperamide, pectin, somatostatin, or oral antibiotics can be used singly or in combination to control the diarrhea. The presence of blood in the stool is always an ominous sign and indicates rejection until proven otherwise.

Serum tests are important in assessing injury to the liver (bilirubin concentration, aspartate aminotransferase concentration, and alanine aminotransferase concentration), but no such tests exist for intestinal grafts. Serum markers for nutritional adequacy and anabolic status (circulating levels of transferrin, albumin, and retinoic acid) are of limited value, whereas specific tests of the absorptive ability of the graft are good measures of overall function. Assessment of small bowel function relies on absorption studies of D-xylose and tacrolimus and on the quantitation of fat in the stool. Most patients develop satisfactory absorption curves for D-xylose within the first postoperative month, and absorption continues to improve over time. Abnormal results obtained after 1 month always should prompt an aggressive search for underlying pathology, especially rejection. The maintenance of satisfactory tacrolimus whole blood trough levels of 15 to 20 ng/mL on oral therapy alone is a good indicator of adequate absorption. In our patients, evidence of good absorptive function occurs at a mean of 28 days after transplantation and tends to be delayed longer in recipients of multivisceral grafts.[33] The excretion of fat in the stool has been abnormal in almost all patients. However, clinical steatorrhea has not been a problem.

Radiologic evaluations by standard barium gastrointestinal examination are valuable in assessing mucosal pattern and motility and are performed routinely after the first postoperative week. A normal mucosal pattern is expected. Intestinal transit time is around 2 hours. Intestinal graft rejection, when mild, can be suspected when evidence of mucosal edema exists. Severe rejection, with exfoliation of the mucosa, ablates the normal mucosal pattern and can be seen as segments of "tubulized" intestine and strictures (Fig. 236-5).

COMPLICATIONS

Before a description of the variety of potential complications, it is important to have a general perspective on the care of these patients. Comprehensive management of intestinal recipients requires a multidisciplinary approach by surgeons, anesthesiologists, nurses, critical care physicians, pathologists, and a host of internal medicine subspecialists. Easy access to diagnostic and therapeutic modalities, including mechanical

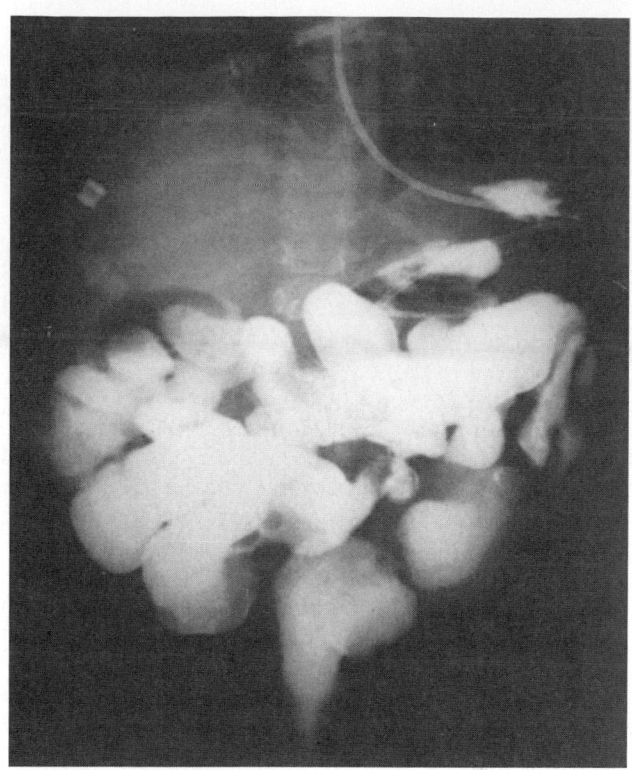

FIGURE 236–5. Severely damaged allograft intestine in a recipient of a liver-small bowel after multiple episodes of rejection. Diffuse tubulized gut, strictures, and significant distention of the native duodenum are seen.

ventilation, hemodialysis, bronchoscopy, gastrointestinal endoscopy, thromboelastography, percutaneous cholangiography, ultrasonography, invasive and noninvasive contrast radiography, and sophisticated hemodynamic monitoring systems is paramount.

More important than the above, however, is vigilance about patient care and attention to detail, on the part of both physicians and nurses. Problems in these patients can originate from a multiplicity of sources. Several assumptions can be made in these patients based on our experience:

1. Preoperative deterioration of physical performance status predisposes to various organ system failures that persist in the postoperative period even though allograft function may be acceptable.
2. Transplant cases are labor-intensive and patients require aggressive respiratory therapy, nutritional and antibiotic support, fluid management, and nursing care, often for prolonged periods in the intensive care unit.
3. Immunotherapy doses in patients with multivisceral transplants tend to be higher than in patients with single organ transplants.
4. The majority of patients develop episodes of infection and rejection after transplantation, often concomitantly. Any subjective complaints or objective abnormalities should be vigorously pursued until a cause is found or until the symptoms resolve.

GRAFT REJECTION

Intestinal allograft rejection can manifest as an array of symptoms that include fever, abdominal pain, distention,

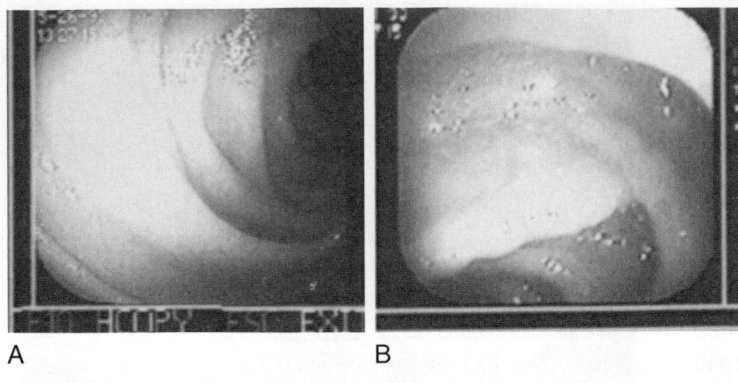

A   B

FIGURE 236–6. (*A*) Normal endoscopic appearance of transplanted small intestine. (*B*) Moderate acute cellular rejection of an intestinal allograft demonstrating diffuse edema and focal erythema.

nausea, vomiting, and a sudden increase in stomal output. The stoma may become edematous, erythematous, and friable. Gastrointestinal bleeding can occur in cases of severe uncontrollable rejection in which ulcerations and sloughing of the intestinal mucosa occur. Septic shock or acute respiratory distress syndrome may develop. Bacterial or fungal translocation can occur during intestinal allograft rejection due to disruption of the intestinal mucosal barrier. Gut decontamination must be instituted during these episodes.[34]

Endoscopically, the transplanted intestinal mucosa loses its velvety appearance. It may become hyperemic or dusky as well as hypoperistaltic. Erythema may be focal or diffuse. The mucosa becomes friable, and diffuse ulcerations appear (Fig. 236-6).

Histologically, there is variable presence of edema in the lamina propria and villous blunting. However, the presence of mononuclear cell infiltrates and cryptitis with apoptosis and regeneration are necessary for establishing the diagnosis of rejection. Neutrophils, eosinophils, and macrophages may be seen traversing the muscularis mucosa.[35,36] The degree of epithelial and crypt cell damage varies. Complete mucosal sloughing and crypt destruction are seen in grafts with severe rejection. The mucosal surface is partially replaced by inflammatory pseudomembranes and granulation tissue (Fig. 236-7). This may precipitate continuous blood loss as well as intermittent septic episodes from the damaged intestine.

Chronic rejection has been observed in patients with persistent intractable rejection episodes. Clinically progressive weight loss, chronic diarrhea, intermittent fever, and gastrointestinal bleeding dominate the presentation. Histologically, villous blunting, focal ulcerations, epithelial metaplasia, and scant cellular infiltrate are present on endoscopic mucosal biopsy specimens. Full-thickness intestinal biopsies show obliterative thickening of intestinal arterioles.

Historically, the incidence of acute intestinal allograft rejection during the first 90 days after transplantation was 92% in isolated small bowel recipients and 66% in recipients of composite grafts, suggesting that the liver is "protective" for the intestine, as is seen experimentally.[37,38] Interestingly, the incidence of acute liver allograft rejection in recipients of composite grafts is 43%, which is similar to that seen after isolated liver transplantation.[30] However, the rate of acute rejection has steadily decreased to current levels of approximately 30% with the use of a preconditioning protocol.

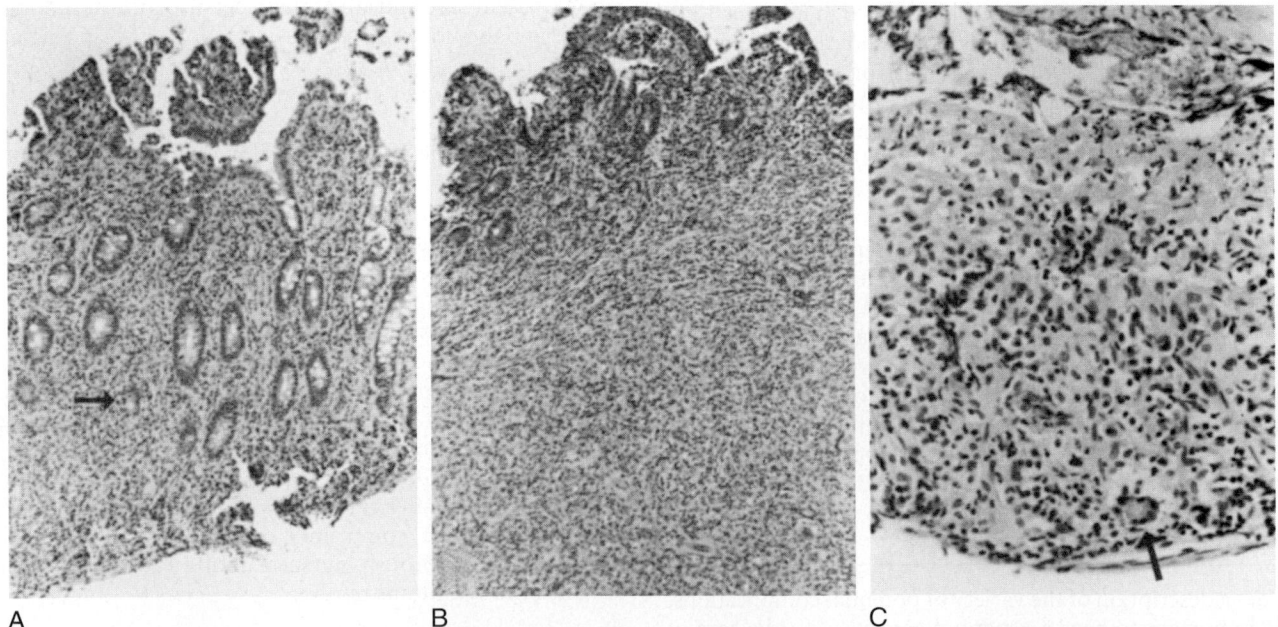

A   B   C

FIGURE 236–7. Acute cellular rejection. (*A*) Endoscopic biopsy sample obtained 14 days after transplantation showed widening of the lamina propria with increased mononuclear cells, which were often cuffed around small vessels and infiltrating the crypt epithelium (*arrow*; hematoxylin and eosin, original magnification ×140). (*B*) The reaction was more intense in biopsies that contained lymphoid nodules and where blastogenesis, focal ulcerations, congestion, and neutrophil plugging of capillaries were also seen (moderate acute cellular rejection; hematoxylin and eosin, original magnification ×140). (*C*) Uncontrolled acute rejection eventually resulted in widespread mucosal destruction; the mucosa was replaced by granulation tissue. Note the overlying inflammatory pseudomembrane (*arrow*; hematoxylin and eosin, original magnification ×350).

Lower overall immunosuppression has subsequently allowed a concomitant reduction in Epstein-Barr virus and cytomegalovirus disease, especially in pediatric recipients.

Mild graft rejection is treated initially with intravenous methylprednisolone, and with a methylprednisolone taper in cases of moderate rejection. The tacrolimus trough levels in whole blood should reach 15 to 25 ng/mL, with the drug administered by either the oral or the intravenous route. OKT3 is used when rejection has progressed with a steroid taper; however, it should be entertained as the initial therapeutic agent in cases of severe mucosal injury and crypt damage. The use of cyclophosphamide/mycophenolate mofetil induction therapy or bone marrow augmentation had no beneficial effect on the frequency of rejection.[30,36]

POSTOPERATIVE HEMORRHAGE

Coagulopathy is more often an intraoperative problem that relates to liver dysfunction, qualitative and quantitative platelet defects, and fibrinolysis.[38] Intraoperative bleeding is further promoted by vascularized adhesions due to previous surgery and portal hypertension. Temporary graft reperfusion coagulopathy mediated by plasminogen activators from the graft may occur.[39] Efforts are made to normalize these global aspects of coagulation by the end of the operative procedure so that in the absence of liver dysfunction, the coagulopathy is usually minor in the postoperative period. Postoperative intra-abdominal bleeding is most often a technical problem, arising from vascular anastomoses or extensive, raw peritoneal surfaces. Certainly, coagulation parameters should be normalized, if postoperative bleeding occurs; if bleeding is proved, the origin should be presumed to be surgical and managed as such by early reexploration.

BILIARY COMPLICATIONS

Continuity of the biliary axis is surgically re-established in multivisceral grafts. Correspondingly, these grafts can develop biliary system-related surgical complications (i.e., leaks and obstructions).

Biliary leaks usually occur within the first 2 weeks after transplantation and may herald their presence with bilious drainage from the abdominal wound or drains or merely with unexplained sepsis. The response to external bilious drainage should be immediate exploration with surgical revision of the biliary dehiscence. In the case of unexplained sepsis in any intestinal transplant recipient, all surgical anastomoses should be radiographically inspected (with percutaneous cholangiography), and if leakage is suspected, they should be revised. There is no place for percutaneous diversion of biliary or intestinal leakage in these patients, since both wound healing and antimicrobial immunity are impaired by multimodal immunotherapy.

Biliary obstruction generally follows an anastomotic stricture and is a delayed complication, but any clinical picture that resembles cholangitis or biliary obstruction should be followed with cholangiography to prove patency of the biliary tree, regardless of the timing after transplantation.

VASCULAR COMPLICATIONS

Major arterial thrombosis is a disastrous complication that leads to massive necrosis of the organs correspondingly supplied. Elevation of hepatic enzymes and pallor of the intestinal stoma are accompanied by clinical deterioration, fulminant sepsis, and hepatic coma. Isolated small bowel grafts can be removed with the expectation of patient recovery, but in patients with composite grafts, the event is usually fatal unless early retransplantation can be performed. Patency of the arteries can be rapidly confirmed with Doppler ultrasonographic examination.

Since the superior mesenteric vein–portal vein axis is preserved in the composite grafts, venous outflow thrombosis is less likely to occur in these recipients. Isolated small bowel grafts have an anastomosis of these veins that can occlude. Ascites, stomal congestion, and mesenteric infarction are the ultimate result.

Neither of these problems is associated with subtle clinical signs; diagnosis should be prompt and obvious. In our series, isolated thrombosis of the hepatic artery has occurred in a pediatric recipient of a liver–small bowel graft, with consequent hepatic gangrene. This patient required retransplantation of the liver component of the graft, even though a full liver–small bowel graft was desirable.

Incomplete obstruction of major inflow or outflow vessels may be suspected on biopsy or based on clinical and laboratory evidence of organ dysfunction. Contrast vascular radiographic studies are confirmatory, and the correction is surgical or, in some cases, with balloon dilatation.

GASTROINTESTINAL COMPLICATIONS

Gastrointestinal bleeding after intestinal transplantation is an ominous sign that requires prompt attention. Rejection or infection are the most probable causes and should be immediately diagnosed or ruled out on the basis of enteroscopic biopsy results. The diagnosis of rejection relies not only on histologic evidence but also on the endoscopic appearance of the mucosa (Figs. 236-6 and 236-7). Bleeding from ulcerated Epstein-Barr virus– or cytomegalovirus-induced lesions can be easily differentiated by gross endoscopic examination. Empiric therapy for rejection is not acceptable.

Leakage of either the proximal or the distal gastrointestinal anastomosis can occur in any recipient, but it is more common in pediatric patients than in adults. Any fresh surgical margin, including the native duodenal and colonic stumps and gastrostomy sites, are vulnerable to poor wound healing and subsequent leakage. Presentation is often dramatic (florid sepsis), and confirmation is with radiologic contrast imaging. Surg revision, evacuation of peritoneal soilage, and often reexploration are required to eliminate the contamination effectively. Again, sepsis without an obvious source should prompt the performance of contrast studies to document the integrity of all gastrointestinal anastomoses; if the findings are inconclusive, diagnostic laparotomy is indicated.

Atony of the native stomach and pylorospasm that produce early satiety or vomiting are common and self-limiting. The evolution of motility patterns in the denervated allograft intestine is not fully understood. Hypermotility of the allograft intestine occurs early after transplantation; in the absence of rejection or bacterial overgrowth, it can be controlled with agents such as paregoric, loperamide, or pectin. Sudden changes in intestinal motility, particularly when accompanied by abdominal distention and vomiting in the case of decreased motility, should initiate a search for rejection.

INFECTIONS

Historically, frequency of infectious complications has been high and was responsible for the significant morbidity and mortality initially reported after intestinal transplantation. The high incidence of serious infectious complications was due in part to the relatively high level of immunosuppression required to maintain the graft in these intestinal recipients. Other predisposing factors include the severity of the preoperative liver failure as well as the presence of intra-abdominal, pulmonary, or intravenous line-induced sepsis before transplantation. Also, technically more difficult transplantation procedures with increased operative time, transfusion requirements, and likelihood of reexploration reflect the advanced disease of these patients. Recipients of small bowel grafts have the lowest incidence of complications because of the more elective nature of their operations.

Although current immunosuppressive modifications have decreased the incidence of life-threatening septic complications, the recognition and management of infection is still an important component of the care of these patients. Infectious pathogens include bacteria, fungi, and viruses. Infections are related (in order of frequency) to intravenous lines, the abdominal wound, deep abdominal abscesses, peritonitis, and pneumonia. Bacterial translocation in grafts damaged by rejection illustrates the need for concomitant antirejection and antimicrobial therapy and is a frequent source of infection.

Of the bacterial pathogens, staphylococcal and enterococcal species are common, whereas gram-negative rods usually accompany polymicrobial infections. Not uncommonly, separate sources of infection occur simultaneously, or mixed infections from the same source are present. This leads to multiple antibiotic regimens and sets the stage for the development of resistant organisms. Panresistant enterococcal isolates are an increasing problem. Persistence of a physiologic hyperdynamic state in a patient being treated for proven infection should raise the suspicion of retained phlegmonous material in the abdomen or the possibility of rejection.[40,41]

Fungal infections become problematic after heavy treatment for rejection, massive antibiotic usage, intestinal leaks, and multiple surgical explorations. The authors routinely

TABLE 236–3. PEDIATRIC INTESTINAL TRANSPLANTATION: CYTOMEGALOVIRUS DISEASE BY ERA

Year	Drug	Rate, %
1990-1995	Tacrolimus/steroids	23
1995-1997	Cyclophosphamide	56
1997-1998	Tacrolimus/steroids	11
1998-2001	Daclizumab	4
2002-2003	Thymoglobulin preconditioning protocol	5

employ low-dose amphotericin B prophylaxis in patients with these complications. Established fungal infections require long-term, full-dose antibiotic therapy and reduction of immunotherapy. All persistently septic recipients are potential candidates for moderation of immunosuppressant dosages, if no coexistent cellular rejection is present. However, complete withdrawal of immunosuppression has been impossible in this recipient population owing to a high incidence of rebound rejection, which then mandates augmentation of immunotherapy.

Historically, clinical cytomegalovirus infection has occurred in 36% of intestinal graft recipients and often involves the allograft intestine. The current incidence of cytomegalovirus disease is approximately 5% (Table 236-3). Although the incidence and distribution of disease according to donor and recipient cytomegalovirus serologic status is similar in adults (44%) and children (31%), the clinical course is dramatically better in children. Successful clinical management has been accomplished in 88% of episodes using ganciclovir alone or ganciclovir in combination with cytomegalovirus-specific hyperimmunoglobulin. Immunosuppression is maintained at baseline and reduced only in the face of deteriorating clinical disease, thus decreasing the risk of rebound rejection.[29] A cytomegalovirus-positive donor graft transplanted into a cytomegalovirus-negative recipient is a significant risk factor for cytomegalovirus disease, but monitoring for pp65 antigenemia and preemptive therapy allow the successful use of cytomegalovirus-mismatched organs. Clinical presentation is generally enteritis of variable severity with focal ulcerations and bleeding (Fig. 236-8).

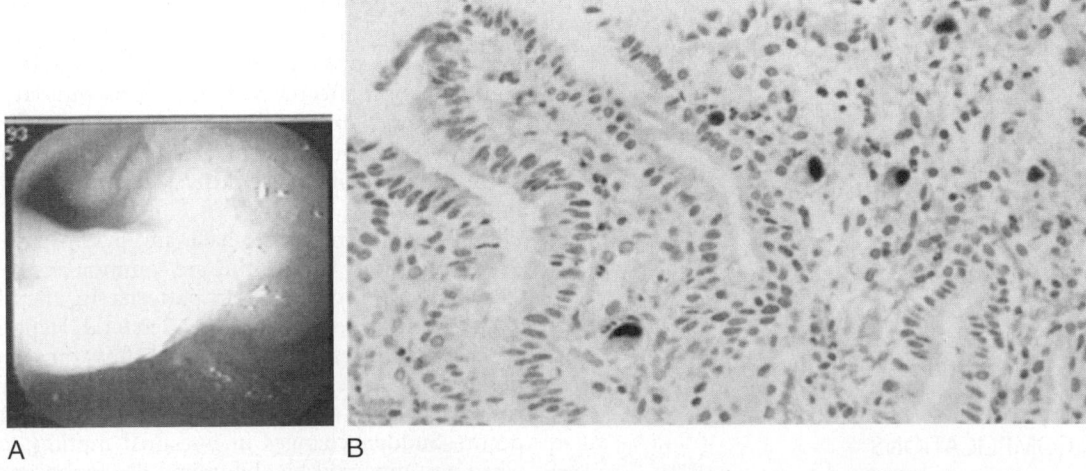

A   B

FIGURE 236–8. (*A*) Endoscopic appearance of cytomegaloviral enteritis is characterized by hyperemic erosions. (*B*) The diagnosis was confirmed histologically by the presence of characteristic inclusions, by staining for viral antigens, or both. Note the focal neutrophilic inflammation (immunoperoxidase for cytomegalovirus antigens, original magnification ×350).

TABLE 236–4. PEDIATRIC INTESTINAL TRANSPLANTATION: PTLD BY ERA

Year	Drug	Rate, %
1990-1995	Tacrolimus/steroids	44
1995-1997	Cyclophosphamide	19
1997-1998	Tacrolimus/steroids	33
1998-2001	Daclizumab	17
2002-2003	Thymoglobulin preconditioning protocol	5

Less commonly, respiratory syncytial virus, adenovirus, and parainfluenza virus infections occur in the pediatric population. All viral infections are opportunistic and have as a common denominator the need for aggressive treatment of rejection episodes in complicated patients with high Acute Physiologic and Chronic Health Evaluation (APACHE) scores.

Post-transplantation lymphoproliferative disease associated with Epstein-Barr virus occurs in 20% of patients, and children (27%) have traditionally been at a significantly higher risk than adults (11%). Presentation varies from totally asymptomatic observations at routine endoscopy to nonspecific intestinal and systemic symptoms to bleeding, lymphadenopathy, and tumors to fulminant disease. Risk factors other than age include the type of graft, splenectomy, and the use of OKT3. Therapy includes the reduction and withdrawal of immunosuppression, antiviral therapy using ganciclovir, acyclovir, and/or hyperimmunoglobulin, rituximab (anti-CD 20 monoclonal antibody), and chemotherapy. Rebound rejection is a significant contributor to mortality.[31,37,42] With current immunosuppressive practice, the post-transplant lymphoproliferative disease rate has decreased to less than 10% (Table 236-4).

GRAFT-VERSUS-HOST DISEASE

Skin changes consistent with graft-versus-host disease were diagnosed by histopathologic criteria and confirmed by immunohistochemical studies visualizing donor cell infiltration into the lesions on two occasions or by flow cytometry detecting elevated donor cell chimerism in peripheral blood. One child died with hereditary IgG and IgM deficiency,[43] and one adult developed a complex chronic graft-versus-host disease in association with post-transplant lymphoproliferative disease. All other cases have been treated with optimization of immunosuppression and limited steroid therapy, if necessary.

PRESENT STATUS AND FUTURE

The causes of graft and patient loss are invariably multifactorial and complex. The evolution of technical and clinical management factors have improved outcome (Fig. 236-9). However, the interplay between the need for high levels of immunosuppression, the high incidence of rejection, and the opportunistic infections consequent to this remain the major stumbling block to further progress.

Accumulated experience has allowed the development of clinical and surgical strategies that benefit a very complex group of patients. Reserved optimism is taken in light of previous experience with intestinal transplantation, as well as the grim outcome for patients not transplanted. Nonetheless, the overall actuarial survival rate at 1 and 5 years is 72% and 48%, respectively, and full nutritional support has been achieved in 91% of surviving patients (see Fig. 236-5). Improved results have been achieved in the pediatric population between 2 and 18 years of age (65% at 5 years).[37]

The transplantation of the isolated intestinal graft provides better patient survival at all follow-up times (see Fig. 236-6). However, because of the higher incidence of rejection with this type of graft, the long-term outcome of all types of grafts (isolated intestine or composite grafts) is similar (Fig. 236-10) and is estimated to be about 50% at 5 years.[31,37]

Improved strategies for immunosuppression have lowered the morbidity rate of transplantation and the concurrent infection rate and may allow for improved survival in the current era of preconditioning with Thymoglobulin.

FIGURE 236–9. Patient and graft survival. (From Abu-Elmagd K, Reyes J, Bond G, et al: Clinical intestinal transplantation: A decade of experience at a single center. Ann Surg 2001;234:404-417.)

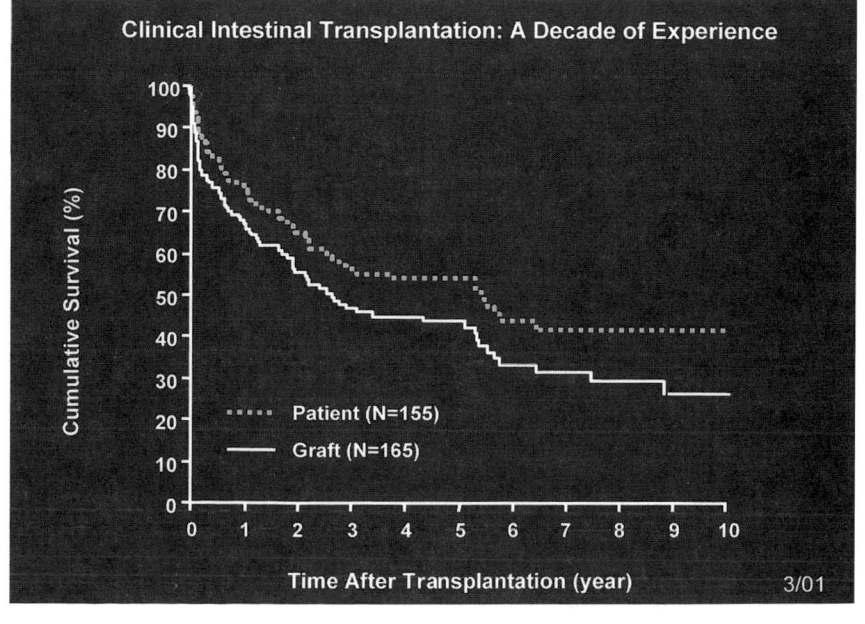

Clinical Intestinal Transplantation: A Decade of Experience

Cumulative Survival (%)

Time After Transplantation (year)

······ Patient (N=155)

—— Graft (N=165)

3/01

The first attempts to treat this condition surgically involved wrapping of the dissected aorta to prevent rupture[4] or treatment of the complications of dissection without definitive repair. This usually resulted in a catastrophic outcome and death. DeBakey and colleagues pioneered the surgical treatment of aortic disease, including dissection, and first reported graft replacement of the dissected aorta as definitive treatment.[5] Aortic graft interposition has become the cornerstone of modern surgical therapy.

The modern approach to acute aortic dissection involves initially controlling blood pressure with vasodilator medications and decreasing the rate of change of aortic pressure with beta blocker drugs, followed by surgical repair in appropriate cases. Improved surgical and anesthetic techniques and improved postoperative monitoring and management have dramatically improved the results of treatment of aortic dissection.

CLASSIFICATION

An understanding and description of aortic dissection are critical for the optimal care of these patients. The first widely used classification system was developed by DeBakey and colleagues and consists of three categories: types I, II, and III.[5,6] Type I involves dissection of the ascending aorta continuing to the descending aorta. Type II involves only the ascending aorta, and type III involves only the descending aortic from the ligamentum arteriosum distally. Subsequently, Daily and associates at Stanford developed a classification system involving only two groups, now known as the Stanford system.[7] In the Stanford classification system (Fig. 237-1), type A dissections involve the ascending aorta, and type B involve the more distal aorta from the innominate artery to more distal regions. There have been many other attempts to classify aortic dissection, but most have been abandoned. Despite the fact that different categories are used, the essential element of a classification system of aortic dissection is involvement of the ascending aorta, regardless of the location of the primary intimal tear and irrespective of the distal extent of the dissection process.[8] This functional classification approach is consistent with the pathophysiology of aortic dissection, considering that involvement of the ascending aorta is the principal predictor of the biologic behavior of the disease process, including the most common fatal complications—rupture with tamponade, congestive heart failure, and myocardial infarction. Moreover, functional classification simplifies diagnosis, because it is easier to accurately identify involvement of the ascending aorta than to determine the exact site of the primary intimal tear or the total extent of propagation of the dissection process.

The Stanford classification system facilitates the clinical decision-making process and definitive patient management. Patients presenting with acute Stanford type A dissections should be treated surgically in essentially all cases, and individuals with Stanford type B dissections are generally treated medically, using surgical intervention or endovascular stent-graft placement only if major complications are present. Generally, aortic dissections are defined as acute if they are diagnosed within 14 days of the onset of presenting symptoms. When dissection is diagnosed more than 14 days after onset, it is classified as chronic. Chronic dissection usually occurs only if the initial diagnosis was incorrect or if the patient suffered mild symptoms and did not seek appropriate medical care.

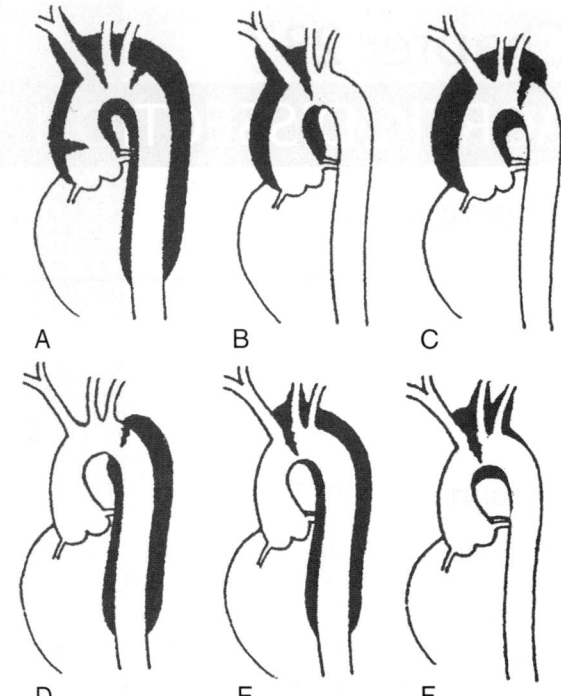

FIGURE 237–1. Schematic illustration of the Stanford classification system of aortic dissections. The three examples in the top row (*A, B,* and *C*) are all type A aortic dissections, involving the ascending aorta. The examples in the bottom row (*D, E,* and *F*) are all examples of type B dissections, in which the ascending aorta is not involved. Note that the aortic arch can be involved in a type B dissection. (From Miller DC: Surgical management of aortic dissections: Indications, perioperative management, and long-term results. In Doroghazi RM, Slater EE [eds]: Aortic Dissection. New York, McGraw-Hill, 1983, p 196.)

Over the past decade, advances in vascular imaging technology have led to the increased recognition of other conditions of the aorta, such as intramural hematoma and penetrating aortic ulcers, as distinct pathologic variants of classic aortic dissection.[9,10] Both these entities are characterized by the lack of a classic intimal flap dividing the aortic lumen into true and false channels. Intramural hematoma can be precipitated by an atherosclerotic ulcer penetrating the aortic wall or can occur spontaneously without intimal disruption after rupture of a vasa vasorum. Intramural hematoma can involve the ascending aorta (type A) as well as the descending aorta (type B). Although it is possible, an intramural hematoma rarely evolves into an aortic dissection.[11] Penetrating atherosclerotic ulcers occur most commonly in the descending thoracic aorta. Distinguishing intramural hematoma or penetrating aortic ulcer from aortic dissection is important, because the prognosis and management of these lesions can differ.[12,13]

CLINICAL FINDINGS

Aortic dissection can be seen in all age groups, although the majority of cases occur in men aged 50 to 80 years. Dissection in patients younger than 40 years is generally an acute type A dissection and occurs in those with Marfan's syndrome or a similar connective tissue disorder. On rare occasions, women during the last trimester of pregnancy or during delivery present with acute aortic dissection, presumably due to hormone-induced weakness of the aortic connective tissue and the markedly increased intra-aortic pressure that often occurs during delivery. There is a male predominance, with an estimated male-to-female ratio of approximately 2:1. The exact incidence of aortic dissection is difficult to ascertain, because in many cases the diagnosis is not made before death. Indeed, the delayed recognition of acute aortic dissection is a frequent cause of malpractice suits. In one series, acute aortic dissection was found in 1% to 2% of autopsies.[14] Recently, it has been estimated that the incidence of acute aortic dissection in the United States might be as high as 10 to 20 or more cases per million population per year.[15] Most aortic dissections (two thirds) are of the ascending Stanford type A, versus the more distal Stanford type B. Most surgeons and physicians incorrectly believe that ruptured abdominal aortic aneurysms are more common than aortic dissections; however, the former just tend to be diagnosed correctly more often than the latter are.

Left untreated, most patients suffering an acute aortic dissection die, generally within the first 24 to 48 hours. Death may occur due to rupture of the dissected aorta into the pericardial space, leading to tamponade and cardiovascular collapse; proximal extension, leading to severe, acute aortic insufficiency and heart failure; or acute myocardial infarction if the dissection involves the ostia of the coronary arteries. It has been estimated that 40% of patients with dissection involving the ascending aorta die immediately or before reaching the hospital, and more than 67% die within the first 24 hours. In addition, patients may die as a result of occlusion of major aortic branches supplying the cerebral or visceral circulation, causing massive stroke or visceral ischemia and severe metabolic acidosis. In contrast, among patients with Stanford type B dissections (distal aortic arch or descending thoracic aorta), 75% are alive 1 month after the onset of symptoms.

Patients with untreated acute type B dissection can expire from acute aortic rupture or from occlusion of one of several major aortic branches, resulting in ischemic injury to vital abdominal organs or the brain. However, comparative studies have determined that in most cases of type B aortic dissection, survival is better with medical treatment alone (aggressive antihypertensive therapy) than with urgent surgical repair or aortic replacement. After acute aortic dissection, the false lumen remains patent in most cases, depending on the presence of distal reentry sites. When the false lumen remains patent, the aorta is prone to progressive expansion over time, necessitating the need for close long-term follow-up.

The most consistent clinical condition associated with aortic dissection is arterial hypertension. In patients with aortic dissection, the prevalence of arterial hypertension varies between 45% and 80%[16-19] and is highest in patients with acute type B dissection (Table 237-1). Hypertension may lead to smooth muscle degeneration in the aortic wall, which may predispose to aortic dissection. Connective tissue disorders such as Marfan's or Ehlers-Danlos syndrome are associated with an increased risk of aortic dissection. Although both these conditions are relatively rare, they are frequently associated with acute dissection. In fact, aortic rupture or dissection is a frequent cause of death in patients with Marfan's syndrome or other connective tissue disorders.[20] Severe aortic atherosclerosis has been associated with a slight increase in the incidence of aortic dissection, but if dissection occurs, its extent seems to be more limited.

The risk of perioperative and late postoperative dissection[21] is also increased in patients with a bicuspid aortic valve or aortic coarctation, presumably due impaired connective

TABLE 237–1. CONDITIONS ASSOCIATED WITH AORTIC DISSECTION

Hypertension
Aortic valve and congenital aortic disorders
   Bicuspid aortic valve
   Coarctation of the aorta
Connective tissue disorders
   Marfan's syndrome
   Cystic medial necrosis
   Ehlers-Danlos syndrome
   Turner's syndrome
Pregnancy
Atherosclerosis
Relapsing polychondritis
Giant cell arteritis
Syphilis
Cocaine abuse
Iatrogenic
   Insertion of intra-aortic balloon pump
   Cardiac catheterization or angioplasty
   Aortic or femoral arterial cannulation for cardiopulmonary bypass

tissue integrity. In addition, aortic dissection is more common in patients with Turner's syndrome and inflammatory disorders of the aorta, such as syphilis or giant cell arteritis. Aortic dissection is a rare complication of cardiac catheterization and other percutaneous diagnostic and therapeutic interventional techniques involving manipulation of catheters inside the thoracic aorta. Unfortunately, most veteran cardiac surgeons have experienced cases of intraoperative aortic dissection due to a clamp injury of the ascending aorta or a dissection initiating at the arterial cannulation site, especially when femoral arterial cannulation is performed. One of the cardiovascular complications of cocaine use is acute aortic dissection, and this diagnosis should be considered in drug abusers presenting with acute chest pain.[22,23] Aortic dissection in this setting occurs as a result of sudden severe hypertension secondary to catecholamine release.

PATHOLOGIC FINDINGS

Most surgeons and pathologists believe that the initiating event in aortic dissection is a tear in the intima of the aortic wall that allows blood to enter, leading to separation of the medial layers of the aorta. The primary intimal tear causes communication between the true aortic lumen and the false lumen. Few aortic dissections lack an identifiable intimal tear. Indeed, most extensive aortic dissections have multiple reentry sites. Intramural hematoma due to rupture of an intramural vessel is another potential initiating event, although this cause of dissection is less frequent. Dissections usually propagate antegrade in a spiral manner but may also extend in a retrograde fashion. The rate of increase of aortic systolic pressure and absolute blood pressure and the integrity and strength of the aortic wall determine the rate and extent of progression of the dissection. Ironically, distal progression of the dissection may be limited by extensive atherosclerotic disease, because the layers of the aorta are more tightly fused. Younger patients presenting with acute dissection frequently have involvement of the entire thoracic and abdominal aorta. Reentry into the true lumen may allow decompression of the false lumen and may maintain perfusion to distal organs. This is the rationale behind surgical and percutaneous techniques of fenestration for the treatment of malperfusion syndromes associated with aortic dissection.

Organ or limb ischemia or malperfusion may occur when the dissection process compromises blood flow to various aortic branches. Malperfusion usually occurs when flow is impaired due to vascular compression of the true lumen by the false lumen, extravascular compression of abdominal viscera or vessels, or occlusion of a branch artery by a dissection flap. The pattern of involvement of branches of the thoracic and abdominal aorta is variable and often leads to confusion regarding the correct diagnosis.

PRESENTATION

Severe chest pain of a sudden nature is the most common presenting symptom of aortic dissection. The pain is typically abrupt and severe at onset and is often described as "tearing" and "the worst pain I have ever experienced." This is especially true for patients who have never experienced childbirth. With type A dissections, the pain tends to be in the anterior chest and similar to that observed with myocardial infarction. Type B dissections classically cause midscapular pain, although this can be quite variable; this variability may lead to an incorrect diagnosis. Migration of pain and constant pain suggest continued expansion or progression. Differentiating the chest pain of acute aortic dissection from that of other causes, such as acute myocardial ischemia, esophageal reflux disease, pericarditis, chest trauma, or abdominal pathology, is critical in the initial evaluation of these patients to allow prompt, correct management. On occasion, acute dissection can be painless, although this presentation is uncommon and is often the case in patients presenting with chronic dissection. A relative minority of patients with acute aortic dissection present with signs of cardiac and other organ system involvement.[17-19,24-26] Other clinical manifestations may include stroke, paraplegia, upper or lower extremity ischemia, and anuria or abdominal pain due to renal or mesenteric ischemia. These latter findings portend a grave prognosis.

DIAGNOSIS

The diagnosis of aortic dissection requires a strong index of suspicion by the evaluating physician. If the acute, sudden onset of chest pain cannot be attributed to myocardial infarction or ischemia, pericarditis, or traumatic chest injury, the diagnosis of acute dissection must be considered. Even in cases of acute myocardial infarction, the diagnosis of aortic dissection should still be entertained, especially if the patient develops migrating chest or back pain, leg ischemia, syncope, or other neurologic symptoms that may be related to vascular compromise. Physical findings often include a disparity in blood pressure measurements between the right and left arms or between the arms and legs, or a diminished pulse in one of the limbs. After the diagnosis is suspected, rapid confirmation or exclusion of aortic dissection is critical for optimal care. Until quite recently, aortic angiography was considered the gold standard for the diagnosis of acute dissection because other methods, such as computed tomography and echocardiography, were untested or fraught with artifactual findings. However, improved computed tomography-angiography, transesophageal echocardiography (TEE), and magnetic resonance imaging (MRI) techniques are at least as accurate as aortic angiography and are usually far more rapidly obtained. The selection of the diagnostic method depends on which technique is most accurate and can be most quickly obtained in the treating hospital. In general, the procedure of choice is TEE because it can be obtained rapidly and the cardiologist is often already involved in the patient's care. The type of dissection (i.e., Stanford type A or B), the extent of dissection, the presence or absence of hemodynamically significant aortic valve regurgitation, and the presence or absence of pericardial effusion can all be determined using TEE.

Although the chest radiograph is neither sensitive nor specific for the diagnosis of dissection, some findings may be suggestive. These findings include the presence of a widened upper mediastinum, blunting of the aortic knob, and pleural effusion. The electrocardiogram (ECG), though neither specific nor sensitive, can help establish the need for concomitant coronary revascularization if the dissection involves the coronary arteries or if the patient suffers from ordinary coronary artery disease. Elderly male patients often present with ECG changes during acute aortic dissection, even if no direct coronary involvement is present. This phenomenon is likely related to concomitant coronary artery disease. Coronary angiography is rarely performed unless there is clear compromise of myocardial perfusion. However, when the patient has a clear history of coronary artery disease and is hemodynamically stable, consideration should be given to performing coronary angiography before repairing a type A aortic dissection. Moderate coronary occlusive disease can generally be treated percutaneously in the catheterization laboratory after aortic surgery. When hemodynamic instability is present, the patient should proceed directly to the operating room on an emergent basis, unless acute rupture is strongly suspected or confirmed and no operating room or staff is currently available.

Computed tomography (CT) is noninvasive and easy to perform and can usually be obtained without delay. Owing to major technologic advances, acquisition of a large number of thin-slice images is possible within minutes using ultrafast CT scanners. Further, modern computer technology allows complex reconstruction of high-quality images. The diagnosis of aortic dissection requires the identification of two distinct lumens separated by an intimal flap.[27] Contrast-enhanced CT scanning has a sensitivity of 82% to 100% and a specificity between 90% and 100%.[17,27-32] Disadvantages include the need for intravenous contrast and the presence of artifacts, although the latter is now less of a problem than in the past.

MRI is also noninvasive and does not require the use of contrast material. MRI produces high-quality images of the aorta in multiple planes and allows clear delineation of the entire aorta, localization of the intimal tear, delineation of aortic branch artery involvement, and diagnosis of a pericardial effusion, suggestive of aortic rupture. As with CT scanning, the criterion used to diagnose acute aortic dissection with MRI is the identification of two lumens separated by an intimal flap. MRI is associated with sensitivity and specificity rates of 95% to 100%.[17,27,29-32] In urgent circumstances, MRI may not be immediately available, and this approach should not be performed in patients with pacemakers, defibrillators, or other metallic implants. In addition, the relatively long time necessary for image acquisition in hemodynamically compromised patients is a potential drawback to using MRI to make or confirm the diagnosis of aortic dissection.

Transthoracic echocardiography has a limited role in the diagnosis of aortic dissection because the images produced are not optimal. TEE is the main method used in most centers for the diagnosis of acute aortic dissection. High-resolution imaging of the heart and the thoracic aorta is possible with TEE because of the close proximity of the esophagus and the thoracic aorta. TEE can provide information regarding aortic valve function, flow characteristics within the true and false lumens, adequacy of coronary perfusion, and estimates of left ventricular size and function. Importantly, TEE can be performed in the emergency room, ICU, or operating room. Even if the diagnosis of acute aortic dissection has been confirmed with another imaging modality, TEE can aid in the preoperative, intraoperative, and postoperative assessment of cardiac and valvular function and the extent of residual disease .

TREATMENT

In general, all patients with acute type A aortic dissections should be considered for emergency surgical repair of the ascending aorta to prevent life-threatening conditions or complications.[6,8,15-17,19,25,33-35] Patients with acute type A dissection presenting with irreversible stroke or other severe malperfusion syndromes,[8,18,36] those with debilitating systemic diseases such as metastatic cancer with a life expectancy of less than 1 year, or those older than 80 years with multiple major complications may be considered for medical management. It should be recognized, however, that patients treated nonoperatively are not likely to survive very long. The presence of acute hemiplegia alone should not be considered an absolute contraindication to early surgical intervention,[36] because many of these patients recover significant neurologic function after surgery. However, patients presenting with hypotension, massive stroke, anuria, and acidosis suggestive of mesenteric ischemia should be considered nonoperative cases. Patients presenting with acute type A intramural hematoma are managed identically to those with acute type A aortic dissection.[9,11,37] However, some authors believe that medical therapy is indicated for selected patients with uncomplicated acute type A intramural hematoma when the ascending aorta is not excessively dilated.[38-40] If a patient with acute type A intramural hematoma is treated medically, close observation is mandatory. Serial imaging studies should be obtained over several days.

As soon as the diagnosis of acute type A aortic dissection is suspected, intensive monitoring must be initiated. An arterial line, central venous catheter, and urinary catheter should be inserted. Antihypertensive treatment is a major part of the initial management of patients with acute type A or type B dissection before and after surgical correction (Table 237-2). Generally, patients with acute severe hypotension or other evidence of rupture or impending rupture should be taken to the operating room emergently, and attempts at pericardial drainage should be avoided.

The primary goal of surgical treatment for patients with acute type A dissection is to replace the ascending aorta to prevent aortic rupture or proximal extension of the process, with resultant tamponade or severe heart failure. Ideally, the primary intimal tear should be completely resected, and the dissected aortic layers reconstituted proximally and distally to obliterate the false lumen and reestablish normal perfusion to distal organs. When aortic valve regurgitation is present, aortic valve competence is restored either by reconstructing the sinuses of Valsalva and the aortic root or by resuspending the valve commissures. These approaches are possible in the majority of cases.[41] Complete aortic root replacement with

TABLE 237-2. INITIAL MEDICAL MANAGEMENT FOR PATIENTS WITH ACUTE AORTIC DISSECTION

Drug	Dosage
Metoprolol	5-10 mg slow i.v. bolus until SBP <120 mm Hg and HR <70 bpm; repeat as needed
Esmolol	500 µg/kg/min i.v. for 1 min, followed by 30-50 µg/kg/min for 5 min; titrate to maintain SBP <120 mm Hg systolic and HR <70 bpm
Labetalol	0.25 mg/kg i.v. over 2 min; 40-80 mg q10min up to 300 mg; continuous i.v. infusion to maintain SBP <120 mm Hg and HR <70 bpm
Sodium nitroprusside	1-8 µg/kg/min i.v. to maintain SBP <120 mm Hg; should be used in conjunction with a beta blocker (metoprolol, esmolol, labetalol)

bpm, beats per minute; HR, heart rate; SBP, systolic blood pressure.

reimplantation of the coronary ostia using either a composite valve graft or a valve-sparing technique should be considered if the aortic root is severely damaged by the dissection process, the patient has Marfan's syndrome or another connective tissue disorder, severe annuloaortic ectasia is present, or the valve needs to be replaced for other reasons, such as aortic stenosis.[42-44] In selected cases, aortic valve replacement and supracoronary aortic graft replacement may be used to treat acute type A aortic dissections, if the aortic root is not destroyed by the dissection. Excellent surgical technique needs to be used to prevent excessive bleeding, continued dissection, and residual coronary ischemia or aortic valve insufficiently. Aprotinin or ε-aminocaproic acid (Amicar) can be administered to decrease bleeding. Some centers avoid using aprotinin when hypothermic circulatory arrest is contemplated. When necessary, reinforcement of the dissected aortic layers is facilitated by reapproximation of the dissection flap to the aortic wall using strips of Teflon felt or bovine pericardium. Biologic glue composed of purified bovine serum albumin and 10% glutaraldehyde was recently approved in the United States (BioGlue, CryoLife Inc., Kennesaw, GA). Biologic glue is easy to use and decreases blood loss,[45] but cases have been reported in which use of a large amount of glue has resulted in the development of false aneurysms, graft dehiscence, and full-thickness aortic necrosis. Most modern woven vascular grafts are not plagued by excessive bleeding and are easy to use.

In the past 10 years, the use of hypothermic circulatory arrest has been advocated to allow careful inspection of the aortic arch and performance of an "open" distal aortic anastomosis in cases of acute type A dissection.[46,47] The construction of a completely hemostatic distal anastomosis is easier in the absence of an aortic cross-clamp. However, profound circulatory arrest increases the risk of neurologic injury, especially if the distal anastomosis cannot be performed in a rapid manner.

A midline sternotomy incision is used to repair acute type A dissections. Arterial cannulation can be performed via the right axillary artery or either femoral artery. Cardiopulmonary bypass is then established. If the patient has severe aortic insufficiency, a vent is inserted into the left ventricle through the right superior pulmonary vein to prevent distention. I place a single venous cannula, although some suggest bicaval cannulation. The use of retrograde blood cardioplegia facilitates the operative procedure, although supplemental antegrade cardioplegia can be delivered directly into the coronary arteries.

Patients with dissection-related destruction of the aortic root should undergo composite valve graft root replacement or valve-sparing aortic root replacement using the David reimplantation method, with complete or near-complete excision of the sinuses of Valsalva. Alternatively, resuspension of the aortic valve and preservation of the sinuses can be performed if the aortic root is not destroyed. If the aortic valve is markedly abnormal or cannot be satisfactorily repaired, separate valve and supracoronary aortic graft replacement is a reasonable alternative in selected patients, but the supracoronary aortic arch should be resected as extensively as possible to prevent pseudoaneurysm formation.

In up to a third of patients, the primary intimal tear is located in the aortic arch or descending aorta, a condition that is associated with a poorer prognosis.[47-50] These tears should be resected if possible, but such resection is often not feasible without combining arch or distal aortic resection with ascending aortic repair. Elderly patients often do not tolerate such extensive surgery and sustain major complications. In addition, reentry tears may occur in the distal aorta, precluding establishment of a totally intact, normally perfused aorta at the end of the operation. Although failure to include the arch in the repair may increase the need for subsequent aortic reoperation and reduce long-term survival, most cardiovascular surgeons simply treat the most critical portion of the aorta (i.e., the ascending segment) in these cases and leave the remainder of the aorta alone in an effort to end up with a viable patient. This strategy is especially reasonable for very elderly patients or those with major comorbid conditions. Although infrequently encountered, patients with chronic type A or type B dissection may need surgical repair if an aortic false aneurysm or progressive aortic enlargement has developed. In some case, it is difficult to distinguish between acute and chronic type A aortic dissection. In these cases, urgent repair should be undertaken. Aortic dilatation due to significant aortic valve insufficiency is an indication for operation. In asymptomatic patients, surgical intervention is generally recommended when the diameter of the ascending aorta is greater than 55 to 60 mm, depending on the size of the normal native aorta (50 mm in patients with Marfan's syndrome), or if the documented rate of expansion is greater than 5 to 10 mm over 1 year.[51]

With optimal medical and surgical methods, patients with aortic dissection have a mortality of 5% to 30% in the best centers.[17,19,33,46,48,52-58] These relatively low early mortality rates are due to advances in early diagnosis, surgical techniques, and myocardial protection. In the Stanford experience, the overall survival rates for patients with acute type A dissections at 1, 5, and 10 years were 67%, 55%, and 37%, respectively.[18] For patients with chronic type A dissections, the survival was 76%, 65%, and 45%, respectively. For patients with acute type A dissections, late survival for discharged patients was 91%, 75%, and 51% at 1, 5, and 10 years, respectively, compared with 93%, 79%, and 54% for those with chronic type A dissections. One third of the late deaths were cardiac related, and many (10% to 20%) were due to complications related to extension of the dissection or dilatation of the dissected aortic segment.

The treatment of Stanford type B dissections is generally medical, with aggressive antihypertensive and beta blocker therapy and close long-term observation for progressive dilatation (see Table 237-2). Generally, beta blockade is initiated, and a vasodilator drug such as sodium nitroprusside is added later for blood pressure control. Pure vasodilator drugs should be avoided as an initial treatment, because reflex tachycardia and increased cardiac contractility may actually increase the change in aortic pressure and, at least theoretically, exacerbate the dissection process. Alternatively, one of the newer antihypertensive agents, such as nicardipine or fenoldopam, may be considered. Initial medical monitoring and management should take place in an ICU in most cases, because a rapid and significant reduction in blood pressure and heart rate is the hallmark of optimal care. Blood pressure monitoring with an automatic blood pressure cuff apparatus may be sufficient if severe hypertension is not evident, the patient remains hemodynamically stable, and only a low dose of medication is required to control changes in aortic pressure. If the blood pressure and heart rate cannot be rapidly controlled, or if the patient does not rapidly become pain free, becomes hemodynamically unstable, or develops symptoms of associated malperfusion, an arterial monitoring line is mandatory, and early reimaging of the aorta should be considered. If the patient remains stable and pain free, he or she may be monitored outside the ICU after 24 to 48 hours. An imaging study (usually CT scan or MRI) should be obtained before discharge as a baseline study.

Because surgical management of type B dissections is associated with very high mortality and morbidity, and because the results of medical management tend to be similar to or better than the outcome after urgent surgical intervention, a nonoperative approach is taken in the vast majority of cases. Surgery through a lateral left thoracotomy is indicated for complications related to malperfusion or for chronic, severe pain indicative of dilatation, impending rupture, or progressive dissection. However, most of the complications related to malperfusion can be treated with catheter-based fenestration procedures or stent grafting,[59] and these patients do not require surgical therapy. Stenting of the thoracic aorta is still in its infancy, and no approved devices are currently available. Continued pain, new neurologic findings, and malperfusion syndromes not correctable with catheter-based fenestration or stent grafting may require surgical intervention. Cardiopulmonary bypass is generally used in these cases, cannulating the femoral artery and left atrium or both the femoral artery and vein. Cardiopulmonary bypass is usually instituted using total bypass, with or without profound hypothermic circulatory arrest. Alternatively, partial cardiopulmonary bypass (or isolated left heart bypass) can be used, depending on the surgeon's preference. Although, in theory, the use of cardiopulmonary bypass should lessen the incidence of postoperative paraplegia, the results of descending aortic surgery using total or partial cardiopulmonary bypass (or isolated left heart bypass) or a non–cardiopulmonary bypass approach are similar in most series.

LONG-TERM FOLLOW-UP

Close medical follow-up and careful periodic surveillance using appropriate imaging are critical to the optimal long-term management of postsurgical type A aortic dissection patients and those with type B dissection. It is mandatory for patients with aortic dissections to undergo routine imaging for as long as they live. Following operative repair, serial CT or MRI scans of the thoracic and abdominal aorta are essential to detect complications related to aortic dissection; these scans should be performed at 3- to 6-month intervals for the first year and then every year thereafter. An echocardiogram may also be performed annually to evaluate the aortic root and aortic valve function, especially if aortic root reconstruction was performed. The hallmark of the long-term management of patients who have suffered aortic dissection is the aggressive control of arterial blood pressure, regardless of whether they have undergone surgical repair.

ANNOTATED REFERENCES

Daily PO, Trueblood HW, Stinson EB, et al: Management of acute aortic dissections. Ann Thorac Surg 1970;10:237-247.

The most frequently used classification system for aortic dissections was developed by Daily and associates at Stanford University. This system of classification, now known as the Stanford classification, involves only two groups. Type A dissections involve the ascending aorta, and type B involve the more distal aorta from the innominate artery to more distal regions.

David TE, Feindel CM: An aortic valve-sparing operation for patients with aortic incompetence and aneurysm of the ascending aorta. J Thorac Cardiovasc Surg 1992;103:617-621.

This paper discusses the treatment of aortic dissection involving the aortic root. If the aortic root is severely damaged by the dissection process, the patient has Marfan's syndrome or another connective tissue disorder, severe annuloaortic ectasia is present, or the valve needs to be replaced for other reasons (e.g., aortic stenosis), a valve-sparing technique may be appropriate.

Gillinov AM, Lytle BW, Kaplon RJ, et al: Dissection of the ascending aorta after previous cardiac surgery: Differences in presentation and management. J Thorac Cardiovasc Surg 1999;117:252-260.

The risk of perioperative and late postoperative dissection is discussed in the paper, as are many other associated pathologic findings, such as bicuspid aortic valve, aortic coarctation, and Turner's syndrome. Aortic dissection as a rare complication of cardiac catheterization and other percutaneous diagnostic and therapeutic interventional techniques is also examined.

Miller DC: Surgical management of aortic dissections: Indications, perioperative management, and long-term results. In Doroghazi RM, Slater EE (eds): Aortic Dissection. New York, McGraw-Hill, 1983, pp 193-243.

This chapter provides an excellent overview of the clinical features, surgical and medical management, and outcomes after aortic dissection.

Yacoub MH, Gehle P, Chandrasekaran V, et al: Late results of a valve-preserving operation in patients with aneurysms of the ascending aorta and root. J Thorac Cardiovasc Surg 1998;115:1080-1090.

This paper presents the late results of a valve-preserving operation in patients with aneurysms of the ascending aorta and root.

Chapter 238

SPLANCHNIC ISCHEMIA

Jeroen J. Kolkman • Robert H. Geelkerken

KEY POINTS

1. Nonocclusive mucosal or mesenteric ischemia (NOMI) is **a common disorder** in intensive care patients and **can be detected with tonometry.**

2. NOMI is best **treated by aggressive volume resuscitation and avoidance of alpha-adrenergic drugs.**

3. **Abnormal tonometry** is the earliest and best indicator of NOMI; normalization of tonometry seems to be a good endpoint of volume resuscitation.

4. **Tonometry is ideal for ICUs with less experienced clinicians and residents,** as it identifies the early and nonresolved phases of NOMI; experienced intensivists often have the clinical skills to recognize NOMI based on the patient's presentation.

5. **NOMI is the extreme adaptation of blood flow distribution in all types of circulatory stress.**

6. **Angiography** is the gold standard for delineating vessel anatomy, as well as providing a route for treatment with medication, dilatation, and stent placement; it is therefore **the method of choice for critically ill patients suspected of having splanchnic ischemia.**

7. Multivessel chronic splanchnic ischemia has an accelerated "final course" and a high infarction rate; therefore, **analysis and treatment should not be delayed.**

8. **Enteral nutrition** improves splanchnic perfusion in most patients; it can provoke an infarction in extreme low-flow conditions, however, and **should therefore be used cautiously.**

9. **Colonoscopy** is the gold standard for diagnosing early mucosal ischemic colitis; **laparotomy** is the gold standard for diagnosing transmural or gangrenous ischemic colitis.

Vascular disorders of the splanchnic circulation are usually asymptomatic but can occasionally be catastrophic. Therefore, early diagnosis and treatment have important clinical implications. There is much confusion regarding terminology. The generally used term *mesenteric ischemia* indicates ischemia in the region supplied only by the mesenteric arteries, for example, the small and large bowel. The official *Medical Subject Headings* term *splanchnic circulation* denotes all the vascular beds supplied by the celiac, superior mesenteric, and inferior mesenteric arteries, including those in the stomach, liver, pancreas, and spleen, as well as those in the large and small intestines. *Splanchnic ischemia* is the preferred term.

Splanchnic artery stenosis is common, but splanchnic ischemia is supposedly rare due to abundant collateral circulation. Moreover, the diagnosis is often overlooked, as indicated by the long delay before the condition is diagnosed in many cases and the large variation in reported prevalence among centers. A simple diagnostic test is unavailable. For the intensivist, patients with chronic occlusive splanchnic ischemia are few, but these patients may have a prolonged and complicated course in the ICU. Nonocclusive mucosal or mesenteric ischemia (NOMI) is quite common in critically ill patients. NOMI is also called "intramucosal ischemia" and is characterized by mucosal acidosis.

PHYSIOLOGY, ANATOMY, AND PATHOPHYSIOLOGY

NORMAL BLOOD FLOW

The goal of perfusion of any organ is to support normal cellular functions by delivering a sufficient amount of oxygen to meet metabolic demands. During ischemia, the amount of oxygen available to the organ is insufficient to maintain aerobic processes. Typically, cells attempt to defend the production of adenosine triphosphate (ATP), the "energy currency" of metabolism, by increasing the rate of anaerobic glycolysis. Depending on the degree and duration of ischemia, this process may result in tissue necrosis, ischemia-reperfusion damage, increased mucosal permeability, and bacterial translocation. This complicated process results from at least six factors: (1) impaired blood supply via the main vessels, (2) reduced blood oxygen and hemoglobin content, (3) maldistribution of blood flow in the bowel wall, (4) countercurrent exchange of oxygen within the mucosa from the bases to the tips of the villi, (5) mismatching of metabolism and perfusion within the mucosa, and (6) alterations in the cell's capacity to use oxygen.

MAIN VESSELS

The arterial blood supply of the gastrointestinal (GI) tract comes from three arteries: celiac artery (CA), superior mesenteric artery (SMA), and inferior mesenteric artery (IMA). The CA supplies the stomach, liver, part of the pancreas, and the proximal part of the duodenum. The SMA supplies the distal part of the duodenum, the entire small bowel, the ascending colon, and the proximal part of the transverse colon. The IMA, the smallest of the three vessels, supplies the metabolically less active distal colon. Branches of these arteries enter the bowel wall to form two plexuses within the serosa and the submucosa. Finally, arterioles penetrate the muscular layer toward the mucosa. At the mucosal villi, they branch into an extensive network of capillaries and venules, which permits diffusional shunting of oxygen via a countercurrent mechanism.

Numerous collaterals exist between the main arteries. The first collaterals are enlargements of normally small arteries or embryonic remnants (Buhler's arc) connecting the CA and SMA in the region of the pancreas and duodenal bulb. Other collaterals connect the SMA and the IMA (Riolan's artery or marginal artery of Drummond). Additionally, the aforementioned plexuses in the bowel wall form a large collateral network. Still, even with this large collateral reserve, the superficial layers of the mucosa are very susceptible to the development of ischemia. This susceptibility is due to the countercurrent arteriovenous exchange of oxygen that starts at the base of the villus; when the blood flow rate is low, oxygen may be depleted before the villus tip is reached.[1-3]

During fasting basal conditions, approximately 20% of the cardiac output goes through the splanchnic vasculature. The flow doubles after a meal. Blood draining from the bowel enters the mesenteric veins and finally the portal vein. The liver, therefore, receives its blood supply from two sources: venous blood from the portal vein, and arterial blood from the hepatic artery, a branch of the CA, or, in 25% of cases, the SMA. This dual blood supply renders the liver relatively protected against ischemia. However, in cases of multivessel occlusion or stenosis of both the CA and the SMA, both sources are involved, and severe liver ischemia can ensue.

REGULATION OF BOWEL WALL BLOOD FLOW

Vasoconstrictors

Catecholamines have differing effects on the splanchnic blood flow; alpha$_1$-adrenergic receptor stimulation leads to vasoconstriction, whereas beta$_2$-adrenergic and dopamine receptor stimulation leads to vasodilation. The relation between the renin-angiotensin axis and splanchnic perfusion is less uniform, although angiotensin II acts as a key splanchnic vasoconstrictor during low flow.[4] The main splanchnic vasoconstrictor is endothelin-1.[5,6] Two main endothelin-1 receptor types have been described: ET_A and ET_B. Activation of ET_A, which is expressed in the mucosa, submucosa, and muscularis of the bowel wall, leads to vasoconstriction; ET_A is stimulated early when the effective circulating volume is low.[5]

Vasodilators

The main splanchnic vasodilators are nitric oxide (NO) and prostaglandins. NO has paradoxical effects on GI perfusion and mucosal integrity. Normally, low levels of NO are produced by the endothelium to sustain perfusion by promoting local vasodilation. In pathologic circumstances, such as circulatory shock or sepsis, a large amount of NO is produced and acts as a free radical, similar to oxygen free radicals, and is extremely toxic. In an animal model of hemorrhagic shock, inhibition of NO production is beneficial.[7] Locally formed prostaglandins act as mucosal vasodilators, especially during low-flow states or following mucosal injury. Inhibition of cyclo-oxygenase, as with nonsteroidal anti-inflammatory drugs, diminishes this vasodilatory response and renders the GI mucosa more susceptible to the effects of circulatory shock.[8]

LOW-FLOW CONDITIONS

All the previously mentioned receptors and messengers act to balance perfusion with metabolic demand on a moment-to-moment basis. During circulatory shock, blood flow distribution changes due to constriction and dilation of different vascular beds. When circulating volume is decreased, relative blood flow to the heart increases and brain perfusion is maintained, but perfusion of skeletal muscles, skin, and gut is reduced. Splanchnic vasoconstriction occurs early and profoundly,[9] even before systemic hemodynamic instability arises.[10] Splanchnic vasoconstriction can be triggered by different shock states and by the direct effects of vasoactive medications or nicotine or cocaine abuse. GI ischemia occurs only when blood flow is reduced to less than 50% of the basal rate.[11-13]

During splanchnic hypoperfusion, blood flow within the bowel wall is unevenly distributed among the different layers. In general, the mucosa is protected at the expense of the serosal layers.[14] Still, the surface of the mucosa is most vulnerable to ischemia, owing to countercurrent diffusional shunting of oxygen. Even within the mucosal layer, blood flow is unevenly distributed. Thus, mismatches between metabolic demand and oxygen delivery can be caused by several microcirculatory disturbances and shunting.[15-17] When global perfusion is compromised the patchy distribution of flow can be observed among different villi and within individual villi. These phenomena help explain why, in some studies, mucosal blood flow measurements are within the normal range despite evidence of mucosal ischemia. Thus, for the (early) detection of ischemia, flow measurements alone do not suffice. This combination of ischemia and normal vessel anatomy has given rise to the term "NOMI."

ISCHEMIC DAMAGE: THE CRUCIAL ROLE OF REPERFUSION

After the onset of ischemia, three different processes can be distinguished. In acute arterial occlusion, these processes occur sequentially; in nonocclusive ischemia, they occur simultaneously and remittently.

Ischemic Phase

The immediate effect of reduced oxygen utilization is ATP depletion. One of the consequences of ATP depletion is derangement of the tight junctions between adjacent enterocytes, leading to the formation of "cracks" in the mucosal lining. Also, key membrane-bound pumps are deprived of energy; as a consequence, electrolytes and water enter the cells, which swell and, if the process continues, eventually die. Both mechanisms lead to reduced intestinal epithelial barrier function and the movement of bacteria across the bowel wall from the lumen into the systemic compartment (bacterial translocation).[18] During cellular hypoxia, the enzyme xanthine dehydrogenase is converted to xanthine oxidase (XO), which is harmless at this stage, because XO needs oxygen as a substrate. Finally, tissue necrosis triggers an inflammatory response, resulting in cytokine release. The effects of the ischemic phase are localized and can remain clinically undetected for many hours (closed compartment). The condition may be silent until reperfusion initiates a systemic inflammatory response or transmural gangrene occurs.

Local Effects of Reperfusion

After flow is restored—for example, as a result of the partial dissolution of an embolus—oxygen enters the ischemic tissue. In a reaction catalyzed by XO, oxygen forms reactive oxygen species (ROS) that can damage proteins and DNA.[19] The damage to mucosa, blood vessels, and submucosal tissues is intensified and spreads to adjacent regions by diffusion of the small ROS molecules. Locally present ROS scavengers, including glutathione, catalase, and superoxide dismutase, can neutralize ROS, but their efficacy is limited.

Systemic Effects of Reperfusion

Reperfusion delivers toxic products, including XO, proinflammatory cytokines, and activated neutrophils, into the systemic circulation.[20] In animal studies, liver and lung damage has been attributed to activated neutrophils coming from reperfused ischemic bowel.[19] Therefore, reperfusion leads to amplification and spreading of the ischemic damage.

DIAGNOSTIC METHODS

DETECTION OF STENOSIS

Duplex ultrasonography of the splanchnic arteries is widely used as a screening test for splanchnic artery stenosis and is 80% to 90% accurate in experienced hands. Measurement of the flow velocity at the origin of the CA and the SMA grades the severity of the stenosis. In 10% to 15% of patients, it is difficult to visualize the main vessels because of overlying (gastric) air. This technique does not permit assessment of the smaller vessels, and the success of the technique is highly operator dependent. These limitations make it unsuitable for almost all critically ill patients.

Magnetic resonance angiography (MRA) of the splanchnic vessels has gained popularity. MRA has the advantage of enabling a 360-degree view of the vessels and, in the future, may become a functional test by permitting the measurement of flow or oxygen saturation in the portal vein. Its main disadvantages are relatively low spatial resolution, a tendency to exaggerate the degree of stenosis, and lack of utility for assessing the status of collateral vessels. At this time, MRA is used mainly as a screening test in patients with chronic abdominal complaints.

Intra-arterial digital subtraction angiography of the splanchnic vessels is still the gold standard for the assessment of vascular anatomy, stenosis, and collateral circulation. Moreover, this technique allows the performance of endovascular procedures in the same session, including infusion of papaverine and angioplasty or stenting of stenoses. The combination of high diagnostic accuracy and the possibility of intervention makes angiography the procedure of choice in patients suspected of having symptomatic splanchnic stenoses, especially in those with imminent or ongoing infarction. In acute splanchnic infarction, angiography serves as a guide for endovascular or operative revascularization.

INSPECTION OF MUCOSA AND SEROSA

Endoscopy has great potential to detect ischemia, because the earliest ischemic changes in the bowel wall appear in the superficial mucosal layers.[13] Endoscopy is used mostly to diagnose ischemic colitis, for which it is the procedure of choice. It should be stressed that the endoscopic appearance may be difficult to interpret, especially with an imperfectly rinsed bowel; therefore, preparation with an enema using 2 to 4 L of water is advisable. Differentiation of ischemic colitis from inflammatory bowel disease can be difficult. During the first days, ischemic colitis closely resembles ulcerative colitis; later, it may be indistinguishable from Crohn's disease. Endoscopy can show even the earliest stages of mucosal ischemia; as a rule, it cannot distinguish between mucosal and transmural ischemia or gangrene, however. The latter (irreversible) condition can be detected only by inspecting the serosal side of the bowel. Therefore, laparoscopy or laparotomy is indicated when colonic gangrene is clinically suspected.

LABORATORY TESTS

In general, hematologic tests are of limited use for the detection of ischemia. Classic parameters, such as the leukocyte count and arterial lactate level, are of limited value because they lack sensitivity as well as specificity. Various parameters have been successfully used in animal models, including the intestinal fatty acid binding protein and D-lactate,[21,22] but clinical data are scarce.[23,24]

TONOMETRY

Tonometry of the GI tract has the unique potential to detect ischemia regardless of flow or metabolism. Tonometry is based on the general physiologic principle that, during ischemia, anaerobic metabolism leads to the increased production of acids, which are buffered locally by bicarbonate ion, leading to increased carbon dioxide tension (P_{CO_2}) in the tissue. This relation between ischemia and increased P_{CO_2} has been observed in all ischemic models and all animals studied. It can be measured conveniently using a nasogastric tonometry catheter (Fig. 238-1). In the early days, tonometry was expressed as a compound parameter, pHi, that was based on blood gas and luminal P_{CO_2} values. This can be calculated using the Henderson-Hasselbalch equation and luminal P_{CO_2} and blood bicarbonate, resulting in a value for pHi. A pHi below 7.32 may indicate ischemia. More recently, this parameter has been abandoned for the P_{CO_2} gradient. The gradient is the difference between the intraluminal and arterial P_{CO_2}. In the stomach, the normal gastric-arterial P_{CO_2} gradient is below 0.9 kPa (7 mm Hg).[25] A low pHi, referred to as mucosal acidosis, corresponds with a high P_{CO_2} gradient.[12] Tonometry has been used extensively in critically ill patients suspected of having NOMI in the ICU, but it has been used by only a few groups for the evaluation of occlusive disorders.

Nonocclusive Mucosal or Mesenteric Ischemia

Because splanchnic ischemia is one of the earliest events in circulatory stress and typically begins at a stage when all other systemic parameters are still within the normal range, it has been referred to as "the canary of the body,"[26] a reference to the birds that were once used in coal mines to detect

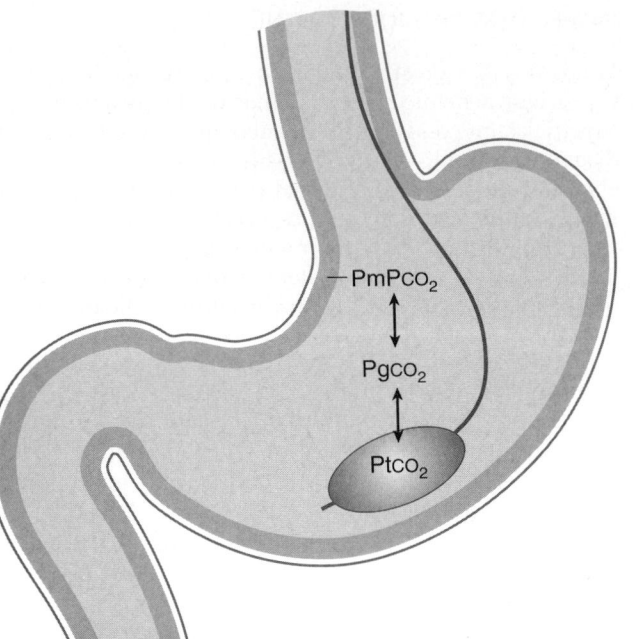

FIGURE 238–1. Tonometry of intraluminal partial pressure of carbon dioxide (Pco_2). The Pco_2 can be measured from a specialized balloon-tipped catheter placed in the stomach or in the small or large bowel. Because CO_2 diffuses rapidly over different membranes, the mucosal Pco_2 ($PmPco_2$) equals the gastric lumen Pco_2 ($Pgco_2$). Because the tonometer balloon is CO_2 permeable as well, the tonometric Pco_2 ($Ptco_2$) ultimately reflects mucosal values. This $Ptco_2$ is measured from air aspirated and inflated automatically into the balloon using a modified capnograph (Tonocap, Datex-Engström). (Modified from Kolkman JJ, Mensink PB: Non-occlusive mesenteric ischemia: A common disorder in gastroenterology and intensive care. Best Pract Res Clin Gastroenterol 2003;17:457-473.)

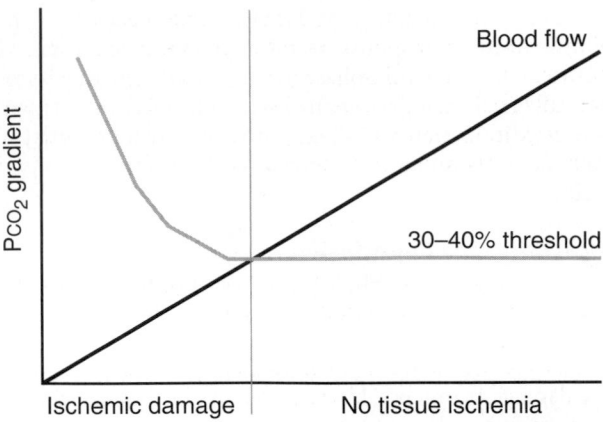

FIGURE 238–2. Blood flow, ischemia, and luminal partial pressure of carbon dioxide (Pco_2). Reduction of the splanchnic blood flow to approximately 50% does not increase the luminal Pco_2 or cause tissue damage. Further reduction below approximately 30% of basal blood flow causes a gradual increase in luminal Pco_2 and characteristic ischemic tissue changes. The blood flow is indicated by the solid line; the tonometric Pco_2 by the gray line. The vertical line indicates the anaerobic threshold of the tissue. (Modified from Kolkman JJ, Mensink PB: Non-occlusive mesenteric ischemia: A common disorder in gastroenterology and intensive care. Best Pract Res Clin Gastroenterol 2003;17:457-473.)

toxic levels of gas. Tonometry may be "a good, inexpensive and relatively early warning of impending trouble."[27] The unique ability of tonometry to measure ischemia per se sets it apart from all other diagnostic methods.[12] Indeed, when blood flow is gradually reduced, the Pco_2 gradient remains normal until the blood flow decreases to less than 50% of basal flow and then increases sharply (Fig. 238-2).[13,25] The Pco_2 gradient is very specific for mucosal ischemia and is less influenced by other systemic factors.

Despite these characteristics that make tonometry an almost ideal diagnostic test for ischemia, it is not widely used. There are three main reasons for tonometry's lack of acceptance into regular critical care practice. First, tonometry acquired a reputation for being a laborious, time-consuming, and error-prone technique. Second, many methodologic issues remained unresolved, including the need for acid suppression and the potential for confounding by food intake. Three, there was a lack of evidence that tonometry-based ischemia detection led to therapeutic interventions that improved outcomes. Most of these issues have been addressed. The use of acid suppression and measurement on an empty stomach improve the accuracy and reproducibility. The use of air tonometry (Tonocap device) instead of the error-prone fluid tonometry approach permits accurate measurement with minimal effort in the clinical setting. This may also be possible with the recently introduced sublingual tonometry,

which showed good correlation with gastric values in severe ischemia in animal models and ICU patients.[28,29] The toughest problem that hindered the wide-scale use of tonometry was the scarcity of studies that convincingly showed that treatment aimed directly at improving mucosal perfusion—that is, normalizing tonometric indices—actually improved survival. Studies in trauma patients clearly show advantages,[30,31] but in more complicated problems such as sepsis, the value of tonometry remains less clear. Still, based on all the available data from published clinical studies, it is evident that gastric or sigmoid tonometry is the only proven diagnostic tool for detecting ischemia at an early and reversible stage. Tonometry may also be the ideal parameter for guiding fluid resuscitation, because a wide Pco_2 gradient is the earliest and best indicator of insufficient intravascular volume and NOMI. Thus, normalization of this parameter seems to be a good endpoint during volume resuscitation.

Occlusive Splanchnic Ischemia

Because a large number of patients with splanchnic stenoses have no ischemia and remain asymptomatic, tonometry might be useful to distinguish asymptomatic and symptomatic splanchnic disease. For this purpose, gastric tonometry was used after a test meal, with variable success,[32-34] probably owing to buffering and dilution effects of the test meal.[35] Performing gastric tonometry during exercise as a provocative maneuver enabled the detection of ischemia. With gastric exercise tonometry, patients with asymptomatic stenoses can be distinguished from those with ischemic symptoms.[36]

Splanchnic ischemia can be detected by performing prolonged tonometry for 24 hours using the Tonocap device (with potent suppression of gastric acid production by intravenous administration of omeprazole) and standardized meals. This 24-hour tonometry permits the measurement of postprandial and fasting Pco_2 levels; following meals, gastric and small bowel Pco_2 gradients may increase up to 5 to 6 kPa

(35 mm Hg). During ischemia, gradients of 8 kPa (60 mm Hg) or greater can be found. Some patients with abdominal pain during fasting had these elevated P_{CO_2} gradients for hours, indicating imminent bowel infarction. Especially in critically ill patients, long-term tonometry is a promising way to assess tissue oxygenation.

CLINICAL PRESENTATION

Splanchnic vascular disorders encompass a spectrum of acute and chronic occlusive, nonocclusive, and aneurysmal disorders affecting the vessels of the abdominal viscera. Acute splanchnic ischemia can be caused by arterial embolism, arterial and venous thrombosis, arterial stenoses, or NOMI. For the intensivist, NOMI is the most common problem; it is discussed first. The discussion of occlusive ischemia focuses on the different, and often underappreciated, clinical, diagnostic, and treatment issues, with special emphasis on ICU care.

NONOCCLUSIVE MUCOSAL OR MESENTERIC ISCHEMIA

Critically Ill Patients and Major Operations

In gastroenterology and surgery, NOMI is considered a rare disorder that can lead to ischemic colitis[37] or acute splanchnic infarction.[38] NOMI is generally regarded as being caused by certain drugs or underlying cardiovascular and renal diseases; its widespread occurrence in ICU patients is not mentioned in the cited reviews. NOMI is caused by reduced splanchnic blood flow despite normal arteries. It can be considered an extension of the normal splanchnic vascular response to decreased intravascular blood volume. Major operations are often associated with splanchnic ischemia, a complication with adverse prognostic significance.[39,40] Similarly, in acute pancreatitis, gastric mucosal ischemia is associated with a poor prognosis.[41] NOMI may be more than an epiphenomenon; increased gut-derived cytokine and endotoxin levels have been detected in patients with this syndrome.[42,43] NOMI may be a key factor in the pathogenesis of multiple organ failure syndrome. For example, endotoxemia can cause mucosal microcirculatory disturbances, contributing to hypovolemia-induced vasoconstriction.[44] As mentioned earlier, gut-derived cytokines and other factors can have negative effects as well.

Hemodialyis Patients

In hemodialysis patients, NOMI is quite common[45]; it may lead to bowel infarction in 2%, with a 45% mortality rate.[46] Not surprisingly, the onset of NOMI is associated with hypotension, often during hemodialysis. Thus, close monitoring and prevention of hypotension are crucial to avoid this problem.[46]

Medications

Many drugs have been implicated as causative agents in NOMI. Nonsteroidal anti-inflammatory drugs affect the integrity of the GI mucous and bicarbonate layer and reduce mucosal perfusion. Alpha-adrenergic agents, such as epinephrine and dopamine, reduce GI perfusion, whereas predominantly beta-adrenergic agents, such as dobutamine and dopexamine, tend to sustain mucosal perfusion. Conflicting data have been reported from studies evaluating the effects of vasoactive drugs, including dobutamine, norepinephrine, and dopexamine, on GI mucosal perfusion.[47-52] On balance, however, avoidance of alpha-adrenergic agents seems prudent.

ISCHEMIC COLITIS

Ischemic colitis is a well-defined disease. It is a nonocclusive disorder in most cases, and angiograms are almost invariably normal.[37,38] Most cases of spontaneous ischemic colitis are not preceded by shock states, as has been suggested; most cases are discovered as a result of unexpected findings at endoscopy performed to evaluate patients with abdominal cramps, diarrhea, or blood loss (Table 238-1). Because the course of spontaneous left-sided ischemic colitis is benign, patients rarely come to the attention of the intensivist.

In contrast, ischemic colitis following aortic surgery is frequently seen in the ICU. It was observed in 20% to 27% of patients after conventional open repair of ruptured abdominal aortic aneurysms and was associated with an overall mortality rate of 48%.[53-56] After elective aortic surgery, sigmoid ischemia is reported in less than 2% of patients.[57] The main factors inducing postoperative left-sided ischemic colitis seem to be preoperative shock, massive blood loss, and persisting hemodynamic instability. In these patients, the IMA is usually already occluded or surgically ligated; thus, ischemic colitis may be partially occlusive in nature.[54] With the introduction of endovascular stent placement for the elective management

TABLE 238–1. CLINICAL FEATURES OF ISCHEMIC COLITIS

Localization	Cause	History	Angiography	Course	Mortality (%)
Right-sided (3)*	Spontaneous (3)	Chronic splanchnic syndrome (1) None (2)	SMA stenosis (1) SMA and CA stenosis (2)	Operated and recovered (1) Died from bowel gangrene (2)	67
Left-sided (19)	Spontaneous (11)	Cardiovascular history (5) Trigger event or hypotension (0) None (6)	Normal angiogram (2) No angiogram done (9)	Died from gangrenous colitis (3) Operated and recovered from gangrene (1) Resolved spontaneously (7)	27
	Postoperative(8)	After acute aortic surgery (7) After elective aortic surgery (1)	No angiogram done (8)	Recovered without operation (5) Operated and recovered from gangrenous colon (1) Died from ischemic colitis (2)	25

*Numbers in parentheses indicate the number of patients, based on 22 patients presenting with ischemic colitis in Enschede, Netherlands, between 1998 and 2001.
CA, celiac artery; SMA, superior mesenteric artery.

of abdominal aortic aneurysms or the treatment of acute ruptured aneurysms, the mortality rate, ICU stay, and incidence of ischemic colitis after abdominal aortic aneurysm repair have decreased dramatically.[58-60]

Left- versus Right-Sided Ischemic Colitis

An important clinical distinction should be made between left-sided ischemic colitis (discussed earlier) and right-sided ischemic colitis.[61] Right-sided ischemic colitis is a symptom of acute SMA occlusion and, consequently, acute splanchnic infarction. To improve the prognosis, this entity requires immediate treatment. Our preference is to perform angiography first in order to plan the appropriate revascularization approach or embolectomy and thereby avoid "blind" laparotomy. The time between the onset of acute small bowel ischemia and irreversible gangrene is only 6 to 8 hours. If the presenting symptom is gangrene, the prognosis is very poor (see Table 238-1).

OCCLUSIVE ISCHEMIA

The incidence of asymptomatic splanchnic stenosis, so-called chronic splanchnic disease, ranges from 8% to 70% in populations with other manifestations of atherosclerotic disease and is comparable to the incidence of carotid atherosclerosis. Nevertheless, symptomatic occlusive splanchnic ischemia, or chronic splanchnic syndrome, is relatively rare, accounting for only 4 or 5 cases per 100,000 population yearly.[62] Acute splanchnic ischemia is also rare, although it currently accounts for 0.36% of all hospital admissions because of the aging of Western societies and the greater availability of diagnostic and therapeutic options.

Causes, Risk Factors, and Disease Associations

External compression by the arcuate ligament of the diaphragm is the predominant cause of single-vessel CA stenosis in young adults. Atherosclerosis is the main cause of single-vessel SMA or IMA occlusive disease and multivessel disease. The latter is defined as stenoses or occlusions in more than one main splanchnic artery. Information on the natural history of splanchnic artery occlusive disease is scarce. Using serial duplex ultrasound scans, it was demonstrated that visceral artery atherosclerotic stenoses progress in approximately 20% of patients per year. This progression of lesions is especially important in multivessel chronic splanchnic disease, which carries a considerable risk for acute splanchnic infarction.[63]

Single-Vessel Chronic Occlusive Ischemia

Patients with a single splanchnic vessel stenosis, most often involving the CA, typically complain of chronic abdominal discomfort that usually occurs after meals or exercise. About 50% of these patients suffer from weight loss because they fear eating. Complications are rare, and the risk of infarction or mortality is low. Although the importance of single-artery stenosis has been debated, in our own series, roughly 80% of patients benefited from treatment by revascularization or stent placement (paper in preparation). Because these patients are generally in good health, they rarely need prolonged ICU treatment, even after surgery.

Multivessel Chronic Occlusive Ischemia

Patients with two or three stenoses in the main arteries supplying the GI tract almost invariably suffer from pain after meals and weight loss, which may be severe. In many patients, an epigastric bruit, often considered a classic sign, is absent. Complaints generally persist for many years and eventually seem to lessen because patients grow accustomed to the pain and it becomes part of their lives. In the end stage of the disease, the pattern of complaints can become extremely atypical and may be dominated by a sensation of abdominal fullness or loss of appetite.

Untreated, progressive multivessel splanchnic disease results in bowel infarction. The time frame for treatment is extremely narrow, because irreversible damage or gangrene develops within 8 to 12 hours after the onset of ischemia. Ischemia may remain clinically silent for several hours or even days, as long as the necrotic segment remains without perfusion.[13] With reperfusion or perforation of gangrenous bowel, multiple organ dysfunction syndrome develops rapidly, and death usually ensues within days.

Acute Occlusive Ischemia and Splanchnic Infarction

Acute splanchnic ischemia is defined as the sudden cessation of splanchnic mucosal perfusion. In 75% of patients with acute splanchnic artery occlusion, an embolus in the SMA is present. The prognosis depends on the cause of the infarction and ranges from approximately 32% for venous thrombosis and 54% for arterial embolism to 70% to 80% for acute arterial thrombosis and nonocclusive ischemia. The overall survival after acute mesenteric ischemia has improved over the past 4 decades.[64]

Unexpected Occlusive Splanchnic Ischemia in the ICU

As mentioned earlier, many patients with splanchnic stenoses remain undiagnosed or have no complaints whatsoever. During major abdominal surgery or inflammatory disorders such as pancreatitis or cholecystitis, however, the increased metabolic demand related to this stress may precipitate ischemia with vascular stenoses. Thus, this diagnosis should be considered in patients with known atherosclerotic disease or risk factors for it and a prolonged or unusually complicated course related to acute cholecystitis or acute pancreatitis. The diagnosis also should be suspected when the histopathology of surgical specimens suggests ischemic injury. Complications that can be caused by splanchnic ischemia include ischemic hepatitis, acalculous cholecystitis, and ischemic pancreatitis. In these patients, revascularization, preferably by endovascular stent placement, may dramatically improve the clinical course within days.

TREATMENT

NONOCCLUSIVE MUCOSAL OR MESENTERIC ISCHEMIA

The key factors for successful treatment of NOMI include (Table 238-2):

1. High index of suspicion and readiness for aggressive intervention.
2. Fluid resuscitation to restore the proper balance between metabolic demand and perfusion.
3. Prevention of reperfusion damage.
4. Recognition and avoidance of NOMI-inducing medications.

TABLE 238–2. TREATMENT OPTIONS IN SPLANCHNIC ISCHEMIA

NOMI

Aggressive volume resuscitation, ideally with normalized tonometry as endpoint

Avoid alpha-adrenergic drugs* when possible

Chronic Occlusive Ischemia

Determine risk for infarction (angiography, clinical assessment, tonometry)

High risk:

Intravenous fluids

Avoid aggressive nutrition

Volume resuscitation

Revascularization (stents preferred) within days

Low risk:

Avoid dehydration

Nutritional measures

Preoperative analysis (cardiac and pulmonary)

Choice of surgery (antegrade or retrograde, single or two vessel) or stent

Bowel Infarction (Acute Splanchnic Infarction)

Urgent angiography and urgent laparotomy (order may vary)

Aggressive volume replacement

Consider intra-arterial papaverine after angiography

Revascularization (stent, embolectomy, surgery)

Consider removing first 500 mL of portal blood after revascularization (to prevent ischemia-reperfusion damage)

Assess bowel viability after revascularization; resect necrotic bowel

Avoid leaving too much borderline viable bowel (ongoing ischemia-reperfusion damage)

Weigh risk of parenteral nutrition dependency against insufficient bowel resection

Postoperative

Maintain optimal fluid status

Avoid alpha-adrenergic drugs* when possible

Ischemic Colitis

Right-sided (ascending colon):

Urgent angiography; to be treated as (imminent) bowel infarction

Aggressive volume resuscitation

Consider laparotomy

Left-sided:

Treat as for NOMI

Angiography generally not indicated

Consider endoscopy:

    Unstable, fever, or signs of sepsis >48 days after surgery

    Consider in all urgent cases

Consider laparotomy and partial colectomy:

    Persistent sepsis, fever, hemodynamic instability

    Proven ischemic colitis (endoscopy) despite NOMI treatment

    Diarrhea, protein losses >14 days after surgery

*For example, epinephrine and dopamine.

NOMI, nonocclusive mucosal or mesenteric ischemia.

The first step toward successful treatment is early detection of mucosal ischemia. Tonometric monitoring is advocated for this purpose.[37] By using gastric tonometry as an endpoint for fluid resuscitation, rapid optimization of intravascular volume can be achieved.[65-67] Volume overload can worsen NOMI owing to increased intraperitoneal pressure and the development of abdominal compartment syndrome.[68]

Vasoactive agents are often used in the resuscitation of hypotensive patients. Dopexamine and dobutamine generally improve intestinal mucosal perfusion, whereas epinephrine and dopamine tend to compromise splanchnic perfusion,[47,48] although some studies reported opposite effects.[69] Norepinephrine has variable effects on splanchnic perfusion.[47,70] In any case, treatment with catecholamines should be started only after sufficient fluid resuscitation has been achieved. Treatment with angiotensin-converting enzyme inhibitors was effective in animal studies[71] but in only one of two clinical studies.[72,73] Endothelin antagonists, which block the final common pathway of splanchnic vasoconstriction, are promising new drugs, but clinical data are not available. Finally, there are small inconclusive studies on the use of prostaglandins in animal sepsis models[74] and in septic shock patients.[75]

Early institution of enteral nutrition may improve perfusion, in addition to having salutary immunologic and nutritional effects. The mechanisms responsible for mucosal vasodilation due to enteral nutrition are autoregulatory responses driven by the metabolic demands associated with absorption of food in the lumen.[76] However, in extreme low- or no-flow states, enteral nutrition can be harmful and provoke infarction; it should therefore be used cautiously.[77] Treatment of reperfusion damage is a promising but clinically unproven approach. Several new compounds,[78-80] as well as established drugs such as N-acetylcysteine[81] and vitamin E,[82] have been used in animal models to reduce damage induced by ischemia-reperfusion. The best-known ROS scavenger, N-acetylcysteine, increases intracellular glutathione levels and increases NO release,[83] leading to vasodilation of small blood vessels. In some studies, administration of N-acetylcysteine early in sepsis was associated with improved hemodynamic parameters[84] and splanchnic ischemia.[85] However, data from clinical studies are lacking.

ISCHEMIC COLITIS

In most cases, left-sided ischemic colitis resolves spontaneously with only fluid resuscitation and antibiotics; endoscopic bowel decompression should be considered if the colon is markedly dilated. Surgery is restricted to patients with transmural irreversible ischemia, but the occurrence of this complication is associated with a poor prognosis. Some experts advocate routine repetitive sigmoidoscopy to evaluate high-risk patients after acute aortic surgery, especially those with severe preoperative shock or requiring a large volume of intravenous fluids.[86] After aortic surgery, repeated colonoscopy should also be considered in patients with persistent hemodynamic instability lasting longer than 48 hours. At endoscopy, ischemic colitis is graded in four categories: grade 0, normal mucosa; grade 1, mucosal edema; grade 2, deep mucosal ulcers; grade 3, gangrene. Grade 3 or progressive grade 2 ischemia is an indication for laparotomy and subtotal colon resection. Angiography is rarely indicated in these patients. Treatment is aggressive fluid resuscitation, antibiotics, and bowel decompression, if indicated.

Chronic Single-Vessel Disease

The majority of patients with single-vessel disease have no comorbidities. Complications are extremely rare, and the operative course is usually uneventful. These patients are rarely encountered by the intensivist.

Chronic Multivessel Disease

Many patients with multivessel disease have severe comorbidities and have lost a considerable amount of weight (often >15 kg). The risk of bowel infarction is high. Therefore, these patients are likely to come to the attention of the intensivist. This consultation could start during the preoperative assessment when treatment choices are made. The treatment options in these patients are many, partly because solid clinical evidence regarding efficacy and risk is lacking.[87] Restoration of blood flow can be achieved with three different treatment strategies.

First, antegrade multivessel autologous revascularization is suitable for patients in relatively good clinical condition, without severe weight loss or comorbidities. This approach yields excellent long-term results with regard to patency and clinical response.[88,89] The downside of this approach is that it uses a supraceliac aortic clamp technique, resulting in at least 15 to 20 minutes of ischemia affecting the bowel, legs, and kidneys. For patients in poor clinical condition, this approach is too risky; the hemodynamic instability and other adverse effects of lower-body reperfusion may not be well tolerated.

Second, retrograde revascularization can be performed by making a long bypass from the common iliac artery or the distal aorta to either the common hepatic artery or the SMA. This procedure is preferred in patients with major comorbid conditions or very low body weight when primary stenting is not an option. It is better tolerated because the aortic cross-clamp is positioned distal to the renal arteries. The main disadvantage of this procedure is that the long bypass graft has a greater risk of kinks, thrombosis, or stenosis and, consequently, an increased likelihood of occluding, leading to a recurrence of symptoms or even splanchnic organ infarction.

Third, percutaneous transluminal angioplasty with stent placement can be performed via the femoral artery in the groin or the brachial artery. The former approach is suboptimal for proper positioning of the stent at the origin of the CA, which makes a sharp angle with the aorta. The brachial artery approach carries a higher risk of local complications, including neural damage, hemorrhage, and pseudoaneurysm formation. Percutaneous transluminal angioplasty alone has proved to have a short patency rate in these arteries; therefore, stent placement is obligatory. During the perioperative period, adequate volume replacement and avoidance of alpha-adrenergic drugs are crucial.

ACUTE OCCLUSIVE ISCHEMIA

Acute splanchnic ischemia should be considered when patients present with acute severe abdominal pain and there is no other obvious diagnosis. The classic presentation is pain out of proportion to physical findings. If untreated, acute splanchnic ischemia ultimately results in bowel necrosis within 6 to 8 hours. Two points are often underappreciated in the treatment of patients with acute occlusive splanchnic ischemia. First, many of these patients have periods of severe splanchnic vasoconstriction and NOMI as well. In acute splanchnic occlusion, for example, concurrent splanchnic vasoconstriction may worsen ischemia. As a rule, NOMI should be considered in all patients with occlusive disease. Second, ischemia-reperfusion damage is often neglected. In the surgical management of acute splanchnic ischemia with

bowel gangrene, many recommend not resecting parts of intestine with marginal viability at the initial procedure and performing a routine "second-look" procedure 24 hours after the first operation and resecting additional intestine then, if necessary. This approach is advocated to save as much bowel length as possible. However, many of these patients eventually die from multiple organ dysfunction syndrome, presumably related to ischemia-reperfusion–induced inflammation in areas of bowel with borderline ischemia. We currently prefer an alternative approach that involves restoration of blood flow, followed by removal of all nonvital bowel. In our experience, this reduces postoperative problems but results in more patients with short bowel syndrome. Initially, many of these patients will be dependent on parenteral nutrition; however, with intestinal adaptation, which may take up to 1 year, most can resume enteral nutrition. Restoration of complete, but adjusted,[90] enteral nutrition can be expected in patients with a remaining small bowel length greater than 50 cm with an intact ileocecal valve, or 100 cm without an ileocecal valve.[91] The quality of life of these patients is relatively good and comparable to that of hemodialysis patients.[92] In the future, small bowel transplantation may become an option, with a current 1-year transplant survival of 60%, according to the international Intestinal Transplant Registry. Therefore, treatment should at least be considered, even in patients with necrotic small bowel.

ACUTE ON CHRONIC SPLANCHNIC ISCHEMIA

The course of patients with multivessel chronic splanchnic syndrome is initially stable or slowly progressive. Ultimately, these patients become severely cachectic. The end stage of the disease is rapidly progressive. Bowel infarction develops in up to 30% of patients after 1 year and in 60% after 4 years of follow-up.[63] The prognosis for these patients is very poor; mortality is 80% once bowel infarction develops.[38,64] Therefore, symptomatic patients with severe bowel pain and weight loss and multivessel disease should be analyzed and treated in a matter of days to weeks. During the time leading up to the revascularization procedure, maintenance of adequate intravascular volume is essential.

Although it seems reasonable to start feeding these patients preoperatively, this approach can have dismal effects in patients with minimal blood flow to the bowel and may actually precipitate acute bowel infarction. Although the use of parenteral nutrition may reduce the risk of bowel infarction, it can provoke liver ischemia. This is probably caused by the increased energy expenditure required to metabolize nutrients in the liver, which already has severely compromised perfusion because flow from the portal vein and hepatic artery is impaired due to occlusive disease involving the CA and SMA. These patients show extreme increases in gastric and jejunal PCO_2 for several hours following polymeric feeding.[93] Treatment should begin as soon as possible, and feeding should be restarted immediately after treatment. Endovascular treatment is the preferred approach. Reconstructive surgery is risky, and despite prolonged ICU care afterward, many patients still have a fatal outcome.

ACUTE SPLANCHNIC INFARCTION

After the onset of pain in acute splanchnic ischemia, infarction ensues within 6 to 8 hours. Emergency revascularization is the main goal of treatment. Angiography can be useful for stenting of the CA or SMA and eventually for removing an SMA embolus by Fogerty catheter. In the case of NOMI, papaverine (30 to 60 mg/h for 4 hours maximum) or prostaglandin E_1 (bolus 0.020 mg, then 0.060 mg/h for up to 72 hours) can be administered by selective SMA catheterization to diminish arterial spasm.[94] Angiography is essential to provide the surgeon with guidelines for revascularization during laparotomy. Again, maintenance of intravascular volume and avoidance of alpha-adrenergic drugs are essential.

ANNOTATED REFERENCES

Hamilton-Davies C, Mythen N, Salmon LB, et al: Comparison of commonly used clinical indicators of hypovolaemia with gastrointestinal tonometer. Intensive Care Med 1997;23:276-281.

This small study in six healthy volunteers showed that hemorrhage induces early and profound NOMI at a stage when all hemodynamic measures, including stroke volume, heart rate, and blood pressure, and arterial lactate are still normal—a clear demonstration that tonometry can be used as an "early warning system."

Knichwitz G, Rotker J, Mollhoff T, et al: Continuous intramucosal P_{CO_2} measurement allows the early detection of intestinal malperfusion. Crit Care Med 1998;26:1550-1557.

This study in pigs clearly showed that tonometry does not measure flow but only the onset of ischemia, as changes occur only after 50% or greater flow reduction. Also, this paper points out the importance of the closed compartment and open compartment phases of splanchnic ischemia.

Kolkman JJ, Otte JA, Groeneveld AB: Gastrointestinal luminal P_{CO_2} tonometry: An update on physiology, methodology and clinical applications. Br J Anaesth 2000;84:74-86.

All available data on tonometry are reviewed, with a special emphasis on measurement accuracy. This article analyzes all earlier flaws in methodology, as well as the potential of this technique.

MacDonald PH: Ischaemic colitis. Best Pract Res Clin Gastroenterol 2002; 16:51-61.

An overview of the pathophysiology, diagnosis, and treatment options for ischemic colitis, which can be occlusive or nonocclusive in nature.

van Bockel JH, Geelkerken RH, Wasser MN: Chronic splanchnic ischaemia. Best Pract Res Clin Gastroenterol 2001;15:99-119.

An extensive review of the clinical presentation, diagnosis, and treatment options in chronic splanchnic ischemia. The discussion of surgical treatment is especially thorough.

Chapter 239

ABDOMINAL COMPARTMENT SYNDROME

Zsolt Balogh • Frederick A. Moore

KEY POINTS

1. It is essential to distinguish intra-abdominal hypertension from abdominal compartment syndrome (ACS). The difference between them is **the presence of organ dysfunction in ACS, which makes it a life-threatening condition.**

2. Intra-abdominal pressure **(IAP) should be monitored in all shock resuscitation patients,** regardless the cause of the shock (e.g., burn, sepsis, trauma, hypovolemia).

3. Presently, the safest and **most feasible way to monitor IAP** is the intravesical technique.

4. ACS can occur without abdominal pathology or injury **(secondary ACS).**

5. To date, the **best-characterized ACS** group is postinjury ACS.

6. Because the **outcome of ACS is very poor,** even with early decompression, prevention, prediction, and surveillance are key.

7. Postinjury primary and secondary **ACS can be accurately predicted** 6 hours after hospital admission with adequate monitoring.

8. In the future, awareness of the predictors of ACS, fine-tuning of shock resuscitation, and abundant monitoring should **decrease the incidence of ACS.**

9. **Solving the problem of managing the open abdomen** will be the next decade's challenge.

DEFINITIONS

Intra-Abdominal Pressure. To date, the most common way to measure intra-abdominal pressure (IAP) is the intravesical technique via a urinary catheter (often referred to as urinary bladder pressure).[1] The mean value of IAP in hospitalized nontrauma patients is 6.5 mm Hg (range, 0.2 to 16.2 mm Hg).[2] In critically ill ICU patients or trauma patients with shock and subsequent resuscitation, IAP is typically higher (12 to 16 mm Hg).[3]

Intra-Abdominal Hypertension. Intra-abdominal hypertension is defined as IAP 10 mm Hg or greater that persists without the characteristic pathophysiology of abdominal compartment syndrome (see Pathophysiology section). Intra-abdominal hypertension is graded as follows: grade I,

IAP 10 to 15 mm Hg; grade II, IAP 16 to 25 mm Hg; grade III, IAP 26 to 35 mm Hg; and grade IV, IAP greater than 35 mm Hg.[4] This grading system, however, does not take into account the duration of hypertension. Unless the patient's physiologic response to intra-abdominal hypertension is known, these numbers should not drive therapeutic interventions.

Abdominal Compartment Syndrome. Abdominal compartment syndrome (ACS) is defined as the combination of (1) IAP greater than 25 mm Hg, (2) progressive organ dysfunction (urinary output <1 mL/kg/h, $PaO_2/FiO_2 <150$, peak airway pressure >45 cm H_2O, or cardiac index <3 L/min/m^2 despite resuscitation), and (3) improved organ function after decompression. ACS is classified as primary if intra-abdominal injuries are present and secondary if no intra-abdominal injuries are present.[5]

Damage Control. Patients undergoing laparotomy for major abdominal bleeding are at risk for entering a vicious circle of acidosis, hypothermia, and coagulopathy; selected patients benefit from an abbreviated laparotomy ("damage-control" strategy).[6,7] The goals are to quickly control bleeding and prevent further contamination or spillage from hollow viscus perforations. The abdomen is temporarily closed without fascial approximation, and the patient is triaged to the ICU, where resuscitation can be optimized and the "vicious circle" physiology corrected. Damage control has saved the lives of severely injured patients who otherwise would have died. Nevertheless, use of damage control has created new challenges for clinicians, including recognition and management of ACS, management of the open abdomen, and early multiple organ failure (MOF).

Decompressive Laparotomy. The midline abdominal fascia is completely opened. This increases abdominal volume and thus decreases IAP. An interposition material (e.g., opened intravenous fluid bag [Bogota bag], synthetic mesh, or vacuum-assisted closure system) is attached to the fascial or skin edges to prevent bowel evisceration. This procedure can be performed at the bedside in the ICU or in the operating room, but the latter is preferred if ongoing bleeding (as the cause of ACS) is anticipated.

HISTORICAL PERSPECTIVE

ACS is an increasingly recognized and investigated critical care topic. A literature search, however, reveals that IAP measurement and intra-abdominal hypertension and ACS-related pathophysiology were investigated and described more than 150 years ago in both animal and human studies.[8,9] Initially, IAP was thought to be negative (subatmospheric), but by the beginning of the 20th century, animal studies verified that IAP is generally positive and, if it is significantly increased, can cause cardiac failure.[10] These laboratory observations had little impact on clinical practice until the 1950s, when pediatric surgeons recognized the catastrophic consequences of acutely closing large congenital abdominal defects. Silo closure with gradual reduction of the abdominal defect was recommended to prevent fulminant organ failures.[11] In the 1980s, vascular surgeons described ACS after abdominal aortic aneurysmorrhaphy. Additionally, they described the present technique of IAP measurement and used high IAP as a criterion for re-exploration.[1] However, it was not until the 1990s, when trauma surgeons adopted the liberal use of the damage-control strategy, that sufficient numbers of patients were available to define the epidemiology and pathophysiology of this previously rare and elusive complication.[12-15] Early observational case descriptions and retrospective series allowed for the development of appropriate prospective epidemiologic characterization. These clinical observations stimulated laboratory investigations, which have revealed some surprising and potentially important immunologic consequences of decompressive laparotomy of ACS after traumatic shock resuscitation (i.e., it may serve as a "second hit" in the systemic inflammatory response that causes early MOF).[15] Parallel with these advances in the understanding of postinjury ACS is the recognition that ACS occurs in a variety of clinical scenarios, such as extreme constipation,[16] ovarian hyperstimulation,[17] noninvasive ventilation,[18] pancreatitis,[19] and severe burns.[20]

INTRA-ABDOMINAL PRESSURE MEASUREMENT

Clinical examination of the abdomen is inaccurate for determining the presence of intra-abdominal hypertension.[21,22] A standardized measurement of IAP is fundamental to the definition of intra-abdominal hypertension and ACS. IAP has been measured in virtually all parts of the abdominal cavity. The intravesical technique using a standard urinary catheter seems to be the most reliable and least invasive method. The rationale is that IAP is transmitted to the urinary bladder, which serves as a pressure transducer when filled with 50 mL of normal saline. The pressure is conducted by the fluid in the bladder to fluid in the urinary catheter, which is clamped during the interval when pressure is being measured. The pressure in the catheter tubing can be measured by inserting a sterile needle into the sample port of the catheter tube. Alternatively, a T-piece with three-way stopcock can be inserted into the catheter tube, connecting one limb to a strain-gauge pressure transducer.[23] The intravesical technique has been shown to correlate well with IAP measured directly using a laparoscopic insufflator.[24] The vesical route is more accurate than the use of rectal and gastric probes, which tend to provide different readouts, depending on the position of the patient.[24] Animal studies have shown that the pressure in the inferior vena cava correlates well with the vesical pressure,[25] but the inferior vena caval and direct peritoneal routes are more invasive. The urinary bladder pressure technique for IAP measurement was originally described by Kron and colleagues[1] and validated by Iberti and associates.[26] The technique was simplified by Sugrue and coworkers, who described the insertion of a T-connector into the drainage tubing.[23] This modification eliminated the need for multiple needle insertions into the sample port and minimized the risk of needle-stick injury and microbial contamination of the bladder. The steps of IAP measurement are as follows:

1. The patient is positioned supine.
2. A T-piece with a three-way stopcock is placed between the urinary catheter and the drainage tubing.
3. The T-piece is connected to the bedside monitor, using a strain-gauge pressure transducer placed to the midaxillary line.
4. The urinary tubing is emptied and clamped distal to the T-piece.
5. Sterile normal saline (50 mL) is instilled into the bladder via the three-way stopcock.
6. The transducer is zeroed.
7. The pressure is recorded on the bedside monitor.
8. The clamp is opened, and 50 mL is subtracted from the patient's urinary output for the hour to account for the instillation of normal saline.

The pressure is preferably measured in kPa, but many publications report results as cm H_2O, potentially causing confusion (1 mm Hg = 1.36 cm H_2O; 1 kPa = 7.5 mm Hg).

This technique is relatively simple and can be performed in any ICU where a pressure transducer is available. Unfortunately, obtaining an accurate measurement requires about 7 minutes of nursing time, limiting the frequency with which measurements can be obtained. Even when personnel are highly aware of the possible consequences of ACS, screening measurements of IAP are rarely obtained more often than every 4 hours. ACS can develop 4 to 6 hours after ICU admission in patients who are at high risk.[3] The standard protocol for intermittent measurements of IAP does not provide information about the duration of intra-abdominal hypertension. To address these shortcomings (labor intensity, intermittent nature), a continuous IAP measurement technique was developed and is currently being validated. The IAP can be continuously measured without clamping the tubing and filling the bladder with 50 mL of normal saline. For this new method, a standard three-way catheter is inserted, and the pressure transducer is connected to the saline-filled irrigation port. Once the set-up is zeroed, the continuous IAP trace can be monitored without any further intervention or interference with the urine flow or tubing; this is the Balogh-Sugrue technique.[27]

PATHOPHYSIOLOGY

The pathophysiologic effects of increased pressure in a closed body compartment are well described in other regions (e.g., tension pneumothorax, pericardial tamponade, increased intracranial pressure, extremity compartment syndromes) and are taught in the basic medical curriculum. The abdominal cavity is a "neglected" compartment (see Historical Perspective). The volume of the abdominal cavity is limited by its least tensile component, the fascia. Increased pressure can be due to an increase in the volume of the abdominal contents or to a decrease in the volume of the "container" (Table 239-1). After IAP increases to greater than 20 mm Hg, the abdominal cavity is on the steep portion of its pressure-volume curve, and, as a result, small increases in content volume or decreases in cavity volume can cause dramatic increases in IAP. This is when close monitoring of IAP (preferably continuously) and organ function is essential for timely intervention.

TABLE 239-1. CAUSES OF INTRA-ABDOMINAL HYPERTENSION AND ABDOMINAL COMPARTMENT SYNDROME

Increased Abdominal Contents	Decreased Abdominal Volume
Ascites	Reduction of large long-standing hernia
Hemoperitoneum	
Visceral edema	Direct closure of large, long-standing abdominal wall defect
Abdominal packs	
Peritonitis	Circumferential abdominal wall burn
Retroperitoneal edema (pancreatitis)	Continuous positive-pressure ventilation
Large pelvic, retroperitoneal hematoma	Retroperitoneal edema (pancreatitis)
Intestinal obstruction	Large pelvic, retroperitoneal hematoma
Ileus	
Gastric distention (esophageal ventilation)	
Abdominal aortic aneurysm	
Severe constipation	
Large abdominal tumor (chronic)	
Morbid obesity (chronic)	
Pregnancy (chronic)	

PATHOPHYSIOLOGIC RESPONSE OF SPECIFIC ORGANS

Cerebral Perfusion. Increased IAP forces the diaphragm cephalad, thus decreasing the size of the thoracic cavity and causing intrathoracic pressure to increase. High intrathoracic pressure increases jugular venous pressure and impedes venous return from the brain. This effect can increase intracranial pressure and, consequently, decrease cerebral blood flow.[28-30] The effect of intra-abdominal hypertension on intracranial pressure is especially relevant in severe blunt trauma, because head and abdominal injuries frequently coexist.

Cardiac Function. Increased IAP impedes venous return to the heart, causing sequestration of blood in the lower extremities. High intrathoracic pressure increases central venous pressure and pulmonary capillary wedge pressure but does not increase right or left ventricular end-diastolic volume. In other words, when intrathoracic pressure is increased, central venous and pulmonary capillary wedge pressures are not reliable indices for assessing the adequacy of preload. Simultaneously, left ventricular afterload increases owing to increased systemic vascular resistance. Increased intrathoracic pressure can increase right ventricular afterload, potentially leading to right ventricular failure and dilation, with consequent leftward displacement of the ventricular septum and impairment of left ventricular filling.[31-34] Cardiac failure with elevated pulmonary capillary wedge pressure, increased systemic vascular resistance, and decreased cardiac index is a typical finding in profound intra-abdominal hypertension and defines ACS. The cardiac index usually does not respond to fluid challenges, which can be detrimental if the underlying cause (ACS) is not treated. The cardiac index's response to decompression is predictive of outcome; patients who survive have a significantly greater increase in cardiac index after decompression than do those who subsequently die.[3]

Respiratory Function. Increased IAP pushes the diaphragms into the thoracic cavity. Thoracic compliance decreases, and increased airway pressure is required for mechanical ventilation. Additionally, functional residual capacity decreases, and ventilation-perfusion mismatching increases, leading to impaired oxygenation.[34,35] In the setting of massive resuscitation, these changes can be misinterpreted as being caused by acute lung injury. Historically, ACS was diagnosed by the presence of a firm abdomen in the setting of oliguria and increased airway pressures. Although airway pressure promptly decreases in response to abdominal decompression, this finding does not differentiate survivors from nonsurvivors.[3] The peak airway pressure is an important parameter to monitor during attempted primary fascial closure after laparotomy when ACS is a possible complication.

Renal Function. Oliguria or anuria despite aggressive fluid resuscitation is a typical sign of ACS. Mechanisms responsible for decreased renal function include direct compression of the renal parenchyma, decreased perfusion of the kidneys due to decreased cardiac index, and increased water and sodium retention due to activation of the renin-angiotensin system.[36-38] The usual threshold for defining acute oliguria—urinary output less than 0.5 mL/kg per hour—should be used cautiously and considered in the context of the magnitude of the resuscitation. Among patients who require massive resuscitation, the index of suspicion for ACS should be high when urinary output is less than 1 mL/kg per hour.

Gut Function. Increased IAP impairs splanchnic perfusion by decreasing the cardiac index and increasing splanchnic vascular resistance. When severe, tissue ischemia can result.[39-42] Intestinal perfusion can be assessed objectively using gastric tonometry. Decreased gastric intramural pH (pHi), increased gastric regional partial pressure of carbon dioxide (P_{CO_2}), and a wide gap between gastric regional P_{CO_2} and end-tidal P_{CO_2} are all indicators of impaired abdominal visceral perfusion. Combined with urinary bladder pressure measurements, the newer semicontinuous tonometers are an excellent adjunct for the early identification of impending ACS.[3] Moreover, the physiologic response to decompression can be evaluated by assessing changes in pHi and related parameters using gastric tonometry.[3]

Extremity Perfusion. Increased IAP increases femoral venous pressure, increases peripheral vascular resistance, and reduces femoral artery blood flow by as much as 65%.[43]

Microcirculation. Laboratory studies have shown that decompression of ACS causes circulating neutrophils to increase CD11b adhesion receptor expression.[44] Decompression of ACS is also associated with the release of cytokines into the portal circulation and increased lung permeability, similar in degree to that seen after hemorrhagic shock and resuscitation.[44,45] Moreover, when ACS decompression is appropriately sequenced with hemorrhagic shock, it can serve as a "second hit" (i.e., ACS decompression 8 hours after hemorrhagic shock causes more intense acute lung injury than does ACS decompression 2 or 18 hours after shock).[44-46]

CLASSIFICATION

ACS can be classified based on the duration of the syndrome, the presence or absence of intraperitoneal pathology, and the cause of the raised IAP (Table 239-2).

ACUTE VERSUS CHRONIC

The pathophysiologic responses described earlier are usually acute phenomena in critically ill or injured patients.

TABLE 239–2. CLASSIFICATION OF ABDOMINAL COMPARTMENT SYNDROME

Basis of Classification	Subcategories
Time frame	Acute
	Chronic
Relation to peritoneal cavity	Primary
	Secondary
Etiology	Trauma
	Burn
	Postoperative
	Pancreatitis
	Bowel obstruction
	Ileus
	Abdominal aortic aneurysm
	Oncologic
	Gynecologic

However, the organ dysfunctions characterizing ACS can be present for long periods (chronic intra-abdominal hypertension or ACS) in certain clinical conditions, such as morbid obesity, chronic constipation, and pregnancy. In morbid obesity, chronic headaches and tinnitus are features of persistently increased intracranial pressure. The symptoms markedly improve when a special device is used to apply negative pressure to the abdomen to decrease IAP.[47]

PRIMARY VERSUS SECONDARY

Irrespective of cause, the presence of intraperitoneal pathology defines primary ACS. A typical case is one in which the damage-control paradigm was followed and perihepatic packing, combined with temporary closure of the abdominal wall, was used to tamonade bleeding from the liver.[48] As time progressed, intra-abdominal bleeding and bowel edema (secondary to resuscitation) caused the volume of the intra-abdominal contents to increase, precipitating ACS. Recognition of this problem has prompted trauma surgeons to leave the abdominal incision open after many damage-control procedures, reducing but not eliminating the risk of ACS. Primary ACS can also occur in patients who fail non-operative management of abdominal organ injuries because of ongoing bleeding.[49]

Secondary ACS typically occurs in the setting of severe shock requiring massive resuscitation (whole body ischemia-reperfusion injury) in the absence of intraperitoneal pathology or injury.[5] Because there is no abdominal cause, secondary ACS is a more elusive diagnosis, and recognition is often delayed.[5,50] Typical causes are hypovolemic shock related to multiple open extremity fractures, unstable pelvic fractures, penetrating chest injuries,[51] and severe burns.[52] Secondary ACS can also develop during resuscitation for septic shock.[53]

ETIOLOGIC

Classification of ACS based on the underlying cause is highly relevant, because the underlying disease process and its treatment are contributing factors in the pathophysiology of the syndrome.

EPIDEMIOLOGY

INCIDENCE

Because of different definitions and different study populations, the reported incidence of ACS is inconsistent. In the trauma literature of the mid-1990s, the reported incidence among high-risk patients undergoing laparotomy varied from 3% to 36%.[15] Fietsam and colleagues reported a 4% incidence of ACS in patients undergoing operation with primary fascial closure for ruptured abdominal aortic aneurysms.[54] Malbrain prospectively investigated medical ICU patients and documented the incidence of ACS at 2%.[55]

Another issue is that the epidemiology of ACS changes as treatment strategies evolve. For example, Meldrum and associates[4] and Balogh and coworkers[3] studied similar traumatic shock populations, and both reported that the incidence of ACS was 14%. These two studies, however, were performed 6 years apart. In the earlier series reported by Meldrum, only primary ACS was considered and liberal use of the open abdomen was just starting. In contrast, in the series described by Balogh 6 years later, the abdomen was initially left open in virtually all cases of damage-control laparotomy (Bogota bag closure), and this strategy was associated with a decreased incidence of primary ACS. However, the previously unrecognized problem of secondary ACS was now an equally prevalent clinical entity.

If intra-abdominal hypertension is used as a surrogate for ACS, the incidence is higher but similarly inconsistent. Sugrue and colleagues reported that the incidence of intra-abdominal hypertension among general surgical patients undergoing laparotomy was 33% to 81%, depending on the definition (20 mm Hg or 18 mm Hg).[23,38] In a study of medical patients, Malbrain reported that the incidence of intra-abdominal hypertension was only 18%, despite using a liberal cutoff value (12 mm Hg).[55] Using a cutoff value of 20 mm Hg, Balogh and coworkers reported a 39% incidence of intra-abdominal hypertension in a cohort of patients with severe traumatic shock.[56] Ivatury and associates reported that the incidence of intra-abdominal hypertension was 32% among patients with life-threatening penetrating abdominal trauma.[42]

OUTCOME

Full-blown ACS with organ dysfunction was once uniformly fatal. With more timely diagnosis and treatment, roughly half of afflicted patients are now surviving. With decompressive laparotomy, organ dysfunction typically improves transiently, but most patients who survive more than 48 hours progress into MOF.[3,53] A fundamental problem is differentiating incomplete resuscitation from early organ failure. ACS and MOF appear to be closely linked. In our series, ACS was a surprisingly early event (occurring, on average, 12 hours after hospital admission) and was shown to be a strong independent predictor for subsequent MOF and death.

PREDICTION AND DIAGNOSIS

Epidemiologic studies carried out during the 1990s clearly documented that ACS is a significant clinical problem.[15] Additionally, more recent studies indicate that, despite early recognition and decompression, the outcome remains poor for patients with ACS. Thus, early and accurate prediction is important, because it allows us to recognize the population at risk and concentrate our preventive efforts on decreasing the incidence of ACS.[3,51,57] The urinary bladder pressure measurement is a widely accepted, inexpensive, and simple monitoring tool for ACS. However, organ dysfunction associated with ACS can occur when IAP is less than 25 mm Hg, and some patients with IAP greater than 25 mm Hg do not develop any symptoms. Not surprisingly, trauma surgeons are reluctant to make decisions regarding decompression based only on measurements of IAP.[58] Potential risk factors for ACS include severe hemorrhagic shock, damage-control laparotomy, fascial closure after damage-control laparotomy, high abdominal trauma index, high injury severity score, and decreased pHi.[42,59] Studies of secondary ACS have identified resuscitation fluid volume thresholds that warrant the monitoring of urinary bladder pressure. Maxwell and colleagues recommended monitoring when the resuscitation volume exceeds 10 L of crystalloid fluid or 10 U of packed red blood cells.[5] Ivy and associates suggested that the trigger to initiate urinary bladder pressure monitoring should be greater than 0.25 L/kg of crystalloid resuscitation.[20,52] Biffl and coworkers reported that both these cutoffs are ineffective and recommended the following thresholds: 6 L or more of crystalloid resuscitation or 6 U or more of packed red blood cells in a 6-hour period in patients with a base deficit greater than 10 mEq/L, especially if a vasopressor agent is required.[53]

More recent studies from general surgical, burn, and trauma populations have tried to identify the independent risk factors for ACS. For example, McNelis and coworkers performed a case-control study of 22 patients with ACS (diagnosed by elevated IAP and peak airway pressure) and 22 general surgical patients without ACS, and created a predictive equation[60]: $P = 1/(1 + e^{-z})$, where $z = -18.6763 + 0.1671$ (peak airway pressure) $+ 0.0009$ (24-hour fluid balance). In our experience, postinjury ACS occurs most frequently during the first 12 hours after injury, and waiting for a 24-hour fluid balance entails too much delay. By this time, most susceptible patients already exhibit the full-blown syndrome.[3,51] Postinjury ACS recognized after 24 hours is lethal.[5,50] Additionally, two prospective studies of trauma patients failed to identify predictors for ACS, possibly because the study populations were either too heterogeneous or too homogeneous. In a study of unselected trauma patients requiring ICU admission (mean injury severity score 18), Hong and colleagues found that only 2% of the patients developed intra-abdominal hypertension and only 1% developed ACS.[61] In a review of patients undergoing damage-control laparotomy (mean injury severity score 29), Raeburn and associates found that the incidence of ACS was 36%.[62] Both of these groups failed to identify independent predictors of ACS.

From a prediction modeling perspective, patients requiring traumatic shock resuscitation are an ideal group to study. They are at substantial risk for ACS, the time of insult is defined, and the subsequent treatment (resuscitation) can be standardized. We therefore performed a multiple logistic regression analysis on a prospective database of major torso trauma patients who required shock resuscitation.[3] Given the early occurrence of postinjury ACS, we focused our prediction models on the first 6 hours after hospital admission. We developed two prediction models: emergency department (ED) model (0 to 3 hours; i.e., all patients had an initial diagnostic workup and clinical laboratory results and were discharged from the ED) and ICU model (0 to 6 hours; i.e., all patients were admitted to the ICU, and their first physiologic monitor and clinical laboratory measurements on a standardized resuscitation protocol were available). Our goals were to identify the independent risk factors that may be causative and to build prediction models that could identify high-risk patients early during resuscitation so that standard care could be modified to prevent or improve the outcome of patients at risk for ACS.

As described earlier, patients with postinjury ACS are not a homogeneous group. Primary and secondary ACS patients develop the same symptoms and predecompression physiology, but their injury patterns, resuscitation times, and hospital stays are different. We therefore hypothesized that predictors of ACS would be different for these two groups. The variables used in the multivariate prediction models included demographic parameters, shock severity, injury severity, interventions, hospital times, crystalloid and blood volumes, and vital signs. In the ICU, they also included initial pulmonary artery catheter readings, mechanical ventilator settings and response parameters, gastric tonometry data, and blood gas, clinical chemistry, and coagulation results. Among these variables, those listed in Table 239-3 were found to be independent risk factors for ACS. The primary ACS predictors at ICU admission (low temperature, low hemoglobin concentration, high base deficit) are all indicators of the "vicious circle" physiology, the reason that damage-control surgery is elected. The secondary ACS predictors (high crystalloid infusion volume, impaired renal function) suggest that the process is strongly related to the current standard of care in the United States (i.e., crystalloid resuscitation). The receiver operator characteristic analysis showed that ACS can be predicted with 0.88 accuracy at the time of ED discharge and, surprisingly, with 0.99 accuracy 1 hour after ICU admission with adequate monitoring. The use of these predictors together (even without urinary bladder pressure measurements) permits very early detection of the impaired physiologic findings that are characteristic of ACS. Because the predictors of ACS include both physiologic measurements and resuscitative interventions, this model should perform

TABLE 239–3. INDEPENDENT PREDICTORS OF POSTINJURY PRIMARY AND SECONDARY ABDOMINAL COMPARTMENT SYNDROME

		ED Model			ICU Model		
	Independent Predictors	Odds Ratio	95% CI	Independent Predictors	Odds Ratio	95% CI
Primary ACS	To OR <75 min	103	10->999	Temp ≤34°C	23	1.4-378
	Crystalloids ≥3 L	70	10-478	GAP_{CO_2} ≥16	54	2.2->999
				Hb ≤8/dL	206	7.4->999
				BD ≥12 mEq/L	4	1.4-840
Secondary ACS	Crystalloids ≥3 L	16	1.7-144	GAP_{CO_2} ≥16	>999	>999->999
	No urgent surgery	0.3	0.07-0.9	Crystalloids ≥7.5 L	39	3-470
	PRBC ≥3 U	5.6	1.0-31	UO ≤150 mL	64	6-750

ACS, abdominal compartment syndrome; BD, arterial base deficit; CI, confidence interval; ED, emergency department; GAP_{CO_2}, carbon dioxide gap; Hb, hemoglobin concentration; ICU, intensive care unit; OR, operating room; PRBC, packed red blood cells; Temp, temperature; UO, urine output.

better in clinical situations during ongoing resuscitation than do arbitrary urinary bladder pressure and organ dysfunction thresholds.[4] The ED model (≈3 hours after admission) is very sensitive (overinclusive), which minimizes the chance of missing ACS patients; the ICU model (≈6 hours after hospital admission) is very specific and can pinpoint individuals at highest risk.

TREATMENT

NONSURGICAL METHODS

Support of early organ dysfunction by traditional ICU interventions is often necessary in patients with impending ACS but may aggravate the underlying pathophysiology. For example, ventilator strategies to increase mean airway pressure to improve oxygenation (e.g., high levels of positive end-expiratory pressure) directly increase intra-abdominal hypertension by pushing down on the diaphragm. Additionally, increased mean airway pressure increases intrathoracic pressure, impeding venous outflow from the abdominal cavity. This promotes more gut edema with ongoing crystalloid resuscitation, another intervention that is often used in patients with impending ACS. Seminal papers in the mid-1990s advocated hypervolemic resuscitation to ameliorate cardiac and renal dysfunction. The concept was that increased IAP elevates pulmonary capillary wedge pressure but not preload, and fluid should be administered to increase left ventricular end-diastolic volume to improve the cardiac index.[63] This approach seems to be harmful, according to the most recent evidence.[56,64] Patients with similar demographic characteristics, injuries, and shock severity without impending ACS responded very well to preload-directed resuscitation and increased the cardiac index appropriately.[64] However, patients with impending ACS did not respond with increased cardiac index, despite vigorous crystalloid infusion. Vigorous attempts to increase preload (especially with crystalloid infusions) in patients with intra-abdominal hypertension have a detrimental effect on outcome (futile crystalloid cycle) (Fig. 239-1).

Theoretically, other nonsurgical interventions may have beneficial effects, but their efficacy is unproved. Colloids and albumin could mobilize interstitial fluids into the vascular space, and muscle relaxants might have a salutary effect by decreasing the tension in the abdominal wall.[52,65] Continuous external application of negative abdominal pressure with a suction device shows promise in morbidly obese patients with cerebral symptoms secondary to chronic ACS.[48]

PERCUTANEOUS METHODS

If intra-abdominal hypertension or ACS is caused by acute or chronic fluid collection, symptoms can be relieved by percutaneous drainage. Recent case reports described the successful drainage of abdominal fluid in burn patients with secondary ACS and the drainage of blood in nonoperatively managed liver injuries.[65-67] The major limitation of the technique is that it is applicable only when a significant amount of fluid is causing increased IAP. This technique will not work and might be dangerous when extensive bowel edema or retroperitoneal hematoma is the dominant contributing factor.

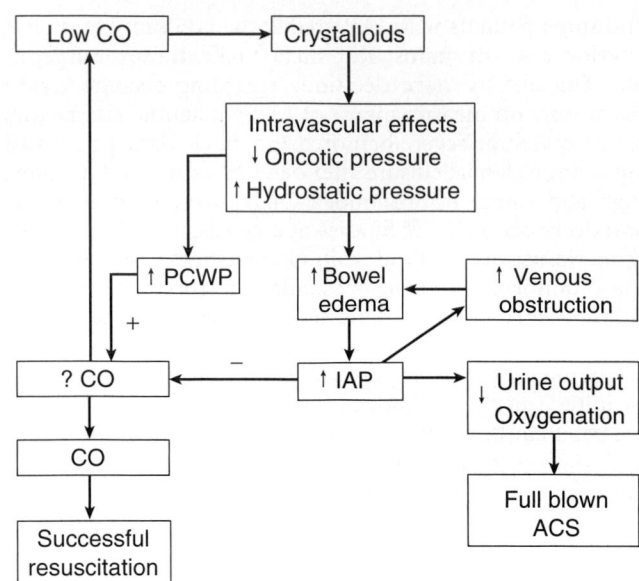

FIGURE 239–1. Futile crystalloid preloading. ACS, abdominal compartment syndrome; CO, cardiac output; IAP, intra-abdominal pressure; PCWP, pulmonary capillary wedge pressure; ↑, increased; ↓, decreased; +, positive effect; –, negative effect.

SURGICAL DECOMPRESSION

Surgical decompression remains the primary recommended intervention. Decompression is achieved by opening the midline fascia (avascular plane) along its full length. Virtually all reports describe a very good physiologic response to decompression, but this does not necessarily translate into better outcomes. The best predictors of survival are postdecompression improvement in cardiac index and urine output.[3,51] The decision to undertake surgical decompression is a difficult one, because it results in a chronically open abdomen that is associated with numerous hazards. Several case series have shown that early decompression is associated with better outcomes. However, in those studies, "late" decompression was often carried out days after the initial signs of ACS. If decompression is carried out within 12 hours of hospital admission, timing has no significant effect on outcome.[3,51] Patients with ACS are in critical condition and require mechanical ventilation and other forms of organ support. Any unnecessary intrahospital transportation of these patients can be detrimental. Thus, if no other intra-abdominal surgical intervention is needed, decompression can be performed at the bedside in the ICU.

MANAGEMENT OF THE OPEN ABDOMEN

Decompressive laparotomy results in an open abdomen, because the incision should not be closed until the risk of recreating ACS by closing the fascia diminishes. After abdominal decompression, temporary abdominal closure is applied to the wound to keep the fascia open. Several methods (towel clips, Bogota bag, synthetic mesh, vacuum-assisted closure) are available, and none has proved to be superior to the others. It is advantageous for the ICU specialist to understand each of these methods and discuss them with the surgical team. The key goals of temporary abdominal closure are as follows: prevent evisceration, allow enough room for swelling of the abdominal contents, control peritoneal fluids, prevent contamination, and preserve the fascia and skin for possible later closure or reconstruction. Open abdomen management has multiple complications and long-term morbidity. Fistulas, abdominal infections, and intra-abdominal collections are common, and the end result is usually a large abdominal wall defect. Recent experience with a vacuum-assisted closure device (VAC, Kinetic Corporation Inc., San Antonio, TX) is very promising, and use of this approach may improve the management of the open abdomen.[68,69]

PREVENTION, SURVEILLANCE, AND FUTURE DIRECTIONS

Prospective data suggest that the mortality rate for ACS, even with early decompression and resuscitation, is very high. In addition, early favorable physiologic responses to decompression do not necessarily translate into improved outcomes.[3] Accordingly, prevention of ACS is paramount. The avoidance of fascial closure after high-risk laparotomy reduces the incidence of MOF and mortality.[59] In the operating room, monitoring for increases in peak airway pressures during the attempted fascial closure is valuable in the absence of IAP measurement. In the ICU, all patients with severe shock and subsequent resuscitation (whole body ischemia-reperfusion injury), regardless of the cause (burn, trauma, sepsis, or hypovolemia), benefit from IAP monitoring, which is a simple, noninvasive tool.

ACS is strongly associated with the magnitude and quality of resuscitation.[3,5,50-53,56,64] Uncontrolled, goal-oriented resuscitation of trauma victims, chasing supranormal values for oxygen delivery, is harmful.[56] To eliminate uncontrolled resuscitation, treatment of the underlying cause of shock is crucial. Timely hemorrhage control and elimination of septic foci should happen simultaneously. There is increasing evidence that Ringer's lactate solution is proinflammatory, and use of this agent is an independent predictor of postinjury ACS.[70] During burn and trauma resuscitation, crystalloid limits should be implemented, and after reaching them, alternative resuscitation fluids should be used. The best resuscitation fluid during impending ACS has yet to be determined.

In postinjury primary ACS, correction of the vicious circle of coagulopathy, acidosis, and hypothermia should be an early goal. Abbreviated laparotomy saves lives, but the tight abdominal packing increases the risk of ACS. The use of topical hemorrhage control techniques (e.g., fibrin sealants) offers a workable solution.[71] When abnormalities in respiratory and renal function are identified, ACS should be included in the differential diagnosis and is an easily excludable cause if IAP measurements are performed. A direct effect of ACS is impaired abdominal visceral perfusion. Gastric tonometry is a relatively noninvasive monitor for intra-abdominal hypertension. A high gastric regional P_{CO_2} (>60 mm Hg) and a wide gap between gastric and end-tidal P_{CO_2} (>16 mm Hg) are important indicators and predictors of ACS. With the availability of continuous IAP measurement, the abdominal perfusion pressure (mean arterial pressure minus IAP) can be easily monitored at the bedside. The value of this variable needs to be prospectively validated.

ACS can occur in a wide range of critically ill patients. With increased awareness of ACS, focused monitoring, the application of temporary abdominal closure methods, and fine-tuned resuscitation, the incidence of primary ACS should decrease. Secondary ACS represents failure of resuscitation (over-resuscitation, neglected hemorrhage control, or nonexistent monitoring for ACS) and is a problem that can be eliminated. The occurrence of secondary ACS in burn and shock or trauma ICUs should be considered a negative performance indicator.

The future of open abdomen management is less clear. The number of patients being managed with an open abdomen will likely increase as awareness of ACS increases. Presumptive decompression to prevent ACS is an attractive concept, but without validated accurate predictors, this could lead to increased morbidity secondary to fistulas, infections, abscesses, large abdominal wall defects, and extended hospitalization. Despite encouraging results with the vacuum-assisted closure technique, decompressive laparotomy should not be viewed as a definitive solution.

ANNOTATED REFERENCES

Balogh Z, McKinley BA, Cox CS Jr, et al: Abdominal compartment syndrome: The cause or effect of postinjury multiple organ failure. Shock 2003;20:483-492.

This article summarizes the present knowledge on postinjury ACS, including cause, pathomechanism, individual organ responses, and decompression. It focuses on the most recent findings about the relationship between shock resuscitation and ACS. The authors review the growing evidence that ACS is a second hit in the development of multiple organ failure and provide guidelines for prevention and therapy.

Balogh Z, McKinley BA, Holcomb JB, et al: Both primary and secondary abdominal compartment syndrome can be predicted early and are harbingers of multiple organ failure. J Trauma 2003;54:848-861.

This is a comprehensive paper on the epidemiology, outcome, and prediction of postinjury primary and secondary ACS. The study population consisted of 188 patients from the prospective shock-trauma resuscitation database, with strict inclusion criteria and standardized resuscitation with bedside computerized decision support. The distinct characteristics of primary and secondary ACS are described based on the results of uni- and multivariate analysis. Multivariate prediction models show that the syndrome can be predicted during the first few hours after hospital admission.

Ivy ME, Atweh NA, Palmer J, et al: Intra-abdominal hypertension and abdominal compartment syndrome in burn patients. J Trauma 2000;49:387-391.

This is a prospective evaluation of patients with high-percentage burns, in whom secondary ACS is a frequent complication. The authors recommend IAP measurements after 0.25-L/kg crystalloid resuscitation and report a high success rate using conservative management of ACS in burn patients.

Malbrain ML: Abdominal pressure in the critically ill: Measurement and clinical relevance. Intensive Care Med 1999;25:1453-1458.

This prospective clinical study describes the incidence of intra-abdominal hypertension and ACS in a general medical ICU.

McNelis J, Soffer S, Marini CP, et al: Abdominal compartment syndrome in the surgical intensive care unit. Am Surg 2002;68:18-23.

This prospective clinical study describes the incidence of ACS in a mixed surgical ICU.

Saggi BH, Sugerman HJ, Ivatury RR, Bloomfield GL: Abdominal compartment syndrome. J Trauma 1998;45:597-609.

This excellent comprehensive review is a good place to start to understand the concept of intra-abdominal hypertension and ACS.

Sugrue M, Bauman A, Jones F, et al: Clinical examination is an inaccurate predictor of intraabdominal pressure. World J Surg 2002;26:1428-1431.

This prospective clinical study concluded that physical examination is a poor way to determine the presence of intra-abdominal hypertension. The authors strongly support routine IAP measurements.

Chapter 240
THROMBOLYTICS

Joel Edward Barbato • Edith Tzeng

KEY POINTS

1. **Thrombolytics** comprise a diverse group of compounds that convert plasminogen to plasmin.

2. **Thrombolytic therapy** is indicated within 6 hours of the onset of acute myocardial infarction, especially in patients who are not eligible for primary angioplasty.

3. **Patients with acute ischemic stroke** receive the greatest long-term benefit from thrombolytic therapy when receiving treatment within 3 hours of the onset of symptoms.

4. **The role of thrombolytics in pulmonary embolus** is controversial and confined largely to use in those patients with hemodynamic instability.

5. **Urokinase and tissue plasminogen activator** are commonly used in the management of acute peripheral occlusion and most benefit those patients with occlusions of less than 14 days and those patients with previous extremity bypasses.

6. **Thrombolytic therapy requires intensive monitoring and follow-up radiography.** Fibrinogen levels should be monitored every 6 to 8 hours and the patient closely monitored for signs of major hemorrhage.

Thrombolytic agents comprise a diverse group of compounds that lyse thrombus. In the formation of thrombus, fibrin provides the scaffolding for the clot. After the initiation of the coagulation cascade, fibrinolytic mechanisms are activated to prevent unchecked thrombosis. The fibrinolytic process begins with the cleavage of plasminogen to plasmin, an enzyme that catalyzes the lysis of fibrin (Fig. 240-1). Thrombolytic agents function by promoting the conversion of plasminogen to active plasmin. The different thrombolytic agents vary in their specificity for fibrin (i.e., specificity to the degradation of fibrin rather than its precursor fibrinogen), their metabolic half-life, and their antigenicity (Table 240-1).

DRUGS

STREPTOKINASE

Streptokinase was first identified as a product that possessed fibrinolytic properties in the 1930s[1] and was the first compound used clinically as a thrombolytic drug.[2] It is produced by beta-hemolytic streptococcal bacteria. Despite its name, streptokinase is not an enzyme. Rather, it complexes with plasminogen in a 1:1 stoichiometric relationship. This complex then converts plasminogen to plasmin, consuming two plasminogen molecules in the process. One of the major drawbacks to the clinical use of streptokinase is its antigenicity. Allergic reactions occur in 2% to 5% of patients receiving the drug.[3] It also has a very short half-life (approximately 20 minutes). Anistreplase (APSAC) is a modified form of streptokinase that has a substantially longer half-life but still can cause allergic reactions (see Fig. 240-1).

UROKINASE

Urokinase is a thrombolytic protein that was initially isolated from human urine and has been used clinically for over 30 years. The drug is isolated from human fetal renal tissue cultures and, unlike streptokinase, enzymatically cleaves plasminogen. During the 1980s and early 1990s, urokinase was the primary thrombolytic agent used clinically for the treatment of graft thrombosis and peripheral arterial occlusion. In 1999, urokinase was removed from the U.S. market after questions were raised by the Food and Drug Administration (FDA) regarding the safety of this product.[4] It was reintroduced in the United States in late 2002 after rigorous testing showed it to be free of human pathogens. Prourokinase, also known as single-chain urokinase-type plasminogen activator (scu-PA), is a single-chain precursor molecule of urokinase that is converted into two-chain urokinase by hydrolysis. It is relatively fibrin specific like tissue plasminogen activator and has low antigenicity.

TISSUE PLASMINOGEN ACTIVATOR

Tissue plasminogen activator (t-PA) was first isolated in 1981.[5] It is a naturally occurring protein synthesized by human vascular endothelial cells. Commercially available preparations are manufactured using recombinant technologies, as first described by Pennica and colleagues.[6] A number of different recombinant variants are available, including alteplase (rt-PA, approved by the FDA in 1987) and duteplase, as well as other forms of the tissue-type plasminogen activators: reteplase (r-PA), tenecteplase (TNK-tPA), and lanoteplase (n-PA). Recombinant t-PAs have the advantage of being nonantigenic and fibrin specific and avoid the risks associated with products isolated from cultured human tissues.

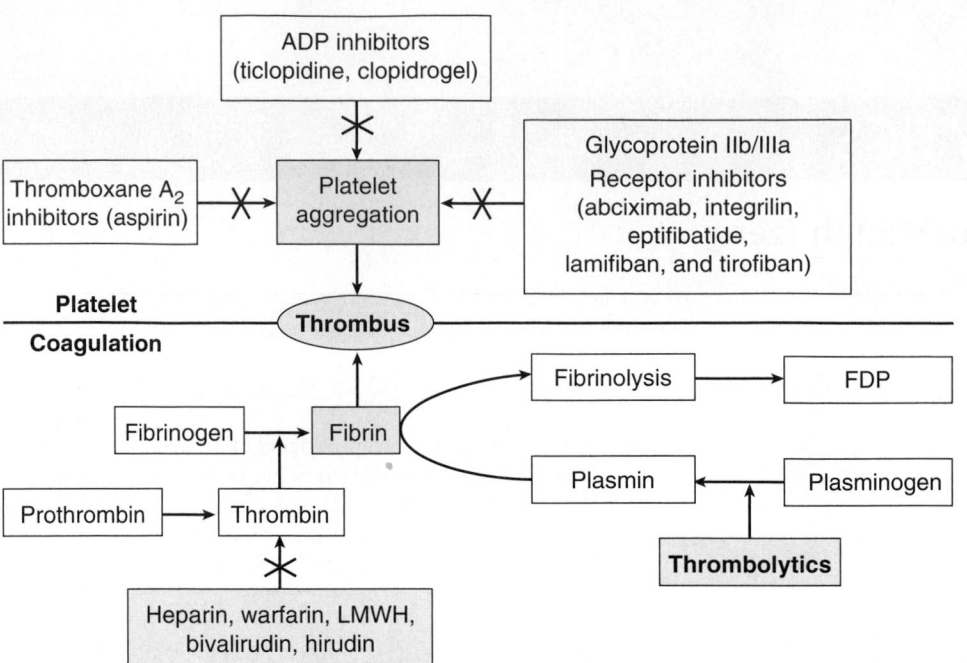

FIGURE 240–1. Components of thrombus formation and actions of various antithrombotic and thrombolytic agents. FDP, fibrin degradation products; LMWH, low molecular weight heparin.

OTHER AGENTS

In addition to streptokinase, urokinase, t-PA, and their derivatives, a number of other compounds have been developed and investigated. These include vampire bat plasminogen activator (derived from the saliva of the vampire bat), fibrolase (from the venom of the southern copperhead snake), and staphylokinase (from *Staphylococcus aureus*). Data regarding the use of these compounds are relatively limited, however, and they are rarely used clinically.

CLINICAL INDICATIONS

MYOCARDIAL INFARCTION

The use of lytic therapy for the treatment of acute myocardial infarction (AMI) was first attempted in the 1950s.[7] The rationale for this therapy was that reestablishing coronary blood flow in an acutely thrombosed vessel would reduce infarct size and mortality. Indeed, a meta-analysis of 33 randomized trials in 1985 demonstrated a 22% reduction in mortality with the use of thrombolytics in AMI, and the findings from this study prompted further investigation into lytic therapy for MI.[8] A followup meta-analysis done almost a decade later aggregated the results from over 58,000 patients treated with thrombolytics.[9] The analysis revealed a time-dependent reduction in mortality of 30 per 1000 treated patients when lysis was initiated within 6 hours of the onset of symptoms. Only four hemorrhagic strokes occurred per 1000 patients treated, most of which occurred within the first 2 days. Numerous studies since have been performed to evaluate the efficacy of different lytic agents, dosing strategies, routes of administration, and adjunctive therapies for the rapid restoration of antegrade flow in thrombosed coronary arteries.

Currently accepted guidelines for lytic therapy in AMI were outlined by the American College of Chest Physicians in the 2001 Sixth Consensus Conference and the American College of Cardiology/American Heart Association in their 1999 and 2002 guideline updates.[10-12] The treatment algorithm is summarized in Figure 240-2. Unfortunately, the value of thrombolytic agents for the management of unstable angina remains unproven. Currently, there is no role for lytic therapy in acute coronary syndromes in the absence of

TABLE 240–1. SUMMARY OF PROPERTIES OF COMMONLY USED THROMBOLYTICS

	Streptokinase	Urokinase	Tissue Plasminogen Activator (t-PA)
Source	Group C *Streptococcus*	Human fetal kidney	Recombinant
Lytic Generation	First	First (prourokinase— second)	Second (non-alteplase t-PAs—third)
Variants	Anistreplase [APSAC] (half-life 70-120 min)	Prourokinase	Alteplase, duteplase, reteplase (r-PA), tenecteplase (TNK-tPA), lanoteplase (n-PA)
Molecular Weight (kD)	47	35-55	63-70
Half-Life (min)	18-23	14-20	3-4
Metabolism	Hepatic	Hepatic	Hepatic
Antigenicity	Yes	No	No
Fibrin Specificity	Minimal	Moderate	Moderate
Plasminogen Binding	Indirect	Direct	Direct

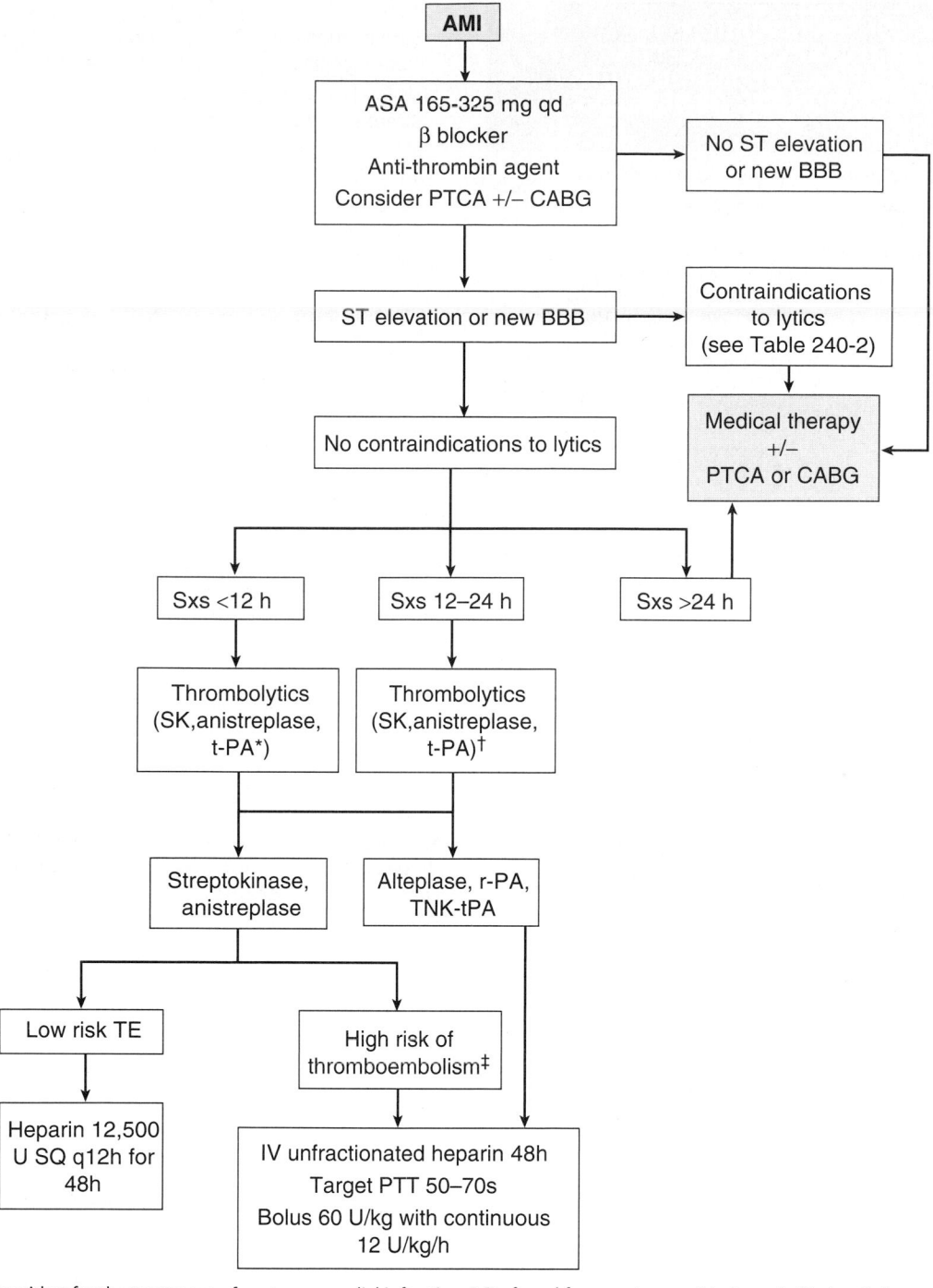

FIGURE 240–2. Algorithm for the treatment of acute myocardial infarction. *, Preferred for symptoms < 6 h; †, grade 2b data[11]; ‡, anterior myocardial infarction, existing heart failure, previous embolus, atrial fibrillation, left ventricular thrombus; AMI, acute myocardial infarction; BBB, bundle branch block; PTCA, percutaneous transluminal coronary angioplasty; CABG, coronary artery bypass grafting; Sxs, signs and symptoms; PTT, partial thromboplastin time; SK, streptokinase; SQ, subcutaneous; TE, thromboembolism. (Adapted from 1999/2002 ACC/AHA Guideline Update and 2001 ACCP Consensus Conference.[11,12])

ST-segment elevation in two or more contiguous leads or without new-onset bundle branch block. Contraindications to lytic therapy in the setting of AMI are summarized in Table 240-2.

The timing of diagnosis and institution of thrombolytic therapy is critical.[13,14] Patients with AMI treated with thrombolytic agents more than 4 hours after the onset of symptoms have 30-day and 6-month mortality rates that are two to three times higher than those for patients who receive lytic therapy within 2 hours of the onset of symptoms.[15] Eighty-two percent of patients treated within 2 hours have return of normal cardiac wall motion whereas only 46% of those treated within 2 to 5 hours of the onset of symptoms have return of normal wall motion.[16] The LATE (Late Assessment of Thrombolytic Efficacy) study reported 1-year mortality rates of 17.6% versus 15.8% in those patients treated with rt-PA at greater than 3 hours versus less than 3 hours, respectively, after the onset of symptoms.[17] So critical is the timing of the initiation of treatment that prehospital administration of thrombolytics has been advocated in select patients with ST-segment elevations on an electrocardiogram.[18,19]

TABLE 240–2. CONTRAINDICATIONS TO THROMBOLYTIC THERAPY IN THE SETTING OF ACUTE MYOCARDIAL INFARCTION (WITH ST-SEGMENT ELEVATION AND/OR NEW BUNDLE BRANCH BLOCK)

Absolute Contraindications	Relative Contraindications
>24 hours since onset of symptoms	12 to 24 hours since onset of symptoms
Prior intracranial hemorrhage	Age > 75 years
Stroke within past year	Systolic blood pressure > 180 mm Hg or diastolic blood pressure > 110 mm Hg
Intracranial neoplasm	Bleeding disorder
Active bleeding	Prior allergic reaction to thrombolytics
Suspected aortic dissection	Pregnant or lactating
	Prolonged cardiopulmonary resuscitation (>10 min)

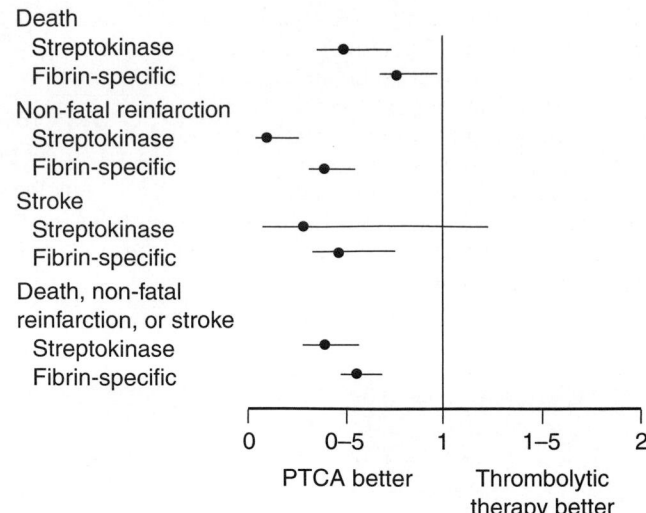

FIGURE 240–3. Short-term clinical outcomes in patients treated with PTCA versus thrombolytic therapy. Odds ratios with 95% confidence intervals. (Reprinted with permission from Keeley EC, Boura JA, Grines CL: Primary angioplasty versus intravenous thrombolytic therapy for acute myocardial infarction: A quantitative review of 23 randomised trials. Lancet 2003;361:13-20.)

There are few data to suggest that one thrombolytic drug is more effective than another in the setting of AMI. Early studies focused on the use of streptokinase, demonstrating 18% and 25% reductions in mortality at 3 and 5 weeks, respectively, in the ISIS-2[4] and GISSI studies.[20] The efficacy of t-PA was studied in the GUSTO-1 trial, which examined four dosing regimens for the treatment of an MI in over 40,000 patients.[21] This study utilized "accelerated" t-PA dosing, wherein two thirds of the total dose was administered in the first 30 minutes rather than over 3 hours, and demonstrated a modest but significant reduction in 30-day mortality (6.3%) with accelerated t-PA dosing as compared with streptokinase (7.4%) or a combination of t-PA and streptokinase (7.0%). A subsequent meta-analysis of this approach, however, failed to validate the survival advantage.[22]

It is now recognized that adjunctive therapies, such as aspirin and antithrombin agents, improve the results of lytic therapy. As fibrinolytic therapies strip fibrin from the occluding thrombus, the exposed underlying thrombin can initiate platelet aggregation and subsequently result in re-thrombosis.[23] Therefore, some form of antithrombin strategy is warranted. Heparin can be infused to keep the activated partial thromboplastin time (aPTT) between 50 and 70 seconds. If heparin-induced thrombocytopenia is suspected, then use direct thrombin inhibitors (hirudin or bivalirudin).[24] Another development has been the introduction of glycoprotein IIb/IIIa receptor blockers such as abciximab (ReoPro), eptifibatide (Integrilin), and tirofiban (Aggrastat).[25-27] Despite some promising early results,[28] a randomized trial has yet to demonstrate a reduction in mortality with combination therapy.[29-31]

Recently, a large meta-analysis was performed that examined 7739 patients with ST-segment elevation randomized to either thrombolytic agents (76% receiving fibrin-specific lytics) or primary percutaneous transluminal coronary angioplasty (PTCA).[32] Short-term (4 to 6 week) mortality in the PTCA group was 7% as compared with 9% in the group that received lytic therapy (P = .0003). The group treated with primary PTCA had lower rates for nonfatal reinfarction (3% vs. 7%) and stroke (1% vs. 2%) as part of a follow-up to a smaller study.[33] The short-term results of this meta-analysis are summarized in Figure 240-3.

The potential advantages of angioplasty over thrombolysis[34-37] as primary therapy for AMI must be tempered by the recognition that angioplasty results are highly dependent on the volume of cases at a given treatment center. Moreover, comparisons to lytic therapy often use historical data before the era of accelerated dosing regimens and adjunctive treatment with antiplatelet and antithrombin agents. Lytic therapy also may be advantageous in critically ill patients who are unable to be transported to cardiac catheterization facilities or in those who have other contraindications to PTCA. Ultimately, the ideal treatment for some patients may involve combinations of angioplasty, reduced-dose thrombolytic therapy, antithrombotic agents, and antiplatelet agents.

STROKE

Stroke is the third leading cause of death in the United States, affecting over 700,000 people per year. Strokes are a major source of morbidity and mortality among hospitalized patients.[38] Most strokes are caused by thromboemboli from a variety of sources.[39] Traditional therapy for ischemic stroke has focused on the use of anticoagulation and antiplatelet agents. More recently, the efficacy of thrombolytic therapy for the treatment of stroke has been clearly shown. Intravenous administration of t-PA was approved for use by the FDA for the treatment of acute ischemic stroke in 1996. It remains the only therapy proven to reduce morbidity in the setting of acute ischemic stroke. Similar to the treatment of AMI, the efficacy of thrombolytic agents is highly time dependent and there is little demonstrable benefit when lytic treatment is initiated more than 3 hours after the onset of symptoms.[40] Efficacy is greater when lytic treatment is administered within 90 minutes.[40]

The concept of utilizing "clot-busting" therapies for ischemic stroke blossomed in 1995 when a study by the National Institute of Neurological Disorders and Stroke (NINDS) on rt-PA in acute ischemic stroke was published.[41] This trial consisted of two parts. Part I enrolled 291 patients and examined the clinical efficacy of t-PA. Treatment with this agent failed to demonstrate an improvement in neurologic function after 24 hours of treatment compared with placebo. At 3 months, however, patients treated with t-PA showed significant improvements in four different functional outcomes measurements as assessed by the National Institutes of Health Stroke Scale (NIHSS). Part II of this study assessed the long-term outcomes of t-PA treatment. Those patients who received t-PA were 30% more likely to have minimal residual disability or to have returned to baseline functional status. Unfortunately, patients treated with t-PA suffered a greater incidence of intracerebral hemorrhage (6.4% vs. 0.6% in the placebo group, P < .001) at 36 hours. Subsequent studies have shown similar rates of intracranial hemorrhage after lytic therapy. Nevertheless, mortality at 3 months was not significantly different (17% vs. 21%, P = .30). The beneficial effects of lytic therapy were also apparent at 1 year after the stroke.[42]

These encouraging results provided the impetus for subsequent trials examining the efficacy of different thrombolytic agents as well as different routes of administration (intravenous vs. intra-arterial). The early studies included the European Cooperative Acute Stroke Study (ECASS-I),[43] ECASS-II,[44] and the ATLANTIS trials.[45,46] All of these trials used intravenous t-PA administration and emphasized the importance of early treatment. These studies showed that the benefit of thrombolytic therapy was lost if it was administered beyond the 3-hour window previously established by the NINDS trial. The use of streptokinase in the setting of ischemic stroke has been largely abandoned because early placebo-controlled trials revealed increased rates of early mortality and intracranial bleeding.[47-49]

The only drug and route of administration currently approved by the FDA for the treatment of ischemic stroke is intravenous t-PA. However, prourokinase and the intra-arterial route of administration are also used in the setting of established clinical protocols. Intravenous delivery has both practical and theoretical disadvantages. One disadvantage is the inability to effectively lyse the internal carotid artery or the middle cerebral artery.[50] Intravenous administration does not permit mechanical thrombectomy. After confirmation by head CT of ischemic stroke (i.e., not associated with hemorrhage), patients are typically treated by intravenous administration of t-PA at a dose of 0.9 mg/kg with 10% of the total dose given as an initial bolus and the remainder infused over 60 minutes.[51]

As mentioned, intra-arterial administration of lytics is gaining popularity for the treatment of ischemic stroke. This method requires that patients be imaged by a neuro-interventional radiologist, who places an intra-arterial catheter into the thrombosed vessel. The thrombolytic agent is then infused through the catheter directly into the target vessel. Direct intra-arterial delivery has been shown to be effective in limited studies. The Prolyse in Acute Cerebral Thromboembolism (PROACT II) study[52] randomized 180 patients with occlusions of the middle cerebral artery to either intra-arterial pro-urokinase plus heparin or heparin alone. Intra-arterial administration of pro-urokinase improved the modified Rankin score to 2 or less in over 40% of patients, whereas heparin infusion alone improved the score in only 25%. Also, pro-urokinase was associated with significantly higher vessel recanalization rates (66% vs. 18%, P < .0001). Pro-urokinase is not yet available for general use, but rt-PA and its variants are frequently administered in intra-arterial fashion.[53,54] One obvious drawback to the

TABLE 240–3. CONTRAINDICATIONS FOR THROMBOLYTIC THERAPY IN ISCHEMIC STROKE

Contraindications	Relative Contraindications
Symptom duration > 6 hours	Symptom duration of 3 to 6 hours
Intracranial hemorrhage	Witnessed seizure
Evidence of active bleeding	Gastrointestinal or urinary
Platelet count < 100,000/mm³	hemorrhage within 3 weeks
Elevated partial thromboplastin time or International Normalized Ratio (>1.7)	Recent lumbar puncture Noncompressible arterial puncture site
Prior stroke, head trauma, or intracranial surgery within 3 months	Systolic blood pressure > 185 mm Hg or diastolic blood pressure > 110 mm Hg
Rapidly improving or only minor symptoms	Mass effect or hypodensity of > {1/3} middle cerebral artery distribution on head CT
Known arteriovenous malformation or intracranial aneurysm	Glucose < 50 mg/dL or > 400 mg/dL

intra-arterial approach is the time required to assemble an interventional radiology team and position the infusion catheter. Nevertheless, intra-arterial infusion offers the added advantage of delivering higher local concentrations of thrombolytic agent with much lower systemic drug levels.

Standard contraindications to intravenous thrombolytic therapy in acute ischemic stroke are similar to the exclusion criteria utilized in the NINDS study (Table 240-3). Although attempts have been made to stratify the benefit of lytic therapy based on stroke subtype, there are no conclusive data to support this practice and the time required to determine the type of stroke may contribute to costly delays in the initiation of therapy.[55] Blood pressure should be tightly controlled, ideally being maintained below 180/105 mm Hg. Antithrombotic agents should also be withheld for 24 hours owing to the risk of intracranial hemorrhage. A number of adjunctive therapies, including mechanical thrombectomy,[56] glycoprotein IIb/IIIa inhibitors,[57] and ultrasound,[58,59] have shown promise in improving recanalization rates.

PULMONARY EMBOLISM

Pulmonary emboli are not only a major source of morbidity and mortality in hospitalized patients, accounting for up to 15% of in-hospital deaths, but also are a surprisingly under-recognized source of cardiovascular collapse.[60-62] Heparinization with an initial bolus of 80 U/kg followed by 18 U/kg/h to maintain the aPTT at two to three times normal has been the standard of care for pulmonary embolization since anticoagulation was first shown to be beneficial in 1960.[63] Unfortunately, despite the proven efficacy of systemic heparin in this setting, a significant proportion of patients will have incomplete resolution of their occlusion with subsequent organization of the thrombus and obliteration of the pulmonary artery.[64-66] Accordingly, thrombolytic therapy for pulmonary embolism continues to be controversial. Also unresolved is the question of whether thrombolytic treatment should be delivered locally or systemically.

One of the initial studies that investigated the use of lytic therapy for pulmonary embolism was the Urokinase Pulmonary Embolism Trial (UPET).[64] This prospective trial randomized 160 patients to either urokinase followed by heparin or heparin alone. Although transient hemodynamic improvement was achieved, no differences were evident with regard to mortality or perfusion scan past 5 days. Nonetheless, the UPET and the subsequent Urokinase-Streptokinase Embolism Trial (USET) demonstrated improvements in small vessel patency at 2 weeks and 1 year compared with anticoagulation alone.[67,68] Seven-year follow-up of this cohort of patients suggested the risk of pulmonary hypertension was decreased by thrombolysis, presumably because lytic therapy achieved superior clot dissolution and decreased the risk of subsequent pulmonary embolism.[69]

Currently, the only patients who clearly benefit from lytic therapy are those with hemodynamic instability due to massive pulmonary emboli. Other patients who may benefit are those with right ventricular dysfunction or those with refractory hypoxemia in the setting of documented pulmonary embolism. The intravenous route of administration is most commonly used. The only trial to compare direct pulmonary artery infusion to intravenous infusion was by Verstraete and associates.[70] The study failed to show a benefit of pulmonary artery infusion. In addition, the time required to place a pulmonary artery catheter can further delay treatment and increase the risk of bleeding from a central venous puncture. On the other hand, local catheterization permits mechanical lysis, which has been shown to benefit selected patients.[71] FDA-approved regimens for acute pulmonary emboli are listed in Table 240-4.

Most agree that the drug of choice is intravenously administered t-PA.[72] Unlike patients treated for AMI, patients treated with thrombolytic agents for acute pulmonary embolism are generally not heparinized. However, systemic heparinization should begin on completion of thrombolysis, maintaining the aPTT at 1.5 to 2.5 times control. After the acute treatment of pulmonary emboli, patients should be maintained on anticoagulation for a minimum of 3 months, keeping the International Normalized Ratio at 2.5 or greater.[73] Major hemorrhagic complications occur in approximately 12% of patients irrespective of the lytic agent used.[74]

DEEP VENOUS THROMBOSIS

The formation of deep venous thrombosis (DVT) is surprisingly common in acutely ill patients, occurring in as many as 30% of ICU patients, despite prophylaxis with pneumatic compression devices and/or various prophylactic anticoagulation regimens.[75] ICU patients are at especially high risk for DVT because they often have indwelling central venous catheters. Central venous catheterization can increase the incidence of DVT by 5% to 30% depending on the site of insertion, type of catheter, duration of placement, and presence or absence of infection.[76-80] Acute occlusion of the deep venous system can lead to acute sequelae, such as venous gangrene (phlegmasia cerulea dolens), as well as long-term consequences, including recurrent venous thrombosis and post-phlebitic syndrome.[81-83]

The treatment of DVT, therefore, focuses both on the prevention of pulmonary embolism as well as the dissolution of the clot to prevent development of post-phlebitic syndrome, which is characterized by persistent pain, edema, discoloration, and ulceration. A number of randomized clinical studies have demonstrated the efficacy of both streptokinase and rt-PA compared with heparin alone in this setting.[84-87] These studies reported partial lysis in 70% and complete lysis in 28% of patients treated with thrombolytic therapy as compared with only 24% and 4%, respectively, in patients treated with heparin alone.[72] Meta-analyses of the available data indicated that systemic streptokinase is 3.7 times more likely[88] and t-PA is 7 times more likely[89] to lead to thrombolysis than is anticoagulation alone.

Exact indications for thrombolytic therapy are unclear. The patients who are most likely to benefit include those patients with a first occurrence of iliofemoral DVT (<10 days old) who are at low risk for major bleeding complications.[90] Others have advocated lytic therapy for young patients with primary upper extremity DVT either due to effort thrombosis (Paget-Schroetter syndrome) or idiopathic factors.[91] Most investigations have utilized a locoregional approach with infusions from a distal peripheral vein (e.g., a pedal vein). Another approach involves catheter-directed infusions that offer the advantage of requiring lower total doses of lytic agents with fewer systemic side effects as well as the ability to use angioplasty to dilate underlying venous stenoses.[92,93] Both systemic and catheter-directed thrombolysis have been shown to be effective in nonrandomized studies.[95] However, there is no clear-cut benefit for catheter-directed thrombolysis[84,94] and, therefore, either approach is acceptable.

ACUTE PERIPHERAL ARTERIAL OCCLUSION

Acute peripheral arterial occlusion (APAO) is a highly morbid condition that leads to amputation in 10% to 30% of cases and is associated with a mortality rate as high as 15% at 30 days.[95] Occlusive events generally arise either from dissection, trauma, local thrombosis, or embolus. Traumatic occlusion or disruption of the vessel almost always warrants surgical exploration and repair. A variety of noninvasive maneuvers, however, have been developed for the treatment of thromboembolic disease. Differentiating between in situ thrombosis and embolus as the etiology of the arterial occlusion can be extremely challenging if not impossible in up to 15% of cases.[95] In the Thrombolysis or Peripheral Arterial Surgery (TOPAS) trial, thrombosis (85%) was much more common than embolism (15%).[96,97]

Thrombolysis has become a popular means of treating acute arterial occlusion in certain settings. This approach has been performed since the 1950s.[3] Formerly, lytic therapy was administered intravenously but was associated with prohibitively high bleeding risks. Since the early 1970s, however, catheter-directed infusion has become the standard of care.[98] More recently, the development of multi-side-hole catheters (as compared with the older end-hole catheters) has improved the effectiveness of lytic therapy. Although streptokinase was the first agent used for acute arterial occlusion, multiple studies indicate that urokinase and t-PA are more effective for this indication and have fewer bleeding complications.[99-101] Before its removal from the U.S. market, urokinase was the predominant thrombolytic agent utilized in the treatment of acute arterial occlusion. Currently, t-PA and its

TABLE 240–4. FDA APPROVED REGIMENS FOR THE TREATMENT OF PULMONARY EMBOLISM

Drug	Systemic Administration
Streptokinase	250,000 U over 30 minutes followed by 100,000 U/h for 24 hours
Urokinase	4400 U/kg over 10 minutes followed by 4400 U/kg/h for 12-24 hours
t-PA (alteplase)	100 mg over 2 hours

derivatives have supplanted urokinase as the drug of choice for APAO. t-PA has been shown to have similar safety and efficacy profiles as urokinase when using "low dose" (≤ 2 mg/h, usually beginning at 0.5 mg/h) regimens with adjunctive heparin infusions to maintain the aPTT at 1.5 times baseline. With this regimen, over 60% of patients have complete resolution and 30% have partial resolution within 24 hours of initiating treatment.[102] An advisory panel recommended either weight-based dosing (0.001 to 0.02 mg/kg/h) or non–weight-based dosing (0.12 to 2.0 mg/h) with total doses not to exceed 40 mg.[103] They also recommended subtherapeutic heparin infusions to maintain the aPTT at between 1.25 and 1.5 times control values. Infusions should be discontinued approximately an hour before removing the arterial sheath and systemic heparin restarted 4 hours after the sheath is pulled.

In general, patients who are candidates for thrombolysis include those with symptoms of acute occlusion of less than 14 days, thromboemboli not accessible to embolectomy catheters, and a thrombosed popliteal artery aneurysm with little or no runoff (minimizing the risk of embolism after lysis). In addition, lytic therapy is indicated for patients who are poor surgical candidates. In addition to previously stated general contraindications to thrombolytic therapy, intracardiac thrombus should be considered a relative contraindication because there is an elevated risk of subsequent embolization in these patients.[104]

It is important to understand that thrombolytics in the setting of APAO is part of a multifaceted approach, often involving additional endovascular techniques and/or surgical intervention. There are several well-controlled trials examining initial surgical versus lytic therapy. The Rochester trial compared initial surgery with urokinase in severely threatened limbs (mean symptom duration, 2 days) in 114 patients.[105] Limb salvage rates in the two groups were identical (82%) at 12 months, whereas mortality was significantly lower in the patients treated with urokinase (16% with urokinase vs. 42% with surgery). The Surgery or Thrombolysis for the Ischemic Lower Extremity (STILE) trial examined 393 patients randomized to either primary surgery or one of two lytic therapies (rt-PA or urokinase).[106] At 30 days, limb loss rates were similar (5% with lytic therapy vs. 6% with surgery) and mortality rates were similar (4% vs. 5%, respectively). One of the major contributions of this study involved subgroup analyses[107,108] that demonstrated a greater benefit of lytic therapy in those patients with graft occlusion rather than native vessel occlusion and in those patients with acute ischemia of less than 2 weeks' duration. Finally, the TOPAS trial investigated recombinant urokinase versus surgery in 544 patients.[96] Although it failed to demonstrate an amputation-free survival benefit at 1 year (68% and 69% in the urokinase and surgical groups, respectively), it did show that over 30% of the patients treated with urokinase were not only alive without amputation but also had nothing more than a percutaneous procedure at 6 months. Therefore, a significant number of patients were able to avoid surgical intervention safely with the use of lytic therapy.

The most commonly employed technique for peripheral arterial thrombolysis involves direct catheter-mediated infusion into the thrombosed segment. In the proximal femoral and iliac arteries the contralateral femoral artery is accessed. In superficial femoral, popliteal, and tibial vessels the ipsilateral femoral artery is preferred. Once the catheter is positioned above the thrombus, a number of different techniques can be employed, including constant infusions and "pulse spray" modifications. A variety of catheter types can be used (end-hole or multi-side hole). Lytic therapy can be combined with mechanical thrombolysis. In addition, combining modalities such as antiplatelet therapy with thrombolytic agents hastens the dissolution of the thrombus but is associated with an increased risk of hemorrhage.[109] The overall hemorrhagic complication rate is approximately 5% with alteplase.[110]

Thrombolytic therapy is still not considered to be the standard of care for treatment of acute peripheral arterial occlusion. Lytic therapy, however, may prove to be a useful tool for treating patients who are poor candidates for surgery. These include patients too sick to safely undergo extremity revascularization and those with distal thromboemboli that are not amenable to surgical extraction or bypass. Thrombolysis also may benefit selected patients who present with less than 2 weeks of symptoms. Thrombolytic therapy may be the best approach for patients with occlusion of bypass grafts rather than native vessels. Furthermore, thrombolysis can open run-off vessels that are not initially patent to permit subsequent revascularization. It also unveils an offending plaque as the cause of the thrombosis. This plaque can be treated using angioplasty or surgical approaches (Fig. 240-4). Finally, thrombolysis may allow a more gradual reperfusion of an ischemic limb and reduce the metabolic derangements associated with ischemia/reperfusion. The use of lytic agents is contraindicated for treating of early postoperative thrombosis or in limbs with irreversible ischemia.

OTHER APPLICATIONS

In addition to the just-listed indications for lytic therapy, other common indications include the treatment of thrombosed dialysis grafts or central venous catheters. Vascular access complications are the single greatest source of morbidity among patients receiving hemodialysis, accounting for 15% of all hospitalizations.[111] Whereas the ultimate goal is to recognize and treat a graft before it clots, thrombolytics can play an important role once the graft has occluded. A number of techniques have been utilized for the acutely thrombosed graft, including mechanical thrombectomy, surgical revision, and pharmacologic thrombolysis. A technique that has gained popularity recently is called "lyse and wait." This method avoids the need for mechanical devices or pulse-spray catheters and shortens lysis times to approximately 45 minutes as compared with 65 minutes for the pulse-spray technique.[112] It involves placing a mixture of urokinase (250,000 IU) and heparin (5000 U) into the graft (or, alternatively, injecting 2 to 5 mg of rt-PA into the graft and administering 5000 U of heparin systemically).[113] After lysis, the arterial plug is removed and the venous anastomosis is dilated. With this technique, Cynamon and coworkers reported that 98% of patients have successful restoration of graft flow and function with 1- and 3-month patency rates of 80% and 55%, respectively.[112] Nevertheless, surgical thrombectomy remains the standard of care and achieved superior patency rates in a recent meta-analysis,[114] presumably because anastomotic revision is performed concurrently. As for occluded central venous catheters, the Advisory Panel on Catheter-Directed Thrombolytic Therapy in 2000 recommended a 2-mg (1 mg/mL) aliquot of alteplase for each occluded lumen for up to 2 hours.[103] This therapy can

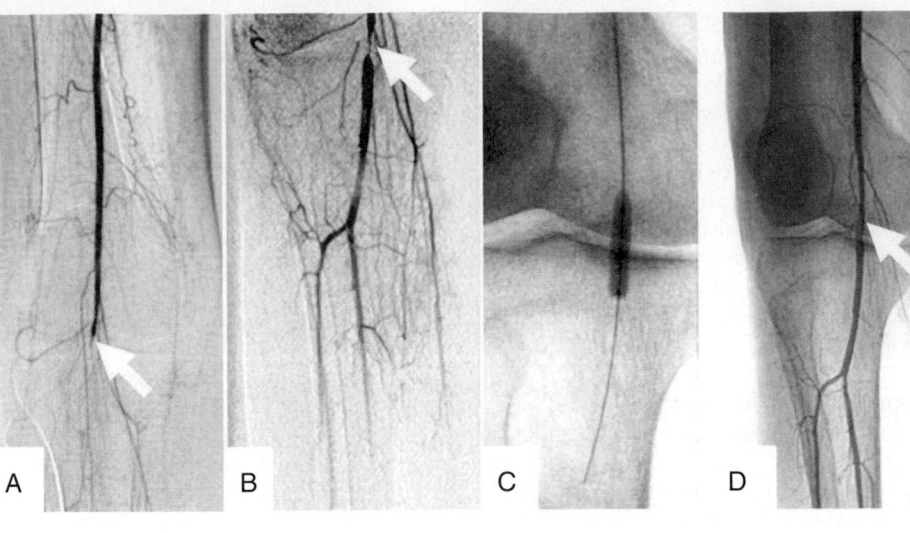

FIGURE 240–4. Successive angiograms demonstrating occluded popliteal artery (*arrow,* **A**) treated with thrombolytics. After thrombolysis, a focal popliteal artery stenosis was identified (*arrow,* **B**) with patent distal vessels. This area was subsequently subjected to balloon angioplasty (**C**). After thrombolysis and angioplasty, the result is a patent popliteal artery (*arrow,* **D**) with good distal arterial flow.

be repeated a second time if necessary. This regimen has proven to be both safe (≤1% bleeding risk) and efficacious (≈90% patency after two treatments) in multiple studies.[115-118]

MANAGEMENT/LABORATORIES

During administration of lytic agents, circulating plasminogen and fibrinogen concentrations decrease. Fibrinogen is degraded as part of the fibrinolytic process, reaching nadir values between 5 and 7 hours after the institution of therapy.[119] These values return to baseline in most patients within 48 hours of discontinuation of therapy. Likewise, circulating plasminogen levels begin to decrease immediately after initiating streptokinase and urokinase infusions; the decrease is greater with streptokinase as it complexes with plasminogen in a 1:1 relationship. Despite being relatively fibrin specific, the second- and third-generation lytic agents (recombinant t-PAs, APSAC, and pro-urokinase) still interact with circulating fibrinogen and therefore decrease circulating fibrinogen levels. Fibrin degradation products are a reliable indicator of the activity of the fibrinolytic system because the only source in humans is the degradation of fibrinogen or fibrin by plasmin.

Most advocate monitoring fibrinogen levels every 6 to 8 hours during lytic therapy, decreasing the dose or discontinuing the infusion if levels drop below 100 mg/dL. In addition to monitoring the fibrinolytic system, daily or every-other-day monitoring of the platelet count should be performed. rt-PA has been associated with thrombocytopenia in as many as 10% of patients whereas thrombocytopenia occurred in less than 1% of patients receiving streptokinase.[120-122] Selected patients should be typed for blood products. If bleeding does occur, thrombolytic infusion should be discontinued and blood products (fresh frozen plasma or cryoprecipitate) administered as necessary to correct the patient's hypocoagulable state.

CONCLUSION

Despite evidence in strong support of the use of thrombolytic agents in a variety of occlusive vascular disorders, relatively few patients ultimately receive this treatment. With increasing data supporting the safety and efficacy of thrombolytic therapy, however, use of this treatment modality increased substantially over the past decade.[123] One of the challenges in the coming years will be to more clearly define the patients who will benefit most, both in terms of reducing mortality and preventing hemorrhagic complications. Evolution in technologies, including diagnostic modalities, mechanical "clot busters," and adjuvant therapies, will undoubtedly expand the indications for lytic therapy in all the aforementioned areas.

ANNOTATED REFERENCES

Arcasoy SM, Vachani A: Local and systemic thrombolytic therapy for acute venous thromboembolism. Clin Chest Med 2003;24:73-91.
> *An excellent review of the current state of thrombolytic treatment of acute deep venous thrombosis and pulmonary embolus. It summarizes the results of the important trials and gives dosing recommendations for both indications.*

Keeley EC, Boura JA, Grines CL: Primary angioplasty versus intravenous thrombolytic therapy for acute myocardial infarction: A quantitative review of 23 randomised trials. Lancet 2003;361:13-20.
> *This meta-analysis summarizes the results of those trials comparing the use of lytics in acute myocardial infarction either with primary angioplasty or lytic therapy. It concludes that there is an overall benefit in the use of primary percutaneous thrombolytic coronary angioplasty.*

Kwiatkowski TG, Libman RB, Frankel M, et al: Effects of tissue plasminogen activator for acute ischemic stroke at one year. National Institute of Neurological Disorders and Stroke Recombinant Tissue Plasminogen Activator Stroke Study Group. N Engl J Med 1999;340:1781-1787.
> *This is a follow-up study to the landmark NINDS study published in 1995 examining the use of lytics in the treatment of acute ischemic stroke. This study documented a functional improvement in those patients treated with t-PA within 3 hours of symptom onset compared with treatment with placebo, although no change in mortality was documented.*

Ohman EM, Harrington RA, Cannon CP, et al: Intravenous thrombolysis in acute myocardial infarction. Chest 2001;119(1 Suppl):253S-277S.
> *This summary statements gives an excellent overview of the pharmacology of the various available lytic drugs and their use in the treatment of acute myocardial infarction. In addition, it summarizes the many articles that attempt to define which patients most benefit from lytics and the dosing regimens utilized.*

Ouriel K, Veith FJ, Sasahara AA: A comparison of recombinant urokinase with vascular surgery as initial treatment for acute arterial occlusion of the legs. Thrombolysis or Peripheral Arterial Surgery (TOPAS) Investigators. N Engl J Med 1998;338:1105-1111.
> *Randomized, multicenter trial examining intra-arterial urokinase versus surgery for acute (<14 days) arterial occlusion. This trial, along with the Rochester and STILE trials provide the cornerstone for the argument supporting the use of lytics in acute peripheral arterial occlusion.*

Chapter 241

ATHEROMATOUS EMBOLIZATION

Yasir Abu-Omar • David P. Taggart

Atherosclerosis and its thromboembolic complications are a leading cause of mortality and morbidity, contributing to half of all deaths in the Western world. It is a progressive disorder that usually remains clinically silent until it causes end-organ damage resulting in stroke, ischemic heart disease, and peripheral vascular insufficiency.

The distribution of atherosclerosis is characteristic, affecting the aorta more extensively than the peripheral vessels. The abdominal aorta is more widely involved than the thoracic aorta. Lower limb vessels are more frequently affected than upper limb vessels. The renal, pulmonary, and mesenteric vessels are the least susceptible.

As recently as the 1950s, nearly half of strokes were thought to result from cerebral vasospasm. Fisher subsequently stressed the etiologic importance of emboli from atherosclerotic plaques in the carotid artery.[1] Although embolization from the heart and major vessels accounts for a large number of ischemic cerebrovascular accidents, the cause of a significant proportion remains undetermined.[2] In those cases, the source is thought to be mainly embolic in origin.

The pathophysiology of atheromatous embolization is considered in this chapter, followed by a discussion of the general principles of the prevention and management.

PATHOPHYSIOLOGY

ATHEROSCLEROSIS

The process of atherosclerosis begins as early as childhood or adolescence, developing slowly over many years. Its effects rarely manifest before the fourth of fifth decade of life. Risk factors for atherosclerosis include hypertension, diabetes, smoking, and elevated serum cholesterol concentration.

Atherosclerosis affects mainly large and medium-size arteries. Intravascular sites of blood turbulence favor the development of atherosclerotic lesions. Initial changes in arterial wall morphology result in the formation of fatty streaks that consist of lipid-engorged macrophages in the arterial intima. Progression of such precursor lesions occurs secondary to an inflammatory process initiated by endothelial injury and dysfunction. A detailed account is given in a review by Ross.[3] Briefly, insufficient nitric oxide production results in increased adhesion and aggregation of platelets. Up-regulation in the endothelial expression of adhesion molecules and selectins leads to the accumulation of monocytes and T lymphocytes. These cells become activated and produce growth factors, cytokines, and chemokines. Smooth muscle cells migrate from the media into the intima and proliferate. In time, these lesions develop into raised fibrous plaques consisting of a fibrous cap covering a core containing necrotic material, lipids, and cholesteryl esters. This advanced plaque forms the basis on which the complicated plaque develops, consisting of fissures, erosions, or ulceration. This may lead to thrombosis or embolism and ensuing clinical manifestations.

ATHEROMATOUS EMBOLIZATION

Atheromatous embolization is a descriptive term for embolization of any atheromatous material. Atheroembolization refers to the dislodgment of vascular plaque material that contains cholesterol crystals, red blood cells, and fibrin.[4] This "cholesterol emboli" syndrome consists of renal failure, skin lesions, blue toes, and neurologic manifestations. It may develop spontaneously (due to plaque rupture) or following the use of thrombolytics or anticoagulants,[5] or it may result from arterial manipulation (during surgical procedures, cardiac catheterization, or insertion of an intra-aortic balloon pump).[6] Disruption of vascular plaque results in the release of cholesterol crystals. These crystals cause downstream vascular obstruction and initiate an inflammatory process, leading to lymphocytic and mononuclear cell infiltration. Biopsy specimens of affected organs (e.g., skin, kidney) are usually diagnostic.

PLAQUE MORPHOLOGY AND EMBOLIC RISK

Severe atherosclerosis of the ascending aorta appears to be the most important morphologic indicator of an increased risk of atheromatous embolization. The French Aortic Plaque in Stroke group identified a plaque thickness of 4 mm or greater as an independent predictor of recurrent embolization.[7,8] The odds ratio for plaques thickness less than 1 mm was 1.0 (i.e., no increase in risk); for plaques 1 to 3.9 mm, it was 3.9; and for plaques 4 mm or greater, it was 13.8. Ulceration and calcification occurred more frequently in plaques at least 4 mm thick. In this study, the presence of ulceration did not significantly increase the risk of vascular events in plaques 4 mm thick or greater. The absence of calcification, however, was associated with a significant increase in risk (relative risk 10.3, compared with 5.7 for those with calcification). Another study reported an association between the presence of ulceration in aortic plaques and an increased rate of cryptogenic stroke.[9] Ulceration and increased size of aortic plaques seem to be markers of severe generalized atherosclerosis and therefore predict a higher risk for thromboembolic complications.

MACROEMBOLIZATION AND MICROEMBOLIZATION

Emboli can be divided into macroemboli and microemboli. The former occlude arteries larger than 200 μm in diameter, whereas the latter occlude smaller arteries, arterioles, and capillaries.[10] The clinical manifestations of each vary. Whereas macrocmboli may result in overt clinical presentations (e.g., stroke, peripheral ischemia), microemboli tend to be more occult in their manifestations of end-organ injury or dysfunction (e.g., renal injury, neuropsychological impairment). Their clinical impact depends on the number and nature of microemboli. Embolization may arise spontaneously, or it may be related to vascular interventions and cardiovascular surgery.

CLINICAL CONSEQUENCES

CEREBRAL

As the prevalence of aortic atherosclerotic disease increases with age, so does the rate of atheromatous embolization. Postmortem studies indicate that it affects 20% of patients in the fifth decade of life and 80% in the eighth decade.[11] Emboli from the atherosclerotic aorta may result in stroke or transient ischemic attack, and the clinical manifestations of these conditions vary, depending on the cerebrovascular territory affected; the middle cerebral artery is the most frequent site of arterial embolism. Stroke has profound effects, and outcomes from acute stroke are measured in terms of survival, functional independence, and financial cost. Survival after stroke is significantly poorer than after myocardial infarction or most cancers; 1-year survival is about 70%.[12] Stroke is the leading cause of disability in developed countries, and its economic impact is huge, accounting for 5% to 6% of health care and social services budgets in the United Kingdom.[13]

Cholesterol emboli are an important and frequently unrecognized cause of stroke.[14,15] Microembolization is a recognized cause of more subtle, sometimes subclinical neurologic injury. Most frequently, this injury is manifested by

subtle changes in cognitive function that may be evident only with detailed neuropsychological testing.[16,17] Although this more subtle impairment may appear trivial, its importance has increased in recent years, particularly in patients undergoing cardiac surgery.

CARDIAC

Atherosclerotic cardiovascular disease is the leading cause of death in developed countries. Every year, it results in more than 19 million deaths worldwide, and coronary heart disease accounts for the majority of those.[18] Myocardial infarction is a consequence of diseased coronary arteries as part of the overall systemic picture of atherosclerosis. Most acute coronary syndromes are due to plaque rupture. Distal embolization of cholesterol and atheromatous material may be important in the pathogenesis of some acute coronary syndromes.[19] The occurrence of distal coronary embolization in the setting of acute coronary syndromes has been followed using serum levels of cardiac troponins to detect small degrees of myocardial necrosis. The clinical importance of distal coronary embolization, as defined by serum troponins, is its predictive value for future cardiac events.[20] Embolization following percutaneous coronary interventions is well recognized, and elevations in cardiac troponins are seen in up to 44% of patients undergoing intervention.[21,22]

PERIPHERAL

Peripheral emboli most frequently lodge in the lower extremities. Cholesterol atheroembolization may be subclinical or it may result in systemic effects. Although renal, neurologic, and cutaneous manifestations tend to dominate the clinical picture, involvement of most organs has been reported. Atheromatous material can be identified in the pancreas, intestine, and spleen. Symptoms and presentation depend on the site of dislodgment. Embolization into the renal arteries results in renal ischemia and can lead to renal impairment or failure.[23] Renal involvement characteristically worsens over a 2- to 4-week period following the acute event, and renal biopsy is diagnostic.[24]

Involvement of the cutaneous vessels leads to livedo reticularis and the "blue toe" syndrome, whereas retinal emboli result in visual symptoms.[25] Other reported effects include small bowel bleeding[26] and renal transplant failure.[27]

DIAGNOSIS AND SCREENING

Asymptomatic atherosclerotic disease may be discovered incidentally. The clinical presentation of atheromatous embolization varies, depending on the site affected. Full clinical assessment and screening of patients presenting with embolic complications are essential in guiding management and prevention strategies.

Diagnosis of the cholesterol embolization syndrome relies on clinical findings in patients with atherosclerotic disease and recent vascular intervention. Because different organs can be involved, the clinician should maintain a high index of suspicion.

Many modalities have been used for the purpose of imaging atherosclerotic plaques; some are used routinely in clinical practice, whereas others are reserved for research purposes. The most commonly used techniques are described here.

X-RAY ANGIOGRAPHY

X-ray angiography is an invasive procedure that allows assessment of the vascular lumen by providing a measure of the degree of stenosis and by identifying plaque disruption, thrombosis, and calcification. However, it provides no information about the vessel wall or the components of the atherosclerotic plaque. Despite these shortcomings, angiography is still regarded as the gold standard for imaging coronary, carotid, and peripheral arterial disease.[28]

SURFACE AND TRANSESOPHAGEAL ULTRASONOGRAPHY

Measurement of carotid and aortic wall thickness, as well as qualitative and quantitative assessment of atherosclerotic plaques, can be accomplished using ultrasonography. The North American Symptomatic Carotid Endarterectomy Trial and the Asymptomatic Carotid Artery Stenosis Study have shown that the degree of stenosis and its hemodynamic consequences are important in the development of stroke.[29,30] High-resolution, real-time, B-mode ultrasonography with Doppler flow imaging is currently considered the modality of choice for imaging the carotid arteries.[31]

Transesophageal echocardiography (TEE) is a quick, safe, and minimally invasive procedure that can be used in different settings, ranging from the operating theater to the bedside. It is regarded as the procedure of choice for the detection, assessment, and characterization of thoracic aortic atherosclerosis. Imaging using the transthoracic approach is also possible, but at the expense of significant loss of resolution compared with the transesophageal technique. TEE can reliably detect intimal thickening, ulceration, calcification, and the presence of mobile components within the aortic plaque. As outlined earlier, the French Aortic Plaque in Stroke investigators used TEE to assess aortic plaque thickness in patients with stroke and reported that increased plaque thickness was associated with a significant increase in stroke risk.[7,8] Katz and colleagues used a five-grade ranking system for the severity of aortic atherosclerosis assessed using TEE in 130 patients undergoing cardiac surgery with cardiopulmonary bypass: grade 1, normal aorta; grade 2, flat intimal thickening; grade 3, protruding atheroma in the aortic lumen (<5 mm); grade 4, protruding atheroma (>5 mm); and grade 5, atheroma with a mobile thrombus.[32] Patients with grade 5 lesions had the highest risk of stroke. Logistic regression identified aortic arch atheroma as the only variable that was predictive of stroke, with an odds ratio of 5.8. Another study of 315 coronary artery bypass graft (CABG) patients undergoing intraoperative TEE also reported a significant increase in the risk of stroke in patients with aortic arch intimal thickening greater than 5 mm.[33]

It is no surprise that patients with the highest-risk carotid lesions also have high-risk aortic plaques. Assessment of the carotid arteries as well as the aorta is prudent in the evaluation of atherosclerotic patients who have suffered embolic events.

INTRAOPERATIVE EPIAORTIC ULTRASONOGRAPHY

Epiaortic ultrasonography involves intraoperative imaging of the ascending aorta using a sterile-sheathed transducer. This technique is noninvasive and has been used in the context of cardiac surgery to detect areas of ascending aortic atherosclerosis.[34] It allows modification of the surgical technique in an attempt to reduce potential embolic complications. The main disadvantage of this technique is suboptimal imaging of the aortic arch. Intraoperative epiaortic ultrasonography can therefore be used to complement the information obtained about the aortic arch with TEE.

TRANSCRANIAL DOPPLER ULTRASONOGRAPHY

Transcranial Doppler ultrasonography can be used to detect and quantify cerebral microemboli. Ultrasound probes are placed bilaterally on the temple overlying the middle cerebral vessels. Emboli cause an increase in the reflected ultrasound, causing high-intensity transient signals. These signals are the footprints of microemboli, which may consist of air, fat, atheromatous material, or platelet-fibrin emboli.

Transcranial Doppler can reliably detect high-intensity transient signals intraoperatively and has been used extensively in the context of cardiac and carotid surgery. During cardiac surgery, microemboli can be detected following intraoperative aortic manipulation (aortic cannulation and application and removal of aortic cross-clamp), as well as during cardiopulmonary bypass.[35,36] High-intensity transient signals have also been identified in patients with symptomatic carotid artery stenosis[37] and in those with aortic atherosclerosis.[38] They are a common phenomenon in patients with acute stroke, and their detection may continue for several days after the acute event.[39] Their presence is a significant independent predictor of early recurrence of stroke.[40]

Transcranial Doppler is a simple, user-friendly technique that can be performed at the patient's bedside as well as in the operating theater. It can provide valuable information intraoperatively on cerebral blood velocity, which is closely related to flow, and microembolic load, allowing for intraoperative technical modifications. A major limitation of the technique is an inadequate acoustic window in 5% to 20% of individuals.[41] Until recently, it was generally not possible to reliably reject artifacts closely resembling microembolic signals, generated by movement, or to distinguish between gaseous and particulate microemboli. With the availability of multirange multifrequency Doppler systems and automatic artifact rejection, differentiation between solid and gaseous microemboli has become possible with high sensitivity and specificity.[42,43] We recently reported a significant reduction in intraoperative cerebral microembolism, as well as a reduction in the proportion of solid microemboli, with avoidance of cardiopulmonary bypass and minimal manipulation of the ascending aorta during cardiac surgery.[36]

COMPUTED TOMOGRAPHY

Computed tomography can be used to image the aorta and quantify aortic wall calcification. Contrast-enhanced computed tomography has been proposed as a valuable method for following the progression or regression of atherosclerotic disease.[44] The main advantage over TEE is the ability to completely image the thoracic and abdominal aorta.

MAGNETIC RESONANCE IMAGING

Magnetic resonance imaging (MRI) can be used to image atherosclerotic plaques in aortic,[45] carotid,[46] peripheral,[47] and coronary arterial disease.[48] Its major strength is its ability to determine plaque morphology. Using a range of techniques, MRI can provide valuable information on the composition of the atherosclerotic plaque by identifying the three main factors that determine plaque stability: presence of a lipid core, thickness of the fibrous cap, and inflammation within the cap. MRI allows the identification of high-risk unstable plaques and thus guides intervention and therapy.[49] Magnetic resonance angiography has high sensitivity and specificity and can be used to image the aorta and the carotid, renal, and other peripheral vessels. Evolving magnetic resonance techniques include intravascular[50] and transesophageal[51] MRI.

MRI is a powerful noninvasive tool with high spatial resolution that can be used clinically without exposing the patient to the risks of ionizing radiation. However, it is expensive, and its major use is for experimental and research purposes.

VASCULAR MANIPULATION AND EMBOLIC EVENTS

CARDIAC SURGERY

Stroke, transient ischemic attack, and peripheral embolization are potential complications following cardiac surgery. Atheroembolism results in a variety of clinical manifestations and is fatal in about 20% of patients.[52] Stroke affects 3% of CABG patients,[53,54] 8% of those undergoing isolated valve surgery, and up to 11% of those undergoing combined CABG and valve procedures.[55] The risk of perioperative stroke increases with advancing age, and those with concomitant cardiovascular risk factors are at highest risk.[56] In addition, it has been shown that female gender is independently associated with a significantly higher risk of perioperative stroke.[54] Embolization from the atheromatous aorta is the single most important etiologic factor for stroke. This risk arises during intraoperative manipulation of the aorta, including cannulation for cardiopulmonary bypass, application and removal of the aortic cross-clamp for administration of cardioplegia, and use of side clamps for anastomosis of the proximal end of the graft to the aorta.[57] Roach and colleague showed that atherosclerosis of the ascending aorta is the strongest independent predictor of perioperative stroke, with an odds ratio of 4.5.[53]

The functional impact of stroke is enormous; adverse cerebral outcomes after coronary bypass surgery are associated with a 10-fold increase in mortality and substantial increases in the length of hospitalization and in the use of intermediate- or long-term care facilities.[57] New diagnostic and therapeutic strategies must be developed to lessen such injury.

CARDIAC CATHETERIZATION AND PERIPHERAL VASCULAR INTERVENTION

Aortic manipulation during cardiac catheterization procedures or intra-aortic balloon pumping may cause embolization from aortic atheroma. In a report comparing 59 patients with atherosclerotic aortic debris undergoing transfemoral cardiac catheterization with 71 control patients, an embolic event occurred in 17% of the patients with atherosclerotic aortas, compared with 3% of controls.[58] Among the patients requiring intra-aortic balloon pumping, 5 out of 10 patients with atherosclerotic aortas had embolic events, compared with none of the 12 patients in the control group. When a transbrachial approach was used in patients with atherosclerotic aortas, none of 11 patients suffered an embolic event. Patients with mobile aortic atheromas, identified using TEE, are at highest risk of catheter-related embolization.[58]

Cholesterol embolization can complicate cardiac catheterization. Because it is commonly asymptomatic, the exact incidence is uncertain and depends mainly on the detection criteria used (clinical or pathologic). Cholesterol can be identified in the lumen of affected arterioles in up to 12% of patients following cardiac catheterization.[59] A recent prospective multicenter study reported cholesterol embolization in 1.4% of patients following cardiac catheterization.[6] The diagnostic criteria used in this study was based on evidence of peripheral cutaneous involvement or renal dysfunction. The syndrome occurred more frequently in patients with generalized atherosclerosis. Interestingly, the authors identified preprocedural elevation of C-reactive protein as an independent predictor of cholesterol embolization, suggesting involvement of an inflammatory process.

PREVENTION AND MANAGEMENT

Treatment of atheromatous embolization depends on the clinical manifestation. General measures include identification and modification of risk factors. Patients with the clinical syndrome of cholesterol embolization have a generally poor prognosis, particularly when there is evidence of visceral and renal involvement. Supportive management with blood pressure control and, if necessary, renal replacement therapy is indicated. Strategies for the general prevention and management of atheromatous embolization are discussed here.

ANTIPLATELETS, ANTICOAGULANTS, AND ANTITHROMBOTICS

Because thrombi can develop on and embolize from atherosclerotic plaques, it seems logical to use antiplatelet agents or anticoagulants to prevent these thromboembolic complications. There have been reports, however, linking the atheroemboli syndrome with anticoagulation in patients with atherosclerosis. Although three studies reported a reduction in the risk of stroke with anticoagulation,[60-62] these studies were not randomized and did not include long-term follow-up. It is over the long term that the potential risks of warfarin therapy may become evident. In addition, anticoagulation in these patients has been linked with the cholesterol embolization syndrome.[63]

Antiplatelet therapy has been used for many years in patients with atherosclerotic disease to prevent a range of coronary and cerebrovascular events.[64] The Antithrombotic Trialists' Collaboration published a major meta-analysis of more than 200,000 patients, assessing the effect of antiplatelet therapy in patients with various manifestations of atherosclerosis. This meta-analysis found a significant reduction in the rate of stroke, myocardial infarction, and vascular death.[65]

Aspirin is the most commonly used antiplatelet agent. It inhibits thromboxane-dependent platelet activation. Thienopyridines, including clopidogrel and ticlopidine, act by blocking adenosine diphosphate–dependent activation of platelets. There is evidence that thienopyridine derivatives are modestly but significantly more effective than aspirin in preventing serious vascular events in patients at high risk, but there is uncertainty about the size of the additional benefit.[65] The thienopyridines are also associated with less gastrointestinal hemorrhage and upper gastrointestinal upset compared with aspirin, but have a higher incidence of skin rash and diarrhea.[66] The risk of the latter is greater with ticlopidine than with clopidogrel.[12] Ticlopidine, but not clopidogrel, is associated with neutropenia and thrombotic thrombocytopenic purpura.[12,66] In the Clopidogrel in Unstable Angina to Prevent Recurrent Events (CURE) trial, a long-term benefit was observed with the use of both clopidogrel and aspirin in high-risk patients (unstable angina and non–Q wave myocardial infarction).[67]

Activation of platelets leads to a conformational change in glycoprotein IIb/IIIa, the major fibrinogen receptor on platelets. Intravenous glycoprotein IIb/IIIa inhibitors (e.g., abciximab) are generally reserved for the high-risk setting of percutaneous coronary intervention.

Dextran has antiplatelet and intravascular volume expansion effects. Lennard and colleagues observed that post-operative or perioperative administration of 10% dextran 40 reduces the rate of microembolic signals detected by transcranial Doppler after carotid endarterectomy.[68,69] Dextran, however, may interfere with the crossmatching of blood, cause bleeding, renal failure, or occasionally acute allergic reactions.

Aspirin should be used routinely in all patients with atherosclerotic disease, unless there are specific contraindications. Clopidogrel might be an appropriate alternative in such circumstances.

STATINS

There is a clear association between elevated levels of plasma cholesterol and atherosclerotic disease. Statins, or 3-hydroxy-3-methylglutaryl coenzyme A (HMG-CoA) reductase inhibitors, reduce the hepatocyte cholesterol content and increase the expression of low-density lipoprotein cholesterol receptors, resulting in a drop in serum low-density lipoprotein cholesterol. In addition, it has become evident that statins possess cholesterol-independent or pleiotropic effects. These include improvement of endothelial function by increasing the bioavailability of nitric oxide, reduction of vascular inflammation, and plaque stabilization.[70] Statins are widely used in the primary and secondary prevention of ischemic heart disease. A meta-analysis of randomized, placebo-controlled, double-blind trials with statins reported a 30% reduction in stroke risk with statin therapy.[71] Another meta-analysis of data pooled from more than 49,000 patients treated with statins in 28 trials reported a relative risk of stroke of 0.76 in statin-treated patients.[72] Tunick and associates showed that statin therapy was independently and significantly protective against the occurrence of embolic events (risk ratio 0.39) in patients with severe thoracic aortic plaque.[73]

Plaque size reduction, stabilization, and prevention of plaque thrombosis may be the mechanisms leading to a reduction in atheromatous embolization. Patients with widespread atherosclerosis are at an increased risk of coronary and cerebrovascular morbidity, and it seems reasonable to use statins in this setting.

MINIMAL AORTIC MANIPULATION

The use of smaller arterial catheters during cardiac catheterization may help reduce the risk of embolization.[74]

Reduction of embolization during cardiac surgery is possible with modifications to the operative technique. Avoidance of intraoperative aortic manipulation is most important.[57] This can be achieved in patients undergoing CABG by not using cardiopulmonary bypass, which obviates the need for aortic cannulation and cross-clamping.[75] The use of composite arterial grafts (bilateral internal thoracic artery grafts with the radial artery anastomosed to the internal thoracic artery)[76,77] avoids the need for proximal aortic anastomosis requiring a side clamp. In addition, there is a potential survival advantage with arterial grafts. Off-pump surgery has been shown to result in a significant reduction in the risk of stroke in patients with atheromatous aortas.[78] Kim and colleagues reported a 0% stroke rate in 222 patients undergoing off-pump CABG with a "no-touch" technique.[79] We routinely adopt a strategy of off-pump total arterial revascularization using composite arterial grafts and avoidance of aortic manipulation, particularly in high-risk patients. In addition, we reported a significant reduction in cerebral microembolization with avoidance of cardiopulmonary bypass and aortic manipulation.[36] A strategy for the prevention of embolization in cardiac surgery is summarized in Table 241-1.

SCREENING WITH ECHOCARDIOGRAPHY AND ULTRASONOGRAPHY

As previously outlined, patients with mobile atheromas in the aortic lumen have the highest incidence of perioperative stroke.[32] TEE has confirmed the association between aortic atherosclerosis and perioperative stroke, providing a means of identifying patients at highest risk[32,80] and allowing for modification of surgical techniques to minimize embolic complications.

There is an association between atherosclerosis of the ascending aorta, detected using epiaortic ultrasonography, and increased postoperative neurologic morbidity.[34,81,82] In a study of more than 1900 patients undergoing cardiac surgery, detection of atherosclerosis of the ascending aorta using epiaortic ultrasonography was identified as an independent predictor of long-term neurologic morbidity and mortality.[34] A comparison of intraoperative TEE and epiaortic ultrasonography demonstrated that the former underestimates the presence and severity of aortic atherosclerosis.[83] Modification of surgical technique based on intraoperative epiaortic ultrasonography may reduce the frequency of stroke and neurobehavioral changes related to atheromatous embolization.[11,84]

TABLE 241–1. PREVENTION OF EMBOLIZATION DURING CARDIAC SURGERY IN PATIENTS WITH ATHEROSCLEROSIS

Establish the patient's preoperative risk factors
Image the ascending aorta and arch preoperatively
Assess the carotid arteries
Assess the ascending aorta using intraoperative epiaortic ultrasonography
Use evidence-based decisions to reflect the operative technique
Decide on the site and risk of cannulation
Avoid repeated aortic clamping
Consider no-touch aortic techniques
Perform off-pump surgery with composite arterial grafting when possible

SURGICAL TREATMENT

The treatment of patients with symptomatic carotid atherosclerosis is well established. The European Carotid Surgery Trial and North American Symptomatic Carotid Endarterectomy Trial investigators reported a clear benefit of carotid endarterectomy in the prevention of stroke in patients with high-grade, recently symptomatic carotid stenosis.[29,85] This benefit is offset by the surgical risk of the procedure. The perioperative stroke and death rate for patients with high-grade stenosis was 8% at 30 days in the European trial and 6% in the North American trial. These rates are acceptable, given that the absolute risk reduction from surgery was 10% and 17%, respectively. However, for patients with asymptomatic carotid disease, the risk-to-benefit ratio is narrower, and carotid endarterectomy is currently recommended only for high-grade carotid stenosis (70% to 99%).

In recent years, there has been an increasing interest in endovascular intervention for carotid stenosis with angioplasty and stenting. The technology is evolving rapidly. A multicenter randomized trial of endovascular versus surgical treatment in patients with carotid stenosis showed no difference in the major risks and effectiveness at stroke prevention.[86]

The management of patients with recurrent embolic events due to aortic atherosclerotic disease can be problematic. Aortic arch endarterectomy in patients with severe aortic atherosclerosis has been reported.[87-89] This procedure is performed using deep hypothermic circulatory arrest and is associated with significant perioperative morbidity and mortality. However, it has been shown to result in a significant reduction in the rate of embolic events. As with any major surgical intervention, the risks and merits of the procedure have to be carefully weighed, and it should be carried out by a surgeon with adequate experience in aortic surgery. Aortic endarterectomy is recommended only in carefully selected patients with recurrent systemic emboli from diffuse aortic atherosclerosis, especially those with mobile plaques, that is refractory to conservative management.

CONCLUSION

Patients with atherosclerotic disease should be given an antiplatelet agent and a statin. Imaging of the ascending aorta, aortic arch, and carotid arteries is recommended in those at high risk for atheromatous embolization. Minimizing or completely avoiding aortic manipulation in these patients is recommended. Surgical treatment may be considered in carefully selected patients with recurrent embolization secondary to advanced atherosclerotic aortic disease.

ANNOTATED REFERENCES

Amarenco P, Cohen A, Tzourio C, et al: Atherosclerotic disease of the aortic arch and the risk of ischemic stroke. N Engl J Med 1994;331:1474-1479.

This prospective, case-controlled study by the French Aortic Plaque in Stroke group involved 250 patients with ischemic stroke. It found that increasing plaque thickness was associated with an increased risk of stroke, especially with plaques greater than 4 mm thick.

Bucher HC, Griffith LE, Guyatt GH: Effect of HMG CoA reductase inhibitors on stroke: A meta-analysis of randomized, controlled trials. Ann Intern Med 1998;128:89-95.

This meta-analysis of more than 49,000 participants treated with statins from 28 trials reported that the risk ratio for nonfatal and fatal stroke with HMG-CoA reductase inhibitors was 0.76 (95% confidence interval 0.62 to 0.92). It also demonstrated an overall reduction in the rate of death from coronary heart disease, as well as a reduction in overall mortality with HMG-CoA reductase inhibitors.

Cohen A, Tzourio C, Bertrand B, et al: Aortic plaque morphology and vascular events: A follow-up study in patients with ischemic stroke. FAPS Investigators. French Study of Aortic Plaques in Stroke. Circulation 1997; 96:3838-3841.

This study of 334 patients aged 60 years and older reported that in those with brain infarction, the risk associated with aortic plaque thickness of 4 mm or greater was markedly increased by the absence of plaque calcification.

Collaborative meta-analysis of randomised trials of antiplatelet therapy for prevention of death, myocardial infarction, and stroke in high risk patients. BMJ 2002;324:71 86.

This large meta-analysis of more than 200,000 patients reported that aspirin is protective in most patients at increased risk of occlusive vascular events, including those with acute myocardial infarction or ischemic stroke; unstable or stable angina; previous myocardial infarction, stroke, or cerebral ischemia; peripheral arterial disease; and atrial fibrillation.

Davila-Roman VG, Murphy SF, Nickerson NJ, et al: Atherosclerosis of the ascending aorta is an independent predictor of long-term neurologic events and mortality. J Am Coll Cardiol 1999;33:1308-1316.

In this study of more than 1900 patients undergoing cardiac surgery, atherosclerosis of the ascending aorta, as defined intraoperatively using ultrasonography, was shown to be an independent predictor of long-term neurologic morbidity and mortality. There was a greater than threefold increase in the incidence of both neurologic events and mortality as the severity of the atherosclerosis increased from normal or mild to severe.

Chapter 242

PRESSURE ULCERATION

Courtney H. Lyder

Pressure ulceration is a major risk factor for critically ill adults. Presently, approximately 1 million adults have pressure ulcers, with an annual treatment cost of over 1.3 billion dollars.[1] Reported incidence rates are 0.4% to 38% for hospitals, 2.2% to 23.9% for long-term care facilities, and 0% to 17% for home care.[2] Pressure ulcer incidence rates in critical care units range from 8% to 79%.[2] Thus, pressure ulcers occur much more commonly in critical care units than other sites of care within the health care system.

PREVENTION

Pressure ulcers develop when capillaries supplying the skin and subcutaneous tissues are compressed enough to impede perfusion, leading ultimately to tissue necrosis. Normal blood pressure within capillaries ranges from 20 to 40 mm Hg; 32 mm Hg is considered to be the average. Thus, keeping the external pressure less than 32 mm Hg should be sufficient to prevent the development of pressure ulcers. However, capillary blood pressure may be less than 32 mm Hg in critically ill patients owing to hemodynamic instability and comorbid conditions; thus, even less pressure may be sufficient to induce ulceration in this group of patients. Pressure ulcers can develop within 2 to 6 hours.[3,4] Therefore, it is essential to accurately identify risk factors for pressure ulcer formation and intervene appropriately in a timely fashion to prevent ulcerations in the highly vulnerable ICU population.

Preventing pressure ulcers in critically ill adults remain challenging; however, the basic principles of prevention include risk assessment, skin care, modification of mechanical loading, nutrition, and use of proper support surfaces. When all of these components are implemented, the incidence of pressure ulcers may decrease.[5,6]

RISK FACTORS

Numerous risk factors have been identified for pressure ulcer development, including age 70 years or older, male gender, white race, current smoking history, low body mass index, impaired mobility, altered mental status (i.e., confusion), urinary and fecal incontinence, malnutrition, physical restraints, malignancy, diabetes mellitus, cerebrovascular accident, pneumonia, heart failure, fever, sepsis, hypotension, renal failure, dry scaly skin, history of pressure ulcers, anemia, lymphopenia, and hypoalbuminemia.[7-10] Neural and endothelial control of blood flow is often impaired during acute illness, making the critically ill adult more susceptible to ischemic organ damage (e.g., pressure ulcers).[11]

Given the abundant number of risk factors that are associated with pressure ulcer development, various risk scales have been developed. The two most widely used risk scales are the Norton Scale[12] and the Braden Scale.[13] Both tools use broad clinical categories to identify patients at risk for pressure ulcers. The Norton Scale has five subscales: physical condition, mental condition, activity, mobility, and incontinence. The total score ranges from 5 (high risk) to 20 (low risk). The Norton Scale has a sensitivity of 73% to 92% and a specificity of 61% to 94%. The Braden Scale is composed of six subscales: sensory perception, moisture, activity, mobility, nutrition, and friction and shear. The total score ranges from 6 (high risk) to 23 (low risk). The Braden Scale has a sensitivity of 83% to 100% and specificity of 64% to 77%. Thus, both tools have a tendency to overpredict ulceration. Because neither tool has been validated in every critical care setting, optimal cutoff scores may differ dependent on the specific critical care unit population. Thus, titration of preventive measures based on level of risk (high vs. low) is essential to decrease costs and the burden placed on patients and staff.[4]

SKIN CARE

The goal of skin care is to maintain the skin integrity. The skin should be assessed daily, paying particular attention to the anatomic areas most vulnerable for ulceration. These areas are the heels of the feet and the skin over the coccyx, sacrum, and femoral trochanters.[2] The skin should be assessed and cleansed with warm water and a mild cleansing agent to minimize irritation and drying. Moisturizing creams should be applied if the skin appears dry. Massaging erythematous bony prominences is not recommended, because this practice does improve perfusion and can increase skin damage.[1] Excessive moisture (owing to perspiration or incontinence) should be avoided, because macerated skin is at higher risk for ulceration.

REPOSITIONING

Patients unable to independently shift weight should be repositioned in bed every 2 hours and every hour while sitting in a chair. However, when reactive hyperemia lasting more than 5 minutes is noted, the frequency of repositioning should be increased. Prolonged reactive hyperemia has been noted to be a precursor to the development of pressure ulcers.[14] Ideally, the head of the bed should be at the lowest degree of elevation consistent with the patient's medical condition to decrease friction and shear forces. When a patient is on a ventilator the head of the bed should be elevated to decrease the incidence of ventilator-associated pneumonia. Thus, clinicians should pay close attention to properly align these patients to decrease the potential for sliding in the bed. The national pressure ulcer guidelines suggest that the head of the bed should be elevated above 30 degrees to decrease friction and shear forces unless medically contraindicated.

SUPPORT SURFACES

Support surfaces do not relieve pressure; rather, they redistribute pressure. The Centers for Medicare and Medicaid Services have divided support surfaces into three categories for reimbursement purposes. Each classification of support surfaces has advantages and disadvantages (Table 242-1). The majority of critically ill patients are placed on dynamic surfaces. Although these surfaces are more effective in redistributing pressure, some of their adverse effects include dehydration, sensory deprivation, and loss of muscle strength. Data are lacking to support the view that different support surfaces are better (or worse) for preventing or healing pressure ulcers. Thus, patients who are at low risk for pressure ulcer development should receive pressure reducing overlays (e.g., solid foams or gel overlays) whereas patients at

high risk for pressure ulcers should receive more dynamic support surfaces (e.g., alternating air mattresses or low air-loss beds).

MANAGEMENT

Once ulceration has occurred, it is necessary to assess and document the ulcer location, area (length and width), depth, drainage, tissue type present in wound bed (necrotic, sloughed tissue, granulation tissue), and presence of cellulitis. It is also important to stage the ulcer, because most experts agree that the stage should dictate the treatment plan. The most common staging system used is the four-stage system developed by the National Pressure Ulcer Advisory Panel (Table 242-2).

WOUND BED PREPARATION

Wound bed preparation is a recent concept in the healing of chronic ulcers. The goal of wound bed preparation is to provide the ulcer with an optimal environment for healing. The optimal wound bed is one that is highly vascularized with minimal exudate. The three main principles are débridement, bacterial balance, and control of exudates.

There is no optimal débridement method. Thus, the best method for débridement is determined by the absence or presence of infection, the amount of devitalized tissue present, and economic considerations for the patient and institution. There are five types of débridement: mechanical, autolytic, enzymatic, sharp, and biosurgical. Mechanical débridement uses application of wet-to-dry gauzes. The gauze adheres to the necrotic tissue. On removal of the gauze dressing, necrotic tissue is removed. The problem with mechanical débridement is that healthy granulation tissue may be removed along with the devitalized tissue, thereby delaying wound healing. Autolytic débridement involves the use of semi-occlusive (transparent film) dressings and occlusive dressings (hydrocolloids or hydrogels) to create an environment that promotes the breakdown the necrotic tissue by the body's own enzymes. Enzymatic débridement uses proteolytic enzymes (i.e., papain, collagenase, and trypsin) to remove necrotic tissue. Although, enzymatic débridement is an effective method for débridement, it is slower than the other approaches and can be costly. Sharp débridement entails the use of a scalpel or laser and is probably the most effective type. Sharp débridement always should be considered when the patient is suspected of having cellulitis

TABLE 242–1. SELECTED CHARACTERISTICS FOR CLASSES OF SUPPORT SURFACES

Performance characteristics	Air fluidized (high air loss)	Low air loss	Alternating air (dynamic)	Static flotation (air or water)	Foam	Standard hospital mattress
Increased support area	Yes	Yes	Yes	Yes	Yes	No
Low moisture retention	Yes	Yes	No	No	No	No
Reduced heat accumulation	Yes	Yes	No	No	No	No
Shear reduction	Yes	?	Yes	Yes	No	No
Pressure reduction	Yes	Yes	Yes	Yes	Yes	No
Dynamic	Yes	Yes	Yes	No	No	No
Cost per day	High	High	Moderate	Low	Low	Low

Reprinted from Bergstrom N, Bennett MA, Carlson CE, et al: Treatment of Pressure Ulcers, Clinical Practice Guideline No. 15, December, 1994, U.S. Department of Health and Human Services, Public Health Service, Agency for Health Care Policy and Research, AHCPR publication No. 95-0652.

TABLE 242–2. NATIONAL PRESSURE ULCER STAGING SYSTEM

Pressure ulcer stage	Definitions
Stage I	An observable pressure-related alteration of intact skin whose indicators, as compared with the adjacent or opposite area on the body, may include changes in one or more of the following: skin temperature (warmth or coolness), tissue consistency (firm or boggy feel), and/or sensations (pain, itching). The ulcer appears as a defined area of persistent redness in lightly pigmented skin, whereas, in darker skin tones, the ulcer may appear with persistent red, blue, or purple hues.
Stage II	Partial-thickness skin loss involving epidermis or dermis, or both. The ulcer is superficial and presents clinically as an abrasion, blister, or shallow crater.
Stage III	Full-thickness skin loss involving damage or necrosis of subcutaneous tissue, which may extend down to but not through underlying fascia. The ulcer presents clinically as a deep crater, with or without undermining of adjacent tissue.
Stage IV	Full thickness skin loss with extensive destruction, tissue necrosis, or damage to muscle bone or supporting structures (e.g., tendon, joint capsule).

or sepsis. Finally, biosurgery (maggot therapy) is an effective and relatively quick method of débridement. This type of débridement is especially effective when sharp débridement might expose bones, joints, or tendons.

Managing the bacterial burden is an important consideration in wound bed preparation. All pressure ulcers are colonized by a variety of bacteria. Healing is compromised if the colony count exceeds 10^5 or 10^6 organisms per gram. Certain strains of bacteria will impede healing when even fewer organisms are present in the ulcer. Clinical signs of infection include presence of a malodorous, purulent exudate, excessive drainage, bleeding in the ulcer, and pain. Treatment using silver-impregnated dressings or topical silver sulfadiazine will decrease the bacterial burden.

Exudate management is the last major concept in wound bed preparation. Excessive exudate impairs ulcer healing and may damage healthy surrounding tissue. Exudates are best managed by selecting the appropriate dressing. Currently, more than 300 different dressings are available for treating pressure ulcers. The dressings can be classified as gauze, petroleum-based nonadherent gauze, transparent films, hydrocolloids, foam islands, alginates, hydrogels, composites, and combinations (Table 242–3). Regardless of the type of dressing selected, the goal should be to keep the pressure ulcer moist. Because no dressing is likely to promote healing of all pressure ulcers within an ulcer classification, a careful assessment of the pressure ulcer, needs of the patient, and environmental factors is essential.[13] Wet-to-dry gauze dressings are a form of débridement and should only be used for managing necrotic wounds. Once healthy granulation tissue is observed, another type of dressing should be used.

The use of negative pressure therapy (Vacuum Assisted Closure, KCI, Inc, San Antonio, TX 78230) should be considered for highly exudative pressure ulcers. Negative pressure therapy removes excessive exudate from the ulcer, increases local blood flow, and promotes formation of granulation tissue.[15] Negative pressure therapy should not be used if osteomyelitis is present or suspected or in the presence of eschar, exposed blood vessels, or organs.

NUTRITION

Positive nitrogen balance is essential for healing of pressure ulcers. Correcting malnutrition is important to promote healing of ulcers. Data are lacking to suggest that vitamins and minerals supplements help to promote healing of pressure ulcers healing or prevent their development.[16-18]

MONITORING HEALING

The Pressure Ulcer Scale for Healing (PUSH)[19] and the Pressure Sore Status Tool (PSST)[20] are both valid and reliable tools for assessing healing of pressure ulcers. The PUSH tool requires less time to complete, because it has only three items whereas the PSST tool has 13 elements. Both tools use a numerical indicator to determine healing; the lower the score, the more healing that has occurred. Both tools are usually used on a weekly basis.

SURGICAL REPAIR

Less than 5% of pressure ulcers require surgically intervention. However, if surgery is indicated, then direct closure, skin grafting, skin flaps, musculocutaneous flaps, and free flaps are the most common operative procedures.

TABLE 242–3. PRESSURE ULCER DRESSING CLASSIFICATION SELECTION

Dressing classification	Partial-thickness (Stages I and II)	Full-thickness (Stages III and IV)	Light/Moderate excavated	Heavy excavated
Transparent films	X		X (Light drainage only)	
Hydrocolloids	X	X (As a secondary dressing)	X	X
Alginates	X (Stage II only)	X		X
Foams	X (Stage II only)	X	X (Moderate drainage only)	X
Composites	X (Stage II only)	X	X (Moderate drainage only)	X
Hydrogels	X (Stage II with dry wound bed only)	X (Dry wound beds only)		
Hydrofibers		X		X
Anti-recalcitrant dressings		X	X	X

Prophylactic ischiectomy should be avoided because there is an increased probability of a perineal ulcers and urethral fistulas.

ADJUNCTIVE THERAPIES

Most adjunctive therapies have not been rigorously studied. Moreover, many adjunctive therapies are not reimbursed, resulting in additional costs to the patient. Therefore, before one is selected, the mechanism for reimbursement should be considered. The most promising adjunctive therapies include electrical stimulation, topical application of growth factors, use of skin equivalents, and hyperbaric oxygen.

ANNOTATED REFERENCES

Bergstrom N, Allman RM, Carlson CE, et al: Pressure Ulcers in Adults: Prediction and Prevention. Clinical Guidelines No. 3, Rockville, MD, U.S. Department of Health and Human Services, Public Health Service, Agency for Health Care Policy and Research. May 1992. AHCPR publication No. 95-0047.

This is a comprehensive guideline to the prediction and prevention of pressure ulcers. Although this document is over 12 years old, the recommendations remain extremely relevant to current practice. There are numerous useful algorithms, validated assessment tools, practical treatment approaches, and helpful glossary.

Bergstrom N, Bennett MA, Carlson CE, et al. Treatment of Pressure Ulcers. Clinical Guidelines No. 15, Rockville, MD, U.S. Department of Health and Human Services, Public Health Service, Agency for Health Care Policy and Research. December 1994. AHCPR publication No. 95-0652.

This is a comprehensive guideline to the assessment and management of pressure ulcers. As in other guidelines from this agency, the strength of the evidence supporting recommendations is provided. There are numerous useful algorithms, validated assessment tools, practical treatment approaches, and a helpful glossary.

Brem H, Lyder C: Protocol for successful treatment of pressure ulcers. Am J Surg 2004;188(1A Suppl):9-11.

A comprehensive 11-step detailed protocol for the treatment of pressure ulcers is described. Some of these steps include (1) recognizing that every patient with limited mobility is at risk for pressure ulcers, (2) targeted assessments of specific anatomic locations, (3) objective measurement of pressure ulcers, (4) mechanical débridement of all nonviable tissue, (5) establishing a moist wound-healing environment, (6) elimination of drainage and cellulites and (6) biologic therapy for patients whose ulcers fail to heal.

Carlson EV, Kemp MG, Shott S: Predicting the risk of pressure ulcers in critically ill patients. Am J Crit Care1999;8:262-269.

The purpose of this prospective study was to examine Braden subscales in predicting pressure ulcers in critically ill patients and to investigate how often the Braden scale should be completed to assess the risk of critical ill patients for developing pressure ulcers. A total of 136 adult patients without pressure ulcers from the medical and surgical intensive care units and the noninvasive respiratory care unit were assessed using the Braden scale. A total of 36 pressure ulcers, most commonly on the sacrum or coccyx and the heels (15 stage 1, 20 stage 2, 1 stage 3), developed in 17 patients (12%). In 14 (82%) of the 17, the ulcers developed within 72 hours of admission to the ICU. The risk for pressure ulcers increased as the mean sensory perception (P = .01) and the mean total Braden (P = .046) scores decreased. The mean sensory perception scores obtained at 12 and 36 hours after admission also had a significant relationship to the risk for pressure ulcers (P = .03). Thus, these researchers concluded that patients in ICUs have an increased risk for pressure ulcers.

Lyder C: Pressure ulcer prevention and management. JAMA 2003;289: 223-226.

This brief article reviews current medical thinking on the comprehensive principles of pressure ulcer prevention and treatment. Guidance is provided on how to select appropriate dressings and support surfaces for patients. A brief discussion on current adjunctive therapies for recalcitrant pressure ulcers is presented.

Chapter 243

MANAGEMENT OF PAIN, ANXIETY, AND DELIRIUM

Eric B. Milbrandt • E. Wesley Ely

Pain, anxiety, and delirium are extremely common in the ICU, where they are often underappreciated and inadequately treated due to fear of adverse effects or addiction. Unrelieved pain, anxiety, and delirium contribute to patient distress, evoke the stress response, complicate the management of lifesaving devices, and may negatively affect outcome. Ensuring patient comfort and safety is a universal goal that has been endorsed by national medical societies[1] and oversight bodies such as the Center for Medicare and Medicaid Services, the Joint Commissions for the Accreditation of Healthcare Organizations,[2] and the Leapfrog Organization. Recently, a panel of experts in this field developed clinical practice guidelines for the sustained use of sedatives and analgesics in critically ill adults.[1] Using a systematic and evidence-based approach, these guidelines established the standard of care for the management of pain, anxiety, and delirium in the ICU (Fig. 243-1). In our discussion of this topic, we build on the framework established by these experts.

GENERAL PRINCIPLES

The primary goal of pain, anxiety, and delirium management is to ensure patient comfort while preventing overmedication and its attendant complications. There are several general principles that should be followed in achieving this goal. The first is routine and objective assessment using valid and reliable measures of pain, anxiety, and delirium. Scales to measure these conditions are now available, providing a common language for providers to quantify their degree and to record the response to therapy. Further, these scales can be used to assign a specific target for goal-directed delivery of sedatives

and analgesics, an approach that has been shown to improve patient comfort, shorten duration of mechanical ventilation, and reduce length of stay.[3-6] It is important to frequently reassess and adjust these targets, based on the condition of the patient. For example, a targeted sedation level of "unresponsive" might be an appropriate goal early in the course of acute respiratory distress syndrome but inappropriate in the recovery phase during attempts at weaning from mechanical ventilation.[7] Nonpharmacologic interventions, such as proper positioning of patients and equipment, fracture stabilization, and noise reduction, should always be attempted first. When nonpharmacologic means are insufficient, pharmacologic interventions should be instituted using standardized, nurse-driven protocols whenever possible, because these have been shown to improve outcome.[3-6] It is important to keep in mind that pain must always be addressed first; unrelieved pain can be the underlying cause of anxiety, agitation, and delirium. Intermittent dosing and daily interruption of continuous infusions are important techniques that can be used to prevent systemic drug accumulation.[8] They can be challenging to institute, but careful attention to patient selection and avoidance of "overawakening" can prevent complications while improving outcome.

PAIN

Pain is an unpleasant sensory and emotional experience associated with actual or potential tissue damage.[9] Pain is a frequent occurrence in critically ill patients for a variety of reasons, including surgical incisions, invasive devices and procedures, nursing care, and prolonged immobility.[10,11] Unrelieved pain may actually be harmful, evoking increased catecholamine release, myocardial ischemia, increased catabolism, hypercoagulability, immunosuppression, agitation, and anxiety.[1,7] Long-term effects such as post-traumatic stress disorder also may be seen.[12] Unfortunately, pain is often undertreated because of concerns about the adverse effects and addiction potential of opiates[13] and because caregivers sometimes lack the necessary skills for proper pain assessment and treatment.[1]

ASSESSMENT

In order to be recognized and treated, pain must be routinely and objectively assessed.[14] In the ICU, we have instruments that measure temperature, blood pressure, oxygen saturation, airway pressures, and other physiologic parameters, but the most valid and reliable indicator of pain is the

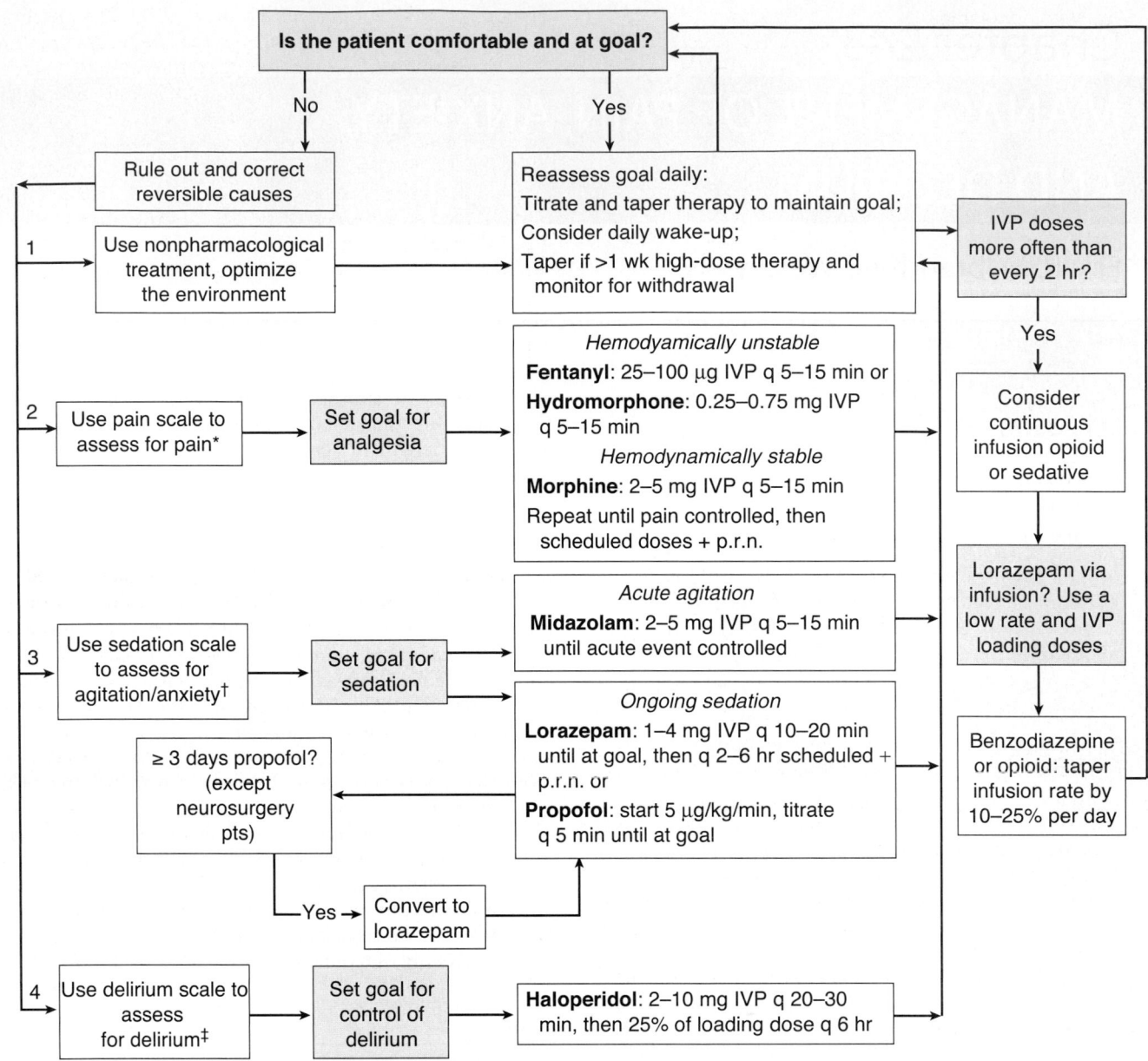

Is the patient comfortable and at goal?

No → **Rule out and correct reversible causes**

Yes → **Reassess goal daily:**
Titrate and taper therapy to maintain goal;
Consider daily wake-up;
Taper if >1 wk high-dose therapy and monitor for withdrawal

IVP doses more often than every 2 hr?

1 — **Use nonpharmacological treatment, optimize the environment**

2 — **Use pain scale to assess for pain*** → **Set goal for analgesia**

Hemodyamically unstable
Fentanyl: 25–100 μg IVP q 5–15 min or
Hydromorphone: 0.25–0.75 mg IVP q 5–15 min
Hemodynamically stable
Morphine: 2–5 mg IVP q 5–15 min
Repeat until pain controlled, then scheduled doses + p.r.n.

Yes → **Consider continuous infusion opioid or sedative**

3 — **Use sedation scale to assess for agitation/anxiety†** → **Set goal for sedation**

Acute agitation
Midazolam: 2–5 mg IVP q 5–15 min until acute event controlled

Lorazepam via infusion? Use a low rate and IVP loading doses

Ongoing sedation
Lorazepam: 1–4 mg IVP q 10–20 min until at goal, then q 2–6 hr scheduled + p.r.n. or
Propofol: start 5 μg/kg/min, titrate q 5 min until at goal

≥ 3 days propofol? (except neurosurgery pts)

Yes → **Convert to lorazepam**

Benzodiazepine or opioid: taper infusion rate by 10–25% per day

4 — **Use delirium scale to assess for delirium‡** → **Set goal for control of delirium**

Haloperidol: 2–10 mg IVP q 20–30 min, then 25% of loading dose q 6 hr

*Numeric rating scale or other pain scale.

†Ricker Sedation-agitation scale or other sedation scale.

‡Confusion Assessment Method for the ICU.

FIGURE 243–1. Algorithm for the sedation and analgesia of mechanically ventilated patients. IVP, intravenous push; p.r.n., as needed. (Modified from Jacobi J, Fraser GL, Coursin DB, et al: Clinical practice guidelines for the sustained use of sedatives and analgesics in the critically ill adult. Crit Care Med 2002;30:124.)

patient's self-report.[15] Information about pain, including location, quality, and intensity, should be elicited routinely as part of the patient's vitals signs and recorded on the flowsheet. Intensity can be objectively measured using tools such as the visual analog scale or numeric rating scale (Fig. 243-2A and B).[16] The visual analog scale is 10-cm horizontal line with the words "no pain" and "worst pain" at opposite ends. Patients rate the intensity of their pain by indicating the point on the line that corresponds to their rating. The numeric rating scale asks patients to assign a number between 0 and 10 to the pain, with 0 being no pain and 10 being the worst pain imaginable.

It is not uncommon for ICU patients to be unable to communicate with caregivers owing to endotracheal intubation or altered mental status. During such times, behavioral and physiologic indicators must be used to assess pain intensity. Examples of pain-related behaviors include facial expressions, restlessness, and lacrimation; physiologic indicators include tachycardia, hypertension, and tachypnea.[13] Unfortunately, these indicators are nonspecific and somewhat subjective in nature. As a result, clinicians are likely to underestimate and undertreat pain. The FACES scale[17] (see Fig. 243-2C) was developed to objectify the use of facial expression as a measure of pain intensity. It shows moderate

Visual analog scale

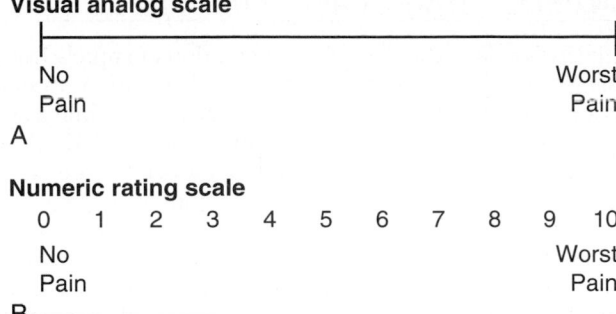

No Pain — Worst Pain

A

Numeric rating scale

0 1 2 3 4 5 6 7 8 9 10

No Pain — Worst Pain

B

FACES* scale

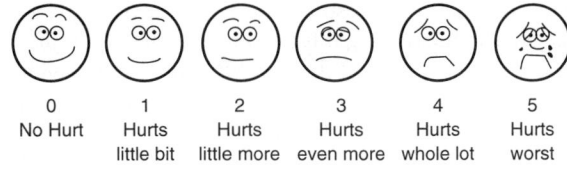

0	1	2	3	4	5
No Hurt	Hurts little bit	Hurts little more	Hurts even more	Hurts whole lot	Hurts worst

C

FIGURE 243–2. Examples of commonly used pain intensity scales. *A,* Visual analog scale. *B,* Numeric rating scale. *C,* FACES scale. (*C,* From Wong DL, Hockenberry-Eaton M, Wilson D, et al: Wong's Essentials of Pediatric Nursing, 6th ed. St Louis, Mosby, 2001, p 1301.)

correlation with different levels of pain and is most highly correlated in patients with severe pain.[18,19]

MANAGEMENT

In managing pain, nonpharmacologic methods should be attempted first. These include patient repositioning, injury stabilization, removal of noxious or irritating stimuli, and application of heat or cold.[1] When nonpharmacologic approaches are insufficient to provide analgesia (as is often the case), local, regional, or systemic therapy is indicated.

Local and Regional Approaches

Local infusions of anesthetics such as lidocaine or bupivacaine are useful adjuncts that can reduce or eliminate the need for systemic analgesia.[13] Local infusions are particularly helpful for pain associated with operative incisions and may prove useful for alleviating pain associated with other invasive procedures that are commonly performed in the ICU (e.g., tube thoracostomy). Analgesia may last up to 24 hours when a long-acting local anesthetic such as bupivacaine 0.25% is used. Epinephrine-containing agents should be avoided because of the possibility of reduced blood flow and delayed wound healing.

Regional blockade of nerves or nerve plexus provides analgesia for a large area of the body without the sedative effects of systemic analgesia. Intercostal blocks can be used to manage pain due to thoracic or upper abdominal trauma or surgery and can improve respiratory mechanics and reduce the risk of pulmonary compromise.[20] Although intercostal nerves can be blocked anywhere along their course, the usual technique is to inject 3 to 5 mL of local anesthetic, such as 0.25% bupivacaine, with a blunt 22-gauge needle into the intercostal nerve sheath at the angle of the rib approximately 8 to 10 cm lateral to the posterior midline, where the paraspinous muscles attach to the ribs.[13,21] Intercostal blocks have the advantage of providing analgesia without sedation or respiratory depression. Placement of an intercostal block carries the risk of pneumothorax and may need to be

repeated once the initial effect wears off.[22] Paravertebral blocks are useful for managing pain related to unilateral thoracic or abdominal procedures. With this technique, a short, beveled spinal needle is inserted 2 to 3 cm lateral to the spinous process and advanced at a 90-degree angle to the skin plane.[22-24] Upon striking the vertebral transverse process, the needle is angled superiorly and walked 1 to 1.5 cm over the top of the process until loss of resistance to saline or air is felt. A bolus of local anesthetic, such as 10 to 20 mL of 0.5% bupivacaine, is then administered.[24] Paravertebral blockade carries the risk of inadvertent epidural blockade. Interpleural catheters can be used to provide thoracic and upper abdominal analgesia; however, the sensory blockade achieved may not be dense enough to improve pulmonary function, and care must be taken to avoid accumulating toxic doses of local anesthetic.[13] Blockade of the brachial plexus, lumbar plexus, or femoral nerve may prove beneficial for the relief of pain involving an extremity and can facilitate nursing care, such as dressing changes and frequent turning.[25-27] These nerve blocks are generally well tolerated and may provide pain relief when systemic opioids have failed.

Epidural analgesia is a regional technique that has become increasingly popular for the management of pain related to labor and delivery, as well as pain from abdominal, thoracic, or lower extremity operative procedures.[28] With this method, a catheter is placed in the thoracic or lumbar epidural space through a hollow needle. Opiates, such morphine or fentanyl, may be infused as the sole agent, although local anesthetics, such as bupivacaine, are often infused in combination with opiates to take advantage of their synergistic analgesic effects. This may reduce the spinal opiate requirement and the occurrence of opiate-related side effects. However, it carries the added risk of side effects due to the local anesthetic, specifically, hypotension, motor weakness, and inability to ambulate.

When an opiate is given epidurally, its lipid solubility is directly related to its speed of onset, extent of dermatomal spread, and duration of effect.[13] Morphine is highly hydrophobic and thus has a long onset of action, significant dermatomal spread, and extended duration of action. Because of this property, it has a tendency to cause adverse effects such as respiratory depression. Morphine is typically given as a single dose of 1 to 6 mg, although continuous infusions of 0.1 to 1 mg/h may also be used. Fentanyl is highly lipophilic, with a rapid onset, a short duration of action, and a tendency to stay localized. Because of its short duration of action, fentanyl is typically given as a continuous infusion at doses of 0.5 to 1 µg/kg per hour.

Possible adverse effects of epidural opiates include respiratory depression, urinary retention, nausea, vomiting, pruritus, and headache. Respiratory depression is greatest with morphine and is temporally biphasic. Early respiratory depression is caused by systemic absorption, whereas late events occur due to rostral spread through the cerebrospinal fluid to the central nervous system respiratory centers.[21] Respiratory depression can be reversed with intravenous naloxone, and infusions of 5 µg/kg per hour have been used prophylactically.[29] Epidural catheters should be used with extreme caution in patients who are receiving low-molecular-weight heparin because of reports of epidural hematoma formation resulting in long-term or permanent paralysis.[30]

Systemic Therapy

It is generally accepted that pain is easier to prevent than to treat. Therefore, when administering analgesics, it is important to give them in sufficient quantities to relieve pain and to prevent pain from returning to severe pretreatment levels. Intramuscular dosing should be avoided because it results in unnecessary discomfort. Scheduled intermittent doses or continuous infusions are preferred over an as-needed approach to ensure consistent analgesia, prevent breakthrough pain, and avoid treatment delays. In patients who are able to participate in their care, patient-controlled analgesia can permit even greater pain relief by allowing the patient to self-administer analgesics without the delay of having to notify the nurse. As noted earlier, systemic analgesics should be administered as part of a goal-directed sedation and analgesia protocol.

Systemic therapies include nonsteroidal anti-inflammatory drugs and acetaminophen, but opioids are more commonly used because they provide dose-related pain relief without a ceiling effect. Opioids also provide some degree of anxiolysis but should not be used primarily for this indication, as benzodiazepines are more effective. Although they are the mainstay of analgesia in the ICU, opioids have a number of adverse effects. Respiratory depression and decreased gastrointestinal motility are commonly seen, although their impact can be reduced through proper airway and ventilator management and stimulant laxative use, respectively. Hypotension can also result, particularly in patients who are hypovolemic and cannot tolerate the reduction in systemic vascular resistance caused by opiates. Hypotension can also be due to histamine release, a phenomenon more prevalent with morphine than with other opiate analgesics. Other side effects include pruritus, flushing, urinary retention, and delirium.

The opiate analgesics most commonly used in the ICU are morphine and fentanyl. Other opioid analgesics are available; however, because of their cost, pharmacokinetic characteristics, lack of analgesic potency, or side effects, they are not routinely used. When morphine is injected intravenously, the peak effect occurs within 15 to 20 minutes, and analgesia lasts 2 to 4 hours. Morphine is given in doses of 2 to 5 mg i.v. every 5 to 15 minutes until the pain is controlled and then 0.01 to 0.15 mg/kg i.v. on a scheduled basis every 1 to 2 hours, with extra doses available as needed for breakthrough pain.[1] Continuous infusions may also be used; the usual dose ranges from 0.07 to 0.5 mg/kg per hour. Morphine is characterized by hepatic metabolism and renal excretion, so its effects can be prolonged in patients with renal or hepatic impairment. When given as a bolus injection, morphine causes vasodilatation and histamine release, so it should be used with caution in patients with hemodynamic instability. Fentanyl is a synthetic opioid with a rapid onset (5 to 15 minutes) and a short duration of action (30 to 60 minutes). Because of its short half-life, it is usually given by continuous infusion. Loading doses of 25 to 100 μg are given every 5 to 15 minutes until the pain is controlled; then infusion rates of 0.7 to 10 μg/kg per hour are used.[1] Because it causes less histamine release than morphine and does not undergo renal elimination, it is the preferred opioid analgesic in hemodynamically unstable patients or those with renal insufficiency.

With patient-controlled analgesia, a loading dose of analgesic is given, and then the pump is set to deliver subsequent medication doses on demand. A lockout time interval is used to prevent premature dosing. For added safety, 1-hour and 4-hour total dosage limits may also be set. For morphine, doses of 0.5 to 3 mg with a lockout period of 5 to 12 minutes are typically used.[31] With fentanyl, doses of 10 to 20 μg with a 5- to 10-minute lockout period are used.

ANXIETY, AGITATION, AND SEDATION

Anxiety is a diffuse and unpleasant emotion of apprehension that is not associated with a specific threat. Agitation is a state of anxiety accompanied by extreme arousal, irritability, and motor restlessness. Both are very common in the ICU, where they have a variety of causes, including excessive stimulation, pain, dyspnea, delirium, inability to communicate, sleep deprivation, and underlying anxiety disorders. Anxiety can be present without agitation, as evidenced by anxious patients who become fearful and withdrawn. Unrelieved anxiety can be a significant source of physical and psychological stress for patients both during an acute event and in the long term, when unpleasant, frightening memories and post-traumatic stress disorder may result.[32] Left untreated, agitation can become life threatening if it leads to the removal of lifesaving devices such as endotracheal tubes and intravascular lines. Like pain, anxiety and agitation require a systematic approach in their assessment and treatment.

ASSESSMENT

It is clear that the use of a defined sedation target for the provision of protocol-based, goal-directed sedation and analgesia reduces patient discomfort and improves outcome.[3,4,6] There are many scales available for the assessment of sedation and agitation, including the Ramsay scale,[33] Riker sedation-agitation scale,[34] motor activity assessment scale,[35] and Richmond agitation-sedation scale (RASS).[36] Each has good reliability and validity among adult ICU patients and can be used to set targets for goal-directed therapy. The 7-point Riker sedation-agitation scale has excellent interrater reliability (kappa = 0.92) and is highly correlated (r^2 = 0.83 to 0.86) with other scales. However, only the RASS has been shown to detect variations in the level of consciousness over time or in response to changes in sedative and analgesic drug use.[1,37] The RASS is a 10-point scale with discrete criteria to distinguish levels of agitation and sedation (Table 243-1). It involves a set of three steps to evaluate patients. First, the patient is observed to see whether he or she is alert, restless, or agitated (0 to +4). If the patient is not spontaneously alert, his or her name is called and the duration of eye contact is measured (−1 to −3). If there is no eye contact with verbal stimulation, the patient's shoulder is shaken or the sternum is rubbed, and the response is noted (−4 to −5). This assessment takes less than 20 seconds and was found to correlate well with other measures of sedation (e.g., Glasgow coma scale, bispectral electroencephalography, neuropsychiatric ratings).

MANAGEMENT

The management of anxiety, agitation, and sedation follows the same general principles outlined at the beginning of this chapter—goal-directed, protocol-based management with intermittent dosing or daily interruption of continuous infusions. Before administering sedative agents, it is important to search for an underlying cause (e.g., hypoxemia, hypoglycemia, hypotension, drug withdrawal), especially when a previously calm patient becomes anxious or agitated. If pain is present, an analgesic should be the initial sedative choice. Once pain has been addressed, benzodiazepines and propofol are the drugs most often used.

Benzodiazepines bind to γ-aminobutyric acid receptors in the central nervous system, thereby providing sedation, anxiolysis, hypnosis, muscle relaxation, anticonvulsant

TABLE 243–1. RICHMOND AGITATION-SEDATION SCALE (RASS)

+4	Combative	Combative, violent, immediate danger to staff
+3	Very agitated	Pulls or removes tubes or catheters; aggressive
+2	Agitated	Frequent nonpurposeful movement; fights ventilator
+1	Restless	Anxious, apprehensive, but movements not aggressive or vigorous
0	Alert and calm	
−1	Drowsy	Not fully alert, but has sustained (>10 sec) awakening (eye opening/contact) to voice
−2	Light sedation	Drowsy, briefly (<10 sec) awakens to voice or physical stimulation
−3	Moderate sedation	Movement or eye opening (but no eye contact) to voice
−4	Deep sedation	No response to voice, but movement or eye opening to physical stimulation
−5	Unarousable	No response to voice or physical stimulation

Procedure for RASS Assessment

1. Observe patient.
   a. Is patient alert, restless, or agitated?   (Score 0 to +4)
2. If not alert, state patient's name and instruct to open eyes and look at speaker.
   b. Does patient awaken, with sustained eye opening and contact?   (Score −1)
   c. Does patient awaken, with eye opening and contact, but not sustained?   (Score −2)
   d. Does patient fail to awaken (no eye contact), but has eye opening or movement in response to voice?   (Score −3)
3. Physically stimulate patient by shaking shoulder or rubbing sternum.
   e. No response to voice, but response (movement) to physical stimulation.   (Score −4)
   f. No response to voice or physical stimulation.   (Score −5)

From Sessler et al: Am J Respir Crit Care Med 2002;166:1338-1344; Ely EW, Truman B, Shintani A, et al: Monitoring sedation status over time in ICU patients: Reliability and validity of the Richmond agitation-sedation scale (RASS). JAMA 2003;289:2983-2991.

activity, and amnesia.[38] These agents do not relieve pain, but their anxiolytic and amnestic properties may improve pain tolerance by moderating the anticipatory pain response.[39] Benzodiazepines vary considerably in their pharmacology, and patient-specific factors such as advanced age, drug or alcohol use, and organ dysfunction make their potency, onset, and duration of action even more unpredictable. These drugs can cause hypotension when given in bolus doses, particularly in hemodynamically unstable patients. Benzodiazepine-induced anxiolysis can decrease sympathetic vascular tone, leading to hypotension. By reducing inhibitions, benzodiazepines sometimes paradoxically increase agitation and aggressiveness. Benzodiazepines can also cause delirium, so their use in treating hyperactive delirium can be counterproductive.

Of the benzodiazepines that are currently available, diazepam, midazolam, and lorazepam are the preferred agents in the ICU. The onset of action of diazepam is 2 to 5 minutes, making it useful for rapidly sedating acutely agitated patients. However, its long half-life makes prolonged sedation a risk with repeated use, particularly in patients with renal or hepatic dysfunction. To control acute agitation, diazepam is given in doses of 2 to 6 mg every 5 to 15 minutes until the event is controlled. Continuous infusions are not recommended. Midazolam is also useful for acute agitation because it has a rapid onset (2 to 5 minutes) and a short duration of action. It is given as bolus injections of 2 to 5 mg every 5 to 15 minutes. When used for long-term sedation (>48 to 72 hours), it tends to produce unpredictable awakening times, especially in patients who are obese, have low serum albumin concentrations, or have renal failure.[1] Lorazepam has a slower onset of action (5 to 20 minutes), making it less helpful for acute agitation. However, it is less lipid soluble and has no active metabolites, making it the preferred agent for long-term administration in most critically ill patients according to the 2002 Society for Critical Care Medicine guidelines. Intermittent doses of 1 to 4 mg are given every 2 to 6 hours, or continuous infusions may be used.

Propofol is an intravenous anesthetic with an unknown mechanism of action. It has proven utility as a sedating agent in the ICU due to its rapid onset (1 to 2 minutes) and short duration of action (2 to 8 minutes). It is the preferred sedative when rapid awakening is important, such as for neurologic assessment or pending extubation.[1] When used for long-term sedation (>48 to 72 hours), propofol has not been shown to reduce the duration of mechanical ventilation or ICU length of stay.[40]

Propofol can cause significant hypotension by decreasing preload and causing myocardial depression.[41] Propofol is provided as a lipid emulsion that provides 1.1 kcal/mL from fat. Therefore, it must be counted as a calorie source and can occasionally cause hypertriglyceridemia.[1] Strict aseptic technique and frequent infusion tubing changes are necessary, because propofol can support the growth of bacteria and fungi.[42] High-dose continuous infusions have been associated with lactic acidosis in children (doses >66 µg/kg/min)[43] and metabolic acidosis, arrhythmias, and cardiac arrest in adults (doses >83 µg/kg/min).[44,45] Consequently, providers should consider alternative sedative agents for any patient receiving high-dose propofol infusions who develops unexplained metabolic acidosis, arrhythmia, or cardiac failure.

DELIRIUM

Delirium is an acute, fluctuating change in mental status, with inattention and altered levels of consciousness. Delirium is a tangible sign of cerebral insufficiency or acute cognitive dysfunction. It should be thought of as a form of organ dysfunction, much like shock and hypoxemia are manifestations of cardiovascular and pulmonary dysfunction, respectively. Delirium has myriad causes, including pain and anxiety, medications, toxic and metabolic changes, and the effects of critical illness itself. Also known as acute encephalopathy[46] or ICU psychosis,[47] it occurs in as many as 80% of mechanically ventilated ICU patients and is associated with increased length of stay, medical complications, and poor outcomes, including increased 6-month mortality.[48-52] ICU delirium frequently goes unrecognized because the majority of patients manifest hypoactive delirium instead of the more visible hyperactive subtype.[53-58] Even when ICU

Linking Sedation and Delirium Monitoring:
A Two Step Approach to Assess Consciousness

<u>Step One</u>: Sedation Assessment

The Richmond Agitation and Sedation Scale: The RASS

+4	Combative	Combative, violent, immediate danger to staff
+3	Very agitated	Pulls or removes tube(s) or catheter(s); aggressive
+2	Agitated	Frequent nonpurposeful movement, fights ventilator
+1	Restless	Anxious, apprehensive but movements not aggressive or vigorous
0	Alert and calm	
–1	Drowsy	Not fully alert, but has sustained awakening to voice (eye opening & contact > 10 sec)
–2	Light sedation	Briefly awakens to voice (eye opening & contact < 10 sec)
–3	Moderate sedation	Movement or eye opening to voice (but no eye contact)
–4	Deep sedation	No response to voice, but movement or eye opening to physical stimulation
–5	Unarousable	No response to voice or physical stimulation

If RASS is -4 or -5, then **Stop** and **Reassess** patient at later time

If RASS is above - 4 (-3 through +4) then **Proceed to Step 2**

Sessler et al., AJRCCM 2002;166:1338-44

Ely et al., JAMA 2003;289:2983-91

<u>Step Two</u>: Delirium Assessment

> **Feature 1**: Acute onset of mental status changes
> or a fluctuating course

And

> **Feature 2**: Inattention

And

| **Feature 3**: Disorganized Thinking | OR | **Feature 4**: Altered Level of Consciousness |

= DELIRIUM

FIGURE 243–3. Linking sedation and delirium monitoring: a two-step approach to assess consciousness. (From Sessler CN, et al. The Richmond Agitation-Sedation Scale: Validity and reliability in adult intensive care unit patients. Am J Respir Crit Care Med 2002;166:1338-1344; and Ely EW, Truman B, Shintani A, et al: Monitoring sedation status over time in ICU patients: Reliability and validity of the Richmond agitation-sedation scale [RASS]. JAMA 2003;289:2983-2991.)

delirium is recognized, most clinicians consider it an expected event that is often iatrogenic and without consequence.[59] The risk factors, causes, and outcomes of delirium are discussed in greater detail in Chapter 2 of this text.

ASSESSMENT

Until recently, there was no valid and reliable way to assess delirium in critically ill patients, many of whom are nonverbal owing to sedation or mechanical ventilation. The confusion assessment method for the ICU (CAM-ICU) is a delirium measurement tool that was developed by a team of specialists in critical care, psychiatry, neurology, and geriatrics (Fig. 243-3).[48-52] Administered by nurses, it takes only 1 to 2 minutes to conduct and is 98% accurate for detecting delirium, compared with a full assessment by a geriatric psychiatrist. With the CAM-ICU, delirium is diagnosed when patients demonstrate acute-onset mental status change or fluctuating course, inattention, and either disorganized thinking or altered level of consciousness. With the advent of the CAM-ICU, national guidelines now recommend routine delirium assessment in all critically ill patients.[1]

MANAGEMENT

As with the management of anxiety and agitation, pharmacologic therapy should be attempted only after correcting any contributing factors (e.g., pain, anxiety, sleep disturbance, environmental stimuli, delirium-causing drugs) or underlying physiologic abnormalities (e.g., hypoxia, hypoglycemia, metabolic derangements, shock). After such concerns have been addressed, patients who manifest delirium should be treated with a traditional antipsychotic medication (e.g., haloperidol). When given intravenously, these medications exert a calming effect, flattening the affect and diminishing psychomotor agitation without suppressing the respiratory drive or affecting hemodynamics. They achieve this effect by blocking dopamine receptors in the central nervous system. With acute delirium, haloperidol is given in doses of 2 to 10 mg i.v. every 20 to 30 minutes until the delirium is controlled, then 25% of the total loading dose is administered every 6 hours.[1] The dose should be tapered over several days. Despite their favorable safety profile, antipsychotics can cause extrapyramidal reactions, neuroleptic malignant syndrome, and QT interval prolongation, leading to torsades de pointes. These side effects are thought to be dose related, leading some to question the safety of the rapid-loading approach and to opt instead for a more conservative strategy of no more than 20 mg/day.[60]

CONCLUSION

Pain, anxiety, and delirium are common events in the ICU, where their occurrence is associated with adverse outcomes. Using a systematic management approach that follows the general principles outlined in this chapter can maximize patient comfort while reducing the likelihood of overmedication and its attendant complications.

ANNOTATED REFERENCES

Brook AD, Ahrens TS, Schaiff R, et al: Effect of a nursing-implemented sedation protocol on the duration of mechanical ventilation. Crit Care Med 1999;27:2609-2615.

This single-center randomized, controlled trial in mechanically ventilated medical ICU patients showed that protocol-directed sedation can reduce the duration of mechanical ventilation, the ICU and hospital lengths of stay, and the need for tracheostomy among critically ill patients with acute respiratory failure.

Ely EW, Inouye SK, Bernard GR, et al: Delirium in mechanically ventilated patients: Validity and reliability of the confusion assessment method for the intensive care unit (CAM-ICU). JAMA 2001;286:2703-2710.

This prospective study established the validity and reliability of the CAM-ICU, a delirium assessment tool that is administered by nurses, takes only 1 to 2 minutes to conduct, and is 98% accurate for detecting delirium.

Jacobi J, Fraser GL, Coursin DB, et al: Clinical practice guidelines for the sustained use of sedatives and analgesics in the critically ill adult. Crit Care Med 2002;30:119-141.

These guidelines, which were developed by a panel of experts in the field using a systematic and evidence-based approach, established the standard of care for the management of pain, anxiety, and delirium in the ICU.

Kress JP, Pohlman AS, O'Connor MF, Hall JB: Daily interruption of sedative infusions in critically ill patients undergoing mechanical ventilation. N Engl J Med 2000;342:1471-1477.

This randomized, controlled trial in adult mechanically ventilated ICU patients showed that daily interruption of sedative infusions decreased the duration of mechanical ventilation, ICU length of stay, and rates of diagnostic testing to assess changes in mental status.

Mascia MF, Koch M, Medicis JJ: Pharmacoeconomic impact of rational use guidelines on the provision of analgesia, sedation, and neuromuscular blockade in critical care. Crit Care Med 2000;28:2300-2306.

This single-center before-and-after study in a mixed medical-surgical ICU showed that the introduction of guideline-based analgesia, sedation, and neuromuscular blockade was associated with significantly reduced direct drug costs, ventilator time, length of stay, and use of neuromuscular blockers.

Chapter 244

BURNS

Robert L. Sheridan

KEY POINTS

1. Burn care can be divided into four clinical phases: (a) initial evaluation and resuscitation, (b) initial wound excision and biologic closure, (c) definitive wound closure, and (d) rehabilitation and reconstruction.

2. Post-resuscitation physiology is characterized by high cardiac output, reduced afterload, moderate fever, and muscle metabolism.

3. Burn units and burn operating rooms need to be engineered to maintain high ambient temperature to avoid hypothermia and energy loss.

4. The burn-specific secondary survey must often be completed in the ICU.

5. Monitoring and early identification of extremity ischemia secondary to overlying eschar or tight compartments is essential.

6. The wound should not distract examiners from a thorough and complete patient evaluation.

7. No standard resuscitation formula is accurate in an individual patient. Patients must be resuscitated using resuscitation endpoints.

8. Patients with inhalation injuries typically have normal chest radiographs and near-normal gas exchange and compliance early. Over the 3 to 7 days after injury, significant pulmonary dysfunction may occur.

9. The best way to reduce burn wound pain is prompt wound closure.

10. Exposure of the globe must be anticipated and managed to preserve vision.

11. Early nutritional support is essential in light of post-resuscitation physiologic changes. This is ideally accomplished enterally, but parenteral support is also safe when properly administered.

12. Physical and occupational therapy should begin from the outset of burn care.

13. Intensive care management of the patient should proceed throughout operations.

14. Patients with toxic epidermal necrolysis have both a cutaneous and a visceral wound.

Over the past few decades, survival and quality of life have improved markedly for victims of serious burns. A better understanding of injury physiology and realization that the natural history of burns can be changed by prompt surgery led to these improvements.[1] Maintenance of patients with serious burns through the physiologic trial of staged wound closure is an essential component of this success. Many aspects of burn critical care are unique to this disease process.[2]

PHASES OF BURN CARE

Successful management of patients with serious burns requires both effective initial resuscitation as well as development of an overall plan for acute-phase hospitalization. Commonly, this overall plan can be considered to have four phases (Table 244-1).[3] The first phase, from day 1 through 3, the initial evaluation and resuscitation phase, focuses on complete evaluation and accurate fluid resuscitation. The second phase, initial wound excision and biologic closure, describes changes in the natural history of the disease, which include progressive wound sepsis and systemic inflammation and infection. This phase entails a series of staged operations that are completed during the first few days after injury. The third phase, definitive wound closure, requires that temporary wound covers be replaced with definitive covers and that small complex wounds, such as those of the face and hands, are addressed. The final stage of care is rehabilitation and reconstruction. Although rehabilitation begins during resuscitation, it becomes much more time consuming and involved near the end of the acute stay. Return to work, school, and community is the major objective of the entire acute hospitalization.

PHYSIOLOGY OF BURN INJURY

Serious burns are associated with a stereotypical sequence of physiologic changes. Anticipation of these metabolic aberrations facilitates optimal support (see Table 244-1). During the first 1 or 2 days after a serious burn, patients require substantial hemodynamic support.[4] If the patient is successfully resuscitated, a hyperdynamic and hypermetabolic state typically ensues. This later phase, characterized by high cardiac output, reduced afterload, fever, and muscle catabolism, must be supported by provision of adequate quantity and quality of substrates.

RESUSCITATION PHASE

The massive fluid resuscitation required by burn patients is unique in medicine. It is secondary to a diffuse but transient

TABLE 244-1. THE FOUR PHASES OF BURN CARE, WITH PHYSIOLOGIC CHANGES AND OBJECTIVES

Phase and Timing	Physiologic Changes	Objectives
1: Initial evaluation and resuscitation, 0 to 72 h	Massive capillary leak	Accurate fluid resuscitation and thorough evaluation
2: Initial wound excision and biologic closure, days 1-7	Hyperdynamic and catabolic state with high risk of infection	Exactly identify and remove all full-thickness wounds and achieve biologic closure
3: Definitive wound closure, day 7–week 6	Continued catabolic state and risk of non-wound septic events	Replace temporary with definitive covers and close small complex wounds
4: Rehabilitation, reconstruction, and reintegration, day 1 through discharge	Waning catabolic state and recovering strength	Initially to maintain range of motion and reduce edema; subsequently to strengthen and facilitate return to home, work, school

capillary leak driven by poorly characterized mediators.[5] The clinical result is extravasation of fluids, electrolytes, and even moderate-sized colloid molecules into both burned and unburned soft tissues to a degree not seen in other disease processes. Since the 1930s a variety of resuscitation formulas have been developed, based on burn and patient size. However, this remains an area of clinical art, with no formula being reliably accurate for all patients.[2] Besides burn size and patient size, a variety of other factors have an impact on resuscitation requirements. These include delay in initiation of resuscitation, inhalation injury, patient age, baseline cardiovascular health, and the depth and vapor transmission characteristics of the wound itself.[6]

Burns under 15% generally do not require a formal fluid resuscitation program. As burn size increases, the physiologic aberrations increase in intensity, explaining the escalating volume requirements. Formulas do not predict accurately the needs of individual patients.[7] Optimal burn resuscitation requires hourly re-evaluation of resuscitation endpoints with titration of volume infusions. In essence, the formula chosen will only help to initiate resuscitation and roughly guide planning of volume needs. Of the many resuscitation formulas

available, the modified Brooke protocol (Table 244-2) is representative. All formulas have their adherents, and all are useful if employed as rough guidelines only, while monitoring physiologic resuscitation endpoints.

HYPERDYNAMIC PHASE

Typically, there is a very noticeable decline in intravenous volume requirements 18 to 30 hours after injury. It is assumed that this is because the capillary leak has "sealed" in well-resuscitated patients. After this hypodynamic period, a systemic hypermetabolic state predictably develops and is sustained in surviving patients until it slowly regresses, well after wound closure.[8] This state is characterized by high cardiac output, low peripheral vascular resistance, fever, and increased protein flux. In patients not well supported with protein substrate, this increased protein flux will be associated with significant muscle catabolism. Although the basic biology is not well understood, the post-resuscitation physiologic state is assumed to be caused by inflammatory mediators and augmented release of the counter-regulatory hormones, cortisol, catecholamines, and glucagon.[9] These hormonal changes

TABLE 244–2. THE MODIFIED BROOKE RESUSCITATION FORMULA

0-24 Hours

Adults and children >10 kg:
Lactated Ringer's: 2-4 mL/kg/% burn/24 h (first half in first 8 h)
Colloid: none*

Children <10 kg:
Lactated Ringer's: 2-3 mL/kg/% burn/24 h (first half in first 8 h)
Lactated Ringer's with 5% dextrose: 4 mL/kg/h
Colloid: none

24-48 Hours

All patients:
Crystalloid: To maintain urine output. If silver nitrate is used, sodium leaching will mandate continued isotonic crystalloid. If other topical is used, free water requirement is significant. Serum sodium should be monitored closely. Nutritional support should begin, ideally by the enteral route.
Colloid: (5% albumin in lactated Ringer's):
    0-30% burn: none
    30-50% burn: 0.3 mL/kg/% burn/24 h
    50-70% burn: 0.4 mL/kg/% burn/24 h
    >70% burn: 0.5 mL/kg/% burn/24 h

*Increasingly, early colloid infusion (generally 5% albumin) is being used in patients with very large burns, particularly if they are young or resuscitation is not going smoothly.
Note: The Modified Brooke formula is a common consensus formula that, like other formulas, is only useful in individual patients if adjusted to physiologic endpoints. Like all resuscitative formulas it is a helpful starting point. However, a quality resuscitation requires the bedside presence of a physician capable of regularly evaluating resuscitation endpoints.

are triggered by a combination of wound- and gut-released bacteria and their byproducts, pain, foci of infection, and some degree of evaporative heat loss.

A central component of burn critical care is to ensure adequate support of the hypermetabolic state. This is done by providing accurate fluid repletion, adequate supplies of metabolic substrates, control of environmental temperature, and competent pain control. Early identification and excision of necrotic skin and soft tissue with immediate biologic closure of the resulting wounds truncates the hypermetabolic physiologic state and is the most effective way to avoid the deleterious consequences of prolonged hypermetabolism.[10]

Burn critical care requires control of the patient's environmental temperature. Burn patients have enormous and invisible evaporative water and energy losses if they are maintained in the typical cool, dry air of a general hospital.[11] Burn units and burn operating rooms need to be engineered to maintain high ambient temperature and humidity to avoid the difficult problem of hypothermia and excessive energy loss.

INITIAL EVALUATION AND BURN-SPECIFIC SECONDARY SURVEY

Burn patients often spend many hours in transport before reaching the location of definitive care, and their initial evaluation and management must be completed outside the burn unit setting. Often, when patients arrive in the ICU where definitive care will be rendered, a complete burn-specific secondary survey has not been completed.[12] It is essential for the intensivist to have a familiarity with these issues so that burn-related pathology and coexisting injuries are not overlooked. Evaluations should follow the format taught by the Advanced Trauma Life Support course. All seriously burned patients should be approached as having potential multiple trauma.[13]

INITIAL EVALUATION

The primary survey of the burn patient differs little from that of the trauma patient, although there are a few important differences worthy of emphasis. First among these differences is a sensitivity to the fact that progressive mucosal edema may compromise airway patency in the early hours after burns. This is especially true in young children because of their much smaller airway.[14] Progressive stridor or hoarseness should prompt visualization and/or intubation of the airway. Ideally, this need is anticipated before the crisis stage, so that proper equipment and personnel can be gathered, facilitating smooth tube placement. The facial and airway edema that is so common makes the burn patients airway among the most challenging to control. Re-intubation can be exceedingly difficult, if not impossible, after airway edema has progressed, making accidental extubation a potentially lethal complication. Security of the endotracheal tube should be regularly assessed. A twill-tie harness is a reliable method of securing the endotracheal tube (Fig. 244-1). Secure, reliable vascular access is essential for burn resuscitation. This usually requires central venous access. Sometimes it is best to wait until volume depletion has been corrected with peripheral lines to more safely place central venous, or especially arterial, catheters.

BURN-SPECIFIC SECONDARY SURVEY

In parallel with the trauma secondary survey, a burn-specific secondary survey will identify many of the unique insults associated with this type of injury. This survey should begin with a through history. At this time, the best opportunity exists to elicit important points of medical history and mechanism of injury. Important points include details of the injury mechanism, neurologic status at the scene, extrication time, and tetanus immune status. Highlights of the burn-specific secondary survey are described in the following paragraphs.

The ocular and otolaryngologic examination should begin with palpation of the head and face for signs of coincident blunt or penetrating trauma. The globes should be examined early, prior to the development of facial and eyelid edema, which will limit examination (Fig. 244-2).[15] Serious globe burns impart a clouded appearance to the cornea, and fluorescein staining will detect more subtle injuries. Tarsorrhaphy is virtually never indicated acutely, because lid edema will generally provide excellent globe coverage even in the presence of serious lid burns. Pressure on the burned ear and occiput is avoided. Topical mafenide

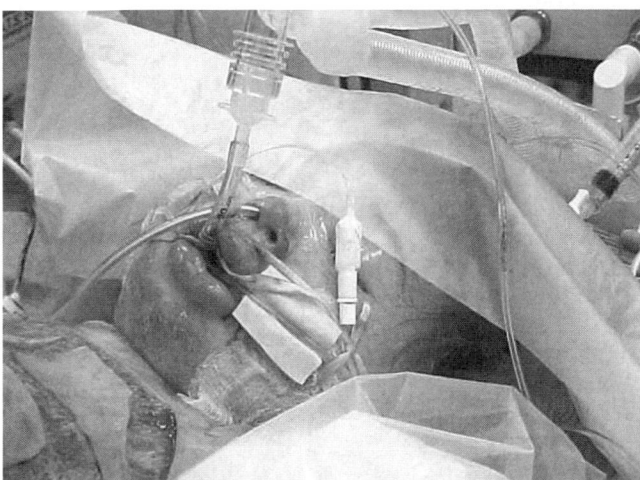

FIGURE 244-1. A twill-tie harness is a reliable way of securing the endotracheal tube. Protective pads may reduce injury to the oral commissures. Tube security should be regularly assessed, because re-intubation can be very difficult in this setting.

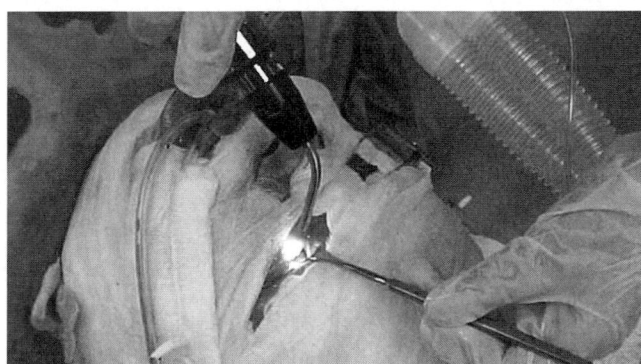

FIGURE 244-2. The globes should be examined early, before the development of facial and eyelid edema that will limit examinations. Serious globe burns impart a clouded appearance to the cornea, and fluorescein staining will detect more subtle injuries. Tarsorrhaphy is virtually never indicated acutely, because lid edema will generally provide excellent globe coverage even in the presence of serious lid burns.

acetate is applied, as it will penetrate the relatively avascular underlying cartilage.[16] Signs of inhalation injury, such as carbonaceous debris and singed nasal hairs, are noted on examination of the nose and throat. Ties securing endotracheal and nasogastric tubes should be checked so that pressure on the nasal septum or oral commissures is avoided.

The initial neurologic evaluation centers on exclusion of coincident neurologic injury and control of pain and anxiety. Even if arriving alert and oriented, patients with serious burns typically become obtunded over the succeeding hours and days, if only because of the effects of pain medications and sleep deprivation. It is therefore important to exclude central nervous system trauma if the mechanism of injury is either unknown or consistent with such trauma. There should be a low threshold for ordering a computed tomographic scan of the head and spine, based on mechanism of injury. Pain and anxiety management should begin during the initial evaluation, within limits of safety.[17] Good pain control may have physiologic, as well as the obvious psychologic benefits. In the emergency setting, this is best done with incremental administration of small doses of narcotics and benzodiazepines. When caring for paralyzed or obtunded patients, it is important to make sure there is no pressure on peripheral nerves, so that neuropathies are avoided. Finally, those burned in structural fires should be assessed for carbon monoxide (CO) exposure by history, neurologic examination, and determination of a carboxyhemoglobin level, because selected patients with significant exposure may benefit from hyperbaric oxygen treatment.[18]

The cervical spine and neck should be assessed for trauma, based on mechanism of injury. Extremely deep circumferential neck burns may require escharotomy to facilitate normal venous drainage of the head.

The chest wall should be assessed for compliance and symmetrical air movement. Patients with deep near-circumferential or circumferential chest wall burns may require escharotomy to facilitate ventilation (Fig. 244-3). If properly performed, escharotomy of the torso markedly enhances compliance.

Most patients are hypovolemic at the time of presentation and respond promptly to volume administration. Some patients, especially the elderly, will have previously unsuspected myocardial disease that may become clinically important during the stress of resuscitation. Some data also exist to support the existence of a myocardial depressant factor in some patients with very extensive injuries.[19] Patients who do not respond as expected to calculated resuscitation volumes may benefit from invasive monitoring, pulmonary artery catheterization, or cardiac ultrasonography.

Genitourinary evaluation is limited in this setting. The foreskin should be reduced over the bladder catheter so that paraphimosis is not the result of progressive edema during resuscitation.

Burned extremities should be examined, based on mechanism of injury, for other trauma. It can sometimes be difficult to identify fractures in this setting, so liberal use of radiography is appropriate. Fractured and burned extremities are initially stabilized with external splints, prior to placement of external fixators.

Perhaps the most important component of the evaluation of the extremities is to identify those extremities at risk for loss of perfusion with progressive edema during resuscitation and to develop an effective monitoring plan. Resuscitation-associated edema can cause profound limb ischemia secondary

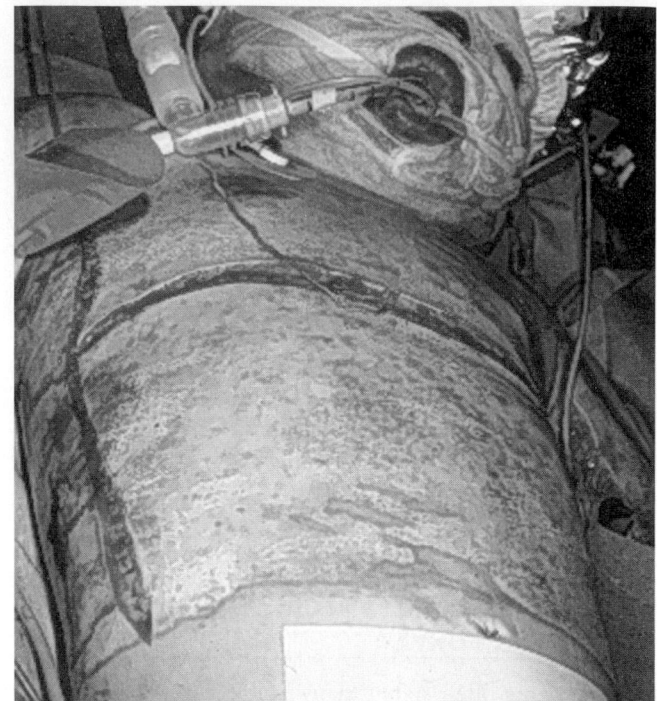

FIGURE 244–3. Patients with deep near-circumferential or circumferential chest wall burns may require escharotomy to facilitate ventilation. If properly performed, escharotomy of the torso will markedly enhance compliance.

to swelling under a circumferential eschar or within inelastic muscle compartments. This complication is seen in patients who have suffered deep extremity burns (especially if circumferential) or high-voltage electrical injuries. Low pressure flow in the extremity should be monitored, commonly using a Doppler probe to demonstrate flow in the palmar arch or digital vessels, because capillary perfusion pressure is only one third the mean arterial pressure monitored in larger vessels. Prompt identification of ischemic extremities is essential, so that escharotomy (Fig. 244-4) or fasciotomy (Fig. 244-5) can be effected in a timely manner.[20]

The wound should not be allowed to interfere with complete evaluation of the patient. Wounds are assessed for

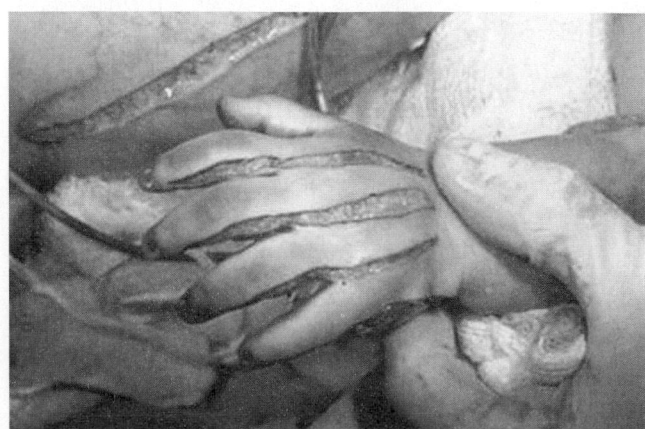

FIGURE 244–4. Properly performed escharotomy will result in immediate improvement in extremity blood flow.

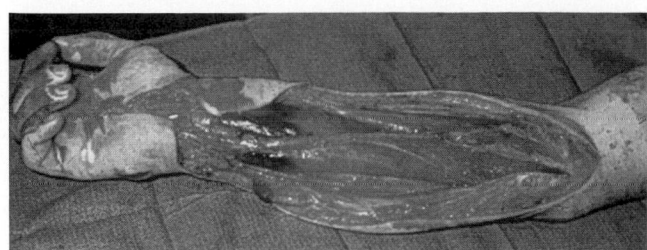

FIGURE 244-5. Fasciotomy will release pressure in edematous muscle compartments.

TABLE 244–3. AGE-SPECIFIC RESUSCITATION ENDPOINTS

Resuscitation Endpoint	Resuscitation Target
Sensorium	Comfortable, arousable
Physical examination	Warm extremities, full peripheral pulses
Urine output	Infants: 1-2 mL/kg/h; children: 0.5-1 mL/kg/h; all others: 0.5 mL/kg/h
Base deficit	Less than 2
Systolic blood pressure	Infants: 60 to 70 mm Hg
	Children: 70 to 90 ı (twice age in years) mm Hg
	Adolescents and adults: 90 to 120 mm Hg

Note: Age-specific resuscitation endpoints should be assessed regularly throughout burn resuscitation and infusions adjusted up or down in 10% to 20% increments to meet the needs of the individual patient.

extent using a Lund-Browder or other burn diagram, depth by visual examination, and the presence of circumferential components that may require decompression to ensure adequate perfusion. Typically, wounds are underestimated in depth on initial evaluation.

Carboxyhemoglobin and arterial blood gas determinations and screening baseline laboratories are part of the initial evaluation. Chest radiographs are useful to document proper placement of catheters and tubes and the absence of chest trauma. Inhalation injuries typically do not cause early radiographic changes.

Abuse or neglect should be considered when evaluating all burns, not just those in young children. Approximately 20% of burns in young children are reported to state authorities for investigation, but abuse occurs in all age groups.[21] Burns can also be a result of domestic violence or other interpersonal assaults. Often this determination is not made until the patient has been admitted to the ICU. Suspicious cases should be filed with appropriate state agencies. Documentation of the stated injury circumstances and of the wounds is essential. Wound photography is ideal (Fig. 244-6).

FLUID RESUSCITATION

In the first 1 or 2 hours after a large burn, patients experience little change in intravascular volume or hemodynamics. In fact,

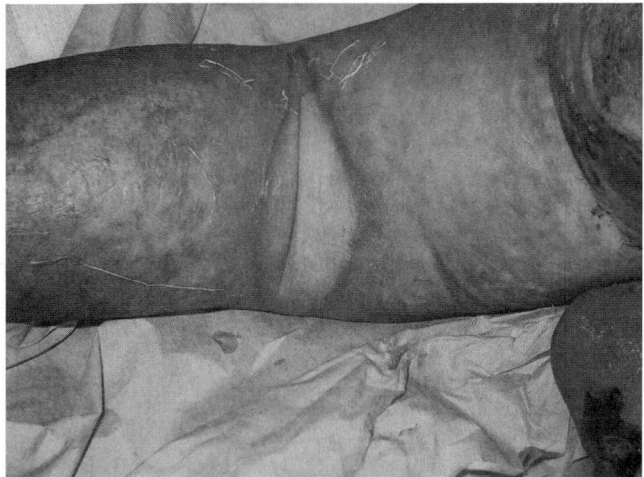

FIGURE 244–6. Suspicious cases should be filed with appropriate state agencies. Documentation of the stated injury circumstances and of the wounds is essential. Wound photography is ideal. Note the flexor-sparing pattern here.

patients are often remarkably alert during this period. In the hours that follow, however, the wound releases mediators that are absorbed into the systemic circulation. In addition, stress-related hormones are secreted and reactive oxygen species are formed on reperfusion of marginally perfused tissues. These and perhaps other factors trigger a diffuse loss of capillary integrity, resulting in extravasation of fluids, electrolytes, and even moderate-sized colloid molecules into soft tissues, including tissues that are distant from the burn. This "capillary leak" abates 18 to 24 hours later. This remarkable physiologic phenomenon explains the unique resuscitation needs of patients who have sustained large burns. A large number of formulas have been developed to predict resuscitation requirements. None of these is reliable in predicting the needs of specific patients because multiple variables impact resuscitation requirement besides burn size. These variables include burn depth, vapor transmission characteristics of the wound, patient age and cardiovascular health, resuscitation delay, environmental temperature and humidity, and presence or absence of concomitant inhalation injury. Numerous formulas have been promulgated to roughly guide resuscitation efforts. None is accurate in every patient.[6,22] A common consensus formula is the modified Brooke formula, which is summarized in Table 244-2.

Inaccurate fluid resuscitation will cause significant morbidity. Formulas are so inherently inaccurate that resuscitation should be guided by the hourly re-evaluation of clinical endpoints. Formulas can only help determine initial volume infusion rates and roughly predict 24-hour volume requirements. Resuscitation endpoints are summarized in Table 244-3. Measured oxygen delivery and consumption have been used as adjunctive resuscitation guides but are not necessary in the vast majority of patients.

BURN CRITICAL CARE ISSUES

Patients with serious burns require a high level of intensive care to survive their injuries. These issues are generally similar to those of "non-burned" patient, with several important differences.

AIRWAY ISSUES

Dangerous and frightening emergencies in the seriously burned involve the airway. Although evaluation and control of the airway are part of the initial evaluation, concerns extend throughout the period of intensive care. Endotracheal tube security should be part of the regular re-evaluation of every patient in the burn ICU, because re-intubation after unplanned extubation can be incredibly difficult in burn patients because of facial and hypopharyngeal edema.[23]

INHALATION INJURY

Inhalation injury remains a clinical diagnosis.[24] A history of closed-space fire, the presence of singed nasal hairs and facial burns, and carbonaceous sputum support the diagnosis of inhalation injury. Fiberoptic bronchoscopy can be useful in equivocal cases, as can technetium scanning. However, in the large majority of patients, the diagnosis is made by history and physical examination. The initial chest radiograph is almost always normal. Gas exchange and compliance are similarly almost always normal, until the endobronchial mucosa sloughs several days later, occluding small airways and leading to subsegmental atelectasis and respiratory insufficiency.

Five clinical consequences commonly occur in patients with inhalation injury: acute upper airway obstruction, bronchospasm, small airway occlusion, pulmonary infection, and respiratory failure.[25] The early complications, occurring during the first day, are airway obstruction and bronchospasm. Airway edema and obstruction are managed with endotracheal intubation. Bronchospasm from aerosolized irritants can be particularly intense during the first 24 to 48 hours and is managed with in-line nebulization beta-adrenergic agonists with infrequent use of intravenous bronchodilators, such as terbutaline or low-dose epinephrine infusions. Ventilatory strategies should be designed to minimize automatic positive end-expiratory pressure in this setting.

After 3 to 5 days, and with the sloughing of necrotic endobronchial debris, pulmonary toilet commonly becomes an increasing problem. Subsegmental atelectasis occurs, and shunting becomes an increasing problem. Bronchoscopy to aid pulmonary toilet can help to clear the airways.

Depending on how it is defined, as many as 50% of patients with inhalation injury will develop pulmonary infection. The differentiation between pneumonia (lobar involvement) and tracheobronchitis (purulent infection of the denuded tracheobronchial tree) is often difficult, but this difference is not really clinically important. Anyone who has fever and newly purulent sputum should be treated with antibiotics, guided by sputum cultures. Pulmonary toilet is particularly important in these patients.

Respiratory failure is unfortunately common in patients with inhalation injury. Patients are well managed with a pressure-limited ventilation strategy based on permissive hypercapnia.[26] Those who fail this can sometimes benefit from investigational modes of support, such as inhaled nitric oxide or extracorporeal oxygenation.[27,28]

CARBON MONOXIDE AND CYANIDE EXPOSURE

Patients injured in structural fires are commonly exposed to high levels of CO. Although an obtunded state in this clinical setting can be due to other causes, such as intoxication, trauma, or anoxia, hyperbaric oxygen (HBO) has been reported to improve the prognosis of patients who have suffered very severe CO exposure.[18] There are controlled data both supporting[29] its use and refuting the utility of HBO,[30] so clinical judgment must be brought to bear in the decision whether to use this form of therapy in individual patients.

CO binds and inactivates heme-containing enzymes, such as hemoglobin and the cytochromes. The binding of CO and hemoglobin forms carboxyhemoglobin, which does not deliver oxygen, resulting in acute physiologic anemia, much like an isovolemic hemodilution. A serum carboxyhemoglobin level of 50% is similar to an isovolemic hemodilution to 50% of the baseline hemoglobin concentration. This level of carboxyhemoglobin results in unconsciousness, implying that other mechanisms are also involved in the pathophysiology of CO injury. CO binding to the cytochrome system in the mitochondria probably interferes with oxygen utilization. Approximately 10% of patients with severe CO exposure have been reported to develop severe delayed neurologic sequelae.[31]

There are two practical treatment options: 100% normobaric oxygen or HBO, generally at 2 to 3 atm for 90 minutes. There are well-designed clinical studies both supporting and refuting the utility of HBO for CO poisoning.[29,30] Proponents cite a decreased incidence of delayed neurologic sequelae in those treated with HBO. In patients with very severe CO poisoning, with either very high carboxyhemoglobin levels or neurologic impairment not otherwise explainable, then HBO is probably warranted if it can be safely administered.

Commonly recommended HBO treatment is 2 or 3 atm for 90 minutes, with three 10-minute "air breaks" (breathing of pressurized room air rather than pressurized oxygen) to decrease the incidence of seizures. Most treatments are delivered in monoplace chambers, making it more risky to attempt treatment in unstable patients. Other relative contraindications are wheezing or air trapping, which increase the risks of pneumothorax or gas embolism, and high fever, which increases the risk of seizures. Before placement in the chamber, endotracheal tube balloons should be filled with saline to avoid balloon compression–associated air leaks and upper body central venous cannulation should be avoided if possible to avoid sudden enlargement of an occult pneumothorax during decompression.[32]

Hydrogen cyanide is detected in the smoke from many structural fires and in the serum of some burn patients. At a high enough concentration, cyanide causes failure of oxygen utilization at the cytochrome level with a secondary unexplained metabolic acidosis. Cyanide poisoning can be treated with amyl nitrate and sodium thiosulfate.[33] However, cyanide is rapidly metabolized in resuscitated patients, making specific treatment generally not necessary or useful.

PAIN AND ANXIETY MANAGEMENT

Undertreatment of pain and anxiety was very common in the past, and burn intensivists need to pay particular attention to this issue. Reasons for undertreatment are related to the extraordinary drug doses required to adequately address pain in seriously burned patients and consequent fear of respiratory depression, addiction, and litigation. The opiate and benzodiazepine tolerance of patients with large open wounds is truly remarkable.[34] Once wounds are closed, drug needs rapidly decrease and addiction is rare. The best way to eliminate burn pain is prompt wound closure.

Unfortunately, control of pain and anxiety is very difficult in burn patients. Successful management is greatly aided by a set of guidelines. One such program addresses four clinical states: intubated acute, nonintubated acute, chronic acute, and reconstructive patients.[35] Within each clinical state are separate guidelines for background pain, background anxiety, procedural pain, procedural anxiety, and transition to the next clinical state. Guidelines seem most effective when they use a limited formulary and emphasize dose ranging based on the regular assessment of objective efficacy. Attention to the issue has physiologic as well as the obvious psychological benefits. Reduced secretion of catecholamines may decrease systemic hypermetabolism. Treatment-related acute stress is reduced.[36]

OCULAR EXPOSURE

Contraction of burned eyelids and facial skin can cause exposure of the globe in the days or weeks after burns.[15] If unchecked, this will result in exposure and then desiccation of the globe with secondary keratitis and corneal ulceration. Infected corneal ulcers rapidly lead to globe perforation because the cornea is almost avascular and tolerates desiccation and infection very poorly. When minimal or moderate, globe exposure can be managed with frequent ocular lubrication. Acute eyelid release should be done promptly, if exposure is severe or keratitis does not resolve with lubrication over a few days.

PERIPHERAL NEUROPATHIES

Peripheral neuropathies are more common than is usually appreciated in burn patients.[37,38] They can be caused by direct thermal damage to peripheral nerves or by the many metabolic disturbances seen during acute burn care. A minority of these lesions are caused by constricting eschar, compartment syndrome, or improperly filled splints. Extremities at risk should be monitored for compartment syndrome and constricting eschar. These issues are best addressed surgically as early as possible. Heavily sedated patients, or those under general anesthesia in the operating room, should be examined to make sure that traction and pressure injuries are avoided.

GASTROINTESTINAL ISSUES

Curling's ulcers were a common cause of massive upper gastrointestinal bleeding in the past. This is now an infrequent occurrence with better resuscitation, which decreases splanchnic ischemia. The routine use of prophylactic gastric alkalinization also has been important. Patients with serious burns should be treated with empirical histamine-receptor blockers and/or antacids until they are tolerating tube feedings and are at low enough risk that this therapy can reasonably be stopped.

Calculous or acalculous cholecystitis in the critically ill burn patient is easily missed and can be the cause of significant illness. Fevers are often assumed to be secondary to the wound. Cholestatic blood chemistry values and modest clinical jaundice are identical to the changes that typify hepatic insufficiency. If untreated, gangrenous cholecystitis, associated with peritonitis and sepsis, can result. Diagnosis is generally easily made by bedside ultrasonography. Treatment can be either laparoscopic or open cholecystectomy. In the critically ill patient, percutaneous transhepatic drainage is a very reasonable alternative.[39]

Although uncommon, pancreatitis is a reported complication seen in patients with very large burns.[40] Like cholecystitis, it is easily missed until the condition is far advanced. Abdominal distention and ileus, with tenderness in those who are conscious, should prompt measurements of serum amylase and lipase concentrations as well as appropriate abdominal imaging in selected cases. Most patients can be treated with bowel rest, although pseudocysts and abscesses have been reported in this population.

Bowel ischemia and necrosis are complications seen generally in those with prolonged burn shock, often part of a delayed resuscitation syndrome. These complications present as ileus and then peritonitis. Bowel necrosis is lethal unless operated on promptly. It is a frequently reported autopsy finding in patients dying of burns.[41,42]

Superior mesenteric artery syndrome is a rare occurrence but should be seriously considered in patients with major weight loss during the acute phase of injury, who develop intractable vomiting in the recovery phase of their illness. It is caused by compression of the duodenum in the angle between the aorta and superior mesenteric artery.[43] Diagnosis is by barium swallow, and treatment is by a combination of parenteral nutrition and tube feedings past the point of obstruction, if possible.

Finally, it is easy to miss more common abdominal pathology in the setting of burns. Appendicitis can be a lethal complication first diagnosed at autopsy. Constipation from narcotic use and inactivity is common and is ideally prevented with a bowel regimen.

NUTRITIONAL SUPPORT

Burn patients need accurate energy and protein support. Underfeeding and overfeeding have adverse sequelae. Ideally, tube feedings are begun during resuscitation.[44] Most patients do well with continuous intragastric tube feedings, although some require post-pyloric feedings.[45] Enteral nutritional support can be started through a nasogastric sump tube so that gastric residuals can be used to help determine tolerance of the feedings initially.[46] Parenteral support is useful during periods when ileus is likely or during the perioperative period. Burn patients are very catabolic and therefore do not tolerate prolonged periods of fasting.

Goals for nutritional support for burned patients are controversial. There are a variety of formulas designed to predict these needs, but actual requirements vary widely and unpredictably in individual patients. Consensus recommendations are as follows: approximately 2.5 g/kg/day of protein should be provided and the caloric load should be between 1.5 and 1.7 times the calculated basal metabolic rate or 1.3 to 1. 5 times the measured (by indirect calorimetry) resting energy expenditure.[47,48] Nutritional support should be adjusted through the illness based on specific endpoints. Serial physical examination, quality of wound healing, nitrogen balance, and indirect calorimetry can be integrated to assess the adequacy of support and to help fine-tune the predictions of nutritional equations.

INFECTIOUS DISEASE ISSUES

Through loss of skin, necrosis of the endobronchial epithelium, and invasive devices, serious burns impair the host's physical barriers to bacteria while interfering with immune function. Therefore, burn patients are prone to virulent

TABLE 244-4. TOPICAL AGENTS USED IN WOUND MANAGEMENT

Agent	Characteristics
Silver sulfadiazine	Painless on application, fair to poor eschar penetration, no metabolic side effects, broad antibacterial spectrum
Mafenide acetate	Painful on application, excellent eschar penetration, carbonic anhydrase, inhibitor, broad antibacterial spectrum
0.5% Silver nitrate	Painless on application, poor eschar penetration, leaches electrolytes, broad spectrum (including fungi)

infectious complications. Anticipation of these infections will help to minimize infectious morbidity and mortality.

Historically, wound sepsis has been the great killer in burn units, and burn wound infections remain surprisingly common today.[49] The diagnosis of wound sepsis is generally clinical, based on signs and symptoms of systemic infection, along with changes in the appearance of the wounds. The diagnosis can be supported by wound biopsy and quantitative cultures, but both of these diagnostic techniques are infamously inaccurate, making a clinical diagnosis the most reliable.[50]

The best way to prevent wound sepsis is to identify and excise deep burns within the first few days after injury and to close the resulting wounds. Topical agents are only an adjunct to this effort and cannot, on their own, be relied on to prevent wound sepsis. Topical agents can delay the onset of wound sepsis in deep wounds. They can also serve to minimize desiccation and colonization of healing wounds. There are several agents in wide general use; the most common are listed in Table 244-4. All have specific advantages and disadvantages. Use of aqueous silver nitrate commonly promotes development of hyponatremia and hypokalemia. Use of mafenide acetate, which inhibits carbonic anhydrase, leads the development of metabolic acidosis, making it more difficult to use permissive hypercapnia for the management of patients with severe respiratory failure. Silver sulfadiazine application leads to large losses of free water across the burn wound eschar.

Antibiotic use must be focused. Too liberal empirical use will lead to the development of resistant organisms. Burn physiology, in the absence of infection, includes fever and a hyperdynamic circulation. When systemic infection is suspected, a careful physical examination and wound inspection should be done and cultures taken, particularly of blood, urine, and sputum. If the patient is hypotensive or otherwise unstable, then it is reasonable to start a short course of empirical antibiotic treatment while awaiting return of blood cultures. Clinical deterioration of the burn patient is most often related to infection.

Infection control practices should be routine and relatively rigid in burn units. This patient population has a high incidence of infection in general, and resistant bacterial species are very common. Universal precautions should be practiced in all patients. The use of prophylactic antibiotics is not advised.[51]

PREVENTION AND RECOGNITION OF COMPLICATIONS

Some common burn complications are itemized in Table 244-5. Optimally, complications should be diagnosed

TABLE 244–5. COMMON COMPLICATIONS IN BURN PATIENTS

Cardiovascular

- Endocarditis and suppurative thrombophlebitis are intravascular infections that typically present as fever and bacteremia without signs of local infection.
- Hypertension occurs in up to 20% of children and is best managed with beta-adrenergic blockers.
- Venous thromboembolic complications are so infrequent in patients with large burns that routine prophylaxis is not currently routine. Iatrogenic catheter insertion complications are minimized by meticulous technique.

Pulmonary

- Carbon monoxide intoxication, which is best managed acutely with effective ventilation with pure oxygen, can be associated with delayed neurologic sequelae.
- Pneumonia may occur with or without antecedent inhalation injury and is treated with pulmonary toilet and antibiotics.
- Respiratory failure may occur early post injury secondary to inhalation of noxious chemicals or later in the course secondary to sepsis or pneumonia.

Neurologic

- Transient delirium occurs in up to 30% of patients and generally resolves with supportive therapy when the possibility of anoxia, metabolic disturbance, and structural lesions is eliminated by appropriate studies.
- Seizures most commonly result from hyponatremia or abrupt benzodiazepine withdrawal.
- Peripheral nerve injuries occur from direct thermal injury, compression from compartment syndrome or overlying inelastic eschar, major metabolic disturbances, or improper splinting techniques.
- Delayed peripheral nerve and spinal cord deficits develop weeks or months after high-voltage injury secondary to small-vessel injury and demyelinization.

Hematologic

- Neutropenia and thrombocytopenia, as well as disseminated intravascular coagulation, are common indicators of impending sepsis and should prompt appropriate investigations.
- Global immunologic deficits associated with burn injury contribute to a high rate of infectious complications.

Renal

- Early acute renal failure follows inadequate perfusion during resuscitation or myoglobinuria.
- Late renal failure complicates sepsis and multiorgan failure or the use of nephrotoxic agents.

TABLE 244–5. COMMON COMPLICATIONS IN BURN PATIENTS—cont'd

Adrenal

- Acute adrenal insufficiency secondary to hemorrhage into the gland presents as hypotension, fever, hyponatremia, and hyperkalemia.

Otolaryngologic

- Auricular chondritis secondary to bacterial invasion of cartilage results in rapid loss of viable tissue and is prevented by the routine use of topical mafenide acetate on all burned ears.
- Sinusitis and otitis media can be caused by transnasal instrumentation and are treated by relocation of tubes, antibiotics, and judicious surgical drainage.
- Complications of endotracheal intubation include nasal alar and septal necrosis, vocal cord erosions and ulcerations, tracheal stenosis, and tracheoesophageal and tracheoinnominate artery fistulas. The occurrence of such complications is minimized by compulsive attention to tube position, avoidance of oversized tubes, and attention to cuff pressures.

Gastrointestinal

- Hepatic dysfunction, secondary to transient hepatic blood flow deficits and manifested as transaminase elevations, is extremely common during resuscitation from large burns and resolves with volume restitution. Late hepatic failure, beginning with elevations of cholestatic chemistries and progressing through coagulopathy and frank failure, complicates sepsis and multiorgan failure.
- Pancreatitis, beginning with amylase and lipase elevations and ileus and progressing through hemorrhagic pancreatitis, is generally coincident with splanchnic flow deficits early and sepsis-induced organ failures later in the hospital course.
- Acalculous cholecystitis can present as sepsis without localized symptoms or signs accompanied by rising cholestatic chemistries. A standard radiographic evaluation can be followed by bedside percutaneous cholecystostomy in unstable patients.
- Gastroduodenal ulceration secondary to splanchnic flow deficits that degrade mucosal defenses is extremely common and often life threatening if routine histamine-receptor blockers and antacids are not administered.
- Intestinal ischemia, which can progress to infarction, is secondary to inadequate resuscitation and splanchnic flow deficits.

Ophthalmologic

- Ectropia, from progressive contraction of burned ocular adnexa, results in exposure of the globe. This requires acute eyelid release. Tarsorrhaphy is rarely helpful, more often resulting in injury to the tarsal plate as contraction forces pull out tarsorrhaphy sutures.
- Corneal ulceration, which develops after initial epithelial injury or later exposure secondary to ectropion, can progress to full-thickness corneal destruction if secondary infection occurs. This is prevented by careful globe lubrication with topical antibiotics in the former case and acute lid release in the later.
- Symblepharon, or scarring of the lid to the denuded conjunctiva after chemical burns or corneal epithelial defects complicating toxic epidermal necrolysis, is prevented by daily examination and adhesion disruption with a fine glass rod.

Genitourinary

- Urinary tract infections are minimized by maintaining bladder catheters only when absolutely required and are treated with appropriate antibiotics. Neither catheterization nor colonic diversion is required for management of perineal and genital burns.
- *Candida* cystitis occurs in those patients treated with bladder catheters and broad-spectrum antibiotics. Catheter change and amphotericin irrigation for 5 days is generally successful. If infections are recurrent, the upper tracts should be screened ultrasonographically.

Musculoskeletal

- Burned exposed bone is generally débrided with a dental drill until viable cortical bone is reached, which is then allowed to granulate and is autografted. Patients whose overall condition and wounds are appropriate are managed with local or distant flaps.
- Fractured and burned extremities are best immobilized with external fixators while overlying burns are grafted. Burn patients with coincident fractures in unburned extremities benefit from prompt internal fixation.
- Heterotopic ossification develops weeks after injury, is seen most commonly around deeply burned major joints such as the triceps tendon, and presents as pain and decreased range of motion. Most patients respond to physical therapy, but some require excision of heterotopic bone to achieve full function.

Soft Tissue

- Hypertrophic scar formation is a major cause of long-term functional and cosmetic deformities seen in burn patients. This poorly understood process is heralded by a secondary increase in neovascularity between 9 and 13 weeks after epithelialization. Management options include grafting of deep dermal and full-thickness wounds, compression garments, judicious steroid injections, topical silicone products, and scar release and resurfacing procedures.

Note: Systematic reassessment of seriously ill burn patients facilitates timely detection of complications. It is the very rare burn patient who does not experience complications during their care, particularly while in the intensive care unit. Unfortunately, many common burn complications are obscured by the fevers and hyperdynamic physiology that accompany a large burn.

early, through regular careful physical examinations, aided by a high degree of suspicion.

REHABILITATION THERAPY IN THE BURN INTENSIVE CARE SETTING

Good burn care is extremely multidisciplinary. Physical and occupational therapists should be involved from the outset and strategies implemented to avoid common contractures that will otherwise interfere with recovery later (Table 244-6). Typically, physical therapy includes passive movement of all joints through an appropriate range of motion and static positioning in ways that minimize the risk of deformity. Involvement of physical and occupational therapists escalates as patients progress toward recovery; many hours of treatment are required each day after wound closure. Burn patients will have a much harder time with subsequent

TABLE 244–6. COMMON CONTRACTURES AND PREVENTION STRATEGIES USEFUL IN THE ICU

Anatomic Area	Common Contracture	ICU Preventive Splinting and Positioning Strategy
Neck	Flexion	Daily range of motion exercises and extension splinting and conformers, split mattress
Shoulder	Adduction	Daily range of motion exercises and abduction splinting with axillary splints or troughs
Elbow	Flexion and extension	Daily range of motion exercises and alternating extension and flexion splints
Wrist	Flexion and extension	Daily range of motion exercises and splinting in functional position (20 degrees of extension)
Metacarpophalangeal joints	Extension	Daily range of motion exercises and splinting in functional position (metacarpophalangeal joints at 70 to 90 degrees of flexion, all interphalangeal joints in extension, first web space open, wrist at 20 degrees of extension)
Hips	Flexion	Daily range of motion exercises and extension splints and prone positioning (if tolerated)
Knees	Flexion	Daily range of motion exercises and knee splints and knee immobilizers
Ankles	Extension	Daily range of motion exercises and neutral splints
Metatarsophalangeal joints	Extension	Daily range of motion and splinting in functional position, rocker-bottom shoes

rehabilitation if therapeutic efforts are ignored during the period of protracted critical illness.[12,52]

It is helpful for physical and occupational therapists to be involved in operative planning. Therapists need to be aware of the sequence of planned operations, because these events will impact therapy plans, splinting strategies, and ability to mobilize joints. Therapists may also use range-of-motion exercising in selected patients after induction of anesthesia to better distinguish between physical limitations and anxiety-induced resistance.

INTRAOPERATIVE CRITICAL CARE

Often, burn patients must be subjected to stressful operative procedures to excise and close wounds, even during periods of critical illness and hemodynamic instability. They can only survive these interventions if critical care efforts are continued during the operations. There must be continuous communication between the surgical and anesthesia teams during surgery. Each team must understand what the other is doing and is about to do, so it can anticipate its own next interventions.

Intrahospital transports from the protected environment of the ICU to the operating room must be carefully planned, and skilled people need to accompany the patient during transport. Burn patients have huge evaporative heat losses that can rapidly render them hypothermic, unless the operating room is kept warm and core temperature is continuously monitored. Hypothermia promotes development of coagulopathy, which can complicate these operations. The intensive care team should be involved in operative events.

SPECIAL INJURY CONSIDERATIONS

Several "non-burn" illnesses and injuries are commonly referred to burn units because they benefit from its unique set of surgical and critical care resources. The most common illnesses are toxic epidermal necrolysis and purpura fulminans. The most common injuries involve electrical, chemical, tar, and soft tissue trauma and soft tissue infections.

ELECTRICAL INJURY

Exposures can be somewhat arbitrarily divided into low- (household 110 to 220 volts), intermediate- (220 to 1000 volts),

and high-voltage (greater than 1000 volts). Patients with good contact to low and intermediate voltages commonly have severe local wounds but rarely suffer systemic consequences, such as compartment syndromes or rhabdomyolysis.[53] Patients with good contact to high voltages commonly have compartment syndromes, myocardial injury, fractures of the long bones and spine, and free pigment in the plasma that may cause renal failure if not promptly cleared.[54,55] These patients also suffer from electrical soft tissue burns, flash burns, and burns from clothing ignition. Many such patients have also suffered blunt trauma during the incident.

After high-voltage injury, cardiac monitoring is a good idea for 24 to 72 hours. Urine should be examined for myoglobin after placement of a bladder catheter. Fluid resuscitation should be started based on surface burn size, but this usually does not correlate well with deep tissue injury, so resuscitation must be closely monitored and titrated to the patient's physiology. Compartment syndromes are common, and this should be considered. Compartments at risk should undergo serial re-examination and should be decompressed in the operating room when an evolving compartment syndrome is suspected. Wounds associated with the injury are excised and closed in the following days with a combination of skin grafts and flaps.

COLD INJURY

Cold injuries often generate wounds best managed in the burn unit. The wounds are generally managed conservatively initially. Necrotic tissue is excised when demarcation is clear, and the resulting wounds are grafted. These patients very often suffer coincident hypothermia, which must be managed, often in the ICU.

CHEMICAL AND TAR INJURY

Chemical injuries can be associated with both local and systemic effects. Poison control centers should be consulted, particularly as regards systemic toxicities. It is essential to protect staff from exposure to the chemicals during removal. Most agents can be irrigated off with tap water for 30 minutes, although some, particularly alkaline substances, may take longer. When the "soapy feeling" that alkaline substances often impart to the gloved finger is gone, or when litmus paper indicates a neutral pH, irrigation may be stopped.

Hydrofluoric acid, especially in concentrated form, may result in severe acute hypocalcemia, because the fluoride anion strongly binds divalent cations.[56] Subeschar injection of 10% calcium gluconate and/or immediate excision of the wound may be lifesaving. Elemental metals, such as solid lithium or sodium, can ignite on contact with water or air and should therefore be covered with oil. White phosphorus, a component of many munitions, will also ignite on contact with air, and wound particles are ideally covered with wet cloth or gauze. There are a number of road-surfacing materials that are viscous and heated up to 700°F for application. They are designed to stay solid in the hot sun on dark pavement. When these materials splash road workers, the wounds should be quickly cooled by tap water irrigation. Wounds should be soaked in a lipophilic solvent after cooling. They should then be débrided and grafted as indicated by burn depth, which is often quite deep.

TOXIC EPIDERMAL NECROLYSIS

The cause of toxic epidermal necrolysis remains a mystery. For unclear immunologic reasons, epidermal-dermal bonding is disrupted to a variable degree. Frequently there is an influenza-like prodrome and usually there is a drug exposure that is believed to trigger the syndrome (commonly anticonvulsants or nonsteroidal anti-inflammatory agents). All mucosal surfaces are affected to some degree. Most patients are only affected slightly, whereas others are affected to a large degree. These patients have a life-threatening condition and are often referred to burn units for care.[57,58]

Seriously affected patients with toxic epidermal necrolysis have both a cutaneous and a visceral wound, caused by slough of the skin and of surfaces lined by mucosa or conjunctiva (Fig. 244-7). The cutaneous wound usually begins first. The severity of the skin and of the mucosal sloughs are not directly related. Although the skin slough is what heralds the disease, and is what brings most patients to the attention of burn programs, it is generally the easier of the two wounds to manage, with topical antimicrobials and biologic dressings.[59] The visceral wound is much more problematic. Conjunctival sloughing threatens the globe.[60] Pulmonary involvement leads to respiratory failure.[61] Gastrointestinal sloughing may lead to bleeding and bacterial translocation. Clinical outcomes have been best when these patients are managed in burn units.[62] The utility of intravenous gamma-globulin in toxic epidermal necrolysis remains controversial and is not considered a standard of care.[63]

PURPURA FULMINANS

Patients with meningococcal and other bacterial septic lesions may develop a syndrome in which soft tissues are rendered ischemic by spotty small-vessel thrombosis. It has been theorized that thrombosis is caused by transient protein C deficiency, which occurs when the liver ceases production of clotting proteins secondary to the septic event.[64] Protein C is an anticoagulant protein that helps maintain control of the process of clotting and has the shortest half-life of the clotting factors (about 6 hours). Patients with purpura fulminans present with organ failures and acute new deep wounds, often heralded by an ominous rash in the affected distribution. These patients are often referred promptly to burn units for care of organ failures associated with large soft tissue wounds.[65]

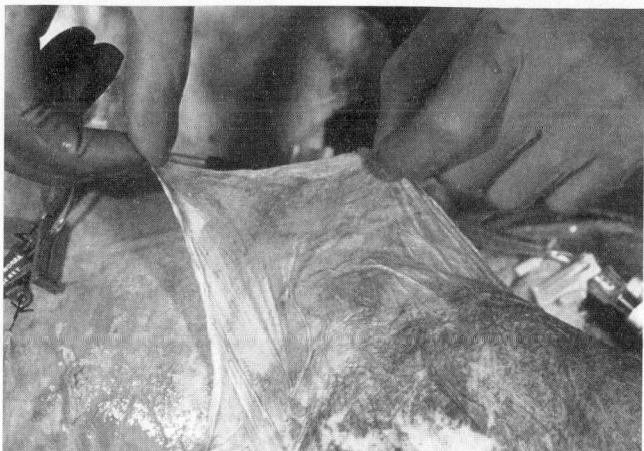

FIGURE 244–7. The cause of toxic epidermal necrolysis remains a mystery. This patient has both a cutaneous and a visceral wound.

SOFT TISSUE INFECTIONS

Patients with serious soft tissue infections share many characteristics of burn patients, often having wounds requiring complex surgical care with associated sepsis-induced organ failures. Such patients are increasingly managed in burn programs. Early diagnosis is perhaps the most important component of management, and some patients require operative exploration of severely swollen extremities with severe cellulitis if physical examination and soft tissue radiography are not diagnostic. Involved tissues should be widely resected. An early "second-look" procedure is often a very wise idea. With resection of involved tissue, sepsis-induced organ failures often quickly improve.

CONCLUSION

Serious burns present a unique set of challenges to the ICU team that crosses multiple disciplines. However, outcome data support the contention that most survivors of serious burns can have a very satisfying long-term quality of life.[66] A successful outcome requires a coordinated effort by intensive care, surgical, nursing, and rehabilitation therapy professionals during what is often a technically demanding, but ultimately rewarding, ICU stay.

ANNOTATED REFERENCES

Hollingsed TC, Saffle JR, Barton RG, et al: Etiology and consequences of respiratory failure in thermally injured patients. Am J Surg 1993;166:592–596.
  These authors emphasize that respiratory failure is very common in patients with serious burns and is not always a direct result of inhalation injury but may be secondary to systemic factors such as sepsis.

Peck MD, Weber J, McManus A, et al: Surveillance of burn wound infection: A proposal for definitions: J Burn Care Rehabil 1998;19:386–389.
  These authors have addressed the problem of multiple sets of definitions for burn wound infection that vary between various programs. They propose a set of standardized definitions that will improve the ability to compare infection surveillance data from various burn programs.

Sax EG, Stoddard F, Courtney D, et al: Relationship between acute morphine and course of PTSD in children with burns. J Am Acad Child Adolesc Psychiatry 2001;40:915–921.
  These authors were able to document a strong inverse statistically significant relationship between total morphine dose and PTSD symptoms, implying that proper pain control during the acute phase of burns will directly reduce psychiatric morbidity after recovery.

Sheridan RL: Burn care: Results of technical and organizational progress. JAMA 2003;290:719–722.

This reference reviews major organizational changes that have occurred in burn care over the past decades and also highlights some of the technical changes that have contributed to the improved outcomes that are now more routinely seen. It is stressed that this is a result of both technical and organizational progress in burn care.

Sheridan RL, Hinson MI, Liang MH, et al: Long-term outcome of children surviving massive burns. JAMA 2000;283:69–73.

These authors studied long-term outcome at an average of 15 years after injury in 80 young adults who had survived massive burns as children. They were able to show that the long-term quality of life was very satisfying for the large majority.

Chapter 245

THORACIC TRAUMA

Daniel Herzig • Walter L. Biffl

KEY POINTS

INITIAL ASSESSMENT

1. The initial management of seriously injured patients should follow the tenets of the American College of Surgeons Committee on Trauma **Advanced Trauma Life Support Course.**

2. The critical determinants of survival following thoracotomy in the emergency department are the mechanism of injury and the patient's condition at the time of thoracotomy. **Blunt trauma patients should have vital signs, and penetrating trauma patients should have some signs of life** to optimize outcome.

PLEURAL SPACE

1. "Prophylactic" tube thoracostomy is not necessary for **occult pneumothoraces,** even in the setting of positive-pressure ventilation.

2. Needle decompression, when performed, should be done in the **midaxillary line in the fifth intercostal space** to maximize the risk-benefit ratio.

3. **Prophylactic antibiotics for tube thoracostomy** should not be given for longer than 24 hours.

4. **Chest tube removal algorithms** should include lung expansion, drainage less than 2 mL/kg per day, and 6- to 12-hour water seal drainage.

5. High-volume chest tube output that abruptly decreases should raise the suspicion of **caked hemothorax.**

CHEST WALL INJURY

1. **Rib fractures in elderly patients** are associated with significant morbidity and mortality.

2. Treatment of flail chest is strictly supportive, recognizing that the **primary cause of respiratory compromise is the accompanying pulmonary contusion.**

3. **Sternal fractures from the "seat-belt syndrome"** infrequently have significant associated injuries.

LUNG INJURY

1. **Treatment of pulmonary contusion is strictly supportive,** with mechanical ventilation, tube thoracostomy, and antibiotics used only when indicated.

2. **Pulmonary tractotomy results in favorable morbidity and mortality rates** compared with lung resection for trauma.

TRACHEOBRONCHIAL INJURY

1. **Bronchoscopy** should be performed for cervical subcutaneous emphysema, pneumomediastinum, or pneumothorax with a persistent air leak.

ESOPHAGEAL INJURY

1. **Contrast esophagography followed by esophagoscopy** improves the sensitivity of either test alone and should be performed in the cervical esophagus.

2. **Primary repair is usually inadvisable after 24 hours.**

CARDIAC INJURY

1. **Blunt cardiac injury is commonly diagnosed,** but cardiac enzymes, echocardiography, and nuclear medicine studies are not predictive of the uncommon but life-threatening complications of **ventricular dysrhythmias and cardiac pump failure.**

2. Clinical decisions should be based on the **initial electrocardiogram.**

3. Echocardiography is most useful in identifying **pericardial tamponade or intracardiac injuries.**

4. All patients in shock who have **penetrating chest injuries between the right midclavicular line and left anterior axillary line** should be considered to have a cardiac injury until proved otherwise.

5. **Ultrasonography and central venous pressure monitoring** are critical adjuncts in diagnosing

pericardial tamponade, as the classic findings of Beck's triad are present in very few patients.

TRANSMEDIASTINAL PENETRATING TRAUMA

1. **Helical computed tomography scanning** is useful in delineating the trajectory of potential transmediastinal gunshot wounds, allowing a truncated and cost-effective workup in stable, asymptomatic patients.

THORACIC GREAT VESSEL INJURY

1. A reasonable operative approach to unstable patients can be inferred from the **chest radiograph and the location of wounds.**

2. Blunt thoracic aortic injury should be suspected in any patient with **severe energy transfer, regardless of mechanism.**

3. **Helical computed tomography is an excellent screening test** and should be considered even in the face of a normal chest radiograph if there is severe energy transfer.

4. Once aortic injury is diagnosed, the **systolic blood pressure and heart rate should be controlled with a rapidly reversible beta-blocking agent.**

5. During aortic repair, it is safest **to provide distal circulation via a bypass circuit.**

6. The subgroup of patients with brain injuries or severe thoracic injuries may best be served by **delayed operation or nonoperative management.**

Thoracic trauma is responsible for approximately 20% of all trauma-related deaths and is second only to head trauma as the primary cause of death at injury scenes. For patients who arrive at the emergency department (ED) alive, rapid diagnosis and treatment of potentially life-threatening injuries are required to prevent death during the "golden hour" of initial resuscitation. However, many thoracic injuries that are not immediately life threatening still have the potential for significant morbidity and mortality. The following is an overview of the diagnosis and management of thoracic trauma.

INITIAL ASSESSMENT

PRIMARY SURVEY

The Advanced Trauma Life Support Course of the American College of Surgeons Committee on Trauma[1] provides the basic tenets for the management of all injured patients. The initial treatment of seriously injured patients consists of a primary survey, resuscitation, secondary survey, diagnostic evaluation, and definitive care. Although the concepts are presented in a sequential fashion, in reality, they often proceed simultaneously. The process begins with the primary survey,

designed to identify and treat conditions that constitute an immediate threat to life. The primary survey includes a stepwise evaluation of the "ABCs": airway, with cervical spine protection; breathing, and circulation.

Trauma to the larynx, trachea, or bronchus may complicate or preclude airway control, but the more typical threats to maintaining a patent airway are neurologic injury, facial injury, and foreign body obstruction. In contrast, thoracic trauma more commonly causes life-threatening breathing (e.g., pneumothorax, hemothorax, pulmonary contusion) and circulation (e.g., tension pneumothorax, pericardial tamponade) problems. These must be identified and treated rapidly.

RESUSCITATIVE THORACOTOMY

Some trauma victims who arrive in extremis may be candidates for resuscitative thoracotomy in the ED. The primary objectives of the procedure are to (1) release pericardial tamponade, (2) control intrathoracic hemorrhage, (3) control bronchovenous air embolism or bronchopleural fistula, (4) perform open cardiac massage, and (5) temporarily occlude the descending thoracic aorta to redistribute limited blood flow to the brain and myocardium and attenuate subdiaphragmatic hemorrhage.[2] The critical determinants of survival following this procedure are the mechanism of injury and the patient's condition at the time of thoracotomy. The best outcomes are seen in adult patients with isolated cardiac injuries who present to the ED with detectable blood pressure; survival averages 35% in large series. For penetrating noncardiac injuries, the salvage rate is 15% for patients who present with vital signs and 10% if only signs of life (i.e., pupillary activity, spontaneous respirations, narrow complex cardiac activity) are present. Resuscitative thoracotomy is least beneficial in the treatment of blunt injury or in the absence of signs of life, with only 1% to 2% of patients surviving.[2]

The value of thoracotomy in the resuscitation of a patient in profound shock but not yet dead is unquestioned. Its indiscriminate use, however, renders it a low-yield, high-risk, and high-cost procedure. Based on our experience and that reflected in the current literature, we have formulated a decision algorithm for the resuscitation of moribund trauma patients (Fig. 245-1). Patients arriving in extremis following blunt injury undergo thoracotomy only if they have vital signs—that is, a palpable pulse or obtainable blood pressure. Penetrating trauma victims in extremis undergo thoracotomy if any signs of life (pupillary reactivity, respiratory effort, narrow QRS complex) are present. If, upon opening the chest, there is no cardiac activity and no blood in the pericardium, the patient is declared dead. All other patients are treated according to the injury. Pericardial tamponade is decompressed, and bleeding from cardiac wounds is controlled. Suspected air embolism is treated by the application of a pulmonary hilar cross-clamp, vigorous cardiac massage, and aortic root and left ventricular aspiration for air. Intrathoracic hemorrhage is controlled. Cardiovascular collapse from suspected intra-abdominal hemorrhage is temporized by occluding the descending thoracic aorta. Those patients with intra-abdominal hemorrhage who respond to occlusion of the thoracic aorta and have a systolic blood pressure above 70 mm Hg, as well as all other surviving patients, are rapidly transported to the operating room for definitive treatment of their injuries.

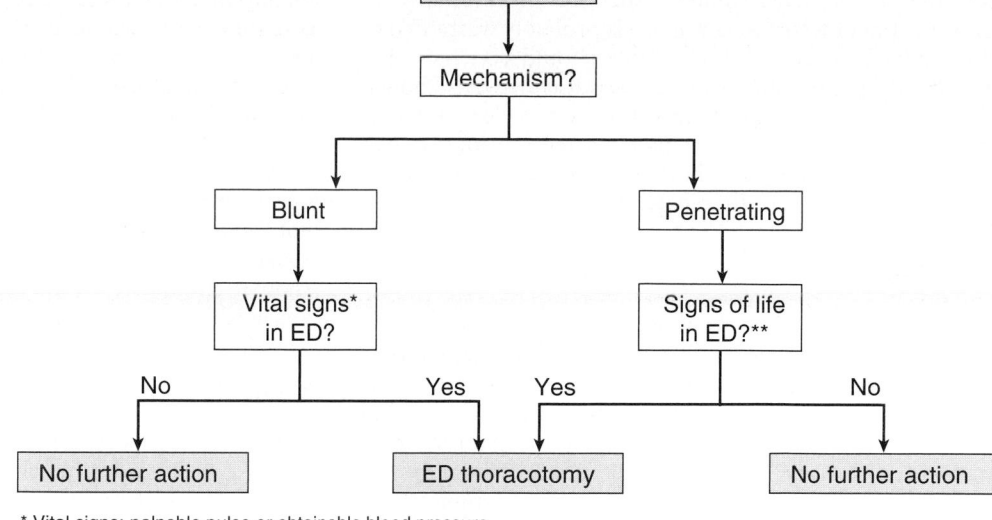

FIGURE 245–1. Algorithm for emergency department thoracotomy. Vital signs consist of a palpable pulse or obtainable blood pressure. Signs of life consist of pupillary activity, respiratory effort, or narrow complex QRS complex. ED, emergency department; SBP, systolic blood pressure.

* Vital signs: palpable pulse or obtainable blood pressure

**Signs of life: pupillary activity, respiratory effort, or narrow complex QRS complex

PLEURAL SPACE

PNEUMOTHORAX

Pneumothorax is a common sequela of thoracic trauma. Visceral pleural disruption, due to penetrating trauma, blunt shearing, or lacerations from fractured bones, allows air to enter the pleural space as negative intrapleural pressure is created during inspiration. Physical findings include decreased breath sounds, hyperresonance to percussion, and decreased expansion of the chest wall on the affected side. If not relieved, a simple pneumothorax may progress to a tension pneumothorax, especially if the patient is receiving positive-pressure ventilation. In this setting, the mediastinal structures are shifted away from the affected side. In addition to the mechanical impediment to gas exchange, venous return to the heart is impaired due to vena caval distortion, and shock ensues. Immediate decompression is mandatory and can be lifesaving (see Tube Thoracostomy, later).

An open pneumothorax, also called a "sucking chest wound," results from a full-thickness chest wall wound. If the wound diameter exceeds two thirds of the tracheal diameter, negative intrapleural pressure associated with inspiratory effort results in air entering the pleural space preferentially through the wound. Because of the large hole, there is little chance of tension pneumothorax. However, this can be immediately life threatening because it prevents pulmonary gas exchange. It is immediately managed by an occlusive dressing secured on three sides, to prevent sucking of more air but allowing egress of the pnemothorax until definitive wound closure and tube thoracostomy can be performed.

With the growing use of thoracoabdominal computed tomography (CT) in the evaluation of trauma patients, small pneumothoraces that are not seen on plain radiographs are often discovered. The treatment of these so-called occult pneumothoraces is not as well defined as the treatment of the usual pneumothorax. Generally, they do not require treatment but should be monitored for progression. The notion of "prophylactic" tube thoracostomy in the setting of positive-pressure ventilation has been challenged, but vigilance is critical.[3]

TUBE THORACOSTOMY

Tube thoracostomy is the definitive treatment for most pneumothoraces, as well as hemothoraces (see later). The procedure is not difficult and can be performed rapidly, but care must be taken to avoid transdiaphragmatic–lung parenchymal–extrapleural–interlobar fissure placement, as well as kinking. The optimal position is posterior, to facilitate dependent drainage of blood, and directed to the apex of the pleural cavity. Although large-bore (36 Fr.) tubes are typically chosen in the ED, the tube size can be individualized. Small-diameter tubes, which cause less discomfort for the patient, can certainly evacuate air and are adequate to drain most small to moderate hemothoraces.

If tube thoracostomy is not immediately available, the chest can be decompressed with a large-bore needle as a temporizing measure in the setting of tension pneumothorax. Although many texts promote decompression via the second intercostal space in the midclavicular line, injuries to the great vessels have been described as a result of this procedure. Further, catheters may be misdirected or kinked in the pectoralis major muscle, rendering them ineffective (often unbeknownst to the clinician). Our preference is to insert the needle through the fifth intercostal space in the midaxillary line. This site allows rapid, reliable entry into the pleural space, and the risk of great vessel injury is essentially nil.

The major morbidity related to tube thoracostomy is infectious (pneumonia, empyema), reported in 1% to 20% of patients. Some investigators have proposed routine prophylactic antibiotics to prevent such morbidity, but this is controversial, and the available literature does not allow definitive conclusions.[4,5] The Eastern Association for the Surgery of Trauma Practice Management Guidelines Work Group recently suggested that level III evidence favors prophylactic administration of a first-generation cephalosporin for 24 hours.[6] Our institution is presently participating in a multicenter trial of the Western Trauma Association to try to definitively answer this question.

Pneumothoraces and air leaks should be resolved before removal of the tube, and ideally, drainage should be less than

2 mL/kg per day. After 12 to 24 hours without an air leak, the tube may be removed while on suction. However, a 6- to 12-hour trial of water seal drainage is probably warranted to observe for an occult air leak.[7] Tubes should be removed at maximal deep inspiration with a Valsalva maneuver, although recurrent pneumothorax may still occur in 6% to 8% of patients.[8] More than 20% of patients require longer than 3 days to resolve an air leak; their hospital course may be expedited by the use of thoracoscopy.[9]

HEMOTHORAX

Hemothorax can range from small and asymptomatic to massive and immediately life threatening. A small hemothorax can be difficult to appreciate on a chest radiograph. In the upright position, blunting of the costophrenic angle requires 200 to 250 mL of blood, and in a supine patient, there may be only subtle haziness of the affected hemithorax. Hemothoraces should generally be drained by tube thoracostomy. However, as with occult pneumothoraces, hemothoraces that are asymptomatic and seen only on CT scan can be managed expectantly. A massive hemothorax is usually the result of a major vascular injury and is life threatening. Indications for thoracotomy include the immediate return of 1500 mL of blood via tube thoracostomy or continued output of 250 mL/h for 2 to 3 consecutive hours. A hemodynamically unstable patient with more than 800 mL of blood from the chest should undergo thoracotomy, if other sites of bleeding have been excluded. The clinician should be wary of an initial high-volume output that is followed by an abrupt decrease in volume. In this case, a repeat chest radiography should be obtained to rule out a "caked hemothorax." A second tube may need to be inserted, but if the hemothorax is not being evacuated, thoracoscopy or thoracotomy is indicated. Hemothoraces associated with massive blunt chest wall trauma can pose special challenges. Ongoing bleeding suggests the need for thoracotomy, but a large incision may compound the bleeding, and diffuse bleeding from bone and soft tissue disruption may prove difficult to control. In this setting, one might consider arteriography with embolization of intercostal bleeders in a hemodynamically stable patient.

CHEST WALL INJURY

RIB FRACTURE

Rib fractures are estimated to occur in 10% of patients presenting for evaluation by trauma services. Ziegler and Agarwal reported that more than 90% of patients with rib fractures had associated injuries, and half of these patients required ICU care.[10] In their series, the overall mortality of patients presenting with rib fractures was 12%. Multiple rib fractures, fractures of the first or second rib, and scapular fractures signify higher-energy injuries and should prompt a search for associated intra-abdominal injury or thoracic vascular injury.

Single rib fractures in young patients are generally of little consequence; however, rib fractures in elderly patients can lead to diminished pulmonary function with potentially disastrous infectious complications. Patients over the age of 65 have two- to fivefold increases in morbidity and mortality compared with younger patients with similar injuries.[11,12] Bulger and colleagues found that for each additional rib fracture in the elderly, mortality increases by 19%, and the

risk of pneumonia increases by 27%.[12] A key factor in the management of these patients is pain control to facilitate coughing and clearance of secretions. Epidural catheters have proved to be efficacious and superior to patient-controlled analgesia in this regard and may also modify the immune response.[13,14] Rib blocks may provide immediate relief in the ED or ICU while awaiting epidural catheter placement. Bupivacaine or a lidocaine-bupivacaine mixture may be injected into the intercostal bundle (with care taken not to inject intravascularly) of the fractured ribs and those above and below them. An intercostal catheter provides another alternative, in the event that an epidural catheter is unavailable or contraindicated.[15]

FLAIL CHEST

Two or more ribs fractured in two or more places produce a flail segment of the chest wall. This segment moves paradoxically—inward during inspiration, outward during expiration—because it is detached from the chest wall and thus susceptible to the forces of intrapleural pressure. The mechanical effects on respiration are related to the size of the flail segment. However, a more important cause of respiratory compromise following flail chest injury is the pulmonary contusion that invariably accompanies it. Treatment is supportive, including supplemental oxygen, analgesia, and pulmonary toilet. Endotracheal intubation with positive-pressure ventilation is sometimes necessary. Surgical stabilization of the flail segment is not routinely performed, as its benefits are marginal.[16]

STERNAL FRACTURE

Early series of sternal fractures described the "steering wheel syndrome" (rapid deceleration, with impact of the sternum on the steering wheel) as the most common cause of sternal fracture. In these series, associated blunt cardiac injury (see later) was common; thus, sternal fractures were thought to be harbingers of significant occult thoracic injury. More recently, however, sternal fractures have been reported more commonly with the "seat-belt syndrome" (in conjunction with three-point, or bandolier, seat belts). Because the elements of deceleration and steering wheel impact are no longer prominent, associated injuries are relatively infrequent.[17,18] Stable patients without dyspnea, electrocardiographic abnormalities, or significantly displaced fractures can be safely discharged from the ED. Rest and analgesia are adequate treatment.

LUNG INJURY

PULMONARY CONTUSION

Pulmonary contusion is a common problem, occurring in 15% to 20% of patients with injury severity scores greater than 15 and in a majority of patients sustaining major chest trauma. The injury may result from a direct blow, shearing or bursting at gas-liquid or high-density–low-density interfaces, or the transmission of a shock wave. The pathophysiologic changes fundamentally include hemorrhage with surrounding edema, with a broad range of severity up to "hepatization" of the lung. The clinical result is hypoxia, hypercarbia, and increased work of breathing due to ventilation-perfusion mismatching and decreased pulmonary compliance. Pulmonary contusions may not appear radiographically on initial presentation, although they are usually seen by 6 hours after the injury; CT of the chest is more sensitive at diagnosing early pulmonary contusions. Treatment is supportive, including supplemental oxygen, pain control, pulmonary toilet, and judicious fluid management. There is no role for either routine antibiotics or steroid therapy.[19] Intubation and mechanical ventilation are employed only as necessary. The degree of pulmonary dysfunction usually peaks at 72 hours and generally resolves within 7 days in the absence of associated nosocomial pneumonia. An admission PaO_2/FiO_2 ratio less than 250 is the best indicator of poor outcome.[20]

Post-traumatic pulmonary pseudocysts are cavitary lesions that occur in approximately 3% of lung parenchymal injuries.[21] They may be asymptomatic or associated with mild, nonspecific symptoms and are often noted incidentally on the chest radiograph. Most resolve spontaneously within 2 to 4 months. However, surgical intervention is indicated for infection, bleeding, and rupture. The lesion can be distinguished from an abscess by CT-guided aspiration.[22] If infected, catheter drainage may be required for definitive management.

PULMONARY LACERATION

Penetrating trauma, blunt shearing, or the ends of fractured bones can cause pulmonary laceration and parenchymal disruption. The typical clinical presentation is a hemopneumothorax. Bleeding is usually self-limited, and the vast majority of these injuries are definitively managed by tube thoracostomy alone. Of the 10% of patients requiring thoracotomy, approximately 20% need lung resection. Historically, this group has experienced high morbidity and mortality, with mortality following pneumonectomy approaching 100%. In 1994, Wall and colleagues introduced the concept of pulmonary tractotomy as a nonresectional means of managing penetrating lung injuries.[23] It is indicated for deep through-and-through injuries that do not involve central hilar vessels or airways. The wound tract is exposed by passing clamps (as originally described) or a stapling device (our preference) through the wound and dividing the bridge of lung tissue. Air leaks and bleeding points are sutured, and the wound tract is left open. The literature contains mixed reports of the success of this approach, but the morbidity and mortality compare favorably with those associated with anatomic resections.[24]

TRACHEOBRONCHIAL INJURY

Tracheobronchial injuries are uncommon but should be excluded in the presence of cervical subcutaneous emphysema, pneumomediastinum, or pneumothorax with a persistent air leak. Although CT may reveal some injuries, the preferred diagnostic test is bronchoscopy. Laryngotracheal injuries often require tracheostomy as an adjunct to repair. Tracheal stenosis is a common late complication. Tracheal injuries can usually be repaired primarily, or by resection and reanastomosis, without tracheostomy. Cervical incisions are employed, with partial or complete sternotomy as needed. If additional length is required for tracheal resection, thoracotomy may be necessary to release a bronchus. Absorbable monofilament sutures are preferred, and late stenosis is uncommon. Bronchial injuries may be repaired, but severe disruptions or associated vascular injuries may necessitate pneumonectomy or lobectomy. Postive end-expiratory pressure is avoided postoperatively.[25]

ESOPHAGEAL INJURY

Blunt-force mechanisms may cause a sudden rise in intraluminal pressure, or the upper esophagus may be crushed between the trachea and a vertebral body; however, esophageal injury is usually the result of penetrating trauma. Pneumomediastinum should raise the suspicion of this injury. Evaluation of the esophagus is also an important component of the workup of potential transmediastinal penetrating injuries (see later). Esophagoscopy has been reported to have 100% sensitivity for thoracic esophageal injuries.[26,27] However, in an awake, asymptomatic patient, barium esophagography is easier to obtain and may be adequate by itself. It should be noted that contrast esophagography followed by esophagoscopy improves the sensitivity of either test alone. Because the cervical esophagus is difficult to reliably evaluate, both studies are generally warranted. The evaluation should be expeditious, because delays in definitive care are associated with increased morbidity and mortality.[28] If the injury is identified within 24 hours, it can usually be treated with debridement, primary repair, and drainage. Injuries identified after 24 hours are better treated with debridement and drainage, cervical esophagostomy, and feeding tube placement.[29]

CARDIAC INJURY

BLUNT CARDIAC INJURY

The term *blunt cardiac injury* (BCI) is preferable to terms such as *myocardial* or *cardiac contusion* or *concussion*. Modifiers such as "with electrocardiographic or enzyme changes," "with complex arrhythmia," "with cardiac failure," "with coronary thrombosis," or "with septal or free wall rupture" may be added. BCI most commonly results from motor vehicle crashes (80% to 90%) but can occur following virtually any trauma to the chest. A wide spectrum of cardiac injuries may result, ranging from immediately fatal to occult and inconsequential. The threat of immediate decompensation mandates that trauma care providers be quick to recognize and treat cardiac injuries.

Cardiac Rupture. Cardiac rupture is the most severe form of BCI; 80% to 90% of ruptures are lethal within minutes. Cardiac rupture may result from direct-impact force to the heart or pressure transmitted via venous channels; deceleration with lacerations at junctions between fixed and mobile structures (e.g., atriocaval disruptions); myocardial contusion, with subsequent necrosis and rupture; and broken ribs or sternum penetrating the heart. The most common chambers ruptured are the right atrium and ventricle, followed by the left atrium and then the left ventricle.[30,31] A coexistent pericardial laceration allows free hemorrhage into the pleural or peritoneal cavity. Those who reach the hospital alive typically have a pericardial effusion and may develop pericardial tamponade. A characteristic mill-wheel murmur, the bruit de moulin, may be heard.

Pericardial Injury. Pericardial tears may result from direct thoracic impact or from an acute increase in intra-abdominal pressure. The tears most commonly occur on the left (64%), paralleling the phrenic nerve; the diaphragmatic surface (18%), right pleuropericardium (9%), and mediastinum (9%) are the next most frequent sites.[30] Herniation of the heart through a large tear may be associated with significant cardiac dysfunction. A pericardial rub may be detected on physical examination. The chest radiograph may demonstrate pneumopericardium, displacement of the heart, or bowel gas in the chest. Echocardiography or CT may be required to confirm the injury. In a stable patient, a subxiphoid pericardial window should be performed, followed by sternotomy in the presence of hemopericardium or a visible pericardial tear. An unstable patient may require ED thoracotomy. Pericardial lacerations should be repaired, but large holes that cannot be closed primarily should be left widely open to prevent future cardiac herniation. A late complication is the postpericardiotomy syndrome, manifested by fever, chest pain, pericardial effusion, a pericardial rub, and electrocardiographic abnormalities; this is adequately treated with anti-inflammatory agents.

Valvular Injury. Lethal cardiac trauma involves the valves in approximately 5% of patients. The most commonly injured valve is the aortic, followed by the mitral, tricuspid, and pulmonary. The aortic cusps may be lacerated or avulsed when a sudden increase in intrathoracic pressure leads to a concomitant increase in aortic pressure. The result is often acute, severe cardiac failure, but a mild injury may present with syncope or anginal symptoms.[32] Violent compression of the heart in early systole, during isovolumetric contraction, may tear mitral valve leaflets but more commonly ruptures the papillary muscles or chordae tendineae. Acute heart failure may ensue, and a holosystolic murmur of mitral regurgitation is heard.[33] Tricuspid valve injuries are rare; they usually occur in the subvalvular area following compression in late diastole. They are generally of less hemodynamic consequence than aortic or mitral valve injuries are. However, endocarditis and hepatic dysfunction from chronic venous congestion have been reported. Cardiac catheterization and echocardiography are used to confirm the diagnosis. Most valve injuries are amenable to supportive care until other injuries have been stabilized. Valve repair is generally preferred over valve replacement, when feasible.[34]

Septal Injury. Septal injuries are found in 5% to 7% of patients dying from blunt trauma. Ventricular septal ruptures are much more common than atrial septal injuries; they usually occur in the muscular portion near the apex. Characteristic physical findings include a systolic thrill and a harsh holosystolic murmur heard best at the left sternal edge and radiating to the right, but the symptoms may be delayed for hours or days as the defect enlarges. Atrioventricular conduction abnormalities may also be present, simulating myocardial ischemia, and severe hypoxemia may result from an acute left-to-right shunt. Prompt echocardiography is indicated to establish the diagnosis; cardiac catheterization may be needed.

Small septal defects may heal primarily, allowing expectant management with periodic follow-up. Surgical repair— either primary or with a patch graft—is indicated if the patient is hemodynamically compromised or has a left-to-right shunt with a shunt ratio of 2:1 or greater. Repair of the defect is delayed for several weeks, if possible.[35]

Coronary Artery Injury. Direct injuries to coronary arteries are rare. The left anterior descending artery is most susceptible (76% of cases), followed by the right coronary artery (12%) and the circumflex coronary artery (6%). The sequela of coronary artery dissection or thrombosis is myocardial infarction, with ischemic consequences dependent on the vessel and level of injury. Cardiac catheterization is indicated, and therapeutic angioplasty or stenting may be performed occasionally; however, the usual treatment is medical. Recanalization of arteries is frequently reported, but surgical revascularization or repair of delayed complications related to infarction, such as ventricular pseudoaneurysms, may be indicated.[36]

Coronary artery laceration may result in pericardial tamponade, as well as myocardial ischemia. The decision whether to ligate or reconstruct lacerated vessels can be difficult. A nondominant right coronary artery can probably be ligated, but the resultant dysrhythmias may be extremely resistant to treatment. The left anterior descending and circumflex coronary arteries cannot be ligated proximally without causing a large infarct. Reconstruction requires cardiopulmonary bypass, which is frequently poorly tolerated in the early postinjury period and requires systemic anticoagulation. Intraluminal shunts offer a means of minimizing ischemic time while planning elective reconstruction.

Diagnosis, Monitoring, and Treatment

The frequency of the diagnosis of BCI depends on the diagnostic criteria, which may include specific electrocardiographic abnormalities (e.g., ventricular dysrhythmias, atrial fibrillation, sinus bradycardia, bundle branch block), cardiac enzyme elevation, or evidence of cardiac dysfunction on echocardiography or nuclear medicine studies. Unfortunately, none of these tests is predictive of the uncommon but life-threatening complications of ventricular dysrhythmias and cardiac pump failure.[37,38] The pivotal issue is to identify patients at risk and have them in a setting where the complication can be identified and treated.

Our practice guidelines for monitoring patients with suspected BCI are depicted in Figure 245-2. BCI should be suspected in all individuals who sustain major chest trauma. The initial evaluation should include an electrocardiogram (ECG) as part of the secondary survey. Patients with shock from any cause, ischemic changes on the ECG, or significant dysrhythmias are admitted to the ICU. If angina or ischemic ECG changes are noted, the "rule out myocardial infarction" protocol is followed. Nonspecific ECG findings are rarely associated with significant BCI, and patients may be discharged after 24 hours of cardiac monitoring if no new symptoms occur. Patients with significant blunt chest trauma who are being admitted for associated injuries should have cardiac monitoring for 24 hours. A subset of patients may not require admission for other injuries. These patients can be safely discharged from the ED if ECGs at presentation and at 8 hours are normal, and if a troponin I level at 8 hours is less than 1.5 ng/mL.[39]

Dysrhythmias are treated by pharmacologic suppression. The management of cardiogenic shock from cardiac pump failure includes early placement of a pulmonary artery catheter to optimize fluid administration and inotropic support. An echocardiogram may be indicated to exclude septal or free wall rupture, valvular disruption, or pericardial tamponade. Patients with refractory cardiogenic shock may require placement of an intra-aortic balloon pump to decrease myocardial work and enhance coronary perfusion. Patients who sustain significant BCI can have operative procedures under general anesthesia with a low incidence of

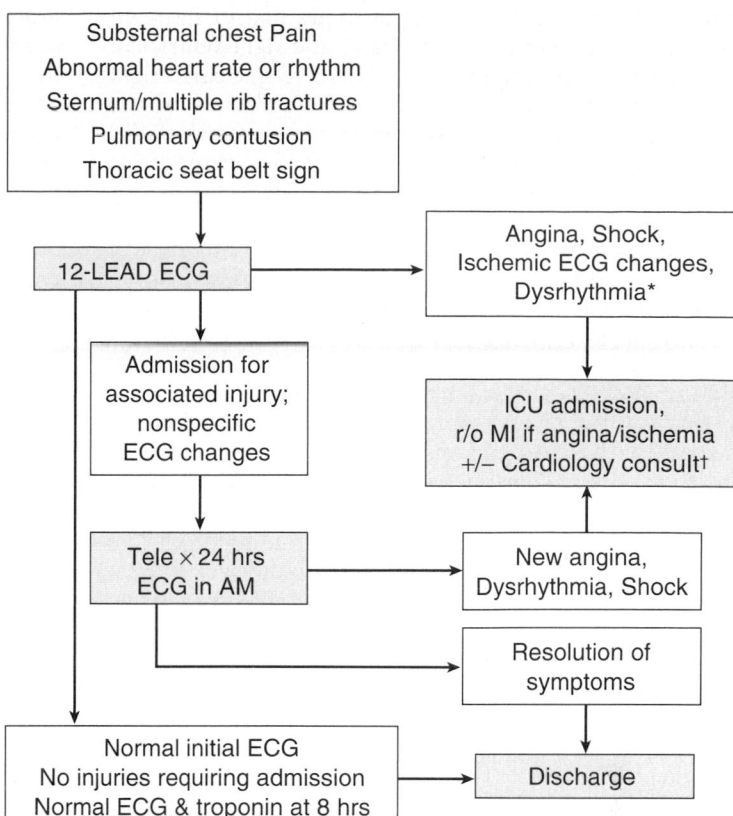

FIGURE 245–2. Evaluation for suspected blunt cardiac injury: blunt chest trauma with substernal chest pain, abnormal heart rate or rhythm, sternum or multiple rib fractures, pulmonary contusion, thoracic seat-belt sign. Ischemic changes consist of ST elevation or depression or T-wave inversion in two leads. Dysrhythmia consists of frequent premature atrial or ventricular contractions, heart block, new atrial fibrillation, or bundle branch block. Echocardiogram may be indicated in selected patients with unexplained or refractory shock, new murmur, or clinical suspicion of pericardial effusion or tamponade. ECG, electrocardiogram; MI, myocardial infarction.

*Ischemic changes: ST elevation/depression, T wave inversion in ≥ 2 leads; Dysrhythmia: Frequent premature atrial/ventricular contractions, heart block, new atrial fibrillation/bundle branch block
†Echocardiogram may be indicated in selected patients with unexplained or refractory shock, new murmur, or clinical suspicion of pericardial effusion/tamponade

cardiac complications; however, they should have close hemodynamic monitoring in the early postinjury period.

Commotio cordis is a distinct entity in which "virtually instantaneous cardiac arrest is produced by nonpenetrating chest blows in the absence of heart disease or identifiable morphologic injury to the chest wall or heart."[40] In a series of 70 cases, Maron and colleagues reported a 90% mortality rate in a young (mean age, 12 years) population of patients.[40] An experimental model demonstrated that ventricular fibrillation is reproducibly triggered by a precisely timed blow during a narrow window within the repolarization phase of the cardiac cycle (15 to 30 msec before the peak of the T wave). Heart block may be produced by a blow during the QRS complex.[41]

PENETRATING CARDIAC INJURY

Cardiac penetration is rapidly lethal in 90% of gunshot wounds and up to 50% of stab wounds. The most important factors for survival are rapid transport to the trauma center, early diagnosis, and immediate treatment. Patients arriving in extremis after penetrating chest trauma should undergo ED thoracotomy. All patients in shock with penetrating chest injuries between the right midclavicular line and left anterior axillary line should be considered to have a cardiac injury until proved otherwise.[42] The right ventricle, with its maximal anterior exposure, is at greatest risk, followed by the left ventricle, right atrium, and left atrium. Multiple cardiac structures are involved in a third of patients. Stab wounds are more commonly associated with tamponade, while gunshot wounds generally bleed freely into the chest.

Repair of cardiac injuries can be accomplished through either a median sternotomy or a thoracotomy incision. In a hemodynamically compromised patient, left anterior thoracotomy with transsternal extension is used for definitive repair. Otherwise, in a hemodynamically stable patient, sternotomy is generally preferred. A limitation of sternotomy is access to posterior injuries or associated aortic or esophageal injuries. In any case, control of hemorrhage is the first priority. Satinsky clamps are useful in isolating atrial or caval injuries, whereas small ventricular lacerations are controlled digitally. Larger wounds may occasionally require insertion of a Foley catheter with temporary balloon occlusion of the wound to facilitate repair, being careful not to extend the injury.[43] Wounds that are too large for balloon occlusion are occasionally salvageable using temporary caval inflow occlusion.[44]

PERICARDIAL TAMPONADE

Potential pericardial tamponade should be suspected in all patients sustaining penetrating injuries to the anterior chest wall. Pericardial tamponade can be a two-edged sword: although it may limit initial blood loss, it can prove fatal by restricting diastolic filling of the heart.[45] As blood leaks out of the injured heart, it accumulates in the pericardial sac. Because the pericardium is not acutely distensible, the pressure in the pericardial sac rises to match that of the injured chamber. When this pressure approaches that of the right atrium, right atrial filling is impaired, and right ventricular preload is reduced; ultimately, this leads to decreased right ventricular output. Increased intrapericardial pressure also impedes myocardial blood flow, which leads to subendocardial and later subepicardial ischemia, with a further reduction of cardiac output. This vicious cycle may progress insidiously with injury to low-pressure conduits, or it may occur precipitously with a ventricular wound. Acute tamponade of as little as 100 mL of blood within the pericardial sac can produce life-threatening hemodynamic compromise.

Early diagnosis is key, because these patients may appear deceptively hemodynamically stable; however, only a small additional hemopericardium may cause abrupt cardiac arrest. Compensatory responses, including catecholamine-mediated tachycardia and vasoconstriction, can transiently stabilize the hemodynamic status of the patient. Similarly, vigorous fluid administration may improve the patient's vital signs. The classic findings of Beck's triad (hypotension, distended neck veins, and muffled heart sounds) are present in less than 10% of patients; furthermore, Kussmaul's sign (neck vein swelling with inspiration) and pulsus paradoxus (systolic blood pressure drop with inspiration) are not reliable indicators of acute tamponade. In fact, neck veins may not become distended until hypovolemia is corrected. Thus, the surgeon must have a high index of suspicion for pericardial tamponade.

In the setting of suspected pericardial tamponade, ultrasonography in the ED, using subxiphoid and parasternal views (or formal echocardiography, if immediately available), is extremely helpful if the findings are positive. If so, the patient should be transported immediately to the operating room for sternotomy. However, if ultrasonography is equivocal, a central venous pressure line should be inserted promptly. Persistently elevated central venous pressure in a patient with thoracic trauma should prompt consideration of ultrasound-guided pericardiocentesis or subxiphoid pericardial window. If the pericardial ultrasonography is positive and there will be any delay in getting to the operating room, pericardiocentesis should be done even if the patient appears hemodynamically stable, because subclinical myocardial ischemia can lead to sudden lethal dysrhythmias. The pericardial tap should be performed with a pigtail catheter to allow repeated aspiration during preparation for thoracotomy. In the setting of shock, evacuation of as little as 15 mL of blood may dramatically improve the patient's hemodynamic profile. Pericardiocentesis is successful in decompressing tamponade in approximately 80% of cases; most failures are due to clotted blood within the pericardium. Although a subxiphoid pericardial window can be created under local anesthesia in the ED, hemorrhage may be difficult to control if an injury is found. If pericardiocentesis is unsuccessful and the patient remains severely hypotensive (systolic blood pressure <70 mm Hg), ED thoracotomy should be performed.

TRANSMEDIASTINAL PENETRATING TRAUMA

Transmediastinal trajectory of a bullet should be considered in the setting of (1) entry and exit wounds on opposite sides of the thorax, (2) a single entry wound with the bullet ending up on the opposite side of the thoracic cavity or in close proximity to the mediastinum, or (3) multiple gunshot wounds to the thorax. Significant injury, especially to the heart or great vessels, often results in prehospital death or hemodynamic instability. There is little controversy regarding the management of unstable patients: they should have emergent thoracotomy. However, stable patients may harbor occult injuries to critical mediastinal structures (heart, great vessels, trachea, esophagus). Consequently, patients have routinely been submitted to a battery of invasive diagnostic tests: echocardiography or subxiphoid pericardial window, arch aortography, bronchoscopy, esophagoscopy, and esophagography.[46] The last two have been employed together to improve on the sensitivity of each test individually. This array of tests can be expensive and time-consuming. Further, only a small percentage of hemodynamically stable, asymptomatic patients have clinically significant injuries.[47]

Helical CT of the chest has proved useful in demonstrating the trajectory of missiles in the thorax.[48,49] In the setting of a potential transmediastinal gunshot wound, a CT scan may confirm a trajectory remote from the mediastinum, obviating further testing. A proven transmediastinal trajectory mandates further evaluation. However, rather than performing all the aforementioned tests, the investigation can be tailored to the specific clinical scenario. For example, trajectory near the pericardium warrants echocardiography or pericardial window. If CT suggests aortic or great vessel injury, arteriography should follow (see later). Bronchoscopy is indicated for pneumomediastinum, respiratory distress, or bronchopleural fistula or massive air leak. The esophagus is evaluated as outlined earlier. Our current approach to evaluating these patients is outlined in Figure 245-3.

THORACIC GREAT VESSEL INJURY

Patients with penetrating injuries to extrapericardial thoracic great vessels usually succumb in the field; however, an occasional patient arrives with a contained hematoma. Early chest radiography is critical to identify hemothorax, as well as a widened mediastinum. Patients who are hemodynamically unstable should be taken directly to the operating room; those in extremis should undergo ED thoracotomy. A reasonable approach can be inferred from the chest radiograph and the location of the wounds. If the patient has a left hemothorax, a left anterolateral thoracotomy in the third or fourth interspace should be performed. Patients with a right hemothorax should likewise be approached via a right anterolateral thoracotomy. Unstable patients with injuries near the sternal notch may have large mediastinal hematomas or may have lost blood externally. These patients should be explored via a median sternotomy with cervical extension, similar to a penetrating zone I neck wound. Hemorrhage should be controlled digitally until the vascular injury is delineated. In a hemodynamically stable patient, angiography can facilitate a more directed approach. Recent series suggest that clinical assessment may be adequate to detect injuries, obviating arteriography in cases in which the suspicion is based on periclavicular trajectory alone.[50,51] However, it must be remembered that collateral flow around the shoulder girdle can result in palpable pulses, even in the presence of a significant proximal injury.

Blunt thoracic great vessel injuries require tremendous force, because the aortic arch branch arteries are protected by strong musculoskeletal tissues. Traction and compression forces are responsible for most injuries. After the aortic isthmus (see later), the most commonly injured artery in the chest is the innominate artery. The clinical presentation is

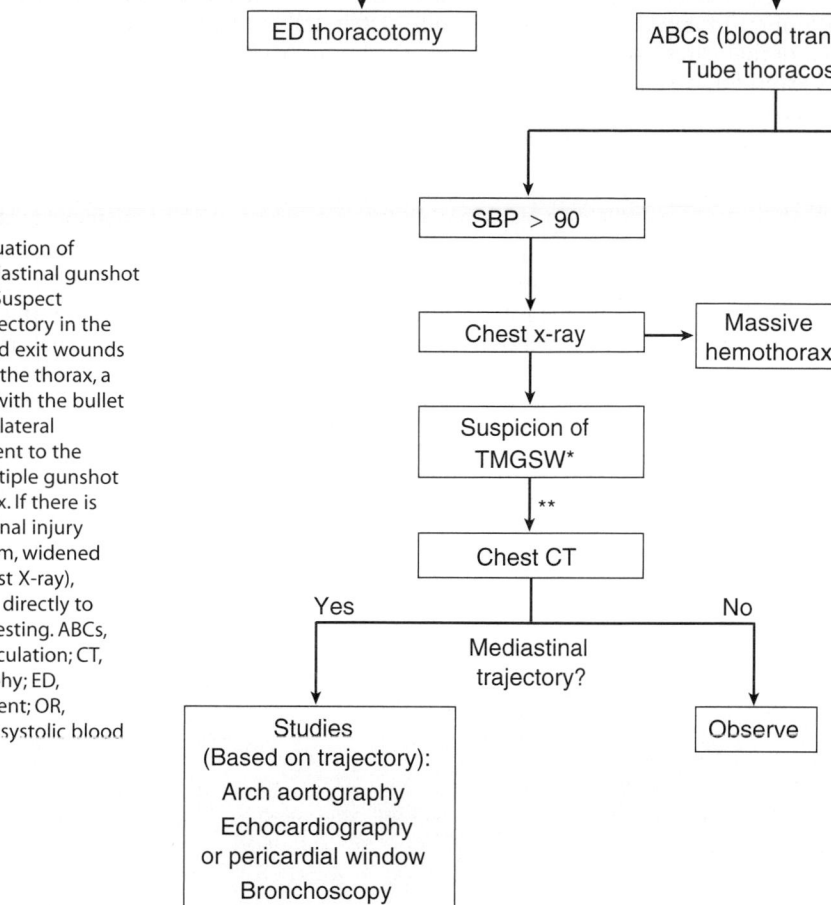

FIGURE 245–3. Evaluation of suspected transmediastinal gunshot wounds (TMGSWs). Suspect transmediastinal trajectory in the presence of entry and exit wounds on opposite sides of the thorax, a single entry wound with the bullet located in the contralateral hemithorax or adjacent to the mediastinum, or multiple gunshot wounds to the thorax. If there is evidence of mediastinal injury (pneumomediastinum, widened mediastinum on chest X-ray), consider proceeding directly to invasive diagnostic testing. ABCs, airway, breathing, circulation; CT, computed tomography; ED, emergency department; OR, operating room; SBP, systolic blood pressure.

*Suspect transmediastinal trajectory in the presence of:
Entry and exit wounds on opposite sides of the thorax
Single entry wound with missile in contralateral hemithorax or adjacent to mediastinum
Multiple gunshot wounds to the thorax.
** If evidence of mediastinal injury (pneumomediastinum, widened mediastinum) consider proceeding directly to invasive diagnostic testing.

less dramatic than that of penetrating injuries, with the typical signs and symptoms related to arterial insufficiency. Until CT-angiography and magnetic resonance angiography are better studied, arteriography remains the gold standard for diagnosis.

A median sternotomy, with appropriate extension, is used for exposure of the innominate, proximal right carotid, proximal right subclavian, and proximal left carotid arteries. The proximal left subclavian artery presents a unique challenge. Because it arises from the aortic arch posteriorly, it is not readily approached via a median sternotomy. A left posterolateral thoracotomy provides excellent exposure to the descending thoracic aorta but severely limits access to other structures. The best option is to create a full-thickness flap of the upper chest wall. This is accomplished with a third or fourth interspace anterolateral thoracotomy for proximal control, a supraclavicular incision, and a median sternotomy

that links the two horizontal incisions. If necessary, the ribs can be transected laterally, allowing the flap to be folded laterally, but this is rarely required. This incision has been referred to as an open-book or trapdoor thoracotomy. The midportion of the subclavian artery is accessible via a supraclavicular skin incision.

The great vessels are rather fragile and can be easily torn during dissection or crushed with a clamp. For this reason, injuries adjacent to the aortic arch are oversewn, and a graft is inserted onto a new location on the arch. The graft is then sewn to the distal artery without tension. Nonoperative management of nonocclusive peripheral arterial injuries has proved successful, and there are limited data supporting similar management within the thorax for certain patients. Similarly, those lesions associated with severe neurologic injuries are usually managed nonoperatively. However, pseudoaneurysms and all symptomatic injuries should be treated operatively.[52] Experience with intravascular stenting is growing but is still limited; its role remains to be defined.

BLUNT THORACIC AORTIC INJURY

Perhaps the most feared occult injury in trauma surgery is a tear of the thoracic aorta. The mechanism of aortic tears is believed to be primarily a shearing force. The tear usually occurs just distal to the left subclavian artery, where the aorta is tethered by the ligamentum arteriosum. In 5% of cases, the tear occurs in the ascending aorta, in the transverse arch, or at the diaphragm. An estimated 85% of thoracic aortic injuries are fatal at the injury scene. A multicenter report from the American Association for the Surgery of Trauma (AAST) analyzed 274 accident-scene survivors of blunt thoracic aortic injury.[53] Motor vehicle crashes accounted for 81% of the injuries, with frontal impact in 72%, lateral impact in 24%, and rear impact in 4%. Two additional series also documented substantial numbers of torn thoracic aortas following lateral-impact crashes: 57 of 165 (35%) autopsy cases reported by Burkhart and colleagues,[54] and 48 of 97 (50%) cases reviewed by Katyal and colleagues.[55] Thus, the surgeon should suspect this injury whenever there is significant energy transfer, regardless of directionality.

Chest radiograph is considered the initial screening tool for determining whether further investigation is needed for blunt aortic injury. Commonly associated radiographic findings include mediastinal widening, obscured aortic knob, deviation of the left mainstem bronchus (downward) or nasogastric tube (rightward), and opacification of the aortopulmonary window (Fig. 245-4A). In the AAST multicenter study,[53] widening of the mediastinum on the anteroposterior chest radiograph was present in 85% of cases. However, 7% of patients with torn aortas had normal chest radiographs. Dyer and colleagues reported normal initial radiographs in 13% of patients.[56] Thus, additional investigations are warranted in the setting of significant energy transfer. Thoracic aortography was previously considered the gold standard for diagnosis (see Fig. 245-4C). However, helical CT scan is now well accepted as an excellent screening test (see Fig. 245-4B).[56-58] When hematoma adjacent to the thoracic aorta is considered a positive finding, CT's sensitivity for aortic injury is 100% in large series. Some authors advocate omitting the aortogram and operating on the basis of CT alone, but this is up to the individual surgeon. Transesophageal echocardiography is portable and fairly sensitive and specific; however, it is highly operator dependent and is not reliable for visualizing the ascending or transverse

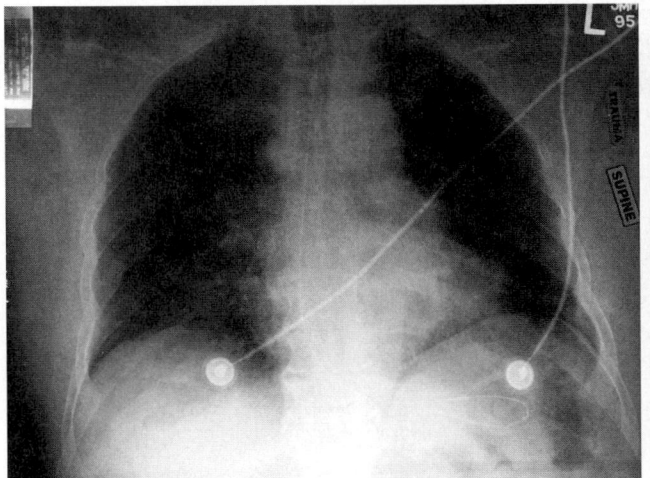

A

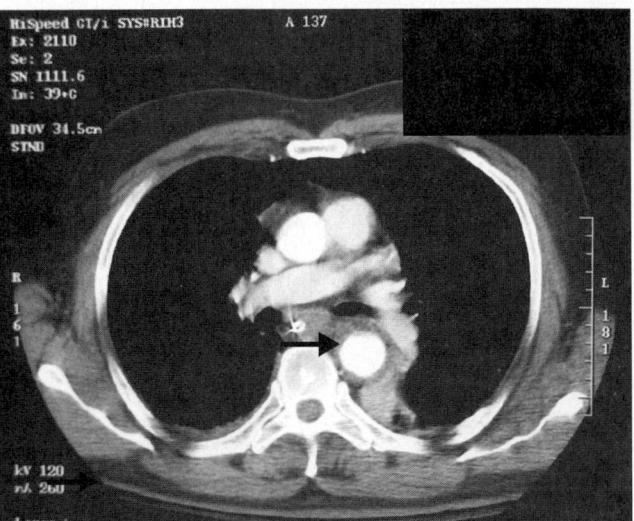

B

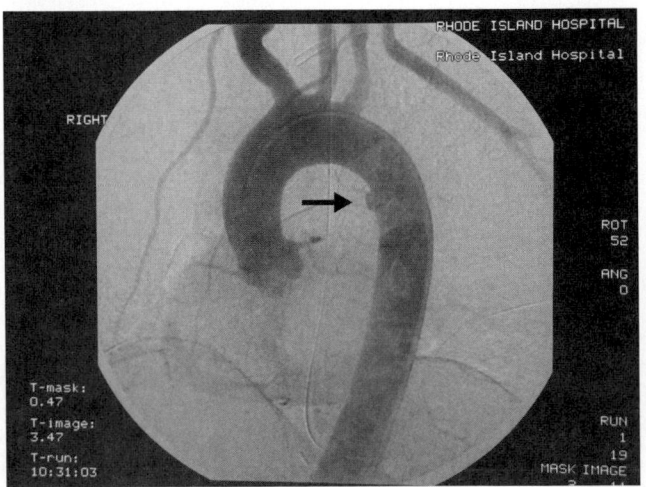

C

FIGURE 245–4. Images from a patient with a descending thoracic aortic injury. *A,* Anteroposterior chest radiograph. Note the widened mediastinum and widened left paratracheal stripe, indistinct aortic knob, and slight depression of the left mainstem bronchus. *B,* Helical CT scan of the chest. Note the periaortic hematoma *(arrow). C,* Digital subtraction arteriogram of the aortic arch. Note the pseudoaneurysm in the common location, distal to the left subclavian artery *(arrow).*

aorta or its branches. It has been supplanted by CT, and its primary role may be in following small intimal injuries that are managed nonoperatively. Intravascular ultrasonography is another tool with a poorly defined role.

Once aortic injury is diagnosed, the systolic blood pressure and heart rate should be controlled (target <100 mm Hg, <100 beats/min) with a rapidly reversible beta-blocking agent to reduce aortic shear pressure.[57] Repair of the descending thoracic aorta has been associated with some controversy, with respect to both who should repair it and how it should be accomplished. At present, both thoracic and trauma surgeons are managing these injuries. With respect to technique, a primary concern has been the occurrence of paraplegia from ischemic injury of the spinal cord. Conceptually, two techniques have been advocated. The simpler technique, often referred to as "clamp and sew," is accomplished with the application of vascular clamps proximal and distal to the aortic injury. Razzouk and colleagues have successfully employed this technique in the majority of their patients over a 25-year period.[59] However, this method results in transient hypoperfusion of the spinal cord distal to the clamps, as well as of abdominal organs. In the AAST study,[53] the paraplegia incidence was 1.6% in patients with cross-clamp times less than 30 minutes, but 12% if the time was greater than 30 minutes. A 20-year meta-analysis found a 19% incidence of paraplegia associated with this method and noted that average cross-clamp times were over 40 minutes.[60] The alternative approach is to provide some method for maintaining spinal perfusion during cross-clamping. Two techniques have been used to accomplish this goal—one passive, and one active. Passive shunting uses a temporary extra-anatomic route around the clamps. A heparin-impregnated tube, the Gott shunt, was specifically designed for this purpose. However, blood flow to the distal aorta is inadequate; consequently, this technique is no longer used. With the availability of centrifugal pumps that do not require systemic anticoagulation, the current preferred method is to use either active partial left heart bypass (siphoning blood from the left heart and pumping it to the distal aorta) or full bypass, such as femoral-femoral bypass. The former can be a significant benefit in a patient with multiple injuries, particularly in those with intracranial

hemorrhage. However, occasional small cerebral infarcts have occurred; thus, heparin is administered unless contraindicated. The injury may be primarily repaired, or a graft may be inserted. A large, multicenter trial suggested that polytetrafluoroethylene is the preferred graft material for aortic replacement, given its long-term patency and apparent resistance to infection.[61] Recently, endovascular stents have been used for aortic tears. Numerous case reports can be found, but their long-term outcome remains to be clarified. Injuries that are amenable to stenting may be similarly treated nonoperatively. The subgroup of patients with brain injuries or severe thoracic injuries may be best served by delayed operation or nonoperative management.[57,62] Beta blockade is usually administered as a precaution against rupture.

ANNOTATED REFERENCES

Biffl WL, Moore EE, Johnson JL: Emergency department thoracotomy. In Moore EE, Feliciano DV, Mattox KL (eds): Trauma, 5th ed. New York, McGraw-Hill, 2004.
A comprehensive review of the literature on ED thoracotomy. It also provides detailed discussions and descriptions of the procedures.

Dyer DS, Moore EE, Ilke DN, et al: Thoracic aortic injury: How predictive is mechanism and is chest computed tomography a reliable screening tool? A prospective study of 1561 patients. J Trauma 2000;48:673-683.
A large study that examined the specificity of helical CT scanning and established it as an excellent screening tool. It also identified the shortcomings of chest radiographs and the importance of clinical suspicion.

Fabian TC, Richardson JD, Croce MA, et al: Prospective study of blunt aortic injury: Multicenter trial of the American Association for the Surgery of Trauma. J Trauma 1997;42:374-380.
A comprehensive, multicenter data review. This paper discusses all aspects of managing blunt thoracic aortic trauma, with a database that allows conclusions and practice guidelines.

Moon MR, Luchette FA, Gibson SW, et al: Prospective, randomized comparison of epidural versus parenteral opioid analgesia in thoracic trauma. Ann Surg 1999;229:684-692.
This trial demonstrated the superiority of epidural analgesia over parenteral opioids in pain control associated with thoracic trauma. In addition, it documented an attenuated immune response to injury.

Wall MJ, Hirshberg A, Mattox KL: Pulmonary tractotomy with selective vascular ligation for penetrating injuries to the lung. Am J Surg 1994;168:665-669.
The original description of pulmonary tractotomy.

Chapter 246

ABDOMINAL TRAUMA

Vaishali Dixit Schuchert • Andrew B. Peitzman

KEY POINTS

1. **Repeat the initial evaluation** of the patient starting with the primary survey.

2. **Always suspect abdominal injury,** even in the presence of normal results of studies.

3. **Early communication with the trauma surgeon is essential.**

4. It is not always important to establish a specific anatomic diagnosis; **at times an operation serves both diagnostic and therapeutic purposes.**

5. **The unstable patient should not leave the ICU** for abdominal or head CT or other diagnostic tests.

In the management of trauma patients, several key principles must be understood. First, minute-to-minute management must be guided by both the patient's anatomic injuries and hemodynamic stability. Thus, for example, a grade III splenic injury can be safely managed nonoperatively if the patient is hemodynamically stable but urgent exploratory laparotomy is required if the patient is hypotensive or requires massive resuscitation to maintain normal blood pressure. Second, certain injuries infrequently occur in isolation; rather, they occur as a component of a pattern of injuries. Third, the trauma patient admitted to the ICU generally has multiple injuries, any one of which is a potential threat to life or limb. Prioritization of the management of these injuries must be based on the most immediate threat to life or limb. For example, if the patient is hemodynamically unstable or is hypoxemic despite substantial respiratory support, it is not appropriate to perform computed tomography (CT) to exclude cervical spine injury. Fourth, the "damage control" approach mandates that critically injured and hemodynamically unstable patients should be taken to the ICU postoperatively for further stabilization and management.[1-4] Abdominal vascular injuries and major hepatic injuries are the abdominal injuries most often requiring a "damage control" approach. Fifth, the intensivist should always repeat the primary and secondary surveys on new admissions to the ICU with the knowledge that 10% of injuries in trauma patients are detected after admission.[5,6]

Head trauma and hemorrhagic shock are the most common causes of death in trauma patients. The most common etiology of hemorrhagic shock is intra-abdominal bleeding. Late deaths occur from intra abdominal sepsis, most often from hollow viscus injuries. A large proportion of multiply injured patients admitted to the ICU will have either known or suspected abdominal injuries. Often these injuries have been definitively addressed in the operating room. On the other hand, the stable patient with blunt solid organ injury is often managed nonoperatively in the ICU. Missed or delayed diagnosis and treatment of abdominal injuries are common causes of preventable deaths in the trauma population, particularly at inexperienced trauma centers or hospitals without a formal trauma program. The evaluation of the abdomen, as well as the ICU management of abdominal injuries and complications, is the focus of this chapter.

INITIAL ASSESSMENT OF THE TRAUMA PATIENT

The four major steps in the initial assessment and treatment of the trauma patient, whether in the emergency department or the ICU, are primary survey, resuscitation, secondary survey, and definitive care (Table 246-1).[6] The goal of the primary survey in the multiply injured patient is identification and immediate treatment of emergent life-threatening injuries. The airway must be secured, generally in a patient with the potential for having cervical spine injury. Thus, the cervical spine must be immobilized while the patient is intubated. Tension pneumothoraces and significant hemothoraces must be recognized and treated. Adequate circulation and perfusion must be restored. In the patient with active hemorrhage in the chest or abdomen, control of bleeding generally occurs in the operating room. Delaying operative control of ongoing hemorrhage in an attempt to stabilize an actively bleeding patient will fail and increase mortality.[7,8] The primary survey, followed by the secondary survey, generally occurs as part of evaluation in the trauma resuscitation area of the emergency department. The trauma team should proceed to the secondary survey only when the patient has been stabilized based on treatment in the primary survey and resuscitation phases. Furthermore, if a patient deteriorates hemodynamically or fails to respond to seemingly adequate therapy, whether in the trauma bay, the operating room, or the ICU, the initial assessment should be repeated, starting with the primary survey.

In the awake patient, the airway can best be assessed by having the patient speak. A patient able to speak clearly almost always has a stable airway. Hoarseness may indicate an upper airway injury and should prompt an urgent evaluation by an otolaryngologist. Pooled saliva or secretions suggest inability to protect the airway and a risk for aspiration. The indications for orotracheal intubation in the trauma patient

TABLE 246–1. INITIAL ASSESSMENT OF THE TRAUMA PATIENT

Primary Survey

- Identify and treat immediate threats to life.
- Stabilize patient before continuing to the secondary survey.
- Secure airway, treat ventilatory problems, and restore adequate circulation and perfusion.

Resuscitation Phase

- Establish at least two large-bore intravenous lines.
- Resuscitate to specific endpoints (restore blood pressure, ensure adequate urine output, reverse lactic acidosis).

Secondary Survey

- Perform detailed head-to-toe examination of the patient.
- Order radiographic studies.

Definitive Care

- Move the patient from the emergency department to the operating room or ICU as quickly as possible.

include impaired airway protection, increased work of breathing, hypoventilation, refractory hypoxia, and inability to properly assess or manage the patient owing to other factors such as pain, agitation, or intoxication. It is important to assess the airway in the already intubated patient as well. Even small movements of an endotracheal tube during transfer or moving the patient can dislodge the endotracheal tube.

After the airway is secured, breathing must be assessed. Breathing can be compromised by chest wall injury (e.g., rib fractures, flail chest), pneumothorax or hemothorax, or pulmonary parenchymal injury and pulmonary contusion. Physical examination may be unreliable; when possible, a chest radiograph is obtained. In the unstable patient, it is sometimes necessary to perform urgent tube thoracostomy without the benefit of a chest radiograph. Insertion of a thoracostomy tube in these circumstances is both diagnostic and potentially therapeutic.

The multiply injured patient who arrives to the ICU and becomes unstable after initial resuscitation usually has a derangement in circulation. Assessment includes feeling the pulse to determine rate as well as quality and inspection of the distal extremities for warmth, color, and capillary refill. Other signs of impaired perfusion include oliguria and altered mental status. Even with normal vital signs, a substantial portion (up to 75%) of trauma patients in the ICU are hypoperfused.[9-11] Biochemical indices of perfusion, such as base deficit or blood lactate level, should be determined to assess global perfusion.[9-13] The hemodynamically unstable trauma patient is bleeding until proved otherwise. Adequate intravenous access must be obtained, ideally using two large-bore antecubital lines. If necessary, an 8-French introducer can be placed percutaneously into the femoral vein using the Seldinger technique. Triple-lumen catheters do permit adequate flow rates for resuscitating trauma patients. Resuscitation should be started using warmed crystalloid solution or packed red blood cells if the patient is profoundly hypotensive or has failed to respond to crystalloid resuscitation.[14,15] In the unstable patient, transfusion of non-crossmatched blood is often necessary until crossmatched blood becomes available. While instituting these therapeutic maneuvers, attempts should be made to identify and treat the source of bleeding. Major hemorrhage can be external

(visible) or internal (occult). Sources of major blood loss due to trauma include open fractures, scalp lacerations, penetrating vascular injuries, intraperitoneal injuries, retroperitoneal sources (generally due to pelvic fractures in blunt trauma), and fractures of the long bones. The gastrointestinal tract is rarely the source for blood loss acutely in the trauma victim. Although significant blood loss is possible from extremity fractures or even scalp lacerations, it must be assumed that the life-threatening blood loss is from the thorax or abdomen. A completely normal chest radiograph will exclude significant intrathoracic bleeding. Although hypotension that is unresponsive to fluid resuscitation is generally due to ongoing bleeding, cardiac tamponade, tension pneumothorax, and (rarely) neurogenic shock can be the cause. These diagnoses should be considered, but only with the recognition that ongoing hemorrhage or inadequate volume resuscitation is much more likely to be the basis for persistent or recurrent hypotension. The approach taken to evaluate the abdomen as the source of blood loss differs depending on the hemodynamic status of the trauma patient and the mechanism of injury. Because penetrating and blunt abdominal trauma are managed differently, they will be discussed separately.

PENETRATING ABDOMINAL INJURY

Any penetrating wound from the nipple line anteriorly or scapular tip posteriorly to the buttocks inferiorly can produce an intraperitoneal injury.

GUNSHOT WOUNDS

After a rapid primary survey, the entire body must be carefully inspected by rolling the patient on both sides. Special attention should be paid to hidden areas, such as skin folds, body creases, axillae, and the perineum. The number of wounds should be noted. Plain radiographs of the chest, abdomen, and pelvis assist in the evaluation by accounting for bullets and aiding in attempts to estimate the trajectory of the bullets. Management of the trauma patient with truncal gunshot wounds will be determined by the structures likely to be in the path of the bullet. It is important to remember that bullets do not always follow straight courses but can ricochet off bony structures and that trajectory is impossible to determine with complete confidence. The number of external wounds plus the number of bullets found inside the body must equal an even number; an odd number means that a bullet has not been found and other body cavities are at risk. Patients with gunshot wounds that violate the peritoneal cavity, irrespective of vital signs, require immediate exploratory laparotomy. The likelihood of finding injuries requiring operative repair for abdominal gunshot wound is 80% to 95%.[16] The hypotensive patient with an abdominal gunshot wound generally has a major vascular injury and ideally should bypass the emergency department and undergo initial evaluation and resuscitation in the operating room. On rare occasion, in the stable patient with an apparently tangential, extraperitoneal gunshot wound, obtaining an abdominal CT may be appropriate to confirm a tangential, superficial tract.[17]

STAB WOUNDS

Unlike gunshot wounds, the likelihood of finding an injury that requires operative repair in a patient with an anterior abdominal stab wound is only 25% to 33%.[18] Immediate exploration is mandated by hypotension, evisceration, or signs of peritoneal irritation. In the absence of these signs, selective management is justified, provided that a surgeon and operating room are immediately available if the patient's condition changes. Of anterior abdominal stab wounds, one third are extraperitoneal, one third violate the peritoneum but do not produce a visceral injury requiring repair, and one third are intraperitoneal with visceral injury requiring repair.[18] Local wound exploration consists of enlarging the original stab wound under local anesthesia to assess for fascial penetration. If the fascia is breached, laparotomy or diagnostic peritoneal lavage (DPL) may be performed in the trauma resuscitation area. The criteria for positive DPL for stab wounds are fewer than for blunt trauma; the presence of 1000 to 10,000 red blood cells per milliliter of fluid and that of bile, bacteria, or enteric matter are criteria for a positive DPL when the test is used to evaluate abdominal stab wounds.[19-22] In the stable patient with a reliable abdominal examination, the surgeon may elect to perform serial examinations (selective management). The need for exploratory laparotomy is suggested by changes in vital signs (especially temperature or heart rate), development of abdominal tenderness, decreased urine output, or increased leukocyte count. The only role for abdominal CT is for the evaluation of back or flank stab wounds in stable patients, when there is a low suspicion for visceral injury. A triple-contrast (oral, intravenous, and rectal) CT scan is 97% accurate in these injuries.[20,21]

BLUNT ABDOMINAL INJURY

At most hospitals (including trauma centers), blunt injury is seen much more commonly than penetrating injury. In rural or suburban communities, 95% of trauma patients have blunt injury. At urban trauma centers, the incidence of penetrating trauma is higher but the majority of patients admitted (generally 70% to 80%) have blunt mechanisms of injury. Management and decision-making in patients with blunt abdominal injury is often more difficult than it is for patients with penetrating trauma. Most patients with blunt abdominal trauma are the victims of motor vehicle crashes, although crush injuries, sports-related injuries, falls, and assaults account for a fair number of admissions. Patients with blunt abdominal injuries requiring ICU care generally have injuries involving multiple systems, including the central nervous system, thoracic organs, or major long bones. These patients are generally intubated, are unresponsive, and have the potential for injury anywhere. Identification and prioritization of care for all of the injuries is a major challenge in the ICU management of blunt trauma patients.

As mentioned earlier, ongoing hemorrhage is the most likely cause of persistent or recurrent hemodynamic instability despite initial attempts at crystalloid resuscitation. In these patients, once the primary survey has been completed, an aggressive search must be made to find and stop the source of bleeding. The source of bleeding is usually in the thorax or the abdomen. The chest is evaluated by chest radiograph or, on occasion, tube thoracostomy and/or thoracotomy, which serve both diagnostic and therapeutic purposes if the patient is in extremis.

Careful, repeated physical examination is critical for the evaluation of blunt abdominal injury. The initial goal is not to diagnose a specific abdominal organ injury but rather to determine whether there are signs and symptoms that indicate a need for immediate laparotomy. If an awake patient is complaining of abdominal pain, the clinician's index of suspicion for serious abdominal injury should be high. However, the absence of pain or tenderness, especially in the presence of other distracting injuries, does not exclude the possibility of significant intra-abdominal injury. Evaluation of the abdomen in blunt trauma is challenging; physical examination fails to detect significant injury in 45% of patients.[23] These patients are often unconscious, inebriated, or distracted by pain originating from other injuries. Seatbelt marks or other external signs of trauma may be evidence that substantial energy has been imparted and there is a high risk for internal injuries. Twenty to 30% of patients with lap-belt marks have associated mesenteric or intestinal injuries.[24] Thirty percent of patients with lumbar Chance fractures have associated bowel or mesenteric injuries.[24] Because physical examination alone is unreliable so frequently in the evaluation of blunt abdominal injury, diagnostic tests have a key role in the management of these patients.[17,19-32] Which diagnostic tests, if any, are warranted is largely determined by the patient's hemodynamic status. If the patient is in extremis, the best strategy may be immediate transfer to the operating room for placement of bilateral chest tubes and exploratory laparotomy. There is no role for plain abdominal radiographs in the evaluation of blunt abdominal trauma. The FAST exam (Focused Abdominal Sonography in Trauma) has been utilized in Europe and Japan for decades and has become the first-line diagnostic test at many trauma centers in the United States. FAST has a sensitivity and specificity of 70% to 95%.[25,26] The technique involves directing the ultrasound probe in four regions: (1) the subxiphoid location to determine whether there is fluid in the pericardial space and to make a rough assessment of cardiac contractility and filling; (2) the right upper quadrant; (3) the splenorenal recess; and (4) the pelvis. Any fluid seen between the liver and kidney, between the spleen and kidney, or in the pelvis outside the bladder is presumed to be blood. The goal with FAST is to visualize intraperitoneal blood; the examination is not reliable enough to be used for identification of specific organ injuries. The FAST is routinely performed in the trauma resuscitation area as an adjunct to the secondary survey. It can be performed rapidly at the bedside regardless of the patient's hemodynamic status; it is noninvasive and relatively inexpensive; and it can be repeated as necessary. Accuracy depends on the skill of the sonogram operator. Because children can have solid organ injuries without hemoperitoneum, the false-negative rate with FAST is higher in the pediatric age group.[33] There also can be false-negative test results with thoracic spine or pelvic fractures. FAST is technically more difficult and often limited in obese patients or in the setting of subcutaneous emphysema.

CT of the abdomen and pelvis is the diagnostic modality of choice for the stable blunt trauma patient. The major main reason not to obtain a CT scan is hemodynamic instability; hemodynamically unstable patients should not be placed in the radiology department for CT scan or any radiographic study. CT has been reported to be 92% to 98% accurate in the assessment of blunt abdominal injury.[28,29] Unlike FAST and DPL, CT is both sensitive and specific. Both hemoperitoneum and its source can be identified; specific organ injuries can be graded. In addition, CT permits evaluation of retroperitoneal structures, including the kidneys, major blood vessels (e.g., aorta and inferior vena cava), and the bony pelvis. CT has revolutionized the management of solid abdominal organ injury; the majority of blunt injuries to the spleen, liver, and kidneys are currently managed nonoperatively in trauma centers. A blush of intravenous contrast agent indicates active extravasation from a bleeding vessel and is a strong predictor of failure of nonoperative management.[34] By using interventional radiologic approaches, it is often possible to control arterial bleeding in association with pelvic fractures, hepatic injury, or, in selected cases, splenic injury. Technical disadvantages of CT are the need to transport the patient to the radiology suite or other area, the time involved in transfer and scanning, and the risks associated with infusion of intravenous contrast agents. Hollow viscus, diaphragmatic, and pancreatic injuries are frequently missed by CT, at least when the scan is initially performed.

DPL has an accuracy of 98% for detection of hemoperitoneum.[30] As with FAST, DPL can determine the presence of intraperitoneal blood but not its source. DPL, although used less often since the widespread adoption of the FAST, still has a role in the evaluation of the unstable patient. DPL is generally performed in the trauma resuscitation area for the evaluation of multiply injured patients who are too unstable for transport to the CT scanner. A positive FAST obviates the need to perform a DPL in the unstable patient; the next step in the care of these patients is immediate laparotomy. A negative FAST, however, does not exclude intra-abdominal bleeding. DPL also has a selective role in the evaluation of abdominal stab wounds. It is also an appropriate test for patients with blunt trauma requiring an emergency operation for another injury, such as immediate evacuation of an intracranial mass lesion (subdural or epidural hematoma). The technique for performing DPL involves a mini-laparotomy with placement of the lavage catheter into the peritoneal cavity, directed toward the pelvis. The return of 10 mL of gross blood is a positive result. If the DPL is grossly negative, 1 L of warmed saline is instilled into the abdominal cavity. This fluid is then drained back into the intravenous fluid bag by gravity. The effluent lavage fluid is sent to the laboratory for analysis. Laboratory criteria for positive DPL in blunt trauma are more than 100,000 RBCs/mm³, more than 500 WBCs/mm³, or the presence of food particles, bile, or bacteria. The most obvious disadvantage to DPL is that it is an invasive procedure. DPL is highly accurate, but one fourth of the patients with positive DPL have injuries that result in a nontherapeutic laparotomy.[21,22] In addition, DPL may yield false-negative results (4% to 5%) with retroperitoneal, hollow viscus, or diaphragmatic injuries. This technique, similar to FAST, does not identify specific injuries but answers the question: does the patient have intraperitoneal blood?

SPECIFIC ORGAN INJURIES

DIAPHRAGM

Diaphragmatic injuries due to penetrating trauma are very difficult to diagnose.[31] Penetrating thoracoabdominal wounds, particularly on the left side, can produce small diaphragmatic defects that are a cause for internal hernias with entrapped bowel that become apparent years later. If the trajectory suggests the possibility of diaphragmatic injury, then appropriate evaluation should be carried out. In the stable patient with a thoracoabdominal penetrating injury, laparoscopy may be a useful technique.[32]

With blunt diaphragmatic injury, the chest radiograph is diagnostic in 25% of patients and shows an obscured left hemidiaphragm in 25% to 50% of cases, but is often normal.[35] If the diaphragm is injured, it may be difficult or impossible to pass a nasogastric tube owing to herniation of the stomach into the chest. Alternatively, the nasogastric tube may be observed above the left hemidiaphragm on the chest radiograph. The majority of diaphragmatic injuries are associated with other significant intra-abdominal injuries. Diaphragmatic injuries occur more commonly on the left side than the right side. A normal CT scan of the chest or abdomen does not preclude a diaphragmatic injury. Diaphragmatic injury is acutely repaired via exploratory laparotomy, because of the high likelihood of associated abdominal injury. When diagnosed late, diaphragmatic injuries can be repaired through the thorax.

STOMACH, SMALL BOWEL, AND COLON

The stomach, small bowel, and colon are often involved in gunshot injuries. The small bowel is the most commonly injured organ in cases of penetrating abdominal trauma. These injuries are usually diagnosed intraoperatively because the vast majority of gunshot wounds to the abdomen result in laparotomy. Bowel injuries from blunt trauma are extremely difficult to diagnose. Injury to the bowel can be present despite initially normal findings by abdominal CT, FAST, and routine laboratory studies. The possibility of hollow viscus injury always should be considered when evaluating patients with blunt trauma to the abdomen or multiple trauma, particularly if examination reveals lap-belt marks or a Chance fracture. Injuries that violate the mucosa should be repaired primarily. Devitalized segments must be débrided, sometimes necessitating a formal bowel resection and anastomosis. In the case of a colonic injury, the degree of intra-abdominal contamination and the presence or absence of shock should guide operative management (repair vs. resection and colostomy).[36]

RECTUM

Gross blood on rectal examination signifies a rectal injury, whether from penetrating or blunt injury. Blunt rectal injury generally occurs in association with a pelvic fracture. Rectal injuries are challenging from a management standpoint. The four "Ds" of operative management are divert (diverting colostomy), distal washout, drainage (wide presacral drainage), and definitive repair (repair the hole itself). Postoperative issues include stoma care and the change in lifestyle for the patient. The risk of pelvic sepsis, particularly in association with a pelvic fracture, is high. Any pelvic fracture that leads to perforation of skin or (rectal or vaginal) mucosa is by definition an open fracture. Open pelvic fractures account for only 5% of cases but 50% of mortality.

PANCREAS

Most pancreatic injuries are caused by penetrating trauma. Blunt injury to the pancreas is usually the result of a crush injury (e.g., steering wheel, handle bars, blunt weapons). The vast majority of pancreatic injuries are associated with other intra-abdominal injuries. Because of the anatomic location of the pancreas there is a strong association between pancreatic injury and injury to major blood vessels (e.g., aorta, inferior vena cava, portal vein). In part due to its retroperitoneal location, injury to the pancreas is often difficult to diagnose. Measurements of serum amylase concentration are neither sensitive nor specific. Physical examination, FAST, and CT are often unrevealing. Mechanism of injury and associated intra-abdominal injuries may provide the best clues to the presence of a pancreatic injury. Endoscopic retrograde cholangiopancreatography (ERCP) may delineate a major pancreatic ductal injury in the stable patient not requiring laparotomy for other injuries. The appropriate management of major pancreatic injury, especially when there is disruption of the pancreatic duct, is operative.[37,38] The presence or absence of a major ductal injury should guide operative management. Devitalized tissue must be débrided. If the major duct is intact, wide drainage is sufficient. Formal resection may be necessary with ductal injury. Wide local drainage with closed suction drains is paramount in either case. This approach converts the uncontrolled leakage of tissue-destructive pancreatic secretions into a controlled pancreatic fistula, which usually can be managed conservatively.

DUODENUM

Most duodenal injuries are associated with other intra-abdominal injuries, and penetrating trauma is the most common mechanism. The second portion of the duodenum is the most frequently injured segment. Findings on CT suggestive of duodenal injury include paraduodenal hematoma, retroperitoneal or intraperitoneal air, or leakage of contrast agent outside the lumen. An upper gastrointestinal contrast study may aid in the diagnosis of duodenal injury, if this diagnosis is suspected in a stable patient. The diagnosis of duodenal injury is most commonly made at the time of laparotomy carried out for the treatment of associated injuries. On abdominal exploration, the presence of bile staining, retroperitoneal air, or a central (zone I) retroperitoneal hematoma suggests duodenal injury. Operative management varies depending on the location and degree of injury. Most duodenal injuries are amenable to primary closure. As with any injury, any devitalized tissue must be débrided. Extensive injuries may require pyloric exclusion and gastrojejunostomy. Repairs will require protective tubes to keep the duodenum decompressed; placement of a gastric tube connected to suction is always necessary. Retrograde tubes in the jejunum may be employed for further decompression of the duodenal closure. A feeding jejunostomy tube is often placed at the time of operative repair.

LIVER

The liver is the most commonly injured intra-abdominal organ. In the patient stable enough to undergo CT, liver injury is easily identified. Up to 80% of patients with liver injuries can be treated nonoperatively. The key factor determining whether operation is needed is the presence or absence of hemodynamic stability. Patients with major liver injuries generally arrive hemodynamically unstable and require urgent laparotomy. Patients with liver injuries, who are stable enough to undergo CT, generally can be managed nonoperatively.[39-41] Nonoperative management typically consists of ICU admission, bed rest, serial measurements of hemoglobin concentration, aggressive correction of any coagulation defects, and serial abdominal examination. The presence of a contrast blush on CT suggests ongoing bleeding and identifies patients who are likely to fail nonoperative management. Angioembolization is rapidly becoming the first line of treatment for liver injuries that fail nonoperative management; this modality is also useful in the postoperative management of patients with major hepatic injury.[42,43] Operative management may involve simply packing the abdomen to tamponade bleeding, performing hepatorrhaphy with cautery or suture, or carrying out extensive débridement and resection. Closed suction drains are placed around injuries greater than grade III for potential bile leaks (Table 246-2). As many as 25% of patients with liver injuries that are initially managed nonoperatively will require a subsequent intervention for a complication.[42] These complications include bile leak, biloma, abscess, hemobilia, and, less commonly, bleeding. The vast majority (85%) of these complications can be managed with endoscopic retrograde cholangiopancreatography and stent placement, angiography and embolization, or percutaneous drain placement.[42]

SPLEEN

The spleen is commonly injured in blunt trauma. Left upper quadrant pain and referred pain to the left shoulder (Kehr's sign) may be elicited from awake and communicative patients. Twenty-five percent of patients with left lower rib

TABLE 246–2. LIVER INJURY SCALE (1994 REVISION)

Grade*	Type of Injury	Description of Injury	AIS-90
I	Hematoma	Subcapsular, < 10% surface area	2
	Laceration	Capsular tear, < 1 cm parenchymal depth	2
II	Hematoma	Subcapsular, 10% to 50% surface area; intraparenchymal hematoma < 10 cm in diameter	2
	Laceration	Capsular tear 1 to 3 cm parenchymal depth, < 10 cm in length	2
III	Hematoma	Subcapsular, > 50% surface area or expanding; ruptured subcapsular or parenchymal hematoma; intraparenchymal hematoma > 10 cm or expanding	3
	Laceration	Parenchymal depth > 3 cm	3
IV	Laceration	Parenchymal disruption involving 25% to 75% hepatic lobe or 1 to 3 Couinaud's segments	4
V	Laceration	Parenchymal disruption involving > 75% of hepatic lobe or > 3 Couinaud's segments within a single lobe	5
	Vascular	Juxtahepatic venous injuries (i.e., retrohepatic vena cava/central major hepatic veins)	5
VI	Vascular	Hepatic avulsion	6

*Advance one grade for multiple injuries up to grade III.
AIS, Abbreviated Injury Score.
From Peitzman A, Rhodes M, Schwab CW, et al: Trauma Manual, 2nd ed. Philadelphia, Lippincott Williams & Wilkins, 2002.

fractures have a splenic injury. In stable patients, CT allows identification and grading of a splenic injury. As with liver injury, only hemodynamically stable patients should be considered for nonoperative management. In the unstable patient, FAST or DPL may be positive for hemoperitoneum, often owing to splenic injury. Over 90% of children with blunt splenic injury are candidates for nonoperative management.[44] The failure rate (i.e., need for delayed laparotomy) in children with splenic injury managed nonoperatively is less than 2%.[45-47] Unlike adults, children with blunt splenic injury can be managed nonoperatively irrespective of the grade of splenic injury or the quantity of blood in the peritoneum. Sixty-five to 85 percent of adult patients with splenic injuries can be successfully treated nonoperatively. Again, hemodynamic stability is the key criterion for nonoperative management. In adults, the risk factors for failure of nonoperative management include increasing grade of splenic injury, increasing hemoperitoneum, contrast blush on abdominal CT, and age older than 55 years (this factor is controversial) (Table 246-3).[46] The failure rate of nonoperative management of blunt splenic injury in adults is 10% overall. The failure rates by grade are as follows: grade I (5%), grade II (10%), grade III (20%), grade IV (33%), and grade V (75%).[45-47] Hemodynamic instability mandates immediate laparotomy. There is an increasing role for angioembolization in the management of patients with splenic injuries and failure of nonoperative management. Patients rendered asplenic should be immunized against *Streptococcus pneumoniae* (using Pneumovax, 0.5 mL i.m.), *Hemophilus influenzae* (Act HIB, 0.5 mL i.m.), and *Neisseria meningitidis* (MenomuneACYW-135, 0.5 mL i.m.). It is currently recommended that Pneumovax be administered every 5 to 10 years post splenectomy in adult patients.

GENITOURINARY

Hematuria is the hallmark of genitourinary injury. Macroscopic hematuria mandates further evaluation of the genitourinary tract. Microscopic hematuria should prompt further testing in any patient with physical findings suggestive of injury or a mechanism of injury consistent with genitourinary injury. Physical findings include penetrating injuries in proximity to the genitourinary tract structures, lower rib fractures, flank ecchymosis or tenderness, spine fractures, hypotension, or multiple injuries. Straddle injuries (associated with risk for urethral injury) or high-energy impact injuries (i.e., motor vehicle crash) are likely to produce a genitourinary injury. Microscopic hematuria in a child younger than age 15 years warrants further work-up. Blood at the urethral meatus should prompt cystourethrography before Foley catheterization. Pubic rami fractures in males are a relative indication for performing a cystourethrogram in the trauma resuscitation area. Similarly, the finding of gross hematuria on initial catheterization or voiding in any multiply injured trauma patient should prompt immediate cystography. Abdominal and pelvic CT with intravenous contrast medium enhancement is the modality of choice for diagnosing renal trauma.

RETROPERITONEAL HEMATOMA

The retroperitoneum is divided into three zones.[48] All retroperitoneal hematomas in penetrating trauma require exploration. In blunt trauma, zone II (lateral) and zone III (pelvic) hematomas should not be explored unless they are expanding or pulsatile. Zone I (central) hematomas should be explored in cases of blunt injury; 65% will have associated visceral injury (aorta or branches, inferior vena cava, pancreas, or duodenum).[48]

ICU MANAGEMENT

Admission to the ICU after initial resuscitation in the trauma bay or operating room necessitates reevaluation of the patient. This is best accomplished by repeating the primary survey, then moving on to the secondary (head-to-toe) survey. This reevaluation is vital for several reasons. During transport to the ICU, monitoring of the patient is perfunctory and tubes and lines sometimes become dislodged. In addition, a substantial amount of time has elapsed since the initial primary survey. The secondary survey may have been interrupted by more pressing issues, such as the urgent need for operation. The decision to move the patient to the ICU may have been made because of a decline in clinical status (e.g., development of acidosis, hypothermia, and/or coagulopathy). It is important to reemphasize that 10% of trauma patients have injuries that are missed during the initial evaluation. Furthermore, up to 25% of abdominal injuries are undetected at the time of presentation. A rapid but thorough primary

Grade*	Injury Type	Description of Injury	AIS-90
I	Hematoma	Subcapsular, < 10% surface area	2
	Laceration	Capsular tear, < 1 cm parenchymal depth	2
II	Hematoma	Subcapsular, 10% to 50% surface area; intraparenchymal hematoma, < 5 cm in diameter	2
	Laceration	Capsular tear, 1 to 3 cm parenchymal depth that does not involve a trabecular vessel	2
III	Hematoma	Subcapsular, > 50% surface area or expanding; ruptured subcapsular or parenchymal hematoma; intraparenchymal hematoma, ≥ 5 cm or expanding	3
	Laceration	Parenchymal depth > 3 cm or involving trabecular vessels	3
IV	Laceration	Laceration involving segmental or hilar vessels producing major devascularization (>25% of spleen)	4
V	Laceration	Completely shattered spleen	5
	Vascular	Hilar vascular injury that devascularizes spleen	5

TABLE 246–3. SPLEEN INJURY SCALE (1994 REVISION)

*Advance one grade for multiple injuries up to grade III.
AIS, Abbreviated Injury Score.
From Peitzman A, Rhodes M, Schwab CW, et al: Trauma Manual, 2nd ed. Philadelphia, Lippincott Williams & Wilkins, 2002.

and secondary survey on ICU admission may identify problems before they become life threatening.

ICU MANAGEMENT AFTER "DAMAGE CONTROL" LAPAROTOMY

Patients may arrive in the ICU after "damage control" laparotomy, most often with penetrating abdominal vascular or major hepatic injuries. "Damage control" refers to urgent abdominal exploration with the basic goal of controlling massive bleeding and preventing ongoing peritoneal contamination.[1-4] Patients often arrive in the ICU with hypothermia, acidosis, and coagulopathy. After "damage control" surgery, the next goal is to warm the patient and correct acidosis and coagulopathy with a plan to return to the operating room for definitive resection and/or reconstruction, as needed. Warming blankets and a warm room are essential and should be ready before the patient's arrival to the ICU. All intravenous fluids should be warmed. The gases in the ventilator system should be warmed as well. Rarely, invasive techniques for active rewarming are required to rapidly achieve normothermia. These techniques include peritoneal lavage or lavage through tube thoracostomies with warm saline, hemodialysis, or cardiopulmonary bypass. Acidosis is generally the result of global hypoperfusion and/or anemia and should be corrected by restoring intravascular volume and circulating hemoglobin concentration. Failure to correct acidosis or coagulopathy should alert the clinician to the possibility of ongoing bleeding, which may require urgent, early return to the operating room in 20% of these critically ill patients.[1-4] The intensivist caring for these patients must maintain a high index of suspicion for surgical bleeding and should alert the trauma surgeon of any concerns. Crush injuries can lead to acidosis secondary to rhabdomyolysis, but muscle necrosis is an uncommon cause of early acidosis. Coagulopathy results from both hypothermia and acidosis. Clotting factors function best at normal values for temperature and pH. Standard coagulation studies (prothrombin time, partial thromboplastin time) are likely to be normal, because the assays are performed at 37°C in the laboratory. Coagulopathy also occurs from dilution of platelets and clotting factors after massive blood transfusion. Platelets should be replenished in proportion to the transfusion of packed red cells. Recommended indications for platelet transfusion include a platelet count less than 20,000/mm³ or less than 50,000/mm³ in high-risk patients (patients with solid viscus injury, major pelvic fracture, or intracranial hemorrhage), impaired platelet function, and massive transfusion (greater than 15 units of packed red blood cells). Clotting factors should be replaced based in part on total blood loss, but abnormalities do not follow a linear relationship based on blood loss. Recommended indications for replacement therapy with thawed fresh frozen plasma include ongoing bleeding secondary to coagulopathy (documented or presumed), elevated prothrombin time or partial thromboplastin time in a patient with intracranial hemorrhage, major pelvic fracture, or solid viscus injury or anticipated transfusion of greater than 10 units of packed red blood cells. Calcium is a required clotting factor that is bound by citrate, a preservative in packed red blood cells, and must be replaced aggressively. Calcium replacement therapy should be based on frequently measured ionized calcium levels. Finally, a consumptive coagulopathy may occur in the presence of a large retroperitoneal hematoma or fulminant disseminated intravascular coagulation. The treatment of disseminated intravascular coagulation is supportive and should focus on treatment of the underlying etiology.

In most cases of "damage control," the abdomen is left open with plans to return to the operating room in 24 to 48 hours. Several trips to the operating room may be necessary before closure of the abdominal wall is possible. At every exploration, bleeding and gastrointestinal spillage are managed and devitalized tissue is débrided. Once definitive repair of specific structures and reestablishment of bowel continuity is achieved, definitive closure of the abdomen is undertaken.

In the "damage control" approach, laparotomy pads are usually left in the abdomen as packing in areas associated with high risk for bleeding, such as the pelvis, around the liver, and around the spleen. Packing serves to tamponade low pressure venous vessels, thereby controlling hemorrhage. After the initial damage control procedure, segments of intestine may have been resected with the open ends stapled closed rather than re-anastomosed to restored continuity of the gastrointestinal tract. Generally, the fascia is not closed, because definitive closure of the abdomen is deferred until the final operation. To prevent evisceration and minimize spillage of ascites, several techniques have been developed. The skin may be closed with a running suture if there is enough mobility of the skin. Under most circumstances, edema in all tissues precludes this type of closure and other devices are used. The "Bogota bag" closure is a product of the creativity of a surgical resident in Colombia, who used a sterilized intravenous fluid bag as a bridge to temporarily close the abdominal wall and prevent evisceration.[49] This closure affords the advantage of providing a "window" to the underlying bowel but frequently leaks ascites, creating problems for dressing the wound. The "Vac-Pack" closure is the fastest approach. This closure consists of placing a nonstick surface, such as a bowel bag, on the viscera. Suction drains are sandwiched between two sterile blue towels.[50] A large, clear, occlusive dressing covers the entire abdomen. The drains are connected to wall suction. When done properly, taking pains to prevent any air leaks in the system, the entire dressing "vacuum packs" the abdomen. This approach provides a clean, easy-to-maintain temporary closure.

Postoperative care of the multiply injured patient presents ongoing challenges to the intensivist. Unlike the postoperative general surgical patient in whom the problem or insult has been definitively addressed, the trauma patient has other injuries that may not be recognized yet.

Patients arriving to the ICU from the trauma resuscitation area or from the operating room having undergone extra-abdominal operations can be particularly challenging to manage. Often these patients do not have any documented abdominal injuries. A negative reading of an initial abdominal CT can lull the caregiver into not considering the abdomen as a site of significant injury. However, even when the initial CT is completely normal, hollow viscus, diaphragmatic, or pancreatic injuries can still be present. The clinician must remain vigilant for unrecognized abdominal trauma when taking care of patients with multiple injuries.

It is common for the intensivist to assist in the nonoperative management of known abdominal trauma. Most solid organ (liver, spleen, and kidney) injuries are managed nonoperatively.[39,41,45,46] Patients requiring immediate operation for solid organ injuries are those with other proven or suspected intra-abdominal injuries, hemodynamic instability, hilar injuries evident by CT, or a "blush" of extravascular intravenous contrast agent, suggesting ongoing active bleeding. Most patients with diagnosed kidney, liver, or splenic lacerations are admitted to the ICU for serial physical examinations, serial measurements of laboratory parameters, and strict bed rest. Hemoglobin concentration is followed using serial determinations. Coagulation parameters, such as platelet count, prothrombin time, and ionized calcium concentration, are optimized. Changes in hemodynamic status, including tachycardia, warrant reassessment by the clinician and evaluation for bleeding. Changes in the physical examination or hemodynamic status or a requirement for blood transfusion must be communicated promptly to the trauma surgeon. Any clinical deterioration may necessitate immediate angiography with embolization or operation.

Delayed complications from either known or unsuspected intra-abdominal injuries generally manifest as sepsis. The possibility of missed hollow viscus injury is a major concern during the nonoperative management of patients with a solid viscus injury. The success rate is high, in large part because of the low incidence of blunt hollow viscus injuries (<1%) in patients with blunt abdominal trauma.[51,52] However, when solid organ injuries are identified, the risk of hollow viscus injury increases. Thus, 6% of patients with one solid organ injury will have an associated hollow viscus injury; 22% of patients with two solid organ injuries will have a hollow viscus injury; and more than one third of patients with three solid organ injuries will have a hollow viscus injury.[53] Any work-up for the cause of fever in the patient with multiple injuries must take into consideration the possibility of abdominal sepsis.

ABDOMINAL COMPARTMENT SYNDROME

Abdominal compartment syndrome (ACS) occurs in up to 10% of trauma patients. It is defined as symptomatic organ dysfunction that results from an increase in intra-abdominal pressure.[54] ACS most commonly develops in trauma patients requiring massive volume resuscitation. The clinical manifestations that should alert the clinician to the possibility of ACS are a tense distended abdomen, increased requirements for mechanical ventilation, high airway pressures, and progressively worsening oliguria. Increased intra-abdominal pressure also adversely affects cardiac output, venous return, and mesenteric perfusion. Physical examination is often unreliable in these patients. In addition, central filling pressures (central venous pressure and pulmonary artery pressures) are often normal in the setting of ACS. The cardiac output will be low if the patient is hypovolemic, but it may be normal or elevated in euvolemic or hypervolemic patients.[54] Diagnosis is aided by the measurement of intravesical pressure.[54] This measurement is performed by instilling 50 to 100 mL of sterile normal saline into the bladder with the Foley drainage tube clamped. Intravesical pressure is measured by inserting a needle attached to a pressure transducer into the aspiration port of the Foley catheter. Conversion to a three-way Foley catheter facilitates making repeated measurements. The transducer is zeroed at the level of the pubic symphysis. This technique may be unreliable in the presence of pelvic fractures, morbid obesity, pregnancy, or a neurogenic bladder. In general, a bladder pressure greater than 25 mm Hg almost always signifies ACS in the appropriate clinical setting. However, no absolute value of bladder pressure makes the diagnosis of ACS in all patients. The trauma surgeon should be alerted if there is any concern about impending ACS. The only definitive management of ACS is operative decompression leaving the abdomen open ("Vac-Pack" closure). Despite a heightened awareness of the syndrome, mortality remains high. Most patients do not die as a direct result of ACS. Rather, ACS is a marker that identifies the critically ill trauma patient with severe physiologic derangements.

ANNOTATED REFERENCES

Demetriades D, Velmahos G: Indications for laparotomy. In Moore EE, Feliciano DV, Mattox KL (eds): Trauma. New York, McGraw-Hill, 2004, p 593.
  A resource chapter for indications for laparotomy.

Frankel HL, Boone DC, Peitzman AB: Abdominal trauma. In Peitzman AB, Rhodes M, Schwab CW, et al (eds): The Trauma Manual, 2nd ed. Philadelphia, Lippincott Williams & Wilkins, 2002, p 236.
  An overview of the approach to abdominal injury in a concise, easy-to-understand handbook.

Peitzman AB, Heil B, Rivera L, et al: Blunt splenic injury in adults: Multi-institutional study of the Eastern Association for the Surgery of Trauma. J Trauma 2000;49:177.
  A multicenter review of 1488 adult patients with blunt splenic injury. Predictors of successful nonoperative management are described.

Richardson JD, Franklin GA, Lukan JK, et al: Evolution in the management of hepatic trauma: A 25-year perspective. Ann Surg 2000;232:324.
  An important review of the changes in management of hepatic trauma over 25 years, with a marked shift toward nonoperative management. The mortality for bleeding from major hepatic injury has declined in part because of better trauma care but also because many of the major hepatic injuries are now managed without operation.

Shapiro MB, Jenkins DH, Schwab CW, et al: Damage control: Collective review. J Trauma 2000;49:969.
  A review of the key principles in damage control in the management of critically ill trauma patients.

Chapter 247

PELVIC AND MAJOR LONG BONE FRACTURES

Anatole Besman • Orlando Kirton

KEY POINTS

1. Most deaths in patients with pelvic fracture are from head injury, nonpelvic hemorrhage, pulmonary injury, thromboembolic complications, and multiple organ system failure.

2. Hemorrhage from unstable pelvic fractures can be minimized by early re-approximation and stabilization of the pelvic ring. If this is unsuccessful, angiography with embolization can be helpful.

3. Approximately 15% of seriously injured motor vehicle passengers presenting to a level I trauma center have femur fractures.

4. Associated injuries occur in more than 80% of patients and are responsible for more than 90% of deaths in patients with femur fracture.

5. Infection can manifest as an acute complication of fracture, with gas gangrene, or necrotizing fasciitis, a life-threatening infection. Treatment generally consists of debridement and antibiotic therapy.

6. Tetanus can result from any open fracture, but patients who have had farming accidents are at particularly high risk. Diagnosis relies on clinical recognition. Treatment consists of supportive care, surgical debridement, passive immunization, and antibiotics.

7. Diagnosis of compartment syndrome can be made on clinical grounds when the compartment is tense on physical examination, severe pain is present with passive motion, the compartment is tender throughout, and sensory nervous function is impaired.

8. Treatment of rhabdomyolysis involves aggressive intravenous fluid therapy to avoid the accumulation of myoglobin in the renal tubules and aiding the clearance of hyperkalemia.

9. It is estimated that 5000 deaths occur annually due to fat embolism syndrome after pathologic fracture, traumatic fracture, and orthopedic surgery combined.

10. The diagnosis of fat embolism syndrome is based on the presence of the classic triad of respiratory compromise, mental status changes, and petechial rash in the setting of long bone fractures or orthopedic surgery. Treatment is supportive.

11. A number of risk factors for thromboembolic disease have been identified, including long bone and pelvic fractures, age older than 40, immobility, blood transfusion, multiple trauma, head injury, spine fracture, spinal cord injury, and high injury severity score.

12. Signs and symptoms may be present in only 1.5% of patients diagnosed with deep vein thrombosis by venography.

13. Because of its low cost, noninvasive nature, and high accuracy, color-flow duplex ultrasonography has become the test of choice for deep vein thrombosis.

14. Treatment of deep vein thrombosis and pulmonary embolism usually starts with full anticoagulation using unfractionated heparin transitioning to sodium warfarin after a period.

15. Fifty percent of deaths caused by pulmonary embolism occur within the first hour. After that, patients are at a 2.5% to 10% risk of dying when treated adequately and at a 30% risk of death when untreated.

Pelvic and long bone fractures have serious local and systemic consequences for the trauma victim. Familiarity with the sequelae of serious orthopedic injuries is essential for the successful management of these patients in the ICU.

PELVIC FRACTURE

Pelvic fractures are present in about 10% of patients presenting to a level I trauma center after blunt trauma.[1] The incidence of pelvic fracture is highest after motorcycle crash, pedestrian trauma caused by a motor vehicle, falls from height greater than 15 feet, and motor vehicle crash, in that order.[1] The overall mortality rate for pelvic fracture is from 7% to almost 14%, rising to nearly 30% with severe or open fractures.[1-3] However, less than 3% of patients die as a direct result of hemorrhage from the pelvic fracture itself.[1-3] Most deaths in patients with pelvic fracture are from head injury, nonpelvic hemorrhage, pulmonary injury, thromboembolic complications, or multiple organ system failure.[1-4] There is a high incidence of solid and hollow organ injury and other skeletal trauma in patients with pelvic fracture due to the powerful forces involved.[1,2,4] More then 90% of patients with a pelvic fracture have other associated injuries, including gastrointestinal injuries (5%) and abdominal injuries

(16.5%).[1,2] Risk factors for associated abdominal injury include motor vehicle crash, fall greater than 15 feet, and pelvis Abbreviated Injury Severity Score greater than 3.[1,4] Overall Injury Severity Score and mortality is correlated with the severity of the pelvic fracture, although death is usually the result of associated injuries rather than the fracture itself.[3]

Complications occur in roughly one third of patients. Infections are the most common complication (15.7%), followed by respiratory complications (9.3%), hematologic complications (5.5%), and thromboembolic complications (3.4%).[5] Cardiac complications occur in about 2.5% of patients.[5] Patients with unstable pelvic fractures are at significantly greater risk of complications than those with stable fractures.[5,6] The mean transfusion requirement for patients with pelvic fracture is 8 units of packed red blood cells but can be much greater.[5] The degree of hemorrhage is highly dependent on the type of fracture. Complete dissociation of the posterior pelvis has the highest degree of hemorrhage and connected mortality.[7] Significant hemorrhage often occurs from other sites, such as the abdomen or thorax, as well. Less than 1% of all patients with pelvic fractures have hypotension based on blood loss attributable to the fracture itself.[5,8] Nevertheless, 12% of patients with open pelvic fractures die as direct result of hemorrhage.[6]

Hemorrhage from unstable pelvic fractures can be minimized by early re-approximation and stabilization of the pelvic ring. Stabilization can be accomplished with external fixation devices such as the Browner clamp or expediently with as simple an appliance as a bed sheet wrapped tightly around the pelvis. If external pelvic fixation is unsuccessful at restoring hemodynamic stability after initial resuscitation and other sources of ongoing hemorrhage have been ruled out, angiography to evaluate and treat pelvic arterial bleeding is indicated. Pelvic arterial disruption is responsible for hemorrhage in less than 5% of all cases of pelvic fracture.[8-10] A blush of contrast identified on pelvic computed tomography (CT) scan is evidence for arterial bleeding and is an indication for angiography.[8]

LONG BONE FRACTURE

The most studied and serious long bone fracture is fracture of the femur. Approximately 15% of seriously injured motor vehicle passengers presenting to a level I trauma center have femur fractures.[11] Eight percent to 10% of these patients have bilateral fractures.[11,12] The mortality rate for unilateral fracture is 10% to 12%.[11,12] Mortality increases to 26% to 33% with bilateral fractures and is 20% in patients older than 65 year of age.[11-13] As in pelvic fractures, death is more closely connected with the severity of associated injuries rather than the fracture itself.[11-13] Predictably, other injuries are responsible for more than 90% of deaths in patients with femur fracture.[14]

Associated injuries occur in more than 80% of patients with femur fracture.[14] Blunt trauma patients who present with femur fracture have a higher incidence of abdominal, thoracic, and skeletal injuries compared with patients without femur fracture.[11,12] Those with bilateral fractures have an increased incidence of head injury, requirement for laparotomy, and pelvic fracture as compared with those with a unilateral femur fracture.[11,12]

The risk of complications, including acute respiratory distress syndrome (ARDS), pneumonia, and fat embolism syndrome, in the multiply injured patient with femur fracture can be markedly decreased by early operative fixation within 24 hours.[15,16] Early operative repair also results in decreased ICU length of stay, hospital stay, cost, and risk of mortality.[15,16]

Although hemorrhage is a feared complication of femur fracture, a study of isolated femur fracture found that blood loss from the fracture itself is insufficient to cause hypotension.[17] Of 100 patients with isolated femur fractures, only 24% were in class I or II shock. None were in class III or IV shock. Nevertheless, hemorrhage is the cause of death in a significant proportion of patients with femur fracture, an indication of the importance of other sites of hemorrhage in these patients.[12] In addition, special attention must be paid to avoid occult hypoperfusion (nonhypotensive shock), which is associated with an increased incidence of complications, especially infections, in patients with femur fracture.[18] Hemorrhage from long bone fractures is best managed by early stabilization. Stabilization can be initiated with traction splints such as a Hare traction splint for femur fractures or closed reduction and splinting for other fracture sites.

LOCAL COMPLICATIONS

INFECTION

Infection can manifest as an acute complication in the setting of both long bone and pelvic fractures. Acute infection of a fracture hematoma or fracture repair can manifest with cutaneous signs such as erythema, warmth, and induration. However, if the infected site is deep to the fascia, infection may manifest with systemic signs such as leukocytosis and fever without cutaneous signs.[19] Diagnosis can be achieved using CT, magnetic resonance imaging, three-phase bone scan, or radiolabeled white blood cell scans. Plain radiographs are less useful; findings are often delayed until 10 to 21 days after the onset of infection.[20] The most common causative organism is *Staphylococcus aureus*, but infection may be due to many other organisms, including *Pseudomonas aeruginosa* and Enterobacteriaceae.[7,19] Generally, these infections take a week or more to manifest.

Treatment depends on the organism or organisms present. The best option in high-risk open fractures remains prophylactic antibiotics tailored to provide coverage against both gram-positive and gram-negative organisms. One common regimen consists of a first-generation cephalosporin (e.g., cefazolin, 1 g intravenously immediately then every 8 hours) and an aminoglycoside (e.g., tobramycin, 7 g/kg body weight intravenously immediately, then every 24 hours) administered for 72 hours starting prior to surgery. For established infections, the mainstay of treatment is debridement of devitalized and infected bone and soft tissue followed by antibiotic therapy tailored to operative culture results. Hyperbaric oxygen has been used as an adjunct to therapy for osteomyelitis, but convincing data showing efficacy are lacking.[19,21]

Gas gangrene, or necrotizing fasciitis, can appear within the first 24 hours after fracture or operative repair. These fulminant, necrotizing infections usually occur in the setting of open fracture with extensive soft tissue injury requiring debridement and are especially likely if there is a delay in treatment. The causative organism is *Clostridium perfringens* in 10% of cases, with synergistic multiple organisms including *Streptococcus*, anaerobes, and coliform bacteria causing the remainder.[7,19] Findings can include skin changes, purulent or "dishwater" wound drainage, and profound shock due to vasodilatation. Treatment is aggressive surgical debridement of necrotic tissue, which may require amputation, and broad-spectrum antibiotics or high-dose penicillin. Hyperbaric oxygen also can be used in conjunction with surgical and pharmacologic treatment. Prophylaxis consists of early treatment of open fractures with thorough debridement of all devitalized tissue. Despite treatment, gas gangrene often results in fatality due to the severe septic manifestations of this infection.[7,19,20]

Tetanus can result from any open fracture, but patients with fractures caused by farming accidents are at particularly high risk. Symptoms, caused by *Clostridium tetani* toxin, occur 1 to 2 weeks after injury and are often fatal. The case fatality rate is about 60%.[7] Presenting symptoms include trismus, difficulty swallowing, restlessness, and headache. The syndrome progresses to convulsions and asphyxia. Muscle spasm and convulsions are caused by excitation of spinal motor neurons. Diagnosis relies on clinical recognition, as cultures are positive in only one third of cases.[7,19]

Prophylaxis consists of 0.5 mL adsorbed tetanus toxoid administered intramuscularly on presentation for all patients with traumatic wounds, including open fractures, who have not received a booster within the last 5 years. High-risk patients, such as those involved in farming accidents or with neglected wounds, are candidates for tetanus immunoglobulin (250 units administered by deep intramuscular injection). Antibiotics are not adequate prophylaxis. Treatment of diagnosed tetanus infection consists of sedation, supportive care, including airway management with intubation or a surgical airway, surgical debridement of the infected wound, passive immunization with tetanus immunoglobulin (recommended doses vary from 500 IU to 10,000 IU administered intramuscularly), and antibiotics (metronidazole 500 mg administered intravenously every 8 hours).[7,19]

COMPARTMENT SYNDROME

Compartment syndrome is a potentially devastating complication that arises in the setting of either open or closed fracture. Tissue edema and bleeding raise the pressure in the fixed volume of a fascial compartment, which impedes blood flow, especially in arterioles and capillaries, resulting in tissue ischemia. The degree of tissue necrosis depends on the pressure within the compartment, the duration of time during which compartment pressure is elevated, and the sensitivity of specific tissues to ischemia. Nervous tissue demonstrates functional abnormalities after 30 minutes of ischemia with irreversible loss of function occurring after 12 to 24 hours. Muscle, on the other hand, does not exhibit functional effects for 2 to 4 hours and irreversible loss of function occurs after 4 to 12 hours. Capillary permeability also increases, resulting in further tissue edema.[7,22]

The most common location for compartment syndrome after fracture is the anterior compartment of the leg. This complication usually results from closed tibia fracture. As many as 17% of patients with a tibia fracture secondary to a motor vehicle crash develop a compartment syndrome.[22] Compartment syndrome of the thigh can develop after open or closed fracture and may develop after operative treatment of the fracture. Compartment syndrome of the arm, buttock, and foot are also possible after fracture. Risk factors associated with developing compartment syndrome include the severity of the fracture and associated soft tissue injury, the use of compressive devises such as military antishock trousers or tourniquets, and systemic hypotension.[7,22,23]

Diagnosis of compartment syndrome can be made on clinical grounds. The diagnosis is established when the compartment is tense on physical examination, severe pain is present with passive motion, the compartment is tender throughout, and sensory nervous function is impaired. Loss of distal pulses is often the last manifestation of compartment syndrome. By the time pulses and distal perfusion are diminished, extensive necrosis of tissues within the compartment already may be present. It is important to be aware that compartment syndrome can occur both acutely and after operative fixation of a fracture. The diagnosis must be made early before permanent tissue damage has occurred. Serial examinations are critical to monitor for compartment syndrome in patients at risk.[7,22]

Measurement of compartment pressure is an additional way to confirm the diagnosis. Measurements are not necessary when the diagnosis is clear on clinical grounds. They are useful when the physical examination is limited because the patient is unresponsive due to head injury or sedation. Compartment pressure values ranging from 30 to 45 mm Hg have been recommended as the threshold for triggering surgical intervention.[22] Compartment pressures are measured by placement of a sterile needle connected to a pressure transducer into each compartment. Alternatively, commercial devices such as the Stryker compartment monitor (Stryker, Kalamazoo, Michigan) are available that accomplish the same task.

Treatment is by urgent, complete surgical fasciotomy to open all affected compartments. Care must be taken to adequately open the skin because it may constrict the compartment, even if the fascia has been opened. Fasciotomy can be performed in the ICU if the patient is too unstable to be transported to the operating room. Complete fasciotomy within 12 hours of onset results in a normal functional outcome in 68% of cases, whereas delay decreases the likelihood of successful outcome to 8%.[24]

Once the compartment has been opened, wash-out of the metabolic products of the ischemic compartment occurs. It is critical to closely monitor acid-base status, serum potassium concentration, serum myoglobin concentration, fluid status, and renal function. Adequate hydration and monitoring of serum electrolyte levels are critical to successful postoperative care of these patients. The clinician must also be aware of the high incidence of infection at the fasciotomy site.[23,24]

RHABDOMYOLYSIS

Rhabdomyolysis can occur for several reasons after skeletal trauma. The most obvious reason is direct injury to muscles surrounding the fracture site. Direct injury to skeletal muscle tissue is especially likely when the mechanism of injury resulted in transfer of a great deal of energy; an example is a motor vehicle crash. Second, rhabdomyolysis can occur secondary to compression of tissues for a prolonged period after the injury. The compression causes an ischemic injury to the involved muscle. Lastly, rhabdomyolysis can result from compartment syndrome due to a fracture. Again, the mechanism involves compression of circulation resulting in an ischemic injury. All three mechanisms of rhabdomyolysis can be exacerbated by hemorrhagic shock.[25,26]

The systemic effects of rhabdomyolysis are the result of anaerobic metabolism and cell lysis. Lactic acid release can lead to systemic acidosis, especially if volume replacement is inadequate. Potassium and myoglobin are released by the lysed myocytes. Hyperkalemia can lead to life-threatening cardiac arrhythmias. Intravenous calcium should be used with caution in this setting because it can rapidly combine with phosphate anions, leading to precipitation of calcium salts if hyperphosphatemia from muscle necrosis is present. Elevated serum myoglobin levels can cause direct renal tubular damage, leading to acute renal failure.

The successful treatment of rhabdomyolysis involves aggressive intravenous fluid therapy to maximize tubular flow rate, avoiding the accumulation of myoglobin in the renal tubules and aiding the clearance of hyperkalemia. Administration of iron-chelating agents such as desferriox-amine (standard dosage for rhabdomyolysis not established) and alkalinization of the urine using sodium bicarbonate as 50% of the resuscitation fluid (150 mEq dissolved in 1 L of 5% dextrose solution) or a carbonic anhydrase inhibitor such as acetazolamide is recommended by some experts. Ultimately, acute renal failure may necessitate hemofiltration or hemodialysis.[25,27-29] In our institution, we aim to maintain a urine output of 1 mL/kg/hr using intravenous fluids and follow serial serum and urine myoglobin levels. We have had good success in avoiding acute renal failure without the use of urine alkalinization or iron-chelating agents.

FAT EMBOLISM SYNDROME

Pathophysiology

Fat embolism syndrome occurs when marrow fat particles embolize to the pulmonary and systemic circulation via injured veins in the setting of acute fracture or fracture repair. Larger particles lodge in the pulmonary circulation, whereas smaller particles (7-10 μM) will pass through to the systemic circulation. In experimental models of fat embolism syndrome and autopsy series of blunt-trauma patients, the degree of fat embolization, the severity of pulmonary compromise, and deaths attributable to fat embolism syndrome correlate with the severity of and the number of fractures.[30-32] Other causes of systemic embolization include intrapulmonary shunts and patent foramen ovale.[33]

Beyond simple occlusion of capillaries, liberation of free fatty acids is thought to be pathophysiologically significant through the activation of inflammatory processes and/or direct toxicity to lung capillaries and pneumocytes. Histamine and serotonin are also released, exacerbating pulmonary dysfunction and causing bronchospasm and vasospasm.[19,24,30,34,35]

Epidemiology

Estimates of the number of patients with fractures who develop the pulmonary, skin, and neurologic manifestations of fat embolism syndrome vary between 0.5% and 20%.[7,19,35] The incidence of fat embolism syndrome increases to 5% to 35% after multiple fractures.[7,19] The mortality rate is about 10% and death is usually due to severe pulmonary dysfunction and multiple organ system failure and severe neurologic dysfunction.[7,19,35-37] It is estimated that 5000 deaths occur annually due to fat embolism syndrome after pathologic fractures, traumatic fractures, and orthopedic surgery.[34]

Clinical Manifestations

The clinical diagnosis of fat embolism syndrome is based on the presence of the classic triad of respiratory compromise, mental status changes, and petechial rash in the setting of long bone fractures or orthopedic surgery involving long bone manipulation. In patients with long bone fractures, 60% manifest symptoms within 24 hours of injury and 85% within 48 hours.[7,19] Severity can vary from subclinical to subacute clinically apparent symptoms to fulminant acute symptoms.[38] Subclinical emboli probably occur in nearly all patients with long bone fractures or intramedullary manipulation.[7,39] The subacute course is associated with mild respiratory dysfunction and mild neurologic manifestations or cardiovascular compromise. Supportive care is usually adequate in these cases. The fulminant variety can involve any of the following: rapidly progressive ARDS, complete cardiovascular collapse, or deep coma, possibly resulting in death.[40]

Some degree of respiratory compromise is always present and is often the most severe and life-threatening of the manifestations of fat embolism syndrome.[33,41] In trauma patients, it may be difficult to distinguish fat embolism syndrome from other causes for compromised pulmonary function. Indeed, the cause of respiratory compromise in multitrauma patients with significant long bone fractures can be multifactorial, including fat embolism syndrome, direct pulmonary/thoracic cavity trauma, and ischemia reperfusion injury and systemic activation of the inflammatory response. Isolated long bone fracture, however, is sufficient to cause all of the respiratory as well as the cardiac manifestations of fat embolism syndrome.[30]

The cardiovascular effects of fat embolism syndrome are mainly attributable to partial occlusion of pulmonary arterial flow resulting in acute pulmonary hypertension and increased right ventricular afterload. The cardiovascular effects of fat embolism syndrome vary in severity from sinus tachycardia to reversible hypotension to irreversible profound shock due to right heart failure resulting in death.[19,24,30,34] Changes on the electrocardiogram include sinus tachycardia, bradycardia, other arrhythmias, and ST segment changes.[19,24,38] Treatment is supportive with inotropic agents to increase contractility of the right ventricle to overcome the adverse effect of increased afterload. Increasing preload with intravenous fluids is usually not helpful and can lead to overdistention of an already overloaded right ventricle. To make matters worse, increased right heart pressure resulting from pulmonary hypertension can cause a closed foramen ovale to open, contributing to systemic embolization.[34]

Central nervous system manifestations of varying degrees are present in 70% to 80% of patients with fat embolism syndrome.[33,41] These findings can vary from mild confusion or restlessness to profound coma resulting in death.[7,40] Most commonly, agitation, confusion, and lethargy not attributable to hypoxia are encountered.[24,35,38] Patients also can develop focal changes, such as hemiplegia, due to cerebral ischemia.[24] The more severe neurologic outcomes are often attributed to paradoxical emboli through a patent foramen ovale, although massive systemic embolization with profound coma and petechial hemorrhage of the brain in the absence of a patent foramen ovale can occur.[32,33,42]

Petechial rash is present in 40% to 70% of cases and is usually present on the chest, neck, and axilla, although less often the rash appears on mucous membranes or the conjunctiva.[32,35,38,41] Retinal changes also can be observed and include microinfarcts, cotton-wool spots, and flame-like hemorrhages.[7,33,38] Petechial rash is usually a late sign of fat embolism syndrome. The petechial rash is attributed to capillary occlusion or distention by fat globules.[38] Although it appears late and is often not present, when it does appear it can greatly aid in the definitive diagnosis.

Diagnosis

Many laboratory abnormalities are encountered in cases of fat embolism syndrome, but none is specific. These laboratory findings include decreased PaO_2 with decreased or increased PCO_2, thrombocytopenia, slowly decreasing hematocrit, increased fibrin split products, and decreased fibrinogen.[35,38]

Bronchoalveolar lavage has been advocated as a more specific test to diagnose fat embolism syndrome. The percentage of alveolar macrophages laden with fat droplets in the bronchoalveolar lavage fluid as determined by fat stains is elevated in patients with fat embolism syndrome. This finding may be helpful in confirming suspected cases of fat embolism syndrome, although precise diagnostic criteria have not been established. False-positive results are seen in patients with long bone fractures and after orthopedic procedures without clinical evidence of fat embolism syndrome.[39,43,44]

Findings on chest CT scan include patchy ground-glass or nodular opacities and thickening of the interlobar septa. The differential diagnosis of these findings includes pulmonary contusion and aspiration. Because they most often occur 24 hours or more after injury, they can usually be differentiated from contusion, which should be evident earlier. CT findings in more severe cases of fat embolism syndrome include more extensive bilateral patchy airspace consolidation; similar abnormalities also can be seen on the chest radiograph.[36,45] Occasionally, CT imaging also reveals large emboli lodged in the femoral veins, inferior vena cava, or the proximal pulmonary circulation.[46]

Treatment

The mainstay of treatment for fat embolism syndrome is supportive. The pulmonary manifestations often respond to supplemental oxygen. However, more severe cases of fat embolism syndrome develop into ARDS and multiple organ system failure, requiring prolonged mechanical ventilation. Cardiac dysfunction is due to increased pulmonary resistance, and shock due to fat embolism syndrome may require inotropic support. There is no specific treatment for the neurologic symptoms of fat embolism syndrome other than eliminating and treating other potential causes such as hypoxia. Rare cases of severe neurologic dysfunction that result in profound coma can be irreversible and result in death.

The most important treatment of fat embolism syndrome is prevention. In the setting of traumatic fracture, prevention is achieved by providing early fixation. Multiple experimental and clinical studies clearly show that early fracture fixation (within 24 hours) decreases both the pulmonary and the cardiac effects of fat embolism syndrome when compared with delayed (greater than 24 hours) fixation and nonoperative treatment.[19,24,30,47-49] There is also some suggestion that fixation within 10 hours may be even more beneficial.[50]

Trials of intravenous alcohol, low-molecular-weight dextran, hypertonic glucose, and heparin have shown these agents to be ineffective in the treatment of fat embolism syndrome. Prophylactic administration of corticosteroids may be beneficial.[7,24,35,51] Two reasonable regimens are methylprednisolone (30 mg/kg administered intravenously on admission and then repeated in 4 hours) or methylprednisolone (1 g IV initially followed by two more 1 g doses at 8-hour intervals).[7,19] Other investigators have shown a reduction in

the incidence of fat embolism syndrome, reduced severity of hypoxia, and reduced incidence of hypoxia following lower prophylactic doses of methylprednisolone, ranging from 7.5 to 10 mg/kg repeated up to 12 times. Pulmonary hypertension has not been shown to improve, however.[7,24,34,52]

THROMBOEMBOLISM

Pathophysiology

Venous injury, stasis, and hypercoagulability can all contribute to the risk of thromboembolism after pelvic or long bone fractures.[7] Embolic thrombi to the pulmonary circulation or systemic circulation (paradoxical embolization) can originate in the deep veins of the thigh, pelvis, or upper extremity. Calf vein thrombosis, in general, does not embolize but extends to involve more proximal deep veins 20% to 25% of the time.[7]

Risk Factors

A number of risk factors for thromboembolic disease, including femur, tibia, and pelvic fractures, have been identified in trauma patients. Other identified risk factors include age older than 40 years, immobility, blood transfusion, multiple trauma, head injury, spinal fracture, spinal cord injury, and high injury severity score.[19,38,53-58] However, a systematic review of the literature by the Eastern Association for the Surgery of Trauma (EAST) found that only spinal fractures and spinal cord injuries were consistently shown to be associated with a higher risk of deep vein thrombosis.[59] Despite these data, most trauma and orthopedic surgeons regard the risk of thromboembolic disease in trauma patients with long bone or pelvic fractures as real.[19]

Prophylaxis

Elevation of the affected extremity and passive motion exercises increase lower extremity venous flow rates and reduce deep vein thrombosis.[19] Lower extremity sequential compression devices decrease the incidence of deep vein thrombosis by up to 90% in orthopedic patients.[19] Compression devices placed on the foot have also been shown to decrease the incidence of deep vein thrombosis in patients undergoing orthopedic surgery for elective indications or trauma.[19] These devices are useful when the anatomy of injury and surgery precludes the placement of sequential compression devices on the leg.[19] Similar improvements in the thromboembolism rate have been seen in the surgical ICU population.[60] In the multitrauma population, some studies have shown sequential compression device use to be equivalent to low-dose heparin whereas other studies have shown no improvement in thromboembolic events when compared to no prophylaxis.[58] Despite the conflicting data in the literature, the use of sequential compression devices continues to be a main way to provide thromboembolism prophylaxis in the skeletal trauma population because of its low cost, ease of use, and inherent safety. The salutary effects of sequential compression devices are thought to include improved venous flow and activation of endogenous antithrombotic mechanisms. The anticoagulant effects of sequential compression devices decrease minutes after discontinuing the device, emphasizing the importance of continuous therapy.[59,60] Because of its low cost, noninvasive nature, and high accuracy, color-flow duplex ultrasonography has become the test of choice for deep vein thrombosis.[61,62]

Low-dose unfractionated heparin (5000 U IV two to three times daily) decreases the incidence of thromboembolic events when compared with placebo in various populations of acutely ill patients. These studies have included orthopedic and nonorthopedic critically ill and noncritically ill patients. Overall reduction in thromboembolic rates are on the order of two- to threefold.[59,60] However, multiple studies of trauma and orthopedic patients, including two meta-analyses, have failed to show significant improvement in the rate of thromboembolic events when low-dose unfractionated heparin is compared to placebo.[19,59]

The literature on low-molecular-weight heparin is more convincing. Several studies have shown that treatment with low-molecular-weight heparin decreases the incidence of thromboembolism and has an excellent safety profile in patients with hip fracture or multisystem trauma.[19,53] Moreover, studies have also shown that low-molecular-weight heparin (enoxaparin 30 mg SQ every 12 hours) provides superior venous thromboembolism prophylaxis when compared to low-dose unfractionated heparin (5000 U SQ every 12 hours) in the trauma population.[59,60,63]

Several studies have shown improved efficacy using combined sequential compression devices and low-dose unfractionated heparin or low-molecular-weight heparin therapy when compared to either therapy alone in stroke, cardiac surgery, and neurosurgery populations.[61] Other studies, however, have shown no difference between combined and single-modality therapy.[59] Further study of the fracture population is needed.

Treatment

Treatment of deep vein thrombosis and pulmonary embolism in patients with orthopedic injuries or multiple trauma involves a balance between the risk of bleeding and thromboembolic disease. Although virtually all pulmonary emboli arise from deep vein thrombosis in the thigh, pelvis, or upper extremity, calf vein thrombosis tends to propagate into the proximal veins, meaning that treatment should be to avoid embolic phenomena.[64-67] Treatment of deep vein thrombosis and pulmonary embolism usually starts with full anticoagulation using unfractionated heparin. Once therapeutic heparinization has been achieved for an average of 72 hours, treatment with sodium warfarin is begun. Patients are usually kept on bedrest for this period to prevent embolic events.[64-67] Alternative therapy includes low-molecular-weight heparin.

Inferior vena cava filters are generally reserved for patients who have failed anticoagulation, exhibit embolic phenomena or propagation of clot while on full anticoagulation, or are inappropriate candidates for systemic anticoagulation.[60,68]

Prognosis

More than 50% of deaths caused by pulmonary embolism occur within the first hour. After the first hour, patients are at a 2.5% to 10% risk of dying when treated adequately. Inadequate treatment carries a 30% risk of death.[38]

ANNOTATED REFERENCES

Bone LB, Johnson KD, Weigelt J, Scheinberg R: Early versus delayed stabilization of femoral fractures: A prospective randomized study. J Bone Joint Surg Am 1989;71:336-340.
> *This prospective randomized study examined the timing of operative stabilization of femoral fractures in 178 patients. The authors showed that when fracture fixation was delayed in multiply injured patients, the incidence of pulmonary complications was higher, the length of hospitalization was longer, the number of days in the ICU was greater, and the cost of hospitalization was greater.*

Crowl AC, Young JS, Kahler DM, et al: Occult hypoperfusion is associated with increased morbidity in patients undergoing early femur fracture fixation. J Trauma 2000;48:260-267.
> *This retrospective study of 177 patients with femur fracture compared the incidence of complications between those with occult hypoperfusion (elevated lactate level with normal vital signs) at the time of fracture fixation to those without (normal lactate level and vital signs). The group with occult hypoperfusion had a significantly higher incidence of postoperative complications (50%) versus those without (20%; P < .01).*

Demetriades D, Karaiskakis M, Toutouzas K, et al: Pelvic fractures: Epidemiology and predictors of associated abdominal injuries and outcomes. J Am Coll Surg 2002;195:1-10.
> *This retrospective study of 1545 patients with pelvic fractures identifies risk factors associated with coexisting intra-abdominal injury including motor vehicle crash as mechanism, Abbreviated Injury Severity Score 4 or higher, and age older than 55 years. The rate of mortality attributable directly to pelvic fracture was only 0.8% whereas the overall mortality rate was 13.5%.*

Fabian TC, Hoots AV, Stanford DS, et al: Fat embolism syndrome: Prospective evaluation in 92 fracture patients. Crit Care Med 1990;18:42-46.
> *This prospective observational study examined 92 consecutive patients admitted to a level I trauma center with long bone or pelvic fracture. This descriptive study found a rate of fat embolism syndrome of at least 11% among these patients, but it may be much higher if patients with coexisting lung injury are included. The associated mortality rate was 10%.*

Geerts WH, Jay RM, Code KI, et al: A comparison of low-dose heparin with low-molecular-weight heparin as prophylaxis against venous thromboembolism after major trauma. N Engl J Med 1996;335:701-707.
> *A prospective, randomized study of 344 adult trauma patients comparing unfractionated heparin to enoxaparin in the prophylaxis of deep-vein thrombosis. This study found a 30% reduction in risk with the use of 30 mg of enoxaparin versus 5000 U of heparin administered subcutaneously every 12 hours. The risk of major bleeding was not significantly different.*

Chapter 248

PEDIATRIC TRAUMA

Bradley Peterson • Susan Duthie

KEY POINTS

1. Trauma systems and trauma centers improve outcome, and pediatric trauma centers improve outcome for children, especially for those with severe traumatic brain injury.

2. An inclusive system is the right system for pediatric trauma patients, and the pediatric critical care physician should have a significant role.

3. **Injuries to the airway in children can be rapidly life threatening.** Small airway diameter combined with penetrating or blunt injury to the neck can produce rapid airway compromise. The majority of penetrating airway injuries in children occur in adolescent males.

4. Mortality rate for thoracic trauma (rare in children) can exceed 40% when a **combination of head, chest, and abdominal injuries** is present.

5. Traumatic injury to the heart and great vessels is significantly less common in pediatric patients than in adults. **Most injuries are the result of blunt trauma,** with penetrating injury being rare and carrying a higher mortality rate.

6. More than 90% of abdominal trauma in children is the result of blunt trauma, with penetrating trauma accounting for only 5% to 10% of injuries. **The gold standard for the evaluation of children with blunt abdominal trauma** is computed tomography with intravenous contrast.

7. Pelvic fractures are a marker of significant trauma. Mortality varies from 10% to 50% and is often due to the **high rate of associated injuries.** The most common mechanisms are fall, crush, and motor vehicle accidents.

8. **Genitourinary trauma is common** and occurs in 12% of injuries in children. It rarely results in death; when death occurs, it is usually due to **associated injuries.**

9. Approximately 5% of all **spinal cord injuries** occur in the pediatric age group. Common causes in the youngest children include falls and motor vehicle accidents. Inflicted trauma has been identified as a significant mechanism of injury in young children. For older children, common causes of spinal injuries are sports and other recreational activities, such as bicycle riding.

10. An estimated 300 children and youths die each year from **traumatic brain injury;** 29,000 are hospitalized, and 400,000 are treated in hospital emergency departments. Traumatic brain injury is caused by linear and inertial forces resulting in an impact injury. This is the primary injury. It includes hematomas, lacerations, and axonal shearing and is often referred to as irreparable. Secondary injury refers to the injury that occurs after impact. It is considered both preventable and potentially reversible. An aggressive management strategy is indicated as it is associated with improved outcomes.

11. **Trauma can result in lung injury and respiratory failure, the most severe of which is acute respiratory distress syndrome** (ARDS). ARDS management in pediatrics focuses on minimizing iatrogenic lung injury and on adjuncts to mechanical ventilation.

Injury is the leading cause of medical expenditure for children age 5 to 14 years. In addition, traumatic injury accounts for approximately 300,000 childhood hospitalizations per year and, in the year 2000, was responsible for more deaths in the 1- to 14-year age group than all natural causes combined.

This chapter focuses on trauma-related topics from the viewpoint of a pediatric critical care physician.

TRAUMA SYSTEMS AND TRAUMA CENTERS

Many studies support the concept that trauma systems and trauma centers improve outcome and that pediatric trauma centers improve outcome for children, especially for those with severe traumatic brain injury. The "Guidelines for the Acute Medical Management of Severe Traumatic Brain Injury in Infants and Children and Adolescents," published in 2003, found sufficient evidence to set seven guidelines for pediatric management. One of the guidelines states, "In a metropolitan area pediatric patients with severe traumatic brain injury (TBI) should be transported directly to pediatric trauma center if available." An accompanying option states, "Pediatric patients with severe TBI should be treated in a pediatric trauma center or in an adult trauma center with added qualifications for pediatric treatment." These guidelines have been endorsed by six medical societies, including the American Association for the Surgery of Trauma and the Society of Critical Care. Over the last 3 decades, due to heroic efforts by the American College of Surgery (ACS), many trauma systems with designated adult and pediatric trauma centers have been developed. The ACS program provides verification of trauma centers by an excellent outside review process. To date, the ACS has verified 13 level 1 pediatric trauma centers. The ACS delineates recommended equipment, staffing, policies, and procedures. Important to the trauma center is a designated trauma director and an active morbidity and mortality conference that is attended by all physician members of the trauma team.

TRAUMA TEAMS

Trauma teams are essential to the trauma center. A trauma team refers to all who care for the trauma patient from resuscitation through discharge. Members of the trauma team include the trauma surgeons, emergency department physicians and nurses, critical care physicians and nurses, respiratory therapists, subspecialty surgeons, radiologists, rehabilitation team, social workers, and clergy. A trauma team requires strong hospital commitment and support. To function optimally, multiple policies and procedures that are understood and respected by all members need to be in place. The resuscitation team is usually led by a surgeon and performs best when led by an attending trauma surgeon. The prepared trauma team improves performance in resuscitation as well as outcome of the patient.[1]

ROLE OF PEDIATRIC CRITICAL CARE PHYSICIANS

The role of the intensivist in the care of trauma patients has been debated for decades. In 1986, Meyer and Trunkey argued that, in most instances, optimal care of seriously injured patients requires "participation between trauma surgeons and critical care specialists, as well as trauma and critical care services. With proper leadership and systems to ensure effective communication between such services, these goals can be achieved. Important secondary goals, in education and research, can also be achieved by such methods."[1] Such attitudes of collaboration and inclusiveness were not always apparent in the 1990s. An editorial in the *Journal of Trauma* stated, "the American Association for the Surgery of Trauma ratifies the position of the American College of Surgeons Committee on Trauma that the trauma surgeon is and must be responsible for the comprehensive management of the injured patient in the critical care unit, including hemodynamic monitoring, ventilator management, nutrition, and posttraumatic complications."[2] A letter to the editor responding to the editorial stated, "Except for a nod to a team effort, the tenor of your editorial would imply that the trauma surgeon and only the trauma surgeon has all the necessary skills in all areas to care for the multiply injured patient to the exclusion of all others."[3] A reply to the letter stated that the intent of the editorial was not meant to be exclusive and that collaborative participation with all specialties was important. Such debates led to feelings of noncollaboration and exclusion among critical care physicians.

In 1991, the American College of Surgeons Committee on Trauma recommended that an "inclusive" trauma system be developed.[4] Atweh advocated that the concept of the inclusive trauma system be broadened to include all phases of injury, as well as all the disciplines involved with injuries.[5] In 1999, the president of the American Association for the Surgery of Trauma stated, "it is interesting to note who actually provides much of the minute-to-minute and day-to-day care of patients

in many trauma centers. The busier the trauma center, the more likely the care is provided by nonsurgeons: anesthesiologists, emergency physicians, critical care doctors of various stripes. . . . Clearly these workers are needed to manage patients."[6] Cooper wrote, "What we do know, however, is that trauma systems and trauma centers that make special provision for the needs of children achieve better outcomes than those that don't."[7] He went on to say that the reason for this is more likely to be the specialized system than the surgeon per se and to recommend the development of a fully inclusive trauma system. In October 2002, the Trauma System Agenda for the Future, coordinated through the American Trauma Society, stated that trauma requires a multidisciplinary approach, hospital physicians of all specialties should be included, and appropriate use of all members of the trauma team must be planned.[8] The most recent version of "Resources for Optimal Care of the Injured Patient" states, "appropriately trained surgical and medical trained specialists may staff the pediatric critical care unit."[8a]

An inclusive system is the right system for pediatric trauma patients, and the pediatric critical care physician should have a significant role. The pediatric critical care physician has the most training and experience in life-support therapies for children, including mechanical ventilation, hemodynamic support, renal replacement therapies, and prevention and treatment of secondary brain injury. As an example, data from San Diego Children's Hospital (unpublished) show that during an 18-month period, 80 trauma patients required mechanical ventilation. During the same period, 904 nontrauma patients required mechanical ventilation. The critical care physician is also in the critical care unit on a minute-to-minute basis. Statistical studies have shown better outcomes for children in critical care units directed and attended by critical care physicians.[9] In our system, the critical care physician and the trauma surgeon conduct daily rounds together, including all trauma patients in the pediatric ICU. All patients are discussed on a daily basis with a neurosurgeon as well. This has built mutual respect, contributed to better patient care, and promoted a good working environment. Inclusive attitudes, teamwork, leadership, standard protocols and policies, an ongoing review of the system, and monthly morbidity and mortality conferences all contribute to the quality of the pediatric trauma center and better patient outcomes.

INITIAL RESUSCITATION

Resuscitation of the pediatric trauma patient follows the ABCs (airway, breathing, circulation) of Advanced Trauma Life Support (ATLS) and Pediatric Advanced Life Support (PALS) guidelines. Additional discussion of pediatric resuscitation is provided in Chapter 59 on pediatric neurointensive care. Resuscitation begins in the field with emergency medical service personnel and continues at the trauma center with the designated trauma team.

Upon arrival, the airway is assessed for patency and maintainability. The airway may need to be secured if the patient has experienced head, thoracic, abdominal, or airway trauma. Adequate airway control must be obtained while maintaining cervical spine immobilization. These patients are at risk for aspiration secondary to absent or diminished laryngeal reflexes and delayed gastric emptying. Most trauma patients should be orally intubated with direct cricoid pressure.

Many pharmacologic agents are available for rapid-sequence intubation, similar to adult resuscitation. Doses are adjusted for patient weight. The reason for intubation as well as the type of injuries present dictate the medications used. Endotracheal tube placement should be confirmed by auscultation of the abdomen and both sides of the chest, by checking the position at the lips, and by palpation of the cuff in the suprasternal notch. Placement should also be confirmed by end-tidal carbon dioxide monitoring and by radiography. The patient's heart rate, blood pressure, oxygen saturation, color, and perfusion should be continuously monitored. Once the airway is secure, ventilation should be evaluated. If unequal breath sounds are noted, and the endotracheal tube is in the correct position, a hemothorax, pneumothorax, or plugging of a large bronchus may be present. Tracheal deviation, though rare, may help with the diagnosis of tension pneumo- or hemothorax. Breath sounds are transmitted easily in children, and a simple pneumothorax is often not apparent until a chest radiograph is obtained. Tube thoracostomies are placed as needed. Flail chest is rare in pediatrics owing to the flexibility of the rib cage. Ventilation should be maintained with 100% oxygen during resuscitation.

After successful airway establishment and ventilation, the circulation must be assessed. Direct pressure should be applied to any site of active hemorrhage. Pulses, perfusion, capillary refill, heart rate and rhythm, and blood pressure should be evaluated. Intravenous access, preferably two large-bore catheters, must be obtained rapidly for volume resuscitation. Subgaleal, intra-abdominal, intrathoracic, or fracture-related hemorrhage may be life threatening. Heart rate is the most sensitive indicator of hypovolemia in pediatric trauma patients. Young children preserve blood pressure despite losing as much as 25% of their intravascular blood volume.[10,11] Thready pulses and altered mental status are evident with loss of 30% to 45% of blood volume. Volume resuscitation begins with crystalloid at 20 mL/kg with further volume boluses based on the patients status. Blood products may be necessary to stabilize patients with hemorrhagic shock. Hypertonic (3%) saline has been shown to effectively restore intravascular volume while also decreasing cerebral edema and may be used as a bolus of 5 to 10 mL/kg. Blood products should be warmed, because pediatric patients are at high risk for hypothermia. Hypotension contributes to secondary injury to the brain and other vital organs and must be treated aggressively. In rare cases, vasoactive agents may be necessary in the resuscitation room. Trauma victims who are pulseless at the scene have an almost uniformly fatal outcome.[11,12] Prolonged, heroic resuscitative efforts should be avoided in these patients. Patients who have a pulse at the scene but arrest on route or in the emergency department have a slightly better prognosis, and resuscitation should be attempted. Most cardiac arrest associated with blunt trauma is a result of multisystem injuries, including severe brain injury.[13] Open chest resuscitation should be considered only in the rare case of penetrating chest trauma, as it has been shown to be of no benefit in blunt trauma.

The neurologic examination should focus on the level of alertness, Glasgow Coma Scale (GCS) score, pupillary response, focal signs of spinal cord injury, and signs of increased intracranial pressure (ICP). Subjects with a GCS score of 8 or less or with a waning mental status should be intubated using rapid-sequence intubation. Noncontrast head computed tomography (CT) should be performed immediately.

All trauma patients are undressed and exposed for a full examination. Children rapidly lose heat and should be warmed with lights and blankets.

A secondary survey with full physical examination and radiographs, as needed, should follow the primary survey and stabilization. Once the patient is stabilized and resuscitation is complete, the team decides on a disposition.

SPECIFIC INJURIES AND CRITICAL CARE MANAGEMENT

NECK INJURIES

Injuries to the airway in children can be rapidly life threatening. Small airway diameter combined with penetrating or blunt injury to the neck can produce rapid airway obstruction. Children are at greater risk than are adults for spinal and major vascular injury from neck trauma. Death from airway injury may occur due to disruption of the airway at any level.

Clinically, the neck is divided into three anatomic zones, and management of traumatic airway injuries largely depends on which zone contains the injury. Zone 1 extends from the level of the clavicles up to the cricoid cartilage. Injuries to this area may involve the apex of the lung; trachea; subclavian, carotid, and jugular vessels; thoracic duct; esophagus; vagus nerve; and thyroid gland. Patients suffering zone 1 injuries typically exhibit hypotension, because the great vessels are often injured. Zone 2 encompasses the area from the cricoid to the mandible. Injuries to this area are the easiest to detect. Active bleeding can be reduced by direct pressure. The previous approach of mandatory operative management for zone 2 penetrating injury has been replaced by one of selective surgical exploration of wounds after clinical, endoscopic, and radiographic evaluation. Zone 3 extends from the angle of the mandible to the base of the skull. The oropharynx, jaw, and teeth are located within this area. Mandibular fractures in children manifest as malocclusion of the biting surfaces of the teeth and are usually associated with dental injuries. Injury to the chin associated with tympanic membrane perforation or hemotympanum is associated with an occult fracture of the mandible. Orotracheal intubation is not usually problematic in children with mandibular fractures unless there is copious oral hemorrhage. The neck is further divided into anterior and posterior regions. The anterior region contains the oropharynx, trachea, esophagus, and major vascular structures. The posterior neck contains the spine, spinal cord, and large neck muscles.

Penetrating neck and airway injuries occur less frequently in children than in adults. The majority of penetrating airway injuries in children occur in adolescent males.[14] Because major structures of the airway, central nervous system, and digestive and vascular systems are contained within the neck, penetrating injuries can be lethal owing to the anatomic structures injured. Wounds from sharp objects or bullets may injure the major vascular structures in the neck, the trachea, or the esophagus. As a result, penetrating wounds to the face and neck are more likely to require surgical intervention than blunt injuries are. Extensive damage to deep tissues may not be apparent on examination of the wound site. Stab wounds typically produce linear tissue injury that follows a predictable path from the entrance wound into the deeper tissue. Bullet injuries may produce unpredictable tissue damage as the result of deflection and shattering of the projectile throughout the neck. Penetrating injury to any of the major systems usually results in rapid airway compromise and shock.

Penetrating injury to the esophagus may not be immediately apparent but can produce delayed morbidity due to mediastinitis. Investigation of anterior neck injuries that involve the trachea should always include evaluation of the esophagus for perforation. Esophageal perforation should be suspected if fever, elevated white blood cell count, and subcutaneous air in the neck occur in the days following a traumatic neck injury. Management of the perforation requires prompt surgical repair of the esophagus, drainage of the surrounding soft tissue infection, and intravenous antibiotics.

Although less common than penetrating injuries, blunt neck injuries can be associated with life-threatening airway disruption.[15] This injury is frequently missed in the presence of concurrent head, face, and thoracic injuries. Also associated with blunt neck trauma are injuries to the cervical spine, esophagus, lungs, and great vessels. Mortality rates of up to 30% are reported for children with these injuries, and half these children die of tracheobronchial rupture within 1 hour of the injury.[16]

Blunt laryngeal trauma in children is uncommon and frequently unrecognized. The pediatric larynx is characterized by features related to immaturity. Its small diameter, funnel shape, and elastic structure result in significantly greater respiratory problems after trauma compared with adults. Due to its high, anterior position in the neck, the larynx of a child is relatively sheltered by the mandible.[17] Greater cricothyroid pliability decreases the incidence of fractures, but surrounding tissue edema or blood in the lumen may rapidly produce respiratory difficulties because of the smaller diameter of the airway. The clinical presentation of laryngeal injury in children includes frank respiratory distress with hoarseness, stridor, and palpable subcutaneous emphysema.[15] Radiographs of the chest and neck may show subcutaneous emphysema as well. The diagnosis of blunt laryngeal trauma in children is based on history, physical examination, and radiographic studies, followed by flexible or rigid bronchoscopy. CT of the neck adds little to the diagnosis of laryngeal injury. Once a laryngeal injury is suspected, rigid endoscopy in the operating suite should be used to secure the airway, as well as delineate and repair the injury. Although adult patients with laryngeal injury frequently undergo an awake tracheostomy under local anesthesia, this is not routine in children. Careful placement of an endotracheal tube below the level of injury provides an airway, but this may be difficult to accomplish. Difficulties in securing the airway usually reflect a lack of appreciation of the injury. Typical problems include hematoma and airway distortion, bleeding into the airway, or passage of the endotracheal tube into the mediastinum.[18]

THORACIC INJURIES

Thoracic trauma, though rare in children, accounts for 5% to 10% of admissions to trauma centers. In isolation, it carries a 5% mortality rate. This increases fivefold when there is concomitant head or abdominal injury and can exceed 40% when a combination of head, chest, and abdominal injuries is present.[19] Potentially life-threatening injuries such as airway obstruction, tension pneumothorax, massive hemothorax, open pneumothorax, flail chest, and cardiac tamponade must be corrected immediately. The last three injuries are relatively uncommon in the pediatric population. Young children have a significantly more flexible thoracic cage than adults do. As a result, compression of intrathoracic organs with blunt trauma may lead to significant parenchymal injuries in the absence of rib fractures. Thus, pulmonary contusions, rather than broken ribs, are far more common in children. In isolation, a broken rib is rarely associated with increased morbidity or mortality.[20] An isolated first rib fracture, however, is a potential sign of child abuse[21] or may be associated with significant thoracic injury. Multiple rib fractures should alert the clinician to look for underlying injuries in the thoracic cavity. Further radiographic evaluation, such as CT or angiography, may be warranted to complete the diagnostic evaluation. Numerous studies have demonstrated that the presence of multiple rib fractures has an approximate 40% mortality rate, often due to the presence of associated multisystem injury.[22] Supportive care is the mainstay of rib fracture management. Appropriate analgesia is necessary to promote deep inspiratory effort and prevent atelectasis. Intercostal nerve blocks may be helpful but are rarely necessary.

Trauma to the intrathoracic trachea and bronchi is fortunately rare, as 50% of pediatric patients die within 1 hour of tracheobronchial disruption.[23] Pneumothorax and subcutaneous emphysema are common findings, but rib fractures are not common. Failure of tube thoracostomy to re-expand the lung and the continued presence of a large air leak denote a tracheal or bronchial disruption. If the site of tracheal or bronchial disruption is within the chest cavity, the endotracheal tube tip should be placed distal to the disruption. This may require bronchoscopy. Selective intubation of the undisrupted mainstem bronchus, followed by one-lung ventilation until the proper resources can be obtained for control of the damaged bronchus, may be required. This must be done rapidly and with great care to avoid extending the tracheal injury. Once the injury is repaired, the patient may benefit from a low-tidal-volume ventilation strategy.

Pulmonary contusion may occur with or without the presence of overlying rib fractures or chest wall injury. Symptoms include tachypnea, dyspnea, cyanosis, hemoptysis, and respiratory failure. The initial chest radiograph may not demonstrate this injury, and repeat x-rays may be necessary to reveal the infiltrates. Excessive fluid administration should be avoided. Mechanical ventilation may be necessary. Acute respiratory distress syndrome (ARDS) is uncommonly associated with pulmonary contusion, but it may develop. In rare cases, there may be severe pulmonary hypertension.

In children, the mediastinum is less fixed than in adults, and the physiologic consequences of tension pneumothoraces may become evident rapidly. Each hemithorax can hold 40% of a child's blood volume. A chest tube large enough to drain the entire hemithorax, without clotting or occluding, is necessary. Surgical exploration for hemostasis may be required if the initial chest tube output is 20 mL/kg or greater than 3 to 4 mL/kg per hour.[24] Inadequate evacuation leads to lung entrapment from a fibrothorax and predisposes the patient to chronic atelectasis. Penetrating injuries may require thoracotomy in the operating room. Anterior penetrating injuries below the nipple line and posterior penetrating injuries below the tip of the scapula warrant the exclusion of intra-abdominal injuries.

Other thoracic injuries include traumatic asphyxia and chylothorax. Traumatic asphyxia is caused by sudden, severe compression of the chest and upper abdomen and is characterized by craniofacial and cervical cyanosis, edema, and petechiae. Subconjunctival and thoracic wall petechiae also occur. There may be associated respiratory distress, cardiac arrest, and cerebral edema with raised ICP. Retinal hemorrhage, blindness, and orbital compartment syndrome have also been reported.[25] Traumatic chylothorax is rare in children but has been reported with blunt and penetrating injury and with child abuse.

CARDIAC AND AORTIC INJURIES

Traumatic injury to the heart and great vessels is significantly less common in pediatric patients than in adults. Most injuries are the result of blunt trauma; penetrating injuries are rare and carry a higher mortality rate.

Myocardial contusion results from blunt force injury to the chest. The vast majority of pediatric patients with myocardial contusions have multisystem trauma; pulmonary contusion is the most common coexisting injury, found in 50% of patients.[26] Hemodynamically significant myocardial contusion is relatively rare in pediatric patients and may present with arrhythmia or ventricular dysfunction. The majority of arrhythmias occur within 24 hours. In a study of 184 pediatric patients with blunt cardiac injury, no hemodynamically stable patient who presented with normal sinus rhythm subsequently developed an arrhythmia or cardiac failure.[26] However, there have been case reports of delayed arrhythmia occurring up to 6 days later.

The diagnostic evaluation of myocardial contusion is controversial and is usually based on a series of tests in the appropriate clinical setting. In pediatrics, testing may include a combination of cardiac enzyme determinations, electrocardiography, and echocardiography. Creatine kinase-MB and cardiac troponin I elevation following blunt trauma has been used to diagnose contusion. Cardiac troponin I is highly specific for the myocardium, but creatine kinase-MB may be elevated with injury to skeletal muscle. Elevation of troponin I occurs within 4 hours of injury and peaks within 24 hours. The significance of elevation in a hemodynamically stable patient is unclear, and determination may not be necessary in these patients.[27,28] An admission 12-lead electrocardiogram (ECG) is recommended in all patients. Echocardiography may show wall motion abnormalities or ventricular dysfunction. In a small pediatric study, echocardiography was diagnostic of cardiac injury in patients with hemodynamic instability or abnormal chest radiographs who had nondiagnostic ECG and creatine kinase-MB.[29]

In addition to myocardial contusion, structural damage such as traumatic ventriculoseptal defect, valve injury, ventricular rupture, or aneurysm may occur with blunt chest trauma. The management of all blunt cardiac injury is largely supportive, with operative intervention as needed for significant structural damage. Continuous ECG monitoring is recommended.

Commotio cordis is an unusual event but is much more common in pediatric patients, with 80% of victims younger than 18 years and 50% younger than 14 years. Blunt trauma to the chest with the impact centered over the heart results in immediate cardiac arrest. It is thought that the narrow anteroposterior diameter of the chest, in conjunction with the increased compliance of the chest wall in pediatric patients, allows a chest wall blow to be transmitted to the underlying heart. Many but not all cases occur during sports-related activity.[30] Blunt chest trauma leads to cardiovascular collapse, with ventricular tachyarrhythmia being the most common arrhythmia. Unlike myocardial contusion, there is no evidence of myocardial injury on autopsy. The survival rate is low, even with prompt resuscitation.[30,31]

Blunt aortic injury is an extremely uncommon pediatric injury; however, as in adults, it is potentially lethal. The aortic arch is relatively fixed, and the descending aorta is more mobile, making it susceptible to shearing forces during horizontal and vertical deceleration. Three reasons for the rarity of blunt aortic injury in pediatric patients have been proposed. First, most adult thoracic aortic injuries are the result of the driver of a vehicle impacting the steering wheel, with a large force being imparted over a small area. This mechanism does not occur in pediatric patients. Second, blunt trauma in children is often the result of pedestrian-automobile accidents, allowing the force of impact to be widely distributed over the body surface area.[32] Third, the breaking stress of the thoracic aorta is inversely related to age.[33] The breaking stress of the thoracic aorta is decreased, however, in connective tissue disease such as Ehlers-Danlos syndrome and Marfan's syndrome. One of our rare cases of blunt aortic injury occurred in a young child with a connective tissue disorder.

Diagnosis of thoracic aortic injury is similar in children and adults. The pattern of chest x-ray findings is similar, although one study found that depression of the left mainstem bronchus is not as common in pediatric patients. Angiography remains the gold standard for the diagnosis of thoracic aortic injury.[34] Helical CT is becoming an important diagnostic tool and, when performed properly, has a sensitivity and specificity similar to that of angiography.[35] Transesophageal echocardiography may also have a role in diagnosis, although its place is less clear. As in adults, successful management of these potentially lethal injuries depends on prompt recognition and treatment.

ABDOMINAL INJURIES

More than 90% of abdominal trauma in pediatrics is the result of blunt trauma; penetrating trauma accounts for only 5% to 10% of injuries. After initial resuscitation, evaluation of specific injuries begins. It is important to know the mechanism of trauma to appreciate the potential abdominal injuries. A nasogastric or orogastric tube as well as a Foley catheter should be placed during abdominal evaluation, because dilatation of the stomach and bladder can cause significant pain, interfering with the examination. Inspection of the abdomen may reveal external evidence of trauma, suggestive of an underlying injury. Evaluation of abdominal tenderness is important but may be an unreliable finding in a child with lower rib fractures, contusion or soft tissue injury to the abdominal wall, or pelvic fracture. Auscultation with absent bowel sounds indicates ileus and may suggest underlying gastrointestinal (GI) injury. The pelvis should be examined by compression. Rectal examination should always be performed. If there is blood at the urethral meatus, perineal hematoma, or pelvic instability, a serious pelvic injury should be suspected. Hematuria is indicative of genitourinary injury.

The initial evaluation of children with abdominal trauma includes radiographs of the chest, abdomen, and pelvis. Focused abdominal sonography for trauma is an excellent initial study of the peritoneum and pericardium.[36-38] The gold standard for the evaluation of children with blunt abdominal trauma is CT with intravenous contrast. It gives reliable information about solid organ injuries, the presence of abnormal fluid, the presence of pneumoperitoneum and the retroperitoneal space. Further, organ blood flow and contrast extravasation can be observed. The detection of a hollow viscus injury is more difficult. Diagnostic peritoneal lavage is a sensitive test to detect bleeding and a perforated hollow viscus in blunt abdominal trauma; however, its use in pediatrics is limited, owing to the success of nonoperative management of solid organ injuries. Diagnostic peritoneal lavage may be indicated in children who have an emergent operative neurologic injury and require immediate assessment of the abdominal cavity.

Penetrating injury is rare in pediatrics. Virtually all gunshot wounds to the abdomen and lower chest should be treated by mandatory laparotomy. Stab wounds below the nipple line and above the inguinal ligament can be managed selectively by local wound exploration, peritoneal lavage, CT scan, and frequent serial physical examinations to determine the need for laparotomy.

Liver

Signs and symptoms of hepatic injury include pain and tenderness, abrasions, and contusion of the abdominal wall. Signs of peritonitis are frequently present due to hemoperitoneum. Most isolated liver injuries can be managed nonoperatively. Selective angiography and embolization may control bleeding without the need for operative repair. Operation, however, may be required for hemodynamic instability, continued transfusion requirement, or other associated injuries. The decision to operate is based on the child's physiologic status and not the graded classification of injury.[36] Complications of hepatic injury include hemobilia, abscess, biliary fistula, and bile peritonitis. The potential for delayed bleeding is higher in hepatic than in splenic injury.

Spleen

The spleen is the organ most frequently injured in blunt abdominal trauma. Ecchymosis, pain, and tenderness over the left upper quadrant are suggestive of splenic injury. Left shoulder pain may be present as a result of diaphragmatic irritation. Abdominal CT is recommended to determine the extent of injury as well as the presence of hemoperitoneum and other associated injuries.

Nonoperative management is preferable and is similar to the nonoperative management of liver injuries. Angiography and selective embolization should be considered in patients with active bleeding seen on CT.[39] Surgical management may be necessary in patients who are hemodynamically unstable, require continued transfusions, or have other associated abdominal injuries. A variety of surgical techniques are available to control bleeding, often without a total splenectomy. In patients requiring total splenectomy, there is a risk of post-splenectomy sepsis. In patients splenectomized for trauma, sepsis develops in 1.5%, with a mortality rate of 50%. Post-splenectomy sepsis may occur at any time, but the risk is greatest in the first 5 years of life.

Duodenum and Pancreas

The duodenum and pancreas are considered as a unit because they share a blood supply and are connected in the retroperitoneum. For these reasons, managing pancreaticoduodenal injuries is complicated. The most common cause of injury is blunt midepigastrium trauma from a blow, automobile crash, or bicycle handlebar. The diagnosis of pancreaticoduodenal injuries can be achieved using chemical markers and imaging studies. Serum amylase and lipase are indicators of pancreatic injury, but amylase levels may be elevated due to injuries to other organs, including the salivary glands. Ultrasonography and CT are the preferred imaging studies to delineate the pancreas. A duodenal perforation can be diagnosed using upper GI studies with water-soluble contrast or CT scan with oral contrast, in which free air or extravasation may be seen.

Most pancreatic injuries are mild.[40] They can be managed nonoperatively with nasogastric decompression and parenteral nutrition. When the patient's condition improves, nasogastric drainage can be discontinued and oral intake begun. Serial enzyme levels and ultrasonography should be performed to identify complications. Patients with severe pancreatic injury may require surgical repair or endoscopic placement of pancreatic duct stents.

Several complications may occur after pancreatic injury, including pleural effusion, bile duct obstruction, and pancreatic pseudocyst. Pancreatic pseudocyst occurs in one third of patients.

Most duodenal injuries are lacerations that can be treated by simple débridement and primary repair. For extensive duodenal injuries in which more than 50% of the circumference is affected, the blood supply is compromised, or bile duct–pancreatic injury is present, an aggressive surgical approach may be necessary. Duodenal hematoma results from blunt abdominal trauma associated with rapid deceleration or from a direct blow to the upper abdomen. It may present a day or more after injury as vomiting or a large amount of nasogastric drainage. It is easily diagnosed by ultrasonography or upper GI studies. The resultant intestinal occlusion should be treated by nasogastric decompression and parenteral nutrition until the obstruction resolves. If it fails to resolve within 3 weeks, an operation should be considered.

Small Intestine

Hollow viscus injuries are far less common than solid organ injuries in pediatric abdominal trauma patients. Nevertheless, bowel injury may result from even mild abdominal trauma. The mechanism of injury is either compression or shear forces resulting from rapid deceleration. There are two points of fixation to the retroperitoneum that frequently lead to transections: the ligament of Treitz and the cecum. Handlebar blows or direct blows to the abdomen compress the bowel against the vertebral column, resulting in intestinal perforation. In the lap-belt complex, contusions or abrasions of the abdominal wall and lumbar spine injury are associated with bowel perforation.

Identification of patients with a bowel injury may be challenging. Obtaining a detailed history of the mechanism of injury may prevent a delay in diagnosis and late complications. Detection of peritoneal signs may be difficult owing to distracting pain from the abdominal wall and back injury. If there is also a solid organ injury, peritoneal signs and symptoms may be interpreted as solely from the associated hemoperitoneum. There is no completely reliable imaging study available to detect intestinal injury. CT may show nonspecific findings suggestive of bowel injury. Serial clinical examinations and repeat CT scanning are important to diagnose injury in a timely fashion. Diagnostic peritoneal lavage may also play a role. Patients should receive nothing by mouth until a bowel injury is no longer suspected.

Diaphragm

Diaphragmatic rupture is the consequence of direct blunt trauma over the lower thorax and abdomen. The injury is most frequent on the left side. Contusion or abrasions of the upper abdomen, bowel sounds in the chest, and respiratory distress are the classic findings of a traumatic diaphragmatic rupture. A chest radiograph may show bowel and the naso-gastric tube in the thorax. The diagnosis may be confirmed by upper GI studies, ultrasonography, or CT. Laparotomy allows proper repair of the diaphragmatic defect and assessment of other organs.

Damage Control and Abdominal Compartment Syndrome

If the child is hemodynamically unstable despite aggressive resuscitation, a laparotomy for damage control may be required.[41] In the presence of the lethal triad of hypothermia, acidosis, and coagulopathy, an immediate definitive surgical repair is unnecessary.[42,43] The damage-control approach has three stages.[44] The first stage is the initial laparotomy, the goal being to prevent ongoing damage by controlling hemorrhage and fecal contamination. Abdominal packing and temporary closure of the wounds with loose retention sutures may be required.[45] Definitive surgical repair is postponed until the patient is stabilized. The second stage is carried out in the ICU with the goals of rewarming, correcting the coagulopathy, and restoring acid-base balance. An abdominal compartment syndrome may develop during the second phase.[46] The intra-abdominal pressure may be increased by edema, tissue swelling, ascites, and ongoing bleeding. The high pressure may cause cardiorespiratory and renal deterioration. Elevation of the diaphragm produces basilar atelectasis and restriction of lung inflation, which makes ventilation difficult. Increased abdominal pressure can also cause hypoperfusion of the abdominal contents, leading to renal failure and ischemic bowel injury with resultant bacterial translocation. Increased abdominal pressure also may decrease venous return and therefore cardiac output. Treatment of abdominal compartment syndrome is urgent and may require a peritoneal drain or opening of the abdominal wound and the placement of a prosthetic silo.[47] The third stage involves definitive surgery once the patient is stabilized. Packs are removed, tissues are debrided, bowel anastomoses are performed, and fractures are reduced. Most injured patients are not candidates for damage-control surgery. Unstable pediatric patients with severe abdominal injury benefit from this staged approach, which is designed to allow medical resuscitation and to avoid continued hypothermia, acidosis, and coagulopathy.

GENITOURINARY INJURIES

Genitourinary trauma is common and occurs in 12% of injuries in children. It rarely results in death, but when death does occur, it is usually due to associated injuries. The unique characteristics of a child's anatomy predispose to genitourinary trauma. The kidneys are proportionally larger, the abdominal musculature underdeveloped, and the ribs less ossified. In addition, the underdeveloped renal capsule and Gerota's fascia increase the likelihood of laceration, hemorrhage, and urine extravasation.

The mechanism of injury is usually blunt force (98%) and has a high association with pelvic trauma. Preexisting renal disease (neoplasms and duplicated collecting systems) predisposes to renal injury and is found in 20% of cases of documented renal trauma. Findings suggestive of genitourinary trauma include flank or abdominal tenderness, perineal injury, blood at the urinary meatus, mobile or displaced prostate, and gross hematuria.

Renal injuries are classified according to severity. Parenchymal injuries not involving the collecting system or renal vessels constitute 85% of renal injuries (grades I to III). Injuries to the collecting system or renal vessels account for 10% of renal injuries (grade IV), and the most severe injuries (grade V), including a shattered or devascularized kidney, constitute 5% of renal injuries.

Treatment goals for pediatric renal trauma include preserving kidney tissue and minimizing patient morbidity. Minor injuries rarely require surgery and are treated expectantly. Limited hospitalization with decreased activity until hematuria has resolved is all that is necessary. Imaging at 6 to 8 weeks following discharge is recommended.

Surgical intervention should be reserved for patients with major injuries and hemodynamic instability from persistent bleeding. An imaging study (CT) or intraoperative intravenous pyelogram should be performed to assess the contralateral kidney before undertaking renal exploration. Controversy exists over the management of major injuries in patients who have normal vital signs. Even in the case of urine extravasation without urethral injury, expectant treatment with frequent imaging studies at 5- to 7-day intervals is recommended. Nonoperative management of pediatric renal trauma has become the preferred approach in managing blunt renal injuries.

Penetrating renal injuries secondary to gunshot wounds should be explored because of the high incidence of associated injuries. Surgical treatment for stab wounds with suspected renal involvement should be based on the severity of hemorrhage and both the clinical and imaging evidence suggesting intra-abdominal injury.

Renovascular injuries generally occur in patients who have sustained life-threatening multisystem injuries. The mechanism of renovascular injury is thought to be deceleration with initial injury and arterial thrombosis. This occurs more frequently on the left side. The diagnosis is established with either contrast-enhanced CT or arteriography. Successful revascularization depends on the length of renal ischemia, the extent of vascular injuries, and the extent of associated injuries. Renal vein injuries are repaired in most cases. Repair of penetrating renal artery injuries is most successful if the ischemic time is less than 8 hours. Blunt arterial injuries are associated with the lowest rate of renal preservation and are most often treated by nephrectomy when they are unilateral.

PELVIC FRACTURES

Pelvic fractures are a marker for significant trauma and are often associated with other injuries. Pelvic fractures occur in approximately 2% of all blunt abdominal injuries, and 20% of those with pelvic fractures have intra-abdominal injuries. Mortality varies from 10% to 50% and is often due to associated injuries. The most common mechanisms are falls, crush injuries, and motor vehicle accidents. Clinically, the diagnosis is suggested by pain with anterior or lateral compression of the pelvis. Other findings may include perineal ecchymosis, blood at the urinary meatus or on the rectal examination, disruption of the rectal wall with mass effect due to bony fragments, or displacement of the prostate.

Evaluation of pelvic trauma begins with a pelvic radiograph and should include CT. Morbidity is lower in children than in adults. Treatment usually consists of bed rest, immobilization, and blood loss replacement. Severe injuries with significant blood loss may require prompt intervention and immobilization to minimize blood loss, including application of a pneumatic device (MAST garment), wrapping the pelvis with a bed sheet, or application of an external fixation device. Selective embolization can also provide hemostasis.

SPINAL INJURIES

Approximately 5% of all spinal cord injuries occur in the pediatric age group. Common causes in young children include falls and motor vehicle accidents. Recently, inflicted trauma, including gunshot wounds in urban areas, has been identified as a significant mechanism of injury for this age group.[48] For older children, sports and other recreational activities, such as bicycle riding, have greater etiologic importance.

The head and neck anatomy of a young child resembles that of a "bobble-head" doll, with a relatively large head resting on a small, highly flexible neck. To maintain neutral cervical alignment during the transport and initial resuscitation of a child at risk for a spinal injury, a support is often placed under the thorax to achieve torsal elevation, in addition to the use of an appropriately sized cervical collar. Alternatively, a board with an occipital recess may be used for this purpose.[49]

The initial assessment dictates the need for imaging studies. An awake, communicative child without midline cervical tenderness, intoxication, decreased level of consciousness, focal neurologic deficit, or a painful distracting injury does not require spinal imaging studies. Children younger than 9 years who fail to meet these criteria, including all children age 2 years or younger, require lateral and anteroposterior cervical radiographs. For children older than 9 years who fail to meet these initial criteria, an open-mouth odontoid image should also be obtained. Any child with abnormalities noted on these initial studies or a neurologic deficit consistent with a spinal cord injury requires further imaging studies, including CT and magnetic resonance imaging (MRI) of the spine. The role of these imaging studies in children with normal initial studies is controversial.[50] There is a paucity of evidence in the literature to support their use, as well as that of flexion-extension radiographs, in the setting of a normal neutral lateral cervical radiograph in a child. These studies may be necessary, however, in a child with a normal radiograph who remains comatose or has persistent tenderness.

Prospective, randomized, multicenter trials of pharmacologic agents for the treatment of acute spinal cord injury in children younger than 13 years have not been carried out. However, data from adult studies have been extrapolated and are commonly used to dictate management schemes in children. Methylprednisolone is administered within 3 hours of injury as an initial intravenous bolus of 30 mg/kg to run over 15 minutes, followed by an infusion of 5.4 mg/kg per hour to run over 23 hours.[51] If the initial administration is between 3 and 8 hours after injury, the infusion is continued for 48 hours. Methylprednisolone treatment is not initiated more than 8 hours after injury.[52]

In a child with a spinal cord injury, emphasis is placed on the maintenance of optimal physiologic homeostasis. Because of loss of sympathetic tone, intravenous pressor agents are frequently required in addition to crystalloid and colloid solutions to maintain age-appropriate blood pressure and cardiac output. Intubation may be necessary with high cervical spine injuries because of respiratory compromise. Avoidance of unnecessary neck manipulation is essential.

After initial resuscitation and the identification of spinal injuries, urgent neurosurgical and orthopedic consultation is indicated. Closed reduction and initial stabilization of these injuries are frequently performed in the ICU. Halo rings can be placed with acceptably low morbidity in the ICU setting, even in infants; they can be attached to weighted traction mechanisms for closed reduction, if necessary, and converted to halo jackets to maintain alignment. The need for and timing of internal surgical stabilization should be discussed in the context of the child's concomitant multisystem issues.

CLOSED HEAD INJURIES

It is estimated that each year 300 children and youths die from TBI; 29,000 are hospitalized, and 400,000 are treated in hospital emergency departments at a cost of more than $10 billion.[53] TBI is caused by linear and inertial forces resulting in an impact injury.[54] This is the primary injury. It includes hematomas, lacerations, and axonal shearing and is often referred to as irreparable. Secondary injury refers to the injury that occurs after impact. It is considered both preventable and potentially reversible. Pathologic alterations in respiratory, hemodynamic, and cellular function occur, which may lead to secondary injury and cell death. The pathways to neuron death include inadequate oxygen and nutrient supply secondary to hypoxia and decreased cerebral blood flow. Decreased cerebral blood flow can occur secondary to hypotension, decreased cardiac output, raised ICP, and cerebrovascular dysregulation, including endothelial dysfunction, vasospasm, and microthrombus formation. Elevated ICP occurs secondary to mass lesions, cerebral edema, and increases in cerebrospinal fluid volume and cerebral blood volume. Other pathways to neuron death include excitotoxicity, energy failure, inflammation, oxidative stress, and apoptosis. Present therapies are directed primarily at supporting oxygenation, blood pressure, and cardiac output and at controlling ICP.[55]

After an exhaustive literature review, the "Guidelines for the Acute Medical Management of Severe Traumatic Brain Injury in Infants, Children, and Adolescents"[56] found insufficient evidence to support any standards of care, but sufficient evidence to support seven guidelines for care: transfer of children in a metropolitan area with severe TBI to a pediatric trauma center, avoidance of hypoxia, correction of hypotension, maintenance of cerebral perfusion pressure greater than 40 mm Hg in children, a recommendation against the continuous infusion of propofol for either sedation or the control of intracranial hypertension, a warning against the use of corticosteroids, and a recommendation against the prophylactic use of antiseizure medication. Evidence was sufficient to support 17 care options and a flow diagram.

Initial stabilization requires support of the ABCs. The airway must be maintained and breathing supported to prevent hypoxemia and hypercarbia. Hyperoxia and brief aggressive hyperventilation are indicated during the initial resuscitation if the clinical examination reveals signs of herniation or acute neurologic deterioration. Normotension or mild hypertension and mild hypervolemia are indicated to support cardiac output and cerebral blood flow. Fluid administration, sedation, and vasoactive agents must be judiciously administered. Hypertonic saline may be advantageous as a resuscitation fluid for patients with shock, especially those with raised ICP. All children with a suspected head injury, a history of loss of consciousness, an altered level of consciousness, focal neurologic signs, evidence of a depressed or basilar skull fracture, a bulging fontanelle, or persistent headache and vomiting should have CT of the head.[54] Surgery is indicated for significant mass lesions. ICP monitoring is indicated for patients with a GCS score less than 8. Even with a normal CT scan, 10% to 15% of patients with a GCS score less than 8 have elevated ICP. A physician may also choose to monitor ICP in certain conscious patients whose CT scans indicate a high potential for decompensation or in patients in whom neurologic examination is precluded by sedation or anesthesia. Physicians should be aware that in a few patients with normal CT findings and elevated ICP, the only symptoms are moderate to severe headaches, vomiting, and lethargy.

ICP monitoring with a ventricular catheter, an external strain gauge transducer, or a catheter tip pressure transducer is considered accurate and reliable. Ventriculostomy allows cerebrospinal fluid drainage in addition to ICP monitoring and appears to decrease the magnitude of other therapies needed. In patients with a significant cerebral contusion, an ICP monitor on the same side may more accurately reflect the ICP near the contusion.

ICP in children and adolescents should be kept less than 20 mm Hg. In young infants with open fontanelles and sutures and in older children with large diastatic skull fractures, controlling the ICP at less than 15 mm Hg may be wise.

The guidelines recommend a cerebral perfusion pressure greater than 40 mm Hg in children with TBI. It may be better to maintain cerebral perfusion pressure according to an age-related continuum between 45 and 70 mm Hg.

Initial treatment for elevated ICP includes mild hyperventilation with partial pressure of carbon dioxide (PCO_2) 35 to 40 mm Hg, sedation and analgesia, ventriculostomy drainage, and muscle relaxants. Sedation can be accomplished with low-dose fentanyl 1 to 2 μg/kg per hour, intermittent doses of benzodiazapines or barbiturates, or a low continuous infusion such as pentobarbital or sodium thiopental at 1 mg/kg per hour. If ICP is not controlled, a repeat CT should be obtained and hyperosmolar therapy begun. Osmolar agents include mannitol and hypertonic saline. Hypertonic saline appears to have several advantages over mannitol.[55] A continuous infusion of hypertonic saline allows consistent control of osmolality, potentially minimizing the frequency and magnitude of ICP spikes.[57] Hypertonic saline supports mean arterial pressure and cardiac output. It also has beneficial vasoregulatory properties and may have beneficial effects on the immune and inflammatory responses.[55] The guidelines have found sufficient evidence to include hypertonic saline as an option under hyperosmolar therapy and to regard it as first-tier therapy. Recommendations for osmotherapy include mannitol (also as a first-tier therapy) given as a bolus (0.25 to 1 g/kg) if serum osmolarity is less than 320 mOsm/L, and hypertonic saline (3%) administered as a continuous infusion (0.1 to 1 mL/kg/h). The appropriate dose is the minimum dose required to keep the ICP less than 20 mmHg. The dose may be increased if serum osmolarity is less than 360 mOsm/L.

High-dose barbiturate therapy, hyperventilation to a PCO_2 less than 30 mm Hg, moderate hypothermia, and decompressive craniectomy are regarded as second-tier therapies. It is prudent to obtain a repeat CT of the head each time a significant increase in medical therapy is required. In adults with severe TBI, an aggressive management strategy has been associated with a lower mortality rate, with no significant difference in functional status at discharge among survivors.[58]

ORGAN FAILURE

ACUTE RESPIRATORY DISTRESS SYNDROME

Trauma can result in lung injury and respiratory failure, the most severe of which is ARDS. Post-traumatic respiratory failure results from both direct and indirect injury to the respiratory system. Direct injuries include aspiration of gastric contents, near drowning, smoke inhalation, and pulmonary contusion. Lung injury also occurs indirectly as a consequence of systemic insults such as shock, sepsis, massive transfusion, fat embolism syndrome, or the systemic inflammatory response syndrome (SIRS). ARDS is an acute and progressive respiratory disease of a noncardiac nature associated with diffuse bilateral pulmonary infiltrates and hypoxemia. The definition includes a ratio of arterial oxygen tension (PaO_2) to inspired oxygen fraction (FiO_2) less than 200.

The pathologic findings in ARDS are the result of a complex sequence of cellular and biochemical changes that lead to damage of the endothelial membranes. The specific roles and relative importance of leukocytes, complement activation, prostaglandin release, oxygen radicals, and other mediators of vascular damage are not completely understood. Neutrophils are thought to be an important mediator. This is supported by clinical findings of transient leukopenia in ARDS patients and increased numbers of neutrophils in lung tissue and bronchoalveolar lavage fluid. Blunt trauma enhances the migratory capacity of neutrophils in response to interleukin-8, potentially increasing the risk of ARDS.[59]

The incidence and outcome of ARDS in the pediatric trauma population have not been well studied. In a series of 1989 pediatric trauma patients over an 8-year period with blunt trauma (79%), penetrating trauma (12%), and burns (9%), the overall risk of ARDS was 14%, with a mortality rate of 24%. In those patients with burns, all intubated patients developed ARDS, and the mortality rate was 42%.[60] In a study of adult patients with severe head injury, those patients who developed acute lung injury had a significant increase in mortality (38% versus 15%) and a worse neurologic outome.[61] In our trauma practice, ARDS is seen most often in association with SIRS in patients with severe TBI, often as cerebral edema is improving (unpublished data).

ARDS management in pediatrics has focused on minimizing iatrogenic lung injury and on adjuncts to mechanical ventilation. Both oxygen and mechanical ventilation can be injurious to the lung. Oxygen causes oxidative damage and absorptive atelectasis, with chronic exposure to high inspired concentrations of oxygen creating a pathologic picture indistinguishable from ARDS. In both animal and human studies, toxic reactions to oxygen occur commonly with the use of FiO_2 greater than 0.5, and these effects worsen when excessive oxygen is used for longer than 24 hours. Mechanical ventilation also causes lung injury due to increased shear forces applied in the terminal airways. The higher the tidal volumes used to ventilate patients, the greater the stresses and the larger the risk of secondary lung injury. These stresses on the terminal airways and pulmonary endothelium incite pulmonary edema, surfactant dysfunction, decreased compliance, hyaline membrane formation, and impairment of gas exchange.

Ventilatory strategies focus on decreasing iatrogenic lung injury by limiting oxygen concentration and by using high-frequency or oscillatory ventilation. Permissive hypercapnia (allowing PCO_2 45 to 60 mm Hg or higher) is also practiced when the patient's condition allows. The strategy of "low-stretch" ventilation has been shown to decrease morbidity and mortality in pediatric ARDS.[62,63] Additional support for low-volume, low-pressure ventilation comes from the National Institutes of Health ARDS Network trial comparing 6 mL/kg versus 12 mL/kg tidal volumes in patients with ARDS. Mortality in the low-tidal-volume group was 31.3%, versus a mortality of 39.8% in the higher-tidal-volume group.[64] Paulson and colleagues used a high-rate, low-tidal-volume (3 to 5 mL/kg) strategy on 53 children with severe ARDS and had a survival rate of 89%.[62] Hypercapnia is well tolerated, except in patients with head injury with intracranial hypertension or those with severe pulmonary hypertension. In addition to low-stretch ventilation strategies, helium-oxygen mixtures are being used to improve gas exchange at lower peak pressures. For patients who fail support with mechanical ventilation, some centers are using extracorporeal membrane oxygenation support, with mixed results. There are many other adjuncts to ventilation that may decrease the morbidity and mortality of ARDS. These adjuncts include prone positioning, inhaled nitric oxide (NO), surfactant, steroids, immunomodulation, anti-inflammatory agents, and immunonutrition.

Prone positioning has been used to improve oxygenation in ARDS patients. The improvement may be a result of the redistribution of ventilation or lung perfusion with improved ventilation-perfusion matching. However, prospective randomized trials have not yet been conducted on the effect of prone positioning on the outcome in ARDS. Prone positioning is possible in patients with a wide variety of injuries as well as support lines. If it is not possible, a roto-bed with rotation to 45 degrees can be used with similar benefit.

Inhaled NO has potent pulmonary vasodilatory effects and is potentially useful in ARDS, because increased pulmonary vascular resistance and increased pulmonary shunt are common in this disease. Dellinger and coworkers conducted a randomized trial of inhaled NO versus placebo in 177 patients with ARDS.[65] Although an acute increase in PaO_2 was observed in 60% of patients receiving NO versus 24% of placebo-treated patients, this did not confer any advantage in overall survival. Several other randomized studies of inhaled NO have had similar results.[66] The use of inhaled NO delivered during high-frequency oscillatory ventilation in patients with ARDS resulted in a significant increase in arterial oxygenation.[67]

SHOCK

Shock in children sustaining trauma is most commonly a direct result of hemorrhage, but it can occasionally be the result of tension pneumothorax, spinal cord injury, cardiac tamponade, myocardial contusion, or sepsis. Direct tissue injury and hemorrhage play roles in early shock, while inflammation and altered immune function can result in SIRS, multiple organ failure, and septic shock later in the course.

Children and adults respond differently to hemorrhagic shock. Children have remarkable compensatory mechanisms in response to hypovolemia. Children maintain cardiac output by increasing the heart rate more than the stroke volume. Hypotension is a relatively late sign of traumatic shock in children; therefore, relying on hypotension as an indicator for fluid resuscitation can be deleterious. Tachycardia and signs of end-organ hypoperfusion, such as altered mental status, cool distal extremities, and decreased urine output, may be the primary clinical signs of shock in an injured child.

The focus of therapy for shock in an injured child should be on the restoration and maintenance of adequate oxygen delivery and organ perfusion. Hemodynamic monitoring of central venous pressure and direct arterial blood pressure, as well as cardiac output, may be necessary. In addition, clinical parameters such as base deficit,[68] serum lactate,[69] and measured creatinine clearance are useful indirect measures of adequate end-organ perfusion and may have prognostic value.[68,70] Appropriate therapy of early shock resulting from trauma can alleviate the development of SIRS and multiple organ failure later. Resuscitation with hypertonic saline in two animal models of trauma and hemorrhagic shock was shown to attenuate neutrophil-mediated organ injury; specifically, this occurred in the lung, where much of the inflammation of SIRS occurs, and in the intestine, which is believed to be a major source of neutrophil activation following ischemia.[71,72] There may also be a role for stress-dose steroids following hemorrhagic shock, because sustained adrenal impairment is frequently seen and may be related to the inflammatory consequences and vasopressor dependency of hemorrhagic shock.[73]

The tissue ischemia and hypoperfusion associated with shock result in alteration of cellular function due to oxygen and nutrient deficiency, eventually leading to activation of inflammatory mediators. A current model of SIRS and multiple organ failure in trauma patients is the "two-hit hypothesis." This initial hit is the shock-resuscitation or ischemia-reperfusion phase, which activates neutrophils, making them more susceptible to an exaggerated immune response to late inflammatory stimuli, the second hit.[74,75] Barbiturates and hypothermia, both used to treat severely head injured patients, suppress neutrophil function, increase infectious risks, and may contribute to the late inflammatory stimuli leading to SIRS and multiple organ failure. It may be that severe head injury with release of cytokines itself triggers SIRS. The inflammatory mediator response to trauma that leads to SIRS and multiple organ failure has been proposed as a "three-level model," with mediators acting at the levels of cells, organs, and the organism. Immune modulation has been the focus of current research in trauma with regard to the late sequelae of SIRS and multiple organ failure.[76]

RENAL FAILURE

Renal failure in pediatric trauma patients early in the hospital course is most often due to organ injury from initial shock or from primary injury to the kidney, its vasculature, or urinary outflow tract. Anatomic reasons for renal insufficiency should be delineated by radiographic evaluation. One kidney is sufficient for adequate function; therefore, clinically evident renal failure requires injury to both kidneys or shock.

Renal failure that develops during the course of hospitalization is most commonly secondary to SIRS and multiple organ dysfunction syndrome. In addition, rhabdomyolysis, contrast nephropathy from imaging studies, or nephrotoxicity from medications may occur. Abdominal compartment syndrome and renal vein thrombosis also can lead to renal failure. High-dose mannitol, 0.25 gm/kg/hour as an infusion over 58 ± 28 hours, has been associated with renal failure.[77] This is thought to be secondary to renal vasoconstriction. There is also concern that hypernatremia can cause renal failure. However, in studies using hypertonic saline for control of intracranial hypertension, renal failure did not occur unless SIRS with multiple organ failure was also present.[57]

Signs and symptoms of acute renal failure are due to the accumulation of urea, electrolyte derangements, and volume overload. The first clinical features may be oliguria, hyperkalemia, and elevations in blood urea nitrogen (BUN) and creatinine. The laboratory evaluation of acute renal failure should include measurements of BUN, creatinine, electrolytes with phosphate, magnesium, and calcium, urinalysis, and urine electrolytes. Creatinine clearance should be measured to estimate glomerular filtration rate. Daily 4-hour creatinine clearances are helpful in detecting early changes in renal perfusion and function. Microscopy is necessary to differentiate hemoglobinuria or myoglobinuria from hematuria, and additional tests such as creatine phosphokinase can aid in the confirmation of crush injuries threatening renal function.

Prevention of acute renal failure includes aggressive resuscitation from shock and continued maintenance of cardiac output and organ perfusion pressure. In addition, minimizing and monitoring of nephrotoxic drugs may be helpful. Many agents have been used to prevent and treat acute ischemic or nephrotoxic renal injury. They include furosemide, mannitol, calcium channel blockers, and dopamine, most without benefit.[78] Although diuretic therapy may convert oliguric to nonoliguric acute renal failure, there is no evidence that patient outcome is improved. Prehydration and prophylaxis with theophylline or N-acetylcysteine has been shown to reduce the risk of contrast nephropathy and may be of benefit for children undergoing contrast scans who already have or are otherwise predisposed to develop renal failure.[79] The use of "renal-dose" dopamine has a controversial history marked by conflicting studies. A large randomized, controlled trial in adults concluded that it did not confer clinically significant protection from renal dysfunction.[80] Definitive studies on renal-dose dopamine are lacking in children. Fenoldopam, a selective dopaminergic agent and more potent renal vasodilator than dopamine, has shown some promise in the prevention and treatment of acute renal failure in adults.[81,82]

Early institution of renal replacement therapy in the face of acute renal failure decreases morbidity.[83] Peritoneal dialysis is an excellent modality for infants and children, although trauma patients may have contraindications. Continuous venovenous hemofiltration dialysis is an excellent choice in a high-acuity or head injured patient requiring a steady hyperosmolar state for control of ICP. It offers the benefit of constant and gentle manipulation and control of intravascular volume, electrolytes, dialyzable molecules, and serum osmolarity.[84] The development of regional anticoagulation with citrate-induced hypocalcemia has increased the efficacy and safety of continuous venovenous hemofiltration dialysis, especially in children at risk for bleeding from systemic anticoagulation.

SPECIAL CONSIDERATIONS

IMAGING

Spine Trauma

- Injuries in young children commonly involve C1, C2, and C3. In older children and adolescents, the injury pattern is similar to that in adults, predominantly involving the mid and lower spine.[85]
- The lateral radiograph is the most important view, especially in children younger than 5 years. The false-negative rate for a single cross-table lateral view is 21% to 26%; therefore, additional views or preferably CT scans should be used liberally.[85] If a patient has severe head trauma, consideration should be given to extending the examination to include the cervical spine, because associated fractures are common. Occasionally, no osseous abnormality is seen despite neurologic deficits (SCIWORA).
- Predental space up to 5 mm is normal.

- To confirm pseudosubluxation of C2 on C3, or C3 on C4, use the posterior cervical line. If the posterior cervical line misses the anterior cortex of the C2 spinous process by 2 mm or more, the subluxation is pathologic. A normal posterior cervical line does not exclude underlying ligamentous injury at C2–C3.[85]
- Above the glottis, soft tissue thickness of 7 mm or more is considered abnormal; below the glottis, a measurement of 14 mm should be considered abnormal.[86]
- A distance of 6 mm or more between the lateral mass of C1 and the odontoid process is suggestive of ligamentous disruption of the transverse ligament.
- Posterior tilting of the odontoid is a common normal finding; however, anterior tilting is abnormal and suggests injury.
- When evaluating for atlanto-occipital dislocation, a gap of more than 5 mm between the occipital condyles and the condylar surface of the atlas is highly suggestive of craniocervical injury. A line drawn along the posterior aspect of the clivus toward the odontoid should intersect the odontoid.[85]
- Wedged C3 vertebral body is a normal phenomenon in infants and young children.
- The most common injury of the thoracolumbar spine is a flexion injury. This often results in anterior compression fractures. The more severe the injury, the greater the likelihood of posterior ligamentous injury. It is very important to look for abnormalities of the disc space, widening of the interspinous distance and neural foramina, and fractures of the spinous process and neural arch.
- Transverse fracture of the vertebral body with anterior or lateral dislocation of the upper half of the fractured vertebra is called a Chance fracture and is common in lap-belt injuries. Associated abdominal injuries, especially to the bowel, are common.

Head Trauma

- The type and site of skull fracture are important. Fractures traversing the paranasal sinuses and mastoid can lead to complications such as meningitis, pneumocephalus, and cerebrospinal fluid leak. Depressed fractures commonly have dural tears and brain injury. Fractures that traverse vascular structures, such as the middle meningeal artery, dural sinuses, and carotid and vertebral arteries, are important to recognize because of the possibility of underlying vascular injury.
- Acute subdural hematoma has a crescent shape and is generally hyperdense; however, approximately 40% are heterogeneous owing to unclotted blood or cerebrospinal fluid.
- Diffuse axonal injury tends to occur in the lobar white matter (especially at the gray-white matter interface), corpus callosum, and dorsolateral aspect of the upper brainstem. Gradient-echo magnetic resonance sequences are sensitive for evaluation.
- CT often finds more contusions 24 to 48 hours after the initial CT scan. In 20% of contusions, delayed hemorrhage occurs in what were thought to be nonhemorrhagic contusions on initial CT.
- A common place for subarachnoid hemorrhage to accumulate is in the interpeduncular fossa. Fluid attenuated inversion recovery magnetic resonance sequences are very sensitive for subarachnoid hemorrhage.
- Manifestations of nonaccidental trauma include multiple, complex, or depressed skull fractures; subdural hematomas

of varying ages; bilateral subdural hematomas; cortical contusions; diffuse axonal injury; retinal hemorrhages; and cerebral ischemia or infarction.[87]

Thoracic Trauma

- Anterior or lateral rib fractures over the lower thoracic region may be associated with splenic or hepatic injury. Fractures of the first three ribs should raise the suspicion of great vessel injury. Low posterior rib fractures may be associated with renal injury.
- Sternal fractures are frequently associated with underlying cardiac injury.[86]
- Radiographs usually underestimate the full extent of pulmonary trauma.
- Tears of the right mainstem and distal left bronchus give rise to pneumothorax. Tears of the trachea and left mainstem bronchus usually cause pneumomediastinum and widening of the mediastinum if bleeding occurs.

Abdominal Trauma

- Indirect indications of organ injury on radiographs include elevation of the diaphragm, obliteration of fat planes, free intraperitoneal air or trapped air (retroperitoneal air), mass effect, thumb-printing of bowel owing to intramural hematoma, fractures, portal venous gas, and hemoperitoneum.
- Hypoperfusion complex is seen in patients presenting in shock who seem to respond to initial resuscitation. Mortality is approximately 85%. Constant findings on CT include marked, diffuse bowel dilatation; intense contrast enhancement (bowel wall, mesentery, kidneys), and small-caliber inferior vena cava and aorta.
- Plain film findings associated with splenic injury include medial displacement of the stomach, displacement of the splenic flexure, elevation of the left hemidiaphragm, scoliosis of the spine with concavity on the left, sentinel loops in the left upper quadrant, left pleural effusions or atelectasis, and rib fractures.
- Periportal tracking is seen in up to 22% cases of hepatic injury, which is due to dissecting blood, bile, or dilated lymphatics. Hemoperitoneum is common in liver laceration owing to the inability of liver vessels to contract.
- Technetium-labeled N-substituted iminodiacetic acid compound (HIDA) scans are very useful in evaluating for possible bile leak in a patient with persistent free fluid in the abdomen after liver injury.
- Pancreatic injury is difficult to visualize on initial CT scans.
- Trauma to the duodenum may include duodenal rupture, intramural tears, or intramural hematoma. The usual site of perforation is along the posterior duodenal wall.[86]
- CT findings of bowel injury in blunt abdominal trauma include hypodense free fluid (85%), particularly in an interloop location due to perforation; focal bowel wall thickening (>3 cm); focal discontinuity of bowel; sentinel clot adjacent to bowel; streaky, hyperattenuating mesentery; mesenteric hematoma; hyperdense contrast enhancement of injured bowel; pneumoperitoneum; and extravasation of contrast.[88]

Genitourinary Trauma

- CT findings of renal injury are as follows. For contusion: focal patchy enhancement or striated nephrogram. For laceration: irregular, linear, hypodense parenchymal abnormalities. For shattered kidney: multiple separated fragments, some of which may not enhance owing to a lack of perfusion. For subcapsular hematoma: superficial crescentic hypodense area compressing adjacent parenchyma. For segmental arterial injury: wedge-shaped perfusion defect. For devascularized kidney: diffuse lack of enhancement of kidney. For renal vein thrombosis: persistent nephrogram on delayed images and renal swelling.[88] Delayed images are essential in the evaluation of renal trauma.
- Blunt trauma to the ureteropelvic junction is associated with transverse process fractures (30%).
- In infants and young children, a full bladder becomes an abdominal organ as it arises out of the pelvis and is more prone to injury because it is not as protected as the adult urinary bladder.
- CT cystography is highly accurate as an adjunct to routine abdominopelvic CT in the trauma setting. It obviates the need for a separate study with conventional cystography, which entails additional cost and more radiation exposure.

INFECTIOUS DISEASE AND IMMUNOLOGY

A child who sustains trauma is susceptible to infection in several ways. The trauma itself may destroy the barriers of skin and mucosa, allowing both pathogenic and nonpathogenic organisms the opportunity to establish a productive infection. In addition, significant immune dysfunction occurs following trauma; both nonspecific and specific abnormalities have been described in cellular and humoral responses, as well as in macrophage and neutrophil function.[89-91] More recent investigations provide data on cytokines and other mediators and molecular markers of inflammation, both circulating and cell surface.[92,93] These abnormalities of immune dysfunction can be categorized under two basic mechanisms: hyperactive systemic proinflammatory processes, and depression of cell-mediated immunity. Hyperactive proinflammatory responses may be ultimately deleterious to a child, leading to SIRS, multiple organ dysfunction syndrome, and death. Hyperactive proinflammatory response may be the result of priming the trauma patient for an exaggerated response to a second inflammatory stimulus, referred to as the two-hit hypothesis. Differences in the characteristics of immune dysfunction appear to be a function of the type of trauma (e.g., head injury, blunt trauma, burn injury) and appear to change over time after trauma to reflect changes in the acute activation seen immediately after the injury, with subsequent evolution into immune suppression.[91] Many of the abnormalities may be directly correlated with the severity of injury.[90] Infections occurring within approximately 5 to 7 days of admission are more likely to represent inoculation at the time of trauma, whereas infections occurring after the first week of trauma reflect nosocomial pathogens present in the trauma center.

Empiric therapy of the pediatric trauma patient on admission to the ICU is not well studied. Extrapolation from prospective, controlled surgical studies in adults has provided some support for empirical, prophylactic therapy, with the selection of antibiotics designed to provide reasonable coverage against anticipated pathogens. However, each trauma case should be evaluated individually for the types of organisms likely to cause infection, with empirical antibiotic therapy tailored to the location and severity of injury. No published data exist on the benefits or risks of empirical therapy for fungi or multiply resistant environmental bacteria in soil-contaminated injuries; therefore, extremely broad-spectrum antibiotic and antifungal agent prophylaxis is usually not recommended. Cultures obtained at the time of admission and surgical closure of open wounds can help the trauma team evaluate the child for infection later in the hospital course. Tetanus immunization should be considered in a child with devitalized, ischemic, and denervated tissues that have been inoculated by soil, or with deep tissue injury by foreign objects that have been in contact with soil.

Nosocomial infections of indwelling vascular catheters, surgically implanted foreign bodies, the lung, the urinary tract, and injured tissues are all well recognized, with therapy targeted to the organisms prevalent in the ICU. Gram stained exudates and cultures can assist in providing information on the types and susceptibilities of the nosocomial pathogens causing infection. Providing sufficiently broad coverage empirically to achieve a high likelihood of success may both improve patient outcomes and decrease the emergence of certain antibiotic-resistant organisms. The definitive selection of antibiotics and a decision on the duration of therapy should be based on the isolated or suspected pathogens and the child's response to therapy. A poor response to broad-spectrum therapy despite the use of antimicrobial agents active against the isolated pathogens suggests either a hidden focus of infection, which may require further investigation and possible surgical intervention, or additional antibiotic-resistant pathogens not originally isolated. Lack of response to therapy may also be related to noninfectious causes of clinical instability. Therapy should not be continued indefinitely, because subsequent colonization and infection by antibiotic-resistant bacteria or yeast are likely to occur. Once antimicrobial therapy is discontinued, careful observation for relapse or recurrence of infection is essential.

Several therapies have been suggested to obviate the consequences of immune dysfunction in trauma patients. Circulating granulocyte colony-stimulating factor has been shown to be highest on postinjury day 1 and then quickly declines to near normal values by postinjury day 3.[94] In addition, plasma from trauma patients suppresses bone marrow colony growth of granulocyte-monocyte precursors for up to 2 weeks after injury.[95] Administration of filgrastim in neutropenic, septic, and head injured patients has resulted in improved generation and function of neutrophils.[96] Prophylactic use in patients with TBI showed a dose-dependent decrease in the frequency of bacteremia.[97] Because there is a complex relationship between the neuroendocrine and immune systems, many studies have explored hormonal therapies to improve T-cell and macrophage function. Potential therapeutic agents after trauma include dehydroepiandrosterone and prolactin and metoclopramide. In addition, hypertonic saline may improve T-cell function and possibly prevent the exaggerated proinflammatory response leading to lung injury.

COAGULOPATHIES

Trauma is a potent activator of the inflammatory response, and a growing body of literature describes the relationship among inflammatory cytokines, endothelial function, and coagulation through cellular and molecular signaling.[98] A severely injured child is at risk for impaired hemostasis as well as pathologic thrombosis.

Activation of the coagulation cascade is proportional to the stimulus. Local thrombus formation by a discrete injury is protective by inhibiting local bleeding, and pathologic thrombosis is normally impeded by anticoagulant mechanisms. Massive activation of the coagulation axis can overwhelm the counterbalancing mechanisms, leading to deep venous thrombosis locally or microvascular thrombosis systemically. The latter culminates in varying degrees of clotting factor consumption and pathologic and protective thrombolysis and may ultimately result in disseminated intravascular coagulopathy (DIC). The microangiopathic thrombosis of DIC can also contribute to hemolytic anemia, ARDS, and organ failure remote to the site of traumatic injury. The epidemiology of injuries in children puts them at increased risk for trauma-induced DIC because the brain and liver release strong procoagulant thromboplastins. Indeed, the likelihood of coagulopathy has an inverse relationship to the presenting GCS score.[99]

The evaluation and treatment of physiologic derangements that promote bleeding are necessary in an injured child. Although definitive evaluation by laboratory assays may not be available immediately, early suspicion of coagulopathy based on clinical history, physical examination, and medical interventions may be lifesaving in a traumatically injured child.

Even in the absence of a coagulopathy at presentation, it is necessary to prevent iatrogenic coagulation disturbances. Dilutional coagulopathy can occur with the administration of as little as one unwarmed blood volume. After one to two blood volumes, platelets can be halved, and the activated partial thromboplastin time and prothrombin time can be doubled. In an injured child receiving blood products, coagulation studies should be sent early. As volume resuscitation continues, these studies should be checked frequently to refine blood product administration. Hypothermia may contribute to coagulopathy during resuscitation and should be prevented.

If a patient has normal coagulation values but continues to bleed diffusely, an underlying bleeding diathesis should be considered. Von Willebrand's disease is the most common congenital bleeding disorder and has traditionally been assessed by a bedside bleeding time. However, uncertainty about the sensitivity, reliability, and predictive value of the bleeding time has led to a decline in its use. A platelet function assay, PFA-100, has been compared with bleeding time and is considered a superior screening test for primary hemostasis disorders.[100]

Although the overall physiology of coagulation in children is nearly identical to that of adults, there are some special considerations in injured children. The neonate's relatively immature liver and initial nutritional state increase the likelihood that vitamin K–dependent clotting factors will be decreased. Nonaccidental trauma in infants and children frequently includes occult head injuries and the release of potent thromboplastins. Young children may have a yet undiagnosed congenital bleeding disorder. Compared with adults, the relative health of the cardiopulmonary and renal systems allows children to tolerate significant hypovolemia and large-volume resuscitation that may result in a dilutional coagulopathy. The medical disorders and medications that can promote bleeding in adults also apply to children, although most are far less prevalent in the pediatric population.

In the ICU, patients are at increased risk of pathologic thrombosis secondary to endothelial damage and indwelling central catheters. Traumatic and pharmacologic paralysis, in addition to bed rest, contribute to venous stasis. Although the risk of deep venous thrombosis and thromboembolic disease is lower in prepubertal children than in adults, it is more prevalent than previously recognized.[101,102] Hypercoagulable states occur across the age spectrum, and children with nephrotic syndrome, inherited forms of thrombophilia, and some rheumatologic disorders are at increased risk for pathologic clot formation. Prophylaxis with low-dose heparin or automated venous compression stockings should be used in appropriate patients.

NUTRITION

Nutritional support of critically injured children is extremely important and is based on knowledge gained from research in critically ill adult and pediatric patients, as well as physiologic differences between pediatric and adult patients. A key difference is the requirement for maintenance of growth and development. Pediatric patients' resting basal metabolic rate is approximately 50% higher than adults'. In addition, pediatric patients have lower energy stores than adults.

A state of hypermetabolism is well documented in adult patients after major traumatic injury and surgical stress. Similar data also exist in critically ill pediatric patients and pediatric trauma patients. Following an extensive review of the literature, the "Guidelines for the Acute Medical Management of Severe Traumatic Brain Injury in Infants, Children, and Adolescents" lists as a treatment option the replacement of 130% to 160% of resting metabolism after TBI in pediatric patients.[56] Patients who are paralyzed or in barbiturate coma have a lower resting metabolic rate and require fewer calories.

The enteral route is preferable, and much research has been performed related to the benefits of enteral versus parenteral nutrition. In a meta-analysis, benefits of enteral nutrition included lower risk of infection and reduction in hospital length of stay.[103] Other proposed benefits include preservation of intestinal mucosal integrity, with decreased bacterial translocation, and decrease in multiple organ failure. Enteral feeding is also more cost-effective than parenteral nutrition in pediatric patients.[104] There are many adult studies supporting the initiation of enteral feeding within 24 to 72 hours of ICU admission.

Owing to impaired GI motility in critically ill trauma patients, enteral feeding may be poorly tolerated. Gastric emptying is often delayed following severe head injury. In addition, many of the medications used during the treatment of traumatically injured patients may affect GI motility. Narcotics, benzodiazepines, and catecholamines can adversely affect feeding tolerance. Barbiturates decrease GI motility, and severe gastroparesis has been described. Many patients with severe head injury requiring barbiturate coma do not tolerate full enteral nutrition.

Large gastric residual volume, associated with lack of tolerance of gastric feeding, may increase the incidence of aspiration pneumonia and has been associated with higher ICU mortality in adults.[105] Continuous gastric infusion of formula, addition of prokinetic agents, or transpyloric feeding may improve feeding tolerance. In some pediatric trauma patients, enteral feeding is unrealistic. It is clear that the most important action is to provide nutritional support as soon as feasible, with the decision of enteral versus parenteral support individualized to the patient.

Two special topics deserve mention. First, although there are no data regarding the effect of immune-enhancing diets in pediatric patients, in adults, supplementation of arginine, glutamine, nucleotides, and omega-3-fatty acids has been used to improve outcome. These special formulations show promise with respect to decreased length of stay and decreased infectious complications.[106-108] Second, control of blood glucose levels in adult surgical ICU patients has been shown to have an important beneficial effect. Tight glucose control with insulin significantly reduced morbidity and mortality in these patients.[109] Similar studies have not been performed in pediatric patients.

SEDATION AND PAIN

Injured children commonly require analgesia and anxiolysis during therapy and management of various injuries. There are myriad drugs that can be safely used to provide appropriate levels of analgesia and anxiolysis.

In addition to providing pain relief and anxiolysis, sedatives and analgesics may reduce elevated ICP, facilitate mechanical ventilation, prevent shivering, provide anticonvulsant activity, and minimize long-term psychological trauma from untreated pain and stress.[56] The importance of restoring and maintaining circulating intravascular volume before administering sedatives cannot be overstated, as children may be "surviving" on endogenous catecholamine release, thereby barely maintaining adequate blood pressure and tissue perfusion. The administration of even small doses of any sedative in this situation may precipitate cardiovascular collapse and cardiac arrest. Empirical treatment of presumed hypovolemia should precede administration of sedatives in an acutely injured child.

In the initial setting of evaluating an acutely injured child, small doses of narcotics such as fentanyl, given in incremental doses (0.5 µg/kg per dose, up to 1 to 2 µg/kg) titrated to effect, can be useful in both providing analgesia and allowing a more detailed examination. A child with painful injuries (e.g., fractures, multiple abrasions) is often more cooperative and allows a more thorough examination after receiving adequate analgesia. Concerns about "masking" the presence of intra-abdominal injury are unfounded, as the cooperation achieved from the analgesia outweighs the difficulty in examining an agitated, screaming child who is experiencing acute pain. It is rarely necessary to administer benzodiazepines or other anxiolytic drugs in the acute setting of pediatric trauma, provided adequate analgesia is given. In a mechanically ventilated patient, benzodiazepine (midazolam, diazepam, lorazepam) administration by intermittent dosing or by continuous infusion is commonly used to provide anxiolysis.

A variety of short-acting drugs can be used to provide hypnosis and loss of consciousness for endotracheal intubation. A detailed analysis of the advantages and disadvantages of these drugs is beyond the scope of this chapter.

Sodium thiopental (4 to 6 mg/kg) is commonly used in a hemodynamically stable child in this setting because it is rapid acting (30 to 60 seconds) and can be used to treat elevated ICP. Further, sodium thiopental (1 to 2 mg/kg every 15 to 30 minutes) can be used following successful intubation to maintain unconsciousness during transport to the ICU, operating room, or radiology department. The use of thiopental for sedation for radiographic procedures in a nonintubated, spontaneously breathing patient should be reserved for elective situations in fasted patients, and it should be administered by an anesthesiologist.[56]

Except for inducing general anesthesia, the use of propofol for critically injured children is controversial and, in fact, is rarely necessary in the acute setting. A poorly defined syndrome of metabolic acidosis and myocardial failure has been reported after giving propofol by continuous infusion in the critical care setting. Nevertheless, many pediatric intensivists use propofol for short intervals, especially during the weaning of narcotic-dependent children from mechanical ventilation.

INFLICTED TRAUMA

Abuse is a common cause of traumatic injury in infants and young children.[110,111] Nationally, it is estimated that 1200 children died due to abuse or neglect in 2000, a rate of 1.71 per 100,000 children. Children younger than 12 months accounted for 43.7% of these fatalities, and 85% were younger than 6 years. Recognition of inflicted injury is important to ensure appropriate care, prevent recurrence of abuse, protect siblings, and comply with reporting mandates.

A delay in seeking care is common in children with abusive injuries. Injury history may be absent, incomplete, or inconsistent with physical findings or the developmental capability of the child. Domestic violence is common in families of abused children. Children with inflicted injuries that have more subtle findings and patients with intact families are more likely to be misdiagnosed as accidentally injured. This may have serious repercussions, including further injury and death.[112] Children with abusive injuries have worse outcomes than those with accidental injuries, with higher severity and mortality rates and higher patient costs.[113] Having a high index of suspicion for nonaccidental trauma is critical in assessing an infant that presents with lethargy, apnea, cyanosis, mottling, poor perfusion, or seizures without an obvious history of trauma.

Evaluation of children with inflicted injury should reflect the occult nature of many abusive injuries. The constellation of subdural hematoma, traction-type metaphyseal (bucket-handle) fractures of long bones, posterior rib fractures, and retinal hemorrhages are characteristic of inflicted injuries in infants. Although TBI is the leading cause of morbidity and mortality in abused children, some head injuries may not be easily diagnosed clinically.[114] Therefore, a nonambulatory infant with any type of abusive injury should have CT or magnetic resonance imaging studies of the brain performed. The sudden deceleration with forceful striking of the head against a surface is an important mechanism responsible for inflicted brain injuries in children. Hypoxic-ischemic insults and other mechanisms also appear to play a role. Subdural hemorrhage, classically localized at the parieto-occipital convexity or posterior interhemispheric fissure, is the most consistent autopsy finding in shaking-impact syndrome. Subdural hematoma results from rotational deceleration forces that cause shearing of bridging cortical veins. Retinal hemorrhages are present in the majority of children with inflicted injuries, but their absence does not rule out abuse. In addition, not all retinal hemorrhages are due to abuse. Infrequently, accidental head injuries may cause retinal hemorrhages.[115] Therefore, an evaluation by a pediatric ophthalmologist is recommended in all children with suspected abusive head injury. A skeletal survey should be done in all children with serious injury due to abuse. Screening for abdominal trauma is also important, either through imaging or laboratory studies. A psychosocial evaluation is critical in families of children with inflicted injuries. This is to help support the family during a time of crisis; evaluate for other comorbid factors such as domestic violence, substance abuse, and mental illness; comply with mandated reporting requirements; and help interface with investigative and protective agencies.

A multidisciplinary team is optimal for treating children with inflicted injuries. The team should consist of the treating staff, a medical social worker, and a child abuse pediatrician.

REHABILITATION

Once life-threatening conditions have been ameliorated and the medical condition stabilized, the pediatric trauma patient should be assessed for the restoration of maximal functional independence. It is the role of the pediatric physiatrist and rehabilitation medicine team to identify, assess, and promote the maximum restoration of physical, cognitive, and psychosocial functioning in each patient. Members of the rehabilitation team, including occupational therapists, physical therapists, speech therapists, social workers, and schoolteachers, provide their expertise in returning the patient to maximum independent function. As a first step, it is important to identify the patient's functional deficits and subsequent level of disability and handicap as they relate to the patient's home, community, and school settings.

The rehabilitation process should begin early in the patient's critical care stay, because physical and occupational modalities may limit the adverse physiologic effects of prolonged immobilization. For instance, muscles lose their flexibility and bulk, resulting in diminished strength and endurance. Joints become stiff and contracted, and skin breaks down, creating pressure ulcers. Interventions include passive joint range of motion, isometric strengthening, and appropriate bed positioning. Orthotic devices placed at joints (e.g., elbows and ankles), in a neutral position, limit contracture formation. Speech and occupational therapists can evaluate oral motor function to assess safe swallowing and feeding, decreasing the patient's risk of aspiration. The dietitian evaluates the patient's nutritional status, providing recommendations for appropriate diet and caloric intake. The social worker and child life specialist provide the patient and family members with emotional and educational support during the patient's acute critical care stabilization.

It is through the collaborative efforts of the pediatric trauma team and the pediatric rehabilitation team that the survivor of a pediatric trauma maximizes functional independence and has a successful discharge home.

BRAIN DEATH AND ORGAN DONATION

The first definition of irreversible coma as a criterion for death, as well as the criteria for diagnosis, was published in 1968 by an ad hoc committee of the Harvard Medical School. In 1981, the President's Commission for the Study of Ethical Problems in Medicine and Biomedical and Behavioral Research published a report titled "Defining Death: Medical, Legal, and Ethical Issues in the Determination of Death," which summarized medical practice for the determination of cardiorespiratory and neurologic death. A summary of the guidelines was published in the medical literature. These guidelines provided a conceptual definition of brain death and left the criteria for determination up to accepted medical standards. In addition, it established common ground for law related to the diagnosis of brain death. In 1987, the American Academy of Pediatrics published guidelines for the determination of brain death in pediatric patients,[116] with specifications for physical examination, observation period, and confirmatory laboratory testing. These guidelines have attempted to define the clinical determination of irreversible cessation of all brain function to the best of medical ability. The need to define brain death was fueled by improvements in the intensive care of critically ill patients, as well as advances in solid organ transplantation. There is continued debate by experts regarding whether patients who have been determined to be brain dead by current guidelines have irreversible loss of all brain function. In addition, controversy exists regarding whether brain death should be defined as loss of higher brain function and not loss of all brain function.[117]

Trauma patients represent a large percentage of those who are declared brain dead in a pediatric ICU and therefore a large pool of potential organ donors. There continues to be a wide gap between the number of organs available for transplantation and the number of patients needing transplants, with more than 80,000 patients currently awaiting transplantation in the United States. Improvement in consent for organ donation is one way to decrease this gap. Despite widespread acceptance of, and support for, organ donation among the general public, only 40% to 60% of families give consent for donation. Consent rates for donation are improved when the family understands the concept of brain death and when the understanding occurs before the request for donation (decoupling). In addition, the consent rate is maximized when the requester has specialized training or is a member of the organ procurement organization. In pediatric trauma patients, the involvement of the attending physician in the request process may also have a beneficial effect on consent rates.[118]

In an effort to increase organ donation, federal regulations were issued in 1998 governing how potential organ donors should be identified and approached.[119] All hospitals must have an agreement with an organ procurement organization (OPO) and must notify the organization of patient deaths. The procurement organization then determines the patient's suitability for organ donation. In addition, the hospital must have an agreement with a tissue bank and eye bank to coordinate tissue and eye donation. The family of every potential donor must be informed of the option to donate organs or tissues.

Until recently, virtually all organ donors were declared brain dead before organ procurement. In the early 1990s, the University of Pittsburgh introduced a protocol for non-heart-beating cadaveric donation. There is controversy regarding the ethics of these protocols; however, it appears that the general public supports the use of non-heart-beating donors once the decision to remove life support has been made.[120] Recommendations for non-heart-beating donation have been proposed by the Society of Critical Care Medicine, including recommendations for pediatric patients.[121]

Victims of child abuse represent a special subset of pediatric patients. The documentation of injuries in child abuse cases is extremely important and has significant legal ramifications. The medical examiner plays a key role in determining whether legally deceased child abuse victims may be released for organ procurement. The medical examiner may prohibit organ procurement if there is concern that the process will alter forensic evidence. Implementation of procedures to fully document the state of the abdominal cavity and the extent of abdominal injuries in the operating room before procurement may facilitate release for donation.

Documentation may be performed by the transplant surgeon or the medical examiner.[122,123]

BURNOUT

Much attention has been given to trauma team composition and member qualifications, the roles and responsibilities of members, policies and procedures, and who should lead the team. Burnout of team members, as well as the qualities of an effective leader, however, are seldom referred to in the trauma literature.

The burnout rate is 30% to 40% for the medical profession, including trauma surgeons, general surgeons, emergency physicians, pediatric critical care specialists, social workers, and nurses. Two major contributing factors to burnout in pediatric intensivists include needing to argue to get things accomplished and the feeling that one's work is not valued by patients, colleagues, administrators, and nurses. A survey of surgical residents reported a high degree of dissatisfaction with trauma medicine as a career. Reasons for dissatisfaction included the belief that trauma was becoming a nonoperative specialty (81% of respondents) and dislike of working with other specialists, including neurosurgeons and orthopedic surgeons (77%).

Even physicians who are not burned out are subject to frustrations, many of which relate to personal conflicts, fragmented personal relationships, breakdown of communication, undermining of teamwork, and a system where physicians work separately—often working against each other rather than working together. Reducing these types of frustration may lead not only to less burnout and greater job satisfaction but also better outcomes for patients.[124]

ANNOTATED REFERENCES

Bayir H, Kochanek PM, Clark RS: Traumatic brain injury in infants and children: Mechanisms of secondary damage and treatment in the intensive care unit. Crit Care Clin 2003;19:529-549.

No specific pharmacologic therapies are available for the treatment of TBI in patients. More detailed knowledge regarding the dominant pathophysiologic mechanisms associated with TBI-excitotoxicity, CBF dysregulation, oxidative stress, and programmed cell death will lead to development of more efficacious therapies—a potent agent targeting a single dominant pathway, a broad-spectrum intervention such as hypothermia, or, more likely, a combination of therapies. Meanwhile, practitioners must offer meticulous supportive neurointensive care using clinically proven therapies aimed at minimizing cerebral swelling for the management of pediatric patients who are victims of TBI.

Bliss D, Silen M: Pediatric thoracic trauma. Crit Care Med 2002;30 (11 Suppl):S409-S415.

Thoracic injuries in children remain a source of substantial morbidity and mortality. Disparate problems such as rib fractures, lung injury, hemothorax, pneumothorax, mediastinal injuries, and others may present in isolation or in combination with one another. Differences in pulmonary functional residual capacity, blood volume, chest wall and spinal soft-tissue mobility, and cardiac function all have to be carefully evaluated.

Mazzola CA, Adelson PD: Critical care management of head trauma in children. Crit Care Med 2002;30(11 Suppl):S393-S401.

Trauma is the leading cause of morbidity and mortality in the pediatric population, and traumatic injury causes > 50% of all childhood deaths. Significant mortality rates have been reported for children with traumatic brain injury. Although children have better survival rates as compared with adults with traumatic brain injury, the long-term sequelae and consequences are often more devastating in children due to their age and developmental potential.

Proctor MR: Spinal cord injury. Crit Care Med 2002;30(11 Suppl):S489-S499.

This article discusses the types of injuries seen in children with an emphasis an acute management and clearance of the cervical spine. Treatment options and long-term issues are also discussed.

Chapter 249

MANAGEMENT OF THE BRAIN-DEAD ORGAN DONOR

Robert Chavko • Akhtar S. Khan • Joseph M. Darby

KEY POINTS

1. Because the **supply of cadaveric organ donors is limited and their ICU management is complex,** a multidisciplinary, well-coordinated, and institutionally supported approach to management is essential to ensure the maintenance of the current supply and to increase the future supply of organs and tissues that are suitable for transplantation.

2. **Early identification of the potential organ donor,** the diagnosis and certification of brain death, life support and resuscitation, family support, and coordination of care with the local organ procurement organization (OPO) are the essential elements in the process leading to the successful procurement of organs and tissues from the potential donor.

3. All patients admitted to the ICU with an obviously **lethal brain insult or injury** should be considered potential organ donors unless they have been determined to be medically ineligible by the OPO or the family has refused consent to donation after brain death has been certified.

4. **Physiologic changes occurring during and after the evolution of brain death** that result in the loss of physiologic homeostasis as well as complications associated with life support may lead to hemodynamic instability, cardiac arrest, infectious complications, and the loss of the potential organ donor.

5. **Hemodynamic instability in the potential organ donor after brain death** manifests principally as hypotension as a result of infarction of brainstem vasomotor centers, volume depletion from diabetes insipidus, and myocardial injury that may occur during the catecholamine storm that precedes brain death.

6. **Hormonal changes occurring after brain death** and potentially influencing hemodynamic stability of the organ donor include reductions in circulating antidiuretic hormone and thyroid hormones.

7. The **inherent instability of the potential organ donor** necessitates that the principal goal of ICU management be the maintenance of vital organ function under conditions in which hypotension, diabetes insipidus, hypothermia, cardiac arrhythmias, electrolyte disturbances, metabolic acidosis, pulmonary edema, and cardiac arrest all threaten the viability of the transplantable organs.

8. The **keys to successful ICU management of the potential organ donor** include a dedicated multidisciplinary team approach that is focused on the anticipation of complications, appropriate physiologic monitoring, aggressive life support, with frequent reassessment and titration of therapy.

9. **The greatest danger to the viability of transplantable organs is hypotension,** which is treated with liberal volume expansion and vasopressors balanced to minimize the adverse effects of vasopressors on organ flow while reducing the risk of pulmonary edema from too vigorous fluid resuscitation.

10. Although controversial, **"hormonal resuscitation"** of the potential organ donor including the use of thyroid hormones, vasopressin, and insulin is considered by the United Network for Organ Sharing to be an integral component of the critical pathway for donor management.

11. **Family refusal to consent to donation remains the most important problem** that reduces the available pool of actual organ donors in the United States, necessitating federal regulations that require hospitals to notify the local OPO of all imminent and actual deaths, offer all potential donors the option to donate, and also require that any request for organ donation be made by an OPO representative or "designated requestor."

12. **Interventions that appear to improve the likelihood of a successful request for organ donation** include the provision of a private setting for family members, involvement of an on-site organ procurement coordinator, separation of the notification of brain death from the request for donation, race-specific requestors, and an institutional commitment to improving the education of staff and the processes pertinent to the potential organ donor.

Approximately 77% of all organs transplanted in the United States are obtained from cadaver donors, most of whom are brain dead at the time of organ procurement.[1] Although the numbers are increasing, a very small percentage of these donors are non–heartbeating donors when organs are procured after the termination of life support and death is certified by standard cardiopulmonary criteria. Whereas the pool of actual potential brain-dead organ donors has grown steadily over the past decade, the rate of growth is still inadequate to meet the demands of an ever-increasing pool of patients who are awaiting organ transplants. The nature of the donor supply emphasizes the central role that the ICU and ICU management of the potential organ donor plays in maintaining and increasing the current supply of donor organs.

Because of the inherent instability of the potential organ donor and the implications for family members, successful outcomes in this complex process of care require a multidisciplinary, well-coordinated, and institutionally supported approach. For the intensivist and other physicians attending to the patient with a catastrophic brain injury or insult, optimal management requires knowledge of pathophysiology and treatment strategies. It is also worth mentioning that care of the brain-dead donor entails substantial time commitment from the intensivist and other members of the ICU team to establish and confirm brain death, provide resuscitation, maintain ongoing cardiac and pulmonary support, provide emotional support for the family, and coordinate care with the local OPO.[2] Finally, it is important to emphasize that the process of requesting and obtaining consent for organ donation is challenging and time consuming. This aspect of the organ-procurement process requires commitment, experience, knowledge, and judgment on the part of the participating physicians.[3] The diagnosis and certification of brain death is discussed in Chapter 256.

RECOGNITION OF THE POTENTIAL ORGAN DONOR

In the past, one of the major impediments to achieving maximum utilization of the potential organ donor pool has been the failure to recognize the potential donor after admission to the hospital. Federal legislation in the United States has mandated notification of the local OPO of all imminent deaths.[4] This approach has helped to increase the number of patients who are recognized as potential organ donors.[5,6] However, to optimize the number of organs successfully procured from appropriate donors, it is essential that ICU personnel identify catastrophically brain-injured patients as early as possible after ICU admission and recognize their potential as organ donors in case therapy directed at sustaining life proves to be futile. Early identification will help to ensure that the ICU staff maintains vigilance in all aspects of supportive care and provides the necessary support of the family. Prompt notification of the OPO can reduce the time necessary to evaluate the potential donor should patient progress to brain death and can also provide a preliminary assessment of medical eligibility. Delayed recognition of patients as potential organ donors may result in missed opportunities for organ procurement as a consequence of hemodynamic instability, cardiac arrest, inadequate resuscitation, infectious complications, or dissatisfaction with care on the part of family members.[7-10]

The typical brain-dead organ donor has sustained a catastrophic brain insult or injury that is manifested clinically by coma, impairment in brainstem reflexes, massive brain swelling, and/or refractory intracranial hypertension. Of the 6182 cadaveric organ donors in 2002, death was caused by cardiovascular accident/stroke in 42%, head injury in 42%, and anoxia in 12%.[11] Comatose patients in these diagnostic categories are at risk for progressing to brain death and should be considered potentially eligible organ donors.

DONOR ACCEPTANCE CRITERIA

Donor and organ acceptance criteria are not yet standardized and continue to evolve. Each local OPO is required to have acceptance criteria. Despite the lack of universal standards, general medical criteria that usually exclude potential donors from further consideration are infectious diseases and disseminated malignancies. Viral hepatitis, encephalitis, AIDS, active cytomegalovirus infection, systemic herpesvirus infections, active tuberculosis, and untreated syphilis generally exclude potential donors from further consideration. However, there is some variability in practice regarding serologic evidence of hepatitis and cytomegalovirus infection. In the past, bacterial and fungal sepsis were considered contraindications to organ donation. Recent data, however, indicate that the risk of transmission of these infections to recipients receiving prophylactic antibiotics is negligible.[12,13] Malignancies localized to the skin, central nervous system, or cervix are generally not cause for exclusion from organ donation.

There is a general tendency to consider the elderly as ineligible as potential donors. A number of factors, including aging of the population, the limited availability of donor organs, the increased demand for organs, and the decreasing number of younger donors with traumatic brain injury, militate against using chronologic age of the organ donor as a firm donor acceptance criterion. Recent trends in the relaxation of donor age criteria have resulted in an increase in the average donor age; the percentage of organ donors older than age 65 now approaches 10%.[11] Increasingly, organs previously considered to be too marginal for transplantation are now being transplanted. In consideration of these trends, age should not be used to exclude a potential donor without first consulting the local OPO. Ultimately, medical eligibility of the donor and the suitability of individual organs will be determined by the local OPO and transplant surgeons. A focused diagnostic evaluation of donor organ function and serologic testing for compatibility is typically performed by the OPO after consent for donation has been obtained.

PATHOPHYSIOLOGY OF BRAIN DEATH

The potential organ donor is at high risk for instability as a direct consequence of the loss of physiologic homeostatic mechanisms that are dependent on functioning of the central nervous system. Hemodynamic instability and cardiac arrest after brain death accounts for the loss of as many as 25% of potential donors.[8,10,14,15] Optimal care of the potential organ donor in the ICU therefore requires an understanding of the basic pathophysiologic changes that occur during the evolution of brain death and the subsequent changes that become apparent during the somatic life-support phase following brain death. The vast majority of patients progressing to brain death deteriorate in a similar fashion, but the cause of the neurologic insult, rate of rise in intracranial pressure, and type and intensity of prior treatment may account for some variability in physiologic patterns observed.

Comprehensive physiologic investigations of humans before, during, and after brain death are not available, and, thus, much of our knowledge of the basic physiology of brain death is derived from experimental models.[16-22] All catastrophic brain insults leading to brain death result in a progressive rise in intracranial pressure and a decline in cerebral perfusion pressure and cerebral blood flow. The endpoint of this process is brain herniation and infarction. As intracranial hypertension worsens and herniation develops, circulating catecholamine levels and sympathetic tone are high. Once complete brain infarction occurs, catecholamine levels decline and central vasomotor control, respiratory drive, and the important regulatory influences of the hypothalamic-pituitary axis are lost. Some of the variability in the physiologic responses during and after brain death in animal models and humans may be explained on the basis of differences in the mechanism and rate of rise in intracranial pressure.

CARDIOVASCULAR CHANGES

The cardiovascular changes occurring during and after the evolution of brain death are important not only in terms of their impact on hemodynamic stability but also because there can be important influences on cardiac and other organ function after transplantation. Hypertension and tachycardia preceding brain death and hypotension after death are characteristic features in most donors. Progressive increases in intracranial pressure are associated with increased arterial pressure. Vagal effects during this phase can cause bradycardia, sinus arrest, or atrioventricular dissociation. As intracranial hypertension worsens and the brainstem becomes ischemic, adrenergic stimulation is augmented, further exacerbating arterial hypertension and leading to increases in left atrial and pulmonary capillary wedge pressure. Cardiac output usually increases early in the course of herniation because of the surge in the release of catecholamines from the sympathoadrenal axis. However, in some cases, left ventricular function can deteriorate, leading to a decline in cardiac output. Pulmonary edema is observed in some models (neurogenic pulmonary edema) as elevation of left atrial pressure and redistribution of blood into the pulmonary circuit disrupts the pulmonary capillary epithelium. As catecholamine levels continue to rise, sinus tachycardia, supraventricular and ventricular arrhythmias, and ischemic changes on the electrocardiogram (ECG) can occur; this phase typically last for 15 to 30 minutes.[16,23-25] It is during this phase of extreme hypertension and tachycardia that myocardial injury is thought to occur. The mechanism is thought to be direct release of catecholamines from sympathetic nerve endings, because myocardial injury can be prevented by sympathectomy but not adrenalectomy.[17,24] Findings from clinical studies corroborate experimental data and indicate that myocardial injury is a prominent feature in patients with catastrophic intracranial injuries.[26-28] Treatment with beta-blockers or calcium channel blockers can reduce myocardial injury in experimental models.[24,25,29-31]

Total infarction of the vasomotor centers in the brainstem causes an abrupt loss of sympathetic tone and usually results in sudden hypotension. This finding generally indicates that brain death is imminent or has occurred. Circulating catecholamine levels decline after brain death has occurred. Subsequently, heart rate is determined by the intrinsic automaticity of the heart. In addition, heart rate may be modulated by catecholamines that are infused to maintain arterial pressure. Typical heart rates in potential donors range from 70 to 150 beats/min.[32,33]

The myocardial injury that sometimes occurs during the evolution of brain death can result in right and/or left ventricular dysfunction. Myocardial damage can adversely impact the hemodynamic stability of the donor and organ function in the recipient.[34-39] A variety of mechanisms have been postulated to explain cardiac dysfunction, including myocardial ischemia, myocardial infarction, and impaired myocardial metabolism.[16,25,29,40] Only a few hemodynamic studies of human brain-dead organ donors have been carried out. The data reveal considerable variability in cardiac index (average: 2.9 to 5.0 L/min/M²) and systemic vascular resistance (332 to 2500 dynes/sec/cm⁵).[33,41,42] Echocardiographic studies of potential donors have revealed impaired left ventricular function (ejection fraction < 50%) in 15% to 40% of potential donors.[38,43] Left ventricular stroke work index (calculated using data obtained by thermodilution) is greater than 30 g • m/M² in 96%.[44]

HORMONAL CHANGES

Infarction of the hypothalamic-pituitary axis during the course of brain death impairs the release of arginine vasopressin (antidiuretic hormone) from the posterior pituitary. As a consequence, potential donors usually manifest signs and laboratory features of diabetes insipidus (DI). The onset of DI suggests imminent brain death or that brain death has occurred and commonly contributes to problems with hemodynamic stability and fluid and electrolyte balance after brain death. Polyuria, signaling the onset of DI, may be absent because of hypovolemia or acute renal failure. The absence of DI after brain death is well recognized and is likely due to preserved circulation to the pituitary gland.

Many studies have documented a reduction in circulating thyroid hormones after brain death.[16,20,40,45-51] It has been suggested that reduced circulating thyroid hormone levels shift anaerobic myocardial metabolism, resulting in hemodynamic instability. Some studies have suggested that thyroid hormone supplementation can reverse metabolic abnormalities, stabilize hemodynamics, reduce vasopressor requirements, and improve cardiac and renal function.[7,50-54] Although there are conflicting data in the literature,[45,46,48,55-59] hormonal resuscitation of the organ donor has been adopted as a management strategy by the United Network for Organ Sharing (UNOS) as a component of its critical pathway for donor management.[60]

Most animal models have demonstrated reductions in both adrenocorticotropic hormone and cortisol after brain death. Human studies have been somewhat inconsistent, showing either normal or low levels of cortisol.[55,56,61-64] In one clinical study, adrenal reserve was assessed using the cosyntropin-stimulation test.[65] The data from this study suggest that brain-dead patients have relative adrenal insufficiency when compared with similarly injured but viable controls. Seeking to improve or preserve pulmonary function, some donor management strategies administer high doses of corticosteroids to potential donors, but the effect of this therapy on hemodynamic stability remains uncertain.

Patients with catastrophic brain injuries are commonly hyperglycemic as a result of the hormonal stress responses, catecholamine administration, and relative insulin resistance. Glucose intolerance has been demonstrated in brain-dead humans after brain death; however, synthesis and release of insulin is preserved.[66,67]

ELECTROLYTE AND ACID-BASE CHANGES

A variety of electrolyte and acid-base disturbances commonly occur in brain-dead patients. These derangements are a result of the hormonal perturbations induced by brain death and/or various therapeutic interventions. In any case, electrolyte and acid-base abnormalities can increase the risk of cardiovascular instability.[9,10,68] The most common electrolyte problems are hypernatremia, hypokalemia, hypomagnesemia, and hypophosphatemia. Hypernatremia occurs as a consequence of DI and the associated losses of solute-free water via the kidneys. The tendency for these patients to develop hypernatremia is further exacerbated by prior therapeutic interventions, notably administration of mannitol or hypertonic saline, in the (failed) effort to control intracranial hypertension. Polyuria, the effects of endogenous or exogenous catecholamines, hypocapnia, and insulin all can contribute to the development of hypokalemia. Solute-induced diuresis and respiratory alkalosis contribute to the development of hypomagnesemia and hypophosphatemia. Hyponatremia, hyperkalemia, and ionized hypocalcemia are sometimes observed in brain-dead patients, but these abnormalities are less frequent than the ones discussed earlier.

The most common acid-base disturbance after brain death is metabolic acidosis. Lactic acidosis is almost universally present,[40,47,58,69,70] although a hyperchloremic component may be present secondary to resuscitation using fluids containing relatively high chloride concentrations (e.g., normal or hypertonic saline solutions) and renal compensation for induced hypocapnia. The etiology of hyperlactatemia is likely multifactorial. Possible factors include hypovolemia, reduced cardiac output, hypothermia, respiratory alkalosis, and metabolic changes associated with high catecholamine levels.

COAGULOPATHY

Abnormalities of coagulation may be present in potential donors as a result of prior use of anticoagulants, of dilution and consumption of factors with hemorrhagic shock, or of disseminated intravascular coagulation secondary to the release of tissue factor after gunshot wounds to the brain.[71,72] Coagulation and platelet function also can be impaired as a consequence of hypothermia, a common problem in potential donors. Blood coagulation disorders are relevant to the management when ongoing hemorrhage threatens hemodynamic stability or disseminated intravascular coagulation impairs organ system function.

TEMPERATURE REGULATION

Hypothermia is common after brain death. The mechanisms responsible for the development of hypothermia include destruction of hypothalamic and mesencephalic thermoregulation centers in the brain, resuscitation with cold fluids and blood, exposure, and reduced metabolism. Hypothermia is

present in the majority of potential organ donors[73]; body temperatures after brain death range from 31°C to 34°C.[74,75] Hypothermia can have detrimental effects on the function of the heart and other organ systems in the potential donor.[39,76] Hyperthermia can occur during herniation, and fever also can occur after brain death in those who develop infections.

ICU MANAGEMENT OF THE ORGAN DONOR

Despite the inherent instability of the brain-dead potential organ donor, when given appropriate supportive care, organ function can be maintained at a level that will permit acquisition of organs suitable for transplantation even when care is extended considerably beyond the first few days of ICU admission. The key to successful management is anticipation of complications, frequent reassessment, and titration of therapy. Care must be provided in an ICU environment by a staff that is motivated, knowledgeable, and experienced. Once a patient has been determined to be a potential donor, aggressive physiologic support must continue up to the time of organ procurement unless or until medical ineligibility has been determined or the family refuses to consent to donation.

Complications that can occur after brain death and threaten the viability of organs include hypotension, diabetes insipidus, hypothermia, cardiac arrhythmias, electrolyte disturbances, metabolic acidosis, pulmonary edema, and cardiac arrest.[9,10,47,77] The maintenance of vital organ function and prevention and treatment of complications are the principal goals of supportive care of the donor. A substantial amount of skill is required in balancing the need to maintain perfusion of vital organs while avoiding the potentially deleterious effects of the supportive interventions such as mechanical ventilation, vasopressors, and excessive fluid administration. Routine care applicable to many critically ill patients such as proper body position, turning, pulmonary toilet, nasogastric decompression, and stress ulcer prophylaxis are also important and should be standard. The eyes should be lubricated and closed to prevent desiccation and infection, and contaminated resuscitation lines and tubes should be removed or replaced, especially if care of the donor is anticipated to extend beyond 1 to 2 days. Antibiotic therapy is administered for clinically obvious infections or contaminated wounds. Measures to prevent exposure and to maintain body temperature with blankets also should be employed.

Whereas the intensivist is best suited to manage these complex patients before the certification of brain death, the local OPO and its coordinators are also skilled and generally assume medical management after certification of death. Standardized protocols, clinical pathways, and order sets help to minimize variability in management.

MONITORING

Once it has been determined that a patient has suffered a lethal brain insult, invasive hemodynamic monitoring of arterial and central venous pressures should be established or continued. Such monitoring is essential for recognizing the onset of brain death (sudden hypotension) and for the proper titration of fluids and vasopressors. Routine pulmonary artery catheterization is not warranted but should

TABLE 249–1. PHYSIOLOGIC ENDPOINTS IN THE POTENTIAL ORGAN DONOR

Systolic blood pressure ≥90 mm Hg
Mean arterial pressure ≥60 mm Hg
Central venous pressure ≤12 mm Hg
Pulmonary capillary wedge pressure ≤12 mm Hg
Cardiac index >2.5 L/min/M²
Left ventricular stroke work index >15 g.m/M²
Urine output >1 and <4 mL/kg/h
Core temperature >35°C
Hematocrit ≥25%
Oxygen saturation >95%
pH 7.35-7.45

be considered if the potential donor is unresponsive to fluid challenges or if the clinical conditions are complicated by the acute respiratory distress syndrome (ARDS), severe myocardial contusion, or pre-existing heart failure. Insertion of a pulmonary artery catheter also may be warranted to help determine if a donor's heart is suitable for transplantation because a low left ventricular stroke work index was reported to be predictive of a poor outcome after transplant.[44] A recent consensus conference also recommended that monitoring using a pulmonary artery catheter be employed when caring for potential donors with an ejection fraction less than 45% as determined by echocardiography.[78] Other parameters that should be monitored routinely include core temperature, arterial oxygen saturation (pulse oximetry), hourly urine output, and urinary specific gravity (if polyuria is present). Laboratory parameters that should be assessed repetitively include arterial blood gases, serum electrolyte concentrations, serum glucose concentration, and hematocrit. Physiologic endpoints that provide for adequate organ perfusion while minimizing fluid overload are shown in Table 249-1.

HEMODYNAMIC AND CARDIOVASCULAR SUPPORT

Severe hypertension occurring during early herniation has the potential to produce impaired cardiopulmonary function after brain death and threaten the ongoing perfusion of organs in the donor after brain death. However, the use of antihypertensive agents also has the potential to produce profound hypotension once herniation occurs. Because controlled trials have not been performed, it is difficult to know whether treatment of hypertension in the organ donor is beneficial. However, careful titration of a short-acting beta blocker (e.g., esmolol) during the sympathetic storm associated with brain death might be beneficial in minimizing catecholamine-related myocardial injury and should be considered.[30,31,79] Potent vasodilators such as sodium nitroprusside should not be used to manage brain-dead organ donors.

Hypotension and impaired blood flow to vital tissues pose the greatest danger to the viability of transplantable organs. These problems occur in the vast majority of organ donors. Once hypotension occurs, attendance by a physician skilled in resuscitation is necessary until circulating blood volume is optimized and adequate perfusion pressure re-established. Intravascular volume expansion is the most important component of the interventions that are used to establish and maintain hemodynamic stability after brain death. Data have also shown that positive fluid balance in the organ

donor is a significant factor affecting survival in heart transplant recipients.[80] Commonly, it is necessary to infuse several liters of fluid to restore adequate blood pressure, especially if DI has gone untreated or if there is ongoing bleeding. Fluid resuscitation can have deleterious effects on lung and heart function, if filling pressures exceed recommended endpoints; thus, these parameters should be carefully monitored.[17,81,82] Lactated Ringer's solution is preferable to isotonic saline to expand plasma volume when hypernatremia and metabolic acidosis are present. Colloids and blood are used to supplement crystalloid volume resuscitation and treat anemia if more aggressive volume expansion is needed.

Occasionally, an organ donor will spontaneously maintain adequate blood pressure after brain death has occurred. One possible explanation for this observation may be that a gradual rather than an explosive rise in intracranial pressure tends to preserve upper cervical spinal sympathetic pathways.[22] The vast majority of organ donors, however, require some form of vasopressor support. Most authorities recommend using dopamine (at doses ≤10 µg/kg/min) as the preferred vasopressor. Data, however, suggest that epinephrine might have a better safety profile than either dopamine or norepinephrine, especially with regard to effects on renal perfusion.[83] Although the best choice for vasopressor in reference to objective measures of post-transplant organ function remains unclear, the vasopressor doses should be titrated carefully, so that the lowest infusion rate that will achieve and maintain hemodynamic stability is employed.

If there is an unsatisfactory response to volume loading and low doses of vasopressors, consideration should be given to placement of a pulmonary artery catheter to further evaluate preload and cardiac function. Additional volume expansion or a second vasopressor (e.g., norepinephrine) may be required to support blood pressure. A low-dose infusion of vasopressin (0.04 to 0.1 U/min) may be helpful in enhancing responsiveness of the vasculature to catecholamines and allow for a reduction in the dose or discontinuation of dopamine or norepinephrine.[84,85] Dobutamine or epinephrine may be used if the cardiac index is low despite restoration of circulating blood volume. A trial of sodium bicarbonate is warranted in donors with hemodynamic instability and severe metabolic acidosis. If oliguria is present after adequate volume resuscitation and restoration of adequate perfusion pressure, loop diuretics or mannitol should be given to establish urine flow, which is an important factor influencing post-transplant kidney function.[86] An algorithm for the management of hypotension is shown in Figure 249-1.

Some data suggest that therapy with thyroxine and other hormones can improve hemodynamic stability, reduce vasopressor requirements, and improve post-transplant organ function.[50-54,87] Accordingly, "hormonal resuscitation" of the potential organ donor is now considered by UNOS and other groups to be an integral component of the critical pathway for donor management.[60] The recommended hormone replacement regimen includes administration of triiodothyronine (T_3) (3-µg bolus followed by a 3-µg/h infusion), vasopressin (1 U bolus followed by 0.5 to 4 U/h infusion), and insulin (1 U/h titrated to maintain glucose at 120 to 180 mg/dL). When T_3 is not available, thyroxine (T_4) can be administered (20-µg bolus followed by 10-µg/hr infusion). Methylprednisolone (15 mg/kg) is also included in the critical pathway because of its potentially beneficial effects on the lungs. Although other studies have shown no benefits with hormonal replacement,[46,56,88,89] preliminary data

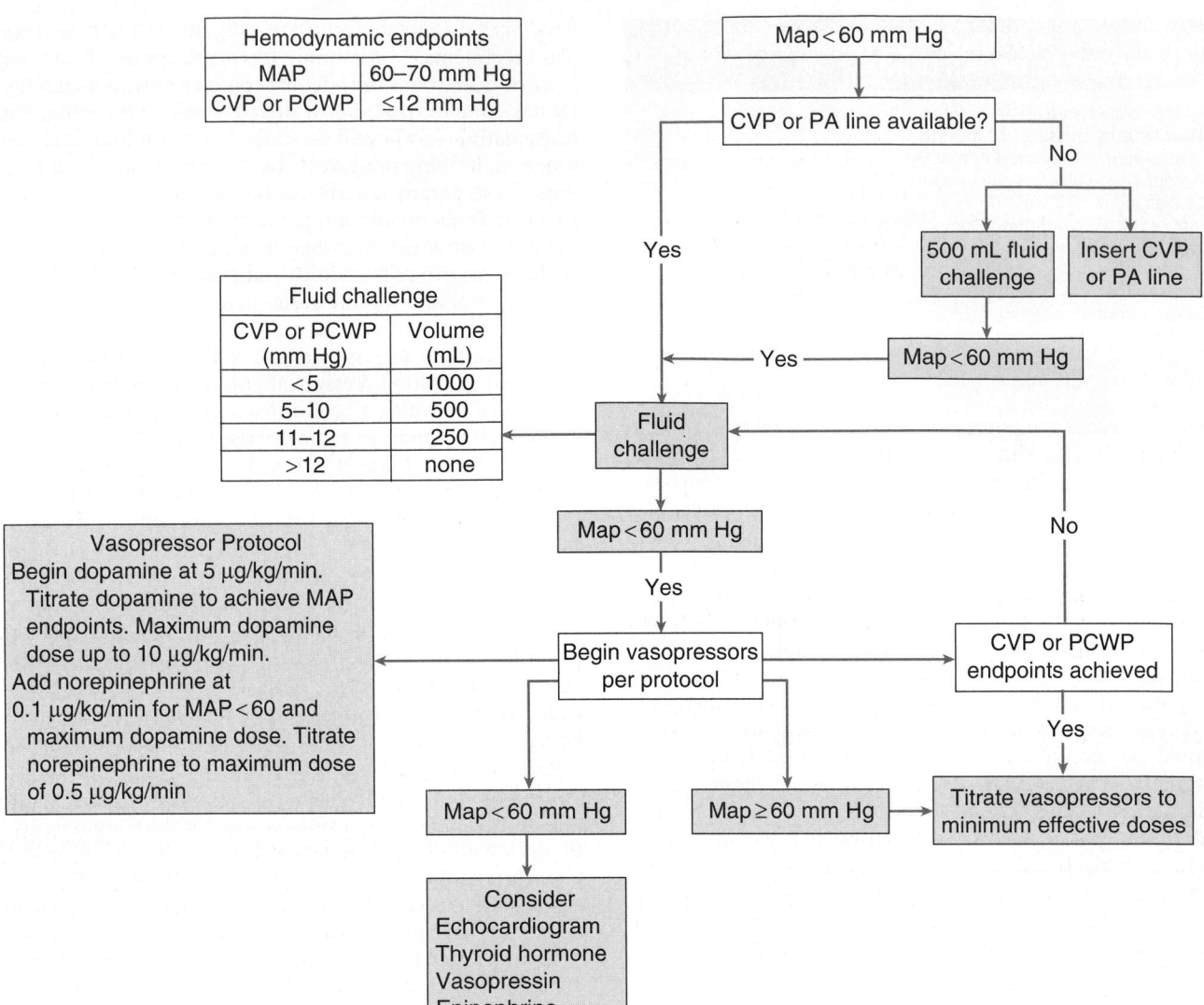

FIGURE 249–1. Algorithm for the management of hypotension in the potential organ donor. MAP, mean arterial pressure; CVP, central venous pressure; PCWP, pulmonary capillary wedge pressure; PA, pulmonary artery.

regarding the use of the UNOS pathway suggest that there is an improvement in the number of donor organs recovered.[87] Furthermore, a retrospective review of a large number of donors in the UNOS database suggests that hormone replacement therapy is associated with an increase in the number of organs recovered.[90] Although these data are not high quality and donors can be successfully managed without hormonal therapy, many OPOs are now routinely employing it. Controlled trials of hormone replacement therapy are necessary to firmly establish the efficacy of this approach in influencing donor hemodynamics and posttransplant function.

A need for antiarrhythmic therapy is uncommon in the potential donor during the evolution of and following brain death. The decision to treat cardiac rhythm disturbances is generally based on their impact on hemodynamic stability. Supraventricular or ventricular tachycardias occurring during the catecholamine storm of herniation often resolve without specific therapy after brain death has occurred. However, the cautious use of beta blockade may be indicated as previously noted to minimize myocardial injury. Once brain death

has occurred, bradyarrhythmias will not respond to atropine. Therefore, clinically and hemodynamically significant bradycardia should be treated with epinephrine or cardiac pacing. Cardiopulmonary arrest is not a contraindication to organ donation. Thus, vigorous resuscitative interventions should be employed using standard techniques if cardiac arrest occurs in the potential donor.

RESPIRATORY SUPPORT

Ventilatory support in the potential donor should provide for adequate arterial oxygenation and near-normal acid-base balance while minimizing the potential adverse effects of positive-pressure ventilation on hemodynamics or lung structure and function. Many organ donors have been hyperventilated for management of intracranial hypertension, but once brain death has occurred, minute volume should be normalized to help facilitate hemodynamic stability. The only exception to this guideline is that some degree of hyperventilation may be useful to control blood pH when the potential donor has severe metabolic acidosis. Additional volume resuscitation and administration of intravenous sodium bicarbonate may be helpful to allow normalization of minute ventilation when acidosis is present. Oxygen is administered in the lowest concentration compatible with an arterial saturation of greater than 95% while using low positive end-expiratory pressure levels (5 to 8 cm H_2O). In the presence of poor lung compliance or high airway resistance in the absence of reversible obstruction, pressure-controlled ventilation along with reversal of the inspiratory/expiratory ratio should be considered to maintain adequate tissue oxygenation.[91] If the lungs have been excluded from consideration for procurement, it is preferable to use a higher FiO_2 rather than a higher mean airway pressure to maintain adequate arterial oxygenation.

Aggressive pulmonary toilet regimens have been successful in increasing the number of lungs that are suitable for transplantation.[92,93] Interventions include bronchoscopy, chest physiotherapy, lavage and suction, diuresis for increased central venous pressure, and antibiotics for established pulmonary infections. Although there are no randomized controlled trials, several studies indicate that high doses of methylprednisolone (15 mg/kg) increase donor lung recovery.[93-95] Routine bronchoscopy is often performed by the transplant team before procurement of the lungs. Bronchoscopy should also be considered by the donor management team when there is refractory atelectasis or there is a need to remove foreign bodies or blood clots.

FLUIDS, ELECTROLYTES, AND ACID-BASE BALANCE

Once ICU management has shifted to organ donor support, fluid therapy is focused on volume resuscitation and the restoration of normal water and electrolyte balance. The type of maintenance fluid selected will depend in part on the presence and severity of electrolyte disorders (e.g., hypernatremia or hypokalemia). Typically, 5% dextrose in 0.2% or 0.45% saline with added potassium is infused at a rate of 100 to 125 mL/h to meet basal fluid and electrolyte requirements. The presence of ongoing losses or pre-existing deficits determines the need for additional fluid and electrolyte supplements.

Perhaps the biggest challenge encountered is the management of DI, which typically is manifested by the sudden onset of polyuria (urine output > 4 mL/kg/h), low urinary specific gravity (SG < 1.005), low urinary osmolality (Uosm < 100 mOsm/kg), high plasma osmolality (Posm > 295 mOsm/kg), and increasing serum sodium concentration. Hormone replacement with vasopressin, volume expansion, and correction of hypernatremia and associated electrolyte losses are the main priorities in management. The simplest strategy for vasopressin replacement is to use desmopressin, 1 to 2 µg intravenously every 8 to 12 hours, as needed to control polyuria. Polyuria may persist after administration of desmopressin as a consequence of a salt diuresis from previously administered crystalloids. Alternatively, low doses of vasopressin (0.5 to 3 U/h) can be infused to control polyuria and enhance hemodynamic stability, especially when prolonged donor support is required (> 24 h). Continuous vasopressin infusion is a component of the previously noted hormonal resuscitation regimen. The use of vasopressin should be judicious, because use of this agent can cause splanchnic vasoconstriction, reducing hepatic and pancreatic blood flow. When severe hypernatremia is present,

free water deficits can be estimated using standard formulas and rapidly replaced with a hypotonic fluid such as 5% dextrose or 0.2% saline. If there are ongoing and excessive urinary losses, those losses can be replaced every 1 to 2 hours with crystalloid solutions approximating the same concentration of electrolytes lost in the urine as determined by urinary electrolyte measurement. To prevent a "vicious cycle" of perpetuating polyuria by replacement of all urinary losses, partial volumetric replacement of urinary losses is reasonable until urinary output has declined to less than 200 to 250 mL/h.

In addition to interventions directed at maintaining sodium and water balance, additional supplements of potassium, phosphate, and magnesium are also usually required to maintain normal electrolyte balance. Because hyperglycemia may cause or contribute to polyuria and associated electrolyte losses, glucose should be monitored and hyperglycemia controlled with intravenous insulin to keep the glucose concentration less than 200 mg/dL.

HYPOTHERMIA

Mild to moderate hypothermia is common and may predispose the organ donor to hemodynamic instability, cardiac arrhythmias, bleeding, acidosis, and impairment in organ function. Core temperature should be maintained at or above 35°C. In most cases, simple measures such as external warming blankets, heated humidified air (39°C to 41°C), and increasing room temperature are effective in establishing and maintaining adequate core body temperature. If there are active resuscitative efforts under way because of hemorrhage, blood products and resuscitation fluids should be warmed. For potential donors with severe or profound hypothermia, more aggressive measures including the use of partial cardiopulmonary bypass should be considered.[96]

HEMATOLOGIC SUPPORT

Transfusion of blood components is generally reserved for unstable donors with active hemorrhage. In those donors who are not bleeding there is a general recommendation to maintain the hematocrit at or above 25%, but there are no firm data to recommend one transfusion threshold as being better than another. Because overall oxygen consumption after brain death is relatively low, there is likely no systemic benefit to be gained by aggressive red cell transfusions for otherwise stable donors. When disseminated intravascular coagulation is clearly evident and there is no active bleeding, anticoagulation with heparin may be of some benefit in preserving organ function.

ANTIBIOTIC THERAPY

The overall incidence of infectious complications and the value of using prophylactic antibiotics in organ donors are unknown. Studies have indicated that the rates of bacteremia in the potential donor range from 5% to 7.5%; most isolates are gram positive.[12,13,97] Overt or occult pulmonary infection also may be present.[98,99] It is generally recommended that antibiotic therapy be employed in donors with obvious infection or in potential lung donors with purulent sputum. However, because the risk of transmission of bacterial infections to transplant recipients receiving perioperative antibiotics is so low, antimicrobial prophylaxis in the potential donor does not seem warranted at this time.

STANDARDIZED THERAPY FOR THE ORGAN DONOR

There are currently no evidence-based guidelines that address the ICU management of the cadaveric organ donor. Furthermore, because the number of potential organ donors is relatively small, individual hospitals and physicians may not gain enough experience to maintain a consistent approach in management. These factors can contribute to variability or inconsistency in management. In an effort to standardize the approach to management of the potential donor, UNOS has published a critical pathway for management, which includes recommendations for hormonal therapy.[60] Initial data using this pathway have suggested that it may increase the number of transplanted organs.[87] In an effort to minimize variability, our institution designed and implemented a standardized order set that permits nursing staff to intervene on behalf of the potential donor to establish and maintain physiologic stability after brain death up to the time of organ procurement (Fig. 249-2). Hormonal resuscitation may be employed at the discretion of the physician or OPO.

1. Notify ICU staff physician or ICU staff physician on call, social service, pastoral care, and organ procurement organization.

2. Consult ICU physician for arterial and central venous line placements.

3. Discontinue all antihypertensives, anticonvulsants, sedatives, barbiturates, and neuromuscular blockers. Continue all previously ordered antibiotics.

4. Monitor vital signs per ICU standards, urine output and urinary specific gravity hourly.

5. NG to low continuous suction.

6. Lubricate eyes q 2 h and tape eyes closed if necessary.

7. Maintain head of bed elevated at 30 degrees.

8. Convective air warming blanket. Warm and maintain 36°–37°C

9. Verify and document neuromuscular function with nerve stimulator.

10. Labs: stat electrolytes, magnesium, phosphate, glucose, hematocrit, platelet count, PT/PTT, and ABGs

11. Monitor: Na^+, K^+, hematocrit, and glucose q 2 h

12. ABG 30 min after each ventilator adjustment

13. Maintenance fluids: Add KCl 30 mEq/L. Infuse at 125 mL/h. No added KCl if $K^+ > 5$ mEq/L.

$Na^+ \le 150$:	D5W/0.45% NaCl
$Na^+ > 150$:	D5W/0.2% NaCl

14. Urinary replacement fluid (hourly): replace all urine output in excess of 250 mL/h with 0.2% saline + KCl 10 mEq/L

15. Free water (5% dextrose) replacement every 2 h based on measured serum sodium. Infuse over 2 h.

Na^+ 150–155:	500 mL
Na^+ 156–160:	1000 mL
Na^+ 161–165:	1500 mL
Na^+ 166–170:	2000 mL

16. Fluid bolus therapy (hourly) with Ringer's lactate. Maximum bolus volume 5 L.

CVP < 5 mm Hg:	1000 mL
CVP 5–10 mm Hg:	500 mL
CVP 11–12 mm Hg:	250 mL

17. Electrolyte replacement

$K^+ = 2.5–3.0$: KCl	20 mEq/h × 2
$K^+ = 3.1–3.5$: KCl	20 mEq/h × 1
$K^+ = 3.6–4.0$: KCl	10 mEq/h × 1
$Mg^{+2} < 2.0$: $MgSO_4$	6 g IV over 4 h
$PO_4 < 1.5$: KPO_4	15 mmol IV over 4 h

18. Transfuse blood products

Hematocrit < 25%:	2 U pRBC
Platelet count < 50 K:	6 U platelets
PT > 18 seconds:	2 U FFP

19. DDAVP 2 µg IV q 8 h prn hourly urine output > 500 mL/h or > 250 mL/h for 2 consecutive hours with urinary SG < 1.005.

20. Sliding scale regular insulin SQ q 4 h prn

Glucose 150–200:	5 units
Glucose 201–250:	10 units
Glucose 251–300:	15 units
Glucose 301–350:	20 units
Glucose > 250:	Notify MD

21. Vasopressors (check): titrate to MAP 60–65 mm Hg

☐ Dopamine infusion: 5 µg/kg/min
  Max dose = 10 µg/kg/min

☐ Norepinephrine infusion: 0.1 µg/kg/min
  Max dose = 0.5 µg/kg/min

☐ Vasopressin infusion: 0.04 U/min

22. Notify physician:

MAP sustained < 60 mm Hg
Temperature < 32°C
Heart rate < 45 or > 120 bpm
Urine output < 50 mL/h
Arterial saturation < 90%
pH < 7.35 or > 7.45
Hematocrit ≤ 21%
Glucose > 350 mg%
$Na^+ > 170$ mEq/L
$K^+ < 2.5$ or > 5.5 mEq/L
Maximum 5 L fluid boluses

FIGURE 249–2. Physician's orders after brain death.

NUTRITION SUPPORT

The typical organ donor spends less than 72 hours in the ICU before organ procurement. Consequently, the role of nutritional support for the organ donor has not been investigated extensively. In one review nutritional issues were outlined that might be important in favorably influencing post-transplant function of the liver, heart, and kidneys.[100] Whereas definitive recommendations regarding the composition and value of any nutritional support regimen in the organ donor cannot be made, it is reasonable to begin a balanced nutrition support regimen in the potential organ donor when extended life support is expected. In contrast to the typical critically ill patient, metabolic rate is lower in brain-dead donors. Resting energy expenditure is 25% to 30% lower than the basal metabolic rate.[101] Therefore, when nutrition support is administered, caloric intake should be adjusted downward.

CONSENT AND COORDINATION WITH THE ORGAN PROCUREMENT ORGANIZATION

Optimum medical management of the potential organ donor is essential to the success of transplantation. Of the recognized impediments to organ donation, however, the refusal of families to consent to donation remains the most important problem that reduces the available pool of actual organ donors in the United States.[102] Despite the fact that the majority of Americans would be willing to donate the organs of a loved one after death,[103,104] consent rates for eligible donors are typically less than 50%.[102,105,106] A number of factors have been recognized to influence the family's decision to donate (Table 249-2).[106-111]

TABLE 249–2. FACTORS POTENTIALLY INFLUENCING THE DECISION TO DONATE ORGANS

Patient or Family

Signed donor card or advanced directive
Prior expressed wishes of patient
Socioeconomic status
Educational level
Religious beliefs
Racial and ethnic background
Knowledge and understanding of brain death
Beliefs and attitudes toward organ donation
Family satisfaction with care provided
Family disputes
Grief and denial reactions
Concerns about bodily disfigurement
Uncertainty in funeral arrangements

Health Care Personnel and Institution

Experience, knowledge, and attitudes of personnel
Manners and approach of physicians
Involvement of the organ procurement organization
Cooperation of unit personnel with organ procurement
    organization/organ procurement coordinator
Emotional support of the family
Hospital facilities
Provision of privacy
Explanation of brain death and its implications
Timing of the request for donation
Separation of brain death notification from request
Location of the request

In an effort to reduce the number of organ donors lost as a result of failed identification and problems emerging during the request for organ donation, the Health Care Financing Administration has established regulations that address these problems.[4] These regulations require hospitals to notify the local OPO of all imminent and actual deaths and offer all potential donors the option to donate. These regulations also require that any request for organ donation be made by an OPO representative or "designated requestor." A designated requestor is an individual who has completed a course offered or approved by the local OPO. The course generally is focused on methods for approaching potential donor families and requesting organ or tissue donation. Although these regulations do not prohibit physicians who are not designated requestors from approaching families, they do require the presence of the OPO representative unless the physician is a designated requestor. There is no prohibition of the physician's discussing organ donation when family members initiate the discussion.

Interventions that appear to improve the likelihood of a successful request for organ donation include the provision of a private setting for family members, involvement of an on-site organ procurement coordinator (OPC), separation of the notification of brain death from the request for donation, race-specific requestors, and an institutional commitment to improving the education of staff and the processes pertinent to the potential organ donor.[5,112-121] The process leading to the request for organ donation begins once it is clear that the patient has suffered from a catastrophic and obviously lethal brain injury. In recognition of the complexity of the process, the emotional responses of the family, and the need for privacy and cohesion, the family should be provided with a private location separated from the families of other critically ill patients in the unit. Visitation rules should be relaxed. Support for the family must be provided in a multidisciplinary effort to meet all of the family's needs. Individuals providing this support should include the bedside nurse, the intensivist, the attending physician (if different from the intensivist), the social worker, clergy, and, later, the on-site OPC. The local OPO should be notified of the potential donor as early as possible. Nonessential personnel who are unfamiliar with the issues surrounding the management of potential donors should relinquish responsibilities to more experienced personnel. No patient in the category described should be excluded as a potential donor nor should a discussion of withdrawal of life support take place until the OPO has had an opportunity to properly evaluate the patient's status as a potential donor.

After the family has been gathered and isolated, the responsible physician along with other support personnel should explain the nature and severity of the injury or insult. A summary of the clinical situation should be provided, including a history of the diagnostic and therapeutic efforts that have been undertaken. The prognosis should be explained in clear and unequivocal terms. Often, it is helpful to show and explain the results of imaging studies that demonstrate the severity of the brain insult. Depending on the response of the family, it is prudent to inform the family that there is an expectation that the patient will likely progress to the point of brain death and that further interventions directed at the brain insult are futile. If the patient is already clinically brain dead, a thorough explanation of brain death to family members at this point is reasonable, depending on their knowledge and degree of medical sophistication.

Once brain death is certified, it is important to avoid using terms that might cause confusion between ongoing efforts to provide physiologic support of the donor with those interventions that are usually intended to sustain life under ordinary circumstances. If the patient has not been certified dead, the family should be informed that a process of formal brain death certification will take place and that they will be notified when certification of death by neurologic criteria has been completed. The family should be allowed time to digest the information provided to them. Other members of the team can help support family members through their grief responses as the physician returns to supporting the potential donor and/or certifying brain death.

Once the patient progresses to brain death and death has been legally certified, the physician must inform the family that brain death has been declared. The use of radionuclide studies confirming brain death may help families understand and accept death[15] and may also have a positive influence on the decision to donate organs.[122] Around the time that this inevitably upsetting news is presented, it is important that members of the support team be available for the family. Perhaps the most important principle guiding the process at this point in time is to ensure that any request for or discussion of organ donation be separated in time from the notification that the patient has been declared dead. The amount of time transpiring between the notification of death and the request for consent to organ donation varies depending on the family's needs or the physiologic stability of the potential donor. Often, it is not possible to separate these issues because the family may inquire about procedures subsequent to brain death certification. If it appears that the family needs to discuss post-mortem options at this time, it is reasonable to offer the option of organ donation (if the physician is a designated requestor) or to introduce the on-site OPC. If such inquiries are not made, the family should be informed that post-mortem options will be discussed at a later time. If family members indicate that the patient was predesignated as an organ donor or they make an unsolicited request for organ donation, then it is appropriate at this time to involve the on-site OPC to discuss issues surrounding organ donation with the family.

Although a timely request for donation after brain death is desirable, consideration for the individual family members and their response to the death may necessitate a delay until it is judged that they are best able to comprehend and respond to the request. At that time, the physician should return to the family and explain the option of organ donation if the local OPO has determined that the patient is medically eligible. Introduction and involvement of the OPC at this stage of the process will help ensure that the all questions surrounding the process of organ procurement are answered. Sensitivity to the family's psychosocial, religious, and cultural needs all need to be taken into consideration at the time of request for organ donation is made. Continued multidisciplinary involvement of the ICU team will help to ensure that these needs are met. The OPC's prior experience in dealing with grieving families can be invaluable in obtaining an affirmative response to the request for donation. If the family indicates a desire to donate, the OPC typically remains with the family to obtain formal written consent and answer any further questions the family may have regarding the timing and coordination of the process and discuss issues related to postmortem care. After consent is obtained, the OPC coordinates the acquisition of additional diagnostic testing as well as notification of the coroner and transplant surgeons. The OPC also commonly provides assistance or assumes full responsibility for physiologic management of the donor after death.

If, after a thorough discussion with the family, there is unequivocal refusal for organ donation, then the decision of the family should be accepted and respected while preparations are made to withdraw mechanical ventilation and other forms of physiologic support. If there is uncertainty or dispute among family members, it is reasonable to allow them more time for discussion. The family should then be reapproached by the physician and OPC to help resolve issues pertinent to the option of organ donation.

ANNOTATED REFERENCES

Darby JM, Stein K, Grenvik A, et al: Approach to management of the heart-beating brain dead organ donor. JAMA 1989;261:2222-2228.

Although it has been over a decade since it was originally published, this paper provides a comprehensive and still relevant review of all aspects of the management of the potential organ donor, including donor identification criteria, the diagnosis of brain death, and the physiologic basis for ICU management of the potential donor.

Power BM, Van Heeren PV: The physiological changes associated with brain death: Current concepts and implications for the treatment of the brain dead organ donor. Anesth Intensive Care 1995;23:26-36.

The authors of this paper present an excellent review of the pathophysiology of brain death, the effects on specific organ systems, and the relevance of these changes to management of the potential organ donor.

Rosendale JD, Kauffman HM, McBride MA, et al: Aggressive pharmacologic donor management results in more transplanted organs. Transplantation 2003;75:482-487.

Based on the UNOS database, this paper retrospectively reviews the outcome with respect to the number of transplanted organs in a large number of brain-dead organ donors and the potential influence of "hormonal resuscitation" added to a standardized clinical pathway for management. The data suggested that "hormonal resuscitation" increased the yield and also emphasized that standardized management strategies are important to successful organ procurement.

Williams MA, Lipsett PA, Rushton CH, et al: The physician's role in discussing organ donation with families. Crit Care Med 2003;31:1568-1573.

This paper was written by the AMA Council on Scientific Affairs in response to federal legislation requiring the use of "designated requestors" in the complex process of obtaining consent for organ donation from families of potential organ donors. The authors outline the major issues of concern to the physician in this end-of-life process, emphasizing not only the importance of physician involvement but also calling for improved training of physicians and collaboration with organ procurement organizations.

Zaroff JG, Rosengard BR, Armstrong WF, et al: Consensus conference report: Maximizing use of organs recovered from the cadaver donor: Cardiac recommendations. Circulation 2002;106:836-841.

This paper is unique because it is the first evidenced-based review of any aspect of organ donor evaluation and management. Whereas the main focus of the paper and the consensus recommendations are directed toward evaluation and management of the cardiac donor, other important aspects of donor management are discussed, including recommendations for future scientific investigations.

Chapter 250

NON-HEARTBEATING ORGAN DONATION (DONATION AFTER CARDIAC DEATH)

Lawrence Scott Wilner • Michael A. DeVita

KEY POINTS

1. In the early years of transplantation, before "brain death" was described and accepted, organs for transplantation were procured from patients whose death was certified according to traditional cardiopulmonary criteria. This process is called non-heartbeating donation. Now the preferred and less ambiguous term is **donation after cardiac death (DCD).**

2. For "brain-dead" donors, it is possible to obtain donor organs that are virtually free of warm ischemia—**one of the two most important physiologic obstacles in organ transplantation (the other is immune rejection).**

3. When improved outcomes were demonstrated with organs from brain-dead donors, **DCD was abandoned for medical—and *not ethical*—reasons.**

4. In the early 1990s, **DCD was reintroduced into clinical practice *to accommodate the wishes of terminally ill patients (or their families).***

5. Although the number of transplants resulting from DCD remains comparatively small at this time, **most organizations that have offered an opinion endorse DCD as an ethical and potentially effective strategy to increase the supply of donor organs.**

6. Despite this endorsement, many hospitals and organ procurement organizations have not undertaken DCD in part because of debate regarding its potential to improve organ availability.

7. An important step in the process of DCD is **early recognition and appropriate management of patients with the potential to become organ donors.**

8. It is essential that caregivers treat **individuals being removed from life-sustaining technology with the primary goal of excellent palliative care and a secondary goal of facilitating organ donation.**

9. DCD is logistically complicated. It requires planning and interdisciplinary coordination. The United Network for Organ Sharing (UNOS) has now published **a comprehensive *Critical Pathway for DCD*** that can guide the development of local protocols and procedures.

10. The certification of death in patients being removed from life-sustaining technology is a central medical and ethical issue with regard to DCD. However, **there is no consensus on a specific "*required asystolic time*" that must be observed before certification of death.** Nevertheless, a specific institutional policy is required to ensure consistency of practice. There does appear to be a consensus that at least 2 but not more than 5 minutes is required.

11. Current data demonstrate that **outcomes for transplantation of kidneys—by far the most commonly utilized organ from DCD cadavers—are now essentially equivalent for both brain-dead and DCD organs.** Liver and whole pancreas transplants have also been successfully performed using DCD organs, but the limited number of these cases makes relative outcomes more difficult to assess.

12. Heart and lung transplantation using organs from DCD donors remains incompletely realized.

HISTORY

A familiarity with the history of transplantation is vital to understanding non-heartbeating organ donation in its proper context. Transplantation is a relatively new science. The first successful transplantation of a solid human organ, a kidney, took place in 1954. Over the intervening 50 years, clinical practice has progressed to the point that transplantation of each of the vital solid internal organs is now common practice. Transplantation has indeed "emerged from being an experimental procedure undertaken by patients brave enough to seek a cure for their illnesses, to a discipline to which patients with end-stage organ failure are now routinely referred."[1] Such dramatic progress undeniably represents one of the foremost successes of modern medicine.[2]

Advances in transplantation have not been achieved easily, and a number of formidable challenges have been confronted along the way. A prime example is the management of rejection. Circumventing the natural tendency of the organ recipient to attack "foreign" tissue has been a central concern from the beginning of clinical transplantation. In this context, it is clear why the first successful procedure involved identical twins as donor and recipient. Of course, the use of genetically identical individuals as donor and recipient, while useful as a proof-of-principle strategy, is not a practical option when dealing with large populations. Instead, a predictable and reproducible way to modulate host defenses was required. The resulting research revolutionized our understanding of molecular immunology and paved the way for a continuing stream of new anti-rejection therapies.

Another obstacle to transplantation is organ damage caused by ischemia. Cessation of blood flow deprives tissues of oxygen and cripples metabolism—possibly irreversibly—at the cellular level. Ischemia in the context of transplantation is often conceptually divided into a warm period (organ temperature > 70°F) and a cold period. Warm ischemia begins with the loss of blood flow to a donor organ before its actual removal from the donor's body. Cold ischemia begins when the donor organ is flushed with a chilled preservative solution (either before or after removal from the donor's body) and ends with the restoration of normothermic circulation in the body of the recipient.[3,4] Certainly other factors, such as the potential for transmitting infectious agents or the seeds of neoplastic disease, can affect the suitability of a donated organ in a given case, but the greatest general risk remains ischemia.

An inadequate supply of suitable donor organs is the single most vexing issue that keeps solid organ transplantation from achieving its full potential for relieving suffering and improving survival for patients with end-stage renal, hepatic, pulmonary, cardiac, or endocrine pancreatic failure. Over time, attempts to address this problem have prompted landmark—and often controversial—developments on the intersecting frontiers of clinical medicine, bioethics, and health care policy.

In the earliest years of transplantation, the vast majority of organs available for donation came from patients whose death was certified according to traditional, cardiopulmonary, criteria.[5] Because the hearts and lungs of these patients no longer functioned (so-called non-heartbeating donors, now also referred to as donors after cardiac death [DCD]), and because the initial organ harvest techniques were somewhat unsophisticated and based largely on autopsy practices, ischemia was often prolonged and many early transplants failed.[6] At about the same time, physicians gained the ability to maintain physiologic bodily function in patients with little hope of neurologic recovery from severe insults to the central nervous system. And so a new philosophical debate began over the fundamental meaning of life and human identity in this context,[7] culminating in the emergence of a new concept: brain death. This new concept was introduced at a CIBA Foundation meeting in England in 1965 and subsequently endorsed with formal diagnostic criteria by Harvard Medical School in 1968.[8] Acceptance of this medically, philosophically, and legally novel concept changed the practice of transplantation. The ability to certify death while perfusion of the body with oxygenated blood continued enabled surgeons to procure organs for transplantation with minimal warm ischemia.[9] When early experience with the organs transplanted from these so-called heartbeating donors demonstrated superior outcomes, the use of non-heartbeating donors declined and was subsequently abandoned.[8] Consequently, an entire generation of transplant surgeons and other medical specialists was trained knowing only heartbeating organ donation.[10]

As transplantation outcomes improved, the procedure became increasingly common over the next two decades. To some degree, transplantation became a victim of its own accomplishments[11] because "success bred demand, and this demand… outpaced supply."[12] The gap between supply and demand arose in part from an unforeseen conflict between public health initiatives. On the one hand, transplantation's "irresistible utilitarian appeal"[13] facilitated large-scale efforts at public education, and society "accepted and largely endorsed the transplantation enterprise."[14] Simultaneously, however, numerous statutory changes in the areas of gun control, automobile safety (air bags, seat belts, lower "legal alcohol" limits), and helmet use by motorcyclists reduced traumatic fatalities among young, previously healthy patients and inadvertently decreased the number of potential organ donors in the process.[15,16] Ironically, increasing clinical expertise itself also contributed to the supply gap, by causing an expansion in the list of indications for transplantation.[13] This supply gap continued to widen over time despite growing public awareness of the situation,[17-19] increasingly proactive measures to increase the organ supply (examples include "required notification" of family members of the donation option; "required response" to the question of donation preferences to obtain a driver's license; and "opting out" of legal mandates presuming consent to donate organs), and investigation of xenotransplantation (the use of non-human organs).

In 1993, The University of Pittsburgh Medical Center introduced the nation's first institutional policy to permit and regulate non-heartbeating organ donation.[20] The need for such a policy arose when several patients and families asked to participate in organ donation after a previously elected withdrawal of life sustaining treatment; this was a request that fell outside the parameters of donation policies and guidelines then in effect.[21] Of necessity, the policy therefore became the first detailed and concrete model for the use of cardiopulmonary criteria to determine death for the purposes of organ procurement.[22] Despite the fact that non-heartbeating organ donation was commonplace in the early years of transplantation, and was abandoned in the early 1970s for technical, rather than ethical, reasons,[12,23] the so-called Pittsburgh Protocol proved to be ethically quite controversial. Whereas some observers took issue with the policy, describing it in such vivid terms as "ghoulish" and "macabre"[17] and even questioning whether the donors might not yet actually be dead at the time of procurement,[24] others suggested that the widespread reinstatement of non-heartbeating organ donation might help solve the ever-worsening organ shortage.[21] Such conflicting views have kept non-heartbeating organ donation a subject of debate ever since.

After more than a decade of ongoing scrutiny, several issues regarding non-heartbeating organ donation remain unresolved. The ultimate impact of non-heartbeating donation on the number of organs available for transplantation, although potentially large, remains unclear.[25] And whereas ethical questions regarding non-heartbeating organ donation persist, the process is believed to accommodate the needs of dying patients as well as those awaiting transplantation[8] and to be worthy of the same public understanding as current practices surrounding heartbeating organ donation.[26] A variety of organizations, including the Society of Critical Care Medicine (SCCM),[27] the United Network for Organ Sharing (UNOS), and the Institute of Medicine (IOM),[5]

TABLE 250–1. U.S. OPOS—DECEASED DONORS AND NON-HEARTBEATING DONORS, 1993-2002

Year of recovery	Deceased donors	NHBD	NHBD as percentage of total donors	OPOs with at least 1 NHBD
1993	4,861	42	0.86%	13
1994	5,099	57	1.11%	22
1995	5,362	64	1.20%	22
1996	5,417	71	1.31%	21
1997	5,478	78	1.43%	19
1998	5,794	75	1.29%	16
1999	5,825	87	1.49%	20
2000	5,986	119	1.98%	30
2001	6,082	169	2.77%	33
2002	6,184	188	3.04%	29

From UNOS, personal communication. Based on UNOS OPTN data as of March 14, 2003. Data subject to change due to future data submission or correction.

have endorsed the concept and issued relevant guidelines. The remainder of this chapter focuses on the practical application of those guidelines by reviewing the current state of practice of non-heartbeating organ transplantation.

EPIDEMIOLOGY

The use of organs from non-heartbeating donors is not a new phenomenon. Some of the controversy surrounding its resurgence stems from debate over whether it would translate into increased numbers of donor organs and shortened waiting lists.[3,5,8,9,28-32] In an effort to answer some of these questions, UNOS has been collecting information on organs procured via non-heartbeating donation from the regional organ procurement organizations (OPOs) since 1994.[33]

Much of this information—stored as part of Unet, the comprehensive UNOS database for all organ transplantation activity in the United States since 1986—is public domain and is available online at both a searchable website, *www.unos.org*, and in annual reports from UNOS.[34] Table 250-1 demonstrates that the annual number of non-heartbeating organ donors has increased steadily for the better part of a decade. Although there is no documented correlation with this trend, it is interesting to note that during this same period there has been a change in the typical deceased donor, from

a young person dying as a result of devastating head trauma toward a typically older patient who dies of a neurovascular insult.[34] The 188 non-heartbeating organ donors in 2002 represented just over 3% of all donors that year. The number of OPOs that recovered organs from non-heartbeating donors in a given year has also risen overall, although not as steadily, from 13 in 1993 to a high of 33 in 2001. Not shown in the table, but cited in the annual report,[34] is the fact that during this same time period 43 of the OPOs participated in at least one non-heartbeating donor procurement (for comparison purposes, there are currently 59 OPOs in the United States). Overall experience with non-heartbeating organ donation is also steadily increasing at transplant centers, as shown in Table 250-2. Finally, Table 250-3 shows the steady annual rise in the total number of kidneys and livers recovered and transplanted, as well as the improving yield of organs per donor and the increasing percentage of recovered organs that are ultimately successfully transplanted.

TABLE 250–2. TRANSPLANT CENTER EXPERIENCE WITH NON-HEARTBEATING ORGAN DONATION, 2000-2002

	No. of Transplant Centers		
No. of Non-heartbeating Donors	2000	2001	2002
0	230	198	187
1	61	71	74
2	10	12	18
3	2	10	7
4	5	0	5
5	0	1	4
6	2	3	0
7	0	1	1
8	0	1	0
Total No. of centers with at least 1 non-heartbeating donor	80	99	109

From UNOS, personal communication. Based on UNOS OPTN data as of March 14, 2003. Data subject to change due to future data submission or correction.

TABLE 250–3. RECOVERY AND TRANSPLANTATION OF NON-HEARTBEATING DONOR ORGANS, 2000-2002

		Year Recovered		
		2000	2001	2002
Number of Donors		119	169	188
Kidneys recovered	Total*	225	321	363
	Average†	1.89	1.9	1.93
Kidneys transplanted	Total	177	253	308
	Average	1.49	1.5	1.64
Livers recovered	Total	54	92	102
	Average	0.45	0.54	0.54
Livers transplanted	Total	39	69	80
	Average	0.33	0.41	0.43
Organs recovered	Total	288	429	490
	Average	2.42	2.54	2.61
Organs transplanted	Total	221	332	400
	Average	1.86	1.96	2.13
Organs transplanted as percentage of organs recovered		76%	77%	82%

*Total = cumulative number of organs annually.
†Average = ratio of (total organs) to (number of donors per year).
Note: Total for organs transplanted is greater than the sum of total kidneys transplanted and total livers transplanted, reflecting transplantation of other organs not shown in this table.
From UNOS, personal communication. Based on UNOS OPTN data as of March 14, 2003. Data subject to change due to future data submission or correction.

TABLE 250–4. OPO EXPERIENCE WITH NON-HEARTBEATING ORGAN DONATION, 1999-2001

No. NHBDs per OPO	No. of OPOs (Total No. of NHBDs)		
	1999	2000	2001
1-5	16 (41)	23 (46)	25 (60)
6-10	3 (23)	4 (29)	2 (17)
>10	1 (24)	3 (47)	6 (93)
Total	20 (88)	30 (122)	33 (170)
NHBDs as % of donors	1%-8%	<1%-16%	<1%-15%

From UNOS, personal communication. Based on UNOS OPTN data as of August 16, 2002. Data subject to change due to future data submission or correction.

TABLE 250–5. CAUSE OF DEATH FOR ORGAN DONORS, NON-HEARTBEATING VERSUS HEARTBEATING

Etiology of Donor Death	Non-heartbeating (n, %)	Heartbeating (n, %)
Motor vehicle accident	5 (27.8)	135 (39.8)
Intracranial hemorrhage	4 (22.2)	110 (32.4)
Gunshot wound	2 (11.1)	39 (11.5)
Anoxic injury	4 (22.2)	25 (7.4)
Fall	3 (16.7)	22 (6.5)
Tumor	0 (0.0)	6 (1.8)
Other	0 (0.0)	2 (0.6)
Total	18 (100)	339 (100)

From D'Alessandro AM, Odorico JS, Knechtle SJ, et al: Simultaneous pancreas-kidney (SPK) transplantation from controlled non-heartbeating donors (NHBDs). Cell Transplant 2000;9:889-893.

Another trend is that the population of *potential* organ donors is not evenly distributed across the United States.[34] Because the procurement and distribution of organs is largely geographically based, and because not all of the OPOs are performing non-heartbeating organ donation, not every OPO has had equivalent experience with the process of non-heartbeating organ donation. For example, as Table 250-4 shows, a limited number of OPOs account for a large number of the non-heartbeating donations occurring each year. This same trend is shown at the national level in Figure 250-1, which demonstrates the considerable regional variation in the distribution of non-heartbeating donors. Among the OPOs handling the largest numbers of non-heartbeating donors in 2001, these cases represented an average of 10% of their procurements for the year.[34]

In addition to the UNOS statistics, there is instructive epidemiologic data in the published results from individual transplant centers. Table 250-5 shows statistics reported by the University of Wisconsin, reflecting their experience with simultaneous kidney-pancreas transplantation over a 6½-year period. These data suggest that the nature of the terminal insult is similar in patients who ultimately become organ donors, whether or not brain death results. In other words, a serious injury should alert clinicians to the possibility that the patient may be a candidate for organ donation even if brain death criteria are not met. Additional findings

of interest, drawn from the same patient population and shown in Table 250-6, include the similarity of age distribution and the equivalent gender mix among the two donor populations. As indicated, the only statistically significant difference between the two groups was the warm ischemia time; this difference, of course, is expected.

The general applicability of the findings obtained by studying a particular type of transplant procedure at a single center is suggested by the very similar observations resulting from a comprehensive analysis of several years' worth of renal transplantation data from the UNOS database.[33] The data in Table 250-7, comparing the non-heartbeating donors of 229 kidneys between 1994 and 1996 to the heartbeating donors of 8718 kidneys during the same period of time, show parallel similarities for age and gender distribution for the two groups of donors. Also apparent from this table is the relative under-representation of minorities between both groups of donors, an observation that has been noted previously by multiple authors.[15,35]

Ultimately, only time will tell whether improved recognition of the potential non-heartbeating donor, as exemplified by the preceding data, will translate into greater numbers of organs being made available for transplantation. To date, estimates of the numeric potential of non-heartbeating organ donation have varied.[25] UNOS projects that roughly 600 more donors, and at least 1200 more organs, could be recovered annually in the United States if each of the 59 OPOs was as active as the most prolific of their counterparts

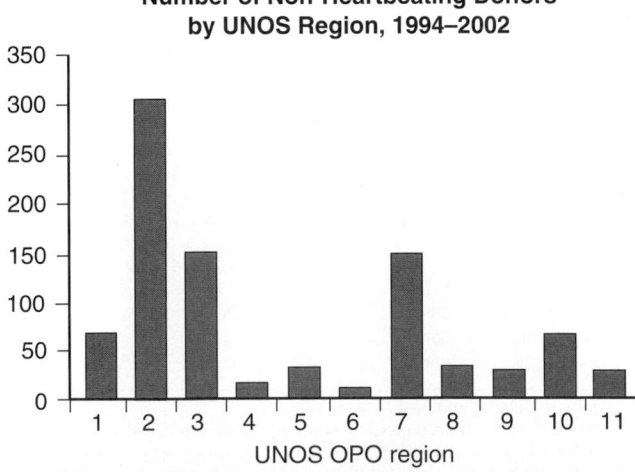

Number of Non-Heartbeating Donors by UNOS Region, 1994–2002

FIGURE 250–1. Cumulative regional distribution of non-heartbeating organ donors. (Courtesy of the United Network for Organ Sharing. Based on OPTN Data as of March 14, 2003. Data subject to change due to future data submission or correction.)

TABLE 250–6. ORGAN DONOR CHARACTERISTICS, NON-HEARTBEATING VERSUS HEARTBEATING

Donor Characteristics	Non-heartbeating	Heartbeating
Age (yr)	31.8	30.8
Gender (M/F)	1.6/1	1.6/1
Glucose (mg/dL)	176.6	190.4
Creatinine (mg/dL)	0.96	1.01
Warm ischemic time (min)	14.8	0.0*
Cold ischemic time (h)		
Pancreas	16.3	15.8
Kidney	17.4	17.0

*P < .001
From D'Alessandro AM, Odorico JS, Knechtle SJ, et al: Simultaneous pancreas-kidney (SPK) transplantation rom controlled non-heartbeating donors (NHBDs). Cell Transplant 2000;9:889-893.

TABLE 250–7. ORGAN DONOR CHARACTERISTICS, NON-HEARTBEATING VERSUS HEARTBEATING

Characteristic	Non-heartbeating	Heartbeating	P Value
Age (yr)	35 ± 17	33 ± 18	0.08
Height (cm)	170 ± 16	167 ± 21	0.01
Weight (kg)	73.4 ± 24.2	69.8 ± 23.0	0.07
Creatinine (mg/dL)	1.3 ± 2.9	1.3 ± 1.9	0.28
Male sex (%)	66	63	0.24
White race (%)	86	77	
Black race (%)	5	12	<0.001
Other race (%)	9	11	

From Cho YW, Terasaki PI, Cecka JM, et al: Transplantation of kidneys from donors whose hearts have stopped beating. N Engl J Med 1998;338:221-225.

with respect to non-heartbeating organ procurement.[34] In considering these estimates, and weighing the potential utility of non-heartbeating organ donation, it is sobering to view them against the background of these final statistical trends and epidemiologic truths:[34]

- Despite a substantial increase in cadaveric organ donation over the past decade, the number of patients waiting for organs continues to rise. As of this writing, the waiting list numbers more than 82,000.
- The number of kidneys from heartbeating donors has declined over the past few years, but the total number of cadaveric kidney donations has been held steady by a 40% rise in the number of non-heartbeating donor kidneys. The waiting list for kidneys continues to grow, and waiting times are getting longer. Only 20% of listed patients have received a kidney in a given year since 1998.

IDENTIFICATION OF THE POTENTIAL NON-HEARTBEATING DONOR

An important initial step in the process of non-heartbeating organ transplantation is the recognition of patients with the potential to be suitable donors. By convention, four types of potential non-heartbeating donors are recognized according to a scheme developed at a conference in The Netherlands in 1994. As shown in Table 250-8, the Maastricht Classification defines potential donors by the particular circumstances under which their cardiovascular death occurs.[9,36,37] A distinction is recognized between those donors whose cardiopulmonary failure—and subsequent

TABLE 250–8. THE MAASTRICHT CLASSIFICATION FOR NON-HEARTBEATING ORGAN DONATION

Category	Description	Condition
1	Cardiac arrest outside the hospital, no resuscitation attempted	Uncontrolled
2	Cardiac arrest followed by unsuccessful resuscitation, either inside or outside a hospital	Uncontrolled
3	Cardiac arrest after planned withdrawal of life support technology	Controlled
4	Cardiac arrest in a brain-dead patient awaiting organ procurement	Uncontrolled

From Koostra G, Daemen JHC, Oomen APA: Categories of non-heartbeating donors. Transplant Proc 1995;27:2893-2894.

organ procurement—is "uncontrolled" and therefore emergent in nature (categories 1, 2, and 4), and those donors whose death by cardiopulmonary criteria occurs in a "controlled" and planned manner (category 3).[21] These different types of donation raise different issues with respect to the management of the donor, the technical processes of the procurement, the ethical issues that may arise, and the potential outcome of the transplant.

Procurement of organs from non-heartbeating donors under uncontrolled conditions is technically possible,[38] but it remains relatively uncommon.[8] One significant potential difficulty is the need to minimize organ ischemia in the presence of an unanticipated cardiac arrest. Critical decisions must be made quickly to preserve organ viability. In situations in which a patient's wishes regarding organ donation are unknown, crucial time may pass—and transplant suitability may decline—while attempts are made to locate family members to discuss consent. In response to this dilemma, some institutions have developed protocols whereby category 1 or 2 non-heartbeating donors presenting to the emergency department undergo placement of vascular and/or intraperitoneal catheters and are infused with cold organ preservation solution *before* formal consent for procurement is available.[39,40] If consent is subsequently granted, procurement and donation go forward; if consent is refused, the catheters are removed and the deceased patient is moved to the morgue. Justification for such protocols stems from the presumption of consent, the desire to maintain the opportunity to donate organs,[10] and the idea that the procedures are relatively minimally invasive and straightforward.[6] These protocols have generated debate on ethical grounds[41,42] and remain controversial.

A second difficulty with uncontrolled non-heartbeating organ donation is evidence to suggest that the practice lacks support by a majority of public opinion across racial lines.[35] A third problem is that significant logistical resources are required to maintain such a program. In the case of at least one transplant center, these practical demands have proven insurmountable despite both clinical success with uncontrolled non-heartbeating organ donation and an innovative and progressive community-centered approach to the ethical questions.[43] For these—and perhaps other—reasons, to our knowledge, there are no OPOs with active programs for the uncontrolled recovery of organs from non-heartbeating donors in the United States at this time.[44] In the rare category 4 circumstance, the patient has already been declared dead using whole brain criteria but subsequently loses circulation. If resuscitation fails, rapid procurement may still occur.

More common is the category 3 non-heartbeating organ donor, whose death occurs in a controlled setting. It is vital for the intensive care practitioner to be familiar with the kinds of diagnoses and clinical circumstances that may qualify a patient as a controlled non-heartbeating donor. The success of non-heartbeating organ donation depends in large degree on the identification of potential donors whose death is expected to be rapid—typically occurring over less than 60 minutes—and predictable.[8] In practice, they are patients in whom withdrawal of life-sustaining treatment or pharmacologic support of the cardiovascular system is being planned.[8] As shown in Figure 250-2, the UNOS Critical Pathway for DCD, typical patients may have the following characteristics: absent or hyperactive respiratory drive, lack of adequate respiratory muscle strength, severe hypoxemia, or inadequate circulation in the absence of inotropic or vasopressor drugs. Such patients are usually supported by ventilators or mechanical circulatory assistance such as ventricular-assist devices (VAD) or intra-aortic balloon pumps.[8] Often, but not necessarily, they are patients who have suffered a severe neurologic insult.[5,32] Conscious ventilator or VAD-dependent patients occasionally decide to discontinue their support devices and request that their organs subsequently be donated.[23,45] They, too, may be reasonable donor candidates if rapid physiologic deterioration and death are expected soon after withdrawal of life-sustaining treatment. Potential controlled non-heartbeating organ donors are subject to the same general medical considerations and screening processes as all other organ donors, as previously described elsewhere.[46,47]

Identification of the potential non-heartbeating donor relies on experienced clinicians' best judgment of a patient's ability to tolerate the combination of withdrawal of life support and the administration of palliative therapies.[8] Currently, attention has been focused on identifying clinical factors that suggest a high likelihood of death within 60 minutes (within 30 minutes for some programs) of withdrawal of life-sustaining therapy. Accurate predictive indices would enable OPOs to more readily identify potential organ donors, help minimize the financial impact and resource drain of failed donation for hospitals, and prevent any unnecessary stress and disappointment for families during a psychologically vulnerable time. To that end, a recent abstract[48] has suggested a decision rule incorporating four simple, readily obtainable clinical criteria: (1) requirement for vasopressors to support arterial blood pressure, (2) absence of primary brain injury, (3) history of 6 or more days on mechanical ventilation, and (4) respiratory rate less than 20 breaths/min (in the absence of mechanical ventilatory support). When two or more of the proposed indicators were present, the rule accurately predicted death within 60 minutes (after life-supporting treatments were withdrawn) with a sensitivity of 81% and a specificity of 78% in the study population. Larger follow-up studies are needed to create reliable criteria to guide both potential non-heartbeating organ donation as well as facilitate end-of-life care.

ETHICAL PRINCIPLES FOR DONOR MANAGEMENT

Appropriate management of the non-heartbeating organ donor requires the integration of several fundamental principles. These principles share a common thread of protecting the rights and interests of the donor as an individual and specifically attempt to prevent the care of the organ from superseding the care of the dying patient.

The first of these "doctrines" is commonly referred to as the "dead donor rule." This term, widely cited by ethicists and policymakers alike, has never actually been codified by law.[49] In essence, the dead donor rule encompasses two complementary ideas: first, that patients must be dead before the initiation of organ procurement; and second, that organ procurement itself must not be the cause of the donor's death. The purpose of such a rule is to protect patients and prevent the perception that transplantation medicine is "preying upon" sick people. Debate has raged over the question of whether non-heartbeating donors are in fact dead at the time of procurement, and concern has been voiced that patients are being "sacrificed" for their organs.[24]

However, the prevailing opinion is that if appropriate death determination occurs, then this concern is mitigated.

The second core concept in non-heartbeating organ transplantation is that a person's status as a critically ill *patient* takes precedence over his or her potential as a *donor*. In other words, the needs of the patient "trump" the needs of the organ donation process, and appropriate care of the dying patient must always be the primary goal.[50] This merits explicit mention because inherent in the process of non-heartbeating organ transplantation there is "a possible conflict between the interests of dying patients (potential donors) and the interests of persons waiting for organs (potential recipients)."[13] This concept is important, because studies have documented fear among the lay public that their likelihood of receiving aggressive life support might be compromised by consenting to organ donor status.[18,35] Indeed, "perhaps the greatest obstacle to public policy change with respect to non-heartbeating organ donation is the public perception that the transplant community is too willing to draw the boundary between life and death wherever it happens to maximize the chances for organ procurement."[51] In a practical sense, these concepts are manifest in two analogous practices designed to maintain maximum separation between terminal care of the patient and the organ transplantation process. The first practice is that "as a general rule two discussions—whether to forego life-sustaining therapy and whether to donate organs—must be made separately and on their own individual merit."[8] Ideally, discussion regarding withdrawing life-sustaining treatment should come first, so as not to be biased by the issue of transplantation.[5]

The second practical application of this concept of separation is a clear division of responsibility among members of the health care team, such that no provider participates in more than one phase of the process. Thus, the discussion of withdrawing life-sustaining treatment, the accompanying terminal care of the patient, and the actual pronouncement of death are supervised by critical care physicians, whereas procurement of organs, actual transplant surgery, and subsequent clinical management of the recipient are handled by the transplant surgeon (see Fig. 250-2). These safeguards help validate the claim that non-heartbeating organ donation protocols are "not designed or intended to take organs, but rather, under an extremely limited set of circumstances, to make possible donation."[31]

The question of "code status" in this context may seem at first to be paradoxical, because non-heartbeating donors by their very nature will have their life support withdrawn and be allowed—in fact, expected—to die without further attempts at resuscitation. Things may be more complicated in practice, as exemplified by the following situation. Suppose that a patient has decided to withdraw life-sustaining treatment, has expressed a wish to be a non-heartbeating donor, has been properly evaluated, and has provided consent. If this patient has a sudden cardiac arrest before the planned withdrawal of life support, then what should be done? On the one hand, it has been argued that instituting resuscitation at this point would be inappropriate on multiple levels.[30] First, this patient—by virtue of a prior decision to withdraw life support—has already effectively accepted death as an outcome and has refused life-sustaining therapies. Second, the resuscitation may cause pain or harm—a consequence that is inconsistent with the goal of dignified comfort care for a terminally ill patient. And third, attempting to resuscitate this patient amounts to placing treatment

Critical Pathway for Donation after Cardiac Death (DCD)

Patient Name _____

UNOS ID Number _____

Collaborative Practice	Phase I Identification and Referral	Phase II Preliminary Evaluation	Phase III Family Discussion and Consent	Phase IV Comprehensive Evaluation and Donor Management	Phase V Withdrawal of Support/ Pronouncement of Death/ Organ Recovery
The following health care professionals may be involved in the DCD donation process: Check all that apply: ☐ Physician (MD) ☐ Critical Care RN ☐ Nurse Supervisor ☐ Medical Examiner/ Coroner ☐ Respiratory Therapy (RT) ☐ Laboratory ☐ Pharmacy ☐ Radiology ☐ Anesthesiology ☐ OR/Surgery Staff ☐ Clergy ☐ Social Worker ☐ Organ Procurement Coordinator (OPC) ☐ Organ Procurement Organization (OPO)	Prior to withdrawing life support, contact local OPO for any patient who fulfills the following criteria: ☐ Devastating neurologic injury and/or organ failure requiring mechanical ventilatory or circulatory support Following referral, additional evaluation is done collaboratively to determine if death is likely to occur within one hour (or within a specified time frame as determined by caregiving team and OPO) following withdrawal of support Patient conditions might include the following: ☐ **Ventilator dependent for respiratory insufficiency:** apneic or severe hypopneic; tachypnea ≥ 30 breaths/min after DC ventilator ☐ **Dependent on mechanical circulatory support** (LVAD; RVAD; V-A ECMO; Pacemaker with unassisted rhythm < 30 beats per minute.	**Physician** ☐ Supportive of withdrawal of care and has communicated grave prognosis to family ☐ Review DCD procedure with OPC ☐ Will be involved in withdrawal/pronounce-ment ☐ Family and/or care giving team initiate conversation about withdrawal of support ☐ Will designate a person to be involved with withdrawal and/or pronouncement **Family** ☐ Has received grave prognosis ☐ Understands prognosis ☐ In conjunction with care giving team, decide to withdraw support **Patient** ☐ Age _____ ☐ Weight _____ ☐ Height _____ ☐ ABO _____ ☐ Medical Hx _____ ☐ Surgical Hx _____ ☐ Social Hx _____ ☐ Death likely < 1 hour following withdrawal (determined collaboratively by evaluating: injury, level of support, respiratory drive assessment)	☐ Support services offered to family ☐ OPC/Hospital Staff approach family about donation options ☐ Legal next-of-kin (NOK) fully informed of donation options and recovery procedures ☐ Legal NOK grants consent for DCD following withdrawal of support ☐ Family offered opportunity to be present during withdrawal of support ☐ OPC obtains _____ Witnessed consent from legal NOK for DCD _____ Signed consent _____ Time _____ Date _____ Detailed med/soc history Notification of donation ☐ Hospital supervisor ☐ ME/coroner notified ☐ ME/Coroner and releases for donation _____ ME/Coroner has restrictions *Stop Pathway if—* ☐ *Family, ME/Coroner denies consent* ☐ *Patient determined to be unsuitable candidate for DCD*	☐ MD, in collaboration with OPO, implements management guidelines. ☐ Establish location and time of withdrawal of support ☐ Review plan for withdrawal to include: –Pronouncing MD (should be in attendance for duration of withdrawal of support, determination of death, and may not be a member of the transplant team) –Comfort care –Extubation and discontinuation of ventilator support –Establish plan for continued supportive care if pt survives > one hour or predetermined time interval after withdrawal of support ☐ Notify OR/anesthesia _____ Review patient's clinical course, withdrawal plan and potential organ recovery procedures _____ Schedule OR time ☐ Notify recovery teams ☐ Prepare patient for transport to pre-arranged area for withdrawal of support	☐ Withdrawal occurs in _____ OR _____ ICU _____ Other ☐ Family present for withdrawal of support _____ yes _____ no ☐ OR/Room prepared and equipment set up ☐ Transplant team in the OR (not in attendance during withdrawal) ☐ Caregiving team present ☐ Administration of pre-approved medication (e.g. Heparin/Regitine) ☐ **Withdrawal of support according to hospital/MD practice guidelines** _____ Time _____ Date ☐ **Vital signs are monitored and recorded every minute [See attached sheet]** ☐ **Pt pronounced dead and appropriate documentation completed** _____ Time _____ Date _____ MD ☐ **Transplant Team initiates surgical recovery** at prescribed time following pronouncement of death ☐ Allocation of organs per

FIGURE 250–2. Critical pathway for donation after cardiac death (DCD). (Courtesy of the United Network for Organ Sharing.)

Critical Pathway for
Donation after Cardiac Death (DCD)

Patient Name _____
UNOS ID Number _____

		Patient progresses to brain death during evaluation – refer to brain dead pathway	OPTN/UNOS policy
	☐ **Severe disruption in oxygenation:** PEEP ≥ 10 and SaO$_2$ ≤ 92%; FiO$_2$ ≥ .50 and SaO$_2$ ≤ 92%; V-V ECMO ☐ **Dependent upon pharmacologic circulatory assist:** Norephinephrine, epinephrine, or phenylephrine ≥ 0.2 ug/kg/min; Dopamine ≥ 15 mg/kg/min ☐ **IABP and inotropic support:** IABP 1:1 and dobutamine or dopamine ≥ 10 ug/kg/min and CI ≤ 2.2 L/min/M2; IABP 1:1 and CI ≤ 1.5 L/min/M2	☐ Patient transported to prearranged area ☐ Note: should the clinical situation require premortum femoral cannulation, the following should be reviewed: -family consent or understanding -MD inserting cannula -Time and location of cannula insertion -If death does not occur, determine if cannula should be removed	☐ ***If cardiac death not established within 1 hour or predetermined time interval after withdrawal of support—Stop Pathway. Patient moved to predetermined area for continuation of supportive care.*** ☐ Post Mortem care administered
Labs/Diagnostics	☐ ABO ☐ Electrolytes ☐ LFTs ☐ PT/PTT ☐ CBC with Diff ☐ Beta HCG (female pts) ☐ ABG	Repeat full panel of labs additionally: ☐ Serology Testing infectious disease profile ☐ Blood cultures × 2 ☐ UA & Urine culture ☐ Sputum Culture ☐ Tissue typing	
Respiratory	☐ Maintain ventilator support ☐ Pulmonary toilet PRN ☐ Respiratory drive assessment RR _____ VT _____ VE _____ NIF _____ Minutes off ventilator _____	☐ ABGs as requested ☐ Notify RT of location and time of withdrawal of support	☐ Transport with mechanical ventilation using lowest FiO$_2$ possible while maintaining the SaO$_2$ > 90%

FIGURE 250–2. Cont'd

Critical Pathway for
Donation after Cardiac Death (DCD)

Patient Name _____

UNOS ID Number _____

Treatments/Ongoing Care	Maintain standard nursing care to include: ☐ Vital signs q 1 hour ☐ I & O q 1 hour	☐ Hemodynamics while off ventilator HR _____ BP _____ SaO$_2$ _____	☐ Post mortem care at conclusion of case
Medications		☐ Provide medications as directed by MD in consult with OPC	☐ Heparin and other medications prior to withdrawal of support
Optimal Outcomes	The potential DCD donor is identified and a referral is made to the OPO.	The donor is evaluated and found to be a suitable candidate for donation.	The family is offered the option of donation and their decision is supported.	Optimal organ function is maintained, withdrawal of support plan is established, and personnel prepared for potential organ recovery.	Death occurs within one hour of withdrawal of support and all suitable organs and tissues are recovered for transplant.

This work supported by HRSA contract 231-00-0115.

of the organ(s) above treatment of the patient (because a non-donor patient who arrests while awaiting withdrawal of life support would be allowed to die). On the other hand, there is an argument to be made that resuscitation might be appropriate in this instance.[52] If we want to abide by this patient's request that his organs be made available for transplantation, then resuscitation under these circumstances could be justified. Indeed, failing to attempt to accommodate this patient's wish might even be construed as a disservice to the patient. The arguments favoring resuscitation are supported if specific informed consent for such measures is obtained ahead of time. To date, there appears to be no national standard or consensus on the question of resuscitation for the non-heartbeating donor awaiting the withdrawal of life-sustaining treatment. For the time being, this issue is left to the discretion of individual centers.

END OF LIFE MANAGEMENT FOR POTENTIAL DONOR PATIENTS

In recent years, there has been increased recognition of the importance of good end-of-life care even in the ICU.[53] The SCCM has issued recommendations on the subject,[54] specific protocols have been described in the literature,[55-57] and the topic is covered in depth elsewhere in this textbook (see Chapter 255). The dying patient who also wishes to be a non-heartbeating organ donor presents a special challenge, requiring care that is not only comparable to that afforded to all dying patients but also sensitive to the concerns described in the preceding section. To that end, the SCCM has also offered recommendations particular to non-heartbeating organ donation.[27] These guidelines, supplemented by reports of the experience at some transplant centers[22,39] and the pathway put forth by UNOS (see Fig. 250-2), provide direction for intensivists caring for patients who wish to become non-heartbeating donors. It is vital that all health care providers involved in this process be comfortable with, and knowledgeable about, their specific role.[58]

The first issue to be considered is the use of analgesics and anxiolytics. It is regrettable when any patient dies in pain, regardless of the setting, because it is usually possible to provide every patient a dignified and painless death.[54] Indeed, pain relief may be the single most important objective in the final hours of life.[8] There is firm ethical, legal, and medical justification for using opioids and benzodiazepines (among other agents) to relieve anxiety, pain, and suffering.[54] Each dose of these medications should be provided either to relieve symptoms or prevent symptoms that are believed to be imminent. Doses should be titrated to fulfill these goals, because some patients require huge doses whereas others may require none. Past requirements provide a useful guide to the medication range the patient may require. Doses must be chosen with the understanding that comforting medications may have unintended, unwanted, but not unexpected side effects, for example, hypotension or respiratory depression. The perception that the use of medications to enhance patient comfort may amount to "euthanizing" patients can be particularly problematic where non-heartbeating donation is concerned because of the added benefit of a rapid death to donated organs.[22,59] There is a consensus that "medications given to provide comfort are reasonable, even if they might hasten death" but "no medication whose purpose is to hasten death should be given to the patient."[27]

Of course this approach should apply equally to all dying patients, whether or not they are to become non-heartbeating donors, and failure to attend to potential non-heartbeating donors' comfort is considered to be less-than-optimal end of life care.

A second issue in the withdrawal of life-sustaining care is the setting. The SCCM endorses hospital policies "that explicitly allow and encourage the continuous presence of family and friends at the bedside," suggests that "a private room is the environment most conducive to emotional and physical intimacy and should be identified as a goal for excellent care of the dying," and recommends that "whenever possible and within reason, withdrawal of life support should be timed to allow for the arrival of family members who must travel long distances."[54] These considerations take on particular importance in the case of the non-heartbeating donor, who must be in the operating room within a very short period of time after death if organ procurement is to go forward. Thus, there will be little time for the family to say extended goodbyes or grieve at the bedside. There is perhaps some irony in this dilemma, in the sense that patients may opt for withdrawal of life support as the means to a dignified and natural death, only to have that choice undermined somewhat by the desire for non-heartbeating donation and its attendant constraints on the process.[60] Attempts to balance these competing needs have evolved over time.

The initial University of Pittsburgh policy called for the withdrawal of care to occur in the operating room, which offered the advantage of minimizing the need to transport the patient after death and permitting the prepping and draping of the patient before to death.[8] This protocol was denounced for subjecting the patient to "a desolate, profanely 'high tech' death" surrounded by "masked, gowned, and gloved strangers."[17] The initial experience in Pittsburgh found some truth to the proposition that presence of family at the patient's bedside at the time of death may be more important to patients and families than organ donation or location of death. When three of the first four families approached about non-heartbeating donation agreed to consent only if they could be physically present at the time of death,[22] the Pittsburgh policy was changed to allow families into the operating room or to move the withdrawal of care to an operating room "holding" area. The area selected for withdrawal of support should allow family members to be present, accommodate the necessary monitors and equipment, and be close enough to the operating room to allow rapid transport immediately after death.[61] A review of recent policies from some other transplant centers and OPOs suggests that, whereas practice appears to vary somewhat in this regard, the family's need to be present and involved in the dying process is widely cited and respected.[5]

A final consideration in the withdrawal of life-sustaining treatment in the case of a non-heartbeating organ donor is logistics. Careful coordination of numerous personnel, equipment, and resources is absolutely vital to the success of the process. At the University of Pittsburgh Medical Center, the necessary steps are conceptually divided into three key areas and a simple checklist is used to ensure that appropriate preparations are in place before the patient is ever transported to the selected area for withdrawal of life-sustaining treatment. The first area of emphasis is the medical record. Three items are required. First, an attending intensivist's note is necessary to document the decision to withdraw life support and institute comfort measures, the consensus of other physicians caring for the patient with this decision, and absence of neuromuscular blocking agents and apnea-inducing medications. Second, a formal Ethics Consult Service note is necessary. Third, there must be a signed consent for organ donation.

The second area of emphasis is necessary notifications and communication. This section of the checklist requires documentation that the patient and family have been fully informed and have had their questions answered. This section also requires that all appropriate personnel—including a hospital administrator, transplant coordinator, clergy, the on-call anesthesiologist, operating room coordinator, nursing and respiratory staff, as well as the patient's primary care physician—have been notified of the planned events.

The third area of emphasis relates to necessary equipment and supplies. The checklist directs that appropriate intravenous access must be in place, that a portable ventilator must be available, and that a special supply cart—akin to a "crash cart"—is available and stocked with a charged oxygen tank, a two-channel cardiac monitor, and adequate supplies of appropriate sedatives and narcotics. While the specific steps required will vary with the policies and protocols of individual institutions, it is the methodical approach to preparation and the emphasis on careful documentation that merits emphasis here.

DETERMINATION OF DEATH

The determination of death by cardiopulmonary criteria has been a controversial issue. Historically speaking, the diagnosis of death has long been a difficult matter.[62] To this day, there are no universally recognized cardiopulmonary criteria for the certification of death.[21] In contrast, the neurologic criteria for death, after some prolonged debate, have become much better codified and accepted. Interestingly, most major medical textbooks are silent on the subject of appropriate cardiopulmonary criteria for the declaration of death, even though death is declared in hospitals most often based on cessation of cardiac and pulmonary function.[63]

The essential quandary in determining cardiopulmonary death in non-heartbeating organ donation is one of timing.[13] Because the actual tolerable limits of warm ischemia are not well defined and may vary from one clinical situation to the next,[6,11] there is a logical presumption in favor of minimizing warm ischemic time as much as possible. Concern arises because circulatory collapse is a process that takes time, and the precise onset of warm ischemia is difficult to delineate.[64] Clearly, it begins no later than when death occurs, but more often organ compromise begins much earlier,[3,65] probably about the time that systolic blood pressure decreases to less than 80 mm Hg or the arterial oxygen saturation decreases to less than 80%. As a result of the need to minimize ischemia, there is a strong incentive to procure organs as quickly as possible[5,13,63] and to certify death as soon as reasonable. This forces an important question: how soon after circulation, respiration, and responsiveness cease can death be certified?[11]

The recognition of a so-called required asystolic time is perhaps the single most contentious issue in all of the debate surrounding non-heartbeating organ donation.[5,49] The obvious significance of this issue, plainly stated, is that "the longer you wait the more uncertainty there is about the organs, and the shorter you wait the more uncertainty [there is

about] whether the person is really dead or not.[13] Interestingly, this subject had not previously received much attention, because to a large degree it was not clinically important; there was never any sense of urgency to certify the death of a "no-code" patient, and the actual interval between cardiac arrest and pronouncement could extend for hours.[63]

From a legal standpoint, the 1980 Uniform Determination of Death Act establishes that death is determined when there is irreversible cessation of circulatory and respiratory function.[66] The authors of the act specifically framed it as a legal standard for establishing death and readily admitted that it lacked accompanying medical criteria. Therefore, medical professionals must determine acceptable practices, informed by new scientific information, diagnostic tools, and technology. The act's introduction of the term *irreversible* represented a departure from the previous common law standard for determining death: "the cessation of all vital functions, traditionally demonstrated by an absence of spontaneous respiratory and cardiac functions." Thus, a situation was created whereby the legal determination of death became dependent on the *irreversible* loss of cardiopulmonary function, independent of any medical convention for the limits of reversibility.[67] Consensus has yet to be reached on the question of the point in time at which this standard of irreversibility is attained.[63]

To maintain criteria for cardiopulmonary death that are "immune" to serial displacement by advancing clinical science, some have suggested that it might be helpful to consider the question to be context dependent because "the irreversibility of cardiac arrest (and death) hinges on whether resuscitation will be attempted."[62] The question is thus reformulated to explore whether the morally relevant time of death is reached when death is certain despite all **possible** medical intervention or whether death is assured once all ethically **permissible** remedies have been utilized.[45] It does seem logical that once a principled decision is made not to correct a loss of function, that loss becomes irreversible.[42]

Historically, there have been little data relating to the patterns of electrical and mechanical activity generated by the dying human heart.[21] No study has ever documented the spontaneous return of circulation after more than 65 seconds of combined circulatory and respiratory arrest.[62] The University of Pittsburgh's protocol concludes that death may be determined after 2 minutes of pulselessness, apnea, and unresponsiveness, because the likelihood of subsequent autoresuscitation becomes "vanishingly small,"[20] a conclusion supported by existing (although scant) literature. However, this standard has not been universally applied.

When the Institute of Medicine first reviewed non-heartbeating organ donation, it found highly variable organ procurement policies, running the gamut from ignoring the issue of required waiting times after loss of circulation, respiration, and responsiveness, to imposing intervals of up to 10 minutes. This led to a call for further empirical research and an interim recommendation for a 5-minute asystolic interval. Little new research had been published by the time of the Institute of Medicine's revisiting of these issues several years later; thus, it's second report offered no new recommendations on asystolic time and more explicitly suggested the need for additional studies.[5]

As of this writing, there are now at least two published reports that bear directly on the likelihood of the spontaneous reversal of cardiac arrest in patients withdrawn from life support in conjunction with non-heartbeating organ donation.[21,68] Both studies are retrospective chart reviews and are underpowered from a statistical standpoint. Still, neither study found any evidence of autoresuscitation using asystolic observation intervals ranging from 2 to 5 minutes. This finding—coming directly from the clinical context of non-heartbeating organ donation—adds weight to the older data and supports the SCCM's determination that "there is no ethically or physiologically important distinction between the two minute observation period utilized by the University of Pittsburgh, the five minutes recommended by the IOM, and, for example, ten minutes."[27] Whereas the asystolic interval to be observed remains a matter of institutional policy, it seems prudent to recommend that each center establish specific criteria that it will use. In addition, physicians should document that the patient has met them before beginning organ procurement procedures. Highly sensitive methodologies to document the absence of circulation, such as intra-arterial pressure monitoring or echocardiography, may be helpful because of the short observation time.[62]

A final logistic issue is the management of patients who die too slowly to be suitable for donation.[21] Most programs disqualify patients from donation if they are still alive 1 hour after discontinuing life support.[5] For this reason, contingency plans should be in place so that these patients receive appropriate ongoing end of life care (see Fig. 250-2).

ORGAN PROCUREMENT

Because every organ from a non-heartbeating donor suffers some degree of unavoidable warm ischemic damage,[69] several aggressive methodologies to protect organ viability have been developed. These techniques bring back into vivid focus familiar questions arising from the dead donor rule, the need to protect the rights of the dying patient, and the impulse to employ aggressive maneuvers in the name of a perceived greater good.

There are several premortem strategies to improve organ function post transplant. The first is the use of anticoagulants such as heparin to prevent vascular thrombosis during the low flow state before and after death as well as to promote the patency of the circulation for postmortem perfusion with organ preservation solution.[70] The second is the use of vasodilators, such as phentolamine, chlorpromazine, or trifluoperazine, which are thought to prevent the agonal vasospasm induced by hypoxia and surging catecholamine levels.[3,71] A third is the placement of large-bore arterial and venous catheters[72-74] to enable the single most important element of ischemic injury protection: cooling the organs to slow ongoing cellular metabolism.[9]

Frequently, these interventions are used together for additive effect.[75] These interventions are not part of the usual end of life care, and so some could consider them objectionable.[76] In addition, these measures by their very nature might pose specific risks to the dying patient—namely, bleeding in the case of heparin, hypotension in the case of the vasodilators, and pain or vascular injury from catheter placement. These latter concerns seem intuitively plausible, although scientific proof of their validity is lacking.[77] In sorting through these issues, the SCCM and IOM, among others,[42] have agreed that the use of these medications and devices is acceptable as long as they cause no significant harm to the patient, and family consent is obtained wherever practical. That they are of no direct benefit to the patient is

balanced by the fact that they improve the likelihood that a patient's wish—organ donation—will ultimately be realized.[5,27]

The desire to protect the option to donate organs after death has led some centers to perform catheterization and cold perfusion presumptively in cases of uncontrolled death when the patient's wishes are unknown.[37,39,78] This has caused a considerable amount of controversy,[41] even though the patients are technically already dead at the time these measures are initiated. Less controversy has been raised by other procurement strategies implemented after death, such as whole-body external cooling,[64] cold intraperitoneal lavage,[3,6,79] and the use of portable bypass[80] and extracorporeal membrane oxygenation technologies.[81]

A glimpse of the complexities that may lie ahead can be seen in the emerging idea of ischemic preconditioning. It has been known for some time that a brief ischemic challenge to myocardial tissue can trigger protective mechanisms that improve the ability to compensate during later insults.[82] The prearranged timing of the withdrawal of cardiopulmonary support in non-heartbeating donation in theory lends itself to instituting such pretreatment in a synchronized way. For example, counterintuitive as it may sound, this effect has already been demonstrated with phenylephrine in an animal model of non-heartbeating cardiac transplant.[83] It seems inevitable that transplant physicians will want to use other agents effective in brain-dead donors or experimental models in human non-heartbeating donors.[84,85]

OUTCOMES

There are perceived advantages of using organs from brain-dead donors based on both theoretical concerns[6,9,78,79] and early clinical experience suggesting more favorable results than could be obtained with non-heartbeating donor organs. The very question of differential outcomes itself raises additional issues, including the right of a potential recipient to such data[27] and whether a recipient should be afforded the prerogative to decline an organ based on the nature of the donor without penalty vis-à-vis candidacy or waiting-list status. As these questions have accumulated over the decade since non-heartbeating organ donation was reintroduced in this country, a growing body of evidence has emerged to suggest that outcomes for some transplants are comparable for cadaver organs from non-heartbeating and brain-dead donors.

Virtually all accumulated experience with organs from non-heartbeating donors comes from kidney, and to a lesser extent liver, transplantation. Suboptimal organ function—either primary nonfunction (PNF) or delayed graft function (DGF)—is a threat to kidney transplantation from non-heartbeating donors, because the metabolically active renal cortex is exquisitely sensitive to warm ischemia.[28] Indeed, as many as 35% of all kidneys procured from non-heartbeating donors have not been transplanted.[86] For those organs that are transplanted, some degree of DGF, typically manifested as acute tubular necrosis,[87] may be the "cost paid" for using kidneys from non-heartbeating donors.[16,88] This "cost" can be significant, both literally and figuratively, as DGF contributes to longer hospital stays, difficulty in diagnosing acute rejection, and problems dosing immunosuppressive drugs.[89] Still, with improvements in organ preservation techniques[86,90] it is now clear from a growing number of studies that the outcomes for kidneys transplanted from non-heartbeating donors are essentially equivalent to those

TABLE 250–9. CADAVERIC KIDNEY AND LIVER TRANSPLANTS PERFORMED: 1996-2001 KAPLAN-MEIER GRAFT SURVIVAL RATES

Organ	DCD Donor?	No. of Transplants	Year Post Transplant	No. Functioning	Survival Rate*
Kidney	No	40,886	1	31,130	88.5
			2	22,950	83.4
			3	15,951	78.0
	Yes	779	1	531	88.1
			2	351	82.7
			3	232	77.9
Liver	No	23,466	1	16,809	81.0
			2	12,364	76.4
			3	8,789	72.8
	Yes	168	1	103	77.0
			2	63	69.7
			3	41	67.0

*Survival rates are within 95% confidence intervals in each instance.
From UNOS, personal communication. Based on UNOS OPTN data as of March 14, 2003. Data subject to change due to future data submission or correction.

from brain-dead donors for periods of up to 10 years, despite a higher initial incidence of DGF.[6,9,29,65,71,91,92]

The outcome data for hepatic and pancreatic transplantation using organs from non-heartbeating donors is less extensive and less definitive. Transplantation of organs other than kidneys from non-heartbeating donors is uncommon. Only about 150 livers and 25 pancreata were transplanted from non-heartbeating donors in the United States during the years between 1993 and 2000.[93]

There are considerations that make the use of non-heartbeating hepatic donors particularly challenging. For example, high physiologic stress levels in patients with prolonged ICU stays may cause depletion of hepatic glycogen stores in the donor and threaten graft viability in the recipient.[94] Also, variant anatomy in the celiac trunk can add a considerable degree of difficulty to in situ dissection of the liver and pancreas under the time constraints of a non-heartbeating procurement.[93] Early results of liver transplants involving non-heartbeating donors were mixed, producing 1-year graft and patient survival rates that were substantially lower compared with brain-dead donors. Morbidity rates were higher as well.[10,79] Recent studies have yielded more promising results. Some centers with small caseloads have reported universal patient and graft survival in the short run without any major complications,[95] whereas larger programs have reported patient survival and complication rates comparable to cases involving brain-dead donors. However, these programs also report higher rates of PNF and lower rates of allograft survival for organs from non-heartbeating donors than brain-dead donors.[3]

With respect to pancreatic transplantation, much of the limited available outcome data for non-heartbeating donor organs is derived from cases of simultaneous pancreas-kidney (SPK) procedures. The emerging data suggest that non-heartbeating donors are a practical source of organs for SPK, yielding pancreatic graft and patient survival rates in keeping with those for brain-dead donors.[32,96] It is worth noting that there is no theoretical reason that the same techniques used in SPK could not be applied to isolated pancreatic transplantation.[32] More clinical experience will determine whether outcomes in such cases would be equally promising.

Cumulative UNOS outcomes data on renal and hepatic non-heartbeating organ transplantation, reflecting both graft survival and patient survival, are depicted in Tables 250-9 and 250-10, respectively.

TABLE 250–10. CADAVERIC KIDNEY AND LIVER TRANSPLANTS PERFORMED: 1996-2001 KAPLAN-MEIER PATIENT SURVIVAL RATES

Organ	DCD Donor?	No. of Transplants	Year Post Transplant	No. Functioning	Survival Rate*
Kidney	No	40,866	1	32,444	94.3
			2	24,138	91.7
			3	16,888	88.8
	Yes	779	1	554	94.7
			2	374	91.7
			3	248	90.9
Liver	No	23,466	1	16,809	86.8
			2	12,364	82.9
			3	8,789	79.8
	Yes	168	1	103	85.3
			2	63	79.0
			3	41	75.9

*Survival rates are within 95% confidence intervals in each instance.
From UNOS, personal communication. Based on UNOS OPTN data as of March 14, 2003. Data subject to change due to future data submission or correction.

FUTURE DIRECTIONS

Notwithstanding the success with kidneys, livers, and pancreata as described earlier, there are still a number of unmet challenges in the transplantation of organs from non-heartbeating donors.

One frontier where progress has been slower is thoracic transplantation. First, the heart and lungs are difficult to utilize when procured from non-heartbeating donors because nonfunction of these organs is more difficult to treat than is pancreas or kidney nonfunction.[65,84,85,97] With regard to pulmonary transplantation, the problem is ischemia/reperfusion injury, which is difficult both to predict and to treat in the recipient.[98] Whereas there is a firm foundation from research using animal models to support the use of lungs from non-heartbeating donors,[99-101] there are only a handful of recent reports in the literature describing use of the procedure in humans.[10,102] There are even fewer reports of cardiac transplants involving non-heartbeating donors, despite a growing body of expertise with ischemic and pharmacologic preconditioning in experimental systems.[83,97] Given the technical complexies, it is understandable that there is some hesitation about pursuing cardiac transplantation from non-heartbeating donors on a larger scale. Other barriers include ethical and psychosocial concerns about the reasonability and "palatability" of transplanting the heart of a donor after cardiac death. It may seem counterintuitive to some to ascertain death in one patient using cardiac nonfunction as one criterion and then use that same heart to restore health in another patient. Nevertheless, cardiac transplantation from a non-heartbeating donor is technically possible. The first human cardiac transplant nearly 40 years ago was made possible using a non-heartbeating donor heart, which, rather poetically, started and functioned well after a single electrical shock.[103]

A second area of likely future growth is transplantation of organs from pediatric non-heartbeating donors. As is true with transplantation in the adult population, the number of pediatric organs available for transplantation is insufficient to meet the demand and consideration has been given to the use of non-heartbeating donors.[7] However, to date there is little published literature on the subject. Still, a fair bit of groundwork has been done, including development of criteria for screening potential donors,[7] as well as study of the nature of terminal events in pediatric patients after the withdrawal of life support.[104] Additional consideration has also been given to some unique aspects of potential pediatric non-heartbeating donation, including the psychological importance of a parent being able to physically hold and comfort a dying child,[5] a practice that could make non-heartbeating donation more difficult. Only time will tell how society at large will react to the idea of the pediatric non-heartbeating donor and whether the ethical framework that guides adult non-heartbeating donation will be sufficient to respond to the concerns that will inevitably arise. Figure 250-3 shows the limited numbers of pediatric non-heartbeating donors reported to UNOS to date, in comparison to the steadily increasing total number of non-heartbeating organ transplants annually.

There are a number of other questions concerning non-heartbeating organ donation that cannot yet be answered. First, what, if any, increase in available donor organs can reasonably be expected by promoting the utilization of non-heartbeating donors?[29] Second, what is the potential impact of non-heartbeating donation—or the failure to accomplish it—on families, health care providers, and the community at large?[5,105,106] Third, what are the monetary costs of non-heartbeating organ transplantation relative to the costs associated with brain-dead donors, and what might account for any differences?[5] Fourth, how, if at all, will non-heartbeating organ donation affect public trust in the health care system and the organ procurement network specifically?[60] This is particularly important in light of some early studies suggesting public distrust of organ transplantation generally[107] and non-heartbeating organ donation specifically.[108] Answers to these and other questions can presumably be found through the same combination of multidisciplinary research and reasoned public discourse

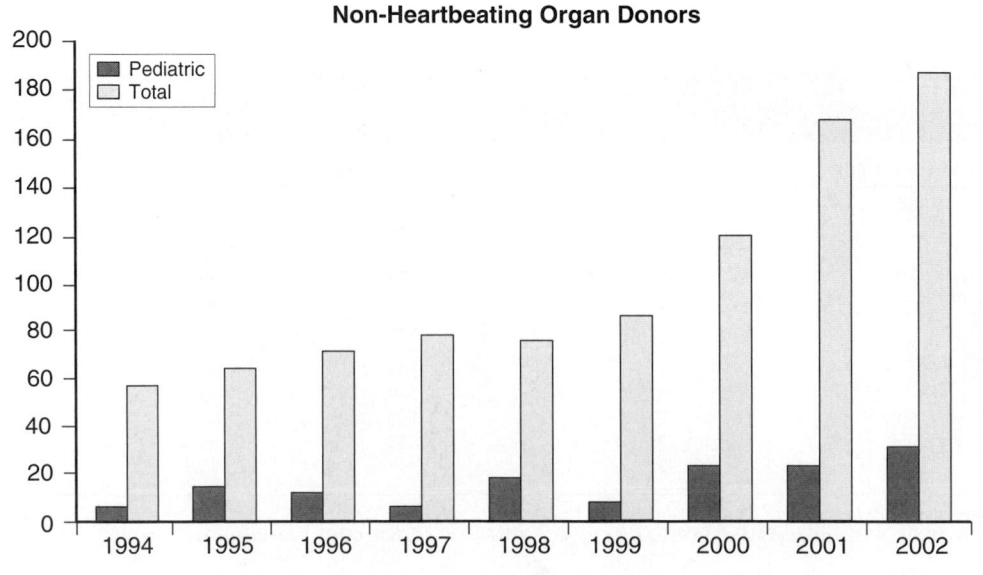

Annual Number of Pediatric and Total Non-Heartbeating Organ Donors

FIGURE 250–3. Pediatric and total non-heartbeating donors, 1994-2002. (Courtesy of the United Network for Organ Sharing. Based on OPTN Data as of March 14, 2003. Data subject to change due to future data submission or correction.)

that has already brought non-heartbeating organ donation back from historical obscurity to a prominent place in contemporary clinical practice.

CONCLUSION

Non-heartbeating organ donation represents a unique link between transplantation's dramatic history and its unwritten future. From the time of the first human organ transplant in 1954 until the widespread clinical implementation of the neurologic criteria for death in the early 1970s, non-heartbeating organ donation was central to the development of clinical transplantation before falling out of favor for technical reasons. When it was reintroduced in the 1990s, in response to the wish of some terminally ill patients to donate their organs for transplantation, the practice generated a considerable amount of ethical debate. The resulting "calculus of values"[8] suggests that non-heartbeating organ donation—when conducted according to established principles—is an acceptable and worthwhile endeavor. Over this same period of time, transplantation has made significant clinical advances but has been plagued by an ever-growing shortage of donor organs. This shortage is projected to worsen as the baby boom generation ages, making organ donation an increasingly important issue in the years ahead.[109] While some technical challenges remain, mounting evidence now suggests that non-heartbeating organ donation is practical for most organs and is increasing in frequency, albeit slowly. As experience grows, attitudes change, and outcomes continue to improve, that trend may accelerate. Thus, it is possible—but by no means certain—that non-heartbeating organ donation may yet have a significant impact on the number of organs available for transplantation. Those numbers aside, non-heartbeating organ donation ultimately succeeds or fails on a case-by-case basis and in every instance demands the involvement of a well-informed and capable intensivist at the bedside.

ACKNOWLEDGMENT

The authors gratefully acknowledge the assistance of Franki L. Chabalewski, RN, MS, of the United Network for Organ Sharing, in providing figures, tables, and statistics.

ANNOTATED REFERENCES

DeVita MA, Snyder JV, Arnold RM, et al: Observations of withdrawal of life-sustaining treatment from patients who became non-heart-beating organ donors. Crit Care Med 2000;28:1709-1712.

This retrospective study reviews 5 years of observational data from a major transplant medical center, describing the terminal events of patients who were withdrawn from life-sustaining treatment and subsequently became donors after cardiac death. The analysis supports the adequacy of a 2-minute interval of asystole to certify death in this circumstance and highlights the need for consistent and accurate clinical record keeping for these purposes.

Ethics Committee, American College of Critical Care Medicine, Society of Critical Care Medicine: Position Paper: Recommendations for nonheart-beating organ donation. Crit Care Med 2001;29:1826-1831.

This leading article provides a concise topical review of the subject of non-heartbeating organ donation, with particular attention to relevant history, terminology, ethics, death certification, and appropriate care of patients with the potential to become donors, as well as their families. The authors conclude with 16 material recommendations to guide the practice of non-heartbeating organ donation.

Institute of Medicine: Non-Heart-Beating Organ Transplantation: Medical and Ethical Issues in Procurement. Washington, DC, National Academy Press, 1997.

This landmark report on the state of non-heartbeating organ donation reveals considerable variation in then-current procedures among hospitals and organ procurement organizations. In an effort to ensure consistency in the care of patients with the potential to donate organs and sustain public trust in the transplantation enterprise, seven specific recommendations are made to guide subsequent policy development.

The United Network for Organ Sharing, and United States Department of Health and Human Services, Health Resources and Services Administration, Office of Special Programs, Division of Transplantation: UNOS Home page. Copyright 2004. http://www.unos.org. Accessed January 27, 2004.

The UNOS website provides a gateway to a wealth of online resources. In addition to the Key Clinical Pathway for Donation After Cardiac Death presented in this textbook, publicly accessible content includes continuously updated transplant waiting list data, news releases, annual reports, national, regional, and state transplant statistics, policy statements, public discussion forums, and links to other transplant-related websites.

Youngner SJ, Arnold RM: Ethical, psychosocial, and public policy implications of procuring organs from non-heart-beating cadaver donors. JAMA 1993;269:2769-2774.

Stemming from a conference to review the so-called Pittsburgh Protocol (the nation's first comprehensive institutional policy on procuring organs from patients following the withdrawal of life-sustaining treatment), this early exploration of the inherent complexities of non-heartbeating organ donation remains among the most comprehensive reviews of the subject.

Section XV

ETHICAL AND END-OF-LIFE ISSUES

Chapter 251

BEYOND TECHNOLOGY: CARING FOR THE CRITICALLY ILL

Phillip D. Levin • Charles L. Sprung

KEY POINTS

1. Ethical issues in intensive care center around the patient, the family, and the ICU as a location.

2. There are no "right answers" to ethical issues: different people may view similar issues in very different ways.

3. Huge variations in ethical practice are found in different cultures.

4. Tolerance, communication, and patience are vital.

5. Most patients and their families are ultimately satisfied with their ICU experience.

Over the past half century, intensive care has grown from the position of a fledgling specialty to occupy a central role in hospital medicine. Intensive care has changed the natural history of many disease processes and has also allowed other specialties to progress with the performance of ever more challenging procedures in sicker and sicker patients. Over the past decades, however, this progress has been accompanied by increasingly complex ethical, moral, and social questions. These questions can be broadly divided into those that relate to the patient's treatment, those that relate to the patient's family or surrogates, and those that relate to the ICU as a location, although they are all interrelated to some degree. In this chapter, a brief overview of the main issues relating to these three elements is introduced (prior to in-depth discussion in the following chapters) and the concepts of diversity and satisfaction are elucidated. Diversity is relevant because it is important to appreciate that diverse groups of people will view ethical or moral issues in very different ways, whereas an examination of patient and family satisfaction with their ICU experience might provide indications as to areas where care has been deficient and might be improved.

THE PATIENT—WHEN THE OUTCOME IS POOR

The predominant intensive care dilemma relating to the patient concerns "end-of-life care." Prior to the 1980s the accepted aim of intensive care was to stave off death for as long as possible in the hope that the patient would eventually recover. Although patients did die, typically they did so only after full care, including cardiopulmonary resuscitation (CPR). Gradually it became clear that some patients had no chance of recovery, that is, that they were going to die either in the ICU or in hospital after an ICU admission despite all attempts at treatment. Empirically, physicians believed they were able to identify a proportion of these patients early in their ICU course. It also became clear that other ICU patients entered a chronic state where their lives could only be preserved within an ICU or that they recovered to some extent but not to a level of functional independence (e.g., after severe head injury). Many patients, their families/surrogates, and physicians viewed these outcomes as worse than death. As a result, questions began to arise regarding the justification for continuing life support measures for these patients. Should interventions that were of no avail and yet invasive be continued, or should the process of dying be allowed to proceed unhampered? Voices were raised suggesting that when quality of life could not be ensured or restored, or when maintaining life was no longer possible, dignity and humanity would suggest that palliative care should replace active treatment. Once resources began to be restricted, their allocation to such patients was also questioned. Various terms arose to describe treatments that, although they may have had an effect on the patient, would not change the final poor outcome. These terms included *futile, nonbeneficial,* and *undesirable.* The limitation or cessation of such treatments became widely accepted, even if it led to or hastened the patient's death.[1]

The limitation of undesirable treatments can take one of three main avenues: treatment may be either withheld or withdrawn, or steps may be taken to actively shorten the dying process.[2] Withholding treatment implies not administering a treatment considered to be nonbeneficial. An example might be not starting dialysis for a patient with renal failure but no hope of recovery or a "do not resuscitate" order, whereby CPR will not be performed in the event of a cardiac arrest. Withdrawal of treatment (but not care) implies the removal of a treatment modality. Examples include cessation of inotropes or ventilation. Steps that actively shorten the dying process (considered by some to be akin to euthanasia)[2] might include the administration of a drug (such as potassium chloride or a muscle relaxant to a nonventilated patient) that will directly end the patient's life. Gray zones exist between the borders of these definitions. For example, after the withdrawal of ventilation by extubation, morphine and midazolam might be administered to reduce suffering and agonal breathing. These drugs will, however, also depress ventilation and may possibly shorten the dying process.

It must be noted that huge diversity exists in practices relating to end of life care. Diversity exists both in the practices of physicians and in the expectations of patients and families, and both within and between individual countries. In a study from Europe these variations were emphasized. Data were collected concerning end-of-life care for 4248 patients who died in 37 ICUs located in 17 European countries. Life-sustaining treatment was limited to some degree for 76% of all patients who died. Withdrawal of life support was more common in Northern European countries than in Southern European countries (performed prior to 47% vs. 18% of deaths, respectively). The time taken from admission until limitation of life support was also shorter (median 1.6 vs. 5.7 days, Northern vs. Southern Europe), while in parallel the performance of CPR was rarer (10% vs. 30%) in Northern European countries. An attempt was made to correlate these differences with physicians' religion (with the finding that Catholic, nonaffiliated, or Protestant physicians limited life-sustaining interventions more frequently than their Jewish, Greek Orthodox, or Moslem colleagues); however, these religious variations may be indistinguishable from the regional variations and are thus difficult to interpret.[2] So, even between the closely linked countries of Europe, geographic variation influences end-of-life practice to a significant degree.

Variations in end-of-life practice have been found in many other studies relating to different countries and regions. In the United States, for example, a study of 5910 patients who died in 131 ICUs showed that limitation of life-sustaining treatment was performed before the death of 71% of patients.[3] When the incidence rates for each type of limitation were compared across the different centers contributing to the study, however, large variations were discovered: full resuscitation including CPR was performed for between 4% and 79% of patients at different centers, whereas treatments were withheld for between 0% and 67% and withdrawn for 0% to 79%. Similarly, in a study from Canada, 1361 ICU nurses and physicians were asked to determine the appropriate level of care in 12 patient vignettes. In only one case was there greater than 50% agreement between the participants.[4] Great variation exists in practices relating to end-of-life care in North America.

These data also suggest that country of residence is not sufficient to fully explain the variations in attitudes of medical staff to end-of-life care. Indeed, many other aspects of a physician's life and practice have been associated with differences in willingness to limit life-supporting therapies. For example, physicians in certain specialties (e.g., cardiology),[5,6] in nonacademic practice,[7] or who are older[8] have been shown to be less aggressive in the limitation of such care.

Variability in attitudes toward end-of-life care is not limited to the ICU staff. Similar variability has been demonstrated in the expectations of patients, their families, and the general public, which likewise, are not defined by geographic borders. The following anthropologic study of four ethnic subgroups within the United States attempts to illustrate and explain some of the differences in approach. African Americans, European Americans, Korean Americans, and Mexican Americans were interviewed regarding their attitudes toward life-support measures in general (i.e., for others) and for themselves.[9] Korean Americans had the most positive general attitude toward life support; that is, these interviewees

believed that life support should be continued under most circumstances for others but paradoxically showed a low personal desire to have these measures performed for themselves. In-depth interviews revealed a strong concept of family obligation, which obligation would mandate continuation of therapy for a different family member while the interviewees would be happy to have therapy limited for themselves. African American interviewees revealed the opposite. They had a positive view toward personal life support but were willing to forgo life-sustaining treatment in general. These respondents were described as understanding the inevitability of death but lacking trust in institutionalized medicine. They expressed the view that life support should be attempted (thinking physicians might be mistaken or unwilling to initiate therapy due to financial considerations) and if it was unsuccessful, then the therapy could be stopped. European American interviewees were negative in both their general and personal attitudes toward life support. They expressed fears of being functionally limited or a burden to their families and would prefer death to these outcomes.

Attitudes in Hong Kong and Japan have been described and are different still. Traditional Chinese society has been described as having less emphasis on individual rights, self-expression, and self-determination than Western society.[10] The traditional Chinese family might therefore want to protect their loved ones and not burden them with the truth regarding their poor prognosis. Similarly, 97% of Japanese interviewees in Japan were of the opinion that the patient's family should be informed of the patient's poor prognosis (in a scenario of gastric cancer), but only 63% thought that the patient should be informed. Exposure to American culture in the United States seemed to alter these views: whereas 93% of English-speaking Japanese Americans (presumed to be more acculturated to American culture than the Japanese in Japan) agreed that the family should be informed, the proportion who believed that the patient should know his diagnosis increased to 95%, perhaps in line with American views of patient autonomy.[11]

Over the past 50 years, population movement and immigration have resulted in large and varied ethnic communities' living side by side, particularly in larger cities. The result of this is that an ICU physician or nurse may well encounter— and be expected to communicate with—patients and families from entirely different and possibly unfamiliar cultures and at very difficult times in the lives of patients/families. The ICU personnel may view life, injury, and death in one way, whereas the patient and their family may view these events in quite another. The ICU team may expect patient autonomy, whereas the family may object. Language may be a significant barrier. Differences in expectations regarding the goals of ICU admission may also be considerable. Because the ICU team is providing a service to the patient and the family, it would seem reasonable to expect that the team adapt to the patient's or family's expectation. Such adaptation may not be easy, and setting limits to it may represent a considerable challenge. A paradox could even appear—the patient expecting the physician to make treatment decisions without his or her involvement while the physician feels bound by patient autonomy. Indeed, can patient autonomy extend to the abrogation of that autonomy? In any event, understanding and accepting cultural diversity may help create a calmer and more objective outlook at these difficult times.

THE FAMILY—DIFFICULT DECISIONS, AUTONOMY, AND PATERNALISM

In light of the previous discussion, it should be clear that views concerning life and death are by no means uniform. For example, some patients may be willing to pursue life after injury leading to quadriplegia whereas others would prefer to die. Physicians, patients, and their families may be equally divided on such a qualitative decision. The next main dilemma to be discussed then concerns the process of decision making.

"Autonomy" is defined as "liberty to follow one's will, personal freedom," and this is the pre-eminent value in health care today, at least in North America. Autonomy suggests that the patient should be able to determine the course of his or her therapy and that physicians should act as consultants who share their knowledge. Unfortunately, as a result of either their illness or injury, the majority of intensive care patients are not able to communicate clearly and only a minority will have prepared a "living will" describing their wishes for life-sustaining therapy.[12] Even if a living will has been prepared, it might not be sufficiently descriptive, leaving doubt as to the patient's needs under particular circumstances. For example, a living will might indicate that ventilation would be inappropriate. The patient presents to the emergency department with pulmonary edema. Should continuous positive airway pressure via a mask be used to help the patient recover from this transient episode? And who should decide? Practically (in the ICU), the vast majority of decisions regarding philosophy of care result from an interaction of some description between the patient's surrogates and the ICU physicians.

Most patients would want a surrogate to represent them[13] and would want this to be a family member,[14,15] frequently a spouse.[15] Indeed, classically the patient's autonomy is extended to his closest family. These family members may have discussed care requirements with the patient in the past (although this is not common) or at least may share the commonality of cultural milieu. Unfortunately when examined empirically there is little evidence that family members are able to speak accurately for the patient. Agreement between the patient and his or her surrogate has been found to range between 50% and 88%,[16-20] although rarely is agreement more likely than chance.[19] Similarly, even when children knew what their elderly parents would have wanted, in only 46% of cases were they willing to abide by these requests.[17] In addition, the decision-making ability of families may not be optimal under the stresses of a sudden ICU admission for a loved one. High prevalences of anxiety and depression (69.1% and 35.4%, respectively) have been found among family members of ICU patients,[21] whereas their understanding of the implications of critical disease is not always perfect.[22] Families may also perceive ICU admission as more stressful than the patients report themselves (after recovery).[23] Despite these caveats, it is widely accepted that the patient's immediate and close family will act as surrogates in decision making.

In North America, family involvement in decision making is almost universal,[24] although the opinions of family members are not universally respected. In a survey of 879 U.S. physicians, 96% of whom had withheld or withdrawn life-sustaining treatments, 25% had withheld and 23% had withdrawn treatments without the family's consent; 14% and 12%, respectively, without their knowledge; and 3% despite their objection. In contrast, therapy had been continued by 34% despite the request by family members that it be terminated.[25] This is not to suggest that physicians have a better understanding of the patient's needs than family—agreement between the views of the physicians and patients regarding priorities in end-of-life care ranges from 47% to 72%, never being better than chance.[19,26,27]

The role of the family varies among countries and cultures. For example, in Spain, 28% of families were not involved in the end-of-life decision-making process and in 3% their requests were disregarded.[28] In France, families participated in the decision-making process on only 17% to 44% of occasions.[29,30] In Hong Kong and Japan, cultural values may dictate that the patient be protected from bad news and difficult life-and-death decisions. In these cases, no discussion might take place at all or the family might conduct end-of-life discussions to the exclusion of the patient, even in the event that the patient is able to be included.

Although the principles of autonomy would suggest a hierarchy of decision making, beginning with the patient, followed by the proxy, and ending with the physician, clearly this does not always occur. The divergence from this utopia may even be inevitable to some degree, because defining the limits for involvement in the decision-making process for both the physician and the patient/family is not simple. Choosing the correct type of enteral nutrition for an ICU patient is clearly a medical decision that the physician might make alone. The decision to use mechanical ventilation indefinitely in a terminal neurologic condition such as amyotrophic lateral sclerosis on the other hand is very personal and should be made by the patient. Between these extremes lie the shades of gray, where the treatment plan is based on a negotiation of some description between the main protagonists—the patient (when possible), the surrogate, and the ICU team. Individual personality, philosophy, beliefs, and experience will determine the course that such negotiations take and the relative involvement or weight of each party.

Unfortunately, the process by which decisions are reached is not always smooth and not infrequently leads to conflict. Indeed, 44% of all conflicts between the ICU team and family members of patients admitted to seven U.S. ICUs for longer than 1 week concerned end-of-life care, and in 85% of these conflicts the family was interested in more aggressive care than the ICU team was suggesting.[31] End-of-life care issues also accounted for 57% of the conflicts observed within families and 7% of conflicts within the IUC team.[31] An additional study examining conflict arising from end-of life-discussions only found that conflict occurred equally between ICU staff and family and within the ICU team, both occurring in 48% of cases, whereas conflict within families occurred in 24% of cases.[32] Some of the less desirable techniques for conflict resolution have been described previously—ignoring the family's wishes or not informing them of their options. Fortunately, the most common path taken in the resolution of conflict is negotiation (in one study, 71% of physicians said they would choose this path).[33] If differences cannot be resolved by direct negotiation, the use of an ethics consultant has been advocated. An ethics consultant is a third party, not necessarily a physician, who conducts discussions with the ICU team and the patient or the family to elucidate values and bridge gaps in a nonconfrontational manner.[34] Although reported to be useful,[35] ethics consultations have not found widespread use. When no accommodation can be reached between physicians and patients/families, the courts have been used (by both parties) as final arbiters.[36,37]

THE ICU—RESTRICTED SPACE, MANY PATIENTS, LIMITED FINANCES

The main dilemma facing the ICU as a location is resource allocation. Patients are frequently denied ICU care despite this care being appropriate, owing to lack of space.[38] Patients who require ICU care but do not receive it do not do well.[39,40] So, when two patients require ICU care but only one bed is available, who is to be admitted?

Prognostic scoring systems have been suggested as a tool to help. However, many of these scoring systems require data from the first 24 hours of ICU care to reach a value, and all have been validated on groups of patients. For example, a group of patients with a poor prognostic score might be expected to have a 90% mortality. For the individual patient within that group, it is not possible to say whether he or she will be among the 90% who will die or the 10% who will survive. Society has not determined a percentage point for expected survival below which intensive care is thought not to be appropriate; and many patients, their surrogates, and their physicians would be willing to endure or suggest ICU care even when the chances of survival are small.[41] Thus, even a very poor prognostic score might not help decide whether to admit a particular patient. Surveys have also shown that poor prognosis does not deter physicians from admitting patients to the ICU.[38,42] Patient characteristics, such as age, sex, and economic or social standing seem entirely inappropriate for determining which patient to admit, so, unfortunately, no clear help is available in this aspect of decision making.

Alternative solutions to the problem of lack of space could include increasing the number of ICU beds or increasing the efficiency of use of existing beds. Increasing bed space requires increased funding and is associated with problems of its own. If funding to ICU is increased from a fixed budget, then funding for some other aspect of the hospital's function will have to be decreased, engendering a direct comparison between the importance of the ICU patients and the dialysis or radiotherapy patient, for example. Increased overall funding for the hospital is a societal issue, often meaning that government funding from another field has to be reduced. Furthermore, the presence of more ICU beds might not alleviate the pressure on them, as more beds might simply mean a lowering of the requirement for ICU admission in a particular institution and leave the ICU as full as ever.

Increasing bed efficiency implies making better use of the facilities that already exist. In an attempt to create a model for bed usage, the concept of a triage chain has been suggested.[43] This chain starts when the patient refers himself or herself or is referred to the hospital; it continues through the referral by the emergency department physician to the ICU, through ICU admission, ICU discharge, and then ward discharge. If flow along this chain could be improved, for example, if patients do not remain in the ICU waiting for bed space on the ward, then the efficiency of ICU bed usage could be improved. Care must be taken with this concept, however, because premature discharge from the ICU may be associated with increased patient mortality on the ward.[44]

The cost of ICU care in itself is a source of dilemma. Take, for example, a new treatment available to the ICU physician—activated protein C. As the first drug proven to change the outcome of septic shock, this drug has raised much interest. Unfortunately, its cost is high (approximately $8000 for the 72-hour course). This cost is perhaps of most interest to the hospital administration. However, the acceptability (or inevitability) that the use of this new drug should be limited only because of its high cost is debatable. Indeed, with increasing patient awareness of therapeutic options, the ICU team members may find themselves having to explain an administrative policy concerning drug administration not based on medical indication alone.

So, having described the seemingly endless diversity, dilemmas, and difficulties that face the ICU team, the patient, and the family, it might be expected that patient and surrogate satisfaction with their ICU experience is low. This is not the case.

PATIENT SATISFACTION

Patients' satisfaction with their ICU experiences has been addressed in three main ways: by descriptive studies, directed questionnaires, and assessments of willingness to undergo ICU care again. A common factor to many of these studies is that approximately one third of ICU patients have no recollection at all of their ICU admission.[45,46]

Descriptive studies reveal both negative and positive comments about ICU experiences.[45,47,48] Statements such as "The place was very upsetting. Like a war zone. I remember hearing a man making animal noises" are balanced by "the staff made me feel safe," and "this made me feel very safe and secure." Overall, however, 81% of the patients who were interviewed were extremely pleased that resuscitative equipment had been used, and 80% would be willing to undergo further ICU treatment under all circumstances.[45] A directed questionnaire examined recollection of ventilation after 1 year. The majority of these patients recalled no pain or discomfort (78.2%) and would be willing to undergo ventilation again (86.5%).[49] The additional use of chemical paralysis did not seem to have a major effect.[50] Similarly, when a patient group was asked whether they would be willing to go through intensive care again, the majority (up to 70%) would be willing,[41,51] even if only for a month of further survival.[41] If, however, levels of outcome were added to the question, then willingness to undergo mechanical ventilation decreased—if the outcome was described as a permanent vegetative state only 30% of a group of ICU survivors would agree to readmission to the ICU.[52]

Directed questionnaires also provide more specific details of the ICU experience. Stressful events in the ICU included pain, inability to sleep, having tubes in the nose or mouth, being unable to talk, and lack of control.[23,53-55] Stress was also associated with the presence of an endotracheal tube.[46] Interestingly, when patients' experiences were compared to the perception of these experiences by family and physicians, both overestimated the "stress scores."[23]

These studies do suffer from some common limitations. As mentioned earlier, many ICU patients have no recollection of their stay in an ICU. All the studies are based on interviews with patients who have survived their ICU admission in a sufficiently good functional state to be able to answer sometimes complex questions. This implies a degree of patient selection. For those who have survived ICU and are being interviewed by a researcher associated with the ICU, an element of gratitude might also bias the responses. For the studies performed long after ICU admission, memories might not be reliable. The studies also obviously do not describe the experiences of patients who have died.

In general, however, it seems that most patients are satisfied with their ICU experience (provided that they survive it in a good functional state) and would be willing to undergo such care once again. A hint is given that families see ICU care as more traumatic than patients see it.

FAMILY SATISFACTION

Ironically, family satisfaction is much more complex to assess than patient satisfaction. Many earlier studies attempted to analyze and describe the needs of families of ICU patients. The need for hope, the need to receive adequate and honest information, and the feeling that the hospital staff members were concerned about the patient were, for example, described as important.[56] However, a correlation between meeting these needs and family satisfaction is elusive. Families may be satisfied despite not having their needs met or dissatisfied despite attempts to meet their needs.

Multiple tools have been developed and validated in an attempt to quantify family satisfaction.[57-60] These tools are based on questionnaires including areas such as assurance (the need to feel hope for a desired outcome), information (the need for consistent realistic and timely information), proximity (the need for personal contact and physical proximity to the patient), support (the need for resources and support systems), and comfort (the need for family members personal comfort).[57] Use of one such tool[60] revealed a high overall satisfaction score of 84.3/100. The highest scoring elements in this study were nursing skill and competence, the compassion and respect given to a patient, and pain management. Communication with physicians and the physical conditions in the waiting room were the least satisfactory.[61] In the same study a regression analysis was performed that found that higher family satisfaction was associated with higher ratings for information provided by the ICU staff; courtesy, compassion, and respect; and the amount and level of care provided. Azoulay and associates found that increased satisfaction was associated with a higher nurse-to-patient ratio, with information being provided by a junior physician and with involvement of the family physician. Interestingly, being of French descent (and presumably co-cultural with the ICU team) was also associated with increased satisfaction. In contrast, contradictory information, poor acquaintance with the ICU team members, and a low desired to allowed time ratio in discussions with the ICU team were associated with decreased satisfaction.[62] These authors also found that approximately half of the families did not understand their family member's diagnosis or its implications[22] whereas an increased understanding was associated with improved satisfaction.[63]

The families of patients who have died may represent a subgroup with respect to satisfaction measures and have been investigated separately. These families also describe discussion regarding end of life care as difficult (40% to 48%

perceived conflict with the medical staff)[32,64]; however, their overall rating of satisfaction with the ICU care remained high (70% to 90%).[65] Dissatisfaction was reported among those families who had received notification of their family member's death over the telephone (rather than face to face) and among those whose family member had died suddenly.

Perhaps the conclusions reached by these studies are not surprising—family satisfaction is more likely when staff are competent and caring, respectful, courteous and compassionate, and well acquainted to the family and when they devote time to communication and explanation in person. Achieving these objectives is not always easy within the confines of busy schedules.

In this chapter we attempted to present a number of the major ethical, moral, and social issues of contemporary intensive care and some of the dilemmas that lie behind them. The concept of diversity has been introduced to show that attitudes toward these issues vary considerably from person to person, from city to city, and from country to country. It has been suggested that tolerance and communication are key elements to coping with diversity at times of stress and emotional turmoil. Finally, data have been presented showing that the large majority of both patients and their families are able to express satisfaction with their ICU experience despite the difficulties and suffering that they may have encountered therein.

ANNOTATED REFERENCES

Azoulay E, Pochard F, Chevret S, et al, French FAMIREA Group: Meeting the needs of intensive care unit patient families: A multicenter study. Am J Respir Crit Care Med 2001;163:135-139.
> A multicenter prospective observational study of satisfaction among family members of ICU patients. Seven factors associated with satisfaction were identified, and the suggestion is made that investment in these areas might improve satisfaction.

Blackhall LJ, Frank G, Murphy ST, et al: Ethnicity and attitudes towards life sustaining technology. Soc Sci Med 1999;48:1779-1789.
> A questionnaire-based survey of attitudes concerning end of life care among four American ethnic subgroups. The study showed marked differences in personal and general attitudes to life-sustaining treatments across the four groups, and in-depth interviews provide some insight into possible explanations.

Helft PR, Siegler M, Lantos J: The rise and fall of the futility movement. N Engl J Med 2000;343:293-296.
> A review describing the development of the futility concept. The article addresses four main areas as they relate to futility: definitions, empirical assessment, autonomy, and resolution of disputes.

Sprung CL, Cohen SL, Sjokvist P, et al: End-of-life practices in European intensive care units: The Ethicus Study. JAMA 2003;290:790-797.
> A large prospective observational study of end of life practices in European ICUs. The article shows that limitation of treatment before death was common with an overall incidence of 72.6% (including withholding therapy 38%, withdrawing 33%). Marked variability from country to country is described, with Southern Europe being in general more conservative in its practices than Northern Europe.

Studdert DM, Mello MM, Burns JP, et al: Conflict in the care of patients with prolonged stay in the ICU: Types, sources, and predictors. Intensive Care Med 2003;29:1489-1497.
> A multicenter prospective observational study investigating conflict in the ICU. The majority of conflict arose between the ICU team and the family (accounting for 57% of 248 conflicts studied) and concerned end of life care. Conflict also arose within the ICU team and within families. Multiple risk factors for conflict were examined in a multivariate regression analysis.

Chapter 252

RESOURCE ALLOCATION IN THE INTENSIVE CARE UNIT

Gordon D. Rubenfeld

KEY POINTS

1. **Allocation of resources is synonymous with rationing** and is an inevitable part of medical practice.

2. **Clinicians often use a variety of euphemisms,** including triage, optimization, prioritization, and cost-effective care, to obscure what are essentially allocation decisions.

3. **Clinical decisions based solely on the evidence of risk, benefit, or patient utility are not rationing decisions** because they do not incorporate cost or availability.

4. **Clinicians may implicitly incorporate cost or availability** into their judgments of the evidence of risk or benefit in an attempt to avoid an explicit decision incorporating cost.

5. **Allocation can occur at the macrolevel,** where decisions affect populations of patients, **or at the microlevel,** where decisions affect individual identifiable patients.

6. **Cost-effectiveness analysis** is a quantitative methodology that applies a utilitarian approach to allocate resources to maximize the benefit to a population for any specified cost.

7. **Cost is difficult to measure** in complex endeavors such as providing medical care.

8. **Claims of the ability to reduce costs** by reducing length of stay, ordering fewer tests, or failing to admit patients who will likely die should be examined critically.

Two truisms of economics are that the supply of goods and services is finite and that the supply will be insufficient to meet all demands. The tension between supply and demand for food, water, energy, education, and other goods and services creates economies. All societies must determine how goods and services will be allocated to individuals. Although the term *rationing* connotes a specific process of allocation during circumstances of severe resource limitation (rationing coupons to allocate gasoline during World War II, for example, or one's daily ration of water on a life raft), rationing is just an emotionally laden synonym for *resource allocation*. In this chapter, the terms are used interchangeably.

Market-based economies allocate many resources on the basis of ability to pay, but other strategies exist (Table 252-1).[1] In developed nations, some goods and services—for example, health care and education—are treated differently from luxury goods and are allocated by society using criteria other than an individual's ability to pay. Regardless of the strategy ultimately used, decisions to allocate medical resources are fundamentally identical to decisions to allocate other resources. Because medical resources are finite, it is impossible to provide every effective treatment in every case in which it might offer benefit and the patient desires the care. That does not mean that clinicians are aware on a daily basis of the burden of this reality. Sometimes the decisions are explicit, with immediate repercussions—for example, the selection of one patient to receive a heart transplant when several might benefit from the sole available organ, or the decision to admit one patient to the last ICU bed when several critically ill patients could benefit from ICU admission. More frequently, the decisions are subtle and occur even when the supply of therapy is not absolutely limited—for example, the decision to use cheaper antibiotics, sedatives, imaging modalities, or operative procedures when more expensive options might be beneficial. Finally, allocation decisions can be completely implicit and almost hidden. For example, the decision to build an ambulatory care clinic instead of adding ICU beds has profound implications for the delivery of critical care services, but individual clinicians are largely unaware of it.

Although common and necessary, allocation decisions are stigmatized in medicine. Such decisions bring two major ethical principles into conflict: the principle of beneficence guides clinicians to act solely in their patients' best interests, while the principle of justice directs clinicians to act fairly.[2] This conflict may explain why euphemisms are frequently used to describe decisions that essentially involve the rationing of resources. For example, "triage," "optimization," "prioritization," "cost-effective care," and "basic health care" all indicate some form of allocation decision.[3-5] The purpose of this chapter is to explore these decisions in their many guises as they occur in critical care and to offer some guidance to clinicians for constructing processes for allocating resources in their ICU.

ALLOCATION VERSUS EVIDENCE-BASED MEDICINE

Decisions based solely on evidence of the efficacy of medical care are *not* rationing decisions. There is no medical obligation

TABLE 252–1. STRATEGIES FOR ALLOCATING RESOURCES

Principle	Definition
Autocracy	To each according to the will of one
Democracy	To each according to the will of the majority
Equality	To each according to an equal share
Lottery	To each according to an equal chance
Capitalism	To each according to their ability to buy
Personal worth	To each according to their contribution to the community
Utilitarianism	To each so that the utility of the community is maximized

to provide and no societal obligation to pay for care that is harmful or ineffective. In fact, clinicians use special terms to describe interventions that fall into these categories, including "futile," "not standard of care," "medically inappropriate," "wasteful," or "experimental."[5,6] For example, an intensivist who decides not to transfuse a critically ill patient with a hematocrit of 27 is *not* rationing blood, even though blood is an expensive and limited resource; in this case, there is evidence that a transfusion would be of no benefit and might even be harmful.[7] Likewise, the decision not to use human growth hormone, an expensive medication, in a chronically critically ill patient is not a rationing decision, because this treatment has been shown to be ineffective and may be harmful.[8]

Unfortunately, assessments of benefit and harm are not as straightforward as the terms would suggest, and the line between effective, ineffective, and experimental treatment often lies in the eyes of the individual clinician. Decision science has taught us that medical decision-making is a complex process that frequently obscures the true rationale of the choice.[9] In fact, judgments allegedly based solely on objective evidence of safety and benefit often incorporate a variety of subjective values and biases.[10] These may include the value the clinician assigns to being wrong; the value assigned to trying to "rescue" a patient in imminent danger of death; the clinician's tolerance for uncertainty; the impact of the decision on the clinician's finances; biases about the patient's race, gender, functional status, or age; and the cost or availability of the resource.[11] The transition from statements that summarize the evidence of benefit to recommendations that incorporate cost and other values is often very subtle. For example, the authors of a recent systematic review of colloid resuscitation in critical care conclude that "there is no evidence from randomized controlled trials that resuscitation with colloids reduces the risk of death compared to crystalloids in patients with trauma, burns and following surgery."[12] This is a statement of their summary of the evidence of efficacy of colloid therapy. Like many treatments in critical care, the evidence neither supports nor completely refutes the use of colloids as resuscitation fluids in the critically ill. However, the authors conclude, "As colloids are not associated with an improvement in survival, and as they are more expensive than crystalloids, it is hard to see how their continued use in these patient types can be justified outside the context of randomized controlled trials." Whereas the first statement may be a fair summary of the evidence, the recommendation against using colloids in the second sentence is not based solely on the evidence. It incorporates an implicit rationing strategy that pays only for treatments that have demonstrated benefit in a certain way. Although one might conclude from

the authors' review that colloid resuscitation is experimental or that its benefit is likely to be small, the reasoning for recommending against its use is based on the cost of the treatment. Presumably, if colloid fluids were the same price as crystalloids, the authors might reach different conclusions, even though the cost does not change the evidence of efficacy.

The preceding example shows how assessments of cost can creep into recommendations for therapy even without a formal discussion of allocation. Because clinicians and payers may be reluctant to admit that they are incorporating cost or availability into the rationale for a decision, they may find decisions based on futility or appropriateness less ethically problematic than those based on rationing. In fact, these judgments may implicitly contain assessments of cost by incorporating cost into the definition. When is there sufficient evidence to move a treatment or diagnostic device from experimental care to standard care? When is there sufficient evidence, absent evidence of outright harm, that a treatment is ineffective as opposed to not yet of proven efficacy? These decisions are frequently made by consensus bodies using subjective or poorly characterized criteria. The evidence threshold tends to be higher for treatments that are risky or expensive or for which there is no alternative. Conversely, the threshold for accepting a treatment as "standard" is lower if it is inexpensive and safe and offers the potential of rescuing a patient in imminent danger of dying. For example, consider the decision to elevate the head of the bed of mechanically ventilated patients to prevent ventilator-associated pneumonia. This is an inexpensive and safe treatment to offer patients. It might take less evidence to convince clinicians to use this treatment than to use kinetic beds or topical prophylactic antibiotics, which are more expensive and may raise safety issues. Therefore, the cost of an intervention may be incorporated into the assessment of whether it is a standard of care.

These judgments are further complicated by the motivation of the decision-maker. It would be difficult for an insurance company that is assessing whether a specific therapy is experimental or standard of care to be unbiased, because its decision will affect its profits. Alternatively, surgeons who developed a procedure may be committed to its benefits in a way that compromises an objective evaluation. The complexity of the assessment of efficacy and cost highlights the importance of making allocation decisions as objective, explicit, and public as possible. Because medical decisions are so complex, and because decisions in the ICU are further complicated by their immediacy and the severity of patients' illnesses, it is essential that clinicians understand their own motivations and the evidence supporting their decisions and have a process in place for allocating resources.

ALLOCATION STRATEGIES

Allocation decisions are usually separated into macro-allocation decisions (involving groups of people and usually made at a managerial or health policy level) and micro-allocation decisions (made at the bedside and involving specific cases). A hospital's decision not to hire additional ICU nurses is a macro-allocation decision; a nurse-manager's decision to allocate a specific patient to share a nurse in the ICU rather than to receive 1:1 nursing is a micro-allocation decision. This chapter is concerned primarily with bedside, or micro-allocation, decisions that clinicians make on a routine basis. There is an important interaction between micro- and macro-allocation decisions, because macro-allocation decisions ultimately affect individuals, and macro-allocation regulations are an effective rationing strategy (Table 252-2).

There are a number of approaches to allocating resources (see Table 252-1). Although they are all feasible, they are not all equally ethical. The principles of equality, fairness, justice, and due process make some strategies less acceptable. The principle of utilitarianism directs resource allocation to maximize the "utility" or benefit to the greatest number of people for any given amount of resources. To the extent that utility can be determined by measuring patient outcomes such as health-related quality of life, and to the extent that we can estimate the effects of medical treatments on utility, theoretically, we can calculate exactly which set of medical treatments to pay for to maximize the benefit to the population. These studies are called cost-effectiveness analyses and are the quantitative embodiment of utilitarianism. Allocating medical resources through cost-effectiveness analysis has important limitations. First, medical cost-effectiveness analysis cannot tell how much money to allocate to medical as opposed to other goods and services; it can only determine how to maximize health outcomes for a selected outlay of resources. Second, cost-effectiveness analysis may not fully account for some factors that society values. For example, cost-effectiveness analysis routinely treats all human lives as equally valuable; however, society often places a high value on saving identifiable lives in imminent danger of death, and it may not value additional years of life in the elderly as highly as additional years of life in the young.[13] Cost-effectiveness and other utility-based allocation strategies fail to account for the value society places on rescuing lives in imminent peril—a not uncommon occurrence in the ICU.[14] Standard economic analyses may not value equal distribution as much as optimal distribution and, to this end, may discriminate in settings that society finds unacceptable.[15] Finally, cost-effectiveness analysis is a mathematical technique that generates comparative outcomes for populations of patients. It is meaningless to speak of a treatment as being "cost-effective" in an individual.

The primary value of cost-effectiveness analysis as an allocation tool is the ability to *compare* various strategies.[16] For example, one can compare the cost-effectiveness of captopril versus no captopril in survivors of myocardial infarction with the use of fluoxetine versus imipramine for major depression to decide whether to use captopril, fluoxetine, both, or neither. Cost-effectiveness analysis provides a ruler, in terms of dollars per life-year or dollars per quality-adjusted life-year (QALY), that allows different treatments for different diseases to be compared. The crucial data that must be available to make these comparisons is information on the treatments' effect on survival or health-related quality of life. Unfortunately, in critical care, the number of treatments shown to improve survival or health-related quality of life is small. Although we have data on strategies to reduce gastrointestinal bleeding, duration of mechanical ventilation, and catheter-related infections, none of these interventions has been shown to affect QALYs.[17-19] Therefore, the cost-effectiveness analyses for these interventions are expressed as, for example, dollars per gastrointestinal bleed prevented.[20] These ratios cannot be used to compare a treatment to prevent gastrointestinal bleeding with a treatment for myocardial infarction, because the latter is expressed in dollars per QALY. Cost-effectiveness analyses with non-QALY denominators can be helpful in bedside rationing decisions when the intervention is shown to be equally or more effective and *reduces cost*. For example, special beds in the ICU both prevent decubitus ulcers and reduce the overall cost of care, even when the cost of the bed is factored in. Therefore, the cost-effectiveness ratio (expressed in dollars per decubitus ulcer prevented) is a negative number.[21]

ILLUSORY COST SAVINGS

Since the earliest days of intensive care, technologic, workforce, and organizational innovations have been proposed as

TABLE 252–2. ALLOCATION DECISIONS AT DIFFERENT LEVELS

Decision-Maker	Decision	Rationale
Nonallocation Decision		
Physician	Not to use human growth hormone in chronically critically ill patients	Evidence of harm in critically ill patients
President of insurance company	Not to offer routine chest computed tomography screening for lung cancer	Lack of sufficient evidence of benefit
Health care official	Not to offer basic medical coverage to all people in the country	Endorses goals other than equal access to health care, for example, the importance of choice or the value of free market
Macro-allocation Decision		
Physician	Not to admit routine post–coronary artery bypass patients to ICU	Limited ICU beds better used for patients with more severe illness
President of insurance company	Not to increase reimbursement for septic shock when new, expensive drug is approved	Hopes to limit cost of care for patients to increase profitability of insurance company
Health care official	To capitate reimbursement for hospital care	By providing single fee for all care, hopes to limit costs so that increased outpatient services can be provided
Micro-allocation Decision		
Physician	Not to admit a debilitated, elderly man with urosepsis to the ICU, despite a request by the patient's primary care physician	The patient is moribund, and the intensivist believes that the ICU's resources can be used to better effect on other patients
President of insurance company	Denial of claim to pay for prostacyclin infusion for pulmonary hypertension	Treatment specifically not covered by contractual arrangement with insured patient
Health care official	Not applicable	Not applicable

opportunities to reduce the exorbitant cost of critical care. In 1973, an optimistic author wrote, "[the] more promising approaches to cost reduction are all in an early stage of development now. Both deprofessionalization of the ICU by wider use of allied health personnel, and the automation of therapeutic functions are just beginning to be applied."[22] Despite the implementation of both these measures, there is little evidence that cost increases in hospital or ICU care have been curbed by technologic innovation. In fact, the opposite has occurred. This is not surprising, because technologic innovation in other areas of health care, though often associated with better outcomes, is rarely a source of cost savings.

Cost analyses are problematic in medical care, and critical investigators must be able to identify cost savings that are real and that will appear in their budgets from savings in indirect costs that will be accrued elsewhere.[23] There are several common, but problematic, arguments about cost reduction in critical care: (1) that reduced ICU length of stay will reduce the cost of care in the ICU, (2) that ordering fewer tests will reduce the cost of care in the ICU, and (3) that fewer admissions of futile-care patients will save money. It is important to recognize that not all calculated cost savings will be realized at the ICU or hospital level.

ICU costs are frequently inferred from length of stay. For example, in a cost-effectiveness analysis of antibiotic-coated catheters, the authors assigned a cost of $9738 to a catheter-related bloodstream infection.[24] Epidemiologic studies show that patients with catheter-related infections spend more time in the hospital, even after controlling for severity of illness.[25] The cost of a catheter-related infection is, in part, derived by simply multiplying the estimated number of extra days spent in the hospital by the cost (based on hospital charges) of a day in the ICU or ward. In fact, we do not really know whether using antibiotic-coated catheters shortens ICU length of stay, because the randomized trials demonstrating that they prevent infection were not sufficiently powered or did not show a reduction in mortality or length of stay.[19] Even if antibiotic-coated catheters do reduce length of stay, money "saved" by reducing length of stay is a different kind of money from that used to buy the catheters. By reducing length of stay, the ICU will be able to care for more patients, but they will be sicker and more expensive patients.

Identifying treatments for specific conditions in the ICU that reduce overall costs, even if they have no effect on QALYs, is extremely useful to the intensivist who must allocate resources. Implementing economically dominant strategies is an easy allocation decision, because they reduce costs but do not worsen patient outcomes. However, predicting the actual effect of any decision on actual costs in an ICU or hospital is complex, because each hospital performs cost accounting and budgeting in idiosyncratic ways. The effect of different payer mixes, contracts for nursing and respiratory therapist labor, allocation of indirect costs, and whether the ICU budget is fixed or grows with the number of patients served all influence whether allocation decisions accrue savings that can be appreciated at the ICU level. For example, the drug acquisition costs of once-daily medications are frequently higher than the costs of medications given more frequently. However, there are labor costs associated with administering medication more frequently that may offset the costs of the once-daily medication. Unfortunately, unless changing to once-daily medication

reduces the workload to the point where it is feasible to actually fire a nurse, there will be little realized savings. This is because labor costs are not infinitely scaleable. Even if there is 15% less work to do, it may not be possible to hire 15% fewer nursing hours. Patients who need 1:1 nursing care will continue to need this level of care regardless of whether the nurses are administering once-daily medication or not. It may be that changing medication routines improves care by using nursing time more efficiently, but this may not be reflected in a cost reduction. A reasonable criterion to consider for a proposed cost-saving intervention is whether it will reduce the number of staff that need to be hired or whether it can reduce acquisition costs for equipment or medications. If it will not, then cost savings are not likely to be realized in the ICU.

The cost estimate used in many cost-effectiveness analyses assumes that every day in the ICU costs the same. This is certainly true for what the hospital charges, but it is not true in reality. The first few days in the hospital and ICU are generally far more expensive than the last days.[26] Patients are more likely to require active interventions and closer nursing care in the early days in the ICU. Clearly, interventions that reduce ICU length of stay cannot reduce early days in the ICU; they simply eliminate later lower-cost days. This is rarely accounted for in cost analyses. This was validated at the national level as U.S. health care costs peaked during a period when hospital inpatient days declined by 40%.[27] Therefore, standard cost analyses overestimate cost savings likely to be realized by reducing length of stay.

Reducing test ordering in the ICU has been offered as a technique for cost reduction. This, too, is a perfectly reasonable option on clinical grounds. Overtesting yields increased false-positive results, which may lead to clinical complications in search of diseases that never existed. However, the actual cost reduction at the ICU level achieved by limiting test ordering is likely to be overestimated in a simple charge-based analysis. The actual marginal cost of performing the 101st arterial blood gas once the analyzer has been purchased and the technician has been paid to perform 100 arterial blood gases is minimal. If reductions in test ordering are of sufficient magnitude to staff the laboratory with fewer people or to forgo purchasing new equipment, then significant cost reductions can be realized. In fact, depending on how indirect costs in the hospital are allocated, it is possible that a reduction in test ordering will place the clinical laboratory under considerable budgetary constraints. Fewer tests may reduce the amount of money the laboratory director receives to cover staff costs, which may not decrease in the same proportion as test ordering.

Patients may be admitted to the ICU even when they have a negligible chance of survival. It seems reasonable to assume that if these patients receive care outside the ICU, the resources that would have been expended without benefit in the ICU will be saved. On its face, this appears to be the sort of painless cost saving that intensivists should look for. Unfortunately, a careful analysis of the potential savings from limiting care at the end of life shows that such care accounts for a relatively small amount of overall health care spending, that implementing these strategies may worsen overall health outcomes by affecting the care that nonterminal patients receive, and that care would have to be withheld from young patients (some of whom would have had prolonged survival) to achieve any savings.[28]

STRATEGIES FOR BEDSIDE ALLOCATION OF RESOURCES IN THE INTENSIVE CARE UNIT

Ultimately, allocation decisions occur at the bedside in the ICU. A number of studies demonstrate that under settings of restricted access to ICU beds, physicians allocate these beds on the basis of severity of illness. In these situations, the average severity of illness in the ICU increases, as it does on the hospital ward.[29] Unfortunately, these decisions are also driven by arbitrary factors, including patient age and gender, reimbursement, and physician power in the institution.[30] It is important that clinicians plan in advance for such difficult decisions so that their deliberations are explicit, open, and guided by principles, rather than ad hoc case-by-case decisions.

CASE 1: ADMISSION AND DISCHARGE CRITERIA

The Last ICU Bed. An intensivist is responsible for an eight-bed mixed medical-surgical ICU in a large community hospital that is currently near capacity. Within minutes, she receives two calls: one from the emergency room, where a 17-year-old has been admitted with severe diabetic keto-acidosis and altered mental status, but who is not intubated; and one from a hospital resident who has an 83-year-old severely demented patient on the ward who has developed acute respiratory failure and will soon require mechanical ventilation. There is only one open ICU bed, and none of the existing patients can be moved.

Perhaps the most difficult decision an ICU physician faces is the allocation of the ICU itself.[31] Although this is a wrenching decision and has generated a literature devoted to triaging the last ICU bed, there is little evidence to indicate how frequently this occurs in actual practice. Mobile technology, flexible nursing staffing, and the availability of postanesthesia, emergency room, and step-down beds may make the ritual of allocating the last ICU bed more a theoretical concern than an actual one. Deciding who gets the last ICU bed is particularly difficult because identifiable patients are affected by an explicit decision. The decision is further complicated by the almost complete lack of data on the actual benefit of ICU care in specific conditions compared with care on the ward. Few question that ICU outcomes are superior, but the relative benefit of ICU care and monitoring in specific conditions is completely unknown. Finally, the decisions must be made rapidly. Although a transplant committee also allocates a fixed resource—organs for transplantation—it can deliberate for weeks to prioritize recipients. The intensivist must allocate an ICU bed within minutes or hours.

The two most important steps in allocating the last ICU bed are to prevent the situation from occurring in the first place and to develop guidelines for managing the problem when it does occur. Strategies to prevent the last ICU bed phenomenon include staffing sufficiently for the anticipated volume of elective surgery, or stopping planned surgery if sufficient ICU beds are not available. It includes arranging flexible nursing and monitoring options to care for critically ill patients in other environments that are not physically located in the ICU. Individual clinician biases and training can have a strong effect on the perception of the value of

various life-sustaining treatments in the ICU.[32] To minimize the effect of these influences and maintain fair and equitable access to intensive care services, admission and discharge criteria should be public, explicit, evidence based, and fair. Public and explicit criteria allow all clinicians in the hospital to be aware of the policy. To the extent possible, decisions should be evidence based or, in the absence of evidence, should appeal to national policy statements or local consensus.[33]

Resolution. The intensivist went to the emergency room, evaluated the patient with diabetic ketoacidosis, placed arterial and central venous catheters, and arranged to have a nurse from the ICU float to the emergency department during the night to care for the patient there. The patient with acute respiratory failure from the floor was intubated and admitted to the ICU's last bed.

CASE 2: TECHNOLOGY PURCHASE

Bedside Laboratory Testing. An intensivist is considering purchasing a point-of-care testing system to allow him to do arterial blood gases as well as certain chemistries and coagulation tests at the ICU bedside. The salesperson has data showing that the cost of performing the tests at the bedside is 40% less than the hospital laboratory charges, saving money for the patient and potentially making money for the ICU. Further, the salesperson presents data that the rapid turnaround of bedside testing leads to faster clinical decisions and a 1-day reduction in ICU stay. The reduction in length of stay, argues the salesperson, pays for the cost of the testing system in 18 months.

Arguments that better technology will ultimately lead to cost reductions have been promulgated since the beginning of intensive care.[22] When a purchase is being made primarily because it will save money or, at worst, be cost-neutral, there are two important considerations for the intensivist: Does the cost saving involve shifting fixed costs? To what extent does the cost analysis rely on savings from reduced nursing time or fewer ICU days? As noted previously, calculations that fail to take into account the proper cost perspective, rely on shifting fixed costs, and/or rely on reduced labor time or ICU days to demonstrate cost savings may overestimate actual cost savings.

None of the preceding discussion relates to the potential benefits of new technology. If clinicians believe that the evidence supports better patient outcomes from the technology and that it merits implementation regardless of economic consequences, this is not a resource allocation decision. However, technologic innovation is rarely cheap, and the medical industry usually tries to persuade clinicians that the novel technology not only is better but also saves money.

Resolution. The intensivist met with the director of the clinical laboratory. At this hospital, the laboratory's budget is directly tied to the volume of tests performed. If the ICU started to perform its own tests, the clinical laboratory would not be able to continue to provide its services. The ICU and laboratory directors instituted a quality-improvement intervention to decrease stat lab turnaround time with existing technology.

When a clinical laboratory charges $100 to perform an arterial blood gas, this is not because the reagents, analyzer rental, and 7 minutes of technician time to perform the test cost $100. Most of the costs reflected by this charge involve the fixed costs of maintaining a 24-hour-a-day, 7-day-a-week laboratory, including quality controls, managerial costs, government reporting, and the laboratory's portion of janitorial and other services in the hospital. If the ICU switches to a point-of-care system and reduces the number of laboratory tests by 30%, none of these fixed costs will disappear. Unless the reduction in testing is so significant that the laboratory director can fire a technician or sell some machinery, the overall costs of running the laboratory will not be affected by the ICU's switch to point-of-care testing. If these fixed cost savings cannot be realized, the laboratory director must still meet the budget demands of the laboratory in the face of reduced testing. The point-of-care approach appears to be less expensive because the fixed costs of maintaining an entire laboratory are not bundled into the purchase of the testing device, not because the tests themselves are fundamentally less expensive.

CONCLUSION

Allocation of resources in medicine is an unavoidable process. Clinicians do have control over whether these decisions are implicit or explicit, whether they are made after open discourse or with no discussion, and whether the decisions are informed by the available literature. Clinicians in the ICU may, in fact, face fewer implicit allocation decisions than their colleagues in other areas because of the imminent risk of death in the ICU and the value society places on protecting those lives. In fact, there is relatively little empirical evidence of how often intensive care services are allocated. The effect of different interventions on actual costs varies, depending on local factors such as reimbursement and indirect cost allocation. Allocating ICU beds is the most challenging allocation decision most intensivists will face. The best time to handle these situations is before they occur. Public, explicit triage, and discharge criteria that are developed in collaboration with ICU users (emergency department, surgery,

oncology) well in advance of the actual decisions are essential for fair and efficient use of intensive care resources.

ANNOTATED REFERENCES

Hadorn DC: Setting health care priorities in Oregon: Cost-effectiveness meets the rule of rescue. JAMA 1991;265:2218-2225.

A rigorous application of cost-utility analysis fails to capture the value we place on saving identifiable lives. Whether this value is rational and whether it should be perpetuated are important questions; however, this analysis shows why rescue must be considered in any attempt to prioritize health care spending.

Luce JM, Rubenfeld GD: Can health care costs be reduced by limiting intensive care at the end of life? Am J Respir Crit Care Med 2002;165:750-754.

Challenges the notion that significant reductions in ICU costs can be achieved by limiting intensive care at the end of life. The authors argue that while there are many very good ethical and medical reasons not to continue care for patients in the ICU when their prognosis is grim, the cost savings from these decisions are not likely to be enormous.

Marshall MF, Schwenzer KJ, Orsina M, et al: Influence of political power, medical provincialism, and economic incentives on the rationing of surgical intensive care unit beds. Crit Care Med 1992;20:387-394.

An interesting and honest analysis of what happened when ICU beds were in scarce supply without an explicit plan for their allocation. The power and income generation of individual surgical attending physicians drove ICU allocation decisions.

Mehlman MJ: The legal implications of health care cost containment. A symposium: Health care cost containment and medical technology: A critique of waste theory. Case Western Reserve Law Review 1986;36:778-877.

A scholarly analysis that brings rigor to terminology used loosely by medical professionals.

Reinhardt UE: Spending more through "cost control": Our obsessive quest to gut the hospital. Health Aff (Millwood) 1996;15:145-154.

A leading health economist challenges the notion that reducing hospital length of stay will reduce overall health care expenditures. Data from the United States show that marked reductions in hospital length of stay were not associated with a reduction in the rate of growth of medical expenditures. Instead, the author argues that costs were merely shifted from the hospital to other settings.

Chapter 253

ETHICAL ISSUES IN THE INTENSIVE CARE UNIT

Thomas A. Bledsoe • Mitchell M. Levy

KEY POINTS

1. Ethics in medical care is based on four fundamental principles: beneficence, nonmaleficence, autonomy, and justice.

2. In the United States, competent patients have the right to make their own decisions about health care.

3. The process of making known one's wishes regarding future care is called advance care planning.

4. In the absence of an advance directive, a surrogate decision-maker attempts to make medical decisions for a patient using substituted judgment. When no specific information is available about a patient, decision-makers apply a "reasonable-person" standard and sometimes resort to a "best-interest" standard.

5. Discussions about advance directives should be rooted in the patient's values and goals for medical care, as well as the appropriateness of specific interventions.

6. Shared decision-making is a process that combines patient autonomy and physician judgment.

THE FOUNDATIONS OF ETHICS IN CRITICAL CARE

Ethics in critical care is based on four fundamental principles: (1) beneficence, or the physician's obligation to do good for patients; (2) nonmaleficence, or the duty to avoid harm; (3) autonomy, or respect for patients' right to self-determination; and (4) justice, or the fair allocation of health care resources. The first three principles form the basis of the physician-patient relationship and provide the ethical imperative for physicians to act in the best interests of their patients. The relative importance of these three principles differs from country to country, but physicians' responsibility to their patients is common to all cultures.

GOALS OF CARE AND MEDICAL DECISION-MAKING

SURROGATE DECISION-MAKING

Modern medicine has embraced the concept of shared decision-making between patients and their physicians

based on the principle of autonomy.[1,2] This approach is often more complicated in the ICU, because patients are frequently too ill or otherwise impaired to make meaningful contributions to decisions about their care. Increasingly, decisions are made in the ICU to withdraw care,[3] and conflicts are common between physicians' practices and patients' wishes.[4] In the ICU, as in other medical situations, patients have an ethical (and in many places, a legal) right to determine the goals of their medical care. An individual patient's wishes regarding future care in the case of his or her incapacity may be made known in advance of a serious medical illness. The process by which patients, with or without the assistance and participation of their physicians, family members, or other close personal relations, plan for future medical care is called advance care planning.[5] In general, the results of these deliberations are known as advance directives; defined broadly, they may be verbal or written and may be quite specific or very general. In this process, the patient determines what kind of care he or she would want in the setting of some hypothetical (or anticipated) situation and makes known his or her wishes regarding future medical care. The advance directive helps direct medical care in case of the patient's incapacity and comes into play only if the patient is unable to make his or her current wishes known.[6] For example, a patient who awakens after a surgical procedure and is deemed competent (see below) is asked outright about his or her wishes, and the advance directive is no longer necessary.

Advance directives have ethical authority in whatever form (including verbal), as long as the directive was promulgated within the requirements of informed consent (see below). Unfortunately, the reliability of a specific advance directive as "authentic representations of autonomous patient choices" is often suspect.[7] Advance directives specific enough to guide day-to-day clinical decision-making in the ICU are rare; more commonly, the ICU physician is left to work with a surrogate to make decisions for a patient who is too sick to participate in decisions.

For medical decisions in which patient factors play a large role, the physician must have a surrogate decision-maker with whom to discuss goals of care and treatment options. There are two questions that must be answered: Who may and should act as surrogate? How should the surrogate make decisions for the ill patient?

In some cultures, physicians often turn to the "next of kin" for surrogate decision-making. However, the legal status of surrogates varies from country to country, and this individual may have no legal or ethical grounds for assuming this role. Even in cultures in which surrogate decision-making is valued, there is often no designated hierarchy of surrogates. In those cultures in which such a hierarchy has been determined by law, a typical sequence might be (1) spouse, (2) eldest child, (3) next child, (4) parent, (5) sibling. In addition to legal standing, the surrogate should have some moral standing to act as such. For example, a surrogate specifically named in an advance directive document or verbally designated by the patient as the preferred surrogate would have this standing. In fact, some would argue that this is the single most important question for a patient who is sick enough to warrant ICU care ("If you become too sick to speak for yourself, who would you want to make medical decisions for you?").[8] In surveys about advance directives and surrogates, patients and well individuals typically name their spouses or other immediate family members as their preferred surrogates. These individuals frequently (though not always) have a shared value system. Interestingly, when asked whether they would prefer that their advance directives be followed no matter what or that their care be discussed with their chosen surrogate, a majority of patients would cede authority to the surrogate.[9]

In many cultures, surrogate decision-making is not considered acceptable. Even in this paternalistic approach, it is incumbent on the physician to collect information from those who know the patient well in an attempt to collectively determine what this patient would prefer in terms of medical care and then balance that information with the physician's judgment as to the best course of therapy. This shared decision-making model is now viewed as the most appropriate in many cultures, including North America and Europe.

In the United States, advance directives allow patients to make their wishes for future care known, either formally or informally. These directives may also designate a specific surrogate decision-maker who then has ethical and possibly legal standing (if the appropriate statutory document is properly executed) to make medical decisions for the patient. In the absence of advance directives, the legally appointed surrogate—or, in the absence of such a surrogate, those who know the patient well—make decisions for the patient using substituted judgment based on their knowledge of the patient. When no specific information is available about a patient, the decision-makers apply a "reasonable-person" standard—that is, what a reasonable person would prefer in the clinical situation at hand—and sometimes resort to a "best-interest" standard.

ADVANCE DIRECTIVES

As noted, in the United States, advance directives are formal or informal instructions to health care providers, family members, or others involved in a patient's care regarding treatment that may be required while the patient is unable to participate in medical decision-making. The earliest form of advance directive was the "living will." Classically, the living will is restricted in terms of both scope and applicability. Living wills are usually reserved for patients with terminal illnesses and are typically restricted to statements about forgoing medical treatments that would "only prolong my dying"; they typically make explicit statements about the acceptability of discontinuing intravenous fluids and artificial nutrition if death is imminent and there is no significant hope for recovery. They usually do not provide instructions in case of nonterminal illness and typically do not name a surrogate.

A more generally useful legal document is one that gives statutory authority to an individual to make medical decisions for a patient in case of incapacity. This document is sometimes referred to as a "durable power of attorney for health care." Similar to a durable power of attorney that provides legal decision-making authority for financial and other matters in case of incapacity, this document provides legal standing to a named surrogate with regard to health care decisions. These documents typically provide an opportunity for an individual to give general information about health care preferences in a variety of situations. Some also provide an opportunity for the person to make a statement about quality of life and the kind of life that would and would not be worth living. Preferences for organ donation, wishes for spiritual care, and even funeral arrangements are sometimes included.

Additionally, a number of advisory documents have been developed, including "values histories" and the medical directive, developed by Linda and Ezekiel Emanuel.[10] These documents may present a series of increasingly dire scenarios and ask about overall preferences ("do everything possible to prolong life," "continue aggressive care but reevaluate often," "keep me comfortable but do not provide care that prolongs my life"), or they may ask more general questions about what makes the person's life "worth living." It is hoped that this information will be helpful to a surrogate who must decide whether to continue supportive care in the case of irreversible injury or damage or even to continue disease-oriented care in the case of critical illness and impaired decision-making capacity.

For a variety of reasons, advance directives have not achieved wide popularity. When they exist, they are often not specific enough to provide meaningful guidance.[11] Even when a detailed directive exists, a question often remains about whether the individual was adequately informed. For example, a patient's advance directive says that she would *never* want to be on "life support," but when she is asked about mechanical ventilation in the case of reversible respiratory failure from pneumonia, she says of course she would want that. Thus, following a legally executed advance directive without verifying what was meant by the patient and whether the written wishes apply to the current illness is often quite problematic. It could, in fact, result in a preventable death in a patient who, with proper education, would wish to be treated.

A more limited form of advance directive, known as a "code status," is sometimes sought on admission to the hospital, and especially on admission to the ICU. A code status is an advance directive that is specifically limited to a patient's (or surrogate's) preferences regarding cardiopulmonary resuscitation (CPR) and other measures in the event of cardiopulmonary arrest. In many hospitals and other health care institutions, as a matter of policy, any patient who suffers cardiac arrest is treated with interventions designed to attempt to reverse the life-threatening derangement, including CPR, electrical defibrillation, and intubation and mechanical ventilatory support. Because a patient who suffers a cardiopulmonary arrest will die in a very short time without interventions, the discussion about code status is as much about how a patient wishes to die as it is about whether he or she wishes to live. Tomlinson and Brody distinguish three distinct rationales for a "do not resuscitate" (DNR) status[12]: (1) CPR has such a low likelihood of producing the desired outcome that it is effectively "futile," (2) there would be an unacceptable quality of life after CPR, and (3) there is already an unacceptable quality of life, and cardiopulmonary arrest would be a welcome deliverance. A decision about CPR may not give much useful information about a patient's preferences regarding other aspects of his or her illness. A patient may choose aggressive disease-oriented measures well into a severe illness but still choose to forgo resuscitation in the event of an arrest. This approach may be voiced in a statement such as, "I want to fight this thing with all I have, but when it is my time, I want to go quickly without suffering." Such a statement would be an opportunity to address resuscitation status, in addition to addressing overall goals of care (see later). Many ICU patients who are actively receiving intensive disease-oriented care have a DNR code status. Such a directive may save surrogates and family members from the emotionally difficult task of removing life-supporting care. A patient's acceptance of a DNR status may signify acceptance of the limits of medical science; refusal of a DNR status in the setting of progressive, irreversible illness may be an indication that the patient has an incomplete and perhaps unrealistic understanding of the illness. Further discussion, addressing knowledge deficits or unspoken fears, may increase the likelihood that the patient's true wishes will be followed.

A common error when discussing code status is the failure to address post-resuscitation issues. Patients who undergo CPR will most likely be incapacitated for at least a period of time after the resuscitation, even in the best scenarios. There is also a significant risk of permanent brain injury after cardiopulmonary arrest and resuscitation. Thus, it would be prudent for the patient to name a preferred surrogate as well.

Any discussion of advance directives should attempt to answer at least three questions: (1) In the event of cardiac arrest, do you want the health care team to attempt resuscitation? (2) If you became incapacitated, who do you want to make decisions for you? (3) If you were left significantly impaired after an attempt at resuscitation, would you want us to discontinue life-sustaining care? Preferences for resuscitation are best understood in the context of an individual's values, beliefs, relationships, and culture.[7]

Many problematic end-of-life issues can be traced to a focus on interventions ("Would you wish to be intubated?") without an adequate exploration of values ("What do you value about your life? What are the things that make your life worth living?"). It is also a mistake to think about advance directives as an issue limited to end-of-life situations. Advance directives are really just part of informed consent for any treatment, and discussion of advance directives is an important aspect of good medical care.

INFORMED DECISION-MAKING (INFORMED CONSENT)

In the United States, autonomy is one of the core principles that define the relationship between doctor and patient. Autonomy requires respect for the values and wishes of the individual. An individual patient's autonomy is best respected when decision-making takes place through informed consent. Without adequate information, the power of reason, and freedom of choice, patients' decisions cannot be said to be autonomous. Informed consent (or, more accurately, informed decision-making) is a decision-making model designed to safeguard the autonomy of vulnerable patients.

Brock discussed the basic requirements for informed consent and identified three critical elements: the person giving consent must be competent, informed, and able to make a decision free from coercion.[13] Competence has several critical elements.[14] First, the decision-maker must be capable

of understanding relevant information, which involves both memory and mental processing. Second, it requires the ability to attend to and retain information, the ability to manipulate information, and the ability to foresee consequences. A third element is the ability to formulate and communicate choice. Some standards of competency strengthen this requirement by demanding the ability to communicate a *stable* choice (in this case, ambivalence may be a sign of incompetence).

To adequately participate in medical decision-making, patients must have enough information to weigh the risks and benefits of various medical interventions. In the past, the standard for being "informed" was the standard practice of other physicians in the community.[15] Subsequently, "informed" came to mean what a "reasonable person would want to know." Because the main point of informed consent is to respect the rights and values of individuals, it is most appropriate to address this issue in terms of what a particular patient needs to know.[16] In general, patients need to know about the illness and its natural history to make informed decisions about medical care. They need information about the effectiveness of treatment, the risks of treatment, and the likelihood of success with treatment. This information must be presented in a way that is understandable to the patient, at an appropriate educational level, and in the patient's language. Whether enough information has been transmitted can be assessed at the most basic level by simply asking a patient whether he or she has any questions. Brock writes of "informed understanding" and notes that this "permits an informed exercise in self-determination and promotes a decision most in accord with the patient's well-being."[13] In addition, this approach values autonomy.

The decision must also be voluntary, that is, free of coercion. The decision-maker must have the freedom to accept or refuse the intervention or test being proposed. Consent given as a result of undue coercion is generally not valid.

Informed consent in the ICU raises some special issues. First, as mentioned earlier, the decision-maker is often a surrogate rather than the patient. The surrogate decision-maker should have access to all relevant information that the patient would need to make informed decisions; however, the surrogate should not routinely be given confidential information *simply because the patient is no longer competent.* An example may be helpful in illustrating this point. An HIV-positive patient in the ICU has designated a family member as his surrogate; however, the family is unaware of his HIV status. The ICU physician believes that a central line is indicated for continued care and seeks informed consent from the family member. In this case, it may be possible to obtain true informed consent for the procedure without divulging the patient's HIV status. Alternatively, a decision about a test or treatment specifically related to the patient's HIV status may require that this information be divulged to the surrogate for her to make an informed decision.

The adequacy of a properly designated surrogate is usually assumed but should be questioned in two situations. The first is when the surrogate acts in contrast to the patient's known wishes. Anyone who knows that the surrogate's directions conflict with the patient's expressed wishes has an obligation to work with the surrogate to come to a treatment decision more in keeping with the patient's wishes or to seek outside assistance from the hospital ethics committee or the hospital's legal department. The second situation occurs when there is doubt about the surrogate's competence, specifically, his or her ability to retain and process information. Again, the ethics committee or the risk management department can be of help in this situation.

In summary, ethics in critical care are founded on the same four primary directives common to all disciplines of medicine. Critical care decision-making presents special challenges because these decisions often involve the life or death of patients who are unable to participate in the decision-making process. Although the balance between physician and patient responsibility for decision-making may vary across cultures, the primary directive for physicians to act in the best interest of their patients is universal.

ANNOTATED REFERENCES

Applebaum PS, Grisso T: Assessing patients' capacities to consent to treatment. N Engl J Med 1988;319:1635-1638.

This paper outlines four tasks that a patient must be able to execute to be considered competent: communicating a choice, understanding relevant information, appreciating the current situation and its consequences, and manipulating information rationally.

Brock DW: Informed consent. In Regan T, VandeVeer D (eds): Health Care Ethics. Philadelphia, Temple University Press, 1987, pp 98-126.

In this chapter, Brock outlines with great clarity the ethical and practical considerations underlying the doctrine of informed consent.

Brock DW: Surrogate decision making for incompetent adults: An ethical framework. Mt Sinai J Med 1991;58:388-392.

An excellent overview of a philosophically sound approach to surrogate decision-making.

Burns JP, Edwards J, Johnson J, et al: Do-not-resuscitate order after 25 years. Crit Care Med 2003; 31:1543-1550.

A review of the development, implementation, and present standing of the DNR order. Emphasizes the usefulness of the DNR order to clarify a patient's wishes with regard to end-of life care.

Cantor NL: My annotated living will. Law Med Health Care 1990;18:115-119.

This is an excellent example of an annotated advance directive.

Prendergast T: Advance care planning: Pitfalls, progress, promise. Crit Care Med 2001;29(Suppl):N34-N39.

Review of the (largely disappointing) literature on the usefulness of advance directives, but makes the point that "preferences for care are not fixed but emerge in a clinical context from a process of discussion and feedback within the network of the patient's most important relationships."

Chapter 254

ETHICAL CONTROVERSIES IN PEDIATRIC CRITICAL CARE

Jeffrey P. Burns • Robert D. Truog

KEY POINTS

1. The majority of deaths in the pediatric intensive care unit (PICU) occur following the withholding or withdrawal of life-sustaining treatments. This fact heightens the importance of competence in end-of-life decision-making and palliative patient management by all practitioners of pediatric critical care medicine.

2. In the United States, there is consensus in the law and bioethics communities that parents have the authority to determine the best interests of their children and to make decisions in accord with their own values. However, critical care providers must be thoroughly familiar with their legal and ethical duties to their pediatric patients, independent of parental viewpoints about life-sustaining treatments.

3. National guidelines advocate that children should participate in decision-making commensurate with their development, they should provide assent to care whenever reasonable, and they should not be excluded from decision-making without persuasive reasons.

4. According to national guidelines, the optimal dose of sedatives and analgesics to administer to a dying patient for symptom relief can be determined only by increasing the dose until the symptoms are relieved.

5. Most recent commentary states that because neuromuscular blocking agents have no sedative or analgesic properties, the initiation of these agents when life-sustaining treatment is withdrawn is morally indefensible.

6. Attending physicians must affirm that the requesting physician has the right to request organ donation or an autopsy by virtue of his or her involvement in the care of the patient and relationship with the family. Renewed educational efforts on best consent practices for organ donation and autopsy are needed.

7. Although still a controversial subject, the Council on Ethical and Judicial Affairs of the American Medical Association recently concluded that performing procedures on the newly dead for teaching purposes should be allowed, but only in the context of a structured training sequence completed under close supervision, and only after permission from family members has been obtained.

Advances in pediatric critical care medicine in the last 25 years have led to ethical issues of profound concern to all practitioners. One of the most striking changes is that the majority of deaths in the pediatric intensive care unit (PICU), as is true for adult and neonatal ICUs, occur following the withholding or withdrawal of life-sustaining treatments.[1] For this reason, many troubling issues in the PICU revolve around end-of-life decision-making and palliative patient management. In this chapter, we explore both issues.

DECISION-MAKING IN THE PEDIATRIC INTENSIVE CARE UNIT

THE ROLE OF PARENTS AND PHYSICIANS

Who should make the final decision about treatment for a child in the PICU? In the United States, the clear consensus in the fields of ethics and the law is that a competent adult patient has the right to refuse all forms of medical therapy, including life-sustaining treatment, even if it is certain that such a refusal will hasten death.[2] A similar moral and legal consensus holds that parents have the authority to determine the best interests of their children and to make decisions in accord with their own values.[3] However, pediatric health care providers also have legal and ethical duties to their patients, independent of parental desires or proxy consent.[3]

How can one objectively assess whether a decision is within the range of acceptable ethical choices for a child? More than 20 years ago, a widely respected decision-making framework for children in the PICU context was published by the President's Commission for the Study of Ethical Problems in Medicine and Biomedical and Behavioral Research.[4] The commission proposed five considerations for determining a child's "best interests" and therefore the appropriate approach when weighing different treatment options: (1) the amount of suffering and the potential for relief, (2) the severity of dysfunction and the potential for restoration of function, (3) the expected duration of life, (4) the potential for personal satisfaction and enjoyment of life, and (5) the possibility of developing a capacity for self-determination. The commission then advocated applying these criteria based on an assessment of the proposed treatment plan as clearly beneficial, ambiguous or uncertain, or futile. The commission concluded that in most circumstances, the child's parents should be the final decision-makers on all medical decisions (Table 254-1). The Committee on Bioethics of the American Academy of Pediatrics has similarly recommended great deference to patents' informed decisions.[5]

The President's Commission also concluded, reflecting the legal consensus in this area, that parental authority must

TABLE 254–1. DECISION-MAKING IN THE PEDIATRIC INTENSIVE CARE UNIT

Physician's Assessment of Treatment Option	Parents Prefer to Accept Treatment	Parents Prefer to Forgo Treatment
Clearly beneficial	Provide treatment	Provide treatment (during review process)
Ambiguous/uncertain	Provide treatment	Forgo treatment
Futile	Provide treatment (unless provider prefers not to)	Forgo treatment

occasionally be superseded by clinicians when it is determined that the parents' decisions are at odds with the societal consensus about a child's interests or when parents' actions produce certain risk or harm to the child. If life-threatening choices are not involved, or if the risk of substantial harm is minimal, courts have generally respected the decisions of the parents, even though physicians may have disagreed strongly. In some states, parents are legally permitted to refuse standard immunizations for religious reasons.[6] As the potential threat to the child increases, however, and as the benefits of treatment become more certain, actions to override parental choices are not only legally supportable but also mandatory, in most jurisdictions. Numerous court opinions have upheld the notion, first pronounced in the 1944 Supreme court case of *Prince v. Massachusetts*, that a parent may make a martyr of himself because of religious convictions, "but he is not free to make a martyr of his child."[7]

SEEKING THE CHILD'S ASSENT

The prevailing consensus is that patients should participate in treatment decisions to the extent of their decision-making capacity. The President's Commission advocated this perspective when it noted, "Determining whether a patient lacks capacity to make a particular health care decision requires assessing the patient's capability to understand information relevant to the decision, to communicate with care givers about it, and to reason about relevant alternatives against a background of reasonably stable personal values and life goals."[4] Restricting medical decision-making only to patients who fulfill the legal definition of competency would infringe on the autonomy of many individuals with decisional capacity, such as adolescents.

Around the age of 7 years, children develop an increasing capacity to understand, process, and make decisions about their care. For children this age and older, it becomes increasingly important for clinicians to obtain the child's assent whenever appropriate. As a matter of policy, the American Academy of Pediatrics has stated, "Patients should participate in decision-making commensurate with their development; they should provide assent to care whenever reasonable. Parents and physicians should not exclude children and adolescents from decision-making without persuasive reasons."[3] It defines "assent" to include at least the following elements:

1. Helping the patient achieve a developmentally appropriate awareness of the nature of his or her condition.
2. Telling the patient what he or she can expect with tests and treatments.
3. Making a clinical assessment of the patient's understanding of the situation and the factors influencing how he or she

is responding (including whether there is inappropriate pressure to accept testing or therapy).
4. Soliciting an expression of the patient's willingness to accept the proposed care. Regarding this final point, "no one should solicit a patient's views without intending to weigh them seriously. In situations in which the patient will have to receive medical care despite his or her objection, the patient should be told that fact and should not be deceived."[3]

Although children cannot give consent for treatment (only a person who has reached the age of majority can give consent in the eyes of the law), in almost all cases they should be approached for their "assent." Accordingly, many consent forms include a section for documenting the assent of the child. Most states also recognize "emancipated minors" as having decisional capacity for health care matters. For example, minors who are married or who are serving in the armed forces may be designated as emancipated. In addition, some states have a "mature minor" doctrine that allows a judge to decide that an individual adolescent is mature enough to make a particular decision.[8]

BABY DOE REGULATIONS

Perhaps the most controversial and misunderstood regulations on decision-making about life-sustaining treatments in pediatrics are the so-called Baby Doe regulations. Baby Doe was an infant with Down's syndrome and tracheo-esophageal fistula born in Bloomington, Indiana, in 1982. His parents declined corrective surgery on the grounds that he would never achieve a "minimally acceptable quality of life," and the child subsequently died. The case generated public controversy. Following a number of appeals, the final Baby Doe regulations, often referred to as the "Final Rule," were passed by Congress as the 1984 Amendments to the Child Abuse Prevention and Treatment Act.[9] This legislation required all states to create a regulatory system to investigate cases in which medically indicated treatment is withheld from handicapped infants, or risk the withholding of federal funding for children's services. It also stipulated that "the withholding of medically indicated treatment from a disabled infant with a life-threatening condition" by parents or providers would be considered medical neglect. The legislation then outlined three medical conditions that would justify the withholding of otherwise required treatment: "The term 'withholding of medically indicated treatment' means the failure to respond to the infant's life threatening conditions by providing treatment (including appropriate nutrition, hydration, and medication) which, in the treating physician's reasonable medical judgment, will be most likely to be effective in ameliorating or correcting all such conditions, except that the term does not include the failure to provide treatment (other than appropriate nutrition, hydration, or medication) to an infant when, in the treating physician's reasonable medical judgment any of the following circumstances apply: (1) the infant is chronically and irreversibly comatose; (2) the provision of such treatment would merely prolong dying, not be effective in ameliorating or correcting all of the infant's life-threatening conditions, or otherwise be futile in terms of survival of the infant; or (3) the provision of such treatment would be virtually futile in terms of survival of the infant and the treatment itself under such circumstances would be inhumane."[9]

Many argue that the Baby Doe regulations are not helpful in decision-making for infants because of the ambiguity of the term "appropriate." Regardless of how one interprets the intentions of the legislation, this is not a commonly recommended framework for ethical end-of-life decision-making for pediatric patients. Rather, it is viewed as a regulatory statute without common clinical application.

DETERMINING FUTILITY

Few issues have provoked as much controversy as the notion of futility. Who should determine when a situation is futile? Helft and colleagues noted that discussions of futility can be grouped into four categories: attempts to define medical futility, attempts to resolve the debate with the use of empirical data, discussions that cast the debate as a struggle between the autonomy of patients and the autonomy of physicians, and attempts to develop a process for resolving disputes over futility.[10]

In pediatrics, a widely publicized futility case was that of Baby K.[11] Baby K was born in Virginia in the early 1990s with anencephaly. Baby K's mother demanded that physicians provide mechanical ventilation for her daughter during multiple hospitalizations for aspiration pneumonia. The clinicians refused, stating that mechanical ventilation could not reverse the anencephalic infant's malformation and therefore was not indicated. Her mother responded by saying that she understood the medical facts about anencephaly and the natural history of the malformation, "but the value of this kind of life is God's secret." All parties concerned agreed about the facts of the case, but these "medical facts" were valued differently. In such a situation, whose values should predominate? Can patients or their surrogates demand care that clinicians believe goes against their professional conscience? In the case of Baby K, a federal appeals court ruled that the hospital was required to provide care to any patient seeking emergency treatment, as dictated by the Emergency Medical Treatment and Active Labor Act. However, this question remains largely unresolved in our society, for several reasons.

First, in practice, situations of true futility are difficult to define. The first definition proposed in the literature stated that "when physicians conclude (either through personal experience, experiences shared with colleagues, or consideration of published empiric data) that in the last 100 cases a medical treatment has been useless, they should regard that treatment as futile. If a treatment merely preserves permanent unconsciousness or cannot end dependence on intensive medical care, the treatment should be considered futile."[12] Yet this and other attempts to define futility are seen as inherently flawed by critics of the concept, because each patient's situation is unique. In addition, there is no universal agreement among physicians on how to define futility. Second, people's opinions of the value of life may differ, as in the case of Baby K. For instance, whereas some may value the preservation of life at all costs, others may conclude that the quality of life is so poor that death is the preferred outcome. Or some may see hope in an extremely small chance of success ("hoping for a miracle"), whereas others see a prolongation of the dying process.[13] Who is right?

The Society for Critical Care Medicine (SCCM) states that treatments should be defined as futile only when they will "not accomplish their intended goal."[14] Moreover, this official position on futility states that "treatments that are extremely unlikely to be beneficial, are extremely costly, or are of uncertain benefit may be considered inappropriate and hence inadvisable, but should not be labeled futile. Futile treatments constitute a small fraction of medical care. Thus, employing the concept of futile care in decision-making will not primarily contribute to a reduction in resource use. Nonetheless, communities have a legitimate interest in allocating medical resources by limiting inadvisable treatments." This approach advocates that the local community draft procedures to be followed in cases of dispute, with broad input from the community, instead of ad hoc attempts at the bedside to define and resolve differences over futility. This policy goes on to state, "communities should seek to do so using a rationale that is explicit, equitable, and democratic; that does not disadvantage the disabled, poor, or uninsured; and that recognizes the diversity of individual values and goals. Policies to limit inadvisable treatment should have the following characteristics: (a) be disclosed in the public record; (b) reflect moral values acceptable to the community; (c) not be based exclusively on prognostic scoring systems; (d) articulate appellate mechanisms; and (e) be recognized by the courts." These sentiments have also been supported by the Bioethics Committee of the American Academy of Pediatrics.[15]

ISSUES IN END-OF-LIFE CARE

ANALGESIA

Perhaps the most comprehensive and authoritative document on this issue comes from the Ethics Committee of the SCCM, which writes, "These agents should be titrated to effect, and the dose should not be limited solely on the basis of 'recommended' or 'suggested' maximal doses. In most cases, patients who do not respond to a given dose of an opioid or benzodiazepine will respond if the dose is increased—there is no theoretical or practical maximal dose."[16] Other experts have expressed similar recommendations: "The optimal dose of morphine for relief of pain or dyspnea is determined by increasing the dose until the patient responds. Patients who have not previously received opioids should initially be given low doses, which should be rapidly increased until symptoms are relieved. For patients with particularly severe or acute symptoms, rapid titration requires that an experienced clinician be at the bedside."[17]

However, assuming that one can externally validate the "appropriate" administration of sedation and analgesia in this setting, determining when to do so is likely to be difficult. There is no constellation of patient signs, symptoms, or pain scores that meets a universally accepted threshold for treatment, let alone the extent of treatment to be given. Regardless of the dosing scheme required to effectively treat pain and suffering, it should be standard medical practice to thoroughly document the observable signs and symptoms of suffering and the rationale behind the regimen chosen to treat those symptoms.

AGGRESSIVE PALLIATIVE CARE

The ethical principle that is relevant to this issue is the doctrine of double effect.[18] This doctrine states that when an action has two effects, one of which is inherently good and the other of which is inherently bad, it can be justified if four conditions are met. First, the action in itself must be good or at least morally indifferent. Second, the agent must intend only the good effect and not the bad effect. That is, the bad effect is foreseen, not intended; it is allowed, not sought. For example, in the case of administering morphine to a terminally ill patient, the physician must intend only the relief of the patient's pain and suffering. Respiratory depression and the potential for an earlier death are foreseen complications, but they are not sought. Third, the bad effect cannot be a means to the good effect. For example, if a physician administers a bolus of potassium chloride, the bad effect (death) becomes the means to the good effect (relief from suffering). (By contrast, morphine does not depend on the side effect of death in order to effectively relieve pain.) Fourth, the good that is intended must outweigh the bad that is permitted. For instance, in the case of a patient whose death is imminent, the benefit of pain relief clearly outweighs the risk of death.

Whether double-effect reasoning is a necessary or sufficient determinant of morally permissible behavior by clinicians providing terminal care is much disputed. Critics argue that the principle is not morally relevant or logically valid, for it relies on an overly simplistic notion of intent that is impossible to verify externally, and it may have the paradoxical effect of constraining some clinicians from providing adequate medication for relief of suffering because of the fear of violating the principle's absolute prohibition against intentionally causing death. They maintain that the fundamental ethical justification for care is based on the patient's informed consent, not the intentions of clinicians. Still others assert that those who appeal to the moral cover of double-effect reasoning are really engaging in disingenuous hair-splitting, a form of rationalization for a practice that is really surreptitious euthanasia.[19,20]

Viable alternatives to double-effect reasoning in guiding the care of patients dying in the ICU are limited. Most terminally ill patients on life support, whether child or adult, lack decisional capacity; therefore, voluntary consent is not an option. Further, a rapid decline in patient comfort is common when life support is withdrawn from the critically ill. The sedation and analgesia adequate for a patient receiving mechanical ventilation are usually inadequate to treat the air hunger experienced when controlled ventilation is removed from dying patients without severe neurologic injuries. Double-effect reasoning provides a defensible rationale for escalating doses of these medications among practitioners who support neither euthanasia nor allowing patients to die with untreated suffering.[1]

The Supreme Court of the United States has also commented on this issue. Writing for the majority, Chief Justice Rehnquist wrote in the 1997 case of *Vacco v. Quill*, "It is widely recognized that the provision of pain medication is ethically and professionally acceptable even when the treatment may hasten the patient's death if the medication is intended to alleviate pain and severe discomfort, not to cause death."[21]

NEUROMUSCULAR BLOCKADE

Is it acceptable to administer a neuromuscular blockade to a dying patient for the sole purpose of making the process of ventilator withdrawal easier for the family? Neuromuscular blocking agents, used to reduce ventilator-patient asynchrony and minimize oxygen consumption by eliminating patient movement, have no sedative or analgesic properties. Given this, many believe that administering these agents as the ventilator is being withdrawn is morally indefensible.[16,17,22] Some argue that minimizing the distress of the patient's family is an important consideration, and given the certainty of the patient's death following the withdrawal of mechanical ventilation, regardless of muscle relaxation, these clinicians believe that initiating neuromuscular blockade at the time of withdrawal is acceptable.[23,24] However, others believe that the patient's well-being always takes precedence over family interests.[22] Neuromuscular blockade potentially masks symptoms of patient suffering and therefore interferes with the clinician's primary obligation to ensure that a dying patient does not experience untreated suffering. Such an action also does not allow for the chance that the patient might survive without mechanical ventilation when there is some degree of prognostic uncertainty.

What should be done when a patient is experiencing the effects of residual neuromuscular blockade and the family decides to withdraw mechanical ventilation? The Ethics Committee of the SCCM has taken the position that efforts should be made to allow the restoration of neuromuscular function before withdrawing mechanical ventilation from patients who have previously been receiving therapeutic neuromuscular blockade. A similar position has been advocated by other experts in the field.[16,17,22]

Some experts believe that only in very limited circumstances is it morally justified to withdraw mechanical ventilation from a patient who is still experiencing the effects of residual neuromuscular blocking agents that were given as part of appropriate management before the decision to forgo life-sustaining treatment was made. If the attempt to reverse neuromuscular blockade is to be more than a charade, the patient must regain sufficient function to potentially sustain life and manifest symptoms of unnecessary pain or suffering. Yet, in some critically ill patients with multiple organ failure, drug clearance may be prolonged and unpredictable, and restoration of full neuromuscular function may take many days or weeks, even with routine neuromuscular monitoring and attempts at pharmacologic reversal. In this instance, the reasons for waiting for the restoration of neuromuscular function must be balanced against the added suffering and continued use of life-sustaining treatments, possibly long after the family and clinicians have concluded that the burdens outweigh the benefits. Open discussion with the family and among the caregivers should be undertaken, followed by clear documentation in the chart of decisions regarding the restoration of neuromuscular function.[3,22]

FAMILY PRESENCE AT RESUSCITATION ATTEMPTS

The official position of the Guidelines 2000 for Cardiopulmonary Resuscitation and Emergency Cardiovascular Care is that "family members should be given the option of being present at resuscitation attempts, but they will require support and specific attention during the resuscitation." This statement stems from surveys that have found that most people would like to be present during the attempted resuscitation of a loved one, especially when it is a child. If family members are present, a clinician must be in attendance to meet the unexpected needs of the family, which may stretch the limited resources of the resuscitation team.[25,26]

ETHICAL CONCERNS AFTER DEATH

ORGAN DONATION

Organ donation rates continue to be inadequate. For example, it is frequently noted that 86% of the general public claims to support organ and tissue donation but only 40% to 50% of those approached grant consent for donation.[27,28] Rocheleau reviewed the research in this area and found that the reasons for denying consent can be grouped into eight broad categories: donor characteristics, distrust of the medical community, religious beliefs, fear of mutilation, concern regarding the use of organs, lack of knowledge about the deceased's wishes, misunderstanding of brain death, and the bereaved family's emotional state.[29]

The questions of who should approach the family about potential organ donation, when to broach the subject, and what should be said have been simplified by federal regulations issued in 1998.[30] One of the requirements is that a hospital must have an agreement with an organ procurement organization, under which it contacts the organization in a timely manner about individuals who die or whose death is imminent in the hospital. The organ procurement organization then determines the individual's medical suitability for donation. Hospitals are also required to have an agreement with at least one tissue bank and one eye bank for tissue and eye referrals. The regulations require hospitals to collaborate with the organ procurement organization in notifying the families of potential donors of their donation options and to work cooperatively with such organizations and tissue and eye banks in educating hospital staff on donation issues, reviewing death records to improve the identification of potential donors, and maintaining potential donors during the testing and placement of organs.

Who should approach the family and request organ donation? The Centers for Medicare and Medicaid Services has answered this question by stating: "Ideally, the organ procurement organization [OPO] and hospital will decide together how and by whom the family will be approached. If possible, the organ procurement organization representative and a designated requestor (such as someone from the hospital staff who has established a rapport with the family) should approach the family together. Research has shown that the highest consent rates occur when the OPO and hospital staff approach the family together. However, in the event that collaboration is not possible, the hospital decides who approaches the family to provide information, discuss the family's options, and request donation. The hospital may choose to have an organ procurement coordinator from the organization approach the family or may choose to have a 'designated requestor' approach the family."[31]

Previous research revealed the importance of discussing specific topics when asking for donation. Siminoff and colleagues found that discussing funeral arrangements and related issues (particularly open-casket services) was associated with favorable responses to donation requests.[32,33] Gallagher also documented that all major religions have stated support for donation.[34]

AUTOPSY

How well informed are families and clinicians about the actual autopsy procedure? Rosenbaum and colleagues conducted a study of current autopsy consent practices in U.S. teaching hospitals by examining autopsy consent forms and surveying the chief residents at those institutions to assess their knowledge and attitudes.[35] More than half the chief residents surveyed reported that they were not knowledgeable about the actual procedures used in the removal of organs or about the tests done on routine autopsies. In addition, although the consent forms used by 85% of the institutions surveyed contained at least 7 of the 10 elements of autopsy consent recommended by the College of American Pathologists, only 7% of forms contained (or were accompanied by) the recommended educational materials for the family and the physician. Moreover, physicians who are poorly educated about autopsies are likely to misinform families and potentially generate medicolegal issues, and several studies reveal that they are also more likely not to request autopsies.

Problems with autopsy consent have caused major scandals in other countries. For example, the failure to obtain adequate permission for autopsy led to major revisions in British medical practice. In September 1999, the president-elect of the British Paediatric Cardiac Association commented that the Alder Hey Children's Hospital in Liverpool had "probably the biggest and best collection" of hearts in the country, triggering a public outcry in the media about whether these organs had been retained with permission. Upon investigation, it was determined that the organs of 3500 children had been removed without parental knowledge or consent and that more than 100,000 organs had been retained by hospitals across England.[36-38] In response to this, the Royal College of Pathologists issued new guidelines for the retention of tissues and organs at autopsy in Britain.[38] These guidelines give relatives the right to refuse permission for organs of the deceased to be used for research, examination, or education. They also recommend that hospitals and medical schools provide training for doctors and other health care staff in obtaining autopsy permission. The updated consent form allows families to limit the extent of the autopsy; agree or refuse to allow organs to be taken for further examination; have tissue or organs disposed of lawfully and respectfully by the hospital or taken away for personal burial; and donate tissue, fluids, or organs for research for an unlimited period.[38]

Rosenbaum and colleagues proposed similar changes in the autopsy consent process. They argued that the autopsy procedure at teaching hospitals continues to be an essential component of clinical care. They further recommended that essential elements of the autopsy consent process include the following components[35]:

1. Resident physicians receive education on the autopsy procedure; limitations to the procedure; and the storage, use, and disposition of organs.
2. Clinicians learn to ask open-ended questions, such as: What are the most important results you would hope to receive from an autopsy? What are the most important concerns that you have about autopsy? Clinicians may not be able to learn all the nuances of different cultural and religious beliefs, but such questions will help elicit these concerns.
3. To accompany and reinforce the educational process, written material should be created and perhaps attached to the consent form to promote self-education before obtaining consent.
4. Teaching physicians must affirm that the requesting physician has the right to request an autopsy by virtue of

his or her involvement in the care of the patient and relationship with the family.

5. It must clearly be communicated to the family that the organs will be kept by the hospital.

PRACTICING PROCEDURES ON NEWLY DECEASED PATIENTS

Is it ethical to practice resuscitation procedures on newly deceased patients? The use of the newly dead to teach procedures is widely practiced in training institutions. One study reported that 39% of training programs in emergency and critical care medicine use newly dead patients to teach various resuscitation procedures (e.g., endotracheal intubation, central catheter placement, pericardiocentesis). Few of these programs obtain either verbal or written consent from the families.[39]

Whether to seek permission from the deceased's relatives has been an issue of intense debate. Some argue that a "don't ask, don't tell" policy is justified. Advocates argue that it is ethically justifiable to perform practice procedures on the newly dead without permission from the family because these procedures cannot harm the deceased, there is substantial social benefit to be gained, and families could not realistically be expected to discuss consent at such a difficult time.[40,41]

Others argue that practicing procedures on newly deceased patients is ethical only when permission is obtained from the family.[39] They believe that although seeking permission from family members to practice resuscitation procedures may cause them additional stress, this does not justify practicing on the dead without consent. They note that the same arguments were advanced more than 100 years ago by physicians trying to explain why they did not seek permission to perform autopsies. Opponents of the surreptitious use of this teaching technique argue that it will further deteriorate the public's trust in the medical profession and ultimately cause more harm than good.

The presumption that it is impractical to require permission to practice procedures on newly deceased patients is not supported by a review of the literature. The only two studies in the literature that examined this concern have found that many families will give permission if asked. McNamara and coworkers found that 26 of 44 families of newly deceased patients (59%) gave permission to perform wire-guided

retrograde intubation in an emergency department setting. The investigators noted that permission was obtained "despite the lack of a prior relationship with the family by the persons requesting consent." Permission was obtained more frequently in unexpected deaths than expected deaths (77% versus 41%, $P = 0.03$).[41] These results are similar to those reported by Benfield and associates, who found that 73% of parents gave permission for the use of their newly deceased children to teach intubation skills in a neonatal ICU, including several parents who consented to the intubation procedures but not an autopsy.[42]

A position statement from the Council on Ethical and Judicial Affairs of the American Medical Association concluded that performing procedures on the newly dead should be allowed, but only in the context of a structured training sequence completed under close supervision, and only after permission from family members has been obtained.[43]

ANNOTATED REFERENCES

American Academy of Pediatrics Committee on Bioethics: Guidelines on forgoing life-sustaining medical treatment. Pediatrics 1994;93:532-536.

> *The official position of the American Academy of Pediatrics on the forgoing of life-sustaining treatment.*

Burns JP, Mitchell C, Outwater KM, et al: End-of-life care in the pediatric intensive care unit after the forgoing of life-sustaining treatment. Crit Care Med 2000;28:3060-3066.

> *The largest observational study of death in the PICU following the withholding or withdrawal of life-sustaining treatments. This study reports on the attitudes and practices of physicians and nurses who provide palliative care. The discussion section has a detailed examination of the doctrine of double effect and the use of neuromuscular blockade in this setting.*

Meisel A, Snyder L, Quill T: American College of Physicians–American Society of Internal Medicine End-of-Life Care Consensus Panel. Seven legal barriers to end-of-life care: Myths, realities, and grains of truth. JAMA 2000;284:2495-2501.

> *An excellent review of common misperceptions about the law in this area.*

Rosenbaum GE, Burns J, Johnson J, et al: Autopsy consent practice at US teaching hospitals: Results of a national survey. Arch Intern Med 2000; 160:374-380.

> *A survey of chief residents' knowledge of the autopsy procedure and a constructive outline for an educational program to improve the consent process.*

Truog RD, Cist AF, Brackett SE, et al: Recommendations for end-of-life care in the intensive care unit: The Ethics Committee of the Society of Critical Care Medicine. Crit Care Med 2001;29:2332-2348.

> *A detailed set of recommendations on how to care for ICU patients following the withholding or withdrawal of life-sustaining treatment covering a wide range of issues, not simply what medications to administer.*

Chapter 255

END-OF-LIFE ISSUES IN THE INTENSIVE CARE UNIT

Nicholas S. Ward • Mitchell M. Levy

KEY POINTS

1. Unlike in previous decades, **more and more people are dying in hospitals and ICUs as opposed to home.** Studies now show that the vast majority of patients who die in the hospital do so only after some limitation has been placed on their care. Other studies show that ICUs, and even physicians, can vary greatly in the frequency with which they limit or withdraw care.

2. **Many studies have tried to demonstrate what accounts for the variability in end-of-life practices.** Various patient characteristics, such as ethnicity, and physician characteristics, such as community-versus university-based status, may impact these decisions, but the data are unclear at this time.

3. Currently, **most decisions to limit care are not made by the patient.** This raises new problems regarding surrogate decision-making. Clearly identifying one legal surrogate can be difficult, and most state laws give few specifics about who can qualify as a surrogate decision-maker. Usually, the decision to limit care is made by the health care team in association with the family.

4. One of the greatest barriers to delivering optimal end-of-life care is the **ability to predict patient outcomes.** Two common instruments that aid in this are severity scores and published outcome data. However, both are fraught with potential error and should not automatically be relied on as accurate predictors of morbidity and mortality.

5. Throughout the world, cultures and people differ in their beliefs about how important medical decisions should be made. Some favor a decision-making model in which the physician makes the majority of the decisions—often referred to as **medical paternalism.** Recently, the United States has been characterized by a model that favors the patient (or surrogate) as the primary decision-maker—referred to as **patient autonomy.** Both systems have advantages as well as drawbacks, and a physician must consider which system is considered "normal" by the patient.

In the last century, the process of dying changed dramatically. Previously, doctors simply did all they could for a patient and when their treatments failed, the patient died, almost always at home. However, with the advent of more sophisticated medical technologies, even patients with severe organ failure can be kept alive. Unfortunately, with this progress has come a new set of complex medical and societal issues.

In the United States, about 80% of people now die in health care facilities (60% in acute care facilities),[1] despite the fact that about 90% of Americans polled say that they would prefer to die at home.[2] This disparity is caused by two factors. One is that many people die while undergoing treatments meant to postpone death—treatments that are often futile. The other reason is that many families are unable to care for a dying person or are uncomfortable having a loved one die at home. The net result of this is that most people will die in a hospital or other health care facility, and many of them will undergo high levels of medical care before death. A recent study showed that about 20% of Americans will die in an ICU or be admitted to an ICU just before death.[3]

Two conclusions can be drawn from the preceding information. One is that a tremendous amount of health care is being delivered to dying patients. This has been reflected in several studies, such as that of Cher and Lenert, which showed that a relatively large percentage of Medicare expenditures goes to treat patients in the last weeks of their lives.[4] The other conclusion is that doctors have to learn a new set of skills that were not necessary in the past. They need to be able to recognize patients who are going to die despite medical care and help decide which of the almost limitless supply of medical therapies available are appropriate and which are not. They need to guide their patients through a maze of medical options in an attempt to balance preservation of life with quality of life—a daunting task, to say the least. This chapter reviews some of the major medical, ethical, and legal issues involved in making these end-of-life decisions.

HOW ARE CRITICALLY ILL PATIENTS DYING?

In 1995, a landmark study in end-of-life issues was published. This was the first large-scale attempt to define how people die in American ICUs. In a two-part study involving 4301 critically ill ICU patients, the investigators examined multiple aspects of end-of-life care and found major short-comings in current practice. Only 47% of the time did the physician know when a patient wanted to avoid cardiopulmonary resuscitation (CPR), and the incidence of dying with moderate or severe pain was 50%.[5]

More insight into the dying experience came in subsequent studies that showed that the vast majority of ICU deaths occur only after a decision to limit care has been made.[6-8] In two important studies, Prendergast and coworkers helped define how patients die in ICUs.[9] In their first study, they compared deaths in their ICU from two periods, 1987 to 1988 and 1992 to 1993, to determine how often CPR was performed before death and how often limits were placed on care before death. Their data showed that the incidence of CPR before death had declined from 49% to 10% and that the incidence of withholding or withdrawing therapy had increased from 51% to 90% of all ICU deaths.

In an effort to benchmark their data with the rest of the country, the same investigators then did a large follow-up study 1 year later. They collected data from more than 6000 patient deaths occurring in 131 ICUs in 38 states over a 6-month period and analyzed the data for the incidence of various limits on care. They found that, on average, only 25% of patients dying in ICUs were given CPR before death. About 70% of patients had some restriction on care, and almost 50% of patients had some medical therapy withheld or withdrawn before death.[6]

The other striking piece of data to emerge from this study was the degree of variability that existed among ICUs. The incidence of patients dying with full aggressive measures ranged from 4% in one ICU to 79% in another. Likewise, the incidence of withdrawing medical support ranged from 0% to 79%, depending on the ICU. These data clearly show that although the overall practice of limiting care in ICUs is common, there is tremendous variability from place to place in end-of-life care.

Interestingly, in 2003, another study examined deaths in 31 ICUs in 17 European countries and found many similarities. Overall, the percentage of patients dying with some limits on care was 72.6%, which was very similar to studies done in the United States. Like in the American studies, there was also tremendous variability in practices among the different ICUs, with rates of CPR before death ranging from 5% to almost 50%.[10]

WHAT ACCOUNTS FOR VARIABILITY IN PRACTICES?

It should not be surprising that there is so much variability in a practice as multidimensional as end-of-life care. Even the standard practice of medicine varies from institution to institution. The decision to limit or not limit care is generally a complex one that may reflect the personal biases of both physician and patient. Many attempts have been made to find patterns among different types of physicians and patients that can explain the variation. For example, one study showed that university-based physicians are more likely than community-based physicians to write do-not-resuscitate (DNR) orders and withhold or withdraw care.[11] A similar study showed that patients without private physicians in the ICU were more likely to undergo active withdrawal of care.[12] Unfortunately, studies like this are meaningless unless one knows the contexts in which these decisions were made.

Withholding care from a terminally ill patient may reflect a weaker physician-patient relationship or a stronger one based on the patient's wishes.

Other studies have sought to explain variation by culture, race, or religion.[13-17] Although such factors may play a role in these important decisions, and there may be some general trends in decision patterns, there is enough variation even within these studies to indicate that one cannot generalize this information to a given individual. Physicians need to be cognizant of the fact that their patients may have markedly different views of optimal end-of-life care, regardless of their culture, religion, or race.

WHO DECIDES?

SURROGATE DECISION-MAKING

As stated earlier, the vast majority of people will die with some limit on care in place, whether in or out of an ICU. Unfortunately, the patient rarely participates in these decisions. Most studies show that someone else makes the decision to limit a dying patient's care 60% to 70% of the time.[8,18] Only about 15% to 20% of patients have advance directives when they are admitted to a hospital, and even when they exist, advance directives are often inadequate to handle anything but the most obvious treatment decisions. Therefore, the burden of these difficult decisions falls to a proxy (a legal delegation) or a surrogate (a nonlegal delegation). Most often, this is a family member.

The process of surrogate decision-making is fraught with problems. Although most would agree that family or friends of the patient are the best people to make such decisions, several studies have shown that patients rarely discuss specific treatment options with their proxies, and surrogate decisions correlate poorly with what the patient would actually want done.[19,20] Further, in a study by Hare and colleagues, it was shown that surrogates often place greater emphasis on certain aspects of dying, such as pain and suffering, than patients do; patients are more concerned with burdening their families and the amount of time left to live.[19]

LEGAL ISSUES

In the United States, all 50 states now recognize the legality of a patient's right to refuse medical care, although there remains some controversy and confusion about specific issues. The legal issues involved in proxy decision-making can also be a source of great confusion. Perhaps realizing that it is impossible to account for the many possible family and social relationships involved, most states have few laws dealing with the issue of medical surrogates and have purposely kept the codes vague and malleable (thoroughly reviewed in reference 21). Most states accept a properly drafted written advance directive as sufficient legal guidance to limit care. Unfortunately, most advance directives or living wills are too vague in their language, using phrases such as "terminal illness" and "little chance of recovery," which are subject to interpretation. Diseases such as chronic obstructive pulmonary disease and congestive heart failure may be considered terminal illnesses by some people but not by others. Some people may consider diseases such as early-stage lung cancer not imminently terminal.

Nevertheless, these directives can be of great help. They can help prevent futile or unwanted care when no other surrogate is available. More often, they are useful in family decision-making when dealing with an unconscious patient facing potentially futile care. The previously stated wishes of the patient in an advance directive can help assuage feelings of guilt or uncertainty regarding end-of-life decisions. They can also be helpful when there is disagreement between surrogates about a course of action. Because a surrogate, by definition, is an agent representing what the patient would decide if he or she were able, the advance directive can be a helpful guide.

Sometimes advance directives can be a source of discord, such as when the written directive differs from what a surrogate decides. In most states, the law recognizes a properly drafted and witnessed directive as the legal opinion that should be followed; however, many physicians are wary of ignoring the requests of a living surrogate, especially if it is a spouse or other close family member. In situations like this, attempts should be made to build consensus among all parties before making any decision. Most state laws regarding written advance directives also allow for some flexibility in the physician's obligation to follow them. They often state that if a physician feels that the directive is of questionable validity or if he or she feels ethically unable to follow the directive, it is not binding.

PREDICTING OUTCOMES

A central problem complicating end-of-life decisions is the difficulty of predicting outcomes in critically ill patients. The combination of multiple coinciding medical problems and rapidly changing clinical status can make this a very difficult task. Essentially, three tools are available to a physician when trying to determine the prognosis of a critically ill patient: published outcomes, severity scores, and personal experience. All these can be helpful, yet all have limitations.

SEVERITY SCORES

Severity scores have been available for almost 3 decades, and much has been learned in that time. In most severity score algorithms, data are collected during the first 24 hours of admission and are then used to compile a score that, theoretically, predicts the risk of death during hospitalization. These scoring systems were developed by reviewing data from thousands of ICU patients and employing logistic regression models to choose some important input variables. Other variables were simply chosen based on presumed clinical value. These scores were then validated prospectively on patients.

Unfortunately, there are several problems with these systems. First, they make predictions based on hospital outcomes at the time of their creation. Thus, as medical treatments improve, the scores need to be updated. In the 1970s, for example, acute respiratory distress syndrome (ARDS) had a mortality rate approaching 80%; thus, its presence might justifiably increase a patient's severity score. These days, ARDS has about a 40% mortality. Thus, a severity scoring system using the diagnosis of ARDS, or even components of the diagnosis such as hypoxemia, would need to be adjusted. Some commercially available proprietary severity scoring systems, such as the Acute Physiology and Chronic Health Evaluation (APACHE III), are updated and revalidated on a regular basis to avoid this problem, but many that are widely used today, such as APACHE II, are based on patient data collected as much as 2 or 3 decades ago.

Another problem with using severity scores is that most models derive their predictions from factors present at or shortly after admission to the ICU and do not provide updated mortality estimates as the patient's condition changes. Further, severity scores often give intermediate mortality estimates such as 60% instead of a clear yes or no answer. Even these numbers are subject to confidence intervals. Perhaps the most glaring problem of using severity scores is that they say nothing about morbidity, disability, or survival after hospitalization. These factors are often just as important as risk of death in making end-of-life decisions. A patient may accept a 30% chance of survival if it were followed by a high quality of life, but not accept a 70% chance of survival if it were likely to entail a poor quality of life.

OUTCOME DATA

Many of the same problems encountered with severity scores characterize the use of outcome data as well. Although published outcome studies are an essential tool for clinicians in predicting a course of illness, they suffer from two major problems. One is that the population studied for a particular illness may not share the same characteristics as a particular patient. For example, in a large, multicenter clinical trial of a new therapy for sepsis, the mortality rate in the control (untreated) population was 31%.[22] It is important to note, however, that this trial excluded patients with conditions such as renal failure, liver failure, pancreatitis, acquired immunodeficiency syndrome (AIDS), and a variety of other comorbid conditions, thus limiting the usefulness of these data for prognostic purposes.

Another problem with using outcome data is the rapidity with which therapies can change and improve. In four published studies by different authors between 1981 and 2000 examining the mortality of *Pneumocystis carinii* pneumonia in ICU patients, the mortality decreased from 86% to approximately 50%.[23] Similar changes in outcome over time have been reported with a variety of other illnesses, such as ARDS, as treatments have improved.

PATIENT AUTONOMY VERSUS MEDICAL PATERNALISM

A central problem with the end-of-life decision-making process is defining the role of the physician. Usually the physician's role is a combination of educator and adviser, but this is not always the case. In the past, physicians were more likely to dictate courses of action or treatment plans for their patients, a concept referred to as *medical paternalism*. In many parts of the world to this day, medical decisions are made this way with little input from the patient or family. In these cultures, patients are often comfortable with this kind of decision-making. More recently in the United States, the concept of *patient autonomy* has dictated medical decision-making. In the extreme form of patient autonomy, the physician's role is only to educate the patient about the problem and offer available treatment plans, along with their risks and benefits. The patient then independently chooses a course of action. Many physicians use this model of practice today, or something similar to it, believing that it empowers patients and frees them from physician bias.

In contrast to this philosophy, many physicians and patients believe that the physician is obliged to recommend a course of action. The physician thus offers several possible courses of action but makes specific recommendations. This model is often referred to as *shared decision-making* and may well represent an ideal blending of the autonomous and paternalistic approach. In this model, caregivers do their best to understand the wishes of their patients. This is accomplished through a process of genuine listening to family members and eliciting their understanding of the wishes of their loved one, then combining that knowledge with the clinician's best guess about the likely prognosis and outcome. Through this process, a clinician can proactively offer an opinion about the appropriate course of therapy. Ultimately, it is up to each individual physician to determine the degree of involvement warranted in end-of-life decisions.

CONCLUSION

It is clear that the process of dying in America is changing rapidly. Although the physician has always had an important role in the dying process, that role has changed. Today's physician not only must be adept at administering comfort measures but also must decide when to initiate those measures rather than other therapies aimed at restoring health. Because the dying process now involves the health care system more and more, physicians need to have good end-of-life skills. Failure to address these issues will result in patients getting more futile care at the expense of their own comfort and increased costs to the health care system.

ANNOTATED REFERENCES

Cook DJ, Guyatt GH, Jaeschke R, et al: Determinants in Canadian health care workers of the decision to withdraw life support from the critically ill. JAMA 1995;273:703-708.
This prospective study identifies several factors that influence the decision to withdraw life support. The most important factors were likelihood of surviving the current episode, likelihood of long-term survival, premorbid cognitive function, and patient age.

Curtis JR, Rubenfeld GR: Managing Death in the ICU. Oxford University Press, New York, 2000.
This comprehensive textbook has contributions from many authors and includes practical suggestions for end-of-life care, as well as philosophical pieces.

Danis M, Federman D, Fins JJ, et al: Incorporating palliative care into critical care education: Principles, challenges, and opportunities. Crit Care Med 1999;27:2005-2013.
This well-written overview describes the fundamental principles of palliative care in the ICU and offers concrete suggestions for building an educational curriculum.

Danis M, Mutran E, Garrett JM: A prospective study of the impact of patient preferences on life-sustaining treatment and hospital cost. Crit Care Med 1996;24:1811-1817.
In this prospective study, patients were asked about life-support preferences and then followed for 6 months. Of interest, there was no significant association between patient desire for life support and the use of these therapies.

Johnson D, Wilson M, Cavanaugh B, et al: Measuring the ability to meet family needs in an intensive care unit. Crit Care Med 1998;26:266-271.
A survey instrument was used to identify the top needs of families of critically ill patients. Continuity of caregiver communication was identified as a priority.

Keenan SP, Busche KD, Chen LM, et al: A retrospective review of a large cohort of patients undergoing the process of withholding or withdrawal of life support. Crit Care Med 1997;22:1020-1025.
This retrospective chart review compared the withholding or withdrawal of life support in community versus teaching hospitals and found no significant difference.

Prendergast TJ, Luce JM: Increasing incidence of withholding and withdrawal of life support from the critically ill. Am J Respir Crit Care Med 1997; 155:15-20.
This important prospective study describes how patients die in ICUs and documents a dramatic increase in the practice of limiting some form of life-support measures in several hospitals over a 5-year period.

SUPPORT principal investigators: A controlled trial to improve care for seriously ill hospitalized patients: The Study to Understand Prognoses and Preferences for Outcomes and Risks of Treatments (SUPPORT). JAMA 1996;274:1591-1598.
In two consecutive 2-year periods, a prospective observational study documented major shortcomings in communication, the frequency of aggressive treatment, and the characteristics of death in the hospital; an intervention study using a nurse to facilitate communication and clinical care of the dying demonstrated essentially no improvement in outcomes.

Chapter 256

DETERMINATION OF DEATH BY NEUROLOGIC CRITERIA

Teresa L. Smith • Thomas P. Bleck

KEY POINTS

1. After certain prerequisites are met, there are three essential components to the determination of death by neurologic criteria: irreversible coma or unresponsiveness; absence of brainstem reflexes; apnea.

2. Patients being examined for a determination of death by neurologic criteria will all be on ventilatory assistance. The gag response can be difficult to determine in patients with endotracheal tubes in place.

3. Demonstration of lack of intracranial flow on angiography can be used to confirm death by neurologic criteria.

4. The determination of death by neurologic criteria has some differences in children.

5. Local laws and regulations should be understood before a determination of death by neurologic criteria is made.

Determination of death by neurologic criteria is a clinical diagnosis. After certain prerequisites are met, there are three essential components to the determination: irreversible coma or unresponsiveness, absence of brainstem reflexes, and apnea. Before the diagnosis is made, it is essential to rule out alternative causes of the patient's neurologic status, including hypothermia, drug-induced coma, and severe metabolic disarray.

PREREQUISITES

Determination of death can be made in patients who continue to have cardiac function during mechanical ventilation in the appropriate clinical scenario. A clear irreversible cause must be known based on history, brain imaging, or cerebrospinal fluid examination. Determination of death by neurologic criteria cannot be made in patients with a temperature below 32°C or in those who may have drug intoxications or poisoning without a confirmatory study indicating the absence of intracranial blood flow. If neuromuscular junction blocking agents have been administered, electrical stimulation should be performed to document the presence of transmission at the neuromuscular junction. Severe acid-base, electrolyte, or endocrine abnormalities also may not be present.

UNRESPONSIVENESS

The examination shows that the patient has no eye movements or motor response to verbal or noxious stimulation, with the exception of spinally mediated responses. Standard points of pressure application for administration of noxious stimuli are nailbeds, supraorbital nerve, and temporomandibular joint.[1]

ABSENCE OF BRAINSTEM REFLEXES

PUPILLARY RESPONSE

Pupillary responsiveness should be assessed using a bright flashlight. Using an ophthalmoscope allows for magnification of the iris and pupil so that even a subtle response can be detected. Pupils are usually mid-position (4-6 cm in diameter); rarely, they may be more dilated if spinal sympathetic pathways are intact.

FACIAL SENSATION AND MOTOR RESPONSE

A very gentle stimulus such as a wisp of cotton should be gently touched to the cornea of each eye individually. We prefer to use a small squirt of saline from the small plastic containers used for saline administration during airway suctioning, as the saline will not harm the cornea. In patients with a diagnosis of death by neurologic criteria, no blink will be induced. There can be no grimace to painful stimuli or jaw reflex.

GAG AND COUGH REFLEXES

Patients being examined for a determination of death by neurologic criteria will all be on ventilatory assistance. The gag response can be difficult to determine in patients with endotracheal tubes in place. The endotracheal tube itself should not be maneuvered to stimulate a gag response, as this could lead to tracheal damage; a tongue blade should be used instead. Cough in response to deep bronchial suctioning should be sought. Absence of these responses is required for a determination of death by neurologic criteria.

ASSESSMENT OF EYE MOVEMENTS

Cervico-Ocular Reflexes ("doll's-eyes maneuver"; only performed in the absence of cervical instability). With the eyes held open, the head should be briskly turned from side to side (mid-position to 90 degrees), looking for any eye movements. If an endotracheal tube is in place, it should be moved together with the head movements to avoid tracheal damage or unplanned extubation. No eye movements occur in patients with a diagnosis of death by neurologic criteria. The term *doll's eyes* refers to the expected horizontal movement in the direction opposite to the head movement, indicating that the brainstem centers for conjugate horizontal gaze are functional but the cerebral cortex is not controlling them. However, the likelihood of inaccurate use of this term is so great that it should be avoided.

Vestibulo-Ocular Reflexes ("cold calorics"). Once the absence of the cervico-ocular reflex is determined, or in circumstances in which it cannot be tested due to cervical instability, caloric testing should be performed. First, the tympanic membranes are examined for perforations and to ensure that no obstructions are present. The caloric test is sufficiently important, however, that it should proceed when death by neurologic criteria is being proved even if a perforation is present. The head of the bed should be elevated to 30 degrees. Ice cold water, 50 mL, should be placed in a syringe. Soft tubing connected to the syringe (for instance, from a butterfly intravenous line) should be inserted into the external auditory canal, and the water irrigated into the ear while the patient's eyelids are held open. In cases of coma with intact brainstem pathways, the eyes should deviate toward the side of the cold water instillation. Absence of any eye movement will be present in a case of death by neurologic criteria. The eyes should be scrutinized for 1 minute after the cessation of ice water irrigation. After 5 minutes, the identical procedure should be repeated for the opposite ear.

APNEA TESTING

Before a formal apnea test is conducted, the patient should have fulfilled all of the previously discussed criteria for death by neurologic criteria. Severe chronic obstructive pulmonary disease or morbid obesity should not be present. Care should be taken to ensure that the patient has a systolic blood pressure of at least 90 mm Hg, has an adequate intravascular volume, and is treated with vasopressin if diabetes insipidus is suspected.

The patient should be preoxygenated to a PaO_2 exceeding 200 mm Hg. The ventilator should be disconnected, and 100% oxygen at a rate of 6 L/min placed at the carina or delivered directly into the trachea. Alternatively, 10 cm continuous positive airway pressure may be used. Maximal respiratory drive is believed to occur with a $PaCO_2$ of 60 mm Hg, which should occur within 8 minutes after disconnection.[1] The patient is observed during this period for respiratory movements, and the electrocardiographic monitor examined for signs of respiratory artifact. If an arterial blood gas assessment shows a $PaCO_2$ exceeding 60 mm Hg with continued apnea, the diagnosis of death by neurologic criteria is completed. The pH is the major determinant of respiratory drive, and if the patient's baseline $PaCO_2$ is markedly abnormal, the equivalent change in the arterial pH should be employed.

If cardiac arrhythmias, hypotension, or arterial desaturation ensue, apnea testing is abandoned, and a confirmatory test must then be performed.

CONFIRMATORY TESTING

If apnea testing is not possible or cannot be completed, or if specific brainstem function testing is not possible, a confirmatory test must be performed. Numerous tests are available. Ranked from highest to lowest sensitivities, they are angiography, electroencephalography, transcranial Doppler echography, technetium-99m hexamethylpropyleneamineoxime (^{99m}Tc-HMPAO) brain scan (single photon emission computed tomography), and somatosensory evoked potentials.[2]

Cerebral Angiography. Demonstration of lack of intracranial flow on angiography can be used to confirm death by neurologic criteria. Internal carotid artery flow usually stops shortly after the carotid bifurcation.[3] Vertebral flow usually stops at the atlanto-occipital junction.

Electroencephalography. Confirmation of death by neurologic criteria can be made by establishing electrocerebral silence by electroencephalography (EEG). Since the EEG is affected by the same confounding factors as the physical examination (hypothermia and sedative drugs), it should be used only when such confounding factors have been disproved. Tracings are performed for at least 30 minutes with these settings: sensitivity greater than 2 μV/mm, high-frequency filter greater than 30 Hz, low-frequency filter less than 1 Hz, interelectrode impedance less than 10,000 Ohms, and a minimum of eight scalp electrodes placed at least 10 cm apart. Guidelines for the minimal technical criteria for using EEG in confirming the diagnosis of death by neurologic criteria are available.[4]

Transcranial Doppler Blood Flow Velocity Measurement. Transcranial Doppler echography can also be used to confirm death by neurologic criteria. Early transcranial Doppler findings include oscillating flow signifying nearly equal forward and reverse flow, followed by small systolic spike pattern suggesting lack of diastolic flow from severely increased intracranial pressure, and finally no signal. Because the absence of the transcranial Doppler signal can be due to technical difficulties, extracranial oscillating flow can be helpful when no signal is detected intracranially. Sensitivity and specificity for detecting death by neurologic criteria have been found to be 91.3% and 100%, respectively, when compared with the EEG.[5] Guidelines for the use of transcranial Doppler in confirming the diagnosis of death by neurologic criteria include two separate examinations at least 30 minutes apart demonstrating bilateral oscillating flow or systolic spikes in conjunction with bilateral common carotid artery, internal carotid artery, and vertebral artery oscillating flow.[6]

Single Photon Emission Computed Tomography. Single photon emission computed tomography with ^{99m}Tc-HMPAO can be used to document absent intracranial flow as noted by absent uptake of the tracer, which is administered 15 to 20 minutes prior to the scan.[7] This gives the appearance of an "empty skull."

Somatosensory Evoked Potentials. Somatosensory evoked potentials are useful in predicting outcome in patients who are comatose. N20 potentials are typically absent in those who have a diagnosis of death by neurologic criteria but are also absent in 15% to 20% of those who are comatose but do not have the diagnosis of death by neurologic criteria.

Other Tests. Magnetic resonance angiography and computed tomography angiography can show absence of intracranial flow, but experience with these modalities is limited.

CHILDREN

The determination of death by neurologic criteria has some differences in children. For those between 7 days and 2 months of age, two examinations and EEGs should be performed at least 48 hours apart. For those 2 months to 1 year of age, a second examination and EEG are required 24 hours after the first, unless a radionuclide angiographic study fails to visualize cerebral vessels. For those older than 1 year, a repeat examination after 12 hours is typically recommended. In the case of hypoxic-ischemic cause, a longer period of observation is often recommended, unless a confirmatory test is performed.[8]

REGIONAL RULES AND LAWS

Unfortunately, there has been no standardization of legal determination of death by neurologic criteria internationally or even among the states in the United States. The basis for laws concerning the determination of death by neurologic criteria in most states is the Uniform Determination of Death Act, which indicates that death can be determined by irreversible lack of all brain function made in accordance with accepted medical standards. In 1995, the American Academy of Neurology published guidelines for the determination of death by neurologic criteria.[2] Individual institutions and some states have required additional standards to these guidelines. Local laws and regulations should be understood before a determination of death by neurologic criteria is made.

ANNOTATED REFERENCES

American Electroencephalographic Society: Guidelines three: Minimum technical standards for EEG recording in suspected cerebral death. J Clin Neurophysiol 1994;11:10-13.
> Guidelines for the determination of brain death in children. Pediatrics 1987;80:298-300.

The Quality Standards Subcommittee of the American Academy of Neurology: Practice parameters for determining brain death in adults (summary statement). Neurology 1995;45:1012-1014.
> These provide guidelines for determining death by neurologic criteria.

Section XVI

ORGANIZATION, MANAGEMENT, AND EDUCATION

Chapter 257

BUILDING BEDSIDE COLLABORATIVE PRACTICE

Connie Jastremski • Maurene A. Harvey

KEY POINTS

1. As care has become more complex for the critically ill patient, mechanisms to integrate complex behavior into a functional whole have become increasingly important. Accordingly, **harmonious and efficient integration of personnel** and their respective tasks in critical care is an important goal to ensure optimal delivery of intensive care.

2. **Organizational structures and process impact patient care outcomes.** These processes include open communication and collegial relationships among members of the care team, especially nurses and physicians.

3. **Important components of collaborative practice** include trust, communication, role negotiation, competence, accountability, and conflict resolution.

4. **Five characteristics** of the multidisciplinary collaborative approach to ICU care include:

   a. Medical and nursing directors with authority and co-responsibility for ICU management

   b. Nursing, respiratory therapy, and pharmacy collaboration with medical staff in a team approach to care

   c. Use of standards, protocols, and guidelines to ensure consistent approach to medical, nursing, and technical issues

   d. Dedication to coordination and communication for all aspects of ICU management

   e. Emphasis on practitioner certification, research, education, ethical issues, and patient advocacy

5. A detailed description of the multidisciplinary approach to critical care practice has been further outlined by the **American College of Critical Care Medicine** (ACCM) in its recommendations for services and personnel required to perform critical care medicine for adults.

6. A **strong ongoing commitment from hospital administration** and the nursing, medicine, pharmacy, and respiratory therapy departments is essential for the continued development of the collaborative practice model.

7. Multiple published articles have stated that the presence of a team of health care professionals from various disciplines working in concert **may improve efficiency, outcomes of care, and the costs of care for the ICU patients.**

8. Collaborative practice teams serve as the vehicle to **facilitate the outcomes management process.**

9. Collaboration allows all members of the health care team to participate fully in care delivery by **bringing their unique knowledge and skills to the process.**

As we entered the 21st century, health care was faced with its greatest challenges to date. In 1999 the Institute of Medicine (IOM) reported the in-depth study, "To Err is Human, Building a Safer Health Care System," which mandated action for needed change to improve health care safety.[1,2] The aging of the population has strained the health care system and has produced a greater demand for critical care services. Over 5 million patients are admitted annually to an ICU in the United States. At the same time that demand appears to be rising there are fewer critical care practitioners, physicians, nurses, and others to provide the necessary care, with the prediction that the problem will only become worse in the future. Health care professionals are very concerned about fragmented impersonal care related to being asked to do more with less.[3] We now operate in an increasingly sophisticated environment in which specialization and communication have dominant influences on human activity. As the division of labor increases in our society, mechanisms to integrate complex behavior into a functional whole become increasingly important. Accordingly, harmonious and efficient integration of personnel and their respective tasks in the critical care environment is an important goal to ensure optimal delivery of intensive care. In this chapter, we explore the traditional hierarchy of medical care and present-day barriers to collaborative practice in critical care, data that support the improvement in outcomes in a collaborative environment, techniques to implement collaborative practice, and the need to collaborate beyond the medical team and include families.

HISTORICAL PERSPECTIVE

Hospitals have traditionally been places where departments of professionals have had their own ways of functioning, frequently in isolation and without the understanding of or cooperation with other departments. The result of this system of care has often been the delivery of fragmented, inefficient, costly, and potentially harmful care.[4] The inertia displayed by the health care system to adopt collaborative practice seems rooted in the trusteeship for health care that has been assumed by physicians,[5] who traditionally have directed all aspects of care in a vertical hierarchy in which communication and planning are unidirectional. This arrangement has fostered conflict among other health care team professionals, who have operated under a restricted scope of activities and have been dependent on physicians' directives for providing various aspects of care (Fig. 257-1).

Recent changes in practice environments, however, have led to greater recognition and reliance on the knowledge, expertise, and services of the other practitioners in the ICU, especially professional nurses. In fact, patients are often admitted to hospitals because they require nursing care. One of the biggest secrets in U.S. health care today is that the medical care of our most vulnerable patients is being managed by nurses.[6] In addition, as nurses and other care professionals involved in critical care (e.g., respiratory therapists, pharmacists, and dieticians) have developed distinctive identities through parallel research and professional activities, their contributions have ever more affected patient management. This evolution has necessitated the development of integrated health care practices and the sharing of knowledge across the disciplines. Moreover, as society assumes a larger role in shaping health care policy, health care providers find themselves under increasing economic and regulatory pressure to provide comprehensive, efficient, effective, and safe care. Both regulatory and accrediting agencies, including the Joint Commission on the Accreditation of Healthcare Organizations (JCAHO), have increased their emphasis on the importance of collaboration to obtain quality outcomes of care. Although the need for a smoothly functioning team effort is self-evident in the critical care setting, several factors can hamper the achievement of harmonious coordination of care in the ICU.

We are in the midst of a revolution that is permanently altering how health care is delivered and how its quality is assessed. There is now an emphasis in the United States on primary preventive and holistic care, and the impact of the managed care efforts has substantially altered the roles and philosophies of many health care professionals. The patients who are actually admitted to the hospital today are acutely ill and require intense care in shorter hospitalizations.

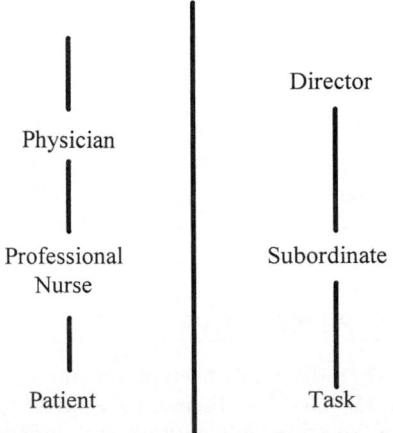

FIGURE 257–1. Traditional, hierarchical medical model of care.

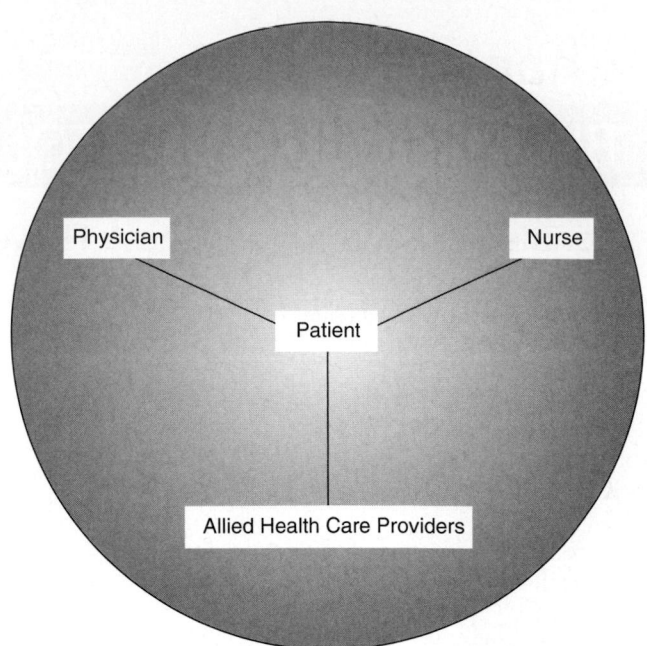

FIGURE 257–2. Collaborative or horizontal medical model of care.

Outcomes research, patient autonomy and advocacy, and a heightened awareness of ethical issues have eroded the paternalistic image of the physicians, and many physicians feel a loss of autonomy in practice today. Increasing numbers of physicians are now employed, and the distinction between ambulatory practice and the services provided in hospitals continues to shape the economics and careers of health care professionals. The impact of managed care and the third-party payers has affected bedside decision making as caregivers struggle to observe fiscal restraint without compromising quality of care.[7] This struggle appears to be exacerbated in the critical care environment.

Clinicians and managers in a variety of health care delivery organizations are convinced that organizational structures and processes affect patient care outcomes.[8] These processes include open communication among members of the care team, especially nurses and physicians, and collegial relationships. The flow of information between health care providers of different degrees of status (e.g., between nurses and physicians) is of particular relevance to effective teamwork (collaboration) in the ICU, because research has shown that individuals lower in a hierarchy often are not asked for relevant information that only they have.[9,10] The emphasis in collaborative practice is on the provision of care to patients. Collaborative practice can be described as the practice of forming partnerships to provide the care needed by the patients (Fig. 257-2).[11] The need to collaborate in the delivery of care has also been fostered by the widespread development and use of clinical pathways that require positive interprofessional relationships, respect for the contributions of other team members, problem-solving skills, and partnering for quality outcomes.

COMPONENTS OF COLLABORATIVE PRACTICE

In the broadest sense, collaboration is defined as working together.[3,12] Important components of the collaborative process include trust, communication, role negotiation, competence, accountability, and conflict resolution. Baggs identifies six critical elements in collaborative practice between physicians and nurses[3,11,13]:

1. Cooperation
2. Assertiveness
3. Shared decision making
4. Communication
5. Joint planning
6. Coordination

The development of collaboration using these essential factors has a natural history, beginning with the movement away from practice in isolation toward practice in concert with other health care providers. Increasing contact favors open communication, which is essential for staff development. Increasing contact can automatically lead to greater collaboration and communications whether or not they are consciously pursued. Communication is much more likely to be optimal, however, when it reflects a deliberate effort to identify and clarify goals and to focus efforts on patient outcomes.[14] Through the exchange of ideas and expertise, practitioners become familiar with the nature and scope of one another's practice. In this way each practitioner is better able to assess individual competence. Once clinical expertise is demonstrated, trust can be established and negotiation of new roles for all care team members in the critical care environment is possible.

Collaboration focuses on trying to reach agreements among divergent opinions to accomplish mutual goals. Weiss suggests that the conflicts between nurses and physicians are due to the overlapping nature of their domains and the lack of clarification of their respective roles.[14] Both professions have dependent, independent, and interdependent roles in the ICU. Adding to the difficulty of achieving agreement, doctors and nurses use different methods to resolve conflict. When resolving differences, physicians tend to bargain or negotiate and nurses avoid, accommodate, or compete.[15] It appears that collaboration in the ICU is difficult owing to the inherent differences in the nature and roles of the care providers, especially physicians and nurses.

MILESTONES IN NURSE-PHYSICIAN COLLABORATION

In the late 1960s and early 1970s, the social dimension of the nurse-physician was explored in many studies.[3,15,16] Physicians clearly had a dominant position in the hospital environment and both nurses' and physicians' behavior at the time preserved this order. In response to emerging interest in collaboration in 1972, the American Medical Association and the American Nurses Association formed the National Joint Practice Commission (NJPC) to identify factors that would promote close working relationships.[17,18] The NJPC identified five essential prerequisites to effect a collaborative practice environment: communication, competence, accountability, trust, and administrative support.[18]

In 1977, under the guidance of the NJPC, a demonstration project was developed in which clinical elements incorporating the prerequisites were introduced simultaneously into certain hospital settings. Several years after the practice environments were restructured, participants were surveyed about their preferences in practice models. Although objective measures of performance were not obtained, general support was expressed for collaborative practice and satisfaction with patient outcomes was high among those involved in the demonstration project.[19]

Following the NJPC's lead, the Society of Critical Care Medicine (SCCM) and the American Association of Critical Care Nurses (AACN) established a task force to identify factors necessary to foster collaboration in the intensive care environments. The task force, named the Interorganization Liaison Group (ILG), developed a position paper on joint practice in the ICU that was subsequently adopted by both parent organizations. The statement was released in 1982 (Table 257-1) and has been periodically revisited for revision and reaffirmation of the position. The statement stressed the importance of physician and nurse autonomy in their

---

TABLE 257–1. JOINTLY APPROVED SOCIETY OF CRITICAL CARE MEDICINE/AMERICAN ASSOCIATION OF CRITICAL CARE NURSES POSITION STATEMENT—1982

Principles:

1. Responsibility and accountability for effective functioning of critical care unit must be vested in physician and nurse directors who are on an equal decision-making level.
2. These directors must be appropriately prepared and educated. In addition to competence in patient management, they need knowledge and experience in the following areas: management principles, resource management, and skills in interpersonal relationships (including conflict resolution).
3. The organizational structure of a critical care unit must ensure that physicians are autonomous when dealing with issues that affect medical practice.
4. The organizational structure of a critical care unit must ensure that nurses are autonomous when dealing with issues that affect nursing practice.
5. Some aspects of patient care require interdependence between physicians and nurses. These aspects must be identified and addressed jointly.
6. Every critically ill person requires medical and nursing care. The services of additional disciplines may also be required in specific situations. To provide a holistic approach, the care delivered by other health team members must be coordinated by the physician and nurse directors.
7. Unit support services must be organized to enable the directors to optimally carry out their primary responsibilities in the practice of their respective disciplines (i.e., patient care).
8. The directors are accountable for the evaluation of the quality and efficiency of care and the financial provision of that care. They must develop a unit-specific system for the evaluation of care on a timely basis.
9. The directors are responsible for creating and maintaining an environment in which individuals have opportunities to realize their potential.
10. Close collaboration between the directors is essential for successful management. This collaboration can be enhanced by daily rounds, weekly meetings, and other means that will ensure continuous, open communication.

respective fields and of accountability of all health care professionals. The statement also affirmed that nurse and physician directors of a unit should have equal authority in the organization of critical care units.[20] These societies continue to explore various practice models as part of their ongoing commitment to problem solving in the issues facing critical care practitioners. The final revision of the joint position statement was published in 1994.[21] The original ILG no longer exists, but a new group that includes the American College of Chest Physicians (ACCP) and the American Thoracic Society (ATS) has continued to work on improving collaboration. These organizations are joining forces now to establish programs with the intensivist-led expert multidisciplinary team as the core component.[6]

Endorsement of a multidisciplinary approach to critical care also came from a consensus conference held at the National Institutes of Health (NIH) in Washington, DC, in 1983.[22] Collegial practice was supported at all levels, and the conference attendees recommended that the organizational structure of an ICU promote collaboration. In addition, as was mentioned earlier, the JCAHO has recognized the value of integrated practice and has endorsed collaboration, especially in the area of patient care and quality improvement.

COMPONENTS OF COLLABORATION

Certain components must exist if a collaborative model is to be successful. Collaboration is about relationships—so many of the elements of a good friendship, marriage, or partnership also promote collaboration.

Trust is the most important characteristic of a collaborative relationship.[3] The ability to trust by the members of the multidisciplinary team will allow for open discussion of issues. There must also be the element of respect for each member and for his or her profession and recognition of each member's knowledge and judgment. The recognition of the skills and knowledge of all of the members of the team will allow for decision making in a collaborative manner. In a collaborative practice, responsibility is shared, so that goal setting and decision making occur jointly. No member will always get his or her way, but an understanding is established to achieve the best outcome for the patients. The collaborative partners must be good listeners and must possess effective communication skills so that discussion and decision making are enhanced.

In a collaborative practice environment, authority and autonomy for decision making are given to the professional with the expertise. Structures and processes must be in place to ensure that autonomy is preserved. Administrative support is necessary to allow for the decision-making model to work successfully. Collegiality and cohesiveness will supercede competition in a patient-focused collaborative practice.

Competence is another critical component of collaboration. Incompetence destroys trust and respect, and undermines independent thinking, thus preventing collaboration.[3] All members of the multidisciplinary team should demonstrate their competence during shared decision making but also demonstrate flexibility so as not to block collaboration. Flexibility is also inherent in negotiation and compromise and does contribute to the overall sense of the collaboration effort.

Carlson and his colleagues outline five characteristics of the multidisciplinary, collaborative approach to ICU care[1,23]:

1. Medical and nursing directors with authority and co-responsibility for ICU management
2. Nursing, respiratory therapy, and pharmacy collaboration with medical staff in a team approach
3. Use of standards, protocols, and guidelines to ensure a consistent approach to medical, nursing, and technical issues
4. Dedication to coordination and communication for all aspects of ICU management
5. Emphasis on practitioner certification, research, education, ethical issues, and patient advocacy

GOALS OF COLLABORATION

There are multiple goals in a collaborative practice model. The most important goal is to provide superior patient care by utilizing the unique expertise of all of the professionals on the multidisciplinary team. Many studies have demonstrated improved patient outcomes.[24-32] Interdisciplinary collaboration affects patient outcomes in part because trust and respect between and among professional staff enhance communication about patient issues, affect the authority of nursing and physician directors to manage the unit as they think best, and increase staff retention.[32]

Productivity is enhanced by the improved communication among the staff caring for the critically ill. In Henneman and colleagues' study on a collaborative approach to weaning, the ability of the nurses and respiratory therapists to work together in managing the patient plan of care was highlighted as one reason for the reduced duration of mechanical ventilation.[27,28] Everyone on the collaborative team works together, which increases productivity across the disciplines and decreases repetition across the disciplines. There is a more efficient use of personnel in the collaborative practice model. Cost savings may also be achieved as a result of collaborative quality improvement efforts in the ICU. Many studies have reported reduction in the length of stay in various patient populations, including neonates and mechanically ventilated patients.[26-29,32-37]

In 1986, Knaus and his colleagues described the outcomes from different ICUs in 13 major medical centers. One finding of this sentinel work was that the units where staff, particularly the nursing staff, were organized in a collaborative practice model had higher staff satisfaction and nurse retention than units without collaboration.[32] This finding was validated by the AACN in their Demonstration Project conducted in 1988.[24] Mitchell and her team found that in the ideal ICU, nurses had a great deal of autonomy regarding care of the patients and they were part of a collaborative practice team. Staff satisfaction is highest when staff members are recognized for the knowledge and skill they bring to the care of the patients. Along with recognition comes a trust and communication system with a great deal of respect for all of the care providers on the team.

Two tragic medication errors at the Dana-Farber Cancer Institute (DCFI) in 1995 forced this world-renowned center to reexamine and create systems and processes to improve the delivery of care and the commitment to safety. It was recognized early in their work that patient safety cannot be accomplished without an interdisciplinary collaborative approach.[30] Multidisciplinary patient safety rounds, regular multidisciplinary meetings to address patient care and practice standards, and creation of a culture of collaborative care improved the care at that institution. The need to address error and risk in health care came to light after the IOM report of 1999 that stated that as many as 98,000 people die in hospitals each year as a result of medical errors that could have been prevented.[33] Creating an environment within the health care system to ensure the safest collaborative care model is the responsibility of every nurse, physician, pharmacist, and administrator. The second IOM report, "Crossing the Quality Chasm,"[34] highlights the importance of the commitment to high quality system improvement through creation of a culture of strong interdisciplinary collaborative practice.[30]

IMPLEMENTING COLLABORATIVE PRACTICE

Collaborative practices do not arise spontaneously but grow out of commitment to a cooperative enterprise and dedication to common goals. These themes must be anchored in an organizational and managerial structure that facilitates team building.[36] The organizational factors identified by the NJPC that contribute to collaboration include primary nursing and clear definitions of the unit's environment. That is, each unit must identify the patient population it serves best and strive to minimize care for patients who do not "match" the facilities and expertise of the unit.

Organizational characteristics and managerial methods have been related to productivity, quality, and other patient outcomes. As previously cited, Knaus and others found that specific management features, including an intensivist in the ICU and the presence of a team of health care professionals from various disciplines working in concert, resulted in improved patient and staff outcomes. A detailed description of this multidisciplinary approach to critical care practice have been further outlined by the American College of Critical Care Medicine (ACCM) in their recommendations for services and personnel required to provide critical care medicine to adults.[1]

Defining the nature of the population served is a key consideration in the implementation of primary nursing in a critical care setting. If patient needs are accurately characterized, then nursing requirements can be assessed, mechanisms can be developed to adjust to changing patient acuity, and teams can be created that have the necessary skills to care for the patients. Controlled access through clearly articulated admission and discharge criteria helps to define unit goals and preserve unit integrity.

Managerial factors can be divided into two broad categories: (1) programming and (2) feedback mechanisms. Programming involves standardization of work and skills (i.e. development of protocols and procedures) to enable the organization to respond to routine situations in a predictable manner. Through the development of stereotypical responses, a high level of staff coordination and cooperation can be achieved.

Feedback mechanisms become important when novel situations are encountered. In the ICU environment, much patient instability and uncertainty about outcomes often exist. In these instances, preprogrammed responses, such as care maps or pathways, cannot be relied on to cover all contingencies. Thus, the organizational structure must allow for discretionary activity, means for self-adjustment, and development. Standardization of knowledge and skills are important first steps in this process. Dedication to coordination of care and communication in all aspects of ICU management contribute to improved patient outcomes.[1]

Incorporating the collaborative team concepts into the day-to-day activities of critical care units continues to be a challenge. The mere fact that work groups recognize the need to collaborate does not ensure that they will possess the skills and qualities needed to achieve collaboration. Nursing staff, medical staff, pharmacists, respiratory therapists, and families must all become a part of the collaborative effort in the ICU. In the process of developing the collaborative framework, the team members must discuss the issues surrounding the change in culture collaborative practice brings. The team needs shared vision and values and must determine how conflicts will be resolved. The collaborative partners will define the practice model that will guide the teams' standards of care, protocol development, and day-to-day caring for patients.

Other significant steps to improve collaboration that were endorsed by the NJPC include integration of the patient practice committees, an integrated medical record, and creation of joint care review panels.[17] Implementation of an integrated medical record obviates physician, nurse, and respiratory documentation all being on separate notes. Of course, computerization and point of care charting are facilitating the attainment of an integrated medical record. The ability to understand how everyone on the team views the patient and documents the procedures being completed in patient care and other information needed to plan care improves and expedites treatment.

The next step in implementation is the adoption of independent, clinical decision making, which allows the nursing staff, pharmacists, and respiratory therapists to take full advantage of their clinical skills. Areas in which independent assessment and judgment may be employed must be clearly delineated. Practice policies should be developed by the team and should reflect the appropriate evidenced-based practices for each of the disciplines on the team in keeping with legislated practice boundaries. Although many ICUs currently have routine multidisciplinary rounds, some are simply designed to meet the JCAHO requirements or to focus on cost containment. In units with a culture that embraces collaboration, these rounds encourage a team approach to outcomes established for the patient.

A strong ongoing commitment from hospital administration and the nursing, medicine, pharmacy, and respiratory departments is essential for the continued development of the collaborative practice model. Such commitment may take the form of seminars and workshops that define areas of competence, update skills, or stress concepts of professional practice. Support can also be demonstrated through the creation of practice committees, like the ICU committee, composed of all disciplines represented in the care of the critically ill patient charged to monitor the team relationships and to develop strategies that support the collaborative practice. Through ongoing self-examination, these groups develop a certain structure, definition, and direction that deflects attention from the individual discipline to the team members to sharpen the focus of health care delivery in the unit.

The model can be also be strengthened through collaborative record review in which members of the collaborative team scrutinize care provided to the patients. This is an expansion from the original NJPC recommendation of nurse-physician joint review. This form of collaboration affords an opportunity to develop formal and informal clinical case conferences with a multidisciplinary focus to examine all aspects of care for patients chosen for discussion and facilitates the development of group competence.

Despite the belief that collaboration in care is better for staff, patients, and the organization there are many barriers to successful implementation of collaborative practice. These barriers can be divided into three categories: problems with attitude, behavior, or the system.[3]

Attitude problems in any of the partners on the collaborative team can create dysfunction within the team and make collaboration very difficult. Chauvinism can create real trust issues and loss of mutual respect. The member who believes that he or she is the only one who can make a decision or who must control all of the patient care decisions is not a team player, and the collaboration will stop in this situation. Defensive attitudes are generally related to inexperience or immaturity and can stop communication. Acting out with anger or hostility can be related to feeling threatened by members of the team. Each of these attitudes will inevitably block the collaborative efforts because the recipients of any of these attitudes will become frustrated and stop participating.

If a team member demonstrates unilateral, isolated, and independent action as the normal way of behaving, then collaboration will not happen. These behaviors exclude the other team members from planning and therefore are not mutual or shared. Domineering or exploitative behaviors block open communication, which creates a poor collaborative environment. The inability of a team member to handle stress will be seen by other team members as blocking collaboration, especially if the team member is acting out.

A common system barrier to collaboration comes from the way in which various members of the collaborative team, including the administrator, have been socialized and educated in their respective professions. Most professionals are not taught to collaborate with people in other professional roles. There may be little mutual understanding of the roles and the impact each professional has on patient outcomes. A lack of mutual respect for all team members can be a barrier to collaboration. Another system barrier can exist if the administration is not supportive of collaborative practice. It may fail to recognize the importance of a group of professionals working together to improve patient outcomes and may discourage team meetings. It is essential that administration supports collaboration; otherwise, these efforts will fail. The barriers to collaboration are multiple and complex. If attitude, behavioral, or system barriers are allowed to persist, collaborative practice will not be successful and care in the ICU may be negatively impacted. Mechanisms need to be established to evaluate the culture and environment, with particular attention to the barriers that may be preventing sustained collaboration.

OUTCOMES OF COLLABORATIVE PRACTICE

PATIENT OUTCOMES

Multiple published articles have stated that the presence of a team of health care professionals from various disciplines, working in concert, may improve efficiency, outcome, and the cost of care for the ICU patients.[1,8,21-30,33,38-42] It has become very evident over the years that collaborative practice improves team effectiveness, which also impacts patient outcomes positively. The best known data on collaboration and patient outcome were published by Knaus and his colleagues

and suggested that collaboration between physicians and nurses in an ICU had a positive effect on patient outcomes, including a decreased mortality rate.[32] The AACN Demonstration Project reported that nurse/physician collaboration was one of the factors influencing both patient care cost and effectiveness.[24] Including patients and families as a part of the team is also associated with better patient outcomes and improved satisfaction with the care received.[42,43]

NURSE OUTCOMES

In collaborative practice, nurses enjoy a heightened professionalism and participate as equals in decision making. According to the ACCM, the medical director and nursing director have authority and co-responsibility for the ICU management and collaborate in the education, structure, and evaluation of the collaborative team.[1] This leadership role is empowering to all ICU nurses. With increased confidence comes increased autonomy in practice. Studies that reviewed factors affecting nursing retention have demonstrated that collaborative practice ranks high among the qualities that nurses deem important because of increased job satisfaction.[46,47] Collaboration allows nurses to work more effectively and productively as a part of a multidisciplinary team and to work under more consistently applied policies and standards. Collaboration also affords nurses increased opportunities for collaborative education and research. Finally, collaboration tends to enhance resolution of ethical dilemmas.[3]

PHYSICIAN OUTCOMES

Collaborative practice benefits physicians in many of the same ways it does nurses. Collaboration enhances physician productivity and efficiency. There is increased job satisfaction reported by physicians who work in a collaborative practice unit, with decreased stress, tension, and turnover reported.[3] Through enhanced interprofessional communication, physicians have an increased understanding of what the roles of the other care providers in the ICU contribute to the patient outcomes. As for the nurses, dealing with ethical dilemmas is easier with the open communications fostered in the collaborative environment.

ADMINISTRATOR OUTCOMES

The administrator also benefits from a collaborative practice model in critical care. Health care costs are known to be lower owing to reduced patient lengths of stay, increased productivity, and fewer patient complications. Decreased staff turnover due to a more satisfied workforce is another administrative benefit of collaboration. Increased patient and family satisfaction is another desirable outcome for the administration because this fosters a better community image and less litigation. Administrators are encouraged to come to some of the collaborative multidisciplinary rounds to observe the effectiveness of the team and to learn the complexities of care in the ICU.

COLLABORATIVE PRACTICE IN ACTION

COLLABORATIVE WEANING TEAMS

Weaning patients from long-term mechanical ventilation can be challenging for the ICU staff. Patients who require prolonged mechanical ventilation are generally sicker and have more comorbidities than do patients who wean more rapidly.[27] In 1991, Cohen and coworkers described the beneficial effect of a multidisciplinary ventilator management team on the outcomes of ICU patients.[47] The study examined a separate team that only followed mechanically ventilated patients, an approach that is not feasible in an era of cost containment and staff shortages. Henneman and colleagues, in 2001, published a study that used a true collaborative approach to weaning in a medical ICU and demonstrated a decrease in the length of stay and duration of mechanical ventilation—thus patient outcomes were optimized. In the model the plan was developed in a collaborative format and carried out by the respiratory therapists and ICU nurses.[27]

ACUTE STROKE TEAM

Stroke is a common and serious disease in the United States, with over 500,000 new cases per year and 150,000 deaths annually. Alberts and his colleagues conducted a national survey of major stroke program directors to determine the presence of an acute stroke team, their staffing, operational features, and utilization.[26] The results showed that such teams were common. Most of the teams were lead by a neurologist or neurosurgeon, 73% had nurses, and all had some combination of other practitioners. These multidisciplinary teams appear to increase the use of acute stroke therapies. The researchers believe that further studies are needed to determine the impact of the stroke care team on the costs of care and the impact of this approach on patients who are cared for in hospitals that lack neurologists and/or neurosurgeons.[26]

COLLABORATIVE PRACTICE IN THE NEONATAL ICU

Pollack and the NIH-District of Columbia Neonatal Network studied the health outcomes in eight acute care neonatal ICUs in Washington, DC, by examining organizational and management characteristics from 1994 to 1997. The study included selected physiologic and treatment outcomes that were collected on neonates in the eight units in the network. An organizational assessment was done by survey of nurses, physicians, and respiratory therapists in the neonatal ICUs using the Shortell instrument. Their findings were similar to those of Mitchell and Shortell.[8] Within their framework, organizational processes such as interdisciplinary collaboration and reciprocity positively affect patient outcomes.[31]

OUTCOMES MANAGEMENT

Collaborative practice teams (CPT) serve as the vehicle to facilitate the outcomes management process. Outcomes management is the use of outcomes assessment information to enhance clinical and financial quality outcomes through integration of best practice and service.[48] The aim of the CPT is to ensure that quality, cost-effective, research-based care is provided to patients throughout the continuum of care. Many of the CPTs achieve their goals and objectives through the performance-improvement process. The outcomes management process involves identifying values, determining the desirable outcomes for the patient population, analyzing system and care processes, implementing process and outcome improvement, and re-evaluating the outcomes

and variances.[48] Rogowski and coworkers used a multidisciplinary collaborative quality improvement model to examine patient care costs and resource utilization in neonatal ICUs. The ICUs formed their own teams and defined the outcomes project in which they wanted to be involved (e.g., infection or chronic lung disease). The results of their work demonstrated that a cost savings was associated with the collaborative quality improvement work.[27a]

COLLABORATING WITH PATIENTS AND FAMILIES

The needs of the ICU patients and their families have been addressed over the years in multiple nursing studies.[49-52] Despite the wealth of evidence supporting involvement of families in the care of their loved one, the biggest mistake an ICU can make is to view the family as bothersome intruders. All members of the collaborative team must acknowledge the role of the family in the care process.[43] Including families on patient rounds is one example of collaborating with the family in a different way. Active participation in the loved one's decision making and care when faced with a life-threatening illness is expected by today's educated consumer.[52] In any setting, an infrastructure that supports the patient, family, and staff is essential. Components of any program must include communication of guidelines clearly and succinctly, to all family members and other visitors; a formal family communication such as a family meeting that may or may not include the patient, depending on the condition of the patient; and a consistency of approach to collaboration with the patient and family.

COLLABORATIVE PRACTICE AT THE END OF LIFE

In response to the perceived need for greater interdisciplinary cooperation in the management of the terminally ill, practitioners at Wayne State University developed the Comprehensive Supportive Care Team in 1985 that has become a model for caring for the patient at the end of life.[53,54] The team consists of a clinical nurse specialist and a limited number of rotating physicians who in collaboration provide broad support for terminally ill patients and their families. Over the years the team has demonstrated their value to several thousand patients. Moreover, by identifying the special needs of this group of patients, costly care has been curtailed, resulting in better resource utilization.[55]

COLLABORATION FOR PATIENT SAFETY

The risk of adverse events caused by medication errors or equipment malfunction is higher in the ICU, because the number of medical patients received is twice that seen in general care areas. In addition, most require mechanical support of normal bodily functions.[30] Creating an environment within the health care system to ensure safe care is the responsibility of all who work in the hospital. Collaborative models for error prevention are very powerful ways to protect the patients. Practice teams should be established to examine the areas of high risk and to design strategies to reduce the risk for error. For example, the addition of the critical care pharmacist to the collaborative team can reduce preventable adverse drug events and associated costs caused primarily by prescribing practitioners. In one study, pharmacist intervention during prescribing decreased the rate of preventable adverse drug events from 10.4 to 3.5 per 1000 patient days.[56]

CONCLUSION

The ICU is a dynamic environment that requires coordinated efforts to optimize patient outcomes. Through conscientiously applied principles of collaboration, medicine, nursing, and other health care professional practices can be integrated while preserving the interests of each group. In today's health care environment, working together gives bedside practitioners a stronger voice in ensuring that patients receive the best possible care.

Concrete steps that can be taken to implement this practice model have been outlined by the NPJC, the Interorganization Liaison group, and others. The effectiveness of these policies and techniques has been demonstrated in numerous settings and can be expected to be a common feature of future hospital environments, as providers explore way to control costs and implement best practices.

We predict that collaborative practice will continue to evolve and become more robust. Even hospitals seeking magnet recognition for their nursing service must demonstrate a high level of collaborative practice throughout the organization.[57] Collaboration allows all members of the health care team to participate fully in care delivery by bringing their unique knowledge and skills to the process. According to the organizational theorist Peter Senge, the more complex the process, the more collaboration is needed.[58] Critical care delivery requires the talents of all involved in the care to be focused on the patient and on the goal of improving the patient's outcome. Collaboration is the best way to bring the team of providers together to improve outcomes.

ANNOTATED REFERENCES

Brilli RJ, Spevets A, Branson RD, et al: Critical care delivery in the intensive care unit: Defining clinical roles and the best practice model. Crit Care Med 2001;29:2007-2019.

This article is the consensus report of two task forces of the Society of Critical Care Medicine (SCCM). It represents the work of 31 health care professionals and practitioners, including statisticians and representatives from industry, pharmacy, nursing, and respiratory care and physicians who are involved in the practice of critical care. This report suggests that the best practice in critical care is collaborative practice with a multidisciplinary team.

Connor M, Ponte PR, Conway J: Multidisciplinary approaches to reducing error and risk in the patient care setting. Crit Care Nurs Clin North Am 2002;13:359-367.

After two significant medication errors at Dana-Farber Cancer Institute a multidisciplinary team was assembled, including nurses, administrators, physicians, and other clinical staff, to examine the systems that allowed these errors to occur. Clinician communication and cooperation was determined to be a priority to prevent error. One outcome was the birth of multidisciplinary safety rounds. The lesions learned at the Dana-Farber Cancer Institute can be translated to other organizations.

Henneman E, Dracup K, Ganz T, et al: Using a collaborative weaning plan to decrease duration of mechanical ventilation, length of stay in the intensive care unit for patients receiving long-term ventilation. Am J Crit Care 2002;11:132-140.

A collaborative weaning plan was introduced into the medical ICU of a large tertiary care center to attempt to impact the length of stay of long-term mechanically ventilated patients. The study did show that the collaborative approach to the patients' care positively impacted the outcomes: decrease length of ICU stay, decreased duration of mechanical ventilation, and decreased ICU costs for care. This is one of the outcome studies that has demonstrated the importance of collaborative practice in the ICU.

Miccolo MA, Spanier AH: Critical care management in the 1990s: Making collaborative practice work. Crit Care Clin 1993;9:443-453.

This article describes the need for collaboration in critical care even back in the early 1990s. The authors actually give a "how to" approach to building a critical care collaboration in the ICU. Their description of the barriers to collaboration allow the reader to plan for the implementation in their own ICUs. This is an excellent article for practitioners ready to begin collaborative practice in their ICUs.

Pollack MM, Koch MA: The NIH-District of Columbia Neonatal Network. Association of outcomes with organizational characteristics of neonatal intensive care units. Crit Care Med 2003;31:1620-1629.

The study is a first step in investigating the link between managerial performance and clinical outcomes. The findings of the study include the notion that organizational processes such as interdisciplinary collaboration and reciprocity affect patient outcomes because trust and respect between and among the professional staff enhance communication about patient issues; affect the authority of staff directors to manage the unit as they think best, and increase staff retention. Collaborative practice has a positive impact on the outcomes in the neonatal ICUs studied.

Chapter 258

THE PURSUIT OF PERFORMANCE EXCELLENCE

Josh Ettinger • Joel Ettinger • Peter J. Pronovost • Thomas G. Rainey

KEY POINTS

1. The Baldrige program provides a construct and framework for systematic approaches to achieving excellence in organizational performance.

2. Four characteristics differentiate high-performing organizations from average ones in terms of work processes: work is done systematically, systematic approaches are fully deployed throughout the organization, there are ongoing cycles of improvement, and all processes are aligned and integrated.

3. Seven categories of criteria serve as the focus and road map for leaders to achieve role-model performance. These categories are tightly interrelated and provide actionable guidance by identifying existing work process strengths and opportunities for improvement.

4. The Baldrige criteria provide a thoughtful and systematic approach to ensuring attentiveness to patient and family drivers of satisfaction and that segmented needs and expectations are integrated throughout the strategic planning process, action plan designs, and overall work processes.

5. The framework provides the ability to empower, motivate, and inspire the workforce to achieve its potential and deliver care that meets the needs of patients and families, rooted in best-care practices and aligned with the strategic objectives, mission, vision, and values of the unit or organization.

Those interested in running an average ICU need not read this chapter. Those who are willing to make the commitment to strive for world-class performance—even set the bar for ICU performance, with all its complexities—should read on. There is a dearth of literature that directly addresses how leaders of ICUs can create a system that empowers, innovates, achieves continuous and breakthrough improvements, astutely develops and deploys strategy, distinctly focuses on patient satisfaction, and delivers care at the highest possible clinical competency.

Organizations resemble a living being—an organism—with numerous parts, systems, and processes all operating to produce the whole entity. In health care, the different functional units in a hospital make up the actual operating unit—the hospital—itself. Each functional unit in a hospital is its own business, so to speak, and they are linked in a number of ways; in terms of operation, however, each is a separate unit that lives and breathes according to its ability to produce and remain sustainable. Using the Baldrige National Quality Program as a framework (Fig. 258-1), this chapter provides guidance on how to manage the ICU as its own business within the context of the larger hospital system.

For years, the Baldrige program has been the hallmark and standard for high levels of organizational performance and excellence in manufacturing and service industries. Since the program began in 1988, the stock performance of publicly traded Baldrige organizations has outperformed the S&P 500 in most years, by as much as six to one. Organizations around the world have adopted the Baldrige criteria as a framework for improving organizational performance practices, capabilities, and results. Since health care was added as a category in the Baldrige program in 1999, three organizations have been recognized for achieving record-setting levels of excellence, performance, and results, which has increased the health care community's awareness of and push toward the adoption of the Baldrige criteria.

The criteria have proved to be an effective tool on the macro-organizational level, and they can also be used in a smaller health care setting, such as a division, department, or functional unit. Specifically, the Baldrige criteria can be used in hospital ICUs, which care for the sickest patients and consume resources at an equivalent intensity. For example, most ICUs lack intensivist staff, an intervention associated with a 30% reduction in hospital mortality, and they demonstrate inefficient organization. Patients are suffering unnecessary morbidity and mortality and incurring high costs. The need to improve is urgent.

Yet change in the ICU is not easy. An ICU is arguably the most hazardous and complex area of the hospital. Sick patients, multiple caregivers, power struggles, and financial conflicts all make ICU change difficult. ICU leaders can use the Baldrige framework to improve ICU clinical and economic performance. This framework is goal directed and measurement driven.

Briefly, the Baldrige health care criteria are built on four integrated components:

1. Organizational profile
2. Eleven core values and concepts
3. Seven categories of criteria for high performance
4. Differentiation of high performance versus average performance

The first integrated component, the organizational profile, is a brief description of how the organization operates, its customers and their expectations, critical success

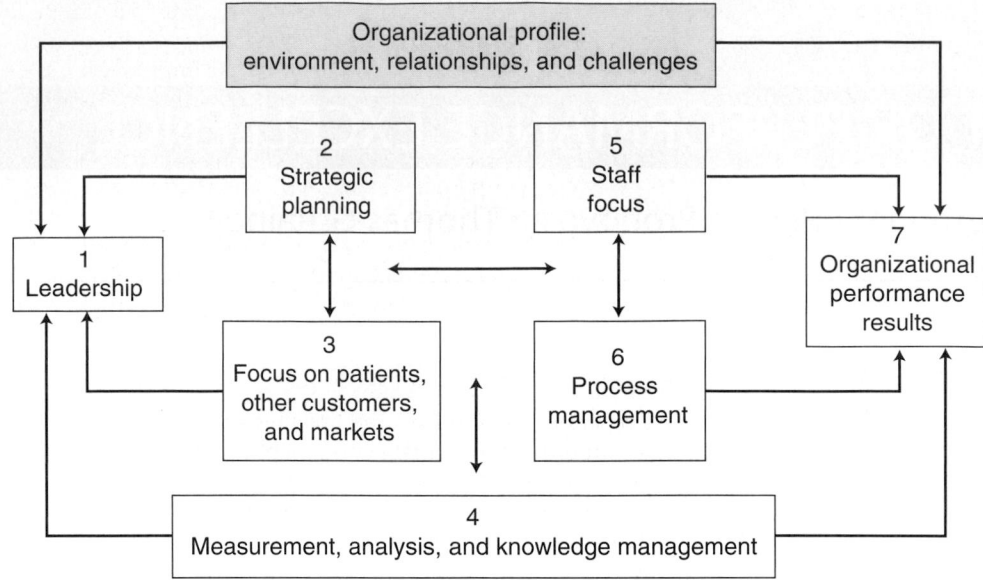

Organizational profile:
environment, relationships, and challenges

2
Strategic
planning

5
Staff
focus

1
Leadership

7
Organizational
performance
results

3
Focus on patients,
other customers,
and markets

6
Process
management

4
Measurement, analysis, and knowledge management

FIGURE 258–1. Baldrige health care criteria for performance excellence framework: a systems perspective.

factors, and key challenges. Although this component was created for an organization, it can easily be translated into a departmental profile.

The second integrated component of the Baldrige framework consists of 11 interrelated core values and concepts that have strong cultural enrichment implications. Over time, they have been validated to be embedded in high-performing organizations:

1. Visionary leadership
2. Patient-focused excellence
3. Organizational and personal learning
4. Valuing of staff and partners
5. Agility
6. Focus on the future
7. Managing for innovation
8. Management by fact
9. Social responsibility and community health
10. Focus on results and the creation of value
11. Systems perspective

The seven categories of health care criteria for performance excellence, which constitute the third integrated component, serve as the locus of role-model performance. The criteria are presented as a series of questions that ask how an organization's approaches to work are designed and managed so that they are systematic (repeatable), deployed throughout the entity, continuously improved, and aligned and integrated across the company. The criteria present direct actionable guidance by identifying existing strengths and opportunities for improvement. The seven categories are as follows:

1. Leadership
2. Strategic planning
3. Focus on patients, other customers, and markets
4. Measurement, analysis, and knowledge management
5. Staff focus
6. Process management
7. Organizational performance results

The scoring guidelines serve as the fourth component of the national quality framework. These guidelines describe

progressive thresholds of differentiated performance in terms of how work is done and what results are achieved. Four characteristics differentiate high-performing organizations from average ones. Work must be:

1. Systematic (i.e., repeatedly done in the way it is designed to be done).
2. Fully deployed (i.e., the work is done systematically everywhere it is supposed to be done—all sites, departments, units, staff).
3. Evaluated via ongoing cycles of improvement (improvement is built into how work is done).
4. Aligned and integrated (i.e., consistent, connected, harmonized to achieve maximum efficiency).

High-performing organizations differentiate the results of their critical success factors from those of lesser organizations based on (1) whether current results are good; (2) how results trend over time (i.e., show consistently better performance); (3) how trended results compare with competitor or industry averages; and (4) how trended results compare with best-in-industry performance.

How does all this relate to ICUs? ICUs across the country are struggling with increased complexity; higher costs; more errors; staffing shortages; staff, customer, and patient satisfaction; and low morale. The human-service purpose of ICUs is far too precious for ICU quality to become increasingly debilitated—a sign of leadership failure. Industry experts must find a road map that can guide the pursuit of sustained excellence. The objective is to move higher and higher in the realm of excellence.

Next, we provide an overview of each of the Baldrige criteria, using a selection of the key ideas in the seven categories, and provide examples of how they can be applied in the ICU to achieve world-class performance and excellence.* It is important to remember that the Baldrige program is not an improvement tool like Six Sigma or the Toyota Production System. Rather, it is a framework that provides guidelines and a structure that go *beyond* conformance to standards,

---

*The Baldrige criteria are elaborate, and a full presentation is beyond the scope of this chapter. A complete guide to the criteria can be found at www.baldrige.org.

differing from requirements such as those of the Joint Commission on Accreditation of Healthcare Organizations. Baldrige asks fundamental questions that will help lead and guide organizations toward the highest levels of performance excellence.

THE BALDRIGE INTENSIVE CARE UNIT

CATEGORY 1: LEADERSHIP

The leadership category provides insight on how leaders can guide their organizations to high levels of performance. It analyzes how clinical and nonclinical leaders use values, directions, and performance expectations, as well as a focus on patients, other customers, staff empowerment, innovation, and continuous improvement, as vehicles to secure systematic action. In the Baldrige framework, leadership is not just an organizational chart of positions. It is also a system—a set of leadership behaviors that move and align the organization toward specific goals and objectives. Using the unit's mission, vision, and values (as they relate to the whole organization), the leadership system orchestrates a systematic approach to communicating and deploying key organizational requirements and expectations throughout the entire workforce by providing a single, unifying purpose to all actions.

The criteria for leadership are instructive as they relate to ICUs and are likely very different from the current approach. Within the ICU, opportunities exist for the leadership team to become a leadership system and promote a unit that is systematic in its actions and fully deployed across all areas, ensures consistency of care across boundaries, incorporates and supports continuous cycles of improvement, and strategically aligns with the overall goals and objectives of the hospital.

To illustrate this point, the following example is offered: One ICU used a multidisciplinary leadership group to set and deploy the values, short- and long-term directions, and performance expectations throughout the unit. This team consisted of the intensivist, physician leader, functional administrator, and nursing supervisor. The multidisciplinary leadership group used a variety of tools and methods to communicate the values and directions of the unit, such as cascading employee development plans that correlated from the top down the ICU's goals and objectives and detailed how each employee would contribute to the achievement of those goals. Another method was a formal orientation training session and biannual education days led by the unit leaders that gathered nursing, physician, and other disciplines together in a room, communicating and learning.

Consistent with the Baldrige criterion that asks how leaders review performance and translate their reviews into continuous, breakthrough improvement and opportunities for innovation, the multidisciplinary leadership group met every month to review performance—using metrics that specifically correlated with the strategic goals and objectives. For example, the multidisciplinary leadership group, through its strategic planning process, identified teamwork and communication as an area for improvement as it related to patient safety and employee satisfaction (two strategic objectives set by the multidisciplinary leadership group). Using a cultural assessment tool to obtain the facts (*management by fact* is a Baldrige core value), it was discovered that over the past year, the ICU had a decrease in nurse satisfaction and an increase in nurse assessment of patient safety. After drill-down sessions with the doctors, nurses, pharmacists, patients, and

others, the multidisciplinary leadership group learned that communication between the nurses and the physicians was lacking and that patients were suffering—all impacting job satisfaction. In addition, the ICU was experiencing an unprecedented level of turnover. As a result, the multidisciplinary leadership group added to each employee's job description the requirement to participate in quarterly teamwork and communication training, and special tests of change (intervention) were implemented. Performance expectations were then set, communicated, and reinforced to all employees in the ICU through use of their work cascade plans and compensation.

Important to the performance expectations for the unit, the multidisciplinary leadership group set a goal to increase employee empowerment, learning, continuous improvement, and innovation. Critical to this goal was the creation of improvement teams that were supported by the ICU leadership in terms of time, finances, and other resources. Through the strategic planning process, the multidisciplinary leadership group learned that the staff felt that their efforts to change and improve patient care consumed large amounts of time, and that these efforts were neither supported nor appreciated by senior leadership. The stress level and complexity of the ICU environment contributed to staff turnover and dissatisfaction. The multidisciplinary leadership group realized that the creation of conduits for the staff to change, innovate, and improve processes that decreased complexity and raised satisfaction levels needed to occur rapidly. The leadership group put together a multidisciplinary action team, using the Plan-Do-Study-Act method of improvement,[†] to design systems that would empower and motivate the staff to change and innovate. These were then presented to the multidisciplinary leadership group and were initiated and tracked for performance.

CATEGORY 2: STRATEGIC PLANNING

This category deals with how the ICU establishes its strategic objectives and how those objectives are deployed throughout the unit. The ICU leadership system incorporates a number of internal and external inputs to create a yearly plan, with both short- and long-term goals for the unit. These goals must align with the mission, vision, and values of the unit and hospital in order to communicate a constancy of purpose. When the leadership team meets to discuss the strategic plan, it needs to consider the following elements: How is the strategic plan developed, communicated, prioritized, benchmarked, and measured? In addition, how does the ICU's strategic planning process incorporate the following:

- Patient needs and expectations?
- The competitive environment and collaborative opportunities within the community?
- Technology and other innovations that might affect ICU services?
- Strengths and weaknesses of the unit?
- Changes in the local, regional, or national environment?

To illustrate this concept, the following example is offered: ICU leaders organize a plan that answers the question, What do we want to do, and how do we get there? The ICU's

---

[†]The Plan-Do-Study-Act model uses the following questions and tests interventions in a rapid cycle, collecting enough data to make a judgment: (1) What are we trying to accomplish? (2) How will we know that a change is an improvement? (3) What changes can we make that will result in improvement?

mission, vision, and values drive the entire decision-making and strategic planning process. Based on the mission, the multidisciplinary leadership group uses the yearly strategic planning process to identify the unit's key objectives and goals (ensuring organizational alignment), key customer groups and segments, measurement strategies, staff-related issues, and action plans linked to strategic objectives. Organizational alignment is achieved through a variety of mechanisms, most importantly, a systematic approach to constant and continuous information exchange between the hospital senior leadership and the ICU leadership team. Providing this singular vision and cascading effect allowed the staff—at all levels of the ICU—to perform tasks linked with the purpose and goals of the entire organization. Each year, this process is updated according to key customer feedback, performance analysis, organizational position, competitive data, and industry standards and trends. Integral to this process is the implementation of actionable measures of the strategic objectives. For example, part of the ICU's mission is "to eliminate all preventable harm to the patient." Bloodstream infections were identified by data analysis as one area of preventable risk for cardiac patients. After the multidisciplinary leadership group discovered that bloodstream infection was an area of concern (and benchmarked their results against local competitors, national averages, and best in class), its prevention became a key strategic objective for the following year, and action plans were designed to create systems that would lower and move to eliminate these infections.

Crucial to this process is how the ICU communicates the strategic plan to the entire unit. In our example, the ICU provided every team member with a laminated color card listing the unit's strategic objectives, along with the mission, vision, and values. In addition, each employee was issued a cascade plan to guide work processes, goal setting, and professional development. These cascade plans list and strategically link and align the objectives of the hospital, the ICU, and the individual. The cascade plan is used quarterly as a performance assessment tool.

CATEGORY 3: FOCUS ON PATIENTS, OTHER CUSTOMERS, AND MARKETS

These criteria address how the ICU determines the needs and expectations of patients, families, colleagues, referring physicians, clinical departments, and regulatory bodies. It asks the question: How does the ICU leadership segment its patients with the goal of building meaningful relationships to acquire, satisfy, and secure their confidence, loyalty, and positive referral? Of course, most patients who end up in the ICU do not want to be there; however, by segmenting the patient population, it is possible to customize care to improve outcomes and eliminate inefficiencies. The following description details how a Baldrige ICU might operate using a few of the principles in category 3.

The ICU is a complex place dealing with complex patients and processes. The challenge for ICU leadership is to determine how to ensure consistency of practice in the midst of this complexity. Key to this effort is the need for the ICU to identify the types of patients (and their families) for whom they typically provide services, segment them according to needs and expectations, and then tailor health care services to meet their particular needs. For example, cardiac ICUs see

a variety of patient types, but most can be broken into two large segments: short term and long term. Within these segments are subgroups of patients, ranging from those recovering from coronary artery bypass grafts to those requiring ventricular assist devices. Care plans can be implemented that are customized to deliver the best outcomes for each of these groups and are consistent with the unit's goals and directions. Patients requiring ventricular assist devices tend to require prolonged ICU stays as they await replacement hearts. Therefore, the ICU team develops a plan to coordinate resources efficiently to meet the needs and expectations of this long-term patient cohort. Similarly, the short-term patient cohort can be segmented according to needs and expectations to better use the unit's resources. For example, medications most frequently used by the short-term patient group can be trended over time for predictability. These medications can then be located in a locked cart at the patient's bedside, reducing the need for the nurse to use the highly complex medication dispensing and delivery process. Numerous studies have identified substantial inefficiencies in the medication system. Use of data to track and predict trends in medication usage can allow unit staff to work more effectively and better serve the needs of patients.

Medically, the talented professionals working in the ICU know what is best for the patient; however, the question remains: What do the patient and family need and expect in order to have a positive experience? To some, this might seem of limited significance, considering the condition of most ICU patients. Yet there needs to be a way to determine these additional requirements. ICUs need to incorporate systems for gathering this information and applying it to the delivery of care. For example, one approach might be to follow up on the ICU experience by having a nurse from the ICU speak with the patient or family after transfer to the step-down unit. The information gained could be analyzed for trends and fed into a prioritization system for planning and implementation. The ICU can also proactively use quarterly focus groups, information sessions, and information gleaned from medical associations to elicit key knowledge to design care that is both medically optimal and patient driven.

In 2002, the Institute of Medicine recommended six tenets of the 21st-century health care system. One of these is a focus on patient-centered care and involvement of the patient and family in the care plan. This concept, though intuitively right, is difficult in practice, especially in the ICU setting. Notwithstanding, it is vital to the success of the ICU to make concerted efforts to identify the key requirements of their patients by segment and then build care plans around those requirements. Without this input, it is unlikely that a given ICU will reach levels of world-class performance and excellence. Through leadership, role-model behavior, and appropriate and effective communication, the workforce will feel empowered to incorporate the information gathered from the different patient segments and deliver care that is deemed appropriate based on the medical evidence and the wants and needs of the patient.

Inherent in the requirements of this category is a clear and distinct focus on determining the requirements, expectations, preferences, and key elements of satisfaction for ICU patients. That information is then used by the team to work effectively toward unit alignment and toward incorporating these elements into the design and delivery of health care services.

CATEGORY 4: MEASUREMENT, ANALYSIS, AND KNOWLEDGE MANAGEMENT

Now that the ICU has set its leadership system, created its strategic goals and objectives, and gathered and used key patient data to set action plans and work processes, a structure of measurement and analysis is needed to evaluate the effectiveness of the strategy and work system in place.

How does one measure performance, analyze performance, and use benchmarking information? How does one make certain that everyone in the chain of delivery of ICU care has all the necessary information when they need it, and that it is in the correct form and accurate, so that the next clinical decision, diagnostic test, or treatment can be carried out in a timely manner? How does one make certain that clinical information is available rapidly on request, given the life-and-death reality of intensive care? And, in the interest of achieving high ICU performance, how does one make certain that the sharing of knowledge is a cherished part of the culture and is actively (versus passively) managed?

This section of the Baldrige criteria describes how the ICU measures key indicators to track performance, continuously aligns unit goals, and identifies opportunities for improvement. In addition to measurement, this section addresses how the ICU manages this knowledge, transfers information to staff and patients, and shares best practices. ICU leadership needs to be sure that its measurement system is tracking the indicators that have been identified as key to the success of the organization and the unit. Without a measurement system that can assess the various levels of performance and match them to goals in all the key areas, it is difficult to achieve and deliver world-class health care. This is demonstrated through the following examples.

The ICU's key measures cascade down from the hospital's overall goals, which in this example fall into four categories: clinical performance, patient (customer) satisfaction, operational performance, and financial performance (Table 258-1). When the multidisciplinary leadership group set the vision and purpose for the unit, it selected three or four leading indicators within each segment that directly related to the goals and objectives of the unit.

The key measures are made clear to all members of the unit, including the front-line workers. A true communication plan and understanding are critical to creating an environment where the nurses, physicians, and other staff on the floor understand why they are performing a certain task and how their actions translate into the goals and objectives of the unit and the entire hospital. This alignment creates a mechanism by which the ICU leadership can review performance and goals and develop timely and meaningful action plans.

Another example is offered: The multidisciplinary leadership group set a goal of zero catheter-related infections. Data reviewed at the monthly leadership meeting revealed that the incidence of bloodstream infections in the ICU was increasing on a weekly basis and that the rate of infection was well above that of best-in-class. The multidisciplinary leadership group identified this as an opportunity for improvement and elected to convene a team to reduce the number of bloodstream infections. This group used the Plan-Do-Study-Act model for improvement and began a course of rapid testing, incorporating innovation and established best practices from other units within the hospital and from the industry. As part of this process, the multidisciplinary leadership group communicated to the entire unit that reducing the number of bloodstream infections was a key strategic objective and would be reviewed each month. The bloodstream infection reduction team used the weekly infection control data collected, and implemented interventions, such as a catheter checklist on line carts, universal presuctioning, and training on teamwork and communication for the nurses and physicians. Continuous cycles of improvement were implemented, and the bloodstream infection trend data demonstrated a progressive reduction. Work systems and processes related to catheter insertions became standardized in the unit and were ultimately communicated through the organization via a new policy and monitored for adherence.

It is also important for ICU leaders to consider how they manage the knowledge assets contained with the ICU. Baldrige defines knowledge assets as "the accumulated intellectual resources . . . it's the knowledge possessed by your organization and employees in the form of information, ideas, learning, understanding, memory, insights, cognitive and technical skills, and capabilities." ICU leaders who are committed not only to high performance but also to distinctive performance should learn how to manage the unique knowledge of their units. For example, in an academic setting, fellows and residents move in and out of different ICUs, bringing new knowledge, skills, and insights; however, there is also the potential for the erosion of existing best practices through lack of knowledge in some key areas. This is particularly important in today's health care industry, where nurse turnover is high and hospitals are losing valuable staff.

TABLE 258–1. KEY MEASURES OF INTENSIVE CARE UNIT PERFORMANCE

Strategic Objectives	Metric	One-Year Goal	Three- to Five-Year Goal
Clinical	Mortality	Reduce 20%	Reduce an additional 20%
	Infections	Zero bloodstream infections	Maintain at zero
	Use of evidence for sepsis patients	100% of patients	Develop quality measures for transfusion
	Use of ventilator bundle	100% of patients	100% of patients
	Rate of adverse drug events	Zero	Zero
Customer	Positive staff satisfaction (%)	Improve 30%	Improve each year by 10%
	Positive patient satisfaction (%)	Improve by 20%	Improve each year by 10%
Operational	Canceled surgery	Zero	Maintain at zero
	Length of stay	Reduce 30%	Reduce an additional 20%
	Rate of diverted cases	Reduce 50%	Zero
	Use of agency nurses	Zero	Zero
Financial	Operating margin	5%	7% (reinvest in quality)
	Drug costs	Reduce 30%	Reduce an additional 15%

A mechanism to maintain this knowledge, communicate it, and share it across the organization is vital to an ICU moving toward high performance.

Another aspect of this section of the Baldrige criteria is to measure what the ICU is doing, as outlined in the strategic plan. Without a measurement system that is continuously reviewed and incorporated into improvement and action-plan designs, it will be difficult for the ICU to determine whether it is meeting its stated goals or improving. Once the ICU has implemented a measurement system that provides actionable information, the next focus is creating work systems for the employees that allow them to reach their full potential and meet and exceed the goals and objectives of the ICU.

CATEGORY 5: STAFF FOCUS

All results are lagging indicators of how well the staff performs. ICUs that do not emphasize maintaining a workforce that is skilled, trained, satisfied, motivated, and safe should expect undistinguished performance. Integral to achieving the desired levels of performance and excellence, as identified by the ICU's strategic objectives, is the way work systems and staff learning enable *all* levels of the ICU staff to achieve their full potential. This category of the Baldrige framework focuses on how the leadership, effectively ensures that the enormous talent that resides within the health care team can achieve its extraordinary potential. Specifically, it involves ensuring a process for the organization and management of work, staff performance management, staff education, training, development, and motivation, as well as maintenance of a work environment that is safe and secure. All these factors are determinants of staff satisfaction, relationship building, and loyalty, and they need to be considered to ensure a high-performing unit. We cannot provide examples and mechanisms for each of these items; however, the paragraphs that follow offer some insight into a few of the key components of this category.

The ICU is an exceedingly complex environment, where issues such as patient safety, liability, and staff turnover are key. To that end, it is important to create an environment, through work system design, that reduces the risk of mistakes and increases the sense of purpose and vision. Research in aviation and in the health care setting has linked teamwork and communication directly to safety, outcomes, and high performance.[1] This research revealed a sizable disconnect between the nursing and physician staffs with respect to their evaluation of teamwork and communication in the ICU. This indicates a lack of continuity in thought, objectives, purpose, and unity among key stakeholders in the delivery of health services. For an ICU leadership team, these results should spur action to make improvements, bringing understanding and a shared vision not only of the purpose of the unit but also of communication expectations and work processes. Clearly, in this example, there are real and tangible differences of perception between nurses and physicians. Reducing ambiguity in this highly complex and risk-prone area can lead to increased levels of safety for both staff and patients.

In the traditional and hierarchical world of health care, a work design that allows the staff to achieve the highest levels of performance while promoting collaboration, initiative, empowerment, and innovation needs to be the goal if the patients are the true customers. So the question remains: How is this accomplished? Using the Baldrige criteria in their entirety is one way of achieving this end. This framework involves a set of characteristics of high-performing organizations inclusive of thematic linkages throughout all process of an ICU: specifically, how is work performed so that it is systematic (repeatable based on how it is designed to be done), fully deployed, continuously improved, and aligned with other care provided to the patient, as well as ensuring that the work is aligned with the mission, vision, values, and strategic objectives of the ICU?

Taking this a step further, and using the example of bloodstream infections, we can examine how teamwork and communication have helped reduce the number of catheter-related infections through the alignment of goals and objectives. After the multidisciplinary leadership group identified bloodstream infections as a strategic priority and funneled it through a working team, concerns arose regarding the nursing staff's ability to intervene when physicians broke standard protocol for catheter insertion. A number of nurses reported situations in which they had tried to intervene, only to have the physician ignore their observations and proceed with central catheter placement that did not follow proper protocol, thus exposing the patient to increased risk for a bloodstream infection. It became clear that the work systems and environment within the ICU allowed physician authority to trump the experience and patient-specific knowledge of the nursing staff, resulting in unsafe practices. Using this feedback, the multidisciplinary leadership group deployed multidisciplinary training on the tools and methodologies of teamwork and communication, such as situational awareness and safety briefings. In addition, the leadership group wrote a new policy that required physicians to stop and listen to the nursing staff if a potential for a bloodstream infection was observed, or be subject to corrective actions. The policy was that they monitored for adherence and staff performance. The result of this endeavor empowered the nursing staff to be supported and feel comfortable intervening when patient safety might be at risk and reinforce the established safe practice.

This category of the Baldrige criteria allows ICU leadership and staff to examine how its work systems contribute to the achievement of the ICU's objectives. The vision and goals of the unit may seem unattainable because the processes that have been created through tradition do not align performance and process such that the ultimate vision is realized. Using the criteria, the ICU can systematically create work processes that support the mission, vision, and overall goals of the unit.

CATEGORY 6: PROCESS MANAGEMENT

Up to this point, we have addressed ICU performance related to its leadership, strategic planning, patient relationships, access to information and knowledge, and human resource management—all in the context of high performance. Now we address the bottom line: How do we "make" ICU care? It is time to think differently about how ICU care creates value. The Baldrige criteria focus on the creation of *value* in every step of health care design, improvement, and ongoing management. The criteria provide ICU leaders with a structure and discipline to think through their delivery processes to ensure that all steps create value, as measured by effective diagnosis and elimination of disease to the extent that the art and science of medicine allow. What care delivery management system can ensure that value is always created, outcomes do not suffer, performance levels do not decline, and safety prevails? Process management is the focal point for ICU high performance. It provides guidance on how the ICU identifies, designs, improves, and manages its health care services to achieve results when trended over time to approach, demonstrate, or sustain world-class performance. It obligates ICU leaders to clarify how these processes are continuously improved to achieve better performance, improved cycle times, reduction of waste, reduced variability, and, of course, improved clinical outcomes. Leaders are guided through a series of questions that ask how health care is designed and managed in ways that are systematic and fully deployed, incorporate ongoing cycles of improvement, and are aligned and integrated with other processes and operations involved in the care and support of ICU patients. These criteria for performance excellence are the key to avoid being just average.

For example, it is important for the ICU multidisciplinary leadership group to create work systems that deliver care based on the needs of all ICU constituents—patients, physicians, nurses, pharmacists, and so forth—and align with the goals and objectives of the unit. The question needs to be asked: How do our processes create value for those we serve and how do we know we have been successful? Using this mantra as a guide, the multidisciplinary leadership group in our ICU example aligned the work processes with the unit to continuously meet the expectations of each ICU customer segment. This involved a number of approaches; however, the ultimate deliverable was a system of work designed to achieve the key requirements (categories 2 and 3) identified in the ICU strategic plan. Data indicated that the lack of clarity around a given patient care plan was causing increased errors and longer stays. Using the goal of reducing harm and improving teamwork and communication among the unit's health care professionals (as stated in the strategic plan), the multidisciplinary leadership group tested and implemented an evidence-based tool developed by Pronovost and colleagues that incorporates a multidisciplinary team approach to making rounds.[2] During these rounds, a daily goals sheet is used to communicate the care plan for the particular patient to the multidisciplinary team, consisting of physicians, nurses, pharmacists, and others. The use of this tool over time led to a reduction in length of stay and adverse drug events, and both nurse and physician teamwork and satisfaction scores have improved. This mechanism is guided by several criteria in this category dealing with the inclusion of patient expectations, testing to prevent errors, and achieving better performance by reducing variation in care. Unexplained and avoidable variation in care is one of the principal causes of failure in health care process and outcomes.

The complexity of ICU care demands that its leaders employ methods of excellence at a greater intensity compared with other health care venues. The application of the Baldrige criteria, designed to enable any operating unit to achieve distinctive performance, is greatest in the ICU. Otherwise, we are left largely with less effective methods of management and improvement that have demonstrated, thus far, the inability to fully leverage the extraordinary talent that resides within.

CATEGORY 7: HEALTH CARE RESULTS

In the end, the results of a given ICU are the ultimate measure of its performance. Now that the ICU has defined its mission, vision, and values; set strategic objectives; become relentlessly patient-focused; established methods to ensure that all ICU staff have the required information and knowledge; and created work processes that inspire the staff and add value to the patient, it is paramount that the ICU use the data it collects (on its key objectives) as a feedback

loop or mechanism to continuously review its performance and achieve the identified goals outlined in the strategic plan. Selecting measures and having a system or process for making the data actionable allow the ICU to constantly implement corrective strategies when an area for improvement is identified. This category does not deal with the deployment of key processes; rather, and quite simply, it involves the unit's ability to effectively align its mission, vision, and values and meet its stated goals and objectives as compared with both the competition and best-in-class benchmarks.

CONCLUSION

ICUs are places of emotion, extraordinary science, compassion, and sometimes high drama in the conflict between disease and injury and the will to live. Optimally, they are designed to enable the uniquely talented professionals who dedicate their careers to healing at the highest levels. Yet experience has proved with alarming frequency that the enormous and sometimes even heroic good that is accomplished is marred by what could or should have been done. Patients enter our ICUs trusting that we will do what is needed, correctly and with compassion. There is only one standard of care acceptable—no excuses are permitted. The Baldrige program, the nation's formally adopted approach to excellence, is not just another improvement tool. Rather, it is a framework of systematic elements that are woven together to achieve the singular aim of excellence (Table 258-2). The Baldrige framework inspires leaders to create the culture through which every employee involved in the care of the very ill performs to his or her potential. It sets forth the

TABLE 258–2. SEVEN CATEGORIES OF HEALTH CARE CRITERIA FOR PERFORMANCE EXCELLENCE AND RELATED KEY QUESTIONS

Categories	Key Questions
1. Leadership	How does the ICU senior leadership guide the unit through its governance system and organizational performance reviews?
2. Strategic planning	How does the ICU establish its strategic objectives and action plans, and how are they deployed and measured across the unit?
3. Focus on patients, other customers, and markets	How does the ICU determine patient requirements, expectations, and preferences, and how does the ICU build relationships with its patients to increase satisfaction and loyalty?
4. Measurement, analysis, and knowledge management	How does the ICU select, gather, analyze, manage, and improve its measurement system, and how is this knowledge shared, transferred, and communicated throughout the unit?
5. Staff focus	How does the ICU's work system, staff learning, and staff motivation enable all staff to develop and utilize their full potential in alignment with the unit's strategic objectives, goals, and action plans?
6. Process management	How does the ICU's process management system, including both key processes and support processes, create value for the patient and staff?
7. Organizational performance results	How do the ICU's results compare to competitors and industry benchmarks over time? are they reflective of the ICU's strategic objectives?

foundation through which leaders of ICUs can track and achieve results that are comprehensive, balanced, and presented in the context of true world-class performance. It probes the leadership structure to consider how key elements of organizational success are accomplished, how they are systematically deployed throughout the unit, how continuous improvement is a system property, and how all the work is aligned with the unit's mission, vision, and values.

ICUs are endowed with extensive human and technologic resources. The first question every ICU leader must ask is: Are we performing at the highest possible level? If the answer is no, then the obligation—not the option—is to achieve it and then sustain it.

ANNOTATED REFERENCES

Langley J, Nolan T, Nolan K, et al: The Improvement Guide. Jossey Bass, 1996.
This book outlines a simple methodology for rapid cycle improvement, providing tools and giving relevant examples.

National Institute for Standards and Technology: Health Care Criteria for Performance Excellence. NIST, 2003. Available at www.baldrige.org.
This guide provides the actual Baldrige criteria used by the national program and organizations.

Pronovost PJ, Angus DC, Dorman T, et al: Physician staffing patterns and clinical outcomes in critically ill patients: A systematic review. JAMA 2002; 288:2151-2162.
This article analyzes patient outcomes in the ICU as they relate to different staffing models.

Pronovost P, Berenholtz S, Dorman T, et al: Improving communication in the ICU using daily goals. J Crit Care 2003;18:71-75.
This article explains the impact and utility of a health care intervention called a daily goals sheet on patient safety, team communication, and length of stay.

Thomas EJ, Sherwood GD, Helmreich RL: Lessons from aviation: Teamwork to improve patient safety. Nurs Econ 2003;21:241-243.
This article examines the history and results of teamwork and communication in the aviation industry and provides similar data for the health care industry. More specifically, it cites the role teamwork and communication play in patient safety.

Chapter 259

SEVERITY OF ILLNESS INDICES AND OUTCOME PREDICTION: DEVELOPMENT AND EVALUATION

Thomas L. Higgins

And he will manage the cure best who has foreseen what is to happen from the present state of matters....[1]

KEY POINTS

1. **Stratification of outcome** based on **risk factors** is necessary when comparing outcomes obtained by different institutions, intensive care teams, and treatment strategies.

2. Although **mortality** is readily defined and easily captured, it is insufficient as the sole measure of clinical outcome and does not capture other important endpoints such as complications, quality of life, or costs.

3. **Administrative data** are plentiful but are typically less reliable than carefully collected **clinical information.** The quality of administrative databases can be improved by including laboratory information.

4. Most outcome stratification models are developed by **univariate analysis** of independent variables against a chosen outcome and then refined using **multivariate techniques.**

5. Model performance is assessed by measuring **discrimination** (typically by ROC-curve area) and **calibration** (typically by goodness-of-fit procedures).

6. The **standardized mortality ratio** is created by dividing observed by expected mortality rates. Values less than 1.0, if statistically significant, indicate performance better than expected.

7. The **Acute Physiology and Chronic Health Evaluation (APACHE-II and APACHE-III),** the **Mortality Probability Models (MPM),** and the **Simplified Acute Physiology Score (SAPS)** are well-developed, prospectively validated models useful in general critical care units. Customized models are necessary for highly specialized ICUs or when evaluating population subsets.

8. Outcome predictions are intended for **groups, not individuals.** Mortality probability estimates range from 0.0 to 1.0, but an individual patient will either live or die. Mortality predictions also vary depending on when the data were temporally collected. Use of scoring systems to direct therapeutic choices has not been adequately studied.

BACKGROUND

Predicting outcome is a time-honored duty of physicians, dating back at least to the time of Hippocrates. The need for a quantitative approach to outcome prediction, however, is more recent. Although the patient or family members will still want to know the prognosis, there is increasing pressure to measure and report medical care outcomes and to adjust these outcomes for the presenting condition of the patient. In today's highly competitive health care environment, such information may be used to award contracts for care, and public dissemination of outcome results is increasingly frequent. Information of variable quality[2] is readily available on the Internet. While the Center for Medicare and Medicaid Services (formally HCFA, the Health Care Financing Administration) no longer releases comparisons of hospital mortality rates, comparative information is available from sites such as www.healthcarechoices.org and www.health-scope.org.[3,4] Local and regional initiatives[5] to assess quality of care are also common. Some of these "report cards" specifically address the performance of intensive care units adjusting outcomes with risk stratification systems, so it is essential that the clinician understand these systems and how they may properly be applied. A focus on performance assessment, however, may detract from other potential uses for risk stratification, including more precise risk-benefit decisions, prognostication, resource allocation, efficient assessment of new therapy and technology, and modifications to individual patient management based on severity of illness.

Prognostication based on clinical observation is affected by memory of recent events, inaccurate estimation of the relative contribution of multiple factors, false beliefs, and human limitations such as fatigue.[6] An outcome prediction model, on the other hand, will always produce the same estimate from a given dataset and will correctly value the importance of relevant data. In an environment in which clinical judgment may later be reviewed for financial or legal issues, an objective prediction of outcome becomes especially important. Yet, even the best risk stratification tools can generate misleading data when misapplied.[7] Discussed in this chapter are the methods by which models are developed, the application of commonly used models in clinical practice, and common reasons why observed outcome may not match predicted outcome in the absence of differences in the quality of care.[8]

Well-established general methods for stratifying clinical outcomes by the presenting condition of the patient include the ASA Physical Status Classification[9] and the Glasgow

Coma Scale (GCS).[10] ICU-specific systems typically adjust for patient physiology, age, and chronic health condition; and they may also assess admitting diagnosis, location before ICU admission or transfer status, cardiopulmonary resuscitation before admission, surgical status, and use of mechanical ventilation. An ideal approach to comparing outcomes would use variables that characterize a patient's *initial* condition, can be statistically and medically related to outcome, are easy to collect, and are independent of treatment decisions.

OUTCOME OF INTEREST

Mortality is a commonly chosen outcome because it is easily defined and readily available. Mortality is insufficient as the sole outcome measure, however, because it does not reflect important issues such as return to work, quality of life, or even costs, because early death results in a lower cost than prolonged hospitalization. There is poor correlation between hospital rankings based on death and those based on other complications.[7,11] ICU length of stay is difficult to use as a proxy for quality of care, because the frequency of distribution is usually skewed and mean length of stay is always higher than median owing to long-stay outliers.[12] Morbidities, such as myocardial infarction, prolonged ventilation, stroke or other central nervous system complications, renal failure, and serious infection, can be difficult to collect accurately, and administrative records may not reflect all relevant events.[8] There is also little standardization on how morbidity should be defined.

Other potential endpoints include ICU or hospital length of stay, resource use, return to work, quality of life, and 1- or 5-year survival. Patient satisfaction is an outcome highly valued by purchasers of health care, but it is subjective[13] and requires substantial effort to accomplish successfully.[14] Evaluation of ICU performance may require a combination of indicators, including severity of illness and resource utilization.[15-17]

DATABASES AND DEFINITIONS

The quality of a risk stratification system depends on the database on which it was developed. Outcome analysis can either be retrospective, relying on existing medical records or administrative databases, or developed prospectively from data collected concurrently with patient care. Retrospective studies using existing data are quicker and less expensive to conduct but may be compromised by missing data,[8] imprecise definitions, interobserver variability,[18] and changes in medical practice over time.[19]

Data derived from discharge summaries or insurance claims do not always capture the presence of comorbid disease[20] and may be discordant with data that are clinically collected.[21] Because some administrative discharge reports truncate the number of reportable events, diagnoses may be missed, and this coding bias is most apparent in severely ill patients.[12] Coding errors and use of computer programs to optimize diagnosis-related group reimbursement can also reduce the validity of claims-derived data. Augmentation of administrative data with laboratory values improves model performance.[22]

A variety of methods can confirm the accuracy of the database, such as re-abstraction of a sample of charts by personnel blinded to the initial results and comparison to an independent database. Kappa analysis is a method for quantifying the rate of discrepancies between measurements (values) of the same variable in different databases (i.e., original and re-abstracted). A kappa value of 0 represents no (or random) agreement and 1.0 is perfect agreement, but it must be interpreted in light of the prevalence of the factor being abstracted.[23]

MODEL DEVELOPMENT

Once data integrity is ensured, there are a number of possible approaches to relating outcome to presenting condition. The empirical approach is to use a large database and to subject the data to a series of statistical manipulations (Table 259-1). Typically, death, a specific morbidity, and resource consumption are chosen as outcomes (dependent variables). Factors (independent variables) that are thought to affect outcome are then evaluated against a specific outcome using univariate tests (chi-square, Fisher's exact, or Student t-test) to establish the magnitude and significance of any relationship.

The independent variables should reflect patient condition independent of therapeutic decisions. Measured variables such as "cardiac index" or "hematocrit" are preferred over "use of inotropes" or "transfusion given" because the criteria for intervention may vary by provider or hospital. Widely used models rely on measured physiologic variables (heart rate, blood pressure, and neurologic status) and laboratory values (serum creatinine level and white blood cell count). In addition, variables are included that reflect age, physiologic reserve, and chronic health status. Items chosen for inclusion in a scoring system should be readily available and clinically relevant to clinicians involved in the care of these patients, and variables that lack both clinical and statistical bearing on outcome should not be included. This requirement may necessitate specialized scoring systems for patient populations (pediatric, burn and trauma, and possibly acute myocardial infarction patients) exhibiting different characteristics than the general ICU population. For example, left ventricular ejection fraction and reoperative status are important predictors of outcome in the cardiac surgical population but are not routinely measured or not directly

TABLE 259–1. STEPS IN DEVELOPING A SEVERITY-OF-ILLNESS MODEL

Precisely define outcome(s) of interest.
Identify and define candidate predictor variables.
Collect data and ensure its accuracy (reabstraction, kappa analysis).
Examine continuous variables and transform or dichotomize as necessary.
Perform univariate analysis (chi-square, Fisher's exact, Student t-test) against outcome(s).
Perform multivariate analysis (multiple logistic regression, neural nets, Bayesian, others).
Examine for and adjust for interactions.
Develop score or equation that relates independent variables to outcome.
Test calibration of model (goodness of fit).
Test discrimination of model (ROC C-statistic, sensitivity and specificity).
Validate model with independent data, split sample, or jackknife techniques.
Obtain external validation in new setting.
Publish in peer-reviewed journal.

TABLE 259–2. TWO-BY-TWO CONTINGENCY TABLE EXAMINING RELATIONSHIP OF MOF AFTER OPEN HEART SURGERY (OUTCOME) TO A HISTORY OF CHF (PREDICTOR) IN 3830 PATIENTS*

Predictor Variable: History of CHF	Outcome Variable: MOF	
	Yes	*No*
Yes	121	846
No	166	2697

*The odds ratio is defined by cross-multiplication (121 × 2697) ÷ (846 × 166). The odds ratio of 2.3 indicates patients with CHF are 2.3 times as likely to develop postoperative organ system failure as those without prior CHF. This univariate relationship can then be tested by chi-square for statistical significance.
Data from Higgins TL, Estafanous FG, Loop FD, et al: ICU admission score for predicting morbidity and mortality risk after coronary artery bypass grafting. Ann Thorac Surg 1997;64:1050-1058.
CHF, congestive heart failure; MOF, multiple organ failure.

relevant to other population groups.[24] If the independent variable is dichotomous (yes/no, male/female), a two-by-two table can be constructed to examine the odds ratio and a chi-square test performed to assess significance (Table 259-2). If multiple variables are being considered, the level of significance is generally set smaller than $P = .05$, using a multiple comparison (e.g., Bonferroni) correction[25] to determine a more appropriate P value.

If the independent variable under consideration is a continuous variable (e.g., age) a Student's t-test is one appropriate choice for statistical comparison. With continuous variables, consideration must be given to the possibility that the relationship of the variable to outcome is not linear. Figure 259-1 demonstrates the relationship of ICU admission serum bicarbonate to mortality outcome in cardiac surgical patients[26] where the data points have been averaged with adjacent values to produce a locally weighted smoothing scatterplot graph.[27] Serum bicarbonate values above 22 mmol/L at ICU admission imply a relatively constant risk. Below this value, the risk of death rises sharply. Analysis of this locally weighted smoothing scatterplot graph suggests

two ways for dealing with the impact of serum bicarbonate on mortality. One would be to make admission bicarbonate a dichotomous variable (i.e., >22 mEq or <22 mEq). The other would be to transform the data via a logarithmic equation to make the relationship more linear. Cubic splines analysis,[28] another statistical smoothing technique, may also be used to assign weight to physiologic variables.

Univariate analysis assesses the forecasting ability of variables without regard to possible correlations or interactions between variables. Linear discriminant and logistic regression techniques[29] can evaluate and correct for overlapping influences on outcome. For example, a history of congestive heart failure (CHF) and depressed left ventricular ejection fraction are both known to be predictors of poor outcome in patients presenting for cardiac surgery.[30] As might be expected, there is considerable overlap between the population with CHF and those with low ejection fraction. The multivariate analysis in this specific instance eliminates history of CHF as a variable and retains only measured ejection fraction in the final equation.

Because linear discriminant techniques require certain assumptions about data, logistic techniques are more commonly utilized. Subjecting the data to multiple logistic regression will produce an equation with a constant, a beta coefficient and standard error, and an odds ratio that represents each term's effect on outcome. Table 259-3 displays the results of the logistic regression used in the Mortality Probability Model II (MPM-II) ICU admission model. There are 15 variable terms and a constant term, each with a beta value that, when multiplied by presence or absence of a factor, becomes part of the calculation of mortality probability using a logistic regression equation. The odds ratios reflect the relative risk of mortality if a factor is present. The challenge in building a model is to include sufficient terms to deliver reliable prediction while keeping the model from being cumbersome to use or too closely fitted to its unique development population. Generally accepted practice is to limit the number of terms in the logistic regression model to 10% of the number of patients having the outcome of interest to avoid "overfitting" the model to the developmental dataset. In a

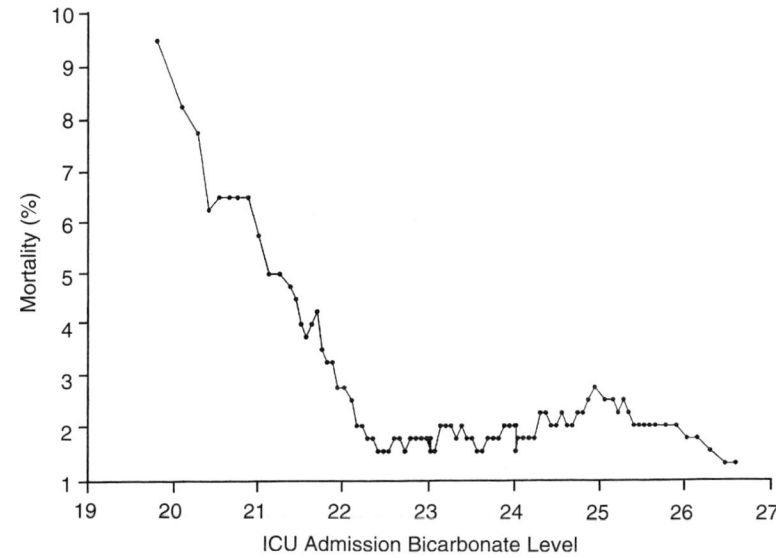

FIGURE 259–1. A locally weighted smoothing scatterplot (LOWESS) analysis of the relationship between ICU admission bicarbonate level (*x*-axis) and mortality (*y*-axis). Individual patient data are grouped and averaged with surrounding data to produce a smooth plot. In this instance, the mortality rate appears to be stable with admission bicarbonate levels of 22 mmol/L and above but rises rapidly with lower values. Admission bicarbonate level of less than 21 mmol/L was given prognostic weight in the model that used these data. (From Higgins TL, Estafanous FG, Loop FD, et al: ICU admission score for predicting morbidity and mortality risk after coronary artery bypass grafting. Ann Thorac Surg 1997;64: 1050-1058.)

TABLE 259–3. VARIABLES IN THE MPM0* WITH THEIR ESTIMATED COEFFICIENTS, STANDARD ERRORS, ADJUSTED ODDS RATIOS, AND 95% CONFIDENCE INTERVALS FOR THE ADJUSTED ODDS RATIOS

Variable	β (SE)	Estimate Adjusted Odds Ratio (95% Confidence Interval)
Constant	−5.46836	Not applicable
Physiology		
Coma or deep stupor	1.48592 (0.079)	4.4 (3.8-5.2)
Heart rate ≥150 beats/min	0.45603 (0.145)	1.6 (1.2-2.1)
Systolic blood pressure ≤90 mm Hg	1.06127 (0.079)	2.9 (2.5-3.4)
Chronic diagnoses		
Chronic renal insufficiency	0.91906 (0.105)	2.5 (2.0-3.1)
Cirrhosis	1.13681 (0.126)	3.1 (2.4-4.0)
Metastatic neoplasm	1.19979 (0.098)	3.3 (2.7-4.0)
Acute diagnoses		
Acute renal failure	1.48210 (0.089)	4.4 (3.7-5.2)
Cardiac dysrhythmias	0.28095 (0.068)	1.3 (1.2-1.5)
Cerebrovascular incident	0.21338 (0.089)	1.2 (1.0-1.5)
Gastrointestinal bleeding	0.39653 (0.094)	1.5 (1.2-1.8)
Intracranial mass effect	0.86533 (0.088)	2.4 (2.0-2.8)
Other		
Age (10-year odds ratio)	0.03057 (0.002)	1.4 (1.3-1.4)
CPR before admission	0.56995 (0.112)	1.4 (1.3-1.4)
Mechanical ventilation	0.79105 (0.056)	2.2 (2.0-2.5)
Nonelective surgery	1.19098 (0.074)	3.3 (2.8-3.8)

*MPM$_0$ indicates Mortality Probability Model system admission model.
Reprinted from Lemeshow S, Teres D, Klar J, et al: Mortality Probability Model (MPM II) based on an international cohort of intensive care unit patients. JAMA 1993;270:2478-2486.

population of 500 patients with a mortality rate of 30%, there will be 150 deaths. Fifteen (10% of 150) would be the upper limit to the number of terms that could reasonably be included in a logistic regression model for this sample size without overfitting. It is important to identify interaction between variables that may be additive, subtractive (canceling), or synergistic and thus require additional terms in the final model.

Data envelopment analysis is an emerging nonparametric technique that determines the relationship between outcomes and inputs on the basis of efficiency. Unlike logistic regression, which finds the best average equation for a population, data envelopment analysis focuses on the high-performing outliers rather than looking for central tendencies.[31] To date, data envelopment analysis has been used primarily in business with only limited application in medicine.[32]

The patient's diagnosis is an important determinant of outcome,[19] but conflicting philosophies exist on how disease status should be addressed by a severity adjustment model. One approach is to define principal diagnostic categories and add a weighted term to the logistic regression equation for each illness. This approach acknowledges the different impact of physiologic derangement by diagnosis. For example, patients with diabetic ketoacidosis have markedly altered physiology but a low expected mortality; a patient with an expanding abdominal aneurysm may show little physiologic abnormality and yet be at high risk for death or morbidity. Too many diagnostic categories, however, may result in too few patients in each category to allow statistical analysis for a typical ICU, and such systems are difficult to use without sophisticated software.

The other approach is to ignore disease status and assume that factors such as age, chronic health status, and altered physiology will suffice to explain outcome in large groups of patients. This method avoids issues with inaccurate labeling of illness in patients with multiple problems and the need

for lengthy lists of coefficients but could result in a model that is more dependent on having an "average" case mix.[33,34] Regardless of the specific approach, age and comorbidities (metastatic or hematologic cancer, immunosuppression, and cirrhosis) are given weight in the popular ICU models to help account for the patient's physiologic reserve or ability to recover from acute illness.

VALIDATION AND TESTING MODEL PERFORMANCE

Models may be validated on an independent dataset or by other methods such as jack-knife or boot-strap validation.[35] Two criteria are important in assessing model performance. *Calibration* refers to how well the model tracks outcomes across its relevant range. A model may be very good at predicting good outcome in healthy patients and poor outcomes in very sick patients yet unable to distinguish outcome for patients in the middle range. The Hosmer-Lemeshow goodness-of-fit test[36] assesses calibration by stratifying the data into categories (usually deciles) of risk. The number of patients with an observed outcome is compared with the number of predicted outcomes at each risk level. If the observed and expected outcomes are very close at each level across the range of the model, the sum of chi-squares will be low, indicating good calibration. The *P* value for the Hosmer-Lemeshow goodness-of-fit *increases* with better calibration and should be nonsignificant (i.e., >.05).

The second measurement of model performance is *discrimination*, or how well the model predicts the correct outcome. A classification table (Table 259-4) displays four possible outcomes that define sensitivity and specificity of a model with a binary (died/survived) prediction and outcome. Sensitivity (the true-positive rate) and specificity (the true-negative rate, or 1 − the false-positive rate) are measures

TABLE 259–4. CLASSIFICATION TABLE

Predicted Outcome	Actual Outcome	
	Died	Survived
Died	a	c
Survived	b	d
True-positive ratio = a/(a + b) (sensitivity)		
False-positive ratio = c/(c + d)		
True-negative ratio = d/(c + d) (specificity)		
False-negative ratio = b/(a + b)		
Accuracy (total correct prediction) = (a + d)/a + b + c + d		

Adapted from Ruttiman VE: Severity of illness indices: Development and evaluation. In Shoemaker WC (ed): Textbook of Critical Care Medicine, 2nd ed. Philadelphia, WB Saunders, 1989.

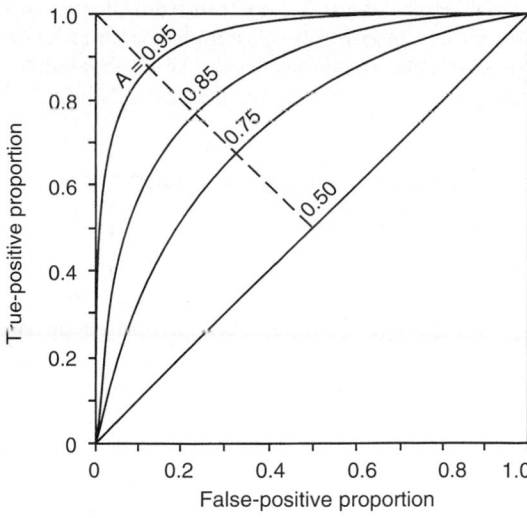

FIGURE 259–2. Relative operating characteristic (ROC) curves. A coin toss gives an ROC of 0.5. In models that discriminate outcome, an increasing area under the curve, also called the C-statistic, is enclosed. (From Swets JA: Measuring the accuracy of diagnostic systems. Science 1988;240:1285-1294.)

of discrimination but will vary according to the decision point chosen to distinguish between outcomes when a model produces a continuous range of possibilities. The sensitivity and specificity of a model when using 50% as the decision point will differ from that using 95% as the decision point. The classification table can be recalculated for a range of outcomes by choosing various decision points: for example, 10%, 25%, 50%, 75%, and 95% mortality risk. At each decision point, the true-positive rate (proportion of observed deaths predicted correctly) and the false-negative (proportion of survivors incorrectly predicted to die) and overall correct classification rate can be presented. The C-statistic, or area under a receiver-operating characteristic (ROC) curve, is a convenient way to summarize sensitivity and specificity at all possible decision points.[37,38] A graph of the true-positive proportion (sensitivity) against the false-positive proportion (1 – specificity) across the range of the model produces the ROC curve (Fig. 259-2). A model with equal probability of producing the correct or incorrect result (e.g., flipping a coin) will produce a straight line at a 45-degree angle that encompasses half of the area (0.5) under the "curve." Models with better discrimination will incorporate increasingly more area under the curve to a theoretical maximum of 1.0. Most ICU models have ROC areas of 0.8 to 0.9 in the development set, although the ROC area usually decreases when models are applied prospectively to new datasets. The ROC analysis is valid only if the model has first been shown to calibrate well.

A model may discriminate and calibrate well on its development dataset yet fail when applied to a new population. Discrepancies in performance can relate to differences in surveillance strategies and definitions[39] and can occur when a population is skewed by an unusual number of patients having certain risk factors, as could be seen in a specialized ICU.[33] Large numbers of low-risk ICU admissions will result in poor predictive accuracy for the entire ICU population.[40] The use of sampling techniques (i.e., choosing to collect data randomly on 50% of patients rather than all patients) also appears to bias results.[43] Models can also deteriorate over time, owing to changes in medical practice. These explanations should be considered before concluding that quality of care is different between the original and later applications of a model.[41]

SCORING SYSTEMS

Logistic regression provides a statistically sound way to express the relationship between independent and dependent variables but requires the use of a computer or programmable calculator. It is possible to use either the beta coefficients or the odds ratios from the logistic regression results to assign integer values based on relative importance of independent variables to create a score that can be calculated by hand at the bedside. The validity of a simplified score can be confirmed by subjecting the clinical score to the same discrimination and calibration tests as the multiple logistic regression models.[30]

STANDARDIZED MORTALITY RATIO

Application of a severity of illness scoring system involves comparison of observed outcomes with those predicted by the model. The standardized mortality ratio is defined as observed divided by expected mortality and is generally expressed as a mean value ±95% confidence intervals, which will depend on the number of patients in the sample. Standardized mortality ratio values of 1.0 (+ the confidence interval) indicate that the mortality rate, adjusted for presenting illness, is at the expected level. Standardized mortality ratio values significantly lower than 1.0 indicate performance better than expected. Small differences in scores, as could be caused by consistent errors in scoring elements, timing of data collection, or sampling rate, have been shown to cause important changes in the standardized mortality ratio.[42,43]

MODELS BASED ON PHYSIOLOGIC DERANGEMENT

Three widely utilized general-purpose ICU outcome systems are based on physiology: the Acute Physiology and Chronic Health Evaluation (APACHE-I, APACHE-II,[44] APACHE-III[45]), the Mortality Probability Model (MPM-I,[46] MPM-II,[47] including MPM_0 and MPM_{24}), and the Simplified Acute Physiology Score (SAPS-I,[48] SAPS-II,[49] SAPS III completed data collection in late 2002 and is in development). These models are all based on the premise that as illness increases, patients will exhibit greater deviation from physiologic normal for a variety of common parameters such as heart rate, blood pressure, neurologic status, and laboratory values. Risk is also assigned for advanced age and chronic illness.

ACUTE PHYSIOLOGY AND CHRONIC HEALTH EVALUATION

APACHE II was developed from data on 5815 medical and surgical ICU patients at 13 hospitals between 1979 and 1982. Severity of illness is assessed with 12 routine physiologic measurements plus the patient's age and previous health status.[44] Scoring is based on the most abnormal measurements during the first 24 hours in the ICU, and the maximum score is 71 points, although more than 80% of patients have scores of 29 or less.[44] Although the developers consider APACHE II to have significant limitations based on its age,[50] it is still in widespread use. APACHE II was developed on a database of medical and surgical patients that excluded patients undergoing coronary artery bypass grafting and coronary care, burn, and pediatric patients. The authors note that "it is crucial to combine the APACHE II score with a precise description of disease" and provide coefficients to adjust the score for 29 non-operative and 16 postoperative diagnostic categories.[44] They also caution that disease-specific mortality predictions be derived from at least 50 patients in each diagnostic category. These appropriate precautions have not always been observed in application of APACHE II.

Another common misunderstanding is to use APACHE II, calibrated for unselected ICU admissions, to assess outcome in a patient sample selected by other criteria, such as severe sepsis. The Acute Physiology Score from APACHE III or a specifically developed model predicting 28-day mortality in sepsis are preferable for risk stratification of septic patients.[51] APACHE II does not control for pre-ICU management, which could restore a patient's altered physiology and lead to a lower score and thus underestimate a patient's true risk. In a study of 235 medical patients scored with APACHE II, actual mortality was the same as predicted mortality only for patients admitted directly from the emergency department.[52] The mortality rate was higher than predicted for transfers from hospital floors, step-down units, or other hospitals. Inclusion of data from the period before ICU admission increases severity of illness scores and thus increases estimated mortality risk, and this effect is greatest with medical patients and emergency admissions.[53] Failure to consider the source of admission could thus lead to erroneous conclusions about the quality of medical care.[52,53]

APACHE III, published in 1991,[45] addresses many of the limitations of APACHE II, including the impact of treatment time and location before ICU admission. The number of separate disease categories was increased from 45 to 78. APACHE III was developed on a representative national database of 17,440 patients at 40 hospitals, including 14 tertiary facilities that volunteered for the study and 26 randomly chosen hospitals. The database is continuously expanded, and adjustments to coefficients keep the data relevant to current practice. Weighting of variables is accomplished by multivariate logistic regression. Compared with APACHE II, the ranges of physiologic "normal" are narrower with APACHE III and deviations are asymmetrically weighted to be more clinically relevant. Interactions between variables were considered, and five new variables (blood

urea nitrogen, urine output, serum albumin, bilirubin, and glucose) were added, and serum potassium and bicarbonate were dropped from the score. Information was also collected on 34 chronic health conditions, of which seven (AIDS, hepatic failure, lymphoma, solid tumor with metastasis, leukemia/multiple myeloma, immunocompromised state, and cirrhosis) were significant in predicting outcome.

APACHE III scoring ranges from 0 to 299, and a five-point increase represents a significant increase in risk of hospital death. In addition to the APACHE III *score*, which provides an initial risk estimate, there is an APACHE III *predictive equation* that uses the APACHE III score and proprietary reference data on disease category and treatment location before ICU admission to provide individual risk estimates for ICU patients. Customized models are available for patient populations (e.g., cardiac surgical patients) excluded from the APACHE II system. Overall correct classification at a 50% cut-point for mortality risk is 88.2%, with an ROC area of 0.90, significantly better than APACHE II.[45] Sequential APACHE III scoring can update the risk estimate daily, allowing for real-time decision support, for example, predicting likelihood of ICU interventions over the next 24-hour period. The single most important factor determining daily risk of hospital death is the updated APACHE III score, but the *change* in the APACHE III score, the admission diagnosis, the age and chronic health status of the patient, and prior treatment are also important. A predicted risk of death in excess of 90% on any of the first 7 days is associated with a 90% mortality rate. APACHE III scores also can be tied to predictions for ICU mortality, length of stay, need for interventions, and nursing workload.

Detailed instructions for calculating an APACHE III *score* (Table 259-5) are readily available.[45] The regression coefficients and detailed definitions for calculating predicted risk of hospital mortality are proprietary and require subscription to a software-based clinical information system. The APACHE system is now marketed by Cerner, a medical informatics company, and integrated systems allow automated data capture from bedside monitors and laboratory systems, thus reducing the data collection burden and facilitating real-time use of risk predictions.

MORTALITY PROBABILITY MODELS (MPM)

The original MPM was developed on 755 patients at Baystate Medical Center using multiple logistic regression to assign weights to variables predicting hospital mortality.[46] The MPM II models were developed on an international sample of 12,610 patients and then validated on a subsequent sample of 6514.[47] MPM, like APACHE II, excludes pediatric, burn, coronary, and cardiac surgical patients and estimates hospital mortality risk based partly on physiologic derangement, using a smaller number of variables. MPM II uses data obtained at ICU admission (MPM_0) and also at the end of the first 24-hour period (MPM_{24}) versus APACHE II or SAPS, which are scored using the most abnormal data obtained during the first 24 hours. The admission model (see Table 259-3) contains 15 variables; the 24-hour model (MPM_{24}) uses 5 of the 15 MPM0 variables plus 8 additional variables. Age and chronic health status are included within both MPM_0 and MPM_{24}. While APACHE generates a score and then with additional information converts that score into

TABLE 259–5. COMPONENTS OF THE APACHE III SCORE

Acute Physiology Score (0 to 252 points)	Points
Mean blood pressure	0 to 23
Respiratory rate adjusted for mechanical ventilation	0 to 18
Temperature	0 to 20
Pulse	0 to 17
Neurologic status	0 to 48
24-Hour urine output	0 to 15
Hematocrit	0 to 3
White blood cell count	0 to 19
Arterial pH adjusted for P_{CO_2}	0 to 12
Arterial P_{O_2} or $A_aD_{O_2}$ if ventilated	0 to 15
Serum sodium	0 to 4
Serum albumin	0 to 11
Serum glucose	0 to 9
Serum creatinine	0 to 10
Blood urea nitrogen	0 to 12
Serum bilirubin	0 to 16

Age, in Years (0 to 24 points)	
≤44	0
45-59	5
60-64	11
65-69	13
70-74	16
75-84	17
≥85	24

Chronic Health Condition* (0 to 23 points)	
AIDS	23
Hepatic failure	16
Lymphoma	13
Metastatic cancer	11
Leukemia/multiple myeloma	10
Immunosuppression	10
Cirrhosis	4

*Excluded for elective surgery patients.
Adapted from Knaus WA, Wagner DP, Draper EA, et al: The APACHE III Prognostic System. Risk prediction of hospital mortality for critically ill hospitalized adults. Chest 1991;100:1619-1636.

a probability estimate of survival, MPM directly calculates a probability of survival from the available data. Because this involves a logistic regression equation, it is difficult to accomplish at bedside without a computer or programmable calculator. The MPM_{24} variables account for differences in patients who remain in the ICU for 24 hours or longer versus those who die early or recover rapidly. This line of reasoning has been further extended to create 48- and 72-hour models.[54] Additional variables in MPM_{24}, MPM_{48}, and MPM_{72} but not MPM_0 are prothrombin time, urine output, creatinine, arterial oxygenation, continuing coma or deep stupor, confirmed infection, mechanical ventilation, or intravenous vasoactive drug therapy. Probability of death increases at 48 and 72 hours even if the MPM variables and coefficients are unchanged, implying that mortality risk is increasing in patients whose clinical profile remains unchanged over time.[54] MPM_{48} and MPM_{72} adjust for this observation by changing the β_0 (constant term) in the MPM_{24} equation. The most important difference between MPM and other systems is that the MPM_0, with the exception of information related to CPR, produces a probability estimate that is available at ICU presentation and is independent of ICU treatment. MPM does not require specifying a diagnosis, which can be an advantage in complex ICU patients but may also make it more susceptible to error with

changes in case mix.[33] MPM II calibrates well and has ROC areas of 0.837 for the admission model and 0.844 for the MPM_{24}. Unlike APACHE III, which is periodically updated, MPM II is based on aging data and may require recalibration to fit current medical practice.

SIMPLIFIED ACUTE PHYSIOLOGY SCORES I AND II

SAPS was developed on a population of 679 consecutive patients admitted to eight multidisciplinary ICUs in France and, like the APACHE systems, uses the most abnormal values collected during the first 24 hours after ICU admission. SAPS II was developed on 13,152 patients at 137 adult medical or surgical ICUs in Europe and North America, overlapping with the MPM II dataset. Like MPM and APACHE II, SAPS excludes burn patients, patients younger than 18 years, coronary care patients, and cardiac surgery patients. The outcome measure for SAPS II is vital status at hospital discharge. Seventeen variables are used in the SAPS II model: 12 physiologic variables, age, type of admission, and the presence of AIDS, metastatic cancer, or hematologic malignancy (Table 259-6). The area under the ROC curve is 0.88 in the developmental sample and 0.86 in the validation sample, with good performance measured by goodness-of-fit testing. Like MPM, the SAPS II can be scored without specifying a primary diagnosis and can be fully implemented from published information. Also like MPM II, the SAPS II model may have drifted out of calibration over time. The SAPS III project has recently collected data from more than 18,000 patients in 320 international ICUs, and a revised model is under development.

SPECIALIZED MODELS

APACHE II, MPM, and SAPS, while useful for general medical/surgical ICUs, exclude patients younger than age 18, burn patients, coronary care, and cardiac surgical patients. Murphy-Filkins and colleagues[33] have demonstrated that performance of severity of illness models deteriorates when critical values are reached for individual scoring variables, as might be seen in a highly specialized ICU. Twenty percent of the patients in the MPM II database were aged 75 or older. If this percentage of elderly patients is experimentally increased, at 42% elderly patients the model becomes unstable. Similar changes are seen if the proportion of patients with cardiac dysrhythmias, cerebrovascular disease, intracranial mass effects, coma, cardiopulmonary resuscitation before ICU admission, emergency admission, or gastrointestinal bleeding rise above their individual critical values. Thus, severity-of-illness scoring systems should be used with caution when units become highly specialized to care for subsets of patients. The European Consensus Conference recommends that severity indices be validated and customized if needed when applied to a new setting such as a particular country or specialized type of ICU.[17]

To address this problem, specific models have been developed for pediatric,[55] trauma,[56,57] and cardiac surgical populations.[26,58] The cardiac surgical population differs from the general ICU population because admission physiology data can be misleading in a population routinely subjected to hypothermia, hemodilution, and deliberate control of hemodynamics by the operating room team. Important

TABLE 259–6. VARIABLES AND DEFINITION FOR SAPS II

Variable	Definition	Points
Age	Age (in years) at last birthday	0 to 18
Heart rate	Use the worst value in 24 h, either low or high heart rate: if it varied from cardiac arrest (11 points) to extreme tachycardic (7 points), assign 11 points.	0 to 11
Systolic blood pressure	Use the same method as for heart rate: e.g., if it varied from 60 mm Hg to 205 mm Hg, assign 13 points.	0 to 13
Body temperature	Use the highest temperature.	0 to 3
Pao_2/Fio_2	If ventilated or continuous pulmonary artery pressure, use the lowest value of the ratio.	0 to 11
Urinary output	If the patient is in the intensive care unit for <24 h, make the calculation for 24 h: e.g., 1 L in 8 h = 3 L in 24 h	0 to 11
Serum urea or serum urea nitrogen level	Use the highest value in mmol/L for serum urea and in mg/dL for serum urea nitrogen	0 to 10
WBC count	Use the worst (high or low) WBC count	0 to 3
Serum potassium level	Use the worst (high or low) value in mmol/L	0 to 3
Serum sodium level	Use the worst (high or low) value in mmol/L	0 to 5
Serum bicarbonate level	Use the lowest value in mEq/L	0 to 6
Bilirubin level	Use the highest value in μmol/L or mg/dL	0 to 9
Glasgow Coma Scale	If the patient is sedated, record the estimated Glasgow Coma Scale score before sedation.	0 to 26
Type of admission	Unscheduled surgical* scheduled surgical†, or medical‡	8, 0, or 6
AIDS	Yes, if HIV-positive with clinical complications such as *Pneumocystis carinii* pneumonia, Kaposi's sarcoma, lymphoma, tuberculosis, or *Toxoplasma* infection	17
Hematologic malignancy	Yes, if lymphoma, acute leukemia, or multiple myeloma	10
Metastatic cancer	Yes, if proven metastatic by surgery, CT, or any other method	9

*Patients added to operating room schedule within 24 hours of the operation.
†Patient whose surgery was scheduled at least 24 hours in advance.
‡Patients having no surgery within 1 week of admission to intensive care unit.
SAPS, Simplified Acute Physiology Score; Fio₂, fraction of inspired oxygen; WBC, white blood cells; AIDS, acquired immunodeficiency syndrome; HIV, human immuno-deficiency virus; CT, computed tomography.
Adapted from Le Gall J-R, Lemeshow S, Saulnier F: A new Simplified Acute Physiology Score (SAPS II) based on a European/North American Multicenter study. JAMA 1993;270:2957-2963.

variables for predicting outcome in cardiac surgery include ventricular function, coronary anatomy, and heart valve pathology and reoperation status.[24] The Cooperative CABG Database Project, analyzing 172,000 patients, identified seven core variables (urgency of operation, age, prior heart surgery, gender, ejection fraction, percent stenosis of the left main coronary artery, and number of major coronary arteries with greater than 70% stenosis) to be predictive of mortality.[58] An additional 13 variables influence outcome to a lesser extent. These variables include recent angioplasty or myocardial infarction, history of angina, ventricular arrhythmias, CHF, mitral regurgitation, and coexisting diseases such as diabetes, cerebral vascular disease, peripheral vascular disease, chronic obstructive pulmonary disease, and renal dysfunction. At least 10 cardiac surgical models exist; head-to-head comparisons have demonstrated international differences in sensitivity and specificity and marked discrepancies in individual patient prediction.[59,60] In addition, the independent variables predicting morbidity do not perfectly overlap those predicting mortality or length of stay, suggesting that multiple risk scores may be required to best predict various outcomes. The preoperative cardiac surgical models are useful for evaluating the results of an entire hospitalization but do not specifically address the ICU component of care. Operating room events can neutralize or amplify preoperative risk, depending on such events as reopening the chest, hemodynamic management in an emergency patient, and the degree of myocardial protection. In 5000 patients

undergoing CABG, eight risk factors available at ICU admission appeared to predict hospital mortality and an additional five factors also predict morbidity.[26] These 13 mortality or morbidity variables, identified by logistic regression, are available in a clinical score (Table 259-7) that can be used in patients undergoing isolated coronary artery bypass grafting alone, or combined with a valve or carotid procedure. A modified APACHE III has also been successfully used for cardiac surgical patients in a prospective multicenter study of 2435 patients.[61] Independent predictors of hospital mortality included the APACHE score, age, emergency or reoperation status, the number of bypass grafts, and the gender of the patient. Risk prediction for cardiac surgical patients is incorporated into the APACHE III software package.

COMPARISONS BETWEEN MODELS

A number of papers compare the performance of the three general prognostic systems.[62-69] Based on a review of published articles, Lemeshow and Le Gall[70] concluded in 1994 that the newer models (APACHE III, MPM II, and SAPS II) reported performance sufficient to justify use in assessing prognosis, comparing ICU performance, and in stratifying patients for clinical trials. Castella and colleagues[67] compared APACHE II and III, SAPS I and II, and MPM I and II in a multicenter, multinational study of 14,745 patients in 137 ICUs (Table 259-8). None of the older models calibrated well, but

TABLE 259–7. INTENSIVE CARE UNIT RISK STRATIFICATION SCORE FOR CARDIAC SURGERY

Variable	Value
Preoperative Factors	
Small body size BSA <1.72 M²	1
Prior heart operation	
One	1
Two or more	2
History of operation or angioplasty for peripheral vascular disease	3
Age ≥70 y	3
Preoperative creatinine ≥1.9 mg/dL	4
Preoperative albumin <3.5 mg/dL	5
Intraoperative Factors	
CPB time ≥160 min	3
Use of IABP after CPB	7
ICU Admission Physiology	
A-a O₂ gradient ≥250 mm Hg	2
Heart rate ≥100 beats/min	3
Cardiac index <2.1 L/min/M²	3
CVP ≥18 mm Hg	4
Arterial bicarbonate <21 mmol/L	4

A-a, alveolar-atrial; BSA, body surface area; CPB, cardiopulmonary bypass; CVP, central venous pressure; IABP, intra-aortic balloon pump.
Reprinted from Higgins TL, Estafanous FG, Loop FD, et al: ICU admission score for predicting morbidity and mortality risk after coronary artery bypass grafting. Ann Thorac Surg 1997;64:1050-1058.

the revised systems were consistently superior to their earlier versions, as judged by both ROC area and goodness of fit. The newer systems all posted adequate discrimination. This study evaluated patients from the same database used for the development of SAPS II and MPM II. Even though comparisons were made using a subset of 4685 patients not part of the development samples, the data collection techniques and definitions would have been identical, a situation unlikely to be replicated by others.

Moreno and Morais[71] compared the performance of SAPS II with APACHE II in an independent database of 1094 patients in 19 Portuguese ICUs. Discrimination by ROC analysis was better for SAPS II, but neither model calibrated well by Hosmer-Lemeshow goodness-of-fit testing. In a comparison of the APACHE systems in 1144 British ICU patients, APACHE II had better calibration but APACHE III had better discrimination.[72] Hospital mortality was higher than predicted with either model,

agreement being best in respiratory patients and worst in trauma patients. The authors note that differences in trauma care infrastructure between the United States and the United Kingdom might account for some of this discrepancy. APACHE II had superior risk estimates for surgical patients.

Table 259-9 summarizes the results of nine recent studies in which two or more of the risk-adjustment models were applied to a specific regional population. There is no consistent pattern to accuracy-of-outcome prediction (discrimination), with examples of observed mortality higher than predicted, lower than predicted, as predicted, or predicted differently by different systems. There is no consistent leader in calibration; it tends to be poor in many studies. Ratios of observed to expected mortality rates are influenced by case mix as well as quality of care,[73] which argues for caution when using ratios such as the standardized mortality ratio for quality of care comparisons. Application of APACHE III to an Australian ICU underestimated mortality in a population that was younger, more male, and had more comorbidities than the APACHE III developmental set. Agreement was closer when Australian results were compared with the APACHE U.S. database or when the APACHE III model adjusted for hospital characteristics.[74] This suggests that cross-hospital comparisons for quality assessment require adjustment for hospital characteristics as well as patient severity of illness.

USES FOR SEVERITY-OF-ILLNESS INDICES

There are four major applications for severity-of-illness scoring systems:

1. Performance assessment
2. Predicting and planning resource utilization
3. Clinical research
4. Individual patient management

QUALITY IMPROVEMENT AND BENCHMARKING (PERFORMANCE ASSESSMENT)

Meaningful evaluation for ICU performance must consider both severity of illness of the patient population and characteristics of the institution. Benchmarking refers to the

TABLE 259–8. COMPARISON OF SEVERITY MODELS ON A COMMON DATA SET

	Discrimination ROC Area	Calibration GOF (H Statistic)	Sample Size
APACHE II*	0.853	< .0001	12,899
APACHE III	0.848	Not available	12,899
MPM₀I	0.766	< .0001	4,605
MPM₀II	0.805	0.0143	4,605
MPM₂₄I	0.815	< .0001	4,101
MPM₂₄II	0.833	.0247	4,101
SAPS I	0.784	Not applicable	4,605
SAPS II*	0.847	.1019	4,605

*Discrimination and calibration assessed on probability estimate, not score.
†Lower P value implies poor fit. For example, the newer MPM₂₄ at P = .0247 calibrates than the original MPM₂₄ at P < .0001. All P values approach significance due to the size of the database.
Adapted from Castella X, Artigas A, Bion J, Kari A: A comparison of severity of illness scoring systems for intensive care unit patients: Results of a multicenter, multinational study. The European/North American Severity Study Group. Crit Care Med 1995;23:1327-1335.

TABLE 259–9. SITE SPECIFIC APPLICATION OF SEVERITY SCORING MODELS

Study	Country	Systems	Findings Good Discrimination
Arabi, et al.[107]	Saudi Arabia = 969	APACHE II MPM II$_0$ and II$_{24}$ SAPS II	Predicted mortality similar to that observed for all systems (SMR 1.0 to 1.09) Calibration best with MPM II$_{24}$ Discrimination best with MPM II$_0$ followed by MPM II$_{24}$, APACHE II and SAPS; all ROC >0.79
Capuzzo, et al.[64]	Italy Single center n = 1,721	APACHE II SAPS II	ROC area >0.8 both models Mortality in high-risk patients overpredicted by SAPS II and underpredicted by APACHE II
Katsaragakis, et al.[108]	Greece Single center n = 661	APACHE II SAPS II	Good discrimination, but poor calibration with both models Better performance with APACHE II
Livingston, et al.[69]	Scotland 22 centers n = 10,393	APACHE II APACHE III UK APACHE II MPM II$_0$ MPM II$_{24}$	Discrimination adequate (ROC areas 0.74 to 0.795) Observed mortality significantly different than predicted by all systems APACHE II had best calibration followed by MPM II$_{24}$ and SAPS II
Markgraf, et al.[66]	Germany Single center n = 2,661 to 2,795	APACHE II APACHE III SAPS II	Observed mortality higher than predicted by any model Worst discrepancy with trauma, respiratory, neurologic, and renal disease Best calibration with APACHE II ROC area >0.8 all models
Moreno, et al.[68]	Europe 89 centers n = 16,060	MPM II$_0$ SAPS II	Discrimination adequate (ROC 0.822 for SAPS II, 0.785 for MPM$_0$) Both models overestimated risk of death Large variations across subgroups of patients
Nouira, et al.[109]	Tunisia 3 centers n = 1325	APACHE II MPM II$_0$ and II$_{24}$ SAPS II	Observed mortality higher than predicted except with MPM$_0$ Good discrimination, poor calibration for all models
Patel, et al.[41]	United States Single VA medical center n = 302	APACHE II MPM II SAPS II	Predicted mortality for all three scoring systems within 95% CI of predicted ROC area 0.672 to 0.702
Tan et al[110]	China (Hong Kong) Single center n = 1064	APACHE II SAPS II	Discrimination good (ROC area 0.87 to 0.88) but calibration poor Both models overpredict mortality

process of comparing an individual unit's performance either against established case mix–adjusted standards, with similar ICUs, or with the units' own data over time. Benchmarking is not for morbidity and mortality outcomes alone, and severity adjustment has been successfully used to explain variations in cost[75] and ICU length of stay.[76] Outlier length-of-stay status is only partially predicted by severity of illness, and factors such as long ward stays before ICU admission and absence of an intensivist-directed multidisciplinary care team increase length of stay.[77]

The mortality rate for patients transferred to a hospital is higher than that of nontransferred patients,[78] and this has implications in profiling hospital quality.[79] Medical patients transferred from another hospital have higher acute physiology scores but, even after adjustment for case mix and severity of illness, experience longer hospital and ICU lengths of stay and have more than twice the risk of hospital mortality compared with directly admitted patients.[7] The authors of these studies suggest that a referral hospital with a 25% transfer rate would suffer a penalty when undergoing profiling and that public policy should take this into account to reduce the disincentive for tertiary-care centers to accept these patients.

PREDICTING AND PLANNING RESOURCE UTILIZATION

The Therapeutic Intervention Scoring System (TISS) was developed as a method for quantifying patient care and severity of illness.[80] As a prognostic measure it was supplanted by the newer scoring systems once it was realized that application of technology depended on local availability and local practice. The TISS score does reflect ICU workload and costs[81] and has been used to measure nursing workload.[82] TISS is available in an abbreviated version[83] and can also be correlated to APACHE III scores. APACHE III and SAPS II have also been applied to measuring severity of illness in intermediate-care units. By extension, risk prediction systems can be used to guide patient selection for critical care in graded settings, depending on initial presentation.[84,85]

USE OF SEVERITY INDICES IN CLINICAL RESEARCH

Existing databases and severity adjustment make possible hypothesis-generating observations and conclusions about therapeutic choices in situations where randomized, prospective evaluations might not be permitted or funded. For prospective studies, severity scoring indices can be used to "risk stratify" the population before randomization, thus reducing the number of patients and cost of clinical trials.[86] Clinical studies have also used scoring systems as part of inclusion criteria and to demonstrate that control and study groups have similar disease burden. Representative examples of this approach include risk stratification for comparison of different antibiotic regimens[87] and anticytokine therapies.[88] Acute physiologic abnormalities are important prognostic factors influencing outcome in patients meeting criteria for severe sepsis.[51] Correlations have been noted between the MPM_0 II sepsis score[89] and interleukin-6 plasma levels and between APACHE III scores and plasma levels of tumor necrosis factor-sR, interleukin-6, and C-reactive protein.[90] Nonsurvivors have significantly higher MPM II or APACHE III scores at any time during sepsis.

USES OF SEVERITY ADJUSTMENT FOR INDIVIDUAL PREDICTIONS

The difficulty in using scoring systems for individuals arises from attempts to apply a probability estimate, which may range from 0 to 1, to an individual for whom the result will be 0 *or* 1. No model is accurate enough to predict that a given patient will certainly survive or invariably die, so the use of scoring systems alone to direct or withhold therapy is not recommended. It is unlikely that any score calculated within 24 hours of ICU admission could ever perfectly predict outcome, because the patient's individual response to therapy clearly plays a role. APACHE III could not independently predict survival in 114 patients with perforated gastrointestinal viscus and only the development of overt multiple organ failure predicted death.[91] Sequential prognostic estimates, an approach explored by both APACHE[92] and MPM,[54] may improve prognosis by incorporating response to therapy, but this application of scoring systems should not create a vicious cycle in which a declining risk of survival could precipitate withdrawal or limitation of care. Objective predictions of the need for next-day life support are used by APACHE III to guide triage and discharge decisions.[93]

Use of scoring systems to guide therapy has not been well studied. The package insert for recombinant human activated protein C (rhAPC) suggests the use of APACHE scores greater than 25 as one possible criterion for drug administration. This recommendation is based in part on post-hoc subgroup analysis of PROWESS trial[94] patients showing that patients with higher APACHE II scores were more likely to benefit from this therapy than those with lower scores. Problems with limiting administration of this agent to patients with low severity include wide variability in severity score between those obtained at ICU admission versus at the time of drug administration.[95] Because the APACHE II score is weighted for age and chronic health status, younger patients and those with less chronic disease burden will have lower scores for an equal amount of physiologic derangement. The Australian study quoted earlier[74] indirectly suggests that younger, healthier patients may be improperly categorized. An efficient emergency department may well stabilize the patients and lower the APACHE score before arrival in the ICU.[96] These same general concerns would apply to many situations in which a severity score could be used to decide on ICU admission or to administer or withhold therapeutic interventions for an individual patient. Sequential prediction, as used by APACHE III for bed triage function, may be preferable to a single point estimate.

Objectively calculated severity scores are not necessarily more accurate than physician or nurse intuition when dealing with individual patients. APACHE II has been compared to clinical assessment by nurses and housestaff working in the ICU.[97] Sensitivity, specificity, correct prediction, and area under the ROC curve were compared, and no significant differences were noted between ROC areas for APACHE II versus nurses, fellows, residents, or interns. Accurate prognosis may be most difficult for patients with the highest risk of death. A recent multicenter study addressing the issue of medical futility found that divergent judgments on patient prognosis by doctors and nurses increased with higher SAPS II scores and longer ICU stays.[98]

APACHE, SAPS, and MPM scores are specific, having better than 90% ability to predict survival, but are relatively insensitive in predicting death. Such information should not be taken as a rationale to rely on clinical judgment and forego the use of formal scoring. The existing severity indices, despite their flaws, do provide useful, objective information that can guide individual prognosis and triage decisions, bearing in mind that patient autonomy and medical ethics may ultimately dictate a different plan.

PITFALLS IN THE APPLICATION OF SEVERITY OF ILLNESS INDICES

Like any tool, severity-of-illness indices can be misused. The use (and abuse) of databases for profiling ICUs and/or individual physicians is growing, despite flaws in administrative databases and problems identified with application of statistical models.[20,21,33,99,100] Assuming a properly developed model is applied, potential pitfalls in application fall into four major categories: data collection and entry errors,[101] misapplication of the model, especially related to case mix,[33] use of mortality as the sole criterion of outcome, and failure to account for sample size and chance variability when reporting results (Table 259-10). Determination of the diagnosis is prone to bias.[102] Models that assess performance using a patient's condition at 24 hours are not truly independent of treatment. If the characteristics of patients are markedly different from a general population's, the resulting case mix will alter model performance.[33] Less obvious is the fact that all models start the clock with ICU admission, the timing of which is not standardized,[103] and frequently are influenced by local conditions such as ICU bed availability. Intensive care units also do not function in isolation in the process of care,[104] and the recent trend toward aggressive use of step-down facilities and off-site chronic ventilation and rehabilitation units raises the question of whether hospital mortality is valid when patients may be transferred alive, but still technology-dependent, to other facilities. The issue of lead-time bias (pre-ICU stabilization) has been mentioned earlier; assessment is further complicated for patients with multiple ICU admissions.[105,106] Which ICU stay, for example, should be counted for a patient who has ICU observation after an uneventful vascular procedure and then develops complications requiring ICU readmission on the fifth postoperative day? It is increasingly necessary to evaluate the performance of an ICU *system*, which includes pre-ICU,

TABLE 259–10. POTENTIAL PITFALLS IN THE APPLICATION AND REPORTING OF SEVERITY-ADJUSTED OUTCOME

Data Collection and Entry

Inclusion of ineligible patients
Missing variables and data management errors
Substitution of available for properly timed data
Transcription and data entry errors
Wrong diagnosis selected
Administrative data may not reflect clinical condition
Deliberate "gaming" of the system

Models

Case-mix differences (critical threshold exceeded)
Application to subsets of development population
Changes in weighting over time
Small clinical changes can translate into large risk increments
    when continuous data are categorized.
Lead-time bias

Outcomes

Insufficient range of outcomes reported
Use of proxy outcomes that inadequately reflect true status
Patient lost to follow-up
Change variability masquerading as true difference
Relationships of scores to resource utilization and costs reflect
    observed practice, not ideal

Reporting

Confidence intervals not reported
Inadequate sample size
Physician of record misidentified
Computational errors
Misapplication of group data to individuals
Misinterpretation of statistical significance as clinical significance

ICU, and post-ICU care. Rules for starting times and endpoints of evaluation need to be better defined.[103,104]

CONCLUSION

APACHE III, MPM II, and SAPS II are highly developed, prospectively validated tools useful for comparison of ICU performance in the care of groups of patients. Specialized models are available for burn, trauma, sepsis, cardiac surgical, and pediatric patients. When used as intended, these models allow stratification of patients for performance assessment, utilization management, clinical research, and dissemination of outcome results. Important implementation considerations include careful data collections, appropriate matching of the model and the population under study, and use of proper sample sizes and confidence intervals in reporting results.

None of the models can ever perfectly predict the outcome for an individual patient. However, this limitation is true of almost any test utilized in medicine and need not preclude the use of prognostic estimates for clinical decision support. Work now under way on sequential probability estimates and customized models may increase the acceptance of objective measurements in defining potentially ineffective care. Physicians must be alert to the limitations of severity-adjustment models in performance-based assessment, because case-mix differences, inadequate sample sizes, or systemic errors in data collection can generate erroneous conclusions about the quality of care.

ANNOTATED REFERENCES

Knaus WA, Wagner DP, Draper EA et al: The APACHE III Prognostic System—Risk prediction of hospital mortality for critically ill hospitalized adults. Chest 1991;100:1619-1636.

Knaus and colleagues were among the first to recognize the importance of prognostic scoring systems and have continuously refined the APACHE system over the past quarter century. This article details the development of APACHE-III, currently one of the most widely used models.

Glance LG, Osler TM, Dick A: Rating the quality of intensive care units: Is it a function of the intensive care unit scoring system? Crit Care Med 2002;30:1976-1982.

APACHE-II, SAPS-II, and MPM-II showed fair to moderate agreement in identifying ICU quality outliers. Most units in the 32-hospital database were judged to be high-performing, raising questions about the utility of these dated models to be useful for current benchmarking.

Murphy-Filkins RL, Teres D, Lemeshow S, Hosmer DW: Effect of changing patient mix on the performance of an intensive care unit severity-of-illness model: How to distinguish a general from a specialty intensive care unit. Crit Care Med 1996;24:1968-1973.

The authors artificially manipulated a database to create conditions in which generalized models would fail. This article points out the importance of using customized models when a unit or patient population differs substantially from "average" conditions.

Tunnell RD, Millar BW, Smith GB: The effect of lead time bias on severity of illness scoring, mortality prediction, and standardized mortality ratio in intensive care: A pilot study. Anaesthesia 1998;53:1045-1053.

This small study carefully evaluated the effect of including data prior to ICU admission on outcome predictions using APACHE-II, APACHE-III, and SAPS-II. Temporal differences in data collection will change standardized mortality ratios, and the effect is most pronounced in medical patients and emergency admissions.

Zimmerman JE, Alzola C, Von Rueden KT: The use of benchmarking to identify top performing critical care units: A preliminary assessment of their policies and practices. Crit Care 2003;18:76-86.

Clinical data from 359,715 patients in 108 intensive care units was used to validate APACHE-III for benchmarking mortality, ICU and hospital length of stay, and percentage of low-risk monitor patients. Availability of alternative care areas, efficient throughput, and use of protocols were characteristics of better-performing units.

Chapter 260

EVALUATING PEDIATRIC CRITICAL CARE

Anthony D. Slonim • Murray M. Pollack

KEY POINTS

SAFETY

1. Medical errors and patient safety are particularly important aspects of evaluating pediatric critical care practice.

2. Medical errors can be classified in a variety of ways. The Institute of Medicine categorizes common patient-related errors as diagnostic errors, preventive errors, procedural errors, and errors in treatment. This classification scheme is particularly relevant to the pediatric intensive care unit (PICU).

EFFECTIVENESS

1. Effective clinical practice is dependent on evidence-based principles that incorporate research evidence, clinical expertise, and patient values to achieve the best outcomes for critically ill pediatric patients.

2. Providers are not always successful in incorporating these principles into their practice. However, the use of standardized protocols and guidelines can be effective in reducing variability and improving patient care.

EQUITY

1. The provision of care to critically ill pediatric patients should be free from discrimination based on personal attributes or ability to pay. Maintaining this objectivity is necessary if children are to receive access to the important technologic advances that PICUs can provide.

2. Disparities based on race and insurance status are two examples of inequities in the provision of critical care services. Identifying and reducing these disparities are important means of improving care.

TIMELINESS

1. Families of critically ill pediatric patients deserve timely explanations of the care their children are receiving.

2. Children hospitalized in the PICU should receive timely care provided by trained critical care practitioners around the clock.

PATIENT CENTEREDNESS

1. Families' satisfaction with the care provided in the PICU is an important outcome measure. This satisfaction is not wholly dependent on the outcome of the child. Rather, it depends on the health care team's attention to communication, parent-provider partnerships, and end-of-life care.

EFFICIENCY

1. Each ICU's value is increased by its ability to achieve selected measures of outcome while keeping costs to a minimum.

Assessment of the clinical services provided to critically ill children is an important aspect of intensive care medicine. Over the past 20 to 30 years, increased attention has been paid to the issues of quality in health care, beginning with the seminal work by Donabedian, which identified the components of structure, process, and outcome required for a careful analysis of this issue.[1] The most recent attempts to characterize health care quality and move the health care system toward performance measures include a major effort by the Institute of Medicine (IOM). Its report titled *Crossing the Quality Chasm* recommends "Six Aims for Improvement."[2] These aims, which relate to the fundamental changes that must made to improve health care services, are:

- Safety
- Effectiveness
- Equity
- Timeliness
- Patient-centeredness
- Efficiency

The IOM model is the prevailing paradigm for evaluating the provision of clinical services. In this chapter, the evaluation of pediatric critical care services is reviewed, with attention to each of these aims. The existing evidence supporting clinical practice in the pediatric intensive care unit (PICU), its gaps, and the resulting opportunities to drive the quality research agenda in the future are also considered.

SAFETY

The IOM's report on medical errors and patient safety highlighted the problem of iatrogenic injury in hospitalized inpatients.[3] As a result, the federal government and regulatory agencies, as well as health care organizations and providers, have begun to focus on reducing medical errors as a means of improving patient safety in hospitals. In the IOM's report on health care quality, safety was included as one of the six aims intended to reduce the harm associated with the delivery of health care.[2] Adverse patient occurrences are inevitable in the high-risk environment of the PICU,[4-6] but interventions aimed at reducing these adverse events can be designed once one understands the types of errors and the circumstances that contribute to them.

CLASSIFICATION OF MEDICAL ERRORS

Several different classification schemes for medical errors have been developed, each addressing the issue from a different perspective. In an early attempt to categorize medical complications, Brennan and colleagues classified adverse events in medical practice as operative and nonoperative.[7] The usefulness of this classification system is derived from its simplicity and reproducibility. McClead and Menke created a classification system for the neonatal ICU that includes both the investigation of complications associated with new or unproven technologies and the study of "human error," which continues to have relevance in current patient safety efforts.[8-10] The identification of "critical incidents" is another approach to improving the quality of care.[11] Underlying this conceptual approach is a belief that these incidents provide opportunities for the health care team to make system improvements. With the increased computerization of health care, several classification schemes have used administrative data sets to analyze medical errors in children. Two prevailing epidemiologic approaches that use International Classification of Diseases codes have been published for pediatrics,[12,13] and one of these has been applied to medical errors in the neonatal ICU population.[14] The IOM used the definitions of Brennan and colleagues to categorize medical errors based on their diagnosis, treatment, or prevention (Table 260-1).[3] A residual "other" category consists of medical errors that arise from communication or equipment failures or are otherwise related to a "systems" problem (see Table 260-1). Each of these categories has particular relevance for the evaluation of pediatric critical care services.

Diagnostic Errors

The autopsy has been used as a tool to detect missed diagnoses that may have had antemortem clinical relevance for practitioners.[15] Therefore, it may be a useful technique to enhance quality assurance programs in medical care. Diagnostic errors uncovered at autopsy are classified as "major errors," those that involved a primary cause of death, or "class 1 errors," which likely affected patient outcome in a more general way.[15] In a systematic literature review that evaluated 53 autopsy series, the median rates of major errors and class 1 errors were 23.5% and 9.0%, respectively.[15]

In three single-institution studies of critically ill adult patients, autopsies revealed diagnoses that would have

TABLE 260-1. INSTITUTE OF MEDICINE CLASSIFICATION OF MEDICAL ERRORS

Diagnostic errors
    Delay or error in diagnosis
    Failure to apply appropriate tests
    Use of outmoded tests
    Failure to act on results of tests or monitoring
Treatment errors
    Error in the performance of a procedure, surgery, or test
    Error in administering a treatment
    Error in the dosage or method of use of a drug
    Avoidable delay in treatment or responding to a test result
    Inappropriate (not indicated) care
Preventive errors
    Failure to provide prophylactic treatment
    Inadequate monitoring and treatment
Other errors
    Failure to communicate
    Equipment failure
    Other system failure

changed antemortem management and affected outcome in 10% to 27% of cases.[16-18] In a single-institution trauma series, the rate of missed injuries resulting in death was considerably lower (3%).[19] In children, the rate of missed diagnoses that affected outcome was estimated as 7% in one study.[20] In a pediatric emergency department series, the correct diagnosis was made in 85% of patients, and no class 1 errors were identified.[21] In the PICU, one study identified major diagnostic errors that would have affected outcome in 5% of patients; in an additional 25% of cases, there were missed diagnoses that were not believed to be clinically meaningful.[22] Importantly, iatrogenic injury was a major subset of these missed diagnoses, occurring 17% of the time.[22] Thus, autopsy remains an important tool for identifying diagnostic errors and deaths related to iatrogenic injury.

Treatment Errors

Medication Errors. The administration of medications is one of the most frequent types of treatment for critically ill children. There is a high risk of medication errors and adverse drug events in the PICU setting, and this is a well-studied type of treatment error. In one study of pediatric inpatients, the rate of medication error was approximately 5.7%.[23] Adverse drug events are common among hospitalized children and occur more often and have more importance in those with greater disease burdens, who may also have increased opportunities for exposure to medication errors.[23,24] PICUs are important locations for these adverse events to occur.[23,25] In addition, specific classes of medications may be more prone to errors.[26,27] Specific investigations of high-risk drug classes such as sedatives, vasoactive infusions, and parenteral nutrition have been performed.[26,28,29] One useful and cost-effective strategy to improve the rate of medication errors in the PICU is to have a unit-based pharmacist.[30] On average, the clinical pharmacist was found to intervene approximately 35 times per 100 patient-days. The most frequent interventions were to adjust dosages (28%) and to provide drug information (26%).[30] The availability of practitioners with specific expertise (such as a unit-based pharmacist) who can contribute to the management decisions of the critical care team is becoming increasingly important in the provision of high-quality critical care services.

Nosocomial Infection. Acquired infections are important contributors to morbidity and mortality in the

PICU population.[31-33] The Joint Commission on Accreditation of Healthcare Organizations now considers nosocomial infection contributing to a patient's death a reportable sentinel event.[34] Recent efforts have expanded our knowledge of the incidence, prevalence, risk factors, and costs of nosocomial infections in critically ill pediatric patients.[31-33,35-38] The median rate of bloodstream infections is 13.9 per 1000 patient-days.[31] Consistent observations among studies demonstrate that the most common sites for nosocomial infection are the bloodstream (28% to 41%), lower respiratory tract (21% to 22.7%), and urinary tract (13% to 15%).[32,33,35] The microbiology typically includes coagulase-negative staphylococcal species and aerobic gram-negative bacilli, depending on the source of the infection.[32,33] Risk factors for nosocomial infection in the PICU include severity of illness, postoperative status, and device use.[39-42] Nosocomial infections are associated with increased resource use and cost.[36] In one study investigating the costs of nosocomial bloodstream infections, each case was associated with an attributable cost of $46,000 and an attributable PICU and hospital length of stay of 14.6 and 21.1 days, respectively.[36]

Specific investigations into the types of nosocomial infection (e.g., urinary tract, pneumonia),[43] specific organisms (e.g., influenza, respiratory syncytial virus, methicillin-resistant *Staphylococcus aureus*),[44,45] specific PICU patient populations (e.g., cardiac surgery, burns),[46,47] and specific procedures (e.g., mechanical ventilation, extracorporeal membrane oxygenation)[48,49] have been performed. These studies provide insight for the development of directed strategies to reduce nosocomial infection rates and their associated morbidity and mortality in PICUs. These strategies include more stringent infection control policies, reduction of colonization with resistant organisms, and scheduled rotation of prescribed antibiotics.[50-53]

Procedures. Interventional procedures are an important component of pediatric critical care practice. They allow the intensivist to address each failing organ system and provide a means of compensation until recovery occurs. Although these procedures may be lifesaving, they are also associated with risk.

ICUs are noted for their variability in patient care. This variability in clinical care practices exists both within and between pediatric and adult ICUs.[54,55] Because accidental extubation has potentially lethal effects, it is a good starting point for discussing patient safety practices related to ICU procedures. Accidental extubation is a familiar, frequent occurrence in many ICUs, regardless of their practice structure (e.g., adult or pediatric, medical or surgical, teaching or nonteaching).[56-63] Accidental extubation can occur in any intubated critically ill patient and contributes significantly to risk.[56-63] Efforts to reduce the accidental extubation rate in ICUs might involve addressing the high level of variability in the processes of care. For example, despite many years of study and numerous reports, there is no standardized, accepted method (e.g., taping methods, restraint use, sedation protocols) for maintaining a patient who is mechanically ventilated and therefore at risk for accidental extubation. Optimal methods of securing endotracheal tubes and maintaining the safety of intubated patients could be shared among different ICUs. This would help reduce variability and ensure the safety of patients with respiratory failure.

Preventive Errors

One major component of preventive errors is the failure to provide prophylactic treatment.[2] In the ICU environment, considerable evidence has been accumulated regarding prophylaxis for gastrointestinal stress ulcers, deep venous thrombosis, pressure ulcers, and other adverse events.[64-67] Intensive care providers must balance the risks and benefits of such care in the ICU setting.

Efforts have been made to address prophylactic care more broadly. For example, the PRIMACORP study was initiated to determine whether the prophylactic, postoperative use of milrinone in pediatric cardiac surgery patients improves the outcome associated with low cardiac output syndrome.[68] Another example of a prophylactic intervention is the "tunneling" of femoral central venous catheters.[69] This intervention is safe and effective in reducing the colonization of these catheters in critically ill pediatric patients.

Other Errors

The PICU environment may be an independent contributor to patient safety or the lack thereof. The IOM highlights communication errors, equipment failures, and system failures as components of an unsafe environment.[3] Equipment failures are an obvious and often unavoidable problem related to patient safety. However, communication failures and system failures can enhance the likelihood of errors and require further explanation.[3]

Clinical microsystems are small, discrete, yet functional front-line units that provide health care to patients.[70-72] These microsystems operate within the hierarchy of the larger macrosystem to provide care.[73] For example, the microsystem that cares for a congenital heart disease patient after surgery may include the patient's parents, nurse, intensivist, cardiologist, cardiac surgeon, respiratory therapist, and social worker. These people's interactions with the patient may be structured within a pathway or care guideline to provide optimal care for the patient. However, dynamic changes in the patient's condition, such as the need for emergent cardiac catheterization, may require that additional expertise or resources be drawn from the other microsystems within the PICU or from the macrosystem of the hospital.[73] Two characteristics of these microsystems contribute to the likelihood of errors. The first is complexity, or the degree to which system components are specialized and interdependent. Complex systems are more prone to errors. The second characteristic is coupling. Tightly coupled systems have no buffer, and sequences are fixed, whereas loosely coupled systems can tolerate delays or variations in sequencing.

Studies of patient safety and medical errors in the PICU environment must account for the hospital characteristics that might influence the occurrence of errors, their reporting,[2] or the types of patients cared for in these settings. Such factors include patient volume, location, and teaching status, all of which can influence the microsystem. For example, PICUs are likely to be sited in hospitals where children with complex medical problems receive care. However, with the expansion of PICUs beyond academic medical centers into the community, integrated and specialized services may not be immediately available. These voids may jeopardize the timely delivery of some services to critically ill children and adversely affect their care.

EFFECTIVENESS

Evidence-based practice incorporates the best research evidence with clinical expertise and patient values to achieve the best outcomes for patients.[2] The clinical practice of critical care medicine is highly variable among practitioners and institutions.[54,55] An opportunity to reduce the variability in care is provided by the implementation of practice guidelines.[74-76]

Private, governmental, and subspecialty organizations have developed numerous guidelines to reduce unnecessary variability in care. The American Academy of Pediatrics and the Society for Critical Care Medicine have developed guidelines and policy statements to help improve the care of critically ill children.[75,77] These guidelines are heterogeneous with respect to their creation. At one extreme, results from randomized controlled trials are incorporated into the care guidelines; at the other extreme, the consensus of a group of practitioners is all that is required.[75] This is important, because the success of any practice guideline is dependent on its ability to influence physician decision-making.[74-77]

One major effort to improve the care of critically ill children with traumatic brain injury has been accomplished.[77] Several important components of these guidelines are worth mentioning, because they will ultimately contribute to the guidelines' acceptance by practitioners of critical care medicine. First, the guidelines are grounded in the existing evidence base from randomized controlled trials.[78] Second, when the evidence did not exist, the authors assembled a multidisciplinary group of clinicians and researchers to reach consensus regarding treatment options. This was done to minimize bias by any one group of practitioners or any one discipline.[78] Third, and perhaps most important, the guidelines are considered a work in progress that helps identify current deficiencies, from a data perspective, so that future research initiatives can be used to further support these guidelines.[78] This effort benefited from the contributions of clinicians from a number of professional societies, all with the intent of creating the best guidelines for children with traumatic brain injury. It is hoped that the multidisciplinary nature of this effort will lead to the acceptance of these guidelines and ultimately an improved outcome for children with traumatic brain injury. Further, this methodology may provide an approach that can be extrapolated to other problems encountered in critically ill pediatric patients.

EQUITY

Achieving equity in health care quality means ensuring impartial care for populations and individuals that is free from bias related to race, ethnicity, insurance status, income, or gender.[2] This bias may be manifested at two independent levels. First, discrimination may be targeted at the population level before the patient actually reaches a health care provider.[2] These problems are primarily ones of restricted access to health care. Second, once patients have accessed health care services, they may receive differential treatment based on personal characteristics.[2] In its most overt form, this is called discrimination.

Distributive justice is linked to equity, and this is the term applied to fairness in the distribution of limited resources and benefits. It would seem that in the ICU, with its unique patient base, inequities related to personal characteristics would be minimized.[79] The allocation of scarce ICU resources has traditionally been reserved for those with more severe illness.[79] However, there are examples of inequitable distribution of ICU resources for patients with the same severity of illness but racial or insurance status differences.[79]

INSURANCE STATUS

Insurance status differences affect access to outpatient physicians, hospital services, and procedures. These differences also affect physicians' practice patterns and thereby influence resource use and outcome for adult primary care and critical care patients alike.[80-87]

For example, one study found that in critically ill adults with *Pneumocystis carinii* pneumonia, the performance of diagnostic tests was correlated with insurance status.[83] In another study, patients with private insurance received pulmonary artery catheters in greater proportions than did other ICU patients.[87] Adult Medicaid and Medicare patients undergoing liver transplantation experienced higher costs and longer lengths of stay than did patients with commercial insurance.[84] Among adults admitted to a trauma ICU, operative procedures and ICU care were less likely to be provided to Medicaid patients than to those with private insurance.[88] Another study of trauma patients demonstrated a delay in access to rehabilitative services for the noncommercially insured.[85]

Insurance status differences apply not only to different types of insurance but also to the method of administering the insurance.[86,89] For example, the care delivered under a managed care arrangement is expected to be different from that delivered in a non–managed care environment.[89] However, these differences in care do not necessarily mean that one type of care is worse; it may simply be different.[89] In a comparison of managed care versus non–managed care hospital admissions in Massachusetts and Florida, there were no differences in the admission rates to ICUs. The length of stay was found to be somewhat less in Massachusetts for managed care patients, which was attributed to a relatively constrained supply of ICU beds.[89] For patients with respiratory failure requiring mechanical ventilator support, managed care patients actually received more procedures and were more costly to care for during their ICU stays. However, their mortality rates and lengths of stay were lower than those of a similar cohort of commercially insured patients.[90] This example provides evidence that managed care is not synonymous with a reduction in appropriate care. These examples also demonstrate how the aims of the IOM paradigm are not isolated, but rather overlap. The aims of equity and efficiency are both operative when evaluating quality in managed care.

Inequities in access to health care exist for children as well as adults, especially for outpatient services.[91-94] For example, insurance status was associated with access to a primary care provider, provision of immunizations and innovative technologies, and access to health care during nighttime hours.[91-97] Lack of access to needed services may be responsible for delayed disease presentation and avoidable morbidity,[98,99] which may lead to more severe illness and longer hospital stay.[98,99] This is consistent with the observation that patients from lower socioeconomic status have more severe illness on admission to the PICU.[100]

There are limited data describing the relationship of insurance status to resource utilization or outcome in specific subgroups of critically ill pediatric patients, including neonates and medical and surgical patients.[101-108] The interhospital transfer of pregnant women and sick newborns covered by Medicaid is higher than that among commercially insured patients.[106] Newborns with Medicaid were also more likely to be born prematurely and to have more severe illness than commercially insured newborns.[106] In another study, Medicaid-insured newborns were sicker and had higher resource use than did commercially insured newborns.[107] However, sick newborns without insurance received fewer inpatient services than did either Medicaid or commercially insured patients.[107] In one study, publicly insured premature neonates were 50% more likely to be subjected to medical errors.[14] As discussed earlier, managed care penetration can influence the availability of technologic interventions in health care.[104] Managed care is positively associated with the adoption of high-intensity neonatal ICUs in a given market to care for the sickest patients, but slower adoption of midlevel care units.[104]

Insurance status differences in critically ill pediatric medical patients have also been demonstrated. After adjusting for illness severity, children with acute, severe asthma who were insured by Medicaid received mechanical ventilation more often and for longer durations and had longer PICU and hospital stays than did commercially insured or managed care patients.[108] Children with Medicaid who were hospitalized with diabetic ketoacidosis experienced coma more often and had longer lengths of stay than did their commercially insured counterparts.[103]

Similar differences, based on insurance status, can be found among critically ill pediatric surgical patients. Postoperative congenital heart disease patients with Medicaid had higher mortality rates than did commercially insured children.[102] Medicaid patients experienced complicated appendicitis, including perforation or abscess formation, more often than did other patients,[108] and they had longer stays. Observed mortality rates among uninsured children with head trauma were higher than those among privately or publicly insured children.[105]

In 1997, a major effort to reduce the health care inequities for children without insurance led to the State Children's Health Insurance Program, which was designed to provide insurance coverage for low-income children.[109-111] This program has been successful in reducing the number of uninsured children.[109] However, states differed in their strategies for implementing the program, and as a result, related improvements in health care performance are still awaiting documentation.[110] This is important, because inequities in care related to insurance status continue to be documented, even among the sickest children requiring ICU admission.[109-111] These differences among uninsured, publicly insured, and commercially insured patients may lead to differences in the observed quality of health care. In addition, managed care has altered the way health care is delivered for publicly and privately insured patients alike.[111] The effects of these differences on the health status of children also remains to be determined.[111]

RACE

The IOM was charged with assessing the extent of racial disparities in health care, identifying the factors contributing to the inequities, and recommending policies and practices to eliminate them.[112] The integration of national efforts to address racial disparities in health care and the work being accomplished in health care quality provides opportunities to improve the equity of delivered health care services to minority populations.[113]

Racial differences in health care are evident for adult and pediatric patients alike.[112-147] These differences affect access to health care services and outcomes.[112-147] Primary care and mental health services for children and adults are different based on race.[117,121,124,127,131,134] Preventive services, such as immunizations, are also offered differently based on race and ethnicity.[136] When children have special medical needs or disabilities, the inequality becomes even more dramatic.[118,135]

Intensivists have reason to be concerned about these findings. When racial differences in survival were investigated, blacks had a higher rate of age-adjusted, gender-specific mortality than whites did.[147] Importantly, there is increasing divergence between white and black mortality rates.[147] Minority children and their families perceive differences in their care, treatment, and relationships with providers.[116]

A number of studies have addressed the topic of racial disparities in adult ICUs.[138-143] These reports fall into the major categories of disease presentation, outcome, and limitations of care.[138-143] In a series of patients experiencing stroke, black patients had a somewhat higher initial stroke severity compared with white patients; however, this difference did not totally account for the differences in morbidity and mortality.[142] One explanation for this may be related to differential processes used by practitioners in caring for black and white patients. One single-institution study on the association between race and ICU mortality demonstrated that black patients had a nearly three times higher likelihood of dying.[139] In a large multi-institutional cohort of ICU patients, race had no effect on severity-adjusted survival.[140] Small differences were noted in the severity-adjusted length of stay and resource use between the races, which may represent variations in the provision of care.[140] One consistent finding from the ICU literature involves end-of-life care; each of three studies found a higher likelihood of lack of aggressive care among black patients.[138,141,143] Unmeasured differences related to the patients, their religion, education, or physician may be as likely as race to account for the differences in these studies, however.[140]

The literature regarding racial disparities in critically ill children is not nearly as well established. In a 25-year study of mortality associated with congenital heart disease, black patients had a nearly 20% higher mortality rate than white patients did.[130] For pediatric patients requiring single-ventricle palliation for congenital heart disease, there was considerably more variation in the age of palliation in black babies than in white babies in a single-institution study. Black pediatric patients with renal failure are less likely than white patients to be wait-listed for kidney transplantation.[115] However, in a study of low-birth-weight infants, there were no survival differences between white and black babies.[114]

Race has been used as a proxy for a number of other socio-economic factors.[145] It has become evident, however, that if meaningful information is to be gained by including racial variables in research, reliable and valid definitions need to be used.[145] Race is a relatively nonspecific term that incorporates biologic, social, and cultural components, which are more than mere physical descriptors and are not consistently considered in the definition.[145] As a result, when comparing outcome measures—whether vitality outcomes such as mortality or resource use outcomes such as length of stay—it may be inappropriate to conclude that race is the explanatory variable.[145]

TIMELINESS

Timeliness is a marker of the adequacy of processes in the ICU environment to achieve acceptable outcomes.[148]

The IOM report characterizes timeliness in two distinctive ways.[2] First, the report uses a "customer service" focus by addressing such issues as waiting times in offices and emergency departments and for diagnostic testing or surgery. The suggestion is that health care providers' inattention to the flow of patients demonstrates a lack of respect for patients and their families.[2] The second focus extends beyond customer satisfaction to include patient outcomes, which are particularly germane to ICUs. The ICU is a valuable resource for critically ill patients, and if ICU resources, which are in limited supply, are not available when patients need them, adverse outcomes are possible. In this section, we explore how these two foci of timeliness can be demonstrated as quality concerns in pediatric critical care.

CUSTOMER SATISFACTION

The ICU is a highly technical, state-of-the-art environment that can provide minute-to-minute changes in care, as physiologic derangements become apparent. Many families, though aware of the intensity and sophistication of the PICU, may not be attuned to the attention to detail and rapid response that often contribute to the care of their children. They simply want their children returned to them in a healthy state. The hospitalization of pediatric patients with critical illnesses is a frightening and stressful event for both patient and family. One opportunity to allay the anxiety associated with these circumstances is to provide timely and effective communication in a clear, honest, and direct manner.[149-151]

OUTCOMES

In the prehospital arena, a coordinated emergency medical system that can provide timely transportation is essential. Practitioners in this setting should be competent in the pediatric skills that are essential to provide effective care in a timely manner at the scene of an accident or other emergency.[152-154] Transportation of a child to a regional center with the necessary resources is an important component in the continuum of care.

The organizational and structural components of pediatric trauma centers and PICUs have been associated with quality care. Pediatric patients treated at pediatric trauma centers have a lower proportion of missed injuries compared with those treated at adult trauma centers.[155,156] Similarly, pediatric patients treated in PICUs rather than adult ICUs have a significantly lower mortality rate, especially among the most seriously ill children. These PICU outcomes have been associated with specific care factors and may be related to the experience and competency of the physician, nursing, and technical staff.[157] The presence of pediatric intensivists and pediatric critical care fellows improves the timeliness of intervention and has a positive impact on outcome.[158] Unfortunately, many critically ill children with ultimately fatal outcomes may not receive this high level of care, owing, in part, to delays in diagnosis or treatment.[155,159,160]

Why do PICUs have better outcomes? The ICU is a complex, dynamic, tightly coupled system. Therefore, multiple processes and personnel must interact to provide high-quality, error-free care. To accomplish this, ICUs depend on the multidisciplinary critical care team. These organized work groups are essential to the provision of highly complex care and to the smooth flow of patient processes that will decrease the "cycle time," or time from PICU admission to PICU discharge.[2] A central component that affects team functioning is communication among team members.[161-163] Communication and collaboration at the nurse-physician interface are important parts of providing high-quality critical care. This is discussed in greater detail in Chapter 261. When practitioners participate in an open dialogue and exchange opinions about a patient's condition, timely interventions can be made that improve patient outcome.[163,164]

Another component of effective critical care is the surveillance for potential problems. The presence of an intensivist who can anticipate physiologic derangements and institute diagnostic testing or therapeutic interventions before such problems become obvious allows the provision of timely care. The access to timely care is as important as the effectiveness of that care.

PATIENT CENTEREDNESS

Accompanying the rapid growth of medical literature for professionals is a similar expansion in the amount of health care information available to patients and their families.[2] This availability of information leads to more knowledgeable patients who demand to participate actively in health care decision-making.[2] As a result, patients' and families' needs have become the focal point of the health care experience. The IOM's aim of patient centeredness helps characterize the interactions between practitioners and their patients.[2] A number of terms, including *empathy*, *compassion*, *needs*, and *respect*, encompass the qualities of patient centeredness and reflect the focus of attention on the patient.[2] Additional components that help establish priority areas for the care of individual patients include the provision of information, communication, and education; attention to physical comfort; emotional support by relieving fear and anxiety; and the involvement of family and friends.[2] These characteristics constitute what is known as service quality; in contrast, clinical quality is the clinical expertise offered by critical care practitioners. The Healthcare Advisory Board identified several broad types of service problems in specialty care (Table 260-2), which are also relevant to the PICU.

SATISFACTION WITH CARE

Admission to the PICU, especially when emergent and unexpected, is an anxiety-provoking and fearful experience for patients and their families.[165,166] For parents, the anxiety is generated from the lack of parental control; the appearance and discomfort of the child, both emotionally and physically; and the difficulty in communicating with staff.[165] The age of the parents and their ability to focus on problems and participate in care are associated with an ability to cope with a critically ill child.[167] Coping strategies for parents also include an ability to be supported by the PICU health care team. A variety of needs, including emotional, physical, and spiritual, have to be addressed by this support system.[168] This can be accomplished by providing accurate information, allowing ready access to the child, and encouraging parents' participation in their child's care.[165,168] For hospitalized children, anxiety and stress may manifest themselves in behavior problems, especially in those with repeated or prolonged

TABLE 260-2. SERVICE PROBLEMS IN SPECIALTY CARE

Speed of service
  Delay in care or excessive waiting time
  Lack of explanation for delay
Coordination of care
  Organization of the environment
  Availability of appropriate person to answer questions
Respect and courtesy
  Staff courtesy
  Treatment with respect and dignity
Understanding of treatment
  Information regarding symptoms, medications, and treatments
    provided
  Patient or family included in decisions
  Adequate explanations provided
  Patient and family listened to
Trust in the provider
Availability of the provider
  Psychosocial support

From Advisory Board Company: Service Innovations in Specialty Care: Enhancing Patient Satisfaction with Diagnosis and Treatment Selection. Washington DC, Advisory Board Company, 1998.

hospitalizations, those who are critically ill, and those with underlying mood or psychological disorders.[169]

If family members perceive that emotional support is inadequate, their satisfaction with the experience and, more important, their long-term viability and cohesion as a family unit are at risk.[170] Most families are satisfied with the care their children receive in the PICU and are particularly complimentary about the skill and competence of the nursing staff, as well as the compassion and respect shown toward their children, especially with regard to pain management.[171] Attention to adequate pain and anxiety control is an essential component of the care of critically ill pediatric patients.[172-174] Pain control addresses a fundamental need and is a compassionate practice that helps allay parents' anxiety and improve coping.[171] The environment of the waiting area and the frequency of physician communication were both identified as detracting from parents' satisfaction with the PICU experience.[171] The family's ability to function after the ICU admission of a child is dependent not only on their satisfaction but also on the severity of the child's illness, the duration of the hospitalization, and the location of the hospital.[170]

The PICU is a microsystem within a larger organization of care; as such, it presents an opportunity to analyze the degree of patient centeredness as a broad indicator of health care quality.[175] Patients and their parents are positioned to provide information to clinicians regarding these highly personal aspects of care.[176] In a multi-institutional study investigating processes of care in pediatric hospitals, parents reported problems with more than 25% of the health care processes.[177] The two most common problems were lack of adequate information and lack of coordination of care.[177] These problems were exaggerated in academic health centers, which had a higher rate of problems overall and in the area of coordination of care.[177] Front-line staff may be able to solicit information from parents regarding process deficiencies, with the intent of identifying necessary changes that can be implemented quickly.[178] In addition, validated and reliable surveys investigating satisfaction with ICU care are available to assist providers.[179]

OPPORTUNITIES FOR IMPROVEMENT

Communication

In the highly technical environment of the ICU, parents' knowledge may be particularly lacking, making communication especially relevant. For example, practitioners in the ICU are familiar with the machines, interventions, alarms, and responses. With experience, these practitioners learn to maintain a sense of calm even in the face of a crisis. Parents of critically ill children are new to the environment, however, and an explanation of the various pieces of equipment and the routine sights and sounds may help them settle in. In addition, because of tubes and catheters, as well as bruising and edema, the child's appearance may be alarming. It is thus paramount to ensure that discussions with parents are adequate. This is particularly relevant in relation to informed consent. In one study of patients receiving extracorporeal membrane oxygenation, only a minority of parents of nonsurvivors had a recollection that death was discussed before the child was placed on bypass.[180] Parents also had a sense of relief when first seeing the child alive on bypass. More than 90% of nonsurvivors' families felt comforted by follow-up contact after the child's death.[180]

Parent-Provider Partnerships

A partnership between members of the PICU team and parents of critically ill children can minimize the pressures of the situation and allow the family to cope more effectively.[181,182] Studies have found that an increased family presence is becoming more common, owing to open visitation and the practice of permitting families to be present during medical procedures and other particularly stressful times,[183-186] including during lifesaving procedures such as cardiopulmonary resuscitation.[187] A multidisciplinary team approach helps ensure coordination of care and facilitate communication, particularly if the parents are considered to be members of the health care team.[188] Teams ultimately improve the quality of care provided.[189]

Creating an environment that eases isolation and enhances a sense of family is important for patients, their families, and caregivers. Closed-circuit televisions may help alleviate the tediousness of waiting and provide a distraction during the long hours that parents often spend with their children.[190] Creating an environment that includes family photographs, special toys, and familiar voices on a tape recorder can minimize the seclusion that families often perceive and can help open avenues of communication, allowing parents to express their concerns and thus enhance their ability to cope.[191] One of the more difficult times for families is transitioning from the high-intensity care of the ICU to the ward, especially if the child's care has been especially intense or prolonged.[192] Parents develop a degree of familiarity with the technology and are used to the high nurse-to-patient ratios. They may have come to know and trust the PICU nurses. Most families have mixed emotions about transferring to the ward. Although it implies that the child's health is improving, it also means, in many instances, a new care team, a new location, and less intensive nursing care.

End-of-Life Care

Regardless of the cause, the death of a child tests parents' ability to function as a family unit; in fact, the death of a child is often associated with divorce and financial ruin.

Sudden pediatric deaths are often associated with a greater intensity of early and late grief than are deaths following a chronic illness. The parents' coping styles and the compassion of PICU staff can predict the intensity of short-term grief.[193] In addition, the adequacy of information provided by staff can help predict the intensity of long-term grief.[193]

Parents place a high priority on quality of life when making decisions about limiting care in the ICU.[194] However, acute disease was found to be the predominant reason for placing restrictions on care.[195] In one large multi-institutional study, the categories of restrictions were fairly evenly divided among do-not-resuscitate (DNR) orders (39%), additional limitations beyond DNR orders (27%), and withdrawal of medical intervention (34%).[195] Parents and staff tend to agree significantly more often than do other family members about decisions to withdraw support.[194]

Providers

The provision of patient-centered care can be one of the most rewarding professional experiences in pediatric critical care practice. However, a syndrome of emotional exhaustion, depersonalization, and reduced professional accomplishment constitutes what is known as professional burnout.[196] This problem applies to ICU nurses and physicians alike. Identifying and addressing this syndrome are important.[197]

EFFICIENCY

Economics demands that health care resources be delivered in a cost-effective and efficient manner while not jeopardizing the quality of care.[198] The achievement of specific outcome goals is a measure of an ICU's quality. Costs vary with outcome measures. Mortality rates, efficiency rates, lengths of stay, rates of nosocomial infection and readmission, and the presence of a teaching program all impact expenses and reimbursement.[199] Quality at a given level of cost determines the value of a commodity. In this case, the commodity is ICU care.[199]

The value of an individual ICU is increased by its ability to achieve selected measures of outcome while keeping costs to a minimum. This is concordant with the concept of efficiency as an aim in the IOM's current model of health care quality.[2] Intensive care services are a commodity, and those units providing quality care at a reasonable cost, as judged by efficiency and a similar patient mix, will be most appealing. Less efficient ICUs will need to optimize efficiency or have cost-containment strategies imposed on them.[199]

MACROECONOMICS

From a macroeconomic perspective, PICUs have experienced a dramatic increase in the number of available beds.[199] A single PICU study using two different costing methods demonstrated that personnel and infrastructure are the most important contributors to total cost.[200] As older, more established ICUs reduce their capital expenditures, the marginal cost of each successive admission is lower, and profit margins are higher. Successive admissions are also more effective because the demand for ICU services will be greater with fewer beds. Stated a different way, increasing the supply of ICU beds increases the total costs associated with more recent capital outlays and thereby makes the practice of critical care less efficient from an economic perspective.[199]

MICROECONOMICS

From a microeconomic perspective, patients who are sicker require more services in the ICU, stay longer, are more likely to die, and cost more to be treated.[201,202] This is not new information. However, to balance the issues of cost and quality, ICUs should identify same-strata "best practices" ICUs with similar cost drivers (e.g., severity of illness) and operate under a philosophy of "targeted benchmarking" to achieve comparability up to a specified level.[203] To accomplish this, clinical scoring systems are frequently used to control for case-mix variables (physiology, diagnoses, and so forth) and thus allow for standardized comparisons. Length of stay has become a standard in benchmarking ICU performance and quality, and reducing length of stay is one method of reducing cost, although, as a variable itself, length of stay is subject to differences in measurement.[204,205] The standardized length of stay ratio is that of observed to predicted length of stay and is an indicator of resource use, adjusted for severity.[206] The standardized length of stay ratio can be used to compare a particular unit's performance over time, but it can also be used to determine whether a particular ICU's resource use is above or below that of similar ICUs.[206]

Another method of assessing the efficiency of resource use in the ICU is to evaluate unique ICU therapies,[207-213] that is, those that are best delivered in the ICU, such as mechanical ventilation and vasoactive infusions.[209] Individual ICUs and physicians differ in their monitoring strategies, so monitoring technologies should not be classified as unique therapies.[209] The benefits of this approach are that it allows physicians to determine the proportion of "low-risk" monitor-only patients[213] and compare the number of "high-risk" critical care patients requiring unique ICU therapies. As alluded to earlier, excess bed capacity leads to a higher ratio of monitored to high-risk patients and reduces the efficiency of the ICU.[213] Opportunities to evaluate admission and discharge criteria as well as throughput issues, resulting from the inability to transfer ICU patients because of a high hospital occupancy rate, may serve to improve an individual ICU's efficiency.

USING A BUSINESS MODEL

ICUs differ considerably in their use of resources.[198] Physicians also differ in their practice patterns and how they influence the use of resources.[214] However, there are opportunities to affect the structural components of the ICU and achieve efficiencies in the process of care. A recent patient safety recommendation was to have 24-hour intensivist coverage for ICUs.[215] This recommendation is based on the premise that an intensivist-led model of critical care practice will lead to improvements in care.[215] The majority of PICUs with on-site physician staffing have been providing this level of care for many years. In this way, pediatric critical care differs from many adult ICUs, where critical care is practiced from remote locations after once-daily rounds.

There are other opportunities to improve efficiency by invoking a business model. Concentrating on the ICU's design and staffing patterns may help improve outcomes and efficiency.[216] An intelligently designed ICU will facilitate the work of all members of the ICU team while optimizing patient and family safety and comfort. Staffing patterns for physicians and nurses both on rounds and for the remainder of their shifts are important considerations.[217,218] Staffing patterns in which patient assignments are on opposite ends of the ICU create excess work and rework. In addition, it invokes concerns regarding patient safety. For physicians, finding the right balance of team size and composition on rounds will optimize quality and improve efficiency in workflow.

Organizational characteristics, including the concept of a critical care team,[203,209,218,219] that can improve coordination and collaboration in care are associated with both positive outcomes and improved efficiency. ICUs with medical directors who act in the role of manager to improve resource use, especially in high-occupancy institutions, are a key component of this team concept.[220,221] Consistent admission, discharge, and triage policies and procedures are process components that also contribute to an efficient ICU. Reducing variability in care by streamlining care and implementing guidelines and pathways for ICU patients is another example of a process mechanism to improve efficiency. Simply improving the awareness of cost in the culture of the ICU is an easy way of reducing waste and achieving cost containment.

CONCLUSION

Use of the six aims of quality is a good approach for evaluating the current state of pediatric critical care. Critically ill or injured children benefit by these intermittent assessments, which ensure that the discipline of pediatric critical care is keeping pace with the broader medical literature. It also provides a framework for addressing deficiencies in the evidence base through future research initiatives.

ANNOTATED REFERENCES

Institute of Medicine Committee on Quality of Health Care in America: Crossing the Quality Chasm: A New Health System for the 21st Century. Washington, DC, National Academies Press, 2001.

This document provides a contemporary review of quality in health care. It is useful in its own right because of its framework based on the six aims of quality. In addition, it is highly referenced, providing an overview of the evaluation of health care services.

Kohn LT, Corrigan JM, Donaldson MS (eds): Institute of Medicine Committee on Quality of Health Care in America: To Err Is Human: Building a Safer Health System. Washington, DC, National Academies Press, 2000.

This is the sentinel publication about medical errors in health care. It provides a thorough literature review, background on the problem of iatrogenic injury, and a framework for professionals and the lay public to understand the circumstances in which medical errors occur and what needs to be done to prevent them.

Pollack MM, Patel KM, Ruttimann UE: PRISM III: An updated pediatric risk of mortality score. Crit Care Med 1996;24:743-752.

The authors have developed a physiology-based method of assessing severity of illness using data available in the first 12 hours of care. It illustrates the method of adjusting mortality rates for severity of illness to measure the effectiveness of PICU care.

Ruttimann UE, Patel KM, Pollack MM: Length of stay and efficiency in pediatric intensive care units. J Pediatr 1998;133:79-85.

This article outlines a method for estimating length of stay based on data available in the first 24 hours and illustrates how it can be used for benchmarking. This is a key component of quality of care evaluations, especially for efficiency and timeliness measures.

Smedley BD, Stith AY, Nelson AR: Institute of Medicine Committee on Understanding and Eliminating Racial and Ethnic Disparities in Healthcare: Unequal Treatment: Confronting Racial and Ethnic Disparities in Health Care. Washington, DC, National Academies Press, 2002.

Racial and ethnic disparities have become a major concern in health care. This IOM report adds a contextual element to the problem by providing an assessment method, identifying interventions, and proposing solutions.

Chapter 261

KEY ISSUES IN CRITICAL CARE NURSING

Franco A. Carnevale

KEY POINTS

1. **Studies of critical care nurses' expertise** have demonstrated that this expertise is highly sophisticated and consists predominantly of experientially acquired knowledge, rather than learning from books and classrooms.

2. **The development of observational pain rating methods is necessary** in the critical care setting because this population is incapable of self-report.

3. Improvements in the pharmacologic management of pain and discomfort have contributed to **the increased incidence of withdrawal reactions.**

4. **Studies of critical care nurses' clinical judgment of pain** report that nurses demonstrate a sophisticated balancing of patients' analgesic needs against other competing needs.

5. Given the significant responsibility that nurses have conventionally held toward the care of basic needs, such as skin care, the nursing literature has devoted particular attention to **the prevention and care of pressure ulcers.**

6. **The Braden Scale** is a highly regarded scoring system for predicting the risk of pressure ulcers.

7. Nursing research has consistently demonstrated **a strong interest in the psychosocial aspects of critical illness.**

8. A significant number of critically ill patients endure **profound psychological trauma.**

9. Families of critically ill patients are **not "visitors."**

10. **Critical care nurses can experience moral distress** because they frequently find themselves in situations in which they do not have the power to do what they believe should be done.

Prevailing issues in critical care nursing are reviewed in this chapter. Topics are examined that have particular importance for nurses as well as topics that have broad multidisciplinary appeal. Special focus is placed on contributions from nursing research. The reader is invited to delve further into the nursing literature by examining the numerous excellent critical care nursing journals and textbooks that are currently available, as well as CINAHL (Cumulative Index to Nursing and Allied Health Literature), the nursing literature database (a "nursing Medline").

CRITICAL CARE NURSING KNOWLEDGE AND SKILL DEVELOPMENT

Patricia Benner is said to have revolutionized our understanding of clinical expertise in nursing. In her landmark book *From Novice to Expert: Excellence and Power in Clinical Nursing Practice*, Benner related the Dreyfus Model of Skill Acquisition to her study of nursing expertise.[1] This model was originally developed through a study of skill development among nonclinicians (e.g., chess players and airline pilots). Benner and her colleagues have recently directed their analysis specifically to critical care nursing.[2]

Benner has challenged the prevailing "top-down" view of clinical expertise that believes clinicians acquire theoretical and empirical knowledge from books, journals, and classrooms and then *apply* this to practice. Rather, she demonstrated that such a form of practice is characteristic of *novices*. Lacking an experiential base to draw on, novices refer to their formal learning as well as various "rules of thumb" to help them sort through clinical problems.

An *expert*, however, will have acquired a rich store of clinical cases. This serves as a "bottom-up" foundation that enables expert nurses to rapidly discern what is meaningful in a clinical scenario without having to go through a stepwise linear algorithm-like process. Therefore, expert critical care nurses (as well as other clinicians) are able to "think in action." Expert *know-how* enables experienced nurses to readily identify patterns in a presenting case by immediately referring to numerous comparable cases—directly inferring hypotheses about the likely problem, the gravity of the situation, and how it should be managed. As the expert proceeds to manage the situation, the patient's response presents further cues that can either confirm the nurses' initial interpretation or generate new probable hypotheses.

Some have argued that Benner's conception of skill acquisition is also relevant to medicine.[3] A recent study demonstrated that critical care physicians employ a similar mode of thinking in their practice of diagnostic reasoning.[4]

Concurrent with this management of a specific case, Benner and her associates further described how an expert nurse also monitors and limits potential hazards in the highly technological critical care environment, fosters teamwork, and initiates preventive and corrective management of systems breakdown.[2] These functions are commonly performed without the nurse necessarily being consciously aware of the reasoning that underlies them.

This experienced-based view of nursing expertise raises important implications for nursing education and management. First, this suggests that the extent to which clinical expertise can be acquired from books or in a classroom is highly limited. The development of complex clinical judgment requires naturalistic exposure to numerous "real life" cases. Although some useful learning can be acquired through formal educational methods, such as formal lectures and readings, Benner's framework favors an apprenticeship model of nursing education. A tailored program of clinical experiences, with access to expert guidance, will most effectively foster the development of expert knowledge and skill among critical care nurses.

Second, this calls for management approaches that recognize the complexity of clinical expertise and the significant investment required to develop it. Expert nurses do not simply perform tasks that are prescribed by physicians or protocols. Expert nurses bring sophisticated knowledge and judgment that is essential toward the early and effective management of patient as well as unit problems. This implies that skilled critical care nurses should be regarded as essential resources.

Administrators need to exercise extreme caution toward decisions aiming to reduce costs that rely on strategies such as "de-skilling" (i.e., relying on less qualified health professionals to perform nursing work), "casualization" (i.e., reducing the number of full-time staff to rely on casual, typically less experienced, staff that can be called in ad hoc), or "downsizing" (i.e., dismissing skilled staff to reduce staffing levels).

Any strategy that diminishes or fragments the depth of critical care nursing expertise will fundamentally diminish the strength of a critical care service.[5] Cho and associates have demonstrated that efforts to reduce nursing staffing levels can significantly increase levels of patient morbidity. A 1-hour decrease of worked nursing hours per patient was associated with a 8.9% increased probability of patients acquiring pneumonia.[6]

CLINICAL TOPICS

Critical care nurses are concerned about the same issues as physicians and other allied professionals. Some nurses have emerged across disciplines as respected leaders because of their impressive research work on selected critical care problems, such as prone positioning in patients with acute lung injury[7] and infant pain.[8]

The remainder of this chapter is devoted to a review of a small number of topics that nurses are particularly concerned about. These address key problems that have especially perplexed nursing practice and captured the research attention of nurses. Although the following discussion primarily highlights nursing contributions to these problems, this does not intend to dismiss the importance of related research in other disciplines. Space constraints limit the number of topics that can be reviewed, but the few subjects that are presented deliberately span a wide range of domains.

PAIN AND DISCOMFORT

It is likely that most nurses would describe pain and discomfort as their most challenging clinical problems. The constancy and proximity of nurses' bedside relationship with their patients heightens their attentiveness to these problems. Unresolved pain and discomfort can take a deep toll on nurses. This is partly attributable to nursing's traditional commitment to the promotion of comfort and caring.[9,10]

Although significant advances have been made over the years in developing effective pharmacologic agents for managing these problems, pain and discomfort commonly persist.[11,12]

One factor that has limited successful management of these problems is the challenge involved in their evaluation.[13] Outside of the critical care setting, pain management has benefited from systematic measurement and documentation. Widely accepted pain measures, such as the Visual Analogue Scale or numeric rating scales, rely on patient self-report. Self-report is typically not accessible in critical care, given patients' diminished level of consciousness. Thus, observational methods are most appropriate for this population. A significant body of experience exists in pediatrics with the utilization of observational pain measures, such as the Faces Pain Scale[14] and the Children's Hospital of Eastern Ontario Pain Scale: CHEOPS.[15] However, most of the research on these has been conducted outside of critical care settings.

An overall "comfort" measurement tool that has established some reliability and validity for critically ill adults is the Ramsay Scale.[16] This is a six-level sedation scale, three levels for when the patient is awake and three levels for when the patient is asleep: 1—anxious, agitated, or restless; 2—cooperative, oriented, or tranquil; 3—responds to commands only; 4—asleep, brisk response to light touch on cheek or loud auditory stimulus; 5—sluggish response; and 6—no response. In pediatric critical care, the COMFORT Scale has demonstrated impressive merits.[17] This consists of eight behavioral and physiologic parameters, including alertness, calmness/agitation, respiratory response, physical movement, blood pressure, heart rate, muscle tone, and facial tension. Each parameter is measured along a five-point rating scale and summed to provide a total score that ranges from 8 to 40. Some work with this tool has indicated that physiologic parameters such as blood pressure and heart rate have weak validity as indicators of discomfort.[18] Although these signs are commonly and intuitively associated with patient discomfort, these are also affected by numerous other phenomena within the critical care setting, such as cardiovascular dysfunction.

Overall improvements in pharmacologic management of pain and discomfort have contributed to a more recent concern: withdrawal reactions.[19] In the pediatric setting, such reactions are associated with tremors, jitteriness, irritability, gagging, vomiting, feeding problems, and inconsolable crying.[20] This problem is complicated by the absence of any accepted instruments for systematically measuring withdrawal among the critically ill, although the Neonatal Abstinence Scoring System (developed for monitoring withdrawal in infants born to substance-dependent mothers) is an exception.[21]

Reliable and valid measures are especially needed for evaluating withdrawal reactions because the successful management of this problem is frequently limited by caregiver disagreements about what signs constitute withdrawal reactions, as opposed to pain, distress, or agitation. Overly rapid weaning can precipitate a constellation of phenomena such as acute pain, excessive agitation, "ICU psychosis," as well as withdrawal reactions. Given the typically multifaceted determinants of patient discomfort in critical care, one research team has recommended that the term *adverse reactions to weaning* be employed in this context (rather than *withdrawal reactions*).[20]

Although some guidelines have been published that indicate recommended rates of weaning, very little empirical research has established the optimal rate for reducing opioid and benzodiazepine infusions, balancing the need to rapidly extubate patients (and therefore minimize ventilation-related morbidities) with the prevention of withdrawal reactions. Some evidence suggests that there does not exist one optimal weaning rate. This will need to be tailored to the length of time the patient has been receiving such infusions, whereby 20% *daily weaning* is optimal for patients receiving continuous infusions for 1 to 3 days, 13% to 20% for 4 to 7 days of infusions, 8% to 13% for 1 to 2 weeks, 8% for 2 to 3 weeks, and 2% to 4% for more than 4 weeks of infusions.[22]

Cumbersome decisional processes further complicate the management of pain and discomfort in critical care. A common occurrence in a university setting is for the intensivist to direct house staff and nurses to wean a patient's sedation and analgesia overnight so the patient will be ready for extubation in the morning. However, such weaning can trigger significant discomfort, whereby the house staff and nurses can enter into disputes over how to balance the need to wean with the need to maintain patient comfort, through a series of repeated adjustments in infusion rates and ad hoc bolus doses.

In their study of critical care nursing judgment in the management of pain, Stannard and colleagues reported that nurses demonstrated a sophisticated balancing of patients' analgesic needs against other competing needs.[23] A less cumbersome pain and discomfort management process can be established through the use of a sedation protocol or standing orders that "transfer" some decisional autonomy to nurses. A protocol can authorize nurses to modify sedation and analgesia infusion rates and bolus administration according to a prescribed target level of patient comfort.

For example, Alexander and associates reported on a sedation protocol used in pediatric critical care where the COMFORT Scale was used to measure patients' level of comfort.[24] The physician's prescription specifies a target COMFORT Scale range for the patient, which the nurse can then use as a guideline for modifying the administration of sedation and analgesia. This study reported that patient comfort was managed effectively, while facilitating the decision-making process.

Finally, the nursing literature has devoted some attention toward the use of nonpharmacologic means for managing pain and discomfort, such as massage, relaxation exercises, transcutaneous electrical nerve stimulation (TENS), acupuncture, guided imagery, and hypnosis, among others.[25-26] However, these techniques have undergone very little clinical research investigation within critical care. In light of major adverse effects associated with pharmacologic agents as well as their limitations in fully ensuring patient comfort, these adjunctive measures should be further developed for the critically ill.

PRESSURE ULCERS

Given the significant responsibility that nurses have conventionally held toward the care of basic needs, such as skin care, the nursing literature has devoted particular attention to the prevention and care of pressure ulcers.

In their study of iatrogenic problems, Cho and associates reported that pressure ulcers had the greatest impact on length of stay (i.e., a 1.84-fold increase).[6] Documented prevalence rates vary from 7.1% to 11.1%.[27-29] Jiricka and colleagues have reported that prevalence rates are even higher among the critically ill.[30] This is attributable to the greater likelihood of immobility and reduced skin perfusion.

The principal extrinsic causes of pressure ulcers are pressure, friction, and shear. Therefore, preventive strategies are directed toward the minimization of these extrinsic forces. Although over 200 pressure-relieving devices are commercially available, there is a paucity of controlled clinical trials that examine their efficacy.[31]

A body of literature is emerging that is effectively identifying the sites of pressure ulcers and the relative significance of various risk factors. This will help build a base of evidence from which clinical trials can be designed. This literature has led to the development of scoring systems for predicting the risk of pressure ulcers. A highly regarded system is the Braden Scale.[32] This scale has six subscales: mobility, activity, friction and shear, sensory perception, skin moisture, and nutrition, providing a total score that ranges from 6 to 23 points (high scores indicate less risk). A Braden score of 16 has demonstrated a high degree of sensitivity and specificity in predicting pressure ulcer formation in critically ill adults. This tool has recently been adapted and validated for the pediatric critical care population.[33]

Whereas pressure ulcers in adults predominantly appear on the lower body (sacrum, ischium, and heels), these are more common on the upper body of children (occiput and ears). This is attributable to the proportional differences in body weight distribution between these age groups. A 27% rate of pressure ulcer incidence has been reported in critically ill children, 57% of which were identified on their second day in the ICU.[34] Particularly disturbing was that an additional 27 ulcers were identified that were caused by medical devices, such as oximetry probes, BiPAP masks, and endotracheal tubes.

It is remarkable that wide disparities of preventive measures are currently practiced, including some high-cost pressure-relieving mattresses.[31,35] These include some aids that are largely regarded as ineffective, such as synthetic sheepskins.[34] Although a substantial amount of evidence has examined this problem outside of critical care, systematic evaluations of management strategies are required to understand their efficacy among the critically ill.

PSYCHOSOCIAL ISSUES IN CRITICALLY ILL PATIENTS AND THEIR FAMILIES

Nursing has consistently demonstrated a strong interest in psychosocial aspects of illness. In critical care, nurses have directed some of the most respected psychosocial research. A number of studies have examined the psychological impact of critical illness on *patients*, whereas others have concentrated on their *families*. Nursing investigations of these populations include a significant number of *qualitative* studies. Although most nursing research employs quantitative methods, nurses have conducted a large proportion of qualitative studies within the health sciences.

Patients

It is apparent that a significant number of critically ill patients endure profound psychological trauma. Many patients develop delirium or "ICU psychosis."[36,37] One group of patients, examined up to 8 weeks after their discharge from an ICU, reported "experiences of chaos," feelings of extreme instability, vulnerability, and fear, as well as prolonged inner tension.[38] It was found that even trivial events could trigger changes in their feelings of fear or inner tension. The caring behaviors of nurses provided an important degree of security and comfort. Hupcey reported that the overarching need of critically ill patients is the need to feel safe.[39]

A number of studies suggest that some of these patients exhibit manifestations of post-traumatic stress disorder (PTSD).[40-42] In an investigation of the experiences of patients through their transfer out of ICU, patients exhibited feelings of significant despondency and apprehension.[43] These findings highlight the need for greater attentiveness to the needs of these highly vulnerable adults.

McKinley and colleagues[44] have developed a tool for assessing anxiety in critically ill patients: the Faces Anxiety Scale. This single-item tool requires patients to select one of five drawings of faces. The scale exhibits minimal subject burden, while eliciting self-reports more often than other self-report scales.

Among psychological studies of critically ill children, Rennick and associates have reported that children who were younger, more severely ill, and underwent more invasive procedures demonstrated more medical fears, a lower sense of control over their health, and ongoing post-traumatic stress responses up to 6 months after discharge.[41] In a long-term follow-up study of critically ill children, significant dispositional and mental function changes were reported.[45,46] Parental accounts and clinical evaluations suggested that these children were profoundly transformed by their critical illness, for variable lengths of time. Papathanassoglou and Patiraki reported similar observations among critically ill adults.[47]

Families

Many studies of families of the critically ill can be traced to Molter's examination of family needs.[48] Following Molter's introduction of the *Critical Care Family Needs Inventory*, several studies have systematically investigated the needs of these families. This body of research has demonstrated that families need honest, clear, and timely information, liberal "visiting" policies, and competent and compassionate care for their family member.[48-51] "Hope" has been described as the most frequently used method of coping,[52] which has complex implications for how clinicians portray the patient's outlook. The latter report also indicated that families identified the provision of information, emotional support, and the competence and manner of the nurse as helpful nursing interventions. A large body of research has also documented the needs, stressors, and coping strategies of families of critically ill children.[53-56]

Carnevale[46,57] has described a *family systems* model for understanding the experiences of families of critically ill patients. Drawing on family therapy theory, this model recognizes families as constellations of interrelationships among members, including the critically ill patient. Variable levels of attachments or conflicts that continually change over time characterize these ties (Figs. 261-1 and 261-2). Space constraints do not permit an additional discussion of death and dying in critical care, although some relevant issues will be discussed in the ethics review in the next section.

Any significant event that affects one member of a family system will necessarily affect the entire family constellation. A common feature that appears to characterize the response of families of critically ill children is a deeply motivated attempt to recapture life as it was before the need for critical care.[46] Although, it is plausible that families of critically ill adults have similar responses, this requires further study. This work suggests that the quality of the *patient's* experience through his/her critical illness is intimately intertwined with the quality of the *family's* experience. For example, efforts to preserve family integration—through the rigorous promotion of family presence and participation in the care of the patient—help satisfy numerous family needs, while also profoundly comforting the patient's deepest stresses. Generally, what is good for the family tends to be good for the patient and vice versa.

These findings highlight a central problem in the conventional ICU view of families as "visitors." Units commonly have visiting policies and visitors' rooms. Families are not visitors. Rather, they are spouses, partners, parents, children, siblings, and grandparents, among others. Each family member can help foster a sense of continuity for the patient. Meanwhile, they are personally adapting to the new reality that confronts him or her. This enables the patient and family to carry on as congruently as possible—fostering family cohesion within the resources that are available to it. These views can also be extended to the significant friends of the patient.

Therefore, ICUs should promote the implementation of family support and follow-up programs to help alleviate patient and family distress. Some data have demonstrated that such programs can be highly effective.[58,59]

ETHICAL DILEMMAS IN CRITICAL CARE NURSING

In an anonymous survey of 852 critical care nurses in the United States, Asch reported that 16% stated they had either performed euthanasia or assisted in suicide, following the requests of patients or family members.[60] Several informant quotes were provided that suggested these nurses were quite frustrated with the physicians they were working with, whom they described as detached and insensitive to patients' suffering. The paper implies that these frustrated nurses unilaterally took matters into their own hands, to do what they thought was right for the patient. Following the release of this paper and the understandable media attention that followed, many hospital centers turned to their critical care nurses to examine whether such practices were performed within their own institution. Although the practice of euthanasia or assisted suicide was clearly illegal and therefore unacceptable within the study's jurisdictions, many of the controversies that ensued missed the central phenomenon highlighted by the study: these nurses attempted to report serious problems in their units that placed them in significant ethical binds.

Nurses are autonomous professionals who bear responsibility for patient well-being (albeit within a multidisciplinary team context). Nurses practice according to a professional code of ethics (which may vary somewhat across regions) that requires them to do everything that they can to ensure that patient needs are adequately met. Bioethicist Tristam Englehardt[61] outlined that

> Nurses are caught between physicians, on the one hand, who are authorities regarding scientific and technological knowledge and are in authority, and patients, on the other hand, who give authority for health care endeavors. Nurses are often placed, as a result, in ambiguous circumstances regarding which side is authorizing them to do what.

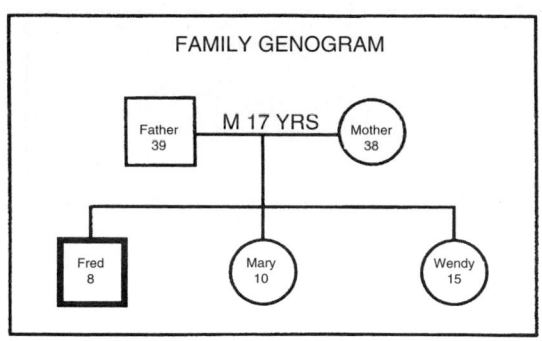

FAMILY GENOGRAM

FIGURE 261-1. Diagrams showing the various relational shifts that were experienced by the family of an 8-year-old boy with multiple trauma. The number of straight lines between persons indicate the strength of attachment in the relationship, whereas the number of irregular lines represent the intensity of conflict.

Prior to accident   PICU (2 days)

PICU (5 weeks)   PICU (2 weeks)

Home (3 months)   Home (3 years)

Critical care nurses frequently find themselves in a moral bind in which they judge that the current medical plan conflicts with their appraisal of the wishes or needs of the patient. This can create moral distress among nurses, as they find themselves in a situation where they do not have the power to do what they believe should be done.[62]

The Manitoba, Canada, government recently commissioned an inquest into a series of pediatric cardiac deaths in which there was suspicion regarding a surgeon's competence. The inquest report recognized that the nurses held important insights into the unfolding situation and were inadequately "heard" by their organization.[63] The report highlighted that nurses bear a responsibility to ensure patients are protected from harms and risks and that the organization is responsible for creating mechanisms that can facilitate the inclusion of nurses in clinical and administrative decisions. One such mechanism can include the creation of a nursing ethics committee, where nurses can feel free to examine nursing-specific concerns.[64]

This "in between" viewpoint of nurses (between the patient and the physician) can help shed new light on a number of ethical dilemmas in critical care and foster new

strategies for resolving them. For example, one study examined the controversy over the practice of judging some critical care interventions as *futile* under certain conditions (e.g., cardiopulmonary resuscitation in a patient with a very grave prognosis) and can therefore be unilaterally withheld or withdrawn by the critical care team.[65] This study highlighted that such conflicts are rarely related to an intervention's actual futility (i.e., whether or not it will achieve its intended purpose) but about fundamental disparities in the beliefs and values of the various persons involved in the conflict. Therefore, ethically sensitive strategies should aim to address these differences, through reciprocal discussions and negotiations that seek to reconcile the disparities, rather than asserting declarations of futility.

Chambers-Evans has illuminated the particular difficulties involved in being a surrogate decision-maker (i.e., a family member making decisions for a critically ill patient).[66] She has proposed a model that promotes *shared* decision-making. This ensures that the surrogate's intimate understanding of the patient's wishes and interests are adequately considered while diminishing the surrogate's moral burden associated with feeling solely responsible for the life and

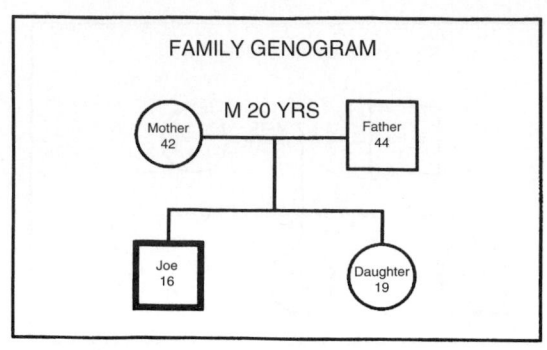

FAMILY GENOGRAM

M 20 YRS

Mother 42 — Father 44

Joe 16 — Daughter 19

Prior to accident

PICU (1 day)

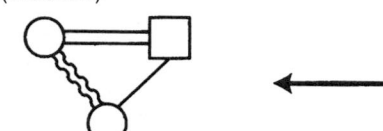

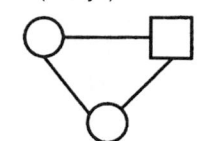

FIGURE 261-2. Diagrams demonstrating the profound relational transitions that followed the death of a family member.

Home (2 months)

Home (6 days)

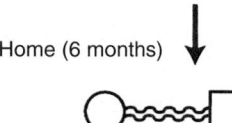

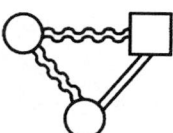

Home (6 months)

Home (14 months)

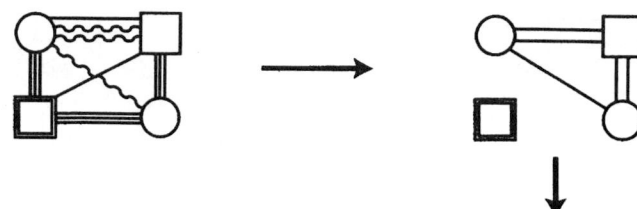

death of their loved one. Finally, some nurses have examined the impact of family presence during resuscitation.[67-68] This work suggests that there is an increasing recognition of the merits of family presence, although priorities for further research are outlined. In sum, nursing perspectives on ethical issues in critical care both foster an awareness of the particular moral binds of nurses and illuminate new insights into the multidisciplinary management of prevalent ethical problems.

CONCLUSION

Knaus and associates demonstrated that the mortality outcomes of a critical care unit are not a function of the level of technology that the unit possesses, its university-teaching status, or a closed (vs. open) unit.[69] Rather, outcomes are strongly associated with the strength of the interdisciplinary collaboration that is practiced within the unit.

The aim of this chapter was *not* to assert that nurses possess privileged knowledge or views about critical care. Rather, the aim was to highlight that critical care nurses offer (along with other practitioners) a rich body of clinical and research knowledge as well as shared professional responsibility for patient and family outcomes. The quality of critical care services can be strengthened through the recognition of the potential and actual contributions of critical care nursing.

ANNOTATED REFERENCES

Benner P, Hooper-Kyriakidis P, Stannard D: Clinical Wisdom and Interventions in Critical Care: A Thinking-in-Action Approach. Philadelphia, WB Saunders, 1999.

> *This is an extensive study of expertise among critical care nurses. This demonstrates that in addition to employing complex experience-based patient management judgment, an expert nurse also monitors and limits potential hazards, fosters teamwork, and initiates preventive and corrective management of systems breakdown.*

Cho SH, Ketefian S, Barkauskas VH, et al: The effects of nurse staffing on adverse events, morbidity, mortality, and medical costs. Nurs Res 2003;52:71-79.

> *This study reported that efforts to reduce nursing staffing levels can significantly increase levels of patient morbidity: A one-hour decrease of worked nursing hours per patient was associated with an 8.9% increased probability of patients acquiring pneumonia.*

Stannard D, Puntillo K, Miaskowski C, et al: Clinical judgment and management of postoperative pain in critical care patients. Am J Crit Care 1996;5:433-441.

> *This examination of critical care nurses' clinical judgment in the management of pain reported that nurses demonstrated a sophisticated balancing of patients' analgesic needs against other competing needs: A less cumbersome management process can be established through the use of a sedation*

protocol or standing orders that "transfer" some decisional autonomy to nurses.

Bergstrom N, Braden BJ, Laguzza A, et al: The Braden Scale for predicting pressure sore risk. Nurs Res 1987;36:205-210.
The Braden Scale is a highly regarded scoring system for predicting the risk of pressure ulcers. The scale has six subscales (mobility, activity, friction and shear, sensory perception, skin moisture, and nutrition), providing a total score that ranges from 6 to 23 points (high scores indicate less risk); a score of 16 has demonstrated a high degree of sensitivity and specificity in predicting pressure ulcer formation in critically ill adults.

Rodney P, Starzomski R: Constraints on the moral agency of nurses. Can Nurse 1993;89:23-26.
This paper discusses how critical care nurses frequently find themselves in a moral bind in which they judge the current medical plan conflicts with their appraisal of the patients' wishes or needs. This can create moral distress among nurses, as they find themselves in a situation in which they do not have the power to do what they believe should be done.

Chapter 262

TRANSPORT MEDICINE

Richard Orr • John Cole • Kimberly Roth

KEY POINTS

1. Patients are often subjected to a high-risk moving environment with limited resources and few monitoring capabilities. The goal during transport should be to provide the same or better quality of care than the patient had before transport.

2. A retrieval system has a responsibility to the referral community to provide accessible tertiary care. The components include a communications center, administrative staff, appropriately trained team members, reliable equipment, and education and safety programs.

3. A hospital should not transfer a patient until the patient has been appropriately stabilized, the patient consents to transfer after being informed of the risks of transfer, and the referring physician certifies that the medical benefits expected from the transfer outweigh the risks. The transferring hospital must provide care and stabilization within its capability; copies of the medical records and imaging studies must accompany the patient; the receiving facility must have available space and qualified personnel and have agreed to accept the patient; and the transport must be made by *qualified* personnel.

4. Underutilization of an acquired skill often leads to fear on the part of the provider and an aversion to performing an intervention during a time of crisis. A busy emergency medical services system with 50 active, advanced, life support providers would be expected to have one pediatric bag-valve-mask case every 1.7 years, one pediatric intubation every 3.3 years, and one intraosseous cannulation every 6.7 years!

5. The current paradigm of transport must shift if we are to realize improved outcomes in the critically ill who require transport to a critical care center. We must abandon the current paradigm of "scoop and run" as a means of initiating care. We must adopt a system whereby goal-directed therapy begins in the prehospital arena and continues throughout the critical care continuum.

Critically ill patients often need to be moved either within an institution for special procedures or between hospitals when a referring physician believes that a patient could benefit from such a transfer. Despite the numerous advances in health care, transport of the critically ill is often a neglected area of critical care and emergency medicine. Although major decisions are made daily with regard to the mode of travel and the staffing of transports, there is still little research to support the validity of this decision-making process. Patients are often subjected to a high-risk moving environment with limited resources and few monitoring capabilities. The goal during transport should be to provide the same or better quality care than the patient had before transport. Therefore, physicians throughout the critical care continuum must take an active role in designing the transport segments and maintaining quality assurance, if optimal care is to be provided.[1] (Please note that transport issues important to the management of mass casualties in disasters are addressed in Chapter 263.)

OUT-OF-HOSPITAL TRANSPORT

PREHOSPITAL OPTIONS

Current day emergency medical services (EMS) are focused on rapid transport from the scene to the nearest emergency department or trauma center that can render appropriate care. The transport team should be able to immediately recognize a critically ill or injured patient and be trained in advanced procedures. Patient management is usually limited to supporting the airway, breathing, and circulation. Rapid assessment, stabilization, and transport are the goals for the transport team in the prehospital setting. Airway management utilizing rapid sequence intubation is a common procedure performed by air medical crews. The transport team should also be able to perform a needle thoracostomy if indicated, control active bleeding, and establish venous access. Other procedures should be kept to a minimum.

Appropriate utilization of resources (air vs. ground units) for the transport of injured patients has been a subject of study and debate since the inception of air medical transport. The transport of trauma patients directly from the scene should be supported by on-line medical control or pre-approved protocols based on the factors of time, distance, geography, patient stability, and local resources. The National Association of Emergency Medical Service Physicians (NAEMSP) and the American College of Emergency Physicians (ACEP) have each recommended triage guidelines for on-scene helicopter transport.[2] Early retrospective studies were able to show improved outcomes in patients transported by air.[3,4] Defining the types of specific injuries that benefit from air medical transport has been difficult owing to many variables, such as ground transport team skills, variable composition, skill of flight crews, time from injury to arrival at definitive care, and treatment received at the receiving trauma center. A recent multicenter study has demonstrated that helicopter transport was associated with a significant reduction in mortality rates compared with ground transport in victims of blunt trauma.[5] As specialized cardiac and stroke centers have developed, air transport has also begun to be utilized for the rapid transports of these patients directly from the scene. This emerging trend will likely continue and develop similarly to the current system of trauma referral networks for patients directly from the scene of injury or illness.

INTERFACILITY OPTIONS

Most transfers do not involve critically ill patients and can be accomplished safely using local ambulance services. Depending on available resources in the area, a physician may have up to five options.

First, the patient may be transported by private automobile or public transportation. Since the responsibility for the patient rests with the referring physician, this method, devoid of a trained caregiver, should be used only for a patient whose medical condition does not include derangements of the cardiovascular, pulmonary, and central nervous systems and whose medical condition is not likely to deteriorate during transport.

Second, the patient may be transferred by a local EMS under predefined protocols or with specific instructions from a command physician. The advantages of this option are the low cost and the minimal time lapse before the patient can be taken to the receiving hospital. In rural areas, however, this option carries the risk of depleting a large geographic area of valuable medical resources, such as ambulances, emergency medical technicians, and paramedics. In addition, the referring physician, who has little control over the en route phase of the transport, again assumes a significant legal risk. Because of the variable backgrounds of EMS staff, the transferring personnel may not be equipped or trained to provide the necessary care in every situation.

The third option entails the addition of referring hospital staff to a local ambulance service. This option is less costly and possibly faster than the use of a critical care transport team. The legal risk is reduced because the referring physician maintains a tighter control over the patient's treatment during the transfer. Disadvantages of this option include the loss of personnel from the referring hospital and the lack of appropriate portable monitoring equipment.

The fourth option involves the use of a regional critical care transport team, which will not deplete EMS or referring hospital resources. A command physician who is usually based at the institution from which the team originates provides recommendations for management until the team arrives. The team routinely carries equipment to manage virtually any emergency during transfer and has battery-powered portable monitoring devices designed for use in moving environments. Team members are usually specially trained to deal with out-of-hospital emergencies and are acclimated to the stress of working in a moving environment.

Based on the experience of the Korean and Vietnam Wars, air medical transport has become an integral part of regional systems in the United States. The first civilian helicopter EMS program in the United States was established at St. Anthony's Hospital in Denver in 1972.[6] Today, over 300 private, hospital-based, public-service, and military air medical helicopter programs transport over 250,000 patients annually. Helicopter transport significantly reduces transport time. The practical transport range for helicopter transfers is generally 150 miles from its base of operations. For longer distance transports or in poor weather conditions, fixed-wing aircraft are used by many air medical services. Most air medical transport today is done with twin-engine helicopters specifically configured for medical missions. Some flight programs are able to fly instrument-flight-rules missions, allowing transport of patients in weather conditions that previously prevented rotorcraft transport. The flight environment is noisy, making simple procedures such as auscultation of blood pressure and breath sounds difficult or impossible.[7] Therefore, "nonaudible-dependent" monitoring is employed. Most flight crews rely on noninvasive blood pressure monitoring, capnometry, and pulse oximetry to monitor patients in flight. Rotorcraft rarely fly at altitudes more than 2000 feet above ground level. At these altitudes, pressure changes have only a minor impact on the volume of air-filled spaces. Most therapeutic interventions such as endotracheal intubation, chest decompression, intravenous access, and control of bleeding are done before liftoff. Intravenous analgesia, sedation, neuromuscular blockade, vasoactive drugs, and blood products can be given in flight. These interventions must be performed under strict on-line medical direction or preapproved protocols. The perceived disadvantage of a regional retrieval system, especially when air transport is not available, is the delay imposed by round-trip travel time. Personnel may also lack pediatric experience, especially if they are based at a nonpediatric hospital or have minimal exposure to pediatric emergencies.

The fifth option, a specialty team, has all of the advantages of a regional critical care transport team and provides additional expertise in the care of selected patients. Examples include patients requiring left-ventricular assist devices or extracorporeal membrane oxygenation (ECMO) and very young patients who are critically ill. The only disadvantage of this option is that in many areas specialty teams are unavailable.

RESPONSIBILITY OF THE RETRIEVAL SYSTEM

The retrieval system has a responsibility to the referral community to provide accessible tertiary care, including transport. This responsibility begins with a commitment to a formal structure. Optimally, this structure is designed to begin providing intensive care, when necessary, to the patient at the referring institution and to continue appropriate care while en route. Care en route should be similar to the care given in the ICU. The referring community's expectations of the regional center's response to transport requests vary according to the standard of care and the topography for that region. Regardless of its origin, a retrieval system should include a communications center, administrative staff, appropriately trained team members, reliable equipment, and a safety program.

COMMUNICATIONS

The communications center for the retrieval system should be easily accessible to both the referring physician and the transport team.[8,9] It should be staffed around the clock by full-time communication specialists who are trained in handling emergency calls and who have no other distracting duties that would delay a response. The communication specialist should follow a prescribed protocol to minimize the number of calls necessary to organize efforts, notify the appropriate personnel, and arrange all aspects of the transport, so that the referring physician can direct his or her attention to patient care, rather than waste valuable time on the telephone. A detailed log of transport requests, including time, demographic data, diagnosis, and vehicle availability, is kept both for administrative review and for medical-legal documentation. Equipment for direct communication with the center should be available in every transport vehicle. The receiving physician who is responsible for the transport maintains contact with the communications center and with the referring physician. The receiving physician should obtain a brief history of the patient's present illness, a summary of interventions, and recommendations that are tailored to the capabilities of the referring hospital and pertinent to the current problem. This information should be documented on a log that remains a part of the patient's medical record. It is also suggested that the referring physician have a copy of the patient's record and radiographs to accompany the transport team.

STAFFING A RETRIEVAL SYSTEM

The administrative staff of a retrieval system should include, at a minimum, a program director, medical director, transport coordinator, and medical command.[9,10] The program director is responsible for the structure, activities, and organization of the transport system and assumes overall program responsibilities; acts as a liaison between the team and hospital administration; and develops and implements quality management.

The medical director should be a specialist in critical care or emergency medicine and might also have training in a surgical subspecialty (trauma) or in pediatrics (neonatology). He or she must be a licensed physician who is responsible for supervising and evaluating the quality of medical care provided by the transport team and must have educational experience in those areas of medicine that are commensurate with the mission of the retrieval service. The medical director should be experienced in both air and ground transport (as appropriate), should understand patient care capabilities and limitations in the transport environment, and should be educated in infection control, stress recognition and management, and altitude physiology and stressors in the flight environment. The medical director must also be actively involved in quality management, administrative decisions affecting medical care, and the hiring, training, and continuing education of all transport personnel. This person must also orient physicians who provide on-line medical direction in the policies, procedures, and patient care protocols and should act as a liaison to the referral community for teaching and outreach.[9,10] The transport coordinator, usually a nurse or paramedic, collaborates with the medical director in training, protocols, scheduling, data collection, quality management, and marketing. The medical director and transport coordinator should participate in patient transport, whenever possible, to maintain skill and perspective.

A command physician should oversee every transport and provide advice to the referring physician and transport team as necessary. The command physician must be experienced in handling transport calls and in offering management suggestions for the period before the arrival of the transport team. He or she should be knowledgeable about the availability of resources, have authority to accept transferred patients without further consultation, and perform triage as well as activate back-up systems when necessary. Medical control is usually accomplished in one of two ways: on line or off line.[11] On-line medical control is direct real-time voice communication (radio, telephone, cellular telephone, or satellite phone) between the medical control physician and the transport team. The transport team must always know who their command physician is throughout the transport process. Responsibility for medical control will vary based on local practices and the policies of the transport service. Medical control physicians must be experienced in critical care transports to ensure that crews provide appropriate care. For specialized transports, the transport service should have a mechanism in place that affords medical control physicians timely consultation with subspecialists or the receiving physician. Alternatively, the critical care transport team should have the ability to consult with the receiving physician and to provide updates to the receiving facility. During off-line medical control, patient management by the transport team is driven by written protocols or standing orders. There is no direct communication between the team and the medical control physician. The medical director is responsible for developing transport protocols and procedures used for off-line medical control.

Transport crewmembers should be experienced in the care of critically ill patients and able to deal with complex environments with limited resources. They must be highly skilled in airway management, resuscitation, and vascular access. They should have a fundamental knowledge of field priorities and be able to make decisions independently. All team members should have specific training in transport medicine, which includes methods of functioning in a moving environment, aeromedical physiology, and troubleshooting for equipment-related problems.

Medical crew composition represents a broad spectrum of health care providers. Most critical care transport services have a standard crew composition for most transports. More than 70% of the medical flight crews consist of a nurse-paramedic team. Approximately 20% of programs use two nurses, and only 3% of programs use a flight physician. Respiratory therapists are teamed with nurses in a small percentage of programs.[9] Flight nurses typically have extensive experience in the emergency department or the ICU.

Paramedics have experience with critically injured or ill patients in the prehospital setting. Flight physicians are, generally, emergency medicine residents. In a few programs they may be attending physicians or medical directors of flight programs. The use of physicians in these services as flight crew members is indicated when the physician might contribute significantly to the care provided in flight. Studies suggest that specific physician judgment or skill may be required in approximately 25% of transports.[3,12,13]

EQUIPMENT

Equipment taken on transport should be complete and adequate to provide continuing intensive care throughout the trip. Oxygen reserve should be calculated for each patient transported and should be at least twice the amount needed for the expected duration of the trip, in case of delays or equipment malfunction. Portable, compartmentalized equipment packs must be designed for easy access and must be able to withstand the stress of the transport environment. For air medical transport, weight and space restrictions must also be considered in selecting equipment and range of medications. Transport monitors should have battery power that will last beyond the expected duration of transport because of the possibility of unexpected delays or vehicle breakdowns and should be free of movement artifact. Most important, the transport team should be self-sufficient and not dependent on the referring hospital for supplies. All equipment should be routinely checked and maintained after transport by a team member dedicated to that task.

SAFETY

Safety should be a high priority in any transport program. Emergency vehicle operation carries substantial risks, not only to the crew and the patient but also to others in its vicinity. The medical director is responsible for thoroughly researching vendors of air or ground transport services in the areas of maintenance, safety records, experience of drivers and pilots, and reliability of equipment. Written contracts between the institution and the vendor should include specific insurance details. Ambulance drivers should be discouraged from exceeding the speed limit, because there is no evidence that "red-balling" has any positive effect on patient outcome.

Aeromedical transport involves a unique set of safety issues. The four leading causes of accidents are weather, engine failure, collision, and loss of control. Pressure on pilots to fly, competition among aeromedical services within a region, and failure to observe minimal weather standards are among the components contributing to these accidents. For pilots to make sound decisions based on the flight conditions, they must be isolated from patient-care issues. In regions where there are competing aeromedical services, they should act jointly to establish regional safety guidelines, minimal weather standards, and a quality-assurance program that would examine compliance.

Transport team members must have a good understanding of aviation medicine and of how the aeromedical environment affects both the team and the patient. Barometric pressure changes associated with increasing cabin altitude lower alveolar oxygen tension and increase the volume of any entrapped gas (e.g., in the bowel, sinuses, pneumothorax, endotracheal tube cuffs) and may affect intravenous infusion rates. The results of poor eating habits (hypoglycemia), sleep deprivation, and drugs (e.g., alcohol, marijuana, antihistamines) are potentiated by increasing altitude. Vibration can produce fatigue, and accelerating and decelerating forces can produce vertigo. Night vision is decreased above cabin altitudes of 5000 feet. The transport team should be adept at survival techniques for their region and should always be prepared to deal with an off-airport landing. Regular sessions to review safety and emergency procedures for each transport mode should be provided for the transport team members.

RESPONSIBILITIES OF THE REFERRING HOSPITAL

The transfer of patients from one institution to another is regulated by federal statute. The legislation that created the

patient stabilization and transfer requirements for hospitals and physicians was the Consolidated Omnibus Budget Reconciliation Act (COBRA) of 1986, also known as the "anti-dumping law" and its amendment, the Omnibus Reconciliation Act of 1989.[14,15] This is the current legal standard. One of the main objectives of this resolution was to guarantee equal access to emergency treatment to all citizens, regardless of their ability to pay. COBRA attributes responsibility for the patient's transfer to the referring hospital and physician. Violations can result in a number of penalties, including termination of Medicare privileges for the physician and hospital. A hospital can be fined between $25,000 and $50,000 per violation, and a physician can be fined $50,000 per violation. A patient can also sue the hospital for personal injury in civil court. The Emergency Medical Treatment and Labor Act established by the COBRA legislation governs how patients may be transferred from one hospital to another. Hospitals cannot transfer patients unless the transfer is "appropriate," the patient consents to transfer after being informed of the risks of transfer, and the referring physician certifies that the medical benefits expected from the transfer outweigh the risks. Appropriate transfers must meet the following criteria: (1) the transferring hospital must provide care and stabilization within its ability; (2) copies of medical records and imaging studies must accompany the patient; (3) the receiving facility must have available space and qualified personnel and agree to accept the transfer; and (4) the interfacility transport must be made by qualified personnel with the necessary equipment.

Significant advances in therapeutic and diagnostic interventions for critically ill patients have occurred, but often at great cost and limited availability, prompting the need for transport of these patients to tertiary care centers. Emergent interfacility transport should occur after initial stabilization and determination by the referring facility that the patient's needs for care are beyond the scope of local capabilities. Receiving centers should have communication centers that facilitate transfers, outreach teams to provide referring facilities with continuing education, and education programs about regional resources and trauma systems.

Transfer of the critically ill patient occurs with the expectation that care will continue en route to the receiving facility and that complications will be identified and treated. These goals frequently require specialized personnel and equipment. Coordination between referring and receiving institutions and medical direction during transport are measures fundamental to guaranteeing continuation of care and maximal utilization of resources. Interfacility transport can be performed by a transport team from the referring facility, the receiving facility, or by a third party. It is the responsibility of the referring physician, in consultation with the receiving physician, to decide the best mode of transportation (air vs. ground) and to ensure that the transporting personnel have the necessary expertise and equipment to deal with the patient's condition and possible complications. For example, some out-of-hospital–based personnel may not be trained in the use of certain hospital equipment (e.g., drug infusion pumps).

Complete documentation of all patient care records must be sent. This includes results of all therapeutic and diagnostic interventions, copies of all imaging studies performed, and patient consent for transfer. Teleradiology has a role in allowing receiving centers to review a patient's studies before arrival. It is essential that the transport team establish direct communication with both referring and accepting physicians. Communication with the referring physician must detail the following information: (1) identification of the patient and medical history; (2) interventions performed during initial stabilization and the patient's response; (3) pertinent physical examination findings; (4) ongoing therapy; and (5) complications that might occur during transport.

UNIQUE ASPECTS OF PEDIATRIC TRANSPORT

EPIDEMIOLOGY OF PEDIATRIC EMS

The majority of children are transported by EMS providers with variable educational backgrounds and experience. EMS includes all aspects of basic life support (BLS), advanced life support (ALS), and critical care transport where emergency medical personnel are used. EMS encompasses prehospital and interfacility components of transport, including hospital-based specialized teams. A critically ill child in a rural setting might receive care from a basic emergency medical technician and an ambulance driver but in a more organized system have the benefit of a transport team who specialize in pediatric critical care. Currently, there are no national regulations for EMS as they relate to children. Only two states require all the pediatric equipment recommended for BLS ambulances and only five states require all essential pediatric equipment for advanced life support ambulances. Pediatric guidelines for EMS are just beginning to evolve from the various national organizations that represent children.[16]

Less than 10% of all EMS transports nationwide are for infants and children; 12% of those involve advanced life support, and even fewer provide critical care.[17-20] Overall, this translates into three pediatric patients per month for 60% of the nation's paramedics, and fewer than 3% of the nation's paramedics see 15 or more children per month! Seidel and colleagues first described these deficiencies and found that 41% of emergency medical technician training programs offered no more than 10 hours in both didactic and clinical pediatric training, 24% did not carry a complete set of pediatric blood pressure cuffs, and 79% of providers were not equipped with a complete set of pediatric ventilation masks.[17-19] Children were twice as likely to die of trauma in the field compared with adults, and this was attributed to the lack of training in pediatric critical care.[17] Glaeser and coworkers performed a survey of nationally registered EMS providers and found that they receive a median of 16 hours of pediatric didactic instruction out of a total of 358 hours but are not required to take pediatric continuing medical education training. However, 76% of the providers supported a mandate for continuing education in pediatrics.[20] More recently, Macnab determined that "preventable" insults to children occurred more frequently when the transport team had no formal pediatric training. When formal pediatric training was offered as a "hands-on" patient care module for prehospital providers, there was a significant reduction in insults during transport.[21]

SKILL MAINTENANCE AND PROVIDER CONFIDENCE

The logical outcome of limited provider exposure to critically ill children is the problem of maintaining pediatric assessment and interventional skills. Babl and associates demonstrated that in a program with 50 active ALS providers in the current milieu of EMS, each provider would be expected to have one pediatric bag-valve-mask case every 1.7 years, one pediatric intubation every 3.3 years, and one intraosseous cannulation every 6.7 years.[22] Underutilization of an acquired skill often leads to fear on the part of the provider and an aversion to performing an intervention during a time of crisis, especially in infants and children. Reluctance to provide advanced airway management is a good example. Aijian and coworkers examined a population of pediatric patients who had suffered a prehospital cardiopulmonary arrest and determined that endotracheal intubation was attempted only 68% of the time, with only a 64% success rate. In patients younger than 1 year, endotracheal intubation was attempted only 38% of the time, with only a 50% success rate.[23] Losek and colleagues reviewed a series of 1467 children in the prehospital setting and determined that only 78% of endotracheal attempts were successful. Of patients who were pulseless and not breathing at the scene, 93% were successfully intubated. Of those who were judged to be in impending respiratory failure, only 48% were successfully intubated.[24]

With any given scenario in the EMS setting, adult patients are more likely to receive an appropriate intervention compared with a child having the same problem. Gausche and colleagues found that children in the field who were younger than 14 years were more likely to be undertreated as compared with adults (33% vs. 3%), but with discordant overtreatment in placement of intravenous catheters—a procedure with which paramedics are more comfortable.[25] Emergency providers often call on air medical services to transport children because of their presumed expertise and training in pediatric care when compared with local prehospital EMS providers. Air medical services are usually hospital-based or near major medical centers, where providers are given the opportunity to rotate through pediatric units and receive hands-on experience in the care of critically ill children. However, the literature suggests that airway management in children remains a problem even among these "more experienced" providers.[26-28] Additional training in airway management in children and the use of medications (neuromuscular blockade) to facilitate intubation would probably result in a greater success rate.

Despite the time and effort given to the training of EMS personnel, cognitive and interventional skills deteriorate over time, especially when there are few encounters with children in the field. Su and coworkers demonstrated through a randomized controlled trial that the knowledge a paramedic receives through education courses deteriorates rapidly over a 6-month period.[29] Henderson and associates also demonstrated that the ability of a provider to intubate or provide bag-valve-mask ventilation for a child deteriorates significantly over 6 months. The issue of more concern in this study was that 95% of the paramedics who failed attempts at both bag-valve-mask and endotracheal intubation reported confidence and lack of anxiety in their ability to provide these lifesaving procedures in the field.[30]

Finally, referring hospitals are often not equipped to care for critically ill and injured children. Seidel and colleagues demonstrated that many emergency departments were ill-prepared to care for children and suggested that hospital facilities be designated for pediatric emergency care.[17-19] Esposito and coworkers found that frequent errors occur in emergency department management of pediatric trauma, leading to about 9% preventable mortality. They reported a 64% error rate in management of children, including gross violations of basic trauma care.[31] More recently, Athey and associates found that a significant number of critically ill infants and children are still being admitted to hospitals lacking pediatric specialty facilities or expertise. They reported that nearly 10% of all U.S. hospitals without pediatric intensive care facilities admit critically ill and injured children and that 7% of these hospitals routinely admit these children to adult ICUs rather than transferring them to a more appropriate facility. Of the facilities who keep children, few have protocols for obtaining pediatric consultation for emergencies and most did not have appropriately sized equipment to care for these children.[32] Consequently, there are two extremes in handling referrals from these hospitals. The first is to employ a "scoop-and-run" approach with minimal initial care from the emergency department, using inexperienced personnel en route to the tertiary center "to save time." Harrison and colleagues found that children were likely to be transferred significantly more quickly from referring hospitals than were adults with comparably severe injuries.[33] The second is to keep the critically ill child in the adult ICU until irreparable damage to major organ systems has occurred, at which point a transfer is requested.

UNAPPRECIATED DIFFERENCES BETWEEN ADULTS AND CHILDREN

Airway and respiratory difficulties are the most likely causes of pediatric cardiopulmonary arrest and account for over 50% of ICU admissions for children.[34-36] The caregiver on transport should be cognizant of the anatomic and physiologic differences between the respiratory systems of children and adults. Earlier intervention is often required to correct a respiratory problem in a child when compared with an adult patient with a similar respiratory derangement because of these differences. Airway interventions should be planned carefully and performed early in the course of respiratory failure to obviate respiratory crisis during the en route phase of transport.

First, adults differ from children in the site of the major contribution to the total airflow resistance. The upper airway, particularly the nose, accounts for the major portion of total resistance in the adult. Conversely, the peripheral airway resistance in children younger than 5 years is approximately four times higher than in adults or older children.[37] This observation explains the high incidence of lower airway obstructive disease in young children. Respiratory distress in an adult patient can often be ameliorated by performing a few simple upper airway maneuvers during transport, obviating intubation and positive-pressure breathing, at least until the patient arrives at the receiving facility. This approach will not work in an infant or child, and a delay in performing advanced airway management in an effort to save time can lead to a progression of respiratory failure and cardiopulmonary arrest.

Second, infants and small children have more compliant chest walls and weaker cartilaginous support than do older children and adults, leading to several clinical implications.[38,39] The very low elastic recoil pressure of the newborn chest wall raises the risk of lung collapse. Most tidal volume breathing in the infant takes place in the range of the closing capacity of the lung. The relatively high closing capacity is

due to reduced elastic recoil of the lung, raising the subatmospheric pressure in the intrapleural space. This leads to early airway closure in the dependent regions of the lung, particularly when there is disease. In addition, the highly compliant chest wall is at a mechanical disadvantage during breathing because the infant must generate greater pressure and perform more work to move the same tidal volume. When infants are confronted with the need to increase their work of breathing because of lung disease, a certain percentage of them will fatigue and stop breathing.[40] Therefore, aggressive airway intervention and positive-pressure breathing early in the transport process will stop the progression of atelectasis and respiratory failure. In addition, because tidal volume breathing is much more dependent on diaphragmatic function in infants and small children, a nasogastric tube should always be inserted for patients who are intubated and for those with impending respiratory failure.

Third, in an infant the alveolar diameter is half the size of that in an adult, predisposing an infant or small child to alveolar collapse much earlier in the course of respiratory failure.[41] In addition, the adult lung contains anatomic channels that allow ventilation distal to an obstructed airway, also known as "collateral ventilation."[42] Without these pathways for collateral ventilation, the infant and young child are presumably at increased risk for atelectasis and emphysematous changes and ventilation/perfusion mismatching. In addition, infants and children have higher metabolic rates than adults, and hypoxia progresses more quickly during the course of respiratory failure.

Finally, cardiorespiratory compensatory mechanisms are more pronounced in children. For infants and children, blood pressure is preserved during the course of early shock, through increases in systemic vascular resistance. In the authors' experience, goal-directed therapy for shock is either delayed or minimized because caregivers in the transport environment often use blood pressure as a guide to therapy… something they are more accustomed to doing with adult patients.

CHANGING THE TRANSPORT PARADIGM: CAN WE IMPROVE OUTCOME?

Emergency medical services and regional flight teams are essentially focused on the adult population and have been developed to deal primarily with myocardial infarction and trauma, the major causes of morbidity and mortality in adults.[19] They are designed for rapid response and are expected to keep time at the scene to a minimum. EMS personnel are often taught that they are working against a clock (the "golden hour") that begins ticking at the onset of the illness or injury, and that for every minute spent away from the critical care center, the probability of survival diminishes. This golden hour is the driving force for clinical decision making and usually translates into providing minimal care while moving quickly. The concept of the golden hour is often described as having its origin in an article published by Cowley and colleagues in which survival of patients with traumatic injuries markedly improved when they reached the trauma center within 1 hour of their injury or illness.[43] This article was not a study on the outcome of trauma victims but rather a commentary on the success of implementing a helicopter-based program for trauma. The article does, however, contain the following quote taken from

Modern Hospital: "It has been recorded that for every 30 minutes that elapse between the accident and the time the patient gets to definitive care, the mortality rate can be expected to increase threefold."[44] The truth of the matter at the time that article was written was that definitive care rarely was provided until the patient arrived at the trauma unit. Prehospital care at that time consisted of providing supplemental oxygen, a fast-moving vehicle, and minimal resuscitation. Intuitively, under these circumstances, a worse outcome could be expected as prehospital time increased. Interestingly, even during this era, experiences suggested improved survival when stabilization occurred in the field. Military medical experience showed that stabilization in the field markedly improved survival of trauma victims.[45] Field stabilization also improved the outcome of victims requiring cardiopulmonary life support.[46,47] In a landmark article, Rivers and coworkers demonstrated that the initiation of goal-directed therapy in the emergency department setting improved survival for patients with severe sepsis and septic shock.[48] Patients assigned to the early goal-directed therapeutic group also had better central venous oxygen saturations, lower base deficits, and a lower incidence of multisystem organ dysfunction than did those who had "standard therapy" (minimal resuscitation before arrival to the ICU). Han and colleagues published similar results in a pediatric transport study. When community physicians successfully achieved shock reversal through aggressive resuscitation before a transport team arrived, patients had a ninefold increase in their odds of survival. Overall, resuscitation practice was consistent with American College of Critical Care Medicine-PALS guidelines in only 30% of children presenting with septic shock in a community emergency department.[49] This reluctance to treat is typical of the current paradigm of EMS, where the "scoop-and-run" mentality prevails. Caregivers who do provide stabilization before the patient arrives in a critical care unit are often criticized for their efforts because of the popular notion that out-of-hospital stabilization "wastes time" and "delays" definitive therapy that should be rendered at the receiving facility.

The current paradigm of transport must shift if we are to realize improved outcomes in the critically ill who require transport to a critical care center. We must abandon the current paradigm of "scoop and run" through a disjointed system as a means to initiating care on arrival at the critical care center. We must adopt a system whereby goal-directed therapy begins in the prehospital arena and continues throughout the critical care continuum.

IN-HOSPITAL TRANSPORT

Despite the primary focus of transport on prehospital and interfacility settings, in-hospital transport of ICU patients occurs more commonly and is just as life threatening. Problems generally occur when patients are being brought to the ICU from the emergency department or the operating room or when they are on their way from the ICU to another department for special procedures.

STUDIES ON IN-HOSPITAL TRANSPORT

Adult patients who were admitted to the ICU with severe trauma experienced serious physiologic changes in heart rate, blood pressure, respiratory rate, intracranial pressure, or oxygen saturation when they were transported out of the ICU for diagnostic studies.[50-52] Indeck and coworkers reported that one fourth of these patients had their clinical treatment changed within 48 hours of the transport.[53] Mechanically ventilated patients transported out of the ICU experienced cardiovascular changes related to altered ventilation or changes in intracranial pressure, and the incidence of adverse events during such transports out of the ICU correlated with the severity of injury.[50,51] Insel and associates showed that patients transferred from the operating room to the ICU had significant increases in systolic blood pressure and heart rate.[54] Hypoxemia was seen in 15% to 22% of unconscious victims with head trauma transferred from the emergency department to the neurosurgical unit.[50,52] An inadequately managed airway was the major reason for hypoxemia in these patients.[52,55] Other adverse events seen in these patients included arterial hypertension or hypotension and intracranial hypertension.[50] Smith and colleagues reported that 34% of the adults who were transported out of the ICU for diagnostic studies had an equipment-related mishap, and the rate of mishap did not correlate with the duration of transport or type of escort.[56]

Wallen and associates showed that 83% of the transports from the ICU for diagnostic studies had a significant change in heart rate, blood pressure, respiratory rate, or temperature; 16.4% had at least one equipment-related mishap; and 27.3% required at least one major intervention.[57] This study also showed that, of the patients transported from the ICU to the operating room, 63% had a significant change in heart rate, blood pressure, respiratory rate, or temperature; 8% had at least one equipment-related mishap; and 9.1% received at least one major intervention. In all transports, mechanically ventilated patients had a higher incidence of adverse events and required more interventions than did those who were not receiving mechanical ventilation. Severity of illness and the duration of transport were both significantly associated with the occurrence of an adverse event. They also showed that all significant changes in heart rate, blood pressure, respiratory rate, and temperature were due to the transport process itself.

GENERAL PRINCIPLES OF IN-HOSPITAL TRANSPORT

The general principles of in-hospital transport are the same as those for interfacility transport and should ensure patient and personnel safety, minimal mobilization and transfer times, provision of optimal care, and physician accountability. Transfer of critically ill patients to another location should be treated as an extension of intensive care. Because the incidence of adverse events during in-hospital transport is affected by the pretransport severity of illness and time away from the ICU, personnel, equipment, and monitoring should be appropriate and should not result in a degradation of care.[50,51,57]

Adequate medical supervision should be provided during the entire in-hospital transfer. ICU personnel may have a tendency to ignore what happens outside the ICU or to send the least-experienced caregivers on a transfer. The attending physician from the ICU is ultimately responsible for all that occurs during the transport and therefore should be aware of all in-house transports and should be ready to respond to an emergency. In the authors' opinion, a physician member of the critical care team should accompany all patients who are intubated and require mechanical ventilation, as well as those who have instability of the respiratory, cardiovascular, or central nervous system.

Equipment taken on an in-hospital transport should include a portable system that contains everything normally found on a crash cart and an airway compartment complete with suction apparatus, laryngoscopes, endotracheal tubes, bag-valve-mask devices, and medication for emergency intubation. An E-sized oxygen cylinder with a high-pressure regulator, flowmeter, and tubing of sufficient length should accompany all transports and be secured safely to the transport stretcher. Monitoring should include the cardiorespiratory system (electrocardiography, impedance pneumography) at the very least, pulse oximetry for patients in whom oxygen delivery is a potential concern, and the addition of capnography for patients who require mechanical ventilation. Intravascular monitoring should also be continued. It is important to use monitors with reliable batteries in the event of power loss or unexpected delays.

CONCLUSION

Transport is clearly a challenge to the intensivist, who often must make difficult choices in a complex treatment environment. The risk/benefit ratio should always be examined, with specific attention paid to the risk of transport versus the risk of not performing the transfer or procedure. Intensivists must be actively involved in the planning, maintenance, and quality management of transport if optimal care is to be expected. Ensuring patient and personnel safety, keeping transport time to a minimum, providing constant optimal care, and having an accountable physician in charge at all times are general principles that must always be observed. Transport outcomes will not improve until we adopt a system whereby early goal-directed therapy is the driving force rather than "scoop and run."

ANNOTATED REFERENCES

Han YY, Carcillo JA, Dragotta MA, et al: Early reversal of pediatric-neonatal septic shock by community physicians is associated with improved outcome. Pediatrics 2003;12:793-799.

This study demonstrated that when community physicians successfully achieved shock reversal through aggressive resuscitation before a transport team arrived, patients had a ninefold increase in their odds of survival.

Rivers E, Nguyen B, Havstad S, et al: Early goal-directed therapy in the treatment of severe sepsis and septic shock. N Engl J Med 2001;345:1368-1377.

This landmark article demonstrated that early goal-directed therapy in the treatment of septic shock before arrival in the ICU improved survival. Patients assigned to the early goal-directed therapy group had improved central venous oxygen saturations, lower base deficits, and a lower incidence of multisystem organ dysfunction compared with those who had standard therapy.

Seidel JS, Hornbein M, Yoshiyama K, et al: Emergency medical services and the pediatric patient: Are the needs being met? Pediatrics 1984;73:769-772.

This observational study provided a major impetus in the development of the Emergency Medical Services for Children (EMSC) program. It noted that EMS throughout the United States was developed primarily to deal with myocardial infarction and trauma and failed to recognize the special needs of the critically ill child. Children were noted to have a higher death rate in the field than adults, and deaths occurred more commonly in areas where there were no pediatric centers.

Task Force on Interhospital Transport: Guidelines for Air and Ground Transport of Neonatal and Pediatric Transport. Elk Grove Village, IL, American Academy of Pediatrics, 1999.

This document was published by the American Academy of Pediatrics and provides guidelines and education for all health care professionals who provide or supervise patient care and make decisions about the emergency interfacility transport of children. When medically feasible, stabilization of the patient's condition before transport is key to achieving optimal patient outcome and required by the Emergency Medical Treatment and Active Labor Act.

Wallen E, Venkataraman ST, Grosso MJ, et al: Intrahospital transport of critically ill pediatric patients. Crit Care Med 1995;23:1588-1595.

This study showed that serious physiologic deterioration can occur during intrahospital transport of critically ill children. Severity of illness and the duration of transport were associated with the occurrence of adverse events during transport. Team composition and equipment required on transport must be commensurate with the pretransport severity of illness and the anticipated duration of transport.

Chapter 263

DISASTER MEDICINE FOR THE ICU PHYSICIAN

Raghu S. Loganathan • Rakesh Alva • Manoj Karwa • Vladimir Kvetan

KEY POINTS

1. Disaster medicine is a unique specialty that has evolved over the past few years. It shares a common ideal with public health: **"greatest good for the greatest number."** Critical care medicine forms an indispensable part of this science because intensive care physicians not only care for the sickest of the salvageable patients in any hospital but also bring with them their clinical expertise in triage, resuscitation, and help in providing care outside the domains of the unit through mobile ICU teams.

2. **Clear, common, and concise definitions are important** in effective communication and evoking appropriate responses to disaster situations. The concept of functional impact of a disaster on the health care system is paramount while classifying disasters.

3. **It is important to understand the common effects of different natural and manmade disasters to predict their impact on the health care system.** Even though manmade disasters such as terrorist attacks have gained recent attention, the numbers of geophysical disasters such as earthquakes, floods, and hurricanes have remained fairly constant and place the greatest burden on the health care system.

4. Disaster situations present with many unique medical syndromes that require specific therapy. **Knowledge and immediate recognition of different medical syndromes with appropriate interventions is critical to minimizing morbidity and mortality.**

5. **Disaster planning** includes developing action programs to minimize loss of life and damage during a disaster, training health care personnel and civilians, coordinating response efforts, maintaining adequate supplies of equipment and personnel, and rehabilitating the community after the disaster. Knowledge of potential manmade and natural disasters to which the community is prone should be an integral part of the planning process. Common principles involved in the creation of an emergency response plan should be followed and applied from an ICU perspective.

6. With their natural role of caring for critically ill patients, intensivists bring with them unique abilities that can be applied to a disaster situation, such as a **multidisciplinary approach to patient care,** management skills, procedural expertise, and flexible attitudes.

7. **Intensivists can also provide care outside the domains of the ICU through mobile ICU teams and transport of critically ill patients.** Various factors need to be considered in the formation of such teams and in the safe transport of patients.

Natural and manmade disasters have always been a part of life and are occurring with increasing frequency. They create varied degrees of chaos owing to mismatch of resources and needs, and they place a huge burden on health care systems. Restoring an affected society back to its pre-event status requires extraordinary efforts and incurs substantial costs. Thousands of persons are injured physically and emotionally as a result of such events and their effects continue long after worldwide attention has disappeared.

The devastating events of September 11, 2001, in the United States, subsequent acts of bioterrorism, as well as the threat of new and emerging infections have brought new challenges to the field of disaster management and multidisciplinary hazard mitigation. Even though war- and terrorism-related disasters have gathered much attention recently, natural disasters have occurred with increasing frequency over the past decades. This has been attributed to the growth of human populations in geographically disaster-prone areas, rapid industrialization, and increasing exposure to toxic and hazardous materials.[1-3] The United Nations recognized the increasing impact on the world's population and environment of disasters by declaring the 1990s the International Decade for the Reduction of Natural Disasters (IDNDR).

Analysis of the response of different health care systems to major disasters in the past have demonstrated the need for a more clearly identified planning process to attend to the response to multi-hazard events.[4,5] Many disciplines and allied health care professions have been working in an integrated manner in the field of disaster medicine, and this has evolved into a unique multi-specialty over the past decade. Critical care forms an indispensable part of this science as intensivists not only care for the sickest of the salvageable patients in any hospital but also bring with them their clinical expertise in resuscitation, triage, and transportation of the critically ill outside the ICU. This chapter is written from the perspective of the ICU physician and provides a basic understanding of common disaster scenarios and increases awareness of the role of an intensivist in the medical response to disasters.

BACKGROUND

Major disasters occur regularly and cause widespread human death and suffering. Over the past two decades, more than 3 million lives have been lost worldwide to major disasters. A total of 39,073 people were reported killed by disasters alone in 2001, with the decade's annual average of around 62,000. Even though the numbers of geophysical disasters such as earthquakes and volcanic eruptions have remained fairly constant over the past decade, the past 2 years have seen the highest number of weather-related disasters reported over the decade.[6] As populations grow and occupy spaces that are vulnerable to different hazards, disasters will increase in severity and impact. Recent events since the September 2001 terrorism attacks have brought to attention the effects of manmade disasters on the health care system and the need to anticipate and plan for such low-probability, yet catastrophic events. Even though there is basic similarity in the response to various hazardous events, each type of disaster presents responders with unique demands. After any disaster it is the health care system that is burdened with the responsibility to prevent excessive deaths, mitigate suffering, and deal with the overwhelming inadequacy of resources. Over the past few years, disaster medicine has thus grown into a unique specialty to deal with planning and preparing for such cataclysmic events. It shares a common ideal with public health: "greatest good for the greatest number."[3]

A fundamental part of designing a medical response to disasters is to coordinate health care personnel across the hospital system so that they overcome natural differences associated with each group and maximize the efficient use of scarce resources. Because the sickest of all viable patients will require ICU care, critical care physicians can form an invaluable part in this coordination effort. In addition to their usual role of being the caregiver for patients in the ICU, intensivists will be expected to help in triage decisions, transport critically ill patients, and treat the multitude of injured in a rational order. They can also help in integrating various specialties with their normal prototypical roles and even provide essential medical care at the actual site of disasters through mobile ICU teams. Second only to emergency medical services (EMS) personnel and emergency department (ED) physicians (who constitute the first responders), intensivists and trauma surgeons bring with them the flexibility and the required skills to provide an effective medical response to disasters. It is thus important for critical care physicians to be familiar with the basics of disaster management, acquire organizational and leadership skills, practice delivery of unconventional critical care, and be familiar with different disaster-related medical syndromes.

TERMINOLOGY

It is important for physicians and health care personnel to be familiar with basic nomenclature and terminology in disaster medicine. Clear, common, and concise definitions are important to effective communication and evoking appropriate responses to disaster situations. Uniform use of terminology across health care systems provides a basis for physicians in analysis and construction of an effective disaster plan and response.[7] Controversies surrounding the definition of disasters, hazards, and causalities are discussed.

The word "disaster" connotes a subjective assessment that has various meanings to different people and has an inherent bias, depending on the person using it. For example, a local, state, or federal "disaster declaration" implies commitment of financial and other resources. Similarly, a disaster in one community is not necessarily the same to another. Currently there is no uniformly accepted definition for the word "disaster."[7] De Boer recognizes the lack of a meaningful definition for the word and proposes instead the term *medical severity index* (MSI).[8] This term however has not gained sufficient acceptance for routine use. Different modifiers can lead to different definitions of the term *disaster*. They include the etiologic type of disaster, geographic area involved, timing, type of onset of the event, size of the community affected, baseline resources available to the community, and, finally, the physical, psychosocial, and economic injury caused by the event. However, from a health care standpoint, the most important variable that defines a disaster is its functional impact on the health care facility.[7] Despite various attempts that have been made to clear the confusion surrounding the terminology, the issue remains unresolved.[7,9,10] The following are the commonly used definitions in disaster medicine from a health care perspective:

Hazard: an event with the potential to cause catastrophic damage. It may be "naturally" occurring phenomena such as volcano eruptions or "manmade" such as nuclear power plant accidents.[11]

Emergency: a natural or manmade event that significantly disrupts the environment of care (e.g., damage to an organization's buildings due to severe winds, storms, or earthquakes) resulting in disrupted care and treatment (e.g., loss of utilities such as power, water, or telephones due to floods, civil disturbances, accidents, or emergencies within the organization or in its community); or that results in sudden, significantly changed, or increased demand for the organization's services (e.g., bioterrorist attack, building collapse, plane crash in the organization's community). Some emergencies are called "disasters" or "potential injury creating events" (PICEs).[11]

Disaster: a hazardous event causing physical, psychological, social, economic, or even political effects on a scale such that the stricken community needs extraordinary efforts to cope with it, and often outside help or international aid.[9,10,12] Medical disasters form a subset of this category, in which the physical and/or psychosocial injuries exceed the medical response capabilities of the community affected.

PICE System: a new terminology system developed to overcome the differences in disaster nomenclature. This system uses the functional impact on the health care facility as the only determining factor to define an "emergency" or "disaster" situation. It uses four modifiers to effectively communicate the impact caused by the situation on the health care facility. It is described in more detail later.[7]

Multicasualty Incident: a hazardous event that regardless of its size is containable by the local EMS. From an operational standpoint, an event becomes a multicasualty incident when its impact exceeds the day-to-day response routine to the EMS. Significant adjustments within the local response system are required to cope with this demand, without the need to request outside help (Level 1 response).[13,14]

Mass Casualty Incident: a hazardous event that overwhelms the local response capability. It is likely to impose a sustained demand for health services rather than a short, intense peak typical of many smaller-scale disasters. This may require a Level 2 response (neighboring and regional resources are activated) or a Level 3 response (state, interstate, and federal resources are activated in the rescue and recovery process).[14-16]

Casualty: any person suffering physical and/or psychological damage by outside violence leading to death, injuries, or material losses. Again the word has no standard definition and is sometimes used to imply injury, death, or both. It may also bear financial implications because federal reimbursement may be approved only for persons classified as casualties.[7,9,10]

Hazard Vulnerability Analysis (HVA): the identification of potential emergencies and the direct and indirect effects these emergencies may have on the organization's operations and the demand for its services. This concept is described in further detail later in the section on principles of disaster planning.[17]

CLASSIFICATION OF DISASTERS

Just as there is lack of uniformity with disaster medicine terminology, there is wide variation in the classification of disasters. Classifications of disasters are described in the literature based on various modifiers previously mentioned. For example, cause is a simple and common basis on which to classify disasters as "natural" or "manmade" events. Natural disasters arise from forces of nature and include earthquakes, volcanic eruptions, hurricanes, floods, fire, and tornadoes. Manmade disasters are caused by identifiable human causes and may be further classified as complex emergencies (e.g., wars, terrorist attacks) and technologic disasters (e.g., industrial accidents, explosions from hazardous material).[18] Other classifications include those based on onset (acute vs. insidious disasters), predictability, duration, and frequency. Although these methods provide a conceptual perspective, they bear little relevance to the functional impact on the health care system. From a public health perspective, disasters need to be defined by their effect on people and the health care system. The concept of functional impact to the health care system is thus paramount.[7,18]

To create uniformity to address the wide spectrum of situations, a new paradigm has been suggested called the PICE system.[7] The two major aims of this system are to effectively communicate both the operational consequences to a hospital or community and the type and amount of outside assistance needed. Four modifiers for an event are chosen from a standardized group of prefixes and a stage is assigned (Table 263-1). *Column A* (first prefix) describes

TABLE 263–1. PICE NOMENCLATURE

A	B	C
Static	Controlled	Local
Dynamic	Disruptive	Regional
	Paralytic	National
		International

From Koenig KL, Dinerman N, Kuehl AE: Disaster nomenclature—a functional impact approach: The PICE system. Available at http://www.homelandsecurity.org/journal/articles/displayArticle.asp?article=74

TABLE 263–2. PARALYTIC PICE

Destructive	Nondestructive
Bomb explosion	Snow storm
Earthquake	Employee strike
Tornado	Power failure
Civil unrest	Water supply cutoff
HazMat spill	
Fire	
Building collapse	

From Koenig KL, Dinerman N, Kuehl AE: Disaster nomenclature—a functional impact approach: The PICE system. Available at http://www.homelandsecurity.org/journal/articles/displayArticle.asp?article=74

the potential for additional casualties. For example a finite number of persons injured in an airplane crash is a "static event" whereas an ongoing fire is a "dynamic" event. *Column B* (second prefix) describes whether local resources are sufficient ("controlled") or overwhelmed. If they are overwhelmed, the two modifiers "disruptive" and "paralytic" indicate whether they must be simply augmented or totally reconstituted. Paralytic PICE are the most daunting of all situations, and they can be either destructive or nondestructive (Table 263-2). *Column C* describes the extent of geographic involvement. PICE stage refers to the likelihood that outside medical help is required (Table 263-3). This PICE model provides important concepts for disaster planners, researchers, and responders. Using this system, disasters can be described both prospectively and retrospectively. PICE is a valuable tool for use in planning and disaster mitigation. This system, however, needs validation on a wider scale. It may also require further refinement to delineate the type of aid required by an affected community.[7]

Regardless of the type of classification used to categorize disasters, certain unique features are associated with each type of disaster. It is important to understand the common effects of different natural and manmade disasters to predict their impact and plan effectively. Some common disaster situations are reviewed next.

TABLE 263–3. PICE SYSTEM STAGING WITH EXAMPLES

Stage	Projected Need for Outside Help	Status of Outside Help
0	Little to none	Inactive
I	Small	Alert
II	Moderate	Standby
III	Great	Dispatch

Examples of PICE Staging

1. Multiple-vehicle crash in a big city	Static, controlled, local PICE, stage 0
2. Multiple-vehicle crash in a small town	Static, disruptive, local PICE, stage I
3. Los angeles civil disturbance	Dynamic, disruptive, regional PICE, stage II
4. SARS outbreak in China	Dynamic, disruptive, national PICE, stage III

From Koenig KL, Dinerman N, Kuehl AE: Disaster nomenclature—a functional impact approach: The PICE system. Available at http://www.homelandsecurity.org/journal/articles/displayArticle.asp?article=74

NATURAL DISASTERS

EARTHQUAKES

An earthquake can be defined as the shaking of earth caused by waves moving on and below the earth's surface resulting in surface faulting, tremors, vibration, liquefaction, landslides, aftershocks, and/or tsunamis.[19] The vast majority of earthquakes occur around the Pacific plate. A logarithmic scale measuring the magnitude of reverberations produced by an earthquake, called the Richter scale, determines the size of the earthquake. Because the Richter scale does not measure the damage caused, a subjective scale based on the degree of structural damage caused at particular sites, the Modified Mercalli Intensity Scale, is used.[20] Earthquakes are the most devastating and costly of natural phenomena known to occur. Even in countries with modern seismic building codes, the death toll can be great. The Northbridge earthquake in California caused $20 to $30 billion in damage, whereas the Kobe earthquake in Japan produced twice the amount of damage and over 6000 fatalities.[21,22] In less-developed nations the death toll can be astronomical. The high mortality rate associated with earthquakes is primarily attributable to trauma, asphyxia, dust inhalation (acute respiratory distress), or exposure to the environment (e.g., hypo- or hyperthermia). Eighty-five to 95 percent of persons rescued alive from collapsed buildings are rescued in the first 24 to 48 hours, and survival in entrapment rarely lasts longer than 48 hours.[23] National urban search and rescue (USAR) teams generally take 24 hours to deploy and begin operations, whereas international USAR teams require at least 48 hours.[24] Unfortunately most victims that are not extracted within 24 hours from the debris will die. Thus, evidence for need to mobilize large numbers of medical personnel to an earthquake disaster area is unsubstantiated.

Hospitals are the medical providers of choice after an earthquake. An important part of response to an earthquake disaster is an assessment of both the hospital's structural integrity and the need for evacuation. All hospital personnel must respond and prepare for the influx of patients. In the Northbridge earthquake, eight hospitals were forced to evacuate.[25] The first wave of patients presenting to a hospital in the first half hour are likely to be those with minor cuts, bruises, and simple fractures. The later wave of patients presents with serious multiple fractures, internal injuries, exacerbations of respiratory distress, cardiac syndromes, and crush syndrome. There seems to be an increase in the number of cardiac-related complaints and events after an earthquake. Hospital admission data during the Athens earthquake in 1981 showed a 50% increase in cardiac arrests.[26] In the Northbridge earthquake there was a decrease in the incidence of sudden death 6 days after the event (suggesting that many had presented during the event).[27] Usually, there is less demand for blood and blood donations so local and neighboring resources suffice. Demand for health services is concentrated within the first 24 to 76 hours after the event. Three to 5 days after the event the hospital case mix generally returns to normal.[23]

VOLCANIC ERUPTIONS

A volcano is a hill or a mountain built around a vent that connects with reservoirs of molten rock below the earth's surface.[28] Different types of eruptive events occur, including pyroclastic explosions, hot ash releases, lava flows, gas emissions, and glowing avalanches (gas and ash releases). Lava flows tend not to result in high casualties, because they are easily avoidable. The "composite" type of volcanoes are associated with a more violent eruption from within the chimney. These eruptions are associated with air shock waves, rock projectiles (some with high thermal energy), release of noxious gases, pyroclastic flows, and mud flows (lahars). Pyroclastic flows and lahars are often fast moving and are the main cause of damage and deaths from volcanoes, as evidenced by the small eruption of the Nevada del Ruiz in Columbia that killed more than 23,000 people.[29] The release of ash and its subsequent rapid buildup on building structures can be substantial, causing them to collapse within a matter of hours. Ash is also responsible for the clogging of filters and machinery, causing electrical storms and fires, and interfering with communications. Ash is a main cause for respiratory-related syndromes and conjunctival and corneal injury. A variety of toxic gases (e.g., carbon dioxide, hydrogen sulfide, sulfur dioxide, hydrogen chloride, hydrogen fluoride, and carbon monoxide [CO]) are released during eruptions, causing bronchospasm, pulmonary edema, hypoxemia, cellular asphyxiation, topical irritation of skin and other mucosal surfaces, and death. Damage to health infrastructures and water systems can be severe. Problems related to communication (ashes cause serious interference) and transportation (poor visibility and slippery roads) are likely. Depending on the initial assessment, various needs can be anticipated. Reducing the risk for vulnerable groups of being exposed to ash, raising awareness on the risk associated with ash (health and mechanical risk), and maintaining food security conditions over the long term (lava, ash, and acid rain cause damage to crops and livestock) can help minimize suffering.[19,30,31]

HURRICANES, CYCLONES, AND TYPHOONS

The large rotating weather systems that form seasonally over tropical oceans are variously named, depending on the geographic region where they form.[19] They consist of a calm inner portion called the "eye" surrounded by a wall of rain and high-velocity winds. Based on central pressure, wind speed, storm surge, and potential destruction, their severity is graded on a scale of 1 to 5 (Saffir Simpson scale).[32] They are among the most destructive natural phenomena. Cyclones during 1970 and 1991 in Bangladesh claimed 300,000 and 100,000 lives, respectively, due to flooding.[33] The most devastating hurricane ever to hit the United States was in 1900 at Galveston, Texas. It claimed an estimated 8000 to 12,000 lives.[32] The greatest damage to life and property is not from the wind but from secondary events such as storm surges, flooding, landslides, and tornadoes. Ninety percent of all hurricane-related deaths occur from storm surge–related drowning.[34] The most common injury patterns include lacerations (during the cleanup phase), followed by blunt trauma and puncture wounds. Data from Cyclone Tracey of 1975 showed over 145 cyclone-related hospital admissions, 41% being severe lacerations, 35% blunt trauma injury, and 2% blunt abdominal trauma.[35] Late morbidity can be due to post-disaster cleanup accidents (e.g., electrocution), dehydration, wound infection, and outbreaks of communicable disease.[34]

FLOODS

There are three major types of floods: flash floods (caused by heavy rain and dam failures), coastal floods, and river floods. Together, they are the most common type of disasters and account for at least half of all disaster-related deaths.[19,36] In 1887, the Yangtze flood in China claimed 2 million lives. The primary cause of death is drowning, followed by hypothermia and injury due to floating debris. The impact on the health infrastructures and lifeline systems can be massive and may result in food shortages. Interruption of basic public services (e.g., sanitation, drinking water, electricity) may result in outbreak of communicable diseases.[19] Another concern is the increase in both vector-borne diseases (e.g., malaria, St. Louis encephalitis) and displacement of wildlife (e.g., poisonous snakes).[37,38]

LANDSLIDES

Landslides are more widespread than any other geologic event. They are defined as downslope transport of soil and rock resulting from natural phenomena or manmade actions. Landslides can also occur secondary to heavy storms, volcanic eruptions, and earthquakes. Landslides cause high mortality and few injuries. Trauma and suffocation by entrapment are common. Pending an assessment, needs can be anticipated, such as search and rescue, mass casualty management, and emergency shelter for the homeless.[19]

OTHER NATURAL DISASTERS

Tornadoes occur most commonly in the North American Midwest. Over 4115 deaths and 70,000 injuries have been ascribed to them during the years 1950 to 1994. They cause widespread destruction of community infrastructure. Injuries most commonly seen are complex contaminated soft tissue injury (50%), fractures (30%), head injury (10%), and blunt trauma to the chest and abdomen (10%).[39] Firestorms, wildfires, tsunamis, winter storms, and heat waves are other natural phenomena that are capable of creating mass injuries from thermal burns, airway injury, smoke inhalation, heat-related disorders, and hypothermia.

MANMADE DISASTERS

TRANSPORTATION DISASTERS

Transportation accidents can produce injuries and death similar to those seen in major natural disasters. Some of the largest civilian disasters in North America have been related to transportation of hazardous materials.[40] Motor vehicle accidents, railway accidents, airplane crashes, and shipwrecks are some of the common transportation accidents. They cause a wide range of injuries, including multiple trauma, fractures, burns, chemical injuries, hypothermia, dehydration, asphyxiation, and CO inhalation. The hazard risk to a health care facility increases with its proximity to a chemical plant or highway, and such factors should be considered in the emergency preparedness plan of the hospital.

WEAPONS OF MASS DESTRUCTION

Weapons of mass destruction (WMD) are those nuclear, biologic, chemical, incendiary, or conventional explosive agents that pose a potential threat to health, safety, food supply, property, or the environment. Since the devastating terrorist attacks in September 2001 and subsequent intentional release of anthrax spores in the United States, there is growing concern around the world about the possible threat of chemical, biologic, or nuclear weapons used against a civilian population. Compared with the frequency of natural and technology-related disasters, the incidence of use of WMD to cause death and injury is relatively rare. However, biologic and chemical weapons are relatively accessible and WMD are thought to be available to most foreign states and terrorist groups. In response to a WMD incident, health care personnel will be called on to manage unprecedented numbers of casualties in an environment of panic, fear, and paranoia that accompanies terrorism. Because most attacks occur without warning, the local health care system will be the first and most critical interface for detection, notification, rapid diagnosis, and treatment. The best defense in reducing casualties will therefore rest on the ability of medical and public health personnel to recognize symptoms and to provide rapid clinical and epidemiologic diagnosis of an event. This requires that health care providers be well informed of potential biological, chemical, and nuclear agents. They must have a heightened index of suspicion and be able to identify unusual disease patterns to determine whether WMD are the etiologic agents of illness. Physicians will need to practice appropriate surveillance and reporting and develop knowledge of mass decontamination, use of proper personal protection equipment, and safety protocols related to a biologic, chemical, or radiologic event.[41-43] Salient characteristics and brief management strategies of the different WMD are discussed here. Detailed description of individual biologic and chemical agents, diagnosis, postexposure management, vaccination, infection control measures, and use of personal protection equipment is beyond the scope of this chapter. Numerous peer-reviewed articles have been published on different WMD, and readers are referred to these reports. Some of the available resources on the Internet are included in the Appendix at the end of this chapter.

Biologic Weapons

Biologic weapons are WMD that can be either pathogens (disease-causing organisms, such as viruses or bacteria) or toxins (poisons of biologic origin). History has been witness to numerous examples of the devastating impact of these agents, ranging from apocryphal plagues in the past to the more recent intentional release of anthrax in the United States.[44] Compared with other WMD, biologic weapons are characterized by ease of accessibility and dissemination, difficulty in detection because of their slow onset of action, and their ability to cause widespread panic through the fear of contagion. They can be spread through various means, including aerial bombs, aerosol sprays, explosives, and food or water contamination. Multiple factors including particle size of the agent, stability of the agent, wind speed, wind direction, and atmospheric conditions can alter the effectiveness of a delivery system. Based on the ease of dissemination, ability to cause high mortality, public panic and social disruption, and requirement for special action for public health preparedness, the Centers for Disease Control and Prevention (CDC) has classified biologic weapons into three categories (Table 263-4). Category A agents are of particular concern, because they can cause widespread disease through their ease of transmission, result in high mortality

TABLE 263–4. TRIAGE CLASSIFICATION

Groups	Color	Symbol	Type of injury
Priority I (Emergent)	Red	R	CRITICAL: likely to survive if simple* care given within minutes
Priority II (Catastrophic)	Blue	B	CATASTROPHIC: unlikely to survive and/or extensive or complicated care needed within minutes
Priority III (Urgent)	Yellow	Y	URGENT: likely to survive if simple† care given within hours
Priority IV (Nonurgent)	Green	G	MINOR: likely to survive even if care delayed hours to days
Priority V (None)	Black	X‡	Dead

*Simple: Care that does not require unusual equipment or excessive use of time or personnel.
†Assigned THIRD priority (after YELLOWS) when there are so many casualties that if resources are used in vain to try to save BLUE cases, the YELLOWS will needlessly die.
‡The circling of this symbol prevents its being confused with a sloppily written Y.
From Auf der Heide E: Disaster Response: Principles of Preparation and Coordination, St. Louis, CV Mosby, 1989. Full text online edition available at the CDC website through the following hyperlink: http://216.202.128.19/dr/DisasterResponse.nsf/section/chapters?openview&home=flash

rates, cause panic and social disruption, and need special attention during public health preparedness.[42-44] General features that should alert health care providers to the possibility of a bioterrorism-related outbreak include the following[44,45]:

1. A rapidly increasing disease incidence (e.g., within hours or days) in a normally healthy population
2. An epidemic curve that rises and falls during a short period of time
3. An unusual increase in the number of people seeking care, especially with fever, or respiratory or gastrointestinal complaints
4. An endemic disease rapidly emerging at an uncharacteristic time or in an unusual pattern
5. Lower attack rates among people who had been indoors, especially in areas with filtered air or closed ventilation systems, compared with people who had been outdoors
6. Clusters of patients arriving from a single locale and large numbers of rapidly fatal cases
7. Any patient presenting with a disease that is relatively uncommon and has bioterrorism potential (e.g., pulmonary anthrax, tularemia, plague)

The main steps involved in management of a bioterrorist attack are containment, notification, confirmation, and directed antibiotic treatment and prophylaxis. In the event of a suspected bioterrorist attack, the CDC has issued protocols for early notification of local and state public health department agencies.[46] The Association for Professionals in Infection Control and Epidemiology in cooperation with the CDC devised the "Bioterrorism Readiness Plan," with a template for health care facilities to serve as a reference document to facilitate preparation of bioterrorism readiness plans for health care facilities. This tool guides infection-control professionals and health care epidemiologists in the development of practical and realistic response plans for their institutions in the event of a bioterrorism attack.[45] Discussion of individual biologic agents is beyond the scope of this chapter. The reader is referred to our review of bioterrorism and critical care[47] as well as the numerous resources and websites available on the internet (see the Appendix).

Chemical Weapons

Chemical incidents can be defined as accidental or intentional events that threaten to expose or do expose responders and members of the public to a chemical hazard. Agents that have been commonly used as chemical weapons are also used in industrial processes. Most industrial incidents occur at an interface between transport, storage, processing, use, or disposal of hazardous chemicals, where these systems are more vulnerable to failure, error, or manipulation. The catastrophic effect of these agents has been utilized several times in the past for military purposes; and with the proliferation of these weapons, civilian populations are now faced with a significant threat.[48,49] Typically, chemical warfare agents are classified into the following categories.[42,50]

Nerve agents (e.g., tabun, sarin, VX, soman) are organophosphates that inhibit the enzyme anticholinesterase, resulting in overstimulation of both muscarinic and nicotinic receptors. Muscarinic symptoms include lacrimation, bronchorrhea, bronchospasm, miosis, salivation, rhinorrhea, vomiting, and diarrhea. Nicotinic receptor stimulation produces muscle fasciculations, flaccid paralysis, tachycardia, and hypertension. These agents are also capable of producing central nervous system effects (i.e., seizures, coma). Death from these agents is usually from respiratory failure. These agents are extremely toxic and have a rapid effect. Sarin presents as a vapor threat, and the onset of symptoms is within seconds, with a peak effect in 5 minutes. Exposed victims who are asymptomatic after 1 hour are unlikely to be contaminated. VX represents a liquid exposure, with as little as a drop being lethal. The onset to action and death is less than 30 minutes. The cardinal rule in decontaminating patients is to remove and dispose of all articles of clothing. Therapy is directed toward the predominating symptoms. Atropine is used for the relief of muscarinic symptoms, pralidoxime chloride (2-PAM) is used for nicotinic effects, and benzodiazepines are used for the central nervous system manifestations. Most of the care is supportive and includes mechanical ventilation for respiratory failure and treatment of arrhythmias.

Blister agents (e.g., mustard gas, lewisite) cause wounds on the skin and mucosal surfaces. They are capable of causing second-degree burns of the skin within 4 to 8 hours. Airway injury and edema can be severe and are dose dependent. Of concern to the ICU physician is the need for correcting fluid losses and maintaining the airway.

Choking agents (e.g., chlorine gas, phosgene gas) mainly affect the respiratory system, inducing inflammation of the airway and the lung and leading to acute respiratory distress syndrome (ARDS) and death. Treatment is mainly supportive.

Cyanides bind to cytochromes within the mitochondria and inhibit cellular oxygen use. In smaller doses they cause tachypnea, headache, dizziness, anxiety, and vomiting. However, with higher doses, seizures, respiratory arrest, and cardiac arrest occur. They are highly toxic and in sufficient concentrations can cause death within 5 minutes of inhalation. They are most commonly inhaled but also can be absorbed through the skin. Care for the patient is primarily supportive with supplemental oxygen. Specific therapy is with amyl nitrates, sodium nitrite, and sodium thiosulfate.

In general, unlike biologic weapons, disease secondary to release of chemical agents is likely to be more obvious, rapid in onset, and homogeneous. These agents, however, pose serious problems for emergency care providers because of their potential to cause a large number of casualties rapidly and their potential for secondary contamination. Any emergency medical or public health response to a major incident involving a chemical warfare agent will require coordination among local, state, and federal organizations. First responders should be aware of access to specialized local and federal response teams, basic triage, and demarcation of the contaminated area, use of hand-held devices for agent detection and identification, use of personal protective equipment, and knowledge of appropriate medical treatment and antidotes.[48]

Nuclear Weapons and Radiation Accidents

A variety of terrorist applications of radiation exist that could produce varying degrees of damage to public infrastructure and operations, human casualties and illnesses, and, most importantly, fear.

Radiation devices include radionuclides from the health care industries (e.g., brachytherapy, radiation oncology sources). The consequences of the exposure are dose and source dependent. Although not linked to a terrorist event the accidental dispersion of a hospital therapy source in Goiania, Brazil, resulted in the death of 4 of the 249 exposed persons.[51,52]

Radionuclide dispersal devices are also known as "dirty bombs." These have limited nuclear yield but can contaminate a wide area.

Improvised nuclear devices are made of uranium or plutonium constructed by a nongovernmental source and limited by the critical mass of nuclear material. They yield less destructive power than a conventional nuclear warhead but are still capable of contamination effects.

Tactical and strategic nuclear weapons are those that are created by governments and vary in yields from 0.5 kiloton to greater than 1 megaton. Their destructive capacities are enormous, and they contaminate a vast perimeter of space depending on the yield.

Approximately 50% of the energy released from a nuclear bomb is due to the blast and shock waves, giving a majority of the survivors blast-related injuries as well as creating extensive infrastructure damage. About 35% of the energy released is thermal radiation (in orders of tens of millions of degrees), giving rise to high-degree skin burns. Depending on the size of the device and the altitude of detonatation, an electromagnetic pulse is generated with the explosion. This is capable of disrupting all electrical equipment within 20 to

several hundreds of kilometers.[51] The radiation-related energy released from a nuclear detonation is approximately 15% (5% from the initial nuclear radiation and 10% from the residual nuclear radiation), giving rise to external contamination, systemic irradiation, and internal contamination-related illness. Immediate ionizing radiation consists of gamma, beta, neutron, and a small amount of alpha radiation. Residual radiation occurs in the forms of induced radiation and fallout. Induced radiation occurs because of neutron-induced gamma activity of the immediate soil, silicon, manganese, aluminum, zinc, copper, and sodium. The half-lives of the various substances are a few minutes to 15 hours. "Fallout" is the fusion of the various radionuclides generated in the fission reaction with condensation producing a snowflake-like debris that falls to earth. Fallout is a potential form of delayed radiation exposure and can cause internal contamination.[51]

Surviving hospitals and staff near an impact area should serve as a triage center and transport victims to other, unaffected, centers through the notification of the National Disaster Medical System Hospital Activation System. Other agencies that need to be notified include the Federal Bureau of Investigation, Nuclear Regulatory Commission, Department of Energy, and the Department of Defense. Large-scale decontamination should be managed outside the hospital area as far as is possible, but plans for indoor decontamination should also be in place. A radiation emergency area (both in and out of the hospital) would need to be designated with checkpoints nearing the cold zone. Management plans for the safe disposal of human waste and bodies should be in place so as not to increase the exposure risk. Triage of patients should be done on the basis of doing the greatest good for the greatest number. Based on predictive models, isolated irradiation, burns, and blast-related injuries would constitute 40% of injuries. Combined injuries would account for the rest. Attending to trauma victims should take precedence over all other medical issues, because a given patient is not likely to succumb immediately from radiation injury.

Patient care should begin with the use of universal precautions and the use of personal protective equipment. Specific recommendations for decontamination, management of radiation accident area, and hospital preparedness are available at the Radiation Emergency Assistance Center Training Site in Oak Ridge, Tennessee (865-576-3131).[53] Dosimetry readings of the area may help during triage, defining those with systemic irradiation injury (possibly received greater than 450 rad exposure). In determining patient viability, three parameters are of the most use; time of onset of vomiting, the decrease in the absolute lymphocyte count over a 24-hour period, and presence of conventional trauma burns. These parameters were used during the Chernobyl reactor accident in 1986. Victims who are not viable or who have lethal doses of radiation exposure are likely to benefit from supportive/palliative care. Radionuclide-dispersal devices are not associated with the blast injuries or other related trauma from the nuclear bomb. However, they are still capable of externally irradiating and internally contaminating individuals, leading to radiation-induced illnesses. These situations may actually go unnoticed for long periods of time, and identifying the radiation source may be elusive. Identifying such patients, decontaminating them, and treating various complications such as sepsis are likely to involve the ICU physician.

Usually, the prodromal phase would have been completed, and victims are likely to present in the manifest and recovery phases of acute radiation syndrome.[51,54]

Hazardous Materials (HazMat) Disasters

A HazMat is a substance potentially toxic to the environment or living organisms. They are not limited to chemicals but can include various biologic and radiologic materials as well. Disasters from HazMat are relatively rare, but incidents themselves are among the most common in the community. Knowledge of the types of industries that are present in the community would be helpful in developing a potential plan to deal with likely HazMat situations. Management of a HazMat situation requires attention to several key points: identification of the offending agent, appropriate personal protection equipment of responders, prompt containment of the agent, demarcating areas for decontamination (including removal and disposal of clothes and waste from the decontamination), and resuscitation of victims. Injuries secondary to release of hazardous materials can present as chemical burns, inhalational injury, as well as a variety of systemic injuries.[55,56]

Armed Conflict

This continues to be the most preventable and most destructive of manmade disasters in terms of human physical and emotional suffering, economic loss, and environmental destruction. Specific health care issues during these conflicts that are relevant to the intensivist include trauma from blast injuries, projectiles, and crush-related injuries; communicable diseases due to the breakdown of public infrastructure and mass displacement of populations; and burns and radiation-related injury.

MEDICAL DISASTER SYNDROMES

Disaster situations present with many unique medical syndromes that require specific therapy. Treatment of these entities is often difficult owing to a large volume of patients, lack of qualified medical personnel on site, and inadequate supplies and equipment. It is important to emphasize that initial recognition of the medical syndromes, and appropriate intervention are critical to minimizing morbidity and mortality. Appropriate triage, knowledge of field management of each syndrome, flexibility to adapt to each situation, ability to ignore natural differences among different specialties, and recognition of limits of medical care that can be provided in overwhelming situations are key to a good disaster medical response. In the following paragraphs, we discuss commonly encountered medical syndromes in a disaster situation.

BLAST INJURIES

Bombs contain an array of compounds such as nitroglycerin, trinitrotoluene, and others that are encased in a metal or plastic case. Decomposition of the solid or liquid compound into gas leads to massive dissipation of energy and pressure creating a blast wave (shock wave). This destructive effect can be increased by the presence of nuts, nails, and bolts in the casing. Water transmits blast waves more efficiently than air, with the greatest impact being on structures that are the deepest.[35,36] There are four types of blast injuries:

1. *Primary blast injury* is caused solely by the blast wave and almost always affects air-filled structures such as the lung, ear, and gastrointestinal tract. The presence of tympanic membrane rupture may indicate exposure to a high-pressure wave and is thought to correlate with more severe organ injury.
2. *Secondary blast injury* is caused by the rapid acceleration of small fragments caused by the blast injury.
3. *Tertiary blast injury* is a feature of high-energy explosions. They result from the collision of the flying victim against a hard surface.
4. *Miscellaneous blast-related injuries* encompass all other injuries caused by explosions. They include flash burns, inhalation injuries, and blunt trauma.[58-60]

The most common injuries associated with fatality in blast incidents include subarachnoid hemorrhage (66%), fracture of the skull (51%), lung contusion (47%), tympanic membrane rupture (45%), and liver laceration (34%). Unfortunately, the extent of the blast injury cannot be assessed during the course of rapid triage examinations. In the absence of overt trauma, a focused physical examination should include examination for ruptured tympanic membrane, hypopharyngeal contusions, hemoptysis, and auscultation for wheezing. The presence of a ruptured tympanic membrane is almost always an indicator that the patient has been exposed to a blast wave powerful enough to cause serious damage.[59] The thorax is frequently involved in a blast injury, manifesting with wheezing, hemoptysis, pneumothorax, hemothorax, and air embolism. Patients may have myocardial contusion as well. The presentation of serious pulmonary injury may be delayed. Pulmonary barotrauma is the most common fatal primary blast injury. Patients with nonpenetrating lung injury will likely have hypoxia requiring support ranging from oxygen therapy to mechanical ventilation. This may result from pulmonary contusion, systemic air embolism, and disseminated intravascular coagulation. Acute gas embolism, a form of pulmonary barotrauma, is also associated with blast injuries. Air emboli most commonly occlude blood vessels in the brain or spinal cord, resulting in neurologic symptoms that must be differentiated from the direct effect of trauma. Patients thought to have gas embolism require decompression treatment. Administration of 100% oxygen by tight-fitting facemask and left lateral recumbent position may help. Definitive treatment is with the use of hyperbaric oxygen.[59,61] Patients with blast injury of the lung are likely to present with abdominal injuries that are usually more delayed. These include delayed bowel perforation and liver lacerations. The former may warrant exploratory laparotomy.

Blast victims receiving general anesthesia have an increased mortality rate; other forms of local and spinal anesthesia are preferred, and general anesthesia should be deferred, if possible, for 24 to 48 hours. Intensivists should be aware of the increased need for resuscitation equipment, ventilators, and movement in and out of the operating room during such situations. The analysis of 12 urban bombing attacks in Israel revealed that the major bottleneck in the flow of critically injured patients was the unavailability, not of operating rooms, but of shock resuscitation rooms and computed tomographic scanners.[62] Thus, disaster plans should make arrangements to delay imaging for all noncritical patients.

All patients with significant burns, suspected air embolism, radiation or white phosphorus contamination, abdominal signs of contusion/hematoma, or clinical evidence of pulmonary contusion or pneumothorax should be admitted to the hospital. Patients with tympanic membrane rupture and suspected pneumothorax should get some form of chest imaging, and a significant observation period may be warranted. Other investigations must be judiciously ordered, keeping in mind the limited availability of resources in a mass-casualty incident. Screening urinalysis for presence of hematuria, tests for CO poisoning (explosion in a closed space or associated with fire) and cyanide toxicity (due to combustion of plastics), and assessment of acid-base status may be indicated. Use of abdominal computed tomography to rule out intestinal hematomas is not routinely warranted and should be dictated by clinical signs and symptoms. Pregnant patients with blast injuries warrant special consideration, and appropriate consultation is necessary to rule out blast injury to the fetus.[58,59] Supplemental oxygen therapy, maintaining spontaneous respiration, and low positive end-expiratory pressure (PEEP) (if mechanical ventilation is required) are some of the guiding principles in managing pulmonary blast injuries. Routine corticosteroids and antibiotics are not warranted.[58,59] Exposure to white phosphorus explosives (e.g., in hand grenades) deserves special mention. Use of a Wood's light in a darkened resuscitation suite or operating room may help identify white phosphorus light particles in the wound. White phosphorus injury can cause lung injury through irritation and severe hypokalemia and hyperphosphatemia with cardiac arrhythmias and death. External burns should be lavaged with 1% copper sulfate solution. This forms a blue-black cupric phosphide coating and prevents combustion so that the particles can safely be removed.[60]

CRUSH INJURY SYNDROME

Crush injury syndrome refers to systemic manifestations of extensive muscle damage caused by entrapment of victims under collapsed buildings or debris. Reported incidence depends on the type of disaster, ranging from 2% to 40%. Metabolic alterations from the release of muscle constituents into the circulation include myoglobinemia leading to acute renal failure, hyperkalemia, hyperphosphatemia, and disseminated intravascular coagulation. Increased intracellular calcium concentrations appear to be the final common pathway.[58] Muscle damage that occurs is due not only to direct crush injury but also to vascular injury and insufficiency leading to altered compartment pressures and reperfusion injury. Inelastic fascial sheaths encase skeletal muscles in the forearm and lower leg and are particularly vulnerable to dramatic increases in compartment pressures, resulting in compartment syndrome. An intracompartmental pressure in excess of 40 mm Hg lasting longer than 8 hours defines this syndrome. Pressures as high as 240 mm Hg can be seen with crush injuries.[63,64] Compartment syndromes are seen with limb fractures, use of military antishock trousers, pneumatic splints, vascular injuries, and crush injuries. The affected limb may present with severe pain associated with passive stretch or extension, flaccid paralysis, and sensory loss. Capillary refill and peripheral pulses are usually present unless the compartmental pressure equals the diastolic pressure. Diagnosis requires a high degree of clinical suspicion and entails prompt bedside measurement of compartment pressures. A simple and easy method that can be performed in hospital or at field hospital is using an 18-gauge needle attached to a mercury manometer. In an ICU, pressure transducers used to measure central venous pressures can be attached to the 18-gauge needle to obtain the same information.

Compartment syndrome is a surgical emergency and requires urgent fasciotomy. The affected limb is maintained at a level no higher than that of the heart. Fasciotomy on the upper limb is curvilinear on the volar aspect and commences distal to the elbow flexor crease and extends toward the mid-palm. On the thigh, incisions are made on the medial and lateral surfaces and obliquely over the buttocks. The pressures are checked after decompression, and Steri-strips are applied over the incision area.[58] Three to 4 hours after limb tamponade is relieved, hemodynamic instability may occur in an otherwise deceptively stable-looking patient. Release of myoglobin and ensuing reperfusion injury ultimately lead to florid renal failure with severe intravascular hypovolemia. Resulting metabolic acidosis, hyperkalemia, hyperphosphatemia, and hypocalcemia can lead to cardiac arrhythmias and death. Testing of urine with benzidine shows red coloration indicating the presence of myoglobin, and serum shows elevated creatine kinase levels.

Resuscitation of patients with crush injury (any victim crushed or immobilized for more than 4 hours) should begin in the field. After adequate intravenous access is achieved, isotonic fluid replacement with normal saline (rate of 1 to 1.5 L/h) should begin even before the extrication of the crushed limb. If fluid therapy is delayed, the incidence of renal failure increases to 50%; delays of 12 hours are associated with a 100% incidence. Occurrence of renal failure is associated with a 20% to 40% mortality rate. Urinary alkalinization with sodium bicarbonate and mannitol or acetazolamide administration are used to maintain the urine pH greater than 7.5.[65,66] Although this intervention is widely used, there are no prospective randomized controlled trials to support it. Dialysis may be indicated if aggressive fluid resuscitation fails and this may create a huge demand for dialysis machines in disaster situations. Peritoneal dialysis if the abdomen is intact and continuous arteriovenous hemofiltration may be other useful options. The latter option, however, is complicated by hemorrhagic problems related to the use of heparin and immobilization. Life-threatening infections are common after crush injuries and may be increased in the presence of a fasciotomy. In unsalvageable limbs it may be advisable to perform on-field amputations to avoid the systemic effects of a crush injury syndrome.[58] For this purpose ketamine is the anesthetic and analgesic of choice because of its safety profile in the field.[67] Meticulous medical, surgical, and nursing care to the affected extremities is required to obtain good functional recovery.

PARTICULATE HEALTH PROBLEMS

Many disasters result in release of copious particulate matter, causing a wide spectrum of respiratory illnesses, including cough, wheezing, smoke inhalation injury, reactive airways disease, and ARDS. Volcanic eruptions with associated pyroclastic flows and ash fall are some of the most devastating producers of particulate matter. Mortality in these situations arises from suffocation by ash in the upper airways, ARDS, and inhalation burns.[68] The massive building collapse and fires associated with the 2001 World Trade Center terrorist attack caused significant pulmonary complaints among rescue personnel.[69]

Smoke inhalation injury resulting from exposure to noxious products of combustion in fires may account for as many as 75% of fire-related deaths in the United States. The United States has one of the highest fire fatality rates in the developed world, accounting for 2.3 deaths per 100,000 population.[70] The three primary mechanisms that lead to injury in smoke inhalation are thermal damage, asphyxiation, and pulmonary irritation. Combustion utilizes oxygen in the airways and causes a decrease in fraction of inspired oxygen, leading to hypoxemia. Increased CO levels decrease the oxygen-carrying capacity of the blood and cause myocardial depression. Combustion of plastics, polyurethane, wool, silk, nylon, rubber, and paper products can lead to the production of cyanide gas, and this results in anaerobic metabolism and decreased oxygen consumption. Rarely, we may also find methemoglobinemia, which reduces oxygen-carrying capacity.[70] Factors predicting survival in fire fatalities include age (older than 64 years or younger than 5 years) and presence of a physical or cognitive disability.[71] Mortality rate with smoke inhalation alone is about 10% but increases to about 77% in the presence of major burns or respiratory failure. Early deaths are mostly caused by airway compromise or metabolic poisoning.[72,73] Laboratory workup should include co-oximetry; CO, methemoglobin, and cyanide levels (if there is discordance in measured saturation and pulse oximetry readings); blood lactate levels (a level greater than 10 mmol/L that is refractory to restoration of adequate ventilation, oxygenation, and perfusion is considered a surrogate marker of cyanide toxicity) on blood gases; and a calculated alveolar-arterial pressure gradient. Initial blood gas measurements and chest radiograph may be normal. Carboxyhemoglobin level obtained in the emergency department does not correlate with tissue hypoxia or long-term neurologic sequelae, and, ideally, a carboxyhemoglobin level at the scene would be most valuable.[45,49]

Serial bronchoscopy is indicated in the first 18 to 24 hours to assess airway edema and sloughing. Early bronchoscopy can be of diagnostic and therapeutic value, particularly when lobar atelectasis is present. High-flow humidified oxygen is critical to reverse or prevent hypoxemia. About 50% of patients with an inhalation injury require endotracheal intubation, and this number increases in patients who have burn injuries. The need for tracheal intubation is determined by the need to maintain airway patency and pulmonary toilet and to provide positive-pressure ventilation. Positive-pressure ventilation with PEEP increases short-term survival and is associated with decreased tracheobronchial cast formation. Cyanide toxicity (levels > 0.1 mg/L) should be promptly treated using a USA cyanide kit. Recommendations for the use of hyperbaric oxygen in the setting of CO poisoning include CO levels greater than 25% to 30%, neurologic compromise, metabolic acidosis, or electrocardiographic evidence of myocardial ischemia, infarction, or dysrhythmias. Hyperbaric oxygen has been used in cyanide toxicity but has not been proven effective. The role of corticosteroids is controversial and they can be detrimental if given in the presence of cutaneous burns. Empirically administered antibiotics are another issue in dispute. Common pitfalls in the initial management of smoke inhalation are using initial PaO_2 to predict adequacy of oxygenation, placing small-diameter nasotracheal tubes, intubating without applying PEEP, and restricting fluids for concomitant inhalation and burn injury.[70,74]

General measures that could be employed in a field setting include simple airway protection by clearing any particulate matter in the airway, supplemental oxygen, and nebulizer treatment if available. Patients with pre-existing asthma and emphysema should be observed for exacerbations. Critical care specialists should also be familiar with the latest techniques in obtaining a difficult airway in the field.[75]

ACUTE RADIATION SYNDROME

Ionizing radiation can be either charged or uncharged particles (photons). Beta particles are capable of penetrating a few centimeters of tissue. Gamma rays and x-rays are capable of penetrating through tissue and concrete. Gamma, x-ray, and beta radiations are considered low linear energy transfer radiation. Alpha particles have no penetrating power past the keratinized layer of skin but they take on clinical significance if they are internalized by ingestion or inhalation. Neutron emission (e.g., from nuclear reactors, nuclear devices, and industrial moisture detectors) is highly potent radiation that penetrates deep and creates denser ionization trails. Alpha and neutron emissions are considered high linear energy transfer radiation and have significantly more biologic effects than low linear energy transfer radiation by a factor of up to 20.[76,77] When the process of ionization occurs within living tissue it causes breakage in the chemical bonds and the most susceptible target is the cellular DNA. This leads to impaired mitosis and subsequent organ failure. Large doses of radiation are generally considered to cause more biologic destruction than fractionated doses. Systemic radiation illness and lethality from it can result from as little as 450 rad. Precise measurements of the amount of radiation following a nuclear accident will be delayed. Hospital gamma cameras are an invaluable resource for helping determine the exposure in an individual. Higher systemic doses are suggested by shorter onset of prodromal symptoms such as nausea, vomiting, and diarrhea. Serial absolute lymphocyte counts will screen those patients who have psychogenic vomiting.

Acute radiation syndrome has four distinct phases[42,58,76]:

1. *Prodromal phase,* characterized by nausea, vomiting, and diarrhea. Other symptoms of eye burning, abdominal pain, and fever can also occur with higher doses. This phase may last from 0 to 2 days, depending on the dose received.
2. *Latent phase,* in which the patient will have a period of relative well-being due to subsidence of the inflammation. However, ultimately the damaged cells will not be able to repair or regenerate. This may last for 2 to 3 weeks.
3. *Manifest phase,* in which the cellular deficits of various organs affected will become apparent. Mature cells of the skin slough off, revealing an atrophic dermis. Endothelial cells are not replaced, leading to vascular permeability. Mucosal linings slough, causing mucositis and diarrhea. Hematopoietic progenitor cells fail to produce cell lines, leading to anemia, thrombocytopenia, and neutropenia. Fibrosis of the various organ beds develops. This may last for up to 3 weeks.
4. *Recovery phase/death,* in which some stem cells may proliferate and lead to a slow recovery or there will be symptoms of progressive organ failure leading to death.

For radiation syndrome to occur, radiation must be of the penetrating type in a sufficiently large dose (> 0.7 Gy), must be external, and must occur within a short time period.

The disease complex has three syndromes: bone marrow, gastrointestinal, and cardiovascular/central nervous system. Serial absolute lymphocyte counts should be measured immediately on suspicion of exposure (every 3 hours), because lymphocytes are among the most radiosensitive cells and reach nadir within 2 days; platelets reach nadir in 15 to 30 days; and neutrophils at about 30 days. Patients are immunocompromised and susceptible to a wide variety of infections, that of most concern to the intensivist being septic shock.[76] Gastrointestinal syndrome leads to mucosal sloughing, decreased nutrient absorption, and translocation of bacteria and endotoxin. Veno-occlusive disease may also develop if the dose is large enough. Cardiovascular and central nervous system disease develop with doses greater than 5000 rad, and death can occur in as little as 3 days from myocarditis, capillary leak, pulmonary edema, and brain edema. Pneumonitis and subsequent fibrosis can lead to respiratory failure and the need for ventilator support.[77] Treatment of ARS is mainly supportive. If internal contamination is thought to have occurred, then enhancement of excretion and specific antidote therapy are warranted. For inhalational contamination, bronchoalveolar lavage may be warranted; and for ingestion, gastric lavage and purgative management are warranted. Plutonium and transuranic elements can be treated with chelating agents such as calcium or zinc diethylenetriamine pentaacetic acid. Radiocesium can be treated with Prussian blue, which helps in enhancing excretion in feces. Radioiodine exposure can be treated with potassium iodide. Uranium excretion can be enhanced by the alkalinization of urine and with potassium supplementation.[76,77]

PSYCHOLOGICAL TRAUMA

The psychological component in a traumatic event is often overlooked, with the major focus usually being on physical health issues. Studies evaluating the emotional impact from disasters indicate that a majority of victims, first responders, and mortuary volunteers will suffer some form of psychological trauma. Intensivists should be aware that behavioral changes may not be only due to the catastrophic insult but also due to organic causes such as head injury, inability to take pre-disaster psychiatric medications, and toxin or chemical exposure. Groups at risk, such as children, adolescents, and victims who have been exposed to traumatic stressors of bereavement, witnessing death, and situations evoking guilt, fear, or anger, should receive prompt psychiatric and post-traumatic counseling. Interventions such as debriefing, eye movement desensitization and reprocessing, and critical incident stress management may help minimize emotional suffering and morbidity.[78]

OTHER SYNDROMES

Burns, blunt trauma, intra-abdominal injury, head injuries, penetrating trauma, and hypothermia are some of the other disaster syndromes encountered in the field. Specific discussion of these entities is beyond the scope of this chapter, and the reader is referred to other chapters for management details.

DISASTER PREPAREDNESS

For intensivists to be able to deal with a disaster, it is paramount that they be a part of the disaster-planning effort.

Disaster planning includes development of action programs to minimize loss of life and damage during a disaster, provide the greatest good for the greatest number of people, train health care personnel and civilians, coordinate response efforts, maintain adequate supplies of equipment and personnel, and rehabilitate the community after the disaster. Knowledge of potential disasters to which the community is prone should be an integral part of the planning process. Having an understanding of what the resources and capabilities are of the community, hospital, and its ICU on a continual basis and provision for modular expandability are vital for any successful emergency response. The mere existence of a disaster plan does not ensure that the hospital system is actually prepared.[79] The following paragraphs elucidate some of the common issues and misconceptions related to disasters and common principles useful in designing a disaster plan. Subsequently a pragmatic view is presented of the role of the ICU physician in a disaster situation.

COMMON ISSUES AND MISCONCEPTIONS IN DISASTER PLANNING

Most disasters in the United States, fortunately, are not of extraordinary magnitude.[16] Until the more recent terrorist events of September 2001, statistics over the past century reveal only six civilian, peacetime disasters with fatality rates exceeding 1000.[3] Furthermore, some of the largest civilian disasters in North America thus far have been related to hazardous materials accidents.[80] Even though these numbers may not reflect the new threat of domestic terrorism, these statistics do point out that disaster planning does not always require massive mobilization of resources and personnel.

Typically, the hospital nearest to the disaster site will receive the bulk of the casualties. It is thus important to conduct a careful survey of a disaster plan's jurisdiction to identify potential sites (i.e., industries, nuclear reactors, highways) and likely types of hazardous events that could occur in the area. Hospitals in the nearby area receive few disaster victims, and an average have at least 20% of their beds vacant.[40] Disaster plans would thus need to include transfer agreements between hospitals and nearby ICUs to meet bed shortages by activating the National Disaster Medical System Hospital Activation System.[40,79,81]

Very few casualties actually require hospital admission. A study of 29 mass-casualty incidents found that less than 10% of casualties required overnight admission under usual criteria (even though more were admitted because they were involved in the disaster rather than because of severity of their condition).[82] Large numbers of casualties with minor conditions will appear at the nearest hospitals, often on foot or in private vehicles, police cars, buses, taxis, and other non-ambulance forms of transport. Field triage stations are often bypassed, and this in turn causes enormous strain on the emergency department services.[40]

Most of the logistical problems faced in disaster situations are not caused by shortages of medical resources but rather from failure to coordinate their distribution.[79] Convergent volunteerism and altruism can compound the chaos of a disaster scenario. Inexperienced volunteers may not be familiar with the triage system or principles of personal safety, and massive numbers of volunteers can present serious administrative challenges. This results in disorganization and inefficiency.[56] Technical hazard sheets designed by the World Health Organization for most disasters also suggest that medical personnel, blood donors, and blood products should not be sent empirically to a disaster site.[19]

Lack of communication and breakdown of information technology systems during disasters in the past are well documented. Communication is essential not only for notification and mobilization of health care personnel but also for effective overall functioning of the incident command center. Failure to communicate between hospitals in a disaster-affected area can occur, and this in turn leads to overburdening of some hospitals, while the rest remain relatively vacant. In this age of mass media and the Internet, there is also a huge demand for the most up-to-date information. It is therefore crucial that planned and structured communication to the outside world occurs to minimize speculation and dissemination of conflicting messages to the community. Breakdown of major utilities such as power and water supply can cascade to interruption of laboratory, radiology, and other ancillary systems, and back-up plans should be in place to ensure uninterrupted functioning.[16,79,84]

Having a written disaster plan does not necessarily ensure preparedness. The mere existence of a plan can create an illusion of preparedness. Disasters demand multi-organizational, multidisciplinary, and inter-jurisdictional responses, and an effective response can occur in the real world only if there are adequate drills and training.[79] There is also apathy toward planning and preparedness, which stems from the fact that disasters are overall "low-probability events." In times of economic constraints, disaster preparedness competes with priorities of daily living, but failure to prepare may come at a very high cost.[3,81]

PRINCIPLES IN DISASTER PLANNING

Disaster planning for a health care facility is a complex process that can be both expensive and time consuming. This together with a passive attitude toward preparedness makes the entire process highly vulnerable to failure. To design a plan that is simple and cost-effective, it is essential for health care personnel, including intensivists, to have clear and realistic goals that suit individual facility needs and have the flexibility to meet unexpected challenges. Common principles for designing a disaster plan are discussed below. Readers are also referred to various publications and agencies that provide a more comprehensive basis for development and implementation of a disaster plan.[3,11,16,41-43,45,57,81]

Existing Preparedness Requirements
In developing disaster plans, hospitals must take into account the broad national and local requirements imposed by various governmental agencies. Common agencies that are involved in this process include the Centers for Medicare and Medicaid Services (CMS; formerly called the HCFA) and the Joint Commission on Accreditation of Healthcare Organizations (JCAHO). The CMS's conditions for emergency preparedness and services establish minimum requirements for hospitals that participate in Medicare or Medicaid programs. Similarly, JCAHO standards apply to a full range of hospitals from small rural to large urban academic centers and are focused on four main areas: (1) emergency preparedness management plan (Standard EC 4.1); (2) security management plan (Standard EC 2.1); (3) hazardous materials and waste management plan (Standard EC 3.1); and (4) emergency preparedness drills (Standard EC

4.2). Readers are referred to the JCAHO website for the most up-to-date standards for management of environment of care.[11,16]

Hazard Vulnerability Analysis
This is the first step of any disaster plan, with the main aim of identifying potential hazardous events and situations that can occur in or around the health care facility. This process of evaluating and predicting hazard risk is restricted not to geographic events but also to institution-specific variables such as utility failures, local threats of gang-related activity, and presence of a local high-risk industry such as a chemical or nuclear power plant. JCAHO requires a formal, documented hazard vulnerability analysis that is integrated with the emergency management plan, setting priorities among potential emergencies and also defining the hospital's role in the local community-wide emergency plan. The American Society of Healthcare Engineering provides a hazard vulnerability analysis tool that uses three factors to predict the risk: probability of occurrence, risk, and preparedness status with quantitative score. This tool can be modified to each facility's needs and is available on the Internet at www.ashe.org.[11,17]

Incident Command System
The Incident Command System (ICS) is a management system designed to provide the basic architecture of an emergency management response. Major barriers to medical response arise from the lack of coordination among various public and health care agencies and from the lack of operational integration of various medical specialties. The ICS incorporates all these agencies and ensures a cooperative and effective response to a crisis. The concept of ICS resulted from the analysis of the devastating wildfires in Southern California in 1970 and has since been modified and successfully adapted to different disaster situations related to health care facilities.[84-86] The ICS specifies a common terminology and a command structure with five functional sections:

1. *Command:* Unified command staff responsible for overall management of the incident
2. *Operations:* Performs the actual response work under the directives of the command center
3. *Planning:* Gathers relevant information and develops response strategies as the situation progresses
4. *Logistics:* Responsible for facility-wide supplies, equipment, personnel, and services. It also provides for basic services to personnel of the command center.
5. *Finance:* Authorizes expenditures, maintains records, and provides documentation of the incident

There is a designated person who will have the authority to declare an emergency. All personnel involved in the command system should be aware of the exact predetermined location of the command center. The plan should also provide protocols that will guide notification and the sequence of mobilization of these personnel in a disaster situation. The command system must also have independent telephone lines to ensure uninterrupted communication with the external world in a disaster situation. Once initiated, the ICS has a built-in chain of command that would be responsible for triage of patients and allocation of personnel and resources.[3,84]

Triage

Appropriate triage is a vital function during an emergency management response. This is a dynamic process that is not necessarily confined to the disaster site or the emergency department but is carried through several levels of the medical response pathway of a disaster response. Compared with the initial concept based on the management of the most severely injured, modern triage is based on the likelihood of survival in relation to the resources available at the time of the decision.[58,85] Problems that have been usually encountered in the triage process include:

1. Lack of medical direction at the scene. Making triage decisions in a chaotic situation requires skill and experience and can often initially seem confusing and unmanageable. Lessons from the first Persian Gulf War showed that on-field triage was correct only 70% of the time.[87] It is necessary to have experienced physicians entrusted with this job and also to have simple and clear guidelines in this decision-making process. In addition to emergency physicians and trauma surgeons, critical care physicians bring with them the expertise to deal with complex and time-bound situations and are thus well-suited to head a triage team.[84]
2. Lack of interorganizational planning. Dynamic management of the triage process requires interorganizational coordination and flow of information. Up-to-date assessment of medical resources and personnel should be communicated from the command center to the triage site, and similar communication should occur from the scene to the command center. This will allow for rational and appropriate triage based on the availability of resources.
3. Transport of victims from the site by nonambulance vehicles to nearby hospitals.
4. There is no single universally accepted form of triage. Traditionally, triage systems have used color-coded systems to sort out victims in a disaster setting. Different categorization systems and tools have also been used, with an arbitrary selection of colors and codes to indicate each category. The number of categories varies from two to five, with a greater number of categories offering more precision but less simplicity. A commonly used five-color triage system is described in Table 263-4.[3] Similarly different tools and mathematical formulas have been proposed to predict the number of casualties in a mass trauma event and also the hospital capacity to care for critical casualties. These tools are based on disaster statistics from the past and can help in rapid assessment of available resources to guide triage.[3,88]
5. Triage continues from victims in the field to existing patients already in hospitals. Continuous assessment of bed availability including the surge capacity of the hospital, activation of prearranged contracts for patient transfer to nearby hospitals, ease of restrictive policies on the floors (e.g., use of unusual intravenous infusion and ventilators on regular wards), cancellation of nonessential surgeries, and prioritization of laboratory and radiologic procedures are some of the interventions that will directly impact the triage process.[84]

Triage is not a perfect and democratic process and often raises ethical issues. It can be a daunting task because it carries the burden of sorting out victims who are not likely to survive. The definition of "hopeless" or "expected to die" is not absolute and is relative to available resources. Thus, the process must be a continuous one, taking into account resource availability and the caseload of victims being triaged.[89]

Major Utilities, Supplies, and Equipment

Disaster plans and drills should factor in the possibility of internal and external power outages and related disruptions (ventilator and monitoring device failures, communication failures including breakdown of cellular phones, and elevator failures) and water supply and gas supply shortages. The plan should have an up-to-date inventory of all supplies and capabilities of the facility. Number of ventilators in use and its absolute capacity, inventory of various ICU supplies, and vendor lists should be readily available if there is sudden demand for supplies. The disaster plan should allow for at least 2 days worth of supplies. Regular drills will help identify various bottlenecks and will also provide knowledge of the absolute capacity of devices, equipment, and services in a disaster situation. Plans to evacuate critically ill patients to nearby hospitals in the event of failure of backup systems should also be addressed in the process. Since the anthrax attacks and the resulting strain on antibiotic supplies in 2001, more attention has been paid to the national repository of lifesaving pharmaceuticals and medical supplies called the National Pharmaceutical Stockpile Program. This response is a component of the CDC's larger Bioterrorism Preparedness and Response Initiative and is composed of a stockpile of pharmaceuticals, vaccines, medical supplies, and equipment to augment local and state resources in a disaster situation. After a federal decision to deploy, a "push package" will arrive by ground or air in 12 hours or less at any location in the United States. A CDC team accompanying the push package will then determine the amount and type of shipments in the second phase.[90]

Security and Casualty Reception

Security is a major concern during natural or manmade disasters. Desire to seek immediate medical evaluation, panic, and curiosity are some of the forces that place the health care facility and its personnel under enormous strain. Internal and external traffic control, protection of personnel who are involved in the response effort, and strict enforcement of staging and triage areas are key security-related issues. Law enforcement plays a more critical role during terrorist attacks or during bioterrorism, and failure to maintain order will lead to rapid overwhelming of the facility's resources and a disorganized medical response. Because most of the victims will arrive at the hospital by foot or by personal vehicles, provision must be made for a predetermined staging area with adequate mass decontamination facilities and respiratory protective equipment.[11,84]

Communication

Secure communications with backup systems must be established to ensure proper functioning of the ICS and implementing an effective management response. Alternative communication channels such as cellular phones and hand-held two-way radio systems should be in place if usual methods fail. A media liaison officer or spokesperson should be designated to ensure planned and structured communication to the outside world. The plan should also provide guidelines for a specific holding area for media conferences and for the use of neutral terminology in communication.[16,84]

Community-wide Preparedness and Disaster Drills

Mass casualty incidents require hospitals to respond as an individual entity, as a part of a community's health care system, and beyond. Administrators need to develop horizontal and vertical relationships between local and federal governmental agencies and with other nongovernmental organizations that can provide valuable resources during a disaster. Physicians, including intensivists, should understand the limitations and resources available through these agencies and verify if the hospital administration has an established relationship with these agencies. Some of the interventions that will determine a successful emergency management response plan include special funding for the development of disaster plans in the community; testing of alliances between the facility and neighboring hospitals, the EMS system, police, and fire departments; education of the public; and interagency communication drills. In addition to annual community-wide drills, JCAHO now mandates testing the response phase of the disaster plan at least twice a year. This ensures that the plan designed by the facility will not suffer the "paper plan syndrome."[3,11,16]

ISSUES UNIQUE TO THE ICU

The responsibility of caring for the most serious salvageable casualties in natural and manmade disasters will ultimately involve the critical care physician. As opposed to overwhelming shortage of resources, lack of coordination among various agencies and specialties has been often cited as the main contributing factor to an ineffective emergency medical response.[3,11] This response therefore requires the cooperation of not just physicians but also between prehospital medical personnel, nurses, and ancillary services such as radiology and laboratory services. In providing critical care beyond the domains of the ICU, intensivists can function in a role that is consonant with their usual expectations, break down natural barriers between various disciplines, and help them function beyond their prototypical roles. Natural skills of intensivists, such as the ability to organize and manage triage under exceptional circumstances and the ability to improvise in difficult situations and yet provide sustained definitive care, make them ideally suited to lead an effective medical response during disasters. An average ICU typically consumes approximately one third of the hospital resources. A chaotic situation such as a disaster will require continuous assessment and assignment of this valuable component of hospital resources. It is therefore important for critical care physicians to participate in committees and forums involved in formulating a disaster plan and ensure adequate representation in the response to a disaster.[84,91] Common principles involved in the creation of an emergency response plan should be followed and applied from an ICU perspective.[84,91] They include:

1. *Clear role definition and understanding of the overall organization of the emergency response plan.* Based on hazard vulnerability analysis of individual hospitals, different plans for external and internal disasters may exist. Plans may also provide for separate medical and administrative command posts; it is thus crucial for the intensivist to know their exact position in the command structure and provide a leadership role if required.
2. *Knowledge of the usual limit, surge capacity, and absolute limit of ICU resources.* This includes ICU beds, ventilators, oxygen tanks, safety masks, isolation rooms, resuscitation equipment, pharmaceutical supplies, and other essential equipment. Designation of personnel to authorize utilization or limitation of these resources, contacts to vendors, backup system plans in the event of a breakdown of crucial laboratory and radiologic services, description of territories to be covered by the ICU triage team, and transfer agreements between nearby ICUs need to be incorporated in the plan.
3. *Staffing.* On activation of a disaster plan, it is usual to ask all staff currently on duty to remain in the hospital beyond the end of their shift. Templates of schedules for staff members for the initial few days will increase efficiency, reduce post-incident stress and exhaustion, and prevent duplication. Leaders for nursing and ancillary services should be designated, and updated telephone lists should be readily available to command posts.
4. *Communication/security and major utilities.* Direct telephone lines to the ICU, two-way walkie-talkie systems between triage personnel and the command center, waiting area for relatives, specific holding area for the media, designated liaison officer for media relations, guidelines for release of messages to the public, and enforcement of security are vital for execution of a disaster plan. Alternative and backup arrangements for power outages and water and gas supply failures should be made to continue uninterrupted patient care. Disaster drills should specifically address such issues, and intensivists should have ready access to inventory of ventilators, monitoring devices, and essential power-driven equipment that can function in a disrupted environment.
5. *Cooperation between the facility and external agencies.* Notification and coordination between various governmental and nongovernmental organizations and maintaining an up-to-date contact list will ensure timely help that is required in a disaster response. Critical care physicians should also be up-to-date with medical literature pertaining to disasters, organizational issues, triage, recognition and treatment of individual disaster syndromes, decontamination, vaccinations, and use of personal protective equipment. Readers are also referred to various governmental and nongovernmental agencies that can provide valuable help and advice in such chaotic situations (see Appendix).

CRITICAL CARE IN UNCONVENTIONAL SITUATIONS

The concept of the "golden hour" in treating critically ill patients can be applied outside the ICU at the site of a disaster. Studies of earthquakes in Armenia and Costa Rica identified victims whose deaths might have been prevented by timely medical attention in the first few hours after the catastrophe.[92,93] Furthermore, critical injuries such as burns, crush injuries, and blunt trauma require transport to a nearby health care facility for more definitive care. Early treatment and resuscitation of the critically ill in these unconventional situations has led to the expansion of critical care medicine outside its usual high-technology environment to the site of the disaster. The provision of critical care in such conditions can take two forms: mobile/field ICU teams and critical care transport.[84]

MOBILE ICU TEAMS

Since the first response of a civilian critical care team to the earthquake site in Armenia, there have been numerous other examples in medical literature describing extended critical care through mobile ICU teams.[94] The use of mobile ICU teams has not been restricted to disaster settings but has also been used throughout the world during peacetime. Various factors that need to be considered in the formation of ICU teams are discussed next.

Personnel

Based on the anticipated needs of the disaster, appropriate specialists and ancillary personnel are chosen. Mobile ICU teams with different compositions have been used successfully in the past (e.g., the renal dialysis team in the Armenian earthquake in 1988, the burns teams during the pipeline explosion in Ufa in 1989). At least three critical care physicians, a minimum of four nurses for round-the-clock coverage, and paramedics for transport and triage would be necessary to staff the field hospital.[95] Other essential personnel include biomedical engineers (to adapt equipment to local electric standards) and pharmacy support.[84]

Equipment

The kind of equipment to be brought to the site will depend on the number and nature of casualties anticipated.[95] As in case of the chemical gas leak tragedy in Bhopal, India (1984), mechanical ventilators, intubation equipment, oxygen supplies, and pulse oximeters were required to manage inhalational injuries. Similarly, dialysis equipment would be required to deal with crush injuries after an earthquake. Other factors that need to be considered include portability, familiarity to users, and flexibility to adapt to alternative power sources.[84]

Training

Adequate pre-departure training is essential for a coordinated and effective response. In addition, interaction and on-site training ensures effective functioning of a foreign medical unit and allows for the smooth transition of care to local physicians when the foreign team departs.[84]

Casualty Assessment

Studies from the past and more recently the experience of the Israeli defense forces in providing care to earthquake victims in Turkey showed that the effectiveness of mobile ICU teams was limited by time. It sometimes takes 3 days to mobilize such an effort, and crucial time is lost before delivery of intended care.[95,96] Efforts must therefore be made to epidemiologically assess the efficacy of such teams. They should include review of the overall effort and adequacy of the ICU teams, outcome of victims, operational costs, and analysis of the structure and process of the ICU in the field.[84,95,97]

CRITICAL CARE TRANSPORT

Transport forms a vital link in the chain of care for a disaster victim that begins with first responders and culminates at a specialized receiving facility. Transport of victims after a major disaster often occurs in less than ideal conditions; the roads may be blocked, demand very often exceeds supply, and air transport may be impaired by dust clouds, poor visibility, or unavailability of landing areas. The goals of transport are to expedite the movement of patients from the scene of the disaster to definitive care areas, to prevent deterioration in the patient's condition, and to provide ongoing care en route. Common principles involved in the safe transport of patients include:[98,99]

1. Rapid assessment of the severity of injuries, recognition of the need for transport, and anticipation of problems during transport
2. Safe movement of patients in and out of vehicles, continuous monitoring of vital signs, and recognition and treatment of problems encountered during transport
3. Documentation of the events during transport and provision of a detailed report to the admitting personnel

TYPES OF TRANSPORT

Ground Transport

Ground ambulances have the advantage of rapid deployment, high mobility, and lower cost. However, patients and equipment are subject to significant deceleration and vibration forces. Equipment may vary depending on the size of the ambulance and usually includes blood pressure and electrocardiograph monitors, pulse oximeters, ventilators, and, in some cases, modern support devices such as intra-aortic balloon pumps. Gebremichael and colleagues in their experience of transporting 39 patients found that, to minimize the risks associated with transport, the level of care during transport should be at least at the level of the sending hospital's ICU. Mobile ICUs were staffed with a transport team that was composed of an attending critical care physician, a nurse with at least 2 years of critical care experience, a respiratory therapist, and the driver. The transport van was custom built and extensively equipped to provide advanced ventilatory support, invasive and noninvasive hemodynamic monitoring, cardiac pacing and defibrillation, central line and thoracostomy tube placement, airway management including bronchoscopy, and an onboard pharmacy. The majority of these patients were considered candidates for extracorporeal lung assist with extremely poor PaO_2/FIO_2 ratios (<60) and mean FIO_2 requirements more than 0.90. Nineteen of 36 patients transferred were ultimately discharged alive. Thus, by ensuring a level of care similar to that in an ICU during transport, patients with extreme respiratory compromise can be transported safely.[100]

Air Transport

There is growing literature on air transport of critically ill patients since the first medical aeroevacuation in 1870 in the Franco-Prussian war. Air medical transport has since been used in different combat situations in World Wars I and II, the Korean and Vietnam conflicts, and, more recently, in the Persian Gulf wars. Air transport can be via fixed-wing aircraft or helicopter. The choice between the two depends on accessibility of terrain and flight range. In general, helicopters are more effective for transport within 250 miles. Advantages of helicopter transport include vertical takeoff and landing capability. They do not require an airfield for landing and can be deployed to evacuate patients from areas inaccessible to other transport vehicles. Horizontal and decelerative forces are avoided. Disadvantages include short flight range (≤250 to 300 miles), small passenger/patient load capabilities, vibration and noise, limits imposed by weather conditions, and lack of pressurization capability. Airplanes are not restricted by these limits but require both an airfield and more preflight planning. In general, aerial critical care transport is subject to sudden three-dimensional, gravitational, and centrifugal forces, rapid and extreme temperature changes, turbulence and vibration causing monitoring errors and malfunction of equipment, diminished levels of ambient P_{O_2} in the cabin, limited cabin space and electric power, and, finally, limitations in payload (i.e., the weight and bulk of passengers and supplies).[101,102] Another key issue related to air transport is the effect of altitude on oxygenation. Helicopters generally maintain low altitudes, and cabin pressurization is usually not available. In healthy individuals, an elevation of 8000 feet would correspond to a PaO_2 of 55, which is hypoxemia by clinical standards. This would be clearly dangerous to the critically ill patient. By the alveolar gas equation, an increase in FIO_2 from 0.21 to 0.30 should bring PaO_2 back to sea level values in individuals with normal lungs exposed to 8000 feet of altitude. Even though, FIO_2 is typically increased during air transport to compensate for altitude-induced hypoxia, data from animal studies with ARDS have shown that increasing FIO_2 does not always achieve target oxygenation. Increases in PEEP were more reliable than increase in FIO_2 for correcting altitude-induced hypoxia in this model of ARDS.[101] Composition of an ideal air ambulance crew has been much debated. Traditionally, trained nurses, paramedics, or respiratory therapists have been used. Patient mortality has been shown to decrease when a flight physician is present.[103,104]

The decision whether to transport by ground or by air can be a difficult one. Ambulances provide door-to-door service but have to deal with different road surfaces and sudden changes in traffic. Air transport on the other hand is dependent on an ambulance to bring the patient to and from airports and may also be significantly limited by weather. Ehrenwerth and coworkers in their 4-year retrospective review of the transport of 204 critically ill patients showed that the mortality rate was approximately the same for patients brought by air and by ambulance (29.5% vs. 27.3%). All patients survived the trip, and 71% were eventually discharged from the hospital.[102]

MEDICAL CONSIDERATIONS DURING TRANSPORT

Certain medical conditions and equipment may present specific problems during transport, especially in long, high-altitude flights.

Head Injury
Patients with head injuries are exquisitely sensitive to pressure-volume changes, hypoxemia, and gravitational and centrifugal forces. The aim is to maintain normal intracranial pressure, ensure airway control, and provide adequate oxygenation and ventilation. The flight should be pressurized and maintained at low altitude. Management of arterial and central venous access is crucial because an intracranial arterial gas embolus can be devastating with depressurization. Intracranial venous pooling can markedly increase intracranial pressure, causing a precipitous drop in cerebral perfusion during takeoff, landing, and banking turns. The patient must be transported in a head-raised, cross-cabin position if possible. Careful observation is imperative; and if the patient's condition deteriorates as a result of

transport, then the physician must request an emergency landing or a decrease in altitude.[103,105,106]

Spinal Injuries
The patient should be stabilized at the scene with a backboard and cervical collar with sandbags or equivalent device. A nasogastric tube in cases of paralytic ileus (which may worsen due to intraviscus gas expansion) and a Foley catheter to relieve a neurogenic bladder are necessary before air transport. Free-weight traction is undesirable in most ground and air ambulances and should be substituted by traction-free devices.

Thoracoabdominal Trauma
With increasing altitude, intrathoracic air spaces enlarge. To avoid a tension pneumothorax, prophylactic chest tubes may be necessary. Drainage should be via a Heimlich valve unless water-sealed suction is available on board the aircraft.[107] The physician should be prepared to manage the new development of a pneumothorax in flight. For abdominal trauma, a nasogastric tube is essential owing to concerns of intra-abdominal gas expansion, aspiration, and ongoing hemorrhage.

Hemorrhagic Shock
The patient with trauma, uncontrolled hemorrhage, or partially corrected bleeding is particularly sensitive to hypoxia. An acute drop in hemoglobin concentration to 10 g/dL is equivalent to an altitude hypoxia effect of 6000 ft. Such a patient should be stabilized and adequately transfused before flight if prolonged transport is anticipated.

Ocular and Maxillofacial Injuries
The retina is very sensitive to hypoxemia, which should be avoided in case of retinal injuries. Open eye injuries are susceptible to pressure changes.[77] Facial fractures may be associated with injury to the sinuses and subcutaneous emphysema. The swelling may cause pain, local ischemia, and airway obstruction. When transporting patients with wired jaws, wire cutters should be available during transport.[101]

Orthopedic Injuries
Pneumatic splints expand at high altitudes and threaten limb viability. Plaster casts can cause ischemia, and the physician should be able to monitor the limb and split the cast, if necessary. Traction should be from springs rather than free weights. Pelvic fractures may be managed with military anti-shock trousers, but the physician should be aware of changing gas pressures and release air as required during flight.[101]

Burns
The major concerns of transporting patients with complicated burns are airway management and fluid status. Inadequate fluid resuscitation can exacerbate altitude hypoxemia whereas over-resuscitation can cause tissue swelling and airway obstruction. Such patients may benefit from prophylactic intubation, especially if a long transport and extensive fluid shifts are anticipated. Patients with inhalational injury require intubation and PEEP to ensure adequate oxygenation at high altitude.[108]

Other Medical Conditions
Patients with chronic lung disease may be at risk for hypoxemia, and prophylactic intubation with mechanical ventilation

may be indicated. In the patient with heart disease, venous pooling during accelerative and decelerative forces may cause a critical drop in end-diastolic filling, leading to coronary insufficiency and hypotension.

Medical Equipment

Medical equipment that contains gas may be affected by altitude. These devices include orthopedic air splints, pneumatic antishock garments, intravenous reservoirs, blood pressure cuffs, and balloon cuffs of endotracheal tubes, Foley catheters, and suction equipment. Blood pressure cuffs should be forcibly expelled of air and should not be left on the patient's limb between readings. Air in endotracheal tubes and Foley catheter cuffs should be replaced fully or in part by saline to avoid cuff expansion with ensuing tissue compression during high-altitude flight. Mechanical ventilators that are pneumatically driven may need a compressed gas source. Flowmeters that are calibrated at 1 atm may be inaccurate at high altitudes. Electrical power for all essential equipment must be ensured during transport, and an emergency battery pack should be available. Crew members should also remember that regulations for equipment such as color-coding of oxygen cylinders might vary in different countries.[101]

CONCLUSION

Disasters are unique and challenging situations. Understanding characteristics of different disasters, developing an interdisciplinary approach to hazard mitigation, and knowledge of related clinical syndromes are key to an effective medical disaster response. With their natural role of caring for critically ill patients, intensivists bring with them unique abilities that can be applied to a disaster situation such as multidisciplinary approach to patient care, management skills, procedural expertise, and flexible attitudes. In addition, they can also deliver care beyond the domain of the ICU through provision of medical care on the field and transport of critically ill patients. To ensure an integrated and effective response to future disasters, it is necessary for critical care physicians to understand fundamental principles in disaster medicine and participate in the disaster planning process in and out of their usual realm of the ICU.

ANNOTATED REFERENCES

Auf der Heide E: Disaster Response: Principles of Preparation and Coordination, St. Louis, CV Mosby, 1989. Full text online edition available at the CDC website through the following hyperlink: http://216.202.128.19/dr/DisasterResponse.nsf/section/chapters?openview&home=flash.
An excellent resource that includes basic principles and pitfalls in disaster planning and offers valuable assistance to those involved in disaster preparedness, mitigation, and response.

Gans L, Kennedy T: Management of unique clinical entities in disaster medicine. Emerg Med Clin North Am 1996;14:301-330.
A review of various topics including triage, disaster-related injuries, and different disaster syndromes. Intensivists who will be involved in mobile ICU teams will find this particularly useful.

Jarrett DG (ed): Medical Management of Radiological Casualties Handbook, Armed Forces Radiobiology Research Institute, Bethesda, Maryland, 1999. Available at http://www.afrri.usuhs.mil/www/outreach/pdf/2edmmrchandbook.pdf.
This online source not only provides basic explanations and definitions related to radiation syndromes but also offers guidance to those responding both at the scene of an accident and at the hospital.

Karwa M, Bronzert P, Kvetan V: Bioterrorism and critical care. Crit Care Clin 2003;19:279-313.
A recent and clinically useful review of the subject of bioterrorism. It deals with individual biological agents and strategies that can be applied from a critical care perspective in such situations.

Koenig KL, Dinermann N, Kuehl AE: Disaster nomenclature—a functional impact approach: The PICE system. Available at http://www.homelandsecurity.org/journal/articles/displayArticle.asp?article=74.
This paper considers traditional "disaster" nomenclature, which usually focuses on issues other than the functional impact of the crisis, and presents a new concept to describe "disasters" called the PICE system.

APPENDIX A

General Disaster Resources and Websites

1. Agency for Toxic Substances and Disease Registry. Available at http://www.atsdr.cdc.gov/atsdrhome.html
2. Centers for Disease Control and Prevention: Extensive resources for issues regarding bioterrorism. Available at http://www.cdc.gov/. Department of Defense. Available at: http://www.defenselink.mil/
3. Disaster Management Higher Education Project; Emergency Management Institute, Federal Emergency Management Agency. Several academic texts on disaster management are available for free downloading. Available at http://www.fema.gov/emi/ edu/higher.htm
4. Federal Emergency Management Agency. Available at http://www.fema.gov/
5. Federal Response Plan for Disasters; Emergency Support Functions of Various Government Agencies.
   a. Transportation: Primary agency: Department of Transportation (DOT), Contact: 202-366-4000, Available at http://www.dot.gov/
   b. Communications: Primary agency: National Communications System. Available at http://www.ncs.gov/.
   c. Public works and engineering: Primary agency: United States Army Corps of Engineering (CaE), Department of Defense (DaD). Available at http://www.usace.army.mil/ and http://www.defenselink.mil/
   d. Firefighting: Primary agency: United States Forest Service (USFS), Department of Agriculture (USDA). Contact: 202-205-8333. Available at http://www.fs.fed.us/
   e. Information and planning: Primary agency: Federal Emergency Management Agency (FEMA). Contact: 1-800-621-FEMA. Available at http://www.fema.gov/
   f. Mass care: Primary agency: American Red Cross (ARC). Contact: (202) 303-4498. Available at http://www.redcross.org/
   g. Health and medical services. Primary agency: United States Public Health Services (USPHS), Department of Health and Human Services (DHHS). Contact: 202-619-0257. Available at http://www.hhs.gov/disasters/index.shtml.
   h. Urban search and rescue. Primary agency: Federal Emergency Management Agency (FEMA). Available at http://www.fema.gov/
   i. Hazardous materials. Primary agency: Environmental Protection Agency (EPA). Contact: 1-800-424-8802. Available at http://www.epa.gov/ebtpages/emernaturaldisasters.html
   j. Energy: Primary agency: Department of Energy (DOE). Contact: 800-dial-DOE. Available at http://www.energy.gov/engine/content.do?BT_CODE=DOEHOME
6. Health Library for Disasters (HELID). Available at http://www.helid.desastres.net/cgi-bin/library.exe
7. Joint Commission on Accreditation of Healthcare Organizations. Available at http://www.jcaho.org/
8. Medical Chemical and Biological Defense: provides detailed information on chemical and biological agents; also linked to the U.S. Army Medical Research Institute for Chemical Defense Home Page. Available at http://mrmc-www.army.mil/.
9. NBC Medical Defense Information Server. Available at http://www.nbc-med.org/
10. Office of Emergency Preparedness and National Disaster Medical System, part of the Department of Health and Human Services. Available at http://www.oep-ndms.dhhs.gov/
11. Occupational Safety and Health Administration. Hospitals and community emergency response—what you need to know. Publication No. OSHA 3152: a pamphlet about preparedness for chemically contaminated patients. Available at http://www.osha-slc.gov/Publications/OSHA3152/osha3152.html
12. Pan American Health Organization. Available at http://www.paho.org/disasters/
13. Prehospital and Disaster Medicine. Provides links to various international disaster medicine websites. Available at http://pdm.medicine.wisc.edu/links.html

14. Storm Prediction Center at the National Oceanic and Atmospheric Agency. Available at http://www.spc.noaa.gov
15. State Department Counter-Terrorism Coordinator. Available at http://www.state.gov/www/global/terrorism/index.html
16. U.S. Department of Homeland Security. Available at http://www.dhs.gov/dhspublic/theme_home2.jsp
17. World Health Organization (WHO) Handbook for Emergency Related Field Operations. Available at http://www.who.int/disasters/tg.cfm?doctypelD=25.
18. World Health Organization (WHO) Health Library for Disasters. (Downloadable full-text documents.). Available at http://www.helid.desastres.net

Resources for Radiation Accidents

1. Agency for Toxic Substances and Disease Registry (ATSDR). Telephone at 888-422-8737. Provides 24-hour advice. Available at http://www.atsdr.cdc.gov/atsdrhome.html
2. Armed Forces Radiobiological Research Institute, Medical Radiation Assistance Team (MRAT). Page at 800-SKY-PAGE (Pin 801-0338) or telephone at 301-295-0316. Available at http://www.afrri.usuhs.mil
3. Chemical Transportation Emergency Center (CHEMTREC). Telephone at 800-424-9300 (in the District of Columbia 202-483-7616) or 703-527-3887 if outside the continental United States. Available at http://www.chemtrec.org/
4. Conference of Radiation Control Program Directors, Inc. (CRCPD). Telephone at 502-227-4543. Maintains lists of state radiation health contacts for planning purposes. Available at http://www.crcpd.org/
5. International Atomic Energy Agency (IAEA) referral. Available at http://www.iaea.or.at
6. Radiation Emergency Assistance Center Training Site (REACTS). Telephone at 865-481-1000, or page through the operator at Methodist Medical Center, Oak Ridge, Tennessee, at 865-576-3131. Provides medical consultation on radiation accidents. Available at http://www.orau.gov/reacts

Resources for Bioterrorism

1. Centers for Disease Control and Prevention website for bioterrorism. Available at http://www.bt.cdc.gov/

2. Department of Defense Global Emerging Infections Surveillance and Response System. Available at http://www.geis.ha.osd.mil/
3. U.S. Food and Drug Administration: drug preparedness and response to bioterrorism. Available at http://www.fda.gov/cder/drugprepare/default.htm
4. U.S. Army Medical Research Institute of Infectious Disease (USAMRIID). Available at http://www.usamriid.army.mil/

Professional Organizations

1. American College of Emergency Physicians. Available at http://www.acep.org/
2. American Hospital Association, Disaster Readiness. Available at http://www.hospitalconnect.com/aha/key_issues/disaster_readiness/index.html
3. Association for Professionals in Infection Control and Epidemiology (APIC). Available at http://www.apic.org/
4. American Public Health Association. Available at http://www.apha.org/
5. American Society for Microbiology (ASM). Available at http://www.asmusa.org/
6. National Association of EMS Physicians. Available at http://www.naemsp.org/

Institutional Resources

1. Center for Nonproliferation Studies/Monterey Institute for International Studies. Available at http://www.cns.miis.edu/
2. Johns Hopkins Center for Civilian Biodefense Studies. Available at http://www.hopkins-biodefense.org/
3. Saint Louis School of Public Health/Center for the Study of Bioterrorism and Emerging Infections. Available at http://bioterrorism.slu.edu/
4. University Health Sciences, Irvine, Environmental Health and Safety. Available at http://www.ehs.uci.edu/emerg.html

Chapter 264

EVIDENCE-BASED CRITICAL CARE

Mary E. Hartman • John A. Kellum • Derek C. Angus

KEY POINTS

1. **The first step in practicing evidence-based medicine (EBM) is asking a well-constructed clinical question.** Developing a specific, thoughtful question leads to a much more efficient search for the answer. Search results themselves can be used to further refine a question.

2. After the question is formulated, one must consider the type of question that is being asked. **Different types of studies,** based on their size, design, and methodology, provide evidence of differing quality and relevance to a research question.

3. **Randomized clinical trials are the cornerstones** of medical evidence.

4. **The principal alternative approach to the randomized clinical trial involves observation rather than experimentation.** Observational outcomes studies are very powerful tools for addressing many questions that randomized clinical trials cannot address.

5. Another valuable source of information, especially for the busy clinician with limited time for reading and research, is **primary research that has already been summarized and evaluated.** One format for appraising individual studies is the critically appraised topic; another is the systematic literature review.

6. With every clinical question, the clinician must determine which type of study will provide the highest quality evidence for the question. A hierarchy exists for this assessment and is referred to in EBM resources as the **"level of evidence."**

7. **Specialized EBM databases** are available for clinical decision making that yield results much quicker than MEDLINE or PubMed.

8. After a search has yielded some potentially useful evidence, the clinician must critically appraise the information and determine its scientific validity and clinical utility. **For evidence to be useful, it needs to be valid, have clinically important findings, and be applicable to the particular patient.**

9. **The strongest evidence available remains useless until it is effectively applied.** Application of EBM can occur directly at the patient level or be implemented on a larger scale through guidelines and protocols.

10. **Effective practice of EBM** depends on a solid body of evidence in the literature and commitment to its implementation at the practitioner, institution, and regional/national level.

The practice of critical care, like all fields of medicine, is changing constantly, and the pace of change is ever increasing. Among the many forces for change, the rapid increase in information is one of the most important. Although the majority of practitioners do not engage in research themselves, they are consumers of research information and must therefore understand how research is conducted to apply this information to their patients. Fellowship programs in critical care medicine emphasize education in this area to varying degrees. The traditional approach has been to require fellows to actively participate in a research project, either clinical or basic science. However, there has also been a growing interest in instructing fellows in the methods of clinical epidemiology.[1] The practical application of clinical epidemiology is evidence-based medicine (EBM), which Sackett defines as "the conscientious and judicious use of current best evidence in making decisions about the care of individual patients."[2] The clinical practice of EBM involves integrating this evidence with individual physician expertise and patient preferences so that informed, thoughtful medical decisions are made.[3]

However, despite two decades of international support, EBM has not been applied in many disciplines. Traditional explanations for this included the perception that EBM is difficult and time consuming to conduct, that EBM is "cookbook" medicine, and that EBM is a tool of hospital administrators and insurers to cut health care costs and reduce physician choice.[2] While the latter of these concerns has been addressed and is likely no longer relevant, persistent opinion that EBM is difficult and time consuming has prevented its widespread use. In this chapter we present the methodology of EBM and its application in critical care medicine.

ASKING A QUESTION

The first step in practicing EBM is asking a well-constructed clinical question. To benefit the patient and aid the clinician,

TABLE 264–1. FOUR ESSENTIAL ELEMENTS OF A WELL-CONSTRUCTED CLINICAL QUESTION

Patient or problem	Intervention	Comparison intervention (if necessary)	Outcome
Starting with your patient, ask "How would I describe a group of patients similar to mine?" Balance precision with brevity.	Ask "Which main intervention am I considering?" Be specific.	Ask "What is the main alternative to compare with the intervention?" Again, be specific.	Ask "What can I hope to accomplish," or "What could this exposure really affect?"

Focusing clinical questions retrieved from the Centre for Evidence Based Medicine website at http://www.cebm.net/index.asp

clinical questions need to be both directly relevant to patients' problems and constructed in a way that guides an efficient literature search to relevant and precise answers. The Centre for Evidence Based Medicine (CEBM) in Oxford, England, provides an excellent description of the four essential elements of an EBM question, summarized in Table 264-1.

Developing a specific, thoughtful question leads to a much more efficient search for the answer. Search results themselves can be used to further refine a question. For example, too many results may indicate the question is too broad, and too few results often necessitates a broader description of the patient population, intervention, or outcome.

TYPES OF EVIDENCE

After the question is formulated, one must consider the type of question that is being asked. Different types of studies, based on their size, design, and methodology, provide evidence of differing quality and relevance to a research question. For example, is the question about therapy, prevention, etiology, or harm? A randomized controlled trial (RCT) or (better yet) systematic review of RCTs will provide the best evidence for this kind of question. Is the investigator interested in the prevalence of a specific disease or symptom in the general population? If so, a large cohort study will best answer this question.

PRIMARY RESEFARCH

Randomized Clinical Trials

Randomized clinical trials, also referred to as experimental or interventional studies, are the cornerstones of medical evidence. Physicians place considerable faith in the results of randomized control trials.[4,5] This faith is placed with good reason as randomization remains perhaps the best solution to avoid misinterpreting the effect of a therapy in the presence of confounding variables.[6] When participants are randomly allocated to groups, factors other than the variable of interest (e.g., a new therapy for sepsis) that are likely to affect the outcome of interest are usually distributed equally to both groups. For example, with randomization, the number of patients with underlying comorbidity, which may adversely affect outcome, should be similar in each study arm, presuming sample size is appropriate. A special advantage of randomization is that this equal distribution will occur for all variables (excluding the intervention) whether these variables are identified by the researcher or not, thus maximizing the ability to determine the effect of the intervention.

However, RCTs are expensive, difficult, and sometimes unethical to conduct with the consequence that less than 20% of clinical practice is based on the results of RCTs.[7] Moreover, many important questions, such as determining the optimal timing of a new therapy or determining the effects of health care practices, cannot practically be studied by RCTs.

Observational studies

The principal alternative approach to the RCT involves observation rather than experimentation. Prior experience has biased us to favor RCTs, but partly in response to the increasing need to answer questions unanswerable by the RCT, the design and execution of observational outcomes studies have become much more sophisticated.

Observational outcomes studies are very powerful tools for addressing many questions that RCTs cannot address, including measuring the effect of harmful substances (e.g., smoking and other carcinogens), organizational structures (e.g., payer status, open vs. closed ICUs), or geography (e.g., rural vs. urban access to health care). Because of their cost and the regulatory demands on drug and device manufacturers, RCTs are frequently designed as efficacy studies in highly defined patient populations with experienced providers and, therefore, provide little evidence about effectiveness in the "real" world.[8] Alternatively, observational studies can generate hypotheses about the effectiveness of treatments that can be tested using other research methods.[8] Investigators have also explored the effects of different therapies that are already accepted, but used variably, in clinical practice.[9]

There are a number of different kinds of observational studies, each designed to address a different type of clinical question. These include case-control, cross-sectional surveys, and cohort studies. Case-control studies compare a group of patients with a disease or symptom of interest to a selected control group. They have the advantage of being quick and relatively inexpensive to perform and are often the only feasible study method for very rare disorders, or when the lag time between an exposure and the related disease is very long. They can also be conducted with a relatively small number of patients. Cross-sectional studies provide a snapshot of a population at one point in time. They can also be conducted inexpensively and in a short time. Cohort studies prospectively identify an at-risk group (the inception cohort) and follow them through time, recording exposures and development (or not) of the disease under investigation. Cohort studies have a number of strengths, including the ability to match subjects to controls for some confounders, establish the timing and sequence of events, and standardize eligibility criteria and outcome assessments, and they are easier and less expensive to conduct than RCTs.

However, observational studies have several significant limitations. First, the data source must be considered. Observational outcomes studies are often performed on large data sets wherein the data were collected for purposes other than research. This can lead to error owing to either a lack of pertinent information or bias in the information recorded.[10] Second, one must consider how the authors attempt to control for confounding. The measured effect size of a variable on outcome (e.g., the effect of the pulmonary artery catheter on mortality rate) can be confounded by the distribution of other known and unknown variables. More specifically, case-control studies are subject to recall and selection bias, and the selection of an appropriate control group can be difficult. Cross-sectional studies can only establish association (at most), not causality, and are also subject to recall bias. Cohort studies have a number of limitations, including difficulty in finding appropriate controls and difficulty determining whether the exposure being studied is linked to a hidden confounder, and the requirement of large sample size or long follow-up to sufficiently answer a research question can be timely and expensive.

Case reports or Case Series

The last form of primary research is the case report or case series. A case is a published account of a single or small number of patients and their response to a particular therapeutic intervention. The inability to generalize from a case report makes it the weakest form of clinical evidence available. However, case reports may be the only available or practical information in support of a therapeutic strategy, especially in the case of rare diseases, when the evolution of the therapy predates the common use of randomized study designs in medical practice. This is also true for new therapies that have not yet been tested in clinical trials.

Summaries of Primary Research

Another valuable source of information, especially for the busy clinician with limited time for reading and research, is primary research that has already been summarized and evaluated. There are a number of high-quality, peer-reviewed sources of summary information, including those that summarize the results of individual trials and those that combine and summarize the results of multiple trials addressing the same topic. The following is a description of the most common types of literature summaries.

SINGLE STUDY RESULTS—CRITICALLY APPRAISED TOPICS

Determining which studies provide information useful in the care of patients is largely a question of deciding whether a study is valid and, if so, can its results be applied to the patients in question. One format for appraising individual studies is the critically appraised topic (CAT) format that has been popularized as part of EBM. The purpose of the CAT is to evaluate a given study or set of studies using a standardized approach. Studies that address diagnosis, prognosis, etiology, therapy, and cost-effectiveness all have a separate CAT format.[3] An example is shown in Table 264-2 for studies that address therapy. The CAT format for studies on therapy asks several questions intended to address the issues of validity and clinical utility. Studies that fail to achieve these measures are not generally useful, although studies do not necessarily have to fulfill every criterion, depending on the nature of the topic.

TABLE 264–2. CRITICAL APPRAISAL OF THE LITERATURE

Are the results of the study valid?

- Correctly randomized?
- Were all the patients accounted for?
- Was follow-up complete?
- Were patients analyzed according to how they were randomized (i.e., intention to treat)?
- Were all people involved in the study blinded?
- Were the groups similar at the start?
- Were the groups treated equally apart from the experimental intervention?

Are the results clinically useful?

- How large was the treatment effect?
- How precise was the estimate of the treatment effect?
- Are the patients similar to the "norm"?
- Were all clinically important outcomes considered?
- Was a cost-benefit analysis performed?

Adapted from Sackett DL, Straus SE, Richardson WS, et al: Evidence-based Medicine: How to Practice and Teach EBM. London, Harcourt, 2000.

For example, a study that examined the effect of walking once a day for the prevention of stroke would not be expected to include a detailed examination of side effects or a cost-effectiveness analysis. However, a study comparing streptokinase to placebo for treatment of stroke would likely be required to include a detailed examination of side effects and a cost-effectiveness analysis because of the excessive risks and costs associated with such therapy. Similarly, blinding may not always be possible and the effects of the investigators being unblinded can be minimized by separating them from the clinicians making the treatment decisions or by establishing standard treatment protocols that are applied equally to both the study and control groups. Alternatively, a study would be "fatally flawed" if it failed in terms of randomization or was not analyzed as "intention to treat" (Table 264-3). There are a number of other useful tools for assessing study design and for quantifying effect size and cost effectiveness. In general, these are the tools of epidemiology and biostatistics and their discussion is beyond the scope of this chapter. A basic primer and glossary of terms is included in Table 264-3.

SYSTEMATIC REVIEWS OF MULTIPLE STUDIES

A systematic literature review combines the results of multiple studies through the systematic search, assembly, and appraisal of existing primary research on a given subject. Meta-analysis is a type of systematic review that incorporates a quantitative summary of the data, which combines actual data from several small, although high-quality studies. Criteria for reviews to be systematic, as opposed to narrative (see later), are quite explicit. All systematic reviews should start with a four-part (three-part when applicable) question, as described previously. Both the search criteria and inclusion and exclusion criteria should be predefined. The review should combine only RCTs or discuss how and why it is combining different types of evidence. Additionally, the methods section should provide search terms and key words, thus establishing some degree of reproducibility.

The advantages of systematic reviews are that by pooling many studies the power to find a true effect is increased. This is particularly important when many well-done but small

TABLE 264–3. DEFINITIONS AND EQUATIONS

Study Design: The research methodology used. There are basically four categories. From weakest to strongest, these are:
1. Case series.
2. Case-control study.
3. Cohort study.
4. Randomized clinical trial.

Two-by-Two Table:

		Disease/Outcome	
		+	−
Test or Exposure	+	a	b
	−	c	d
	Total	a + c	b + d

For diagnostic tests

Sensitivity: Probability that the test will be (+) when the disease is present. a/a + c
Specificity: Probability that the test will be (−) when the disease is absent. d/b + d
Positive Predictive Value: Probability that the disease is present given a (+) test. a/a + b
Negative Predictive Value: Probability that the disease is absent given a (−) test. d/c + d

For association (with exposure or therapy)

Relative Risk (RR): Estimates the magnitude of an association between exposure and disease (or in the case of therapy, the negative association between treatment and morbid outcome). The relative risk indicates the likelihood of development of disease in the exposed group relative to those who were not exposed (also called risk ratio).

$$RR = \frac{\text{Incidence in exposed group}}{\text{Incidence in unexposed group}} = \frac{a/(a+b)}{c/(c+d)}$$

Relative Risk Reduction (RRR): Expressed as a percentage reduction in events in treated versus untreated groups.
$$RRR = (1 - [a/(a+b)]/[c/(c+d)]) \times 100\%$$
Odds Ratio (OR): For case-control studies, RR cannot be used because participants are selected on the basis of disease, not exposure. The RR can be estimated by the OR, however.

$$OR = \frac{a/c}{b/d} = \frac{ad}{be}$$

Attributable Risk (AR): A measure of association that provides information about the absolute effect of the exposure or the excess risk of disease in those exposed compared with those unexposed.
$$AR = (\text{Incidence in exposed group}) - (\text{Incidence in unexposed group})$$
$$= [a/(a+b)] - [c/(c+d)]$$
Absolute Risk Reduction (ARR): A measure of the treatment effect. Note the order is reversed compared with AR.
$$ARR = [c/(c+d)] - [a/(a+b)]$$
Number Needed to Treat (NNT): The inverse of the ARR: 1/ARR.
$$NNT = 1/[c/(c+d)] - [a/(a+b)]$$

Biostatistics

Type I Error (alpha): A difference between study and control groups is found when in reality there is none. Standard = 5%.
Type II Error (beta): No difference between study and control groups is found when in reality there is a difference. Standard = 20%.

Types of Data

Nominal: Numbers are arbitrary.
Ordinal: Numbers denote rank order only.
Interval: Numbers denote units of equal magnitude and rank order.
Parametric: Interval data in a normal distribution.
Standard Deviation (SD): Measure of the scatter of data in a normally distributed sample; 95.44% of the data will fall within 2 SD of the mean. SD = square root of the variance.
Standard Error of the Mean (SE): SE = SD/√n. Used to calculate confidence intervals but not a measure of scatter. Should not be used in place of SD.
Confidence Interval (CI): The estimated range of values likely to include the true value for the entire population. The standard is 95%.
Power Calculation (1 − β): Statistical power is the ability of an experiment to find a significant difference between groups when in fact one exists. Note: As a increases, so does power. As n is increased, β decreases and power increases; that is, the chance of either a type I or type II error is reduced.
Intention-to-Treat Analysis: All data are analyzed according to what group the subject was assigned to regardless of what treatment the subject actually received: analyzed as randomized

and inconclusive studies have attempted to answer a particular question. Systematic reviews often represent an exhaustive effort to find all related information in a given area. In this regard, they provide an excellent summary of the literature up to the date of the review.

The disadvantage of systematic reviews is that they are only as good as the studies they include and can only be interpreted if all the criteria just mentioned have been met.

Unfortunately, there is considerable variability in the quality and comprehensiveness of systematic reviews that are available. Much of this stems from a lack of commonly accepted methodology for conducting and writing systematic reviews. For example, there are no standard exclusion criteria for studies in systematic reviews. Each author establishes the criteria, which the reader must assess to determine the quality and utility of the review to answer his clinical question.

In addition, there is publication bias. Popular search techniques to identify studies are inherently limited by the fact that unpublished studies are unaccounted for in any review. Issues such as these have led authors to propose the development and maintenance of study registries where all RCTs are registered irrespective of their publication status.[11] This would enable review of smaller studies and those studies published in journals that are not listed in cumulative *Index Medicus*, MEDLINE, and other popular databases in systematic reviews.

NARRATIVE REVIEWS OF MULTIPLE STUDIES

The most common system of non–peer-reviewed pooling of study results is the familiar "review" article or collection of reviews. This textbook is an example of the latter. These articles or chapters combine the information from several primary articles, sometimes a few hundred, in a way that is digestible by the average reader. Reviews may be focused on recent advances, or they may provide a complete tutorial on a given subject. In either case, in the traditional method, known as the narrative review, the methodology is the same: an author, presumably someone knowledgeable of the subject matter, reviews the existing literature in some way, formulates an opinion, and disseminates this opinion along with references to support each argument. This approach is also used in the discussion section of most original articles in which the authors attempt to discuss their findings in the context of the existing literature.

The advantage of narrative reviews is that they provide a detailed qualitative discussion, usually by an expert with years of experience. However, they do have several limitations. The most important of these is that evidence used to support the author's positions is not collected, evaluated, and compared in an organized and reproducible manner. That information is complete or that it is judged in an unbiased manner cannot be assured. Journal articles are often peer reviewed, which provides some limited oversight for completeness and lack of bias, but this is far from perfect. Furthermore, review articles and textbook chapters are not generally subject to vigorous review and therefore may be the least reliable sources of information, particularly current information. For example, by 1988, fifteen studies had been reported on the use of prophylactic lidocaine in acute myocardial infarction. While no single study was definitive, pooled data from the nearly 9000 patients showed that the practice was useless at best. Nonetheless, by 1990 there were still more recommendations for its use than against it appearing in textbooks and review articles.[12]

LEVELS OF EVIDENCE

Randomized control trials and observational studies answer different types of questions. Thus with every clinical question, the clinician must determine which type of study will provide the highest quality evidence for the clinical question. A hierarchy exists for this assessment and is referred to in EBM resources as the "level of evidence." For each type of question, there are 5 levels of evidence, from high-quality level 1 evidence down to low-quality level 5 evidence. In general, the highest-quality evidence consists of systematic reviews and RCTs, although certain types of observational studies answer some questions best. Case reports and expert opinion provide the lowest level of evidence in all settings. A complete reference for the levels of evidence is included in Table 264-4.

TABLE 264–4. LEVELS OF EVIDENCE

Level	Therapy/prevention, etiology/harm	Prognosis	Diagnosis	Differential diagnosis/symptom prevalence study	Economic and decision analyses
1a	SR (with homogeneity*) of RCTs	SR (with homogeneity*) of inception cohort studies; CDR† validated in different populations	SR (with homogeneity*) of Level 1 diagnostic studies; CDR† with 1b studies from different clinical centers	SR (with homogeneity*) of prospective cohort studies	SR (with homogeneity*)of Level 1 economic studies
1b	Individual RCT (with narrow confidence interval‡)	Individual inception cohort study with ≥ 80% follow-up; CDR validated in a single population	Validating** cohort study with good††† reference standards; or CDR tested within one clinical center	Prospective cohort study with good follow-up****	Analysis based on clinically sensible costs or alternatives; systematic review(s) of the evidence; and including multi-way sensitivity analyses
1c	All or none§	All or none case-series	Absolute SpPins and SnNouts††	All or none case-series	Absolute better-value or worse-value analyses††††
2a	SR (with homogeneity*) of cohort studies	SR (with homogeneity*) of either retrospective cohort studies or untreated control groups in RCTs	SR (with homogeneity*) of Level >2 diagnostic studies	SR (with homogeneity*) of 2b and better studies	SR (with homogeneity*) of level > 2 economic studies
2b	Individual cohort study (including low quality RCT; e.g., <80% follow-up)	Retrospective cohort study or follow-up of untreated control patients in an RCT;	Exploratory** cohort study with good reference standards; CDR†	Retrospective cohort study, or poor follow-up	Analysis based on clinically sensible costs or alternatives; limited review(s) of the

Continued

TABLE 264–4. LEVELS OF EVIDENCE—cont'd

Level	Therapy/prevention, etiology/harm	Prognosis	Diagnosis	Differential diagnosis/symptom prevalence study	Economic and decision analyses
		Derivation of CDR[†] or validated on split-sample§§§ only	after derivation, or validated only on split-sample§§§ or databases		evidence, or single studies; and including multi-way sensitivity analyses
2c	"Outcomes" research; ecological studies	"Outcomes" research		Ecological studies	Audit or outcomes research
3a	SR (with homogeneity*) of case-control studies		SR (with homogeneity*) of 3b and better studies	SR (with homogeneity*) of 3b and better studies	SR (with homogeneity*) of 3b and better studies
3b	Individual case-control study		Nonconsecutive study; or without consistently applied reference standards	Nonconsecutive cohort study, or very limited population	Analysis based on limited alternatives or costs, poor quality estimates of data, but including sensitivity analyses incorporating clinically sensible variations.
4	Case-series (and poor quality cohort and case-control studies§§)	Case-series (and poor quality prognostic cohort studies***)	Case-control study, poor or non-independent reference standards	Case-series or superseded reference standard	Analysis with no sensitivity analysis
5	Expert opinion without explicit critical appraisal, or based on physiology, bench research or "first principles"	Expert opinion without explicit critical appraisal, or based on physiology, bench research or "first principles"	Expert opinion without explicit critical appraisal, or based on physiology, bench research or "first principles"	Expert opinion without explicit critical appraisal, or based on physiology, bench research or "first principles"	Expert opinion without explicit critical appraisal, or based on economic theory or "first principles"

Grades of Recommendation

A	Consistent level 1 studies
B	Consistent level 2 or 3 studies *or* extrapolations from level 1 studies
C	Level 4 studies *or* extrapolations from level 2 or 3 studies
D	Level 5 evidence *or* troublingly inconsistent or inconclusive studies of any level

Users can add a minus-sign "–" to denote the level that fails to provide a conclusive answer because of:
- EITHER a single result with a wide confidence interval (such that, for example, an ARR in an RCT is not statistically significant but whose confidence intervals fail to exclude clinically important benefit or harm)
- OR a systematic review with troublesome (and statistically significant) heterogeneity.
- Such evidence is inconclusive and therefore can only generate grade D recommendations.

*By homogeneity we mean a systematic review that is free of worrisome variations (heterogeneity) in the directions and degrees of results between individual studies. Not all systematic reviews with statistically significant heterogeneity need be worrisome, and not all worrisome heterogeneity need be statistically significant. As noted above, studies displaying worrisome heterogeneity should be tagged with a "–" at the end of their designated level.

[†]Clinical Decision Rule. (These are algorithms or scoring systems that lead to a prognostic estimation or a diagnostic category.)

[‡]See earlier for advice on how to understand, rate, and use trials or other studies with wide confidence intervals.

§Met when *all* patients died before the Rx became available, but some now survive on it; or when some patients died before the Rx became available, but *none* now die on it.

§§By poor quality *cohort* study we mean one that failed to clearly define comparison groups and/or failed to measure exposures and outcomes in the same (preferably blinded), objective way in both exposed and nonexposed individuals and/or failed to identify or appropriately control known confounders and/or failed to carry out a sufficiently long and complete follow-up of patients. By poor quality *case-control* study we mean one that failed to clearly define comparison groups and/or failed to measure exposures and outcomes in the same (preferably blinded), objective way in both cases and controls and/or failed to identify or appropriately control known confounders.

§§§Split-sample validation is achieved by collecting all the information in a single tranche, then artificially dividing this into "derivation" and "validation" samples.

[††]An "Absolute SpPin" is a diagnostic finding whose *Specificity* is so high that a *Positive* result rules-*in* the diagnosis. An "Absolute SnNout" is a diagnostic finding whose *Sensitivity* is so high that a *Negative* result rules *out* the diagnosis.

[‡‡]*Good, better, bad,* and *worse* refer to the comparisons between treatments in terms of their clinical risks and benefits.

[†††]*Good* reference standards are independent of the test and applied blindly or objectively to all patients. *Poor* reference standards are haphazardly applied but still independent of the test. Use of a non-independent reference standard (where the "test" is included in the "reference" or where the "testing" affects the "reference") implies a level 4 study.

[††††]Better-value treatments are clearly as good but cheaper, or better at the same or reduced cost. Worse-value treatments are as good and more expensive, or worse and equally or more expensive.

**Validating studies test the quality of a specific diagnostic test, based on prior evidence. An exploratory study collects information and trawls the data (e.g., using a regression analysis) to find which factors are "significant."

***By poor quality prognostic cohort study we mean one in which sampling was biased in favor of patients who already had the target outcome, or the measurement of outcomes was accomplished in < 80% of study patients, or outcomes were determined in an unblinded, nonobjective way, or there was no correction for confounding factors.

****Good follow-up in a differential diagnosis study is > 80%, with adequate time for alternative diagnoses to emerge (e.g., 1 to 6 months, acute; 1 to 5 years, chronic)

From Phillips B, Ball C, Sackett D, et al: Grades of recommendation (n.d.) Retrieved from the Centre for Evidence Based Medicine website at: http://www.cebm.net/index.asp

GATHERING EVIDENCE—THE LITERATURE SEARCH

For most busy critical care physicians, the objective here will be to find the answer as quickly as possible, in as efficient a presentation as possible. MEDLINE, accessed either through Ovid or PubMed, is likely to be the resource most clinicians are familiar and comfortable with. However, MEDLINE can be a low-yield EBM resource because of its large size and broad scope. More specialized databases are available for clinical decision making that yield much more relevant results much more quickly. The best known of these resources is likely the Cochrane Library. Maintained by the Cochrane Collaboration, the Cochrane Library contains a large collection of peer-reviewed systematic reviews on a wide variety of health care interventions.[13] It is thoroughly indexed and easily searched, and the Cochrane Library can be easily accessed via CD-ROM, at a medical library, or directly online. Best Evidence is another widely available electronic database that summarizes both individual studies and systematic reviews.[13] In the past decade a number of EBM journals have been developed, including *ACP Journal Club, Evidence-based Medicine,* and a number of other specialty-specific journals. All of these are summary journals that select and present the best evidence from high-quality studies in a given field.[13] All of these EBM resources, and others, are linked for searching with MEDLINE through a specialty EBM electronic database, called Evidence-based Medicine Reviews (EBMR), which is available at many medical libraries.

Textbooks deserve a final word. Whereas textbooks have considerable appeal because they are well organized and synthesize a large amount of material, they are not a primary source of current information.[13] In general, textbooks are useful for gaining basic background information on a disease or condition but should not used as a primary source of EBM. One notable exception to this recommendation is the *Clinical Evidence.* Compiled and published by the *British Medical Journal* and updated every 6 months, *Clinical Evidence* is an annual compilation in book and CD-ROM format of the best available evidence on the effects of common medical interventions.[13] A more complete list of EBM publications and websites is located in Table 264-5.

APPRAISING EVIDENCE

After a search has yielded some potentially useful evidence, the clinician must critically appraise the information and determine its scientific validity and clinical utility. For a piece of evidence to be useful, it needs to be valid, have clinically important findings, and be applicable to the particular patient. Guides for assessment of validity, like that shown in Table 264-2, exist for different types of studies (e.g., therapy, diagnosis, prognosis) and are presented in detail in *Evidence-based Medicine.*[13] Worksheets to determine whether a study is valid are also available from a number of sources, including the Centre for Evidence Based Medicine and a number of the websites listed in Table 264-4. The importance of the findings again depends on the type of study. For studies on therapy, the clinician must decide if there was a true treatment effect and, if so, how large of an effect. For studies on diagnosis, the characteristics of a test must be presented and the clinician must decide if the test characteristics (sensitivity, specificity, positive and negative predictive values) would make the same test useful for current patient. Again, a number of guides exist

TABLE 264–5. WEB SITES AND OTHER SOURCES OF INFORMATION ON EVALUATING AND USING EVIDENCE IN MEDICINE

Evidence use and appraisal resources on the internet

Centre for Evidence Based Medicine, Oxford: http://cebm.jr2.ox.ac.uk/
The Health Information Research Unit, McMaster University: http://hiru.mcmaster.ca/
The Unit for Evidence-Based Practice and Policy, London: http://www.ucl.ac.uk/openlearning/uebpp/uebpp.htm
Cochrane Collaboration: http://www.cochrane.org/
The ScHARR Guide to Evidence-Based Medicine on the Internet: http://www.sheffield.ac.uk/~scharr/ir/netting/
Oregon Health & Science University Evidence-based Practice Center: http://www.ohsu.edu/epc/
Bandolier, Oxford: http://www.jr2.ox.ac.uk/Bandolier/index.html
Library of the Health Sciences Peoria: http://www.uic.edu/depts/lib/lhsp/resources/ebm.shtml
Evidence-based Medicine Toolkit: http://www.med.ualberta.ca/ebm/ebm.htm

Journals clubs on the internet

Critical care
MCCTP Pittsburgh: http://www.anes.upmc.edu/mcctp
SORAHSN, Ontario: http://ahsn.lhsc.on.ca
PedsCCM EB Journal Club: http://pedsccm.wustl.edu/EBJournal_Club.html

Other
Journal Club on the Web: http://www.journalclub.org/
Health Reviews for Primary Care Providers: http://library.mcphu.edu/resources/reviews/revw_ind.htm
Journal of Family Practice-POEMS: http://www.jfponline.com/

On-line journals

Critical Care Forum: http://ccforum.com/
Evidence-Based Medicine: http://ebm.bmjjournals.com/
ACP Journal Club: http://www.acpjc.org/

Other useful resources

Journal series
Journal of the American Medical Association
  Oxman AD, et al: 1993;270:2093-2095
  Guyatt GH, et al: 1993;270:2598-2601
  Guyatt Gil, et al: 1994;271:59-63
  Jaeschke R, et al: 1994;271:703-707
  Levine MS, et al: 1994;271:1615-1619
  Laupacis A, et al: 1994;272:234-237
  Oxman AD, et al: 1994;272:1367-1371
  Richardson WS, et al: 1995;273:1292-1295
  Richardson WS, et al: 1995;273:1610-1613
  Hayward R, et al: 1995;274:570-574
  Wilson MC, et al: 1995;274:1630-1632
  Guyatt GH, et al: 1995;274:1800-1804
  Naylor CD, et al: 1996;275:554-558
  Naylor CD, et al: 1996;275:1435-1439
Canadian Medical Association Journal
  Oxman AD, et al: 1994;150:1249-1254
  Oxman AD, et al: 1994;150:1417-1423
  Oxman AD, et al: 1994;150:1575-1579
  Oxman AD, et al: 1994;150:1793-1796
  Oxman AD, et al: 1994;150:1971-1973
Critical Care Medicine
  Cook DJ, et al: 1996;24:334-337
  Cook DJ, et al: 1996;24:1757-1768

Book
Sackett DL, et al: Evidence-Based Medicine: How to Practice and Teach EBM, 2nd ed. London, Churchill Livingstone, 2000.

to help physicians make these decisions. *Evidence-based Medicine* discusses these points in great detail and includes pocket-sized note cards that prompt the reader with important criteria for assessing validity and determining the clinical relevance of a study's findings.[13] The last step in appraising a piece of evidence is to determine its applicability in a given clinical situation. This forms the grade of recommendation that a piece of evidence generates. In general, a high-grade recommendation is given when a high-level piece of evidence is directly applicable to the clinical situation. A summary of the grades of recommendation is provided in Table 264-4.

APPLYING EVIDENCE

The strongest evidence available remains useless until it is effectively applied. Application of EBM can occur directly at the patient level or implemented on a larger scale through guidelines and protocols. Although bedside decision making has been the traditional focus of EBM, guidelines and protocols are important means to promote the standardization of care at an institutional or regional level.

BEDSIDE DECISION MAKING

The goal of EBM is to facilitate bedside decision making by placing evidence in the context of clinical judgment and the preferences of the patient.[14] There is often sufficient medical evidence to influence a number of daily decisions. Therefore, the clinician should always ask, "Is my patient receiving the best level of care as indicated by the evidence in the literature? Are there any study protocols or results that could be applied to this patient that currently are not?" Clinicians should also recognize knowledge deficits and be alert for opportunities to formulate EBM questions during daily rounds or routine patient care. Once the evidence is found and deemed useful, it needs to be judiciously applied. Clinicians must use their knowledge and experience to understand how to apply the results of studies to individual patients. Some cases, due to patient- or environment-specific circumstances, may be sufficiently unique to render even good evidence inappropriate. Individual patient or family values and expectations could also direct therapy in one direction when medical evidence and physician judgment would have led it in another.

GUIDELINES AND PROTOCOLS

Perhaps a natural extension of EBM is the desire to standardize care when evidence can be found for treatments or diagnostic procedures that are cost effective. When such therapeutic or diagnostic strategies exist they should be widely applied. A convenient way to ensure this is to develop a protocol or a guideline. Protocols and guidelines are especially useful for common illnesses and procedures and have the advantage of allowing an institution to implement EBM even in the presence of physician lack of expertise in EBM. However, developing and maintaining protocols and guidelines is extremely labor intensive because the EBM criteria for guideline validity are explicit. Sackett states, "We should think of [a guideline] as having two distinct components: first the evidence summary, and second, the detailed instructions for applying that evidence to our patient."[13] The evidence summary consists of a recent review of the literature

both for and against the guideline.[3] The applicability of the guideline in each clinical situation with particular patient and institutional characteristics is assessed in the same manner as other evidence.

PROBLEMS WITH EVIDENCE-BASED MEDICINE IN CRITICAL CARE

Although EBM faces challenges when applied in many fields, there are some unique challenges for its implementation in critical care medicine. These include the difficulty in collecting high-quality evidence on which physicians can base decisions, difficulty in determining what to do when there is a general lack of evidence, and difficulty applying evidence to patient care.

GENERATING EVIDENCE

It is impossible to practice EBM without a body of evidence in the literature. Until recently, there was little strong evidence supporting particular care paradigms in the critically ill. There are now a large number of studies guiding a wide set of critical care problems,[15-20] whereas other elements of care remain largely empirical. Why has our field had such difficulty conducting clinical trials? There are a number of reasons. First, critical illness occurs in a heterogeneous group of patients in whom treatment effects may be small. Narrow selection criteria may introduce bias, and smaller sample sizes may not show an effect. Second, investigators must ensure the novel therapy is tested against "current best methods of care." Since a study will be interpreted in the light of likely treatment patterns at the completion of a trial, rather than the initiation, recent, strong evidence should be promoted in both arms of a trial. But the large number of recent critical care trials combined with the financial and practical difficulties of implementing all of the changes has made "current best methods of care" an evolving process that remains a constantly moving target. Third, the choice of appropriate outcomes continues to be debated in critical care. The historic choice of 28 (or 30) day mortality rate, which has been used as the primary outcome in most critical care trials,[21] has been criticized as arbitrary and incomplete. There is a growing recognition that clinical research needs to define and focus on the outcomes that are most meaningful to patients and society, including quality of life, functional status, freedom from pain and other symptoms, and satisfaction with medical care.[8]

PRACTICING WHEN EVIDENCE IS LACKING

Although the application of EBM has produced very useful information to guide therapy[22] and further research,[23] it has also generated considerable controversy.[24-26] The disagreement is not over recommendation of practices based on sound evidence but, instead, whether these practices should be avoided when evidence is lacking. Thus, clinicians are weary of being told that they and their patients cannot pursue diagnostic and therapeutic choices because there is no evidence that these practices work. In this regard it is important to note one of the basic principles of EBM: "not finding an effect is not the same as finding no effect." Stated differently, the lack of evidence that something works, is not evidence that it does not work. This issue is particularly relevant to critical illness where, by definition, patients are seriously ill and often do not respond to therapy. Should treatment that is possibly effective be withheld from patients with otherwise lethal conditions on grounds that it is unproved?

For new therapies there are already evidence-based standards in place for evaluation and approval.[27] However, numerous therapies are in use in the ICU today without proven efficacy and many others, for which there may be proof in one patient population, are being prescribed in another. Unfortunately, there may be significant barriers to obtaining evidence for these practices. For example, funding agencies and corporations may be unwilling to study therapies that are no longer patented. Furthermore, placebo-controlled studies are often impossible to conduct because clinicians find it unethical to withhold "standard" therapies. Efforts to use "lack of evidence" to justify withholding these therapies should be tempered by these and the following considerations:

1. Are alternatives available that are proven to be effective?
2. Is there evidence that the treatment or procedure is potentially harmful?
3. What is the natural history of the disease being treated?
4. In the case of prophylaxis, what is the risk of developing disease?
5. What is the cost of treatment as well as not treating?

Clinicians routinely grapple with these issues even for therapies that have proven to be effective. The risk-benefit ratio for any therapy is patient specific, and the clinician must judge the probability for benefit or harm to each individual patient. Evidence-based guidelines can be useful in helping clinicians and patients make these decisions, but they cannot take the place of clinical judgment. Treatments that are proven to be useless or even harmful should be avoided unless compelling evidence exists for their use in a specific patient. However, restrictions on existing therapy on the grounds that this therapy is unproven will need to be developed with great caution.

BARRIERS TO APPLYING EVIDENCE

When we see patients we are responsible for applying EBM in the management of their clinical problems. But even when the evidence is strong and the patient is in agreement with the plan, powerful impediments often bar our way.[28] As has been experienced by other specialties, critical care medicine has many logistical barriers to implementing EBM at the level of the clinician or the institution and regionally/nationally.

At the level of the clinician there are a number of potential barriers. First, each step of EBM practice is difficult. For example, generating specific, patient-centered questions is difficult when patients suffer from poorly defined conditions with unknown underlying pathophysiology and uncertain outcome. Because of the relative paucity of available evidence, searching for the right article can be something akin to searching for a needle in a haystack. Second, there are time pressures in clinical practice. This is true both for finding and appraising evidence and for developing the skills of practicing EBM. Whereas this may be true in some circumstances, many non-urgent decisions (e.g., when to restart feeds, ventilator weaning, ulcer prophylaxis) are made in ICUs every day. All of these decisions could benefit from thoughtful consideration of the evidence. And, after an emergent situation, the

clinician (in training) could identify any questions about the course of action taken and review later what evidence exists in such a circumstance. Fortunately, electronic databases are increasingly making this concern less of an issue. Last, clinicians are largely responsible for implementing EBM on their own initiative. If they lack the skills or confidence to apply best evidence to their patient care, nothing will change.

At the institutional level, commitment to practicing EBM requires both philosophical and financial support. Regular revision of institutional guidelines and protocols is time consuming to conduct and expensive to implement. And, full implementation of best care practices may require changes in the array of clinical services available to patients. The purchase of new medical technology or establishing new clinical units can be very expensive. In the current health care environment, many hospitals are likely to be hesitant about such expenses, especially if the evidence is relatively young and the practice not firmly established.

Regionally and/or nationally, implementing EBM requires enormous resources in the effort to continually educate physicians and insurers and to update policies. State and federal governments need to consider medical education requirements and how compliance with policies and guidelines will be defined and enforced. Effective strategies to communicate policy changes and updates in guidelines must also be developed. Because regional and national systems are responsible for socially and geographically diverse health care environments, the aforementioned issues must be adaptable to local needs and circumstances.

Although the obstacles are significant, we are not without resources to overcome them. Paralleling the evolution of EBM has been research into how evidence can be implemented into practice—so-called implementation research.[29] Understanding how individuals and institutions absorb evidence and implement change has, in select cases, translated into fundamental improvements in health care. And, we have learned much about barriers to research transfer through our failed attempts to modify behavior. Success in modifying a discrete aspect of medical practice has invariably been achieved through multidisciplinary strategies that meld concepts and techniques from epidemiology, education, marketing, psychology, sociology, and economics.

PERSPECTIVES ON THE FUTURE

There can be little doubt that the recent social upheaval in medicine has fueled interest in EBM. Throughout the past three decades, hospitals have steadily increased charges to patients to maintain revenues. However, the emphasis in the future, and already a growing force, will be on increasing efficiency.[30,31] This latter goal will require the sophisticated tools available though clinical epidemiology and health services research. In this way, evidenced-based initiatives can be seen as the outgrowth of the quality improvement initiatives of this decade.[32] However, the medical literature is for clinicians and not for hospital administrators.[33,34] Physicians caring for patients remain the target audience for most reviews and editorials written today, and physicians continue to be in control of the vast majority of clinical practice. Unfortunately, this traditional arrangement is being eroded not only by the demands of hospitals, governments, and third-party payers but also by the sheer amount of information now available to all parties. The dissemination and evaluation of this information has become an increasingly difficult undertaking.

Clinicians are being asked to justify their practice as never before.

A frequent misunderstanding about reviewing evidence is the notion that the methodology is fixed. Indeed, the current EBM methodology has serious limitations that are perhaps most evident in its application in the ICU. Evidence appraisal must evolve to solve these problems, and the techniques will need to be further refined and improved. However, these same problems exist across the entire spectrum of clinical research in the ICU today. Unless a better way is found to identify the correct patients, much larger trials than currently performed will be needed. In addition, economic pressures demand that we determine not only efficacy but also effectiveness and cost. Solutions to the first problem limit our ability to solve the second. Approaches to measure effectiveness require even larger trials and may therefore force us to include observational outcomes studies and simulation models in our current methodology toolset. Although well established in other fields, these methods have played little role in critical care medicine research to date. By further refining our techniques for evaluating and applying evidence we may be able to realize a goal of Sir William Osler "to blend the art of medicine with the science of probability."

CONCLUSION

Clinicians are required to effectively identify and interpret the evidence in their fields. It is much easier to teach a physician how to use the tools of clinical epidemiology and biostatistics than to teach a non-physician medicine. With clinician leadership, efforts to improve the practice of medicine can succeed, and not just from a financial standpoint. The techniques for identifying, evaluating, and applying evidence are not panaceas. They are, like the medical literature itself, only tools for clinicians to use to provide the best care for their patients. Experience and consensus are equally as important and will still have a role in modern decision analysis. Evidence is no more or less important than these, although it is by definition more objective. Is EBM a tool of clinicians or a leash held by hospital administrators, insurance companies, and government bureaucracies? It is likely to be both; however, in the hands of the clinician it can be much more powerful and accurate.

ANNOTATED REFERENCES

Cook DJ, Sibbald WJ, Vincent JL, Cerra FB: Evidence based critical care medicine: What is it and what can it do for us? Evidence Based Medicine in Critical Care Group. Crit Care Med 1996;24:334-337.
> *This is the first article in a series entitled "Evidence Based Critical Care Medicine" that demonstrates how an EBM approach can be used at the bedside. It summarizes the rationale for EBM and its applications and future developments and suggests several methods for intensivists to use EBM in their practice and teaching.*

Evidence-Based Medicine Working Group: Evidence-based medicine: A new approach to teaching the practice of medicine. JAMA 1992;268:2420-2425.
> *A practical guide to implementing EBM in a training program. It includes a discussion of the typical barriers to implementing EBM, identifies the solutions to these barriers, and discusses the necessary paradigm shifts that need to occur in most training programs for better implementation. Hands-on guidance is included for both residents and their teachers.*

Sackett DL, Straus SE, Richardson WS, et al: Evidence-Based Medicine: How to Practice and Teach EBM. London, Harcourt, 2000.
> *A comprehensive introduction to EBM and its practice.*

Internet Sources

Centre for Evidence Based Medicine, Oxford: http://cebm.jr2.ox.ac.uk/
The Health Information Research Unit, McMaster University: http://hiru.mcmaster.ca/
The Unit for Evidence-Based Practice and Policy, London: http://www.ucl.ac.uk/openlearning/uebpp/uebpp.htm
Cochrane Collaboration: http://www.cochrane.org/
The ScHARR Guide to Evidence-Based Medicine on the Internet: http://www.sheffield.ac.uk/~scharr/ir/netting/
> Excellent web sites dedicated to evidence-based medicine information. All are regularly updated and have links to many other resources.

Chapter 265

TEACHING CRITICAL CARE

Paul Rogers

Teaching success should be measured in terms of student performance, not the activities of the teacher. Delivering a carefully organized PowerPoint presentation, supervising problem-based workshops, or providing bedside clinical tutorials does not mean one has taught. Unless the learner has acquired new cognitive or psychomotor skills, teaching has not occurred.[1] An effective teacher takes responsibility for ensuring that students learn. If the teacher's perception is that providing a lecture or any instructional methodology fulfills this obligation, then the teacher is serving as "the" educational resource. The focus of this model is on what the teacher did and not on what the learner learned.

Stritter described a different model, one that is focused on the student.[1] In this model the teacher assumes responsibility for the learner's success and creates an environment conducive to learning by managing the educational resources. The teacher as a "manager" creates specific educational objectives, motivates students, utilizes various educational strategies, evaluates learning, and provides effective feedback to ensure the learner achieves all the educational objectives.[1]

The goal of this chapter is to provide a detailed description of each of these steps, from creating educational objectives to providing feedback, so that the teacher can apply the concepts, whether organizing and presenting a 1-hour lecture, a 1-day workshop, a 1-month elective, or a 1-year curriculum.

CREATING EDUCATIONAL OBJECTIVES

Educational objectives outline the skills and behaviors that the student, resident, or fellow will be able to demonstrate after the teacher has completed a lecture, daily bedside instruction, 1-month elective, or fellowship training. Objectives should be developed for every instructional activity because they are a road map. They guide the teacher in developing an appropriate curriculum, they set unambiguous expectations for the learner, and they serve as a reference for evaluation and feedback.[2,3]

Developing educational objectives involves three steps.[2,3] First, using action verbs (e.g., defines, explains, demonstrates, identifies, summarizes, evaluates) the instructor describes a specific behavior that the learner must perform to show the achievement of the objective. An objective such as "teaches concepts of airway management" is not adequate because it defines what the teacher is doing and does not clearly describe what the learner should be demonstrating. Therefore, it neither serves as a road map for the teacher or the student nor does it identify a clear behavior that the teacher can evaluate.

Second, the teacher should describe the conditions under which the behaviors are to occur. For example "given a scenario using human simulation, the student will evaluate the airway and demonstrate effective bag-mask ventilation" or "given a patient with sleep apnea the fellow will outline a plan for management of the difficult airway." Finally, the criteria for acceptable performance should accompany the objective, that is, "bag-mask ventilation will be followed by successful laryngotracheal intubation within 30 seconds."

Bloom and Krathwohl developed a classification of educational objectives to assess three domains: cognitive, affective, and psychomotor.[4,5] Objectives related to acquisition of knowledge are described in the cognitive domain, objectives related to the demonstration of attitudes and values are described in the affective domain, and objectives related to the acquisition of skills are described in the psychomotor domain.[4,5]

When teaching students a specific clinical skill, for example, how to manage a patient with hypotension, the teacher must first establish that the learner has first mastered the lower cognitive domains, knowledge, and comprehension. Learners will not be able to initiate an appropriate treatment for hypotension or evaluate effectiveness of treatment unless they can first list the causes of hypotension and describe the effect of preload on stroke volume. The teacher must be able to identify where learners are in the cognitive domain and help them reach the higher domains such as synthesis and judgment. To accomplish this, the teacher needs to develop

that more effective learning occurs when the educational experience provides interactive clues similar to situations in which the learning is applied.[18] In other words, teaching management of unstable patients in a simulated environment, providing instruction, and evaluating learning is more effective than didactic sessions.

What initially began as computerized software with a separate torso apparatus has evolved into complex whole-body computerized mannequins with a functional mouth and airway, allowing bag-mask ventilation and intubation.[19,20] The chest wall expands and relaxes; there are heart and breath sounds, and real-time display of physiologic variables including electrocardiogram, noninvasive blood pressure, temperature, and pulse oximetry. The human simulator has individual operator controls for upper airway obstruction, tongue edema, trismus, and reduced cervical range of motion. These computerized human simulators require trainees to integrate cognitive and psychomotor learning along with multisensory contextual cues to aid in recall and application in clinical settings.[21,22] This type of simulation has been successfully incorporated into curricula to teach management of obstetrical emergencies, management of difficult airway in operating room, crisis management in the operating room,[20,23] and management of unstable patients for critical care medicine trainees. Examples of learning objectives for third-year medical students, fourth-year medical students, and critical care medicine fellows using the simulator are listed in Tables 265-4 to 265-6. Note, all objectives are written in terms of behaviors the student must perform, thus giving the teacher clear guidelines for evaluation.

In addition to providing the learner with the opportunity to practice specific scenarios such as those outlined in Table 265-5, the simulator can be used to teach crisis management skills.[24] Gaba and colleagues recognized the similarities that airline pilots and physicians face during crisis situations.[24] To bring order to the chaos that often accompanies a crisis, the team leader, whether he or she is an airline pilot or a physician, must demonstrate specific behaviors to effectively manage the situation. The leader must clearly identify himself or herself as the leader and be exempt from any responsibility other than providing orders. For example, when team leaders become involved with other activities, such as inserting intravenous catheters or performing laryngotracheal intubation, they lose oversight of the entire crisis. The leader must demonstrate effective communication skills by assigning specific responsibilities to specific team members. Identifying the nurse who will administer 1 L of normal saline wide open is more effective than asking someone to start some fluids. The leader should identify the essential members and ask nonessential personnel to step back. Finally, the team leader needs to "close the loop" by asking members to report when a specific task has been completed.

Studies of anesthesiology residents have demonstrated that training using simulation technology can improve performance in a simulated crisis,[25] although no study has unequivocally demonstrated improvement in actual patient outcomes.

EVALUATION

Evaluation is an essential component of any education curriculum and should address whether the goals and objectives of the course were met. When developing an assessment tool it is important to define what is being tested (the educational objective), define the behavior that indicates the task has been performed, select the testing method, and determine the acceptable standard for performance.[26] Some goals, including acquisition of knowledge, can be evaluated using written examinations or multiple-choice questionnaires. However, written examinations do not evaluate higher cognitive skills, such as evaluation, and cannot predict if the learner has become clinically competent and can exercise safe clinical judgment. Written examinations lack validity unless they are simply evaluating knowledge.[26] In addition, they tend to reinforce surface or superficial learning by rewarding students for memorizing facts for recall.

Chart-stimulated recalls are utilized to evaluate the student's higher cognitive capabilities. Whereas multiple-choice questions evaluate knowledge, the chart-stimulated recall requires the students to defend the workup, evaluation, diagnosis, and treatment of specific cases. As with other examinations, there must be predefined scoring rules and those conducting the oral review must be trained on how to administer and score the examinations.[27]

Performance-based examinations can be utilized to assess clinical competency, psychomotor skills, and judgment.[28] An example of a performance-based examination is the Objective Structured Clinical Examinations (OSCE), which were developed by Harden and colleagues[29] in 1975. The examinations consist of several "clinical stations," each with its own specific educational objectives. The OSCE requires the learner to recall knowledge, outline a treatment plan, interpret a study such as an electrocardiogram, or perform a specific motor skill.

These examinations are reliable and valid[30-32] and have been utilized to assess competency following medical school

---

TABLE 265–4. LEARNING OBJECTIVES FOR THIRD-YEAR CRITICAL CARE MEDICINE COURSE

Respiratory Distress

- Evaluate a simulated patient in respiratory distress (tachypneic and hypoxemic).
- Initiate appropriate oxygen therapy.
- Evaluate effectiveness of therapeutic intervention.
- Demonstrate effective bag-mask ventilation.
- Insert intravenous line for resuscitation.
- Evaluate patient for potentially difficult airway.

Cardiovascular

- Evaluate a patient with hypotension.
- Initiate therapy for a patient with hypotension (initiate intravenous fluids).
- Order appropriate diagnostic tests for evaluation of a patient with hypotension.
- Evaluate effectiveness of therapeutic intervention.
- Evaluate a patient with sinus tachycardia, develop a differential diagnosis, and order appropriate diagnostic tests.

Arrhythmias

- Evaluate a patient with sinus tachycardia, develop a differential diagnosis, and order appropriate diagnostic tests.
- Demonstrate defibrillation of ventricular fibrillation and pulseless ventricular tachycardia.
- Demonstrate airway management and cardiovascular resuscitation for simulated patients with ventricular fibrillation, ventricular tachycardia, pulseless electrical activity, and asystole.

TABLE 265–5. LEARNING OBJECTIVES FOR FOURTH YEAR CRITICAL CARE MEDICINE COURSE

Scenario	Educational Objective	Correct Response	Typical Response before Training	Consequences
1. An 82-year-old man with coronary artery disease was receiving patient-controlled analgesia after a hip replacement. He is unresponsive and hypoventilating.	Administer correct dose of naloxone.	• Mix 400 µg with 9 mL NS for a concentration of 40 µg/mL. • Administer 1 mL at a time.	• Administer 1 ampule, 400 µg i.v. push.	• Patient wakens hypertensive with chest pain and shortness of breath • ST segment changes are evident on rhythm strip.
2. Patient with shortness of breath; respiratory rate in 30s, refractory hypoxemia on 100% O_2 via facemask. Able to improve saturation with synchronized bag-mask ventilation but is is unable to open his mouth.	Prepare patient for intubation	• Call for help. • Crash cart at bedside. • Provide bag-mask ventilation. • Ensure all equipment is available. • Ensure adequate intravenous line is present. • Assess airway for difficulty before sedation/paralysis.	• Not calling for assistance • Not having necessary equipment • Not evaluating airway • Not ensuring adequate IV access	• Unable to intubate after sedation • Oxygen saturation falls. • Patient develops bradycardia.
3. Patient is unresponsive and without a pulse.	Assume team leader position.	• Assume leadership role. • Assign responsibilities. • Provide specific instructions. • Assess response to interventions. • Evaluate outcome.	• Becomes involved in obtaining arterial blood gas or inserting an intravenous line. • Provides nonspecific instructions (i.e., "Someone start fluid").	• The response is disorganized. • Instructions are not carried out.
4. Patient develops stable atrial fibrillation in a nonmonitored area.	Rate control in monitored environment	• Transfer to a monitored environment where staff can manage any complications.	• Administer rate-controlling agent on the medical ward. • Students often prepare to electrically cardiovert with the patient awake. • Often administer etomidate to cardiovert without preparing for airway management.	• Patient becomes hypotensive. • If intravenous access has not been established, the patient remains hypotensive.
5. Postoperative day 1, nurse calls you to bedside to evaluate a patient whose tracheotomy tube falls out.	Successful reinsertion of tracheotomy tube	• If the patient is stable, call ENT and insert with direct visualization using bronchoscopy. • If patient is unstable, intubate orally.	• Reinsert tracheotomy tube into false passages.	• Tracheotomy tube placed in subcutaneous tissue. • Patient develops hypoxemia and respiratory distress. • Patient develops bradycardia.
6. Patient unresponsive with sinus bradycardia and hypoxemia	Perform bag-mask ventilation.	• Increase oxygen saturation. • Administer epinephrine at 10 µg. • Secure airway.	• Administer 1 mg epinephrine	• Patient develops chest pain, tachycardia to 200 beats/min, and hypertension.

TABLE 265–6. LEARNING OBJECTIVES FOR CRITICAL CARE MEDICINE FELLOWS

1. Assess the patient's airway.
2. Immediately call for help and follow the difficult airway algorithm if difficulty is anticipated.
3. Have primary and secondary airway strategies available (at least one supraglottic and one subglottic strategy).
4. Demonstrate good head position (sniffing position).
5. Check oxygen source and ensure connection of tubing to oxygen source.
6. Ensure two good peripheral intravenous lines are available and functional.
7. Demonstrate one- and two-hand bag-mask ventilation.
8. Use oropharyngeal or nasopharyngeal airway.
9. Establish working suction (check it yourself).
10. Check laryngoscope blades (have size 3 and 4 Mac and Miller blades available).
11. Have at least two sizes of endotracheal tubes available (recommended sizes: 7.0 and 8.0).
12. Check the balloon of the endotracheal tube.
13. Have stylet and CO_2 detector ready.
14. Have medications (etomidate [0.3 mg/kg] and succinylcholine [1 to 1.5 mg/kg] ready in the room).
15. Have 2 ampules of Neo-Synephrine and 250 mL of D_5W in the room in the event of hypotension.

electives, for surgical and emergency medicine internships, and for licensure to practice by the Medical Council of Canada.[31-34]

Some potential disadvantages of OSCEs are that they are labor intensive, they fail to simulate reality because they are broken down into separate stations, and students must rely on the person giving the examination for physical findings or response to treatment.

These limitations can be overcome using the human simulator, which allows the teacher to evaluate a student's cognitive and psychomotor skills in real time. Checklists should be developed, and all observers participating in the evaluation should prospectively agree on what constitutes a successful performance (interrater reliability).[35,36] Because students receive immediate feedback, their analytic and evaluative skills can be assessed and, when necessary, they can be instructed how to perform the task appropriately. Both computer-controlled simulators and OSCEs have been shown to be better than written examinations in predicting if students can solve clinical problems.[37] Gaba and colleagues have shown that technical skills can be assessed reliably from videotapes of the learner's performance on the simulator; however, behavioral skills, such as clinical decision making, were less reliably assessed.[24]

Probably the most common method of assessing clinical competency is to evaluate the learner's performance in real-life clinical situations. Several evaluation tools can be utilized in this environment. Global rating scales are used to evaluate patient care, knowledge application, interpersonal, and communication skills. These evaluations are typically conducted in retrospect and are used to summarize a performance at the end of a clinical rotation. This type of rating has the potential to be highly subjective; and if those performing the evaluation have not been trained, the results may reflect evaluation bias and lose validity.[27]

Psychomotor skills such as evaluation of airway management, bag-mask ventilation, intubation, central catheter insertion, and chest tube insertion are evaluated with procedure logs. Checklists should include the specific behaviors that need to be demonstrated to achieve a satisfactory evaluation.[27] An example of a procedure log for intubation is demonstrated in Table 265-7.

Communication and interpersonal skills can be evaluated by peers, staff, and families using 360-degree reviews and patient surveys. The 360-degree review is a tool that is completed by those individuals (nurses, respiratory therapists, families) working with the learner. The difficulty with this review is making sure staff understand the intent of each question, coordinating the distribution and collecting the completed examination reviews.[27]

Finally, patient surveys are used to obtain feedback on communication, interpersonal skills, and professionalism. They are reliable if there are 20 to 40 patient responses per student, which limits the use of this tool.[27]

PROVIDING EFFECTIVE FEEDBACK

The final step in being a manager of learning is to effectively utilize feedback to enhance learning. Too often feedback is used to fulfill an administrative function. It is provided as a summative report once the rotation is complete. When feedback is utilized effectively it enhances affective learning, and when utilized inappropriately or done poorly it can inhibit learning.[38]

Students want feedback: they want to know how they are performing and how their performance can be improved. Most students, however, report inadequate feedback during their training.[35] Explanations for lack of feedback include a teacher's concerns that the feedback will result in unintended

TABLE 265–7. RESPIRATORY SUPPORT

	Yes	No	N/A	Comments
Equipment Preparation				
1. Assembles equipment correctly				
2. Ensures suction is available				
Drugs				
1. Provides adequate/appropriate use of muscle relaxants				
2. Provides adequate/appropriate use of sedative drugs				
3. Provides adequate/appropriate use of topical anesthetics				
Ventilation				
1. Ensures oxygen flow to bag				
2. Preoxygenates patient to 100%				
3. Provides adequate coordination of bag-mask support with spontaneous effort by patient				
4. Provides effective mask seal				
5. Provides effective ventilation by bag-mask				
6. Demonstrates appropriate use of naso- or oropharyngeal airway				
Intubation				
1. Demonstrates appropriate head positioning				
2. Provides cricoid pressure used				
3. Verifies endotracheal tube placement				
Complications				
1. Prolonged laryngoscopy complications				
2. Number of intubation attempts _____				
3. Esophageal intubation (duration in minutes ____)				
4. Bleeding from lip, mouth, nose				
5. Dental injury				
6. Failed intubation				

consequences, will damage the student-teacher relationship, or will result in students evaluating the teacher as having performed poorly. None of these consequences will occur if the feedback is delivered correctly. Formative feedback is the only way to ensure the success of students, telling them what they have done well and, if necessary, what they need to do to achieve an educational objective. Without effective formative feedback, the behaviors go uncorrected and the student develops a system of self-validation: "I did well because no one told me otherwise."

For feedback to effectively change behavior without causing unintended consequences, several rules should be followed. First, all feedback should be based on how the student performed regarding a specific goal and/or objective of the program.[38] This is another reason that teachers must develop clear educational goals. They serve not only as the framework for the curriculum but also as a reference for feedback. If feedback is provided in the context of specific performance, there should be no untoward consequence.[38] For example, if the goal is for the learner to demonstrate effective bag-mask ventilation with appropriate chest excursion and adequate oxygen saturation, then the goal was either achieved or it was not. This is a statement based on an objective and is not a personal affront unless the feedback contains judgmental language. Therefore, it is important not to tell the student he or she did a "terrible job." Second, feedback must include a description of how to succeed. In the example presented, if the patient was not effectively ventilated, the teacher should suggest repositioning the head, inserting an oral airway, and performing two-person bag-mask ventilation so that there is a better seal with the mask. Third, the specific behavior that the learner demonstrated should be addressed and not just interpreted.[38] If students are late to rounds, do not assume they do not care or are lazy. Stating the expectation that rounds begin at 7 AM and the expectation is to be prepared by then assigns no judgment. Fourth, for feedback to be effective, it should be an expected component of the learning tools.[38] Students should be informed during orientation that they will receive daily feedback on their performance of the stated goals and objectives. Without successfully implementing feedback, the model of teaching described by Irby is incomplete.[9]

In conclusion, a teacher who begins every educational session with clear objectives, creates an environment where students want to learn, applies different educational strategies, evaluates learning, and provides formative feedback will help his or her students to successfully achieve the educational objectives. These guidelines are applicable for developing a bedside teaching session, a 1-month rotation, or a year-long curriculum for critical care medicine fellows.

ANNOTATED REFERENCES

Bloom BS: Taxonomy of educational objectives. In A Committee of College and University Examiners (eds): The Classification of Educational Goals, Handbook 1/Cognitive Domain. New York, Longman, 1956, pp 120-200.
   Bloom's taxonomy is a description of cognitive objectives arranged from the lowest level of cognitive function, knowledge, to the highest, judgment. Faculty must ensure students have mastered the lower domain before they can expect the learner to comprehend, apply, analyze, synthesize, and judge.

Ende J: Feedback in clinical medical education. JAMA 1983;250:777-781.
   This review discusses the formative functions of feedback, rather than the administrative function. Formative feedback is provided to the learner to help him or her successfully achieve the educational goals. It is based on student behaviors, not faculty interpretation of behaviors, and must be accompanied by a description of how to succeed.

Irby DM: What clinical teachers in medicine need to know. Acad Med 1994;69:333-342.
   There are a variety of instructional activities. Whereas didactic sessions are the most common, they are the least effective, because adult learners prefer interactive learning that allows them to defend clinical decision-making.

Mager RF: Preparing Instructional Objectives. Palo Alto, CA, Fearson, 1962.
   Educational objectives should be developed for every instructional activity. They guide the teacher in curriculum development, set unambiguous goals, and serve as a reference for feedback. Educational objectives should describe the exact behavior learners must demonstrate to successfully achieve the goal.

Rogers PL, Jacob H, Rashwan AS, et al: Quantifying learning in medical students during a critical care medicine elective: A comparison of three evaluation instruments. Crit Care Med 2001;29:1268-1273.
   Evaluation is an essential component of any curriculum. The most common evaluative tool is written examination; however, this study showed that written examinations were not as good as performance examinations in predicting if students could manage complex clinical situations.

INDEX

Note: Page numbers followed by f indicate figures; those followed by t indicate tables; those followed by b indicate boxed material.